P9-BYQ-569

Brunner & Suddarth's

Textbook of
MEDICAL-SURGICAL NURSING

First Canadian Edition

Rene A. Day, PhD, RN

Professor
Faculty of Nursing, University of Alberta
Edmonton, Alberta

Pauline Paul, PhD, RN

Associate Professor
Faculty of Nursing, University of Alberta
Edmonton, Alberta

Bev Williams, PhD, RN

Associate Professor
Faculty of Nursing, University of Alberta
Edmonton, Alberta

Suzanne C. Smeltzer, RN, EdD, FAAN

Professor and Director, Nursing Research
Villanova University College of Nursing
Villanova, Pennsylvania

Brenda G. Bare, RN, MSN

Associate Administrator Patient Care Services/
   Chief Nurse Executive
Inova Mount Vernon Hospital
Alexandria, Virginia

Lippincott Williams & Wilkins
a Wolters Kluwer business
Philadelphia · Baltimore · New York · London
Buenos Aires · Hong Kong · Sydney · Tokyo

Senior Acquisitions Editor: Pete Darcy
Senior Managing Editor: Helen Kogut
Editorial Assistant: Marivette Torres
Senior Production Editor: Debra Schiff
Director Nursing Production: Helen Ewan
Senior Managing Editor / Production: Erika Kors
Art Director: Joan Wendt
Illustration Coordinator: Brett MacNaughton
Manufacturing Coordinator: Karin Duffield
Indexer: Coughlin Indexing Services, Inc.
Compositor: Circle Graphics
Printer: R. R. Donnelley

First Canadian Edition

9 8 7 6 5 4 3 2

ISBN 13: 978-0-7817-9130-4
ISBN 10: 0-7817-9130-8

Care has been taken to confirm the accuracy of the information presented and to describe generally accepted practices. However, the authors, editors, and publisher are not responsible for errors or omissions or for any consequences from application of the information in this book and make no warranty, express or implied, with respect to the content of the publication.

The authors, editors, and publisher have exerted every effort to ensure that drug selection and dosage set forth in this text are in accordance with the current recommendations and practice at the time of publication. However, in view of ongoing research, changes in government regulations, and the constant flow of information relating to drug therapy and drug reactions, the reader is urged to check the package insert for each drug for any change in indications and dosage and for added warnings and precautions. This is particularly important when the recommended agent is a new or infrequently employed drug.

Some drugs and medical devices presented in this publication have Food and Drug Administration (FDA) clearance for limited use in restricted research settings. It is the responsibility of the health care provider to ascertain the FDA status of each drug or device planned for use in his or her clinical practice.

LWW.com

Contributors

Contributors to the First Canadian Edition

Eric Bone, MA
Senior Planner, Emergency Preparedness
Capital Health
Edmonton, Alberta
> Chapter 72: Disaster, Mass Casualty, Epidemics/Pandemics,
> and Terrorism Nursing

Madeleine Buck, BScN, RN
Faculty Lecturer
School of Nursing, McGill University
Montreal, Quebec
> Chapter 6: Homeostasis, Stress and Adaptation
> Chapter 7: Individual and Family Considerations Related to Illness
> Chapter 9: Genetics Perspectives in Nursing
> Chapter 14: Fluid and Electrolytes: Balance and Distribution
> Chapter 15: Shock and Multisystem Failure

Jaeyoung Choi, MScN, RN
PhD Student
Faculty of Nursing, University of Alberta
Edmonton, Alberta
> Chapter 12: Health Care of the Older Adult

Jean Chow, PhD, RN
Assistant Professor
Faculty of Nursing, University of Calgary
Calgary, Alberta
> Chapter 46: Assessment and Management of Female Physiologic Processes
> Chapter 47: Management of Patients With Female Reproductive
>   Disorders
> Chapter 48: Assessment and Management of Patients With
>   Breast Disorders

Alexander M. Clark, PhD, RN
Assistant Professor
Faculty of Nursing, University of Alberta
Edmonton, Alberta
> Chapter 26: Assessment of Cardiovascular Function
> Chapter 27: Management of Patients With Dysrhythmias
>   and Conduction Problems
> Chapter 28: Management of Patients With Coronary
>   Vascular Disorders
> Chapter 29: Management of Patients With Structural, Infectious,
>   and Inflammatory Cardiac Disorders
> Chapter 30: Management of Patients With Complications From
>   Heart Disease

Cynthia Cummings-Winfield, BScN, RN, CON(C)
Coordinator—Nursing Research and Professional Practice Development
Cross Cancer Institute
Edmonton, Alberta
> Chapter 16: Oncology: Nursing Management in Cancer Care
> Chapter 17: End-of-Life Care

Rene A. Day, PhD, RN
Professor
Faculty of Nursing, University of Alberta
Edmonton, Alberta
> Chapter 3: Critical Thinking, Ethical Decision Making, and the
>   Nursing Process
> Chapter 5: Health Assessment
> Chapter 7: Individual and Family Considerations Related to Illness
> Chapter 9: Genetics Perspectives in Nursing
> Chapter 46: Assessment and Management of Female Physiologic Processes
> Chapter 68: Management of Patients With Musculoskeletal Disorders
> Chapter 72: Disaster, Mass Casualty, Epidemics/Pandemics, and
>   Terrorism Nursing
> Appendix B: Diagnostic Studies and Interpretation

Bernadette Dodd, BScN, RN
Recipient Transplant Coordinator
University of Alberta Hospital
Edmonton, Alberta
> Chapter 39: Assessment and Management of Patients With
>   Hepatic Disorders

Glenn Donnelly, PhD, RN, ENC(C)
Assistant Professor
College of Nursing, University of Saskatchewan
Saskatoon, Saskatchewan
> Chapter 71: Emergency Nursing

Lynne Esson, BSN, RN
Lecturer
The University of British Columbia School of Nursing
Vancouver, British Columbia
> Chapter 60: Assessment of Neurologic Function
> Chapter 61: Management of Patients With Neurologic Dysfunction
> Chapter 62: Management of Patients With Cerebrovascular Disorders

Bonnie Friesen, MN, RN
Senior Instructor
Faculty of Nursing, University of Calgary
Calgary, Alberta
> Chapter 66: Assessment of Musculoskeletal Function
> Chapter 67: Musculoskeletal Care Modalities
> Chapter 68: Management of Patients With Musculoskeletal Disorders
> Chapter 69: Management of Patients With Musculoskeletal Trauma

Cathy Giblin, MS, RN
Regional Manager, Nursing Affairs
Capital Health
Edmonton, Alberta
> Chapter 72: Disaster, Mass Casualty, Epidemics/Pandemics, and
>   Terrorism Nursing
> Appendix A: Understanding Clinical Pathways

Audrey Groeneveld, MN, RN
Infection Control Practitioner, Capital Health and
Associate Faculty, Faculty of Nursing, University of Alberta
Edmonton, Alberta
Chapter 70: Management of Patients With Infectious Diseases

Jean Groft, MN, RN
PhD Student
Faculty of Nursing, University of Alberta and
Lecturer
School of Health Sciences, University of Lethbridge
Lethbridge, Alberta
Chapter 52: Management of Patients With HIV Infection and AIDS

Janice A. Lander, PhD, RN
Professor
Faculty of Nursing, University of Alberta
Edmonton, Alberta
Chapter 13: Pain Management

Linda Larsen, MN, RN
Clinical Nurse Specialist, Bone and Joint Health Program
Rockyview Hospital, Calgary Health Region
Calgary, Alberta
Chapter 66: Assessment of Musculoskeletal Function
Chapter 67: Musculoskeletal Care Modalities
Chapter 68: Management of Patients With Musculoskeletal Disorders
Chapter 69: Management of Patients With Musculoskeletal Trauma

Deborah Michalyk, RN
Project Manager
Capital Health
Edmonton, Alberta
Appendix A: Understanding Clinical Pathways

Judy Mill, PhD, RN
Associate Professor
Faculty of Nursing, University of Alberta
Edmonton, Alberta
Chapter 52: Management of Patients With HIV Infection and AIDS

Jill Milne, PhD, RN
Postdoctoral Fellow (2004-2005)
Faculty of Nursing, University of Alberta
Edmonton, Alberta
Chapter 43: Assessment of Renal and Urinary Tract Function
Chapter 44: Management of Patients With Upper or Lower Urinary Tract Dysfunction
Chapter 45: Management of Patients With Urinary Disorders
Chapter 49: Assessment and Management of Problems Related to Male Reproductive Processes

F. Margaret Milner, MN, RN
Research Manager
Faculty of Nursing, University of Alberta
Edmonton, Alberta
Chapter 57: Management of Patients With Burn Injury

Evelyn Myles, BScN, RN
Clinical Nurse Specialist, Adult Rehabilitation
Glenrose Rehabilitation Hospital
Edmonton, Alberta
Chapter 11: Principles and Practices of Rehabilitation

Joe Noon, PhD, RN
Associate Professor
Faculty of Nursing, University of Alberta
Edmonton, Alberta
Chapter 31: Assessment and Management of Patients With Vascular Disorders and Problems of Peripheral Circulation
Chapter 32: Assessment and Management of Patients With Hypertension
Chapter 33: Assessment and Management of Patients With Hematologic Disorders

Colleen M. Norris, PhD, RN
Assistant Professor
Faculty of Nursing, University of Alberta
Edmonton, Alberta
Chapter 26: Assessment of Cardiovascular Function
Chapter 27: Management of Patients With Dysrhythmias and Conduction Problems
Chapter 28: Management of Patients With Coronary Vascular Disorders
Chapter 29: Management of Patients With Structural, Infectious, and Inflammatory Cardiac Disorders
Chapter 30: Management of Patients With Complications From Heart Disease

Joanne K. Olson, PhD, RN
Professor
Faculty of Nursing, University of Alberta
Edmonton, Alberta
Chapter 2: Community-Based Nursing Practice

Kärin Olson, PhD, RN
Associate Professor
Faculty of Nursing, University of Alberta
Edmonton, Alberta
Chapter 16: Oncology: Nursing Management in Cancer Care
Chapter 17: End-of-Life Care

Pauline Paul, PhD, RN
Associate Professor
Faculty of Nursing, University of Alberta
Edmonton, Alberta
Chapter 1: Health Care Delivery and Nursing Practice
Chapter 8: Perspectives in Transcultural Nursing

Wanda Pierson, PhD, RN
Chairperson
Nursing Department, Langara College
Vancouver, British Columbia
Chapter 50: Assessment of Immune Function
Chapter 51: Management of Patients With Immunodeficiency
Chapter 53: Assessment and Management of Patients With Allergic Disorders
Chapter 54: Assessment and Management of Patients With Rheumatic Disorders
Chapter 65: Management of Patients With Oncologic or Degenerative Neurologic Disorders

Christy Raymond, MEd, BScN, RN
Coordinator
School of Nursing, Grant MacEwan College
Edmonton, Alberta
Chapter 18: Preoperative Nursing Management
Chapter 19: Intraoperative Nursing Management
Chapter 20: Postoperative Nursing Management

Chapter 34: Assessment of Digestive and Gastrointestinal Function
Chapter 35: Management of Patients With Oral and Esophageal Disorders
Chapter 36: Gastrointestinal Intubation and Special Nutritional Modalities
Chapter 37: Management of Patients With Gastric and Duodenal Disorders
Chapter 38: Management of Patients With Intestinal and Rectal Disorders

Carolyn J. M. Ross, PhD, RN
Associate Professor
Faculty of Nursing, University of Alberta
Edmonton, Alberta
Chapter 21: Assessment of Respiratory Function
Chapter 22: Management of Patients With Upper Respiratory Tract Disorders
Chapter 23: Management of Patients With Chest and Lower Respiratory Tract Disorders
Chapter 24: Management of Patients With Chronic Obstructive Pulmonary Disease
Chapter 25: Respiratory Care Modalities

Shannon M. Spenceley, MN, RN
PhD Student
Faculty of Nursing, University of Alberta
Edmonton, Alberta
Chapter 10: Chronic Illness

Tracey Stephen, MN, RN
Sessional Instructor
Faculty of Nursing, University of Alberta
Edmonton, Alberta
Chapter 55: Assessment of Integumentary Function
Chapter 56: Management of Patients With Dermatologic Problems
Chapter 58: Assessment and Management of Patients With Eye and Vision Disorders
Chapter 59: Assessment and Management of Patients With Hearing and Balance Disorders

Lorraine A. Watson, PhD, RN
Associate Professor
Faculty of Nursing, University of Calgary
Calgary, Alberta
Chapter 41: Assessment and Management of Patients With Diabetes Mellitus

Bev Williams, PhD, RN
Associate Professor
Faculty of Nursing, University of Alberta
Edmonton, Alberta
Chapter 4: Health Education and Health Promotion
Chapter 39: Assessment and Management of Patients With Hepatic Disorders
Chapter 40: Assessment and Management of Patients With Biliary Disorders
Chapter 42: Assessment and Management of Patients With Endocrine Disorders

Donna M. Wilson, PhD, RN
Professor
Faculty of Nursing, University of Alberta
Edmonton, Alberta
Chapter 12: Health Care of the Older Adult

Linda J. Youell, MHSA, RN
Director—Undergraduate Services
Faculty of Nursing, University of Alberta
Edmonton, Alberta
Chapter 11: Principles and Practices of Rehabilitation

Susan Young, MN, RN
Clinical Nurse Specialist, Critical Care, Burns and Neurosciences
University of Alberta Hospital
Edmonton, Alberta
Chapter 63: Management of Patients With Neurologic Trauma
Chapter 64: Management of Patients With Neurologic Infections, Autoimmune Disorders, and Neuropathies

Contributors to the 10th Edition

Sandra M. Annesi, MSN, RN
Assistant Professor
Nursing Program
Daytona Beach Community College
DeLand, Florida
Chapter 25: Respiratory Care Modalities

Judith C. Bautch, PhD, RN, CS
Professor
Department of Nursing, Winona State University
Winona, Minnesota
Chapter 54: Assessment and Management of Patients With Rheumatic Disorders

Jo Ann Brooks-Brunn, DNS, RN, FAAN, FCCP
Assistant Professor
Thoracic Surgery
Pulmonary and Critical Care Medicine
Indiana University School of Medicine
Indianapolis, Indiana
Chapter 23: Management of Patients With Chest and Lower Respiratory Tract Disorders
Chapter 24: Management of Patients With Chronic Obstructive Pulmonary Disease

Jacqueline Fowler Byers, PhD, RN, CNAA
Associate Professor
School of Nursing
University of Central Florida
Orlando, Florida
Chapter 21: Assessment of Respiratory Function

Kim Cantwell-Gab, BSN, RN, CVN, RVT, RDMS
Vascular Surgery Nurse Specialist
Department of Surgery
Division of Vascular Surgery
University of Washington School of Medicine
Seattle, Washington
Chapter 31: Assessment and Management of Patients With Vascular Disorders and Problems of Peripheral Circulation

Patricia E. Casey, MSN, RN
Director, Regional Cardiovascular Program
Kaiser Permanente Mid-Atlantic Region
Rockville, Maryland
  *Chapter 27: Management of Patients With Dysrhythmias
    and Conduction Problems*
  Chapter 28: Management of Patients With Coronary Vascular Disorders
  *Chapter 29: Management of Patients With Structural, Infectious,
    and Inflammatory Cardiac Disorders*
  *Chapter 30: Management of Patients With Complications
    From Heart Disease*

Jill Cash, MSN, APRN, BC
Family Nurse Practitioner
Southern Illinois OB-GYN Associates, SC
Carbondale, Illinois
  *Chapter 59: Assessment and Management of Patients With Hearing
    and Balance Disorders*

Linda Carman Copel, PhD, RN, CS, CGP, DAPA
Associate Professor
Villanova University College of Nursing
Villanova, Pennsylvania
  Chapter 4: Health Education and Health Promotion
  Chapter 6: Homeostasis, Stress, and Adaptation
  Chapter 7: Individual and Family Considerations Related to Illness

Juliet Corbin, RNC, DNS, FNP
Lecturer
School of Nursing
San Jose State University
San Jose, California
  Chapter 10: Chronic Illness

Susanna G. Cunningham, PhD, RN, FAAN, FAHA
Professor
Department of Biobehavioral Nursing and Health Systems
University of Washington School of Nursing
Seattle, Washington
  *Chapter 32: Assessment and Management of Patients
    With Hypertension*

Lana Currance, BSN, RN, CCRN
Chief Nursing Officer
National Medical Response System
Colorado 2 DMAT/Central U.S. NMRT-Weapons of
  Mass Destruction
Parker, Colorado
  Chapter 72: Terrorism, Mass Casualty, and Disaster Nursing

Margaret A. Degler, MSN, RN, CRNP, CUNP
Director, Continence Program
West Office of the Center for Urologic Care of Berks County, P.C.
West Reading, Pennsylvania
  Chapter 12: Health Care of the Older Adult
  Chapter 43: Assessment of Renal and Urinary Tract Function
  *Chapter 44: Management of Patients With Upper or Lower Urinary
    Tract Dysfunction*
  Chapter 45: Management of Patients With Urinary Disorders

Nancy E. Donegan, MPH, BS, RN
Director, Infection Control
Washington Hospital Center
Washington, D.C.
  Chapter 70: Management of Patients With Infectious Diseases

Phyllis Dubendorf, MSN, RN, CS-ACNP
Lecturer, Acute Care Nurse Practitioner Program
School of Nursing
University of Pennsylvania
Philadelphia, Pennsylvania
  Chapter 61: Management of Patients With Neurologic Dysfunction

Eleanor Fitzpatrick, MSN, RN, CRNP, CCRN
Clinical Nurse Specialist
Surgical ICU/Intermediate Surgical ICU
Thomas Jefferson University Hospital
Philadelphia, Pennsylvania
  *Chapter 39: Assessment and Management of Patients With
    Hepatic Disorders*
  *Chapter 40: Assessment and Management of Patients With Biliary
    Disorders*

Mary Beth Flynn, MS, RN
CNS/Clinical Educator
University of Colorado Hospital
Clinical Faculty
University of Colorado Health Science Center
Denver, Colorado
  Chapter 15: Shock and Multisystem Failure

Kathleen K. Furniss, MSN, APN-C
Nurse Practitioner, Women's Health
Women's Health Initiative
University of Medicine and Dentistry of New Jersey and Associates in
  Women's Health Care
Newark, New Jersey
  *Chapter 46: Assessment and Management of Female
    Physiologic Processes*
  *Chapter 47: Management of Patients With Female
    Reproductive Disorders*

Paula Graling, MSN, RN, CNS
Clinical Nurse Specialist
Perioperative Services
Inova Fairfax Hospital
Falls Church, Virginia
  Chapter 18: Preoperative Nursing Management
  Chapter 19: Intraoperative Nursing Management
  Chapter 20: Postoperative Nursing Management

Randolph E. Gross, MS, RN, CS, AOCN
Clinical Nurse Specialist
Evelyn H. Louder Breast Center
Memorial Sloan-Kettering Cancer Center
New York, New York
  *Chapter 48: Assessment and Management of Patients
    With Breast Disorders*

Doreen Grzelak, MSN, RN, AOCN
Operations Manager
Medical Imaging Center
Department of Radiology
Reston Hospital Center
Reston, Virginia
  *Chapter 35: Management of Patients With Oral and Esophageal
    Disorders*
  *Chapter 37: Management of Patients With Gastric and Duodenal
    Disorders*

Janice L. Hinkle, PhD, RN, CNRN
Assistant Professor
Villanova University College of Nursing
Villanova, Pennsylvania
Chapter 5: Health Assessment
Chapter 62: Management of Patients With Cerebrovascular Disorders
Chapter 65: Management of Patient With Oncologic and Degenerative Neurologic Disorders

Ryan R. Iwamoto, MN, ARNP, AOCN
Oncology Clinical Coordinator
Genentech BioOncology, Inc.
South San Francisco, California
Nurse Practitioner
Department of Radiation Oncology
Virginia Mason Medical Center
Clinical Instructor
University of Washington and Seattle University
Seattle, Washington
Chapter 49: Assessment and Management of Problems Related to Male Reproductive Processes

Joyce Young Johnson, PhD, RN, CCRN
Assistant Chair
Department of Nursing
Georgia Perimeter College
Clarkston, Georgia
Chapter 1: Health Care Delivery and Nursing Practice
Chapter 2: Community-Based Nursing Practice
Chapter 3: Critical Thinking, Ethical Decision Making, and the Nursing Process
Chapter 8: Perspectives in Transcultural Nursing

Rhonda Kyanko, MS, RN
Nursing Education Coordinator
National Rehabilitation Hospital
Washington, DC
Chapter 11: Principles and Practices of Rehabilitation

Pamela J. LaBorde, MSN, RN
Clinical Nurse Specialist, Patient Care Services
University of Arkansas Medical Sciences Center
Little Rock, Arkansas
Formerly, Clinical Nurse Specialist, Burn Unit
Orlando Regional Medical Center
Orlando, Florida
Chapter 57: Management of Patients With Burn Injury

Dale Halsey Lea, MPH, RN, CGC, APGN, FAAN
Assistant Director
Southern Maine Regional Genetics Services
Foundations for Blood Research
Scarborough, Maine
Chapter 9: Genetics Perspectives in Nursing Practice

Dorothy B. Liddel, MSN, RN, ONC
Associate Professor (Retired)
Department of Nursing
Columbia Union College
Takoma Park, Maryland
Chapter 66: Assessment of Musculoskeletal Function
Chapter 67: Musculoskeletal Care Modalities
Chapter 68: Management of Patients With Musculoskeletal Disorders
Chapter 69: Management of Patients With Musculoskeletal Trauma

Martha V. Manning, MSN, RN
Nurse Clinician
Inova Emergency Care Center at Fairfax
Fairfax, Virginia
Chapter 34: Assessment of Digestive and Gastrointestinal Function
Chapter 38: Management of Patients With Intestinal and Rectal Disorders

Barbara J. Maschak-Carey, MSN, RN, CDE
Clinical Nurse Specialist
Department of Endocrinology, Diabetes and Metabolism
University of Pennsylvania Health System
Philadelphia, Pennsylvania
Chapter 41: Assessment and Management of Patients With Diabetes Mellitus

Agnes Masny, MPH, MSN, RN, CRNP
Research Associate/Nurse Practitioner
Population Science Division, Family Risk Assessment Program
Fox Chase Cancer Center
Philadelphia, Pennsylvania
Chapter 9: Genetics Perspectives in Nursing

Lou Ann McGinty, MSN, RN
Nurse Science Clinical Specialist
Capitol Health System
Trenton, New Jersey
Chapter 64: Management of Patients With Neurologic Infections, Autoimmune Disorders, and Neuropathies

Nancy A. Morrissey, PhD, RN,C
Patient Care Director
Mental Health and Behavioral Center
Inova Alexandria Hospital
Alexandria, Virginia
Chapter 36: Gastrointestinal Intubation and Special Nutritional Modalities

Martha A. Mulvey, CNS,C
Advanced Practice Nurse
Neurosciences
University of Medicine and Dentistry of New Jersey, University Hospital
Newark, New Jersey
Chapter 14: Fluids and Electrolytes: Balance and Distribution

Victoria Navarro, MAS, MSN, RN
Director of Clinical Services
Wilmer Eye Institute
The Johns Hopkins Medical Institutions
Baltimore, Maryland
Chapter 58: Assessment and Management of Patients With Eye and Vision Disorders

Donna Nayduch, MSN, RN-CS, CCRN
Trauma Regional Director
Banner Health
Greeley, Colorado
Chapter 71: Emergency Nursing
Chapter 72: Terrorism, Mass Casualty, and Disaster Nursing

Kathleen Nokes, PhD, RN, FAAN
Professor
Hunter-Bellevue School of Nursing
New York, New York
Chapter 52: Management of Patients With HIV Infection and AIDS

Janet A. Parkosewich, MSN, RN, CCRN
Cardiac Clinical Nurse Specialist
Department of Patient Services
Yale-New Haven Hospital
New Haven, Connecticut
Chapter 26: Assessment of Cardiovascular Function

Anne Gallagher Peach, MSN, RN
Chief Operating Officer
M.D. Anderson Cancer Center Orlando
Orlando, Florida
Chapter 22: Management of Patients With Upper Respiratory
Tract Disorders

JoAnne Reifsnyder, PhD, RN, AOCN
Postdoctoral fellow, Psychosocial Oncology
School of Nursing
University of Pennsylvania
Philadelphia, Pennsylvania
Chapter 17: End-of-Life Care

Susan A. Rokita, MS, RN, CRNP
Nurse Coordinator, Cancer Center
Oncology Clinical Nurse Specialist
Milton S. Hershey Medical Center of Pennsylvania State University
Hershey, Pennsylvania
Chapter 16: Oncology: Nursing Management in Cancer Care

Al Rundio, PhD, RN, ANP
Associate Professor
Medical College of Pennsylvania/Hahnemann University
College of Nursing and Health Professions
Philadelphia, Pennsylvania
Chapter 50: Assessment of Immune Function
Chapter 51: Management of Patients With Immunodeficiency
Chapter 53: Assessment and Management of Patients
With Allergic Disorders

Catherine Sackett, BS, RN, CANP
Ophthalmic Research Nurse Practitioner
Wilmer Eye Institute
Retinal Vascular Center
The Johns Hopkins Medical Institutions
Baltimore, Maryland
Chapter 58: Assessment and Management of Patients With Eye
and Vision Disorders

Linda Schakenbach, MSN, RN, CNS, CCRN, COCN, CWCN, CS
Clinical Nurse Specialist, Critical Care
Inova Alexandria Hospital
Alexandria, Virginia
Chapter 27: Management of Patients With Dysrhythmias
and Conduction Problems
Chapter 28: Management of Patients With Coronary
Vascular Disorders
Chapter 29: Management of Patients With Structural, Infectious,
and Inflammatory Cardiac Disorders

Margaret A. Spera, NP, APRN
Nurse Practitioner
Family Medical Associates

Ridgefield, Connecticut
Assistant Clinical Professor
Yale University School of Nursing
New Haven, Connecticut
Chapter 60: Assessment of Neurologic Function

Cindy Stern, MSN, RN
Cancer Network Coordinator
University of Pennsylvania Cancer Center
University of Pennsylvania Health System
Philadelphia, Pennsylvania
Chapter 16: Oncology: Nursing Management in
Cancer Care

Christine Tea, MSN, RN, CNA
Patient Care Director
Main OR Perioperative Services
Inova Fairfax Hospital
Falls Church, Virginia
Chapter 18: Preoperative Nursing Management
Chapter 19: Intraoperative Nursing Management
Chapter 20: Postoperative Nursing Management

Mary Laudon Thomas, MS, RN, AOCN
Hematology Clinical Nurse Specialist
Veterans' Administration, Palo Alto Health Care System
Palo Alto, California
Chapter 33: Assessment and Management of Patients
With Hematologic Disorders

Dorraine Day Watts, PhD, RN
Interim Director of Research and Education
Inova Health System
Falls Church, Virginia
Chapter 63: Management of Patients With Neurologic Trauma

Joan Webb, MSN, RN
Instructor
College of Nursing
Widener University
Chester, Pennsylvania
Chapter 40: Assessment and Management of Patients
With Biliary Disorders
Chapter 42: Assessment and Management of Patients
With Endocrine Disorders

Joyce S. Willens, PhD, RN
Assistant Professor
College of Nursing
Villanova University
Villanova, Pennsylvania
Chapter 13: Pain Management

Iris Woodard, BSN, RN-CS, ANP
Nurse Practitioner
Department of Dermatology
Kaiser Permanente
Springfield, Virginia
Chapter 55: Assessment of Integumentary Function
Chapter 56: Management of Patients With Dermatologic Problems

Preface

*I*n the 21st century, nurses face a future characterized by changes comparable to those of no preceding century:

- Science and technology have made the world smaller by making it more accessible.
- Mass communication is more widespread, and information is now just an instant away and very easy to obtain.
- Economies are more global than regional.
- Industrial and social changes have made world travel and cultural exchange common.

Today's nurses enter a realm of opportunities and challenges for providing high-quality, evidence-based care in traditional as well as new and innovative health care settings. The rapid changes in health care mandate that nurses be prepared to provide or plan care across a continuum of settings–from hospital or clinic, to home, to community agencies or hospice settings–and during all phases of illness. Recent research has indicated that nurses make significant contributions to the health care outcomes of patients who are hospitalized. Therefore, today's nurses must be prepared to identify patients' short- and long-term needs quickly and to collaborate effectively with patients and families, other members of the health care team, and community agencies to create a seamless system of care. The continued emphasis on health promotion and disease and injury prevention efforts to keep well people healthy and to promote a higher level of well-being among those with acute and chronic illnesses requires today's nurses to assist patients in adopting healthy lifestyles and strategies. As well, the focus of nurses' care may be the individual, families, groups, or entire communities.

In preparing for those vast opportunities and responsibilities, today's nurses must be well informed and up-to-date, not only in nursing knowledge and skills but also in research findings, scientific advances, and the ethical dilemmas inherent in many areas of clinical practice. More than ever, today's nurses need to think critically, creatively, and compassionately.

ABOUT THE FIRST CANADIAN EDITION

The first Canadian edition is based on *Brunner & Suddarth's Textbook of Medical-Surgical Nursing*, which was designed to provide today's nursing students with an understanding of the nurse's role in health and illness within evolving practice environments and across the spectrum of health and illness. New chapters on genetics; end-of-life care; and mass casualty, disaster, and terrorism nursing are included. A goal of the Canadian edition is to continue to provide balanced attention to the art and science of adult medical-surgical nursing. It addresses nursing care issues from a physiological, pathophysiological, psychosocial, and spiritual context and assists the reader to identify priorities of care from that context.

Canadian experts examined each chapter and changed the following as needed: drug names, names of tests and procedures, spelling, laboratory values to SI units, and other measurements that needed to be metric. Wherever possible, the Contributors replaced American citations/references with Canadian ones, American research studies with Canadian research studies, and provided Canadian epidemiological content. Nursing practice or procedures that were not used in Canada were changed and updated.

This first Canadian edition includes new and updated material to reflect the differences in practice in terms of: the health care system, community health, ethics, culture, epidemiology, pain management, gerontology, end-of-life care, infection control, nursing and medical management, pharmacology, diagnostics tests and investigations, patient teaching/discharge, equipment and procedural guidelines, disaster and pandemic planning, as well as support groups and web resources specific to Canada. The 2005 version of the North American Nursing Diagnosis Association (NANDA) and the 2004 versions of the Nursing Interventions Classification (NIC) and the Nursing-Sensitive Outcomes Classification (NOC) are included in Chapter 3.

NANDA, NIC, NOC: LINKS, LANGUAGES, AND CONCEPT MAPS

Although *Brunner & Suddarth's Textbook of Medical-Surgical Nursing* has long used nursing diagnoses developed by the North American Nursing Diagnosis Association (NANDA), this edition presents the links between the NANDA diagnoses and the Nursing Interventions Classification (NIC) and Nursing-sensitive Outcomes Classification (NOC). The opening page of each unit presents a concept map illustrating these three classification systems and their relationships. Each unit's concept map is accompanied by a case study and a chart presenting examples of actual NANDA, NIC, and NOC terminologies related to the case study. This material is included to introduce the reader to the NIC and NOC language and classifications and bring them to life in the clinical realm. Faculty and students alike may use some of the issues presented in the case studies as a springboard for developing their own concept maps.

RECENT NURSING RESEARCH AND OTHER FEATURES

Nursing Research Profiles included in the chapters identify the implications and applications of recent nursing research findings for nursing practice. The chapters also include charts and text detailing special considerations in caring for the elderly patient and for those with disabilities.

TEACHING TOOLBOX

Each chapter opens with Learning Objectives and a Glossary. Throughout the text the reader will find Nursing Alerts as well as specialized charts focusing on

- Physiology/Pathophysiology
- Risk Factors
- Assessment
- Plans of Nursing Care
- Pharmacology

- Home Care
- Patient Education
- Health Promotion
- Ethics and Related Issues
- Guidelines
- Gerontological Considerations
- Genetics in Nursing Practice

Illustrations, photographs, charts, and tables supplement the text and round out the applied-learning experience. Each chapter concludes with Critical Thinking Exercises, References and Selected Readings, and a list of specialized Resources and Websites.

MANY MORE OF THE LATEST RESOURCES

Additional learning tools that accompany *Brunner & Suddarth's Textbook of Medical-Surgical Nursing* are available for Canadian instructors and students who use this Canadian edition. These tools offer visual, tactile and auditory reinforcement and include:

- **CD-ROM** to help students test their knowledge and enhance their understanding of medical-surgical nursing. The CD includes 500 self-study questions organized by unit; 3000 bonus NCLEX-style questions; 3-D animated illustrations that explain common disease processes; and interactive clinical simulations.
- **Instructor's Resource CD-ROM** to help facilitate classroom preparation, with an instructor's manual, test generator, and searchable image collection, among other features.
- Supplemental cartridges for Learning Management Systems including **Blackboard, WebCT** and **Desire to Learn** and any SCORM 2004 compliant system.
- **thePoint Website** – Get connected at http://thePoint.lww. com/CanadianMedSurg.

Acknowledgments

We gratefully acknowledge our Canadian contributors who took on the challenge of "Canadianizing" *Brunner & Suddarth's Textbook of Medical-Surgical Nursing*. At the Faculty of Nursing, University of Alberta, we thank Leona Laird and Alice Da Silva for their often daily assistance in sending materials to contributors and then the revised chapters and page proofs to Lippincott Williams & Wilkins. We especially want to acknowledge the role L. Wayne Day played as Project Manager, his skills in locating websites and references and in keeping the three of us on track.

Rene A. Day, PhD, RN
Pauline Paul, PhD, RN
Bev Williams, PhD, RN

With great appreciation and respect, the authors acknowledge Lillian S. Brunner, ScD, LittD, MSN, RN, FAAN, and Doris S. Suddarth, MSN, BSNE, RN. The foundation and expertise that they provided for this textbook for many years and the mentoring that they provided to us during earlier editions continue to support us as we strive toward the development of a textbook that encourages students and practitioners of nursing to strive toward excellence in providing skillful and compassionate nursing care.

The authors also gratefully acknowledge the contributions of Janice L. Hinkle, PhD, RN, and Linda Schakenbach, MSN, RN, to this tenth edition of *Brunner and Suddarth's Textbook of Medical-Surgical Nursing*. They have authored chapters of the textbook and guided many contributors in writing and developing chapters throughout the textbook. We greatly appreciate the nursing expertise and experience and the spirit of inquiry that they bring to this tenth edition.

Suzanne C. O'Connell Smeltzer, EdD, RN, FAAN
Brenda G. Bare, MSN, RN

How to use

Brunner & Suddarth's
Textbook of Medical-Surgical Nursing
10th edition

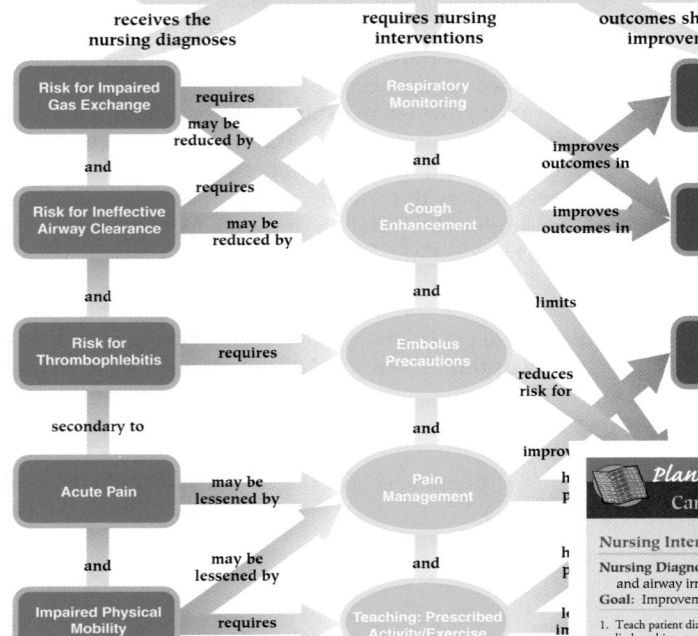

The patient recovering from abdominal surgery with reluctance to move and a history of smoking

receives the nursing diagnoses → requires nursing interventions → outcomes should show improvement in

- Risk for Impaired Gas Exchange — requires / may be reduced by → Respiratory Monitoring
- and
- Risk for Ineffective Airway Clearance — requires / may be reduced by → Cough Enhancement
- and
- Risk for Thrombophlebitis — requires → Embolus Precautions
- secondary to
- Acute Pain — may be lessened by → Pain Management
- and
- Impaired Physical Mobility — may be lessened by / requires → Teaching: Prescribed Activity/Exercise

and → Respiratory Monitoring — improves outcomes in → Anxiety Control
and → Cough Enhancement — improves outcomes in → Respiratory Status: Gas Exchange
and → limits → Pain Level
reduces risk for
improv...

◄ **Concept Maps**—with NANDA, NIC, and NOC illustrate reality-based clinical scenarios for the visual learner.

▼ **Plans of Nursing Care**—illustrate applications of the nursing process to diseases and disorders.

Plan of Nursing Care
Care of the Patient With COPD (Continued)

Nursing Interventions	Rationale	Expected Outcomes
Nursing Diagnosis: Ineffective breathing pattern related to shortness of breath, mucus, bronchoconstriction, and airway irritants **Goal:** Improvement in breathing pattern		
1. Teach patient diaphragmatic and pursed-lip breathing.	1. Helps patient prolong expiration time and decreases air trapping. With these techniques, patient will breathe more efficiently and effectively.	• Practices pursed-lip and diaphragmatic breathing and uses them when short of breath and with activity
2. Encourage alternating activity with rest periods. Allow patient to make some decisions (bath, shaving) about care based on tolerance level.	2. Pacing activities permits patient to perform activities without excessive distress.	• Shows signs of decreased respiratory effort and paces activities • Uses inspiratory muscle trainer as prescribed
3. Encourage use of an inspiratory muscle trainer if prescribed.	3. Strengthens and conditions the respiratory muscles.	
Nursing Diagnosis: Self-care deficits related to fatigue secondary to increased work of breathing and insufficient ventilation and oxygenation **Goal:** Independence in self-care activities		
1. Teach patient to coordinate diaphragmatic breathing with activity (eg, walking, bending).	1. This will allow the patient to be more active and to avoid excessive fatigue or dyspnea during activity.	• Uses controlled breathing while bathing, bending, and walking
2. Encourage patient to begin to bathe self, dress self, walk, and drink fluids. Discuss energy conservation measures.	2. As condition resolves, patient will be able to do more but needs to be encouraged to avoid increasing dependence.	• Paces activities of daily living to alternate with rest periods to reduce fatigue and dyspnea • Describes energy conservation strategies
3. Teach postural drainage if appropriate.	3. Encourages patient to become involved in own care. Prepares patient to manage at home.	• Performs same self-care activities as before • Performs postural drainage correctly
Nursing Diagnosis: Activity intolerance due to fatigue, hypoxemia, and ineffective breathing patterns		
...tioned consume... additional bur...gh regular, graded ...ups become ...he patient can do ...hort of breath. ...e cycle of		• Performs activities with less shortness of breath • Verbalizes need to exercise daily and demonstrates an exercise plan to be carried out at home • Walks and gradually increases walking time and distance to improve physical condition • Exercises both upper and lower body muscle groups
...ialization, anxiety, depression, lower activity level,		
...ls will promote a ...plishment rather ...lessness.	• Expresses interest in the future • Participates in the discharge plan • Discusses activities or methods that can be performed to ease shortness of breath
2. Encourage activity to level of symptom tolerance.	2. Activity reduces tension and decreases degree of dyspnea as patient becomes conditioned.	• Uses relaxation techniques appropriately • Expresses interest in a pulmonary rehabilitation program

(continued)

Chart 16-5
Home Care Checklist • Chemotherapy Administration

At the completion of the home care instruction, the patient or caregiver will be able to:	Patient	Caregiver
• Demonstrate how to administer the chemotherapy agent in the home.	✓	✓
• Demonstrate safe disposal of needles, syringes, IV supplies, or unused chemotherapy medications.	✓	✓
• List possible side effects of chemotherapeutic agents.	✓	✓
• List complications of medications necessitating a call to the nurse or physician.	✓	✓
• List complications of medications necessitating a visit to the emergency department.	✓	✓
• List names and telephone numbers of resource personnel involved in care (ie, home care nurse, infusion services, IV vendor, equipment company).	✓	✓
• Explain treatment plan (protocol) and importance of upcoming visits to physician.	✓	✓

▲ **Home Care Checklists**—include guidelines on goals and management of home-based patients.

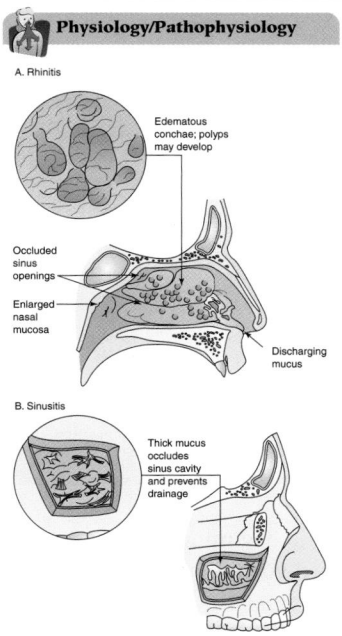

▲ **Pathophysiology Displays**—utilize illustrations and algorithms to demonstrate processes.

---

 chart 17-6 • ASSESSMENT

Nursing Assessment of Symptoms Associated With Terminal Illness

- How is this symptom affecting the patient's life?
- What is the meaning of the symptom to the patient? To the family?
- How does the symptom affect physical functioning, mobility, comfort, sleep, nutritional status, elimination, activity level, and relationships with others?
- What makes the symptom better?
- What makes it worse?
- Is it worse at any particular time of the day?
- What are the patient's expectations and goals for managing the symptom? The family's?
- How is the patient coping with the symptom?
- What is the economic effect of the symptom and its management?

Adapted from Jacox, A., Carr, D. B., & Payne, R. (1994). *M cancer pain.* Rockville, MD: AHCPR.

▲ **Assessment Displays**—provide clinical features of diseases and disorders and include guidelines for assessing health history and exam findings.

---

 chart 16-4 • PHARMACOLOGY

Investigational Antineoplastic Therapies and Clinical Trials

Evaluation of the effectiveness and toxic potential of promising new modalities for preventing, diagnosing, and treating cancer is accomplished through clinical trials. Before new chemotherapy agents are approved for clinical use, they are subjected to rigorous and lengthy evaluations to identify beneficial effects, adverse effects, and safety.

- *Phase I* clinical trials determine optimal dosing, scheduling, and toxicity.
- *Phase II* trials determine effectiveness with specific tumor types and further define toxicities. Participants in these early trials are most often those who have not responded to standard forms of treatment. Because phase I and II trials may be viewed as last-chance efforts, patients and families are fully informed about the experimental nature of the trial therapies. Although it is hoped that investigational therapy will effectively treat the disease, the purpose of early phase trials is to gather information concerning maximal tolerated doses, adverse effects, and effects of the antineoplastic agents on tumor growth.
- *Phase III* clinical trials establish the effectiveness of new medications or procedures as compared with conventional approaches. Nurses may assist in the recruitment, consent, and education processes for patients who participate. In many cases, nurses are instrumental in monitoring adherence, assisting patients to adhere to the parameters of the trial, and documenting data describing patients' responses. The physical and emotional needs of patients in clinical trials are addressed in much the same way as those of patients who receive standard forms of cancer treatment.
- *Phase IV* testing further investigates medications in terms of new uses, dosing schedule, and toxicities.

Pharmacology Charts—review ▶ recent or common drug therapies with discussion of clinical trials where appropriate.

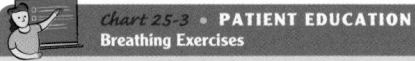 **chart 25-3** • PATIENT EDUCATION

Breathing Exercises

General Instructions
- Breathe slowly and rhythmically to exhale completely and empty the lungs completely.
- Inhale through the nose to filter, humidify, and warm the air before it enters the lungs.
- If you feel out of breath, breathe more slowly by prolonging the exhalation time.
- Keep the air moist with a humidifier.

Diaphragmatic Breathing
Goal: To use and strengthen the diaphragm during breathing
- Place one hand on the abdomen (just below the ribs) and the other hand on the middle of the chest to increase the awareness of the position of the diaphragm and its function in breathing.
- Breathe in slowly and deeply through the nose, letting the abdomen protrude as far as possible.
- Breathe out through pursed lips while tightening (contracting) the abdominal muscles.
- Press firmly inward and upward on the abdomen while breathing out.
- Repeat for 1 minute; follow with a rest period of 2 minutes.
- Gradually increase duration up to 5 minutes, several times a day (before meals and at bedtime).

Pursed-Lip Breathing
Goal: To prolong exhalation and increase airway pressure during expiration, thus reducing the amount of trapped air and the amount of airway resistance.
- Inhale through the nose while counting to 3—the amount of time needed to say "Smell a rose."
- Exhale slowly and evenly against pursed lips while tightening the abdominal muscles. (Pursing the lips increases intratracheal pressure; exhaling through the mouth offers less resistance to expired air.)
- Count to 7 while prolonging expiration through pursed lips—the length of time to say "Blow out the candle."
- While sitting in a chair:
  Fold arms over the abdomen.
  Inhale through the nose while counting to 3.
  Bend forward and exhale slowly through pursed lips while counting to 7.
- While walking:
  Inhale while walking two steps.
  Exhale through pursed lips while walking four or five steps.

---

 chart 21-8

Risk Factors for Hypoventilation

- Limited neurologic impulses transmitted from the brain to the respiratory muscles, as in spinal cord trauma, cerebrovascular accidents, tumours, myasthenia gravis, Guillain-Barré syndrome, polio, and drug overdose
- Depressed respiratory centres in the medulla, as with anesthesia and drug overdose
- Limited thoracic movement (kyphoscoliosis), limited lung movement (pleural effusion, pneumothorax), or reduced functional lung tissue (chronic pulmonary diseases, severe pulmonary edema)

◀ **Risk Factor Charts**—outline factors that may impair health (eg, carcinogens, environmental factors), and offer preventive measures to sidestep them.

 Gerontologic Considerations

Factors Contributing to Urinary Tract Infection in Older Adults

- High incidence of chronic illness
- Frequent use of antimicrobial agents
- Presence of infected pressure ulcers
- Immobility and incomplete emptying of bladder
- Use of a bedpan rather than a commode or toilet

Gerontologic ▶ **Considerations**— provide specific information relevant to the older population.

◀ **Patient Education Boxes**—provide suggestions on such topics as self-care, or how to cope with health challenges.

! **NURSING ALERT** It is the responsibility of all nurses, and particularly perianesthesia and perioperative nurses, to be aware of latex allergies, necessary precautions, and products that are latex-free (Meeker & Rothrock, 1999). Hospital staff are also at risk for developing a latex allergy secondary to repeated exposure to latex products.

▲ Nursing Alerts—offer brief tips for clinical practice and red-flag warnings to help students avoid common mistakes.

Glossary

adaptation: a change or alteration designed to assist in adapting to a new situation or environment
adrenocorticotropic hormone (ACTH): a hormone produced by the anterior lobe of the pituitary gland that stimulates the secretion of cortisone and other hormones by the adrenal cortex
antidiuretic hormone (ADH): a hormone secreted by the posterior lobe of the pituitary gland that constricts blood vessels, elevates blood pressure, and reduces the excretion of urine
catecholamines: any of the group of amines (such as epinephrine, norepinephrine, or [...] that serve as neurotransmitters [...] itive and behavioral strate- [...] anage the stressors that tax a [...] urces
[...]nge in the appearance of a [...]sure to chronic irritation [...]: the group of steroid hor- [...]as cortisol, that are produced

by the adrenal cortex; they are involved in carbohydrate, protein, and fat metabolism and have anti-inflammatory properties
gluconeogenesis: the formation of glucose, especially by the liver from noncarbohydrate sources such as amino acids and the glycerol portion of fats
guided imagery: use of the imagination to achieve relaxation or direct attention away from uncomfortable sensations or situations
homeostasis: a steady state within the body; the stability of the internal environment
hyperplasia: an increase in the number of new cells
hypoxia: inadequate supply of oxygen to the cell
infectious agents: biologic agents, such as viruses, bacteria, rickettsiae, mycoplasmas, fungi, protozoa, and nematodes, that cause disease in people
inflammation: a localized, protective reaction of tissue to injury, irritation, or infec-

tion, manifested by pain, redness, heat, swelling, and sometimes loss of function
metabolic rate: the speed at which some substances are broken down to yield energy for bodily processes and other substances are synthesized
metaplasia: a cell transformation in which a highly specialized cell changes to a less specialized cell
negative feedback: feedback that decreases the output of a system
positive feedback: feedback that increases the output of a system
steady state: a stable condition that does not change over time, or when change in one direction is balanced by change in an opposite direction
stress: a disruptive condition that occurs in response to adverse influences from the internal or external environments
vasoconstriction: the narrowing of a blood vessel

▲ Glossary—at the beginning of every chapter, helps students learn vocabulary.

◀ Nursing Research Profiles—contain research samples with purpose of research, study sample, and design and findings, and implications for use in evidence-based nursing.

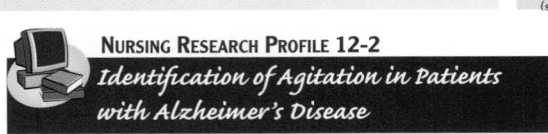

NURSING RESEARCH PROFILE 12-2
Identification of Agitation in Patients with Alzheimer's Disease

Whall, A. L., Black, M. E. A., Yankou, D. J., et al. (1999). Nurse aides' identification of onset and level of agitation in late stage dementia patients. *American Journal of Alzheimer's Disease, 14,* 202–206.

Purpose
Nursing assistants provide the majority of care to patients in nursing homes. They are vital links in the early identification, and therefore in the treatment, of agitation in patients with Alzheimer's disease. Nurses' aides (NAs) are sometimes characterized as unwilling or unable to manage patients' agitation. This study examines the process by which nurses' aides can successfully identify this agitation.

Design
NAs from five different nursing homes owned by the same corporate entity were asked to participate in the study. Criteria to participate included being employed for at least 1 year. (Rese[...] demonstrates that NAs who remain at a facility longer than 1 usually have a commitment to those they serve.) The NAs di[...] receive any additional wages and were only promised a letter t[...] dicate that they had participated in the study. Each NA receive[...] proximately 1 hour of training via audio tapes and conversation[...] nurse experts. Each NA was then paired with a nurse expert t[...] sess his or her skill at appropriately identifying levels of agitati[...] patients with late-stage Alzheimer's disease.

Conclusions
This study demonstrated that NAs with a minimum of 1 ye[...] employment did an excellent job in acquiring new observa[...] skills with only 1 hour of training and positive reinforcement[...] letter noting their participation in this study. The NAs' assess[...] of signs of agitation agreed with that of the nurse expert more[...] 90% of the time. All the NAs involved reported gaining helpf[...] sights in managing agitated behavior as a result of participati[...] the study.

Implications f[...]
The results of th[...] observe and repo[...] session using adu[...] of their input in [...] servation and rep[...] agitation from ir[...]

Chart 22-7 • Ethics and Related Issues

Situation
A 68-year-old attorney was diagnosed with cancer of the larynx 8 years ago. He was treated successfully with radiation therapy, resulting in an altered voice quality. Recently, he has complained of shortness of breath and difficulty swallowing. In the past few months, he also has noticed a marked change in his voice and physical condition, which he attributed to "winter colds."

After a complete physical exam and an extensive diagnostic workup and biopsy, it is determined that the cancer has recurred at a new primary site. His health care provider recommends surgery (a total laryngectomy) and chemotherapy as the best options. The patient states that he is not willing to "lose my voice and my livelihood" but instead will "take my chances." He has also expressed concern about his quality of life after surgery. His family has approached you about trying to convince him to have surgery.

Dilemma
The patient's right to refuse treatment conflicts with the family's wishes and recommendation from his health care provider.

Discussion
1. Is the patient making a decision based upon all pertinent information concerning his health status, treatment, options, risk/benefits, and long-term prognosis?
2. What arguments can be made to support the patient's decision to forego treatment?
3. What arguments can be made to question the patient's decision to forego treatment?

Chart 25-15
GUIDELINES FOR Care of the Patient Being Weaned From Mechanical Ventilation

NURSING INTERVENTIONS	RATIONALE
1. Assess patient for weaning criteria: Vital capacity—10 to 15 mL/kg Maximum inspiratory pressure (MIP) at least −20 cm H₂O Tidal volume—7 to 9 mL/kg Minute ventilation—6 L/min Rapid/shallow breathing index—below 100 breaths/minute/L PaO₂ greater than 60 mm Hg with FiO₂ less than 40%	1. Careful assessment of multiple weaning indices helps to determine readiness for weaning. When the criteria have been met, the patient's likelihood of successful weaning increases.
2. Monitor activity level, assess dietary intake, and monitor results of laboratory tests of nutritional status.	2. Reestablishing independent spontaneous ventilation can be physically exhausting. It is crucial that the patient have enough energy reserves to succeed. Providing periods of rest and recommended nutritional intake can increase the likelihood of successful weaning.
3. Assess the patient's and family's understanding of the weaning process and address any concerns about the process. Explain that the patient may feel short of breath initially and provide encouragement as needed. Reassure the patient that he or she will be attended closely and that if the weaning attempt is not successful, it can be tried again later.	3. The weaning process can be psychologically tiring; emotional support can help promote a sense of security. Explaining that weaning will be attempted again later helps reduce the sense of failure if the first attempts are unsuccessful.
4. Implement the weaning method prescribed: A/C, IMV, SIMV, PSV, PAV, CPAP, or T-piece.	4. The prescribed weaning method should reflect the patient's individualized criteria for weaning and weaning history. By having different methods to choose from, the physician can select the one that best fits the patient.
5. M[...] al signs, pulse oximetry, ECG, and respiratory pattern [...] or the first 20 to 30 minutes and every 5 minutes after [...] eaning is complete.	5. Monitoring the patient closely provides ongoing indications of success or failure.
[...] patent airway; monitor arterial blood gas levels and [...] function tests. Suction the airway as needed.	6. These values can be compared to baseline measurements to evaluate weaning. Suctioning helps to reduce the risk of aspiration and maintain the airway.
[...] tion with the physician, terminate the weaning process [...] actions occur. [...] n, systolic blood pressure increase of 20 mm Hg, a [...] xygen saturation to less than 90%, respiratory rate [...] r greater than 20 breaths/minute, ventricular dys- [...] atigue, panic, cyanosis, erratic or labored breathing, [...] chest movement.	7. These signs and symptoms indicate an unstable patient at risk for hypoxia and ventricular dysrhythmias. Continuing the weaning process can lead to cardiopulmonary arrest.
[...] ng process continues, measure tidal volume and minute [...] very 20 to 30 minutes; compare with the patient's [...] s, which have been determined in collaboration [...] ysician.	8. These values help to determine if weaning is successful and should be continued.
[...] ychological dependence if the physiologic parameters [...] ning is feasible and the patient still resists.	9. Psychological dependence is a common problem after mechanical ventilation. Possible causes include fear of dying and depression from chronic illness. It is important to address this issue before the next weaning attempt.

▲ Procedure Guidelines Charts—offer nursing activities and rationales for important skills.

◀ Ethics and Related Issues—showcase brief scenarios and present possible ethical dilemmas for discussion.

Contents

Brunner & Suddarth's

Textbook of

MEDICAL-SURGICAL NURSING

First Canadian edition

Unit 1

Basic Concepts in Nursing

Applying Concepts from NANDA, NIC, and NOC

A nurse working in an urgent care clinic that serves an economically depressed urban area notes a high incidence of elderly patients with dehydration and heatstroke in the summer months. The nurse verifies the observations by accessing data about hospital admissions for dehydration and heatstroke. The nurse determines that many of the admitted patients live in the area served by the clinic, and that many of the patients live alone and have other chronic illnesses. The nurse sees the need for a plan that includes a community response to this problem. The plan includes arranging an education program about the prevention of dehydration; a community support buddy system in which neighbors or volunteers call or visit homebound elders during critical periods in the summer; and economic support to air condition the senior citizens' centre. The concept map illustrates some of the diagnoses, interventions, and outcomes the nurse uses to guide the plan of care.

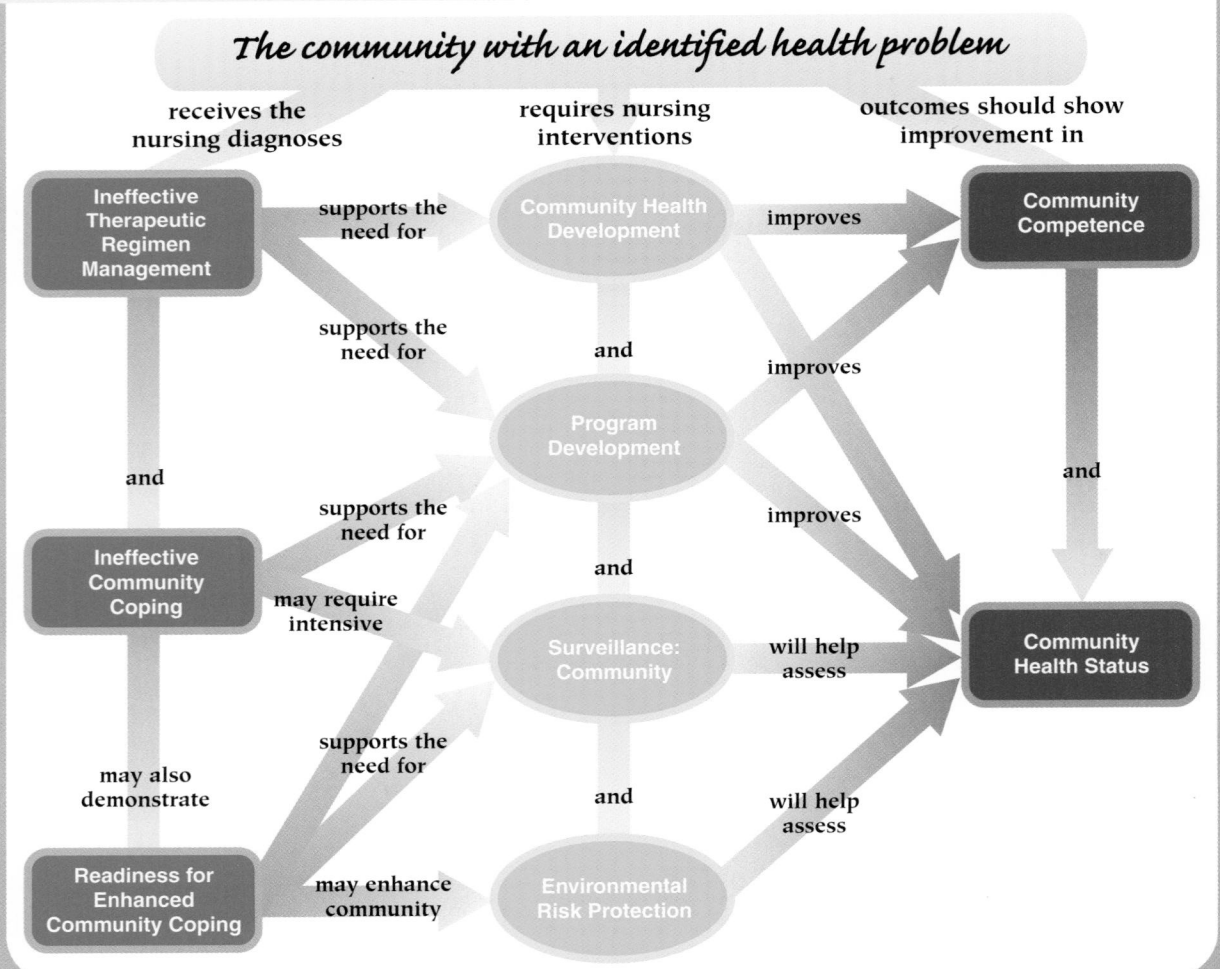

The community with an identified health problem

receives the nursing diagnoses

requires nursing interventions

outcomes should show improvement in

Ineffective Therapeutic Regimen Management

supports the need for

Community Health Development

improves

Community Competence

supports the need for

Program Development

improves

and

and

Ineffective Community Coping

supports the need for

improves

may require intensive

Surveillance: Community

will help assess

Community Health Status

may also demonstrate

supports the need for

and

will help assess

Readiness for Enhanced Community Coping

may enhance community

Environmental Risk Protection

Nursing Classifications and Languages

NANDA
Nursing Diagnoses

Ineffective Community Therapeutic Regimen Management— Pattern of regulating and integrating into community processes programs for treatment of illness and the sequelae of illness that are unsatisfactory for meeting health-related goals

Ineffective Community Coping— A pattern of community activities for adaptation and problem solving that is unsatisfactory for meeting the demands or needs of the community

Readiness for Enhanced Community Coping—Pattern of community activities for adaptation and problem solving that is satisfactory for meeting the demands or needs of the community but can be improved for management of current and future problems/stressors

NIC
Nursing Interventions*

Community Health Development—Facilitating members of a community to identify a community's health concerns, mobilize resources, and implement solutions

Program Development— Planning, implementing, and evaluating a coordinated set of activities designed to enhance wellness, or to prevent, reduce or eliminate one or more health problems of a group or community

Surveillance: Community— Purposeful and ongoing acquisition, interpretation, and synthesis of data for decision making in the community

Environmental Risk Protection— Preventing and detecting disease and injury in populations at risk from environmental hazards

NOC
Nursing Outcomes†

Return to functional baseline status, stabilization of, or improvement in

Community Competence—The ability of a community to collectively problem solve to achieve goals

Community Health Status—The general state of well-being of a community or population

NANDA, North American Nursing Diagnosis Association; NIC, Nursing Interventions Classification; NOC, Nursing Outcomes Classification

*Iowa Intervention Project © 2000. In McCloskey, J. C., & Bulechek, G. M. (2000). *Nursing interventions classification (NIC)* (3rd ed.). St. Louis: Mosby.

†Iowa Outcomes Project © 2000. In Johnson, M., Maas, M., & Moorhead, S. (2000). *Nursing outcomes classification (NOC)* (3rd ed.). St. Louis: Mosby.

Health Care Delivery and Nursing Practice

Adapted by Pauline Paul

LEARNING OBJECTIVES

On completion of this chapter, the learner will be able to:

1. Define health, wellness, and health promotion.
2. Recognize and define the principles of the Canada Health Act.
3. Define primary health care and define the principles of primary health care.
4. Describe factors causing significant changes in the health care delivery system and their impact on the health care field and the nursing profession.
5. Describe the practitioner, leadership, and research roles of the nurse.
6. Describe nursing care delivery models.
7. Discuss expanded nursing roles.

*O*rganized nursing in Canada began in the seventeenth century with the settlement by France of the parts of North America that were then known as Acadia and New France. The provision of nursing care was one of the first services offered to settlers and Aboriginal people alike. For example, only 27 years after the foundation of Quebec City, the Augustinian Sisters had founded the Hôtel-Dieu de Québec, the first hospital of New France. After the British North America Act of 1867, Roman Catholic nursing sisters continued to play an instrumental role in the development of nursing and health care in every region of the country. For example, the Grey Nuns of Montreal spearheaded the creation in the late 1800s and early 1900s of an impressive network of hospitals across the Canadian Prairies. Although in the twenty-first century religious orders no longer play a predominant role in health care delivery, their legacy is alive and well through new generations of nurses and through the institutions they created and once managed. The nurses of today continue to be essential to the delivery and organization of health care services.

The Health Care Industry and the Nursing Profession

Although the delivery of nursing care has been affected by changes occurring in the health care system, the definition of nursing has continued to distinguish nursing care and identify the major aspects of nursing care.

NURSING DEFINED

Since the time of Florence Nightingale, who wrote in 1858 that the goal of nursing was "to put the patient in the best condition for nature to act upon him," nursing leaders have described nursing as both an art and a science. However, the definition of nursing has evolved over time. The International Council of Nurses (ICN) states:

> Nursing encompasses autonomous and collaborative care of individuals of all ages, families, groups and communities, sick or well and in all settings. Nursing includes the promotion of health, prevention of illness, and the care of the ill, disabled and dying people. Advocacy, promotion of safe environment, research, participation in shaping health policy and in patient and health systems management, and education are also key nursing roles (ICN, 2005).

The Canadian Nurses Association (CNA) defines nursing practice as "a dynamic, caring, helping relationship in which the nurse assists the client to achieve and maintain optimal health" (CNA, 1987, p. iii). Because the regulation of health care professionals is under provincial jurisdiction, the provincial nursing associations, or colleges as they are most often called, regulate individual nurses. Registered nurses have the responsibility to adhere to the *Canadian Nurses Association Code of Ethics for Registered Nurses* (CNA, 2002) and to adhere to the nursing practice standards of their provincial/territorial jurisdiction.

Understanding the needs of health care consumers and the health care delivery system, including the forces that affect nursing and health care delivery, will provide a foundation for examining the delivery of nursing care.

THE PATIENT/CLIENT: CONSUMER OF NURSING AND HEALTH CARE

The central figure in health care services is, of course, the patient. The term *patient,* which is derived from a Latin verb meaning "to suffer," has traditionally been used to describe those who are recipients of care. The connotation commonly attached to the word is one of dependence. For this reason, many nurses prefer to use the term *client,* which is derived from a Latin verb meaning "to lean," connoting alliance and interdependence. For the purposes of this book, the term *patient* will be used throughout, but with the understanding that either term is acceptable.

The patient who seeks care for a health problem or problems (increasing numbers of people have multiple health problems) is also an individual, a member of a family, and a citizen of the community. Patients' needs vary depending on their problem, associated circumstances, and past experiences. One of the nurse's important functions in health care delivery is to identify the patient's immediate needs and take measures to address them.

The Patient's Basic Needs

Certain needs are basic to all people and require satisfaction accordingly. Such needs are addressed on the basis of priority, meaning that some needs are more pressing than others. Once an essential need is met, the person experiences a need on a higher level. Approaching needs according to priority reflects Maslow's hierarchy of needs (Fig. 1-1).

Maslow's Hierarchy

Maslow ranked human needs as follows: physiologic needs; safety and security; belongingness and affection; esteem and self-respect; and self-actualization, which includes self-fulfillment, desire to

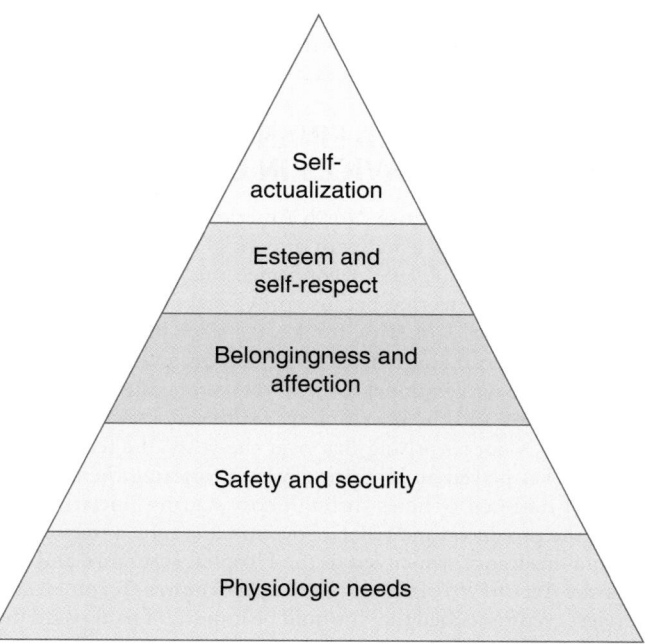

FIGURE 1-1 This scheme of Maslow's hierarchy of human needs shows how a person moves from fulfillment of basic needs to higher levels of needs, with the ultimate goal being integrated human functioning and health.

know and understand, and aesthetic needs. Lower-level needs always remain, but a person's ability to pursue higher-level needs indicates that he or she is moving toward psychological health and well-being. Such a hierarchy of needs is a useful organizational framework that can be applied to the various nursing models for assessment of a patient's strengths, limitations, and need for nursing interventions.

HEALTH CARE IN TRANSITION

Changes occurring in health care delivery and nursing are the result of societal, economic, technological, scientific, and political forces that have evolved throughout the 20th and into the 21st century. Among the most significant changes are shifts in population demographics, particularly the increase in the aging population and the cultural diversity of the population; changing patterns of diseases; increased technology; increased consumer expectations; the high costs of health care and changes in health care financing; and other health care reform efforts. These changes have led to institutional restructuring, staff downsizing, increased outpatient care services, decreased lengths of hospital stay, and more care being provided in the community and in the home. Such changes are having a dramatic influence on where nurses practice, with an increasing trend for nurses to provide health care in community and home settings. Indeed, these changes have a dynamic influence on our view of health and illness and therefore affect the focus of nursing and health care.

As an increasing proportion of the population reaches age 65 years and older, and with the shift in disease patterns from acute illnesses to chronic illnesses, the traditional disease management and care focus of the health care professions has expanded. There is growing concern about emerging infectious diseases and trauma. The health care focus must centre more on prevention, health promotion, and management of chronic conditions than in previous times. This shift in focus coincides with a nationwide emphasis on cost control and resource management directed toward providing cost-efficient and cost-effective health care services to the population as a whole.

ORGANIZATION AND FINANCING OF HEALTH CARE SERVICES IN CANADA

The passage of the British North American Act of 1867 made health care in Canada a matter of provincial jurisdiction, and the Constitutional Act of 1982 reconfirmed this division of power. In practice, it means that because provincial governments have this constitutional authority, it takes considerable efforts to obtain the provincial and federal consensus necessary to establish policies that have a national scope. However, because Canadians see health care and the provision of health care services as a key priority, it is not surprising that over the years, the federal government has played an increasing role in fostering the development of national policies through cost-sharing initiatives. In 1955, the provincial and federal governments agreed to establish hospital insurance, which led to the Hospital Insurance and Diagnostic Act of 1957. In 1964, the Royal Commission on Health Services recommended that it would be important to also add the provision of medical services to the national program. This recommendation led to the passage of the Medical Care Act of 1968. Although all provincial governments entered into these partnerships, the development in the following decades of provincial variations, such as the introduction of extra-billing and users fees,

concerned federal authorities and brought about the Canada Health Act of 1984 (Ross-Kerr, 2003).

The Canada Health Act

The Canada Health Act stipulates that health care insurance plans must be publicly administered, universal, comprehensive, accessible, and portable. Providing an exhaustive definition of these principles is beyond the scope of this chapter, but in brief, the plan must be operated and administered on a nonprofit basis by a public authority responsible to the provincial government; 100% of the insured individuals in a province are entitled to the services that are provided under this plan; the plan must insure all services offered by hospitals and physicians and, where permitted, by other health care professionals; these services must be reasonably accessible; and when moving from one province to another, or when temporarily absent from their province (but within Canada), residents must be continued to be covered (Health Canada, 1992). Current issues related to the financing of health care services are further addressed in the section of this chapter on economic pressures.

HEALTH

How health is perceived depends on how health is defined. In the preamble to its constitution, the World Health Organization (WHO) defines health as a "state of complete physical, mental, and social well-being and not merely the absence of disease and infirmity" (Hood & Leddy, 2002). Such a definition of health does not allow for any variation in degrees of wellness or illness. On the other hand, the concept of a health–illness continuum allows for a greater range in describing a person's health status. By viewing health and illness on a continuum, it is possible to consider a person as having neither complete health nor complete illness. Instead, a person's state of health is ever-changing and has the potential to range from high-level wellness to extremely poor health and imminent death. The model of the health–illness continuum makes it possible to view a person as simultaneously possessing degrees of both health and illness.

The limitations of the WHO definition of health are clear in relation to chronic illness and disability. A chronically ill person cannot meet the standards of health as established by the WHO definition. However, when viewed from the perspective of the health–illness continuum, people with chronic illness or disability can be understood as having the potential to attain a high level of wellness, if they are successful in meeting their health potential within the limits of their chronic illness or disability.

WELLNESS

Wellness has been defined as being equivalent to health. Cookfair (1996) indicated that wellness "includes a conscious and deliberate approach to an advanced state of physical, psychological, and spiritual health and is a dynamic, fluctuating state of being" (p. 149). Leddy and Pepper (1998) contended that wellness is indicated by the capacity of the person to perform to the best of his or her ability, the ability to adjust and adapt to varying situations, a reported feeling of well-being, and a feeling that "everything is together" and harmonious. With this in mind, it becomes evident that the goal of health care providers is to promote positive changes that are directed toward health and well-being. The fact that the sense of wellness has a subjective aspect emphasizes the importance of recognizing and responding to patient individuality and diversity in health care and nursing.

HEALTH PROMOTION

In Canada, the 1974 report *A New Perspective on the Health of Canadians*, also commonly known as the Lalonde Report, brought to the forefront the concept of health promotion. This report suggested that medical care was not the most important determinant of health and that changes in lifestyle and environment would play the greatest role in improving the health of populations. During the 1970s, strategies for health promotion were focussed on health education and mass communication. However, some Canadian and American authors became critical of the health education model and argued that a more social view of health was needed (O'Neil & Pederson, 1994).

The World Health Organization and Canada played a central role in creating a new vision of health promotion that clearly recognizes that social factors are paramount to the health of populations. In 1986, Canada hosted the first international conference on health promotion at which was promulgated the Ottawa Charter for Health Promotion. In this charter, health promotion is defined as:

> …. the process of enabling people to increase control over, and to improve, their health. To reach a state of complete physical, mental, social well being, an individual or group must be able to identify and to realize aspirations, to satisfy needs, and to change or cope with the environment. Health is therefore seen as a resource for everyday life, not the objective of living. Health is a positive concept emphasizing social and personal resources, as well as physical capacities. Therefore, health promotion is not just the responsibility of the health sector, but goes beyond healthy lifestyles to well being (WHO, 1986, p.1).

The "new" health promotion recognizes that a series of factors known as determinants of health have a profound impact on the health of individuals and populations. These factors are income and social status, social support networks, employment and working conditions, education, physical environment, social environment, biology and genetic endowment, personal health practices and coping skills, healthy child development, health services, gender, and culture (Public Health Agency of Canada, 2003).

PRIMARY HEALTH CARE

The primary health care (PHC) model, first introduced by the Alma-Ata Declaration of 1978, is important in the Canadian context, especially because there is a renewed interest by governments, who see it as a way to sustain our publicly funded health care system (Ogilvie & Reutter, 2003). It is also very congruent with the Principles of the Canada Health Act. Primary health care is defined as:

> Essential health care based on acceptable methods made universally accessible to individuals and families in the community through their full participation and at a cost that the community and country can afford to maintain at every stage of their development in the spirit of self-reliance and self-determination. It forms an integral part of both the country's health system, of which it is the central function and main focus, and of the overall social and economic development of the community. It is the first level of contact of individuals, the family and community with the national health system bringing health care as close as possible to where people live and work, and constitutes the first element of a continuing health care process (WHO, 1988, p. 8).

Primary health care is based on five principles which are seen as essential if a nation wishes to improve the health of its population: services must be accessibility to the population, this population must be involved in the planning and operation of services, intersectoral and interdisciplinary collaboration are essential because determinants of health cannot be addressed by one type of provider alone and by only the health care sector, technologies must be adapted to the given context, and a focus on health promotion and prevention of illness and injury must be present (Ogilvie & Reutter, 2003; Vollman, Anderson, & McFarlane, 2004).

Influences on Health Care Delivery

The health care delivery system is rapidly changing as the population and its health care needs and expectations change. The shifting demographics of the population, the increase in chronic illnesses and disability, the greater emphasis on economics, and technological advances have resulted in changing emphases in health care delivery and in nursing.

POPULATION DEMOGRAPHICS

Changes in the population in general are affecting the need for and the delivery of health care. The 2001 Canadian census data indicated that there were 30,007,094 people in the country (Statistics Canada, 2001). This population expansion is attributed in part to improved public health services and improved nutrition.

Not only is the population increasing, but the composition of the population is also changing. The decline in birth rate and the increase in life span attributed to improved health care have resulted in fewer school-age children and more senior citizens, most of whom are women. Much of the population resides in urban areas, with a steady migration of minority groups to the inner cities and a migration of middle-class people to suburban areas. Homelessness is an increasing problem, particularly in urban areas. The population has become more culturally diverse as increasing numbers of people from different national backgrounds enter the country. Because of such population changes, the need for health care for specific age groups, for women, and for a diverse group of people within specific geographic locations is bringing new challenges that must be addressed using a multisectoral approach.

Aging Population

The elderly population in Canada has increased significantly and will continue to grow in future years. "In 2001, one Canadian in eight was aged 65 years or over. By 2026, one Canadian in five will have reached 65" (Health Canada, 2002, p.1). In 1995, there were 3.5 million senior citizens in Canada; it is estimated that by 2021 this segment of the population will reach 6.9 million. The number of very old Canadians has also increased significantly. "In 2001, over 430,000 Canadians were 85 years of age or older—more than twice as many as in 1981, and more than twenty times as many as in 1921" (Health Canada, 2002, p. 3).

Although older Canadians view their health as good, more than one in four has long-term health problems that restrict their activities. "In 1996-97, activity limitations affected slightly more than one fifth of seniors aged 65 to 74, but nearly half of seniors aged 85 or more" (Health Canada, 2002, p. 9). The conditions of elderly women, who represent 70% of seniors aged 85 and above (Health Canada, 2002), are frequently underdiagnosed and untreated. Providing health services to older people requires a comprehensive approach. As the Canadian population continues to age, it will become increasingly imperative to provide services that make it easier for older people to remain in their home and continue to have fulfilling lives.

Cultural Diversity

An appreciation for the diverse characteristics and needs of individuals from varied ethnic and cultural backgrounds is important in health care and nursing. In the 1996 census, 44% of the Canadian population reported at least one ethnic origin other than British, French, or Canadian (Leman, 1999). It has also been projected that by 2016, visible minorities will constitute close to 20% of the population (Beaujot, 2004). As the cultural composition of the population changes, it becomes increasingly important to address cultural considerations in the delivery of health care. Patients from diverse sociocultural groups bring to the health care setting different health care beliefs, values, and practices, as well as different risk factors for some disease conditions and unique reactions to treatment. These factors significantly affect the way an individual responds to health care problems or illness, to those who provide the care, and to the care itself. Unless these factors are understood and respected by health care providers, the care delivered may be ineffective and health care outcomes may be negatively affected.

Culture is defined as learned patterns of behaviour, beliefs, and values that can be attributed to a particular group of people. Included among the many characteristics that distinguish cultural groups are the manner of dress, language spoken, values, rules or norms of behaviour, gender-specific practices, economics, politics, law and social control, artefacts, technology, dietary practices, and health beliefs and practices.

Health promotion, illness prevention, causes of sickness, treatment, coping, caring, dying, and death are part of the health-related component of every culture. Every person has a unique belief and value system that has been shaped at least in part by his or her cultural environment. This belief and value system is very important and guides the individual's thinking, decisions, and actions. It provides direction for interpreting and responding to illness and to health care.

To promote an effective nurse–patient relationship and positive outcomes of care, nursing care must be culturally competent, appropriate, and sensitive to cultural differences. All attempts should be made to help the individual retain his or her unique cultural characteristics. Providing special foods that have significance and arranging for special religious observances may enable the patient to maintain a feeling of wholeness at a time when he or she may feel isolated from family and community.

Knowing the cultural and social significance that particular situations have for each patient helps the nurse avoid imposing a personal value system when the patient has a different point of view. In most cases, cooperation with the plan of care is greatest when communication among the nurse, the patient, and the patient's family is directed toward understanding the situation or the problem and respecting each other's goals.

CHANGING PATTERNS OF DISEASE

During the past 50 years, the health problems of Canadians have changed significantly. Many infectious diseases have been controlled or eradicated; others, such as tuberculosis, acquired immunodeficiency syndrome (AIDS), and sexually transmitted diseases, are on the rise. An increasing number of infectious agents are becoming resistant to antibiotic therapy as a result of widespread inappropriate use of antibiotics. Therefore, conditions that were once easily treated have become complex and more life-threatening than ever before.

Noncommunicable diseases are the main cause of disease in Canada (Centre for Chronic Disease and Prevention Control of the Public Health Agency of Canada, 2005). The chronicity of illnesses and disability is increasing because of the lengthening life span of Canadians and the expansion of successful treatment options for conditions such as cancer, human immunodeficiency virus (HIV) infection, and spina bifida; many people with these conditions live decades longer than in earlier years. Because the majority of health problems seen today are chronic in nature, many people are learning to protect and maximize their health within the constraints of chronic illness and disability.

As chronic conditions increase, health care broadens from a focus on cure and eradication of disease to include the prevention or rapid treatment of exacerbations of chronic conditions. Nursing, which has always encouraged patients to take control of their conditions, plays a prominent role in the current focus on management of chronic illness and disability.

ADVANCES IN TECHNOLOGY AND GENETICS

Advances in technology and genetics have occurred with greater frequency during the past several decades than in all other periods of civilization. Sophisticated techniques and devices have revolutionized surgery and diagnostic testing, making it possible to perform many procedures and tests on an outpatient basis. Increased knowledge and understanding of genetics has resulted in expanded screening, diagnostic testing, and treatments for a variety of conditions. This is also an era of sophisticated communication systems that connect most parts of the world, with the capability of rapid storage, retrieval, and dissemination of information. Such scientific and technological advances are themselves stimulating brisk change as well as swift obsolescence in health care delivery strategies. The advances in technology and genetics have raised many ethical issues for the health care system, health care providers, and society.

ECONOMIC PRESSURES

In the 1990s, the continuing rise in health care expenditures pushed governments to find ways to reduce spending and consider reforms. This period was marked in many provinces by downsizing and restructuring. It is in this context that provincial and federal governments engaged in studies about the health care system, which resulted in the publication of major reports such as the Romanow Report (Commission on the Future of Health Care in Canada, 2002), the Kirby Report (Standing Senate Committee, 2002), and the Mazankowski Report (Alberta Premier's Advisory Council, 2001), to name a few. These reports and the need to find innovative solutions have continued to fuel the debate about the financing of health care services and the extent to which it may be advantageous or disadvantageous to contract out or privatize some of the services.

DEMAND FOR QUALITY CARE

The general public has become increasingly interested in and knowledgeable about health care and health promotion. This awareness has been stimulated by television, newspapers, magazines, and other communications media and by political debate.

The public desires care that is both personalized and delivered in a timely manner. Over the last three decades, new systems of quality insurance and delivery have gradually emerged. Three of them—continuous quality improvement and evidence-based practice, clinical pathways and care mapping, and case management—are discussed in more detail.

Continuous Quality Improvement and Evidence-Based Practice

Seeking to ensure the quality of patient care, Canadian hospitals have adopted over time various methods aimed at improving quality. The adoption of these methods has also been linked with the aim of meeting accreditation standards. Since 1958, the Canadian Council on Health Services Accreditation, formerly known as the Canadian Council on Hospital Accreditation, has the mandate to provide accreditation programs. In the 1970s and the 1980s, the presence of a QA program was one of its standards of accreditation. Although well intentioned, QA programs were found to have limitations including, for example, their cost-effectiveness and their department-specific focus, which limited opportunities for interdisciplinary involvement to solve problems needing the involvement of more than a single discipline. In light of this, in the early 1990s, attention shifted from achieving predetermined standards to using processes of continuous quality improvement (Cummings, 2003).

Continuous quality improvement (CQI) emphasizes the importance of improving the care processes used by organizations, that improvement must be continuous, that customers must be the focus, that leaders must be committed, that staff education is essential to ensure a motivated workforce, and that cultural transformation is a long-term proposition. In contrast with QA, which was department and disciplinary focused, CQI is system-wide and interdisciplinary. The principles of quality improvement are recognized in the current accreditation standards of the Canadian Council on Health Services Accreditation (Cummings, 2003).

If care is to be of the best possible quality and continuously improve, it follows that practice must be based on evidence. In other words, health professionals must incorporate the latest research findings in their practice. However, it is increasingly recognized that health professionals face challenges in locating and using research findings. This is why research on knowledge utilization and knowledge transfer is such a growing field of research and why The Centre for Knowledge Transfer was created. This centre is a partnership between l'Université Laval and the Universities of Manitoba, Saskatchewan, and Alberta.

Clinical Pathways and Care Mapping

First developed in the United States, the use of clinical pathways, or care mapping, is increasingly common in Canada. Clinical pathways serve as an interdisciplinary care plan and as the tool for tracking a patient's progress toward achieving positive outcomes within specified time frames. Clinical pathways have been developed for certain diagnoses (eg, open heart surgery, pneumonia with comorbidity, fractured hip), for high-risk patients (eg, those receiving chemotherapy), and for patients with certain common health problems (eg, diabetes, chronic pain). Using current literature and expertise, pathways identify best care. The pathway indicates key events, such as diagnostic tests, treatments, activities, medications, consultation, and education, that must occur within specified times for the patient to achieve the desired and timely outcomes.

Nurses providing direct care have an important role in the development and use of clinical pathways through their participation in researching the literature and then developing, piloting, implementing, and revising clinical pathways. In addition, nurses monitor outcome achievement and document and analyze variances. Examples of clinical pathways can be found in Appendix A.

Care mapping, multidisciplinary action plans (MAPs), clinical guidelines, and algorithms are other evidence-based practice tools that are used for interdisciplinary care planning. These tools are used to move patients toward predetermined outcome markers using phases and stages of the disease or condition. Algorithms are used more often in an acute situation to determine a particular treatment based on patient information or response. Care maps, clinical guidelines, and MAPs (the most detailed of all tools) provide coordination of care and education through hospitalization and after discharge (Cesta & Falter, 1999).

Because care mapping and guidelines are used for conditions in which the patient's progression often defies prediction, specific time frames for achieving outcomes are excluded. Patients with highly complex conditions or multiple underlying illnesses may benefit more from care mapping or guidelines than from clinical pathways, because the use of outcome markers (rather than specific time frames) is more realistic in such cases.

Through case management and the use of clinical pathways or care mapping, patients and the care they receive are continually assessed from preadmission to discharge—and in many cases after discharge in the home care and community settings. These tools are used in hospitals and alternative health care delivery systems to facilitate the effective and efficient care of large groups of patients. The resultant continuity of care, effective utilization of services, and cost containment are expected to be major benefits for society and for the health care system.

Case Management

Case management is a prominent method for coordinating health care services to ensure cost-effectiveness, accountability, and quality care. Case management has been defined as interventions "… undertaken to facilitate access to, and integration of, services, including assessment, planning, coordination, delivery, and monitoring of the services that are provided to individuals and families" (Smith, Smith, Newhook, et al., 2006, p. 92). The case management process dates back to the public health programs of the early 1900s, in which public health nursing played a dominant role. Over the years, the process has varied in form and function, but the basic theme has remained. The premise of case management is that the responsibility for meeting patient needs rests with one individual or team whose goals are to provide the patient and family with access to required services, to ensure coordination of these services, and to evaluate how effectively these services are delivered.

Since the 1980s, case management has become prominent in American hospitals. In Canada, case management is primarily used for care delivered in the community, such as home care services, and it is expanding as the shift to community-based care continues. Nurses or other members of the health care team (eg, occupational therapists or social workers) serve as case managers. Case managers may cumulate a variety of roles, depending on the way in which services are organized in a health region. Case managers may be responsible for the care of individual clients or groups of clients, and they may also have responsibility at the level of program, organizations, or service-delivery systems. A case manager may serve as clinical expert, facilitator, coordinator, liaison, supporter, educator, researcher, negotiator, monitor, advocate, and manager (Smith, Smith, Newhook, et al., 2006).

Roles of the Nurse

As stated earlier, nursing is the diagnosis and treatment of human responses to health and illness and therefore focuses on a broad array of phenomena. There are three major roles assumed by the nurse when caring for patients. These roles are often used in concert with one another to provide comprehensive care.

The professional nurse in institutional, community-based or public health, and home care settings has three major roles: the practitioner role, which includes teaching and collaborating; the leadership role; and the research role. Although each role carries specific responsibilities, these roles relate to one another and are found in all nursing positions. These roles are designed to meet the immediate and future health care and nursing needs of consumers who are the recipients of nursing care.

PRACTITIONER ROLE

The practitioner role of the nurse involves those actions that the nurse takes when assuming responsibility for meeting the health care and nursing needs of individual patients, their families, and significant others. This role is the dominant role of nurses in primary, secondary, and tertiary health care settings and in home care and community nursing. It is a role that can be achieved only through use of the nursing process, the basis for all nursing practice. The nurse helps patients meet their needs through direct intervention, by teaching patients and family members to perform care, and by coordinating and collaborating with other disciplines to provide needed services.

LEADERSHIP ROLE

The leadership role of the nurse has traditionally been perceived as a specialized role assumed only by those nurses who have titles that suggest leadership and who are the leaders of large groups of nurses or related health care professionals. However, the constant fluctuation of health care delivery demands and consumers requires a broader definition of nursing leadership, one that identifies the leadership role as inherent within all nursing positions. The leadership role of the nurse involves those actions the nurse executes when assuming responsibility for the actions of others that are directed toward determining and achieving patient care goals.

Nursing leadership is a process involving four components: decision making, relating, influencing, and facilitating. Each of these components promotes change and the ultimate outcome of goal achievement. Basic to the entire process is effective communication, which determines the accomplishment of the process. Leadership in nursing is a process in which the nurse uses interpersonal skills to effect change in the behaviour of others. The components of the leadership process are appropriate during all phases of the nursing process and in all settings.

RESEARCH ROLE

The research role of the nurse was traditionally viewed as one carried out only by academicians, nurse scientists, and graduate nursing students. Today, participation in the research process is also considered to be a responsibility of nurses in clinical practice.

The primary task of nursing research is to contribute to the scientific base of nursing practice. Studies are needed to determine the effectiveness of nursing interventions and nursing care. Through such research efforts, the science of nursing will grow and a scientifically based rationale for making changes in nursing practice and patient care will be generated. Evidence-based practice will be facilitated, with a resultant increase in the quality of patient care.

Nurses who have preparation in research methods can use their research knowledge and skills to initiate and implement timely, relevant studies. This is not to say that nurses who do not initiate and implement nursing research studies do not play a significant role in nursing research. Every nurse has valuable contributions to make to nursing research and a responsibility to make these contributions. All nurses must constantly be alert for nursing problems and important issues related to patient care that can serve as a basis for the identification of researchable questions.

Those nurses directly involved in patient care are often in the best position to identify potential research problems and questions. Their clinical insights are invaluable. Nurses also have a responsibility to become actively involved in ongoing research studies. This participation may involve facilitating the data collection process, or it may include actual collection of data. Explaining the study to other health care professionals or to patients and their families is often of invaluable assistance to the nurse who is conducting the study.

Above all, nurses must use research findings in their nursing practice. Research for the sake of research alone is meaningless. As stated previously, evidence-based practice requires the inclusion of valid research. Only with the use and evaluation of research findings in nursing practice will the science of nursing be furthered. Research findings can be substantiated only through use, validation, replication, and dissemination. Nurses must continually be aware of studies that are directly related to their own area of clinical practice and critically analyze those studies to determine the applicability of their conclusions and the implications for specific patient populations. Relevant conclusions and implications can be used to improve patient care.

Models of Nursing Care Delivery

Nursing care can be carried out through a variety of organizational methods. The model of nursing care used varies greatly from one facility to another and from one set of patient circumstances to another. A review of *selected* models provides a background for understanding models of nursing care deliveries that may be encountered in practice. It must be understood that health care agencies may use elements of a variety of models in the actual delivery of care.

TEAM NURSING

Team nursing was developed in the 1950s "…to ease the pressure of nursing shortages following WWII and to find ways of integrating auxiliary health care personnel trained by the military during the war into the civilian system" (Smith, Smith, Boechler, et al., 2006, p. 215). It involved the use of a team leader and team members to provide various aspects of nursing care to a group of patients. In team nursing, medications might be given by one nurse, whereas baths and physical care are given by nursing assistants under the supervision of a nurse team leader. Skill mixes include registered nurses (RNs), often as team leaders; licensed practical nurses (LPNs); and nursing assistants or unlicensed aides. As part of the current emphasis on cost containment in health care agencies, variations of team nursing are sometime used. There has been little substantiation, however, that team nursing is cost effective. As noted by Smith, Smith, Boechler and colleagues (2006), the use of different workers to provide different aspects of the care of one patient may lead to fragmentation.

PRIMARY NURSING

Primary nursing (not to be confused with primary health care; see earlier in this chapter) refers to individualized care provided by the same nurse throughout the period of care. It was developed in the 1960s and 1970s as the number of baccalaureate-prepared nurses was increasing and work satisfaction for RNs was an important issue in that period of shortages. This model reduces fragmentation of care and provides a more holistic approach to care (Smith, Smith, Boechler, et al., 2006). This type of nursing allows the nurse to give direct patient care rather than manage and supervise the functions of others who provide direct care to patients.

The primary nurse accepts total 24-hour responsibility for a patient's nursing care. Nursing care is directed toward meeting all of the individualized patient needs. The primary nurse is responsible and accountable for involving the patient and family directly in all facets of care and has autonomy in making decisions in this regard. When the primary nurse is not on duty, associate nurses provide care to the patient using the plan of care designed by the primary nurse (Manthey, 2003). This process promotes continuity of care and collaborative efforts directed toward quality patient care.

The long-term survival of primary nursing as it is currently designed is uncertain. As cost-containment measures continue and patient acuity increases, staffing ratios of patients to nurses are increasing. Many nursing service departments and agencies are meeting the increased workload demands by making modifications in their approach to primary nursing or by reverting to team or functional systems for delivering care. Others are changing their staffing mix and redesigning their models of practice to accommodate nurse-extender roles.

COMMUNITY-BASED NURSING AND COMMUNITY HEALTH– PUBLIC HEALTH NURSING

Canadian nurses have always played a vital role in the provision of services to the community. At different times in our history, religious nursing orders, public health nurses, district nurses, members of the Victorian Order of Nurses, and home care nurses have provided nursing services in the community. Although community health nursing (CH), public health nursing (PH), and community-based nursing such as home care may be discussed together and aspects of care in each type do overlap, there are distinctions among these terms. Confusion exists regarding the differences, and the similar settings may blur these distinctions (Hunt, 2000; Kovner, 2001). The central idea of CH-PH nursing is that nursing intervention can promote wellness, reduce the spread of illness, and improve the health status of groups of citizens. CH-PH nursing practice is concerned with the general and comprehensive care of the community at large, with emphasis on primary, secondary, and tertiary prevention. Nurses in these settings have traditionally focused on health promotion, maternal and child health, and chronic care.

Community-based nursing occurs in a variety of settings within the community and is directed toward individuals and families

(Hunt, 2000). It includes home health care nursing. Most community-based and home health care is directed toward specific patient groups with identified needs; these needs usually relate to illness, injury, or disability resulting most often from advanced age or chronic illness. However, both community-based and CH-PH nurses are now expanding to meet the needs of many groups of patients with a variety of problems and needs. Home health care will be a major aspect of community-based care discussed throughout this text. Home health care services are provided by community-based programs and agencies for specific populations (eg, the elderly, ventilator-dependent patients).

As trends continue toward shortened hospital stays and increased use of outpatient health care services, the need for nursing care in the home and community setting has increased dramatically. Because nursing services are being provided outside as well as within the hospital, nurses have a choice of practicing in a variety of health care delivery settings. These settings include acute care medi-centres, ambulatory care settings, community health centres, CLSCs (Centre local de services communautaires of Quebec), home care services, and home care agencies.

The numbers and kinds of agencies that provide care in the home and community have expanded because of the expanding needs of patients requiring care. Home health care nurses are challenged because patients are discharged from acute care institutions to their homes and communities early in the recovery process and with more complex needs. Many are elderly, and many have multiple medical and nursing diagnoses and multisystem health problems that require acute and intensive nursing care. Medical technologies such as ventilatory support and intravenous or parenteral nutrition therapy, once limited to acute care settings, have been adapted to the home care setting.

As a result, the community-based setting is becoming an increasingly important area of nursing practice. Home care nursing requires advanced knowledge and skills in general nursing practice, with emphasis on community health and acute medical-surgical nursing. Also required are high-level assessment skills, critical thinking, and decision-making skills in a setting where other health care professionals are not available to validate observations, conclusions, and decisions.

Home care nurses often function as acute care nurses in the home, providing "high-tech, high-touch" services to patients with acute health care needs. In addition, they are responsible for patient and family teaching and for contacting community resources and coordinating the continuing care of the patient. For these reasons, the scope of medical-surgical nursing encompasses not only the acute care setting within the hospital but also the acute care setting as it expands into the community and the home. Throughout this textbook, emphasis is placed on the home health care needs of patients, with particular attention given to the teaching, self-care management, and health maintenance needs of patients and their families.

Advanced Nursing Practice

Professional nursing is adapting to meet changing health needs and expectations. One such adaptation is through advanced nursing practice, which has developed to better respond to the needs of the population. The nurse who functions in an advanced practice role provides direct care to patients through independent practice, practice within a health care agency, or collaboration with a physician. Specialization has evolved within the expanded roles of nursing as a result of the recent explosion of technology and knowledge.

Nurses may receive advanced education in such specialties as family, critical care, coronary care, respiratory care, oncologic care, maternal and child health care, neonatal intensive care, rehabilitation, trauma, rural health, and gerontologic nursing, to name just a few. With the expanded role of the nurse, various titles have emerged that attempt to specify the functions as well as the educational preparation of nurses, although functions are less distinct than in previous years. In medical-surgical nursing, the most significant of these titles are *nurse practitioner* and *clinical nurse specialist,* and the more recent title of *advanced practice nurse,* which encompasses both NPs and CNSs.

The International Council of Nurses defines a nurse practitioner as "a registered nurse who has acquired the expert knowledge base, complex decision-making skills and clinical competencies for expanded practice, the characteristics of which are shaped by the context and/or country in which s/he is credentialed to practice" (ICN, 2002, p.1). In Canada, the level of education required to work as a nurse practitioner varies from province to province. Increasingly, however, nurse practitioners are prepared at the master's level. The Canadian Institute for Health Information (2003) estimated that in 2002, there were 912 nurse practitioners in Canada.

Nurses who worked in remote northern areas were among the first nurses to practice in an advanced practice role, well before the advent of the term nurse practitioner. In the more populated southern areas of the country, the introduction of nurse practitioners remains relatively new, and this form of nursing practice is certainly not as common as in the United States.

Clinical nurse specialists are normally prepared at the master's level. They define their role as having five major components: clinical practice, education, management, consultation, and research. CNSs practice in a variety of settings, including the community and the home, although most practice in acute care settings.

With advanced practice roles has come a continuing effort by professional nursing organizations to define more clearly the practice of nursing. Provincial legislations regulating nursing practice have had to be amended or clarified to make room for some of these roles. Although there are variations from province to province, it is clear that the health care system is increasingly seeking to employ nurses in advanced practice roles.

In general, initial care, ambulatory health care, and anticipatory guidance are all becoming increasingly important in nursing practice. Advanced practice roles enable nurses to function interdependently with other health care professionals and to establish a more collegial relationship with physicians. As changes in health care continue, the role of advanced practice nurses, especially in primary care settings, is expected to increase in terms of scope, responsibility, and recognition.

INTERDISCIPLINARY PRACTICE

Throughout this chapter, we have explored key concepts related to health, health care, and nursing. As the unique competencies of nurses are becoming more clearly articulated, there is increasing evidence that nurses provide certain health care services distinct to the profession. However, it should be clear, particularly if one takes into account health promotion, the determinants of health, and the principles of primary health care, that nurses must be actively engaged in interdisciplinary practice and contribute to intersectoral activities. The importance of interdisciplinary practice has been well recognized by the Canadian Nurses Association and by provincial regulatory bodies, who include it in their documents outlining competencies of registered nurses and new graduates of nursing programs.

 Critical Thinking Exercises

1. Your clinical assignment is on a cardiac care step-down nursing unit in an acute care hospital. Identify a patient care issue (eg, family support) that could be improved. Describe the mechanism that is available within the hospital to address such quality improvement issues.

2. You are planning the discharge of an elderly patient who has several chronic medical conditions. A case manager has been assigned to this patient. How would you explain the role of the case manager to the patient and her husband?

REFERENCES AND SELECTED READINGS
Books
Alberta Premier's Advisory Council on Health. (2001). *A framework for reform: Report of the Premier's Advisory Council on Health.* Edmonton: Author.

American Nurses Association. (1995). *Nursing's social policy statement.* Washington, DC: Author.

American Nurses Association. (1991). *Nursing's agenda for health care reform.* Kansas City, MO: Author.

Beaujot, R. P. (2004). Immigration and demographic structures. In E. Cameron (Ed.), *Multiculturalism & immigration in Canada: An introductory reader* (pp. 193–206). Toronto, ON: Canadian Scholars Press Inc.

Canadian Institute for Health Information. (2003). *Workforce trends of registered nurses in Canada, 2002.* Ottawa, ON: Author.

Canadian Nurses Association. (1987). *A definition of nursing practice: Standards for nursing practice.* Ottawa, ON: Author.

Canadian Nurses Association. (2002). *Canadian Nurses Association code of ethics for registered nurses.* Ottawa, ON: Author.

Cookfair, J. M. (1996). *Nursing care in the community.* St. Louis: Mosby–Year Book.

Commission on the Future of Health Care in Canada. (2002). *Building on values: The future of health care in Canada.* Saskatoon: Author.

Cummings, G. (2003). Quality of care: From quality assurance to continuous quality improvement. In J. C. Ross-Kerr & M. J. Wood (Eds.), *Canadian nursing issues and perspectives* (4th ed., pp. 177–194). Toronto, ON: Mosby.

Health Canada. (1992). *Canada Health Act annual report.* Ottawa, ON: Author.

Health Canada, Division of Aging and Seniors. (2002). *Canada's aging population.* Ottawa, ON: Author.

Hood, L., & Leddy, S. K. (2002). *Leddy & Pepper's conceptual bases of professional nursing* (5th ed.). Philadelphia: Lippincott Williams & Wilkins.

Hunt, R. (2000). *Readings in community-based nursing.* Philadelphia: Lippincott Williams & Wilkins.

Krozok, C., & Scoggins, A. (2001). *Patient rights . . . amended to comply with JCAHO standards.* Glendale, CA: CINAHL Information Systems.

National League for Nursing. (1977). *Nursing's role in patients' rights.* New York: Author.

Ogilvie, L., & Reutter, L. (2003). Primary health care: Complexities and possibilities from a nursing perspective. In J. C. Ross-Kerr & M. J. Wood (Eds.), *Canadian nursing issues and perspectives* (4th ed., pp. 441–465). Toronto, ON: Mosby.

O'Neil, M., & Pederson, A. (1994). Two analytical paths for understanding Canadian development in health promotion. In A. Perderson, M. O'Neil, & I. Rootman (Eds.), *Health promotion in Canada.* (pp. 40–55). Toronto, ON: W.B. Saunders.

Ross-Kerr, J. C. (2003). Issues in the organization and financing of health care. In J. C. Ross-Kerr & M. J. Wood (Eds.), *Canadian nursing issues and perspectives* (4th ed., pp. 254–268). Toronto, ON: Mosby.

Smith, D. L., Smith, J. E., Boechler, V., et al. (2006). Structure and organization of nurses' work. In J. M. Hibberd & D. L. Smith (Eds.),

Nursing leadership and management in Canada. (3rd ed., pp. 199–237). Toronto, ON: Elsevier Canada.

Smith, D. L., Smith, J. E., Newhook, C., et al. (2006). Continuity of care, service integration, and case management. In J. M. Hibberd and D. L. Smith (Eds.), *Nursing leadership and management in Canada.* (3rd ed., pp. 81–112). Toronto, ON: Elsevier Canada.

The Standing Senate Committee on Social Affairs, Science and Technology. (2003). *Reforming health protection and promotion in Canada: Time to act.* Ottowa: Author.

Vollman, A. R., Anderson, E. T., & McFarlane, J. (2004). *Canadian community as partner.* Philadelphia: Lippincott Williams & Wilkins.

World Health Organization. (1986). *Ottawa charter for health promotion.* Geneva: Author.

World Health Organization. (1988). *From Alma-Ata to the year 2000. Reflections at the midpoint.* Geneva: Author.

Journals

Boyd, L. (2000). Advanced practice nursing today. *RN, 63*(9), 57–62.

Centre for Chronic Disease Prevention and Control of the Public Health Agency of Canada. (2005). *Integrated approach to chronic disease.* Available at: http://www.pahc-aspc.gc.ca/ccdpc-cpcmc/index_e.html. Retrieved September 15, 2005.

Cesta, T. G., & Falter, E. J. (1999). Case management. *American Journal of Nursing, 99*(5), 48–51.

International Council of Nurses. (n.d.). *The ICN definition of nursing.* Available at: http//www.icn.ch/abouticn.htm. Retrieved June 15, 2005.

International Council of Nurses. (2002). ICN announces position on advanced nursing roles. Available at: http://www.icn/ch/pr19_02.htm. Retrieved June 15, 2005.

Klenner, S. (2000). Mapping out a clinical pathway. *RN, 63*(6), 33–36.

Kovner, C. (2001). Counting nurses: What is community health-public health nursing? *American Journal of Nursing, 101*(1), 59–60.

Leman, M. (1999). *Canadian multiculturalism.* Available at: http://www.parl.gc.ca/information/library/PRBpubs/963-e.htm.

Manthey, M. (2003). Aka primary nursing. [Guest editorial.] *Journal of Nursing Administration, 33*(7/8), 369–370.

Public Health Agency of Canada. (2003). *What determines health?* Available at: http://www.phac-aspc.gc.ca/phdd/determinants/index.html. Retrieved January 14, 2006.

Smith-Campbell, B. (2000). Across to health care: Effects of public funding of the uninsured. *Journal of Nursing Scholarship, 32*(3), 295–300.

Statistics Canada. (2005). *2001 Census of Canada.* Available at: http://www.12.statcan.ca/english/census01/home/index.cfm. Retrieved January 14, 2006.

RESOURCES AND WEBSITES

Canadian Nurses Association/Association des infirmières et infirmiers du Canada, 50 Driveway, Ottawa, ON K2P 1E2; www.cna-nurses.ca.

Health Canada, Division of Aging and Seniors; http://www.hc-sc.gc.ca/seniors-aines.

The Centre for Knowledge Transfer; http://www.ckt-ctc.ca.

Community-Based Nursing Practice

Adapted by Joanne K. Olson

LEARNING OBJECTIVES

On completion of this chapter, the learner will be able to:

1. Discuss the changes in the health care system that have increased the need for medical-surgical nurses to practice in community-based settings.

2. Compare the differences and similarities between community-based and hospital nursing.

3. Describe the discharge planning process in relation to home care preparation.

4. Explain methods for identifying community resources and making referrals.

5. Discuss how to prepare for a home health care visit and how to conduct the visit.

6. Identify personal safety precautions a home care nurse should take when making home visits.

7. Describe the various types of nursing functions provided in ambulatory care facilities, in occupational health and school nursing programs, and to the homeless.

*T*he changes that have occurred in the health care system in the past two decades have increased the need for care in ambulatory settings and in the home. These changes have created a demand for highly skilled and well-prepared nurses to provide community-based care.

The Growing Need for Community-Based Health Care

The delivery of community health care occurs within the Canadian health care system, also known as *Medicare.* This system reflects the values that define Canadian culture: social justice, equity, and community. Guided by the *Canada Health Act,* passed in 1984, the system is based on the fundamental principle that all members of Canadian society, including the most vulnerable, are entitled to health care. Within the Canadian health care system, there has recently been a trend toward more health care being delivered within communities. This shift is partly due to ongoing implementation of a long-held Canadian belief that health promotion services are a critical component of the country's health care system. The more recent factors contributing to this trend are earlier hospital discharge, hospital bed closures, and an increase in the technology that makes home care more possible (Falk-Rafael & Coffey, 2005).

As more health care delivery shifts into the community, more nurses are working in a variety of public health and community-based settings. These settings include public health departments, ambulatory health clinics, long-term care facilities, prenatal and well-baby clinics, hospice agencies, industrial settings (as occupational nurses), homeless shelters and clinics, nursing centres, home health agencies, urgent care centres, same day surgical centres, short-stay facilities, and patients' homes.

Nurses in these settings often deliver care without direct on-site supervision or the support of other health care personnel. They must be self-directed, flexible, adaptable, and tolerant of various lifestyles and living conditions. Expertise in independent decision making, critical thinking, assessment, and health education, and competence in basic nursing care are essential to function effectively in the community-based setting (Brown, 2000; Pierson, 1999).

Community-based nursing is a philosophy of care of individuals and families. The care is provided in a community as the individual or family move among various kinds of service providers outside of hospitals (Hunt, 2000). Although the phrase "community-based nursing" is often interchanged with "community health nursing," a distinction should be made. The phrase "community health nursing" has generally been equated to "public health nursing." Public health nursing is a specialty focused on total populations, although care may be given to individuals. Community-based nursing is broader and may incorporate community health–public health nursing; it is focused on individuals and families rather than total populations. Community-based nursing also includes home health nursing, school health nursing, and a host of other nursing services provided to individuals and groups in the community (Fig. 2-1).

COMMUNITY-BASED CARE

Community-based nursing practice focuses on promoting and maintaining the health of individuals and groups, preventing and minimizing the progression of disease, and improving quality of life (Hunt, 2000). Although nursing interventions used by public health nurses may involve individuals, families, or small groups, the

FIGURE 2-1 Community-based nursing takes many forms and focuses. Here the nursing focus is on wellness and the nursing setting is industry. When enlightened employers offer flu vaccines or other health services, the whole community benefits.

central focus remains promotion of health and prevention of disease in the entire community. The actions of community health nurses may include provision of direct care to patients and families as well as political advocacy to secure resources for aggregate populations (eg, the aged population). The community health nurse may function as an epidemiologist, a case manager for a group of patients, a coordinator of services provided to an aggregate of patients, an occupational health nurse, a school nurse, a visiting nurse, or a parish nurse. (In parish nursing, the members of the religious community—the parish—are the recipients of care.) The commonality of these various roles is that the nurse maintains a focus on community needs as well as on the needs of the individual patient. Community-based care is generally focused on the individual or family; although efforts may be undertaken to improve the health of the whole community, the individual or family unit is the main focus. The primary concepts of community-based nursing care are self-care and preventive care within the context of culture and community. Two other important concepts are continuity of care and collaboration (Hunt, 2000). Some community-based nursing fields have become specialties in their own right, such as school health nursing and home health nursing.

Primary, secondary, and tertiary levels of preventive care are used by nurses in community-based practice. The focus of primary prevention is on health promotion and prevention of illness or disease, including interventions such as teaching regarding healthy lifestyles (Hunt, 2000). Secondary prevention centres on health maintenance and is aimed at early detection and prompt intervention to prevent or minimize loss of function and independence; it includes interventions such as health screening and health risk appraisal. Tertiary prevention focuses on minimizing deterioration and improving quality of life. Tertiary care may include rehabilitation to assist patients in achieving their maximum potential by working through their physical or psychological challenges (Hunt, 2000).

HOME HEALTH CARE

Home health care is becoming one of the largest practice areas for nurses. Because of the high acuity level of patients, nurses with acute care and high-technology experience are in demand in this field. Tertiary preventive nursing care, which focuses on rehabilitation and restoring maximum health function, is a major goal for home care nurses, although primary and secondary prevention are also included in care. Health care visits may be intermittent or periodic, and telephonic case management may be used to promote communication with home care consumers.

Home care nursing is a unique aspect of community-based nursing. Home care visits are made by nurses who work for home care agencies, public health agencies, and visiting nurse associations; by nurses who are employed by hospitals; and by parish nurses who voluntarily work with the members of their religious communities to promote health. Such visits may also be part of the responsibilities of school nurses, clinic nurses, or occupational health nurses. The type of nursing services provided to patients in their homes varies from agency to agency. Nurses working for home care or hospice agencies make home visits to provide skilled nursing care, follow-up care, and teaching to promote health and prevent complications. Clinic nurses may conduct home visits as part of patient follow-up. Public health, parish, and school nurses may make visits to provide anticipatory guidance to high-risk families and follow-up care to patients with communicable diseases. Many home care patients are acutely ill, and many have chronic health problems and disabilities, requiring nurses to provide more education and monitoring to the patient and family to facilitate compliance.

Holistic care is provided in the home through the collaboration of a multidisciplinary team that includes professional nurses; home health aides; social workers; physical, speech, and occupational therapists; and the physician (Touchard & Berthelot, 1999). The team provides health and social services with oversight of the total health care plan by a case manager, clinical nurse specialist, or nurse practitioner.

Basic home care services are provided to Canadians through programs operated by territorial or provincial governments. The basic services covered may vary from province to province. Private payment or insurance coverage is therefore sometimes required to cover costs not publicly funded.

The elderly are the most frequent users of home care services. To be eligible for service, the patient must be acutely ill, homebound, and in need of skilled nursing services. Nursing care includes skilled assessment of the patient's physical, psychological, social, and environmental status. Nursing interventions may include intravenous therapy and injections (Fig. 2-2), parenteral nutrition, venipuncture, catheter insertion, pressure ulcer treatment, wound care, ostomy care, and patient and family teaching. The nurse instructs the patient and family in skills and self-care strategies and in health maintenance and promotion activities (eg, nutritional counselling, exercise programs, stress management).

Some nurses manage and evaluate patient care for seriously ill patients who have complex, labile conditions and are at high risk for rehospitalization. The nurse serves as a case manager and monitors the delivery of care provided to patients in their homes.

Hospital and Community-Based Nursing

Providing nursing care in a patient's home is different from providing care in a hospital. Patients must sign a release form to stay and receive treatment in a hospital. They have little control over what happens to them, and they are expected to comply with the hospital's rules, regulations, and schedule of activities. They sleep in the hospital's beds and often wear hospital gowns or clothes. They are given care, treatments, baths, and medications at times that are usually determined by institutional schedules rather than convenience for the patient. Although hospitalized patients may select meals from a daily menu, there is a limited choice in the type of food they are offered. Family members and friends visit during the hospital's visiting hours.

FIGURE 2-2 Intravenous therapy is one of the types of skilled nursing care that may be provided in the home. Courtesy Good Samaritan Certified Home Health Agency, Babylon, New York.

By contrast, the home care nurse is considered a guest in the patient's home and needs permission to visit and give care. The nurse has minimal control over the lifestyle, living situation, and health practices of the patients he or she visits. This lack of full decision-making authority can create a conflict for the nurse and lead to problems in the nurse–patient relationship. To work successfully with patients, no matter what the setting, it is important for the nurse to be nonjudgmental and to convey respect for the patient's beliefs, even if they differ sharply from the nurse's. This can be difficult when a patient's lifestyle involves activities that the nurse considers harmful or unacceptable, such as smoking, use of alcohol, drug abuse, or overeating.

The cleanliness of a patient's home may not meet the standards of a hospital. Although the nurse can provide teaching points about maintaining clean surroundings, the patient and family determine whether they will implement the nurse's suggestions. The nurse must accept the reality of the situation and deliver the care required regardless of the sanitary conditions of the surroundings.

The kind of equipment and the supplies or resources that usually are available in acute care settings are often unavailable in the patient's home. The nurse has to learn to improvise when providing care, such as when changing a dressing or catheterizing a patient in a regular bed that is not adjustable and lacks a bedside table (Johnson, Smith-Temple, & Carr, 1998).

Infection control is as important in the home as it is in the hospital, but it can be more challenging and requires creative approaches. As in any situation, it is important to cleanse one's hands before and after giving direct patient care, even in a home that does not have running water. If aseptic technique is required, the nurse must have a plan for implementing this technique before going to the home. This applies also to standard precautions, transmission-based precautions, and disposal of bodily secretions and excretions.

If injections are given, the nurse should use a closed container to dispose of syringes. Injectable and other medications must be kept out of the reach of children during visits and must be stored in a safe place if they are to remain in the house. Nurses who perform invasive procedures need to be up-to-date with their immunizations, including hepatitis B and tetanus.

The home environment often has more distractions than a hospital. The home can be filled with background noise and crowded with people and objects. A nurse may have to request that the television be turned down during the visit or that the patient move to a more private place to be interviewed.

Friends, neighbors, or family members may ask the nurse about the patient's condition. A patient has a right to confidentiality, and information should be shared only with the patient's permission. If the nurse carries the patient's medical record into the house, it must be put in a secure place to prevent it from being picked up by others or misplaced.

Discharge Planning for Home Care

To prepare for early hospital discharge and the possible need for follow-up care in the home, discharge planning begins with the patient's admission. Several different personnel or agencies may be involved in the planning process. In hospitals, social workers or nurses may serve as the discharge planners. Some home care agencies have liaison nurses who work with discharge planners to ensure that the patient's needs are met when he or she is released from the hospital. Professionals in ambulatory health care settings may refer patients for home care services to prevent hospitalization. Public health nurses care for patients referred for anticipatory guidance with high-risk families, for case finding, and for follow-up treatment (eg, patients with communicable diseases). Parish nurses may have patients referred, or they may be contacted directly by members of the parish community who need guidance or referrals related to physical or psychosocial health care concerns (Palmer, 2001).

The development of a comprehensive discharge plan requires collaboration with professionals at both the referring agency and the home care agency, public health agency, or other community resource. The process involves identifying the patient's needs and developing a thorough plan to meet them. Communication with and cooperation of the patient and family are essential.

Community Resources and Referrals

Home health nurses and public health nurses act as case managers. After assessing the patient's needs, they may make referrals to other team members, such as home health aides and social workers. They work collaboratively with the health team and the agency or person who referred the patient for service. Continuous coordinated care among all health care providers involved in the patient's care is essential to avoid duplication of effort by the various personnel caring for the patient.

Home care and public health nurses are responsible for providing the patient and family with information about other community resources that are available to meet their needs. During the initial and subsequent visits, they help patients identify these community services and encourage the patient and family to contact the appropriate agencies. When appropriate, the nurse makes the initial contact (Pierson, 1999).

A community-based nurse needs to be knowledgeable about community resources available to patients as well as services provided by local agencies, eligibility requirements, and any possible charges for the services. Most communities have directories of health and social service agencies that the nurse can consult. These directories need to be continually updated as resources change. If a community does not have a resource booklet, the agency may develop one for its staff. It should include the commonly used community resources that patients need, the costs of the services, and eligibility requirements. The patient's place of worship or parish may serve as an important resource for services. The telephone book is often a useful resource for helping patients identify the locations of grocery and drug stores, banks, health care facilities, ambulances, physicians, dentists, pharmacists, social service agencies, and senior citizens programs.

Preparing for a Home Visit

Most agencies have a policy manual that states their philosophy and procedures and defines the services they provide. Becoming familiar with these policies is an essential step before initiating a home visit. It is also important to know the agency's policies and the state law regarding what actions to take if the nurse finds a patient dead, encounters an abusive situation in the family, or determines that a patient cannot safely remain at home.

Before making a home visit, the nurse should review the patient's referral form and other pertinent data concerning the patient. It may be necessary to contact the referring agency if the purpose for the referral is unclear or if important information is missing.

The first step is to call the patient to obtain permission to visit, schedule a time for the visit, and verify the address. This initial phone conversation provides an opportunity to introduce oneself, identify the agency, and explain the reason for the visit.

If a patient does not have a telephone, the nurse should see whether those who made the referral have a number where a phone message can be left for the patient. If an unannounced visit must be made to a patient's home, the nurse should ask permission to come in before entering the house. Explaining the purpose of the referral at the outset and setting up the times for future visits before leaving are also recommended approaches.

Most agencies provide nurses with bags that contain standard supplies and equipment needed during home visits. It is important to keep the bag properly supplied and to bring any additional items that might be needed for the visit. Patients usually do not have the medical supplies they need for treatment.

Conducting a Home Visit

PERSONAL SAFETY PRECAUTIONS

Personal safety in community-based nursing practice begins even before making a home visit. Preparation prior to the visit involves personal preparation, agency preparation, and vehicle preparation. Attention to personal safety continues during implementation of the home visit when the nurse attends to environmental surveillance and anticipates responses to situations. A useful tool assessing knowledge and skills about home safety was developed at the University of Alberta in Edmonton (Skillen, Olson, & Gilbert, 2003).

Whenever a nurse makes a home visit, the agency should know the nurse's schedule and the locations of the visits. The nurse should learn about the neighbourhood and obtain directions for reaching the expected destination. A plan of action should always be established in case of emergencies.

Nurses are not expected to disregard their personal safety in an effort to make or complete home visits. If nurses encounter dangerous situations during visits, they should return to their agencies and contact their supervisors or law enforcement officials, or both. Suggested precautions to take when making a home visit are presented in Chart 2-1.

INITIAL HOME VISIT

The first visit sets the tone for subsequent visits and is a crucial step in establishing the nurse–patient relationship. The situations encountered can vary depending on numerous factors. Patients

Chart 2-1 Safety Precautions in Home Health Care

- Learn, or preprogram a cellular phone with the telephone numbers of the agency, police, and emergency services.
- Let the agency know your daily schedule and the telephone numbers of your patients so that you can be located if you do not return when expected.
- Know where the patient lives before leaving to make the visit and carry a map for quick referral.
- Keep your car in good working order and have sufficient gas in the tank.
- Park the car near the patient's home and lock it during the visit.
- Do not drive an expensive car or wear expensive jewelry when making visits.
- Know the regular bus schedule and know the routes when using public transportation or walking to the patient's house.
- Carry agency identification and have enough change to make telephone calls in case you get lost or have problems. Most agencies provide cellular phones for their nurses so that the agency can contact the nurse, and so that the nurse can contact the agency in case of an emergency or unexpected situation.
- When making visits in high-crime areas, visit with another person rather than alone.
- Schedule visits only during daylight hours.
- Never walk into a patient's home uninvited.
- If you do not feel safe entering a patient's home, leave the area.
- Become familiar with the layout of the house, including exits from the house.
- If a patient or family member is intoxicated, hostile, or obnoxious, reschedule the visit and leave.
- If a family is having a serious argument or abusing the patient or anyone else in the household, reschedule the visit, contact your supervisor, and report the abuse to the appropriate authorities.

may be in pain and unable to care for themselves. Families may be overwhelmed and doubt their ability to care for their loved one. They may not understand why the patient was sent home from the hospital before being totally rehabilitated. They may not comprehend what home care is or why they cannot have 24-hour nursing services. It is critical that the nurse try to convey an understanding of what the patient and family are experiencing and how the illness is affecting their lives.

During the initial home visit, which usually lasts less than an hour, the patient is evaluated and a plan of care is established to be followed or modified on subsequent visits. The nurse informs the patient of the agency's practices, policies, and hours of operation.

The initial assessment includes evaluating the patient, the home environment, the patient's self-care abilities or the family's ability to provide care, and the patient's need for additional resources. Identifying possible hazards, such as cluttered walk areas, potential fire risks, air or water pollution, or inadequate sanitation facilities, is also part of the initial assessment.

Documentation considerations for home visits follow fairly specific regulations. The patient's needs and the nursing care given are documented accurately. The medical diagnosis and specific detailed information on the functional limitations of the patient are usually part of the documentation. The goals and the actions appropriate for attaining them need to be identified. Ex-

pected outcomes of the nursing interventions must be stated in terms of patient behaviours and must be realistic and measurable. They must reflect the nursing diagnosis or the patient's problems and must specify those actions that are expected to solve the patient's problems.

DETERMINING THE NEED FOR FUTURE VISITS

While conducting an assessment of the patient's situation, the nurse evaluates the need for future visits and the frequency with which those visits may need to be made. To make these judgments, the nurse may find it helpful to consider the following factors:

- *Current health status:* How well is the patient progressing? How serious are the present signs and symptoms? Has the patient shown signs of progressing as expected, or does it seem that recovery will be delayed?
- *Home environment:* Are worrisome safety factors apparent? Are family or friends available to provide care, or is the patient alone?
- *Level of self-care abilities:* Is the patient capable of self-care? What is the patient's level of independence? Is the patient ambulatory or bedridden? Does the patient have sufficient energy or is he or she frail and easily fatigued?
- *Level of nursing care needed:* What level of nursing care does the patient require? Does the care require basic skills or more complex interventions?
- *Prognosis:* What is the expectation for recovery in this particular instance? What are the chances that complications may develop if nursing care is not provided?
- *Patient education needs:* How well has the patient or family grasped the teaching points made? Is there a need for further follow-up and retraining? What level of proficiency does the patient or family show in carrying out the necessary care?
- *Mental status:* How alert is the patient? Are there signs of confusion or thinking difficulties? Does the patient tend to be forgetful or have a limited attention span?
- *Level of adherence:* Is the patient following the instructions provided? Does the patient seem capable of doing so? Are the family members helpful in this regard, or are they unwilling or unable to assist in caring for the patient as expected?

With each subsequent visit, these same factors are evaluated to determine the continuing health needs of the patient. As progress is made and the patient, with or without the help of significant others, becomes more capable of self-care and more independent, the need for home visits may decline.

CLOSING THE VISIT

As the visit comes to a close, it is important to summarize the main points of the visit for the patient and family and to identify expectations for future visits or patient achievements. The following points should be considered at the end of each visit:

- What are the main points the patient or family should remember from the visit?
- What positive attributes have been noted about the patient and the family that will give them a sense of accomplishment?

- What were the main points of the teaching plan or the treatments needed to ensure that the patient and family understand what they must do? A written set of instructions should be left with the patient or family, provided they can read and see (alternative formats include video or audio recordings). Printed material should be in the patient's primary language and in large print when indicated.
- Whom should the patient or family call in case they need to contact someone immediately? Are current emergency telephone numbers readily available? Is telephone service available or can an emergency cell phone service be provided?
- What signs of complications should be reported immediately?
- What is the day and time of the next visit? Will a different nurse make the visit? How frequently will visits be made, and for how long (if determinable at this time)?

Other Community-Based Health Care Settings

AMBULATORY SETTINGS

Ambulatory health care is provided for patients in community or hospital-based settings. The types of agencies that provide ambulatory health care are medical clinics, ambulatory care units, urgent care centres, cardiac rehabilitation programs, mental health centres, student health centres, community outreach programs, and nursing centres. Neighbourhood health centres provide services to patients who live in a geographically defined area. The centres may operate in freestanding buildings, storefronts, or mobile units. Agencies may provide ambulatory health care in addition to other services, such as offering an adult day care or health program. The kinds of services offered and the patients served depend on the agency's mission.

Nursing responsibilities in ambulatory health care settings include providing direct patient care, conducting patient intake screenings, treating patients with acute or chronic illnesses or emergency conditions, referring patients to other agencies for additional services, teaching patients self-care activities, and offering health education programs that promote health maintenance. A useful tool for the community-based nurse might be the classification scheme developed by the Visiting Nurses Association of Omaha, which contains patient-focused problems that are in one of four domains: environmental, psychosocial, physiologic, and health-related behaviours (Cookfair, 1996).

Nurses also work as clinic managers, direct the operation of clinics, and supervise other health team members. Nurse practitioners, educated in primary care, often practice in ambulatory care settings with a focus on gerontology, pediatrics, family or adult health, or women's health. Nurses can play an important part in facilitating the function of the ambulatory care facility.

OCCUPATIONAL HEALTH PROGRAMS

In Canada, health and safety standards in the workplace are legislated by provincial and territorial governments (Chadwick & Doyle, 2005). The legislated standards are directed at creating safer and healthier work conditions. It is in an employer's interest to try to provide a safe working environment, because the result is reduced costs associated with employee absenteeism, hospitalization, and disability.

Occupational nurses may work in solo units in an industrial setting, or they may serve as consultants on a limited or part-time basis. They may also be members of an interdisciplinary team composed of a variety of health care workers such as nurses, physicians, exercise physiologists, health educators, counselors, nutritionists, safety engineers, and industrial hygienists. The occupational health nurse functions in several ways and may provide direct care to employees who become ill or injured, conduct health education programs for company staff members, or set up health programs aimed at establishing specific health behaviours, such as eating properly and getting enough exercise. The nurse must also be knowledgeable about government regulations pertaining to occupational health and familiar with other pertinent legislation. The occupational health nurse may monitor employees' hearing, vision, blood pressure, or blood glucose levels (Capriotti, Kirby, & Smeltzer, 2000). Exposures to radiation, infectious diseases, and toxic substances are also tracked and reported to government agencies as required.

SCHOOL HEALTH PROGRAMS

School health programs provide valuable services for students and may also serve the school's community. School-age children and adolescents with health problems are at major risk for underachieving or failing in school. The leading health problems of elementary-school children are injuries, infections (including influenza and pneumonia), malnutrition, dental disease, and cancer. The leading problems for high-school students are alcohol and drug abuse, injuries, homicide, pregnancy, sexually transmitted disease, sports injuries, dental disease, and mental and emotional problems. Ideally, school health programs have an interdisciplinary health team consisting of physicians, nurses, dentists, social workers, counselors, school administrators, parents, and students. Many school nurses have baccalaureate degrees, and advanced practice nurses are ideally suited to provide the primary care in these settings. Some school nurse programs provide community care.

The roles of the school nurse are care provider, health educator, consultant, and counselor. The school nurse collaborates with students, parents, administrators, and other health and social service professionals regarding a student's health problems. Nurses perform health screenings, give basic care for minor injuries and complaints, administer medications, monitor the immunization status of students and families, and identify children with health problems. They need to be knowledgeable about government regulations affecting school-age children, such as ordinances for excluding students from school because of communicable diseases or parasites such as lice or scabies.

The school nurse is also a health education consultant for teachers. In addition to providing information on health practices, teaching health classes, or participating in the development of the health education curriculum, the school nurse educates the teacher and class when one of the students has a special problem, a disability, or a disease such as hemophilia or acquired immunodeficiency syndrome (AIDS).

CARE FOR THE HOMELESS

No exact figures exist on the number of homeless people in Canada. However, homelessness is a growing problem, especially in Canadian cities. It is estimated that in Canada's 11 largest cities, approximately 11,000 people sleep in shelters each night (Malloy & Stamler, 2005; Murphy, 2000). The homeless population includes increasing numbers of women with children (often victims of abuse) and elderly people. The homeless are a heterogeneous group, including members of dysfunctional families, the unemployed, and those who cannot find affordable housing. A large number of homeless persons, about 85%, are chronically mentally ill or abuse alcohol or other drugs (Walker, 1998). Some are temporarily homeless as a result of catastrophic natural disasters.

The homeless often have difficulty affording or gaining access to health care. Because of numerous obstacles, they seek health care late in the course of a disease and deteriorate more quickly than other patients. Many of the health problems they experience are related in large part to their living situations. Street life exposes homeless persons to the extremes of hot and cold environments and compounds their health risks.

Homeless persons have high rates of trauma, tuberculosis, upper respiratory tract infections, poor nutrition and anemia, lice, scabies, peripheral vascular problems, sexually transmitted diseases, dental problems, arthritis, hypothermia, skin disorders, and foot problems. Common chronic health problems of the homeless include diabetes, hypertension, heart disease, AIDS, and mental illness. These problems are made more difficult by living on the street and by being discharged to a transitory, homeless situation in which follow-up is unlikely (Hunter, Crosby, Ventura, & Warkentin, 1997; Walker, 1998). Homeless persons who live in shelters frequently encounter overcrowded, unventilated quarters that provide an ideal environment for the spread of communicable diseases such as tuberculosis.

Community-based nurses who work with the homeless must be nonjudgmental, patient, and understanding. They must be proficient in dealing with many different kinds of people who have a wide variety of health problems and needs. Nursing interventions are aimed at attempting to obtain health care services for the homeless and evaluating the health care needs of those who reside in the shelters.

 Critical Thinking Exercises

1. Recall a difficult discharge planning situation in which you have been involved. Evaluate the effectiveness of the processes used to accomplish the goals. What changes could have been made that would have improved the processes and the outcomes?

2. A homeless young mother was referred for follow-up home care after discharge from the hospital. During the nurse's initial visit, to the homeless shelter, the patient's daughter asks how often visits will be made and for how long. What assessment criteria would you use to develop answers to these questions? What factors affect the patient's eligibility for home care services versus ambulatory health services?

REFERENCES AND SELECTED READINGS

Books

Chadwick, S. L. & Doyle, B. (2005). Environmental and occupational health. In L. L Stamler & L. Yiu (Eds.), *Community health nursing: A Canadian perspective* (pp. 173–186). Toronto, ON: Pearson.

Cookfair, J. M. (1996). *Nursing care in the community* (2nd ed.). St. Louis: Mosby–Year Book.

Falk-Rafael, A. & Coffey, S. (2005). Financing, policy, and politics of health care delivery. In L. L Stamler & L. Yiu (Eds.), *Community health nursing: A Canadian perspective* (pp. 17–34). Toronto, ON: Pearson.

Hunt, R. (2000). *Readings in community-based nursing.* Philadelphia: Lippincott, Williams & Wilkins.

Johnson, J. Y., Smith-Temple, A. J., & Carr, P. (1998). *Nurses' guide to home health procedures.* Philadelphia: Lippincott-Raven.

Malloy, P. M. & Stamler, L. L. (2005). Poverty and homelessness. In L. L. Stamler & L. Yiu (Eds.), *Community health nursing: A Canadian perspective* (pp. 283–290).

Murphy, B. (2000). *On the street: How we created homelessness.* Winnipeg, MB: J. G. Shillingford.

Olson, J. K. & Clark, M. B. (2000). *Nursing within a faith community: Promoting health in times of transition.* Thousand Oaks, CA: Sage.

Steward, M. (Ed.). (2000). *Community nursing: Promoting Canadians' health* (2nd ed.). Toronto, ON: W. B. Saunders Canada.

Journals

Allison, D. M. (1997). The nurse practitioner and culturally diverse populations. *Nurse Practitioner Forum, 8*(1), 4.

Brown, S. (2000). The legal pitfalls of home care. *RN, 63*(11), 75–80.

Capriotti, T., Kirby, L. G., & Smeltzer, S. C. (2000). Unrecognized high blood pressure: A major public health issue for the workplace. *AAOHN J, 48*(7), 338–343.

Hunter, J. K., Crosby, F., Ventura, M. R., & Warkentin, L. (1997). Factors limiting evaluation of health care programs for the homeless. *Nursing Outlook, 45*(2), 224–228.

Palmer, J. (2001). Parish nursing: Connecting faith and health. *Reflections on Nursing Leadership, 27*(1), 17–19.

Pierson, C. L. (1999). APNs in home care. *American Journal of Nursing, 99*(10), 22–23.

Skillen, D. L., Olson, J. K., & Gilbert, J. A. (2003). Promoting personal safety in community health: Four educational strategies. *Nurse Educator, 28*(2), 89–94.

Touchard, B., & Berthelot, K. (1999). Collaborative home practice: Nursing and occupational therapy ensure appropriate medication administration. *Home Healthcare Nurse, 17*(1), 45–51.

Walker, C. (1998). Homeless people and mental health: A nursing concern. *American Journal of Nursing, 98*(11), 26–32.

RESOURCES AND WEBSITES

Canadian Association for Parish Nursing Ministry (CAPNM); www.capnm.ca.

Canadian Nurses Association; www.can-nurses.ca.

Canadian Occupational Health Nurses Association (COHNA); www.cohna-aciist.ca.

Canadian Public Health Association; www.cpha.ca.

Centers for Disease Control and Prevention (CDC), 1600 Clifton Road, Atlanta, GA 30333; (800) 311-3435; http://www.cdc.gov.

Community Health Nurses Association of Canada (CHNAC); www.communityhealthnursescanada.ca.

Health Canada, Centre for Infectious Disease Prevention and Control; www.hc-sc.gc.ca/pphb-dgspsp/centres_e.html#cidpc.

Critical Thinking, Ethical Decision Making, and the Nursing Process

Adapted by Rene A. Day

LEARNING OBJECTIVES

On completion of this chapter, the learner will be able to:

1. Define the characteristics of critical thinking and critical thinkers.
2. Describe the critical thinking process.
3. Define ethics and nursing ethics.
4. Identify several ethical dilemmas common to the medical-surgical area of nursing practice.
5. Specify strategies that can be helpful to nurses in ethical decision making.
6. Describe the components of the nursing process.
7. Describe the nursing process.
8. Develop a plan of nursing care for a patient using strategies of critical thinking.

In today's health care arena, the nurse is faced with increasingly complex issues and situations resulting from advanced technology, greater acuity of patients in hospital and community settings, an aging population, and complex disease processes, as well as ethical and cultural factors. Traditionally, nurses have used a problem-solving approach in planning and providing nursing care. Today the decision-making part of problem solving has become increasingly complex and requires critical thinking.

Definition of Critical Thinking

Critical thinking is a multidimensional skill, a cognitive or mental process or set of procedures. It involves reasoning and purposeful, systematic, reflective, rational, outcome-directed thinking based on a body of knowledge, as well as examination and analysis of all available information and ideas. Critical thinking leads to the formulation of conclusions and the most appropriate, often creative, decisions, options, or alternatives (Ignatavicius, 2001; Prideaux, 2000).

Critical thinking includes metacognition, the examination of one's own reasoning or thought processes while thinking, to help strengthen and refine thinking skills (Wilkinson, 2001). Independent judgments and decisions evolve from a sound knowledge base and the ability to synthesize information within the context in which it is presented. Nursing practice in today's society mandates the use of high-level critical thinking skills within the nursing process. Critical thinking enhances clinical decision making, helping to identify patient needs and to determine the best nursing actions that will assist the patient in meeting those needs.

Scheffer and Rubenfeld (2000) identified distinctive characteristics of critical thinkers in nursing as having confidence, contextual perspective, creativity, flexibility, inquisitiveness, intellectual integrity, intuition, open-mindedness, perseverance, and reflection.

Nursing education programs are expected by accreditation bodies to prepare graduates who have developed critical thinking skills (Canadian Association of University Schools of Nursing, 1995). In responding to this expectation, several questions come to mind. The initial questions are: What is critical thinking in the context of nursing? Do we need a discipline-specific definition of critical thinking or a discipline-neutral definition? The American Philosophical Association, through extensive rounds of discussion among over 40 critical thinking experts, came to the conclusion that a discipline-neutral definition was possible and was useful (1990). The next question relates to how to teach/learn critical thinking skills. Active participation in learning (eg, problem-based learning) is one strategy to develop students' critical thinking skills and dispositions (Day & Williams, 2000; see Nursing Research Profile 3-1). In addition, students and faculty members can learn to ask questions that lead to more complex levels of critical thinking (Profetto-McGrath, Smith, Day, et al., 2004). The final question is: How do we measure students' levels of critical thinking? While the Watson-Glaser Critical Thinking Appraisal Test (1980) has been used in nursing for many years, researchers have concluded that the test is not sensitive enough to pick up changes in critical thinking and that it is too general to be useful in nursing education (McMillan, 1987). Newer tests (based on the American Philosophical Association's consensus statement) include measurement of critical thinking skills (Facione, 1991) and two developed by Facione and Facione, dispositions to be a critical thinker (1992), and a holistic rubric that can be used to examine critical thinking through presentations or written assignments (1994). The Holistic Critical Thinking Scoring Rubric is available for educational purposes from Insight Assessment online at www.insightassessment.com/HCTSR.html. Examples of research in nursing education using tools developed by Facione and Facione include critical thinking skills and dispositions of baccalaureate nursing students in a traditional lecture-based format (Profetto-

---

NURSING RESEARCH PROFILE 3-1

Development of Critical Thinking Through Problem-Based Learning: A Pilot Study

Day, R. A., & Williams, B. (2000). Journal on Excellence in College Teaching, 11(2–3), 203–226.

Purpose
The purpose of the study was to determine if the critical thinking skills and dispositions of year-one nursing students (in a 4-year baccalaureate program) in a problem-based learning (PBL) curriculum would change by the end of year one.

Study Sample and Design
Year-one nursing students were invited to complete the California Critical Thinking Skill Test (CCTST) and the California Critical Thinking Dispositions Inventory (CCTDI) at the beginning of the academic year (pre-test, September) and at the end of the year (post-test, March). They also provided a copy of a scholarly paper on the topic "There is no such thing as an accident." The Holistic Critical Thinking Scoring Rubric (HCTSR) was used to analyze evidence of critical thinking in the papers. For the CCTST, 27 students completed both pre- and post-tests. For the CCTDI, 21 students completed the pre- and post-tests. Seventy-eight students provided a scholarly paper for the analysis using the HCTSR.

Findings
Despite the small sample size, year-one baccalaureate nursing students' critical thinking scores and dispositions did increase over the

first year in a PBL curriculum. For critical thinking skills (CCTST), the Total, Evaluation, and Induction scores increased significantly (p = 05). Critical thinking disposition scores showed significant increases for Truth-seeking and Self-confidence (p = .05). Using the HCTSR, 6% of student papers were scored as level 1 (biased interpretations, closed-minded, and ignored other points of view), 59% of papers were scored as level 2 (misinterpreted evidence, made false conclusions), 24% of papers were scored at level 3 (could evaluate other points of view and demonstrated fair-mindedness), and 10% were at level 4 (interpreted evidence accurately and analyzed and evaluated other points of view).

Nursing Implications
The HCTSR can be used to evaluate nursing students' levels of critical thinking demonstrated in written work. Through opportunities to work with real nursing situations in a group setting using a problem-based approach, nursing students increase their dispositions to be critical thinkers (truth-seeking, open-minded, analytical and systematic, self-confident, inquisitive, and mature) and their critical thinking skills (analysis, evaluation, inference, deduction, and induction). These dispositions and skills can then be applied to the care of patients in the clinical setting.

McGrath, 2003), in a problem-based learning format (Day & Williams, 2000), and with practicing nurses (Profetto-McGrath, Hesketh, Lang, et al., 2003).

Critical Thinking Process

RATIONALITY AND INSIGHT

Critical thinking is systematic and organized. The skills involved in critical thinking are developed over time through effort, practice, and experience. Skills needed in critical thinking include interpretation, analysis, evaluation, inference, explanation, and self-regulation (Ignatavicius, 2001; American Philosophical Association, 1990). Critical thinking requires background knowledge and knowledge of key concepts as well as standards of good thinking (Prideaux, 2000). The critical thinker uses reality-based deliberation to validate the accuracy of data and the reliability of sources, being mindful of and questioning inconsistencies. Interpretation is used to determine the significance of data that are gathered, and analysis is used to identify patient problems indicated by the data. The nurse uses inference to draw conclusions. Explanation is the justification of actions or interventions used to address patient problems and to help a patient move toward desired outcomes. Evaluation is the process of determining whether outcomes have been or are being met, and self-regulation is the process of examining the care provided and adjusting the interventions as needed (Ignatavicius, 2001).

Critical thinking is also reflective, involving metacognition, active evaluation, and refinement of the thinking process. The critical thinker considers the possibility of personal bias when interpreting data and determining appropriate actions. The critical thinker must be insightful and have a sense of fairness and integrity, the courage to question personal ethics, and the perseverance to strive continuously to minimize the effects of egocentricity, ethnocentricity, and other biases on the decision-making process (Alfaro-LeFevre, 1999).

COMPONENTS OF CRITICAL THINKING

Certain cognitive or mental activities can be identified as key components of critical thinking. When thinking critically, a person will do the following:

- Ask questions to determine the reason why certain developments have occurred and to see whether more information is needed to understand the situation accurately.
- Gather as much relevant information as possible to consider as many factors as possible.
- Validate the information presented to make sure that it is accurate (not just supposition or opinion), that it makes sense, and that it is based on fact and evidence.
- Analyze the information to determine what it means and to see whether it forms clusters or patterns that point to certain conclusions.
- Draw on past clinical experience and knowledge to explain what is happening and to anticipate what might happen next, acknowledging personal bias and cultural influences.
- Maintain a flexible attitude that allows the facts to guide thinking and takes into account all possibilities.
- Consider available options and examine each in terms of its advantages and disadvantages.
- Formulate decisions that reflect creativity and independent decision making.

Critical thinking requires going beyond basic problem solving into a realm of inquisitive exploration, looking for all relevant factors that affect the issue, and being an "out-of-the-box" thinker. It includes questioning all findings until a comprehensive picture emerges that explains the phenomenon, possible solutions, and creative methods for proceeding (Wilkinson, 2001). Critical thinking in nursing practice results in a comprehensive patient plan of care with maximized potential for success.

CRITICAL THINKING IN NURSING PRACTICE

Using critical thinking to develop a plan of nursing care requires considering the human factors that might influence the plan. The nurse interacts with the patient, family, and other health care providers in the process of providing appropriate, individualized nursing care. The culture, attitude, and thought processes of the nurse, the patient, and others will affect the critical thinking process from the data-gathering stage through the decision-making stage; therefore, aspects of the nurse-patient interaction must be considered (Wilkinson, 2001). Nurses must use critical thinking skills in all practice settings—acute care, ambulatory care, extended care, and in the home and community. Regardless of the setting, each patient situation is viewed as unique and dynamic. The unique factors that the patient and nurse bring to the health care situation are considered, studied, analyzed, and interpreted. Interpretation of the information presented then allows the nurse to focus on those factors that are most relevant and most significant to the clinical situation. Decisions about what to do and how to do it are then developed into a plan of action.

Fonteyn (1998) identified 12 predominant thinking strategies used by nurses, regardless of their area of clinical practice:

- Recognizing a pattern
- Setting priorities
- Searching for information
- Generating hypotheses
- Making predictions
- Forming relationships
- Stating a proposition ("if–then")
- Asserting a practice rule
- Making choices (alternative actions)
- Judging the value
- Drawing conclusions
- Providing explanations

Fonteyn further identified other, less prominent thinking strategies the nurse might use:

- Pondering
- Posing a question
- Making assumptions (supposing)
- Qualifying
- Making generalizations

These thought processes are consistent with the characteristics of critical thinking and cognitive activities discussed earlier. Fonteyn asserted that exploring how these thinking strategies are used in various clinical situations, and practicing using the strategies, might assist the nurse–learner in examining and refining his or her own thinking skills.

Because developing the skill of critical thinking takes time and practice, critical thinking exercises are offered throughout this book as a means of practicing one's ability to think critically. Additional exercises can be found in the study guide that accompanies the text. The questions listed in Chart 3-1 can serve as a guide in working through the exercises, although it is important to remember that each situation is unique and calls for an approach that fits the particular circumstances being described.

Ethical Nursing Care

In the complex modern world, we are surrounded by ethical issues in all facets of our lives. Consequently, there has been a heightened interest in the field of ethics, in an attempt to gain a better understanding of how these issues influence us. Specifically, in health care the focus on ethics has intensified in response to controversial developments, including advances in technology and genetics, as well as diminished health care and financial resources.

Today, sophisticated technology can prolong life well beyond the time when death would have occurred in the past. Expensive experimental procedures and medications are available for attempting to preserve life, even when such attempts are likely to fail. The development of technological support has had an influence on all stages of life. For example, the prenatal period has been influenced by genetic screening, in vitro fertilization, the harvesting and freezing of embryos, and prenatal surgery. In the early stages of life, premature infants are given a chance for survival by the use of technical support. Children and adults who would have died as a result of organ failure are living longer because of organ transplantation. Technological advances have also contributed to an increase in the average life expectancy. These advances in technology, however, have been a mixed blessing. Questions have been raised about whether, and under what circumstances, it is appropriate to use such technology. Although many individuals are afforded a better quality of life, others face extended suffering as a result of efforts to prolong life, usually at great expense. Ethical issues also surround those practices or policies that seem to allocate health care resources unjustly on the basis of age, race, gender, disability, or social mores.

Domain of Nursing Ethics

The ethical dilemmas a nurse may encounter in the medical-surgical arena are numerous and diverse. An awareness of underlying philosophical concepts will help the nurse to reason through these dilemmas. Basic concepts related to moral philosophy, such as ethics terminology, theories, and approaches, are included in this chapter. Understanding the role of the professional nurse in ethical decision making will assist nurses in articulating their ethical positions and in developing the skills needed to make ethical decisions.

ETHICS VERSUS MORALITY

The terms *ethics* and *morality* are used to describe beliefs about right and wrong and to suggest appropriate guidelines for action. In essence, ethics is the formal, systematic study of moral beliefs, whereas morality is the adherence to informal personal values. Because the distinction between the two is slight, they are often used interchangeably.

ETHICS THEORIES

One classic theory in ethics is teleologic theory or consequentialism, which focuses on the ends or consequences of actions. The most well-known form of this theory, utilitarianism, is based on the concept of "the greatest good for the greatest number." The choice of action is clear under this theory, because the action that maximizes good over bad is the correct one. The theory poses difficulty when one must judge intrinsic values and determine whose good is the greatest. Additionally, the question must be asked whether good consequences can justify any amoral actions that might be used to achieve them.

Another theory in ethics is the deontologic or formalist theory, which argues that moral standards or principles exist independently of the ends or consequences. In a given situation, one or more moral principles may apply. The nurse has a duty to act based on the one relevant principle, or the most relevant of several moral principles. Problems arise with this theory when personal and cultural biases influence the choice of the most primary moral principle.

APPROACHES TO ETHICS

Two approaches to ethics are metaethics and applied ethics. An example of metaethics (understanding the concepts and linguistic terminology used in ethics) in the health care environment

Chart 3-1

The Inquiring Mind: Critical Thinking in Action

Throughout the critical thinking process, a continuous flow of questions evolves in the thinker's mind. Although the questions will vary according to the particular clinical situation, certain general inquiries can serve as a basis for reaching conclusions and determining a course of action.

When faced with a patient situation, it is often helpful to seek answers to some or all of the following questions in an attempt to determine those actions that are most appropriate:

- What relevant assessment information do I need, and how do I interpret this information? What does this information tell me?
- To what problems does this information point? Have I identified the most important ones? Does the information point to any other problems that I should consider?
- Have I gathered all the information I need (signs/symptoms, laboratory values, medication history, emotional factors, mental status)? Is anything missing?
- Is there anything that needs to be reported immediately? Do I need to seek additional assistance?
- Does this patient have any special risk factors? Which ones are most significant? What must I do to minimize these risks?
- What possible complications must I anticipate?
- What are the most important problems in this situation? Do the patient and the patient's family recognize the same problems?
- What are the desired outcomes for this patient? Which have the highest priority? Does the patient see eye to eye with me on these points?
- What is going to be my first action in this situation?
- How can I construct a plan of care to achieve the goals?
- Are there any age-related factors involved, and will they require some special approach? Will I need to make some change in the plan of care to take these factors into account?
- How do the family dynamics affect this situation, and will this have an affect on my actions or the plan of care?
- Are there cultural factors that I must address and consider?
- Am I dealing with an ethical problem here? If so, how am I going to resolve it?
- Has any nursing research been conducted on this subject?

would be analysis of the concept of informed consent. Nurses are aware that patients must give consent before surgery, but sometimes a question arises as to whether the patient is truly informed. Delving more deeply into the concept of informed consent would be a metaethical inquiry.

Applied ethics is the term used when questions are asked of a specific discipline to identify ethical problems within that discipline's practice. Various disciplines use the frameworks of general ethical theories and moral principles and apply them to specific problems within their domain. Common ethical principles that apply in nursing include autonomy, beneficence, confidentiality, double effect, fidelity, justice, nonmaleficence, paternalism, respect for people, sanctity of life, and veracity. Brief definitions of these important principles can be found in Chart 3-2.

Nursing ethics may be considered a form of applied ethics because it addresses moral situations that are specific to the nursing profession and patient care. Some ethical problems that affect nursing may also apply to the broader area of bioethics and health care ethics. However, the nursing profession is a "caring" rather than a predominantly "curing" profession; therefore, it is imperative that one not equate nursing ethics solely with medical ethics, because the medical profession has a "cure" focus. Nursing has its own professional code of ethics.

A third way to talk about ethics is as relational ethics. According to Bergum and Dossetor (2005), "the focus of relational ethics is on people (whole persons) and the quality of the commitment between them. These commitments are experienced in a relational or ethical space which stimulates a fundamental shift in how to think about health ethics" (pp. 8–9). The focus becomes asking the ethical question, rather than trying to solve the ethical problem. Another way to look at relational ethics is about "nurturing of another person, the nurturing of the self, and the nurturing of the relationship" (Bergum & Dossetor, p. 16). Health professionals give of themselves and demonstrate a willingness and respect to meet another's needs. In examining a relationship, we can ask the following questions: What is being said? What is meant here? What is another way to look at the issue? What has been missed or overlooked? What else can be said? What about the silences? (Bergum & Dossetor, pp. 18–19). Cameron describes asking, "How are you?" in a genuine way to open up an ethical space for dialogue (2004, p. 61). This question "...turns us back to who we are and calls us yet again to be more deeply attentive to the other" (p. 61).

ETHICAL SITUATIONS

Many situations exist in health care in which ethical analysis is needed. The Code of Ethics for Registered Nurses provides the following information:

> In their practice, nurses constantly face situations involving ethics. These can be described in several ways. Description allows nurses to name their source of discomfort, a first step in addressing these

---

Chart 3-2   Common Ethical Principles

The following common ethical principles may be used to validate moral claims.

Autonomy
This word is derived from the Greek words *autos* ("self") and *nomos* ("rule" or "law"), and therefore refers to self-rule. In contemporary discourse it has broad meanings, including individual rights, privacy, and choice. Autonomy entails the ability to make a choice free from external constraints.

Beneficence
Beneficence is the duty to do good and the active promotion of benevolent acts (eg, goodness, kindness, charity). It may also include the injunction not to inflict harm (see nonmaleficence).

Confidentiality
Confidentiality relates to the concept of privacy. Information obtained from an individual will not be disclosed to another unless it will benefit the person or there is a direct threat to the social good.

Double Effect
This is a principle that may morally justify some actions that produce both good and evil effects.

All four of the following criteria must be fulfilled:

1. The action itself is good or morally neutral.
2. The agent sincerely intends the good and not the evil effect (the evil effect may be foreseen but is not intended).
3. The good effect is not achieved by means of the evil effect.
4. There is proportionate or favourable balance of good over evil.

Fidelity
Fidelity is promise keeping; the duty to be faithful to one's commitments. It includes both explicit and implicit promises to another person.

Justice
From a broad perspective, justice states that like cases should be treated alike. A more restricted version of justice is *distributive justice,*

which refers to the distribution of social benefits and burdens based on various criteria that may include the following:

    Equality
    Individual need
    Individual effort
    Societal contribution
    Individual merit
    Legal entitlement

Retributive justice is concerned with the distribution of punishment.

Nonmaleficence
This is the duty not to inflict harm as well as to prevent and remove harm. Nonmaleficence may be included within the principle of beneficence, in which case nonmaleficence would be more binding.

Paternalism
Paternalism is the intentional limitation of another's autonomy, justified by an appeal to beneficence or the welfare or needs of another. Under this principle, the prevention of evils or harm takes precedence over any potential evils caused by interference with the individual's autonomy or liberty.

Respect for Persons
Respect for persons is frequently used synonymously with *autonomy.* However, it goes beyond accepting the notion or attitude that people have autonomous choice, to treating others in such a way that enables them to make the choice.

Sanctity of Life
This is the perspective that life is the highest good. Therefore, all forms of life, including mere biologic existence, should take precedence over external criteria for judging quality of life.

Veracity
Veracity is the obligation to tell the truth and not to lie or deceive others.

ethical situations. Everyday ethics [is] the way nurses approach their practice and reflect on the ethical commitment to the people they serve. It involves the nurses' attention to common ethical events such as protecting a person's physical privacy. Ethical violations [involve] neglecting fundamental nursing obligations in a situation where the nurse knows that the action or lack of action is not appropriate. Ethical dilemmas [are] situations arising when equally compelling ethical reasons both for and against a particular course of action are recognized and a decision must be made, for example, caring for a young teenager who is refusing treatment. Ethical distress [occurs in] situations in which nurses cannot fulfill their ethical obligations and commitments (i.e. their moral agency), or they fail to pursue what they believe to be the right course of action, or fail to live up to their own expectation of ethical practice, for one or more of the following reasons: error in judgement, insufficient personal resolve or other circumstances truly beyond their control (Webster & Baylis, 2000). They may feel guilt, concern or distaste as a result. Moral residue is "… that which each of us carries with us from those times in our lives when in the face of ethical distress we have seriously compromised ourselves or allowed ourselves to be compromised" (Webster & Baylis, 2000, p. 218). Moral residue may, for example, be an outcome for some nurses who are required to implement behaviour modification strategies in the treatment of mentally ill persons (Mitchell, 2001). Ethical uncertainty arises when one is unsure what ethical principles or values to apply or even what the moral problem is (Jameton, 1984). Nurses may experience ethical situations differently. Regardless of this, the code provides guidelines for reflection and guides to action, and is intended to assist nurses through these experiences. Naming situations can be a turning point from which nurses can begin to address difficult situations. For example, dealing with ethical distress and moral residue can often lead to "defining moments" in one's career (e.g., if the nurse determines that this specific situation shall not occur again), thus allowing for positive outcomes to emerge from a difficult experience (Canadian Nurses Association, 2002a, pp. 5–6.).

For example, a patient tells a nurse that if he is dying he wants everything possible done. The surgeon and family have made the decision not to tell the patient he is terminally ill and not to resuscitate him if he stops breathing. (Canadian Healthcare Association, Canadian Medical Association, Canadian Nurses Association, et al., 1995). From an ethical perspective, patients should be told the truth about their diagnoses and should have the opportunity to make decisions about treatments. Ideally, this information should come from the physician, with the nurse present to assist the patient in understanding the terminology and to provide further support, if necessary. An ethical problem exists because of the competing claims of the family and physician, who wish to spare the patient distress, and the nurse, who wishes to be truthful with the patient as the patient has requested. If the patient's competency were questionable, an ethical dilemma would exist because no dominant principle would be evident. The nurse could experience ethical distress if the hospital threatens disciplinary action or job termination if the information is disclosed without the agreement of the physician or the family, or both.

It is essential that nurses freely engage in dialogue concerning ethical situations, even though such dialogue is difficult for everyone involved. Improved interdisciplinary communication is supported when all members of the health care team can voice their concerns and come to an understanding of the ethical situation. The use of an ethics consultant or consultation team could be helpful to assist the health care team, patient, and family to identify the ethical dilemma and possible approaches to the dilemma. The nurse should be familiar with agency policy supporting patient self-determination and resolution of ethical issues. The nurse should be an advocate for patient rights in each situation (Trammelleo, 2000).

TYPES OF ETHICAL PROBLEMS IN NURSING

As a profession, nursing is accountable to society. Such accountability is often spelled out in a patient's bill of rights. Currently, the Canadian Nurses Association (CNA) and the Canadian Federation of Nurses Unions are considering a Canadian patient's bill of rights that could include statements about the right to access emergency care, the right to subsidized travel to emergency hospital treatment, and the right of patients who are dying to decide where they want care. Included in Chart 3-3 is one example of a patient's bill of rights (British Columbia Nurses Union, 2004). Nursing has further defined its standards of accountability through a formal code of ethics that explicitly states the profession's values. The Code of Ethics for Registered Nurses (Chart 3-4), established by the Canadian Nurses Association (2002), is structured around eight primary values that are central to nursing practice. A specific responsibility statement is included with each value. The code is an ideal framework for nurses to use in ethical decision making.

Ethical issues have always affected the role of the professional nurse. The accepted definition of professional nursing has inspired a new advocacy role for nurses. The International Council of Nurses (2005) states, "Nursing encompasses autonomous and collaborative care of individuals of all ages, families, groups and communities, sick or well and in all settings. Nursing includes the promotion of health, prevention of illness, and the care of ill, disabled and dying people. Advocacy, promotion of a safe environment, research, participation in shaping health policy and in patient and health systems management, and education are also key nursing roles." This definition supports the claim that nurses must be actively involved in the decision-making process regarding ethical concerns surrounding health care and human responses. Efforts to enact this standard may cause conflict in health care settings in which the traditional roles of the nurse are delineated within a bureaucratic structure. If, however, nurses learn to present ethical conflicts within a logical, systematic framework, struggles over jurisdictional boundaries may decrease. Health care settings in which nurses are valued members of the team promote interdisciplinary communication and may enhance patient care. To practice effectively in these settings, nurses must be aware of ethical issues and assist patients in voicing their moral concerns.

The basic ethical framework of the nursing profession is the phenomenon of human caring. Nursing theories that incorporate the biopsychosocial–spiritual dimensions emphasize a holistic viewpoint, with humanism or caring as the core. As the nursing profession strives to delineate its own theory of ethics, caring is often cited as the moral foundation. For nurses to embrace this professional ethos, it is necessary to be aware not only of major ethical dilemmas but also of those daily interactions with health care consumers that frequently give rise to ethical challenges that are not as easily identified. Although technological advances and diminished resources have been instrumental in raising numerous ethical questions and controversies, including life-and-death issues, nurses should not ignore the many routine situations that involve ethical considerations. Some of the most common issues faced by nurses today include confidentiality, use of restraints, trust, refusing care, the practice environment, and end-of-life concerns.

Confidentiality

We all need to be aware of the confidential nature of information obtained in daily practice. (Alberta Association of Registered Nurses, 2001; Canadian Dental Association, Canadian Medical Association,

Chart 3-3 Patient's Bill of Rights

Preamble

As Registered Nurses and Registered Psychiatric Nurses, we are committed to giving the best possible health care service and advocating for British Columbians when we see their health care needs not being met.

We believe that residents of British Columbia have the right to an effective publicly funded and publicly administered health care system consistent with the Canada Health Act.

We believe residents of British Columbia have the right to timely access to care appropriate to their needs from appropriately qualified health care professionals. We also believe residents both in the hospital and the community setting have the right to choose their own physician.

We recognize the health care system does not currently have the capacity to meet patients' needs in all cases, and that funding needs to be increased at both the Federal and Provincial level in order to provide better health care. We believe the provincial government should meet with providers and develop an implementation plan to improve the health care system over the next five years.

This document describes the improvements Registered Nurses and Registered Psychiatric Nurses believe are needed in the system, and some of the health care rights the provincial government should be ensuring British Columbians receive.

British Columbia Nurses' Union

Access to Hospital Services

1. Residents of urban and rural communities have a right to access an emergency department within a maximum of half an hour's travel, and 98% of residents in remote communities must be able to access emergency care within 1 hour's travel.
2. Patients who access an emergency department have a right to be immediately assessed (triaged) and, consistent with national standards, assessed/treated immediately if requiring resuscitation, within 15 minutes for emergent cases, and within 30 minutes for urgent cases. Patients requiring hospital admission must not be held in emergency departments for more than 6 hours, and must be discharged, transferred to another hospital, or admitted to a hospital bed within that time frame.
3. Patients have the right to agreed upon maximum wait times for diagnostic, therapeutic, surgical, and rehabilitative treatment, based on whether their condition is life-threatening, urgent, or non-urgent.
4. Residents of British Columbia have the right to an open and transparent public process to establish maximum wait times, which includes input from the public and health care providers.
5. Patients who cannot be provided with emergent hospital treatment in their community have a right to subsidized travel to and from their community, including when their surgery or treatment is cancelled.
6. Patients whose operations are cancelled on the day of their surgery have the right to be re-booked for their operations within 1 month of cancellation.
7. Patients who are being discharged from hospital have the right to have arrangements made to provide them with continuing nursing or rehabilitation care, including the provision of medications and equipment, prior to discharge, and their caregiver(s) have the right to be informed of these arrangements prior to discharge.
8. Palliative patients have the right to decide whether they want to die at home, in a hospice, or in a hospital palliative care bed.
9. Patients who require mental health care in a hospital or mental health institution have the right to access a psychiatric bed within 6 hours of referral.
10. Patients in hospitals and residents in long term care facilities have the right to an environment that is clean and safe, and the right to a choice of meals suitable for their dietary needs with a choice of portion sizes.

Access to Community Services

11. Residents of rural and remote communities have a right to first care in their community by a physician, or where a doctor is not available, a nurse who is authorized to initiate medical evacuation.

12. Parents have a right to subsidized pre-natal teaching. In addition, they have a right to pre-natal care and the right to post-natal nursing follow-up in their homes.
13. Children have a right to fully funded, comprehensive health screening and education programs in their schools. These programs should include immunizations, dental, scoliosis, eye and hearing screening as well as reproductive, nutrition, and preventative health education from a school nurse.
14. Addicted patients have a right to detox and addiction treatment in a treatment centre where they can receive physical and psychological support within 48 hours of them making a decision to detox.
15. Patients who require mental health care in the community have a right to a visit from a mental health nurse within 4 hours in the daytime if referred as an urgent patient, and within 2 days if non-urgent.
16. Patients with persistent, serious mental illness who live outside an institution have the right to a subsidized group home or supportive housing, and fully funded medication and psychotherapy services as required.

Access to Seniors' Care

17. Seniors have the right to home care services, including home support, occupational and physical therapy, and nursing care, to enable them to remain as independent as possible and reside in their home and in their community as long as possible.
18. Seniors have the right to subsidized combination programs that allow older people to remain at home but link them with programs in the community, such as day health centres several times a week, where they receive meals, exercise, and social contact.
19. Seniors who need residential care have the right to access long term care in their community within 90 days of referral. They have the right to a residential facility with 24-hour registered nursing care, medical coverage, and recreational opportunities.
20. Seniors who need supportive housing (assisted living) have the right to access supportive housing in their community within 6 months of referral. They have the right to personal living spaces that allow for independence and privacy within a safe setting with adequate services as well as regular assessment by health care professionals. These forms of housing and care must be publicly regulated to ensure care standards.
21. Seniors in assisted living or long term care facilities have the right to security of tenure so they are only moved after appropriate plans, services, and accommodation have been put in place, and the family and resident have agreed to the plan.
22. Married seniors have the right to live together in the same long-term care or assisted living facility if they both require care.

Access to Information

23. Patients have a right to information about their patient records, their medical condition, and their care. They also have the right to have their personal health information protected from inappropriate use and/or disclosure.
24. Residents of British Columbia have the right to a health care system that is accountable and reports regularly on its performance through various mechanisms such as report cards. Patients have the right to know how well the health authority responsible for their treatment meets its performance contract with the Ministry of Health and how patient outcomes at the hospital to which they are referred compare with those of other hospitals.
25. Patients in hospitals and residents in long term care and their families have the right to know the registered nurse to patient ratio in the facility, the ratio of other health care professionals to patients, and any proven contravention of care standards, which have been reported to regulators.
26. Patients must be provided with complete information about the services available to them and how to access those services.

Chart 3-4   **Canadian Nurses Association Code of Ethics for Registered Nurses**

Nursing Values

- Safe, competent, and ethical care
  Nurses value the ability to provide safe, competent, and ethical care that allows them to fulfill their ethical and professional obligations to the people they serve.
- Health and well-being
  Nurses value health promotion and well-being and assisting persons to achieve their optimum level of health in situations of normal health, illness, injury, disability, or at the end of life.
- Choice
  Nurses respect and promote the autonomy of persons and help them to express their health needs and values and also to obtain desired information and services so they can make informed decisions.
- Dignity
  Nurses recognize and respect the inherent worth of each person and advocate for respectful treatment of all persons.

- Confidentiality
  Nurses safeguard information learned in the context of a professional relationship, and ensure it is shared outside the health care team only with the person's informed consent, or as may be legally required, or where the failure to disclose would cause significant harm.
- Justice
  Nurses uphold principles of equity and fairness to assist persons in receiving a share of health services and resources proportionate to their needs and in promoting social justice.
- Accountability
  Nurses are answerable for their practice, and they act in a manner consistent with their professional responsibilities and standards of practice.
- Quality practice environments
  Nurses value and advocate for practice environments that have the organizational structures and resources necessary to ensure safety, support, and respect for all persons in the work setting.

Reprinted with permission from the Canadian Nurses Association. (2002). Code of ethics for registered nurses (p. 8). © 2002. Ottawa, ON: Author.

Canadian Pharmacists Association, et al., 2000; College of Registered Nurses of Manitoba, 2002). If information is not pertinent to a case, the nurse should question whether it is prudent to record it in the patient's chart. In the practice setting, discussion of the patient with other members of the health care team is often necessary. These discussions should, however, occur in a private area where it is unlikely that the conversation will be overheard.

Another threat to keeping information confidential is the widespread use of computers and the easy access people have to them. This may increase the potential for misuse of information, which may have negative social consequences (Zolot, 1999). For example, laboratory results regarding testing for human immunodeficiency virus (HIV) infection or genetic screening may lead to loss of employment or insurance if the information is disclosed. Because of these possibilities of maleficence (see Chart 3-2) to the patient, sensitivity to the principle of confidentiality is essential.

Restraints

The use of restraints (including physical and pharmacologic measures) is another issue with ethical overtones (Ellerton, 2002). It is important to weigh carefully the risks of limiting a person's autonomy and increasing the risk of injury by using restraints against the risks of not using restraints. Before restraints are used, other strategies, such as asking family members to sit with the patient, should be tried (Rogers & Bocchino, 1999). The Joint Commission on Accreditation of Healthcare Organizations (JCAHO) and the Health Care Financing Administration (HCFA) have designated standards for use in care of patients with restraints; these standards are available on the website listed at the end of this chapter (Schiff, 2001).

Trust Issues

Telling the truth (veracity) is one of the basic principles of our culture. Two ethical dilemmas in clinical practice that can directly conflict with this principle are the use of placebos (nonactive substances used to treat symptoms) and not revealing a diagnosis to the patient. Both involve the issue of trust, which is an essential element in the nurse–patient relationship (Peter & Morgan, 2001).

Placebos may be used in experimental research, where the patient is involved in the decision-making process and is aware that placebos are being used in the treatment regimen. However, the use of a placebo as a substitute for an active drug to show that the patient does not have real symptoms is deceptive. This practice may severely undermine the nurse–patient relationship.

Informing patients of their diagnoses when the family and physician have chosen to withhold information is a common ethical situation in nursing practice. The nursing staff often use evasive comments with the patient as a means to maintain professional relationships with other health practitioners. This area is indeed complex because it challenges the nurse's integrity. Trust and connection with the patient play an important part in optimizing care (Day & Stannard, 1999). Strategies the nurse could consider in this situation include the following:

- Not lying to the patient
- Providing all information related to nursing procedures and diagnoses
- Communicating to the family and physician the patient's requests for information

Families often are unaware of the patient's repeated questions to the nurse. With a better understanding of the situation, families may change their perspective. Finally, although providing the information may be the morally appropriate behaviour, the manner in which the patient is told is important. Nurses must be compassionate and caring while informing patients; disclosure of information merely for the sake of patient autonomy does not convey respect for others.

Refusing to Provide Care

Any nurse who feels compelled to refuse to provide care for a particular type of patient faces an ethical dilemma. The reasons given for refusal range from a conflict of personal values to fear of personal risk of injury. Such instances have increased since the advent of acquired immunodeficiency syndrome (AIDS) as a major health problem. In one survey, the number of nurses who stated they might refuse to care for a patient with AIDS declined over a 10-year period, from 75% to 20%. The number who might refuse to care for a patient with AIDS who was violent or uncooperative, however, rose from 72% to 82% (Ventura, 1999).

There is an ethical obligation to care for all patients (McAlpine, 2001; Registered Nurses Association of British Columbia, 2001). Included under the value of Choice (CNA, 2002a, p. 12) is the following statement: "If nursing care is requested that is contrary to the nurse's personal values, the nurse must provide appropriate care until alternative care arrangements are in place to meet the person's desires." To avoid facing these ethical situations, a nurse can follow certain strategies. For example, when applying for a job, one should ask questions regarding the patient population. If one is uncomfortable with a particular situation, then not accepting the position would be an option. Denial of care, or providing substandard nursing care to some members of our society, is not acceptable nursing practice.

Nursing Practice Environment

The eighth nursing value in the Code of Ethics for Registered Nurses (CNA, 2002a) relates to quality practice environments. Nurses and nurse managers/administrators are expected to advocate for sufficient staff and the material resources necessary to provide "safe and competent care" (CNA, 2002a, p. 17). If a unit is short staffed, nurses are expected to set priorities and to notify patients, families and employers of any changes in nursing care practices (CNA, 2000a, 2001; College of Registered Nurses of Manitoba, 2002). When faced with potential violence to "themselves, others, or property" nurses are justified in taking self-protective action (CNA, 2002a, p. 18; Registered Nurses Association of Nova Scotia, 1996; International Council of Nurses, 2000). Patients expect to be protected from "incompetent, unethical, or unsafe care" (CNA, 2002a, p. 17) and nurses are required to report any such occurrences (whistle-blowing) (CNA, 1999). Nurses can improve their practice environments by working with nursing colleagues and other members of the health care team to ensure that all are treated with respect and support. A goal to work towards is to become a moral community. "A moral community is one where there is coherence between what the agency publicly professes to be their goal and what employees, persons in care, and others witness and participate in (Webster & Baylis, 2000). A moral community for nurses would include, for example, a community in which the development of effective teams was fostered, ethics education opportunities were available, and provision was made for ethics rounds and/or an ethics committee" (CNA, 2002a, p. 18).

End-of-Life Issues

Dilemmas that centre on death and dying are prevalent in medical-surgical nursing practice and frequently initiate ethical discussion (Canadian Nurses Association, 1992; Ellerton, 2000). The dilemmas are compounded by the fact that the idea of curing is paramount in health care. With advanced technology, it may be difficult to accept the fact that nothing more can be done, or that technology may prolong life but at the expense of comfort and quality of life. Focusing on the caring as well as the curing role may assist nurses in dealing with these difficult ethical situations. End-of-life issues are discussed in detail in Chapter 17.

PAIN CONTROL

The use of opioids to alleviate a patient's pain may present a dilemma for nurses. Patients with excruciating pain may require large doses of analgesics. Fear of respiratory depression or unwarranted fear of addiction should not prevent nurses from attempting to alleviate pain for the dying patient or for a patient experiencing an acute pain episode. In the case of the terminally ill patient, for example, the actions may be justified by the principle of double effect (see Chart 3-2). The intent or goal of nursing interventions is to alleviate pain and suffering while promoting comfort. The risk of respiratory depression is not the intent of the actions and should not be used as an excuse for withholding analgesia. However, the patient's respiratory status should be carefully monitored and any signs of respiratory depression reported to the physician. The administration of analgesia should be governed by the patient's needs.

DO-NOT-RESUSCITATE ORDERS

The "do not resuscitate" (DNR) order is a controversial issue. When a patient is competent to make decisions, his or her choice for a DNR order should be honoured, according to the principles of autonomy or respect for the individual (Trammelleo, 2000). However, a DNR order is at times interpreted to mean that the patient requires less nursing care, when actually these patients may have significant medical and nursing needs, all of which demand attention. Ethically, all patients deserve and should receive appropriate nursing interventions, regardless of their resuscitation status (Canadian Healthcare Association, Canadian Medical Association, Canadian Nurses Association, et al., 1995; Moorhouse, 2001).

LIFE SUPPORT

In contrast to the previous situations are those in which a DNR decision has not been made by or for a dying patient. The nurse may be put in the uncomfortable position of initiating life-support measures when, because of the patient's physical condition, they appear futile. This frequently occurs when the patient is not competent to make the decision and the family (or surrogate decision maker) refuses to consider a DNR order as an option. The nurse may be told to perform a "slow code" (ie, not to rush to resuscitate the patient) or may be given a verbal order not to resuscitate the patient; both are unacceptable medical orders. The best recourse for nurses in these situations is to be aware of hospital policy and execution of advance directives. The nurse should communicate with the physician. Discussing the matter with the physician may lead to further communication with the family and to a reconsideration of their decision, especially if they are afraid to let a loved one die with no further efforts to resuscitate (Trammelleo, 2000). Finally, when working with colleagues who are confronting such difficult situations, it helps to talk and listen to their concerns as a way of providing support.

FOOD AND FLUID

In addition to requesting that no heroic measures be taken to prolong life, a dying patient or their family may request that no more food or fluid be administered. Evaluation of harm requires a careful review of the reasons the person or their family has requested the withdrawal of food and hydration. Although the principle of autonomy has considerable merit and is supported by the Code of Ethics for Nurses, there may be situations when the request for withdrawal of food and hydration cannot be upheld. For patients with decreased decision-making capacity, the issues are more complex. Some of these cases have reached courts of law. Although an advance directive may provide some answers, at present there are no firm guidelines to assist nurses in this area.

Many individuals think that food and hydration are basic human needs, not "invasive measures," and therefore should always be maintained. However, some consider food and hydration as means of prolonging suffering. In evaluating this issue, nurses must take into consideration the potential harm as well as the benefit to the patient of either administering or withdrawing sustenance. Research has not supported the belief that withholding fluids results in a painful death due to thirst (Smith, 1997; Zerwekh, 1997).

In some cases, the physician orders that the rate of intravenous fluids be slowed to only the amount needed to keep the vein open as a route for administering medications. In this situation, the nurse's role is to assist the family to understand the change from active treatment to preparing for death.

Preventive Ethics

As previously mentioned, a dilemma refers to a conflict between two alternatives. In such instances, one's moral decision is to choose the lesser evil of the two. However, various preventive strategies are available to help nurses anticipate or avoid certain kinds of ethical dilemmas.

Frequently, dilemmas occur when the health care practitioners are unsure of the patient's wishes because the person is unconscious or too cognitively impaired to communicate directly. One famous U.S. court case in this area of clinical ethics is that of Nancy Cruzan. Cruzan was a young woman involved in a single-car crash, after which she remained in a persistent vegetative state. Her family endured a 3-year legal battle to have her feeding tube removed so that she could be allowed to die. The U.S. Supreme Court decided that a state could require "clear and convincing evidence" of the patient's wishes before withdrawing life support. This ruling and the public response to it served as an impetus for legislation on advance directives, entitled the Patient Self-Determination Act, which became effective in December 1991. The intent of this legislation is to encourage people to prepare advance directives in which they indicate their wishes concerning the degree of supportive care to be provided if they become incapacitated. The regulatory language is quite broad and allows for different institutions to have latitude in implementing the person's directives. This legislation does not require a patient to have an advance directive, but it does require that the patient be informed about them by the staff of the health care facility. Consequently, this is an area where nursing can play a significant role in patient education.

ADVANCE DIRECTIVES

An advance directive is a legal document that specifies a person's wishes prior to illness (and before hospitalization) and provides valuable information that may assist health care providers in decision making (Canadian Healthcare Association, Canadian Medical Association, Canadian Nurses Association, et al., 1995; Canadian Nurses Association, 1998 May). This directive is used only if the person becomes unable to speak for him or herself, and it is revoked if the person regains the ability to make decisions. Whereas one tends to think that the advance directive contains information about treatments that are not to be initiated or maintained, it can also provide the direction that active, potentially life-saving treatment is to occur. An advance directive usually includes the name of a substitute decision maker who has agreed to make decisions that respect the instructions contained within the document. The advance directive is signed and dated by the person developing it and two witnesses. A lawyer is not required to develop a legal advance directive. People are encouraged to distribute copies to their physicians, family members, and, especially, the designated decision maker. The document needs to be readily available when an emergency occurs.

Each province and territory in Canada has advance directive legislation with information on what to include and how to ensure that the directive is legally binding. All advance directives in Canada are about future health care decisions. There are fines or other penalties in place if an advance directive is not followed. Whereas the provinces and territories support the development of advance directives, only 7.4% of all Canadians have actually prepared one (Bravo, Dubois, & Pacquet, 2003). This is an area where nursing can play a significant role in patient education.

The provinces and territories have laws that regulate how individuals can arrange for another person to manage their financial affairs if they become physically unable to do so themselves (power of attorney). This type of power of attorney ends if the signer becomes mentally incompetent. Of more importance is the durable power of attorney in which an individual identifies another person to make health care decisions on his or her behalf. In this type of directive, the person may have clarified his or her wishes concerning a variety of medical situations. The benefit of a durable power of attorney is that it continues even if the signer becomes mentally incompetent.

Institutional ethics committees, which exist in many hospitals to assist practitioners with ethical dilemmas, also aid in preventive ethics. The purpose of these multidisciplinary committees varies among institutions. In some hospitals, the committee exists solely for the purpose of developing policies; in others it may have a strong educational or consultation focus. Because these committees usually comprise individuals with some advanced training in ethics, they are important resources to the health care team, patient, and family. Nurses with a particular interest or expertise in the area of ethics are valuable members of ethics committees and can serve as resources for staff nurses.

The heightened interest in ethical decision making has resulted in many continuing education programs, ranging from seminars or workshops to full-semester courses offered by local colleges or professional organizations. In addition, nursing and medical journals contain articles on ethical issues, and numerous textbooks on clinical ethics or nursing ethics are available. These are valuable resources because they cover the ethical theory and dilemmas of practice in greater depth. The CNA also has publications available to assist nurses with ethical decision making.

Ethical Decision Making

As noted in the preceding discussions, ethical dilemmas are common and diverse in nursing practice. Although the situations vary and experience indicates that there are no clear solutions to these dilemmas, the fundamental philosophical principles are the same, and the process of moral reflection will help nurses to justify their actions. The approach to ethical decision making can follow the steps of the nursing process. Chart 3-5 outlines the steps of an ethical analysis.

Steps of the Nursing Process

The nursing process is a deliberate problem-solving approach for meeting a person's health care and nursing needs. Although the steps of the nursing process have been stated in various ways by different writers, the common components cited are assessment, diagnosis, planning, implementation, and evaluation. The steps are defined as follows:

1. *Assessment:* The systematic collection of data to determine the patient's health status and identify any actual or potential health problems. (Analysis of data is included as part of the assessment. For those who wish to emphasize its importance, analysis may be identified as a separate step of the nursing process.)

Chart 3-5 Steps of an Ethical Analysis

The following are guidelines to assist nurses in ethical decision making. These guidelines reflect an active process in decision making, similar to the nursing process detailed in this chapter.

Assessment
1. Assess the ethical/moral situations of the problem. This step entails recognition of the ethical, legal, and professional dimensions involved.
   a. Does the situation entail substantive moral problems (conflicts among ethical principles or professional obligations)?
   b. Are there procedural conflicts? (For example, who should make the decisions? Any conflicts among the patient, health care providers, family and guardians?)
   c. Identify the significant people involved and those affected by the decision.

Planning
2. Collect information.
   a. Include the following information: the medical facts, treatment options, nursing diagnoses, legal data, and the values, beliefs, and religious components.
   b. Make a distinction between the factual information and the values/beliefs.

c. Validate the patient's capacity, or lack of capacity, to make decisions.
d. Identify any other relevant information that should be elicited.
e. Identify the ethical/moral issues and the competing claims.

Implementation
3. List the alternatives. Compare alternatives with applicable ethical principles and professional code of ethics. Choose either of the frameworks below, or other frameworks, and compare outcomes.
   a. *Utilitarian approach:* Predict the consequences of the alternatives; assign a positive or negative value to each consequence; choose the consequence that predicts the highest positive value or "the greatest good for the greatest number."
   b. *Deontological approach:* Identify the relevant moral principles; compare alternatives with moral principles; appeal to the "higher-level" moral principle if there is a conflict.

Evaluation
4. Decide and evaluate the decision.
   a. What is the best or morally correct action?
   b. Give the ethical reasons for your decision.
   c. What are the ethical reasons against your decision?
   d. How do you respond to the reasons against your decision?

---

2. *Diagnosis:* Identification of the following two types of patient problems:
   a. *Nursing diagnoses:* Actual or potential health problems that can be managed by independent nursing interventions
   b. *Collaborative problems:* "Certain physiologic complications that nurses monitor to detect onset or changes in status. Nurses manage collaborative problems using physician-prescribed and nursing-prescribed interventions to minimize the complications of the events" (Carpenito, 1999, p. 7).
3. *Planning:* Development of goals and outcomes, as well as a plan of care designed to assist the patient in resolving the diagnosed problems and achieving the identified goals and desired outcomes.
4. *Implementation:* Actualization of the plan of care through nursing interventions.
5. *Evaluation:* Determination of the patient's responses to the nursing interventions and the extent to which the outcomes have been achieved.

Dividing the nursing process into distinct steps serves to emphasize the essential nursing actions that must be taken to resolve the patient's nursing diagnoses and manage any collaborative problems or complications. Dividing the process into separate steps is, however, artificial: the process functions as an integrated whole, with the steps being interrelated, interdependent, and recurrent (Fig. 3-1). Chart 3-6 presents an overview of the nursing activities involved in applying the nursing process.

Using the Nursing Process

ASSESSMENT

Assessment data are gathered through the health history and the physical assessment. In addition, ongoing monitoring is crucial to remain aware of patient needs and the effectiveness of the nursing care that the patient receives.

Health History

The health history is conducted to determine the individual's state of wellness or illness and is best accomplished as part of a planned interview. The interview is a personal dialogue between the patient and the nurse that is conducted in order to obtain in-

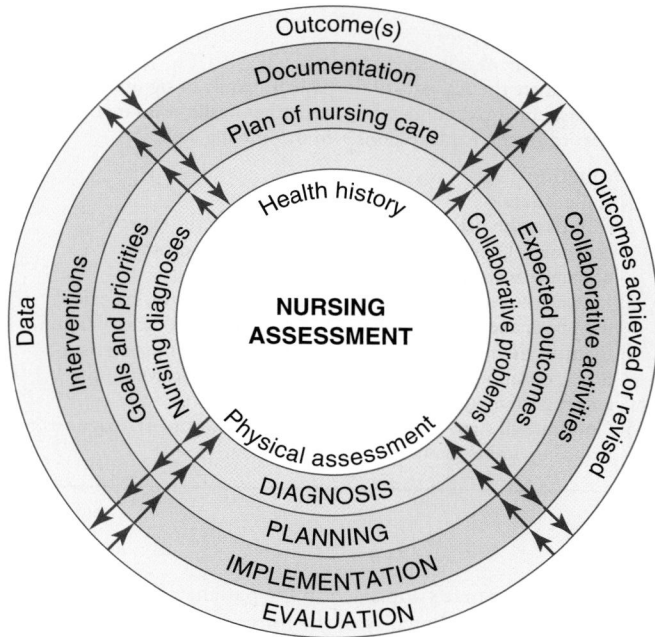

FIGURE 3-1 The nursing process is depicted schematically in this circle. Starting from the innermost circle, nursing assessment, the process moves outward through the formulation of nursing diagnoses and collaborative problems; planning, with setting of goals and priorities in the nursing plan of care; implementation and documentation; and, finally, the ongoing process of evaluation and outcomes.

Chart 3-6 — Steps of the Nursing Process

Assessment
1. Conduct the health history.
2. Perform the physical assessment.
3. Interview the patient's family or significant others.
4. Study the health record.
5. Organize, analyze, synthesize, and summarize the collected data.

Diagnosis
Nursing Diagnosis
1. Identify the patient's nursing problems.
2. Identify the defining characteristics of the nursing problems.
3. Identify the etiology of the nursing problems.
4. State nursing diagnoses concisely and precisely.

Collaborative Problems
1. Identify potential problems or complications that require collaborative interventions.
2. Identify health team members with whom collaboration is essential.

Planning
1. Assign priority to the nursing diagnoses.
2. Specify the goals.
   a. Develop immediate, intermediate, and long-term goals.
   b. State the goals in realistic and measurable terms.
3. Identify nursing interventions appropriate for goal attainment.
4. Establish expected outcomes.
   a. Make sure that the outcomes are realistic and measurable.
   b. Identify critical times for the attainment of outcomes.
5. Develop the written plan of nursing care.
   a. Include nursing diagnoses, goals, nursing interventions, expected outcomes, and critical times.
   b. Write all entries precisely, concisely, and systematically.
   c. Keep the plan current and flexible to meet the patient's changing problems and needs.
6. Involve the patient, family or significant others, nursing team members, and other health team members in all aspects of planning.

Implementation
1. Put the plan of nursing care into action.
2. Coordinate the activities of the patient, family or significant others, nursing team members, and other health team members.
3. Record the patient's responses to the nursing actions.

Evaluation
1. Collect data.
2. Compare the patient's actual outcomes with the expected outcomes. Determine the extent to which the expected outcomes were achieved.
3. Include the patient, family or significant others, nursing team members, and other health care team members in the evaluation.
4. Identify alterations that need to be made in the nursing diagnoses, collaborative problems, goals, nursing interventions, and expected outcomes.
5. Continue all steps of the nursing process: assessment, diagnosis, planning, implementation, and evaluation.

---

formation. The nurse's approach to the patient will largely determine the amount and quality of the information that is received. Achieving a relationship of mutual trust and respect requires the ability to communicate a sincere interest in the patient. Examples of effective therapeutic communication techniques that can be used to achieve this goal are found in Table 3-1.

The use of a health history guide may help in obtaining pertinent information and in directing the course of the interview. A variety of health history formats designed to guide the interview are available, but they must be adapted to the responses, problems and needs of the individual. If a previous history is available, it should be used to reduce the need for the patient to repeat information. An experienced interviewer will develop a comfortable style and format for conducting an interview and will be flexible in adapting the format to suit the individual situation, while still obtaining the essential information. Various frameworks are available for acquiring the assessment data, such as functional health patterns, Maslow's hierarchy of needs, and Erikson's "eight stages of man." The information gathered will relate to the patient's physical, psychological, social, emotional, intellectual, developmental, cultural, and spiritual needs.

In some instances, it may be appropriate for the patient to fill out a health history form. When a form is used, the nurse verifies and clarifies the information provided by the patient and seeks any additional information necessary to identify the individual's nursing needs.

Physical Assessment

A physical assessment should ideally be carried out after the health history. However, depending on the patient's physical and emotional state and the immediate priorities of the situation, the physical assessment may be carried out before or during the health history.

The purpose of the health assessment is to identify those aspects of the patient's physical, psychological, and emotional state that indicate a need for nursing care. It requires the use of sight, hearing, touch, and smell as well as the appropriate interview skills and techniques. Physical examination techniques as well as techniques and strategies for assessing behaviours and role changes are discussed in Chapters 5 and 7.

Other Components of the Database

Additional relevant information should be obtained from the patient's family or significant others, from other members of the health team, and from the patient's health record or chart. Depending on the patient's immediate needs, this information may have been obtained before the health history and the physical assessment were done. Whatever the sequence of events, it is important to use all available sources of pertinent data to complete the nursing assessment.

Recording the Database

After the health history and physical assessment are completed, the information obtained is recorded in the patient's permanent record. This record provides a means of communication among members of the health care team and facilitates coordinated planning and continuity of care. The record fulfills other functions as well:

- It serves as the business and legal record for the health care agency and for the professional staff members who are responsible for the patient's care.
- It serves as a basis for evaluating the quality and appropriateness of care and for reviewing the effective use of patient care services.
- It provides data that are useful in research, education, and short- and long-range planning.

A variety of systems are used for documenting patient care, and each health care agency selects the system that best meets its needs. The types of systems available include the problem-oriented

Table 3-1 • **Therapeutic Communication Techniques**

TECHNIQUE	DEFINITION	THERAPEUTIC VALUE
Listening	Active process of receiving information and examining one's reactions to the messages received	Nonverbally communicates nurse's interest in patient
Silence	Periods of no verbal communication among participants for therapeutic reasons	Gives patient time to think and gain insights, slows the pace of the interaction, and encourages the patient to initiate conversation, while conveying the nurse's support, understanding, and acceptance
Restating	Repeating to the patient what the nurse believes is the main thought or idea expressed	Demonstrates that the nurse is listening and validates, reinforces, or calls attention to something important that has been said
Reflection	Directing back to the patient his or her feelings, ideas, questions, or content	Validates the nurse's understanding of what the patient is saying and signifies empathy, interest, and respect for the patient
Clarification	Asking the patient to explain what he or she means or attempting to verbalize vague ideas or unclear thoughts of the patient to enhance the nurse's understanding	Helps to clarify the patient's feelings, ideas, and perceptions and to provide an explicit correlation between them and the patient's actions
Focusing	Questions or statements to help the patient develop or expand an idea	Allows the patient to discuss central issues and keeps communication goal-directed
Broad openings	Encouraging the patient to select topics for discussion	Indicates acceptance by the nurse and the value of the patient's initiative
Humour	Discharge of energy through the comic enjoyment of the imperfect	Promotes insight by bringing repressed material to consciousness, resolving paradoxes, tempering aggression, and revealing new options; a socially acceptable form of sublimation
Informing	Providing information	Helpful in health teaching or patient education about relevant aspects of patient's well-being and self-care
Sharing perceptions	Asking the patient to verify the nurse's understanding of what the patient is thinking or feeling	Conveys the nurse's understanding to the patient and has the potential to clarify confusing communication
Theme identification	Underlying issues or problems experienced by the patient that emerge repeatedly during the course of the nurse–patient relationship	Allows the nurse to best promote the patient's exploration and understanding of important problems
Suggesting	Presentation of alternative ideas for the patient's consideration relative to problem solving	Increases the patient's perceived options or choices

Adapted from Stuart, G. W., & Laraia, M. T. (2001). *Stuart and Sundeen's principles and practice of psychiatric nursing* (7th ed., pp. 34–35). St Louis: CV Mosby.

health record system, focus charting, patient outcome charting, problem intervention evaluation (PIE) charting, and charting by exception (CBE). In addition, many health care agencies have moved toward computerized documentation systems; these appear to save time, improve the monitoring of quality improvement issues, and make it easier to gain access to patient information. Confidentiality of patient records may be an issue.

DIAGNOSIS

The assessment component of the nursing process serves as the basis for identifying nursing diagnoses and collaborative problems. Soon after the completion of the health history and the physical assessment, the nurse organizes, analyzes, synthesizes, and summarizes the data collected and determines the patient's need for nursing care.

Nursing Diagnosis

Nursing, unlike medicine, does not yet have a complete taxonomy, or classification system, of diagnostic labels. Classification of discrete items into meaningful categories organizes components of knowledge into coherent units of related information. Some reasons for establishing taxonomies are to help identify what is known about a field of study, to discover what gaps in knowledge exist, to provide a common language that enhances communication among colleagues, and to facilitate the coding of standardized information for use in databases. Nursing diagnoses, the first taxonomy created in nursing, have fostered the development of autonomy and accountability in nursing and have helped to delineate the scope of practice. Many state nurse practice acts include nursing diagnosis as a nursing function, and nursing diagnosis is included in the ANA's *Standards of Clinical Nursing Practice* and the standards of many nursing specialty organizations.

The official organization that has assumed responsibility for developing the taxonomy of nursing diagnoses and formulating nursing diagnoses acceptable for study is the North American Nursing Diagnosis Association (NANDA). NANDA has grouped diagnoses according to patterns of human responses (Chart 3-7). The diagnostic labels identified by NANDA have been generally accepted but require further validation, refinement, and expansion based on clinical use and research; they are not yet complete or mutually exclusive, and more investigation is needed to determine their validity and clinical applicability.

NANDA-Approved Nursing Diagnoses 2005–2006

This list represents the NANDA-approved nursing diagnoses for clinical use and testing.

- Activity Intolerance
- Activity Intolerance, Risk for
- Adjustment, Impaired
- Airway Clearance, Ineffective
- Allergy Response, Latex
- Allergy Response, Risk for Latex
- Anxiety
- Anxiety, Death
- Aspiration, Risk for
- Attachment, Risk for Impaired Parent/Infant/Child
- Autonomic Dysreflexia
- Autonomic Dysreflexia, Risk for
- Body Image, Disturbed
- Body Temperature, Risk for Imbalanced
- Bowel Incontinence
- Breastfeeding, Effective
- Breastfeeding, Ineffective
- Breastfeeding, Interrupted
- Breathing Pattern, Ineffective
- Cardiac Output, Decreased
- Caregiver Role Strain
- Caregiver Role Strain, Risk for
- Communication, Impaired Verbal
- Communication, Readiness for Enhanced
- Conflict, Decisional (Specify)
- Conflict, Parental Role
- Confusion, Acute
- Confusion, Chronic
- Constipation
- Constipation, Perceived
- Constipation, Risk for
- Coping, Ineffective
- Coping, Defensive
- Coping, Readiness for Enhanced
- Coping, Ineffective Community
- Coping, Readiness for Enhanced Community
- Coping, Compromised Family
- Coping, Disabled Family
- Coping, Readiness for Enhanced Family
- Death Syndrome, Risk for Sudden Infant
- Denial, Ineffective
- Dentition, Impaired
- Development, Risk for Delayed
- Diarrhea
- Disuse Syndrome, Risk for
- Diversional Activity, Deficient
- Energy Field, Disturbed
- Environmental Interpretation Syndrome, Impaired
- Failure to Thrive, Adult
- Falls, Risk for
- Family Processes, Dysfunctional: Alcoholism
- Family Processes, Interrupted
- Family Processes, Readiness for Enhanced
- Fatigue
- Fear
- Fluid Balance, Readiness for Enhanced
- Fluid Volume, Deficient
- Fluid Volume, Excess
- Fluid Volume, Risk for Deficient
- Fluid Volume, Risk for Imbalanced
- Gas Exchange, Impaired
- Grieving, Anticipatory
- Grieving, Dysfunctional
- Grieving, Risk for Dysfunctional
- Growth and Development, Delayed

- Growth, Risk for Disproportionate
- Health Maintenance, Ineffective
- Health-Seeking Behaviours (Specify)
- Home Maintenance, Impaired
- Hopelessness
- Hyperthermia
- Hypothermia
- Identity, Disturbed Personal
- Incontinence, Functional Urinary
- Incontinence, Reflex Urinary
- Incontinence, Stress Urinary
- Incontinence, Total Urinary
- Incontinence, Urge Urinary
- Incontinence, Risk for Urge Urinary
- Infant Behaviour, Disorganized
- Infant Behaviour, Risk for Disorganized
- Infant Behaviour, Readiness for Enhanced Organized
- Infant Feeding Pattern, Ineffective
- Infection, Risk for
- Injury, Risk for
- Injury, Risk for Perioperative-Positioning
- Intracranial Adaptive Capacity, Decreased
- Knowledge, Deficient (Specify)
- Knowledge, Readiness for Enhanced (Specify)
- Lifestyle, Sedentary
- Loneliness, Risk for
- Memory, Impaired
- Mobility, Impaired Bed
- Mobility, Impaired Physical
- Mobility, Impaired Wheelchair
- Nausea
- Neglect, Unilateral
- Noncompliance
- Nutrition, Imbalanced: Less Than Body Requirements
- Nutrition, Imbalanced: More Than Body Requirements
- Nutrition, Readiness for Enhanced
- Nutrition, Risk for Imbalanced: More Than Body Requirements
- Oral Mucous Membrane, Impaired
- Pain, Acute
- Pain, Chronic
- Parenting, Readiness for Enhanced
- Parenting, Impaired
- Parenting, Risk for Impaired
- Peripheral Neurovascular Dysfunction, Risk for
- Poisoning, Risk for
- Post-Trauma Syndrome
- Post-Trauma Syndrome, Risk for
- Powerlessness
- Powerlessness, Risk for
- Protection, Ineffective
- Rape-Trauma Syndrome
- Rape-Trauma Syndrome: Compound Reaction
- Rape-Trauma Syndrome: Silent Reaction
- Religiosity, Impaired
- Religiosity, Readiness for Enhanced
- Religiosity, Risk for Impaired
- Relocation Stress Syndrome
- Relocation Stress Syndrome, Risk for
- Role Performance, Ineffective
- Self-Care Deficit, Bathing/Hygiene
- Self-Care Deficit, Dressing/Grooming
- Self-Care Deficit, Feeding
- Self-Care Deficit, Toileting
- Self-Concept, Readiness for Enhanced
- Self-Esteem, Chronic Low
- Self-Esteem, Situational Low

(continued)

NANDA-Approved Nursing Diagnoses 2005–2006 (Continued)

- Self-Esteem, Risk for Situational Low
- Self-Mutilation
- Self-Mutilation, Risk for
- Sensory Perception, Disturbed (Specify: Visual, Auditory, Kinesthetic, Gustatory, Tactile, Olfactory)
- Sexual Dysfunction
- Sexuality Pattern, Ineffective
- Skin Integrity, Impaired
- Skin Integrity, Risk for Impaired
- Sleep Deprivation
- Sleep Pattern, Disturbed
- Sleep, Readiness for Enhanced
- Social Interaction, Impaired
- Social Isolation
- Sorrow, Chronic
- Spiritual Distress
- Spiritual Distress, Risk for
- Spiritual Well-Being, Readiness for Enhanced
- Suffocation, Risk for
- Suicide, Risk for
- Surgical Recovery, Delayed
- Swallowing, Impaired

- Therapeutic Regimen Management, Effective
- Therapeutic Regimen Management, Ineffective
- Therapeutic Regimen Management, Readiness for Enhanced
- Therapeutic Regimen Management, Ineffective Community
- Therapeutic Regimen Management, Ineffective Family
- Thermoregulation, Ineffective
- Thought Processes, Disturbed
- Tissue Integrity, Impaired
- Tissue Perfusion, Ineffective (Specify Type: Renal, Cerebral, Cardiopulmonary, Gastrointestinal, Peripheral)
- Transfer Ability, Impaired
- Trauma, Risk for
- Urinary Elimination, Impaired
- Urinary Elimination, Readiness for Enhanced
- Urinary Retention
- Ventilation, Impaired Spontaneous
- Ventilatory Weaning Response, Dysfunctional
- Violence, Risk for Other-Directed
- Violence, Risk for Self-Directed
- Walking, Impaired
- Wandering

NANDA International. (2005). Nursing diagnoses: Definitions & classification 2005-2006. Philadelphia: Author.

Choosing a Nursing Diagnosis

When choosing the nursing diagnoses for a particular patient, the nurse must first identify the commonalities among the assessment data collected. These common features lead to the categorization of related data that reveal the existence of a problem and the need for nursing intervention. The patient's identified problems are then defined in the nursing diagnoses. The most commonly selected nursing diagnoses are compiled and categorized by NANDA in a taxonomy that is updated at least every 2 years. It is important to remember that nursing diagnoses are not medical diagnoses; they are not medical treatments prescribed by the physician; and they are not diagnostic studies. Nursing diagnoses are not the equipment used to implement medical therapy, and they are not the problems that the nurse experiences while caring for the patient. They are the patient's actual or potential health problems that independent nursing actions can resolve. Nursing diagnoses that are succinctly stated in terms of the specific problems of the patient will guide the nurse in the development of the nursing plan of care.

To give additional meaning to the diagnosis, the characteristics and the etiology of the problem must be identified and included as part of the diagnosis. For example, the nursing diagnoses and their defining characteristics and etiology for a patient who has rheumatoid arthritis may include

- Impaired physical mobility related to pain and stiffness with joint movement
- Self-care deficits (bathing/hygiene, dressing/grooming, feeding, toileting) related to fatigue and joint stiffness
- Low self-esteem (chronic, situational, risk for situational) related to loss of independence
- Imbalanced nutrition: Less than body requirements related to fatigue and inadequate food intake

Collaborative Problems

In addition to nursing diagnoses and their related nursing interventions, nursing practice involves certain situations and interventions that do not fall within the definition of nursing diagnoses. These activities pertain to potential problems or complications that are medical in origin and require collaborative interventions with the physician and other members of the health care team. The term *collaborative problem* is used to identify these situations.

A primary focus of the nurse when treating collaborative problems is monitoring the patient for the onset of complications or changes in the status of existing complications. The complications are usually related to the patient's disease process, treatments, medications, or diagnostic studies. The nurse prescribes nursing interventions that are appropriate for managing the complications and implements the treatments prescribed by the physician. Figure 3-2 depicts the differences between nursing diagnoses and collaborative problems. After the nursing diagnoses and collaborative problems have been identified, they are recorded on the plan of nursing care.

PLANNING

Once the nursing diagnoses have been identified, the planning component of the nursing process begins. This phase entails the following:

1. Assigning priorities to the nursing diagnoses and collaborative problems
2. Specifying expected outcomes
3. Specifying the immediate, intermediate, and long-term goals of nursing action
4. Identifying specific nursing interventions appropriate for attaining the outcomes
5. Identifying interdependent interventions

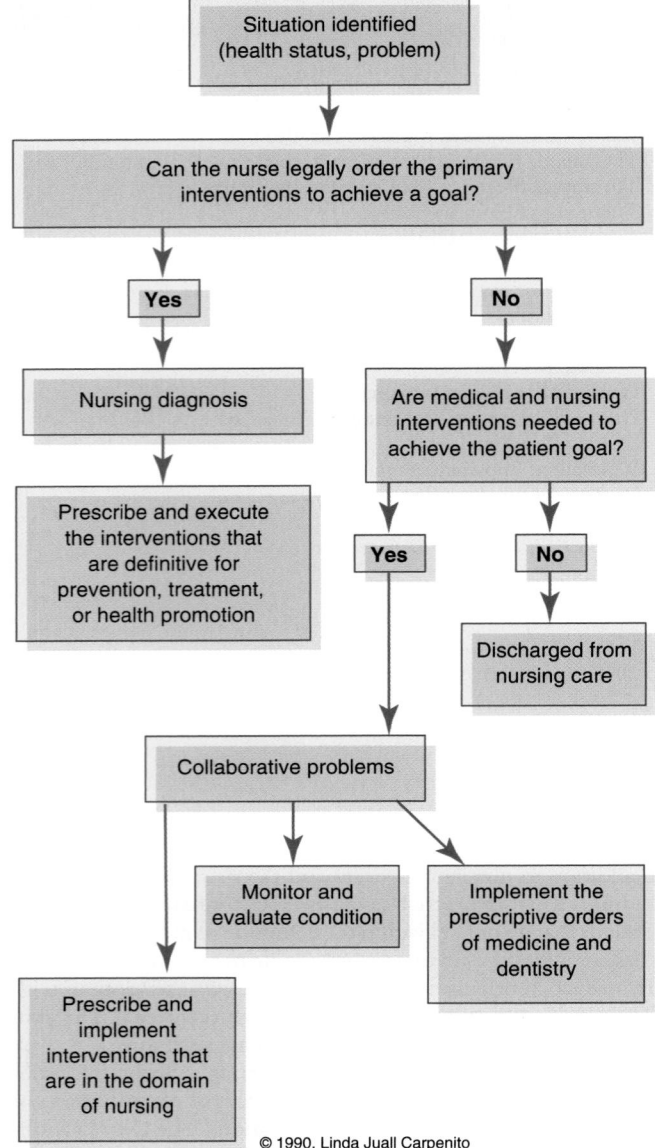

FIGURE 3-2 Differentiating nursing diagnoses and collaborative problems. Source: Carpenito, L. J. (2001). *Nursing diagnosis: Application to clinical practice* (8th ed). Philadelphia: Lippincott Williams & Wilkins. Copyright © 1990, Linda Juall Carpenito.

6. Documenting the nursing diagnoses, collaborative problems, expected outcomes, nursing goals, and nursing interventions on the plan of nursing care
7. Communicating to appropriate personnel any assessment data that point to health needs that can best be met by other members of the health care team

Setting Priorities

Assigning priorities to the nursing diagnoses and collaborative problems is a joint effort by the nurse and the patient or family members. Any disagreement about priorities is resolved in a way that is mutually acceptable. Consideration must be given to the urgency of the problems, with the most critical problems receiving the highest priority. Maslow's hierarchy of needs provides a useful framework for prioritizing problems, with importance being given first to physical needs; once those lower-level needs are met, higher-level needs can be addressed.

Establishing Expected Outcomes

Expected outcomes of the nursing interventions are stated in terms of the patient's behaviours and the time period in which they are to be achieved, as well as any special circumstances related to achieving the outcome (Smith-Temple & Johnson, 2002). These outcomes must be realistic and measurable. The Nursing-Sensitive Outcomes Classification (NOC) (Chart 3-8) and standard outcome criteria for people with specific health problems established by health care agencies are resources for identifying appropriate expected outcomes. These outcomes can be associated with nursing diagnoses and interventions and can be used when appropriate (Aquilino & Keenan, 2000). However, NOC may need to be adapted to establish realistic criteria for the specific patient involved.

The expected outcomes that define the desired behaviour of the patient will be used to measure to what extent progress toward resolving the problem has been made. The expected outcomes also serve as the basis for evaluating the effectiveness of the nursing interventions and for deciding whether additional nursing care is needed or whether the plan of care needs to be revised.

Establishing Goals

After the priorities of the nursing diagnoses and expected outcomes have been established, the immediate, intermediate, and long-term goals and the nursing actions appropriate for attaining the goals are identified. The patient and his or her family are included in establishing goals for the nursing actions. Immediate goals are those that can be reached within a short period. Intermediate and long-term goals require a longer time to be achieved and usually involve preventing complications and other health problems and promoting self-care and rehabilitation. For example, goals for a patient with diabetes and a nursing diagnosis of *deficient knowledge related to the prescribed diet* may be stated as follows:

Immediate goal: Demonstrates oral intake and tolerance of 1500-calorie diabetic diet spaced in three meals and one snack per day
Intermediate goal: Plans meals for 1 week based on diabetic exchange list
Long-term goal: Adheres to prescribed diabetic diet

Determining Nursing Actions

In planning appropriate nursing actions to achieve the desired goals and outcomes, the nurse, with input from the patient and significant others, identifies individualized interventions based on the patient's circumstances and preferences that will address each outcome. Interventions should identify the activities needed and who will carry them out. Determination of interdisciplinary activities is made in collaboration with other health care providers as needed.

The nurse identifies and plans patient teaching and return demonstrations as needed to assist the patient in learning self-care

Chart 3-8   Nursing-Sensitive Outcomes Classification (NOC)

The NOC is a classification of patient outcomes sensitive to nursing interventions. Each outcome is a neutral statement about a variable patient condition, behaviour, or perception coupled with a rating scale. The outcome statement and scale can be used to identify baseline functioning, expected outcomes, and actual outcomes for individual patients. The following table is an example of a nursing-sensitive outcome.

Respiratory Status: Airway Patency (0410)

Domain—Physiologic Health (II)
Class—Cardiopulmonary (E)
Scale(s)—Severely compromised to Not compromised (a) and Severe to None (n)
Definition Open, clear tracheobronchial passages for air exchange

OUTCOME TARGET RATING: Maintain at____   Increase to ___

Respiratory Status: Airway Patency Overall Rating	Severely Compromised 1	Substantially Compromised 2	Moderately Compromised 3	Mildly Compromised 4	Not Compromised 5
Indicators					
041009 Ease of breathing	1	2	3	4	5
041004 Respiratory rate	1	2	3	4	5
041005 Respiratory rhythm	1	2	3	4	5
041006 Moves sputum out of airway	1	2	3	4	5
041010 Moves blockage out of airway	1	2	3	4	5
	Severely	**Substantially**	**Moderate**	**Mildly**	**None**
041002 Anxiety	1	2	3	4	5
041011 Fear	1	2	3	4	5
041003 Choking	1	2	3	4	5
041007 Adventitious breath sounds	1	2	3	4	5

With permission from Moorhead, S., Johnson, M., & Maas, M. (Eds.). (2004). *Nursing outcomes classification [NOC]: Iowa Outcomes Project* (3rd ed.). St. Louis: Mosby–Year Book.

---

activities to be performed. Planned interventions should be ethical and appropriate to the patient's culture, age, and gender. Standardized interventions, such as those found on institutional care plans or in the Nursing Interventions Classification (NIC) (Aquilino & Keenan, 2000; McCloskey & Bulechek, 2000) can be used. Chart 3-9 describes the NIC system and provides an example of an NIC system intervention. It is important to individualize prewritten interventions to promote optimal effectiveness for each patient.

IMPLEMENTATION

The implementation phase of the nursing process involves carrying out the proposed plan of nursing care. The nurse assumes responsibility for the implementation. Performance of interventions, however, may be carried out by the patient and the family, other members of the nursing team, or other members of the health care team as appropriate. The nurse coordinates the activities of all those involved in implementation so that the schedule of activities

Chart 3-9   Nursing Interventions Classification (NIC)

The NIC is a standardized classification of nursing treatments (interventions) that includes independent and collaborative interventions. Intervention labels are terms such as hemorrhage control, medication administration, or pain management. Listed under each intervention are multiple discrete nursing actions that together constitute a comprehensive approach to treatment of a particular condition. Not all actions are applicable to every patient; nursing judgment will determine which actions to implement. The following is an example of a nursing intervention:

Chest Physiotherapy*
Definition: Assisting the patient to move airway secretions from peripheral airways to more central airways for expectoration and/or suctioning
Activities:
  Determine presence of contraindications for use of chest physical therapy

  Determine which lung segment(s) needs to be drained
  Position patient with the lung segment to be drained in uppermost position
  Use pillows to support patient in designated position
  Use percussion with postural drainage by cupping hands and clapping the chest wall in rapid succession to produce a series of hollow sounds
  Use chest vibration in combination with postural drainage, as appropriate
  Use an ultrasonic nebulizer, as appropriate
  Use aerosol therapy, as appropriate
  Administer bronchodilators, as appropriate
  Monitor amount and type of sputum expectoration
  Encourage coughing during and after postural drainage
  Monitor patient tolerance by means of SaO_2, respiratory rhythm and rate, cardiac rhythm and rate, and comfort levels

With permission from Dochterman, G. M, & Bulechek, G. M. (Eds.). (2004). *Nursing interventions classification (NIC)* (4th ed). St. Louis: Mosby.

Plan of Nursing Care

Example of an Individualized Plan of Nursing Care

Mr. John Lee, a 50-year-old management consultant, was admitted to the nursing unit from his physician's office. A routine physical examination 3 months previously had revealed essential hypertension with BP 170/110 and decreased urine creatinine clearance. During the subsequent 3 months the blood pressure elevation did not respond to diet therapy. Mr. Lee admitted that he had not been successful in adhering to the low-sodium, low-cholesterol weight-reduction diet that had been prescribed for him. He stated, "My life is just too busy—I work all hours of the day and night." He indicated that in addition to his work he and his wife share the responsibility for raising their two teenage daughters. He drinks five to seven cups of coffee daily and drinks alcohol only at social occasions. Admission physical examination revealed BP 194/112, P 96, R 20, T 37°C (98.6°F), height 5′10″, weight 210 lbs, and slight edema of the ankles and feet. Mr. Lee stated that his feet are "always puffy at night." There were several darkened areas (2 cm in diameter) on the anterior lower legs bilaterally. A brief hospitalization was planned for thorough evaluation and initiation of therapy. The physician's orders on admission included activity as desired; Lasix, 40 mg bid; monitor vital signs every 4 hours while awake; and 1500 calorie, 1 g sodium, low-cholesterol diet.

Nursing Diagnosis
- Ineffective health maintenance related to hypertension, stress, obesity, and caffeine
- Ineffective coping related to role responsibilities at work and home
- Noncompliance with dietary regimen related to knowledge deficit and lifestyle

Collaborative Problems
1. Ischemic ulcers of lower legs

Goals
Immediate: Gradual decrease in blood pressure
Intermediate: Initiation of lifestyle alterations to decrease stress
Long-term: Alteration of lifestyle to reduce emotional and environmental stressors
      Compliance with dietary regimen
      Absence of ischemic leg ulcers

Nursing Interventions	Expected Outcomes	Outcomes
1. Monitor BP lying, sitting, and standing every 4 h	Experiences no further increase in BP	BP range of 162/112–138/98 since admission No variation greater than 5 mm Hg in systolic or diastolic pressures with position changes No variation between right and left arms Maximum BP from 24 h after admission to time of discharge: 138/98
2. Monitor fluid status: a. I&O	Urinary output adequate in relation to oral intake	Intake: 1850 mL Output: 1685 mL
b. Peripheral edema	No evidence of peripheral edema	Minimal edema of feet late in evening
3. Promote atmosphere conducive to physical and mental rest: a. Encourage alternation of rest and activity	Alternates periods of rest and activity	Rests in bed 1 h in morning and 2 h in afternoon; disconnects phone during rest periods Awake at intervals during night: 8 h of uninterrupted sleep at night after initiation of 30 mg Dalmane at bedtime
b. Encourage limitation of visitors and interactions that are stress-producing	Limits visitors to family in the evenings	Wife and daughters visit 2 h in evening: patient calm and relaxed after visits
	Avoids stress-producing interactions	Wife and daughters aware of need to decrease stress: they consult with patient about regular family activities
4. Assist patient to alter lifestyle to decrease stress a. Discuss relationship between emotional stress and physiologic functioning:	Describes stress as a precursor to alteration in physiologic functioning	Accurately described relationship between stress and hypertension

b. Encourage patient to identify stress-producing stimuli	Identifies lifestyle factors that produce stress	Identified the following stressors:
		    Self-imposed demands of job; unwillingness to refer clients
		    Excessive involvement in daughters' school and recreational activities

(continued)

Plan of Nursing Care

Example of an Individualized Plan of Nursing Care *(Continued)*

Nursing Interventions	Expected Outcomes	Outcomes
c. Encourage patient to identify adjustments necessary to reduce stress	Identifies lifestyle adjustments necessary to reduce stress Discusses lifestyle adjustments with family	Verbalized plans to make more referrals Identified need to decrease work hours to maximum of 8 h per day Consulted with wife and daughters; will alternate with wife in attending daughters' activities; all family members supportive
5. Encourage patient to identify obesity and caffeine as stressors and aggravators of hypertension; request consultation with dietitian and reinforce instructions given	Identifies harmful effects of obesity and caffeine Makes plans for losing weight Makes plans for decreasing caffeine intake	Accurately described effects of obesity and caffeine on blood pressure Plans to go to Weight Watchers; has had success with this program in the past Drinks 1 cup of coffee for breakfast; uses decaffeinated coffee at mid-morning, lunch, and dinner; expressed satisfaction with this plan
6. Assess for ischemic leg ulcers; report changes in darkened spots on legs to physician	Absence of changes in skin integrity on lower extremities	No changes noted in characteristics of skin of lower legs on days 2 and 3
7. Teach foot care: daily inspection and washing, nail care, avoidance of caustic solutions, lubrication of dry skin, avoidance of heat to feet, well-fitting shoes and socks, avoidance of crossing legs	Describes principles and techniques of proper foot care	Discussed importance of proper foot care; demonstrated proper technique of foot care; shoes and socks fit well; does not cross legs when sitting

facilitates the patient's recovery. The plan of nursing care serves as the basis for implementation:

- The immediate, intermediate, and long-term goals are used as a focus for the implementation of the designated nursing interventions.
- While implementing nursing care, the nurse continually assesses the patient and his or her response to the nursing care.
- Revisions are made in the plan of care as the patient's condition, problems, and responses change and when reassignment of priorities is required

Implementation includes direct or indirect execution of the planned interventions. It is focused on resolving the patient's nursing diagnoses and collaborative problems and achieving expected outcomes, thus meeting the patient's health needs.

Included among nursing interventions are assisting with hygienic care; promoting physical and psychological comfort; supporting respiratory and elimination functions; facilitating the ingestion of food, fluids, and nutrients; managing the patient's immediate surroundings; providing health teaching; promoting a therapeutic relationship; and carrying out a variety of therapeutic nursing activities. Judgment, critical thinking, and good decision-making skills are essential in the selection of appropriate scientifically and ethically based nursing interventions. All nursing interventions are patient-focused and outcome-directed and are implemented with compassion, confidence and a willingness to accept and understand the patient's responses.

Although many nursing actions are independent, others are interdependent, such as carrying out prescribed treatments, administering medications and therapies, and collaborating with other health care team members to accomplish specific expected outcomes and to monitor and manage potential complications. Such inter-

dependent functioning is just that—interdependent. Requests or orders from other health care team members should not be followed blindly but should be assessed critically and questioned when necessary. The implementation phase of the nursing process ends when the nursing interventions have been completed.

EVALUATION

Evaluation, the final step of the nursing process, allows the nurse to determine the patient's response to the nursing interventions and the extent to which the objectives have been achieved. The plan of nursing care is the basis for evaluation. The nursing diagnoses, collaborative problems, priorities, nursing interventions, and expected outcomes provide the specific guidelines that dictate the focus of the evaluation. Through evaluation, the nurse can answer the following questions:

- Were the nursing diagnoses and collaborative problems accurate?
- Did the patient achieve the expected outcomes within the critical time periods?
- Have the patient's nursing diagnoses been resolved?
- Have the collaborative problems been resolved?
- Have the patient's nursing needs been met?
- Should the nursing interventions be continued, revised, or discontinued?
- Have new problems evolved for which nursing interventions have not been planned or implemented?
- What factors influenced the achievement or lack of achievement of the objectives?
- Do priorities need to be reassigned?
- Should changes be made in the expected outcomes and outcome criteria?

Objective data that provide answers to these questions are collected from all available sources (eg, patient, family, significant others, and health care team members). These data are included in the patient's record and must be substantiated by direct observation of the patient before the outcomes are recorded.

DOCUMENTATION OF OUTCOMES AND REVISION OF PLAN

Outcomes are documented concisely and objectively. Documentation should relate outcomes to the nursing diagnoses and collaborative problems, describe the patient's responses to the interventions, indicate whether the outcomes were met, and include any additional pertinent data (see Plan of Nursing Care).

The plan of care is subject to change as the patient's needs change, as the priorities of the needs shift, as needs are resolved, and as additional information about the patient's state of health is collected. As the nursing interventions are implemented, the patient's responses are evaluated and documented and the plan of care is revised accordingly. A well-developed, continuously updated plan of care is the greatest assurance that the patient's nursing diagnoses and collaborative problems will be addressed and his or her basic needs will be met.

 Critical Thinking Exercises

1. You are an acute care nurse and you have been assigned to the outpatient unit for the shift. How does the approach to critical thinking differ among nursing practice settings (acute care versus ambulatory care settings)?

2. You have just completed the health history for your assigned patient. How would you identify the patient's nursing diagnoses? Describe the kind of resources that are available to help you with identifying these diagnoses.

3. A terminally ill patient's daughter tells you she is not ready to let her father go. The next day you note a "Do Not Resuscitate" order on the chart. Describe which critical thinking skills you could use to address the issue and to develop a plan of care for the patient and family. How did you integrate your critical thinking into the nursing process? What changes might you make in your plan of care considering the DNR order? What ethical problems or dilemmas might you anticipate?

4. The spouse of your patient tells you information about the patient that the patient has not revealed. How would you determine whether you should communicate this information to the patient's primary nurse?

REFERENCES AND SELECTED READINGS

Books

Alberta Association of Registered Nurses. (2001a). *Working extra hours: Guidelines for registered nurses on fitness to practice and the provision of safe, competent, ethical nursing care.* Edmonton: Author.

Alberta Association of Registered Nurses. (2001b). *Professional boundaries: A discussion paper on expectations for nurse-client relationships.* Edmonton: Author.

Alberta Association of Registered Nurses. (1996). *Ethical decision-making for registered nurses in Alberta: Guidelines and recommendations.* Edmonton: Author.

Alfaro-LeFevre, R. (1999). *Critical thinking in nursing* (2nd ed.). Philadelphia: W. B. Saunders.

American Nurses Association. (2001). *American Nurses Association code of ethics.* Washington: Author.

American Philosophical Association. (1990). Critical thinking: A statement of expert consensus for purposes of educational assessment and instruments. In *The Delphi report: Research findings and recommendations prepared for the Committee on Pre-College Philosophy.* Newark, DE: Author.

Bergum, V., & Dossetor, J. (2005). *Relational ethics. The full measure of respect.* Hagerstown, MD: University Publishing Group.

Bickley, L. S., & Szilagyi, P. G. (2003). *Bates' guide to physical examination and history taking* (8th ed.). Philadelphia: Lippincott Williams & Wilkins.

Bolaria, B. S., & Dickinson, H. (Eds.). (2002). *Health, illness and health care in Canada* (3rd ed.). Scarborough, ON: Nelson Thomas Learning.

Burkhardt, M. A., & Nathaniel, A. K. (1998). *Ethics & issues in contemporary nursing.* Toronto: Delmar Publishers.

Canadian Association of University Schools of Nursing. (1995). *CAUSN statement on baccalaureate education.* Ottawa: Author.

Canadian Dental Association, Canadian Medical Association, Canadian Pharmacists Association, et al. (2000). *Principles for privacy protection of personal health information in Canada.* Ottawa: Authors.

Canadian Healthcare Association, Canadian Medical Association, Canadian Nurses Association, et al. (1995). Joint statement on resuscitative interventions. Ottawa: Authors.

Canadian Home Care Association, Canadian Healthcare Association, Canadian Long Term Care Association, et al. (1994). *Joint statement on advance directives.* Ottawa: Authors.

Canadian Nurses Association. (2002a). *Code of ethics for registered nurses.* Ottawa: Author.

Canadian Nurses Association. (2002b). *Ethical research guidelines for registered nurses* (3rd ed.). Ottawa: Author.

Canadian Nurses Association. (2001a). *Quality professional practice environments for registered nurses.* Ottawa: Author.

Canadian Nurses Association. (2001b). *The role of the nurse in telepractice.* Ottawa: Author.

Canadian Nurses Association, Policy Regulation and Research Division. (2000, September). *Ethics in practice. Working with limited resources: Nurses' moral constraints.* Ottawa: Author.

Canadian Nurses Association, Policy Regulation and Research Division. (1999, November). *Ethics in practice. I see and am silent/I see and speak out: The ethical dilemma of whistleblowing.* Ottawa: Author.

Canadian Nurses Association, Policy Regulation and Research Division. (1998, June). *Ethics in practice. Ethical issues related to appropriate staff mixes.* Ottawa: Author.

Canadian Nurses Association, Policy Regulation and Research Division. (1998, May). *Ethics in practice. Advance directives: The nurse's role.* Ottawa: Author.

Canadian Nurses Association. (1992a). *Privacy of personal health information.* Ottawa: Author.

Canadian Nurses Association. (1992b). *A question of respect: Nurses and end-of-life treatment dilemmas.* Ottawa: Author.

Canadian Nurses Association. (1992c). *The role of the nurse in the use of health care technology.* Ottawa: Author.

Carpenito, L. J. (2001). *Nursing diagnosis: Application to clinical practice* (9th ed.). Philadelphia: Lippincott Williams & Wilkins.

Carpenito, L. J. (1999). *Nursing care plan and documentation.* Philadelphia: Lippincott Williams & Wilkins.

College of Registered Nurses of Manitoba. (2002a). *Professional boundaries for therapeutic relationships.* Winnipeg: Author.

College of Registered Nurses of Manitoba. (2002b). *Working short staffed.* Winnipeg: Author.

Dochterman, G. M., & Bulechek, G. M. (Eds.). (2004). *Nursing interventions classification (NIC)* (4th ed.). St. Louis: Mosby.

Facione, P. A. (1991). *Using the California critical thinking skill test in research, evaluation, and assessment.* Millbrae, CA: California Academic Press.

Facione, P. A., & Facione, N. C. (1992). CCTDI: *A disposition inventory.* Millbrae, CA: California Academic Press.

Facione, P. A., & Facione, N. C. (1994). *Holistic critical thinking scoring rubric.* Millbrae, CA: California Academic Press.

Fonteyn, M. E. (1998). *Thinking strategies for nursing practice.* Philadelphia: Lippincott-Raven.

International Council of Nurses. (2000). *Guidelines on coping with violence in the workplace.* Geneva: Author.

Jameton, A. (1984). *Nursing practice: The ethical issues.* Englewood Cliffs, NJ: Prentice-Hall.

Joint Commission for Accreditation of Hospital Organizations (JCAHO). (1999). *Standards, rights, responsibilities, and ethics.* Oakbrook Terrace, IL: Author.

McCloskey, J. C., & Bulechek, G. M. (Eds.). (2000). *Nursing interventions classification (NIC): Iowa Interventions Project* (2nd ed.). St. Louis: Mosby–Year Book.

Moorhead, S., Johnson, M., & Maas, M. (Eds.). (2004). *Nursing outcomes classification [NOC]: Iowa outcomes project* (3rd ed.). St. Louis: Mosby–Year Book.

NANDA International. (2005). *Nursing diagnoses: Definitions & classification 2005–2006.* Philadelphia: Author.

Registered Nurses Association of British Columbia. (2000). *Advocacy and the registered nurse.* Vancouver: Author.

Registered Nurses Association of British Columbia. (2001). *Nursing practice guidelines: Duty to provide care.* Vancouver: Author.

Registered Nurses Association of Nova Scotia. (1996a). *Violence in the workplace: A resource guide.* Halifax: Author.

Registered Nurses Association of Nova Scotia. (1996b). *Guidelines for telenursing practice.* Halifax: Author.

Smith-Temple, J., & Johnson, J. Y. (2002). *Nurses' guide to clinical procedures* (4th ed.). Philadelphia: Lippincott-Raven.

Storch, J., Rodney, P., & Starzomski, R. (2002). Ethics in health care in Canada. In B. S. Bolaria & H. Dickinson (Eds.), *Health, illness and health care in Canada* (3rd ed., pp. 409–444). Scarborough, ON: Nelson Thomas Learning.

Stuart, G. W., & Laraia, M. T. (2001). *Stuart and Sundeen's principles and practice of psychiatric nursing.* (7th ed.). St. Louis: Mosby.

Watson, G., & Glaser, E. (1980). *Watson-Glaser critical thinking appraisal manual.* San Antonio: The Psychologic Corporation: Harcourt Brace Jovanovich.

Webster, G., & Baylis, F. (2000). Moral residue. In S. B. Rubin & L. Zoloth (Eds.), *Margin of error: The ethics of mistakes in the practice of medicine* (pp. 217–232). Hagerstown, MD: University Publishing Group.

Wilkinson, J. M. (2001). *Nursing process and critical thinking.* New Jersey: Prentice-Hall.

Journals

Asterisks indicate nursing research articles.

Aquilino, M. L., & Keenan, G. (2000). Having our say: Nursing's standardized nomenclatures. *American Journal of Nursing, 100*(7), 33–38.

*Bowles, K. (2000). The relationship of critical-thinking skills and the clinical-judgment skills of baccalaureate nursing students. *Journal of Nursing Education, 39*(8), 373–376.

Bravo, G., Dubois, M. F., & Paquet, M. (2003). Advance directives for health care and research: Prevalence and correlates. *Alzheimer Disease & Associated Disorders, 17*(4), 215–222.

Cameron, B. (2004). Ethical moments in practice: The nursing 'How are you?' revisited. *Nursing Ethics, 11*(1), 53–62.

Canadian Nurses Protective Society (CNPS). (1996, November). Confidentiality of health information: Your client's right. [Entire issue]. *infoLaw 1*(2).

Caplan, R. L., Light, D. W., & Daniels, N. (1999). Benchmarks of fairness: A moral framework for assessing equity. *International Journal of Health Services, 29*(4), 853–869.

Corley, M. C., & Goren, S. (1998). The dark side of nursing: Impact of stigmatizing responses on patients. *Scholarly Inquiry for Nursing Practice 12*(2), 99–122.

Daly, J. M. (1996). A care planning tool that proves what we do. *RN, 59*(6), 26–30.

Day, L. J., & Stannard, D. (1999). Developing trust and connection with patients and their families. *Critical Care Nurse, 19*(3), 66–70.

*Day, R. A., & Williams, B. (2000). Development of critical thinking through problem-based learning: A pilot study. *Journal of Excellence in College Teaching, 11*(2 & 3), 203–226.

Ellerton, M. L. (2002). Client restraints: More than a safety issue. *Canadian Nurse 98*(2), 32–33.

Ellerton, M. L. (2000). When parents and children disagree about care. *Canadian Nurse 96*(7), 35–36.

Haddad, A. (2000). Ethics in action. *RN, 63*(7), 21–22, 24.

Haddad, A. (2001). Ethics in action. *RN, 64*(1), 29–30, 32.

Ignatavicius, D. D. (2001). Six critical thinking skills for at-the-bedside success. *Nursing Management, 32*(1), 37–39.

International Council of Nursing. (2005). *The ICN definition of nursing.* Available at: http://www.icn.ch/definition.htm. Retrieved October 21, 2005.

McAlpine, H. (2001). Refusal to care. *Canadian Nurse 97*(6), 33–34.

McMillan, J. (1987). Enhancing college students' critical thinking: A review of studies. *Research in Higher Education, 26*(1), 3–29.

Mitchell, G. J. (2001). Policy, procedure, and routine: Matters of moral influence. *Nursing Science Quarterly, 14*(2), 109–114.

Moorhouse, A. (2001). When CPR is not an option. *Canadian Nurse 97*(1), 37–38.

Peter, E., & Morgan, K. (2001). Explorations of a trust approach for nursing ethics. *Nursing Inquiry 8*(1), 3–0.

Prideaux, D. (2000). Do you know? *Medical Teacher, 22*(6), 607.

*Profetto-McGrath, J. (2003). The relationship of critical thinking skills and critical thinking dispositions of baccalaureate nursing students. *Journal of Advanced Nursing, 43*(6), 569–577.

*Profetto-McGrath, J., Hesketh, K. L., Lang, S., et al. (2003). A study of critical thinking and research utilization among nurses. *Western Journal of Nursing Research, 25*(3), 322–337.

*Profetto-McGrath, J., Smith, K. B., Day, R. A., et al. (2004). The questioning skills of tutors and students in a context-based baccalaureate nursing program. *Nursing Education Today, 24*(5), 363–372.

Rodney, P., & Starzomski, R. (1993). Constraints on moral agency of nurses. *Canadian Nurse, 89*(9), 23–26.

Rogers, P. D., & Bocchino, N. L. (1999). Restraint-free care: Is it possible? *American Journal of Nursing, 99*(10), 26–33.

Saint-Arnaud, J. (2002). Technologies biomédicales et enjeux éthiques en soins infirmiers: La vie, oui… mais à quell prix?, *infirmière canadienne, 3*(3), 4–8.

*Scheffer, B. K., & Rubenfeld, M. G. (2000). A consensus statement on critical thinking in nursing. *Journal of Nursing Education, 39*(8), 352–359.

Schiff, L. (2001). RN news watch: JCAHO and HCFA now agree on restraint standards. *RN, 64*(1), 14.

Smith, S. A. (1997). Controversies in hydrating the terminally ill patient. *Journal of Intravenous Nursing, 20*(4), 193–200.

Storch, J. (2002). Exposure to body fluids. *Canadian Nurse, 96*(6), 35–36.

Storch, J. (2002). When a client considers surrogacy. *Canadian Nurse 98*(5), 32–33.

Trammelleo, A. D. (2000). Protecting patients' end-of-life choices. *RN, 63*(8), 75, 77, 79.

*Ventura, M. J. (1999). Ethics on the job—A survey: The realities of HIV/AIDS. *RN, 62*(4), 26–30.

Zerwekh, J. V. (1997). Do dying patients really need IV fluids? *American Journal of Nursing, 97*(3), 26–31.

Zolot, J. S. (1999). Computer-based patient records. *American Journal of Nursing, 99*(12), 64–69.

RESOURCES AND WEBSITES

Association of Nurses of Prince Edward Island, 53 Grafton Street, Charlottetown, PE C1A 1K8; (902) 368-3764; fax: (902) 628-1430; e-mail: anpei@pei.aibn.com; http://www.anpei.ca.

Association of Registered Nurses of Newfoundland and Labrador, 55 Military Road, Box 6116, St. John's, NL A1C 5X8; (709) 753-

6040; fax: (709) 753-4940; e-mail: info@arnnl.nf.ca; http://www.anpei.ca.

Canadian Association of Schools of Nursing (CASN); www.casn.ca.

Canadian Council on Health Services Accreditation (CCHSA); www.cchsa.ca.

Canadian Nurses Association (CNA); 50 Driveway, Ottawa, ON K2P 1E2; (613) 237-2133 or 1-800-361-8404; www.cna-aiic.ca.

College and Association of Registered Nurses of Alberta (CARNA); 11620-168 Street, Edmonton, AB T5M 4A6; (780) 451-0043; fax: (780) 452-3276; e-mail: carna@nurses.ab.ca; http://nurses.ab.ca.

College of Nurses of Ontario/Ordre des infirmières et infirmiers de l'Ontario, 101 Davenport Road, Toronto, ON M5R 3P1; 1-800-387-5526 /(416) 928-0900; fax/télécopieur: (416) 928-6507; e-mail/courriel: cno@cnomail.org; http://www.cno.org.

College of Registered Nurses of British Columbia (CRNBC), 2855 Arbutus Street, Vancouver, BC V6J 3Y8; (604) 736-7331; fax: (604) 738-2272; e-mail: info@rnabc.bc.ca; http://www.crnbc.ca.

College of Registered Nurses of Manitoba, 890 Pembina Highway, Winnipeg, MB R3M 2M8; (204) 774-3477; fax: (204) 775-6052; e-mail: info@crnm.mb.ca; http://www.crnm.mb.ca.

College of Registered Nurses of Nova Scotia, Suite 600, Barrington Tower, 94 Barrington Street, Halifax, NS B3J 2A8; 02) 491-9744; fax: (902) 491-9510; e-mail: info@crnns.ca; http://www.crnns.ca.

International Council of Nurses (ICN); www.icn.ch.

International Organization for Standardization (ISO); www.iso.org.

Joint Commission on Accreditation of Healthcare Organizations (JCAHO), One Renaissance Blvd., Oakbrook Terrace, IL 60181; (630) 792-5000; http://www.jcaho.org.

Nurses Association of New Brunswick, 165 Regent Street, Fredericton, NB E3B 7B4; (506) 458-8731; fax/télécopieur: (506) 459-2838; e-mail/courriel: nanb@nanb.nb.ca; http://www.nanb.nb.ca.

Ordre des infirmières et infirmiers du Québec, 4200, boul. Dorchester Ouest, Montréal, QC H3Z 1V4; (514) 935-2501/1-800-363-6048; fax/télécopieur: (514) 935-1799; e-mail/courriel: inf@oiiq.org; http://www.oiiq.org.

Registered Nurses Association of Ontario, 438 University Avenue, Suite 1600, Toronto, ON M5G 2K8; 1-800-268-7199/(416) 599-1925; fax: (416) 599-1926; e-mail: info@rnao.org; http://www.rnao.org.

Registered Nurses Association of the Northwest Territories and Nunavut, Box 2757 Yellowknife, NT X1A 2R1; (867) 873-2745; fax: (867) 873-2336; e-mail: admin@rnantnu.ca; http://www.rnantnu.ca.

Saskatchewan Registered Nurses' Association, 2066 Retallack Street, Regina, SK S4T 7X5; 1-800-667-9945/ (306) 359-4200; fax: (306) 525-0849; e-mail: info@srna.org; http://www.srna.org.

World Health Organization (WHO); www.who.int.

Yukon Registered Nurses Association, 204-4133 4th Avenue, Whitehorse, YT Y1A 1H8; (867) 667-4062; fax: (867) 668-5123; e-mail: yrna@yknet.ca; http://www.yrna.ca.

Health Education and Health Promotion

Adapted by Bev Williams

On completion of this chapter, the learner will be able to:

1. Describe the purposes and significance of health education.
2. Describe the concept of adherence to a therapeutic regimen.
3. Identify variables influencing the elderly person's adherence to a therapeutic regimen.
4. Distinguish the variables that affect learning readiness.
5. Describe strategies that facilitate elderly adults' learning abilities.
6. Describe the relationship of the teaching–learning process to the nursing process.
7. Develop a teaching plan for a patient.
8. Define the concepts of health, wellness, and health promotion.
9. Discuss major health promotion theories.
10. Describe the health promotion principles of self-responsibility, nutrition, stress management, and exercise.
11. Specify the variables that affect health promotion activities for children, young and middle-aged adults, and elderly adults.
12. Describe the role of the nurse in health promotion.

*E*ffective health education lays a solid foundation for individual and community wellness. Teaching is an integral tool that all nurses use to assist patients and families in developing effective health behaviours and in altering lifestyle patterns that predispose people to health risks. Health education is an influential factor directly related to positive patient care outcomes.

Health Education Today

The changes in today's health care environment mandate the use of an organized approach to health education so that patients can meet their specific health care needs. Significant factors for the nurse to consider when planning patient education include the availability of health care outside the conventional hospital setting, the employment of diverse health care providers to accomplish care management goals, and the increased use of alternative strategies rather than traditional approaches to care. The careful consideration of these factors can provide patients with the comprehensive information that is essential for making informed decisions about health care. Demands from consumers for comprehensive information about their health issues throughout the life cycle accentuate the need for holistic health education to occur in every patient–nurse encounter.

The nurse as a teacher is challenged, not only to provide specific patient and family education, but also to focus on the educational needs of communities. Health education is important to nursing care, because it can determine how well individuals and families are able to perform behaviours conducive to optimal self-care.

Teaching, as a function of nursing, is included in all provincial nursing regulations (Canadian Nurses Association, 2005). Health education is an independent function of nursing practice and is a primary responsibility of the nursing profession. All nursing care is directed toward promoting, maintaining, and restoring health; preventing illness; and assisting people to adapt to the residual effects of illness. Many of these nursing activities are accomplished through health education or patient teaching.

Every contact a nurse has with a health care consumer, whether that person is ill or not, should be considered an opportunity for health teaching. Although the person has a right to decide whether or not to learn, the nurse has the responsibility to present information that will motivate the person to recognize the need to learn. Therefore, the nurse must seize opportunities both inside and outside health care settings to facilitate wellness. Educational environments can include homes, hospitals, community health centres, places of business, service organizations, shelters, and consumer action or support groups.

THE PURPOSE OF HEALTH EDUCATION

This emphasis on health education stems in part from the public's right to comprehensive health care, which includes up-to-date health information. It also reflects the emergence of an informed public that is asking more significant questions about health and the health care services it receives. Because of the importance Canadian society places on health and the responsibility each of us has to maintain and promote our own health, members of the health care team, specifically nurses, are obligated to make health education consistently available. Without adequate knowledge and training in self-care skills, consumers cannot make effective decisions about their health.

People with chronic illnesses are among those most in need of health education. As the life span of our population continues to increase, the number of people with such illnesses will also increase. People with chronic illness need health care information to participate actively in and assume responsibility for much of their own care. Health education can help these individuals to adapt to illness, prevent complications, carry out prescribed therapy, and solve problems when confronted with new situations. It can also prevent crisis situations and reduce the potential for rehospitalization resulting from inadequate information about self-care. The goal of health education is to teach people to live life to its healthiest—that is, to strive toward achieving their maximum health potential.

In addition to the public's right to and desire for health education, patient education is also a strategy for reducing health care costs by preventing illness, avoiding expensive medical treatments, decreasing lengthy hospital stays, and facilitating earlier discharge. For health care agencies, offering community wellness programs is a public relations tool for increasing patient satisfaction and for developing a positive image of the institution. Patient education is also a cost-avoidance strategy for those who believe that positive staff–patient relationships avert malpractice suits.

Adherence to the Therapeutic Regimen

One of the goals of patient education is to encourage people to adhere to their therapeutic regimen. Adherence to a therapeutic regimen usually requires that the person make one or more lifestyle changes to carry out specific activities that promote and maintain health. Common examples of behaviours facilitating health include taking prescribed medications, maintaining a healthy diet, increasing daily activities and exercise, self-monitoring for signs and symptoms of illness, practicing specific hygienic measures, seeking

Glossary

adherence: the process of faithfully following guidelines or directions

community: a group of people living in the same geographical area under the same guidelines

feedback: the return of information about the results of input given to a person or a system

health education: a variety of learning experiences designed to promote behaviours that facilitate health

health promotion: the art and science of assisting people to change their lifestyle toward a higher state of wellness

learning: the act of gaining knowledge and skill

learning readiness: the optimum time for learning to occur; usually corresponds to the learner's perceived need and desire to obtain specific knowledge

nutrition: the science that deals with food and nourishment in humans

physical fitness: the condition of being physically healthy as a result of proper exercise and nutrition

reinforcement: the process of strengthening a given response or behaviour to increase

the likelihood that the behaviour will continue

self-responsibility: personal accountability for one's actions or behaviour

stress management: behaviours and techniques used to strengthen a person's resources against stress

teaching: the imparting of knowledge

therapeutic regimen: a routine that promotes health and healing

wellness: a condition of good physical and emotional health sustained by a healthy lifestyle periodic health evaluations, and performing other therapeutic and preventive measures. The fact that many people do not adhere to their prescribed regimens cannot be ignored or minimized; rates of adherence are generally low, especially when the regimens are complex or of long duration.

Nonadherence to prescribed therapy has been the subject of many studies. For the most part, the findings have been inconclusive, and no one predominant causative factor has been found. Instead, a wide range of variables appears to influence the degree of adherence:

- Demographic variables, such as age, gender, race, socioeconomic status, and level of education
- Illness variables, such as the severity of the illness and the relief of symptoms afforded by the therapy
- Therapeutic regimen variables, such as the complexity of the regimen and uncomfortable side effects
- Psychosocial variables, such as intelligence, availability of significant and supportive people (especially family members), attitudes toward health professionals, acceptance or denial of illness, and religious or cultural beliefs
- Financial variables, especially the direct and indirect costs associated with a prescribed regimen

The nurse's success with health education is determined by ongoing assessment of the variables affecting the patient's capacity to adopt specific behaviours, to obtain resources, and to maintain a helpful social environment (Murray & Zentner, 2001). Teaching programs are more likely to succeed if the variables affecting the patient's adherence are identified and considered in the teaching plan.

The problem of nonadherence to therapeutic regimens is a substantial one that must be remedied before patients can achieve their maximum self-care capabilities and health potential. Surprisingly, a patient's need for knowledge has not been found to be a sufficient stimulus for acquiring knowledge and thereby enabling complete adherence to a health regimen. Teaching programs directed toward stimulating patient motivation produce varying degrees of adherence. The variables of choice, establishment of mutual goals, and the quality of the patient–provider relationship directly influence the behavioural changes that can result from patient education (Rankin & Stallings, 2005). These factors are directly linked to motivation for learning.

Using a learning contract can also be a motivator for learning. Such a contract is based on the assessment of patient needs, health care data, and specific, measurable goals (Redman, 2001). A well-designed learning contract is realistic and positive; it also includes measurable goals, with a specific time frame and reward system for goal achievement. The learning contract is recorded in writing and contains methods for ongoing evaluation.

The value of the contract lies in its clarity, specific delineation of what is to be accomplished, and usefulness for evaluating behavioural change. In a typical learning contract, a series of goals is established, beginning with small, easily attainable objectives and progressing to more advanced goals. Frequent, positive **reinforcement** is provided as the person moves from one goal to the next. An example of incremental goals would be a weight reduction program based on losing 1 to 2 kilograms per week rather than one that merely identifies a general goal of losing 15 kilograms.

🍃 Gerontologic Considerations

Nonadherence to therapeutic regimens is a significant problem for elderly people, leading to increased morbidity and mortality and increased cost of treatment. Many nursing home admissions and hospital admissions are linked to nonadherence.

Elderly people frequently have one or more chronic illnesses that are managed with numerous medications and complicated by periodic acute episodes. Elderly people may also have other problems that affect adherence to therapeutic regimens, such as increased sensitivity to medications and their side effects, difficulty in adjusting to change and stress, financial constraints, forgetfulness, inadequate support systems, lifetime habits of self-treatment with over-the-counter medications, visual and hearing impairments, and mobility limitations. To promote adherence among the elderly, time and effort must be taken to assess all variables that may affect health behaviour (Fig. 4-1). The nurse must also consider that cognitive deficiencies may be manifested by the elderly person's inability to draw inferences, apply information, or understand the major teaching points (Eliopoulos, 2000). The patient's strengths and limitations must be assessed in order to use existing strengths to compensate for limitations. Above all, health care professionals must work together to provide continuous, coordinated care; otherwise, the efforts of one health care professional may be negated by those of another.

The Nature of Teaching and Learning

Learning can be defined as acquiring knowledge, attitudes, or skills. Teaching is defined as helping another person to learn. These definitions indicate that the teaching–learning process is an active one, requiring the involvement of both teacher and learner in the effort to reach the desired outcome, a change in behaviour. The teacher does not simply give knowledge to the learner, but instead serves as a facilitator of learning.

In general, there is no definitive theory about how learning occurs and how it is affected by teaching. However, learning can be affected by factors such as readiness to learn, the learning environment, and the teaching techniques employed (Bastable, 2003; Green & Kreuter, 1999).

LEARNING READINESS

One of the most significant factors influencing learning is the person's learning readiness. For adults, readiness is based on culture, personal values, physical and emotional status, and past experiences

FIGURE 4-1 Taking time to teach patients about their medication and treatment program promotes interest and cooperation. Older adults who are actively involved in learning about their medication and treatment program and the expected effects may be more likely to adhere to the therapeutic regimen.

in learning. The teachable moment for an adult occurs when the content and skills being taught are congruent with the task to be accomplished (Redman, 2001).

Culture encompasses values, ideals, and behaviours, and the traditions within each culture provide the framework for solving the issues and concerns of daily living. Because people with different cultural backgrounds hold different values, lifestyles and choices about health care vary. Culture is a major variable influencing readiness to learn because it affects how a person learns and what information can be learned. Sometimes people will not accept health teaching because it conflicts with culturally mediated values. Before beginning health teaching, the nurse must perform an individual cultural assessment instead of relying only on generalized assumptions about a particular culture. A patient's social and cultural patterns must be appropriately incorporated into the teaching–learning interaction. Chart 4-1 describes cultural assessment components to consider when formulating a teaching plan.

An individual's values include beliefs about what are desirable and undesirable behaviours. The nurse must know what value the patient places on health and health care. In clinical situations, patients express their values through the actions performed and the level of knowledge pursued (Andrews & Boyle, 1998). When the nurse lacks knowledge about the cultural values of the patient being instructed, misunderstanding, lack of cooperation, and negative health outcomes may occur (Leininger, 1991). Each person's values and behaviours can be either an asset or a deficit to the readiness to learn. Therefore, no amount of health education will be accepted by patients unless their values and beliefs about health and illness are respected (Davidhizar & Giger, 1998).

Physical readiness is of vital importance, because until a person is physically capable of learning, attempts at teaching and learning may be both futile and frustrating. For example, someone in acute pain will be unable to focus attention away from the pain long enough to concentrate on learning. Likewise, a person who is short of breath will concentrate on breathing rather than on learning.

Emotional readiness also affects the motivation to learn. A person who has not accepted an existing illness or the threat of illness will not be motivated to learn. People who do not accept a therapeutic regimen, or who view it as conflicting with their present lifestyle, may consciously avoid learning about it. Until a person recognizes the need to learn and demonstrates an ability to learn, teaching efforts may be thwarted. However, it is not always wise to wait for a patient to become emotionally ready to learn, because that time might never come unless efforts are made by the nurse to stimulate the individual's motivation.

Illness and the threat of illness are usually accompanied by anxiety and stress. The nurse who recognizes such reactions can use simple explanations and instructions to alleviate these anxieties and provide further motivation to learn. Because learning involves changes in behaviour, it normally produces mild anxiety, which can often be a useful motivating factor.

Emotional readiness can be promoted by creating a warm, accepting, positive atmosphere and by establishing realistic learning goals. When learners achieve success and a feeling of accomplishment, they experience further motivation for participating in additional learning opportunities.

Feedback about progress also motivates learning. Such feedback should be presented in the form of positive reinforcement when learners are successful and in the form of constructive suggestions for improvement when they are unsuccessful.

Experiential readiness refers to past experiences that influence a person's ability to learn. Previous educational experiences and life experiences in general are significant determinants of an individual's approach to learning. A person who has had little or no formal education may not be able to understand the instructional materials presented. A person who has had difficulty learning in the past may be hesitant to try again. Many behaviours required for reaching maximum health potential demand a rather extensive background of knowledge, physical skills, and attitudes. Without this background on which to build, learning may be very difficult and very slow. For example, someone who does not understand the basics of normal nutrition may not be able to understand the restrictions of a specific diet. A person who does not view the desired learning as personally meaningful may reject teaching efforts. A person who is not future-oriented may be unable to appreciate many aspects of preventive health teaching. Experiential readiness is closely related to emotional readiness because motivation tends to be stimulated by an appreciation for the need to learn and by those learning tasks that are familiar, interesting, and meaningful.

Before initiating a teaching–learning program, it is important to assess the learner's physical and emotional readiness to learn, as well as his or her ability to learn what is being taught. This information then becomes the basis for establishing goals that can motivate the person to learn. Involving the learner in the establishment of mutually acceptable goals serves the purpose of encouraging active involvement in the learning process and a willingness to share the responsibility for learning.

THE LEARNING ENVIRONMENT

Although learning can take place without a teacher, most people who are attempting to learn new or altered health behaviours will need the services of a nurse for at least part of the time. The interpersonal interaction between the learner and the nurse who is attempting to meet the individual's learning needs may be formal or informal, depending on the method and techniques of teaching that are found to be most appropriate.

Learning can be optimized by minimizing external variables that interfere with the learning process. For example, the room temperature, lighting, noise levels, and other environmental conditions should be appropriate to the learning situation. Also, the time selected for teaching should be suited to the individual's

Chart 4-1

Cultural Assessment Components to Consider When Formulating a Teaching Plan

When formulating a teaching plan, consider the patient's beliefs about

- Body size, shape, boundaries, and functions
- Beauty and strength
- Value of the mind or brain
- Nature and function of blood
- Diet and nutrition
- Communication
- Gender
- Family and social support
- Physical health and illness
- Mental health and illness
- Pain
- Medicine, herbs, and talismans
- Spirituality or religion
- Where a person's essence or soul lies

Table 4-1 • Teaching People with Disabilities

TYPE OF DISABILITY	TEACHING STRATEGY
Physical or Emotional Disability	Adapt information to accommodate the person's cognitive, perceptual, and behaviour disabilities. Give clear written and oral information. Highlight significant information for easy reference. Avoid medical terminology.
Hearing Impairment	Use slow, directed, deliberate speech. Use sign language if appropriate. Position yourself so that the person can see your mouth if lip reading. Use telecommunication devices for the hearing impaired (TDD). Use written materials and visual aids, such as models and diagrams. Use captioned videos and films. Teach on the side of the "good ear" if unilateral deafness is present.
Visual Impairment	Use optical devices such as a magnifying lens. Use proper lighting and proper contrast of colours on materials and equipment. Use large-print materials. Use Braille materials if appropriate. Convert information to auditory and tactile formats. Obtain audiotapes and talking books. Explain noises associated with procedures, equipment, and treatments. Arrange materials in clockwise pattern.
Learning Disabilities Input disability	If visual perceptual disorder: • Explain information verbally, repeat, and reinforce frequently. • Use audiotapes. • Encourage learner to verbalize information received. If auditory perceptual disorder: • Speak slowly with as few words as possible, repeat, and reinforce frequently. • Use direct eye contact to focus person on task. • Use demonstration and return demonstration such as modeling, role playing, and hands-on experiences. • Use visual tools, written materials, and computers.
Output disability	Use all senses as appropriate. Use written, audiotape, and computer information. Review information and give time to interact and ask questions. Use hand gestures and motions.
Developmental disability	Base information and teaching on developmental stage, not person's age. Use nonverbal cues, gestures, signing, and symbols as needed. Use simple explanations and concrete examples with repetition. Encourage active participation. Demonstrate information and have the person perform return demonstrations.

thorough assessment of each person's level of physiologic and psychological functioning before teaching begins.

Changes in cognition with age may include slowed mental functioning; decreased short-term memory, abstract thinking, and concentration; and slowed reaction time. These changes are often accentuated by the health problems that cause the elderly to seek health care in the first place. Effective teaching strategies include a slow-paced presentation of small amounts of material at a time, frequent repetition of information, and the use of reinforcement techniques, such as audiovisual and written materials and repeated practice sessions. Distracting stimuli should be minimized as much as possible in the teaching environment.

Sensory changes associated with aging also affect teaching and learning. Teaching strategies to accommodate decreased visual acuity include large-print and easy-to-read materials printed on non-glare paper. Because colour discrimination is often impaired, the use of colour-coded or highlighted teaching materials may not be effective. To maximize hearing, the teacher must speak distinctly with a normal or lowered pitch, facing the person so that lip reading can occur as needed. Visual cues often help to reinforce verbal teaching.

Family members should be involved in teaching sessions when possible. They provide another source for reinforcement of material and can help the learner to recall instructions later. They can also provide valuable assessment information about the person's living situation and related learning needs.

When the nurse, the family, and other involved health care professionals work collaboratively to facilitate an elderly person's learning, the chances of success will be maximized. Successful learning for the elderly should result in improved self-care management skills, enhanced self-esteem, and a willingness to learn in future sessions.

The Nursing Process in Patient Teaching

The steps of the nursing process—assessment, diagnosis, planning, implementation, and evaluation—are used when constructing a teaching plan to meet an individual's teaching and learning needs (Chart 4-2).

ASSESSMENT

Assessment in the teaching–learning process is directed toward the systematic collection of data about the person's learning needs, the person's readiness to learn, and the family's learning needs. All internal and external variables that affect the patient's readiness to learn are identified. A learning assessment guide may be used for this purpose. Some of the available guides are very general and are directed toward the collection of general health information, whereas others are specific to common medication regimens or disease processes. Such guides facilitate the assessment but must be adapted to the individual's responses, problems, and needs.

As soon as possible after completing the assessment, the nurse organizes, analyzes, synthesizes, and summarizes the data collected and determines the patient's need for teaching.

NURSING DIAGNOSIS

Formulating nursing diagnoses makes educational goals and evaluations of progress more specific and meaningful. Teaching is an integral intervention implied by all nursing diagnoses, and for some diagnoses education is the primary intervention. Ineffective therapeutic regimen management, Impaired home maintenance, Health-seeking behaviours, and Decisional conflict are examples of nursing diagnoses that direct planning for educational needs. The diagnosis "Deficient knowledge" should be used cautiously, because knowledge deficit is not a human response but a factor relating to or causing the diagnosis (eg, Ineffective therapeutic regimen management related to a deficiency of information about wound care is a more appropriate nursing diagnosis than "Deficient knowledge") (Carpenito, 2002). A nursing diagnosis that relates specifically to the patient's and family's learning needs will serve as a guide in the development of the teaching plan.

PLANNING

Once the nursing diagnoses have been identified, the planning component of the teaching–learning process is established in accordance with the steps of the nursing process:

1. Assigning priorities to the diagnoses
2. Specifying the immediate, intermediate, and long-term goals of learning
3. Identifying specific teaching strategies appropriate for attaining goals

---

A Guide to Patient Education

Assessment
1. Assess the person's readiness for health education.
   a. What are the person's health beliefs and behaviours?
   b. What physical and psychosocial adaptations does the person need to make?
   c. Is the learner ready to learn?
   d. Is the person able to learn these behaviours?
   e. What additional information about the person is needed?
   f. Are there any variables (eg, hearing or visual impairment, cognitive issues, literacy issues) that will affect the choice of teaching strategy or approach?
   g. What are the person's expectations?
   h. What does the person want to learn?
   i. What does the person already know?
2. Organize, analyze, synthesize, and summarize the collected data.

Nursing Diagnosis
1. Formulate the nursing diagnoses that relate to the person's learning needs.
2. Identify the learning needs, their characteristics, and their aetiology.
3. State nursing diagnoses concisely and precisely.

Planning and Goals
1. Assign priority to the nursing diagnoses that relate to the individual's learning needs.
2. Specify the immediate, intermediate, and long-term learning goals established by teacher and learner together.
3. Identify teaching strategies appropriate for goal attainment.
4. Establish expected outcomes.
5. Develop the written teaching plan.
   a. Include diagnoses, goals, teaching strategies, and expected outcomes.
   b. Put the information to be taught in logical sequence.
   c. Write down the key points.
   d. Select appropriate teaching aids.
   e. Keep the plan current and flexible to meet the person's changing learning needs.
6. Involve the learner, family or significant others, nursing team members, and other health care team members in all aspects of planning.

Implementation
1. Put the teaching plan into action.
2. Use language the person can understand.
3. Use appropriate teaching aids and provide Internet resources if appropriate.
4. Use the same equipment that the person will use after discharge.
5. Encourage the person to participate actively in learning.
6. Record the learner's responses to the teaching actions.
7. Provide feedback.

Evaluation
1. Collect objective data.
   a. Observe the person.
   b. Ask questions to determine whether the person understands.
   c. Use rating scales, checklists, anecdotal notes, and written tests when appropriate.
2. Compare the person's behavioural responses with the expected outcomes. Determine the extent to which the goals were achieved.
3. Include the person, family or significant others, nursing team members, and other health care team members in the evaluation.
4. Identify alterations that need to be made in the teaching plan.
5. Make referrals to appropriate sources or agencies for reinforcement of learning after discharge.
6. Continue all steps of the teaching process: assessment, diagnosis, planning, implementation, and evaluation.

4. Specifying the expected outcomes
5. Documenting the diagnoses, goals, teaching strategies, and expected outcomes on the teaching plan

As in the nursing process, the assignment of priorities to the diagnoses should be a joint effort by the nurse and the learner or family members. Consideration must be given to the urgency of the individual's learning needs, with the most critical needs receiving the highest priority.

After the priorities of the diagnoses have been established, the immediate and long-term goals and the teaching strategies appropriate for attaining the goals are identified. Teaching is most effective when the objectives of both the learner and the nurse are in agreement (Lorig, et al., 1996). Learning begins with the establishment of goals that are appropriate to the situation and realistic in terms of the individual's ability and desire to achieve them. Involving the patient and family in establishing goals and subsequently in the planning of teaching strategies promotes their cooperation in the implementation of the teaching plan.

Expected outcomes of teaching strategies can be stated in terms of behaviours of the person, the family, or both. Outcomes should be realistic and measurable, and the critical time periods for attaining them should also be identified. The desired outcomes and the critical time periods will serve as a basis for evaluating the effectiveness of the teaching strategies.

During the planning phase, the nurse must consider the sequence in which the subject matter will be presented in each of the teaching strategies. Critical information (eg, survival skills for the person with diabetes) and material that the person or family identifies to be of particular importance receive high priority. An outline is often helpful for arranging the subject matter and for ensuring that all necessary information is included. Also during this time, appropriate teaching aids to be used in implementing the teaching strategies are prepared or selected.

The entire planning phase of the teaching–learning process is concluded with the formulation of the teaching plan. This teaching plan communicates the following information to all members of the nursing team:

1. The nursing diagnoses that specifically relate to the individual's learning needs and the priorities of these diagnoses
2. The goals of the teaching strategies
3. The teaching strategies, expressed in the form of teaching orders
4. The expected outcomes, which identify the desired behavioural responses of the learner
5. The critical time period within which each outcome is expected to be met
6. The individual's behavioural responses (which must be documented on the teaching plan)

The same rules that apply to writing and revising the plan of nursing care apply to the teaching plan.

IMPLEMENTATION

In the implementation phase of the teaching–learning process, the patient, the family, and other members of the nursing and health care teams carry out the activities outlined in the teaching plan. The nurse coordinates all the activities.

Flexibility during the implementation phase of the teaching–learning process and ongoing assessment of the individual's responses to the teaching strategies support modification of the teaching plan as necessary. Creativity in promoting and sustaining the learner's motivation to learn is essential. New learning needs that may arise after discharge from the hospital or after home care visits have ended should also be taken into account.

The implementation phase is concluded when the teaching strategies have been completed and when the individual's responses to the actions have been recorded. This record serves as the basis for evaluating how well the defined goals and expected outcomes have been achieved.

EVALUATION

Evaluation of the teaching–learning process determines how effectively the person has responded to the teaching strategies and to what extent the goals have been achieved. An important part of the evaluation phase addresses the question, "What can be done to improve the teaching and enhance the learning?" Answers to this question will direct the changes to be made in the teaching plan.

An evaluation must be made of what was done well, and what needs to be changed or reinforced. It cannot be assumed that individuals have learned just because teaching has occurred: learning does not automatically follow teaching. A variety of measurement techniques can be used to identify changes in behaviour as evidence that learning has taken place. These techniques include directly observing the behaviour; using rating scales, checklists, or anecdotal notes to document the behaviour; and indirectly measuring results through oral questioning and written tests. Measurement of actual behaviour (direct measurement) is the most accurate and appropriate technique in many patient teaching situations. Nurses often do comparative analysis using patient admission data as the baseline: selected data points observed during the period when nursing care is given and self-care was initiated are compared with the patient's baseline data.

Some examples of indirect measurements are patient satisfaction surveys, attitude surveys, and instruments that evaluate specific health status variables. All direct measurements should be supplemented with indirect measurements whenever possible. Using more than one measuring technique enhances the reliability of the resulting data and decreases the potential for error from a specific measurement strategy.

Measuring is only the beginning of evaluation. It must be followed by interpreting the data and making value judgments about the learning and teaching. Such evaluation should be conducted periodically throughout the teaching–learning program, at its conclusion, and at varying periods after the teaching has ended.

Evaluation of learning after hospitalization is highly desirable, because the analysis of teaching outcomes must extend into home care. With shortened lengths of hospital stay and with short-stay and same-day surgical procedures, follow-up evaluation in the home is especially important. Coordination of efforts and sharing of information between hospital-based and community-based nursing personnel facilitates post-discharge teaching and home care evaluation.

Evaluation is not the end step in the teaching–learning process, but the beginning of a new patient assessment. The information gathered during evaluation should be used to redirect teaching actions, with the goal of improving the learner's responses and outcomes.

Health Promotion

Health teaching and health promotion are linked by a common goal—to encourage people to achieve as high a level of wellness as possible so that they can live maximally healthy lives and avoid preventable illnesses. The call for health promotion has become a cornerstone in health policy because of the need to control costs and reduce unnecessary sickness and death.

The nation's first health agenda was established in 1974 with the identification of factors that influenced the health of Canadians: human biology, lifestyle, organization of health care, and the social and physical environments in which people live (Lalonde, 1974). The primary challenges facing the Canadian health system were and continue to be reducing inequities, increasing prevention, and enhancing people's capacity to cope. Creating the Health Promotion Framework was the nation's response to dealing with these challenges (Health Canada, 2005). Health promotion is understood to be the process of enabling people to increase control over their health. The three mechanisms considered intrinsic to health promotion are identified as self-care through healthy choices, mutual aid by working together, and environments conducive to health. Focal strategies for achieving health promotion include fostering public participation, strengthening community health services, and coordinating health public policy among various community sectors. The Health Promotion Framework helps Canadians formulate ways of dealing with day-to-day health issues in an effort to achieve health and improve the quality of life of the people and communities of Canada.

Health goals for the nation were first established in 1999 by the Canadian Institute for Health Information. A core set of health indicators relating to the goals correspond to the overall health of the population and major nonmedical determinants of health. The leading health indicators considered to reflect the health of Canadians are outlined in Chart 4-3.

HEALTH AND WELLNESS

The concept of health promotion has evolved because of a changing definition of health and an awareness that wellness exists at many levels of functioning. The definition of health as the mere absence of disease is no longer accepted. Today, health is viewed as a dynamic, ever-changing condition that enables a person to function at an optimum potential at any given time. The ideal health status is one in which people are successful in achieving their full potential regardless of any limitations they might have.

Wellness, as a reflection of health, involves a conscious and deliberate attempt to maximize one's health. Wellness does not just happen; it requires planning and conscious commitment and is the result of adopting lifestyle behaviours for the purpose of attaining one's highest potential for well-being. Wellness is not the

same for every person. The person with a chronic illness or disability may still be able to achieve a desirable level of wellness. The key to wellness is to function at the highest potential within the limitations over which there is no control.

A significant amount of information has shown that people, by virtue of what they do or fail to do, influence their own health. Today, many of the major causes of illness are chronic diseases that have been closely related to lifestyle behaviours (eg, heart disease, lung and colon cancer, chronic obstructive pulmonary diseases, hypertension, cirrhosis, traumatic injury, HIV [human immunodeficiency virus] infection, and acquired immunodeficiency syndrome [AIDS]). Consequently, a person's health status to a large extent is reflective of lifestyle.

HEALTH PROMOTION MODELS

Since the 1950s, many health-promotion models have been constructed to identify health-protecting behaviours and to help explain what makes people engage in these preventive behaviours. A health-protecting behaviour is defined as any behaviour performed by people, regardless of their actual or perceived health condition, for the purpose of promoting or maintaining their health, whether or not the behaviour produces the desired outcome (Downie, Fyfe, & Tannahill, 1990). One framework, the health belief model, was devised to foster understanding of what made some healthy people choose actions to prevent illness while others refused to engage in these protective recommendations (Becker, 1974).

Another model, the resource model of preventive health behaviour (Downie, Fyfe, & Tannahill, 1990), addresses the ways that people use resources to promote health. Nurse educators can use this model to assess how demographic variables, health behaviours, and social and health resources influence health promotion. LaLonde's (1974) health determinants model views human biology, environment, lifestyle, and the health care delivery system as the four determinants of a person's health.

A model for promotion of health, designed by Becker and colleagues (1993), is based on the premise that four variables influence the selection and use of health promotion behaviours. The first variable, demographic and disease factors, includes client characteristics such as age, gender, education, employment, severity of illness or disability, and length of illness. Barriers, the next component, are defined as factors that lead to unavailability or difficulty in gaining access to a specific health promotion alternative. The third variable, resources, encompasses such items as financial and social support. The last variable, perceptual factors, consists of how people view their health status, self-efficacy, and the perceived demands of their illness. The developers of this model conducted research to substantiate that these four variables have a positive correlation with a person's quality of life.

The health promotion model developed by Pender (2002), is based on social learning theory and emphasizes the importance of motivational factors that influence the acquiring and sustaining of health-promotion behaviours. This model explores how cognitive-perceptual factors affect one's view of the importance of health. It also examines perceived control of health, self-efficacy, health status, and the benefits and barriers to health promoting behaviours.

These models, along with other examples that can be found in the health promotion literature, can serve as an organizing framework for clinical work and research that supports the enhancement of health. Further efforts, however, are needed to advance understanding of the health promotion behaviours of families and communities.

Chart 4-3	**Leading Health Indicators to be Used to Measure the Health of the Nation**

1. Physical activity
2. Overweight and obesity
3. Tobacco use
4. Substance abuse
5. Responsible sexual behaviour
6. Mental health
7. Injury and violence
8. Environmental quality
9. Immunization
10. Access to health care

From Canadian Institute for Health Information. (1999). *National consensus conference on population health indicators*. Ottawa, ON: Author.

DEFINITION OF HEALTH PROMOTION

Health promotion can be defined as those activities that assist individuals in developing resources that will maintain or enhance well-being and improve their quality of life. These activities involve a person's efforts to remain healthy in the absence of symptoms and do not require the assistance of a health care team member.

The purpose of health promotion is to focus on a person's potential for wellness and to encourage appropriate alterations in personal habits, lifestyle, and environment in ways that will reduce risks and enhance health and well-being. Health promotion is an active process; that is, it is not something that can be prescribed or dictated. It is up to the individual to decide whether to make the changes that will promote a higher level of wellness. Choices must be made, and only the individual can make these choices.

The concepts of health, wellness, health promotion, and disease prevention have been extensively addressed in the lay literature and news media as well as in professional journals. The result has been a public demand for health information and a response by health care professionals and agencies to provide this information. Health-promotion programs that were once limited to hospital settings have now moved into community settings such as clinics, schools, churches, businesses, and industry. The workplace is quickly becoming an important site for health promotion programs, as employers strive to reduce costs associated with absenteeism, health insurance, hospitalization, disability, excessive turnover of personnel, and premature death.

HEALTH PROMOTION PRINCIPLES

Certain principles underlie the concept of health promotion as an active process: self-responsibility, nutritional awareness, stress reduction and management, and physical fitness.

Self-Responsibility

Taking responsibility for oneself is the key to successful health promotion. The concept of **self-responsibility** is based on the understanding that individuals control their lives. Each of us alone must make those choices that determine how healthy our lifestyle is. As more people recognize the significant effects that lifestyle and behaviour have on health, they may assume responsibility for avoiding high-risk behaviours such as smoking, alcohol and drug abuse, overeating, driving while intoxicated, risky sexual practices, and other unhealthy habits. They may also assume responsibility for adopting routines that have been found to have a positive influence on health, such as engaging in regular exercise, wearing a seat belt, and eating a balanced diet.

A variety of different techniques have been used to encourage people to accept responsibility for their health, ranging from extensive educational programs to reward systems. No one technique has been found to be superior to any other. Instead, self-responsibility for health promotion is very individualized and depends on a person's desires and inner motivations. Health promotion programs are important tools for encouraging people to assume responsibility for their health and to develop behaviours that improve health.

Nutrition

Nutrition as a component of health promotion has become the focus of considerable attention and publicity. A vast array of books and magazine articles address the topics of special diets, natural foods, and the hazards of certain substances, such as sugar, salt, cholesterol, artificial colours, and food additives. Good nutrition has been suggested as the single most significant factor in determining health status and longevity.

Nutritional awareness involves an understanding of the importance of a properly balanced diet that supplies all of the essential nutrients. Understanding the relationship between diet and disease is an important facet of a person's self-care. Some clinicians believe that a healthy diet is one that substitutes "natural" foods for processed and refined ones and reduces the intake of sugar, salt, fat, cholesterol, caffeine, alcohol, food additives, and preservatives.

Chapter 5 contains detailed information about the assessment of an individual's nutritional status. The chapter covers physical signs indicating nutritional status, assessment of food intake (food record, 24-hour recall), comparison of food intake with the dietary guidelines outlined in the Canada Food Guide, and calculation of ideal body weight.

Stress Management

Stress management and stress reduction are important aspects of health promotion. Studies have shown the negative effects of stress on health and a cause-and-effect relationship between stress and infectious diseases, traumatic injuries (eg, motor vehicle crashes), and some chronic illnesses. Stress has become inevitable in contemporary societies in which demands for productivity have become excessive. More and more emphasis is placed on encouraging people to manage stress appropriately and to reduce stress that is counterproductive. Techniques such as relaxation training, exercise, and modification of stressful situations are often included in health promotion programs that deal with stress. Further information on stress management, including health risk appraisal and stress reduction methods such as biofeedback and the relaxation response, can be found in Chapter 6.

Exercise

Physical fitness is another important component of health promotion. Clinicians and researchers (Anspaugh, Hamrick & Rosata, 1994; Edelman & Mandle, 1998) examining the relationship between health and physical fitness have found that a regular exercise program can promote health by improving the function of the circulatory system and the lungs, decreasing cholesterol and low-density lipoprotein concentrations, lowering body weight by increasing kilojoule expenditure, delaying degenerative changes such as osteoporosis, and improving flexibility and overall muscle strength and endurance. On the other hand, exercise can be harmful if it is not started gradually and increased slowly in accordance with the individual's response. An exercise program should be designed specifically for the individual, with consideration given to age, physical condition, and any known cardiovascular or other risk factors. An appropriate exercise program can have a significantly positive effect on the individual's performance capacity, appearance, and general state of physical and emotional health (Nursing Research Profile 4-2).

Health Promotion Throughout the Life Span

Health promotion is a concept and a process that extends throughout the life span. Studies have shown that the health of a child can be affected either positively or negatively by the health practices of the mother during the prenatal period. Therefore, health promotion starts before birth and extends through childhood, adulthood, and old age.

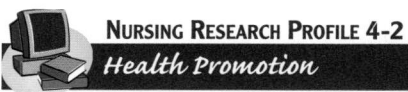

NURSING RESEARCH PROFILE 4-2
Health Promotion

Hays, I., Damuch, T., & Clark, D. (2005). Relationships between exercise self-definitions and exercise participation among urban women in primary care. *Journal of Cardiovascular Nursing, 20*(1), 9–17.

Purpose
The purpose of this study was to explore the relationships between exercise self-definition and participation in a group-based exercise program among middle aged to older women who had at least one cardiovascular risk factor and were leading a mostly sedentary life.

Sample and Study Design
The study was a secondary analysis of selected data from a larger study (exercise referral and older women study, R01-AG15098) designed to evaluate the long-term effectiveness of physician-initiated exercise referral among women receiving primary care. The study targeted women 50 years or older who received primary care from one of two health centres associated with an urban hospital that served low-income adults. 860 women met the age criterion. For budgetary and timeline reasons, enrolment stopped at 500. Of these, 192 completed the baseline telephone survey and 86 completed the 6-month telephone survey. Exercise programs were offered several times a day, Monday through Friday, near the health centre and were free to participants.

Findings
At baseline, participants had moderate total exercise self-definition scores indicating that they were a little to somewhat sure of defining themselves as exercisers. Six-month scores were significantly higher than baseline scores, suggesting that exercise self-definitions strengthened over time and were important in maintaining an exercise program. It is possible that some people will drop out of an exercise program early because their exercise self-definition is not strong enough to influence them to continue or even to start exercising.

Nursing Implications
Nurses might want to consider assessing self-definitions when helping patients initiate and maintain an exercise program. Nurses can offer tools that foster exercise self-definition by raising subconscious thoughts that affect self-views, by reminding participants of exercise behaviours they already do and acknowledging changes in self-definition as they occur. It might also be necessary to correct misconceptions about exercise or address fears of injury.

Health promotion includes health screening. In 2004, the Canadian Task Force on Preventative Health Care and the College of Family Physicians of Canada developed recommendations for periodic health examinations that identify the age groups for which specific screening interventions are appropriate (Canadian Task Force on Preventative Health Care, 2005; The College of Family Physicians of Canada, 2004). Table 4-2 presents the general population guidelines; specific population standards and guidelines have also been recommended.

CHILDREN AND ADOLESCENTS

Health screening has traditionally been an important aspect of childhood health care. The goal has been to detect health problems at an early age so that they can be treated early in a child's life. Today, health promotion goes beyond the mere screening of children for disabilities and includes extensive efforts to promote positive health practices at a very young age. Because health habits and practices are formed early in life, children should be encouraged to develop positive health attitudes. For this reason, more and more

programs are being offered to school-age children and to adolescents to help them develop good health habits. Although the negative results of practices such as smoking, risky sexual activities, alcohol and drug abuse, and poor nutrition are explained in these educational programs, emphasis is also placed on values training, self-esteem, and healthy lifestyle practices. The projects are designed to appeal to a particular age group, with emphasis on learning experiences that are fun, interesting, and relevant.

YOUNG AND MIDDLE-AGED ADULTS

Young and middle-aged adults represent an age group that not only expresses an interest in health and health promotion but also responds enthusiastically to suggestions that show how lifestyle practices can improve health. Adults are frequently motivated to change their lifestyles in ways that are believed to enhance their health and wellness. Many adults who wish to improve their health turn to health-promotion programs to help them make the desired changes in their lifestyles. They respond in overwhelming numbers to programs that focus on topics such as general wellness, smoking cessation, exercise, physical conditioning, weight control, conflict resolution, and stress management. Because of the nationwide emphasis on health during the reproductive years, young adults actively seek programs that address prenatal health, parenting, family planning, and women's health issues.

Programs that provide health screening, such as those that screen for cancer, high cholesterol, hypertension, diabetes, and hearing impairments, are quite popular with this age group. Programs that cover health promotion for people with specific chronic illnesses such as cancer, diabetes, heart disease, and pulmonary disease are also popular. It is becoming more evident that chronic disease and disability do not preclude health and wellness; rather, positive health attitudes and practices can promote optimal health for people who must live with the limitations imposed by their chronic illnesses and disabilities.

Health-promotion programs can be offered almost anywhere in the community. Common sites include local clinics, elementary schools, high schools, community colleges, recreation centres, churches, and even private homes. Health fairs are frequently held in civic centres and shopping malls. The outreach idea for health-promotion programs has served to meet the needs of many adults who otherwise would not avail themselves of opportunities to strive toward a healthier lifestyle.

The workplace has become a centre for health-promotion activity as employers become increasingly concerned about the rising costs of health care insurance to treat illnesses that are related to lifestyle behaviours. They are also concerned about increased absenteeism and lost productivity. For these reasons, many businesses have instituted health-promotion programs in the workplace. Some employ health-promotion specialists to develop and implement the program, and others purchase packaged programs that have already been developed by health care agencies or private health-promotion corporations.

Programs offered at the workplace usually include employee health screening and counselling, physical fitness, nutritional awareness, work safety, and stress management and stress reduction. In addition, efforts are made to promote a safe and healthy work environment. Many large businesses provide exercise facilities for their employees and offer their health-promotion programs to retirees. If employers can show cost-containment benefits from such programs, their dollars will be considered well spent, and more businesses will provide health-promotion programs as a benefit of employment.

Table 4-2 • **Routine Health Promotion Screening for Adults***

TYPE OF SCREENING	SUGGESTED TIME FRAME
Routine health examination	Yearly
Blood chemistry profile	Baseline at age 20, then as mutually determined by patient and clinician
Complete blood count	Baseline at age 20, then as mutually determined by patient and clinician
Lipid profile	Baseline at age 20, all men over 40, all women over 50 or post-menopausal, then every 5 years if asymptomatic
Hemoccult screening	Yearly after age 50
Electrocardiogram	Baseline at age 40, then as mutually determined by patient and clinician
Blood pressure	Yearly, then as mutually determined by patient and clinician
Tuberculosis skin test	Every 2 years or as mutually determined by patient and clinician
Chest x-ray film	For positive PPD results
Breast self-examination	Monthly
Mammogram	Yearly for women over 40, or earlier or more often if indicated
Clinical breast examination	Yearly
Gynecologic examination	Yearly
Pap test	Yearly
Bone density screening	Based on identification of primary and secondary risk factors (prior to onset of menopause, if indicated, then every 1–2 years if abnormal and every 2–3 years if normal)
Nutritional screening	As mutually determined by patient and clinician
Digital rectal examination	Yearly
Sigmoidoscopy	Every 3–5 years after age 50 or as mutually determined by patient and clinician
Prostate examination	Yearly
Prostate-specific antigen	Every 1–2 years after age 50
Testicular examination	Monthly
Skin examination	Yearly or as mutually determined by patient and clinician
Vision screening	Every 2–3 years
Glaucoma	Baseline at age 40, then every 2–3 years until age 70, then yearly
Dental screening	Every 6 months
Hearing screening	As needed
Health risk appraisal	As needed
Adult Immunizations	
Tetanus	Boosters every 10 years
Diphtheria	Boosters every 10 years
Rubella	Given to women of childbearing age if not previously given or if titer is low
Pneumococcal vaccine	Given one time at age 65 or younger if chronic illness or disability is present
Hepatitis B (if not received as a child)	Series of three doses (now, 1 month later, then 5 months after the second date)
Influenza vaccine	Yearly
Lyme disease vaccine, if at risk	Series of three doses (now, 1 month later, and 11 months after the second dose)

*Note: Any of these screenings may be performed more frequently if deemed necessary by the patient or recommended by the health care provider.

ELDERLY ADULTS

Health promotion is as important for the elderly as it is for other age groups. Despite the fact that 80% of people older than 65 years of age have one or more chronic illnesses and about 50% are limited in their activity, the elderly as a group experience significant gains from health promotion. Clinical work indicates that the elderly are very health-conscious and that most view their health positively and are willing to adopt practices that will improve their health and well-being (Ebersole & Hess, 1997; Staab & Hodges, 1996). Although their chronic illnesses and disabilities cannot be eliminated, these adults can benefit from activities that help them maintain independence and achieve an optimal level of health.

Various health-promotion programs have been developed to meet the needs of older Canadians, many of which began within Health Canada. Both public and private organizations continue to

be responsive to health promotion, and more programs that serve the elderly are emerging. Many of these programs are offered by health care agencies, churches, community centres, senior citizen residences, and a variety of other organizations. The activities directed toward health promotion for the elderly are the same as those for other age groups: physical fitness and exercise, nutrition, safety, and stress management.

Implications for Nursing

Nurses, by virtue of their expertise in health and health care and their long-established credibility with consumers, play a vital role in health promotion. In many instances they have initiated health-promotion programs or have participated with other health care personnel in developing and providing wellness services in a variety of settings (Fig. 4-2).

FIGURE 4-2 Teaching aids and demonstrations enhance learning. Here a nurse (*right*) instructs learners during a community health education program. Often generated and developed by nurses, these programs offer the public opportunities to obtain health information about topics ranging from diet, nutrition, and hypercholesterolemia to hypertension, diabetes, cardiopulmonary resuscitation, and others.

As health care professionals, nurses have a responsibility to promote activities that foster well-being, self-actualization, and personal fulfillment. Every interaction with consumers of health care must be viewed as an opportunity to promote positive health attitudes and behaviours.

 Critical Thinking Exercises

1. You are constructing a patient teaching plan for a mid-life woman who has a diagnosis of multiple sclerosis and is at high risk for development of osteoporosis. Describe the health promotion strategies you would develop for this patient. Indicate the possible variables that could influence the patient's willingness or ability to follow the instructions.

2. You are assigned to teach an elderly patient about the cardiac and diabetic medications that she will be taking at home. How would you assess this patient's condition and psychosocial situation to determine how best to instruct her about her medications? How would you modify your teaching plan if the patient was hard of hearing, visually impaired, or unable to read or write?

3. A neighbour tells you that he has heard about a health fair that is being offered at a nearby civic centre. He asks you if you think that he should attend. Describe the reasons you might give for why the neighbour should attend the health fair. He also states that his wife does not need to attend because she is receiving medical care for her arthritis and diabetes. What advice would you offer him about his wife's attending the health fair?

REFERENCES AND SELECTED READINGS

Books

Andrews, M. M., & Boyle, J. S. (1998). *Transcultural concepts in nursing care* (3rd ed.). Philadelphia: Lippincott Williams & Wilkins.

Anspaugh D. J., Hamrick, M. H., & Rosato, F. D. (1994). *Wellness: Concepts and applications* (2nd ed.). St. Louis: Mosby.

Bastable, S. G. (Ed.). (2003). *Nurse as educator: Principles of teaching and learning.* Boston: Jones & Bartlett.

Becker, M. H. (Ed.). (1974). *The health belief model and personal health behavior.* Thorofare, NJ: Charles B. Slack.

Carpenito, L. J. (2002). *Nursing diagnosis: Application to clinical practice.* Philadelphia: Lippincott Williams & Wilkins.

Davidhizar, R. E., & Giger, J. N. (1998). *Canadian transcultural nursing: Assessment and intervention.* St. Louis: C. V. Mosby.

Downie, R. S., Fyfe, C., & Tannahill, A. (1990). *Health promotion: Models and values.* New York: Oxford University Press.

Doyle, E., & Ward, S. (2001). *The process of community health education and promotion.* Palo Alto, CA: Mayfield Publishing.

Ebersole, P., & Hess, P. (1997). *Toward health aging: Human needs and nursing responses* (5th ed.). Philadelphia: Lippincott-Raven.

Edelman, C., & Mandle, C. L. (1998). *Health promotion throughout the lifespan* (4th ed.). St. Louis: C. V. Mosby.

Eliopoulos, C. (2000). *Gerontological nursing* (5th ed.). Philadelphia: Lippincott Williams & Wilkins.

Green, L. W., & Kreuter, M. (1999). *Health promotion planning.* Palo Alto, CA: Mayfield Publishing.

Insel, P. M., & Roth, W. T. (2000). *Core concepts in health.* Palo Alto, CA: Mayfield Publishing.

Kreuter, T. L., Farrell, D., Olevitch, L., Brennan, L., & Rimer, B. K. (2000). *Tailoring health messages: Customizing communication with computer technology.* Mahwah, NJ: Lawrence Erlbaum Associates.

LaLonde, M. (1974). *New perspectives on the health of Canadians: A working document.* Ottawa, Canada: Minister of Supply and Services.

Leininger, M. M. (1991). *Culture care diversity and universality: A theory of nursing.* New York: National League of Nursing.

Lorig, K., Stewart, A., Ritter, P., Gonzalez, V., Laurent, D., & Lynch, J. (1996). *Outcome measures for health education and other health care interventions.* Thousand Oaks, CA: Sage.

Marion, L. N. (1996). *Nursing's vision for primary health care in the 21st century.* Washington, DC: ANA Publications.

Murray, R. B., & Zentner, J. P. (2001). *Nursing assessment and health promotion through the life span* (7th ed.). Englewood Cliffs, NJ: Prentice-Hall.

O'Donnell, M. P. (2001). *Health promotion in the workplace.* Albany, NY: Delmar Publishing.

Pender, N. J. (2002). *Health promotion in nursing practice* (4th ed.). Norwalk, CT: Appleton & Lange.

Rankin, S. H., & Stallings, K. D. (2005). *Patient education: Issues, principles, practices* (5th ed.). Philadelphia: Lippincott Williams & Wilkins.

Redman, B. (2001). *The practice of patient education* (9th ed.). St. Louis: C. V. Mosby.

Staab, A. S., & Hodges, L. C. (1996). *Essentials of gerontological nursing: Adaptation to the aging process.* Philadelphia: Lippincott-Raven.

Whitman, T. L. (Ed.). (1999). *Life-span perspectives on health and illness.* Mahwah, NJ: Lawrence Erlbaum Associates.

Woolf, S. H., Jonas, S., & Lawrence, R. S. (1996). *Health promotion and disease prevention in clinical practice.* Baltimore: Williams & Wilkins.

Journals

Asterisks indicate nursing research articles.

Beauchesne, M. A., & Meservey, P. M. (1999). An interdisciplinary community based educational model. *Journal of Professional Nursing, 15*(1), 38–43.

Becker, H. A., Stuifbergen, A. K., Oh, H., & Hall, S. (1993). The self-rated abilities for health practices scale: A health self-efficacy measure. *Health Values, 17,* 42–50.

Campbell, K. N. (1999). Adult education: Helping adults begin the process of learning. *American Association of Occupational Health Nursing, 47*(1), 31–42.

Canadian Nurses Association. (2005). *Standards and best practices.* Available at: http://www.cna-nurses.ca/CNA/practice/standards/default_e.aspx.

Canadian Task Force on Preventative Health Care. (2005). *Evidence-based clinical prevention.* Available at: http://www.ctfphc.org.

Gray, M., Kanner, S., & Lacey, K. O. (1999). Characteristics of the learner: Children and adolescents. *Diabetes Educator, 25*(6), (Suppl.), 25–33.

Haber, J. (1999). Rx for teaching: Assessing stress. *Home Health Focus, 5*(9), 70–71, 67.

Health Canada. (2005). *Achieving health for all: A framework for health promotion.* Available at: http://hc-sc.gc/english/care/achieving_health.html.

Herje, P. A. (1980). Hows and whys of patient contracting. *Journal of Nursing Education, 5,* 30–34.

Jacubowitz, T. R. (1999). Culturally sensitive care for the elderly. *Nurse Practitioner Forum, 10*(1), 8–11.

Kelleher, C. (1996). Education and training in health promotion: Theory and methods. *Health Promotion International, 11*(1), 47–53.

Lai, S. C., & Cohen, M. N. (1999). Promoting lifestyle changes. *American Journal of Nursing, 99*(4), 63–67.

*Lev, E. L., & Owen, S. V. (1996). A measure of self-care self-efficacy: Strategies used by people to promote health. *Research in Nursing and Health, 19*(5), 421–429.

Lucas, J. A., Orshan, S. A., & Cook, F. (2000). Determinants of health-promoting behaviours among women ages 65 and above living in the community. *Scholarly Inquiry for Nursing Practice, 14*(1), 77–109.

Malone, S. B. (2000). Patient education: Stress management. *Clinical Nurse Specialist, 4*(2), 234–236.

Poss, J. E. (1999). Providing culturally competent care: Is there a role for health promoters? *Nursing Outlook, 47*(1), 30–36.

Robinson, A. W., & Sloan, H. L. (2000). Healthy People 2000: Heart health and old women. *Journal of Gerontological Nursing, 26*(5), 38–45.

Schank, M. J. (1999). Educational innovations—Self-health appraisal: Learning the difficulties of lifestyle change. *Journal of Nursing Education, 38*(1), 10–12.

Schneider, S. L., Richard, M., Huss, K., et al. (1997). Moving health care education into the community. *Nursing Management, 28*(9), 40–43.

Stuifbergen, A. K. (1995). Health-promoting behaviors and quality of life among individuals with multiple sclerosis. *Scholarly Inquiry for Nursing Practice, 9*(1), 31–50.

The College of Family Physicians of Canada. (2004). *The evidence-based preventive care checklist form.* Available at: http://cfpc.ca/English/cfpc/communication/health%20policy/preventive%20care/%20checklist/%20forms.

Wilkinson, J. A. (1999). Understanding patients' health beliefs. *Professional Nurse, 14*(5), 320–322.

RESOURCES AND WEBSITES

Canadian Nurses Association; http://www.cna-nurses.ca/CNA/practice/standards/default_e.aspx.

Canadian Task Force on Preventative Health Care; http://www.ctfphc.org.

Health Canada; http://hc-sc.gc/english/care/achieving_health.html.

The College of Family Physicians of Canada; http://cfpc.ca/English/cfpc/communication/health%20policy/preventive%20care/%20checklist/%20forms.

Health Assessment

Adapted by Rene A. Day

LEARNING OBJECTIVES

On completion of this chapter, the learner will be able to:

1. Describe the components of the health history.
2. Apply interviewing skills and techniques to conduct a successful interview.
3. Describe the physical examination techniques of inspection, palpation, percussion, and auscultation.
4. Apply the techniques of inspection, palpation, percussion, and auscultation to perform physical assessment of the major body systems.
5. Discuss the techniques of measurement of body mass index, anthropometric measurements, biochemical assessment, clinical examination, and assessment of food intake to assess a person's nutritional status.
6. Identify ethical considerations necessary for protecting the individual's rights related to data collected in the health history or physical examination.
7. Describe factors that may contribute to altered nutritional status in high-risk groups such as adolescents and the elderly.
8. Conduct a health history and physical and nutritional assessment of the patient at home.

*T*he ability to assess the patient is one of the most important skills of the nurse, regardless of the practice setting. In all settings where nurses interact with patients and provide care, eliciting a complete health history and using appropriate assessment skills are critical to identifying physical and psychological problems and concerns experienced by the patient. As the first step in the nursing process, patient assessment is necessary to obtain data that will enable the nurse to make a nursing diagnosis, identify and implement nursing interventions, and assess their effectiveness.

The Role of the Nurse in Assessment

The role of the nurse in health assessment includes obtaining the patient's health history and performing a physical assessment. This role can be carried out in a variety of settings, including the acute care setting, clinic or outpatient office, school, long-term care facility, and the home. A growing list of nursing diagnoses is used by nurses to identify and categorize patient problems that nurses have the knowledge, skills, and responsibility to treat independently. All members of the health care team—physicians, nurses, nutritionists, social workers, and others—use their unique skills and knowledge to contribute to the resolution of patient problems by first obtaining a health history and physical examination. Because the focus of each member of the health care team is unique, a variety of health history and physical examination formats have been developed. Regardless of the format, the database obtained by the nurse is complementary to the databases obtained by other members of the health care team and focuses on nursing's unique concern for the patient.

Basic Guidelines for Conducting a Health Assessment

People who seek health care for a specific problem often feel anxious. Their anxiety may be increased by fear about potential diagnoses, possible disruption of lifestyle, and other concerns. With this in mind, the nurse attempts to establish rapport, put the person at ease, encourage honest communication (Fuller & Schaller-Ayers, 2000), make eye contact, and listen carefully to the person's responses to questions about health issues (Fig. 5-1).

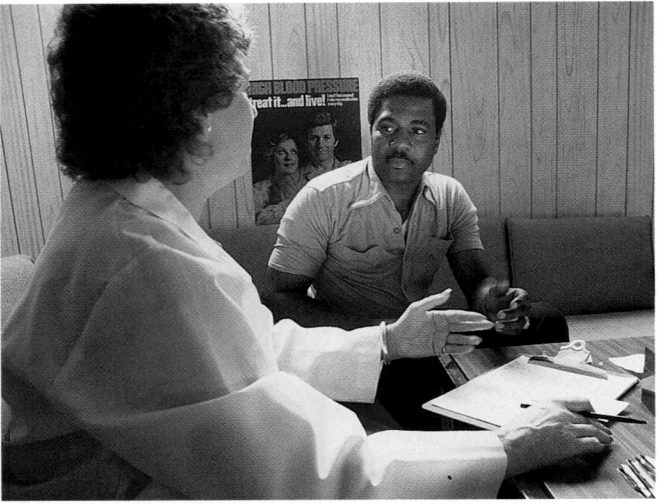

FIGURE 5-1 A comfortable, relaxed atmosphere and an attentive interviewer are essential for a successful clinical interview.

When obtaining the health history or performing the physical examination, the nurse must be aware of his or her own nonverbal communication as well as that of the patient. The nurse takes into consideration the educational and cultural background as well as language proficiency of the patient. Questions and instructions to the patient are phrased in a way that is easily understandable. Technical terms and medical jargon are avoided. In addition, the examiner needs to be aware of the patient's disabilities or impairments (hearing, vision, cognitive, and physical limitations) and takes these into consideration during the history as well as the physical examination. At the end of the assessment, the examiner may summarize and clarify the information obtained and ask if the person has any questions; this provides an opportunity to correct misinformation and add facts that may have been omitted.

Ethical Use of History or Physical Examination Data

A particularly important guideline for use whenever information is elicited from a person through the health history or physical examination is that the person has the right to know why the information is sought and how it will be used. For this reason, it is important to explain what the history and physical examination are, how the information will be obtained, and how it will be used (Fuller & Schaller-Ayers, 2000). It is also important that the individual be aware that the decision to participate is voluntary. A private setting for the history interview and physical examination promotes trust and encourages open, honest communication. After the history collection and examination, the nurse selectively records the data pertinent to the patient's health status. This written record of the patient's history and physical examination findings is then maintained in a secure place and made available only to those health professionals directly involved in the care of the patient. This protects confidentiality and promotes professional conduct.

The Health History

Throughout assessment, and particularly when obtaining the history, attention is focused on the impact of psychosocial, ethnic, and cultural background on the person's health, illness, and health-promotion behaviours. The interpersonal and physical environments, as well as the person's lifestyle and activities of daily living, are explored in depth. Many nurses are responsible for obtaining a detailed history of the person's current health problems, past medical history, family history, and a review of the person's functional status. This results in a total health profile that focuses on health as well as illness and is more appropriately called a health history rather than a medical or a nursing history.

The format of the health history traditionally combines the medical history and the nursing assessment, although formats based on nursing frameworks, such as functional health patterns, have also become a standard. Both the review of systems and patient profile are expanded to include individual and family relationships, lifestyle patterns, health practices, and coping strategies. These components of the health history are the basis of nursing assessment and can be easily adapted to address the needs of any patient population in any setting, institution, or agency.

Combining the information obtained by the physician and the nurse in one health history prevents duplication of information and minimizes efforts on the part of the person to provide this information. This also encourages collaboration among members of the health care team who share in the collection and interpretation of the data (Butler, 1999).

THE INFORMANT

The informant, or the person providing the health history, may not always be the patient, as in the case of a developmentally delayed, mentally impaired, disoriented, confused, unconscious, or comatose patient. The interviewer assesses the reliability of the informant and the usefulness of the information provided. For example, a disoriented patient is often unable to provide a reliable database; people who abuse drugs and alcohol often deny using these substances. The interviewer must make a judgment about the reliability of the information (based on the context of the entire interview), and he or she includes this evaluation in the record.

CULTURAL CONSIDERATIONS

When obtaining the health history, the interviewer takes into account the person's cultural background (Weber & Kelley, 2003). Cultural attitudes and beliefs about health, illness, health care, hospitalization, the use of medications, and the use of complementary therapies are derived from each person's experiences. They vary according to the person's ethnic and cultural background. A person from another culture may have a different view of personal health practices than the health care practitioner.

Similarly, people from some ethnic and cultural backgrounds will not complain of pain, even when it is severe, because outward expressions of pain are considered unacceptable. In some instances they may refuse to take analgesics. Other cultures have their own folklore and beliefs about the treatment of illnesses. All such differences in outlook must be taken into account and accepted when caring for members of other cultures. Attitudes and beliefs about family relationships and the role of women and elderly members of a family must be respected even if those attitudes and beliefs conflict with those of the interviewer.

CONTENT OF THE HEALTH HISTORY

When the patient is seen for the first time by a member of the health care team, the first requirement is a database (except in emergency situations). The sequence and format of obtaining data about the patient vary, but the content, regardless of format, usually addresses the same general topics. One approach includes the following:

- Biographical data
- Reason for seeking health care (chief complaint)
- Present health concern (or present illness)
- Past history
- Family history
- Review of systems
- Patient profile

Biographical Data

Biographical information puts the patient's health history in context. This information includes the person's name, address, age, gender, marital status, occupation, and ethnic origins. Some interviewers prefer to ask more personal questions at this part of the interview, while others wait until more trust and confidence have been established or until the patient's immediate or urgent needs are first addressed. The patient in severe pain or with another urgent problem is unlikely to have a great deal of patience for an interviewer who is more concerned about marital or occupational status than with quickly addressing the problem at hand.

Reason for Seeking Health Care (Chief Complaint)

The reason for seeking health care, or chief complaint, is the issue that brings the person to the attention of the health care provider. At this point it is important to "invite" the person's story (Bickley & Szilagyi, 2003). An open-ended question such as, "What brings you to the health centre today?" encourages the person to discuss concerns and usually elicits the needed information. In answering the next question, "How do you feel about having to seek health care?" the person has the opportunity to express fears and describe previous contact with other health professionals. In the home setting the initial question might be, "How can I help you today?"

Present Health Concern or Illness

The history of the present health concern or illness is the single most important factor in helping the health care team to arrive at a diagnosis or determine the person's needs. The physical examination is helpful but often only validates the information obtained from the history. A careful history assists in correct selection of appropriate diagnostic tests. While diagnostic test results can be helpful, they often support rather than establish the diagnosis.

If the present illness is only one episode in a series of episodes, the entire sequence of events is recorded. For example, a history from a patient whose reason for seeking care is an episode of insulin shock describes the entire course of the diabetes to put the current episode in context. The details of the health concern or present illness are described from onset until the time of contact with the health care team. These facts are recorded in chronological order, beginning with, for example, "The patient was in good health until . . ." or "The patient first experienced abdominal pain 2 months prior to seeking help."

The person is encouraged to describe details of the present health concern or illness. After allowing time for a full response, the health care provider may ask if there is anything else to be added. Then, following the individual's lead, the health care provider asks for clarification of the points raised and for additional information.

The history of the present illness or problem includes such information as the date and manner (sudden or gradual) in which the problem occurred, the setting in which the problem occurred (at home, at work, after an argument, after exercise), manifestations of the problem, and the course of the illness or problem. This includes self-treatment (including complementary therapies), medical interventions, progress and effects of treatment, and the patient's perceptions of the cause or meaning of the problem.

When a symptom is mentioned, the person is again invited to describe all aspects. The interviewer keeps in mind the seven attributes of a symptom (Bickley & Szilagyi, 2003) and follows with specific questions as needed:

- Location
- Quality
- Quantity or severity
- Timing
- Setting in which it occurs
- Remitting or exacerbating factors
- Associated manifestations

Another approach for analyzing signs, symptoms, and concerns is to use a mnemonic ("memory helper") such as COLDSPA (Weber & Kelley, 2003).

- **C**haracter
- **O**nset
- **L**ocation
- **D**uration
- **S**everity
- **P**attern
- **A**ssociated Factors

Following the person's description of a symptom, the interviewer asks specific questions to ensure that all attributes of the symptom in question have been explored. Examples of symptoms include pain, headache, fever, and changes in bowel and urinary habits.

Associated manifestations are symptoms that occur simultaneously with the chief health problem. The presence or absence of such symptoms may shed light on the origin or extent of the problem, as well as on the diagnosis. These symptoms are referred to as significant positive or negative findings and are obtained from a review of systems directly related to the reason for seeking care. For example, if the person reports a vague symptom such as fatigue or weight loss, all body systems are reviewed and included in this section of the history. If, on the other hand, the person's chief complaint is chest pain, only the cardiopulmonary and gastrointestinal systems may be included in the history of the present illness. In either situation, both positive and negative findings are recorded to define the problem further.

Past Health History

A detailed summary of the person's past health is an important part of the database. After determining the general health status, the interviewer may inquire about immunization status and any known allergies to medications or other substances. The dates of immunization are recorded, along with the type of allergy and adverse reactions. The person is asked to provide information, if known, about his or her last physical examination, chest x-ray, electrocardiogram, eye examination, hearing tests, dental checkup, as well as Papanicolaou (Pap) smear and mammogram (if female), digital rectal examination of the prostate gland (if male), and any other pertinent tests. Previous illnesses are then discussed. Negative as well as positive responses to a list of specific diseases are recorded. Dates, or the age of the patient at the time of illness, as well as the names of the primary health care provider and hospital, the diagnosis, and the treatment are also recorded. A history of the following areas is elicited:

- Childhood illness—rubeola, rubella, polio, whooping cough, mumps, chickenpox, scarlet fever, rheumatic fever, strep throat
- Adult illnesses
- Psychiatric illnesses
- Injuries—burns, fractures, head injuries
- Hospitalizations
- Surgical and diagnostic procedures
- Current medications—prescription, over-the-counter, home remedies, complementary therapies
- Use of alcohol and other drugs

If a particular hospitalization or major medical intervention is related to the present illness, the account of it is not repeated; rather, the report refers to the appropriate part of the report, such as "see history of present illness" or "see HPI" on the data sheet.

Family History

The age and health status, or the age and cause of death, of first-order relatives (parents, siblings, spouse, children) and second-order relatives (grandparents, cousins) are elicited to identify diseases that may be genetic in origin, communicable, or possibly environmental in cause. The following diseases are generally included: cancer, hypertension, heart disease, diabetes, epilepsy, mental illness, tuberculosis, kidney disease, arthritis, allergies, asthma, alcoholism, and obesity. One of the easiest methods of recording such data is by using the family tree or genogram (Fig. 5-2). The results of genetic testing or screening, if known, are recorded. See Chapter 9 for a detailed discussion of genetics.

Review of Systems

The systems review includes an overview of general health as well as symptoms related to each body system. Open-ended questions, followed by specific questions as needed, are asked about each of the major body systems in terms of past or present symptoms. Reviewing each body system helps reveal any relevant data. Negative as well as positive answers are recorded. If the patient responds positively to questions about a particular system, the information is analyzed carefully. If any symptoms are mentioned, the seven attributes of a symptom or the mnemonic COLDSPA can be used to collect the required information. If any illnesses were previously mentioned or recorded, it is not necessary to repeat them in this part of the history. Instead, reference is made to the appropriate place in the history where the information can be found.

A review of systems can be organized in a formal checklist, which becomes a part of the health history. One advantage of a checklist is that it can be easily audited and is less subject to error than a system that relies heavily on the interviewer's memory.

Patient Profile

In the patient profile, more biographical information is gathered. A complete composite, or profile, of the patient is critical to an

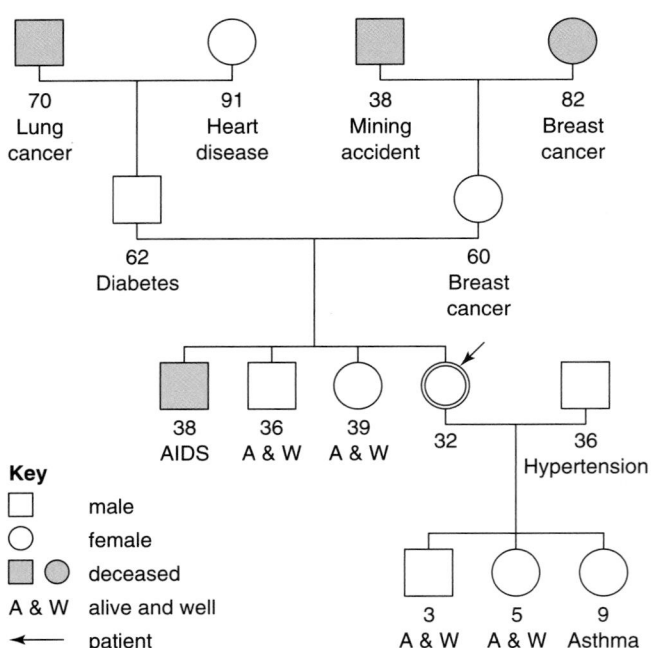

FIGURE 5-2 Diagram (called a genogram) used to record history of family members, including their age and cause of death or, if living, their current health status.

GENETICS IN NURSING PRACTICE

New and exciting discoveries emerging from human genome research are clarifying genetic aspects of health and disease and expanding health opportunities for individuals, families, and communities around the world. These advances call for all nurses to have a heightened awareness of genetics as the core understanding of the mechanisms of disease. Genetics concepts are central to every step of the nursing process.

GENETIC ASPECTS OF HEALTH CARE DELIVERY AND NURSING PRACTICE
Nurses in all areas of practice carry out five main practice activities:
- Help to collect, report, and record genetics information
- Offer genetics information and resources
- Participate in the informed consent process and facilitate informed decision making
- Participate in ongoing management of patients with genetic conditions
- Evaluate and monitor the impact of genetic conditions, testing, and treatment on the individual and family

COMMUNITY-BASED NURSING PRACTICE
Nurses providing community-based care:
- Participate in genetic screening (eg, prenatal screening and newborn screening)
- Provide health care regarding genetic risk factors and management of genetically related disorders in a way that respects the beliefs and concerns of specific ethnic communities
- Educate the public about the contribution of genetics to health and disease
- Engage in dialogue with the public about ethical, legal, and social issues related to genetics discoveries

CRITICAL THINKING AND DECISION MAKING
Nurses use these skills in providing genetic-related health care when they:
- Assess and analyze family history data for genetic risk factors
- Identify those individuals and families in need of referral for genetic testing or counselling
- Ensure the privacy and confidentiality of genetics information

HEALTH EDUCATION AND PROMOTION
Nurses in all settings should be prepared to:
- Inquire about patients' and families' desired health outcomes with regard to genetic-related conditions or risk factors
- Refer patients for genetics services when indicated
- Identify barriers to accessing genetic-related health services
- Offer appropriate genetics information and resources

HEALTH ASSESSMENT
Nurses incorporate a genetics focus into the following health assessments:
- Family history—assess for genetic-related risk factors
- Cultural, social, and spiritual assessment—assess for individual and family perceptions and beliefs around genetics topics
- Physical assessment—assess for clinical features that may suggest a genetic condition is present (eg, unusually tall stature—Marfan syndrome)
- Ethnic background—since many conditions are more common in specific ethnic populations, the nurse gathers information about ethnic background (eg, Tay-Sachs disease in Ashkenazi Jewish populations or thalassemia in Southeast Asian populations)

GENETICS RESOURCES FOR NURSES AND PATIENTS ON THE WEB
Canadian Association of Genetic Counsellors (CAGC) http://www.cagc-accg.ca—a listing of genetic centres across Canada

Canadian Cancer Society http://www.cancer.ca—a source of information on genetic factors/risk and genetic testing

Canadian Directory of Genetic Support Groups http://www.lhsc.on.ca/programs/medgenet—a resource guide for families and professionals

Canadian Genetic Disease Network http://www.cgdn.ca—a group with the stated mission to be the primary catalyst in advancing Canada's scientific and commercial competitiveness in genetic research and the application of genetic discoveries to the prevention, diagnosis, and treatment of human disease

Canadian Organization for Rare Disorders (CORD) http://www.cord.ca—a source of information on over 6,000 rare disorders; links individuals/families with the same rare disorder

Genetic Alliance http://www.geneticalliance.org—an organization that increases the capacity of genetic advocacy groups to achieve their missions and leverages the voices of millions of individuals and families living with genetic conditions

The Genetics Society of Canada (GSC) http://life.biology.mcmaster.ca/GSC—a group that promotes research and communicates the results and implications of genetics to the public

GeneTests http://www.genetests.org—a publicly funded medical genetics information resource developed for physicians, other healthcare providers, and researchers

OMIM Online Mendelian Inheritance in Man http://www.ncbi.nlm.nih.gov/entrez/query.fcgi?db=OMIM—a catalogue of human genes and genetic disorders

---

analysis of the reason for seeking health care and of the person's ability to deal with the problem. A complete patient profile is summarized in Chart 5-1.

The information elicited at this point in the interview is highly personal and subjective. During this stage, the person is encouraged to express feelings honestly and to discuss personal experiences. It is best to begin with general, open-ended questions and to move to direct questioning when specific facts are needed. The patient is often less anxious when the interview progresses from information that is less personal (birthplace, occupation, education) to information that is more personal (sexuality, body image, coping abilities).

A general patient profile consists of the following content areas:

Chart 5-1 **Patient Profile**

Past Events Related to Health
Place of birth
Places lived
Significant childhood/adolescent experiences

Education and Occupation
Jobs held in past
Current position/job
Length of time at position
Educational preparation
Work satisfaction and career goals

Financial Resources
Income
Insurance coverage

Environment
Physical—living arrangements (type of housing, neighbourhood, presence of hazards), work environment (presence of hazards)
Spiritual—extent to which religion is a part of individual's life; religious beliefs related to perception of health and illness; religious practices
Interpersonal—ethnic background (language spoken, customs and values held, folk practices used to maintain health or to cure illness); family relationships (family structure, roles, communication patterns, support system); friendships (quality of relationship)

Lifestyle Patterns
Sleep (time individual retires, hours per night, comfort measures, awakens rested)
Exercise (type, frequency, time spent)
Nutrition (24-hour diet recall, idiosyncrasies, restrictions)

Recreation (type of activity, time spent)
Caffeine (coffee, tea, cola, chocolate)—kind, amount
Smoking (cigarette, pipe, cigar, chewing tobacco [smokeless tobacco], marijuana)—kind, amount per day, number of years, desire to quit
Alcohol—kind, amount, pattern over past year
Drugs—kind, amount, route of administration (includes over-the-counter, complementary, illicit)

Physical or Mental Disability
Presence of a disability (physical or mental)
Effect of disability on function and health access
Accommodations needed to support functioning

Self-Concept
View of self in present
View of self in future
Body image (level of satisfaction, concerns)

Sexuality
Perception of self as a man or woman
Quality of sexual relationships
Concerns related to sexuality or sexual functioning

Risk for Abuse
Physical injury in past
Afraid of partner, caregiver, family

Stress and Coping Response
Major concerns or problems at present
Daily "hassles"
Past experiences with similar problems
Past coping patterns and outcomes
Present coping strategies and anticipated outcomes
Individual's expectations of family/friends and health care team in problem resolution

---

- Past life events related to health
- Education and occupation
- Environment (physical, spiritual, cultural, interpersonal)
- Lifestyle (patterns and habits)
- Presence of a physical or mental disability
- Self-concept
- Sexuality
- Risk for abuse
- Stress and coping response

PAST LIFE EVENTS RELATED TO HEALTH

The patient profile begins with a brief life history. Questions about place of birth and past places of residence help focus attention on the earlier years of life. Personal experiences during childhood or adolescence that have special significance may be elicited by asking, "Was there anything that you experienced as a child or adolescent that would be helpful for me to know about?" The interviewer's intent is to encourage the person to make a quick review of his or her earlier life, highlighting information of particular significance. Although many patients may not recall anything significant, others may share information such as a personal achievement, a failure, a developmental crisis, or an instance of physical or emotional abuse.

EDUCATION AND OCCUPATION

Inquiring about current occupation can reveal much about a person's economic status and educational preparation. A statement

such as, "Tell me about your job" often elicits information about role, job tasks, and satisfaction with the position. Direct questions about past employment and career goals may be asked if the person does not provide this information.

Asking the person what kind of educational requirements were necessary to attain his or her present job is a more sensitive approach to educational background than asking whether he or she graduated from high school. Information about the patient's general financial status may be obtained by questions such as, "Do you have any financial concerns at this time?" or "Sometimes there just doesn't seem to be enough money to make ends meet. Are you finding this true?"

ENVIRONMENT

The person's physical environment and its potential hazards, spiritual awareness, cultural background, interpersonal relationships, and support system are included in the concept of environment.

Physical Environment

Information is elicited about the type of housing (apartment, duplex, single-family) in which the person lives, its location, the level of safety and comfort within the home and neighbourhood, and the presence of environmental hazards (eg, isolation, potential fire risks, inadequate sanitation). The patient's environment takes on special importance if the patient is homeless or living in a homeless shelter or has a disability.

Spiritual Environment

The term "spiritual environment" refers to the degree to which a person thinks about or contemplates his or her existence, accepts challenges in life, and seeks and finds answers to personal questions. Spirituality may be expressed through identification with a particular religion. Spiritual values and beliefs often direct a person's behaviour and approach to health problems and can influence responses to sickness. Illness may create a spiritual crisis and can place considerable stress on a person's internal resources and beliefs. Inquiring about spirituality can identify possible support systems as well as beliefs and customs that need to be considered in planning care. Thus, information is gathered in the following three areas:

- The extent to which religion is a part of the person's life
- Religious beliefs related to the person's perception of health and illness
- Religious practices

The following questions can be used in a spiritual assessment:

- Is religion or God (or a higher being) important to you?
- If yes, in what way?
- If no, what is the most important thing in your life?
- Are there any religious practices that are important to you?
- Do you have any spiritual concerns because of your present health problem?

Interpersonal and Cultural Environment

Cultural influences, relationships with family and friends, and the presence or absence of a support system are all a part of one's interpersonal environment. The beliefs and practices that have been shared from generation to generation are known as cultural or ethnic patterns. They are expressed through language, dress, dietary choices, and role behaviours, in perceptions of health and illness, and in health-related behaviours. The influence of these beliefs and customs on how a person reacts to health problems and interacts with health care providers cannot be underestimated (Fuller & Schaller-Ayers, 2000). For this reason, the health history includes information about ethnic identity (cultural and social) and racial identity (biologic). The following questions may assist in obtaining relevant information:

- Where did your parents or ancestors come from? When?
- What language do you speak at home?
- Are there certain customs or values that are important to you?
- Is there anything special you do to keep in good health?
- Do you have any specific practices for treating illness?

Family Relationships and Support System

An assessment of family structure (members, ages, roles), patterns of communication, and the presence or absence of a support system is an integral part of the patient profile. Although the traditional family is recognized as a mother, a father, and children, many different types of living arrangements exist within our society. "Family" may mean two or more people bound by emotional ties or commitments. Live-in companions, roommates, and close friends can all play a significant role in an individual's support system.

LIFESTYLE

The lifestyle section of the patient profile provides information about health-related behaviours. These behaviours include patterns of sleep, exercise, nutrition, and recreation, as well as personal habits such as smoking and the use of drugs, alcohol, and caffeine. Although most people readily describe their exercise patterns or recreational activities, many are unwilling to report their smoking, alcohol use, and drug use; many deny or understate the degree to which they use such substances. Questions such as, "What kind of alcohol do you enjoy drinking at a party?" may elicit more accurate information than, "Do you drink?" The specific type of alcohol (eg, wine, liquor, beer) and the amount ingested per day or per week (eg, 1 pint of whiskey daily for 2 years) are described.

When alcohol abuse is suspected, additional information may be obtained by using common alcohol screening questionnaires such as the CAGE (Cutting down, Annoyance by criticism, Guilty feelings, and Eye-openers), AUDIT (Alcohol Use Disorders Identification Test), TWEAK (Tolerance, Worry, Eye-opener, Amnesia, Kut down), or SMAST (Short Michigan Alcoholism Screening Test). Chart 5-2 shows the CAGE Questions Adapted to Include Drugs (CAGEAID).

Similar questions can be used to elicit information about smoking and caffeine consumption. Questions about drug use follow naturally after questions about smoking, caffeine consumption, and alcohol use. A nonjudgmental approach will make it easier for the person to respond truthfully and factually. If street names or unfamiliar terms are used to describe drugs, the person is asked to define the terms used.

Investigation of lifestyle should also include questions about complementary and alternative theories such as special diets; the use of prayer, visualization, or guided imagery; massage; medication; herbal products and many others. It is estimated that 25% to 30% of Canadians recently used at least one remedy other than vitamins (Canada Health Monitor, 1997; PricewaterhouseCoopers, 1999; Ramsay, Walker, & Alexander, 1999).

PHYSICAL OR MENTAL DISABILITY

The general patient profile also needs to contain questions about any hearing, vision, cognitive, or physical disability. The presence

---

Chart 5-2 · Assessment

Instrument for Assessing Alcohol or Drug Use

CAGE Questions Adapted to Include Drugs (CAGEAID)*

Have you felt you ought to cut down on your drinking *(or drug use)*?
_____Yes _____No

Have people annoyed you by criticizing your drinking *(or drug use)*?
_____Yes _____No

Have you felt bad or guilty about your drinking *(or drug use)*?
_____Yes _____No

Have you ever had a drink *(or used drugs)* **first thing in the morning to steady your nerves or get rid of a hangover** *(or to get the day started)*?
_____Yes _____No

*Boldface text shows the original CAGE questions; boldface italic text shows modifications of the CAGE questions used to screen for drug disorders. In a general population, two or more positive answers indicate a need for more in-depth assessment.
From Fleming, M. F., & Barry, K. L. (1992). *Addictive Disorders.* St. Louis: Mosby; and Ewing, J. A. (1984). Detecting alcoholism: The CAGE questionnaire. *Journal of the American Medical Association, 252*(14), 1905–1907.

of an obvious physical deformity—for instance, if the patient walks with crutches or needs a wheelchair to get around—needs further investigation. The etiology of the disability should be elicited; the length of time the patient has had the disability and the impact on function and health access are important to assess.

SELF-CONCEPT

Self-concept refers to one's view of oneself, an image that has developed over many years. To assess self-concept, the interviewer might ask the person how he or she views life: "How do you feel about your life in general?" A person's self-concept can be threatened very easily by changes in physical function or appearance or other threats to health. The impact of certain medical conditions or surgical interventions, such as a colostomy or a mastectomy, can threaten body image. Asking, "Do you have any particular concerns about your body?" may elicit useful information about self-image.

SEXUALITY

No area of assessment is more personal than the sexual history. Interviewers are frequently uncomfortable with such questions and ignore this area of the patient profile or conduct a very cursory interview at this point. Lack of knowledge about sexuality and anxiety about one's own sexuality may hamper the interviewer's effectiveness in dealing with this subject (Ross, Channon-Little & Rosser, 2000).

Sexual assessment can be approached at the end of the interview, at the time interpersonal or lifestyle factors are assessed, or it can be a part of the genitourinary history within the review of systems. For instance, it may be easier to approach a discussion of sexuality after a discussion of menstruation. A similar discussion with the male patient would follow questions related to the urinary system.

Obtaining the sexual history provides an opportunity to discuss sexual matters openly and gives the person permission to express sexual concerns to an informed professional. The interviewer must be nonjudgmental and must use language appropriate to the patient's age and background. It is advisable to begin the assessment with a general question concerning the person's developmental stage and the presence or absence of intimate relationships. Such questions may lead to a discussion of concerns related to sexual expression or the quality of a relationship, or to questions about contraception, risky sexual behaviours, and safer sex practices.

Finding out whether a person is sexually active should precede any attempts to explore issues related to sexuality and sexual function. Care should be taken to initiate conversations about sexuality with elderly patients and not to treat them as asexual beings (Miller, Zylstra & Stranridge, 2000). Questions are worded in such a way that the person feels free to discuss his or her sexuality regardless of marital status or sexual preference. Direct questions are usually less threatening when prefaced with such statements as, "Most people feel that . . ." or "Many people worry about. . . ." This suggests the normalcy of such feelings or behaviour and encourages the person to share information that might otherwise be omitted from fear of seeming "different."

If the person answers abruptly or does not wish to carry the discussion any further, then the interviewer should move to the next topic. However, introducing the subject of sexuality indicates to the person that a discussion of sexual concerns is acceptable and can be approached again in the future if so desired. Further discussion of the sexual history is presented in Chapters 46 and 49.

RISK FOR ABUSE

A topic of growing importance in today's society is physical, sexual, and psychological abuse. Such abuse occurs at all ages, to men and women from all socioeconomic, ethnic, and cultural groups (Little, 2000; Marshall, Benton & Brazier, 2000). Few patients, however, will discuss this topic unless they are asked specifically about it. Therefore, it is important to ask direct questions, such as:

- Is anyone physically hurting you?
- Has anyone ever hurt you physically or threatened to do so?
- Are you ever afraid of anyone close to you (your partner, caretaker, or other family members)?

If the person's response indicates that abuse is a risk, further assessment is called for and efforts are made to ensure the person's safety and provide access to appropriate community and professional resources and support systems. Further discussion of domestic violence and abuse is presented in Chapter 46. When questioned directly, elderly patients rarely admit to abuse (Marshall, Benton & Brazier, 2000). Health care professionals should assess for risk factors, such as high levels of stress or alcoholism in caregivers, evidence of violence, high emotions as well as financial, emotional, or physical dependency. Patients who are elderly or disabled are at increased risk for abuse and should be asked about it as a routine part of assessment.

STRESS AND COPING RESPONSES

Each person handles stress differently. How well we adapt depends on our ability to cope. During a health history, past coping patterns and perceptions of current stresses and anticipated outcomes are explored to identify the person's overall ability to handle stress. It is especially important to identify expectations

Gerontologic Considerations

A health history from the elderly patient should be obtained in a calm, unrushed manner. Because of the increased incidence of impaired hearing and sight in the elderly, lighting should be adequate but not glaring, and distracting noises should be kept to a minimum (Miller, Zylstra & Standridge, 2000). The interviewer should assume a position that enables the person to read lips and facial expressions. People who normally use a hearing aid are asked to use it during the interview. The interviewer should also recognize that there is wide diversity among the elderly population and that differences exist in health, gender, income, and functional status (Bakshi & Miller, 1999; Ludwick, Dieckman & Snelson, 1999).

Elderly people often assume that new physical problems are a result of age rather than a treatable illness. In addition, the signs and symptoms of illness in the elderly are often more subtle than those in younger people and may go unreported. Therefore, the interviewer inquires about subtle physical symptoms and recent changes in function and well-being. Special care is taken in obtaining a complete history of medications used, because many elderly people take many different kinds of prescription and over-the-counter medications (Palmer, 1999). Although elderly people may experience a decline in mental function, it should not be assumed that an elderly person is unable to provide an adequate history. Including a member of the family in the interview process, however (ie, spouse, adult child, sibling, or caretaker), may validate information and provide missing details. Further details about assessment of the elderly are provided in Chapter 12.

that the person may have of family, friends, and caregivers in providing financial, emotional, or physical support.

OTHER HEALTH HISTORY FORMATS

The health history format discussed in this chapter is only one possible format that is useful in obtaining and organizing information about a person's health status. Some consider this traditional format to be inappropriate for nurses because it does not focus exclusively on the assessment of human responses to actual or potential health problems. Several attempts have been made to develop an assessment format and database with this focus in mind. One example is the nursing database prototype based on the North American Nursing Diagnosis Association's (NANDA) Unitary Person Framework and its nine human response patterns: exchanging, communicating, relating, valuing, choosing, moving, perceiving, knowing, and feeling. Although there is support in nursing for using this approach, no consensus for its use has been reached.

Groups from the public and private sectors have focused on assessing not only biologic health but also other dimensions of health. These dimensions include physical, functional, emotional, mental, and social health. Modern efforts to assess health status have focused on the manner in which disease or disability affects the patient's functional status—that is, the ability of the person to function and perform his or her usual physical, mental, and social activities. An emphasis on functional assessment is viewed as more holistic than the traditional health or medical history. Instruments to assess health status in these ways may be used by nurses along with their own clinical assessment skills to determine the impact of illness, disease, disability, and health problems on functional status.

Health concerns that are not complex (earache, tonsillectomy) and can be resolved in a short period of time usually do not require the depth or detail that is required when a person is experiencing a major illness or health problem. Additional assessments that go beyond the general patient profile may be used when the patient's health problems are acute and complex or when the illness is chronic. Individuals should be asked about their continuing health promotion and screening practices. Patients who have not been involved in these practices in the past are educated about their importance and are referred to appropriate health care providers.

Regardless of the assessment format used, the nurse's focus during data collection is different from that of the physician and other health team members; however, it complements these approaches and encourages collaboration among the health care providers, as each member brings his or her own expertise and focus to the situation.

Physical Assessment

Physical assessment, or the physical examination, is an integral part of nursing assessment. The basic techniques and tools used in performing a physical examination are described in general in this chapter. The examination of specific systems, including special manoeuvres, is described in the appropriate chapters throughout the book. Because the patient's nutritional status is an important factor in health and well-being, a section on nutritional assessment is included in this chapter.

The physical examination is usually performed after the health history is obtained. It is carried out in a well-lighted, warm area. The patient is asked to undress and draped appropriately so that only the area to be examined is exposed. The person's physical and psychological comfort is considered at all times. Procedures and sensations to expect are described to the patient before each part of the examination. The examiner's hands are washed before and immediately after the examination. Fingernails are kept short to avoid injuring the patient. The examiner wears gloves when there is a possibility of coming into contact with blood or other body secretions during the physical examination.

Taking and recording vital signs is the beginning of the hands-on portion of the physical examination and is a part of every physical examination (Weber & Kelley, 2003). Blood pressure, pulse rate, respiratory rate, and body temperature measurements are obtained and recorded. Acute changes and trends over time are documented; unexpected changes and values that deviate significantly from the patient's normal values are brought to the attention of the patient's primary health care provider. The "fifth vital sign," pain, is also assessed and documented, if indicated.

Fever is an increase in body temperature above what is usual. An oral temperature for most people is an average of 37.0 C; however, some variation is expected. Some individuals' usual temperatures are 36.6 C and others are 37.3 C. There is an expected diurnal variation of a degree or two in body temperature throughout the day, with temperature usually lowest in the morning and rising during the day to between 37.3 and 37.5 C and then decreasing again during the night.

An organized and systematic examination is the key to obtaining appropriate data in the shortest time. Such an approach encourages cooperation and trust on the part of the patient. The individual's health history provides the examiner with a health profile that guides all aspects of the physical examination. Although the sequence of physical examination depends on the circumstances and on the patient's reason for seeking health care, the complete examination usually proceeds as follows:

- Skin
- Head and neck
- Thorax and lungs
- Breasts
- Cardiovascular system
- Abdomen
- Rectum
- Genitalia
- Neurologic system
- Musculoskeletal system

In clinical practice, all relevant body systems are tested throughout the physical examination, not necessarily in the sequence described (Weber & Kelley, 2003). For example, when the face is examined, it is appropriate to check for facial asymmetry and, thus, for the integrity of the seventh cranial nerve; the examiner does not need to repeat this as part of a neurologic examination. When systems are combined in this manner, the patient does not need to change positions repeatedly, which can be exhausting and time-consuming.

A "complete" physical examination is not routine; however, a "complete" physical examination provides baseline data for people who will have ongoing contact with nurses. Examples include persons in rehabilitation, long-term care, or correctional facilities. Many of the body systems are selectively assessed on the basis of the individual's presenting problem. If, for example, a healthy 20-year-old college student requires an examination to play basketball and reports no history of neurologic abnormality, the neurologic assessment is brief. Conversely, a history of transient numbness and diplopia (double vision) usually necessitates a complete neurologic investigation. Similarly, a person with chest pain receives a much more intensive examination of the chest and heart than the person with an earache. In general, the individual's health history guides the examiner in obtaining additional data for a complete picture of the patient's health.

The process of learning physical examination requires repetition and reinforcement in a clinical setting. Only after basic physical assessment techniques are mastered can the examiner tailor the routine screening examination to include thorough assessments of a particular system, including special manoeuvres.

The basic tools of the physical examination are vision, hearing, touch, and smell. These human senses may be augmented by special tools (eg, stethoscope, ophthalmoscope, and reflex hammer) that are extensions of the human senses; they are simple tools that anyone can learn to use well. Expertise comes with practice, and sophistication comes with the interpretation of what is seen and heard. The four fundamental techniques used in the physical examination are inspection, palpation, percussion, and auscultation (Weber & Kelley, 2003).

INSPECTION

The first fundamental technique is inspection or observation. The general survey begins with the first contact with the patient. It is often useful to observe the patient and environment for a moment before introducing oneself. This allows the nurse to notice body posture and facial expressions, such as distress, sadness, or pain, before the patient covers them up (Weber & Kelley, 2003). For example, a patient with a 2-week history of headaches is noticed in the waiting room, holding her head in both hands. These types of "private" observations guide the health care provider in deciding which elements of the physical assessment to include for a specific patient.

Introducing oneself and shaking hands provide opportunities for making contact with the patient. Bickley and Szilagyi (2003) include the following in a general survey:

- Level of consciousness, state of awareness
- General state of health, signs of distress, skin colour
- Body build
- Sexual development
- Posture, motor activity, gait
- Dress, grooming, personal hygiene
- Odours: body, breath
- Facial expressions, manner, affect
- Interaction with people and the environment
- Manner of speech

It is essential to pay attention to the details in observation. Vague, general statements are not a substitute for specific descriptions based on careful observation; for example:

- "The person appears sick." In what way does he or she appear sick? Is the skin pale, jaundiced, or cyanotic; is the person grimacing in pain; is breathing difficult; does he or she have edema? What specific physical features or behavioural manifestations indicate that the person is "sick"?
- These important observations are documented in the patient's chart or health record.

Further detailed observations that should be noted in the initial examination of the patient are posture and stature, body movements, nutrition, and speech pattern.

Posture and Stature

The posture that a person assumes often provides valuable information about the illness. Patients who have breathing difficulties (dyspnea) secondary to cardiac disease prefer to sit and may report feeling short of breath lying flat for even a brief time. People with obstructive pulmonary disease not only sit upright but also may thrust their arms forward and laterally onto the edge of the bed (tripod position) to place accessory respiratory muscles at an optimal mechanical advantage. Those with abdominal pain due to peritonitis prefer to lie perfectly still; even slight jarring of the bed will cause agonizing pain. In contrast, patients with abdominal pain due to renal or biliary colic are often restless and may pace the room. Patients with meningeal irritation may experience head or neck pain on bending the head or flexing their knees.

Body Movements

Abnormalities of body movement may be of two general kinds: generalized disruption of voluntary or involuntary movement, and asymmetry of movement. The first category includes tremors of a wide variety; some tremors may occur at rest (Parkinson's disease), whereas others occur only on voluntary movement (cerebellar ataxia). Other tremors may exist during both rest and activity (alcohol withdrawal syndrome, thyrotoxicosis). Some voluntary or involuntary movements are fine, others quite coarse. At the extreme are the convulsive movements of epilepsy or tetanus and the choreiform (involuntary and irregular) movements of patients with rheumatic fever or Huntington's disease. Other aspects of body movement that are noted on inspection include spasticity, muscle spasms, and an abnormal gait.

Asymmetry of movement, in which only one side of the body is affected, may occur with disorders of the central nervous system (CNS), principally in those patients who have had cerebrovascular accidents (strokes). The patient may have drooping of one side of the face, weakness or paralysis of the extremities on one side of the body, and a foot-dragging gait. Spasticity (increased muscle tone) may also be present, particularly in patients with multiple sclerosis.

Nutrition

Nutritional status is important to note. Obesity may be generalized as a result of excessive intake of calories or may be specifically localized to the trunk in those with endocrine disorders (Cushing's disease) or those who have been taking corticosteroids for long periods of time. Loss of weight may be generalized as a result of inadequate caloric intake or may be seen in loss of muscle mass with disorders that affect protein synthesis. Nutritional assessment is discussed in more detail later in this chapter.

Speech Pattern

Speech may be slurred because of CNS disease or because of damage to cranial nerves. Recurrent damage to the laryngeal nerve will produce hoarseness, as will disorders that produce edema or swelling of the vocal cords. Speech may be halting, slurred, or interrupted in flow in some CNS disorders (eg, multiple sclerosis).

PALPATION

Palpation is a vital part of the physical examination. Many structures of the body, although not visible, may be assessed through the techniques of light and deep palpation (Fig. 5-3). Examples include superficial blood vessels, lymph nodes, the thyroid, the organs of the abdomen and pelvis, and the rectum. When the abdomen is examined, auscultation is performed before palpation and percussion to avoid altering bowel sounds.

FIGURE 5-3 Light palpation technique (*top*) and deep palpation (*bottom*). Photo © Ken Kasper.

FIGURE 5-4 Percussion technique. The middle finger of one hand strikes the terminal phalanx of the middle finger of the other hand, which is placed firmly against the body. If the action is performed sharply, a brief resonant tone will be produced. The clarity of the tone depends on the brevity of the action. The intensity of the tone varies with the force used. Photo © Ken Kasper.

Sounds generated within the body, if within specified frequency ranges, also may be detected through touch. Thus, certain murmurs generated in the heart or within blood vessels (thrills) may be detected. Thrills cause a sensation to the hand much like the purring of a cat. Voice sounds are transmitted along the bronchi to the periphery of the lung. These may be perceived by touch and may be altered by disorders affecting the lungs. The phenomenon is called *tactile fremitus* and is useful in assessing diseases of the chest. The significance of these findings is discussed in the relevant chapters of this book.

PERCUSSION

The technique of percussion (Fig. 5-4) translates the application of physical force into sound. It is a skill requiring practice but one that yields much information about disease processes in the chest and abdomen. The principle is to set the chest wall or abdominal wall into vibration by striking it with a firm object. The sound produced reflects the density of the underlying structure. Certain densities produce sounds as percussion notes. These sounds, listed in a sequence that proceeds from the least to the most dense, are called tympany, hyperresonance, resonance, dullness, and flatness. Tympany is the drumlike sound produced by percussing the air-filled stomach. Hyperresonance is audible when one percusses over inflated lung tissue in someone with emphysema. Resonance is the sound elicited over air-filled lungs. Percussion of the liver produces a dull sound, whereas percussion of the thigh results in flatness.

Percussion allows the examiner to assess such usual anatomic details as the borders of the heart and the movement of the diaphragm during inspiration. One may determine the level of pleural effusion (fluid in the pleural cavity) and the location of a consolidated area caused by pneumonia or atelectasis (collapse) of a lobe of the lung. The use of percussion is described further with disorders of the thorax and abdomen.

AUSCULTATION

Auscultation is the skill of listening to sounds produced within the body created by the movement of air or fluid. Examples include breath sounds, the spoken voice, bowel sounds, cardiac murmurs, and heart sounds. Physiologic sounds may be normal (eg, first and second heart sounds) or pathologic (eg, heart murmurs in diastole, or crackles in the lung). Some normal sounds may be distorted by abnormalities of structures through which the sound must travel (eg, changes in the character of breath sounds as they travel through the consolidated lung of the patient with lobar pneumonia).

Sound produced within the body, if of sufficient amplitude, may be detected with the stethoscope, which functions as an extension of the human ear and channels sound. Two end pieces are available for the stethoscope: the bell and the diaphragm. The bell is used to assess very-low-frequency sounds such as diastolic heart murmurs. The entire surface of the bell's disc is placed lightly on the skin surface to avoid flattening the skin and reducing audible vibratory sensations. The diaphragm, the larger disc, is used to assess high-frequency sounds such as heart and lung sounds and is held in firm contact with the skin surface (Fig. 5-5). Touching the tubing or rubbing other surfaces (hair, clothing) during auscultation is avoided to minimize extraneous noises.

Sound produced by the body, like any other sound, is characterized by intensity, frequency, and quality. *Intensity,* or loudness, associated with physiologic sound is low; thus, the use of the stethoscope is needed. *Frequency,* or pitch, of physiologic sound is in reality "noise" in that most sounds consist of a frequency spectrum as opposed to the single-frequency sounds that we associate with music or the tuning fork. The frequency spectrum may be quite low, yielding a rumbling noise, or comparatively high, producing a harsh or blowing sound. *Quality* of sound relates to overtones that allow one to distinguish between different sounds. Sound

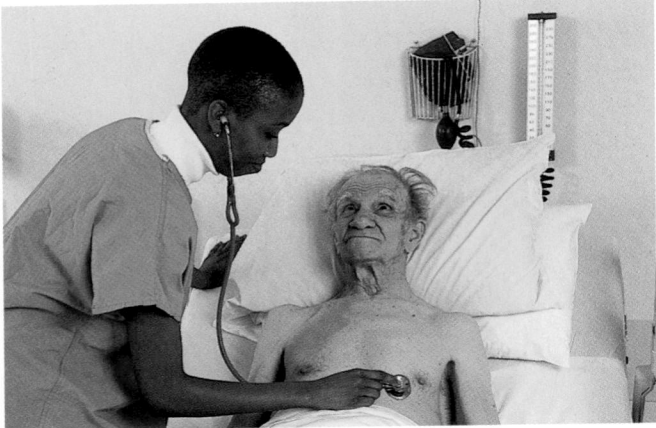

FIGURE 5-5 Technique for auscultating the heart. © B. Proud Photography.

quality enables the examiner to distinguish between the musical quality of high-pitched wheezing and the low-pitched rumbling of a diastolic murmur.

Nutritional Assessment

An additional area of concern that is often integrated into the health history and physical examination is an in-depth nutritional assessment. Nutrition is important to maintain health and to prevent disease and death (Kant, Schatzkin, Graubard & Schairer, 2000; Landi, Onder, Gambassi et al., 2000; Stampfer, Hu & Manson, 2000). Disorders caused by nutritional deficiency, overeating, or eating poorly balanced meals are among the leading causes of illness and death in Canada today. The three leading causes of death are related, in part, to consequences of unhealthy nutrition: cancer, heart disease, and stroke (Statistics Canada, 2005). Other examples of health problems associated with poor nutrition include obesity, osteoporosis, cirrhosis, diverticulitis, and eating disorders. When illness or injury occurs, optimal nutrition is an essential factor in promoting healing and resisting infection and other complications (Braunschweig, Gomez & Sheean, 2000). Assessment of a person's nutritional status provides information on obesity, undernutrition, weight loss, malnutrition, deficiencies in specific nutrients, metabolic abnormalities, the effects of medications on nutrition, and special problems of the hospitalized patient and the person who is cared for in the home and in other community settings.

Certain signs and symptoms that suggest possible nutritional deficiency are easy to note because they are specific. Other physical signs may be subtle and must be carefully assessed. A physical sign that suggests a nutritional abnormality should be pursued further. For example, certain signs that may appear to indicate nutritional deficiency may actually reflect other systemic conditions (eg, endocrine disorders, infectious disease). Others may result from impaired digestion, absorption, excretion, or storage of nutrients in the body.

The sequence of assessment of parameters may vary, but evaluation of nutritional status and physical growth and development includes one or more of the following methods: measurement of body mass index (BMI) and anthropometric measurements; biochemical measurements (albumin, transferrin, prealbumin, retinol-binding protein, total lymphocyte count, electrolyte levels, creatinine/height index); clinical examination findings; and dietary data.

BODY MASS INDEX (BMI)

BMI is a ratio based on body weight and height (Chart 5-3). The obtained value is compared to the established standards; however, trends or changes in values over time are considered more useful than isolated or one-time measurements. BMI (Fig. 5-6) is highly correlated with body fat, but increased lean body mass or a large body frame can also increase the BMI. Individuals who have a BMI below 18.5 are at increased risk for problems associated with poor nutritional status. In addition, a low BMI is associated with higher mortality rates in hospitalized patients and community-dwelling elderly (Landi et al., 2000; Landi, Zuccala, Gambassi, et al., 1999).

People who have a BMI of 18.5 to 24.9 are in a healthy weight range. Those with a BMI between 25.0 and 29.9 are overweight and have an increased risk of developing health problems. People with a BMI of 30.0 to 34.9 are in obese class I (high risk of health problems), while those with a BMI of 35.0 to 39.9 are in obese class II with a very high risk of health problems. Individuals with a BMI of over 40.0 (obese class III) are at extremely high risk of developing health problems. For people who are 65 years or older, the "healthy" weight range may begin above a BMI of 18.5 and may take in part of the "overweight" category (Expert Group on Weight Standards, 1988).

It is important to assess for usual body weight and height. Current weight does not provide information about recent changes in weight. Decreased height may be due to osteoporosis, an important problem related to nutrition, especially in postmenopausal women. A loss of 5 to 8 centimetres of height may indicate osteoporosis.

The patient's height and wrist circumference are useful for determining frame size for comparison with standard charts. Skinfold tests can be taken over the triceps, at the suprailiac region of the abdomen, or the subscapular area to measure subcutaneous fat stores (Weber & Kelley, 2003). The mid-arm circumference is measured halfway between the acromion process and the olecranon process on the nondominant arm to indicate skeletal muscle mass and fat store.

To determine the waist-to-hip ratio, the waist is measured to the nearest 0.5 cm (midway between the lower costal margin and the iliac crest) when the person exhales. The hip is measured midway between the iliac crest and the greater trocanter. Then the waist-to-hip ratio is calculated. If a female's waist-to-hip ratio is greater than 0.80 and male's waist-to-hip ratio is greater than 1.0, the risk of heart attack or stroke is increased three to five times (Weber & Kelley, 2003).

Chart 5-3	**Calculating Body Mass Index (BMI)**

$$BMI = \frac{\text{weight in kilograms}}{(\text{height in metres})^2}$$

Examples: Tom weighs 85 kg and is 180 cm in height (1.80 metres)

$$\frac{85}{(1.8)^2} = \frac{85}{3.2} = \text{BMI of 26.2 (overweight category)}$$

Sharon weighs 60 kg and is 160 cm in height (1.6 metres)

$$\frac{60}{(1.6)^2} = \frac{60}{2.6} = \text{BMI of 23.4 (healthy weight category)}$$

Canada's Guidelines for Healthy Eating (1991) recommend that we all achieve and maintain a healthy body weight by enjoying regular physical activity and healthy eating.

A healthy body weight is different for everyone. In fact, there is a range of body weights that are healthy for each person, depending on how big their body is and on how well it works.

To find out what a healthy weight range is for you, try the Body Mass Index test below.

I am _____ (feet and inches)
or_____ (cm) tall

I weigh _____ (lbs) or _____ (kg).

1. Mark an X at your correct height on the line in box A.
2. Mark an X at your correct weight in box B.
3. Draw a straight line from X in A through the X in B and across to the line under box C.
4. Your Body Mass Index is the number where your line crosses box C.

FIGURE 5-6 Body mass index. (Source: Expert Group on Weight Standards, Health and Welfare Canada)

Waist circumference is useful for people with a body mass index (BMI) in the range 18.5 to 34.9; if a BMI is equal to or greater than 35.0, no additional risk information is gained by doing this measurement. Waist measurement to the nearest 0.5 cm is taken as described above. Men with a waist circumference equal to or greater than 102 cm and women with a waist circumference equal or greater than 88 cm have excess abdominal fat and are at increased risk of developing type 2 diabetes, coronary heart disease, and hypertension (adapted from World Health Organization, 2000).

BIOCHEMICAL ASSESSMENT

Biochemical assessment reflects both the tissue level of a given nutrient and any abnormality of metabolism in the utilization of nutrients. These determinations are made from studies of serum (serum protein, serum albumin and globulin, transferrin, retinol-binding protein, hemoglobin, serum vitamin A, carotene, and vitamin C) and studies of urine (creatinine, thiamine, riboflavin, niacin, and iodine). Some of these tests, while reflecting recent intake of the elements detected, can also identify below-normal levels when there are no clinical symptoms of deficiency (see Table 5-1 for a description of serum protein indices).

Low serum albumin and transferrin levels are often used as measures of protein deficits in adults and are expressed as percentages of normal values. Albumin synthesis depends on normal liver function and an adequate supply of amino acids. Because the body stores a large amount of albumin, the serum albumin level may not decrease until malnutrition is severe; thus, its usefulness in detecting recent protein depletion is limited. Decreased albumin levels may be due to overhydration, liver or renal disease, and excessive protein loss because of burns, major surgery, infection,

Table 5-1 • **Standard Serum Protein Indices**

SERUM PROTEIN	STANDARD RANGE
Albumin	35–50 g/L
Transferrin	2.3–3.2 g/L*
Prealbumin	0.16–0.3 g/L
Retinol-binding protein	26–77 mg/L

From Dudek, S. G. (2001). *Nutrition essentials for nursing practice* (4th ed.). Philadelphia: Lippincott Williams & Wilkins.
*From Jacobs, D. S., DeMott, W. R., & Oxley, D. K. (2001). *Laboratory test handbook.* (5th ed.). Hudson, OH: Lexi-Comp. Inc.

and cancer (Dudek, 2000). Transferrin is a protein that binds and carries iron from the intestine through the serum. Because of its short half-life, decreased transferrin levels respond more quickly to protein depletion than albumin. Serial measurements of these, as well as prealbumin levels, are used to assess the results of nutritional therapy.

Although not available from many laboratories, retinol-binding protein may be a useful means of monitoring acute, short-term changes in protein status.

Reduced total lymphocyte count in people who become acutely malnourished as a result of stress and low-calorie feeding are associated with impaired cellular immunity (Dudek, 2000). Anergy, the absence of an immune response to injection of small concentrations of recall antigen under the skin, may also indicate malnutrition because of delayed antibody synthesis and response.

Serum electrolyte levels provide information about fluid and electrolyte balance and kidney function. The creatinine/height index calculated over a 24-hour period assesses the metabolically active tissue and indicates the degree of protein depletion, comparing expected body mass for height and actual body cell mass. A 24-hour urine sample is obtained, and the amount of creatinine is measured and compared to normal ranges based on the patient's height and gender. Values less than normal may indicate loss of lean body mass and protein malnutrition.

CLINICAL EXAMINATION

The state of nutrition is often reflected in a person's appearance. Although the most obvious physical sign of good nutrition is a normal body weight with respect to height, body frame, and age, other tissues can serve as indicators of general nutritional status and adequate intake of specific nutrients; these include the hair, skin, teeth, gums, mucous membranes, mouth and tongue, skeletal muscles, abdomen, lower extremities, and thyroid gland (Table 5-2). Specific aspects of clinical examination useful in identifying nutritional deficits include oral examination and assessment of skin for turgor, edema, elasticity, dryness, subcutaneous tone, poorly healing wounds and ulcers, purpura, and bruises. The musculoskeletal examination also provides information about muscle wasting and weakness.

DIETARY DATA

The appraisal of food intake considers the quantity and quality of the diet and also the frequency with which certain food items and nutrients are consumed. Commonly used methods of determining individual eating patterns include the food record and the 24-hour food recall, which can help estimate if the food intake is adequate and appropriate. If these methods are used, instructions about measurement and recording food intake are given when the patient's dietary history is obtained.

Food Record

The food record is used most often in nutritional status studies. The person is instructed to keep a record of food actually consumed over a period of time, varying from 3 to 7 days, and to accurately estimate and describe the specific foods consumed. Food records are fairly accurate if the person is willing to provide factual information and able to estimate food quantities.

Table 5-2 • **Physical Signs Indicative of Nutritional Status**

	SIGNS OF GOOD NUTRITION	SIGNS OF POOR NUTRITION
General appearance	Alert, responsive, energetic	Listless, apathetic, appears acutely or chronically ill
Hair	Shiny, lustrous, minimal loss	Dull and dry, brittle, depigmented, easily plucked, thin and sparse
Face	Skin colour uniform; smooth, moist	Skin dark over cheeks and under eyes, skin flaky, face swollen or hollow/sunken cheeks
Eyes	Bright, clear, moist	Eye membranes pale, dry; increased vascularity
Lips	Pink colour, smooth, moist	Edematous, cracks, angular lesions at corners of mouth (cheilosis)
Tongue	Deep red in appearance; surface papillae present	Smooth, edematous, beefy red, atrophic papillae
Teeth	Straight, no crowding, no dental caries, uniform colour	Dental caries, missing teeth, mottled appearance (fluorosis), malpositioned, dentures no longer fit
Gums	Firm, pink colour; margins tight around teeth	Spongy; bleed easily; marginal redness, recession
Thyroid	No enlargement of the thyroid	Thyroid enlargement (simple goitre)
Skin	Smooth, uniform colour; moist, warm	Rough, dry, flaky; edema present; pale, pigmented; lack of fat under skin or excess fat under skin
Nails	Firm, pink	Spoon-shaped, ridged, brittle
Skeleton	Good posture, no malformation	Poor posture, stooped, bending of ribs, bowed legs or knock knees
Muscles	Well developed, firm	Flaccid, poor tone, wasted, underdeveloped
Extremities	No tenderness	Weak and tender, edematous
Abdomen	Flat	Concave or hollowed (scaphoid), protruding
Nervous system	Reflexes present	Decreased or absent ankle and knee reflexes
Weight	Appropriate for height, age, and body build	Overweight or underweight

24-Hour Recall

The 24-hour recall method is, as the name implies, a recall of food intake over a 24-hour period. The person is asked by the interviewer to recall all food eaten during the previous day and to estimate the quantities of the food consumed. Because information does not always represent usual intake, at the end of the interview the patient is asked if the previous day's food intake was a typical one. To obtain supplementary information about the typical diet, the interviewer also asks how frequently the person eats foods from the major food groups.

CONDUCTING THE DIETARY INTERVIEW

The success of the interviewer in obtaining information for dietary assessment depends on effective communication, which requires that good rapport be established to promote respect and trust. The interviewer explains the purpose of the interview. It is conducted in a nondirective and exploratory way, allowing the respondent to express feelings and thoughts while encouraging him or her to answer specific questions. The manner in which questions are asked will influence the respondent's cooperation. Thus, the interviewer must be nonjudgmental and avoid expressing disapproval, either verbally or by facial expression.

Character of General Intake

Several questions may be necessary to elicit the information needed. When attempting to elicit information about the type and quantity of food eaten at a particular time, the interviewer avoids leading questions, such as, "Do you use sugar or cream in your coffee?" Also, assumptions are not made about the size of servings; instead, questions are phrased so that quantities are more clearly determined. For example, to help determine the size of one hamburger eaten, the patient may be asked, "How many servings were prepared with the 0.5 kg or pound of meat you bought?" Another approach to determining quantities is to use food models of known sizes in estimating portions of meat, cake, or pie or to record quantities in common measurements, such as a cup (250 mL) or spoonfulls (1–15 mL), or according to the size of containers (eg, ml or L), when discussing intake of bottled beverages.

In recording a particular combination dish, such as a casserole, it is useful to ask for the ingredients in the recipe, recording the largest quantities first. When recording quantities of ingredients, one notes whether the food item was raw or cooked and the number of servings provided by the recipe. When the client lists the foods for the recall questionnaire, it may be helpful to read back the list of foods and ask if anything was forgotten, such as fruit, cake, candy, between-meal snacks, or alcoholic beverages.

Additional information obtained during the interview should include methods of preparing food, sources available for food (food bank), food-buying practices, vitamin and mineral supplements, and income range.

Cultural and Religious Considerations

An individual's culture determines to a large extent which foods are eaten and how they are prepared and served. Culture and religious practices together often determine if certain foods are prohibited and if certain foods and spices are eaten on certain holidays or at specific family gatherings. Because of the importance of culture and religious beliefs to many individuals, it is important to be sensitive to these factors when obtaining a dietary history. It is, however, equally important not to stereotype individuals and assume that because they are from a certain culture or religious group, they adhere to specific dietary customs.

Culturally sensitive materials, such as food pyramids for Asians and Latin Americans (U.S. Department of Agriculture Food Guide Pyramid) or a food pagoda (The Chinese Nutrition Society, 1999), are available for making appropriate dietary recommendations.

EVALUATING THE DIETARY INFORMATION

After the dietary information has been obtained, the nurse evaluates the patient's dietary intake. If the goal is to determine if the person generally eats a healthful diet, the food intake may be compared to the dietary guidelines outlined in Canada's Food Guide to Healthy Eating (Fig. 5-7). The Food Guide divides foods into four major groups (grain products, vegetables and fruit, milk products, meat and alternatives) and offers recommendations for variety in the diet, proportion of food from each food group, and moderation in eating fats, oils, and sweets. The person's food intake is compared with recommendations for each food group. A revised Food Guide that will reflect cultural and ethnic diversity, aging population, family structure, and the pressures of home and work is expected in Spring 2006.

If the nurse or dietitian is interested in knowing about the intake of specific nutrients, such as vitamin A, iron, or calcium, the patient's food intake is analyzed by consulting a list of foods and their composition and nutrient content. The diet is then analyzed in terms of grams and milligrams of specific nutrients. The total nutritive value is then compared with the recommended dietary allowances that are specific for different age categories, gender, and special circumstances such as pregnancy or lactation (Monsen, 2000). The nurse frequently participates in the nutrition screening of patients and communicates the information to the dietitian and the rest of the team for more detailed assessment and for clinical nutrition intervention.

FACTORS INFLUENCING NUTRITIONAL STATUS IN VARIED SITUATIONS

One sensitive indicator of the body's gain or loss of protein is its nitrogen balance. An adult is said to be in nitrogen equilibrium when the nitrogen intake (from food) equals the nitrogen output (in urine, feces, and perspiration); it is a sign of health. A positive nitrogen balance exists when nitrogen intake exceeds nitrogen output and indicates tissue growth, such as occurs during pregnancy, childhood, recovery from surgery, and rebuilding of wasted tissue. Negative nitrogen balance indicates that tissue is breaking down faster than it is being replaced. In the absence of an adequate intake of protein, the body converts protein to glucose for energy. This can occur with fever, starvation, surgery, burns, and debilitating diseases. Each gram of nitrogen loss in excess of intake represents the depletion of 6.25 g of protein or 25 g of muscle tissue. Therefore, a negative nitrogen balance of 10 g/day for 10 days could mean the wasting of 2.5 kg of muscle tissue as it is converted to glucose for energy.

When conditions that result in negative nitrogen balance are coupled with anorexia (loss of appetite), they can lead to malnutrition. Malnutrition interferes with wound healing, increases susceptibility to infection, and contributes to an increased incidence of complications, longer hospital stay, and prolonged confinement of the patient to bed (Bender, Pusateri, Cook et al., 2000).

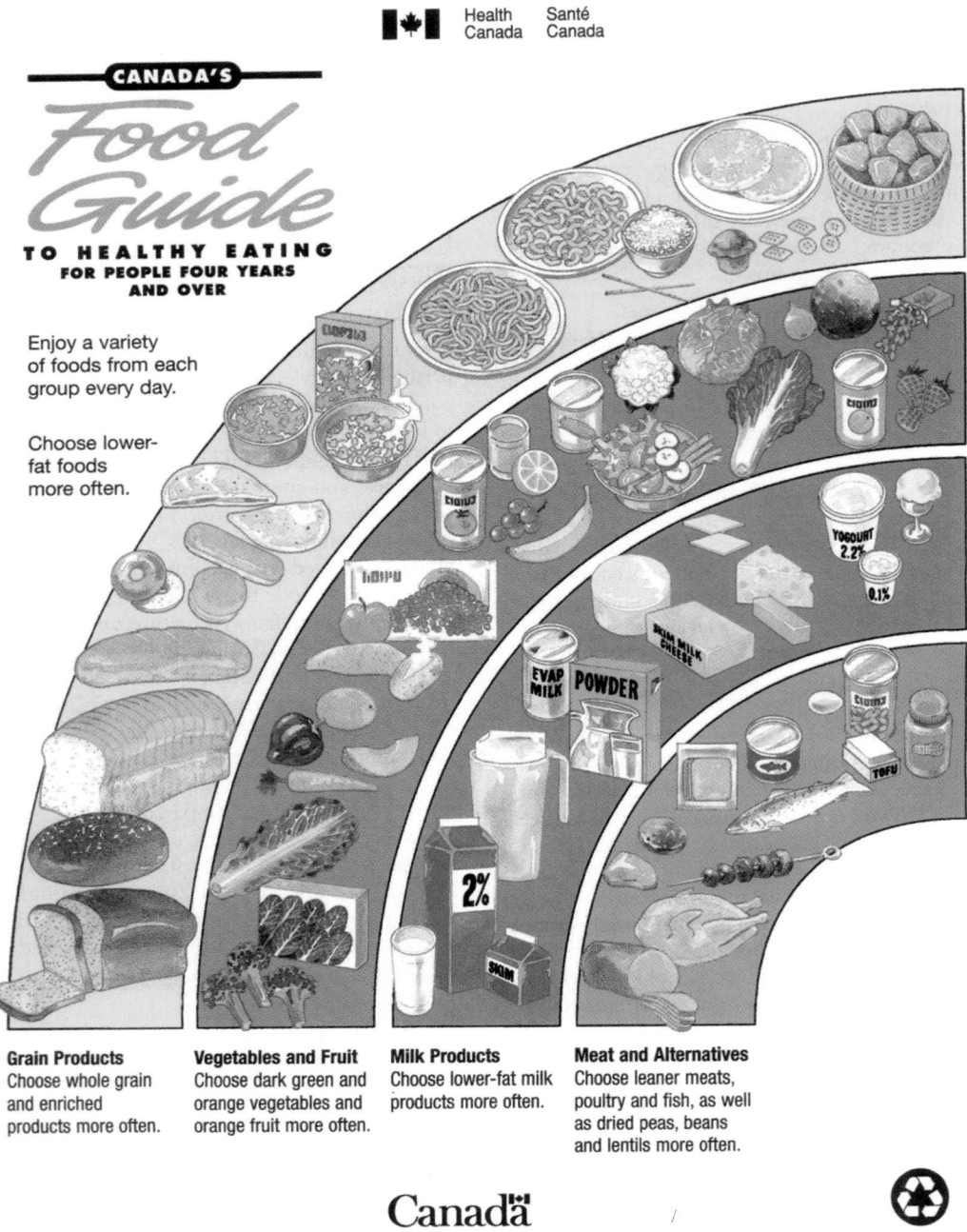

FIGURE 5-7 Canada's Food Guide—Rainbow. (Source: www.hc-sc.gc.ca/hpfb-dgpsa/onpp-bppn/food_guide_rainbow_e.html)

The patient who is hospitalized may have an inadequate dietary intake because of the illness or disorder that necessitated the hospital stay or because the hospital's food is unfamiliar or unappealing (Dudek, 2000; Wilkes, 2000). The person who is cared for at home may feel too sick or fatigued to shop and prepare food or may be unable to eat because of other physical problems or limitations. Limited or fixed incomes or the high costs of medications may result in insufficient money to buy nutritious foods. Patients with inadequate housing or inadequate cooking facilities are unlikely to have an adequate nutritional intake.

Because complex treatments (eg, ventilators, intravenous infusions, chemotherapy) once used only in the hospital setting are now being provided in the home and outpatient settings, nutri-

tional assessment of the patient in these settings is an important aspect of home and community-based care as well as hospital-based care (Dabrowski & Rombeau, 2000; Worthington, Gilbert & Wagner, 2000).

Many medications influence nutritional status by suppressing the appetite, irritating the mucosa, or causing nausea and vomiting. Others may influence bacterial flora in the intestine or directly affect nutrient absorption so that secondary malnutrition results. People who must take many medications in a single day often report feeling too full to eat. The person's use of prescription and over-the-counter medications and their effect on appetite and dietary intake are assessed. Many of the factors that contribute to poor nutritional status are identified in Table 5-3.

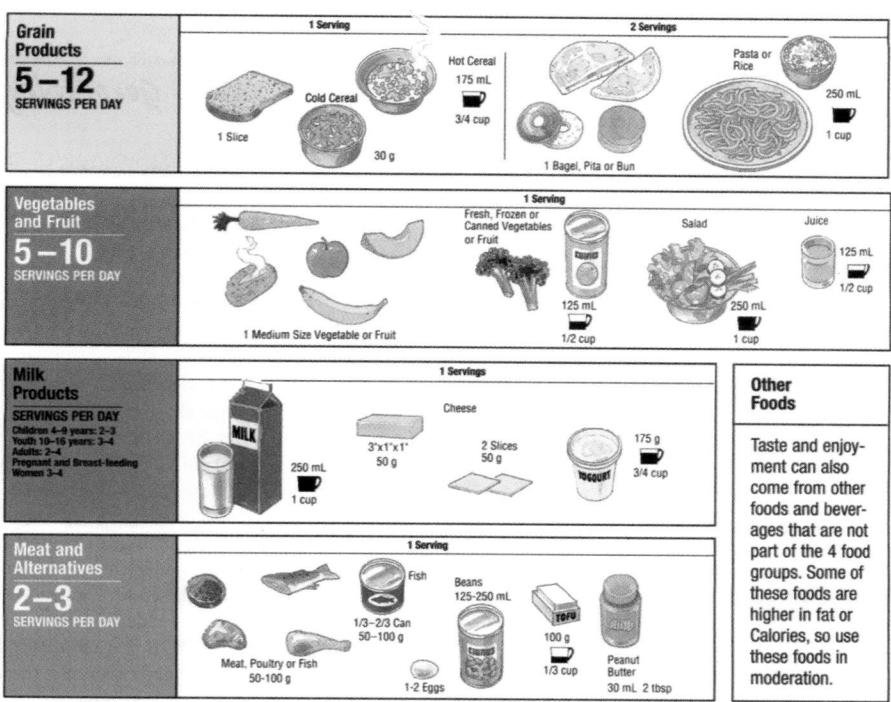

Different People Need Different Amounts of Food

The amount of food you need every day from the 4 food groups and other foods depends on your age, body size, activity level, whether you are male or female and if you are pregnant or breast-feeding. That's why the Food Guide gives a lower and higher number of servings for each food group. For example, young children can choose the lower number of servings, while male teenagers can go to the higher number. Most other people can choose servings somewhere in between.

Consult *Canada's Physical Activity Guide to Healthy Active Living* to help you build physical activity into your daily life.

Enjoy eating well, being active and feeling good about yourself. That's VITALIT

FIGURE 5-7 (Continued)

Table 5-3 • **Factors Associated With Potential Nutritional Deficits**

FACTORS	POSSIBLE CONSEQUENCES
Dental and oral problems (missing teeth, ill-fitting dentures, impaired swallowing or chewing)	Inadequate intake of high-fibre foods
NPO for diagnostic testing	Inadequate caloric and protein intake; dehydration
Prolonged use of glucose and saline IV fluids	Inadequate caloric and protein intake
Nausea and vomiting	Inadequate caloric and protein intake; loss of fluid, electrolytes, and minerals
Stress of illness, surgery, and/or hospitalization	Increased protein and caloric requirement; increased catabolism
Wound drainage	Loss of protein, fluid, electrolytes, and minerals
Pain	Loss of appetite; inability to shop, cook, eat
Fever	Increased caloric and fluid requirement; increased catabolism
Gastrointestinal intubation	Loss of protein, fluid, and minerals
Tube feedings	Inadequate amounts; various nutrients in each formula
Gastrointestinal disease	Inadequate intake and malabsorption of nutrients
Alcoholism	Inadequate intake of nutrients; increased consumption of calories without other nutrients; vitamin deficiencies
Depression	Loss of appetite; inability to shop, cook, eat
Eating disorders (anorexia, bulimia)	Inadequate caloric and protein intake; loss of fluid, electrolytes, and minerals
Medications	Inadequate intake due to medication side effects, such as dry mouth, loss of appetite, decreased taste perception, difficulty swallowing, nausea and vomiting, physical problems that limit shopping, cooking, eating; malabsorption of nutrients
Restricted ambulation or disability	Inability to help self to food, liquids, other nutrients

ANALYSIS OF NUTRITIONAL STATUS

Measurement of BMI, anthropometric measurements, and biochemical, clinical, and dietary data are used together to determine the patient's nutritional status. Often the BMI, anthropometric measurements, biochemical measures, and dietary data provide more information about the patient's nutritional status than the clinical examination; the clinical examination may not detect subclinical deficiencies unless such deficiencies become so advanced that overt signs develop. A low intake of nutrients over a period of time may lead to low biochemical levels and without nutritional intervention may result in characteristic and observable signs and symptoms (see Table 5-2). A plan of action for nutritional intervention is based on the results of the dietary assessment and the patient's profile. To be effective, the plan must meet the patient's need for a balanced diet, maintain or control weight, and compensate for increased nutritional needs.

Adolescent Considerations

Adolescence is a time of critical growth and acquisition of lifelong eating habits, and therefore nutritional assessment and analysis are critical. In the past two decades the percentage of adolescents who are overweight or obese has greatly increased. Despite this, total milk consumption has decreased by 36% compared to prior years (Cavadini, Siega-Riz & Popkin, 2000). Fruit and vegetable consumption is also below the recommended five to ten servings per day.

Adolescent girls are at particular nutritional risk as iron, folate, and calcium intake is below recommended levels (Cavadini, Siega-Riz & Popkin, 2000). Low calcium intake in adolescence sets the stage for osteoporosis in later life. Persons with other nutritional disorders, such as anorexia and bulimia, have a better chance for recovery if these disorders are identified in the adolescent years compared to adulthood (Orbanic, 2001).

Assessment in the Home and Community

Assessment of the person in community settings, including the home, consists of collecting information specific to existing health problems, including the patient's physiologic and emotional status, the community and home environment, the adequacy of support systems or care given by family and other care providers, and the availability of needed resources. In addition, the ability of the individual and family to cope with and address their respective needs is evaluated. The physical assessment in the community and home consists of the same techniques used in the hospital, outpatient clinic, or office setting. Privacy is provided and the person is made as comfortable as possible.

A call made to the patient's home before the first home visit lets the patient know when to expect the home care nurse and also provides the opportunity for the patient's primary caregiver to be available. During the home visit, the nurse's assessment is not limited to physical assessment of the patient. Other aspects of assessment include the home environment, safety factors (eg, smoke alarms, obstacles, safety bars in the bathroom), adequacy of facilities required for the patient's care and recovery, food preparation and storage facilities, bathroom facilities, access to a telephone, and the availability of family and community supports. Because patients may have no family mem-

 Gerontologic Considerations

Between 5% and 10% of community-dwelling elderly are estimated to be malnourished, and the prevalence ranges from 30% to 60% in home-bound or elderly living in retirement homes (Griep, Mets, Colly et al., 2000). Elderly people who are malnourished tend to have longer and more expensive hospital stays than those who are adequately nourished; the risk of costly complications is also increased in those who are malnourished (Bender et al., 2000; Braunschweig, Gomez & Sheean, 2000; Cammon & Hackshaw, 2000).

Inadequate dietary intake in the elderly may result from physiologic changes in the gastrointestinal tract, social and economic factors, drug interactions, disease, excessive use of alcohol, and poor dentition or missing teeth. Malnutrition is a common consequence of these factors and in turn leads to illness and frailty of the elderly. Important aspects of care of the elderly in the hospital, home, outpatient setting, or extended care facility include recognizing risk factors and identifying those at risk for inadequate nutrition (Bender et al., 2000; Cammon & Hackshaw, 2000; Morley, 2000).

Some elderly people take excessive and inappropriate medications; this is referred to as polypharmacy. About 50% of Canadians 65 years and older take three prescriptions daily and consume 40% of all medications, even though they only represent 13% of the Canadian population. In 2004, individuals 80 years or older had an average of 42 prescriptions filled whereas those 59 to 79 years old had 9 filled (MacAuley, 2005). The Beers Criteria contains a list of drugs that may be hazardous to seniors (Fick, Cooper, Wade, et al., 2003). The Canadian Broadcasting Corporation (CBC) reported in April 2005 that "more than a third of all seniors had taken a drug from the Beers list during the past year and that of those seniors who died, a third had been on a Beers-listed drug" (MacAuley, p. 30). The number of adverse reactions increases proportionately with the number of prescribed and over-the-counter medications taken. Age-related physiologic (eg, declining heart, liver, and kidney function) and pathophysiologic changes may alter the metabolism and elimination of many medications. Medications can influence food intake by producing side effects such as nausea, vomiting, decreased appetite, and changes in sensorium (Morley, 2000). They may also interfere with the distribution, utilization, and storage of nutrients. Some foods interfere with the action of medications (eg, grapefruit and Coumadin). Disorders affecting any part of the gastrointestinal tract can alter nutritional requirements and health status in people of any age; however, they are likely to occur quickly and more frequently in the elderly.

Nutritional problems in the elderly often occur or are precipitated by such illnesses as pneumonia and urinary tract infections. Acute and chronic diseases may affect the metabolism and utilization of nutrients, which already are altered by the aging process. Flu and pneumonia immunizations, prompt treatment of bacterial infections, and social programs such as Meals on Wheels may reduce the risk of illness-associated malnutrition.

Even the well elderly may be nutritionally at risk because of decreased odour perception, poor dental health, limited ability to shop and cook, financial hardship, and the fact that they often eat alone (Griep, Mets, Colly, et al., 2000). The effort required to prepare meals can lead to the elderly having "tea and toast" as a meal. Also, reduction in exercise with age without concomitant changes in carbohydrate intake places the elderly at risk for obesity. Nutritional screening in the elderly is a first step in maintaining adequate nutrition and replacing nutrient losses to maintain the individual's health and well being.

bers available to assist them and may live alone in substandard housing or homeless shelters, the nurse needs to be aware of resources available in the community and methods of obtaining those resources for the patient. Figure 5-8 provides an example of a checklist that may be useful in conducting an assessment in the home.

 Critical Thinking Exercises

1. Compare the approach and techniques you would use in assessing a patient who is experiencing severe abdominal pain. How would your approach and technique differ if your patient has dementia? If your patient has dementia and is blind or hard of hearing? If your patient is from a culture with very different values from yours?

2. Your health history and physical examination of an elderly patient alerts you to the possibility of abuse. Explain how you would pursue this further. What assessments are available to assist in assessing this in a more comprehensive manner?

3. You are conducting a health history on a patient who is admitted to the emergency room after he was hit by a car while walking down the centre of a major street at 2200 hours. He is responsive and able to talk and has no apparent major physical injuries. The ambulance crew that brought him to the emergency room tells you that the patient has probably been drinking. How would this history affect your assessment? How would you assess history of alcohol use in an emergency room setting? How would you do so in a patient in a primary care office? Explain the rationale for your responses.

4. Your nutritional assessment reveals that a female adolescent patient has a high fat intake and minimal calcium intake. What dietary recommendations would you make for this client? What dietary instructions would you develop for her if she is a vegetarian?

5. You have received a referral for home care for a 75-year-old patient who has recently had a stroke and who lives alone in a travel trailer. What physical and environmental factors are important to assess on the initial home visit? Identify the elements in the home that would be safety hazards and those that would be safety factors.

Physical Facilities (check all that apply)

Exterior
- ☐ steps_____
- ☐ unsafe steps_____
- ☐ porch_____
- ☐ litter_____
- ☐ noise_____
- ☐ inadequate lighting_____
- ☐ other_____

Interior
- ☐ accessible bathroom_____
- ☐ level, safe floor surface_____
- ☐ number of rooms_____
- ☐ privacy_____
- ☐ sleeping arrangements_____
- ☐ refrigeration_____
- ☐ garbage management _____
- ☐ animals_____
- ☐ adequate lighting_____
- ☐ steps/stairs_____
- ☐ other_____
_____

Safety Hazards found in the patient's current residence (check all that apply)
- ☐ none
- ☐ inadequate floor, roof, or windows
- ☐ inadequate lighting
- ☐ unsafe gas/electric appliances
- ☐ inadequate heating
- ☐ inadequate cooling
- ☐ lack of fire safety devices
- ☐ unsafe floor coverings
- ☐ inadequate stair rails
- ☐ lead-based paint
- ☐ improperly stored hazardous material
- ☐ improper wiring/electrical cords
- ☐ other_____
_____

Safety Factors (check all that apply)
- ☐ smoke/fire detectors_____
- ☐ fire extinguisher_____
- ☐ carbon monoxide detector_____
- ☐ telephone_____
- ☐ placement of electrical cords_____
- ☐ emergency plan_____
_____
- ☐ emergency phone numbers displayed_____
- ☐ safe portable heaters_____
- ☐ obstacle-free paths_____
- ☐ other_____
_____

FIGURE 5-8 Home assessment checklist.

REFERENCES AND SELECTED READINGS

Books and Pamphlets

American Heart Association. (2000). *An eating plan for healthy Americans: Our American Heart Association Diet.* Dallas, TX: Author.

Bickley, L. S., & Szilagyi, P. G. (2003). *Bates' guide to physical examination and history taking* (8th ed.). Philadelphia: Lippincott Williams & Wilkins.

Chandler, F. (Ed.). (2000). *Herbs: Everyday reference for health professionals.* Ottawa: Canadian Pharmacists' Association and Canadian Medical Association.

Critser, G. (2003). *Fatland: How Americans became the fattest people in the world.* New York: Houghton Mifflin.

Dudek, S. G. (2001). *Nutrition essentials for nursing practice* (4th ed.). Philadelphia: Lippincott Williams & Wilkins.

Expert Group on Weight Standards. (1998). *Canadian guidelines for healthy weights: Report of an expert group convened by Health Promotion Directorate, Health Services and Promotion Branch.* Ottawa, ON: Health and Welfare Canada.

Food and Nutrition Board, Institutes of Medicine. (2002). *Dietary reference intakes for energy, carbohydrates, fiber, fat, protein and amino acids (macronutrients): A report of the Panel on Micronutrients, Subcommittees on Upper Reference Levels of Nutrients and Interpretation and Uses of Dietary Reference Intakes, and the Standing Committee on the Scientific Evaluation of Dietary Reference Intakes.* Washington, DC: National Academy Press.

Fuller, J., & Schaller-Ayers, J. (2000). *Health assessment: A nursing approach* (3rd ed.). Philadelphia: Lippincott Williams & Wilkins.

Guiliano, M. (2005). *French women don't get fat: The secret of eating for pleasure.* New York: Knopf.

Health Canada. (2003). *Canadian guidelines for body weight classification in adults.* Ottawa: Minister of Public Works and Government Services.

Health Canada. Office of Nutrition Policy and Promotion. Health Products and Food Branch. (1997). *Canada's food guide to healthy eating.* Ottawa: Author.

Health Canada. Office of Nutrition Policy and Promotion. Health Products and Food Branch. (2003). *Body mass index (BMI) nomogram.* Ottawa: Author.

Kuhn, M. (1999). *Complementary therapies for health care providers.* Philadelphia: Lippincott Williams & Wilkins.

National Institutes of Health, National Heart, Lung and Blood Institute, North American Association for the Study of Obesity. (2000). *The practical guide: Identification, evaluation, and treatment of overweight and obesity in adults.* NIH Publication Number 00-4084. Bethesda, MD: NIH.

Ramsay, C., Walker, M., & Alexander, J. (1999). Alternative medicine in Canada: Use and public attitudes. Public Policy Sources paper No. 21. Vancouver: Fraser Institute.

Ross, M., Channon-Little, L., & Rosser, S. (2000). *Sexual health concerns: Interviewing and history taking for health practitioners* (2nd ed.). Philadelphia: F. A. Davis.

Statistics Canada, Health Statistics Division. (2005). *Selected leading causes of death, by sex (1997).* Ottawa: Author. Available at: http://www40.statcan.ca/l01/cst01/health36.htm.

United States Department of Agriculture, United States Department of Health and Human Services. *Nutrition and your health: Dietary guidelines for Americans* (5th ed). Bull. No. 232:39.

United States Department of Health and Human Services. (2001). *The Surgeon General's call to action to prevent and decrease overweight and obesity.* Rockville, MD: USDHHS, PHS.

Weber, J., & Kelley, J. (2003). *Health assessment in nursing* (2nd ed.). Philadelphia: Lippincott Williams & Wilkins.

World Health Organization. (2000). *Obesity: Preventing and managing the global epidemic. Report of a WHO consultation on obesity.* Geneva: World Health Organization.

Journals

An asterisk indicates a nursing research article.

General Assessment

Andersen, R. E. (2000). The spread of the childhood obesity epidemic. *Canadian Medical Association Journal, 163*(11), 1461–1462.

Bakshi, S., & Miller, D. (1999). Assessment of the aging man. *Medical Clinics of North America, 83*(5), 1131–1149.

Birmingham, C. L., Muller, J. L., Palepu, A., Spinelli, J. J., & Anis, A. H. (1999). The cost of obesity in Canada. *Canadian Medical Association Journal, 160*(4), 483–488.

Butler, R. (1999). The 15-minute geriatric assessment. *Geriatrics, 54*(7), 3.

Canada Health Monitor, Survey No. 16, June-July 1997.

Druss, B. G., & Rosenheck, R. A. (1999). Association between use of unconventional therapies and conventional medical services. *Journal of the American Medical Association, 282,* 651–656.

Evans, V. (2000). Herbs and the brain: Friend or foe? *Journal of Neuroscience Nursing, 32*(4), 229–232.

Fiellin, D. A., Reid, M. C., & O'Connor, P. G. Screening for alcohol problems in primary care: A systematic review. *Archives of Internal Medicine, 160*(13), 1977–1989.

Goolsby, M. (2001). Evaluating acute musculoskeletal complaints. *Journal of the American Academy of Nurse Practitioners, 13*(5), 195–199.

Henderson-Martin, B. (2000). No more surprises: Screening patients for alcohol abuse. *American Journal of Nursing, 100*(9), 26–32.

Isaacson, J. H., & Schorling, J. B. (1999). Screening for alcohol problems in primary care. *Medical Clinics of North America, 83*(6), 1547–1563.

Joudrey, R., & Gough, J. (2003). Student nurses' use and perceptions of alternative medicine: An exploratory study. *Canadian Journal of Nursing Research, 35*(3), 80–93.

Katzmarzyk, P. T., Perusse, L., Malina, R. M., & Bouchard, C. (1999). Seven-year stability of indicators of obesity and adipose tissue distribution in the Canadian population. *American Journal of Clinical Nutrition, 69*(6), 1123–1129.

King, M., Pettigrew, A., & Reed, F. (1999). Complementary, alternative, integrative: Have nurses kept pace with their clients? *MedSurg Nursing, 8*(4), 239–246.

Kushner, R., & Weinsier, R. (2000). Evaluation of the obese patient. *Medical Clinics of North America, 84*(2), 387–399.

Lau, D. C. W. (1999). Call for action: Preventing and managing the expansive and expensive obesity epidemic. *Canadian Medical Association Journal, 160*(4), 503–506.

Little, K. (2000). Screening for domestic violence. *Postgraduate Medicine, 108*(2), 135–141.

Ludwick, R., Dieckman, B., & Snelson, C. (1999). Assessment of the geriatric orthopedic trauma patient. *Orthopedic Nursing,* 13–18.

Marshall, C., Benton, D., & Brazier, J. (2000). Elder abuse: Using clinical tools to identify clues of mistreatment. *Geriatrics, 55*(2), 42–53.

Mathre, M. L. (2001). Therapeutic cannabis: A patient advocacy issue. *American Journal of Nursing, 101*(4), 61–68.

McClennon-Leong, J., & Kerr, J. R. (1999). Alternative health care options in Canada. *Canadian Nurse, 95*(10), 26–28, 30.

Miller, K., Zylstra, R., & Standridge, J. (2000). The geriatric patient: A systematic approach to maintaining health. *American Family Physician, 61*(4), 1089–1104

Palmer, R. (1999). Geriatric assessment. *Medical Clinics of North America, 83*(6), 1503–1520.

PricewaterhouseCoopers. (1999). *HealthInsider: National public opinion survey on health care, 2.*

Walton, J., Miller, J., & Tordecilla, L. (2001). Elder oral assessment and care. *MedSurg Nursing, 10*(1), 37–44.

Nutritional Assessment

Bender, S., Pusateri, M., Cook, A., et al. (2000). Malnutrition: Role of the TwoCal HN med pass program. *MedSurg Nursing, 9*(6), 284–296.

Braunschweig, C., Gomez, S., & Sheean, P. (2000). Impact of declines in nutritional status on outcomes in adult patients hospitalized for more than 7 days. *Journal of the American Dietetic Association, 100*(11), 1316–1322.

Cammon, S., & Hackshaw, H. (2000). Are we starving our patients? *American Journal of Nursing, 100*(5), 43–47.

Cavadini, C., Siega-Riz, A. M., & Popkin, B. (2000). U.S. adolescent food intake trends from 1965 to 1996. *Archives of Diseases of Children, 83*(1), 18–24.

CBC News Online. (April 3, 2005). *Drugs seniors should avoid—The Beers criteria.* Available at: http://www.cbc.ca/news/background/seniors drugs/beers_table_more.html. Retrieved June 21, 2005.

Dabrowski, C., & Rombeau, J. (2000). Practical nutritional management in the trauma intensive care unit. *Surgical Clinics of North America, 80*(3), 921–931.

Dudek, S. (2000). Malnutrition in hospitals: Who's assessing what patients eat? *American Journal of Nursing, 100*(4), 36–43.

Fick, D. M., Cooper, J. W., Wade, W. E., et al. (2003). Updating the Beers criteria for potentially inappropriate medication use in older adults: Results of a US consensus panel of experts. *Archives of Internal Medicine, 163*(22), 2716–2724.

*Griep, M., Mets, T., Colly, K., et al. (2000). Risk of malnutrition in retirement homes elderly persons measured by the "Mini-nutritional assessment." *Journal of Gerontology: Medical Sciences, 55A*(2), M57–M63.

Hensrud, D. (1999). Nutrition screening and assessment. *Medical Clinics of North America, 83*(6), 1525–1543.

Kant, A., Schatzkin, A., Graubard, B., & Schairer, C. (2000). A prospective study of diet quality and mortality in women. *JAMA, 283*(16), 2109–2115.

Kennedy, E., & Davis, C. (2000). Dietary guidelines 2000: The opportunity and challenges for reaching the consumer. *Journal of the American Dietetic Association, 100*(12), 1462–1465.

Landi, F., Onder, G., Gambassi, G., et al. (2000). Body mass index and mortality among hospitalized patients. *Archives of Internal Medicine, 160,* 2641–2644.

Landi, F., Zuccala, G., Gambassi, G., et al. (1999). Body mass index and mortality among older people living in the community. *Journal of the American Geriatrics Society, 47,* 1072–1076.

Monsen, E. (2000). Dietary reference intakes for the antioxidant nutrients: Vitamin C, vitamin E, selenium, and carotenoids. *Journal of the American Dietetic Association, 100*(6), 637–640.

Morley, J. (2000). Management of nutritional problems in subacute care. *Clinics in Geriatric Medicine, 16*(4), 817–829.

Orbanic, S. (2001). Understanding bulimia. *American Journal of Nursing, 101*(3), 35–42.

Stampfer, M., Hu, F., Manson, J., et al. (2000). Primary prevention of coronary heart disease in women through diet and lifestyle. *New England Journal of Medicine, 343*(1), 16–22.

The Chinese Nutrition Society. (1999). Dietary guidelines and the food guide pagoda for Chinese residents: Balanced diet, rational nutrition, and health promotion. *Nutrition Today, 34*(3), 106–115.

Wilkes, G. (2000). Nutrition: The forgotten ingredient in cancer care. *American Journal of Nursing, 100*(4), 46–51.

Worthington, P., Gilbert, K., & Wagner, B. (2000). Parenteral nutrition for the acutely ill. *AACN Clinical Issues, 11*(4), 559–579.

RESOURCES AND WEBSITES

The Alliance of Cannabis Therapeutics, http://marijuana-as-medicine.org/alliance.htm.

American Dietetic Association, 216 W. Jackson Blvd., Suite 800, Chicago, IL 60606; Consumer Nutrition Hotline: 800-366-1655; http://www.eatright.org.

American Heart Association, 7320 Greenville Ave., Dallas, TX 75231; National Centre: 214-373-6300, Nutrition Information: 214-706-1179; http://www.americanheart.org.

Beers criteria; http://www.hgc.sk.ca or http://archiv.ama-assn.org.

BMI chart; http://www.hc-sc.gc.ca/hpfb-dgpsa/onpp-bppn/bmi_chart_java_e.html.

Canada's Food Guide to Healthy Eating; http://www.hc-sc.gc.ca/hpfb-dgpsa/onpp-bppn/food_guide_rainbow_e.html.

Canada's Physical Activity Guide to Healthy Active Living; http://www.phac-aspc.gc.ca/pau-uap/paguide/index.html.

Canadian Association of Genetic Counsellors (CAGC); http://www.cagc-accg.ca; e-mail: lola.cartier@muhc.mcgill.ca.

CARP Canada's Association for the 50 Plus; http://www.50Plus.com; e-mail: carp@50Plus.com; advocacy@50Plus.com (for advocacy issues).

Canadian Cancer Society/Société Canadienne du Cancer, National Office, Suite 200, 10 Alcorn Avenue, Toronto, ON M4V 3B1; 416-961-7223; fax: 416-961-4189; http://www.cancer.ca.

Canadian Diabetes Association, National Life Building, 1400-522 University Ave., Toronto, ON M5G 2R5; http://www.diabetes.ca.

Canadian Directory of Genetic Support Groups; Support Group Directory, Regional Medical Genetics Centre, Children's Hospital of Western Ontario, 800 Commissioner's Road East, London, ON N6C 2V5; 519-685-8453; 1-800-243-8416 (Ontario only); fax: 519-685-8214; http://www.lhsc.on.ca/programs/medgenet.

Canadian Genetic Disease Network, Suite 201, 2150 Western Parkway, Vancouver, BC V6T 1V6; 604-221-7300; fax: 604-221-0778; e-mail: info@cgdn.ca; http://www.cgdn.ca.

Canadian Organization for Rare Disorders (CORD), P.O. Box 814, Coaldale, AB T1M 1M7;403-345-4544; toll free: 1-877-302-7273; fax: 403-345-3948; http://www.cord.ca.

GeneTests, 9725 Third Avenue NE, Suite 602, Seattle, WA 98115, USA 206-616-4033; fax: 206-221-4679; e-mail: genetests@genetests.org; http://www.genetests.org.

Genetic Alliance, 4301 Connecticut Ave. NW, Suite 404, Washington, DC 20008-2369 USA; 202-966-5557; fax: (202) 966-8553; e-mail: info@geneticalliance.org; http://www.geneticalliance.org.

Genetics Society of Canada; http://life.biology.mcmaster.ca/GSC/.

Heart and Stroke Foundation of Canada, 222 Queen Street, Suite 1402, Ottawa, ON K1P 5V9; 613-569-4361; fax: 613-569-3278; http://ww1.heartandstroke.ca.

National Cancer Institute of Canada/Institut National du Cancer du Canada, 10 Alcorn Avenue, Suite 200, Toronto, ON M4V 3B1; 416-961-7223; fax: 416-961-4189; http://www.ncic.cancer.ca.

National Cancer Institute, Cancer Information Service, 9000 Rockville Pike, Bldg. 31, Room 10A-24, Bethesda, MD 20892; 1-800-4-CANCER; http://www.nci.nih.gov, http://www.ncu.nih.gov/hpage/cis.htm.

Nutrition Screening Initiative, P.O. Box 753, Waldorf, MD 20604; 202-625-1662, http://www.fiu.edu/~nutreld/NSI.html.

OMIM Online Mendelian Inheritance in Man; http://www.ncbi.nlm.nih.gov/entrez/query.fcgi?db=OMIM.

Pennsylvania State Nutrition Center, The Pennsylvania State University, Ruth Building, 417 E. Calder Way, University Park, PA 16802; 814-865-6323.

Statistics Canada; http://www.statcan.ca.

Biophysical and Psychosocial Concepts in Nursing Practice

Applying Concepts from NANDA, NIC, and NOC

Mr. Hussein is a 38-year-old man who comes to the emergency department (ED) for treatment of high blood pressure. On his previous visit to the ED he reported chest pressure, feelings of numbness and tingling in his arms, and extreme fearfulness that he was having a heart attack. Even though a myocardial infarction was ruled out and subsequent testing revealed that he had no heart disease, Mr. Hussein continues to have feelings of chest pressure and fear that he is having a heart attack. The only abnormal finding has been an elevation of blood pressure (158/88). The nurse interviews Mr. Hussein, who reveals he is under intense financial pressure. The nurse assesses his compliance with his antihypertensive therapy and suggests interventions to help with Mr. Hussein's anxiety. The concept map illustrates the relationships that exist among selected diagnoses, interventions, and outcomes.

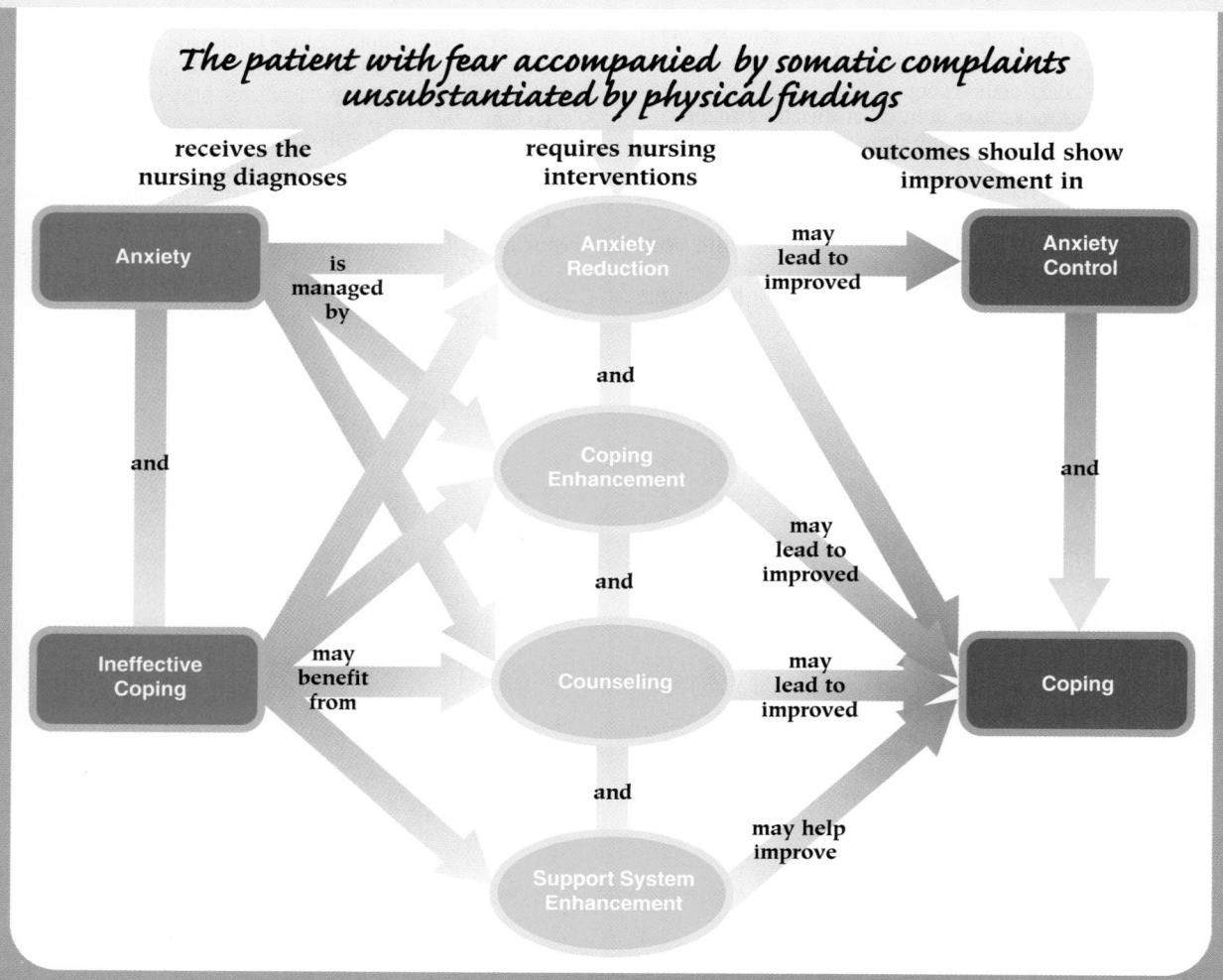

Nursing Classifications and Languages

NANDA
Nursing Diagnoses

Anxiety—Vague uneasy feeling of discomfort or dread accompanied by an autonomic response (the source often nonspecific or unknown to the individual); a feeling of apprehension caused by anticipation of danger. It is an alerting signal that warns of impending danger and enables the individual to take measures to deal with threat.

Ineffective Coping—Inability to perform a valid appraisal of the stressors, inadequate choices of practiced responses, and/or inability to use available resources

NIC
Nursing Interventions*

Anxiety Reduction—Minimizing apprehension, dread, foreboding, or uneasiness related to unidentified source of anticipated danger

Coping Enhancement—Assisting a person to adapt to perceived stressors, changes, or threats that interfere with meeting life demands and roles

Counselling—Use of an interactive helping process focusing on the needs, problems, or feelings of the patient and significant others to enhance or support coping, problem-solving, and interpersonal relationships

Support System Enhancement—Facilitation of support to patient by family, friends, and community

NOC
Nursing Outcomes†

Return to functional baseline status, stabilization of, or improvement in

Anxiety Control—Personal actions to eliminate or reduce feelings of apprehension and tension from an unidentifiable source

Coping—Actions to manage stressors that tax an individual's resources

NANDA, North American Nursing Diagnosis Association; NIC, Nursing Interventions Classification; NOC, Nursing Outcomes Classification

*Iowa Intervention Project © 2000. In McCloskey, J. C., & Bulechek, G. M. (2000). *Nursing interventions classification (NIC)* (3rd ed.). St. Louis: Mosby.

†Iowa Outcomes Project © 2000. In Johnson, M., Maas, M., & Moorhead, S. (2000). *Nursing outcomes classification (NOC)* (3rd ed.). St. Louis: Mosby.

Homeostasis, Stress, and Adaptation

Adapted by Madeleine Buck

LEARNING OBJECTIVES

On completion of this chapter, the learner will be able to:

1. Relate the principles of internal constancy, homeostasis, stress, and adaptation to the concept of steady state.
2. Identify the significance of the body's compensatory mechanisms in promoting adaptation and maintaining the steady state.
3. Identify physiologic and psychosocial stressors.
4. Compare the sympathetic-adrenal-medullary response to stress to the hypothalamic-pituitary response to stress.
5. Describe the general adaptation syndrome as a theory of adaptation to biologic stress.
6. Describe the relationship of the process of negative feedback to the maintenance of the steady state.
7. Compare the adaptive processes of hypertrophy, atrophy, hyperplasia, dysplasia, and metaplasia.
8. Describe the inflammatory and reparative processes.
9. Assess the health patterns of an individual and determine their effects on maintenance of the steady state.
10. Identify ways in which maladaptive responses to stress can increase the risk of illness and cause disease.
11. Identify measures that are useful in reducing stress.
12. Specify the functions of social networks and support groups in reducing stress.

When the body is threatened or suffers an injury, its response may involve functional and structural changes; these changes may be adaptive (having a positive effect) or maladaptive (having a negative effect). The defense mechanisms that the body exhibits determine the difference between adaptation and maladaptation—health and disease.

Stress and Function

Physiology is the study of the functional activities of the living organism and its parts. Pathophysiology is the study of disordered function of the body. Each different body system performs specific functions to sustain optimal life for the organism. Mechanisms for adjusting internal conditions promote the normal steady state of the organism and ultimately its survival. These mechanisms are compensatory in nature and work to restore balance in the body. An example of this restorative effort is the development of rapid breathing (hyperpnea) after intense exercise in an attempt to compensate for an oxygen deficit and excess lactic acid accumulated in the muscle tissue.

Pathophysiologic processes result when cellular injury occurs at such a rapid rate that the body's compensatory mechanisms can no longer make the adaptive changes necessary to remain healthy. An example of a pathophysiologic change is the development of heart failure: the body reacts by retaining sodium and water and increasing venous pressure, which worsens the condition. These pathophysiologic mechanisms give rise to signs that are observed by the patient, nurse, or other health care provider, or symptoms that are reported by the patient. These observations, plus a sound knowledge of physiologic and pathophysiologic processes, can assist in determining the existence of a problem and can guide the nurse in planning the appropriate course of action.

Dynamic Balance: The Steady State

Physiologic mechanisms must be understood in the context of the body as a whole. The person, as a living system, has both an internal and an external environment, between which information

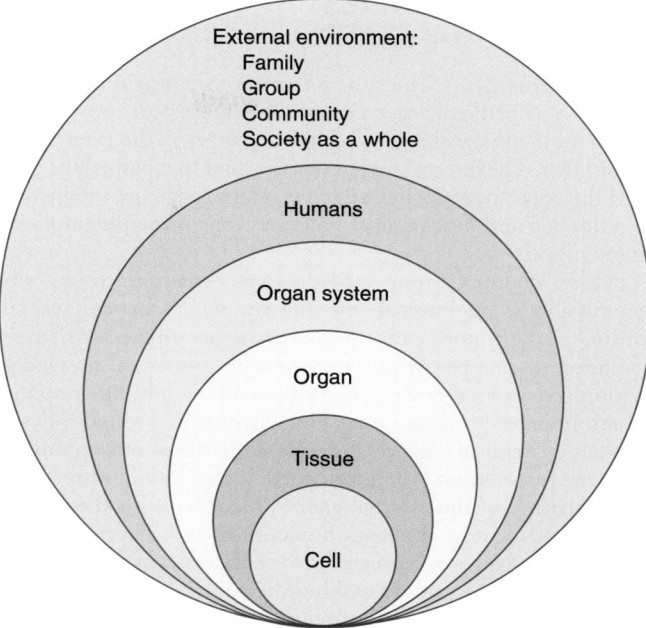

FIGURE 6-1 Constellation of systems. Each system is a subsystem of the larger system (suprasystem) of which it is a part. In this figure the cell is the smallest system, being a subsystem of all other systems.

and matter are continuously exchanged. Within the internal environment each organ, tissue, and cell is also a system or subsystem of the whole, each with its own internal and external environment, each exchanging information and matter (Fig. 6-1). The goal of the interaction of the body's subsystems is to produce a dynamic balance or **steady state** (even in the presence of change), so that all subsystems are in harmony with each other. Four concepts—constancy, homeostasis, stress, and adaptation—enhance the nurse's understanding of steady state.

Glossary

adaptation: a change or alteration designed to assist in adapting to a new situation or environment

adrenocorticotropic hormone (ACTH): a hormone produced by the anterior lobe of the pituitary gland that stimulates the secretion of cortisone and other hormones by the adrenal cortex

antidiuretic hormone (ADH): a hormone secreted by the posterior lobe of the pituitary gland that constricts blood vessels, elevates blood pressure, and reduces the excretion of urine

catecholamines: any of the group of amines (such as epinephrine, norepinephrine, or dopamine) that serve as neurotransmitters

coping: the cognitive and behavioural strategies used to manage the stressors that tax a person's resources

dysplasia: a change in the appearance of a cell after exposure to chronic irritation

glucocorticoids: the group of steroid hormones, such as cortisol, that are produced

by the adrenal cortex; they are involved in carbohydrate, protein, and fat metabolism and have anti-inflammatory properties

gluconeogenesis: the formation of glucose, especially by the liver from noncarbohydrate sources such as amino acids and the glycerol portion of fats

guided imagery: use of the imagination to achieve relaxation or direct attention away from uncomfortable sensations or situations

homeostasis: a steady state within the body; the stability of the internal environment

hyperplasia: an increase in the number of new cells

hypoxia: inadequate supply of oxygen to the cell

infectious agents: biologic agents, such as viruses, bacteria, rickettsiae, mycoplasmas, fungi, protozoa, and nematodes, that cause disease in people

inflammation: a localized, protective reaction of tissue to injury, irritation, or infec-

tion, manifested by pain, redness, heat, swelling, and sometimes loss of function

metabolic rate: the speed at which some substances are broken down to yield energy for bodily processes and other substances are synthesized

metaplasia: a cell transformation in which a highly specialized cell changes to a less specialized cell

negative feedback: feedback that decreases the output of a system

positive feedback: feedback that increases the output of a system

steady state: a stable condition that does not change over time, or when change in one direction is balanced by change in an opposite direction

stress: a disruptive condition that occurs in response to adverse influences from the internal or external environments

vasoconstriction: the narrowing of a blood vessel

HISTORICAL THEORIES OF THE STEADY STATE

Claude Bernard, a 19th-century French physiologist, developed the biologic principle that for life there must be a constancy or "fixity of the internal milieu" despite changes in the external environment. The internal milieu was the fluid that bathed the cells, and the constancy was the balanced internal state maintained by physiologic and biochemical processes. His principle implied a static process.

Later, Walter Cannon used the term *homeostasis* to describe the stability of the internal environment, which, he said, was coordinated by homeostatic or compensatory processes that responded to changes in the internal environment. Any change within the internal environment initiated a "righting" response to minimize the change. These biologic processes sought physiologic and chemical balance and were under involuntary control.

Rene Jules Dubos (1965) provided further insight into the dynamic nature of the internal environment with his theory that two complementary concepts, homeostasis and adaptation, were necessary for balance. Homeostatic processes occurred quickly in response to stress, rapidly making the adjustments necessary to maintain the internal environment. Adaptive processes resulted in structural or functional changes over time. Dubos also emphasized that acceptable ranges of response to stimuli existed and that these responses varied for different individuals: "Absolute constancy is only a concept of the ideal." Homeostasis and adaptation were both necessary for survival in a changing world.

Homeostasis, then, refers to a steady state within the body. When a change or stress occurs that causes a body function to deviate from its stable range, processes are initiated to restore and maintain the dynamic balance. When these adjustment processes or compensatory mechanisms are not adequate, the steady state is threatened, function becomes disordered, and pathophysiologic mechanisms occur. The pathophysiologic processes can lead to disease and may be active during disease, which is a threat to the steady state. Disease is an abnormal variation in the structure or function of any part of the body. It disrupts function and therefore limits the person's freedom of action.

STRESS AND ADAPTATION

Stress is a state produced by a change in the environment that is perceived as challenging, threatening, or damaging to the person's dynamic balance or equilibrium. The person is, or feels, unable to meet the demands of the new situation. The change or stimulus that evokes this state is the stressor. The nature of the stressor is variable; an event or change that will produce stress in one person may be neutral for another, and an event that produces stress at one time and place for one person may not do so for the same person at another time and place. A person appraises and copes with changing situations. The desired goal is **adaptation**, or adjustment to the change so that the person is again in equilibrium and has the energy and ability to meet new demands. This is the process of **coping** with the stress, a compensatory process with physiologic and psychological components.

Adaptation is a constant, ongoing process that requires a change in structure, function, or behaviour so that the person is better suited to the environment; it involves an interaction between the person and the environment. The outcome depends on the degree of "fit" between the skills and capacities of the person, the type of social support available, and the various challenges or stressors being confronted. As such, adaptation is an individual process: each individual has varying abilities to cope or respond. As new challenges are met, this ability to cope and adapt can change, thereby providing the individual with a wide range of adaptive ability. Adaptation occurs throughout the life span as the individual encounters many developmental and situational challenges, especially related to health and illness. The goal of these encounters is to promote adaptation. In situations of health and illness, this goal is realized by optimal wellness.

Because both stress and adaptation may exist at different levels of a system, it is possible to study these reactions at the cellular, tissue, and organ levels. Biologists are concerned mainly with subcellular components or with subsystems of the total body. Behavioural scientists, including many nurse researchers, study stress and adaptation in individuals, families, groups, and societies; they focus on how a group's organizational features are modified to meet the requirements of the social and physical environment in which they exist. Adaptation is a continuous process of seeking harmony in an environment. The desired goals of adaptation for any system are survival, growth, and reproduction.

Stressors: Threats to the Steady State

Each person operates at a certain level of adaptation and regularly encounters a certain amount of change. Such change is expected; it contributes to growth and enhances life. Stressors, however, can upset this equilibrium. A stressor may be defined as an internal or external event or situation that creates the potential for physiologic, emotional, cognitive, or behavioural changes in an individual.

TYPES OF STRESSORS

Stressors exist in many forms and categories. They may be described as physical, physiologic, or psychosocial. Physical stressors include cold, heat, and chemical agents; physiologic stressors include pain and fatigue. Examples of psychosocial stressors are fear of failing an examination and losing a job. Stressors can also occur as normal life transitions that require some adjustment, such as going from childhood into puberty, getting married, or giving birth.

Stressors have also been classified as: (1) day-to-day frustrations or hassles; (2) major complex occurrences involving large groups, even entire nations; and (3) stressors that occur less frequently and involve fewer people. The first group, the day-to-day stressors, includes such common occurrences as getting caught in a traffic jam, experiencing computer downtime, and having an argument with a spouse or roommate. These experiences vary in effect; for example, encountering a rainstorm while one is vacationing at the beach will most likely evoke a more negative response than it might at another time. These less dramatic, frustrating, and irritating events—daily hassles—have been shown to have a greater health impact than major life events because of the cumulative effect they have over time. They can lead to high blood pressure, palpitations, or other physiologic problems (Jalowiec, 1993).

The second group of stressors influences larger groups of people, possibly even entire nations. These include events of history, such as terrorism and war, which are threatening situations when experienced either directly, in the war zone, or indirectly, as through live news coverage. The demographic, economic, and technological changes occurring in society also serve as stressors. The tension produced by any stressor is sometimes a result not only of the change itself, but also of the speed with which the change occurs.

The third group of stressors has been studied most extensively and concerns relatively infrequent situations that directly affect the individual. This category includes the influence of life events such as death, birth, marriage, divorce, and retirement. It also includes the psychosocial crises described by Erikson as occurring in the life cycle stages of the human experience. More enduring chronic stressors have also been placed in this category and may include such things as having a permanent functional disability or coping with the difficulties of providing long-term care to a frail elderly parent.

A stressor can also be categorized according to duration. It may be

- An acute, time-limited stressor, such as studying for final examinations
- A stressor sequence—a series of stressful events that result from an initial event such as job loss or divorce
- A chronic intermittent stressor, such as daily hassles
- A chronic enduring stressor that persists over time, such as chronic illness, a disability, or poverty

STRESS AS A STIMULUS FOR DISEASE

Relating life events to illness (the theoretical approach that defines stress as a stimulus) has been a major focus of psychosocial studies. This can be traced to Adolph Meyer, who in the 1930s observed in "life charts" of his patients a linkage between illnesses and critical life events. Subsequent research revealed that people under constant stress have a high incidence of psychosomatic disease.

Holmes and Rahe (1967) developed life events scales that assign numerical values, called life-change units, to typical life events. Because the items in the scales reflect events that require a change in a person's life pattern, and stress is defined as an accumulation of changes in one's life that require psychological adaptation, one can theoretically predict the likelihood of illness by checking off the number of recent events and deriving a total score. The Recent Life Changes Questionnaire (Tausig, 1982) contains 118 items such as death, birth, marriage, divorce, promotions, serious arguments, and vacations. The events listed include both desirable and undesirable circumstances.

Sources of stress for patients have been well researched (Ballard, 1981; Bryla, 1996; Jalowiec, 1993). People typically experience distress related to alterations in their physical and emotional health status, changes in their level of daily functioning, and decreased social support or the loss of significant others. Fears of immobilization, isolation, loneliness, sensory changes, financial problems, and death or disability increase a person's anxiety level. Loss of one's role or perceived purpose in life can cause intense discomfort. Any of these identified variables plus a myriad of other conditions or overwhelming demands are likely to cause ineffective coping, and a lack of necessary coping skills is often a source of additional distress for an individual. When a person endures prolonged or unrelenting suffering, the outcome is frequently the development of a stress-related illness. Nurses possess the skills to assist people to alter their distressing circumstances and manage their responses to stress.

PSYCHOLOGICAL RESPONSES TO STRESS

After the recognition of a stressor, an individual consciously or unconsciously reacts to manage the situation. This is called the mediating process. A theory developed by Lazarus (1991a) emphasizes cognitive appraisal and coping as important mediators of stress. Appraisal and coping are influenced by antecedent variables that include the internal and external resources of the person.

Appraisal of the Stressful Event

Cognitive appraisal (Lazarus, 1991a; Lazarus & Folkman, 1984) is a process by which an event is evaluated with respect to what is at stake (primary appraisal) and what might and can be done (secondary appraisal). What individuals see as being at stake is influenced by their personal goals, commitments, or motivations. Important factors include how important or relevant the event is to them, whether the event conflicts with what they want or desire, and whether the situation threatens their own sense of strength and ego identity.

As an outcome of primary appraisal, the situation is identified as either nonstressful or stressful. If nonstressful, the situation is irrelevant or benign (positive). A stressful situation may be one of three kinds: (1) one in which harm or loss has occurred; (2) one that is threatening, in that harm or loss is anticipated; and (3) one that is challenging, in that some opportunity or gain is anticipated.

Secondary appraisal is an evaluation of what might and can be done about this situation Actions include assigning blame to those responsible for a frustrating event, thinking about whether one can do something about the situation (coping potential), and determining future expectancy, or whether things are likely to change for better or worse (Lazarus, 1991a, 1991c). A comparison of what is at stake and what can be done about it (a type of risk–benefit analysis) determines the degree of stress.

Reappraisal, a change of opinion based on new information, also occurs. The appraisal process is not necessarily sequential; primary and secondary appraisal and reappraisal may occur simultaneously. Information learned from an adaptational encounter can be stored, so that when a similar situation is encountered again the whole process does not need to be repeated.

The appraisal process contributes to the development of an emotion. Negative emotions such as fear and anger accompany harm/loss appraisals, and positive emotions accompany challenge. In addition to the subjective component or feeling that accompanies a particular emotion, each emotion also includes a tendency to act in a certain way. For example, an unexpected quiz in the classroom might be judged as threatening by unprepared students. They might feel fear, anger, and resentment and might express these emotions outwardly with hostile behaviour or comments.

Lazarus (1991a) expanded his former ideas about stress, appraisal, and coping into a more complex model relating emotion to adaptation. He called this model a "cognitive-motivational-relational theory," with the term *relational* "standing for a focus on negotiation with a physical and social world" (p. 13). A theory of emotion was proposed as the bridge to connect psychology, physiology, and sociology: "More than any other arena of psychological thought, emotion is an integrative, organismic concept that subsumes psychological stress and coping within itself and unites motivation, cognition, and adaptation in a complex configuration" (p. 40).

Coping With the Stressful Event

Coping, according to Lazarus, consists of the cognitive and behavioural efforts made to manage the specific external or internal demands that tax a person's resources and may be emotion-focused or problem-focused. Coping that is emotion focused seeks to make the person feel better by lessening the emotional distress felt. Problem-focused coping aims to make direct changes in the environment so that the situation can be managed more effectively. Both types of coping usually occur in a stressful situation. Even if the situation is viewed as challenging or beneficial, coping efforts may be required to develop and sustain the challenge—that is, to maintain the positive benefits of the challenge and to ward off any threats. In harmful or threatening situations, successful coping reduces or eliminates the source of stress and relieves the emotion it generated.

Appraisal and coping are affected by internal characteristics such as health, energy, personal belief systems, commitments or life goals, self-esteem, control, mastery, knowledge, problem-solving skills, and social skills. The characteristics that have been studied most often in nursing research are health-promoting lifestyles and hardiness. A health-promoting lifestyle buffers the effect of stressors. From a nursing practice standpoint, this outcome—buffering the effect of stressors—supports nursing's goal of promoting health. In many circumstances, promoting a healthy lifestyle is more achievable than altering the stressors.

Hardiness is the name given to a general quality that comes from having rich, varied, and rewarding experiences. It is a personality characteristic composed of control, commitment, and challenge. Hardy people perceive stressors as something they can change and therefore control. To them, potentially stressful situations are interesting and meaningful; change and new situations are viewed as challenging opportunities for growth. Some positive support has been found for hardiness as a significant variable that positively influences rehabilitation and overall improvement after an onset of an acute or chronic illness (Felton, 2000; Williams, 2000).

PHYSIOLOGIC RESPONSE TO STRESS

The physiologic response to a stressor, whether it is a physical stressor or a psychological stressor, is a protective and adaptive mechanism to maintain the homeostatic balance of the body. The stress response is a "cascade of neural and hormonal events that have short- and long-lasting consequences for both brain and body . . .; a stressor is an event that challenges homeostasis, with a disease outcome being looked upon as a failure of the normal process of adaptation to the stress" (McEwen & Mendelson, 1993, p. 101).

The General Adaptation Syndrome

Hans Selye developed a theory of adaptation that profoundly influenced the scientific study of stress. In 1936, Selye, experimenting with animals, first described a syndrome consisting of enlargement of the adrenal cortex; shrinkage of the thymus, spleen, lymph nodes, and other lymphatic structures; and the appearance of deep, bleeding ulcers in the stomach and duodenum. He identified this as a nonspecific response to diverse, noxious stimuli. From this beginning, he developed a theory of adaptation to biologic stress that he named the general adaptation syndrome.

PHASES OF THE GENERAL ADAPTATION SYNDROME
The general adaptation syndrome has three phases: alarm, resistance, and exhaustion. During the alarm phase, the sympathetic "fight-or-flight" response is activated with release of **catecholamines** and the onset of the **adrenocorticotropic hormone (ACTH)**–adrenal cortical response. The alarm reaction is defensive and anti-inflammatory but self-limited. Because living in a continuous state of alarm would result in death, the person moves

into the second stage, resistance. During this stage, adaptation to the noxious stressor occurs, and cortisol activity is still increased. If exposure to the stressor is prolonged, exhaustion sets in and endocrine activity increases. This produces deleterious effects on the body systems (especially the circulatory, digestive, and immune systems) that can lead to death. Stages one and two of this syndrome are repeated, in different degrees, throughout life as the person encounters stressors.

Selye compared the general adaptation syndrome with the life process. During childhood, there are too few encounters with stress to promote the development of adaptive functioning, and the child is vulnerable. During adulthood, the person encounters a number of life's stressful events and develops a resistance or adaptation. During the later years, the accumulation of life's stressors and the wear and tear on the organism again deplete the person's ability to adapt, resistance falls, and eventually death occurs.

LOCAL ADAPTATION SYNDROME
According to Selye's theory, a local adaptation syndrome also occurs. This syndrome includes the inflammatory response and repair processes that occur at the local site of tissue injury. The local adaptation syndrome occurs in small, topical injuries, such as contact dermatitis. If the local injury is severe enough, the general adaptation syndrome is activated as well.

Selye emphasized that stress is the nonspecific response common to all stressors, regardless of whether they are physiologic, psychological, or social. The many conditioning factors in each person's environment account for why different demands are interpreted by different people as stressors. Conditioning factors also account for differences in the tolerance of different people for stress: some people may develop diseases of adaptation, such as hypertension and migraine headaches, while others are unaffected.

Interpretation of Stressful Stimuli by the Brain

Physiologic responses to stress are mediated by the brain through a complex network of chemical and electrical messages. The neural and hormonal actions that maintain homeostatic balance are integrated by the hypothalamus, which is located in the centre of the brain, surrounded by the limbic system and the cerebral hemispheres. The hypothalamus integrates autonomic nervous system mechanisms that maintain the chemical constancy of the internal environment of the body. Together with the limbic system, it also regulates emotions and many visceral behaviours necessary for survival (eg, eating, drinking, temperature control, reproduction, defense, aggression). The hypothalamus is made up of a number of nuclei; the limbic system contains the amygdala, hippocampus, and septal nuclei, along with other structures.

Literature supports the concept that each of these structures responds differently to stimuli, and each has its own characteristic response (Watkins, 1997). The cerebral hemispheres are concerned with cognitive functions: thought processes, learning, and memory. The limbic system has connections with both the cerebral hemispheres and the brain stem. In addition, the reticular activating system, which is a network of cells that forms a two-way communication system, extends from the brain stem into the midbrain and limbic system. This network controls the alert or waking state of the body.

In the stress response, afferent impulses are carried from sensory organs (eye, ear, nose, skin) and internal sensors (baroreceptors, chemoreceptors) to nerve centres in the brain. The response to the perception of stress is integrated in the hypothalamus, which coordinates the adjustments necessary to return to homeostatic balance. The degree and duration of the response varies; major stress evokes both sympathetic and pituitary adrenal responses.

Neural and neuroendocrine pathways under the control of the hypothalamus are also activated in the stress response. First, there is a sympathetic nervous system discharge, followed by a sympathetic-adrenal-medullary discharge. If the stress persists, the hypothalamic-pituitary system is activated (Fig. 6-2).

SYMPATHETIC NERVOUS SYSTEM RESPONSE

The sympathetic nervous system response is rapid and short-lived. Norepinephrine is released at nerve endings that are in direct contact with their respective end organs to cause an increase in function of the vital organs and a state of general body arousal. The heart rate is increased and peripheral **vasoconstriction** occurs, raising the blood pressure. Blood is also shunted away from abdominal organs. The purpose of these activities is to provide better perfusion of vital organs (brain, heart, skeletal muscles).

Blood glucose is increased, supplying more readily available energy. The pupils are dilated, and mental activity is increased; a greater sense of awareness exists. Constriction of the blood vessels of the skin limits bleeding in the event of trauma. The person is likely to experience cold feet, clammy skin and hands, chills, palpitations, and a knot in the stomach. Typically, the person appears tense, with the muscles of the neck, upper back, and shoulders tightened; respirations may be rapid and shallow, with the diaphragm tense.

SYMPATHETIC-ADRENAL-MEDULLARY RESPONSE

In addition to its direct effect on major end organs, the sympathetic nervous system also stimulates the medulla of the adrenal gland to release the hormones epinephrine and norepinephrine into the bloodstream. The action of these hormones is similar to that of the sympathetic nervous system and have the effect of sustaining and prolonging its actions. Epinephrine and norepinephrine are catecholamines that stimulate the nervous system and produce metabolic effects that increase the blood glucose level

Physiology/Pathophysiology

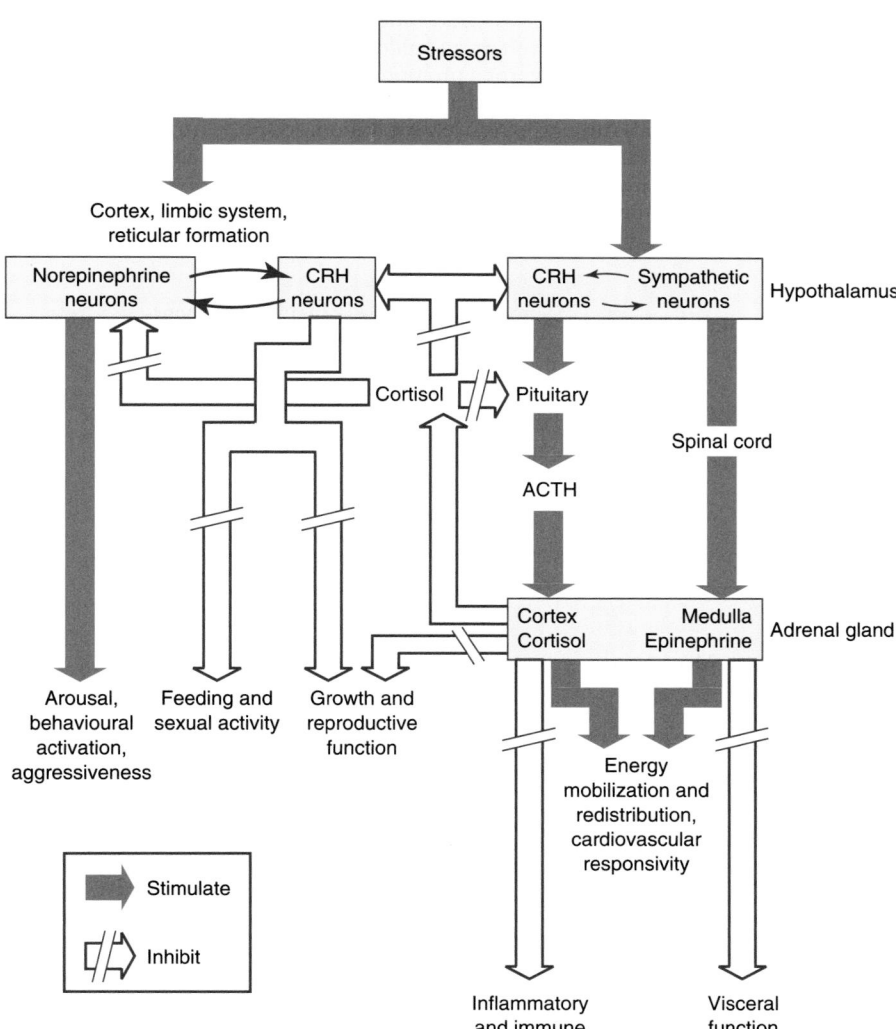

FIGURE 6-2 Integrated responses to stress mediated by the sympathetic nervous system and the hypothalamic–pituitary–adrenocortical axis. The responses are mutually reinforcing, at both the central and peripheral levels. Negative feedback by cortisol also can limit an overresponse that might be harmful to the individual. *Coloured arrows,* stimulation; *open arrows,* inhibition; CRH, corticotropin-releasing hormone; ACTH, adrenocorticotropic hormone. Reproduced with permission from Berne, R. M., & Levy, M. N. (1993). *Physiology.* St. Louis: C. V. Mosby.

and increase the **metabolic rate**. The effect of the sympathetic and adrenal-medullary responses is summarized in Table 6-1. This effect is called the "fight-or-flight" reaction.

HYPOTHALAMIC-PITUITARY RESPONSE

The longest-acting phase of the physiologic response, which is more likely to occur in persistent stress, involves the hypothalamic-pituitary pathway. The hypothalamus secretes corticotropin-releasing factor, which stimulates the anterior pituitary to produce ACTH. ACTH in turn stimulates the adrenal cortex to produce **glucocorticoids**, primarily cortisol. Cortisol stimulates protein catabolism, releasing amino acids; stimulates liver uptake of amino acids and their conversion to glucose (**gluconeogenesis**); and inhibits glucose uptake (anti-insulin action) by many body cells but not those of the brain and heart. These cortisol-induced metabolic effects provide the body with a ready source of energy during a stressful situation. This effect has some important implications. For example, a person with diabetes who is under stress, such as that caused by an infection, needs more insulin than usual. Any patient who is under stress (caused, for example, by illness, surgery, trauma or prolonged psychological stress) catabolizes body protein and needs supplements. Children subjected to severe stress have retarded growth.

The actions of the catecholamines (epinephrine and norepinephrine) and cortisol are the most important in the general response to stress. Other hormones released are **antidiuretic hormone (ADH)** from the posterior pituitary and aldosterone from the adrenal cortex. ADH and aldosterone promote sodium and water retention, which is an adaptive mechanism in the event of hemorrhage or loss of fluids through excessive perspiration. ADH has also been shown to influence learning and may thus facilitate coping in new and threatening situations. Secretion of growth hormone and glucagon stimulates the uptake of amino acids by cells, helping to mobilize energy resources. Endorphins, which are endogenous opiates, increase during stress and enhance the threshold for tolerance of painful stimuli. They may also affect mood and have been implicated in the so-called "high" that long-distance runners experience. The secretion of other hormones is also affected, but their adaptive function is less clear.

IMMUNOLOGIC RESPONSE

Research findings show that the immune system is connected to the neuroendocrine and autonomic systems. Lymphoid tissue is richly supplied by autonomic nerves capable of releasing a number of different neuropeptides that can have a direct effect on leukocyte regulation and the inflammatory response. Neuroendocrine hormones released by the central nervous system and endocrine tissues can inhibit or stimulate leukocyte function. The wide variety of stressors people experience may result in different alterations in autonomic activity and subtle variations in neurohormone and neuropeptide synthesis. All of these possible autonomic and neuroendocrine responses can interact to initiate, weaken, enhance, or terminate an immune response (Watkins, 1997).

The study of the relationships among the neuroendocrine system, the central and autonomic nervous systems, and the immune system and the effects of these relationships on overall health outcomes is called *psychoneuroimmunology*. Because one's perception of events and coping styles determine whether, and to what extent, an event activates the stress response system, and because the stress response affects immune activity, one's perceptions, ideas, and thoughts can have profound neurochemical and immunologic consequences. Multiple studies have demonstrated alteration of immune function in people who are under stress, as evidenced by a decrease in the number of leukocytes, impaired immune response to immunizations, and diminished cytotoxic-

Table 6-1 • **Sympathetic–Adrenal–Medullary Response to Stress**

EFFECT	PURPOSE	MECHANISM
Increased heart rate and blood pressure	Better perfusion of vital organs	Increased cardiac output due to increased myocardial contractility and heart rate; increased venous return (peripheral vasoconstriction)
Increased blood glucose level	Increased available energy	Increased liver and muscle glycogen breakdown; increased breakdown of adipose tissue triglycerides
Mental acuity	Alert state	Increase in amount of blood shunted to the brain from the abdominal viscera and skin
Dilated pupils	Increased awareness	Contraction of radial muscle of iris
Increased tension of skeletal muscles	Preparedness for activity, decreased fatigue	Excitation of muscles; increase in amount of blood shunted to the muscles from the abdominal viscera and skin
Increased ventilation (may be rapid and shallow)	Provision of oxygen for energy	Stimulation of respiratory centre in medulla; bronchodilation
Increased coagulability of blood	Prevention of hemorrhage in event of trauma	Vasoconstriction of surface vessels

ity of natural killer cells (Andersen et al., 1998; Constantino, Secula, Rabin, & Stone, 2000; Glaser & Kiecolt-Glaser, 1997; Pike et al., 1997; Robinson, Matthews, & Witek-Janusek, 2000). Other studies have identified certain personality traits, such as optimism and active coping, as having positive effects on health or specific immune measures (Chalfont & Bennett, 1999; Goodkin et al., 1996; Kennedy, 2000; Sergerstrom, Fahey, Kemeny, & Taylor, 1998). As research continues, this new field of study will continue to uncover to what extent and by what mechanisms people can consciously influence their immunity.

MALADAPTIVE RESPONSES TO STRESS

The stress response, which, as indicated earlier facilitates adaptation to threatening situations, has been retained from our evolutionary past. The "fight-or-flight" response, for example, is an anticipatory response that mobilized the bodily resources of our ancestors to deal with predators and other harsh factors in their environment. This same mobilization comes into play in response to emotional stimuli unrelated to danger. For example, a person may get an "adrenaline rush" when competing over a decisive point in a ball game, or when excited about attending a party.

When the responses to stress are ineffective, they are referred to as *maladaptive*. Maladaptive responses are chronic, recurrent responses or patterns of response over time that do not promote the goals of adaptation. The goals of adaptation are somatic or physical health (optimal wellness); psychological health or having a sense of well-being (happiness, satisfaction with life, morale); and enhanced social functioning, which includes work, social life, and family (positive relationships). Maladaptive responses that threaten these goals include faulty appraisals and inappropriate coping (Lazarus, 1991a).

The frequency, intensity, and duration of stressful situations contribute to the development of negative emotions and subsequent patterns of neurochemical discharge. By appraising situations more adequately and coping more appropriately, it is possible to anticipate and defuse some of these situations. For example, frequent potentially stressful encounters (eg, marital discord) might be avoided with better communication and problem solving, or a pattern of procrastination (eg, delaying work on tasks) could be corrected to reduce stress when deadlines approach.

Coping processes that include the use of alcohol or drugs to reduce stress increase the risk of illness. Other inappropriate coping patterns may increase the risk of illness less directly. For example, people who demonstrate "type A" personality behaviours such as impatience, competitiveness, and achievement orientation and have an underlying hostile approach to life are more prone than others to develop stress-related illnesses. Type A behaviours increase the output of catecholamines, the adrenal-medullary hormones, with their attendant effects on the body.

Other forms of inappropriate coping include denial, avoidance, and distancing. Denial may be illustrated by the woman who feels a lump in her breast but downplays its seriousness and delays seeking medical attention. The intent of denial is to control the threat, but it may also endanger life.

Models of illness frequently cite stress and maladaptation as precursors to disease. A general model of illness, based on Selye's theory, suggests that any stressor elicits a state of disturbed physiologic equilibrium. If this state is prolonged or the response is excessive, it will increase the susceptibility of the person to illness. This susceptibility, coupled with a predisposition in the person

(whether from genetic traits, health, or age), leads to illness. If the sympathetic adrenal-medullary response is prolonged or excessive, a state of chronic arousal develops that may lead to high blood pressure, arteriosclerotic changes, and cardiovascular disease. If the production of the ACTH is prolonged or excessive, behaviour patterns of withdrawal and depression are seen. In addition, the immune response is decreased, and infections and tumours may develop.

Selye (1976) proposed a list of disorders that he called diseases of maladaptation: high blood pressure, diseases of the heart and blood vessels, diseases of the kidney, hypertension of pregnancy, rheumatic and rheumatoid arthritis, inflammatory diseases of the skin and eyes, infections, allergic and hypersensitivity diseases, nervous and mental diseases, sexual derangements, digestive diseases, metabolic diseases, and cancer.

INDICATORS OF STRESS

Indicators of stress and the stress response include both subjective and objective measures. Chart 6-1 lists signs and symptoms that may be observed directly or reported by the person. They are psychological, physiologic, or behavioural and reflect social behaviours and thought processes. Some of these reactions may be coping behaviours. Over time, each person tends to develop a characteristic pattern of behaviour during stress that is a warning that the system is out of balance.

Chart 6-1	**Signs and Symptoms of Stress**

General irritability, hyperexcitation, or depression
Dryness of the throat and mouth
Overpowering urge to cry, scream, or run and hide
Easily fatigued, loss of interest
"Floating anxiety"—do not know exactly why or what
Easily startled
Stuttering or other speech difficulties
Hypermotility: pacing, moving about, cannot sit still
Gastrointestinal signs and symptoms: "butterflies" in the stomach, diarrhea, vomiting
Change in menstrual cycle
Loss of or excessive appetite
Increased use of legally prescribed drugs, such as anxiolytics or antidepressants
Prone to injuries
Disturbed behaviour
Pounding of the heart
Impulsive behaviour, emotional instability
Inability to concentrate or think clearly
Feelings of unreality, weakness, or dizziness
Tension, alertness
Trembling, nervous tics
Nervous laughter
Grinding of teeth
Insomnia, nightmares, or other sleep difficulties
Excessive perspiration
Increased frequency of urination
Muscle tension and migraine headaches
Pain in the neck or lower back
Increased smoking
Alcohol and drug addiction

Based on Selye, H. (1976). *Stress in health and disease.* Stoneham, MA: Butterworths. Reprinted with permission of the publisher.

Laboratory measurements of indicators of stress have helped in understanding this complex process. Among the measures, blood and urine analyses can be used to demonstrate changes in hormonal levels and hormonal breakdown products. Reliable measures of stress include blood levels of catecholamines, corticoids, ACTH, and eosinophils. The serum creatine/creatinine ratio and elevations of cholesterol and free fatty acids can also be measured. Immunoglobulin assays may be determined. With greater attention to neuroimmunology, improved laboratory measures are likely to follow. Increases in blood pressure and heart rate can also be measured.

In addition to using laboratory tests, researchers have developed questionnaires to identify and assess stressors, stress, and coping strategies. Many of these are discussed in the research monograph developed by Barnfather and Lyon (1993), which was based on a synthesis conference held by nurse scientists on the state of the science in stress and coping nursing research. Some examples of the research instruments that nurses commonly use to measure levels of client distress and client functioning can be found in a variety of research reports (Cronquist, Wredding, Norlander, Langius, & Bjorvell, 2000; Starzonski & Hilton, 2000). Miller and Smith (1993) provided a stress audit and a stress profile measurement tool that is available in the popular lay literature.

NURSING IMPLICATIONS

It is important for the nurse to realize that the optimal point of intervention to promote health is during the stage when the individual's own compensatory processes are still functioning. Early identification of both physiologic and psychological stressors remains a major role of the nurse, and information on the interrelationships between physical and emotional health can be found in research journals. The nurse should be able to relate the presenting signs and symptoms of distress to the physiology they represent and identify the individual's position on the continuum of function, from health and compensation to pathophysiology and disease. For example, if an anxious middle-aged woman presented for a checkup and was found to be overweight, with a blood pressure of 130/85 mm Hg, the nurse would counsel her with respect to diet, stress management, and activity. The nurse would also encourage weight loss and discuss the woman's intake of salt (which affects fluid balance) and caffeine (which provides a stimulant effect). The patient and the nurse would identify both individual and environmental stressors and discuss strategies to decrease the lifestyle stress, with the ultimate goal being to create a healthy lifestyle and prevent hypertension and its sequelae.

Stress at the Cellular Level

Pathologic processes may occur at all levels of the biologic organism. If the cell is considered the smallest unit or subsystem (tissues being aggregates of cells, organs aggregates of tissues, and so forth), the processes of health and disease or adaptation and maladaptation can all occur at the cellular level. Indeed, pathologic processes are often described by scientists at the subcellular or molecular level.

The cell exists on a continuum of function and structure, ranging from the normal cell, to the adapted cell, to the injured or diseased cell, to the dead cell (Fig. 6-3). Changes from one state to another may occur rapidly and may not be readily de-

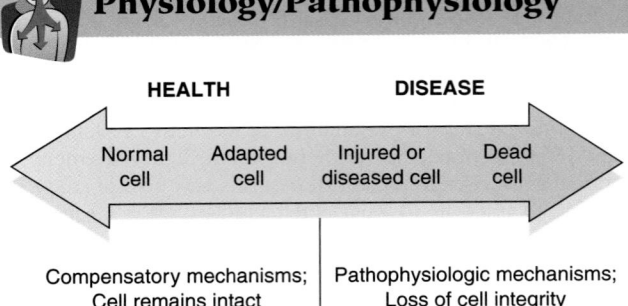

Physiology/Pathophysiology

HEALTH   **DISEASE**

| Normal cell | Adapted cell | Injured or diseased cell | Dead cell |

Compensatory mechanisms; Cell remains intact

Pathophysiologic mechanisms; Loss of cell integrity

FIGURE 6-3 The cell on a continuum of function and structure. Changes in the cell are not as easily discerned as the diagram depicts. The point at which compensation subsides and pathophysiology begins is not clearly defined.

tectable, because each state does not have discrete boundaries, and disease represents an extension and distortion of normal processes. The earliest changes occur at the molecular or subcellular level and are not perceptible until steady-state functions or structures are altered. With cell injury, some changes may be reversible; in other instances, the injuries are lethal. For example, tanning of the skin is an adaptive, morphologic response to exposure to the rays of the sun. If the exposure is continued, however, sunburn and injury occur, and some cells may die, as evidenced by desquamation ("peeling").

Different cells and tissues respond to stimuli with different patterns and rates of response; some cells are more vulnerable to one type of stimulus or stressor than others. The cell involved, its ability to adapt, and its physiologic state are determinants of the response. For example, cardiac muscle cells respond to **hypoxia** (inadequate oxygenation) more quickly than smooth muscle cells do.

Other determinants of cellular response are the type or nature of the stimulus, its duration, and its severity. For example, neurons that control respiration can develop a tolerance to regular, small amounts of a barbiturate, but one large dose may result in respiratory depression and death.

CONTROL OF THE STEADY STATE

The concept of the cell as existing on a continuum of function and structure includes the relationship of the cell to compensatory mechanisms, which occur continuously in the body to maintain the steady state. Compensatory processes are regulated primarily by the autonomic nervous system and the endocrine system, with control achieved through negative feedback.

Negative Feedback

Negative feedback mechanisms throughout the body monitor the internal environment and restore homeostasis when conditions shift out of the normal range. These mechanisms work by sensing deviations from a predetermined set point or range of adaptability and triggering a response aimed at offsetting the deviation. Blood pressure, acid–base balance, blood glucose level, body temperature, and fluid and electrolyte balance are examples of functions regulated through such compensatory mechanisms.

Most of the human body's control systems are integrated by the brain and influenced by the nervous and endocrine systems. Control activities involve detecting deviations from the predetermined reference point and stimulating compensatory responses in the muscles and glands of the body. The major organs affected are the heart, lungs, kidneys, liver, gastrointestinal tract, and skin. When stimulated, these organs alter their rate of activity or the amount of secretions they produce. Because of this, they have been called the "organs of homeostasis or adjustment."

In addition to the responses controlled by the nervous and endocrine systems, local responses consisting of small feedback loops in a group of cells or tissues are possible. The cells detect a change in their immediate environment and initiate an action to counteract its effect. For example, the accumulation of lactic acid in an exercised muscle stimulates dilation of blood vessels in the area to increase blood flow and improve the delivery of oxygen and removal of waste products.

The net result of the activities of feedback loops is homeostasis. A steady state is achieved by the continuous, variable action of the organs involved in making the adjustments and by the continuous small exchanges of chemical substances among cells, interstitial fluid, and blood. For example, an increase in the carbon dioxide concentration of the extracellular fluid leads to increased pulmonary ventilation, which decreases the carbon dioxide level. On a cellular level, increased carbon dioxide raises the hydrogen ion concentration of the blood. This is detected by chemosensitive receptors in the respiratory control centre of the medulla of the brain. The chemoreceptors stimulate an increase in the rate of discharge of the neurons that innervate the diaphragm and intercostal muscles, which increases the rate of respiration. Excess carbon dioxide is exhaled, the hydrogen ion concentration returns to normal, and the chemically sensitive neurons are no longer stimulated.

Positive Feedback

Another type of feedback, **positive feedback**, perpetuates the chain of events set in motion by the original disturbance instead of compensating for it. As the system becomes more unbalanced, disorder and disintegration occur. There are some exceptions to this; blood clotting in humans, for example, is an important positive feedback mechanism.

CELLULAR ADAPTATION

Cells are complex units that dynamically respond to the changing demands and stresses of daily life. They possess a maintenance function and a specialized function. The maintenance function refers to the activities that the cell must perform with respect to itself; specialized functions are those that the cell performs in relation to the tissues and organs of which it is a part. Individual cells may cease to function without posing a threat to the organism. As the number of dead cells increases, however, the specialized functions of the tissues are altered and the individual's health is threatened.

Cells can adapt to environmental stress through structural and functional changes. Some of these adaptations are hypertrophy, atrophy, hyperplasia, dysplasia, and metaplasia (Table 6-2).

Hypertrophy and atrophy lead to changes in the size of cells and hence the size of the organs they form. Compensatory hypertrophy is the result of an enlarged muscle mass and commonly occurs in skeletal and cardiac muscle that experiences a prolonged, increased workload. One example is the bulging muscles of the athlete who engages in body building.

Atrophy can be the consequence of a disease or of decreased use, decreased blood supply, loss of nerve supply, or inadequate nutrition. Disuse of a body part is often associated with the aging

---

Table 6-2 • **Cellular Adaptation to Stressors**

ADAPTATION	STIMULUS	EXAMPLE
Hypertrophy—increase in cell size leading to increase in organ size	Increased workload	Leg muscles of runner Arm muscles in tennis player Cardiac muscle in person with hypertension
Atrophy—shrinkage in size of cell, leading to decrease in organ size	Decrease in: Use Blood supply Nutrition Hormonal stimulation Innervation	Secondary sex organs in aging person Extremity immobilized in plaster cast
Hyperplasia—increase in number of new cells (increase in mitosis)	Hormonal influence	Breast changes of a girl in puberty or of a pregnant woman Regeneration of liver cells New red blood cells in blood loss
Dysplasia—change in the appearance of cells after they have been subjected to chronic irritation	Reproduction of cells with resulting alteration of their size and shape	Alterations in epithelial cells of the skin or the cervix, producing irregular tissue changes that could be the precursors of a malignancy
Metaplasia—transformation of one adult cell type to another (reversible)	Stress applied to highly specialized cell	Changes in epithelial cells lining bronchi in response to smoke irritation (cells become less specialized)

process. Cell size and organ size decrease; structures principally affected are the skeletal muscles, the secondary sex organs, the heart, and the brain.

Hyperplasia is an increase in the number of new cells in an organ or tissue. As cells multiply and are subjected to increased stimulation, the tissue mass enlarges. It is a mitotic response (a change occurring with mitosis), but it is reversible when the stimulus is removed. This distinguishes it from neoplasia or malignant growth, which continues after the stimulus is removed. Hyperplasia may be hormonally induced. An example is the increase in the size of the thyroid gland caused by thyroid-stimulating hormone (secreted from the pituitary gland) when a deficit in thyroid hormone is detected.

Dysplasia is the change in the appearance of cells after they have been subjected to chronic irritation. Dysplastic cells have a tendency to become malignant; dysplasia is seen commonly in epithelial cells in the bronchi of smokers.

Metaplasia is a cell transformation in which a highly specialized cell changes to a less specialized cell. This serves a protective function, because the less specialized cell is more resistant to the stress that stimulated the change. For example, the ciliated columnar epithelium lining the bronchi of smokers is replaced by squamous epithelium. The squamous cells can survive; loss of the cilia and protective mucus, however, can have damaging consequences.

These adaptations allow the survival of the organism. They also reflect changes in the normal cell in response to stress. If the stress is unrelenting, the function of the adapted cell may succumb, and cell injury will occur.

CELLULAR INJURY

Injury is defined as a disorder in steady-state regulation. Any stressor that alters the ability of the cell or system to maintain optimal balance of its adjustment processes will lead to injury. Structural and functional damage then occurs, which may be reversible (permitting recovery) or irreversible (leading to disability or death). Homeostatic adjustments are concerned with the small changes within the body's systems. With adaptive changes, compensation occurs and a steady state is achieved, although it may be at new levels. With injury, steady-state regulation is lost, and changes in functioning ensue.

Causes of disorder and injury in the system (cell, tissue, organ, body) may arise from the external or internal environment (Fig. 6-4) and include hypoxia, nutritional imbalance, physical agents, chemical agents, **infectious agents**, immune mechanisms, genetic defects, and psychogenic factors. The most common causes are hypoxia (oxygen deficiency), chemical injury, and infectious agents. In addition, the presence of one injury makes the system more susceptible to another injury. For example, inadequate oxygenation and nutritional deficiencies make the system vulnerable to infection. These agents act at the cellular level by damaging or destroying

- The integrity of the cell membrane, necessary for ionic balance
- The ability of the cell to transform energy (aerobic respiration, production of adenosine triphosphate)
- The ability of the cell to synthesize enzymes and other necessary proteins
- The ability of the cell to grow and reproduce (genetic integrity)

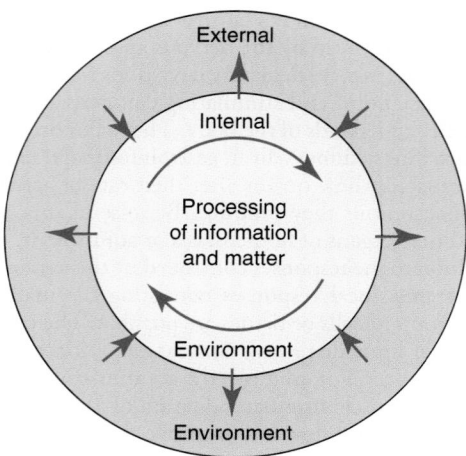

FIGURE 6-4 Influences leading to disorder may arise from the internal environment and the external environment of the system. Excesses or deficits of information and matter may occur, or there may be faulty regulation of processing.

Hypoxia

Inadequate cellular oxygenation (hypoxia) interferes with the cell's ability to transform energy. Hypoxia may be caused by:

- A decrease in blood supply to an area
- A decrease in the oxygen-carrying capacity of the blood (decreased hemoglobin)
- A ventilation/perfusion or respiratory problem that reduces the amount of oxygen available in the blood
- A problem in the cell's enzyme system that makes it unable to use the oxygen delivered to it

The usual cause is ischemia, or deficient blood supply. Ischemia is commonly seen in myocardial cell injury in which arterial blood flow is decreased because of atherosclerotic narrowing of blood vessels. Ischemia also results from intravascular clots (thrombi or emboli) that may form and interfere with blood supply. Thrombi and emboli are common causes of cerebrovascular accidents (strokes). The length of time different tissues can survive without oxygen varies. For example, brain cells may succumb in 3 to 6 minutes, depending on the situation. If the condition leading to hypoxia is slow and progressive, collateral circulation may develop, whereby blood is supplied by other blood vessels in the area. However, this mechanism is not highly reliable.

Nutritional Imbalance

Nutritional imbalance refers to a relative or absolute deficiency or excess of one or more essential nutrients. This may be manifested as undernutrition (inadequate consumption of food or calories) or overnutrition (caloric excess). Caloric excess to the point of obesity overloads cells in the body with lipids. By requiring more energy to maintain the extra tissue, obesity places a strain on the body and has been associated with the development of disease, especially pulmonary and cardiovascular disease.

Specific deficiencies arise when an essential nutrient is deficient or when there is an imbalance of nutrients. Protein deficiencies and avitaminosis (deficiency of vitamins) are typical examples. An energy deficit leading to cell injury can occur if there is insufficient glucose, or insufficient oxygen to transform the glucose into energy. A lack of insulin, or the inability to use insulin, may also prevent glucose from entering the cell from the blood. This occurs in diabetes mellitus, a metabolic disorder that can lead to nutritional deficiency.

Physical Agents

Physical agents, including temperature extremes, radiation, electrical shock, and mechanical trauma, can cause injury to the cells or to the entire body. The duration of exposure and the intensity of the stressor determine the severity of damage.

EXTREMES OF HIGH TEMPERATURE

When a person's temperature is elevated, hypermetabolism occurs and the respiratory rate, heart rate, and basal metabolic rate all increase. With fever induced by infections, the hypothalamic thermostat may be reset at a higher temperature, then return to normal when the fever abates. The increase in body temperature is achieved through physiologic mechanisms. Body temperatures greater than 41°C suggest hyperthermia, because the physiologic function of the thermoregulatory centre breaks down and the temperature soars. This physiologic condition occurs in people with heat stroke. Eventually, the high temperature causes coagulation of cell proteins, and the cells die. The body must be cooled rapidly to prevent brain damage.

The local response to thermal or burn injury is similar. There is an increase in metabolic activity, and, as heat increases, protein is coagulated, enzyme systems are destroyed, and, in the extreme, charring or carbonization occurs. Burns of the epithelium are classified as partial-thickness burns if epithelializing elements remain to support healing. Full-thickness burns lack such elements and must be grafted for healing. The amount of body surface involved determines the prognosis for the patient. If the injury is severe, the entire body system becomes involved, and hypermetabolism develops as a pathophysiologic response.

EXTREMES OF LOW TEMPERATURE

Extremes of low temperature, or cold, cause vasoconstriction. Blood flow becomes sluggish and clots form, leading to ischemic damage in the involved tissues. With still lower temperatures, ice crystals may form, and the cells may burst.

RADIATION AND ELECTRICAL SHOCK

Radiation is used for diagnosis and treatment of diseases. Ionizing forms of radiation may cause injury by their destructive action. Radiation decreases the protective inflammatory response of the cell, creating a favourable environment for opportunistic infections. Electrical shock produces burns as a result of the heat generated when electrical current travels through the body. It may also abnormally stimulate nerves, leading, for example, to fibrillation of the heart.

MECHANICAL TRAUMA

Mechanical trauma can result in wounds that disrupt the cells and tissues of the body. The severity of the wound, the amount of blood loss, and the extent of nerve damage are significant factors in the outcome.

Chemical Agents

Chemical injuries are caused by poisons, such as lye, which has a corrosive action on epithelial tissue, or by heavy metals, such as mercury, arsenic, and lead, each with its own specific destructive action. Many other chemicals are toxic in specific amounts, in certain people, and in distinctive tissues. Excessive secretion of

hydrochloric acid can damage the stomach lining; large amounts of glucose can cause osmotic shifts, affecting the fluid and electrolyte balance; and too much insulin can cause subnormal levels of glucose in the blood (hypoglycemia) and can lead to coma.

Drugs, including prescribed medications, can also cause chemical poisoning. Some individuals are less tolerant of medications than others and manifest toxic reactions at the usual or customary dosages. Aging tends to decrease tolerance to medications. Polypharmacy (taking many medications at one time) also occurs frequently in the aging population and is a problem because of the unpredictable effects of the resulting medication interactions.

Alcohol (ethanol) is also a chemical irritant. In the body, alcohol is broken down into acetaldehyde, which has a direct toxic effect on liver cells that leads to a variety of liver abnormalities, including cirrhosis in susceptible individuals. Disordered liver cell function leads to complications in other organs of the body.

Infectious Agents

Biologic agents known to cause disease in humans are viruses, bacteria, rickettsiae, mycoplasmas, fungi, protozoa, and nematodes. The severity of the infectious disease depends on the number of microorganisms entering the body, their virulence, and the host's defenses (eg, health, age, immune defenses).

Some bacteria, such as those that cause tetanus and diphtheria, produce exotoxins that circulate and create cell damage. Others, such as the gram-negative bacteria, produce endotoxins when they are killed. The tubercle bacillus induces an immune reaction.

Viruses, the smallest living organisms, survive as parasites of the living cells they invade. Viruses infect specific cells. Through a complex mechanism, they replicate within the cells, then invade other cells and continue to replicate. An immune response is mounted by the body to eliminate the viruses, and the cells harbouring the viruses can be injured in the process. Typically, an inflammatory response and immune reaction are the physiologic responses of the body to the presence of infection.

Disordered Immune Responses

The immune system is an exceedingly complex system; its purpose is to defend the body from invasion by any foreign object or foreign cell type, such as cancerous cells. This is a steady-state mechanism, but like other adjustment processes it can become disordered, and cell injury will occur. The immune response detects foreign bodies by distinguishing non-self substances from self substances and destroying the non-self entities. The entrance of an antigen (foreign substance) into the body evokes the production of antibodies that attack and destroy the antigen (antigen–antibody reaction).

The immune system can be hypoactive or hyperactive. When it is hypoactive, immunodeficiency diseases occur; when it is hyperactive, hypersensitivity disorders arise. A disorder of the immune system itself can result in damage to the body's own tissues. Such disorders are labelled autoimmune diseases (see Unit 11).

Genetic Disorders

Genetic defects as causes of disease and their effects on genetic structure are of intense research interest. Many of these defects produce mutations that have no recognizable effect, such as lack of a single enzyme; others contribute to more obvious congenital abnormalities, such as Down syndrome. As a result of the Human Genome Project, patients can be genetically assessed for conditions such as sickle cell disease, cystic fibrosis, hemophilia A and B, breast cancer, obesity, cardiovascular disease, phenylketonuria, and Alzheimer's disease. The availability of genetic information and technology enables health care providers to perform screening, testing, and counselling for patients with genetic concerns. Knowledge obtained from the Human Genome Project has also created opportunities for assessing a person's genetic profile and preventing or treating disease. Diagnostic genetics and gene therapy have the potential to identify and modify a gene before it begins to express traits that would lead to disease or disability.

CELLULAR RESPONSE TO INJURY: INFLAMMATION

Cells or tissues of the body may be injured or killed by any of the agents (physical, chemical, infectious) described earlier. When this happens, an inflammatory response (or inflammation) naturally occurs in the healthy tissues adjacent to the site of injury. **Inflammation** is a defensive reaction intended to neutralize, control, or eliminate the offending agent and to prepare the site for repair. It is a nonspecific response (not dependent on a particular cause) that is meant to serve a protective function. For example, inflammation may be observed at the site of a bee sting, in a sore throat, in a surgical incision, and at a burn site. Inflammation also occurs in cell injury events, such as strokes and myocardial infarctions.

Inflammation is not the same as infection. An infectious agent is only one of several agents that may trigger an inflammatory response. An infection exists when the infectious agent is living, growing, and multiplying in the tissues and is able to overcome the body's normal defenses.

Regardless of the cause, a general sequence of events occurs in the local inflammatory response. This sequence involves changes in the microcirculation, including vasodilation, increased vascular permeability, and leukocytic cellular infiltration (Fig. 6-5). As these changes take place, five cardinal signs of inflammation are produced: redness, heat, swelling, pain, and loss of function.

The transient vasoconstriction that occurs immediately after injury is followed by vasodilation and an increased rate of blood flow through the microcirculation. Local heat and redness result. Next, vascular permeability increases, and plasma fluids (including proteins and solutes) leak into the inflamed tissues, producing swelling. The pain produced is attributed to the pressure of fluids or swelling on nerve endings, and to the irritation of nerve endings by chemical mediators released at the site. Bradykinin is one of the chemical mediators suspected of causing pain. Loss of function is most likely related to the pain and swelling, but the exact mechanism is not completely known.

As blood flow increases and fluid leaks into the surrounding tissues, the formed elements (red blood cells, white blood cells, and platelets) remain in the blood, causing it to become more viscous. Leukocytes (white blood cells) collect in the vessels, exit, and migrate to the site of injury to engulf offending organisms and to remove cellular debris in a process called phagocytosis. Fibrinogen in the leaked plasma fluid coagulates, forming fibrin for clot formation, which serves to wall off the injured area and prevent the spread of infection.

Chemical Mediators

Injury initiates the inflammatory response, but chemical substances released at the site induce the vascular changes. Foremost among these chemicals are histamine and the kinins. Histamine

Physiology/Pathophysiology

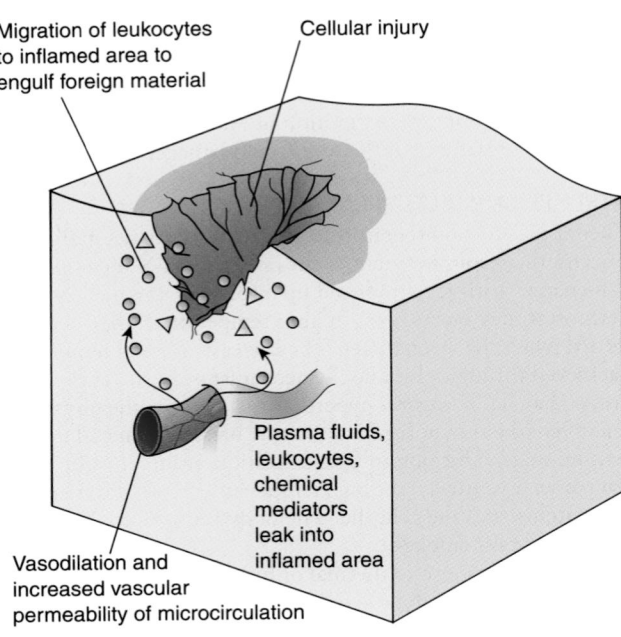

FIGURE 6-5 Inflammatory response. Chemical, physical, infectious, or other factors cause cellular injury. Vasodilation and release of chemical mediators, leukocytes, and proteins occur. Leukocytes remove cellular debris. Fibrinogen and plasma coagulate to prevent spread of infection.

is present in many tissues of the body but is concentrated in the mast cells. It is released when injury occurs and is responsible for the early changes in vasodilation and vascular permeability. Kinins increase vasodilation and vascular permeability; they also attract neutrophils to the area. Prostaglandins, another group of chemical substances, are also suspected of causing increased permeability.

Systemic Response to Inflammation

The inflammatory response is often confined to the site, causing only local signs and symptoms. However, systemic responses can also occur. Fever is the most common sign of a systemic response to injury, and it is most likely caused by endogenous pyrogens (internal substances that cause fever) released from neutrophils and macrophages (specialized forms of leukocytes). These substances reset the hypothalamic thermostat, which controls body temperature, and produce fever. Leukocytosis, an increase in the synthesis and release of neutrophils from bone marrow, may occur to provide the body with greater ability to fight infection. During this process, general, nonspecific symptoms develop, including malaise, loss of appetite, aching, and weakness.

Types of Inflammation

Inflammation is categorized primarily by its duration and the type of exudate produced. It may be acute, subacute, or chronic. Acute inflammation is characterized by the local vascular and exudative changes described earlier and usually lasts less than 2 weeks. An acute inflammatory response is immediate and serves a protective function. After the injurious agent is removed, the inflammation subsides and healing takes place with the return of normal or near-normal structure and function.

Chronic inflammation develops if the injurious agent persists and the acute response is perpetuated. Symptoms are present for many months or years. Chronic inflammation may also begin insidiously and never have an acute phase. The chronic response does not serve a beneficial and protective function; on the contrary, it is debilitating and can produce long-lasting effects. As the inflammation becomes chronic, changes occur at the site of injury and the nature of the exudate becomes proliferative. A cycle of cellular infiltration, necrosis, and fibrosis begins, with repair and breakdown occurring simultaneously. Considerable scarring may occur, resulting in permanent tissue damage.

Subacute inflammation falls between acute and chronic inflammation. It includes elements of the active exudative phase of the acute response as well as elements of repair, as in the chronic phase. The term subacute inflammation is not widely used.

CELLULAR HEALING

The reparative process begins at approximately the same time as the injury and is interwoven with inflammation. Healing proceeds after the inflammatory debris has been removed. Healing may occur by regeneration, in which gradual repair of the defect occurs by proliferation of cells of the same type as those destroyed, or by replacement, in which cells of another type, usually connective tissue, fill in the tissue defect and result in scar formation.

Healing by Regeneration

The ability of cells to regenerate depends on whether they are labile, permanent, or stable. Labile cells multiply constantly to replace cells worn out by normal physiologic processes; these include epithelial cells of the skin and those lining the gastrointestinal tract. Permanent cells include neurons—the nerve cell bodies, not their axons. Destruction of a neuron is a permanent loss, but axons may regenerate. If normal activity is to return, tissue regeneration must occur in a functional pattern, especially in the growth of several axons. Stable cells have a latent ability to regenerate. Under normal physiologic processes, they are not shed and do not need replacement, but if they are damaged or destroyed, they are able to regenerate. These include functional cells of the kidney, liver, and pancreas.

Healing by Replacement

Depending on the extent of damage, tissue healing may occur by primary intention or by secondary intention. In primary intention healing, the wound is clean and dry and the edges are approximated, as in a surgical wound. Little scar formation occurs, and the wound is usually healed in a week. In secondary intention healing, the wound or defect is larger and gaping and has necrotic or dead material. The wound fills from the bottom upward with granulation tissue. The process of repair takes longer and results in more scar formation, with loss of specialized function. People who have recovered from myocardial infarction, for example, have abnormal electrocardiographic (ECG) tracings because the electrical signal cannot be conducted through the connective tissue that has replaced the infarcted area.

The condition of the host, the environment, and the nature and severity of the injury affect the processes of inflammation and repair. Any of the injuries previously discussed can lead to death of the cell. Essentially, the cell membrane becomes impaired, resulting in a nonrestricted flow of ions. Sodium and calcium enter the cell, followed by water, which leads to edema, and energy transformation ceases. Nerve impulses are no longer transmitted; muscles no longer contract. As the cells rupture, lysosomal enzymes that destroy tissues escape, and cell death and necrosis occur.

NURSING IMPLICATIONS

In the assessment of the person who seeks health care, both objective signs and subjective symptoms are the primary indicators of the physiologic processes that are occurring. The following questions are addressed during the assessment:

- Are the heart rate, respiratory rate, and temperature normal?
- What emotional distress may be contributing to the patient's health problems?
- Are there other indicators of steady-state deviation?
- What is the person's blood pressure, height, and weight?
- Are there any problems in movement or sensation?
- Does the person demonstrate any problems with affect, behaviour, speech, cognitive ability, orientation, or memory?
- Are there obvious impairments, lesions, or deformities?

Further signs of change are indicated in diagnostic studies such as computed tomography (CT), magnetic resonance imaging (MRI), and positron emission tomography (PET). Objective evidence can also be obtained from laboratory data, including electrolytes, blood urea nitrogen (BUN), blood glucose, and urinalysis.

In making a nursing diagnosis, the nurse must relate the symptoms or complaints expressed by the patient to the physical signs that are present. Management of specific biologic disorders is discussed in subsequent chapters; however, the nurse can assist any patient to respond to stress-inducing biologic or psychological disorders with stress-management interventions.

Stress Management: Nursing Interventions

Stress or the potential for stress is ubiquitous; that is, it is everywhere and anywhere at once. Anxiety, frustration, anger, and feelings of inadequacy, helplessness, or powerlessness are emotions often associated with stress. In the presence of these emotions, the customary activities of daily living may be disrupted; for example, a sleep disturbance may be present, eating and activity patterns may be altered, and family processes or role performance may be disrupted.

Many nursing diagnoses are possible for patients suffering from stress. One nursing diagnosis related to stress is Anxiety, which is defined as a vague, uneasy feeling, the source of which may be nonspecific or not known to the person. Stress may also be manifested as ineffective coping patterns, impaired thought processes, or disrupted relationships. These human responses are reflected in the nursing diagnoses of Impaired adjustment, Ineffective coping, Defensive coping, and Ineffective denial, all of which indicate poor adaptive responses. Other possible nursing diagnoses include Social isolation, Risk for impaired parenting, Spiritual distress, Readiness for family coping, Decisional conflict, Situational low self-esteem, and Powerlessness, among others. Because human responses to stress are varied, as are the sources of stress, arriving at an accurate diagnosis allows interventions and goals to be more specific and leads to improved outcomes.

Stress management is directed toward reducing and controlling stress and improving coping. Nurses might use these methods not only with their patients but also in their own lives. The need to prevent illness, improve the quality of life, and decrease the cost of health care makes efforts to promote health essential, and stress control is a significant health-promotion goal. Stress-reduction methods and coping enhancements can derive from either internal or external sources. For example, adopting healthy eating habits and practicing relaxation techniques are internal resources that help to reduce stress; developing a broad social network is an external resource that helps reduce stress. Goods and services that can be purchased are also external resources for stress management, and it is much easier for individuals with adequate financial resources to cope with constraints in the environment, because their sense of vulnerability to threat is decreased.

PROMOTING A HEALTHY LIFESTYLE

An individual's personal resources that aid in coping include health and energy. A health-promoting lifestyle provides these resources and buffers or cushions the impact of stressors. Lifestyles or habits that contribute to the risk of illness can be identified through a health risk appraisal.

A health risk appraisal is an assessment method that is designed to promote health by examining an individual's personal habits and recommending changes when a health risk is identified. Health risk questionnaires estimate the likelihood that a person with a given set of characteristics will become ill. It is hoped that if people are provided with this information, they will alter their activities (eg, stop smoking, have periodic screening examinations) to improve their health. Questionnaires typically address the following information:

1. Demographic data: age, sex, race, ethnic background
2. Personal and family history of diseases and health problems
3. Lifestyle choices
   a. Eating, sleeping, exercise, smoking, drinking, sexual activity, and driving habits
   b. Stressors at home and on the job
   c. Role relationships and associated stressors
4. Physical measurements
   a. Blood pressure
   b. Height, weight
   c. Laboratory analyses of blood and urine
5. Participation in high-risk behaviours

The personal information is compared with average population risk data, and the risk factors are identified and weighted. From this analysis, the person's risks and major health hazards are identified. Further comparisons with population data can estimate how many years will be added to the person's life span if the suggested changes are made. However, research so far has not demonstrated that providing people with such information ensures that they will change their habits. The single most important factor for determining health status is social class, and within a social class the research suggests that the major factor influencing health is level of education (Mickler, 1997).

ENHANCING COPING STRATEGIES

McCloskey and Bulechek (1999) identified "coping enhancement" as a nursing intervention and defined it as "assisting a patient to adapt to perceived stressors, changes, or threats that interfere with meeting life demands and roles" (Chart 6-2). The nurse can build on the patient's existing coping strategies, as identified in the health appraisal, or teach new strategies for coping if necessary.

The five predominant ways of coping with illness identified in a review of 57 nursing research studies were as follows (Jalowiec, 1993):

- Trying to be optimistic about the outcome
- Using social support
- Using spiritual resources
- Trying to maintain control either over the situation or over feelings
- Trying to accept the situation

Other ways of coping included seeking information, reprioritizing needs and roles, lowering expectations, making compromises, comparing oneself to others, planning activities to conserve energy, taking things one step at a time, listening to one's body, and using self-talk for encouragement.

The nurse can implement the coping enhancement interventions and explore methods for improving the patient's coping abilities.

TEACHING RELAXATION TECHNIQUES

Relaxation techniques are a major method used to relieve stress. Commonly used techniques include progressive muscle relaxation, the Benson Relaxation Response, and relaxation with guided imagery. The goal of relaxation training is to produce a response that counters the stress response. When this goal is achieved, the action of the hypothalamus adjusts and decreases the activity of the sympathetic and parasympathetic nervous systems. The sequence of physiologic effects and their signs and symptoms are interrupted, and psychological stress is reduced. This is a learned response and requires practice to achieve.

The different relaxation techniques share four similar elements: (1) a quiet environment, (2) a comfortable position, (3) a passive attitude, and (4) a mental device (something on which to focus the attention, such as a word, phrase, or sound).

Progressive Muscle Relaxation

Progressive muscle relaxation involves tensing and releasing the muscles of the body in sequence and sensing the difference in feeling. It is best if the person lies on a soft cushion on the floor, in a quiet room, breathing easily. Someone usually reads the instructions in a low tone and with a slow and relaxed manner, or a tape of the instructions may be played. The person tenses the muscles in the whole body (one muscle group at a time), holds, senses the tension, and then relaxes. As each muscle group is tensed, the person keeps the rest of the body relaxed. Each time the focus is on feeling the tension and relaxation. When the exercise is completed, the whole body should be relaxed (Benson, 1993; Benson & Stark, 1996).

Benson's Relaxation Response

Benson (1993) describes the following steps of the Benson Relaxation Response:

1. Pick a brief phrase or word that reflects your basic belief system.
2. Choose a comfortable position.
3. Close your eyes.
4. Relax your muscles.

Chart 6-2 — Coping Enhancement: Nursing Interventions

Definition

Assisting a patient to adapt to perceived stressors, changes, or threats that interfere with meeting life demands and roles

Activities

Appraise a patient's adjustment to changes in body image as indicated.

Appraise the impact of the patient's life situation on roles and relationships.

Encourage the patient to identify a realistic description of change in role.

Appraise the patient's understanding of the disease process.

Appraise and discuss alternative responses to the situation.

Use a calm, reassuring approach.

Provide an atmosphere of acceptance.

Assist the patient in developing an objective appraisal of the event.

Help the patient to identify the information that he or she is most interested in obtaining.

Provide factual information concerning diagnosis, treatment, and prognosis.

Provide the patient with realistic choices about certain aspects of care.

Encourage an attitude of realistic hope as a way of dealing with feelings of helplessness.

Evaluate the patient's decision-making ability.

Seek to understand the patient's perspective of a stressful situation.

Discourage decision making when the patient is under severe stress.

Encourage gradual mastery of the situation.

Encourage patience in developing relationships.

Encourage relationships with persons who have common interests and goals.

Encourage social and community activities.

Encourage the acceptance of limitations in others.

Acknowledge the patient's spiritual/cultural background.

Encourage the use of spiritual resources if desired.

Explore the patient's previous achievements of success.

Explore the patient's reasons for self-criticism.

Confront the patient's ambivalent (angry or depressed) feelings.

Foster constructive outlets for anger and hostility.

Arrange situations that encourage the patient's autonomy.

Assist the patient in identifying positive responses from others.

Encourage the identification of specific life values.

Explore with the patient previous methods of dealing with life problems.

Introduce the patient to persons (or groups) who have successfully undergone the same experience.

Support the use of appropriate defense mechanisms.

Encourage verbalization of feelings, perceptions, and fears.

Discuss the consequences of not dealing with guilt and shame.

Encourage the patient to identify his or her own strengths and abilities.

Assist the patient in identifying appropriate short- and long-term goals.

Assist the patient in breaking down complex goals into small, manageable steps.

Assist the patient in examining available resources to meet the goals.

Reduce stimuli in the environment that could be misinterpreted as threatening.

Appraise the patient's needs and desires for social support.

Assist the patient to identify available support systems.

Determine the risk of the patient's inflicting self-harm.

Encourage family involvement as appropriate.

Encourage the family to verbalize their feelings about the ill family member.

Provide appropriate social skills training.

Assist the patient to identify positive strategies to deal with limitations and manage needed lifestyle or role changes.

Assist the patient to solve problems in a constructive manner.

Instruct the patient in the use of relaxation techniques as needed.

Assist the patient to grieve and to work through the losses of chronic illness and/or disability if appropriate.

Assist the patient to clarify misconceptions.

Encourage the patient to evaluate his or her own behaviour.

Reproduced with permission from McCloskey, J. C., & Bulechek, G. M. (1999). *Nursing intervention classification* (NIC) (3rd ed.) St. Louis: Mosby–Year Book.

---

5. Become aware of your breathing, and start using your selected focus word.
6. Maintain a passive attitude.
7. Continue for a set period of time.
8. Practice the technique twice daily.

This response combines meditation with relaxation. Along with the repeated word or phrase, a passive attitude is essential. If other thoughts or distractions (noises, the pain of an ailment) occur, Benson recommends not fighting the distraction but simply continuing to repeat the focus phrase. The time of day is not important, but the exercise works best on an empty stomach.

Relaxation With Guided Imagery

Simple **guided imagery** is the "purposeful use of imagination to achieve relaxation or direct attention away from undesirable sensations" (McCloskey & Bulechek, 1999, p. 506). The nurse helps the person select a pleasant scene or experience, such as watching the ocean or dabbling the feet in a cool stream. This image serves as the mental device in this technique. As the person sits comfortably and quietly, the nurse guides the individual to review the scene, trying to feel and relive the imagery with all of the senses. A tape recording may be made of the description of the image, or commercial tape recordings for guided imagery and relaxation can be used.

Other relaxation techniques include meditation, breathing techniques, massage, Reiki, music therapy, biofeedback, and the use of humour.

EDUCATING ABOUT STRESS MANAGEMENT

Two commonly prescribed nursing educational interventions— providing sensory information and providing procedural information (eg, preoperative teaching)—have the goal of reducing stress and improving the patient's coping ability. This preparatory education includes giving structured content, such as a lesson in childbirth preparation to expectant parents, a review of cardiovascular anatomy to the cardiac patient, or a description of sensations the patient will experience during cardiac catheterization. These techniques may alter the person–environment relationship such that something that might have been viewed as harmful or a threat will now be perceived more positively. Giving patients information also reduces the emotional response so that they can concentrate and solve problems more effectively (Calvin & Lane, 1999; Millo & Sullivan, 2000).

ENHANCING SOCIAL SUPPORT

The nature of social support and its influence on coping have been studied extensively with a variety of groups: immigrant women (Neufeld, Harrison, Stewart, Hughes, & Spitzer, 2002), women as caregivers (Neufeld & Harrison, 2003), men and women (Hibberd, Neufeld, & Harrison, 1996), and men as caregivers (Neufeld & Harrison, 1998). Social support can be defined as "interactions with family members, friends, peers, and health professionals that communicate information, esteem, practical aid, or emotional help. When these communications are perceived as supportive, they may enhance coping, moderate the impact of stressors, and promote health and self-care" (Stewart, 1993, p. 7). The construct of social support includes the dimensions of structure, function and appraisal.

The structure of social support consists primarily of lay sources such as family, friends, coworkers, and peer support groups, but can include health professionals (Stewart, 2000). Health professionals may offer specific support and facilitate lay support.

The dimension of function includes four types of resources: affirmational, emotional, instrumental (practical), and informational (House & Kahn, 1985). Affirmational includes positive feedback, whereas emotional is about encouragement and reassurance. Instrumental relates to practical assistance such as transportation and meals. Informational, which is about the acquisition of essential knowledge, often comes from health professionals and may include referrals. From research of self-help groups, Stewart (1995) concluded that family members provide practical (instrumental) support, spouses or partners provide emotional support, and peers provide affirmational support because of their first-hand knowledge. Health professionals were seen as educators and provided informational support.

When appraising social support, it may be viewed as available or delivered and received. An individual needs to be aware that help is required and be willing to accept help. The ideal situation is when support occurs in both directions (to the individual and to the social network) and that reciprocity and advocacy are present (Finfgeld-Connett, 2005). People who are ill may experience nonreciprocal relationships and may feel indebted. In the same way, family members may be in a nonreciprocal relationship and be overwhelmed by a sense of obligation. Individuals may report low support; this can be an absence of supportive relationships or one in which there is conflict. An important aspect of appraisal is to consider the duration of the support. Support can continue, increase or decrease over time, and may be seen as supportive or as a conflict or burden. The longer a situation or a stressor continues (for example, additional hospitalizations, or many months on a waiting list for surgery), the less support there may be. Nurses can assess a person's perception of the quality and presence of effective relationships. People who are loners; those with health problems such as tuberculosis, alcoholism, or HIV; or those from disadvantaged populations are more at risk for decreased social support. Nursing intervention may include strengthening existing networks and facilitating connections to new resources to compensate for deficiencies in the social network (Finfgeld-Connett, 2005).

It is also important that nurses assess family members and friends of the person who are in the role of caregiver, in terms of the support they need. Here the nurse may provide informational resources but the affirmational and emotional support may be even more critical. In other situations it is the nurses themselves who require support. Those working with disadvantaged populations or in areas like palliative care may be at increased risk of burnout.

Effective social support "moderates the impact of stress on health outcomes and influences health status, health behaviour and the use of health services" (Stewart, 2000, p. 3). This use of others helps the person to maintain self-esteem and mastery of their situation.

Thus, social networks assist with management of stress by providing the individual with

- A positive social identity
- Emotional support
- Material aid and tangible services
- Access to information
- Access to new social contacts and new social roles

RECOMMENDING SUPPORT AND THERAPY GROUPS

Support groups exist especially for people in similar stressful situations. Groups have been formed by parents of children with leukemia, people with ostomies, mastectomy patients, and those with other kinds of cancer or other serious diseases, chronic illnesses, and disabilities. There are groups for single parents, substance abusers and their family members, and victims of child abuse. Professional, civic, and religious support groups are active in many communities. There are also encounter groups, assertiveness training programs, and consciousness-raising groups to help people modify their usual behaviours in their transactions with their environment. Being a member of a group with similar problems or goals has a releasing effect on a person that promotes freedom of expression and exchange of ideas.

As previously noted, a person's psychological and biologic health, internal and external sources of stress management, and relationships with the environment are predictors of health outcomes. These factors are directly related to the health patterns of the individual. The nurse has a significant role and responsibility in identifying the health patterns of the person receiving care. If those patterns are not achieving physiologic, psychological, and social balance, the nurse is obligated, with the assistance and agreement of the patient, to seek ways to promote balance.

Although this chapter has presented some physiologic mechanisms and perspectives on health and disease, the way that one copes with stress, the way one relates to others, and the values and goals held are also interwoven into those physiologic patterns. To evaluate a patient's health patterns and to intervene if a problem exists requires a total assessment of the person. Specific problems and their nursing management are addressed in greater depth in other chapters.

 Critical Thinking Exercises

1. Think about a patient who has survived a major motor vehicle crash and is hospitalized for severe burns, a fractured hip, and multiple lacerations and abrasions. Identify the actual and potential physical, physiological, and psychosocial stressors evident from this person's trauma. Determine nursing strategies to reduce or alleviate these stressors.

2. A 50-year-old woman is diagnosed with osteoporosis after sustaining a rib fracture. The nurse is evaluating the coping style of the woman. What indications would the nurse note in her interactions and follow-up care for this patient that demonstrate that the woman uses problem-focused coping and emotion-focused coping?

3. Select a patient to whom you are assigned who has an acute illness or injury. Describe the manner in which homeostasis has been maintained or disrupted and the compensatory mechanisms that are evident. How does the patient's medical treatment support the compensatory mechanisms? How do you determine the nursing interventions that are appropriate for promoting the healing process?

4. A family composed of two parents, two adolescent male sons, and the maternal grandfather explore with the nurse their health promotion needs. The family's health history reveals that the mother has adult-onset diabetes; the father has coronary artery disease; the sons are somewhat overweight; and the grandfather has mild congestive heart failure. The family has ample resources for making changes in their lifestyle. What interventions would the nurse initiate to promote a healthier lifestyle for this family?

REFERENCES AND SELECTED READINGS

Books

Andreoli, T. E. (Ed.). (1997). *Cecil essentials of medicine* (4th ed.). Philadelphia: W. B. Saunders.

Barnfather, J. S., & Lyon, B. L. (Eds.). (1993). *Stress and coping: State of the science and implications for nursing theory, research and practice.* Indianapolis: Sigma Theta Tau International Inc.

Benson, H. (1993). The relaxation response. In D. Goleman & J. Gurin (Eds.), *Mind-body medicine: How to use your mind for better health* (pp. 125–148). Yonkers, NY: Consumer Reports Books.

Benson, H., & Proctor, W. (1984). *Beyond the relaxation response.* New York: Berkley Books.

Benson, H., & Stark, M. (1996). *Timeless healing.* New York: Scribner.

Copel, L. C. (2000). *Nurse's clinical guide: Psychiatric and mental health care* (2nd ed.). Springhouse, PA: Springhouse.

Dubos, R. (1965). *Man adapting.* New Haven, CT: Yale University Press.

Fauci, A. (Ed.). (1998). *Harrison's principles of internal medicine* (14th ed.). New York: McGraw-Hill.

Guyton, A. C. (1996). *Human physiology: Mechanisms of disease* (6th ed.). Philadelphia: W. B. Saunders.

Guyton, A. C. (1995). *Textbook of medical physiology* (9th ed.). Philadelphia: W. B. Saunders.

House, J. S., & Kahn, R. L. (1985). Measures and concepts of social support. In S. Cohen & S. L. Syme (Eds.), *Social support and health* (pp. 83–108). Orlando, FL: Academic Press.

Jalowiec, A. (1993). Coping with illness: Synthesis and critique of the nursing literature from 1980–1990. In J. S. Barnfather & B. L. Lyon (Eds.), *Stress and coping: State of the science and implications for nursing theory, research and practice.* Indianapolis: Sigma Theta Tau International Inc.

Lazarus, R. S. (1991a). *Emotion and adaptation.* New York: Oxford University Press.

Lazarus, R. S. (1993). Why we should think of stress as a subset of emotion. In L. Goldberger & S. Breznitz (Eds.), *Handbook of stress* (2nd ed.). New York: The Free Press.

Lazarus, R. S., & Folkman, S. (1984). *Stress, appraisal, and coping.* New York: Springer Publishing Co.

McCloskey, J. C., & Bulechek, G. M. (Eds.). (1999). *Nursing interventions classification (NIC)* (2nd ed.). St. Louis: Mosby–Year Book.

McEwen, B., & Mendelson, S. (1993). Effects of stress on the neurochemistry and morphology of the brain: Counterregulation versus damage. In I. Goldberger & S. Breznitz (Eds.), *Handbook of stress* (2nd ed.). New York: The Free Press.

Mickler, M. (1997). *Community organizing and community building for health.* New Brunswick, NJ: Rutgers University Press.

Miller, L. H., & Smith, A. D. (1993). *The stress solution.* New York: Pocket Books.

Neufeld, A., & Harrison, M. J. (2000). Family caregiving: Issues in gaining access to support. In M. J. Stewart (Ed.), *Chronic conditions and caregiving in Canada: Social support strategies* (pp. 247–273). Toronto: University of Toronto Press.

North American Nursing Diagnosis Association. (2000). *NANDA nursing diagnoses: Definitions and classifications.* Philadelphia: Author.

Selye, H. (1976). *The stress of life.* (Rev. ed.). New York: McGraw-Hill.

Stewart, M. J. (1993). *Integrating social support in nursing.* Newberry Park, CA: Sage.

Stewart, M. J. (Ed.). (1995). *Community nursing: Promoting Canadians' health* (2nd ed.). Toronto: W. B. Saunders.

Stewart, M. J. (Ed.). (2000). *Chronic conditions and caregiving in Canada: Social support strategies.* Toronto: University of Toronto Press.

Stewart, M. J., & Langille, L. (2000). A framework for social support assessment and intervention in the context of chronic conditions and caregiving. In M. J. Stewart (Ed.), *Chronic conditions and caregiving in Canada: Social support strategies* (pp. 3–28). Toronto: University of Toronto Press.

Watkins, A. (Ed.). (1997). *Mind-body medicine: A clinician's guide to psychoneuroimmunology.* New York: Churchill Livingstone.

Journals

Asterisks indicate nursing research articles.

*Almberg, B., Grafstrom, M., & Winblad, B. (1997). Major strain and coping strategies as reported by family members who care for aged demented relatives. *Journal of Advanced Nursing, 26*(4), 683–691.

Anderson, B. L., Farrar, W. B., Golden-Kreutz, D., et al. (1998). Stress and immune responses after surgical treatment for regional breast cancer. *Journal of National Cancer Institute, 90*(1), 30–36.

Baird, C. L. (2000). Living with hurting and difficulty doing: Older women with osteoarthritis. *Clinical Excellence for Nurse Practitioners, 4*(4), 231–237.

Ballard, A. (1981). Identification of environmental stressors for patients in a surgical intensive care unit. *Issues in Mental Health Nursing, 11*(3), 89–100.

Biondi, M., Peronti, M., Pacitti, F., Pancheri, P., Pacifici, R., Altieri, I., Paris, L., & Zuccaro, P. (1994). Personality, endocrine and immune changes after eight months in healthy individuals under normal daily stress. *Psychotherapy and Psychosomatics, 62*(3–4), 176–184.

Black, P. H. (1994). Central nervous system–immune system interactions: Psychoneuroendocrinology of stress and its immune consequences. *Antimicrobial Agents and Chemotherapy, 38*(1), 1–6.

*Brillhart, B., & Johnson, K. (1997). Motivation and the coping process of adults with disabilities: A qualitative study. *Rehabilitation Nursing, 22*(5), 249–256.

Bryla, C. M. (1996). The relationship between stress and the development of breast cancer: A literature review. *Oncology Nursing Forum, 23*(3), 441–448.

Calvin, R. L., & Lane, P. L. (1999). Perioperative uncertainty and state anxiety of orthopedic surgical patients. *Orthopaedic Nursing, 18*(6), 61–66.

Chalfont, L., & Bennett, P. (1999). Personality and coping: Their influence on affect and behavior following myocardial infarction. *Coronary Health Care, 3*(3), 110–116.

Clements, K., & Turpin, G. (2000). Life events exposure, physiological reactivity, and psychological strain. *Journal of Behavioral Medicine, 23*(1), 73–94.

*Coe, M., & Neufeld, A. (1999). Male caregivers' use of formal support. *Western Journal of Nursing Research, 21*(4), 568–588.

Cohen, J. I. (2000). Stress and mental health: A biobehavioral perspective. *Issues in Mental Health Nursing, 21*(2), 185–202.

*Collins, M. A. (1996). The relation of work stress, hardiness, and burnout among full-time hospital staff nurses. *Journal of Nursing Staff Development, 12*(2), 81–85.

*Constantino, R. E., Sekula, L. K., Rabin, B., & Stone, C. (2000). Negative life experiences, depression, and immune function in abused and non-abused women. *Biological Research in Nursing, 1*(3), 190–198.

Cronquist, A., Wredding, R., Norlander, R., Langius, A., & Bjorvell, H. (2000). Perceived discomfort and related coping phenomenon in patients undergoing percutaneous transluminal coronary angioplasty. *Coronary Health Care, 4*(3), 123–129.

*Fallon, M., Gould, D., & Wainwright, S. P. (1997). Stress and quality of life in the renal transplant patient: A preliminary investigation. *Journal of Advanced Nursing, 25*(3), 562–570.

*Felton, B. S. (2000). Resilience in a multicultural sample of community-dwelling women older than age 85. *Clinical Nursing Research, 9*(2), 102–103.

*Finfgeld-Connett, D. (2005). Clarification of social support. *Journal of Nursing Scholarship,* First Quarter 2005, 4–9.

*Fudge, H., Neufeld, A., & Harrison, M. J. (1997). Social networks of women caregivers. *Public Health Nursing, 14*(1), 20–27.

Glaser, R., & Kiecolt-Glaser, J. K. (1997). Chronic stress modulates the virus-specific immune response to latent herpes simplex virus type 1. *Annals Behavioral Medicine, 19*(2), 78–82.

Goodkin, K., Feaster, D. J., Tuttle, R., Blaney, N. T., Kumar, M., Baum, M. K., Shapshak, P., & Fletcher, M. A. (1996). Bereavement is associated with time-dependent decrements in cellular immune function in asymptomatic human immunodeficiency virus type 1-seropositive homosexual men. *Clinics in Diagnostic Laboratory Immunology, 3*(1), 109–180.

*Hagerty, B. M., Williams, R. A., Coyne, J. C., & Early, M. R. (1996). Sense of belonging and indicators of social and psychological functioning. *Archives of Psychiatric Nursing, 10*(4), 235–244.

*Harrison, M. J., & Neufeld, A. (1997). Women's experience of barriers to support while caregiving. *Health Care for Women International, 18,* 591–602.

*Harrison, M. J., Neufeld, A., & Kushner, K. (1995). Women in transition: Access and barriers to social support. *Journal of Advanced Nursing, 21,* 858–864.

*Heinrich, M., Neufeld, A., & Harrison, M. J. (2003). Perceptions of formal support: Caregivers' strategies to maintain preservative caregiving. *Canadian Journal of Nursing Research, 35*(4), 39–56.

Heitzman, C. A., & Kaplan, R. M. (1998). Assessment of methods for measuring social support. *Health Psychology, 7,* 75–109.

*Hibberd, J. M., Neufeld, A., & Harrison, M. J. (1996). Gender differences in the support networks of caregivers. *Journal of Gerontological Nursing, 22*(9), 15–23.

Holmes, T. H., & Rahe, R. H. (1967). The social readjustment rating scale. *Journal of Psychosomatic Research, 11,* 213–218.

*Kennedy, J. W. (2000). Women's inner balance: A comparison of stressors, personality traits, and health problems by age groups. *Journal of Advanced Nursing, 31*(3): 639–650.

*Langford, C. P., Bowsher, J., Maloney, J. P., & Lillis, P. P. (1997). Social support: A conceptual analysis. *Journal of Advanced Nursing, 25*(1), 95–100.

Lazarus, R. S. (1991b). Cognition and motivation in emotion. *American Psychologist, 46*(4), 352–367.

Lazarus, R. S. (1991c). Progress on a cognitive-motivational-relational theory of emotion. *American Psychologist, 46*(8), 819–834.

*Mahat, G. (1997). Perceived stressors and coping strategies among individuals with rheumatoid arthritis. *Journal of Advanced Nursing, 25*(6), 1144–1150.

Matthews, K. A., Caggiula, A. R., McAllister, C. G., et al. (1995). Sympathetic reactivity to acute stress and immune response in women. *Psychosomatic Medicine, 57*(6), 564–571.

*Millio, M. E., & Sullivan, K. (2000). Patients with operable esophageal cancer: Their experience of information giving in a regional thoracic unit. *Journal of Clinical Nursing, 9*(2), 236–246.

Morse, D. L. (2000). Continuing care extra: Relocation stress is real. *American Journal of Nursing, 100*(8), 24A–24D.

*Morse, S. R., & Fife, B. (1998). Coping with a partner's cancer, adjustment at four stages of the illness trajectory. *Oncology Nursing Forum, 25*(4), 751–760.

*Neufeld, A., & Harrison, M. J. (1995). Reciprocity and social support in caregivers' relationships: Variations and consequences. *Qualitative Health Research, 5,* 349–366.

*Neufeld, A., & Harrison, M. J. (1998). Men as caregivers: Reciprocal relationships or obligation? *Journal of Advanced Nursing, 28*(5), 959–968.

*Neufeld, A., & Harrison, M. J. (2003). Unfulfilled expectations and negative interactions: Nonsupport in relationships of women caregivers. *Journal of Advanced Nursing, 41*(4), 323–331.

*Neufeld, A., Harrison, M. J., Stewart, M. J., Hughes, K., & Spitzer, D. (2002). Immigrant women: Making connections to community resources. *Qualitative Health Research, 12*(6), 751–768.

Pike, J. L., Smith, T. L., Hauger, R. L., et al. (1997). Chronic life stress alters sympathetic, neuroendocrine, and immune responsivity to an acute psychological stressor in humans. *Psychosomatic Medicine, 59*(4), 447–457.

Robinson, F. P., Matthews, H. L., Witek-Janusek, L. (2000). Stress reduction and HIV disease: A review of intervention studies using a psychoimmunology framework. *Journal of the Association of Nurses in AIDS Care, 11*(2), 87–96.

*Ryan, M. C. (1996). Loneliness, social support and depression as interactive variables with cognitive status: testing Roy's model. *Nursing Science Quarterly, 9*(3), 107–114.

Schrader, K. A. (1996). Stress and immunity after traumatic injury: The mind–body link. *AACN Clinical Issues in Critical Care Nursing, 7*(3), 351–358.

Seers, K., & Carrol, D. (1998). Relaxation techniques for acute pain management: A systematic review. *Journal of Advanced Nursing, 27*(3), 466–475.

Sergerstrom, S. C., Fahey, J. L., Kemeny, M. E., & Taylor, S. E. (1998). Optimism is associated with mood, coping, and immune change in response to stress. *Journal of Perspectives in Social Psychology, 74*(6), 1646–1655.

Smith, L. L. (2000). Cytokine hypothesis of overtraining: A physiological adaptation to excessive stress? *Medicine and Science in Sports and Exercise, 32*(2), 317–331.

*Spitzer, D., Neufeld, A., Harrison, M. J., Hughes, K., & Stewart, M. J. (2003). "My wings have been cut, where can I fly?" Gender, migration and caregiving: Chinese and South Asian Canadian Perspectives. *Gender and Society, 17*(2), 267–286.

*Starzonski, R., & Hilton, A. (2000). Patient and family adjustment to kidney transplantation with and without an interim period of dialysis. *Nephrology Nursing Journal, 27*(1), 17, 18, 21–33, 52.

Stewart, M. J., Ellerton, M. L., Hart, G., Hirth, A., Mann, K., Meagher-Stewart, D., et al. (1997). Insights from a nursing research program on social support. *Canadian Journal of Nursing Research, 29*(3), 93–110.

Tausig, M. (1982). Measuring life events. *Journal of Health and Social Behavior, 23*(1), 52–64.

Wells-Federman, C. (1996). Awakening the nurse healer within. *Holistic Nursing Practice, 10*(2), 13–29.

*Williams, A. M. (2000). Distress and hardiness: A comparison of African Americans and white caregivers. *Journal of National Black Nurses Association, 11*(1), 21–26.

*Wineman, N. M. (1990). Adaptation to multiple sclerosis: The role of social support, functional disability, and perceived uncertainty. *Nursing Research, 39,* 294–299.

RESOURCES AND WEBSITES

American Academy of Experts in Traumatic Stress; http://www.info@crisisinfo.net.

Individual and Family Considerations Related to Illness

Adapted by Madeleine Buck and Rene A. Day

LEARNING OBJECTIVES ●

On completion of this chapter, the learner will be able to:

1. Describe the holistic approach to sustaining health and well-being.
2. Discuss the concepts of emotional well-being and emotional distress.
3. Identify variables that influence the ability to cope with stress and that are antecedents to emotional disorders.
4. Explain the concepts of anxiety, posttraumatic stress disorder, depression, loss, and grief.
5. Describe a framework for understanding death and dying.
6. Assess the impact of illness on the patient's family and on family functioning.
7. Determine the role of the nurse in identifying substance abuse problems and in assisting the family to cope.
8. Explore the concept of spirituality and address the spiritual needs of patients.
9. Identify nursing actions that promote effective coping for both the patient and the family.

*W*hen people experience threats to their health, they seek out various care providers for the purpose of maintaining or restoring health. In recent years, both the patient and the family have become more involved participants in health care and health promotion activities. At the same time, greater numbers of consumers and practitioners have recognized the interconnectedness of mind, body, and spirit in sustaining well-being and overcoming or coping with illness. This holistic approach to health and wellness and the increased consumer involvement reflect a renewed emphasis on the concepts of choice, healing, and patient–practitioner partnerships. The holistic perspective focuses not only on promoting well-being but also on understanding how one's emotional state contributes to health and illness. By using this knowledge, people are better able to prevent the reoccurrence or exacerbation of problems and to develop strategies to improve their future health status.

Holistic Approach to Health and Health Care

Since the 1980s, the use of holistic therapies has increased. A survey on the use of **holistic health** practices reported that about 34% of the 1539 respondents in a U.S. national random sample of adults older than 18 years of age (732 women and 807 men) had consulted with at least one holistic health care practitioner within the past year. The study further noted that although many of the people were also seeing a traditional health care provider, 72% did not inform the physician that they were obtaining holistic treatment (Eisenberg et al., 1993). Canadian surveys reported that 25% to 33% of Canadians were using at least one complementary remedy other than vitamins (Canada Health Monitor, 1997; PricewaterhouseCoopers, 1999; Ramsay, Walker, & Alexander, 1999) along with medical care (Druss & Rosenheck, 1999). It is imperative for nursing students and nurses to be knowledgeable about **complementary therapies** and their effectiveness and to be able to assess and discuss the use of such therapies with clients in all settings (Joudrey & Gough, 2003; McClennon-Leong & Kerr, 1999). Some of the most commonly used complementary therapies are listed in Chart 7-1.

For some people, the holistic approach is viewed as a way to capitalize on personal strengths and recultivate the values and beliefs about health that were common before the age of technological innovations and the sophistication of biomedical science. A lack of focus on the individual patient, the family, and the environment by some health care providers has created feelings of disillusionment and depersonalization in many patients. The cost of illness, especially chronic illness care, continues to escalate and accounts for

Chart 7-1 Common Complementary and Alternative Therapies

- Alternative medical systems including acupuncture, Ayurveda, homeopathic medicine, and naturopathic medicine
- Mind-body interventions including meditation, certain uses of hypnosis, dance, music, art therapy and prayer
- Biologically based therapies including herbal, special dietary, orthomolecular, and individual biological therapies
- Manipulative and body-based methods including chiropractic and osteopathy
- Energy therapies including Qi gong, Reiki, and therapeutic touch

Reprinted with permission from Dossey, B. M., Guzzetta, C., & Keegan, L. (2002). *Holistic nursing: A handbook for practice.* Gaithersburg, MD: Aspen Publications.

an increasing percentage of health care dollars. At the same time, patient satisfaction with the health care received has decreased.

Active participation of the patient and family in promoting health supports the self-care model historically embraced by the nursing profession. This model is congruent with the philosophy that seeks to balance and integrate the use of crisis medicine and advanced technology with the influence of the mind and spirit on healing. A holistic approach to health reconnects the traditionally separate approaches to mind and body. Factors such as the physical environment, economic conditions, sociocultural issues, emotional state, interpersonal relationships, and support systems can work together or alone to influence health. The connections among physical health, emotional health, and spiritual well-being must be understood and considered when providing health care. It is the nurse's conceptual integration of the physiologic health condition with the emotional and social context, along with the tasks and developments of the patient's life stage, that allows for the development of a holistic plan of nursing care.

The Brain and Physical and Emotional Health

Research on brain structure and function, neurochemical messenger systems (neurotransmitters), and brain–body connections suggests fundamental, delicate, two-way relationships between the brain's environment and mood, behaviour, and resistance to disease (Cohen & Herbert, 1996). One focus of brain research has been to identify and integrate traditional medical and psy-

Glossary

anxiety: an emotional state characterized by feelings of apprehension, discomfort, restlessness, or worry

bereavement: feelings, thoughts, and responses that occur after a loss

complementary therapies: used as an adjunct to traditional health modalities; they typically influence the effects of stress, anxiety, depression, and other physical and emotional states

depression: state in which a person feels sad, distressed, and hopeless, with little to no energy for normal activities

faith: belief and trust in a God or higher power

family: a group whose members are related by reciprocal caring, mutual responsibilities, and loyalties

grief: a universal response to any loss

holistic health: promotion of the total health of mind, body, and spirit

homeopathic medicine: a system of medicine that promotes healing of the whole person by stimulating the natural healing processes within the person

mental disorder: a state in which a person has deficits in functioning, has a distorted sense of self or the world, is unable to sustain relationships, or cannot handle stress or conflict effectively

mental health: a state in which a person can meet basic needs, assume responsibilities, sustain relationships, resolve conflicts, and grow throughout life

posttraumatic stress disorder (PTSD): the development of severe anxiety-type symptoms after the experience of a traumatic life event

substance abuse: a maladaptive pattern of drug use that causes physical and emotional harm with the potential for disruption of daily life chiatric knowledge with new psychobiologic and psychoneuroimmunologic data. Researchers in the field of psychobiology study the biologic basis of mental disturbances and have established some relationships between mental disorders and changes in the structure and function of the brain. Researchers in the field of psychoneuroimmunology study the connections between the emotions, stress, the central nervous system, the neuroendocrine system, and the immune system and have established compelling evidence that psychosocial variables can affect the functioning of the immune system. In the article "Emotions, morbidity and mortality: New perspectives from psychoneuroimmunology," the authors provide an excellent overview of the knowledge nurses need about this rapidly evolving area of investigation (Kiecolt-Glaser, McGuire, Robles, & Glaser, 2002).

As this neuroscientific research continues, data about neurotransmitters and the functioning of the brain will augment existing understanding of emotions, intelligence, memory, and many aspects of general body functioning. In the future, an accepted definition of mental illness may well include biologic information. By enhancing the biologic knowledge base about the brain and nervous system, scientists establish the foundation for breakthroughs in the treatment of both symptoms and illnesses.

These findings suggest that the health care community ought to place as much emphasis on emotional health as it places on physiologic health and ought to recognize how biologic, emotional, and societal problems combine to affect individual patients, families, and communities. Some problems that nurses and other health care providers must address include **substance abuse**, homelessness, family violence, eating disorders, trauma, and chronic **mental health** conditions such as anxiety and depression. Nurses in all settings encounter patients with mental health problems and have an integral role in helping to achieve the national goals by recognizing and treating emotional distress and promoting emotional health.

In May of 2004, the Canadian Mental Health Association (CMHA) presented to the Senate Standing Committee on Social Affairs, Science, and Technology. The submission "Working Together Toward a Pan-Canadian Strategy on Mental Health/Mental Illness for the People of Canada" contains five recommendations requiring action:

- Develop and implement a Pan-Canadian National Strategy on Mental Health/Mental Illness.
- Respond to the Premier's Council's commitment to community mental health.
- Ensure that children and youth, Aboriginals, women, and new immigrants are included in the national strategy.
- Ensure that suicide is addressed as part of the national strategy.
- Commit to increasing the capacity of the voluntary sector in the mental health community to participate in public policy development. (Canadian Mental Health Association, 2004)

Since 1998, the Canadian Alliance for Mental Illness and Mental Health (CAMIMH) has worked to advise on a national mental health policy; to speak for the consumer, family, community, and professional organizations; and to improve services and supports for persons facing mental illness or mental health obstacles. Goals are presented in Chart 7-2.

Emotional Health and Emotional Distress

The concept of emotional health encompasses a person's ability to function as comfortably and productively as possible. Typically, people who are mentally healthy are satisfied with them-

Chart 7-2 **Goals of the Canadian Alliance for Mental Illness and Mental Health**

A. Public Education and Awareness

Goal A1: Reduce the stigma associated with mental illnesses in Canadian society.

Goal A2: Increase public knowledge and awareness about effective practices in the fields of mental illness and mental health.

B. National Policy Framework

Goal B1: Ensure that the impact on mental illness and mental health is considered in the development and implementation of every federal policy and legislative initiative.

Goal B2: Establish and adopt national guidelines or benchmarks for key outcome areas of a desired mental health system and for mental health promotion.

Goal B3: Develop collaborative and cooperative partnerships that will enhance systems of care and mental health promotion opportunities.

Goal B4: Strengthen consumer and family participation in national policy development affecting mental illness services and supports as well as mental health promotion.

Goal B5: The federal government recognizes consumer and family self-help as a significant and vital mental health resource.

Goal B6: Encourage and facilitate the piloting, testing and dissemination of information about new and innovative models of delivering mental illness/health services based on effective practices.

Goal B7: Develop a national mental illness and mental health human resource plan to the year 2005.

C. Research

Goal C1: Establish and support a national research agenda.

Goal C2: Establish and implement a public education and awareness strategy to support comprehensive and sufficient research funding and value research.

Goal C3: Strengthen the voluntary fundraising sector so that it demonstrates a unified commitment and enhanced support for mental illness/health research.

Goal C4: Increase the cadres of new mental illness and mental health researchers.

Goal C5: Create a more supportive environment for Canadian researchers in mental illness and mental health research.

Goal C6: Ensure that mental illness and mental health research informs policy development in all areas of health.

Goal C7: Increase the involvement of consumers, other stakeholders and their organizations, and the voluntary sector in the development, implementation, and dissemination of the knowledge acquired through enhanced mental illness and mental health research.

D. National Data/Information System

Goal D1: Create a national public health surveillance and reporting program in collaboration with other stakeholders, including the Centre for Chronic Disease Prevention and Control of Health Canada.

From Canadian Alliance for Mental Illness and Mental Health. (2004). Available at: http://www.phac-aspc.gc.ca/publicat/miic-mmac/.

selves and their life situations. In the usual course of living, emotionally healthy people focus on activities geared to meet their needs and attempt to accomplish personal goals while concurrently managing everyday challenges and problems. Often, people must work hard to balance their feelings, thoughts, and behaviours to alleviate emotional distress, and much energy is used to change, adapt, or manage the obstacles inherent in daily living. A mentally healthy person accepts reality and has a positive sense of self. Emotional health is also manifested by having moral and humanistic values and beliefs, having satisfying interpersonal relationships, doing productive work, and maintaining a realistic sense of hope (Chart 7-3).

When people have unmet emotional needs or distress, they experience an overall feeling of unhappiness. As tension escalates, security and survival are threatened. How different people respond to these troublesome situations reflects their level of coping and maturity. Emotionally healthy people endeavour to meet the demands of distressing situations while still facing the typical issues that emerge in their lives. The ways in which people respond to uncomfortable stimuli reflect their exposure to various biologic, emotional, and sociocultural experiences.

When stress interferes with a person's ability to function comfortably and inhibits the effective management of personal needs, that person is at risk for emotional problems. The use of ineffective and unhealthy methods of coping is manifested by dysfunctional behaviours, thoughts, and feelings. These behaviours are aimed at relieving the overwhelming stress, even though they may cause further problems.

Coping ability is strongly influenced by biologic or genetic factors, physical and emotional growth and development, family and childhood experiences, and learning. Typically, a person reverts to the strategies observed early in life that were used by family members, caregivers, and others to solve conflict. If these strategies were not adaptive, the person exhibits a range of painful and nonproductive behaviours. Dysfunctional behaviour in one person not only seriously affects that person's emotional health but can also put others at risk for injury or death. As these destructive behaviours are repeated, a cyclic pattern becomes evident: impaired thinking, negative feelings, and more dysfunctional actions that prevent the person from meeting the demands of daily living (Chart 7-4).

No universally accepted definition of what constitutes an emotional disorder exists. But many views and theories share in common the idea that a number of variables can interfere with emotional growth and development and impede successful adaptation to the environment. Most clinicians have adopted the statement from the American Psychiatric Association's *Diagnostic and Statistical Manual of Mental Disorders (DSM-IV TR)*, which defines the term **mental disorder** as a group of behavioural or psychological symptoms or a pattern that manifests itself in significant distress, impaired functioning, or accentuated risk of enduring severe suffering or possible death (American Psychiatric Association,

Chart 7-4   Characteristics Associated With Mental Disorders

- Severe anxiety
- Severe depression
- Ineffective coping mechanisms
- Extreme feelings of helplessness or powerlessness
- Maladaptive ways of dealing with stress
- Uncomfortable with self and others
- Lack of pleasure from living
- Extreme negative thoughts, feelings, and behaviours
- Disorganized or disturbed thoughts
- Inability to accept reality
- Personality traits that contribute to dysfunctional behaviours
- Desire to hurt self or others
- History of traumatic experience
- Inability to satisfy basic needs
- Lack of a support system
- Physiologic problems resulting from severe, unrelenting stress

2000, p. xxi). Risk factors for mental health problems are listed in Chart 7-5.

Patients seen in medical-surgical settings often struggle with psychosocial issues of anxiety, depression, loss, and grief. Abuse, addiction, chemical dependency, body image disturbances, and eating disorders are a few examples of health situations that require extensive physical and emotional care to restore optimal functioning. The dual challenge for the health team is to understand how the patient's emotions influence current physiologic conditions and to identify the best care for the patient experiencing underlying emotional and spiritual distress.

Family Health and Distress

The **family** plays a central role in the life of the patient and is a major part of the context of the patient's life. It is within families that people grow, are nurtured, attain a sense of self, cultivate beliefs and values about life, and progress through life's developmen-

Chart 7-5   Risk Factors for Mental Health Problems

Risk Factors That Cannot Be Changed
Age
Gender
Genetic background
Family history

Risk Factors That Can Be Changed
Marital status
Family environment
Housing problems
Poverty or economic difficulties
Physical health
Nutritional status
Stress level
Social environment and activities
Exposure to trauma
Alcohol and drug use
Environmental toxins or other pollutants
Availability, accessibility, and cost of health services

Chart 7-3   Characteristics Associated With Mental Health

- Positive sense of self
- Satisfying interpersonal relationships
- Wide range of appropriate emotions
- Love and care for self and others
- Realistic and responsible behaviour
- Effective coping skills
- Ability to negotiate and resolve conflict
- Cooperative and interdependent in working with others
- Engagement in rewarding, productive work
- Adaptable to the daily challenges of life
- Finds meaning and purpose in life
- Has hopes and dreams
- Knowledge of personal strengths and areas needing improvement
- Sense of humour
- Respect for the rights and differences of others

Chart 7-6 Adult Developmental Tasks

Developmental stage and associated tasks can have an impact on how individuals cope with illness.

Young Adult
Establish independence
Establish lifestyle
Develop career
Develop intimate relationships
Marry and start a family

Middle Adult
Establish financial security
Prepare for retirement
Launch children
Refocus on marital relationship
Support growing children and aging parents

Older Adult
Adapt to retirement and alteration in role
Adapt to declining physical stamina
Review life's accomplishments
Prepare for death

tal stages (Chart 7-6). The family is also the first source for socialization and teaching about health and illness. The family prepares the person with strategies for balancing closeness with separateness and togetherness with individuality. A major role of the family is to provide physical and emotional resources to maintain health and a system of support in times of crises, such as in periods of illness. Educating families has been shown to add to their resiliency, adaptation, and adjustment to life stressors (Friedman, 1998).

When a family member becomes ill, all members of the family are affected. Depending on the nature of the health problem, family members may need to make several adaptations to their existing lifestyles or even restructure their lifestyles.

Health problems often have an impact on the family's ability to function. Five family functions described by Wright and Leahey (2000) are viewed as essential to the individual's and family's growth. The first function, management, involves the use of power, decision making about resources, establishment of rules, provision of finances, and future planning—responsibilities assumed by the adults of the family. The second function, boundary setting, makes clear distinctions between the generations and the roles of adults and children within the family structure. Communication is the third function that is important to individual and family growth; healthy families have a full range of clear, direct, and meaningful communication among their members. The fourth function is education and support. Education involves modeling skills for living a physically, emotionally, and socially healthy life; support is manifested by actions that tell family members they are cared about and loved. Family support promotes health and is seen as a critical factor in coping with crises and illness situations. The final function is socialization. Families transmit culture and the acceptable behaviours needed to perform adequately in the home and in the world.

NURSING IMPLICATIONS

There are many degrees of family functioning. The nurse assesses family functioning to determine how the family will cope with the impact of the health condition. If the family is chaotic or disorganized, promoting coping skills becomes a priority in the plan of care. The family with preexisting problems may require additional assistance before participating fully in the current health

situation. In performing a family assessment, the nurse must evaluate the present family structure and function. Areas of appraisal include demographic data, developmental information (keeping in mind that family members can be in several different developmental stages simultaneously), family structure, family functioning, and coping abilities. The role that the environment plays in family health is also assessed.

Interventions with family members are based on strengthening coping skills through direct care, communication skills, and education. Healthy family communication has a strong influence on the quality of family life and can help the family to make appropriate choices, consider alternative strategies, or persevere through complex circumstances. Within a family system, for example, the identified patient may be undergoing extensive surgery for cancer while the partner has cardiac disease, the adolescent has a fractured humerus, and the child has type 1 diabetes. In this situation, there are multiple health concerns along with competing developmental tasks and needs. Despite the obvious concerns of the family members, both individually and collectively, a crisis may or may not be present. This family may be coping effectively; alternatively, the family may be in crisis or may manifest a chronic inability to handle the situation. The health team conducts a careful and comprehensive family assessment, develops interventions tailored to handle the stressors, implements the specified treatment protocols, and facilitates the construction of social support systems.

The use of existing family strengths, resources, and education is augmented by therapeutic family interventions. The nurse's primary goals are to maintain and improve the patient's present level of health and to prevent physical and emotional deterioration. Next, the nurse intervenes in the cycle that the illness creates: patient illness, stress for other family members, generation of potential for illness in other family members, and additional stress for the patient.

Helping the family members handle the myriad stressors that bombard them daily involves working with family members to develop coping skills. In a 1994 study, Burr and associates identified seven traits that enhance coping of family members under stress. Communication skills and spirituality were the most useful traits. Cognitive abilities, emotional strengths, relationship capabilities, willingness to use community resources, and individual strengths and talents were also associated with effective coping. As nurses work with families, they must not underestimate the impact that their therapeutic interactions, educational information, positive role modeling, provision of direct care, and corrective teaching have on promoting health.

Without the active support of the family members and the health team, the potential for using maladaptive coping mechanisms increases. Often, denial and blaming of individuals occur. Sometimes, physiologic illness, emotional withdrawal, and physical distancing are the results of severe family conflict, violent behaviours, or addiction to drugs and alcohol. Substance abuse is sometimes the outcome for family members who view their ability to cope or solve problems as impossible. Often, people engage in these dysfunctional behaviours when faced with difficult or problematic situations.

Anxiety

All people experience some degree of **anxiety** (a tense emotional state) as they face new, challenging, or threatening life situations. In clinical settings, fear of the unknown, unexpected news about one's health, and any impairment of bodily functions engenders anxiety. Although a mild level of anxiety can mobilize people to take a position, act on the task that needs to be done, or learn to

NURSING RESEARCH PROFILE 7-1
Anxiety and Coping Behaviours

Dropkin, M. J. (2001). Anxiety, coping strategies, and coping behaviors in patients undergoing head and neck cancer surgery. *Cancer Nursing, 24*(2), 143–148.

Purpose

This research study described the relationships between preoperative anxiety and the use of coping strategies, and between postoperative self-care and resocialization behaviours, in patients who have facial disfigurement or dysfunction as a result of head and neck cancer surgery.

Study Sample and Design

The sample for this descriptive correlational study consisted of 75 participants (53 men and 22 women) who were about to sustain facial disfigurement and dysfunction as an outcome of head and neck surgery. Subjects were requested to complete the State Trait Anxiety Inventory and the Ways of Coping Questionnaire before their surgery and the Coping Behaviours Score and the Disfigurement/Dysfunction Scale afterward.

Findings

The results of the study revealed no significant correlations between preoperative anxiety and the percentage of problem-focused coping strategies used to handle disfiguring surgery. A high level of anxiety was present, which was equivalent to the anxiety of people admitted to a psychiatric treatment centre for an acute anxiety reaction. Although there was low use of problem-focused coping strategies before the surgery, postoperative coping behaviours occurred early in the recovery period. Scores indicated that severe functional impairment was present immediately after surgery. The anxiety scores for these patients decreased over time, but there was no significant correlation between disfigurement/dysfunction and anxiety. The level of anxiety was negatively correlated with self-care after surgery on the fourth and fifth postoperative days. These findings indicate that anxiety is decreased by the performance of self-care behaviours in the early postoperative period.

Nursing Implications

For the nurse caring for a postoperative patient who is undergoing head and neck surgery, it is important to recognize that early participation in self-care behaviours is associated with reduced anxiety in these patients. This relationship between anxiety and self-care increases over time. Therefore, nurses need to facilitate self-care activities in this population, because this intervention can help to promote positive postoperative outcomes.

Chart 7-7 • ASSESSMENT

Assessing Signs and Symptoms of Anxiety

Physiologic Symptoms
Appetite change
Headaches
Muscle tension
Fatigue or lethargy
Weight change
Cold and flu symptoms
Digestive upsets
Grinding teeth
Palpitations
Hypertension
Restlessness
Difficulty sleeping
Skin irritations
Injury prone
Increased use of any alcohol
  or drugs

Emotional Symptoms
Forgetfulness
Low productivity
Feeling dull
Poor concentration
Negative attitude
Confusion
Whirling mind
No new ideas
Boredom
Negative self-talk
Anxiety

Frustration
Depression
Crying periods
Irritability
Worrying
Feeling discouraged
Nervous laughter

Relational Symptoms
Isolation
Intolerance
Resentment
Loneliness
Lashing out
"Clamming up"
Nagging
Distrust
Few friends
No intimacy
Using people

Spiritual Symptoms
Emptiness
Loss of meaning
Doubt
Unforgiving attitude
Martyrdom
Loss of direction
Cynicism
Apathy

alter lifestyle habits, a more severe level can be almost paralyzing. Anxiety that escalates to a near panic state can be incapacitating. When patients receive unwelcome news about results of diagnostic studies, they are sure to experience anxiety. Different patients manifest the physiologic, emotional, and behavioural signs and symptoms of anxiety in various ways (Nursing Research Profile 7-1).

NURSING IMPLICATIONS

Early clinical observations of guilt or anxiety are an essential component of nursing care (Chart 7-7). A high level of anxiety in a patient will probably exacerbate physiologic distress. For example, a postoperative patient who is in pain may discover that anxiety intensifies the sensation of pain. A patient newly diagnosed with type 2 diabetes may be worried and fearful and therefore unable to focus on or complete essential self-care activities. The possibility of developing somatic symptoms is high in any patient who is experiencing moderate to severe anxiety.

The *DSM-IV TR* (2000) lists general medical conditions that cause anxiety. They include endocrine diseases, such as hypothyroidism, hyperthyroidism, hypoglycemia, and hyperadrenocorticism; cardiovascular conditions, such as cardiac dysrhythmia, congestive heart failure, and pulmonary emboli; respiratory problems, such as pneumonia, asthma, and chronic obstructive pulmonary disease; and neurologic conditions, such as encephalitis and neoplasms.

Every nurse must be vigilant about the patient who worries excessively and demonstrates deterioration in emotional, social, or occupational functioning. If participation in the therapeutic regimen (eg, administration of insulin) becomes a problem because of extreme anxiety, nursing interventions must be immediately initiated. Caring strategies emphasize ways for the patient to verbalize feelings and fears and to identify sources of anxiety. The need to teach and promote effective coping abilities and the use of relaxation techniques are the priorities of care. In some cases, antianxiety medication may be prescribed. Chart 7-8 provides a list of basic nursing principles that are useful for assisting patients to manage severe anxiety. Chapter 6 presents additional information about stress and the relaxation response.

Posttraumatic Stress Disorder

In medical-surgical settings, especially in emergency departments, burn units, and rehabilitation centres, nurses care for extremely anxious patients who have experienced devastating events that are typically considered to be outside the realm of normal human experience. Many of these patients suffer from **posttraumatic stress disorder (PTSD)**. PTSD has been described as a condition that

Chart 7-8
GUIDELINES FOR Managing Anxiety

- Listen actively and focus on having the patient discuss personal feelings.
- Use positive remarks and focus on the positive aspects of life in the "here and now."
- Use appropriate touch (with patient permission) to demonstrate support.
- Discuss the importance of safety and the patient's overall sense of well-being.
- Explain all procedures, policies, diagnostic studies, medications, treatments, or protocols for care.
- Explore coping strategies and work with the patient to practice and use them effectively (eg, breathing, progressive relaxation, visualization, imagery).
- Use distraction as indicated to relax and prevent self from being overwhelmed.

generates waves of anxiety, anger, aggression, depression, and suspicion that threaten the person's sense of self and interfere with daily functioning. Specific examples of events that place a person at risk for PTSD are rape, family violence, torture, terrorism, fire, earthquake, and military combat. Patients who have suffered a traumatic event are often frequent users of the health care system by virtue of their extensive injuries, the various treatment modalities that they require, and the overall emotional and physical difficulties experienced.

The physiologic responses noted in people who have been severely traumatized include increased activity of the sympathetic nervous system, increased plasma catecholamine levels, and increased urinary epinephrine and norepinephrine levels. It has been postulated (Gelles, 1997; Gelles & Loseke, 1993) that people with PTSD lose the ability to control their response to stimuli. The resulting excessive arousal can increase overall body metabolism and trigger emotional reactivity. In this situation, the nurse would observe that the patient has difficulty sleeping, has an exaggerated startle response, and is excessively vigilant.

Older people are more susceptible to the physical effects of trauma and the effects of PTSD because of the increased neural inactivation associated with aging. It has also been speculated that when people have a preexisting tendency to become extremely anxious, their vulnerability to PTSD increases (Nursing Research Profile 7-2).

Symptoms of PTSD can occur hours to years after the trauma is experienced. Acute PTSD is defined as the experience of symptoms for less than a 3-month period. Chronic PTSD is defined as the experience of symptoms lasting longer than 3 months. In the case of delayed PTSD, up to 6 months may elapse between the trauma and the manifestation of symptoms (American Psychiatric Association, 2000). For more information see Chart 7-9.

Retired General Romeo D'Allaire (now Senator D'Allaire) was the Forces Commander of United Nations troops in Rwanda. Despite his pleas for more troops to avert disaster, he was ignored by the international community and a genocide occurred in which over 800,000 people were killed. In his book *Shake Hands With the Devil: The Failure of Humanity in Rwanda*, he describes how upon returning to Canada, his mental health deteriorated, culminating in suicide attempts, a diagnosis of posttraumatic stress disorder (PTSD), a medical discharge from the armed forces, and dozens of therapy sessions and medications (D'Allaire, 2003).

NURSING RESEARCH PROFILE 7-2
Posttraumatic Stress Disorder

Hampton, M. R., & Frombach, I. (2000). Women's experience of traumatic stress in cancer treatment. *Health Care of Women International, 21*(1), 67–76.

Purpose
A review of literature revealed that few articles in health care journals acknowledge that women's and men's experiences in the health care setting may often be different. The purpose of this study was to examine gender differences in the prevalence and predictors of cancer-related posttraumatic stress disorder (PTSD) in a group of cancer patients.

Study Sample and Design
A total of 225 consecutive patients going to a local cancer clinic were invited to complete a questionnaire packet. The final sample size included 87 patients (59 women and 28 men). Subjects completed the Impact of Events Scale (to measure PTSD), the Appraisal of Life Threat and Treatment Intensity Scale (to differentiate between trauma related to cancer treatment and cancer diagnosis), Ways of Coping—Cancer Version (to measure coping strategies commonly used by cancer patients), and the Meaning of Illness Scale (to assess the meaning the patients constructed out of their experience and three measures of social support).

Findings
The symptoms of PTSD were significantly higher for women than for men ($p > .05$). Major predictors of PTSD for women were perceived intensity of the cancer treatment, problems with health care professionals, and a cognitive avoidance in their coping style. The only predictor of increased PTSD in men was behavioural avoidance. The women reported significantly higher ($p > .05$) levels of treatment intensity, many more types of treatments and number of treatments, and more difficulties with health care professionals. It was further reported by the women that the interpersonal and relational facets of their illnesses were more stressful and were the most difficult aspects of having cancer. Men indicated that their stress was associated with the work role and loss of finances.

Nursing Implications
Some women find the experience of cancer treatment to be very difficult. The intensity of the treatment may place women at risk for development of PTSD. Overall, women need support from health care professionals, additional control over their treatment, opportunity to tell their stories and concerns, support groups, and access to complementary therapies. Having psychosocial resources available could assist in the prevention of, assessment for, and interventions with patients encountering cancer-related PTSD.

Romeo D'Allaire became the "public face" of PTSD when he was found inebriated on a park bench in Ottawa. He publicly talks about this episode on radio and television to help people understand more about PTSD. He describes how he walked around Ottawa and bought a bottle of scotch. "And I walked to the—to the park, sat on the bench, and I was reliving my mission. The booze was—I mean I was just drinking it like that out of the bottle. And I was just like any other rubby-dub or person who is left homeless, screaming and yelling and crying and drinking. I was screaming for them to kill me."

NURSING IMPLICATIONS

It is often thought that the incidence of PTSD is very low in the overall population; when high-risk groups are studied, however, the results indicate that more than 50% of study participants have

Chart 7-9 • ASSESSMENT

Assessing Physiologic and Psychological Indicators of PTSD

Physiologic Indicators
Dilated pupils
Headaches
Sleep pattern disturbances
Tremors
Elevated blood pressure
Tachycardia or palpitations
Diaphoresis with cold, clammy skin
Hyperventilation
Dyspnea
Smothering or choking sensation
Nausea, vomiting, or diarrhea
Stomach ulcers
Dry mouth
Abdominal pain
Muscle tension or soreness
Exhaustion

Psychological Indicators
Anxiety
Anger
Depression
Fears or phobias
Survivor guilt
Hypervigilance
Nightmares or flashbacks
Intrusive thoughts about the trauma
Impaired memory
Dissociative states
Restlessness or irritability
Strong startle response
Substance abuse
Self-hatred
Feelings of estrangement
Feelings of helplessness, hopelessness, or powerlessness
Lack of interest in life
Inability to concentrate
Difficulty communicating, caring, and expressing love
Problems with relationships
Sexual problems ranging from acting out to impotence
Difficulty with intimacy
Inability to trust
Lack of impulse control
Aggressive, abusive, or violent behaviour, including suicide
Thrill-seeking behaviours

Copel, L. C. (2000). *Nurse's clinical guide: Psychiatric and mental health care* (2nd ed.). Springhouse, PA: Springhouse.

PTSD (McCann & Pearlman, 1990). Therefore, it is important that nurses consider which of their patients are at risk for PTSD and be knowledgeable about the common symptoms associated with it.

The sensitivity and caring of the nurse creates the interpersonal relationship necessary to work with patients who have PTSD. These patients are physically compromised and are struggling emotionally with situations that are outside the realm of normal human experience—situations that violate the commonly held perceptions of human social justice. Treatment of patients with PTSD includes several essential components: establishing a trusting relationship, addressing and working through the trauma experience, and providing education about the coping skills needed for recovery and self-care. The patient's progress can be influenced

by the ability to cope with the various aspects of both the physical and the emotional distress.

Depression

Depression is a common response to health problems and is an often underdiagnosed problem in the patient population. People may become depressed as a result of injury or illness; may be suffering from an earlier loss that is compounded by a new health problem; or they may seek health care for somatic complaints that are bodily manifestations of depression.

Clinical depression is distinguished from everyday feelings of sadness by its duration and severity. Most people occasionally feel down or depressed, but these feelings are short-lived and do not result in impaired functioning. Clinically depressed people usually have had signs of a depressed mood or a decreased interest in pleasurable activities for at least a 2-week period. An obvious impairment in social, occupational, and overall daily functioning occurs in some people. Others function appropriately in their interactions with the outside world by exerting great effort and forcing themselves to mask their distress. Sometimes they are successful at camouflaging their depression for months or years and astonish family members and others when they finally succumb to the problem.

Many people experience depression but seek treatment for somatic complaints. The leading somatic complaints of patients struggling with depression are headache, backache, abdominal pain, fatigue, malaise, anxiety, and decreased desire or problems with sexual functioning (Stuart & Laraia, 2000). These sensations are frequently manifestations of depression. The depression is undiagnosed about half of the time and masquerades as physical health problems (Carson, 1999). People with depression also exhibit poor functioning and high rates of absenteeism from work and school.

Specific symptoms of clinical depression include feelings of sadness, worthlessness, fatigue, and guilt and difficulty concentrating or making decisions. Changes in appetite, weight gain or loss, sleep disturbances, and psychomotor retardation or agitation are also common. Often, patients have recurrent thoughts about death or suicide or have made suicide attempts (American Psychiatric Association, 2000). A diagnosis of clinical depression is made when a person presents with at least five of nine diagnostic criteria for depression. Chart 7-10 lists these criteria (American Psychiatric Association, 2000). Unfortunately, only one of three depressed people is properly diagnosed and appropriately treated.

Chart 7-10
Diagnostic Criteria for Depression Based on the DSM-IV TR

A person experiences at least five out of nine characteristics, with one of the first two symptoms present most of the time.
1. Depressed mood
2. Loss of pleasure or interest
3. Weight gain or loss
4. Sleeping difficulties
5. Psychomotor agitation or retardation
6. Fatigue
7. Feeling worthless
8. Inability to concentrate
9. Thoughts of suicide or death

American Psychiatric Association. (2000). *Diagnostic and statistical manual of mental disorders (DSM IV-TR)* (4th ed.). Washington, DC: Author.

Number of Suicide Deaths 1998					
AGE GROUP					
<15 years	15–24 years	25–44 years	45–64 years	65+ years	TOTAL
46	562	1596	1,038	457	3,699

Suicide deaths account for 2% of all deaths in Canada. This figure is likely an underestimation due to difficulty in determining if the death was intentional, and by use of the term "undetermined." The stigma about suicide may also influence what is indicated on the death certificate. Men have about four times the number of suicides than do women. Men's attempts (often by firearms or hanging) are more often fatal. Women tend to select methods, such as an overdose of pills, where there is a chance of being rescued and resuscitated. For young men (15–24 years), suicide is a major cause of death (26.3% of all deaths). Rates for men were high in those 15 to 44 years old, higher yet in those 70 to 74 years old, with the highest rate in men for those aged 80 years and older (Health Canada, 2002).

Persons of Aboriginal origin have three to six times the rate of suicide as the general population. Teenagers and young adults have the highest rates. Government policies and a history of sending children away from their communities to residential schools have led to conflicting ideas of the value of Aboriginal culture. Contributing factors for suicide include sexual abuse, family violence, substance abuse, poverty, and access to firearms (Health Canada, 2002).

The rates for attempted suicide are very difficult to quantify because most cases are treated in the community. In 1999, women were 1.5 times more likely than men to be hospitalized for a suicide attempt. This held across age groups except that men older than age 70 had higher hospitalization rates. The group with the highest hospitalization rate for attempted suicide was young women between 15 and 19 years of age (Health Canada, 2002).

The teenage years present the challenging developmental tasks of identity formation, acceptance by peers, and independence from family. For some, the loss of relationships and pressure to excel scholastically conflict with family or peers, and a lack of coping skills places teenagers at increased risk for suicide. At the other end of the age continuum are seniors who experience the loss of friends and life partners through illness and death. Seniors see the loss of physical and mental abilities, may have undiagnosed depression, are faced with their own mortality, and are preparing for death. Some make the choice of managing their own death by suicide (Health Canada, 2002).

When patients make statements that are self-deprecating, express feelings of failure, or are convinced that things are hopeless and will not improve, they may be at risk for suicide. Risk factors for suicide include the following:

- Age younger than 20 or older than 45 years, especially older than 65 years
- Gender—women make more attempts, men are more successful
- Dysfunctional family—members have experienced cumulative multiple losses and possess limited coping skills
- Family history of suicide
- Severe depression
- Severe, intractable pain

- Chronic, debilitating medical problems
- Substance abuse
- Severe anxiety
- Overwhelming problems
- Severe alteration in self-esteem or body image
- Lethal suicide plan

NURSING IMPLICATIONS

Because any loss in function, change in role, or alteration in body image is a possible antecedent to depression, nurses in all settings encounter patients who are depressed or who have thought about suicide. Depression is suspected if changes in the patient's thoughts or feelings and a loss of self-esteem are noted. See Chart 7-11 for a list of risk factors for depression. Depression can occur at any age, and it is diagnosed more frequently in women than in men. For elderly patients, the nurse should be aware that decreased mental alertness and withdrawal-type responses may be indicative of depression. Consultation with a psychiatric nurse to assess and differentiate between dementia-like symptoms and depression is often helpful.

For all patients, talking about their fears, frustration, anger, and despair can help alleviate a sense of helplessness and facilitate the process of obtaining the necessary treatment. Helping patients learn to cope effectively with conflict, interpersonal problems, and grief, and encouraging patients to discuss actual and potential losses may hasten their recovery from depression. Patients can also be helped to identify and decrease negative self-talk and unrealistic expectations and shown how negative thinking contributes to depression. Because physical health and self-care activities are adversely affected by depression, nurses should monitor patients for the onset of new problems. All patients with depression should be evaluated to determine whether they would benefit from antidepressant therapy.

In addition to the measures cited previously for helping patients manage depression, research studies indicate a reduction in distress when anxiety and depression are treated with psychoeducational programs, the establishment of support systems, and counselling (Devine & Westlake, 1995). Referrals to psychoeducational programs can be instrumental in helping patients and their families understand depression, treatment options, and coping strategies. (In crisis situations, it is better to refer the patient to a psychiatrist, psychiatric nurse specialist, or crisis centre.) Explaining to patients that depression is a medical illness and not a sign of personal weakness, and that effective treatment will allow them to feel better and stay emotionally healthy, is an important aspect of care (Stuart & Laraia, 2000).

Chart 7-11
Risk Factors for Depression

Family history
Stressful situations
Female gender
Prior episodes of depression
Onset before age 40 years
Medical comorbidity
Past suicide attempts
Lack of support systems
History of physical or sexual abuse
Current substance abuse

Several Canadian nursing research intervention studies on coping skills training have been conducted. These include a randomized trial of a cognitive intervention for acutely ill men who are HIV positive (Côté & Pepler, 2002) and nursing approaches to reduce psychological distress in men and women who were recovering from myocardial infarctions (Cossette, Frasure-Smith, & Lespérance, 2002). Other studies of social support with different patient groups are also of relevance (see Chapter 6).

Substance Abuse

Some people use mood-altering substances in an attempt to cope with life's challenges. A person who abuses substances has an inability to make healthy decisions and to solve problems effectively. Typically, people who abuse substances are unable to identify and implement adaptive behaviours and use illegally obtained drugs, prescribed or over-the-counter medications, and alcohol alone or in combination with other drugs in an ineffective attempt to cope with the pressures, strains, and burdens of life. Over time, physiologic, emotional, cognitive, and behavioural problems develop as a result of continuous substance use. These problems cause distress for the individual, the family, and the community. Some people may respond to personal illness or the illness of a loved one by using substances to decrease emotional pain.

NURSING IMPLICATIONS

Substance abuse is encountered in all clinical settings. Intoxication and withdrawal are two common substance abuse problems. Often, the nurse sees patients who have experienced trauma as a result of inebriation. Other patients who are active substance abusers enter the primary care setting with a diagnosis other than that of substance abuse. Many do not disclose the extent of their substance use. The patient's use of denial or lack of knowledge about the devastating effects of psychoactive substances can be detected by the nurse who performs a substance use assessment (Chart 7-12). In addition, the nurse can incorporate tools into the assessment that enable drug use to be detected. Examples of such instruments are the CAGE Questionnaire (Ewing, 1984), the Michigan Alcohol Screening Test (Selzer, 1971), and the Addiction Severity Index (McLellan, Kushner, Metzger, & Peters, 1992). The CAGE Questions Adapted to Include Drugs (CAGEAID) is presented in Chapter 5, Chart 5-2.

Health professionals are in pivotal positions for identifying a substance abuse problem, instituting treatment protocols, and making follow-up referrals. Because substance abuse severely affects the family, the nurse helps the family members confront the situation, decrease their enabling behaviours, and motivate the person to obtain treatment.

Caring for codependent family members is another nursing priority. A codependent person tends to manifest unhealthy patterns in relationships with others. Codependents struggle with a need to be needed, an urge to control others, and a willingness to remain involved and suffer with a person who has a drug problem.

The family may approach the health care team to help set limits on the dysfunctional behaviour of a person who abuses substances. At these times, a therapeutic intervention is organized for the purpose of confronting the patient about substance use and the need to obtain drug or alcohol treatment. The nurse or other knowledgeable addiction counsellor helps the family present the addicted person with a realistic perspective about the problem, their concerns about and caring for the person, and a specific plan for treatment. This therapeutic intervention works on the premise that honest and caring confrontation can break through the person's denial of the addiction. If the person refuses to participate in the designed plan, the family members define the consequences and state their commitment to follow through with them. This intervention is empowering to the family and usually provides the structure needed to secure treatment.

Even with treatment, however, patients may experience relapse. Nurses work with patients and their families to prevent relapse and to be prepared if relapse occurs. Relapse is considered a part of the illness process and therefore must be viewed and addressed in the same way that chronic illness is treated.

The nurse who is working with a patient and family struggling with an addiction must dispel the myth that addiction is a defect in character or a moral fault. Views on substance abuse vary within our society. A person's background may help determine whether he or she uses drugs, what drugs are used, and when they are used (Copel, 2000). The combination of variables, such as values and beliefs, family and personal norms, spiritual convictions, and conditions of the current social environment, predisposes a person to the possibility of drug use, motivation for treatment, and continual recovery (Copel, 2000). It has also been said that a person's attitude, especially toward alcohol, reflects the overall beliefs and attitudes of that individual's culture (Giger & Davidhizar, 1999).

Loss and Grief

Loss is a part of the life cycle. All people experience loss in the form of change, growth, and transition. The experience of loss is painful, frightening, and lonely, and it triggers an array of emotional responses (Chart 7-13). People may vacillate between denial, shock, disbelief, anger, inertia, intense yearning, loneliness, sadness, loss of control, depression, and spiritual despair (Brewster, 1999).

In addition to normal losses associated with life cycle stages there are the potential losses of health, a body part, self-image, self-esteem, and even one's life. When loss is not acknowledged or there are multiple losses, anxiety, depression, and health problems may occur. Likewise, people with physical health problems, such as diabetes, acquired immunodeficiency syndrome (AIDS), cardiac conditions, gastrointestinal disorders, disabilities, and neurologic impairments, tend to respond to these illnesses with feelings of **grief**.

People grieve in different ways, and there is no time line for completing the grief process. The time of grieving often depends

---

Chart 7-12 • ASSESSMENT

Assessing Substance Abuse

- Past and recurrent use of the substance
- Patient's view of substance use as a problem
- Age when first used and last used substance
- Length and duration of use of substance
- Preferred method of use of substance
- Amount of substance used
- How substance is procured
- Effect of or reaction to substance
- All attempts to cease or decrease substance use

Chart 7-13 • ASSESSMENT

Assessing Signs and Symptoms of Grieving

Physiologic Signs and Symptoms
Heart rate changes
Blood pressure alterations
Gastrointestinal disturbances
Chest discomfort
Shortness of breath
Weakness
Appetite changes
Sleep problems
Vague, but distressing, physical symptoms

Emotional Symptoms
Sadness
Depression
Anger
Social withdrawal
Loneliness
Apathy
Longing for who or what was lost
Blaming of self or others
Questioning of beliefs

Behavioural Symptoms
Slow movements
Forgetfulness
Purposeless activity
Crying
Sighing
Lack of interest
Easily distracted from tasks

Chart 7-14   Caring for the Bereaved

- Have contact physically (with the patient's permission) and emotionally with the person.
- Assess where the person is in the grieving process.
- Demonstrate genuine compassion and caring.
- Give permission to grieve and normalize the grieving process.
- Mention the loss or the deceased person's name.
- Encourage the person to talk about the relationship he or she had with the deceased person.
- Understand that people need to talk about the events and feelings around the death and will repeat themselves.
- Tell the person to expect mood swings, pain, and various life changes.
- Focus on clarifying and using coping skills.
- Allow the person to take a break from grieving and focus on self-care.
- Encourage sources of comfort such as religion or nature.
- Identify secondary losses and unfinished business.
- Acknowledge that there will be eventual recovery.
- Discuss the anniversary phenomenon.
- Encourage medical or psychiatric care as needed.

---

on the significance of the loss, the length of time the person was known and loved, the anticipation of or preparation for the loss, the person's emotional stability and maturity, and the person's coping ability (Arnold & Boggs, 1999).

Regardless of the duration of the grieving process, there are two basic goals: (1) healing the self, and (2) recovering from the loss. Other factors that influence grieving are the type of loss, life experiences with various changes and transitions, religious beliefs, cultural background, and personality type (Kemp, 2000). Some patients may resort to abuse of prescription medications, illegal drugs, or alcohol if they find it difficult to cope with the loss; the grief process is then complicated by the use of addictive substances.

NURSING IMPLICATIONS

Nurses identify patients and family members who are grieving and work with them to accomplish the four major tasks of the grief process: (1) acceptance of the loss, (2) acknowledgment of the intensity of the pain, (3) adaptation to life after the loss, and (4) cultivation of new relationships and activities (Worden, 1982). Chart 7-14 outlines nursing care activities useful for those who are bereaved.

Another responsibility of the nurse is to assess and differentiate between grief and depression by knowing the common thoughts, feelings, physical or bodily reactions, and behaviours associated with grief compared with depression (see Chart 7-14). The physical response to grief includes the sensation of somatic distress, a tightness in the throat followed by a choking sensation or shortness of breath, the need to sigh, an empty feeling inside

the abdomen, lack of muscle power, and intense disabling distress. Grief can further debilitate an already compromised patient and can have a strong impact on family functioning.

Death and Dying

Coping with death, one's own or a loved one's, is considered the ultimate challenge. The idea of death is threatening and anxiety-provoking to many people. Kubler-Ross (1975, p. 1) stated, "The key to the question of death unlocks the door of life. . . . For those who seek to understand it, death is a highly creative force." Common fears of dying people are fear of the unknown, pain, suffering, loneliness, loss of the body, and loss of personal control.

In recent years, the process of dying has changed as advances have been made in the care of chronically and terminally ill patients. Technological innovations and modern therapeutic treatments have prolonged the life span, and many deaths are now the result of chronic illnesses that result in physiologic deterioration and subsequent multisystem failure.

Preparation for an impending death can precipitate the experience of anticipatory grieving. Although anticipatory grief can have positive effects on later grief, this does not hold true for all people. For some family members, anticipatory grief is seen as a risk factor for poor early **bereavement** adjustment (Levy, 1991). The nurse must be aware of the uniqueness and individuality inherent in the grieving process and work to meet the needs of those involved in the best way possible.

DEATH AND DYING FRAMEWORKS

Various frameworks for understanding the concept of grief and the stages of death and dying may be useful to the nurse. The stages of bereavement described by Bowlby (1961) are protest, disorganization, and reorganization. Kubler-Ross (1975) conceptualized five stages of grieving: denial, anger, bargaining, depression, and acceptance. Often, the dying person and the survivors do not experience these responses in an orderly or linear fashion;

rather, there is random movement between all the stages for differing periods of time. Another model for successful grieving, proposed by Engel (1964), is shock and disbelief, development of awareness, and restitution. The themes common to almost all models of grieving are periods of avoidance, confrontation, and acceptance (Cooley, 1992).

Another framework for understanding the individuality of the dying process is provided by the "patterns of living while dying" described by Martocchio (1982). There are four identified patterns of living based on the clinical trajectories of dying people. The first is referred to as peaks and valleys or periods of hope and periods of depression. Despite the hopeful times, there is still an overall movement toward decline and death. The second pattern is one described as distinct but descending plateaus. This course also reflects a downward trend with progressive debilitation and eventual death. The third pattern is a clear downward slope with many physiologic parameters indicating that death is imminent. This pattern is often observed in the critical care unit when people and families have no time to prepare for the death. The last pattern is a downward slant that reveals a crisis event, such as a severe cerebral hemorrhage with almost no hope of recovery. Often, a patient in this pattern is being maintained on life support systems. The nurse should recognize that a person may experience one or more of these living–dying patterns.

NURSING IMPLICATIONS

Nursing care involves providing comfort, maintaining safety, addressing physical and emotional needs, and teaching coping strategies to terminally ill patients and their families. More than ever, the nurse must explain what is happening to the patient and the family and be a confidante who listens to them talk about dying. Hospice care, attention to family and individual psychosocial issues, and symptom and pain management are all part of the nurse's responsibilities. The nurse must also be concerned with ethical considerations and quality-of-life issues that affect dying people. Of utmost importance to the patient is assistance with the transition from living to dying, maintaining and sustaining relationships, finishing well with the family, and accomplishing what needs to be said and done.

The nurse is the consistent link in promoting understanding of the patient's disease and the dying process and in making the event more manageable for the patient and family, who will require assistance to resolve problems and proceed through the grief work. Retaining as much control as possible during the process of dying allows the patient and family to make as much sense as possible out of an overwhelming situation. In the hospital, in long-term care facilities, and in home settings, the nurse explores choices and end-of-life decisions with the patient and family. Referrals to home care and hospice services, as well as specific referrals appropriate for the management of the situation, are initiated. The nurse is also an advocate for the dying person and works to uphold that person's rights. An advance directive allows the patient to exercise the right to have a "good" death or to die with dignity. Additional information about end-of-life care is presented in Chapter 17.

Spirituality and Spiritual Distress

Spirituality is defined as connectedness with self, others, a life force, or God that allows people to experience self-transcendence and find meaning in life. Spirituality helps people discover a pur-

pose in life, understand the vicissitudes of life, and develop their relationship with God or a Higher Power. Within the framework of spirituality, a person discovers truths about the self, about the world, and about concepts such as love, compassion, wisdom, honesty, commitment, imagination, reverence, and morality. Often, spiritual behaviour is expressed through sacrifice, self-discipline, and spending time in activities that focus on the inner self or the soul. Religion and nature are two vehicles that people use to connect themselves with God or a Higher Power; however, bonds to religious institutions, beliefs, or dogma are not required to experience the spiritual sense of self. **Faith,** considered the foundation of spirituality, is a belief in something that a person cannot see (Carson, 1999). The spiritual part of a person views life as a mystery that unfolds over the lifetime, encompassing questions about meaning, hope, relatedness to God, acceptance or forgiveness, and transcendence (Byrd, 1999; Sheldon, 2000; Sussman, Nezami, & Mishra, 1997).

A strong sense of spirituality or religious faith can have a positive impact on health (Dunn & Horgas, 2000; Kendrick & Robinson, 2000; Matthews & Larson, 1995). Spirituality is also a component of hope, and, especially during chronic, serious, or terminal illness, patients and their families often find comfort and emotional strength in their religious traditions or spiritual beliefs. At other times, illness and loss can cause a loss of faith or meaning in life and a spiritual crisis. The nursing diagnosis of spiritual distress is applicable to those who have a disturbance in the belief or value system that provides strength, hope, and meaning in life.

NURSING IMPLICATIONS

Spiritually distressed patients (or family members) may show despair, discouragement, ambivalence, detachment, anger, resentment, or fear. They may question the meaning of suffering, life, and death, and express a sense of emptiness. The nurse assesses spiritual strength by inquiring about the person's sense of spiritual well-being, hope, and peacefulness. Have spiritual beliefs and values changed in response to illness or loss? The nurse assesses current and past participation in religious or spiritual practices and notes the patient's response to questions about spiritual needs—grief, anger, guilt, depression, doubt, anxiety, or calmness—to help determine the patient's need for spiritual care. Another simple assessment technique is to inquire about the patient's and family's desire for spiritual support.

For nurses to provide spiritual care, they must be open to being present and supportive when patients experience doubt, fearfulness, suffering, despair, or other difficult psychological states of being. Interventions that foster spiritual growth or reconciliation include being fully present; listening actively; conveying a sense of caring, respect, and acceptance; using therapeutic communication techniques to encourage expression; suggesting the use of prayer, meditation, or imagery; and facilitating contact with spiritual leaders or performance of spiritual rituals (Sumner, 1998; Sussman, 2000).

Patients with serious, chronic, or terminal illnesses face physical and emotional losses that threaten their spiritual integrity. During acute and chronic illness, rehabilitation, or the dying process, spiritual support can stimulate patients to regain or strengthen their connections with their inner selves, their loved ones, and their God or Higher Power to transcend suffering and find meaning. Nurses can alleviate distress and suffering and enhance wellness by meeting their patients' spiritual needs.

Critical Thinking Exercises

1. A 55-year old man tells the nurse that he is not going to be a part of a clinical drug investigation. He states, "I may not get the drug. I may end up with a placebo. I'm going to try some alternative methods. I feel like traditional medicine is letting me down." How does the nurse handle this situation? What assessment data need to be collected and discussed with other members of the health care team?

2. The nurse is working with a family to develop therapeutic interventions for a family member who has a cocaine and alcohol addiction problem. One family member tells the nurse she will never be able to support the plan decided on by the rest of the family. How would you approach this person? What strategies would be useful for this person and for the entire family?

3. The family of a man who is dying from lung cancer tells the hospice nurse that they are overwhelmed by the hopelessness of their father's situation. What can the nurse do to provide guidance and find hope within terminal illness? How does the nurse assist this family to meet their emotional, social, and spiritual needs?

REFERENCES AND SELECTED READINGS
Books

Aiken, L. (2000). *Dying, death, and bereavement* (4th ed.). Mahwah, NJ: Lawrence Erlbaum.

American Psychiatric Association. (2000). *Diagnostic and statistical manual of mental disorders (DSM IV)* (4th ed.). Washington, DC: Author.

Arnold, E., & Boggs, K. (1999). *Interpersonal relationships: Professional communication skills for nurses* (3rd ed.). Philadelphia: W. B. Saunders.

Barry, P. D. (1998). *Mental health and mental illness* (6th ed.). Philadelphia: Lippincott-Raven.

Bowlby, J. (1961). *Attachment and loss* (Vol. 1). New York: Basic Books.

Boyd-Franklin, N., & Bry, B. H. (2001). *Reaching out in family therapy.* New York: Guilford Press.

Brewster, S. (1999). *To be an anchor in the storm: A guide for families and friends.* New York: Sealpress.

Burr, W., Klein, S., Burr, R., Doxey, C., Haeker, B., Holman, T., Martin, P., McClure, R., Parrish, S., Stuart, D., Taylor, A., & White, M. (1994). *Reexamining family stress: New theory and research.* Thousand Oaks, CA: Sage.

Burr, W., et al. (1993). *Family science.* Pacific Grove, CA: Brooks/Cole.

Carson, V. B. (1999). *Mental health nursing: The nurse-patient journey* (2nd ed.). St. Louis, MO: Mosby.

Chandler, F. (Ed.). (2000). *Herbs: Everyday reference for health professionals.* Ottawa: Canadian Pharmacists' Association & Canadian Medical Association.

Clark, M. B., & Olson, J. K. (2000). *Nursing within a faith community: Promoting health in times of transition.* Thousand Oaks, CA: Sage Publications.

Copel, L. C. (2000). *Nurse's clinical guide: Psychiatric and mental health care* (2nd ed.). Springhouse, PA: Springhouse.

D'Allaire, R. (2003). *Shake hands with the devil: The failure of humanity in Rwanda.* Toronto: Random House of Canada.

Feldman, R. (2000). *Development across the life span* (2nd ed.). Upper Saddle River, NJ: Prentice Hall.

Friedman, M. M. (1998). *Family nursing: Research, theory, and practice* (4th ed.). Stamford, CT: Appleton & Lange.

Gelles, J. (1997). *Intimate violence in families.* Thousands Oaks, CA: Sage.

Gelles, J., & Loseke, D. (Eds.) (1993). *Current controversies on family violence.* Newbury Park, CA: Sage.

Giger, J. N., & Davidhizar, R. E. (1999). *Transcultural nursing: Assessment and intervention* (3rd ed.). St. Louis: C. V. Mosby.

Health Canada. (2002). Suicidal behaviour. In *A report on mental illnesses in Canada.* Ottawa: Author. Available at www.phac-aspc.gc.ca/publicat/miic-mmac/chap_7_e.html. Retrieved June 21, 2005.

Keegan, L. (2001). *Healing with complementary and alternative therapies.* Albany, NY: Delmar.

Kemp, C. (2000). *Terminal illness.* Philadelphia: Lippincott Williams & Wilkins.

Kubler-Ross, E. (1975). *Death: The final stage of growth.* Englewood Cliffs, NJ: Prentice-Hall.

Kuhn, M. A. (1999). *Complementary therapies for health care providers.* Philadelphia, Lippincott Williams & Wilkins.

Luckmann, J. (1999). *Transcultural communication in nursing.* Albany, NY: Delmar.

Martocchio, B. C. (1982). *Living while dying.* Bowie, MD: Robert J. Brady.

Matthews, D. A., & Larson, D. B. (1995). *The faith factor: An annotated bibliography of clinical research on spiritual subjects* (Vol. 3). Rockville, MD: National Institute for Health Care Research.

McCann, I. J., & Pearlman, L. A. (1990). *Psychological trauma and the adult survivor.* New York: Brunner/Mazel.

McDowell, D. M., & Spitz, H. I. (1999). *Substance abuse: From principles to practice.* Philadelphia: Brunner/Mazel.

Murray, R. B., & Zentner, J. P. (2001). *Health assessment and promotion strategies through the life span* (7th ed.). Stamford, CT: Appleton & Lange.

Nowinski, J. K. (1998). *Family recovery and substance abuse.* Thousand Oaks, CA: Sage.

Ramsay, C., Walker, M., & Alexander, J. (1999). *Alternative medicine in Canada: Use and public attitudes.* Public Policy Sources paper No. 21. Vancouver: Fraser Institute.

Rice, F. P. (2001). *Human development: A lifespan approach* (4th ed.). Upper Saddle River, NJ: Prentice Hall.

Rice, V. H. (Ed.). (2000). *Handbook of stress, coping, and health: Implications for nursing research, theory, and practice.* Thousand Oaks, CA: Sage.

Roach, S. S., & Nieto, B. C. (1998). *Healing and the grief process.* Albany, NY: Delmar.

Simmie, S., & Nunes, J. (2000). *The last taboo: A survival guide to mental health care in Canada.* Toronto: McClelland & Stewart.

Stanhope, M., & Lancaster, J. (1999). *Community and public health nursing* (7th ed.). St. Louis: C. V. Mosby.

Stewart, M. J. (1993). *Integrating social support in nursing.* Newberry Park, CA: Sage.

Stewart, M. J. (Ed.). (1995). *Community nursing: Promoting Canadians' health* (2nd ed.). Toronto: W. B. Saunders.

Stewart, M. J. (Ed.). (2000). *Chronic conditions and caregiving in Canada: Social support strategies.* Toronto: University of Toronto Press.

Stewart, M. J., & Langille, L. (2000). A framework for social support assessment and intervention in the context of chronic conditions and caregiving. In M. J. Stewart (Ed.), *Chronic conditions and caregiving in Canada: Social support strategies* (pp. 3–28). Toronto: University of Toronto Press.

Stuart, G. W., & Laraia, M. T. (2000). *Principles and practice of psychiatric nursing* (7th ed.). St. Louis: C. V. Mosby.

Tucker, J. A., Donovan, D. M., & Marlatt, G. A. (2001). *Changing additive behavior.* NY: Guilford.

U.S. Department of Health & Human Services (1993). *Clinical practice guidelines Agency for Health Care Policy and Research: Number 5. Depression in clinical care: Vol. 1. Detection and diagnosis.* Rockville, MD: U.S. Government Printing Office.

U.S. Department of Health & Human Services (1993). *Clinical practice guidelines Agency for Health Care Policy and Research: Number 5. Depression in primary care: Vol. 2. Treatment of major depression.* Rockville, MD: U.S. Government Printing Office.

U.S. Department of Health & Human Services, Public Health Service, Agency for Health Care Policy and Research. (1993). *Depression in* primary care: Vol. 1. Detection and diagnosis. Clinical Practice Guideline. (AHCPR Publication No. 93-0550). Rockville, MD: U.S. Government Printing Office.

U.S. Department of Health & Human Services, Public Health Service, Agency for Health Care Policy and Research. (1993) *Depression in primary care: Vol. 2, Treatment of major depression.* Clinical Practice Guideline. (AHCPR Publication No. 93-0551). Rockville, MD: U.S. Government Printing Office.

Worden, W. (1982). *Grief counseling and grief therapy: A handbook for the mental health practitioner.* New York: Springer Publishing.

Wright, L. M., & Leahey, M. (2000). *Nurses and families: A guide to family assessment and intervention.* Philadelphia, PA: Davis.

Journals

Asterisks indicate nursing research articles.

General

Canadian Mental Health Association. (2004). *Working together toward a pan-Canadian strategy on mental health/mental illness for the people of Canada.* Available at: http://www.cmha.ca/bins/content_page.asp?cid=5-221. Retrieved June 6, 2005.

Cohen, S., & Herbert, T. (1996). Health psychology: Psychological factors and physical disease from the perspective of human psychoneuroimmunology. *Annual Review of Psychology, 47,* 113–142.

Devine, E. C., & Westlake, S. K. (1995). The effects of psychoeducational care provided to adults with cancer: Metaanalysis of 116 studies. *Oncology Nursing Forum, 22*(9), 1369–1376.

Eisenberg, D., Kessler, R., Foster, C., Norlock, F., Calkins, D., & Delbanco, T. (1993). Unconventional medicine in the United States: Prevalence, costs, and patterns of use. *New England Journal of Medicine, 328,* 246–252.

Kiecolt-Glaser, J. K., McGuire, L., Robles, T. F., & Glaser, R. (2002). Emotions, morbidity, and mortality: New perspectives from psychoneuroimmunology. *Annual Review of Psychology, 53*(1), 83–107.

Alternative Therapies

Boutin, P. D., Buchwald, D., Robinson, L., & Collier, A. C. (2000). Use of alternative and complementary therapies among outpatients and physicians at a municipal hospital. *Journal of Alternative and Complementary Medicine, 6*(4), 353–343.

Canada Health Monitor. (1997). Survey No. 16, June-July.

Canadian Medical Association. (2000). *Natural health products: Ensuring safety, quality and efficacy. Response to the Office of Natural Health Products (ONHP) regarding its preliminary consultation on a proposed regulatory framework for natural health products.* Available at: http://www.cma.ca/index.cfm/ci_id/3103/la_id/1.htm. Retrieved June 6, 2005.

Canadian Nurses Association. (1999). Complementary therapies–Finding the right balance. *Nursing Now, 6,* 1–4. Available at http://cna-aiic.ca/CNA/documents/pdf/publications/ComplimentaryTherapies_July1999_e.pdf. Retrieved June 6, 2005.

Druss, B. G., & Rosenheck, R. A. (1999). Association between use of unconventional therapies and conventional medical services. *Journal of the American Medical Association, 282,* 651–656.

Joudrey, R., & Gough, J. (2003). Student nurses' use and perceptions of alternative medicine: An exploratory study. *Canadian Journal of Nursing Research, 35*(3), 80–93.

McClennon-Leong, J., & Kerr, J. R. (1999). Alternative health care options in Canada. *Canadian Nurse, 95*(10), 26–28, 30.

PricewaterhouseCoopers. (1999). *HealthInsider: National public opinion on health care, 2.*

Sparber, A., Wootton, J. C., Bauer, L., Curt, G., Eisenberg, D. M., Levin, T., & Steinberg, S. M. (2000). Use of complementary medicine by adult patients participating in HIV/AIDS clinical trials. *Journal of Alternative and Complementary Medicine, 6*(5), 415–422.

Wolsho, P., Ware, L., Kutner, J., Lin, C., Albertson, G., Cyran, L., Schilling, L., & Anderson, R. J. (2000). Alternative/complementary medicine: Wider usage than generally appreciated. *Journal of Alternative and Complementary Medicine, 6*(4), 321–326.

Wynia, M. K., Eisenberg, D. M., & Wilson, I. B. (1999). Physician-patient communication about complementary and alternative medical therapies: A survey of physicians caring for patients with human immunodeficiency virus infection. *Journal of Alternative and Complementary Medicine, 5*(5), 447–456.

Coping

Backer, J. H. (2000). Stressors, social support, and coping and health dysfunction in individuals with Parkinson's disease. *Journal of Gerontological Nursing, 26*(11), 6–16.

Cossette, S., Frasure-Smith, N., & Lespérance, F. (2002). Nursing approaches to reducing psychological distress in men and women recovering from myocardial infarction. *International Journal of Nursing Studies, 39*(5), 479–494.

Côté, J. K., & Pepler, C. (2002). A randomized trial of a cognitive coping intervention for acutely ill HIV-positive men. *Nursing Research, 51*(4), 237–244.

Dzurec, L. C. (2000). Fatigue and relatedness in inordinately tired women. *Journal of Gerontological Nursing, 32*(4), 339–345.

Finfgeld-Connett, D. (2005). Clarification of social support. *Journal of Nursing Scholarship,* First Quarter 2005, 4–9.

King, K. B., Zewic, J. J., Kimble, L. P., & Rowe, M. A. (1998). Optimism, coping, and long-term recovery from coronary artery surgery in women. *Research in Nursing & Health, 21*(1), 15–26.

Morse, S. R., & Fife, B. (1998). Coping with a partner's cancer: Adjustment at four stages of the illness trajectory. *Oncology Nursing Forum, 25*(4), 751–760.

Schnoll, R. A., Harlow, L. L., & Brower, L. (2000). Spirituality, demographic and disease factors, and adjustment to cancer. *Cancer Practice: A Multidisciplinary Journal of Cancer Care, 8*(6), 298–304.

Twibell, R. S. (1998). Family coping during critical illness. *Dimensions in Critical Care Nursing, 17*(2), 100–112.

Depression

Martin, A. C. (2000). Major depressive illness in women: Assessment and treatment in the primary care setting. *Nurse Practitioner Forum, 11*(3), 179–186.

National Institute of Mental Health. (1992). *Depression awareness, recognition, treatment fact sheet.* DHHS Publication No. [ADM] 92-1680. Rockville, MD: Government Printing Office.

Rasmussen, J. (2000). Treating depression: The continuing challenge of achieving long term recovery. *Mental Health Care and Learning Disabilities, 3*(9), 295–308.

Rogers, J. C., & Holm, M. B. (2000). Daily living skills and habits of older women with depression. *Occupational Therapy Journal of Research, 20*(Suppl. 1), 68S–85S.

Grief, Death, and Dying

Conrad, N. L. (1985). Spiritual support for the dying. *Nursing Clinics of North America, 20*(2), 415–425.

Cooley, M. E. (1992). Bereavement care: A role for nurses. *Cancer Nursing, 15*(2), 125–129.

Fauri, D. P., Ettner, B., & Kovacs, P. T. (2000). Bereavement services in acute care settings. *Death Studies, 24*(1), 51–64.

Engel, G. (1964). Grief and grieving. *American Journal of Nursing, 64*(7), 93–96.

Hallgrinsdottir, E. M. (2000). Accident and emergency nurses' perceptions of caring for families. *Journal of Clinical Nursing, 9*(4), 611–619.

Katz, J., Sedell, M., & Komaromy, C. (2000). Death in homes: Bereavement needs of residents, relatives, and staff. *International Journal of Palliative Nursing, 6*(6), 274–279.

Levy, L. H. (1991). Anticipatory grief: Its measurement and proposed reconceptualization. *Hospice Journal, 7*(4), 1–28.

Nishimoto, P. (1996). Venturing into the unknown: Cultural beliefs about death and dying. *Oncology Nursing Forum, 23*(6), 889–894.

Posttraumatic Stress Disorder

Ellensweig-Tepper, D. (2000). Trauma group therapy for the adolescent female client. *Journal of Child and Adolescent Psychiatric Nursing, 13*(1), 17–28.

McGrath, P. (1999). Posttraumatic stress and the experience of cancer: A literature review. *Journal of Rehabilitation, 65*(3), 17–23.

Miller, J. L. (2000). Post-traumatic stress disorder in primary care. *Journal of the American Academy of Nurse Practitioners, 12*(11), 475–485.

Spirituality

Buijs, R., & Olson, J. (2001). Parish nurses influencing determinants of health. *Journal of Community Health Nursing, 18*(1), 13–23.

Byrd, E. K. (1999). Spiritual care matters: Application of helping theories and faith in the lives of persons with disabilities. *Journal of Religion, Disability, and Health, 3*(1), 3–13.

Chandler, E. (1999). Spirituality. *Hospice Journal, 14*(3/40), 63–74.

Clark, M. B., & Olson, J. K. (2001). A partnership that matters: Collaborative interdisciplinary ministry among parish nurses and faith group leaders. *Journal of Health Care Chaplaincy, 11*(2), 27–40.

Dunn, K. S., & Horgas, A. L. (2000). The prevalence of prayer as a spiritual self-care modality in elders. *Journal of Holistic Nursing, 18*(4), 337–351.

Dyson, J., Cobb, M. & Forman, D. (1997). The meaning of spirituality: A literature review. *Journal of Advanced Nursing, 26*(6), 1183–1188.

Haln, M. A., Myers, R. N., & Bennetts, P. (2000). Providing spiritual care to cardiac patients: Assessment and implications for practice. *Critical Care Nurse, 20*(4), 54–56, 58, 64, 66–72.

Havranek, J. E. (1999). The role of spirituality in the rehabilitation process. *Journal of Religion, Disability, and Health, 3*(2), 15–35.

*Humphreys, J. (2000). Spirituality and distress in sheltered battered women. *Scholarly Inquiry for Nursing Practice, 14*(2), 115–141.

Kendrick, K. D., & Robinson, S. (2000). Spirituality: Its relevance and purpose for clinical nursing in a new millennium. *Journal of Clinical Nursing, 9*(5), 701–705.

Langer, N. (2000). The importance of spirituality in later life. *Gerontology and Geriatric Education, 20*(3), 41–50.

Olson, J. K., Simington, J. A., & Clark, M. B. (1998). Educating parish nurses. *Canadian Nurse, 94*(8), 40–44.

Sheldon, T. E. (2000). Spirituality as a part of nursing. *Journal of Hospice and Palliative Care, 2*(3), 101–108.

Sherwood, G. D. (2000). The power of nurse-client encounters interpreting spiritual themes. *Journal of Holistic Nursing, 18*(2), 159–175.

Simington, J., & Olson, J. (1995). Parish nursing in Alberta. *AARN Newsletter, 51*(8), 16.

Simington, J., Olson, J., & Douglass, L. (1996). *Promoting well-being within a parish. Canadian Nurse, 92*(1), 20–24.

Sumner, C. H. (1998). Recognizing and responding to spiritual distress. *American Journal of Nursing, 98*(1), 26–30.

Sussman, D. (2000). A spiritual approach: Nurses and chaplains team up to provide pastoral care. *Healthweek, 5*(17), 12.

Sussman, S., Nezami, E., & Mishra, S. (1997). On operationalizing spiritual experience for health promotion research and practice. *Alternative Therapies in Clinical Practice, 4*(4), 120–125.

Treloar, L. L. (2000). Integration of spirituality into health care practice by nurse practitioners. *Journal of American Academy of Nurse Practitioners, 12*(7), 280–285.

Substance Abuse

Ewing, J. A. (1984). Detecting alcoholism: The CAGE questionnaire. *Journal of American Medical Association, 252*(14), 1906.

McLellan, A. T., Kushner, H., Metzger, D., & Peters, R. (1992). The fifth edition of the addiction severity index. *Journal of Substance Abuse Treatment, 9*(3), 199–213.

Sedlak, C. A., Dokery, M. O., Estok, P. J., & Zeller, R. A. (2000). Alcohol use in women 65 years of age and older. *Health Care of Women International, 21*(7), 567–581.

Selzer, M. L. (1971). The Michigan alcoholism screening test: The quest for a new diagnostic instrument. *American Journal of Psychiatry, 127,* 1653–1658.

Sturn, R., & Sherbourne, C. D. (2000). Data points: Managed care and unmet need for mental health and substance abuse care in 1998. *Psychiatric Services, 51*(2), 177.

RESOURCES AND WEBSITES

Agencies
Canadian Institutes of Health Research–Institute of Neurosciences, Mental Health and Addiction; http://www.cihr-irsc.gc.ca/institutes/inmha.

Centers for Disease Control and Prevention; http://www.cdc.gov.

Health Canada, Mental Health; http://www.hc-sc.gc.ca/hppb/mental health/mhp/index.html; http://www.hc-sc.gc.ca/english/lifestyles/mental_health.html.

Aging
Alzheimer Society of Canada; http://www.alzheimer.ca.

Canadian Association on Gerontology; http://www.cagacg.ca/whoweare/200_e.php.

Public Health Agency of Canada; http://www.phac-aspc.gc.ca/seniors-aines/index_pages/publications_e.htm#stats.

Anxiety
Anxiety Disorders Association of Canada; http://www.anxietycanada.ca.

Bereavement
The Compassionate Friends of Canada, Inc.; http://www.tcfcanada.net.

Eating Disorders
The National Eating Disorder Information Centre; http://www.nedic.ca.

Mental Health
Canadian Association for the Mentally Ill; http://www.cami.org.

Canadian Health Network; http://www.canadian-health-network.ca/1mental_health.html.

The Canadian Mental Health Association, 8 King Street East, Suite 810, Toronto, ON M5C 1B5; 416-484-7750; fax: 416-484-4617; e-mail: info@cmha.ca; http://www.cmha.ca; some pages from this website of particular interest are: *Mental Health Priorities of the Voluntary Sector*; http://www.cmha.ca/bins/content_page.asp?cid=2-49&lang=1; *Working Together Toward a Pan-Canadian Strategy on Mental Health/Mental Illness for the People of Canada*; http://www.cmha.ca/bins/content_page.asp?cid=5-221; *Your Education–Your Future* (a comprehensive Canadian guide for college and university students with psychiatric disabilities); http://www.cmha.ca/youreducation/.

Canadian Psychiatric Association; http://www.cpa-apc.org.

Canadian Psychiatric Research Foundation; http://www.cprf.ca.

Canadian Psychological Association; http://www.cpa.ca.

National Network for Mental Health; http://www.nnmh.ca.

Schizophrenia Society of Canada; http://www.schizophrenia.ca.

The Mood Disorders Society of Canada; http://www.mooddisorders canada.ca.

Posttraumatic Stress Disorder
Veteran Affairs Canada; http://www.vac-acc.gc.ca/clients/sub.cfm?source=forces/stress.

Substance Abuse
Centre for Addiction and Mental Health; http://www.camh.net.

Alcoholics Anonymous; http://www.alcoholics-anonymous.org.

Al-Anon/Alateen; http://www.al-anon.org.

Canadian Assembly of Narcotics Anonymous; http://www.canaacna.org.

Cocaine Anonymous (CA) in Canada; http://www.theagapecenter.com/CA/Canada.htm.

Perspectives in Transcultural Nursing

Adapted by Pauline Paul

LEARNING OBJECTIVES

On completion of this chapter, the learner will be able to:

1. Apply transcultural nursing principles, concepts, and theories when providing nursing care to patients (individuals, families, groups, and communities).

2. Develop strategies for planning, providing, and evaluating culturally competent nursing care for patients from diverse backgrounds.

3. Critically analyze the influence of culture on nursing care decisions and actions for patients.

4. Identify key components of cultural assessment for self and patients.

*I*n the health care delivery system, as in society, the nurse interacts with people of similar and diverse cultural backgrounds. People may have similar or different frames of reference and varied preferences regarding their health and health care needs. Acknowledging and adapting to the cultural needs of the patient and significant others is an important component of nursing care. To plan and deliver culturally competent care, the nurse must understand the definitions of culture and cultural competence and the various aspects of culture that should be explored for each patient.

Definitions of Culture

The concept of culture and its relationship to the health care beliefs and practices of patients and their families and friends provide the foundation for transcultural nursing. This awareness of culture in the delivery of nursing care has been described in different ways, including respect for cultural diversity, culturally sensitive or comprehensive care, and culturally competent or appropriate nursing care (American Association of Colleges of Nursing, 1996; Giger & Davidhizar, 1999; Spector, 2000), or culturally congruent nursing care (Leininger, 2001). Two commonly discussed concepts are cultural diversity and culturally competent care.

The term *culture* was initially defined by the British anthropologist Sir Edward Tylor in 1871 as the knowledge, belief, art, morals, laws, customs, and any other capabilities and habits acquired by humans as members of society. During the past century, and especially during recent decades, hundreds of definitions of culture have been offered that integrate the themes stated by Tylor and the themes of ethnic variations of a population based on race, nationality, religion, language, physical characteristics, and geography (Spector, 2000). To fully appreciate the impact of culture, aspects such as disabilities, gender, social class, physical appearance (eg, weight, height), ideologies (political views), or sexual orientation must be integrated into the definition of culture as well (Gooden, Porter, Gonzalez, & Mims, 2001).

Madeleine Leininger, founder of the specialty called transcultural nursing, indicates that culture involves learned and transmitted knowledge about values, beliefs, rules of behaviour, and lifestyle practices that guide designated groups in their thinking and actions in patterned ways (2001). Giger and Davidhizar (1999) state that transcultural nursing is a practice based on the differences and similarities between cultures in relation to health, health care, and illness, with consideration of patient values, beliefs, and practices. Further, culture develops over time as a result of "imprinting the mind through social and religious structures and intellectual and artistic manifestations" (p. 3).

The concept of ethnic culture has four basic characteristics:

- It is learned from birth through language and socialization.
- It is shared by members of the same cultural group, and it includes an internal sense and external perception of distinctiveness.
- It is influenced by specific conditions related to environmental and technical factors and to the availability of resources.
- It is dynamic and ever-changing.

With the exception of the first characteristic, culture related to age, physical appearance, lifestyle, and other less frequently acknowledged aspects also adhere to the above characteristics.

Cultural diversity has also been defined in a number of ways. Often, skin colour, religion, and geographic area are the only elements used to identify diversity, with ethnic minorities being considered the primary sources of cultural diversity. As stated earlier, however, there are several other possible sources of cultural diversity. In addition, to truly acknowledge the cultural differences that may influence health care delivery, the nurse must recognize the influence of his or her own culture and cultural heritage (Krumberger, 2000).

Culturally competent nursing care has been defined as effective, individualized care that considers cultural values, is culturally aware and sensitive, and incorporates cultural skills (Hunt, 2000; Krumberger, 2000; Wilkinson, 2001). Culturally competent care is a dynamic process that requires comprehensive knowledge of culture-specific information and an awareness of, and sensitivity to, the effect that culture has on the care situation. It requires the nurse to integrate cultural knowledge, awareness of his or her own cultural perspective, and the patient's cultural perspectives into the plan of care (Giger & Davidhizar, 1999). Exploring one's own cultural beliefs and how they might conflict with the beliefs of the patients being cared for is a first step toward becoming culturally competent (Krumberger, 2000). Understanding the diversity within cultures, such as subcultures, is also important.

BILINGUALISM, MULTICULTURALISM, SUBCULTURES, AND MINORITIES

Canada is a bilingual and multicultural nation. The Official Languages Act of 1969 established that French and English are Canada's two official languages. In 1971, Prime Minister Trudeau introduced Canada's first official policy on multiculturalism, "Multiculturalism within a Bilingual Framework" (Esses, V.M., & Gardner, R.C., 1996). In 1988, The Canadian Multiculturalism Act was proclaimed, thus making multiculturalism a defining characteristic of Canadian society (Department of Canadian Heritage, 1999).

> "Multiculturalism" in Canada refers to the presence and persistence of diverse racial and ethnic minorities who define themselves as different and who wish to remain so. Ideologically, multiculturalism consists of a relatively coherent set of ideas and ideals pertaining to the celebration of Canada's cultural mosaic. Multiculturalism at the policy level is structured around the management of diversity through formal initiatives in the federal, provincial, and municipal domains. Finally, multiculturalism is the process by which racial and ethnic minorities compete with central authorities for achievement of certain goals and aspirations (Leman, 1999, p.1).

Aboriginal Canadians (status Indians, non-status Indians, Métis, and Inuit) and Canadians of French and British origins are considered the founding nations of Canada. Through immigration, Canada has welcomed people of varied origins who have also contributed to making this country one of the most culturally and ethnically diverse nations in the world.

Although culture is a universal phenomenon, it takes on specific and distinctive features for a particular group, since it encompasses all of the knowledge, beliefs, customs, and skills acquired by the members of that group. When such groups function within a larger cultural group, they are referred to as subcultures.

The term *subculture* is used for relatively large groups of people who share characteristics that enable them to be identified as a distinct entity. Examples of Canadian subcultures based on ethnicity (ie, subcultures with common traits such as physical characteristics, language, or ancestry) include Native Canadians, French Canadians, and Eastern European Canadians. Each of these subcultures can be further divided. For example, Native Canadians include diverse groups such as Mohawk, Cree, and Blackfoot, to name only a few.

Subcultures may also be based on religion (eg, Anglican, Greek Orthodox, Judaism), occupation (eg, nurses, physicians, other members of the health care team), or shared disability or illness (eg, the Deaf community). In addition, subcultures may be based on age (eg, infants, children, adolescents, adults, older adults), gender (eg, male, female); sexual orientation (eg, homosexual or bisexual men and women), or geographic location (eg, Newfoundlanders, Québécois, Westerners).

The nurse should also be sensitive to the intraracial applications of cultural competence. Tensions between subcultures within a designated group could add to the complexity of planning culturally competent care. Some members of one ethnic subculture may be offended or angered if mistaken for members of a different subculture. Similarly, if the attributes of one subculture are mistakenly generalized to a patient belonging to a different subculture, extreme offense could result, as well as inappropriate care planning and implementation (Fields, 2000). It is crucial that nurses refrain from culturally stereotyping a patient in an attempt to be culturally competent. Instead, the patient or significant others should be consulted regarding personal values, beliefs, preferences and cultural identification. This strategy is also applicable for members of nonethnic subcultures.

The term *minority* refers to a group of people whose physical or cultural characteristics differ from the majority of people in a society. At times, minorities may be singled out or isolated from others in society or treated in different or unequal ways. The concept of "minority" varies widely and must be understood within a specific context. For example, men may be considered a minority within the nursing profession, but they constitute a majority within the field of medicine. Similarly, while francophones are the minority in Canada, they are the majority in Québec. Who constitutes a minority or a majority may also change over time; therefore, the minority of today could be the majority of tomorrow. Finally, because the term minority may connote inferiority, attention needs to be paid to ensure that it is used appropriately and in the right context.

Transcultural Nursing

Transcultural nursing, a term sometimes used interchangeably with cross-cultural, intercultural, or multicultural nursing, refers to a formal area of study and practice that focuses on the cultural care (caring) values, beliefs, and practices of individuals and groups from a particular culture (Giger & Davidhizar, 1999). The underlying focus of transcultural nursing is to provide culture-specific and culture-universal care that promotes the well-being or health of individuals, families, groups, communities, and institutions (Giger & Davidhizar, 1999; Leininger, 2001). When culturally appropriate care is provided, all individuals, and the community or institution at large, benefit. When the care is delivered beyond the nurse's national boundaries, the term international or transnational nursing is often used.

Although many nurses, anthropologists, and others have written about the cultural aspects of nursing and health care, Leininger (2001) developed a comprehensive research-based theory called Culture Care Diversity and Universality. The goal of the theory is to provide culturally congruent nursing care to improve care for people of different or similar cultures. This means promoting recovery from illness, preventing conditions that would limit the patient's health or well-being, or facilitating a peaceful death in ways that are culturally meaningful and appropriate. Nursing care needs to be tailored to fit the patient's cultural values, beliefs, and lifestyle.

Leininger's theory includes providing culturally congruent nursing care (meaningful, beneficial, and satisfying health care tailored to fit the patient's cultural values) through culture care

accommodation and culture care restructuring (Fig. 8-1). *Culture care accommodation* refers to those professional actions and decisions that a nurse makes in his or her care to help people of a designated culture achieve a beneficial or satisfying health outcome. *Culture care restructuring* or repatterning refers to those professional actions and decisions that help patients reorder, change, or modify their lifestyles toward new, different, or more beneficial health care patterns. At the same time, the patient's cultural values and beliefs are respected, and a better or healthier lifestyle is provided. Other terms and definitions that provide further insight into culture and health care include the following:

- *Acculturation* is the process by which members of a cultural group adapt to or learn how to take on the behaviours of another group.
- *Cultural blindness* is the inability of a person to recognize his or her own values, beliefs, and practices and those of others because of strong ethnocentric tendencies (the tendency to view one's own culture as superior to others).
- *Cultural imposition* is the tendency to impose one's cultural beliefs, values, and patterns of behaviour on a person or persons from a different culture.
- *Cultural taboos* are those activities governed by rules of behaviour that are avoided, forbidden, or prohibited by a particular cultural group.

Cultural Effectiveness and Competent Nursing Care

To be culturally effective, care must include a partnership between the nurse and the client. Cultural effectiveness is necessary to ensure accurate assessment, needs, and goals. (Canadian Nurses Association, 2000). *Culturally competent or congruent nursing care* refers to the complex integration of attitudes, knowledge, and skills (including assessment, decision making, judgments, critical thinking, and evaluation) that enables the nurse to provide care in a culturally sensitive and appropriate manner. Agency and institutional policies are important to achieve culturally competent care.

Policies that promote culturally competent care establish flexible regulations pertaining to visitors (number, frequency, and length of visits), provide translation services for non–English-speaking or non–French-speaking patients, and train staff to provide care for patients with different cultural values (Suro, 2000). Culturally competent policies also recognize the special dietary needs of patients from selected cultural groups and create an environment in which the traditional healing, spiritual, and religious practices of patients are respected and encouraged.

Giger and Davidhizar (1999) created an assessment model to guide the nurse in exploring cultural phenomena that might affect nursing care. They identified communication, space, time orientation, social organization, environmental control, and biologic variations as relevant phenomena (Giger & Davidhizar, 1999). This model has been used in various patient care settings to provide data essential to the provision of culturally competent care.

CROSS-CULTURAL COMMUNICATION

Establishing an environment of culturally congruent care and respect begins with effective communication, which occurs not only through words, but also through body language and other cues, such as voice, tone, and loudness. Nurse–patient interactions, as well as communications among members of a multicultural health care team, are dependent on the ability to understand and be understood.

FIGURE 8-1 Leininger's Sunrise Model depicts theory of cultural care diversity and universality. From Leininger, M. M. (Ed.). (2001). *Culture care diversity and university: A theory of nursing.* New York: New York: National League for Nursing Press.

Approximately 150 different languages are spoken in Canada, with French accounting for the largest percentage after English. Obviously, nurses cannot become fluent in all languages, but certain strategies for fostering effective cross-cultural communication are necessary when providing care for patients who are not fluent in English or French. Cultural needs should be considered when choosing an interpreter; fluency in varied dialects, for instance, is beneficial (Suro, 2000). The interpreter's voice quality, pronunciation, use of silence, use of touch, and use of nonverbal communication should also be assessed (Giger & Davidhizar, 1999).

During illness, patients of all ages tend to regress, and the regression often involves language skills. Chart 8-1 summarizes suggested strategies for overcoming language barriers. The nurse should also assess how well the patient and family have understood what has been said. The following cues may signal lack of effective communication:

- Efforts to change the subject. This could indicate that the patient does not understand what you are saying and is attempting to talk about something more familiar.

- Absence of questions. Paradoxically, this often means that the listener is not grasping the message and therefore has difficulty formulating questions to ask.
- Inappropriate laughter. A self-conscious giggle may signal poor comprehension and may be an attempt to disguise embarrassment.
- Nonverbal cues. Although a blank expression may signal poor understanding, among some Asian Canadians it may reflect a desire to avoid overt expression of emotion. Similarly, avoidance of eye contact may be a cultural expression of respect for the speaker; some Native Canadians and Asian Canadians use this gesture.

Culturally Mediated Characteristics

Nurses should be aware that patients act and behave in a variety of ways, in part because of the influence of culture on behaviours and attitudes. However, although certain attributes and attitudes are frequently associated with particular cultural groups, as described

---

> ### Chart 8-1 Overcoming Language Barriers
>
> - Greet the patient using the last or complete name. Avoid being too casual or familiar. Point to yourself and say your name. Smile.
> - Proceed in an unhurried manner. Pay attention to any effort by the patient or family to communicate.
> - Speak in a low, moderate voice. Avoid talking loudly. Remember that there is a tendency to raise the volume and pitch of your voice when the listener appears not to understand. The listener may perceive that you are shouting and/or angry.
> - Organize your thoughts. Repeat and summarize frequently. Use audiovisual aids when feasible.
> - Use short, simple sentence structure and speak in the active voice.
> - Use simple words, such as "pain" rather than "discomfort." Avoid medical jargon, idioms, and slang. Avoid using contractions, such as don't, can't, won't.
> - Use nouns repeatedly instead of pronouns. *Example:* Do not say: "He has been taking his medicine, hasn't he?" Do say: "Does Sukhi take medicine?"
> - Pantomime words (use gestures) and simple actions while verbalizing them.
> - Give instructions in the proper sequence. *Example:* Do not say: "Before you rinse the bottle, sterilize it." Do say: "First, wash the bottle. Second, rinse the bottle."
> - Discuss one topic at a time, and avoid giving too much information in a single conversation. Avoid using conjunctions. *Example:* Do not say: "Are you cold and in pain?" Do say (while pantomiming/gesturing): "Are you cold?" "Are you in pain?"
> - Validate whether the person understands by having him or her repeat instructions, demonstrate the procedure, or act out the meaning.
> - Use any words you know in the person's language. This indicates that you are aware of and respect the patient's primary means of communicating.
> - Try a third language. Many Indo-Chinese speak French. Europeans often know three or four languages. Try Latin words or phrases, if you are familiar with the language.
> - Ask who among the patient's family and friends could serve as an interpreter. Be aware of culturally based gender and age differences and diverse socioeconomic, educational, and tribal/regional differences when choosing an interpreter.
> - Obtain phrase books from a library or bookstore, make or purchase flash cards, contact hospitals for a list of interpreters, and use both formal and informal networking to locate a suitable interpreter. Although they are costly, some telecommunication companies provide translation services.

in the following pages, it is important to remember that not all people from the same cultural background share the same behaviours and views. Although the nurse who fails to consider a patient's cultural preferences and beliefs is considered insensitive and possibly indifferent, the nurse who assumes that all members of any one culture act and behave in the same way runs the risk of stereotyping people. The best way to avoid stereotyping is to view each patient as an individual and to find out the patient's cultural preferences. A thorough culture assessment using a culture assessment tool or questionnaire (see later discussion) is very beneficial.

SPACE AND DISTANCE

People tend to regard the space in their immediate vicinity as an extension of themselves. The amount of space they need between themselves and others to feel comfortable is a culturally determined phenomenon.

Because nurses and patients usually are not consciously aware of their personal space requirements, they frequently have difficulty understanding different behaviours in this regard. For example, one patient may perceive the nurse sitting close to him or her as an expression of warmth and care; another patient may perceive the nurse's act as a threatening invasion of personal space. Research reveals that people from the United States, Canada, and Great Britain require the most personal space between themselves and others, whereas those from Latin America, Japan, and the Middle East need the least amount of space and feel comfortable standing close to others.

If patients appear to position themselves too close or too far away, the nurse should consider cultural preferences for space and distance. Ideally, patients should be permitted to assume a position that is comfortable to them in terms of personal space and distance. Because a significant amount of communication during nursing care requires close physical contact, the nurse should be aware of these important cultural differences and consider them when delivering care (Davidhizar, Dowd, & Newman-Giger, 1999).

EYE CONTACT

Eye contact is also a culturally determined behaviour. Although most nurses have been taught to maintain eye contact when speaking with patients, some people from certain cultural backgrounds may interpret this behaviour differently. Some Asians, Native Canadians, Indo-Chinese, and Arabs, for example, may consider direct eye contact impolite or aggressive, and they may avert their own eyes when talking with nurses and others whom they perceive to be in positions of authority. Some Native Canadians stare at the floor during conversations, a cultural behaviour conveying respect and indicating that the listener is paying close attention to the speaker. Some Hispanic patients maintain downcast eyes as a sign of appropriate deferential behaviour toward others on the basis of age, gender, social position, economic status, and position of authority. Being aware that whether a person makes eye contact may be a result of the culture from which they come will help the nurse understand a patient's behaviour and provide an atmosphere in which the patient can feel comfortable.

TIME

Attitudes about time vary widely among cultures and can be a barrier to effective communication between nurses and patients. Views about punctuality and the use of time are culturally determined, as is the concept of waiting. Symbols of time, such as watches, sunrises, and sunsets, represent methods for measuring the duration and passage of time (Giger & Davidhizar, 1999; Spector, 2000).

For most health care providers, time and promptness are extremely important. For example, nurses frequently expect patients to arrive at an exact time for an appointment, despite the fact that the patient is often kept waiting by health care providers who are running late. Health care providers are likely to function according to an appointment system in which there are short intervals of perhaps only a few minutes. For patients from some cultures, however, time is a relative phenomenon, with little attention paid to the exact hour or minute. Some Hispanic people, for example, consider time in a wider frame of reference and make the primary distinction between day and night. Time may also be determined according to traditional times for meals, sleep, and other activities or events. For people from some cultures, the present is of the greatest importance, and time is viewed in broad ranges rather than in terms of a fixed hour. Being flexible in regard to schedules is the best way to accommodate these differences.

Value differences also may influence a person's sense of priority when it comes to time. For example, responding to a family matter may be more important to a patient than meeting a scheduled health care appointment. Allowing for these different views is essential in maintaining an effective nurse-patient relationship. Scolding or acting annoyed at a patient for being late undermines the patient's confidence in the health care system and might result in further missed appointments or indifference to health care suggestions.

TOUCH

The meaning people associate with touching is culturally determined to a great degree. In some cultures (eg, Hispanic, Arab), male health care providers may be prohibited from touching or examining certain parts of the female body. Similarly, it may be inappropriate for females to care for males. Among many Asian Canadians, it is impolite to touch a person's head because the spirit is believed to reside there. Therefore, assessment of the head or evaluation of a head injury requires alternative approaches. The patient's culturally defined sense of modesty must also be considered when providing nursing care. For example, some Jewish and Islamic women believe that modesty requires covering their head, arms, and legs with clothing.

COMMUNICATION

Many aspects of care may be influenced by the diverse cultural perspectives held by the health care providers, patient, family, or significant others. One example is the issue of informed consent and full disclosure. In general, a nurse may argue that patients have the right to full disclosure about their disease and prognosis and may feel that advocacy means working to provide that disclosure. Family members of some cultural backgrounds may believe it is their responsibility to protect and spare the patient, their loved one, the knowledge of a terminal illness. Similarly, patients may, in fact, not want to know about their condition and may expect their family members to "take the burden" of that knowledge and related decision-making (Kudzma, 1999). The nurse should not decide that the family or patient is simply wrong or that the patient must know all details of his or her illness. Similar concerns may be noted when patients refuse pain medication or treatment because of cultural beliefs regarding pain or belief in divine intervention or faith healing. Determining the most appropriate and ethical approach to patient care requires an exploration of the cultural aspects of these situations. Self-examination by the nurse and recognition of one's own cultural bias and world view, as discussed earlier, will play a major part in helping the nurse to resolve cultural and ethical conflicts. The nurse must promote open dialogue and work with the patient, family, physician, and other health care providers to reach the culturally appropriate solution for the patient.

OBSERVANCE OF HOLIDAYS

People from all cultures celebrate civil and religious holidays. Nurses should familiarize themselves with major holidays for members of the cultural groups they serve. Information about these important celebrations is available from various sources, including religious organizations, hospital chaplains, and patients themselves. Routine health appointments, diagnostic tests, surgery,

and other major procedures should be scheduled to avoid those holidays a patient identifies as significant. Efforts should also be made to accommodate patients and family or significant others, when not contraindicated, as they perform holiday rituals in the health care setting.

DIET

The cultural meanings associated with food vary widely but usually include one or more of the following: relief of hunger; promotion of health and healing; prevention of disease or illness; expression of caring for another; promotion of interpersonal closeness among individuals, families, groups, communities, or nations; and promotion of kinship and family alliances. Food may also be associated with solidification of social ties; celebration of life events (eg, birthdays, marriages, funerals); expression of gratitude or appreciation; recognition of achievement or accomplishment; validation of social, cultural, or religious ceremonial functions; facilitation of business negotiations; and expression of affluence, wealth, or social status.

Culture determines which foods are served and when they are served, the number and frequency of meals, who eats with whom, and who is given the choicest portions. Culture also determines how foods are prepared and served; how they are eaten (with chopsticks, hands, or fork, knife, and spoon); and where people shop for their favorite food items (eg, ethnic grocery stores, specialty food markets).

Religious practices may include fasting (eg, Mormons, Roman Catholics, Buddhists, Jews, Muslims), abstaining from selected foods at particular times (eg, Roman Catholics abstain from meat on Ash Wednesday and on Fridays during Lent), and considerations for medications (eg, Muslims may prefer to use non-pork-derived insulin). Practices may also include the ritualistic use of food and beverages (eg, Passover dinner, consumption of bread and wine during religious ceremonies). Chart 8-2 summarizes some dietary practices of selected religious groups.

Many groups tend to feast, often in the company of family and friends, on selected holidays. For example, many Christians eat large dinners on Christmas and Easter and consume other traditional high-calorie, high-fat foods, such as seasonal cookies, pastries, and candies. These culturally-based dietary practices are especially significant in the care of patients with diabetes, hypertension, gastrointestinal disorders, and other conditions in which diet plays a key role in the treatment and health maintenance regimen.

BIOLOGIC VARIATIONS

Along with psychosocial adaptations, nurses must also consider the physiologic impact of culture on patient response to treatment, particularly medications. Data have been collected for many years regarding differences in the effect some medications have on persons of diverse ethnic or cultural origins. Genetic predispositions to different rates of metabolism cause some patients to be prone to overdose reactions to the "normal dose" of a medication, while other patients are likely to experience a greatly reduced benefit from the standard dose of the medication. An antihypertensive agent, for example, may work well for a white male client within a 4-week time span but may take much longer to work or not work at all for an African-American male patient with hypertension. General polymorphism—variation in response to medications resulting from patient age, gender, size, and body composition—has long been acknowledged by the health care community (Kudzma, 1999). Culturally competent medication administration requires

Chart 8-2 · Prohibited Foods and Beverages of Selected Religious Groups

Hinduism
All meats
Animal shortenings

Islam
Pork
Alcoholic products and beverages (including extracts, such as vanilla and lemon)
Animal shortenings
Gelatin made with pork, marshmallow, and other confections made with gelatin

Judaism
Pork
Predatory fowl
Shellfish and scavenger fish (eg, shrimp, crab, lobster, escargot, catfish). Fish with fins and scales are permissible.
Mixing milk and meat dishes at same meal
Blood by ingestion (eg, blood sausage, raw meat). Blood by transfusion is acceptable.
Note: Packaged foods will contain labels identifying kosher ("properly preserved" or "fitting") and pareve (made without meat or milk) items.

Mormonism (Church of Jesus Christ of Latter-Day Saints)
Alcohol
Tobacco
Beverages containing caffeine stimulants (coffee, tea, colas, and selected carbonated soft drinks)

Seventh-Day Adventism
Pork
Certain seafood, including shellfish
Fermented beverages
Note: Optional vegetarianism is encouraged.

---

that consideration of ethnicity and related factors such as values and beliefs regarding the use of herbal supplements, dietary intake, and genetic factors can affect the effectiveness of treatment and compliance with the treatment regimen (Giger & Davidhizar, 1999; Kudzma, 1999).

COMPLEMENTARY AND ALTERNATIVE THERAPIES

Complementary therapies, also referred to as alternative therapies when they replace Western medicine, can be defined as "… all of the medicine systems that are outside mainstream conventional Western medicine" (York University Centre for Health Studies, 1999, p. 275). Numerous frameworks can be used to group these therapies. In Canada, the York University Centre for Health Studies (1999) proposed that therapies can be classified as follows:

- *Nutritional:* therapies in which food, diet, and nutritional supplements are used. Some examples are macrobiotic diets, minerals, and vitamins.
- *Herbal/botanical:* therapies in which herbs are used. Some examples are naturopathy, North American Native tradition, and Ayurveda.
- *Physical:* therapies that include touch, manipulation or exercise. Some examples are osteopathy, chiropractic, massage, reflexology, acupressure, Tai Chi, and Yoga.

- *Energy or life-force:* therapies based on manipulation of energy. Some examples are acupuncture, reiki, therapeutic touch, and Qi gong.
- *Psychological and mind/body control:* therapies that act at the psychological level. Some examples are meditation, hypnosis, and imagery and music therapies.
- *Pharmacologic and biologic treatments:* therapies in which pharmacologic or biologic products are used. Some examples are anti-oxidizing agents, chelation therapy, and cell treatment.

A patient may choose to seek an alternative to conventional medical or surgical therapies. Many of these alternative therapies are becoming widely accepted as feasible treatment options. Therapies such as acupuncture and herbal treatments may be recommended by a patient's physician to address aspects of a condition that are unresponsive to conventional medical treatment or to minimize side effects associated with conventional medical therapy. Alternative therapy used to supplement conventional medicine may be referred to as *complementary therapy.*

Physicians and advanced practice nurses may work in collaboration with an herbalist or with a spiritualist or shaman to provide a comprehensive treatment plan for the patient. Out of respect for the way of life and beliefs of patients from different cultures, it is often necessary that the healers and health care providers respect the strengths of each approach (Palmer, 2001). Complementary therapy is becoming more common as health care consumers become more aware of what is available through information in printed media and on the Internet.

As patients become more informed, they are more likely to participate in a variety of therapies in conjunction with their conventional medical treatments. The nurse needs to assess each patient for use of complementary therapies, remain alert to the danger of conflicting treatments, and be prepared to provide information to the patient regarding treatment that may be harmful. The nurse must, however, be accepting of the patient's beliefs and right to control his or her own care. As a patient advocate, the nurse facilitates the integration of conventional medical, complementary, and alternative medical therapies.

Causes of Illness

Three major views, or paradigms, attempt to explain the causes of disease and illness: the biomedical or scientific view, the naturalistic or holistic perspective, and the magico-religious view.

BIOMEDICAL OR SCIENTIFIC

The biomedical or scientific world view prevails in most health care settings and is embraced by most nurses and other health care providers. The basic assumptions underlying the biomedical perspective are that all events in life have a cause and effect, that the human body functions much like a machine, and that all of reality can be observed and measured (eg, blood pressures, PaO_2 levels, intelligence tests). One example of the biomedical or scientific view is the bacterial or viral explanation of communicable diseases.

NATURALISTIC OR HOLISTIC

The second way that some cultures explain the cause of illness is through the naturalistic or holistic perspective, a viewpoint that is found among many Native Canadians, Asians, and others.

According to this view, the forces of nature must be kept in natural balance or harmony.

One example of a naturalistic belief, held by many Asian groups, is the yin/yang theory, in which health is believed to exist when all aspects of a person are in perfect balance or harmony. Rooted in the ancient Chinese philosophy of Taoism (which translates as "The Way"), the yin/yang theory proposes that all organisms and objects in the universe consist of yin and yang energy. The seat of the energy forces is within the autonomic nervous system, where balance between the opposing forces is maintained during health. Yin energy represents the female and negative forces, such as emptiness, darkness, and cold, whereas the yang forces are male and positive, emitting warmth and fullness. Foods are classified as cold (yin) or hot (yang) in this theory and are transformed into yin and yang energy when metabolized by the body. Cold foods are eaten when the person has a hot illness (eg, fever, rash, sore throat, ulcer, infection), and hot foods are eaten with a cold illness (eg, cancer, headache, stomach cramps, colds). The yin/yang theory is the basis for Eastern or Chinese medicine and is embraced by some Asian Canadians.

Many Hispanic and Arab groups also embrace the hot/cold theory of health and illness. The four humours of the body—blood, phlegm, black bile, and yellow bile—regulate basic bodily functions and are described in terms of temperature and moisture. The treatment of disease consists of adding or subtracting cold, heat, dryness, or wetness to restore the balance of these humours. Beverages, foods, herbs, medicines, and diseases are classified as hot or cold according to their perceived effects on the body, not their physical characteristics. According to the hot/cold theory, the individual as a whole, not just a particular ailment, is significant. Those who embrace the hot/cold theory maintain that health consists of a positive state of total well-being, including physical, psychological, spiritual, and social aspects of the person.

According to the naturalistic world view, breaking the laws of nature creates imbalances, chaos, and disease. People who embrace the naturalistic paradigm use metaphors such as "the healing power of Nature." From the perspective of the Chinese, for example, illness is seen, not as an intruding agent, but as a part of life's rhythmic course and an outward sign of disharmony within.

MAGICO-RELIGIOUS

The third major way in which people view the world and explain the causes of illness is the magico-religious world view. This view's basic premise is that the world is an arena in which supernatural forces dominate and that the fate of the world and those in it depends on the action of supernatural forces for good or evil. Examples of magical causes of illness include belief in voodoo or witchcraft among some Haitian Canadians and others from Caribbean countries. Faith healing is based on religious beliefs and is most prevalent among selected Christian religions, including Christian Science, while various healing rituals may be found in many other religions, such as Roman Catholicism and Mormonism (Church of Jesus Christ of Latter Day Saints).

Of course, it is possible to hold a combination of world views, and many patients offer more than one explanation for the cause of their illness. As a profession, nursing largely embraces the scientific or biomedical world view, but some aspects of holism have begun to gain popularity, including a wide variety of techniques for managing chronic pain, such as hypnosis, therapeutic touch, and biofeedback. Belief in spiritual power is also held by many nurses who credit supernatural forces with various unexplained phenomena related to patients' health and illness states.

Regardless of the view held and whether the nurse agrees with the patient's beliefs in this regard, it is important to be aware of how people view their illness and their health and to work within this framework to promote patients' care and well-being.

Folk Healers

Several cultures believe in folk or indigenous healers. The nurse may find some Hispanic patients, for instance, turning to a curandero or curandera, espiritualista (spiritualist), yerbo (herbalist), or sabador (healer who manipulates bones and muscles). Some Haitian Canadian patients may seek assistance from a voodoo priest. Native Canadian patients may seek assistance from a shaman or medicine man or woman. Patients of Asian descent may mention that they have visited herbalists, acupuncturists, or bone setters. Several cultures have their own healers, most of whom speak the native tongue of the patient, make house calls, and cost significantly less than healers practicing in the conventional medical health care system.

People seeking complementary and alternative therapies have expanded the practices of folk healers beyond their traditional populations, so the nurse needs to ask patients about participation with folk healers regardless of their cultural background. It is best not to disregard a patient's belief in a folk healer or try to undermine trust in the healer. To do so may alienate and drive the patient away from receiving the care prescribed. A nurse should make an effort to accommodate the patient's beliefs while also advocating the treatment proposed by health science.

Cultural Assessment

Cultural nursing assessment refers to a systematic appraisal or examination of individuals, families, groups, and communities in terms of their cultural beliefs, values, and practices. The purpose of such an assessment is to provide culturally competent care (Giger & Davidhizar, 1999). In an effort to establish a database for determining a patient's cultural background, nurses have developed cultural assessment tools or modified existing assessment tools (Spector, 2000; Leininger, 2001) to ensure that transcultural considerations are included in the plan of care. Giger and Davidhizar's (1999) model has been used to design nursing care from health promotion to nursing skills activities (Giger & Davidhizar, 1999; Smith-Temple & Johnson, 2002). The information presented in this chapter and the following general guidelines can be used to direct the nurse's assessment of culture and its influence on a patient's health beliefs and practices.

- What is the patient's country of origin? How long has the patient lived in this country? What is the primary language and literacy level?
- What is the patient's ethnic background? Does he or she identify strongly with others from the same cultural background?
- What is the patient's religion, and how important is it to his or her daily life?
- Does the patient participate in cultural activities such as dressing in traditional clothing and observing traditional holidays and festivals?
- Are there any food preferences or restrictions?
- What are the patient's communication styles? Is eye contact avoided? How much physical distance is maintained? Is the patient open and verbal about symptoms?

- Who is the head of the family, and is he or she involved in decision making about the patient?
- What does the patient do to maintain his or her health?
- What does the patient think caused the current problem?
- Has the advice of traditional healers been sought?
- Have complementary therapies been utilized?
- What kind of treatment does the patient think will help? What are the most important results he or she hopes to get from this treatment?
- Are there religious rituals related to health, sickness, or death that the patient observes?

Additional Cultural Considerations: Know Thyself

Because the nurse–patient interaction is the focal point of nursing, nurses should consider their own cultural orientation when conducting assessment of the patient and the patient's family and friends.

- Know your own cultural attitudes, values, beliefs, and practices.
- Regardless of "good intention," everyone has cultural "baggage" that ultimately results in ethnocentrism.
- In general, it is easier to understand those whose cultural heritage is similar to our own, while viewing those who are unlike us as strange and different.
- Maintain a broad, open attitude. Expect the unexpected. Enjoy surprises.
- Avoid seeing all people as alike; that is, avoid cultural stereotypes, such as "all Chinese like rice" or "all Italians eat spaghetti."
- Try to understand the reasons for any behaviour by discussing commonalities and differences.
- If a patient has said or done something that you do not understand, ask for clarification. Be a good listener. Most patients will respond positively to questions that arise from a genuine concern for and interest in them.
- If at all possible, speak the patient's language (even simple greetings and social courtesies will be appreciated). Avoid feigning an accent or using words that are ordinarily not part of your vocabulary.
- Be yourself. There are no right or wrong ways to learn about cultural diversity.

The Future of Transcultural Nursing Care

Until recently, the majority of Canadian immigrants were of European origin. In the last two decades, more Asians and Middle Easterners than Europeans have immigrated to Canada (Canadian Nurses Association, 2000). In 1991, visible minorities constituted 9.7% of the population; it has been projected that by 2016 they will constitute close to 20% of the population (Beaujot, 2004). As indicated previously, the concept of culturally competent care applies to health care institutions, which must develop culturally sensitive policies and provide an atmosphere that fosters the provision of culturally competent care by nurses. Those nurses, who reflect the multicultural complexion of our society, must learn to acknowledge and adapt to diversity among their colleagues in the workplace (Davidhizar, Dowd, & Newman-Giger, 1999). In addition, educational institutions must prepare nurses to deliver culturally competent care. Nursing programs,

therefore, are exploring creative ways to promote cultural competence in nursing students, including offering multicultural health studies in their curricula (Spector, 2000).

An additional issue related to the provision of culturally competent care is the diversity of the health care delivery workforce. As the population becomes more culturally diverse, efforts to increase the number of ethnic minority nurses must continue and accelerate. Efforts must be made to facilitate the recruitment and successful program completion of ethnic minority nursing students.

With increasing frequency, nurses will be expected to provide culturally competent care for patients. Nurses must work effectively with patients, one another, and other health care team members whose ancestry reflects the multicultural complexion of contemporary society in increasing numbers. Cultural diversity remains one of the foremost issues in health care today.

 Critical Thinking Exercises

1. You are assigned to care for a hospitalized young male adult whose cultural background is very different from yours. Describe how you would assess his cultural beliefs and practices in developing a plan of nursing care. Explain why it is important to examine your own feelings about his cultural beliefs and practices.

2. An elderly East-Indian Canadian female patient who does not speak English is hospitalized after elective surgery. Even though she is progressing well and her discharge has been planned, her family insists on staying with her for as many hours as possible, refusing to leave when visiting hours are over. How can you help the nursing staff to explore the meaning of the family's behaviour and to understand their own feelings about this behaviour? Devise a strategy that you think will help resolve this situation.

3. You are preparing to discharge an elderly patient who is of foreign origin. The record indicates that she does not speak English and lives alone in a neighbourhood where most of the residents are from the same ethnic background as herself. Describe how you would plan discharge teaching to ensure that you can communicate with the patient and family to promote the necessary follow-up care. Explore other aspects of the patient's and family's background that you would want to assess to determine the need for referral to a home health care agency.

REFERENCES AND SELECTED READINGS
Books

American Academy of Nursing, Subpanel on Cultural Competence in Nursing. (1995). *Promoting cultural competence in and through nursing education.* New York: Author.

American Association of Colleges of Nursing. (1996). *Diversity Task Force Report, October 1996.* Washington, D.C.: Author.

Andrews, M. M., & Boyle, J. S. (1999). *Transcultural concepts in nursing care* (3rd ed.). Philadelphia: J. B. Lippincott.

Beaujot, R. P. (2004). Immigration and demographic structures. In E. Cameron (Ed.), *Multiculturalism & immigration in Canada: An introductory reader* (pp. 193–206). Toronto: Canadian Scholars' Press Inc.

Department of Canadian Heritage. (1999). *10th annual report on the operation of The Canadian Multiculturalism Act, 1997–1998.* Ottawa: Author. Available at: http://www.pch.gc.ca.

Giger, J. N., & Davidhizar, R. E. (1999). *Transcultural nursing: Assessment and intervention* (3rd ed.). St. Louis: C. V. Mosby.

Health Canada. (2001). *Perspectives on complementary and alternative health care: A collection of papers prepared for Health Canada.* Ottawa, ON: Author.

Hunt, R. (2000). *Readings in community-based nursing.* Philadelphia: Lippincott Williams & Wilkins.

Kuhn, M. A. (1999). *Complementary therapies for health care providers.* Philadelphia: Lippincott Williams & Wilkins.

Leininger, M. M. (Ed.). (2001). *Culture care diversity and universality: A theory of nursing.* New York: National League for Nursing Press.

Leman, M. (1999). *Canadian multiculturalism.* Ottawa: Library of Parliament. Available at: http://www.parl.gc.ca/information/library/PRBpubs/936-e.htm.

Smith-Temple, J., & Johnson, J. Y. (2002). *Nurse's guide to clinical procedures.* (4th ed.). Philadelphia: Lippincott Williams & Wilkins.

Spector, R. E. (2000). *Cultural diversity in health and illness.* New Jersey: Prentice-Hall.

Sugunasiri, S. (2001). *Towards multicultural growth. A look at Canada from classical racism to neomulticulturalism.* Toronto, ON: Village Publishing House.

Wilkinson, J. M. (2001). *Nursing process and critical thinking.* New Jersey: Prentice-Hall.

York University Centre for Health Studies. (1999). *Complementary and alternative health practices and therapies: A Canadian overview.* Toronto, ON: Author.

Journals

Buerhaus, P. I., & Auerbach, D. (1999). Slow growth in the United States of the number of minorities in the RN workforce. *Image: Journal of Nursing Scholarship, 31*(2), 179–183.

Canadian Nurses Association. (2000). Cultural diversity—changes and challenges. *Nursing Now–Issues and Trends in Canadian Nursing, 7,* 1–4. Available at: http://www.cna-nurses.ca/CNA/documents/pdf/publications/CulturalDiversity_February2000_e.pdf.

Davidhizar, R., Dowd, S., & Newman-Giger, J. (1999). Managing diversity in the health care workplace. *Health Care Supervisor, 17*(3), 51–62.

Esses, V. M., & Gardner, R. C. (1996). Multiculturalism in Canada: Context and Current Status. *Canadian Journal of Behavioural Science, 28* (3), 145–154.

Fields, C. D. (2000). Choosing cultural competence over diaspora division. *Black Issues in Higher Education, 17*(16), 6.

Gonzalez, R. I., Gooden, M. B., & Porter, C. P. (2000). Eliminating racial and ethnic disparities in health care. *American Journal of Nursing, 100*(3), 56–58.

Gonzalez, R. (1999). Washington Watch: ANA advocates more diversity in nursing. *American Journal of Nursing, 99*(11), 24.

Gooden, M. B., Porter, C. P., Gonzalez, R. I., & Mims, B. L. (2001). Rethinking the relationship between nursing and diversity. *American Journal of Nursing, 101*(1), 63, 65.

Krumberger, J. M. (2000). Critical care close-up. *RN, 63*(4), 24AC2–24AC3.

Kudzma, E. C. (1999). Culturally competent drug administration. *American Journal of Nursing, 99*(8), 46–51.

Leininger, M. M. (1988). Leininger's theory of nursing: Cultural care diversity and universality. *Nursing Science Quarterly, 1*(4), 152–159.

National Institutes of Health, National Center for Complementary and Alternative Medicine (n.d.). *Major domains of complementary & alternative medicine.* Available at: http://nccam.nih.gov/fcp/classify/. Accessed September 8, 2001.

Palmer, J. (2001). Respecting tradition in healing. *Reflections on Nursing Leadership, 27*(2), 30–31.

Suro, R. (2000). Beyond economics. *American Demographics, 22*(2), 48–55.

RESOURCES AND WEBSITES

Organizations

Aboriginal Nurses Association of Canada, 56 Sparks Street, Suite 502, Ottawa, ON K1P 5A9;613-724-4677; http://www.anac.on.ca/contactus.html.

Canadian Council for Refugees; http:/www.net/~ccr/history.html.

Council on Nursing and Anthropology, c/o Dr. Mildred Roberson, Nursing and Health Sciences, Salisbury State University, Salisbury, MD 21801.

National Institutes of Health, National Center for Complementary and Alternative Medicine, 6707 Democracy Blvd., Suite 2000, Bethesda, MD 20892-5475; 1-888-644-6226; fax 1-866-464-3616; http://nccam.nih.gov. Accessed 9/8/01.

Office of Minority Health, U.S. Department of Health and Human Services, P.O. Box 37337, Washington, DC 20013-7337; 1-800-444-6472; http://www.omhrc.gov. No cost for accessing database, information specialists, resource network, and publications on major health problems affecting African Americans, Hispanics, Native Americans, and Asian/Pacific Islanders.

Transcultural Nursing Society, c/o Madonna University College of Nursing and Health, 36600 Schoolcraft Road, Livonia MI 48150-1173; 888-432-5470.

Translation Services

AT&T Language Line Services; 1-800-752-6096. Provides written and oral translation in 140 languages.

Genetics Perspectives in Nursing

Adapted by Madeleine Buck and Rene A. Day

LEARNING OBJECTIVES

On completion of this chapter, the learner will be able to:

1. Describe the role of the nurse in integrating genetics in nursing care.
2. Conduct a genetics-based assessment.
3. Identify the common patterns of inheritance of genetic disorders.
4. Identify ethical issues in nursing related to genetics.

^Human **genome** discoveries have ushered in a new era of medicine, *genomic medicine,* which recognizes that multiple genes work in concert with environmental influences to cause disease. Genomic medicine aims to improve predictions about individuals' susceptibility to diseases, the time of onset for those diseases, their extent and eventual severity, and which treatments or medications are likely to be most effective or harmful (Billings, 2000). Already, new gene-based strategies for disease detection, management, and treatment have been created, allowing health professionals to tailor care to an individual's particular genetic make-up.

To meet the challenges of genomic medicine, nurses need to understand the new technologies and treatments of gene-based health care. Nurses also must recognize that they are a vital link between patients and health care services; patients often turn to nurses first with questions about family history of risk factors, genetics information, and genetic tests and interpretations. Incorporating genetics into nursing means bringing a genetics framework to health assessments, planning, and interventions that supports identification of and response to individuals' changing genetics-related health needs (Lea, Williams, Jenkins, et al., 2000).

Nurses must learn to recognize patterns of inheritance when obtaining family and medical histories and understand when it is appropriate to consider new gene-based testing and treatment options. This chapter offers a foundation for the clinical applications of genetics principles in medical and surgical nursing, outlines the nurse's role in genetic counselling and evaluation, addresses important ethical issues, and provides genetics resources for nurses and patients.

A Framework for Integrating Genetics Into Nursing Practice

Nursing's unique contribution to genomic medicine is its philosophy of holism. Nurses are ideally positioned to incorporate genetics into their assessments, planning, and interventions for patients at different ages and stages across the lifespan and in all settings. The holistic view that characterizes nursing takes into account each person's intellectual, physical, spiritual, social, cultural, biopsychologic, ethical, and esthetic experiences while

Glossary

allele: any one of two or more alternate forms of a gene at the same location. An allele for each gene is inherited from each parent.

autosome: a single chromosome from any of the 22 pairs of chromosomes not involved in sex determination (XX or XY)

carrier: person who is heterozygous; possessing two different alleles of a gene pair

chromosome: microscopic structures in the cell nucleus that contain genetic information and are constant in number in a species (eg, humans have 46 chromosomes)

deoxyribonucleic acid (DNA): the primary genetic material in humans consisting of nitrogenous bases, a sugar group, and phosphate combined into a double helix

diploid: the number of chromosomes normally present in somatic cells. For humans, that number is 46.

dominant: a genetic trait that is normally expressed when a person has a gene mutation on one of a pair of chromosomes and the "normal" form of the gene is on the other chromosome

genetics: the scientific study of heredity; how specific traits or predispositions are transmitted from parents to offspring

genome: the total genetic complement of an individual genotype

genomics: the study of the human genome, including gene sequencing, mapping, and function

genotype: the genes and the variations therein that a person inherits from his or her parents

haploid: the number of chromosomes present in egg or sperm (gametes); in humans, this is 23

Human Genome Project: an international research effort aimed at identifying and

characterizing the order of every base in the human genome

meiosis: the reduction division of diploid egg or sperm (germ cells) resulting in haploid gametes (having 23 chromosomes each)

mitosis: cell division occurring in somatic cells that normally results in daughter cells with the same number of chromosomes—46 (diploid)

monosomy: missing one of a chromosome pair in normally diploid cells (for example, 45,X females have only one X chromosome)

mutation: a heritable alteration in the genetic material

nondisjunction: the failure of a chromosome pair to separate appropriately during meiosis, resulting in abnormal chromosome numbers in reproductive cells (gametes) or cells

nucleotide: a nucleic acid "building block" composed of a nitrogenous base, a five-carbon sugar, and a phosphate group

pedigree: a diagrammatic representation of a family history

penetrance: the percentage of individuals known to carry the gene for a trait who actually manifest the condition. For example, a trait with 90% penetrance will not be manifested by 10% of persons possessing the gene.

phenotype: a person's entire physical, biochemical, and physiological makeup, as determined by the individual's genotype and environmental factors

polymorphism: a genetic variation with two or more alleles that is maintained in a population

population screening: the application of a test or inquiry to a group to determine if

individuals in the group have an increased likelihood of a genetic condition or a mutation in a specific gene (eg, cholesterol screening for hypercholesterolemia)

predisposition testing: testing that is used to determine the likelihood that a healthy person with or without a family history of a condition will develop the disorder. Having the gene mutation would indicate that the person has an increased susceptibility to the disorder, but this is not a diagnosis. One example is DNA mutation testing for hereditary breast/ovarian cancer.

prenatal screening: testing that is used to identify if a fetus is at risk for a birth defect such as Down syndrome or spina bifida (eg, multiple marker maternal serum screening in pregnancy)

presymptomatic testing: genetic testing that is used to determine whether persons with a family history of a disorder, but no current symptoms, have the gene mutation. An example of this would be Huntington disease.

recessive: a genetic trait that is expressed only when a person has two copies of a mutant autosomal gene or a single copy of a mutant X-linked gene in the absence of another X chromosome

transcription: the process of transforming information from DNA into new strands of messenger RNA

trisomy: the presence of one extra chromosome in an otherwise diploid chromosome complement—for example, trisomy 21 (Down syndrome)

variable expression: variation in the degree to which a trait is manifested; clinical severity

X-linked: located on the X chromosome

addressing genetics information, gene-based testing, diagnosis, and treatments. Thus, knowledge about genetics is basic to nursing practice (Lea, Anderson & Monsen, 1998).

A framework for integrating genetics into nursing practice includes a philosophy of care that recognizes when genetics factors are playing a role or could play a role in an individual's health. This means using family history and the results of genetics tests effectively, informing patients about genetics concepts, understanding the personal and societal impact of genetics information, and valuing the privacy and confidentiality of genetics information.

A person's response to genetics information, genetic testing, or conditions may be either disabling or empowering. Genetics information may stigmatize individuals if it affects how they view themselves or how others view them. Nurses can help individuals and families understand the genetic aspect of themselves and learn how genetic traits and conditions are passed on within families and how genetic and environmental factors influence health and disease (Lea, Anderson & Monsen, 1998; Peters et al., 1999).

Nurses facilitate communication among family members, the health care system, and community resources; they offer valuable support by virtue of their continuity of care with patients and families. All nurses should be able to recognize when a client is asking a question related to genetics information and should know how to obtain genetics information by gathering family

and health histories and conducting physical and developmental assessments. Being able to recognize a genetics concern allows the nurse to provide appropriate genetics resources and support to individuals and families (Lea, Jenkins & Francomano, 1998).

Key to nurses' genetics framework is the awareness of one's attitudes, experience, and assumptions about genetics concepts and how these are manifested in one's own practice. Chart 9-1 offers insights on how nurses can conduct periodic self-assessments.

Genetics Concepts

Scientists and philosophers have long speculated about heredity and developed theories to explain how traits are transmitted to offspring. Developments in technology and research have accelerated progress in our understanding of genetics, allowing scientists to better understand relatively rare diseases such as phenylketonuria (PKU) or hemophilia that are related to mutations of a single gene inherited in families. New technologies and tools allow scientists to characterize inherited metabolic variations that interact over time and lead to common diseases such as cancer, heart disease, and dementia. This transition from **genetics** to **genomics** highlights how our understanding of single genes and their individual functions has evolved to understanding how

---

Chart 9-1   **Examining Our Own Attitudes, Experiences, and Assumptions**

Self-knowledge is one of the cornerstones to providing quality nursing care, and as practitioners, our attitudes and experiences have an impact on clinical practice. These attitudes emerge from social, cultural, and religious experiences in one's personal life. Awareness of our own values, beliefs, and cultural perceptions not only is important to the nurse–patient relationship, but it is also the first step in developing a genetics framework.

Periodic self-assessment can help maintain an effective framework as nurses update genetics knowledge and practice. Nurses can develop an awareness of their own attitudes, experiences, and assumptions about genetics concepts by considering the following:

- *One's family's beliefs or values about health.* What are your family, religious, or cultural beliefs about the cause of illness? How have your values or biases influenced your understanding of genetic conditions?
- *One's philosophical, theologic, cultural, and ethical perspectives related to health.* How would these attitudes influence your own use of genetics information or services? What experiences have you had with people from different social, cultural, religious, or ethnic groups? How would you deliver genetics information to individuals from different social, cultural, or ethnic groups? Can you recognize when personal values or biases may affect or interfere with the delivery of genetics information?
- *One's level of genetics expertise.* Can you recognize the limitations of your own genetics experience and know when to refer patients for further genetics work-up?
- *One's experience with birth defects, chronic illnesses, and genetic conditions.* Do you have a family member or friend who has a genetic condition or disorder? Has your experience been that

genetic disorders are disabling or empowering? Do you view a parent "at fault" for having a baby born with a birth defect or genetic condition? Do you advocate for fair access and other rights for individuals who have birth defects, genetic conditions, or other disabilities?

- *One's view of DNA (the most basic concept of who we are, since our genetic makeup is unlike that of any other person except an identical twin).* What are your assumptions about DNA? For example, do you assume that the genetic component of "the self" is a defective self? As another example, healthy carriers of genetic alterations that predispose them to develop certain diseases in the future now belong to a new class of "at risk" individuals. A person who is "at risk" is not ill at present, but may not remain well as long as the "average" person. Is it good to know that you are "at risk" or is this information that should not be identified or revealed because of the risk of potential discrimination?
- *One's beliefs about reproductive options.* What are your beliefs regarding reproductive options such as prenatal diagnosis and pregnancy termination? How might these influence your care of a patient who holds different beliefs?
- *One's view of genetic testing and engineering.* Do you see genetic testing and engineering—the ability to eliminate or enhance certain traits—as a way to create an "ideal genetic self"?
- *One's approach to patients with disabilities.* How are your attitudes made apparent in your practice and practice settings? For example, do you have access to TTY machines and/or interpreters for those who have hearing impairment? Are your intake procedures adapted to meet the needs of an individual with disabilities?

Sources: National Coalition of Health Professional Education in Genetics (2001). *Core competencies;* http://www.nchpeg.org; Kenan, R. (1996). The at-risk health status and technology: A diagnostic invitation and the gift of knowing. *Social Science and Medicine, 42*(11), 1545–1553; Peters, J. A., Djurdjinovic, L. & Baker, D. (1999). The genetic self: The Human Genome Project, genetic counseling and family therapy. *Families, Systems & Health, 17*(1), 5–25.

multiple genes act and control biologic processes. Most health conditions are now believed to be the result of a combination of genetic and environmental influences and interactions (Billings, 2000).

GENES AND THEIR ROLE IN HUMAN VARIATION

Genes are central components of human health and disease. Work on the **Human Genome Project** (an international research effort to map and sequence the human genome in its entirety) has shown how basic human genetics is to human development, health, and disease. Knowledge that specific genes are associated with specific genetic conditions makes diagnosis possible, even in the unborn. Research continues to demonstrate how many common conditions have genetic causes. Many more associations between genetics, health, and disease will likely be identified as scientists complete and refine human genome mapping and sequencing.

Genes and Chromosomes

A person's unique genetic constitution, called a **genotype**, is made up of some 30,000 to 40,000 genes. A person's **phenotype**, the observable characteristics of his or her genotype, includes physical appearance and other biologic, physiologic, and molecular traits. Environmental influences modify every individual's phenotype, even those with a major genetic component.

Human growth, development, and disease occur as a result of both genetic and environmental influences and interactions. The contribution of genetic factors may be large or small. For example, in a person with cystic fibrosis or PKU, the genetic contribution is significant. In contrast, the genetic contribution underlying a person's response to infection may be less so.

An individual gene is conceptualized as a unit of heredity. A gene is composed of a segment of **deoxyribonucleic acid (DNA)** that contains a specific set of instructions for making the protein or proteins needed by body cells for proper functioning. Genes regulate both the types of proteins made and the rate at which proteins are produced. The structure of the DNA molecule is referred to as the double helix. The essential components of the DNA molecule are sugar-phosphate molecules and pairs of nitrogenous bases. Each **nucleotide** contains a sugar (deoxyribose), a phosphate group, and one of four nitrogenous bases: adenine (A), cytosine (C), guanine (G), and thymine (T). DNA is composed of two-paired strands, each made up of a number of nucleotides. The strands are held together by hydrogen bonds between pairs of bases (Fig. 9-1).

Genes are packaged and arranged in a linear order within **chromosomes**, which are located in the cell nucleus. In humans, 46 chromosomes occur in pairs in all body cells except oocytes (eggs) and sperm, which each contain only 23 chromosomes. Twenty-two pairs of chromosomes, called **autosomes**, are the same in females and males. The 23rd pair is referred to as the sex chromosomes. A female has two X chromosomes, while a male has one X and one Y chromosome. At conception, each parent normally gives one chromosome of each pair to his or her children. As a result, children receive half of their chromosomes from their fathers and half from their mothers (Fig. 9-2).

Careful examination of DNA sequences from many individuals shows that these sequences have multiple versions in a pop-

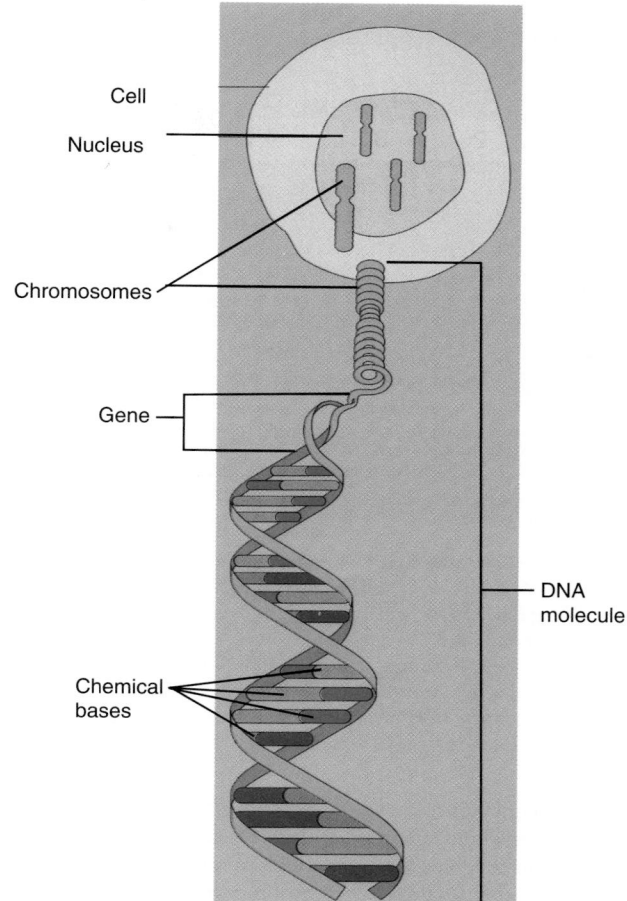

FIGURE 9-1 DNA that carries the instructions that allow cells to make proteins is made up of four chemical bases. Tightly coiled strands of DNA are packaged in units called chromosomes, housed in the cell's nucleus. Working subunits of DNA are known as genes. From the National Institutes of Health and National Cancer Institute. (1995). *Understanding gene testing* (NIH Pub. No. 96-3905). Washington, DC: U.S. Department of Human Services.

ulation. These different versions, or sequence variations, are called **alleles**. Sequences found in many forms are said to be polymorphic, meaning that there are at least two common forms of a particular gene.

Cell Division

The human body grows and develops through a process of cell division. Mitosis and meiosis, two distinctly different types of cell division, contribute to these processes.

Mitosis is the process of cell division involved in cell growth, differentiation, and repair. During mitosis, the chromosomes of each cell duplicate. The result is two cells, called daughter cells, each containing the same number of chromosomes as the parent cell. The daughter cells are said to be **diploid** because they contain 46 chromosomes in 23 pairs. Mitosis occurs in all cells of the body except oocytes (eggs) and sperm.

Meiosis, in contrast, occurs only in reproductive cells and is the process by which oocytes and sperm are formed. During meiosis a reduction in the number of chromosomes takes place,

FIGURE 9-2 Each human cell contains 23 pairs of chromosomes, which can be distinguished by size and by unique banding patterns. This set is from a male, since it contains a Y chromosome. Females have two X chromosomes. From the National Institutes of Health and National Cancer Institute. (1995). *Understanding gene testing* (NIH Pub. No. 96-3905). Washington, DC: U.S. Department of Human Services.

resulting in oocytes or sperm that contain half the usual number or 23 chromosomes. Oocytes and sperm are referred to as **haploid** because they contain a single copy of each chromosome, compared to the usual two chromosomes in all other body cells. During the initial phase of meiosis, paired chromosomes come together in preparation for cell division, portions cross over, and an exchange of genetic material occurs. This event, called recombination, creates greater diversity in the makeup of oocytes and sperm.

During meiosis, a pair of chromosomes may fail to separate completely, creating a sperm or oocyte that contains either two copies or no copy of a particular chromosome. This sporadic event, called **nondisjunction**, can lead to either a trisomy or a monosomy. Down syndrome is an example of **trisomy**. An individual with Down syndrome has three number 21 chromosomes. Turner syndrome is an example of **monosomy**. Girls who have Turner syndrome usually have a single X chromosome, causing them to have short stature and infertility (Lashley, 1998).

Gene Mutations

Within each cell, many intricate and complex interactions regulate and express human genes. Gene structure and function, **transcription** and translation, and protein synthesis are all involved. Alterations in gene structure and function and the process of protein synthesis may influence a person's health. Changes in gene structure, called **mutations**, permanently change the sequence of DNA, which in turn can alter the nature and type of proteins made (Fig. 9-3).

Some gene mutations have no significant effect on the protein product made, while others cause partial or complete changes. How a protein is altered and its importance to proper body functioning determine the mutation's impact. Gene mutations may occur in hormones or enzymes or important protein products, thereby having significant implications for health and disease.

Sickle cell anemia is an example of a genetic condition caused by a small gene mutation that affects protein structure, producing hemoglobin S. A person who inherits two copies of the hemoglobin S gene mutation has the condition sickle cell anemia and experiences the symptoms of severe anemia and thrombotic organ damage resulting from hypoxia (Lashley, 1998; Lea, 2000).

Other gene mutations may be larger, such as a deletion (loss), insertion (addition), duplication (multiplication), or rearrangement (translocation) of a longer DNA segment. Duchenne muscular dystrophy, an inherited form of muscular dystrophy, is an example of a genetic disorder caused by structural gene mutations such as deletions or duplications in the dystrophin gene. Another type of gene mutation, called a triplet or trinucleotide repeat, involves the expansion of more than the usual number of a triplet

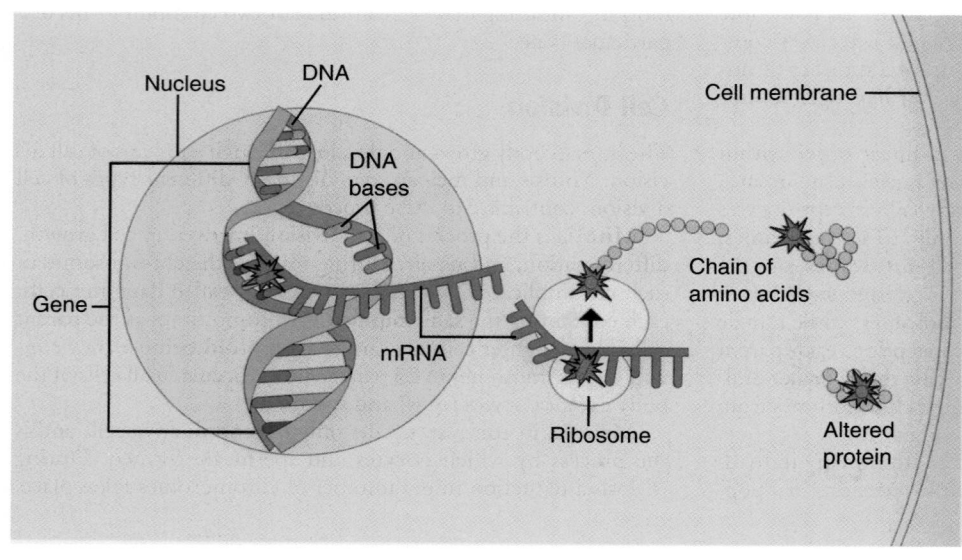

FIGURE 9-3 When a gene contains a mutation, the protein encoded by that gene will be abnormal. Some protein changes are insignificant, others are disabling. From the National Institutes of Health and National Cancer Institute. (1995). *Understanding gene testing* (NIH Pub. No. 96-3905). Washington, DC: U.S. Department of Human Services.

repeat sequence within a gene. Myotonic dystrophy, Huntington disease, and fragile X syndrome are examples of conditions caused by this type of gene mutation.

Gene mutations may be inherited or acquired. Inherited or germ-line gene mutations are present in the DNA of all body cells and are passed on in reproductive cells from parent to child. Germ-line mutations are passed on to all daughter cells when body cells replicate (Fig. 9-4). The gene that causes Huntington disease is one example of a germ-line mutation.

Spontaneous gene mutations take place in individual oocytes or sperm at the time of conception. These mutations are not inherited in other family members. A person who carries the new "spontaneous" mutation, however, may pass on the gene mutation to his or her children. Achondroplasia, Marfan syndrome, and neurofibromatosis type 1 are examples of genetic conditions that may occur in a single family member as a result of spontaneous mutation.

Acquired mutations take place in somatic cells and involve changes in DNA that occur after conception, during a person's lifetime. Acquired mutations develop as a result of cumulative changes in body cells other than reproductive cells (Fig. 9-5). Somatic gene mutations are passed on to the daughter cells derived from that particular cell line.

Gene mutations occur in the human body all the time. Cells have built-in mechanisms by which they can recognize mutations in DNA, and in most situations they correct the change before it is passed on by cell division. However, over time, body cells may lose their ability to repair damage from gene mutations, causing an accumulation of genetic changes that may ultimately result in diseases such as cancer and possibly other conditions of aging, such as Alzheimer's disease (Lashley, 1998).

Genetic Variation

Sorting out the genetic components of complex conditions (eg, heart disease, diabetes, common cancers, psychiatric disorders) that result from the interaction of environment, lifestyle, and the small effects of many genes is ongoing. New studies of genetic variation in humans are underway to develop a map of common DNA variants. Genetic variations occur among individuals of all populations. **Polymorphisms** and single nucleotide polymorphisms (SNPs, pronounced "snips") are the terms used for common genetic variations that occur most frequently throughout the human genome. Some SNPs may contribute directly to a trait or disease expression by altering function. SNPs are becoming increasingly important for the discovery of DNA sequence variations that affect biologic function. Such knowledge will allow clinicians to subclassify diseases and adapt therapies to the individual patient (Collins, 1999; Collins & McKusick, 2001). For example, a polymorphism or SNP can alter a protein or enzyme activity and can thus affect drug efficacy and safety when it occurs in proteins that are targets of medication regimens or that are involved in drug transport or drug metabolism (McCarthy & Hilfiker, 2000; Schafer & Hawkins, 1998).

INHERITANCE PATTERNS IN FAMILIES

Nursing assessment of patients' health includes obtaining and recording family history information. Family history evaluation in the form of a **pedigree** is a first step in establishing the pattern of inheritance. Nurses must become familiar with mendelian patterns of inheritance and pedigree construction and analysis to be able to help identify individuals and families who may benefit from further genetic counselling, testing and therapeutics (Lea, Jenkins & Francomano, 1998; Lea, 2000).

Mendelian conditions are genetic conditions that are inherited in families in fixed proportions among generations. Named after Gregor Mendel, mendelian conditions result from gene mutations present on one or both chromosomes of a pair. An individual gene inherited from one or both parents can cause a mendelian inherited condition. Mendelian conditions are classified according to their pattern of inheritance in families: autosomal dominant, autosomal recessive, and **X-linked**. The terms **dominant** and **recessive** refer to the trait, genetic condition, or phenotype, but not to the genes or alleles that cause the observable characteristics (Thompson et al., 2001).

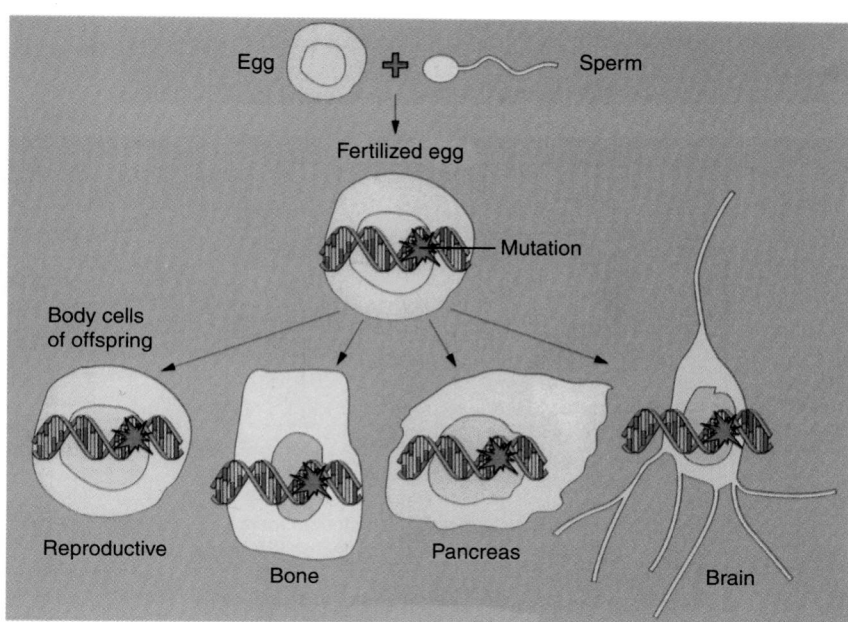

FIGURE 9-4 Hereditary mutations are carried in the DNA of the reproductive cells. When reproductive cells containing mutations combine to produce offspring, the mutation will be present in all of the offspring's body cells. From the National Institutes of Health and National Cancer Institute. (1995). *Understanding gene testing* (NIH Pub. No. 96-3905). Washington, DC: U.S. Department of Human Services.

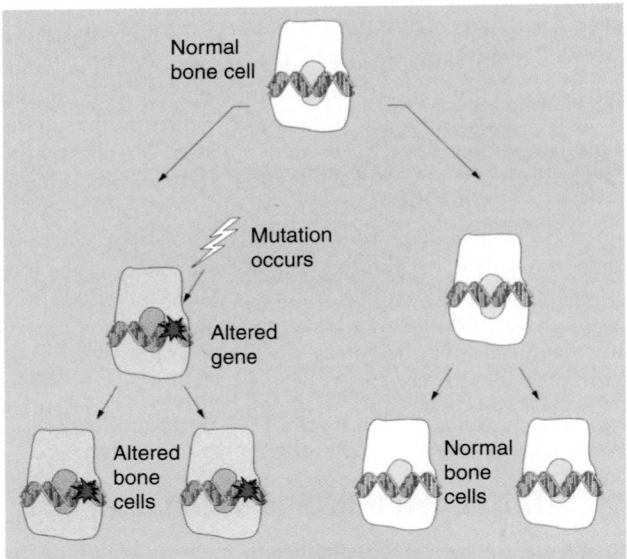

FIGURE 9-5 Acquired mutations develop in DNA during a person's lifetime. If the mutation arises in a body cell, copies of the mutation will exist only in the descendants of that particular cell. From the National Institutes of Health and National Cancer Institute. (1995). *Understanding gene testing* (NIH Pub. No. 96-3905). Washington, DC: U.S. Department of Human Services.

Autosomal Dominant Inheritance

Autosomal dominant inherited conditions affect female and male family members equally and follow a vertical pattern of inheritance in families (Fig. 9-6). An individual who has an autosomal dominant inherited condition carries a gene mutation for that condition on one chromosome of a pair. Each of that individual's offspring has a 50% chance of inheriting the gene mutation for the condition and a 50% chance of inheriting the normal version of the gene. Offspring who do not inherit the gene mutation for the dominant condition will not develop the condition and do not have an increased chance for having chil-

dren with the same condition (Fig. 9-7). Table 9-1 presents characteristics and examples of different patterns of inherited conditions.

Autosomal dominant inherited conditions often present with varying degrees of severity among affected family members and persons. Some individuals with the condition may have significant symptoms, while others may have only mild ones. This characteristic is referred to as **variable expression**; it results from the influences of genetic and environmental factors on clinical presentation.

Another phenomenon observed in autosomal dominant inheritance is **penetrance**, the percentage of persons known to have a particular gene mutation who actually show the trait. Penetrance is observed in conditions such as achondroplasia, in which nearly 100% of persons with the gene mutation typically display traits of the disease. In some conditions, the presence of a gene mutation does not invariably mean that a person will have or develop an autosomal inherited condition. For example, a woman who has the BRCA1 hereditary breast cancer gene mutation has a lifetime risk for breast cancer up to 80%, not 100%. This quality, known as incomplete penetrance, indicates the probability that a given gene will produce disease. In other words, a person may inherit the gene mutation that causes an autosomal dominant condition but may not have any of the observable physical or developmental features of that condition. However, these individuals carry the gene mutation and still have a 50% chance of passing the gene for the condition to each of their children. One of the effects of incomplete penetrance is that the gene appears to "skip" a generation, thus leading to errors in interpreting family history and in genetic counselling. Examples of other genetic conditions with incomplete penetrance include otosclerosis (40%) and retinoblastoma (80%) (Lashley, 1998).

FIGURE 9-7 In dominant genetic disorders, if one affected parent has a disease-causing allele that dominates its normal counterpart, each child in the family has a 50% chance of inheriting the disease allele and the disorder. From the National Institutes of Health and National Cancer Institute. (1995). *Understanding gene testing* (NIH Pub. No. 96-3905). Washington, DC: U.S. Department of Human Services.

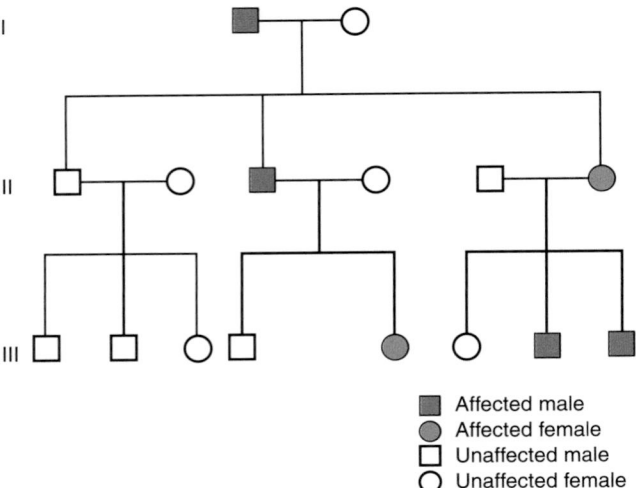

FIGURE 9-6 Three-generation pedigree illustrating autosomal dominant inheritance.

Table 9-1 • Patterns of Mendelian Inheritance

CHARACTERISTICS	EXAMPLES
Autosomal Dominant Inherited Conditions	
Vertical transmission in families	Hereditary breast/ovarian cancer syndrome
Males and females equally affected	Familial hypercholesterolemia
Variable expression among family members and others with condition	Hereditary non-polyposis colorectal cancer
	Huntington disease
Reduced penetrance (in some conditions)	Marfan syndrome
Advanced paternal age associated with sporadic cases	Neurofibromatosis
Autosomal Recessive Inherited Conditions	
Horizontal pattern of transmission seen in families	Cystic fibrosis
Males and females equally affected	Galactosemia
Associated with consanguinity (genetic relatedness)	Phenylketonuria
Associated with particular ethnic groups	Sickle cell anemia
	Tay-Sachs disease
	Canavan disease
X-Linked Recessive Inherited Conditions	
Vertical transmission in families	Duchenne muscular dystrophy
Males predominantly affected	Hemophilia A and B
	Wiscott-Aldrich syndrome
	Protan and Deutran forms of colour blindness
Multifactorial Inherited Conditions	
Occur as a result of genetic and environmental factors combining	Congenital heart defects
May recur in families	Cleft lip and/or palate
Inheritance pattern does not demonstrate the characteristic pattern of inheritance seen with other mendelian inherited conditions	Neural tube defects (anencephaly and spina bifida)
	Diabetes mellitus
	Osteoarthritis
	High blood pressure

Adapted from Lea, D. H., Jenkins, J. F., & Francomano, C. A. (1998). *Genetics in clinical practice: New directions for nursing and health care.* Sudbury, MA: Jones & Bartlett; Lea, D. H. (2002). Genetics. In Maher, A. B., Salmond, S. W., & Pellino, T. A. (Eds.) *Orthopaedic nursing.* Philadelphia: W. B. Saunders.

Autosomal Recessive Inheritance

The pattern of inheritance in autosomal recessive inherited conditions differs from that of autosomal dominant inherited conditions in that it is more horizontal than vertical, with relatives of a single generation tending to have the condition (Fig. 9-8). Genetic conditions inherited in an autosomal recessive pattern are frequently seen among particular ethnic groups and tend to occur more often in children of parents who are related by blood, such as first cousins (see Table 9-1).

In autosomal recessive inheritance, each parent carries a gene mutation on one chromosome of the pair and the normal working copy of the gene on the other chromosome. The parents are said to be **carriers** of the particular gene mutation. Unlike an individual with an autosomal dominant inherited condition, a carrier of a gene mutation for a recessive inherited condition does not have symptoms of the genetic condition. When two carrier parents have children together, they have (with each of their pregnancies) a 25% chance of having a child who inherits the gene mutation from each parent and who will have the condition (Fig. 9-9).

X-Linked Inheritance

X-linked conditions may be inherited in families in recessive or dominant patterns (see Table 9-1). In both, the gene mutation is located on the X chromosome. All males inherit an X chromosome from their mother and a Y chromosome from their father for a normal sex constitution of 46,XY. Since males have only one X chromosome, they do not have a counterpart for its genes as do females.

This means that a gene mutation on their X chromosome is expressed when present in one copy. A female, on the other hand, inherits one X chromosome from each parent for a normal sex constitution of 46,XX. A female may be a carrier of a gene mutation or affected if the condition results from a gene mutation causing a dominant X-linked condition. Either the X chromosome that

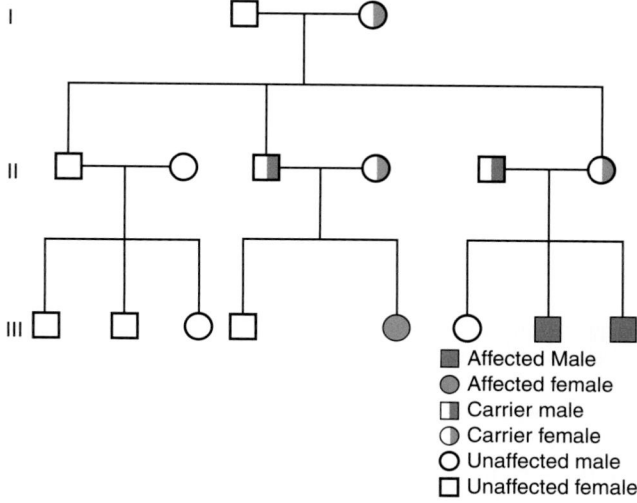

■ Affected Male
● Affected female
◧ Carrier male
◐ Carrier female
○ Unaffected male
□ Unaffected female

FIGURE 9-8 Three-generation pedigree illustrating autosomal recessive inheritance.

Carrier father Carrier mother

Normal son   Carrier daughter   Carrier son   Affected daughter

FIGURE 9-9 In diseases associated with altered recessive genes, both parents—though disease-free themselves—carry one normal allele and one altered allele. Each child has one chance in four of inheriting two altered alleles and developing the disorder; one chance in four of inheriting two normal alleles; and two chances in four of inheriting one normal and one altered allele, and being a carrier like both parents. From the National Institutes of Health and National Cancer Institute. (1995). *Understanding gene testing* (NIH Pub. No. 96-3905). Washington, DC: U.S. Department of Human Services.

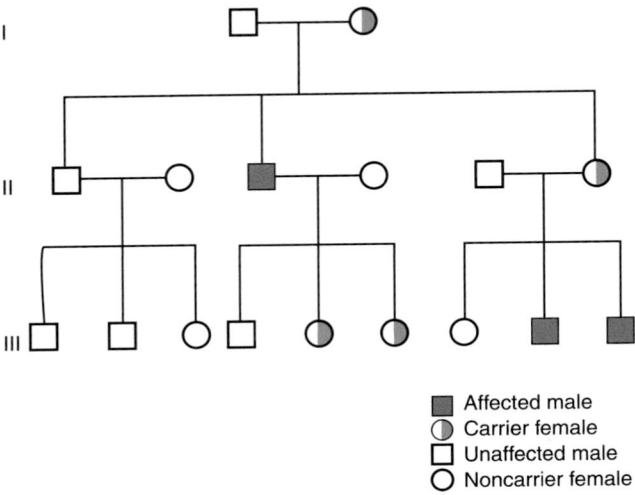

■ Affected male
◑ Carrier female
□ Unaffected male
○ Noncarrier female

FIGURE 9-10 Three-generation pedigree illustrating X-linked recessive inheritance.

a female receives from her mother or the X chromosome she receives from her father may be passed on to her sons, and this is a random occurrence.

The most common pattern of X-linked inheritance is that in which a female is a carrier for a gene mutation on one of her X chromosomes. This is referred to as X-linked recessive inheritance. In X-linked recessive inherited conditions, a female carrier has a 50% chance to pass on the gene mutation to a son, who would be affected, or to a daughter, who would be a carrier like her mother (Fig. 9-10).

Nontraditional Inheritance Patterns

Although mendelian inherited conditions present with a specific pattern of inheritance in some families, many diseases and traits do not follow these simple patterns. A variety of factors influence how a gene performs and is expressed. Different mutations in the same gene can produce variable symptoms in different individuals, as is the case with cystic fibrosis. Different mutations in several genes can lead to the identical outcome, as observed with Alzheimer's disease. Some traits involve the simultaneous mutation in two or more genes. A recently observed phenomenon, imprinting, can determine which pair of genes (the mother's or the father's) will be silenced or activated. This form of inheritance has been observed in Angelman syndrome, a severe form of mental retardation and ataxia (Thompson et al., 2001).

Another example is Tourette syndrome (TS), which was identified in 1885. It is described as autosomal dominant but is sex in-

fluenced. No gene has been identified yet and a definite mendelian inheritance pattern has not been established (Bradley, Daroff, Fenichel, & Jankovic, 2004). Individuals with TS have a 50% chance of passing the disorder to offspring, but not equally to boys and girls. Boys are three times more likely to have TS than girls. Varying symptoms will be seen in family members; most will not require treatment.

Tourette syndrome is considered a neurochemical imbalance disorder with no special pattern of onset or progression. There is no test for TS. Diagnosis is made on the basis of onset before 18 years (usually about 6 to 7 years); presence of tics (involuntary muscle movements) and vocalizations (yelps, sniffing, throat clearing, repeating words [echolalia] or socially inappropriate words [coprolalia]); and the waxing and waning of symptoms (Tourette Syndrome Foundation of Canada website, 2005).

Of interest are associated conditions that also have a neurochemical basis. Attention-deficit hyperactive disease (ADHD) occurs in one half of the boys with TS and one third of the girls with TS and occurs eight times more often than in the general population. Symptoms of ADHD may be the first symptom of TS. Learning disabilities affect one half of the boys and one quarter of the girls with TS. Obsessive-compulsive disorder (OCD) affects 30% of people with TS versus 3% of the general population. People with TS may be generally at risk for other disorders such as depression or substance abuse (National Institute of Neurological Disorders, 2005).

Multifactorial and Complex Genetic Conditions

Many birth defects and common health conditions such as heart disease, high blood pressure, cancer, osteoarthritis, and diabetes occur as a result of interactions of multiple gene mutations and environmental influences, and thus are called multifactorial or complex conditions (see Table 9-1). Multifactorial conditions may cluster in families but do not present with the characteristic pattern of inheritance seen in families having mendelian inherited conditions (Fig. 9-11). Neural tube defects, such as spina bifida and anencephaly, are examples of multifactorial genetic conditions (Chart 9-2).

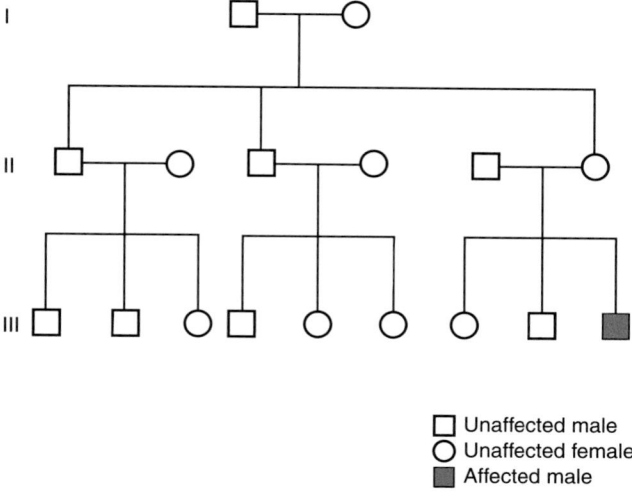

□ Unaffected male
○ Unaffected female
■ Affected male

FIGURE 9-11 Three-generation pedigree illustrating multifactorial conditions.

CHROMOSOMAL DIFFERENCES AND GENETIC CONDITIONS

Differences in the number or structure of chromosomes are a major cause of birth defects, mental retardation, and malignancies. Chromosomal differences are present in approximately 1 in every 160 live-born infants and are the cause of greater than 50% of all spontaneous first-trimester pregnancy losses (Lashley, 1998; Thompson et al., 2001). Chromosomal differences most com-

monly involve an extra or missing chromosome. This is called aneuploidy. Whenever there is an extra or missing chromosome, there is always associated mental or physical disability to some degree.

Down syndrome, or trisomy 21, is a common chromosomal condition that occurs with greater frequency in pregnancies of women who are 35 years or older. A person who has trisomy 21 Down syndrome has a complete extra number 21 chromosome, which causes a particular facial appearance and increased risk for congenital heart defects, thyroid and vision problems, and mental retardation. Other examples of chromosomal differences include trisomy 13 and 18, both more severe than Down syndrome, and conditions involving extra or missing sex chromosomes (eg, Turner syndrome, in which females have only one X chromosome instead of the usual two) (Lashley, 1998).

Chromosomal differences may also involve a structural rearrangement within or between chromosomes. These are less common than chromosomal conditions in which there is an extra or missing chromosome, but occur in 1 in every 500 newborns (Thompson et al., 2001). People who carry "balanced" chromosome rearrangements have all of their chromosomal material, but it is rearranged. A person who carries a balanced chromosomal rearrangement has an increased risk for spontaneous pregnancy loss and for having children with an unbalanced chromosomal arrangement that may result in physical or mental disabilities. Known carriers are therefore offered prenatal counselling and testing.

Chromosome studies may be needed at any age, depending upon the indication. Two common indications are for confirmation of a suspected diagnosis such as Down syndrome, and for a history of two or more unexplained pregnancy losses. Chromosome studies are accomplished by obtaining a tissue sample (eg, blood, skin, amniotic fluid), preparing and staining the chromosomes,

---

Chart 9-2 **Neural Tube Defects or Other Congenital Abnormalities and Folic Acid**

Most neural tube defects (NTD) are caused by both genetic and environmental influences that combine during the third to fourth week following conception, leading to incomplete closure of the neural tube (Jones, 1997). The incidence of NTD in Canada in 1997 was 7.5 per 10,000 total births (Kohut & Rusen, 2002). Rates were higher in Quebec and Newfoundland (40 per 10,000 total births each) than in western Canada (British Columbia at 16 per 10,000 total births) (Chambers, Popkin, Arnold, et al., 1994; Hall, Friedman, Kenna, et al., 1988). Women from ethnic groups such as Celtic (Little & Elwood, 1992), and Sikh (Baird, 1983), and those from Northern China (Berry, Li, Erickson, et al., 1999) are more at risk of having a child with NTD.

A folic acid supplement taken prior to pregnancy and for the first three months of the pregnancy will reduce the risk of NTD but will not eliminate it (MRC Vitamin Study Research Group, 1991). Taking folic acid will also reduce the number of other congenital abnormalities such as heart defects (Cziezel, 1993), urinary tract anomalies (Li, Daling, Mueller, et al., 1995), oral facial cleft (Hayes, Werler, Willett, & Mitchell, 1996), limb defects (Shaw, O'Malley, Wasserman, et al., 1995), and pyloric stenosis (Cziezel, 1993).

Canadian Folic Acid Treatment Guidelines
1. For women who could become pregnant:
   Folic acid: 400 μg (0.4 mg)–1000 μg (1.0 mg) daily
   Caution: If taken as part of a multivitamin, take only one dose per day.

2. For women in intermediate- or high-risk categories (previous neural tube–affected pregnancy, three-generational history of NTD in either the male or female partner, insulin-dependent diabetes, treatment of epilepsy with valproic acid or carbamazepine):
   Folic acid: 4000 μg (4 mg)–5000 μg (5 mg) alone
   Caution:
   • Take only after checking Vitamin B_{12} level.
   • Do not take a multivitamin due to risk of excessive Vitamin A.

The following health teaching for women who could become pregnant should occur at all visits with nurses and other health professionals:
   • Maintain a healthy diet by following Canada's Food Guide to Healthy Eating (see Chapter 5).
   • Eat folic acid–rich foods such as broccoli, spinach, peas, Brussels sprouts, corn, beans, lentils, and oranges (raw is preferable).
   • Eat folic acid–enriched foods such as white flour, pasta, and cornmeal.
   • Know the benefits of taking an appropriate dose of folic acid.
   Caution:
   • Rare allergic responses to folic acid include redness, rash, itching, general malaise, and bronchospasm.
   • There is a risk for interaction of folic acid with medications such as hyperthyroid/thiazide combinations, digoxin, thyroid hormones, tetracycline, and thiazide diuretics.

From Wilson et al. (2003). The use of folic acid for the prevention of neural tube defects and other congenital anomalies. SOGC Clinical Practice Guidelines No. 138. *Journal of Obstetrics & Gynaecology Canada: JOGC, 25*(11), 959–973.

and analyzing them under a microscope. The microscopic study of chromosomes is called cytogenetics and is an area that is rapidly evolving. Today, cytogenetics is used with new molecular techniques such as fluorescent in situ hybridization (FISH), which permits more detailed examination of chromosomes. FISH is useful to detect small abnormalities, including characterizing chromosomal rearrangements (Thompson et al., 2001).

Clinical Applications of Genetics

One of the most immediate applications of new genetics discoveries is the development of genetic tests that can be used to detect a trait, diagnose a genetic condition, and identify people who have a genetic predisposition to a disease such as cancer or heart disease. Another emerging application is pharmacogenetics. Pharmacogenetics involves the use of genetic testing to identify genetic variations that relate to the safety and efficacy of medications and gene-based treatments, so that individualized treatment and management plans can be developed. Future applications may include the use of gene chips to map a person's individual genome for genetic variations that may lead to disease. Nurses will be involved in caring for patients who are undergoing genetic testing and gene-based treatments. Knowledge of the clinical applications of modern genetics technologies will prepare nurses to inform and support patients, and to provide high-quality genetics-related health care.

GENETIC TESTING

Genetic tests provide information leading to the diagnosis of inherited conditions or other conditions with a known genetic contribution. Genetic testing involves the use of specific laboratory analyses of chromosomes, genes, or gene products (eg, enzymes, proteins) to learn whether a genetic alteration related to a specific disease or condition is present in an individual. Genetic testing can be DNA-based, chromosomal or biochemical.

There are several important uses for genetic testing, as identified by the Secretary's Advisory Committee on Genetic Testing (SACGT, 2000). Prenatal testing includes all three types of genetic testing (DNA-based, chromosomal and biochemical) and is widely used for prenatal screening and diagnosis of such conditions as Down syndrome. Carrier testing is used to determine carrier status, helping couples or individuals learn whether they carry a recessive allele for an inherited condition (eg, cystic fibrosis, sickle cell anemia, or Tay-Sachs disease) and thus risk passing it on to their children. Genetic testing is also used widely in newborn screening, and in Canada is made available for an increasing number of genetic conditions. Each province determines which tests will be done. For example, in Alberta newborns are tested for PKU, biotinidase deficiency, and thyroid (TSH). Since most babies leave hospital about 24 hours after delivery, newborn metabolic screening tests are coordinated by community health nurses. Diagnostic testing is used to detect the presence or absence of a particular genetic alteration or allele to identify or confirm a diagnosis of a disease or condition in an affected individual—for example, myotonic dystrophy and fragile X syndrome. In the near future, genetic tests will be increasingly used to identify a person's predisposition to disease and to design specific and individualized treatment and management plans. Examples of current uses of genetic tests are shown in Table 9-2.

Nurses will increasingly participate in genetic testing, especially in the areas of patient education, ensuring informed health choices and consent, advocating for privacy and confidentiality with regard

---

Table 9-2 • **Genetic Tests: Examples of Current Uses**

PURPOSE OF GENETIC TEST	TYPE OF GENETIC TEST
Carrier Testing	
Cystic fibrosis	DNA analysis
Tay-Sachs disease	Hexosaminidase A activity testing and DNA analysis
Canavan disease	DNA analysis
Sickle cell anemia	Hemoglobin electrophoresis
Thalassemia	Complete blood count and hemoglobin electrophoresis
Prenatal Diagnosis—amniocentesis is often performed when there is a risk for a chromosomal or genetic disorder:	
Risk for Down syndrome	Chromosomal analysis
Risk for cystic fibrosis	DNA analysis
Risk for Tay-Sachs disease	Hexosaminidase A activity testing and/or DNA analysis
Risk for open neural tube defect	Protein analysis
Diagnosis	
Down syndrome	Chromosomal analysis
Fragile X syndrome	DNA analysis
Myotonic dystrophy	DNA analysis
Presymptomatic Testing	
Huntington disease	DNA analysis
Myotonic dystrophy	DNA analysis
Susceptibility Testing	
Hereditary breast/ovarian cancer	DNA analysis
Hereditary non-polyposis colorectal cancer	DNA analysis

to genetic test results, and assisting patients to understand the complex issues involved in genetic testing (Lea & Williams, 2002).

GENETIC SCREENING

Genetic screening, in contrast to genetic testing, is a broader concept and applies to testing of populations or groups independent of a positive family history or symptom manifestation. Genetic screening, as defined in 1975 by the Committee for the Study of Inborn Errors of Metabolism of the National Academy of Sciences (SACGT, 2000), has several major aims. One is management; that is, identifying people with treatable genetic conditions that could prove dangerous to their health if left untreated. An example of this is screening of newborns. A second aim is to provide reproductive options to people with a high probability of having children with severe, untreatable diseases and for whom genetic counselling, prenatal diagnosis, and other reproductive options could be helpful and of interest. This is illustrated by the screening of individuals of Ashkenazi Jewish descent for conditions such Tay-Sachs disease and Canavan disease. A third aim is screening pregnant women to detect birth defects such as neural tube defects and Down syndrome using multiple marker screening. Genetic screening may also be used for public health purposes to determine the incidence and prevalence of a birth defect, or to investigate the feasibility and value of new genetic testing methods.

Most commonly genetic screening occurs in prenatal and newborn programs that involve nurses in various roles and settings. However, it is anticipated that genetic screening will expand in the future to include adult-onset conditions such as cancer, heart disease, diabetes, and hemochromatosis. Table 9-3 gives examples of genetic screening applications.

In the future, population-based (widespread) genetic screening will be applied to help identify people who are predisposed to develop conditions such as breast and colon cancer and heart disease. Nurses will be expected to participate in explaining genetics concepts such as risk and genetic predisposition, supporting informed health decisions and opportunities for prevention and early intervention, and protecting patients' privacy (Lea & Williams, 2002).

TESTING AND SCREENING FOR ADULT-ONSET CONDITIONS

Adult-onset conditions are disorders with a genetic component that are manifested in later life. Often symptoms or clinical manifestations occur only in late adolescence or adulthood, and disease is clearly observed to run in families. Some of these conditions are attributed to specific genetic mutations following either autosomal dominant inheritance or autosomal recessive inheritance. However, the majority of adult-onset conditions are considered to be multifactorial (polygenetic) in nature (eg, heart disease, diabetes, arthritis). Nursing assessment for adult-onset conditions is based on the family history and the identification of diseases or clinical manifestations associated with adult-onset conditions. Knowledge of adult-onset conditions and their genetic basis (ie, mendelian versus multifactorial conditions) influences the nursing considerations for genetic testing. Table 9-4 describes adult-onset conditions, their age of onset, pattern of inheritance, genes involved, and testing availability.

If a single gene accounts for an adult-onset condition in a symptomatic individual, diagnostic testing is used to confirm a diagnosis to assist in the plan of care and management. Diagnostic testing for adult-onset conditions is most frequently used with autosomal dominant conditions, such as Huntington disease or Factor V Leiden thrombophilia, and autosomal recessive conditions, such as hemochromatosis. In families with known adult-onset conditions or with a confirmed genetic mutation in an affected family member, **presymptomatic testing** provides asymptomatic individuals with information about having a genetic mutation and about the likelihood of developing the disease. Huntington disease has served as the model for presymptomatic testing because the presence of the genetic mutation predicts disease onset and progression. Although preventive measures are not yet available for Huntington disease, the genetics information enables health care providers to develop a clinical, supportive, and psychological plan of care. Presymptomatic testing is considered for families with a known adult-onset condition in which either a positive or negative result will affect medical management or in

Table 9-3 • **Applications for Genetic Screening**

TIMING OF SCREENING	PURPOSE	EXAMPLES
Preconception screening	For autosomal recessive inherited genetic conditions that occur with greater frequency among individuals of certain ethnic groups	Cystic fibrosis—all couples, but especially Northern European Caucasian, and Ashkenazi Jewish Tay-Sachs disease—Ashkenazi Jewish Sickle cell anemia—African American, Puerto Rican, Mediterranean, Middle Eastern Alpha-thalassemia—Southeast Asian, African American
Prenatal screening	For genetic conditions that are common and for which prenatal diagnosis is available when a pregnancy is identified at increased risk	Neural tube defects—spina bifida, anencephaly Down syndrome Other chromosomal abnormalities—trisomy 18
Newborn screening	For genetic conditions for which there is specific treatment	Phenylketonuria (PKU) Galactosemia Homocystinuria Biotinidase deficiency

Table 9-4 • **Adult-Onset Disorders**

CLINICAL DESCRIPTION	AGE OF ONSET	GENETIC INHERITANCE	TEST AVAILABILITY
Early-onset familial Alzheimer's disease Progressive dementia, memory failure, personality disturbance, loss of intellectual functioning associated with cerebral cortical atrophy, beta-amyloid plaque formation and intraneuronal neurofibrillary tangles	<60–65 years and often before 55	A.D.	Presymptomatic
Late-onset familial Alzheimer's disease Progressive dementia, cognitive decline	>60–65 years		Presymptomatic
Frontotemporal dementia with parkinsonism—linked to chromosome 17 Dementia and/or parkinsonism. Slowly progressive behavioural changes, language disturbances and/or extrapyramidal signs and symptoms, rigidity, bradykinesia, and saccadic eye movements	40–60 years	A.D.	Research
Huntington disease Widespread degenerative brain change with progressive motor loss both voluntary and involuntary disability, cognitive decline, chorea (involuntary movements) at later stage, psychiatric disturbances	Mean age 35–44 years	A.D.	Diagnostic and presymptomatic
Neuromuscular disorders **Spinocerebellar ataxia type 6** Slowly progressive cerebellar ataxia, dysarthria, and nystagmus	Mean age 43–52 years	A.D.	Diagnostic and presymptomatic
Spinocerebellar ataxia type 1 Ataxia, dysarthria, and bulbar dysfunction	Mean age 30–40 years	A.D.	Diagnostic and presymptomatic
Spinocerebellar ataxia type 2 Slow saccadic eye movement, peripheral neuropathy, decreased deep tendon reflexes, dementia	Mean age 30–40 years	A.D.	Diagnostic and presymptomatic
Spinocerebellar ataxia type 3 Progressive cerebellar ataxia and variety of other neurologic symptoms including dystonic-rigid syndrome, parkinsonian syndrome or combined dystonia and peripheral neuropathy	Mean age 30s	A.D.	Diagnostic and presymptomatic
Mild myotonic muscular dystrophy Cataracts and myotonia or muscle wasting and weakness, frontal balding, and ECG changes (heart block or arrhythmia), diabetes mellitus in 5% of all cases	20–70 years	A.D. with variable penetrance	Research
Amyotrophic lateral sclerosis (ALS) Progressive loss of motor function with predominantly lower motor neuron manifestations	50–70 years	Both A.D. and A.R.	Research
Hematologic conditions **Hereditary hemochromatosis** High absorption of iron by GI mucosa resulting in excessive iron storage in liver, skin, pancreas, heart, joints and testes. Abdominal pain, weakness, lethargy, weight loss are early symptoms. Untreated individuals can present with skin pigmentation, diabetes mellitus, hepatic fibrosis or cirrhosis, heart failure, dysrhythmias or arthritis.	40–60 in males; after menopause in females	A.R.	Diagnostic and presymptomatic
Factor V Leiden thrombophilia Poor anticoagulant response to activated protein C with increased risk for venous thromboembolism and risk for increased fetal loss during pregnancy	30s; during pregnancy in females	A.D.	Diagnostic and presymptomatic
Polycystic kidney disease dominant Most common genetic disease in humans. Manifests with renal cysts, liver cysts, and occasionally intracranial and aortic aneurysm and hypertension. Loss of glomerular filtration can lead to kidney failure.	Variable onset—all carriers have detectable disease by ultrasound at age 30	A.D.	Diagnostic and presymptomatic
Diabetes mellitus type II Insulin resistance and impaired glucose tolerance	Variable onset—most often >30	M.F.	Research

(continued)

Table 9-4 • **Adult-Onset Disorders** (Continued)

CLINICAL DESCRIPTION	AGE OF ONSET	GENETIC INHERITANCE	TEST AVAILABILITY
Cardiovascular disease			
Familial hypercholesterolemia. Elevated LDL levels leading to coronary artery disease, xanthomas and corneal arcus.	40–50 years	A.D.	Research
Hyperlipidemia			
Elevated low-density lipoproteins and triglycerides associated with premature coronary disease and peripheral vascular disease	30–40 years		Diagnostic and research
Alpha-1 antitrypsin deficiency			
60–70% small airway and alveolar wall destruction, emphysema especially at bases, COPD	35 yr/smoker 45 yr/nonsmk	M.F. in A.R. fashion	Diagnostic and presymptomatic
Oncology conditions			
Multiple endocrine neoplasia (MEN 2a)	Early adulthood	A.D.	Diagnostic and presymptomatic
(Familial medullary thyroid cancer) Medullary thyroid cancer, pheochromocytoma and parathyroid abnormalities			
Breast cancer			
BRCA1, BRCA2 hereditary breast/ovarian cancer	30–70 years often <50 years	A.D.	Predisposition
Breast, ovarian, prostate and colon (BRCA1)			
Breast, ovarian and other cancer (BRCA2)			Predisposition
Hereditary non-polyposis colorectal cancer			
Colorectal, endometrial, bladder, gastric, biliary and renal cell cancers as well as atypical endometrial hyperplasia and uterine leiomyosarcoma	<50 years	A.D.	Predisposition
Li-Fraumeni syndrome			
Soft tissue sarcoma, breast cancer, leukemia, osteosarcoma, melanoma, and other cancers, often including colon, pancreas, adrenal cortex and brain	Often <40 years	A.D.	Predisposition and research
Cowden syndrome			
Breast, non-medullary (papillary or follicular) thyroid cancer. Breast fibroadenomas and noncancerous thyroid nodules or goitre. Multiple buccal mucosa papillomas (cobblestone-line papules), facial trichilemmomas, gastrointestinal polyps. High arched palate, thickened furrowed tongue, megaloencephaly and pectus excavatum.	40–50 years for cancer Teens–20s for mucocutaneous lesions	A.D.	Predisposition and research

A.R. = autosomal recessive; A.D. = autosomal dominant; M.F. = multifactorial.
From Cummings, J. L., Vinters, H. V., Cole, G. M., & Khachaturiar, Z. S. (1998). Alzheimer's disease: Etiologies, pathophysiology, cognitive reserve and treatment opportunities. *Neurology, 51(Suppl),* 2–17; Dik, M. G., Jonker, C., Comijs, H. C., Bouter, L. M., Twisk, J. W., van Kamp, G. J., & Deeg, D. J. (2001). Memory complaints and APOE-epsilon4 accelerate cognitive decline in cognitively normal elderly. *Neurology, 57*(12), 2217–2222; Durr, A., & Brice, A. (2000). Clinical and genetic aspects of spinocerebellar degeneration. *Current Opinions in Neurology, 13*(4), 407–413; GeneTests GeneClinics. (2001). Web site: http://www.genetest.org; Larkin, K., & Fardaei, M. (2001). Myotonic dystrophy—a multigene disorder. *Brain Research Bulletin 2001, 56*(3–4), 389–395; Lindor, N. M., Greene, M. H. and the Mayo Familial Cancer Program. (1998). The concise handbook of familial cancer syndromes. *Journal of the National Cancer Institute, 90*(14), 1039–1071; McIntyre, E. A., & Walker, M. (2002). Genetics of type 2 diabetes and insulin resistance: Knowledge from human studies. *Clinical Endocrinology, 57*(3), 303–311; Pizzuti, A., Friedman, D. L., & Coskey, C. T. (1993). The myotonic dystrophy gene. *Archives of Neurology, 50*(11), 1173–1179; Ridker, P. M., Miletich, J. P., Buring, J. E., Ariyo, A. A., Price, D. T., Manson, J. E., & Hill, J. A. (1998). Factor V Leiden mutation as a risk factor for recurrent pregnancy loss. *Annals of Internal Medicine, 128*(12), 1000–1003; Rogaeva, E. (2002). The solved and unsolved mysteries of the genetics of early-onset Alzheimer's disease. *Neuromolecular Medicine, 2*(1), 1–10; Rosso, S. M., & van Swieten, J. C. (2002). New developments in frontotemporal dementia and parkinsonism linked to chromosome 17. *Current Opinions in Neurology, 15*(4), 423–428.

which earlier treatment of a condition is more beneficial than treatment at a later stage. Presymptomatic testing is therefore offered for several adult-onset conditions, such as cancer, thrombophilia, and antitrypsin deficiency.

In the absence of a single disease-causing gene, it is thought that multiple genes are related to the onset of most adult diseases. These susceptibility genes modify or influence the development and severity of disease. Most susceptibility testing is conducted in the research setting to identify candidate genes for disease, such as Alzheimer's, psychiatric conditions, heart disease, hypertension, and hypercholesterolemia. For some diseases, the interaction of several genes and other environmental or metabolic events affect disease onset and progression. Susceptibility testing can help to distinguish variations within the same disease or response to treatment. For example, no single gene is associated with osteoporosis. Several polymorphisms on candidate genes related to the vitamin D receptor, estrogen and androgen receptors, cytokine production and its associated stimulation of osteoclasts, and collagen type 1-alpha 1 are under study to predict bone mineral density and fracture risk. Some susceptibility genes may predict treatment response. For example, individuals can present with similar clinical signs and symptoms of asthma but have different responses to treatment. Susceptibility testing can help classify the asthma as sensitive or resistant to treatment with corticosteroids.

Population screening, the use of genetic testing for large groups or whole populations, to identify late-onset conditions is under development. Currently population screening is offered in some ethnic groups to identify cancer-predisposing genes. For example, Ashkenazi Jewish individuals (Jews of Eastern European origin) have a greater chance of having inherited a specific genetic mutation in the BRCA1 or BRCA2 genes. Individuals with one of these BRCA mutations have approximately a 56% risk for breast cancer, 16% risk for ovarian cancer, and 16% risk for prostate cancer by age 70 (Struewing et al., 1997). Therefore, identifying one of these mutations allows the patient the options of cancer screening as well as other medical management such as chemoprevention or prophylactic mastectomy or oophorectomy in carriers. Population screening is being explored for other adult-onset conditions such as type 2 diabetes and hereditary hemochromatosis (iron overload disorder). For a test to be considered for population screening, there must be: (1) sufficient information about gene distribution within populations, (2) accurate prediction about the development and progression of disease, and (3) appropriate medical management for asymptomatic individuals with a mutation (U.S. Preventive Services Task Force, 1996).

Nursing Considerations for Adult-Onset Conditions

Nurses must be alert for family histories that indicate multiple generations (autosomal dominant inheritance) or multiple siblings (autosomal recessive inheritance) affected with the same condition, or onset of disease earlier than expected in the general population (eg, multiple generations with early-onset hyperlipidemia). Possible adult-onset conditions are discussed with other members of the health care team for appropriate resources and referral.

Information about diagnostic testing is often introduced as part of a diagnostic work-up. The nurse supports the patient in making decisions related to genetic testing and provides referrals for appropriate education and counselling about the adult-onset condition prior to genetic testing. The nurse addresses the patient's questions or concerns about the benefits and limitations of genetic testing for the individual and the impact on the family. When testing is completed, the nurse provides support for individuals newly diagnosed with an adult-onset condition and provides teaching about the meaning and implications of the test results.

Once a mutation for an adult-onset condition is identified in a family, at-risk family members can be referred for **predisposition testing**. If the patient is found to be the mutation carrier, the nurse provides the patient with information about the risk to other family members. As part of that discussion, the nurse assures the patient that his or her test results are private and confidential and will be shared with others, including family members, only with the patient's permission. If the patient is an unaffected family member, the nurse discusses inheritance and the risk of developing the disease, provides support for the decision-making process, and offers referral for genetics services.

Nursing Care and Interventions in Genetic Counselling and Evaluation

The genetic counselling and evaluation process often involves additional genetic testing and procedures and subsequent decisions for patients and families with regard to reproduction, fertility, testing of children, and management options such as prophylactic surgery. Genetic counselling and evaluation services are traditionally offered at various stages: prenatal or perinatal, newborn or neonatal, childhood, adolescence, and adulthood. Nurses have

responsibilities in each of these areas for assessment and providing psychosocial interventions and accurate information as the family members consider their genetic testing and treatment options. In all of these areas, the nurse considers the patient in the context of the family.

When individuals or family members are considering genetic testing, whether it is for prenatal, newborn, childhood or adult-onset conditions, the nurse provides accurate information as they consider their options. For prenatal testing, this would include information and support for subsequent decisions regarding the pregnancy in the event of a prenatal diagnosis of a genetic condition in the fetus. When a genetic diagnosis such as Down syndrome or hereditary breast or ovarian cancer is made, families need information about the range and severity of potential problems, the proportion of individuals with milder aspects of the condition, management options, support organizations, and current understanding of the long-term prognosis (Williams & Lea, 2003).

Decision-making support is an important nursing intervention in many genetic counselling situations. Examples include when a woman or couple considers the options regarding termination of a pregnancy or when individuals are considering presymptomatic testing for conditions such as Huntington disease or predisposition testing for hereditary cancers. The nurse helps the individual and family to acquire information about options, identifies the pros and cons of each option, helps the individual and family to explore their values and beliefs, respects each person's right to receive or not to receive information, and helps the individual to explain the decision to others (McCloskey & Bulechek, 2000).

Other essential components of nursing care and genetic counselling include teaching and an intervention called "coping enhancement." Teaching is needed, for example, when a new genetic diagnosis is made. The family will need information about the range of possible health outcomes in this condition, treatment options, and (in the case of prenatal diagnosis of a genetic condition) management options regarding continuing or ending the pregnancy. "Coping enhancement" involves "assisting a person to adapt to perceived stressors, changes or threats that interfere with meeting life demands and roles" (McCloskey & Bulechek, 2000, p. 234). Coping enhancement is essential throughout the entire genetic counselling, evaluation, and testing process. Indicators of patient knowledge, decision-making, and coping outcomes have been developed (Johnson, Maas, & Moorhead, 2000), and the nurse can use these indicators when documenting nursing care provided to families.

INDIVIDUALIZING GENETIC PROFILES

Information about genes and their variations is helping researchers to identify genetic differences that predispose some individuals or groups to disease and that affect their responses to treatment. The use of individualized genetics information to predict predisposition to common diseases will take considerable time to develop. However, genetic tests for non-disease genes (ie, polymorphisms in detoxifying enzymes, cell or drug receptor variations, or other inherited polymorphisms related to metabolism) are underway. These genetic tests for individual variations or inherited polymorphisms are called genetic profiles. One major effort of genetic profiling is focused on enzyme metabolism. Several polymorphisms related to enzyme metabolism have been identified in the cytochrome P450 family, long known to affect drug metabolism. There are three subcategories of genetic profiles that describe population differences in enzyme metabolism genotypes. These are based on an individual's genetic make-up for the metabolism of medications or other exogenous compounds into inactive or active metabolites (Norton, 2001b).

The field of pharmacogenetics (the study of gene variations in drug response) is rapidly advancing the way nurses will administer and manage drug treatments. Drug metabolism involves enzyme activity, controlled by genes, for absorption, distribution, and excretion. A single base change, SNPs (single nucleotide polymorphisms), in genes activated for enzyme activity can cause either decreased or increased drug metabolism. Genetic testing for these SNPs will provide a genetic profile, classifying patients according to their drug metabolism type. The SNP classifications of drug metabolism are effective metabolizers (having the expected metabolism), poor metabolizers (lacking the ability to metabolize effectively), and ultra-rapid or rapid metabolizers (having extremely rapid metabolism of drug compounds). Poor metabolizers are most likely to have adverse events due to the prolonged bioavailability of the drug, while ultra-rapid metabolizers have insufficient drug response. Efficient metabolizers can receive the standard expected drug dosage, whereas poor metabolizers need lower doses and ultra-rapid metabolizers need higher doses to obtain a therapeutic effect (Roses, 2000). For example, poor metabolizers of antipsychotic agents are more likely to have oversedation and require dose modification to achieve an expected therapeutic response (Scordo & Spina, 2002).

DNA tests to identify patient-specific genetic profiles will be a treatment priority to assist in planning and evaluating treatment outcomes, to prevent adverse effects, and to improve therapies. Nurses therefore will need to know how polymorphisms affect a patient's susceptibility to disease and treatment response. Understanding the effect of polymorphisms on protein and enzyme function and their distribution in specific populations will be needed for health promotion. Since nurses will provide information about genetic profiles, they will need to know about the impact of genetics on treatment.

Applications of Genetics in Nursing Practice

Nursing practice in genetics-related health care blends the principles of human genetics with nursing care in collaboration with other professionals, including genetics specialists, to foster health improvement, maintenance, and restoration. In any practice setting, nurses will carry out five main activities in genetics-related nursing practice: help collect and interpret relevant family and medical histories; identify patients and families who need further genetic evaluation and counselling and refer them to appropriate genetics services; offer genetics information and resources to patients and families; collaborate with genetics specialists; and participate in the management and coordination of care of patients with genetic conditions. Genetics-related nursing practice includes the care of patients who have genetics conditions, persons who may be predisposed to develop or pass on genetic conditions, and persons who are seeking genetics information and referral for additional genetics services (Lea, Williams, Jenkins, et al., 2000).

Nurses support patients and families with genetics-related health concerns by ensuring that their health choices are informed ones and by advocating for the privacy and confidentiality of genetics information and for equal access to genetic testing and treatments. *The Scope and Standards of Genetics Clinical Nursing Practice,* developed by the International Society of Nurses in Genetics (ISONG, 1998) and published by the American Nurses Association, delineates roles and responsibilities for nurses in providing genetics health care.

GENETICS AND HEALTH ASSESSMENT

Assessment of a person's genetics-related health status is an ongoing process. The nurse collects information that can help identify individuals and families who have actual or potential genetics-related health concerns or who may benefit from further genetics information, counselling, testing, and treatment. This process can begin before conception and continue throughout the lifespan. Nurses evaluate family and past medical histories, including prenatal history, childhood illnesses, developmental history, adult-onset conditions (if adult), past surgeries, treatments, and medications; this information may relate to the genetic condition at hand or being considered. (See Chap. 5 for more information on assessing past medical history.) The nurse also identifies the patient's ethnic background and conducts a physical assessment to gather pertinent genetics information. The assessment also includes the patient's culture, spiritual beliefs, and ancestry. Genetics-related health assessment always includes determining a patient's or family's understanding of actual or potential health concerns related to genetics and understanding how these issues are communicated within a family (ISONG, 1998; Lea, Jenkins & Francomano, 1998).

Family History Assessment

Nurses in any practice setting continuously assess genetic family history to identify the presence of a genetic trait, inherited condition, or predisposition. A questionnaire (Chart 9-3) is often used to identify genetic conditions for which further information, education, testing, or treatment can be offered. In consultation and collaboration with other health care providers and specialists, the nurse can then determine whether further genetic testing and evaluation should be offered for the trait or condition in question. A detailed and accurate family history provides the most complete genetics health information. The family history should include at least three generations, as well as information about the current and past health status of all family members, including the age of onset of any illnesses and cause of death and age at death. The nurse also inquires about medical conditions known to have a heritable component and for which genetic testing may be offered. The nurse obtains information about the presence of birth defects, mental retardation, familial traits, or similarly affected family members (Lashley, 1998; Lea, Jenkins & Francomano, 1998).

The nurse also considers the presence of genetic relatedness (consanguinity) among family members when assessing the risk for genetic conditions in couples or families. For example, when obtaining a preconception or prenatal family history, the nurse asks whether the prospective parents have common ancestors (ie, they are first cousins). This is important to know because individuals who share ancestors have more genes in common than those who are unrelated, thus increasing their chance for having children with an autosomal recessive inherited condition such as cystic fibrosis. The number of shared genes depends upon the degree of relationship. A parent and child, for example, share half of their genes, while first cousins share one in eight of their genes. Ascertaining genetic relatedness gives the nurse the opportunity to offer additional genetic counselling and evaluation. It may also serve as an explanation for families who have a child or individual with a rare autosomal recessive inherited condition (Lea, Jenkins & Francomano, 1998).

When the assessment of family history reveals that the patient has been adopted, genetics-based health assessment becomes more challenging. The nurse and health care team should make

Chart 9-3   Primary Genetic Family History Screening Questionnaire

Question 1

If you, yourself, have, or if a family member in either your family or the family of your partner has, or ever has had, one of the following please circle the check mark under SELF or PARTNER and write in the exact relationship of that person to SELF or PARTNER, i.e., child (born or unborn), partner, sibling, grandparent, cousin, aunt or uncle, niece or nephew.

Condition	Self	Partner	Relationship
Birth defect name?_____	✓	✓	_____
Cancer name?_____	✓	✓	_____
High cholesterol	✓	✓	_____
Cleft lip/cleft palate	✓	✓	_____
Cystic fibrosis (CF)	✓	✓	_____
Down syndrome (DS)	✓	✓	_____
Fragile X syndrome	✓	✓	_____
Gastroschisis (opening in belly at birth)	✓	✓	_____
Hearing loss/deafness (not from aging)	✓	✓	_____
Heart problem (from birth)	✓	✓	_____
Heart disease (early onset)	✓	✓	_____
Hemophilia (slow clotting/heavy bleeding)	✓	✓	_____
Infant death (before one year of age)	✓	✓	_____
Inherited health problems	✓	✓	_____
Kidney problems (other than infection)	✓	✓	_____
Miscarriages	✓	✓	_____
Mental retardation	✓	✓	_____
Muscular weakness (muscular dystrophy)	✓	✓	_____
Pregnancy termination (due to birth defect) _____	✓	✓	_____
Sickle cell anemia	✓	✓	_____
Skin or nerve tumour	✓	✓	_____
Spina bifida (opening in spine, at birth)	✓	✓	_____
Stillbirths	✓	✓	_____
Stroke at an early age (called thrombosis)	✓	✓	_____
Thalassemia	✓	✓	_____
Visual loss/blindness (not from aging)	✓	✓	_____

Note: If you have checked any of these conditions, please talk with your nurse about a genetics referral for counselling and evaluation.

Do you have any other medical problems or issues that are of concern to you?

(Please circle one)   Yes   No

If you circled Yes, please tell your nurse, who may be able to help you or be able to find appropriate support/help for you.

Patient name _____

Date of birth _____

Name of person filling out the form (if different from patient) _____

Relationship to patient _____

Date form filled out _____

Nurse name _____

Date patient seen _____

_____

Courtesy of the Foundation for Blood Research.

all efforts to help the patient obtain as much information as possible about his or her biological parents, including their ethnic backgrounds.

Questions regarding reproductive history (eg, history of miscarriage or stillbirth) are included in genetic family history health assessments to identify possible chromosomal conditions. The nurse also inquires about any history of family members with inherited conditions or birth defects; maternal health conditions such as type 1 diabetes, seizure disorder, or maternal PKU, which may increase the risk for birth defects in children; and exposure to alcohol or other drugs during pregnancy. Maternal age is also noted: women who are 35 years or older who are considering

pregnancy and childbearing or who are already pregnant should be offered prenatal diagnosis (eg, testing through amniocentesis) because of the association between advancing maternal age and chromosomal abnormalities such as Down syndrome (Lea, Jenkins & Francomano, 1998).

Ancestry and Ethnicity Assessment

Assessing ancestry and ethnicity helps identify individuals and groups who could benefit from genetic testing for carrier identification, prenatal diagnosis, and susceptibility testing. For example, carrier testing for sickle cell anemia is routinely offered to individuals of African-American heritage, while carrier testing for Tay-Sachs disease and Canavan disease is offered to individuals of Ashkenazi Jewish descent. Professional organizations such as the American College of Obstetrics and Gynecology (ACOG, 2001) recommend that relevant racial and ethnic populations be offered carrier testing. Recently, ACOG and the American College of Medical Genetics (ACMG) recommended that all couples, particularly those of Northern European and Ashkenazi Jewish ancestry, be offered carrier screening for cystic fibrosis (ACOG, 2001). Ideally, carrier testing is offered before conception to allow persons who are carriers to make reproductive decisions. Prenatal diagnosis is offered and discussed when both partners of a couple are found to be carriers.

Inquiring about a patient's ethnic background is also important when assessing for susceptibilities to adult-onset conditions such as hereditary breast or ovarian cancer. For example, a specific BRCA1 cancer-predisposing gene mutation seems to occur more frequently in women of Ashkenazi Jewish descent. Therefore, asking about ethnicity can help identify persons with an increased risk for certain cancer gene mutations (American Medical Association, 2001).

The nurse assesses ancestry and ethnic background to identify individuals who may have an underlying genetic condition that may affect the safety and efficacy of certain medications or treatments. For example, glucose-6-phosphate dehydrogenase deficiency (G6PD) is a common enzyme abnormality that affects millions of people throughout the world, especially those of Mediterranean, Southeast Asian, African, Middle Eastern, and Near Eastern origin. G6PD is transmitted as a gene mutation on the X chromosome. Individuals with a severe deficiency have chronic hemolytic anemia, while others with a milder deficiency develop hemolytic anemia upon exposure to peroxide-producing drugs, infection, exposure to naphthalene in mothballs, or ingestion of the fava (broad) bean (Lashley, 1998).

Assessment of ancestry and ethnic background is also important when considering drug metabolism. The ability to metabolize and eliminate certain medications depends upon acetylation in the liver by the enzyme N-acetyltransferase. Many different versions (polymorphisms) of the gene that codes for N-acetyltransferase exist, and these polymorphisms vary among ethnic groups. This is an important consideration, for example, when isoniazid (INH) is prescribed for the treatment of tuberculosis. Patients who are rapid or ultra-rapid metabolizers have a significantly higher risk for developing isoniazid-induced hepatitis; this is especially true for persons of Chinese and Japanese descent (Lashley, 1998).

Physical Assessment

Physical assessment may provide clues that a particular genetic condition is present in an individual and family. Family history assessment may offer initial guidance regarding the particular area for physical assessment. For example, a family history of familial hypercholesterolemia would alert the nurse to assess family members for symptoms of hyperlipidemias (xanthomas, corneal arcus, abdominal pain of unexplained origin). As another example, a family history of neurofibromatosis type I, an inherited condition involving tumours of the central nervous system, would prompt the nurse to carry out a detailed assessment of closely related family members. Skin findings such as café-au-lait spots, axillary freckling, or tumours of the skin (neurofibromas) would warrant referral for further evaluation, including genetic evaluation and counselling (Lea, Jenkins & Francomano, 1998).

When a genetic condition is suspected as a result of a family history or physical assessment, the nurse, in collaboration with the health care team, may initiate further discussion and evaluation. Providing genetics information, offering and discussing genetic tests, and suggesting a referral to a geneticist may be performed (Chart 9-4).

Cultural, Social, and Spiritual Assessment

When collecting and discussing genetics information, the nurse needs to assess the patient's and family's cultural, social, and spiritual orientations. The nurse also needs to consider the patient's views about the significance of a genetic condition and its effect on self-concept, as well as the patient's perception of the role of genetics in health and illness, reproduction, and disability. Patients' social and cultural backgrounds determine their interpretations and values about information obtained from genetic testing and evaluation and thus influence their perceptions of health, illness, and risk. Family structure and decision-making and educational background contribute in the same way (Lea, Jenkins & Francomano, 1998).

Assessing a patient's beliefs, values, and expectations regarding genetic testing and information helps the nurse to provide appropriate information about the specific genetics topic. In some

Chart 9-4 · Indications for Making a Genetic Referral

Prepregnancy and Prenatal
- Maternal age of 35 years or greater at expected time of delivery
- Previous child with a chromosome problem
- Positive AFP profile screening test
- Previous child with a birth defect or family history of birth defects
- Pregnancy history of two or more unexplained miscarriages
- Maternal conditions such as diabetes, epilepsy, or alcoholism
- Exposures to certain medications or drugs during pregnancy
- Family history of mental retardation

Pediatric
- Positive newborn screening test
- One or more major birth defects
- Unusual (dysmorphic) facial features
- Developmental delay/mental retardation
- Suspicion of a metabolic disorder
- Unusually tall or short stature, or growth delays
- Known chromosomal abnormality

Adult
- Mental retardation without a known cause
- Unexplained infertility or multiple pregnancy losses
- A personal or family history of thrombotic events
- Adult-onset conditions such as hemochromatosis, hearing loss, visual impairment
- Family history of an adult-onset neurodegenerative disorder (eg, Huntington disease)
- Features of a genetic condition such as neurofibromatosis (café-au-lait spots, neurofibromas on the skin), Marfan syndrome (unusually tall stature, dilation of the aortic root), others

Cancer History
- A personal or family history of cancer with a known or suspected inherited predisposition (eg, early-onset breast cancer, colon cancer, ovarian cancer, retinoblastoma)
- Several family members affected by cancer
- A family member with cancer at an unusually young age
- A family member with an unusual type of cancer

cultures, for example, individuals believe that health means the absence of symptoms and that the cause of illness is supernatural. Patients with these beliefs may initially reject suggestions for pre-symptomatic or carrier testing. However, by including resources such as family, cultural, and religious community leaders when providing genetics-related health care, the nurse can help ensure that patients receive information in a way that transcends social, cultural, and economic barriers (Lea, Jenkins & Francomano, 1998).

Psychosocial Assessment

Psychosocial assessment is an essential nursing component of the genetics health assessment (Chart 9-5). After conducting an initial psychosocial assessment, the nurse will be aware of the potential impact of new genetic information on the patient and family and how they may cope with this information.

GENETIC COUNSELLING AND EVALUATION SERVICES

As the contribution of genetics to the health–illness continuum is recognized, the process of genetic counselling is expected to become a responsibility of all health care professionals in clinical practice. Nurses are obvious and natural providers of genetics services because they are aware of a patient's personal and family history. They assess patients' health and make referrals for specialized diagnosis and treatment. They offer anticipatory guidance by explaining the purpose and goals of a referral. They collaborate with primary care providers and specialists in giving supportive and follow-up counselling. They coordinate follow-up and case management.

Genetics Services

Genetics services provide genetics information, education, and support to patients and families with genetics-related health concerns. Genetics professionals, including medical geneticists, genetics counsellors, and advanced practice nurses in genetics, provide specific genetics services to patients and families who are referred by their primary health care providers. A team approach is often used by genetics specialists to obtain and interpret complex family history information, evaluate and diagnose genetic conditions, interpret and discuss complicated genetic test results,

support patients throughout the evaluation process, and offer resources for additional professional and family support. Patients participate as team members and decision-makers throughout the process. Genetics services encompass an evaluation and communication process by which individuals and their families come to learn and understand relevant aspects of genetics, to make informed health decisions, and to receive support as they integrate personal and family genetics information into daily living (Lea, Jenkins & Francomano, 1998).

Genetic counselling may take place over an extended period and may entail more than one counselling session, which may include other family members. This allows patients and families to learn and understand genetics information, to receive support and guidance in decision-making, and to obtain comprehensive and coordinated care if they have specific genetic conditions or concerns. The components of genetic counselling are outlined in Chart 9-6. Genetic counselling may be offered at any point during the lifespan, although genetic counselling issues are often relevant to the life stage in which counselling is sought. Some examples are presented in Chart 9-7 (Lea, Jenkins & Francomano, 1998).

Nursing Role in Genetic Counselling

Patients seek genetic counselling for a variety of reasons and at different stages of life. Some are seeking preconception or prenatal information; others are referred following the birth of a child with a birth defect or suspected genetic condition; still others are seek-

Chart 9-6 **Components of Genetic Counselling**

Information and Assessment Sources
- Reason for referral
- Family history
- Medical history/records
- Relevant test results and other medical evaluations
- Social and emotional concerns
- Relevant cultural, educational, and financial factors

Analysis of Data
- Family history
- Physical examination as needed
- Additional laboratory testing and/or procedures (eg, echocardiogram, ophthalmology or neurologic examination)

Communication of Genetic Finding
- Natural history of disorder
- Pattern of inheritance
- Reproductive and family health issues and options
- Testing options
- Management and treatment issues

Counselling and Support
- Identify individual and family questions and concerns.
- Identify existing support systems.
- Provide emotional and social support.
- Refer for additional support and counselling as indicated.

Follow-Up
- Written summary to referring primary care providers and family
- Coordination of care with primary care providers and specialists
- Additional discussions of test results and/or diagnosis

Lea, D. H., Jenkins, J. F., & Francomano, C. A. (1998). *Genetics in clinical practice: New directions for nursing and health care.* Sudbury, MA: Jones & Bartlett.

Chart 9-5 • ASSESSMENT

Psychosocial Genetic Health Assessment

The nurse assesses:
- Educational level and understanding of the genetic condition or concern in the family.
- Desired goals and health outcomes in relation to genetic condition or concern.
- Family rules regarding disclosure of medical information (eg, some families may not reveal a history of diseases such as cancer or mental illness during the family history assessment).
- Family rules, boundaries, and cultural practices as well as personal preferences about knowing medical information.
- Past coping mechanisms and social support.
- Ability to make an informed decision (eg, is the patient under stress from family situations, acute or chronic illness, or medications that may impair the ability to make an informed decision).

Chart 9-7   Genetic Counselling Across the Lifespan

Prenatal Issues
- Understanding prenatal screening and diagnosis testing
- Implications of reproductive choices
- Potential for anxiety and emotional distress
- Effects on partnership, family and parental–fetal bonding

Newborn Issues
- Understanding newborn screening results
- Potential for disrupted parent–newborn relationship upon diagnosis of a genetic condition
- Parental guilt
- Implications for siblings and other family members
- Coordination and continuity of care

Pediatric Issues
- Caring for children with complex medical needs
- Coordination of care
- Potential for impaired parent–child relationship
- Potential for social stigmatization

Adolescent Issues
- Potential for impaired self-image and decreased self-esteem
- Potential for altered perception of family
- Implications for lifestyle and family planning

Adult Issues
- Potential for ambiguous test results
- Identification of a genetic susceptibility or diagnosis without an existing cure ("therapeutic gap")
- Effect on marriage, reproduction, parenting, and lifestyle
- Potential impact on insurability and employability

Lea, D. H., Jenkins, J. F., & Francomano, C. A. (1998). *Genetics in clinical practice: New directions for nursing and health care.* Sudbury, MA: Jones & Bartlett.

ing information for themselves or their families because of the presence or family history of a genetic condition. Regardless of the timing or setting, genetic counselling is offered to all patients who have questions about genetics and their health. In collaboration with the health care team, the nurse considers referring for genetic counselling any patient in whose family a heritable condition exists and who asks questions such as, "What are my chances for having this condition? Is there a genetic test that will tell me? Is there a genetic treatment or cure? What are my options?" (Lea, Jenkins & Francomano, 1998).

Nurses refer clients, collaborate with genetics specialists, and participate in genetic counselling when they carry out the following activities:

- Provide appropriate genetic information before, during, and in follow-up to genetic counselling
- Help gather relevant family and medical history information
- Offer support to patients and families throughout the genetic counselling process
- Coordinate genetics-related health care with relevant community and national support resources

These activities, carried out in collaboration with patients and families, help ensure that they receive the most benefit from genetic counselling (Lea, Jenkins & Francomano, 1998; Lea, Williams, Jenkins, et al., 2000).

RESPECTING PATIENTS' RIGHTS
Respecting the patient's right to self-determination—that is, supporting decisions that reflect the patient's personal beliefs, values,

and interests—is a central principle of how nurses provide genetics information and counselling. Genetics specialists and nurses participating in genetic counselling make every attempt to respect the patient's ability to make autonomous decisions. A first step in providing such nondirective counselling is recognizing one's own values (see Chart 9-1) and how communication of genetics information may be influenced by those values.

Confidentiality of genetics information and respect for privacy are other essential principles underlying genetic counselling. The patient has the right to have testing without having the results divulged to anyone, including insurers or physicians. Some patients pay for testing themselves so that insurers will not learn of the test; others use a different name for testing to protect their privacy.

All genetics specialists, including nurses who participate in the genetic counselling process and those with access to individuals' genetic information, must honour the patient's desire for confidentiality. Genetics information should be kept from family members, insurance companies, employers, and schools if the patient desires, even if keeping the information confidential is difficult. The nurse may want to disclose genetics information to family members who could experience significant harm if they do not know such information. However, the patient may have other views and may wish to keep this information from the family, resulting in an ethical dilemma for both patient and nurse. The nurse must honour the patient's wishes while explaining to the patient the potential benefit this information may have to other family members (ISONG, 2002).

PROVIDING PRECOUNSELLING INFORMATION
Preparing the patient and family, promoting informed decision-making, and obtaining informed consent are essential in genetic counselling. The nurse assesses the patient's capacity and ability to give voluntary consent. This includes assessment of factors that may interfere with informed consent such as hearing and language deficits, impaired intelligence, and the effects of medication. The nurse makes sure that the individual's decision to undergo testing is not affected by coercion, persuasion, or manipulation. Because information may need to be repeated over time, the nurse offers follow-up discussion as needed (Bove et al., 1997).

The genetics service to which the nurse refers a patient or family for genetic counselling will ask the nurse to provide background information for evaluation. Genetics specialists need to know the reason for referral, the patient's or family's reason for seeking genetic counselling, and potential genetics-related health concerns. The nurse may refer a family with a new diagnosis of hereditary breast or ovarian cancer, for example, to obtain more information or counselling or to discuss the likelihood of developing the disease and the implications for other family members. The family may have concerns about confidentiality and privacy. Using the nursing assessment, the genetics specialists tailor the genetic counselling to respond to these concerns.

With the patient's permission, the nurse may also provide to the genetics specialists the relevant test results and medical evaluations. The nurse needs to obtain permission from the patient and, if applicable, from other family members to retrieve, review, and transfer medical records that document the genetic condition of concern. In some situations, evaluation of more than one family member may be necessary to establish a diagnosis of a genetic disorder. The nurse can prepare the family for this assessment by explaining that the medical information and evaluation are necessary to ensure that appropriate information and counselling (including risk interpretation) are provided.

The nurse will be asked to provide information about the emotional and social status of the patient and family. Genetics specialists will want to know the coping skills of a family that has recently learned of the diagnosis of a genetic disorder. They will want to be aware of the types of genetics information being sought. The nurse helps to identify cultural and other issues that may influence how information is provided and by whom. For patients with hearing loss, for example, an interpreter's services may have to be arranged. The genetics professional, after determining these issues with the nurse, prepares for the genetic counselling and evaluation with these relevant issues in mind (Lea, Jenkins & Francomano, 1998).

PREPARING THE PATIENT FOR GENETIC EVALUATION

Before the genetic counselling appointment, the nurse discusses with the patient and family the type and nature of family history information that will be collected during the consultation. Family history collection and analysis are comprehensive and focus on information that may be relevant to the specific genetic concern in question. Although targeted to each genetic counselling situation, such analysis always includes assessment for any other potentially inherited conditions for which testing and preventive and treatment measures may be offered.

A physical examination performed by the medical geneticist may be needed to identify specific clinical features that are diagnostic of a genetic condition. The examination also helps to identify whether additional laboratory tests are needed to clarify the diagnosis of a genetic disorder. The detailed physical examination generally involves assessment of all body systems, with a focus on specific physical characteristics considered for diagnosis. The nurse describes the diagnostic evaluations that are part of a genetics consultation and explains their purposes (Lashley, 1998; Lea, Jenkins & Francomano, 1998).

COMMUNICATING GENETICS INFORMATION TO THE PATIENT

After the family history and physical examination are completed, the genetics team reviews the information gathered before beginning genetic counselling with the patient and family. The genetics specialists meet with the patient and family to discuss their findings. When information from family and medical histories and examination confirms the presence of a genetic condition in a family, the genetics specialist discusses with the patient the natural history of the condition, the pattern of inheritance, and the implications of the genetic condition for reproductive and general health. When appropriate, the genetic specialists discuss and describe relevant testing and management options. The nurse assesses the patient's understanding of the genetic consultation and clarifies information given by the specialists.

PROVIDING SUPPORT

The genetics team provides support throughout the counselling session and makes every effort to elicit individual and family concerns. The genetics specialist uses principles of active listening to interpret patient concerns and emotions, seek and provide feedback, and demonstrate understanding of those concerns. When needed, the genetics specialist suggests referral for additional social and emotional support. The genetics specialist discusses pertinent patient and family concerns and needs with the nurse and primary health care team so that they can provide additional support and guidance (Lea, Jenkins & Francomano, 1998). The nurse assesses the patient's understanding of the information given during the counselling session, clarifies information, answers questions, assesses the patient's reactions, and identifies supports.

Providing Follow-Up After Genetic Evaluation

In follow-up to genetic evaluation and counselling, the genetics specialists prepare a written summary of the evaluation and counselling session and, with the patient's permission, send this summary to the primary health care provider as well as all other providers and participants in the patient's care, as identified by the family. The consultation summary outlines the results of family history and physical and laboratory assessments, provides a discussion of the specific diagnosis (when made), reviews the inheritance and associated risk of recurrence for the patient and family, presents reproductive and general health options, and makes recommendations for further testing and management. The summary is also sent to the patient and a copy is retained in the patient's medical records. The nurse has an important role in reviewing the summary with the patient and family and identifying information, education, and counselling for which follow-up genetic counselling may be useful (Lea, Jenkins & Francomano, 1998; Lea & Williams, 2002; Lea & Smith, 2002).

Follow-up genetic counselling is always offered to patients and families, as some may need more time to understand and discuss the specifics of a genetic test or diagnosis or wish to review reproductive options again later when pregnancy is being considered. Follow-up genetic counselling is also offered to clients when further evaluation and counselling of extended family members is recommended (Lea, Jenkins & Francomano, 1998).

As part of follow-up, nurses can educate patients about where to find information about genetics issues. Some resources that provide the most up-to-date and reliable genetics information are available on the Internet. Several of these are listed at the end of the chapter.

Ethical Issues

With recent advances in genetics, nurses must consider their responsibilities in handling genetics information and potential ethical implications such as informed decision-making, privacy and confidentiality of genetics information, and access to and justice in health care. The ethical principles of autonomy, fidelity, and veracity are also important.

Ethical questions relating to genetics occur in various settings and at all levels of nursing practice. At the level of direct patient care, nurses participate in providing genetics information, testing, and gene-based therapeutics. They provide patient care based on the values of self-determination and personal autonomy. Patients should be as fully involved as possible in the planning and implementation of their own health care; to do so, patients need appropriate, accurate, and complete information given at such a level and in such a form that they and their families can make well-informed personal, medical, and reproductive health decisions. Nurses, as the most accessible health care professionals, are invaluable in the informed consent process. Nurses can help patients clarify values and goals, assess understanding of information, protect the patient's rights, and support their decisions. Nurses can advocate for patient autonomy in health decisions. ISONG's Position Statement "Informed Decision-Making and Consent" (2000) provides support and guidance for nurses who are helping patients who are considering genetic testing.

Nurses need to ensure the privacy and confidentiality of genetics information derived from such sources as the family history, genetic tests, and other genetics-based interventions. Many Canadians are increasingly concerned about threats to their personal privacy. Nurses must be aware of the potential ethical issues related to the privacy and confidentiality of genetics information, including conflicts between an individual's privacy versus the family's need for genetics information. ISONG's Position Statement "Privacy and Confidentiality of Genetic Information" (2002) is a useful resource.

An ethical foundation provides nurses with a holistic framework for handling ethical issues with integrity. It also supplies the basis for communicating genetics information to a patient, to a family, to other care providers, to community agencies and organizations, and to society as a whole. In addition, it provides support for nurses facing clinical situations that involve ethical dilemmas. Principle-based ethics offers moral guidelines that nurses can use to justify their nursing practice. The emphasis is on ethical principles of beneficence (to do good) and non-maleficence (to do no harm), as well as autonomy, justice, fidelity, veracity, to help solve ethical dilemmas that may arise in clinical care. Respect for persons is the ethical principle underlying all nursing care. With an ethical foundation that is based on these principles and that incorporates the values of caring, nurses can promote the kind of thoughtful discussions that are useful when patients and families are facing genetics-related health and reproductive decisions and consequences (Scanlon & Fibison, 1995; ISONG, 2000).

 Critical Thinking Exercises

1. Your patient, age 53, is recovering from a right mastectomy. She underwent a left mastectomy for breast cancer at age 45. Her daughter, age 31, expresses concern about her own breast cancer risk, telling you that her sister and maternal grandmother have also had breast cancer. What pattern of inheritance is suggested in this family? What genetics information would you provide to this woman?

2. A 48-year-old man is admitted to your medical unit with a new diagnosis of liver cancer. He says he is worried about his children, an 18-year-old boy and a 15-year-old girl: "I don't want them to get this, too." Your nursing assessment reveals a past history of arthritis and diabetes and a family history of "iron overload" in the patient's 40-year-old brother. What adult-onset condition does this history suggest? What nursing action would you take?

3. Your patient has three daughters, ages 25, 30, and 32, and one son, age 22. He also has four sisters, two of whom were diagnosed with breast cancer in their early 40s and chose to have BRCA gene mutation testing. Both were found to carry a BRCA1 gene mutation. The patient's daughters learn of these results and want to be tested to learn of their status. The patient does not want to be tested and tells the nurse at a routine check-up, "I don't want to have testing. I have a right not to be tested, and I don't want to know if I carry that cancer gene. I care about my daughters, but I am afraid to find out for them." How might you respond to the patient? What would you say if one of the patient's daughters calls you and asks for your help? What are the counselling issues for this daughter that are unique to this situation?

REFERENCES AND SELECTED READINGS

Books

American College of Obstetricians and Gynecologists (ACOG). (2001). *Preconception and prenatal carrier screening for cystic fibrosis: Clinical and laboratory guidelines.* Washington, DC: Author.

American Medical Association. (2001). *Identifying and managing hereditary risk for breast and ovarian cancer.* Chicago: Author.

Bradley, W. G., Daroff, R. B., Fenichel, G. M., & Jankovic, J. (2004). *Neurology in clinical practice* (Vols. 1 & 2). Philadelphia: Elsevier.

Canadian Nurses Association. (2002). *Code of ethics for registered nurses.* Ottawa: Author. Available at: http://www.cna-nurses.ca/cna/documents/pdf/publications/CodeofEthics2002_e.pdf.

Gardiner, R. R. M., & Sutherland, G. R. (1996). *Chromosome abnormalities and genetic counseling* (2d ed.). New York: Oxford University Press.

Haerle, T. (Ed.). (1992). *Children with Tourette syndrome. A parents' guide.* Rockville, MD: Woodbine.

Hartl, D., & Jones, E. W. (1998). *Genetics principles and analysis* (4th ed.). Sudbury, MA: Jones & Bartlett Publishing.

Hughes, S. (1996). *What makes Ryan tick?* Duarte, CA: Hope Press.

ISONG. (1998). *Statement on the scope and standards of genetics clinical nursing practice.* Washington, DC: American Nurses Association.

Iowa Intervention Project. (2000). *Nursing interventions classification* (3rd ed.). St Louis: Mosby.

Iowa Outcomes Project. (2000). *Nursing outcomes classification* (2d ed.) St. Louis: Mosby.

Johnson, M., Maas, M. L., & Moorhead, S. (Eds.) (2000). *Nursing interventions classification.* St. Louis: C.V. Mosby.

Lashley, F. R. (1998). *Clinical genetics in nursing practice* (2d ed.). New York: Springer.

Lea, D. H. (2002). Genetics. In Maher, A. B., Salmond, S. W., & Pellino, T. A. (Eds.) *Orthopaedic nursing.* Philadelphia: W. B. Saunders.

Lea, D. H., Jenkins, J. F., & Francomano, C. A. (1998). *Genetics in clinical practice: New directions for nursing and health care.* Sudbury, MA: Jones & Bartlett.

Lea, D. H., & Smith, R. S. (2002). *Genetics resource guide: A handy reference for public health nurses.* Scarborough, ME: Foundation for Blood Research.

McCloskey, J. C. & Bulechek, G. M. (Eds.). (2000). *Nursing interventions classification (NIC): Iowa Intervention Project* (3rd ed.). St. Louis: C. V. Mosby.

National Academy of Science, Committee for the Study of Inborn Errors of Metabolism. (1975). *Genetic Screening.* Washington, DC: National Academy of Sciences.

National Institute of Neurological Disorders. (2005). *Tourette fact sheet.* Available at: http://www.ninds.nig.gov/disorders/tourette/detail.

National Institutes of Health, National Cancer Institute. (1995). *Understanding gene testing.* Washington, DC: U.S. Department of Health and Human Services, NIH Pub. No. 9603905.

Rimoin, D., Connor, J. M., & Pyeritz, R. (2002). *Emery-Rimoin principles and practice of medical genetics* (4th ed.). New York: Churchill-Livingstone.

Scanlon, C., & Fibison, W. (1995). *Managing genetic information: Implications for nursing practice.* Washington, DC: American Nurses Association.

Secretary's Advisory Committee on Genetic Testing (SACGT). (2000). National Institutes of Health. A public consultation of oversight of genetic tests. Bethesda, MD. Available from http://www4.od.nih.gov/oba/sacgt.htm.

Thompson, M. W., McInnes, R. R., & Willard, H. F. (2001). *Thompson and Thompson's genetics in medicine* (6th ed.). Philadelphia: W. B. Saunders.

U.S. Preventive Services Task Force. (1996). *Guide to clinical preventive services* (2d ed.). Baltimore: Williams & Wilkins.

Williams, J. K., & Lea, D. H. (2003). *Genetic issues for perinatal nurses* (2d ed.). White Plains, NY: March of Dimes.

Journals

ACOG Committee on Genetics. (1996). Screening for Tay-Sachs disease. *International Journal of Gynaecology & Obstetrics, 52*(3), 311–312.

ACOG Committee on Genetics. (1999). Screening for Canavan disease. *International Journal of Gynaecology & Obstetrics, 65*(1), 91–92.

ACOG Committee on Genetics. (2001). Genetic screening for hemoglobinopathies. *International Journal of Gynaecology & Obstetrics, 74*(3), 309–310.

American College of Medical Genetics/American Society of Human Genetics Huntington Disease Genetic Testing Working Group. (1998). ACMG/ASHG statement. Laboratory guidelines for Huntington disease genetic testing. *American Journal of Human Genetics, 62*(5), 1243–1247.

American Society of Clinical Oncology. (1996). Statement of the American Society of Clinical Oncology: Genetic testing for cancer susceptibility. *Journal of Clinical Oncology, 14*(5), 1730–1736.

Anderson, G., Monsen, R. B., Prows, C. A., Tinley, S., & Jenkins, J. (2000). Preparing the nursing profession for participation in a genetic paradigm in health care. *Nursing Outlook, 48*(1), 23–27.

Baird, P. A. (1983). Neural tube defects in the Sikhs. *American Journal of Medical Genetics, 16*(1), 49–56.

Bartsch, H., Nair, U., Risch, A., et al. (2000). Genetic polymorphism of CYP genes, alone or in combination, as a risk modifier of tobacco-related cancers. *Cancer Epidemiology, Biomarkers and Prevention, 9*(1), 3–28.

Berry, R. J., Li, Z., Erickson, D., Li, S., Moore, C. A., Wang, H., et al. (1999). Prevention of neural-tube defects with folic acid in China. *New England Journal of Medicine, 341*(20), 1485–1490.

Billings, P. R. (2000). Applying advances in genetic medicine: Where do we go from here? *Healthplan, 41*(6), 32–35.

Bove, C. M., Fry, S. T., & MacDonald, D. J. (1997). Presymptomatic and predisposition genetic testing: Ethical and social considerations. *Seminars in Oncology Nursing, 13*(2), 135–140.

Brookes, A. J. (1999). The essence of SNPs. *Gene, 234*(2), 177–186.

Burke, W. (2002). Genetic testing. *New England Journal of Medicine, 347*(23), 1867–1875.

Burke, W., Thomson, E., Khoury, M. J., et al. (1998). Hereditary hemochromatosis: gene discovery and its implications for population-based screening. *Journal of the American Medical Association, 280*(2), 172–178.

Canadian Paediatric Society (CPS), Bioethics Committee. (2003). Guidelines for genetic testing of healthy children. *Paediatrics & Child Health. 8*(1), 42–45. Available at: http://www.cps.ca/English/statements/B/b03-01.htm.

Chambers, K., Popkin, J., Arnold, W., Irwin, B., & Hall, J. G. (1994). Neural tube defects in British Columbia [29]. *Lancet, 343*(8895), 489–490.

Collins, F. S. (1999). Medical and societal consequences of the Human Genome Project. *New England Journal of Medicine, 341*(1), 28–37.

Collins, F. S., & McKusick, V. A. (2001). Implications of the Human Genome Project for medical science. *Journal of the American Medical Association, 285*(5), 540–544.

Cox, N. J., Frigge, M., Nicolae, D. L., et al. (1999). Loci on chromosomes 2 (NIDDM1) and 15 interact to increase susceptibility to diabetes in Mexican Americans. *Nature Genetics, 21*(2), 213–215.

Czeizel, A. E. (1993). Prevention of congenital abnormalities by periconceptional multivitamin supplementation. *British Medical Journal, 306*, 1645–1648.

Evans, W. E. & McLeod. (2003). Drug therapy: Pharmacogenomics—Drug disposition, drug targets, and side effects. *New England Journal of Medicine, 348*(6), 538–549.

Evans, W. E., & Relling, M. V. (1999). Pharmacogenomics: Translating functional genomics into rational therapeutics. *Science, 286*(5439), 487–491

Feetham, S. (1999). Families and the genetic revolution. Implications for primary healthcare, education, and research. *Families, Systems & Health, 17*(1), 27–43.

FitzGerald, M. G., MacDonald, D. J., Krainer, M., et al. (1996). Germline BRCA1 mutations in Jewish and non-Jewish women with early-onset breast cancer. *New England Journal of Medicine, 334*(3), 143–149.

Ghosh, S., Watanabe, R. M., Valle, T. T., et al. (2000). The Finland-United States Investigation of Non-insulin-dependent Diabetes Mellitus Genetics (FUSION) Study. I. An autosomal genome scan for genes that predispose to type 2 diabetes. *American Journal of Human Genetics, 67*(5), 1174–1185.

Guttmacher, A. E. & Collins, F. S. (2002). Genomic medicine—a primer. *New England Journal of Medicine, 347*(19), 1512–1520.

Hall, J. G., Friedman, J. M., Kenna, B. A., Popkin, J., Jawanda, M., & Arnold, W. (1988). Clinical, genetic, and epidemiological factors in neural tube defects. *American Journal of Human Genetics, 43*(6), 827–837.

Hall, J., & Solehdin, M. (1998). Folic acid for the prevention of congenital anomalies. *European Journal of Pediatrics, 157*, 445–450.

Hanis, C. L., Boerwinkle, E., Chakraborty, R., et al. (1996). A genome-wide search for human non-insulin-dependent (type 2) diabetes genes reveals a major susceptibility locus on chromosome 2. *Nature Genetics, 13*(2), 161–166.

Hayes, C., Werler, M. M., Willett, W. C., & Mitchell, A. A. (1996). Case-control study of periconceptional folic acid supplementation and oral clefts. *American Journal of Epidemiology, 143*, 1229–1234.

ISONG. (2002). Position statement. Privacy and confidentiality of genetic information: The role of the nurse. *MedSurg Nursing, 11*(2), 103. Position statement available on-line: http://www.globalreferrals.com/privacy.htm.

ISONG. (2000). Position statement. Informed decision-making and consent: The role of nursing. *International Society of Nurses in Genetics Newsletter, 11*(3), 7–8. Position statement available on-line: http://www.globalreferrals.com/consent.htm.

ISONG. (2002). Position statement. Genetic counselling for vulnerable populations: The role of nursing. *MedSurg Nursing, 11*(6), 305.

Jones, K. L. (1997). *Smith's recognizable patterns of human malformation* (5th ed.). Philadelphia: W.B. Saunders.

Khoury, M. J., McCabe, L. L., & McCabe, E. R. B. (2003). Population screening in the age of genomic medicine. *New England Journal of Medicine, 348*(1), 50–58.

Kohut, R., & Rusen, I. D. (2002). *Congenital anomalies in Canada. Health Canada: A perinatal health report 2002.* Ottawa: Ministry of Public Works and Government Services Canada.

Lea, D. H., Anderson, G., & Monsen, R. B. (1998). A multiplicity of roles for genetic nursing: Building toward holistic practice. *Holistic Nursing Practice, 12*(3), 77–87.

Lea, D. H. & Williams, J. K. (2002). Genetic testing and screening. *American Journal of Nursing, 102*(7), 36–50.

Lea, D. H., Williams, J. K., Jenkins, J., Jones, S., & Calzone, K. (2000). Genetic health care: Creating interdisciplinary partnerships with nursing in clinical practice. *National Academies of Practice Forum, 2*(3), 177–186.

Lea, D. H. (2000). A clinician's primer in human genetics: What nurses need to know. *Nursing Clinics of North America, 35*(3), 583–614.

Li, D. K., Daling, J. R., Mueller, B. A., Hickok, D. E., Fantel, A. G., & Weiss, N. S. (1995). Periconceptional multivitamin use in relation to the risk of congenital urinary tract anomalies.[see comment]. *Epidemiology, 6*(3), 212–218.

Little, J., & Elwood, J. M. (1992). Epidemiology and control of neural tube defects. In J. Little & J. M. Elwood (Eds.), *Monograph in epidemiology and biostatistics* (Vol. 20). Oxford: Oxford University Press.

McCarthy, J. J., & Hilfiker, R. (2000). The use of single-nucleotide polymorphism maps in pharmacogenomics. *Nature Biotechnology, 18*(5), 505–508.

McKinnon, W. C., Baty, B. J., Bennett, R. L., et al. (1997). Predisposition genetic testing for late-onset disorders in adults. A position paper of the National Society of Genetic Counselors. *Journal of the American Medical Association, 278*(15), 1217–1220.

MRC Vitamin Study Research Group. (1991). Prevention of neural tube defects: Results of the Medical Research Council vitamin study. *Lancet, 338*, 131–137.

Nebert, D. W., & Dieter, M. Z. (2000). The evolution of drug metabolism. *Pharmacology, 61*(3), 124–135.

Norton, R. M. (2001*a*). Clinical pharmacogenomics: Applications in pharmaceutical R&D. *Drug Discovery Today, 6*(4), 180–185.

Norton, R. M. (2001*b*). Pharmacogenomics: Pharmacogenomics and individualized drug therapy. *Medscape Pharmacotherapy* (http://www.medscape.com).

Peters, J. L., Djurdjinovic, L., & Baker, D. (1999). The genetic self: The Human Genome Project, genetic counseling and family therapy. *Families, Systems & Health, 17*(1), 5–25.

Regaldo, A. (1999). Inventing the pharmacogenomics business. *American Journal of Health Systems Pharmacology, 56*(1), 40–50.

Roses, A. (2000). Pharmacogenetics and future drug development and delivery. *Lancet, 355*(9212), 1358–1361.

Sachidanandam, R., Weissman, D., Schmidt, S. C., et al. (2001). A map of human genome sequence variation containing 1.42 million single nucleotide polymorphisms. *Nature, 409*(6822), 928–933.

Schafer, A. J., & Hawkins, J. R. (1998). DNA variation and the future of human genetics. *Nature Biotechnology, 16,* 33–39.

Scordo, M. G., & Spina, E. (2002). Cytochrome P450 polymorphisms and response to antipsychotic therapy. *Pharmacogenomics, 3*(2), 201–218.

Shaw, G. M., O'Malley, C. D., Wasserman, C. R., Tolarova, M. M., & Lammer, E. J. (1995). Maternal periconceptional use of multivitamins and reduced risk for conotruncal heart defects and limb deficiencies among offspring. *American Journal of Medical Genetics, 59*(4), 536–545.

Struewing, J. P., Abeliovich, D., Peretz, T., et al. (1996). The carrier frequency of the BRCA1 185delAG mutation is approximately 1 percent in Ashkenazi Jewish individuals. *Nature Genetics, 12*(1), 198–200.

Struewing, J. P., Hartge, P., Wacholder, S., et al. (1997). The risk of cancer associated with specific mutations of BRCA1 and BRCA2 among Ashkenazi Jews. *New England Journal of Medicine, 336*(20), 1401–1408.

Summers, A. (2001). Genetics and the Canadian Paediatric Surveillance Program. *Paediatrics and Child Health, 6*(5). Available at: http://www.pulsus.com/Paeds/06_05/summ_ed.htm.

Wald, N., Sneddon, J., Densem, J., Frost, C., & Stone, R. (1991). Prevention of neural tube defects: Results of the Medical Research Council vitamin study. *Lancet, 338*(8760), 131–137.

Weinshilboum, R. (2003). Genomic medicine: Inheritance and drug response. *New England Journal of Medicine, 348*(6), 529–537.

Wilson, R. D., Davies, G., Désilets, V., Reid, G. J., Summers, A., Wyatt, P., et al. (2003). The use of folic acid for the prevention of neural tube defects and other congenital anomalies. SOGC Clinical Practice Guidelines No. 138. *Journal of Obstetrics & Gynaecology Canada: JOGC, 25*(11), 959–973.

RESOURCES AND WEBSITES

Biologics and Genetic Therapies Directorate (BGTD) of Health Canada, Director's General Office, HPB Building # 7, (A.L. 0702E), Tunney's Pasture, Ottawa, ON K1A 0L2; (613) 946-7264; fax: (613) 946-5214; http://www.hc-sc.gc.ca/hpfb-dgpsa/bgtd-dpbtg/index_e.html.

Canadian Association of Genetic Counsellors (CAGC); http://www.cagc-accg.ca; e-mail: lola.cartier@muhc.mcgill.ca.

Canadian Cancer Society/Société canadienne du cancer, National Office, Suite 200, 10 Alcorn Avenue, Toronto, ON M4V 3B1 416-961-7223; fax: 416-961-4189; http://www.cancer.ca.

Canadian Directory of Genetic Support Groups; Support Group Directory, Regional Medical Genetics Centre, Children's Hospital of Western Ontario, 800 Commissioner's Road East, London ON N6C 2V5; 519-685-8453; 1-800-243-8416 (Ontario only); fax: 519-685-8214; e-mail: Database Administrator; http://www.lhsc.on.ca/programs/medgenet.

Canadian Genetic Disease Network, Suite 201, 2150 Western Parkway, Vancouver, BC V6T 1V6; 604-221-7300; fax: 604-221-0778; e-mail: info@cgdn.ca; http://www.cgdn.ca.

Canadian Organization for Rare Disorders (CORD), P.O. Box 814, Coaldale, AB T1M 1M7; 403-345-4544; toll free: 1-877-302-7273; fax: 403-345-3948; http://www.cord.ca.

Gene Clinics, University of Washington School of Medicine, 9725 Third Avenue NE, Suite 610, Seattle, WA 98115; (206) 221-4674; fax (206) 221-4679; e-mail: geneclinics@geneclinics.org; http://www.geneclinics.org.

GeneTests, 9725 Third Avenue NE, Suite 602, Seattle, WA 98115, USA; 206-616-4033; fax: 206-221-4679; e-mail: genetests@genetests.org; http://www.genetests.org.

Genetic Alliance, 4301 Connecticut Ave. NW, Suite 404, Washington, DC 20008-2369 USA; 202-966-5557; fax: (202) 966-8553; e-mail: info@geneticalliance.org; http://www.geneticalliance.org.

Genetics Society of Canada; http://life.biology.mcmaster.ca/GSC/.

International Society of Nurses in Genetics, Inc. (ISONG), Executive Director Eileen Rawnsley, 7 Haskins Road, Hanover, NH 03755; (603) 643-5706; fax (603) 643-3169; e-mail: Eileen.Rawnsley@valleynet; http://www.nursing.creighton.edu/isong/.

National Coalition for Health Professional Education in Genetics (NCHPEG); 2630 W. Joppa Rd., Suite 320, Lutherville, MD 21093; (410) 583-0600; http://www.nchpeg.org.

National Organization for Rare Disorders, Inc. (NORD), P.O. Box 8923, New Fairfield, CT 06812-8923; (203) 746-6518; fax (203) 746-6481; e-mail: orphan@rarediseases.org.

National Cancer Institute (NCI), Public Inquiries Office, Building, 31, Room 10A03, 31 Center Drive, MSC 2580, Bethesda, MD 20892-2580; (301) 435-3848; http://www.nci.nih.gov.

Online Mendelian Inheritance in Man (OMIM), National Center for Biotechnology Information, National Library of Medicine, Building 38A, Room 8N805, Bethesda, MD 20894; (301) 496-2475; fax (301) 480-9241; http://www.ncbi.nlm.nih.gov/Omim.

The Canadian Paediatric Surveillance Program (CPSP); https://www.pulsus.com/Paeds/06_05/summ_ed.htm.

Tourette Syndrome Foundation of Canada, #206, 194 Jarvis Street, Toronto, ON M5B 2B7; 416-861-8398; 1-800-361-3120; fax: (416) 861-2472; e-mail: tsfc@tourette.ca; https://www.tourette.ca.

Tourette Syndrome Association, Inc., 42-40 Bell Boulevard, Bayside, NY 11331-2820, USA; 718-224-2999; fax: 718-279-9596; e-mail: ts@tsa-usa.org; http://www.tsa-usa.org.

Chronic Illness

Adapted by Shannon Spenceley

LEARNING OBJECTIVES

On completion of this chapter, the learner will be able to:

1. Define "chronic conditions."
2. Identify factors related to the increasing incidence of chronic conditions.
3. Describe characteristics of chronic conditions and implications for people with chronic conditions and for their families.
4. Describe the phases of chronic conditions.
5. Apply the nursing process to the care of the patient with chronic conditions.

*C*hronic health problems affect people of all ages—they occur in the very young, the middle-aged, and the very old. Chronic conditions do, however, increase in frequency with age, and elderly people often have multiple chronic disorders (Broemeling, Watson, & Black, 2005; Public Health Agency of Canada, 2005). Chronic illnesses are found in all socioeconomic, ethnic, cultural, and racial groups; certain diseases, however, occur more frequently in some groups than in others (Losos, 2002). For example, the prevalence of diabetes among Aboriginal Canadians is three to five times the national average (Health Canada, 2000, 2002). Poverty, cultural, or language barriers, and social or geographic isolation often act as barriers to receiving preventive screening measures such as mammography, cervical screening, and routine check-ups (Gupta, Roos, Walld, Traverse, & Dahl, 2003; Hislop et al., 2003; Spenceley, in press). Although some chronic conditions have little effect on quality of life, others have a considerable effect because of related disability (Kopec & Schultz, 2003). Certain conditions require advanced technology for survival, as in the late stages of amyotrophic lateral sclerosis or end-stage renal disease. Some people with chronic health conditions and disability function independently with only minor inconvenience to their everyday lives; others require frequent and close monitoring or placement in long-term care facilities.

The Phenomenon of Chronicity

Although each chronic condition has its own specific physiologic characteristics, chronic conditions do share common qualities. Many chronic conditions, for example, have pain and fatigue as associated symptoms. Some degree of disability is usually present in severe or advanced chronic illness, limiting the patient's participation in activities (Crimmins, Kim, & Hagedorn, 2003). Many chronic conditions require therapeutic regimens to keep them under control. Unlike the term "acute," which implies a curable and relatively short disease course, *chronic* describes a long disease course and conditions that may be incurable. It is this characteristic of duration that often makes managing chronic conditions so difficult for those who must live with them.

Psychological and emotional reactions of people to acute and chronic conditions and changes in their health status are described in detail in Chapter 7. People who develop chronic conditions may react with shock, disbelief, depression, anger, resentment, or a number of other emotions. How people react and cope with chronic conditions is usually similar to how they react to other events in their lives, depending, in part, on their understanding of the condition and their perceptions of its potential impact on their own and their family's lives. Adjustment to chronic illness is affected by various factors:

- Personality before the illness
- Unresolved anger or grief from the past
- Suddenness, extent, and duration of lifestyle changes necessitated by the illness
- Family and individual resources for dealing with stress
- Stages of individual/family life cycle
- Previous experience with illness and crises
- Codependency in family systems (Lewis, 1998)

Psychological, emotional, and cognitive reactions to chronic conditions are likely to occur at the initial onset, but they may also recur if symptoms worsen or recur after a period of remission. Symptoms associated with chronic illnesses are often unpredictable, and some are perceived as crisis events by people and their families, who must contend with both the uncertainty of chronic illness and the changes it brings to their lives. This chapter describes some of the problems of living with chronic conditions and offers a guide to nursing assessment and intervention when providing care to people with chronic illness.

DEFINITION OF CHRONIC CONDITIONS

Chronic conditions are health problems requiring ongoing management over a period of years, even decades. Considered from this perspective, "chronic conditions" cover a broad array of what could appear on the surface as disparate health problems. Chronic conditions include the following:

- Noncommunicable diseases (eg, cardiovascular disease, cancer, and diabetes)
- Persistent communicable diseases (eg, HIV/AIDS)
- Certain mental disorders (eg, depression and schizophrenia)
- Ongoing impairments in structure (eg, amputations, blindness, and joint disorders)

(World Health Organization, 2005)

Management of such conditions includes learning to live with symptoms and/or disabilities and coming to terms with changes brought about by having a chronic condition. It also consists of carrying out the lifestyle alterations and self-care regimens that are designed to keep symptoms under control and to prevent complications. Chronic illness, when viewed through a subjective lens, is far more than simply a matter of functional impairments or discomforts. Although often viewed as a "factual clinical event" (Thorne, 1999, p. 398) from the perspective of the world of health care, chronic illness takes on significance and meaning in the lives of people because of its psychosocial construction and the way in which it transforms identities, changes role relationships, and disrupts the living of life (Thorne, 1999).

PREVALENCE AND CAUSES OF CHRONIC CONDITIONS

Chronic conditions occur in people of every age group, socioeconomic level, and culture. In 2002, an estimated 16 million Canadians had at least one chronic disease. As shown in Figure 10-1, five of the six most costly diagnostic categories of illness in Canada are constituted by chronic diseases, including cardiovascular illness, musculoskeletal disease, cancer, respiratory disease, and nervous system diseases (Health Canada, 1998). Cardiovascular disease is the leading cause of death in Canada at 36% and the most costly diagnostic category, accounting for 11.6% (18.5 billion dollars) of the total cost of illness classifiable by diagnostic category (Health Canada, 1998). There are a number of factors that contribute to the rising costs of chronic disease in Canada, including our aging population, longer life with chronic disease, rising drug and treatment costs, economic inflation, and new technology (Harvey, Hook, Kozyniak, & Selvanathan, 2002).

Not every chronic condition is disabling; many people living with a chronic condition do not experience significant limitations (Wilkins & Park, 1996). Many chronic diseases, however, are severe enough to cause major disability. Such limitations are not limited to adults: an estimated 30.3% of Canadian children aged 6 to 11 have one or more chronic physical health conditions or impairments, while 3.6% have activity-limiting conditions or impairments (McDougall et al., 2004). People with limitations due to disability or pain may experience difficulty with the expectations of their medical regimen (Riegel & Carlson, 2002; Wilson, Hutchison, & Holzemer, 2002), problems with activities of daily

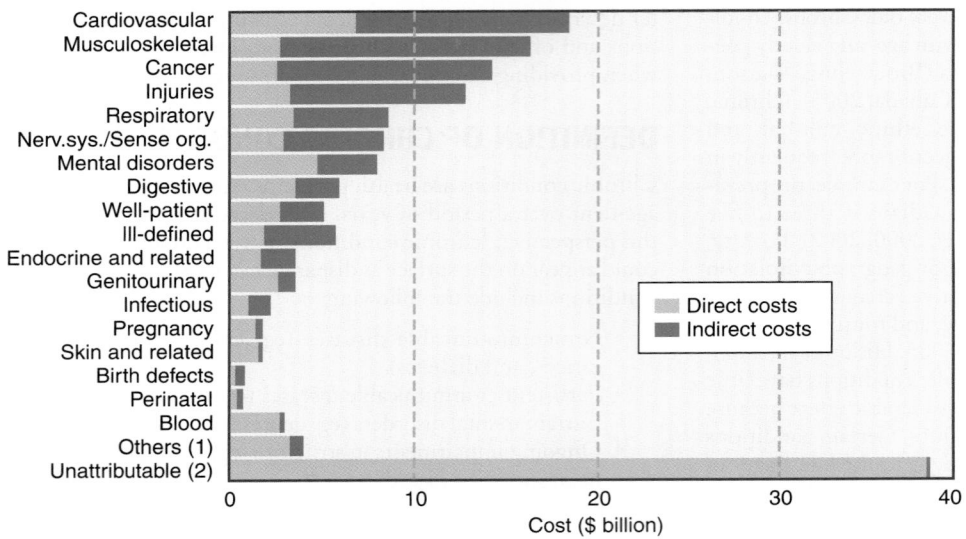

Direct and Indirect Costs by Diagnostic Category in Canada,* 1998

Cost ($ billion)

*Based on total cost of illness of $159.4 billion

(1) Refers to data for which coding is not provided (for diagnostic categories), or data that are grouped because of small counts.

(2) Refers to data that could not be coded by ICD-9 code.

FIGURE 10-1 Direct and indirect costs by diagnostic category in Canada, 1998. Source: *Economic burden of illness in Canada.* Public Health Agency of Canada, 1998. Reproduced with the permission of the Minister of Public Works and Government Services Canada, 2005.

living, emotional distress, and difficulty meeting social expectations (Dewar, White, Posade, & Dillon, 2003).

Chronic conditions have become the major cause of health-related problems in developed countries. Developing countries are also experiencing an increase in chronic conditions, giving these countries the dual burden of trying to eradicate infectious diseases while learning to manage chronic conditions (World Health Organization, 2005). Some of the reasons that chronic diseases are becoming more prevalent globally include the following:

- Lower infant mortality, and increases in life expectancy due to successful public health measures, medical advances, and technology
- Improved screening and diagnostic procedures, and aggressive management of acute conditions
- Tendency for the development of single or multiple chronic diseases with advancing age
- Lifestyle factors and consumption patterns: poor nutrition, obesity, tobacco use, physical inactivity, unmanaged psychosocial stress, unsafe sexual practices

(Harvey et al., 2002; World Health Organization, 2005)

Recently, much greater emphasis has been placed upon the adoption of healthy lifestyles, beginning in childhood. This is not a new idea in Canada; in fact, Lalonde's *A New Perspective on the Health of Canadians,* an influential Canadian health policy document (Lalonde, 1974), framed health or disease as the result of lifestyle choices and self-imposed risks. Although the "new perspective" emphasized that a variety of factors constitute the "health field" (social and physical environments, health care services, biology, and lifestyle), lifestyle choices and risks have received the most attention in relation to chronic disease. Epp's Framework for Health Promotion (Epp, 1986) and the 1986 Ottawa Charter for Health Promotion (World Health Organization, 1986) also emphasized the importance of enhancing personal skills and knowledge in relation to health and the development of community and individual capacities in maintaining good health and preventing chronic disease. Although many chronic diseases can be prevented or post-

poned, factors that place people at significantly higher risk for developing any number of chronic diseases remain prevalent. Many chronic diseases share common risk factors; a significant lowering of chronic disease risk would be achieved if the prevalence of these risk factors could be decreased. Two thirds of Canadians have at least one modifiable risk factor for chronic disease: smoking, physical inactivity, poor nutritional habits, or obesity. The Advisory Committee on Population Health (2002) reported on the prevalence of these risk factors:

- *Smoking:* Among Canadian adults, smoking rates have declined, with current statistics showing that approximately 21% of Canadians aged 15 or over are current smokers. Smoking rates are highest among young adults; 32% of women and men aged 20 to 24 report being current smokers. Smoking is a major risk factor for respiratory diseases, cardiovascular diseases, and several forms of cancer.
- *Unhealthy diet:* Overconsumption of dietary fats and underconsumption of dietary fibre are risk factors for several cancers and cardiovascular disease. Diets containing substantial amounts of a variety of vegetables and fruits may reduce the overall incidence of cancer by over 20%. Improved diets can reduce coronary heart disease and stroke mortality by at least 20% and diabetes mortality by at least 30%.
- *Physical inactivity:* 49% of Canadians over the age of 12 are physically inactive (Statistics Canada, 2002). Lack of physical activity is a risk factor for many diseases and conditions, including cardiovascular disease, several common cancers, diabetes, and osteoporosis.
- *Overweight and obesity:* Over half of Canadians are overweight, 14.7% of adults are obese (Katzmarzyk & Janssen, 2004), and obesity in children is increasing substantially. Obesity is an important risk factor for coronary heart disease, diabetes, and some cancers.

It has been noted, however, that while assisting people with making healthier individual lifestyle choices is sure to have some positive effect on the prevalence of chronic disease, it is equally important to acknowledge that most chronic diseases are also linked to underlying societal conditions and factors such as personal resources and life chances. Indeed, most risk factors and chronic illnesses are most likely to be experienced by low-income or disadvantaged groups (Ontario Public Health Association, 2004).

The Characteristics of Chronic Conditions

It is sometimes difficult to understand how lives are changed, often forever, because of chronic conditions. Perhaps it is this difficulty that underlies the common tendency for health professionals to focus on treating the illness while overlooking the person and family living with the condition. In all illnesses, but even more so with chronic conditions, the illness cannot be separated from the life as lived (Thorne, 1999; Thorne & Paterson, 2001). Chronic illness is something that people must live with on a daily basis. The focus of nursing is on human responses to disruption in health (Morse, 1997). Therefore, effective nursing care is premised upon seeking to understand the meaning of the chronic illness to the person living with it (Cumbie, Conley, & Burman, 2004; Thorne, 1999). There are, however, some characteristic patterns to the chronic illness experience that are important to understand:

1. Managing chronic illness involves much more than managing medical problems. There may be emotional, psychological, and social distress encountered in living for long periods of time with an illness, including threats to identity, role changes, an altered concept of self (Morse, 1997; Thorne, 1999), and episodes of depression (Patten, Jacobs, Reimer, & Metz, 2002). This means that continuous adaptation and accommodation are called for, depending upon age and situation in life (Price, 1996; Sidell, 1997). Each significant change or decrease in functional ability requires further physical, emotional, psychological, and social adaptation for patients and their families (Benbow & Koopman, 2003; Carroll, 1998; Lewis, 1998; Miller, 1999; Tappan, Williams, Fishman, & Theris, 1999), adaptation that is greatly assisted by effective and supportive communication with health care providers (Thorne, Con, McGuiness, McPherson, & Harris, 2004).

2. Chronic conditions usually involve many different phases over the course of a person's lifetime. There can be acute periods, stable and unstable periods, flare-ups, and remissions. Each phase brings its own challenges, priorities, and problems. Sometimes the illness is in the foreground, a perspective that is focused upon the suffering, loss, or burden associated with the illness. At other times, wellness takes the foreground, and the person experiences an opportunity to take a step back from the illness and focus on the emotional, spiritual, and social aspects of life, rather than on the disease (Thorne & Paterson, 2001; Thorne, Paterson, & Russell, 2003).

3. An important component of chronic disease management is adherence to therapeutic regimens. It has been noted that nonadherence to a prescribed treatment plan or management regimen increases the risk of developing complications, or accelerating the disease process. However, it is important to remember that disease management regimens are only one part of a life lived with chronic disease, and that the complexities, demands, and priorities of life can create challenges to adherence (Cicutto, Brooks, & Henderson, 2004). Knowledge about how to manage a chronic illness develops over time as people live life with the

illness (Paterson & Thorne, 2000b) and requires a great deal of anticipatory thinking and planning (Paterson & Thorne, 2000a). It is not unusual for people to discontinue taking medications or to alter dosages because of side effects that are more disturbing or disruptive than the illness symptoms. People also frequently cut back on regimens they consider overly time-consuming, fatiguing, or costly (Cagle, Appel, Skelly, & Carter-Edwards, 2002; Schoenberg & Drungle, 2001).

4. One chronic disease can lead to the development of other chronic conditions. Diabetes, for example, can eventually lead to neurological and vascular changes that may result in hypertension, cardiovascular disease, cerebrovascular disease, peripheral vascular disease, kidney disease, and visual impairment (Health Canada, 2002).

5. Chronic illness affects the whole family. Family life can be dramatically altered as a result of role reversals, role conflicts (Miller, 2000), loss of income, time spent managing illness, decrease in family socialization activities, and the costs of treatment (Cagle et al., 2002; Hunt, Pugh, & Valenzuela, 1998). Stress and caretaker fatigue are common with severe chronic conditions, and the whole family rather than just the individual needs care (Morgan, Semchuk, Stewart, & D'Arcy, 2002; Neufeld, Query, & Drummond, 2001).

6. The major responsibility for the everyday management of chronic illness falls upon the shoulders of chronically ill people and their families. In today's health care system, especially in the case of chronic conditions, self-care has increasingly become a major part of the role of the person or family. The home, rather than the hospital, is the centre of care in chronic conditions, since this is where the day-to-day management occurs. Hospitals, clinics, doctor's offices, nursing homes, health centres, and community agencies become adjuncts or back-up services to that daily home management.

7. Learning to manage chronic conditions is a developmental process of trial and error, discovery, and a "fine tuning of understanding related to the meaning of self-care decisions" (Thorne, Paterson, & Russell, 2003, p. 1341). Health care professionals can share knowledge about the medical management of the condition, avoidance of complications, and control of symptoms. Teaching about the disease, however, is not the same as living with the disease. Each person must discover how her or his own body reacts under varying conditions—for example, what it is like to be hypoglycemic, what activities are likely to bring on angina, and how these or other conditions can best be prevented and managed. Over time, people living with such conditions develop considerable knowledge about how to best manage their life with chronic disease and about their own unique responses to various aspects of disease management.

8. Managing chronic conditions is a collaborative process. The medical, social, emotional, and psychological challenges associated with chronic disease tend to be complex, especially in severe conditions. The management of chronic conditions, therefore, is best served through the collaboration of many different health professionals, in ongoing partnership with people and their families, with the goal of providing the resources, services, and support required for self-management at home. There is a growing acknowledgment that the focus of self-care must be on living life well with chronic disease, and that trusting, respectful partnerships with health care providers constitute an important resource for self-care support (Thorne & Paterson, 2001).

9. As shown in Figure 10-1, the management of chronic conditions is expensive (Health Canada, 1998). Billions of dollars in direct and indirect costs are spent every year on health care for people with chronic conditions. The costs are incurred from hospitalizations, physician services, medications, and productivity losses related to premature short- and long-term disability, or death. Overall health care costs are not likely to decrease until there is a substantial downward trend in the incidence of chronic conditions and the costs of chronic health care.

10. Chronic conditions raise difficult ethical issues for the patient, health care professionals, and society. No easy solutions exist to problems such as how to establish cost controls, how to allocate scarce resources (eg, organs for transplantation), how to determine what constitutes quality of life, and when to terminate life support. People living with chronic conditions, their families, and society respond to ethical issues according to their own moral standards and definitions of quality of life.

11. Living with chronic illness means living with uncertainty (LeFort, 2000; Mishel, 1999). Although health care professionals have some notion about the usual progression of a chronic disease such as Parkinson's disease, so many specific variables enter into each case that no one can predict with certainty an individual's illness course (that is, how the person will respond to treatment and how quickly or even whether a disease will progress). Even when a person is "in remission" or "disease-free," he or she experiences a lingering doubt and dread that the illness will reactivate (Mahon & Casperson, 1997).

THE PROBLEMS OF MANAGING CHRONIC CONDITIONS

Chronic conditions have implications for everyday living and management problems for individuals and their families as well as for society at large. Most importantly, efforts should be directed at preventing chronic conditions since many chronic conditions can be traced, at least in part, to unhealthy lifestyle choices or behaviours such as smoking and overeating. Thus, changes in lifestyle can result in the prevention of some chronic conditions, or at least a delay in their onset until a later age. Because of the tendency of some people to resist change, however, facilitating healthy lifestyles is one of the major challenges facing nurses today.

Once a chronic condition has occurred, the focus shifts from disease prevention to managing symptoms and staying well by avoiding complications (eg, eye problems in the person with diabetes) and the development of other acute illnesses (eg, pneumonia in a person with chronic obstructive lung disease). Quality of life, often overlooked by health professionals in their approach to care of people with chronic conditions, is also important. Health-promoting behaviours, such as exercise, are essential to quality of life in people who have chronic illnesses and disabilities because they help to maintain functional status (Westby, Wade, Rangno, & Berkowitz, 2000). See Nursing Research Profile 10-1 for more information.

Although coworkers, extended family, and health care professionals are affected by the problems of people with chronic illnesses, the problems of living with chronic conditions are most acutely experienced by people living with these conditions, and their immediate families. It is they who feel the greatest impact with lifestyle changes that directly affect quality of life. Nurses provide direct care, especially during acute episodes, but they also provide the teaching and mobilize the resources and other supports that enable

NURSING RESEARCH PROFILE 10-1
Health-Related Hardiness and Chronic Illness

Martin, J. C., Engle, V. F., & Graney, M. J. (1999). Determinants of health-related hardiness among urban older African-American women with chronic illness. *Holistic Nursing Practice, 13*(3), 62–70.

Purpose
Although statistics demonstrated that older African American women experience earlier, more frequent, and more severe limitations from chronic illnesses than any other older adult group, African American women who live beyond the age of 85 usually live longer than their Anglo-American counterparts. Health-related hardiness (HRH), defined as a set of personality characteristics that buffer negative stressful effects associated with living with chronic illness, has been suggested as one factor that contributes to these statistics. The purpose of this study was to identify and quantify the relationship between HRH and function, self-assessed health, morbidity, and health behaviours in urban, older African American women with chronic illness.

Study Sample and Design
A correlational design was used to obtain data about demographic characteristics and the variables of interest among chronically ill older African American women. Questionnaires and structured interviews were used to obtain the data from women during routine appointments at the outpatient clinic of a large urban hospital. Instruments included the Health-Related Hardiness Scale (HRHS), Self-Assess Health (SAH) instrument, Sickness Impact Profile (SIP), and Health Habits Scale. Demographic data obtained included age, education, and marital status of the women.

Findings
The mean age of the sample of 100 women was 68.8 ± 8.6 years. They had a mean of four medical diagnoses and five prescribed daily medications. Hypertension and osteoarthritis were the most common chronic illnesses reported; they occurred in 90% and 74% of the women, respectively. Analysis of data revealed that the women had high levels of HRH, little functional impairment, moderate ratings of the state of their own health, multiple chronic illnesses and use of multiple daily medications, and frequent participation in health behaviours. Significant correlations were found between HRH and years of education and HRH and SIP, which measures the impact of illness on function and performance of activities of daily living. Upon analysis by stepwise multiple linear regression, HRH was best predicted by years of education and function as measured by the SIP.

Nursing Implications
The findings of this study (ie, high levels of HRH, little impairment in function, average levels of self-assessed health, and frequent practice of health behaviours) support the existence of hardiness in older African American women. These findings increase understanding of hardiness as an important variable related to health. Further research is needed to identify factors that will facilitate health promotion and health protection among this group of women.

people to integrate their illness into their lives and maintain quality of life despite their illness (Michael, 1996). To understand what nursing care is needed, it is important to appreciate the complexity of the issues that people with chronic illness and their families contend with and manage on a daily basis. Some of the challenges of living with chronic conditions include the following:

- Alleviating and managing symptoms
- Psychologically adjusting to and physically accommodating disabilities

- Preventing and managing crises and complications
- Carrying out regimens as prescribed
- Validating individual self-worth and family functioning
- Managing threats to identity
- Normalizing individual and family life as much as possible
- Living with altered time, social isolation, and loneliness
- Establishing the networks of support and resources that can enhance quality of life
- Returning to a satisfactory way of life after an acute debilitating episode (another myocardial infarction or stroke) or reactivation of a chronic condition
- Dying with dignity and comfort

IMPLICATIONS FOR NURSING

Working with people with chronic illness or disability requires dealing with the medical aspects of their disorder, and working with the whole person, physically, emotionally, and socially (Dean, 1999). This holistic approach to care requires nurses to draw upon their entire repertoire of knowledge and skills, including knowledge from the social sciences, psychology in particular. People often respond to illness, health teaching, and regimens in ways that are different from the expectations of health care providers. Although quality of life is usually affected by chronic illness, especially if the illness is severe (Kopec & Schultz, 2003), an individual's perceptions of what constitutes quality of life often drives management behaviours. Nurses and other health care professionals need to recognize this, even though it may be difficult to see people make choices and decisions about lifestyles and disease management that we may think are unwise. Individuals have the right to receive care without fearing ridicule or refusal of treatment.

As stated previously, chronic conditions have a course, although that course might be too uncertain to predict with any degree of accuracy. An illness course can be thought of as a trajectory—a course—that can be managed or shaped over time to some extent through planned and supported illness management strategies (Robinson, Bevil, Arcangelo et al., 2001; Corbin, 1998). The trajectory of an illness can also be divided into phases that enable more precise thinking about a person's condition. This enables the nurse to put the present situation into the context of what might have happened to the person in the past—that is, the life factors and understandings that might have influenced the present state of the illness. In this way, nurses can more accurately assess the underlying issues and problems.

Each phase of chronic illness brings with it different problems, both medical and psychosocial. The needs of a person who has had a stroke and is a good candidate for rehabilitation, for example, are very different from those of a person with terminal cancer. By thinking in terms of phases, and where the person may be in relation to these phases, nurses can target their care more specifically to each person. Not every chronic condition is necessarily life-threatening, and not every person passes through each possible phase of a chronic condition.

PHASES OF CHRONIC ILLNESS

There are a number of theoretical frameworks that are useful in understanding the human experience of chronic illness. Paterson's Shifting Perspectives Model (Paterson, 2001, 2003) facilitates an understanding of chronic illness as lived according to people's needs and situations, rather than according to predictable stages or phases. Miller (2000) framed chronic illness as an experience that challenges one's perceptions of power—with power defined as the ability to provide and care for self, direct others regarding self-care, and retain the status of ultimate decision maker regarding care.

One of the best known models of chronic illness is Corbin and Strauss' Chronic Illness Trajectory Model (Corbin, 1998; Corbin & Cherry, 1997; Strauss & Corbin, 1988). In this model, the progress of chronic conditions is conceptualized in nine different phases (Chart 10-1):

1. The **pretrajectory phase** describes the stage at which the person is at risk for developing a chronic condition because of genetic factors or lifestyle behaviours that increase susceptibility to chronic illness.
2. The **trajectory phase** is characterized by the onset of symptoms or disability associated with a chronic condition. Since symptoms are being evaluated and diagnostic tests are performed, this phase is often accompanied by uncertainty as the person awaits a diagnosis. Nursing care often involves preparing people for diagnostic tests and offering emotional support.
3. The **stable phase** of the trajectory indicates that symptoms and disability are being managed adequately. Although the person is doing well, nursing care is still important at this time to support positive behaviours and to offer ongoing monitoring.

Chart 10-1 Phases in the Trajectory Model of Chronic Illness

- **Pretrajectory:** Genetic factors or lifestyle behaviours that place an individual or community at risk for the development of a chronic condition
- **Trajectory onset:** Appearance of noticeable symptoms; includes period of diagnostic workup and announcement of diagnosis; may be accompanied by biographic limbo as person begins to discover and cope with implications of diagnosis
- **Stable:** Illness course and symptoms are under control; biography and everyday life activities are being managed within limitations of illness; illness management centred in the home
- **Unstable:** Period of inability to keep symptoms under control or reactivation of illness; biographic disruption and difficulty in carrying out everyday life activities; adjustments being made in regimen, with care usually taking place at home
- **Acute:** Severe and unrelieved symptoms or the development of illness complications necessitating hospitalization or bed rest to bring illness course under control; biography and everyday life activities temporarily placed on hold or drastically cut back
- **Crisis:** Critical or life-threatening situation requiring emergency treatment or care; biography and everyday life activities suspended until the crisis passes
- **Comeback:** Gradual return to an acceptable way of life within limits imposed by disability or illness; involves physical healing, stretching limitations through rehabilitative procedures, psychosocial coming to terms, and biographic reengagement with adjustments in everyday life activities
- **Downward:** Illness course characterized by rapid or gradual physical decline accompanied by increasing disability or difficulty in controlling symptoms; requires biographic adjustment and alterations in everyday life activities with each major downward step
- **Dying:** Final days or weeks before death; characterized by gradual or rapid shutting down of body processes, biographic disengagement and closure, and relinquishment of everyday life interests and activities

4. The **unstable phase** is characterized by an exacerbation of illness symptoms, development of complications, or reactivation of an illness in remission. During this phase, a person's everyday activities may be temporarily disrupted because symptoms are not well controlled. There may also be more diagnostic tests and a trial of new regimens until some degree of control over symptoms is achieved. During this time of uncertainty, people often look to nurses for guidance and support.

5. The **acute phase** is characterized by sudden onset of severe or unrelieved symptoms or complications that require hospitalization for their management. This phase may require major modification of the person's usual activities for a period of time. Nurses are intensely involved in the care of the chronically ill person during this period, providing direct care and emotional support to the person and family members.

6. The **crisis phase** is characterized by a critical or life-threatening situation that requires emergency treatment or care. During this phase people and their families depend upon the skill, knowledge, and support of nurses and other professionals to stabilize their conditions.

7. The **comeback phase** is the period in the trajectory marked by recovery after an acute period. It includes learning to live with or to overcome disabilities and a return to an acceptable way of life within the limitations imposed by the chronic condition. Although aspects of care may shift to other health care providers during the rehabilitative phase, the role of nurses as organizers of care and collaborators in the recovery is essential.

8. The **downward phase** marks the worsening of a condition. Symptoms and disability continue to progress despite attempts to gain some control through treatment and management regimens. A downward turn does not necessarily mean imminent death; the downward trend can be arrested and an illness restabilized. Since people are not yet acute or dying but usually are living at home during this time, their contact with nurses is often limited. The supportive presence of nurses is needed, however, because of adjustment issues. Nurses working in clinics and physicians' offices can play an important role in helping people understand and come to terms with what is happening to them.

9. The **dying phase** is characterized by the gradual or rapid decline in the trajectory despite efforts to halt the disorder or slow the decline through illness management; it is characterized by failure of life-maintaining body functions. During this phase nurses provide direct and supportive care to individuals and their families through hospice programs.

Nursing Management

Nursing care of people living with chronic conditions is varied and occurs in an assortment of settings. It can include provision of direct care or supportive care. Such care is often provided in the clinic or physician's office, the hospital, or the home, depending on the status of the illness.

Examples of direct care may include assessing the patient's physical status, providing wound care, managing and overseeing medication regimens, and performing other technical tasks. The availability of this type of nursing care is one of the main reasons patients can remain at home and return to a somewhat normal life after an acute episode of illness.

Because much of the day-to-day responsibility for managing chronic conditions rests with the individual and family, nurses often provide supportive care unless the person is hospitalized. Supportive care may include ongoing monitoring, teaching, counselling, serving as an advocate, making referrals, coordinating services, mobilizing resources, and case-managing. Providing supportive care is just as important as the performance of technical care. For example, through ongoing monitoring that might take place either in the home or a nursing clinic, such as a heart failure clinic, a nurse might detect impending complications, such as signs of heart failure. The nurse might detect these signs before they are noticeable to the person and could make a referral (call the physician or consult the medical protocol in a clinic) for medical evaluation, thereby preventing a lengthy and costly hospitalization.

CARE BY PHASE: APPLYING THE NURSING PROCESS

The focus of care for people with chronic conditions is determined by the unique needs of the person and family and the particular phase of illness. Care is organized by the nursing process, incorporating assessment, diagnosis, planning, implementation, and evaluation.

Step 1: Identifying the Trajectory Phase

The first step is assessment of the person to determine the specific phase (see Chart 10-1). Assessment enables the nurse to identify the specific medical, social, and psychological problems likely to be encountered in a phase. For instance, the problems associated with having an acute myocardial infarction are very different from those likely to be encountered with the same person, 10 years later, dying at home of heart failure. The kinds of direct care, referrals, teaching, and emotional support needed in each situation are different as well.

Step 2: Establishing Goals

Once the phase of illness has been identified for a specific person, along with the specific medical problems and related social and psychological issues, the next step involves establishing the goals of care. The establishment of goals must be a collaborative effort with the person, family, and nurse working together, for the attainment of a goal is unlikely if it is primarily the nurse's goal. The following are two examples of goals to be determined collaboratively, then written in the language of the nursing process.

An elderly man with severe progressive COPD reports increasing difficulty breathing, even with the oxygen level set at 2 litres/min. This interferes with his ability to carry out activities of daily living and has decreased his quality of life. He asks the nurse for help. The nursing diagnosis for this problem might be "Activity intolerance related to less than adequate intake of oxygen secondary to lung disease," and the mutually agreed upon goal of care might be to increase his ability to care for himself. Nursing interventions related to this goal might include teaching him how to pace his activities and helping him to obtain assistance with the most demanding activities of daily living.

In another example, a 45-year-old woman with moderately advanced multiple sclerosis (MS) is hospitalized with a severe bladder infection. She reports that she has problems with self-catheterization because of her disability and that she has difficulty obtaining and consuming adequate fluids during the day. The nursing diagnosis for this problem might be "Toileting self-care deficit (in bladder care) related to decreased functional ability secondary to MS," and the mutual outcomes of care might be to develop strategies to facilitate the self-catheterization process and increase daily fluid intake.

Step 3: Establishing a Plan to Achieve Desired Outcomes

Once goals have been established, the next step consists of establishing a realistic and mutually agreed upon plan for achieving them and identifying specific criteria that can be used to assess progress. A plan of care for the man with COPD who complains of a decreased ability to care for himself, for example, might include assisting him to prioritize his activities of daily living so he can carry out those that are most important to him before he becomes too short of breath and tired. It might also include exploring how he feels about having someone assist him at home on a regular basis and, if he agrees to having help, checking on the availability and any costs associated with such services. In many cases, people with chronic illness perceive someone helping them as a threat to their independence and self-esteem, the first step to a nursing home or rehabilitation centre. Therefore, they may be resistant to someone coming into their home to help them. Criteria to measure progress toward goal attainment and strategies to accomplish the goals might include the following:

- At the end of the first care session, the person with COPD will be able to prioritize activities of daily living and agree to look over an information sheet and list of community support services provided by the nurse.
- By the second session, he will report that he is pacing his activities and is therefore better able to carry out important self-care activities. He will also report that he has read the information provided by the nurse about available services.
- By the third session, he will have compiled a list of the self-care activities that are difficult for him to carry out and for which assistance would be beneficial.
- By the fourth session, he will have made arrangements for assistive services for 2 hours each morning. If he is unable to make the arrangements, then the nurse would suggest that the family or someone else make them. The goal is to enable him to meet basic self-care needs and improve quality of life, thereby having enough time and energy available for other activities. People with chronic illness-related disabilities often feel that they have lost a great deal of control over what happens to them; any activities that they can do for themselves, therefore, enhance psychological well being.
- By the fifth home visit, he will report that all self-care needs are met either by self-pacing of activities or through the assistance of a home support worker.

A plan of care for the woman with MS might be to develop techniques for carrying out self-catheterization within the limitations imposed by her disability and to increase her daily fluid intake to six to eight 8-oz glasses of fluid per day. Indicators that the desired goal has been achieved may include the following:

- By the end of the first care session, the individual and the nurse will identify which steps in the self-catheterization procedure are causing the most difficulty. The woman will also be able to list three strategies for improving her intake of fluids.
- By the end of the second session, she will report that she is performing self-catheterization using the strategies suggested by the nurse for improving her technique. She will also report that she has increased her fluid intake by three glasses.

- By the end of the third session, she will report that she can perform self-catheterization three out of four times without difficulty and that her fluid intake is now up to six to eight 8-oz glasses a day.
- By the end of the fourth session, she will be ready for discharge with the confidence that she is competent in performing self-catheterization and obtaining adequate fluid intake despite the physical limitations imposed by her illness.

Step 4: Identifying Factors That Facilitate or Hinder Attainment of Goals

The next step involves identifying environmental, social, and psychological factors that might interfere with or facilitate achieving the goal. In the case of the man with COPD, for example, not having sufficient resources could prevent him from seeking additional support services. The nurse might want to explore carefully the issue of resources with him and, if there are financial constraints, enlist the services of a social worker, with his consent, to explore possible community resources. Since he is having trouble breathing, the nurse should determine whether he is also having difficulty cooking and eating, and whether he is losing weight because of insufficient caloric intake to meet his nutritional needs. If cooking is a problem, then the nurse might look into community resources such as Meals on Wheels. If he is losing weight, then the nurse should advise him to eat frequent small meals to lessen the fatigue associated with eating and to supplement meals with high-protein drinks.

In the case of the patient with MS, the nurse might want to explore the extent of the physical limitations, how rapidly the MS seems to be progressing, when during the day she has the most difficulty doing the catheterization, and whether that difficulty might be related to fatigue. If fatigue is a factor, the nurse might explore whether she would consider having a home health aide to help her with some of her self-care activities. This would enable her to conserve her energy for social activities and personal care, such as self-catheterization. The nurse would also discuss with her the reasons she is not taking in an adequate amount of fluids. If she is too busy or tired to make frequent trips to the sink or refrigerator to get fluids, the nurse might help her develop strategies for saving time and energy. For example, she could attach a bottle of water to her wheelchair or walker and carry it around with her, or strategically place bottles of water or other liquids around the house to increase their accessibility. The nurse might also explore with her the types of caffeine-free fluids that she enjoys drinking.

Step 5: Implementing Interventions

The fifth step is the intervention phase. Possible interventions include providing direct care, serving as an advocate, teaching, counselling, making referrals, and case-managing (arranging for resources). For example, if the man with COPD reports after prioritizing his activities of daily living that showering each morning is the most important self-care activity for him, then having a home health aide come early in the morning to help with the shower may be the best arrangement. The home health aide could also help with breakfast, make the bed, and straighten up the house. In this way, the man would use less energy doing these mundane tasks. After showering and dressing, he might also want to plan a daily rest period, such as sitting down with a crossword puzzle or reading, that might help him overcome some of his sense of breathlessness and feel more rested.

If spasms or tremors are interfering with the ability of the woman with MS to catheterize herself, then the nurse would want to review the medications she is taking; if, for instance, she is taking antispasmodics, the self-catheterizations could be timed to coincide with the peak medication levels. In an effort to encourage an increased fluid intake, the nurse might want to help the woman build into her daily routine a set time in the morning and afternoon, allowing for flexibility, to take an herbal tea or juice break that would increase the amount of fluids ingested and also provide a rest period. While it is important for a person with MS to maintain a sense of independence and accomplishment, it is equally important to learn to recognize his or her limits, through such signs as fatigue, and to manage them through proper planning.

Physicians prescribe therapies, such as medications and diet, and give directions for how much, when, and how they are to be used. Nurses, however, by virtue of their broad knowledge base, are equipped to help people develop the strategies needed to live with both the symptoms and therapies associated with chronic conditions. It is important to work individually with each individual and family to identify the best ways to integrate their treatment regimens into their daily living activities. In chronic illness management, two tasks are of key importance: (1) incorporating disease-management regimens into life in a way that controls symptoms, keeps the disease stable, and is manageable within one's life context; and (2) addressing the psychological, social, and emotional issues that often accompany chronic disease and that can potentially hinder one's ability to self-care and live well.

Diagnosis and medical treatment by physicians are important aspects of chronic illness care, but they are only part of the disease management picture. Other essential components include teaching, counselling, supporting, problem-solving, arranging, and case-managing in collaboration with people living with chronic disease, with the goal of enabling people to live well with their disease and preserve autonomy and independence (Kralik, Koch, Price, & Howard, 2004). Saving the life of a person with an acute myocardial infarction in the ICU, for example, is a positive outcome, but he or she will likely relapse if not supported in making the lifestyle changes necessary to reduce the probability of another heart attack. Seeking to understand the person's perspective on illness management, and supporting his or her efforts to make sense of treatment regimens and to live life well within the limits of his or her disabilities is one of the most important aspects of health care delivery—and nursing care—for people living with chronic illness and for their families.

Step 6: Evaluating the Effectiveness of Interventions

The final step is evaluating the effectiveness of interventions. In chronic illness, maintaining the stability of the condition while at the same time preserving the person's control over his or her life and a sense of identity and accomplishment are the primary goals. Success may be defined, however, as merely making progress toward a goal when an individual finds it difficult to implement rapid and drastic changes in the way that he or she does things. Nurses cannot expect that the sedentary person with high blood pressure, for example, is going to develop a sudden passion for exercise. Nor can they expect that working people can easily rearrange their day to accommodate time-consuming regimens such as special diets or complex medication schedules. Bringing about change takes time, patience, creativity, encouragement, respect, and trust from the nurse. Validation by the nurse for each small increment toward goal accomplishment is important for enhancing self-esteem and reinforcing behaviours. If no progress is made or if progress toward goals seems slow, it may be necessary to redefine the goals or the time frame. The person may not be ready to progress toward the goals or may be ambivalent about the illness, its treatments, or both (Chin, Polonsky, Thomas & Nerney, 2000). Other conditions such as depression may also interfere with the person's ability to carry out regimens and make lifestyle changes.

Nurses must also realize that some people will not choose to change. Some people, for example, are unwilling to give up smoking despite advanced COPD. Nor is it unusual to find people with the diagnosis of diabetes failing to adhere to their diabetic diets. When people are having difficulty carrying out regimens or are reluctant to change their lifestyles, nurses should not feel that this is a failure on their part. This chronic illness management relationship is a partnership, and decision making is shared. Ultimately, however, the responsibility for management resides with the person living with the disease.

Promoting Home and Community-Based Care

TEACHING SELF-CARE

Since chronic conditions are so costly to individuals, families, and society, one of the major goals of nursing in the 21st century should be the prevention of chronic conditions and the care of people with them. This requires promoting healthy lifestyles and encouraging the use of safety and disease-prevention measures, such as wearing seat belts and obtaining immunizations. Prevention should also begin early in life and continue throughout the life span.

Teaching is one of the most significant aspects of nursing care and may make the difference in the ability of people and their families to adapt to chronic health conditions. Well-informed, educated people are more likely to be concerned about their health and do what is necessary to maintain it. They are also more likely to manage symptoms, recognize the onset of complications, and seek health care early: knowledge is the key to making informed choices and decisions during all phases of the chronic illness trajectory (Bodenheimer, Wagner, & Grumbach, 2002).

Despite the importance of health education, the nurse must recognize that persons recently diagnosed with serious chronic conditions and their families may need time to grasp the significance of their condition and its effect on life. Teaching should be planned carefully so that it provides information that is important to the person's well-being at the time, without being overwhelming.

The nurse who cares for people with chronic conditions in the hospital, clinic, or home should assess each person's knowledge about the illness and its management; the nurse cannot assume that a patient with a long-standing chronic condition has the knowledge necessary to manage the condition. Learning needs change as the trajectory phase and his or her personal situation changes. It is also important to remember, however, that those living with chronic disease are often the best experts. Engaging in shared decision making and practicing in authentic, respectful partnership with people as they continue to learn their self-care has been described as facilitative of the evolution of self-care knowledge (Thorne & Paterson, 2001).

CONTINUING CARE

Chronic illness management is a collaborative process between the person with the illness, the family, nurse, and other health care professionals. Collaboration is not limited to hospital settings; rather, it is important in all settings and throughout the illness trajectory (Corbin & Cherry, 2001). Keeping an illness stable over time requires careful and continued monitoring of symptoms and attention to management regimens. Detecting problems early and assisting people to develop appropriate management strategies can make a significant difference in outcomes.

Most chronic conditions are managed in the home. Therefore, care and teaching during hospitalization should focus on what the person needs to know about the condition in order to manage once discharged to home. Nurses in all settings should be aware of the resources and services available in a community and should make the arrangements (before hospital discharge if the person is hospitalized) necessary to secure those resources and services. When appropriate, home care services are contacted directly. The home care nurse will reassess how the person and family are adapting to the chronic condition and its treatment and will continue or revise the plan of care accordingly.

Because chronic conditions occur worldwide and the world is increasingly interconnected, nurses should think beyond the individual level to the community and global levels. In terms of illness prevention and health promotion, this entails wide-ranging efforts to assess people for risk factors for chronic illness (eg, blood pressure and diabetes screening, stroke risk assessments) and group teaching related to illness prevention and management.

Also, in terms of factors operating in the societal context, there are many considerations at the level of health policy that require the attention of health care professionals interested in improving population health and reducing the incidence and impact of chronic illness. The Canadian Nurses Association Code of Ethics states that nurses should "recognize the need to address organizational, social, economic and political factors influencing health" (Canadian Nurses Association, 2002), and take all steps consistent with the role of the professional registered nurse to advocate for healthy policy. Good public health policy requires an understanding of the broad determinants of health, and includes, but goes beyond, policies that support healthy behaviours such as non-smoking, exercise, and good nutrition to address socioenvironmental risk factors such as poverty, poor working conditions, and educational disadvantage (Reutter & Duncan, 2002). While it is not realistic to expect all registered nurses to become policy experts or activists, it is realistic to expect nurses to be able to assess, identify, and articulate the impact of some of these broader factors and capitalize upon opportunities to effect policy change through professional or advocacy organizations (Malone, 2005).

NURSING CARE FOR SPECIAL POPULATIONS WITH CHRONIC ILLNESS

When providing care and teaching, the nurse must consider a variety of factors (eg, age, gender, culture, and ethnicity) that influence susceptibility to chronic illness and the ways people respond to chronic disorders. Certain populations, for example, tend to be more susceptible to certain chronic conditions. Populations at high risk for specific conditions can be targeted for special teaching and monitoring programs. People of different cultures and genders tend to respond to illness differently; being aware of these differences is extremely important (Denton, Prus, & Walters, 2004; Thorne, McCormick, & Carty, 1997). For cultures in which the ill person relies heavily on family support, families must be involved and made part of the nursing care plan. As Canada becomes more multicultural and ethnically diverse, and as the general population ages, nurses need to be aware of how an individual's culture and age facilitate or hinder chronic illness management, and nurses should be prepared to adapt the care they give accordingly (Anderson, 1998; Mok, Lai, & Zhang, 2004).

 Critical Thinking Exercises

1. A 25-year-old graduate student is diagnosed with fibromyalgia after several years of visiting physicians and being told that her symptoms were "all in your mind." Due to chronic fatigue and pain, she often missed days from school and eventually withdrew from school. Her husband is not very supportive because he too thinks the disease is "in her head." How would you help this woman learn to cope with her condition and the damages to her self-esteem? How would you involve her husband in the process?

2. A 19-year-old has been recently diagnosed with diabetes. He is very active in sports and involved with his peers. He says that he is not interested in learning about his condition, refuses to learn to give insulin injections to himself, and eats whatever he wants. How would you approach goal setting and establishing a plan of care with this young adult? What developmental issues will you consider in your teaching?

3. An 85-year-old woman is about to be discharged from the hospital after an acute episode of heart failure. How would the teaching and planning for discharge be different from that of a 45-year-old going home after an acute myocardial infarction?

4. A 43-year-old Aboriginal woman tells you that she is always thirsty and has frequent yeast infections. She also tells you that she has not had a Pap smear or any kind of physical examination since her last child was born 8 years ago because she lives a full day's travel from the health clinic, has no reliable means of transportation, and no one to care for her four children while she is away. What would you tell this woman? How would you advise her to obtain health care?

5. A 45-year-old Indo-Canadian woman with multiple sclerosis in remission has been advised by her doctor to start a regular exercise program. She asks why she should do exercise since eventually her disease is only going to get worse anyway. She works and has three teenage children at home. How would you explain to her the relationship between health-promotion activities and quality of life? How might you go about establishing with her an exercise plan? How might her family become involved in helping her?

REFERENCES AND SELECTED READINGS

Books

Advisory Committee on Population Health. (2002). *Advancing integrated prevention strategies in Canada: An approach to reducing the burden of chronic diseases.* Ottawa, ON: Health Canada.

Broemeling, A., Watson, D., & Black, C. (2005). *Chronic conditions and co-morbidity among residents of British Columbia.* Vancouver, BC: Centre for Health Services and Policy Research.

Corbin, J. (2001). Introduction and overview: Chronic illness and nursing. *Chronic illness: Research and theory for nursing practice.* New York: Springer Publishing Co.

Corbin, J., & Cherry, J. (1997). Caring for the chronically ill elderly in the community. In L. Swanson & T. Tripp-Reiner (Eds.). *Advances in gerontological nursing* (Vol. 2). New York: Springer.

Corbin, J., & Cherry J. (2001). Epilogue: A proactive model of health care. In R. Hyman & J. Corbin (Eds.). *Chronic illness: Research and theory for nursing practice* (pp. 294–299). New York: Springer.

Crimmins, E. M., Kim, J. K., & Hagedorn, A. (2003). Health expectancy: An indicator of successful aging and a measure of the impact of chronic disease and disability. In L.W. Poon, S. H. Gueldner, & B. M. Sprouse (Eds.), *Successful aging and adaptation with chronic diseases* (pp. 70–82). New York: Springer.

Health Canada. (1998). *Economic burden of illness in Canada.* Report No. H21-136/1998E. Ottawa ON: Population and Public Health Branch.

Health Canada. (2000). *Diabetes among Aboriginal people (First Nations, Inuit, Metis) in Canada: The evidence.* Report No. 0-662-29976-0. Ottawa, ON: Author.

Health Canada. (2002). *Diabetes in Canada.* Ottawa, ON: Population and Public Health Branch.

Health Canada. (2003). *Chronic disease surveillance in Canada: A background paper.* Report No. 0-662-67114-7. Ottawa, ON: Population and Public Health Branch, Health Surveillance Coordination Division.

Lalonde, M. (1974). *A new perspective on the health of Canadians: A working document.* Ottawa, ON: Government of Canada.

Losos, J. (2002). *Promotion and protection of health and well-being of the population: Vision of federal/national roles.* Ottawa, ON: University of Ottawa Institute of Population Health.

Lubkin, I. M. & Larson, P. D. (2002). *Chronic illness: Impact and interventions* (5th ed.). Sudbury, MA: Jones & Bartlett.

Miller, J. F. (2000). *Coping with chronic illness: Overcoming powerlessness* (3rd ed.). Philadelphia: F.A. Davis

Raphael, D. (2004). *Social determinants of health: Canadian perspectives.* Toronto, ON: Canadian Scholar's Press.

Robinson, L., Bevil, C., Arcangelo, V., Reifsnyder, J. A., Rothman, N., & Smeltzer, S. (2001). Operationalizing the Corbin and Strauss Trajectory Model for elderly clients with chronic illness. In R. Hyman & J. Corbin (Eds.). *Chronic illness: Research and theory for nursing practice.* New York: Springer.

Strauss, A., & Corbin, J. (1988). *Shaping a new health care system.* San Francisco: Jossey-Bass.

Woog, P. (Ed.). (1992). *The chronic illness trajectory framework.* New York: Springer.

Journals

Asterisks indicate nursing research articles.

*Anderson, J. M. (1998). Speaking of illness: Issues of first generation Canadian women—implications for patient education and counselling. *Patient Education and Counselling, 33*(3), 197–207.

*Benbow, C. & Koopman, W. J. (2003). Clinic based needs assessment of individuals with multiple sclerosis and significant others: Implications for program planning—psychological needs. *Rehabilitation Nursing, 28*(4), 109–116.

Bodenheimer, T., Wagner, E. H. &., & Grumbach, K. (2002). Improving primary care for patients with chronic illness. *Journal of the American Medical Association, 288*(14), 1775–1779.

Cagle, C. S., Appel, S., Skelly, A. H., & Carter-Edwards, L. (2002). Midlife African-American women with type 2 diabetes: Influence on work and the multi-caregiver role. *Ethnicity & Disease, 12*(4), 555–566.

Canadian Nurses Association. (2002). *Code of ethics for registered nurses.* Available at: http://www.cna-aiic.ca/cna/documents/pdf/publications/codeofethics2002_e.pdf. Retrieved May 13, 2005.

Carroll, L. W. (1998). Understanding chronic illness from the patient's perspective. *Radiologic Technology, 70*(1), 37–41.

Chin, M. H., Polonsky, R. S., Thomas, V. D., & Nerney, M. P. (2000). Developing a conceptual framework for understanding illness and attitudes in older, urban African Americans with diabetes. *Diabetes Education, 26*(3), 439–449.

Cicutto, L., Brooks, D., & Henderson, K. (2003). Self-care issues from the perspective of individuals with chronic obstructive pulmonary disease. *Patient Education and Counselling, 55*, 168–176.

Corbin, J. M. (1998). The Corbin and Strauss chronic illness trajectory model: An update. *Scholarly Inquiry for Nursing Practice, 12*(1), 33–41.

Corbin, J., & Strauss, A. (1991). A nursing model for chronic illness management based upon the trajectory framework. *Scholarly Inquiry for Nursing Practice, 5*(3), 155–174.

*Cumbie, S. A., Conley, V. M., & Burman, M. E. (2004). Advanced practice nursing model for comprehensive care with chronic illness. *Advances in Nursing Science, 27*(1), 70–80.

Dean, P. R. (1999). Personal perception of chronic illness. *Home Care Provider, 4*(2), 54–57.

Denton, M., Prus, S., & Walters, V. (2004). Gender differences in health: A Canadian study of the psychosocial, structural and behavioural determinants of health. *Social Science & Medicine, 58*(12), 2585–2600.

Dewar, A., White, M., Posade, S., & Dillon, W. (2003). Using nominal group technique to assess chronic pain, patients' perceived challenges and needs in a community health region. *Health Expectations, 6*(1), 44–52.

Epp, J. (1986). *Achieving health for all: A framework for health promotion.* Available at: http://www.hc-sc.gc.ca/english/care/achieving_health.html. Retrieved November 10, 2004.

Gupta, S., Roos, L. L., Walld, R., Traverse, D., & Dahl, M. (2003). Delivering equitable care: Comparing preventive services in Manitoba. *American Journal of Public Health, 93*(12), 2089–2092.

Harvey, D., Hook, E., Kozyniak, J., & Selvanathan, M. (2002). *Building the case for the prevention of chronic disease.* Available at: http://www.apcd.mb.ca/apcd/research.asp. Retrieved October 12, 2002.

*Hislop, T. G., Deschamps, M., Teh, C., Jackson, C., Tu, S., Yasui, Y. et al. (2003). Facilitators and barriers to cervical cancer screening among Chinese Canadian women. *Canadian Journal of Public Health, 94*(1), 68–73.

*Hough, E. S., Brumitt, G. A., & Templin, T. N. (1999). Social support, demands of illness, and depression in chronically ill urban women. *Health Care for Women International, 20*(4), 349–362.

Hunt, L. M., Pugh, J., & Valenzuela, M. (1998). How patients adapt diabetes self-care recommendations in everyday life. *Journal of Family Practice, 46*(3), 207–215.

Katzmarzyk, P. & Janssen, I. (2004). The economic costs associated with physical inactivity and obesity in Canada: An update. *Canadian Journal of Applied Physiology, 29*(1), 90–115.

Kopec, J. & Schultz, S. (2003). Impact of chronic conditions. *Health Reports, 14*(4), 41–56.

*Kralik, D., Koch, T., Price, K., & Howard, N. (2004). Chronic illness self-management: Taking action to create order. *Journal of Clinical Nursing, 13*, 259–267.

*Lefort, S. M. (2000). A test of Braden's self-help model in adults with chronic pain. *Journal of Nursing Scholarship, 32*(2), 153–160.

Lewis, K. S. (1998). Emotional adjustment to a chronic illness. *Lippincott's Primary Care Practice, 2*(1), 38–51.

*Mahon, D. & Casperson, D. (1997). Exploring the psychosocial meaning of recurrent cancer: a descriptive study. *Cancer Nursing, 20*(3), 178–186.

Malone, R. E. (2005). Assessing the policy environment. *Policy, Politics & Nursing Practice, 6*(2), 135–143.

*Martin, J. C., Engle, V. F., & Graney, M. J. (1999). Determinants of health-related hardiness among urban older African-American women with chronic illness. *Holistic Nursing Practice, 13*(3), 62–70.

McDougall, J., King, G., De Wit, D., Miller, L., Hong, S., Offord, D. et al. (2004). Chronic physical health conditions and disability among Canadian school-aged children: A national profile. *Disability & Rehabilitation, 26*(1), 35–45.

*Michael, S. R. (1996). Integrating chronic illness into one's life: a phenomenological inquiry. *Journal of Holistic Nursing, 14*(3), 251–267.

Miller, M. (1999). Clinical sidebar. *Image: Journal of Nursing Scholarship, 31*(2), 125.

Mishel, M. H. (1999). Uncertainty in chronic illness. *Annual Review of Nursing Research, 17*, 269–294.

*Mok, E., Lai, C., & Zhang, A. (2004). Coping with chronic renal failure in Hong Kong. *International Journal of Nursing Studies, 41*(2), 205–213.

*Morgan, D., Semchuk, K., Stewart, N., & D'Arcy, C. (2002). Rural families caring for a relative with dementia: Barriers to use of formal services. *Social Science & Medicine, 55*(7), 1129–1142.

*Morse, J. (1997). Responding to threats to integrity of self. *Advances in Nursing Science, 19*(4), 21–36.

National Advisory Council on Aging. (1999). *1999 and beyond: Challenges of an aging Canadian society.* Available at: http://www.naca-ccnta.ca/publications_e.htm. Retrieved April 15, 2005.

*Neufeld, S., Query, B., & Drummond, J. (2001). Respite care users who have children with chronic conditions: Are they getting a break? *Journal of Pediatric Nursing, 16*(4), 234–244.

Nodhturft, V., Schneider, J. M., Hebert, P. et al. (2000). Chronic disease self-management: improving health outcomes. *Nursing Clinics of North America, 35*(2), 507–518.

Ontario Public Health Association. (2004). *Orientation to health in Ontario.* Available at: http://www.hhrc.net/pdfs/orientation_section3.pdf. Retrieved April 21, 2005.

*Paterson, B. & Thorne, S. (2000a). Developmental evolution of expertise in diabetes self-management. *Clinical Nursing Research, 9*(4), 402–419.

*Paterson, B. & Thorne, S. (2000b). Expert decision making in relation to unanticipated blood glucose levels. *Research in Nursing & Health, 23*(2), 147–157.

Patten, S., Jacobs, P., Reimer, P., & Metz, L. (2002). Major depressive disorder and health care costs in multiple sclerosis. *International Journal of Psychiatry in Medicine, 32*(2), 167–178.

*Price, B. (1996). Illness careers: the chronic illness experience. *Journal of Advanced Nursing, 24*(2), 275–279.

Public Health Agency of Canada. (2005). *Publications: Age related chronic diseases.* Available at: http://www.phac-aspc.gc.ca/seniors-aines/index_pages/publications_e.htm#age. Retrieved April 25, 2005.

Reutter, L. & Duncan, S. (2002). Preparing nurses to promote health-enhancing public policies. *Policy, Politics & Nursing Practice, 3*(4), 294–305.

*Riegel, B. & Carlson, B. (2002). Facilitators and barriers to heart failure self-care. *Patient Education & Counselling, 46*(4), 287–295.

*Saiki-Craighill, S. (1997). The children's sentinels: mothers and their relationships with health professionals in the context of Japanese health care. *Social Science and Medicine, 44*(3), 291–300.

Schoenberg, N. E. & Drungle, S. C. (2001). Barriers to non-insulin dependent diabetes mellitus (NIDDM) self-care practices among older women. *Journal of Aging & Health, 13*(4), 443–466.

Sidell, N. L. (1997). Adult adjustment to chronic illness: a review of the literature. *Health and Social Work, 22*(1), 5–11.

*Spenceley, S. (in press). A systematic review of access to health services by chronically ill Canadians. *Western Journal of Nursing Research.*

Statistics Canada. (2002). *Health indicators, volume 2: Health behaviors—physical activity.* Report No. 82-221-XIE. Available at: http://www.statcan.ca/english/freepub/82-221-XIE/01002/nonmed/behaviors3.htm. Retrieved April 15, 2005.

*Tappan, R. M., Williams, C., Fishman, S., & Theris, T. (1999). Persistence of self in advanced Alzheimer's disease. *Image: Journal of Nursing Scholarship, 31*(2), 121–125.

*Thorne, S. E. (1999). The science of meaning in chronic illness. *International Journal of Nursing Studies, 36*(5), 397–404.

*Thorne, S., Con, A., McGuinness, L., McPherson, G., & Harris, S. R. (2004). Health care communication issues in multiple sclerosis: An interpretive description. *Qualitative Health Research, 14*(1), 5–22.

*Thorne, S., McCormick, J., & Carty, E. (1997). Deconstructing the gender neutrality of chronic illness and disability. *Health Care Women International, 18*(1), 1–16.

*Thorne, S. E. & Paterson, B. L. (2000). Two decades of insider research: What we know and don't know about chronic illness experience. *Annual Review of Nursing Research, 18*, 3–25.

*Thorne, S. E. & Paterson, B. L. (2001). Health care professional support for self-care management in chronic illness: Insights from diabetes research. *Patient Education & Counselling, 42*(1), 81–90.

*Thorne, S., Paterson, B., & Russell, C. (2003). The structure of everyday self-care decision making in chronic illness. *Qualitative Health Research, 13*(10), 1337–1352.

Westby M., Wade J., Rangno K., & Berkowitz J. (2000). A randomized controlled trial to evaluate the effectiveness of an exercise program in women with rheumatoid arthritis taking low dose prednisone. *Journal of Rheumatology, 27*(7), 1674–1680.

Wilkins, K. &. Park, E. (1996). Chronic conditions, physical limitations and dependency among seniors living in the community. *Health Reports, 8*(3), 7–15.

*Wilson, H. S., Hutchinson, S. A., & Holzemer, W. L. (2002). Reconciling incompatibilities: A grounded theory of HIV medication adherence and symptom management. *Qualitative Health Research, 12*(10), 1309–1322.

World Health Organization. (1986). *Ottawa charter for health promotion.* Available at: http://www.who.int/hpr/NPH/docs/ottawa_charter_hp.pdf.

World Health Organization. (2005). *Observatory on health care for chronic conditions.* Available at: http://www.who.int/chronic_conditions/why/en/index.html. Retrieved April 10, 2005.

RESOURCES AND WEBSITES

Alliance for the Prevention of Chronic Disease; http://www.apcd.mb.ca

Chronic Disease Management in British Columbia; http://www.hlth.gov.bc.ca/cdm/

Chronic Disease Prevention Alliance of Canada; http://www.chronicdiseaseprevention.ca

Health Canada. Commission on the Future of Health Care in Canada (Romanow Commission website); http://www.hc-sc.gc.ca/english/care/romanow/index1.html

Health in Action: Alberta Health Living Network; http://www.health-in-action.org/content.asp?catid=37&rootid=7

Public Health Agency of Canada—Canadian Health Network website; http://www.canadian-health-network.ca

Public Health Agency of Canada—Centre for Chronic Disease Prevention and Control; http://www.phac-aspc.gc.ca/ccdpc-cpcmc/index_e.html

Public Health Agency of Canada—Chronic Diseases in Canada online journal access; http://www.phac-aspc.gc.ca/publicat/cdic-mcc/index.html.

Principles and Practices of Rehabilitation

Adapted by Linda J. Youell and Evelyn Myles

LEARNING OBJECTIVES

On completion of this chapter, the learner will be able to:

1. Describe the goals of rehabilitation.
2. Discuss the interdisciplinary approach to rehabilitation.
3. Identify emotional reactions exhibited by patients with disabilities.
4. Use the nursing process as a framework for care of patients with self-care deficits, impaired physical mobility, impaired skin integrity, and altered patterns of elimination.
5. Describe nursing strategies appropriate for promoting self-care through activities of daily living.
6. Describe nursing strategies appropriate for promoting mobility and ambulation and the use of assistive devices.
7. Describe risk factors and related nursing measures to prevent development of pressure ulcers.
8. Incorporate bladder training and bowel training into the plan of care for patients with bladder and bowel problems.
9. Describe the significance of continuity of care from the health care facility to the home or extended care facility for patients who need rehabilitative assistance and services.

*R*ehabilitation is a dynamic, health-oriented process that assists an ill person or a person with **disability** (restriction in performance or function in everyday activities) to achieve the greatest possible level of physical, mental, spiritual, social, and economic functioning. The rehabilitation process helps the patient achieve an acceptable quality of life with dignity, self-respect, and independence and is designed for people with physical, mental, or emotional disabilities. During rehabilitation—sometimes called habilitation—the patient adjusts to the disability by learning how to use resources and to focus on existing abilities. In **habilitation**, abilities, not disabilities, are emphasized.

Rehabilitation is an integral part of nursing because every major illness or injury carries the threat of disability or **impairment**, which involves a loss of function or an abnormality. The principles of rehabilitation are basic to the care of all patients, and rehabilitation efforts should begin during the initial contact with a patient. The goal of rehabilitation is to restore the patient's ability to function independently or at a preillness or preinjury level of functioning as quickly as possible. If this is not possible, the aims of rehabilitation are maximal independence and a quality of life acceptable to the patient. Realistic goals based on individual patient assessment are established with the patient to guide the rehabilitation program.

Rehabilitation services are required by more people than ever before because of advances in technology that save or prolong the lives of seriously ill, injured, and disabled patients. Increasing numbers of patients who are recovering from serious illnesses or injuries are returning to their homes and communities with ongoing needs. Every patient, regardless of age, gender, ethnic group, socioeconomic status, or diagnosis, has a right to rehabilitation services (Chart 11-1).

Approximately 1 in 8 Canadians has some form of disability, and 1 in 20 has a severe disability (Government of Canada, 2004). A person is considered to have a disability, such as a restriction in performance or function in everyday activities, if he or she has difficulty talking, hearing, seeing, walking, climbing stairs, lifting or carrying objects, performing activities of daily living, doing school work, or working at a job. A severe disability is present if a person is unable to perform one or more activities, uses an assistive device for mobility, or needs help from another person to accomplish basic activities. Individuals are also considered severely disabled if they receive federal benefits based on an inability to work.

Approximately 3.6 million Canadians are affected by some form of disability, and this number is expected to increase in the com-

---

Chart 11-1 • Ethics and Related Issues

Are All Persons Entitled to Rehabilitation?

Situation

You work in an area populated by the poor and homeless. Community violence often creates life-threatening and disabling conditions in members of the population. After a victim of violence has been saved and stabilized, the health care team identifies rehabilitation needs. You are concerned about your patient's inability to perform self-care and to demonstrate safe mobility skills.

Dilemma

As a health care provider, you are concerned about the community as a whole; costs to the community, and the values of the community. You are also aware of socio-economic factors; you recognize costs to your patient when treatment is provided or not provided.

Discussion

Who determines the length of stay and level of care? Who will take care of patients who need longer-term rehabilitation but services are not readily available? Is rehabilitation a basic health care need?

---

ing decades due to the aging of the population. More than half of persons with disabilities are women, irrespective of age. On average, women also live longer, making them more likely to develop age-related chronic conditions that lead to disability. Canada's aboriginal population experiences more than one and a half times the disability rate of the non-aboriginal population (Government of Canada, 2004).

Persons with disabilities may need any of three types of disability supports: "individual supports (aids and devices or more sophisticated **assistive technology,** help needed for everyday **activities of daily living,** home modifications); supports for informal caregivers; and inclusive environments (transportation, information in multiple formats)" (Government of Canada, 2004, p. 15.).

Supporting Persons With Disabilities

For years, people with disabilities have been discriminated against in employment, public accommodations, and public and private services including health care. The needs of the disabled in health care settings produce many challenges to health care providers: how to communicate effectively if there are communication deficits, the

---

Glossary

activities of daily living (ADLs): Self-care activities including bathing, grooming, dressing, eating, toileting, and bowel and bladder care.

assistive technology: Any item, piece of equipment, or product system—whether acquired commercially, off the shelf, modified, or customized—that is used to improve the functional capabilities of individuals with disabilities.

disability: Restriction or lack of ability to perform an activity in a normal manner; the consequences of impairment in terms of an individual's functional performance and ac-

tivity. Disabilities represent disturbances at the level of the person (eg, bathing, dressing, communication, walking, grooming).

habilitation: Making able; learning new skills and abilities to meet maximum potential.

impairment: Loss or abnormality of psychological, physiologic, or anatomic structure or function at the organ level (eg, dysphagia, hemiparesis); an abnormality of body structure, appearance, and organ or system function resulting from any cause.

inclusion: Providing persons with disabilities opportunities like those of all

Canadians to participate fully in all daily activities—at home, at school, at work, and in the community.

instrumental activities of daily living (IADLs): Complex aspects of independence including meal preparation, grocery shopping, household management, finances, and transportation.

pressure ulcers: Breakdown of the skin due to prolonged pressure and insufficient blood supply, usually at boney prominences.

rehabilitation: Making able again; relearning skills or abilities or adjusting existing functions.

additional physical demands for mobility, and time required to provide assistance with self-care routines during hospitalization. Physicians and nurses may not know the specific needs of individuals with disability and may fail to provide services for them. For example, an obstetrician may advise a woman with a spinal cord injury not to become pregnant because the physician lacks experience and knowledge in this area of care. The physician and nurses caring for an expectant woman with disability may not know specific transfer techniques to help her onto an examining table or how to advise her on bowel, bladder, and skin care issues during pregnancy. Before labour and delivery, the medical team needs to be educated about the special needs of a woman with a cervical spinal cord injury in regard to management of autonomic hyperreflexia (also known as autonomic dysreflexia). Often, the person with disability must educate the health care professionals.

Because of unfavourable interactions with health care providers, including negative attitudes, insensitivity, and lack of knowledge, people with disability may avoid seeking medical intervention or health promotion programs and activities. For this reason, and because the number of individuals with disability is increasing, nurses must acquire knowledge and skills and be accessible to assist these individuals in maintaining a high level of wellness.

Nurses are in key positions to influence the architectural design of health care settings and the selection of equipment that promotes ease of access and health. Padded examination tables that can be raised or lowered make transfers easier for the disabled. Birthing chairs benefit women with disability during yearly pelvic examinations and Pap smears and for urologic evaluations. Ramps, grab bars, and raised and padded toilet seats benefit many persons who have orthopedic disabilities and need routine physical examination and monitoring (eg, bone density measurements). Just as people without disability should have regular screening tests, such as mammography or testicular and prostate examinations, so should people with disability. The health care professionals who provide these screening and monitoring procedures are in a position to influence decisions about how equipment and procedures can be adapted to meet the special needs of their patients, whether these needs are cognitive, motor, or communicative.

Nurses can provide expert health promotion education classes that are targeted to the disabled. Classes on nutrition and weight management are extremely important to individuals who are wheelchair dependent and need assistance with transfers. Safe sex classes are needed by adolescents and young adults who have spinal cord or traumatic brain injury, because the threats of acquired immunodeficiency syndrome (AIDS) and unplanned pregnancy exist for these populations just as they do for the population in general. Other healthy behaviours about which neurologically disabled persons need education include avoiding alcohol and non-prescription medications while taking antispasmodic and anti-seizure medications. Nurses should teach all stroke survivors and patients with diabetes how to monitor their own blood pressure or glucose levels. The warning signs and symptoms of stroke, heart attack, and cancer, as well as how to access help, should also be taught to all disabled persons.

As active members of society, people with disabilities are no longer an invisible minority. An increased awareness of the needs of people with disabilities will bring about changes to improve their access and accommodate their needs. Modification of the physical environment permits access to public and private facilities and services, including health care, and nurses can serve as advocates for the disabled to eliminate discriminatory practices.

The Government of Canada is committed to advancing the **inclusion** of people with disabilities. In its 2004 report *Advanc-*

ing the Inclusion of Persons With Disabilities, the federal government outlined six areas of inclusion toward which it is working: disability supports, skills development and learning, employment, income, capacity of the disability community, and health and well-being (Government of Canada, 2004).

Focus of Rehabilitation

Disability can occur at any age and may result from an acute incident, such as stroke or trauma, or from the progression of a chronic condition, such as arthritis or multiple sclerosis. A person with disability experiences many losses, including loss of function, independence, social role, status, and income. A patient and his or her family members experience a range of emotional reactions to these losses. The reactions may progress from disorganization and confusion to denial of the disability, grief over the lost function or body part, depression, anger, and, finally, acceptance of the disability. The reactions may subside over time and may recur at a later time, especially if chronic illness is progressive and results in increasing losses. Not all patients experience all of the stages, although most do exhibit grief. Patients who exhibit grief should not be blithely encouraged to "cheer up." The nurse should show a willingness to listen to the patient talk about the disability and should understand that grief, anger, regret, and resentment are all part of the healing process. See the accompanying Gerontologic Considerations box for concerns unique to older adults.

The patient's preexisting coping abilities play an important role in the adaptation process: one patient may be particularly independent and determined, while another may be dependent and seem to lack personal power. One goal of rehabilitation is to help the patient gain a positive self-image through effective coping. The nurse must recognize different coping abilities and identify when the patient is not coping well or not adjusting to the disability (Nursing Research Profile 11-1). The patient and family may benefit from participating in a support group or talking with a mental health professional to achieve this goal. Refer to Chapter 6 for a detailed discussion of adaptive and maladaptive responses to illness.

The Rehabilitation Team

Rehabilitation is a creative, dynamic process that requires a team of professionals working together with the patient and the family. The team members represent a variety of disciplines, with

---

Gerontologic Considerations
Concerns of Older Adults Facing Disability

- Loss of independence, which is a source of self-respect and dignity
- Increased potential for discrimination or abuse
- Increased social isolation
- Added burden on spouse who may also have impaired health
- Less access to community services and health care
- Less access to religious institutions
- Increased vulnerability to declining health secondary to other disorders, reduced physiologic reserve, or preexisting impairments of mobility and balance
- Fears and doubts about ability to learn or relearn self-care activities, exercises, and transfer and independent mobility techniques
- Inadequate support system for successful rehabilitation

NURSING RESEARCH PROFILE 11-1
Older Adults and Disability

Cataldo, J. (2001). The relationship of hardiness and depression to disability in institutionalized older adults. *Rehabilitation Nursing 26*(1), 28–33.

Purpose
Depression has been linked with disability in several studies of older adults. Hardiness is a personality characteristic that is a buffer in the stress and depression dynamic and increases a person's capability of having a positive psychological reaction to a stressor. Hardiness only partially explains the variance of depression since the hardiest of individuals may become depressed. This study tested two hypotheses: (1) After accounting for the effects of physiologic factors (physical status and length of stay [LOS]), hardiness will significantly contribute to the explanation of disability in a sample of institutionalized elderly people; (2) after accounting for the effects of physical health status, LOS, and hardiness, depression will significantly contribute to the explanation of disability in a sample of institutionalized older people.

Study Sample and Design
A culturally diverse group of 33 women and 25 men ranging in age from 60 to 93 years participated in a 45-minute interview. Hardiness was measured with the Health-Related Hardiness Scale (HRHS) which had 34 items on a 6-point Likert-type scale. The instrument had two dimensions: commitment/challenge and control. High scores indicated higher hardiness. Depression was measured with the Zung Self-Rating Depression Scale (ZSDS), a 22-item screening inventory. High scores indicated a high level of depressive symptomatology. Physical health status was measured with the Clinical Response Scale (CRS), a 56-item generic health index. The items were scored using data from the participants' medical records in a 1-month period. Higher scores indicated worsened health status. LOS data were collected from the facility's computerized system with day of admission being day 1. Disability was measured by the Barthel Activities of Daily Living Index, which had 10 variables related to self-care and mobility. A high score indicated independence, and a low score indicated disability.

Findings
Both hypotheses were supported. The psychological variables of hardiness and depression contributed more than did health status and LOS to explain disability in a sample of elderly nursing home residents. LOS and physical health status accounted for 14.7% of the variance in disability. Hardiness explained 10.5% of the variance, and depression accounted for an additional 7.4% of the variance in disability.

Nursing Implications
Nurses need to guide older persons with disability to develop hardiness. Nurses can encourage them to view the disability as a challenge and to make a commitment to life. The nurse can assist older individuals with disability to take control of their life circumstances (ie, become actively involved in pain management and all daily decision making). Because the level of disability is not exclusively the result of physiologic factors, the nurse should suggest treatment of depression in the older adult with disability.

each health professional making a unique contribution. Each health professional assesses the patient and identifies patient needs within the discipline's domain. Rehabilitative goals are set. Each health professional assesses the patient, identifies patient needs within the discipline's domain, and sets rehabilitative goals. Team members hold group sessions at frequent intervals to collaborate, evaluate progress, and modify goals as needed to facilitate reha-

bilitation and to promote independence, self-respect, and an acceptable quality of life for the patient.

The patient is the key member of the rehabilitation team. He or she is the focus of the team effort and the one who determines the final outcomes of the process. The patient participates in goal setting, in learning to function using remaining abilities, and in adjusting to living with disabilities.

The patient's family is also incorporated into the team. The family is a dynamic system, so disability of one member affects the other family members. Only by incorporating the family into the rehabilitation process can the family system adapt to the change in one of its members. The family provides ongoing support, participates in problem solving, and learns to provide necessary ongoing care (Nursing Research Profile 11-2).

The rehabilitation nurse develops a therapeutic and supportive relationship with the patient and the family. The nurse always emphasizes the patient's assets and strengths, positively reinforcing his or her efforts to improve self-concept and self-care abilities. During nurse–patient interactions, the nurse actively listens, encourages, and shares the patient's successes.

Using the nursing process, the nurse develops a plan of care designed to facilitate rehabilitation, restore and maintain optimum health, and prevent complications. The nurse helps the patient identify strengths and past successes and develop new goals. Coping with the disability, self-care, mobility, skin care, and bowel and bladder management are frequently areas for nursing intervention. The nurse assumes the roles of caregiver, teacher, counsellor, patient advocate, and consultant. The nurse is often the case manager responsible for coordinating the total rehabilitative plan, collaborating with and coordinating the services provided by all members of the health care team, including the home care nurse, who is responsible for directing the patient's care after return to the home.

Other members of the rehabilitation team may include a physician, nurse practitioner, physiatrist, physical therapist, occupational therapist, speech-language therapist, psychologist, psychiatric liaison nurse, social worker, vocational counsellor, orthotist or prosthetist, rehabilitation engineer, and sex counsellor or therapist.

Areas of Specialty Practice

Although rehabilitation is a component of every patient's care, there are specialty rehabilitation programs established in general hospitals, free-standing rehabilitation hospitals, and outpatient facilities. The Canadian Council on Health Services Accreditation (CCHSA) and the Commission for the Accreditation of Rehabilitation Facilities (CARF) set standards for these programs and monitor compliance with them.

Specialty rehabilitation programs often meet the needs of patients with neurologic disabilities. Stroke recovery programs and traumatic brain injury rehabilitation emphasize cognitive remediation: assisting patients to compensate for memory, perceptual, judgment, and safety deficits as well as teaching self-care and mobility skills. Other goals include assisting patients to swallow food safely and to communicate effectively. In addition to stroke and brain injury, other neurologic disorders treated include multiple sclerosis, Parkinson's disease, amyotrophic lateral sclerosis, and nervous system tumours.

The number of spinal cord injury rehabilitation programs has increased since World War II. Integral components of the programs include understanding the effects and complications of spinal cord injury; neurogenic bowel and bladder management; sexuality and

NURSING RESEARCH PROFILE 11-2

Caregivers

Secrest, J. (2000). Transformation of the relationship: The experience of primary support persons of stroke survivors. *Rehabilitation Nursing* 25(3), 93–99.

Purpose

Most stroke survivors live at home. Effective rehabilitation must include the primary support person (PSP). Nurses teach and counsel the PSP during acute hospitalization, during the rehabilitation phase, and in the home. Understanding the experience of stroke from the PSP's perspective can help nurses design effective interventions for the PSP. The purpose of this study was to investigate the quality, or nature, of life experienced by PSPs of stroke survivors.

Study Sample and Design

The study sample consisted of 8 women and 2 men between the ages of 40 to 72 years. Criteria for inclusion in the study were that (1) the participant was the PSP of a stroke survivor whose stroke occurred at least 6 months previously, and who had completed inpatient rehabilitation and was living at home and (2) the participant was willing and able to articulate the experience. The study design sought to attain a first-person description of the PSP experience. The single interview item was, "Please describe specific experiences you've had since your [significant other's] stroke that stands out for you." The researchers "bracketed" or identified potential biases about the phenomenon being studied so that they would not unduly influence the course of the study. The interview was transcribed verbatim and analyzed by members of the research group.

Findings

Participants rarely spoke of themselves as individuals. Experiences described were in relation to others. They expressed concern about being able to sustain their role over time. Time permeated the interviews: the length of time the couples had been married; changes in the stroke survivor's perception of time; and memory as it is of past time. Memory loss in the stroke survivor was perceived as a loss of an important aspect of the relationship. Other themes emerged. Life was perceived by the PSPs as being fragile. They experienced vigilance as they watched over the stroke victim. The PSP's vigilance did not diminish over time because they were aware of life's fragility and had an increased responsibility in the relationship. A weighty responsibility and a sense of loss were recurrent throughout the transcripts. All participants described the experience of a transformed relationship. The quality was different, but all of the relationships remained intact.

Nursing Implications

Nurses need to assess the pre-stroke relationship of the patient and PSP in order to prepare the PSP for the future. This will enable the nurse to negotiate goals, teach, and counsel the PSP more effectively. Attendance at support groups specifically for the PSP should be encouraged. Nurses are key individuals to organize and maintain support groups. PSPs need permission to focus on themselves, grieve their losses, and find support for their added responsibilities.

---

male fertility enhancement; self-care, including prevention of skin breakdown; bed mobility and transfers; and driving with adaptive equipment. The programs also focus on vocational assessment, training, and reentry into employment and the community.

Orthopedic rehabilitation programs provide comprehensive services to traumatic or nontraumatic amputee patients, patients undergoing joint replacements, and patients with arthritis. Learning to be independent with a prosthesis or a new joint is a major

goal of the program. Pain management, energy conservation, and joint protection are other goals.

For patients who have had myocardial infarction, cardiac rehabilitation begins during the acute hospitalization and continues on an outpatient basis. Emphasis is placed on monitored, progressive exercise; nutritional counselling; stress management; and sexuality.

Patients with restrictive or chronic obstructive pulmonary disease or ventilator dependency may be admitted to pulmonary rehabilitation programs. Respiratory therapists help the patient achieve more effective breathing patterns. The programs also teach energy conservation techniques, self-medication, and home airway management.

Comprehensive pain management programs are available for sufferers of chronic pain, especially low back pain. These programs focus on alternative pain treatment modalities, exercise, supportive counselling, and vocational evaluation.

A comprehensive burn rehabilitation program may serve as a step-down unit from an intensive care burn unit. Although rehabilitation strategies are implemented immediately in acute care, a program focused on progressive joint mobility, self-care, and ongoing counselling is imperative for the burn patient.

Children are not exempt from the need for specialized rehabilitation. Pediatric rehabilitation programs meet the needs of children with developmental and acquired disabilities, including cerebral palsy, spina bifida, traumatic brain injuries, and spinal cord injuries.

As in all areas of nursing practice, nurses practicing in the area of rehabilitation must be skilled and knowledgeable about care of patients with substance abuse. For all individuals with disability, including adolescents, the nurse must assess actual or potential substance abuse. Almost 15 million Americans use illicit drugs; approximately 58 million engage in binge or heavy drinking of alcohol; and about 30% of the population uses nicotine products. In Canada, 13.6% of all Canadians are considered high-risk drinkers (8.9% of women drinkers, 25.1% of men drinkers). The use of illicit drugs is generally limited to cannabis only. About 28.7% of Canadians report using only cannabis during their lifetime, and 11% used only cannabis during the past year. Although about 1 in 6 Canadians has used an illicit drug other than cannabis in their lifetime, few have used these drugs during the past year (Health Canada, 2004).

Parental alcoholism is one of the strongest predictors of substance abuse. Alcohol abuse rates for people with disability may be twice as high as the general population. Forty to eighty percent of spinal cord injuries are related to substance abuse, and 40% to 80% of all traumatic brain injured patients are intoxicated at the time of injury (U.S. Department of Health and Human Services, 2000).

Substance abuse is a critical issue in rehabilitation, especially for disabled individuals who are attempting to gain employment via vocational rehabilitation. Treatment for alcoholism and drug dependencies includes a thorough physical and psychosocial evaluation; detoxification; counselling; medical treatment; psychological assistance for the patient and family; treatment of any coexisting psychiatric illness; and referral to community resources for social, legal, spiritual, or vocational assistance. Length of treatment and the rehabilitation process depends on the individual's needs. Self-help groups are also encouraged, although attendance in such groups (eg, Alcoholics Anonymous, Narcotics Anonymous) poses various challenges for the person who has neurologic deficits, is confined to a wheelchair, or must adapt to encounters with able-bodied attendees who may not understand disability.

All specialty areas of rehabilitation require implementation of the nursing process as described in this chapter.

Assessment of Functional Abilities

Comprehensive assessment of functional capacity is the basis for developing a rehabilitation program. Functional capacity measures a person's ability to perform activities of ADLs and IADLs. ADLs include activities performed to meet basic needs, such as personal hygiene, dressing, toileting, eating, and moving. IADLs include activities that are necessary for independent living, such as the ability to shop for and prepare meals, use the telephone, clean, manage finances, and travel.

The nurse observes the patient performing specific activities (eg, eating, dressing) and notes the degree of independence; the time taken; the patient's mobility, coordination, and endurance; and the amount of assistance required. Good joint motion, muscle strength, cardiovascular reserve, and an intact neurologic system are also carefully assessed, because functional ability depends on these factors as well. Observations are recorded on a functional assessment tool. These tools provide a way to standardize assessment parameters and supply a scale or score against which improvements may be measured. They also clearly communicate the patient's level of functioning to all members of the rehabilitation team. Rehabilitation staff use these tools to provide an initial assessment of the patient's abilities and to monitor the patient's progress in independence.

One of the most frequently used tools to assess the patient's level of independence is the Functional Independence Measure (FIM). The FIM is a minimum data set, measuring 18 items. The self-care items measured are eating, bathing, grooming, dressing upper body, dressing lower body, toileting, bladder management, and bowel management. The FIM addresses transfers and the ability to ambulate and climb stairs and also includes communication and social cognition items. A WeeFIM instrument is used for children. For both children and adults, scoring is based on a seven-point scale with items used to assess the patient's level of independence.

Occupational therapists in Canada use the Canadian Occupational Performance Measure (COPM) as an individualized, client-centred measure to detect change in a client's self-perception of occupational performance over time (Law et al., 1998). There are many other assessment tools designed to evaluate function in persons with specific disabling conditions.

In addition to the detailed functional assessment, the nurse assesses the patient's physical, mental, emotional, spiritual, social, and economic status. Secondary problems related to the disability, such as muscle atrophy and deconditioning, are assessed, as are residual strengths unaffected by disease or disability. Other areas that require nursing assessment include potential for altered skin integrity, altered bowel and bladder control, and sexual dysfunction.

NURSING PROCESS: THE PATIENT WITH SELF-CARE DEFICITS IN ACTIVITIES OF DAILY LIVING

ADLs are those self-care activities that the patient must accomplish each day to meet personal needs. ADLs include personal hygiene/bathing, dressing/grooming, feeding, and toileting. Many patients are unable to perform such activities easily. An ADL program is started as soon as the rehabilitation process begins, because the ability to perform ADLs is frequently the key to independence, return to the home, and reentry into the community.

Assessment

The nurse must observe and assess the patient's ability to perform ADLs to determine the level of independence in self-care and the need for nursing intervention. The activity of bathing requires obtaining bath water and utensils, washing, and drying the body after bathing. Dressing requires getting clothes from the closet, putting on and taking off clothing, and fastening the clothing. Self-feeding requires using utensils to bring food to the mouth, and chewing and swallowing the food. The activity of toileting includes removing clothing to use the toilet, cleansing oneself, and readjusting clothing. Grooming activities include combing hair, brushing teeth, shaving or applying makeup, and washing the hands. Patients who can sit up and raise their hands to their head can begin self-care activities.

In addition, the nurse needs to be aware of the patient's medical conditions, the effect that they have on the ability to perform ADLs, and the family's involvement in the patient's ADLs. This information is valuable in setting goals and developing the plan of care to maximize self-care.

Nursing Diagnosis

Based on the assessment data, major nursing diagnoses for the patient may include the following:

- Self-care deficit: bathing/hygiene, dressing/grooming, feeding, toileting

Planning and Goals

The major goals of the patient include bathing/hygiene independently or with assistance, using adaptive devices as appropriate; dressing/grooming independently or with assistance, using adaptive devices as appropriate; feeding independently or with assistance, using adaptive devices as appropriate; and toileting independently or with assistance, using adaptive devices as appropriate. Another goal is that the patient with a self-care deficit expresses satisfaction with the extent of independence in self-care activities.

Nursing Interventions

FOSTERING SELF-CARE ABILITIES

To learn methods of self-care effectively, the patient must be motivated. An "I'd rather do it myself" attitude is encouraged. The nurse must also help the patient identify the safe limits of independent activity; knowing when to ask for assistance is particularly important.

The nurse teaches, guides, and supports the patient who is learning or relearning how to perform self-care activities. Consistency in instructions and assistance given by health care providers facilitates the learning process. Recording the patient's performance provides data for evaluating progress and may be used as a source for motivation and morale building (Chart 11-2).

Often, a simple manoeuvre requires concentration and the exertion of considerable effort on the part of the patient with a disability; therefore, self-care techniques need to be adapted to

> ### Chart 11-2 • PATIENT EDUCATION
> **Teaching About Activities of Daily Living**
>
> 1. Define the goal of the activity with the patient. Be realistic. Set short-term goals that can be accomplished in the near future.
> 2. Identify several approaches to accomplish the task (eg, there are several ways to put on a given garment).
> 3. Select the approach most likely to succeed.
> 4. Specify the approach on the patient's care plan and the patient's level of accomplishment on the progress notes.
> 5. Identify the motions necessary to accomplish the activity (eg, to pick up a glass, extend arm with hand open; place open hand next to glass; flex fingers around glass; move arm and hand holding glass vertically; flex arm toward body).
> 6. Focus on gross functional movements initially, and gradually include activities that use finer motions (eg, buttoning clothes, eating with a fork).
> 7. Encourage the patient to perform the activity up to maximal capacity within the limitations of the disability.
> 8. Monitor the patient's tolerance.
> 9. Minimize frustration and fatigue.
> 10. Support the patient by giving appropriate praise for effort put forth and for acts accomplished.
> 11. Assist the patient to perform and practice the activity in real-life situations.

accommodate the individual patient's lifestyle. There is usually more than one way to accomplish a self-care activity, so common sense and a little ingenuity may promote increased independence. For example, a person who cannot quite reach his or her head may be able to do so by leaning forward. Encouraging the patient to participate in a support group may also help the patient to discover inventive or creative solutions to self-care problems.

RECOMMENDING ASSISTIVE DEVICES

If the patient has difficulty in performing an ADL, an adaptive or assistive device (self-help device) may be useful. A large variety of assistive devices are available commercially or can be fabricated by the nurse, the occupational therapist, the patient, or the family. The nurse should be alert to "gadgets" coming on the market and evaluate their potential for usefulness. Of course, the nurse must exercise professional judgment and caution in recommending devices, because unscrupulous vendors have marketed unnecessary, overly expensive, or useless items to patients in the past.

A wide selection of computerized assistive devices is available, or devices can be designed to help individual patients with severe disabilities to function more independently. The Government of Canada Website (see Resources list) offers a computerized listing of commercially available aids and equipment for patients with disabilities.

HELPING THE PATIENT ACCEPT LIMITATIONS

If the patient has a severe disability, independent self-care may be an unrealistic goal; in this situation, the rehabilitation nurse teaches the patient how to direct his or her own care. The patient may require a personal attendant to perform ADLs. Family members may not be appropriate for providing bathing/hygiene, dressing/grooming, feeding, and toileting assistance, and a spouse may have difficulty providing bowel and bladder care for the patient and maintaining the role of sexual partner. If a personal caregiver is needed, the disabled person or family members must learn how

to manage an employee effectively. The nurse assists the patient in accepting self-care dependency. Independence in other areas, such as social interaction, should be emphasized to promote positive self-concept.

Evaluation

EXPECTED PATIENT OUTCOMES

Expected patient outcomes may include:

1. Demonstrates independent self-care in bathing/hygiene or with assistance, using adaptive devices as appropriate
   a. Bathes self at maximal level of independence
   b. Uses adaptive devices effectively
   c. Reports satisfaction with level of independence in bathing/hygiene
2. Demonstrates independent self-care in dressing/grooming or with assistance, using adaptive devices as appropriate
   a. Dresses/grooms self at maximal level of independence
   b. Uses adaptive devices effectively
   c. Reports satisfaction with level of independence in dressing/grooming
   d. Demonstrates increased interest in appearance
3. Demonstrates independent self-care in feeding or with assistance, using adaptive and assistive devices as appropriate
   a. Feeds self at maximal level of independence
   b. Uses adaptive and assistive devices effectively
   c. Demonstrates increased interest in eating
   d. Maintains adequate nutritional intake
4. Demonstrates independent self-care in toileting or with assistance, using adaptive and assistive devices as appropriate
   a. Toilets self at maximal level of independence
   b. Uses adaptive and assistive devices effectively
   c. Indicates positive feelings regarding level of toileting independence
   d. Experiences adequate frequency of bowel and bladder elimination
   e. Does not experience incontinence, constipation, urinary tract infection, or other complications

NURSING PROCESS: THE PATIENT WITH IMPAIRED PHYSICAL MOBILITY

Patients who are ill or injured are frequently placed on bed rest or have their activities limited. Problems commonly associated with immobility include weakened muscles, joint contracture, and deformity. Each joint of the body has a normal range of motion; if the range is limited, the functions of the joint and of the muscles that move the joint are impaired, and painful deformities may develop. Nurses must identify patients at risk for such complications.

Another problem frequently seen in rehabilitation nursing is an altered ambulatory/mobility pattern. The patient with a disability may be either temporarily or permanently unable to walk independently and unaided. The nurse assesses the mobility of the patient and designs care that promotes independent mobility within the prescribed therapeutic limits.

If a person is not able to exercise and move the joints through their full range of motion, contractures may develop. A contracture is a shortening of the muscle and tendon that leads to deformity and limits joint mobility. When the contracted joint is moved, the patient experiences pain; in addition, more energy is required to move when joints are contracted and deformed.

Assessment

At times, a patient's mobility is restricted because of pain, paralysis, loss of muscle strength, systemic disease, an immobilizing device (eg, cast, brace), or prescribed limits to promote healing. Assessment of the patient's mobility includes positioning, ability to move, muscle strength and tone, joint function, and the prescribed mobility limits. The nurse may need to collaborate with the physical therapist or other team members to assess mobility.

During position change, transfer, and ambulation activities, the nurse assesses the patient's abilities, the extent of disability, and residual capacity for physiologic adaptation. The nurse observes for orthostatic hypotension, pallor, diaphoresis, nausea, tachycardia, and fatigue.

If a patient is not able to ambulate without assistance, the nurse assesses ability to balance, transfer, and use assistive devices (eg, crutches, walker). Crutch walking requires a high energy expenditure and produces considerable cardiovascular stress, so older people with reduced exercise capacity, decreased arm strength, and problems with balance because of old age and multiple diseases may be unable to use them. A walker is more stable and may be a better choice for such patients. The nurse assesses the patient's ability to use various devices that promote mobility. If a patient uses an orthosis, an external appliance that provides support, prevents or corrects deformities, and improves function, the nurse monitors the patient for effective use and potential problems associated with its use.

Nursing Diagnosis

Based on the assessment data, major nursing diagnoses for the patient may include the following:

- Impaired physical mobility
- Activity intolerance
- Risk for injury
- Risk for disuse syndrome
- Impaired walking
- Impaired wheelchair mobility
- Impaired bed mobility

Planning and Goals

The major goals of the patient may include absence of contracture and deformity, maintenance of muscle strength and joint mobility, independent mobility, and increased activity tolerance.

Nursing Interventions

POSITIONING TO PREVENT MUSCULOSKELETAL COMPLICATIONS

Deformities and contractures can often be prevented by proper positioning. Maintaining correct body alignment when the patient is in bed is essential regardless of the position selected. During each contact with the patient, the nurse evaluates the patient's position and assists the patient to achieve proper positioning and alignment. The most common positions that a patient assumes in bed are supine (dorsal), side-lying (lateral), and prone. The nurse helps the patient assume these positions and supports the body in correct alignment with pillows (Chart 11-3). At times, a splint (eg, wrist or hand splint) may be fabricated by the occupa-

tional therapist to support a joint and prevent deformity. The nurse must ensure proper use of the splint and provide skin care.

Preventing External Rotation of the Hip

Patients who are in bed for any period of time may develop external rotation deformity of the hip because the ball-and-socket joint of the hip has a tendency to rotate outward when the patient lies on his or her back. A trochanter roll extending from the crest of the ilium to the midthigh prevents this deformity; with correct placement, it serves as a mechanical wedge under the projection of the greater trochanter.

Preventing Footdrop

Footdrop is a deformity in which the foot is plantar flexed (the ankle bends in the direction of the sole of the foot). If the condition continues without correction, the patient will not be able to hold the foot in a normal position and will be able to walk only on his or her toes, without touching the ground with the heel of the foot. The deformity is caused by contracture of both the gastrocnemius and soleus muscles. Damage to the peroneal nerve or loss of flexibility of the Achilles tendon may result in footdrop.

 NURSING ALERT Prolonged bed rest, lack of exercise, incorrect positioning in bed, and the weight of bedding that forces the toes into plantar flexion are factors that contribute to footdrop.

To prevent this disabling deformity, the patient is positioned to sit at 90 degrees in a wheelchair with feet on the footrests or flat on the floor. When the patient is supine in bed, padded splints or protective boots are used to keep the feet at right angles to the legs. Frequent skin inspection of the feet must also be performed to determine whether positioning devices have created any unwanted pressure areas.

The patient is encouraged to perform the following ankle exercises several times each hour: dorsiflexion and plantar flexion of the feet, flexion and extension (curl and stretch) of the toes, and eversion and inversion of the feet at the ankles. The nurse provides frequent passive range-of-motion exercises if the patient is unable to perform active exercises.

MAINTAINING MUSCLE STRENGTH AND JOINT MOBILITY

Optimal function depends on the strength of the muscles and joint motion, and active participation in ADLs promotes maintenance of muscle strength and joint mobility. Range-of-motion exercises and specific therapeutic exercises may be included in the nursing plan of care.

Performing Range-of-Motion Exercises

Range of motion is movement of a joint through its full range in all appropriate planes (Chart 11-4). To maintain or increase the motion of a joint, range-of-motion exercises are initiated as soon as the patient's condition permits. The exercises are planned for the individual to accommodate the wide variation in the degrees of motion that people of varying body builds and age groups can attain (Chart 11-5).

Range-of-motion exercises may be active (performed by the patient under supervision of the nurse), assisted (with the nurse helping if the patient is unable to do the exercise independently), or passive (performed by the nurse). Unless prescribed otherwise, a joint should be moved through its range of motion three times, at least twice a day. The joint to be exercised is supported, the

Chart 11-3   Positioning a Patient in Bed

Supine (Dorsal) Position
1. Align the head with the spine, both laterally and anteroposteriorly.
2. Position the trunk to minimize hip flexion.
3. Flex the arms at the elbow and rest the hands against the lateral abdomen.
4. Extend the legs with a small, firm support under the popliteal area.
5. Support the heels off the mattress with a small pillow or towel roll at the ankles.
6. Point the toes straight up using protective boots to prevent footdrop.
7. Place trochanter rolls under the greater trochanters to prevent external rotation of the hip.

Side-Lying (Lateral Position)
1. Align the head with the spine, and support it with a pillow.
2. Properly align the body; avoid twisting at the shoulders, waist, or hips.
3. Flex shoulders and elbows and support the upper arm with a pillow.
4. Position the uppermost hip joint slightly forward and support the leg in a position of slight abduction by a pillow.
5. Place and support the feet in neutral dorsiflexion.
6. Support the back with a pillow.

Prone (on Abdomen) Position
1. Turn the head laterally and align it with the rest of the body.
2. Abduct and externally rotate the arms at the shoulder joint; flex the elbows.
3. Place a small, flat support under the pelvis, extending from the level of the umbilicus to the upper third of the thigh.
4. Maintain the lower extremities in a neutral position.
5. Suspend the toes over the edge of the mattress.

Note: Side rails of bed are down for photographic purposes; they should remain raised if the patient is at risk for falling.

bones above the joint are stabilized, and the body part distal to the joint is moved through the range of motion of the joint. For example, the humerus must be stabilized while the radius and ulna are moved through their range of motion at the elbow joint.

The joint should not be moved beyond its free range of motion; the joint is moved to the point of resistance and stopped at the point of pain. If muscle spasms are present, the joint is moved slowly to the point of resistance. Gentle, steady pressure is then applied until the muscle relaxes, and the motion is continued to the joint's final point of resistance.

To perform assisted or passive range-of-motion exercises, the patient must be in a comfortable supine position with arms at the sides and knees extended. Good body posture is maintained during the exercises. The nurse also uses good body mechanics during the exercise session.

Range-of-Motion Terminology

Abduction: movement away from the midline of the body

Adduction: movement toward the midline of the body

Flexion: bending of a joint so that the angle of the joint diminishes

Extension: the return movement from flexion; the joint angle is increased

Rotation: turning or movement of a part around its axis

Internal: turning inward, toward the centre

External: turning outward, away from the centre

Dorsiflexion: movement that flexes or bends the hand back toward the body or the foot toward the leg

Palmar flexion: movement that flexes or bends the hand in the direction of the palm

Plantar flexion: movement that flexes or bends the foot in the direction of the sole

Pronation: rotation of the forearm so that the palm of the hand is down

Supination: rotation of the forearm so that the palm of the hand is up

Opposition: touching the thumb to each fingertip on same hand

Inversion: movement that turns the sole of the foot inward

Eversion: movement that turns the sole of the foot outward

Performing Therapeutic Exercises

Therapeutic exercises are prescribed by the physician and performed with the assistance and guidance of a physical therapist or nurse. Research is also underway to develop computerized robots with gentle, compliant behaviour that could be used in the home setting for upper-extremity exercises (Krebs, 2000).

The patient should have a clear understanding of the goal of the prescribed exercise. Written instructions about the frequency, duration, and number of repetitions, as well as simple line drawings of the exercise, help to ensure adherence to the exercise program.

Exercise, when performed correctly, assists in maintaining and building muscle strength, maintaining joint function, preventing deformity, stimulating circulation, developing endurance, and promoting relaxation. Exercise is also valuable in helping to restore motivation and the well-being of the patient. Weight-bearing exercises may slow the bone loss that occurs with disability. There are five types of exercise: passive, active-assistive, active, resistive, and isometric. The description, purpose, and action of each of these exercises are summarized in Table 11-1.

PROMOTING INDEPENDENT MOBILITY

When the patient's condition stabilizes and the physical condition permits, the patient is assisted to sit up on the side of the bed and then to stand. The patient's tolerance of this activity is assessed. Orthostatic (postural) hypotension may develop when the patient assumes a vertical position. Because of inadequate vasomotor reflexes, blood pools in the splanchnic (visceral) area and in the legs, resulting in inadequate cerebral circulation. If indicators of orthostatic hypotension (eg, drop in blood pressure, pallor, diaphoresis, nausea, tachycardia, dizziness) are present, the activity is stopped, and the patient is assisted to a supine position in bed.

Some disabilities, such as spinal cord injury, acute brain injury, and other conditions that require extended periods in the recumbent position, prevent patients from assuming an upright position at the bedside. Several strategies can be used to assist a patient to assume a 90-degree sitting position. First, a reclining wheelchair with elevating leg rests allows a slow and controlled progression from a supine position to a 90-degree sitting position. A tilt table, a board that can be tilted in 5- to 10-degree increments from a horizontal to a vertical position, may also be used. The tilt table promotes vasomotor adjustment to positional changes and helps the patient with limited standing balance and limited weight-bearing activities to avoid the decalcification of bones and low bone mass associated with disuse syndrome and lack of weight-bearing exercise.

Elastic compression stockings are used to prevent venous stasis. For some patients, a compression garment (leotard) or snug-fitting abdominal binder and elastic compression bandaging of the legs are needed to prevent venous stasis and ensuing orthostatic hypotension. When the patient is standing, the feet are protected with a pair of properly fitted shoes. Extended periods of standing are avoided because of venous pooling and pressure on the soles of the feet. The nurse monitors the patient's blood pressure and pulse and observes for signs of orthostatic hypotension and cerebral insufficiency (eg, the patient reports feeling faint and weak), which suggest intolerance of the upright position. If the patient does not tolerate the upright position, the nurse should recline the patient and elevate the patient's legs.

Assisting the Patient With Transfer

A transfer is movement of the patient from one place to another (eg, bed to chair, chair to commode, wheelchair to tub). As soon as the patient is permitted out of bed, transfer activities are started. The nurse assesses the patient's ability to participate actively in the transfer and determines in conjunction with an occupational therapist or physical therapist the required adaptive equipment to promote independence and safety. A lightweight wheelchair with brake extensions, removable and detachable arm rests, and leg rests minimizes structural obstacles during the transfer. Tub seats or benches make transfers in and out of tubs easier and safer. Raised, padded commode seats may also be warranted for patients who must avoid flexing the hips greater than 90 degrees when transferring to a toilet.

It is important that the patient maintain muscle strength and, if possible, perform push-up exercises to strengthen the arm and shoulder extensor muscles. The push-up exercise requires the patient to sit upright in bed; a book is placed under each of the patient's hands to provide a hard surface, and the patient is instructed to push down on the book, raising the body. The nurse should encourage the patient to raise and move the body in different directions by means of these push-up exercises.

The nurse or physical therapist teaches the patient how to transfer. There are several methods of transferring from the bed to the wheelchair when the patient is unable to stand, and the technique chosen should be appropriate for the patient, considering his or her abilities and disabilities. It is helpful for the nurse to demonstrate the technique. If the physical therapist is involved in teaching the patient to transfer, the nurse and the physical therapist must collaborate so that consistent instructions are given to the patient. During transfer, the nurse assists and coaches the patient. Figure 11-1 shows weight-bearing and non–weight-bearing transfer.

If the patient's muscles are not strong enough to overcome the resistance of body weight, a polished lightweight board (transfer board, sliding board) may be used to bridge the gap between the bed and the chair. The patient slides across on the board with or without assistance from a caregiver. This board may also be used to transfer the patient from the chair to the toilet or bathtub bench.

Chart 11-5   **Performing Range-of-Motion Exercises**

Abduction of shoulder. Move arm from side of body to above the head, then return arm to side of body or neutral position (adduction).

Forward flexion of shoulder. Move arm forward and upward until it is alongside of head.

Flexion of elbow. Bend elbow, bringing forearm and hand toward shoulder, then return forearm and hand to neutral position (arm straight).

Internal rotation of shoulder. With arm at shoulder height, elbow bent at a 90-degree angle, and palm toward feet, turn upper arm until palm and forearm point backward.

Pronation of forearm. With elbow at waist and bent at a 90-degree angle, turn hand so that palm is facing down.

Wrist extension.

External rotation of shoulder. With arm at shoulder height, elbow bent at a 90-degree angle, and palm toward feet, turn upper arm until the palm and forearm point forward.

Supination of forearm. With elbow at waist and arm bent at a 90-degree angle, turn hand so that palm is facing up.

Flexion of wrist. Bend wrist so that palm is toward forearm. Straighten to a neutral position.

Ulnar deviation. Move hand sideways so that the side of hand on which the little finger is located moves toward forearm.

Extension of fingers.

Internal-external rotation of hip. Turn leg in an inward motion so that toes point in. Turn leg in an outward motion so that toes point out.

(continued)

Chart 11-5 **Performing Range-of-Motion Exercises (Continued)**

Radial deviation. Move hand sideways so that side of hand on which thumb is located moves toward forearm.

To perform abduction-adduction of hip, move leg outward from the body as far as possible, as shown. Return leg from abducted position to neutral position and across the other leg as far as possible.

Hyperextension of hip. Place the patient in a prone position, and move leg backward from the body as far as possible.

Thumb opposition. Move thumb out and around to touch little finger.

Flexion of the hip and the knee. Bend hip by moving the leg forward as far as possible. Return leg from the flexed position to the neutral position.

Dorsiflexion of foot. Move foot up and toward the leg. Then move the foot down and away from the leg (plantar flexion).

Inversion and eversion of foot. Move foot so that sole is facing outward (eversion). Then move foot so that sole is facing inward (inversion).

Flexion of toes. Bend the toes toward the ball of foot.

Extension of toes. Straighten toes and pull them toward the leg as far as possible.

The nurse should make sure that the patient's fingers do not curl around the edge of the board during the transfer, because the weight of the patient's body can crush them as the patient moves across the board. Safety is a primary concern during a transfer:

- Wheelchairs and beds must be locked before the patient transfers.
- Detachable arm and foot rests are removed to make getting in and out of the chair easier.
- One end of the transfer board is placed under the patient's buttocks and the other end on the surface to which the transfer is being made (eg, the chair).

- The patient is instructed to lean forward, push up with his or her hands, and then slide across the board to the other surface.

The nurse frequently assists weak and incapacitated patients out of bed. The nurse supports and gently assists the patient during position changes, protecting the patient from injury. The nurse avoids pulling on the weak or paralyzed upper extremity, to prevent dislocation of the shoulder. The patient is assisted to move toward the stronger side (Chart 11-6).

In the home setting, getting in and out of bed and performing chair, toilet, and tub transfers are difficult for patients with weak musculature and loss of hip, knee, and ankle motion. A

Table 11-1 • **Therapeutic Exercises**

	DESCRIPTION	PURPOSES	ACTION
Passive	An exercise carried out by the therapist or the nurse without assistance from the patient	To retain as much joint range of motion as possible; to maintain circulation	Stabilize the proximal joint and support the distal part; move the joint smoothly, slowly, and gently through its full range of motion; avoid producing pain.
Active-assistive	An exercise carried out by the patient with the assistance of the therapist or the nurse	To encourage normal muscle function	Support the distal part, and encourage the patient to take the joint actively through its range of motion; give no more assistance than is necessary to accomplish the action; short periods of activity should be followed by adequate rest periods.
Active	An exercise accomplished by the patient without assistance; activities include turning from side to side and from back to abdomen and moving up and down in bed	To increase muscle strength	When possible, active exercise should be performed against gravity; the joint is moved through full range of motion without assistance; make sure that the patient does not substitute another joint movement for the one intended.
Resistive	An active exercise carried out by the patient working against resistance produced by either manual or mechanical means	To provide resistance to increase muscle power	The patient moves the joint through its range of motion while the therapist resists slightly at first and then with progressively increasing resistance; sandbags and weights can be used and are applied at the distal point of the involved joint; the movements should be performed smoothly.
Isometric or muscle setting	Alternately contracting and relaxing a muscle while keeping the part in a fixed position; this exercise is performed by the patient	To maintain strength when a joint is immobilized	Contract or tighten the muscle as much as possible without moving the joint, hold for several seconds, then let go and relax; breathe deeply.

rope attached to the headboard of the bed enables the patient to pull toward the centre of the bed, and the use of a rope attached to the footboard facilitates getting in and out of bed. The height of a chair can be raised with cushions on the seat or with hollowed-out blocks placed under the chair legs. Grab bars can be attached to the wall near the toilet and tub to provide leverage and stability.

Preparing for Ambulation

Regaining the ability to walk is a prime morale builder. However, to be prepared for ambulation—whether with brace, walker, cane, or crutches—the patient must strengthen the muscles required. Exercise, therefore, is the foundation of preparation. The nurse and physical therapist instruct and supervise the patient in these exercises.

For ambulation, the quadriceps muscles, which stabilize the knee joint, and the gluteal muscles are strengthened. To perform quadriceps-setting exercises, the patient contracts the quadriceps muscle by attempting to push the popliteal area against the mattress and at the same time raising the heel. The patient maintains the muscle contraction until a count of five and relaxes for a count of five. The exercise is repeated 10 to 15 times hourly. Exercising the quadriceps muscles prevents flexion contractures of the knee.

In gluteal setting, the patient contracts or "pinches" the buttocks together to the count of five, relaxes for the count of five, and repeats 10 to 15 times hourly. If ambulatory aids (ie, walker, cane, crutches) are to be used, the muscles of the upper extremities are exercised and strengthened. Push-up exercises are useful. While in a sitting position, the patient raises the body by pushing the hands against the chair seat or mattress. The patient should be encouraged to do push-up exercises while in a prone position also. Pull-up exercises done on a trapeze while lifting the body are also effective

for conditioning. The patient is taught to raise the arms above the head and then lower them in a slow, rhythmic manner while holding weights. Gradually, the weight is increased. The hands are strengthened by squeezing a rubber ball.

Typically, the physical therapist designs exercises to help the patient develop the sitting and standing balance, stability, and coordination needed for ambulation. After sitting and standing balance are achieved, the patient uses parallel bars. Under the supervision of the physical therapist, the patient practices shifting weight from side to side, lifting one leg while supporting weight on the other, and then walking between the parallel bars.

A patient who is ready to begin ambulation must be fitted with the appropriate ambulatory aid, instructed about the prescribed weight-bearing limits (eg, non–weight-bearing, partial weight-bearing ambulation), and taught how to use the aid safely. The nurse continually assesses the patient for stability and adherence to weight-bearing precautions and protects the patient from falling. The nurse provides contact guarding by holding on to a gait belt that the patient wears around the waist. The patient should wear sturdy, well-fitting shoes and be advised of the dangers of wet or highly polished floors and throw rugs. The patient should also learn how to ambulate on inclines, uneven surfaces, and stairs.

Ambulating With Crutches

Patients who are prescribed partial weight-bearing or non–weight-bearing ambulation may use crutches. The nurse or physical therapist should determine whether crutches are appropriate for the patient, because good balance, adequate cardiovascular reserve, strong upper extremities, and erect posture are essential for crutch walking. Ambulating a functional distance (at least the length of a room or house) or manoeuvreing stairs on crutches requires signif-

FIGURE 11-1 Methods of patient transfer from the bed to a wheelchair. The wheelchair is in a locked position. Coloured areas indicate non–weight-bearing body parts. (**A**) Weight-bearing transfer from bed to chair. The patient stands up, pivots until his back is opposite the new seat, and sits down. (**B**) (*Left*) Non–weight-bearing transfer from chair to bed. (*Right*) With legs braced. (**C**) (*Left*) Non–weight-bearing transfer, combined method. (*Right*) Non–weight-bearing transfer, pull-up method.

icant arm strength, because the arms must bear the patient's weight. Muscle groups important for crutch walking include the following:

- Shoulder depressors—to stabilize the upper extremity and prevent shoulder hiking
- Shoulder adductors—to hold the crutch top against the chest wall
- Arm flexors, extensors, and abductors (at the shoulder)—to move crutches forward, backward, and sideways
- Forearm extensors—to prevent flexion or buckling; important in raising the body for swinging gait
- Wrist extensors—to enable weight bearing on hand pieces
- Finger and thumb flexors—to grasp the hand piece

Chart 11-6   Assisting the Patient Out of Bed

Technique for Moving the Patient to the Edge of the Bed
1. Move head and shoulders of patient toward the edge of the bed.
2. Move feet and legs to the edge of the bed. (The patient is now in a crescent position, which gives good range of motion to the lateral trunk muscles.)
3. Place both arms well under the patient's hips. Next, tighten (set) the muscles of your back and abdomen.
4. Straighten your back while moving the patient toward you.

Technique for Sitting Patient on the Edge of the Bed
1. Place arm and hand under the patient's shoulders.
2. Instruct the patient to push into the bed with the elbow while you lift the patient's shoulders with one arm and swing the legs over the edge of the bed with the other. (Gravity pulls the legs downward, which aids in raising the patient's trunk.)

Technique for Assisting Patient to Stand
1. Position the patient's feet so that they will be well grounded.
2. Face the patient while firmly grasping each side of the patient's rib cage with your hands.
3. Push your knee against one knee of the patient.
4. Rock the patient forward to a standing position. (Your knee is pushed against the patient's knee as he or she comes to the standing position.)
5. Ensure that the patient's knees are "locked" (in full extension) while standing. (Locking the patient's knees is a safety measure for those who are weak or have been in bed for some time.)
6. Give the patient enough time to establish balance.
7. Pivot the patient into a sitting position in the chair.

Preparing the Patient to Walk With Crutches

Preparatory exercises are prescribed to strengthen the shoulder girdle and upper extremity muscles. Meanwhile, crutches need to be adjusted to the patient before the patient begins ambulating. To determine the approximate crutch length, the patient may be measured standing or lying down. A standing patient is positioned against the wall with the feet slightly apart and away from the wall. Then a distance of 5 cm (2 inches) is marked on the floor, out to the side from the tip of the toe; 15 cm (6 inches) is measured straight ahead from the first mark, and this point is marked on the floor. Next, 5 cm (2 inches) is measured below the axilla to the second mark for the approximate crutch length.

If the patient has to be measured while lying down, he or she is measured from the anterior fold of the axilla to the sole of the foot, and then 5 cm (2 inches) is added. If the patient's height is used, 40 cm (16 inches) is subtracted to obtain the approximate crutch length. The hand piece should be adjusted to allow 20 to 30 degrees of flexion at the elbow. The wrist should be extended and the hand dorsiflexed. A foam rubber pad on the underarm piece is used to relieve pressure of the crutch on the upper arm and thoracic cage. For safety, crutches should have large rubber tips, and the patient should wear firm-soled shoes that fit well.

Teaching Crutch Walking

The nurse or physical therapist explains and demonstrates to the patient how to use the crutches. The patient learns standing balance by standing on the unaffected leg by a chair. To help the patient maintain balance, the nurse holds the patient near the waist or uses a transfer belt.

The patient is taught to support his or her weight on the hand pieces. (For patients who are unable to support their weight through the wrist and hand because of arthritis or fracture, platform crutches that support the forearm and allow the weight to be borne through the elbow are available.) If weight is borne on the axilla, the pressure of the crutch can damage the brachial plexus nerves, producing "crutch paralysis."

For maximum stability, the patient first assumes the tripod position by placing the crutches about 20 to 25 cm (8 to 10 inches) in front and to the side of his or her toes (Fig. 11-2). (This base of support is adjusted according to the height of the patient; a tall person requires a broader base of support than does a short person). In this position, the patient learns how to shift weight and maintain balance.

Before teaching crutch walking, the nurse or therapist determines which gait will be best for the patient. The selection of the crutch gait depends on the type and severity of the disability and on the patient's physical condition, arm and trunk strength, and body balance. The patient should be taught two gaits so that he or she can change from one to another. Shifting crutch gaits relieves fatigue, because each gait requires the use of a different combination of muscles (if a muscle is forced to contract steadily without relaxing, the circulation of the blood to that part is decreased). A faster gait can be used when walking an uninterrupted distance, and a slower gait can be used for short distances or in crowded places. The more common gaits are the four-point, the three-point, the two-point, and the swinging-to and swinging-through gaits. The sequence of movements for each of these gaits is depicted in Chart 11-7.

The nurse walks with the patient who is just learning how to ambulate with crutches, holding him or her at the waist as needed for balance. During this time, the nurse protects the patient from falls and continually assesses the patient's stability and stamina, since prolonged periods of bed rest and inactivity affect a patient's

FIGURE 11-2   Crutch walking. The tripod position for basic crutch stance.

strength and endurance. Sweating and shortness of breath are indications that crutch-walking practice should be stopped and the patient permitted to rest.

Teaching Manoeuvreing Techniques

Before a patient is considered to be independent in crutch walking, he or she needs to learn to sit in a chair, stand from sitting, and go up and down stairs.

To sit down:
1. Grasp the crutches at the hand pieces for control.
2. Bend forward slightly while assuming a sitting position.
3. Place the affected leg forward to prevent weight-bearing and flexion.

To stand up:
1. Move forward to the edge of the chair with the strong leg slightly under the seat.
2. Place both crutches in the hand on the side of the affected extremity.
3. Push down on the hand piece while raising the body to a standing position.

To go down stairs:
1. Walk forward as far as possible on the step.
2. Advance crutches to the lower step. The weaker leg is advanced first and then the stronger one. In this way, the stronger extremity shares with the arms the work of raising and lowering the body weight.

To go up stairs:
1. Advance the stronger leg first up to the next step.
2. Advance the crutches and the weaker extremity. Note that the strong leg goes up first and comes down last. A memory device for the patients is, "Up with the good, down with the bad."

Chart 11-7   Crutch Gaits

Shaded areas are weight-bearing. Arrow indicates advance of foot or crutch. (Read chart from bottom, starting with beginning stance.)

4 POINT GAIT	2 POINT GAIT	3 POINT GAIT	SWING TO	SWING THROUGH
• Partial weight bearing both feet • Maximal support provided • Requires constant shift of weight	• Partial weight bearing both feet • Provides less support • Faster than a 4 point gait	• Non-weight bearing • Requires good balance • Requires arm strength • Faster gait • Can use with walker	• Weight bearing both feet • Provides stability • Requires arm strength • Can use with walker	• Weight bearing • Requires arm strength • Requires coordination/balance • Most advanced gait
4. Advance right foot	4. Advance right foot and left crutch	4. Advance right foot	4. Lift both feet/swing forward/land feet next to crutches	4. Lift both feet/swing forward/land feet in front of crutches
3. Advance left crutch	3. Advance left foot and right crutch	3. Advance left foot and both crutches	3. Advance both crutches	3. Advance both crutches
2. Advance left foot	2. Advance right foot and left crutch	2. Advance right foot	2. Lift both feet/swing forward/land feet next to crutches	2. Lift both feet/swing forward/land feet in front of crutches
1. Advance right crutch	1. Advance left foot and right crutch	1. Advance left foot and both crutches	1. Advance both crutches	1. Advance both crutches
Beginning stance	Beginning stance	Beginning stance	Beginning stance	Beginning stance

AMBULATING WITH A WALKER

A walker provides more support and stability than a cane or crutches. There are two types of walkers: pick-up walkers and rolling walkers. A pick-up walker (one that has to be picked up and moved with each step forward) does not permit a natural walking pattern and is useful for patients who have poor balance or limited cardiovascular reserve or who cannot use crutches. A rolling walker allows automatic walking and is used by patients who cannot lift or who inappropriately carry a pick-up walker. The height of the walker is adjusted to the patient. The patient's arms resting on the walker hand grips should exhibit 20 to 30 degrees of flexion at the elbows. The patient should wear sturdy, well-fitting shoes. The nurse walks with the patient, holds him or her at the waist as needed for balance, continually assesses the patient's stability, and protects the patient from falls.

The patient is instructed to ambulate with a pick-up walker as follows:

1. Push off a chair or bed to come to a standing position. Never pull yourself up using the walker.
2. Hold the walker on the hand grips for stability.
3. Lift the walker, placing it in front of you while leaning your body slightly forward.
4. Walk into the walker, supporting your body weight on your hands when advancing your weaker leg, permitting partial weight bearing or non–weight bearing as prescribed.
5. Balance yourself on your feet.
6. Lift the walker, and place it in front of you again. Continue this pattern of walking.
7. Remember to look up as you walk.

USING A CANE

A cane helps the patient walk with greater balance and support and relieves the pressure on weight-bearing joints by redistributing weight. Quad canes (four-footed canes) provide more stability than straight canes. To fit the patient for a cane, the patient is instructed to flex the elbow at a 30-degree angle, hold the handle of the cane about level with the greater trochanter, and place the tip of the cane 15 cm (6 inches) lateral to the base of the fifth toe. Adjustable canes make individualization easy. The cane should be fitted with a gently flaring tip that has flexible, concentric rings; the tip with its concentric rings provides optimal stability, functions as a shock absorber, and enables the patient to walk with greater speed and less fatigue.

The cane is held in the hand opposite the affected extremity. In normal walking, the opposite leg and arm move together (reciprocal motion); this motion is to be carried through in walking with a cane. The patient is taught to ambulate with a cane as follows:

Cane–foot sequence:
1. Hold the cane in the hand opposite the affected extremity to widen the base of support and to reduce the stress on the involved extremity. If the patient for some reason is unable to use the cane in the opposite hand, the cane may be used on the same side.
2. Advance the cane at the same time the affected leg is moved forward.
3. Keep the cane fairly close to the body to prevent leaning.
4. Bear down on the cane when the unaffected extremity begins the swing phase.

To go up and down stairs using the cane:
1. Step up on the unaffected extremity.
2. Place the cane and affected extremity up on the step.
3. Reverse this procedure for descending steps ("up with the good, down with the bad").

As for all patients beginning ambulation with an ambulatory aid, the nurse continually assesses the patient's stability and protects the patient from falls. The nurse accompanies the patient, holding him or her at the waist as needed for balance. The patient is assessed for tolerance of walking, and rest periods are provided as needed.

ASSISTING THE PATIENT WHO USES AN ORTHOSIS OR PROSTHESIS

Orthoses and prostheses are designed to facilitate mobilization and to maximize the patient's quality of life. An orthosis is an external appliance that provides support, prevents or corrects deformities, and improves function. Orthoses include braces, splints, collars, corsets, or supports that are designed and fitted by an orthotist or prosthetist. Static orthoses (no moving parts) are used to stabilize joints and prevent contractures. Dynamic orthoses are flexible and are used to improve function by assisting weak muscles. A prosthesis is an artificial body part; it may be internal, such as an artificial knee or hip joint, or external, such as an artificial leg or arm.

In addition to learning how to apply and remove the orthosis and manoeuvre the affected body part correctly, rehabilitation patients must learn how to properly care for the skin that comes in contact with the appliance. Skin problems or **pressure ulcers** may develop if the device is applied too tightly or too loosely, or if it is adjusted improperly. The nurse instructs the patient to clean and inspect the skin daily, to make sure the brace fits snugly without being too tight, to check that the padding distributes pressure evenly, and to wear a cotton garment without seams between the orthosis and the skin.

If the patient has had an amputation, the nurse promotes tissue healing, uses compression dressings to promote residual limb shaping, and minimizes contracture formation. A permanent prosthetic limb cannot be fitted until the tissue has healed completely and the residual limb shape is stable and free of edema. The nurse also helps the patient cope with the emotional issues surrounding loss of a limb and encourages acceptance of the prosthesis. The prosthetist, the nurse, and the physician collaborate to provide instructions related to skin care and care of the prosthesis.

Evaluation

EXPECTED PATIENT OUTCOMES
Expected patient outcomes may include:

1. Demonstrates improved physical mobility
   a. Maintains muscle strength and joint mobility
   b. Does not develop contractures
   c. Participates in exercise program
2. Transfers safely
   a. Demonstrates assisted transfers
   b. Performs independent transfers
3. Ambulates with maximum independence
   a. Uses ambulatory aid safely
   b. Adheres to weight-bearing prescription
   c. Requests assistance as needed
4. Demonstrates increased activity tolerance
   a. Does not experience episodes of orthostatic hypotension
   b. Reports absence of fatigue with ambulatory efforts
   c. Gradually increases distance and speed of ambulation

NURSING PROCESS: THE PATIENT WITH IMPAIRED SKIN INTEGRITY

An estimated 1.5 to 3 million patients develop pressure ulcers annually (Mayo Clinic Rochester, 2001). Both prevention and treatment of pressure ulcers are costly in terms of health care dollars and quality of life for patients at risk. Because the cost in terms of pain and suffering for a person with a pressure ulcer cannot be quantified, all possible efforts should be made to prevent skin breakdown.

Patients confined to bed for long periods, patients with motor or sensory dysfunction, and patients who experience muscular atrophy and reduction of padding between the overlying skin and the underlying bone are prone to pressure ulcers. Pressure ulcers are localized areas of infarcted soft tissue that occur when pressure applied to the skin over time is greater than normal capillary closure pressure, which is about 32 mm Hg. Critically ill patients have a lower capillary closure pressure and are at greater risk for pressure ulcers. The initial sign of pressure is erythema (redness of the skin) caused by reactive hyperemia, which normally resolves in less than 1 hour. Unrelieved pressure results in tissue ischemia or anoxia. The cutaneous tissues become broken or destroyed, leading to progressive destruction and necrosis of underlying soft tissue, and the resulting pressure ulcer is painful and slow to heal.

Assessment

Immobility, impaired sensory perception or cognition, decreased tissue perfusion, decreased nutritional status, friction and shear forces, increased moisture, and age-related skin changes all contribute to the development of pressure ulcers.

IMMOBILITY

When a person is immobile and inactive, pressure is exerted on the skin and subcutaneous tissue by objects on which the person rests, such as a mattress, chair seat, or cast. The development of pressure ulcers is directly related to the duration of immobility: if pressure continues long enough, small vessel thrombosis and tissue necrosis occur, and a pressure ulcer results. Weight-bearing bony prominences are most susceptible to pressure ulcer development because they are covered only by skin and small amounts of subcutaneous tissue. Susceptible areas include the sacrum and coccygeal areas, ischial tuberosities (especially in people who sit for prolonged periods), greater trochanter, heel, knee, malleolus, medial condyle of the tibia, fibular head, scapula, and elbow (Fig. 11-3).

IMPAIRED SENSORY PERCEPTION OR COGNITION

Patients with sensory loss, impaired level of consciousness, or paralysis may not be aware of the discomfort associated with prolonged pressure on the skin and, therefore, may not change their position themselves to relieve the pressure. This prolonged pressure impedes blood flow, reducing nourishment of the skin and underlying tissues. A pressure ulcer may develop in a short period.

DECREASED TISSUE PERFUSION

Any condition that reduces the circulation and nourishment of the skin and subcutaneous tissue (altered peripheral tissue perfusion) increases the risk of pressure ulcer development. Patients with diabetes mellitus experience an alteration in microcirculation. Similarly, patients with edema have impaired circulation and poor nourishment of the skin tissue. Obese patients have

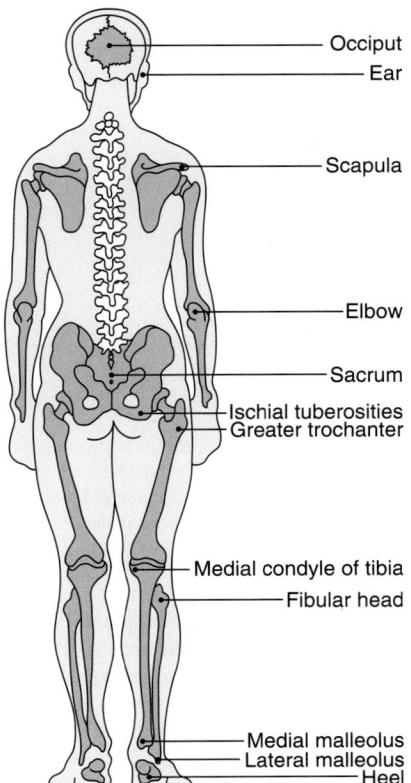

FIGURE 11-3 Areas susceptible to pressure ulcers.

large amounts of poorly vascularized adipose tissue, which is susceptible to breakdown.

ALTERED NUTRITIONAL STATUS

Nutritional deficiencies, anemias, and metabolic disorders also contribute to pressure ulcer development. Anemia, regardless of its cause, decreases the blood's oxygen-carrying ability and predisposes a patient to pressure ulcer formation. Patients who have low protein levels or who are in a negative nitrogen balance experience tissue wasting and inhibited tissue repair. Serum albumin is a sensitive indicator of protein deficiency; serum albumin levels of less than 35 g/L are associated with hypoalbuminemic tissue edema and increased risk of pressure ulcers. Specific nutrients, such as vitamin C and trace minerals, are needed for tissue maintenance and repair.

FRICTION AND SHEAR

Mechanical forces also contribute to the development of pressure ulcers. Friction is the resistance to movement that occurs when two surfaces are moved across each other. Shear is created by the interplay of gravitational forces (forces that push the body down) and friction. When shear occurs, tissue layers slide over one another, blood vessels stretch and twist, and the microcirculation of the skin and subcutaneous tissue is disrupted. Evidence of deep tissue damage may be slow to develop and may present through the development of a draining tract. The sacrum and heels are most susceptible to the effects of shear. Pressure ulcers from friction and shear occur when the patient slides down in bed (Fig. 11-4) or when the patient is moved or positioned improperly (eg, dragged up in bed). Spastic muscles and paralysis increase the patient's vulnerability to pressure ulcers related to friction and shear.

FIGURE 11-4 Mechanical forces contribute to pressure ulcer development. As the person slides down or is improperly pulled up in bed, *friction* resists this movement. *Shear* occurs when one layer of tissue slides over another, disrupting microcirculation of skin and subcutaneous tissue.

INCREASED MOISTURE

Prolonged contact with moisture from perspiration, urine, feces, or drainage produces maceration (softening) of the skin. The skin reacts to the caustic substances in the excreta or drainage and becomes irritated. Moist, irritated skin is more vulnerable to pressure breakdown. Once the skin breaks, the area is invaded by microorganisms (eg, streptococci, staphylococci, *Pseudomonas aeruginosa, Escherichia coli*), and infection occurs. Foul-smelling infectious drainage is present. The lesion may enlarge and allow a continuous loss of serum, which may further deplete the body of essential protein needed for tissue repair and maintenance. The lesion may continue to enlarge and extend deep into the fascia, muscle, and bone, with multiple sinus tracts radiating from the pressure ulcer. With extensive pressure ulcers, systemic infections may develop, frequently from gram-negative organisms.

Gerontologic Considerations

In older adults, the skin has diminished epidermal thickness, dermal collagen, and tissue elasticity. The skin is drier as a result of diminished sebaceous and sweat gland activity. Cardiovascular changes result in decreased tissue perfusion. Muscles atrophy, and bone structures become prominent. Diminished sensory perception and reduced ability to reposition oneself contribute to prolonged pressure on the skin. Therefore, the older adult is more susceptible to pressure ulcers, which cause pain and suffering and reduce quality of life (Agency for Health Care Policy and Research [AHCPR], 1994).

ADDITIONAL RISK FACTORS

In assessing the patient for potential risk for pressure ulcer development, the nurse assesses the patient's mobility, sensory perception, cognitive abilities, tissue perfusion, nutritional status, friction and shear forces, sources of moisture on the skin, and age. The nurse

- Assesses total skin condition at least twice a day
- Inspects each pressure site for erythema
- Assesses areas of erythema for blanching response
- Palpates the skin for increased warmth
- Inspects for dry skin, moist skin, breaks in skin
- Notes drainage and odour
- Evaluates level of mobility
- Notes restrictive devices (eg, restraints, splints)
- Evaluates circulatory status (eg, peripheral pulses, edema)

- Assesses neurovascular status
- Determines presence of incontinence
- Evaluates nutritional and hydration status
- Reviews the patient's record for laboratory studies, including hematocrit, hemoglobin, electrolytes, albumin, transferrin, and creatinine
- Notes present health problems
- Reviews current medications

Scales such as the Braden or Norton scale may be used to facilitate systematic assessment and quantification of a patient's risk for pressure ulcer, although the nurse needs to recognize that the reliability of these scales is not well established. They tend to overestimate those at risk and may promote unwarranted use of costly preventive equipment. See Chart 11-8 for a list of risk factors for development of pressure ulcers.

If a pressure area is noted, the nurse notes its size and location and may use a grading system to describe its severity (see Chart 11-9). Generally, a stage I pressure ulcer is an area of nonblanchable erythema, tissue swelling, and congestion, and the patient complains of discomfort. The skin temperature is elevated because of the increased vasodilation. The redness progresses to a dusky, cyanotic blue-grey appearance, which is the result of skin capillary occlusion and subcutaneous weakening.

A stage II pressure ulcer exhibits a break in the skin through the epidermis or the dermis. An abrasion, blister, or shallow crater may be seen. Necrosis occurs along with venous sludging and thrombosis and edema with cellular extravasation and infiltration.

A stage III pressure ulcer extends into the subcutaneous tissues. Clinically, a deep crater with or without undermining of adjacent tissues is noted.

A stage IV pressure ulcer extends into the underlying structures, including the muscle and, possibly, the bone. The skin lesion may appear insignificant when in reality, beneath the small surface ulcer is a large undermined area of necrotic tissue.

The appearance of purulent drainage or foul odour suggests an infection. With an extensive pressure ulcer, deep pockets of infection are often present. Drying and crusting of exudate may be present. Infection of a pressure ulcer may advance to osteomyelitis, pyarthrosis (pus formation within a joint cavity), sepsis, and septic shock.

Nursing Diagnosis

Based on the assessment data, the nursing diagnoses may include the following:

- Risk for impaired skin integrity
- Impaired skin integrity (related to immobility, decreased sensory perception, decreased tissue perfusion, decreased

Chart 11-8

Risk Factors for Developing Pressure Ulcers

Prolonged pressure on tissue
Immobility, compromised mobility
Loss of protective reflexes, sensory deficit/loss
Poor skin perfusion, edema
Malnutrition, hypoproteinemia, anemia, vitamin deficiency
Friction, shearing forces, trauma
Incontinence of urine or feces
Altered skin moisture: excessively dry, excessively moist
Advanced age, debilitation
Equipment: casts, traction, restraints

...

Chart 11-9 • ASSESSMENT

Assessing Pressure Ulcer Stages

Stage I
- Area of erythema
- Erythema does not blanch with pressure
- Skin temperature elevated
- Tissue swollen and congested
- Patient complains of discomfort
- Erythema progresses to dusky blue-grey

Stage II
- Skin breaks
- Abrasion, blister, or shallow crater
- Edema persists
- Ulcer drains
- Infection may develop

Stage III
- Ulcer extends into subcutaneous tissue
- Necrosis and drainage continue
- Infection develops

Stage IV
- Ulcer extends to underlying muscle and bone
- Deep pockets of infection develop
- Necrosis and drainage continue

From Weber, J. W., & Kelley, J. (2002). *Health assessment in nursing* (2nd ed.). Philadelphia: Lippincott Williams & Wilkins. Maklebust and Sieggreen (2001) list two additional stages of pressure ulcers and these are referenced in some Canadian wound care guidelines. **Stage V:** Closed pressure ulcer lined with chronic fibrosis and extending down into the structures. Presents as intact skin with a small open sinus tract. Feels boggy to the touch. **Stage X** or **N** (unstageable): True depth of a pressure ulcer, where the wound bed is partially or completely covered with necrotic tissue, cannot be determined; therefore, the wound cannot be staged.

---

nutritional status, friction and shear forces, increased moisture, or advanced age)

Planning and Goals

The major goals for the patient may include relief of pressure, improved mobility, improved sensory perception, improved tissue perfusion, improved nutritional status, minimized friction and

shear forces, dry surfaces in contact with skin, and healing of pressure ulcer, if present.

Nursing Interventions

RELIEVING PRESSURE

Frequent changes of position are needed to relieve and redistribute the pressure on the patient's skin and to prevent prolonged reduced blood flow to the skin and subcutaneous tissues. This can be accomplished by teaching the patient to change position or by turning and repositioning the patient. The patient's family members should be taught how to position and turn the patient at home to prevent pressure ulcers. Shifting weight allows the blood to flow into the ischemic areas and helps the tissues recover from the effects of pressure. Thus, the patient should be cared for as follows:

- Turned and repositioned at 1-hour to 2-hour intervals
- Encouraged to shift weight actively every 15 minutes

POSITIONING THE PATIENT

The patient should be positioned laterally, prone, and dorsally in sequence unless a position is not tolerated or is contraindicated. The recumbent position is preferred to the semi-Fowler's position because of increased supporting body surface area in this position. In addition to regular turning, there should be small shifts of body weight, such as repositioning of an ankle, elbow, or shoulder. The skin is inspected at each position change and assessed for temperature elevation. If redness or heat is noted or if the patient complains of discomfort, pressure on the area must be relieved.

Another way to relieve pressure over bony prominences is the bridging technique, accomplished through the correct positioning of pillows. Just as a bridge is supported on pillars to allow traffic to move underneath, so can the body be supported by pillows to allow for space between bony prominences and the mattress. A pillow or commercial heel protector may be used to support the heels off the bed when the patient is supine. Placing pillows superior and inferior to the sacrum relieves sacral pressure. Supporting the patient in a 30-degree side-lying position avoids pressure on the trochanter. In the aging patient, frequent small shifts of body weight may be effective. Placing a small rolled towel or sheepskin under a shoulder or hip will allow a return of blood flow to the skin in the area on which the patient is sitting or lying. The towel or sheepskin is moved around the patient's pressure points in a clockwise fashion.

USING PRESSURE-RELIEVING DEVICES

At times, special equipment and beds may be needed to help relieve the pressure on the skin. These are designed to provide support for specific body areas or to distribute pressure evenly.

Patients sitting in wheelchairs for prolonged periods should have wheelchair cushions fitted and adjusted on an individualized basis, using pressure measurement techniques as a guide to selection and fitting. The aim is to redistribute pressure away from areas at risk for ulcers, but no cushion is able to eliminate excessive pressure completely. The patient should be reminded to shift weight frequently and to rise for a few seconds every 15 minutes while sitting in a chair (Fig. 11-5).

Static support devices (such as high-density foam, air, or liquid mattress overlays) distribute pressure evenly by bringing more of the patient's body surface into contact with the supporting surface. Gel-type flotation pads and air-fluidized beds reduce pressure. The weight of a body floating on a fluid system is evenly distributed over the entire supporting surface (according to Pascal's law). Therefore, as the patient's body sinks into the fluid, additional surface becomes available for weight bearing, body weight per unit area is decreased, and there is less pressure on the body parts.

Soft, moisture-absorbing padding is also useful because the softness and resilience of padding provides for more even distribution of pressure and the dissipation and absorption of moisture, along with freedom from wrinkles and friction. Bony prominences may be protected by gel pads, sheepskin padding, or soft foam rubber beneath the sacrum, the trochanters, heels, elbows, scapulae, and back of the head when there is pressure on the sites.

FIGURE 11-5 Wheelchair push-up to prevent ischial pressure ulcers. These push-ups should become an automatic routine (every 15 minutes) for the person with paraplegia. The person should stay up, out of contact with the seat for several seconds. The wheels are kept in the locked position during the exercise.

Specialized beds have been designed to prevent pressure on the skin. Air-fluidized beds float the patient. Dynamic support surfaces, such as low air-loss pockets, alternately inflate and deflate sections to change support pressure for very high-risk patients who are critically ill and debilitated and cannot be repositioned to relieve pressure. Oscillating or kinetic beds change pressure by means of rocking movements of the bed that redistribute the patient's weight and stimulate circulation. These beds are frequently used with patients who have injuries due to multiple trauma.

IMPROVING MOBILITY

The patient is encouraged to remain active and is ambulated whenever possible. When sitting, the patient is reminded to change positions frequently to redistribute weight. Active and passive exercises increase muscular, skin, and vascular tone. Activity stimulates circulation, which relieves tissue ischemia, the forerunner of pressure ulcers. For the patient at risk for pressure ulcers, turning and exercise schedules are essential: repositioning must occur around the clock.

IMPROVING SENSORY PERCEPTION

The nurse helps the patient recognize and compensate for altered sensory perception. Depending on the origin of the alteration (eg, decreased level of consciousness, spinal cord lesion), specific interventions are selected. Strategies to improve cognition and sensory perception may include stimulating the patient to increase awareness of self in the environment, encouraging the patient to participate in self-care, or supporting the patient's efforts toward active compensation for loss of sensation (eg, a paraplegic patient lifting up from the sitting position every 15 minutes). When decreased sensory perception exists, the patient and caregiver are taught to inspect potential pressure areas visually every morning and evening, using a mirror if necessary, for evidence of pressure ulcer development.

IMPROVING TISSUE PERFUSION

Exercise and repositioning improve tissue perfusion. Massage of erythematous areas is avoided because damage to the capillaries and deep tissue may occur.

> **NURSING ALERT** Avoid massaging reddened areas, because this may increase the damage to already traumatized skin and tissue.

In patients who have evidence of compromised peripheral circulation (eg, edema), positioning and elevation of the edematous body part to promote venous return and diminish congestion improve tissue perfusion. In addition, the nurse or family must be alert to environmental factors (eg, wrinkles in sheets, pressure of tubes) that may contribute to pressure on the skin and diminished circulation and remove the source of pressure.

IMPROVING NUTRITIONAL STATUS

The patient's nutritional status must be adequate, and a positive nitrogen balance must be maintained, because pressure ulcers develop more quickly and are more resistant to treatment in patients with nutritional disorders. A high-protein diet with protein supplements may be helpful. Iron preparations may be necessary to raise the hemoglobin concentration so that tissue oxygen levels can be maintained within acceptable limits. Ascorbic acid (vitamin C) is necessary for tissue healing. Other nutrients associated with healthy skin include vitamin A, B vitamins, zinc, and sulfur. With balanced nutrition and hydration, the skin is able to remain healthy, and damaged tissues can be repaired (Table 11-2).

To assess nutritional status response to therapeutic strategies, the nurse monitors the patient's hemoglobin, albumin, and body weight weekly. Nutritional assessment is described in further detail in Chapter 5.

REDUCING FRICTION AND SHEAR

Shear occurs when the patient is pulled, is allowed to slump, or moves by digging heels or elbows into the mattress. Raising the head of the bed by even a few centimeters increases the shearing force over the sacral area; therefore, the semireclining position is avoided in patients at risk. Proper positioning with adequate support is also important when a patient is sitting in a chair. Polyester sheepskin pads are thought to reduce shear and friction and may be used with at-risk patients.

> **NURSING ALERT** To avoid shearing forces when repositioning the patient, the nurse lifts and avoids dragging the patient across a surface.

MINIMIZING IRRITATING MOISTURE

Continuous moisture on the skin must be prevented by meticulous hygienic measures. Perspiration, urine, stool, and drainage must be removed from the skin promptly. The soiled skin should be washed immediately with mild soap and water and blotted dry with a soft towel. The skin may be lubricated with a bland lotion to keep it soft and pliable. Drying agents and powders are avoided. Topical barrier ointments (eg, petroleum jelly) may be helpful in protecting the skin of patients who are incontinent.

Absorbent pads that wick moisture away from the body should be used to absorb drainage. Patients who are incontinent need to be checked *regularly* and have their wet incontinence pads and linens changed promptly. Their skin needs to be cleansed and dried promptly.

PROMOTING PRESSURE ULCER HEALING

Regardless of the stage of the pressure ulcer, the pressure on the area must be eliminated, because the ulcer will not heal until all pressure is removed. The patient must not lie or sit on the pressure ulcer, even for a few minutes. Individualized positioning and turning schedules must be written in the plan of nursing care and followed meticulously.

In addition, inadequate nutritional status and fluid and electrolyte abnormalities must be corrected to promote healing. Wounds that drain body fluids and protein place the patient in a catabolic state and predispose to hypoproteinemia and serious secondary infections. Protein deficiency must be corrected to heal the pressure ulcer. Carbohydrates are necessary to "spare" the protein and to provide an energy source. Vitamin C and trace elements, especially zinc, are necessary for collagen formation and wound healing.

Table 11-2 • **Nutritional Requirements to Promote Healing of Pressure Ulcers**

NUTRIENT	RATIONALE	RECOMMENDED AMOUNT
Protein	Tissue repair	1.25–1.50 g/kg/day
Calories	Spare protein Restore normal weight	30–35 calories/kg/day
Water	Maintain homeostasis	1 mL/calorie fed or 30 mL/kg/day
Multivitamin	Promote collagen formation	1 daily
Vitamin C	Promote collagen synthesis Support integrity of capillary wall	500–1000 mg daily
Zinc sulfate	Cofactor for collagen formation and protein synthesis Normal lymphocyte and phagocyte response	220 mg daily
Vitamin A	*Caution:* An excess can cause an excessive inflammatory response that could impair healing	—

Stage I Pressure Ulcers

To permit healing of stage I pressure ulcers, the pressure is removed to allow increased tissue perfusion, nutritional and fluid and electrolyte balance are maintained, friction and shear are reduced, and moisture to the skin is avoided.

Stage II Pressure Ulcers

Stage II pressure ulcers have broken skin. In addition to measures listed for stage I pressure ulcers, a moist environment, in which migration of epidermal cells over the ulcer surface occurs more rapidly, should be provided to aid wound healing. The ulcer is gently cleansed with sterile saline solution. Use of a heat lamp to dry the open wound is avoided, as is use of antiseptic solutions that damage healthy tissues and delay wound healing. Semipermeable occlusive dressing, hydrocolloid wafers, or wet saline dressings are helpful in providing a moist environment for healing and in minimizing the loss of fluids and proteins from the body.

Stage III and IV Pressure Ulcers

Stage III and IV pressure ulcers are characterized by extensive tissue damage. In addition to measures listed for stage I, these advanced draining, necrotic pressure ulcers must be cleaned (débrided) to create an area that will heal. Necrotic, devitalized tissue favours bacterial growth, delays granulation, and inhibits healing. Wound cleaning and dressing are uncomfortable; therefore, the nurse must prepare the patient for the procedure by explaining what will occur and administering prescribed analgesia.

Débridement may be accomplished by wet-to-damp dressing changes, mechanical flushing of necrotic and infective exudate, application of prescribed enzyme preparations that dissolve necrotic tissue, or surgical dissection. If an eschar covers the ulcer, it is removed surgically to ensure a clean, vitalized wound. Exudate may be absorbed by dressings or special hydrophilic powders, beads, or gels. Cultures of infected pressure ulcers are obtained to guide selection of antibiotic therapy.

After the pressure ulcer is clean, a topical treatment is prescribed to promote granulation. New granulation tissue must be protected from reinfection, drying, and damage, and care should be taken to prevent pressure and further trauma to the area. Dressings, solutions, and ointments applied to the ulcer should not disrupt the healing process. Multiple agents and protocols are used to treat pressure ulcers, but consistency is an important key to success. Objective evaluation of the pressure ulcer (eg, measurement of the pressure ulcer, inspection for granulation tissue) for response to the treatment protocol must be made every 4 to 6 days. Taking photographs at weekly intervals is a reliable strategy for monitoring the healing process, which may take weeks to months to complete.

Surgical intervention is necessary when the ulcer is extensive, when potential complications (eg, fistula) exist, and when the ulcer does not respond to treatment. Surgical procedures include débridement, incision and drainage, bone resection, and skin grafting.

PREVENTING RECURRENCE

Recurrence of pressure ulcers should be anticipated; therefore, active, preventive intervention and frequent continuing assessments are essential. The patient's tolerance for sitting or lying on the healed pressure area is increased gradually by increasing the time that pressure is allowed on the area in 5- to 15-minute increments. The patient is taught to increase mobility and to follow a regimen of turning, weight shifting, and repositioning. The patient teaching plan includes instruction on strategies to reduce the risk for development of pressure ulcers and methods to detect, inspect, and minimize pressure areas. Early recognition and intervention are keys to long-term management of potential impaired skin integrity.

Evaluation

EXPECTED PATIENT OUTCOMES

Expected patient outcomes may include:

1. Maintains intact skin
   a. Exhibits no areas of nonblanchable erythema at bony prominences
   b. Avoids massage of bony prominences
   c. Exhibits no breaks in skin
2. Limits pressure on bony prominences
   a. Changes position every 1 to 2 hours
   b. Uses bridging techniques to reduce pressure
   c. Uses special equipment as appropriate
   d. Raises self from seat of wheelchair every 15 minutes
3. Increases mobility
   a. Performs range-of-motion exercises
   b. Adheres to turning schedule
   c. Advances sitting time as tolerated
4. Sensory and cognitive ability improved
   a. Demonstrates improved level of consciousness
   b. Remembers to inspect potential pressure ulcer areas every morning and evening
5. Demonstrates improved tissue perfusion
   a. Exercises to increase circulation
   b. Elevates body parts susceptible to edema
6. Attains and maintains adequate nutritional status
   a. Verbalizes the importance of protein and vitamin C in diet
   b. Eats diet high in protein and vitamin C
   c. Maintains hemoglobin, electrolyte, albumin, transferrin, and creatinine levels at acceptable levels
7. Avoids friction and shear
   a. Avoids semireclining position
   b. Uses sheepskin pad and heel protectors when appropriate
   c. Lifts body instead of sliding across surfaces
8. Maintains clean, dry skin
   a. Avoids prolonged contact with wet or soiled surfaces
   b. Keeps skin clean and dry
   c. Uses lotion to keep skin lubricated
9. Experiences healing of pressure ulcer
   a. Avoids pressure on area
   b. Improves nutritional status
   c. Participates in therapeutic regimen
   d. Demonstrates behaviours to prevent new pressure ulcers
   e. States early indicators of pressure ulcer development

NURSING PROCESS: THE PATIENT WITH ALTERED ELIMINATION PATTERNS

Urinary and bowel incontinence or constipation and impaction are problems that often occur in disabled patients. Incontinence curtails a person's independence, causing embarrassment and isolation. It occurs in up to 15% of the community-based elderly population, and almost half of nursing home residents are bowel or bladder incontinent or both. In addition, constipation may be a problem for patients with disabilities. Complete and predictable evacuation of the bowel is the goal. If a bowel routine is not established, the person may experience abdominal distention; small, frequent oozing of stool; or impaction.

Urinary and bowel constipation and impaction are particularly dangerous for a spinal cord patient with an injury above T6. Autonomic hyperreflexia (dysreflexia) is a potentially life-threatening condition involving the autonomic nervous system and is caused by a variety of stimuli, including bladder or bowel fullness.

Assessment

Urinary incontinence can be classified as urge, reflex, stress, functional, or total incontinence (AHCPR, 1996). Urge incontinence is involuntary elimination of urine associated with a strong perceived need to void. Reflex (neurogenic) incontinence is associated with a spinal cord lesion that interrupts cerebral control, resulting in no sensory awareness of the need to void. Stress incontinence is associated with weakened perineal muscles that permit leakage of urine when intra-abdominal pressure is increased (eg, with coughing or sneezing). Functional incontinence refers to incontinence in patients with intact urinary physiology who experience mobility impairment, environmental barriers, or cognitive problems and are unable to reach and use the toilet before soiling themselves. Total incontinence occurs in patients who are unable to control excreta because of physiologic or psychological impairment; management of the excreta is the focus of nursing care. Urinary incontinence may result from multiple causes, including urinary tract infection, detrusor instability, bladder outlet obstruction or incompetence, neurologic impairment, bladder spasm or contracture, and inability to reach the toilet in time.

The health history is used to explore bladder and bowel function, symptoms associated with dysfunction, physiologic risk factors for elimination problems, perception of micturition and defecation cues, and functional toileting abilities. Previous and current fluid intake and voiding patterns may be helpful in designing the plan of nursing care. A record of times of voiding and amounts voided is kept for at least 48 hours. In addition, episodes of incontinence and associated activity (eg, coughing, sneezing, lifting), fluid intake time and amount, and medications are recorded. This record is analyzed and used to determine patterns and relationships of incontinence to other activities and factors.

The ability to get to the bathroom, manipulate clothing, and use the toilet are important functional factors that may be related to incontinence. Related cognitive functioning (perception of need to void, verbalization of need to void, and ability to learn to control urination) must also be assessed. In addition, the nurse reviews the results of the diagnostic studies (eg, urinalysis, urodynamic tests, postvoiding residual volumes). See the accompanying Gerontologic Considerations box for factors that affect the older adult.

Bowel incontinence and constipation may result from multiple causes, such as diminished or absent sphincter control, cognitive or perceptual impairment, neurogenic factors, diet, and immobility. The origin of the bowel problem must be determined.

The nurse assesses the patient's normal bowel patterns, nutritional patterns, use of laxatives, gastrointestinal problems (eg, colitis), bowel sounds, anal reflex and tone, and functional abilities. The character and frequency of bowel movements are recorded and analyzed.

Nursing Diagnosis

Based on the assessment data, major nursing diagnoses for the patient may include the following:

Gerontologic Considerations
Factors That Alter Elimination Patterns in the Older Adult

Decreased bladder capacity
Decreased muscle tone
Increased residual volumes
Delayed perception of elimination cues
Use of medications that alter elimination patterns, such as diuretics (increase volume of urine produced), sedatives (alter bladder sensitivity to cues), and adrenergics or anticholinergics (cause urinary retention)
Functional immobility
Sedentary lifestyle

- Impaired bowel elimination
- Impaired urinary elimination

Planning and Goals

The major goals of the patient may include control of urinary incontinence or urinary retention, control of bowel incontinence, and regular elimination patterns.

Nursing Interventions

PROMOTING URINARY CONTINENCE

After the nature of the urinary incontinence has been identified, a nursing plan of care is developed based on analysis of the assessment data. Various approaches to promotion of urinary continence have been designed. Most approaches attempt to condition the body to control urination or to minimize the occurrence of unscheduled urination. Selection of the approach depends on the cause and type of the patient's incontinence. For the program to be successful, the patient's participation and desire to avoid incontinence episodes are crucial, and an optimistic attitude with positive feedback for even slight gains is essential for success. Accurate recording of intake and output and of the response to selected strategies is essential for evaluation.

At no time should the fluid intake be restricted to decrease the frequency of urination. Sufficient fluid intake (2000 to 3000 mL/day according to patient needs) must be ensured. To optimize the likelihood of voiding as scheduled, measured amounts of fluids may be administered about 30 minutes before voiding attempts. In addition, most of the fluids should be consumed before evening to minimize the need to void frequently during the night.

The goal of bladder training is to restore the bladder to normal function. Bladder training can be used with cognitively intact patients experiencing urge incontinence. A voiding and toileting schedule is formulated based on analysis of the assessment data. The schedule specifies times for the patient to try to empty the bladder using a bedpan, toilet, or commode. Privacy should be provided during voiding efforts. The interval between voiding times in the early phase of the bladder training period is short (90 to 120 minutes). The patient is encouraged not to void until the specified voiding time. Voiding success and episodes of incontinence are recorded. As the patient's bladder capacity and control increase, the interval is lengthened. Usually, there is a temporal relationship between drinking, eating, exercising, and voiding. The alert patient can participate in recording intake, activity, and voiding and can plan the schedule to achieve maximum continence. Barrier-free access to the toilet and modification of clothing can help the patient with functional incontinence to achieve self-care in toileting and continence.

Habit training is used to try to keep the patient dry by strict adherence to a toileting schedule and may be successful with stress, urge, or functional incontinence. In the case of a confused person, the caregiver takes the person to the toilet according to the schedule before involuntary voiding occurs. Simple cuing and consistency promote success. Periods of continence and successful voidings are positively reinforced.

Biofeedback is a system through which the patient learns consciously to contract excretory sphincters and control voiding cues. Cognitively intact patients who have stress or urge incontinence may gain bladder control through biofeedback.

Pelvic floor exercises (Kegel exercises) strengthen the pubococcygeus muscle. The patient is instructed to tighten pelvic floor muscles for 4 seconds ten times, and this is repeated four to six times a day. Stopping and starting the stream during urination is recommended to increase control. Daily practice is essential. These exercises are helpful for cognitively intact women who experience stress incontinence.

Suprapubic tapping or stroking of the inner thigh may produce voiding by stimulating the voiding reflex arc in patients with reflex incontinence. This method is not always effective, however, because of detrusor–sphincter dyssynergy. As the bladder reflexively contracts to expel urine, the bladder sphincter reflexively closes, producing a high residual urine volume and an increased incidence of urinary tract infection.

Intermittent self-catheterization is an appropriate alternative for managing reflex incontinence, urinary retention, and overflow incontinence due to an overdistended bladder. The emphasis of patient teaching is on regular emptying of the bladder rather than sterility. Disabled patients reuse and clean catheters with bleach or hydrogen peroxide solutions or soap and water and may use a microwave oven to sterilize catheters. Aseptic intermittent catheterization technique is required in health care institutions because of the potential for bladder infection from resistant organisms. Intermittent self-catheterization may be difficult for patients with limited mobility, dexterity, or vision; however, family members can be taught the procedure.

Indwelling catheters are avoided if at all possible because of the high incidence of urinary tract infections with their use. Short-term use may be needed during treatment of severe skin breakdown due to continued incontinence. Patients with disability who are unable to perform intermittent self-catheterization may elect to use a suprapubic catheter for long-term bladder management. Suprapubic catheters are easier to maintain than indwelling catheters. A fluid intake of 3000 mL/day must be encouraged.

External catheters (condom catheters) and leg bags to collect spontaneous voidings are useful for male patients with reflex or total incontinence. The appropriate design and size must be chosen for maximal success, and the patient or caregiver must be taught how to apply the condom catheter and how to provide daily hygiene, including skin inspection. Instruction on emptying the leg bag must also be provided, and modifications can be made for patients with limited hand dexterity. External collection devices for women do exist, but difficulties with fit have precluded widespread use.

Incontinence pads (briefs) are used only as a last resort, because they only manage rather than solve the incontinence problem. Also, they have a negative psychological effect on the patient because many people think of them as diapers. Every effort should

be made to reduce the incidence of incontinence episodes through the other methods that have been described. Incontinence pads may be useful at times for patients with stress or total incontinence to protect clothing, but they should be avoided whenever possible. When incontinence pads are used, they should wick moisture away from the body to minimize contact of moisture and excreta with the skin. Wet incontinence pads must be changed promptly, the skin cleansed, and a moisture barrier applied to protect the skin.

PROMOTING BOWEL CONTINENCE

The goals of a bowel training program are to develop regular bowel habits and to prevent uninhibited bowel elimination. Regular, complete emptying of the lower bowel results in bowel continence. A bowel-training program takes advantage of the patient's natural reflexes. Regularity, timing, nutrition and fluids, exercise, and correct positioning promote predictable defecation.

The nurse records defecation time, character of stool, nutritional intake, cognitive abilities, and functional self-care toileting abilities for 5 to 7 days. Analysis of this record is helpful when designing a bowel program for the patient with fecal incontinence.

Consistency in implementing the plan is essential. A regular time for defecation is established, and attempts at evacuation should be made within 15 minutes of the designated time daily. Natural gastrocolic and duodenocolic reflexes occur about 30 minutes after a meal; therefore, after breakfast is one of the best times to plan for bowel evacuation. If the patient had a previously established habit pattern at a different time of day, however, it should be followed.

The anorectal reflex may be stimulated by rectal suppository (eg, glycerin) or by mechanical stimulation (eg, digital stimulation with a lubricated gloved finger or anal dilator). Mechanical stimulation should be used only in patients with disability who have no voluntary motor function and no sensation as a result of injuries above the sacral segments of the spinal cord, such as quadriplegic, high paraplegic, or severely brain-injured patients. The technique is not effective in patients who do not have an intact sacral reflex arc (eg, those with flaccid paralysis). Mechanical stimulation, suppository insertion, or both should be initiated about 30 minutes before the scheduled bowel elimination time, and the interval between stimulation and defecation is noted for subsequent modification of the bowel program. Once the bowel routine is well established, stimulation with a suppository may not be necessary.

The patient should assume the normal squatting position (knees higher than the hips) and be in a private bathroom for defecation if at all possible, although a padded commode chair or bedside toilet is an acceptable alternative. Seating time is limited in patients who are at risk for skin breakdown. Bedpans should be avoided. A patient with disability who is unable to sit on a toilet should be positioned on the left side with legs flexed and the head of the bed elevated 30 to 45 degrees to increase intra-abdominal pressure. Protective padding is placed behind the buttocks. When possible, the patient is instructed to bear down and to contract the abdominal muscles. Massaging the abdomen from right to left facilitates movement of feces in the lower tract.

PREVENTING CONSTIPATION

The record of bowel elimination, character of stool, food and fluid intake, level of activity, bowel sounds, medications, and other assessment data are reviewed to develop the plan of care. Multiple approaches may be used to prevent constipation. The diet should be well balanced and should include adequate intake of high-fibre foods (vegetables, fruits, bran) to prevent hard stools and to stimulate peristalsis. Fluid intake should be between 2 and 3 L/day unless contraindicated. Prune juice or fig juice (120 mL) taken 30 minutes before a meal once daily is helpful to some cases when constipation is a problem. Physical activity and exercise are encouraged, as is self-care in toileting. The patient is encouraged to respond to the natural urge to defecate. Privacy during toileting is provided. Stool softeners, bulk-forming agents, mild stimulants, and suppositories may be prescribed to stimulate defecation and to prevent constipation.

Evaluation

EXPECTED PATIENT OUTCOMES
Expected patient outcomes may include:

1. Demonstrates control of bowel and bladder function
   a. Experiences no episodes of incontinence
   b. Avoids constipation
   c. Achieves independence in toileting
   d. Expresses satisfaction in level of bowel and bladder control
2. Achieves urinary continence
   a. Uses therapeutic approach appropriate to type of incontinence
   b. Maintains adequate fluid intake
   c. Washes and dries skin after episodes of incontinence
3. Achieves bowel continence
   a. Participates in bowel program
   b. Verbalizes need for regular time for bowel evacuation
   c. Modifies diet to promote continence
   d. Uses bowel stimulants as prescribed and needed
4. Experiences relief of constipation
   a. Uses high-fibre diet, fluids, and exercise to promote defecation
   b. Responds to urge to defecate

Disability and Sexuality Issues

An important issue confronting the patient with a disability, and a vital component of self-concept, is sexuality. Sexuality involves not only biologic sexual activity but also one's concept of masculinity or femininity. It affects the way a person reacts to others and is perceived by them, and it is expressed not only by physical intimacy but also by caring and emotional intimacy.

Sexuality problems faced by patients with disabilities include limited access to information about sexuality, lack of opportunity to form friendships and loving relationships, impaired self-image, and low self-esteem. The person with a disability may have physical and emotional difficulties that interfere with sexual activities. For example, diabetes and spinal cord injury may affect the ability to have an erection. The patient who has suffered a heart attack or stroke may fear having a life-threatening event (eg, another heart attack or stroke) during sexual activity. He or she may fear loss of bowel or bladder control during intimate moments. Changes in desire for sex and in the quality of sexual activities can occur for the patient and the partner, who may be too involved as the caregiver to have desire and energy for sexual activities.

Unfortunately, society and some health care providers contribute to these problems by ignoring patients' sexuality and by viewing disabled persons as asexual. Health care providers' own discomfort and lack of knowledge related to sexuality issues prevent them from providing the patient with disability and his or her partner interventions that promote healthy intimacy. Nurses caring for persons with disability must recognize and address sexual issues in order to promote feelings of self-worth, which are essential to total rehabilitation. The nurse should give the patient "permission" to discuss sexuality concerns and show a willingness to listen and help the patient overcome these concerns. The nurse also has a key role to provide appropriate patient education about how specific disabilities affect sexual function. For example, arthritis produces fatigue and morning stiffness, making planned afternoon sex a better alternative; spinal cord injury impairs erections and ejaculations; and traumatic brain injury may produce an increased or decreased interest in sexual behaviour. Classes, books, movies, and support groups are useful tools to help patients learn about sexuality and disability. When open discussion and education about disability and sexuality do not result in a patient's achieving his or her sexuality goals, the nurse should refer the patient for ongoing counselling with a sex counsellor or therapist. The patient may need training in communication and in social and assertiveness skills to develop desired relationships.

Fatigue

People with disabilities frequently experience fatigue. Physical and emotional weariness may be caused by discomfort and pain associated with a chronic health problem, deconditioning associated with prolonged periods of bed rest and immobility, impaired motor function requiring excessive expenditure of energy to ambulate, and the frustrations of performing ADLs. Ineffective coping with the disability, unresolved grief, and depression can also contribute to fatigue. The patient can use coping strategies to manage the psychological impact of the disability and pain management techniques to control the associated discomforts (see Chapter 13 for a discussion of pain management). In addition, the nurse can teach the patient to manage fatigue through priority setting and energy-conserving techniques. Special teaching strategies for patients with disabilities are included in Chart 11-10.

Home and Community-Based Care

An important goal of rehabilitation is to assist the person to return to the home environment after learning to manage the disability. A referral system maintains continuity of care when the patient is transferred to the home or to an extended care facility. The plan for discharge is formulated when the patient is first admitted to the hospital, and discharge plans are made with the patient's functional potential in mind.

The patient's support system (family, friends) is assessed. The attitudes of family and friends toward the patient, the disability, and the return home are important in making a successful transition to home. Not all families are able to carry on the arduous programs of exercise, physical training, and personal care that a patient may need. They may not have the resources or stability to care for a severely disabled family member. Even a stable family may be overwhelmed by the physical, emotional, economic, and energy strains of a disabling condition in their family member. Members of the rehabilitation team must not judge the family

Chart 11-10 • PATIENT EDUCATION
Learning to Cope With Disabilities

The following points may be useful in teaching patients how to reduce their energy output and conserve their strength to achieve a meaningful lifestyle.

Take Control of Your Life
- Face the reality of your disability.
- Emphasize areas of strength.
- Remain outward looking.
- Seek inventive ways to tackle problems.
- Share concerns and frustrations.
- Maintain and improve general health.
- Plan for recreation.

Have Well-Defined Goals and Priorities
- Keep priorities in order; eliminate nonessential activities.
- Plan and pace your activities.

Organize Your Life
- Plan each day.
- Organize work.
- Perform tasks in steps.
- Distribute heavy work throughout the day or week.

Conserve Energy
- Rest before undertaking difficult tasks.
- Stop the activity before fatigue occurs.
- Continue with an exercise conditioning program to strengthen muscles.

Control Your Environment
- Try to be well organized.
- Keep possessions in the same place, so that they can be found with a minimum of effort.
- Store equipment (personal care, crafts, work) in a box or basket.
- Use energy-conservation and work-simplification techniques.
- Keep work within easy reach and in front of you.
- Use adaptive equipment, self-help aids, and labour-saving devices.
- Recruit assistance from others; delegate when necessary.
- Take safety precautions.

but rather should provide supportive interventions that help them attain their highest level of function.

The family needs to know as much as possible about the patient's condition and care so that they do not fear the patient's return home. The nurse develops methods for coping with problems that may arise with the patient and family. A skill checklist individualized for the patient and family can be developed to make certain that the family is proficient in assisting the patient with certain tasks. See Chart 11-11 for an example of a home care checklist.

Complementary Therapies

Individuals with disabilities may seek a variety of different therapies. For some, therapeutic horseback riding influences the whole body and has a profound effect on all body systems. Pet therapy and canine companion programs have reduced stress and promoted coping for many disabled persons. Some animals including simian monkeys can pick up the phone, retrieve small assistive devices, assist with drinking beverages, or assist with activating emergency calls. The "working" animals provide companionship as well as physical assistance for elderly persons and persons with disability who may live alone.

Nurses can also encourage persons with disability to take advantage of community programs. T'ai chi classes improve muscle strength, balance, and coordination and can help to prevent falls in the elderly. Disabled persons, including wheelchair users, can participate in T'ai chi classes for improved balance, coordination, muscle strength and control, and a sense of well-being.

Daily journal writing has helped depressed individuals and their families overcome many emotionally draining reactions to adverse circumstances. Nurses are instrumental in teaching patients and family members this cost-effective technique. Relaxation exercises can also be taught by the nurse and encouraged in all settings, including the hospital, rehabilitation setting, outpatient areas, and the home.

Follow-Up Care

The home care nurse may visit the patient in the hospital, interview the patient and family, and review the ADL sheet to learn which activities the patient can perform. This helps ensure continuity of care and that the patient does not regress but instead maintains the independence gained while in the hospital or rehabilitation setting. The family may need to purchase, borrow, or improvise needed equipment, such as safety rails, a raised toilet seat or commode, or a tub bench. Ramps may need to be built or doorways widened to achieve full access.

Family members are taught how to use equipment and are given a copy of the equipment manufacturer's instruction booklet, the names of resource people, lists of equipment-related supplies, and locations where they may be obtained. A written summary of the care plan is included in family teaching.

A network of support services and communication systems may be required to enhance opportunities for independent living. The nurse uses collaborative, administrative skills to coordinate these activities and to pull together the network of care. The nurse also provides skilled care, initiates additional referrals when indicated, and serves as the patient's advocate and counsellor when obstacles are encountered. The nurse continues to reinforce prior teaching and helps the patient to set and achieve attainable goals. The degree to which the patient adapts to the home and community environment depends on the confidence and self-esteem developed during the rehabilitation process and on the acceptance, support, and reactions of the family, employer, and community members.

There is a growing trend toward independent living by people with severe disabilities, either alone or in groups that share resources. Preparation for independent living should include training in managing a household and working with personal care attendants as well as training in mobility. The goal is integration into the community—living and working in the community with accessible housing, employment, public buildings, transportation, and recreation.

Agencies are available to provide services to assist people with disability in obtaining the help they need to engage in gainful employment. These services include diagnostic, medical, and mental health services. Counselling, training, placement, and follow-up services are available to help people with disabilities select and attain jobs.

If the patient is transferred to an extended care facility, the transition is planned to promote continued progress. Independence gained continues to be supported, and progress is fostered. Adjustment to the extended care facility is facilitated through communication. The family is encouraged to visit, to be involved, and to take the patient home on weekends and holidays if possible.

Chart 11-11
Home Care Checklist • Managing the Therapeutic Regimen at Home

At the completion of the discharge teaching, the patient or caregiver will be able to:	Patient	Caregiver
• State the impact of disability on physiologic functioning.	✓	✓
• State changes in lifestyle necessary to maintain health.	✓	✓
• State the name, dose, side effects, frequency, and schedule for all medications.	✓	✓
• State how to obtain medical supplies after discharge.	✓	✓
• Identify durable medical equipment needs, proper usage, and maintenance necessary for safe utilization:	✓	✓

[ ] Wheelchair—manual/power
[ ] Cushion
[ ] Grab bars
[ ] Sliding board
[ ] Mechanical lift
[ ] Raised padded commode seat
[ ] Padded commode wheelchair
[ ] Bedside toilet
[ ] Crutches
[ ] Walker
[ ] Prosthesis
[ ] Orthosis
[ ] Specialty bed

	Patient	Caregiver
• Demonstrate usage of adaptive equipment for activities of daily living:	✓	✓

[ ] Long-handled sponge
[ ] Reacher
[ ] Universal cuff
[ ] Plate mat and guard
[ ] Rocker-knife, spork, weighted utensils
[ ] Special closures for clothing
[ ] Other

	Patient	Caregiver
• Demonstrate mobility skills:	✓	✓

[ ] Transfers: bed to chair; in and out of toilet and tub; in and out of car
[ ] Negotiate ramps, curbs, stairs
[ ] Assume sitting from supine position
[ ] Turn side to side in bed
[ ] Manoeuvre wheelchair; manage arm and leg rests; lock brakes
[ ] Ambulate safely using assistive devices
[ ] Range-of-motion exercises
[ ] Muscle-strengthening exercises

	Patient	Caregiver
• Demonstrate skin care:	✓	✓

[ ] Inspect bony prominences every morning and evening
[ ] Identify stage I pressure ulcer and actions to take if present
[ ] Change dressings for stage II to IV pressure ulcers
[ ] State dietary requirements to promote healing of pressure ulcers
[ ] Demonstrate pressure relief at prescribed intervals
[ ] State sitting schedule
[ ] Demonstrate adherence to bed turning schedule, bed positioning, and use of bridging techniques
[ ] Apply and wear protective boots at prescribed times
[ ] Demonstrate correct wheelchair sitting posture
[ ] Demonstrate techniques to avoid friction and shear in bed
[ ] Demonstrate proper hygiene to maintain skin integrity

	Patient	Caregiver
• Demonstrate bladder care:	✓	✓

[ ] State schedule for voiding, toileting, and catheterization
[ ] Identify relationship of fluid intake to voiding and catheterization schedule
[ ] State how to perform pelvic floor exercises
[ ] Demonstrate clean self-intermittent catheterization and care of catheterization equipment
[ ] Demonstrate indwelling catheter care
[ ] Demonstrate application of external condom catheter
[ ] Demonstrate application, emptying, and cleaning of urinary drainage bag
[ ] Demonstrate application of incontinence pads and performing perineal hygiene
[ ] State signs and symptoms of urinary tract infection
[ ] State signs and symptoms of autonomic hyperreflexia (dysreflexia)

	Patient	Caregiver
• Demonstrate bowel care	✓	✓

[ ] State optimum dietary intake to promote evacuation
[ ] Identify schedule for optimum bowel evacuation
[ ] Demonstrate techniques to increase intra-abdominal pressure; Valsalva manoeuvre; abdominal massage; leaning forward
[ ] Demonstrate techniques to stimulate bowel movements: ingesting warm liquids; digital stimulation; insertion of suppositories
[ ] Demonstrate optimum position for bowel evacuation: on toilet with knees higher than hips; left side in bed with knees flexed and head slightly elevated
[ ] Identify complications and corrective strategies for bowel retraining: constipation, impaction, diarrhea, hemorrhoids, rectal bleeding, anal tears
[ ] State signs and symptoms of autonomic hyperreflexia (dysreflexia)

(continued)

Chart 11-11

Home Care Checklist • **Managing the Therapeutic Regimen at Home (Continued)**

	Patient	Caregiver

• Identify community resources for peer and family support
   [ ] Identify phone numbers for disabled support groups
   [ ] State meeting locations and times
	✓	✓

• Demonstrate how to access transportation
   [ ] Identify locations of wheelchair accessibility for public buses or trains
   [ ] Identify phone numbers for private wheelchair van
   [ ] Contact Division of Motor Vehicles for handicapped parking permit
   [ ] Contact Division of Motor Vehicles for driving test when appropriate
   [ ] Identify resources for adapting private vehicle with hand controls or wheelchair lift
	✓	✓

• Identify vocational rehabilitation resources
   [ ] State name and phone number of vocational rehabilitation counsellor
   [ ] Identify educational opportunities that may lead to future employment
	✓	✓

• Identify community resources for recreation
   [ ] State local recreation centres that offer programs for the disabled
   [ ] Identify leisure activities that can be pursued in the community
	✓	✓

• Identify the need for health promotion and screening activities		

Critical Thinking Exercises

1. The patient who has just been admitted to your unit in the rehabilitation hospital is a 58-year-old woman who is recovering from a stroke. She has paralysis on one side, but speech is intact. In discussing the patient's level of functioning with the physical rehabilitation team, describe the kinds of self-care activities that you would assess in developing a rehabilitation plan for the patient.

2. An elderly man who has lost his leg as a result of diabetes is to be discharged to his home, where he will be cared for by his family. The family members are particularly concerned about how to prevent pressure ulcers, because the patient is a diabetic and will be confined primarily to a wheelchair. Describe the instructions you would give them. How might your teaching strategies differ if family members converse primarily in their native tongue, which is not English?

3. You are caring for a young man who has sustained a traumatic brain injury and multiple fractures in a motor vehicle crash. He is ready to return home to continue rehabilitation as an outpatient. You accompany the physical and occupational therapist to assess the patient's home environment in anticipation of his discharge. Compare the types of safety factors that might be considered if the patient lives in a single-story house, in a two-story house, in a two-room apartment in a high-rise building, or on a farm.

REFERENCES AND SELECTED READINGS

Books

Agency for Health Care Policy and Research, Public Health Service, U.S. Department of Health and Human Services. Panel for the Prediction and Prevention of Pressure Ulcers in Adults. (1992). *Pressure ulcers in adults: Prediction and prevention.* Clinical Practice Guideline, Number 3. AHCPR Publication No. 92-0047. Rockville, MD: Author.

Agency for Health Care Policy and Research, Public Health Service, U.S. Department of Health and Human Services. (1994). *Treatment of pressure ulcers.* Clinical Practice Guideline, Number 15. AHCPR Publication No. 95-0652. Rockville, MD: Author.

Agency for Health Care Policy and Research. Public Health Service, U.S. Department of Health and Human Services. Urinary Incontinence Guideline Panel. (1996). *Urinary incontinence in adults: Clinical practice guideline.* AHCPR Pub. No. 96-0682. Rockville, MD: Author.

Alexander, T., Hiduke, R., & Stevens, K. (1999). *Rehabilitation nursing policy and procedure manual* (2nd ed.). Rehabilitation Institute of Chicago. Chicago, IL: McGraw-Hill.

Association of Rehabilitation Nurses. (2000). *Standards and scope of rehabilitation nursing practice.* Glenview, IL: Author.

Association of Rehabilitation Nurses. (2000). *The specialty practice of rehabilitation nursing: A core curriculum* (4th ed.). Skokie, IL: Author.

Association of Rehabilitation Nurses. (1995). *Twenty-one rehabilitation nursing diagnoses: A guide to interventions and outcomes.* Glenview, IL: Author.

Association of Rehabilitation Nurses. (1996). *Scope and standards of advanced clinical practice in rehabilitation nursing.* Glenview, IL: Author.

Association of Rehabilitation Nurses. (1997). *Advanced practice in rehabilitation nursing: A core curriculum.* Glenview, IL: Author.

Derstine, J., & Hargrove, S. (2000). *Comprehensive rehabilitation nursing.* St. Louis, MO: W.B. Saunders.

Dittmar, S., & Gresham, G. (1997). *Functional assessment and outcome measures for the rehabilitation health professional.* Gaithersburg, MD: Aspen.

Easton, K. (1999). *Gerontological rehabilitation nursing.* St. Louis, MO: W. B. Saunders.

Edwards, P., Hertzberg, D., Hays, S., & Youngblood, N. (1999). *Pediatric rehabilitation nursing.* St. Louis, MO: W. B. Saunders.

Government of Canada. (2004). *Advancing the inclusion of persons with disabilities—A Government of Canada report.* Ottawa: Office of Disability Issues, Social Development Canada. Available: www.sdc.gc.ca. Retrieved August 29, 2005.

Health Canada. (November 2004). *Canadian Addiction Survey (CAS): A national survey of Canadians' use of alcohol and other drugs. Prevalence of use and related harms.* Ottawa: Canadian Centre on Substance Abuse. Available: www.ccsa.ca. Retrieved August 29, 2005.

Hess, C. (1999). *Wound care* (3rd ed.). Springhouse, PA: Springhouse.

Hoeman, S. (1996). *Rehabilitation nursing: Process and application* (2nd ed.). St. Louis, MO: Mosby.

Jans, L., & Stoddard, S. (1999). *Chartbook on women and disability in the United States.* Washington, DC: U.S. National Institute on Disability and Rehabilitation Research.

Krasner, D., & Kane, D. (1997). *Chronic wound care: A clinical source book for healthcare professionals* (2nd ed.). Wayne, PA: Health Management Publications, Inc.

Law, M., Baptiste, S., Carswell, A., McColl, M. A., Polatajko, H., & Pollock, N. (1998). *Canadian occupational performance measure* (2nd ed., rev.). Ottawa, ON: CAOT Publications ACE.

Maklebust, J., & Sieggreen, M. (2001). *Pressure ulcers: Guidelines for prevention and management* (3rd ed.). Philadelphia: Springhouse.

Morrison, M. (2001). *The prevention and treatment of pressure ulcers.* St. Louis, MO: Mosby.

Newman, D. (1999). *The urinary incontinence sourcebook.* Chicago: Lowell House.

Sipski, M., & Alexander, C. (1997). *Sexual function in people with disability and chronic illness: A health professional's guide.* Gaithersburg, MD: Aspen.

Sussman, C., & Bates-Jenson, B. (1998). *Wound care: A collaborative practice manual for physical therapists and nurses.* Gaithersburg, MD: Aspen.

U.S. Census Bureau (1997). *Americans with disabilities, 1997: Household Economic Studies Current Population Reports.* Washington, DC: U.S. Government Printing Office.

U.S. Department of Health and Human Services. (2000, December 14). *HHS Fact Sheet. Substance Abuse—A National Challenge: Prevention, Treatment and Research at HHS.* Washington, DC: U.S. Government Printing Office.

U.S. Department of Justice. (1996). *A guide to disability rights laws.* Washington, DC: U.S. Government Printing Office.

Journals

Asterisks indicate nursing research articles.

Akdolun, N., & Terakye, G. (2001). Sexual problems before and after myocardial infarction: Patients' needs for information. *Rehabilitation Nursing, 26*(4), 152–159.

Beitz, J. (2001). Overcoming barriers to wound care: a systems perspective. *Ostomy/Wound Management, 47*(3), 56–64.

*Cataldo, J. (2001). The relationship of hardiness and depression to disability in institutionalized older adults. *Rehabilitation Nursing, 26*(1), 28–33.

Daly, M. (2000). Rehabilitation in the therapeutic riding arena. *Rehabilitation Nursing, 25*(5), 167–168.

Government of Canada. References related to assistive devices. Available: www.at-links.gc.ca/as/. Retrieved December 19, 2005.

Gray, M. (2000). Urinary retention: management in the acute care setting: Part 1. *American Journal of Nursing, 100*(7), 40–48.

Gray, M. (2000). Urinary retention: management in the acute care setting: Part 2. *American Journal of Nursing, 100*(8), 36–44.

Henderson-Martin, B. (2000). No more surprises: Screening patients for alcohol abuse. *American Journal of Nursing, 100*(9), 26–33.

Hood, P. (2000). Handicapped parking. *American Journal of Nursing, 100*(9), 11.

Krebs, H. (2000). Increasing productivity and quality of care: Robot-aided neuro-rehabilitation. *Journal of Rehabilitation Research and Development, 37*(6), 639–652.

*Masayuki, I. (2000). Prediction of functional outcome after stroke rehabilitation. *American Journal of Physical Medicine and Rehabilitation, 79*(6), 513–518.

Mayo Clinic Rochester (2001). *Geriatric Medicine.* Pressure ulcers: Prevention and management. Available at: http://www.mayo.edu/geriatrics-rst/PU-ToC.html. Retrieved August 15, 2001.

*Missik, E. (2001). Women and cardiac rehabilitation: Accessibility issues and policy recommendations. *Rehabilitation Nursing, 26*(4), 141–147.

Modlin, S. (2001). From puppy to service dog: Raising service dogs for the rehabilitation team. *Rehabilitation Nursing, 26*(1), 12–17.

Patel, C. (2000). Vacuum-assisted wound closure. *American Journal of Nursing, 100*(12), 45–48.

Pryor, J. (2000). Creating a rehabilitative milieu. *Rehabilitation Nursing, 25*(4), 141–144.

*Secrest, J. (2000). Transformation of the relationship: The experience of primary support persons of stroke survivors. *Rehabilitation Nursing, 25*(3), 93–99.

Smeltzer, S. C. (2000). Viewpoint: Double jeopardy. The health care system slights women with disabilities. *American Journal of Nursing, 100*(8), 11.

Smith, C., & Holcroft, C. (2000). Journal writing as a complementary therapy for reactive depression: A rehabilitation teaching program. *Rehabilitation Nursing, 25*(5), 170–176.

Sperazza, L. (2001). Rehabilitation options for patients with low vision. *Rehabilitation Nursing, 26*(4), 148–151.

Sullivan, M., & Sharts-Hopko, N. (2000). Preventing the downward spiral: Osteoporosis and MS. *American Journal of Nursing, 100*(8), 26–33.

Thompson, J. (2000). A practical guide to wound care. *RN, 63*(1), 48–58.

Wolf, S., & Barnhardt, H. (1996). Reducing frailty and falls in older persons: An investigation of T'ai chi and computerized balance training. *Journal of American Geriatrics Society, 44,* 489–497.

RESOURCES AND WEBSITES

Agency for Healthcare Research and Quality (formerly the Agency for Health Care Policy and Research), 2101 East Jefferson Street, Suite 501; Rockville, MD 20852; 1-800-358-9295; http://www.ahrq.gov.

American Society of Addiction Medicine, 4601 North Park Avenue, Arcade Suite 101, Chevy Chase, MD 20815; 1-301-656-3920; http://www.asam.org.

Assistive Technology Industry Association, 526 Davis Street, Suite 217; Evanston, IL 60201; 1-877-687-2842/847-969-1282; http://www.atia.org.

Association of Rehabilitation Nurses, 4700 W. Lake Avenue, Glenview, IL 60025-1485; 1-800-229-7530; fax 1-847-375-4710; http://www.rehabnurse.org.

Canine Companions for Independence, PO Box 446, Santa Rosa, CA 95402-0446; 1-800-572-2275; http://www.caninecompanions.org.

Council for Disability Rights, 205 West Randolph, Suite 1650, Chicago, IL 60606; 1-312-444-9484; http://www.disabilityrights.org.

National Centre for Health Statistics, Division of Data Services, Hyattsville, MD 20782-2003; 1-301-458-4636; http://www.cdc.gov/nchs.

National Council on Alcoholism and Drug Dependence, Inc., 20 Exchange Place, Suite 2902, New York, NY 10005; 1-212-269-7797; http://www.ncadd.org.

National Council on Disability, 1331 F Street, NW, Suite 1050, Washington, DC 20004; 1-202-272-2004; http://www.ncd.gov.

National Institute on Disability and Rehabilitation Research (NIDRR), Office of Special Education and Rehabilitation Research, U.S. Department of Education, Washington, DC 20202; 1-202-205-9151; http://www.ed.gov/offices/OSERS/NIDRR.

National Rehabilitation Information Center (NARIC), 1010 Wayne Avenue, Suite 800, Silver Spring, MD 20910; 1-800-346-2742; http://www.naric.com.

Rehabilitation Accreditation Commission, 4891 E. Grant Road, Tucson, AZ 85712.

Sexuality and Information and Education Council of the U.S. (SIECUS), 130 West 42nd Street, Suite 350, New York, NY 10036-7802; 1-212-819-9770; http://www.siecus.org.

Substance Abuse Resources and Disability Issues, Wright State University School of Medicine, Dayton, Ohio 45435; 1-937-259-1384; http://www.med.wright.edu.

U.S. Census Bureau, 4700 Silver Hill Road, Suitland, MD 20746; 1-301-457-4608; http://www.census.gov.

U.S. Department of Health and Human Services, 200 Independence Avenue SW, Washington, DC 20201; 1-202-690-6343; http://www.hhs.gov.

Health Care of the Older Adult

Adapted by Donna Wilson and Jaeyoung Choi

LEARNING OBJECTIVES

On completion of this chapter, the learner will be able to:

1. Describe the aging Canadian population based on demographic trends and statistical data.

2. Discuss the potential economic effect of the large aging population in Canada on health care.

3. Identify major legal issues relevant to the care of older people.

4. Compare and contrast the physiologic aspects of aging with those of middle-age adults.

5. Describe the significance of preventive health care and health promotion for the elderly.

6. Identify the important physical and mental health problems of aging and their effects on the functioning of older people and their families.

7. Identify the major geriatric syndromes and their effects on the individual patient.

8. Specify nursing implications related to medication therapy in older people.

9. Examine the concerns of older people and their families in the home and community, in the acute care setting, and in long-term care facilities.

10. Identify the resources available to allow older adults to receive medical and nursing services in their own homes.

Aging, the normal process of time-related change, begins at or before birth and continues throughout life. In the year 2000, 13% of the Canadian population, or 3.8 million Canadians, were seniors (65 years of age or older) (Statistics Canada, n.d.). This segment of the Canadian population has been and will continue to grow more rapidly than the rest of the population (Fig. 12-1). In 1981, only 10% of the Canadian population were seniors, as compared with a projected 19% or 7 million persons in 2021 (Statistics Canada, 2001). In 2041, when the entire large baby-boom generation (those born between 1946 and 1966) has reached old age, 25%—or 9 million—of all Canadians will be seniors. Rapid aging within the present senior population is also occurring, with seniors aged 85 and older being the fastest-growing population group in Canada. Currently, 1 of every 10 seniors is aged 85 or older; these people are often designated as the oldest-old or the frail elderly (Rockwood et al., 2004). Although the vast majority of seniors report they are in good to excellent health (Clarke, Marshall, Ryff, & Rosenthal, 2000), persons in the oldest-old age range typically have health care or other needs (Health Canada, 2002). As this population grows, health professionals will be challenged to design strategies that address their needs. Unfortunately, ageism is so prevalent in Canadian society that many believe ill health is common to all seniors. People who live into old age should be considered physically and socio-emotionally hardy individuals (Magai, Consedine, King, & Gillespie, 2003). Many of the health conditions affecting seniors today can be better managed, limited, and even prevented. Older individuals are more likely to maintain good health and functional independence when appropriate community-based support is available.

Overview of Aging

DEMOGRAPHICS OF AGING

According to many sources that use census data and other vital statistics information collected by Statistics Canada, life expectancy, the average number of years that a person can expect to live, has increased considerably over the past century. Since 1920, life expectancy has increased by 7 years for men and 13 years for women (Canada Online, n.d.). Using 2002 mortality data, the current life expectancy for both sexes was calculated as 79.7 years (Canada Online, n.d.). However, the life expectancy for women was 82.1 years and 77.2 years for men, a gap of 4.9 years. This gap helps explain why there are more older women than men, and why more older women than men live alone. Currently, 57% of all Canadian seniors are female, while 70% of all persons aged 85 and older are female (Health Canada, 2002). Although this gender-based age gap is currently quite large, it has been narrowing in recent years as more men are reaching older ages. For instance, from 1997 to 2002 life expectancy improved by 5.8 years for men, while only improving 3.3 years for women (Canada Online, n.d.).

The vast majority of seniors in Canada do not live in nursing homes, just as the vast majority of seniors do not receive any formal home care services (MacKnight et al., 2003). Although most seniors are disability free for all but the last 2 to 4 years of life (Division of Aging and Seniors, 2001), with women more often disabled because they live longer (Martel & Belanger, 2000), a considerable number of seniors receive informal caregiving support from their family (Cranswick, 1997, 1999). A cross-Canada survey revealed that one in six older men and one in four older women living in the community received ongoing assistance of various types from their family, friends, or neighbours (Wilkins & Park, 1996). Most often this support is with instrumental activities of daily living, such as grocery shopping, driving, housework, and other strenuous or complex activities (Lafreniere, Carriere, Martel, & Belanger, 2003). Less often this support is for activities of daily living, such as bathing and dressing (Chen & Wilkins, 1998). Unfortunately, not all seniors have someone who can provide the help they need, which puts these persons much more at risk of illness, and thus at risk of hospitalization (Canadian Institute of Health Information, 2004a) or admission to a nursing home (Lafreniere et al., 2003). Family caregiver support may be less common in the future because of a major reduction in fertility since 1966 (Health Canada, 2002). Baby-boomers have produced,

Glossary

ageism: a bias against older people based solely on their chronologic age, without consideration of their functional status

dehydration: condition resulting from excessively low levels of fluid in the body; occurs when fluid output exceeds fluid intake

delirium: an acute, confused state that begins with disorientation but, if not immediately evaluated, can progress to changes in level of consciousness, irreversible brain damage, and sometimes death

dementia: broad term for a syndrome characterized by a general decline in higher brain functioning, such as reasoning, with a pattern of eventual decline in ability to perform even basic activities of daily living, such as toileting and eating

depression: the most common disorder affecting adults, it is a mental health condition marked by negative affect which lasts 2 or more weeks. It is more common among older adults who suffer from multiple chronic illnesses or losses

elder abuse: the physical or emotional harm arising from the mistreatment or neglect of an elderly person by any other person

geriatrics: the study of old age that includes the physiology, pathology, diagnosis, and management of the disorders and diseases of older adults

gerontology: the combined biologic, psychologic, and sociologic study of older adults within their environment

gerontologic/geriatric nursing: the field of nursing that specializes in the nursing process as it relates to the assessment, nursing diagnosis, planning, implementation, and evaluation of older adults in all environments including acute, intermediate, and skilled care as well as within the community

life expectancy: the average number of years that a person is expected to live

life span: the maximum number of years an individual can be expected to live in the absence of disease or life-threatening trauma

orientation: a term that refers to a person's ability to recognize who and where he or she is in a time continuum; used to evaluate an individual's basic cognitive status

polypharmacy: the use of multiple medications each day, a situation which is common to older persons who have several chronic illnesses

presbycusis: the decreased ability to hear high-pitched tones that naturally begins in midlife as a result of irreversible inner ear changes

presbyopia: the decrease in visual accommodation that occurs with advancing age

urinary incontinence: the unplanned loss of urine, which affects up to 50% of community-residing older adults and approximately 75% to 85% of nursing home residents

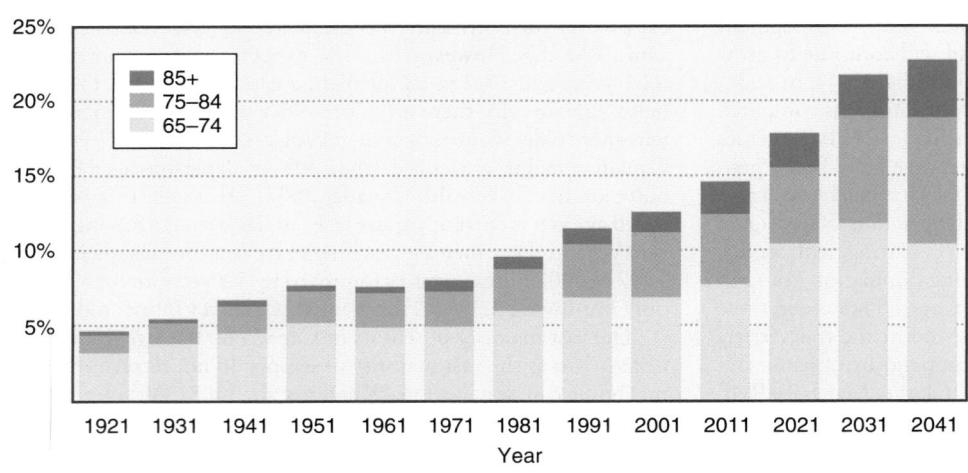

FIGURE 12-1   Source: Health Canada. (2002). *Canada's aging population.* Ottawa: Minister of Public Works and Government Services Canada.

on average, fewer than half the number of children than did their parents, the cohort that created the baby-boom generation.

Although most older adults enjoy good health, surveys such as the National Population Health Survey and the Canadian Study of Health and Aging reveal that nearly 60% of Canadians aged 15 and older have one or more chronic health problems (Schultz & Kopec, 2004). With aging, the prevalence of most chronic health conditions increases, as does the prevalence of physical problems and the dependency arising with these health problems (Martel & Belanger, 2000). It is remarkable, however, that one mid-1990s survey found only one in six older men and one in four older women

living in the community had a physical limitation or disability (Wilkins & Park, 1996). A 2001 survey similarly found that only 15% of surveyed Canadians of all ages had some form of a disability, with mobility difficulties the most common; all disabilities were more common and severe with aging (Profile of disability, 2004). Regardless, Shields (2004) found that only 7% of Canadian seniors aged 85 or older used a wheelchair, although an additional 32% used another mobility assist device, such as a cane. Among the persons who used an assistive device, half indicated they used it because of an illness or disease, one quarter used it because of normal aging, and one in five used it because of a past injury.

People over the age of 65 who have more than one chronic illness and those with marked physical disability are much more likely to receive formal home care services (Wilkins & Park, 1998) or to be institutionalized in a nursing home (Canadian Institute for Health Information, 2004a). The most commonly reported chronic health problems among community-dwelling adults, from most common to least common, are nonfood allergies (reported by 22.3%), back problems, arthritis or rheumatism, high blood pressure, migraine headaches, asthma, food allergies, heart disease, diabetes, urinary incontinence, stroke, and Alzheimer's disease (Schultz & Kopec, 2004). Many other chronic conditions are also problematic for seniors, such as vision and hearing loss. Among seniors, the most problematic chronic health conditions are Alzheimer's disease, stroke, epilepsy, bowel problems, urinary incontinence, and lung disorders (Schultz & Kopec, 2004). The three most common causes of death among older persons are cardiovascular (heart and stroke) disease, death, cancer, and all others (Table 12-1). These three categories are responsible for 83% of all deaths among seniors. A much more serious concern, is that seniors often have comorbidities that together lead to death (Hodgson, 2002). For instance, a senior citizen may experience the simultaneous effects of cancer, congestive heart failure, diabetes, and renal failure, along with the effects of chemotherapy and other treatments. With autopsies rarely done now, the health care provider who completes the death certificate must judge the primary cause of death from among many probable causes. Secondary causes of death are listed on the death certificate, but it is the primary cause of death that is normally used to create the statistics that lead to new health policies and programs.

Table 12-1 • **Cause of Death in Canada, 2000**

PRIMARY CAUSE OF DEATH (2000)	UNDER AGE 65 # (%)	65 YEARS OF AGE OR OLDER # (%)	TOTAL # (%)
Cardiovascular	9,574 (19.7)	66,661 (39.4)	76,235 (35.0)
Cancer	18,394 (37.9)	45,693 (27.0)	64,087 (29.5)
Respiratory	1,556 (3.2)	16,169 (9.5)	17,725 (8.1)
Digestive	1,927 (4.0)	6,212 (3.7)	8,139 (3.7)
Accidents, Injury, Suicide	8,817 (18.1)	4,413 (2.6)	13,230 (6.1)
Infectious and Parasitic	1,142 (2.3)	1,967 (1.2)	3,109 (1.5)
Congenital	806 (1.7)	114 (0.1)	920 (0.4)
All other	6,381 (13.1)	27,949 (16.5)	34,330 (15.7)
Total	48,597 (100.0)	169,178 (100.0)	217,775 (100.0)

Source: Statistics Canada 2000 mortality data, purchased through an NHRDP research grant and a University of Alberta research grant, with data also analyzed by D. M. Wilson. June 2005.

HEALTH CARE COSTS OF AGING

Some fear that there will be an unsustainable increase in the demand for health care with population aging, particularly because Canada has universal access and no user fees for medically necessary health care (Department of Justice, 1984). Three important trends and their impacts are becoming evident, however. The first trend is improved health and well-being into old age (Canadian Institute for Health Information, 2004a). One important study revealed Canadian seniors today are healthier than seniors twenty years ago (Chen & Millar, 2000). This may help explain why there has been a reduction in the number of nursing home beds across Canada. Nursing home beds numbered 188,357 in the year 2001/2002, as compared with a high of 201,009 in 1991/92 (Residential care facilities, 2004). Other researchers are indicating that improved population health is not only already responsible for greater longevity, but also a higher quality of life among older adults (Swanson, Tripp-Reimer, & Buckwalter, 2001). Improved health into old age could not only reduce the length of disability and thus dependency, but also the possibility of developing acute or chronic health problems.

The second trend is improved health care services. Despite some concern that health technology advances and new medications are increasing the cost of health care (as noted in the Mazankowski or Premier's Advisory Council on Health report of 2001 [Premier's Advisory Council on Health, 2001]), these developments and advances are having profound effects through reducing the need for and use of health care services. The Canadian Institute for Health Information is a key organization in Canada for noting health care trends and outcomes. Their 2004 report clearly indicates hospital admission rates and nursing home admission rates are declining. In addition, hospital and nursing home stays are shorter.

The third major change is a shift of care from more expensive inpatient care settings to outpatient hospital or community care settings (Canadian Institute for Health Information, 2004a). One example of this is a reduction in the number of surgeries across Canada and the fact that over half of all of the surgeries in Canada now are done on a day surgery basis (Canadian Institute for Health Information, 2004a). Having surgical patients arrive for surgery, receive their surgery, and return home on the same day is beneficial in many respects. One of the most apparent benefits is a substantial reduction in hospital costs, since day surgery patients do not receive nursing and other inpatient care services over a number of days both pre- and postoperatively. Hospital access is also improved, making inpatient beds more available for persons who need care for more than 1 day. Other less apparent benefits include more rapid postoperative recovery and a reduced risk of acquiring an infection or experiencing an adverse event in hospital (Baker et al., 2004). Eye surgery is a prime example of the shift from inpatient to outpatient care, with cataract surgery the most commonly performed surgery among Canadian seniors (Hadjistavropoulos, Snider, & Hadjistavropoulos, 2001).

Despite improvements in health care services and the health care system, much more could be done to improve population health and well-being, particularly to enhance the probability of longevity among Canadians and to ensure a higher quality of life in old age. Some of these efforts need to be aimed at seniors, while others need to be aimed at younger persons, because chronic illnesses are normally acquired when younger and are carried into old age (Health in mid-life, 1999). Most chronic health problems begin in the working-age years following years of minimal exercise, inadequate sleep, poor nutrition, high-risk habits and stress-reduction behaviours such as smoking, and workplace hazards such as repetitive motion injuries (World Health Organization, 2001). Unless these personal health hazards are mitigated at retirement, declining health throughout the senior years is all but inevitable (Swanson, Tripp-Reimer, & Buckwalter, 2001). For instance, diabetes affects 4.5% of all adult Canadians now, and although new adult-onset cases are more often reported among seniors (Millar & Young, 2003), diabetes is largely a manifestation of lifelong dietary and exercise habits. Reducing the incidence of diabetes and also improving its daily management are critical health promotion imperatives for reducing the many serious complications that can arise from diabetes. Hospitalization rates are more than double (18% compared with 8% admitted each year) for adults who have diabetes (Millar & Young, 2003). Health promotion programs for seniors can be very effective, as illustrated by influenza vaccination programs (Fletcher, 2002). In 2000–2001, two out of every three seniors in Canada were vaccinated against influenza as compared with half in 1996–1997 (Johansen et al., 2004). The most common reason for not having a flu shot was not believing it was necessary, yet complications of influenza are a common cause of hospitalization and death among seniors (Menec, Black, MacWilliam, & Aoki, et al., 2003). The much higher demand for health care during the winter months is due in part to influenza (Squires, Pelletier, Zabchuk, Winchester, & Tam, 2001).

It is also important to note that seniors are highly appropriate candidates for all three forms of health promotion: primary (ie, preventing exposure of an entire population to risk factors), secondary (ie, eliminating the risks known to be affecting the health of individuals), and tertiary (ie, restoring health after illness). The relevance of tertiary health promotion for seniors has been shown by a large 2-year study involving Canadian seniors. This study found that 14% had developed some irreversible dependency while 32% had both lost and regained their independence (Martel, Belanger & Berthelot, 2002). Five risk factors for lost independence were found: advanced old age, female gender, history of stroke, a smoking habit, and physical inactivity. The majority of these risk factors are clearly amenable to primary and secondary health promotion efforts. Unfortunately, few Canadian seniors are physically active (Chen & Millar, 2001). The smoking rate among seniors is declining, although illnesses from long-term exposure to tobacco continue to be a major health problem in Canada (Illing & Kaiserman, 2004).

Although health care costs and health services utilization are normally thought to be higher for older persons than younger persons, some research is showing that younger persons are high users of health care. Seniors who were admitted to hospital had longer stays, which may be an outcome of an unmet need for formal home care because they have greater transportation and other difficulties in accessing health care (Chen & Hou, 2002). One other factor, low income, has been repeatedly identified as a key variable in higher health services utilization (Canadian Institute for Health Information, 2004a). Low income also contributes to poor diets, higher stress levels, and many other factors that predispose people to ill health (Finlayson, 2002). Approximately 20% of seniors live at or below Statistics Canada's low-income cut-off (Public Health Agency of Canada, n.d.). Some seniors are not eligible for the retirement pension funds that can be obtained through applying to the Canada Pension Plan, and many more have only these funds as a source of secure income in old age. In reality, only a small proportion of younger or older persons are high users of hospitals (Wilson & Truman, 2002) or other health services (Reid, et al., 2003). High users of health care typically suffer from multiple severe health problems (Randhowa & Riley, 1995).

ETHICAL AND LEGAL ISSUES AFFECTING THE OLDER ADULT

Loss of rights, victimization, and other grave problems face the person who has made no plans for personal and property management in the event of disability or death. The advice and services of a competent attorney regarding financial and personal issues can preserve future autonomy and self-determination. The nurse as an advocate can encourage the older person to prepare advance directives for future decision making in the event of incapacitation (Patterson et al., 1997).

A power of attorney is a legal agreement that authorizes a designated person to act in specific, outlined circumstances on behalf of the signer. Each province or territory has laws that govern this process and also govern what can be authorized. A power of attorney is normally only developed for legal and financial matters, and only when the signer would have difficulty taking care of these matters. This is a form of voluntary guardianship, usually involving a trusted family member or friend, which is freely granted by the signer. Older persons may arrange a power of attorney in advance of traveling out of country or when they develop a temporary or permanent physical disability that makes it difficult for them to pay bills. In most instances, a power of attorney is invalidated if the signer becomes mentally incompetent through illness or injury. A durable power of attorney is a similar legal agreement that continues even after mental incompetence has occurred, while a springing power of attorney only comes into effect if mental incompetence occurs. These both end if the signer recovers mental competency, the signer revokes it, or the signer dies (Chart 12-1). A legal document that only comes into effect upon death is a will. A will stipulates who will be gifted with the deceased person's belongings, such as money and property. Unfortunately, only about half of all Canadian adults develop a will and even fewer develop an enduring power of attorney. Each province or territory has a public trustee who is responsible for protecting the financial interests of vulnerable persons by administering the estate of dependent adults, deceased persons, and minors who have no one else to act for them.

In a trust, a person designates someone or an organization to manage his or property or a sum of money, and stipulates how these valuables are to be managed.

If no advance arrangement has been made, and the older person appears unable to make decisions, *anyone* can petition the court for a competency hearing. If the court rules that the person is incompetent, the judge will appoint a guardian—a third party who is given powers by the court to assume responsibility for making financial or personal decisions for that person. There are two kinds of guardians: private and public. Private guardians are normally valued and trusted family members or friends. All provinces and territories have developed an office of the public guardian, with the public guardian becoming responsible for a person's personal or nonfinancial matters if mental incompetence has occurred and no other guardian or guardians have been appointed. Because such a court action strips away the normal rights of a person to make personal or health care decisions, a potential for great harm exists. Safeguards include the following: (1) the older person must be given notice, (2) he or she must be given an opportunity to be legally represented, and (3) medical testimony can be cross-examined.

An advance directive is a formal legal document that contains a person's instructions for future health care or health care preferences (living will). Such documents are used only in the event that individuals cannot competently speak for themselves. Advance directives often state that certain treatments should not be initiated or when health care is to be withdrawn, but they can also indicate that

Chart 12-1 • Ethics and Related Issues

Should a family member, who is a primary informal caregiver, continue to care for an older relative who wants to stay at home, or is there a point when placing that person in a nursing home is both ethically and legally appropriate?

Situation

Mrs. A is an 83-year-old widow who has always lived in her own home. Her husband passed away 4 years previously. She has four children—three married sons and one divorced daughter—with two living in the same city as she does. She has become weak in the past year and is a bit forgetful, with her daughter now visiting on a daily basis to help her. Her daughter is 60 and works full time; she has a son living with her who is attending university. He has had emotional difficulties because he was laid off unexpectedly and recently separated from his wife. Mrs. A has a will, but no living will or advance directive, nor have any guardianship or related legal issues been addressed. She has said repeatedly that she wants to stay at home for the rest of her life, that she never wants to be admitted to a nursing home.

Dilemma

Mrs. A's daughter has developed diabetes and has found it increasingly difficult to manage her full schedule of work and other responsibilities. She talked with her brothers and their wives and learned they are only able to provide some financial support to pay for part-time help. Mrs. A needs help now with her daily bath, dressing and undressing, and meals. She recently left her stove on and caused a small fire in the kitchen.

Discussion

- What arguments would you offer against arranging for a nursing home placement?
- What arguments would you offer for arranging for a nursing home placement?
- Are there other alternatives that should be explored?

Resources for this case situation: Canadian Institute for Health Information. (2004a). *How healthy are Canadians? 2004 Annual Report.* Ottawa: Author; Hagen, B. (2001). Nursing home placement: Factors affecting caregivers' decisions to place family members with dementia. *Journal of Gerontological Nursing, 27*(2), 44–53; Levin, H. G., & Levitt, Z. A. (2003). Capacity assessment for admission to long-term care: A double-edged sword. *Geriatrics and Aging, 6*(6), 45–46; and Morgan, D. G., Semchuk, K. M., Stewart, N. J., & D'Arcy, C. (2002). Rural families caring for a relative with dementia: Barriers to use of formal services. *Social Science & Medicine, 55*(7), 1129–1142.

aggressive ongoing treatment is to be used to sustain life. Advance directives also normally contain the name of a proxy or substitute decision maker who would either ensure that the stated health care instructions are respected and acted upon, or make health care decisions based on the stated health care preferences. Each province and territory has unique legislation that governs how these documents are developed to ensure that they are legally binding and also what can be stated in an advance directive. Alberta's *Personal Directives Act* of 2000 states that people who are not to be involved in health care decision making can be named. Furthermore, this Act stipulates that a lawyer is not needed to develop a legal advance directive. The directive instead should be signed and dated, with two witnesses then signing and dating the document. What is common across all the provinces and territories is that advance directives are for future health care decisions; they only come into force when the maker is unable to take part in health care decisions, and they are no longer valid if the maker regains this ability.

Advance directive legislation is currently present in all Canadian provinces and territories. Most provinces and territories have also sought to educate the public about advance directives and to ensure that advance directives are used as required. All persons who make an advance directive are encouraged to distribute copies of this document to their physicians and to any person who is named as a proxy or substitute decision maker. Fines or other penalties may result if an advance directive is not adhered to. People are also encouraged to ensure that the most current copy of their advance directive is readily available for use or carefully distributed to ensure that it can be used in an emergency situation. Because only a small proportion (7.4%) of Canadians actually develop an advance directive (Bravo, Dubois, & Paquet, 2003), some health care professionals and organizations routinely ask about health care preferences. Care plans made at nursing home admission are one example. Verbal directives given by both mentally competent and incompetent persons can also impact health care decisions. The nurse is often in a position to hear verbal directives and also to learn when advance directives are not being complied with. Patient advocacy is required in both instances (Blondeau et al., 2000). Patient advocacy can be difficult, as verbal directives are not legally binding and surrogates are ultimately responsible for all decisions made.

NURSING CARE OF OLDER ADULTS

Geriatrics, the study of old age, includes the physiology, pathology, diagnosis, and management of the diseases of older adults. The broader field of **gerontology,** or the study of the aging process, draws from the biologic, psychological, and sociologic sciences. Because hospitalized patients are being discharged to home "sicker and quicker" and because of rapid population aging, nurses in all settings, including hospital, home care, rehabilitation, and outpatient settings, need to be knowledgeable about geriatric nursing principles and skilled in meeting the needs of elderly persons.

Gerontologic or **geriatric nursing** is the field of nursing that specializes in the care of the elderly. The Canadian Gerontological Nursing Association (1996) *Standards of Practice* are very useful for all nurses who provide care for elderly persons. These standards are complementary to other Canadian nursing standards of practice and codes of ethics for nurses. The nurse gerontologist can be either a specialist or a generalist offering comprehensive nursing care to older persons by combining the basic nursing process of assessment, diagnosis, planning, implementation, and evaluation with a specialized knowledge of aging. Currently, graduates from all nursing programs at universities and colleges, as well as master's or doctorally prepared advanced practice nurses (clinical nurse specialists or nurse practitioners) care for older adults.

Gerontological nursing is provided in acute care hospitals, rehabilitative and mental health hospitals, nursing homes and other residential care facilities, public health clinics and other community care settings, and the home. Its goals include promoting and maintaining functional status and helping older adults to identify and use their strengths to achieve optimal independence. The nurse helps the older person to maintain dignity and maximum autonomy despite physical, social, and psychological losses. The nurse who becomes certified in gerontologic nursing has specialized knowledge in the acute and chronic changes specific to older people. The use of advanced practice nurses (APNs) in long-term care has proved to be very effective: when APNs using current scientific knowledge about clinical problems interface with nursing home staff, significantly less deterioration in affect and overall health issues has been demonstrated (Ryden et al., 2000).

Because old age is a normal occurrence that encompasses all experiences of life, care and concern for the elderly cannot be limited to one discipline, but is best provided through a cooperative effort. An interdisciplinary team, through comprehensive geriatric assessment, can combine expertise and resources to provide insight into all aspects of the aging process. Nurses collaborate with the interdisciplinary team to obtain non-nursing services and provide a holistic approach to care.

Normal Age-Related Changes and Health Promotion Activities

Intrinsic aging (from within the person) refers to those changes caused by the normal aging process that are genetically programmed and essentially universal within a species. Universality is the major criterion used to distinguish normal from abnormal aging. Extrinsic aging results from influences outside the person. Illness and disease, air pollution, and sunlight are examples of extrinsic factors that may hasten the aging process and that can be eliminated or reduced through effective health promotion.

Cellular and extracellular changes of old age cause a change in physical appearance and a decline in function. Measurable changes in shape and body makeup occur. The body's ability to maintain homeostasis becomes increasingly diminished with cellular aging, and organ systems cannot function at full efficiency because of cellular and tissue deficits. Cells become less able to replace themselves, and they accumulate a pigment known as lipofuscin. A degradation of elastin and collagen causes connective tissue to become stiffer and less elastic.

The well-being of an aged person depends on physical, mental, social, and environmental factors. A total assessment includes an evaluation of all major body systems, social and mental status, and the ability of the person to function independently. Table 12-2 summarizes the signs and symptoms of age-related changes in the functioning of body systems and suggested nursing interventions.

PHYSICAL ASPECTS OF AGING

Cardiovascular System

Cardiovascular disease is the leading cause of death in the aged. The heart valves become thicker and stiffer, and the heart muscle and arteries lose their elasticity. Calcium and fat deposits accumulate within arterial walls, and veins become increasingly tortuous. Although function is maintained under normal circumstances, the cardiovascular system has less reserve and responds less efficiently to stress. The maximum cardiac output decreases by about 25% from age 20 to age 80. Under conditions of stress, both the maximum cardiac output and the maximum HR diminish gradually. The relationship between maximum HR and age is as follows:

$$\text{Normal maximum HR for age} = 220 - \text{age in years}$$

Hypertension has been shown to be a serious risk factor at all ages for cardiovascular disease and stroke. A diagnosis of hypertension is made only after it has been confirmed by at least two subsequent readings. In older people, hypertension is classified as follows:

Isolated systolic hypertension: the systolic reading exceeds 140 mm Hg, and the diastolic measurement is normal or near normal (less than 90 mm Hg)
Primary hypertension: the diastolic pressure is greater than or equal to 90 mm Hg regardless of the systolic pressure
Secondary hypertension: hypertension that can be attributed to an underlying cause

Table 12-2 • **Health Promotion:**
Age-Related Changes in Body Systems and Health Promotion Strategies

CHANGES	SUBJECTIVE AND OBJECTIVE FINDINGS	HEALTH PROMOTION STRATEGIES
Cardiovascular System Decreased cardiac output; diminished ability to respond to stress; heart rate and stroke volume do not increase with maximum demand; slower heart recovery rate; increased blood pressure	Complaints of fatigue with increased activity Increased heart rate recovery time Normal BP ≤140/90 mm Hg	Exercise regularly; pace activities; avoid smoking; eat a low-fat, low-salt diet; participate in stress-reduction activities; check blood pressure regularly; medication compliance; weight control
Respiratory System Increase in residual lung volume; decrease in vital capacity; decreased gas exchange and diffusing capacity; decreased cough efficiency	Fatigue and breathlessness with sustained activity; impaired healing of tissues as a result of decreased oxygenation; difficulty coughing up secretions	Exercise regularly; avoid smoking; take adequate fluids to liquefy secretions; receive yearly influenza immunization; avoid exposure to upper respiratory tract infections
Integumentary System Decreased protection against trauma and sun exposure; decreased protection against temperature extremes; diminished secretion of natural oils and perspiration	Skin appears thin and wrinkled; complaints of injuries, bruises, and sunburn; complaints of intolerance to heat; bone structure is prominent; dry skin	Avoid solar exposure (clothing, sunscreen, stay indoors); dress appropriately for temperature; maintain a safe indoor temperature; shower preferable to tub bath; lubricate skin
Reproductive System *Female:* Vaginal narrowing and decreased elasticity; decreased vaginal secretions *Male:* Decreased size of penis and testes *Male and female:* Slower sexual response	*Female:* Painful intercourse; vaginal bleeding following intercourse; vaginal itching and irritation; delayed orgasm *Male:* Delayed erection and achievement of orgasm	May require vaginal estrogen replacement; gynecology/urology follow-up; use a lubricant with intercourse
Musculoskeletal System Loss of bone density; loss of muscle strength and size; degenerated joint cartilage	Height loss; prone to fractures; kyphosis; back pain; loss of strength, flexibility, and endurance; joint pain	Exercise regularly; eat a high-calcium diet; limit phosphorus intake; take calcium and vitamin D supplements as prescribed
Genitourinary System *Male:* Benign prostatic hyperplasia	Urinary retention; irritative voiding symptoms including frequency, feeling of incomplete bladder emptying, multiple nighttime voidings	Seek referral to urology specialist; have ready access to toilet; wear easily manipulated clothing; drink adequate fluids; avoid bladder irritants (eg, caffeinated beverages, alcohol, artificial sweeteners); pelvic floor muscle exercises, preferably learned via biofeedback; consider urologic workup
Female: Relaxed perineal muscles, detrusor instability (urge incontinence), urethral dysfunction (stress urinary incontinence)	Urgency/frequency syndrome, decreased "warning time," bathroom mapping; drops of urine lost with cough, laugh, position change	Wear easily manipulated clothing; drink adequate fluids; avoid bladder irritants (eg, caffeinated beverages, alcohol, artificial sweeteners); pelvic floor muscle exercises, preferably learned via biofeedback; consider urologic workup
Gastrointestinal System Decreased salivation; difficulty swallowing food; delayed esophageal and gastric emptying; reduced gastrointestinal motility	Complaints of dry mouth; complaints of fullness, heartburn, and indigestion; constipation, flatulence, and abdominal discomfort	Use ice chips, mouthwash; brush, floss, and massage gums daily; receive regular dental care; eat small, frequent meals; sit up and avoid heavy activity after eating; limit antacids; eat a high-fibre, low-fat diet; limit laxatives; toilet regularly; drink adequate fluids
Nervous System Reduced speed in nerve conduction; increased confusion with physical illness and loss of environmental cues; reduced cerebral circulation (becomes faint, loses balance)	Slower to respond and react; learning takes longer; becomes confused with hospital admission; faintness; frequent falls	Pace teaching; with hospitalization, encourage visitors; enhance sensory stimulation; with sudden confusion, look for cause; encourage slow rising from a resting position

(continued)

Table 12-2 ● **Health Promotion:**
Age-Related Changes in Body Systems and Health Promotion Strategies (Continued)

CHANGES	SUBJECTIVE AND OBJECTIVE FINDINGS	HEALTH PROMOTION STRATEGIES
Special Senses		
Vision: Diminished ability to focus on close objects; inability to tolerate glare; difficulty adjusting to changes of light intensity; decreased ability to distinguish colours	Holds objects far away from face; complains of glare; poor night vision; confuses colours	Wear eyeglasses, use sunglasses outdoors; avoid abrupt changes from dark to light; use adequate indoor lighting with area lights and nightlights; use large-print books; use magnifier for reading; avoid night driving; use contrasting colours for colour coding; avoid glare of shiny surfaces and direct sunlight
Hearing: Decreased ability to hear high-frequency sounds	Gives inappropriate responses; asks people to repeat words; strains forward to hear	Recommend a hearing examination; reduce background noise; face person; enunciate clearly; speak with a low-pitched voice; use nonverbal cues
Taste and smell: Decreased ability to taste and smell	Uses excessive sugar and salt	Encourage use of lemon, spices, herbs

Cardiovascular dysfunction may manifest as congestive heart failure, coronary artery disease, arteriosclerosis, hypertension, intermittent claudication (leg pain caused by walking), peripheral vascular disease, orthostatic hypotension, dysrhythmias, cerebrovascular accidents (strokes), angina, or myocardial infarction (heart attack).

Heart failure (HF) is a major cause of morbidity and mortality among Canadian seniors. Older patients often present with different symptoms than those seen in younger patients. Typically, younger persons present for care with the symptoms of exertional dyspnea, orthopnea, and peripheral edema, whereas older patients typically report fatigue, nausea, and abdominal discomfort. In the younger population, men are more prone to HF, but in the elderly population far greater numbers of women develop it. Depending on its cause, HF can require various forms of therapy. The current standard therapy for HF includes diuretics, angiotensin-converting enzyme inhibitors (ACE inhibitors), and digoxin; although digoxin may only be indicated in persons with atrial fibrillation or advanced symptoms of heart failure (Heart Failure Society of America, 1999). Other common medications include beta-blockers, anticoagulant or antiplatelet drugs, cholesterol-lowering drugs, and antiarrhythmic drugs. Drug therapy has been shown to reduce the symptoms of heart failure, improve quality of life, and slow the progression of heart failure for reduced morbidity and mortality. Unfortunately, only half of all Canadians diagnosed with heart failure are alive in five years; 85% of these persons are aged 65 or older at the time of diagnosis (Lee et al., 2004).

Cardiovascular health can be promoted by regular exercise, proper diet, weight control, regular blood pressure measurements, stress management, and smoking cessation. To avoid light-headedness, fainting, and possible falls caused by orthostatic hypotension, the older person should be counselled to rise slowly (from a lying, to a sitting, to a standing position); to avoid straining when having a bowel movement; and to consider having five or six small meals each day, rather than three, to minimize the hypotension that can occur after a large meal. Extremes in temperature should be avoided, including hot showers and whirlpool baths. Yard work should be limited to no more than 20 minutes on hot summer days. Exposure to wind or cold weather also should be avoided because of the risk of dizziness or falling associated with slower adjustments of blood pressure. If an individual experiences dependent edema as the day progresses, the use of elastic compression stockings helps to minimize venous pooling.

Respiratory System

Age-related changes in the respiratory system affect lung capacity and function and include increased anteroposterior chest diameter, osteoporotic collapse of vertebrae resulting in kyphosis (increased convex curvature of the spine), calcification of the costal cartilages and reduced mobility of the ribs, diminished efficiency of the respiratory muscles, increased lung rigidity, and decreased alveolar surface area. Increased rigidity or loss of elastic recoil in the lung results in increased residual lung volume and decreased vital capacity. Gas exchange and diffusing capacity are also diminished. Decreased cough efficiency, reduced ciliary activity, and increased respiratory dead space make the older person more vulnerable to respiratory infections.

Health promotion activities that help elderly persons maintain adequate respiratory function include regular exercise, appropriate fluid intake, pneumococcal vaccination, yearly influenza immunizations, and avoidance of people who are ill. As with people of all ages, smoking cessation and frequent hand hygiene are prudent health practices. Hospitalized older adults should be frequently reminded to cough and take deep breaths, particularly postoperatively, because their decreased lung capacity and decreased cough efficiency predispose them to respiratory infections and atelectasis.

Integumentary System

The functions of the skin include protection, temperature regulation, sensation, and excretion. With aging, changes occur that affect the function and appearance of the skin. The epidermis and dermis become thinner. Elastic fibres are reduced in number, and collagen becomes stiffer. Subcutaneous fat diminishes, particularly in the extremities. Decreased numbers of capillaries in the skin result in diminished blood supply. These changes cause a loss of resiliency and wrinkling and sagging of the skin. Hair pigmentation decreases, resulting in gradual greying. The skin becomes drier and susceptible to irritations because of decreased activity of the sebaceous and sweat glands. These changes in the integument reduce tolerance to extremes of temperature and to exposure to the sun.

Strategies to promote healthy skin function include avoiding excess exposure to the sun, using a lubricating skin cream, not using strong soaps, avoiding long hot showers and soaks in the tub, and maintaining adequate fluid intake. The average fluid intake per day for adults is 1.6 litres, with an additional 700 millilitres of fluid gained through ingested foods (Innvista, n.d.).

Reproductive System

Ovarian production of estrogen and progesterone ceases with menopause. The onset of menopause is typically around 51 years of age, and although menopause is a process lasting a number of years, the vast majority of senior women are postmenopausal. Changes occurring in the female reproductive system include thinning of the vaginal wall, along with a narrowing in size and a loss of elasticity; decreased vaginal secretions, resulting in vaginal dryness, itching, and decreased acidity; involution (atrophy) of the uterus and ovaries; and decreased pubococcygeal muscle tone, resulting in a relaxed vagina and perineum. These changes contribute to vaginal bleeding and painful intercourse.

In older men, the penis and testes decrease in size, and levels of androgens diminish. Erectile dysfunction may develop with concomitant cardiovascular disease, neurologic disorders, diabetes, or even respiratory disease, which limits exercise tolerance.

Sexual desire and activity decline but do not disappear. The use of water-based lubricants can help prevent painful intercourse. Local estrogen replacement intravaginally enhances vaginal tissue without the risks and side effects of oral estrogen. Several modalities are available for treatment of erectile dysfunction, which is linked to cardiovascular, neurologic, endocrine, or occasionally psychological dysfunction. The use of vacuum penile pumps, local injection or placement of vasostimulating medication into the urethral opening, and use of an oral medication, sildenafil citrate (Viagra), have all proved effective for some patients. Sildenafil citrate is contraindicated in patients who are taking oral nitrates.

If significant sexual dysfunction is present, referral to a gynecologist or urologist is warranted. For both men and women, maintenance of a daily physical exercise routine promotes enhanced sexual performance.

Genitourinary System

The genitourinary system continues to function adequately in older people, although there is a decrease in kidney mass, primarily because of a loss of nephrons. Changes in kidney function include a decreased filtration rate, diminished tubular function with less efficiency in resorbing and concentrating the urine, and a slower restoration of acid–base balance in response to stress. Older women often suffer from stress or urge incontinence, or both. Benign prostatic hyperplasia (enlarged prostate gland), which is a common finding in older men, causes a gradual increase in urine retention and overflow incontinence. Prostate cancer, a slow-growing cancer, is most often seen in men older than 70 years of age. Kidney and bladder cancers are most frequently seen after the age of 50 years. Smoking is known to be a primary causative agent of these carcinomas.

Adequate consumption of fluids is important to reduce the risk of bladder infections and urinary incontinence. Other healthy habits include having ready access to toilet facilities and voiding every 2 to 3 hours while awake. Avoidance of bladder-irritating substances—such as caffeinated, carbonated, and acidic beverages, Nutra-sweet, and alcohol—will greatly reduce urinary urgency and frequency. Water intake should be increased to avoid concentrated urine, which causes urinary urgency.

Pelvic floor exercises, first described by Kegel (1948), can also be extremely useful in reducing the symptoms of stress and urge incontinence. Teaching the patient how to do the exercises begins with identifying the pubococcygeus muscle, which is the same muscle used to hold back flatus or to voluntarily stop the flow of urine without contracting the abdomen, buttocks, or inner thigh muscles. The pelvic muscles are first tightened and then relaxed, maintaining a 5-second contraction with 10-second rest intervals. This exercise should be routinely practiced for 30 to 80 repetitions each day; additional repetitions are discouraged because of the risk of fatigue of the muscle. Because achieving better muscle control takes at least several months to accomplish, the elderly person is encouraged to consistently perform the exercises. To maintain pubococcygeus muscle control, these daily exercises must continue indefinitely. The use of biofeedback to confirm the correct execution of these exercises increases their effectiveness significantly.

As menopause approaches, a woman's circulating estrogen decreases, and, as a result, the pelvic floor is deprived of its needed blood supply and nutrients. This causes increasing stress and urge incontinence. Through the use of biofeedback-assisted pelvic muscle exercise, an individual can successfully regain bladder function. These exercises are also recommended for men with dribbling incontinence related to prostatectomy. The nurse instructs the patient to tighten the rectal sphincter until the penis and testes slightly lift. Frequent repetition produces the desired muscle tone.

Constipation can be a major factor contributing to urinary incontinence. The patient is encouraged to eat a high-fibre diet, drink adequate fluids, and increase mobility to promote regular bowel function.

Urinary tract infections are prevalent in older women. The reasons include the effects of decreased estrogen, which shortens the urethral length, allowing easier passage of bacteria into the bladder; less overall fluid consumption, which causes a concentrated urine in which bacteria can proliferate; and the introduction of bacteria from the rectum as a result of poor bathroom hygiene secondary to impaired mobility and joint changes. Limited range of motion of the arm and limited hand dexterity often result in a woman's cleansing the perineal area in a back-to-front motion, causing bacteria such as *Escherichia coli* to be introduced to the urethral meatus and thus into the bladder (Degler, 2000b).

Gastrointestinal System

The older adult is at increased risk for impaired nutrition. Periodontal disease leading to tooth decay and loss of teeth is common. Salivary flow diminishes, and the older person may experience a dry mouth. A preference for sweet and salty foods results from a decrease of taste receptors. Major complaints often centre on feelings of fullness, heartburn, and indigestion. Gastric motility may decrease, resulting in delayed emptying of stomach contents. Diminished secretion of acid and pepsin reduces the absorption of iron, calcium, and vitamin B_{12}. Absorption of nutrients in the small intestine also appears to diminish with age. The function of the liver, gallbladder, and pancreas is generally maintained, although absorption and tolerance to fat may decrease. The incidence of gallstones and common bile duct stones increases progressively with advancing years.

Difficulty in swallowing, or dysphagia, affects between 10% and 50% of adults in acute care hospitals, and as many as 66% of nursing home residents (Dietitians in Canada, 2005). It is a serious condition that can be life-threatening. It results from interruption or dysfunction of neural pathways, such as can occur with stroke. It may also develop from dysfunction of the striated and smooth muscles of the gastrointestinal tract in up to 50% of patients with Parkinson's disease and in those with conditions such as multiple sclerosis, poliomyelitis, and amyotrophic lateral sclerosis (Lou Gehrig's disease). Aspiration of food or fluid is the most serious complication and can occur in the absence of coughing or choking (Galvan, 2001).

Constipation is common in aged people. When mild, the symptoms involve abdominal discomfort and flatulence, but more serious consequences include fecal impaction that contributes to diarrhea around the impaction, fecal incontinence, and obstruction. Predisposing factors for constipation include lack of dietary bulk, prolonged use of laxatives, the use of some medications, inactivity, insufficient fluid intake, and excessive dietary fat. Another factor may be ignoring the urge to defecate.

Gastrointestinal health promotion practices include receiving regular dental care; eating small, frequent meals; avoiding heavy activity after eating; eating a high-fibre, low-fat diet; ingesting an adequate amount of fluids; establishing regular bowel habits; and avoiding the use of laxatives and antacids. Understanding that there is a direct correlation between loss of smell and taste perception and food intake helps caregivers to intervene to maintain elderly patients' health.

Nutritional Health

The social, psychological, and physiologic functions of eating influence the dietary habits of the aged person. Decreased physical activity and a slower metabolic rate reduce the number of calories needed by the older adult to maintain an ideal weight. Apathy, immobility, depression, loneliness, poverty, inadequate knowledge, lack of oral health, and lack of taste discrimination also contribute to suboptimal nutrient intake. Budgetary constraints and physical limitations may impair food shopping and meal preparation. Education regarding healthy versus "empty-calorie" foods is helpful.

Health promotion teaching includes encouraging a diet that is low in sodium and saturated fats and high in vegetables, fruits, and fish. The older adult requires a variety of foods to maintain balanced nutrition. No more than 20% to 25% of dietary calories should be consumed as fat. Reducing salt intake is also advocated, because sodium reduction has been shown to correct hypertension in some people. Protein intake should remain the same in later adulthood as in earlier years. Carbohydrates, a major source of energy, should supply the diet with 55% to 60% of the daily calories. Simple sugars should be avoided and complex carbohydrates encouraged. Potatoes, whole grains, brown rice, and fruit provide the person with minerals, vitamins, and fibre and should be encouraged. Drinking 1.6 litres of fluid or more per day is recommended, unless contraindicated by a medical condition. A multivitamin each day may be needed by seniors who are unable to absorb ingested nutrients or who do not follow Canada's *Food Guide to Healthy Eating* recommendations (Canada's Food Guide, 1997).

Sleep

Sleep disturbances frequently occur in older people, affecting more than 50% of adults 65 years of age or older. The elderly often experience variations in their normal sleep–wake cycles, and the lack of quality sleep at night often creates the need for napping during the day. Laboratory screening can help to rule out disease processes that might be affecting an older person's ability to sleep at night. If a spouse notes excessive snoring, a sleep study is indicated to rule out sleep apnea. The nurse can recommend prudent sleep hygiene behaviours such as avoiding daytime napping, eating a light snack before bedtime, and decreasing the overall time in bed to adjust for the fewer hours of sleep needed than when the patient was younger (Grandjean & Gibbons, 2000).

Musculoskeletal System

A gradual, progressive decrease in bone mass begins before the age of 40 years. Excessive loss of bone density results in osteoporosis, which affects both older men and women but is most prevalent in postmenopausal women. It is also seen in older men who are receiving hormone treatments for prostate cancer. A higher incidence is found among northern Europeans and Asians. Its typical form is associated with inactivity, inadequate calcium intake, loss of estrogens, and a history of cigarette smoking. The danger of fracture as a result of bone reabsorption is especially high for the dorsal portion of the vertebra, humerus, radius, femur, and tibia. A loss of height occurs in later life as a result of osteoporotic changes of the spine, kyphosis (excessive convex curvature of the spine), and flexion of the hips and knees. These changes negatively affect mobility, balance, and internal organ function (Fig. 12-2).

The muscles diminish in size and lose strength, flexibility, and endurance with decreased activity and advanced age. Back pain is common. Beginning in middle age, the cartilage of joints progressively deteriorates. Degenerative joint disease is found in everyone past the age of 70 years.

FIGURE 12-2 Kyphosis, or hunchback, is a form of advanced osteoporosis.

Calcium supplements, vitamin D, fluoride, and weight-bearing exercises are often prescribed for the person who is at high risk for or already has osteoporosis. Although osteoporosis cannot be reversed, the disease process can be slowed. A bone density test is the gold standard to assess for osteoporosis. Once it is diagnosed and treatment begun, yearly follow-up determinations of the bone density level are indicated. For skeletal health, the nurse can recommend the following (Scheiber & Torregrosa, 2000):

- A high calcium intake, 1500 mg/day. Dairy products and dark green vegetables are excellent sources, as are soups and broths made with a soup bone and cooked with added vinegar to leach calcium from the bone. Calcium supplements can be recommended to ensure that the daily calcium intake is adequate.
- A higher intake of vitamin D_3 (cholecalciferol), 800 IU per day for men and women over age 50, is needed in Canada due to inadequate ultraviolet exposure to stimulate vitamin D synthesis in the skin, especially from October to March (Brown & Josse, 2002).
- A low-phosphorus diet. A calcium-to-phosphorus ratio of 1:1 is ideal; red meats, cola drinks, and processed foods that are low in calcium and high in phosphorus are avoided.
- Weight-bearing exercise. The pull of muscle insertions on the long bones strengthens the muscles and retards calcium resorption.
- Reduction of caffeine and alcohol. This assists in stopping further demineralization and renal excretion of calcium.
- Smoking cessation.
- Selective estrogen receptor modulators, such as raloxifene (Evista), preserve bone mineral density without estrogenic effects on the uterus. This medication is indicated for both prevention and treatment of osteoporosis. Although hormone replacement therapy (HRT) has been the mainstay of therapy for perimenopausal women, recent studies have demonstrated greater risks than previously recognized (Chen, Weiss, Newcomb, Barlow & White, 2002).
- The bisphosphate drugs (e.g., Fosamax, Actonel). These drugs bind to mineralized bone surfaces to inhibit osteoclastic activity and promote bone formation.

Muscle strength and flexibility can be enhanced greatly through a program of regular exercise, even for seniors with chronic illnesses or disabilities (Paterson et al., 2004). The axiom "use it or lose it" is very relevant when considering the physical capacity of aged people. The nurse plays an important role by encouraging older adults to participate in a regular exercise program. Regular exercise increases the strength and efficiency of heart contractions, improves oxygen uptake by cardiac and skeletal muscles, reduces fatigue, increases energy, and reduces cardiovascular risk factors. Muscle endurance, strength, and flexibility—all outcomes of regular exercise—also help to promote independence and psychological well-being. Aerobic exercises are the foundation of programs of cardiovascular endurance conditioning. A physical examination by a physician or nurse practitioner may be necessary before initiating an exercise program, and older persons may need to perform exercises in moderation and use short rests to avoid undue fatigue. Swimming and brisk walking are often recommended because they are managed easily and usually are enjoyed by the older person.

Information about the nature and time course of menopause-associated bone loss through early markers may be used to help to preserve bone and thus stop the natural sequelae of osteoporosis. A nurse-led research team used frequent sequential serum markers to confirm these changes and found a correlation with elevated alkaline phosphatase (ALP) and concentrations of follicle-stimulating hormone as a marker for vitamin K status. Therefore, perimenopausal women with elevated ALP can be targeted for health promotion to preserve bone density (Lukacs, 2000). Further information about osteoporosis is presented in Chapter 68.

Nervous System

The structure and function of the nervous system change with advanced age, and a reduction in cerebral blood flow accompanies nervous system changes. The loss of nerve cells contributes to a progressive loss of brain mass, and the synthesis and metabolism of the major neurotransmitters are also reduced. Because nerve impulses are conducted more slowly, older people take longer to respond and react. The autonomic nervous system performs less efficiently, and postural hypotension, which causes the person to lose consciousness or feel lightheaded on standing up quickly, may occur. Cerebral ischemia with related lightheadedness may interfere with mobility and safety. The nurse advises the person to allow a longer time to respond to a stimulus and to move more deliberately. Homeostasis is more difficult to maintain, but in the absence of pathologic changes, the older person functions adequately and retains cognitive and intellectual abilities.

Mental function is threatened by physical or emotional stresses. A sudden onset of confusion may be the first symptom of an infection or change in physical condition (pneumonia, urinary tract infection, medication interactions, dehydration, and others).

A slowed reaction time places the older person at risk for falls and injuries, including driving errors. Although seniors drive less and many voluntarily stop driving, Canadians over the age of 70 have a higher collision per kilometre rate than younger persons (Canada Safety Council, n.d.). The injury and mortality rates from motor vehicle accidents, however, are lower for persons aged 65 and older than some other age groups (Transport Canada, n.d.). Illnesses and medications may be the reason for unsafe senior drivers (DriveABLE, n.d.). Family members and other persons who witness unsafe driving, as well as physicians and persons who are trained to assess driving ability (normally occupational therapists), can recommend to the transport or motor vehicle licensing authority of each province or territory that a driver's license be suspended or revoked. The loss of a driver's licence can have a severe impact on seniors.

Sensory System

Sensory losses with old age affect all sensory organs and can be devastating to the person who cannot see to read or watch television, hear conversation well enough to communicate, or discriminate taste well enough to enjoy food.

SENSORY LOSSES VERSUS SENSORY DEPRIVATION

Sensory losses can often be helped by assistive devices such as glasses and hearing aids. In contrast, sensory deprivation is the absence of stimuli in the environment or the inability to interpret existing stimuli (perhaps as a result of a sensory loss). This deprivation can lead to boredom, confusion, irritability, disorientation, and anxiety. Meaningful sensory stimulation offered to the older person is often helpful in correcting this problem. One sense can substitute for another in observing and interpreting stimuli. The nurse can enhance sensory stimulation in the environment with colours, pictures, textures, tastes, smells, and sounds. The stimuli are most meaningful if they are interpreted to the older person and if they are changed often. Cognitively impaired persons respond well to touch and to familiar music.

VISION

As new cells form on the outside surface of the lens of the eye, the older central cells accumulate and become yellow, rigid, dense, and cloudy, leaving only the outer portion of the lens elastic enough to change shape (accommodate) and focus at near and far distances. As the lens becomes less flexible, the near point of focus gets farther away. This condition, **presbyopia**, usually begins in the fifth decade of life, and requires the wearing of reading glasses to magnify objects. In addition, the yellowing, cloudy lens causes light to scatter and makes the older person sensitive to glare. The ability to discern blue from green decreases. The pupil dilates slowly and less completely because of increased stiffness of the muscles of the iris, so the older person takes longer to adjust when going to and from light and dark environments or settings and needs brighter light for close vision. Although pathologic visual conditions are not part of normal aging, the incidence of eye disease (most commonly cataracts, glaucoma, diabetic retinopathy, and age-related macular degeneration) increases in older people.

The majority (82%) of older persons aged 65 or older experience visual problems, ranging from minor difficulties to serious impairments (Millar, 2004). Yearly eye examinations are recommended. Uncorrectable problems, such as age-related macular degeneration, are more common in persons aged 80 or older (Millar, 2004). Diabetes, glaucoma, and cataracts are the most common reasons for vision impairment in seniors; eye surgery is often required to preserve vision (Millar, 2004). The use of sunglasses and/or hats to shade the eyes is also important for eye health. Optical aids to magnify print and large-print books are available when visual problems persist.

HEARING

Presbycusis, a loss of the ability to hear high-frequency tones attributed to irreversible inner ear changes, occurs in midlife. Older people are often unable to follow conversation because tones of high-frequency consonants (letters f, s, th, ch, sh, b, t, p) all sound alike. Hearing loss may cause the older person to respond inappropriately, misunderstand conversation, and avoid social interaction. This behaviour may be erroneously interpreted as confusion. Wax buildup or other correctable problems may also be responsible for major hearing difficulties. A properly prescribed and fitted hearing aid may be useful in reducing hearing deficits.

TASTE AND SMELL

Of the four basic tastes (sweet, sour, salty, and bitter), sweet tastes are particularly dulled in older people. Blunted taste may contribute to the preference for salty, highly seasoned foods, but herbs, onions, garlic, and lemon should be encouraged as substitutes for salt to flavor food.

PSYCHOSOCIAL ASPECTS OF AGING

Successful psychological aging is reflected in the older person's ability to adapt to physical, social, and emotional losses and to achieve contentment, serenity, and life satisfactions. Because changes in life patterns are inevitable over a lifetime, the older person needs resiliency and coping skills when confronting stresses and change. A positive self-image enhances risk taking and participation in new, untested roles.

Although attitudes toward old people differ in ethnic subcultures, a subtle theme of **ageism**—prejudice or discrimination against older people—predominates in our society. It is often based on stereotypes, simplified and often untrue beliefs that reinforce society's negative image of the aged person. Elderly people make up an extremely heterogeneous group, yet negative stereotypes are attributed to all of them.

Fear of aging and the inability of many to confront their own aging process may trigger ageist beliefs. Retirement and perceived nonproductivity are also responsible for negative feelings, since the younger working person may see the older person as not contributing to society and draining economic resources. This negative image is so common that the elderly themselves often believe it. Only through an understanding of the aging process and respect for each person as an individual can the myths of aging be dispelled. If the elderly are treated with dignity and encouraged to maintain autonomy, the quality of their lives will improve.

Stress and Coping in the Older Adult

Coping patterns and the ability to adapt to stress are developed over the course of a lifetime and remain consistent later in life. Experiencing success in younger adulthood helps a person develop a positive self-image that remains solid through even the adversities of old age. A person's abilities to adapt to changes, make decisions, and respond predictably are also determined by past experiences. A flexible, well-functioning person will probably continue as such. Losses may accumulate within a short period of time, however, and become overwhelming. The older person will often have fewer choices and diminished resources to deal with stressful events. Common stressors of old age include normal aging changes that impair physical function, activities, and appearance; disabilities from chronic illness; social and environmental losses related to loss of income and decreased ability to perform previous roles and activities; and the deaths of significant others. Many older adults rely strongly on their spiritual beliefs for comfort during stressful times.

Developmental Theories of Aging

Erikson (1963) theorized that a person's life consists of eight stages, each stage representing a crucial turning point in the **life span** stretching from birth to death with its own developmental conflict to be resolved. According to Erikson, the major developmental task of old age is to either achieve ego integrity or suffer despair. Achieving ego integrity requires accepting one's lifestyle, believing that one's choices were the best that could be made at a particular time, and being in control of one's life. Despair results when an older person feels dissatisfied and disappointed with his or her life, and would live differently if given another chance.

Havighurst (1972) also suggested a list of developmental tasks that occur during a lifetime. The tasks of the older person include adjusting to retirement after a lifetime of employment with a possible reduction of income, decreases in physical strength and health, the death of a spouse, establishing affiliation with one's age group, adapting to new social roles in a flexible way, and establishing satisfactory physical living arrangements.

Combining the concepts of both Erikson and Havighurst suggests the following developmental tasks for the older adult: (1) maintenance of self-worth, (2) conflict resolution, (3) adjustment to the loss of dominant roles, (4) adjustment to the deaths of significant others, (5) environmental adaptation, and (6) maintenance of optimal levels of wellness.

Sociologic Theories of Aging

Sociologic theories of aging attempt to predict and explain the social interactions and roles that contribute to the older adult's successful adjustment to old age. The activity theory proposes that life satisfaction in normal aging requires maintaining the active lifestyle of middle age (Havighurst, 1972). The continuity theory proposes that successful adjustment to old age requires continuing life patterns across a lifetime (Atchley, 1989; Neugarten, 1961). Continuity and a connection to the past are maintained through a continuation of well-established habits, values, and interests that are integral to the person's present lifestyle.

COGNITIVE ASPECTS OF AGING

Cognition can be affected by many variables, including sensory impairment, physiologic health, environment, and psychosocial influences. Older adults may experience temporary changes in cognitive function when hospitalized or admitted to nursing homes, rehabilitation facilities, and other institutions. These changes are related to differences in environment or in medical therapy, or to alteration in role performance.

Intelligence

When intelligence test scores from people of all ages are compared (cross-sectional testing), test scores for older adults show a progressive decline beginning in midlife. Research has shown, however, that environment and health have a considerable influence on scores and that certain types of intelligence (eg, spatial perceptions and retention of nonintellectual information) decline, whereas other types do not (problem-solving ability based on past experiences, verbal comprehension, mathematical ability). Cardiovascular health, a stimulating environment, high levels of education, occupational status, and income all appear to have a positive effect on intelligence scores in later life.

Learning and Memory

The ability to learn and acquire new skills and information decreases in the older adult, particularly after the seventh decade of life. Despite this, many older people continue to learn and participate in varied educational experiences. Motivation, speed of performance, and physical status all are important influences on learning.

The components of memory, an integral part of learning, include short-term memory (5 to 30 seconds), recent memory (1 hour to several days), and long-term memory (lifetime). Acquisition of information, registration (recording), retention (storing), and recall (retrieval) are essential components of the memory process. Sensory losses, distractions, and disinterest interfere with acquiring and recording information. Age-related loss occurs more frequently with short-term and recent memory; in the absence of a pathologic process, this is called benign senescent forgetfulness. A nurse considers the process by which older adults learn when he or she uses the following strategies:

- Supplies mnemonics to enhance recall of related data
- Encourages ongoing learning
- Links new information with familiar information
- Uses visual, auditory, and other sensory cues
- Encourages learners to wear prescribed glasses and hearing aids
- Provides glare-free lighting
- Provides a quiet, nondistracting environment
- Sets short-term goals with input from the learner
- Keeps teaching periods short
- Paces learning tasks according to the endurance of the learner
- Encourages verbal participation by learners
- Reinforces successful learning in a positive manner

ENVIRONMENTAL ASPECTS OF AGING

About 95% of the elderly live in the community, as compared with 5% who live in a nursing home (MacKnight et al., 2003). Advanced physical dependency and dementia are the most common reasons for institutionalization. The 2001 Canadian census revealed that 23% of men and 35% of women aged 85 and older lived in nursing homes (Statistics Canada, n.d). The proportion of seniors, even among the oldest-old seniors, who live in nursing homes has been declining for a number of decades. Most community-dwelling seniors live in their own residence, either with a spouse or alone. A considerable and growing proportion of community-dwelling seniors live alone (29%), with older women twice as likely to live alone as older men (35% compared with 16%) (Statistics Canada, 2001). In 2001, only 35% of Canadian women aged 65 or older lived with a spouse or partner as compared with 61% of senior men. Census data also revealed 12% to 13% of older people live with one of their adult children and 6.5% live with a grandchild.

Living Arrangement Options

Ideally, older persons do best in their own, familiar environment. But adjustments to the environment may be required to allow the older adult to remain in his or her own home or apartment. Sometimes, in order to enable them to remain in their own home, an older adult or couple seek out family members who might be willing to live in the home, or agree to board someone in exchange for completion of household chores (Che-Alford & Stevenson, 1998).

Sometimes older adults or couples agree to move in with adult children. This can be a rewarding experience as the children, their parents, and the grandchildren interact and share household responsibilities. It can also be stressful, depending on the family dynamics. Adult children and their older parents may also choose to pool their financial resources by moving into a house that has an attached "in-law suite." This arrangement provides security for the older adult along with privacy for both families.

Retirement communities are becoming more popular, with older people now having the option to move into one of the many types of supportive living options. Moving to a community-care setting specifically designed to support seniors, particularly if a need for assistance develops, is a much more appealing option than being forced through ill health to move into a nursing home. There are many excellent nursing homes, but nursing homes typically only provide total care near the end of life. This level of care is not needed or desired by most seniors. Older people are aware that they may need increasing assistance over time, with many making housing and other living arrangements in advance (Che-Alford & Stevenson, 1998). Many different community-care options currently exist in Canada, including lodges, group homes, seniors' apartment or condominium complexes, supportive housing, retirement facilities, and assisted living (Public Health Agency of Canada, n.d.). These are private options, as opposed to nursing homes, which are considered public because of specific government regulation and public funding. Web-based or print guidelines exist to help seniors choose among these options (ie, Canadian Health Network, Veterans Affairs Canada, CBC News, and The Care Guide).

Assisted living facilities are an option when physical or cognitive changes require at least minimal supervision. Assisted living allows for a degree of independence while providing minimal nursing assistance (eg, administration of medication and coordination of scheduled and acute care medical assistance). Other services, such as laundry, cleaning, and meals, may also be included.

Although widely considered a public or government responsibility, nursing homes in Canada are not always government owned and operated. Regardless, nursing homes are subject to provincial or territorial nursing home and other standards, such as health care accreditation standards, and all are subsidized through government funding. Approximately three quarters of the total cost of nursing home care is met through government funding. The portion paid by government addresses the cost of the nursing care and other health care services in nursing homes, as required by the *Canada Health Act* since these are "extended health care services." Nursing home residents pay the residential care or "hotel" costs, the same costs they would incur if they paid for rent or utilities elsewhere. This residential care cost is also paid by persons in hospitals who must wait many weeks or months for a nursing home to become available, because nursing homes have high (96 to 99%) occupancy rates. These long stays in hospital are a serious issue, because these beds are consequently not available for persons who are acutely ill. Also, there are risks for long-stay seniors because of the greater probability of acquiring a hospital superbug and experiencing a medical or other error (Baker et al., 2004). An increasing number of nursing homes are offering subacute care, which permits earlier hospital discharge. Some nursing homes also offer day care programs, palliative care programs, and respite care programs. These programs provide short-term care for seniors, which may be needed by family caregivers who work, need a vacation, or must renovate their home to accommodate a wheelchair.

Life Care Planning

A life care plan is an individualized document that outlines what has been assessed with regard to current and future health care and living arrangement needs (National Advisory Council on Aging, 2003). All persons upon admission to a nursing home have a life care plan or nursing care plan developed (Chart 12-2). Many community-based seniors develop their own life care plan, although most of these are not in written form. Bravo and colleagues' (2003) study of community-living seniors in Quebec found that 42.3% had an informal advance directive for health care. These were more common among older persons, women, and persons who had known someone with a cognitive impairment. Receiving a diagnosis of a serious life-limiting illness is a common reason for life care planning. Life planning provides valuable information regarding factors that can radically affect a senior's health care and quality of life. Life care plans are helpful when life circumstances change.

The Role of the Family

Planning for care and understanding the psychosocial issues confronting the older person must be accomplished within the context of the family. If dependency needs occur, the spouse often assumes the role of primary caregiver. In the absence of the surviving spouse, an adult child usually assumes caregiver responsibilities and may eventually need help in providing care and support. Two common myths are that adult children and their aged parents are socially alienated and that adult children abandon their parents when health and other dependency problems arise. Extensive

---

Chart 12-2   Life Care Plan Components

Medical history
Social history
Family issues
Vocational/educational history
Projected medical evaluations
Projected physical and occupational therapy needs
Future medical care and medications
Therapeutic supplies
Personal items
Diagnostic testing
Medical equipment and supply needs
Recreational equipment
Aids for independent function
Home/facility care
Transportation needs
Architectural renovations
Potential medical complications
Compromised financial status

Adapted with permission from Schuman, J. (2001). Old concept, new trends: A primer on life care planning. *Long-Term Care Interface, 2,* 28.

---

research refutes both of these beliefs. The family is an important source of support for older people (Fig. 12-3). Approximately 80% of elderly persons today have living children. A high proportion of elderly persons live near one or more of their children, and it is common for family members to move so that they can live in close proximity (Cranswick, 1999). Even when children and their parents do not live close to each other, the majority of seniors in Canada are in contact with their children at least once a month.

Social attitudes and cultural values often dictate that adult children should provide services and financial support and assume the burden of care if their aged parents are unable to care for themselves. Illness creates special problems for people who live

FIGURE 12-3 Families are an important source of psychosocial and physical support for elders and youngsters alike. Caring interaction among grandchildren, grandparents, and other family members typically contributes to the health of all.

alone. If community agencies or adult children are unable to provide care, elders are at high risk for institutionalization.

Regardless of the amount of responsibility and love an adult child exhibits toward dependent elderly parents, strains can develop if care continues for a long period. Research exploring the relationship between aged parents and their adult children shows that the quality of the parent–child relationship changes with the poor health of the parent. Under certain circumstances of high risk, strains in intergenerational relationships can result in elder abuse (Hoban & Kearney, 2000; Phillips, 2000).

Elder abuse is an active or passive act or behaviour that is harmful to the elderly person. Such behaviour includes physical violence, personal neglect, financial exploitation, violation of rights, denial of health care, and self-inflicted abuse. Dauvergne (2003) found, through the 1999 General Social Survey, that 7% of seniors experienced emotional abuse, 1% experienced financial abuse, and 1% experienced physical or sexual violence, with 37% sustaining minor injury and 2% suffering major physical injury or death. Most often their children or their spouse were the abuser(s) (Canadian Network for the Prevention of Elder Abuse, n.d.; National Clearinghouse on Family Violence, n.d.; World Health Organization, 2002). Preventive action should be taken when strains are evident, before elder abuse occurs. Interdisciplinary team members can be enlisted to help the caregiver develop self-awareness, increased insight, and an understanding of the aging process. At the same time, community resources may be useful for both the aged person and the caregiver (Canadian Network for the Prevention of Elder Abuse, n.d.; National Clearinghouse on Family Violence, n.d.; World Health Organization, 2002).

Community Support Services

Many community supports exist that help the older person maintain independence. Informal sources of help, such as family, friends, the mail carrier, church members, and neighbors, can all keep an informal watch. Government and non-government organizations perform many community services, including telephone reassurance, friendly visitors, home repair services, and home-delivered meals. Homemaker and chore services can be obtained at an hourly rate through these agencies or through local community nursing services. If a person is unable to pay, these services may be subsidized through local and state funds.

Other community support services are available to help the older person outside the home. Senior centres have social and health promotion activities, and some provide a nutritious noontime meal. Adult day care facilities offer daily nursing care and social opportunities; these services also enable family members to carry on daily activities while the older person is at the day care centre.

Home Health Care

Home care is an option for shortening hospital stays and preventing hospitalization, particularly among frail or chronically ill seniors. Home care may also be palliative, with end-of-life care support provided to enable a senior to die at home or to stay at home as long as possible. Even though formal home care services are listed as one of the "extended health care services" in the *Canada Health Act,* home care services vary considerably by province or territory. Many studies have indicated that formal home care services are inadequate in Canada. One study that used a provincial home care database found that only one in five persons who died in that province had received home care, only half of all seniors admitted to nursing homes had received home care, home care recipients typically received less than 1 hour of home care each

day, and home care was normally received for only a few weeks or months at a time (Wilson & Truman, 2004a, 2004b).

Home care services have been increasing; however (Wilson et al., in press) this increase has been relatively minimal, in terms of dollars for health care and the availability of services. The Commission on the Future of Health Care (2002) recommended both a national home care program and substantial increases in government funding for home care in their final report entitled *Building on Values. The Future of Health Care in Canada.* Home care services (such as basic personal care provided by nursing aides, registered nurse care, and other specialized care from respiratory therapists, physical therapists, or others) are particularly important for seniors, because these services not only can enable earlier discharge from hospital, but can also prevent the need for hospital or nursing home admission. Home care services are often credited with stabilizing and improving the health of seniors. Formal home care services, such as respite care, can also reduce the burden of responsibility and hours of care for informal caregivers (Hodgetts, Pullman, & Goto, 2003). A 1996 General Social Survey revealed that 83% of Canadian women and 89% of men who provided 7.5 hours or more each week to a senior felt they were burdened by this care (Frederick & Fast, 1999). A more recent General Social Survey revealed that Canadian women caregivers provide an average of 29.6 hours of informal care each month, while caregiving men provide 16.1 hours of care each month (Stobert & Cranswick, 2004). This same survey revealed that 16% of younger Canadians (aged 45 to 64) provided informal care to their parents or their spouse's parents (Stobert & Cranswick, 2004). One of every 12 seniors (8%) also provided informal care for a contemporary who was restricted by long-term disabilities, commonly physical limitations. This study and many others have found that women are the most frequent informal care providers. The 1998 General Social Survey revealed that 6 of every 10 hours of informal care were provided by women (Zukewich, 2003). Although considerable concern exists about this burden and the effect of this burden on the health and well-being of informal caregivers, many positives may also occur through providing care to a family member or friend (Koop & Strang, 2003).

Safety and Comfort in the Home Environment

Injuries have serious mortality and morbidity implications for older people. One third of seniors fall each year, with one quarter of these falls resulting in serious injuries, such as fractures (An Inventory of Canadian Programs, 2001). Many seniors never fully recover from these injuries. A recent Ontario study found 41% of seniors living at home restricted their social outings and physical activities because of falling (Fletcher & Hirdes, 2004). The nurse can encourage lifestyle and environmental changes that older adults and their families can adopt. Adequate lighting with minimal glare and shadow can be achieved through the use of small area lamps, indirect lighting, sheer curtains to diffuse direct sunlight, dull rather than shiny surfaces, and nightlights. Sharply contrasting colours can be used to mark the edges of stairs. Grab bars by the tub and toilet are useful. Loose clothing, improperly fitting shoes, scatter rugs, small objects, and pets create hazards and increase the risk of falls. A person functions best in familiar settings if furniture and objects remain as unchanged as is safely possible.

Hospice Palliative Care Services

Hospice palliative care is a dignified and effective alternative to curative or treatment-oriented care when a person nears the end of life. Hospice palliative care, as defined on the Canadian Hospice

Palliative Care Association's website, is "care that aims to relieve suffering and improve the quality of living and dying" (Canadian Hospice Palliative Care Association, n.d.). All hospitals, nursing homes, and home care agencies today provide comfort-oriented end-of-life care to dying persons, although this care is usually provided by nurses and physicians who have not specialized in hospice palliative care. End-of-life care as defined as the final stage preceding death is typically only 1 to 3 days in duration (Hall, Schroeder, & Weaver, 2002), although some people have longer dying processes (Wilson, 2002a).

The first hospice palliative care programs were initiated in Canadian hospitals in the mid-1970s. Hospice palliative care has since branched into the community, generally in the form of comprehensive multidisciplinary programs that provide care across a continuum of care settings. A few freestanding hospices also exist in Canada. Although the proportion of dying Canadians needing specialized hospice palliative care has never been established, only approximately 5% of the 220,000 persons who die each year receive such care (Special Senate Committee, 2000). These persons are typically younger and are experiencing physically or emotionally difficult dying processes. The need for additional specialized hospice palliative care programs has been evident for some time now (Brazil et al., 2003), as reflected in both the 1995 Special Senate Committee report *Of Life and Death,* completed in response to a request for the legalization of assisted suicide in Canada, and their subsequent 2000 report *Quality End-of-Life Care: The Right of Every Canadian.* End-of-life care issues primarily impact seniors, as three of every four persons who die each year in Canada are 65 years of age or older (Northcott & Wilson, 2002). In 2000, only 2% of all deaths involved young persons (birth to age 21 inclusive), while 20% of all deaths involved people aged 86 or older (Figure 12-4). One major development in 2004 was the passing of national legislation, *Employment Insurance (EI) Compassionate Care Benefits.* Compassionate care benefits (or lost wages) may be received for a maximum of 6 weeks by a primary informal caregiver who is absent from work and providing care or support to a family member who is considered at risk of dying within 26 weeks. For further discussion of hospice care and services see Chapter 17.

Nurses are in a unique position to facilitate early discussions about a patient's wishes and goals at the end of life. Too often, discussion regarding end-of-life care is postponed until a crisis situation occurs, making it difficult or impossible for the patient to be an active participant in the discussion. Nurses can assist the patient and family with identifying available options and initiating conversation about preparing an end-of-life plan (Norlander & McSteen, 2000).

PHARMACOLOGIC ASPECTS OF AGING

Although almost all Canadians take one or more prescribed medications each year, older people generally use one or more on a daily basis (Canadian Institute for Health Information, 2004a). Canadian seniors purchase 45% of all prescription drugs sold, yet they comprise only 13% of the population (Health Canada, 2002). The most common prescription medications used by seniors are heart or blood pressure medications (45% and 35% of older men and women, respectively) and pain relievers (33% and 30% of older women and men, respectively), followed by diuretics, stomach remedies, and laxatives (Health Canada, 2002). Rising concern over the use of medications by seniors is evident in Canada (Bronskill et al., 2004). Medications have improved the health and well-being of older people by alleviating symptoms of discomfort, treating chronic illnesses, and curing infectious processes. Problems commonly occur, however, because of medication interactions, multiple medication effects, multiple medication use (**polypharmacy**), and noncompliance. Combinations of prescription medications and some over-the-counter medications further complicate the problem.

Any medication is capable of altering nutritional status, which, in the elderly, may already be compromised by a marginal diet or

FIGURE 12-4 Age at death in Canada (2000). Source: Statistics Canada 2000 mortality data, purchased through an NHRDP research grant and a University of Alberta research grant, with data also analyzed by D. M. Wilson.

by chronic disease and its treatment. Medications can depress the appetite, cause nausea and vomiting, irritate the stomach, cause constipation or diarrhea, and decrease absorption of nutrients. In addition, they can alter electrolyte balance and carbohydrate and fat metabolism. A few examples of medications capable of altering the nutritional status are antacids, which produce thiamine deficiency; cathartics, which diminish absorption; antibiotics and phenytoin, which reduce utilization of folic acid; and phenothiazines, estrogens, and corticosteroids, which increase food intake and cause weight gain.

Altered Pharmacokinetics

Pharmacokinetics is the study of the actions of medications in the body, including the processes of absorption, distribution, metabolism, and excretion. Variability in these processes in older people (Table 12-3) is caused, in part, by a reduced capacity of the liver and kidneys to metabolize and excrete the medications and

by lowered efficiency of the circulatory and nervous systems in coping with the effect of certain medications. Many medications and their metabolites are excreted by the kidney. With advanced age, body weight, total body water, lean body mass, and plasma albumin (protein) all decrease, while body fat increases. Consequently, agents that are highly protein-bound have fewer binding sites and higher pharmacologic activity, whereas fat-soluble agents have more binding sites, and therefore enhanced storage and delayed elimination.

Nursing Implications

The nurse administering medications to older people must be aware of the following:

- Medications removed from the body primarily by renal excretion remain in the body for a longer time in people with decreased renal function. Often dosages must be reduced,

---

Table 12-3 • **Altered Drug Responses in Older People**

AGE-RELATED CHANGES	EFFECT OF AGE-RELATED CHANGE	APPLICABLE MEDICATIONS
Absorption		
Reduced gastric acid; increased pH (less acid)	Rate of drug absorption—possibly delayed	
Reduced gastrointestinal motility; prolonged gastric emptying	Extent of drug absorption—not affected	
Distribution		
Decreased albumin sites	Serious alterations in drug binding to plasma proteins (the unbound drug gives the pharmacologic response); highly protein-bound medications have fewer binding sites, leading to increased effects and accelerated metabolism and excretion	Selected highly protein-binding medications: Oral anticoagulants (warfarin) Oral hypoglycemic agents (sulfonylureas) Barbiturates Calcium channel blockers Furosemide (Lasix) Nonsteroidal anti-inflammatory drugs (NSAIDs) Sulfonamides Quinidine Phenytoin (Dilantin)
Reduced cardiac output	Decreased perfusion of many bodily organs	
Impaired peripheral blood flow	Decreased perfusion	
Increased percentage of body fat	Proportion of body fat increases with age, resulting in increased ability to store fat-soluble medications; this causes drug accumulation, prolonged storage, and delayed excretion	Selected fat-soluble medications: Barbiturates Diazepam (Valium) Lidocaine Phenothiazines (antipsychotics) Ethanol Morphine
Decreased lean body mass	Decreased body volume allows higher peak levels of medications	
Metabolism		
Decreased cardiac output and decreased perfusion of the liver	Decreased metabolism and delay of breakdown of medications, resulting in prolonged duration of action, accumulation, and drug toxicity	All medications metabolized by the liver
Excretion		
Decreased renal blood flow; loss of functioning nephrons; decreased renal efficiency	Decreased rates of elimination and increased duration of action; danger of accumulation and drug toxicity	Selected medications with prolonged action: Aminoglycoside antibiotics Cimetidine (Tagamet) Chlorpropamide (Diabinase) Digoxin Lithium Procainamide

because overdosage and medication toxicity at usual therapeutic dosages are common.

- Medications with a narrow safety margin (eg, digitalis glycosides) must be administered cautiously.
- A decline in cardiac output may decrease the delivery rate to the target organ or storage tissue.
- The circulatory and central nervous systems of older people are less able to cope with the effects of certain medications, even when blood levels are normal.
- Idiosyncratic or unusual responses to medications may manifest as toxic reactions and complications.
- As a result of a slowing metabolism, medication levels may increase in the tissues and plasma, leading to prolonged medication action.
- Many elderly people have multiple medical problems that require treatment with one or more medications. The possibility of interactions between medications is further magnified if the older person is also taking one or more over-the-counter medications.
- A high-fibre diet and the use of psyllium (Metamucil) or other laxatives may accelerate gastrointestinal transport and reduce absorption of medications taken concurrently.
- If, for any reason, a patient is not dependable about taking medication, the nurse must be sure that the pill or capsule is actually swallowed and not retained between the cheeks and the gums or teeth.

Teaching self-administration of medication requires asking the patient questions and requesting return demonstrations to ensure that learning has occurred. Sensory and memory losses, as well as decreased manual dexterity, can affect the patient's ability to carry out instructions properly, and the teaching plan will need to be adjusted to meet each patient's needs. The following steps taken by the nurse can help the patient to manage his or her medications and improve compliance:

- Explain the action, side effects, and dosage of each medication.
- Write out the medication schedule.
- Encourage the use of standard containers without safety lids (if there are no children in the household).
- Suggest the use of a multiple-day, multiple-dose medication dispenser to help patients adhere to the medication schedule (Fig. 12-5).
- Destroy old, unused medications.
- Review the medication schedule periodically.
- Discourage the use of over-the-counter medications and herbal agents without consulting a health professional.
- Encourage the patient to take all medications, including over-the-counter medications, with him or her regularly when visiting the primary health care provider.

FIGURE 12-5 Commercially available, multiple-dose, multiple-day medication dispensers, such as this one, help older people to follow complex medication regimens safely at home.

Physical Health Problems in Older Populations

GERIATRIC SYNDROMES: MULTIPLE PROBLEMS WITH MULTIPLE ETIOLOGIC FACTORS

The frail elderly frequently experience multiple problems, or syndromes. Illness, whether acute or chronic, generally results from several factors rather than from a single cause. When combined with a decrease in host resistance, these factors lead to illness or injury. Although the problems may have developed slowly, the onset of symptoms is often acute. Furthermore, the presenting symptoms may appear in other body systems before becoming apparent in the affected system. The term "frail" is used to describe those elders who are at highest risk for adverse health outcomes or geriatric syndromes. There are no standard clinical criteria for frailty. According to the most widely agreed on definition, frail people are those who are most vulnerable to significant problems because they meet one or more of the following conditions:

- Being 85 years of age or older
- Being unable to perform IADLs or ADLs independently
- Suffering from multiple chronic diseases

As with specific illnesses, geriatric syndromes are never a normal consequence of aging. Early intervention can prevent further complications and help to maximize the quality of life for many older people (Hazzard et al., 1999).

Impaired Mobility

The causes of decreased mobility are many and varied. Common causes are Parkinson's disease, diabetic neuropathy, cardiovascular compromise, osteoarthritis, osteoporosis, and sensory deficits. Environmental barriers and iatrogenic factors are also significant. Elderly patients should be encouraged to stay as active as possible to avoid the downward spiral of immobility. During illness, bed rest should be kept to a minimum, because even brief periods of bed rest quickly lead to deconditioning and, consequently, to a wide range of complications. When bed rest cannot be avoided, the patient should perform active range-of-motion and strengthening exercises with the unaffected extremities, and the nurse should perform passive range-of-motion exercises on the affected extremities. Frequent position changes help offset the hazards of immobility. Both the staff and the patient's family can assist in maintaining the current level of mobility (Tappen, Roach, Applegate, & Stowell, 2000).

Dizziness

Older people frequently seek help for dizziness, which presents a particular challenge because there are so many possible internal and external causes. For many, the problem is further complicated because of an inability to differentiate between the true dizziness (a sensation of disorientation in relation to position) and vertigo (a spinning sensation). Other similar sensations include near-syncope and disequilibrium. The causes for these sensations range in severity from minor, as in a buildup of ear wax, to severe, as in dysfunction of the cerebral cortex, cerebellum, brain stem, proprioceptive receptors, or the vestibular system. Even a minor reversible cause, such as an ear wax impaction, can result in a loss of balance and a subsequent fall and injury. Because of the many predisposing factors, nurses should seek to identify potentially treatable factors related to the dizziness. This impairment reduction strategy may reduce the vulnerability of older persons to injury (Tinetti, Williams, & Gill, 2000).

Falls and Falling

Falling is a common and preventable source of mortality and morbidity in older adults. As the major cause of trauma in the elderly, falls are not often fatal but do threaten health and the quality of life. Normal and pathologic consequences of aging that contribute to increased falls include visual changes such as loss of depth perception, susceptibility to glare, loss of visual acuity, and difficulty in light accommodation. Neurologic changes include loss of balance, dizziness, loss of position sense, and delayed reaction time (Ruckenstein, 2001). Cardiovascular changes may result in cerebral hypoxia and postural hypotension. Cognitive changes include confusion, loss of judgment, and impulsive behaviour. Musculoskeletal changes include altered posture and decreased muscle strength. Use of many medications, medication interactions, and alcohol precipitate falls by causing drowsiness, incoordination, and postural hypotension. Osteoporosis-related fractures can have a negative effect on the individual's ability to maintain an independent living arrangement (Peterson, 2001).

Overall, elderly women who fall sustain a greater degree of injury than do elderly men. The most common fracture occurring from a fall is hip fracture resulting from the combined comorbidities of osteoporosis and the condition or situation that provoked the fall. Studies have shown that elderly people who fall experience a greater decline in their ability to perform ADLs and social activities, have a greater chance of being institutionalized, and use more health care services than elderly people who do not fall (Division of Aging and Seniors, 2002).

In institutionalized elderly people, restraints in the form of physical modalities (lap belts; geriatric chairs; vest, waist, and jacket restraints) and chemical modalities (medications) are known to precipitate many of the injuries they were meant to prevent. Documented injuries and deaths resulting from these restraints include strangulation, vascular and neurologic damage, pressure ulcers, skin tears, fractures, increased confusion, and significant emotional trauma. The time required to supervise restrained patients adequately is better used addressing the unmet need that provoked the behaviour that resulted in the use of restraint. Because of the overwhelming negative consequences of restraint use, the accrediting agencies of nursing homes and acute care facilities now maintain stringent guidelines concerning their use.

Urinary Incontinence

Urinary incontinence can be acute, developing during an illness, or it can develop chronically over a period of years. The older patient often does not report this very common problem unless specifically asked. Transient causes may be attributed to *d*elirium and dehydration; *r*estricted mobility and restraints; *i*nflammation, infection, and impaction; and *p*harmaceuticals and polyuria (use the acronym DRIP to remember them). Once identified, the causative factor can be eliminated. Established incontinence may be a result of neurologic or structural abnormalities (Degler, 2000b).

The pelvic floor serves as the supporting mechanism or "hammock" for the bladder, uterus, and rectum. It may have become weakened as a result of pregnancy, labour and delivery, prior pelvic surgeries, or work that required prolonged standing or lifting. Dysfunction of the pelvic floor can be greatly improved with Kegel exercises. Other measures that help prevent episodes of incontinence include having quick access to toilet facilities and wearing clothing that can be unfastened easily. Incontinence pads may be needed.

The patient with this problem should be urged to seek help from appropriate health personnel, because incontinence can be as emotionally devastating as it is physically debilitating. Nurses who specialize in behavioural approaches to urinary incontinence management are particularly successful in assisting an individual either to regain continence or to significantly improve the level of continence. Although medications such as anticholinergics may decrease some of the symptoms of urge incontinence (detrusor instability), their side effects (dry mouth, slowed gastrointestinal motility, and confusion) may make them inappropriate choices for the elderly. Various surgical procedures are also used to manage urinary incontinence, particularly stress urinary incontinence.

Detrusor hyperactivity with impaired contractility is a type of urge incontinence that is seen predominantly in the elderly population. In this variation of urge incontinence, the patient has absolutely no warning that he or she is about to lose urine. When toileted, the patient often voids only a small volume of urine or none at all, then experiences a large volume of incontinence after leaving the bathroom. The nursing staff should be familiar with this form of incontinence and should not show disapproval to the patient. Many patients with dementia suffer from this type of incontinence because both incontinence and dementia are a result of dysfunction in similar areas of the brain. Prompted, timed voiding can be of assistance to these individuals, although clean intermittent catheterization is the preferred management.

ACQUIRED IMMUNODEFICIENCY SYNDROME IN OLDER ADULTS

According to the Centre for Infectious Disease Prevention and Control (2004), 8.3% of the 56,000 Canadians who have received a positive HIV test since 1985 (when testing began) were age 50 and older at the time of diagnosis. HIV drug and treatment advances are helping many younger HIV-infected adults live to old age. The most common AIDS-indicator disease in the older person is *Pneumocystis carinii* pneumonia. Wasting syndrome and HIV encephalopathy are also common in older HIV-infected people. Survival time is significantly shorter in older patients than in younger patients with AIDS (Ory & Mack, 1998).

Common Mental Health Problems in Older Populations

Older adults are less likely than younger people to seek treatment for mental health symptoms, so health professionals are challenged to recognize, assess, refer, collaborate, treat, and support those older adults who exhibit noticeable changes in intellect or affect. In a community setting, the nurse may be the only health care provider who has contact with the person. Symptoms should not be dismissed as age-related changes; a thorough assessment may reveal a treatable, reversible physical or mental condition.

DEPRESSION

Depression is the most common affective or mood disorder of old age and is often responsive to treatment. Its classification and diagnosis vary according to the number, severity, and duration of symptoms. Depression disrupts quality of life, increases the risk of suicide, and becomes self-perpetuating. It may also be an early sign of a chronic illness or the result of physical illness. Signs of depression include feelings of sadness, fatigue, diminished memory and concentration, feelings of guilt or worthlessness, sleep disturbances, appetite disturbances with excessive weight loss or gain, restlessness, impaired attention span, and suicidal ideation.

Although depression among the elderly is widespread, it is often undiagnosed and untreated. Attentive clinical evaluation is essential. Geriatric depression and symptoms of dementia often overlap, so cognitive impairment may be a result of depression rather than dementia. When depression and medical illnesses coexist, as they often do, neglect of the depression can retard physical recovery. Symptoms might be secondary to a medication interaction or an undiagnosed physical condition. Assessing the patient's mental status, including assessing for depression, is vital and must not be overlooked (Charts 12-3 and 12-4).

Depressive illness in late life should be vigorously treated with antidepressants. Psychosocial approaches have also been found to be effective. Selective serotonin reuptake inhibitors, such as paroxetine (Paxil), are clinically useful and exhibit rapid action with a low occurrence of adverse effects. Tricyclic antidepressants, specifically nortriptyline (Aventyl), desipramine (Norpramin), and doxepin (Sinequan), are also clinically effective for depression. Anticholinergic, cardiac, and orthostatic side effects, as well as interactions with other medications, require that these agents be used with care: the dosage must be managed carefully to relieve symptoms

Chart 12-3 Mini-Mental State Examination

Maximum Score

Orientation
5 What is the (year) (season) (date) (day) (month)?
5 Where are we (state) (county) (city) (hospital) (floor)?

Registration
3 Name three objects: One second to say each. Then ask the patient all three after you have said them. Give one point for each correct answer. Repeat them until he learns all three. Count trials and record number. Number of trials: _____.

Attention and calculation
5 Begin with 100 and count backwards by 7 (stop after five answers). Alternatively, spell "world" backwards.

Recall
3 Ask for the three objects repeated above. Give one point for each correct answer.

Language
2 Show a pencil and a watch, and ask subject to name them.
1 Repeat the following: "No 'if's,' 'and's,' or 'but's.'"
3 A three-stage command: "Take a paper in your right hand; fold it in half, and put it on the floor."
1 Read and obey the following: (Show subject the written item.) CLOSE YOUR EYES.
1 Write a sentence.
1 Copy a design (complex polygon as in Bender-Gestalt).
30 Total score possible

Reprinted from Folstein, M. F., Folstein, S., & McHugh, P. R. (1975). Mini-mental state: A practical method for grading the cognitive state of patients for the clinician. *Journal of Psychiatric Research, 12,* 189–198. With permission from Pergamon Press Ltd, Headington Hill Hall, Oxford OX3 OBW, UK.

Chart 12-4 Geriatric Depression Scale

Choose the best answer for how you felt this past week.

*1.	Are you basically satisfied with your life?	YES	NO
2.	Have you dropped many of your activities and interests?	YES	NO
3.	Do you feel that your life is empty?	YES	NO
4.	Do you often get bored?	YES	NO
*5.	Are you hopeful about the future?	YES	NO
6.	Are you bothered by thoughts you can't get out of your head?	YES	NO
*7.	Are you in good spirits most of the time?	YES	NO
8.	Are you afraid that something bad is going to happen to you?	YES	NO
*9.	Do you feel happy most of the time?	YES	NO
10.	Do you often feel helpless?	YES	NO
11.	Do you often get restless and fidgety?	YES	NO
12.	Do you prefer to stay at home, rather than going out and doing new things?	YES	NO
13.	Do you frequently worry about the future?	YES	NO
14.	Do you feel you have more problems with memory than most?	YES	NO
*15.	Do you think it is wonderful to be alive now?	YES	NO
16.	Do you often feel downhearted and blue?	YES	NO
17.	Do you feel pretty worthless the way you are now?	YES	NO
18.	Do you worry a lot about the past?	YES	NO
*19.	Do you find life very exciting?	YES	NO
20.	Is it hard for you to get started on new projects?	YES	NO
*21.	Do you feel full of energy?	YES	NO
22.	Do you feel that your situation is hopeless?	YES	NO
23.	Do you think that most people are better off than you are?	YES	NO
24.	Do you frequently get upset over little things?	YES	NO
25.	Do you frequently feel like crying?	YES	NO
26.	Do you have trouble concentrating?	YES	NO
*27.	Do you enjoy getting up in the morning?	YES	NO
28.	Do you prefer to avoid social gatherings?	YES	NO
*29.	Is it easy for you to make decisions?	YES	NO
*30.	Is your mind as clear as it used to be?	YES	NO

Score: _____ *(Number of "depressed" answers)*

Norms
Normal: 5 ± 4
Mildly depressed: 15 ± 6
Very depressed: 23 ± 5

*Appropriate (nondepressed) answers = yes; all others = no.

Yesavage, J., et al. (1983). Development and validation of a geriatric screening scale: A preliminary report. *Journal of Psychiatric Research, 17* (1), 37–49. Reprinted with permission from Pergamon Press Ltd., Headington Hill Hall, Oxford OX3 OBW, UK.

and at the same time avoid medication toxicity. It may take 4 to 6 weeks for symptoms to recede, so the nurse should offer explanations and encouragement during this period.

Alcohol abuse related to depression is significant in the elderly population. Alcohol-related problems in older people often remain hidden, however, since many older adults deny their habit when questioned. Alcohol abuse is especially dangerous in the older person because of changes in renal and liver function as well as the probability of side effects in interactions with prescriptive medications (Adams, Atkinson, Ganz, & O'Conner, 2000).

DELIRIUM

Delirium, often called acute confusional state, begins with confusion and progresses to disorientation. The patient may experience an altered level of consciousness ranging from stupor to excessive activity. Thinking is disorganized, and the attention span is characteristically short. Hallucinations, delusions, fear, anxiety, and paranoia may also be evident. Because of the acute and unexpected onset of symptoms and the unknown underlying cause, delirium is a medical emergency. Delirium occurs secondary to a number of causes, including physical illness, medication or alcohol toxicity, dehydration, fecal impaction, malnutrition, infection, head trauma, lack of environmental cues, and sensory deprivation or overload. Older adults are particularly vulnerable to acute confusion because of their decreased biologic reserve and the large number of medications that many take. The nurse must recognize the grave implications of the acute symptoms and report them immediately. If the delirium goes unrecognized and the underlying cause is not treated, permanent, irreversible brain damage or death can follow. Delirium is sometimes mistaken for dementia (see Table 12-4 for a comparison of dementia and delirium).

Therapeutic interventions vary, depending on the reason for the symptoms. Because medication interactions and toxicity are often implicated, nonessential medications should be stopped. Nutritional and fluid intake should be supervised and monitored. The environment should be quiet and calm. To increase **orientation** and provide familiar environmental cues, the nurse encourages family members or friends to touch and talk to the patient. It is important to question the family carefully about the patient's prior cognitive state. Ongoing mental status assessments using this baseline are helpful in evaluating responses to treatment and to the hospital or extended care facility admission.

THE DEMENTIAS: MULTI-INFARCT DEMENTIA AND ALZHEIMER'S DISEASE

Dementias affect 8% of older Canadians, with an additional 16% exhibiting mild cognitive impairment (National Advisory Council on Aging, 2004). Many dementias are not diagnosed (Sternberg, Wolfson & Baumgarten, 2000). The risk of **dementia** increases greatly throughout the senior years, with one in three persons aged 85 and older diagnosed with dementia—this rate is 20 times higher than for those 65 to 69 years old (Canadian Study of Health and Aging, 2002). Women, who typically live longer, are much more likely to develop a dementia (Hill et al., 1997). In 1991, women accounted for 68% of dementias. Advanced dementia is a common reason for nursing home admission, following a patterned decline in cognitive and functional status (Njegovan et al., 2001). Death often occurs 8 to 10 years after the first symptoms of memory loss, with death often due to secondary infections (National Advisory Council on Aging, 2004). In order for a diagnosis of dementia to be made, at least two domains of altered function must exist—memory and at least one of the following: language, perception, visuospatial function, calculation, judgment, abstraction, and problem-solving (Mayo Foundation for Medical Education and Research [Mayo], 2001).

Symptoms are usually subtle in onset and often progress slowly until they are obvious and devastating. The changes characteristic of dementia fall into three general categories: cognitive, functional, and behavioural. Reversible causes of dementia include alcohol abuse, medication use (polypharmacy), psychiatric disorders, and normal-pressure hydrocephalus. The three most common

nonreversible dementias are Alzheimer's disease, multi-infarct dementia, and mixed Alzheimer's and multi-infarct dementia. Of all dementias, 65% are associated with Alzheimer's disease (Veterans Affairs Canada, n.d.). Multi-infarct dementia (vascular dementia) is the next most common cause. Less common causes of dementia are Parkinson's disease, AIDS-related dementia, Pick's disease, and bovine spongiform encephalopathy ("mad cow" disease) or Creutzfeldt-Jakob disease.

Dementia is characterized by an uneven, downward decline in mental function. Multi-infarct dementia is sometimes confused with Alzheimer's disease, paranoia, or delirium because of its unpredictable clinical course. The diagnosis can be even more difficult if the patient is suffering from both Alzheimer's disease and multi-infarct dementia.

Multi-infarct, or vascular dementia, has the following defining characteristics:

- There must be evidence of dementia.
- There must be evidence of cerebrovascular disease (by history, clinical examination, or brain imaging).
- The two disorders must be reasonably related.

Alzheimer's disease is a progressive, irreversible, degenerative neurologic disease that begins insidiously and is characterized by gradual losses of cognitive function and disturbances in behaviour and affect. Alzheimer's disease is not found exclusively in the elderly; in 1% to 10% of cases, its onset occurs in middle age. A family history of Alzheimer's disease and the presence of Down syndrome are two established risk factors for Alzheimer's disease. If family members have at least one other relative with Alzheimer's disease, then a familial component, which nonspecifically includes both environmental triggers and genetic determinants, is said to exist. Genetic studies show that autosomal-dominant forms of Alzheimer's disease are associated with early onset and early death.

In 1987, chromosome 21 was first implicated in early-onset familial Alzheimer's disease. Soon after, the gene coding for amyloid precursor protein (*APP*) was also found to be on chromosome 21. Not until 1991 was an actual mutation in association with familial Alzheimer's disease found in the *APP* gene of chromosome 21. For those with this gene, onset of Alzheimer's disease began in their 50s. Only a few of the cases of familial Alzheimer's disease have been found to involve this genetic mutation. In 1992, chromosome 14 was found to contain an unidentified mutation also linked to familial Alzheimer's disease. Since 1995, molecular biologists have been discovering even more-specific genetic information about the various forms of Alzheimer's disease, including genetic differences between early- and late-onset Alzheimer's disease. These genetic differences are helping to pinpoint risk factors associated with the disease, although the genetic indicators are not specific enough to be used as reliable diagnostic markers (Mayo, 2001).

Pathophysiology

Specific neuropathologic and biochemical changes are found in patients with Alzheimer's disease. These include neurofibrillary tangles (a tangled mass of nonfunctioning neurons) and senile or neuritic plaques (deposits of amyloid protein, part of a larger protein, *APP*) in the brain. This neuronal damage occurs primarily in the cerebral cortex and results in decreased brain size. Similar changes are found to a lesser extent in the normal brain tissue of older adults. Cells that use the neurotransmitter acetylcholine are the ones principally affected by this disease. Biochemically, the enzyme active in producing acetylcholine, which is specifically involved in memory processing, is decreased.

Table 12-4 • **Summary of Differences Between Dementia and Delirium**

	DEMENTIA		DELIRIUM
	Alzheimer's Disease (AD)	Multi-Infarct Dementia	
Etiology	Familial (genetic [chromosomes 14, 19, 21]) Sporadic	Cardiovascular (CV) disease Cerebrovascular disease Hypertension	Drug toxicity and interactions; acute disease; trauma; chronic disease exacerbation Fluid and electrolyte disorder
Risk factors	Advanced age; genetic factor	Preexisting CV disease	Preexisting cognitive impairment
Occurrence	50%–60% of dementias	20% of dementias	20% of hospitalized older people
Onset	Slow	Often abrupt Follows a stroke or transient ischemic attack	Rapid, acute onset A harbinger of acute medical illness
Age of onset (yr)	Early onset AD: 30s–65 Late onset AD: 65+ Most commonly: 85+	Most commonly 50–70 yr	Any age, but predominantly in older persons
Gender	Males and females equally	Predominantly males	Males and females equally
Course	Chronic, irreversible; progressive, regular, downhill	Chronic, irreversible Fluctuating, stepwise progression	Acute
Duration	2–20 yr	Variable; years	Lasts 1 day to 1 month
Symptom progress	Onset insidious. *Early*—mild and subtle *Middle and late*—intensified Progression to death (infection or malnutrition)	Depends on location of infarct and success of treatment; death due to underlying CV disease	Symptoms are fully reversible with adequate treatment; can progress to chronicity or death if underlying condition is ignored
Mood	Early depression (30%)	Labile: mood swings	Variable
Speech/language	Speech remains intact until late in disease *Early*—mild anomia (cannot name objects); deficits progress until speech lacks meaning; echoes and repeats words and sounds; mutism.	May have speech deficit/aphasia depending on location of lesion	Fluctuating; often cannot concentrate long enough to speak
Physical signs	*Early*—no motor deficits *Middle*—apraxia [70%] (cannot perform purposeful movement) *Late*—Dysarthria (impaired articulation) *End stage*—loss of all voluntary activity; positive neurologic signs	According to location of lesion: focal neurologic signs, seizures Commonly exhibits motor deficits	Signs and symptoms of underlying disease
Orientation	Becomes lost in familiar places (topographic disorientation) Has difficulty drawing three-dimensional objects (visual and spatial disorientation) Disorientation to time, place, and person—with disease progression		May fluctuate between lucidity and complete disorientation to time, place, and person
Memory	Loss is an early sign of dementia; loss of recent memory is soon followed by progressive decline in recent and remote memory		Impaired recent and remote memory; may fluctuate between lucidity and confusion
Personality	Apathy, indifference, irritability *Early disease*—social behaviour intact; hides cognitive deficits *Advanced disease*—disengages from activity and relationships; suspicious; paranoid delusions caused by memory loss; aggressive; catastrophic reactions		Fluctuating; cannot focus attention to converse; alarmed by symptoms (when lucid); hallucinations; paranoid
Functional status, activities of daily living	Poor judgment in everyday activities; has progressive decline in ability to handle money, use telephone, function in home and workplace		Impaired
Attention span	Distractable; short attention span		Highly impaired; cannot maintain or shift attention
Psychomotor activity	Wandering, hyperactivity, pacing, restlessness, agitation		Variable; alternates between high agitation, hyperactivity, restlessness, and lethargy
Sleep–wake cycle	Often impaired; wandering and agitation at nighttime		Takes brief naps throughout day and night

Several theories are currently being tested to explain what predisposes an individual to develop the plaques and neurotangles that can be seen at autopsy on biopsy of the brains of Alzheimer's patients (Mayo, 2001). Scientists continue to increase their understanding of the complex ways in which aging and genetic and nongenetic factors affect and damage brain cells over time and eventually lead to Alzheimer's disease. Researchers have recently discovered how and why amyloid plaques form and cause neuronal death, as well as the possible relationship between various forms of tau protein and impaired function, which leads to neuronal death. The major role of tau protein is to regulate the assembly and stability of neurons. Researchers are also beginning to discover the roles of inflammation and oxidative stress and the contribution of brain infarctions to the disease (Alzheimer's Disease Education and Referral Center, 1999).

Clinical Manifestations

In the early stages of Alzheimer's disease, forgetfulness and subtle memory loss occur. The patient may experience small difficulties in work or social activities but has adequate cognitive function to hide the loss and can function independently. Depression may occur at this time. With further progression of the disease, the deficits can no longer be concealed. Forgetfulness is manifested in many daily actions. These patients may lose their ability to recognize familiar faces, places, and objects and may get lost in a familiar environment. They may repeat the same stories because they forget that they have already told them. Trying to reason with the person and using reality orientation only increase the patient's anxiety without increasing function. Conversation becomes difficult, and there are word-finding difficulties. The ability to formulate concepts and think abstractly disappears; for instance, the patient can interpret a proverb only in concrete terms. The patient is often unable to recognize the consequences of his or her actions and will therefore exhibit impulsive behaviour. For example, on a hot day, the patient may decide to wade in the city fountain fully clothed. The patient has difficulty with everyday activities, such as operating simple appliances and handling money.

Personality changes are also usually evident. The patient may become depressed, suspicious, paranoid, hostile, and even combative. Progression of the disease intensifies the symptoms: speaking skills deteriorate to nonsense syllables, agitation and physical activity increase, and the patient may wander at night. Eventually, assistance is needed for most ADLs, including eating and toileting, since dysphagia occurs and incontinence develops. The terminal stage, in which the patient is usually immobile and requires total care, may last for months or years. Occasionally, the patient may recognize family or caretakers. Death occurs as a result of complications such as pneumonia, malnutrition, or dehydration.

Assessment and Diagnostic Findings

The health history, including medical history; family history; social and cultural history; medication history, and the physical examination, including functional and mental health status, are key in the diagnosis of probable Alzheimer's disease. Diagnostic tests, including complete blood count, the Venereal Disease Research Laboratory (VDRL) test for syphilis, HIV testing, chemistry profile, and vitamin B_{12} and thyroid hormone levels, as well as screening with electroencephalography (EEG), computed tomography (CT), magnetic resonance imaging (MRI), and examination of the cerebrospinal fluid may all refute or support a diagnosis of probable Alzheimer's disease.

Depression can closely mimic early-stage Alzheimer's disease and coexists in many patients. A depression scale is helpful in screening for underlying depression. Tests for cognitive function, such as the Mini-Mental State Examination (see Chart 12-3) and the clock-drawing test, are useful for screening. CT and MRI scans of the brain are useful for excluding hematoma, brain tumour, stroke, normal-pressure hydrocephalus, and atrophy but are not reliable in making a definitive diagnosis of Alzheimer's disease. Infections, physiologic disturbances such as hypothyroidism, Parkinson's disease, and vitamin B_{12} deficiency can produce cognitive impairment that may be misdiagnosed as Alzheimer's disease. Biochemical abnormalities can be excluded through examination of the blood and cerebrospinal fluid, but the findings are not specific enough to make the diagnosis. A diagnosis of "probable Alzheimer's disease" is made when the medical history, physical examination, and laboratory tests have excluded all known causes of other dementias. The diagnosis can be confirmed only by cerebral biopsy (Mayo, 2001).

Medical Management

In 1993, the first medication for treatment of the symptoms of Alzheimer's disease, tacrine hydrochloride (Cognex), was approved (in the United States). This agent enhances acetylcholine uptake in the brain, thus maintaining memory skills for a period of time. Because this medication can cause liver toxicity, patients must be closely monitored. It was not until early 1997 that donepezil (Aricept), a second medication in this category of acetylcholinesterase inhibitors, was introduced. In 2000, a third medication in this class, rivastigmine (Exelon) was introduced after completion of research trials conducted in more than 70 countries. These two newer preparations have far fewer side effects, although they continue to require ongoing monitoring. They vary in their level of effectiveness from patient to patient, due in part to their window of effectiveness, which in general is limited to the early stages of dementia (Fillit, 2000).

Nursing Management

Although Alzheimer's disease is the focus of this nursing management discussion, the interventions described apply to all patients with dementia, regardless of the cause. Nursing interventions are aimed at maintaining the patient's physical safety; reducing anxiety and agitation; improving communication; promoting independence in self-care activities; providing for the patient's needs for socialization, self-esteem, and intimacy; maintaining adequate nutrition; managing sleep pattern disturbances; and supporting and educating family caregivers. Research has demonstrated that when the nurse can provide such support, older adults are able to maintain higher levels of perceived and actual health (Forbes, 2001).

SUPPORTING COGNITIVE FUNCTION

As the patient's cognitive ability declines, the nurse provides a calm, predictable environment that helps the person interpret his or her surroundings and activities. Environmental stimuli are limited, and a regular routine is followed. A quiet, pleasant manner of speaking, clear and simple explanations, and use of memory aids and cues help to minimize confusion and disorientation and give the patient a sense of security. Prominently displayed clocks and calendars may enhance orientation to time. Colour-coding the doorway may help the patient who has difficulty locating his or her room. Active participation may help the patient to maintain cognitive, functional, and social interaction abilities for a longer period. Physical activity and communication have

NURSING RESEARCH PROFILE 12-1
The Effect of Conversation on Functional Mobility

Tappen, R., Roach, K., Applegate, E. B., & Stowell, P. (2000). Effect of a combined walking and conversation intervention on functional mobility of nursing home residents with Alzheimer's disease. *Alzheimer Disease and Associated Disorders, 14,* 196–201.

Purpose
Motor loss becomes evident in the later stages of Alzheimer's disease, leading to gait disturbances that predispose the individual to falls and subsequent injuries. The purpose of this study was to assess the effect of a combination of exercise and conversation, compared with walking-only exercise and conversation-only treatments, on the functional mobility of frail nursing home residents with Alzheimer's disease.

Design
A repeated-measures three-group design was used. Sixty-five nursing home residents with Alzheimer's disease were randomly assigned to one of three treatment groups: walking only, having conversation only, or walking and conversing with the study nurses. Treatments were given for 30 minutes three times a week for 16 weeks. The residents' functional mobility was measured before initiation of the treatments and after 16 weeks of intervention. At the end of the intervention period, descriptive statistics, the Student *t* test, analysis of variance (ANOVA) and the chi square test were used to compare the three groups.

Conclusions
As expected, the ambulation function of the participants in the "conversation only" group dropped dramatically. Those participants who were assisted to walk without conversation demonstrated a dramatic drop in ambulation function as well. Of all three groups, the least decline occurred in ambulation function over time in the group of participants with whom the nurses carried on a conversation while these participants were being assisted to walk. This information suggests that while attempting to maintain physical function in the patient with Alzheimer's disease, the nurse can best achieve this goal if socialization is incorporated into exercise sessions.

Implications for Practice
This study demonstrated that assisted walking with conversation can contribute to maintenance of functional mobility in institutionalized patients with Alzheimer's disease. Staff caring for these patients can promote patients' acceptance of assisted walking through the use of effective communication strategies.

Based on a drawing by Rachel A. Degler.

---

also been demonstrated to slow some of the cognitive decline of Alzheimer's disease (Nursing Research Profile 12-1).

PROMOTING PHYSICAL SAFETY
A safe environment allows the patient to move about as freely as possible and relieves the family of constant worry about safety. To prevent falls and other injuries, all obvious hazards are removed. Nightlights are helpful. The patient's intake of medications and food is monitored. Smoking is allowed only with supervision. A hazard-free environment allows the patient maximum independence and a sense of autonomy. Because of a short attention span and forgetfulness, wandering behaviour can often be reduced by gently persuading or distracting the patient. Restraints are avoided because they may increase agitation. Doors leading from the house must be secured. Outside the home, all activities must be supervised to protect the patient, and the patient should wear an identification bracelet or neck chain in case he or she becomes separated from the caregiver.

REDUCING ANXIETY AND AGITATION
Despite profound cognitive losses, the patient will, at times, be aware of his or her rapidly diminishing abilities. The patient will need constant emotional support that reinforces a positive self-image. When losses of skills occur, goals are adjusted to fit the patient's declining ability.

The environment should be kept uncluttered, familiar, and noise free. Excitement and confusion can be upsetting and may precipitate a combative, agitated state known as a catastrophic reaction (overreaction to excessive stimulation). During such a reaction, the patient responds by screaming, crying, or becoming abusive (physically or verbally). This may be the patient's only way of expressing an inability to cope with the environment. When this occurs, it is important to remain calm and unhurried. Measures such as listening to music, stroking, rocking, or distraction may quiet the patient. Frequently, the patient forgets what triggered the reaction. Structuring of activities is also helpful. Becoming familiar with the patient's predicted responses to certain stressors helps caregivers to avoid similar situations.

By the time most older persons with dementia have progressed to the late stages of the disease, they typically reside in nursing homes and are predominantly cared for by nurses' aides. Dementia education for caregivers is imperative to minimize patient agitation and is very effectively taught by advanced practice nurse specialists (Nursing Research Profile 12-2).

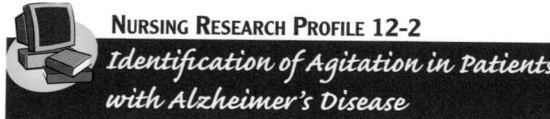

NURSING RESEARCH PROFILE 12-2

Identification of Agitation in Patients with Alzheimer's Disease

Whall, A. L., Black, M. E. A., Yankou, D. J., et al. (1999). Nurse aides' identification of onset and level of agitation in late stage dementia patients. *American Journal of Alzheimer's Disease, 14,* 202–206.

Purpose

Nursing assistants provide the majority of care to patients in nursing homes. They are vital links in the early identification, and therefore in the treatment, of agitation in patients with Alzheimer's disease. Nurses' aides (NAs) are sometimes characterized as unwilling or unable to manage patients' agitation. This study examines the process by which nurses' aides can successfully identify this agitation.

Design

NAs from five different nursing homes owned by the same corporate entity were asked to participate in the study. Criteria to participate included being employed for at least 1 year. (Research demonstrates that NAs who remain at a facility longer than 1 year usually have a commitment to those they serve.) The NAs did not receive any additional wages and were only promised a letter to indicate that they had participated in the study. Each NA received approximately 1 hour of training via audio tapes and conversation with nurse experts. Each NA was then paired with a nurse expert to assess his or her skill at appropriately identifying levels of agitation in patients with late-stage Alzheimer's disease.

Conclusions

This study demonstrated that NAs with a minimum of 1 year of employment did an excellent job in acquiring new observation skills with only 1 hour of training and positive reinforcement via a letter noting their participation in this study. The NAs' assessment of signs of agitation agreed with that of the nurse expert more than 90% of the time. All the NAs involved reported gaining helpful insights in managing agitated behaviour as a result of participation in the study.

Implications for Practice

The results of this study support the ability of NAs to accurately observe and report agitated behaviour as a result of a brief training session using adult learning principles that stressed the importance of their input into the training and learning objectives. Early observation and reporting of agitated behaviour is important to prevent agitation from increasing to the level of physical aggression.

IMPROVING COMMUNICATION

To promote the patient's interpretation of messages, the nurse remains unhurried and reduces noises and distractions. The nurse uses clear, easy-to-understand sentences to convey messages, because the patient frequently forgets the meaning of words or has difficulty organizing and expressing thoughts. Lists and simple written instructions can serve as reminders to the patient and are often helpful. Sometimes, the patient can point to an object or use nonverbal language to communicate. Tactile stimuli, such as a hug or a hand pat, are usually interpreted as signs of affection, concern, and security.

PROMOTING INDEPENDENCE IN SELF-CARE ACTIVITIES

Pathophysiologic changes in the brain make it difficult for a person with Alzheimer's disease to maintain physical independence. The nurse should help the person remain functionally independent for as long as possible. One way to do this is to simplify daily activities by organizing them into short, achievable steps so that the patient experiences a sense of accomplishment. Frequently,

an occupational therapist can suggest ways to simplify tasks or recommend adaptive equipment. Direct patient supervision is sometimes necessary, but maintaining personal dignity and autonomy is important for the person with Alzheimer's disease. He or she is encouraged to make choices when appropriate and to participate in self-care activities as much as possible.

PROVIDING FOR SOCIALIZATION AND INTIMACY NEEDS

Because socialization with old friends can be comforting, visits, letters, and phone calls are encouraged. Visits should be brief and nonstressful; limiting visitors to one or two at a time helps to reduce overstimulation. Because recreation is important, the person is encouraged to enjoy simple activities. Realistic goals that provide satisfaction are appropriate. Hobbies and activities such as walking, exercising, and socializing can improve the quality of life. The nonjudgmental friendliness of a pet may provide a lonely person with stimulation, comfort, and contentment. Care of the pet by the patient can also provide a satisfying activity and an outlet for energy.

Alzheimer's disease does not eliminate the need for intimacy. The patient and his or her spouse may or may not continue to enjoy sexual activity. The spouse should be encouraged to talk about any sexual concerns, and sexual counselling may be suggested if necessary. Simple expressions of love, such as touching and holding, are often meaningful.

PROMOTING ADEQUATE NUTRITION

Mealtime can be a pleasant, social occasion or a time of upset and distress, so it should be kept simple and calm, without confrontations. The patient will prefer familiar foods that look appetizing and taste good. To avoid the patient's "playing" with the food, one dish is offered at a time. Food is cut into small pieces to prevent choking. Liquids may be easier to swallow if they are converted to gelatin. Hot food and beverages are served warm, but the temperature of the foods should be checked to prevent burns.

When lack of coordination interferes with self-feeding, adaptive equipment is helpful. Some patients may do well eating with their fingers. If this is the case, an apron or a smock, rather than a bib, is used to protect clothing. As deficits progress, it may be necessary to feed the patient. Forgetfulness, disinterest, dental problems, incoordination, overstimulation, and choking can all serve as barriers to good nutrition.

PROMOTING BALANCED ACTIVITY AND REST

Many patients with Alzheimer's disease exhibit sleep disturbances, wandering, and behaviours that may be deemed inappropriate. These behaviours are most likely to occur when there are underlying physical or psychological needs that are unmet. It is imperative that caregivers seek to learn the needs of the patient who is exhibiting this type of behaviour, because further health decline can ensue if the source of the problem is not corrected. Adequate sleep and physical exercise are essential. If sleep is interrupted or the patient is unable to fall asleep, music, warm milk, or a back rub may help the person relax. During the day, the patient should be given sufficient opportunity to participate in exercise activities, because a regular pattern of activity and rest will enhance nighttime sleep. Long periods of daytime sleeping are discouraged.

SUPPORTING HOME AND COMMUNITY-BASED CARE

The emotional burden placed on the family of a patient with Alzheimer's disease is enormous. The physical health of the patient is often very stable, and the mental degeneration is gradual. Because the diagnosis is not specific, the family may cling to the hope that the diagnosis is incorrect and that the person will improve if he or she tries harder. Aggression and hostility exhibited by the patient are often misunderstood by the caregiver or family, who feel unappreciated, frustrated, and angry. Feelings of guilt, nervousness, and worry contribute to caregiver fatigue, depression, and family dysfunction. In some cases caregivers themselves can become so fatigued as a result of the stress of caregiving that elder neglect or abuse can occur. This has been documented in home situations as well as institutions. If elder neglect or abuse of any kind—including physical, psychological, sexual, or financial abuse—is suspected, the police or another local adult protective service organization must be notified; the role of the nurse is not to prove the neglect or abuse, but to report it (Department of Justice Canada, n.d.).

The multiple needs of family caregivers have been addressed by many organizations, including the Alzheimer's Society of Canada. This national organization is a coalition of family members and professionals who share the goals of family support and service, education, research, and advocacy. Support groups are often grass-roots organizations that are run by volunteers who are experienced as Alzheimer's caregivers. Respite services allow informal caregivers time for needed activities such as sleep, shopping, and housework.

The nurse must be sensitive to the highly emotional issues that the family is confronting. Support and education of the caregivers are essential components of care. The family may also benefit from joining a support group where they can meet others who are experiencing similar problems.

The Older Adult in an Acute Care Setting: Altered Responses to Illness

The elderly person entering the acute care setting is at increased risk for complications, infections, and functional decline. The interdisciplinary team and nursing staff can help avert negative outcomes by being knowledgeable about the physiologic and psychological responses of older adults to acute illnesses and by planning and implementing preventive measures. In addition to the interventions discussed in the following paragraphs, general nursing measures that can be taken to avoid complications in the older adult include careful and frequent assessment of vital signs, mental status, fluid balance, and skin integrity; prompt identification and treatment of complications; promotion of independent self-care and mobility; assistance with frequent position changes and deep-breathing exercises; alertness to possible medication reactions; and assistance with ADLs and toileting.

INCREASED SUSCEPTIBILITY TO INFECTION

Infectious diseases present a significant threat of morbidity and mortality to older people, in part because of the blunted response of host defenses caused by a reduction in both cell-mediated and humoral immunity (see Chapters 50 and 51). Age-related loss of physiologic reserve and chronic illnesses also contribute to increased susceptibility. Pneumonia, urinary tract infections, tuberculosis (TB), gastrointestinal infections, and skin infections are some of the commonly occurring infections in older people.

The effects of influenza and pneumococcal infections on older people are also significant. Not only are they a potential cause of death, but they also cause much suffering for seniors. Community-acquired pneumonia is a major reason for health services utilization by seniors, particularly during the winter months (Crighton, Moineddin, Mamdani, & Ushur, 2004).

The influenza vaccine is prepared yearly to adjust for the specific immunologic characteristics that are present in the influenza viruses at that time. It is an inactivated preparation that should be taken annually in the fall. The pneumococcal vaccine has 23 type-specific capsular polysaccharides. Protection lasts 4 years or longer. Both of these injections can be received at the same time in separate injection sites. The nurse should urge older people to receive these vaccines. All health care providers working with older people or high-risk chronically ill people should also be immunized.

Although rare, TB is an infectious concern of aging; some seniors were exposed when younger to the tuberculosis bacilli, and this germ can reactivate in old age. Nursing home residents are prime candidates for TB. Of all 1,555 new active and relapsed TB cases reported in 2002, 66% were in persons who were born outside of Canada (Public Health Agency of Canada, 2004). A large proportion of seniors were born outside of Canada and many travelled to areas of the world where TB is common. Respiratory TB is the most common form of TB, followed by lymphatic TB.

ALTERED PAIN AND FEBRILE RESPONSES

Many altered physical, emotional, and systemic reactions to disease are attributed to age-related changes in older people. Useful and reliable physical indicators of illness in young and middle-aged people cannot be relied on for the diagnosis of potential life-threatening problems in older adults. The response to pain in older people may be lessened because of reduced acuity of touch, alterations in neural pathways, and diminished processing of sensory data. Research has demonstrated the absence of chest pain in many older adults experiencing a myocardial infarction. Hiatal hernia or upper gastrointestinal distress is often responsible for chest pain in elderly people. Acute abdominal conditions, such as mesenteric infarction and appendicitis, often go unrecognized in elderly people because of atypical signs and absence of pain (Kufrovich, 2001).

The baseline body temperature for older people is about −17.2°C lower than it is for younger people. In the event of illness, therefore, the body temperature of an older person may not reach a sufficient elevation to qualify as a traditionally defined "fever." A temperature of 37.8°C, in combination with systemic symptoms, may signal infection. A temperature of 38.3°C is almost certainly a serious infection that needs prompt attention. A blunted fever in the face of an infection often indicates a poor prognosis. Elevations in temperature rarely exceed 39.5°C. The nurse must be alert to other subtle signs of infection: mental confusion, increased respirations, tachycardia, and changed facial appearance and colour.

ALTERED EMOTIONAL IMPACT

The emotional component of illness in older people may differ from that in younger people. Many elderly people equate good health with the absence of old age. "You are as old as you feel" is a belief of many. An illness that requires hospitalization or a change in lifestyle is an imminent threat to well-being. Admission to the hospital is often feared and actively avoided. Economic concerns and fear of becoming a burden to the family often lead to high anxiety in older people. The nurse must recognize the implications of fear, anxiety, and dependency in elderly patients. Autonomy and independent decision making are encouraged. A positive and confident demeanor in the nurse and the family promote a positive mental outlook in the elderly patient. In addition to anxiety and fear, older people are at high risk for disorientation, confusion, change in level of consciousness, and other symptoms of delirium if they are admitted to the hospital.

ALTERED SYSTEMIC RESPONSE

The effect of illness on an aged person has far-reaching repercussions. The decline in organ function that occurs in every system of the aging body eventually forces one or more body systems to function at full capacity. Illness places new demands on body systems that have little or no reserve to meet this crisis. Homeostasis, the ability of the body to maintain an internal balance of function and chemical composition, is jeopardized. The older person may be unable to respond effectively to an acute illness or, if a chronic health condition is present, he or she may be unable to sustain appropriate responses over a long period. Furthermore, the older person's ability to respond to definitive treatment is impaired. These altered responses reinforce the need for the nurse to monitor all of the older adult's body system functions closely, being alert to signs of impending systemic complication.

 Critical Thinking Exercises

1. Mrs. C., a 64-year-old woman, arrives at the presurgical admission unit for her scheduled toe amputation; she has chronic arterial insufficiency, secondary to diabetes, with a history of chronic atrial fibrillation. As you review the list of medications that she has brought with her, you discover that she has listed, "Coumadin 3 mg per day", and "Warfarin 1 mg per day." As you question her, she reports that her physician provided a new prescription for her anticoagulation at her preoperative visit last week. She was unaware that Coumadin and warfarin were the same medication and continued on the Coumadin while starting the "new" prescription. What will your first action be?

2. You are working for a home health agency and making regular visits to an 85-year-old widow who recently moved in with her daughter because of declining health. On your first visit since her move, you noted a bruise on the patient's hip. She stated that she had bumped into a chair on the way to the bathroom. On the next visit, you find her in dirty clothing. She stated that the washing machine was broken and her daughter was waiting for the repairman. Today as you visit with the patient, there is a cut on her arm and more bruises. She confides that her daughter is overworked and sometimes gets a bit "impatient" as she is providing care for her. Describe the most appropriate plan of action.

3. As a charge nurse in a skilled nursing facility, your daily assessment of Mr. Jones, a 75-year-old man with late-stage Alzheimer's disease, normally finds him to be medically stable, with a pleasant but confused affect. When you assess him today, his vital signs continue to be stable; however, he angrily yells at you when you speak to him, he is notably agitated, and he cries with pain as he is attempting to void. Based on your understanding of the altered response to acute infection in the elderly, what assessment parameters would you evaluate? What plan of action would you initiate?

REFERENCES AND SELECTED READINGS

Books

Abraham, I. L., & Fulmer, T. (1999). *Geriatric nursing protocols for best practice.* New York: Springer.

Abrams, W. B., Beers, M. H., & Berkow, R. (2000). *Merck manual of geriatrics* (3rd ed.). Whitehouse Station, NJ: Merck & Co.

Alzheimer's Disease Education and Referral (ADEAR) Center. (1999). *Progress report on Alzheimer's Disease.* Silver Springs, MD: U.S. Department of Health and Human Services, Public Health Service, National Institutes of Health, National Institutes of Aging. NIH Pub. No. 99-4664. http://www.alzheimers.org/pubs/prog99.htm.

Burke, M. M., & Laramie, J. A. (2000). *Primary care of the older adult: A multidisciplinary approach.* St. Louis: Mosby.

Canadian Gerontological Nursing Association. (1996). *Standards of practice.* Ottawa: Author.

Canadian Institute for Health Information. (2004a). *How healthy are Canadians? 2004 Annual Report.* Ottawa: Author.

Canadian Institute for Health Information. (2004b). *Preliminary provincial and territorial government health expenditure estimates 1974–1975 to 2004–2005.* Ottawa: Author.

Canadian Lung Association. (2000). *Canadian tuberculosis standards* (5th ed.) Ottawa: Author.

Canadian Nurses Association. (2000). *Position statement. End-of-life issues.* Ottawa: Author.

Canadian Nurses Association. (2002). *Position statement. Code of ethics for Registered Nurses.* Ottawa: Author.

Centre for Infectious Disease Prevention and Control. (2004). *HIV and AIDS in Canada. Surveillance report to June 30, 2004.* Available at: www.phac-aspc.gc.ca/publicat/aids-sida/haic-vsac0604/index.html.

Commission on the Future of Health Care in Canada. (2002). *Building on values. The future of health care in Canada. Final report.* Ottawa: Author.

Costa, P. T. Jr., Williams, T. F., Somerfield, M., et al. (1996, November). *Recognition and initial assessment of Alzheimer's disease and related dementias: Clinical practice guideline no. 19.* (AHCPR Publication No. 97-0702). Rockville, MD: U.S. Department of Health and Human Services, Public Health Service, Agency for Health Care Policy and Research.

Department of Justice Canada. (1984). *Canada health act.* Available at: http://www.laws.justice.gc.ca/en/c-6/17077.html. Retrieved June 15, 2005.

Division of Aging and Seniors, Public Health Agency of Canada. (2001). *An inventory of Canadian programs for the prevention of falls among seniors living in the community.* Ottawa: Author.

Division of Aging and Seniors. Health Canada. (2002). *Healthy aging. Prevention of unintentional injuries among seniors.* Ottawa: Minister of Public Works and Government Services Canada.

Ebersole, P., & Hess, P. (2001). *Geriatric nursing and healthy aging.* St. Louis: Mosby.

Eliopoulos, C. (2000). *Gerontological nursing* (5th ed.). Philadelphia: Lippincott Williams & Wilkins.

Erikson, E. H. (1963). *Childhood and society* (2nd ed.). New York: W. W. Norton.

Fantl, J. A., Newman, D. K., Colling, J., et al. (1996, March). *Managing acute and chronic urinary incontinence: Clinical practice guideline.* Quick Reference Guide for Clinicians No. 2, 1996 Update. (AHCPR Pub. No. 96-0686). Rockville, MD: U.S. Department of Health and Human Services, Public Health Service, Agency for Health Care Policy and Research.

Gallo, J. J., Fulmer, T., Paveza, G. J., & Reichel, W. (2000). *Handbook of geriatric assessment* (3rd ed.). Gaithersburg, MD: Aspen.

Ham, R. J., & Warshaw G. (2001). *Primary care geriatrics: A case-based approach* (4th ed.). St. Louis: Mosby–Year Book.

Havighurst, R. J. (1972). *Developmental tasks and education* (3rd ed.). New York: McKay.

Hazzard, W. R., Blass, J. P., Ettinger, W. H. Jr., Halter, J. B., & Ouslander, J. G. (1999). *Principles of geriatric medicine and gerontology* (4th ed.). New York: McGraw-Hill.

Health Canada. (2002). *Best practices treatment and rehabilitation for seniors with substance use problems.* Ottawa: Author.

Health Services Research on Aging. (2000, January). *Building on biomedical and clinical research. Translating research into practice fact sheet.* (AHRQ Publication No. 00-P012). Rockville, MD: Agency for Healthcare Research and Quality. Available at: http://www.ahrq.gov/research/tripage.htm.

Heart Failure Society of America. (1999). *HFSA guidelines for management of patients with heart failure caused by left ventricular systolic dysfunction–Pharmacological approaches.* Saint Paul, MN: Author.

Hogstel, M. O. (2001). *Gerontology: Nursing care of the older adult.* Albany: Delmar Publishing.

Holmes, D., Teresi, J. A., & Ory, M. (2000). *Special care units: Research and practice in Alzheimer's disease,* Vol. 4. New York: Springer.

Kane, R. L., Ouslander, J. G., & Abrass, I. B. (1999). *Essentials of clinical geriatrics* (4th ed.). New York: McGraw-Hill.

Lueckenotte, A. G. (2000). *Gerontologic nursing* (2nd ed.). St. Louis: Mosby–Year Book.

Mezey, M. D., Berkman, B. J., & Callahan, C. (2000). *The encyclopedia of elder care: the comprehensive resource on geriatric and social care.* New York: Springer.

National Advisory Council on Aging. (2004). *The NACA position on Alzheimer disease and related dementias.* Ottawa: Author.

Noelker, L. S., & Harel, Z. (2000). *Linking quality of long term care and quality of life.* New York: Springer.

Northcott, H. C., & Wilson, D. M. (2002). *Dying and death in Canada.* Aurora, ON: Garamond.

Premier's Advisory Council on Health. (2001). *A framework for reform.* Edmonton, AB: Author.

Public Health Agency of Canada. (2004). *Tuberculosis in Canada: 2002.* Available at: www.phac-aspc.gc.ca/publicat/tbcan02/index.html. Retrieved December 15, 2005.

Roach, S. S. (2000). *Introductory gerontological nursing.* Philadelphia: Lippincott Williams & Wilkins.

Schmidt Luggen, A., Meiner, S. E., & National Gerontological Nursing Association (2000). *NGNA: Core curriculum for gerontological nursing* (2nd ed.). St. Louis: Mosby.

Silin, P. S. (2001). *Nursing homes: The family's journey.* Baltimore: Johns Hopkins University Press.

Social Development Canada. (2005). *Employment insurance (EI) compassionate care benefits.* Available at: http://www.sdc.gc.ca/en/ei/types/compassionate_care.shtml. Retrieved December 15, 2005.

Special Senate Committee on Euthanasia and Assisted Suicide. (1995). *Of life and death—Final report.* Ottawa: Author.

Special Senate Committee of the Standing Senate Committee on Social Affairs, Science and Technology, Subcommittee to update "Of Life and Death." (2000). *Quality end-of-life care: The right of every Canadian.* Ottawa: Author.

Strumpf, N. E., Evans, L. K., Wagner, J., & Patterson, J. (1992). *Reducing restraints: Individualized approaches to behavior. A teaching guide.* Huntingdon Valley, PA: Geriatric Research and Training Center.

Swanson, E. A., Tripp-Reimer, T., & Buckwalter, K. (Eds.). (2001). *Health promotion and disease prevention in the older adult.* New York: Springer.

Takano-Stone, J., Wyman, J. F., & Salisbury, S. S. (1999). *Clinical gerontological nursing: A guide to advanced practice* (2nd ed.). Philadelphia: W. B. Saunders.

Watson, R. R. (2000). *Handbook of nutrition in the aged* (3rd ed.). Boca Raton, FL: CRC Press.

World Health Organization. (2001). *Health and aging. A discussion paper.* Geneva: Author.

World Health Organization. (2002). *The Toronto declaration on the global prevention of elder abuse.* Geneva: Author.

Zang, S. M., & Allender, J. A. (1999). *Home care of the elderly.* Philadelphia: Lippincott Williams & Wilkins.

Journals

Asterisks indicate nursing research articles.

Adams, W., Atkinson, R., Ganz, S. B., & O'Connor, P. G. (2000). Alcohol problems in the elderly. *Patient Care for the Nurse Practitioner, 3,* 68–89.

Alzheimer Society of Canada. (n.d.). *What's new.* Available at: www.alzheimer.ca/english/index.php.

*Anderson, M. A., Helms, L. B., Hanson, K. S., & DeVilder, N. W. (1999). Unplanned hospital readmissions: A home care perspective. *Nursing Research, 48,* 299–307.

Annual report on the Canada Health Act. (n.d.). Available at: http://www.hc-sc.gc.ca/hcs-sss/alt_formats/hpb-dgps/pdf/pubs/cha-lcs-ar-ra/2003-04-fed_e.pdf.

Atchley, R. C. (1989). Continuity theory of normal aging. *Gerontologist, 29,* 183–190.

Baker, C. R., Norton, P. G., Flintoft, V., Blais, R., Brown, A., Cox, J. et al. (2004). The Canadian Adverse Events Study: The incidence of adverse events among hospital patients in Canada. *Canadian Medical Association Journal, 170*(11), 1678-1686.

*Blondeau, D., Lavoie, M., Valois, P., Keyserlink, E. W., Hebert, M., & Martineau, I. (2000). The attitudes of Canadian nurses towards advance directives. *Nursing Ethics: An International Journal for Health Care Professionals, 7*(5), 399–411.

Bravo, G., Dubois, M. F., & Paquet, M. (2003). Advance directives for health care and research: Prevalence and correlates. *Alzheimer Disease & Associated Disorder, 17*(4), 215–222.

Brazil, K., Bedard, M., Willison, K., & Hode, M. (2003). Caregiving and its impact on families of the terminally ill. *Aging & Mental Health, 7*(5), 376–382.

Bronskill, S. E., Anderson, G. M., Sykora, K., Wodchis, W. P., Gill, S., Shulman, K. I., et al. (2004). Neuroleptic drug therapy in older adults newly admitted to nursing homes: Incidence, dose, and specialist contact. *Journal of the American Geriatrics Society, 52*(5), 749–755.

Brown, J., & Josse, R. G. (2002). 2002 Clinical practice guidelines for the diagnosis and management of osteoporosis in Canada. *Canadian Medical Association Journal, 167*(Suppl. 10), S1–S34.

Canada Online. (n.d.). *Life expectancy and death statistics for Canada.* Available at: http://canadaonline.about.com/od/statistics/a/lifedeathstats.htm.

Canada Safety Council. (n.d.). *Safety and the aging driver.* Available at: www.safety-council.org/info/seniors/safedriv.html.

Canada's Food Guide to Healthy Eating. (1997). Available at: www.hc-sc.gc.ca/hpfb-dgpsa/onpp-bppn/food_guide_rainbow_e.html.

Canadian Association on Gerontology. (n.d.). *Who we are.* Available at: www.cagacg.ca/whoweare/200_e.php.

Canadian Hospice Palliative Care Association. (n.d.). Available at: www.chpca.net/home.htm.

Canadian Network for the Prevention of Elder Abuse. (n.d.). Available at: www.cnpea.ca.

Canadian Study of Health and Aging. (2002). *Study results.* Available at: http://csha.ca/r_study_results.asp. Retrieved June 15, 2005.

*Capezuti, E., Strumpf, N., Evans, L. K., et al. (1999). Outcomes of nighttime physical restraint removal for severely impaired nursing home residents. *American Journal of Alzheimer's Disease, 14,* 157–164.

Carriere, G. (2004). Use of hospital emergency rooms. *Health Reports, 16*(1), 35–40.

Che-Alford, J., & Stevenson, K. (1998). Older Canadians on the move. *Canadian Social Trends, 48*(Spring), 15–18.

Chen, C. L., Weiss, N. S., Newcome, P., Barlow, W., & White, E. (2002). Hormone replacement therapy in relation to breast cancer. *JAMA, 287*(6), 734–741.

Chen, J., & Hou, F. (2002). Unmet needs for health care. *Health Reports, 13*(2), 23–34.

Chen, J., & Millar, W. J. (2001). Starting and sustaining physical activity. *Health Reports, 12*(4), 33–43.

Chen, J., & Millar, W. (2000). Are recent cohorts healthier than their predecessors? *Health Reports, 11*(4), 9–23.

Chen, J., & Wilkins, R. (1998). Seniors' needs for health-related personal assistance. *Health Reports, 10*(1), 39-21–32.

Clarke, P. J., Marshall, V. M., Ryff, C. D., & Rosenthal, C. J. (2000). Well-being in Canadian seniors: Findings from the Canadian Study of Health and Aging. *Canadian Journal on Aging, 19*(2), 139–159.

Cranswick, K. (1997). Canada's caregivers. *Canadian Social Trends, 55*(Spring), 2–6.

Cranswick, K. (1999). Help close at hand: Relocating to give or receive care. *Canadian Social Trends, 55*(Winter), 11–13.

Crighton, E. J., Moineddin, R., Mamdani, M., & Ushur, R. E. (2004). Influenza and pneumonia hospitalizations in Ontario: A time-series analysis. *Epidemiology & Infection, 132*(6), 1167–1174.

Dauvergne, M. (2003). Family violence against seniors. *Canadian Social Trends, 68*(Spring), 10–14.

Degler, M. (2000a). Caring for the caregiver. Protocol Driven Healthcare Incorporated. Available at: http://www.MyBladder.com.

Degler, M. (2000b). Reversible causes of urinary incontinence. Protocol Driven Healthcare Incorporated. Available at: http://www.MyBladder.com.

Department of Justice Canada. (n.d.). *Abuse of older adults: A fact sheet from the Department of Justice Canada.* Available at: http://Canada.justice.gc.ca/en/ps/fm/adultsfs.html.

Dietitians in Canada. (2005). *The role of the registered dietitian in dysphagia assessment and treatment. A discussion paper.* Available at: www.dietitians.ca/news/highlights_positions.asp.

Dolinar, T. M., Eisdorfer, C., & Perersen, R. (2001). Strategies for early diagnosis. *Patient Care for the Nurse Practitioner, 4,* 12–22.

DriveABLE. (n.d.). *Assessments for medically at-risk drivers.* Available at: www.driveable.com.

Fillet, H. (2000). Improving the quality of managed care for patients with mild to moderate Alzheimer's disease. *CBS HealthWatch by Medscape.* Cliggott Publishing Co., Division of SCP/Cliggott Communications. Available at: http://www.healthwatch.medscape.com.

Finlayson, M. (2002). Changes predicting long-term care among the oldest-old. *Gerontologist, 42*(4), 443–453.

*Fletcher, M. (2002). Vaccination time: Coalition urges flu shot for widespread health protection. *Canadian Nurse, 98*(9), 9.

Fletcher, P. C., & Hirdes, J. P. (2004). Restriction in activity associated with fear of falling among community-based seniors using home care services. *Age & Ageing, 33*(3), 273–279.

*Forbes, D. A. (2001). Enhancing mastery and sense of coherence: Important determinants of health in older adults. *Geriatric Nursing, 22,* 29–32.

Frederick, J. A., & Fast, J. E. (1999). Elder care in Canada: Who does how much? *Canadian Social Trends, 54*(Autumn), 26–30.

*Galvan, T. J. (2001). Dysphagia: Going down and staying down. *American Journal of Nursing, 101,* 37–42.

*Grandjean, C. K., & Gibbons, S. W. (2000). Assessing ambulatory geriatric sleep complaints. *The Nurse Practitioner, 25,* 25–39.

Hadjistavropoulos, H. D., Snider, B. S., & Hadjistavropoulos, T. (2001). Anxiety in older persons waiting for cataract surgery: Investigating the contributing factors. *Canadian Journal on Aging, 20*(1), 97–111.

*Hagen, B. (2001). Nursing home placement: Factors affecting caregivers' decisions to place family members with dementia. *Journal of Gerontological Nursing, 27*(2), 44–53.

Hall, P., Schroder, C., & Weaver, L. (2002). The last 48 hours of life in long-term care: A focused chart audit. *Journal of the American Geriatrics Society, 50*(3), 501–506.

Havighurst, R. J. (1968). Personality and patterns of aging. *Gerontologist, 8,* 20–23.

Health care/self care. (2001). *Health Reports, 12*(3), 33–39.

Health in mid-life. (1999). *Health Reports, 11*(3), 35–44.

*Hill, G. B., Forbes, W. F., Lindsay, J., & McDowell, I. (1997). Life expectancy and dementia in Canada: The Study of Health and Aging. *Chronic Diseases in Canada, 18*(4). Available online at: www.phac-aspc.gc.ca/publicat/cdic-mcc/18-4/c_e.html.

Hoban, S., & Kearney, K. (2000). Elder abuse and neglect: It takes many forms—If you're not looking, you may miss it. *American Journal of Nursing, 100,* 49–50.

Hodgetts, D., Pullman, D., & Goto, A. (2003). Narrating the negative consequences of elder care and familial obligations in Atlantic Canada. *Journal of Community and Applied Social Psychology, 13*(5), 378–390.

*Hodgson, N. A. (2002). Epidemiological trends of cancer in older adults. *Journal of Gerontological Nursing, 28*(4), 34–43.

Illing, E. M. M., & Kaiserman, M. J. (2004). Mortality attributable to tobacco use in Canada and its regions, 1998. *Canadian Journal of Public Health, 95*(1), 38–44.

Innvista. (n.d.). *Water.* Available at: www.innvista.com/health/nutrition/diet/water.htm.

Johansen, H., Nguyen, K., Mao, L., Mancous, R., Gao, R., & Nair, C. (2004). Influenza vaccination. *Health Reports, 15*(2), 33–43.

Joint statement on preventing and resolving ethical conflicts involving health care providers and persons receiving care. (1998). Available at: www.consciencelaws.org/Conscience-Policies-Papers/PPPMedicalOrg06.html.

Kegel, A. H. (1948). Progressive resistance exercise in the functional restoration of the perineal muscles. *American Journal of Obstetrics and Gynecology, 56,* 238–248.

*Koop, P. M., & Strang, V. R. (2003). The bereavement experience following home-based family caregiving for persons with advanced cancer. *Clinical Nursing Research, 12*(2), 127–144.

Lafreniere, S. A., Carriere, Y., Martel, L., & Belanger, A. (2003). Dependent seniors at home—formal and informal help. *Health Reports, 14*(4), 31–40.

Lee, D., Johansen, H., Gong, Y., Hall, R., Tu, J., & Cox, J. (2004). Regional outcomes of heart failure in Canada. *Canadian Journal of Cardiology, 20*(6), 599–607.

Levin, H. G., & Levitt, Z. A. (2003). Capacity assessment for admission to long-term care: A double-edged sword. *Geriatrics and Aging, 6*(6), 45–46.

*Lukacs, J. L., & Reame, N. E. (2000). Concentrations of follicle-stimulating hormone correlate with alkaline phosphatase and a marker for vitamin K status in the perimenopause. *Journal of Women's Health and Gender-Based Medicine, 9,* 731–739.

MacKnight, C., Beattie, B. L., Bergman, H., Dalziel, W. B., Feightner, J., Goldlist, B., et al. (2003). Response to the Romano Report: The Canadian Geriatrics Society. *Geriatrics Today: Journal of the Canadian Geriatrics Society, 6*(1), 11–15.

Magai, C., Consedine, N. S., King, A. R., & Gillespie, M. (2003). Physical hardiness and styles of socioemotional functioning in later life. *Journals of Gerontology Series B–Psychological Sciences & Social Sciences, 58*(5), 269–279.

Martel, L., & Belanger, A. (2000). Dependence-free life expectancy in Canada. *Canadian Social Trends, 58*(Autumn), 26–29.

Martel, L., Belanger, A., & Berthelot, J. (2002). Loss and recovery of independence among seniors. *Health Reports, 13*(4), 35–48.

Mayo Foundation for Medical Education and Research. (2001). *Dementia: Epidemiology.* Geriatric Medicine. Community Internal Medicine Division. Available at: http://www.mayo.edu/geriatrics-rst/Dementia.I.html.

Menec, V. H., Black, C., MacWilliam, L., & Aoki, F. Y. (2003). The impact of influenza-associated respiratory illnesses on hospitalizations, physician visits, emergency room visits, and mortality. *Canadian Journal of Public Health, 94*(1), 59–63.

Millar, W. J. (2004). Vision problems among seniors. *Health Reports, 16*(1), 45–48.

Millar, W. J., & Young, T. K. (2003). Tracking diabetes: Prevalence, incidence and risk factors. *Health Reports, 14*(3), 35–47.

Morgan, D. G., Semchuk, K. M., Stewart, N. J., & D'Arcy, C. (2002). Rural families caring for a relative with dementia: Barriers to use of formal services. *Social Science & Medicine, 55*(7), 1129–1142.

National Advisory Council on Aging. (2003). Caring for aging parents. *Expression. Bulletin of the National Advisory Council on Aging, 16*(3), 1–8.

National Clearinghouse on Family Violence. (n.d.). Abuse of older adults. Available at: www.phac-aspc.gc.ca/ncfv-cnivf/familyviolence/age_e.html.

*Naylor, M., Brooten, D., Campbell, R., et al. (1999). Comprehensive discharge planning and home follow-up of hospitalized elders. *Journal of the American Medical Association, 281,* 613–620.

Njegovan, V., Hing, M. M., Mitchell, S. L., & Molnar, F. J. (2001). The hierarchy of functional loss associated with cognitive decline in older persons. *Journals of Gerontology Series A–Biological Sciences & Medical Sciences, 56*(10), M638–643.

*Norlander, L., & McSteen, K. (2000). The kitchen table discussion: A creative way to discuss end-of-life issues. *Home Healthcare Nurse, 18,* 532–540.

Patient Self-Determination Act (PSDA). (1990). *Omnibus Budget Reconciliation Act.* Title IV, Sec. 4206. Congress Record 12368, ct 26.

Paterson, D. H., Govindasamy, D., Vidmar, M., Cunningham, D. A., & Koval, J. J. (2004). Longitudinal study of determinants of dependence in an elderly population. *Journal of the American Geriatrics Society, 52*(10), 1632–1638.

*Patterson, C., Molloy, D. W., Guyatt, G. H., Bedard, M., North, J., Hassard, J., et al. (1997). Systematic implementation of an advance health care directive in the community. *Canadian Journal of Nursing Administration, 10*(2), 96–108.

*Pentz, C., & Wilson, A. (2000). Ensuring the quality of OASIS data: One agency's plan. *Home Healthcare Nurse, 19,* 38–42.

*Peterson, J. A. (2001). Osteoporosis overview. *Geriatric Nursing, 22,* 17–23.

*Phillips, L. R. (2000). Domestic violence and aging women. *Geriatric Nursing, 21,* 188–193.

Profile of disability in 2001. (2004). *Canadian Social Trends, 72*(Spring), 14–18.

Public Health Agency of Canada. (n.d.). *Aging and seniors.* Available at: www.phac-aspc.gc.ca/seniors-aines/index_pages/publications_e.htm#stats.

Public Health Agency of Canada. (n.d.). *Canada's physical activity guide to healthy active living for older adults.* Available at: www.phac-aspc.gc.ca/pau-uap/paguide/older/.

Randhawa, J., & Riley, R. (1995). Trends in hospital utilization, 1982–83 to 1992–93. *Health Reports, 7*(1), 41–9, 46–53.

Reid, R., Evans, R., Barer, M., Sheps, S., Kerluke, K., McGrail, K., et al. (2003). Conspicuous consumption: Characterizing high users of physician services in one Canadian province. *Journal of Health Services & Research Policy, 8*(4), 215–224.

Residential care facilities, 1999/2000 to 2001/02. (2004). *Health Reports, 15*(2), 47–50.

*Resnick, B. (2001). Promoting health in older adults: A four-year analysis. *Journal of the American Academy of Nurse Practitioners, 13,* 23–33.

Rockwood, K., Howlett, S. E., MacKnight, C., Beattie, B. L., Bergman, H., Hebert, R., et al. (2004). Prevalence, attributes, and outcomes of fitness and frailty in community-dwelling older adults: Report from the Canadian Study of Health and Aging. *Journals of Gerontology Series A–Biological Sciences & Medical Sciences, 59*(12), 1310–1317.

Ruckenstein, M. J. (2001). The dizzy patient: How you can help. *Consultant, 41,* 29–34.

*Ryden, M. B., Snyder, M., Gross, C. R., et al. (2000). Value-added outcomes: The lure of advanced practice nurses in long-term care facilities. *Gerontologist, 40,* 654–662.

*Schafer, S. L. (2001). Prescribing for seniors: It's a balancing act. *Journal of the American Academy of Nurse Practitioners, 13,* 108–112.

Scheiber, L. B., & Torregrosa, L. (2000). Osteoporosis: What to tell postmenopausal women about prevention and therapy. *Consultant, 40,* 1021–1028.

Schultz, S. E., & Kopec, J. A. (2004). Impact of chronic conditions. *Health Reports, 14*(4), 41–50.

Shields, M. (2004). Use of wheelchairs and other mobile support devices. *Health Reports, 15*(3), 37–43.

Snyder, M., & Olson, J. (1996). Music and hand massage interventions to produce relaxation and reduce aggressive behaviors in cognitively impaired elders: A pilot study. *Clinical Gerontologist, 17*(1), 64–69.

Squires, S. G., Pelletier, L., Zabchuk, P., Winchester, B., & Tam, T. (2001). Influenza in Canada—1999–2000 season. *Canada Communicable Disease Report, 27*(1), 1–9.

Statistics Canada. (2001). *Online census data.* Available at: www12.statcan.ca/English/census01/Products/Analytic/companion/fam/canada.cfm.

Statistics Canada. (n.d.). *Canada's seniors: A growing population.* Available at: www.phac-aspc.gc.ca/seniors-aines/pubs/factoids/2001/pdf/no01_e.pdf.

Sternberg, S. A., Wolfson, C., & Baumgarten, M. (2000). Undetected dementia in community-dwelling older people: The Canadian Study of Health and Aging. *Journal of the American Geriatrics Society, 48*(11), 1430–1434.

Stobert, S., & Cranswick, K. (2004). Who does what for whom? *Canadian Social Trends, 74*(Autumn), 2–6.

*Tappen, R., Roach, K., Applegate, E. B., & Stowell, P. (2000). Effect of a combined walking and conversation intervention on functional mobility of nursing home residents with Alzheimer disease. *Alzheimer Disease and Associated Disorders, 14,* 196–201.

Transport Canada. (n.d.). *Canadian motor vehicle traffic collision statistics: 2003.* Available at: http://www.tc.gc.ca/roadsafety/tp/tp3322/2003/page4.htm.

Vastag, B. (2002). Hormone replacement therapy falls out of favor with expert committee. *JAMA, 287*(15), 1923–1926.

Veterans Affairs Canada. (n.d.). *Dementia and Alzheimer disease.* Available at: http://www.vac-acc.gc.ca/clients/sub.cfm?source=health/dementia&CFID=233789&CFTOKEN=19455649.

*Whall, A. L., Black, M. E. A., Yankou, D. J., et al. (1999). Nurses aides' identification of onset and level of agitation in late stage dementia patients. *American Journal of Alzheimer's Disease, 14,* 202–206.

*Wilkins, K., & Park, E. (1996). Chronic conditions, physical limitations and dependency among seniors living in the community. *Health Reports, 8*(3), 7–15.

*Wilkins, K., & Park, E. (1998). Home care in Canada. *Health Reports, 10*(1), 29–37.

*Wilson, D. M. (2002a). The duration and degree of end-of-life dependency of home care clients and hospital inpatients. *Applied Nursing Research, 15*(2), 81–86.

*Wilson, D. M. (2002b). Making a case for home care. *Canadian Nurse Journal, 98*(1), 8–9.

*Wilson, D. M. & Truman, C. D. (2002). Addressing myths about end-of-life care: Research into the use of acute care hospitals over the last five years of life. *Journal of Palliative Care, 18*(1), 29–38.

*Wilson, D. M., & Truman, C. D. (2004a). Evaluating institutionalization by comparing the use of health services before and after admission to a long-term-care facility. *Evaluation & the Health Professions, 27*(3), 219–236.

*Wilson, D. M., & Truman, C. D. (2004b). Long-term-care residents. Concerns identified by population and care trends. *Canadian Journal of Public Health, 95*(5), 382–386.

*Wilson, D. M., Truman, C. D., Huang, J., Sheps, S., Thomas, R., & Noseworthy, T. (in press). The possibilities and realities of home care. *Canadian Journal of Public Health.*

Zukewich, N. (2003). Unpaid informal caregiving. *Canadian Social Trends, 70*(Autumn), 14–18.

RESOURCES AND WEBSITES

Alzheimer Society of Canada, 20 Eglinton Avenue West, Suite 1200, Toronto, ON M4R 1K8; (416) 488-8772; toll-free: 1-800-616-8816 (valid only in Canada); www.alzheimer.ca.

Canadian Association on Gerontology, 329 March Road, Suite 232, Box 11, Ottawa, ON K2K 2E1; (613) 271-1083; www.cagacg.ca.

The Canadian Continence Foundation, PO Box 30, Victoria Branch, Westmount, QC H3Z 2V4; (514) 488-8379; consumer help line: 1-800-265-9575; www.continence-fdn.ca.

Canadian Gerontological Nursing Association; www.cgna.net.

Canadian Hospice Palliative Care Association, Annex B, Saint-Vincent Hospital, 60 Cambridge Street North, Ottawa, ON K1R 7A5; 613-241-3663 or 1-800-668-2785; hospice palliative care info line: 1-877-203-4636; www.chpca.net.

The Canadian Lung Association, 3 Raymond Street, Suite 300, Ottawa, ON K1R 1A3; 613-569-6411; www.lung.ca.

Canadian National Institute for the Blind (CNIB), National Office, 1929 Bayview Avenue, Toronto, ON M4G 3E8; 416-486-2500; www.cnib.ca.

Canadian Network for the Prevention of Elder Abuse; www.cnpea.ca.

ElderWeb (Canada); www.elderweb.com/?PageID=1191.

National Advisory Council on Aging; www.naca-ccnta.ca/naca_main_e.htm.

National Clearinghouse on Family Violence; www.phac-aspc.gc.ca/ncfv-cnivf/familyviolence/bilingual.htm.

Veteran Affairs Canada; 1-866-522-2122 (English); 1-866-522-2022 (French); www.vac-acc.gc.ca.

Unit 3

Concepts and Challenges in Patient Management

Applying Concepts from NANDA, NIC, and NOC

Mr. Brandon is a 43-year-old man who sustained a back injury in a work-related incident. He reports severe shooting pains in his lower back and both buttocks. Mr. Brandon is not a candidate for surgery and has undergone physical therapy with little improvement in his pain. He reports that the pain makes it impossible for him to return to his former job, work around the house, or obtain enjoyment from leisure activities. He has been referred to a pain clinic for management. The concept map illustrates the relationships that exist among selected nursing diagnoses, interventions, and outcomes for the patient with chronic pain.

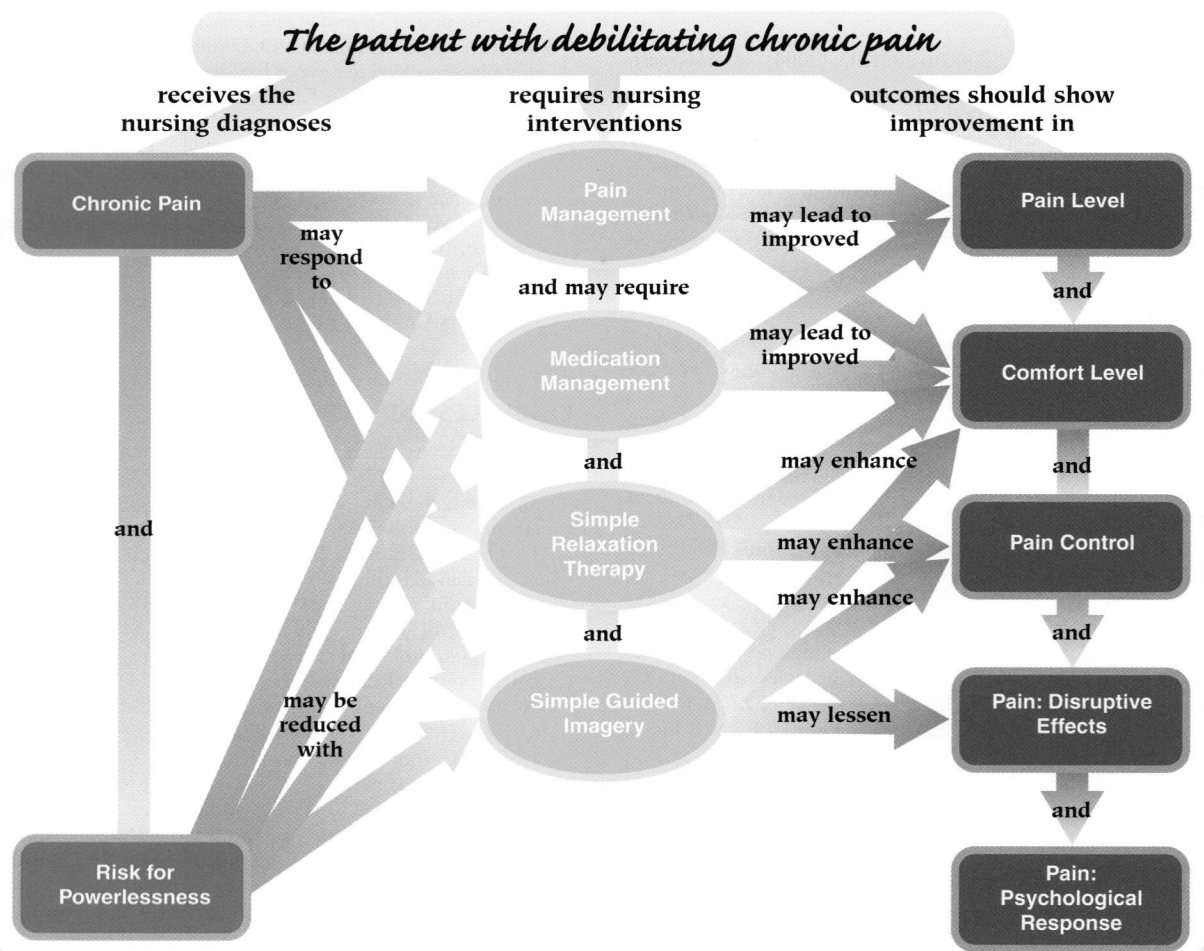

The patient with debilitating chronic pain

Nursing Classifications and Languages

NANDA
Nursing Diagnoses

Chronic Pain—Unpleasant sensory and emotional experience arising from actual or potential tissue damage or described in terms of such damage; sudden or slow onset of any intensity from mild to severe, constant or recurring, without an anticipated or pre-dictable end and a duration of greater than 6 months

Risk for Powerlessness—At risk for perceived lack of control over a situation and/or one's ability to significantly affect an outcome

NIC
Nursing Interventions*

Pain Management—Alleviation of pain or reduction in pain to a level of comfort that is acceptable to the patient

Medication Management—Facilitation of safe and effective use of prescribed or over-the-counter medicine

Simple Relaxation Therapy—Use of techniques to encourage and elicit relaxation for the purpose of decreasing undesirable signs and symptoms such as pain, muscle tension, or anxiety

Simple Guided Imagery—Purposeful use of imagination to achieve relaxation and/or direct attention away from undesirable sensations

Emotional Support—Provision of reassurance, acceptance, and encouragement during times of stress

Self-Esteem Enhancement—Assisting a patient to increase his or her personal judgment of self-worth

NOC
Nursing Outcomes†

Return to functional baseline status, stabilization of, or improvement in

Pain Level—Severity of reported or demonstrated pain

Comfort Level—Extent of physical and psychological ease

Pain Control—Personal actions to control pain

Pain: Disruptive Effects—Observed or reported disruptive effects of pain on emotions and behaviour

Pain: Psychological Response—Cognitive and emotional responses to physical pain

NANDA, North American Nursing Diagnosis Association; NIC, Nursing Interventions Classification; NOC, Nursing Outcomes Classification.

*Iowa Intervention Project © 2000. In McCloskey, J. C., & Bulechek, G. M. (2000). *Nursing interventions classification (NIC)* (3rd ed.). St. Louis: Mosby.

†Iowa Outcomes Project © 2000. In Johnson, M., Maas, M., & Moorhead, S. (2000). *Nursing outcomes classification (NOC)* (3rd ed.). St. Louis: Mosby.

Pain Management

Adapted by Janice A. Lander

LEARNING OBJECTIVES

On completion of this chapter, the learner will be able to:

1. Differentiate between acute pain, procedural pain, chronic pain, and cancer pain.
2. Describe the negative consequences of pain.
3. Describe the pathophysiology of pain.
4. Describe factors that can alter the perception of pain.
5. Demonstrate appropriate use of pain measurement instruments.
6. Explain the physiologic basis of pain relief interventions.
7. Explain the impact of aging on pain.
8. Discuss when opioid tolerance may be a problem.
9. Identify appropriate pain relief interventions for selected groups of patients.
10. Compare the various types of neurosurgical procedures used to treat intractable pain.
11. Develop a plan to prevent and treat the adverse effects of opioid analgesic agents.
12. Use the nursing process as a framework for the care of patients with pain.

$\mathcal{P}$**ain** is an unpleasant sensory and emotional experience associated with actual or potential tissue damage (Merskey & Boduk, 1994). It is the most common reason for seeking health care. It occurs with many disorders, diagnostic tests, and treatments. It disables and distresses more people than any single disease. Since nurses spend more time with the patient in pain than do other health care providers, nurses need to understand the pathophysiology of pain, the physiologic and psychological consequences of acute and chronic pain, and the methods used to treat pain. Nurses encounter patients in pain in a variety of settings, including hospitals, primary care, community, public health, and continuing care settings. Thus, they must have the knowledge and skills to assess pain, to implement pain relief strategies, and to evaluate the effectiveness of these strategies, regardless of setting.

The Fifth Vital Sign

Pain management is considered such an important part of care that the American Pain Society coined the phrase "Pain: The 5th Vital Sign" (Campbell, 1995) to emphasize its significance and to increase the awareness among health care professionals of the importance of effective pain management. Calling pain the fifth vital sign suggests that the assessment of pain should be as automatic as taking a patient's blood pressure and pulse.

Pain assessment and management are mandated by the Canadian Council on Health Services Accreditation (CCHSA). The CCHSA (2005) has incorporated specific actions to meet the standard for pain management. The standards for assessing and managing pain include regular pain assessments, use of standardized clinical pain measures, being knowledgeable about pain-management strategies, and receiving continuing education about evidence-based pain-management strategies. Pain management is considered to be an issue of patient safety. Safe and effective pain management results in optimum outcomes for patients. These standards reflect the importance of pain management.

The nurse collaborates with other health care professionals while administering most pain relief interventions, evaluating their effectiveness, and serving as patient advocate when the intervention is ineffective. In addition, the nurse serves as an educator to the patient and family, teaching them to manage the pain relief regimen themselves when appropriate.

The International Association for the Study of Pain definition mentioned earlier encompasses the multidimensional nature of pain (Merskey & Boduk, 1994). A broad definition of pain is "whatever the person says it is, existing whenever the experiencing person says it does" (McCaffery & Beebe, 1989, p.7). This definition emphasizes the highly subjective nature of pain and pain management. The patient is the best authority on the existence

Glossary

addiction: a neurobiological disorder influenced by genetic, psychosocial, and environmental factors. It refers to drugs or substances and is distinguished by compulsive use, inability to control use, and obsessive need to have the drug or substance despite its harmful effects.

adjuvant analgesic: a drug whose initial use was for another disorder but which later was found to be beneficial for pain. Examples are antidepressants and anticonvulsants.

agonist: a substance that when combined with the receptor produces the drug effect or desired effect. Endorphins and morphine are agonists on the opioid receptors.

algogenic: causing pain

allodynia: pain resulting from a nonpainful stimulus such as a breeze or light touch of clothing.

antagonist: a substance that blocks or reverses the effects of the agonist by occupying the receptor site without producing the drug effect. Naloxone (Narcan) is an opioid antagonist.

breakthrough pain: a sudden and temporary increase in pain occurring in a patient being managed with opioid analgesia

dependence: occurs when a patient who has been taking opioids experiences a withdrawal syndrome when the opioids are discontinued; often occurs with opioid tolerance and does not indicate an addiction

endorphins and enkephalins: morphinelike substances produced by the body. Primarily found in the central nervous system, they have the potential to reduce pain.

multimodal therapy: using more than one method or modality concurrently for controlling pain to obtain greater benefits and fewer side effects. This may also be referred to as balanced analgesia.

nociception: activation of sensory transduction in nerves by thermal, mechanical, or chemical energy impinging on specialized nerve endings. The nerves involved convey information about tissue damage to the central nervous system.

nociceptor: a receptor preferentially sensitive to a noxious stimulus

non-nociceptor: nerve fibre that usually does not transmit pain

opioid: a morphine-like compound that produces bodily effects including pain relief, sedation, constipation, and respiratory depression. This term is preferred over **narcotic**.

pain: an unpleasant sensory and emotional experience resulting from actual or potential tissue damage

pain threshold: the point at which a stimulus is perceived as painful. This term refers to induction of pain for research purposes in a laboratory setting. Pain is induced by various stimuli (eg, mechanical or thermal).

pain tolerance: the maximum intensity of a stimulus that a person is prepared to tolerate. This term refers to induction of pain for research purposes in a laboratory setting.

patient-controlled analgesia (PCA): self-administration of analgesic agents by a patient instructed about the procedure

phantom limb pain and sensation: the sense that an amputated body part is still present. Phantom sensations are experienced almost universally by people who have had amputations and many people suffer from phantom pain. These sensations arise because of damage to peripheral nerves above the site of the amputation.

placebo effect: a beneficial effect in a patient that arises from the patient's positive expectations about the treatment. The effect of any intervention, whether inactive or therapeutic, can be enhanced by positive expectations.

prostaglandins: chemical substances that increase the sensitivity of pain receptors by enhancing the pain-provoking effect of bradykinin

referred pain: pain perceived as coming from an area different from that in which the pathology is occurring. An example would be the perception of left arm or jaw pain in a person having a myocardial infarction.

sensitization: a heightened response seen after exposure to a noxious stimulus. Response to the same stimulus is to feel more pain.

tolerance: occurs when a person who has been taking opioids becomes less sensitive to their analgesic properties (and usually side effects). Characterized by the need for increasing doses to maintain the same level of pain relief of pain. Therefore, validation of the existence of pain is based on the patient's report that it exists.

Although it is important to believe the patient who reports pain, it is equally important to be alert to patients who deny pain in situations where pain would be expected. A nurse who suspects pain in a patient who denies it should explore with the patient the reason for suspecting pain, such as the fact that the disorder or procedure is usually painful or that the patient grimaces when moving or avoids movement. Exploring why the patient may be denying pain is also helpful. Some people deny pain because they fear the treatment that may result if they report or admit pain. Others deny pain for fear of becoming addicted to various medications including **opioids** (previously referred to as narcotics).

Types of Pain

Pain is categorized according to its duration and etiology. Four basic categories of pain are generally recognized: acute pain, procedural pain, chronic (noncancer) pain, and cancer-related pain.

ACUTE PAIN

Usually of recent onset and commonly associated with a specific injury, acute pain indicates that damage or injury has occurred. Pain is significant in that it draws attention to its existence and teaches the person to avoid similar potentially painful situations. If no lasting damage occurs and no systemic disease exists, acute pain usually decreases along with healing. For purposes of definition, acute pain can be described as lasting from days to months. In a situation where healing is expected in weeks and the patient continues to suffer pain, it should be considered chronic and treated with interventions used for chronic pain. Waiting for the full 3- to 6-month time frame in this example could cause needless suffering.

PROCEDURAL PAIN

Procedural pain is brief, intense pain that arises from diagnostic, therapeutic, and preventive procedures. It lasts from seconds to hours. If significant tissue damage occurs, procedural pain may become acute pain. One of the most common sources of procedural pain is needle puncture associated with venipuncture, intravenous cannulation, parenteral drug administration, and lumbar puncture. Wound débridement and wound cleansing also can cause pain, as can many other procedures.

CHRONIC (NONCANCER) PAIN

Chronic pain is classified as noncancer or cancer-related. Chronic noncancer pain was referred to as chronic nonmalignant pain or chronic benign pain in the past but now is referred to simply as chronic pain. Chronic pain is pain that has persisted beyond the expected tissue healing time or pain caused by an underlying disease.

Although acute pain may be a useful signal that something is wrong, chronic pain usually becomes a problem in its own right. Chronic pain may be defined as pain that lasts for 6 months or longer, although 6 months is arbitrary. An episode of pain may assume the characteristics of chronic pain before 6 months have elapsed, or some types of pain may remain primarily acute in nature for longer than 6 months. Nevertheless, after 6 months, most pain experiences are accompanied by problems related to the pain itself. Chronic pain serves no useful purpose. If it persists, it may become the patient's primary disorder.

The nurse may come in contact with patients with chronic pain when they are admitted to the hospital for treatment or when they are seen out of the hospital. Frequently the nurse is called on in community-based settings to assist patients in managing pain.

CANCER-RELATED PAIN

Pain associated with cancer may be acute or chronic. Pain resulting from cancer is so ubiquitous that after fear of dying, it is the second most common fear of newly diagnosed cancer patients (Lema, 1997). In Canada, 70% to 90% of people with cancer will have moderate to severe pain at some time during their illness. Although effective pain interventions are widely available in Canada, many Canadians will suffer needlessly from cancer pain because of poor management. Pain in the patient suffering from cancer can be directly associated with the cancer (eg, bony infiltration with tumour cells or nerve compression), a result of cancer treatment (eg, surgery or radiation), or not associated with the cancer (eg, trauma). Most pain associated with cancer, however, is a direct result of tumour involvement. An approach to cancer pain management is illustrated in Figure 13-1. This three-step approach illustrates the types of analgesic medications used for various levels of pain.

CLASSIFICATION OF CHRONIC PAIN SYNDROMES

It is useful to categorize chronic pain syndromes according to pathophysiology. Three main categories are nociceptive, neuropathic, and a mixed type. Chronic nociceptive pain, which arises from constant stimulation of pain receptors and signals tissue damage in the skin, bone, joints, or viscera, has an aching or throbbing quality to it. Arthritis pain and fibromyalgia are good examples of chronic nociceptive pain.

FIGURE 13-1 The World Health Organization three-step ladder approach to relieving cancer pain. Analgesic regimens are based on pain reported as ranging from mild to moderate to severe. Various opioid and nonopioid medications may be combined with other medications to control pain.

Neuropathic pain is triggered by nerve damage or malfunction of peripheral and central nervous systems resulting in abnormal signalling. The problem may begin with an injury or may be due to nerve compression by tumours, nerve inflammation by infection or nerve impairment from systemic diseases such as diabetes. The pain often has a burning, tingling or piercing quality. **Allodynia,** which is pain arising from a nonpainful stimulus such as a breeze or light touch of clothing or bedding, is also characteristic of neuropathic pain. Examples include post-herpetic neuralgia, diabetic neuropathy and **phantom limb pain.**

Some chronic pain syndromes are both nociceptive and neuropathic. These syndromes are classified as mixed. Migraine pain is a good example. For more information on chronic pain syndromes, see Chart 13-1.

Harmful Effects of Pain

Regardless of its nature, pattern, or cause, pain that is inadequately treated has harmful effects beyond the suffering it causes. For example, unrelieved pain impairs the postoperative patient's ability to sleep (Raymond, Nielsen, Lauigne et al., 2001). Zalon (1997) found that the most common response to severe pain in frail, elderly postoperative women was to lie absolutely still, a response likely to result in postoperative complications.

Chart 13-1   **Pain Syndromes**

Nociceptive Pain Syndromes
Nociceptors are the pain receptors that respond to tissue damage. They transmit signals along the peripheral nerves and spinal cord to the brain. Visceral pain is nociceptive pain that involves the organs.

Arthritis Pain
Various rheumatic diseases, such as osteoarthritis and rheumatoid arthritis, cause arthritis pain, which is characterized by joint pain and stiffness. Osteoarthritis is a degenerative joint disease that typically affects the weight-bearing joints. It typically affects older adults. Rheumatoid arthritis is an inflammatory disease that affects both weight-bearing and non–weight-bearing joints. It can begin in childhood or in young to middle adulthood. Treatment includes use of NSAIDs and physiatric techniques such as heat and cold.

Fibromyalgia (Fibrositis)
Fibromyalgia, a chronic pain syndrome characterized by generalized musculoskeletal pain, trigger points, stiffness, fatigability, and sleep disturbances, is aggravated by stress and overexertion. The disease primarily affects young women. Treatment consists of NSAIDs, trigger point injections with local anesthetics, tricyclic antidepressants, stress reduction, and regular exercise.

Hemiplegia-Associated Shoulder Pain
Hemiplegia-associated shoulder pain is a pain syndrome that affects as many as 80% of stroke patients. It may result from stretching of the shoulder joint due to the uncompensated pull of gravity on the impaired arm. It may be preventable with functional electrical stimulation of involved shoulder muscles.

Neuropathic Pain Syndromes
Neuropathic pain is caused by a malfunction in the nerves, spinal cord, or brain. It may follow injury or be caused by illness and exposure to chemicals or drugs. In some cases, the origin of the neuropathic pain is unknown. The following conditions are among those associated with neuropathic pain: diabetes, cancer, multiple sclerosis, stroke, HIV and AIDS, amputation, spinal injury, herpes zoster, and alcoholism. Neuropathic pain syndromes are characterized by tingling or numbness that evolves to become burning, crushing, or squeezing pain. Those affected by neuropathic pain may be significantly incapacitated. Tricyclic antidepressants and antiepileptic drugs are used as adjuvants to the analgesics for the treatment of neuropathic pain. The latter suppresses hyperexcitability of the nerves.

Reflex Sympathetic Dystrophy (RSD)
Reflex sympathetic dystrophy occurs after a relatively minor trauma. Characterized by unexplained diffuse burning pain, usually in the periphery of an extremity, RSD is accompanied by weakness, skin colour and temperature changes relative to the other extremity, limited range of motion, hyperesthesia, hypoesthesia, edema, altered hair growth, and sweating (Janig, 2001). Currently, regional sympathetic blockade and regional IV bretylium offer promise for relief. Tricyclic antidepressants may be tried as well.

Postmastectomy Pain Syndrome (PMP)
Postmastectomy pain syndrome (PMP) occurs after mastectomy with node dissection but is not necessarily related to the continuation of disease. Characterized by the sensation of constriction accompanied by a burning, prickling, or numbness in the posterior arm, axilla, or chest wall, PMP is often aggravated by movement of the shoulder, resulting in a frozen shoulder from immobilization (Miaskowski & Dibble, 1995).

Peripheral Neuropathy
Peripheral neuropathy is caused by damage to peripheral nerves and is an outcome of many diseases. Common causes are endocrine and nutritional disorders (eg, diabetes and alcoholism), infection (herpes zoster and AIDS), and cancer. In many cases, the etiology of peripheral neuropathy is unknown. The features of peripheral neuropathy include weakness, paresthesia, numbness, and burning pain. Walking and standing become difficult because the patient is unable to identify the position of the joint. Patients risk injury from falls and from inability to feel the development of pressure sores.

AIDS-Related Pain
As AIDS progresses, so do problems that produce increasing amounts of pain, such as neuropathy, esophagitis, headaches, postherpetic pain, and abdominal, back, bone, and joint pain. Pain relief interventions are individualized and may consist of NSAIDs, long-lasting opioids, such as fentanyl patches, and topical lidocaine. Tricyclic antidepressants may provide comfort in neuropathic and postherpetic pain.

Postherpetic Neuralgia
As immunity for chickenpox (varicella zoster virus) progressively declines over time, the risk of herpes zoster (or shingles) increases. Shingles is an outcome of the reactivation of the dormant virus. It is characterized by a vesicular skin rash over a sensory nerve pathway, often on the trunk or face. It tends to occur in older adults, and 50% of them will go on to have complications such as postherpetic neuralgia. If antiviral drugs (eg, famciclovir) are administered soon after onset of symptoms, the severity and duration of shingles can be reduced. Administration of a zoster vaccine to older adults has been found to reduce incidence of shingles and postherpetic neuralgia (Oxman, Levin, Johnson et al, 2005). After a 3-year follow-up, the number needed to treat is 62 (need to treat 62 with the vaccine in order to prevent one case of shingles). As the follow-up continues, the value of vaccination in preventing shingles could be expected to increase.

Mixed Pain Syndromes
The pain is both neuropathic and nociceptive. At one time, these syndromes were referred to as idiopathic.

Migraine
This is characterized by pulsating severe headache lasting from a few hours to days. Headaches can occur in clusters and be accompanied by nausea, vomiting, or photophobia. In recent years, drugs have been developed to put an early end to the headache (eg, sumatriptan). However, they are not effective for all people.

EFFECTS OF ACUTE PAIN

Unrelieved acute pain can affect the pulmonary, cardiovascular, gastrointestinal, endocrine, and immune systems. The stress response ("neuroendocrine response to stress") that occurs with trauma also occurs with other causes of severe pain. The widespread endocrine, immunologic, and inflammatory changes that occur with stress can have significant negative effects. This is particularly harmful in patients compromised by age, illness, or injury. The stress response generally consists of increased metabolic rate and cardiac output, impaired insulin response, increased production of cortisol, and increased retention of fluids (see Chap. 6 for details about the stress response). The stress response may increase the patient's risk for physiologic disorders (eg, myocardial infarction, pulmonary infection, thromboembolism, and prolonged paralytic ileus). The patient with severe pain and associated stress may be unable to take a deep breath and may experience increased fatigue and decreased mobility. Although these effects may be tolerated by a young, healthy person, they may hamper recovery in an elderly, debilitated, or critically ill person. Effective pain relief may result in a faster recovery and improved outcomes.

EFFECTS OF PROCEDURAL PAIN

Poorly managed procedural pain has adverse and often long-lasting physiological and psychological effects. Some evidence exists that severe uncontrolled procedural pain will lead to sensitization to noxious stimuli. Newborn infants who were circumcised without the benefit of an anesthetic had a heightened pain response to immunization administered months after the circumcision (Taddio, Goldbach, Ipp, & Koren, 1995).

Poorly managed procedural pain can give rise to a cycle of pain, anxiety, and fear that ultimately may lead to avoidance of the procedure. Adults will often acknowledge that they dread the anxiety, not the pain, associated with the procedure. At its extreme, people will avoid medical and dental care out of fear that the dreaded procedure awaits them. Poorly managed pain may lead to catastrophizing in vulnerable individuals. This is a negative cognitive response marked by preoccupation with the pain stimulus, inflation of its potential threat, and a sense of helplessness. For example, an adult with a wood splinter in his eye may refuse to go to the Emergency Department out of an irrational belief that health care professionals are waiting to carry out all of the needle procedures he has avoided for years.

It takes less effort for health professionals to prevent procedural pain and its adverse effects than to manage or treat long-term procedural anxiety. Fortunately, many interventions have been developed to minimize procedural pain.

EFFECTS OF CHRONIC PAIN

Like acute pain, chronic pain also has adverse effects. Suppression of the immune function associated with chronic pain may promote tumour growth. Also, chronic pain often results in depression and disability. Although health care providers express concern about the large quantities of opioid medications required to relieve chronic pain in some patients, it is safe to use large doses of these medications to control progressive chronic pain. In fact, failure to administer adequate pain relief may be unsafe because of the consequences of unrelieved pain (Jovey, Ennis, Gardner-Nix et al, 2003).

Regardless of how the patient copes with chronic pain, pain for an extended period can result in disability. Patients with a number of chronic pain syndromes report depression, anger, and fatigue

(Meuser, Pietruck, Radruch et al., 2001; Raymond, Nielsen, Lauigne et al., 2001). The patient may be unable to continue the activities and interpersonal relationships he or she engaged in before the pain began. Disabilities may range from curtailing participation in physical activities to being unable to take care of personal needs, such as dressing or eating. The nurse needs to understand the effects of chronic pain on the patient and family and needs to be knowledgeable about pain-relief strategies and appropriate resources to assist effectively with pain management.

Pathophysiology of Pain

The sensory experience of pain depends on the interaction between the nervous system and the environment. The processing of noxious stimuli and the resulting perception of pain involve the peripheral and central nervous systems.

PAIN TRANSMISSION

Among the nerve mechanisms and structures involved in the transmission of pain perceptions to and from the area of the brain that interprets pain are nociceptors, or pain receptors, and chemical mediators. **Nociceptors** are receptors that are preferentially sensitive to a noxious stimulus. Nociceptors are also called pain receptors, but the former term is preferred.

Nociceptors

Nociceptors are free nerve endings in the skin that respond only to intense, potentially damaging stimuli. Such stimuli may be mechanical, thermal, or chemical in nature. The joints, skeletal muscle, fascia, tendons, and cornea also have nociceptors that have the potential to transmit information about stimuli that produce pain. However, the large internal organs (viscera) do not contain nerve endings that respond only to painful stimuli. Pain originating in these organs results from intense stimulation of receptors that have other purposes. For example, inflammation, stretching, ischemia, dilation, and spasm of the internal organs all cause an intense response in these multipurpose fibres and can cause severe pain.

Nociceptors are part of complex multidirectional pathways. These nerve fibres branch very near their origin in the skin and send fibres to local blood vessels, mast cells, hair follicles, and sweat glands. When these fibres are stimulated, histamine is released from the mast cells, causing vasodilation. Nociceptors respond to high-intensity mechanical, thermal, and chemical stimuli. Some receptors respond to only one type of stimuli; others, called polymodal nociceptors, respond to all three types of stimuli. These highly specialized neurons transfer the mechanical, thermal, or chemical stimulus into electrical activity or action potentials.

The cutaneous fibres located more centrally further branch and communicate with the paravertebral sympathetic chain of the nervous system and with large internal organs. As a result of the connections between these nerve fibres, pain is often accompanied by vasomotor, autonomic, and visceral effects. In a patient with severe acute pain, for example, gastrointestinal peristalsis may decrease or stop.

Peripheral Nervous System

A number of **algogenic** (pain-causing) substances that affect the sensitivity of nociceptors are released into the extracellular tissue as a result of tissue damage. Histamine, bradykinin, acetylcholine, serotonin, and substance P are chemicals that increase the transmission of pain. The transmission of pain is also referred to as **nociception**. **Prostaglandins** are chemical substances thought to increase the sensitivity of pain receptors by enhancing the pain-provoking effect of bradykinin. These chemical mediators also cause vasodilation and increased vascular permeability, resulting in redness, warmth, and swelling of the injured area.

Once nociception is initiated, the nociceptive action potentials are transmitted by the peripheral nervous system (Porth, 2002). The first-order neurons travel from the periphery (skin, cornea, visceral organs) to the spinal cord via the dorsal horn. There are two main types of fibres involved in the transmission of nociception. Smaller, myelinated Aδ (A delta) fibres transmit nociception rapidly, which produces the initial "fast pain." Type C fibres are larger, unmyelinated fibres that transmit what is called second pain. This type of pain has dull, aching, or burning qualities that last longer than the initial fast pain. The type and concentration of nerve fibres to transmit pain vary by tissue type.

If there is repeated C fibre input, a greater response is noted in dorsal horn neurons, causing the person to perceive more pain. In other words, the same noxious stimulus produces hyperalgesia, and the person reports greater pain than was felt at the first stimulus. For this reason, it is important to treat patients with analgesic agents when they first feel the pain. Patients require less medication and experience more effective pain relief if analgesics are administered before the patient becomes sensitized to the pain.

Chemicals that reduce or inhibit the transmission or perception of pain include **endorphins** and **enkephalins**. These morphine-like neurotransmitters are endogenous (produced by the body). They are examples of substances that reduce nociceptive transmission when applied to certain nerve fibres. The term "endorphin" is a combination of two words: endogenous and morphine. Endorphins and enkephalins are found in heavy concentrations in the central nervous system, particularly the spinal and medullary dorsal horn, the periaqueductal grey matter, hypothalamus, and amygdala. Morphine and other opioid medications act at receptor sites to suppress the excitation initiated by noxious stimuli. The binding of opioids to receptor sites is responsible for the effects noted after their administration. Each receptor (mu, kappa, delta) responds differently when activated. Table 13-1 summarizes the classification and action of opioid receptors.

Central Nervous System

After tissue injury occurs, nociception (the neurologic transmission of pain impulses) to the spinal cord via the Aδ and C fibres continues. The fibres enter the dorsal horn, which is divided into laminae based on cell type. The laminae II cell type is commonly referred to as the substantia gelatinosa. In the substantia gelatinosa are projections that relay nociception to other parts of the spinal cord (Fig. 13-2).

Nociception continues from the spinal cord to the reticular formation, thalamus, limbic system, and cerebral cortex. Here nociception is localized and its characteristics become apparent to the person, including the intensity. The involvement of the reticular formation, limbic, and reticular activating systems is responsible for the individual variations in the perception of noxious stimuli. Individuals may report the same stimulus differently based on their anxiety, past experiences, and expectations. This is a result of the conscious perception of pain.

For pain to be consciously perceived, neurons in the ascending system must be activated. Activation occurs as a result of input from the nociceptors located in the skin and internal organs. Once activated, the inhibitory interneuronal fibres in the dorsal horn inhibit or turn off the transmission of noxious stimulating information in the ascending pathway.

Descending Control System

The descending control system is a system of fibres that originate in the lower and midportion of the brain (specifically the periaqueductal grey matter) and terminate on the inhibitory interneuronal fibres in the dorsal horn of the spinal cord. This system is probably always somewhat active; it prevents continuous transmission of information as painful, partly through the action of the endorphins. As nociception occurs, the descending control system is activated to inhibit pain.

Cognitive processes may stimulate endorphin production in the descending control system. The effectiveness of this system is illustrated by the effects of distraction. The distractions of visitors or a favourite TV show may increase activity in the descending control system. Therefore, the person who has visitors may not report pain because activation of the descending control system results in less noxious or painful information being transmitted to consciousness. Once the distraction by the visitors ends, activity in the descending control system decreases, resulting in increased perception of pain.

The interconnections between the descending neuronal system and the ascending sensory tract are called inhibitory interneuronal fibres. These fibres contain enkephalin and are primarily activated through the activity of **non-nociceptor** peripheral fibres (fibres that normally do not transmit information about pain) in the same receptor field as the pain receptor, and descending fibres, grouped together in a system called descending control. The enkephalins

---

Table 13-1 • **Opioid Receptor Classification and Action**

ORGAN EFFECT	μ	κ	δ
Eye: Pupil	Miosis	Miosis	Mydriasis
Lung: Respiratory rate	Stimulation, then depression	No change	Stimulation
Heart: Rate	Bradycardia	No change	Tachycardia
Body: Temperature	Hypothermia	No change	Unknown
Affect	Indifference	Sedation	Dysphoria
Gastrointestinal system	Constipation	No effects	Nausea

μ = mu; κ = kappa; δ = delta

Willens, J. S. (1994). Pain management in the trauma patient. In V. D. Cardona, P. D. Hurn, P. J. B. Mason, A. M. Scanlon, & S. W. Veise-Berry (Eds.), *Trauma nursing from resuscitation through rehabilitation* (2nd ed., pp 325–362). Philadelphia: W. B. Saunders. With permission of W. B. Saunders. Copyright 1994 by W. B. Saunders.

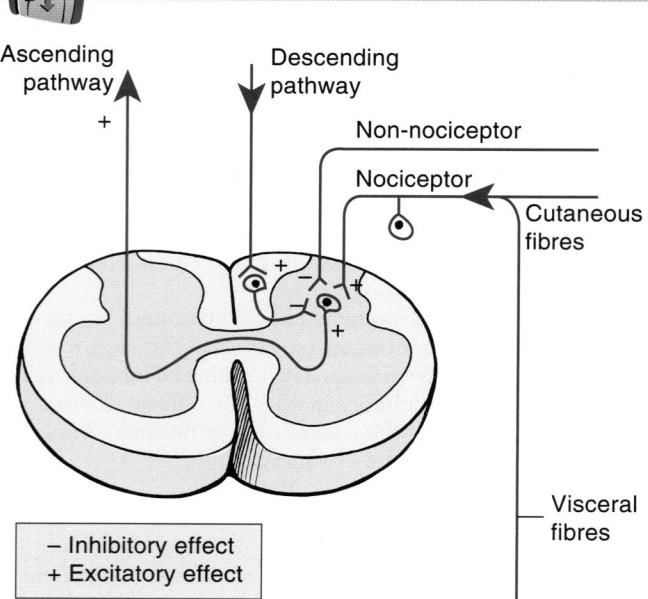

Physiology/Pathophysiology

Ascending pathway

Descending pathway

Non-nociceptor

Nociceptor

Cutaneous fibres

Visceral fibres

− Inhibitory effect
+ Excitatory effect

FIGURE 13-2 Representative nociception system, showing ascending and descending sensory pathways of the dorsal horn.

and endorphins are thought to inhibit pain impulses by stimulating the inhibitory interneuronal fibres, which in turn reduce the transmission of noxious impulses via the ascending system (Puig & Montes, 1998).

The classic gate control theory of pain, described by Melzack and Wall in 1965, was the first to clearly articulate the existence of a pain-modulating system (Melzack, 1996). This theory proposes that stimulation of the skin evokes impulses that are then transmitted by three systems located in the spinal cord. The substantia gelatinosa in the dorsal horn, the dorsal column fibres, and the central transmission cells act to influence nociceptive impulses. The noxious impulses are influenced by a "gating mechanism." Melzack and Wall proposed that stimulation of the large-diameter fibres inhibits the transmission of pain, thus "closing the gate." Conversely, when smaller fibres are stimulated, the gate is opened. The gating mechanism is influenced by nerve impulses that descend from the brain. This theory proposes a specialized system of large-diameter fibres that activate selective cognitive processes via the modulating properties of the spinal gate. Figure 13-3 shows a schematic representation of a gate control system and nociceptive pathways.

The gate control theory was important because it was the first theory to suggest that psychological factors play a role in the perception of pain. The theory guided research toward the cognitive-behavioural approaches to pain management. This theory helps to explain how interventions such as distraction and music therapy provide pain relief.

Melzack (1996) extended the gate control theory after carefully analyzing phantom limb pain. He proposed that a large, widespread network of neurons exists that consists of loops between the thalamus and cortex and between the cortex and the limbic system. Melzack labelled this network the neuromatrix. As information is processed in the neuromatrix, a characteristic pattern emerges. This pattern, referred to as the neurosignature, is a continuous outflow

from the neuromatrix. Ultimately, the neurosignature output, with a constant stream of input and varying patterns, produces the feelings of the whole body with constantly changing qualities.

Melzack (1996) theorized that in the absence of modulating inputs from the missing limb, the active neuromatrix produces a neurosignature pattern that is perceived as pain. The neuromatrix theory highlights the role of the brain in sustaining the experience of pain. Some researchers have criticized this theory as not adding to the understanding of how psychological factors influence pain (Keefe, Lefebvre & Starr, 1996). While the neuromatrix theory might explain unusual pain phenomena, its contribution to understanding pain management remains to be seen.

FACTORS INFLUENCING THE PAIN RESPONSE

A person's pain experience is influenced by a number of factors, including past experiences with pain, anxiety, culture, age, gender, and expectations about pain relief. These factors may increase or decrease the person's perception of pain, increase or decrease ability to withstand pain, and affect responses to pain.

Past Experience

It is tempting to expect that a person who has had multiple or prolonged experiences with pain would be less anxious and more tolerant of pain than one who has had little pain. For most people, however, this is not true. Often, the more experience a person has had with pain, the more frightened he or she is about subsequent painful events. This person may be less able to deal with pain; that is, he or she wants relief from pain sooner and before it becomes severe. This reaction is more likely to occur if the person has received inadequate pain relief in the past. A person with repeated pain experiences may have learned to fear the escalation of pain and its inadequate treatment. Once a person experiences severe pain, that person knows just how severe it can be. Conversely, someone who has never had severe pain may have no fear of such pain.

The way a person responds to pain is a result of many separate painful events during a lifetime. For some, past pain may have been constant and unrelenting, as in prolonged or chronic and persistent pain. The individual who has pain for months or years may become irritable, withdrawn, and depressed.

The undesirable effects that may result from previous experience point to the need for the nurse to be aware of the patient's past experiences with pain. If pain is relieved promptly and adequately, the person may be less fearful of future pain and better able to tolerate it.

Anxiety and Depression

Although it is commonly believed that anxiety will increase pain, this is not necessarily true. Perhaps because of measurement problems, research has demonstrated no consistent relationship between anxiety and pain, nor has research shown that preoperative stress reduction training reduces postoperative pain (Keogh, Ellery, Hunt et al., 2001; Rhudy & Meagher, 2000). Postoperative anxiety is most related to preoperative anxiety and postoperative complications. However, anxiety that is relevant or related to the pain may increase the patient's perception of pain. For example, a patient who was treated 2 years ago for breast cancer and now has hip pain may fear that the pain indicates metastasis. In this case, the anxiety may result in increased pain. Anxiety that is unrelated to the pain

Physiology/Pathophysiology

FIGURE 13-3 A schematic representation of the gate control system and aspects of the nociceptive system. The nervous system is made up of stimulatory and inhibitory fibres. For example, stimulation of the nociceptor will result in the transmission of an impulse that will be interpreted as pain. When it is stimulated it will stimulate transmission at the next fibre junction (represented as +>-). The interneuronal fibre is an inhibitory neuron (->>-). When it is stimulated it, in turn, inhibits or shuts off transmission at the next junction. So a placebo has a (+) stimulatory effect on the descending control system, which has a stimulatory effect (+) on the interneuronal fibre, which has an inhibitory effect (−) on the ascending control system. A topical anesthetic has an inhibitory effect (−) on nerve transmission at the nociceptor level and a spinal anesthetic has the same impact (−) on the ascending nociceptive fibres.

may distract the patient and may actually decrease the perception of pain. For example, a mother who is hospitalized with complications from abdominal surgery and is anxious about her children may perceive less pain as her anxiety about her children increases.

The routine use of antianxiety medications to treat anxiety in someone with pain may prevent the person from reporting pain because of sedation and may impair the patient's ability to take deep breaths, get out of bed, and cooperate with the treatment plan. The most effective way to relieve pain is by directing the treatment at the pain rather than at the anxiety.

Just as anxiety is associated with pain because of concerns and fears about the underlying disease, depression is associated with chronic pain and unrelieved cancer pain. In chronic pain situations, depression is associated with major life changes due to the limiting effects of the pain, specifically unemployment. Longer durations of pain are associated with an increased incidence of depression (Wall, 1999). Unrelieved cancer pain drastically interferes with the patient's quality of life, and relieving the pain may go a long way toward treating the depression.

Learned Responses

Beliefs about pain and how to respond to it differ in society. Early in childhood, individuals learn from those around them what responses to pain are acceptable or unacceptable. For example, a child may learn that a sports injury is not expected to hurt as much as a comparable injury caused by a motor vehicle crash. The child also learns what stimuli are expected to be painful and what behavioural responses are acceptable. These beliefs vary from one social group to another; therefore, people from different cultures who experience the same intensity of pain may not report it or respond to it in the same ways.

Many studies have examined the cultural aspects of pain. Inconsistent results, methodologic weaknesses or flaws (Lasch, 2000), and failure of many researchers to carefully distinguish ethnicity, culture, and race make it difficult to interpret the findings of many of these studies. Factors that help to explain differences in a cultural group include age, gender, education level, and income. In addition, the degree to which a patient identifies with a culture influences the degree to which he or she will adopt new health behaviours or cling to traditional health beliefs and practices. Other factors that affect a patient's response to pain include his or her interaction with the health care system and provider factors (Lasch, Wilkes, Montuori et al., 2000).

The nurse's values may differ from those of other cultures. The nurse's expectations and values may include avoiding exaggerated expressions of pain, such as excessive crying and moaning, seeking immediate relief from pain, and giving complete descriptions of the pain. A patient's expectations may be to moan and complain about pain, to refuse pain relief measures that do not cure the cause of the pain, or to use adjectives such as "unbearable" in describing the pain. A patient from another background may behave in a quiet, stoic manner rather than express the pain loudly. The nurse must react to the person's pain perception and not to the pain behaviour because the behaviour is different from his or her own culture.

Recognizing one's values and learning how these values differ from those of others help the nurse to avoid evaluating the patient's behaviour on the basis of one's own expectations and values. A nurse who recognizes differences will have a greater understanding of the patient's pain and will be more accurate in assessing pain and behavioural responses to pain, as well as more effective in relieving the pain.

The main issues to consider when caring for patients of a different background are:

- What does the illness mean to the patient?
- Are there culturally or socially based stigmas related to this illness or pain?
- What is the role of the family in health care decisions?
- Are traditional pain-relief remedies used?
- What is the role of stoicism?
- Are there culturally or socially determined ways of expressing and communicating pain?
- Does the patient have any fears about the pain?
- Has the patient seen or does the patient want to see a traditional healer?

Nurses need to avoid stereotyping patients and provide individualized care rather than assuming that a patient of a particular background will exhibit more or less pain. In addition to avoiding stereotyping, health care providers need to individualize the amount of medications or therapy according to the information provided by the patient. Nurses need to recognize that stereotypes exist and become sensitive to how stereotypes negatively affect care. Patients in turn must be instructed about how and what to communicate about their pain.

Age

Age has long been the focus of research on pain perception and pain tolerance, and again the results have been inconsistent. For example, although some researchers have found that older adults require a higher intensity of experimental pain than do younger adults before they report pain (Washington, Gibson & Helme, 2000), others have found no differences in responses of younger and older adults (Edwards & Fillingim, 2000). Other researchers have found that elderly patients (older than 65 years of age) reported significantly less pain than younger patients (Li, Greenwald, Gennis et al., 2001). Experts in the field of pain management have concluded that if pain perception is diminished in the elderly person, it is most likely secondary to a disease process (eg, diabetes) rather than to aging (American Geriatrics Society, 1998). More research is needed in the area of aging and its effects on pain perception to understand what the elderly are experiencing.

NURSING RESEARCH PROFILE 13-1

Impact of Preoperative Education on Pain Outcomes After Coronary Artery Bypass Graft Surgery

Watt-Watson, J., Stevens, B., Katz, J., et al. (2004). Impact of preoperative education on pain outcomes after coronary artery bypass graft surgery. *Pain, 109*(1–2), 3–85.

Purpose
Many postoperative coronary artery bypass graft (CABG) surgery patients receive inadequate analgesia and experience unrelieved pain. Educating patients about postoperative pain relief prior to admission for surgery may help them to decrease their postoperative pain. This study evaluated the effectiveness of reducing postoperative pain and related activity interference by educating patients undergoing CABG surgery prior to admission to the hospital. Patients were educated by receiving a self-study booklet entitled *Pain Relief After Surgery* during the preadmission information session.

Study Sample and Design
This randomized controlled trial used a computer-generated randomization table to distribute the 346 male and 60 female (n = 406) participants to either the study or the control group. The target population consisted of elective-surgery patients undergoing their first, uncomplicated CABG surgery and who were able to understand, speak, and read English. Five outcomes were measured: interference with activities using the Interference Subscale of the Brief Pain Inventory; pain using the McGill Pain Questionnaire–Short Form; analgesics prescribed and administered as recorded in the patient's chart; concerns about seeking help and taking analgesics using a portion of the Barriers Questionnaire; and patient satisfaction using three numerically rated scale questions (0–10) from the American Pain Society–Patient Outcome Questionnaire. Gender related subgroup analyses were carried out for each outcome. Data were analysed using intention-to-treat protocols.

Findings
Educating patients about postoperative pain relief prior to admission for surgery had no clinical effect on the pain management out-

comes measured in this study. The preoperative pain relief education changed neither patients' analgesic intake nor their postoperative pain ratings. A large proportion of the study population still experienced moderate to severe pain on the day they were released from the hospital, and presumably then dealt with this pain at home. Gender played some role in patients' preparation for surgery, postoperative pain-related interference with activities, and recovery time. Almost all the women who received the educational booklet read it before their surgeries, whereas only two-thirds of the men who received it read the booklet. Further, women reported much higher pain-related interference scores and stayed in the hospital two days longer on average than did men. Notably, both study groups received inadequate pain relief, and only 33% of the prescribed dose of analgesics on average. On the fourth day after surgery, most patients reported the main reason for not taking analgesics was experiencing the analgesic side effect of constipation.

Nursing Implications
Nurses are in a position to dramatically improve the rate and quality of recovery in postoperative CABG surgery patients, and must:
- Ensure that postoperative CABG surgery patients receive prophylactic stool softeners and laxatives to prevent constipation.
- Administer analgesics preventatively in postoperative CABG surgery patients to ensure pain remains very mild such that patients can breathe deeply and move about.
- Remind patients of the therapeutic and personal benefits of pain relief, and encourage patients to honestly report their pain and request analgesics when their pain increases from mild.

Although many elderly people seek health care because of pain, others are reluctant to seek help even when in severe pain because they consider pain to be part of normal aging. Assessment of pain in older adults may be difficult because of the physiologic, psychosocial, and cognitive changes that often accompany aging. In one study, as many as 93% of nursing home residents reported being in pain daily for the past 6 months (Weiner, Peterson, Ladd et al., 1999). Unrelieved pain contributes to the problems of depression, sleep disturbances, delayed rehabilitation, malnutrition, and cognitive dysfunction (Miaskowski, 2000).

The way an older person responds to pain may differ from the way a younger person responds. Because elderly people have a slower metabolism and a greater ratio of body fat to muscle mass than younger people, smaller doses of analgesic agents may be sufficient to relieve pain, and these doses may be effective longer (Buffum & Buffum, 2000). Elderly patients deal with pain according to their lifestyle, personality, and cultural background, as do younger adults. Many elderly people are fearful of addiction and, as a result, will not report that they are in pain or ask for pain medication. Others fail to seek care because they fear that the pain may indicate serious illness or they fear loss of independence.

Elderly patients must receive adequate pain relief after surgery or trauma. When an elderly person becomes confused after surgery or trauma, the confusion is often attributed to medications, which are then discontinued. However, confusion in the elderly may be a result of untreated and unrelieved pain or lack of sleep because of pain. In some cases postoperative confusion clears once the pain is relieved. Judgments about pain and the adequacy of treatment should be based on the patient's report of pain and pain relief rather than on age.

Gender

Researchers have studied gender differences in diseases associated with pain, in pain levels, and in responses to pain. The prevalence of many conditions associated with pain is higher for women than men. For example, women are more likely to experience migraine, osteoarthritis, rheumatoid arthritis, and fibromyalgia than men (Unruh, 1996). The results about pain levels and responses have been inconsistent. In one study, women tended to report higher levels of pain than men and reported their highest intensity of pain during the day, while men reported the highest intensity at night (Morin, Lund, Villarroel et al., 2000). Kelly (1998) reported no gender differences in pain.

Riley, Robinson, Wade et al. (2001) compared pain intensity, pain unpleasantness, and pain-related emotions (depression, anxiety, frustration, fear, and anger) in men and women who were asked to rate their experiences with chronic pain. Women had higher pain intensity, pain unpleasantness, frustration, and fear compared to men. Robinson, Riley, Meyers et al. (2001) reported that men and women are socialized to respond differently and differ in their expectations relative to pain perception. In a study of responses of men and women to chronic pain and anxiety, Edwards, Auguston and Fillingim (2000) noted no difference between genders regarding pain and depression. There was, however, a difference in anxiety and gender, with men being more anxious about their pain.

The pharmacokinetics and pharmacodynamics of opioids differ in men and women and have been attributed to hepatic metabolism, where the microsomal enzyme activity differs (Vallerand & Polomano, 2000). Genetic factors play a role in the varied responses to nonsteroidal anti-inflammatory drugs (NSAIDs) seen in men and women (Buffum & Buffum, 2000).

Expectation

A patient's positive expectations about treatment may increase the effectiveness of a medication or other intervention. Often the more cues the patient receives about the intervention's effectiveness, the more effective it will be. A person who is informed that a medication is expected to relieve pain is more likely to experience pain relief than one who is told that a medication is unlikely to have any effect.

A **placebo effect** is an example of positive expectation. It is a beneficial effect in a patient that arises from the patient's positive expectations about the treatment. The effect of any intervention, whether inactive or therapeutic, can be enhanced by positive expectations. The placebo effect results from the natural (endogenous) production of endorphins in the descending control system. It is a true physiologic response that can be reversed by naloxone, an opioid antagonist (Wall, 1999).

Researchers have shown that different verbal instructions given to patients about therapies affect patient behaviour and significantly reduce opioid intake. Pollo and colleagues (2001) studied the effect of information and expectations in patients who had undergone thoracotomy. Patients in three groups were given an intravenous infusion of normal saline solution and could receive a dose of analgesic on request. One group was given no information about the analgesic effect of the regimen; one group was informed that the infusion received could be an analgesic or a placebo; the third was told that the infusion was a powerful analgesic. Although the three groups did not differ in reported level of pain, the group told that the infusion was a powerful analgesic used less opioid than the other two groups (Pollo, Amanzio, Arslanina et al., 2001.)

A meta-analysis of 114 published research studies comparing placebo with no treatment showed similar results (Hrobjartsson & Gotzsche, 2001). The studies analyzed investigated many clinical conditions; 27 of the 114 trials involved the treatment of pain. Other clinical conditions in the studies included obesity, asthma, hypertension, insomnia, and anxiety. Pain was the only condition in which a placebo effect was demonstrated.

Nurses will occasionally be asked to give a placebo (a tablet or injection with no active ingredients) to a patient complaining of pain. Placebos should not be used to assess or manage pain in any patient regardless of age or diagnosis. Placebos are to be reserved for research investigations where they are used to separate the effect of positive expectation from the effect of the treatment under investigation. A research subject is apprised of the chances of receiving a placebo when participating in a study. A patient receiving clinical care trusts that health care professionals are providing the best treatment and not practicing deception. The Canadian Nurses Association *Code of Ethics* includes a statement that nurses have a responsibility to provide competent and ethical care to patients (Canadian Nurses Association, 2002). Informing patients that they are receiving an effective treatment when they have been given a placebo violates that code (Chart 13-2).

Nursing Assessment of Pain

The highly subjective nature of pain makes pain assessment and management challenges for every clinician. The report of pain is a social transaction; thus, assessment and management of pain require a good rapport with the person in pain. In assessing a patient with pain, the nurse reviews the patient's description of the pain and other factors that may influence pain (eg, previous experience, anxiety, and age) as well as the person's response to pain relief strategies. Documentation of the pain level as rated on a

Chart 13-2 • Ethics and Related Issues

Ethical Administration of Placebos

Because of misperceptions about placebos and the placebo effect, keep in mind some specific principles and guidelines:
- A placebo effect is not an indication that the person does not have pain; rather, it is a true physiologic response.
- Placebos (tablets or injections with no active ingredients) should never be used to test the person's truthfulness about pain or as the first line of treatment.
- A positive response to a placebo (eg, reduction in pain) should never be interpreted as an indication that the person's pain is not real.
- A patient should never be given a placebo as a substitute for an analgesic medication. Although a placebo can produce analgesia, patients receiving a placebo may report that their pain is relieved or that they feel better simply to avoid disappointing the nurse.

pectations and misconceptions about pain (Chart 13-4). A person who understands that pain relief not only contributes to comfort but also hastens recovery is more likely to request or self-administer treatment appropriately.

CHARACTERISTICS OF PAIN

The factors to consider in a complete pain assessment are the intensity, timing, location, quality, personal meaning, aggravating and alleviating factors, and pain behaviours. The pain assessment begins by observing the patient carefully, noting the patient's overall posture and presence or absence of overt pain behaviours and asking the person to describe, in his or her own words, the specifics of the pain. The words used to describe the pain may point toward the etiology. For example, the classic description of chest pain that results from a myocardial infarction includes pressure or squeezing on the chest. A detailed history should follow the initial description of pain.

pain scale becomes part of the patient's medical record, as does a record of the pain relief obtained from interventions.

Pain assessment includes determining what level of pain relief the acutely ill patient believes is needed to recover quickly or improve function, or what level of relief the chronically or terminally ill patient requires to maintain comfort (Chart 13-3). Part of a thorough pain assessment is to understand the patient's ex-

Intensity

The intensity of pain ranges from none to mild discomfort to excruciating. There is no correlation between reported intensity and the stimulus that produced it. To understand variations, the nurse can ask about the present pain intensity as well as the least and the worst pain intensity. Various tools and surveys are helpful to patients trying to describe pain intensity. Examples of pain scales appear in Figure 13-4.

Chart 13-3   Pain at the End of Life

Pain is one of the most feared symptoms at the end of life. Most patients will experience pain as a terminal illness progresses. The inadequate treatment of cancer pain has been well documented (Agency for Health Care Policy and Research, 1994), and in the Study to Understand Prognoses and Preferences for Outcomes and Risks of Treatments (SUPPORT) (1995) investigators noted that nearly 40% of severely chronically ill and older patients who died in hospitals suffered moderate to severe pain in the last 3 days of life. The suffering caused by unrelieved pain touches all aspects of quality of life (activity, appetite, sleep) and can weaken an already fatigued person. Psychologically, unrelieved pain can create anxiety, and depression, negatively affect relationships, and promote thoughts of suicide.

Current barriers to pain management include lack of education and fear of addiction.

Need for Education
Ferrell et al. (2000) noted that of 45,683 nursing text pages reviewed, 902 were related to pain at the end of life. The end-of-life content constituted 2% of text pages, while the pain content represented only 0.5%. The researchers concluded that more specific content is needed to assist in educating students about pain and pain at the end of life.

Addiction Fears
The fear of addiction plays a role even at the end of life. Family members may be hesitant to assist the patient in pain management for fear of the social stigma of addiction. This causes needless pain and suffering.

Other Issues
Pain management at the end of life differs little from general pain management. Patients still require comprehensive pain assessment and pain management, even though assessment may be hampered by confusion, delirium, or unconsciousness. Caregivers are taught to observe for signs of restlessness or facial expressions as a "proxy" indicator of pain.

Analgesic agents should be titrated to find the most effective dose and the best tolerated route. The nurse and family members should assess the effectiveness of the current pain therapy. If the pain is not relieved, a larger dose of medication may be necessary. If the pain continues, another medication may be needed or the patient should be given a different analgesic. The titration process requires frequent assessment to effectively manage pain. The analgesic agent or treatment should be appropriate for the type of pain. For example, neuropathic pain, usually described as burning, tingling, numbness, shooting, stabbing or electric, requires a different treatment approach compared to acute pain.

Nonpharmacologic approaches, such as guided imagery and relaxation, can be used to decrease pain and help the patient cope. Careful patient positioning and environmental control are other methods to increase patient comfort.

In the last few days of life the patient may become restless, which is an indicator of pain. The need to increase the opioid to provide pain relief and the respiratory effects of opioids are considered in decision making. However, comfort should be a priority in the case of a person who clearly is at the end of life, where cure is no longer the goal.

Side effects from analgesics must be managed as in other painful conditions. Tolerance to constipation is rare. Thus, a careful bowel regimen involving diet, bowel stimulants, stool softeners, and/or osmotic agents, must be instituted. Vigilance in the assessment, management, and treatment evaluation of other side effects is similar to that included in previous discussions.

Careful assessment and management of pain at the end of life can make a "good" death possible. Education of health care providers and the family can help patients realize the goal of adequate pain relief throughout the dying process.

Timing

Sometimes the etiology of pain can be determined when time aspects are known. Therefore, the nurse inquires about the onset, duration, relationship between time and intensity, and whether there are changes in rhythmic patterns. The patient is asked if the pain began suddenly or increased gradually. Sudden pain that rapidly reaches maximum intensity is indicative of tissue rupture, and immediate intervention is necessary. Pain from ischemia gradually increases and becomes intense over a longer time. The chronic pain of arthritis illustrates the usefulness of determining the relationship between time and intensity, because people with arthritis usually report that pain is worse in the morning.

Location

The location of pain is best determined by having the patient point to the area of the body involved. Some general assessment forms have drawings of human figures, and the patient is asked to shade in the area involved. This is especially helpful if the pain radiates (**referred pain**). The shaded figures are helpful in determining the effectiveness of treatment or change in the location of pain over time.

Quality

The nurse asks the patient to describe the pain in his or her own words without offering clues. For example, the patient is asked to describe what the pain feels like. Sufficient time must be allowed for the patient to describe the pain and for the nurse to carefully record all words that are used. If the patient cannot describe the quality of the pain, words such as burning, aching, throbbing, or stabbing can be offered. It is important to document the exact words used to describe the pain and which words were suggested by the nurse conducting the assessment. The words used by the patient can indicate the cause of the pain. A good example is pain described as burning or tingling, which suggests neuropathy.

Personal Meaning

Patients experience pain differently, and the pain experience can mean many different things. It is important to ask how the pain has affected the person's daily life. Some people can continue to work or study, while others may be disabled. The patient is asked if the family or finances have been affected. For others, the recurrence of pain may mean worsening of the disease, such as the spread of cancer. The meaning attached to the pain experience helps the nurse understand how the patient is affected and assists in planning treatment.

Aggravating and Alleviating Factors

The nurse asks the patient what if anything makes the pain worse and what makes it better and asks specifically about the relationship between activity and pain. This helps detect factors associated with pain. For example, in a patient with advanced metastatic cancer, pain with coughing may signal spinal cord compression. The nurse ascertains whether environmental factors influence pain since they may easily be changed to help the patient. For example, making the room warmer may help the patient relax and may improve the patient's pain. Finally, the patient is asked if pain is influenced by or affects the quality of sleep. Factors associated with pain can significantly affect pain intensity and the quality of life.

   Knowledge of alleviating factors assists the nurse in developing a treatment plan. Therefore, it is important to ask about the patient's use of medication (prescribed and over the counter) and the amount and frequency. In addition, the nurse asks if herbal

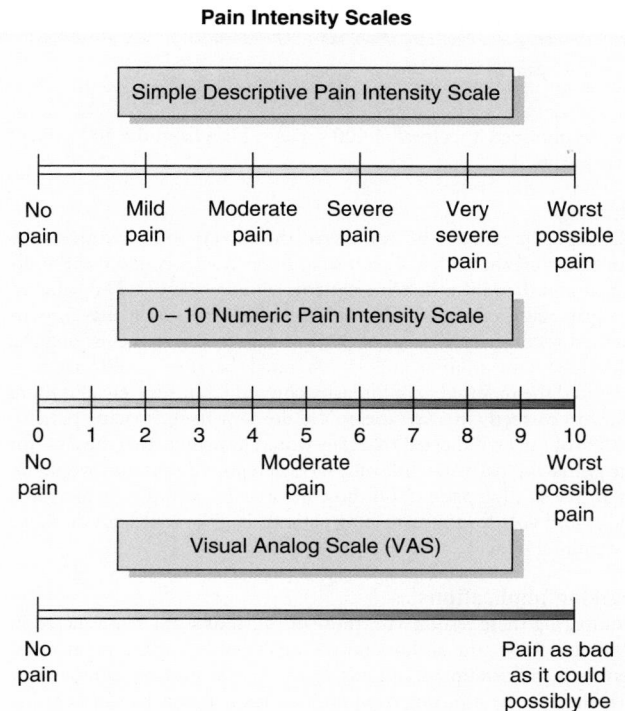

FIGURE 13-4 Examples of unidimensional pain intensity scales.

remedies, nonpharmacologic interventions, or alternative therapies have been used with success. This information assists the nurse in determining teaching needs.

Pain Behaviours

When experiencing pain, people express pain with many different behaviours. These nonverbal and behavioural expressions of pain are not consistent or reliable indicators of the quality or intensity of pain, and they should not be used to determine the presence of or the degree of pain experienced. Patients may grimace, cry, rub the affected area, guard the affected area, or immobilize it. Others may moan, groan, grunt, or sigh. Not all patients exhibit the same behaviours, and there may be different meanings associated with the same behaviour.

Sometimes in the nonverbal patient, pain behaviours are used as a proxy to assess pain. It is unwise to make judgments and formulate treatment plans based on behaviours that may or may not indicate pain. In the case of an unconscious person, pain should always be assumed to be present and treated. All patients have a right to adequate pain management.

Physiologic responses to pain, such as tachycardia, hypertension, tachypnea, pallor, diaphoresis, mydriasis, hypervigilance, and increased muscle tone, are related to stimulation of the autonomic nervous system. These responses are short-lived as the body adapts to the stress. These physiologic signs could be the result of a change in the patient's condition, such as the onset of hypovolemia. Using physiologic signs to indicate pain is unreliable. Although it is important to observe for any and all pain behaviours, the absence of these behaviours does not indicate an absence of pain.

INSTRUMENTS FOR ASSESSING THE PERCEPTION OF PAIN

Only the patient can accurately describe and assess his or her pain. Clinicians consistently underestimate a patient's level of pain (McCaffery & Ferrell, 1997; McCaffery, Ferrell & Pasaro, 2000; Puntillo, Miaskowski, Kehrle et al., 1997; Thomas et al., 1998). Therefore, a number of pain assessment instruments have been developed to assist in the assessment of a patient's perception of pain (see Fig. 13-4). Such instruments may be used to document the need for intervention, to evaluate the effectiveness of the intervention, and to identify the need for alternative or additional interventions if the initial intervention is ineffective in relieving the pain. For a pain assessment instrument to be useful, it must require little effort on the part of the patient, be easy to understand and use, be easily scored, and be sensitive to small changes in the characteristic being measured. Figure 13-5 shows a pain assessment algorithm that can be used at the time of assessment to direct clinical decisions for pain management.

Visual Analogue Scales

Visual analogue scales (VAS; see Fig. 13-4) are useful in assessing the intensity of pain. One version of the scale includes a horizontal 10-cm line, with anchors (ends) indicating the extremes of pain. The person is asked to place a mark indicating where the current pain lies on the line. The left anchor usually represents "none" or "no pain," whereas the right anchor usually represents "severe" or "worst possible pain." To score the results, a ruler is placed along the line and the distance the person marked from the left or low end is measured and reported in millimeters or centimeters.

NURSING RESEARCH PROFILE 13-2
Pain Assessment and Titration of Analgesic Agents

McCaffery, M., Ferrell, B. R., & Pasero, C. (2000). Nurses' personal opinions about patients' pain and their effect on recorded assessments and titration of opioid doses. *Pain Management Nursing, 1*(3), 79–87.

Purpose
Nurses have a key role in pain assessment and management in all areas of clinical practice. Although previous studies have identified lack of knowledge about pain management as a factor contributing to undertreatment of pain, little is known about their personal opinions related to pain management. This study was conducted to explore how nurses' personal opinions about pain intensity influence their decisions about pain assessment and about titration of the prescribed opioid to relieve severe pain.

Study Sample and Design
In this descriptive study, surveys were distributed as a pretest to a convenience sample of nurses attending pain conferences before receiving any information on pain. Data were collected at 20 locations throughout the United States. The surveys presented two vignettes describing patients with postoperative pain. The patients were identical except for their behaviour; one patient was smiling and joking while the other remained quiet in bed and grimaced. Nurses were asked to identify their personal opinions about both patients' reported pain intensity, what they would document in the patient record, and what opioid dose they would administer. Patients in both vignettes rated their pain as 8 on a scale of 0 to 10, indicating inadequate pain management and ineffective opioid doses to relieve the severe pain. In both vignettes, it was made clear that increasing the opioid dose would be safe and appropriate. Completed surveys were returned by 1,276 nurses. Of these, a random sample of 100 surveys from each section of the coun-

try was obtained for a total of 400 surveys. Data from the 400 surveys were analyzed.

Findings
Although the nurses who completed the surveys indicated that they would record the patients' pain as 8, fewer nurses believed the smiling patient than the grimacing patient. More nurses (78.3%) believed the grimacing patient's pain intensity and 90% would have documented it correctly. A total of 39% of nurses reported believing the patient who was smiling, and 85.5% stated that they would have documented the reported pain intensity correctly. Nurses were also more likely to correctly increase the opioid dose for the grimacing patient; 62.5% of nurses indicated that they would have increased the dose for the grimacing patient, while only 47.3% reported that they would do so for the smiling patient. Of those nurses who would have increased the opioid dose for the grimacing patient, 16.3% would not do so for the smiling patient.

Nursing Implications
Comparing these results with those of previous studies conducted in 1990 and 1995, the authors noted considerable improvement in assessment and titration of opioids. However, the findings demonstrate that there is a continuing need for education about the different patient responses to pain and the importance of the patient's report of the intensity of pain. More education is needed to address nurses' responsibilities for opioid titration.

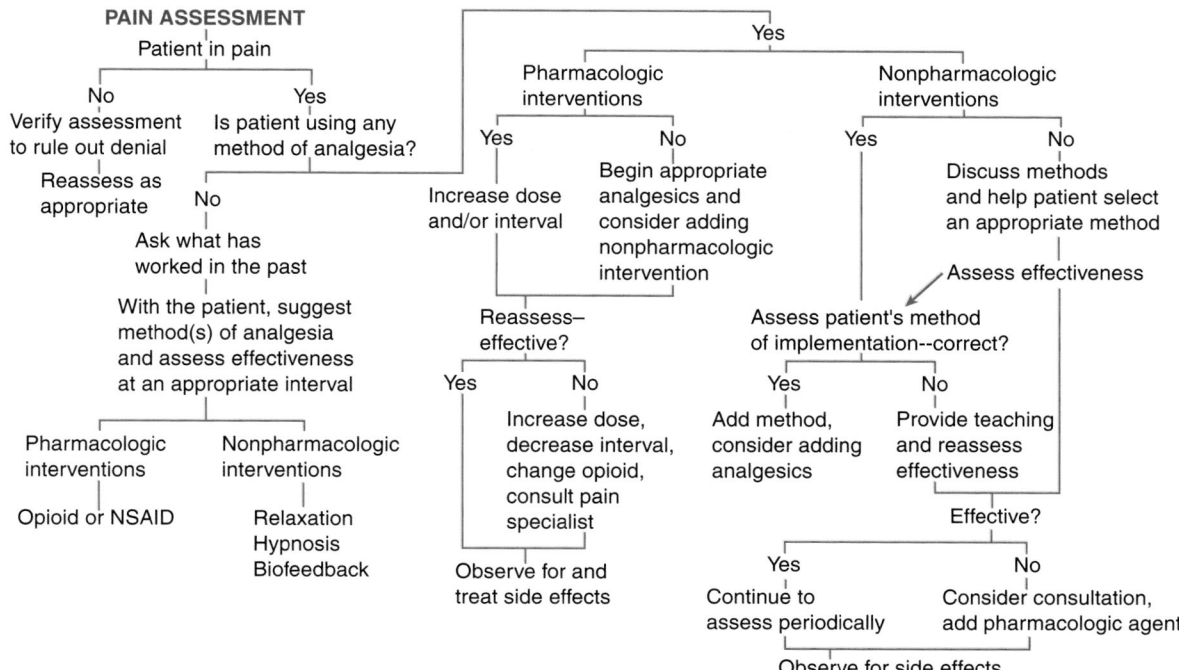

FIGURE 13-5 Pain assessment algorithm. Redrawn with permission from Salerno, E., & Willens, J. S. (1996). *Pain management handbook: An interdisciplinary approach.* St. Louis: C. V. Mosby.

Some patients (eg, children, elderly patients, and visually or cognitively impaired patients) may find it difficult to use an unmarked VAS. In those circumstances, ordinal scales (simple descriptive pain intensity scale, or 0 to 10 numeric pain intensity scale) may be used. With a little ingenuity on the nurse's part, many difficulties that patients have with simple pain instruments can be overcome. For example, a visually impaired person can complete a VAS if the 10-cm line is printed with high contrast or embossed.

Faces Pain Scale, Revised

Used for pediatric patients, this instrument has a series of simple, sketched faces depicting expressions that range from contented to obvious distress. The patient is asked to point to the face that most closely resembles the pain intensity felt. In using faces scales to rate pain, children's ratings may be affected by factors besides pain. Some faces depicting severe pain may be interpreted as angry faces by children. Some faces scales illustrate attributes like gender or age in the sketched faces and those attributes may influence ratings when children wish to set themselves apart or be like the child represented by the face. Figure 13-6 shows the Faces Pain Scale, Revised (Hicks, van Baeyer, Spafford et al., 2001; Hunter, McDowell, Hennessy et al., 2000).

Guidelines for Using Pain Assessment Scales

Using a written scale to assess pain may not be possible if the person is seriously ill, is in severe pain, or has just returned from surgery. In these cases, the nurse can ask the patient, "On a scale of 0 to 10, 0 being no pain and 10 being pain as bad as it can be, how bad is your pain now?" For patients who have difficulty with a 0 to 10 scale, a 0 to 5 scale may be tried. Whichever scale is used, it should be used consistently. Most patients usually can respond without difficulty. Ideally, the nurse teaches the patient how to

use the pain scale before the pain occurs (eg, before surgery). The patient's numerical rating is documented and used to assess the effectiveness of pain relief interventions.

If the person does not speak English or cannot communicate clearly information needed to manage pain, an interpreter, translator, or family member familiar with the person's method of communication should be consulted and a method established for pain assessment. Often a chart can be constructed with English words on one side and the foreign language on the other. The patient can then point to the corresponding word to tell the clinician about the pain.

When a person with pain is cared for at home by family caregivers or the home care nurse, a pain scale may help in assessing the effectiveness of the interventions, if the scale is used before and after the interventions are administered. Scales that address the location and pattern of pain may be useful to the home care nurse in identifying new sources or sites of pain in the chronically or terminally ill patient and in monitoring changes in the patient's level of pain. The patient and family caregivers can be taught to use a pain assessment scale to assess and manage the patient's pain. The home care nurse who sees the patient only at intervals may thus benefit from consulting the patient's or family's written record of the pain scores to evaluate how effective the pain management strategies have been over time.

On occasion, a person will deny having pain when most people in similar circumstances would report significant pain. For example, it is not uncommon for a patient recovering from a total joint replacement to deny feeling "pain," but on further questioning will readily admit to having a "terrible ache, but I wouldn't call it pain." From then on, when evaluating this person's pain, the nurse would use the patient's words rather than the word "pain."

The scales illustrated in Figures 13-4 and 13-6 are unidimensional. They measure pain intensity only and therefore provide a

0   2   4   Fold here   6   8   10

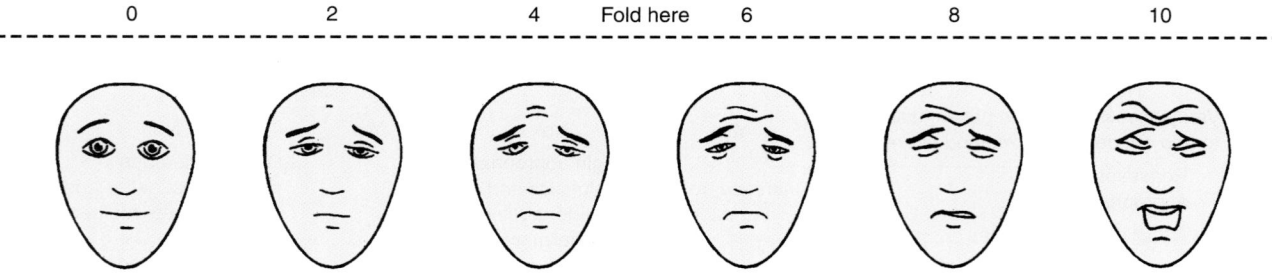

FIGURE 13-6 Faces Pain Scale—Revised. This pain scale is especially suited for helping children describe pain. Instructions for using this scale follow: **"These faces show how much something can hurt. This face** (*point to left-most face*) **shows *no pain*. The faces show more and more pain** (*point to each from left to right*) **up to this one** (*point to right-most face*). It shows *very much pain*. Point to the face that shows how much you hurt (right now). Score the chosen face *0, 2, 4, 6* or *10*, counting left to right, so *0* = no pain and *10* = very much pain. Do not use words like happy or sad. This scale is intended to measure how children feel inside, not how their face looks. From the *Pediatric Pain Sourcebook*. Original copyright © 2001. Used with permission of the International Association for the Study of Pain and the Pain Research Unit, Sydney Children's Hospital, Randwick NSW 2031, Australia.

narrow picture of the pain experience. They do not provide information about pain duration, frequency or quality, and impact of pain. Thus, they offer a very narrow assessment of pain. Nurses in the acute care setting could broaden the assessment by asking for a report of pain interference with sleep or activity.

Chronic pain assessment instruments are multidimensional. They assess the sensory, emotional, social, and financial aspects of pain. The Brief Pain Inventory, Memorial Pain Assessment Card, and the McGill Pain Questionnaire are examples.

NURSE'S ROLE IN PAIN MANAGEMENT

Before discussing what the nurse can do to intervene in the patient's pain, the nurse's role in pain management is reviewed. The nurse helps relieve pain by administering pain-relieving interventions (including both pharmacologic and nonpharmacologic approaches), assessing the effectiveness of those interventions, monitoring for adverse effects, and serving as an advocate for the patient when the prescribed intervention is ineffective in relieving pain. In addition, the nurse serves as an educator to the patient and family to enable them to manage the prescribed intervention themselves when appropriate.

Identifying Goals for Pain Management

The information the nurse obtains from the pain assessment is used to identify goals for managing the pain. The goals identified are shared or validated with the patient. One goal may be elimination of the pain. For many, however, this expectation may be unrealistic. Other goals may include a decrease in the intensity, duration, or frequency of pain, and a decrease in the negative effects the pain has on the patient. For example, pain may have a negative effect by interfering with sleep and thereby hampering recovery from an acute illness or decreasing appetite. In such instances, the goals might be to sleep soundly and to take adequate nutrition. Chronic pain may affect the person's quality of life by interfering with work or interpersonal relationships. Thus, a goal may be to decrease time lost from work or to increase the quality of interpersonal relationships.

To determine the goal, a number of factors are considered. The first is the severity of the pain, as judged by the patient. The second factor is the anticipated harmful effects of pain. A high-

risk patient is at much greater risk for the harmful effects of pain than a young healthy patient. The third factor is the anticipated duration of the pain. In patients with pain from a disease such as cancer, the pain may be prolonged, possibly for the remainder of the patient's life. Therefore, interventions will be needed for some time and should not detract from the patient's quality of life. A different set of interventions is required if the patient is likely to have pain for only a few days or weeks.

In a study of the dying experience, family members of 2,451 people who had died were interviewed (Lynn, Teno, Phillips et al., 1997). Of these patients, 55% were conscious during their last 3 days of life. Of the conscious patients, 4 in 10 were considered by their family members to be in severe pain most of the time. These findings strongly suggest that pain relief for dying patients should be a primary goal.

The goals for the patient may be accomplished by pharmacologic or nonpharmacologic means, but most success will be achieved with a combination of both. In the acute stages of illness, the patient may be unable to participate actively in relief measures, but when sufficient mental and physical energy is present, the patient may learn self-management techniques to relieve the pain. Thus, as the patient progresses through the stages of recovery, a goal may be to increase the patient's use of self-management pain relief measures.

Establishing the Nurse–Patient Relationship and Teaching

A positive nurse–patient relationship and teaching are key to managing analgesia in the patient with pain, because open communication and patient cooperation are essential to success. A positive nurse–patient relationship characterized by trust is essential. By conveying to the patient the belief that he or she has pain, the nurse often helps reduce the patient's anxiety. Acknowledging to the patient, "I know that you have pain" often eases the patient's mind. Occasionally, patients who fear that no one believes the reported pain feel relieved when they know that the nurse can be trusted to believe the pain exists.

Teaching is equally important, because the patient or family may be responsible for managing the pain at home and preventing or managing side effects. Teaching patients about pain and strategies to relieve it may reduce pain in the absence of other pain relief measures and may enhance the effectiveness of the pain relief measures used.

The nurse also provides information by explaining how pain can be controlled. The patient is informed, for example, that pain should be reported in the early stages. When the patient waits too long to report pain, **sensitization** may occur and the pain may be so intense that it is difficult to relieve. The phenomenon of sensitization is important in effective pain management. Since a heightened response is seen after exposure to a noxious stimulus, the response to that stimulus will be greater, causing the person to feel more pain. When health care providers assess and treat pain before it becomes severe, sensitization is diminished or avoided, and thus less medication is needed.

Providing Physical Care

The patient in pain may be unable to participate in the usual activities of daily living or to perform usual self-care and may need assistance to carry out these activities. The patient is usually more comfortable when physical and self-care needs have been met and efforts have been made to ensure as comfortable a position as possible. A fresh gown and change of bed linens, along with efforts to make the person feel refreshed (eg, brushing teeth, combing hair), often increase the level of comfort and improve the effectiveness of the pain relief measures.

Providing physical care to the patient also gives the nurse (in acute, long-term, and home settings) the opportunity to perform a complete assessment and to identify problems that may contribute to the patient's discomfort and pain. Appropriate and gentle physical touch during care may be reassuring and comforting. If treatments such as fentanyl (an opioid analgesic) patches or intravenous or intraspinal catheters are used, the skin around the patch or catheter should be assessed for integrity during physical care.

Managing Anxiety Related to Pain

Anxiety may affect a patient's response to pain. The patient who anticipates pain may become increasingly anxious. Teaching the patient about the nature of the impending painful experience and the ways to reduce pain often decreases anxiety; a person who is experiencing pain will use previously learned strategies to reduce anxiety and pain. Learning about measures to relieve pain may lessen the threat of pain and give the person a sense of control.

What the nurse explains about the available pain relief measures and their effectiveness may also affect the patient's anxiety level. The patient's anxiety may be reduced by explanations that point out the degree of pain relief that can be expected from each measure. For example, the patient who is informed beforehand that an intervention may not eliminate pain completely is less likely to become anxious when a certain amount of pain persists. Anxiety resulting from anticipation of pain or the pain experience itself may often be managed effectively by establishing a relationship with the patient and by patient teaching.

A patient who is anxious about pain may be less tolerant of the pain, which in turn may increase the anxiety level. To prevent the pain and anxiety from escalating, the anxiety-producing cycle must be interrupted. Low levels of pain are easier to reduce or control than are more intense levels. (This concept of sensitization was previously discussed.) Consequently, pain relief measures should be used before pain becomes severe. Many patients believe that they should only request pain relief measures when they can no longer withstand the pain, making it difficult for medications to provide relief. Therefore, it is important to explain to all patients that pain relief or control is more successful if such measures begin before the pain becomes unbearable.

Pain Management Strategies

Reducing pain to a "tolerable" level was once considered the goal of pain management. However, even patients who have described pain relief as adequate often report disturbed sleep and marked distress because of pain. In view of the harmful effects of pain and inadequate pain management, the goal of tolerable pain has been replaced by the goal of relieving the pain. Pain management strategies include both pharmacologic and nonpharmacologic approaches. These approaches are selected on the basis of the patient's requirements and goals. Appropriate analgesic medications are used as prescribed. They are not considered a last resort to be used only when other pain relief measures fail. Any intervention is most successful if initiated before pain sensitization occurs, and the greatest success is usually achieved if several interventions are applied simultaneously.

PHARMACOLOGIC INTERVENTIONS

Managing a patient's pain pharmacologically is accomplished in collaboration with the physician or other primary care provider, the patient, and often the family. The physician or nurse practitioner prescribes specific medications for pain or may insert an intravenous line for administering analgesic medications. Alternatively, an anesthesiologist may insert an epidural catheter for their administration. However, it is the nurse who maintains the epidural, assesses its effectiveness, and reports if the intervention is ineffective or produces side effects.

The pharmacologic management of pain requires close collaboration and effective communication among health care providers. In the home setting, it is often the family who manages the patient's pain and assesses the effectiveness of pharmacologic interventions, while it is the home care nurse who evaluates the adequacy of pain relief strategies and the family's ability to manage the pain. The home care nurse reinforces teaching and ensures communication among the patient, family care providers, physician, pharmacist, and other health care providers involved in the patient's care.

Premedication Assessment

Before administering any medication, the nurse asks the patient about allergies to medications and the nature of any previous allergic responses. True allergic or anaphylactic responses to opioids are rare, but it is not uncommon for a patient to report an allergy to one of the opioids. On further examination, the nurse often learns that the extent of the allergy was "itching" or "nausea and vomiting." These responses are not allergies; rather, they are side effects that, when necessary, can be managed while the patient's pain is relieved. The patient's description of responses or reactions should be documented and reported before administering the medication.

The nurse obtains the patient's medication history (eg, current, usual, or recent use of prescription or over-the-counter medications or herbal agents), along with a history of health problems. Certain medications or conditions may affect the analgesic medication's effectiveness or the metabolism and excretion of analgesic agents. Before administering analgesic agents, the nurse should assess the patient's pain status, including the intensity of current pain, changes in pain intensity after the previous dose of medication, and side effects of the medication.

Gerontologic Considerations Related to Analgesic Agents

Physiologic changes in older adults require that analgesic agents be administered with caution. Drug interactions are more likely to occur in older adults because of the higher incidence of chronic illness and the increased use of prescription and over-the-counter medications.

Absorption and metabolism of medications are altered in elderly patients because of decreased liver, renal, and gastrointestinal function. In addition, changes in body weight, protein stores, and distribution of body fluid alter the distribution of medications in the body. As a result, medications are not metabolized as quickly and blood levels of the medication remain higher for a longer period. Elderly patients are more sensitive to medications and at an increased risk for drug toxicity (American Geriatrics Society, 2002). Before administering analgesic agents to elderly patients, the nurse needs to obtain a thorough medication history and consult with the pharmacist to identify potential drug interactions.

Opioid and nonopioid analgesic medications can be given effectively to elderly patients but must be used cautiously because of the increased susceptibility to depression of both the nervous and the respiratory systems. Although there is no reason to avoid most opioids simply because a person is elderly, meperidine should be avoided because its active and neurotoxic metabolite, normeperidine, is more likely to accumulate in the elderly. In addition, because of decreased binding of meperidine by plasma proteins, blood concentrations of the medication twice those found in younger patients may result. In many cases, the initial dose of analgesic medication prescribed for an elderly patient may be the same as that for a younger person, or slightly smaller than the normal dose, but because of slowed metabolism and excretion related to aging, the safe interval for subsequent doses may be longer (or prolonged). As always, the best guide to pain management and administration of analgesic agents in all patients regardless of age is what the patient says. The elderly patient may obtain more pain relief for a longer time than a younger patient. As a result, smaller, less frequent doses may be required.

Approaches for Using Analgesic Agents

Medications are most effective when the dose and interval between doses are individualized to meet the patient's needs. The only safe and effective way to administer analgesic medications is by asking the patient to rate the pain and by observing the response to medications.

MULTIMODAL INTERVENTIONS

Pharmacologic interventions are most effective when a multimodal or balanced analgesia approach is used. **Multimodal analgesia** refers to use of more than one form of analgesia concurrently to obtain more pain relief with fewer side effects. Pharmacologic and nonpharmacologic forms of analgesia can be combined. Three general categories of analgesic agents are opioids, NSAIDs, and local anesthetics. These agents work by different mechanisms. Using two or three types of agents simultaneously can maximize pain relief while minimizing the potentially toxic effects of any one agent. When one agent is used alone, it usually must be used in a higher dose to be effective. In other words, although it might require 15 mg morphine to relieve a certain pain, it may take only 8 mg morphine plus 30 mg ketorolac (an NSAID) to relieve the same pain.

PRO RE NATA (PRN)

In the past, the standard method used by most nurses and physicians in administering analgesics was to administer the analgesic *pro re nata* (PRN), or "as needed." The standard practice was for the nurse to wait for the patient to complain of pain and then administer the analgesic. As a result, many patients remained in pain because they did not know they needed to ask for medication or waited until the pain became intolerable.

By its very nature, the PRN approach to analgesia leaves the patient sedated or in severe pain much of the time. To receive pain relief from an opioid analgesic, the serum level of that opioid must be maintained at a minimum therapeutic level (Fig. 13-7). By the time the patient complains of pain, the serum opioid level is below the therapeutic level. From the time the patient requests pain medication until the nurse administers the medication, the patient's serum level continues to fall. The lower the serum opioid level, the more difficult it is to achieve the therapeutic level with the next dose. The only way to ensure significant periods of analgesia, using this method, is to give doses large enough to produce periods of sedation.

PREVENTIVE APPROACH

Currently, a preventive approach to relieving pain by administering analgesic agents is considered the most effective strategy because a therapeutic serum level of medication is maintained. With the preventive approach, analgesic agents are administered at set intervals so that the medication acts before the pain becomes severe and before the serum opioid level falls to a subtherapeutic level.

Administering analgesic medication on a time basis, rather than on the basis of the patient's report of pain, prevents the serum drug level from falling to subtherapeutic levels. An example of this would be giving the patient the prescribed morphine or the prescribed NSAID (ibuprofen) every 3 hours rather than waiting until the patient complains of pain. If the patient's pain is likely to occur around the clock or for a great portion of a 24-hour period, a regular around-the-clock schedule of administering analgesics may be indicated. Even if the analgesic is prescribed PRN, it can be administered on a preventive basis before the patient is in severe pain, as long as the prescribed interval between doses is observed. The preventive approach reduces the peaks and troughs in the serum level and provides more pain relief for the patient with fewer adverse effects.

Smaller doses of medication are needed with the preventive approach because the pain does not escalate to a level of severe intensity. Thus, a preventive approach may result in the administration of less medication over a 24-hour period, thereby helping prevent tolerance to analgesic agents and decreasing the severity of side effects (eg, sedation and constipation). Better pain control can be achieved with a preventive approach, reducing the amount of time the patient spends in pain.

In using the preventive approach, the nurse assesses the patient for sedation before administering the next dose. The goal is to provide analgesics before the pain becomes severe. It may be necessary to decrease the dosage of the opioid analgesic so that the patient receives pain relief with less sedation.

INDIVIDUALIZED DOSAGE

The dosage and the interval between doses should be based on the patient's requirements rather than on an inflexible standard or routine. People metabolize and absorb medications at different rates and experience different levels of pain. Therefore, one dose of an opioid medication given at specified intervals may be effective for one patient but ineffective for another.

Because of the fear of causing respiratory depression, health care providers tend to prescribe and administer inadequate dosages of opioid agents to treat acute pain or chronic pain (Chart 13-5).

FIGURE 13-7 Relationship of mode of delivery of analgesic to serum analgesic level. *Top:* intramuscular (IM) and intravenous patient-controlled analgesia (PCA); *bottom:* transdermal (TD) and transmucosal (•).

However, even prolonged administration of opioid agents is associated with an extremely low incidence (less than 1%) of addiction.

Therefore, the effects of opioid analgesic medications must be monitored, especially when the first dose is given or when the dose is changed or given more frequently. The time, date, the patient's pain rating (scale of 0 to 10), the analgesic agent, other pain relief measures, side effects, and patient activity are recorded.

Chart 13-5 • Ethics and Related Issues

Inadequate Pain Management

Situation
When taking over the care of ethnic minority patients at the change of shift from a particular colleague, you usually find these patients to be in a great deal of pain. Your nonsystematic observations have led you to conclude these patients receive only a small portion of the analgesics prescribed for them. You have heard a nurse colleague state a belief that people of certain ethnic groups have "no pain tolerance" and are "just looking for drugs."

Dilemma
Racial biases are difficult to change and deal with. To confront this nurse may not alter the behaviour but will certainly disrupt the working relationships on the unit. It would be easier to look the other way. On the other hand, you believe that the nurse is giving inadequate and unethical care to selected patients and placing them at greater risk for postoperative complications.

Discussion
• What information would you need to collect before acting?
• From whom could you seek counsel?
• Are the two aspects of the dilemma equally important?

When the first dose of an analgesic is administered, the nurse needs to record a pain rating score, blood pressure, and respiratory and pulse rates (all of which are considered "vital signs"). If the pain has not decreased in 30 minutes (sooner if an intravenous route is used) and the patient is reasonably alert and has a satisfactory respiratory status, blood pressure, and pulse rate, then some change in analgesic is indicated. Although the dose of analgesic medication is safe for this patient, it is ineffective in relieving the pain. Therefore, another dose of medication may be indicated. In such instances, the nurse consults with the physician to determine what further action is warranted.

PATIENT-CONTROLLED ANALGESIA
Used to manage postoperative pain as well as chronic pain, **patient-controlled analgesia** (PCA) allows patients to control the administration of their own medication within predetermined safety limits. This approach can be used with continuous infusions of opioid analgesic agents by intravenous, subcutaneous, or epidural routes. PCA can be used in the hospital or home setting.

The PCA pump permits the patient to self-administer continuous infusions of medication (basal rates) safely and to administer extra medication (bolus doses) with episodes of increased pain or painful activities. A PCA pump is electronically controlled by a timing device. Patients experiencing pain can administer small amounts of medication directly into their intravenous, subcutaneous, or epidural catheter by pressing a button. The pump then delivers a preset amount of medication.

The PCA pump also can be programmed to deliver a constant, background infusion of medication or basal rate and still allow the patient to administer additional bolus doses as needed. The timer can be programmed to prevent additional doses from being administered until a specified time period has elapsed (lock-out time) and until the first dose has had time to exert its maximal effect. Even if the patient pushes the button multiple times in rapid succession, no additional doses are released. If another dose is required at the end of the delay period, the button must be pushed again to receive the dose. Patients who are controlling their own opioid administration usually become sedated and stop pushing the button before any significant respiratory depression occurs. Nevertheless, assessing respiratory status remains a role for the nurse.

A continuous infusion plus bolus doses may be more effective with some patients (eg, cancer patients and postoperative patients), especially those who require uninterrupted sleep.

Patients who use PCA achieve better pain relief (Walder, Schafer, Henzi et al., 2001) and often require less pain medication than those who are treated in the standard PRN fashion. Because the patient can maintain a near-constant level of medication, the periods of severe pain and sedation that occur with the traditional PRN regimen are avoided.

To initiate PCA or any analgesics used at home or in the hospital, it is important to avoid playing "catch-up." Pain should be brought under control before PCA starts, often by the use of an initial, larger bolus dose or loading dose. Then, after control is achieved, the pump is programmed to deliver small doses of medication at a time. If the patient with severe pain has a low serum level of opioid analgesic because of an inadequate basal rate, it is difficult to regain control with the small doses available by pump. Before the PCA pump is used, repeated bolus doses of an intravenous opioid may be administered as prescribed over a short time until the pain is relieved. Then PCA is initiated. If pain control is not achieved with the maximal dose of medication prescribed, further prescriptions are obtained. The goal is to achieve a minimum therapeutic level of analgesia and to allow the patient to maintain that level by using the PCA pump. The patient is instructed not to wait until the pain is severe before pushing the button to obtain a bolus dose. The patient is also reminded not to become so distracted by an activity or visitor that he or she forgets to self-administer a prescribed dose of medication. One potential drawback to distraction is that a patient who is using a PCA pump may not self-administer any analgesic during the time of effective distraction. When distraction ends suddenly (eg, the movie ends or the visitors leave), the patient may be left without a therapeutic serum opioid level. When intermittent distraction is used for pain relief, a continuous low-level background infusion of opioid through the PCA pump may be prescribed so that when the distraction ends, it will not be necessary to try to catch up.

If PCA is to be used in the patient's home, the patient and family are taught about the operation of the pump and the side effects of the medication and strategies to manage them.

CONTINUOUS INFUSION

Portable syringe drivers and pumps can be used to administer small pulses of an opioid analgesic to either an intrathecal catheter or a subcutaneous or intravenous line at a set rate and dose. Portable syringe drivers are small, lightweight devices. They are practical and less expensive than pumps, but are limited in terms of their use compared to pumps. Pumps are more expensive, but can be programmed for several different functions. The use of these devices in continuous infusion is beneficial for patients whose dose is too high to be practically served by oral opioids or who cannot take oral opioids due to difficulty swallowing, nausea, vomiting, bowel obstruction, or the presence of a feeding tube. Continuous infusion is sometimes combined with the patient-controlled bolus. The pump can be programmed to deliver small pulses of an opioid at a set rate and dose, yet allow for patient-controlled administration of additional bolus doses of opioid as necessary when breakthrough pain occurs.

 NURSING ALERT Nurses and family members are encouraged to push the button for patients who are receiving bolus doses without continuous infusion. It is especially important to do so when patients are asleep to ensure their sleep is undisturbed by pain.

RESERVOIRS

Physical reservoirs can be used to hold specific quantities of an analgesic for long-term administration via either an intrathecal catheter or a subcutaneous or intravenous line. Reservoirs can be contained within a pouch or bag worn externally by the patient, or they can be implanted subcutaneously. Implanted reservoirs are of particular use in patients whose cancer has invaded the CNS. Patients with an implanted reservoir must be carefully monitored for bacterial infection.

Local Anesthetic Agents

Local anesthetics work by blocking nerve conduction. They can be applied directly to the site of injury (eg, a topical anesthetic spray for sunburn) or injected into tissues surrounding the selected nerve fibres. They can also be administered through an epidural catheter.

LOCAL INFILTRATION

Local infiltration is the injection of an anesthetic to the tissues surrounding the selected nerve fibre. Local anesthetic agents have been successful in reducing the pain associated with thoracic or upper abdominal surgery when injected by the surgeon intercostally. However, infiltrated local anesthetic agents are rapidly absorbed into the bloodstream, resulting in decreased availability at the surgical or injury site and an increased anesthetic level in the blood, increasing the risk of toxicity. Therefore, a vasoconstrictive agent (eg, epinephrine or phenylephrine) is added to the anesthetic agent to decrease its systemic absorption and to maintain its concentration at the surgical or injury site.

TOPICAL ADMINISTRATION

Commonly used topical anesthetics include lidocaine, prilocaine and amethocaine (Tetracaine) in various combinations. LET (lidocaine, epinephrine, and Tetracaine) is for use on broken skin, and therefore is used when suturing lacerations. A liposomal formulation of lidocaine (Maxilene) is for use on mucous membranes, whereas LET is not. EMLA (eutectic mixture or emulsion of local anesthetics) and Ametop are used with unbroken skin (eg, venipuncture and IV cannulation). Trials are underway on a topical anesthetic cream that, once applied, dries to form a peel-away film (S-Caine Peel). Such a product would not require an occlusive dressing, and may eventually become available in Canada for dermatologic surgery. The various combinations of topical anesthetics affect the absorption time and occurrence of vasoconstriction. These two characteristics can affect the wait time needed before performing the procedure and the success of the procedure. For example, EMLA requires a wait time of 60 to 90 minutes for anesthesia to occur and causes vasoconstriction, which may make it difficult to find the vein. EMLA has been effective in preventing the pain associated with administering infiltrated local anesthetics for procedures such as lumbar punctures or the insertion of intravenous lines.

INTRASPINAL ADMINISTRATION

Intermittent or continuous administration of local anesthetic agents through an epidural catheter has been used for years to produce anesthesia during surgery. Although the administration of local anesthetic agents in the spinal canal is still largely confined to acute pain, such as postoperative pain and pain associated with labour and delivery, the epidural administration of local anesthetic agents for pain management is increasing.

A local anesthetic agent administered through an epidural catheter is applied to tissues in the epidural space surrounding the spinal cord. The anesthetic agent can be administered continuously in low doses, intermittently on a schedule, or on demand as the patient requires it, and is often combined with the epidural administration of opioids. Surgical patients treated with this combination experience fewer complications after surgery, ambulate sooner, and have shorter hospital stays than patients receiving standard therapy (Correll, Viscusi, Grunwald et al., 2001).

Opioid Analgesic Agents

Opioids can be administered by various routes, including oral, intravenous, subcutaneous, intraspinal, intranasal, rectal, and transdermal routes. The goal of administering opioids is to relieve pain and improve quality of life; therefore, the route of administration, dose, and frequency of administration are determined on an individual basis. Factors that are considered in determining the route, dose, and frequency of medication include the characteristics of the pain (eg, its expected duration and severity), the overall status of the patient, the patient's response to analgesic medications, and the patient's report of pain. Although the oral route is usually preferred for administering opioids, oral opioids must be given frequently enough and in large enough doses to be effective. Opioid analgesic agents given orally, particularly extended-release formulations, may provide a more consistent serum level than those given intramuscularly. There are several benefits to a consistent serum level of opioid analgesic. First, pain relief is more consistent, continuous, and longer lasting. Second, spikes in serum level, which increase the risks of respiratory depression and sedation and may cause problems in patients with addictive behaviour, are avoided.

If the patient is expected to require opioid analgesic agents at home, the patient's and the family's ability to administer opioids as prescribed is considered in planning. Steps are taken to ensure that the medication will be available to the patient.

With the administration of opioids by any route, side effects must be considered and anticipated. Anticipating side effects and taking steps to minimize them increase the likelihood that the patient will receive adequate pain relief without interrupting therapy to treat these effects.

RESPIRATORY DEPRESSION AND SEDATION

Respiratory sedation is the most serious adverse effect of opioid analgesic agents administered by intravenous, subcutaneous, or epidural routes. However, it is relatively rare because doses administered through these routes are small and tolerance to respiratory depressant effects increases if the opioid dose is increased slowly. The risk of respiratory depression increases with age and the concomitant use of other opioids or other central nervous system depressants. The risk of respiratory depression also increases when the catheter is placed in the thoracic area and when the intra-abdominal or intrathoracic pressure is increased. Despite the risks associated with their use, intravenous and epidural opioids are considered safe, with the risks related to epidural administration no greater than those related to intravenous or other systemic routes of administration.

The patient receiving opioids by any route must be assessed frequently for changes in respiratory status. Specific notable changes are decreasing respiratory rate or shallow respirations. Sedation, which may occur with any method of administering opioids, is

most likely to occur when the opioid doses are increased. However, the patient often develops tolerance quickly, so that in a short time the patient is no longer sedated by the dose that initially caused sedation.

The patient at risk for sedation must be monitored closely for changes in respiratory status. Increasing the time between doses or reducing the dose temporarily, as prescribed, usually prevents deep sedation from occurring. The patient is also at risk for other problems associated with sedation and immobility, such as pressure sores. The nurse must initiate strategies to prevent such problems.

NAUSEA AND VOMITING

Nausea and vomiting frequently occur with opioid use. Usually these effects occur some hours after the initial injection. Patients, especially postoperative patients, may not think to tell the nurse that they are nauseated, particularly if the nausea is mild. However, the patient receiving an opioid should be assessed for nausea and vomiting, which may be triggered by a position change and may be prevented by having the patient change positions slowly. Adequate hydration and the administration of antiemetic agents may decrease the incidence. Opioid-induced nausea and vomiting often subside within a few days.

CONSTIPATION

Constipation, a common side effect of opioid use, may become so severe that the patient is forced to choose between relief of pain and relief of constipation. This situation can occur in patients after surgery and in patients receiving large doses of opioids to treat cancer-related pain. Preventing constipation must be a high priority in all patients receiving opioids. Whenever a patient receives opioids, a bowel regimen should begin at the same time. Tolerance to this side effect does not occur; rather, it persists even with long-term use of opioids.

Several strategies may help prevent and treat opioid-related constipation. Mild laxatives and a high intake of fluid and fibre may be effective in managing mild constipation. Unless contraindicated, a mild laxative and a stool softener should be administered on a regular schedule. Continued severe constipation, however, often requires the use of a stimulating cathartic agent, such as senna derivatives (Senokot) or bisacodyl (Dulcolax). Oral laxatives and stool softeners may prevent constipation; rectal suppositories may be used if oral agents fail (Plaisance & Ellis, 2002).

INADEQUATE PAIN RELIEF

One factor commonly associated with ineffective pain relief is an inadequate dose of opioid. This is most likely to occur when the caregiver underestimates the patient's pain or the route of administration is changed without the differences in absorption and action being considered. As a result, the patient receives doses too small to be effective and, possibly, too infrequently to relieve pain. For example, if opioid delivery is changed from the intravenous route to the oral route, the oral dose must be approximately three times greater than that given parenterally to provide relief. Because of differences in absorption of orally administered opioids among individuals, the patient must be assessed carefully to ensure that the pain is relieved.

Table 13-2 lists opioids and dosages that are equivalent to morphine. In general, no recalculation needs to be done when switching from one brand of an agent to another brand of the same medication, with the exception of extended-release oral morphine. Currently, several brands of extended-release morphine are commonly used by cancer patients. Although these agents come in the same dosage form and contain the same drug, they are not considered therapeutically equivalent because they employ different release

Table 13-2 • **Equianalgesic Conversion Table**

DRUG	TIME TO ONSET (MINUTES)	TIME TO PEAK (MINUTES)	DURATION (HOURS)	HALF-LIFE (HOURS)	EQUIANALGESIC DOSES	
					IV or IM (Mg)	Oral (mg)
codeine	10 to 30	30 to 60	4 to 6	3	120	200
fentanyl	7 to 8	No data	1 to 2	1.5 to 6	0.1	N/A
hydrocodone	No data	No data	4 to 8	3.3 to 4.5	No data	30
hydromorphone	15 to 30	30 to 60	4 to 5	2 to 3	1.3 to 1.5	7.5
levorphanol	No data	No data	6 to 8	12 to 16	2	4
meperidine	No data	No data	2 to 4	3 to 4	75	300
methadone	30 to 60	30 to 60	4 to 6	15 to 30	10	10 to 20
morphine	15 to 60	30 to 60	3 to 7	1.2 to 2	10	30 to 60
oxycodone	15 to 30	60	4 to 6	N/A	No data	20 mg
oxymorphone	5 to 10	30 to 60	3 to 6	N/A	1	10

Source: Texas Children's Cancer Center. (n.d.). *Equianalgesic conversion guide.* Available at: http://www.childcancerpain.org/content.cfm?content=pharm19 and Global RPh.com. (n.d.) *Narcotic analgesic dosage conversion chart.* Available at: http://www.globalrph.com/narcotic.htm.

mechanisms. Patients who need to switch brands should be monitored carefully both for overdose and for inadequate pain relief.

OTHER EFFECTS OF OPIOIDS

During the health history, when asked about drug allergies, patients with previous hospital experience (especially for surgery) may report that they are "allergic" to morphine. This report should be thoroughly investigated. Commonly, this "allergy" will be described as itching only. Pruritus (itching) is a frequent problem associated with opioids administered through any route, but it is not an allergic reaction. Itching can be relieved by administering prescribed antihistamines. In the event of an adverse reaction to a particular opioid, the physician may replace the drug with a different opioid analgesic to ensure the patient continues to receive effective treatment for pain.

A number of factors may influence the safety and effectiveness of opioid administration. Opioid analgesic agents are primarily metabolized by the liver and excreted by the kidney. Therefore, metabolism and excretion of analgesic medications will be impaired in patients with liver or kidney disease, increasing the risk of cumulative or toxic effects. In addition, normeperidine, a metabolite of meperidine, may rapidly or unexpectedly accumulate to toxic levels. This is more likely to occur in patients with impaired kidney function and may result in seizures in susceptible patients.

Patients with untreated hypothyroidism are more susceptible to the analgesic effects and side effects of opioids. In contrast, patients with hyperthyroidism may require larger doses for pain relief. Patients with a decreased respiratory reserve from disease or aging may be more susceptible to the depressant effects of opioids and must be carefully monitored for respiratory depression.

Dehydrated patients are at increased risk for the hypotensive effects of opioids. Patients who become hypotensive after the administration of an opioid should be kept recumbent and rehydrated unless fluids are contraindicated. Patients who are dehydrated are also more likely to experience nausea and vomiting with opioid use. Rehydration usually relieves these symptoms.

Patients receiving certain other medications, such as monoamine oxidase (MAO) inhibitors, phenothiazines, or tricyclic antidepressants, may have an exaggerated response to the depressant effects of opioids. Patients taking these medications should receive small doses of opioids and must be monitored closely. Continued pain in these patients indicates that a therapeutic level of the analgesic has not been achieved. The patient must be monitored for sedation even if an analgesic effect has not been obtained. The use of additional nonopioid analgesic medications may be considered for these patients.

TOLERANCE AND ADDICTION

There is no maximum safe dosage of opioids, nor is there any easily identifiable therapeutic serum level. Both the maximal safe dosage and therapeutic serum level are relative and individual. **Tolerance** (the need for increasing doses of opioids to achieve the same therapeutic effect) will develop in almost all patients taking opioids over an extended period. Patients requiring opioids over a long term, especially cancer patients, will need increasing doses to relieve pain. After the first few weeks of therapy, the patient's dosing requirements usually level off. Patients who become tolerant to the analgesic effects of large doses of morphine may obtain pain relief by switching to a different opioid or adding an adjuvant such as a tricyclic antidepressant. Symptoms of physical *dependence* may occur when the opioids are discontinued; dependence often occurs with opioid tolerance and does not indicate an addiction.

NURSING ALERT Although patients may need increasing levels of opioids, they are not addicted. Physical tolerance usually occurs in the absence of addiction. Tolerance to opioids is common and becomes a problem primarily in terms of delivering or administering the medication (eg, how to administer very large doses of morphine a day to a patient). On the other hand, addiction is rare and should never be the primary concern of the nurse caring for a patient in pain.

Addiction is a behavioural pattern of substance use characterized by a compulsion to take the drug primarily to experience its psychic effects. Fear that patients will become addicted or dependent on opioids has contributed to inadequate treatment of pain. This fear is commonly expressed by health care providers as well as patients and results from lack of knowledge about the low risk of addiction.

In an often-cited classic study (Porter & Jick, 1980) of more than 11,000 patients receiving opioids for a medical indication, only four patients without a history of substance abuse could be identified as becoming addicted. Addiction following therapeutic opioid administration is so negligible that it should not be a consideration when caring for the patient in pain. Thus, patients and health care providers should be dissuaded from withholding pain medication because of concerns about addiction.

Nonsteroidal Anti-inflammatory Drugs

NSAIDs are thought to decrease pain by inhibiting cyclo-oxygenase (COX), the rate-limiting enzyme involved in the production of prostaglandin from traumatized or inflamed tissues. There are two types of COX (COX-1 and COX-2), and the effects of inhibiting each are different. COX-1 is involved with mediating prostaglandin formation involved in the maintenance of physiologic functions. Two such functions include platelet aggregation through the provision of thromboxane precursors, and increased mucosal flow. Together, these two functions prevent ischemia and promote mucosal integrity. Therefore, inhibiting COX-1 will result in the undesirable effects of gastric ulceration, bleeding, and renal damage. COX-2 mediates prostaglandin formation that results in symptoms of pain, inflammation, and fever. Thus, inhibition of COX-2 produces desirable effects.

Two common over-the-counter NSAIDs are aspirin and ibuprofen, and they inhibit both COX-1 and COX-2. Aspirin is infrequently used to treat major acute or chronic pain because it causes frequent and severe side effects. Ibuprofen, however, is effective in relieving mild to moderate pain and has a low incidence of adverse effects. In 1999, the first COX-2–selective inhibitors (simply referred to as COX-2 inhibitors) became available for use in Canada. Since then, these drugs (eg, rofecoxib, valdecoxib) have been highly prescribed and used. Concerns about adverse effects of COX-2 inhibitors, including an increased risk of experiencing a heart attack or stroke, led to the withdrawal of rofecoxib in 2004 and the suspension of valdecoxib in 2005. However, two COX-2 inhibitors, meloxicam and celecoxib, are still available in Canada. Current research on COX-2 inhibitors is focussed on combining COX-2 inhibitors with other drugs that will counteract the adverse effects of the COX-2 inhibitor.

NSAIDs are very helpful in treating arthritic diseases and may be especially powerful in treating cancer-related bone pain. They have been effectively combined with opioids to treat postoperative and other severe pain. The use of an NSAID with an opioid relieves pain more effectively than the opioid alone. In such cases, the patient may obtain pain relief with less opioid and fewer side effects. It has been shown that intraoperative administration of NSAIDs results in improved postoperative pain control following laparoscopic surgery and in some cases shorter hospital stays (McLaughlin, 1994).

A regimen of a fixed-dose, time-contingent NSAID (eg, every 4 hours) and a separately administered fluctuating dose of opioid may be effective in managing moderate to severe cancer pain. In more severe pain, the opioid dose will also be fixed, with an additional fluctuating dose as needed for **breakthrough pain** (a sudden increase in pain despite the administration of pain-relieving medications). These regimens result in better pain relief with fewer opioid-related side effects.

Most patients tolerate NSAIDs well. However, those with impaired kidney function may require a smaller dose and must be monitored closely for side effects. Patients taking NSAIDs bruise easily because NSAIDs have some anticoagulant effect. Moreover, NSAIDs may compete with other medications, such as warfarin, for serum proteins, thereby increasing the effects of the other medications. High doses or prolonged use can irritate the stomach and in some cases result in gastrointestinal bleeding as well. Thus, monitoring the patient for gastrointestinal bleeding is indicated.

Adjuvant Therapy

Adjuvant therapy is the use of two or more drugs to treat a particular condition: the main effect of only one of the drugs is to treat the condition, whereas the other drug(s) work to increase the therapeutic effect of (or potentiate) the original drug. In the treatment of pain, tricyclic antidepressants and anticonvulsants are used to potentiate the effects of opioid analgesics. By using these adjuvants, patients may experience better pain treatment with lower doses of opioids. In addition, a tricyclic antidepressant may improve the quality of sleep and further decrease pain. When indicated, tricyclic antidepressant agents, such as amitriptyline or imipramine, are prescribed in doses considerably smaller than those generally used for depression. The patient needs to know that a therapeutic effect may not occur before 3 weeks. Anticonvulsants such as phenytoin, carbamazepine, or pregabalin also are used in doses lower than those prescribed for seizure disorders. Because a variety of medications can be tried, the nurse should be familiar with the possible side effects and should teach the patient and family how to recognize these effects. The patient perspective of treatment must be considered when an **adjuvant analgesic** is used. Patients may be reluctant to take a tricyclic antidepressant or an anticonvulsant because of a perceived associated stigma, or simply because they do not believe their condition warrants the use of such drugs. It is important to clarify with patients the intended adjuvant benefit of these medications.

ROUTES OF ADMINISTRATION

The route selected for administering an analgesic agent (Table 13-3) depends on the patient's condition and the desired effect of the medication. Analgesic agents can be administered by parenteral, oral, rectal, transdermal, transmucosal, intraspinal, or epidural routes. Each method of administration has advantages and disadvantages. The route chosen should be based on the patient's needs.

Parenteral Route

Parenteral administration (intramuscular, intravenous, or subcutaneous) of the analgesic medication produces effects more rapidly than oral administration, but these effects are of shorter duration. Parenteral administration may be indicated if the patient is not permitted oral intake or is vomiting.

Medication administered by the intramuscular route enters the bloodstream more slowly than medication given intravenously

Table 13-3 • **Administration Routes for Analgesics**

ROUTE	SITE
Parenteral	Intramuscular (IM) Intravenous (IV) Subcutaneous (SC)
Gastrointestinal	Oral (PO) Rectal (PR)
Transdermal	Skin
Transmucosal	Oral mucosa Intranasal mucosa Bronchial mucosa
Epidural Intraspinal	Epidural space Spinal canal

and is metabolized slowly. The rate of absorption may be erratic; it depends on the site selected and the amount of body fat. Intramuscular injections of volumes greater than 2 mL are very painful and may not be an appropriate route for administering analgesics.

The intravenous route is an alternative to intramuscular injection for many but not all analgesic medications. The intravenous route is the preferred parenteral route in most acute care situations because it is much more comfortable for the patient. In addition, peak serum levels and pain relief occur more rapidly and reliably. Because it peaks rapidly (usually within minutes) and is metabolized quickly, an appropriate intravenous dose will be smaller and prescribed at shorter intervals than an intramuscular dose.

Intravenous opioids may be administered by IV push or slow push (eg, over a 5- to 10-minute period) or by continuous infusion with a pump. Continuous infusion provides a steady level of analgesia and is indicated when pain occurs over a 24-hour period (eg, after surgery for the first day or so, or in a patient with prolonged cancer pain who cannot take medication by other routes). The dose of analgesic agent is calculated carefully to relieve pain without producing respiratory depression and other side effects.

The subcutaneous route for infusion of opioid analgesic agents is used for patients with severe pain such as cancer pain; it is particularly useful for patients with limited intravenous access who cannot take oral medications, and patients who are managing their pain at home. The dose of opioid that can be infused through this route is limited because of the small volume that can be administered at one time into the subcutaneous tissue. However, this route is often an effective and convenient way to manage pain.

Oral Route

If the patient can take medication by mouth, oral administration is preferred over parenteral administration because it is easy, noninvasive, and not painful. Severe pain can be relieved with oral opioids if the doses are high enough. The oral route of administration is recommended by the Canadian Pain Society for treating chronic pain.

In terminally ill patients with prolonged pain, doses may gradually be increased as the disease progresses and causes more pain or as the person builds up a tolerance to the medication. If these higher doses are increased gradually, they usually provide additional pain relief without producing respiratory depression or sedation. When a change is made in either the route of administration or the analgesic used, it is important to ensure that the new dose will produce the same analgesic effects as (be equianalgesic to) the replaced dose (see Table 13-2.) Changes that result in a smaller analgesic effect may result in a withdrawal reaction and the recurrence of pain.

Rectal Route

The rectal route of administration may be indicated in patients who cannot take medications by any other route. The rectal route may also be indicated for patients with bleeding problems, such as hemophilia. The onset of action of opioids administered rectally is unclear but is delayed compared with other routes of administration. Similarly, the duration of action is prolonged.

Topical Route

The topical route of administration is used primarily for minor pain due to wounds, burns, insect bites, sutures or procedural pain. Use of topical anesthesia in children is especially important because it can prevent the development of procedural anxiety due to painful experiences. Topically administered drugs usually do not penetrate deeply into the tissues, but rather are contained within the epidermal and dermal layers. Anesthetic agents administered topically are incorporated into either a cream or a patch. Skin to which cream formulations are applied must be covered with an occlusive dressing, whereas patches combining the drug within an occlusive dressing do not require an additional dressing. Occlusive dressings are designed to lose their adhesive ability when stretched horizontally to the skin. This results in a painless dressing removal for the patient.

Transdermal Route

The transdermal route has been used to achieve a consistent opioid serum level through absorption of the medication via the skin. This route is most often used for cancer patients who are at home or in hospice care and who have been receiving oral sustained-release morphine. Fentanyl is the only commercially available transdermal medication. The preparation is a patch consisting of a reservoir containing the medication and a membrane.

When the transdermal system is first applied to the skin, the fentanyl, which is fat-soluble, binds to the skin and fat layers. Then it is slowly and systemically absorbed. Therefore, there is a delay in effect while the dermal layer is being saturated. A drug reservoir actually forms in the upper layer of skin. This results in a slowly rising serum level and a slow tapering of the serum level once the patch is removed. Because it takes 12 to 24 hours for the fentanyl levels to gradually increase from the first patch, the last dose of sustained-release morphine should be given at the same time the first patch is applied (Donner et al., 1996). Transdermal fentanyl is associated with slightly less constipation than oral opioids. Absorption is increased in the febrile patient. A heating pad should never be applied to the area where the patch is applied because heat can increase the release rate of fentanyl and increase the risks of side effects such as respiratory depression. Transdermal fentanyl is much more expensive than sustained-release morphine but less costly than methods that deliver parenteral opioids.

Once it is determined that switching from other routes of morphine administration to the patch is appropriate, the correct dosage for the patch must be calculated. If the patient uses an opioid other than morphine, conversion to milligrams of oral morphine is the first step. After determining how many milligrams of morphine (or morphine equivalents) the patient has been using over 24 hours, an initial dose of transdermal fentanyl can be calculated.

Pasaro (1997) suggests one method of calculating the initial dose of fentanyl: the patient's daily dose of morphine is divided by two. Thus, the equivalent of 400 mg morphine used per day would be equivalent to 200 g fentanyl per hour. Patients switched from morphine to fentanyl need to be assessed not only for pain and potential side effects but also for dependence, reflected by withdrawal symptoms, which may consist of shivering, a feeling of coldness, sweating, headache, and paresthesia (Puntillo, Casella et al., 1997). Patients may require short-acting opioids for breakthrough pain before the systemic fentanyl level reaches a therapeutic level.

These conversions and the conversion-type table in the transdermal fentanyl packet insert should be used only to establish the initial dose of fentanyl when the patient switches from oral morphine to fentanyl (and not vice versa). These tables and equations are not meant to be used to determine the dosages of oral morphine for a patient who has been receiving transdermal fentanyl. Many patients will not achieve satisfactory analgesia from the initial dose of transdermal fentanyl and will require an increase in their fentanyl dose to treat breakthrough pain. If the table or equation is used incorrectly to calculate a morphine dose, there is a risk of overdose. If the patient requires a change from transdermal fentanyl back to oral or intravenous morphine (as in the case of surgery), the patch should be removed and intravenous morphine supplied on an assessed need basis.

Before applying a new patch, the patient should be carefully checked for any older, forgotten patches. These should be discarded. Patches should be replaced every 72 hours.

Intraspinal and Epidural Routes

Infusion of opioids or local anesthetic agents into the subarachnoid space (intrathecal space or spinal canal) or epidural space has been used for effective control of pain in postoperative patients and those with chronic pain unrelieved by other methods. A catheter is inserted into the subarachnoid or the epidural space at the thoracic or lumbar level for administration of opioid or anesthetic agents (Fig. 13-8). With intrathecal administration, the medication infuses directly into the subarachnoid space and cerebrospinal fluid, which surrounds the spinal cord. With epidural administration, medication is deposited in the dura of the spinal canal and diffuses into the subarachnoid space. It is believed that pain relief from intraspinal administration of opioids is due to the existence of opioid receptors in the spinal cord.

Infusion of opioids and local anesthetic agents through an intrathecal or epidural catheter results in pain relief with fewer side effects, including sedation, than with systemic analgesia. Adverse effects associated with intraspinal administration include spinal headache resulting from loss of spinal fluid when the dura is punctured. This is more likely to occur in younger (less than 40 years of age) patients. The dura must be punctured with the intrathecal route, and dural puncture may occur inadvertently with the epidural route. When dural puncture inadvertently occurs, spinal fluid seeps out of the spinal canal. The resultant headache is likely to be more severe with an epidural needle because it is larger than a spinal needle, and therefore more spinal fluid escapes.

Although respiratory depression generally peaks 6 to 12 hours after epidural opioids are administered, it can occur earlier or up to 24 hours after the first injection. Depending on the lipophilicity (affinity for body fat) of the opioid injected, the time frame for respiratory depression can be short or long. Morphine is hydrophilic, and the time for peak effect is longer compared to fentanyl, which is a lipophilic opioid. All patients should be monitored closely for at least the first 24 hours after the first injection, longer if changes in respiratory status or level of consciousness occur. Opioid antagonist agents such as naloxone must be available for intravenous use if respiratory depression occurs.

The patient is also observed for urinary retention, pruritus, nausea, vomiting, and dizziness. Precautions must be taken to avoid infection at the catheter site and catheter displacement. Only medications without preservatives should be administered into the subarachnoid or epidural space because of the potential neurotoxic effects of preservatives.

During surgery, intrathecal opioids are used almost exclusively after a spinal anesthetic agent is administered. For patients undergoing large abdominal surgical procedures, especially those at risk for postoperative complications, a combination of a general inhaled anesthetic agent for the surgery and a local epidural anesthetic agent and epidural opioids administered after surgery results in excellent pain control with fewer postoperative complications.

Patients who have persistent, severe pain that fails to respond to other treatments, or those who obtain pain relief only with the risk of serious side effects, may benefit from medication administered by a long-term intrathecal or epidural catheter. After the physician tunnels the catheter through the subcutaneous tissue and places the inlet (or port) under the skin, the medication is injected through the skin into the inlet and catheter, which delivers the medication directly into the epidural space. The medication may need to be injected several times a day to maintain an adequate level of pain relief.

In patients who require more frequent doses or continuous infusions of opioid analgesic agents to relieve pain, an implantable infusion device or pump may be used to administer the medication continuously. The medication is administered at a small, constant dose at a preset rate into the epidural or subarachnoid space. The reservoir of the infusion device stores the medication for slow release and needs to be refilled every 1 or 2 months, depending on the patient's needs. This eliminates the need for repeated injections through the skin.

> **NURSING ALERT** An epidural catheter inserted for pain control is usually managed by the nurse. Baseline information necessary to provide safe and effective pain control includes the level or site of catheter insertion, the medications (eg, local anesthetic agents or opioids) that have been administered, and the medications anticipated in the future. The infusion rate is increased with caution when anesthetic agents are combined with opioids. Sensory deficits can occur and patients must be assessed frequently. An infusion with a lower concentration of anesthetic agent allows for administration of a greater concentration of the opioid with a lower risk of sensory deficits.

A

B

FIGURE 13-8 Placement of intraspinal catheters for administration of analgesic medications: (**A**) intrathecal route, (**B**) epidural route.

NURSING MANAGEMENT OF SIDE EFFECTS

Headache resulting from spinal fluid loss may be delayed. Therefore, the nurse needs to assess regularly for headache after either type of catheter is placed. Should headache occur, the patient should remain flat in bed and should be given large amounts of fluids (provided the medical condition allows), and the physician should be notified. An epidural blood patch may be carried out to reduce leakage of spinal fluid.

Cardiovascular effects (hypotension and decreased heart rate) may result from relaxation of the vasculature in the lower extremities. Therefore, the nurse assesses frequently for decreases in blood pressure, pulse rate, and urine output.

For patients experiencing opioid-related pruritus, the physician may prescribe diphenhydramine (Benadryl).

PROMOTING HOME AND COMMUNITY-BASED CARE

The patient who receives epidural analgesic agents at home and the family must be taught how to administer the prescribed medication using sterile technique and how to assess for infection. The patient and family also need to learn how to recognize side effects and what to do about them. Although respiratory depression is uncommon, urinary retention may be a problem, and patients and families must be prepared to deal with it if it occurs. Implanted analgesic delivery systems can be safely and confidently used at home only if health care personnel are available for consultation and, possibly, intervention on short notice.

ALTERNATIVE OR COMPLEMENTARY APPROACHES

Although pain medication is the most powerful pain relief tool available to nurses, it is not the only one. Nonpharmacologic nursing activities can assist in relieving pain with usually low risk to the patient. Although such measures are not a substitute for medication, they may be all that is necessary or appropriate to relieve episodes of pain lasting only seconds or minutes. In instances of severe pain that lasts for hours or days, combining nonpharmacologic interventions with medications may be the most effective way to relieve pain.

Physiatric Techniques

People suffering chronic, debilitating pain are often desperate. Often they will try anything, recommended by anyone, at any price. Information about an array of potential therapies can be found on the Internet and in the self-help section of the bookstore. Therapies specifically recommended for pain from these sources include but are not limited to chelation, therapeutic touch, music therapy, herbal therapy, reflexology, magnetic therapy, electrotherapy, polarity therapy, acupressure, emu oil, pectin therapy, aromatherapy, homeopathy, and macrobiotic dieting. Many of these "therapies" (with the exception of macrobiotic dieting) are probably not harmful. However, they have yet to be proven effective by the standards used to evaluate the effectiveness of medical and nursing interventions. The National Institutes of Health has established an office to examine the effectiveness of alternative therapies.

The Canadian Institutes of Health Research placed a priority on investigating the effectiveness of alternative therapies. Despite the lack of scientific evidence that these therapies are effective, a patient may find any one of them helpful via the placebo response. It is important when caring for a patient who is using or considering using untested therapies (often referred to as alternative therapies) not to diminish the patient's hope and potential placebo response.

This must be weighed against the professional nurse's responsibility to protect the patient from costly and potentially harmful and dangerous therapies that the patient is not in a position to evaluate scientifically.

Problems arise when patients do not find relief but are deprived of conventional therapy because the alternative therapy "should be helping," or when patients abandon conventional therapy for alternative therapy. In addition, few alternative therapies are free. Desperate patients may risk financial ruin seeking alternative therapies that do not work.

The nurse's role is to help the patient and family understand scientific research and how that differs from anecdotal evidence. Without diminishing the placebo effects the patient may receive, the nurse encourages the patient to assess the effectiveness of the therapy continually using standard pain assessment techniques. In addition, the nurse encourages the patient using alternative therapies to combine them with conventional therapies and to discuss this use with the physician.

CUTANEOUS STIMULATION AND MASSAGE

The gate control theory of pain proposes that the stimulation of fibres that transmit nonpainful sensations can block or decrease the transmission of pain impulses. Several nonpharmacologic pain relief strategies, including rubbing the skin and using heat and cold, are based on this theory.

Massage, which is generalized cutaneous stimulation of the body, often concentrates on the back and shoulders. A massage does not specifically stimulate the non-pain receptors in the same receptor field as the pain receptors, but it may have an impact through the descending control system (see earlier discussion). Massage also promotes comfort because it produces muscle relaxation.

ICE AND HEAT THERAPIES

Ice and heat therapies may be effective pain relief strategies in some circumstances; however, their effectiveness and mechanism of action need further study. Proponents believe that ice and heat stimulate the non-pain receptors in the same receptor field as the injury.

For greatest effect, ice should be placed on the injury site immediately after injury or surgery. Ice therapy after joint surgery can significantly reduce the amount of analgesic medication required subsequently. Ice therapy may also relieve pain if applied later. Care must be taken to assess the skin prior to treatment and to protect the skin from direct application of the ice. Ice should be applied to an area for no longer than 20 minutes at a time. This prevents the rebound phenomenon that occurs as the body attempts to warm up, rendering the treatment useless. Long applications of ice may result in frostbite or nerve injury. Both ice and heat therapy must be applied carefully and monitored closely to avoid injuring the skin. Neither therapy should be applied to areas with impaired circulation or used with patients with impaired sensation.

Application of heat increases blood flow to an area and contributes to pain reduction by speeding healing. Both dry and moist heat may provide some analgesia, but their mechanisms of action are not well understood. Application of heat to inflamed joints, for example, may provide temporary comfort, but increasing the intra-articular temperature may impair healing (Oosterveld & Rasker, 1994a, 1994b).

NEUROSTIMULATION PROCEDURES

Neurostimulation is the use of a device containing electrodes and a battery to administer tiny therapeutic electrical pulses to neural material, thereby reducing acute or chronic pain. Because the device emits electrical pulses, it is sometimes referred to as a "pain pacemaker." The battery pack for the device may be implanted beneath the surface of the skin or it may be worn externally by the patient. Neurostimulation can be applied directly to the spinal cord (spinal stimulation) or to peripheral areas of the body either using electrodes placed against the skin (transcutaneous electrical nerve stimulation [TENS]) or using electrified acupuncture needles (percutaneous electrical nerve stimulation [PENS]). Neurostimulation causes paresthesia or the production of abnormal sensation; pain sensation is replaced by a tingling sensation. Neurostimulation may work by stimulating the body to produce opioid peptides including enkephalins, dynorphins, and endorphins (Kukushkin et al, 2003). Neurostimulation has been found to be effective in reducing many types of pain including chronic noncancer pain, neuropathic pain, spinal pain, chronic mixed spinal and neuropathic pain, intractable pain of the trunk or limbs, visceral pain, low back pain, myofascial and arthritic pain, sympathetically mediated pain, postoperative pain, refractory angina, and the pain associated with peripheral vascular disease and reflex sympathetic dystrophy. By using neurostimulation, patients may be able to decrease their dose of analgesic drugs and still achieve pain control. Pain from peripheral neuropathies and phantom limb pain do not respond as well to neurostimulation as do the types previously listed.

Transcutaneous Electrical Nerve Stimulation. TENS uses a battery-operated unit with electrodes applied to the skin to produce a tingling, vibrating, or buzzing sensation in the area of pain. It has been used in both acute and chronic pain relief and is thought to decrease pain by stimulating the non-pain receptors in the same area as the fibres that transmit the pain. This mechanism is consistent with the gate control theory of pain and explains the effectiveness of cutaneous stimulation when applied in the same area as an injury. For example, when TENS is used in a postoperative patient, the electrodes are placed around the surgical wound.

Another possible explanation for the effectiveness of TENS is the placebo effect (the patient expects it to be effective). In a review of the literature, Carroll, Tramer, McQuay et al. (1996) found that in 15 of 17 studies with randomized control group designs, TENS was ineffective in relieving postoperative pain. In 17 of 19 studies that did not use this design, the authors of these studies concluded that TENS had a positive analgesic effect. The review of these studies suggests that a placebo effect may explain the effectiveness of TENS.

Percutaneous Electrical Nerve Stimulation. PENS is the application of neurostimulation to peripheral sensory nerves via acupuncture-like needle electrodes inserted into the soft tissues. PENS is effective in relieving deep muscles pain, particularly chronic lower back pain.

ACUPUNCTURE

An alternative therapy for treating pain is acupuncture, which involves the insertion of extremely thin needles into soft tissues. The locations of needle insertion are specific, and the technique is reputed to replace pain with sensations of warmth, tingling, or pressure.

COGNITIVE BEHAVIOURAL TECHNIQUES

Pain is a complex phenomenon with sensory and emotional dimensions. Cognitive behavioural techniques specifically deal with the emotional cognitive, affective, and behavioural components of pain. These techniques can be used alone or in combination with pharmacologic interventions. They are useful for procedural pain. Relaxation and cognitive restructuring are examples of cognitive behavioural techniques.

RELAXATION TECHNIQUES

Distraction. This technique helps relieve both acute and chronic pain (Johnson & Petrie, 1997). Distraction, which involves focusing the patient's attention on something other than the pain, may be the mechanism responsible for other effective cognitive techniques. Distraction is thought to reduce the perception of pain by stimulating the descending control system, resulting in fewer painful stimuli being transmitted to the brain. The effectiveness of distraction depends on the patient's ability to receive and create sensory input other than pain. Distraction techniques may range from simple activities, such as watching TV or listening to music, to highly complex physical and mental exercises. Pain relief generally increases in direct proportion to the person's active participation, the number of sensory modalities used, and the person's interest in the stimuli. Therefore, the stimulation of sight, sound, and touch is likely to be more effective in reducing pain than is the stimulation of a single sense.

Visits from family and friends are effective in relieving pain. Watching an action-packed movie on a large screen with "Surround-Sound" through headphones may be effective (provided the person finds it acceptable). Others may benefit from games and activities (eg, chess) that require concentration. Not all patients obtain pain relief with distraction, especially those in severe pain. With severe pain, the patient may be unable to concentrate well enough to participate in complex physical or mental activities.

Skeletal Muscle Relaxation. It is believed to reduce pain by relaxing tense muscles that contribute to the pain. Considerable evidence supports relaxation as effective in relieving chronic low back pain (NIH Technology Assessment Panel, 1995). Few studies, however, support its effectiveness in reducing postoperative pain. This may be due to the relatively small role skeletal muscles play in postoperative pain, or to the need for the patient to practice the relaxation technique for it to be effective. Practicing the technique may not be possible when it is taught only once, immediately before surgery. A patient who already knows a technique for relaxing may only need to be reminded to use it to reduce or prevent increased pain.

A simple relaxation technique consists of abdominal breathing at a slow, rhythmic rate. The patient may close both eyes and breathe slowly and comfortably. A constant rhythm can be maintained by counting silently and slowly with each inhalation ("in, two, three") and exhalation ("out, two, three"). When teaching this technique, the nurse may count out loud with the patient at first. Slow, rhythmic breathing may also be used as a distraction technique. Relaxation techniques, as well as other noninvasive pain relief measures, may require practice before the patient becomes skilled in using them.

Almost all people with chronic pain can benefit from some method of relaxation. Regular relaxation periods may help to combat the fatigue and muscle tension that occur with and increase chronic pain.

Guided Imagery. Guided imagery uses one's imagination in a special way to achieve a specific positive effect. Guided imagery for relaxation and pain relief may consist of combining slow, rhythmic breathing with a mental image of relaxation and comfort. The nurse instructs the patient to close the eyes and breathe slowly in and out. With each slowly exhaled breath, the patient imagines muscle tension and discomfort being breathed out, carrying away pain and tension and leaving behind a relaxed and comfortable body. With each inhaled breath, the patient imagines healing energy flowing to the area of discomfort.

If guided imagery is to be effective, it requires a considerable amount of time to explain the technique and time for the patient to practice it. Usually, the patient is asked to practice guided imagery for about 5 minutes, three times a day. Several days of practice may be needed before the intensity of pain is reduced. Many patients begin to experience the relaxing effects of guided imagery the first time they try it. Pain relief can continue for hours after the imagery is used. The patient needs to be informed that guided imagery may work only for some people. Guided imagery should be used only in combination with all other forms of treatment that have demonstrated effectiveness.

Hypnosis. Hypnosis has been effective in relieving pain or decreasing the amount of analgesic agents required in patients with acute and chronic pain and may promote pain relief in particularly difficult situations (eg, burns). The mechanism by which hypnosis acts is unclear. Its effectiveness depends on the hypnotic susceptibility of the individual (Farthing, Venturino, Brown et al., 1997). In some cases, hypnosis may be effective in the first session, with effectiveness increasing in additional sessions. In other cases, hypnosis does not work at all. Usually, hypnosis must be induced by a specially skilled person (a psychologist or a nurse with specialized training in hypnosis). Sometimes patients learn to perform self-hypnosis.

Surgical Techniques

In some situations, especially with long-term and severe intractable pain, usual pharmacologic and nonpharmacologic methods of pain relief are ineffective. In those situations, neurologic and neurosurgical approaches to pain management may be considered. Intractable pain refers to pain that cannot be relieved satisfactorily by the usual approaches, including medications. Such pain usually is the result of malignancy (especially of the cervix, bladder, prostate, and lower bowel), but it may occur in other conditions, such as postherpetic neuralgia, trigeminal neuralgia, spinal cord arachnoiditis, and uncontrollable ischemia and other forms of tissue destruction.

Neurologic and neurosurgical methods available for pain relief include (1) stimulation procedures (intermittent electrical stimulation of a tract or centre to inhibit the transmission of pain impulses), (2) administration of intraspinal opioids (see previous discussion), and (3) interruption of the tracts conducting the pain impulse from the periphery to cerebral integration centres. The latter are destructive or ablative procedures, and their effects are permanent. Ablative procedures are used when other methods of pain relief have failed.

INTERRUPTION OF PAIN PATHWAYS

As described above, stimulation of a peripheral nerve, the spinal cord, or the deep brain using minute amounts of electricity and a stimulating device is used if all other pharmacologic and nonpharmacologic treatments fail to provide adequate relief. These treatments are reversible. If they need to be discontinued, the nervous system continues to function. Treatments that interrupt the pain pathways, however, are permanent.

Pain-conducting fibres can be interrupted at any point from their origin to the cerebral cortex. Some part of the nervous system is destroyed, resulting in varying amounts of neurologic deficit and incapacity. In time, pain usually returns as a result of either regeneration of axonal fibres or the development of alternative pain pathways.

Destructive procedures used to interrupt the transmission of pain include cordotomy and rhizotomy. These procedures are offered if the patient is thought to be near the end of life and will

have an improved quality of life as an outcome (Linderoth & Meyerson, 2002). Often these procedures can provide pain relief for the duration of a patient's life. The use of other methods to interrupt pain transmission is waning since the use of intraspinal therapies and newer pain management treatments are available.

Cordotomy. This procedure is the division of certain tracts of the spinal cord (Fig. 13-9). It may be performed percutaneously, by the open method after laminectomy, or by other techniques. Cordotomy is performed to interrupt the transmission of pain (Hodge & Christensen, 2002). Care must be taken to destroy only the sensation of pain, leaving motor functions intact.

Rhizotomy. During a rhizotomy, nerve roots are destroyed where they enter the spinal cord. A lesion is made in the dorsal root to destroy neuronal dysfunction and reduce nociceptive input. With the advent of microsurgical techniques, the complications are few, with mild sensory deficits and mild weakness (Fig. 13-10).

NEUROSTIMULATION PROCEDURES

Electrical stimulation, or neuromodulation, is a method of suppressing pain by applying controlled low-voltage electrical pulses to the different parts of the nervous system. Electrical stimulation is thought to relieve pain by blocking painful stimuli (the gate control theory). There are brain-stimulating techniques in which electrodes are implanted in the periventricular area of the posterior third ventricle, allowing the patient to stimulate this area to produce analgesia.

Spinal Cord Stimulation. In this technique used for the relief of chronic, intractable pain, ischemic pain, and pain from angina, a surgically implanted device allows the patient to apply pulsed

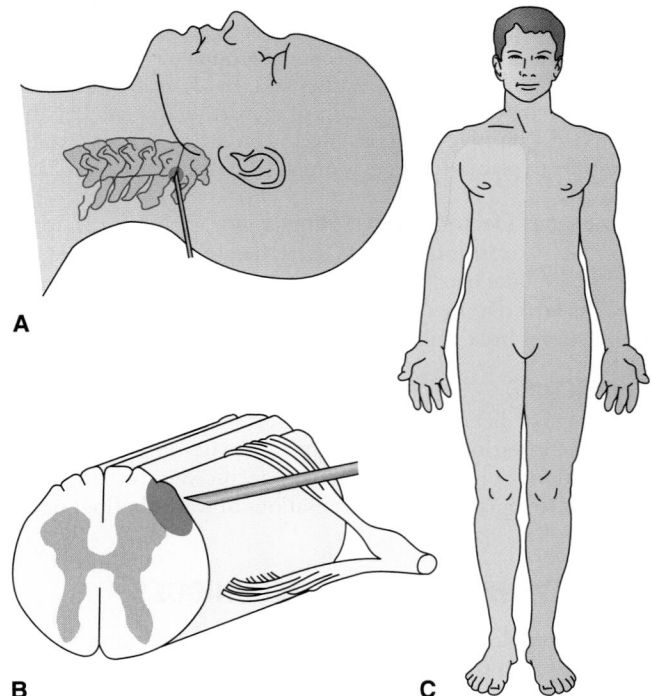

FIGURE 13-9 (**A**) Site of percutaneous C1–C2 cordotomy. (**B**) Lesion produced by percutaneous C1–C2 cordotomy. (**C**) Extent of analgesia produced by left C1–C2 percutaneous cordotomy.

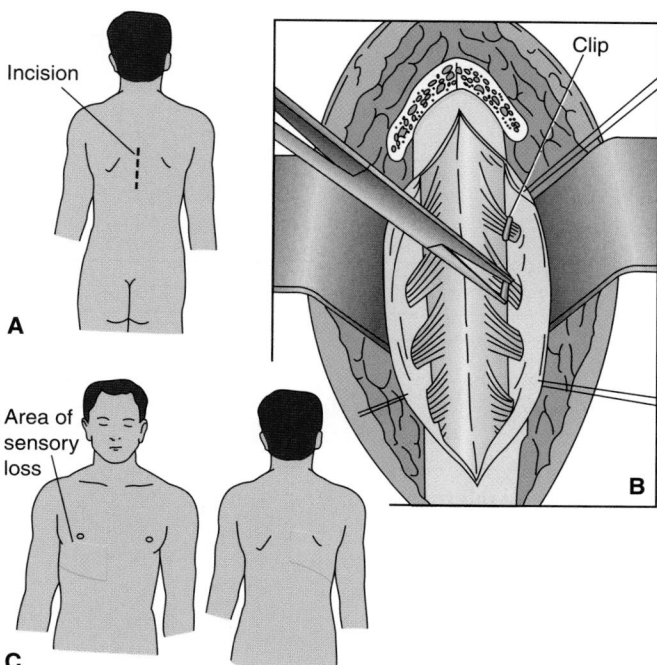

FIGURE 13-10 A rhizotomy may be performed surgically, percutaneously, or chemically, depending on a patient's condition and needs. The procedure is usually done to relieve severe chest pain, for example, from lung cancer. In (**A**) a surgical rhizotomy, (**B**) the spinal roots are divided and banded with a clip to form a lesion and subsequent (**C**) loss of sensation. Adapted with permission from Loeser, J. D. (ed.) (2000). *Bonica's management of pain* (3rd ed.). Philadelphia: Lippincott Williams & Wilkins.

electrical stimulation to the dorsal aspect of the spinal cord to block pain impulses (Linderoth & Meyerson, 2002). (The largest accumulation of afferent fibres is found in the dorsal column of the spinal cord.) The dorsal column stimulation unit consists of a radiofrequency stimulation transmitter, a transmitter antenna, a radiofrequency receiver, and a stimulation electrode. The battery-powered transmitter and antenna are worn externally; the receiver and electrode are implanted. A laminectomy is performed above the highest level of pain input, and the electrode is placed in the epidural space over the posterior column of the spinal cord. (The placement of the stimulating systems varies.) A subcutaneous pocket is constructed over the clavicular area or some other site for placement of the receiver. The two are connected by a subcutaneous tunnel. Careful patient selection is necessary, and not all patients receive total pain relief.

Deep Brain Stimulation. It is performed for special pain problems when the patient does not respond to the usual techniques of pain control. With the patient under local anesthesia, electrodes are introduced through a burr hole in the skull and inserted into a selected site in the brain, depending on the location or type of pain. After the effectiveness of stimulation is confirmed, the implanted electrode is connected to a radiofrequency device or pulse-generator system operated by external telemetry. It is used in neuropathic pain that may occur with damage or injury that occurred following stroke, brain or spinal cord injuries, or phantom limb pain. Use of deep brain stimulation has decreased and may be related to improved pain control and intraspinal therapies (Rezai & Lozano, 2002).

Nursing Interventions. With each of these procedures, patients are provided with written and verbal instructions about their expected effect on pain and on possible untoward consequences. The patient is monitored for specific effects of each method of pain intervention, both positive and negative. The specific nursing care of patients who undergo neurologic and neurosurgical procedures for the relief of chronic pain depends on the type of procedure performed, its effectiveness in relieving the pain, and the changes in neurologic function that accompany the procedure. After the procedure, the patient's pain level and neurologic function are assessed. Other nursing interventions that may be indicated include positioning, turning and skin care, bowel and bladder management, and interventions to promote patient safety. Pain management remains an important aspect of nursing care with each of these procedures.

PROMOTING HOME AND COMMUNITY-BASED CARE

In preparing the patient and family to manage pain at home, the patient and family need to be taught and guided about what type of pain or discomfort to expect, how long the pain is expected to last, and when the pain indicates a problem that should be reported. Preparation is particularly important considering that many surgical procedures are done in day surgery. The person who has experienced acute pain as a result of injury, illness, procedure, or surgery will probably receive one or more prescriptions for analgesic medication. Analgesic prescriptions should be given before the date of day surgery as patients and their families may not be able to stop to fill the prescription on the way home after surgery.

Teaching Patients Self-Care

The patient and family need to understand the purpose of each medication, the appropriate time to use it, the associated side effects, and the strategies that can be used to prevent these problems. The patient and family often need reassurance that pain can be successfully managed at home.

Inadequate control of pain at home is a common reason people seek health care or are readmitted to the hospital. When chronic pain exists, anxiety and fear are often intensified at the time the patient is about to return home. The patient and family are instructed about the techniques for assessing pain, using pain assessment tools, and administering pain medications. These instructions are given verbally and in writing (Chart 13-6).

Opportunities are provided for the patient and family members to practice administering the medication until they are comfortable and confident with the procedure. They are instructed about the risks of respiratory and central nervous system depression associated with opioids and ways to assess for these complications. If the medications cause other predictable effects, such as constipation, the instructions include measures for preventing and treating the problem, as described earlier. Steps are taken to ensure that the needed medications are available from the local pharmacy so that the patient receives the medication when required.

Education for patients and families must stress the need for keeping analgesic agents away from children, who might mistake them for candy. Elderly patients may become lax about this because no children live in the home, but visiting children can be

Chart 13-6 • PATIENT EDUCATION
At-Home Pain Management Plan

Pain control plan for
_____

At home, I will take the following medicines for pain control:

Medicine	How to take	How many	How often	Comments
_____	_____	_____	_____	_____
_____	_____	_____	_____	_____
_____	_____	_____	_____	_____

Medicines that you may take to help treat side effects:

Side effect	Medicine	How to take	How many	How often	Comments
_____	_____	_____	_____	_____	_____
_____	_____	_____	_____	_____	_____

Constipation is a very common problem when taking opioid medications. To prevent this from occurring, do the following:
- Increase fluid intake (8 to 10 glasses of fluid).
- Exercise regularly.
- Increase fibre in the diet (bran, fresh fruits, vegetables).

When this occurs, do the following:
- Use a mild laxative, such as milk of magnesia, if no bowel movement in 3 days.
- Take _____ every day at _____ (time) with a full glass of water.
- Use a glycerin suppository every morning (this may help make a bowel movement less painful).

Nondrug pain control methods:
_____
_____

Additional instructions:
_____
_____
_____

Important phone numbers:
Your doctor _____   Your nurse _____
Your pharmacy _____   Emergencies _____
Call your doctor or nurse immediately if your pain increases or if you have a new pain. Also call your doctor early for refill of pain medicines. Do not let your medicines get below 3 or 4 days' supply.

_____

Agency for Health Care Policy and Research. (1994). *Management of cancer pain.* Clinical Practice Guidelines. Rockville, MD: Agency for Health Care Policy and Research, Public Health Service, U.S. Department of Health and Human Services.

placed at risk. Additionally, analgesic agents must be kept away from other family members who may take them inadvertently.

Ongoing Care

If the patient is to receive analgesics by parenteral or intraspinal routes at home, a referral to a home care nurse is indicated. The home care nurse makes a home visit to assess the patient and to determine if the pain management program is being implemented and if the technique for injecting or infusing the analgesic agent is being carried out safely and effectively. If the patient has an implanted infusion pump in place, the nurse examines the condition of the pump or injection site and may refill the reservoir with medication as prescribed or may supervise family members in the procedure. Any change in the patient's need for analgesic medications is assessed. In collaboration with the physician, the nurse then assists the patient and family in modifying the medication dose. These efforts enable the patient to obtain adequate pain relief while remaining at home and with family.

As tolerance develops, ever-increasing amounts of opioids are needed. It is important to assure the patient and family that slowly increasing doses will not cause an increased risk of respiratory depression and central nervous system depression, because the patient will become tolerant to these effects also. However, the patient will not become tolerant to the constipating effects of opioids and will require increased efforts to prevent constipation.

EVALUATING PAIN MANAGEMENT STRATEGIES

An important aspect of caring for the patient in pain is reassessing the pain after the intervention has been implemented. The measure's effectiveness is based on the patient's assessment of pain, as reflected in pain assessment tools. If the intervention was ineffective, the nurse needs to consider other measures. If these are ineffective, the pain relief goals need to be reassessed in collaboration with the physician. The nurse serves as a patient advocate in obtaining additional pain relief.

Plan of Nursing Care
Care of the Patient With Pain

Nursing Interventions	Rationale	Expected Outcomes
Nursing Diagnosis: Pain **Goal:** Relief of pain or decrease in intensity of pain		
1. Reassure patient that you know pain is real and will assist him or her in dealing with it.	1. Fear that pain will not be accepted as real increases tension and anxiety and decreases pain tolerance.	• Reports relief that pain is accepted as real and that he or she will receive assistance in pain relief
2. Use pain assessment scale to identify intensity of pain.	2. Provides baseline for assessing changes in pain level and evaluating interventions	• Reports lower intensity of pain and discomfort after interventions implemented
3. Assess and record pain and its characteristics: location, quality, frequency, and duration.	3. Data assist in evaluating pain and pain relief and identifying multiple sources and types of pain.	• Reports less disruption from pain and discomfort after use of intervention
4. Administer multimodal analgesics as prescribed to promote optimal pain relief.	4. Analgesics are more effective if administered early in pain cycle. Simultaneous use of analgesics that work on different portions of the nociceptive system will provide greater pain relief with fewer side effects.	• Uses pain medication as prescribed • Identifies effective pain relief strategies • Demonstrates use of new strategies to relieve pain and reports their effectiveness
5. Readminister pain assessment scale.	5. Permits assessment of effectiveness of analgesics and identifies need for further action if ineffective	• Experiences minimal side effects of analgesics without interruption to treat side effects
6. Document severity of patient's pain on chart.	6. Assists in demonstrating need for additional analgesic or alternative approach to pain management	• Increases interactions with family and friends
7. Obtain additional prescriptions as needed.	7. Inadequate pain relief results in an increased stress response, suffering, and prolonged hospitalizations.	
8. Identify and encourage patient to use strategies that have been successful with previous pain.	8. Encourages use of pain relief strategies familiar to and accepted by patient	
9. Teach patient additional strategies to relieve pain and discomfort: distraction, relaxation, cutaneous stimulation, etc.	9. Use of these strategies along with analgesia may produce more effective pain relief.	
10. Instruct patient and family about potential side effects of analgesics and their prevention and management.	10. Anticipating and preventing side effects enable the patient to continue analgesics without interruption because of side effects.	

Reassessments

After interventions have had a chance to work, the patient is asked to rate the intensity of pain. This assessment is repeated at appropriate intervals after the intervention and compared with the previous rating. These assessments indicate the effectiveness of the pain relief measures and provide a basis for continuing or modifying the plan of care. See the accompanying Plan of Nursing Care for more information.

Evaluation

EXPECTED PATIENT OUTCOMES
Expected patient outcomes may include:

1. Achieves pain relief
   a. Rates pain at a lower intensity (on a scale of 0 to 10) after intervention
   b. Rates pain at a lower intensity for longer periods
2. Patient or family administers prescribed analgesic medications correctly
   a. States correct dose of medication
   b. Administers correct dose using correct procedure
   c. Identifies side effects of medication
   d. Describes actions taken to prevent or correct side effects
3. Uses nonpharmacologic pain strategies as recommended
   a. Reports practice of nonpharmacologic strategies
   b. Describes expected outcomes of nonpharmacologic strategies
4. Reports minimal effects of pain and minimal side effects of interventions
   a. Participates in activities important to recovery (eg, drinking fluids, coughing, ambulating)
   b. Participates in activities important to self and to family (eg, family activities, interpersonal relationships, parenting, social interaction, recreation, work)
   c. Reports adequate sleep and absence of fatigue and constipation

Critical Thinking Exercises

1. An 82-year-old woman with cancer has been admitted to a skilled care facility from her home. Her son reports that his mother has become increasingly forgetful and is now unable to manage her medication regimen. He says that she would forget when she took her antidepressant pills and Oxy-Contin. She was so "doped up" that he couldn't bear to see her that way. She is being treated for cancer pain. Two weeks after admission, a pain assessment reveals a pain intensity of 8 on a 0 to 10 scale; she is refusing to get out of bed. Her son is with her and does not want the nurse to give the breakthrough medication or call the physician to titrate the OxyContin for maximal pain relief. Describe the strategies you would use to provide adequate pain management for this patient and the physiologic factors that need to be considered. Identify strategies that you would use to educate her son about her need for pain management. Identify the ethical issues involved in this situation.

2. A 45-year-old patient has just returned from the postanesthesia care unit (PACU) after a laparoscopic chole-cystectomy. She has a history of rheumatoid arthritis for which she takes celecoxib (Celebrex) 200 mg bid. She rates her pain intensity from the recent surgery as a 6 (on a 0 to 10 scale) and is complaining of severe pain in multiple joints. Discuss the factors contributing to the pain that this patient is experiencing. What would be the best approach to manage her pain? Analyze the effect of her rheumatoid arthritis and joint pain on her postoperative pain and its management.

3. A 62-year-old man is receiving epidural infusions of an opioid for intractable pain. He will be discharged home, where his daughter will assist in his pain management. Describe the teaching required for the man and his daughter. What side effects should they observe for, and what actions should they take if they occur? How would you modify your discharge teaching plan if the patient lived alone?

4. A 35-year-old patient with a history of heroin use is admitted to the hospital with multiple stab wounds following an altercation. Two days after extensive surgery to repair his wounds, he reports severe, unrelenting pain and reports that the medication he is receiving (ie, an opioid) is ineffective in diminishing his pain. Several staff members believe that he does not have severe pain and only wants more medication because of his history of drug abuse. Describe how you would address pain relief in this patient, and provide rationale for your actions. How would you address the views of the staff members who believe that the patient should not receive additional medication?

REFERENCES AND SELECTED READINGS

Books

Agency for Health Care Policy and Research, Public Health Service, Department of Health and Human Services. (1992). *Acute pain management: Operative or medical procedures and trauma*. Clinical Practice Guidelines. (AHCPR 92-0032). Washington, DC: U.S. Government Printing Office.

Agency for Health Care Policy and Research, Public Health Service, Department of Health and Human Services. (1994). *Management of cancer pain: Adults*. Clinical Practice Guidelines (AHCPR 94-0592). Washington, DC: U.S. Government Printing Office.

American Cancer Society (2001). *American Cancer Society's guide to pain control: Powerful methods to overcome cancer pain*. Atlanta: American Cancer Society.

American Pain Society. (1999). *Principles of analgesic use in the treatment of acute pain and chronic cancer pain* (4th ed.). Skokie, IL: Author.

Benjamin, L. J., Dampier, C. D., Jacox, A., et al. (1999). *Clinical practice guideline for the management of acute and chronic pain in sickle cell disease*. American Pain Society Clinical Practice Guidelines series, No 1. Glenview, IL: American Pain Society.

Bonica, J. J. (2000). *The management of pain* (3d ed.). Philadelphia: Lea & Febiger.

Fillingim, R. B. (2000). *Sex, gender, and pain. Progress in pain research and management*, Vol. 17. Seattle: IASP Press.

Freeman, L. W., & Lawlis, G. F. (2001). *Mosby's complementary and alternative medicine: A research-based approach*. St. Louis: Mosby.

Gatchel, R. J., & Turk, D. C. (Eds.). (1999). *Psychosocial factors in pain*. New York: Guiliford.

Harden, R. N., Baron, R., & Janig, W. (2001). *Complex regional pain syndrome. Progress in pain research and management*, Vol. 22. Seattle: IASP Press.

Hodge, C. J., & Christensen, M. (2002). Anterolateral cordotomy. In K. J. Burchiel (Ed.). *Surgical management of pain*. New York: Thieme.

Janig, W. (2001). CRPS-I and CRPS-II: A strategic view. In R. N. Harden, R. Baron, & W. Janig (Eds.). *Complex regional pain syndrome. Progress in pain research and management*, 22. Seattle: IASP Press.

Joint Commission on Accreditation of Healthcare Organizations. (2003). *Hospital accreditation standards*. Oakbrook Terrace, IL: JCAHO.

Kuhn, M. A. (1999). *Complementary therapies for health care providers*. Philadelphia: Lippincott Williams & Wilkins.

Linderoth, B. & Meyerson, B. A. (2002). Spinal cord stimulation: Mechanisms of action. In K. Burchiel (Ed.). *Surgical management of pain*. New York: Thieme.

McCaffery, M., & Pasaro, C. (1999). *Pain: Clinical manual for nursing practice* (2d ed.). St. Louis: Mosby.

Merskey, H., & Bogduk, N. (Eds.). (1994). *Classification of chronic pain* (2nd ed). International Association for the Study of Pain Taskforce on Taxonomy. Seattle: IASP Press, pp. 209–214.

National Institutes of Health. *Integration of behavioral and relaxation approaches into the treatment of chronic pain and insomnia*. NIH Technology Assessment Statement, Oct. 16–18, 1995.

Porth, C. M. (2002). *Pathophysiology: Concepts of altered health states* (6th ed.). Philadelphia: Lippincott Williams & Wilkins.

Rezai, A. R., & Lozano, A. M. (2002). Deep brain stimulation for chronic pain. In K. J. Burchiel (Ed.). *Surgical management of pain*. New York: Thieme.

Salerno, E., & Willens, J. S. (1996). *Pain management handbook: An interdisciplinary approach*. St. Louis: C. V. Mosby.

Wall, P. D., & Melzack, R. (Eds). (1999). *Textbook of pain* (4th ed.). New York: Churchill Livingstone.

Wall, P. D. (1999). Introduction. In P. D. Wall & R. Melzack (Eds.). *Textbook of pain*. New York: Churchill-Livingstone, pp. 1–8.

Journals

Asterisks indicate nursing research articles.

Altmaier, E. M., Lehmann, T. R., Russell, D. W., et al. (1992). The effectiveness of psychological interventions for the rehabilitation of low back pain: A randomized controlled trial evaluation. *Pain, 49*(3), 329–335.

American Geriatrics Society Panel on Persistent Pain in Older Persons. (2002). The management of persistent pain in older persons. *Journal of the American Geriatrics Society*. 50, 1–20.

American Medical Association. (2005). *Medical policy: Electrical nerve stimulation, transcutaneous, percutaneous*. Available at: https://provider.bcbsga.com/provider/medpolicy/policies/anesthesia_pain_manag/elec_nerve_stim_TENS_PENS.html. Retrieved June 6, 2005.

American Society of Pain Management Nurses. (1996). ASPMN position statement: Use of placebos for pain management. Available at: http://www.aspmn.org/html/Psplacebo.htm. Retrieved January 8, 2002.

Anderson, R., Saiers, J. H., Abram, S., & Schlicht, C. (2001). Accuracy in equianalgesic dosing: Conversion dilemmas. *Journal of Pain and Symptom Management, 21*(5), 397–406.

Brookoff, D. (2000). Chronic pain: 1. A new disease? *Hospital Practice, 35*(7), 42–59.

Buffum, M., & Buffum, J. C. (2000). Nonsteroidal anti-inflammatory drugs in the elderly. *Pain Management Nursing, 1*(2), 40–50.

Campbell, J. (1995). Pain: The fifth vital sign. Presidential Address. American Pain Society, Nov. 11, 1995, Los Angeles.

Canadian Nurses Association. (2002). *Code of ethics for registered nurses.* Available at: http://www.nurses.info/law_for_nurses_ethics.htm. Retrieved June 17, 2005.

Canadian Pain Society. (2001). *Patient pain manifesto.* Available at: http://www.canadianpainsociety.ca/cont-ang/4nouvelles-manifeste.htm. Retrieved June 17, 2005.

Canadian Pain Society. (2005). *W5 story on opioid addiction one-sided.* Available at: http://www.canadianpainsociety.ca/formulaires/PressReleaseCPSJan142005.pdf. Retrieved June 17, 2005.

Carroll, D., Tramer, M., McQuay, H., et al. (1996). Randomization is important in studies with pain outcomes: Systematic review of transcutaneous electrical nerve stimulation in acute postoperative pain. *British Journal of Anaesthesia, 77*(6), 798–803.

Cleeland, C. S., Gonin, R., Baez, L., et al. (1997). Pain and treatment of pain in minority patients with cancer. *Annals of Internal Medicine, 127*(9), 813–816.

*Conner, M., & Deane, D. (1995). Patterns of patient-controlled analgesia and intramuscular analgesia. *Applied Nursing Research, 8*(2), 67–92.

Correll, D. J., Viscusi, E. R., Grunwald, Z., & Moore, J. H. (2001). Epidural analgesia compared with intravenous morphine patient-controlled analgesia: Postoperative outcome measures after mastectomy with immediate TRAM flap breast reconstruction. *Regional Anesthesia Pain Medicine, 26*(5), 444–449.

Donner, B., Zenz, M., Tryba, M., & Strumpf, M. (1996). Direct conversion from oral morphine to transdermal fentanyl: A multicenter study in patients with cancer pain. *Pain, 64*(3), 527–534.

Douglas, D. B. (1999). Hypnosis: Useful, neglected, available. *American Journal of Hospice and Palliative Care, 16*(5), 665–670.

DuPen, A. R., DuPen, S., Hansberry, J., et al. (2000). An educational implementation of a cancer pain algorithm for ambulatory care. *Pain Management Nursing, 1*(4), 116–128.

Edwards, R., Augustson, E. M., & Fillingim, R. (2000). Sex-specific effects of pain related anxiety on adjustment to chronic pain. *Clinical Journal of Pain, 16*(1), 46–53.

Edwards, R. R., & Fillingim, R. B. (2000). Age-associated differences in responses to noxious stimuli. *Journal of Gerontology Series A: Biological Science & Medical Science, 56*(3), M180–185.

eMedicine.com. (2005). Transcutaneous electrical nerve stimulation. Available at: http://www.emedicine.com/pmr/topic206.htm. Retrieved June 6, 2005.

Farthing, G. W., Venturino, M., Brown, S. W., & Lazar, J. D. (1997). Internal and external distraction in the control of cold-pressor pain as a function of hypnotizability. *International Journal of Clinical & Experimental Hypnosis, 45*(4), 433–446.

Fenstermaker, R. A. (1999). Neurosurgical invasive techniques for cancer pain: A pain specialist's view. *Current Review of Pain, 3*(3), 190–197.

Ferrell, B. A. (1995). Pain evaluation and management in the nursing home. *Annals of Internal Medicine, 123*(9), 681–687.

*Ferrell, B., Virani, R., Grant, M., & McCaffery, M. (2000). Analysis of pain content in nursing textbooks. *Journal of Pain and Symptom Management, 19*(3), 216–228.

Foley, K. M. (1999). Advances in cancer pain. *Archives of Neurology, 56*(4), 413–417.

Foster, N. E., Baxter, F., Walsh, D. M., et al. (1996). Manipulation of transcutaneous electrical nerve stimulation variables has no effect on two models of experimental pain in humans. *Clinical Journal of Pain, 12*(4), 301–310.

Fries, B. E., Simon, S. E., Morris, J. N., et al. (2001). Pain in U.S. nursing homes: validating a pain scale for the minimum data set. *Gerontologist, 41*(2), 173–179.

Gatchel, R. D., Polatin, P. B., Mayer, T. G., & Carcy, P. D. (1994). Psychopathology and the rehabilitation of patients with chronic low back pain disability. *Archives of Physical Medicine and Rehabilitation, 75*(6), 666–670.

Global RPh.com. (n.d). *Narcotic analgesic dosage conversion chart.* Available at: http://www.globalrph.com/narcotic.htm. Retrieved June 8, 2005.

Gordon, D. B., Pellino, T. A., Enloe, M. G., & Foley, D. K. (2000). A nurse-run inpatient pain consultation service. *Pain Management Nursing, 1*(2), 29–33.

Gordon, D. B., & Ward, S. E. (1995). Correcting patient misconceptions about pain. *American Journal of Nursing, 95*(7), 43–45.

Groves K. (2003). An introduction to the Micrel Micropump MP Daily portable syringe driver. *International Journal of Palliative Nursing, Nov 9*(11), 468–473.

Hodkinson, J. (2005). Implantable technology for pain management. *Anaesthesia and Intensive Care Medicine, 6*(2), 61–65. Available at: http://www.extenza-eps.com/extenza/contentviewing/viewJournal.do?journalId=265.

Holleran, R. S. (2002). The problem of pain in emergency care. *Nursing Clinics of North America, 37*(1), 67–78.

Hicks, C. L., von Baeyer, C. L., Spafford, P. A., et al. (2001). The Faces Pain Scale-Revised: Toward a common metric in pediatric pain measurement. *Pain, 93*(2), 173–183.

Hrobjartsson, A., & Gotzsche, P. C. (2001). Is placebo powerless? An analysis of clinical trials comparing placebo with no treatment. *New England Journal of Medicine, 344*(21), 1594–1602.

Hunter, M., McDowell, L., Hennessy, R., & Cassey, J. (2000). An evaluation of the Faces Pain Scale with young children. *Journal of Pain and Symptom Management, 20*(2), 122–129.

Janig, W. (2001). CRPS-I and CRPS-II: A strategic view. In Harden, R. N., Baron, R., & Janig, W. (Eds.). *Complex regional pain syndrome. Progress in pain research and management,* Vol. 22. Seattle: IASP Press.

Johnson, M. H., & Petrie, S. M. (1997). The effects of distraction on exercise and cold presser tolerance for chronic low back pain sufferers. *Pain, 69*(1–2), 43–48.

Jovey, R., Ennis, J., Gardner-Nix J., et al. (2003). Use of opioid analgesics for the treatment of chronic noncancer pain—a consensus statement and guidelines from the Canadian Pain Society, 2002. *Pain Research & Management, 8*(Suppl A), 3A–28A.

Keefe, F. J., Lefebvre, J. C., & Starr, K. R. (1996). From the gate control theory to the neuromatrix: Revolution or evolution? *Pain Forum, 5*(2), 143–146.

Keefe, F. J., & Williams, D. A. (1990). A comparison of coping strategies in chronic pain in patients in different age groups. *Journal of Gerontology, 45*(4), 161–165.

Kelly, A. M. (1998). Does the clinically significant difference in visual analog scale pain scores vary with gender, age, or cause of pain? *Academy of Emergency Medicine, 5*(11), 1086–1090.

Keogh, E., Ellery, D., Hunt, C., & Hannent, I. (2001). Selective attentional bias for pain-related stimuli amongst fearful individuals. *Pain, 91*(1–2), 91–100.

*Knapp-Spooner, C., Karlik, B. A., Pontieri-Lewis, V., & Yarcheski, A. (1995). Efficacy of patient-controlled analgesia in women cholecystectomy patients. *International Journal of Nursing Studies, 32*(5), 434–442.

Kosier, M., & Minkler, P. (1999). Nursing management of patients with an implanted Ommaya reservoir. *Clinical Journal of Oncology Nursing, Apr 3*(2), 63–67.

Krames, E. (2002). Implantable devices for pain control: Spinal cord stimulation and intrathecal therapies. Best practice & research. *Clinical Anaesthesiology, 16*(4), 619–649.

Kukushkin, M. L., Meizerov, E. E., Grafova, V. N., et al. (2003). Peculiarities of the development of analgesic effect during transcutaneous dynamic stimulation. *Bulletin of Experimental Biology & Medicine. 135*(3), 228–230.

Lamberg, L. (1999). Patients in pain need round-the-clock care. *Journal of the American Medical Association, 281*(8), 689–692.

Lasch, K. E. (2000). Culture, pain and culturally sensitive pain care. *Pain Management Nursing, 1*(3), S1, 16–22.

Lasch, K. E., Wilkes, G., Montuori, L. M., et al. (2000). Using focus group methods to develop multicultural cancer patient education materials. *Pain Management Nursing, 1*(4), 129–138.

Li, S. F., Greenwald, P. W., Gennis, P., et al. (2001). Effect of age on acute pain perception of a standardized stimulus in the emergency department. *Annals of Emergency Medicine, 38*(6), 644–647.

Loeb, J. L. (1999). Pain management in long-term care. *American Journal of Nursing, 99*(2), 48–52.

Lynn, J., Teno, J. M., Phillips, R. S., et al. (1997). Perceptions by family members of the dying experience of older and seriously ill patients. *Annals of Internal Medicine, 126*(2), 97–106.

*Malek, C. J. (1996). Pain management: Documenting the decision-making process. *Nursing Case Management, 1*(2), 64–74.

Mayer, D. M., Torma, L., Byock, I., & Norris, K. (2001). Speaking the language of pain. *American Journal of Nursing, 101*(2), 44–49.

McCaffery, M., & Ferrell, B. R. (1997). Nurses' knowledge of pain assessment and management: How much progress have we made? *Journal of Pain Symptom Management, 14*(3), 175–188.

*McCaffery, M., Ferrell, B. R., & Pasaro, C. (2000). Nurses' personal opinions about patients' pain and their effect on recorded assessments and titration of opioid doses. *Pain Management Nursing, 1*(3), 79–87.

McCaffery, M., & Pasero, C. (2001). Stigmatizing patients as addicts. *American Journal of Nursing, 101*(5), 77–79.

McCracken, L. M., & Iverson, G. L. (2001). Predicting complaints of impaired cognitive functioning in patients with chronic pain. *Journal of Pain and Symptom Management, 21*(5), 392–396.

*McNeill, J. A., Sherwood, G. D., Starck, P. L., & Nieto, B. (2001). Pain management outcomes for hospitalized Hispanic patients. *Pain Management Nursing, 2*(4), 25–36.

Medical Advanced Pain Specialists (MAPS). (1998). Implantable therapies for intractable pain: Implantable devices and back pain. Available at: http://www.painphysicians.com/nl_summer98a.html. Retrieved June 6, 2005.

Melzack, R. (1996). Gate control theory: On the evolution of pain concepts. *Pain Forum, 5*(1), 128–138.

Meuser, T., Pietruck, C., Radruch, L., Stute, P., Lehmann, K. A., & Grond, S. (2001). Symptoms during cancer pain treatment following WHO guidelines: A longitudinal follow-up study of symptom prevalence, severity and etiology. *Pain, 93*(3), 247–257.

Miaskowski, C. (2000). The impact of age on a patient's perception of pain and ways it can be managed. *Pain Management Nursing, 1*(3), S1, 2–7.

*Miaskowski, C., & Dibble, S. L. (1995). The problem of pain in outpatients with breast cancer. *Oncology Nursing Forum, 22*(5), 791–797.

Morin, C., Lund, J. P., Villarroel, T., et al. (2000). Differences between the sexes in post-surgical pain. *Pain, 85*(1–2), 79–85.

National Institutes of Health. (1997). Acupuncture. *NIH Consensus Statement, 15*(5), 1–34.

NIH Technology Assessment Panel on Integration of Behavioral and Relaxation Approaches into the Treatment of Chronic Pain and Insomnia. (1995). Integration of behavioral and relaxation approaches into the treatment of chronic pain and insomnia. *Journal of the American Medical Association, 276*(4), 313–318.

North, R., & Levy R. (1994). Consensus conference on the neurosurgical management of pain. *Neurosurgery, 34*(4), 756–760.

Oosterveld, F. G. & Rasker, J. J. (1994a). Effects of local heat and cold treatment on surface and articular temperature of arthritic knees. *Arthritis & Rheumatism, 37*(11), 1578–582.

Oosterveld, F. G. & Rasker, J. J. (1994b). Treating arthritis with locally applied heat or cold. *Seminars in Arthritis & Rheumatism, 24*(2), 82–90.

Osiri, M., Brosseau, L., McGowan, J, et al. (2005). Transcutaneous electrical nerve stimulation for knee osteoarthritis. *Cochrane Database of Systematic Reviews, April*(2). Available from: http://www.cochrane.org/cochrane/revabstr/AB002823.htm.

Oxman, M., Levin, M., Johnson, G., et al. (2005). A vaccine to prevent herpes zoster and postherpetic neuralgia in older adults. *New England Journal of Medicine, 352*(22), 2271–2284.

Pain Control Network PSC. (2001). Drug infusion pumps. Available at: http://yp.bellsouth.com/sites/paincontrolnetwork/page6.html. Retrieved June 6, 2005.

Panke, J. T. (2002). Difficulties in managing pain at the end of life. *American Journal of Nursing, 102*(7), 26–33.

Pasaro, C. L. (1997). Using the Faces scale to assess pain. *American Journal of Nursing, 97*(7), 19–20.

Pasaro, C., & McCaffery, M. (2001). The lidocaine patch. *American Journal of Nursing, 101*(3), 22–23.

Pasaro, C., & McCaffery, M. (2001). Selective COX-2 inhibitors. *American Journal of Nursing, 101*(4), 55–56.

Pasaro, C., & McCaffery, M. (2002). Monitoring sedation *American Journal of Nursing, 102*(2), 67–69.

Pasaro, C. (2002). Subcutaneous opioid infusion. *American Journal of Nursing, 102*(7), 61–62.

Pasaro, C., & Montgomery, R. (2002). Intravenous fentanyl. *American Journal of Nursing, 102*(4), 73–76.

Peloso, P. M. (2000). NSAIDs: A Faustian bargain. *American Journal of Nursing, 100*(6), 34–39.

Perez, R. S. G. M., Kwakkel, G., Zuurmond, W. W. A., & de Lange, J. J. (2001). Treatment of reflex sympathetic dystrophy (CRPS type I): A research synthesis of 21 randomized clinical trials. *Journal of Pain and Symptom Management, 21*(6), 511–526.

Perin, M. L. (2000). Corticosteroids for cancer pain. *American Journal of Nursing, 100*(4), 15–16.

Plaisance, L., & Ellis, J. A. (2002). Opioid-induced constipation. *American Journal of Nursing, 102*(3), 72–73.

Pollo, A., Amanzio, M., Arslanina, A., et al. (2001). Response expectancies in placebo analgesia and their clinical relevance. *Pain, 93*(1), 77–84.

Porter, J., & Jick, H. (1980). Addiction rare in patients treated with narcotics. *New England Journal of Medicine, 302*(2), 123.

Puig, M. M., & Montes, A. (1998). Opioids: From receptors to clinical application. *Current Review of Pain, 2*(4), 243–241.

*Puntillo, K., Casella, W., & Reid, M. (1997). Opioid and benzodiazepine tolerance and dependence: Application of theory to critical care practice. *Heart & Lung, 26*(4), 317–324.

*Puntillo, K. A., Miaskowski, C., Kehrle, K., et al. (1997). Relationship between behavioral and physiological indicators of pain, critical care patients' self-reports of pain, and opioid administration. *Critical Care Medicine, 25*(7), 1159–1166.

Raymond, I., Nielsen, T. A., Lauigne, G., et al. (2001). Quality of sleep and its daily relationship to pain intensity in hospitalized adult burn patients. *Pain, 92*(3), 381–388.

The Richeimer Pain Institute. (2000). Spinal pumps and stimulants for chronic pain. Available at: http://www.helpforpain.com/arch2000sep.htm. Retrieved June 6, 2005.

Rhiner, M., & Kedziera, P. (1999). Managing breakthrough pain. A new approach. *American Journal of Nursing, 99*(3), Supplement, 1–12.

Rhudy, J. L., & Meagher, M. W. (2000). Fear and anxiety: Divergent effects on human pain thresholds. *Pain, 84*(1), 65–75.

Riley, J. L., Robinson, M. E., Wade, J. B., et al. (2001). Sex differences in negative emotional response to chronic pain. *Journal of Pain, 2*(6), 354–359.

Robinson, M. E., Riley, J. L., Meyers, C. D., et al. (2001). Gender role expectations of pain. Relationship to sex differences in pain. *Journal of Pain, 2*(5), 251–257.

Siegal, T., Pfeffer, M., & Steiner I. (1988.) Antibiotic therapy for infected Ommaya reservoir systems. *Neurosurgery, Jan 22*(1 Pt 1), 97–100.

*Simpson, T., Lee, E. R., & Cameron, C. (1996). Relationships among sleep dimensions and factors that impair sleep after cardiac surgery. *Research in Nursing & Health, 19*(3), 213–223.

Slaughter, A., Pasaro, C., & Manworren, R. (2002). Unacceptable pain levels. *American Journal of Nursing, 102*(5), 75–77.

Spine-health.com. (2004). Transcutaneous electrical nerve stimulators (TENS). Available at: http://www.spine-health.com/topics/conserv/electro/el02.html. Retrieved June 6, 2005.

SUPPORT Principal Investigators. (1995). A controlled trial to improve care for seriously ill hospitalized patients: The study to understand prognoses and preferences for outcomes and risks of treatments (SUPPORT). *Journal of the American Medical Association, 274*(20), 1591–1598.

Taddio, A., Goldbach, M., Ipp, M., et al. (1995). Effect of neonatal circumcision on pain responses during vaccination in boys. *Lancet, 345,* 291–292.

Texas Children's Cancer Center. (n.d.). *Equianalgesic conversion guide.* Available at: http://www.childcancerpain.org/content.cfm?content=pharm19. Retrieved June 8, 2005.

Thomas, T., Robinson, C., Champion, D., et al. (1998). Prediction and assessment of the severity of post-operative pain and of satisfaction with management. *Pain, 75*(2–3), 177–185.

Tucker, K. L. (2001). Deceptive placebo administration. *American Journal of Nursing, 101*(8), 55–56.

Unruh, A. (1996). Gender variations in clinical pain experience. *Pain, 65*(2, 3), 123–167.

Unruh, A. M., Ritchie, J., & Merskey, H. (1999). Does gender affect appraisal of pain and pain coping strategies? *Clinical Journal of Pain, 15*(1), 31–40.

Uomoto, J. M., & Esselman, P. C. (1993). Traumatic brain injury and chronic pain: Differential types and rates by head injury severity. *Archives of Physical Medicine and Rehabilitation, 74*(1), 61–64.

Vallerand, A. H., & Polomano, R. C. (2000). The relationship of gender to pain. *Pain Management Nursing, 1*(3, suppl), 8–15.

Walker, B., Shafer, M., Henzi, I. & Tramer, M. R. (2002). Efficacy and safety of patient-controlled opioid analgesia for postoperative pain. A quantitative systematic review. *Acta Anaesthesiology Scandinavia, 45*(7), 795–804.

*Ward, S. E., Berry, P. E., & Misiewicz, H. (1996). Concerns about analgesia among patients and family caregivers in a hospice setting. *Research in Nursing & Health, 19*(3), 205–211.

Washington, L. L., Gibson, S. J., & Helme, R. D. (2000). Age-related differences in endogenous analgesic response to repeated cold water immersion in human volunteers. *Pain, 89*(1), 89–96.

Watt-Watson, J., Stevens, B., Katz J, et al. (2004). Impact of preoperative education on pain outcomes after coronary artery bypass graft surgery. *Pain, 109*(1-2), 73–85.

*Watt-Watson, J., Garfinkel, P., Gallop, R., et al. (2000). The impact of nurses' empathetic responses on patients' pain management in acute care. *Nursing Research, 49*(4), 191–200.

Weiner, D., Peterson, B., Ladd, K., McConnell, E., & Keefe, F. (1999). Pain in nursing home residents: An exploration of prevalence, staff

perspectives, and practical aspects of measurement. *Clinical Journal of Pain, 15*(2), 92–101.

*Zalon, M. L. (1997). Pain in frail, elderly women after surgery. *Image: Journal of Nursing Scholarship, 29*(1), 21–26.

RESOURCES AND WEBSITES

American Academy of Pain Management, 13947 Mono Way #A, Sonora, CA 95370; (209) 533-9744; http://www.aapainmanage.org.

American Chronic Pain Association, P.O. Box 850, Rocklin, CA 95677; (800) 533-3231; http://www.theacpa.org.

American Pain Foundation, 201 N. Charles Street, Suite 710, Baltimore, MD 21201; (888) 615-7246; http://www.painfoundation.org.

American Pain Society, 4700 W. Lake Street, Glenview, IL 60025; (847) 375-4715; http://www.ampainsoc.org.

American Society of Pain Management Nurses, 7794 Grow Drive, Pensacola, FL 32514; (222) 34ASPMN; fax (850) 484-8762; http://www.aspmn.org.

The Canadian Council on Health Services Accreditation (CCHSA); www.cchsa.ca.

Canadian Institutes of Health Research; www.cihr-irsc.gc.ca.

Canadian Neuropathy Association; www.canadianneuropathyassociation.org.

Canadian Pain Society/Société Canadienne de la Douleur; www.canadianpainsociety.ca.

International Pain Foundation, 909 NE 43rd St., Room 306, Seattle, WA 98105-6020; (206) 547-6409; fax (206) 547-1703; http://dasnetO2.dokkyomed.ac.ip/IASPM/IASP.html; e-mail: IASP@locke.hs.washington.ed.

Last Acts: an initiative for care and caring at the end of life. Includes "Innovations in End-of-Life Care," an international journal and on-line forum: http://www.lastacts.org.

National Hospice Organization, Suite 901, 1901 N. Moore St., Arlington, VA 22209; (703) 243-5900; http://www.nho.org.

North American Chronic Pain Association of Canada; http://www.chronicpaincanada.org.

"Pain Control," a monthly column in American Journal of Nursing.

Tame the Pain: information for chronic pain sufferers; Metronic Inc., USA; http://www.tamethepain.co.uk.

Fluid and Electrolytes: Balance and Distribution

Adapted by Madeleine Buck

LEARNING OBJECTIVES

On completion of this chapter, the learner will be able to:

1. Differentiate between osmosis, diffusion, filtration, and active transport.
2. Describe the role of the kidneys, lungs, and endocrine glands in regulating the body's fluid composition and volume.
3. Identify the effects of aging on fluid and electrolyte regulation.
4. Plan effective care of patients with the following imbalances: fluid volume deficit and fluid volume excess; sodium deficit (hyponatremia) and sodium excess (hypernatremia); potassium deficit (hypokalemia) and potassium excess (hyperkalemia).
5. Describe the etiology, clinical manifestations, management, and nursing interventions for the following imbalances: calcium deficit (hypocalcemia) and calcium excess (hypercalcemia); magnesium deficit (hypomagnesemia) and magnesium excess (hypermagnesemia); phosphorus deficit (hypophosphatemia) and phosphorus excess (hyperphosphatemia); chloride deficit (hypochloremia) and chloride excess (hyperchloremia).
6. Explain the role of the lungs, kidneys, and chemical buffers in maintaining acid–base balance.
7. Compare metabolic acidosis and alkalosis with regard to causes, clinical manifestations, diagnosis, and management.
8. Compare respiratory acidosis and alkalosis with regard to causes, clinical manifestations, diagnosis, and management.
9. Interpret arterial blood gas measurements.
10. Demonstrate a safe and effective procedure of venipuncture.
11. Describe measures used for preventing complications of intravenous therapy.

$\mathcal{F}$luid and electrolyte balance is a dynamic process that is crucial for life. Potential and actual disorders of fluid and electrolyte balance occur in every setting, with every disorder, and with a variety of changes that affect well people (eg, increased fluid and sodium loss with strenuous exercise and high environmental temperature; inadequate intake of fluid and electrolytes) as well as those who are ill.

Fundamental Concepts

The nurse needs to understand the physiology of fluid and electrolyte balance and acid–base balance to anticipate, identify, and respond to possible imbalances in each. The nurse also must use effective teaching and communication skills to help prevent and treat various fluid and electrolyte disturbances.

AMOUNT AND COMPOSITION OF BODY FLUIDS

Approximately 60% of a typical adult's weight consists of fluid (water and electrolytes). Factors that influence the amount of body fluid are age, gender, and body fat. In general, younger people have a higher percentage of body fluid than older people, and men have proportionately more body fluid than women. Obese people have less fluid than thin people because fat cells contain little water.

Body fluid is located in two fluid compartments: the intracellular space (fluid in the cells) and the extracellular space (fluid outside the cells). Approximately two thirds of body fluid is in the intracellular fluid (ICF) compartment and is located primarily in the skeletal muscle mass.

The extracellular fluid (ECF) compartment is further divided into the intravascular, interstitial, and transcellular fluid spaces. The intravascular space (the fluid within the blood vessels) contains plasma. Approximately 3 L of the average 6 L of blood volume is made up of plasma. The remaining 3 L is made up of erythrocytes, leukocytes, and thrombocytes. The interstitial space contains the fluid that surrounds the cell and totals about 11 to 12 L in an adult. Lymph is an example of interstitial fluid. The transcellular space is the smallest division of the ECF compartment and contains approximately 1 L of fluid at any given time. Examples of transcellular fluid are cerebrospinal, pericardial, synovial, intraocular, and pleural fluids; sweat; and digestive secretions.

Body fluid normally shifts between the two major compartments or spaces in an effort to maintain an equilibrium between the spaces. Loss of fluid from the body can disrupt this equilibrium. Sometimes fluid is not lost from the body but is unavailable for use by either the ICF or ECF. Loss of ECF into a space that does not contribute to equilibrium between the ICF and the ECF is referred to as a third-space fluid shift, or "third spacing" for short.

An early clue of a third-space fluid shift is a decrease in urine output despite adequate fluid intake. Urine output decreases because fluid shifts out of the intravascular space; the kidneys then receive less blood and attempt to compensate by decreasing urine output. Other signs and symptoms of third spacing that indicate an intravascular fluid volume deficit include increased heart rate, decreased blood pressure, decreased central venous pressure, edema, increased body weight, and imbalances in fluid intake and output (I&O). Third-space shifts occur in ascites, burns, peritonitis, bowel obstruction, and massive bleeding into a joint or body cavity.

Electrolytes

Electrolytes in body fluids are active chemicals (cations, which carry positive charges, and anions, which carry negative charges). The major cations in body fluid are sodium, potassium, calcium, magnesium, and hydrogen ions. The major anions are chloride, bicarbonate, phosphate, sulfate, and proteinate ions.

These chemicals unite in varying combinations. Therefore, electrolyte concentration in the body is expressed in terms of millimole per litre (mmol/L) a measure of chemical activity, rather than in terms of milligrams (mg), a unit of weight. More specifically, a millimole is defined as 1/1000 of a mole, which is the amount in grams numerically equivalent to the molecular (or atomic) weight of a substance. In a solution, cations and anions are equal in mmol/L.

Electrolyte concentrations in the ICF differ from those in the ECF, as reflected in Table 14-1. Because special techniques are

Glossary

acidosis: an acid–base imbalance characterized by an increase in H$^+$ concentration (decreased blood pH). A low arterial pH due to reduced bicarbonate concentration is called metabolic acidosis; a low arterial pH due to increased PCO$_2$ is respiratory acidosis

active transport: physiologic pump that moves fluid from an area of lower concentration to one of higher concentration; active transport requires adenosine triphosphate (ATP) for energy

alkalosis: an acid–base imbalance characterized by a reduction in H$^+$ concentration (increased blood pH). A high arterial pH with increased bicarbonate concentration is called metabolic alkalosis; a high arterial pH due to reduced PCO$_2$ is respiratory alkalosis

diffusion: the process by which solutes move from an area of higher concentration to one of lower concentration; does not require expenditure of energy

hydrostatic pressure: the pressure created by the weight of fluid against the wall that contains it. In the body, hydrostatic pressure in blood vessels results from the weight of fluid itself and the force resulting from cardiac contraction.

hypertonic solution: a solution with an osmolality higher than that of serum

hypotonic solution: a solution with an osmolality lower than that of serum

isotonic solution: a solution with the same osmolality as serum and other body fluids. Osmolality falls within normal range for serum (280–300 mOsm/kg).

osmolality: the number of osmoles (the standard unit of osmotic pressure) per kilogram of solution. Expressed as mOsm/kg. Used more often in clinical practice than the term *osmolarity* to evaluate serum and urine. In addition to urea and glucose, sodium contributes the largest number of particles to osmolality.

osmolarity: the number of osmoles, the standard unit of osmotic pressure per litre of solution. It is expressed as milliosmoles per litre (mOsm/L); describes the concentration of solutes or dissolved particles.

osmosis: the process by which fluid moves across a semipermeable membrane from an area of low solute concentration to an area of high solute concentration; the process continues until the solute concentrations are equal on both sides of the membrane.

tonicity: the measurement of the osmotic pressure of a solution; another term for osmolality

ELECTROLYTES	mmol/L
Extracellular Fluid (Plasma)	
Cations	
Sodium (Na)	142
Potassium (K)	5
Calcium (Ca++)	5
Magnesium (Mg++)	2
Total cations	154
Anions	
Chloride (Cl⁻)	103
Bicarbonate (HCO₃⁻)	26
Phosphate (HPO₄⁻)	2
Sulfate (SO₄⁻)	1
Organic acids	5
Proteinate	17
Total anions	154
Intracellular Fluid	
Cations	
Potassium (K⁺)	150
Magnesium (Mg++)	40
Sodium (Na⁺)	10
Total cations	200
Anions	
Phosphates and sulfates	150
Bicarbonate (HCO₃⁻)	10
Proteinate	40
Total anions	200

Table 14-1 • **Approximate Major Electrolyte Content in Body Fluid**

REGULATION OF BODY FLUID COMPARTMENTS

Osmosis and Osmolality

When two different solutions are separated by a membrane that is impermeable to the dissolved substances, fluid shifts through the membrane from the region of low solute concentration to the region of high solute concentration until the solutions are of equal concentration; this diffusion of water caused by a fluid concentration gradient is known as **osmosis** (Fig. 14-1A). The magnitude of this force depends on the number of particles dissolved in the solutions, not on their weights. The number of dissolved particles contained in a unit of fluid determines the osmolality of a solution, which influences the movement of fluid between the fluid compartments. **Tonicity** is the ability of all the solutes to cause an osmotic driving force that promotes water movement from one compartment to another (Porth, 2002). The control of tonicity determines the normal state of cellular hydration and cell size. Sodium, mannitol, glucose, and sorbitol are effective osmoles (capable of affecting water movement). Three other terms are associated with osmosis: osmotic pressure, oncotic pressure, and osmotic diuresis.

- Osmotic pressure is the amount of hydrostatic pressure needed to stop the flow of water by osmosis. It is primarily determined by the concentration of solutes.
- Oncotic pressure is the osmotic pressure exerted by proteins (eg, albumin).
- Osmotic diuresis occurs when the urine output increases due to the excretion of substances such as glucose, mannitol, or contrast agents in the urine.

Diffusion

Diffusion is the natural tendency of a substance to move from an area of higher concentration to one of lower concentration (see Fig. 14-1B). It occurs through the random movement of ions and molecules. Examples of diffusion are the exchange of oxygen and carbon dioxide between the pulmonary capillaries and alveoli and the tendency of sodium to move from the ECF compartment, where the sodium concentration is high, to the ICF, where its concentration is low.

Filtration

Hydrostatic pressure in the capillaries tends to filter fluid out of the vascular compartment into the interstitial fluid. Movement of water and solutes occurs from an area of high hydrostatic pressure to an area of low hydrostatic pressure. Filtration allows the kidneys to filter 180 L of plasma per day. Another example of filtration is the passage of water and electrolytes from the arterial capillary bed to the interstitial fluid; in this instance, the hydrostatic pressure is furnished by the pumping action of the heart.

Sodium–Potassium Pump

As stated earlier, the sodium concentration is greater in the ECF than in the ICF, and because of this, sodium tends to enter the cell by diffusion. This tendency is offset by the sodium–potassium pump, which is located in the cell membrane and actively moves sodium from the cell into the ECF. Conversely, the high intracellular potassium concentration is maintained by pumping potassium into the cell. By definition, **active transport** implies that

required to measure electrolyte concentrations in the ICF, it is customary to measure the electrolytes in the most accessible portion of the ECF, namely the plasma.

Sodium ions, which are positively charged, far outnumber the other cations in the ECF. Because sodium concentration affects the overall concentration of the ECF, sodium is important in regulating the volume of body fluid. Retention of sodium is associated with fluid retention, and excessive loss of sodium is usually associated with decreased volume of body fluid.

As shown in Table 14-1, the major electrolytes in the ICF are potassium and phosphate. The ECF has a low concentration of potassium and can tolerate only small changes in potassium concentrations. Therefore, release of large stores of intracellular potassium, typically caused by trauma to the cells and tissues, can be extremely dangerous.

The body expends a great deal of energy maintaining the high extracellular concentration of sodium and the high intracellular concentration of potassium. It does so by means of cell membrane pumps that exchange sodium and potassium ions. Normal movement of fluids through the capillary wall into the tissues depends on **hydrostatic pressure** (the pressure exerted by the fluid on the walls of the blood vessel) at both the arterial and the venous ends of the vessel and the osmotic pressure exerted by the protein of plasma. The direction of fluid movement depends on the differences in these two opposing forces (hydrostatic versus osmotic pressure).

In addition to electrolytes, the ECF transports other substances, such as enzymes and hormones. It also carries blood components, such as red and white blood cells, throughout the body.

FIGURE 14-1 (**A**) Osmosis: movement of fluid to area of high solute concentration and eventual equalization of solute concentration. (**B**) Diffusion: movement of fluid and solutes and equalization of solute concentration.

energy must be expended for the movement to occur against a concentration gradient.

ROUTES OF GAINS AND LOSSES

Water and electrolytes are gained in various ways. A healthy person gains fluids by drinking and eating. In patients with some disorders, fluids may be provided by the parenteral route (intravenously or subcutaneously) or by means of an enteral feeding tube in the stomach or intestine.

 NURSING ALERT When fluid balance is critical, all routes of gain and all routes of loss must be recorded and all volumes compared. Organs of fluid loss include the kidneys, skin, lungs, and gastrointestinal (GI) tract.

Kidneys

The usual daily urine volume in the adult is 1 to 2 L. A general rule is that the output is approximately 1 mL of urine per kilogram of body weight per hour (1 mL/kg/h) in all age groups.

Skin

Sensible perspiration refers to visible water and electrolyte loss through the skin (sweating). The chief solutes in sweat are sodium, chloride, and potassium. Actual sweat losses can vary from 0 to 1,000 mL or more every hour, depending on the environmental

temperature. Continuous water loss by evaporation (approximately 600 mL/day) occurs through the skin as insensible perspiration, a nonvisible form of water loss. Fever greatly increases insensible water loss through the lungs and the skin, as does loss of the natural skin barrier (through major burns, for example).

Lungs

The lungs normally eliminate water vapor (insensible loss) at a rate of approximately 400 mL every day. The loss is much greater with increased respiratory rate or depth, or in a dry climate.

GI Tract

The usual loss through the GI tract is only 100 to 200 mL daily, even though approximately 8 L of fluid circulates through the GI system every 24 hours (called the GI circulation). Because the bulk of fluid is reabsorbed in the small intestine, diarrhea and fistulas cause large losses. In healthy people, the daily average intake and output of water are approximately equal (Table 14-2).

LABORATORY TESTS FOR EVALUATING FLUID STATUS

Osmolality reflects the concentration of fluid that affects the movement of water between fluid compartments by osmosis. Osmolality measures the solute concentration per kilogram in blood and urine. It is also a measure of a solution's ability to create os-

Table 14-2 • Average Daily Intake and Output in an Adult

INTAKE		OUTPUT	
Oral liquids	1,300 mL	Urine	1,500 mL
Water in food	1,000 mL	Stool	200 mL
Water produced by metabolism	300 mL	Insensible	
		Lungs	300 mL
		Skin	600 mL
Total gain*	2,600 mL	Total loss*	2,600 mL

*Approximate volumes

motic pressure and affect the movement of water. Serum osmolality primarily reflects the concentration of sodium. Urine osmolality is determined by urea, creatinine, and uric acid. When measured with serum osmolality, urine osmolality is the most reliable indicator of urine concentration. Osmolality is reported as millimoles per litre of water (mmol/L).

Osmolarity, another term that describes the concentration of solutions, is also measured in millimoles per litre. The term "osmolality," however, is used more often in clinical practice. Normal serum osmolality is 280 to 300 mmol/L, and normal urine osmolality is 250 to 900 mmol/L. Sodium predominates in ECF osmolality and holds water in this compartment.

Factors that increase and decrease serum and urine osmolality are identified in Table 14-3. Serum osmolality may be measured directly through laboratory tests or estimated at the bedside by doubling the serum sodium level or by using the following formula:

$$2(Na^+) + BUN + GLUCOSE = \text{Approximate value of serum osmolality}$$

The calculated value usually is within 10 mmol of the measured osmolality.

Urine specific gravity measures the kidneys' ability to excrete or conserve water. The specific gravity of urine is compared to the weight of distilled water, which has a specific gravity of 1.000. The normal range of specific gravity is 1.010 to 1.025. Urine specific gravity can be measured at the bedside by placing a calibrated hydrometer or urinometer in a cylinder of approximately 20 mL of urine. Specific gravity can also be assessed with a refractometer or dipstick with a reagent for this purpose. Specific gravity varies inversely with urine volume; normally, the larger the volume of urine, the lower the specific gravity. Specific gravity is a less reliable indicator of concentration than urine osmolality; increased glucose or protein in urine can cause a falsely high specific gravity. Factors that increase or decrease urine osmolality are the same for urine specific gravity.

Blood urea nitrogen (BUN) is made up of urea, an end product of metabolism of protein (from both muscle and dietary intake) by the liver. Amino acid breakdown produces large amounts of ammonia molecules, which are absorbed into the bloodstream. Ammonia molecules are converted to urea and excreted in the urine. The normal BUN is 3.5–7 mmol/L. The BUN level varies with urine output. Factors that increase BUN include decreased renal function, GI bleeding, dehydration, increased protein intake, fever, and sepsis. Those that decrease BUN include end-stage liver disease, a low-protein diet, starvation, and any condition that results in expanded fluid volume (eg, pregnancy).

Creatinine is the end product of muscle metabolism. It is a better indicator of renal function than BUN because it does not vary with protein intake and metabolic state. The normal serum creatinine is approximately 60–130 mmol/L; however, its concentration depends on lean body mass and varies from person to person. Serum creatinine levels increase when renal function decreases.

Hematocrit measures the volume percentage of red blood cells (erythrocytes) in whole blood and normally ranges from 0.44 to 0.52 for males and 0.39 to 0.47 for females. Conditions that increase the hematocrit value are dehydration and polycythemia; those that decrease hematocrit are overhydration and anemia.

Urine sodium values change with sodium intake and the status of fluid volume (as sodium intake increases, excretion increases; as the circulating fluid volume decreases, sodium is conserved). Normal urine sodium levels range from 50 to 220 mmol/24 h. A random specimen usually contains more than 40 mmol/L of sodium. Urine sodium levels are used to assess volume status and are useful in the diagnosis of hyponatremia and acute renal failure.

HOMEOSTATIC MECHANISMS

The body is equipped with remarkable homeostatic mechanisms to keep the composition and volume of body fluid within narrow limits of normal. Organs involved in homeostasis include the kidneys, lungs, heart, adrenal glands, parathyroid glands, and pituitary gland.

Kidney Functions

Vital to the regulation of fluid and electrolyte balance, the kidneys normally filter 170 L of plasma every day in the adult, while excreting only 1.5 L of urine. They act both autonomously and in response to blood-borne messengers, such as aldosterone and antidiuretic hormone (ADH). Major functions of the kidneys in maintaining normal fluid balance include the following:

- Regulation of ECF volume and osmolality by selective retention and excretion of body fluids
- Regulation of electrolyte levels in the ECF by selective retention of needed substances and excretion of unneeded substances

Table 14-3 • Comparison of Serum and Urine Osmolality

FLUID	FACTORS INCREASING OSMOLALITY	FACTORS DECREASING OSMOLALITY
Serum (275–300 mmol/L)	Free water loss Diabetes insipidus Sodium overload Hyperglycemia Uremia	SIADH Renal failure Diuretic use Adrenal insufficiency
Urine (250–900 mmol/L)	Fluid volume deficit SIADH HF Acidosis	Fluid volume excess Diabetes insipidus

SIADH, syndrome of inappropriate antidiuretic hormone; HF, heart failure.

- Regulation of pH of the ECF by retention of hydrogen ions
- Excretion of metabolic wastes and toxic substances

Given these functions, it is readily apparent that renal failure will result in multiple fluid and electrolyte problems. Renal function declines with advanced age, as do muscle mass and daily exogenous creatinine production. Thus, high-normal and minimally elevated serum creatinine values may indicate substantially reduced renal function in the elderly.

Heart and Blood Vessel Functions

The pumping action of the heart circulates blood through the kidneys under sufficient pressure to allow for urine formation. Failure of this pumping action interferes with renal perfusion and thus with water and electrolyte regulation.

Lung Functions

The lungs are also vital in maintaining homeostasis. Through exhalation, the lungs remove approximately 300 mL of water daily in the normal adult. Abnormal conditions, such as hyperpnea (abnormally deep respiration) or continuous coughing, increase this loss; mechanical ventilation with excessive moisture decreases it. The lungs also have a major role in maintaining acid–base balance. Changes from normal aging result in decreased respiratory function, causing increased difficulty in pH regulation in older adults with major illness or trauma.

Pituitary Functions

The hypothalamus manufactures ADH, which is stored in the posterior pituitary gland and released as needed. ADH is sometimes called the water-conserving hormone because it causes the body to retain water. Functions of ADH include maintaining the osmotic pressure of the cells by controlling the retention or excretion of water by the kidneys and by regulating blood volume (Fig. 14-2).

Adrenal Functions

Aldosterone, a mineralocorticoid secreted by the zona glomerulosa (outer zone) of the adrenal cortex, has a profound effect on fluid balance. Increased secretion of aldosterone causes sodium retention (and thus water retention) and potassium loss. Conversely, decreased secretion of aldosterone causes sodium and water loss and potassium retention.

Cortisol, another adrenocortical hormone, has only a fraction of the mineralocorticoid potency of aldosterone. When secreted in large quantities, however, it can also produce sodium and fluid retention and potassium deficit.

Parathyroid Functions

The parathyroid glands, embedded in the thyroid gland, regulate calcium and phosphate balance by means of parathyroid hormone (PTH). PTH influences bone resorption, calcium absorption from the intestines, and calcium reabsorption from the renal tubules.

Other Mechanisms

Changes in the volume of the interstitial compartment within the ECF can occur without affecting body function. The vascular compartment, however, cannot tolerate change as readily and must be carefully maintained to ensure that tissues receive adequate nutrients.

BARORECEPTORS

The baroreceptors are small nerve receptors that detect changes in pressure within blood vessels and transmit this information to the central nervous system. They are responsible for monitoring the circulating volume, and they regulate sympathetic and parasympathetic neural activity as well as endocrine activities. They are categorized as low-pressure and high-pressure baroreceptor systems. Low-pressure baroreceptors are located in the cardiac atria, particularly the left atrium. The high-pressure baroreceptors are nerve endings in the aortic arch and in the carotid sinus. Another high-pressure baroreceptor is located in the afferent arteriole of the juxtaglomerular apparatus of the nephron.

As arterial pressure decreases, baroreceptors transmit fewer impulses from the carotid sinuses and the aortic arch to the vasomotor centre. A decrease in impulses stimulates the sympathetic nervous system and inhibits the parasympathetic nervous system. The outcome is an increase in cardiac rate, conduction, and contractility and in circulating blood volume. Sympathetic stimulation constricts renal arterioles; this increases the release of aldosterone, decreases glomerular filtration, and increases sodium and water reabsorption.

RENIN–ANGIOTENSIN–ALDOSTERONE SYSTEM

Renin is an enzyme that converts angiotensinogen, an inactive substance formed by the liver, into angiotensin I. Renin is released by the juxtaglomerular cells of the kidneys in response to decreased renal perfusion. Angiotensin-converting enzyme (ACE) converts angiotensin I to angiotensin II. Angiotensin II, with its vasoconstrictor properties, increases arterial perfusion pressure and stimulates thirst. As the sympathetic nervous system is stimulated, aldosterone is released in response to an increased release of renin. Aldosterone is a volume regulator and is also released as serum potassium increases, serum sodium decreases, or adrenocorticotropic hormone increases.

ADH AND THIRST

ADH and the thirst mechanism have important roles in maintaining sodium concentration and oral intake of fluids. Oral intake is controlled by the thirst centre located in the hypothalamus. As serum concentration or osmolality increases or blood volume decreases, neurons in the hypothalamus are stimulated by intracellular dehydration; thirst then occurs, and the person increases oral intake of fluids. Water excretion is controlled by ADH, aldosterone, and baroreceptors, as mentioned previously. The presence or absence of ADH is the most significant factor in determining whether the urine that is excreted is concentrated or dilute.

OSMORECEPTORS

Located on the surface of the hypothalamus, osmoreceptors sense changes in sodium concentration. As osmotic pressure increases, the neurons become dehydrated and quickly release impulses to the posterior pituitary, which increases the release of ADH. ADH travels in the blood to the kidneys, where it alters permeability to water, causing increased reabsorption of water and decreased urine output. The retained water dilutes the ECF and returns its concentration to normal. Restoration of normal osmotic pressure provides feedback to the osmoreceptors to inhibit further ADH release (see Fig. 14-2).

RELEASE OF ATRIAL NATRIURETIC PEPTIDE

Atrial natriuretic peptide (ANP) is released by cardiac cells in the atria of the heart in response to increased atrial pressure. Any dis-

Physiology/Pathophysiology

```
                              ↓ Blood volume
                              ↑ Serum osmolality

           Stimulates                                              Stimulates
    Concentrated                 (↑Thirst and water intake)
    urine excreted                  ECF volume deficit

  ↑ ADH production              ↓ Arterial B/P
   in hypothalamus              (stimulates baroreceptors)
   (osmoreceptors)

                               ↑ Sympathetic discharge
Inhibits
    Diuresis results            ↓ Renal perfusion

                        ↓H₂O and Na⁺          Renin release (↓GFR)
                        filtered by kidney    (promotes peripheral vasoconstriction)    ↑ ADH release into
                                                                                        bloodstream from storage
                                               ↑ Angiotensin I and II                   in posterior pituitary

  ↑ Blood volume                               ↑ Aldosterone by
  ↓ Serum osmolality                            adrenal cortex                          ↑ Reabsorption of H₂O by
                                                                                        distal tubule of kidneys
                              ↓Na⁺ and H₂O excretion by kidneys

                              ↑ Blood pressure                    ↓ Urine excretion

                    ↑ Circulating volume of H₂O and Na⁺ (loss of K⁺)
```

FIGURE 14-2 Fluid regulation cycle.

order that results in volume expansion or increased cardiac filling pressures (eg, high sodium intake, heart failure, chronic renal failure, atrial tachycardia, or use of vasoconstrictor agents) will increase the release of ANP. The action of ANP is the direct opposite of the renin–angiotensin–aldosterone system and decreases blood pressure and volume (Fig. 14-3). The ANP measured in plasma is normally 20–77 ng/L. This level increases in acute heart failure, paroxysmal atrial tachycardia, hyperthyroidism, subarachnoid hemorrhage, and small cell lung cancer. The level decreases

in chronic heart failure and with the use of medications such as urea (Ureaphil) and prazosin (Minipress).

 Gerontologic Considerations

Normal physiologic changes of aging, including reduced renal and respiratory function and reserve and alterations in the ratio of body fluids to muscle mass, may alter the responses of an elderly person to fluid and electrolyte changes and acid–base disturbances. In

Physiology/Pathophysiology

FIGURE 14-3 Role of atrial natriuretic peptide (ANP) in maintenance of fluid balance.

addition, the frequent use of medications in older adults can affect renal and cardiac function and fluid balance, thereby increasing the likelihood of fluid and electrolyte disturbances. Routine procedures, such as the vigorous administration of laxatives before colon x-ray studies, may produce a serious fluid volume deficit, necessitating the use of intravenous (IV) fluids to prevent hypotension and other effects of hypovolemia.

Alterations in fluid and electrolyte balance that may produce minor changes in young and middle-aged adults have the potential to produce profound changes in older adults, accompanied by a rapid onset of signs and symptoms. In other elderly patients, the clinical manifestations of fluid and electrolyte disturbances may be subtle or atypical. For example, fluid deficit may cause confusion in the elderly person, whereas in young and middle-aged people the first sign commonly is increased thirst. Rapid infusion of

an excessive volume of IV fluids may produce fluid overload and cardiac failure in the elderly patient. These reactions are likely to occur more quickly and with the administration of smaller volumes of fluid than in healthy young and middle-aged adults because of the decreased cardiac reserve and reduced renal function that accompany aging.

Increased sensitivity to fluid and electrolyte changes in the elderly patient requires careful assessment, with attention to intake and output of fluids from all sources and to changes in daily weight; careful monitoring of side effects and interactions of medications; and prompt reporting and management of disturbances. Additional gerontologic considerations relating to specific fluid and electrolyte disturbances are discussed later in this chapter.

Fluid Volume Disturbances

FLUID VOLUME DEFICIT (HYPOVOLEMIA)

Fluid volume deficit (FVD) occurs when loss of extracellular fluid volume exceeds the intake of fluid. It occurs when water and electrolytes are lost in the same proportion as they exist in normal body fluids, so that the ratio of serum electrolytes to water remains the same. Fluid volume deficit (hypovolemia) should not be confused with the term *dehydration*, which refers to loss of water alone with increased serum sodium levels. FVD may occur alone or in combination with other imbalances. Unless other imbalances are present concurrently, serum electrolyte concentrations remain essentially unchanged.

Pathophysiology

FVD results from loss of body fluids and occurs more rapidly when coupled with decreased fluid intake. FVD can develop from inadequate intake alone if the decreased intake is prolonged. Causes of FVD include abnormal fluid losses, such as those resulting from vomiting, diarrhea, GI suctioning, and sweating, and decreased intake, as in nausea or inability to gain access to fluids (Beck, 2000).

Additional risk factors include diabetes insipidus, adrenal insufficiency, osmotic diuresis, hemorrhage, and coma. Third-space fluid shifts, or the movement of fluid from the vascular system to other body spaces (eg, with edema formation in burns or ascites with liver dysfunction), also produce FVD.

Clinical Manifestations

FVD can develop rapidly and can be mild, moderate, or severe, depending on the degree of fluid loss. Important characteristics of FVD include acute weight loss; decreased skin turgor; oliguria; concentrated urine; postural hypotension; a weak, rapid heart rate; flattened neck veins; increased temperature; decreased central venous pressure; cool, clammy skin related to peripheral vasoconstriction; thirst; anorexia; nausea; lassitude; muscle weakness; and cramps.

Assessment and Diagnostic Findings

Laboratory data useful in evaluating fluid volume status include BUN and its relation to the serum creatinine concentration. A volume-depleted patient has a BUN elevated out of proportion to the serum creatinine level (a ratio greater than 20:1). The cause of hypovolemia may be determined through the health history and physical examination. The BUN can be elevated due to dehydration or decreased renal perfusion and function. Also, the hematocrit level is greater than normal because the red blood cells become suspended in a decreased plasma volume.

Serum electrolyte changes may also exist. Potassium and sodium levels can be reduced (hypokalemia, hyponatremia) or elevated (hyperkalemia, hypernatremia).

- Hypokalemia occurs with GI and renal losses.
- Hyperkalemia occurs with adrenal insufficiency.
- Hyponatremia occurs with increased thirst and ADH release.
- Hypernatremia results from increased insensible losses and diabetes insipidus.

Urine specific gravity is increased in relation to the kidneys' attempt to conserve water and decreased with diabetes insipidus. Urine osmolality is greater than 450 mmol/kg, since the kidneys try to compensate by conserving water. Normal values for these tests are listed in Table 14-4.

 Gerontologic Considerations

Elderly patients have special nursing care needs because of their propensity for developing fluid and electrolyte imbalances (Beck,

TEST	USUAL REFERENCE RANGE (SI UNITS)
Serum sodium	135–145 mmol/L
Serum potassium	3.5–5.3 mmol/L
Total serum calcium	2.15–2.5 mmol/L
Serum magnesium	0.72–0.95 mmol/L
Serum phosphorus	0.87–1.45 mmol/L
Serum chloride	97–107 mmol/L
Carbon dioxide content	22–30 mmol/L
Serum osmolality	280–300 mmol/kg H_2O
Blood urea nitrogen (BUN)	1.8–7.1 mmol/L
Serum creatinine	44–97 mmol/L 53–105 mmol/L
BUN to creatinine ratio	—
Hematocrit	Volume fraction: 0.42–0.52 Volume fraction: 0.35–0.47
Serum glucose	3.9–5.8 mmol/L
Serum albumin	3.5–5.0 g/L
Urinary sodium	75–220 mmol/day
Urinary potassium (intake-dependent)	25–123 mmol/day
Urinary chloride	110–250 mmol/24 h
Urine specific gravity	1.016–1.022
Urine osmolality	250–900 mmol/kg H_2O
Urinary pH	4.5–8.0 <5–6

Table 14-4 • **Laboratory Values Used In Evaluating Fluid and Electrolyte Status in Adults**

2000; Kugler & Hustead, 2000). Fluid balance in the elderly patient is often marginal at best because of certain physiologic changes associated with the aging process. Some of these changes include reduction in total body water (associated with increased body fat content and decreased muscle mass); reduction in renal function, resulting in decreased ability to concentrate urine; decreased cardiovascular and respiratory function; and disturbances in hormonal regulatory functions. Although these changes are viewed as normal in the aging process, they must be considered when the elderly person becomes ill because age-related changes predispose the person to fluid and electrolyte imbalances. These physiologic changes must be considered during assessment of the elderly patient as well as before initiating treatment for fluid and electrolyte imbalances.

Assessment of the elderly patient should be modified somewhat from that of younger adults. For example, skin turgor is less valid in the assessment of elderly patients because their skin has lost some of its elasticity; therefore, other assessment measures (eg, slowness in filling of veins of the hands and feet) become more important in detecting FVD. In the elderly patient, skin turgor is best tested over the forehead or the sternum, because alterations in skin elasticity are less marked in these areas. As in any patient, skin turgor should be monitored serially to detect subtle changes.

The nurse should perform a functional assessment of the aged person's ability to determine fluid and food needs and to obtain adequate intake. For example, is the patient mentally clear? Is the patient able to ambulate and use both arms and hands to reach fluids and foods? Is the patient able to swallow? All of these questions have a direct bearing on how patients will be able to meet their own need for fluids and foods. During an elderly patient's hospital stay, the nurse must provide fluids for any patient who is unable to carry out self-care activities.

Another concern is that some elderly patients deliberately restrict their fluid intake to avoid embarrassing episodes of incontinence. In this situation, the nurse also identifies interventions to deal with the incontinence, such as encouraging the patient to wear protective clothing or devices, carry a urinal in the car, or pace fluid intake to allow access to toilet facilities during the day. Elderly people without cardiovascular or renal dysfunction should be reminded to drink adequate fluids.

Medical Management

When planning the correction of fluid loss for the patient with FVD, the health care provider considers the usual maintenance requirements of the patient and other factors (such as fever) that can influence fluid needs. When the deficit is not severe, the oral route is preferred, provided the patient can drink. When fluid losses are acute or severe, however, the IV route is required. Isotonic electrolyte solutions (eg, lactated Ringer's or 0.9% sodium chloride) are frequently used to treat the hypotensive patient with FVD because they expand plasma volume. As soon as the patient becomes normotensive, a hypotonic electrolyte solution (eg, 0.45% sodium chloride) is often used to provide both electrolytes and water for renal excretion of metabolic wastes. These and additional fluids are listed in Table 14-5.

Accurate and frequent assessments of intake and output, weight, vital signs, central venous pressure, level of consciousness, breath sounds, and skin colour should be performed to determine when therapy should be slowed to avoid volume overload. The rate of

Table 14-5 • **Selected Water and Electrolyte Solutions**

SOLUTION	COMMENTS
Isotonic Solutions	
0.9% NaCl (isotonic, also called normal saline) Na⁺ 154 mmol/L Cl⁻ 154 mmol/L (308 mmol/L) Also available with varying concentrations of dextrose (the most frequently used is a 5% dextrose concentration)	• An isotonic solution that expands the extracellular fluid volume, used in hypovolemic states, resuscitative efforts, shock, diabetic ketoacidosis, metabolic alkalosis, hypercalcemia, mild Na^+ deficit • Supplies an excess of Na^+ and Cl^-; can cause fluid volume excess and hyperchloremic acidosis if used in excessive volumes, particularly in patients with compromised renal function, heart failure, or edema • Not desirable as a routine maintenance solution, as it provides only Na^+ and Cl^- (and these are provided in excessive amounts) • When mixed with 5% dextrose, the resulting solution becomes hypertonic in relation to plasma and, in addition to the above described electrolytes, provides 170 calories/L • Only solution that may be administered with blood products
Lactated Ringer's solution (Hartmann's solution) Na⁺ 130 mmol/L K⁺ 4 mmol/L Ca⁺⁺ 3 mmol/L Cl⁻ 109 mmol/L Lactate (metabolized to bicarbonate) 274 mmol/L Also available with varying concentrations of dextrose (the most common is 5% dextrose)	• An isotonic solution that contains multiple electrolytes in roughly the same concentration as found in plasma (note that solution is lacking in Mg^{++}): provides 9 calories/L • Used in the treatment of hypovolemia, burns, fluid lost as bile or diarrhea, and for acute blood loss replacement • Lactate is rapidly metabolized into HCO_3^- in the body. Lactated Ringer's solution should not be used in lactic acidosis because the ability to convert lactate into HCO_3^- is impaired in this disorder. • Not to be given with a pH > 7.5, as bicarbonate is formed as lactate breaks down, causing alkalosis • Should not be used in renal failure because it contains potassium and can cause hyperkalemia • Similar to plasma
5% dextrose in water (D₅W) No electrolytes 50 g of dextrose	• An isotonic solution that supplies 170 calories/L and free water to aid in renal excretion of solutes • Used in treatment of hypernatremia, fluid loss, and dehydration • Should not be used in excessive volumes in the early postoperative period (when ADH secretion is increased due to stress reaction) • Should not be used solely in treatment of fluid volume deficit, because it dilutes plasma electrolyte concentrations • Contraindicated in head injury because it may cause increased intracranial pressure • Should not be used for fluid resuscitation as it can cause hyperglycemia • Should be used with caution in patients with renal or cardiac disease because of risk of fluid overload • Electrolyte-free solutions may cause peripheral circulatory collapse, anuria in patients with sodium deficiency, and increased body fluid loss. • Converts to hypotonic solution as dextrose is metabolized by body. Over time, D_5W without NaCl can cause water intoxication (intracellular FVE) as the solution is hypotonic.
Hypotonic Solutions	
0.45% NaCl (half-strength saline) Na⁺ 77 mmol/L Cl⁻ 77 mmol/L (154 mmol/L) Also available with varying concentrations of dextrose (the most common is a 5% concentration)	• Provides Na^+, Cl^-, and free water • Free water is desirable to aid the kidneys in elimination of solute. • Lacking in electrolytes other than Na^+ and Cl^- • When mixed with 5% dextrose, the solution becomes slightly hypertonic to plasma and in addition to the above-described electrolytes provides 170 calories. • Used to treat hypertonic dehydration, Na^+ and Cl^- depletion, and gastric fluid loss • Not indicated for third-space fluid shifts or increased intracranial pressure • Administer cautiously, as it can cause fluid shifts from vascular system into cells, resulting in cardiovascular collapse and increased intracranial pressure.
Hypertonic Solutions	
3% NaCl (hypertonic saline) Na⁺ 513 mmol/L Cl⁻ 513 mmol/L (1,026 mmol/L)	• Highly hypertonic solution used only in critical situations to treat hyponatremia • Must be administered slowly and cautiously, as it can cause intravascular volume overload and pulmonary edema • Supplies no calories • Assists in removing intracellular fluid excess
5% NaCL (hypertonic solution) Na⁺ 855 mmol/L Cl⁻ 855 mmol/L (1,710 mmol/L)	• Highly hypertonic solution used to treat symptomatic hyponatremia • Administered slowly and cautiously, as it can cause intravascular volume overload and pulmonary edema • Supplies no calories
Colloid Solutions Dextran 40 in NS or 5% D₅W	• Colloid solution used as volume/plasma expander for intravascular part of ECF • Affects clotting by coating platelets and decreasing ability to clot • Remains in circulatory system for 6 hours • Used to treat hypovolemia in early shock to increase pulse pressure, cardiac output, and arterial blood pressure • Improves microcirculation by decreasing RBC aggregation • Contraindicated in hemorrhage, thrombocytopenia, renal disease, and severe dehydration

fluid administration is based on the severity of loss and the patient's hemodynamic response to volume replacement.

If the patient with severe FVD is not excreting enough urine and is therefore oliguric, the health care provider needs to determine whether the depressed renal function is the result of reduced renal blood flow secondary to FVD (prerenal azotemia) or, more seriously, to acute tubular necrosis from prolonged FVD. The test used in this situation is referred to as a fluid challenge test. During a fluid challenge test, volumes of fluid are administered at specific rates and intervals while the patient's hemodynamic response to this treatment is monitored (ie, vital signs, breath sounds, sensorium, central venous pressure, urine output).

A typical example of a fluid challenge involves administering 100 to 200 mL of normal saline solution over 15 minutes. The goal is to provide fluids rapidly enough to attain adequate tissue perfusion without compromising the cardiovascular system. The response by a patient with FVD but normal renal function will be increased urine output and an increase in blood pressure and central venous pressure.

Shock can occur when the volume of fluid lost exceeds 25% of the intravascular volume, or when fluid loss is rapid. Shock and its causes and treatment are discussed in detail in Chapter 15.

Nursing Management

To assess for FVD, the nurse monitors and measures fluid intake and output at least every 8 hours, and sometimes hourly. As FVD develops, body fluid losses exceed fluid intake. This loss may be in the form of excessive urination (polyuria), diarrhea, vomiting, and so on. Later, after FVD fully develops, the kidneys attempt to conserve needed body fluids, leading to a urine output of less than 30 mL/h in an adult. Urine in this instance is concentrated and represents a healthy renal response. Daily body weights are monitored; an acute loss of 0.5 kg represents a fluid loss of approximately 500 mL. (One litre of fluid weighs approximately 1 kilogram.)

Vital signs are closely monitored. The nurse observes for a weak, rapid pulse and postural hypotension (ie, a drop in systolic pressure exceeding 15 mm Hg when the patient moves from a lying to a sitting position). A decrease in body temperature often accompanies FVD, unless there is a concurrent infection.

Skin and tongue turgor is monitored on a regular basis. In a healthy person, pinched skin immediately returns to its normal position when released. This elastic property, referred to as turgor, is partially dependent on interstitial fluid volume. In a person with FVD, the skin flattens more slowly after the pinch is released. When FVD is severe, the skin may remain elevated for many seconds. Tissue turgor is best measured by pinching the skin over the sternum, inner aspects of the thighs, or forehead.

 NURSING ALERT The skin turgor test is not as valid in elderly people as in younger people because skin elasticity decreases with age; therefore, other assessment parameters must be considered.

Evaluating tongue turgor, which is not affected by age, may be more valid than evaluating skin turgor. In a normal person, the tongue has one longitudinal furrow. In the person with FVD, there are additional longitudinal furrows and the tongue is smaller,

because of fluid loss. The degree of oral mucous membrane moisture is also assessed; a dry mouth may indicate either FVD or mouth breathing.

Urinary concentration is monitored by measuring the urine specific gravity. In a volume-depleted patient, the urinary specific gravity should be above 1.020, indicating healthy renal conservation of fluid.

Mental function is eventually affected in severe FVD as a result of decreasing cerebral perfusion. Decreased peripheral perfusion can result in cold extremities. In patients with relatively normal cardiopulmonary function, a low central venous pressure is indicative of hypovolemia. Patients with acute cardiopulmonary decompensation require more extensive hemodynamic monitoring of pressures in both sides of the heart to determine if hypovolemia exists.

PREVENTING FVD

To prevent FVD, the nurse identifies patients at risk and takes measures to minimize fluid losses. For example, if the patient has diarrhea, diarrhea control measures should be implemented and replacement fluids administered. These measures may include administering antidiarrheal medications and small volumes of oral fluids at frequent intervals.

CORRECTING FVD

When possible, oral fluids are administered to help correct FVD, with consideration given to the patient's likes and dislikes. Also, the type of fluid the patient has lost is considered, and attempts are made to select fluids most likely to replace the lost electrolytes. If the patient is reluctant to drink because of oral discomfort, the nurse assists with frequent mouth care and provides nonirritating fluids. The patient may be offered small volumes of fluids at frequent intervals rather than a large volume all at once. If nausea is present, antiemetics may be needed before oral fluid replacement can be tolerated.

If the patient cannot eat and drink, the nurse may need to administer fluid by an alternative route (enteral or parenteral) prescribed to prevent renal damage related to prolonged FVD.

FLUID VOLUME EXCESS (HYPERVOLEMIA)

Fluid volume excess (FVE) refers to an isotonic expansion of the ECF caused by the abnormal retention of water and sodium in approximately the same proportions in which they normally exist in the ECF. It is always secondary to an increase in the total body sodium content, which, in turn, leads to an increase in total body water. Because there is isotonic retention of body substances, the serum sodium concentration remains essentially normal.

Pathophysiology

FVE may be related to simple fluid overload or diminished function of the homeostatic mechanisms responsible for regulating fluid balance. Contributing factors can include heart failure, renal failure, and cirrhosis of the liver. Another contributing factor is consumption of excessive amounts of table or other sodium salts. Excessive administration of sodium-containing fluids in a patient with impaired regulatory mechanisms may predispose him or her to a serious FVE as well (Beck, 2000).

Clinical Manifestations

Clinical manifestations of FVE stem from expansion of the ECF and include edema, distended neck veins, and crackles (abnormal lung sounds). Other manifestations include tachycardia; increased blood pressure, pulse pressure, and central venous pressure; increased weight; increased urine output; and shortness of breath and wheezing.

Assessment and Diagnostic Findings

Laboratory data useful in diagnosing FVE include BUN and hematocrit levels. In FVE, both of these values may be decreased because of plasma dilution. Other causes for abnormalities in these values include low protein intake and anemia. In chronic renal failure, both serum osmolality and the sodium level are decreased due to excessive retention of water. The urine sodium level is increased if the kidneys are attempting to excrete excess volume. Chest x-rays may reveal pulmonary congestion. Hypervolemia occurs when aldosterone is chronically stimulated (ie, cirrhosis, heart failure, and nephrotic syndrome). Urine sodium levels, therefore, will not rise in these conditions.

Medical Management

Management of FVE is directed at the causes. When the fluid excess is related to excessive administration of sodium-containing fluids, discontinuing the infusion may be all that is needed. Symptomatic treatment consists of administering diuretics and restricting fluids and sodium.

PHARMACOLOGIC THERAPY

Diuretics are prescribed when dietary restriction of sodium alone is insufficient to reduce edema by inhibiting the reabsorption of sodium and water by the kidneys. The choice of diuretic is based on the severity of the hypervolemic state, the degree of impairment of renal function, and the potency of the diuretic. Thiazide diuretics block sodium reabsorption in the distal tubule, where only 5% to 10% of filtered sodium is reabsorbed. Loop diuretics, the prototype being furosemide (Lasix), can cause a greater loss of both sodium and water because they block sodium reabsorption in the ascending limb of the loop of Henle, where 20% to 30% of filtered sodium is normally reabsorbed. Generally, thiazide diuretics, the prototype being hydrochlorothiazide (HydroDIURIL), are prescribed for mild to moderate hypervolemia and loop diuretics for severe hypervolemia.

Electrolyte imbalances may result from the effect of the diuretic. Hypokalemia can occur with all diuretics except those that work in the last distal tubule of the nephrons (eg, spironolactone). Potassium supplements can be prescribed to avoid this complication. Hyperkalemia can occur with diuretics that work in the last distal tubule, especially in patients with decreased renal function. Hyponatremia occurs with diuresis due to increased release of ADH secondary to reduction in circulating volume. Decreased magnesium levels occur with administration of loop and thiazide diuretics due to decreased reabsorption and increased excretion of magnesium by the kidney.

Azotemia (increased nitrogen levels in the blood) can occur with FVE when urea and creatinine are not excreted due to decreased perfusion by the kidneys and decreased excretion of wastes. High uric acid levels (hyperuricemia) can also occur from increased reabsorption and decreased excretion of uric acid by the kidneys.

HEMODIALYSIS

When renal function is so severely impaired that pharmacologic agents cannot act efficiently, other modalities are considered to remove sodium and fluid from the body. Hemodialysis or peritoneal dialysis may be used to remove nitrogenous wastes and control potassium and acid–base balance, and to remove sodium and fluid. Continuous renal replacement therapy may also be considered. See Chapter 44 for discussion of these treatment modalities.

NUTRITIONAL THERAPY

Treatment of FVE usually involves dietary restriction of sodium. An average daily diet not restricted in sodium contains 6 to 15 g of salt, whereas low-sodium diets can range from a mild restriction to as little as 250 mg of sodium per day, depending on the patient's needs. A mild sodium-restricted diet allows only light salting of food (about half the amount as usual) in cooking and at the table, and no addition of salt to commercially prepared foods that are already seasoned. Of course, foods high in sodium must be avoided. It is the sodium salt, sodium chloride, rather than sodium itself that contributes to edema. Therefore, patients need to read food labels carefully to determine salt content.

Because about half of ingested sodium is in the form of seasoning, seasoning substitutes can play a major role in decreasing sodium intake. Lemon juice, onions, and garlic are excellent substitute flavorings, although some patients prefer salt substitutes. Most salt substitutes contain potassium and must therefore be used cautiously by patients taking potassium-sparing diuretics (eg, spironolactone, triamterene, amiloride). They should not be used at all in conditions associated with potassium retention, such as advanced renal disease. Salt substitutes containing ammonium chloride can be harmful to patients with liver damage.

In some communities, the drinking water may contain too much sodium for a sodium-restricted diet. Depending on its source, water may contain as little as 1 mg or more than 1,500 mg per litre. Patients may need to use distilled water when the local water supply is very high in sodium. Also, patients on sodium-restricted diets should be cautioned to avoid water softeners that add sodium to water in exchange for other ions, such as calcium.

Nursing Management

To assess for FVE, the nurse measures intake and output at regular intervals to identify excessive fluid retention. The patient is weighed daily and acute weight gain is noted. An acute weight gain of 0.9 kg represents a gain of approximately 1 L of fluid. The nurse also needs to assess breath sounds at regular intervals in at-risk patients, particularly when parenteral fluids are being administered. The nurse monitors the degree of edema in the most dependent parts of the body, such as the feet and ankles in ambulatory patients and the sacral region in bedridden patients. The degree of pitting edema is assessed by pressing firmly with the thumb for 5 seconds over the shins, behind each medial malleolus, and on the dorsum of the feet (Bickley & Szilagyi, 2003). The depth of any depression is measured plus the time needed for the depression to refill. The edema is graded on a four-point scale (Dillon, 2004):

+1: 2-mm depression that rapidly disappears
+2: 4-mm depression that disappears in 15–20 seconds
+3: 6-mm depression that disappears after 1 minute or more (extremity appears edematous)

+4: 8-mm depression that disappears after 2–3 minutes (very marked edema of the extremity is visible)

The extent of peripheral edema is monitored by measuring the circumference of the legs with a metric tape measure at four locations: the forefoot, the smallest circumference above the ankle, the largest circumference of the calf, and the midthigh (above the patella with the knee straight). Both legs are compared, and a 1-cm or greater difference above the ankle or a 2-cm or greater difference at the calf usually indicates edema (Bickley & Szilagi, 2003).

PREVENTING FVE

Specific interventions vary somewhat with the underlying condition and the degree of FVE. Most patients, however, require sodium-restricted diets in some form, and adherence to the prescribed diet is encouraged. The patient is instructed to avoid over-the-counter medications without first checking with a health care provider because these substances may contain sodium. When fluid retention persists despite adherence to a prescribed diet, hidden sources of sodium, such as the water supply or use of water softeners, should be considered.

DETECTING AND CONTROLLING FVE

Detecting FVE is of primary importance before the condition becomes critical. Interventions include promoting rest, restricting sodium intake, monitoring parenteral fluid therapy, and administering appropriate medications.

Some patients benefit from regular rest periods, as bed rest favours diuresis of edema fluid. The mechanism is probably related to diminished venous pooling and the subsequent increase in effective circulating blood volume and renal perfusion. Sodium and fluid restriction should be instituted as indicated. Because most patients with FVE require diuretics, the patient's response to these agents is monitored. The rate of parenteral fluids and the patient's response to these fluids are also closely monitored. If dyspnea or orthopnea is present, the patient is placed in a semi-Fowler's position to promote lung expansion. The patient is turned and positioned at regular intervals because edematous tissue is more prone to skin breakdown than normal tissue.

Because conditions predisposing to FVE are likely to be chronic, the patient is taught to monitor his or her response to therapy by documenting fluid intake and output and body weight changes. The importance of adhering to the treatment regimen is emphasized.

TEACHING PATIENTS ABOUT EDEMA

Because edema is a common manifestation of FVE, patients need to recognize its symptoms and importance. The nurse gives special attention to edema when teaching patients with FVE. Edema can occur from increased capillary fluid pressure, decreased capillary oncotic pressure, or increased interstitial oncotic pressure, thus expanding the interstitial fluid compartment. Edema can be localized (eg, in the ankle, as in rheumatoid arthritis) or generalized (as in cardiac and renal failure). Severe generalized edema is called anasarca.

Edema occurs when there is a change in the capillary membrane, increasing the formation of interstitial fluid or decreasing the removal of interstitial fluid. Sodium retention is a frequent cause of the increased extracellular fluid volume. Burns and infection are examples of conditions associated with increased inter-

stitial fluid volume. Obstruction to lymphatic outflow, a plasma albumin level less than 15 to 20 g/L, or a decrease in plasma oncotic pressure contributes to increased interstitial fluid volume. The kidneys retain sodium and water when there is decreased extracellular volume as a result of decreased cardiac output from heart failure. A thorough medication history is necessary to identify any medications that may cause edema, such as nonsteroidal anti-inflammatory drugs (NSAIDs), estrogens, corticosteroids, or antihypertensives.

Ascites is a form of edema in which fluid accumulates in the peritoneal cavity; it results from nephrotic syndrome or cirrhosis. Patients commonly report shortness of breath and a sense of pressure because of pressure on the diaphragm.

Edema usually affects dependent areas. It can be seen in the ankles, sacrum, scrotum, or the periorbital region of the face. Pitting edema is so named because a pit forms after a finger is pressed into edematous tissue. In pulmonary edema, the amount of fluid in the pulmonary interstitium and the alveoli increases. Manifestations include shortness of breath, increased respiratory rate, diaphoresis, and crackles and wheezing on auscultation of the lungs.

Decreased hematocrit resulting from hemodilution, arterial blood gas results indicative of respiratory **alkalosis** and hypoxemia, and decreased serum sodium and osmolality from retention of fluid may occur with edema. BUN and creatinine levels increase, urine specific gravity decreases as the kidneys attempt to excrete excess water, and the urine sodium level drops due to increased aldosterone production.

The goal of treatment is to preserve or restore the circulating intravascular fluid volume. In addition to treating the cause, other treatments may include diuretic therapy, restriction of fluids and sodium, elevation of the extremities, application of elastic compression stockings, paracentesis, dialysis, or continuous arteriovenous hemofiltration in cases of renal failure or life-threatening fluid volume overload.

Electrolyte Imbalances

Disturbances in electrolyte balances occur in clinical practice and must be corrected for the patient's health and safety. Table 14-6 summarizes the major fluid and electrolyte imbalances that are described in the text. An example of an electrolyte imbalance is an altered sodium balance.

SIGNIFICANCE OF SODIUM

Sodium is the most abundant electrolyte in the ECF; its concentration ranges from 135–145 mmol/L. Consequently, sodium is the primary determinant of ECF osmolality. Decreased sodium is associated with parallel changes in osmolality. The fact that sodium does not easily cross the cell wall membrane, plus its abundance or high concentration, accounts for its primary role in controlling water distribution throughout the body. In addition, sodium is the primary regulator of ECF volume. A loss or gain of sodium is usually accompanied by a loss or gain of water. Sodium also functions in establishing the electrochemical state necessary for muscle contraction and the transmission of nerve impulses.

Sodium imbalance occurs frequently in clinical practice and can develop under simple and complex circumstances. Sodium deficit and excess are the two most common sodium imbalances.

Table 14-6 • **Major Fluid and Electrolyte Imbalances**

IMBALANCE	CONTRIBUTING FACTORS	SIGNS/SYMPTOMS AND LABORATORY FINDINGS
Fluid volume deficit (hypovolemia)	Loss of water and electrolytes, as in vomiting, diarrhea, fistulas, fever, excess sweating, burns, blood loss, gastrointestinal suction, and third-space fluid shifts; and decreased intake, as in anorexia, nausea, and inability to gain access to fluid. Diabetes insipidus and uncontrolled diabetes mellitus also contribute to a depletion of extracellular fluid volume.	Acute weight loss, decreased skin turgor, oliguria, concentrated urine, weak rapid pulse, capillary filling time prolonged, low central venous pressure (CVP), ↓ blood pressure, flattened neck veins, dizziness, weakness, thirst and confusion, ↑ pulse, muscle cramps. *Labs indicate:* ↑ hemoglobin and hematocrit, ↑ serum and urine osmolality and specific gravity, ↓ urine sodium, ↑ BUN and creatinine
Fluid volume excess (hypervolemia)	Compromised regulatory mechanisms, such as renal failure, heart failure, and cirrhosis; and overzealous administration of sodium-containing fluids. Prolonged corticosteroid therapy, severe stress, and hyperaldosteronism augment fluid volume excess.	Acute weight gain, edema, distended jugular veins, crackles, and elevated CVP, shortness of breath, ↑ blood pressure, bounding pulse and cough. *Labs indicate:* ↓ hemoglobin and hematocrit, ↓ serum and urine osmolality, ↓ urine sodium and specific gravity
Sodium deficit (hyponatremia) Serum sodium <135 mmol/L	Loss of sodium, as in use of diuretics, loss of GI fluids, renal disease, and adrenal insufficiency. Gain of water, as in excessive administration of D_5W and water supplements for patients receiving hypotonic tube feedings; disease states associated with SIADH such as head trauma and oat-cell lung tumour; and medications associated with water retention (oxytocin and certain tranquilizers). Hyperglycemia and heart failure cause a loss of sodium.	Anorexia, nausea and vomiting, headache, lethargy, confusion, muscle cramps and weakness, muscular twitching, seizures, papilledema, dry skin, ↑ pulse, ↓ BP *Labs indicate:* ↓ serum and urine sodium, ↓ urine specific gravity and osmolality
Sodium excess (hypernatremia) Serum sodium >145 mmol/L	Water deprivation in patients unable to drink at will, hypertonic tube feedings without adequate water supplements, diabetes insipidus, heatstroke, hyperventilation, and watery diarrhea. Excess corticosteroid, sodium bicarbonate, and sodium chloride administration, and salt water near-drowning victims.	Thirst, elevated body temperature, swollen dry tongue and sticky mucous membranes, hallucinations, lethargy, restlessness, irritability, focal or grand mal seizures, pulmonary edema, hyperreflexia, twitching, nausea, vomiting, anorexia, ↑ pulse, and ↑ BP. *Labs indicate.* ↑ serum sodium, ↓ urine sodium, ↑ urine specific gravity and osmolality
Potassium deficit (hypokalemia) Serum potassium <3.5 mmol/L	Diarrhea, vomiting, gastric suction, corticosteroid administration, hyperaldosteronism, carbenicillin, amphotericin B, bulimia, osmotic diuresis, alkalosis, starvation, diuretics, and digoxin toxicity	Fatigue, anorexia, nausea and vomiting, muscle weakness, polyuria, decreased bowel motility, ventricular asystole or fibrillation, paresthesias, leg cramps, ↓ BP, ileus, abdominal distention, hypoactive reflexes, *ECG:* flattened T waves, prominent U waves, ST depression, prolonged PR interval.
Potassium excess (hyperkalemia) Serum potassium >5.0 mmol/L	Pseudohyperkalemia, oliguric renal failure, use of potassium-conserving diuretics in patients with renal insufficiency, metabolic acidosis, Addison's disease, crush injury, burns, stored bank blood transfusions, and rapid IV administration of potassium	Vague muscular weakness, tachycardia → bradycardia, dysrhythmias, flaccid paralysis, paresthesias, intestinal colic, cramps, irritability, anxiety. *ECG:* tall tented T waves, prolonged PR interval and QRS duration, absent P waves, ST depression.
Calcium deficit (hypocalcemia) Serum calcium <2.15 mmol/L	Hypoparathyroidism (may follow thyroid surgery or radical neck dissection), malabsorption, pancreatitis, alkalosis, vitamin D deficiency, massive subcutaneous infection, generalized peritonitis, massive transfusion of citrated blood, chronic diarrhea, decreased parathyroid hormone, and diuretic phase of renal failure	Numbness, tingling of fingers, toes, and circumoral region; positive Trousseau's sign and Chvostek's sign; seizures, carpopedal spasms, hyperactive deep tendon reflexes, irritability, bronchospasm, anxiety, impaired clotting time, ↓ prothrombin, *ECG:* prolonged QT interval and lengthened ST.
Calcium excess (hypercalcemia) Serum calcium >2.55 mmol/L	Hyperparathyroidism, malignant neoplastic disease, prolonged immobilization, overuse of calcium supplements, vitamin D excess, oliguric phase of renal failure, acidosis, corticosteroid therapy, thiazide diuretic use, increased parathyroid hormone, and digoxin toxicity	Muscular weakness, constipation, anorexia, nausea and vomiting, polyuria and polydipsia, hypoactive deep tendon reflexes, lethargy, deep bone pain, pathologic fractures, flank pain, and calcium stones. *ECG:* shortened QT interval, bradycardia, heart blocks.
Magnesium deficit (hypomagnesemia) Serum magnesium <0.72 mmol/L	Chronic alcoholism, hyperparathyroidism, hyperaldosteronism, diuretic phase of renal failure, malabsorptive disorders, diabetic ketoacidosis, refeeding after starvation, parenteral nutrition, chronic laxative use, diarrhea, acute myocardial infarction, heart failure, decreased serum K^+ and Ca^{++} and certain pharmacologic agents (such as gentamicin, cisplatin, and cyclosporine)	Neuromuscular irritability, positive Trousseau's and Chvostek's signs, insomnia, mood changes, anorexia, vomiting, increased tendon reflexes, and ↑ BP. *ECG:* PVCs, flat or inverted T waves, depressed ST segment.

(continued)

Table 14-6 • **Major Fluid and Electrolyte Imbalances** (Continued)

IMBALANCE	CONTRIBUTING FACTORS	SIGNS/SYMPTOMS AND LABORATORY FINDINGS
Magnesium excess (hypermagnesemia) Serum magnesium >0.95 mmol/L	Oliguric phase of renal failure (particularly when magnesium-containing medications are administered), adrenal insufficiency, excessive IV magnesium administration, and DKA	Flushing, hypotension, drowsiness, hypoactive reflexes, depressed respirations, cardiac arrest and coma, diaphoresis. *ECG:* tachycardia → bradycardia, prolonged PR interval and QRS.
Phosphorus deficit (hypophosphatemia) Serum phosphorus <0.80 mmol/L	Refeeding after starvation, alcohol withdrawal, diabetic ketoacidosis, respiratory alkalosis, ↓ magnesium, ↓ potassium, hyperparathyroidism, vomiting, diarrhea, hyperventilation, vitamin D deficiency associated with malabsorptive disorders, burns, acid–base disorders, parenteral nutrition, and diuretic use	Paresthesias, muscle weakness, bone pain and tenderness, chest pain, confusion, cardiomyopathy, respiratory failure, seizures, tissue hypoxia, and increased susceptibility to infection
Phosphorus excess (hyperphosphatemia) Serum phosphorus >1.45 mmol/L	Acute and chronic renal failure, excessive intake of phosphorus, vitamin D excess, respiratory acidosis, hypoparathyroidism, volume depletion, leukemia/lymphoma treated with cytotoxic agents, increased tissue breakdown, rhabdomyolysis	Tetany, tachycardia, anorexia, nausea and vomiting, muscle weakness, signs and symptoms of hypocalcemia
Chloride excess (hyperchloremia) Serum chloride >108 mmol/L	Excessive sodium chloride infusions with water loss, head injury (sodium retention), hypernatremia, renal failure, corticosteroid use, dehydration, severe diarrhea (loss of bicarbonate), respiratory alkalosis, administration of diuretics, overdose of salicylates, Kayexalate, acetazolamide, phenylbutazone and ammonium chloride use, hyperparathyroidism, metabolic acidosis	Tachypnea, lethargy, weakness, deep rapid respirations, decline in cognitive status, decreased cardiac output, dyspnea, tachycardia, pitting edema, dysrhythmias, coma *Labs indicate:* increased serum chloride, increased serum sodium, decreased serum pH, decreased serum bicarbonate, normal anion gap, increased urinary chloride level
Chloride deficit (hypochloremia) Serum chloride <96 mmol/L	Addison's disease, reduced chloride intake or absorption, untreated diabetic ketoacidosis, chronic respiratory acidosis, excessive sweating, vomiting, gastric suction, diarrhea, sodium and potassium deficiency, metabolic alkalosis, loop, osmotic, or thiazide diuretic use, overuse of bicarbonate, rapid removal of ascitic fluid with a high sodium content, intravenous fluids that lack chloride (dextrose and water), draining fistulas and ileostomies, heart failure, cystic fibrosis	Agitation, irritability, tremors, muscle cramps, hyperactive deep tendon reflexes, hypertonicity, tetany, slow, shallow respirations, seizures, dysrhythmias, coma *Labs indicate:* ↓ serum chloride, ↓ serum sodium, ↑ pH, ↑ serum bicarbonate, ↑ total carbon dioxide content, ↓ urine chloride level

SODIUM DEFICIT (HYPONATREMIA)

Hyponatremia refers to a serum sodium level that is below normal (less than 135 mmol/L). Plasma sodium concentration represents the ratio of total body sodium to total body water. A decrease in this ratio can occur from a low quantity of total body sodium with a lesser reduction in total body water, normal total body sodium content with excess total body water, and an excess of total body sodium with an even greater excess of total body water. However, a hyponatremic state can be superimposed on an existing FVD or FVE.

Sodium may be lost by way of vomiting, diarrhea, fistulas, or sweating, or it may be associated with the use of diuretics, particularly in combination with a low-salt diet. A deficiency of aldosterone, as occurs in adrenal insufficiency, also predisposes the patient to sodium deficiency.

Dilutional Hyponatremia

In water intoxication (dilutional hyponatremia), the patient's serum sodium level is diluted by an increase in the ratio of water to sodium. This causes water to move into the cell, so that the patient develops an ECF volume excess. Predisposing conditions for this type of hyponatremia include syndrome of inappropriate antidiuretic hormone (SIADH), hyperglycemia, and increased water intake through the administration of electrolyte-poor parenteral fluids, the use of tap-water enemas, or the irrigation of nasogastric tubes with water instead of normal saline solution.

Water may be gained abnormally by the excessive parenteral administration of dextrose and water solutions, particularly during periods of stress. It may also be gained by compulsive water drinking (psychogenic polydipsia).

SIADH

The basic physiologic disturbances in SIADH are excessive ADH activity, with water retention and dilutional hyponatremia, and inappropriate urinary excretion of sodium in the presence of hyponatremia. SIADH can be the result of either sustained secretion of ADH by the hypothalamus or production of an ADH-like substance from a tumour (aberrant ADH production).

Conditions associated with SIADH include oat-cell lung tumours, head injuries, endocrine and pulmonary disorders, physiologic or psychological stress, and the use of medications such as oxytocin, cyclophosphamide, vincristine, thioridazine, and amitriptyline. SIADH is discussed in more detail in Chapter 42.

Clinical Manifestations

Clinical manifestations of hyponatremia depend on the cause, magnitude, and speed with which the deficit occurs. Poor skin turgor, dry mucosa, decreased saliva production, orthostatic fall in blood pressure, nausea, and abdominal cramping occur. Neurologic changes, including altered mental status, are probably related to the cellular swelling and cerebral edema associated with hyponatremia. As the extracellular sodium level decreases, the cellular fluid becomes relatively more concentrated and pulls water into the cells (Fig. 14-4). In general, patients with an acute decrease in serum sodium levels have more severe symptoms and higher mortality rates than do those with more slowly developing hyponatremia.

Features of hyponatremia associated with sodium loss and water gain include anorexia, muscle cramps, and a feeling of exhaustion. When the serum sodium level drops below 115 mmol/L, signs of increasing intracranial pressure, such as lethargy, confusion, muscle twitching, focal weakness, hemiparesis, papilledema, and seizures, may occur.

Assessment and Diagnostic Findings

Regardless of the cause of hyponatremia, the serum sodium level is less than 135 mmol/L; in SIADH it may be quite low, such as 100 mmol/L or less. Serum osmolality is also decreased, except in azotemia or ingestion of toxins. When hyponatremia is due primarily to sodium loss, the urinary sodium content is less than 20 mmol/L, suggesting increased proximal reabsorption of sodium secondary to ECF volume depletion; the specific gravity is low, such as 1.002 to 1.004. When hyponatremia is due to SIADH, however, the urinary sodium content is greater than 20 mmol/L and the urine specific gravity is usually over 1.012. Although the patient with SIADH retains water abnormally and thus gains body weight, there is no peripheral edema; instead, fluid accumulates inside the cells. This phenomenon is sometimes manifested as "fingerprinting" when the finger is pressed over a bony prominence, such as the sternum.

Medical Management

The key to treating hyponatremia is assessment; this includes the speed with which hyponatremia occurred rather than relying only on the patient's actual serum sodium value (Fall, 2000).

SODIUM REPLACEMENT

The obvious treatment for hyponatremia is careful administration of sodium by mouth, nasogastric tube, or the parenteral route. For patients who can eat and drink, sodium is easily replaced, because sodium is consumed abundantly in a normal diet. For those who cannot consume sodium, lactated Ringer's solution or isotonic saline (0.9% sodium chloride) solution may be prescribed. Serum sodium must not be increased by greater than 12 mmol/L in 24 hours, to avoid neurologic damage due to osmotic demyelination. This condition may occur when the serum sodium concentration is overcorrected (above 140 mmol/L) too rapidly or in the presence of hypoxia or anoxia (Pirzada & Imran, 2001). It may produce lesions in the pons that cause paraparesis, dysarthria, dysphagia, and coma. Table 14-5 describes the components of selected water and electrolyte solutions. The usual daily sodium requirement in adults is approximately 100 mmol, provided there are no abnormal losses.

In SIADH, the administration of hypertonic saline solution alone cannot change the plasma sodium concentration. Excess sodium would be excreted rapidly in a highly concentrated urine. With the addition of the diuretic furosemide (Lasix), urine is not concentrated and isotonic urine is excreted to effect a change in water balance. In patients with SIADH, in whom water restriction is difficult, lithium or demeclocycline can antagonize the osmotic effect of ADH on the medullary collecting tubule.

WATER RESTRICTION

In a patient with normal or excess fluid volume, hyponatremia is treated by restricting fluid to a total of 800 mL in 24 hours. This is far safer than sodium administration and is usually effective. When neurologic symptoms are present, however, it may be necessary to administer small volumes of a hypertonic sodium solution, such as 3% or 5% sodium chloride. Incorrect use of these fluids is extremely dangerous because 1 L of 3% sodium chloride solution contains 513 mmol of sodium, and 1 L of 5% sodium chloride solution contains 855 mmol of sodium. If edema exists alone, sodium is restricted; if edema and hyponatremia occur together, both sodium and water are restricted.

> **NURSING ALERT** Highly hypertonic sodium solutions (3% and 5% sodium chloride) should be administered only in intensive care settings under close observation, because only small volumes are needed to elevate the serum sodium level from a dangerously low value. These fluids are administered slowly and in small volumes, and the patient is monitored closely for fluid overload. The purpose is to relieve acute manifestations of cerebral edema and to prevent neurologic complications rather than to correct the sodium concentration specifically. Along with the sodium solution, the patient may receive a loop diuretic to prevent ECF volume overload and to increase water excretion.

Nursing Management

The nurse needs to identify patients at risk for hyponatremia so that they can be monitored. Early detection and treatment of this disorder are necessary to prevent serious consequences. For patients at risk, the nurse monitors fluid intake and output as well as daily body weights. Abnormal losses of sodium or gains of water are noted. GI manifestations, such as anorexia, nausea, vomiting, and abdominal cramping, are also noted. The nurse must be particularly alert for central nervous system changes, such as lethargy, confusion, muscle twitching, and seizures. In

FIGURE 14-4 Effect of extracellular sodium level on cell size.

general, more severe neurologic signs are associated with very low sodium levels that have fallen rapidly because of fluid overloading. Serum sodium levels are monitored very closely in patients at risk for hyponatremia; when indicated, urinary sodium levels and specific gravity are also monitored.

Hyponatremia is a frequently overlooked cause of confusion in elderly patients. The elderly are at increased risk for hyponatremia because of changes in renal function and subsequent decreased ability to excrete excessive water loads. Administration of medications causing sodium loss or water retention is a predisposing factor.

DETECTING AND CONTROLLING HYPONATREMIA

For patients experiencing abnormal losses of sodium who can consume a general diet, the nurse encourages foods and fluids with a high sodium content. For example, broth made with one beef cube contains approximately 900 mg of sodium; 250 mL of tomato juice contains approximately 700 mg of sodium. The nurse also needs to be familiar with the sodium content of parenteral fluids (see Table 14-5).

> **! NURSING ALERT** When administering fluids to patients with cardiovascular disease, the nurse assesses for signs of circulatory overload (eg, cough, dyspnea, puffy eyelids, dependent edema, or weight gain in 24 hours). The lungs are auscultated for crackles. Extreme care is taken when administering highly hypertonic sodium (eg, 3% or 5% sodium chloride) fluids, because these fluids can be lethal if infused carelessly.

For patients taking lithium, the nurse observes for lithium toxicity, particularly when sodium is lost by an abnormal route. In such instances, supplemental salt and fluid are administered. Because diuretics promote sodium loss, patients taking lithium are instructed not to use diuretics without close medical supervision. For all patients on lithium therapy, adequate salt intake should be ensured.

Excess water supplements are avoided in patients receiving isotonic or hypotonic enteral feedings, particularly if abnormal sodium loss occurs or water is being abnormally retained (as in SIADH). Actual fluid needs are determined by evaluating fluid intake and output, urine specific gravity, and serum sodium levels.

RETURNING SODIUM LEVEL TO NORMAL

When the primary problem is water retention, it is safer to restrict fluid intake than to administer sodium. Administering sodium to a patient with normovolemia or hypervolemia predisposes the patient to fluid volume overload. As stated previously, the nurse must monitor patients with cardiovascular disease very closely.

In severe hyponatremia, the aim of therapy is to elevate the serum sodium level only enough to alleviate neurologic signs and symptoms. It is generally recommended that the serum sodium concentration be raised no higher than 125 mmol/L with a hypertonic saline solution.

SODIUM EXCESS (HYPERNATREMIA)

Hypernatremia is a higher-than-normal serum sodium level (exceeding 145 mmol/L) (Adrogue & Madias, 2000a). It can be caused by a gain of sodium in excess of water or by a loss of water in excess of sodium. It can occur in patients with normal fluid volume or in those with FVD or FVE. With a water loss, the patient loses more water than sodium; as a result, the serum sodium

concentration increases and the increased concentration pulls fluid out of the cell. This is both an extracellular and intracellular FVD. In sodium excess, the patient ingests or retains more sodium than water.

Pathophysiology

A common cause of hypernatremia is fluid deprivation in unconscious patients who cannot perceive, respond to, or communicate their thirst (Adrogue & Madias, 2000a). Most often affected in this regard are very old, very young, and cognitively impaired patients. Administration of hypertonic enteral feedings without adequate water supplements leads to hypernatremia, as does watery diarrhea and greatly increased insensible water loss (eg, hyperventilation, denuding effects of burns).

Diabetes insipidus, a deficiency of ADH from the posterior pituitary gland, leads to hypernatremia if the patient does not experience, or cannot respond to, thirst or if fluids are excessively restricted. Less common causes are heat stroke, near-drowning in sea water (which contains a sodium concentration of approximately 500 mmol/L), and malfunction of either hemodialysis or peritoneal dialysis proportioning systems. IV administration of hypertonic saline or excessive use of sodium bicarbonate also causes hypernatremia.

Clinical Manifestations

The clinical manifestations of hypernatremia are primarily neurologic and are presumably the consequence of cellular dehydration (Adrogue & Madias, 2000a). Hypernatremia results in a relatively concentrated ECF, causing water to be pulled from the cells (see Fig. 14-4). Clinically, these changes may be manifested by restlessness and weakness in moderate hypernatremia and by disorientation, delusions, and hallucinations in severe hypernatremia. Dehydration (resulting in hypernatremia) is often overlooked as the primary reason for behavioural changes in the elderly patient. If hypernatremia is severe, permanent brain damage can occur (especially in children). Brain damage is apparently due to subarachnoid hemorrhages that result from brain contraction.

A primary characteristic of hypernatremia is thirst. Thirst is so strong a defender of serum sodium levels in healthy people that hypernatremia never occurs unless the person is unconscious or is denied access to water. Unfortunately, ill people may have an impaired thirst mechanism. Other signs include a dry, swollen tongue and sticky mucous membranes. Flushed skin, peripheral and pulmonary edema, postural hypotension, and increased muscle tone and deep tendon reflexes are additional signs and symptoms of hypernatremia. Body temperature may rise mildly but returns to normal when the hypernatremia is corrected.

Assessment and Diagnostic Findings

In hypernatremia, the serum sodium level exceeds 145 mmol/L and the serum osmolality exceeds 295 mmol/L. The urine specific gravity and urine osmolality are increased as the kidneys attempt to conserve water (provided the water loss is from a route other than the kidneys) (Fall, 2000).

Medical Management

Hypernatremia treatment consists of a gradual lowering of the serum sodium level by the infusion of a hypotonic electrolyte solution (eg, 0.3% sodium chloride) or an isotonic nonsaline solution (eg, dextrose 5% in water [D_5W]). D_5W is indicated when water needs to be replaced without sodium. Many clinicians consider a hypotonic sodium solution to be safer than D_5W because it allows a gradual reduction in the serum sodium level and thereby decreases the risk of cerebral edema. It is the solution of choice in severe hyperglycemia with hypernatremia. A rapid reduction in the serum sodium level temporarily decreases the plasma osmolality below that of the fluid in the brain tissue, causing dangerous cerebral edema. Diuretics also may be prescribed to treat the sodium gain.

There is no consensus about the exact rate at which serum sodium levels should be reduced. As a general rule, the serum sodium level is reduced at a rate no faster than 0.5 to 1 mmol/L to allow sufficient time for readjustment through diffusion across fluid compartments. Desmopressin acetate (DDAVP) may be prescribed to treat diabetes insipidus if it is the cause of hypernatremia.

Nursing Management

As in hyponatremia, fluid losses and gains are carefully monitored in patients at risk for hypernatremia. The nurse should assess for abnormal losses of water or low water intake and for large gains of sodium, as might occur with ingestion of over-the-counter medications with a high sodium content (such as Alka-Seltzer). Also, it is important to obtain a medication history because some prescription medications have a high sodium content. In addition, the nurse notes the patient's thirst or elevated body temperature and evaluates it in relation to other clinical signs. The nurse monitors for changes in behaviour, such as restlessness, disorientation, and lethargy.

PREVENTING HYPERNATREMIA

The nurse attempts to prevent hypernatremia by offering fluids at regular intervals, particularly in debilitated patients unable to perceive or respond to thirst. If fluid intake remains inadequate, the nurse consults with the physician to plan an alternate route for intake, either by enteral feedings or by the parenteral route. If enteral feedings are used, sufficient water should be administered to keep the serum sodium and BUN within normal limits. As a rule, the higher the osmolality of the enteral feeding, the greater the need for water supplementation.

For patients with diabetes insipidus, adequate water intake must be ensured. If the patient is alert and has an intact thirst mechanism, merely providing access to water may be sufficient. If the patient has a decreased level of consciousness or other disability interfering with adequate fluid intake, parenteral fluid replacement may be prescribed. This therapy can be anticipated in patients with neurologic disorders, particularly in the early postoperative period.

CORRECTING HYPERNATREMIA

When parenteral fluids are necessary for managing hypernatremia, the nurse monitors the patient's response to the fluids by reviewing serial serum sodium levels and by observing for changes in neurologic signs. With a gradual decrease in the serum sodium level, the neurologic signs should improve. As stated in the discussion on management, too-rapid reduction in the serum sodium level renders the plasma temporarily hypo-osmotic to the fluid in the brain tissue, causing movement of fluid into brain cells and dangerous cerebral edema (Adrogue & Madias, 2000a).

SIGNIFICANCE OF POTASSIUM

Potassium is the major intracellular electrolyte; in fact, 98% of the body's potassium is inside the cells. The remaining 2% is in the ECF, and it is this 2% that is important in neuromuscular function. Potassium influences both skeletal and cardiac muscle activity. For example, alterations in its concentration change myocardial irritability and rhythm. Under the influence of the sodium–potassium pump and based on the body's needs, potassium is constantly moving in and out of cells. The normal serum potassium concentration ranges from 3.5–5.5 mmol/L, and even minor variations are significant. Potassium imbalances are commonly associated with various diseases, injuries, medications (diuretics, laxatives, antibiotics), and special treatments, such as parenteral nutrition and chemotherapy (Cohn et al., 2000).

To maintain potassium balance, the renal system must function because 80% of the potassium is excreted daily from the body by way of the kidneys; the other 20% is lost through the bowel and in sweat. The kidneys are the primary regulators of potassium balance and accomplish this by adjusting the amount of potassium that is excreted in the urine. As serum potassium levels increase, so does the potassium level in the renal tubular cell. A concentration gradient occurs, favouring the movement of potassium into the renal tubule with the loss of potassium in the urine. Aldosterone also increases the excretion of potassium by the kidney. Because the kidneys do not conserve potassium as well as they conserve sodium, potassium may still be lost in urine in the presence of a potassium deficit.

POTASSIUM DEFICIT (HYPOKALEMIA)

Hypokalemia (below-normal serum potassium concentration) usually indicates an actual deficit in total potassium stores. Hypokalemia may occur in patients with normal potassium stores; however, when alkalosis is present, a temporary shift of serum potassium into the cells occurs (see discussion of alkalosis later in this chapter).

As stated earlier, hypokalemia is a common imbalance (Gennari, 1998). GI loss of potassium is probably the most common cause of potassium depletion. Vomiting and gastric suction frequently lead to hypokalemia, partly because potassium is actually lost when gastric fluid is lost, but more so because potassium is lost through the kidneys in association with metabolic alkalosis. Because relatively large amounts of potassium are contained in intestinal fluids, potassium deficit occurs frequently with diarrhea. Intestinal fluid may contain as much potassium as 30 mmol/L. Potassium deficit also occurs from prolonged intestinal suctioning, recent ileostomy, and villous adenoma (a tumour of the intestinal tract characterized by excretion of potassium-rich mucus).

Alterations in acid–base balance have a significant effect on potassium distribution. The mechanism involves shifts of hydrogen and potassium ions between the cells and the ECF. Hypokalemia can cause alkalosis, and in turn alkalosis can cause hypokalemia. For example, hydrogen ions move out of the cells in alkalotic states to help correct the high pH, and potassium ions move in to maintain an electrically neutral state. (This is discussed further in the section on acid–base balance.)

Hyperaldosteronism increases renal potassium wasting and can lead to severe potassium depletion. Primary hyperaldosteronism is seen in patients with adrenal adenomas. Secondary hyperaldosteronism occurs in patients with cirrhosis, nephrotic syndrome, heart failure, and malignant hypertension (Wilcox, 1999).

Potassium-losing diuretics, such as the thiazides (eg, chlorothiazide [Diuril] and polythiazide [Renese]), can induce hypokalemia, particularly when administered in large doses to patients with inadequate potassium intake. Other medications that can lead to hypokalemia include corticosteroids, sodium penicillin, carbenicillin, and amphotericin B (Cohn et al., 2000; Gennari, 1998).

Because insulin promotes the entry of potassium into skeletal muscle and hepatic cells, patients with persistent insulin hypersecretion may experience hypokalemia, which is often the case in patients receiving high-carbohydrate parenteral fluids (as in parenteral nutrition).

Patients who are unable or unwilling to eat a normal diet for a prolonged period are at risk for hypokalemia. This may occur in debilitated elderly people, alcoholics, and patients with anorexia nervosa. In addition to poor intake, people with bulimia frequently suffer increased potassium loss through self-induced vomiting and laxative and diuretic abuse.

Magnesium depletion causes renal potassium loss and must be corrected first; otherwise, urine loss of potassium will continue. Penicillins may produce renal potassium loss by acting as poorly reabsorbable anions and thus increasing distal sodium delivery and sodium-potassium loss.

Clinical Manifestations

Potassium deficiency can result in widespread derangements in physiologic function. Severe hypokalemia can cause death through cardiac or respiratory arrest. Clinical signs rarely develop before the serum potassium level has fallen below 3 mmol/L unless the rate of fall has been rapid. Manifestations of hypokalemia include fatigue, anorexia, nausea, vomiting, muscle weakness, leg cramps, decreased bowel motility, paresthesias (numbness and tingling), dysrhythmias, and increased sensitivity to digitalis (Gennari, 1998). If prolonged, hypokalemia can lead to an inability of the kidneys to concentrate urine, causing dilute urine (resulting in polyuria, nocturia) and excessive thirst. Potassium depletion depresses the release of insulin and results in glucose intolerance.

Assessment and Diagnostic Findings

In hypokalemia, the serum potassium concentration is less than the lower limit of normal. Electrocardiographic (ECG) changes can include flat T waves and/or inverted T waves, suggesting ischemia, and depressed ST segments (Fig. 14-5). An elevated U wave is specific to hypokalemia. Hypokalemia increases sensitivity to digitalis, predisposing the patient to digitalis toxicity at lower digitalis levels. Metabolic alkalosis is commonly associated with hypokalemia. This is discussed further in the section on acid–base disturbances.

The source of the potassium loss is usually evident from a careful history. When this is not the case, however, and the etiology of the loss is unclear, a 24-hour urinary potassium excretion test can be performed to distinguish between renal and extrarenal loss. Urinary potassium excretion exceeding 20 mmol/24 h with hypokalemia suggests that renal potassium loss is the cause.

Medical Management

If hypokalemia cannot be prevented by conventional measures such as increased intake in the daily diet, it is treated with oral or IV replacement therapy (Gennari, 1998). Potassium loss must be corrected daily; administration of 40 to 80 mmol/day of potas-

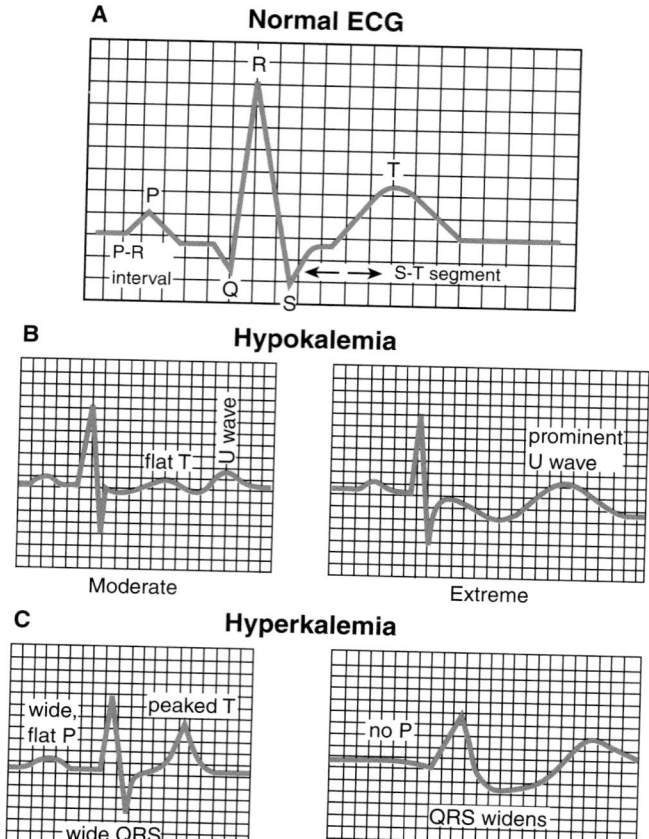

FIGURE 14-5 Effect of potassium on ECG. (**A**) Normal tracing. (**B**) Hypokalemia: serum potassium level below normal. Figure on *left* illustrates flattening of the T wave and the appearance of a U wave. Figure on *right* illustrates further flattening with prominent U wave. (**C**) Hyperkalemia: serum potassium level above normal. Figure on *left* illustrates moderate elevation with wide, flat P wave, wide QRS complex, and peaked T wave. Figure on *right* illustrates ECG changes seen with extreme potassium elevation: widening of QRS complex and absence of P wave.

sium is adequate in the adult if there are no abnormal losses of potassium.

For patients at risk for hypokalemia, a diet containing sufficient potassium should be provided. Dietary intake of potassium in the average adult is 50 to 100 mmol/day. Foods high in potassium include fruits (especially raisins, bananas, apricots, and oranges), vegetables, legumes, whole grains, milk, and meat.

When dietary intake is inadequate for any reason, the physician may prescribe oral or IV potassium supplements (Gennari, 1998). Many salt substitutes contain 50 to 60 mmol of potassium per teaspoon and may be sufficient to prevent hypokalemia.

 NURSING ALERT Oral potassium supplements can produce small bowel lesions; therefore, the patient must be assessed for and cautioned about abdominal distention, pain, or GI bleeding.

When oral administration of potassium is not feasible, the IV route is indicated. The IV route is mandatory for patients with severe hypokalemia (eg, a serum level of 2 mmol/L). Although potassium chloride is usually used to correct potassium deficits, the physician may prescribe potassium acetate or potassium phosphate.

Nursing Management

Because hypokalemia can be life-threatening, the nurse needs to monitor for its early presence in patients at risk. Fatigue, anorexia, muscle weakness, decreased bowel motility, paresthesias, and dysrhythmias are signals that warrant assessing the serum potassium concentration. When available, the ECG may provide useful information. For example, patients receiving digitalis who are at risk for potassium deficiency should be monitored closely for signs of digitalis toxicity, because hypokalemia potentiates the action of digitalis. Physicians usually prefer to keep the serum potassium level above 3.5 mmol/L in patients receiving digitalis medications such as digoxin.

PREVENTING HYPOKALEMIA

Measures are taken to prevent hypokalemia when possible (Gennari, 1998). Prevention may involve encouraging the patient at risk to eat foods rich in potassium (when the diet allows). Sources of potassium include fruit and fruit juices (bananas, melon, citrus fruit), fresh and frozen vegetables, fresh meats, and processed foods. When hypokalemia is due to abuse of laxatives or diuretics, patient education may help alleviate the problem. Part of the health history and assessment should be directed at identifying problems amenable to prevention through education. Careful monitoring of fluid intake and output is necessary because 40 mmol of potassium is lost for every litre of urine output. The ECG is monitored for changes, and arterial blood gas values are checked for elevated bicarbonate and pH levels.

CORRECTING HYPOKALEMIA

Great care should be exercised when administering potassium, particularly in older adults, who have lower lean body mass and total body potassium levels and therefore lower potassium requirements. Additionally, with the physiologic loss of renal function with advancing years, potassium may be retained more readily in older than in younger people.

ADMINISTERING IV POTASSIUM

Potassium should be administered only after adequate urine flow has been established. A decrease in urine volume to less than 20 mL/h for 2 consecutive hours is an indication to stop the potassium infusion until the situation is evaluated. Potassium is primarily excreted by the kidneys; therefore, when oliguria occurs, potassium administration can cause the serum potassium concentration to rise dangerously.

 NURSING ALERT Potassium is never administered IV push or intramuscularly. IV potassium must be administered using an infusion pump to avoid replacing potassium too quickly.

Each health care facility has its own standard of care, which should be consulted; however, IV potassium should not be administered faster than 20 mmol/h or in concentrations greater than 30 to 40 mmol/L unless hypokalemia is severe, because this can cause life-threatening dysrhythmias. When prepared for IV infusions, the fluid should be agitated well to prevent bolus doses that can result when the potassium concentrates at the bottom of the IV container.

 NURSING ALERT Stocking premixed 100-mL minibags of 20 mmol KCl is a safe alternative to adding a vial of KCl to an IV bag. The KCl must be well distributed to prevent it from pooling at the insertion site at the bottom of the bag and causing a life-threatening elevation of the serum potassium level.

When potassium is administered through a peripheral vein, the rate of administration must be decreased to avoid irritating the vein and causing a burning sensation during administration. In general, concentrations greater than 60 mmol/L are not administered in peripheral veins because venous pain and sclerosis may occur. For routine maintenance needs, potassium is suitably diluted and administered at a rate no faster than 10 mmol/h. In critical situations, more concentrated solutions (such as 40 mmol/L) may be administered through a central line. Even in extreme hypokalemia, however, potassium should be administered no faster than 20 to 40 mmol/h (suitably diluted). In such a situation, the patient must be monitored by ECG and observed closely for other signs and symptoms, such as changes in muscle strength.

POTASSIUM EXCESS (HYPERKALEMIA)

Hyperkalemia (greater-than-normal serum potassium concentration) seldom occurs in patients with normal renal function. Like hypokalemia, hyperkalemia is often due to iatrogenic (treatment-induced) causes. Although less common than hypokalemia, hyperkalemia is usually more dangerous because cardiac arrest is more frequently associated with high serum potassium levels.

A variation of hyperkalemia, pseudohyperkalemia has a number of causes The most common causes are the use of a tight tourniquet around an exercising extremity while drawing a blood sample and hemolysis of the sample before analysis. Other causes include marked leukocytosis (white blood cell count exceeding 2.0×10^{11}/L) or thrombocytosis (platelet count exceeding 1.0×10^{12}/L), drawing blood above a site where potassium is infusing, and familial pseudohyperkalemia, where potassium leaks out of the red blood cells while the blood is awaiting analysis. Failure to be aware of these causes of pseudohyperkalemia can lead to aggressive treatment of a nonexistent hyperkalemia, resulting in serious lowering of serum potassium levels. Thus, measurements of grossly elevated levels should be verified.

The major cause of hyperkalemia is decreased renal excretion of potassium. Thus, significant hyperkalemia is commonly seen in patients with untreated renal failure, particularly those in whom potassium levels rise as a result of infection or excessive intake of potassium in food or medications. In addition, patients with hypoaldosteronism and Addison's disease are at risk for hyperkalemia because these conditions are characterized by deficient adrenal hormones, leading to sodium loss and potassium retention.

Medications have been identified as a probable contributing factor in more than 60% of hyperkalemic episodes. Medications commonly implicated are potassium chloride, heparin, ACE inhibitors, captopril, NSAIDs, and potassium-sparing diuretics. In most such cases, potassium regulation is compromised by renal insufficiency (Perazella, 2000).

Although a high intake of potassium can cause severe hyperkalemia in patients with impaired renal function, hyperkalemia rarely occurs in people with normal renal function. For all patients, however, improper use of potassium supplements predisposes them to hyperkalemia, especially when salt substitutes are used. Not all patients receiving potassium-losing diuretics require potassium supplements, and patients receiving potassium-conserving diuretics should not receive supplements.

> ![] **NURSING ALERT** Potassium supplements are extremely dangerous when patients have impaired renal function and thus decreased ability to excrete potassium. Even more dangerous is the IV administration of potassium to such patients, as serum levels can rise very quickly. Aged (stored) blood should not be administered to patients with impaired renal function because the serum potassium concentration of stored blood increases as the storage time increases, a result of red blood cell deterioration. It is possible to exceed the renal tolerance of any patient with rapid IV potassium administration, as well as when large amounts of oral potassium supplements are ingested.

In **acidosis**, potassium moves out of the cells into the ECF. This occurs as hydrogen ions enter the cells, a process that buffers the pH of the ECF (acidosis is discussed later in this chapter). An elevated extracellular potassium level should be anticipated when extensive tissue trauma has occurred, as in burns, crushing injuries, or severe infections. Similarly, it can occur with lysis of malignant cells after chemotherapy.

Clinical Manifestations

The most important consequence of hyperkalemia is its effect on the myocardium. Cardiac effects of an elevated serum potassium level are usually not significant below a concentration of 7 mmol/L, but they are almost always present when the level is 8 mmol/L or greater. As the plasma potassium level rises, disturbances in cardiac conduction occur. The earliest changes, often occurring at a serum potassium level greater than 6 mmol/L, are peaked, narrow T waves; ST-segment depression; and a shortened QT interval. If the serum potassium level continues to rise, the PR interval becomes prolonged and is followed by disappearance of the P waves. Finally, there is decomposition and prolongation of the QRS complex (see Fig. 14-5). Ventricular dysrhythmias and cardiac arrest may occur at any point in this progression.

Severe hyperkalemia causes skeletal muscle weakness and even paralysis, related to a depolarization block in muscle. Similarly, ventricular conduction is slowed. Although hyperkalemia has marked effects on the peripheral nervous system, it has little effect on the central nervous system. Rapidly ascending muscular weakness leading to flaccid quadriplegia has been reported in patients with very high serum potassium levels. Paralysis of respiratory and speech muscles can also occur. Additionally, GI manifestations, such as nausea, intermittent intestinal colic, and diarrhea, may occur in hyperkalemic patients.

Assessment and Diagnostic Findings

Serum potassium levels and ECG changes are crucial to the diagnosis of hyperkalemia, as discussed above. Arterial blood gas analysis may reveal metabolic acidosis; in many cases, hyperkalemia occurs with acidosis.

Medical Management

An immediate ECG should be obtained to detect changes. Shortened repolarization and peaked T waves are seen initially. It is prudent as well to obtain a repeat serum potassium level from a vein without an IV infusion containing potassium to verify results.

In nonacute situations, restriction of dietary potassium and potassium-containing medications may suffice. For example, eliminating the use of potassium-containing salt substitutes in the patient taking a potassium-conserving diuretic may be all that is needed to deal with mild hyperkalemia.

Prevention of serious hyperkalemia by the administration, either orally or by retention enema, of cation exchange resins (eg, Kayexalate) may be necessary in patients with renal impairment. Cation exchange resins cannot be used if the patient has a paralytic ileus because intestinal perforation can occur. Kayexalate can bind with other cations in the GI tract and contribute to the development of hypomagnesemia and hypocalcemia; it may also cause sodium retention and fluid overload (Karch, 2002).

EMERGENCY PHARMACOLOGIC THERAPY

When serum potassium levels are dangerously elevated, it may be necessary to administer IV calcium gluconate. Within minutes after administration, calcium antagonizes the action of hyperkalemia on the heart. Infusion of calcium does not reduce the serum potassium concentration but immediately antagonizes the adverse cardiac conduction abnormalities. Calcium chloride and calcium gluconate are not interchangeable: calcium gluconate contains 4.5 mmol of calcium and calcium chloride contains 13.6 mmol of calcium; therefore, caution must be used.

Monitoring the blood pressure is essential to detect hypotension, which may result from the rapid IV administration of calcium gluconate. The ECG should be continuously monitored during administration; the appearance of bradycardia is an indication to stop the infusion. The myocardial protective effects of calcium are transient, lasting about 30 minutes. Extra caution is required if the patient has been "digitalized" (received accelerated dosages of a digitalis-based cardiac glycoside to reach a desired serum digitalis level rapidly) because parenteral administration of calcium sensitizes the heart to digitalis and may precipitate digitalis toxicity.

IV administration of sodium bicarbonate may be necessary to alkalinize the plasma and cause a temporary shift of potassium into the cells. Also, sodium bicarbonate furnishes sodium to antagonize the cardiac effects of potassium. Effects of this therapy begin within 30 to 60 minutes and may persist for hours; however, they are temporary.

IV administration of regular insulin and a hypertonic dextrose solution causes a temporary shift of potassium into the cells. Glucose and insulin therapy has an onset of action within 30 minutes and lasts for several hours.

Beta-2 agonists also move potassium into the cells and may be used in the absence of ischemic cardiac disease. These stopgap measures only temporarily protect the patient from hyperkalemia. If the hyperkalemic condition is not transient, actual removal of potassium from the body is required; this may be accomplished by using cation exchange resins, peritoneal dialysis, hemodialysis or other forms of renal replacement therapy.

Nursing Management

Patients at risk for potassium excess, for example those with renal failure, should be identified so they can be monitored closely for signs of hyperkalemia. The nurse observes for signs of muscle weakness and dysrhythmias. The presence of paresthesias is noted, as are GI symptoms such as nausea and intestinal colic. For patients at risk, serum potassium levels are measured periodically.

Elevated serum potassium levels may be erroneous; thus, highly abnormal levels should always be verified. To avoid false reports of hyperkalemia, prolonged use of a tourniquet while drawing the blood sample is avoided, and the patient is cautioned not to exercise the extremity immediately before the blood sample is obtained. The blood sample is delivered to the laboratory as soon as possible, because hemolysis of the sample results in a falsely elevated serum potassium level.

PREVENTING HYPERKALEMIA

Measures are taken to prevent hyperkalemia in patients at risk, when possible, by encouraging the patient to adhere to the prescribed potassium restriction. Potassium-rich foods to be avoided include coffee, cocoa, tea, dried fruits, dried beans, and whole-grain breads. Milk and eggs also contain substantial amounts of potassium. Conversely, foods with minimal potassium content include butter, margarine, cranberry juice or sauce, ginger ale, gumdrops or jellybeans, hard candy, root beer, sugar, and honey.

CORRECTING HYPERKALEMIA

As stated earlier, it is possible to exceed the tolerance for potassium in any person if it is administered rapidly by the IV route. Therefore, great care should be taken to monitor potassium solutions closely, paying close attention to the solution's concentration and rate of administration. When potassium is added to parenteral solutions, the potassium is mixed with the fluid by inverting the bottle several times. Potassium chloride should never be added to a hanging bottle because the potassium might be administered as a bolus (potassium chloride is heavy and settles to the bottom of the container).

It is important to caution patients to use salt substitutes sparingly if they are taking other supplementary forms of potassium or potassium-conserving diuretics. Also, potassium-conserving diuretics, such as spironolactone (Aldactone); potassium supplements; and salt substitutes should not be administered to patients with renal dysfunction. Most salt substitutes contain approximately 50–60 mmol of potassium per teaspoon.

SIGNIFICANCE OF CALCIUM

More than 99% of the body's calcium is located in the skeletal system; it is a major component of bones and teeth. About 1% of skeletal calcium is rapidly exchangeable with blood calcium; the rest is more stable and only slowly exchanged. The small amount of calcium located outside the bone circulates in the serum, partly bound to protein and partly ionized. Calcium plays a major role in transmitting nerve impulses and helps to regulate muscle contraction and relaxation, including cardiac muscle. Calcium is instrumental in activating enzymes that stimulate many essential chemical reactions in the body, and it also plays a role in blood coagulation. Because many factors affect calcium regulation, both hypocalcemia and hypercalcemia are relatively common disturbances.

The normal total serum calcium level is 2.1–2.6 mmol/L. It exists in plasma in three forms: ionized, bound, and complexed. About 50% of the serum calcium exists in an ionized form that is physiologically active and important for neuromuscular activity and blood coagulation. The normal ionized serum calcium level is 1.1–1.3 mmol/L and is the only form that is physiologically and clinically significant. Less than half of the plasma calcium is bound to serum proteins, primarily albumin. The remainder is combined with nonprotein anions: phosphate, citrate, and carbonate.

Calcium is absorbed from foods in the presence of normal gastric acidity and vitamin D. Calcium is excreted primarily in the feces, the remainder in urine. The serum calcium level is controlled by PTH and calcitonin. As ionized serum calcium decreases, the parathyroid glands secrete PTH. This event then increases calcium absorption from the GI tract, increases calcium reabsorption from the renal tubule, and releases calcium from the bone. The increase in calcium ion concentration suppresses PTH secretion. When calcium increases excessively, the thyroid gland secretes calcitonin. It briefly inhibits calcium reabsorption from bone and decreases the serum calcium concentration.

CALCIUM DEFICIT (HYPOCALCEMIA)

Hypocalcemia (lower-than-normal serum concentration of calcium) occurs in a variety of clinical situations. A patient may have a total body calcium deficit (as in osteoporosis) but a normal serum calcium level. Elderly people with osteoporosis, who spend an increased amount of time in bed, are at increased risk for hypocalcemia as bed rest increases bone resorption.

Several factors can cause hypocalcemia. Primary hypoparathyroidism results in this disturbance, as does surgical hypoparathyroidism. The latter is far more common. Not only is hypocalcemia associated with thyroid and parathyroid surgery, but it can also occur after radical neck dissection and is most likely in the first 24 to 48 hours after surgery. Transient hypocalcemia can occur with massive administration of citrated blood (as in exchange transfusions in newborns), because citrate can combine with ionized calcium and temporarily remove it from the circulation.

Inflammation of the pancreas causes the breakdown of proteins and lipids. It is thought that calcium ions combine with the fatty acids released by lipolysis, forming soaps. As a result of this process, hypocalcemia occurs and is common in pancreatitis. It has also been suggested that hypocalcemia might be related to excessive secretion of glucagon from the inflamed pancreas, resulting in increased secretion of calcitonin (a hormone that lowers serum calcium).

Hypocalcemia is common in patients with renal failure because these patients frequently have elevated serum phosphate levels. Hyperphosphatemia usually causes a reciprocal drop in the serum calcium level. Other causes of hypocalcemia include inadequate vitamin D consumption, magnesium deficiency, medullary thyroid carcinoma, low serum albumin levels, alkalosis, and alcohol abuse. Medications predisposing to hypocalcemia include aluminum-containing antacids, aminoglycosides, caffeine, cisplatin, corticosteroids, mithramycin, phosphates, isoniazid, and loop diuretics.

Osteoporosis is associated with prolonged low intake of calcium and represents a total body calcium deficit, even though serum calcium levels are usually normal. This disorder occurs in many Canadians and is most common in postmenopausal women. It is characterized by loss of bone mass, causing bones to become porous and brittle and therefore susceptible to fracture. See Chapter 68 for further discussion of osteoporosis.

Clinical Manifestations

Tetany is the most characteristic manifestation of hypocalcemia and hypomagnesemia. Tetany refers to the entire symptom complex induced by increased neural excitability. These symptoms are due to spontaneous discharges of both sensory and motor fibres in peripheral nerves. Sensations of tingling may occur in the tips of the fingers, around the mouth, and less commonly in the feet. Spasms of the muscles of the extremities and face may occur. Pain may develop as a result of these spasms.

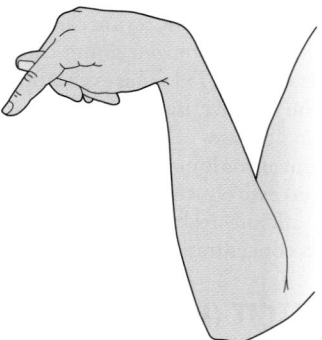

FIGURE 14-6 Trousseau's sign. Ischemia-induced carpal spasm can occur with hypocalcemia or hypomagnesemia.

Trousseau's sign (Fig. 14-6) can be elicited by inflating a blood pressure cuff on the upper arm to about 20 mm Hg above systolic pressure; within 2 to 5 minutes, carpopedal spasm (an adducted thumb, flexed wrist and metacarpophalangeal joints, extended interphalangeal joints with fingers together) will occur as ischemia of the ulnar nerve develops. Chvostek's sign consists of twitching of muscles supplied by the facial nerve when the nerve is tapped about 2 cm anterior to the earlobe, just below the zygomatic arch.

Seizures may occur because hypocalcemia increases irritability of the central nervous system as well as of the peripheral nerves. Other changes associated with hypocalcemia include mental changes such as depression, impaired memory, confusion, delirium, and even hallucinations. A prolonged QT interval is seen on the ECG due to prolongation of the ST segment; a form of ventricular tachycardia called torsades de pointes may occur.

Assessment and Diagnostic Findings

When evaluating serum calcium levels, one must consider several other variables, such as the serum albumin level and arterial pH. Because abnormalities in serum albumin levels may affect interpretation of the serum calcium level, it may be necessary to calculate the corrected serum calcium if the serum albumin level is abnormal. For every decrease in serum albumin of 10 g/L below 40 g/L, the total serum calcium level is underestimated by approximately 0.02 mmol/L. The following is a quick method to calculate the corrected serum calcium level:

Corrected total serum calcium concentration (mmol/L)

$$= \text{measured total serum Ca}^{++} \text{ level (mmol/L)} + 0.02\,\frac{\text{mmol/L}}{\text{g/L}}$$
$$\times\,(40\ \text{g/L} - \text{measured serum albumin [g/L]})$$

An example of the calculation needed to obtain the corrected total serum calcium level is as follows:

A patient's reported serum albumin level is 25 g/L; the reported serum calcium level is 2.63 mmol/L.

Corrected total serum calcium concentration

$$= 2.63\ \text{mmol/L} + 0.02\,\frac{\text{mmol/L}}{\text{g/L}} \times (40\ \text{g/L} - 25\ \text{g/L})$$
$$= 2.63\ \text{mmol/L} + 0.02\,\frac{\text{mmol/L}}{\text{g/L}} \times 15\ \text{g/L}$$
$$= 2.63\ \text{mmol/L} + 0.3\ \text{mmol/L}$$
$$= 2.93\ \text{mmol/L}$$

Clinicians often ignore a low serum calcium level in the presence of a similarly low serum albumin level. The ionized calcium level is usually normal in patients with reduced total serum calcium levels and concomitant hypoalbuminemia. When the arterial pH increases (alkalosis), more calcium becomes bound to protein. As a result, the ionized portion decreases. Symptoms of hypocalcemia may occur with alkalosis. Acidosis (low pH) has the opposite effect—that is, less calcium is bound to protein and thus more exists in the ionized form. However, relatively small changes in serum calcium levels occur in these acid–base abnormalities.

Ideally, the laboratory should measure the ionized level of calcium. In many laboratories, however, only the total calcium level is reported; thus, concentration of the ionized fraction must be estimated by simultaneous measurement of the serum albumin level. PTH levels are decreased in hypoparathyroidism. Magnesium and phosphorus levels need to be assessed to identify possible causes of decreased calcium.

Medical Management

Acute symptomatic hypocalcemia is life-threatening and requires prompt treatment with IV administration of calcium (Marx, 2000). Parenteral calcium salts include calcium gluconate, calcium chloride, and calcium gluceptate. Although calcium chloride produces a significantly higher ionized calcium level than calcium gluconate, it is not used as often because it is more irritating and can cause sloughing of tissue if it infiltrates. Too-rapid IV administration of calcium can cause cardiac arrest, preceded by bradycardia. IV calcium administration is particularly dangerous in patients receiving digitalis-derived medications because calcium ions exert an effect similar to that of digitalis and can cause digitalis toxicity, with adverse cardiac effects. IV calcium should be diluted in D_5W and given as a slow IV bolus or a slow IV infusion using a volumetric infusion pump. The IV site must be observed often for any evidence of infiltration because of the risk for sloughing of tissues with calcium infusions. A 0.9% sodium chloride solution should not be used with calcium because it will increase renal calcium loss. Solutions containing phosphates or bicarbonate should not be used with calcium because they will cause precipitation when calcium is added. The nurse must clarify with the physician which calcium salt to administer, because calcium gluconate yields 4.5 mmol of calcium and calcium chloride provides 13.6 mmol of calcium. Calcium can cause postural hypotension; therefore, the patient is kept in bed for IV replacement and blood pressure is monitored.

Vitamin D therapy may be instituted to increase calcium absorption from the GI tract. Aluminum hydroxide, calcium acetate, or calcium carbonate antacids may be prescribed to decrease elevated phosphorus levels before treating hypocalcemia for the patient with chronic renal failure. Increasing the dietary intake of calcium to at least 1,000 to 1,500 mg/day in the adult is recommended (eg, milk products; green, leafy vegetables; canned salmon; sardines; fresh oysters). Because hypomagnesemia can also cause tetany, if the tetany responds to IV calcium, then a low magnesium level is explored as a possible cause in chronic renal failure.

Nursing Management

It is important to observe for hypocalcemia in patients at risk. Seizure precautions are initiated when hypocalcemia is severe. The status of the airway is closely monitored because laryngeal stridor can occur. Safety precautions are taken, as indicated, if confusion is present.

People at high risk for osteoporosis are instructed about the need for adequate dietary calcium intake; if not consumed in the diet, calcium supplements should be considered. Also, the value of regular weight-bearing exercise in decreasing bone loss should be emphasized, as should the effect of medications on calcium balance. For example, alcohol and caffeine in high doses inhibit calcium absorption, and moderate cigarette smoking increases urinary calcium excretion. Additional teaching topics may involve discussion of medications such as alendronate (Fosamax), risedronate (Actonel), raloxifene (Evista), and calcitonin to reduce the rate of bone loss. Teaching also addresses strategies to reduce risk for falls.

CALCIUM EXCESS (HYPERCALCEMIA)

Hypercalcemia (excess of calcium in the plasma) is a dangerous imbalance when severe; in fact, hypercalcemic crisis has a mortality rate as high as 50% if not treated promptly.

The most common causes of hypercalcemia are malignancies and hyperparathyroidism. Malignant tumours can produce hypercalcemia by a variety of mechanisms. The excessive PTH secretion associated with hyperparathyroidism causes increased release of calcium from the bones and increased intestinal and renal absorption of calcium. Calcifications of soft tissue occur when the calcium–phosphorus product exceeds 5.65 (serum calcium [mmol/L] × serum phosphorus [mmol/L]) (Marx, 2000).

Bone mineral is lost during immobilization, sometimes causing elevation of total (and especially ionized) calcium in the bloodstream. Symptomatic hypercalcemia from immobilization, however, is rare; when it does occur, it is virtually limited to people with high calcium turnover rates (eg, adolescents during a growth spurt). Most cases of hypercalcemia secondary to immobility occur after severe or multiple fractures or spinal cord injury.

Thiazide diuretics may cause a slight elevation in serum calcium levels because they potentiate the action of PTH on the kidneys, reducing urinary calcium excretion. The milk-alkali syndrome can occur in patients with peptic ulcer treated for a prolonged period with milk and alkaline antacids, particularly calcium carbonate. Vitamin A and D intoxication, as well as the use of lithium, can cause calcium excess.

Clinical Manifestations

As a rule, the symptoms of hypercalcemia are proportional to the degree of elevation of the serum calcium level. Hypercalcemia reduces neuromuscular excitability because it suppresses activity at the myoneural junction. Symptoms such as muscle weakness, incoordination, anorexia, and constipation may be due to decreased tone in smooth and striated muscle. Cardiac standstill can occur when the serum calcium level is about 4.5 mmol/L. The inotropic effect of digitalis is enhanced by calcium; therefore, digitalis toxicity is aggravated by hypercalcemia.

Anorexia, nausea, vomiting, and constipation are common symptoms of hypercalcemia. Dehydration occurs with nausea, vomiting, anorexia, and calcium reabsorption at the proximal renal tubule. Abdominal and bone pain may also be present. Abdominal distention and paralytic ileus may complicate severe hypercalcemic crisis. Excessive urination due to disturbed renal tubular function produced by hypercalcemia may be present. Se-

vere thirst may occur secondary to the polyuria caused by the high solute (calcium) load. Patients with chronic hypercalcemia may develop symptoms similar to those of peptic ulcer because hypercalcemia increases the secretion of acid and pepsin by the stomach.

Confusion, impaired memory, slurred speech, lethargy, acute psychotic behaviour, or coma may occur. The more severe symptoms tend to appear when the serum calcium level is approximately 4 mmol/L or above. However, some patients become profoundly disturbed with serum calcium levels of only 3 mmol/L. These symptoms resolve as serum calcium levels return to normal after treatment.

Hypercalcemic crisis refers to an acute rise in the serum calcium level to 4.3 mmol/L or higher. Severe thirst and polyuria are characteristically present. Other findings may include muscle weakness, intractable nausea, abdominal cramps, obstipation (very severe constipation) or diarrhea, peptic ulcer symptoms, and bone pain. Lethargy, confusion, and coma may also occur. This condition is very dangerous and may result in cardiac arrest.

Assessment and Diagnostic Findings

The serum calcium level is greater than 2.55 mmol/L. Cardiovascular changes may include a variety of dysrhythmias and shortening of the QT interval and ST segment. The PR interval is sometimes prolonged. The double-antibody PTH test may be used to differentiate between primary hyperparathyroidism and malignancy as a cause of hypercalcemia: PTH levels are increased in primary or secondary hyperparathyroidism and suppressed in malignancy. X-rays may reveal the presence of osteoporosis, bone cavitation, or urinary calculi. The Sulkowitch urine test analyzes the amount of calcium in the urine; in hypercalcemia, dense precipitation is observed due to hypercalciuria.

Medical Management

Therapeutic aims in hypercalcemia include decreasing the serum calcium level and reversing the process causing hypercalcemia. Treating the underlying cause (eg, chemotherapy for a malignancy or partial parathyroidectomy for hyperparathyroidism) is essential.

PHARMACOLOGIC THERAPY

General measures include administering fluids to dilute serum calcium and promote its excretion by the kidneys, mobilizing the patient, and restricting dietary calcium intake. IV administration of 0.9% sodium chloride solution temporarily dilutes the serum calcium level and increases urinary calcium excretion by inhibiting tubular reabsorption of calcium. Administering IV phosphate can cause a reciprocal drop in serum calcium. Furosemide (Lasix) is often used in conjunction with administration of a saline solution; in addition to causing diuresis, furosemide increases calcium excretion.

Calcitonin can be used to lower the serum calcium level and is particularly useful for patients with heart disease or renal failure who cannot tolerate large sodium loads. Calcitonin reduces bone resorption, increases the deposit of calcium and phosphorus in the bones, and increases urinary excretion of calcium and phosphorus. Although available in several forms, calcitonin derived from salmon is commonly used. Skin testing for allergy to salmon calcitonin is necessary before the hormone is administered. Systemic allergic reactions are possible since this hormone is a protein; resistance to the medication may develop later because of antibody formation. Calcitonin is administered by intramuscular injection rather than subcutaneously because patients with hypercalcemia have poor perfusion of subcutaneous tissue.

For patients with cancer, treatment is directed at controlling the condition by surgery, chemotherapy, or radiation therapy. Corticosteroids may be used to decrease bone turnover and tubular reabsorption for patients with sarcoidosis, myelomas, lymphomas, and leukemias; patients with solid tumours are less responsive. The bisphosphonates inhibit osteoclast activity. Pamidronate (Aredia) is the most potent of these agents and is given IV; it causes a transient, mild pyrexia, decreased white blood cell count, and myalgia. Etidronate (Didronel) is another bisphosphonate that is given IV, but its action is slower. Mithramycin, a cytotoxic antibiotic, inhibits bone resorption and thus lowers the serum calcium level. This agent must be used cautiously because it has significant side effects, including thrombocytopenia, nephrotoxicity, rebound hypercalcemia when discontinued, and hepatotoxicity. Inorganic phosphate salts can be administered orally or by nasogastric tube (in the form of Fleet Phospho-soda), rectally (as retention enemas), or IV. IV phosphate therapy is used with extreme caution in the treatment of hypercalcemia because it can cause severe calcification in various tissues, hypotension, tetany, and acute renal failure.

Nursing Management

It is important to monitor for hypercalcemia in patients at risk. Interventions such as increasing patient mobility and encouraging fluids can help prevent hypercalcemia, or at least minimize its severity. Hospitalized patients at risk for hypercalcemia are encouraged to ambulate as soon as possible; outpatients and those cared for in their homes are informed of the importance of frequent ambulation.

When encouraging oral fluids, the nurse considers the patient's likes and dislikes. Fluids containing sodium should be administered unless contraindicated by other conditions, because sodium favours calcium excretion. Patients are encouraged to drink 2.5 to 3.5 litres of fluid daily. Adequate fibre should be provided in the diet to offset the tendency for constipation. Safety precautions are taken, as necessary, when mental symptoms of hypercalcemia are present. The patient and family are informed that these mental changes are reversible with treatment. Increased calcium potentiates the effects of digitalis; therefore, the patient is assessed for signs and symptoms of digitalis toxicity. ECG changes (premature ventricular contractions, paroxysmal atrial tachycardia, and heart block) can occur; therefore, the cardiac rate and rhythm are monitored for any abnormalities.

SIGNIFICANCE OF MAGNESIUM

Next to potassium, magnesium is the most abundant intracellular cation. It acts as an activator for many intracellular enzyme systems and plays a role in both carbohydrate and protein metabolism. Magnesium balance is important in neuromuscular function. Because magnesium acts directly on the myoneural junction, variations in the serum concentration of magnesium affect neuromuscular irritability and contractility. For example, an excess of magnesium diminishes the excitability of the muscle cells, whereas a deficit increases neuromuscular irritability and contractility. Magnesium produces its sedative effect at the neuromuscular junction, probably by inhibiting the release of the neurotransmitter acetylcholine. It also increases the stimulus threshold in nerve fibres.

Magnesium exerts effects on the cardiovascular system, acting peripherally to produce vasodilation. Magnesium is thought to have a direct effect on peripheral arteries and arterioles, which results in a decreased total peripheral resistance. Magnesium disorders include hypomagnesemia and hypermagnesemia.

MAGNESIUM DEFICIT (HYPOMAGNESEMIA)

Hypomagnesemia refers to a below-normal serum magnesium concentration. The normal serum magnesium level is 0.72 to 0.95 mmol/L. Approximately one third of serum magnesium is bound to protein; the remaining two thirds exists as free cations (Mg^{++}). Like calcium, it is the ionized fraction that is primarily involved in neuromuscular activity and other physiologic processes. As with calcium levels, magnesium levels should be evaluated in combination with albumin levels. Low serum albumin levels decrease total magnesium.

Hypomagnesemia is a common yet often overlooked imbalance in acutely and critically ill patients. It may occur with withdrawal from alcohol and administration of tube feedings or parenteral nutrition.

An important route for magnesium loss is the GI tract. Loss of magnesium from the GI tract may occur with nasogastric suction, diarrhea, or fistulas. Because fluid from the lower GI tract has a higher concentration of magnesium (10–14 mmol/L) than fluid from the upper tract (1–2 mmol/L), losses from diarrhea and intestinal fistulas are more likely to induce magnesium deficit than are those from gastric suction. Although magnesium losses are relatively small in nasogastric suction, hypomagnesemia will occur if losses are prolonged and magnesium is not replaced through IV infusion. Because the distal small bowel is the major site of magnesium absorption, any disruption in small bowel function, as in intestinal resection or inflammatory bowel disease, can lead to hypomagnesemia.

Alcoholism is currently the most common cause of symptomatic hypomagnesemia in Canada. Hypomagnesemia is particularly troublesome during treatment of alcohol withdrawal. Therefore, the serum magnesium level should be measured at least every 2 or 3 days in patients going through withdrawal from alcohol. The serum magnesium level may be normal on admission but fall as a result of metabolic changes, such as the intracellular shift of magnesium associated with IV glucose administration.

During nutritional repletion, the major cellular electrolytes move from the serum to newly synthesized cells. Thus, if the enteral or parenteral feeding formula is deficient in magnesium content, serious hypomagnesemia will occur. Because of this, serum magnesium levels should be measured at regular intervals in patients who are receiving parenteral nutrition and enteral feedings, especially those who have undergone a period of starvation. Other causes of hypomagnesemia include the administration of aminoglycosides, cyclosporine, cisplatin, diuretics, digitalis, and amphotericin and the rapid administration of citrated blood, especially to patients with renal or hepatic disease. Magnesium deficiency often occurs in diabetic ketoacidosis, secondary to increased renal excretion during osmotic diuresis and shifting of magnesium into the cells with insulin therapy. Other contributing causes are sepsis, burns, and hypothermia.

Clinical Manifestations

Clinical manifestations of hypomagnesemia are largely confined to the neuromuscular system. Some of the effects are due directly to the low serum magnesium level; others are due to secondary changes in potassium and calcium metabolism. Symptoms do not usually occur until the serum magnesium level is less than 0.5 mmol/L.

Among the neuromuscular changes are hyperexcitability with muscle weakness, tremors, and athetoid movements (slow, involuntary twisting and writhing). Others include tetany, generalized tonic-clonic or focal seizures, laryngeal stridor, and positive Chvostek's and Trousseau's signs (see earlier discussion in this chapter), which occur, in part, because of accompanying hypocalcemia.

Magnesium deficiency can disturb the ECG by prolonging the QRS, depressing the ST segment, and predisposing to cardiac dysrhythmias, such as premature ventricular contractions, supraventricular tachycardia, torsades de pointes (a form of ventricular tachycardia), and ventricular fibrillation. Increased susceptibility to digitalis toxicity is associated with low serum magnesium levels. This is important because patients receiving digoxin are also likely to be receiving diuretic therapy, predisposing them to renal loss of magnesium.

Hypomagnesemia may be accompanied by marked alterations in mood. Apathy, depression, apprehension, and extreme agitation have been noted, as well as ataxia, dizziness, insomnia, and confusion. At times, delirium, auditory or visual hallucinations, and frank psychoses may occur.

Assessment and Diagnostic Findings

On laboratory analysis, the serum magnesium level is less than 0.62 mmol/L. Hypomagnesemia is frequently associated with hypokalemia and hypocalcemia. About 25% of magnesium is protein-bound, principally to albumin. A decreased serum albumin level can, therefore, reduce the measured total magnesium concentration; however, it does not reduce the ionized plasma magnesium concentration. ECG evaluations reflect magnesium, calcium, and potassium deficiencies, tachydysrhythmias, prolonged PR and QT intervals, widening QRS, ST segment depression, flattened T waves, and a prominent U wave. Torsades de pointes is associated with a low magnesium level. Premature ventricular contractions, paroxysmal atrial tachycardia, and heart block may also occur. Urinary magnesium levels may be helpful in identifying causes of magnesium depletion and are measured after a loading dose of magnesium sulfate is administered. Two newer diagnostic techniques (nuclear magnetic resonance spectroscopy and the ion selective electrode) are sensitive and direct means to measure ionized serum magnesium levels.

Medical Management

Mild magnesium deficiency can be corrected by diet alone. Principal dietary sources of magnesium are green leafy vegetables, nuts, legumes, whole grains, and seafood. Magnesium is also plentiful in peanut butter and chocolate. When necessary, magnesium salts can be administered orally to replace continuous excessive losses. Diarrhea is a common complication of excessive ingestion of magnesium. Patients receiving parenteral nutrition require magnesium in the IV solution to prevent hypomagnesemia. IV administration of magnesium sulfate must be given by an infusion pump and at a rate not to exceed 150 mg/min. A bolus dose of magnesium sulfate given too rapidly can produce cardiac arrest. Vital signs must be assessed frequently during magnesium administration to detect changes in cardiac rate or rhythm, hypotension, and respiratory distress. Monitoring urine output is essential before, during, and after magnesium administration; the physician is notified if urine volume decreases to less than 100 mL over 4 hours. Calcium gluconate must be readily available to treat hypocalcemic tetany or hypermagnesemia.

Overt symptoms of hypomagnesemia are treated with parenteral administration of magnesium. Magnesium sulfate is the most commonly used magnesium salt. Serial magnesium concentrations can be used to regulate the dosage.

Nursing Management

The nurse should be aware of patients at risk for hypomagnesemia and observe for its signs and symptoms. Patients receiving digitalis are monitored closely because a deficit of magnesium can predispose them to digitalis toxicity. When hypomagnesemia is severe, seizure precautions are implemented. Other safety precautions are instituted, as indicated, if confusion is observed.

Because difficulty in swallowing (dysphagia) may occur in magnesium-depleted patients, the ability to swallow should be tested with water before oral medications or foods are offered. Dysphagia is probably related to the athetoid or choreiform (rapid, involuntary, and irregular jerking) movements associated with magnesium deficit. To determine neuromuscular irritability, the nurse needs to assess and grade deep tendon reflexes (see Chap. 60 for discussion of assessment and grading reflexes).

Teaching plays a major role in treating magnesium deficit, particularly that resulting from abuse of diuretic or laxative medications. In such cases, the nurse can instruct the patient about the need to consume magnesium-rich foods. For patients experiencing hypomagnesemia from abuse of alcohol, the nurse can provide teaching, counselling, support, and possible referral to alcohol abstinence programs or other professional help.

MAGNESIUM EXCESS (HYPERMAGNESEMIA)

Hypermagnesemia is a greater-than-normal serum concentration of magnesium. A serum magnesium level can appear falsely elevated when blood specimens are allowed to hemolyze or are drawn from an extremity with a tourniquet that was applied too tightly.

By far the most common cause of hypermagnesemia is renal failure. In fact, most patients with advanced renal failure have at least a slight elevation in serum magnesium levels. This condition is aggravated when such patients receive magnesium to control seizures or inadvertently take one of the many commercial antacids that contain magnesium salts.

Hypermagnesemia can occur in a patient with untreated diabetic ketoacidosis when catabolism causes the release of cellular magnesium that cannot be excreted because of profound fluid volume depletion and resulting oliguria. An excess of magnesium can also result from excessive magnesium administered to treat hypertension of pregnancy and to lower serum magnesium levels. Increased serum magnesium levels can also occur in adrenocortical insufficiency, Addison's disease, or hypothermia. Excessive use of antacids (eg, Maalox, Riopan, Mylanta) and laxatives (Milk of Magnesia) also increases serum magnesium levels.

Clinical Manifestations

Acute elevation of the serum magnesium level depresses the central nervous system as well as the peripheral neuromuscular junction. At mildly elevated levels, there is a tendency for lowered blood pressure because of peripheral vasodilation. Nausea, vomiting, soft tissue calcifications, facial flushing, and sensations of warmth may also occur. At higher magnesium concentrations, lethargy, difficulty speaking (dysarthria), and drowsiness can occur. Deep tendon reflexes are lost, and muscle weakness and paralysis may develop. The respiratory centre is depressed when serum magnesium levels exceed 5 mmol/L. Coma, atrioventricular heart block, and cardiac arrest can occur when the serum magnesium level is greatly elevated and not treated.

Assessment and Diagnostic Findings

On laboratory analysis, the serum magnesium level is greater than 0.95 mmol/L. ECG findings may include a prolonged PR interval, tall T waves, and a widened QRS. ECG findings demonstrate a prolonged QT interval and atrioventricular blocks.

Medical Management

Hypermagnesemia can be prevented by avoiding the administration of magnesium to patients with renal failure and by carefully monitoring seriously ill patients who are receiving magnesium salts. In patients with severe hypermagnesemia, all parenteral and oral magnesium salts are discontinued. In emergencies, such as respiratory depression or defective cardiac conduction, ventilatory support and IV calcium are indicated. In addition, hemodialysis with a magnesium-free dialysate can reduce the serum magnesium to a safe level within hours. Loop diuretics and 0.45% sodium chloride (half-strength saline) solution enhance magnesium excretion in patients with adequate renal function. IV calcium gluconate (10 mL of a 10% solution) antagonizes the neuromuscular effects of magnesium.

Nursing Management

Patients at risk for hypermagnesemia are identified and assessed. When hypermagnesemia is suspected, the nurse monitors the vital signs, noting hypotension and shallow respirations. The nurse also observes for decreased patellar reflexes and changes in the level of consciousness. Medications that contain magnesium are not given to patients with renal failure or compromised renal function, and patients with renal failure are cautioned to check with their health care providers before taking over-the-counter medications. Caution is essential when preparing and administering magnesium-containing fluids parenterally because available parenteral magnesium solutions (eg, 2-mL ampules or 50-mL vials) differ in concentration.

SIGNIFICANCE OF PHOSPHORUS

Phosphorus is a critical constituent of all the body's tissues. It is essential to the function of muscle and red blood cells, the formation of adenosine triphosphate (ATP) and 2,3-diphosphoglycerate, and the maintenance of acid–base balance, as well as to the nervous system and the intermediary metabolism of carbohydrate, protein, and fat. The normal serum phosphorus level is 0.8–1.5 mmol/L and may be as high as 1.94 mmol/L in infants and children. Serum phosphorus levels are presumably greater in children because of the high rate of skeletal growth. Phosphorus is the primary anion of the ICF. About 85% of phosphorus is located in bones and teeth, 14% in soft tissue, and less than 1% in the ECF. Phosphorus is critical to nerve and muscle function and provides structural support to bones and teeth. Phosphorus levels decrease with age.

PHOSPHORUS DEFICIT (HYPOPHOSPHATEMIA)

Hypophosphatemia is a below-normal serum concentration of inorganic phosphorus. Although it often indicates phosphorus deficiency, hypophosphatemia may occur under a variety of circumstances in which total body phosphorus stores are normal. Conversely, phosphorus deficiency is an abnormally low content of phosphorus in lean tissues and may exist in the absence of hypophosphatemia.

Hypophosphatemia may occur during the administration of calories to patients with severe protein-calorie malnutrition. It is most likely to occur with overzealous intake or administration of simple carbohydrates. This syndrome can be induced in anyone with severe protein-calorie malnutrition (eg, patients with anorexia nervosa or alcoholism, or elderly debilitated patients unable to eat). As many as 50% of patients hospitalized because of chronic alcoholism have hypophosphatemia.

Marked hypophosphatemia may develop in malnourished patients who receive parenteral nutrition if the phosphorus loss is not adequately corrected. Other causes of hypophosphatemia include prolonged intense hyperventilation, alcohol withdrawal, poor dietary intake, diabetic ketoacidosis, and major thermal burns. Low magnesium levels, low potassium levels, and hyperparathyroidism related to increased urinary losses of phosphorus contribute to hypophosphatemia. Respiratory alkalosis can cause a decrease in phosphorus because of an intracellular shift of phosphorus.

Excess phosphorus binding by antacids containing magnesium, calcium, or albumin may decrease the phosphorus available from the diet to amounts below that required to maintain serum phosphorus balance. The degree of hypophosphatemia depends on the amount of phosphorus in the diet compared to the dose of antacid. Vitamin D regulates intestinal ion absorption; therefore, a deficiency of vitamin D may cause decreased calcium and phosphorus levels, which may lead to osteomalacia (softened, brittle bones).

Clinical Manifestations

Most of the signs and symptoms of phosphorus deficiency appear to result from a deficiency of ATP, 2,3-diphosphoglycerate, or both. ATP deficiency impairs cellular energy resources; diphosphoglycerate deficiency impairs oxygen delivery to tissues.

A wide range of neurologic symptoms may occur, such as irritability, fatigue, apprehension, weakness, numbness, paresthesias, confusion, seizures, and coma. Low levels of diphosphoglycerate may reduce the delivery of oxygen to peripheral tissues, resulting in tissue anoxia. Hypoxia then leads to an increase in respiratory rate and respiratory alkalosis, causing phosphorus to move into the cells and potentiating hypophosphatemia.

It is thought that hypophosphatemia predisposes a person to infection. In laboratory animals, hypophosphatemia is associated with depression of the chemotactic, phagocytic, and bacterial activity of granulocytes.

Muscle damage may develop as the ATP level in the muscle tissue declines. Clinical manifestations are muscle weakness, muscle pain, and at times acute rhabdomyolysis (disintegration of striated muscle). Weakness of respiratory muscles may greatly impair ventilation. Hypophosphatemia also may predispose a person to insulin resistance and thus hyperglycemia. Chronic loss of phosphorus can cause bruising and bleeding from platelet dysfunction.

Assessment and Diagnostic Findings

On laboratory analysis, the serum phosphorus level is less than 0.80 mmol/L in adults. When reviewing laboratory results, the nurse should keep in mind that glucose or insulin administration causes a slight decrease in the serum phosphorus level. PTH levels are increased in hyperparathyroidism. Serum magnesium may decrease due to increased urinary excretion of magnesium. Alkaline phosphatase is increased with osteoblastic activity. X-rays may show skeletal changes of osteomalacia or rickets.

Medical Management

Prevention of hypophosphatemia is the goal. In patients at risk for hypophosphatemia, serum phosphate levels should be closely monitored and correction initiated before deficits become severe. Adequate amounts of phosphorus should be added to parenteral solutions, and attention should be paid to the phosphorus levels in enteral feeding solutions.

Severe hypophosphatemia is dangerous and requires prompt attention. Aggressive IV phosphorus correction is usually limited to patients whose serum phosphorus levels fall below 0.3 mmol/L and whose GI tract is not functioning. Possible dangers of IV phosphorus administration include tetany from hypocalcemia and metastatic calcification from hyperphosphatemia. The rate of phosphorus administration should not exceed 10 mmol/h, and the site should be carefully monitored because tissue sloughing and necrosis can occur with infiltration. In less acute situations, oral phosphorus replacement is usually adequate.

Nursing Management

The nurse identifies patients at risk for hypophosphatemia and monitors for it. Because malnourished patients receiving parenteral nutrition are at risk when calories are introduced too aggressively, preventive measures involve gradually introducing the solution to avoid rapid shifts of phosphorus into the cells.

For patients with documented hypophosphatemia, careful attention is given to preventing infection because hypophosphatemia may alter the granulocytes. In patients requiring correction of phosphorus losses, the nurse frequently monitors serum phosphorus levels and documents and reports early signs of hypophosphatemia (apprehension, confusion, change in level of consciousness). If the patient experiences mild hypophosphatemia, foods such as milk and milk products, organ meats, nuts, fish, poultry, and whole grains should be encouraged. With moderate hypophosphatemia, supplements such as Fleet Phospho-soda (815 mg phosphorus/5 mL) may be prescribed (Metheny, 2000).

PHOSPHORUS EXCESS (HYPERPHOSPHATEMIA)

Hyperphosphatemia is a serum phosphorus level that exceeds normal. Various conditions can lead to this imbalance, but the most common is renal failure. Other causes include chemotherapy for neoplastic disease, hypoparathyroidism, respiratory acidosis or diabetic ketoacidosis, high phosphate intake, profound muscle necrosis, and increased phosphorus absorption. The primary complication of increased phosphorus is metastatic calcification (soft tissue, joints, and arteries), which results when the calcium–magnesium product (calcium × magnesium) exceeds 7 mmol/L.

Clinical Manifestations

An elevated serum phosphorus level causes few symptoms. Symptoms that do occur usually result from decreased calcium levels and soft tissue calcifications. The most important short-term consequence is tetany. Because of the reciprocal relationship between phosphorus and calcium, a high serum phosphorus level tends to cause a low serum calcium concentration. Tetany can result, causing tingling sensations in the fingertips and around the mouth. Anorexia, nausea, vomiting, muscle weakness, hyperreflexia, and tachycardia may occur.

The major long-term consequence is soft tissue calcification, which occurs mainly in patients with a reduced glomerular filtration rate. High serum levels of inorganic phosphorus promote precipitation of calcium phosphate in nonosseous sites, decreasing urine output, impairing vision, and producing palpitations.

Assessment and Diagnostic Findings

On laboratory analysis, the serum phosphorus level exceeds 1.5 mmol/L in adults. Serum phosphorus levels are normally higher in children, presumably because of the high rate of skeletal growth. The serum calcium level is useful also for diagnosing the primary disorder and assessing the effects of treatments. X-ray studies may show skeletal changes with abnormal bone development. PTH levels are decreased in hypoparathyroidism. BUN and creatinine levels are used to assess renal function.

Medical Management

When possible, treatment is directed at the underlying disorder. For example, hyperphosphatemia may be related to volume depletion or respiratory or metabolic acidosis. In renal failure, elevated PTH production contributes to a high phosphorus level and bone disease. Measures to decrease the serum phosphate level in these patients include vitamin D preparations such as calcitol (Rocaltrol, in oral preparation), Calcijex (for IV administration), or paricalcitol (Zemplar). Vitamin D does not increase the serum calcium, thus permitting more aggressive treatment of hyperphosphatemia with calcium-binding antacids, phosphate-binding gels or antacids, restriction of dietary phosphate, and dialysis.

Nursing Management

The nurse monitors patients at risk for hyperphosphatemia. When a low-phosphorus diet is prescribed, the patient is instructed to avoid phosphorus-rich foods such as hard cheese, cream, nuts, whole-grain cereals, dried fruits, dried vegetables, kidneys, sardines, sweetbreads, and foods made with milk. When appropriate, the nurse instructs the patient to avoid phosphate-containing substances such as laxatives and enemas that contain phosphate. The nurse also teaches the patient to recognize the signs of impending hypocalcemia and to monitor for changes in urine output.

SIGNIFICANCE OF CHLORIDE

Chloride, the major anion of the ECF, is found more in interstitial and lymph fluid compartments than in blood. Chloride is also contained in gastric and pancreatic juices and sweat. Sodium and chloride in water make up the composition of the ECF and assist in determining osmotic pressure.

The serum level of chloride reflects a change in dilution or concentration of the ECF and does so in direct proportion to sodium. Aldosterone secretion increases sodium reabsorption, thereby increasing chloride reabsorption. The choroid plexus, where cerebrospinal fluid forms in the brain, depends on sodium and chloride to attract water to form the fluid portion of the cerebrospinal fluid. Bicarbonate has an inverse relationship with chloride. As chloride moves from plasma into the red blood cells (called the chloride shift), bicarbonate moves back into the plasma. Hydrogen ions are formed, which then help to release oxygen from hemoglobin. When the level of one of these three electrolytes (sodium, bicarbonate, or chloride) is disturbed, the other two will be affected as well.

CHLORIDE DEFICIT (HYPOCHLOREMIA)

Chloride control depends on the intake of chloride and the excretion and reabsorption of its ions in the kidneys. Chloride is produced in the stomach as hydrochloric acid; a small amount of chloride is lost in the feces. Chloride-deficient formulas, salt-restricted diets, GI tube drainage, and severe vomiting and diarrhea are risk factors for hypochloremia. As chloride decreases (usually because of volume depletion), sodium and bicarbonate ions are retained by the kidney to balance the loss. Bicarbonate accumulates in the ECF, which raises the pH and leads to hypochloremic metabolic alkalosis.

Clinical Manifestations

The signs and symptoms of hypochloremia are those of acid–base and electrolyte imbalances. The signs and symptoms of hyponatremia, hypokalemia, and metabolic alkalosis may also be noted. Metabolic alkalosis is a disorder that results in a high pH and a high serum bicarbonate level as a result of excess alkali intake or loss of hydrogen ions. With compensation, the $PaCO_2$ increases to 50 mm Hg. Hyperexcitability of muscles, tetany, hyperactive deep tendon reflexes, weakness, twitching, and muscle cramps may result. Hypokalemia can cause hypochloremia, resulting in cardiac dysrhythmias. In addition, because low chloride levels parallel low sodium levels, a water excess may occur. Hyponatremia can cause seizures and coma.

Assessment and Diagnostic Findings

The normal serum chloride level is 96–106 mmol/L. Inside the cell, the chloride level is 4 mmol/L. In addition to the chloride level, sodium and potassium levels are also evaluated because these electrolytes are lost along with chloride. Arterial blood gas analysis identifies the acid–base imbalance, which is usually metabolic alkalosis. The urine chloride level, which is also measured, decreases in hypochloremia.

Medical Management

Treatment involves correcting the cause of hypochloremia and contributing electrolyte and acid–base imbalances. Normal saline (0.9% sodium chloride) or half-strength saline (0.45% sodium chloride) solution is administered IV to replace the chloride. The physician may reevaluate whether patients receiving diuretics (loop, osmotic, or thiazide) should discontinue these medications or change to another diuretic.

Foods high in chloride are provided; these include tomato juice, salty broth, canned vegetables, processed meats, and fruits. A patient who drinks free water (water without electrolytes) or bottled water will excrete large amounts of chloride; therefore, this kind of water should be avoided. Ammonium chloride, an acidifying agent, may be prescribed to treat metabolic alkalosis; the dosage depends on the patient's weight and serum chloride level. This agent is metabolized by the liver, and its effects last for about 3 days.

Nursing Management

The nurse monitors intake and output, arterial blood gas values, and serum electrolyte levels, as well as the patient's level of consciousness and muscle strength and movement. Changes are reported to the physician promptly. Vital signs are monitored and respiratory assessment is carried out frequently. The nurse teaches the patient about foods with high chloride content.

CHLORIDE EXCESS (HYPERCHLOREMIA)

Hyperchloremia exists when the serum level exceeds 106 mmol/L. Hypernatremia, bicarbonate loss, and metabolic acidosis can occur with high chloride levels. Hyperchloremic metabolic acidosis is also known as normal anion gap acidosis (see discussion in Acid–Base Disturbances section of this chapter). It is usually caused by the loss of bicarbonate ions via the kidney or the GI tract with a corresponding increase in chloride ions. Chloride ions in the form of acidifying salts accumulate and acidosis occurs with a decrease in bicarbonate ions.

Clinical Manifestations

The signs and symptoms of hyperchloremia are the same as those of metabolic acidosis, hypervolemia, and hypernatremia. Tachypnea; weakness; lethargy; deep, rapid respirations; diminished cognitive ability; and hypertension occur. If untreated, hyperchloremia can lead to a decrease in cardiac output, dysrhythmias, and coma. A high chloride level is accompanied by a high sodium level and fluid retention.

Assessment and Diagnostic Findings

The serum chloride level is 108 mmol/L or greater, the serum sodium level is greater than 145 mmol/L, the serum pH is less than 7.35, the serum bicarbonate level is less than 22 mmol/L, and there is a normal anion gap of 8–12 mmol/L. Urine chloride excretion increases.

Calculation of the serum anion gap is important in analyzing acid–base disorders. The sum of all negatively charged electrolytes (anions) equals the sum of all positively charged electrolytes (cations) with several anions that are not routinely measured leading to an anion gap. It is based primarily on three electrolytes: sodium, chloride, and bicarbonate or serum CO_2. A low anion gap may be attributed to hypoproteinemia, while an elevated anion gap can be due to metabolic acidosis.

Medical Management

Correcting the underlying cause of hyperchloremia and restoring electrolyte, fluid, and acid–base balance are essential. Lactated Ringer's solution may be prescribed to convert lactate to bicarbonate in the liver, which will increase the base bicarbonate level and correct the acidosis. Sodium bicarbonate may be given IV to increase bicarbonate levels, which leads to the renal excretion of chloride ions as bicarbonate and chloride compete for combination with sodium. Diuretics may be administered to eliminate chloride as well. Sodium, fluids, and chloride are restricted.

Nursing Management

Monitoring vital signs, arterial blood gas values, and intake and output is important to assess the patient's status and the effectiveness of treatment. Assessment findings related to respiratory, neurologic, and cardiac systems are documented and changes discussed with the physician. The nurse teaches the patient about the diet that should be followed to manage hyperchloremia.

Acid–Base Disturbances

Acid–base disturbances are commonly encountered in clinical practice. Identification of the specific acid–base imbalance is important in identifying the underlying cause of the disorder and in determining appropriate treatment (Kraut & Madias, 2001).

Plasma pH is an indicator of hydrogen ion (H^+) concentration. Homeostatic mechanisms keep pH within a normal range (7.35–7.45). These mechanisms consist of buffer systems, the kidneys, and the lungs. The H^+ concentration is extremely important: the greater the concentration, the more acidic the solution and the lower the pH. The lower the H^+ concentration, the more alkaline the solution and the higher the pH. The pH range compatible with life (6.8–7.8) represents a tenfold difference in H^+ concentration in plasma.

BUFFER SYSTEMS

Buffer systems prevent major changes in the pH of body fluids by removing or releasing H^+; they can act quickly to prevent excessive changes in H^+ concentration. Hydrogen ions are buffered by both intracellular and extracellular buffers. The body's major extracellular buffer system is the bicarbonate-carbonic acid buffer system. This is the system that is assessed when arterial blood gases are measured. Normally, there are 20 parts of bicarbonate (HCO_3^-) to one part of carbonic acid (H_2CO_3). If this ratio is altered, the pH will change. It is the ratio of HCO_3^- to H_2CO_3 that is important in maintaining pH, not absolute values. Carbon dioxide (CO_2) is a potential acid; when dissolved in water, it becomes carbonic acid ($CO_2 + H_2O = H_2CO_3$). Thus, when CO_2 is increased, the carbonic acid content is also increased, and vice versa. If either bicarbonate or carbonic acid is increased or decreased so that the 20:1 ratio is no longer maintained, acid–base imbalance results.

Less important buffer systems in the ECF include the inorganic phosphates and the plasma proteins. Intracellular buffers include proteins, organic and inorganic phosphates, and, in red blood cells, hemoglobin.

Kidneys

The kidneys regulate the bicarbonate level in the ECF; they can regenerate bicarbonate ions as well as reabsorb them from the renal tubular cells. In respiratory acidosis and most cases of metabolic acidosis, the kidneys excrete hydrogen ions and conserve bicarbonate ions to help restore balance. In respiratory and metabolic alkalosis, the kidneys retain hydrogen ions and excrete bicarbonate ions to help restore balance. The kidneys obviously cannot compensate for the metabolic acidosis created by renal failure. Renal compensation for imbalances is relatively slow (a matter of hours or days).

Lungs

The lungs, under the control of the medulla, control the CO_2 and thus the carbonic acid content of the ECF. They do so by adjusting ventilation in response to the amount of CO_2 in the blood. A rise in the partial pressure of CO_2 in arterial blood ($PaCO_2$) is a powerful stimulant to respiration. Of course, the partial pressure of oxygen in arterial blood (PaO_2) also influences respiration. Its effect, however, is not as marked as that produced by the $PaCO_2$.

In metabolic acidosis, the respiratory rate increases, causing greater elimination of CO_2 (to reduce the acid load). In metabolic alkalosis, the respiratory rate decreases, causing CO_2 to be retained (to increase the acid load).

ACUTE AND CHRONIC METABOLIC ACIDOSIS (BASE BICARBONATE DEFICIT)

Metabolic acidosis is a clinical disturbance characterized by a low pH (increased H^+ concentration) and a low plasma bicarbonate concentration. It can be produced by a gain of hydrogen ion or a loss of bicarbonate (Swenson, 2001). It can be divided clinically into two forms, according to the values of the serum anion gap: high anion gap acidosis and normal anion gap acidosis. The anion gap reflects normally unmeasured anions (phosphates, sulfates, and proteins) in plasma. Measuring the anion gap is essential in analyzing acid–base disorders correctly. The anion gap can be calculated by either one of the following equations:

$$\text{Anion gap} = Na^+ + K^+ - (Cl^- + HCO_3^-)$$
$$\text{Anion gap} = Na^+ - (Cl^- + HCO_3^-)$$

Potassium is often omitted from the equation because of its low level in the plasma; thus, the second equation is used more often than the first.

The normal value for an anion gap is 8 to 12 mmol/L without potassium in the equation. The normal value for the anion gap if including potassium in the equation is 12 to 16 mmol/L. The unmeasured anions in the serum normally account for less than 16 mmol/L of the anion production. An anion gap greater than 16 mmol/L suggests excessive accumulation of unmeasured anions. An anion gap occurs because not all electrolytes are measured. More anions are left unmeasured than cations.

Normal anion gap acidosis results from the direct loss of bicarbonate, as in diarrhea, lower intestinal fistulas, ureterostomies, and use of diuretics; early renal insufficiency; excessive administration of chloride; and the administration of parenteral nutrition without bicarbonate or bicarbonate-producing solutes (eg, lactate).

Normal anion gap acidosis is also referred to as hyperchloremic acidosis. A reduced or negative anion gap is primarily caused by hypoproteinemia. Disorders that cause a decreased or negative anion gap are rare compared to those related to an increased or high anion gap (Rose & Post, 2001).

High anion gap acidosis results from excessive accumulation of fixed acid. If it is increased to 30 mmol/L or more, then a high anion gap metabolic acidosis is present regardless of what the pH and the HCO_3^- are. High ion gap occurs in ketoacidosis, lactic acidosis, the late phase of salicylate poisoning, uremia, methanol or ethylene glycol toxicity, and ketoacidosis with starvation. The hydrogen is buffered by HCO_3^-, causing the bicarbonate concentration to fall. In all of these instances, abnormally high levels of anions flood the system, increasing the anion gap above normal limits.

Clinical Manifestations

Signs and symptoms of metabolic acidosis vary with the severity of the acidosis. They may include headache, confusion, drowsiness, increased respiratory rate and depth, nausea, and vomiting. Peripheral vasodilation and decreased cardiac output occur when the pH falls below 7. Additional physical assessment findings include decreased blood pressure, cold and clammy skin, dysrhythmias, and shock (Swenson, 2001).

Chronic metabolic acidosis is usually seen with chronic renal failure. The bicarbonate and pH decrease slowly; thus, the patient is asymptomatic until the bicarbonate is approximately 15 mmol/L or less.

Assessment and Diagnostic Findings

Arterial blood gas measurements are valuable in diagnosing metabolic acidosis (Swenson, 2001). Expected blood gas changes include a low bicarbonate level (less than 22 mmol/L) and a low pH (less than 7.35). The cardinal feature of metabolic acidosis is a decrease in the serum bicarbonate level. Hyperkalemia may accompany metabolic acidosis as a result of the shift of potassium out of the cells. Later, as the acidosis is corrected, potassium moves back into the cells and hypokalemia may occur. Hyperventilation decreases the CO_2 level as a compensatory action. As stated previously, calculation of the anion gap is helpful in determining the cause of metabolic acidosis. An ECG will detect dysrhythmias caused by the increased potassium.

Medical Management

Treatment is directed at correcting the metabolic defect (Swenson, 2001). If the problem results from excessive intake of chloride, treatment is aimed at eliminating the source of the chloride. When necessary, bicarbonate is administered if the pH is less than 7.1 and the bicarbonate level is less than 10. Although hyperkalemia occurs with acidosis, hypokalemia may occur with reversal of the acidosis and subsequent movement of potassium back into the cells. Therefore, the serum potassium level is monitored closely and hypokalemia is corrected as acidosis is reversed.

In chronic metabolic acidosis, low serum calcium levels are treated before treating chronic metabolic acidosis to avoid tetany resulting from an increase in pH and a decrease in ionized calcium. Alkalyzing agents may be given if the serum bicarbonate level is less than 12 mmol/L. Treatment modalities may also include hemodialysis or peritoneal dialysis.

ACUTE AND CHRONIC METABOLIC ALKALOSIS (BASE BICARBONATE EXCESS)

Metabolic alkalosis is a clinical disturbance characterized by a high pH (decreased H^+ concentration) and a high plasma bicarbonate concentration. It can be produced by a gain of bicarbonate or a loss of H^+ (Khanna & Kurtzman, 2001).

Probably the most common cause of metabolic alkalosis is vomiting or gastric suction with loss of hydrogen and chloride ions. The disorder also occurs in pyloric stenosis, in which only gastric fluid is lost. Gastric fluid has an acid pH (usually 1–3); therefore, loss of this highly acidic fluid increases the alkalinity of body fluids. Other situations predisposing to metabolic alkalosis include those associated with loss of potassium, such as diuretic therapy that promotes excretion of potassium (eg, thiazides, furosemide), and excessive adrenocorticoid hormones (as in hyperaldosteronism and Cushing's syndrome).

Hypokalemia produces alkalosis in two ways: (1) the kidneys conserve potassium, and thus H^+ excretion increases; and (2) cellular potassium moves out of the cells into the ECF in an attempt to maintain near-normal serum levels (as potassium ions leave the cells, hydrogen ions must enter to maintain electroneutrality). Excessive alkali ingestion from antacids containing bicarbonate or from using sodium bicarbonate during cardiopulmonary resuscitation can also cause metabolic alkalosis.

Chronic metabolic alkalosis can occur with long-term diuretic therapy (thiazides or furosemide), villous adenoma, external drainage of gastric fluids, significant potassium depletion, cystic fibrosis, and the chronic ingestion of milk and calcium carbonate.

Clinical Manifestations

Alkalosis is primarily manifested by symptoms related to decreased calcium ionization, such as tingling of the fingers and toes, dizziness, and hypertonic muscles. The ionized fraction of serum calcium decreases in alkalosis as more calcium combines with serum proteins. Because it is the ionized fraction of calcium that influences neuromuscular activity, symptoms of hypocalcemia are often the predominant symptoms of alkalosis. Respirations are depressed as a compensatory action by the lungs. Atrial tachycardia may occur. As the pH increases above 7.6 and hypokalemia develops, ventricular disturbances may occur. Decreased motility and paralytic ileus may also occur.

Symptoms of chronic metabolic alkalosis are the same as for acute metabolic alkalosis, and as potassium decreases, frequent premature ventricular contractions or U waves are seen on the ECG.

Assessment and Diagnostic Findings

Evaluation of arterial blood gases reveals a pH greater than 7.45 and a serum bicarbonate concentration greater than 26 mmol/L. The $PaCO_2$ increases as the lungs attempt to compensate for the excess bicarbonate by retaining CO_2. This hypoventilation is more pronounced in semiconscious, unconscious, or debilitated patients than in alert patients. The former may develop marked hypoxemia as a result of hypoventilation. Hypokalemia may accompany metabolic alkalosis.

Urinary chloride levels may help to identify the cause of metabolic alkalosis if the patient's history provides inadequate information. Metabolic alkalosis is the setting in which urine chloride concentration may be a more accurate estimate of volume than is the urine sodium concentration. Urine chloride concentrations help to differentiate between vomiting or diuretic ingestion or one of the causes of mineralocorticoid excess. Hypovolemia and hypochloremia in patients with vomiting or cystic fibrosis, those receiving nutritional repletion, or those taking diuretics produce urine chloride concentrations less than 25 mmol/L. Signs of hypovolemia are not present and the urine chloride concentration exceeds 40 mmol/L in patients with mineralocorticoid excess or alkali loading; these patients usually have expanded fluid volume. The urine chloride concentration should be less than 15 mmol/L when decreased chloride levels and hypovolemia occur.

Medical Management

Treatment of metabolic alkalosis is aimed at reversing the underlying disorder (Khanna & Kurtzman, 2001).

Sufficient chloride must be supplied for the kidney to absorb sodium with chloride (allowing the excretion of excess bicarbonate). Treatment also includes restoring normal fluid volume by administering sodium chloride fluids (because continued volume depletion serves to maintain the alkalosis). In patients with hypokalemia, potassium is administered as KCl to replace both K^+ and Cl^- losses. Histamine-2 receptor antagonists, such as cimetidine (Tagamet) and ranitidine HCl (Zantac), reduce the production of gastric HCl, thereby decreasing the metabolic alkalosis associated with gastric suction. Carbonic anhydrase inhibitors are useful in treating metabolic alkalosis in patients who cannot tolerate rapid volume expansion (eg, patients with heart failure). Because of volume depletion from GI loss, the patient's fluid intake and output must be monitored carefully. Management of chronic metabolic alkalosis is aimed at correcting the underlying acid–base disorder.

ACUTE AND CHRONIC RESPIRATORY ACIDOSIS (CARBONIC ACID EXCESS)

Respiratory acidosis is a clinical disorder in which the pH is less than 7.35 and the $PaCO_2$ is greater than 42 mm Hg. It may be either acute or chronic.

Respiratory acidosis is always due to inadequate excretion of CO_2 with inadequate ventilation, resulting in elevated plasma CO_2 levels and thus elevated carbonic acid (H_2CO_3) levels (Epstein & Singh, 2001). In addition to an elevated $PaCO_2$, hypoventilation usually causes a decrease in PaO_2. Acute respiratory acidosis occurs in emergency situations, such as acute pulmonary edema, aspiration of a foreign object, atelectasis, pneumothorax, overdose of sedatives, sleep apnea syndrome, administration of oxygen to a patient with chronic hypercapnia (excessive CO_2 in the blood), severe pneumonia, and acute respiratory distress syndrome. Respiratory acidosis can also occur in diseases that impair respiratory muscles, such as muscular dystrophy, myasthenia gravis, and Guillain-Barré syndrome.

Mechanical ventilation can be associated with hypercapnia if the rate of effective alveolar ventilation is inadequate. Ventilation is fixed in these patients, and CO_2 may be retained if the rate of CO_2 production is increased.

Clinical Manifestations

Clinical signs in acute and chronic respiratory acidosis vary. Sudden hypercapnia (elevated $PaCO_2$) can cause increased pulse and respiratory rate, increased blood pressure, mental cloudiness, and feeling of fullness in the head. An elevated $PaCO_2$ causes cerebrovascular vasodilation and increased cerebral blood flow, par-

ticularly when it is higher than 60 mm Hg. Ventricular fibrillation may be the first sign of respiratory acidosis in anesthetized patients.

If respiratory acidosis is severe, intracranial pressure may increase, resulting in papilledema and dilated conjunctival blood vessels. Hyperkalemia may result as hydrogen concentration overwhelms the compensatory mechanisms and moves into cells, causing a shift of potassium out of the cell.

Chronic respiratory acidosis occurs with pulmonary diseases such as chronic emphysema and bronchitis, obstructive sleep apnea, and obesity. As long as the $PaCO_2$ does not exceed the body's ability to compensate, the patient will be asymptomatic. However, if the $PaCO_2$ rises rapidly, cerebral vasodilation will increase intracranial pressure; cyanosis and tachypnea will develop. Patients with chronic obstructive pulmonary disease who gradually accumulate CO_2 over a prolonged period (days to months) may not develop symptoms of hypercapnia because compensatory renal changes have had time to occur.

NURSING ALERT When the $PaCO_2$ is chronically above 50 mm Hg, the respiratory centre becomes relatively insensitive to CO_2 as a respiratory stimulant, leaving hypoxemia as the major drive for respiration. Oxygen administration may remove the stimulus of hypoxemia, and the patient develops "carbon dioxide narcosis" unless the situation is quickly reversed. Therefore, oxygen is administered only with extreme caution.

Assessment and Diagnostic Findings

Arterial blood gas evaluation reveals a pH less than 7.35, a $PaCO_2$ greater than 42 mm Hg, and a variation in the bicarbonate level, depending on the duration of the acidosis in acute respiratory acidosis. When compensation (renal retention of bicarbonate) has fully occurred, the arterial pH may be within the lower limits of normal. Depending on the cause of respiratory acidosis, other diagnostic measures would include monitoring of serum electrolyte levels, chest x-ray for determining any respiratory disease, and a drug screen if an overdose is suspected. An ECG to identify any cardiac involvement as a result of chronic obstructive pulmonary disease may be indicated as well.

Medical Management

Treatment is directed at improving ventilation (Epstein & Singh, 2001); exact measures vary with the cause of inadequate ventilation. Pharmacologic agents are used as indicated. For example, bronchodilators help reduce bronchial spasm, antibiotics are used for respiratory infections, and thrombolytics or anticoagulants are used for pulmonary emboli.

Pulmonary hygiene measures are initiated, when necessary, to clear the respiratory tract of mucus and purulent drainage. Adequate hydration (2–3 L/day) is indicated to keep the mucous membranes moist and thereby facilitate the removal of secretions. Supplemental oxygen is used as necessary.

Mechanical ventilation, used appropriately, may improve pulmonary ventilation. Inappropriate mechanical ventilation (eg, increased dead space, insufficient rate or volume settings, high fraction of inspired oxygen [FiO_2] with excessive CO_2 production) may cause such rapid excretion of CO_2 that the kidneys will be unable to eliminate excess bicarbonate quickly enough to prevent alkalosis and seizures. For this reason, the elevated $PaCO_2$ must be decreased slowly. Placing the patient in a semi-Fowler's position facilitates expansion of the chest wall. Treatment of chronic respiratory acidosis is the same as for acute respiratory acidosis.

ACUTE AND CHRONIC RESPIRATORY ALKALOSIS (CARBONIC ACID DEFICIT)

Respiratory alkalosis is a clinical condition in which the arterial pH is greater than 7.45 and the $PaCO_2$ is less than 38 mm Hg. As with respiratory acidosis, acute and chronic conditions can occur.

Respiratory alkalosis is always due to hyperventilation, which causes excessive "blowing off" of CO_2 and, hence, a decrease in the plasma carbonic acid concentration. Causes can include extreme anxiety, hypoxemia, the early phase of salicylate intoxication, gram-negative bacteremia, and inappropriate ventilator settings that do not match the patient's requirements.

Chronic respiratory alkalosis results from chronic hypocapnia, and decreased serum bicarbonate levels are the consequence. Chronic hepatic insufficiency and cerebral tumours are predisposing factors.

Clinical Manifestations

Clinical signs consist of lightheadedness due to vasoconstriction and decreased cerebral blood flow, inability to concentrate, numbness and tingling from decreased calcium ionization, tinnitus, and at times loss of consciousness. Cardiac effects of respiratory alkalosis include tachycardia and ventricular and atrial dysrhythmias (Foster et al., 2001).

Assessment and Diagnostic Findings

Analysis of arterial blood gases assists in the diagnosis of respiratory alkalosis. In the acute state, the pH is elevated above normal as a result of a low $PaCO_2$ and a normal bicarbonate level. (The kidneys cannot alter the bicarbonate level quickly.) In the compensated state, the kidneys have had sufficient time to lower the bicarbonate level to a near-normal level. Evaluation of serum electrolytes is indicated to identify any decrease in potassium as hydrogen is pulled out of the cells in exchange for potassium; decreased calcium, as severe alkalosis inhibits calcium ionization, resulting in carpopedal spasms and tetany; or decreased phosphate due to alkalosis, causing an increased uptake of phosphate by the cells. A toxicology screen should be performed to rule out salicylate intoxication.

Patients with chronic respiratory alkalosis are usually asymptomatic, and the diagnostic evaluation and plan of care are the same as for acute respiratory alkalosis.

Medical Management

Treatment depends on the underlying cause of respiratory alkalosis (Foster et al., 2001). If the cause is anxiety, the patient is instructed to breathe more slowly to allow CO_2 to accumulate or to breathe into a closed system (such as a paper bag). A sedative may be required to relieve hyperventilation in very anxious patients. Treatment for other causes of respiratory alkalosis is directed at correcting the underlying problem.

MIXED ACID–BASE DISORDERS

At times patients can simultaneously experience two or more independent acid–base disorders. A normal pH in the presence of changes in the $PaCO_2$ and plasma HCO_3^- concentration immediately suggests a mixed disorder. The only mixed disorder that cannot occur is a mixed respiratory acidosis and alkalosis, because it is impossible to have alveolar hypoventilation and hyperventilation at the same time. An example of a mixed disorder is the simultaneous occurrence of metabolic acidosis and respiratory acidosis during respiratory and cardiac arrest.

COMPENSATION

Generally, the pulmonary and renal systems compensate for each other to return the pH to normal. In a single acid–base disorder, the system not causing the problem will try to compensate by returning the ratio of bicarbonate to carbonic acid to the normal 20:1. The lungs compensate for metabolic disturbances by changing CO_2 excretion. The kidneys compensate for respiratory disturbances by altering bicarbonate retention and H^+ secretion.

In respiratory acidosis, excess hydrogen is excreted in the urine in exchange for bicarbonate ions. In respiratory alkalosis, the renal excretion of bicarbonate increases, and hydrogen ions are retained. In metabolic acidosis, the compensatory mechanisms increase the ventilation rate and the renal retention of bicarbonate.

In metabolic alkalosis, the respiratory system compensates by decreasing ventilation to conserve CO_2 and raise the $PaCO_2$. Because the lungs respond to acid–base disorders within minutes, compensation for metabolic imbalances occurs faster than compensation for respiratory imbalances. Table 14-7 summarizes compensation effects.

BLOOD GAS ANALYSIS

Blood gas analysis is often used to identify the specific acid–base disturbance and the degree of compensation that has occurred. The analysis is usually based on an arterial blood sample, but when an arterial sample cannot be obtained, a mixed venous sample may be used. Results of arterial blood gas analysis provide information about alveolar ventilation, oxygenation, and acid–base balance. It is necessary to evaluate the serum electrolytes (sodium, potassium, and chloride) and carbon dioxide along with arterial blood gas data as they are often the first sign of an acid–base disorder. The health history, physical examination, previous blood gas results, and serum electrolytes should always be part of the assessment used to determine the cause of the acid–base disorder (Kraut & Madias, 2001). Treatment of the underlying condition usually corrects most acid–base disorders. Table 14-8 compares normal ranges of venous and arterial blood gas values. See also Chart 14-1.

Table 14-7 • **Acid–Base Disturbances and Compensation**

DISORDER	INITIAL EVENT	COMPENSATION
Respiratory acidosis	↑ $PaCO_2$, ↑ or normal HCO_3^-, ↓ pH	Kidneys eliminate H^+ and retain HCO_3^-
Respiratory alkalosis	↓ $PaCO_2$, ↓ or normal HCO_3^-, ↑ pH	Kidneys conserve H^+ and excrete HCO_3^-
Metabolic acidosis	↓ or normal $PaCO_2$, ↓ HCO_3^-, ↓ pH	Lungs eliminate CO_2, conserve HCO_3^-
Metabolic alkalosis	↑ or normal $PaCO_2$, ↑ HCO_3^-, ↑ pH	Lungs ↓ ventilation to ↑ PCO_2, kidneys conserve H^+ to excrete HCO_3^-

Table 14-8 • **Normal Values: Arterial and Venous Blood**

PARAMETER	ARTERIAL SAMPLE	VENOUS SAMPLE
pH	7.35–7.45	7.33–7.41
$PaCO_2$	35–45 mm Hg	35–40 mmHg
Oxygen saturation	93–98%	65–75%
Base excess or deficit	+/– 2 mmol/L	+/– 4 mmol/L
HCO_3^-	22–26 mmol/L	24–28 mmol/L

Parenteral Fluid Therapy

IV fluid administration is performed in the hospital, outpatient diagnostic and surgical settings, clinics, and home to replace fluids, administer medications, and provide nutrients when no other route is available.

PURPOSE

The choice of an IV solution depends on the purpose of its administration. Generally, IV fluids are administered to achieve one or more of the following goals:

- To provide water, electrolytes, and nutrients to meet daily requirements
- To replace water and correct electrolyte deficits
- To administer medications and blood products

IV solutions contain dextrose or electrolytes mixed in various proportions with water. Pure, electrolyte-free water can never be administered IV because it rapidly enters red blood cells and causes them to rupture.

TYPES OF IV SOLUTIONS

Solutions are often categorized as **isotonic, hypotonic,** or **hypertonic,** according to whether their total osmolality is the same as, less than, or greater than that of blood (see the section Laboratory Tests for Evaluating Fluid Status for a discussion of osmolality).

Electrolyte solutions are considered isotonic if the total electrolyte content (anions + cations) is approximately 310 mmol/L. They are considered hypotonic if the total electrolyte content is less than 250 mmol/L and hypertonic if the total electrolyte content exceeds 375 mmol/L. The nurse must also consider a solution's osmolality, keeping in mind that the osmolality of plasma is approximately 300 mmol/L. For example, a 10% dextrose solution has an osmolality of approximately 505 mmol/L.

Chart 14-1 • ASSESSMENT

Arterial Blood Gases

The following steps are recommended to evaluate arterial blood gas values. They are based on the assumption that the average values are:

pH = 7.4
$PaCO_2$ = 40 mm Hg
HCO_3^- = 24 mmol/L

1. *First, note the pH.* It can be high, low, or normal, as follows:
   pH > 7.4 (alkalosis)
   pH < 7.4 (acidosis)
   pH = 7.4 (normal)
   A normal pH may indicate perfectly normal blood gases, *or* it may be an indication of a *compensated* imbalance. A compensated imbalance is one in which the body has been able to correct the pH by either respiratory or metabolic changes (depending on the primary problem). For example, a patient with primary metabolic acidosis starts out with a low bicarbonate level but a normal CO_2 level. Soon afterward, the lungs try to compensate for the imbalance by exhaling large amounts of CO_2 (hyperventilation). As another example, a patient with primary respiratory acidosis starts out with a high CO_2 level; soon afterward, the kidneys attempt to compensate by retaining bicarbonate. If the compensatory mechanism is able to restore the bicarbonate to carbonic acid ratio back to 20:1, full compensation (and thus normal pH) will be achieved.
2. The next step is to determine the primary cause of the disturbance. This is done by evaluating the $PaCO_2$ and HCO_3^- in relation to the pH.
   Example: pH > 7.4 (alkalosis)
   a. If the $PaCO_2$ is < 40 mm Hg, the primary disturbance is respiratory alkalosis. (This situation occurs when a patient hyperventilates and "blows off" too much CO_2. Recall that CO_2 dissolved in water becomes carbonic acid, the acid side of the "carbonic acid–bicarbonate buffer system.")
   b. If the HCO_3^- is >24 mmol/L, the primary disturbance is metabolic alkalosis. (This situation occurs when the body gains too

much bicarbonate, an alkaline substance. Bicarbonate is the basic or alkaline side of the "carbonic acid–bicarbonate buffer system.")

   Example: pH < 7.4 (acidosis)
   a. If the $PaCO_2$ is >40 mm Hg, the primary disturbance is respiratory acidosis. (This situation occurs when a patient hypoventilates and thus retains too much CO_2, an acidic substance.)
   b. If the HCO_3^- is <24 mmol/L, the primary disturbance is metabolic acidosis. (This situation occurs when the body's bicarbonate level drops, either because of direct bicarbonate loss or because of gains of acids such as lactic acid or ketones.)
3. The next step involves determining if compensation has begun. This is done by looking at the value other than the primary disorder. If it is moving in the same direction as the primary value, compensation is underway. Consider the following gases:

pH	$PaCO_2$	HCO_3^-
(1) 7.20	60 mm Hg	24 mmol/L
(2) 7.40	60 mm Hg	37 mmol/L

   The first set (1) indicates acute respiratory acidosis without compensation (the $PaCO_2$ is high, the HCO_3^- is normal). The second set (2) indicates chronic respiratory acidosis. Note that compensation has take place; that is, the HCO_3^- has elevated to an appropriate level to balance the high $PaCO_2$ and produce a normal pH.
4. Two distinct acid–base disturbances may occur simultaneously. These can be identified when the pH does not explain one of the changes.
   Example: Metabolic and respiratory acidosis
   a. pH   7.21   decreased acid
   b. $PaCO_2$ 52   increased acid
   c. HCO_3 13   decreased acid
   This is an example of metabolic and respiratory acidosis.

When administering parenteral fluids, the nurse monitors the patient's response to the fluids, considering the fluid volume, the content of the fluid, and the patient's clinical status.

Isotonic Fluids

Fluids that are classified as isotonic have a total osmolality close to that of the ECF and do not cause red blood cells to shrink or swell. The composition of these fluids may or may not approximate that of the ECF. Isotonic fluids expand the ECF volume. One litre of isotonic fluid expands the ECF by 1 L; however, it expands the plasma by only 0.25 L because it is a crystalloid fluid and diffuses quickly into the ECF compartment. For the same reason, 3 L of isotonic fluid is needed to replace 1 L of blood loss. Because these fluids expand the intravascular space, patients with hypertension and heart failure should be carefully monitored for signs of fluid overload.

D$_5$W

A solution of D$_5$W has a serum osmolality of 252 mmol/L. Once administered, the glucose is rapidly metabolized, and this initially isotonic solution then disperses as a hypotonic fluid, one-third extracellular and two-thirds intracellular. It is essential to consider this action of D$_5$W, especially if the patient is at risk for increased intracranial pressure. During fluid resuscitation, this solution should not be used because it can cause hyperglycemia. Therefore, D$_5$W is used mainly to supply water and to correct an increased serum osmolality. About 1 L of D$_5$W provides fewer than 800 kJ and is a minor source of energy for the body's daily requirements.

NORMAL SALINE SOLUTION

Normal saline (0.9% sodium chloride) solution has a total osmolality of 308 mmol/L. Because the osmolality is entirely contributed by electrolytes, the solution remains within the ECF. For this reason, normal saline solution is often used to correct an extracellular volume deficit. Although referred to as "normal," it contains only sodium and chloride and does not actually simulate the ECF. It is used with administration of blood transfusions and to replace large sodium losses, as in burn injuries. It is not used for heart failure, pulmonary edema, renal impairment, or sodium retention. Normal saline does not supply calories.

OTHER ISOTONIC SOLUTIONS

Several other solutions contain ions in addition to sodium and chloride and are somewhat similar to the ECF in composition. Lactated Ringer's solution contains potassium and calcium in addition to sodium chloride. It is used to correct dehydration and sodium depletion and replace GI losses. Lactated Ringer's solution contains bicarbonate precursors as well. These solutions are marketed, with slight variations, under various trade names.

Hypotonic Fluids

One purpose of hypotonic solutions is to replace cellular fluid, because it is hypotonic as compared with plasma. Another is to provide free water for excretion of body wastes. At times, hypotonic sodium solutions are used to treat hypernatremia and other hyperosmolar conditions. Half-strength saline (0.45% sodium chloride) solution, with an osmolality of 154 mmol/L, is frequently used. Multiple-electrolyte solutions are also available. Excessive infusions of hypotonic solutions can lead to intravascular fluid depletion, decreased blood pressure, cellular edema, and cell damage. These solutions exert less osmotic pressure than the ECF.

Hypertonic Fluids

When normal saline solution or lactated Ringer's solution contains 5% dextrose, the total osmolality exceeds that of the ECF. The dextrose is quickly metabolized, however, and only the isotonic solution remains. Therefore, any effect on the intracellular compartment is temporary. Similarly, with hypotonic multiple-electrolyte solutions containing 5% dextrose, once the dextrose is metabolized, these solutions disperse as hypotonic fluids.

Higher concentrations of dextrose, such as 50% dextrose in water, are administered to help meet caloric requirements. These solutions are strongly hypertonic and must be administered into central veins so that they can be diluted by rapid blood flow.

Saline solutions are also available in osmolar concentrations greater than that of the ECF. These solutions draw water from the ICF to the ECF and cause cells to shrink. If administered rapidly or in large quantity, they may cause an extracellular volume excess and precipitate circulatory overload and dehydration. As a result, these solutions must be administered cautiously and usually only when the serum osmolality has decreased to dangerously low levels. Hypertonic solutions exert an osmotic pressure greater than that of the ECF.

Other IV Substances

When the patient's GI tract is unable to tolerate food, nutritional requirements are often met using the IV route. Parenteral solutions may include high concentrations of glucose, protein, or fat to meet nutritional requirements. The parenteral route may also be used to administer colloids, plasma expanders, and blood products. Examples of blood products include whole blood, packed red blood cells, albumin, and cryoprecipitate; these are discussed in more detail in Chapter 33.

Many medications are also delivered by the IV route, either by infusion or directly into the vein. Because IV medications enter the circulation rapidly, administration by this route is potentially very hazardous. All medications can produce adverse reactions; however, medications given by the IV route can cause these reactions within 15 minutes after administration because the medications are delivered directly into the bloodstream. Administration rates and recommended dilutions for individual medications are available in specialized texts pertaining to IV medications and in manufacturers' package inserts; these should be consulted to ensure safe IV administration of medications.

 NURSING ALERT The nurse must assess the patient for a history of allergic reactions to medications; although this is important when any medication is to be administered, it is even more important with IV administration because the medication is delivered directly into the bloodstream.

Nursing Management of the Patient Receiving IV Therapy

Venipuncture, or the ability to gain access to the venous system for administering fluids and medications, is an expected nursing skill in many settings. This responsibility includes selecting the appropriate venipuncture site and type of cannula and being proficient in the technique of vein entry.

PREPARING TO ADMINISTER IV THERAPY

The Registered Nurses Association of Ontario best practice guideline *Assessment and Device Selection for Vascular Access* contains evidence-based support for nurses related to client assessment and device selection, risk reduction, client education and documentation (RNAO, 2004). Before performing venipuncture, the nurse carries out hand hygiene, applies gloves, and informs the patient about the procedure. Next the nurse selects the most appropriate insertion site and type of cannula for a particular patient. Factors influencing these choices include the type of solution to be administered, the expected duration of IV therapy, the patient's general condition, and the availability of veins. The skill of the person initiating the infusion is also an important consideration.

CHOOSING AN IV SITE

Many sites can be used for IV therapy, but ease of access and potential hazards vary. Veins of the extremities are designated as peripheral locations and are ordinarily the only sites used by nurses. Because they are relatively safe and easy to enter, arm veins are most commonly used (Fig. 14-7). The metacarpal, cephalic, basilic, and median veins as well as their branches are recommended sites because of their size and ease of access. More distal sites should be used first, with more proximal sites used subsequently. Leg veins should rarely, if ever, be used because of the high risk of thromboembolism. Additional sites to avoid include veins distal to a previous IV infiltration or phlebitic area, sclerosed or thrombosed veins, an arm with an arteriovenous shunt or fistula, or an arm affected by edema, in-

FIGURE 14-7 Site selection for peripheral cannulation of veins: anterior (palmar) veins at *left,* posterior (dorsal) veins at *right.*

fection, blood clot, or skin breakdown. The arm on the side of a mastectomy is avoided because of impaired lymphatic flow.

Central veins commonly used by physicians include the subclavian and internal jugular veins. It is possible to gain access to (or cannulate) these larger vessels even when peripheral sites have collapsed, and they allow for the administration of hyperosmolar solutions. Hazards are much greater, however, and may include inadvertent entry into an artery or the pleural space.

Ideally, both arms and hands are carefully inspected before choosing a specific venipuncture site that does not interfere with mobility. For this reason, the antecubital fossa is avoided, except as a last resort. The most distal site of the arm or hand is generally used first so that subsequent IV access sites can be moved progressively upward. The following are factors to consider when selecting a site for venipuncture:

- Condition of the vein
- Type of fluid or medication to be infused
- Duration of therapy
- Patient's age and size
- Whether the patient is right- or left-handed
- Patient's medical history and current health status
- Skill of the person performing the venipuncture

After applying a tourniquet, the nurse palpates and inspects the vein. The vein should feel firm, elastic, engorged, and round, not hard, flat, or bumpy. Because arteries lie close to veins in the antecubital fossa, the vessel should be palpated for arterial pulsation (even with a tourniquet on), and cannulation of pulsating vessels should be avoided. General guidelines for selecting a cannula include:

- Length: 1.9 to 3.175 cm long
- Diameter: narrow diameter of the cannula to occupy minimal space within the vein
- Gauge: 20 to 22 gauge for most IV fluids; a larger gauge for caustic or viscous solutions; 14 to 18 gauge for blood administration and for trauma patients and those undergoing surgery

Hand veins are easiest to cannulate. Cannula tips should not rest in a flexion area (eg, the antecubital fossa) as this could inhibit the IV flow.

SELECTING VENIPUNCTURE DEVICES

Equipment used to gain access to the vasculature includes cannulas, needleless IV delivery systems, and peripherally inserted central catheter or midline catheter access lines.

Cannulas. Most peripheral access devices are cannulas. They have an obturator inside a tube that is later removed. "Catheter" and "cannula" are terms that are used interchangeably. The main types of cannula devices available are those referred to as winged infusion sets (butterfly) with a steel needle or as an over-the-needle catheter with wings, indwelling plastic cannulas inserted over a steel needle, and indwelling plastic cannulas inserted through a steel needle. Scalp vein or butterfly needles are short steel needles with plastic wing handles. These are easy to insert, but because they are small and nonpliable, infiltration occurs easily. The use of these needles should be limited to obtaining blood specimens or administering bolus injections or infusions lasting only a few hours, as they increase the risk for vein injury and infiltration. Insertion of an over-the-needle catheter requires the additional step of advancing the catheter into the vein after venipuncture. Because these devices are less likely to cause infiltration, they are frequently preferred over winged infusion sets.

Plastic cannulas inserted through a hollow needle are usually called intracatheters. They are available in long lengths and are well suited for placement in central locations. Because insertion requires threading the cannula through the vein for a relatively long distance, these can be difficult to insert. The most commonly used infusion device is the over-the-needle catheter. A hollow metal stylet is preinserted into the catheter and extends through the distal tip of the catheter to allow puncture of the vessel, in an effort to guide the catheter as the venipuncture is performed. The vein is punctured and a flashback of blood appears in the closed chamber behind the catheter hub. The catheter is threaded through the stylet into the vein and the stylet is then removed. There are many safety over-the-needle catheter designs available with retracting stylets to protect health care workers from needlestick injuries.

Many types of cannulas are available for IV therapy. Some of the variations in these cannulas include the thickness of the cannula wall (affects rate of flow), the sharpness of the insertion needles (determines needle insertion technique), the softening properties of the cannula (influences the length of time the cannula can remain in place), safety features (minimizes risk of needlestick injuries and blood-borne exposure), and the number of lumens (determines the number of solutions that can be infused simultaneously). Cannula systems that help prevent needlesticks and transmission of blood-borne diseases are discussed below. Most standard peripheral catheters are composed of some form of plastic. Teflon (polytetrafluoroethylene)–coated catheters have less thrombogenic properties and are less inflammatory than polyurethane or PVC. Catheter size for steel needles can range from 27 to 13 gauge. Plastic catheters range in size from 27 to 12 gauge.

To select the ideal product for use, consideration should be given to which product provides the greatest patient satisfaction and offers quality, cost-effective infusion care. All devices should be radiopaque to determine catheter location by x-ray, if indicated. All catheters are thrombogenic and differ only in their degree of thrombus occurrence. Biocompatibility, another characteristic of a catheter, ensures that inflammation and irritation do not occur. Silicone catheters are the most bioinert catheter available today.

Needleless IV Delivery Systems. In an effort to decrease needlestick injuries and exposure to HIV, hepatitis, and other blood-borne pathogens, agencies have implemented needleless IV delivery systems. These systems have built-in protection against needlestick injuries and provide a safe means of using and disposing of an IV administration set (which consists of tubing, an area for inserting the tubing into the container of IV fluid, and an adapter for connecting the tubing to the needle). Numerous companies produce needleless components. IV line connectors allow the simultaneous infusion of IV medications and other intermittent medications (known as a piggyback delivery) without the use of needles (Fig. 14-8). Technology is advancing and moving away from use of the traditional stylet. An example is a self-sheathing stylet that is recessed into a rigid chamber at the hub of the catheter when its insertion is complete. Other designs have placed the stylet at the end of a flexible wire to avoid needlesticks.

Many examples of these devices are on the market. Each institution must evaluate products to determine its own needs based on best practice guidelines and the institution's policies and procedures.

Peripherally Inserted Central Catheter or Midline Catheter Access Lines. Patients who need moderate- to long-term parenteral therapy often receive a peripherally inserted central

A

B

C

FIGURE 14-8 One example of a needleless IV access device (InterLink Syringe Cannula, Baxter Healthcare Corp., Becton Dickinson Division) (**A**) designed to prevent needlesticks and other accidents. After drawing medication into a syringe according to manufacturer's guidelines and swabbing the Y-site intersection with antiseptic, the nurse can insert the syringe-cannula apparatus into the Y site (**B**) and deliver bolus dose medications. If a blood tube holder (**C**) is attached to the cannula, blood can be withdrawn safely without fear of contact or spills.

catheter or a midline catheter. These catheters are also used for patients with limited peripheral access (eg, obese or emaciated patients, IV/injection drug users) who require IV antibiotics, blood, and parenteral nutrition. For these devices to be used, the median cephalic, basilic, and cephalic veins must be pliable (not sclerosed or hardened) and not subject to repeated puncture. If these veins are damaged, then central venous access via the subclavian or internal jugular vein, or surgical placement of an implanted port or a vascular access device, must be considered as an alternative. Table 14-9 compares peripherally inserted central and midline catheter lines.

The principles for inserting these lines are much the same as those for inserting peripheral catheters; however, their insertion should be undertaken only by those who are experienced and specially skilled in inserting IV lines.

The physician prescribes the line and the solution to be infused. Insertion of either line requires sterile technique. The size of the catheter lumen chosen is based on the type of solution, the size of the patient, and the vein to be used. The patient's consent is obtained before use of these catheters. Use of the dominant arm is recommended as the site for inserting the cannula into the superior vena cava to ensure adequate arm movement, which encourages blood flow and reduces the risk of dependent edema.

TEACHING THE PATIENT

Except in emergency situations, a patient should be prepared in advance for an IV infusion. The venipuncture, the expected length of infusion, and activity restrictions are explained. Then the patient should have an opportunity to ask questions and voice concerns. For example, some patients believe they will die if small bubbles in the tubing enter their veins. After acknowledging this fear, the nurse can explain that usually only relatively large volumes of air administered rapidly are dangerous.

PREPARING THE IV SITE

Before preparing the skin, the nurse should ask the patient if he or she is allergic to latex or iodine, products commonly used in preparing for IV therapy. Excessive hair at the selected site may be removed by clipping to increase the visibility of the veins and to facilitate insertion of the cannula and adherence of dressings to the IV insertion site. Because infection can be a major complication of IV therapy, the IV device, the fluid, the container, and the tubing must be sterile. The insertion site is scrubbed with a sterile pad soaked in 10% povidone–iodine (Betadine) or chlorhexidine gluconate solution for 2 to 3 minutes, working from the centre of the area to the periphery and allowing the area to air dry. The site should not be wiped with 70% alcohol because the alcohol negates the effect of the disinfecting solution. (Alcohol pledgets are used for 30 seconds instead, only if the patient is allergic to iodine.) The nurse must perform hand hygiene and put on gloves. Nonsterile disposable gloves must be worn during the venipuncture procedure because of the likelihood of coming into contact with the patient's blood.

PERFORMING VENIPUNCTURE

Guidelines and a suggested sequence for venipuncture are presented in Chart 14-2. For veins that are very small or particularly fragile, modifications in the technique may be necessary. Alternative methods can be found in journal articles or in specialized textbooks of IV therapy. Institutional policies and procedures determine whether all nurses must be certified to perform venipuncture. A nurse certified in IV therapy or an IV team can be consulted to assist with initiating IV therapy.

MAINTAINING THERAPY

Maintaining an existing IV infusion is a nursing responsibility that demands knowledge of the solutions being administered and the principles of flow. In addition, patients must be assessed carefully for both local and systemic complications.

FACTORS AFFECTING FLOW

The flow of an IV infusion is governed by the same principles that govern fluid movement in general.

- Flow is directly proportional to the height of the liquid column. Raising the height of the infusion container may improve a sluggish flow.
- Flow is directly proportional to the diameter of the tubing. The clamp on IV tubing regulates the flow by changing the tubing diameter. In addition, the flow is faster through large-gauge rather than small-gauge cannulas.
- Flow is inversely proportional to the length of the tubing. Adding extension tubing to an IV line will decrease the flow.
- Flow is inversely proportional to the viscosity of a fluid. Viscous IV solutions, such as blood, require a larger cannula than do water or saline solutions.

MONITORING FLOW

Because so many factors influence gravity flow, a solution does not necessarily continue to run at the speed originally set. Therefore, the nurse monitors IV infusions frequently to make sure that the fluid is flowing at the intended rate. The IV container should be marked with tape to indicate at a glance whether the correct amount has infused. The flow rate is calculated when the solution is originally started, then monitored at least hourly. To calculate the flow rate, the nurse determines the number of drops delivered per millilitre; this varies with equipment and is usually printed on the administration set packaging. A formula that can be used to calculate the drop rate is:

gtt/mL of infusion set/60 (min in hr) × total hourly vol = gtt/min

Flushing of a vascular device is performed to ensure patency and prevent the mixing of incompatible medications or solutions. This procedure should be carried out at established intervals, according to hospital policy and procedure, especially for intermittently used catheters. Most manufacturers and researchers (LeDuc, 1997) suggest the use of saline for flushing. The volume of the flush solution should be equal to at least twice the volume capacity of the catheter. The catheter should be clamped before the syringe is completely empty and withdrawn to prevent reflux of blood into the lumen, which could cause catheter clotting.

A variety of electronic infusion devices are available to assist in IV fluid delivery. These devices allow more accurate administration of fluids and medications than is possible with routine gravity-flow setups. A pump is a positive-pressure device that uses pressure to infuse fluid at a pressure of 10 psi. Newer models use a pressure of 5 psi. The pressure exerted by the pump overrides vascular resistance (increased tubing length, low height of the IV container).

Volumetric pumps calculate the volume delivered by measuring the volume in a reservoir that is part of the set and calibrated in mL/h. A controller is an infusion assist device that relies on gravity for infusion; the volume is calibrated in drops/min. A controller

Table 14-9 • **Comparison of Peripherally Inserted Central and Midline Catheters**

	PERIPHERALLY INSERTED CENTRAL CATHETER	MIDLINE CATHETER
Indications	Parenteral nutrition; IV fluid replacement; administration of chemotherapy agents, analgesics, and antibiotics; removal of blood specimens	Parenteral nutrition; IV fluid replacement; administration of analgesics and antibiotics (no solution or medications with a pH <5 or >9 or osmolarity >500 mmol/L); removal of blood specimens
Features	Single- and double-lumen catheters available 40–60 cm long; gauge variable (16–24 g)	Single- and double-lumen catheters available (16–24 g) 7.5–20 cm in length. Can increase two gauges in size as it softens
Material	Radiopaque, polymer (polyurethane), Silastic materials. Flexible.	Silicone, polyurethane and their derivatives
Insertion sites	Venipuncture performed in the antecubital fossa, above or below it into the basilic, cephalic, or axillary veins of the dominant arm. The median basilic is the ideal insertion site.	Venipuncture performed 2–3 fingerbreadths above the antecubital fossa or 1 fingerbreadth below the antecubital fossa into the cephalic, basilic, or median cubital vein
Catheter placement	The tip of the catheter lies in the superior vena cava or the brachiocephalic vein.	Between the antecubital area and the head of the clavicle (tip in axilla region). The tip terminates in the proximal portion of the extremity below axilla and proximal to central veins and is advanced 8–25 cm.
Insertion method	Through-the-needle technique, with or without a guidewire, breakaway needle with introducer or cannula with introducer (peelaway sheath). (A peripherally inserted central catheter can also be used as a midline catheter.) Insertion can be accomplished at the bedside using sterile technique. Arm to be used should be positioned in abduction to 90-degree angle. Consent is required. Catheter may stay in place for up to 12 months or as long as required without complications.	No separate guidewire or introducer is needed. Stiff catheter is passed using the catheter advancement tab. Insertion can be accomplished at the bedside using sterile technique. Arm to be used should be positioned in abduction to 45-degree angle. Consent is required. Catheter may stay in place for 2–4 weeks.
Potential complications	Malposition, pneumothorax, hemothorax, hydrothorax, dysrhythmias, nerve or tendon damage, respiratory distress, catheter embolism, thrombophlebitis, or catheter occlusion. Compared with centrally placed catheters, venipuncture in the antecubital space reduces risk of insertion complications.	Thrombosis, phlebitis, air embolism, infection, vascular perforation, bleeding, catheter transection, occlusion
Contraindications	Dermatitis, cellulitis, burns, high fluid volume infusions, rapid bolus injections, hemodialysis, and venous thrombosis. No clamping of this catheter or splinting of the arm permitted. No blood pressure or tourniquets to be used on extremity where PICC is inserted.	Dermatitis, cellulitis, burns, high fluid volume infusions, rapid bolus injection, hemodialysis, and venous thrombosis. No blood pressure or tourniquet to be used on extremity where midline catheter is placed.
Catheter maintenance	Sterile dressing changes according to agency policy and procedures. Generally, dressing is changed 2 or 3 ×/week or when wet, soiled, or nonocclusive. Line is flushed every 12 hours with 3 mL normal saline followed by heparin 3 mL (100 U/mL) per lumen.	Sterile dressing changes according to policy and procedures. Generally the dressing should be changed 2 or 3 ×/week or when wet, soiled, or nonocclusive. Line is flushed after each infusion or every 12 hours with 5–10 mL normal saline followed by 1 mL of heparin (100 U/mL). Catheter must be anchored securely to prevent its dislodgment.
Postplacement	Chest x-ray needed to confirm placement	Chest x-ray to assess placement may be obtained if unable to flush catheter, if no free flow blood return, if difficulty with catheter advancement, or if guidewire difficult to remove or bent on removal.
Assessment	Daily measurement of arm circumference (10 cm above insertion site) and length of exposed catheter	Daily measurement of arm circumference (10 cm above insertion site) and length of exposed catheter
Removal	Catheter should be removed when no longer indicated for use, if contaminated, or if complications occur. Arm is abducted during removal. Pressure is applied on removal with a sterile dressing and antiseptic ointment to site. Dressing is changed every 24 hours until epithelialization occurs.	Catheter should be removed when no longer indicated for use, if contaminated, or if complications occur. Arm is abducted during removal. Pressure is applied on removal with a sterile dressing and antiseptic ointment to site. Dressing is changed every 24 hours until epithelialization occurs.
Advantages	Reduces cost and avoids repeated venipunctures compared with centrally placed catheters. Decreases incidence of catheter-related infections.	Reduces cost and avoids repeated venipunctures compared with centrally placed catheters. Decreases incidence of catheter-related infections.

Chart 14-2

GUIDELINES FOR Starting an Intravenous Infusion

NURSING ACTION	RATIONALE
Preparation	
1. Verify prescription for IV therapy, check solution label, and identify patient.	1. Serious errors can be avoided by careful checking.
2. Explain procedure to patient.	2. Knowledge increases patient comfort and cooperation.
3. Carry out hand hygiene and put on disposable nonlatex gloves.	3. Asepsis is essential to prevent infection. Prevents exposure of nurse to patient's blood and of patient and nurse to latex.
4. Apply a tourniquet 10–15 cm above the site and identify a suitable vein.	4. This will distend the veins and allow them to be visualized.
5. Choose site. Use distal veins of hands and arms first.	5. Careful site selection will increase likelihood of successful venipuncture and preservation of vein. Using distal sites first preserves sites proximal to the previously cannulated site for subsequent venipunctures. Veins of feet and lower extremity should be avoided due to risk of thrombophlebitis. (In consultation with the physician, the saphenous vein of the ankle or dorsum of the foot may occasionally be used.)
6. Choose IV cannula or catheter.	6. Length and gauge of cannula should be appropriate for both site and purpose of infusion. The shortest gauge and length needed to deliver prescribed therapy should be used.
7. Connect infusion bag and tubing, and run solution through tubing to displace air; cover end of tubing.	7. Prevents delay; equipment must be ready to connect immediately after successful venipuncture to prevent clotting
8. Raise bed to comfortable working height and position for patient; adjust lighting. Position patient's arm below heart level to encourage capillary filling. Place protective pad on bed under patient's arm.	8. Proper positioning will increase likelihood of success and provide comfort for patient.
Procedure	
1. Depending on agency policy and procedure, lidocaine 1% (without epinephrine) 0.1–0.2 mL may be injected locally to the IV site or a transdermal analgesic cream (EMLA) may be applied to the site 60 minutes before IV placement or blood withdrawal. Intradermal injection of bacteriostatic 0.9% sodium chloride may have a local anesthetic effect.	1. Reduces pain locally from procedure and decreases anxiety about pain
2. Question the patient carefully about sensitivity to latex; use blood-pressure cuff rather than latex tourniquet if there is possibility of sensitivity.	2. Reduces risk of allergic reaction
3. Apply a new tourniquet for each patient or a blood pressure cuff 15 to 20 cm above injection site. Palpate for a pulse distal to the tourniquet. Ask patient to open and close fist several times or position patient's arm in a dependent position to distend a vein.	3. The tourniquet distends the vein and makes it easier to enter; it should never be tight enough to occlude arterial flow. If a radial pulse cannot be palpated distal to the tourniquet, it is too tight. A new tourniquet should be used for each patient to prevent the transmission of microorganisms. A blood pressure cuff may be used for elderly patients to avoid rupture of the veins. A clenched fist encourages the vein to become round and turgid. Positioning the arm below the level of the patient's heart promotes capillary filling. Warm packs can promote vasodilation as well.
4. Ascertain if the patient is allergic to iodine. Prepare site by scrubbing with chlorhexidine gluconate or povidone–iodine swabs for 2–3 min in circular motion, moving outward from injection site. Allow to dry. a. If the site selected is excessively hairy, clip hair. (Check agency's policy and procedure about this practice.) b. 70% isopropyl alcohol is an alternative solution that may be used.	4. Strict asepsis and careful site preparation are essential to prevent infection.
5. With hand not holding the venous access device, steady patient's arm and use finger or thumb to pull skin taut over vessel.	5. Applying traction to the vein helps to stabilize it.
6. Holding needle bevel up and at 5°–25° angle, depending on the depth of the vein, pierce skin to reach but not penetrate vein.	6. Bevel-up position usually produces less trauma to skin and vein. A superficial vein needs a smaller cannula angle and a vein deeper in subcutaneous tissue requires a greater cannula angle.
7. Decrease angle of needle further until nearly parallel with skin, then enter vein either directly above or from the side in one quick motion.	7. Two-stage procedure decreases chance of thrusting needle through posterior wall of vein as skin is entered. No attempt should be made to reinsert the stylet because of risk of severing or puncturing the catheter.

(continued)

Chart 14-2

GUIDELINES FOR Starting an Intravenous Infusion (Continued)

NURSING ACTION	RATIONALE

8. If backflow of blood is visible, straighten angle and advance needle. Additional steps for catheter inserted over needle:
  a. Advance needle 0.6 cm after successful venipuncture.
 	
  b. Hold needle hub, and slide catheter over the needle into the vein. Never reinsert needle into a plastic catheter or pull the catheter back into the needle.
  c. Remove needle while pressing lightly on the skin over the catheter tip; hold catheter hub in place.
9. Release tourniquet and attach infusion tubing; open clamp enough to allow drip.
	8. Backflow may not occur if vein is small; this position decreases chance of puncturing posterior wall of vein.
	  a. Advancing the needle slightly makes certain the plastic catheter has entered the vein.
	  b. Reinsertion of the needle or pulling the catheter back can sever the catheter, causing catheter embolism.
	
	  c. Slight pressure prevents bleeding before tubing is attached.
	9. Infusion must be attached promptly to prevent clotting of blood in cannula. After two unsuccessful attempts at venipuncture, assistance by a more experienced health care provider is recommended to avoid unnecessary trauma to the patient and the possibility of limiting future sites for vascular access.

10. Slip a sterile 5 cm × 5 cm gauze pad under the catheter hub. 11. Anchor needle firmly in place with tape. 12. Cover the insertion site with a transparent dressing, bandage, or sterile gauze; tape in place with nonallergenic tape but do not encircle extremity. 13. Tape a small loop of IV tubing onto dressing. 14. Cover the insertion site with a dressing according to hospital policy and procedure. A gauze or transparent dressing may be used. 15. Label dressing with type and length of cannula, date, time, and initials. 16. A padded, appropriate-length arm board may be applied to an area of flexion (neurovascular checks should be performed frequently). 17. Calculate infusion rate and regulate flow of infusion. For hourly IV rate use the following formula: gtt/mL of infusion set/60 (min in hr) × total hourly vol = gtt/min 18. Document site, cannula size and type, the number of attempts at insertion, time, solution, IV rate, and patient response to procedure.	10. The gauze acts as a sterile field. 11. A stable needle is less likely to become dislodged or to irritate the vein. 12. Tape encircling extremity can act as a tourniquet. 13. The loop decreases the chance of inadvertent cannula removal if the tubing is pulled. 14. Transparent dressings allow assessment of the insertion site for phlebitis, infiltration, and infection without removing the dressing. 15. Labelling facilitates assessment and safe discontinuation. 16. Secures cannula placement and allows correct flow rate (neurovascular checks assess nerve, muscle, and vascular function to be sure function is not affected by immobilization) 17. Infusion must be regulated carefully to prevent overinfusion or underinfusion. Calculation of the IV rate is essential for the safe delivery of fluids. Safe administration requires knowledge of the volume of fluid to be infused, total infusion time, and the calibration of the administration set (found on the IV tubing package; 10, 12, 15, or 60 drops to deliver 1 mL of fluid). 18. Documentation is essential to promote continuity of care.

uses a drop sensor to monitor the flow. Factors essential for the safe use of pumps include alarms to signify the presence of air in the IV line and occlusion. The standard for the accurate delivery of fluid or medication via an electronic IV infusion pump is plus or minus 5%. The manufacturer's directions must be read carefully before using any infusion pump or controller, because there are many variations in available models. Use of these devices does not eliminate the need for the nurse to monitor the infusion and the patient frequently.

DISCONTINUING AN INFUSION

The removal of an IV catheter is associated with two possible dangers: bleeding and catheter embolism. To prevent excessive bleeding, a dry, sterile pressure dressing should be held over the site as the catheter is removed. Firm pressure is applied until hemostasis occurs.

If a plastic IV catheter is severed, the loose fragment can travel to the right ventricle and block blood flow. To detect this com-

plication when the catheter is removed, the nurse compares the expected length of the catheter with its actual length. Plastic catheters should be withdrawn carefully and their length measured to make certain that no fragment has broken off.

Great care must be exercised when using scissors around the dressing site. If the catheter clearly has been severed, the nurse can attempt to occlude the vein above the site by applying a tourniquet to prevent the catheter from entering the central circulation (until surgical removal is possible). As always, however, it is better to prevent a potentially fatal problem than to deal with it after it has occurred. Fortunately, catheter embolism can be prevented easily by following simple rules:

- Avoid using scissors near the catheter.
- Avoid withdrawing the catheter through the insertion needle.
- Follow the manufacturer's guidelines carefully (eg, cover the needle point with the bevel shield to prevent severance of the catheter).

MANAGING SYSTEMIC COMPLICATIONS

IV therapy predisposes the patient to numerous hazards, including both local and systemic complications. Systemic complications occur less frequently but are usually more serious than local complications. They include circulatory overload, air embolism, febrile reaction, and infection.

Fluid Overload. Overloading the circulatory system with excessive IV fluids causes increased blood pressure and central venous pressure. Signs and symptoms of fluid overload include moist crackles on auscultation of the lungs, edema, weight gain, dyspnea, and respirations that are shallow and have an increased rate. Possible causes include rapid infusion of an IV solution or hepatic, cardiac, or renal disease. The risk for fluid overload and subsequent pulmonary edema is especially increased in elderly patients with cardiac disease; this is referred to as circulatory overload.

The treatment for circulatory overload is decreasing the IV rate, monitoring vital signs frequently, assessing breath sounds, and placing the patient in a high Fowler's position. The physician is contacted immediately. This complication can be avoided by using an infusion pump for infusions and by carefully monitoring all infusions. Complications of circulatory overload include heart failure and pulmonary edema.

Air Embolism. The risk of air embolism is rare but ever-present. It is most often associated with cannulation of central veins. Manifestations of air embolism include dyspnea and cyanosis; hypotension; weak, rapid pulse; loss of consciousness; and chest, shoulder, and low back pain. Treatment calls for immediately clamping the cannula, placing the patient on the left side in the Trendelenburg position, assessing vital signs and breath sounds, and administering oxygen. Air embolism can be prevented by using a Luer-Lok adapter on all lines, filling all tubing completely with solution, and using an air detection alarm on an IV pump. Complications of air embolism include shock and death. The amount of air necessary to induce death in humans is not known; however, the rate of entry is probably as important as the actual volume of air.

Septicemia and Other Infections. Pyrogenic substances in either the infusion solution or the IV administration set can induce a febrile reaction and septicemia. Signs and symptoms include an abrupt temperature elevation shortly after the infusion is started, backache, headache, increased pulse and respiratory rate, nausea and vomiting, diarrhea, chills and shaking, and general malaise. In severe septicemia, vascular collapse and septic shock may occur. Causes of septicemia include contamination of the IV product or a break in aseptic technique, especially in immunocompromised patients. Treatment is symptomatic and includes culturing of the IV cannula, tubing, or solution if suspect and establishing a new IV site for medication or fluid administration. See Chapter 15 for a discussion of septic shock.

Infection ranges in severity from local involvement of the insertion site to systemic dissemination of organisms through the bloodstream, as in septicemia. Measures to prevent infection are essential at the time the IV line is inserted and throughout the entire infusion. Prevention includes:

- Careful hand hygiene before every contact with any part of the infusion system or patient
- Examining the IV containers for cracks, leaks, or cloudiness, which may indicate a contaminated solution
- Using strict aseptic technique

- Firmly anchoring the IV cannula to prevent to-and-fro motion
- Inspecting the IV site daily and replacing a soiled or wet dressing with a dry sterile dressing. (Antimicrobial agents that should be used for site care include 2% tincture of iodine, 10% povidone–iodine, alcohol, or chlorhexidine, used alone or in combination.)
- Removing the IV cannula at the first sign of local inflammation, contamination, or complication
- Replacing the peripheral IV cannula every 48 to 72 hours, or as indicated
- Replacing the IV cannula inserted during emergency conditions (with questionable asepsis) as soon as possible
- Using a 0.2-micron air-eliminating and bacteria/particulate retentive filter with non-lipid-containing solutions that require filtration. The filter can be added to the proximal or distal end of the administration set. If added to the proximal end between the fluid container and the tubing spike, the filter ensures sterility and particulate removal from the infusate container and prevents inadvertent infusion of air. If added to the distal end of the administration set, it filters air particles and contaminants introduced from add-on devices, secondary administration sets, or interruptions to the primary system.
- Replacing the solution bag and administration set in accordance with agency policy and procedure
- Infusing or discarding medication or solution within 24 hours of its addition to an administration set
- Changing primary and secondary continuous administration sets every 72 hours, or immediately if contamination is suspected
- Changing primary intermittent administration sets every 24 hours, or immediately if contamination is suspected

MANAGING LOCAL COMPLICATIONS

Local complications of IV therapy include infiltration and extravasation, phlebitis, thrombophlebitis, hematoma, and clotting of the needle.

Infiltration and Extravasation. Infiltration is the unintentional administration of a nonvesicant solution or medication into surrounding tissue. This can occur when the IV cannula dislodges or perforates the wall of the vein. Infiltration is characterized by edema around the insertion site, leakage of IV fluid from the insertion site, discomfort and coolness in the area of infiltration, and a significant decrease in the flow rate. When the solution is particularly irritating, sloughing of tissue may result. Closely monitoring the insertion site is necessary to detect infiltration before it becomes severe.

Infiltration is usually easily recognized if the insertion area is larger than the same site of the opposite extremity; however, it is not always so obvious. A common misconception is that a backflow of blood into the tubing proves that the catheter is properly placed within the vein. If the catheter tip has pierced the wall of the vessel, however, IV fluid will seep into tissues as well as flow into the vein. Although blood return occurs, infiltration has occurred as well. A more reliable means of confirming infiltration is to apply a tourniquet above (or proximal to) the infusion site and tighten it enough to restrict venous flow. If the infusion continues to drip despite the venous obstruction, infiltration is present.

As soon as the nurse notes infiltration, the infusion should be stopped, the IV discontinued, and a sterile dressing applied to the site after careful inspection to determine the extent of infiltration. The infiltration of any amount of blood product, irritant, or vesicant is considered the most severe.

The IV infusion should be started in a new site or proximal to the infiltration if the same extremity is used. A warm compress may be applied to the site if small volumes of noncaustic solutions have infiltrated over a long time, and the affected extremity should be elevated to promote the absorption of fluid. If the infiltration is recent, a cold compress may be applied to the area. Infiltration can be detected and treated early by inspecting the site every hour for redness, pain, edema, blood return, coolness at the site, and IV fluid draining from the IV site. Using the appropriate size and type of cannula for the vein prevents this complication. According to the Infusion Nursing Standards of Practice, a standardized infiltration scale should be used to document the infiltration (Alexander, 2000):

0 = No symptoms
1 = Skin blanched, edema less than 2.5 cm in any direction, cool to touch, with or without pain
2 = Skin blanched, edema 2.5 to 15 cm in any direction, cool to touch, with or without pain
3 = Skin blanched, translucent, gross edema greater than 15 cm in any direction, cool to touch, mild to moderate pain, possible numbness
4 = Skin blanched, translucent, skin tight, leaking, skin discoloured, bruised, swollen, gross edema greater than 15 cm in any direction, deep pitting tissue edema, circulatory impairment, moderate to severe pain, infiltration of any amount of blood products, irritant, or vesicant

Extravasation is similar to infiltration, with an inadvertent administration of vesicant or irritant solution or medication into the surrounding tissue. Medications such as dopamine, calcium preparations, and chemotherapeutic agents can cause pain, burning, and redness at the site. Blistering, inflammation, and necrosis of tissues can occur. The extent of tissue damage is determined by the concentration of the medication, the quantity that extravasated, the location of the infusion site, the tissue response, and the duration of the process of extravasation.

The infusion must be stopped and the physician notified promptly. The agency's protocol for extravasation is initiated; the protocol may specify specific treatments, including antidotes specific to the medication that extravasated, and may indicate whether the IV line should remain in place or be removed before treatment. The protocol often specifies that the infusion site be infiltrated with an antidote prescribed after assessment by the physician and application of warm or cold compresses, depending on the medication infusing. This extremity should not be used for further cannula placement. Thorough neurovascular assessments of the affected extremity must be performed frequently.

Reviewing the institution's IV policy and procedures and incompatibility charts and checking with the pharmacist before administering any IV medication, whether given peripherally or centrally, is a prudent way to determine incompatibilities and vesicant potential to prevent extravasation. Careful, frequent monitoring of the IV site, avoiding insertion of IV devices in areas of flexion, securing the IV line, and using the smallest catheter possible that accommodates the vein help minimize the incidence and severity of this complication. In addition, when vesicant medication is administered by IV push, it should be given through a side port of an infusing IV solution to dilute the medication and decrease the severity of tissue damage if extravasation oc-

curs. Extravasation should always be rated as a grade 4 on the infiltration scale.

Phlebitis. Phlebitis is defined as inflammation of a vein related to a chemical or mechanical irritation, or both. It is characterized by a reddened, warm area around the insertion site or along the path of the vein, pain or tenderness at the site or along the vein, and swelling. The incidence of phlebitis increases with the length of time the IV line is in place, the composition of the fluid or medication infused (especially its pH and tonicity), the size and site of the cannula inserted, ineffective filtration, improper anchoring of the line, and the introduction of microorganisms at the time of insertion. The Intravenous Nursing Society has identified specific standards for assessing phlebitis (Alexander, 2000); these appear in Chart 14-3.

Treatment consists of discontinuing the IV and restarting it in another site, and applying a warm, moist compress to the affected site. Phlebitis can be prevented by using aseptic technique during insertion, using the appropriate-size cannula or needle for the vein, considering the composition of fluids and medications when selecting a site, observing the site hourly for any complications, anchoring the cannula or needle well, and changing the IV site according to agency policy and procedures.

Thrombophlebitis. Thrombophlebitis refers to the presence of a clot plus inflammation in the vein. It is evidenced by localized pain, redness, warmth, and swelling around the insertion site or along the path of the vein, immobility of the extremity because of discomfort and swelling, sluggish flow rate, fever, malaise, and leukocytosis.

Treatment includes discontinuing the IV infusion, applying a cold compress first to decrease the flow of blood and increase platelet aggregation followed by a warm compress, elevating the extremity, and restarting the line in the opposite extremity. If the patient has signs and symptoms of thrombophlebitis, the IV line should not be flushed (although flushing may be indicated in

---

Chart 14-3 • ASSESSMENT

Phlebitis

According to the Infusion Nurses Society, documentation of phlebitis should be standardized. Phlebitis should be graded according to the most severe presenting indication

Grade	Clinical Criteria
0	No clinical symptoms
1	Erythema at access site with or without pain
2	Pain at access site Erythema, edema, or both
3	Pain at access site Erythema, edema, or both Streak formation Palpable venous cord (2.5 cm or shorter)
4	Pain at access site with erythema Streak formation Palpable venous cord (longer than 2.5 cm) Purulent drainage

Note: If this scale is not being used in an institution, then the description associated with the number can be used to describe the assessment.
From Infusion Nursing Standards of Practice (2000). *Journal of Intravenous Nursing,* 23(6S), S56–S69.

the absence of phlebitis to ensure cannula patency and to prevent mixing incompatible medications and solutions).

Thrombophlebitis can be prevented by avoiding trauma to the vein at the time the IV is inserted, observing the site every hour, and checking medication additives for compatibility.

Hematoma. Hematoma results when blood leaks into tissues surrounding the IV insertion site. Leakage can result from perforation of the opposite vein wall during venipuncture, the needle slipping out of the vein, and insufficient pressure applied to the site after removing the needle or cannula. The signs of a hematoma include ecchymosis, immediate swelling at the site, and leakage of blood at the site.

Treatment includes removing the needle or cannula and applying pressure with a sterile dressing; applying ice for 24 hours to the site to avoid extension of the hematoma and then a warm compress to increase absorption of blood; assessing the site; and restarting the line in the other extremity if indicated. A hematoma can be prevented by carefully inserting the needle and using diligent care when a patient has a bleeding disorder, takes anticoagulant medication, or has advanced liver disease.

Clotting and Obstruction. Blood clots may form in the IV line as a result of kinked IV tubing, a very slow infusion rate, an empty IV bag, or failure to flush the IV line after intermittent medication or solution administrations. The signs are decreased flow rate and blood backflow into the IV tubing.

If blood clots in the IV line, the infusion must be discontinued and restarted in another site with a new cannula and administration set. The tubing should not be irrigated or milked. Neither the infusion rate nor the solution container should be raised, and the clot should not be aspirated from the tubing. Clotting of the needle or cannula may be prevented by not permitting the IV solution bag to run dry, taping the tubing to prevent kinking and maintain patency, maintaining an adequate flow rate, and flushing the line after intermittent medication or other solution administration. In some cases, a specially trained nurse or physician may inject a thrombolytic agent into the catheter to clear an occlusion resulting from fibrin or clotted blood.

PROMOTING HOME AND COMMUNITY-BASED CARE

Teaching Patients Self-Care. At times, IV therapy must be administered in the home setting, in which case much of the daily management rests with the patient and family. Teaching becomes essential to ensure that the patient and family can manage the IV fluid and infusion properly and avoid complications. Written instructions as well as demonstration and return demonstration help reinforce the key points for all these functions.

Continuing Care. Home infusion therapies cover a wide range of treatments, including antibiotic, analgesic, and antineoplastic medications; blood or blood component therapy; and parenteral nutrition. When direct nursing care is necessary, arrangements can be made to have an infusion nurse visit the home and administer the IV therapy as prescribed. In addition to implementing and monitoring the IV therapy, the nurse carries out a comprehensive assessment of the patient's condition and continues to teach the patient and family about the skills involved in overseeing the IV therapy setup. Any dietary changes that may be necessary because of fluid or electrolyte imbalances are explained or reinforced during such sessions.

Periodic laboratory testing may be necessary to assess the effects of IV therapy and the patient's progress. Blood specimens may be obtained by a laboratory near the patient's home, or a home visit may be arranged to obtain blood specimens for analysis.

The nurse collaborates with the case manager in assessing the patient, family, and home environment; developing a plan of care in accordance with the patient's treatment plan and level of ability; and arranging for appropriate referral and follow-up if necessary. Any necessary equipment may be provided by the agency or purchased by the patient, depending on the terms of the home care arrangements. Appropriate documentation is necessary to assist in obtaining third-party payment for the service provided.

 Critical Thinking Exercises

1. A 40-year-old man with peptic ulcer disease reports vomiting, nausea, dry mucous membranes, and abdominal pain for the last 2 days. His BP is 92/64 and pulse is 120. His laboratory results show a serum sodium level of 125 mmol/L, urine sodium level of 5 mmol/L, and measured serum osmolality of 270 mmol/L. What IV solution do you anticipate will be prescribed for him? Provide a rationale for its use, and discuss the nursing actions relevant to its administration.

2. A 30-year-old woman comes into the emergency department with a temperature of 39.4°C. For the last 4 days she has had a productive cough and has experienced dyspnea increasing in severity. Her serum laboratory results are as follows: WBC $= 20 \times 10^9$, pH $= 7.59$, $PaCO_2 = 26$, $PaO_2 = 40$, $SaO_2 = 80$, $HCO_3 = 20$, $Na^+ = 140$, $K^+ = 4.2$, $Cl^- = 106$, $CO_2 = 20$. What is the acid–base disorder? What treatments and relevant nursing actions related to the underlying disorder and its treatment should the nurse anticipate?

3. A 48-year-old woman reports shortness of breath that has been increasing in the last 3 months so much so that she is no longer able to use her treadmill. She is a nonsmoker. Her chest x-ray is negative. She does not take any medications. Her arterial blood gases are as follows: pH $= 7.41$, $PaCO_2 = 37$ mm Hg, $PaO_2 = 94$ mm Hg, $HCO_3 = 23$ mmHg, pulse oximetry $= 98\%$. What is your interpretation of her blood gas values? What action is indicated by these results?

4. An obtunded 84-year-old man is admitted to the hospital from the nursing home with a high fever. The following clinical data are obtained on admission: temperature 39.4°C; BP 150/90; pulse rate of 110; dry, mucous membranes. Laboratory test results include the following: serum $Na^+ = 184$ mmol/L, urine osmolality $= 640$ mmol/L; urine culture and sensitivity shows pyuria and many bacteria. His peripheral IV at the site of the right dorsal metacarpal vein is infiltrated. What method of administering IV fluids would the nurse anticipate? What factors are probably contributing to his hypernatremia? What nursing actions should be taken in assisting with treatment of this patient's fluid and electrolyte imbalance?

5. A 65-year-old patient with severe, long-standing COPD is admitted to the hospital for treatment of impending renal failure. Explain the effects of his pulmonary disorder on the acid–base disturbances that commonly occur with renal failure. What are the nursing observations and assessment that are indicated because of the occurrence of these two disorders?

REFERENCES AND SELECTED READINGS

Books

Bickley, L. S., & Szilagyi, P. G. (2003). *Bates' guide to physical examination and history taking.* Philadelphia: Lippincott Williams & Wilkins.

Chernecky, C. C., & Berger, B. J. (2001) *Laboratory tests and diagnostic procedures* (3d ed.). Philadelphia: W. B. Saunders.

Dillon, P. M. (2004). *Nursing health assessment: Clinical pocket guide.* Philadelphia: F. A. Davis Company.

Guyton, A. C. (2000). *Textbook of medical physiology* (10th ed.). Philadelphia: W. B. Saunders.

Hankins, J., Lonsway-Waldman, R., Hedrick, C., & Perdue, M. B. (2001). *Infusion therapy in clinical practice* (2d ed.). Philadelphia: W. B. Saunders.

Heitz, U., & Horne, M. (2001). *Pocket guide to fluid, electrolyte, and acid-base balance* (4th ed.). St. Louis: Mosby.

Karch, A. M. (2002). *Lippincott's nursing drug guide.* Philadelphia: Lippincott Williams & Wilkins.

Kee, J., & Paulanka, B. (2000). *Handbook of fluid, electrolyte and acid-base imbalances.* Albany, NY: Delmar Publishers.

Martin, L. (1999). *All you need to know to interpret arterial blood gases* (2d ed.). Philadelphia: Lippincott Williams & Wilkins.

Metheny, N. M. (2000). *Fluid and electrolyte balance: Nursing considerations* (4th ed.). Philadelphia: Lippincott Williams & Wilkins.

Otto, S. E. (2001). *Pocket guide to intravenous therapy* (4th ed.). St. Louis: C. V. Mosby.

Porth, C. M. (2002). *Pathophysiology: Concepts of altered health states* (6th ed.). Philadelphia: Lippincott Williams & Wilkins.

Price, S. A., & Wilson, L. M. (2003). *Pathophysiology. Clinical concepts of disease processes.* St. Louis: Mosby–Year Book.

Registered Nurses Association of Ontario (RNAO). (2004). *Best practice guideline: Assessment and device selection for vascular access.* Available at: http://www.rnao.org/bestpractices/completed_guidelines/BPG_Guide_C4_iv_therap.asp. Retrieved June 6, 2005.

Rose, B., & Post, T. (2001). *Clinical physiology of acid–base and electrolyte disorders* (5th ed.). New York: McGraw-Hill.

Weinstein, S. (2001). *Plumer's principles and practice of intravenous therapy.* Philadelphia: Lippincott Williams & Wilkins.

Journals

Asterisks indicate nursing research articles.

Fluid and Electrolyte Balances

Adrogue, H. J., & Madias, N. E. (2000*a*). Hyponatremia. *New England Journal of Medicine, 342*(21), 1581–1589.

Adrogue, H. J., & Madias, N. E. (2000*b*). Hypernatremia. *New England Journal of Medicine, 342*(20),1493–1499.

Anonymous. (2000). Part 1: Introduction to the International Guidelines 2000 for CPR and ECC: A consensus on science. *Circulation, 102*(8 Suppl), I1–I11.

Beck, L. H. (2000). The aging kidney. Defending a delicate balance of fluid and electrolytes. *Geriatrics, 55*(4), 26–28, 31–32.

Brater, D. C. (1998). Diuretic therapy. *New England Journal of Medicine, 339*(6), 387–395.

Carlstedt, F., & Lind, L. (2001). Hypocalcemic syndromes. *Critical Care Clinics, 17*(1), 139–153, vii–viii.

Castiglione, V. (2000). Emergency: Hyperkalemia. *American Journal of Nursing, 100*(1), 55–56.

Clayton, K. (1997). Cancer-related hypercalcemia: How to spot it, how to manage it. *American Journal of Nursing, 97*(5), 42–49.

Cohn, J. N., Kowey, P. R., Whelton, P. K., & Prisant, L. M. (2000). New guidelines for potassium replacement in clinical practice: A contemporary review by the National Council on Potassium in Clinical Practice. *Archives of Internal Medicine, 160*(16), 2429–2436.

Fall, P. J. (2000). Hyponatremia and hypernatremia. A systematic approach to causes and their correction. *Postgraduate Medicine, 107*(5), 75–82.

Fulop, M. (1998). Algorithms for diagnosing some electrolyte disorders. *American Journal of Emergency Medicine, 16*(1), 76–84.

Gross, P. (2001). Correction of hyponatremia. *Seminars in Nephrology, 21*(3), 269–272.

Gennari, F. J. (1998). Hypokalemia. *New England Journal of Medicine, 339*(7), 451–458.

Goldhill, D. R. (1997). Calcium and magnesium. *Care of the Critically Ill, 13*(3), 112–115.

Kreimeier, U. (2000). Pathophysiology of fluid imbalance. *Critical Care (London), 4,* Suppl 2:S3–S7.

Kugler, J. P., & Hustead, T. (2000). Hyponatremia and hypernatremia in the elderly. *American Family Physician, 61*(12), 3623–3630.

Lee, C. T., Guo, H. R., & Chen, J. B. (2000). Hyponatremia in the emergency department. *American Journal of Emergency Medicine, 18*(3), 264–268.

Lilly, L. L., & Guanci, R. (1997). Persistent potassium problems. *American Journal of Nursing, 97*(6), 14.

Marx, S. J. (2000). Hyperparathyroid and hypoparathyroid disorders. *New England Journal of Medicine, 343*(25), 1863–1875.

Nayback, A. M. (2000). Hyponatremia as a consequence of acute adrenal insufficiency and hypothyroidism. *Journal of Emergency Nursing, 26*(2), 130–133.

Oster, J. R., & Singer, I. (1999). Hyponatremia, hypoosmolality, and hypotonicity. *Archives of Internal Medicine, 159*(4), 333–336.

Perazella, M. A. (2000). Drug-induced hyperkalemia: Old culprits and new offenders. *American Journal of Medicine, 109*(4), 307–314.

Pirzada, N. A., & Ali, I. I. (2001). Central pontine myelinolysis. *Mayo Clinic Proceedings, 76*(5), 559–562.

*Rateau, M. R. (2000). Confusion and aggression in restrained elderly persons undergoing hip repair surgery. *Applied Nursing Research, 13*(1), 50–54.

Schmidt, T. C. (2000). Assessing a sodium and fluid imbalance. *Nursing, 30*(1), 18.

Suhayda, R. & Walton, J. C. (2002). Preventing and managing dehydration. *MedSurg Nursing, 11*(6), 267–278.

Terpstra, T. L., & Terpstra, T. L. (2000). Syndrome of inappropriate antidiuretic hormone: Recognition and management. *MedSurg Nursing, 9*(2). 61–68.

Toto, K. H. (1998). Fluid balance assessment. *Critical Care Nursing Clinics of North America, 10*(4), 383–400.

Wilcox, C. S. (1999). Metabolic and adverse effects of diuretics. *Seminars in Nephrology, 19*(6), 557–568.

Acid–Base Balance

Adrogue, H. E., & Adrogue, H. J. (2001). Acid-base physiology. *Respiratory Care, 46*(4), 328–341.

Epstein, S. K., & Singh, N. (2001). Respiratory acidosis. *Respiratory Care, 46*(4), 366–383.

Foster, G. T., Vaziri, N. D., & Sassoon, C. S. (2001). Respiratory alkalosis. *Respiratory Care, 46*(4), 384–391.

Horne, C., & Derrico, D. (1999). Mastering the art of arterial blood gas measurement. *American Journal of Nursing, 99*(8), 26–32.

Khanna, A., & Kurtzman, N. A. (2001). Metabolic alkalosis. *Respiratory Care, 46*(4), 354–365.

Kraut, J. A., & Madias, N. E. (2001). Approach to patients with acid-base disorders. *Respiratory Care, 46*(4), 392–403.

Sassoon, C. S., & Arruda, J. A. (2001). Acid-base disturbance. *Respiratory Care, 46*(4), 327.

Shoulders-Odom, B. (2000). Using an algorithm to interpret arterial blood gases. *Dimensions of Critical Care Nursing, 19*(1), 36–41.

Swenson, E. R. (2001). Metabolic acidosis. *Respiratory Care, 46*(4), 342–353.

Wallace, L. S. (2000). Using color to simplify ABG interpretation. *MedSurg Nursing, 9*(4), 205–207.

Williams, A. (1998). ABC of oxygen. Assessing and interpreting arterial blood gases and acid-base balance. *British Medical Journal, 317*(7167), 1213–1216.

Wong, F. W. H. (1999). A new approach to ABG interpretation. *American Journal of Nursing, 99*(8), 26–32.

Intravenous Administration

Alexander, M. (2000). Infusion Nursing Standards of Practice. *Journal of Intravenous Nursing, 23*(6), Suppl. S5–S88.

Andrews, C. M. (2002). Emergency: Preventing air embolism. *American Journal of Nursing, 102*(1), 34–36.

Andris, D. A., & Jrzywda, E. A. (1999). Central venous catheter occlusion: Successful management strategies. *MedSurg Nursing, 8*(4), 229–236.

Aschenbrenner, D. A. (2000). Skin preps and protocols. *American Journal of Nursing, 100*(4), 78.

Carlson, K. (1999). Correct utilization and management of peripherally inserted central catheters and midline catheters in the alternate care setting. *Journal of Intravenous Nursing, 22*(6), Suppl. S46–S50.

Driscoll, M., et al. (1997). Inserting and maintaining peripherally inserted central catheters. *MedSurg Nursing, 6*(6), 350–358.

*Fetzer, S. J. (2002). Reducing venipuncture and intravenous insertion pain with eutectic mixture of local anesthetic. A meta-analysis. *Nursing Research, 51*(2), 119–124.

*Fry, C. & Aholt, D. (2001). Local anesthesia prior to the insertion of peripherally inserted central catheters. *Journal of Infusion Nursing, 24*(6), 404–408.

Hadaway, L. C. (1999). Vascular access devices: Meeting patients' needs. *MedSurg Nursing, 8*(5), 296–303.

Intravenous Nurses Society. (1997). Position paper: Midline and midclavicular catheters. *Journal of Intravenous Nursing, 20*(4), 175–178.

Intravenous Nurses Society. (1997). Position paper: Peripherally inserted central catheters. *Journal of Intravenous Nursing, 20*(4), 172–174.

Krzywda, E. A. (1998). Central venous access—catheters, technology, and physiology. *MedSurg Nursing, 7*(3), 132–139.

Kupensky, D. (1998). Applying current research to influence clinical practice. *Journal of Intravenous Nursing, 21*(5), 271–274.

LeDuc, K. (1997) Efficacy of normal saline solution versus heparin solution for maintaining patency of peripheral intravenous catheters in children. *Journal of Emergency Nursing, 23*(4), 306–309.

Macklin, D. (2000). Removing a PICC. *American Journal of Nursing, 100*(1), 52–54.

Millam, D. (2000). On the road to successful venipuncture. *Nursing, 30*(4), 34–48.

Moureau, N., & Zonderman, A. (2000) Does it always have to hurt? Premedications for adults and children for use with intravenous therapy. *Journal of Intravenous Nursing, 23*(4), 213–219.

RESOURCES AND WEBSITES

Canadian Intravenous Nurses Association; PO Box 66572; 685 McCowan Rd., Toronto, ON M1J 3N8; (416) 696-7761; fax: (416) 696-8437; http://www.cina.ca.

Infusion Nurses Society, 220 Norwood Park South, Norwood, MA 02062; (781) 440-9408; http://www.ins1.org.

Shock and Multisystem Failure

Adapted by Madeleine Buck

LEARNING OBJECTIVES

On completion of this chapter, the learner will be able to:

1. Describe shock and its underlying pathophysiology.
2. Compare clinical findings of the compensatory and progressive stages of shock.
3. Describe organ damage that may occur with shock.
4. Compare hypovolemic, cardiogenic, and circulatory shock in terms of causes, pathophysiologic effects, and medical and nursing management.
5. Describe indications for varying types of fluid replacement.
6. Identify vasoactive medications used in treating shock, and describe nursing implications associated with their use.
7. Discuss the importance of nutritional support in all forms of shock.
8. Discuss the role of the nurse in psychosocial support of both the patient experiencing shock and the family.
9. Discuss the syndrome of multiple organ dysfunction.

*S*hock is a life-threatening condition with a variety of underlying causes. It is characterized by inadequate tissue perfusion that, if untreated, results in cell death. The nurse caring for the patient with shock or at risk for shock must understand the underlying mechanisms of shock and recognize its subtle as well as more obvious signs. Rapid assessment and response are essential to the patient's recovery.

Shock can best be defined as a condition in which systemic blood pressure is inadequate to deliver oxygen and nutrients to support vital organs and cellular function (Mikhail, 1999). Adequate blood flow to the tissues and cells requires the following components: adequate cardiac pump, effective vasculature or circulatory system, and sufficient blood volume. When one component is impaired, blood flow to the tissues is threatened or compromised. Without treatment, inadequate blood flow to the tissues results in poor delivery of oxygen and nutrients to the cells, cellular starvation, cell death, organ dysfunction progressing to organ failure, and eventual death.

Significance of Shock

Shock affects all body systems. It may develop rapidly or slowly, depending on the underlying cause. During shock, the body struggles to survive, calling on all its homeostatic mechanisms to restore blood flow and tissue perfusion. Any insult to the body can create a cascade of events resulting in poor tissue perfusion. Therefore, almost any patient with any disease state may be at risk for developing shock.

Nursing care of the patient with shock requires ongoing systematic assessment. Many of the interventions required in caring for the patient with shock call for close collaboration with other members of the health care team and a physician's orders. The nurse must anticipate such orders because they need to be executed with speed and accuracy.

Conditions Precipitating Shock

CLASSIFICATION OF SHOCK

Shock can be classified by etiology and may be described as (1) **hypovolemic shock**, (2) **cardiogenic shock**, or (3) **circulatory** or **distributive shock**. Some authors identify a fourth category, obstructive shock, that results from disorders that cause mechanical obstruction to blood flow through the central circulatory system despite normal myocardial function and intravascular volume.

Examples include pulmonary embolism, cardiac tamponade, dissecting aortic aneurysm, and tension pneumothorax. In this discussion, obstructive disorders are discussed as examples of noncoronary cardiogenic shock. Hypovolemic shock occurs when there is a decrease in the intravascular volume. Cardiogenic shock occurs when the heart has an impaired pumping ability; it may be of coronary or noncoronary origin. Circulatory shock results from a maldistribution or mismatch of blood flow to the cells.

NORMAL CELLULAR FUNCTION

Energy metabolism occurs within the cell, where nutrients are chemically broken down and stored in the form of adenosine triphosphate (ATP). Cells use this stored energy to perform necessary functions, such as active transport, muscle contraction, and biochemical synthesis, as well as specialized cellular functions, such as the conduction of electrical impulses. ATP can be synthesized aerobically (in the presence of oxygen) or anaerobically (in the absence of oxygen). Aerobic metabolism yields far greater amounts of ATP per mole of glucose than does anaerobic metabolism and, therefore, is a more efficient and effective means of producing energy. Additionally, anaerobic metabolism results in the accumulation of the toxic end product lactic acid, which must be removed from the cell and transported to the liver for conversion into glucose and glycogen.

PATHOPHYSIOLOGY

In shock, the cells lack an adequate blood supply and are deprived of oxygen and nutrients; therefore, they must produce energy through anaerobic metabolism. This results in low energy yields from nutrients and an acidotic intracellular environment. Because of these changes, normal cell function ceases (Fig. 15-1). The cell swells and the cell membrane becomes more permeable, allowing electrolytes and fluids to seep out of and into the cell. The sodium-potassium pump becomes impaired; cell structures, primarily the mitochondria, are damaged; and death of the cell results.

Vascular Responses

Oxygen attaches to the hemoglobin molecule in red blood cells, and the blood carries it to body cells. The amount of oxygen that is delivered to cells depends both on blood flow to a specific area and on blood oxygen concentration. Blood is continuously re-

Glossary

anaphylactic shock: circulatory shock state resulting from a severe allergic reaction producing an overwhelming systemic vasodilation and relative hypovolemia

biochemical mediators: messenger substances that may be released by a cell to create an action at that site or be carried by the bloodstream to a distant site before being activated; also called cytokines

cardiogenic shock: shock state resulting from impairment or failure of the myocardium

colloids: intravenous solutions that contain molecules that are too large to pass through capillary membranes

crystalloids: electrolyte solutions that move freely between the intravascular compartment and interstitial spaces

circulatory shock: shock state resulting from displacement of blood volume creating a relative hypovolemia and inadequate delivery of oxygen to the cells; also called distributive shock

hypovolemic shock: shock state resulting from decreased intravascular volume due to fluid loss

neurogenic shock: shock state resulting from loss of sympathetic tone causing relative hypovolemia

septic shock: circulatory shock state resulting from overwhelming infection causing relative hypovolemia

shock: physiologic state in which there is inadequate blood flow to tissues and cells of the body

systemic inflammatory response syndrome (SIRS): overwhelming inflammatory response in the absence of infection causing relative hypovolemia and decreased tissue perfusion

Normal

Effects of shock

FIGURE 15-1 Cellular effects of shock. The cell swells and the cell membrane becomes more permeable, and fluids and electrolytes seep from and into the cell. Mitochondria and lysosomes are damaged, and the cell dies.

cycled through the lungs to be reoxygenated and to eliminate end products of cellular metabolism, such as carbon dioxide. The heart muscle is the pump that propels the freshly oxygenated blood out to the body tissues. This process of circulation is facilitated through an elaborate and dynamic vasculature consisting of arteries, arterioles, capillaries, veins, and venules. The vasculature can dilate or constrict based on central and local regulatory mechanisms. Central regulatory mechanisms stimulate dilation or constriction of the vasculature to maintain an adequate blood pressure. Local regulatory mechanisms, referred to as autoregulation, stimulate vasodilation or vasoconstriction in response to biochemical mediators (also called cytokines) released by the cell, communicating its need for oxygen and nutrients (Jindal, Hollenberg & Dellinger, 2000) A biochemical mediator is a substance released by a cell or immune cells such as polymorphonuclear leukocytes (PMNs) or macrophages; the substance triggers an action at a cell site or travels in the bloodstream to a distant site, where it triggers action.

Blood Pressure Regulation

Three major components of the circulatory system—blood volume, the cardiac pump, and the vasculature—must respond effectively to complex neural, chemical, and hormonal feedback systems to maintain an adequate blood pressure and ultimately perfuse body tissues.

Blood pressure is regulated through a complex interaction of neural, chemical, and hormonal feedback systems affecting both cardiac output and peripheral resistance. This relationship is expressed in the following equation:

Mean arterial blood pressure = cardiac output × peripheral resistance

Cardiac output is determined by stroke volume (the amount of blood ejected at systole) and heart rate. Peripheral resistance is determined by the diameter of the arterioles.

Tissue perfusion and organ perfusion depend on mean arterial pressure (MAP). The MAP is the average pressure at which blood moves through the vasculature. Although true MAP can be calculated only by complex methods, Chart 15-1 displays a convenient formula for clinical use in estimating MAP. MAP should exceed 70 to 80 mm Hg for cells to receive the oxygen and nutrients needed to metabolize energy in amounts sufficient to sustain life (Balk, 2000*a*).

Blood pressure is regulated by the baroreceptors (pressure receptors) located in the carotid sinus and aortic arch. These pressure receptors convey impulses to the sympathetic nervous centre in the medulla of the brain. When blood pressure drops, catecholamines (epinephrine and norepinephrine) are released from the adrenal medulla of the adrenal glands. This increases heart rate and vasoconstriction, thus restoring blood pressure. Chemoreceptors, also located in the aortic arch and carotid arteries, regulate blood pressure and respiratory rate using much the same mechanism in response to changes in oxygen and carbon dioxide concentrations in the blood. These primary regulatory mechanisms can respond to changes in blood pressure on a moment-to-moment basis.

Chart 15-1	**Formula for Estimating Mean Arterial Pressure (MAP)**

$$MAP = \frac{\text{systolic BP} + 2(\text{diastolic BP})}{3}$$

Example: patient's BP = 125/75 mm Hg

$$MAP = \frac{125 + (2 \times 75)}{3}$$

MAP = 92 (rounded to nearest 1/10)

The kidneys also play an important role in blood pressure regulation. They regulate blood pressure by releasing renin, an enzyme needed for the conversion of angiotensin I to angiotensin II, a potent vasoconstrictor. This stimulation of the renin-angiotensin mechanism and resulting vasoconstriction indirectly lead to the release of aldosterone from the adrenal cortex, which promotes the retention of sodium and water. The increased concentration of sodium in the blood then stimulates the release of antidiuretic hormone (ADH) by the pituitary gland. ADH causes the kidneys to retain water further in an effort to raise blood volume and blood pressure. These secondary regulatory mechanisms may take hours or days to respond to changes in blood pressure.

To summarize, adequate blood volume, an effective cardiac pump, and an effective vasculature are necessary to maintain blood pressure and tissue perfusion. When one of the three components of this system begins to fail, the body is able to compensate through increased work by the other two (Fig. 15-2). When compensatory mechanisms can no longer compensate for the failed system, body tissues are inadequately perfused, and shock occurs. Without prompt intervention, shock progresses, resulting in organ dysfunction, organ failure, and death.

Stages of Shock

Some think of the shock syndrome as a continuum along which the patient struggles to survive. A convenient way to understand the physiologic responses and subsequent clinical signs and symptoms is to divide the continuum into separate stages: compensatory, progressive, and irreversible. (Although some authorities identify an initial stage of shock, changes attributed to this stage occur at the cellular level and are generally not detectable clinically.) The earlier that medical management and nursing interventions can be initiated along this continuum, the greater the patient's chance of survival.

Physiology/Pathophysiology

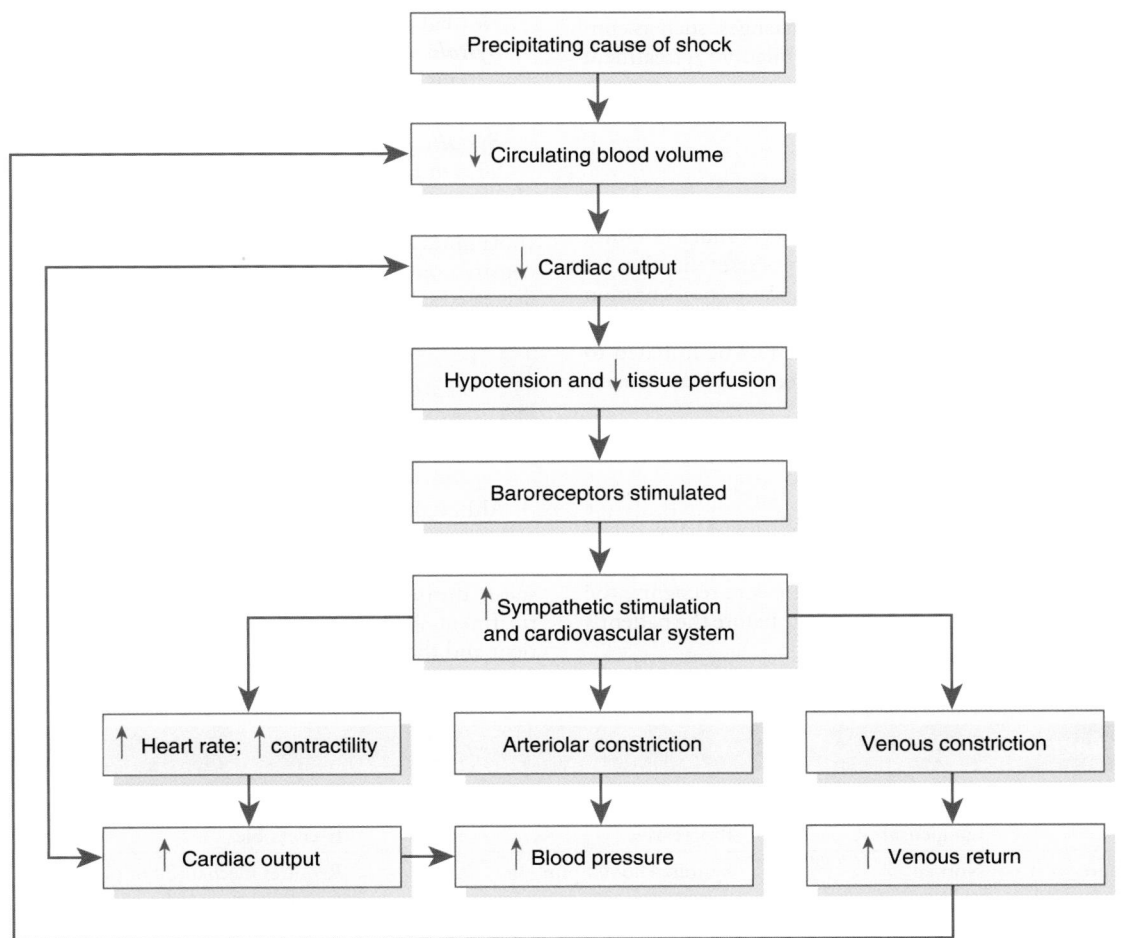

FIGURE 15-2 Compensatory mechanisms for the restoration of circulatory blood volume in shock. Adapted with permission from Jones, K. (1996). Shock. In J. M. Clochesy, C. Breu, et al. (Eds.). *Critical care nursing* (2nd ed.). Philadelphia: W. B. Saunders Company.

COMPENSATORY STAGE

In the compensatory stage of shock, the patient's blood pressure remains within normal limits. Vasoconstriction, increased heart rate, and increased contractility of the heart contribute to maintaining adequate cardiac output. This results from stimulation of the sympathetic nervous system and subsequent release of catecholamines (epinephrine and norepinephrine). The patient displays the often-described "fight or flight" response. The body shunts blood from organs such as the skin, kidneys, and gastrointestinal tract to the brain and heart to ensure adequate blood supply to these vital organs. As a result, the patient's skin is cold and clammy, bowel sounds are hypoactive, and urine output decreases in response to the release of aldosterone and ADH.

Clinical Manifestations

Despite a normal blood pressure, the patient shows numerous clinical signs indicating inadequate organ perfusion (Chart 15-2). The result of inadequate perfusion is anaerobic metabolism and a buildup of lactic acid, producing metabolic acidosis. The respiratory rate increases in response to metabolic acidosis. This rapid respiratory rate facilitates removal of excess carbon dioxide but raises the blood pH and often causes a compensatory respiratory alkalosis. The alkalotic state causes mental status changes, such as confusion or combativeness, as well as arteriolar dilation. If treatment begins in this stage of shock, the prognosis for the patient is good.

Medical Management

Medical treatment is directed toward identifying the cause of the shock, correcting the underlying disorder so that shock does not progress, and supporting those physiologic processes that thus far have responded successfully to the threat. Because compensation cannot be effectively maintained indefinitely, measures such as fluid replacement and medication therapy must be initiated to maintain an adequate blood pressure and reestablish and maintain adequate tissue perfusion.

Nursing Management

Early intervention along the continuum of shock is the key to improving the patient's prognosis. Therefore, the nurse needs to assess systematically those patients at risk for shock to recognize the subtle clinical signs of the compensatory stage before the patient's blood pressure drops.

MONITORING TISSUE PERFUSION

In assessing tissue perfusion, the nurse observes for changes in level of consciousness, vital signs (including pulse pressure), urinary output, skin, and laboratory values. In the compensatory stage of shock, serum sodium and blood glucose levels are elevated in response to the release of aldosterone and catecholamines.

The role of the nurse at the compensatory stage of shock is to monitor the patient's hemodynamic status and promptly report deviations to the physician, assist in identifying and treating the underlying disorder by continuous in-depth assessment of the patient, administer prescribed fluids and medications, and promote patient safety. Vital signs are key indicators of the patient's hemodynamic status; however, blood pressure is an indirect method of monitoring tissue hypoxia. Pulse pressure correlates well to stroke volume, the amount of blood ejected from the heart with systole. Pulse pressure is calculated by subtracting the diastolic measurement from the systolic measurement; the difference is the pulse pressure. Normally, the pulse pressure is 30 to 40 mm Hg (Mikhail, 1999). Narrowing or decreased pulse pressure is an earlier indicator of shock than a drop in systolic blood pressure. Decreased or narrowing pulse pressure, an early indication of decreased stroke volume, is illustrated in the following example:

Systolic blood pressure − diastolic blood pressure = pulse pressure

Normal pulse pressure:

Systolic BP		*Diastolic BP*		*Pulse Pressure*
120 mg Hg	−	80 mm Hg	=	40 mm Hg

Narrowing of pulse pressure:

Systolic BP		*Diastolic BP*		*Pulse Pressure*
90 mm Hg	−	70 mm Hg	=	20 mm Hg

Elevation in the diastolic blood pressure with release of catecholamines and attempts to increase venous return through vasoconstriction is an early compensatory mechanism in response to decreased stroke volume, blood pressure, and overall cardiac output.

 NURSING ALERT By the time blood pressure drops, damage has already been occurring on the cellular and tissue levels. Therefore, the patient at risk for shock must be assessed and monitored closely before the blood pressure falls.

Although treatments are prescribed and initiated by the physician, the nurse usually implements them, operates and troubleshoots equipment used in treatment, monitors the patient's status during treatment, and assesses the immediate effects of treatment. Additionally, the nurse assesses the response of the patient and the family to the crisis and to treatment.

Chart 15-2 • ASSESSMENT

Clinical Findings in Stages of Shock

Finding	Compensatory	Progressive	Irreversible
Blood pressure	Normal	Systolic <80–90 mm Hg	Requires mechanical or pharmacologic support
Heart rate	>100 bpm	>150 bpm	Erratic or asystole
Respiratory status	>20 breaths/min	Rapid, shallow respirations; crackles	Requires intubation
Skin	Cold, clammy	Mottled, petechiae	Jaundice
Urinary output	Decreased	0.5 mL/kg/hr	Anuric, requires dialysis
Mentation	Confusion	Lethargy	Unconscious
Acid–base balance	Respiratory alkalosis	Metabolic acidosis	Profound acidosis

REDUCING ANXIETY

While experiencing a major threat to health and well-being and being the focus of attention of many health care providers, the patient often becomes anxious and apprehensive. Providing brief explanations about the diagnostic and treatment procedures, supporting the patient during those procedures, and providing information about their outcomes are usually effective in reducing stress and anxiety and thus promoting the patient's physical and mental well-being.

PROMOTING SAFETY

Another nursing intervention is monitoring potential threats to the patient's safety, because a high anxiety level and altered mental status typically impair a person's judgment. In this stage, patients who were previously cooperative and followed instructions may now disrupt intravenous lines and catheters and complicate their condition. Therefore, close monitoring is essential.

PROGRESSIVE STAGE

In the progressive stage of shock, the mechanisms that regulate blood pressure can no longer compensate and the MAP falls below normal limits, with an average systolic blood pressure of less than 90 mm Hg (Abraham et al., 2000).

Pathophysiology

Although all organ systems suffer from hypoperfusion at this stage, two events perpetuate the shock syndrome. First, the overworked heart becomes dysfunctional; the body's inability to meet increased oxygen requirements produces ischemia; and biochemical mediators cause myocardial depression (Kumar, Haery & Parrillo, 2000; Price, Anning, Mitchell et al., 1999). This leads to failure of the cardiac pump, even if the underlying cause of the shock is not of cardiac origin. Second, the autoregulatory function of the microcirculation fails in response to numerous biochemical mediators released by the cells, resulting in increased capillary permeability, with areas of arteriolar and venous constriction further compromising cellular perfusion. At this stage, the patient's prognosis worsens. The relaxation of precapillary sphincters causes fluid to leak from the capillaries, creating interstitial edema and return of less fluid to the heart. Even if the underlying cause of the shock is reversed, the breakdown of the circulatory system itself perpetuates the shock state, and a vicious circle ensues.

Assessment and Diagnostic Findings

Chances of survival depend on the patient's general health before the shock state as well as the amount of time it takes to restore tissue perfusion. As shock progresses, organ systems decompensate.

RESPIRATORY EFFECTS

The lungs, which become compromised early in shock, are affected at this stage. Subsequent decompensation of the lungs increases the likelihood that mechanical ventilation will be needed if shock progresses. Respirations are rapid and shallow. Crackles are heard over the lung fields. Decreased pulmonary blood flow causes arterial oxygen levels to decrease and carbon dioxide levels to increase. Hypoxemia and biochemical mediators cause an intense inflammatory response and pulmonary vasoconstriction, perpetuating the pulmonary capillary hypoperfusion and hypoxemia. The hypoperfused alveoli stop producing surfactant and

subsequently collapse. Pulmonary capillaries begin to leak their contents, causing pulmonary edema, diffusion abnormalities (shunting), and additional alveolar collapse. Interstitial inflammation and fibrosis are common as the pulmonary damage progresses (Fein & Calalang-Colucci, 2000). This condition is sometimes referred to as acute respiratory distress syndrome (ARDS), acute lung injury (ALI), shock lung, or noncardiogenic pulmonary edema. Further explanation of ARDS, as well as its nursing management, can be found in Chapter 23.

CARDIOVASCULAR EFFECTS

A lack of adequate blood supply leads to dysrhythmias and ischemia. The patient has a rapid heart rate, sometimes exceeding 150 bpm. The patient may complain of chest pain and even suffer a myocardial infarction. Cardiac enzyme levels (eg, lactate dehydrogenase, CPK-MB, and cTn-I) rise. In addition, myocardial depression and ventricular dilation may further impair the heart's ability to pump enough blood to the tissues to meet oxygen requirements.

NEUROLOGIC EFFECTS

As blood flow to the brain becomes impaired, the patient's mental status deteriorates. Changes in mental status occur as a result of decreased cerebral perfusion and hypoxia; the patient may initially exhibit confusion or a subtle change in behaviour. Subsequently, lethargy increases and the patient begins to lose consciousness. The pupils dilate and are only sluggishly reactive to light.

RENAL EFFECTS

When the MAP falls below 80 mm Hg (Guyton & Hall, 2000), the glomerular filtration rate of the kidneys cannot be maintained, and drastic changes in renal function occur. Acute renal failure (ARF) can develop. ARF is characterized by an increase in blood urea nitrogen (BUN) and serum creatinine levels, fluid and electrolyte shifts, acid–base imbalances, and a loss of the renal-hormonal regulation of blood pressure. Urinary output usually decreases to below 0.5/mL/kg per hour (or below 30 mL per hour) but can be variable depending on the phase of ARF. For further information about ARF, see Chapter 45.

HEPATIC EFFECTS

Decreased blood flow to the liver impairs the liver cells' ability to perform metabolic and phagocytic functions. Consequently, the patient is less able to metabolize medications and metabolic waste products, such as ammonia and lactic acid. The patient becomes more susceptible to infection as the liver fails to filter bacteria from the blood. Liver enzymes (aspartate aminotransferase [AST], formerly serum glutamic-oxaloacetic transaminase [SGOT]; alanine aminotransferase [ALT], formerly serum glutamate pyruvate transaminase [SGPT]; lactate dehydrogenase) and bilirubin levels are elevated, and the patient appears jaundiced.

GASTROINTESTINAL EFFECTS

Gastrointestinal ischemia can cause stress ulcers in the stomach, placing the patient at risk for gastrointestinal bleeding. In the small intestine, the mucosa can become necrotic and slough off, causing bloody diarrhea. Beyond the local effects of impaired perfusion, gastrointestinal ischemia leads to bacterial toxin translocation, in which bacterial toxins enter the bloodstream through the lymph system. In addition to causing infection, bacterial toxins can cause cardiac depression, vasodilation, increased capillary permeability, and an intense inflammatory response with activation of additional biochemical mediators. The net result is interference with healthy cells and their ability to metabolize nutrients (Balk, 2000b; Jindal et al., 2000).

HEMATOLOGIC EFFECTS

The combination of hypotension, sluggish blood flow, metabolic acidosis, and generalized hypoxemia can interfere with normal hemostatic mechanisms. Disseminated intravascular coagulation (DIC) can occur either as a cause or as a complication of shock. In this condition, widespread clotting and bleeding occur simultaneously. Bruises (ecchymoses) and bleeding (petechiae) may appear in the skin. Coagulation times (prothrombin time, partial thromboplastin time) are prolonged. Clotting factors and platelets are consumed and require replacement therapy to achieve hemostasis. Further discussion of disseminated intravascular coagulation appears in Chapter 33.

Medical Management

Specific medical management in the progressive stage of shock depends on the type of shock and its underlying cause. It is also based on the degree of decompensation in the organ systems. Medical management specific to each type of shock is discussed in later sections of this chapter. Although there are several differences in medical management by type of shock, some medical interventions are common to all types. These include use of appropriate intravenous fluids and medications to restore tissue perfusion by (1) optimizing intravascular volume, (2) supporting the pumping action of the heart, and (3) improving the competence of the vascular system. Other aspects of management may include early enteral nutritional support and use of antacids, histamine-2 blockers, or antipeptic agents to reduce the risk of gastrointestinal ulceration and bleeding.

Nursing Management

Nursing care of the patient in the progressive stage of shock requires expertise in assessing and understanding shock and the significance of changes in assessment data. The patient in the progressive stage of shock is often cared for in the intensive care setting to facilitate close monitoring (hemodynamic monitoring, electrocardiographic monitoring, arterial blood gases, serum electrolyte levels, physical and mental status changes), rapid and frequent administration of various prescribed medications and fluids, and possibly intervention with supportive technologies, such as mechanical ventilation, dialysis, and intra-aortic balloon pump.

Working closely with other members of the health care team, the nurse carefully documents treatments, medications, and fluids that are administered by members of the team, recording the time, dosage or volume, and the patient's response. Additionally, the nurse coordinates both the scheduling of diagnostic procedures that may be carried out at the bedside and the flow of health care personnel involved in the patient's care.

PREVENTING COMPLICATIONS

If supportive technologies are used, the nurse helps reduce the risk of related complications and monitors the patient for early signs of complications. Monitoring includes evaluating blood levels of medications, observing invasive vascular lines for signs of infection, and checking neurovascular status if arterial lines are inserted, especially in the lower extremities. Simultaneously, the nurse promotes the patient's safety and comfort by ensuring that

all procedures, including invasive procedures and arterial and venous punctures, are carried out using correct aseptic techniques and that venous and arterial puncture and infusion sites are maintained with the goal of preventing infection. Positioning and repositioning the patient to promote comfort, prevent pulmonary complications, and maintain skin integrity are integral to caring for the patient in shock.

PROMOTING REST AND COMFORT

Efforts are made to minimize the cardiac workload by reducing the patient's physical activity and fear or anxiety. Promoting rest and comfort is a priority in the patient's care. To ensure that the patient gets as much uninterrupted rest as possible, the nurse performs only essential nursing activities. To conserve the patient's energy, the nurse protects the patient from temperature extremes (excessive warmth or shivering cold), which can increase the metabolic rate and subsequently the cardiac workload. The patient should not be warmed too quickly, and warming blankets should not be applied because they can cause vasodilation and a subsequent drop in blood pressure.

SUPPORTING FAMILY MEMBERS

Because the patient in shock is the object of intense attention by the health care team, the family members may feel neglected; however, they may be reluctant to ask questions or seek information for fear that they will be in the way or will interfere with the attention given to the patient. The nurse should make sure that the family is comfortably situated and kept informed about the patient's status. Often, family members need advice from the health care team to get some rest; they are more likely to take this advice if they feel that the patient is being well cared for and that they will be notified of any significant changes in the patient's status. A visit from the hospital chaplain may be comforting to the family and provides some attention to the family while the nurse concentrates on the patient.

IRREVERSIBLE STAGE

The irreversible (or refractory) stage of shock represents the point along the shock continuum at which organ damage is so severe that the patient does not respond to treatment and cannot survive. Despite treatment, blood pressure remains low. Complete renal and liver failure, compounded by the release of necrotic tissue toxins, creates an overwhelming metabolic acidosis. Anaerobic metabolism contributes to a worsening lactic acidosis. Reserves of ATP are almost totally depleted, and mechanisms for storing new supplies of energy have been destroyed. Multiple organ dysfunction progressing to complete organ failure has occurred, and death is imminent. Multiple organ dysfunction can occur as a progression along the shock continuum or as a syndrome unto itself and is further described later in this chapter.

Medical Management

Medical management during the irreversible stage of shock is usually the same as for the progressive stage. Although the patient's condition may have progressed from the progressive to the irreversible stage, the judgment that the shock is irreversible can be made only retrospectively on the basis of the patient's failure to respond to treatment. Strategies that may be experimental (ie, investigational medications, such as antibiotic agents and immunomodulation therapy) may be tried to reduce or reverse the severity of shock.

Nursing Management

As in the progressive stage of shock, the nurse focuses on carrying out prescribed treatments, monitoring the patient, preventing complications, protecting the patient from injury, and providing comfort. Offering brief explanations to the patient about what is happening is essential even if there is no certainty that the patient hears or understands what is being said.

As it becomes obvious that the patient is unlikely to survive, the family needs to be informed about the prognosis and likely outcomes. Opportunities should be provided, throughout the patient's care, for the family to see, touch, and talk to the patient. A close family friend or spiritual advisor may be of comfort to the family in dealing with the inevitable death of the patient. Whenever possible and appropriate, the family should be approached regarding any living will, advance directive, or other written or verbal wishes the patient may have shared in the event that he or she cannot participate in end-of-life decisions. In some cases, ethics committees may assist the family and health care team in making difficult decisions.

During this stage of shock, families may misinterpret the actions of the health care team. They have been told that nothing has been effective in reversing the shock and that the patient's survival is very unlikely, yet the health care team continues to work feverishly on the patient. A distraught, grieving family may interpret this as a chance for recovery when none exists. As a result, family members may become angry when the patient dies. Conferences with all members of the health care team and the family will promote better understanding by the family of the patient's prognosis and the purpose for the measures being taken. During these conferences, it is essential to explain that the equipment and treatments being provided are for the patient's comfort and do not suggest that the patient will recover. Families should be encouraged to express their wishes concerning the use of life-support measures.

Overall Management Strategies in Shock

As described previously and in the discussion of types of shock to follow, management in all types and all phases of shock includes the following:

- Fluid replacement to restore intravascular volume
- Vasoactive medications to restore vasomotor tone and improve cardiac function
- Nutritional support to address the metabolic requirements that are often dramatically increased in shock

Therapies described in this section require collaboration among all members of the health care team to ensure that the manifestations of shock are quickly identified and that adequate and timely treatment is instituted to achieve the best outcome possible.

FLUID REPLACEMENT

Fluid replacement is administered in all types of shock. The type of fluids administered and the speed of delivery vary, but fluids are given to improve cardiac and tissue oxygenation, which in part depends on flow. The fluids administered may include **crystalloids** (electrolyte solutions that move freely between intravascular and interstitial spaces), **colloids** (large-molecule intravenous solutions), or blood components.

Crystalloid and Colloid Solutions

The best fluid to treat shock remains controversial. In emergencies, the "best" fluid is often the fluid that is readily available. Both crystalloids and colloids, as described later, can be given to restore intravascular volume. Blood component therapy is used most frequently in hypovolemic shock.

Crystalloids are electrolyte solutions that move freely between the intravascular compartment and the interstitial spaces. Isotonic crystalloid solutions are often selected because they contain the same concentration of electrolytes as the extracellular fluid and therefore can be given without altering the concentrations of electrolytes in the plasma.

Common intravenous fluids used for resuscitation in hypovolemic shock include 0.9% sodium chloride solution (normal saline) and lactated Ringer's solution (Choi et al., 1999). Ringer's lactate is an electrolyte solution containing the lactate ion, which should not be confused with lactic acid. The lactate ion is converted to bicarbonate, which helps to buffer the overall acidosis that occurs in shock.

A disadvantage of using isotonic crystalloid solutions is that three parts of the volume are lost to the interstitial compartment for every one part that remains in the intravascular compartment. This occurs in response to mechanisms that store extracellular body fluid. Diffusion of crystalloids into the interstitial space necessitates that more fluid be administered than the amount lost (Choi et al., 1999).

Care must be taken when rapidly administering isotonic crystalloids to avoid causing excessive edema, particularly pulmonary edema. For this reason, and depending on the cause of the hypovolemia, a hypertonic crystalloid solution, such as 3% sodium chloride, is sometimes administered in hypovolemic shock. Hypertonic solutions produce a large osmotic force that pulls fluid from the intracellular space to the extracellular space to achieve a fluid balance (Choi et al., 1999; Fein & Calalang-Colucci, 2000). The osmotic effect of hypertonic solutions results in fewer fluids being administered to restore intravascular volume. Complications associated with use of hypertonic saline solution include excessive serum osmolality, hypernatremia, hypokalemia, and altered thermoregulation.

Generally, intravenous colloidal solutions are considered to be plasma proteins, which are molecules that are too large to pass through capillary membranes. Colloids expand intravascular volume by exerting oncotic pressure, thereby pulling fluid into the intravascular space. Colloidal solutions have the same effect as hypertonic solutions in increasing intravascular volume, but less volume of fluid is required than with crystalloids. Additionally, colloids have a longer duration of action than crystalloids because the molecules remain within the intravascular compartment longer.

An albumin solution is commonly used to treat hypovolemic shock. Albumin is a plasma protein; an albumin solution is prepared from human plasma and is heated to reduce its potential to transmit disease. The disadvantages of albumin are its high cost and limited availability, which depends on blood donors. Synthetic colloid preparations, such as hetastarch and dextran solution, are now widely used. Dextran, however, may interfere with platelet aggregation and therefore is not indicated if hemorrhage is the cause of the hypovolemic shock or if the patient has a coagulation disorder (coagulopathy).

 NURSING ALERT With all colloidal solutions, side effects include the rare occurrence of anaphylactic reactions, for which the nurse must monitor the patient closely.

Complications of Fluid Administration

Close monitoring of the patient during fluid replacement is necessary to identify side effects and complications. The most common and serious side effects of fluid replacement are cardiovascular overload and pulmonary edema.

Patients receiving fluid replacement must be monitored frequently for adequate urinary output, changes in mental status, skin perfusion, and changes in vital signs. Lung sounds are auscultated frequently to detect signs of fluid accumulation. Adventitious lung sounds, such as crackles, may indicate pulmonary edema.

Often a right atrial pressure line (also known as a central venous pressure line) is inserted. In addition to physical assessment, the right atrial pressure value helps in monitoring the patient's response to fluid replacement. A normal right atrial pressure value is 4 to 12 mm Hg or cm H_2O. Several readings are obtained to determine a range, and fluid replacement is continued to achieve a pressure within normal limits. Hemodynamic monitoring with arterial and pulmonary artery lines may be implemented to allow close monitoring of the patient's perfusion and cardiac status as well as response to therapy.

VASOACTIVE MEDICATION THERAPY

Vasoactive medications are administered in all forms of shock to improve the patient's hemodynamic stability when fluid therapy alone cannot maintain adequate MAP. Specific medications are selected to correct the particular hemodynamic alteration that is impeding cardiac output. Specific vasoactive medications are prescribed for the patient in shock because they can support the patient's hemodynamic status. These medications help to increase the strength of myocardial contractility, regulate the heart rate, reduce myocardial resistance, and initiate vasoconstriction.

Vasoactive medications are selected for their action on receptors of the sympathetic nervous system. These receptors are known as alpha-adrenergic and beta-adrenergic receptors. Beta-adrenergic receptors are further classified as beta$_1$- and beta$_2$-adrenergic receptors. When alpha-adrenergic receptors are stimulated, blood vessels constrict in the cardiorespiratory and gastrointestinal systems, skin, and kidneys. When beta$_1$-adrenergic receptors are stimulated, heart rate and myocardial contraction increase. When

beta$_2$-adrenergic receptors are stimulated, vasodilation occurs in the heart and skeletal muscles, and the bronchioles relax. The medications used in treating shock consist of various combinations of vasoactive medications to maximize tissue perfusion by stimulating or blocking the alpha- and beta-adrenergic receptors.

When vasoactive medications are administered, vital signs must be monitored frequently (at least every 15 minutes until stable, or more often if indicated). Vasoactive medications should be administered through a central venous line because infiltration and extravasation of some vasoactive medications can cause tissue necrosis and sloughing. An intravenous pump or controller should be used to ensure that the medications are delivered safely and accurately.

Individual medication dosages are usually titrated by the nurse, who adjusts the intravenous drip rates based on the physician's prescription and the patient's response. Dosages are changed to maintain the MAP (usually above 80 mm Hg) at a physiologic level that ensures adequate tissue perfusion.

> **! NURSING ALERT** Vasoactive medications should never be stopped abruptly because this could cause severe hemodynamic instability, perpetuating the shock state.

Dosages of vasoactive medications should be tapered and the patient should be weaned from the medication with frequent monitoring (every 15 minutes) of blood pressure. Table 15-1 presents some of the commonly prescribed vasoactive medications used in treating shock.

NUTRITIONAL SUPPORT

Nutritional support is an important aspect of care for the patient with shock. Increased metabolic rates during shock increase energy requirements and therefore caloric requirements. The patient in shock requires more than 3,000 calories (12,600 kilojoules) daily.

The release of catecholamines early in the shock continuum causes glycogen stores to be depleted in about 8 to 10 hours. Nutritional energy requirements are then met by breaking down lean body mass. In this catabolic process, skeletal muscle mass is broken down even when the patient has large stores of fat or adipose tissue. Loss of skeletal muscle can greatly prolong the recovery

Table 15-1 • Vasoactive Agents Used in Treating Shock

MEDICATION	DESIRED ACTION IN SHOCK	DISADVANTAGES
Sympathomimetics Dobutamine (Dobutrex) Dopamine (Intropin) Epinephrine (Adrenalin) Milrinone (Primacor)	Improve contractility, increase stroke volume, increase cardiac output	Increase oxygen demand of the heart
Vasodilators Nitroglycerine (Tridil) Nitroprusside (Nipride)	Reduce preload and afterload, reduce oxygen demand of heart	Cause hypotension
Vasoconstrictors Norepinephrine (Levophed) Phenylephrine (Neo-Synephrine) Vasopressin (Pitressin)	Increase blood pressure by vasoconstriction	Increase afterload, thereby increasing cardiac workload; compromise perfusion to skin, kidneys, lungs, GI tract

time for the patient in shock. Parenteral or enteral nutritional support should be initiated as soon as possible, with some form of enteral nutrition always being administered. The integrity of the gastrointestinal system depends on direct exposure to nutrients. Additionally, glutamine (an essential amino acid during stress) is important in the immunologic function of the gastrointestinal tract, providing a fuel source for lymphocytes and macrophages. Glutamine can be administered through enteral nutrition (Rauen & Munro, 1998).

Stress ulcers occur frequently in acutely ill patients because of the compromised blood supply to the gastrointestinal tract. Therefore, antacids, histamine-2 blockers (eg, famotidine [Pepcid], ranitidine [Zantac]), and antipeptic agents (eg, sucralfate [Carafate]) are prescribed to prevent ulcer formation by inhibiting gastric acid secretion or increasing gastric pH.

Hypovolemic Shock

In addition to caring for the patient through different stages of shock, the nurse needs to tailor interventions to the type of shock, whether it is hypovolemic, cardiogenic, or circulatory shock.

Hypovolemic shock, the most common type of shock, is characterized by a decreased intravascular volume. Body fluid is contained in the intracellular and extracellular compartments. Intracellular fluid accounts for about two thirds of the total body water. The extracellular body fluid is found in one of two compartments: intravascular (inside blood vessels) or interstitial (surrounding tissues). The volume of interstitial fluid is about three to four times that of intravascular fluid. Hypovolemic shock occurs when there is a reduction in intravascular volume of 15% to 25%. This would represent a loss of 750 to 1,300 mL of blood in a 70-kg person.

Pathophysiology

Hypovolemic shock can be caused by external fluid losses, such as traumatic blood loss, or by internal fluid shifts, as in severe dehydration, severe edema, or ascites (Chart 15-3). Intravascular volume can be reduced both by fluid loss and fluid shifting between the intravascular and interstitial compartments.

The sequence of events in hypovolemic shock begins with a decrease in the intravascular volume. This results in decreased venous return of blood to the heart and subsequent decreased ventricular filling. Decreased ventricular filling results in decreased stroke volume (amount of blood ejected from the heart) and decreased cardiac output. When cardiac output drops, blood pressure drops and tissues cannot be adequately perfused (Fig. 15-3).

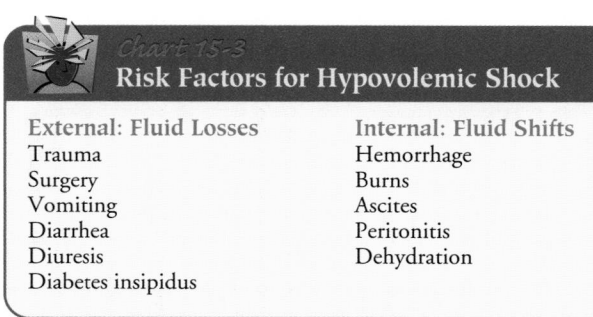

Chart 15-3
Risk Factors for Hypovolemic Shock

External: Fluid Losses	Internal: Fluid Shifts
Trauma	Hemorrhage
Surgery	Burns
Vomiting	Ascites
Diarrhea	Peritonitis
Diuresis	Dehydration
Diabetes insipidus	

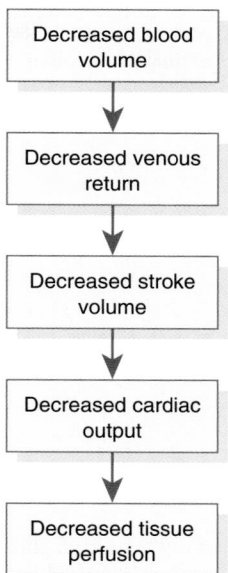

Physiology/Pathophysiology

Decreased blood volume
↓
Decreased venous return
↓
Decreased stroke volume
↓
Decreased cardiac output
↓
Decreased tissue perfusion

FIGURE 15-3 Pathophysiologic sequence of events in hypovolemic shock.

Medical Management

Major goals in treating hypovolemic shock are to (1) restore intravascular volume to reverse the sequence of events leading to inadequate tissue perfusion, (2) redistribute fluid volume, and (3) correct the underlying cause of the fluid loss as quickly as possible. Depending on the severity of shock and the patient's condition, it is likely that efforts will be made to address all three goals simultaneously.

TREATMENT OF THE UNDERLYING CAUSE

If the patient is hemorrhaging, efforts are made to stop the bleeding. This may involve applying pressure to the bleeding site or surgery to stop internal bleeding. If the cause of the hypovolemia is diarrhea or vomiting, medications to treat diarrhea and vomiting are administered as efforts are made simultaneously to identify and treat the cause. In the elderly patient, dehydration may be the cause of hypovolemic shock.

FLUID AND BLOOD REPLACEMENT

Beyond reversing the primary cause of the decreased intravascular volume, fluid replacement (also referred to as fluid resuscitation) is of primary concern. At least two large-gauge intravenous lines are inserted to establish access for fluid administration. Two intravenous lines allow simultaneous administration of fluid, medications, and blood component therapy if required. Because the goal of the fluid replacement is to restore intravascular volume, it is necessary to administer fluids that will remain in the intravascular compartment and thus avoid creating fluid shifts from the intravascular compartment into the intracellular compartment. Table 15-2 summarizes the fluids commonly used in treating shock.

Table 15-2 • **Fluid Replacement in Shock**

FLUIDS	ADVANTAGES	DISADVANTAGES
Crystalloids		
0.9% sodium chloride (normal saline solution)	Widely available, inexpensive	Requires large volume of infusion; can cause pulmonary edema
Lactated Ringer's	Lactate ion helps buffer metabolic acidosis	Requires large volume of infusion; can cause pulmonary edema
Hypertonic saline (3%, 5%, 7.5%)	Small volume needed to restore intra-vascular volume	Danger of hypernatremia
Colloids		
Albumin (5%, 25%)	Rapidly expands plasma volume	Expensive; requires human donors; limited supply; can cause heart failure
Dextran (40, 70)	Synthetic plasma expander	Interferes with platelet aggregation; not recommended for hemorrhagic shock
Hetastarch	Synthetic; less expensive than albumin; effect lasts up to 36 h	Prolongs bleeding and clotting times

Lactated Ringer's and 0.9% sodium chloride solutions are isotonic crystalloid fluids commonly used in treating hypovolemic shock (Jindal et al., 2000). Large amounts of fluid must be administered to restore intravascular volume because isotonic crystalloid solutions move freely between the fluid compartments of the body and do not remain in the vascular system.

Colloids (eg, albumin, hetastarch, and dextran) may also be used. Dextran is not indicated if the cause of the hypovolemic shock is hemorrhage because it interferes with platelet aggregation.

Blood products, also colloids, may need to be administered, particularly when the cause of the hypovolemic shock is hemorrhage. Because of the risk of transmitting bloodborne viruses and the scarcity of blood products, however, these products are used only if other alternatives are unavailable or blood loss is extensive and rapid. Packed red blood cells are administered to replenish the patient's oxygen-carrying capacity in conjunction with other fluids that will expand volume. Current recommendations are to base the need for transfusions on the patient's oxygenation needs, which are determined by vital signs, blood gas values, and clinical appearance rather than using an arbitrary laboratory value. Synthetic forms of blood (ie, compounds capable of carrying oxygen in the same way that blood does) are potential alternatives.

REDISTRIBUTION OF FLUID

In addition to administering fluids to restore intravascular volume, positioning the patient properly assists fluid redistribution. A modified Trendelenburg position (Fig. 15-4) is recommended in hypovolemic shock. Elevating the legs promotes the return of venous blood. Positioning the patient in a full Trendelenburg position, however, makes breathing difficult and therefore is not recommended.

PHARMACOLOGIC THERAPY

If fluid administration fails to reverse hypovolemic shock, then the same medications given in cardiogenic shock are used because unreversed hypovolemic shock progresses to cardiogenic shock (the vicious circle).

If the underlying cause of the hypovolemia is dehydration, medications are also administered to reverse the cause of the dehydration. For example, insulin is administered if dehydration is

secondary to hyperglycemia; desmopressin (DDAVP) is administered for diabetes insipidus, antidiarrheal agents for diarrhea, and antiemetic medications for vomiting.

Nursing Management

Primary prevention of shock is an essential focus of nursing intervention. Hypovolemic shock can be prevented in some instances by closely monitoring patients who are at risk for fluid deficits and assisting with fluid replacement before intravascular volume is depleted. In other circumstances, hypovolemic shock cannot be prevented, and nursing care focuses on assisting with treatment targeted at treating its cause and restoring intravascular volume.

General nursing measures include ensuring safe administration of prescribed fluids and medications and documenting their administration and effects. Another important nursing role is monitoring for signs of complications and side effects of treatment and reporting these signs early in treatment.

FIGURE 15-4 Proper positioning (modified Trendelenburg) for the patient who shows signs of shock. The lower extremities are elevated to an angle of about 20 degrees; the knees are straight, the trunk is horizontal, and the head is slightly elevated.

ADMINISTERING BLOOD AND FLUIDS SAFELY

Administering blood transfusions safely is a vital nursing role. In emergency situations, it is important to obtain blood specimens quickly to obtain a baseline complete blood count and to type and cross-match the blood in anticipation of blood transfusions. The patient who receives a transfusion of blood products must be monitored closely for adverse effects (see Chap. 33).

Fluid replacement complications can occur, often when large volumes are administered rapidly. Therefore, the nurse monitors the patient closely for cardiovascular overload and pulmonary edema. The risk of these complications is increased in the elderly and in patients with pre-existing cardiac disease. Hemodynamic pressure, vital signs, arterial blood gases, hemoglobin and hematocrit levels, and fluid intake and output are among the parameters monitored. The patient's temperature should also be monitored closely to ensure that rapid fluid resuscitation does not precipitate hypothermia. Intravenous fluids may need to be warmed during the administration of large volumes. Physical assessment focuses on observing the jugular veins for distention and monitoring jugular venous pressure. Jugular venous pressure is low in hypovolemic shock; it increases with effective treatment and is significantly increased with fluid overload and heart failure. The nurse needs to monitor cardiac and respiratory status closely and report changes in blood pressure, pulse pressure, heart rate, rhythm, and lung sounds to the physician.

IMPLEMENTING OTHER MEASURES

Oxygen is administered to increase the amount of oxygen carried by available hemoglobin in the blood. A patient who is confused may feel apprehensive with an oxygen mask or cannula in place, and frequent explanations about the need for the mask may reduce some of the patient's fear and anxiety. Simultaneously, the nurse must direct efforts to the safety and comfort of the patient.

Cardiogenic Shock

Cardiogenic shock occurs when the heart's ability to contract and to pump blood is impaired and the supply of oxygen is inadequate for the heart and tissues. The causes of cardiogenic shock are known as either coronary or noncoronary. Coronary cardiogenic shock is more common than noncoronary cardiogenic shock and is seen most often in patients with myocardial infarction. Coronary cardiogenic shock occurs when a significant amount of the left ventricular myocardium has been destroyed (Price et al., 1999). Patients experiencing an anterior wall myocardial infarction are at the greatest risk for developing cardiogenic shock because of the potentially extensive damage to the left ventricle caused by occlusion of the left anterior descending coronary artery (Chart 15-4). Non-coronary causes can be related to

severe metabolic problems (severe hypoxemia, acidosis, hypoglycemia, and hypocalcemia) and tension pneumothorax.

Pathophysiology

In cardiogenic shock, cardiac output, which is a function of both stroke volume and heart rate, is compromised. When stroke volume and heart rate decrease or become erratic, blood pressure drops and tissue perfusion is compromised. Along with other tissues and organs being deprived of adequate blood supply, the heart muscle itself receives inadequate blood. The result is impaired tissue perfusion. Because impaired tissue perfusion weakens the heart and impairs its ability to pump blood forward, the ventricle does not fully eject its volume of blood at systole. As a result, fluid accumulates in the lungs. This sequence of events can occur rapidly or over a period of days (Fig. 15-5).

Clinical Manifestations

Patients in cardiogenic shock may experience angina pain and develop dysrhythmias and hemodynamic instability.

Medical Management

The goals of medical management are to (1) limit further myocardial damage and preserve the healthy myocardium and (2) improve the cardiac function by increasing cardiac contractility, decreasing ventricular afterload, or both (Price et al., 1999). In general, these goals are achieved by increasing oxygen supply to the heart muscle while reducing oxygen demands.

CORRECTION OF UNDERLYING CAUSES

As with all forms of shock, the underlying cause of cardiogenic shock must be corrected. It is necessary first to treat the oxygenation needs of the heart muscle to ensure its continued ability to pump blood to other organs. In the case of coronary cardiogenic shock, the patient may require thrombolytic therapy, angioplasty, or coronary artery bypass graft surgery. In the case of noncoronary cardiogenic shock, the patient may require a cardiac valve replacement or correction of a dysrhythmia. For further explanation of these procedures, refer to Chapters 27 and 28.

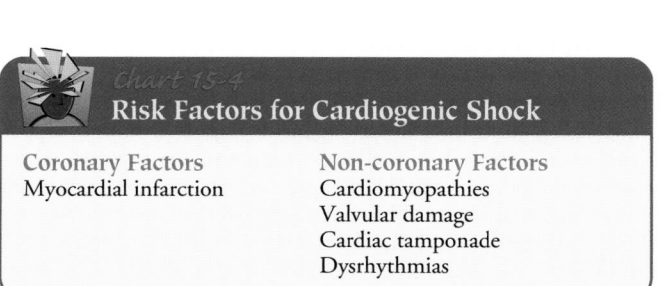

Chart 15-4

Risk Factors for Cardiogenic Shock

Coronary Factors	Non-coronary Factors
Myocardial infarction	Cardiomyopathies
	Valvular damage
	Cardiac tamponade
	Dysrhythmias

Physiology/Pathophysiology

Decreased cardiac contractility

↓

Decreased stroke volume and cardiac output

↓

| Pulmonary congestion | Decreased systemic tissue perfusion | Decreased coronary artery perfusion |

FIGURE 15-5 Pathophysiologic sequence of events in cardiogenic shock.

INITIATION OF FIRST-LINE TREATMENT

First-line treatment of cardiogenic shock involves the following actions:

- Supplying supplemental oxygen
- Controlling chest pain
- Providing selected fluid support
- Administering vasoactive medications
- Controlling heart rate with medication or by implementation of a transthoracic or intravenous pacemaker
- Implementing mechanical cardiac support (intra-aortic balloon counterpulsation therapy, ventricular assist systems, or extracorporeal cardiopulmonary bypass)

Oxygenation. In the early stages of shock, supplemental oxygen is administered by nasal cannula at a rate of 2 to 6 L/min to achieve an oxygen saturation exceeding 90%. Monitoring arterial blood gas values and pulse oximetry values helps to indicate whether the patient requires a more aggressive method of oxygen delivery.

Pain Control. If the patient experiences chest pain, morphine sulfate is administered intravenously for pain relief. In addition to relieving pain, morphine dilates the blood vessels. This reduces the workload of the heart by both decreasing the cardiac filling pressure (preload) and reducing the pressure against which the heart muscle has to eject blood (afterload). Morphine also relieves the patient's anxiety. Cardiac enzyme (CPK-MB and cTn-I) levels are measured, and serial 12-lead electrocardiograms are obtained to assess the degree of myocardial damage.

Hemodynamic Monitoring. Hemodynamic monitoring is initiated to assess the patient's response to treatment. In many institutions, this is performed in the intensive care unit, where an arterial line can be inserted. The arterial line enables accurate and continuous monitoring of blood pressure and provides a port from which to obtain frequent arterial blood samples without having to perform repeated arterial punctures. A multilumen pulmonary artery catheter is inserted to allow measurement of the pulmonary artery pressures, myocardial filling pressures, cardiac output, and pulmonary and systemic resistance. For more information, see Chapter 30.

PHARMACOLOGIC THERAPY

Vasoactive medication therapy consists of multiple pharmacologic strategies to restore and maintain adequate cardiac output. In coronary cardiogenic shock, the aims of vasoactive medication therapy are improved cardiac contractility, decreased preload and afterload, or stable heart rate.

Because improving contractility and decreasing cardiac workload are opposing pharmacologic actions, two classifications of medications may be administered in combination: sympathomimetic agents and vasodilators. Sympathomimetic medications increase cardiac output by mimicking the action of the sympathetic nervous system through vasoconstriction, resulting in increased preload, and by increasing myocardial contractility (inotropic action) or increasing the heart rate (chronotropic action). Vasodilators are used to decrease preload and afterload, thus reducing the workload of the heart and the oxygen demand. Medications commonly combined to treat cardiogenic shock include dobutamine, dopamine, and nitroglycerin (see Table 15-1).

Dobutamine. Dobutamine (Dobutrex) produces inotropic effects by stimulating myocardial beta receptors, increasing the strength of myocardial activity and improving cardiac output. Myocardial alpha-adrenergic receptors are also stimulated, resulting in decreased pulmonary and systemic vascular resistance (decreased afterload). Dobutamine enhances the strength of cardiac contraction, improving stroke volume ejection and overall cardiac output (Jindal et al., 2000; Price et al., 1999).

Nitroglycerin. Intravenous nitroglycerin (Tridil) in low doses acts as a venous vasodilator and therefore reduces preload. At higher doses, nitroglycerin causes arterial vasodilation and therefore reduces afterload as well. These actions, in combination with medium-dose dopamine, increase cardiac output while minimizing cardiac workload. Additionally, vasodilation enhances blood flow to the myocardium, improving oxygen delivery to the weakened heart muscle (Price et al., 1999).

Dopamine. Dopamine (Intropin) is a sympathomimetic agent that has varying vasoactive effects depending on the dosage. It may be used with dobutamine and nitroglycerine to improve tissue perfusion. Low-dose dopamine (0.5 to 3.0 μg/kg/min) increases renal and mesenteric blood flow, thereby preventing ischemia of these organs because shock causes blood to be shunted away from the kidneys and the mesentery. This dosage, however, does not improve cardiac output. Medium-dose dopamine (4 to 8 μg/kg/min) has sympathomimetic properties and improves contractility (inotropic action) and slightly increases the heart rate (chronotropic action). At this dosage, dopamine increases cardiac output and therefore is desirable. High-dose dopamine (8 to 10 μg/kg/min) predominantly causes vasoconstriction, which increases afterload and thus increases cardiac workload. Because this effect is undesirable in patients with cardiogenic shock, dopamine dosages must be carefully titrated. Once the patient's blood pressure stabilizes, low-dose dopamine may be continued for its effect of promoting renal perfusion in particular. In severe metabolic acidosis, which occurs in the later stages of shock, dopamine's effectiveness is diminished. To maximize the effectiveness of any vasoactive agent, metabolic acidosis must first be corrected. The physician may prescribe intravenous sodium bicarbonate to treat the acidosis (Jindal et al., 2000).

Other Vasoactive Medications. Additional vasoactive agents that may be used in managing cardiogenic shock include norepinephrine (Levophed), epinephrine (Adrenalin), milrinone (Primacor), amrinone (Inocor), vasopressin (Pitressin), and phenylephrine (Neo-Synephrine). Each of these medications stimulates different receptors of the sympathetic nervous system. A combination of these medications may be prescribed, depending on the patient's response to treatment. All vasoactive medications have adverse effects, making specific medications more useful than others at different stages of shock. Diuretics such as furosemide (Lasix) may be administered to reduce the workload of the heart by reducing fluid accumulation (see Table 15-1).

Antiarrhythmic Medications. Antiarrhythmic medication is also part of the medication regimen in cardiogenic shock. Multiple factors, such as hypoxemia, electrolyte imbalances, and acid–base imbalances, contribute to serious cardiac dysrhythmias in all patients with shock. Additionally, as a compensatory response to decreased cardiac output and blood pressure, the heart rate increases beyond normal limits. This impedes cardiac output further by shortening diastole and thereby decreasing the time for ventricular filling. Consequently, antiarrhythmic medications are required to stabilize the heart rate. For a full discussion of cardiac dysrhythmias as well as commonly prescribed medications, see Chapter 27. General principles regarding the administration of vasoactive medications are discussed later in this chapter.

Fluid Therapy. In addition to medications, appropriate fluid is necessary in treating cardiogenic shock. Administration of fluids must be monitored closely to detect signs of fluid overload. Incremental intravenous fluid boluses are cautiously administered to determine optimal filling pressures for improving cardiac output. A fluid bolus should never be given quickly because rapid fluid administration in patients with cardiac failure may result in acute pulmonary edema.

MECHANICAL ASSISTIVE DEVICES

If cardiac output does not improve despite supplemental oxygen, vasoactive medications, and fluid boluses, mechanical assistive devices are used temporarily to improve the heart's ability to pump. Intra-aortic balloon counterpulsation is one means of providing temporary circulatory assistance (see Chap. 30). A polyurethane balloon catheter is inserted percutaneously through the common femoral artery and advanced into the descending thoracic aorta. The balloon catheter is connected to a console containing a gas-filled pump. The timing of the balloon inflation is synchronized electrocardiographically with the beginning of diastole, and the balloon deflation occurs just before systole. The goals of intra-aortic balloon counterpulsation include the following:

- Increased stroke volume
- Improved coronary artery perfusion
- Decreased preload
- Decreased cardiac workload
- Decreased myocardial oxygen demand (Kumar et al., 2000)

Other means of mechanical assistance include left and right ventricular assist devices and total artificial hearts. These devices are electrical pumps or pumps driven by air. They assist or replace the ventricular pumping action of the heart. Human heart transplantation may be the only option remaining for a patient who has cardiogenic shock and who cannot be weaned from mechanical assistive devices. (Mechanical assistive devices and heart transplantation are discussed in Chap. 30.)

Another short-term means of providing cardiac or pulmonary support to the patient in cardiogenic shock is through an extracorporeal device similar to the cardiopulmonary bypass (CPB) used in open-heart surgery. The CPB system requires systemic anticoagulation, arterial and venous cannulation of the femoral artery and vein, and connection to a centrifugal, oxygenated pump. The catheter tip is advanced into the right atrium. This system lowers left and right ventricular pressures, reducing the workload and oxygen needs of the heart. Complications of CPB include coagulopathies, myocardial ischemia, infection, and thromboembolism. CPB is used only in emergency situations until definitive treatment, such as heart transplantation, can be initiated.

Nursing Management

PREVENTING CARDIOGENIC SHOCK

In some circumstances, identifying patients at risk early and promoting adequate oxygenation of the heart muscle and decreasing cardiac workload can prevent cardiogenic shock. This can be accomplished by conserving the patient's energy, promptly relieving angina, and administering supplemental oxygen. Often, however, cardiogenic shock cannot be prevented. In such instances, nursing management includes working with other members of the health care team to prevent shock from progressing and to restore adequate cardiac function and tissue perfusion.

MONITORING HEMODYNAMIC STATUS

A major role of the nurse is monitoring the patient's hemodynamic and cardiac status. Arterial lines and electrocardiographic monitoring equipment must be maintained and functioning properly. The nurse anticipates the medications, intravenous fluids, and equipment that might be used and is ready to assist in implementing these measures. Changes in hemodynamic, cardiac, and pulmonary status are documented and reported promptly. Additionally, adventitious breath sounds, changes in cardiac rhythm, and other abnormal physical assessment findings are reported immediately.

ADMINISTERING MEDICATIONS AND INTRAVENOUS FLUIDS

The nurse has a critical role in safe and accurate administration of intravenous fluids and medications. Fluid overload and pulmonary edema are risks because of ineffective cardiac function and accumulation of blood and fluid in the pulmonary tissues. The nurse documents and records medications and treatments that are administered as well as the patient's response to treatment.

The nurse needs to be knowledgeable about the desired effects as well as the side effects of medications. For example, it is important to monitor the patient for decreased blood pressure after administering morphine or nitroglycerin. The patient receiving thrombolytic therapy must be monitored for bleeding. Arterial and venous puncture sites must be observed for bleeding and pressure must be applied at the sites if bleeding occurs. Neurologic assessment is essential after the administration of thrombolytic therapy to assess for the potential complication of cerebral hemorrhage associated with the therapy. Intravenous infusions must be observed closely because tissue necrosis and sloughing may occur if vasopressor medications infiltrate the tissues. Urine output, BUN, and serum creatinine levels are monitored to detect decreased renal function secondary to the effects of cardiogenic shock or its treatment.

MAINTAINING INTRA-AORTIC BALLOON COUNTERPULSATION

The nurse plays a critical role in caring for the patient receiving intra-aortic balloon counterpulsation (see Chap. 30). The nurse makes ongoing timing adjustments of the balloon pump to maximize its effectiveness by synchronizing it with the cardiac cycle. The patient is at great risk for circulatory compromise to the leg on the side where the catheter for the balloon has been placed; therefore, the nurse must frequently check the neurovascular status of the lower extremities.

ENHANCING SAFETY AND COMFORT

Throughout care, the nurse must take an active role in safeguarding the patient, enhancing comfort, and reducing anxiety. This includes administering medication to relieve chest pain, preventing infection at the multiple arterial and venous line insertion sites, protecting the skin, and monitoring respiratory function. Proper positioning of the patient promotes effective breathing without decreasing blood pressure and may also increase the patient's comfort while reducing anxiety.

Brief explanations about procedures that are being performed and the use of comforting touch often provide reassurance to the patient and family. Families are usually anxious and benefit from opportunities to see and talk to the patient. Explanations of treatments and the patient's response to them are often comforting to family members.

Circulatory Shock

Circulatory or distributive shock occurs when blood volume is abnormally displaced in the vasculature—for example, when blood volume pools in peripheral blood vessels. The displacement of blood volume causes a relative hypovolemia because not enough blood returns to the heart, which leads to subsequent inadequate tissue perfusion. The ability of the blood vessels to constrict helps return the blood to the heart. Thus, the vascular tone is determined both by central regulatory mechanisms, as in blood pressure regulation, and by local regulatory mechanisms, as in tissue demands for oxygen and nutrients. Therefore, circulatory shock can be caused either by a loss of sympathetic tone or by release of biochemical mediators from cells.

The varied mechanisms leading to the initial vasodilation in circulatory shock further subdivide this classification of shock into three types: (1) **septic shock**, (2) **neurogenic shock**, and (3) **anaphylactic shock**.

The different types of circulatory shock cause variations in the pathophysiologic chain of events and are explained here separately. In all types of circulatory shock, massive arterial and venous dilation allows blood to pool peripherally. Arterial dilation reduces systemic vascular resistance. Initially, cardiac output can be high in circulatory shock, both from the reduction in afterload (systemic vascular resistance) and from the heart muscle's increased effort to maintain perfusion despite the incompetent vasculature secondary to arterial dilation. Pooling of blood in the periphery results in decreased venous return. Decreased venous return results in decreased stroke volume and decreased cardiac output. Decreased cardiac output, in turn, causes decreased blood pressure and ultimately decreased tissue perfusion. Figure 15-6 presents the pathophysiologic sequence of events in circulatory shock.

SEPTIC SHOCK

Septic shock is the most common type of circulatory shock and is caused by widespread infection (Chart 15-5). Despite the increased sophistication of antibiotic therapy, the incidence of septic shock has continued to rise during the past 60 years. It is the most common cause of death in noncoronary intensive care units in the United States and the 13th leading cause of death in the U.S. population (Balk, 2000a). Elderly patients are at particular risk for sepsis because of decreased physiologic reserves and an aging immune system (Balk, 2000a; Vincent & Ferreira, 2000). Toxic shock syndrome, a specific form of septic shock, is described in Chapter 47.

Nosocomial infections (infections occurring in the hospital) in critically ill patients most frequently originate in the bloodstream, lungs, and urinary tract (in decreasing order of frequency) (Richards, Edwards, Culver et al., 1999). The source of infection is an important determinant of the clinical outcome. The greatest risk of sepsis occurs in patients with bacteremia (bloodstream) and pneumonia (Simon & Trenholme, 2000). Other infections that may progress to septic shock include intra-abdominal infections, wound infections, bacteremia associated with intravascular catheters (Eggimann & Pittet, 2001), and indwelling urinary catheters. Additional risk factors that contribute to the growing incidence of septic shock are the increased awareness and identi-

Physiology/Pathophysiology

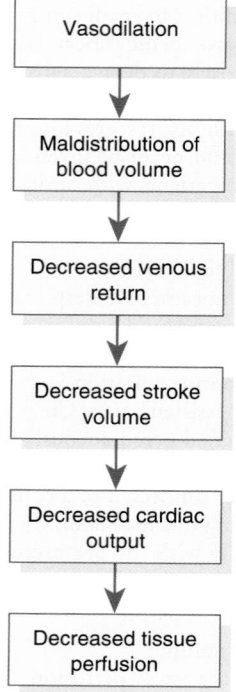

FIGURE 15-6 Pathophysiologic sequence of events in circulatory shock.

fication of septic shock; the increased number of immunocompromised patients (due to malnutrition, alcoholism, malignancy, and diabetes mellitus); the increased incidence of invasive procedures and indwelling medical devices; the increased number of resistant microorganisms; and the increasingly older population (Balk, 2000a). The incidence of septic shock can be reduced by débriding wounds to remove necrotic tissue and carrying out infection control practices, including the use of meticulous aseptic technique, properly cleaning and maintaining equipment, and using thorough hand-hygiene techniques.

The most common causative microorganisms of septic shock are the gram-negative bacteria; however, there is also an increased

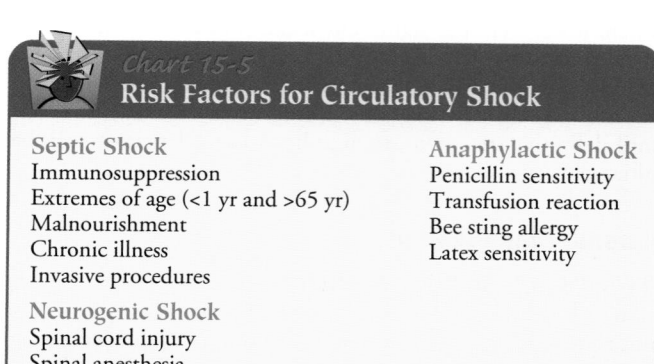

Chart 15-5
Risk Factors for Circulatory Shock

Septic Shock	Anaphylactic Shock
Immunosuppression	Penicillin sensitivity
Extremes of age (<1 yr and >65 yr)	Transfusion reaction
Malnourishment	Bee sting allergy
Chronic illness	Latex sensitivity
Invasive procedures	

Neurogenic Shock
Spinal cord injury
Spinal anesthesia
Depressant action of medications
Glucose deficiency

incidence of gram-positive bacterial infections. Currently, gram-positive bacteria are responsible for 50% of bacteremic events (Simon & Trenholme, 2000). Other infectious agents such as viruses and funguses also can cause septic shock.

When a microorganism invades body tissues, the patient exhibits an immune response. This immune response provokes the activation of biochemical mediators associated with an inflammatory response and produces a variety of effects leading to shock. Increased capillary permeability, which leads to fluid seeping from the capillaries, and vasodilation are two such effects that interrupt the ability of the body to provide adequate perfusion, oxygen, and nutrients to the tissues and cells.

Septic shock typically occurs in two phases. The first phase, referred to as the hyperdynamic, progressive phase, is characterized by a high cardiac output with systemic vasodilation. The blood pressure may remain within normal limits. The heart rate increases, progressing to tachycardia. The patient becomes hyperthermic and febrile, with warm, flushed skin and bounding pulses. The respiratory rate is elevated. Urinary output may remain at normal levels or decrease. Gastrointestinal status may be compromised as evidenced by nausea, vomiting, diarrhea, or decreased bowel sounds. The patient may exhibit subtle changes in mental status, such as confusion or agitation.

The later phase, referred to as the hypodynamic, irreversible phase, is characterized by low cardiac output with vasoconstriction, reflecting the body's effort to compensate for the hypovolemia caused by the loss of intravascular volume through the capillaries. In this phase, the blood pressure drops and the skin is cool and pale. Temperature may be normal or below normal. Heart and respiratory rates remain rapid. The patient no longer produces urine, and multiple organ dysfunction progressing to failure develops.

Systemic inflammatory response syndrome (SIRS) presents clinically like sepsis. The only difference between SIRS and sepsis is that there is no identifiable source of infection. SIRS stimulates an overwhelming inflammatory immunologic and hormonal response, similar to that seen in septic patients. Despite an absence of infection, antibiotic agents may still be administered because of the possibility of unrecognized infection. Additional therapies directed to the support of the patient with SIRS are similar to those for sepsis. If the inflammatory process progresses, septic shock may develop.

Medical Management

Current treatment of septic shock involves identifying and eliminating the cause of infection. Specimens of blood, sputum, urine, wound drainage, and invasive catheter tips are collected for culture using aseptic technique.

Any potential routes of infection must be eliminated. Intravenous lines are removed and reinserted at other body sites. Antibiotic-coated intravenous central lines may be placed to decrease the risk of invasive line-related bacteremia in high-risk patients, such as the elderly (Eggimann & Pittet, 2001). If possible, urinary catheters are removed. Any abscesses are drained and necrotic areas débrided.

Fluid replacement must be instituted to correct the hypovolemia that results from the incompetent vasculature and inflammatory response. Crystalloids, colloids, and blood products may be administered to increase the intravascular volume.

PHARMACOLOGIC THERAPY

If the infecting organism is unknown, broad-spectrum antibiotic agents are started until culture and sensitivity reports are received (Simon & Trenholme, 2000). A third-generation cephalosporin plus an aminoglycoside may be prescribed initially. This combination works against most gram-negative and some gram-positive organisms. When culture and sensitivity reports are available, the antibiotic agent may be changed to one that is more specific to the infecting organism and less toxic to the patient.

Research efforts show promise for improving the outcomes of septic shock. Although past treatments focused on destroying the infectious organism, emphasis is now on altering the patient's immune response to the organism. The cell walls of gram-negative bacteria contain a lipopolysaccharide, an endotoxin released during phagocytosis (Abraham et al., 2001). Endotoxin and/or gram-positive cell wall products interact with inflammatory biochemical mediators, initiating an intense inflammatory response and systemic effects that lead to shock. Current research focuses on the development of medications that will inhibit or modulate the effects of biochemical mediators, such as endotoxin and procalcitonin (Bernard, Vincent, Laterre, et al., 2001). The focus on immunotherapy in treating septic shock is expected to shed light on how the cellular response to infection leads to shock.

Recombinant human activated protein C (APC), or drotrecogin alfa (Xigris), has recently been demonstrated to reduce mortality in patients with severe sepsis (Bernard, Artigas, Dellinger et al., 2001). It was approved by Health Canada (Therapeutic Products Directorate) in 2003 for treatment of adults with severe sepsis and resulting acute organ dysfunction who are at high risk of death. It acts as an antithrombotic, anti-inflammatory, and profibrinolytic agent. Its most common serious side effect is bleeding. Therefore, it is contraindicated in patients with active internal bleeding, recent hemorrhagic stroke, intracranial surgery, or head injury.

NUTRITIONAL THERAPY

Aggressive nutritional supplementation is critical in the management of septic shock because malnutrition further impairs the patient's resistance to infection. Nutritional supplementation should be initiated within the first 24 hours of the onset of shock (Mizock, 2000). Enteral feedings are preferred to the parenteral route because of the increased risk of iatrogenic infection associated with intravenous catheters; however, enteral feedings may not be possible if decreased perfusion to the gastrointestinal tract reduces peristalsis and impairs absorption.

Nursing Management

The nurse caring for any patient in any setting must keep in mind the risks of sepsis and the high mortality rate associated with septic shock. All invasive procedures must be carried out with aseptic technique after careful hand hygiene. Additionally, intravenous lines, arterial and venous puncture sites, surgical incisions, traumatic wounds, urinary catheters, and pressure ulcers are monitored for signs of infection in all patients. The nurse identifies patients at particular risk for sepsis and septic shock (ie, elderly and immunosuppressed patients or patients with extensive trauma or burns or diabetes), keeping in mind that these high-risk patients may not develop typical or classic signs of infection and sepsis. Confusion, for example, may be the first sign of infection and sepsis in elderly patients.

When caring for the patient with septic shock, the nurse collaborates with other members of the health care team to identify the site and source of sepsis and the specific organisms involved. Appropriate specimens for culture and sensitivity are often obtained by the nurse.

Elevated body temperature (hyperthermia) is common with sepsis and raises the patient's metabolic rate and oxygen consumption. Fever is one of the body's natural mechanisms for fighting infections. Thus, an elevated temperature may not be treated unless it reaches dangerous levels (more than 40°C) unless the patient is uncomfortable. Efforts may be made to reduce the temperature by administering acetaminophen or applying hypothermia blankets. During these therapies, the nurse monitors the patient closely for shivering, which increases oxygen consumption. Efforts to increase comfort are important if the patient experiences fever, chills, or shivering.

The nurse administers prescribed intravenous fluids and medications, including antibiotic agents and vasoactive medications to restore vascular volume. Because of decreased perfusion to the kidneys and liver, serum concentrations of antibiotic agents that are normally cleared by these organs may increase and produce toxic effects. Therefore, the nurse monitors blood levels (antibiotic agent, BUN, creatinine, white blood count) and reports increased levels to the physician.

As with other types of shock, the nurse monitors the patient's hemodynamic status, fluid intake and output, and nutritional status. Daily weights and close monitoring of serum albumin levels help determine the patient's protein requirements.

NEUROGENIC SHOCK

In neurogenic shock, vasodilation occurs as a result of a loss of sympathetic tone. This can be caused by spinal cord injury, spinal anesthesia, or nervous system damage. It can also result from the depressant action of medications or lack of glucose (eg, insulin reaction or shock).

Neurogenic shock may have a prolonged course (spinal cord injury) or a short one (syncope or fainting). It is characterized by dry, warm skin rather than the cool, moist skin seen in hypovolemic shock. Another characteristic is bradycardia, rather than the tachycardia that characterizes other forms of shock.

Medical Management

Treatment of neurogenic shock involves restoring sympathetic tone either through the stabilization of a spinal cord injury or, in the instance of spinal anesthesia, by positioning the patient properly. Specific treatment of neurogenic shock depends on its cause. Further discussion of managing the patient with a spinal cord injury is presented in Chapter 63. If hypoglycemia (insulin shock) is the cause, glucose is rapidly administered. Hypoglycemia and the insulin reaction are described further in Chapter 41.

Nursing Management

It is important to elevate and maintain the head of the bed at least 30 degrees to prevent neurogenic shock when a patient is receiving spinal or epidural anesthesia. Elevation of the head of the bed helps to prevent the spread of the anesthetic agent up the spinal cord. In suspected spinal cord injury, neurogenic shock may be prevented by carefully immobilizing the patient to prevent further damage to the spinal cord.

Nursing interventions are directed toward supporting cardiovascular and neurologic function until the usually transient episode of neurogenic shock resolves. Applying elastic compression stockings and elevating the foot of the bed may minimize pooling of blood in the legs. Pooled blood increases the risk for thrombus formation. Therefore, the nurse needs to check the patient daily for any redness, tenderness, warmth of the calves, and positive Homans' sign (calf pain on dorsiflexion of the foot). To elicit Homans' sign, the nurse lifts the patient's leg, flexing it at the knee and dorsiflexing the foot. If the patient complains of pain in the calf, the sign is positive and suggestive of deep vein thrombosis.

Administering heparin or low-molecular-weight heparin (Lovenox) as prescribed, applying elastic compression stockings, or initiating pneumatic compression of the legs may prevent thrombus formation. Performing passive range of motion of the immobile extremities helps promote circulation.

Patients who have experienced a spinal cord injury may not report pain caused by internal injuries. Therefore, in the immediate postinjury period, the nurse must monitor the patient closely for signs of internal bleeding that could lead to hypovolemic shock.

ANAPHYLACTIC SHOCK

Anaphylactic shock is caused by a severe allergic reaction when a patient who has already produced antibodies to a foreign substance (antigen) develops a systemic antigen–antibody reaction. This process requires that the patient has previously been exposed to the substance. An antigen–antibody reaction provokes mast cells to release potent vasoactive substances, such as histamine or bradykinin, that cause widespread vasodilation and capillary permeability. Anaphylactic shock occurs rapidly and is life-threatening. Because anaphylactic shock occurs in patients already exposed to an antigen who have developed antibodies to it, it can often be prevented. Therefore, patients with known allergies need to understand the consequences of subsequent exposure to the antigen and should wear medical identification that lists their sensitivities. This could prevent inadvertent administration of a medication that would lead to anaphylactic shock. Additionally, the patient and family need instruction about emergency use of medications to treat anaphylaxis.

Medical Management

Treatment of anaphylactic shock requires removing the causative antigen (eg, discontinuing an antibiotic agent), administering medications that restore vascular tone, and providing emergency support of basic life functions. Epinephrine is given for its vasoconstrictive action. Diphenhydramine (Benadryl) is administered to reverse the effects of histamine, thereby reducing capillary permeability. These medications are given intravenously. Nebulized medications, such as albuterol (Proventil), may be given to reverse histamine-induced bronchospasm.

If cardiac arrest and respiratory arrest are imminent or have occurred, cardiopulmonary resuscitation is performed. Endotracheal intubation or tracheotomy may be necessary to establish an airway. Intravenous lines are inserted to provide access for administering fluids and medications. Anaphylaxis and specific chemical mediators are discussed further in Chapter 53.

Nursing Management

The nurse has an important role in preventing anaphylactic shock: assessing all patients for allergies or previous reactions to antigens (eg, medications, blood products, foods, contrast agents, latex) and communicating the existence of these allergies or reactions to others. Additionally, the nurse assesses the patient's understanding of previous reactions and steps taken by the patient and family to prevent further exposure to antigens. When new allergies are identified, the nurse advises the patient to wear or carry identification that names the specific allergen or antigen.

When administering any new medication, the nurse observes the patient for an allergic reaction. This is especially important with intravenous medications. Allergy to penicillin is one of the most common causes of anaphylactic shock. Patients who have a penicillin allergy may also develop an allergy to similar medications. For example, they may react to cefazolin sodium (Ancef) because it has a similar antimicrobial action of attaching to the penicillin-binding proteins found on the walls of infectious organisms. Previous adverse drug reactions increase the risk that an elderly patient will develop an undesirable reaction to a new medication. If the elderly patient reports an allergy to a medication, the nurse must be aware of the risks involved in the administration of similar medications.

In the hospital and outpatient diagnostic testing sites, the nurse must identify patients at risk for anaphylactic reactions to contrast agents (radiopaque, dye-like substances that may contain iodine) used for diagnostic tests. These include patients with a known allergy to iodine or fish or those who have had previous allergic reactions to contrast agents. This information must be conveyed to the staff at the diagnostic testing site, including x-ray personnel.

The nurse must be knowledgeable about the clinical signs of anaphylaxis, must take immediate action if signs and symptoms occur, and must be prepared to begin cardiopulmonary resuscitation if cardiorespiratory arrest occurs. In addition to monitoring the patient's response to treatment, the nurse assists with intubation if needed, monitors the hemodynamic status, ensures intravenous access for administration of medications, administers prescribed medications and fluids, and documents treatments and their effects.

Community health and home care nurses whose role includes administering medications, including antibiotic agents, in the patient's home or other settings must be prepared to administer epinephrine subcutaneously or intramuscularly in the event of an anaphylactic reaction.

After recovery from anaphylaxis, the patient and family require an explanation of the event. Further, the nurse provides instruction about avoiding future exposure to antigens and administering emergency medications to treat anaphylaxis (see Chap. 53).

Multiple Organ Dysfunction Syndrome

Multiple organ dysfunction syndrome (MODS) is altered organ function in an acutely ill patient that requires medical intervention to support continued organ function. The disorder can be further categorized as primary or secondary MODS.

Pathophysiology

Primary MODS is the result of direct tissue insult, which then leads to impaired perfusion or ischemia. Secondary MODS is most often a complication of septic shock or SIRS. However, MODS may be a complication of any form of shock because of inadequate tissue perfusion. As previously described, in shock all organ systems suffer damage from a lack of adequate perfusion that can result in organ failure. A syndrome of sequential organ failure has been further observed. The exact mechanism that triggers this syndrome is unknown.

Although various causes of MODS have been identified, including dead or injured tissue, infection, and perfusion deficits, it is not yet possible to predict which patients will develop MODS. This is partly because much of the organ damage occurs at the cellular level and therefore cannot be directly observed or measured. The organ failure usually begins in the lungs and is followed by failure of the liver, gastrointestinal system, and kidneys (Balk, 2000b). Advanced age, malnutrition, and coexisting diseases appear to increase the risk of MODS in an acutely ill patient.

Clinical Manifestations

The clinical course of MODS follows one of two patterns. In both patterns, there is an initial event that results in low blood pressure. The cause of the drop in blood pressure is treated, and the patient appears to respond. In the first pattern of MODS (primary MODS), which occurs most often when the initiating event is a pulmonary one such as lung injury, the patient experiences respiratory compromise that necessitates intubation. This usually occurs within 72 hours of the initiating event. Respiratory failure leads rapidly to MODS, resulting in a mortality rate of 30% to 75% (Fein & Calalang-Colucci, 2000).

In secondary MODS, the pattern is more insidious. It occurs most often in the patient with septic shock and progressively unfolds over about 1 month. The patient also experiences respiratory failure and requires intubation. The patient remains hemodynamically stable for about 7 to 14 days. Despite this apparent stability, the patient exhibits a hypermetabolic state characterized by hyperglycemia (elevated blood glucose level), hyperlacticacidemia (excess of lactic acid in the blood), and polyuria (excessive urinary output). The metabolic rate is 1.5 to 2 times basal metabolic rate. Infection is usually present, and skin breakdown begins to occur. During this stage, there is a severe loss of skeletal muscle mass (autocatabolism). If the hypermetabolic phase can be reversed, patients may survive with some damage to affected organ systems (Mizock, 2000). If the hypermetabolic process cannot be halted and cells do not receive adequate oxygen and nutrients, irreversible organ failure and death occur.

If the hypermetabolic phase cannot be reversed, MODS progresses and is characterized by jaundice, hyperbilirubinemia (liver failure), and oliguria progressing to anuria (renal failure), often requiring dialysis. The patient becomes less hemodynamically stable and begins to require vasoactive medications and fluid support. Because of a lack of consistent definitions to describe organ failure, the exact incidence of MODS is hard to define (Balk, 2000b; Vincent & Ferreira, 2000). However, it is reasonable to say that the onset of organ dysfunction is an ominous prognostic sign; the more organs that fail, the worse the outcome.

Medical Management

Prevention remains the top priority in managing MODS. Elderly patients are at increased risk of MODS because of the lack of physiologic reserve associated with aging and the natural degenerative process, especially immune compromise (Balk, 2000b). Early detection and documentation of initial signs of infection are essential in managing elderly patients with MODS. Subtle changes in mentation and a gradual rise in temperature are early warning signs. Other patients at risk of MODS are those with chronic illness, malnutrition, immunosuppression, and surgical or traumatic wounds.

If preventive measures fail, treatment measures to reverse MODS are aimed at (1) controlling the initiating event, (2) promoting adequate organ perfusion, and (3) providing nutritional support.

Nursing Management

The general plan of nursing care for the patient with MODS is the same as that for the patient in septic shock. Primary nursing interventions are aimed at supporting the patient and monitoring organ perfusion until primary organ insults are halted. Providing information and support to family members is a critical role of the nurse in caring for patients with MODS. Addressing end-of-life decisions is an important role of the health care team to ensure that supportive therapies are congruent with the patient's wishes.

 ### Gerontologic Considerations

The population as a whole is aging: the most rapidly growing population group consists of people over 65 years of age. The physiologic changes associated with aging, coupled with pathologic and chronic disease states, place the older individual at increased risk of developing a state of shock and possibly MODS. Medications such as beta-blocking agents (metoprolol [Lopressor]) used to treat hypertension may mask tachycardia, a primary compensatory mechanism to increase cardiac output, during hypovolemic states. The aging immune system may not mount a truly febrile response (temperature more than 40°C), but an increasing trend in body temperature should be addressed. The heart does not function well in hypoxemic states, and the aging heart may respond to decreased myocardial oxygenation with dysrhythmias that may be misinterpreted as a normal part of the aging process. Lastly, changes in mentation may be inappropriately misinterpreted as dementia. The older individual with a sudden change in mentation should be aggressively treated for the presence of infection and organ hypoperfusion. The elderly patient can overcome shock states if signs and symptoms are treated early with aggressive and supportive therapies. Nurses play an essential role in assessing and interpreting subtle changes in the older patient's response to illness.

PROMOTING COMMUNICATION

The nurse encourages frequent and open communication about treatment modalities and options to ensure that the patient's wishes regarding medical management are met. For patients who survive MODS, communicating the goals of rehabilitation and informing the patient of progress toward those goals are essential, as the massive loss of skeletal muscle mass makes rehabilitation a long, slow process. A strong nurse–patient relationship built on effective communication will provide needed encouragement during this phase of recovery.

PROMOTING HOME AND COMMUNITY-BASED CARE

Teaching Patients Self-Care. The patient who experiences and survives shock may have been unable to get out of bed for an extended period of time and is likely to have a slow, prolonged recovery. The patient and family are instructed about strategies to prevent further episodes of shock by identifying the factors implicated in the initial episode. In addition, the patient and family require instruction about assessments needed to identify the complications that may occur after the patient is discharged from the hospital. Depending on the type of shock and its management, the patient or family may require instruction about treatment modalities such as emergency administration of medications, intravenous therapy, parenteral nutrition, skin care, exercise, and ambulation. The patient and family are also instructed about the need for gradual increases in ambulation and

other activity. The need for adequate dietary intake is another crucial aspect of teaching.

Continuing Care in the Home and Community. Because of the physical toll associated with recovery from shock, the patient may be cared for in an extended care facility or rehabilitation setting after hospital discharge. Alternatively, a referral may be made for home care. The home care nurse assesses the patient's physical status and monitors recovery. The nurse also assesses the adequacy of treatments that are continued at home and the ability of the patient and family to cope with these treatments. The patient is likely to require close medical supervision until complete recovery occurs. The home care nurse reinforces the importance of continuing medical care and assists the patient and family to identify and mobilize community resources.

 ## Critical Thinking Exercises

1. A new nurse on your medical unit tells you that she believes a patient with a myocardial infarction is going into shock. She does not know if the patient is experiencing anaphylactic shock related to a medication he received or cardiogenic shock due to his cardiac disorder. How would you differentiate between anaphylactic and cardiogenic shock, and what medical treatments would you anticipate?

2. An elderly man is admitted from a nursing home with a recent onset of confusion and combative behaviour. You know that sudden changes in mental status may be an early sign of sepsis in the elderly. How would you assess this patient for the possibility of septic shock, and how would the management of the elderly patient differ from that of a younger patient?

3. While driving through a rural area, you see a crash and stop to help. Two passengers who have been removed from the cars by passersby are seriously injured. One is bleeding profusely; the other is clutching his abdomen and chest because of severe pain. Describe the type of shock that is most likely in each of these individuals. What actions would you take at the scene to prevent shock or prevent it from progressing?

4. A patient who has used a wheelchair for the last 10 years because of a spinal cord injury was burned when her clothing caught fire as she prepared dinner. Her burns are extensive but limited to her upper body. What types of shock are possible in this patient? What therapy directed at prevention or treatment of shock would you anticipate? Describe the rationale for the therapies that you have identified. How would this patient's disability affect management?

REFERENCES AND SELECTED READINGS

Books

Baldwin, K. M., Davey, S. S., Morris, S. E., & Burger, M. (1998). Shock, multiple organ dysfunction syndrome, and burns in adults. In K. L. McCance & S. E. Huether (Eds.), *Pathophysiology: The biologic basis for disease in adults and children* (3d ed.). St. Louis: Mosby.

Guyton, A. C., & Hall, J. E. (Eds). (2000). *Textbook of medical physiology* (10th ed.). Philadelphia: W. B. Saunders

Harvey, M. A. (1998). Systemic inflammatory response syndrome and multiorgan dysfunction syndrome. In M. R. Kinney, S. B. Dunbar, J. A. Brooks-Brunn, N. Molter, & J. M. Vitello-Cicciu (Eds.), *AACN's clinical reference for critical care nursing* (4th ed.). St. Louis: Mosby.

McKinley, M. G. (2001). Shock. In M. L. Sole, M. L. Lamborn & J. C. Hartshorn (Eds.), *Introduction to critical care nursing* (3d ed.). Philadelphia: W. B. Saunders.

Rauen, C. A., & Munro, N. (1998). Shock. In M. R. Kinney, S. B. Dunbar, J. A. Brooks-Brunn, N. Moleter, & J. M. Vitello-Cicciu (Eds.), *AACN's clinical reference for critical care nursing* (4th ed.). St. Louis: Mosby.

Journals

Abraham, E., Matthay, M. A., Dinarello, C. A., et al. (2000). Consensus conference definitions for sepsis, septic shock, acute lung injury, and acute respiratory distress syndrome: Time for a reevaluation. *Critical Care Medicine, 28* (1), 232–235.

Balk, R. A. (2000a). Severe sepsis and septic shock: Definitions, epidemiology, and clinical manifestations. *Critical Care Clinics, 16*(2), 179–192.

Balk, R. A. (2000b). Pathogenesis and management of multiple organ dysfunction or failure in severe sepsis and septic shock. *Critical Care Clinics, 16*(2), 337–351.

Bernard, G. R., Vincent, J. L., Laterre, R. F., et al. (2001). Efficacy and safety of recombinant human activated protein C for severe sepsis. *New England Journal of Medicine, 344*(10), 699–707.

Bernard, G., Artigas, A., Dellinger, P., et al. (2001). Clinical expert roundtable discussion (session 3) at the Margaux Conference on Critical Illness: The role of activated protein C in severe sepsis. *Critical Care Medicine, 29*(7): Suppl 1:S75–S77.

Bochud, P. Y., Glauser, M. P., & Calandra, T. (2001) International Sepsis Forum. Antibiotics in sepsis. *Intensive Care Medicine, 27,* Suppl 1:S33–48.

Choi, P. T., Yip, G., Quinonez, L. G., & Cook, D. J. (1999). Crystalloids vs colloids in fluid resuscitation: A systematic review. *Critical Care Medicine, 27*(1), 200–209.

Eggimann, P., & Pittet, D. (2001). Catheter-related infections in intensive care units: An overview with special emphasis on prevention. *Advances in Sepsis, 1*(1), 2–13.

Fein, A. M., & Calalang-Colucci, M. G. (2000). Acute lung injury and acute respiratory distress syndrome in sepsis and septic shock. *Critical Care Clinics, 16*(2), 289–313.

International Sepsis Forum. (2001). Guidelines for the management of severe sepsis and septic shock. *Intensive Care Medicine, 27,* Suppl 1:S1–134.

Jindal, N., Hollenberg, S. M., & Dellinger, R. P. (2000). Pharmacologic issues in the management of septic shock. *Critical Care Clinics, 16*(2), 233–248.

Kirschenbaum, L. A., Astiz, M. E., Rackow, E. C., et al. (2000). Microvascular response in patients with cardiogenic shock. *Critical Care Medicine, 28*(5), 1290–1294.

Kumar, A., Haery, C., & Parrillo, J. E. (2000). Myocardial dysfunction in septic shock. *Critical Care Clinics, 16*(2), 251–281.

Manns, B. J., Lee. H., Doig, C. J., et al. (2002). An economic evaluation of activated protein C treatment for severe sepsis. *New England Journal of Medicine, 347*(13), 993–1000.

Matthay, M. A. (2001). Severe sepsis: A new treatment with both anticoagulant and anti-inflammatory properties. *New England Journal of Medicine, 344*(10), 759–762.

Matot, I., & Sprung, C. L. (2001). Definition of sepsis. *Intensive Care Medicine, 27,* Suppl 1:S3–9.

Mikhail, J. (1999). Resuscitation endpoints in trauma. *AACN Clinical Issues, 10*(1), 10–21.

Mizock, B. A. (2000). Metabolic derangements in sepsis and septic shock. *Critical Care Clinics, 16*(2), 319–333.

Price, S., Anning, P. B., Mitchell, J. A., & Evans, T. W. (1999). Myocardial dysfunction in sepsis: Mechanisms and therapeutic implications. *European Heart Journal, 20*(10), 715–724.

Richards, M. J., Edwards, J. R., Culver, D. H., & Gaynes, R. P. (1999). Nosocomial infections in medical intensive care units in the United States. *Critical Care Medicine, 27*(5), 887–892.

Rivers, E., Nguyen, B., Savstad, S., et al. (2001). Early goal-directed therapy in the treatment of severe sepsis and septic shock. *New England Journal of Medicine, 345*(19), 1368–1377.

Simon, D., & Trenholme, G. (2000). Antibiotic selection for patients with septic shock. *Critical Care Clinics, 16*(2), 215–229.

Vincent, J. L., & Ferreira, F. L. (2000). Evaluation of organ failure: We are making progress. *Intensive Care Medicine, 26*(6), 1023–1024.

Vincent, J. L. (2001). International Sepsis Forum. Hemodynamic support in septic shock. *Intensive Care Medicine, 27,* Suppl 1:S80–92.

RESOURCES AND WEBSITES

Health Canada; www.hc-sc.gc.ca/english/index.html.
Health Products and Food Branch; www.hc-sc.gc.ca/hpfb-dgpsa/index_e.html.
Therapeutic Products Directorate; www.hc-sc.gc.ca/hpfb-dgpsa/tpd-dpt/index_e.html.

Oncology: Nursing Management in Cancer Care

Adapted by Kärin Olson and Cynthia Cummings-Winfield

LEARNING OBJECTIVES

On completion of this chapter, the learner will be able to:

1. Compare the structure and function of the normal cell and the cancer cell.
2. Differentiate between benign and malignant tumours.
3. Identify agents and factors that have been found to be carcinogenic.
4. Describe the significance of health education and preventive care in decreasing the incidence of cancer.
5. Differentiate among the purposes of surgical procedures used in cancer treatment, diagnosis, prophylaxis, palliation, and reconstruction.
6. Describe the roles of surgery, radiation therapy, chemotherapy, bone marrow transplantation, and other therapies in treating cancer.
7. Describe the special nursing needs of patients receiving chemotherapy.
8. Describe common nursing diagnoses and collaborative problems of patients with cancer.
9. Use the nursing process as a framework for care of patients with cancer.
10. Describe the concept of hospice in providing care for patients with advanced cancer.
11. Discuss the role of the nurse in assessment and management of common oncologic emergencies.

Cancer nursing practice covers all age groups and nursing specialties and is carried out in a variety of health care settings, including the home, community, acute care institutions, and rehabilitation centres. The scope, responsibilities, and goals of cancer nursing, also called **oncology** nursing, are as diverse and complex as those of any nursing specialty. Because many people associate cancer with pain and death, nurses need to identify their own reactions to cancer and set realistic goals to meet the challenges inherent in caring for patients with cancer.

In addition, the cancer nurse must be prepared to support the patient and family through a wide range of physical, emotional, social, cultural, and spiritual crises. Chart 16-1 identifies major areas of responsibility for nurses caring for patients with cancer.

Epidemiology

Although cancer affects every age group, most cancers occur in people older than 65 years of age. Overall, the incidence of cancer is higher in men than in women and higher in industrialized sectors and nations.

In 2004, 145,500 Canadians were diagnosed with a cancer affecting one of various body sites (Fig. 16-1). Cancer is second only to cardiovascular disease as a leading cause of death in Canada. In 2004, 68,300 Canadians died of a malignant process. In order of frequency, the leading causes of cancer deaths were lung, colorectal, and prostate cancer in men and lung, breast, and colorectal cancer in women (Canadian Cancer Society, 2004).

Pathophysiology of the Malignant Process

Cancer is a disease process that begins when an abnormal cell is transformed by the genetic mutation of the cellular DNA. This abnormal cell forms a clone and begins to proliferate abnormally, ignoring growth-regulating signals in the environment surrounding the cell. The cells acquire invasive characteristics, and changes occur in surrounding tissues. The cells infiltrate these tissues and gain access to lymph and blood vessels, which carry the cells to other areas of the body. This phenomenon is called **metastasis** (cancer spread to other parts of the body).

Cancer is not a single disease with a single cause; rather, it is a group of distinct diseases with different causes, manifestations, treatments, and prognoses.

PROLIFERATIVE PATTERNS

During the life span, various body tissues normally experience periods of rapid or proliferative growth that must be distinguished from malignant growth activity. Several patterns of cell growth exist: **hyperplasia, metaplasia, dysplasia, anaplasia,** and **neoplasia** (see Glossary).

Cancerous cells are described as **malignant** neoplasms. They demonstrate uncontrolled cell growth that follows no physiologic demand. Benign and malignant growths are classified and named by tissue of origin, as described in Table 16-1.

Benign and malignant cells differ in many cellular growth characteristics, including the method and rate of growth, ability to metastasize or spread, general effects, destruction of tissue,

Glossary

alopecia: hair loss

anaplasia: cells that lack normal cellular characteristics and differ in shape and organization with respect to their cells of origin; usually, anaplastic cells are malignant.

biologic response modifier (BRM) therapy: use of agents or treatment methods that can alter the immunologic relationship between the tumor and the host to provide a therapeutic benefit

biopsy: a diagnostic procedure to remove a small sample of tissue to be examined microscopically to detect malignant cells

brachytherapy: delivery of radiation therapy through internal implants

cancer: a disease process whereby cells proliferate abnormally, ignoring growth-regulating signals in the environment surrounding the cells

carcinogenesis: process of transforming normal cells into malignant cells

chemotherapy: use of drugs to kill tumor cells by interfering with cellular functions and reproduction

control: containment of the growth of cancer cells

cure: prolonged survival and disappearance of all evidence of disease so that the patient has the same life expectancy as anyone else in his or her age group

cytokines: substances produced by cells of the immune system to enhance production and functioning of components of the immune system

dysplasia: bizarre cell growth resulting in cells that differ in size, shape, or arrangement from other cells of the same type of tissue

extravasation: leakage of medication from the veins into the subcutaneous tissues

grading: identification of the type of tissue from which the tumor originated and the degree to which the tumor cells retain the functional and structural characteristics of the tissue of origin

hyperplasia: increase in the number of cells of a tissue; most often associated with periods of rapid body growth

malignant: having cells or processes that are characteristic of cancer

metaplasia: conversion of one type of mature cell into another type of cell

metastasis: spread of cancer cells from the primary tumor to distant sites

myelosuppression: suppression of the blood cell–producing function of the bone marrow

nadir: lowest point of white blood cell depression after therapy that has toxic effects on the bone marrow

neoplasia: uncontrolled cell growth that follows no physiologic demand

neutropenia: abnormally low absolute neutrophil count

oncology: field or study of cancer

palliation: relief of symptoms associated with cancer

radiation therapy: use of ionizing radiation to interrupt the growth of malignant cells

stomatitis: inflammation of the oral tissues, often associated with some chemotherapeutic agents

staging: process of determining the size and spread, or metastasis, of a tumor

thrombocytopenia: decrease in the number of circulating platelets; associated with the potential for bleeding

tumor-specific antigen (TSA): protein on the membrane of cancer cells that distinguishes the malignant cell from a benign cell of the same tissue type

vesicant: substance that can cause tissue necrosis and damage, particularly when extravasated

xerostomia: dry oral cavity resulting from decreased function of salivary glands

Chart 16-1   Responsibilities of the Nurse in Cancer Care

- Support the idea that cancer is a chronic illness that has acute exacerbations rather than one that is synonymous with death and suffering.
- Assess own level of knowledge relative to the pathophysiology of the disease process.
- Make use of current research findings and practices in the care of the patient with cancer and his or her family.
- Identify patients at high risk for cancer.
- Participate in primary and secondary prevention efforts.
- Assess the nursing care needs of the patient with cancer.
- Assess the learning needs, desires, and capabilities of the patient with cancer.
- Identify nursing problems of the patient and the family.
- Assess the social support networks available to the patient.
- Plan appropriate interventions with the patient and the family.
- Assist the patient to identify strengths and limitations.
- Assist the patient to design short-term and long-term goals for care.
- Implement a nursing care plan that interfaces with the medical care regimen and that is consistent with the established goals.
- Collaborate with members of a multidisciplinary team to foster continuity of care.
- Evaluate the goals and resultant outcomes of care with the patient, the family, and members of the multidisciplinary team.
- Reassess and redesign the direction of the care as determined by the evaluation.

and ability to cause death. These differences are summarized in Table 16-2. The degree of anaplasia (lack of differentiation of cells) ultimately determines the malignant potential.

CHARACTERISTICS OF MALIGNANT CELLS

Despite their individual differences, all cancer cells share some common cellular characteristics in relation to the cell membrane, special proteins, the nuclei, chromosomal abnormalities, and the rate of mitosis and growth. The cell membranes are altered in cancer cells, which affects fluid movement in and out of the cell. The cell membrane of malignant cells also contains proteins called **tumour-specific antigens** (for example, carcinoembryonic antigen and prostate-specific antigen), which develop as they become less differentiated (mature) over time. These proteins distinguish the malignant cell from a benign cell of the same tissue type. They may be useful in measuring the extent of disease in a person and in tracking the course of illness during treatment or relapse. Malignant cellular membranes also contain less fibronectin, a cellular cement. They are therefore less cohesive and do not adhere to adjacent cells readily.

Typically, nuclei of cancer cells are large and irregularly shaped (pleomorphism). Nucleoli, structures within the nucleus that house ribonucleic acid (RNA), are larger and more numerous in malignant cells, perhaps because of increased RNA synthesis. Chromosomal abnormalities (translocations, deletions, additions)

Leading Sites of New Cancer Cases and Deaths—2004 Estimates*

Cancer Cases by Site and Sex

Male

Prostate
20,100 (27%)

Lung & bronchus
11,900 (16%)

Colon & rectum
10,400 (14%)

Urinary bladder
3,700 (5%)

Non-Hodgkin's lymphoma
3,300 (4%)

Melanoma
2,300 (3%)

Kidney
2,600 (3%)

Oral cavity
2,100 (3%)

Leukemia
2,300 (3%)

Pancreas
1,600 (2%)

Female

Breast
21,200 (30%)

Lung & bronchus
9,800 (14%)

Colon & rectum
8,800 (12%)

Body of the uterus
3,800 (5%)

Non-Hodgkin's lymphoma
2,900 (4%)

Melanoma
1,950 (3%)

Ovary
2,300 (3%)

Thyroid
2,100 (3%)

Pancreas
1,700 (2%)

Urinary bladder
1,250 (2%)

Cancer Deaths by Site and Sex

Male

Lung
10,700 (30%)

Prostate
4,200 (12%)

Colon & rectum
4,500 (12%)

Pancreas
1,600 (4%)

Non-Hodgkin's lymphoma
1,550 (4%)

Leukemia
1,300 (4%)

Esophagus
1,200 (3%)

Urinary bladder
1,150 (3%)

Kidney
950 (3%)

Female

Lung
8,200 (26%)

Breast
5,200 (16%)

Colon & rectum
3,900 (12%)

Pancreas
1,700 (5%)

Ovary
1,550 (5%)

Non-Hodgkin's lymphoma
1,350 (4%)

Leukemia
930 (3%)

Body of the uterus
700 (2%)

Brain
690 (2%)

Multiple myeloma
580 (2%)

*Excludes basal and squamous cell skin cancers.

Percentages may not total 100% due to rounding.

FIGURE 16-1   Estimated leading sites of cancer incidences and deaths, Canadian Cancer Society. (2004).

GENETICS IN NURSING PRACTICE—Concepts and Challenges in Patient Management

Cancer is a genetic disease. Every phase of carcinogenesis is affected by multiple genetic mutations. Some of these mutations are inherited (present in germ-line cells), but most (90%) are somatic mutations that are acquired mutations in specific cells.

EXAMPLES OF CANCERS INFLUENCED BY GENETIC FACTORS
- Cowden syndrome
- Familial adenomatous polyposis
- Familial melanoma syndrome
- Hereditary breast and ovarian cancer
- Hereditary non-polyposis colon cancer
- Neurofibromatosis type 1
- Retinoblastoma

NURSING ASSESSMENTS
FAMILY HISTORY
- Obtain information about both maternal and paternal sides of family.
- Obtain cancer history of at least three generations.
- Look for clustering of cancers that occur at earlier ages, multiple primary cancers in one individual, cancer in paired organs, and two or more close relatives with the same type of cancer suggestive of hereditary cancer syndromes.

PHYSICAL ASSESSMENT
- Physical findings that may predispose the patient to cancer, such as multiple colonic polyps, suggestive of a polyposis syndrome
- Skin findings, such as atypical moles, that may be related to familial melanoma syndrome

- Multiple café au lait spots, axillary freckling, and two or more neurofibromas associated with neurofibromatosis type I
- Facial trichilemmomas, mucosal papillomatosis, multi-nodular thyroid goitre or thyroid adenomas, macrocephaly, fibrocystic breasts and other fibromas or lipomas related to Cowden syndrome

MANAGEMENT ISSUES SPECIFIC TO GENETICS
- Assess patient's understanding of genetic factors related to his or her cancer.
- Refer for cancer risk assessment when a hereditary cancer syndrome is suspected so that patient and family can discuss inheritance, risk with other family members and availability of genetic testing.
- Offer appropriate genetics information and resources.
- Assess patient's understanding of genetics information.
- Provide support to patient and families with known genetic test results for hereditary cancer syndromes.
- Participate in the management and coordination of risk-reduction measures for those with known genetic mutations.

RESOURCES AND WEBSITES
Canadian Association of Provincial Cancer Agencies www. capca.ca— listing and links to provincial agencies.

Canadian Cancer Society www.cancer.ca—provincial divisions accessible on main page of Canada-wide site.

Canadian Lung Association www.lung.ca/diseases/cancer lungs.html—Lung Association has a section on cancer.

---

and fragility of chromosomes are commonly found when cancer cells are analyzed.

Mitosis (cell division) occurs more frequently in malignant cells than in normal cells. As the cells grow and divide, more glucose and oxygen are needed. If glucose and oxygen are unavailable, malignant cells use anaerobic metabolic channels to produce energy, which makes the cells less dependent on the availability of a constant oxygen supply.

INVASION AND METASTASIS

Malignant disease processes have the ability to allow the spread or transfer of cancerous cells from one organ or body part to another by invasion and metastasis. Patterns of metastasis can be partially explained by circulatory patterns and by specific affinity for certain malignant cells to bind to molecules in specific body tissue.

Invasion, which refers to the growth of the primary tumour into the surrounding host tissues, occurs in several ways. Mechanical pressure exerted by rapidly proliferating neoplasms may force fingerlike projections of tumour cells into surrounding tissue and interstitial spaces. Malignant cells are less adherent and may break off from the primary tumour and invade adjacent structures. Malignant cells are thought to possess or produce specific destructive enzymes (proteinases), such as collagenases (specific to collagen), plasminogen activators (specific to plasma), and lysosomal hydro-

lyses. These enzymes are thought to destroy surrounding tissue, including the structural tissues of the vascular basement membrane, facilitating invasion of malignant cells. The mechanical pressure of a rapidly growing tumour may enhance this process.

Metastasis is the dissemination or spread of malignant cells from the primary tumour to distant sites by direct spread of tumour cells to body cavities or through lymphatic and blood circulation. Tumours growing in or penetrating body cavities may shed cells or emboli that travel within the body cavity and seed the surfaces of other organs. This can occur in ovarian cancer when malignant cells enter the peritoneal cavity and seed the peritoneal surfaces of such abdominal organs as the liver or pancreas.

Metastatic Mechanisms

Lymph and blood are key mechanisms by which cancer cells spread. Angiogenesis, a mechanism by which the tumour cells are ensured a blood supply, is another important process.

LYMPHATIC SPREAD
The most common mechanism of metastasis is lymphatic spread, which is transport of tumour cells through the lymphatic circulation. Tumour emboli enter the lymph channels by way of the interstitial fluid that communicates with lymphatic fluid. Malignant cells also may penetrate lymphatic vessels by invasion. After

Table 16-1 • Tumours and Tissue Types

TISSUE TYPE	BENIGN TUMOURS	MALIGNANT TUMOURS
Epithelial		
Surface	Papilloma	Squamous cell carcinoma
Glandular	Adenoma	Adenocarcinoma
Connective		
Fibrous	Fibroma	Fibrosarcoma
Adipose	Lipoma	Liposarcoma
Cartilage	Chondroma	Chondrosarcoma
Bone	Osteoma	Osteosarcoma
Blood vessels	Hemangioma	Hemangiosarcoma
Lymph vessels	Lymphangioma	Lymphangiosarcoma
Lymph tissue		Lymphosarcoma
Muscle		
Smooth	Leiomyoma	Leiomyosarcoma
Striated	Rhabdomyoma	Rhabdomyosarcoma
Neural Tissue		
Nerve cell	Neuroma	Neuroblastoma
Glial tissue	Glioma (benign)	Glioblastoma, astrocytoma, medulloblastoma, oligodendroglioma
Nerve sheaths	Neurilemmoma	Neurilemmal sarcoma
Meninges	Meningioma	Meningeal sarcoma
Hematologic		
Granulocytic		Myelocytic leukemia
Erythrocytic		Erythrocytic leukemia
Plasma cells		Multiple myeloma
Lymphocytic		Lymphocytic leukemia or lymphoma
Monocytic		Monocytic leukemia
Endothelial Tissue		
Blood vessels	Hemangioma	Hemangiosarcoma
Lymph vessels	Lymphangioma	Lymphangiosarcoma
Endothelial lining		Ewing's sarcoma

Reproduced with permission from Porth, C. M. (2002). *Pathophysiology: Concepts of altered health states* (6th ed.). Philadelphia: Lippincott Williams & Wilkins.

Table 16-2 • Characteristics of Benign and Malignant Neoplasms

CHARACTERISTICS	BENIGN	MALIGNANT
Cell characteristics	Well-differentiated cells that resemble normal cells of the tissue from which the tumor originated	Cells are undifferentiated and often bear little resemblance to the normal cells of the tissue from which they arose
Mode of growth	Tumour grows by expansion and does not infiltrate the surrounding tissues; usually encapsulated	Grows at the periphery and sends out processes that infiltrate and destroy the surrounding tissues
Rate of growth	Rate of growth is usually slow	Rate of growth is variable and depends on level of differentiation; the more anaplastic the tumour, the faster its growth
Metastasis	Does not spread by metastasis	Gains access to the blood and lymphatic channels and metastasizes to other areas of the body
General effects	Is usually a localized phenomenon that does not cause generalized effects unless its location interferes with vital functions	Often causes generalized effects, such as anemia, weakness, and weight loss
Tissue destruction	Does not usually cause tissue damage unless its location interferes with blood flow	Often causes extensive tissue damage as the tumour outgrows its blood supply or encroaches on blood flow to the area; may also produce substances that cause cell damage
Ability to cause death	Does not usually cause death unless its location interferes with vital functions	Usually causes death unless growth can be controlled

Reproduced with permission from Porth, C. M. (2002). *Pathophysiology: Concepts of altered health states* (6th ed.). Philadelphia: Lippincott Williams & Wilkins.

entering the lymphatic circulation, malignant cells either lodge in the lymph nodes or pass between lymphatic and venous circulation. Tumours arising in areas of the body with rapid and extensive lymphatic circulation are at high risk for metastasis through lymphatic channels. Breast tumours frequently metastasize in this manner through axillary, clavicular, and thoracic lymph channels.

HEMATOGENOUS SPREAD

Another metastatic mechanism is hematogenous spread, by which malignant cells are disseminated through the bloodstream. Hematogenous spread is directly related to the vascularity of the tumour. Few malignant cells can survive the turbulence of arterial circulation, insufficient oxygenation, or destruction by the body's immune system. In addition, the structure of most arteries and arterioles is far too secure to permit malignant invasion. Those malignant cells that do survive this hostile environment are able to attach to endothelium and attract fibrin, platelets, and clotting factors to seal themselves from immune system surveillance. The endothelium retracts, allowing the malignant cells to enter the basement membrane and secrete lysosomal enzymes. These enzymes then destroy surrounding body tissues and thereby allow implantation.

ANGIOGENESIS

Malignant cells also have the ability to induce the growth of new capillaries from the host tissue to meet their needs for nutrients and oxygen. This process is referred to as angiogenesis. It is through this vascular network that tumour emboli can enter the systemic circulation and travel to distant sites. Large tumour emboli that become trapped in the microcirculation of distant sites may further metastasize to other sites. Research into ways to prevent angiogenesis is ongoing.

Carcinogenesis

Malignant transformation, or **carcinogenesis**, is thought to be at least a three-step cellular process: initiation, promotion, and progression.

In *initiation,* the first step, initiators (carcinogens), such as chemicals, physical factors, and biologic agents, escape normal enzymatic mechanisms and alter the genetic structure of the cellular DNA. Normally, these alterations are reversed by DNA repair mechanisms, or the changes initiate programmed cellular suicide (apoptosis). Occasionally, cells escape these protective mechanisms, and permanent cellular mutations occur. These mutations usually are not significant to cells until the second step of carcinogenesis.

During *promotion,* repeated exposure to promoting agents (co-carcinogens) causes the expression of abnormal or mutant genetic information even after long latency periods. Latency periods for the promotion of cellular mutations vary with the type of agent and the dosage of the promoter as well as the innate characteristics of the target cell.

Cellular oncogenes, present in all mammalian systems, are responsible for the vital cellular functions of growth and differentiation. Cellular proto-oncogenes are present in cells and act as an "on switch" for cellular growth. Similarly, cancer suppressor genes "turn off" or regulate unneeded cellular proliferation. When the suppressor genes become mutated, rearranged, or amplified or lose their regulatory capabilities, malignant cells are allowed to reproduce. The p53 gene is a tumour suppressor gene that is frequently mutated in many human cancers. This gene regulates whether cells will repair or die after DNA damage. Mutant p53 gene is associated with a poor prognosis and may be associated with determining response to treatment. Once this genetic expression occurs in cells, the cells begin to produce mutant cell populations that are different from their original cellular ancestors.

Progression is the third step of cellular carcinogenesis. The cellular changes formed during initiation and promotion now exhibit increased malignant behaviour. These cells now show a propensity to invade adjacent tissues and to metastasize. Agents that initiate or promote cellular transformation are referred to as carcinogens.

ETIOLOGY

Certain categories of agents or factors implicated in carcinogenesis include viruses and bacteria, physical agents, chemical agents, genetic or familial factors, dietary factors, and hormonal agents.

Viruses and Bacteria

Viruses as a cause of human cancers are hard to determine because viruses are difficult to isolate. Infectious causes are considered or suspected, however, when specific cancers appear in clusters. Viruses are thought to incorporate themselves in the genetic structure of cells, thus altering future generations of that cell population—perhaps leading to a cancer. For example, the Epstein-Barr virus is highly suspect as a cause in Burkitt's lymphoma, nasopharyngeal cancers, and some types of non-Hodgkin's lymphoma and Hodgkin's disease.

Herpes simplex virus type II, cytomegalovirus, and human papillomavirus types 16, 18, 31, and 33 are associated with dysplasia and cancer of the cervix. The hepatitis B virus is implicated in cancer of the liver; the human T-cell lymphotropic virus may be a cause of some lymphocytic leukemias and lymphomas; and the human immunodeficiency virus (HIV) is associated with Kaposi's sarcoma. The bacterium *Helicobacter pylori* has been associated with an increased incidence of gastric malignancy, perhaps secondary to inflammation and injury of gastric cells.

Physical Agents

Physical factors associated with carcinogenesis include exposure to sunlight or radiation, chronic irritation or inflammation, and tobacco use.

Excessive exposure to the ultraviolet rays of the sun, especially in fair-skinned, blue- or green-eyed people, increases the risk for skin cancers. Factors such as clothing styles (sleeveless shirts or shorts), use of sunscreens, occupation, recreational habits, and environmental variables, including humidity, altitude, and latitude, all play a role in the amount of exposure to ultraviolet light.

Exposure to ionizing radiation can occur with repeated diagnostic x-ray procedures or with radiation therapy used to treat disease. Fortunately, improved x-ray equipment appropriately minimizes the risk for extensive radiation exposure. Radiation therapy used in disease treatment or exposure to radioactive materials at nuclear weapon manufacturing sites or nuclear power plants is associated with a higher incidence of leukemias, multiple myeloma, and cancers of the lung, bone, breast, thyroid, and other tissues. Background radiation from the natural decay processes that produce radon has also been associated with lung cancer. Homes with high levels of trapped radon should be ventilated to allow the gas to disperse into the atmosphere.

Chemical Agents

About 75% of all cancers are thought to be related to the environment. Tobacco smoke, thought to be the single most lethal chemical carcinogen, accounts for at least 30% of cancer deaths (Heath & Fontham, 2001). Smoking is strongly associated with cancers of the lung, head and neck, esophagus, pancreas, cervix, and bladder. Tobacco may also act synergistically with other substances, such as alcohol, asbestos, uranium, and viruses, to promote cancer development.

Chewing tobacco is associated with cancers of the oral cavity and primarily occurs in men younger than 40 years of age. Many chemical substances found in the workplace have proved to be carcinogens or co-carcinogens. The extensive list of suspected chemical substances continues to grow and includes aromatic amines and aniline dyes; pesticides and formaldehydes; arsenic, soot, and tars; asbestos; benzene; betel nut and lime; cadmium; chromium compounds; nickel and zinc ores; wood dust; beryllium compounds; and polyvinyl chloride.

Most hazardous chemicals produce their toxic effects by altering DNA structure in body sites distant from chemical exposure. The liver, lungs, and kidneys are the organ systems most often affected, presumably because of their roles in detoxifying chemicals.

Genetic and Familial Factors

Almost every cancer type has been shown to run in families. This may be due to genetics, shared environments, cultural or lifestyle factors, or chance alone. Genetic factors play a role in cancer cell development. Abnormal chromosomal patterns and cancer have been associated with extra chromosomes, too few chromosomes, or translocated chromosomes. Specific cancers with underlying genetic abnormalities include Burkitt's lymphoma, chronic myelogenous leukemia, meningiomas, acute leukemias, retinoblastomas, Wilms' tumour, and skin cancers, including malignant melanoma.

Approximately 5% to 10% of cancers of adulthood and childhood display a familial predisposition. Inherited cancer syndromes, such as premenopausal breast cancer, tend to occur at an early age and at multiple sites in one organ or pair of organs. In cancers with a familial predisposition, individuals may develop multiple cancers; commonly, two or more first-degree relatives share the same cancer type. Cancers associated with familial inheritance include retinoblastomas, nephroblastomas, pheochromocytomas, malignant neurofibromatosis, and breast, ovarian,

endometrial, colorectal, stomach, prostate, and lung cancers. In 1994, the BRCA-1 gene was identified; it is linked to breast and ovarian cancer syndrome. The BRCA-2 gene, which has also been identified, is associated with early-onset breast cancer (Nogueira & Appling, 2000). Work continues to identify other specific genes related to cancer incidence (Greco, 2000).

Dietary Factors

Dietary factors are thought to be related to 35% of all environmental cancers (Heath & Fontham, 2001). Dietary substances can be proactive (protective), carcinogenic, or co-carcinogenic. The risk for cancer increases with long-term ingestion of carcinogens or co-carcinogens or chronic absence of proactive substances in the diet.

Dietary substances associated with an increased cancer risk include fats, alcohol, salt-cured or smoked meats, foods containing nitrates and nitrites, and a high caloric dietary intake. Food substances that appear to reduce cancer risk include high-fibre foods, cruciferous vegetables (cabbage, broccoli, cauliflower, Brussels sprouts, kohlrabi), carotenoids (carrots, tomatoes, spinach, apricots, peaches, dark-green and deep-yellow vegetables), and possibly vitamins E and C, zinc, and selenium.

Obesity is associated with endometrial cancer and possibly postmenopausal breast cancers. Obesity may also increase the risk for cancers of the colon, kidney, and gallbladder.

Hormonal Agents

Tumour growth may be promoted by disturbances in hormonal balance either by the body's own (endogenous) hormone production or by administration of exogenous hormones. Cancers of the breast, prostate, and uterus are thought to depend on endogenous hormonal levels for growth. Diethylstilbestrol (DES) has long been recognized as a cause of vaginal carcinomas. Oral contraceptives and prolonged estrogen replacement therapy are associated with increased incidence of hepatocellular, endometrial, and breast cancers, whereas they appear to decrease the risk for ovarian and endometrial cancers. The combination of estrogen and progesterone appears safest in decreasing the risk for endometrial cancers. Hormonal changes with reproduction are also associated with cancer incidence. Increased numbers of pregnancies are associated with a decreased incidence of breast, endometrial, and ovarian cancers.

ROLE OF THE IMMUNE SYSTEM

In humans, malignant cells are capable of developing on a regular basis. Some evidence indicates, however, that the immune system can detect the development of malignant cells and destroy them before cell growth becomes uncontrolled. When the immune system fails to identify and stop the growth of malignant cells, clinical cancer develops.

Patients who for various reasons are immunoincompetent have been shown to have an increased incidence of cancer. Organ transplant recipients who receive immunosuppressive therapy to prevent rejection of the transplanted organ have an increased incidence of lymphoma, Kaposi's sarcoma, squamous cell cancer of the skin, and cervical and anogenital cancers. Patients with immunodeficiency diseases, such as AIDS, have an increased incidence of Kaposi's sarcoma, lymphoma, and rectal and head and neck cancers. Some patients who have received alkylating chemotherapeutic agents to treat Hodgkin's disease have an increased incidence of secondary malignancies. Autoimmune diseases, such as rheumatoid arthritis and Sjögren's syndrome, are associated with increased cancer development. Finally, age-related changes, such as declining organ function, increased incidence of chronic diseases, and diminished immunocompetence, may contribute to an increased incidence of cancer in older people.

Normal Immune Responses

Normally, an intact immune system has the ability to combat cancer cells in several ways. Usually, the immune system recognizes as foreign certain antigens on the cell membranes of many cancer cells. These antigens are known as tumour-associated antigens (also called tumour cell antigens) and are capable of stimulating both cellular and humoural immune responses.

Along with the macrophages, T lymphocytes, the soldiers of the cellular immune response, are responsible for recognizing tumour-associated antigens. When T lymphocytes recognize tumour antigens, other T lymphocytes that are toxic to the tumour cells are stimulated. These lymphocytes proliferate and are released into the circulation. In addition to possessing cytotoxic (cell-killing) properties, T lymphocytes can stimulate other components of the immune system to rid the body of malignant cells.

Certain lymphokines, which are substances produced by lymphocytes, are capable of killing or damaging various types of malignant cells. Other lymphokines can mobilize other cells, such as macrophages, that disrupt cancer cells. Interferon (IFN), a substance produced by the body in response to viral infection, also possesses some antitumour properties. Antibodies produced by B lymphocytes, associated with the humoural immune response, also defend the body against malignant cells. These antibodies act either alone or in combination with the complement system or the cellular immune system.

Natural killer (NK) cells are a major component of the body's defense against cancer. NK cells are a subpopulation of lymphocytes that act by directly destroying cancer cells or by producing lymphokines and enzymes that assist in cell destruction.

Immune System Failure

How is it, then, that malignant cells can survive and proliferate despite the elaborate immune system defense mechanisms? Several theories suggest how tumour cells can evade an apparently intact immune system. If the body fails to recognize the malignant cell as different from "self" (non-self or foreign), the immune response may not be stimulated. When tumours do not possess tumour-associated antigens that label them as foreign, the immune response is not alerted. The failure of the immune system to respond promptly to the malignant cells allows the tumour to grow too large to be managed by normal immune mechanisms.

Tumour antigens may combine with the antibodies produced by the immune system and hide or disguise themselves from normal immune defense mechanisms. These tumour antigen–antibody complexes can suppress further production of antibodies. Tumours are also capable of changing their appearance or producing substances that impair usual immune responses. These substances not only promote tumour growth but also increase the patient's susceptibility to infection by various pathogenic organisms. As a result of prolonged contact with a tumour antigen, the patient's body may be depleted of the specific lymphocytes and no longer able to mount an appropriate immune response.

Abnormal concentrations of host suppressor T lymphocytes may play a role in developing cancers. Suppressor T lymphocytes normally assist in regulating antibody production and diminishing immune responses when they are no longer required. Low levels of serum antibodies and high levels of suppressor cells have been found in patients with multiple myeloma, a cancer associated with hypogammaglobulinemia (low amounts of serum antibodies). Carcinogens, such as viruses and certain chemicals, including chemotherapeutic agents, may weaken the immune system and ultimately enhance tumour growth.

Detection and Prevention of Cancer

Nurses and physicians have traditionally been involved with tertiary prevention, the care and rehabilitation of the patient after cancer diagnosis and treatment. In recent years, however, cancer organizations, clinicians, and researchers have placed greater emphasis on primary prevention and screening for cancer. Primary prevention is concerned with reducing the risks of cancer in healthy people. Screening involves early detection of cancer and therefore earlier intervention, with improved health outcomes.

PRIMARY PREVENTION

By acquiring the knowledge and skills necessary to educate the community about cancer risk, nurses in all settings play a key role in cancer prevention. Assisting patients to avoid known carcinogens is one way to reduce the risk for cancer. Another way involves adopting dietary and various lifestyle changes that epidemiologic and laboratory studies show influence the risk for cancer. Several clinical trials have been undertaken to identify medications that may help to reduce the incidence of certain types of cancer. Recently, a breast cancer prevention study supported by the National Cancer Institute was conducted at multiple medical centres throughout the United States. The results of this study indicated that the medication tamoxifen can reduce the incidence of breast cancer by 49% in postmenopausal women identified as at high risk for breast cancer (Fisher et al., 1998). Nurses can use their teaching and counselling skills to encourage patients to participate in cancer prevention programs and to promote healthful lifestyles.

SCREENING

The evolving understanding of the role of genetics in cancer cell development has contributed to prevention and screening efforts. Individuals who have inherited specific genetic mutations have an increased susceptibility to cancer. For example, individuals who have familial adenomatosis polyposis have an increased risk for colon cancer. Women in whom the BRCA-1 and BRCA-2 genes have been identified have an increased risk for breast and ovarian cancer. To provide individualized education and recommendations for continued surveillance and care in high-risk populations, nurses need to be familiar with ongoing developments in the field of genetics and cancer (Greco, 2000). Many centres across the country are offering innovative cancer risk evaluation programs that provide in-depth screening and follow-up for individuals who are found to be at high risk for cancer.

Numerous factors, such as race, cultural influences, access to care, physician–patient relationship, level of education, income, and age, influence the knowledge, attitudes, and beliefs people have about cancer. These factors also influence the type of health-promoting behaviours they practice.

Public awareness about health-promoting behaviours can be increased in a variety of ways. Health education and health maintenance programs are sponsored by community organizations such as churches, senior citizen groups, and parent–teacher associations. Although primary prevention programs may focus on the hazards of tobacco use or the importance of nutrition, secondary prevention programs may promote breast and testicular self-examination and Papanicolaou (Pap) tests. Many organizations conduct cancer screening events that focus on cancers with the highest incidence rates or those that have improved survival rates if diagnosed early, such as breast or prostate cancers. These events offer education and examinations such as mammograms, digital rectal examinations, and prostate-specific antigen blood tests for minimal or no cost. Programs of this nature are often targeted to individuals who lack access to health care or cannot afford to participate on their own.

Similarly, nurses in all settings can develop programs that identify risks for patients and families and that incorporate teaching and counselling into all educational efforts, particularly for patients and families with a high incidence of cancer. The Canadian Cancer Society has developed a public education program, "Seven Steps to Health," that integrates diet, exercise, and general health habit tips that people can follow to reduce their risk for cancer (Chart 16-2). Nurses and physicians can encourage individuals to comply with detection efforts as suggested by the Canadian Cancer Society (Table 16-3).

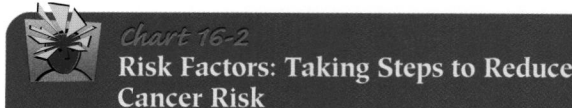

Chart 16-2

Risk Factors: Taking Steps to Reduce Cancer Risk

The following are the "Seven Steps to Health":
1. Be a nonsmoker and avoid secondhand smoke.
2. Eat 5–10 servings of vegetables and fruit a day. Choose high-fibre, lower-fat foods. If you drink alcohol, limit your intake to 1–2 drinks a day.
3. Be physically active on a regular basis; this will also help you maintain a healthy body weight.
4. Protect yourself and your family from the sun.
5. Follow cancer screening guidelines.
6. Visit your doctor or dentist if you notice any change in your normal state of health.
7. Follow health and safety instructions at home and at work when using, storing, and disposing of hazardous materials.

Adapted from the Canadian Cancer Society. (2004). *Seven steps to health.* Available at: http://www.cancer.ca/ccs/internet/standardpf/0,3182,3172_12959_langId-en,00.html.

Diagnosis of Cancer and Related Nursing Considerations

A cancer diagnosis is based on assessment for physiologic and functional changes and results of the diagnostic evaluation. Patients with suspected cancer undergo extensive testing to (1) determine

Table 16-3 • **Canadian Cancer Society Recommendations for Early Detection of Cancer in Asymptomatic, Average-Risk People***

SITE	GENDER	AGE	EVALUATION	FREQUENCY
Colon/rectum	M/F	50 and older	Fecal occult blood test	Every 2 years
Prostate	M	50 and older	Discuss potential benefits of prostate-specific antigen (PSA) testing and digital rectal examination (DRE) with physician	
Skin	M/F	All ages	Watch skin for changes in birthmarks or moles, any new skin growths, sores that don't heal, or patches of skin that bleed, ooze, swell, itch, or become red and bumpy	
Testicles	M	15 and older	Testicular self-examination (TSE)	Regularly
Breast	F	40-49	Clinical breast examination (CBE)	Every 2 years
			Breast self-examination (BSE)	Regularly
			Discuss risks and benefits of mammography with physician	
		50–69	CBE	Every 2 years
			BSE	Regularly
			Mammography	Every 2 years
		70 and older	CBE	Every 2 years
			BSE	Regularly
			Discuss risks and benefits of mammography with physician	
Cervix	F	Women who are sexually active Women who are no longer sexually active should continue to have this test	Pap test	1–3 years, depending on provincial guidelines

*See the Canadian Cancer Society's website (http://www.cancer.ca) for more detailed recommendations for each cancer type.

the presence of tumour and its extent, (2) identify possible spread (metastasis) of disease or invasion of other body tissues, (3) evaluate the function of involved and uninvolved body systems and organs, and (4) obtain tissue and cells for analysis, including evaluation of tumour stage and grade. The diagnostic evaluation is guided by information obtained through a complete history and physical examination. Knowledge of suspicious symptoms and of the behaviour of particular types of cancer assists in determining which diagnostic tests are most appropriate (Table 16-4).

A patient undergoing extensive testing is usually fearful of the procedures and anxious about the possible test results. The nurse can help relieve fear and anxiety by explaining the tests to be performed, the sensations likely to be experienced, and the patient's role in the test procedures. The nurse encourages the patient and family to voice their fears about the test results, supports the patient and family throughout the test period, and reinforces and clarifies information conveyed by the physician. The nurse also encourages the patient and family members to communicate and share their concerns and to discuss their questions and concerns with each other.

TUMOUR STAGING AND GRADING

A complete diagnostic evaluation includes identifying the stage and grade of the tumour. This is accomplished before treatment begins to provide baseline data for evaluating outcomes of therapy and to maintain a systematic and consistent approach to ongoing diagnosis and treatment. Treatment options and prognosis are determined on the basis of staging and grading.

Staging determines the size of the tumour and the existence of metastasis. Several systems exist for classifying the anatomic extent of disease. The TNM system is frequently used. In this system, T refers to the extent of the primary tumour, N refers to lymph node involvement, and M refers to the extent of metastasis (Chart 16-3). A variety of other staging systems are used to describe the extent of cancers, such as central nervous system cancers, hematologic cancers, and malignant melanoma, that the TNM system does not describe appropriately. Staging systems also provide a convenient shorthand notation that condenses lengthy descriptions into manageable terms for comparisons of treatments and prognoses.

Grading refers to the classification of the tumour cells. Grading systems seek to define the type of tissue from which the tumour originated and the degree to which the tumour cells retain the functional and histologic characteristics of the tissue of origin. Samples of cells to be used to establish the grade of a tumour may be obtained through cytology (examination of cells from tissue scrapings, body fluids, secretions, or washings), biopsy, or surgical excision.

This information assists the health care team to predict the behaviour and prognosis of various tumours. The tumour is assigned

---

Table 16-4 • **Imaging Tests Used to Detect Cancer**

TEST	DESCRIPTION	DIAGNOSTIC USES
Tumor marker identification	Analysis of substances found in blood or other body fluids that are made by the tumor or by the body in response to the tumor	Breast, colon, lung, ovarian, testicular, prostate cancers
Magnetic resonance imaging (MRI)	Use of magnetic fields and radiofrequency signals to create sectioned images of various body structures	Neurologic, pelvic, abdominal, thoracic cancers
Computed tomography (CT scan)	Use of narrow beam x-ray to scan successive layers of tissue for a cross-sectional view	Neurologic, pelvic, skeletal, abdominal, thoracic cancers
Fluoroscopy	Use of x-rays that identify contrasts in body tissue densities; may involve the use of contrast agents	Skeletal, lung, gastrointestinal cancers
Ultrasonography (ultrasound)	High-frequency sound waves echoing off body tissues are converted electronically into images; used to assess tissues deep within the body	Abdominal and pelvic cancers
Endoscopy	Direct visualization of a body cavity or passageway by insertion of an endoscope into a body cavity or opening; allows tissue biopsy, fluid aspiration and excision of small tumors; both diagnostic and therapeutic	Bronchial, gastrointestinal cancers
Nuclear medicine imaging	Uses intravenous injection or ingestion of radioisotope substances followed by imaging of tissues that have concentrated the radioisotopes	Bone, liver, kidney, spleen, brain, thyroid cancers
Positron emission tomography (PET scan)	Computed cross-sectional images of increased concentration of radioisotopes in malignant cells provide information about biologic activity of malignant cells; help distinguish between benign and malignant processes and responses to treatment	Lung, colon, liver, pancreatic, breast, esophagus cancers; Hodgkin's and non-Hodgkin's lymphoma and melanoma
Radioimmunoconjugates	Monoclonal antibodies are labelled with a radioisotope and injected intravenously into the patient; the antibodies that aggregate at the tumor site are visualized with scanners	Colorectal, breast, ovarian, head and neck cancers; lymphoma and melanoma

Chart 16-3

TNM Classification System

T The extent of the primary tumour
N The absence or presence and extent of regional lymph node metastasis
M The absence or presence of distant metastasis

The use of numerical subsets of the TNM components indicates the progressive extent of the malignant disease.

Primary Tumour (T)
TX Primary tumour cannot be assessed
T0 No evidence of primary tumour
Tis Carcinoma in situ
T1, T2, T3, T4 Increasing size and/or local extent of the primary tumour

Regional Lymph Nodes (N)
NX Regional lymph nodes cannot be assessed
N0 No regional lymph node metastasis
N1, N2, N3 Increasing involvement of regional lymph nodes

Distant Metastasis (M)
MX Distant metastasis cannot be assessed
M0 No distant metastasis
M1 Distant metastasis

Green, F., et al. (Eds) (2002). *AJCC cancer staging manual* (6th ed.). New York: Springer-Verlag.

a numeric value ranging from I to IV. Grade I tumours, also known as well-differentiated tumours, closely resemble the tissue of origin in structure and function. Tumours that do not clearly resemble the tissue of origin in structure or function are described as poorly differentiated or undifferentiated and are assigned grade IV. These tumours tend to be more aggressive and less responsive to treatment than well-differentiated tumours.

Management of Cancer

Treatment options offered to cancer patients should be based on realistic and achievable goals for each specific type of cancer. The range of possible treatment goals may include complete eradication of malignant disease (**cure**), prolonged survival and containment of cancer cell growth (**control**), or relief of symptoms associated with the disease (**palliation**).

The health care team, the patient, and the patient's family must have a clear understanding of the treatment options and goals. Open communication and support are vital as the patient and family periodically reassess treatment plans and goals when complications of therapy develop or disease progresses.

Multiple modalities are commonly used in cancer treatment. A variety of therapies, including surgery, radiation therapy, chemotherapy, and biologic response modifier (BRM) therapy, may be used at various times throughout treatment. Understanding the principles of each and how they interrelate is important in understanding the rationale and goals of treatment.

SURGERY

Surgical removal of the entire cancer remains the ideal and most frequently used treatment method. The specific surgical approach, however, may vary for several reasons. Diagnostic surgery is the definitive method of identifying the cellular characteristics that influence all treatment decisions. Surgery may be the primary method of treatment, or it may be prophylactic, palliative, or reconstructive.

Diagnostic Surgery

Diagnostic surgery, such as a **biopsy**, is usually performed to obtain a tissue sample for analysis of cells suspected to be malignant. In most instances, the biopsy is taken from the actual tumour. The three most common biopsy methods are the excisional, incisional, and needle methods.

Excisional biopsy is most frequently used for easily accessible tumours of the skin, breast, upper and lower gastrointestinal tract, and upper respiratory tract. In many cases, the surgeon can remove the entire tumour and surrounding marginal tissues as well. This removal of normal tissue beyond the tumour area decreases the possibility that residual microscopic disease cells may lead to a recurrence of the tumour. This approach not only provides the pathologist who stages and grades the cells with the entire tissue specimen but also decreases the chance of seeding the tumour (disseminating cancer cells through surrounding tissues).

Incisional biopsy is performed if the tumour mass is too large to be removed. In this case, a wedge of tissue from the tumour is removed for analysis. The cells of the tissue wedge must be representative of the tumour mass so that the pathologist can provide an accurate diagnosis. If the specimen does not contain representative tissue and cells, negative biopsy results do not guarantee the absence of cancer.

Excisional and incisional approaches are often performed through endoscopy. Surgical incision, however, may be required to determine the anatomic extent or stage of the tumour. For example, a diagnostic or staging laparotomy, the surgical opening of the abdomen to assess malignant abdominal disease, may be necessary to assess malignancies such as gastric cancer.

Needle biopsies are performed to sample suspicious masses that are easily accessible, such as some growths in the breasts, thyroid, lung, liver, and kidney. Needle biopsies are fast, relatively inexpensive, and easy to perform and usually require only local anesthesia. In general, the patient experiences slight and temporary physical discomfort. In addition, the surrounding tissues are disturbed only minimally, thus decreasing the likelihood of seeding cancer cells. Needle aspiration biopsy involves aspirating tissue fragments through a needle guided into an area suspected of bearing disease. Occasionally, radiologic imaging or magnetic resonance imaging is used to help locate the suspected area and guide the placement of the needle. In some instances, the aspiration biopsy does not yield enough tissue to permit accurate diagnosis. A needle core biopsy uses a specially designed needle to obtain a small core of tissue. Most often, this specimen is sufficient to permit accurate diagnosis.

In some situations, it is necessary to biopsy lymph nodes that are near the suspicious tumour. It is well known that many cancers can spread (metastasize) from the primary site to other areas of the body through the lymphatic circulation. Knowing whether adjacent lymph nodes contain tumour cells helps physicians plan for systemic therapies instead of, or in addition to, surgery in order to combat tumour cells that have gone beyond the primary tumour site. The use of injectable dyes and nuclear medicine imaging can assist the surgeon in identifying lymph nodes (sentinel nodes) that process lymphatic drainage for the involved area. This procedure is used in patients with melanoma and is being used with increasing frequency in patients with cancers of the breast, colon, and vulva, although it is still considered investigational.

The choice of biopsy method is based on many factors. Of greatest importance is the type of treatment anticipated if the cancer diagnosis is confirmed. Definitive surgical approaches include the original biopsy site so that any cells disseminated during the biopsy are excised at the time of surgery. Nutrition and hematologic, respiratory, renal, and hepatic function are considered in determining the method of treatment as well. If the biopsy requires general anesthesia and if subsequent surgery is likely, the effects of prolonged anesthesia on the patient are considered.

The patient and family are given an opportunity to discuss the options before definitive plans are made. The nurse, as the patient's advocate, serves as a liaison between the patient and the physician to facilitate this process. Time should be set aside to minimize interruptions. Time should be provided for the patient to ask questions and for thinking through all that has been discussed.

Surgery as Primary Treatment

When surgery is the primary approach in treating cancer, the goal is to remove the entire tumour or as much as is feasible (a procedure sometimes called debulking) and any involved surrounding tissue, including regional lymph nodes.

Two common surgical approaches used for treating primary tumours are local and wide excisions. Local excision is warranted when the mass is small. It includes removal of the mass and a small margin of normal tissue that is easily accessible. Wide or radical excisions (en bloc dissections) include removal of the primary tumour, lymph nodes, adjacent involved structures, and surrounding tissues that may be at high risk for tumour spread. This surgical method can result in disfigurement and altered functioning. Wide excisions are considered, however, if the tumour can be removed completely and the chances of cure or control are good.

In some situations, video-assisted endoscopic surgery is replacing surgeries associated with long incisions and extended recovery periods. In these procedures, an endoscope with intense lighting and an attached multichip minicamera is inserted through a small incision into the body. The surgical instruments are inserted into the surgical field through one or two additional small incisions, each about 3 cm long. The camera transmits the image of the involved area to a monitor so the surgeon can manipulate the instruments to perform the necessary procedure. This type of procedure is now being used for many thoracic and abdominal surgeries.

Salvage surgery is an additional treatment option that uses an extensive surgical approach to treat the local recurrence of the cancer after a less extensive primary approach is used. A mastectomy to treat recurrent breast cancer after primary lumpectomy and radiation is an example of salvage surgery.

In addition to the use of surgical blades or scalpels to excise the mass and surrounding tissues, several other types of surgical interventions are available. Electrosurgery makes use of electrical current to destroy the tumour cells. Cryosurgery uses liquid nitrogen to freeze tissue to cause cell destruction. Chemosurgery uses combined topical chemotherapy and layer-by-layer surgical removal of abnormal tissue. Laser surgery (*l*ight *a*mplification by *s*timulated *e*mission of *r*adiation) makes use of light and energy aimed at an exact tissue location and depth to vaporize cancer cells. Stereotactic radiosurgery (SRS) is a single and highly precise administration of high-dose radiation therapy used in some types of brain and head and neck cancers. This type of radiation has such a dramatic effect on the target area that the changes are considered to be comparable to more traditional surgical approaches (International Radiosurgery Support Association, 2000). (Radiation therapy is discussed later in this chapter.)

A multidisciplinary approach to patient care is essential during and after any type of surgery. The effects of surgery on the patient's body image, self-esteem, and functional abilities are addressed. If necessary, a plan for postoperative rehabilitation is made before the surgery is performed.

The growth and dissemination of cancer cells may have produced distant micrometastases by the time the patient seeks treatment. Therefore, attempting to remove wide margins of tissue in the hope of "getting all the cancer cells" may not be feasible. This reality substantiates the need for a coordinated multidisciplinary approach to cancer therapy. Once the surgery has been completed, one or more additional (or adjuvant) modalities may be chosen to increase the likelihood of destroying the cancer cells. However, some cancers that are treated surgically in the very early stages are considered to be curable (eg, skin cancers, testicular cancers).

Prophylactic Surgery

Prophylactic surgery involves removing nonvital tissues or organs that are likely to develop cancer. The following factors are considered when electing prophylactic surgery:

- Family history and genetic predisposition
- Presence or absence of symptoms
- Potential risks and benefits
- Ability to detect cancer at an early stage
- Patient's acceptance of the postoperative outcome

Colectomy, mastectomy, and oophorectomy are examples of prophylactic operations. Recent developments in the ability to identify genetic markers indicative of a predisposition to develop some types of cancer may play a role in decisions concerning prophylactic surgeries. Some controversy, however, exists about adequate justification for prophylactic surgical procedures. For example, a strong family history of breast cancer, positive BRCA-1 or BRCA-2 findings, an abnormal physical finding on breast examination such as progressive nodularity and cystic disease, a proven history of breast cancer in the opposite breast, abnormal mammography findings, and abnormal biopsy results may be factors considered in making the decision to proceed with a prophylactic mastectomy (Houshmand, Campbell, Briggs, McFadden & Al-Tweigeri, 2000; Zimmerman, 2002).

Because the long-term physiologic and psychological effects are unknown, prophylactic surgery is offered selectively to patients and discussed thoroughly with the patient and family. Preoperative teaching and counselling, as well as long-term follow-up, are provided.

Palliative Surgery

When cure is not possible, the goals of treatment are to make the patient as comfortable as possible and to promote a satisfying and productive life for as long as possible. Whether the period is extremely brief or lengthy, the major goal is a high quality of life—with quality defined by the patient and family. Honest and informative communication with the patient and family about the goal of surgery is essential to avoid false hope and disappointment.

Palliative surgery is performed in an attempt to relieve complications of cancer, such as ulcerations, obstructions, hemorrhage, pain, and malignant effusions (Table 16-5).

Table 16-5 • Indications for Palliative Surgical Procedures

PROCEDURE	INDICATIONS
Pleural drainage tube placement	Pleural effusion
Peritoneal drainage tube placement (Tenckoff catheter)	Ascites
Abdominal shunt placement (Levine shunt)	Ascites
Pericardial drainage tube placement	Pericardial effusion
Colostomy or ileostomy	Bowel obstruction
Gastrostomy, jejunostomy tube placement	Upper gastrointestinal tract obstruction
Biliary stent placement	Biliary obstruction
Ureteral stent placement	Ureteral obstruction
Nerve block	Pain
Cordotomy	Pain
Venous access device placement (for administering parenteral analgesics)	Pain
Epidural catheter placement (for administering epidural analgesics)	Pain
Hormone manipulation (removal of ovaries, testes, adrenals, pituitary)	Tumours that depend on hormones for growth

Reconstructive Surgery

Reconstructive surgery may follow curative or radical surgery and is carried out in an attempt to improve function or obtain a more desirable cosmetic effect. It may be performed in one operation or in stages. Patients are instructed about possible reconstructive surgical options before the primary surgery by the surgeon who will perform the reconstruction. Reconstructive surgery may be indicated for breast, head and neck, and skin cancers.

The nurse must recognize the patient's needs and the impact that altered functioning and altered body image may have on quality of life. Providing the patient and family with opportunities to discuss these issues is imperative. The needs of the individual must be accurately assessed and validated in each situation for any type of reconstructive surgery.

Nursing Management in Cancer Surgery

The patient undergoing surgery for cancer requires general perioperative nursing care, as described in Unit 4, along with specific care related to the patient's age, organ impairment, nutritional deficits, disorders of coagulation, and altered immunity that may increase the risk for postoperative complications. Combining other treatment methods, such as radiation and chemotherapy, with surgery also contributes to postoperative complications, such as infection, impaired wound healing, altered pulmonary or renal function, and the development of deep vein thrombosis. In these situations, the nurse completes a thorough preoperative assessment for all factors that may affect patients undergoing surgical procedures.

The patient undergoing surgery for the diagnosis or treatment of cancer is often anxious about the surgical procedure, possible findings, postoperative limitations, changes in normal body functions, and prognosis. The patient and family require time and assistance to deal with the possible changes and outcomes resulting from the surgery.

The nurse provides education and emotional support by assessing patient and family needs and exploring with the patient and family their fears and coping mechanisms, encouraging them to take an active role in decision making when possible. When the patient or family asks about the results of diagnostic testing and surgical procedures, the nurse's response is guided by the information the physician previously conveyed to them. The patient and family may also ask the nurse to explain and clarify information that the physician initially provided but that they did not grasp because they were anxious at the time. It is important for the nurse to communicate frequently with the physician and other health care team members to be certain that the information provided is consistent.

After surgery, the nurse assesses the patient's responses to the surgery and monitors for possible complications, such as infection, bleeding, thrombophlebitis, wound dehiscence, fluid and electrolyte imbalance, and organ dysfunction. The nurse also provides for patient comfort. Postoperative teaching addresses wound care, activity, nutrition, and medication information.

Plans for discharge, follow-up and home care, and treatment are initiated as early as possible to ensure continuity of care from hospital to home or from a cancer referral centre to the patient's local hospital and health care provider.

RADIATION THERAPY

In **radiation therapy**, ionizing radiation is used to interrupt cellular growth. More than half of patients with cancer receive a form of radiation therapy at some point during treatment. Radiation may be used to cure the cancer, as in Hodgkin's disease, testicular seminomas, thyroid carcinomas, localized cancers of the head and neck, and cancers of the uterine cervix. Radiation therapy may also be used to control malignant disease when a tumour cannot be removed surgically or when local nodal metastasis is present, or it can be used prophylactically to prevent leukemic infiltration to the brain or spinal cord.

Palliative radiation therapy is used to relieve the symptoms of metastatic disease, especially when the cancer has spread to brain, bone, or soft tissue, or to treat oncologic emergencies, such as superior vena cava syndrome or spinal cord compression.

Two types of ionizing radiation—electromagnetic rays (x-rays and gamma rays) and particles (electrons [beta particles], protons, neutrons, and alpha particles)—can lead to tissue disruption. The most harmful tissue disruption is the alteration of the DNA molecule within the cells of the tissue. Ionizing radiation breaks the strands of the DNA helix, leading to cell death. Ionizing radiation can also ionize constituents of body fluids, especially water, leading to the formation of free radicals and irreversibly damaging DNA. If the DNA is incapable of repair, the cell may die immediately, or it may initiate cellular suicide (apoptosis), a genetically programmed cell death.

Cells are most vulnerable to the disruptive effects of radiation during DNA synthesis and mitosis (early S, G2, and M phases of the cell cycle). Therefore, those body tissues that undergo frequent cell division are most sensitive to radiation therapy. These tissues include bone marrow, lymphatic tissue, epithelium of the gastrointestinal tract, hair cells, and gonads. Slower-growing tissues or tissues at rest are relatively radioresistant (less sensitive to the effects of radiation). Such tissues include muscle, cartilage, and connective tissues.

A radiosensitive tumour is one that can be destroyed by a dose of radiation that still allows for cell regeneration in the normal tissue. Tumours that are well oxygenated also appear to be more sensitive to radiation. In theory, therefore, radiation therapy may be enhanced if more oxygen can be delivered to tumours. In addition, if the radiation is delivered when most tumour cells are cycling through the cell cycle, the number of cancer cells destroyed (cell-killing) is maximal.

Certain chemicals, including chemotherapy agents, act as radiosensitizers and sensitize more hypoxic (oxygen-poor) tumours to the effects of radiation therapy. Radiation is delivered to tumour sites by external or internal means.

External Radiation

If external radiation therapy is used, one of several delivery methods may be chosen, depending on the depth of the tumour. Depending on the amount of energy they contain, x-rays can be used to destroy cancerous cells at the skin surface or deeper in the body. The higher the energy, the deeper the penetration into the body. Kilovoltage therapy devices deliver the maximal radiation dose to superficial lesions, such as lesions of the skin and breast, whereas linear accelerators and betatron machines produce higher-energy x-rays and deliver their dosage to deeper structures with less harm to the skin and less scattering of radiation within the body tissues. Gamma rays are another form of energy used in radiation therapy. This energy is produced from the spontaneous decay of naturally occurring radioactive elements such as cobalt 60. The gamma rays also deliver this radiation dose beneath the skin surface, sparing skin tissue from adverse effects.

Some centres nationwide treat more hypoxic, radiation-resistant tumours with particle-beam radiation therapy. This type of therapy accelerates subatomic particles (neutrons, pions, heavy ions) through body tissue. This therapy, which is also known as high linear energy transfer radiation, damages target cells as well as cells in its pathway.

A few centres are using intraoperative radiation therapy (IORT), which involves delivering a single dose of high-fraction radiation therapy to the exposed tumour bed while the body cavity is open during surgery. Cancers for which IORT is being used include gastric, pancreatic, colorectal, bladder, and cervical cancers and sarcomas. Toxicity with IORT is minimized because the radiation is precisely targeted to the diseased areas, and exposure to overlying skin and structures is avoided.

Internal Radiation

Internal radiation implantation, or **brachytherapy**, delivers a high dose of radiation to a localized area. The specific radioisotope for implantation is selected on the basis of its half-life, which is the time it takes for half of its radioactivity to decay. This internal radiation can be implanted by means of needles, seeds, beads, or catheters into body cavities (vagina, abdomen, pleura) or interstitial compartments (breast). Brachytherapy may also be administered orally as with the isotope I[131], used to treat thyroid carcinomas.

Intracavitary radioisotopes are frequently used to treat gynecologic cancers. In these malignancies, the radioisotopes are inserted into specially positioned applicators after the position is verified by x-ray. These radioisotopes remain in place for a prescribed period and then are removed. Patients are maintained on bed rest and log-rolled to prevent displacement of the intracavitary delivery device. An indwelling urinary catheter is inserted to ensure that the bladder remains empty. Low-residue diets and antidiarrheal agents, such as diphenoxylate (Lomotil), are provided

to prevent bowel movement during therapy, to prevent the radioisotopes from being displaced.

Interstitial implants, used in treating such malignancies as prostate, pancreatic, or breast cancer, may be temporary or permanent, depending on the radioisotopes used. These implants usually consist of seeds, needles, wires, or small catheters positioned to provide a local radiation source and are less frequently dislodged. With internal radiation therapy, the farther the tissue is from the radiation source, the lower the dosage. This spares the noncancerous tissue from the radiation dose.

Because patients receiving internal radiation emit radiation while the implant is in place, contacts with the health care team are guided by principles of time, distance, and shielding to minimize exposure of personnel to radiation. Safety precautions used in caring for the patient receiving brachytherapy include assigning the person to a private room, posting appropriate notices about radiation safety precautions, having staff members wear dosimeter badges, making sure that pregnant staff members are not assigned to this patient's care, prohibiting visits by children or pregnant visitors, limiting visits from others to 30 minutes daily, and seeing that visitors maintain a 6-foot distance from the radiation source.

Radiation Dosage

The radiation dosage is dependent on the sensitivity of the target tissues to radiation and on the tumour size. The lethal tumour dose is defined as that dose that will eradicate 95% of the tumour yet preserve normal tissue. The total radiation dose is delivered over several weeks to allow healthy tissue to repair and to achieve greater cell kill by exposing more cells to the radiation as they begin active cell division. Repeated radiation treatments over time (fractionated doses) also allow for the periphery of the tumour to be reoxygenated repeatedly because tumours shrink from the outside inward. This increases the radiosensitivity of the tumour, thereby increasing tumour cell death.

Toxicity

Toxicity of radiation therapy is localized to the region being irradiated. Toxicity may be increased when concomitant chemotherapy is administered. Acute local reactions occur when normal cells in the treatment area are also destroyed and cellular death exceeds cellular regeneration. Body tissues most affected are those that normally proliferate rapidly, such as the skin, the epithelial lining of the gastrointestinal tract, including the oral cavity, and the bone marrow. Altered skin integrity is a common effect and can include alopecia (hair loss), erythema, and shedding of skin (desquamation). After treatments have been completed, reepithelialization occurs.

Alterations in oral mucosa secondary to radiation therapy include stomatitis, **xerostomia** (dryness of the mouth), change and loss of taste, and decreased salivation. The entire gastrointestinal mucosa may be involved, and esophageal irritation with chest pain and dysphagia may result. Anorexia, nausea, vomiting, and diarrhea may occur if the stomach or colon is in the irradiated field. Symptoms subside and gastrointestinal reepithelialization occurs after treatments are complete.

Bone marrow cells proliferate rapidly, and if bone marrow–producing sites are included in the radiation field anemia, leukopenia (decreased white blood cells [WBCs]), and **thrombocytopenia** (a decrease in platelets) may result. Patients are then at increased risk for infection and bleeding until blood cell counts return to normal. Chronic anemia may occur. Research continues to develop radioprotective agents that can protect normal tissue from radiation damage.

Certain systemic side effects are also commonly experienced by patients receiving radiation therapy. These manifestations, which are generalized, include fatigue, malaise, and anorexia. This syndrome may be secondary to substances released when tumour cells break down. The effects are temporary and subside with the cessation of treatment.

Late effects of radiation therapy may also occur in various body tissues. These effects are chronic, usually produce fibrotic changes secondary to a decreased vascular supply, and are irreversible. These late effects can be most severe when they involve vital organs such as the lungs, heart, central nervous system, and bladder. Toxicities may intensify when radiation is combined with other treatment modalities.

Nursing Management in Radiation Therapy

The patient receiving radiation therapy and the family often have questions and concerns about its safety. To answer questions and allay fears about the effects of radiation on others, on the tumour, and on the patient's normal tissues and organs, the nurse can explain the procedure for delivering radiation and describe the equipment, the duration of the procedure (often minutes only), the possible need for immobilizing the patient during the procedure, and the absence of new sensations, including pain, during the procedure. If a radioactive implant is used, the nurse informs the patient and family about the restrictions placed on visitors and health care personnel and other radiation precautions. Patients also need to understand their own role before, during, and after the procedure. See Chapter 47 for further discussion of radiation treatment for gynecologic cancers.

PROTECTING THE SKIN AND ORAL MUCOSA

The nurse assesses the patient's skin, nutritional status, and general feeling of well-being. The skin and oral mucosa are assessed frequently for changes (particularly if radiation therapy is directed to these areas). The skin is protected from irritation, and the patient is instructed to avoid using ointments, lotions, or powders on the area.

Gentle oral hygiene is essential to remove debris, prevent irritation, and promote healing. If systemic symptoms, such as weakness and fatigue, occur, the patient may need assistance with activities of daily living and personal hygiene. Additionally, the nurse offers reassurance by explaining that these symptoms are a result of the treatment and do not represent deterioration or progression of the disease.

PROTECTING THE CAREGIVERS

When a patient has a radioactive implant in place, nurses and other health care providers need to protect themselves as well as the patient from the effects of radiation. Specific instructions are usually provided by the radiation safety officer from the x-ray department. The instructions identify the maximum time that can be spent safely in the patient's room, the shielding equipment to be used, and special precautions and actions to be taken if the implant is dislodged. The nurse should explain the rationale for these precautions to keep the patient from feeling unduly isolated.

CHEMOTHERAPY

In **chemotherapy**, antineoplastic agents are used in an attempt to destroy tumour cells by interfering with cellular functions and reproduction. Chemotherapy is used primarily to treat sys-

temic disease rather than lesions that are localized and amenable to surgery or radiation. Chemotherapy may be combined with surgery or radiation therapy, or both, to reduce tumour size preoperatively, to destroy any remaining tumour cells postoperatively, or to treat some forms of leukemia. The goals of chemotherapy (cure, control, palliation) must be realistic because they will define the medications to be used and the aggressiveness of the treatment plan.

Cell Kill and the Cell Cycle

Each time a tumour is exposed to a chemotherapeutic agent, a percentage of tumour cells (20% to 99%, depending on dosage) is destroyed. Repeated doses of chemotherapy are necessary over a prolonged period to achieve regression of the tumour. Eradication of 100% of the tumour is nearly impossible, but a goal of treatment is to eradicate enough of the tumour so that the remaining tumour cells can be destroyed by the body's immune system.

Actively proliferating cells within a tumour (growth fraction) are the most sensitive to chemotherapeutic agents. Nondividing cells capable of future proliferation are the least sensitive to antineoplastic medications and consequently are potentially dangerous. The nondividing cells must be destroyed, however, to eradicate a cancer completely. Repeated cycles of chemotherapy are used to kill more tumour cells by destroying these nondividing cells as they begin active cell division.

Reproduction of both healthy and malignant cells follows the cell cycle pattern (Fig. 16-2). The cell cycle time is the time required for one tissue cell to divide and reproduce two identical daughter cells. The cell cycle of any cell has four distinct phases, each with a vital underlying function:

1. G_1 phase—RNA and protein synthesis occur.
2. S phase—DNA synthesis occurs.

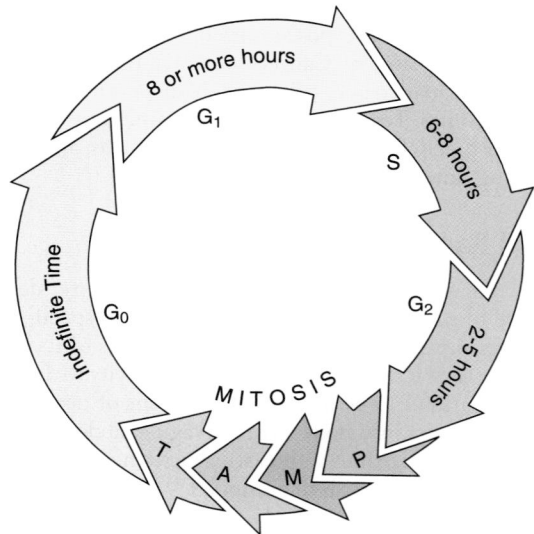

FIGURE 16-2 Phases of the cell cycle extend over the interval between the midpoint of mitosis to the subsequent end point in mitosis in a daughter cell. G_1 is the postmitotic phase during which ribonucleic acid (RNA) and protein synthesis are increased and cell growth occurs. G_0 is the resting, or dormant, phase of the cell cycle. In the S phase, nucleic acids are synthesized and chromosomes replicated in preparation for cell mitosis. During G_2, RNA and protein synthesis occurs as in G_1. (P = prophase, M = metaphase, A = anaphase, T = telophase.) From Porth, C. M. (2002). *Pathophysiology: Concepts of altered health states* (6th ed.) Philadelphia: Lippincott Williams & Wilkins.

3. G_2 phase—premitotic phase; DNA synthesis is complete, mitotic spindle forms.
4. Mitosis—cell division occurs.

The G_0 phase, the resting or dormant phase of cells, can occur after mitosis and during the G_1 phase. In the G_0 phase are those dangerous cells that are not actively dividing but have the potential for replicating. The administration of certain chemotherapeutic agents (as well as administration of some other forms of therapy) is coordinated with the cell cycle.

Classification of Chemotherapeutic Agents

Certain chemotherapeutic agents (cell cycle–specific drugs) destroy cells actively reproducing by means of the cell cycle. Many of these agents are specific to certain phases of the cell cycle. Most affect cells in the S phase by interfering with DNA and RNA synthesis. Others, such as the vinca or plant alkaloids, are specific to the M phase, where they halt mitotic spindle formation.

Chemotherapeutic agents that act independently of the cell cycle phases are termed cell cycle–nonspecific agents. These agents usually have a prolonged effect on cells, leading to cellular damage or death. Many treatment plans combine cell cycle–specific and cell cycle–nonspecific agents to increase the number of vulnerable tumour cells killed during a treatment period.

Chemotherapeutic agents are also classified according to various chemical groups, each with a different mechanism of action. These include the alkylating agents, nitrosureas, antimetabolites, antitumour antibiotics, plant alkaloids, hormonal agents, and miscellaneous agents. The classification, mechanism of action, common drugs, cell cycle specificity, and common side effects of antineoplastic agents are listed in Table 16-6.

Chemotherapeutic agents from each category may be used to enhance the tumour cell kill during therapy by creating multiple cellular lesions. Combined medication therapy relies on medications of differing toxicities and with synergistic actions. Using combination drug therapy also prevents development of drug-resistant mechanisms.

Combining older medications with other agents, such as levamisole, leucovorin, hormones, or interferons (IFN), has shown some benefit in combating resistance of cells to chemotherapeutic agents. Newer investigational agents are being studied for effectiveness in resistant tumour lines. For more information about investigative drugs, see Chart 16-4.

Administration of Chemotherapeutic Agents

Chemotherapeutic agents may be administered in the hospital, clinic, or home setting by topical, oral, intravenous, intramuscular, subcutaneous, arterial, intracavitary, and intrathecal routes. The administration route usually depends on the type of agent, the required dose, and the type, location, and extent of tumour being treated. Guidelines for the administration of chemotherapy have been developed by the Oncology Nursing Society. Patient education is essential to maximize safety if chemotherapy is administered in the patient's home (Chart 16-5).

DOSAGE

Dosage of antineoplastic agents is based primarily on the patient's total body surface area, previous response to chemotherapy or radiation therapy, and major organ function.

SPECIAL PROBLEMS: EXTRAVASATION

Special care must be taken whenever intravenous vesicant agents are administered. **Vesicants** are those agents that, if deposited into the subcutaneous tissue (**extravasation**), cause tissue necrosis and damage to underlying tendons, nerves, and blood vessels. Although the complete mechanism of tissue destruction is unclear, it is known that the pH of many antineoplastic drugs is responsible for the severe inflammatory reaction as well as the ability of these drugs to bind to tissue DNA. Sloughing and ulceration of the tissue may be so severe that skin grafting may be necessary. The full extent of tissue damage may take several weeks to become apparent. Chemotherapeutics classified as vesicants include dactinomycin, epirubicin, amsacrine, melphalan, vinorelbine, paclitaxel, idarubicin, streptozocin, daunorubicin, doxorubicin (Adriamycin), nitrogen mustard, mitomycin, vinblastine, vincristine, and vindesine.

Only specially trained physicians and nurses should administer vesicants. Careful selection of peripheral veins, skilled venipuncture, and careful administration of medications are essential. Indications of extravasation during administration of vesicant agents include the following:

- Absence of blood return from the intravenous catheter
- Resistance to flow of intravenous fluid
- Swelling, pain, or redness at the site

If extravasation is suspected, the medication administration is stopped immediately, and ice is applied to the site (unless the extravasated vesicant is a vinca alkaloid). The physician may aspirate any infiltrated medication from the tissues and inject a neutralizing solution into the area to reduce tissue damage. Selection of the neutralizing solution depends on the extravasated agent. Examples of neutralizing solutions include sodium thiosulfate, and sodium bicarbonate. Recommendations and guidelines for managing vesicant extravasation have been issued by individual medication manufacturers, pharmacies, and the Oncology Nursing Society, and they differ from one medication to the next.

When frequent, prolonged administration of antineoplastic vesicants is anticipated, right atrial Silastic catheters or venous access devices may be inserted to promote safety during medication administration and reduce problems with access to the circulatory system (Figs. 16-3 and 16-4). Complications associated with their use include infection and thrombosis.

TOXICITY

Toxicity associated with chemotherapy can be acute or chronic. Cells with rapid growth rates (eg, epithelium, bone marrow, hair follicles, sperm) are very susceptible to damage, and various body systems may be affected as well.

Gastrointestinal System. Nausea and vomiting are the most common side effects of chemotherapy and may persist for up to 24 hours after its administration. The vomiting centres in the brain are stimulated by (1) activation of the receptors found in the chemoreceptor trigger zone (CTZ) of the medulla; (2) stimulation of peripheral autonomic pathways (gastrointestinal tract and pharynx); (3) stimulation of the vestibular pathways (inner ear imbalances, labyrinth input); (4) cognitive stimulation (central nervous system disease, anticipatory nausea and vomiting); and (5) a combination of these factors.

Medications that can decrease nausea and vomiting include serotonin blockers, such as ondansetron, granisetron, and dolasetron,

Table 16-6 • Antineoplastic Agents

DRUG CLASS AND EXAMPLES	MECHANISM OF ACTION	CELL CYCLE SPECIFICITY	COMMON SIDE EFFECTS
Alkylating Agents busulfan, carboplatin, chlorambucil, cisplatin, cyclophosphamide, dacarbazine, hexamethyl melamine, ifosfamide, melphalan, nitrogen mustard, thiotepa	Alter DNA structure by misreading DNA code, initiating breaks in the DNA molecule, cross-linking DNA strands	Cell cycle–nonspecific	Bone marrow suppression, nausea, vomiting, cystitis (cyclophosphamide, ifosfamide), stomatitis, alopecia, gonadal suppression, renal toxicity (cisplatin)
Nitrosureas carmustine (BCNU), lomustine (CCNU), semustine (methyl CCNU), streptozocin	Similar to the alkylating agents; cross the blood–brain barrier	Cell cycle–nonspecific	Delayed and cumulative myelosuppression, especially thrombocytopenia; nausea, vomiting
Topoisomerase I Inhibitors irinotecan, topotecan	Induce breaks in the DNA strand by binding to enzyme topoisomerase I, preventing cells from dividing	Cell cycle–specific	Bone marrow suppression, diarrhea, nausea, vomiting, hepatotoxicity
Antimetabolites 5-azacytadine, cytarabine, edatrexate fludarabine, 5-fluorouracil (5-FU), FUDR, gemcitabine, hydroxyurea, leustatin, 6-mercaptopurine, methotrexate, pentostatin, 6-thioguanine	Interfere with the biosynthesis of metabolites or nucleic acids necessary for RNA and DNA synthesis	Cell cycle–specific (S phase)	Nausea, vomiting, diarrhea, bone marrow suppression, proctitis, stomatitis, renal toxicity (methotrexate), hepatotoxicity
Antitumor Antibiotics bleomycin, dactinomycin, daunorubicin, doxorubicin (Adriamycin), idarubicin, mitomycin, mitoxantrone, plicamycin	Interfere with DNA synthesis by binding DNA; prevent RNA synthesis	Cell cycle–nonspecific	Bone marrow suppression, nausea, vomiting, alopecia, anorexia, cardiac toxicity (daunorubicin, doxorubicin)
Mitotic Spindle Poisons *Plant alkaloids:* etoposide, teniposide, vinblastine, vincristine (VCR), vindesine, vinorelbine	Arrest metaphase by inhibiting mitotic tubular formation (spindle); inhibit DNA and protein synthesis	Cell cycle–specific (M phase)	Bone marrow suppression (mild with VCR), neuropathies (VCR), stomatitis
Taxanes: paclitaxel, docetaxel	Arrest metaphase by inhibiting tubulin depolymerization	Cell cycle–specific (M phase)	Bradycardia, hypersensitivity reactions, bone marrow suppression, alopecia, neuropathies
Hormonal Agents androgens and antiandrogens, estrogens and antiestrogens, progestins and antiprogestins, aromatase inhibitors, luteinizing hormone–releasing hormone analogs, steroids	Bind to hormone receptor sites that alter cellular growth; block binding of estrogens to receptor sites (antiestrogens); inhibit RNA synthesis; suppress aromatase of P450 system, which decreases estrogen level	Cell cycle–nonspecific	Hypercalcemia, jaundice, increased appetite, masculinization, feminization, sodium and fluid retention, nausea, vomiting, hot flashes, vaginal dryness
Miscellaneous Agents asparaginase, procarbazine	Unknown or too complex to categorize	Varies	Anorexia, nausea, vomiting, bone marrow suppression, hepatotoxicity, anaphylaxis, hypotension, altered glucose metabolism

which block serotonin receptors of the gastrointestinal tract and CTZ, and dopaminergic blockers, such as metoclopramide (Reglan), which block dopamine receptors of the CTZ. Phenothiazines, sedatives, corticosteroids, and histamines are used in combination with serotonin blockers with the more emetogenic chemotherapeutic regimens (Bremerkamp, 2000).

Delayed nausea and vomiting that occur later than 48 to 72 hours after chemotherapy are troublesome for some patients. To minimize discomfort, some antiemetic medications are necessary for the first week at home after chemotherapy. Relaxation techniques and imagery can also help to decrease stimuli contributing to symptoms. Altering the patient's diet to include small

Chart 16-4 • PHARMACOLOGY
Investigational Antineoplastic Therapies and Clinical Trials

Evaluation of the effectiveness and toxic potential of promising new modalities for preventing, diagnosing, and treating cancer is accomplished through clinical trials. Before new chemotherapy agents are approved for clinical use, they are subjected to rigourous and lengthy evaluations to identify beneficial effects, adverse effects, and safety.

- *Phase I* clinical trials determine optimal dosing, scheduling, and toxicity.
- *Phase II* trials determine effectiveness with specific tumor types and further define toxicities. Participants in these early trials are most often those who have not responded to standard forms of treatment. Because phase I and II trials may be viewed as last-chance efforts, patients and families are fully informed about the experimental nature of the trial therapies. Although it is hoped that investigational therapy will effectively treat the disease, the purpose of early phase trials is to gather information concerning maximal tolerated doses, adverse effects, and effects of the antineoplastic agents on tumor growth.
- *Phase III* clinical trials establish the effectiveness of new medications or procedures as compared with conventional approaches. Nurses may assist in the recruitment, consent, and education processes for patients who participate. In many cases, nurses are instrumental in monitoring adherence, assisting patients to adhere to the parameters of the trial, and documenting data describing patients' responses. The physical and emotional needs of patients in clinical trials are addressed in much the same way as those of patients who receive standard forms of cancer treatment.
- *Phase IV* testing further investigates medications in terms of new uses, dosing schedule, and toxicities.

frequent meals, bland foods, and comfort foods may reduce the frequency or severity of these symptoms.

Although the epithelium that lines the oral cavity quickly renews itself, its rapid rate of proliferation makes it susceptible to the effects of chemotherapy. As a result, stomatitis and anorexia are common. The entire gastrointestinal tract is susceptible to mucositis (inflam-

Chart 16-5 Safety in Administering Chemotherapy

Safety recommendations from the Occupational Safety and Health Administration (OSHA), Oncology Nursing Society (ONS), hospitals, and other health care agencies for the preparation and handling of antineoplastic agents follow:

- Use a biologic safety cabinet for the preparation of all chemotherapy agents.
- Wear gloves when handling antineoplastic agents and the excretions of patients who received chemotherapy.
- Wear disposable, long-sleeved gowns when preparing and administering chemotherapy agents.
- Use Luer-Lok fittings on all intravenous tubing used to deliver chemotherapy.
- Dispose of all equipment used in chemotherapy preparation and administration in appropriate, leak-proof, puncture-proof containers.
- Dispose of all chemotherapy wastes as hazardous materials.

When followed, these precautions greatly minimize the risk of exposure to chemotherapy agents.

mation of the mucosal lining), and diarrhea is a common result. Antimetabolites and antitumour antibiotics are the major culprits in mucositis and other gastrointestinal symptoms. Irinotecan is responsible for causing diarrhea, which can be severe in some patients.

Hematopoietic System. Most chemotherapeutic agents cause **myelosuppression** (depression of bone marrow function), resulting in decreased production of blood cells. Myelosuppression decreases the number of WBCs (leukopenia), red blood cells (anemia), and platelets (thrombocytopenia) and increases the risk for infection and bleeding. Depression of these cells is the usual reason for limiting the dose of the chemotherapeutic agents. Monitoring blood cell counts frequently is essential, as is protecting the patient from infection and injury, particularly while the blood cell counts are depressed.

Other agents, called colony-stimulating factors (granulocyte colony-stimulating factor [G-CSF], granulocyte-macrophage colony-stimulating factor [GM-CSF], and erythropoietin [EPO]), can be administered after chemotherapy. G-CSF and GM-CSF stimulate the bone marrow to produce WBCs, especially neutrophils, at an accelerated rate, thus decreasing the duration of neutropenia. The colony-stimulating factors decrease the episodes of infection and the need for antibiotics and allow for more timely cycling of chemotherapy with less need to reduce the dosage. EPO stimulates red blood cell production, thus decreasing the symptoms of chronic administered anemia.

Renal System. Chemotherapeutic agents can damage the kidneys because of their direct effects during excretion and the accumulation of end products after cell lysis. Cisplatin, methotrexate, and mitomycin are particularly toxic to the kidneys. Rapid tumour cell lysis after chemotherapy results in increased urinary excretion of uric acid, which can cause renal damage. In addition, intracellular contents are released into the circulation, resulting in excessive levels of potassium and phosphates (hyperkalemia and hyperphosphatemia) and diminished levels of calcium (hypocalcemia). (See later discussion of tumour lysis syndrome.)

Monitoring blood urea nitrogen, serum creatinine, creatinine clearance, and serum electrolyte levels is essential. Adequate hydration, alkalinization of the urine to prevent formation of uric acid crystals, and the use of allopurinol are frequently indicated to prevent these side effects.

Cardiopulmonary System. Antitumour antibiotics (daunorubicin and doxorubicin) are known to cause irreversible cumulative cardiac toxicities, especially when total dosage reaches 550 mg/m^2. Cardiac ejection fraction (volume of blood ejected from the heart with each beat) and signs of congestive heart failure must be monitored closely. Bleomycin, carmustine (BCNU), and busulfan are known for their cumulative toxic effects on lung function. Pulmonary fibrosis can be a long-term effect of prolonged dosage with these agents. Therefore, the patient is monitored closely for changes in pulmonary function, including pulmonary function test results. Total cumulative doses of bleomycin are not to exceed 400 units.

Reproductive System. Testicular and ovarian function can be affected by chemotherapeutic agents, resulting in possible sterility. Normal ovulation, early menopause, or permanent sterility may result. In men, temporary or permanent azoospermia (absence of spermatozoa) may develop. Reproductive cells may be damaged during treatment, resulting in chromosomal abnormalities in offspring. Banking of sperm is recommended for men before treat-

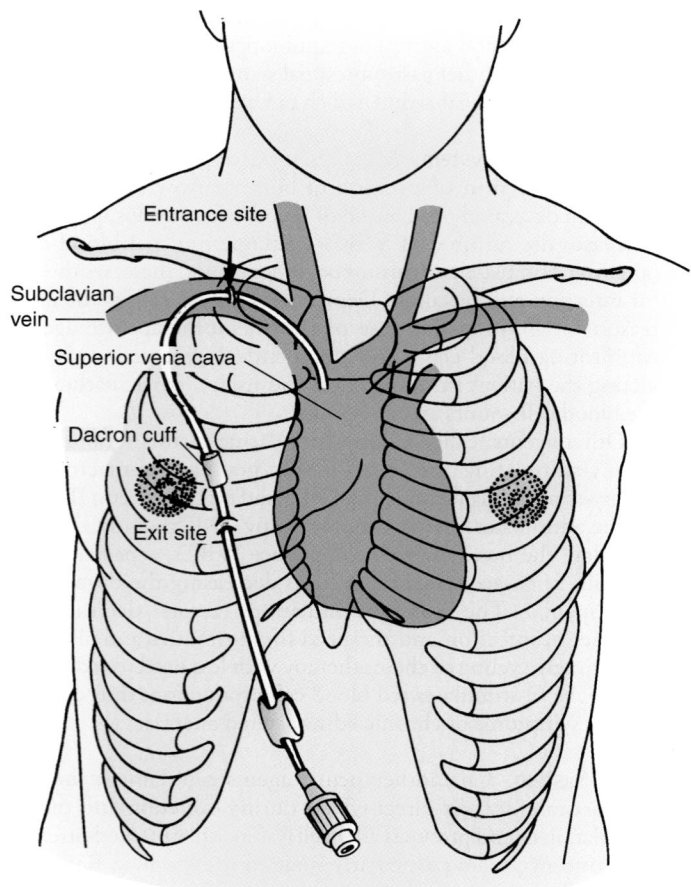

Entrance site

Subclavian vein

Superior vena cava

Dacron cuff

Exit site

FIGURE 16-3 Right atrial catheter. The right atrial catheter is inserted into the subclavian vein and advanced until its tip lies in the superior vena cava just above the right atrium. The proximal end is then tunnelled from the entry site through the subcutaneous tissue of the chest wall and brought out through an exit site on the chest. The Dacron cuff anchors the catheter in place and serves as a barrier to infection.

Self-sealing septum

Skin line

Subcutaneous tissue

Suture

Muscle

Huber needle

Catheter

Fluid flow

Vein

A

B

FIGURE 16-4 Implanted vascular access device. (**A**) A schematic diagram of an implanted vascular access device used for administering medication, fluids, blood products, and nutrition. The self-sealing septum permits repeated puncture by Huber needles without damage or leakage. (**B**) Two Huber needles used to enter the implanted vascular port. The 90-degree needle is used for top-entry ports for continuous infusions.

ments are initiated to protect against sterility or any mutagenic damage to sperm.

Patients and their partners need to be informed about potential changes in reproductive function resulting from chemotherapy. They are advised to use reliable methods of birth control while receiving chemotherapy and not to assume that sterility has resulted.

Neurologic System. The taxanes and plant alkaloids, especially vincristine, can cause neurologic damage with repeated doses. Peripheral neuropathies, loss of deep tendon reflexes, and paralytic ileus may occur. These side effects are usually reversible and disappear after completion of chemotherapy. Cisplatin is also responsible for peripheral neuropathies; hearing loss due to damage to the acoustic nerve can also occur.

Miscellaneous. Fatigue is a distressing side effect for most patients that greatly affects quality of life. Fatigue can be debilitating and last for months after treatment.

Nursing Management in Chemotherapy

The nurse has an important role in assessing and managing many of the problems experienced by the patient undergoing chemotherapy. Because of the systemic effects on normal as well as malignant cells, these problems are often widespread, affecting many body systems.

ASSESSING FLUID AND ELECTROLYTE STATUS
Anorexia, nausea, vomiting, altered taste, and diarrhea put the patient at risk for nutritional and fluid and electrolyte disturbances. Changes in the mucosa of the gastrointestinal tract may lead to irritation of the oral cavity and intestinal tract, further threatening the patient's nutritional status. Therefore, it is important for the nurse to assess the patient's nutritional and fluid and electrolyte status frequently and to use creative ways to encourage an adequate fluid and dietary intake.

MODIFYING RISKS FOR INFECTION AND BLEEDING
Suppression of the bone marrow and immune system is an expected consequence of chemotherapy and frequently serves as a guide in determining appropriate chemotherapy dosage. However, this effect also increases the risk for anemia, infection, and bleeding disorders. Therefore, nursing assessment and care focus on identifying and modifying factors that further increase the patient's risk. Aseptic technique and gentle handling are indicated to prevent infection and trauma. Laboratory test results, particularly blood cell counts, are monitored closely. Untoward changes in blood test results and signs of infection and bleeding must be reported promptly. (see Plan of Nursing Care for more information).

ADMINISTERING CHEMOTHERAPY
The local effects of the chemotherapeutic agent are also of concern. The patient is observed closely during its administration because of the risk and consequences of extravasation (particularly of vesicant agents, which may produce necrosis if deposited in the subcutaneous tissues). Local difficulties or problems with administration of chemotherapeutic agents are brought to the attention of the physician promptly so that corrective measures can be taken immediately to minimize local tissue damage.

IMPLEMENTING SAFEGUARDS
Nurses involved in handling chemotherapeutic agents may be exposed to low doses of the drugs by direct contact, inhalation, and ingestion. Urinalyses of personnel repeatedly exposed to cytotoxic agents demonstrate mutagenic activity. Although not all mutagens are carcinogenic, they can produce permanent inheritable changes in the genetic material of cells.

Although long-term studies of nurses handling chemotherapeutic agents have not been conducted, it is known that chemotherapeutic agents are associated with secondary formation of cancers and chromosome abnormalities. Additionally, nausea, vomiting, dizziness, alopecia, and nasal mucosal ulcerations have been reported in health care personnel who have handled chemotherapeutic agents.

Because of known and potential hazards associated with handling chemotherapeutic agents, the Occupational Safety and Health Administration, Oncology Nursing Society, hospitals, and other health care agencies have developed specific precautions for those involved in the preparation and administration of chemotherapy (Chart 16-5).

BONE MARROW TRANSPLANTATION

Although surgery, radiation therapy, and chemotherapy have resulted in improved survival rates for cancer patients, many cancers that initially respond to therapy recur. This is true of hematologic cancers that affect the bone marrow and solid tumour cancers treated with lower doses of antineoplastics to spare the bone marrow from larger, ablative doses of chemotherapy or radiation therapy.

The role of bone marrow transplantation (BMT) for malignant as well as some nonmalignant diseases continues to grow. Types of BMT based on the source of donor cells include:

1. Allogeneic (from a donor other than the patient): either a related donor (ie, family member) or a matched unrelated donor (national bone marrow registry, cord blood registry)
2. Autologous (from patient)
3. Syngeneic (from an identical twin)

The process of obtaining donor cells has evolved over the years. Donor cells can be obtained by the traditional harvesting of large amounts of bone marrow tissue under general anesthesia in the operating room. A newer method, referred to as peripheral blood stem cell transplant (PBSCT), is gaining widespread use. This method of collection uses apheresis of the donor to collect stem cells for reinfusion. It is considered to be a safer and more cost-effective means of collection than the traditional harvesting of marrow.

Allogeneic BMT, used primarily for disease of the bone marrow, depends on the availability of a human leukocyte antigen–matched donor. This greatly limits the number of transplants possible. An advantage to allogeneic BMT is that the transplanted cells should not be immunologically tolerant of the patient's malignancy and should cause a lethal graft-versus-disease effect to the malignant cells. The recipient must undergo ablative doses of chemotherapy and possibly total body irradiation to destroy all existing bone marrow and malignant disease. The harvested donor marrow is infused intravenously into the recipient and travels to sites in the body where it produces bone marrow and establishes itself. This establishment of the new bone marrow is known as engraftment. Once engraftment is complete (2 to 4 weeks, sometimes longer), the new bone marrow becomes functional and begins producing red blood cells, WBCs, and platelets.

(text continues on page 350)

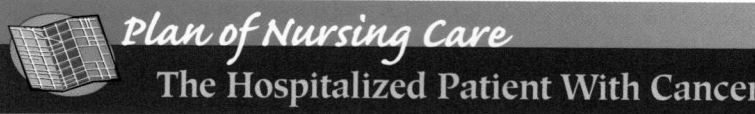

Plan of Nursing Care
The Hospitalized Patient With Cancer

Nursing Interventions	Rationale	Expected Outcomes

Nursing Diagnosis: Risk for infection related to altered immunologic response
Goal: Prevention of infection

Nursing Interventions	Rationale	Expected Outcomes

1. Assess patient for evidence of infection:
 a. Check vital signs daily.
 b. Monitor WBC count and differential each day.
 c. Inspect all sites that may serve as entry ports for pathogens (intravenous sites, wounds, skin folds, bony prominences, perineum, and oral cavity).
2. Report fever ≥38.5°C, chills, diaphoresis, swelling, heat, pain, erythema, exudate on any body surfaces. Also report change in respiratory or mental status, urinary frequency or burning, malaise, myalgias, arthralgias, rash, or diarrhea.
3. Obtain cultures and sensitivities as indicated before initiation of antimicrobial treatment (wound exudate, sputum, urine, stool, blood).
 	
4. Initiate measures to minimize infection.
 a. Discuss with patient and family
  (1) Placing patient in private room if ANC count <1.0 × 10⁹/L.
  (2) Importance of patient avoiding contact with people who have known or recent infection or recent vaccination
 b. Instruct all personnel in careful hand hygiene before and after entering room.
 c. Avoid rectal or vaginal procedures (rectal temperatures, examinations, suppositories; vaginal tampons).
 	
 d. Use stool softeners to prevent constipation and straining.
 e. Assist patient in practice of meticulous personal hygiene.
 f. Instruct patient to use electric razor.
 g. Encourage patient to ambulate in room unless contraindicated.
 h. Avoid fresh flowers and potted plants if ANC <1.0 × 10⁹/L.
 i. Each day: change drinking water, denture cleaning fluids, and respiratory equipment containing water.
5. Assess intravenous sites every day for evidence of infection:
 	
 a. Change intravenous sites every other day if ANC <1.0 × 10⁹/L.
	1. Signs and symptoms of infection may be diminished in the immunocompromised host. Prompt recognition of infection and subsequent initiation of therapy will reduce morbidity and mortality associated with infection.
	
	2. Early detection of infection facilitates early intervention.
	
	3. These tests identify the organism and indicate the most appropriate antimicrobial therapy. Use of inappropriate antibiotics enhances proliferation of additional flora and encourages growth of antibiotic-resistant organisms.
	
	4. Exposure to infection is reduced.
	 a. Preventing contact with pathogens helps prevent infection.
	
	b. Hands are significant source of contamination.
	
	c. Incidence of rectal and perianal abscesses and subsequent systemic infection is high. Manipulation may cause disruption of membrane integrity and enhance progression of infection.
	d. This minimizes trauma to tissues.
	
	e. This prevents skin irritation.
	
	f. Minimizes skin trauma.
	g. Minimizes chance of skin breakdown and stasis of pulmonary secretions.
	h. Fresh flowers and potted plants are also sources of organisms.
	i. Stagnant water is a source of infection.
	
	5. Nosocomial staphylococcal septicemia is closely associated with intravenous catheters.
	 a. Incidence of infection is increased when catheter is in place >72 hr.
		• Demonstrates normal temperature and vital signs.
		• Exhibits absence of signs of inflammation: local edema, erythema, pain, and warmth.
		• Exhibits normal breath sounds on auscultation.
		• Exhibits absence of pathologic bacteria on cultures.
		• Avoids contact with others with infections.
		• Avoids crowds.
		• All personnel carry out hand hygiene after each voiding and bowel movement.
		• Excoriation and trauma of skin are avoided.
		• Trauma to mucous membranes is avoided (avoidance of rectal thermometers, suppositories, vaginal tampons, perianal trauma).
		• Uses recommended procedures and techniques if participating in management of invasive lines or catheters.
		• Uses electric razor.
		• Is free of skin breakdown and stasis of secretions.
		• Adheres to dietary and environmental restrictions.
		• Exhibits no signs of septicemia or septic shock.
		• Exhibits normal vital signs, cardiac output, and arterial pressures when monitored.
		• Demonstrates ability to administer colony-stimulating factor.

(continued)

Plan of Nursing Care
The Hospitalized Patient With Cancer *(Continued)*

Nursing Interventions	Rationale	Expected Outcomes
b. Cleanse skin with chlorhexidine before arterial puncture or venipuncture. c. Change central venous catheter dressings q3 days if ANC >1.0 × 10⁹/L and daily if ANC <1.0 × 10⁹/L. d. Change all solutions and infusion sets q3 days if ANC >1.0 × 10⁹/L and q2 days if ANC <1.0 × 10⁹/L. 6. Avoid intramuscular injections. 7. Avoid insertion of urinary catheters; if catheters are necessary, use strict aseptic technique. 8. Teach patient or family member to administer granulocyte (or granulocyte-macrophage) colony-stimulating factor when prescribed.	b. Chlorhexidine is effective against many gram-positive and gram-negative pathogens. c. Allows observation of site and removes source of contamination. d. Once introduced into the system, microorganisms are capable of growing in infusion sets despite replacement of container and high flow rates. 6. Reduces risk for skin abscesses. 7. Rates of infection *greatly* increase after urinary catheterization. 8. Granulocyte colony-stimulating factor decreases the duration of neutropenia and the potential for infection.	

Nursing Diagnosis: Impaired skin integrity: erythematous and wet desquamation reactions to radiation therapy
Goal: Maintenance of skin integrity

Nursing Interventions	Rationale	Expected Outcomes
1. In erythematous areas: a. Avoid the use of soaps, cosmetics, perfumes, powders, lotions and ointments, deodorants. b. Use only lukewarm water to bathe the area. c. Avoid rubbing or scratching the area. d. Avoid shaving the area with a straight-edged razor. e. Avoid applying hot-water bottles, heating pads, ice, and adhesive tape to the area. f. Avoid exposing the area to sunlight or cold weather. g. Avoid tight clothing in the area. Use cotton clothing. h. Apply Glaxal Base ointment to the area. 2. If wet desquamation occurs: a. Do not disrupt any blisters that have formed. b. Avoid frequent washing of the area. c. Report any blistering. d. Use *prescribed* creams or ointments. e. If area weeps, apply a thin layer of gauze dressing.	1. Care to the affected areas must focus on preventing further skin irritation, drying, and damage g. Allows air circulation to affected area. h. Aids healing. 2. Open weeping areas are susceptible to bacterial infection. Care must be taken to prevent introduction of pathogens. d. Decreases irritation and inflammation of the area. e. Enhances drying.	• Avoids use of soaps, powders, and other cosmetics on site of radiation therapy. • States rationale for special care of skin. • Exhibits minimal change in skin. • Avoids trauma to affected skin region (avoids shaving, constricting and irritating clothing, extremes of temperature, and use of adhesive tape). • Reports change in skin promptly. • Demonstrates proper care of blistered or open areas. • Exhibits absence of infection of blistered and opened areas.

Nursing Diagnosis: Impaired oral mucous membrane: stomatitis
Goal: Maintenance of intact oral mucous membranes

Nursing Interventions	Rationale	Expected Outcomes
1. Assess oral cavity daily. 2. Instruct patient to report oral burning, pain, areas of redness, open lesions on the	1. Provides baseline for later evaluation. 2. Identification of initial stages of stomatitis will facilitate prompt interventions,	• States rationale for frequent oral assessment and hygiene.

(continued)

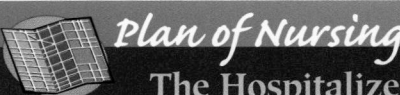

Plan of Nursing Care
The Hospitalized Patient With Cancer *(Continued)*

Nursing Interventions	Rationale	Expected Outcomes

lips, pain associated with swallowing, decreased tolerance to temperature extremes of food, or lack of saliva.
3. Encourage and assist in oral hygiene.
 	
Preventive
  a. Avoid commercial mouthwashes.
 	
  b. Brush with soft toothbrush; use non-abrasive toothpaste after meals and bedtime; floss every 24 h unless painful or platelet count falls below 20×10^9/L.
 	
Mild stomatitis (1-4 lesions, no bleeding, >50% of oral mucosa slightly red)
  c. Use normal saline mouth rinses every 2 h while awake; every 6 h at night.
  d. Use soft toothbrush or toothette.
  e. Remove dentures except for meals; be certain dentures fit well.
  f. Apply lip lubricant.
  g. Avoid foods that are spicy or hard to chew and those with extremes of temperature.
 	
Severe stomatitis (confluent ulcerations with bleeding, >50% of oral mucosa very red)
  h. Obtain mouth swab for culture and sensitivity if infection suspected.
  i. Assess ability to chew and swallow; assess gag reflex.
  j. Use oral rinses as prescribed or place patient on side and irrigate mouth; have suction available (may combine in solution saline, anti-*Candida* agent, such as Mycostatin, and topical anesthetic agent as described below).
  k. Remove dentures.
 	
  l. Use toothette or gauze soaked with solution for cleansing.
  m. Use lip lubricant.
  n. Provide liquid or pureed diet.
 	
  o. Monitor for dehydration.
 	
4. Minimize discomfort.
  a. Consult physician for use of topical anesthetic, such as viscous lidocaine.
 	
  b. Administer systemic analgesics as prescribed.
  c. Perform mouth care as described.
	including modification of treatment as prescribed by physician.
	
	  a. Alcohol content of mouthwashes will dry oral tissues and potentiate breakdown.
	  b. Limits trauma and removes debris.
	
	  c. Assists in removing debris, thick secretions, and bacteria.
	  d. Minimizes trauma.
	  e. Minimizes friction and discomfort.
	
	  f. Promotes comfort.
	  g. Prevents local trauma.
	
	  h. Assists in identifying need for antimicrobial therapy.
	  i. Patient may be in danger of aspiration.
	
	  j. Facilitates cleansing, provides for safety and comfort.
	
	  k. Prevents trauma from ill-fitting dentures.
	  l. Limits trauma, promotes comfort.
	
	  m. Promotes comfort.
	  n. Ensures intake of easily digestible foods.
	  o. Decreased oral intake and ulcerations potentiate fluid deficits.
	
	  a. Alleviates pain and increases sense of well-being; promotes participation in oral hygiene and nutritional intake.
	
	  c. Promotes removal of debris, healing, and comfort.
		• Identifies signs and symptoms of stomatitis to report to nurse or physician.
		• Participates in recommended oral hygiene regimen.
		• Avoids mouthwashes with alcohol.
		• Brushes teeth and mouth with soft toothbrush.
		• Uses lubricant to keep lips soft and non-irritated.
		• Avoids hard-to-chew, spicy, and hot foods.
		• Exhibits clean, intact oral mucosa.
		• Exhibits no ulcerations or infections of oral cavity.
		• Exhibits no evidence of bleeding.
		• Reports absent or decreased oral pain.
		• Reports no difficulty swallowing.
		• Exhibits healing (reepithelialization) of oral mucosa within 5 to 7 days (mild stomatitis).
		• Exhibits healing of oral tissues within 10 to 14 days (severe stomatitis).
		• Exhibits no bleeding or oral ulceration.
		• Consumes adequate fluid and food.
		• Exhibits absence of dehydration and weight loss.

(continued)

Plan of Nursing Care
The Hospitalized Patient With Cancer *(Continued)*

Nursing Interventions	Rationale	Expected Outcomes

Nursing Diagnosis: Impaired tissue integrity: alopecia
Goal: Maintenance of tissue integrity; coping with hair loss

Nursing Interventions	Rationale	Expected Outcomes
1. Discuss potential hair loss and regrowth with patient and family.	1. Provides information so patient and family can begin to prepare cognitively and emotionally for loss.	• Identifies alopecia as potential side effect of treatment.
2. Explore potential impact of hair loss on self-image, interpersonal relationships, and sexuality.	2. Facilitates coping.	• Identifies positive and negative feelings and threats to self-image.
3. Prevent or minimize hair loss through the following:	3. Retains hair as long as possible.	• Verbalizes meaning that hair and possible hair loss have for him or her. • States rationale for modifications in hair care and treatment.
a. Use scalp hypothermia and scalp tourniquets, if appropriate.	a. Decreases hair follicle uptake of chemotherapy (not used for patients with leukemia or lymphoma because tumor cells may be present in blood vessels or scalp tissue).	• Uses mild shampoo and conditioner and shampoos hair only when necessary. • Avoids hair dryer, curlers, sprays, and other stresses on hair and scalp.
b. Cut long hair before treatment.	b–e. Minimizes hair loss due to the weight and manipulation of hair.	• Wears hat or scarf over hair when exposed to sun.
c. Use mild shampoo and conditioner, gently pat dry, and avoid excessive shampooing.		• Takes steps to deal with possible hair loss before it occurs; purchases wig or hairpiece.
d. Avoid electric curlers, curling irons, dryers, clips, barrettes, hair sprays, hair dyes, and permanent waves.		• Maintains hygiene and grooming. • Interacts and socializes with others.
e. Avoid excessive combing or brushing; use wide-toothed comb.		• States that hair loss and necessity of wig are temporary.
4. Prevent trauma to scalp.	4. Preserves tissue integrity.	
a. Lubricate scalp with vitamin A&D ointment to decrease itching.	a. Assists in maintaining skin integrity.	
b. Have patient use sunscreen or wear hat when in the sun.	b. Prevents ultraviolet light exposure.	
5. Suggest ways to assist in coping with hair loss:	5. Minimizes change in appearance.	
a. Purchase wig or hairpiece before hair loss.	a. Wig that closely resembles hair colour and style is more easily selected if hair loss has not begun.	
b. If hair loss has occurred, take photograph to wig shop to assist in selection.	b. Facilitates adjustment.	
c. Begin to wear wig before hair loss.		
d. Wear hat, scarf, or turban.	d. Conceals loss.	
6. Encourage patient to wear own clothes and retain social contacts.	6. Assists in maintaining personal identity.	
7. Explain that hair growth usually begins again once therapy is completed.	7. Reassures patient that hair loss is usually temporary.	

Nursing Diagnosis: Imbalanced nutrition, less than body requirements, related to nausea and vomiting
Goal: Fewer episodes of nausea and vomiting before, during, and after chemotherapy

Nursing Interventions	Rationale	Expected Outcomes
1. Assess the patient's previous experiences and expectations of nausea and vomiting, including causes and interventions used.	1. Identifies patient concerns, misinformation, potential strategies for intervention. Also gives patient sense of empowerment and control.	• Identifies previous triggers of nausea and vomiting. • Exhibits decreased apprehension and anxiety.
2. Adjust diet before and after drug administration according to patient preference and tolerance.	2. Each patient responds differently to food after chemotherapy. A diet containing foods that relieve the patient's nausea or vomiting is most helpful.	• Identifies previously used successful interventions for nausea and vomiting. • Reports decrease in nausea.

(continued)

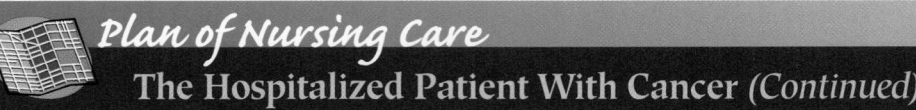

Plan of Nursing Care

The Hospitalized Patient With Cancer *(Continued)*

Nursing Interventions	Rationale	Expected Outcomes
3. Prevent unpleasant sights, odours, and sounds in the environment. 4. Use distraction, music therapy, biofeedback, self-hypnosis, relaxation techniques, and guided imagery before, during, and after chemotherapy. 5. Administer prescribed antiemetics, sedatives, and corticosteroids before chemotherapy and afterward as needed. 6. Ensure adequate fluid hydration before, during, and after drug administration; assess intake and output. 7. Encourage frequent oral hygiene. 8. Provide pain relief measures, if necessary. 9. Assess other causes of nausea and vomiting, such as constipation, gastrointestinal irritation, electrolyte imbalance, radiation therapy, medications, and central nervous system metastasis.	3. Unpleasant sensations can stimulate the nausea and vomiting centre. 4. Decreases anxiety, which can contribute to nausea and vomiting. Psychological conditioning may also be decreased. 5. Administration of antiemetic regimen before onset of nausea and vomiting limits the adverse experience and facilitates control. Combination drug therapy reduces nausea and vomiting through various triggering mechanisms. 6. Adequate fluid volume dilutes drug levels, decreasing stimulation of vomiting receptors. 7. Reduces unpleasant taste sensations. 8. Increased comfort increases physical tolerance of symptoms. 9. Multiple factors may cause nausea and vomiting.	• Reports decrease in incidence of vomiting. • Consumes adequate fluid and food when nausea subsides. • Demonstrates use of distraction, relaxation, and imagery when indicated. • Exhibits normal skin turgor and moist mucous membranes. • Reports no additional weight loss.

Nursing Diagnosis: Imbalanced nutrition: less than body requirements, related to anorexia, cachexia, or malabsorption

Goal: Maintenance of nutritional status and of weight within 10% of pretreatment weight

1. Teach patient to avoid unpleasant sights, odours, sounds in the environment during mealtime. 2. Suggest foods that are preferred and well tolerated by the patient, preferably high-calorie and high-protein foods. Respect ethnic and cultural food preferences. 3. Encourage adequate fluid intake, but limit fluids at mealtime. 4. Suggest smaller, more frequent meals. 5. Promote relaxed, quiet environment during mealtime with increased social interaction as desired. 6. If possible, serve wine at mealtime with foods. 7. Consider cold foods, if desired. 8. Advocate nutritional supplements and high-protein foods between meals. 9. Encourage frequent oral hygiene. 10. Provide pain relief measures. 11. Provide control of nausea and vomiting. 12. Increase activity level as tolerated.	1. Anorexia can be stimulated or increased with noxious stimuli. 2. Foods preferred, well tolerated, and high in calories and protein maintain nutritional status during periods of increased metabolic demand. 3. Fluids are necessary to eliminate wastes and prevent dehydration. Increased fluids with meals can lead to early satiety. 4. Smaller, more frequent meals are better tolerated because early satiety does not occur. 5. A quiet environment promotes relaxation. Social interaction at mealtime increases appetite. 6. Wine often stimulates appetite and adds calories. 7. Cold, high-protein foods are often more tolerable and less odourous than hot foods. 8. Supplements and snacks add protein and calories to meet nutritional requirements. 9. Oral hygiene stimulates appetite and increases saliva production. 10. Pain impairs appetite. 11. Nausea and vomiting increase anorexia. 12. Increased activity promotes appetite.	• Exhibits weight loss no greater than 10% of pretreatment weight. • Reports decreasing anorexia and increased interest in eating. • Demonstrates normal skin turgor. • Identifies rationale for dietary modifications. • Participates in calorie counts and diet histories. • Uses appropriate relaxation and imagery before meals. • Exhibits laboratory and clinical findings indicative of adequate nutritional intake: normal serum protein and transferrin levels; normal serum iron levels; normal hemoglobin, hematocrit, and lymphocyte levels; normal urinary creatinine levels. • Consumes diet high in required nutrients. • Carries out oral hygiene before meals. • Reports that pain does not interfere with meals. • Reports decreasing episodes of nausea and vomiting. • Participates in increasing levels of activity. • States rationale for use of tube feedings or hyperalimentation. • Participates in management of tube feedings or parenteral nutrition, if prescribed.

(continued)

Plan of Nursing Care
The Hospitalized Patient With Cancer *(Continued)*

Nursing Interventions	Rationale	Expected Outcomes
13. Decrease anxiety by encouraging verbalization of fears, concerns; use of relaxation techniques; imagery at mealtime.	13. Relief of anxiety may increase appetite.	
14. Position patient properly at mealtime.	14. Proper body position and alignment are necessary to aid chewing and swallowing.	
15. For collaborative management, provide enteral tube feedings of commercial liquid diets, elemental diets, or blenderized foods as prescribed.	15. Tube feedings may be necessary in the severely debilitated patient who has a functioning gastrointestinal system.	
16. Provide parenteral nutrition with lipid supplements as prescribed.	16. Parenteral nutrition with supplemental fats supplies needed calories and proteins to meet nutritional demands, especially in the nonfunctional gastrointestinal system.	
17. Administer appetite stimulants as prescribed by physician.	17. Although the mechanism is unclear, medications such as megestrol acetate (Megace) have been noted to improve appetite in patients with cancer and HIV infection.	

Nursing Diagnosis: Fatigue
Goal: Increased activity tolerance and decreased fatigue level

1. Encourage several rest periods during the day, especially before and after physical exertion.	1. During rest, energy is conserved and levels are replenished. Several shorter rest periods may be more beneficial than one longer rest period.	• Reports decreasing levels of fatigue. • Increases participation in activities gradually. • Rests when fatigued. • Reports restful sleep.
2. Increase total hours of nighttime sleep.	2. Sleep helps to restore energy levels.	• Requests assistance with activities appropriately.
3. Rearrange daily schedule and organize activities to conserve energy expenditure.	3. Reorganization of activities can reduce energy losses and stressors.	• Reports adequate energy to participate in activities important to him or her (eg, visiting with family, hobbies).
4. Encourage patient to ask for others' assistance with necessary chores, such as housework, child care, shopping, cooking.	4. Conserves energy.	• Consumes diet with recommended protein and caloric intake.
5. Encourage reduced job workload, if possible, by reducing number of hours worked per week.	5. Reducing workload decreases physical and psychological stress and increases periods of rest and relaxation.	• Uses relaxation exercises and imagery to decrease anxiety and promote rest. • Participates in planned exercise program gradually.
6. Encourage adequate protein and calorie intake.	6. Protein and calorie depletion decreases activity tolerance.	• Reports no breathlessness during activities.
7. Encourage use of relaxation techniques, mental imagery, and time for favourite activities.	7. Promotion of relaxation and psychological rest decreases physical fatigue.	• Exhibits acceptable hemoglobin and hematocrit levels.
8. Encourage participation in planned exercise programs.	8. Proper exercise programs increase endurance and stamina.	• Exhibits normal fluid and electrolyte balance.
9. For collaborative management, administer blood products as prescribed.	9. Lowered hemoglobin and hematocrit predispose patient to fatigue due to decreased oxygen availability.	• Reports decreased discomfort. • Exhibits improved mobility.
10. Assess for fluid and electrolyte disturbances.	10. May contribute to altered nerve transmission and muscle function.	
11. Assess for sources of discomfort.	11. Coping with discomfort requires energy expenditure.	
12. Provide strategies to facilitate mobility.	12. Impaired mobility requires increased energy expenditure.	

Nursing Diagnosis: Chronic Pain
Goal: Relief of pain and discomfort

1. Use pain scale to assess pain and discomfort characteristics: location, quality, frequency, duration, etc.	1. Provides baseline for assessing changes in pain level and evaluation of interventions.	• Reports decreased level of pain and discomfort on pain scale.

(continued)

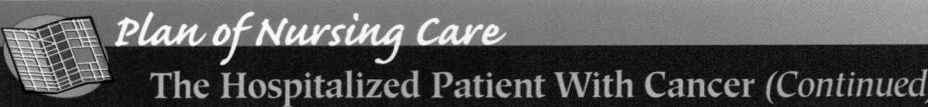

Plan of Nursing Care
The Hospitalized Patient With Cancer *(Continued)*

Nursing Interventions	Rationale	Expected Outcomes
2. Assure patient that you know that pain is real and will assist him or her in reducing it.	2. Fear that pain will not be considered real increases anxiety and reduces pain tolerance.	• Reports less disruption from pain and discomfort.
3. Assess other factors contributing to patient's pain: fear, fatigue, anger, etc.	3. Provides data about factors that decrease patient's ability to tolerate pain and increase pain level.	• Explains how fatigue, fear, anger, etc., contribute to severity of pain and discomfort.
4. Administer analgesics to promote optimum pain relief within limits of physician's prescription.	4. Analgesics tend to be more effective when administered early in pain cycle.	• Accepts pain medication as prescribed. • Exhibits decreased physical and behavioral signs of pain and discomfort in acute pain (no grimacing, crying, moaning; displays interest in surroundings and activities around him).
5. Assess patient's behavioural responses to pain and pain experience.	5. Provides additional information about patient's pain.	• Takes an active role in administration of analgesia.
6. Collaborate with patient, physician, and other health care team members when changes in pain management are necessary.	6. New methods of administering analgesia must be acceptable to patient, physician, and health care team to be effective; patient's participation decreases the sense of powerlessness.	• Identifies additional effective pain relief strategies. • Uses alternative pain relief strategies appropriately.
7. Encourage strategies of pain relief that patient has used successfully in previous pain experience.	7. Encourages success of pain relief strategies accepted by patient and family.	• Reports effective use of new pain relief strategies and decrease in pain intensity.
8. Teach patient new strategies to relieve pain and discomfort: distraction, imagery, relaxation, cutaneous stimulation, etc.	8. Increases number of options and strategies available to patient.	• Reports that decreased level of pain permits participation in other activities and events.

Nursing Diagnosis: Anticipatory grieving related to loss; altered role functioning
Goal: Appropriate progression through grieving process

1. Encourage verbalization of fears, concerns, and questions regarding disease, treatment, and future implications.	1. An increased and accurate knowledge base decreases anxiety and dispels misconceptions.	• The patient and family progress through the phases of grief as evidenced by increased verbalization and expression of grief.
2. Encourage active participation of patient or family in care and treatment decisions.	2. Active participation maintains patient independence and control.	• The patient and family identify resources available to aid coping strategies during grieving.
3. Visit family frequently to establish and maintain relationships and physical closeness.	3. Frequent contacts promote trust and security and reduce feelings of fear and isolation.	• The patient and family use resources and supports appropriately.
4. Encourage ventilation of negative feelings, including projected anger and hostility, within acceptable limits.	4. This allows for emotional expression without loss of self-esteem.	• The patient and family discuss the future openly with each other.
5. Allow for periods of crying and expression of sadness.	5. These feelings are necessary for separation and detachment to occur.	• The patient and family discuss concerns and feelings openly with each other.
6. Involve clergy as desired by the patient and family.	6. This facilitates the grief process and spiritual care.	• The patient and family use nonverbal expressions of concern for each other.
7. Advise professional counselling as indicated for patient or family to alleviate pathologic grieving.	7. This facilitates the grief process.	
8. Allow for progression through the grieving process at the individual pace of the patient and family.	8. Grief work is variable. Not every person uses every phase of the grief process, and the time spent in dealing with each phase varies with every person. To complete grief work, this variability must be allowed.	

Nursing Diagnosis: Disturbed body image and situational low self-esteem related to changes in appearance, function, and roles
Goal: Improved body image and self-esteem

1. Assess patient's feelings about body image and level of self-esteem.	1. Provides baseline assessment for evaluating changes and assessing effectiveness of interventions.	• Identifies concerns of importance. • Takes active role in activities. • Maintains previous role in decision making.

(continued)

Plan of Nursing Care
The Hospitalized Patient With Cancer *(Continued)*

Nursing Interventions	Rationale	Expected Outcomes
2. Identify potential threats to patient's self-esteem (eg, altered appearance, decreased sexual function, hair loss, decreased energy, role changes). Validate concerns with patient.	2. Anticipates changes and permits patient to identify importance of these areas to him or her.	• Verbalizes feelings and reactions to losses or threatened losses. • Participates in self-care activities. • Permits others to assist in care when he or she is unable to be independent.
3. Encourage continued participation in activities and decision making.	3. Encourages and permits continued control of events and self.	• Exhibits interest in appearance and uses aids (cosmetics, scarves, etc.) appropriately.
4. Encourage patient to verbalize concerns.	4. Identifying concerns is an important step in coping with them.	• Participates with others in conversations and social events and activities.
5. Individualize care for the patient.	5. Prevents or reduces depersonalization and emphasizes patient's self-worth.	• Verbalizes concern about sexual partner and/or significant others.
6. Assist patient in self-care when fatigue, lethargy, nausea, vomiting, and other symptoms prevent independence.	6. Physical well-being improves self-esteem.	• Explores alternative ways of expressing concern and affection.
7. Assist patient in selecting and using cosmetics, scarves, hair pieces, and clothing that increase his or her sense of attractiveness.	7. Promotes positive body image.	
8. Encourage patient and partner to share concerns about altered sexuality and sexual function and to explore alternatives to their usual sexual expression.	8. Provides opportunity for expressing concern, affection, and acceptance.	

Collaborative Problem: Potential complication: risk for bleeding problems
Goal: Prevention of bleeding

1. Assess for potential for bleeding: monitor platelet count.	1. Platelet counts of less than 10×10^9/L associated with spontaneous bleeding.	• Signs and symptoms of bleeding are identified.
2. Assess for bleeding:	2. Early detection promotes early intervention.	• Exhibits no blood in feces, urine, or emesis.
		• Exhibits no bleeding of gums or of injection or venipuncture sites.
a. Petechiae or ecchymosis	a. Indicates injury to microcirculation and larger vessels.	• Exhibits no ecchymosis (bruising).
b. Decrease in hemoglobin or hematocrit	b. Indicates blood loss.	• Patient and family identify ways to prevent bleeding.
c. Prolonged bleeding from invasive procedures, venipunctures, minor cuts or scratches		• Uses recommended measures to reduce risk of bleeding (uses soft toothbrush, shaves with electric razor only).
d. Frank or occult blood in any body excretion, emesis, sputum		• Exhibits normal vital signs.
e. Bleeding from any body orifice		• Reports that environmental hazards have been reduced or removed.
f. Altered mental status	f. Indicates neurologic involvement.	• Consumes adequate fluid.
3. Instruct patient and family about ways to minimize bleeding:	3. Patient can participate in self-protection.	• Reports absence of constipation.
a. Use soft toothbrush or toothette for mouth care.	a. Prevents trauma to oral tissues.	• Avoids substances interfering with clotting.
b. Avoid commercial mouthwashes.	b. Contain high alcohol content that will dry oral tissues.	• Absence of tissue destruction.
c. Use electric razor for shaving.	c. Prevents trauma to skin.	• Exhibits normal mental status and absence of signs of intracranial bleeding.
d. Use emery board for nail care.	d. Reduces risk of trauma to nailbeds.	• Avoids medications that interfere with clotting (eg, aspirin).
e. Avoid foods that are difficult to chew.	e. Prevents oral tissue trauma.	• Absence of epistaxis and cerebral bleeding.
4. Initiate measures to minimize bleeding.	4. Preserves circulating blood volume.	
a. Draw all blood for lab work with one daily venipuncture.	a. Minimizes trauma and blood loss.	
b. Avoid taking temperature rectally or administering suppositories and enemas.	b. Prevents trauma to rectal mucosa.	

(continued)

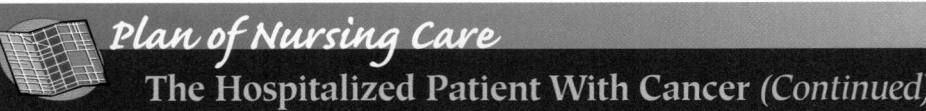

Plan of Nursing Care
The Hospitalized Patient With Cancer (Continued)

Nursing Interventions	Rationale	Expected Outcomes
c. Avoid intramuscular injections; use smallest needle possible.	c. Prevents intramuscular bleeding.	
d. Apply direct pressure to injection and venipuncture sites for at least 5 min.	d. Minimizes blood loss.	
e. Lubricate lips with petrolatum.	e. Prevents skin from drying.	
f. Avoid bladder catheterizations; use smallest catheter if catheterization is necessary.	f. Prevents trauma to urethra.	
g. Maintain fluid intake of at least 3 L/24 h unless contraindicated.	g. Hydration helps to prevent skin drying.	
h. Use stool softeners or increase bulk in diet.	h. Prevents constipation and straining that may injure rectal tissue.	
i. Avoid medications that will interfere with clotting (eg, aspirin).	i. Minimizes risk of bleeding.	
j. Recommend use of water-based lubricant before sexual intercourse.	j. Prevents friction and tissue trauma.	
5. When platelet count is less than 10×10^9/L, institute the following:	5. Platelet count of less than 10×10^9/L is associated with increased of spontaneous bleeding.	
a. Bed rest with padded side rails	a. Reduces risk of injury	
b. Avoidance of strenuous activity	b. Increases intracranial pressure and risk of cerebral hemorrhage.	
c. Platelet transfusions as prescribed; administer prescribed diphenhydramine hydrochloride (Benadryl) or hydrocortisone sodium succinate (Solu-Cortef) to prevent reaction to platelet transfusion.	c. Allergic reactions to blood products are associated with antigen–antibody reaction that causes platelet destruction.	
d. Supervise activity when out of bed.		
e. Caution against forceful nose blowing.	e. Prevents trauma to nasal mucosa and increased intracranial pressure.	

Before engraftment, patients are at a high risk for infection, sepsis, and bleeding. Side effects of the high-dose chemotherapy and total body irradiation can be acute and chronic. Acute side effects include alopecia, hemorrhagic cystitis, nausea, vomiting, diarrhea, and severe stomatitis. Chronic side effects include sterility, pulmonary dysfunction, cardiac dysfunction, and liver disease. Patients receive immunosuppressant drugs, such as cyclosporine, tacrolimus (FK 506), or azathioprine (Imuran), to prevent graft-versus-host disease (GVHD). In allogeneic transplant recipients, GVHD occurs when the T lymphocytes from the transplanted donor marrow become activated and mount an immune response against the recipient's tissues (skin, gastrointestinal tract, liver). T lymphocytes respond in this manner because they view the recipient's tissue as "foreign," immunologically differing from what they recognize as "self" in the donor. GVHD may occur acutely or chronically. The first 100 days or so after allogeneic transplantation are crucial for BMT patients until the immune system and blood-making capacity (hematopoiesis) have recovered sufficiently to prevent infection and hemorrhage. Most acute side effects, such as nausea, vomiting, and mucositis, also resolve in the initial 100 days after transplantation. Patients are also at risk for development of venous occlusive disease (VOD), a vascular injury to the liver from the high-dose chemotherapy occurring in the first 100 days or so after BMT. VOD can lead to acute liver failure and death.

Autologous BMT is considered for patients with disease of the bone marrow who do not have a suitable donor for allogeneic BMT and for patients who have healthy bone marrow but require bone marrow–ablative doses of chemotherapy to cure an aggressive malignancy. Stem cells are collected from the patient and preserved for reinfusion and, if necessary, treated to kill any malignant cells within the marrow. The patient is treated with ablative chemotherapy and, possibly, total body irradiation to eradicate any remaining tumour. The stem cells are then reinfused and engrafted. Until engraftment occurs in the bone marrow sites of the body, the patient is at high risk for infection, sepsis, and bleeding. Acute and chronic toxicities from chemotherapy and radiation therapy may be severe. The risk of VOD is also present after an autologous transplant. No immunosuppressant medications are necessary after autologous BMT because the patient did not receive foreign tissue. A disadvantage of autologous transplantation is the risk that viable tumour cells may remain in the bone marrow despite conditioning regimens (high-dose chemotherapy).

Syngeneic BMT is the least common type of transplantation because it requires an identical sibling for harvest. Syngeneic transplantations result in fewer complications and no marrow rejection because the donor is an identical tissue match to the recipient. The transplantation and collection processes are the same with syngeneic BMT as with allogeneic BMT.

Nursing Management in Bone Marrow Transplantation

Nursing care of patients undergoing BMT is complex and demands a high level of skill. Transplantation nursing can be extremely rewarding yet extremely stressful. The success of BMT is greatly influenced by nursing care throughout the transplantation process.

IMPLEMENTING PRETRANSPLANTATION CARE

All patients must undergo extensive pretransplantation evaluations to assess the current clinical status of the disease. Nutritional assessments, extensive physical examinations and organ function tests, and psychological evaluations are conducted. Blood work includes assessing past antigen exposure (for example, to hepatitis virus, cytomegalovirus, herpes simplex virus, HIV, and syphilis). The patient's social support systems and financial and insurance resources are also evaluated. Informed consent and patient teaching about the procedure and pretransplantation and posttransplantation care are vital.

PROVIDING CARE DURING TREATMENT

Skilled nursing care is required during the treatment phase of BMT when high-dose chemotherapy (conditioning regimen) and total body irradiation are administered. The acute toxicities of nausea, diarrhea, mucositis, and hemorrhagic cystitis require close monitoring and constant attention by the nurse.

Nursing management during the bone marrow or stem cell infusions consists of monitoring the patient's vital signs and blood oxygen saturation; assessing for adverse effects, such as fever, chills, shortness of breath, chest pain, cutaneous reactions, nausea, vomiting, hypotension or hypertension, tachycardia, anxiety, and taste changes; and providing ongoing support and patient teaching.

Throughout the period of bone marrow aplasia until engraftment of the new marrow occurs, patients are at high risk for dying of sepsis and bleeding. Patients require support with blood products and hemopoietic growth factors. Potential infection may be bacterial, viral, fungal, or protozoan in origin. Renal complications arise from the nephrotoxic chemotherapy agents used in the conditioning regimen or those used to treat infection (amphotericin B, aminoglycosides). Tumour lysis syndrome and acute tubular necrosis are also risks after BMT.

GVHD requires skillful nursing assessment to detect early effects on the skin, liver, and gastrointestinal tract. VOD resulting from the conditioning regimens used in BMT can result in fluid retention, jaundice, abdominal pain, ascites, tender and enlarged liver, and encephalopathy. Pulmonary complications, such as pulmonary edema, interstitial pneumonia, and other pneumonias, often complicate the recovery after BMT.

Providing Posttransplantation Care

Ongoing nursing assessment in follow-up visits is essential to detect late effects of therapy in BMT patients. Late complications are those that occur 100 days or more after BMT. Late effects include infections, such as varicella zoster infection, restrictive pulmonary abnormalities, and recurrent pneumonias. Sterility often results. Chronic GVHD involves the skin, liver, intestine, esophagus, eye, lungs, joints, and vaginal mucosa. Cataracts may also develop after total body irradiation.

Psychosocial assessments by nursing staff must be ongoing. In addition to the stressors affecting patients at each phase of the transplantation experience, marrow donors and family members also have psychosocial needs that must be addressed.

CARING FOR THE DONORS

Donors commonly experience mood alterations, decreased self-esteem, and guilt from feelings of failure if the transplantation fails. Family members must be educated and supported to reduce anxiety and promote coping during this difficult time. Family members must also be assisted to maintain realistic expectations of themselves as well as of the patient.

As BMT becomes more prevalent, many moral and ethical issues become apparent, including those related to informed consent, allocation of resources, and quality of life.

HYPERTHERMIA

Hyperthermia (thermal therapy), the generation of temperatures greater than physiologic fever range (above 41.5°C), has been used for many years to destroy tumours in human cancers. Malignant cells may be more sensitive than normal cells to the harmful effects of high temperatures for several reasons. Malignant cells lack the repair mechanisms necessary to repair cell damage by elevated temperatures. Most tumour cells lack an adequate blood supply to provide needed oxygen during periods of increased cellular demand, such as during hyperthermia. Cancerous tumours lack blood vessels of adequate size for dissipation of heat. In addition, the body's immune system may be indirectly stimulated when hyperthermia is used.

Hyperthermia is most effective when combined with radiation therapy, chemotherapy, or biologic therapy. Hyperthermia and radiation therapy are thought to work well together because hypoxic tumour cells and cells in the S phase of the cell cycle are more sensitive to heat than radiation; the addition of heat damages tumour cells so that they cannot repair themselves after radiation therapy. Hyperthermia is thought to alter cellular membrane permeability when used with chemotherapy, allowing for an increased uptake of the chemotherapeutic agent. Hyperthermia may enhance function of immune system cells, such as macrophages and T cells, which are stimulated by many biologic agents.

Heat can be produced by using radiowaves, ultrasound, microwaves, magnetic waves, hot-water baths, or even hot-wax immersions. Hyperthermia may be local or regional, or it may include the whole body. Local or regional hyperthermia may be delivered to a cancerous extremity (for malignant melanoma) by regional perfusion, in which the affected extremity is isolated by a tourniquet and an extracorporeal circulator heats the blood flowing through the affected part. Hyperthermia probes may also be inserted around a tumour in a local area and attached to a heat source during treatment. Chemotherapeutic agents, such as melphalan (Alkeran), may also be heated and instilled into the region's circulating blood. Local or regional hyperthermia may also include infusion of heated solutions into cancerous body organs. Whole-body hyperthermia to treat disseminated disease may be achieved by extracorporeal circulation, immersion of patients in heated water or paraffin, or enclosure in heated suits.

Side effects of hyperthermic treatments include skin burns and tissue damage, fatigue, hypotension, peripheral neuropathies, thrombophlebitis, nausea, vomiting, diarrhea, and electrolyte imbalances. Resistance to hyperthermia may develop during the treatment because cells adapt to repeated thermal insult. Research into the effectiveness of hyperthermia, methods of delivery, and side effects is ongoing.

Nursing Management in Hyperthermia

Although hyperthermia has been used for many years, many patients and their families are unfamiliar with this cancer treatment. Consequently, they need explanations about the procedure, its goals, and its effects. The patient is assessed for adverse effects, and efforts are made to reduce their occurrence and severity. Local skin care at the site of the implanted hyperthermic probes is also required.

BIOLOGIC RESPONSE MODIFIERS

Biologic response modifier (BRM) therapy involves the use of naturally occurring or recombinant (reproduced through genetic engineering) agents or treatment methods that can alter the immunologic relationship between the tumour and the cancer patient (host) to provide a therapeutic benefit. Although the mechanisms of action vary with each type of BRM, the goal is to destroy or stop the malignant growth. The basis of BRM treatment lies in the restoration, modification, stimulation, or augmentation of the body's natural immune defenses against cancer.

Nonspecific Biologic Response Modifiers

Some of the early investigations of the stimulation of the immune system involved nonspecific agents such as Bacille Calmette-Guérin (BCG) and *Corynebacterium parvum*. When injected into the patient, these agents serve as antigens that stimulate an immune response. The hope is that the stimulated immune system will then eradicate malignant cells. Extensive animal and human investigations with BCG have shown promising results, especially in treating localized malignant melanoma. Additionally, BCG is considered to be a standard form of treatment for localized bladder cancer. Use of nonspecific agents in advanced cancer remains limited, however, and research is continuing in an effort to identify other uses and other agents.

Monoclonal Antibodies

Monoclonal antibodies (MoAbs), another type of BRM, became available through technological advances, enabling investigators to grow and produce specific antibodies for specific malignant cells. Theoretically, this type of specificity allows the MoAb to destroy the cancer cells and spare normal cells. The production of MoAbs involves injecting tumour cells that act as antigens into mice. Antibodies made in response to injected antigens can be found in the spleen of the mouse. Antibody-producing spleen cells are combined with a cancer cell that has the ability to grow indefinitely in culture medium and continue producing more antibodies. The combination of spleen cells and the cancer cells is referred to as a hybridoma. From hybridomas that continue to grow in the culture medium, the desired antibodies are harvested, purified, and prepared for diagnostic or therapeutic use (Fig. 16-5). Alternative methods of producing MoAbs using human or genetically engineered sources are under investigation.

FIGURE 16-5 Antibody-producing spleen cells are fused with cancer cells. This process produces cells called hybridomas. These cells, which can grow indefinitely in a culture medium, produce antibodies that are harvested, purified, and prepared for diagnostic or treatment purposes.

MoAbs are being used as aids in diagnostic evaluation. By attaching a radioactive substance to the MoAb, physicians can detect both primary and metastatic tumours through radiologic techniques. This process is referred to as radioimmunodetection. OncoScint (Cytogen Corp., Princeton, NJ) is a U.S. Food and Drug Administration (FDA)-approved MoAb that is used to assist in diagnosing ovarian and colorectal cancers. The use of MoAbs in detecting breast, gastric, and prostate cancers and lymphoma is under investigation. MoAbs are also used in purging residual tumour cells from the bone marrow or peripheral blood of patients who are undergoing BMT for peripheral stem cell rescue after high-dose cytotoxic therapy.

Several MoAbs have been approved for treatment in cancer. Rituximab (Rituxan) is used for the treatment of relapsed or refractory non-Hodgkin's lymphoma (Kosits & Callaghan, 2000). Trastuzumab (Herceptin) is approved as a single agent or given in addition to chemotherapy for the treatment of some types of metastatic breast cancer (Yarbro, 2000). Alemtuzumab (Campath) is used in the treatment of some forms of leukemia (Seeley & DeMeyer, 2002). Gemtuzumab ozogomicin (Mylotarg) is a combination of a MoAb and the antitumour antibiotic calicheamicin, which is used for the treatment of a specific type of acute myeloid leukemia (Sorokin, 2000). Gemtuzumab ozogomicin is an example of immunoconjugate therapy or a "magic bullet" that transports cancer-killing substances to the cancer cells. Ibritumomab-tiuxetan (Zevalin) is another form of immunoconjugate therapy that combines a monoclonal antibody and a radioactive source for the treatment of specific types of non-Hodgkin's lymphoma. The monoclonal antibody delivers the radioactive source to the malignant cells, causing the cells to be destroyed by both radioactivity and normal immune responses (Estes, 2002). Researchers are continuing to explore the development and use of other MoAbs either alone or in combination with other substances such as radioactive materials, chemotherapeutic agents, toxins, hormones, or other BRMs.

Cytokines

Cytokines, substances produced by cells of the immune system to enhance the production and functioning of components of the immune system, are also the focus of cancer treatment research. Cytokines are grouped into families, such as interferons, interleukins, colony-stimulating factors, and tumour necrosis factors (TNFs).

INTERFERON

Interferons (IFNs) are examples of cytokines with both antiviral and antitumour properties. When stimulated, all nucleated cells are capable of producing these glycoproteins, which are classified according to their biologic and chemical properties: IFN-α is produced by leukocytes, IFN-β is produced by fibroblasts, and IFN-γ is produced by lymphocytes.

Although the exact antitumour effects of IFNs have not been thoroughly established, it is thought that they either stimulate the immune system or assist in preventing tumour growth. The antitumour effects are dependent on the type of IFN and the disease for which IFN is being used. IFNs enhance both lymphocyte and antibody production. They also facilitate the cytolytic or cell destruction role of macrophages and natural killer cells. Additionally, IFNs can inhibit cell multiplication by increasing the duration of various phases of the cell cycle.

The effects of IFN have been demonstrated in a variety of malignancies. IFN-α has been approved by the FDA for treating hairy-cell leukemia, Kaposi's sarcoma, chronic myelogenous leukemia, high-grade non-Hodgkin's lymphoma, and melanoma. Other positive responses have been seen in hematologic malignancies and renal carcinomas. IFN-α, IFN-β, and IFN-γ have been approved by the FDA for the treatment of several nonmalignant diseases. IFN is administered through subcutaneous, intramuscular, intravenous, and intracavitary routes. Efforts are underway to establish the effectiveness of IFN for various malignancies in combination with other treatment regimens.

INTERLEUKINS

Interleukins are a subgroup of cytokines known as lymphokines and monokines because they are primarily produced by lymphocytes and monocytes. About 15 different interleukins have been identified. They act by signaling and coordinating other cells of the immune system. The FDA has approved interleukin-2 (IL-2) as a treatment option for renal cell cancer and metastatic melanoma in adults. Originally referred to as T-cell growth factor, IL-2 is known to stimulate the production and activation of several different types of lymphocytes. In addition, IL-2 enhances the production of other types of cytokines and plays a role in influencing both humoural and cell-mediated immunity.

Clinical trials are being conducted on IL-2 as well as other interleukins, such as IL-1, IL-4, and IL-6, for their roles in treating other cancers. Some early-stage clinical trials are assessing the effects of interleukins in combination with chemotherapy. In addition, interleukins are being investigated for their role as growth factors for treating myelosuppression after the use of some forms of chemotherapy.

HEMATOPOIETIC GROWTH FACTORS (COLONY-STIMULATING FACTORS)

Hematopoietic growth factors, also known as colony-stimulating factors, are hormone-like substances naturally produced by cells within the immune system. Hematopoietic growth factors of different types regulate the production of all cells in the blood, including neutrophils, macrophages, monocytes, red blood cells, and platelets. FDA approval of GM-CSF, G-CSF, IL-11, and EPO (Epogen) has contributed significantly to the supportive care of patients with cancer.

Although these agents do not treat the underlying malignancy, they do target the effects of myelotoxic cancer therapies (adversely affecting the bone marrow), such as radiation and chemotherapy. Previously, the myelotoxic or bone marrow suppressive effects of chemotherapy had imposed limits on some chemotherapy agents and contributed to the development of life-threatening infections.

GM-CSF is used to treat the **neutropenia** (decreased numbers of neutrophils in the blood) associated with BMT. G-CSF is used to treat neutropenia associated with chemotherapy for solid tumour malignancies. IL-11 is used to prevent severe thrombocytopenia and reduce the need for platelet transfusions in patients following myelosuppressive therapy for nonmyeloid cancers. EPO is used to treat anemia in cancer patients as well as in patients with chronic renal disease and in patients with HIV infection with zidovudine-induced anemia. Other growth factors, such as macrophage colony-stimulating factor and IL-3, are being investigated.

TUMOUR NECROSIS FACTOR

TNF is a cytokine naturally produced by macrophages, lymphocytes, astrocytes, and microglial cells of the brain. The exact role of TNF is still under investigation. In vitro studies have shown

TNF to stimulate other cells of the immune response; in animal studies it has been shown to have direct tumour-killing activity. Clinical trials using systemic TNF have been halted because of severe toxicities (Pazadur, Coia, Hoskins & Wagman, 2001). Current clinical trials are examining local administration of TNF for patients with sarcomas and melanomas of the extremities.

Retinoids

Retinoids are vitamin A derivatives (retinol, all-*trans*-retinoic acid, and 13-*cis*-retinoic acid) that play a role in growth, reproduction, epithelial cell differentiation, and immune function. All-*trans*-retinoic acid (tretinoin) has been granted FDA approval for treating acute promyelocytic leukemia, a rare form of leukemia. Retinoids are being tested for treating both hematologic cancers and solid tumours and for preventing a variety of cancers (Evans & Kaye, 1999; Kelloff, 2000; Kurie, 1999).

Nursing Management in Biologic Response Modifier Therapy

Patients receiving BRM therapy have many of the same needs as cancer patients undergoing other treatment approaches. However, some BRM therapies are still investigational and considered a last-chance effort by many patients who have not responded to standard treatments. Consequently, it is essential that the nurse assess the need for education, support, and guidance for both the patient and family and assist in planning and evaluating patient care.

MONITORING THERAPEUTIC AND ADVERSE EFFECTS

Nurses need to be familiar with each agent given and the potential effects (Table 16-7). Adverse effects, such as fever, myalgia, nausea, and vomiting, as seen with IFN therapy, may not be life-threatening. However, nurses must be aware of the impact of

---

Table 16-7 • **Side Effects of FDA-Approved Biologic Response Modifiers**

AGENT	SELECTED SIDE EFFECTS
Monoclonal Antibodies	
Rituximab	Allergic/anaphylactic reactions; fever; chills; nausea; headache; abdominal pain; decreased lymphocyte, white blood cell, platelet, and red blood cell counts; back pain; night sweats; itching; cough; infection
Trastuzumab	Allergic/anaphylactic reactions, hypotension, fever, chills, heart failure, stroke, diarrhea, infection, rash, nausea, vomiting, anorexia, insomnia, dizziness, headache, chills, back pain, weakness, rhinitis, pharyngitis, cough
Gemtuzumab	Allergic/anaphylactic reactions; fever; chills; weakness; abdominal pain; headache; dyspnea; epistaxis; cough; tachycardia; hemorrhage; local skin reaction; rash; petechiae; peripheral edema; nausea; vomiting; diarrhea; anorexia; stomatitis; constipation; indigestion; dizziness; decreased platelet, white and red blood cell counts; increased bilirubin, potassium, and LDH values
Alemtuzumab	Allergic/anaphylactic reactions, fever, chills, rash, hives, itching, sweating, nausea, vomiting, diarrhea, stomatitis, abdominal pain, indigestion, infection, headache, dizziness, muscle pain, insomnia, dyspnea, cough, bronchitis/pneumonitis, pharyngitis, fatigue, skeletal pain, anorexia, weakness, peripheral edema, decreased white, platelet, and red blood cell counts
Ibritumomab	Decreased platelets, white blood cell and red blood cell counts, weakness, chills, abdominal pain, fever, difficulty breathing, nausea and vomiting
Cytokines	
Interferon alfa	Flu-like symptoms (fever, chills, weakness, muscle and joint pain, headaches); fatigue; anorexia; mental status changes; rash; pruritus; hair loss; abdominal pain; nausea; constipation; diarrhea; irritation at the injection site; depression; irritability; insomnia; cough; decreased white blood cell, red blood cell, and platelet counts; abnormal liver function values
Interleukin-2	Flu-like symptoms (fever, chills, weakness, muscle and joint pain, headaches); fatigue; anorexia; nausea; vomiting; diarrhea; capillary leak syndrome; edema and fluid retention; hypotension; tachycardia; skin rash; erythema; desquamation; irritation at the injection site; weight gain during therapy due to fluid retention; weight loss after therapy related to anorexia with long-term therapy; decreased white blood cell, red blood cell, and platelet counts; abnormal liver function values
Filgrastim (granulocyte growth factor)	Bone pain, malaise, fever, fatigue, headache, skin rash, weakness
Sargranstim (granulocyte-macrophage growth factor)	Allergic/anaphylactic reaction with first dose, bone pain, fever, fatigue, headache, weakness, chills, skin rash, infection
Epoetin alfa (erythrocyte growth factor)	Fever, fatigue, weakness, bone pain, diarrhea, dizziness, nausea, edema, shortness of breath
Oprelvekin (platelet growth factor)	Edema, fever, headache, rash, chills, bone pain, fatigue, nausea, vomiting, abdominal pain, constipation, rhinitis, cough, arrhythmia, skin discolouration, bleeding, dehydration, amblyopia, dermatitis
Retinoids	
Retinoic acid	Headache, fever, skin and mucous membrane dryness, bone pain, nausea and vomiting, dyspnea, pleural and pericardial effusions, malaise, chills, bleeding, heart failure, mental status changes, depression, abnormal liver function tests

these side effects on the patient's quality of life. Other life-threatening adverse effects (eg, capillary leak syndrome, pulmonary edema, and hypotension) may occur with IL-2 therapy. Nurses must work closely with physicians to assess and manage potential toxicities of BRM therapy. Because of the investigational nature of many of these agents, the nurse will be administering them in a research setting. Accurate observations and careful documentation are essential components of patient assessment and data collection.

PROMOTING HOME AND COMMUNITY-BASED CARE

Teaching Patients Self-Care. Some BRMs, such as IFN, EPO, and G-CSF, can be administered by the patient or family in the home. Nurses teach patients and families, as needed, how to administer these agents through subcutaneous injections. Further, they provide instructions about side effects and assist patients and families to identify strategies to manage many of the common side effects of BRM therapy, such as fatigue, anorexia, and flu-like symptoms.

Continuing Care. Referral for home care is usually indicated to monitor the patient's responses to treatment and continue and reinforce teaching. During home visits, the nurse assesses the patient's and family's technique in administering medications. The nurse collaborates with physicians, third-party payors, and pharmaceutical companies to help patients obtain reimbursement for home administration of BRM therapies. The nurse also reminds patients about the importance of keeping follow-up appointments with the physician and assesses the patient's need for changes in care.

PHOTODYNAMIC THERAPY

Photodynamic therapy, or phototherapy, is an investigational cancer treatment that uses photosensitizing agents, such as porfimer (Photofrin). When administered intravenously, these agents are retained in higher concentrations in malignant tissue than in normal tissue. They are then activated by a light source, usually laser light, which penetrates body tissue. The light-activated agent then creates activated singlet oxygen molecules that are cytotoxic or harmful to body tissue cells. Because most of the photosensitizing agent has been retained in malignant tissue, a selective cytotoxicity can be achieved with minimal destruction to normal tissues.

Cancers treated with phototherapy include esophageal cancers, endobronchial tumours, skin cancers, breast cancers, intraperitoneal tumours, and malignant central nervous system disease. The major side effect of therapy is photosensitivity for 4 to 6 weeks after treatment. Patients must protect themselves from direct and indirect sunlight to prevent skin burns. In addition, local reactions are observed in the area treated. Liver and renal function should also be monitored for transient abnormalities. As with any investigational treatment, emotional support and education are vital to assist the patient and family.

GENE THERAPY

As early as 1914, the somatic mutation theory of cancer suggested that cancer develops as a result of inherited or acquired genetic mutations that lead to a disturbance in the normal chromosomal balance regulating cell growth and reproduction. Technological advances and information gained through in-

tense study of genetics have assisted researchers and clinicians in predicting, diagnosing, and treating cancer. Gene therapy includes approaches that correct genetic defects or manipulate genes to induce tumour cell destruction in the hope of preventing or combating disease. Human germ cell manipulation is considered by many to be controversial and a potential source of bioethical concerns (Frankel & Chapman, 2000).

Although gene therapy is currently investigational, researchers predict it will have a profound impact on medical and health care in the 21st century. More than 100 clinical trials for gene therapy in treating cancer have been initiated. An example of one such trial involves inserting the p53 tumour suppressor gene into cancer cells. Normally this gene is responsible for repairing damaged cells or causing cell death when the cell cannot be repaired. Many types of cancer cells have mutated p53 genes that then lead to uncontrolled cell growth. Insertion of normal p53 genes can lead to either cancer cell death or slowing of tumour growth. This approach has been tested in lung, head and neck, and colon cancers (Wasil & Buchbinder, 2000). In another clinical trial, a "suicide gene" is inserted into tumour cells to facilitate cell death. When the gene for herpes simplex virus thymidine kinase is inserted into malignant cells, those cells become infected with the virus and susceptible to destruction by antiviral drugs, such as ganciclovir. This approach has been tried in treating brain, ovarian, and breast cancers (Fibison, 2000). For more information about investigational therapies, see Chart 16-4.

UNPROVEN AND UNCONVENTIONAL THERAPIES

A diagnosis of cancer evokes many emotions in patients and families, including feelings of fear, frustration, and loss of control. Despite increasing 5-year survival rates with the use of traditional methods of treatment, a significant number of patients use or seriously consider using some form of unconventional treatment. Hopelessness, desperation, unmet needs, lack of factual information, and family or social pressures are major factors that motivate patients to seek unconventional methods of treatment. Although research is scant and accuracy of reporting may be questionable, it is estimated that 30% to 50% of patients with cancer may be using a complementary or alternative method of treatment.

Caring for patients who choose unconventional methods may place members of the health care team in difficult situations professionally, legally, and ethically. Some complementary therapies may interact adversely with standard therapy. Nurses must keep in mind those ethical principles that help guide professional practice, such as autonomy, beneficence, nonmaleficence, and justice.

Unconventional treatments have not yet demonstrated scientifically, in an objective, reproducible way, the ability to cure or control cancer, but a number of studies are in progress. Most unproven cancer treatments can be categorized as machines and devices, drugs and biologicals, metabolic and dietary regimens, or mystical and spiritual approaches.

Machines and Devices

Electrical gadgets and devices are commonly reputed to cure cancers. Most are operated by people with questionable training who report unrealistic and unlikely success stories. Such machines are often decorated with elaborate lights and dials and produce vibrations or other sensations.

Drugs and Biologicals

Medicinal agents, herbs, proteins (such as shark cartilage), mega-vitamins (including vitamin C therapy), immune therapy, vaccines, enzymes, hydrogen peroxide, and sera have been frequent components of fraudulent cancer therapy. These agents have included oral, intravenous, and external medications derived from weeds, flowers, and herbs and the blood and urine of patients and animals. Many of these agents, especially in megadoses, can be toxic and can have untoward interactions with concomitant medications. Herbs commonly used by individuals with cancer include echinacea, essiac, ginseng, green tea, pau d'arco, and hoxsey (Montbriand, 1999). Many of these treatments are costly.

Metabolic and Dietary Regimens

Metabolic and dietary regimens emphasize the ingestion of only natural substances to purify the body and retard cancerous growth. These regimens include the grape diet, the carrot juice diet, garlic, onions, various teas, coffee enemas, and raw liver intake. Laetrile (vitamin B, amygdalin), one of the best-known forms of cancer quackery, was advocated as an agent to kill tumour cells by releasing cyanide, which is especially toxic to malignant cells. The National Cancer Institute, in response to public demand, investigated the effects of laetrile and reported no therapeutic benefits with its use; indeed, many toxic effects (cyanide poisoning, fever, rash, headache, vomiting, diarrhea, and hypotension) were reported. Macrobiotic diets have also been advocated as a cancer treatment to reestablish balance between the major forces in the universe, yin and yang. People who adhere to macrobiotic diets tend to develop vitamin, mineral, and protein deficiencies; experience additional weight loss due to decreased calorie intake; and receive no therapeutic benefits from the diet.

Mystical and Spiritual Approaches

Traditional Chinese medicine attempts to balance chi forces in order to heal the body. Mystical or spiritual approaches to cancer therapy include such techniques as psychic surgery, faith healing, "laying on of hands," prayer groups, and invocation of mystical universal powers to kill cancerous growths. These techniques are difficult to disclaim because they are based on faith.

Nursing Management in Unconventional Therapies

A trusting relationship, supportive care, and promotion of hope in the patient and family are the most effective means of protecting them from fraudulent therapy and questionable cancer cures. Truthful responses given in a nonjudgmental manner to questions and inquiries about unproven methods of cancer treatments may alleviate the fear and guilt on the part of the patient and family that they are not "doing everything we can" to obtain a cure. The nurse may inform the patient and family of the characteristics common to fraudulent therapy so that they will be informed and cautious when evaluating other forms of "therapy." The nurse should encourage any patient who uses unconventional therapies to inform the physician about such use. Knowing this information can help prevent interactions with medications and other therapies that may be prescribed and avoid attributing the side effects of unconventional therapies to prescribed medications.

NURSING PROCESS: THE PATIENT WITH CANCER

The outlook for patients with cancer has greatly improved because of scientific and technological advances. As a result of the underlying disease or various treatment modalities, however, the patient with cancer may experience a variety of secondary problems, such as infection, reduced WBC counts, bleeding, skin problems, nutritional problems, pain, fatigue, and psychological stress.

Assessment

Regardless of the type of cancer treatment or prognosis, many patients with cancer are susceptible to the following problems and complications. An important role of the nurse on the oncology team is to assess the patient for these problems and complications.

INFECTION

In all stages of cancer, the nurse assesses factors that can promote infection. Infection is the leading cause of death in cancer patients. Factors predisposing patients to infection are summarized in Table 16-8. The nurse monitors laboratory studies to detect early changes in WBC counts. Common sites of infection, such as the pharynx, skin, perianal area, urinary tract, and respiratory tract, are assessed frequently. The typical signs of infection (swelling, redness, drainage, and pain), however, may not occur in the immunosuppressed patient due to a diminished local inflammatory response. Fever may be the only sign of infection that the patient exhibits. The nurse also monitors the patient for sepsis, particularly if invasive catheters or infusion lines are in place.

WBC function is often impaired in cancer patients. A decrease in circulating WBCs is referred to as leukopenia or granulocytopenia. There are three types of WBCs: neutrophils, basophils, and eosinophils. The neutrophils, totaling 60% to 70% of all the body's WBCs, play a major role in combating infection by engulfing and destroying infective agents in a process called phagocytosis. Both the total WBC count and the concentration of neutrophils are important in determining the patient's ability to fight infection.

A differential WBC count identifies the relative numbers of WBCs and permits tabulation of polymorphonuclear neutrophils (mature neutrophils, reported as "polys," PMNs, or "segs") and immature forms of neutrophils (reported as bands, metamyelocytes, and "stabs"). These numbers are compiled and reported as the absolute neutrophil count (ANC). The ANC is calculated by the following formula:

$$ANC = \frac{(\text{Total WBC count} \times [\%\text{ segmented neutrophils} + \%\text{ bands}])}{100}$$

For example, if the patient's total WBC count is 6.0×10^9/L, with segmented neutrophils 25% and bands 25%, the ANC would be 3.0×10^9/L.

Neutropenia, an abnormally low ANC, is associated with an increased risk for infection. The risk for infection rises as the ANC decreases and persists. An ANC of less than 1.0×10^9/L reflects a severe risk for infection. **Nadir** is the lowest ANC after myelosuppressive chemotherapy or radiation therapy. Therapies that suppress bone marrow function are called myelosuppressive. Febrile patients who are neutropenic are assessed for infection through cultures of blood, sputum, urine, stool, catheter, or wounds, if appropriate. In addition, a chest x-ray is often included to assess for pulmonary infections.

Table 16-8 • Factors Predisposing Cancer Patients to Infection

FACTORS	UNDERLYING MECHANISMS
1. Impaired skin and mucous membrane integrity	• Loss of body's first line of defense against invading organisms.
2. Chemotherapy	• Many agents cause suppression of bone marrow, resulting in decreased production and function of white blood cells. Chemotherapy agents that cause mucositis impair skin and mucous membrane integrity. Organ damage associated with certain agents may also predispose patients to infection. Organ damage such as pulmonary fibrosis or cardiomyopathy that is associated with certain agents may also predispose patients to infection.
3. Radiation therapy	• Radiation involving sites of bone marrow production may result in bone marrow suppression. May also lead to impaired tissue integrity.
4. Biologic response modifiers	• Some biologic response modifiers may cause bone marrow suppression and organ dysfunction.
5. Malignancy	• Malignant cells may infiltrate the bone marrow and interfere with production of white blood cells and lymphocytes. Hematologic malignancies (leukemias and lymphomas) are associated with impaired function and production of blood cells.
6. Malnutrition	• Results in impaired function and production of cells of the immune response. May contribute to impaired skin integrity.
7. Medications	• Antibiotics disturb the balance of normal flora, allowing them to become pathogenic. This process occurs most commonly in the gastrointestinal tract. Corticosteroids and nonsteroidal anti-inflammatory drugs mask inflammatory responses.
8. Urinary catheter	• Creates port and mechanism of entry for organisms.
9. Intravenous catheter	• Results in impaired skin integrity and site of entry for organisms.
10. Other invasive procedures (surgery, paracentesis, thoracentesis, drainage tubes, endoscopies, mechanical ventilation)	• Creates port of entry and possible introduction of exogenous organisms into the system.
11. Contaminated equipment	• Environmental objects such as stagnant water in oxygen equipment are associated with growth of microorganisms.
12. Age	• Increasing age associated with declining organ function. Also associated with decreased production and functioning of the cells of the immune system.
13. Chronic illness	• Associated with impaired organ function and altered immune responses.
14. Prolonged hospitalization	• Allows increased exposure to nosocomial infection and colonization of new organisms.

BLEEDING

The nurse assesses cancer patients for factors that may contribute to bleeding. These include bone marrow suppression from radiation, chemotherapy, and other medications that interfere with coagulation and platelet functioning, such as aspirin, dipyridamole (Persantine), heparin, or warfarin (Coumadin). Common bleeding sites include skin and mucous membranes; the intestinal, urinary, and respiratory tracts; and the brain. Gross hemorrhage, as well as blood in the stools, urine, sputum, or vomitus (melena, hematuria, hemoptysis, hematemesis), oozing at injection sites, bruising (ecchymosis), petechiae, and changes in mental status, are monitored and reported.

SKIN PROBLEMS

The integrity of skin and tissue is at risk in cancer patients because of the effects of chemotherapy, radiation therapy, surgery, and invasive procedures carried out for diagnosis and therapy. As part of the assessment, the nurse identifies which of these predisposing factors are present and assesses the patient for other risk factors, including nutritional deficits, bowel and bladder incontinence, immobility, immunosuppression, multiple skin folds, and changes related to aging. Skin lesions or ulcerations secondary to the tumour are noted. Alterations in tissue integrity throughout the gastrointestinal tract are particularly bothersome to the patient. Any lesions of the oral mucous membranes are noted, as are their effects on the patient's nutritional status and comfort level.

HAIR LOSS

Alopecia (hair loss) is another form of tissue disruption common to cancer patients who receive radiation therapy or chemotherapy. In addition to noting hair loss, the nurse also assesses the psychological impact of this side effect on the patient and the family.

NUTRITIONAL CONCERNS

Assessing the patient's nutritional status is an important nursing role. Impaired nutritional status may contribute to disease progression, immune incompetence, increased incidence of infection, delayed tissue repair, diminished functional ability, and decreased capacity to continue antineoplastic therapy. Altered nutritional status, weight loss, and cachexia (muscle wasting, emaciation) may be secondary to decreased protein and caloric intake, metabolic or mechanical effects of the cancer, systemic disease, side effects of the treatment, or the emotional status of the patient.

The patient's weight and caloric intake are monitored on a consistent basis. Other information obtained through assessment includes diet history, any episodes of anorexia, changes in appetite, situations and foods that aggravate or relieve anorexia, and medication history. Difficulty in chewing or swallowing is determined and the occurrence of nausea, vomiting, or diarrhea is noted.

Clinical and laboratory data useful in assessing the patient's nutritional status include anthropometric measurements (triceps skin fold and middle-upper arm circumference), serum protein levels (albumin and transferrin), serum electrolytes, lymphocyte count, skin response to intradermal injection of antigens, hemoglobin levels, hematocrit, urinary creatinine levels, and serum iron levels.

PAIN

Pain and discomfort in cancer may be related to the underlying disease, pressure exerted by the tumour, diagnostic procedures, or the cancer treatment itself. As in any other situation involving pain, cancer pain is affected by both physical and psychosocial influences.

In addition to assessing the source and site of pain, the nurse also assesses those factors that increase the patient's perception of pain, such as fear and apprehension, fatigue, anger, and social isolation. Pain assessment scales (see Chap. 13) are useful in assessing the patient's pain level before pain-relieving interventions are instituted and in evaluating their effectiveness.

FATIGUE

Acute fatigue, which occurs after an energy-demanding experience, serves a protective function; chronic fatigue, however, does not. It is often overwhelming, excessive, and not responsive to rest, and it seriously affects quality of life. Fatigue is the most commonly reported side effect in patients who receive chemotherapy and radiation therapy. The nurse assesses for feelings of weariness, weakness, lack of energy, inability to carry out necessary and valued daily functions, lack of motivation, and inability to concentrate. Patients may become less verbal and appear pallid, with relaxed facial musculature. Surprisingly, not all cancer patients experience fatigue. (See Nursing Research Profile 16-1.)

PSYCHOSOCIAL STATUS

Nursing assessment also focuses on the patient's psychological and mental status as the patient and the family face this life-threatening experience, unpleasant diagnostic tests and treatment modalities, and progression of disease. The patient's mood and emotional reaction to the results of diagnostic testing and prognosis are assessed, along with evidence that the patient is progressing through the stages of grief and can talk about the diagnosis and prognosis with the family.

BODY IMAGE

Cancer patients are forced to cope with many assaults to body image throughout the course of disease and treatment. Entry into the health care system is often accompanied by depersonalization. Threats to self-concept are enormous as patients face the realization of illness, possible disability, and death. To accommodate treatments or because of the disease, many cancer patients are forced to alter their lifestyles. Priorities and values change when body image is threatened. Disfiguring surgery, hair loss, cachexia, skin changes, altered communication patterns, and sexual dysfunction are some of the devastating results of cancer and its treatment that threaten the patient's self-esteem and body image. The nurse identifies these potential threats and assesses the patient's ability to cope with these changes.

Diagnosis

NURSING DIAGNOSES

Based on the assessment data, nursing diagnoses of the patient with cancer may include the following:

- Impaired oral mucous membrane
- Impaired tissue integrity
- Impaired tissue integrity: alopecia
- Impaired tissue integrity: malignant skin lesions

NURSING RESEARCH PROFILE 16-1
Cancer-Related Fatigue

Olson, K., Tom, B., Hewitt, J., et al. (2002). Evolving routines: Managing fatigue associated with lung and colorectal cancer. *Qualitative Health Research, 5,* 655–670.

Purpose
Some individuals with advanced cancer develop fatigue while others do not. The purpose of this study was to begin the development of a biobehavioural model that could explain this phenomenon.

Study Sample and Design
This qualitative study used Grounded Theory methods to compare the processes by which individuals who reported fatigue and those who did not report fatigue managed the day-to-day aspects of their cancer experience. Interviews were conducted with 29 individuals who had lung or colorectal cancer before, during and after their treatment. Blood samples and body weight were obtained at the time of each interview.

Findings
A three-stage process, "Evolving Routines," and an adaptive behavioural pattern labelled *gliding* characterized individuals who reported little or no fatigue, even when hemoglobin levels were low. The central component of *gliding* was the identification of something that brought joy (hobbies, family, work) that could be used as an anchor around which to plan treatment and disease-related requirements. Three nonadaptive behavioural patterns (*inertia, disorganization, and overexertion*) characterized individuals who reported fatigue.

Nursing Implications
Nurses can use the behavioural patterns outlined in this study to distinguish between individuals engaged in adaptive and nonadaptive daily routines. Interventions that promote the importance of integrating new requirements related to disease and treatment into routines that includes activities of particular personal significance to patients are expected to result in less fatigue.

- Imbalanced nutrition, less than body requirements
- Anorexia
- Malabsorption
- Cachexia
- Chronic pain
- Fatigue
- Disturbed body image
- Anticipatory grieving

COLLABORATIVE PROBLEMS/ POTENTIAL COMPLICATIONS

Based on the assessment data, potential complications that may develop include the following:

- Infection and sepsis
- Hemorrhage
- Superior vena cava syndrome
- Spinal cord compression
- Hypercalcemia
- Pericardial effusion
- Disseminated intravascular coagulation
- Syndrome of inappropriate secretion of antidiuretic hormone
- Tumour lysis syndrome

See the later section, Oncologic Emergencies, for more information.

Planning and Goals

The major goals for the patient may include management of stomatitis, maintenance of tissue integrity, maintenance of nutrition, relief of pain, relief of fatigue, improved body image, effective progression through the grieving process, and absence of complications.

Nursing Interventions

The patient with cancer is at risk for various adverse effects of therapy and complications. The nurse in all health care settings, including the home, assists the patient and family in managing these problems.

MANAGING STOMATITIS

Stomatitis is characterized by bleeding, ulcers and redness. The severity of stomatitis may be assessed by using the WCCNR stomatitis staging system (Table 16-9).

Stomatitis commonly develops within 5 to 14 days after the patient receives certain chemotherapeutic agents, such as doxorubicin and 5-fluorouracil, and BRMs, such as IL-2 and IFN. As many as 40% of patients receiving chemotherapy experience some degree of stomatitis during treatment. Patients receiving dose-intensive chemotherapy (considerably higher doses than conventional dosing), such as those undergoing BMT, are at increased risk for stomatitis. Stomatitis may also occur with radiation to the head and neck. Stomatitis is characterized by mild redness (erythema) and edema or, if severe, by painful ulcerations, bleeding, and secondary infection. In severe cases of stomatitis, cancer therapy may be temporarily halted until the inflammation decreases.

As a result of normal everyday wear and tear, the epithelial cells that line the oral cavity undergo rapid turnover and slough off routinely. Chemotherapy and radiation interfere with the body's ability to replace those cells. An inflammatory response develops as denuded areas appear in the oral cavity. Poor oral hygiene, existing dental disease, use of other medications that dry mucous membranes, and impaired nutritional status contribute to morbidity associated with stomatitis. Radiation-induced xerostomia (dry mouth) associated with decreased function of the salivary glands may contribute to stomatitis in patients who have received radiation to the head and neck.

Myelosuppression (bone marrow depression) resulting from underlying disease or its treatment predisposes the patient to oral bleeding and infection. Pain associated with ulcerated oral tissues can significantly interfere with nutritional intake, speech, and a willingness to maintain oral hygiene.

Although multiple studies on stomatitis have been published, the optimal prevention and treatment approaches have not been identified. However, most clinicians agree that good oral hygiene that includes brushing, flossing, and rinsing is necessary to minimize the risk for oral complications associated with cancer therapies. Soft-bristled toothbrushes and nonabrasive toothpaste prevent or reduce trauma to the oral mucosa. Oral swabs with spongelike applicators may be used in place of a toothbrush for painful oral tissues. Flossing may be performed unless it causes pain or unless platelet levels are below 20×10^9/L. Oral rinses with saline solution or tap water may be necessary for patients who cannot tolerate a toothbrush. Products that irritate oral tissues or impair healing, such as alcohol-based mouth rinses, are avoided. Foods that are difficult to chew or are hot or spicy are avoided to minimize further trauma. The patient's lips are lubricated to keep them from becoming dry and cracked. Topical anti-inflammatory and anesthetic agents may be prescribed to promote healing and minimize discomfort. Products that coat or protect oral mucosa are used to promote comfort and prevent further trauma. The patient who experiences severe pain and discomfort with stomatitis requires systemic analgesics.

Adequate fluid and food intake is encouraged. In some instances, parenteral hydration and nutrition are needed. Topical or systemic antifungal and antibiotic medications are prescribed to treat local or systemic infections.

MAINTAINING TISSUE INTEGRITY

Some of the most frequently encountered disturbances of tissue integrity, in addition to stomatitis, include skin and tissue reactions to radiation therapy, alopecia, and metastatic skin lesions.

The patient who is experiencing skin and tissue reactions to radiation therapy requires careful skin care to prevent further skin irritation, drying, and damage. The skin over the affected area is handled gently; rubbing and use of hot or cold water, soaps, powders, lotions, and cosmetics are avoided. The patient may avoid tissue injury by wearing loose-fitting clothes and avoiding clothes that constrict, irritate, or rub the affected area. If blistering occurs, care is taken not to disrupt the blisters, thus reducing the risk of introducing bacteria. Moisture- and vapor-permeable dressings, such as hydrocolloids and hydrogels, are helpful in promoting healing and reducing pain. Aseptic wound care is indicated to minimize the risk for infection and sepsis. Topical antibiotics, such as 1% silver sulfadiazine cream (Silvadene), may be prescribed for use on areas of moist desquamation (painful, red, moist skin).

Table 16-9 • **Western Canadian Consortium for Cancer Nursing Research (WCCNR) Stomatitis Staging System**

STAGE	LESIONS	COLOUR	BLEEDING
0	None	Pink >50%	None
1	1-4	Slightly red >50%	None
2	>4	Moderately red >50%	With eating or mouth care
3	Coalescing lesions on 50% or more of the mouth surface	Very red >50%	Spontaneous, fresh bleeding apparent or dried blood on pillow

Directions: Using gloves, a penlight, and a tongue blade, inspect all oral surfaces including the gingiva, tongue, lips, the roof and the floor of the mouth, and the buccal surfaces. Cracks in the lips are not counted as lesions. Add scores for lesions, color, bleeding, and moisture.

Scoring system: 0, normal; 1–4, mild; 5–7, moderate; 8–9, severe.
Western Consortium for Cancer Nursing Research, 1987; Western Consortium for Cancer Nursing Research, 1991; Western Consortium for Cancer Nursing Research, 1998; Olson, K., Hanson, J., Hamilton, H., et al., 2004.

ASSISTING PATIENTS TO COPE WITH ALOPECIA

The temporary or permanent thinning or complete loss of hair is a potential adverse effect of various radiation therapies and chemotherapeutic agents. The extent of alopecia depends on the dose and duration of therapy. These treatments cause alopecia by damaging stem cells and hair follicles. As a result, the hair is brittle and may fall out or break off at the surface of the scalp. Loss of other body hair is less frequent. Hair loss usually begins within 2 to 3 weeks after the initiation of treatment; regrowth begins within 8 weeks after the last treatment. Some patients who undergo radiation to the head may sustain permanent hair loss. Many health care providers view hair loss as a minor problem when compared with the potentially life-threatening consequences of cancer. For many patients, however, hair loss is a major assault on body image, resulting in depression, anxiety, anger, rejection, and isolation. To patients and families, hair loss can serve as a constant reminder of the challenges cancer places on their coping abilities, interpersonal relationships, and sexuality.

The nurse's role is to provide information about alopecia and to support the patient and family in coping with disturbing effects of therapy, such as hair loss and changes in body image. Patients are encouraged to acquire a wig or hairpiece before hair loss occurs so that the replacement matches their own hair. Use of attractive scarves and hats may make the patient feel less conspicuous. Nurses can refer patients to supportive programs offered by the Canadian Cancer Society. Knowledge that hair usually begins to regrow after completing therapy may comfort some patients, although the colour and texture of the new hair may be different.

MANAGING MALIGNANT SKIN LESIONS

Skin lesions may occur with local extension of the tumour or embolization of the tumour into the epithelium and its surrounding lymph and blood vessels. Secondary growth of cancer cells into the skin may result in redness (erythematous areas) or can progress to wounds involving tissue necrosis and infection. The most extensive lesions tend to disintegrate and are purulent and malodourous. In addition, these lesions are a source of considerable pain and discomfort. Although this type of lesion is most often associated with breast cancer and head and neck cancers, it can also occur with lymphoma, leukemia, melanoma, and cancers of the lung, uterus, kidney, colon, and bladder. The development of severe skin lesions is usually associated with a poor prognosis for extended survival.

Ulcerating skin lesions usually indicate widely disseminated disease unlikely to be eradicated. Managing these lesions becomes a nursing priority. Nursing care includes carefully assessing and cleansing the skin, reducing superficial bacteria, controlling bleeding, reducing odour, and protecting the skin from pain and further trauma. The patient and family require assistance and guidance to care for these skin lesions at home. Referral for home care is indicated.

PROMOTING NUTRITION

Most cancer patients experience some weight loss during their illness. Anorexia, malabsorption, and cachexia are examples of nutritional problems that commonly occur in cancer patients; special attention is needed to prevent weight loss and promote nutrition.

Anorexia

Among the many causes of anorexia in the cancer patient are alterations in taste, manifested by increased salty, sour, and metallic taste sensations, and altered responses to sweet and bitter flavors, leading to decreased appetite, decreased nutritional intake, and protein-calorie malnutrition. Taste alterations may result from mineral (eg, zinc) deficiencies, increases in circulating amino acids and cellular metabolites, or the administration of chemotherapeutic agents. Patients undergoing radiation therapy to the head and neck may experience "mouth blindness," which is a severe impairment of taste.

Alterations in the sense of smell also alter taste; this is a common experience of patients with head and neck cancers. Anorexia may occur because the person feels full after eating only a small amount of food. This sense of fullness occurs secondary to a decrease in digestive enzymes, abnormalities in the metabolism of glucose and triglycerides, and prolonged stimulation of gastric volume receptors, which convey the feeling of being full. Psychological distress, such as fear, pain, depression, and isolation, throughout illness may also have a negative impact on appetite. The person may develop an aversion to food because of nausea and vomiting after treatment.

Malabsorption

Many cancer patients are unable to absorb nutrients from the gastrointestinal system as a result of tumour activity and cancer treatment. Tumours can affect the gastrointestinal activity in several ways. They may impair enzyme production or produce fistulas. They secrete hormones and enzymes, such as gastrin; this leads to increased gastrointestinal irritation, peptic ulcer disease, and decreased fat digestion. They also interfere with protein digestion.

Chemotherapy and radiation can irritate and damage mucosal cells of the bowel, inhibiting absorption. Radiation therapy can cause sclerosis of the blood vessels in the bowel and fibrotic changes in the gastrointestinal tissue. Surgical intervention may change peristaltic patterns, alter gastrointestinal secretions, and reduce the absorptive surfaces of the gastrointestinal mucosa, all leading to malabsorption.

Cachexia

Cachexia is common in patients with cancer, especially in advanced disease. Cancer cachexia is related to inadequate nutritional intake along with increasing metabolic demand, increased energy expenditure due to anaerobic metabolism of the tumour, impaired glucose metabolism, competition of the tumour cells for nutrients, altered lipid metabolism, and a suppressed appetite. It is characterized by loss of body weight, adipose tissue, visceral protein, and skeletal muscle. Patients who are cachectic complain of loss of appetite, early satiety, and fatigue. As a result of protein losses they are often anemic and have peripheral edema.

General Nutritional Considerations

Whenever possible, every effort is used to maintain adequate nutrition through the oral route. Food should be prepared in ways that make it appealing. Unpleasant smells and unappetizing-looking foods are avoided. Family members are included in the plan of care to encourage adequate food intake. The patient's preferences, as well as physiologic and metabolic requirements, are considered when selecting foods. Small, frequent meals are provided, with supplements between meals. Patients often tolerate larger amounts of food earlier in the day rather than later, so meals can be planned accordingly. Patients should avoid drinking fluids while eating, to avoid early satiety. Oral hygiene before mealtime often makes meals more pleasant. Pain, nausea, and other symptoms that may interfere with nutrition are assessed and managed. Medications such as corticosteroids or progestational agents such as megestrol acetate have been used successfully as appetite stimulants.

If adequate nutrition cannot be maintained by oral intake, nutritional support via the enteral route may be necessary. Short-term nutritional supplementation may be provided through a nasogastric tube. However, if nutritional support is needed beyond several weeks, a gastrostomy or jejunostomy tube may be inserted. Patients and families are taught to administer enteral nutrition in the home setting.

If malabsorption is a problem, enzyme and vitamin replacement may be instituted. Additional strategies include changing the feeding schedule, using simple diets, and relieving diarrhea. If malabsorption is severe, parenteral nutrition (PN) may be necessary. PN can be administered in several ways: by a long-term venous access device, such as a right atrial catheter, an implanted venous port, or a peripherally inserted central catheter (Fig. 16-6). The nurse teaches the patient and family to care for venous access devices and to administer PN. Home care nurses may assist with or supervise PN in the home.

Interventions to reduce cachexia usually do not prolong survival but may improve the patient's quality of life. Before invasive nutritional strategies are instituted, the nurse should assess the patient carefully and discuss the options with the patient and family. Creative dietary therapies, enteral (tube) feedings, or PN may be necessary to ensure adequate nutrition. Nursing care is also directed toward preventing trauma, infection, and other complications that increase metabolic demands.

RELIEVING PAIN

Of all patients with progressive cancer, more than 75% experience pain (Yarbro, Hansen-Frogge & Goodman, 1999). Although patients with cancer may have acute pain, their pain is more frequently characterized as chronic. (For more information on cancer-related pain, see Chap. 13.) As in other situations involving pain, the experience of cancer pain is influenced by both physical and psychosocial factors.

Cancer can cause pain in various ways (Table 16-10). Pain is also associated with various cancer treatments. Acute pain is linked with trauma from surgery. Occasionally, chronic pain syndromes, such as postsurgical neuropathies (pain related to nerve tissue injury), occur. Some chemotherapeutic agents cause tissue necrosis, peripheral neuropathies, and stomatitis—all potential sources of pain—whereas radiation therapy can cause pain secondary to skin or organ inflammation. Cancer patients may have other sources of pain, such as arthritis or migraine headaches, that are unrelated to the underlying cancer or its treatment.

In today's society, most people expect pain to disappear or resolve quickly, and in fact it usually does. Although controllable, cancer pain is commonly irreversible and not quickly resolved. For many patients, pain is a signal that the tumour is growing and that death is approaching. As the patient anticipates the pain and anxiety increases, pain perception heightens, producing fear and further pain. Chronic cancer pain, then, can be best described as a cycle progressing from pain to anxiety to fear and back to pain again.

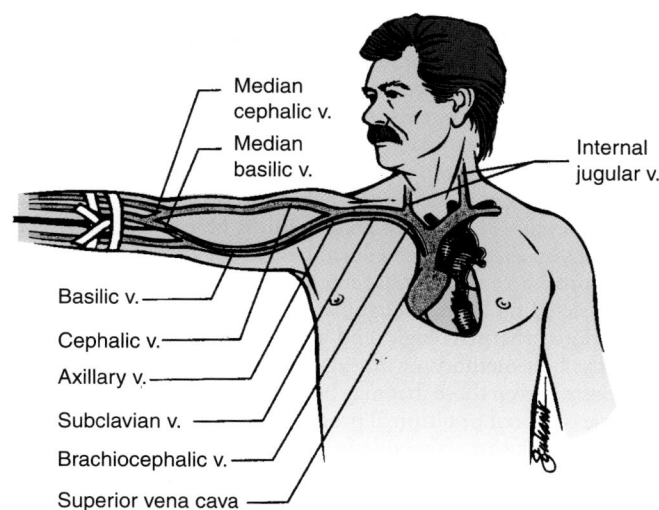

FIGURE 16-6 A peripherally inserted central catheter (PICC) is advanced through the cephalic or basilic vein to the axillary, subclavian, or brachiocephalic vein or the superior vena cava.

Pain tolerance, the point past which pain can no longer be tolerated, varies among people. Pain tolerance is decreased by fatigue, anxiety, fear of death, anger, powerlessness, social isolation, changes in role identity, loss of independence, and past experiences. Adequate rest and sleep, diversion, mood elevation, empathy, and medications such as antidepressants, antianxiety agents, and analgesics enhance tolerance to pain.

Inadequate pain management is most often the result of misconceptions and insufficient knowledge about pain assessment and pharmacologic interventions on the part of patients, families, and health care providers. Successful management of cancer pain is based on thorough and objective pain assessment that examines physical, psychosocial, environmental, and spiritual factors. A multidisciplinary team approach is essential to determine optimal management of the patient's pain. Unlike instances of chronic nonmalignant pain, systemic analgesics play a central role in managing cancer pain.

The World Health Organization (Dalton & Youngblood, 2000) advocates a three-step approach to treating cancer pain (see Chap. 13). Analgesics are administered based on the patient's level of pain. Nonopioid analgesics (eg, acetaminophen) are used for mild pain; weak opioid analgesics (eg, codeine) are used for moderate pain; and strong opioid analgesics (eg, morphine) are used for severe pain. If the patient's pain escalates, the strength of the analgesic medication is increased until the pain

Table 16-10 • Sources of Cancer Pain

SOURCE	DESCRIPTIONS	UNDERLYING CANCER
Bone metastasis	Throbbing, aching	Breast, prostate, myeloma
Nerve compression, infiltration	Burning, sharp, tingling	Breast, prostate, lymphoma
Lymphatic or venous obstruction	Dull, aching, tightness	Lymphoma, breast, Kaposi's sarcoma
Ischemia	Sharp, throbbing	Kaposi's sarcoma
Organ obstruction	Dull, crampy, gnawing	Colon, gastric
Organ infiltration	Distention, crampy	Liver, pancreatic
Skin inflammation, ulceration, infection, necrosis	Burning, sharp	Breast, head and neck, Kaposi's sarcoma

is controlled. Adjuvant medications are also administered to enhance the effectiveness of analgesics and to manage other symptoms that may contribute to the pain experience. Examples of adjuvant medications include antiemetics, antidepressants, anxiolytics, antiseizure agents, stimulants, local anesthetics, radiopharmaceuticals (radioactive agents that may be used to treat painful bone tumours), and corticosteroids.

Preventing and reducing pain help to decrease anxiety and break the pain cycle. This can be accomplished best by administering analgesics on a regularly scheduled basis as prescribed (the preventive approach to pain management), with additional analgesics administered for breakthrough pain as needed and as prescribed.

Various pharmacologic and nonpharmacologic approaches offer the best methods of managing cancer pain. No reasonable approaches, even those that may be invasive, should be overlooked because of a poor or terminal prognosis. Nurses help patients and families to take an active role in managing pain. Nurses provide education and support to correct fears and misconceptions about opioid use. Inadequate pain control leads to suffering, anxiety, fear, immobility, isolation, and depression. Improving a patient's quality of life is as important as preventing a painful death.

DECREASING FATIGUE

In recent years, fatigue has been recognized as one of the most significant and frequent symptoms experienced by patients receiving cancer therapy. Nurses help the patient and family to understand that fatigue is usually an expected and temporary side effect of the cancer process and of many treatments used. Fatigue also stems from the stress of coping with cancer. It does not always signify that the cancer is advancing or that the treatment is failing. Potential sources of fatigue are summarized in Chart 16-6.

Nursing strategies are implemented to minimize fatigue or assist the patient to cope with existing fatigue. Helping the patient to identify sources of fatigue aids in selecting appropriate and individualized interventions. Ways to conserve energy are developed to help the patient plan daily activities. Alternating periods of rest and activity are beneficial. Regular, light exercise may decrease fatigue and facilitate coping, whereas lack of physical activity and "too much rest" can actually contribute to deconditioning and associated fatigue.

Patients are encouraged to maintain as normal a lifestyle as possible by continuing with those activities they value and enjoy. Prioritizing necessary and valued activities can assist patients in planning for each day. Both patients and families are encouraged

> **Chart 16-6** **Sources of Fatigue in Cancer Patients**
>
> Pain, pruritus
> Imbalanced nutrition related to anorexia, nausea, vomiting, cachexia
> Electrolyte imbalance related to vomiting, diarrhea
> Ineffective protection related to neutropenia, thrombocytopenia, anemia
> Impaired tissue integrity related to stomatitis, mucositis
> Impaired physical mobility related to neurologic impairments, surgery, bone metastasis, pain, and analgesic use
> Deficient knowledge related to disease process, treatment
> Anxiety related to fear, diagnosis, role changes, uncertainty of future
> Ineffective breathing patterns related to cough, shortness of breath, and dyspnea
> Disturbed sleep pattern related to cancer therapies, anxiety, and pain

to plan to reallocate responsibilities, such as attending to child care, cleaning, and preparing meals. Patients who are employed full-time may need to reduce the number of hours worked each week. The nurse assists the patient and family in coping with these changing roles and responsibilities.

Nurses also address factors that contribute to fatigue and implement pharmacologic and nonpharmacologic strategies to manage pain. Nutrition counselling is provided to patients who are not eating enough calories or protein. Small, frequent meals require less energy for digestion. Serum hemoglobin and hematocrit levels are monitored for deficiencies, and blood products or EPO are administered as prescribed. Patients are monitored for alterations in oxygenation and electrolyte balances. Physical therapy and assistive devices are beneficial for patients with impaired mobility.

IMPROVING BODY IMAGE AND SELF-ESTEEM

A positive approach is essential when caring for the patient with an altered body image. To help the patient retain control and positive self-esteem, it is important to encourage independence and continued participation in self-care and decision making. The patient should be assisted to assume those tasks and participate in those activities that are personally of most value. Any negative feelings that the patient has or threats to body image should be identified and discussed. The nurse serves as a listener and counselor to both the patient and the family. Referral to a support group can provide the patient with additional assistance in coping with the changes resulting from cancer or its treatment. In many cases, a cosmetologist can provide ideas about hair or wig styling, make-up, and the use of scarves and turbans to help with body image concerns.

Patients who experience alterations in sexuality and sexual function are encouraged to discuss concerns openly with their partner. Alternative forms of sexual expression are explored with the patient and partner to promote positive self-worth and acceptance. The nurse who identifies serious physiologic, psychological, or communication difficulties related to sexuality or sexual function is in a key position to assist the patient and partner to seek further counselling if necessary.

ASSISTING IN THE GRIEVING PROCESS

A cancer diagnosis need not indicate a fatal outcome. Many forms of cancer are curable; others may be cured if treated early. Despite these facts, many patients and their families view cancer as a fatal disease that is inevitably accompanied by pain, suffering, debility, and emaciation. Grieving is a normal response to these fears and to the losses anticipated or experienced by the patient with cancer. These may include loss of health, normal sensations, body image, social interaction, sexuality, and intimacy. The patient, family, and friends may grieve for the loss of quality time to spend with others, the loss of future and unfulfilled plans, and the loss of control over one's own body and emotional reactions.

The patient and family just informed of the cancer diagnosis frequently respond with shock, numbness, and disbelief. It is often during this stage that the patient and family are called on to make important initial decisions about treatment. They require the support of the physician, nurse, and other health care team members to make these decisions. An important role of the nurse is to answer any questions the patient and family have and clarify information provided by the physician.

In addition to assessing the response of the patient and family to the diagnosis and planned treatment, the nurse assists them in framing their questions and concerns, identifying resources and support people (eg, spiritual advisor, counselor), and communicating their concerns with each other. Support groups for patients and families are available through hospitals and various community organizations. These groups provide direct assistance, advice, and emotional support.

As the patient and family progress through the grieving process, they may express anger, frustration, and depression. During this time, the nurse encourages the patient and family to verbalize their feelings in an atmosphere of trust and support. The nurse continues to assess their reactions and provides assistance and support as they confront and learn to deal with new problems.

If the patient enters the terminal phase of disease, the nurse may realize that the patient and family members are at different stages of grief. In such cases, the nurse assists the patient and family to acknowledge and cope with their reactions and feelings. Nurses also assist patients and families to explore preferences for issues related to end-of-life care such as withdrawal of active disease treatment, desire for the use of life support measures, and symptom management. Support, which can be as simple as holding the patient's hand or just being with the patient at home or at the bedside, often contributes to peace of mind. Maintaining contact with the surviving family members after the death of the cancer patient may help them to work through their feelings of loss and grief. See Chapter 17 for further discussion of end-of-life issues.

MONITORING AND MANAGING POTENTIAL COMPLICATIONS

Despite advances in cancer care, infection remains the leading cause of death. In the cancer patient, defense against infection is compromised in many different ways. The integrity of the skin and mucous membrane, the body's first line of defense, is challenged by multiple invasive diagnostic and therapeutic procedures, by adverse effects of radiation and chemotherapy, and by the detrimental effects of immobility.

Impaired nutrition resulting from anorexia, nausea, vomiting, diarrhea, and the underlying disease alters the body's ability to combat invading organisms. Medications such as antibiotics disturb the balance of normal flora, allowing the overgrowth of pathogenic organisms. Other medications can also alter the immune response (see Chap. 50). Cancer itself may be immunosuppressive. Cancers such as leukemia and lymphoma are often associated with defects in cellular and humoural immunity. Advanced cancer can lead to obstruction by the tumour of the hollow viscera (such as the intestines), blood vessels, and lymphatic vessels, creating a favourable environment for proliferation of pathogenic organisms. In some patients, tumour cells infiltrate bone marrow and prevent normal production of WBCs. Most often, however, a decrease in WBCs is a result of bone marrow suppression after chemotherapy or radiation therapy.

The use of the hematopoietic growth factors, also called colony-stimulating factors (see the previous discussion of BRM therapy), has reduced the severity and duration of neutropenia associated with myelosuppressive chemotherapy and radiation therapy. The administration of these factors assists in reducing the risk for infection and, possibly, in maintaining treatment schedules, drug dosages, treatment effectiveness, and the quality of life.

Infection

Gram-positive organisms, such as *Streptococcus* and *Staphylococcus* species, are the most frequently isolated causes of infection. Gram-negative organisms, such as *Escherichia coli* and *Pseudomonas aeruginosa,* and fungal organisms, such as *Candida albicans,* also contribute to the incidence of serious infection.

Fever is probably the most important sign of infection in the immunocompromised patient. Although fever may be related to a variety of noninfectious conditions, including the underlying cancer, any temperature of 38.5°C or higher is reported and dealt with promptly.

Antibiotics may be prescribed to treat infections after cultures of wound drainage, exudate, sputum, urine, stool, or blood are obtained. Patients with neutropenia are treated with broad-spectrum antibiotics before the infecting organism is identified because of the high incidence of mortality associated with untreated infection. Broad-spectrum antibiotic coverage or empiric therapy most often includes a combination of medications to defend the body against the major pathogenic organisms. An important component of the nurse's role is to administer these medications promptly according to the prescribed schedule to achieve adequate blood levels of the medications.

Strict asepsis is essential when handling intravenous lines, catheters, and other invasive equipment. Exposure of the patient to others with an active infection and to crowds is avoided. Patients with profound immunosuppression, such as BMT recipients, may need to be placed in a protective environment where the room and its contents are sterilized and the air is filtered. These patients may also receive low-bacteria diets, avoiding fresh fruits and vegetables. Hand hygiene and appropriate general hygiene are necessary to reduce exposure to potentially harmful bacteria and to eliminate environmental contaminants. Invasive procedures, such as injections, vaginal or rectal examinations, rectal temperatures, and surgery, are avoided. The patient is encouraged to cough and perform deep-breathing exercises frequently to prevent atelectasis and other respiratory problems. Prophylactic antimicrobial therapy may be used for patients who are expected to be profoundly immunosuppressed and at risk for certain infections. The nurse teaches the patient and family to recognize signs and symptoms of infection to report, perform effective hand hygiene, use antipyretics, maintain skin integrity, and administer hematopoietic growth factors when indicated.

Septic Shock

The nurse assesses the patient frequently for infection and inflammation throughout the course of the disease. Septicemia and septic shock are life-threatening complications that must be prevented or detected and treated promptly. Patients with signs and symptoms of impending sepsis and septic shock require immediate hospitalization and aggressive treatment.

Signs and symptoms of septic shock (see Chap. 15) include altered mental status, either subnormal or elevated temperature, cool and clammy skin, decreased urine output, hypotension, dysrhythmias, electrolyte imbalances, and abnormal arterial blood gas values. The patient and family members are instructed about signs of septicemia, methods for preventing infection, and actions to take if infection or septicemia occurs.

Septic shock is most often associated with overwhelming gram-negative bacterial infections. The nurse monitors the blood pressure, pulse rate, respirations, and temperature of the patient with shock every 15 to 30 minutes. Neurologic assessments are carried out to detect changes in orientation and responsiveness. Fluid and electrolyte status is monitored by measuring fluid intake and output and serum electrolytes. Arterial blood gas values and pulse oximetry are monitored to determine tissue oxygenation. The nurse administers intravenous fluids, blood products, and vasopressors as prescribed to maintain the patient's blood pressure and tissue perfusion. Supplemental oxygen is often necessary. Broad-spectrum antibiotics are administered as prescribed to combat the underlying infection (see Chap. 15).

Bleeding and Hemorrhage

Thrombocytopenia, a decrease in the circulating platelet count, is the most common cause of bleeding in cancer patients and is usually defined as a count of less than $100 \times 10^9/L$. When the count falls between $20 \times 10^9/L$ and $50 \times 10^9/L$, the risk for bleeding increases. Counts under $10 \times 10^9/L$ are associated with an increased risk for spontaneous bleeding, for which the patient requires a platelet transfusion. Platelets are essential for normal blood clotting and coagulation (hemostasis).

Thrombocytopenia often results from bone marrow depression after certain types of chemotherapy and radiation therapy. Tumour infiltration of the bone marrow can also impair the normal production of platelets. In some cases, platelet destruction is associated with an enlarged spleen (hypersplenism) and abnormal antibody function that occur with leukemia and lymphoma.

In addition to monitoring laboratory values, the nurse continues to assess the patient for bleeding. The nurse also takes steps to prevent trauma and minimize the risk for bleeding by encouraging the patient to use a soft, not stiff, toothbrush and an electric, not straight-edged, razor. Additionally, the nurse avoids unnecessary invasive procedures (eg, rectal temperatures, intramuscular injections, and catheterization) and assists the patient and family to identify and remove environmental hazards that may lead to falls or other trauma. Soft foods, increased fluid intake, and stool softeners, if prescribed, may be indicated to reduce trauma to the gastrointestinal tract. The joints and extremities are handled and moved gently to minimize the risk for spontaneous bleeding. The nurse may administer IL-11, which has been approved by the FDA (Rust, Wood & Battiato, 1999) to prevent severe thrombocytopenia and to reduce the need for platelet transfusions following myelosuppressive chemotherapy in patients with nonmyeloid malignancies. In some instances, the nurse teaches the patient or family member to administer IL-11 in the home.

Hemorrhage may be related to various underlying abnormalities, such as thrombocytopenia and coagulation disorders. These clinical situations are often associated with the cancer itself or the adverse effects of cancer treatments. Sites of hemorrhage may include the gastrointestinal, respiratory, and genitourinary tracts and the brain. Blood pressure and pulse and respiratory rates are monitored every 15 to 30 minutes when hospitalized patients experience bleeding.

Serum hemoglobin and hematocrit are monitored carefully for changes indicating blood loss. The nurse tests all urine, stool, and emesis for occult blood. Neurologic assessments are performed to detect changes in orientation and behaviour. The nurse administers fluids and blood products as prescribed to replace any losses. Vasopressor agents are administered as prescribed to maintain blood pressure and ensure tissue oxygenation. Supplemental oxygen is used as necessary.

PROMOTING HOME AND COMMUNITY-BASED CARE

Teaching Patients Self-Care

Patients with cancer usually return home from acute care facilities or receive treatment in the home or outpatient area rather than acute care facilities. The shift from the acute care setting also shifts the responsibility for care to the patient and family. As a result, families and friends must assume increased involvement in patient care, which requires teaching that enables them to provide care. Teaching initially focuses on providing information needed by the patient and family to address the most immediate care needs likely to be encountered at home.

Side effects of treatments and changes in the patient's status that should be reported are reviewed verbally and reinforced with written information. Strategies to deal with side effects of treatment are discussed with the patient and family. Other learning needs are identified based on the priorities conveyed by the patient and family as well as on the complexity of care provided in the home.

Technological advances allow home administration of chemotherapy, PN, blood products, parenteral antibiotics, and parenteral analgesics; management of symptoms; and care of vascular access devices. Although home care nurses provide care and support for patients receiving this advanced technical care, the patient and family need instruction and ongoing support that allow them to feel comfortable and proficient in managing these treatments at home. Follow-up visits and telephone calls from the nurse are often reassuring to the patient and family and increase their comfort in dealing with complex and new aspects of care. Continued contact facilitates evaluation of the patient's progress and ongoing needs.

Continuing Care

Referral for home care is often indicated for the patient with cancer. The responsibilities of the home care nurse include assessing the home environment, suggesting modifications in the home or in care to assist the patient and family in addressing the patient's physical needs, providing physical care, and assessing the psychological and emotional impact of the illness on the patient and family.

Assessing changes in the patient's physical status and reporting relevant changes to the physician help to ensure that appropriate and timely modifications in therapy are made. The home care nurse also assesses the adequacy of pain management and the effectiveness of other strategies to prevent or manage the side effects of treatment modalities.

The patient's and family's understanding of the treatment plan and management strategies is assessed, and previous teaching is reinforced. The nurse often facilitates the coordination of patient care by maintaining close communication with all health care providers involved in the patient's care. The nurse may make referrals and coordinate available community resources (eg, local office of the American Cancer Society, home aides, church groups, parish nurses, and support groups) to assist patients and caregivers.

Evaluation

EXPECTED PATIENT OUTCOMES

For specific patient outcomes, see the Plan of Nursing Care. Expected patient outcomes may include:

1. Maintains integrity of oral mucous membranes
2. Maintains adequate tissue integrity
3. Maintains adequate nutritional status
4. Achieves relief of pain and discomfort
5. Demonstrates increased activity tolerance and decreased fatigue
6. Exhibits improved body image and self-esteem
7. Progresses through the grieving process
8. Experiences no complications, such as infection, or sepsis, and no episodes of bleeding or hemorrhage

Cancer Rehabilitation

Many cancer patients, including those who receive primary surgical treatment and adjuvant chemotherapy or radiation therapy, return to work and their usual activities of daily living. These patients may encounter a variety of problems, including changes in their functional abilities and in the attitudes of employers, coworkers, and family members who still view cancer as a terminal, debilitating disease. Nurses play an important role in the rehabilitation of the cancer patient. Both the patient and family are included as part of any rehabilitation effort because cancer affects not only the patient but also the family members. In addition, with the shift away from inpatient care, many families are caring for patients at home. To maximize beneficial outcomes, evaluation of the patient's needs related to cancer rehabilitation begins early in cancer treatment (Table 16-11).

Assessment for body image changes as a result of disfiguring treatments is necessary to facilitate the patient's adjustment to changes in appearance or functional abilities. The nurse can refer the patient and family to a variety of support groups sponsored by the Canadian Cancer Society. Nurses also collaborate with physical, occupational, and enterostomal therapists in improving the patient's abilities in the use of prosthetic and assistive devices, and in altering the home environment as needed.

Table 16-11 • Assessing Patient Needs for Cancer Rehabilitation

AREA OF NEED	FACTORS TO ASSESS
Functional	
Activities of daily living	Mobility
	Cognitive impairment
	Sensory impairments
	Communication barriers
Physiologic	
Nutrition	Need for enteral or parenteral nutrition
Elimination	Alterations in bowel and bladder function
Symptoms related to disease or treatment	Pain
	Nausea, vomiting, diarrhea
	Dyspnea, fatigue
	Skin impairment, alopecia
Psychosocial Resources	
Family	Availability of caregiver, home physical environment
	Availability of private transportation; affordability of transportation
Community	Availability of public transportation; affordability of transportation
	Availability and access to community organizations for assistance and support
Personal	Spiritual concerns
	Family relationships
	Body image
	Coping abilities
	Sexuality
Financial	Job security for patient and family members
	Need for vocational training

Patients often experience distress (eg, pain, nausea) related to the underlying cancer or treatments. These symptoms may interfere with work and quality of life. Nurses assess for these problems and assist the patient in identifying strategies for coping with them. For patients with gastrointestinal disturbances after chemotherapy, altering work hours or receiving treatments in the evenings may prove helpful. Collaboration with physicians and pharmacists is helpful in identifying appropriate interventions.

Nurses collaborate with dietitians to help patients plan meals that will be acceptable and meet nutritional requirements. Nurses are also involved in the ongoing assessment of patients to detect any long-term consequences of cancer treatment.

Recovering cancer patients have reported instances of unfair practices and discrimination in the workplace. Some employers do not understand that different kinds of cancers have different prognoses and different effects on functional ability. As a result, employers may hesitate to hire or continue to employ people with cancer, especially if ongoing treatment regimens require adjustments in work schedules. Employers, coworkers, and families may continue to view the person as "sick" despite ongoing recovery or completion of treatment. Attitudes of coworkers can be a problem when the patient has a communication impairment, as may occur in some head and neck cancers. The patient may benefit from vocational rehabilitation services of the American Cancer Society or other agencies.

Nurses can participate in efforts to educate employers and the public in general to ensure that the rights of patients with cancer are maintained. Whenever possible, nurses assist patients and families to resume preexisting roles. Psychologists and clergy or spiritual advisors are consulted to assist with psychosocial and spiritual concerns. Rehabilitation shifts the focus from what has been lost to what can be done with existing strengths and abilities. In that spirit, nurses encourage patients to regain the highest level of function and independence possible.

Gerontologic Considerations

As a result of an increased life expectancy and an increased risk for cancer with age, nurses are providing cancer-related care for growing numbers of elderly patients. More than 58% of all cancers occur in people older than 65 years of age, and about two thirds of all cancer deaths occur in people 65 years of age and older. Nursing care of this population addresses special needs, including physical, psychosocial, and financial concerns.

Oncology nurses working with the elderly population need to understand the normal physiologic changes that occur with aging. These changes include decreased skin elasticity; decreased skeletal mass, structure, and strength; decreased organ function and structure; impaired immune system mechanisms; alterations in neurologic and sensory functions; and altered drug absorption, distribution, metabolism, and elimination. These changes ultimately influence the elderly patient's ability to tolerate cancer treatment. In addition, many elderly patients have other chronic diseases and associated treatments that may limit tolerance to cancer treatments (Table 16-12).

Potential chemotherapy-related toxicities, such as renal impairment, myelosuppression, fatigue, and cardiomyopathy, may increase as a result of declining organ function and diminished physiologic reserves. The recovery of normal tissues after radiation therapy may be delayed, and the patient may experience more severe adverse effects, such as mucositis, nausea and vomiting, and myelosuppression. Because of decreased tissue healing capacity and declining pulmonary and cardiovascular functioning, the older patient is slower to recover from surgery. Elderly patients are also at increased risk for complications such as atelectasis, pneumonia, and wound infections.

Access to cancer care for elderly patients may be limited by discriminatory or fatalistic attitudes of health care providers, caregivers, and patients themselves. Issues such as the gradual loss of supportive resources, declining health or loss of a spouse, and unavailability of relatives or friends may result in limited access to care and unmet needs for assistance with activities of daily living. In addition, the economic impact of health care may be difficult for those living on fixed incomes.

The nurse must be aware of the special needs of the aging population. Cancer prevention, detection, and screening efforts are directed toward the elderly as well as the younger population. Nurses carefully monitor elderly patients receiving cancer treatments for signs and symptoms of adverse effects. In addition, the elderly patient is instructed to report all symptoms to the physician. It is not uncommon for the elderly patient to delay reporting symptoms, attributing them to "old age." Many elderly people do not want to report illness for fear of losing their independence or financial security. Sensory losses (eg, hearing and visual losses) and memory deficits are considered when planning patient education because they may affect the patient's ability to process and retain information. In such cases, the nurse needs to act as a patient advocate, encouraging independence and identifying resources for support when indicated.

Care of the Patient with Advanced Cancer

The patient with advanced cancer is likely to experience many of the problems previously described, but all to a greater degree. Symptoms of gastrointestinal disturbances, nutritional problems, weight loss, and cachexia make the patient more susceptible to skin breakdown, fluid and electrolyte problems, and infection.

Although not all cancer patients experience pain, those who do commonly fear that it will not be adequately treated. Although treatment at this stage of illness is likely to be palliative rather than curative, prevention and appropriate management of problems can improve the quality of the patient's life considerably. For example, use of analgesia at set intervals rather than on an "as needed" basis usually breaks the cycle of tension and anxiety associated with waiting until pain becomes so severe that pain relief is inadequate once the analgesic is given. Working with the patient and family, as well as with other health care providers, on a pain-management program based on the patient's requirements frequently increases the patient's comfort and sense of control. In addition, the dose of opioid analgesic required is often reduced as pain becomes more manageable and other medications (eg, sedatives, tranquilizers, muscle relaxants) are added to assist in relieving pain.

If the patient is a candidate for radiation therapy or surgical intervention to relieve severe pain, the consequences of these procedures (eg, percutaneous nerve block, cordotomy) are explained to the patient and family, and measures are taken to prevent complications resulting from altered sensation, immobility, and changes in bowel and bladder function.

With the appearance of each new symptom, the patient may experience dread and fear that the disease is progressing. However, one cannot assume that all symptoms are related to the cancer. The new symptoms and problems are evaluated and treated aggressively if possible to increase the patient's comfort and improve quality of life.

Weakness, immobility, fatigue, and inactivity typically occur in the advanced stages of cancer as a result of the tumour, treatment, inadequate nutritional intake, or shortness of breath. The nurse works with the patient to set realistic goals and to provide rest balanced with planned activities and exercise. Other measures include assisting the patient in identifying energy-conserving methods for accomplishing tasks and promoting activities that the patient values the most.

Efforts are made throughout the course of the disease to provide the patient with as much control and independence as desired, but with assurance that support and assistance are available when needed. Additionally, the health care team works with the

---

Table 16-12 • **Age-Related Changes and Their Effects on Patients with Cancer**

AGE-RELATED CHANGES	IMPLICATIONS
Impaired immune system	Use special precautions to avoid infection; monitor for atypical signs and symptoms of infection.
Altered drug absorption, distribution, metabolism, and elimination	Mandates careful calculation of chemotherapy and frequent assessment for drug response and side effects.
Increased prevalence of other chronic diseases	Monitor for effect of cancer or its treatment on patient's other chronic diseases; monitor patient's tolerance for cancer treatment.
Diminished renal, respiratory, and cardiac reserve	Be proactive in prevention of decreased renal function, atelectasis, pneumonia, and cardiovascular compromise.
Decreased skin and tissue integrity; reduction in body mass; delayed healing	Prevent pressure ulcers secondary to immobility. Monitor skin and mucous membranes for changes related to radiation or chemotherapy. Prevent wound infection.
Decreased musculoskeletal strength	Prevent falls; encourage use of hip protectors if indicated.
Decreased neurosensory functioning: loss of vision, hearing, and distal extremity tactile senses	Provide teaching and instructions modified for patient's hearing and vision loss; provide instruction concerning safety and skin care for distal extremities.
Potential changes in cognitive and emotional capacity	Provide teaching and support modified for patient's level of functioning.

patient and family to ascertain and comply with the patient's wishes about treatment methods and care as the terminal phase of illness and death approach.

HOSPICE

For many years, society was unable to cope appropriately with patients in the most advanced stages of cancer, and patients died in acute care settings rather than at home or in facilities designed to meet their needs. The needs of patients with terminal illnesses are best met by a comprehensive multidisciplinary program that focuses on quality of life, palliation of symptoms, and provision of psychosocial and spiritual support for the patient and family when cure and control of the disease are no longer possible. The concept of hospice, which originated in Great Britain, best addresses these needs. Most important, the focus of care is on the family, not just the patient. Hospice care can be provided in several settings: freestanding, hospital-based, and community or home-based settings.

Because of the high costs associated with maintaining freestanding hospices, care is often delivered by coordinating services provided by both the hospital and community. Although physi-cians, social workers, clergy, dietitians, pharmacists, physical therapists, and volunteers are involved in patient care, nurses are most often the coordinators of all hospice activities. It is essential that home care and hospice nurses possess advanced skills in assessing and managing pain, nutrition, dyspnea, bowel dysfunction, and skin impairments.

In addition, hospice programs facilitate clear communication among family members and health care providers. Most patients and families are informed of the prognosis and are encouraged to participate in decisions regarding pursuing or terminating cancer treatment. Through collaboration with other support disciplines, nurses assist patients and families to cope with changes in role identity, family structure, grief, and loss. Hospice nurses are actively involved in bereavement counselling. In many instances, family support for survivors continues for about 1 year. See Chapter 17 for detailed discussion of end-of-life care.

Oncologic Emergencies

For information about these emergencies, see Table 16-13.

Table 16-13 • Oncologic Emergencies: Manifestations and Management

EMERGENCY	CLINICAL MANIFESTATIONS AND DIAGNOSTIC FINDINGS	MANAGEMENT
Superior Vena Cava Syndrome (SVCS) Compression or invasion of the superior vena cava by tumor, enlarged lymph nodes, intraluminal thrombus that obstructs venous circulation, or drainage of the head, neck, arms, and thorax. Typically associated with lung cancer, SVCS can also occur with lymphoma and metastases. If untreated, SVCS may lead to cerebral anoxia (because not enough oxygen reaches the brain), laryngeal edema, bronchial obstruction, and death.	*Clinical* Gradually or suddenly impaired venous drainage giving rise to • Progressive shortness of breath (dyspnea), cough, and facial swelling • Edema of the neck, arms, hands, and thorax and reported sensation of skin tightness and difficulty swallowing • Possibly engorged and distended jugular, temporal, and arm veins • Dilated thoracic vessels causing prominent venous patterns on the chest wall • Increased intracranial pressure, associated visual disturbances, headache, and altered mental status *Diagnostic* Diagnosis is confirmed by • Clinical findings • Chest x-ray • Thoracic CT scan • MRI Intraluminal thrombosis is identified by venogram.	*Medical* • Radiation therapy to shrink tumor size and relieve symptoms • Chemotherapy for radiation-resistant tumor (eg, lymphoma or small cell lung cancer) or when the mediastinum has been irradiated to maximum tolerance • Anticoagulant or thrombolytic therapy for intraluminal thrombosis • Surgery (less common), eg, vena cava bypass graft (synthetic or autologous) to redirect blood flow around the obstruction • Supportive measures such as oxygen therapy, corticosteroids, and diuretics *Nursing* • Identify patients at risk for SVCS. • Monitor and report clinical manifestations of SVCS. • Monitor cardiopulmonary and neurologic status. • Facilitate breathing by positioning the patient properly. This helps to promote comfort and reduce anxiety produced by difficulty breathing resulting from progressive edema. • Promote energy conservation to minimize shortness of breath. • Monitor the patient's fluid volume status and administer fluids cautiously to minimize edema. • Assess for thoracic radiation-related problems such as dysphagia (difficulty swallowing) and esophagitis. • Monitor for chemotherapy-related problems, such as myelosuppression. • Provide postoperative care as appropriate.

(continued)

Table 16-13 • **Oncologic Emergencies: Manifestations and Management** (Continued)

EMERGENCY	CLINICAL MANIFESTATIONS AND DIAGNOSTIC FINDINGS	MANAGEMENT
Spinal Cord Compression Potentially leading to permanent neurologic impairment and associated morbidity and mortality, compression of the cord and its nerve roots may result from tumor, lymphomas, or intervertebral collapse. The prognosis depends on the severity and rapidity of onset. About 70% of compressions occur at the thoracic level, 20% in the lumbosacral level, and 10% in the cervical region. Metastatic cancers (breast, lung, kidney, prostate, myeloma, lymphoma) and related bone erosion are associated with spinal cord compression.	*Clinical* • Local inflammation, edema, venous stasis, and impaired blood supply to nervous tissues • Local or radicular pain along the dermatomal areas innervated by the affected nerve root (eg, thoracic radicular pain extends in a band around the chest or abdomen) • Pain exacerbated by movement, coughing, sneezing, or the Valsalva manoeuvre • Neurologic dysfunction, and related motor and sensory deficits (numbness, tingling, feelings of coldness in the affected area, inability to detect vibration, loss of positional sense) • Motor loss ranging from subtle weakness to flaccid paralysis • Bladder and/or bowel dysfunction depending on level of compression (above S2, overflow incontinence; from S3 to S5, flaccid sphincter tone and bowel incontinence) *Diagnostic* • Percussion tenderness at the level of compression • Abnormal reflexes • Sensory and motor abnormalities • MRI, myelogram, spinal cord x-rays, bone scans, and CT scan	*Medical* • Radiation therapy to reduce tumor size to halt progression and corticosteroid therapy to decrease inflammation and swelling at the compression site • Surgery only if symptoms progress despite radiation therapy or if vertebral fracture leads to additional nerve damage • Chemotherapy as adjuvant to radiation therapy for patients with lymphoma or small cell lung cancer • *Note:* Despite treatment, patients with poor neurologic function before treatment are less likely to regain complete motor and sensory function; patients who develop complete paralysis usually do not regain all neurologic function. *Nursing* • Perform ongoing assessment of neurologic function to identify existing and progressing dysfunction. • Control pain with pharmacologic and non-pharmacologic measures. • Prevent complications of immobility resulting from pain and decreased function (eg, skin breakdown, urinary stasis, thrombophlebitis, and decreased clearance of pulmonary secretions). • Maintain muscle tone by assisting with range-of-motion exercises in collaboration with physical and occupational therapists. • Institute intermittent urinary catheterization and bowel training programs for patients with bladder or bowel dysfunction. • Provide encouragement and support to patient and family coping with pain and altered functioning, lifestyle, roles, and independence.
Hypercalcemia In patients with cancer, hypercalcemia is a potentially life-threatening metabolic abnormality resulting when the calcium released from the bones is more than the kidneys can excrete or the bones can reabsorb. It may result from: • Bone destruction by tumor cells and subsequent release of calcium • Production of prostaglandins and osteoclast-activating factor, which stimulate bone breakdown and calcium release • Tumors that produce parathyroid-like substances that promote calcium release • Excessive use of vitamins and minerals and conditions unrelated to cancer, such as dehydration, renal impairment, primary hyperparathyroidism, thyrotoxicosis, thiazide diuretics, and hormone therapy	*Clinical* Fatigue, weakness, confusion, decreased level of responsiveness, hyporeflexia, nausea, vomiting, constipation, polyuria (excessive urination), polydipsia (excessive thirst), dehydration, and dysrhythmias *Diagnostic* Serum calcium level exceeding 2.74 mmol/L	*Medical* See Chapter 14. *Nursing* • Identify patients at risk for hypercalcemia and assess for signs and symptoms of hypercalcemia. • Educate patient and family; prevention and early detection can prevent fatality. • Teach at-risk patients to recognize and report signs and symptoms of hypercalcemia. • Encourage patients to consume 2 to 3 L of fluid daily unless contraindicated by existing renal or cardiac disease. • Explain the use of dietary and pharmacologic interventions such as stool softeners and laxatives for constipation. • Advise patients to maintain nutritional intake without restricting normal calcium intake. • Discuss antiemetic therapy if nausea and vomiting occur. • Promote mobility by emphasizing its importance in preventing demineralization and breakdown of bones.

(continued)

Table 16-13 • **Oncologic Emergencies: Manifestations and Management (Continued)**

EMERGENCY	CLINICAL MANIFESTATIONS AND DIAGNOSTIC FINDINGS	MANAGEMENT
Pericardial Effusion and Cardiac Tamponade Cardiac tamponade is an accumulation of fluid in the pericardial space. The accumulation compresses the heart and thereby impedes expansion of the ventricles and cardiac filling during diastole. As ventricular volume and cardiac output fall, the heart pump fails, and circulatory collapse develops. With gradual onset, fluid accumulates gradually, and the outer layer of the pericardial space stretches to compensate for rising pressure. Large amounts of fluid accumulate before symptoms of heart failure occur. With rapid onset, pressures rise too quickly for the pericardial space to compensate. Cancerous tumors, particularly from adjacent thoracic tumors (lung, esophagus, breast cancers), and cancer treatment are the most common causes of cardiac tamponade. Radiation therapy of 4,000 cGy or more to the mediastinal area has also been implicated in pericardial fibrosis, pericarditis, and resultant cardiac tamponade. Untreated pericardial effusion and cardiac tamponade lead to circulatory collapse and cardiac arrest.	*Clinical* • Neck vein distention during inspiration (Kussmaul's sign) • Pulsus paradoxus (systolic blood pressure decrease exceeding 10 mm Hg during inspiration; pulse gets stronger on expiration) • Distant heart sounds, rubs and gallops, cardiac dullness • Compensatory tachycardia (heart beats faster to compensate for decreased cardiac output) • Increased venous and vascular pressures *Diagnostic* • ECG helps diagnose pericardial effusion. • In small effusion, chest x-rays show small amounts of fluid in the pericardium; in large effusions, x-ray films disclose "water-bottle" heart (obliteration of vessel contour and cardiac chambers). • ECG and CT scans help diagnose pleural effusions and evaluate effect of treatment. • Narrow pulse pressure • Shortness of breath and tachypnea • Weakness, chest pain, orthopnea, anxiety, diaphoresis, lethargy, and altered consciousness from decreased cerebral perfusion	*Medical* • Pericardiocentesis (the aspiration or withdrawal of the pericardial fluid by a large-bore needle inserted into the pericardial space). In malignant effusions, pericardiocentesis provides only temporary relief; fluid usually reaccumulates. Windows or openings in the pericardium can be created surgically as a palliative measure to drain fluid into the pleural space. Catheters may also be placed in the pericardial space and sclerosing agents (such as tetracycline, talc, bleomycin, 5-fluorouracil, or thiotepa) injected to prevent fluid from reaccumulating. • Radiation therapy or antineoplastic agents, depending on how sensitive the primary tumor is to these treatments. In mild effusions, prednisone and diuretic medications may be prescribed and the patient's status carefully monitored. *Nursing* • Monitor vital signs and oxygen saturation frequently. • Assess for pulsus paradoxus. • Monitor ECG tracings. • Assess heart and lung sounds, neck vein filling, level of consciousness, respiratory status, and skin colour and temperature. • Monitor and record intake and output. • Review laboratory findings (eg, arterial blood gas and electrolyte levels). • Elevate the head of the patient's bed to ease breathing. • Minimize patient's physical activity to reduce oxygen requirements; administer supplemental oxygen as prescribed. • Provide frequent oral hygiene. • Reposition and encourage the patient to cough and take deep breaths every 2 hours. • As needed, maintain patent IV access, reorient the patient, and provide supportive measures and appropriate patient instruction.
Disseminated Intravascular Coagulation (DIC, also called consumption coagulopathy) Complex disorder of coagulation or fibrinolysis (destruction of clots), which results in thrombosis or bleeding. DIC is most commonly associated with hematologic cancers (leukemia); cancer of prostate, GI tract, and lungs; chemotherapy (methotrexate, prednisone, L-asparaginase, vincristine, and 6-mercaptopurine), and disease processes, such as sepsis, hepatic failure, and anaphylaxis. Blood clots form when normal coagulation mechanisms are triggered. Once activated, the clotting cascade continues to consume clotting factors and platelets faster than the body can re-	*Clinical* *Chronic DIC:* Few or no observable symptoms or easy bruising, prolonged bleeding from venipuncture and injection sites, bleeding of the gums, and slow GI bleeding *Acute DIC:* life-threatening hemorrhage and infarction; clinical symptoms of this syndrome are varied and depend on the organ system involved in thrombus and infarction or bleeding episodes *Diagnostic* • Prolonged prothrombin time (PT or protime) • Prolonged partial thromboplastin time (PTT) • Prolonged thrombin time (TT) • Decreased fibrinogen level • Decreased platelet level • Decrease in clotting factors	*Medical* • Chemotherapy, biologic response modifier therapy, radiation therapy, or surgery is used to treat the underlying cancer. • Antibiotic therapy is used for sepsis. • Anticoagulants, such as heparin or antithrombin III, decrease the stimulation of the coagulation pathways. • Transfusion of fresh-frozen plasma or cryoprecipitates (which contain clotting factors and fibrinogen), packed red blood cells, and platelets may be used as replacement therapy to prevent or control bleeding. • Although controversial, antifibrinolytic agents such as aminocaproic acid (Amicar), which is associated with increased thrombus formation, may be used.

(continued)

Table 16-13 • **Oncologic Emergencies: Manifestations and Management** (Continued)

EMERGENCY	CLINICAL MANIFESTATIONS AND DIAGNOSTIC FINDINGS	MANAGEMENT
place them. Clots are deposited in the microvasculature, placing the patient at great risk for impaired circulation, tissue hypoxia, and necrosis. In addition, fibrinolysis occurs, breaking down clots and increasing the circulating levels of anticoagulant substances, thereby placing the patient at risk for hemorrhage.	• Decreased hemoglobin • Decreased hematocrit • Elevated fibrin split products • Positive protamine sulfate precipitation test (thrombin activation test)	*Nursing* • Monitor vital signs. • Measure and document intake and output. • Assess skin colour and temperature; lung, heart, and bowel sounds; level of consciousness, headache, visual disturbances, chest pain, decreased urine output, and abdominal tenderness. • Inspect all body orifices, tube insertion sites, incisions, and bodily excretions for bleeding. • Review laboratory test results. • Minimize physical activity to decrease injury risks and oxygen requirements. • Prevent bleeding; apply pressure to all venipuncture sites, and avoid nonessential invasive procedures; provide electric rather than straight-edged razors; avoid tape on the skin and advise gentle but adequate oral hygiene. • Assist the patient to turn, cough, and take deep breaths every 2 hours. • Reorient the patient, if needed; maintain a safe environment; and provide appropriate patient education and supportive measures.
Syndrome of Inappropriate Secretion of Antidiuretic Hormone (SIADH) The continuous, uncontrolled release of antidiuretic hormone (ADH), produced by tumor cells or by the abnormal stimulation of the hypothalmic–pituitary network, leads to increased extracellular fluid volume, water intoxication, hyponatremia, and increased excretion of urinary sodium. As fluid volume increases, stretch receptors in the right atrium respond by releasing a second hormone, atrial natriuretic factor (ANF). The release of ANF causes increased renal excretion of sodium, which worsens hyponatremia. The most common cause of SIADH is cancer, especially small cell cancers of the lung. Antineoplastics—vincristine, vinblastine, cisplatin, and cyclophosphamide—and morphine also stimulate ADH secretion, which promotes conservation and reabsorption of water by the kidneys. As more fluid is absorbed, the circulatory volume increases, ANF is released, and sodium is actively excreted by the kidneys in compensation.	*Clinical* *Serum sodium levels below 120 mmol/L:* symptoms of hyponatremia including personality changes, irritability, nausea, anorexia, vomiting, weight gain, fatigue, muscular pain (myalgia), headache, lethargy, and confusion. *Serum sodium levels below 110 mmol/L:* seizure, abnormal reflexes, papilledema, coma, and death. Edema is rare. *Diagnostic* • Decreased serum sodium level • Increased urine osmolality • Increased urinary sodium level • Decreased BUN, creatinine, and serum albumin levels secondary to dilution • Abnormal water load test results	*Medical* Fluid intake range limited to 500 to 1,000 mL/day to increase the serum sodium level and decrease fluid overload. If water restriction alone is not effective in correcting or controlling serum sodium levels, demeclocycline is often prescribed to interfere with the antidiuretic action of ADH and ANF. When neurologic symptoms are severe, parenteral sodium replacement and diuretic therapy are indicated. Electrolyte levels are monitored carefully to detect secondary magnesium, potassium, and calcium imbalances. After the symptoms of SIADH are controlled, the underlying cancer is treated. If water excess continues despite treatment, pharmacologic intervention (urea and furosemide) may be indicated. *Nursing* • Maintain intake and output measurements. • Assess level of consciousness, lung and heart sounds, vital signs, daily weight, and urine specific gravity; also assess for nausea, vomiting, anorexia, edema, fatigue, and lethargy. • Monitor laboratory test results, including serum electrolyte levels, osmolality, and blood urea nitrogen, creatinine, and urinary sodium levels. • Minimize the patient's activity; provide appropriate oral hygiene; maintain environmental safety; and restrict fluid intake if necessary. • Reorient the patient and provide instruction and encouragement as needed.
Tumor Lysis Syndrome Potentially fatal complication associated with radiation- or chemotherapy-induced cell destruction of large or rapidly growing cancers such as leukemia, lymphoma, and small cell lung cancer. The release of intracellular contents from the tumor cells, leads to electrolyte imbalances—hyperkalemia,	*Clinical* Clinical manifestations depend on the extent of metabolic abnormalities. • Neurologic: Fatigue, weakness, memory loss, altered mental status, muscle cramps, tetany, paresthesias (numbness and tingling), seizures • Cardiac: Elevated blood pressure, shortened QT complexes, widened QRS waves, dysrhythmias, cardiac arrest	*Medical* • To prevent renal failure and restore electrolyte balance, aggressive fluid hydration is initiated 48 hours before and after the initiation of cytotoxic therapy to increase urine volume and eliminate uric acid and electrolytes. Urine is alkalinized by adding sodium bicarbonate to IV fluid to maintain a urine pH of 7 or more; this prevents renal failure secondary to uric acid precipitation in the kidneys.

(continued)

Table 16-13 • **Oncologic Emergencies: Manifestations and Management** (Continued)

EMERGENCY	CLINICAL MANIFESTATIONS AND DIAGNOSTIC FINDINGS	MANAGEMENT
hypocalcemia, hyperphosphatemia, and hyperuricemia—because the kidneys can no longer excrete large volumes of the released intracellular metabolites.	• GI: Anorexia, nausea, vomiting, abdominal cramps, diarrhea • Renal: Flank pain, oliguria, anuria, renal failure, acidic urine pH *Diagnostic* Electrolyte imbalances identified by laboratory test results	• Diuretic therapy, with a carbonic anhydrase inhibitor or acetazolamide, to alkalinize the urine • Allopurinol therapy to inhibit the conversion of nucleic acids to uric acid • Administration of a cation-exchange resin, such as sodium polystyrene sulfonate (Kayexalate) to treat hyperkalemia by binding and eliminating potassium through the bowel • Administration of hypertonic dextrose and regular insulin temporarily shifts potassium into cells and lowers serum potassium levels. • Administration of phosphate-binding gels, such as aluminum hydroxide, to treat hyperphosphatemia by promoting phosphate excretion in the feces • Hemodialysis when patients are unresponsive to the standard approaches for managing uric acid and electrolyte abnormalities *Nursing* • Identify at-risk patients, including those in whom tumor lysis syndrome may develop up to 1 week after therapy has been completed. • Institute essential preventive measures (eg, fluid hydration and allopurinol). • Assess patient for signs and symptoms of electrolyte imbalances. • Assess urine pH to confirm alkalization. • Monitor serum electrolyte and uric acid levels for evidence of fluid volume overload secondary to aggressive hydration. • Instruct patients to report symptoms indicating electrolyte disturbances.

 Critical Thinking Exercises

1. You are seeing a married couple in their 70s in the clinic for blood pressure checks. What questions regarding cancer screening are appropriate for them? How would you respond if your suggestions for cancer screening are met with the answer that they are too old to worry about cancer? What special considerations are there if the woman has a physical disability that requires her to use a wheelchair?

2. A 54-year-old woman with bone metastases secondary to breast cancer has been admitted to the hospital with a diagnosis of hypercalcemia. Describe the underlying cause of hypercalcemia and the medical and nursing management strategies that are anticipated. What patient monitoring would be essential before and after treatment of hypercalcemia?

3. One of your home care patients, a 42-year-old executive of a major corporation, has a nonresectable malignant brain tumor for which she is receiving radiation therapy. She is being discharged from the hospital and will continue therapy as an outpatient. She and her husband are concerned about her future and survival and are also concerned about the impact of the diagnosis on the couple's 10-year-old twins. She is also concerned about her ability to carry out her executive responsibilities. What assessment by the nurse is indicated at this point, and what actions would be warranted by the nurse to help the patient and her husband deal with their concerns?

4. A 70-year-old man with advanced cancer living at home with his wife has been experiencing increasingly severe pain for which an oral opioid analgesic has recently been prescribed. What nursing assessments are essential for the home care nurse? What teaching will be indicated for the patient and family? How would you modify your teaching if the patient and his wife understand little English?

REFERENCES AND SELECTED READINGS

Books

Abeloff, M. D., Armitage, J. D., Lichter, A., & Niederhuber, J. E. (Eds). (2000). *Clinical oncology* (2nd ed.). Philadelphia: Churchill Livingstone.

Abrahm, J. L. (2000). *A physician's guide to pain and symptom management in cancer patients.* Baltimore: The Johns Hopkins University Press.

Agency for Health Care Policy and Research, Public Health Service, Department of Health and Human Services. (1992). *Acute pain management: Operative or medical procedures and trauma.* Clinical Practice Guideline (AHCPR 92-0032). Washington, DC: U.S. Government Printing Office.

Agency for Health Care Policy and Research, Public Health Service, Department of Health and Human Services. (1994). *Management of cancer pain: adults.* Clinical Practice Guideline (AHCPR 94-0592). Washington, DC: U.S. Government Printing Office.

American Pain Society. (1999). *Principles of analgesic use in the treatment of acute pain and chronic cancer pain: A concise guide to medical practice* (4th ed.). Skokie, IL: American Pain Society.

Barraclough, J. (1999). *Cancer and emotion: A practical guide to psycho-oncology* (3rd ed.). West Sussex: John Wiley and Sons.

Boik, J. (1995). *Cancer and natural medicine: A textbook of basic science and clinical research.* Princeton, MN: Oregon Medical Press.

Canadian Cancer Society. (2004). *Canadian cancer statistics 2004.* Ottawa: Author.

DeVita, V. T., Hellman, S., & Rosenberg, S. A. (Eds.). (1995). *Biologic therapy of cancer* (2nd ed.). Philadelphia: J. B. Lippincott.

Green, F., et al. (2002). *AJCC cancer staging manual* (6th ed.). New York: Springer-Verlag.

Groenwald, S., Hansen-Frogge, M., Goodman, M., & Henke Yarbro, C. (Eds.). (1998). *Comprehensive cancer nursing review* (4th ed.). Boston: Jones and Bartlett.

Heath, C. W., & Fontham, E. (2001). Cancer etiology. In: *Clinical oncology.* Atlanta: American Cancer Society.

Huber, E. B., & Magrath, I. (Eds.) (1998). *Gene therapy in treatment of cancer: Progress and prospects.* New York: Cambridge University Press.

Lenhard, R. E., Osteen, R. T., & Gansler, T. (Eds.). (2001). *Clinical oncology.* Atlanta: American Cancer Society.

Loeser, J. D. (Ed.) (2001). *Bonica's management of pain* (3d ed.). Philadelphia: Lippincott Williams & Wilkins.

Miaskowski, C. (1997). *Oncology nursing: An essential guide for patient care.* Philadelphia: W. B. Saunders.

Pazadur, R., Coia, L. R., Hoskins, W. J., & Wagman, L. D. (Eds.). (2001). *Cancer management: A multidisciplinary approach.* Melville, NY: PRR, Inc.

Perry, M. C. (Ed.). (1997). *The chemotherapy source book* (2nd ed.). Baltimore: Williams & Wilkins.

Ratain, M. J., Tempero, M., & Skosey, C. (2001). *Outline of oncology therapeutics.* Philadelphia: Saunders.

Winningham, M. L., & Barton-Burke, M. (Eds.) (2000). *Fatigue in cancer: A multidisciplinary approach.* Sudbury, MA: Jones & Bartlett.

Yarbro, C., Hansen-Frogge, M., & Goodman, M. (Eds.) (1999). *Cancer symptom management* (2d ed.). Sudbury, MA: Jones & Bartlett.

Yarbro, C. H. (Ed.) (2000). *Cancer: Principles and practice* (5th ed). Sudbury, MA: Jones & Bartlett.

Yokes, E. F., & Golomb, H. M. (Eds.) (1999). *Oncologic therapies.* New York: Springer.

Journals

General

Asterisks indicate nursing research articles.

Balducci, L., & Extermann, M. (2000). Management of cancer in the older person: A practical approach. *The Oncologist, 5*(3), 224–237.

*Berger, A. M., & Farr, L. (1999). The influence of daytime inactivity and nighttime restlessness on cancer-related fatigue. *Oncology Nursing Forum, 26*(10), 1663–1671.

Brown, J. K. (2002). A systematic review of the evidence on symptom management of cancer-related anorexia and cachexia. *Oncology Nursing Forum, 29*(3), 517–532.

Brown, P. A. (1999). Nutrition and cancer. *MedSurg Nursing, 8*(6), 333–345.

Carroll-Johnson, R. M. (Ed.). (2000). Cancer prevention and early detection: Oncology nursing's next frontier. *Oncology Nursing Forum, 27*(9) supplement, 1–63.

Cassileth, B. R. (1999). Evaluating complementary and alternative therapies for cancer patients. *CA: Cancer Journal for Clinicians, 49*(6), 362–375.

Chernecky, C., & Shelton, B. (2001). Pulmonary complications in patients with cancer. *American Journal of Nursing, 101*(5), 24A, 24E, 24G, 24H.

Cunningham, R. S. (Ed.). (2000). Nutrition and cancer. *Seminars in Oncology Nursing, 16*(2), 1–173.

Daniel, B. T. (Ed). (2001). Palliative and supportive care of advanced cancer. *Nursing Clinics of North America, 36*(4), 631–869.

Finley, J. P. (2000). Management of cancer cachexia. *AACN Clinical Issues, 11*(4), 590–603.

Fisher, B., et al. (1998). Tamoxifen for prevention of breast cancer: Report of the National Surgical Adjuvant Breast and Bowel Project P-1 study. *Journal of National Cancer Institute, 90*(18), 1371–1388.

Grant, M., & Kravits, K. (2000). Symptoms and their impact on nutrition. *Seminars in Oncology Nursing, 16*(2), 113–121.

Haisfield-Wolfe, M. E., & Baxendale-Cox, L. (1999). Staging of malignant and cutaneous wounds: A pilot study. *Oncology Nursing Forum, 22*(6), 1055–1064.

*Howell, D., Butler, L., Vincent, L., Watt-Watson, J., & Stearns, N. (2000). Influencing nurses' knowledge, attitudes and practice in cancer pain management. *Cancer Nursing, 23*(1), 55–63.

Houshmand, S. L., Campbell, C. T., Briggs, S. E., McFadden, A. W. J., & Al-Tweigeri, T. (2000). Prophylactic mastectomy and genetic testing: An update. *Oncology Nursing Forum, 27*(10), 1537–1547.

Hsueh, E. C., Hansen, N., & Giulaino, A. E. (2000). Intraoperative lymphatic mapping and sentinel lymph node dissection in breast cancer. *CA: Cancer Journal for Clinicians, 50*(3), 279–291.

International Radiosurgery Support Association (2000). Stereotactic radiosurgery overview. Retrieved from the World Wide Web: http://www.irsa.org/srs.html Jan. 25, 2002.

Jennings, M. (Ed.) (2001). Treatment advances in surgical oncology. *Nursing Clinics of North America, 36*(3), 499–623.

Kelly, L. D. (1999). Nursing assessment and patient management. *Seminars in Oncology Nursing, 15*(4), 282–291.

Kurtz, M. E., Kurtz, J. C., Stommel, M., Given, C. W., & Given, B. (2001). Physical functioning and depression among older persons with cancer. *Cancer Practice, 9*(1), 11–18.

Letizia, M. (2001). Addressing alopecia: Helping patients with cancer deal with hair loss. *American Journal of Nursing, 101*(4), 24LL.

Messner, C., & Patterson, D. (2001). The challenge of cancer in the workplace. *Cancer Practice, 9*(1), 50–51.

Montbriand, M. J. (1999). Past and present herbs used to treat cancer: Medicine, magic, or poison? *Oncology Nursing Forum, 26*(1), 49–59.

Moore, S. (2002). Cutaneous metastatic breast cancer. *Clinical Journal of Oncology Nursing, 6*(5), 255–260

Nail, L. M. (2002). Fatigue in patients with cancer. *Oncology Nursing Forum, 29*(3), 537–546.

Olson, K., Tom, B., Hewitt, J., et al. (2002). Evolving routines: Managing fatigue associated with lung and colorectal cancer. *Qualitative Health Research, 5,* 655–670.

Olson, K., Hanson, J., Hamilton, H., et al. (2004). Assessing the reliability and validity of the revised WCCNR stomatitis staging system for cancer therapy-induced stomatitis. *Canadian Oncology Nursing Journal, 14* (3), 168–174.

*Phillips, M. P., Cohen, M. Z., & Moses, G. (1999). Breast cancer screening and African American women: Fear, fatalism and silence. *Oncology Nursing Forum, 26*(3), 561–571.

Rust, D. M., Wood, L. S., & Battiato, L. A. (1999). Oprelvekin: an alternative treatment for thrombocytopenia. *Clinical Journal of Oncology Nursing, 3*(2), 57–62.

Shih, A., Misakowski, C., Dodd, M. L., et al. (2002). A research review of current treatment for radiation-induced oral mucositis in patients with head and neck cancer. *Oncology Nursing Forum, 29*(7), 1063–1080.

Sonis, S. T., et al. (2001). Oral mucositis and the clinical and economic outcomes of hematopoietic stem-cell transplantation. *Journal of Clinical Oncology, 19*(8), 2201–2205.

Smith, R. A., et al. (2001). American Cancer Society guidelines for the early detection of cancer: Update of early detection guidelines for prostate, colorectal and endometrial cancers. *CA: Cancer Journal for Clinicians, 51*(1), 38–76.

*Sparber, A., Bauer, L., Curt, G., Eisenberg, D., Levin, T., Parks, S., Steinberg, S. M., & Wooten, J. (2000). Use of complementary medicine by adult patients participating in cancer clinical trials. *Oncology Nursing Forum, 27*(4), 623–630.

Western Consortium for Cancer Nursing Research. (1987). Priorities for cancer nursing research: A Canadian replication. *Cancer Nursing, 10* (6), 319–326.

Western Consortium for Cancer Nursing Research. (1991). Development of a staging system for chemotherapy-induced stomatitis. *Cancer Nursing, 14* (1), 6–12.

Western Consortium for Cancer Nursing Research. (1998). Assessing stomatitis: Refinement of the Western Consortium for Cancer Nursing Research (WCCNR) stomatitis staging system. *Canadian Oncology Nursing Journal, 8* (3), 160–162, 165.

Whitman, M. M. (2000). The starving patient: Supportive care for people with cancer. *Clinical Journal of Oncology Nursing, 4*(3), 121–125.

Wilson, R. L. (2000). Optimizing nutrition for patients with cancer. *Clinical Journal of Oncology Nursing, 4*(1), 23–28.

Wojtaszek, C. (2000). Management of chemotherapy-induced stomatitis. *Clinical Journal of Oncology Nursing, 4*(6), 263–270.

Yeager, K. A., Webster, J., Crain, M., Kasow, J., & McGuire, D. B. (2000). Implementation of an oral care standard for leukemia and transplantation patients. *Cancer Nursing, 23*(1), 40–47.

Zimmerman, V. L. (2002). BRCA gene mutations and cancer. *American Journal of Nursing, 102*(8), 28–36.

Biologic Response Modifiers

Buchsel, P. C., Forgey, A., Grape, F. B., & Hamann, S. S. (2002) Granulocyte macrophage colony-stimulating factor: Current practice and novel approaches. *Clinical Journal of Oncology Nursing, 6*(4), 198–205.

Buchsel, P. C., Murph, B. S., & Newton, S. A. (2002). Epoetin alpha: Current and future indications and nursing implications. *Clinical Journal of Oncology Nursing, 6*(5), 261–267.

Capriotti, T. (2001). Monoclonal antibodies: Drugs that combine pharmacology and biotechnology. *MedSurg Nursing, 10*(2), 89–95.

Estes, J. (Ed.) (2002). New approaches to the management of non-Hodgkin's lymphoma. A continuing education activity. *Seminars in Oncology Nursing, 18*(1), supplement, 1–33.

Evans, T. R., & Kaye, S. B. (1999). Retinoids: Present role and future potential. *British Journal of Cancer, 800*(1–2), 1–8.

Kelloff, G. J. (2000). Perspectives on cancer chemoprevention research and drug development. *Advances in Cancer Research, 78*(2000), 199–334.

Kosits, C., & Callaghan, S. (2000). Rituximab: A new monoclonal antibody therapy for non-Hodgkin's lymphoma. *Oncology Nursing Forum, 27*(1), 51–59.

Kurie, J. M. (1999). The biologic basis for the use of retinoids in cancer prevention and treatment. *Current Opinion in Oncology, 11*(6), 497–502.

Moldawer, N., & Carr, E. (2000). The promise of recombinant interleukin-2. *American Journal of Nursing, 100*(5), 35–39.

Peyrot, J. (1999). Herceptin. *Oncology Nursing Forum, 26*(3), 515–516.

Seeley, K. & DeMeyer, E. (2002). Nursing care of patients receiving Campath. *Clinical Journal of Oncology Nursing, 6*(3), 138–143.

Sorokin, P. (2000). Mylotarg approved for patients with CD33+ acute myeloid leukemia. *Clinical Journal of Oncology Nursing, 4*(5), 279–280.

Sorokin, P. (2002). New agents and future directions in biotherapy. *Clinical Journal of Oncology Nursing, 6*(1), 19–24.

Weiner, L. M. (1999). An overview of monoclonal antibody therapy of cancer. *Seminars in Oncology, 26*(4) supplement 12, 41–50.

Yarbro, C. (Ed.). (2000). A new biologic approach for the treatment of metastatic breast cancer. *Seminars in Oncology Nursing, 16*(4) supplement 1, 1–38.

Bone Marrow Transplantation

Alcoser, P. W., & Burchett, S. (1999). Bone marrow transplantation: Immune system suppression and reconstitution. *American Journal of Nursing, 99*(6), 26–31.

Applebaum, F. R. (1996). The use of bone marrow and peripheral blood cell transplantation in the treatment of cancer. *CA: Cancer Journal for Clinicians, 46*(3), 142–164.

Buchsel, P. C., & Kapustay, P. M. (1995). Peripheral stem cell transplantation. *Oncology Nursing Update: Patient Treatment and Support, 2*(2), 1–14.

Buchsel, P. C., et al. (1996). Delayed complications of bone marrow transplantation: An update. *Oncology Nursing Forum, 23*(8), 1267–1291.

Hurley, C. (1997). Ambulatory care after bone marrow or peripheral blood stem cell transplantation. *Clinical Journal of Oncology Nursing, 1*(1), 19–21.

Poliquin, C. M. (1997). Overview of bone marrow and peripheral blood stem cell transplantation. *Clinical Journal of Oncology Nursing, 1*(1), 11–17.

Carcinogenesis and Risk Factors

Foltz, A. T., & Mahon, S. M. (2000). Application of carcinogenesis theory to primary prevention. *Oncology Nursing Forum, 27*(9), supplement, 5–11.

Fraser, M. C., et al. (1997). Familial cancers: Evolving challenges for nursing practice. *Oncology Nursing Update: Patient Treatment and Support, 4*(3), 1–18.

Greco, K. E. (2000). Cancer genetics nursing: Impact of the double helix. *Oncology Nursing Forum, 27*(9), supplement, 29–36.

Kobayashi, A., Miaskowski, C., Wallhagen, M., & Smith-McCune, K. (2000). Recent developments in understanding the immune response to human papilloma virus infection and cervical neoplasia. *Oncology Nursing Forum, 27*(4), 643–651.

Lessick, M., Wickham, R., Chapman, D., et al. (2001). Advances in genetic testing for cancer risk. *MedSurg Nursing, 10*(3), 123–127.

Stillman, J. M., & Stillman, S. D. (1996). Cancer and the workplace. *CA: Cancer Journal for Clinicians, 46*(2), 70–92.

Chemotherapy

Anastasia, P. J. (2000). Effectiveness of oral 5-HT3 receptor antagonists for emetogenic chemotherapy. *Oncology Nursing Forum, 277*(3), 483–493.

Bremerkamp, M. (2000). Mechanisms of action of 5-HT3 receptor antagonists: Clinical overview and nursing implications. *Clinical Journal of Oncology Nursing, 4*(5), 201–207.

Dodd, M. J., Dibble, S. L., Miaskowski, C., et al. (2000). Randomized clinical trial of the effectiveness of 3 commonly used mouthwashes to treat chemotherapy-induced mucositis. *Oral Surgery Oral Medicine Oral Pathology Oral Radiology & Endodontics, 90*(1), 39–47.

Doherty, K. M. (1999). Closing the gap in prophylactic antiemetic therapy: Patient factors in calculating the emetogenic potential of chemotherapy. *Clinical Journal of Oncology Nursing, 3*(3), 113–119.

Line, L. G., Campbell, J. M., & Kinion, E. S. (2001). Infections in patients receiving cytotoxic chemotherapy. *MedSurg Nursing, 10*(2), 61–68.

Rogers, B. B. (2001). Mucositis in the oncology patient. *Nursing Clinics of North America, 36*(4), 745–760.

Schulmeister, L., & Camp-Sorrell, D. (2000). Chemotherapy extravasation from implanted ports. *Oncology Nursing Forum, 27*(3), 531–538.

Gene Therapy

Fibison, W. J. (2000). Gene therapy. *Nursing Clinics of North America, 35*(3), 757–773.

Frankel, M. S., & Chapman, A. R. (2000). Human inheritable genetic modifications: Assessing scientific, ethical, religious and policy issues. *American Association for the Advancement of Science, 1–82.

Johnson, K. J., & Brensinger, J. D. (2000). Genetic counseling and testing: Implications for clinical practice. *Nursing Clinics of North America, 35*(3), 615–626.

Lea, D. H. (2000). A clinician's primer in human genetics. *Nursing Clinics of North America, 35*(3), 583–614.

Nogueira, S. M., & Appling, S. E. (2000). Breast cancer: Genetics, risks and strategies. *Nursing Clinics of North America, 35*(3), 663–669.

Olsen, S. J., & Zawaacki, K. (2000). Hereditary colorectal cancer. *Nursing Clinics of North America, 35*(3), 671–685.

Wasil, T., & Buchbinder, A. (2000). Gene therapy in human cancer: Report of Human Clinical Trials. *Cancer Investigation, 18*(8), 740–746.

Oncologic Emergencies

Barnett, M. L. (1999). Hypercalcemia. *Seminars in Oncology Nursing, 15*(3), 190–201.

Beauchamp, K. A. (1998). Pericardial tamponade: An oncologic emergency. *Clinical Journal of Oncology Nursing, 2*(3), 85–95.

Bucholtz, J. D. (1999). Metastatic epidural spinal cord compression. *Seminars in Oncology Nursing, 15*(3), 150–159.

Ezzone, S. A. (1999). Tumor lysis syndrome. *Seminars in Oncology Nursing, 15*(3), 190–201.

Gardner, C. M. (1999). Cancer-related spinal cord compression. *American Journal of Nursing, 99*(7), 34–35.

Haapoja, I. S., & Blendowski, C. (1999). Superior vena cava syndrome. *Seminars in Oncology Nursing, 15*(3), 183–189.

Holmes Gobel, B. (Ed.). (1999). Oncologic emergencies. *Seminars in Oncology Nursing, 15*(3), 149–234.

Schindler, N., & Vogelzang, R. L. (1999). Superior vena cava: Experience with endovascular stents and surgical treatment. *Surgical Clinics of North America, 79*(3), 683–694.

Terpstra, T. L., & Terpstra, T. L. (2000). Syndrome of inappropriate antidiuretic hormone secretion: Recognition and management. *MedSurg Nursing, 9*(2), 61–68.

Wheeler, A. P., & Gordon, B. R. (1999). Current concepts: Treating patients with severe sepsis. *New England Journal of Medicine, 340*(3), 207–214.

Pain

Chang, H. M. (1999). Cancer pain management. *Medical Clinics of North America, 83*(3), 711–736.

Ciezki, J. P., Komurcy, S., & Macklis, R. M. (2000). Palliative radiotherapy. *Seminars in Oncology, 27*(1), 90–93.

Dalton, J. A. & Youngblood, R. (2000). Clinical application of the WHO analgesic ladder. *Journal of Intravenous Nursing, 23*(2), 118–124.

Easley, M. K., & Elliott, S. (2001). Managing pain at the end of life. *Nursing Clinics of North America, 36*(4), 779–794.

Grossman, S. A., Benditti, C., Payne, R., & Syrjala, K. (1999). NCCN practice guidelines for cancer pain. *Oncology, 13*(11A), 1–4.

Pargeon, K. L., & Hailey, B. J. (1999). Barriers to effective cancer pain management. *Journal of Pain and Symptom Management, 18*(5), 358–368.

Radiation Therapy

Abel, L. J., Blatt, H. J., Stipetich, R. L., et al. (2000). The role of urinary assessment scores in the nursing management of patients receiving prostate brachytherapy. *Clinical Journal of Oncology Nursing, 4*(3), 126–129.

Blackman, A. (1997). Radiation-induced skin alterations. *MedSurg Nursing, 6*(3), 172–175.

Cash, J. C., & Dattoli, M. J. (1997). Management of patients receiving trans-perineal Palladium-103 prostate implants. *Oncology Nursing Forum, 24*(8), 1361–1367.

*Christman, N. J., Oakley, M. G., & Cronin, S. N. (2001). Developing and using preparatory information for women undergoing radiation therapy for cervical or uterine cancer. *Oncology Nursing Forum, 28*(1), 93–98.

Iwamoto, R. R., & Maher, K. E. (2001). Radiation therapy for prostate cancer. *Seminars in Oncology Nursing, 17*(2), 90–100.

Stajduhar, K. I., Neithercut, J., Chu, E., Pham, P., Rohde, J., Sicotte, A., & Young, K. (2000). Thyroid cancer patients' experiences of receiving iodine-131 therapy. *Oncology Nursing Forum, 27*(8), 1213–1218.

*Velji, K., & Fitch, M. (2001). The experience of women receiving brachytherapy for gynecologic cancer. *Oncology Nursing Forum, 28*(4), 743–751.

RESOURCES AND WEBSITES
Patient/Family Support and Education

Alberta Cancer Board; http://www.cancerboard.ab.ca.

American Brain Tumor Association, 2720 River Road, Des Plaines, IL 60018; (847) 827-9910, Fax: (847) 827-9918, Patient Line: (800) 886-2282; http://www.abta.org.

American Cancer Society (ACS), 1599 Clifton Road NE, Atlanta, GA 30329; (800)-ACS-2345 (check your local directory for the unit of division nearest you); http://www.cancer.org.

Atlantic Health Sciences Corporation; http://www.absc.health.nb.ca/.

BC Cancer Agency; http://www.bccancer.bc.ca.

Canadian Breast Cancer Network; http://www.cbcn.ca.

Canadian Cancer Society; http://www.cancer.ca.

Canadian Prostate Cancer Network; http://www.cpcn.org.

Cancer Care, Inc., National Office, 275 7th Ave., New York, NY 10001; Services: (212) 302-2400, (800)-813-HOPE (4673); http://www.info@cancercare.org.

Cancer Care Manitoba; http://www.cancercare.mb.ca.

Cancer Care Ontario; http://www.cancercare.on.ca.

Cancer Care Nova Scotia; http://www.cancercare.ns.ca.

Cancer Information Network: http://www.cancernetwork.com.

CancerNet (a service of the National Cancer Institute): cancernet-staff@mail.nih.gov; http://cancernet.nci.nih.gov/index.html.

CancerSource World Headquarters, 40 Tall Pine Drive, Sudbury, MA 01776; http://www.cancersource.com.

Colorectal Cancer Association of Canada; http://www.ccac-accc.ca.

La Fondation Québécoise du Cancer; http://www.fqc.qc.ca/.

Make Today Count, 1235 East Cherokee Street, Springfield, MO 85804; (407) 885-3324 or (800) 432-2273.

National Alliance of Breast Cancer Organizations (NABCO), 9 East 37th Street, 10th Floor, New York, NY 10016; (888) 806-2226; http://www.nabo.org:80/index.html.

The National Cancer Institute Public Inquiries Office, Building, 31, Room 10A31, 31 Center Drive, MSC 2580, Bethesda, MD 20892-2580; (800)-4-CANCER; http://rex.nci.nih.gov.

National Coalition for Cancer Survivorship, 1010 Wayne Avenue, Suite 770, Silver Spring, MD 20910-5600; (301) 650-9127 or (877) NCCS-YES (877-622-7937); Fax: (301) 565-9670; http://www.cansearch.org.

The National Hospice and Palliative Care Organization, 1700 Diagonal Road, Suite 300, Alexandria, VA 22314; (703) 837-1500; http://info@nhpco.org.

Newfoundland Cancer Treatment and Research Foundation; http://www.nctrf.nf.ca.

Oncolink; the University of Pennsylvania Cancer Center, 3400 Spruce St., Philadelphia, PA 19104; http://www.oncolink.upenn.edu.

Prince Edward Island–Queen Elizabeth Hospital, Oncology Clinic, PO Box 6600, Riverside Drive, Charlottetown, PEI C1A 8T5; (902) 473-4638, fax: (902) 473-4632.

The Quebec Centre for Cancer Control, 1075 Chemin Ste-Foy, 7e etage, Quebec, QC G1S 2M1; (418) 266-405, fax: (418) 266-6938.

Saskatchewan Cancer Agency; http://www.scf.sk.ca.

The Wellness Community, 35 E. Seventh St., Suite 412, Cincinnati, OH 45202; (513) 421-7111, Fax (513) 421-7119, (888)-793-WELL; http://www.wellness-community.org.

End-of-Life Care

Adapted by Kärin Olson and Cynthia Cummings-Winfield

LEARNING OBJECTIVES ●

On completion of this chapter, the learner will be able to:

1. Discuss the historical, legal, and sociocultural perspectives of palliative and end-of-life care.
2. Define palliative care.
3. Compare and contrast the settings where palliative care and end-of-life care are provided.
4. Describe the principles and components of hospice care.
5. Identify barriers to improving care at the end of life.
6. Reflect on personal experience with and attitudes toward death and dying.
7. Apply skills for communicating with terminally ill patients and their families.
8. Provide culturally and spiritually sensitive care to terminally ill patients and their families.
9. Implement nursing measures to manage physiologic responses to terminal illness.
10. Support actively dying patients and their families.
11. Identify components of uncomplicated grief and mourning and implement nursing measures to support the patient and family.

Nursing and End-of-Life Care

One of the most difficult realities that nurses face is that, despite our very best efforts, some patients will die. Although we cannot change this fact, we can have a significant and lasting effect on the way in which patients live until they die, the manner in which the death occurs, and the enduring memories of that death for the families. Nursing has a long history of holistic, person- and family-centred care. There is perhaps no setting or circumstance in which care—that is, attention to human responses—is more important than in caring for the dying patient.

Knowledge about end-of-life decisions and principles of care is essential to supporting patients during decision making and in end-of-life closure in ways that recognize their unique responses to illness and that support their values and goals. Education, clinical practice, and research concerning end-of-life care are evolving, and the need to prepare nurses and other health care professionals to care for the dying has emerged as a priority. At no time in nursing's history has there been a greater opportunity to bring research, education, and practice together to change the culture of dying, bringing much-needed improvement to care that is relevant across practice settings, age groups, cultural backgrounds, and illnesses.

THE CONTEXT FOR DEATH AND DYING

In the past three decades there has been a surge of interest in the care of the dying, with an emphasis on the settings in which death occurs, the technologies used to sustain life, and the challenges of trying to improve end-of-life care. The focus on care of the dying has been motivated by the aging of the population, the prevalence of and publicity surrounding life-threatening illnesses such as cancer and AIDS, and the efforts of health care providers to build a continuum of service that spans the lifetime from birth until death (Lesparre & Matherlee, 1998). Although there are more opportunities than ever before to allow a peaceful death, the knowledge and technologies available to health care providers have made the process of dying anything but peaceful. According to Callahan (1993a), people view death as what happens when medicine fails, an attitude that often places the study of death and improvement of the dying process outside of the focus of modern medicine and health care. Numerous initiatives aimed at improving end-of-life care have been launched in recent years, spurred by a widespread call for substantive change in the way people deal with death.

The Palliative Care Task Force of the Last Acts Campaign (Last Acts, 1997) identified the following as precepts or principles underlying a more comprehensive and humane approach to care of the dying:

- Respecting patients' goals, preferences, and choices
- Attending to the medical, emotional, social, and spiritual needs of the dying person
- Using strengths of interdisciplinary resources
- Acknowledging and addressing caregiver concerns
- Building mechanisms and systems of support

TECHNOLOGY AND END-OF-LIFE CARE

In the last century, chronic, degenerative diseases replaced communicable diseases as the major causes of death. Although technological advances in health care have extended and improved the quality of life for many, the ability of technologies to prolong life beyond the point that some would consider meaningful has raised troubling ethical issues. In particular, the use of technology to sustain life has raised perplexing issues with regard to quality of life, prolongation of dying, adequacy of pain relief and symptom management, and allocation of scarce resources. The major ethical question that has emerged concerning the use of technology to extend life is: Because we can prolong life through a particular intervention, does it necessarily follow that we must do so? In the latter half of the 20th century a "technological imperative" practice pattern among health care professionals emerged, along with an expectation among patients and families that every available means to extend life must be tried.

Decisions to apply every available technology to extend life have contributed to the shift in the place of death from the home to the hospital or extended care facility. In the earlier part of the last century, most deaths occurred at home. Because of this, most families had direct experience "being with" death, providing care to family members at the end of life and mourning for the loss of loved ones. As the place of death shifted to the hospital, families became increasingly distanced from the death experience. By the early 1970s, when hospice care was just beginning in this country, technology had become the expected companion of the critically and terminally ill (Wentzel, 1981). The implications of technological

Glossary

assisted suicide: use of pharmacological agents to hasten the death of a terminally ill patient; illegal in most states

autonomy: self-determination; in the health care context, the right of the individual to make choices about the use and discontinuation of medical treatment

bereavement: period during which mourning for a loss takes place

euthanasia: Greek for "good death;" has evolved to mean the intentional killing by act or omission of a dependent human being for his or her alleged benefit

grief: the personal feelings that accompany an anticipated or actual loss

hospice: a coordinated program of interdisciplinary care and services provided primarily in the home to terminally ill patients and their families

interdisciplinary collaboration: members of diverse health care disciplines jointly plan, implement, and evaluate care

mourning: individual, family, group, and cultural expressions of grief and associated behaviours

palliative care: comprehensive care for patients whose disease is not responsive to cure; care also extends to patients' families

palliative sedation: use of pharmacological agents, at the request of the terminally ill

patient, to induce sedation when symptoms have not responded to other management measures. The purpose is not to hasten the patient's death but to relieve intractable symptoms.

spirituality: personal belief systems that focus on a search for meaning and purpose in life, intangible elements that impart meaning and vitality to life, and a connectedness to a higher or transcendent dimension

terminal illness: progressive, irreversible illness that despite cure-focused medical treatment will result in the patient's death intervention at the end of life continue to be profound, affecting a societal view of death that influences how clinicians care for the dying, how family and friends participate in care, how patients and families understand and choose among end-of-life care options, how families prepare for **terminal illness** and death, and how they heal following the death of a loved one.

SOCIOCULTURAL CONTEXT

Although each individual experiences terminal illness uniquely, such illness is also shaped substantially by the social and cultural contexts in which it occurs. Life-threatening illness, life-sustaining treatment decisions, dying, and death occur in a social environment where illness is largely considered a foe and where battles are either lost or won (Benoliel, 1993). A care/cure dichotomy has emerged in which health care providers may view cure as the ultimate good and care as second best (Benoliel, 1993; Gadow, 1988). In such a model of health or medical care, alleviating suffering is not as valued as curing disease, and patients who cannot be cured feel distanced from the health care team, concluding that when treatment has failed, they too have failed. Patients and families who have internalized the socially constructed meaning of care as second best may fear that any shift from curative goals in the direction of comfort-focused care will result in no care or poorer-quality care, and that the clinicians on whom they have come to rely will abandon them if they withdraw from the battle for cure.

The reduction of patients to their diseases is exemplified in the frequently relayed message in late-stage illness that "nothing more can be done." This all-too-frequently used statement communicates the belief of many clinicians that there is nothing of value to offer patients who are beyond cure. In a care-focused perspective, mind, body, and spirit are inextricable, and treating the body without attending to the other components is considered inadequate to evoke true healing (Upledger, 1989; Wendler, 1996). This expanded notion of healing as care, along with and beyond cure, implies that healing can take place throughout life and outside the boundaries of contemporary medicine. In this expanded definition, healing is transcendent and its boundaries are unlimited, even as body systems begin to fail at the end of life (Byock, 1997).

Clinicians' Attitudes Toward Death

Clinicians' attitudes toward the terminally ill and dying remain the greatest barrier to improving care at the end of life. Kübler-Ross illuminated the concerns of the seriously ill and dying in her seminal work *On Death and Dying,* published in 1969. At that time, it was common for patients to be kept uninformed about life-threatening diagnoses, particularly cancer, and for physicians and nurses to avoid open discussion of death and dying with their patients (Krisman-Scott, 2000; Seale, 1991). Kübler-Ross taught the health care community that having open discussion about life and death issues did not harm patients, and that the patients in fact welcomed such openness. She was openly critical of what she called "a new but depersonalized science in the service of prolonging life rather than diminishing human suffering" (Kübler-Ross, 1969, p. 20). She taught the health care community that healing could not take place in a conspiracy of silence, and that as clinicians break the silence and enter the patient's world, they too can be healed by their struggles and strengths. Her work revealed that, given adequate time and some help in working

through the process, patients could reach a stage of acceptance where they were neither angry nor depressed about their fate (Kübler-Ross, 1969).

Clinicians' reluctance to discuss disease and death openly with patients may stem from their own anxieties about death as well as misconceptions about what and how much patients want to know about their illnesses. In an early study of care of the dying in hospital settings, sociologists Glaser and Strauss (1965) discovered that health care professionals in hospital settings avoided direct communication about dying in hope that the patient would discover it on his or her own. They identified four "awareness contexts," described as the patient's, physician's, family's, and other health care professionals' awareness of the patient's status and their recognition of each other's awareness:

1. Closed awareness: The patient is unaware of his or her terminal state while others are aware. Closed awareness may be characterized by families and health care professionals conspiring to guard the "secret," fearing that the patient would not be able to cope with full disclosure about his or her status, and the patient's acceptance of others' accounts of his or her "future biography" as long as they give him or her no reason to be suspicious.
2. Suspected awareness: The patient suspects what others know and attempts to find out. Suspected awareness may be triggered by inconsistencies in families' and clinicians' communication and behaviour, discrepancies between clinicians' accounts of the seriousness of the patient's illness, or a decline in the patient's condition or other environmental cues.
3. Mutual pretense awareness: The patient, the family, and the health care professionals are aware that the patient is dying but all pretend otherwise.
4. Open awareness: All are aware that the patient is dying and are able to openly acknowledge that reality.

Glaser and Strauss (1965) also identified a pattern of clinician behaviour in which those who feared or were uncomfortable discussing death developed and substituted "personal mythologies" for appraisals of what level of disclosure patients actually wanted. For example, clinicians avoided direct communication with patients about the seriousness of their illness based on their beliefs that (1) patients already knew the truth or would ask if they wanted to know, or (2) patients would subsequently lose all hope, give up, or be psychologically harmed by disclosure.

Glaser and Strauss' findings were published more than 35 years ago, yet their observations remain valid today. Although a growing number of health care providers are becoming comfortable with assessing patients' and families' information needs and disclosing honest information about the seriousness of illness, many still avoid the topic of death in hopes that the patient will ask or find out on his or her own. Despite progress on many health care fronts, those who work with dying patients have identified the persistence of a "conspiracy of silence" about dying (Stanley, 2000, p. 34).

Patient and Family Denial

Denial on the part of the patient and family about the seriousness of terminal illness also has been cited as a barrier to discussion about end-of-life treatment options. Kübler-Ross (1969) was one of the first to examine patient denial and expose it as a useful coping mechanism that enables patients to gain temporary emotional distance from something that is too painful to contemplate fully. Patients who are characterized as being in denial may be using that strategy to preserve important interpersonal relationships, to protect others from the emotional effects of their illness, or to protect themselves because of fears of abandonment.

Connor (1992) studied a small group of terminally ill cancer patients who were characterized by their use of denial as a coping mechanism. Participants in the experimental group were questioned in structured interviews about their perceptions of the most difficult aspects of having cancer and those actions that they or others take that make these difficulties easier or more difficult to bear. They were offered psychosocial intervention that consisted largely of therapeutic communication followed by a postintervention assessment of their use of denial as a defense mechanism. The use of denial by patients in a control group was also assessed, but these patients did not receive the psychosocial intervention. The researcher concluded that terminally ill patients using denial respond favourably to sensitive psychosocial intervention, as indicated by decreased scores on an instrument to measure denial. Connor acknowledged, however, that additional research is needed to gauge the timing of such interventions according to some measure of patient readiness.

In a more recent study, researchers reported that while the majority of a sample of 200 patients with advanced cancer in their final weeks of life were completely aware of their medical prognosis, a combined total of 26.5% were either unaware or only partially aware (Chochinov, Tataryn, Wilson, Ennis & Lander, 2000). Depression was nearly three times greater in those patients who were unaware of their prognosis. The researchers concluded that denial of prognosis is more likely in patients with underlying psychological or emotional distress. Similarly, Chow and colleagues (2001) reported that many patients surveyed about their understanding of palliative radiation therapy for advanced cancer believed that their disease was curable, that the radiation therapy would cure their cancer, or that the therapy would prolong their lives. Importantly, most also reported that they were unfamiliar with the concept of radiation therapy, were not given information, or were not satisfied with the information their physicians had provided. Clearly, further research is needed to examine the complex interplay between patients' misconceptions about advanced illness, their underlying psychological states, and clinicians' persistent lack of candour in discussing treatment expectations and prognosis.

The question of how to communicate with patients in a way that acknowledges where they are on the continuum of acceptance, while providing them with unambiguous information, remains a challenge. Zerwekh (1994) analyzed stories from 32 hospice nurses and concluded that nurses in a hospice setting were adept at interventions deemed important in care of the dying, namely truth telling and encouraging patient **autonomy**. Although she acknowledged that each individual views "truth" differently, she observed that hospice nurses participating in the study used communication skills to assist the patient and family to discuss end-of-life issues. Hospice nurses deliberately spoke about sensitive matters that were usually avoided and gave patients and families truthful representations of their status when patients were in transition from curative to palliative care. Although timing of the questions takes experience, speaking the truth can be a relief to patients and families, enhancing their autonomy by making way for truly informed consent as the basis for decision making.

Assisted Suicide

The assisted suicide debate has aimed a spotlight on the adequacy and quality of end-of-life care. **Assisted suicide** refers to providing another person the means to end his or her own life. Physician-assisted suicide involves the prescription by a physician of a lethal dose of medication for the purpose of ending someone's life (not to be confused with the ethically and legally supported practices of withholding or withdrawing medical treatment in accordance with the wishes of the terminally ill individual).

Judeo-Christian beliefs support the view that suicide is a violation of natural law and the law of God (Helm, 1984; Sorenson, 1991). However, there have recently been calls for the legalization of assisted suicide. Although the preference to take one's own life over awaiting death has been evident through the ages, these recent efforts to legalize assisted suicide underscore the need for changes in the ways individuals with terminal illnesses are cared for and treated at the end of their lives. This is further emphasized by the efforts of groups such as the Hemlock Society to have physician-assisted suicide legalized and the Hemlock Society's publication of information to the public describing methods for ending one's own life when such assistance from physicians is not available.

Although assisted suicide is expressly prohibited in Canada, the calls for legalized assisted suicide have highlighted inadequacies in the care of the dying. In 1990, Dr. Jack Kevorkian, a retired pathologist, assisted a 54-year-old woman with early Alzheimer's disease to end her life using a device that he had devised to allow a patient to control the infusion of a lethal dose of potassium chloride. In 1999, after 130 deaths and nine trials, Kevorkian was convicted on second-degree murder charges in the death of a 52-year-old man with amyotrophic lateral sclerosis and is currently serving a 10- to 25-year prison sentence in Michigan. In a telephone poll conducted the week following the conviction, 55% of respondents disagreed with the verdict (Langer, 1999).

In 1994, voters approved the Oregon Death with Dignity Act, the first such legislative initiative in the United States to pass. This law provides for terminally ill patients' access to physician-assisted suicide under very controlled circumstances. After numerous challenges, a majority of Oregonians voted against an attempted repeal, and the law was implemented in 1997. The most recent challenges to the law included the 1999 federal Pain Relief Promotion Act, a bill designed to derail the implementation of the Oregon law by prohibiting the use of federally controlled substances for physician-assisted suicide, and a 2001 directive from Attorney General John Ashcroft to the Drug Enforcement Agency to track and prosecute physicians who prescribe under the Oregon law. There is an ongoing battle in the courts over this issue, and while Oregon is currently the only state with a statute legalizing physician-assisted suicide, it is likely that the issue will be pursued in the courts and through ballot measures in other states.

Whereas proponents of physician-assisted suicide argue that terminally ill individuals should have a legally sanctioned right to make independent decisions about the value of their lives and the timing and circumstances of their deaths, its opponents argue for greater access to symptom management and psychosocial support for individuals approaching the end of life. Numerous ethical and legal issues have been raised, including voluntariness and authenticity of requests in relation to the mental competence and decision-making capacity of patients who request physician-assisted suicide, the existence of underlying untreated clinical depression or other suffering, and issues of overt or perceived coercion. Assisted suicide is opposed by nursing and medical organizations as a violation of the ethical traditions of nursing and medicine.

Settings for End-of-Life Care: Palliative Care Programs and Hospice

PALLIATIVE CARE

Concerns have grown about the poor quality of life patients experience during progressive illness, broadening the concept of palliative care beyond the hospice (Jones, 1997). **Palliative care** is an approach to care for the seriously ill that has long been a part of cancer care. Both palliative care and hospice have been recognized as important bridges between the compulsion for cure-oriented care and physician-assisted suicide (Saunders & Kastenbaum, 1997). Advocates for improved care for the dying have stated that acceptance, management, and understanding of death should become fully integrated concepts in mainstream health care (Callahan, 1993a; Morrison, Siu, Leipzig et al., 2000). Increasingly, palliative care is being offered to patients with noncancer chronic illnesses, where comprehensive symptom management and psychosocial and spiritual support can enhance the patient's and family's quality of life.

While hospice care is considered by many to be the "gold standard" for palliative care, the term **hospice** is generally associated with palliative care that is delivered at home or in special facilities to patients who are approaching the end of life. Palliative care is conceptually broader than hospice care, defined as the active, total care of patients whose disease is not responsive to treatment (World Health Organization, 1990).

Palliative care emphasizes management of psychological, social, and spiritual problems in addition to control of pain and other physical symptoms. As the definition suggests, palliative care is not care that begins when cure-focused treatment ends. The goal of palliative care is to improve the patient's and family's quality of life, and many aspects of this type of comprehensive, comfort-focused approach to care are applicable earlier in the process of life-threatening disease in conjunction with cure-focused treatment. However, definitions of palliative care, the services that are part of it, and the clinicians who provide it are evolving steadily.

Some would argue that palliative care is no different from comprehensive nursing, medical, social, and spiritual care and that patients should not have to be labelled as "dying" to receive person-focused care and symptom management. In addition to a focus on the multiple dimensions of the illness experience for both patients and their families, palliative care emphasizes the interdisciplinary collaboration that is necessary to bring about the desired outcomes for patients and their families. **Interdisciplinary collaboration** is distinguished from multidisciplinary practice in that the former is based on communication and cooperation among the various disciplines; each member of the team contributes to a single care plan that addresses the needs of the patient and family.

Palliative Care at the End of Life

As discussed above, palliative care is broadly conceptualized as comprehensive, person- and family-centred care when disease is not responsive to treatment. Hospice care is in fact palliative care.

The difference is that hospice care is associated with the end of life, and although it focuses on quality of life, hospice care by necessity usually includes realistic emotional, social, spiritual, and financial preparation for death. In the mid-1970s, when hospice care was introduced, it was more broadly conceived as care that addressed the whole person—physical, social, emotional, and spiritual—and was available to patients earlier in the process of life-threatening illness.

The reasons for late referral to hospice and the underuse of hospice services are complex. They may include values and attitudes of health care providers, the inadequate dissemination of existing knowledge about pain and symptom management, health care providers' difficulties in effectively communicating with terminally ill individuals, and insufficient attention to palliative care concepts in health care providers' education and training.

It is clear that better care for the dying is urgently needed in hospitals, long-term care facilities, home care agencies, and outpatient settings. At the same time, many chronic diseases do not have a predictable "end stage" that fits hospice eligibility criteria, meaning that many patients die after a long, slow, and often painful decline, without the benefit of the coordinated palliative care. The palliative approach to care could benefit many more patients if it were available across settings for care and earlier in the disease process. In an attempt to make this valuable approach to care more widely available, palliative care programs are being developed in other settings for patients who are either not eligible for hospice or are "not ready" to enroll in a formal hospice program. As yet, there is no dedicated reimbursement to providers for palliative care services when they are delivered outside of the hospice setting, making the sustainability of such programs challenging.

HOSPICE CARE

Hospice is not a place, but a concept of care in which the end of life is viewed as a developmental stage. The root of the word hospice is *hospes,* meaning "host." Historically, hospice has referred to a shelter or way station for weary travelers on a pilgrimage (Bennahum, 1996). In the years that followed Kübler-Ross's groundbreaking work, the concept of hospice care as an alternative to depersonalized death in institutions began as a grassroots movement. Her work, and the development of the concept of hospice in England by Dr. Cicely Saunders, resulted in recognition of gaps in the existing system of care for the terminally ill (Amenta, 1986). Hospice care began in response to "noticeable gaps . . . (1) between treating the disease and treating the person, (2) between technological research and psycho-social support, and (3) between the general denial of the fact of death in our society and the acceptance of death by those who face it" (Wentzel, 1981, p. 11). According to Saunders, who founded the world-renowned St. Christopher's Hospice in London (Bennahum, 1996), the principles underlying hospice are as follows:

- Death must be accepted.
- The patient's total care is best managed by an interdisciplinary team whose members communicate regularly with each other.
- Pain and other symptoms of terminal illness must be managed.
- The patient and family should be viewed as a single unit of care.
- Home care of the dying is necessary.
- Bereavement care must be provided to family members.
- Research and education should be ongoing.

Nursing Care of the Terminally Ill Patient

Many patients suffer unnecessarily when they do not receive adequate attention for the symptoms accompanying serious illness. Careful evaluation of the patient should include not only the physical problems but also the psychosocial and spiritual dimensions of the patient's and family's experience of serious illness. This approach contributes to a more comprehensive understanding of how the patient's and family's life has been affected by the illness and will lead to nursing care that addresses the needs in every dimension.

PSYCHOSOCIAL ISSUES

Nurses are responsible for educating patients about the possibilities and probabilities inherent in their illness and their life with the illness, and for supporting them as they conduct life review, values clarification, treatment decision making, and end-of-life closure. The only way to do this effectively is to try to appreciate and understand the illness from the patient's perspective.

Kübler-Ross's (1969) work revealed that patients in the final stages of life can and will talk openly about their experiences, exposing as a myth the view that patients will be harmed by honest discussion with their caregivers about death. Despite the continued reluctance of health care providers to engage in open discussion about end-of-life issues, studies have confirmed that patients want information about their illness and end-of-life choices are not harmed by open discussion about death (McSkimming, Super, Driever et al., 1997; Virmani, Schneiderman & Kaplan, 1994).

At the same time, nurses need to be both culturally aware and sensitive in their approaches to communication with patients and families about death. Attitudes toward open disclosure about terminal illness vary widely among different cultures, and direct communication to the patient about such matters may be viewed as harmful (Blackhall, Murphy, Frank et al., 1995). To provide effective patient- and family-centred care at the end of life, nurses must be willing to set aside their assumptions so that they can discover what type and amount of disclosure is most meaningful to each patient and family within their unique belief systems.

The social and legal evolution of advance directive documents represents some progress in our willingness to both contemplate and communicate our wishes surrounding the end of life (Chart 17-1). Living wills are written documents that allow the individual who is of sound mind to document his or her preferences regarding the use or nonuse of medical treatment at the end of life, specify the preferred setting for care, and communicate other valuable insights into his or her values and beliefs. The addition of a durable medical power of attorney (the appointment and authorization of another individual to make medical decisions on behalf of the person who created the living will when he or she can no longer speak for himself or herself) is an important addition to the "living will." Although these documents are widely available from health care providers, community organizations, bookstores, and the Internet, their underuse reflects society's continued discomfort with openly confronting the subject of death. Further, the existence of a properly executed living will does not reduce the complexity of end-of-life decisions. The living will should not be considered an adequate substitute for ongoing communication between health care provider, patient, and family as the end of life approaches (Lynn, 1991).

Chart 17-1   **Methods of Stating End-of-Life Preferences**

Living will[1] — Also known as a medical directive or advanced directive, the living will is prepared by an individual of sound mind. It documents one's treatment preferences and provides instructions for care in the event that the signer is terminally ill and not able to communicate his or her wishes directly. Currently, only six Canadian provinces (Newfoundland, Nova Scotia, Quebec, Ontario, Manitoba, and Alberta) legally allow living wills.

Durable medical power of attorney[1] — The appointment and authorization of another individual to make medical decision on behalf of the person who created the living will (medical directive, advanced directive), when he or she is no longer able to speak for him or herself.

Power of attorney[2,3] — In Canada, this legal document enables the signer to designate another individual to make financial and legal decision on his or her behalf when he or she is unable to do so. Power of attorney does not give the attorney authority to make health care decisions.

[1] http://www.halifaxlive.com/artman/publish/wills_230305_87651.shtml. Retrieved April 25, 2005.
[2] http://www.publiclegaled.bc.ca/power. Retrieved April 25, 2005.
[3] http://www.cbc.ca/news/background/wills. Retrieved April 25, 2005.

COMMUNICATION

As has been discussed, remarkable strides have been made in the ability to prolong life, but attention to care for the dying lags behind (Callahan, 1993b). On one level, this comes as no surprise. Each of us will eventually face death, and most would agree that one's own demise is a subject he or she would prefer not to contemplate. Indeed, Glaser and Strauss (1965) noted that unwillingness in our culture to talk about the process of dying is tied to our discomfort with the notion of particular deaths—those of our patients' and our own—rather than talking about death in the abstract, which is more comfortable. Finucane (1999) observed that our struggle to stay alive is a prerequisite to being human. Confronting death in our patients uncovers our own deeply rooted fears.

To develop a level of comfort and expertise in communicating with seriously and terminally ill patients and their families, nurses and other clinicians need to first consider their own experiences with and values concerning illness and death. Reflection, reading, and talking with family members, friends, and colleagues can assist the nurse to examine beliefs about death and dying. Talking with individuals from differing cultural backgrounds can assist the nurse to view personally held beliefs through a different lens, and can help to sensitize the nurse to death-related beliefs and practices in other cultures. Discussion with nursing and non-nursing colleagues can also be useful to reveal the values shared by many health care professions and identify diversity in the values of patients in their care. Values clarification and personal death awareness exercises can provide a starting point for self-discovery and discussion.

Skills for Communicating With the Seriously Ill

Nurses need to develop skill and comfort in assessing patients' and families' responses to serious illness and planning interventions that will support their values and choices throughout the continuum of care. Patients and families need ongoing assistance: telling a patient something once is not teaching, and hearing the patient's words is not the same as active listening. Throughout the course of a serious illness, patients and their families will encounter complicated treatment decisions, bad news about disease progression, and recurring emotional responses. In addition to the time of initial diagnosis, lack of response to the treatment course, decisions to continue or withdraw particular interventions, and decisions about hospice care are examples of critical points on the treatment continuum that demand patience, empathy, and honesty from the nurse. Discussing sensitive issues such as serious illness, hopes for survival, and fears associated with death is never easy. However, the art of therapeutic communication can be learned and, like other skills, must be practiced to gain expertise. Similar to other skills, communication should be practiced in a "safe" setting, such as a classroom or clinical skills laboratory with other students or clinicians.

Although communication with each patient and family should be tailored to their level of understanding and values concerning disclosure, general guidelines for the nurse include the following (Addington, 1991):

- Deliver and interpret the technical information necessary for making decisions without hiding behind medical terminology.
- Realize that the best time for the patient to talk may be when it is least convenient for you.
- Being fully present during any opportunity for communication is often the most helpful form of communication.
- Allow the patient and family to set the agenda regarding the depth of the conversation.

Nursing Interventions When the Patient and Family Receive Bad News

Communicating about a life-threatening diagnosis or about disease progression is best accomplished by the interdisciplinary team in any setting—a physician, nurse, and social worker should be present whenever possible to provide information, facilitate discussion, and address concerns. Most importantly, the presence of the team conveys caring and respect for the patient and family. Creating the right setting is particularly important. If the patient wishes to have family present for the discussion, arrangements should be made to have the discussion at a time that is best for the patient and family. A quiet area with a minimum of disturbances should be used. Each clinician who is present should turn off beepers or other communication devices for the duration of the meeting and should allow sufficient time for the patient and family to absorb and respond to the news. Finally, the space in which the meeting takes place should be conducive to seating all of the participants at eye level. It is difficult enough for patients and families to be the recipients of bad news without having an array of clinicians standing uncomfortably over them at the foot of the patient's bed.

After an initial discussion of a life-threatening illness or progression of a disease, patients and their families will have many questions and may need to be reminded of factual information. Coping with news about a serious diagnosis or poor prognosis is an ongoing process. The nurse needs to be sensitive to these ongoing needs and may need to repeat previously provided information or simply be present while the patient and family react emotionally. The most important intervention the nurse can provide is listening empathetically. Seriously ill patients and their families need time and support to cope with the changes brought about by serious illness and the prospect of impending death. The nurse who is able to sit comfortably with another's suffering, time and time again, without judgment and without the need to solve the patient's and family's problems provides an intervention that is a gift beyond measure. Keys to effective listening include the following:

- Resist the impulse to fill the "empty space" in communication with talk.
- Allow the patient and family sufficient time to reflect and respond after asking a question.
- Prompt gently: "Do you need more time to think about this?"
- Avoid distractions (noise, interruptions).
- Avoid the impulse to give advice.
- Avoid canned responses: "I know just how you feel."
- Ask questions.
- Assess understanding—your own and the patient's—by restating, summarizing, and reviewing.

Responding With Sensitivity To Difficult Questions

Patients will often direct questions or concerns to nurses before they have been able to fully discuss the details of their diagnosis and prognosis with the physician or the entire health care team. Using open-ended questions allows the nurse to elicit the patient's and family's concerns, explore misconceptions and needs for information, and form the basis for collaboration with the physician and other team members. For example, the seriously ill patient may ask the nurse, "Am I dying?" The nurse should avoid making unhelpful responses that dismiss the patient's real concerns or defer the issue to another care provider. Nursing assessment and intervention are always possible, even when a need for further discussion with the physician is clearly indicated. Whenever possible, discussions in response to the patient's concerns should occur when the patient expresses a need, although it may be the least convenient time for the nurse (Addington, 1991). Creating an uninterrupted space of just 5 minutes can do much to identify the source of the concern, allay anxieties, and plan for follow-up. For example, in response to the question, "Am I dying?" the nurse could establish eye contact and follow with a statement acknowledging the patient's fears ("This must be very difficult for you") and an open-ended statement or question ("Tell me more about what is on your mind."). The nurse then needs to listen intently, ask additional questions for clarification, and provide reassurance only when it is realistic. In this example, the nurse might quickly ascertain that the patient's question emanates from a need for specific information—about diagnosis and prognosis from the physician, about the physiology of the dying process from the nurse, or perhaps about financial implications for the family from the social worker. The chaplain may also be called upon to talk with the patient about existential concerns.

As a member of the interdisciplinary team caring for the patient at the end of life, the nurse fills an important role in facilitating the team's understanding of the patient's values and preferences, the family dynamics concerning decision making, and the patient's and family's response to treatment and changing health status. Many dilemmas in patient care at the end of life are related to poor communication between team members and the patient and family and failure of team members to communicate effectively with each other. Regardless of the care setting, the nurse can ensure a proactive approach to the psychosocial care of the patient and family. Periodic, structured assessments provide an opportunity for all parties to consider their priorities and plan for an uncertain future. The nurse can assist the patient and family to clarify their values and preferences concerning end-of-life care by using a structured approach. Sufficient time must be devoted to each step, so that the patient and family have time to process new information, formulate questions, and consider their options. The nurse may need to plan several meetings to accomplish the four steps described in Table 17-1.

NURSING RESEARCH PROFILE 17-1
Decision Making at the End of Life

Tilden, V. P., Tolle, S. W., Nelson, C. A., & Fields, J. (2001). Family decision-making to withdraw life-sustaining treatments from hospitalized patients. *Nursing Research, 50*(2), 105–115.

Purpose
Although participation of family members in end-of-life decision making is increasing, little is known about the stress associated with their participation. Further, it is not known how families' reasoning processes compare to those of clinicians. The purpose of this study was to assess factors that affect family stress associated with withdrawal of life-sustaining treatment from their dying, hospitalized relatives. Investigators also compared family members and clinicians on their reasoning about the decision.

Study Sample and Design
A descriptive quantitative study was conducted in four large tertiary-care centres. Family members who had participated in the decision to withdraw life-sustaining treatment from patients who had been unable to make their own decisions were invited to participate.

Seventy-four family members of 51 patients participated in the study and were interviewed for data collection 1 to 2 months after the death of the patient; 65 family members were interviewed again 7 to 8 months later. Clinician data about the families' decision making were obtained from physicians (n = 21) and nurses (n = 24) 2 months after patients' deaths.

The Horowitz Impact of Events Scale and the mental/emotional state scale of the Rand 36-item Health Survey 1.0 was used to measure family stress. The researchers measured the importance of each of three factors (quality of life, patient preference, and prolongation of life) to family and clinician reasoning about treatment decisions by single-item indicators scaled on a 0 to 100-mm visual analog scale (VAS). The VAS scores indicated the likelihood that the respective factors would be considered in reaching a decision.

Findings
High levels of family stress were found 1 month and 7 to 8 months after the death, although stress levels at 7 to 8 months were lower. Patient/family characteristics that were associated with increased stress included the absence of advance directives (ADs), being an ethnic minority, and having a longer commuting distance to the hospital during the decedent's hospitalization. Families were more likely than clinicians to prioritize life prolongation over quality of life, particularly in the absence of an AD. Family members described their participation in decision making about withdrawing life support as one of the most difficult things they had ever had to do.

Nursing Implications
It is important for health care providers to recognize the impact of participation in end-of-life decision making on family members and to support them at this time. The study underscores the importance of assisting families to identify patients' preferences for end-of-life care and the importance of ADs in easing the process for family members. Further research is needed to compare the effect of having a written AD to guide family members versus patients' informal conversations about treatment preferences on family stress levels.

PROVIDING CULTURALLY SENSITIVE CARE AT THE END OF LIFE

Although death, grief, and mourning are universally accepted aspects of living, values, expectations, and practices during serious illness, as death approaches, and following death are culturally bound and expressed. Health care providers may share very similar values concerning end-of-life care and may find that they are inadequately prepared to assess for and implement care plans that support culturally diverse perspectives. Historical mistrust of the health care system and unequal access to even basic medical care may underlie the beliefs and attitudes among ethnically diverse populations (Crawley, Payne, Bolden et al., 2000; Phipps, True & Pomerantz, 2000). In addition, lack of education or knowledge concerning end-of-life care treatment options and language barriers influence decisions among many socioeconomically disadvantaged groups.

Much of the formal structure concerning health care decisions in the United States is rooted in the Western notions of autonomy, truth telling, and the acceptability of withdrawing or withholding life-prolonging medical treatment at the end of life. Yet in many cultures, interdependence is valued over autonomy, leading to decision and communication styles that favour relinquishment of decision making to family members or to a perceived authority figure, such as the physician (Blackhall et al., 1995; Ersek, Kagawa-Singer, Barnes et al., 1998). In addition, there is variation in preference regarding the use of life-prolonging medical treatments such as cardiopulmonary resuscitation and artificially provided nutrition and hydration at the end of life; some groups are less likely to agree with withholding or withdrawing such life support in terminal illness (Caralis, Davis, Wright et al., 1993).

The nurse's role is to assess the values, preferences, and practices of every patient, regardless of ethnicity, socioeconomic status, or background. The nurse can share knowledge about the patient's and family's cultural beliefs and practices with the health care team and facilitate the adaptation of the care plan to accommodate these practices. For example, the nurse may find that a patient prefers to have his eldest son make all of his care decisions. Institutional practices and laws governing informed consent are also rooted in the Western notion of autonomous decision making and informed consent. If a patient wishes to defer decisions to his son, the nurse could work with the team to negotiate informed consent, respecting the patient's right not to participate in decision making and honouring his family's cultural practices (Ersek et al., 1998).

The nurse should assess and document the patient's and family's specific beliefs, preferences, and practices regarding end-of-life care, preparation for death, and after-death rituals. Chart 17-2 identifies topics that the nurse should cover and questions that the nurse may use to elicit the information. The nurse must use judgment and discretion about the timing and setting for eliciting this information. Some patients may wish to have a family member speak for them or because of advanced illness may be un-

Table 17-1 • Discussing End-of-Life Care

STEPS	ACTIONS

1. Initiate discussion	• Establish a supportive relationship with patient and family
	  • State the purposes of the patient/family–health care team conference:
	    • To ensure that the plan of care is consistent with patient and family values and preferences
	    • To find out how best to support this patient and family
	  • Inquire if the patient or family have questions or concerns that they want to express
	• Elicit values and preferences concerning:
	  • Patient and family decision-making roles
	    • How have major decisions been made in the past?
	    • How have treatment/care decisions been made during the course of the illness?
	    • Has the patient appointed a surrogate?
	      • Formal (Durable Power of Attorney)
	      • Informal
	    • How does the patient/family want decisions to be structured from this point on?
	  • Setting for receiving care at the end of life
	    • Home
	    • Home with hospice care
	    • Assisted living or long-term care with/without hospice
	    • Disposition when unable to care for self independently (plan for how and where the patient prefers to receive care when he/she can no longer live independently)
	  • Family involvement in care provision

2. Clarify understanding of the medical treatment plan and prognosis	• Identify what the patient and family understand • Identify gaps in knowledge, need for consultation with other members of the health care team • Use simple, everyday language

3. Identify end-of-life priorities	• Facilitate open discussion about priorities
	  • "What is most important to you now?"
	  • "How can (I/we) best help you to meet your goals?"
	• Allow sufficient time for emotional response

4. Contribute to the interdisciplinary care plan	• Provide guidance and/or referral for understanding medical options
	• Make recommendations for referrals to other disciplines or services (eg, spiritual care, support groups, community resources)
	• Identify need for patient/family teaching
	• Develop a plan for follow-up:
	  • Schedule (frequency, time, place)
	  • Participants
	  • Tasks/assignments
	  • Communication that needs to occur before the next meeting
	  • Family member responsible for coordination

Adapted with permission from Balaban, R. B. (2000). A physician's guide to talking about end-of-life care. *Journal of General Internal Medicine, 15(3)*, 195–200. Oxford: Blackwell Science Ltd.

able to provide information. The nurse should give the patient and family a context for the discussion, such as "It is very important to us to provide care that addresses your needs and the needs of your family. We want to honour and support your wishes, and want you to feel free to tell us how we are doing, and what we could do to better meet your needs. I'd like to ask you some questions; what you tell me will help me to understand and support what is most important to you at this time. You don't need to answer anything that makes you uncomfortable. Is it all right to ask some questions?" The assessment of end-of-life beliefs, preferences, and practices will probably need to be carried out in short segments over a period of time (for example, across multiple days of an inpatient hospital stay or in conjunction with multiple patient visits to an outpatient setting). The novice nurse's discomfort with asking questions and discussing this type of sensitive content can be reduced by prior practice in a classroom or clinical skills laboratory, observation of interviews conducted by experienced nurses, and partnering with an experienced nurse during the first few assessments.

GOAL SETTING IN PALLIATIVE CARE AT THE END OF LIFE

As the treatment goals begin to shift in the direction of comfort care over aggressive disease-focused treatment, symptom relief and patient/family-defined quality of life assume greater prominence in treatment decision making. Patient, family, and clinicians may all be accustomed to an almost automatic tendency to pursue exhaustive diagnostic testing to locate and treat the source of the patient's illness or symptoms. Each decision to withdraw treatment or discontinue diagnostic testing will be an extremely emotional one for the patient and family. They may fear that the support from health care providers on which they have come to rely will be withdrawn along with the treatment.

Chart 17-2 • ASSESSMENT

Nursing Assessment of End-of-Life Care Beliefs, Preferences, and Practices

- *Disclosure/truth telling:* "Tell me how you/your family talk about very sensitive or serious matters."
  - Content: "Are there any topics that you or your family are uncomfortable discussing?"
  - Person responsible for disclosure: "Is there one person in the family who assumes responsibility for obtaining and sharing information?"
  - Disclosure practices regarding children: "What kind of information may be shared with children in your family, and who is responsible for communicating with the children?"
  - Sharing of information within the family or community group: "What kind/how much information should be shared with your immediate family? Your extended family? Others in the community (for example, members of a religious community)?"
- *Decision-making style:* "How are decisions made in your family? Who would you like to be involved in decisions about your treatment or care?"
  - Individual
  - Family-centred
  - Family elder or patriarch/matriarch
  - Deference to authority (such as the physician)
- *Symptom management:* "How would you like us to help you to manage the physical effects of your illness?"
  - Acceptability of medications used for symptom relief
  - Beliefs regarding expression of pain and other symptoms
  - Degree of symptom management desired
- *Life-sustaining treatment expectations:* "Have you thought about what type of medical treatment you/your loved one want(s) as the

end of life is nearing? Do you have an advanced directive (living will and/or durable power of attorney)?"
  - Nutrition/hydration at the end of life
  - Cardiopulmonary resuscitation
  - Ventilator
  - Dialysis
  - Antibiotics
  - Medications to treat infection
- *Desired location of dying:* "Do you have a preference about being at home or in some other location when you die?"
  - Desired role for family members in providing care: "Who do you want to be involved in caring for you at the end of life?"
  - Gender-specific prohibitions: "Are you uncomfortable having either males or females provide your care or your loved one's personal care?"
- *Spiritual/religious practices and rituals:* "Is there anything that we should know about your spiritual or religious beliefs about death? Are there any practices that you would like us to observe as death is nearing?"
- *Care of the body after the death:* "Is there anything that we should know about how a body/your body should be treated after death?"
- *Expression of grief:* "What types of losses have you and your family experienced? How do you and your family express grief?"
- *Funeral and burial practices:* "Are there any rituals or practices associated with funerals or burial that are especially important to you?"
- *Mourning practices:* "How have you and your family carried on after a loss in the past? Are their particular behaviours or practices that are expected or required?"

Throughout the course of the illness, and especially as the patient's functional status and symptoms indicate approaching death, clinicians need to assist the patient and family to weigh the benefits of continued diagnostic testing and disease-focused medical treatment against the burdens of those activities. Patients and their families may be extremely reluctant to forego monitoring that has become routine throughout the illness (such as blood testing, x-rays) but that may contribute little to a primary focus on comfort. Likewise, health care providers from other disciplines may have difficulty discontinuing such diagnostic testing or medical treatment. The nurse should collaborate with other members of the interdisciplinary team to share assessment findings and develop a coordinated plan of care (Fig. 17-1). In addition, the nurse may assist the patient and family to clarify their goals, expected outcomes, and values as they consider treatment options (Chart 17-3). The nurse needs to work with interdisciplinary colleagues to ensure that the patient and family are referred for continuing psychosocial support, symptom management, and assistance with other care-related challenges (eg, arranging for home care or hospice support, referrals for financial assistance).

SPIRITUAL CARE

Attention to the spiritual component of the patient's and family's illness experience is not new within the context of nursing care, yet many nurses lack the comfort or skills to assess and intervene in this dimension. **Spirituality** contains features of religiosity, but the two concepts are not interchangeable (Highfield, 2000). Spir-

ituality involves the "search for meaning and purpose in life and relatedness to a transcendent dimension" (Hermann, 2001, p. 67). For most people, contemplating their own deaths raises many issues, such as the meaning of existence, the purpose of suffering, and the existence of an afterlife. In a survey on spiritual beliefs and the dying process conducted by Gallup for the Nathan Cummings Foundation and Fetzer Institute in 1996 and published in 1997 in the United States, respondents' greatest worries about death included the following:

- The medical matter of greatest worry was the possibility of being vegetable-like for some period of time (73%).
- The emotional matter of greatest worry was not having the chance to say goodbye to someone (73%) or the possibility of having great physical pain before death (67%).
- The practical matter of greatest worry was how family or loved ones will be cared for (65%) or thinking that death will be a cause of inconvenience and stress for those who love them (64%).
- The spiritual matter of greatest worry was not being forgiven by God (56%) or dying when removed or cut off from God or a higher power (51%).

The spiritual assessment is a key component of comprehensive nursing assessment for terminally ill patients and their families. Although the nursing assessment should include religious affiliation, spiritual assessment is conceptually much broader than religion and thus is relevant regardless of the patient's expression of religious

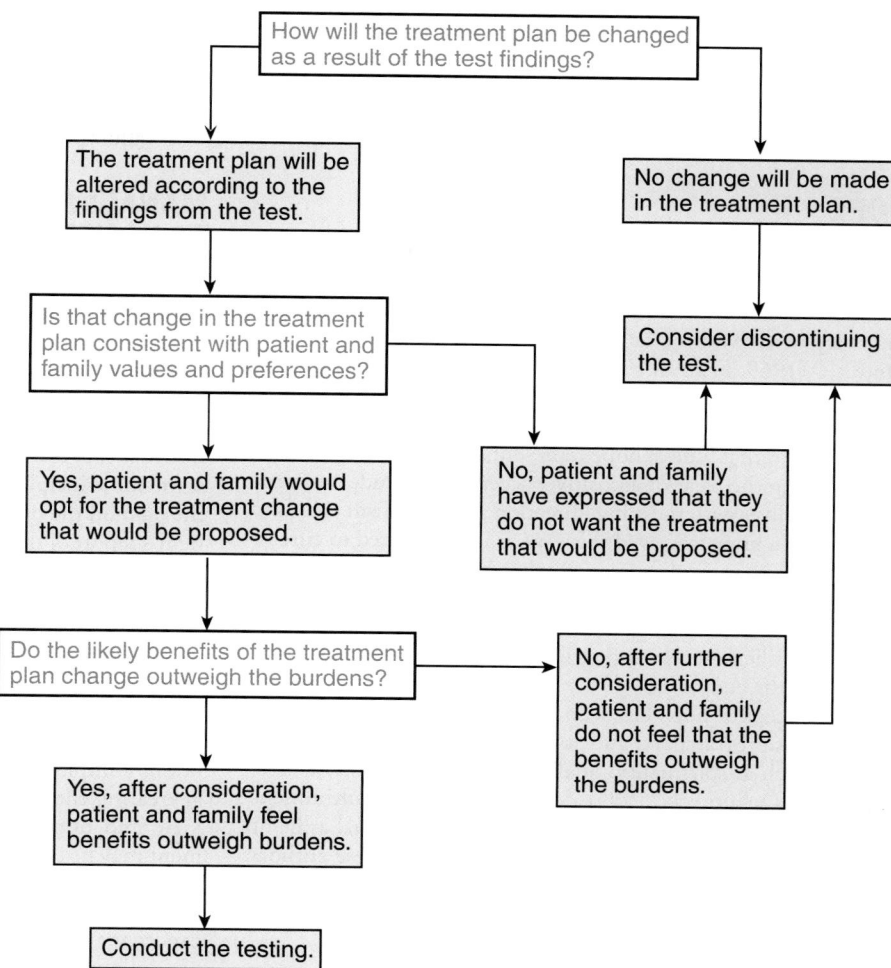

FIGURE 17-1 An algorithm for decision making about diagnostic testing at the end of life.

preference or affiliation. In addition to assessment of the role of religious faith and practices, important religious rituals, and connection to a religious community, the nurse should further explore:

- The harmony or discord between the patient's and family's beliefs
- Other sources of meaning, hope, and comfort
- The presence or absence of a sense of peace of mind and purpose in life

- Spiritually or religiously based beliefs about illness, medical treatment, care of the sick

Maugans (1996) created the useful mnemonic "SPIRIT" to assist health care professionals to include spiritual assessment in their practice:

- *S*piritual belief system
- *P*ersonal spirituality

Chart 17-3 • ASSESSMENT

Nursing Assessment of the Patient and Family Perspective: Goal Setting in Palliative Care

- Patient and family
  - Awareness of diagnosis, illness stage, and prognosis
    - "Tell me your understanding of your illness right now."
  - Values
    - "Tell me what is most important to you as you are thinking about the treatment options available to you/your loved one."
  - Preferences
    - "You've said that being comfortable and pain-free is most important to you right now. Where would you like to receive

care (home, hospital, long-term care facility, doctor's office), and how can I help?"
- Expected/desired outcomes
  - "What are your hopes and expectations for this (diagnostic test [eg, CT scan] or treatment)?"
- Benefits and burdens
  - "Is there a point at which you would say that the testing or treatment is outweighed by the burdens it is causing you (eg, getting from home to the hospital, pain, nausea, fatigue, interference with other important activities)?"

- *I*ntegration and involvement with others in a spiritual community
- *R*itualized practices and restrictions
- *I*mplications for medical care
- *T*erminal events planning

HOPE

Kübler-Ross maintained that hope persisted across every stage of terminal illness, noting that "even the most accepting, the most realistic patients left the possibility open for some cure, for the discovery of a new drug, or the 'last-minute success in a research project' " (1969, p. 139). Viktor Frankl (1984), a survivor of the Holocaust, described a human capacity for optimism that can be maintained in spite of the possibility or even certainty of pain and death. In terminal illness, hope represents patients' imagined future, forming the basis of a positive, accepting attitude and providing their lives with meaning, direction and optimism (Hickey, 1986). When hope is viewed this way, it is not limited to cure of the disease, and instead focuses on what is achievable in the time remaining. Many patients find hope in working on important relationships and creating legacies. The terminally ill patient can be extremely resilient, reconceptualizing hope repeatedly as he or she approaches the end of life.

The concept of hope has been delineated and studied by numerous nurse researchers, and its presence has been related to concepts such as spirituality, quality of life, and transcendence. Morse and Doberneck (1995) defined hope as a multidimensional construct that provides comfort to the individual as he or she endures life threats and personal challenges. These authors identified seven universal components of hope from their study of patients who had survived serious illness:

- Realistic initial assessment of the threat
- Envisioning alternatives and setting goals
- Bracing for negative outcomes
- Realistic assessment of resources
- Solicitation of mutually supportive relationships
- Continuous evaluation for signs reinforcing the goals
- Determination to endure

The nurse can support the patient and family by using effective listening and communication skills and encouraging realistic hope that is specific to the patient's and family's needs for information, expectations for the future, and values and preferences concerning the end of life. It is important for the nurse to engage in self-reflection and identify her or his own biases and fears concerning illness, life, and death. As nurses become more skilled in working with seriously ill patients, they can become less determined to "fix" and more willing to listen, more comfortable with silence, grief, anger, and sadness, and more fully present with patients and their families.

Nursing interventions for enabling and supporting hope include:

- Listening attentively
- Encouraging sharing of feelings
- Providing accurate information
- Encouraging and supporting patient control over his or her circumstances, choices, and environment whenever possible
- Assisting the patient to explore ways for finding meaning in his or her life

- Encouraging realistic goals
- Facilitating effective communication within the family
- Making referrals for psychosocial and spiritual counselling
- Assisting with the development of supports in the home or community when none exist

MANAGING PHYSIOLOGIC RESPONSES TO ILLNESS

Patients approaching the end of life experience many of the same symptoms, regardless of their underlying disease processes. Symptoms in terminal illness may be caused by the disease, either directly (eg, dyspnea due to chronic obstructive lung disease) or indirectly (eg, nausea and vomiting related to pressure in the gastric area), by the treatment for the disease, or by a coexisting disorder that is unrelated to the disease. Chapter 13 presents assessment principles for pain that include identifying the effect of the pain on the patient's life, the importance of believing the patient's report of the pain and its effect, and the importance of systematic assessment of pain. Similarly, symptoms such as dyspnea, nausea, weakness, and anxiety should be as carefully and systematically assessed and managed. Questions that guide the assessment of symptoms are listed in Chart 17-4.

The goals of symptom management at the end of life are to completely relieve the symptom when possible, or to decrease the symptom to a level that the patient can tolerate when it cannot be completely relieved. Medical interventions may be aimed at treating the underlying causes of the symptoms. Pharmacologic and nonpharmacologic methods for symptom management may be used in combination with medical interventions to modify the physiologic causes of symptoms. For example, some patients who develop pleural effusion secondary to metastatic cancer may experience temporary relief of the associated dyspnea following thoracentesis, an invasive medical procedure in which fluid is drained from the pleural space. In addition, pharmacologic management with low-dose oral morphine is very effective in relieving dyspnea, and guided relaxation may reduce the anxiety associated with the sensation of breathlessness. As with pain, the principles of pharmacologic symptom management

Chart 17-4 • ASSESSMENT

Nursing Assessment of Symptoms Associated With Terminal Illness

- How is this symptom affecting the patient's life?
- What is the meaning of the symptom to the patient? To the family?
- How does the symptom affect physical functioning, mobility, comfort, sleep, nutritional status, elimination, activity level, and relationships with others?
- What makes the symptom better?
- What makes it worse?
- Is it worse at any particular time of the day?
- What are the patient's expectations and goals for managing the symptom? The family's?
- How is the patient coping with the symptom?
- What is the economic effect of the symptom and its management?

Adapted from Jacox, A., Carr, D. B., & Payne, R. (1994). *Management of cancer pain.* Rockville, MD: AHCPR.

are the smallest dose of the medication to achieve the desired effect, avoidance of polypharmacy, anticipation and management of medication side effects, and creation of a therapeutic regimen that is acceptable to the patient based on his or her goals for maximizing quality of life.

As with pain management, patients may elect to tolerate higher symptom levels in exchange for greater independence, mobility, alertness, or other priorities. Anticipating and planning interventions for symptoms that have not yet occurred is a cornerstone of end-of-life care. Both patients and family members cope more effectively with new symptoms and exacerbations of existing symptoms when they know what to expect and how to manage it. Hospice programs typically provide "emergency kits" containing ready-to-administer doses of a variety of medications that are useful to treat symptoms in advanced illness. Family members can be instructed to administer a prescribed dose from the emergency kit, often avoiding prolonged suffering for the patient as well as re-hospitalization for symptom management.

Pain

Pain and suffering are among the most feared consequences of cancer (Roth & Breitbart, 1996). Pain is a significant symptom for many cancer patients throughout their treatment and disease course; it results both from the disease and the modalities used to treat it. Numerous studies have indicated that patients with advanced illness, particularly cancer, experience considerable pain (Field & Cassel, 1997; Jacox, Carr, & Payne, 1994). While the means to relieve pain have existed for many years, the continued, pervasive undertreatment of pain has been well documented (American Pain Society, 1999; Jacox et al., 1994). It is estimated that as many of 70% of patients with advanced cancer experience severe pain (Jacox et al., 1994; World Health Organization, 1990). The impact of poorly managed pain on patients' psychological, emotional, social, and financial well-being has attracted considerable research interest, but practice has been slow to change (Spross, 1992).

Patients who have an established regimen of analgesics should continue to receive those medications as they approach the end of life. Inability to communicate pain should not be equated with the absence of pain. While most pain can be managed effectively using the oral route, as the end of life nears patients may be less able to swallow oral medications due to somnolence or nausea. Patients who have been receiving opioids should continue to receive equianalgesic doses via the rectal or sublingual routes. Concentrated morphine solution can be very effectively delivered by the sublingual route, as the small liquid volume is well tolerated even when the patient cannot swallow. As long as the patient continues to receive opioids, a regimen to combat constipation must be implemented. If the patient cannot swallow laxatives or stool softeners, rectal suppositories or enemas may be necessary.

The nurse should teach the family about continuation of comfort measures as the patient approaches the end of life, how to administer analgesics via alternate routes, and how to assess for pain when the patient cannot verbally report pain intensity. Because the analgesics administered orally or rectally are short-acting, typically scheduled as frequently as every 3 to 4 hours around the clock, there is always a strong possibility that the patient approaching the end of life will die in close proximity to the time of analgesic administration. If the patient is at home, family members administering analgesics need to be prepared for this possibility. They will need reassurance that they did not "cause" the death of the patient by administering a dose of analgesic medication (see Chart 13-3).

Dyspnea

Dyspnea is an uncomfortable awareness of breathing that is common in patients approaching the end of life (Brant, 1998). Dyspnea is a highly subjective symptom that often is not associated with visible signs of distress, such as tachypnea, diaphoresis, or cyanosis. Patients with primary lung tumours, lung metastases, pleural effusion, and restrictive lung disease may experience significant dyspnea. Although the underlying cause of the dyspnea can be identified and treated in some cases, the burdens of additional diagnostic evaluation and treatment aimed at the physiological problem may outweigh the benefits. The treatment of dyspnea varies depending on the patient's general physical condition and imminence of death. For example, a blood transfusion may provide temporary symptom relief for the anemic patient earlier in the disease process; however, as the patient approaches the end of life the benefits are typically short-lived or absent.

NURSING ASSESSMENT AND INTERVENTION

As is true in pain assessment and management, the patient's report of dyspnea must be believed. Also like the experience of physical pain, the meaning of the dyspnea to the patient may increase his or her suffering. For example, the patient may interpret increasing dyspnea as a sign that death is approaching. For some patients, sensations of breathlessness may invoke frightening images of drowning or suffocation, and the resulting cycle of fear and anxiety may create even greater sensations of breathlessness. Therefore, the nurse should conduct a careful assessment of the psychosocial and spiritual components of the symptom (see Chart 17-5). Physical assessment parameters include:

- Symptom intensity, distress, and interference with activities (scale of 0 to 10)
- Auscultation of lung sounds
- Assessment of fluid balance
- Measurement of dependent edema (circumference of lower extremities)
- Measurement of abdominal girth
- Temperature
- Skin colour
- Sputum quantity and character
- Cough

To determine the intensity of the symptom and its interference with daily activities, patients can be asked to self-report using a scale of 0 to 10, where 0 is no dyspnea and 10 is the worst imaginable dyspnea. Measurement of the patient's baseline before treatment and subsequent measures during exacerbation of the symptom, periodically during treatment, and whenever the treatment plan changes will provide ongoing objective evidence for the efficacy of the treatment plan. In addition, physical assessment findings may assist in locating the source of the dyspnea and selecting nursing interventions to relieve the symptom. The components of the assessment will change as the patient's condition changes. For example, when the patient who has been on daily weights can no longer get out of bed, the goal of comfort may outweigh the benefit of continued weights. Like other symptoms at the end of life, dyspnea can be managed effectively in the absence of assessment and diagnostic data (ie, arterial blood gases) that are standard when the patient's illness or symptom is reversible.

Nursing management of dyspnea at the end of life is directed toward administering medical treatment for the underlying pathology, monitoring the patient's response to treatment, assisting the patient and family to manage anxiety (which exacerbates dyspnea), altering the perception of the symptom, and conserving energy (Chart 17-5). Pharmacologic intervention is aimed at modifying lung physiology and improving performance as well as altering the perception of the symptom. Bronchodilators and corticosteroids are examples of medications used to treat underlying obstructive pathology, thereby improving overall lung function. Low doses of opioids are very effective in relieving dyspnea, although the mechanism of relief is not entirely clear. Although dyspnea in terminal illness is typically not associated with diminished blood oxygen saturation, low-flow oxygen often provides psychological comfort to the patient and the family, particularly in the home setting.

As discussed above, dyspnea may be exacerbated by anxiety, and anxiety may trigger episodes of dyspnea, setting off a respiratory crisis in which patient and family may panic. For patients receiving care at home, patient and family instruction should include anticipation and management of crisis situations and a clearly communicated emergency plan. Patients and families should be instructed about medication administration, condition changes that should be reported to the physician and nurse, and strategies for coping with diminished reserves and increasing symptomatology as the disease progresses. The patient and family need reassurance that the symptom can be effectively managed at home without the need for activation of the emergency medical services or hospitalization and that a nurse will be available at all times via telephone or to conduct a visit.

Nutrition and Hydration at the End of Life

ANOREXIA

Anorexia and cachexia are common problems in the seriously ill. The profound changes in the patient's appearance and his or her concomitant lack of interest in the socially important rituals of mealtime are particularly disturbing to families. The approach to the problem varies depending on the patient's stage of illness, level of disability associated with the illness, and desires. The anorexia-cachexia syndrome is characterized by disturbances in carbohydrate, protein, and fat metabolism, endocrine dysfunction, and anemia. The syndrome results in severe asthenia (loss of energy). Although causes of anorexia may be controlled for a period of time, progressive anorexia is an expected and natural part of the dying process. Anorexia may be related to or exacerbated by situational variables (eg, the ability to have meals with the family versus eating alone in the "sick room"), progression of the disease, treatment for the disease, or psychological distress. The patient and family should be instructed in strategies to manage the variables associated with anorexia. Table 17-2 summarizes nursing measures and patient and family teaching for managing anorexia.

USE OF PHARMACOLOGIC AGENTS TO STIMULATE APPETITE IN THE TERMINALLY ILL

A number of pharmacologic agents are commonly used to stimulate appetite in anorectic patients. Commonly used medications for appetite stimulation include dexamethasone (Decadron), cyproheptadine (Periactin), megestrol acetate (Megace), and dronabinol (Marinol). Dexamethasone initially increases appetite and may provide short-term weight gain in some patients. However, therapy may need to be discontinued in the patient with a longer life expectancy, as after 3 to 4 weeks corticosteroids interfere with the synthesis of muscle protein. Cyproheptadine may be used when corticosteroids are contraindicated, such as when the patient is diabetic. It promotes mild appetite increase but no appreciable weight gain. Megestrol acetate produces temporary weight gain of primarily fatty tissue, with little effect on protein balance. Because of the time required to see any effect from this agent, therapy should not be initiated if life expectancy is less than 30 days. Finally, dronabinol is a psychoactive compound found in cannabis that may be helpful in reducing nausea and vomiting, appetite loss, pain, and anxiety, thereby improving intake in some patients. However, dronabinol is not as effective as the other agents for appetite stimulation in most patients. Although the use of these agents may cause temporary weight gain, their use is not associated with an increase in lean body mass in the terminally ill. Therapy should be tapered or discontinued after 4 to 8 weeks if there is no response (Wrede-Seaman, 1999).

CACHEXIA

Cachexia refers to severe muscle wasting and weight loss associated with illness. Although anorexia may exacerbate cachexia, it is not the primary cause. Cachexia is associated with changes in metabolism that include hypertriglyceridemia, lipolysis, and accelerated protein turnover, leading to depletion of fat and protein stores (Plata-Salaman, 1997). However, the pathophysiology of cachexia in terminal illness is not well understood. In terminal illness, the severity of tissue wasting is greater than would be expected from reduced food intake alone, and typically increasing appetite or food intake does not reverse cachexia in the terminally ill.

Anorexia and cachexia differ from starvation (simple food deprivation) in several important ways. Appetite is lost early in the process, the body becomes catabolic in a dysfunctional way, and supplementation by gastric feeding (tube feeding) or parenteral nutrition in advanced disease does not replenish lost lean body mass. At one time it was believed that cancer patients with rapidly growing tumours developed cachexia because the

Chart 17-5   Palliative Nursing Interventions for Dyspnea

Decrease Anxiety
- Administer prescribed anxiolytic medications as indicated for anxiety or panic associated with dyspnea.
- Assist with relaxation techniques, guided imagery.
- Provide patient with a means to call for assistance (call bell/light within reach in a hospital or long-term care facility; hand-held bell or other device for home).

Treat Underlying Pathology
- Administer prescribed bronchodilators and corticosteroids (obstructive pathology).
- Administer blood products, erythropoietin as prescribed (typically not beneficial in advanced disease).
- Administer prescribed diuretics and monitor fluid balance.

Alter Perception of Breathlessness
- Administer prescribed oxygen therapy via nasal cannula, if tolerated; masks may not be well tolerated.
- Administer prescribed low-dose opioids via oral route (morphine sulfate is used most commonly).
- Provide air movement in the patient's environment with a portable fan.

Reduce Respiratory Demand
- Teach patient and family to implement energy conservation measures.
- Place needed equipment, supplies, and nourishment within reach.
- For home or hospice care, offer bedside commode, electric bed (with head that elevates).

Table 17-2 • **Measures for Managing Anorexia**

NURSING INTERVENTIONS	PATIENT AND FAMILY TEACHING TIPS
Initiate measures to ensure adequate dietary intake without adding stress to the patient at mealtimes.	Reduce the focus on "balanced" meals; offer the same food as often as the patient desires it.
Assess the impact of medications (eg, chemotherapy, antiretrovirals) or other therapies (radiation therapy, dialysis) that are being used to treat the underlying illness.	Increase the nutritional value of meals. For example, add dry milk powder to milk, and use this fortified milk to prepare cream soups, milkshakes, and gravies.
Administer and monitor effects of prescribed treatment for nausea, vomiting, and delayed gastric emptying.	
Encourage patient to eat when effects of medications have subsided.	Allow and encourage the patient to eat when hungry, regardless of usual meal times.
Assess and modify environment to eliminate unpleasant odours and other factors that cause nausea, vomiting, and anorexia.	Eliminate or reduce noxious cooking odours, pet odours, or other odours that may precipitate nausea, vomiting, or anorexia.
Remove items that may reduce appetite (soiled tissues, bedpans, emesis basins, clutter).	Keep patient's environment clean, uncluttered, and comfortable.
Assess and manage anxiety and depression to the extent possible.	Make mealtime a shared experience away from the "sick" room whenever possible.
	Reduce stress at mealtimes.
	Avoid confrontations about the amount of food consumed.
	Reduce or eliminate routine weighing of the patient.
Position to enhance gastric emptying.	Encourage patient to eat in a sitting position; elevate the head of the patient's bed.
	Plan meals (food selection and portion size) that the patient desires.
	Provide small frequent meals if they are easier for patient to eat.
Assess for constipation and/or intestinal obstruction.	Ensure that patient and family understand that prevention of constipation is essential, even when the patient's intake is minimal.
Prevent and manage constipation on an ongoing basis, even when the patient's intake is minimal.	Encourage adequate fluid intake, dietary fibre, and use of bowel program to prevent constipation.
Provide frequent mouth care, particularly following nourishment.	Assist the patient to rinse after every meal. Avoid mouthwashes that contain alcohol or glycerine, which dry mucous membranes.
Ensure that dentures fit properly.	Weight loss may cause dentures to loosen and cause irritation. Remove them to inspect the gums and to provide oral care.
Administer and monitor effects of topical and systemic treatment for oropharyngeal pain.	Patient's comfort may be enhanced if pain medications given on an as-needed basis for breakthrough pain are administered before mealtimes.

tumour created an excessive nutritional demand and diverted nutrients from the rest of the body. Recent research links cytokines produced by the body in response to a tumour to a complex inflammatory-immune response present in patients whose tumours have metastasized, leading to anorexia, weight loss, and altered metabolism. An increase in cytokines occurs not only in cancer but also in AIDS and many other chronic diseases (Plata-Salaman, 1997).

ARTIFICIAL NUTRITION AND HYDRATION IN TERMINAL ILLNESS

Along with breathing, eating and drinking are essential to survival throughout one's lifetime. As patients near the end of life, their bodies' nutritional needs change, their desire for food and fluid may diminish, and they may no longer be able to use, eliminate, or store nutrients and fluids adequately. Eating, feeding, and sharing meals are important social activities in families and communities, and food preparation and enjoyment are linked to happy memories, strong emotions, and hopes for survival. For the patient with serious illness, food preparation and mealtimes often become battlegrounds where well-meaning family members argue, plead, and cajole to encourage the ill person to eat. It is not unusual for seriously ill patients to lose their appetites entirely, to develop

strong aversions for foods they have enjoyed in the past, or to crave a particular food to the exclusion of all other foods.

Although nutritional supplementation may be an important part of the treatment plan in early or chronic illness, unintended weight loss and dehydration are expected sequelae of progressive illness. As illness progresses, patients, families, and clinicians may believe that without artificial nutrition and hydration, the terminally ill patient will "starve," causing profound suffering and hastened death. However, starvation should not be viewed as the failure to implant tubes for nutritional supplementation or hydration of terminally ill patients with irreversible progression of disease. Studies have demonstrated that terminally ill patients who were hydrated had neither improved biochemical parameters nor improved states of consciousness (Waller, Hershkowitz & Adunsky, 1994). Similarly, survival was not increased when terminally ill patients with advanced dementia received enteral feeding (Meier, Ahronheim, Morris et al., 2001). Further, in patients who are close to death there are beneficial effects to withholding or withdrawing artificial nutrition and hydration, such as decreased urine output and incontinence, decreased gastric fluids and emesis, decreased pulmonary secretions and respiratory distress, and decreased edema and pressure discomfort (Zerwekh, 1987).

As the patient approaches the end of life, families and health care providers should offer the patient what he or she desires and can most easily tolerate. Nurses should instruct the family how to separate feeding from caring by demonstrating love, sharing, and caring by being with the loved one in other ways. Preoccupation with appetite, feeding, and weight loss diverts energy and time that the patient and family could use in other meaningful activities. The following are tips to promote nutrition for the terminally ill patient:

- Offer small portions of favourite foods.
- Do not be overly concerned about a "balanced" diet.
- Cool foods may be better tolerated than hot foods.
- Offer cheese, eggs, peanut butter, mild fish, chicken, or turkey. Meat (especially beef) may taste bitter and unpleasant.
- Add milkshakes, "Instant Breakfast" drinks, or other liquid supplements.
- Add dry milk powder to milkshakes and cream soups to increase protein and calorie content.
- Place nutritious foods at the bedside (fruit juices, milkshakes in insulated drink containers with straws).
- Schedule meals when family members can be present to provide company and stimulation.
- Avoid arguments at mealtime.
- Assist the patient to maintain a schedule of oral care. Rinse the mouth after each meal or snack. Avoid mouthwashes that contain alcohol. Use a soft toothbrush. Treat ulcers or lesions. Make sure dentures fit well.
- Treat pain and other symptoms.
- Offer ice chips made from frozen fruit juices.
- Allow the patient to refuse foods and fluids.

Delirium

Many patients may remain alert, arousable, and able to communicate until very close to death. Others may sleep for long intervals and awaken only intermittently, with eventual somnolence until death. Delirium refers to concurrent disturbances in level of consciousness, psychomotor behaviour, memory, thinking, attention, and sleep-wake cycle (Brant, 1998). In some patients, a period of agitated delirium may precede death, sometimes causing families to be hopeful that the suddenly active patient may be getting better. Confusion may be related to underlying, treatable conditions such as medication side effects or interactions, pain or discomfort, hypoxia or dyspnea, a full bladder or impacted stool. In patients with cancer, confusion may be secondary to brain metastases. Delirium may also be related to metabolic changes, infection, and organ failure.

The patient with delirium may become hypoactive or hyperactive, restless, irritable, and fearful. Sleep deprivation and hallucinations may occur. If treatment of the underlying factors contributing to these symptoms bring no relief, a combination of pharmacologic intervention with neuroleptics or benzodiazepines may be effective in decreasing distressing symptoms. Haloperidol (Haldol) may reduce hallucinations and agitation. Benzodiazepines (eg, lorazepam [Ativan]) can reduce anxiety but will not clear the sensorium and may contribute to worsening cognitive impairment if used alone.

Nursing interventions are aimed at identifying the underlying causes of delirium, acknowledging the family's distress over its occurrence, reassuring them about what is normal, teaching the family how to interact with and ensure safety for the patient with delirium, and monitoring the effects of medications used to treat severe agitation, paranoia, or fear. Confusion may mask the patient's unmet spiritual needs and fears about dying. Spiritual intervention, music therapy, gentle massage, and therapeutic touch may provide some relief. Reducing environmental stimuli, avoiding harsh lighting or very dim lighting (which may produce disturbing shadows), the presence of familiar faces, and gentle reorientation and reassurance are also helpful.

Depression

Clinical depression should not be accepted as an inevitable consequence of dying, nor should it be confused with sadness and anticipatory grieving, which are normal reactions to the losses associated with impending death. Emotional and spiritual support and control of disturbing physical symptoms are appropriate interventions for situational depression associated with terminal illness. The psychological sequelae of cancer pain have been linked to suicidal thought and less frequently to carrying out a planned suicide (Ripamonti, Filiberti, Totis et al., 1999). Cancer patients with advanced disease are especially vulnerable to delirium, depression, suicidal ideation, and severe anxiety (Roth & Breitbart, 1996). Higher levels of debilitation predict higher levels of pain and depressive symptoms, and the presence of pain doubles the likelihood of developing major psychiatric complications of illness (Roth & Breitbart, 1996). Patients and their families must be given space and time to experience sadness and to grieve, but patients should not have to endure untreated depression at the end of their lives. An effective combined approach to clinical depression includes relief of physical symptoms, attention to emotional and spiritual distress, and pharmacologic intervention with psychostimulants, selective serotonin reuptake inhibitors (SSRIs), and tricyclic antidepressants (Block, 2000).

PALLIATIVE SEDATION AT THE END OF LIFE

Effective control of symptoms can be achieved under most conditions, but some patients may experience distressing, intractable symptoms. Although its use remains controversial, **palliative sedation** is offered in some settings to patients who are close to death, who have symptoms that do not respond to conventional pharmacologic and nonpharmacologic approaches, and as a result are experiencing unrelieved suffering. Palliative sedation is distinguished from **euthanasia** or physician-assisted suicide in that the intent of palliative sedation is to palliate the symptoms, not to hasten the patient's death. Palliative sedation is most commonly used when the patient exhibits intractable pain, dyspnea, seizures, or delirium. It is generally considered appropriate in only the most difficult cases. Before implementing palliative sedation, the care team should assess for the presence of underlying and treatable causes of suffering, such as depression or spiritual pain. Finally, patients and families should be fully informed about the use of this treatment and alternatives.

Palliative sedation is accomplished through infusion of a benzodiazepine or barbiturate in doses adequate to induce sleep and eliminate signs of discomfort (Quill & Byock, 2000). The nurse acts as a collaborating member of the interdisciplinary team, providing emotional support to the patient and family, facilitating clarification of values and preferences, and providing comfort-focused physical care. Once sedation has been induced, the nurse will need to continue comfort care, monitor the physiologic effects of the sedation, support the family during the final hours or days of the patient's life, and ensure communication within the care team and between the team and family.

Nursing Care of the Patient Who Is Close to Death

Providing care to the patient who is close to death and being present at the time of death can be one of the most rewarding experiences a nurse can have. Patients and their families are understandably fearful of the unknown, and the approach of death may prompt new concerns or cause previous fears or issues to resurface. It has often been said that as we age and as we approach death, we do not become different people, just more like ourselves. Families that have always had difficulty communicating or in which there are old resentments and hurts may experience heightened difficulty as their loved one nears death. In contrast, the time at the end of life can also afford the family the opportunity to resolve old hurts and learn new ways of being a family. Regardless of the setting, dying patients can be made comfortable, space can be made for their loved ones to remain present when they wish, and the opportunity to experience growth and healing can be facilitated by skilled practitioners. Likewise, regardless of setting, patients' and families' apprehension surrounding the time of death may be diminished if they know what to expect as death nears and how to respond.

EXPECTED PHYSIOLOGIC CHANGES WHEN THE PATIENT IS CLOSE TO DEATH

Observable, expected changes in the body take place as the patient approaches death and organ systems begin to fail. Nursing care measures aimed at patient comfort should be continued: pain medications (administered rectally or sublingually), turning, mouth care, eye care, positioning to facilitate draining of secretions, and measures to protect the skin from incontinence should be continued. The nurse should consult with the physician about discontinuing measures that no longer contribute to patient comfort such as drawing blood, administering tube feedings, suctioning (in most cases), and invasive monitoring. The nurse should prepare the family for the normal, expected changes that accompany the period immediately preceding death. Although the exact time of death cannot be predicted, it is often possible to identify when a patient is very close to death. Hospice programs frequently provide written information for families so they know what to expect and what to do as death nears (Chart 17-6).

If they have been prepared for the time of death, families are less likely to panic and will be better able to be with their loved one in a meaningful way. Noisy, gurgling breathing or moaning is generally most distressing to the family. In most cases, the sounds of breathing at the end of life are related to oropharyngeal relaxation and diminished awareness. Family members may have difficulty believing that the patient is not in pain or that his or her breathing could not be improved by suctioning secretions. Patient positioning and family reassurance are the most helpful responses to these symptoms.

Terminal "Bubbling"

When death is imminent, the patient may become increasingly somnolent and unable to clear sputum or oral secretions, which may lead to further impairment of breathing from pooled and/or dried and crusted secretions. The sound and appearance of the secretions are often more distressing to the family than is the presence of the secretions to the patient. Family distress over the changes in patient condition may be eased by supportive nursing care. Continuation of comfort-focused interventions and reassurance that the patient is not in any distress can do much to ease family concerns. Gentle mouth care with a moistened swab or very soft toothbrush will help to maintain the integrity of the patient's mucous membranes. In addition, gentle oral suctioning, positioning to enhance drainage of secretions, and sublingual or transdermal administration of anticholinergic drugs (Table 17-3) to reduce the production of secretions will provide comfort to the patient and support to the family. Deeper suctioning may cause significant discomfort to the dying patient and is rarely of any benefit, as secretions will reaccumulate rapidly.

THE DEATH VIGIL

Although every death is unique, it is often possible for the experienced clinician to assess that the patient is "actively" or imminently dying and to prepare the family in the final days or hours leading to death. As death nears, the patient may withdraw, sleep for longer intervals, or become somnolent. The family should be encouraged to be with the patient, to speak and reassure him or her of their presence, to stroke or touch him or her, or to lie alongside him or her (even in the hospital or long-term care facility) if they are comfortable with this degree of closeness and can do so without causing discomfort to the patient.

Family members may have gone to great lengths to ensure that their loved one will not die alone. However, despite the best intentions and efforts of families and clinicians, the patient's death may occur at a time when no one is present. In any setting, it is unrealistic for family members to be at the patient's bedside 24 hours a day, and it is not unusual for patients to die when the family has stepped away from the bedside just briefly. Experienced hospice clinicians have observed and reported that some patients appear to "wait" until family members are away from the bedside to die, perhaps to spare their loved ones the pain of being present at the time of death. The nurse can reassure family members throughout the death vigil by being present intermittently or continuously, modeling behaviours (such as touching and speaking to the patient), providing encouragement in relation to family caregiving, providing reassurance about normal physiologic changes, and encouraging family rest breaks. When the patient dies while the family is away from the bedside, the family may express feelings of guilt and profound grief and will need emotional support.

AFTER-DEATH CARE

The time of death is generally preceded by a period of gradual diminishment of bodily functions in which increasing intervals between respirations, a weakened and irregular pulse, diminishing blood pressure, and skin colour changes or mottling may be observed. For the patient who has received adequate management of symptoms and for the family who has received adequate preparation and support, the actual time of death is commonly peaceful and occurs without struggle. The nurse may or may not be present at the time of the patient's death. In many states, the certifying physician may authorize the nurse to make the pronouncement of death and sign the death certificate. The determination of death is made through a physical examination that includes auscultation for the absence of breathing and heart sounds. Immediately upon cessation of vital functions the body will begin to change. The body will become dusky or

Chart 17-6 — Signs of Approaching Death

The person will show less interest in eating and drinking. For many patients, refusal of food is an indication that they are ready to die. Fluid intake may be limited to that which will keep their mouths from feeling too dry.

- What you can do: Offer, but do not force, fluids and medication. Sometimes, pain or other symptoms that have required medication in the past may no longer be present. For most patients, pain medications will still be needed, and can be provided by concentrated oral solutions placed under the tongue or by rectal suppository.

Urinary output may decrease in amount and frequency.

- What you can do: No response is needed unless the patient expresses a desire to urinate and cannot. Call the nurse for advice if you are not sure.

As the body weakens, the patient will sleep more and begin to detach from the environment. He or she may refuse your attempts to provide comfort.

- What you can do: Allow your loved one to sleep. You may wish to sit with him or her, play soft music, or hold hands. Your loved one's withdrawal is normal and is not a rejection of your love.

Mental confusion may become apparent, as less oxygen is available to supply the brain. The patient may report strange dreams or visions.

- What you can do: As he or she awakens from sleep, remind him or her of the day and time, where he or she is, and who is present. This is best done in a casual, conversational way.

Vision and hearing may become somewhat impaired and speech may be difficult to understand.

- What you can do: Speak clearly but no more loudly than necessary. Keep the room as light as the patient wishes, even at night. Carry on all conversations as if they can be heard, since hearing may be the last of the senses to cease functioning. Many patients are able to talk until minutes before death and are reassured by the exchange of a few words with a loved one.

Secretions may collect in the back of the throat and rattle or gurgle as the patient breathes though the mouth. He or she may try to cough, and his or her mouth may become dry and encrusted with secretions.

- What you can do: if the patient is trying to cough up secretions and is experiencing choking or vomiting, call the nurse for assistance.
  Secretions may drain from the mouth if you place the patient on his/her side and provide support with pillows.

Cleansing the mouth with moistened mouth swabs will help to relieve the dryness that occurs with mouth breathing.
Offer water in small amounts to keep the mouth moist. A straw with one finger placed over the end can be used to transfer sips of water to the patient's mouth.

Breathing may become irregular with periods of no breathing (apnea). The patient may be working very hard to breathe and may make a moaning sound with each breath. As the time of death nears, the breathing remains irregular and may become more shallow and mechanical.

- What you can do: Raising the head of the bed may help the patient to breathe more easily. The moaning sound does not mean that the patient is in pain or other distress; it is the sound of air passing over very relaxed vocal cords.

As the oxygen supply to the brain decreases, the patient may become restless. It is not unusual to pull at the bed linens, to have visual hallucinations, or even to try to get out of bed at this point.

- What you can do: Reassure the patient in a calm voice that you are there. Prevent him/her from falling by trying to get out of bed. Soft music or a back rub may be soothing.

The patient may feel hot one moment and cold the next as the body loses its ability to control the temperature. As circulation slows, the arms and legs may become cool and bluish. The underside of the body may darken. It may be difficult to feel a pulse at the wrist.

- What you can do: Provide and remove blankets as needed. Avoid using electric blankets, which may cause burns because the patient cannot tell you if he or she is too warm.
  Sponge the patient's head with a cool cloth if this provides comfort.

Loss of bladder and bowel control may occur around the time of death.

- What you can do: Protect the mattress with waterproof padding and change the padding as needed to keep the patient comfortable.

As people approach death, many times they report seeing gardens, libraries, or family or friends who have died. They may ask you to pack their bags and find tickets or a passport. Sometimes they may become insistent and attempt to do these chores themselves. They may try getting out of bed (even if they have been confined to bed for a long time) so that they can "leave."

- What you can do: Reassure the patient that it is all right; he or she can "go" without getting out of bed. Stay close, share stories, and be present.

Used with permission from the Family Home Hospice of the Visiting Nurse Association of Greater Philadelphia.

---

bluish, waxen-appearing, and cool, blood will darken and pool in dependent areas of the body (such as the back and sacrum if the body is in a supine position), and urine and stool may be evacuated.

Immediately following the death, the family should be allowed and encouraged to spend time with the deceased. Nor-

mal responses of family members at the time of death vary widely and range from quiet expressions of grief to overt expressions that include wailing and prostration. Families' desires for privacy during their time with the deceased should be honoured. Family members may wish to independently manage or assist with care of the body after death. If the death occurs in a

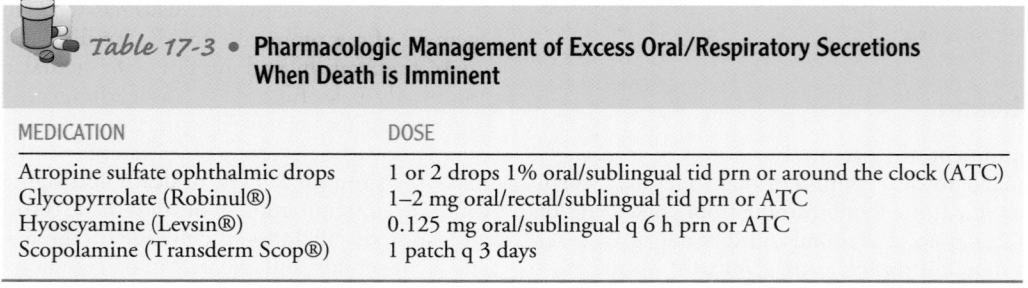

Table 17-3 • **Pharmacologic Management of Excess Oral/Respiratory Secretions When Death is Imminent**

MEDICATION	DOSE
Atropine sulfate ophthalmic drops	1 or 2 drops 1% oral/sublingual tid prn or around the clock (ATC)
Glycopyrrolate (Robinul®)	1–2 mg oral/rectal/sublingual tid prn or ATC
Hyoscyamine (Levsin®)	0.125 mg oral/sublingual q 6 h prn or ATC
Scopolamine (Transderm Scop®)	1 patch q 3 days

Reprinted with permission from ExcelleRx, Inc. (2000). *Hospice Pharmacia Pharmaceutical Care ToolKit* (3rd Ed.). Philadelphia: Author.

long-term care facility, the nurse follows the facility's procedure for preparation of the body and transportation to the facility's morgue. However, the family's needs to remain with the deceased, to wait until other family members arrive before the body is moved, and to perform after-death rituals should be honoured. When an expected death occurs in the home setting, the body is often transported directly to the funeral home by the funeral director.

GRIEF, MOURNING, AND BEREAVEMENT

A wide range of feelings and behaviours are normal, adaptive, and healthy reactions to the loss of a loved one. **Grief** refers to the personal feelings that accompany an anticipated or actual loss. **Mourning** reflects the individual, family, group, and cultural expressions of grief and associated behaviours. **Bereavement** refers to the period of time during which mourning takes place. Both grief reactions and mourning behaviours change over time as the individual learns to live with the loss. Although the pain of the loss may be tempered by the passage of time, recent conceptualizations of loss as an ongoing developmental process maintain that time does not heal the bereaved individual completely (Silverman, 2001); that is, the bereaved do not get over a loss entirely, nor do they return to who they were before the loss. Rather, they develop a new sense of who they are and where they fit in a world that has changed dramatically and permanently.

Anticipatory Grief and Mourning

Denial, sadness, anger, fear, and anxiety are normal grief reactions in the individual with life-threatening illness and those close to him or her. Kübler-Ross (1969) described five common emotional reactions to dying that are applicable to the experience of any loss (Table 17-4). Although useful in understanding the overall experience of the dying process, the stages that Kübler-Ross described have been misinterpreted as following a linear, expected trajectory. Not every patient or family member experiences every stage, many patients never reach a stage of acceptance, and patients and families fluctuate on a sometimes day-to-day basis in their emotional responses. Further, while impending loss stresses the patient, those who are close to him or her, and the functioning of the family unit, awareness of dying also provides a unique opportunity for family members to reminisce, resolve relationships, plan for the future, and say goodbye.

Individual and family coping with the anticipation of death is complicated by the varied and conflicting trajectories that grief and mourning may assume in the family. For example, while the patient may be experiencing sadness while contemplating role changes that have been brought about by the illness, the patient's spouse or partner may be expressing or holding in feelings of anger about the current changes in role and impending loss of the relationship; others in the family may be engaged in denial (eg, "Dad will get better; he just needs to eat more."), fear ("Who will take care of us?" or "Will I get sick too?"), or profound sadness

Table 17-4 • Kübler-Ross's Five Stages of Dying

STAGE	NURSING IMPLICATIONS
Denial: "This cannot be true." Feelings of isolation. May search for another health care professional who will give a more favourable opinion. May seek unproven therapies.	Denial can be an adaptive response, providing a buffer after bad news. It allows time to mobilize defenses, but can be maladaptive when it prevents the patient or family from seeking help and when denial behaviours cause more pain or distress than the illness or interfere with everyday functions. Nurses should assess the patient's and family's coping style, information needs, and understanding of the illness and treatment to establish a basis for empathetic listening, education, and emotional support. Rather than confronting the patient with information he or she is not ready to hear, the nurse can encourage him or her to share fears and concerns. Open-ended questions or statements such as "Tell me more about how you are coping with this new information about your illness" can provide a springboard for expression of concerns.
Anger: "Why me?" Feelings of rage, resentment or envy directed at God, health care professionals, family, others.	Anger can be very isolating, and loved ones or clinicians may withdraw. Nurses should allow the patient and family to express anger, treating them with understanding, respect, and knowledge that the root of the anger is grief over impending loss.
Bargaining: "I just want to see my grandchild's birth, then I'll be ready. . . ." Patient and/or family plead for more time to reach an important goal. Promises are sometimes made with God.	Terminally ill patients are sometimes able to outlive prognoses and achieve some future goal. Nurses should be patient, allow expression of feelings, and support realistic and positive hope.
Depression: "I just don't know how my kids are going to get along after I'm gone." Sadness, grief, mourning for impending losses.	Normal and adaptive response. Clinical depression should be assessed and treated when present. Nurses should encourage the patient and family to express their sadness fully. Insincere reassurance or encouragement of unrealistic hopes should be avoided.
Acceptance: "I've lived a good life, and I have no regrets." Patient and/or family are neither angry nor depressed.	The patient may withdraw as his or her circle of interest diminishes. The family may feel rejected by the patient. Nurses need to support the family's expression of emotions and encourage them to continue to be present for the patient.

and withdrawal. Although each of these behaviours is normal, tension may arise when one or more family members perceive that others are less caring, too emotional, or too detached.

The nurse needs to assess the characteristics of the family system and intervene in a manner that supports and enhances the cohesion of the family unit. Parameters for assessing the family facing life-threatening illness are identified in Chart 17-7. The nurse can patiently guide family members to talk about their feelings and understand them in the broader context of anticipatory grief and mourning. Acknowledging and expressing feelings, continuing to interact with the patient in meaningful ways, and planning for the time of death and bereavement are adaptive family behaviours. Professional support provided by grief counselors in the community, at a local hospital, in the long-term care facility, or associated with a hospice program can help both the patient and family to sort out and acknowledge feelings and make the end of life as meaningful as possible.

Grief and Mourning After Death

When a loved one dies, the family members enter a new phase of grief and mourning as they begin to accept the loss, feel the pain of permanent separation, and prepare to live a life without the deceased. Even if the loved one died after a long illness, preparatory grief experienced during the terminal illness will not preclude the

grief and mourning that follow the death. Following the patient's death after a long or difficult illness, family members may experience conflicting feelings of relief that the loved one's suffering has ended, compounded by guilt and grief related to unresolved issues or the circumstances of death. Grief work may be especially difficult if the patient's death was painful, prolonged, accompanied by unwanted interventions, or unattended. Families who had no preparation or support during the period of imminence and death may have a more difficult time finding a place for the painful memories.

Although some family members may experience prolonged or complicated mourning, most grief reactions fall within a "normal" range. The feelings are often profound, but the bereaved individual eventually reconciles the loss and finds a way to re-engage with his or her life. Grief and mourning are affected by individual characteristics, coping skills, and experiences with illness and death; the nature of the relationship to the deceased; factors surrounding the illness and the death; family dynamics; social support; and cultural expectations and norms. After-death rituals, including preparation of the body, funeral practices, and burial rituals, are socially and culturally significant ways that members of a family begin to accept the reality and finality of death. Preplanning of funerals is becoming increasingly common, and hospice professionals in particular assist families to make plans for death, often involving the patient who may wish to take an active planning role. Preplanning the funeral relieves the family of the decision burden in the intensely emotional period following a death. Uncomplicated grief and mourning are characterized by emotional feelings of sadness, anger, guilt, and numbness; physical sensations such as hollowness in the stomach and tightness in the chest, weakness, and lack of energy; cognitions that include preoccupation with the loss and a sense of the deceased as still present; and behaviours such as crying, visiting places that are reminders of the deceased, social withdrawal, and restless overactivity (Worden, 1991).

In general, the period of mourning is an adaptive response to loss during which the mourner comes to accept the loss as real and permanent, acknowledges and experiences the painful emotions that accompany the loss, experiences life without the deceased, overcomes impediments to adjustment, and finds a new way of living in a world without the loved one. Particularly immediately following the death, the mourner begins to recognize the reality and permanence of the loss by talking about the deceased and telling and retelling the story of the illness and death. Societal norms are frequently at odds with the normal grieving processes of individuals, where time excused from work obligations is typically measured in days and mourners are often expected to get over the loss quickly and get on with life.

In reality, the work of grief and mourning takes time, and avoiding grief work following the death often leads to long-term adjustment difficulties. According to Rando (2000), mourning for a loss involves the "undoing" of psychosocial ties that bind the mourner to the deceased, personal adaptation to the loss, and learning to live in the world without the deceased. Six key processes of mourning allow the individual to accommodate to the loss in a healthy way: recognition of the loss; reaction to the separation, experiencing and expressing the pain of the loss; recollection and re-experiencing the deceased, the relationship, and the associated feelings; relinquishing old attachments to the deceased; readjustment to adapt to the new world without forgetting the old; and reinvestment (Rando, 2000). Similarly, Worden (1991) described four tasks of mourning: acceptance of the reality of the loss, working through the pain of grief, adjusting to the environment in which the deceased is gone, and emotional "relocation" of the deceased in order to move on with life.

Chart 17-7

Assessing Anticipatory Mourning in the Family Facing Life-Threatening Illness

- Family constellation
  - Identify the members who constitute the patient's family.
    - Who is important to the patient?
  - Identify roles and relationships among the family members.
    - Who is the primary caregiver?
    - By what authority is this person the primary caregiver?
- Cohesion and boundaries
  - How autonomous/interdependent are family members?
    - Degree of involvement with each other as individuals and as a family
    - Degree of bonding between family members
    - Degree of "teamwork" in the family
    - Degree of reliance on individual family members for specific tasks/roles
  - How do family members differ in:
    - Personality?
    - World view?
    - Priorities?
  - What are the implicit and explicit expectations or "rules" for behaviour within the family?
- Flexibility and adaptability
  - What is the family's ability to integrate new information?
  - How does the family manage change?
  - How able are the family members to assume new roles and responsibilities?
- Communication
  - What is the style of communication in the family, in terms of:
    - Openness?
    - Directness?
    - Clarity?
  - What are the constraints on communication?
  - What topics are avoided?

Although many individuals complete the work of mourning with the informal support of family and friends, many find that talking with others who have had a similar experience, such as in formal support groups, normalizes the feelings and experiences and provides a framework for learning new skills to cope with the loss and create a new life. Bereavement support groups are often sponsored by hospitals, hospices, and other community organizations. Groups for parents who have lost a child, children who have lost a parent, widows, widowers, and gay men and lesbians who have lost a life partner are some examples of specialized support groups available in many communities. Nursing interventions for those experiencing grief and mourning are identified in Chart 17-8.

Complicated Grief and Mourning

Complicated grief and mourning are characterized by prolonged feelings of sadness and feelings of general worthlessness or hopelessness that persist long after the death, prolonged symptoms that interfere with activities of daily living (anorexia, insomnia, fatigue, panic), or self-destructive behaviours such as alcohol or substance abuse and suicidal ideation or attempts. Complicated grief and mourning require professional assessment and can be treated with pharmacologic and psychological interventions.

Coping With Death and Dying: Professional Caregiver Issues

Whether practicing in the trauma centre, intensive care unit or other acute care setting, home care, hospice, long-term care, or the many locations where patients and their families receive ambulatory services, nurses are closely involved with complex and emotionally laden issues surrounding loss of life. To be most effective and satisfied with the care they provide, nurses need to at-

tend to their own emotional responses to the losses they witness every day. Well before the nurse exhibits symptoms of stress or burnout, he or she should acknowledge the difficulty of coping with others' pain on a daily basis and put healthy practices in place that will guard against emotional exhaustion. In hospice settings, where death, grief, and loss are expected outcomes of patient care, interdisciplinary colleagues rely on each other for support, using meeting time to express frustration, sadness, anger, and other emotions; to learn coping skills from each other; and to speak about how they were affected by the lives of those patients who have died since the last meeting. In many settings, staff members organize or attend memorial services to support families and other caregivers, who find comfort in joining each other to remember and celebrate the lives of patients. Finally, healthy personal habits, including diet, exercise, stress reduction activities (such as dance, yoga, t'ai chi, meditation), and sleep, will help guard against the detrimental effects of stress.

 Critical Thinking Exercises

1. Your patient, age 70, has metastatic prostate cancer and is receiving home care. In the past, he has received transfusions of packed red blood cells to treat anemia associated with bone marrow involvement. He has received only temporary benefit from the transfusions. The patient's wife has asked that her husband's hemoglobin continue to be checked weekly because she is concerned about his increasing weakness and exertional dyspnea. The interdisciplinary team is meeting to discuss the patient's treatment plan. The team consensus is that he is unlikely to live more than a few days or weeks. What additional assessment data are needed to determine the wishes and expectations of the patient? Of the wife? What are the team's options for intervention? What are the pros and cons associated with each option?

2. You are conducting your first home care visit to an 88-year-old woman who has been hospitalized three times in the last 4 months with heart failure. She is short of breath, although she uses oxygen continuously. She is confined to bed and is incontinent and has a stage III pressure ulcer on her coccyx. She is not interested in eating and has lost 30 lb in the last 4 months. She is becoming progressively weaker. Her husband, also 88, has limited mobility due to arthritis. He has a history of colon cancer and has had a colostomy for the last 10 years. Although he tries to take care of her, it is becoming increasingly difficult for him to do so. They have been married for almost 70 years and are very devoted to each other. What assessments would you carry out and what strategies would you implement to (1) relieve some of the patient's symptoms and discomfort, (2) assist her husband in management of her care, and (3) prepare both of them for her inevitable death?

3. You have been assigned to care for a 34-year-old father of three in the end stages of ALS. He was discharged home from the hospital yesterday and is being admitted to the local visiting nurse association's home palliative care program. During the admission assessment, when you ask him about his religion and beliefs as part of the spiritual assessment that is performed at the time of admission, he says to

---

Chart 17-8	**Nursing Interventions for Grief and Mourning**

- Support the expression of feelings.
  - Encourage the telling of the story using open-ended statements or questions (eg, "Tell me about your husband").
  - Assist the mourner to find an outlet for his/her feelings: talking, attending a support group, keeping a journal, finding a safe outlet for angry feelings (writing letters that will not be mailed, physical activity)
- Assess emotional affect and reinforce the normalcy of feelings.
- Assess for guilt and regrets.
  - Are you especially troubled by a certain memory or thought?
  - How do you manage those memories?
- Assess for the presence of social support.
  - Do you have someone to whom you can talk about your husband?
  - Can I help you to find someone you can talk to?
- Assess coping skills.
  - How are you managing day to day?
  - Have you experienced other losses? How did you manage those?
  - Are there things you are having trouble doing?
  - Do you have/need help with specific tasks?
- Assess for signs of complicated grief and mourning and offer professional referral.

you, "I don't go to church anymore and I really don't have time for people who want to talk about religion." Should you respond to his comment? If not, why? If so, what will you say? Should you continue with part or all of a spiritual assessment? Explain your rationale. If you continue with the spiritual assessment, what questions would you use in the assessment? Discuss your plan for follow-up.

REFERENCES AND SELECTED READINGS

Books and Monographs

Addington, T. G. (1991). *Communication and cancer.* Hershey, PA: Central Pennsylvania Oncology Group.

American Pain Society. (1999). *Principles of analgesic use in the treatment of acute pain and cancer pain* (4th ed.). Glenview, IL: Author.

Barnard, D., Towers, A., Boston, P., & Lambrinidou, Y. (2000). *Crossing over: narratives of palliative care.* New York: Oxford.

Bennahum, D. A. (1996). The historical development of hospice and palliative care. In D. C. Sheehan & W. B. Forman (Eds.), *Hospice and palliative care: Concepts and practice* (pp. 1–10). Boston: Jones & Bartlett.

Byock, I. (1997). *Dying well: The prospect for growth at the end of life.* New York: Riverhead.

Callahan, D. (1993*b*). *The troubled dream of life.* New York: Simon & Schuster.

Doyle, D., Hanks, G. W. C., & MacDonald, N. (Eds.). (1998). *Oxford textbook of palliative medicine* (2d Ed.). New York: Oxford.

ExcelleRx, Inc. (2000). *Hospice Pharmacia Pharmaceutical Care ToolKit* (3d Ed.). Philadelphia: Author.

Family Home Hospice of the Visiting Nurse Association of Greater Philadelphia. (1999). *Signs of approaching death.* Philadelphia: Author.

Ferrell, B. R., & Coyle, N. (Eds.). (2001). *Textbook of palliative nursing.* New York: Oxford.

Frankl, V. E. (1984). *Man's search for meaning.* New York: Washington Square.

Gadow, S. (1988). Covenant without cure: Letting go and holding on in chronic illness. In J. Watson & M. A. Ray (Eds.), *The ethics of cure and the ethics of care.* New York: NLN.

George H. Gallup International Institute (1997). *Spiritual beliefs and the dying process.* Princeton, NJ: Author.

Glaser, B. G., & Strauss, A. (1965). *Awareness of dying.* Chicago: Aldine.

Jacox, A., Carr, D. B., & Payne, R. (1994). *Management of cancer pain.* Clinical practice guideline No. 9 (AHCPR Publication No. 94-0592). Washington, DC: Agency for Health Care Policy and Research, United States Department of Health and Human Services, Public Health Service.

Kübler-Ross, E. (1969). *On death and dying.* New York: MacMillan.

Lesparre, M., & Matherlee, K. (1998). *Delivering and financing care at the end of life.* Issue Brief (No. 711). Washington, DC: The George Washington University.

Lynn, J., Schuster, J. L., & Kabcenell, A. (2000). *Improving care for the end of life: A sourcebook for health care managers and clinicians.* New York: Oxford.

Matzo, M. L., & Sherman, D. W. (Eds.). (2001). *Palliative care nursing: Quality care to the end of life.* New York: Springer.

McSkimming, S. A., Super, A., Driever, M. J., Schoessler, M., Franey, S. G., & Fonner, E. (1997). *Living and healing during life-threatening illness.* Portland, OR: Supportive Care of the Dying.

Occupational Home Economics Education Series (1977). Attitudes toward death. In *Care and independent living services for the aging* (Section III-A22). Washington, DC: U.S. Government Printing Office.

Plata-Salaman, C. (1997). Symptoms in terminal illness: A research workshop. Cachexia or wasting: basic perspective [On-line]. Available: http://www.nih.gov/ninr/end-of-life.htm.

Rando, T. A. (2000). Promoting healthy anticipatory mourning in intimates of the life-threatened or dying person. In T. A. Rando (Ed.), *Clinical dimensions of anticipatory mourning* (pp. 307–378). Champaign, IL: Research Press.

Saunders, C., & Kastenbaum, R. (Eds.). (1997). *Hospice care on the international scene.* New York: Springer.

Smith, S. A. (2000). *Hospice concepts: A guide to palliative care in terminal illness.* Champaign, IL: Research Press.

Tilly, J., & Wiener, J. (2001). *Medicaid and end-of-life care.* Washington, DC: Last Acts.

Wentzel, K. B. (1981). *To those who need it most, hospice means hope.* Boston: Charles River.

World Health Organization. (1990). *Cancer pain relief and palliative care: Report of a WHO expert committee.* World Health Organization Technical Report Series, 804, 1–75.

Worden, J. W. (1991). *Grief counseling and grief therapy.* New York: Springer.

Wrede-Seaman, L. (1999). *Symptom management algorithms: A handbook for palliative care.* Yakima, WA: Intellicard.

Journals

Ameling, A., & Povilonis, M. (2002). Spirituality, meaning, mental health, and nursing. *Journal of Psychosocial Nursing and Mental Health Services, 39*(4), 14–20.

Balaban, R. B. (2000). A physician's guide to talking about end-of-life care. *Journal of General Internal Medicine, 15,* 195–200.

Benoliel, J. Q. (1993). The moral context of oncology nursing. *Oncology Nursing Forum (Supplement), 20*(10), 5–12.

Blackhall, L. J., Murphy, S. T., Frank, G., Michel, V., & Azen, S. (1995). Ethnicity and attitudes toward patient autonomy. *Journal of the American Medical Association, 274*(10), 820–825.

Block, S. D. (2000). Assessing and managing depression in the terminally ill patient. *Annals of Internal Medicine, 132*(3), 209–218.

Brant, J. M. (1998). The art of palliative care: Living with hope, dying with dignity. *Oncology Nursing Forum, 25*(96), 995–1004.

Brinson, S. V., & Brunk, Q. (2000). Hospice family caregivers: An experience in coping. *The Hospice Journal, 15*(3), 1–12.

Buchanan, J., Borland, R., Cosolo, W., Millership, R., Haines, I., Zimet, A., & Zalcberg, J. (1996). Patients' beliefs about cancer management. *Supportive Care in Cancer, 4*(2), 110–117.

Callahan, D. (1993*a*). Pursuing a peaceful death. *Hastings Center Report, 23*(4), 33–38.

Campbell, M. L., & Field, B. E. (1991). Management of the patient with do not resuscitate status: Compassion and cost containment. *Heart & Lung, 20*(4), 345–348.

Caralis, P. V., Davis, B., Wright, K., & Marcial, E. (1993). The influence of ethnicity and race on attitudes toward advance directives, life-prolonging treatments and euthanasia. *Journal of Clinical Ethics, 4*(2), 155–165.

Chochinov, H. M., Tataryn, D. J., Wilson, K. G., Ennis, M., & Lander S. (2000). Prognostic awareness and the terminally ill. *Psychosomatics, 41* (6), 500–504.

Chow, E., Anderson, L., Wong, R., et al. (2001). Patients with advanced cancer: A survey of the understanding of their illness and expectations from palliative radiotherapy for symptomatic metastases. *Clinical Oncology, 13*(3), 204–208.

Connor, S. R. (1992). Denial in terminal illness: To intervene or not to intervene. *Hospice Journal, 8*(4), 1–15.

Crawley, L., Payne, R., Bolden, J., Payne, T., Washington, P., & Williams, S. (2000). Palliative and end-of-life care in the African American community. *Journal of the American Medical Association, 284*(19), 2518–2521.

Eiser, A. R., & Weiss, M. D. (2001). The underachieving advance directive: Recommendations for increasing advance directive completion. *American Journal of Bioethics Online, 1*(2). Available: http://www.ajobonline.com/online_carticles/oa03.php.

Ersek, M., Kagawa-Singer, M., Barnes, D., Blackhall, L., & Koenig, B. A. (1998). Multicultural considerations in the use of advance directives. *Oncology Nursing Forum, 25*(10), 1683–1690.

Ferrell, B. R. & Coyle, N. (2002). An overview of palliative nursing care. *American Journal of Nursing, 102*(5), 26–31.

Ferrell, B., Virani, R., Grant, M., Coyne, P., & Uman, G. (2000). Beyond the Supreme Court decision: Nursing perspectives on end-of-life care. *Oncology Nursing Forum, 27*(3), 445–455.

Fetters, M. D., Churchill, L., & Danis, M. (2001). Conflict resolution at the end of life. *Critical Care Medicine, 29*(5), 921–925.

Finucane, T. (1999) How gravely ill becomes dying. *Journal of the American Medical Association, 282*(17), 1670–1672.

Gbrich, C. (2001). The emotions and coping strategies of caregivers of family members with a terminal cancer. *Journal of Palliative Care, 17*(1), 30–36.

Helm, A. (1984). Debating euthanasia: An international perspective. *Journal of Gerontological Nursing, 10*(11), 20–24.

Hermann, C. P. (2001). Spiritual needs of dying patients: A qualitative study. *Oncology Nursing Forum, 28*(91), 67.

Hermann, C., & Looney, S. (2001). The effectiveness of symptom management in hospice patients during the last seven days of life. *Journal of Hospice and Palliative Nursing, 3*(3), 88–96.

Hickey, S. S. (1986). Enabling hope. *Cancer Nursing, 9*, 133–137.

Highfield, M. E. F. (2000). Providing spiritual care to patients with cancer. *Clinical Journal of Oncology Nursing, 4*(3), 115–120.

*Jezuit, D. L. (2000). Suffering of critical care nurses with end-of-life decisions. *MedSurg Nursing, 9*(3). 145–152.

Jones, D. (1997). Issues and trends affecting the nation's hospices. *Caring, 16*(11), 14–24.

Kagawa-Singer, M., & Blackhall, L. J. (2001). Negotiating cross-cultural issues at the end of life. *Journal of the American Medical Association, 286*(23), 2993–3001.

*Kirchhoff, K. T., Spuhler, V., Walker, L. et al. (2000). Intensive care nurses' experiences with end-of-life care. *American Journal of Critical Care 9*(1), 36–42.

Krisman-Scott, M. A. (2000). An historical analysis of disclosure of terminal status. *Journal of Nursing Scholarship, 32*(1), 47–52.

LaDuke, S. (2001). Terminal dyspnea and palliative care. *American Journal of Nursing 101*(11), 26–31.

Langer, G. (1999). Kevorkian verdict unpopular. [Online]. Available: http://abcnews.go.com./sections/us/DailyNews/kevorkian_poll990327.html.

Last Acts Palliative Care Task Force. (1997). Precepts of palliative care [On-line]. Available: http://www.lastacts.org/docs/profprecepts.pdf

Lynn, J. (1991). Why I don't have a living will. *Law, Medicine & Health Care, 19*(1–2), 101–104.

Maugans, T. A. (1996). The SPIRITual history. *Archives of Family Medicine, 5*(1), 11–16.

Meier, D. E., Ahronheim, J. C., Morris, J., Baskin-Lyons, S., & Morrison, S. (2001). High short-term mortality in hospitalized patients with advanced dementia. *Archives of Internal Medicine, 161*, 594–599.

Morrison, R. S., Siu, A. L., Leipzig, R. M., Cassel, C. K., & Meier, D. E. (2000). The hard task of improving care at the end of life. *Archives of Internal Medicine, 160*, 743–747.

Morse, J. M. (2000). On comfort and comforting. *American Journal of Nursing, 100*(9), 34–37.

Morse, J. M., & Doberneck, B. (1995). Delineating the concept of hope. *Image: Journal of Nursing Scholarship, 27*, 283–291.

Patrick, D. L., Engelberg, R. A., & Curtis, J. R. (2001) Evaluating the quality of dying and death. *Journal of Pain and Symptom Management, 22*(3), 717–726.

Phipps, E., True, G., & Pomerantz, S. (2000). Approaches to end-of-life care in culturally diverse communities [On-line]. Available: http://www.lastacts.org/statsite/3770la%5Feln%5Fnewsletter.htm.

Post-White, J., Ceronsky, C., Kreitzer, M. J., Nickelson, K., Drew, D., Mackey, K. W., Koopmeiners, L., & Gutknecht, S. (1996). Hope, spirituality, sense of coherence, and quality of life in patients with cancer. *Oncology Nursing Forum, 23*(10), 1571–1579.

Quill, T. E., & Byock, I. R. (2000). Responding to intractable terminal suffering: The role of terminal sedation and voluntary refusal of foods and fluids. *Annals of Internal Medicine, 132*(5), 408–414.

Raudonis, B. M. (1992). Ethical considerations in qualitative research with hospice patients. *Qualitative Health Research, 2*(2), 238–249.

Ripamonti, C., Filiberti, A., Totis, A., DeConno, F., & Tamburini, M. (1999). Suicide among patients with cancer cared for at home by palliative care teams. *Lancet, 354*(9193), 1877–1878.

Roth, A. J., & Breitbart, W. (1996). Psychiatric emergencies in terminally ill cancer patients. *Hematology/Oncology Clinics of North America, 10*(1), 235–258.

Seale, C. (1991). Communication and awareness about death: A study of a random sample of dying people. *Social Science and Medicine, 32*(8), 943–952.

Silverman, P. R. (2001). Living with grief, rebuilding a world. *Innovations in End-of-Life Care* [On-line serial], 3(3). Available: http://www2.edc.org/lastacts/editorail.asp.

Sorenson, B. F. (1991). Euthanasia: the "good death"? *Surgical Neurology, 35*, 827–830.

Spross, J. A. (1992). Cancer pain relief: An international perspective. *Oncology Nursing Forum, 19*(7), 5–19.

Stanley, K. J. (2000). Silence is not golden: Conversations with the dying. *Clinical Journal of Oncology Nursing, 4*(1), 34–40.

Steinhauser, K. E., Christakis, N. A., Clipp, E. C., McNeilly, M., Grambow, S., Parker, J., & Tulsky, J. A. (2001). Preparing for the end of life: Preferences of patients, families, physicians and other care providers. *Journal of Pain and Symptom Management, 22*(3), 727–737.

SUPPORT Principal Investigators. (1995). A controlled trial to improve care for seriously ill hospitalized patients. *Journal of the American Medical Association, 274*(20), 1591–1598.

Teno, J. M., Fisher, E. S., Hamel, M. B., Coppola, K., & Dawson, N. V. (2002). Medical care inconsistent with patients' treatment goals: Association with 1-year Medicare resource use and survival. *Journal of American Geriatrics Society, 50*(3), 496–500.

Tilden, V. P. (2000). Policy perspectives: Advance directives. *American Journal of Nursing, 100*(12), 49–51.

Tolle, S. W., Tilden, V. P., Rosenfeld, A. G., & Hickman, S. E. (2000). Family reports of barriers to optimal care of the dying. *Nursing Research, 49*(6), 310–317.

Upledger, J. E. (1989). Self-discovery and self-healing. In R. Carlson & B. Shield (Eds.), *Healers on healing* (pp. 67–72). Los Angeles: Tarcher.

Virmani, J., Schneiderman, L. J., & Kaplan, R. M. (1994). Relationship of advance directives to physician-patient communication. *Archives of Internal Medicine, 154*, 909–913.

Waller, A., Hershkowitz, M., & Adunsky, A. (1994). The effects of intravenous fluid infusion on blood and urine parameters of hydration and on state of consciousness in terminally ill patients. *American Journal of Hospice and Palliative Care*, 26–29.

Wendler, M. C. (1996). Understanding healing: A conceptual analysis. *Journal of Advanced Nursing, 24*(4), 836–842.

Wenrich, M. D., Curtis, J. R., Shannon, S. E., Carline, J. D., Ambrozy, D. M., & Ramsey, P. G. (2001). Communicating with dying patients within the spectrum of medical care from terminal diagnosis to death. *Archives of Internal Medicine, 161*(6), 868–874.

Yedidia, M. J., & MacGregor, B. (2001). Confronting the prospect of dying: Reports of terminally ill patients. *Journal of Pain and Symptom Management, 22*(4), 807–819.

Zerwekh, J. V. (1987). Should fluid and nutrition support be withheld from terminally ill patients? *American Journal of Hospice & Palliative Care, 4*(4), 37–38.

Zerwekh, J. (1994). The truth tellers: How hospice nurses help patients confront death. *American Journal of Nursing, 94*(2), 31–34.

Zerwekh, J. V. (1997). Do dying patients really need IV fluids? *American Journal of Nursing, 97*(3), 26–30.

RESOURCES AND WEBSITES

American Academy of Hospice & Palliative Medicine, 4700 West Lake Avenue, Glenview, IL 60025-1485; 847-375-4712; http://www.aahpm.org.

Americans for Better Care of the Dying (ABCD), 4125 Albemarle Street NW, Suite 210, Washington, DC 20016; (202) 895-9485, http://www.abcd-caring.org.

American Hospice Foundation, 2120 L Street NW, Suite 200, Washington, DC 20037; 202-223-0204; Fax 202-223-0208; E-mail: ahf@msn.com; http://www.americanhospice.org/.

Center to Improve Care of the Dying (at George Washington University). Offices located at the RAND Corporation, 1200 South Hayes Street, Arlington, VA 22202-5050; 703-413-1100; http://www.gwu.edu/~cicd/.

Children's Hospice International, 2202 Mount Vernon Avenue, Suite 3C, Alexandria, VA 22301; 800-24-CHILD; http://www.chionline.org.

Choice in Dying, Inc., 1035 30th Street NW, Washington, DC 20016; 202-338-9790; http://www.choices.org.

Compassion in Dying, 6312 SW Capital Highway, Suite 415, Portland, OR 97201; 503-221-9556; http://www.compassionindying.org/.

Department of Pain Medicine and Palliative Care at Beth Israel Medical Center, 1st Avenue at 16th Street, 12 Baird Hall, New York, NY 10003; 212-844-1472; http://www.stoppain.org.

Growthhouse, Inc. (provides information and referral services for agencies working with death and dying issues), San Francisco, CA; 415-863-3045; http://www.growthhouse.org.

HMS Center for Palliative Care (Harvard Medical School), Massachusetts General Hospital, Founders House 606, 55 Fruit Street, Boston, MA 02114; 617-724-9509; http://www.hms.harvard.edu/cdi/pallcare/.

Hospice Association of America, National Association for Home Care, 228 Seventh Street SE, Washington, DC 20003; (202) 547-7424; http://www.nahc.org/.

Hospice Education Institute, 190 Westbrook Road, Essex, CT 06426; (800) 331-1620; http://www.hospiceworld.org/.

Hospice Foundation of America, 2001 S St. NW #300, Washington, DC 20009; (800) 854-3402; http://www.hospicefoundation.org.

Hospice Net, http://www.hospicenet.org/index.html.

Hospice and Palliative Nurses Association (HPNA), Penn Center West One, Suite 229, Pittsburgh, PA 15276; (412) 787-9301; http://www.hpna.org.

Hospice Web (links to other resources), http://www.hospiceweb.com/links.htm.

Innovations in End-of-Life Care (online journal), http://www2.edc.org/lastacts/.

Last Acts Campaign to Improve End-of-Life Care, Located at Partnership for Caring, Inc., 1620 Eye Street NW, Suite 202, Washington, DC 20006; 202-296-8071; http://www.lastacts.org.

Palliative Care Nursing, http://www.palliativecarenursing.net/index.html.

Partnership for Caring: America's Voices for the Dying, National Office, 1620 Eye Street NW, Suite 202, Washington, DC 20006; 202-296-8071; http://www.partnershipforcaring.org.

Project on Death in America, Open Society Institute, 400 West 59th Street, New York, NY 10019; 212-548-0150; http://www.soros.org/death.html.

Supportive Care of the Dying: A Coalition for Compassionate Care, For more information, contact Sylvia McSkimming, PhD, RN, Executive Director c/o Providence Health System, 4805 NE Glisan Street, 2E07, Portland, OR 97213; (503) 215-5053; http://www.careofdying.org.

The Center to Advance Palliative Care at The Mount Sinai School of Medicine, 1255 5th Avenue, Suite C-2, New York, NY, 10029-6574; Main line: (212) 201-2670; http://www.capcmssm.org.

Toolkit of Instruments to Measure End-of-life care (TIME; Dr. Joan Teno at Brown University): http://www.chcr.brown.edu/pcoc/toolkit.htm.

Perioperative Concepts and Nursing Management

Applying Concepts from NANDA, NIC, and NOC

Mr. Ott, a 54-year-old smoker, was admitted to the surgical unit 5 hours ago after colon resection for cancer. He is groggy but easily arousable. He can move all extremities with equal strength, but feels better lying still. In the last 4 hours, 125 mL of greenish material has drained from his nasogastric (NG) tube, which is connected to low intermittent suction. His abdomen is mildly distended; bowel sounds are absent. The large abdominal dressing has a reconstitutable Jackson-Pratt (JP) drain with 30mL of serosanguineous drainage; the dressing's minimal visible drainage has not increased in several hours. A peripheral IV of D5W 1/2NS with 20 mmol/L of KCl is running at 125 mL/h. Mr. Ott has voided 600 mL of clear urine. Vital signs are: Temp 36.1°C; HR 82, B/P 112/70; Resp 12 and shallow. Lung auscultation reveals scattered crackles throughout and a weak cough. After a 50-mg morphine injection, Mr. Ott ranks his pain at 3 out of 10 (down from 7). He is reluctant to use his incentive spirometer for fear of more pain. The concept map illustrates the relationships among the nursing diagnoses, interventions, and outcomes.

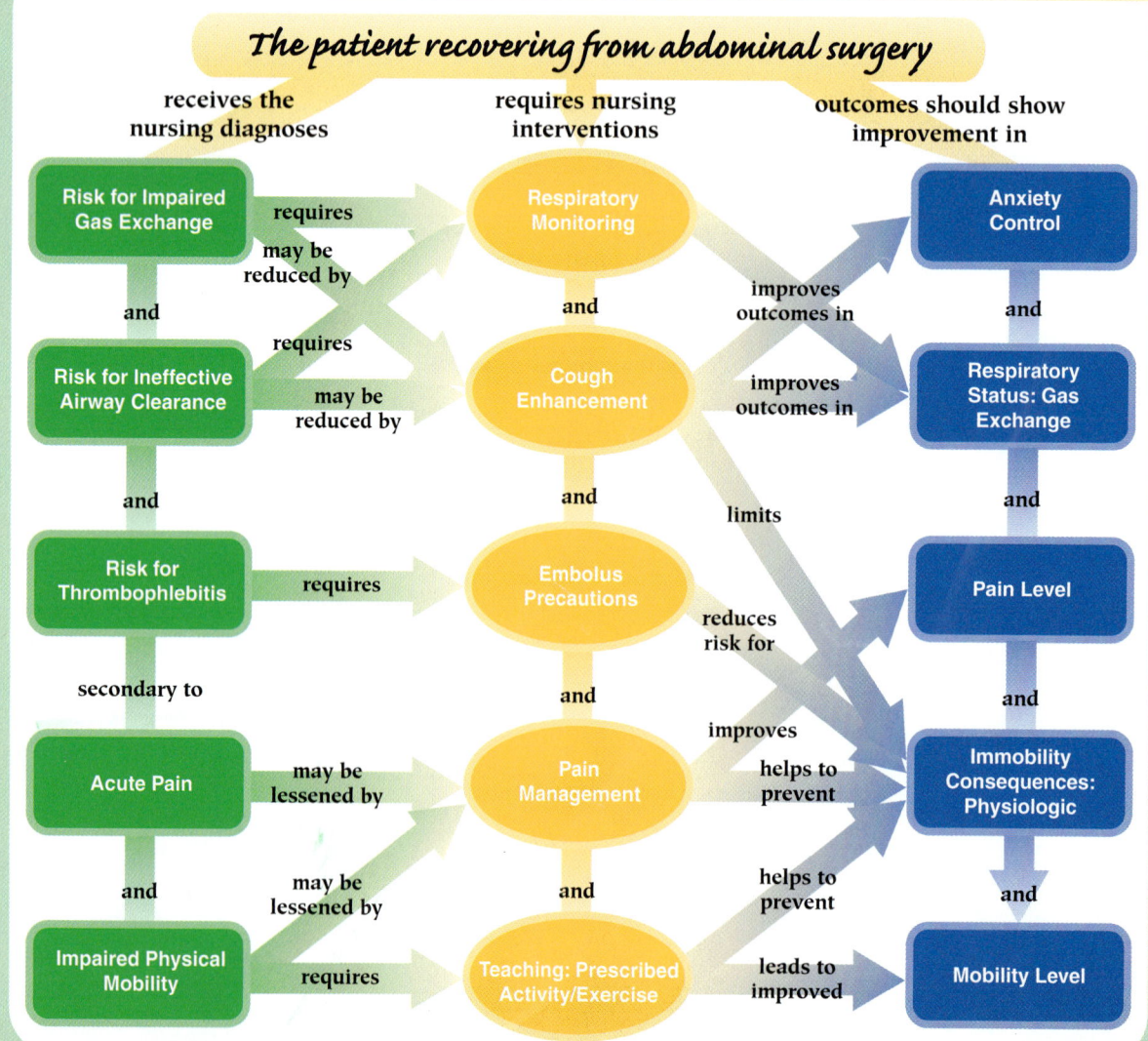

The patient recovering from abdominal surgery

receives the nursing diagnoses — **requires nursing interventions** — **outcomes should show improvement in**

- Risk for Impaired Gas Exchange — requires / may be reduced by — Respiratory Monitoring
- and
- Risk for Ineffective Airway Clearance — requires / may be reduced by — Cough Enhancement — improves outcomes in — Anxiety Control
- and
- Risk for Thrombophlebitis — requires — Embolus Precautions — improves outcomes in — Respiratory Status: Gas Exchange
- secondary to — limits
- Acute Pain — may be lessened by — Pain Management — reduces risk for / improves — Pain Level
- and
- Impaired Physical Mobility — may be lessened by / requires — Teaching: Prescribed Activity/Exercise — helps to prevent / helps to prevent / leads to improved — Immobility Consequences: Physiologic
- and
- Mobility Level

Nursing Classifications and Languages

NANDA
Nursing Diagnoses

Risk for Impaired Gas Exchange—At risk for excess or deficit in oxygenation and/or carbon dioxide elimination at the alveolar-capillary membrane

Risk for Ineffective Airway Clearance—At risk for inability to clear secretions or obstructions from the respiratory tract to maintain a clear airway

Risk for Thrombophlebitis—At risk for clot formation in the deep veins of the legs

Acute Pain—Unpleasant sensory and emotional experience arising from actual or potential tissue damage or described in terms of such damage

Impaired Physical Mobility—Limitation in independent, purposeful physical movement of the body or of one or more extremities

NIC
Nursing Interventions*

Respiratory Monitoring—Collection and analysis of patient data to ensure airway patency and adequate gas exchange

Cough Enhancement—Promotion of deep inhalation by the patient with subsequent generation of high intrathoracic pressures and compression of underlying lung parenchyma for the forceful expulsion of air

Embolus Precautions—Reduction of the risk of embolus in a patient with thrombi or at risk for developing thrombi

Pain Management—Alleviation of pain or reduction in pain to a level of comfort that is acceptable to the patient

Teaching: Prescribed Activity/ Exercise—Preparing a patient to achieve and/or maintain a prescribed level of activity

NOC
Nursing Outcomes†

Return to functional baseline status, stabilization of, or improvement in

Anxiety Control—Personal actions to eliminate or reduce feelings of apprehension and tension from an unidentifiable source

Respiratory Status: Gas Exchange—The alveolar exchange of O_2 or CO_2 to maintain arterial blood gas concentrations; measured on a scale of extremely compromised to not compromised

Pain Level—Severity of reported or demonstrated pain

Immobility Consequences: Physiologic—Extent of compromise in physiologic functioning due to impaired physical mobility

Mobility Level—Ability to move purposefully

NANDA, North American Nursing Diagnosis Association; NIC, Nursing Interventions Classification; NOC, Nursing Outcomes Classification.

*Iowa Intervention Project © 2000. In McCloskey, J. C., & Bulechek, G. M. (2000). *Nursing interventions classification (NIC)* (3rd ed.). St. Louis: Mosby.

†Iowa Outcomes Project © 2000. In Johnson, M., Maas, M., & Moorhead, S. (2000). *Nursing outcomes classification (NOC)* (3rd ed.). St. Louis: Mosby.

Preoperative Nursing Management

Adapted by Christy Raymond

LEARNING OBJECTIVES

On completion of this chapter, the learner will be able to:

1. Define the three phases of the perioperative period.
2. Describe a comprehensive preoperative assessment to identify surgical risk factors.
3. Identify the causes of preoperative anxiety and describe nursing measures to alleviate it.
4. Identify legal and ethical considerations related to informed consent.
5. Describe preoperative nursing measures that decrease the risk for infection and other postoperative complications.
6. Describe the immediate preoperative preparation of the patient.
7. Develop a preoperative teaching plan designed to promote the patient's recovery from anesthesia and surgery, thus preventing postoperative complications.

Surgery, whether elective or emergent, is a stressful, complex event. Today, as a result of advances in surgical techniques and instrumentation as well as in anesthesia, many surgical procedures that were once performed in an inpatient setting now take place in an ambulatory or outpatient setting. Approximately 60% of elective surgeries are now performed in an ambulatory or outpatient setting (Russell, Williams & Bulstrode, 2000). In 2002–2003, Canada recorded over 1.7 million same-day surgeries (Canadian Institute for Health Information, 2004). This is an increase of over 50% from the 1995–1996 statistics. In Canada, waiting times for healthcare, including elective surgeries, is a serious concern for Canadians (Romanow, 2002). In 2002, the Commission on the Future of Health Care in Canada compiled a final report containing recommendations to decrease wait times and increase access to quality health care services, including elective surgeries (Romanow, 2002). This trend has increased the acuity and complexity of surgical patients and procedures. The number of surgical patients admitted for overnight hospital stays is expected to continue to decrease.

In the past, the patient scheduled for elective surgery would be admitted to the hospital at least 1 day before surgery for evaluation and preparation; these activities are now completed before the patient is admitted to the hospital. Today, many patients arrive at the hospital the morning of surgery and go home after recovering in the postanesthesia care unit (PACU) from the anesthesia. Often, surgical patients who require hospital stays are trauma patients, acutely ill patients, patients undergoing major surgery, patients who require emergency surgery, and patients with a concurrent medical disorder. Although each setting offers its own unique advantages for the delivery of patient care, all require a comprehensive preoperative nursing assessment and nursing intervention to prepare the patient and family before surgery.

Today's technology has led to more complex procedures, more complicated microsurgical and laser technology, more sophisticated bypass equipment, increased use of laparoscopic surgery, and more sensitive monitoring devices. Surgery might now involve the transplantation of multiple human organs, the implantation of mechanical devices, the reattachment of body parts, and the use of robots and minimally invasive procedures in the operating room (Mack, 2002). Advances in anesthesia have kept pace with these surgical technologies. More sophisticated monitoring and new pharmacologic agents, such as short-acting anesthetics and more effective antiemetics, have improved postoperative pain management, reduced postoperative nausea and vomiting, and shortened procedure and recovery times.

Pressure to reduce hospital stays and contain costs has resulted in patients undergoing diagnostic **preadmission testing (PAT)** and preoperative preparation before admission to the hospital. Many facilities have a presurgical services department to facilitate testing and to initiate the nursing assessment process, which may focus on patient demographics, health history, and other information pertinent to the surgical procedure. The increasing use of **ambulatory or same-day surgery** means that patients leave the hospital sooner, which increases the need for teaching, discharge planning, preparation for self-care, and referral for home care and rehabilitation services. Competent care of ambulatory or same-day surgical patients requires a sound knowledge of all aspects of perioperative and perianesthesia nursing practice.

Perioperative and Perianesthesia Nursing

The special field known as perioperative and perianesthesia nursing includes a wide variety of nursing functions associated with the patient's surgical experience during the perioperative period. **Perioperative** and perianesthesia nursing addresses the nursing roles relevant to the three phases of the surgical experience: **preoperative**, **intraoperative**, and **postoperative**. As shown in Chart 18-1, each phase begins and ends at a particular point in the sequence of events that constitutes the surgical experience, and each includes a wide range of activities the nurse performs using the nursing process and based on the standards of practice (American Society of PeriAnesthesia Nurses, 2000; Litwack, 1999; Operating Room Nurses Association of Canada, 2003; Quinn, 1999).

PREOPERATIVE PHASE

The **preoperative phase** begins when the decision to proceed with surgical intervention is made and ends with the transfer of the patient onto the operating room table. The scope of nursing activities during this time can include establishing a baseline evaluation of the patient before the day of surgery by carrying out a preoperative interview (which includes not only a physical but also an emotional assessment, previous anesthetic history, and identification of known allergies or genetic problems that may affect the surgical outcome), ensuring that necessary tests have been or will be performed (preadmission testing), arranging appropriate consultative services, and providing preparatory education about recovery from anesthesia and postoperative care. On the day of surgery, patient teaching is reviewed, the patient's identity and the surgical site are verified, informed consent is confirmed, and an intravenous infusion is started. If the patient is going home the same day, the availability of safe transport and the presence of an accompanying responsible adult is verified. Depending on when the preadmission evaluation and testing were done, the nursing activities on the day of surgery may be as basic as performing or updating the preoperative patient assessment and addressing questions the patient or family may have.

Glossary

ambulatory surgery: may include *outpatient (or same-day)* surgery that does not require an overnight hospital stay or *short stay,* with admission to an inpatient hospital setting for less than 24 hours

informed consent: the patient's autonomous decision about whether to undergo a surgical procedure; based on the nature of the condition, the treatment options, and the risks and benefits involved

intraoperative phase: period of time from when the patient is transferred to the operating room table to when he or she is admitted to the postanesthesia care unit (PACU)

perioperative phase: period of time that constitutes the surgical experience; includes the preoperative, intraoperative, and postoperative phases of nursing care

postoperative phase: period of time that begins with the admission of the patient to the PACU and ends after a follow-up evaluation in the clinical setting or home

preadmission testing (PAT): diagnostic testing performed before admission to the hospital

preoperative phase: period of time from when the decision for surgical intervention is made to when the patient is transferred to the operating room table

Chart 18-1 Examples of Perioperative Nursing Activities

Preoperative Phase

Preadmission Testing
1. Initiates initial preoperative assessment
2. Initiates teaching appropriate to patient's needs
3. Involves family in interview
4. Verifies completion of preoperative testing
5. Verifies understanding of surgeon-specific preoperative orders (eg, bowel preparation, preoperative shower)
6. Assesses patient's need for postoperative transportation and care

Admission to Surgical Centre or Unit
1. Completes preoperative assessment
2. Assesses for risks for postoperative complications
3. Reports unexpected findings or any deviations from normal
4. Verifies that operative consent has been signed
5. Coordinates patient teaching with other nursing staff
6. Reinforces previous teaching
7. Explains phases in perioperative period and expectations
8. Answers patient's and family's questions
9. Develops a plan of care

In the Holding Area
1. Assesses patient's status; baseline pain and nutritional status
2. Reviews chart
3. Identifies patient
4. Verifies surgical site and marks site per institutional policy
5. Establishes intravenous line
6. Administers medications if prescribed
7. Takes measures to ensure patient's comfort
8. Provides psychological support
9. Communicates patient's emotional status to other appropriate members of the health care team

Intraoperative Phase

Maintenance of Safety
1. Maintains aseptic, controlled environment
2. Effectively manages human resources, equipment, and supplies for individualized patient care
3. Transfers patient to operating room bed or table
4. Positions the patient
   - Functional alignment
   - Exposure of surgical site
5. Applies grounding device to patient
6. Ensures that the sponge, needle, and instrument counts are correct
7. Completes intraoperative documentation

Physiologic Monitoring
1. Calculates effects on patient of excessive fluid loss or gain
2. Distinguishes normal from abnormal cardiopulmonary data
3. Reports changes in patient's vital signs
4. Institutes measures to promote normothermia

Psychological Support (Before Induction and When Patient Is Conscious)
1. Provides emotional support to patient
2. Stands near or touches patient during procedures and induction
3. Continues to assess patient's emotional status

Postoperative Phase

Transfer of Patient to Postanesthesia Care Unit
1. Communicates intraoperative information
   - Identifies patient by name
   - States type of surgery performed
   - Identifies type of anesthetic used
   - Reports patient's response to surgical procedure and anesthesia
   - Describes intraoperative factors (eg, insertion of drains or catheters; administration of blood, analgesic agents, or other medications during surgery; occurrence of unexpected events)
   - Describes physical limitations
   - Reports patient's preoperative level of consciousness
   - Communicates necessary equipment needs
   - Communicates presence of family and/or significant others

Postoperative Assessment Recovery Area
1. Determines patient's immediate response to surgical intervention
2. Monitors patient's physiologic status
3. Assesses patient's pain level and administers appropriate pain relief
4. Maintains patient's safety (airway, circulation, prevention of injury)
5. Administers medications, fluid, and blood component therapy, if prescribed
6. Provides oral fluids if prescribed for ambulatory surgery patient
7. Assesses patient's readiness for transfer to in-hospital unit or for discharge home based on institutional policy (eg, Alderete score, see Chap. 20)

Surgical Unit
1. Continues close monitoring of patient's physical and psychological response to surgical intervention
2. Assesses patient's pain level and administers appropriate pain relief measures
3. Provides teaching to patient during immediate recovery period
4. Assists patient in recovery and preparation for discharge home
5. Determines patient's psychological status
6. Assists with discharge planning

Home or Clinic
1. Provides follow-up care during office or clinic visit or by telephone contact
2. Reinforces previous teaching and answers patient's and family's questions about surgery and follow-up care
3. Assesses patient's response to surgery and anesthesia and their effects on body image and function
4. Determines family's perception of surgery and its outcome

INTRAOPERATIVE PHASE

The **intraoperative phase** begins when the patient is transferred onto the operating room table and ends when he or she is admitted to the postanesthesia care unit (PACU). In this phase, the scope of nursing activity can include providing for the patient's safety, maintaining an aseptic environment, ensuring proper function of equipment, providing the surgeon with specific instruments and supplies for the surgical field, and completing appropriate documentation. In some instances, the nursing activities can encompass providing emotional support by holding the patient's hand during general anesthesia induction, assisting in positioning the patient on the operating room table using basic principles of body alignment, or acting as scrub nurse, circulating nurse, or registered nurse first assistant (RNFA).

POSTOPERATIVE PHASE

The **postoperative phase** begins with the admission of the patient to the PACU and ends with a follow-up evaluation in the clinical setting or at home. The scope of nursing care covers a wide range of activities during this period. In the immediate postoperative phase, the focus includes maintaining the patient's airway, monitoring vital signs, assessing the effects of the anesthetic agents, assessing the patient for complications, and providing comfort and

GENETICS IN NURSING PRACTICE—Perioperative Nursing

Nurses who are caring for patients undergoing surgery need to take various genetic considerations into account when assessing patients throughout the perioperative experience. For example, surgical outcomes may be altered by genetic conditions that may cause complications with anesthesia, including the following:

- Malignant hyperthermia
- Central core disease (CCD)
- Duchenne muscular dystrophy
- Hyperkalemic periodic paralysis
- King-Denborough

NURSING ASSESSMENTS

PREOPERATIVE FAMILY HISTORY ASSESSMENT

- Obtain a thorough assessment of personal and family history, inquiring about prior problems with surgery or anesthesia with specific attention to complications such as fever, rigidity, dark urine, unexpected reactions.
- Inquire about any history of musculoskeletal complaints, history of heat intolerance, fevers of unknown origin, or unusual drug reaction.
- Assess for family history of any sudden or unexplained death, especially during participation in athletic events.

PHYSICAL ASSESSMENT

- Assess for subclinical muscle weakness.
- Assess for other physical features suggestive of an underlying genetic condition, such as contractures, kyphoscoliosis, and pterygium with progressive weakness.

MANAGEMENT ISSUES SPECIFIC TO GENETICS

- Inquire whether DNA mutation or other genetic testing has been performed on an affected family member.
- If indicated, refer for further genetic counselling and evaluation so that family members can discuss inheritance, risk

to other family members, availability of diagnostic/genetic testing.

- Offer appropriate genetics information and resources.
- Assess patient's understanding of genetics information.
- Provide support to families with newly diagnosed malignant hyperthermia.
- Participate in management and coordination of care of patients with genetic conditions and individuals predisposed to develop or pass on a genetic condition.

GENETICS RESOURCES FOR NURSES AND THEIR PATIENTS ON THE WEB

Canadian Directory of Genetic Support Groups: http://www.lhsc. on.ca/programs/medgenet—resource and guide for families seeking information about genetic disorders

Canadian Organization for Rare Disorders (CORD): http://www. cord.ca—information about support groups for patients and families

Genetic Alliance: http://www.geneticalliance.org—a directory of support groups for patients and families with genetic conditions

Gene Clinics: http://www.geneclinics.org—a listing of common genetic disorders with up-to-date clinical summaries, genetic counselling and testing information

International Council of Nurses http://www.icn.ch/matters genetics.htm—ICN's statement re: genetics and nursing.

National Organization of Rare Disorders: http://www. rarediseases.org—a directory of support groups and information for patients and families with rare genetic disorders

OMIM: Online Mendelian Inheritance in Man: http://www. ncbi.nlm.nih.gov/omim/stats/html—a complete listing of inherited genetic conditions

The Genetics Society of Canada: http://life.biology.mcmaster. ca/GSC—information about genetic research and society initiatives, including links to other genetic-related sites

---

pain relief. Nursing activities then focus on promoting the patient's recovery and initiating the teaching, follow-up care, and referrals essential for recovery and rehabilitation after discharge. Each phase is reviewed in more detail in the three chapters of this unit.

Historically, the perioperative nurse's practice environment has been isolated, consisting of the area behind the double doors of the surgical suite. Although the nursing process guided nursing care, the fundamentals of assessment, diagnosis, planning, intervention, and evaluation were often misunderstood by practitioners unfamiliar with the delivery of surgical care. The United States and Canada each have a nurses association representing perioperative registered nursing practice. The Association of PeriOperative Registered Nurses (AORN) is the organization that is linked to the United States. The Operating Room Nurses Association of Canada (ORNAC) promotes quality perioperative nursing care through establishment of standards and competencies in Canada. From these guidelines, standards, competencies and position statements, the ORNAC has developed a conceptual model to guide nursing practice in the perioperative setting (Fig. 18-1). This model depicts the surgical patient as the focus of nursing practice through a strong foundation of delivering quality perioperative registered nursing care.

Surgical Classifications

Surgery may be performed for various reasons. A surgical procedure may be diagnostic (eg, biopsy or exploratory laparotomy). It may be curative (eg, excision of a tumour or an inflamed appendix) or reparative (eg, multiple wound repair). Surgery may be reconstructive or cosmetic (eg, mammoplasty or a facelift), or it may be palliative (eg, to relieve pain or correct a problem; for instance, a gastrostomy tube may be inserted to compensate for the inability to swallow food). Surgery may also be classified according to the degree of urgency involved: emergent, urgent, required, elective, and optional. These terms are defined in Table 18-1.

Preparation for Surgery

INFORMED CONSENT

Voluntary and written **informed consent** from the patient is necessary before nonemergent surgery can be performed. Such written consent protects the patient from unsanctioned surgery

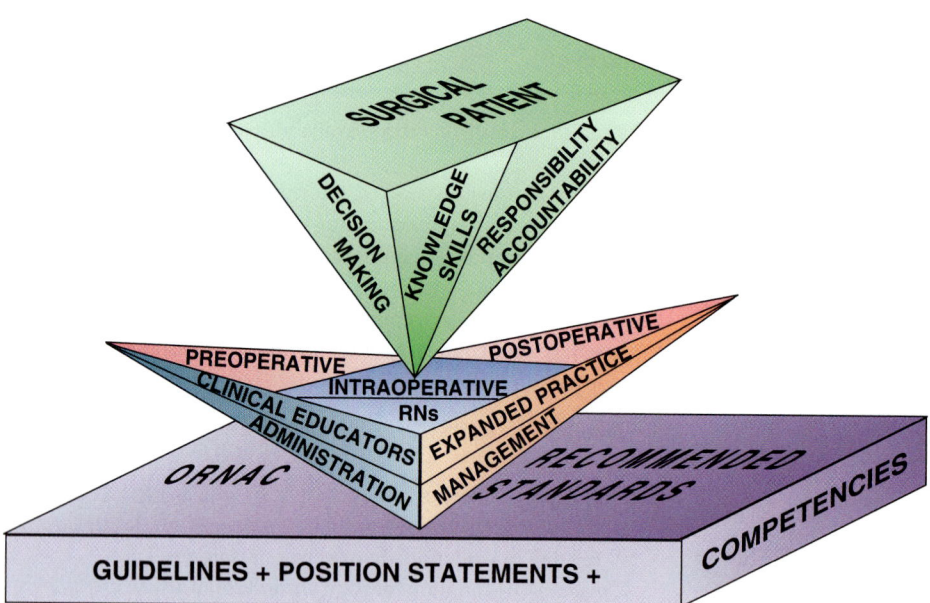

FIGURE 18-1 Conceptual model for perioperative registered nursing practice. © With permission from Operating Room Nurses Association of Canada.

and protects the surgeon from claims of an unauthorized operation. In the best interests of all parties concerned, sound medical, ethical, and legal principles are followed. The nurse may ask the patient to sign the form and may witness the patient's signature. It is the physician's responsibility to provide appropriate information. Chart 18-2 lists the criteria for a valid informed consent.

Many ethical principles are integral to informed consent (see Chap. 3). Before the patient signs the consent form, the surgeon must provide a clear and simple explanation of what the surgery will entail. The surgeon must also inform the patient of the benefits, alternatives, possible risks, complications, disfigurement, disability, and removal of body parts as well as what to expect in the early and late postoperative periods. If the patient needs additional information to make his or her decision, the nurse notifies the physician about this. Also, the nurse ascertains that the consent form has been signed before administering psychoactive premedication, because the consent may not be valid if it was obtained while the patient was under the influence of medications that can affect judgment and decision-making capacity. Informed consent is necessary in the following circumstances:

- Invasive procedures, such as a surgical incision, a biopsy, a cystoscopy, or paracentesis
- Procedures requiring sedation and/or anesthesia (see Chap. 19 for a discussion of levels of sedation and anesthesia)
- A nonsurgical procedure, such as an arteriography, that carries more than slight risk to the patient
- Procedures involving radiation

The patient personally signs the consent if he or she is of legal age and is mentally capable. When the patient is a minor or un-

Table 18-1 • Categories of Surgery Based on Urgency

CLASSIFICATION	INDICATIONS FOR SURGERY	EXAMPLES
I. Emergent—Patient requires immediate attention; disorder may be life-threatening	Without delay	Severe bleeding Bladder or intestinal obstruction Fractured skull Gunshot or stab wounds Extensive burns
II. Urgent—Patient requires prompt attention	Within 24–30 h	Acute gallbladder infection Kidney or ureteral stones
III. Required—Patient needs to have surgery	Plan within a few weeks or months	Prostatic hyperplasia without bladder obstruction Thyroid disorders Cataracts
IV. Elective—Patient should have surgery	Failure to have surgery not catastrophic	Repair of scars Simple hernia Vaginal repair
V. Optional—Decision rests with patient	Personal preference	Cosmetic surgery

---

Chart 18-2 Criteria for Valid Informed Consent

Voluntary Consent

Valid consent must be freely given, without coercion.

Incompetent Patient

Legal definition: individual who is *not* autonomous and cannot give or withhold consent (eg, individuals who are mentally retarded, mentally ill, or comatose)

Informed Subject

Informed consent should be in writing. It should contain the following:

- Explanation of procedure and its risks
- Description of benefits and alternatives
- An offer to answer questions about procedure
- Instructions that the patient may withdraw consent
- A statement informing the patient if the protocol differs from customary procedure

Patient Able to Comprehend

Information must be written and delivered in language understandable to the patient. Questions must be answered to facilitate comprehension if material is confusing.

---

conscious or incompetent, permission must be obtained from a responsible family member (preferably next of kin) or legal guardian. An emancipated minor (married or independently earning his or her own living) may sign his or her own consent form. Agency policy must be followed when obtaining consent from a patient. In an emergency, it may be necessary for the surgeon to operate as a lifesaving measure without the patient's informed consent. Every effort, however, must be made to contact the patient's family. In such a situation, contact can be made by telephone, telegram, fax, or other electronic means.

When the patient has doubts and has not had the opportunity to investigate alternative treatments, a second opinion may be requested. No patient should be urged or coerced to sign an operative permit. Refusing to undergo a surgical procedure is a person's legal right and privilege. However, such information must be documented and relayed to the surgeon so that other arrangements can be made. For example, additional explanations may be provided to the patient and family, or the surgery may be rescheduled.

The consent process can be improved by providing audiovisual materials to supplement discussion, by ensuring that the wording of the consent form is understandable, and by using other strategies and resources as needed to help the patient understand its content.

 NURSING ALERT The signed consent form is placed in a prominent place on the patient's chart and accompanies the patient to the operating room.

ASSESSMENT OF HEALTH FACTORS THAT AFFECT PATIENTS PREOPERATIVELY

The overall goal in the preoperative period is for the patient to have as many positive health factors as possible. Every attempt is made to stabilize those conditions that otherwise hinder a smooth recovery. When negative factors dominate, the risks of surgery and postoperative complications increase.

Before any surgical treatment is initiated, a health history is obtained, a physical examination is performed during which vital signs are noted, and a database is established for future comparisons (Rothrock, 2003). During the physical examination, many factors are considered that have the potential to affect the patient undergoing surgery. Health care providers should be alert for signs of abuse that can occur at all ages and to men and women from all socioeconomic, ethnic, and cultural groups (Little, 2000; Marshall, Benton & Brazier, 2000). Findings need to be reported accordingly (see Chap. 5 for further discussion of signs of abuse).

Blood tests, x-rays, and other diagnostic tests are prescribed when specifically indicated by information obtained from a thorough history and physical examination (King, 2000). These preliminary contacts with the health care team provide the patient with opportunities to ask questions and to become acquainted with those who may be providing care during and after surgery.

Nutritional and Fluid Status

Optimal nutrition is an essential factor in promoting healing and resisting infection and other surgical complications (Braunschweig, Gomez & Sheean, 2000). Assessment of a patient's nutritional status provides information on obesity, undernutrition, weight loss, malnutrition, deficiencies in specific nutrients, metabolic abnormalities, the effects of medications on nutrition, and special problems of the hospitalized patient (Quinn, 1999). Nutritional needs may be determined by measurement of body mass index and waist circumference (Health Canada, 2003; National Institutes of Health, 2000). See Chapter 5 for further discussion of nutritional assessment.

Any nutritional deficiency, such as malnutrition, should be corrected before surgery so that enough protein is available for tissue repair (King, 2000; Russell, Williams & Bulstrode, 2000). The nutrients needed for wound healing are summarized in Table 18-2.

Dehydration, hypovolemia, and electrolyte imbalances can lead to significant problems in patients with comorbid medical conditions or in elderly patients. The severity of fluid and electrolyte imbalances is often difficult to determine. Mild volume deficits may be treated during surgery; however, additional time may be needed to correct pronounced fluid and electrolyte deficits to promote the best possible preoperative condition.

Drug or Alcohol Use

People who abuse drugs or alcohol frequently deny or attempt to hide it. In such situations, the nurse who is obtaining the patient's health history needs to ask frank questions with patience, care, and a nonjudgmental attitude. See Chapter 5 for an assessment of alcohol and drug use.

Because acutely intoxicated persons are susceptible to injury, surgery is postponed in these patients if possible. If emergency surgery is required, local, spinal, or regional block anesthesia is used for minor surgery. Otherwise, to prevent vomiting and potential aspiration, a nasogastric tube is inserted before administering general anesthesia.

The person with a history of chronic alcoholism often suffers from malnutrition and other systemic problems that increase the surgical risk. Additionally, alcohol withdrawal delirium (delirium tremens) may be anticipated up to 72 hours after alcohol withdrawal. Delirium tremens is associated with a significant mortality rate when it occurs postoperatively.

Table 18-2 • Nutrients Important for Wound Healing

NUTRIENT	RATIONALE FOR INCREASED NEED	POSSIBLE DEFICIENCY OUTCOME
Protein	To replace the lean body mass lost during the catabolic phase after stress To restore blood volume and plasma proteins lost through exudates, bleeding from the wound, and possible hemorrhage To replace losses resulting from immobility (increased excretion) To meet the increased needs for tissue repair and resistance to infection	Significant weight loss Impaired/delayed wound healing Shock related to decreased blood volume Edema related to decreased serum albumin Diarrhea related to decreased albumin Anemia Increased risk of infection related to decreased antibodies, impaired tissue integrity Decreased lipoprotein synthesis → fatty infiltration of the liver → liver damage Increased mortality
Calories	To replace losses related to lack of oral intake and hypermetabolism during catabolic phase after stress To spare protein To restore normal weight	Signs and symptoms of protein deficiency due to use of protein to meet energy requirements Extensive weight loss
Water	To replace fluid lost through vomiting, hemorrhage, exudates, fever, drainage, diuresis To maintain homeostasis	Signs, symptoms, and complications of dehydration, such as poor skin turgor, dry mucous membranes, oliguria, anuria, weight loss, increased pulse rate, decreased central venous pressure
Vitamin C	Important for capillary formation, tissue synthesis, and wound healing through collagen formation Needed for antibody formation	Impaired/delayed wound healing related to impaired collagen formation and increased capillary fragility and permeability Increased risk of infection related to decreased antibodies
Thiamine, niacin, riboflavin	Requirements increase with increased metabolic rate	Decreased enzymes available for energy metabolism
Folic acid, vitamin B_{12}	Needed for cell proliferation and therefore tissue synthesis Important for maturation of red blood cells Impaired folic acid synthesis associated with the use of some antibiotics; impaired vitamin B_{12} absorption associated with the use of some antibiotics	Decreased or arrested cell division Megaloblastic anemia
Vitamin A	Important for tissue synthesis, wound healing, and immune function Enhances resistance to infection	Impaired/delayed wound healing related to decreased collagen synthesis; impaired immune function Increased risk of infection
Vitamin K	Important for normal blood clotting Impaired intestinal synthesis associated with the use of antibiotics	Prolonged prothrombin time
Iron	To replace iron lost through blood loss	Signs, symptoms, and complications of iron deficiency anemia, such as fatigue, weakness, pallor, anorexia, dizziness, headaches, stomatitis, glossitis, cardiovascular and respiratory changes, possible cardiac failure
Zinc	Needed for protein synthesis and wound healing Needed for normal lymphocyte and phagocyte response	Impaired/delayed wound healing Impaired immune response

Reproduced with permission from Dudek, S. G. (Ed.). (2001). *Nutrition essentials for nursing practice* (4th ed.). Philadelphia: Lippincott Williams & Wilkins.

Chart 18-3 gives more information about risk factors that may lead to complications.

Respiratory Status

The goal for potential surgical patients is optimal respiratory function. Patients are taught breathing exercises and use of an incentive spirometer if indicated. Because adequate ventilation is potentially compromised during all phases of surgical treatment, surgery is usually postponed when the patient has a respiratory infection. Patients with underlying respiratory disease (eg, asthma, chronic obstructive pulmonary disease) are assessed carefully for current threats to their pulmonary status. Patients' use of medications that may affect recovery is also assessed (King, 2000; Smetana, 1999).

Patients who smoke are urged to stop 2 months before surgery (King, 2000), although many do not do so. These patients should be counselled to stop smoking at least 24 hours prior to surgery. Research suggests that counselling has a positive effect on the patient's smoking behaviour 24 hours preceding surgery, helping reduce the potential for adverse effects associated with smoking such as increased airway reactivity, decreased mucociliary clearance, as well as physiologic changes in the cardiovascular and immune systems (Shannon-Cain, Webster & Cain, 2002).

Chart 18-3
Risk Factors for Surgical Complications

Hypovolemia
Dehydration or electrolyte imbalance
Nutritional deficits
Extremes of age (very young, very old)
Extremes of weight (emaciation, obesity)
Infection and sepsis
Toxic conditions
Immunologic abnormalities
Pulmonary disease
   Obstructive disease
   Restrictive disorder
   Respiratory infection
Renal or urinary tract disease
   Decreased renal function
   Urinary tract infection
   Obstruction
Pregnancy
   Diminished maternal physiologic reserve
Cardiovascular disease
   Coronary artery disease or previous myocardial infarction
   Cardiac failure
   Dysrhythmias
   Hypertension
   Prosthetic heart valve
   Thromboembolism
   Hemorrhagic disorders
   Cerebrovascular disease
Endocrine dysfunction
   Diabetes mellitus
   Adrenal disorders
   Thyroid malfunction
Hepatic disease
   Cirrhosis
   Hepatitis
Preexisting mental or physical disability

Cardiovascular Status

The goal in preparing any patient for surgery is to ensure a well-functioning cardiovascular system to meet the oxygen, fluid, and nutritional needs of the perioperative period. If the patient has uncontrolled hypertension, surgery may be postponed until the blood pressure is under control.

Because cardiovascular disease increases the risk for complications, patients with these conditions require greater-than-usual diligence during all phases of nursing management and care (King, 2000). Depending on the severity of the symptoms, surgery may be deferred until medical treatment can be instituted to improve the patient's condition. At times, surgical treatment can be modified to meet the cardiac tolerance of the patient. For example, in a patient with obstruction of the descending colon and coronary artery disease, a temporary simple colostomy may be performed rather than a more extensive colon resection that would require a prolonged period of anesthesia.

Hepatic and Renal Function

The presurgical goal is optimal function of the liver and urinary systems so that medications, anesthetic agents, body wastes, and toxins are adequately processed and removed from the body.

The liver is important in the biotransformation of anesthetic compounds. Therefore, any disorder of the liver has an effect on how anesthetic agents are metabolized. Because acute liver disease is associated with high surgical mortality, preoperative improvement in liver function is a goal. Careful assessment is made with the help of various liver function tests (see Chap. 39).

Because the kidneys are involved in excreting anesthetic drugs and their metabolites and because acid–base status and metabolism are also important considerations in anesthesia administration, surgery is contraindicated when a patient has acute nephritis, acute renal insufficiency with oliguria or anuria, or other acute renal problems. The exception is surgery that is performed as a lifesaving measure or that is necessary to improve urinary function, as in the case of an obstructive uropathy.

Endocrine Function

The patient with diabetes who is undergoing surgery is at risk for hypoglycemia and hyperglycemia. Hypoglycemia may develop during anesthesia or postoperatively from inadequate carbohydrates or from excessive administration of insulin. Hyperglycemia, which may increase the risk for surgical wound infection, may result from the stress of surgery, which may trigger increased levels of catecholamine. Other risks are acidosis and glucosuria. Although the surgical risk in the patient with controlled diabetes is no greater than in the nondiabetic patient, the goal is to maintain the blood glucose level at less than 67 mmol/L. Frequent monitoring of blood glucose levels is important before, during, and after surgery (see Chap. 41 for discussion of the patient with diabetes undergoing surgery).

Patients who have received corticosteroids are at risk for adrenal insufficiency. Therefore, the use of corticosteroids for any purpose during the preceding year must be reported to the anesthesiologist or anesthetist and surgeon. Additionally, the patient is monitored for signs of adrenal insufficiency.

Patients with uncontrolled thyroid disorders are at risk for thyrotoxicosis (with hyperthyroid disorders) and respiratory failure (with hypothyroid disorders). Therefore, the patient is assessed for a history of these disorders.

Immune Function

An important function of the preoperative assessment is to determine the existence of allergies, including the nature of previous allergic reactions. It is especially important to identify and document any sensitivity to medications and past adverse reactions to these agents. The patient is asked to identify any substances that precipitated previous allergic reactions, including medications, blood transfusions, contrast agents, latex, and food products, and to describe the signs and symptoms produced by these substances. A sample latex allergy screening questionnaire is shown in Figure 18-2.

Immunosuppression is common with corticosteroid therapy, renal transplantation, radiation therapy, chemotherapy, and disorders affecting the immune system, such as acquired immunodeficiency syndrome (AIDS) and leukemia. The mildest symptoms or slightest temperature elevation must be investigated. Because patients who are immunosuppressed are highly susceptible to infection, great care is taken to ensure strict asepsis.

Previous Medication Use

A medication history is obtained from each patient because of the possible effects of medications on the patient's perioperative and perianesthesia course and the possibility of drug interactions (Quinn,

Ask the patient the following questions. Check "Yes" or "No" in the box.	YES	NO
1. Has a doctor ever told you that you are allergic to latex?		
2. Do you have on-the-job exposure to latex?		
3. Were you born with problems involving your spinal cord?		
4. Have you ever had allergies, asthma, hay fever, eczema or problems with rashes?		
5. Have you ever had respiratory distress, rapid heart rate or swelling?		
6. Have you ever had swelling, itching, hives or other symptoms after contact with a balloon?		
7. Have you ever had swelling, itching, hives or other symptoms after a dental examination or procedure?		
8. Have you ever had swelling, itching, hives or other symptoms following a vaginal or rectal examination or after contact with a diaphragm or condom?		
9. Have you ever had swelling, itching, hives or other symptoms during or within one hour after wearing rubber gloves?		
10. Have you ever had a rash on your hands that lasted longer than one week?		
11. Have you ever had swelling, itching, hives, runny nose, eye irritation, wheezing, or asthma after contact with any latex or rubber product?		
12. Have you ever had swelling, itching, hives or other symptoms after being examined by someone wearing rubber or latex gloves?		
13. Are you allergic to bananas, avocados, kiwi or chestnuts?		
14. Have you ever had an unexplained anaphylactic episode?		

Pre-op RN Signature: _____

Patient Name: _____

Procedure: _____

FIGURE 18-2 Example of a latex allergy assessment form. Courtesy of Inova Fairfax Hospital, Falls Church, VA.

1999). Any medication the patient is using or has used in the past is documented, including over-the-counter (OTC) preparations and herbal agents and the frequency with which they are used. Potent medications have an effect on physiologic functions; interactions of such medications with anesthetic agents can cause serious problems, such as arterial hypotension and circulatory collapse.

The potential effects of prior medication therapy are evaluated by the anesthesiologist, who considers the length of time the patient has used the medications, the physical condition of the patient, and the nature of the proposed surgery. Medications that cause particular concern are listed in Table 18-3.

Many patients take self-prescribed or OTC medications in addition to those listed in Table 18-3. Aspirin is a common OTC medication prescribed by physicians or taken independently by patients to prevent myocardial infarction, stroke, and other disorders (Karch, 2002). Because of the effects of aspirin or other

OTC medications and possible interactions with other medications and anesthetic agents, it is important to ask a patient about their use. The information is noted in the patient's chart and conveyed to the anesthesiologist and surgeon.

The use of herbal medications is widespread among patients. Patients with chronic illnesses may be using herbal medications to supplement their prescribed medications or in place of them. Certain herbal medications, such as echinacea, ephedra, garlic (*Allium sativum*), ginkgo, ginseng, kava kava (*Piper methysticum*), St. John's wort (*Hypericum perforatum*), licorice (*Glycyhiza glabra*), and valerian (*Valeriana officinalis*) have been identified as the most commonly used herbal medications that may cause concern during the perioperative period (Ang-Lee, Moss & Yuan, 2001; Kuhn, 1999; Lyons, 2002). Because of the potential effects of herbal medications on coagulation and potential interactions with other medications, the nurse must ask surgical patients ex-

AGENT (GENERIC AND TRADE EXAMPLE)	EFFECT OF INTERACTION WITH ANESTHETICS
Corticosteroids Prednisone (Apo-Prednisone, Deltasone)	Cardiovascular collapse can occur if discontinued suddenly. Therefore, a bolus of corticosteroid may be administered intravenously immediately before and after surgery.
Diuretics Hydrochlorothiazide (Apo-Hydro, HydroDIURIL)	During anesthesia, may cause excessive respiratory depression resulting from an associated electrolyte imbalance
Phenothiazines Chlorpromazine (Largactil, Thorazine)	May increase the hypotensive action of anesthetics
Tranquilizers Diazepam (Diazemuls, Valium)	May cause anxiety, tension, and even seizures if withdrawn suddenly
Insulin	Interaction between anesthetics and insulin must be considered when a patient with diabetes is undergoing surgery.
Antibiotics Erythromycin (Ery-Tab)	When combined with a curariform muscle relaxant, nerve transmission is interrupted and apnea from respiratory paralysis may result.
Anticoagulants Warfarin (Coumadin)	Can increase the risk of bleeding during the intraoperative and postoperative periods; should be discontinued in anticipation of elective surgery. The surgeon will determine how long before the elective surgery the patient should stop taking an anticoagulant, depending on the type of planned procedure and the medical condition of the patient.
Antiseizure Medications Phenytoin (Dilantin)	An intravenous route of medication may need to be administered to keep the patient seizure-free in the intraoperative and postoperative periods.
Monoamine Oxidase (MAO) Inhibitors Phenelzine sulfate (Nardil)	May increase the hypotensive action of anesthetics

Table 18-3 • Medications With the Potential to Affect the Surgical Experience

plicitly about the use of these agents, document their use, and inform the surgical team and anesthesiologist (Brumly, 2000).

NURSING ALERT Because of possible adverse interactions, the nurse must assess and document the patient's use of prescription medications, OTC medications (especially aspirin), and herbal medications. The nurse must clearly communicate this information to the anesthesiologist.

Psychosocial Factors

All patients have some type of emotional reaction before any surgical procedure, be it obvious or hidden, normal or abnormal. For example, preoperative anxiety may be an anticipatory response to an experience the patient views as a threat to his or her customary role in life, body integrity, or life itself. Psychological distress directly influences body functioning. Therefore, it is imperative to identify any anxiety the patient is experiencing.

By taking a careful health history, the nurse elicits patient concerns that can have a bearing on the course of the surgical experience (Quinn, 1999). Undoubtedly, a patient about to undergo surgery is faced with various fears, including fears of the unknown, of death, of anesthesia, pain, or cancer. Concerns about loss of work time, loss of job, increased responsibilities or burden on family members, and the threat of permanent incapacity further contribute to the emotional strain created by the prospect of surgery. Less obvious concerns may occur because of previous experiences with the health care system and people the patient has known with the same condition.

People express fear in different ways. For example, one patient may repeatedly ask a lot of questions, even though answers were given previously. Another person may withdraw, deliberately avoiding communication, perhaps by reading or watching television. Still others may talk about trivialities. Consequently, the nurse must be empathetic, listen well, and provide information that helps alleviate concerns.

An important outcome of the psychosocial assessment is the determination of the extent and role of the patient's support network. The value and reliability of all available support systems are assessed. Other information, such as usual level of functioning and typical daily activities, may assist in the patient's care and rehabilitation plans. Assessing the patient's readiness to learn and determining the best approach to maximize comprehension will provide the basis for preoperative patient education.

Spiritual and Cultural Beliefs

Spiritual beliefs play an important role in how people cope with fear and anxiety. Regardless of the patient's religious affiliation, spiritual beliefs can be as therapeutic as medication. Every attempt must be made to help the patient obtain the spiritual help that he or she requests. Faith has great sustaining power. Thus, the beliefs of each patient should be respected and supported. Some nurses avoid the subject of a clergy visit lest the suggestion alarm the patient. Asking if the patient's spiritual advisor knows about the impending surgery is a caring, nonthreatening approach.

Showing respect for a patient's cultural values and beliefs facilitates rapport and trust. Some areas of assessment include identifying the ethnic group to which the patient relates and the customs and beliefs the patient holds about illness and health care providers. For example, patients from some cultural groups are unaccustomed to expressing feelings openly. Nurses need to consider this pattern of communication when assessing pain. As a sign of respect, people from other cultural groups may not make direct eye contact with others. The nurse needs to know that this lack of eye contact is not avoidance or a lack of interest.

Perhaps the most valuable skill at the nurse's disposal is listening carefully to the patient, especially when obtaining the history. Invaluable information and insights may be gained by engaging in conversation and using communication and interviewing skills. An unhurried, understanding, and caring nurse invites confidence on the part of the patient.

Special Considerations

In the preoperative period, attention needs to be paid to patients with special considerations. These may include the patient who is undergoing ambulatory surgery, the geriatric patient, the patient who is obese, the patient with a disability, and the patient undergoing emergency surgery.

THE AMBULATORY SURGERY PATIENT

The brief time the patient and family spend in the ambulatory setting is an important factor in the preoperative period. The nurse must quickly and comprehensively assess and anticipate the patient's needs and at the same time begin planning for discharge and follow-up home care.

The nurse needs to be sure that the patient and family understand that the patient will go first to the preoperative holding area before going to the operating room for the surgical procedure and then will spend some time in the PACU before being discharged home with the family later that day. Other preoperative teaching content should also be verified (see the section later in this chapter on instructing the ambulatory surgery patient) and reinforced as needed. The nurse should ensure that any plans for follow-up home care are in place if needed (Quinn, 1999).

ELDERLY PATIENTS

The older person undergoing surgery may have a combination of chronic illnesses and health problems in addition to the specific one for which surgery is indicated. Elderly people frequently do not report symptoms, perhaps because they fear a serious illness may be diagnosed or because they accept such symptoms as part of the aging process. Subtle clues alert the nurse to underlying problems.

Health care staff must remember that the hazards of surgery for the aged are proportional to the number and severity of co-existing health problems and the nature and duration of the operative procedure. The underlying principle that guides the preoperative assessment, surgical care, and postoperative care is that the aged patient has less physiologic reserve (the ability of an organ to return to normal after a disturbance in its equilibrium) than the younger patient. Cardiac reserves are lower; renal and hepatic functions are depressed; and gastrointestinal activity is likely to be reduced. Dehydration, constipation, and malnutrition may be evident. Sensory limitations, such as impaired vision or hearing and reduced tactile sensitivity, are often the reasons for falls and burns. Therefore, the nurse must be alert to maintaining a safe environment. Arthritis is common in older people and may affect mobility, making it difficult for the patient to turn from one side to the other or ambulate without discomfort. Protective measures include adequate padding for tender areas, moving the patient slowly, protecting bony prominences from prolonged pressure, and providing gentle massage to promote circulation.

The condition of the mouth is important to assess. Dental caries, dentures, and partial plates are particularly significant to the anesthesiologist or anesthetist because decayed teeth or dental prostheses may become dislodged during intubation and occlude the airway.

An additional area to assess in elderly patients is the preoperative level of activity. Research suggests that elderly patients who had hip replacement surgery and who reported performing greater physical activities (including heavy chores) preoperatively can walk greater distances postoperatively than elderly patients who are less physically active prior to surgery (Whitney & Parkman, 2002).

As the body ages, its ability to perspire decreases. Because decreased perspiration leads to dry, itchy skin, which becomes fragile and is easily abraded, precautions are taken when moving an elderly person. Decreased subcutaneous fat makes older people more susceptible to temperature changes. A lightweight cotton blanket is an appropriate cover when an elderly patient is moved to and from the operating room.

Most elderly people have experienced personal illnesses and possibly life-threatening illnesses of friends and family. Such experiences may result in fears about the surgery and about the future. Providing the patient with an opportunity to express these fears enables the patient to gain some peace of mind and a sense of being understood.

Preoperative pain assessment and teaching are important with elderly patients. It is important for nurses to incorporate pain management information and pain communication skills when teaching elderly persons how to obtain greater postoperative pain relief (McDonald, Freeland, Thomas & Moore, 2001).

Because the elderly patient may have greater risks during the perioperative period, the following are critical: (1) skillful preoperative assessment and treatment, (2) skillful anesthesia and surgery, and (3) meticulous and competent postoperative and postanesthesia management.

OBESE PATIENTS

Like age, obesity increases the risk and severity of complications associated with surgery (National Institutes of Health, 2000). In Canada, over half of individuals are classified as overweight or obese (Tjepkema, 2005). During surgery, fatty tissues are especially susceptible to infection. Additionally, obesity increases technical and mechanical problems related to surgery. Therefore, dehiscence (wound separation) and wound infections are more common. Moreover, the obese patient may be more difficult to care for because of the added weight; the patient tends to breathe poorly when supine, which increases the risk of hypoventilation and postoperative pulmonary complications. In addition, abdominal distention, phlebitis, and cardiovascular, endocrine, hepatic, and biliary diseases occur more readily in obese patients (Dudek, 2001). It has been estimated that for each 30 pounds of excess weight, about 25 additional miles of blood vessels are needed, and this places increased demands on the heart.

PATIENTS WITH DISABILITIES

Special considerations for patients with a mental or physical disability include the need for assistive devices, modifications in preoperative teaching, additional assistance with and attention to positioning or transferring, and the effects of the disability on surgery and anesthesia (Quinn, 1999).

Assistive devices include hearing aids, eyeglasses, braces, prostheses, and other devices. Individuals who are hearing-impaired may need a translator or some alternative communication system perioperatively. If they rely on signing or speech (lip) reading, and if their eyeglasses or contact lenses are removed or if health care staff wear surgical masks, these patients will need an alternative method of communication. These needs must be identified as a factor in the preoperative evaluation and clearly communicated to personnel. Specific strategies for accommodating the patient's needs must be identified ahead of time. Ensuring the safety of assistive devices is important; these devices are expensive and likely to be lost.

Most patients are directed to move from the stretcher to the operating room table and back again. In addition to being unable to see or hear instructions, patients with a disability may be unable to move without special devices or a great deal of assistance. The patient with a disability that affects body position (eg, cerebral palsy, post-polio syndrome, and other neuromuscular disorders) may need special positioning during surgery to prevent pain and injury. Moreover, these patients may be unable to sense whether their extremities are positioned incorrectly.

Patients with respiratory problems related to a disability (eg, multiple sclerosis, muscular dystrophy) may experience difficulties unless the problems are made known to the anesthesiologist or anesthetist and adjustments are made. These factors need to be clearly identified in the preoperative period and communicated to the appropriate personnel.

PATIENTS UNDERGOING EMERGENCY SURGERY

Emergency surgeries are unplanned and occur with little time for preparation (Rothrock, 2003). The unpredictable nature of trauma and emergency surgery poses unique challenges to the nurse throughout the perioperative period.

All of the previously discussed factors that affect patients preparing to undergo surgery apply to these patients, usually in a very condensed time frame. The preoperative assessment may actually coincide with resuscitation efforts in the emergency department (Rothrock, 2003). For the unconscious patient, informed consent and essential information, such as pertinent past medical history and allergies, need to be obtained from a family member, if one is available. A quick visual survey of the patient is essential to identify all sites of injury when the emergency surgery is due to trauma (see Chap. 71 for more information).

The psychological status of the patient undergoing emergency surgery should be assessed quickly if the patient is awake (Rothrock, 2003). The patient may have undergone a very frightening experience and may need extra support and explanation of the surgery.

Preoperative Nursing Interventions

PREOPERATIVE TEACHING

Nurses have long recognized the value of preoperative instruction (Fitzpatrick, 1998). Each patient is taught as an individual, with consideration for any unique concerns or needs; the program of instruction should be based on the individual's learning needs (Quinn, 1999). Multiple teaching strategies should be used (eg, verbal, written, return demonstration), depending on the patient's needs and abilities. Preoperative teaching is initiated as soon as possible. It should start in the physician's office and continue until the patient arrives in the operating room.

When and What to Teach

Ideally, instruction is spaced over a period of time to allow the patient to assimilate information and ask questions as they arise. Frequently, teaching sessions are combined with various preparation procedures to allow for an easy and timely flow of information. The nurse should guide the patient through the experience and allow ample time for questions. Some patients may feel too many descriptive details will increase their anxiety level, and the nurse should respect their wish for less detail.

Teaching should go beyond descriptions of the procedure and should include explanations of the sensations the patient will experience. For example, telling the patient only that preoperative medication will relax him or her before the operation is not as effective as also noting that the medication may result in light-headedness and drowsiness. Knowing what to expect will help the patient anticipate these reactions and thus attain a higher degree of relaxation than might otherwise be expected.

The ideal timing for preoperative teaching is not on the day of surgery but during the preadmission visit when diagnostic tests are performed. At this time, the nurse or resource person answers questions and provides important patient teaching. During this visit, the patient can meet and ask questions of the perioperative nurse, view audiovisuals, receive written materials, and be given the telephone number to call as questions arise closer to the date of surgery. Most institutions provide written instructions (designed to be copied and given to patients) about many types of surgery (Economou & Economou, 1999).

Deep-Breathing, Coughing, and Incentive Spirometers

One goal of preoperative nursing care is to teach the patient how to promote optimal lung expansion and consequent blood oxygenation after anesthesia. The patient assumes a sitting position to enhance lung expansion. The nurse then demonstrates how to take a deep, slow breath and how to exhale slowly. After practicing deep breathing several times, the patient is instructed to breathe deeply, exhale through the mouth, take a short breath, and cough from deep in the lungs (Chart 18-4). The nurse also demonstrates how to use an incentive spirometer, a device that provides measurement and feedback related to breathing effectiveness. In addition to enhancing respiration, these exercises may help the patient to relax.

If there will be a thoracic or abdominal incision, the nurse demonstrates how the incision line can be splinted to minimize pressure and control pain. The patient should put the palms of both hands together, interlacing the fingers snugly. Placing the hands across the incisional site acts as an effective splint when coughing. Additionally, the patient is informed that medications are available to relieve pain and should be taken regularly for pain relief so that effective deep-breathing and coughing exercises can be performed. The goal in promoting coughing is to mobilize secretions so they can be removed. Deep breathing before coughing stimulates the cough reflex. If the patient does not cough effectively, atelectasis (lung collapse), pneumonia, and other lung complications may occur.

Mobility and Active Body Movement

The goals of promoting mobility postoperatively are to improve circulation, prevent venous stasis, and promote optimal respiratory function.

Chart 18-4 • PATIENT EDUCATION
Preoperative Instructions to Prevent Postoperative Complications

Preoperative teaching for patients undergoing surgery includes instruction in breathing and leg exercises used to prevent postoperative complications, such as pneumonia and deep vein thrombosis. These exercises may be performed in the hospital or at home.

Diaphragmatic Breathing
Diaphragmatic breathing refers to a flattening of the dome of the diaphragm during inspiration, with resultant enlargement of the upper abdomen as air rushes in. During expiration, the abdominal muscles contract.

1. Practice in the same position you would assume in bed after surgery: a semi-Fowler's position, propped in bed with the back and shoulders well supported with pillows.
2. With your hands in a loose-fist position, allow the hands to rest lightly on the front of the lower ribs, with your fingertips against lower chest to feel the movement.

Diaphragmatic breathing

3. Breathe out gently and fully as the ribs sink down and inward toward midline.
4. Then take a deep breath through your nose and mouth, letting the abdomen rise as the lungs fill with air.
5. Hold this breath for a count of five.
6. Exhale and let out *all* the air through your nose and mouth.
7. Repeat this exercise 15 times with a short rest after each group of five.
8. Practice this twice a day preoperatively.

Coughing
1. Lean forward slightly from a sitting position in bed, interlace your fingers together, and place your hands across the incisional site to act as a splintlike support when coughing.

Splinting when coughing

2. Breathe with the diaphragm as described under "Diaphragmatic Breathing."
3. With your mouth slightly open, breathe in fully.
4. "Hack" out sharply for three short breaths.
5. Then, keeping your mouth open, take in a quick deep breath and immediately give a strong cough once or twice. This helps clear secretions from your chest. It may cause some discomfort but will not harm your incision.

Leg Exercises
1. Lie in a semi-Fowler's position and perform the following simple exercises to improve circulation.
2. Bend your knee and raise your foot—hold it a few seconds, then extend the leg and lower it to the bed.

Leg exercises

3. Do this five times with one leg, then repeat with the other leg.
4. Then trace circles with the feet by bending them down, in toward each other, up, and then out.
5. Repeat these movements five times.

Foot exercises

Turning to the Side
1. Turn on your side with the uppermost leg flexed most and supported on a pillow.
2. Grasp the side rail as an aid to manoeuvre to the side.
3. Practice diaphragmatic breathing and coughing while on your side.

Getting Out of Bed
1. Turn on your side.
2. Push yourself up with one hand as you swing your legs out of bed.

The nurse explains the rationale for frequent position changes after surgery and then shows the patient how to turn from side to side and how to assume the lateral position without causing pain or disrupting intravenous lines, drainage tubes, or other equipment. Any special position the individual patient will need to maintain after surgery (eg, adduction or elevation of an extremity) is discussed, as is the importance of maintaining as much mobility as possible despite restrictions. Reviewing the process before surgery is helpful because the patient may be too uncomfortable after surgery to absorb new information.

Exercises of the extremities include extension and flexion of the knee and hip joints (similar to bicycle riding while lying on the side). The foot is rotated as though tracing the largest possible circle with the great toe (see illustrations in Chart 18-4). The elbow and shoulder are also put through range of motion. At first, the patient is assisted and reminded to perform these exercises. Later, the patient is encouraged to do them independently. Muscle tone is maintained so that ambulation will be easier.

The nurse should remember to use proper body mechanics and to instruct the patient to do the same. Whenever the patient is positioned, his or her body needs to be properly aligned.

Pain Management

An assessment should include a determination between acute and chronic pain so that the patient may differentiate postoperative pain from a chronic condition. It is at this point that a pain scale should be introduced and its use explained to the patient. Chapter 13 contains several examples of pain scales.

Postoperatively, medications are administered to relieve pain and maintain comfort without increasing the risk for inadequate air exchange. The patient is instructed to take the medication as frequently as prescribed during the initial postoperative period for pain relief. Anticipated methods of administration of analgesic agents for inpatients include patient-controlled analgesia (PCA), epidural catheter bolus or infusion, or patient-controlled epidural analgesia (PCEA). A patient who is expected to go home would receive oral analgesic agents. These are discussed with the patient before surgery, and the patient's interest and willingness to use those methods are assessed. The patient is instructed in use of a pain intensity rating scale to promote effective postoperative pain management.

Cognitive Coping Strategies

Cognitive strategies may be useful for relieving tension, overcoming anxiety, decreasing fear, and achieving relaxation. Examples of such strategies include the following:

- Imagery—The patient concentrates on a pleasant experience or restful scene.
- Distraction—The patient thinks of an enjoyable story or recites a favourite poem or song.
- Optimistic self-recitation—The patient recites optimistic thoughts ("I know all will go well").

Instruction for Ambulatory Surgical Patients

Preoperative education for the same-day or ambulatory surgical patient comprises all the material presented earlier in this chapter as well as collaborative planning with the patient and family for discharge and follow-up home care. The major difference in outpatient preoperative education is the teaching environment (Quinn, 1999).

Preoperative teaching content may be presented in a group meeting, on a videotape, during night classes, at preadmission testing, or by telephone in conjunction with the preoperative interview. In addition to answering questions and describing what to expect, the nurse tells the patient when and where to report, what to bring (insurance card, list of medications and allergies), what to leave at home (jewelry, watch, medications, contact lenses), and what to wear (loose-fitting, comfortable clothes; flat shoes). The nurse in the surgeon's office may initiate teaching before the perioperative telephone contact.

A fasting period of 8 hours or more is recommended for a meal that includes fried or fatty foods or meat (Crenshaw, Winslow &

NURSING RESEARCH PROFILE 18-1
Preoperative Fasting Guidelines

Crenshaw, J., & Winslow, E. (2002). Preoperative fasting: Old habits die hard. *American Journal of Nursing, 102*(5), 36–44.

Purpose
In 1999 the American Society of Anesthesiologists (ASA) made the "NPO after Midnight" rule obsolete with revised practice guidelines that support much more liberal preoperative fasting in healthy adults. This study sought to determine if these guidelines had changed preoperative fasting practices.

Study Sample and Design
This was a descriptive study conducted in a 935-bed medical centre in the United States. The centre did not have a fasting policy. A convenience sample of 155 patients were interviewed about their preoperative fasting, comparing instructed, actual, and ASA-recommended fasting durations for liquids and solids. A semi-structured interview was used by trained staff nurses to collect the data. Subjects were all over 18 years old, admitted to the hospital from home for an elective, nonobstetric or nongastrointestinal surgery. All were in stable condition, had been without an IV infusion for more than 4 hours prior to surgery, were admitted to a noncritical care unit after surgery, and consented to participate. The patients all spoke and understood English; 87% were Caucasian, 7% were African American, and 9.6% were Hispanic, Asian, or of other ethnic origin.

Findings
The patients interviewed fasted from liquids and solids for an average of 12 to 14 hours, with some patients fasting for as long as 20 hours from liquids and 37 hours from solid foods. Ninety-seven percent of the 155 patients fasted from liquids for more than 6 hours. Actual fasting durations were found (using paired t-tests) to be significantly longer than both the instructed fasting durations (mean 10 hours) and the ASA recommendations. Most patients (91%) were instructed to maintain NPO status after midnight. A nurse participated in the preoperative fasting instruction with 63% of the patients. Almost half of the patients rated thirst and worry at a 5 on a 0-to-10 scale.

Nursing Implications
Nurses are an important part of the surgical team and are involved in preoperative fasting instruction with the majority of patients. Therefore, they share the responsibility for recommending excessively long and unnecessary fasting for patients and for patients' lack of understanding of instructions demonstrated in this study. Clear and specific instructions must be given to patients about fasting time for liquids and solids. The rationale for the fasting should also be clearly explained. Patients should be warned that they will feel thirsty and should be taught strategies (as permitted) for coping with thirst, such as brushing teeth, rinsing the mouth, and chewing gum.

Jacobson, 1999). The anesthesiologist may restrict foods and fluids for longer periods of time depending on the patient's fluid status, age, and pulmonary status and the nature of the surgical procedure.

The purpose of withholding food before surgery is to prevent aspiration. Aspiration occurs when food or fluid is regurgitated from the stomach and enters the pulmonary system. Such inhaled material, which is a foreign substance, is irritating and causes an inflammatory reaction that interferes with adequate air exchange. Aspiration is a serious problem, and mortality is high (60% to 70%). If the patient is assessed as being at high risk for aspiration, the anesthesiologist prescribes more stringent food and fluid restrictions. Fluids may be administered intravenously in some patients to ensure an adequate fluid volume when oral fluids are restricted.

PREOPERATIVE PSYCHOSOCIAL INTERVENTIONS

Reducing Preoperative Anxiety

Cognitive strategies useful for reducing anxiety were addressed previously in this chapter. In addition to these strategies, music therapy is an easy-to-administer, inexpensive, noninvasive intervention that can reduce anxiety in the perioperative patient. The patient should be allowed to choose his or her own music and be provided with quiet uninterrupted listening time (White, 2000).

The general preoperative teaching addressed earlier in this section will also help decrease anxiety in many patients. Knowing ahead of time about the possible need for a ventilator, drainage tubes, or other types of equipment will help decrease anxiety in the postoperative period.

Decreasing Fear

During the preoperative assessment the nurse should assist the patient to identify coping strategies that he or she has previously used to decrease fear. The patient benefits from knowing when family and friends will be able to visit after surgery and that a spiritual advisor will be available if desired. Research suggests that hypnosis may be a useful strategy for reducing fear and overcoming the anxiety associated with surgery (Hernandez & Tatarunis, 2000).

Respecting Cultural, Spiritual, and Religious Beliefs

Psychosocial interventions include identifying and showing respect for cultural, spiritual, and religious beliefs. In some cultures, for example, individuals are stoic in regard to pain, whereas others are more expressive. These responses should be recognized as normal for those patients and families and respected by perioperative personnel. When patients decline blood transfusions for religious reasons (Jehovah's Witnesses), this information needs to be clearly identified in the preoperative period, documented, and communicated to the appropriate personnel.

GENERAL PREOPERATIVE NURSING INTERVENTIONS

Managing Nutrition and Fluids

The major purpose of withholding food and fluid before surgery is to prevent aspiration. However, studies demonstrate that in patients who do not have a compromised airway or coexisting diseases or disorders that affect gastric emptying or fluid volume (eg, pregnancy, obesity, diabetes, gastroesophageal reflux, enteral tube feeding, ileus or bowel obstruction), lengthy restriction of fluid and food is unnecessary (Crenshaw & Winslow, 2002; Pandit, Loberg & Pandit, 2000). Until recently, fluid and food were restricted preoperatively overnight and often longer. However, recent review of this practice by the American Society of Anesthesiologists has resulted in new recommendations for persons undergoing elective surgery who are otherwise healthy (ASA Task Force on Preoperative Fasting, 1999). The recommendations depend on the age of the patient and type of food eaten. For example, adults are advised to fast for 8 hours after eating fatty food and 4 hours after ingesting milk products (Crenshaw, Winslow & Jacobson, 1999; Crenshaw & Winslow, 2002).

Preparing the Bowel for Surgery

Enemas are not commonly ordered preoperatively unless the patient is undergoing abdominal or pelvic surgery. In this case, a cleansing enema or laxative may be prescribed the evening before surgery and may be repeated the morning of surgery. The goals of this preparation are to allow satisfactory visualization of the surgical site and to prevent trauma to the intestine or contamination of the peritoneum by feces. Unless the condition of the patient presents some contraindication, the toilet or bedside commode, rather than the bedpan, is used for evacuating the enema if the patient is hospitalized during this time. Additionally, antibiotics may be prescribed to reduce intestinal flora.

Preparing the Skin

The goal of preoperative skin preparation is to decrease bacteria without injuring the skin. If the surgery is not performed as an emergency, the patient may be instructed to use a soap containing a detergent-germicide to cleanse the skin area for several days before surgery to reduce the number of skin organisms; this preparation may be carried out at home.

Generally, hair is not removed preoperatively unless the hair at or around the incision site is likely to interfere with the operation. If hair must be removed, electric clippers are used for safe hair removal immediately before the operation.

IMMEDIATE PREOPERATIVE NURSING INTERVENTIONS

The patient changes into a hospital gown that is left untied and open in the back. The patient with long hair may braid it, remove hairpins, and cover the head completely with a disposable paper cap.

The mouth is inspected, and dentures or plates are removed. If left in the mouth, these items could easily fall to the back of the throat during induction of anesthesia and cause respiratory obstruction.

Jewelry is not worn to the operating room; wedding rings and jewelry of body piercings should be removed to prevent injury (Fogg, 2001). If a patient objects to removing a ring, some institutions allow the ring to be securely fastened to the finger with tape. All articles of value, including assistive devices, dentures, glasses, and prosthetic devices, are given to family members or are labelled clearly with the patient's name and stored in a safe place according to the institution's policy.

All patients (except those with urologic disorders) should void immediately before going to the operating room to promote continence during low abdominal surgery and to make abdominal organs more accessible. Urinary catheterization is performed in the operating room as necessary.

Administering Preanesthetic Medication

The use of preanesthetic medication is minimal with ambulatory or outpatient surgery. If prescribed, it is usually administered in the preoperative holding area. If a preanesthetic medication is administered, the patient is kept in bed with the side rails raised because the medication can cause lightheadedness or drowsiness. During this time, the nurse observes the patient for any untoward reaction to the medications. The immediate surroundings are kept quiet to promote relaxation.

Often, surgery is delayed or operating room schedules are changed, and it becomes impossible to request that a medica-

tion be given at a specific time. In these situations, the preoperative medication is prescribed "on call from operating room." The nurse can have the medication ready to give and administer it as soon as a call is received from the operating room staff. It usually takes 15 to 20 minutes to prepare the patient for the operating room. If the nurse gives the medication before attending to the other details of preoperative preparation, the patient will have at least partial benefit from the preoperative medication and will have a smoother anesthetic and operative course.

Maintaining the Preoperative Record

A preoperative checklist contains critical elements that need to be checked preoperatively (Rothrock, 2003). An example is shown in Figure 18-3. The completed chart accompanies the patient to the operating room with the surgical consent form attached, along with all laboratory reports and nurses' records. Any unusual last-minute

FIGURE 18-3 Preoperative checklist.

observations that may have a bearing on anesthesia or surgery are noted at the front of the chart in a prominent place.

Transporting the Patient to the Presurgical Area

The patient is transferred to the holding area or presurgical suite in a bed or on a stretcher about 30 to 60 minutes before the anesthetic is to be given. The stretcher should be as comfortable as possible, with a sufficient number of blankets to prevent chilling in air-conditioned rooms. A small head pillow is usually provided.

The patient is taken to the preoperative holding area, greeted by name, and positioned comfortably on the stretcher or bed. The surrounding area should be kept quiet if the preoperative medication is to have maximal effect. Unpleasant sounds or conversation should be avoided because a sedated patient who overhears them might misinterpret them.

Patient safety in the preoperative area is a priority. Using a process to verify patient identification, the surgical procedure, and the surgical site maximizes patient safety and allows for early identification and intervention if any discrepancies are identified (Brown, Riippa & Shaneberger, 2001).

> ! **NURSING ALERT** It is important for someone to be with the preoperative patient at all times. Someone must be present to provide reassurance as well as to ensure safety. Facial expression, or the warm grasp of a hand can communicate reassurance nonverbally.

Attending to Family Needs

Most hospitals and ambulatory surgery centres have a waiting room where the family and significant others can wait while the patient is undergoing surgery. This room may be equipped with comfortable chairs, television, telephones, and facilities for light refreshment. Volunteers may remain with the family, offer them coffee, and keep them informed of the patient's progress. After surgery, the surgeon may meet the family in the waiting room and discuss the outcome.

The family and significant others should never judge the seriousness of an operation by the length of time the patient is in the operating room. A patient may be in surgery much longer than the actual operating time for several reasons:

- Patients are routinely transported well in advance of the actual operating time.
- The anesthesiologist often makes additional preparations that may take 30 to 60 minutes.
- The surgeon may take longer than expected with the preceding case, which delays the start of the next surgical procedure.

After surgery, the patient is taken to the PACU to ensure safe emergence from anesthesia.

Family members and significant others waiting to see the patient after surgery should be informed that the patient may have certain equipment or devices (eg, intravenous lines, indwelling urinary catheter, nasogastric tube, oxygen lines, monitoring equipment, and blood transfusion lines) in place when he or she returns from surgery. When the patient returns to the room, the nurse provides explanations regarding the frequent postoperative observations that will be made. However, it is the responsibility of the surgeon, not the nurse, to relay the surgical findings and the prognosis, even when the findings are favourable.

NURSING PROCESS: CARE OF THE PATIENT IN THE PREOPERATIVE PERIOD

Preoperative assessment of the surgical patient involves evaluating the elements addressed in the previous section on the factors that affect the patient undergoing surgery. A variety of patient problems or nursing diagnoses can be anticipated or identified on the basis of the assessment data.

Assessment

During the preoperative phase of care, nursing assessment usually addresses the following parameters:

- Physical condition, including respiratory, cardiac, and other major body systems as discussed earlier in this chapter
- Results of blood tests, x-ray studies, and other diagnostic tests
- Nutritional and fluid status
- Medication use, as previously described
- Psychological preparedness for surgery (anxiety, fear, spiritual and cultural beliefs)
- Special considerations, including the ambulatory surgery patient, gerontologic considerations, obesity, the patient with a disability, or the patient undergoing emergency surgery, as discussed earlier in this chapter

Diagnosis

NURSING DIAGNOSES

Based on the assessment data, major preoperative nursing diagnoses of the surgical patient may include the following:

- Anxiety related to the surgical experience (anesthesia, pain) and the outcome of surgery
- Fear related to perceived threat of the surgical procedure and separation from support system
- Knowledge deficit of preoperative procedures and protocols and postoperative expectations

COLLABORATIVE PROBLEMS/ POTENTIAL COMPLICATIONS

Failure to identify and communicate pertinent preoperative risk factors may lead to complications.

Planning and Goals

The major goals for the preoperative surgical patient may include relief of preoperative anxiety, decreased fear, increased knowledge of perioperative expectations, and absence of preoperative complications.

Nursing Interventions

REDUCING PREOPERATIVE ANXIETY

Specific nursing interventions are discussed in detail under psychosocial interventions and preoperative teaching in the previous sections.

DECREASING FEAR

Nursing management is discussed under psychosocial interventions in the previous section.

PROVIDING PATIENT EDUCATION

Specific nursing interventions pertaining to preoperative patient education are discussed in detail in earlier sections of this chapter.

MONITORING AND MANAGING POTENTIAL COMPLICATIONS

Nursing interventions to prevent preoperative complications include identification and documentation of factors that affect patients preparing to undergo surgery (discussed earlier in this chapter).

Evaluation

EXPECTED PATIENT OUTCOMES

Expected patient outcomes may include:

1. Reports relief of anxiety
   a. Discusses with anesthesiologist concerns related to types of anesthesia and induction
   b. Verbalizes an understanding of the preanesthetic medication and general anesthesia
   c. Discusses last-minute concerns with nurse or physician
   d. Discusses financial concerns with social worker, when appropriate
   e. Requests visit with member of clergy when appropriate
   f. Relaxes quietly after being visited by health care team members
2. Reports that fear is decreased
   a. Discusses fears with health care professionals
   b. Verbalizes an understanding of the location of family members or significant others during procedure
3. Voices understanding of surgical intervention
   a. Participates in preoperative preparation
   b. Demonstrates and describes exercises he or she is expected to perform postoperatively
   c. Reviews information about postoperative care
   d. Accepts preanesthetic medication, if prescribed
   e. Remains in bed once premedicated
   f. Relaxes during transportation to operating room or unit
   g. States rationale for use of side rails
   h. Discusses postoperative expectations
4. Shows no evidence of preoperative complications.

 Critical Thinking Exercises

1. During the preoperative assessment of a man scheduled for hand surgery in an ambulatory setting, you think that the patient's responses indicate that he does not understand the procedure and that he has not made plans for postoperative care. What further assessment and teaching is indicated? What nursing interventions are warranted?

2. A patient with a long history of the use of several herbal supplements is scheduled for major surgery. What effect would this information have on your preoperative care of this patient?

3. Two patients are admitted to the same-day surgery unit for bilateral knee replacements. One patient is a 30-year-old who ambulates with crutches and the other is a 75-year-old who lives alone. How would your assessments, preoperative teaching, and preparation differ for these two patients?

REFERENCES AND SELECTED READINGS

Books

American Society of PeriAnesthesia Nurses. (2000). *Standards of perianesthesia nursing practice.* Thorofare, NJ: ASPAN.

Beyea, S. (Ed.). (2000). *Perioperative nursing data set: The perioperative nursing vocabulary.* Denver: AORN, Inc.

Canadian Institute for Health Information. (2004). *Inpatient hospitalizations continue to decline, same-day surgery visits on the rise, reports CIHI.* Available at: http://secure.cihi.ca/cihiweb/dispPage.jsp?cw_page=media_29oct2004_e. Retrieved December 1, 2005.

Dudek, S. G. (Ed.). (2001). *Nutrition essentials for nursing practice.* Philadelphia: Lippincott Williams & Wilkins.

Economou, S. G., & Economou, T. S. (1999). *Instructions for surgery patients.* Philadelphia: W. B. Saunders.

Fitzpatrick, J. J. (1998). *Encyclopedia of nursing research.* New York: Springer.

Fortunato, N. H. (2000). *Berry & Kohn's operating room technique.* St. Louis: Mosby, Inc.

Health Canada. (2003). *Canadian guidelines for body weight classification in adults.* Ottawa: Author. Available at: http://www.hc-sc.gc.ca/fn-an/nutrition/weights-poids/guide-ld-adult/weight_book_tc-livres_des_poids_tm_e.html.

Karch, A. (Ed.). (2002). *Nursing drug guide.* Philadelphia: Lippincott Williams & Wilkins.

Kuhn, M. (1999). *Complementary therapies for health care providers.* Philadelphia: Lippincott Williams & Wilkins.

Litwack, K. (Ed.). (1999). *Core curriculum for perianesthesia nursing practice.* Philadelphia: W. B. Saunders.

Merli, G., & Weitz, H. (Eds.). (1998). *Medical management of the surgical patient* (2nd ed.). Philadelphia: W. B. Saunders.

Miller, T. A. (Ed.). (1998). *Modern surgical care: Physiologic foundations and clinical applications.* St. Louis: Quality Medical.

National Institutes of Health, National Heart, Lung and Blood Institute, North American Association for the Study of Obesity. (2000). *The practical guide: Identification, evaluation, and treatment of overweight and obesity in adults.* NIH Publication Number 00-4084. Bethesda, MD.

Operating Room Nurses Association of Canada (ORNAC). (2003). *Recommended standards, guidelines, and position statements for perioperative registered nursing practice.* Author.

Quinn, D. M. (Ed.). (1999). *Ambulatory surgical nursing core curriculum.* Philadelphia: W. B. Saunders.

Romanow, R. J. (2002). *Final report: Building on values: The future of health care in Canada.* Ottawa, ON: Commission on the Future of Health Care in Canada. Available at www.hc-sc.gc.ca.

Rothrock, J. C. (2003). *Alexander's care of the patient in surgery* (12th ed). St. Louis: Mosby.

Russell, R., Williams, N., & Bulstrode, C. (Eds.). (2000). *Bailey & Love's short practice of surgery* (23d ed.). New York: Oxford University Press Inc.

Tjepkema, M. (2005). *Adult obesity in Canada: Measured height and weight.* Available at: http://www.statcan.ca/english/research/82-620-MIE/2005001/articles/adults/aobesity.htm. Retrieved December 15, 2005.

Journals

Ambulatory Surgery
Asterisks indicate nursing research articles.

Dunn, D. (1998). Preoperative assessment criteria and patient teaching for ambulatory surgery patients. *Journal of Perianesthesia Nursing, 13*(5), 274–291.

Hession, M. (1998). Factors influencing successful discharge after outpatient laparoscopic cholecystectomy. *Journal of Perianesthesia Nursing, 13*(1), 11–15.

Pandit, S., Loberg, K., & Pandit, U. (2000). Toast and tea before elective surgery? A national survey on current practice. *Anesthesia & Analgesia, 90*(6), 1348–1351.

Yellen, E., & Davis, G. (2001). Patient satisfaction in ambulatory surgery. *AORN Journal, 74*(4), 483–498.

Anesthesia and Surgery

American Society of Anesthesiologists Task Force on Preoperative Fasting (1999). Practice guidelines for preoperative fasting and the use of pharmacologic agents to reduce risk of pulmonary aspiration: Application to healthy patients undergoing elective procedures. *Anesthesiology, 90*(3), 896–905.

Booth, M. (1998). Clinical aspects of CRNA practice: Sedation and monitored anesthesia care. *Nursing Clinics of North America, 31*(3), 667–682.

Braunschweig, C., Gomez, S., & Sheean, P. (2000). Impact of declines in nutritional status on outcomes in adult patients hospitalized for more than 7 days. *Journal of the American Dietetic Association, 100*(11), 1316–1322.

*Crenshaw, J., Winslow, E., & Jacobson, A. (1999). Research for practice: New guidelines for preoperative fasting. *American Journal of Nursing, 99*(4), 49.

Iverson, R. (1999). Sedation and analgesia in ambulatory settings. *Plastic & Reconstructive Surgery, 104*(5), 1559–1564.

Mack, M. (2002). Minimally invasive and robotic surgery. *Journal of the American Medical Association, 285*(5), 568–572.

Perioperative Assessment

Ang-Lee, M., Moss, J., & Yuan, C. (2001). Herbal medicines and perioperative care. *Journal of the American Medical Association, 286*(2), 208–216.

Brown, B., Riippa, M., & Shaneberger, K. (2001). Promoting patient safety through preoperative patient verification. *AORN Journal, 74*(5), 690–694.

Brumly, C. (2000). Herbs and the perioperative patient. *AORN Journal, 72*(5), 783–804.

*Crenshaw, J., & Winslow, E. (2002). Preoperative fasting: Old habits die hard. *American Journal of Nursing, 102*(5), 36–44.

Fogg, D. (2002). Clinical issues: Patient jewelry. *AORN Journal, 74*(2), 249.

Hernandez, A., & Tatarunis, A. (2000). The use of pre-, intra-, and posthypnotic suggestion in anesthesia and surgery. *Clinical Forum for Nurse Anesthetists, 11*(4), 167–72.

King, M. (2000). Preoperative evaluation. *American Family Physician, 62*(2), 387–395.

Little, K. (2000). Screening for domestic violence. *Postgraduate Medicine, 108*(2), 135–141.

Lyons, T. (2002). Herbal medicines and possible anesthesia interactions. *AANA Journal, 70*(1), 47–51.

*McDonald, D., Freeland, M., Thomas, G., & Moore, J. (2001). Testing a preoperative pain management intervention for elders. *Research in Nursing & Health, 24*, 401–409.

Marshall, C., Benton, D., & Brazier, J. (2000). Elder abuse: Using clinical tools to identify clues of mistreatment. *Geriatrics, 55*(2), 42–53.

Miller, K., & Weed, P. (1998). The latex allergy triage or admission tool: An algorithm to identify which patients would benefit from latex precautions. *Journal of Emergency Nursing, 24*(2), 145–152.

Posel, N. (1998). Preoperative teaching in the preadmission clinic. *Journal of Nursing Staff Development, 14*(1), 52–56.

Smetana, G. W. (1999). Preoperative pulmonary evaluation. *New England Journal of Medicine, 340*(12), 937–944.

Shannon-Cain, J., Webster, S., & Cain, B. (2002). Prevalence of and reasons for preoperative tobacco use. *AANA Journal, 70*(1), 33–40.

Tappen, R., Muzic, J., & Kennedy, P. (2001). Preoperative assessment and discharge planning for older adults undergoing ambulatory surgery. *AORN Journal, 464–470.

White, J. (2000). State of the science of music interventions. *Critical Care Nursing Clinics of North America, 12*(2), 219–225.

Whitney, J., & Parkman, S. (2002). Preoperative physical activity, anesthesia, and analgesia: Effects on early postoperative walking after total hip replacement. *Applied Nursing Research, 15*(1), 19–27.

Zambricki, C. (1998). Clinical aspects of the preanesthetic evaluation. *Nursing Clinics of North America, 31*(3), 607–621.

RESOURCES AND WEBSITES

American Academy of Ambulatory Care Nursing, East Holly Ave., Box 56, Pitman, NJ, 08071; (856) 256-2350; (800) AMB-NURS; http://www.aaacn.org.

American Society of PeriAnesthesia Nurses, 10 Melrose Ave., Suite 110, Cherry Hill, NJ 08003-3696; (877) 9696 (toll-free); fax (856) 616-9621; http://www.aspan.org.

Canadian Anesthesiologists' Society, 1 Eglinton Avenue East, Suite 208, Toronto, ON, M4P 3A1; http://www.cas.ca.

Operating Room Nurses Association of Canada (ORNAC); http://www.ornac.ca.

Intraoperative Nursing Management

Adapted by Christy Raymond

On completion of this chapter, the learner will be able to:

1. Describe the interdisciplinary approach to the care of the patient during surgery.
2. Describe the principles of surgical asepsis.
3. Describe various nursing roles as well as the role of the anesthesiologist in the intraoperative phase of care.
4. Identify adverse effects of surgery and anesthesia.
5. Identify the surgical risk factors related to age-specific populations and nursing interventions to reduce those risks.
6. Compare various types of anesthesia with regard to uses, advantages, disadvantages, and nursing responsibilities.
7. Identify the use of the nursing process for optimizing patient outcomes during the intraoperative period.

Anesthesia and surgery place the patient at risk for several complications or adverse events. Consciousness or full awareness, mobility, protective biologic functions, and personal control are totally or partially relinquished by the patient when entering the operating room. Staff from the departments of anesthesia, nursing, and surgery work collaboratively to implement professional standards of care, to control iatrogenic and individual risks, and to promote high-quality patient outcomes.

The Surgical Team

The surgical team consists of the patient, the anesthesiologist, the surgeon, the intraoperative nurses, and the surgical technologists. The anesthesiologist administers the **anesthetic** agent and monitors the patient's physical status throughout the surgery. The surgeon and assistants scrub and perform the surgery. The individual in the scrub role, either a nurse or surgical technologist, provides sterile instruments and supplies to the surgeon during the procedure. The circulating nurse coordinates the care of the patient in the operating room. Care provided by the circulating nurse includes assisting with patient positioning, preparing the patient's skin for surgery, managing surgical specimens, and documenting intraoperative events.

THE PATIENT

As the patient enters the operating room, he or she may feel relaxed and prepared, or fearful and highly stressed. These feelings depend very much on the amount and timing of preoperative sedation and the patient's level of fear and anxiety. Fears about loss of control, the unknown, pain, death, changes in body structure or function, and disruption of lifestyle all may contribute to a generalized anxiety. These fears can increase the amount of anesthetic needed, the level of postoperative pain, and overall recovery time.

The patient is also subject to several risks. Infection, failure of the surgery to relieve symptoms, temporary or permanent complications related to the procedure or the anesthetic, and death are uncommon but potential outcomes of the surgical experience (Chart 19-1). In addition to fears and risks, the patient undergoing sedation and anesthesia temporarily loses both cognitive function and biologic self-protective mechanisms. Loss of pain sense, reflexes, and ability to communicate subjects the intraoperative patient to possible injury.

Chart 19-1

Potential Adverse Effects of Surgery and Anesthesia

Anesthesia and surgery disrupt all major body systems. Although most patients can compensate for surgical trauma and the effects of anesthesia, all patients are at risk during the operative procedure. These risks include the following:

- Cardiac dysrhythmia from electrolyte imbalance or adverse effect of anesthetic agents
- Myocardial depression, bradycardia, and circulatory collapse from toxic levels of local anesthetics
- Central nervous system agitation, seizures, and respiratory arrest from toxic levels of local anesthetics
- Oversedation or undersedation during moderate sedation
- Agitation or disorientation, especially in elderly patients
- Hypoxemia or hypercarbia from hypoventilation and inadequate respiratory support during anesthesia
- Laryngeal trauma, oral trauma, and broken teeth from difficult intubation
- Hypothermia from cool operating room temperatures, exposure of body cavities, and impaired thermoregulation secondary to anesthetic agents
- Hypotension from blood loss or adverse effect of anesthesia
- Infection
- Thrombosis from compression of blood vessels or stasis
- Malignant hyperthermia secondary to adverse effect of anesthesia
- Nerve damage, skin breakdown from prolonged or inappropriate positioning
- Electrical shock or burns
- Laser burns
- Drug toxicity, faulty equipment, and human error

 Gerontologic Considerations

Elderly patients face higher risks from anesthesia and surgery than younger adult patients (Polanczyk et al., 2001). Statistically, perioperative risk increases with each decade over 60 years, often because of the increased incidence of coexisting disease. Modifications tailored to the biologic changes of later life and the application of research findings for this population can reduce the risks.

Biologic variations of particular importance include age-related cardiovascular and pulmonary changes (Townsend, 2002). The

Glossary

anesthesia: a state of narcosis, analgesia, relaxation, and loss of reflexes

anesthesiologist: physician trained to deliver anesthesia and to monitor the patient's condition during surgery

anesthetic: the substance, such as a chemical or gas, used to induce anesthesia

circulating nurse (or circulator): registered nurse who coordinates and documents patient care in the operating room

moderate sedation: use of sedation to depress the level of consciousness without altering the patient's ability to maintain a patent airway and to respond to physical stimuli and verbal commands

restricted zone: area in the operating room where scrub attire and surgical masks are required; includes operating room and sterile core areas

scrub role: registered nurse, licensed practical nurse, or surgical technologist who scrubs and dons sterile surgical attire, prepares instruments and supplies, and hands instruments to the surgeon during the procedure

semirestricted zone: area in the operating room where scrub attire is required; may include areas where surgical instruments are processed

surgical asepsis: absence of microorganisms in the surgical environment to reduce the risk for infection

unrestricted zone: area in the operating room that interfaces with other departments; includes patient reception area and holding area aging heart and blood vessels have decreased ability to respond to stress. Reduced cardiac output and limited cardiac reserve make the elderly patient vulnerable to changes in circulating volume and blood oxygen levels. Excessive or rapid administration of intravenous solutions may cause pulmonary edema. A sudden or prolonged drop in blood pressure may lead to cerebral ischemia, thrombosis, embolism, infarction, and anoxia. Reduced gas exchange can lead to cerebral hypoxia.

The elderly patient needs fewer anesthetics to produce anesthesia and eliminates the anesthetic agent over a longer time than a younger patient. As people age, the percentage of lean body tissue decreases and fatty tissue steadily increases (from age 20 years to 90 years). Anesthetic agents that have an affinity for fatty tissue concentrate in body fat and the brain (Dudek, 2001). Lower doses of anesthetic are appropriate for another reason. The older patient, particularly when malnourished, may have low plasma protein levels. With decreased plasma proteins, more of the anesthetic agent remains free or unbound, and the result is more potent action.

Also in elderly adults, body tissues made up predominantly of water and those with a rich blood supply, such as skeletal muscle, liver, and kidneys, shrink. Reduced liver size decreases the rate at which the liver can inactivate many anesthetics, whereas decreased kidney function slows elimination of waste products and anesthetics. Other factors affecting the elderly surgical patient in the intraoperative period include the following:

- Impaired ability to increase metabolic rate and impaired thermoregulatory mechanisms increase susceptibility to hypothermia.
- Bone loss (25% in women, 12% in men) necessitates careful manipulation and positioning during surgery.
- Reduced ability to adjust rapidly to emotional and physical stress influences surgical outcomes and requires meticulous observation of vital functions.

As expected, mortality is higher with emergency surgery (commonly required for traumatic injuries) than with elective surgery, making continuous and careful monitoring and prompt intervention especially important for older surgical patients (Phippen & Wells, 2000).

Nursing Care

Throughout surgery, nursing responsibilities include providing for the safety and well-being of the patient, coordinating the operating room personnel, and performing scrub and circulating activities. Because the patient's emotional state remains a concern, the care begun by preoperative nurses is continued by the intraoperative nursing staff, who provide the patient with information and realistic reassurance. The nurse supports coping strategies and reinforces the patient's ability to influence outcomes by encouraging his or her active participation in the plan of care.

In the role of patient advocate, intraoperative nurses monitor factors that can cause injury, such as patient position, equipment malfunction, and environmental hazards, and they protect patients' dignity and interests while they are anesthetized. Additional responsibilities include maintaining surgical standards of care, identifying existing patient risk factors, and assisting in modifying complicating factors to help reduce operative risk (Phippen & Wells, 2000).

THE CIRCULATING NURSE

The **circulating nurse** (also known as the **circulator**) must be a registered nurse. He or she manages the operating room and protects the patient's safety and health by monitoring the activities of the surgical team, checking the operating room conditions, and continually assessing the patient for signs of injury and implementing appropriate interventions. The main responsibilities include verifying consent, coordinating the team, and ensuring cleanliness, proper temperature, humidity, and lighting; the safe functioning of equipment; and the availability of supplies and materials. The circulating nurse monitors aseptic practices to avoid breaks in technique while coordinating the movement of related personnel (medical, radiography, and laboratory) as well as implementing fire safety precautions (Phippen & Wells, 2000). The circulating nurse monitors the patient and documents specific activities throughout the operation to ensure the patient's safety and well-being. Nursing activities directly relate to preventing complications and achieving optimal patient outcomes.

THE SCRUB ROLE

Activities of the **scrub role** include performing a surgical hand scrub; setting up the sterile tables; preparing sutures, ligatures, and special equipment (such as a laparoscope); and assisting the surgeon and the surgical assistants during the procedure by anticipating the instruments that will be required, such as sponges, drains, and other equipment (Phippen & Wells, 2000). As the surgical incision is closed, the scrub person and the circulator count all needles, sponges, and instruments to be sure they are accounted for and not retained as a foreign body in the patient. Tissue specimens obtained during surgery must also be labelled by the scrub person and sent to the laboratory by the circulator.

THE SURGEON

The surgeon performs the surgical procedure and heads the surgical team. He or she is a licensed physician (MD), osteopath (DO), oral surgeon (DDS or DMD), or podiatrist (DPM) who is specially trained and qualified. Qualifications may include certification by a specialty board, adherence to accreditation standards, and adherence to hospital standards and admitting practices and procedures (Fortunato, 2000).

THE REGISTERED NURSE FIRST ASSISTANT

The registered nurse first assistant (RNFA) is another member of the operating room staff. Although the scope of practice of the RNFA depends on each institution, the RNFA practices under the direct supervision of the surgeon. RNFA responsibilities may include handling tissue, providing exposure at the operative field, suturing, and providing hemostasis. The entire process requires a thorough understanding of anatomy and physiology, tissue handling, and the principles of **surgical asepsis**. The competent RNFA needs to be aware of the objectives of the surgery, needs to have the knowledge and ability to anticipate needs and to work as a skilled member of a team, and needs to be able to handle any emergency situation in the operating room (Fortunato, 2000; Rothrock, 1999).

THE ANESTHESIOLOGIST

An **anesthesiologist** is a physician specifically trained in the art and science of anesthesiology. The anesthesiologist interviews and assesses the patient prior to surgery, selects the anesthesia, administers it, intubates the patient if necessary, manages any technical problems related to the administration of the anesthetic agent, and supervises the patient's condition throughout the surgical procedure. Before the patient enters the operating room, often at preadmission testing, the anesthesiologist visits the patient to provide information and answer questions. The type of anesthetic to be administered, previous reactions to anesthetics, and known anatomic abnormalities that would make airway management difficult are discussed. Canadian anesthesiologists use the American Society of Anesthesiologists (ASA) Physical Status Classification System to determine the patient's status (Canadian Anesthesiologists' Society, 2004)(Chart 19-2).

When the patient arrives in the operating room, the anesthesiologist reassesses the patient's physical condition immediately prior to initiating anesthesia. The anesthetic is administered, and the patient's airway is maintained either through a laryngeal mask airway (LMA) or an endotracheal tube. During surgery, the anesthesiologist monitors the patient's blood pressure, pulse, and respirations as well as the electrocardiogram (ECG), blood oxygen saturation level, tidal volume, blood gas levels, blood pH, alveolar gas concentrations, and body temperature. Monitoring by electroencephalography is sometimes required. Levels of anesthetics in the body can also be determined; a mass spectrometer can provide instant readouts of critical concentration levels on display terminals. The device also assesses the patient's ability to breathe unassisted and indicates the need for mechanical assistance when ventilation is poor and the patient is not breathing well independently.

Chart 19-2

American Society of Anesthesiologists Physical Status Classification System

Canadian anesthesiologists use the American Society of Anesthesiologists Physical (P) Status Classification System to describe the patient's general status and identify potential risks during surgery. There are five classes of physical status.

- **P 1.** A normally healthy patient
  Example: No systemic abnormality, localized infection without fever, benign tumour, hernia
- **P 2.** A patient with mild systemic disease
  Example: Well-controlled hypertension, well-controlled diabetes mellitus, chronic bronchitis, obesity, age over 80 yr
- **P 3.** A patient with severe systemic disease that is not incapacitating
  Example: Severe disease, compensated heart failure, myocardial infarction more than 6 mo ago, angina pectoris, severe dysrhythmia, cirrhosis, poorly controlled diabetes or hypertension, ileus
- **P 4.** A patient with an incapacitating systemic disease that is a constant threat to life
  Example: Severe heart failure, myocardial infarction less than 6 mo ago, severe respiratory failure, advanced liver or renal failure
- **P 5.** A moribund patient who is not expected to survive for 24 hours with or without operation
  Example: Unconscious patient with traumatic head injury and agonal cardiac rhythm

---

The Surgical Environment

The surgical environment is known for its stark appearance and cool temperature. The surgical suite is behind double doors, and access is limited to authorized personnel. External precautions include adhering to principles of surgical asepsis; strict control of the operating room (OR) environment is required, including traffic pattern restrictions. Policies governing this environment address such issues as the health of the staff; the cleanliness of the rooms; the sterility of equipment and surfaces; processes for scrubbing, gowning, and gloving; and OR attire.

To provide the best possible conditions for surgery, the OR is situated in a location that is central to all supporting services (eg, pathology, radiology, laboratory). The OR has special air filtration devices to screen out contaminating particles, dust, and pollutants. The temperature, humidity, and airflow patterns are controlled (Meeker et al., 1999).

Electrical hazards, emergency exit clearances, and storage of equipment and anesthetic gases are monitored periodically by official entities, such as the Canadian Standards Association. To help decrease microbes, the surgical area is divided into three zones: the **unrestricted zone**, where street clothes are allowed; the **semirestricted zone**, where attire consists of scrub clothes and caps; and the **restricted zone**, where scrub clothes, shoe covers, caps, and masks are worn. The surgeons and other surgical team members wear additional sterile clothing and protective devices during the operation.

The Association of PeriOperative Registered Nurses, formerly known as the Association of Operating Room Nurses (and still abbreviated as AORN), recommends specific practices for those wearing surgical attire to promote a high level of cleanliness in a particular practice setting (AORN, 2002). The Canadian equivalent of the AORN is ORNAC (Operating Room Nurses Association of Canada), which also publishes recommended standards and guidelines (ORNAC, 2003). OR attire includes close-fitting cotton dresses, pantsuits, jumpsuits, and gowns. Knitted cuffs on sleeves and pant legs prevent organisms shed from the perineum, legs, and arms from being released into the immediate surroundings. Shirts and waist drawstrings should be tucked inside the pants to prevent accidental contact with sterile areas and to contain skin shedding. Wet or soiled garments should be changed.

Masks are worn at all times in the restricted zone of the OR. High-filtration masks decrease the risk for postoperative wound infection by containing and filtering microorganisms from the oropharynx and nasopharynx. Masks should fit tightly, should cover the nose and mouth completely, and should not interfere with breathing, speech, or vision. Masks must be adjusted to prevent venting from the sides. Disposable masks have a filtration efficiency exceeding 95%. Masks are changed between patients and should not be worn outside the surgical department. The mask must be either on or off; it must not be allowed to hang around the neck.

Headgear should completely cover the hair (head and neckline, including beard) so that single strands of hair, bobby pins, clips, and particles of dandruff or dust do not fall on the sterile field.

Shoes should be comfortable and supportive. Shoes worn in from the outside must be covered with disposable shoe covers for protection from soiling. Shoe covers are worn one time only and are removed upon leaving the restricted area.

Barriers such as scrub attire and masks do not entirely protect the patient from microorganisms. Upper respiratory tract infections, sore throats, and skin infections in staff and patients are sources of pathogens and must be reported.

> **! NURSING ALERT** Good health is essential for any person in the OR, and any perioperative team member with an infectious disease (eg, an upper respiratory tract infection or infected skin lesion) should not have direct patient contact. Until the infectious process has resolved, the perioperative team member should not work in the OR.

Because artificial fingernails harbour microorganisms and may cause nosocomial infections (Winslow & Jacobson, 2000), a ban on artificial nails by OR personnel is supported by the Centers for Disease Control and Prevention (CDC), AORN, ORNAC, and the Public Health Agency of Canada. Short, natural fingernails are encouraged (Winslow & Jacobson, 2000).

PRINCIPLES OF SURGICAL ASEPSIS

Surgical asepsis prevents the contamination of surgical wounds. The patient's natural skin flora or a previously existing infection may cause postoperative wound infection. Rigourous adherence to the principles of surgical asepsis by OR personnel is the foundation of preventing surgical site infections.

All surgical supplies, any instruments, needles, sutures, dressings, gloves, covers, and solutions that may come in contact with the surgical wound and exposed tissues, must be sterilized before use (Rothrock, 2003; Townsend, 2002). Traditionally, the surgeon, surgical assistants, and nurses prepared themselves by scrubbing their hands and arms with antiseptic soap and water, but this traditional practice is being challenged by research investigating the optimal length of time to scrub and the best preparation to use (Larsen et al., 2001). (See Nursing Research Profile 19-1.)

Surgical team members wear long-sleeved sterile gowns and gloves. Head and hair are covered with a cap, and a mask is worn over the nose and mouth to minimize the possibility that bacteria from the upper respiratory tract will enter the wound. During surgery, the personnel who have scrubbed, gloved, and gowned touch only sterilized objects. Nonscrubbed personnel refrain from touching or contaminating anything sterile.

An area of the patient's skin considerably larger than that requiring exposure during the surgery is meticulously cleansed, and an antimicrobial agent is applied. If hair needs to be removed, it is done immediately prior to the procedure to minimize the risk of wound infection (Townsend, 2002). The remainder of the patient's body is covered with sterile drapes.

Environmental Controls

In addition to the protocols described previously, surgical asepsis requires meticulous cleaning and maintenance of the OR environment. Floors and horizontal surfaces are cleaned frequently with detergent, soap, and water, or a detergent germicide. Sterilizing equipment is inspected regularly to ensure optimal operation and performance.

All equipment that comes into direct contact with the patient must be sterile (Townsend, 2002). Sterilized linens, drapes, and solutions are used. Instruments are cleaned and sterilized in a unit near the operating room. Individually wrapped sterile items are used when additional individual items are needed.

Airborne bacteria are a concern. To decrease the amount of bacteria in the air, standard OR ventilation provides 15 air exchanges per hour (Rothrock, 2003). Staff members shed skin scales, resulting in about 1,000 bacteria-carrying particles (or colony-forming units [CFUs]) per cubic foot per minute. With the standard air exchanges, air counts of bacteria are reduced to 50 to 150 CFUs per cubic foot per minute. The number of personnel and unnecessary physical movements may be restricted to minimize bacteria in the air and achieve an OR infection rate no greater than 3% to 5% in clean, infection-prone surgery.

NURSING RESEARCH PROFILE 19-1

New Techniques for Surgical Hand Preparation

Larsen, E., Aiello, A., Heilman, J., Lyle, C., Cronquist, A., Stahl, J., & Dello-Latta, P. (2001). Comparison of different regimens for surgical hand preparation. *AORN Journal, 73*(2), 412–432.

Purpose

Staff members traditionally perform a lengthy regimen of scrubbing with an antiseptic agent before surgery, mostly due to concerns about reducing the risk for infection. The purpose of this study was to compare the traditional scrubbing technique in the operating room to a waterless hand preparation in terms of antimicrobial effectiveness, effect on skin condition, and time requirements.

Study Sample and Design

This was a 6-week, single-centre, prospective clinical trial. Twenty surgical staff members used the waterless hand preparation for 3 weeks, had a 1-week hiatus, then used the traditional surgical scrub for 3 consecutive weeks. A reference group of five subjects was also included in the study, which was conducted at a 2,000-bed medical centre in three operating suites. The participants were full-time surgical staff members who performed an average of at least 10 scrubs per week and ranged in age from 18 to 65 years of age. The three tools used to measure skin condition consisted of the visual scoring of skin, erythema grading scale, and the hand skin assessment. A total of 13 microbial skin counts were taken of each subject's hands during the study.

Findings

The waterless hand preparation was associated with less skin damage and lower microbial skin counts on days 5 and 19 compared to the traditional scrub. The researchers suggest that a lengthy scrub, as well as the use of a brush or sponge, appears to be counterproductive, causing skin damage and increased skin shedding. The waterless hand preparation protocol had shorter contact time (mean 80.7 seconds) compared to the traditional protocol (mean 145 seconds) and was preferred by the participants. They reported that it was easier, faster, milder on the hands, and conducive to donning gloves.

Nursing Implications

The waterless hand preparation performed better compared to the traditional surgical scrub, but nurses should keep in mind that this was a small study. The results of this study warrant evaluation of this new technique in a larger clinical trial before consideration for widespread implementation.

Some ORs have laminar airflow units. These units provide 400 to 500 air exchanges per hour. When used appropriately, laminar airflow units result in less than 10 CFUs per cubic foot per minute during surgery. The goal for a laminar flow-equipped OR is an infection rate under 1%. An OR equipped with this unit is frequently used for total joint replacement or organ transplant surgery.

Despite all these precautions, wound contamination may occur during surgery but may only become apparent days or weeks later in the form of an incisional infection or abscess. Constant surveillance and conscientious technique in carrying out aseptic practices is necessary to reduce the risk for contamination and infection.

Basic Guidelines for Maintaining Surgical Asepsis

All practitioners involved in the intraoperative phase have a responsibility to provide and maintain a safe environment. Adherence to aseptic practice is part of this responsibility. The eight basic principles of aseptic technique follow:

- All materials in contact with the surgical wound and used within the sterile field must be sterile. Sterile surfaces or articles may touch other sterile surfaces or articles and remain sterile; contact with unsterile objects at any point renders a sterile area contaminated.
- Gowns of the surgical team are considered sterile in front from the chest to the level of the sterile field. The sleeves are also considered sterile from 5 cm above the elbow to the stockinette cuff.
- Sterile drapes are used to create a sterile field. Only the top surface of a draped table is considered sterile. During draping of a table or patient, the sterile drape is held well above the surface to be covered and is positioned from front to back.
- Items should be dispensed to a sterile field by methods that preserve the sterility of the items and the integrity of the sterile field. After a sterile package is opened, the edges are considered unsterile. Sterile supplies, including solutions, are delivered to a sterile field or handed to a scrubbed person in such a way that the sterility of the object or fluid remains intact.
- The movements of the surgical team are from sterile to sterile areas and from unsterile to unsterile areas. Scrubbed persons and sterile items contact only sterile areas; circulating nurses and unsterile items contact only unsterile areas.
- Movement around a sterile field must not cause contamination of the field. Sterile areas must be kept in view during movement around the area. At least 30 cm from the sterile field must be maintained to prevent inadvertent contamination.
- Whenever a sterile barrier is breached, the area must be considered contaminated. A tear or puncture of the drape permitting access to an unsterile surface underneath renders the area unsterile. Such a drape must be replaced.
- Every sterile field should be constantly monitored and maintained. Items of doubtful sterility are considered unsterile. Sterile fields should be prepared as close as possible to the time of use.

HEALTH HAZARDS ASSOCIATED WITH THE SURGICAL ENVIRONMENT

Safety issues in the OR include exposure to blood and body fluids, hazards associated with laser beams, and exposure to latex, radiation, and toxic agents. Internal monitoring of the OR includes the analysis of surface swipe samples and air samples for infectious and toxic agents. In addition, policies and procedures for minimizing exposure to body fluids and reducing the dangers associated with lasers and radiation have been established.

Laser Risks

ORNAC and the Canadian Standards Association has recommended practices for laser safety (Canadian Standards Association, 2001; ORNAC, 2003). While lasers are in use, warning signs should be clearly posted to alert personnel. Among the safety issues are the following: reducing the possibility of exposing the eyes and skin to laser beams, preventing inhalation of the laser plume (smoke and particulate matter), and protecting the patient and personnel from fire and electrical hazards. Because several types of lasers are available for clinical use, perioperative personnel should be familiar with the unique features, specific operation, and safety measures for each type of laser used in the practice setting (Townsend, 2002).

Nurses and other intraoperative personnel working with lasers must have a thorough eye examination before participating in procedures involving lasers. Special protective goggles, specific to the type of laser used in the procedure, are worn. There is controversy about the protection needed to avoid the laser plume and effects of its inhalation. Smoke evacuators are used in some procedures to remove the laser plume from the operative field. In recent years this technology has been applied to protect the surgical team from the hazards associated with the generalized smoke plume generated by standard electrocautery units.

Exposure to Blood and Body Fluids

Since the advent of the acquired immunodeficiency syndrome (AIDS) epidemic, OR attire has changed dramatically. Double gloving is routine, at least in trauma surgery where sharp bone fragments are present. In addition to the routine scrub suit and double gloves, some surgeons wear rubber boots, a waterproof apron, and sleeve protectors. Goggles, or a wrap-around face shield, are worn to protect against splashing when the surgical wound is irrigated or when bone drilling is performed. In hospitals where numerous total joint procedures are performed, a full bubble mask may be used. This mask provides full barrier protection from bone fragments and splashes. Safe ventilation is accomplished through an accompanying hood with a separate air-filtration system.

Latex Allergy

Both the AORN and the American Society of Perianesthesia Nurses (ASPAN) have recommended standards of care for the patient with latex allergy (AORN, 2002; ASPAN, 2000). These recommendations include early identification of the patient with a latex allergy, preparation of a latex allergy supply cart, and maintenance of latex allergy precautions throughout the perioperative period. Due to the increased number of patients with latex allergies, many latex-free products are now available. For safety, manufacturers and hospital material managers need to take responsibility for identifying the latex content in items used by patients and health care personnel. (see Chaps. 18 and 53 for assessment for latex allergy).

> **NURSING ALERT** It is the responsibility of all nurses, and particularly perianesthesia and perioperative nurses, to be aware of latex allergies, necessary precautions, and products that are latex-free (Rothrock, 2003). Hospital staff are also at risk for developing a latex allergy secondary to repeated exposure to latex products.

The Surgical Experience

During the surgical procedure, the patient will need sedation, anesthesia, or a combination of these.

SEDATION AND ANESTHESIA

Sedation and anesthesia have four levels: minimal sedation, moderate sedation, deep sedation, and anesthesia. A surgical procedure may also be performed using anesthetic agents that suspend sensation in parts of the body (local, regional, epidural, or spinal anesthesia).

For the patient, the anesthesia experience consists of having an intravenous line inserted, if it was not inserted earlier; receiving a sedating agent prior to induction with an anesthetic agent; losing consciousness; being intubated, if indicated; and then receiving a combination of anesthetic agents. Typically the experience is a smooth one and the patient has no recall of the events.

Minimal Sedation

The minimal sedation level is a drug-induced state during which the patient can respond normally to verbal commands. Cognitive function and coordination may be impaired, but ventilatory and cardiovascular functions are not affected (JCAHO, 2001; Patterson, 2000a, b).

Moderate Sedation

Moderate sedation is a form of anesthesia that may be produced intravenously. It is defined as a depressed level of consciousness that does not impair the patient's ability to maintain a patent airway and to respond appropriately to physical stimulation and verbal command. Its goal is a calm, tranquil, amnesic patient who, when sedation is combined with analgesic agents, is relatively pain-free during the procedure but able to maintain protective reflexes (JCAHO, 2001; Patterson, 2000a, b). Sedation can be administered by an anesthesiologist, other physician, or nurse. When administered by an anesthesiologist, moderate sedation is referred to as monitored anesthesia care. The medications permitted for use in moderate sedation vary with the credentials of the person administering the sedative. In addition, state departments of health are very specific about who may administer moderate sedation and about the training required for those individuals. These regulations vary greatly from state to state.

Midazolam (Versed) or diazepam (Diazemuls, Valium) is used frequently for intravenous sedation. Other medications used include analgesic agents (eg, morphine, fentanyl) and reversal agonists, such as naloxone (Narcan). A nurse who is knowledgeable and skilled in detecting dysrhythmias, administering oxygen, and performing resuscitation must continuously monitor the patient who receives sedation. The patient receiving this form of anesthesia is never left alone and is closely monitored for respiratory, cardiovascular, and central nervous system depression using such methods as pulse oximetry, ECG, and frequent measurement of vital signs (Patterson, 2000a, b). The level of sedation is monitored by the patient's ability to maintain a patent airway and to respond to verbal commands.

Moderate sedation may be used alone or in combination with local, regional, or spinal anesthesia. Its use is increasing as more surgical procedures and diagnostic studies are performed in ambulatory and same-day settings with the expecta-tion that the patient will be discharged home a few hours after the procedure.

Deep Sedation

Deep sedation is a drug-induced state during which a patient cannot be easily aroused but can respond purposefully after repeated stimulation (JCAHO, 2001). The difference between deep sedation and anesthesia is that the anesthetized patient is not arousable. Deep sedation and anesthesia are achieved when an anesthetic agent is inhaled or administered intravenously. Inhaled anesthetic agents include volatile liquid agents and gases (Aranda & Hanson, 2000; Townsend, 2002). Volatile liquid anesthetics produce anesthesia when their vapors are inhaled. Included in this group are halothane (Fluothane), enflurane (Ethrane), isoflurane (Forane), sevoflurane (Ultrane), and desflurane (Suprane). All are administered with oxygen, and usually with nitrous oxide as well.

Gas anesthetics are administered by inhalation and are always combined with oxygen. Nitrous oxide is the most commonly used gas anesthetic. When inhaled, the anesthetics enter the blood through the pulmonary capillaries and act on cerebral centres to produce loss of consciousness and sensation. When anesthetic administration is discontinued, the vapor or gas is eliminated through the lungs. Table 19-1 lists the advantages, disadvantages, and implications of the different volatile liquid and gas anesthetics.

Anesthesia

General anesthesia consists of four stages, each associated with specific clinical manifestations. When opioid agents (narcotics) and neuromuscular blockers (relaxants) are administered, several of the stages are absent. The anesthesia level consists of general anesthesia and spinal or major regional anesthesia but does not include local anesthesia (JCAHO, 2001). **Anesthesia** is a state of narcosis (severe central nervous system depression produced by pharmacologic agents), analgesia, relaxation, and reflex loss. Patients under general anesthesia are not arousable, even to painful stimuli. They lose the ability to maintain ventilatory function and require assistance in maintaining a patent airway. Cardiovascular function may be impaired as well (JCAHO, 2001).

STAGE I: BEGINNING ANESTHESIA

As the patient breathes in the anesthetic mixture, warmth, dizziness, and a feeling of detachment may be experienced. The patient may have a ringing, roaring, or buzzing in the ears and, though still conscious, may sense an inability to move the extremities easily. During this stage, noises are exaggerated; even low voices or minor sounds seem loud and unreal. For this reason, the nurse avoids making unnecessary noises or motions when anesthesia begins.

STAGE II: EXCITEMENT

The excitement stage, characterized variously by struggling, shouting, talking, singing, laughing, or crying, is often avoided if the anesthetic is administered smoothly and quickly. The pupils dilate, but contract if exposed to light; the pulse rate is rapid, and respirations may be irregular.

Because of the possibility of uncontrolled movements of the patient during this stage, the anesthesiologist must always be assisted by someone ready to help restrain the patient. A strap may be in place across the patient's thighs, and the hands may be secured to an armboard. The patient should not be touched except for purposes of restraint, but restraints should not be applied over the operative site. Manipulation increases circulation to the operative site and thereby increases the potential for bleeding.

Table 19-1 • Inhalation Anesthetic Agents

AGENT	ADMINISTRATION	ADVANTAGES	DISADVANTAGES	IMPLICATIONS/ CONSIDERATIONS
Volatile Liquids				
halothane (Fluothane)	Inhalation; special vaporizer	Not explosive or flammable Induction rapid and smooth Useful in almost every type of surgery Low incidence of postoperative nausea and vomiting	Requires skillful administration to prevent overdosage May cause liver damage May produce hypotension Requires special vaporizer for administration	In addition to observation of pulse and respiration postoperatively, blood pressure must be monitored frequently.
methoxyflurane (Penthrane)	Inhalation; special vaporizer	Nonflammable Seldom causes postoperative nausea and vomiting Analgesic action continues several hours after surgery Excellent muscle relaxation	Requires skillful administration Renal damage may occur. Unpleasant odour	Prolonged postoperative depressant action calls for careful observation by PACU personnel.
enflurane (Ethrane)	Inhalation	Rapid induction and recovery Potent analgesic Not explosive or flammable	Respiratory depression may develop rapidly, along with ECG abnormalities. Not compatible with epinephrine	Observe for possible respiratory depression. Administration with epinephrine may cause ventricular fibrillation.
isoflurane (Forane)	Inhalation	Rapid induction and recovery Muscle relaxants are markedly potentiated.	A profound respiratory depressant	Respirations must be monitored closely and supported when necessary.
sevoflurane (Ultrane)	Inhalation	Rapid induction and excretion; minimal side effects	Coughing and laryngospasm; trigger for malignant hyperthermia	Monitor for malignant hyperthermia.
desflurane (Suprane)	Inhalation	Rapid induction and emergence; rare organ toxicity	Respiratory irritation; trigger for malignant hyperthermia	Monitor for malignant hyperthermia, dysrhythmias.
Gases				
nitrous oxide (N_2O)	Inhalation (semiclosed method)	Induction and recovery rapid Nonflammable Useful with oxygen for short procedures Useful with other agents for all types of surgery	Poor relaxant Weak anesthetic May produce hypoxia	Most useful in conjunction with other agents with longer action Monitor for chest pain, hypertension, and stroke.

STAGE III: SURGICAL ANESTHESIA

Surgical anesthesia is reached by continued administration of the anesthetic vapor or gas. The patient is unconscious and lies quietly on the table. The pupils are small but contract when exposed to light. Respirations are regular, the pulse rate and volume are normal, and the skin is pink or slightly flushed. With proper administration of the anesthetic, this stage may be maintained for hours in one of several planes, ranging from light (1) to deep (4), depending on the depth of anesthesia needed.

STAGE IV: MEDULLARY DEPRESSION

This stage is reached when too much anesthesia has been administered. Respirations become shallow, the pulse is weak and thready, and the pupils become widely dilated and no longer contract when exposed to light. Cyanosis develops and, without prompt intervention, death rapidly follows. If this stage develops, the anesthetic is discontinued immediately and respiratory and circulatory support is initiated to prevent death. Stimulants,

although rarely used, may be administered; narcotic antagonists can be used if overdosage is due to opioids.

During smooth administration of an anesthetic, there is no sharp division between the first three stages, and there is no stage IV. The patient passes gradually from one stage to another, and it is only by close observation of the signs exhibited by the patient that an anesthesiologist can control the situation. The responses of the pupils, the blood pressure, and the respiratory and cardiac rates are probably the most reliable guides to the patient's condition.

METHODS OF ANESTHESIA ADMINISTRATION

Anesthetics produce anesthesia because they are delivered to the brain at a high partial pressure that enables them to cross the blood–brain barrier. Relatively large amounts of anesthetic must be administered during induction and the early maintenance phases because the anesthetic is recirculated and deposited in body tissues. As these sites become saturated, smaller amounts of the anesthetic agent are required to maintain anesthesia because equilibrium or near equilibrium has been achieved between brain, blood, and other tissues.

Anything that diminishes peripheral blood flow, such as vasoconstriction or shock, may reduce the amount of anesthetic required. Conversely, when peripheral blood flow is unusually high, as in the muscularly active or the apprehensive patient, induction is slower and greater quantities of anesthetic are required because the brain receives a smaller quantity of anesthetic.

Inhalation

Liquid anesthetics may be administered by mixing the vapors with oxygen or nitrous oxide–oxygen and then having the patient inhale the mixture (Townsend, 2002). The vapor is administered to the patient through a tube or a mask. The inhalation anesthetic may also be administered through a laryngeal mask (Fig. 19-1), a flexible tube with an inflatable silicone ring and cuff that can be inserted into the larynx (Fortunato, 2000). The endotracheal technique for administering anesthetics consists of introducing a soft rubber or plastic endotracheal tube into the trachea, usually by means of a laryngoscope. The endotracheal tube may be inserted through either the nose or mouth. When in place, the tube seals off the lungs from the esophagus so that if the patient vomits, stomach contents do not enter the lungs.

Intravenous

General anesthesia can also be produced by the intravenous injection of various substances, such as barbiturates, benzodiazepines, nonbarbiturate hypnotics, dissociative agents, and opioid agents (Aranda & Hanson, 2000; Townsend, 2002). These medications may be administered for induction (initiation) or maintenance of anesthesia. They are often used along with inhalation anesthetics but may be used alone. They can also be used to produce moderate sedation. Intravenous anesthetics are presented in Table 19-2.

An advantage of intravenous anesthesia is that the onset of anesthesia is pleasant; there is none of the buzzing, roaring, or dizziness known to follow administration of an inhalation anesthetic. For this reason, induction of anesthesia usually begins with an intravenous agent and is often preferred by patients who have experienced various methods. The duration of action is brief, and the patient awakens with little nausea or vomiting. Thiopental is usually the agent of choice, and it is often administered with other anesthetic agents in prolonged procedures.

Intravenous anesthetic agents are nonexplosive, they require little equipment, and they are easy to administer. The low incidence of postoperative nausea and vomiting makes the method useful in eye surgery because vomiting would increase intraocular pressure and endanger vision in the operated eye. Intravenous anesthesia is useful for short procedures but is used less often for the longer procedures of abdominal surgery. It is not indicated for children, who have small veins and require intubation because of their susceptibility to respiratory obstruction.

A disadvantage of an intravenous anesthetic such as thiopental is its powerful respiratory depressant effect. It must be administered by a skilled anesthesiologist and only when some method of oxygen administration is available immediately in case of difficulty. Sneezing, coughing, and laryngospasm are sometimes noted with its use.

Intravenous neuromuscular blockers (muscle relaxants) block the transmission of nerve impulses at the neuromuscular junction of skeletal muscles. Muscle relaxants are used to relax muscles in abdominal and thoracic surgery, relax eye muscles in certain types of eye surgery, facilitate endotracheal intubation, treat laryngospasm, and assist in mechanical ventilation.

Purified curare was the first widely used muscle relaxant; tubocurarine was isolated as the active ingredient. Succinylcholine was later introduced because it acts more rapidly than curare. Several other agents are also used (Table 19-3). The ideal muscle relaxant has the following characteristics:

- It is nondepolarizing (noncompetitive agent), with an onset and duration of action similar to succinylcholine but without its problems of bradycardia and cardiac dysrhythmias (Townsend, 2002).
- It has a duration of action between those of succinylcholine and pancuronium.
- It lacks cumulative and cardiovascular effects.
- It can be metabolized and does not depend on the kidneys for its elimination.

A. Laryngeal mask   B. Intranasal intubation   C. Oral intubation

FIGURE 19-1 Anesthetic delivery methods: (**A**) laryngeal mask, (**B**) nasal endotracheal catheter (in position), and (**C**) oral endotracheal intubation (tube is in position with cuff inflated).

Table 19-2 • Intravenous Anesthetic Agents

AGENT	ADMINISTRATION	ADVANTAGES	DISADVANTAGES	IMPLICATIONS/CONSIDERATIONS
Tranquilizers and Sedative–Hypnotics				
Benzodiazepines				
midazolam (Versed)	IV	Short acting; has antianxiety, sedative, amnesic, muscle relaxant effects	Increased sensitivity to its effects in chronic obstructive pulmonary disease patients	Monitor respiratory status closely.
diazepam (Diazemuls, Valium)	IV Orally	Preoperative sedation Intraoperative tranquilization during regional anesthesia	Absorbed unpredictably when given IM	IV administration may produce thrombophlebitis (central vein is therefore preferred).
chlordiazepoxide (Librium, Medilium)	IM	Production of hypnosis during anesthetic induction		
droperidol (Inapsine)	IM	Long duration of action	Weak antihistaminic action and α-adrenergic blocking action; inhibition of basic ganglionic dopaminergic pathways may lead to extrapyramidal rigidity resembling parkinsonism	Major tranquilizer Keep IV fluids and vasopressors available to treat hypotension.
lorazepam (Ativan)	IV	Long duration of action	Used with caution in patients with renal and liver impairment	Monitor laboratory values.
Opioids				
morphine (high doses)	IV	Not a myocardial depressant	Can depress arterial blood pressure by decreasing systemic vascular resistance Does not provide good amnesia Does not promote adequate muscular relaxation	Orthostatic hypotension may occur.
meperidine hydrochloride (Demerol, Pethadol)	IV Subcutaneously IM	Prompt onset Because of spasmolytic effect, it is drug of choice for surgery of bile duct, distal colon, and rectum; easily detoxified and excreted	May slow rate of respirations Adverse reactions: dizziness, nausea, and vomiting	In some patients, histamine may be released; treatment is diphenhydramine (Benadryl).

Neuroleptanalgesics

The term *neuroleptanalgesic* refers to the combination of a short-acting synthetic opioid agent (fentanyl) and a butyrophenone (droperidol). Patient becomes very drowsy; responds to voice command, although analgesia is profound. Of significance, the combination produces peripheral vasodilation followed by a decrease in arterial blood pressure. If administered rapidly, it may cause skeletal muscular rigidity and possibly respiratory impairment. These agents are also called narcotic agonist analgesics.

fentanyl (Sublimaze)	IV Transdermally	75–100 times more potent than morphine and about 25% of duration of morphine (IV) Little effect on cardiovascular system	In very high dosage, an α-adrenergic blocking effect Respiratory depression	Short duration of action is due to its more rapid redistribution and more active metabolism by liver than other opioids.
sufentanil (Sufenta)	Injection	Onset extremely rapid		Duration is only about one third that of fentanyl.

Dissociative Agents

When under dissociative analgesia, the patient appears not to be asleep or anesthetized, but rather dissociated from the surroundings.

ketamine (Ketalar; Ketaject)	IV IM	Rapid induction and short action; often used to supplement nitrous oxide Useful when hypotension may be hazardous; can be administered as analgesic or anesthetic	May cause elevated blood pressure and depressed respirations Patient may experience hallucinations. Vomiting and aspiration may occur.	Avoid verbal, visual, or tactile stimulation because this may trigger psychic aberration. Droperidol or diazepam (see below) may eliminate such psychic phenomena. Observe for signs of respiratory depression. Keep resuscitation equipment nearby.

(continued)

Table 19-2 • Intravenous Anesthetic Agents (Continued)

AGENT	ADMINISTRATION	ADVANTAGES	DISADVANTAGES	IMPLICATIONS/CONSIDERATIONS
Barbiturates				
thiopental sodium (Pentothal)	IV injection (or rectal)	Rapid induction Nonexplosive Requires little equipment Low incidence of post-operative nausea and vomiting	Powerful depressant of breathing Poor relaxant May produce coughing, sneezing, and laryngospasm Not useful for children because of small veins	Requires close observation because of potency and rapidity of drug action
methohexital sodium (Brevital)	IV	Rapid onset	Respiratory depression, involuntary muscle movement, seizures; may cause necrosis if IV infiltrates	Monitor respiratory status closely, monitor for seizure activity, ensure IV in vein.
Nonbarbiturate Hypnotics				
etomidate (Amidate)	IV	Few cardiovascular and respiratory effects; useful for frail patients	Transient adrenal suppression; involuntary muscle movements	
propofol (Diprivan)	IV	Rapid induction with minimal excitatory effects; may have antiemetic effect	Myocardial depression; hypotension; pain on injection	Monitor cardiac function and blood pressure closely; contraindicated in patients with allergy to eggs and soybean oil.

Regional Anesthesia

Regional anesthesia is a form of local anesthesia in which an anesthetic agent is injected around nerves so that the area supplied by these nerves is anesthetized. The effect depends on the type of nerve involved. Motor fibres are the largest fibres and have the thickest myelin sheath. Sympathetic fibres are the smallest and have a minimal covering. Sensory fibres are intermediate. Thus, a local anesthetic blocks motor nerves least readily and sympathetic nerves most readily. An anesthetic cannot be regarded as having worn off until all three systems (motor, sensory, and autonomic) are no longer affected.

The patient receiving spinal or local anesthesia is awake and aware of his or her surroundings unless medications are given to produce mild sedation or to relieve anxiety. The nurse must avoid careless conversation, unnecessary noise, and unpleasant odours; these may be noticed by the patient in the OR and may contribute to a negative view of the surgical experience. A quiet environment is therapeutic. The diagnosis must not be stated aloud if the patient is not to know it at this time.

Conduction Blocks and Spinal Anesthesia

There are many types of conduction blocks, depending on the nerve groups affected by the injection. Epidural anesthesia is achieved by injecting a local anesthetic into the spinal canal in the space surrounding the dura mater (Fig. 19-2). Epidural anesthesia also blocks sensory, motor, and autonomic functions, but it is differentiated from spinal anesthesia by the injection site and the amount of anesthetic used. Epidural doses are much higher because the epidural anesthetic does not make direct contact with the cord or nerve roots.

An advantage of epidural anesthesia is the absence of headache that occasionally results from subarachnoid injection. A disadvantage is the greater technical challenge of introducing the anesthetic into the epidural rather than the subarachnoid space. If inadvertent subarachnoid injection occurs during epidural anesthesia and the anesthetic travels toward the head, high spinal anesthesia can result; this can produce severe hypotension and respiratory depression and arrest. Treatment of these complications includes airway support, intravenous fluids, and use of vasopressors. Other types of nerve blocks include:

- Brachial plexus block, which produces anesthesia of the arm
- Paravertebral anesthesia, which produces anesthesia of the nerves supplying the chest, abdominal wall, and extremities
- Transsacral (caudal) block, which produces anesthesia of the perineum and, occasionally, the lower abdomen

Spinal anesthesia is a type of extensive conduction nerve block that is produced when a local anesthetic is introduced into the subarachnoid space at the lumbar level, usually between L4 and L5 (see Fig. 19-2). It produces anesthesia of the lower extremities, perineum, and lower abdomen. For the lumbar puncture procedure, the patient usually lies on the side in a knee–chest position. Sterile technique is used as a spinal puncture is made and the medication is injected through the needle. As soon as the injection has been made, the patient is positioned on his or her back. If a relatively high level of block is sought, the head and shoulders are lowered.

The spread of the anesthetic agent and the level of anesthesia depend on the amount of fluid injected, the speed with which it is injected, the positioning of the patient after the injection, and the specific gravity of the agent. If the specific gravity is greater than that of cerebrospinal fluid (CSF), the agent moves to the dependent position of the subarachnoid space. If the specific gravity is less than that of CSF, the anesthetic moves away from the dependent position. The anesthesiologist controls the spread of the agent. Generally, the agents used are procaine, tetracaine

Table 19-3 • **Neuromuscular Blocking Agents**

MUSCLE RELAXANT	ACTION	ADVANTAGES	DISADVANTAGES	USES AND COMMENTS
Nondepolarizing Neuromuscular Blocking Agents				
tubocurarine chloride (Tubarine)	Peaks at 30–60 min	50%–70% excreted unchanged in 3–6 h	Histamine-like reaction Hypotension Increased airway resistance Skin erythema	Contraindicated with history of allergy, asthma
gallamine (Flaxedil)	20% as potent as curare Lasts 25% shorter time than curare Blocks vagal ganglia in heart	All excreted unchanged	Tachycardia	Used with cyclopropane or halothane
pancuronium bromide (Pavulon)	Similar to curare but 5 times more potent Duration: 60–85 min	Safe; stable Good muscle relaxant Reversible by neostigmine and atropine		Excellent for situations requiring complete relaxation Avoid with myasthenia gravis or renal disease. Avoid with patients sensitive to bromide.
vecuronium bromide (Norcuron)	Blocks depolarization	Facilitates endotracheal intubation; good muscle relaxant	Prolonged dose-related apnea	Related to Pavulon Well tolerated in patients with renal failure
Depolarizing Neuromuscular Blocking Agents				
These mimic the action of acetylcholine at the neuromuscular junction. Acetylcholine is discharged almost immediately on release, then repolarization of muscle takes place. When depolarizing neuromuscular blocking agents are used, skeletal muscle depolarizes.				
succinylcholine (Anectine; Sucostrin)	Onset is rapid: 1 min Duration: 4–8 min	Ideal for endotracheal intubation, fracture reduction; treatment of laryngospasm	Contraindicated in patients with low pseudo-cholinesterase On second IV injection, bradycardia and various dysrhythmias May cause fasciculations of the muscles and pain	Used to treat laryngospasm, status asthmaticus, and toxic reactions to local anesthetic drugs
decamethonium bromide (Syncurine)	Onset: 30–40 sec Duration: 15–20 min	Excreted unchanged by kidney	Some fasciculation of muscle: jaw masseter muscles; posterior calf muscles Difficult to reverse its action	Produces depolarization of end-plate region

(Pontocaine), lidocaine (Xylocaine), and bupivacaine (Marcaine) (Table 19-4).

A few minutes after induction of a spinal anesthetic, anesthesia and paralysis affect the toes and perineum and then gradually the legs and abdomen. If the anesthetic reaches the upper thoracic and cervical spinal cord in high concentrations, a temporary partial or complete respiratory paralysis results. Paralysis of the respiratory muscles is managed by mechanical ventilation until the effects of the anesthetic on the respiratory nerves have worn off.

Nausea, vomiting, and pain may occur during surgery when spinal anesthesia is used. As a rule, these reactions result from manipulation of various structures, particularly those within the abdominal cavity. The simultaneous intravenous administration of a weak solution of thiopental and inhalation of nitrous oxide may prevent such reactions.

Headache may be an after-effect of spinal anesthesia. Several factors are involved in the incidence of headache: the size of the spinal needle used, the leakage of fluid from the subarachnoid space through the puncture site, and the patient's hydration status. Measures that increase cerebrospinal pressure are helpful in relieving headache. These include keeping the patient lying flat, quiet, and well hydrated.

In continuous spinal anesthesia, the tip of a plastic catheter remains in the subarachnoid space during the surgical procedure so that more anesthetics may be injected as needed. This technique allows greater control of the dosage, but there is greater potential for postanesthetic headache because of the large-gauge needle used.

Local Infiltration Anesthesia

Infiltration anesthesia is the injection of a solution containing the local anesthetic into the tissues at the planned incision site. Often it is combined with a local regional block by injecting the nerves immediately supplying the area. The advantages of local anesthesia are as follows:

- It is simple, economical, and nonexplosive.
- Equipment needed is minimal.
- Postoperative recovery is brief.
- Undesirable effects of general anesthesia are avoided.
- It is ideal for short and superficial surgical procedures.

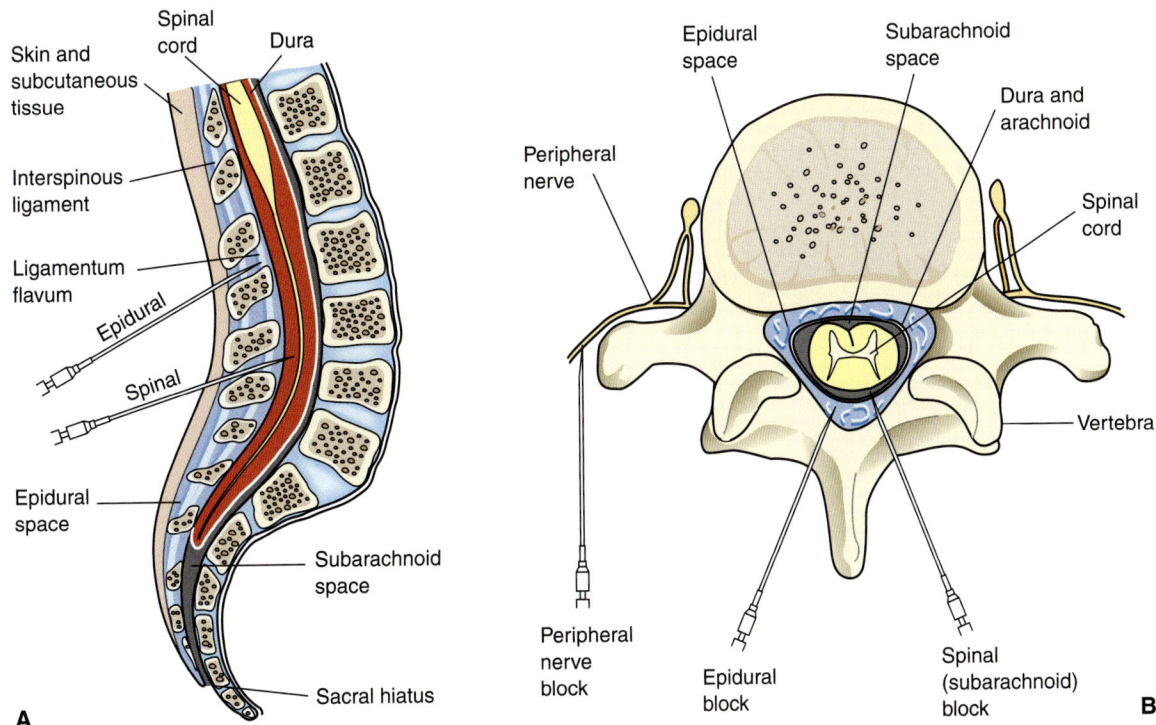

FIGURE 19-2 (**A**) Injection sites for spinal and epidural anesthesia. (**B**) Cross-section of injection sites for peripheral nerve, epidural, and spinal blocks.

Local anesthesia is often administered in combination with epinephrine. Epinephrine constricts blood vessels, which prevents rapid absorption of the anesthetic agent and thus prolongs its local action. Rapid absorption of the anesthetic agent into the bloodstream, which could cause seizures, is also prevented. Types of local anesthetic agents are listed in Table 19-5.

Local anesthesia is the anesthesia of choice in any surgical procedure in which it can be used. However, contraindications include high preoperative levels of anxiety, because surgery with local anesthesia may increase anxiety. A patient who requests general anesthesia rarely does well under local anesthesia. For some surgical procedures, local anesthesia is impractical because of the number of injections and the amount of anesthetic that would be required (breast reconstruction, for example).

The skin is prepared as for any surgical procedure, and a small-gauge needle is used to inject a modest amount of the anesthetic into the skin layers. This produces blanching or a wheal. Additional anesthetic is then injected in the skin until an area the length of the proposed incision is anesthetized. A larger, longer needle then is used to infiltrate deeper tissues with the anesthetic.

The action of the agent is almost immediate, so surgery may begin as soon as the injection is complete. Anesthesia lasts 45 minutes to 3 hours, depending on the anesthetic and the use of epinephrine.

Potential Intraoperative Complications

The surgical patient is subject to several risks. Potential intraoperative complications include nausea and vomiting, anaphylaxis, hypoxia, hypothermia, malignant hyperthermia, and disseminated intravascular coagulopathy.

NAUSEA AND VOMITING

Nausea and vomiting, or regurgitation, may affect patients during the intraoperative period. If gagging occurs, the patient is turned to the side, the head of the table is lowered, and a basin is provided to collect the vomitus. Suction is used to remove saliva and vomited gastric contents. There is no single way to prevent

AGENT	ADVANTAGES OF SPINAL ANESTHESIA (INCLUDES ALL AGENTS)	DISADVANTAGES OF SPINAL ANESTHESIA (INCLUDES ALL AGENTS)
procaine (Novocaine) tetracaine (Pontocaine) lidocaine (Xylocaine, Xylocard)	Easily administered by a physician Inexpensive Minimum of equipment required	Blood pressure may fall rapidly unless monitored carefully and treated with medications such as ephedrine. If the spinal anesthesia ascends to the chest, there may be respiratory distress.
bupivacaine (Marcaine)	Rapid onset Excellent muscular relaxation	Occasionally, postoperative complications occur, such as headache or, rarely, meningitis or paralysis.

Table 19-4 • **Regional Anesthetic Agents**

Table 19-5 • Local Anesthetic Agents

AGENT	ADMINISTRATION	ADVANTAGES	DISADVANTAGES	IMPLICATIONS/ CONSIDERATIONS
lidocaine (Xylocaine) and mepivacaine (Carbocaine)	Topical or injection	Rapid Longer duration of action (compared with procaine) Free from local irritative effect	Occasional idiosyncrasy	Useful topically for cystoscopy Injected for use in dental work and surgery Observe for untoward reactions—drowsiness, depressed respiration.
bupivacaine (Marcaine)	Infiltration Peripheral nerve block Epidural	Duration is 2–3 times longer than lidocaine or mepivacaine	Use cautiously in patients with known drug allergies or sensitivities.	A period of analgesia persists after return of sensation; therefore, need for strong analgesics is reduced.
etidocaine (Duranest)	Infiltration Block			Greater potency and longer action than lidocaine
procaine (Novocaine)	Subcutaneously, intramuscularly, intravenously, or spinal	Low toxicity Inexpensive	Some idiosyncrasies Skin rash Poor stability	Observe for reaction: hypotension, bradycardia, weak pulse. Usually administered with epinephrine, causing vasoconstriction, thereby slowing absorption and prolonging nerve-deadening effect
tetracaine (Pontocaine)	Topical Infiltration Nerve block	Same as procaine	Same as procaine	More than 10 times as potent as procaine Usually administered with epinephrine

nausea and vomiting; an interdisciplinary approach involving the surgeon, anesthesiologist or anesthetist, and nurse is best (Rothrock, 2003).

In some cases, the anesthesiologist administers antiemetics preoperatively or intraoperatively to counteract possible aspiration. If the patient aspirates vomitus, an asthma-like attack with severe bronchial spasms and wheezing is triggered. Pneumonitis and pulmonary edema can subsequently develop, leading to extreme hypoxia. Increasing medical attention is being paid to silent regurgitation of gastric contents, which occurs more frequently than previously realized. The importance of pH in the etiology of acid aspiration is being studied, as is the value of perioperative administration of a histamine-2 receptor antagonist, such as cimetidine (Tagamet), and similar medications (Rothrock, 2003).

ANAPHYLAXIS

Any time a substance foreign to the patient is introduced, there is the potential for an anaphylactic reaction. Because medications are the most common cause of anaphylaxis, intraoperative nurses must be aware of the type and method of anesthesia used as well as the specific agents. An anaphylactic reaction can occur in response to many medications, latex, or other substances. The reaction may be immediate or delayed. Anaphylaxis is a life-threatening acute allergic reaction that causes vasodilation, hypotension, and bronchial constriction (Fortunato, 2000). See Chapters 15 and 53 for more details about the signs, symptoms, and treatment of anaphylaxis.

Fibrin sealants are used in a variety of surgical procedures, and cyanoacrylate tissue adhesives are used to close wounds without the use of sutures (Kassam et al., 2002; Vargas & Reger, 2000). These sealants have been implicated in allergic reactions and anaphylaxis. Although these reactions are rare, the nurse should be alert to the possibility and observe the patient for changes in vital signs and symptoms of anaphylaxis when these products are used.

HYPOXIA AND OTHER RESPIRATORY COMPLICATIONS

Inadequate ventilation, occlusion of the airway, inadvertent intubation of the esophagus, and hypoxia are significant potential problems of general anesthesia. Many factors can contribute to inadequate ventilation. Respiratory depression caused by anesthetic agents, aspiration of respiratory tract secretions or vomitus, and the patient's position on the operating table can compromise the exchange of gases. Anatomic variation can make the trachea difficult to visualize and result in the artificial airway being inserted into the esophagus rather than the trachea. In addition to these dangers, asphyxia caused by foreign bodies in the mouth, spasm of the vocal cords, relaxation of the tongue, or aspiration of vomitus, saliva, or blood can occur. Since brain damage from hypoxia occurs within minutes, vigilant assessment of the patient's oxygenation status is a primary function of the anesthesiologist and the circulating nurse. Peripheral perfusion is checked frequently, and pulse oximetry values are monitored continuously.

HYPOTHERMIA

During anesthesia, the patient's temperature may fall. Glucose metabolism is reduced, and as a result metabolic acidosis may develop. This condition is called hypothermia and is indicated by a core body temperature below normal (36.6°C or lower). Inadvertent hypothermia may occur as a result of a low temperature in the OR, infusion of cold fluids, inhalation of cold gases, open body wounds or cavities, decreased muscle activity, advanced age, or the pharmaceutical agents used (eg, vasodilators, phenothiazines, general anesthetics). Hypothermia may also be intentionally induced in selected surgical procedures (such as cardiac surgeries requiring cardiopulmonary bypass) to reduce the patient's metabolic rate (Finkelmeier, 2000).

Preventing unintentional hypothermia is a major objective. If hypothermia occurs, the goal of intervention is to minimize or reverse the physiologic process. If hypothermia is intentional, the goal is safe return to normal body temperature. Environmental temperature in the OR can temporarily be set at 25° to 26.6°C. Intravenous and irrigating fluids are warmed to 37°C. Wet gowns and drapes are removed promptly and replaced with dry materials because wet linens promote heat loss. Whatever methods are used to rewarm the patient, warming must be accomplished gradually, not rapidly. Conscientious monitoring of core temperature, urinary output, ECG, blood pressure, arterial blood gas levels, and serum electrolyte levels is required.

MALIGNANT HYPERTHERMIA

Malignant hyperthermia is an inherited muscle disorder chemically induced by anesthetic agents (Fortunato-Phillips, 2000; Vermette, 1998). With the mortality rate exceeding 50%, identifying patients at risk for malignant hyperthermia is imperative. Susceptible people include those with strong and bulky muscles, a history of muscle cramps or muscle weakness and unexplained temperature elevation, and an unexplained death of a family member during surgery that was accompanied by a febrile response.

Pathophysiology

During anesthesia, potent agents such as inhalation anesthetics (halothane, enflurane) and muscle relaxants (succinylcholine), may trigger the symptoms of malignant hyperthermia (Fortunato-Phillips, 2000). Stress and some medications, such as sympathomimetics (epinephrine), theophylline, aminophylline, anticholinergics (atropine), and cardiac glycosides (digitalis), can induce or intensify such a reaction as well.

The pathophysiology is related to muscle cell activity. Muscle cells are composed of inner fluid (sarcoplasm) and an outer surrounding membrane. Calcium, an essential factor in muscle contraction, is normally stored in sacs in the sarcoplasm (Fortunato-Phillips, 2000). When nerve impulses stimulate the muscle, calcium is released, allowing contraction to occur. A pumping mechanism returns calcium to the sacs so that the muscle can relax. In malignant hyperthermia, this mechanism is disrupted. Calcium ions are not returned and they accumulate, causing clinical symptoms of hypermetabolism, which in turn increases muscle contraction (rigidity), hyperthermia, and damage to the central nervous system.

Clinical Manifestations

The initial symptoms of malignant hyperthermia are related to cardiovascular and musculoskeletal activity. Tachycardia (heart rate above 150 beats/min) is often the earliest sign. In addition to the tachycardia, sympathetic nervous stimulation leads to ventricular dysrhythmia, hypotension, decreased cardiac output, oliguria, and, later, cardiac arrest. With the abnormal transport of calcium, rigidity or tetanus-like movements occur, often in the jaw. The rise in temperature is actually a late sign that develops rapidly; body temperature can increase 1° to 2°C every 5 minutes (Rothrock, 2003). The temperature can reach or exceed 40°C in a very short time (Fortunato-Phillips, 2000).

Medical Management

Recognizing symptoms early and discontinuing anesthesia promptly are imperative. Goals of treatment are to decrease metabolism, reverse metabolic and respiratory acidosis, correct dysrhythmias, decrease body temperature, provide oxygen and nutrition to tissues, and correct electrolyte imbalance. The Malignant Hyperthermia Association of Canada publishes a treatment protocol that should be posted in the OR or be readily available on a malignant hyperthermia cart.

Although malignant hyperthermia usually presents about 10 to 20 minutes after induction of anesthesia, it can also occur in the first 24 hours after surgery. As soon as the diagnosis is made, anesthesia and surgery are halted and the patient is hyperventilated with 100% oxygen. Dantrolene sodium, a skeletal muscle relaxant, and sodium bicarbonate are administered immediately (Fortunato-Phillips, 2000; Vermette, 1998). Continued monitoring of all parameters is necessary to evaluate the patient's status.

Nursing Management

Although malignant hyperthermia is uncommon, the nurse must identify patients at risk, recognize the signs and symptoms, have the appropriate medication and equipment available, and be knowledgeable about the protocol to follow (Fortunato-Phillips, 2000). This information may be lifesaving.

DISSEMINATED INTRAVASCULAR COAGULOPATHY

Disseminated intravascular coagulopathy is a life-threatening condition characterized by thrombus formation and depletion of select coagulation proteins (Dice, 2000). The exact cause is unknown, but predisposing factors include many conditions that may occur with emergency surgery, such as massive trauma, head injury, massive transfusion, liver or kidney involvement, embolic events, or shock. The signs and symptoms, nursing assessment, and treatment are discussed in Chapter 33.

NURSING PROCESS: THE PATIENT DURING SURGERY

The ORNAC conceptual model for perioperative registered nursing practice is a helpful tool used by nurses in the intraoperative phase of care (see Chap. 18, Fig. 18-1). Phenomena of concern to intraoperative nurses are nursing diagnoses, interventions, and outcomes that surgical patients and their families experience. Additional areas of concern include collaborative problems and expected goals.

Assessment

Nursing assessment of the intraoperative patient involves obtaining data from the patient and the patient's record to identify variables that can affect care and serve as guidelines for developing an individualized plan of patient care. The intraoperative nurse uses the focused preoperative nursing assessment documented on the patient record. This includes assessment of physiologic status (eg, health–illness level, level of consciousness), psychosocial status (eg, anxiety level, verbal communication problems, coping mechanisms), physical status (eg, surgical site, skin condition and effectiveness of preparation; immobile joints), and ethical concerns (Chart 19-3).

Diagnosis

NURSING DIAGNOSES

Based on the assessment data, some major nursing diagnoses may include the following:

- Anxiety related to expressed concerns due to surgery or OR environment
- Risk for perioperative positioning injury related to environmental conditions in the OR
- Risk for injury related to anesthesia and surgery
- Disturbed sensory perception (global) related to general anesthesia or sedation

COLLABORATIVE PROBLEMS/POTENTIAL COMPLICATIONS

Based on the assessment data, potential complications may include the following:

- Nausea and vomiting
- Anaphylaxis
- Hypoxia
- Unintentional hypothermia
- Malignant hyperthermia
- Disseminated intravascular coagulopathy
- Infection

Chart 19-3 • Ethics and Related Issues

To Resuscitate or Not?

Situation
Your hospital has developed a policy, authorized through the medical staff, that allows for patients to have a do-not-resuscitate order (DNR) in place during a surgical procedure. This policy follows the Canadian Anesthesiologists' Society guidelines for DNR in the operating room. You are getting a patient ready for surgery and the anesthesiologist who will be administering the anesthetic writes an order for the DNR to be rescinded during surgery. The physician is refusing to talk to the patient concerning the DNR.

Problem
The patient believes his/her wishes will be followed with regard to resuscitation in the event of a cardiac arrest and the physician does not believe he can administer anesthesia if the DNR is in place.

Discussion
- What are the rights of the patient with regard to advance directives?
- What can you do to advocate for the patient?
- Should you contact the ethics committee of the hospital?
- How do you contact the ethics committee?

Planning and Goals

Goals for care of the patient during surgery include reducing anxiety, preventing positioning injuries, maintaining safety, maintaining the patient's dignity, and avoiding complications.

Nursing Interventions

REDUCING ANXIETY

The OR environment can seem cold, stark, and frightening to the patient, who may be feeling isolated and apprehensive. Introducing yourself, addressing the patient by name warmly and frequently, verifying details, providing explanations, and encouraging and answering questions provide a sense of professionalism and friendliness that can help the patient feel secure. When discussing what the patient can expect in surgery, the nurse uses common, basic communication skills, such as touch and eye contact, to reduce anxiety. Attention to physical comfort (warm blankets, position changes) helps the patient feel more comfortable. Telling the patient who else will be present in the OR, how long the procedure is expected to take, and other details helps the patient prepare for the experience and gain a sense of control.

PREVENTING INTRAOPERATIVE POSITIONING INJURY

The patient's position on the operating table depends on the surgical procedure to be performed as well as on his or her physical condition (Fig. 19-3). The potential for transient discomfort or even permanent injury is clear because many positions are awkward. Hyperextending joints, compressing arteries, or pressing on nerves and bony prominences usually results in discomfort simply because the position must be sustained for a long period (Rothrock, 2003). Factors to consider include the following:

- The patient should be in as comfortable a position as possible, whether asleep or awake.
- The operative field must be adequately exposed.
- An awkward position, undue pressure on a body part, or use of stirrups or traction should not obstruct the vascular supply.
- Respiration should not be impeded by pressure of arms on the chest or by a gown that constricts the neck or chest.
- Nerves must be protected from undue pressure. Improper positioning of the arms, hands, legs, or feet may cause serious injury or paralysis. Shoulder braces must be well padded to prevent irreparable nerve injury, especially when the Trendelenburg position is necessary.
- Precautions for patient safety must be observed, particularly with thin, elderly, or obese patients, or those with a physical deformity (Curet, 2000).
- The patient needs gentle restraint before induction in case of excitement.

The usual position for surgery, called the dorsal recumbent position, is flat on the back. One arm is positioned at the side of the table, with the hand placed palm down; the other is carefully positioned on an armboard to facilitate intravenous infusion of fluids, blood, or medications. This position is used for most abdominal surgeries except for surgery of the gallbladder and pelvis (see Fig. 19-3A).

The Trendelenburg position usually is used for surgery on the lower abdomen and pelvis to obtain good exposure by displacing the intestines into the upper abdomen. In this position, the head and body are lowered. The patient is held in position by padded shoulder braces (see Fig. 19-3B).

A Patient in position on the operating table for a laparotomy. Note the strap above the knees.

B Patient in Trendelenburg position on operating table. Note padded shoulder braces in place. Be sure that brace does not press on brachial plexus.

C Patient in lithotomy position. Note that the hips extend over the edge of the table.

D Patient lies on unaffected side for kidney surgery. Table is broken to spread apart space between the lower ribs and the pelvis. The upper leg is extended; the lower leg is flexed at the knee and the hip joints; a pillow is placed between the legs.

FIGURE 19-3 Positions on the operating table. Captions call attention to safety and comfort features. All surgical patients wear caps to cover the hair completely.

The lithotomy position is used for nearly all perineal, rectal, and vaginal surgical procedures (see Fig. 19-3C). The patient is positioned on the back with the legs and thighs flexed. The position is maintained by placing the feet in stirrups.

The Sims or lateral position is used for renal surgery. The patient is placed on the nonoperative side with an air pillow 12.5 to 15 cm thick under the loin, or on a table with a kidney or back lift (see Fig. 19-3D).

Other procedures, such as neurosurgery or abdominothoracic surgery, may require unique positioning and supplemental apparatus, depending on the operative approach.

PROTECTING THE PATIENT FROM INJURY

One way the nurse protects the patient from injury is by providing a safe environment. A variety of activities are used to address the diverse patient safety issues that arise in the OR. Verifying information, checking the chart for completeness, and maintaining surgical asepsis and an optimal environment are critical nursing responsibilities. Verifying that all required documentation is completed is one of the first functions of the intraoperative nurse. The patient is identified, and the planned surgical procedure and type of anesthesia are verified. It is important to review the patient's record for the following:

- Correct informed surgical consent, with patient's signature
- Completed records for health history and physical examination
- Results of diagnostic studies
- Allergies (including latex)

In addition to checking that all necessary patient data are complete, the perioperative nurse obtains the necessary equipment specific to the procedure. The need for nonroutine medications, blood components, instruments, and other equipment and supplies is assessed, and the readiness of the room, completeness of physical setup, and completeness of instrument, suture, and dressing setups are determined. Any aspects of the OR environment that may negatively affect the patient are identified. These include physical features, such as room temperature and humidity; electrical hazards; potential contaminants (dust, blood, and discharge on floor or surfaces, uncovered hair, faulty attire of personnel, jewelry worn by personnel); and unnecessary traffic. The circulating nurse also sets up and maintains suction equipment in working order, sets up invasive monitoring equipment, assists with insertion of vascular access and monitoring devices (arterial, Swan-Ganz, central venous pressure, intravenous lines), and initiates appropriate physical comfort measures for the patient.

Preventing physical injury includes using safety straps and bed rails and not leaving the sedated patient unattended. Transferring the patient from the stretcher to the OR table requires safe transferring practices. Other safety measures include properly positioning the grounding pad under the patient to prevent electrical burns and shock, removing excess povidone-iodine (Betadine) or other surgical germicide from the patient's skin, and promptly and completely draping exposed areas after the sterile field has been created to decrease the risk for hypothermia.

Nursing measures to prevent injury from excessive blood loss include blood conservation using equipment such as a cell-saver (a device for recirculating the patient's own blood cells) or the administration of blood products (Finkelmeier, 2000). Few patients undergoing an elective procedure require blood transfusion, but those undergoing higher-risk procedures (such as orthopedic or cardiac surgeries) may require an intraoperative transfusion. The circulating nurse should anticipate this need, check that blood has been cross-matched and held in reserve, and be prepared to administer blood (Rothrock, 2003).

SERVING AS PATIENT ADVOCATE

Because the patient undergoing general anesthesia or moderate sedation experiences temporary sensory/perceptual alteration or loss, he or she has an increased need for protection and advocacy. Patient advocacy in the OR entails maintaining the patient's physical and emotional comfort, privacy, rights, and dignity. Patients, whether conscious or not, should not be subjected to excess noise, inappropriate conversation, or, most of all, derogatory comments. As surprising as this sounds, banter in the OR occasionally includes jokes about the patient's physical appearance, job, personal history, and so forth. Cases have been reported in which seemingly deeply anesthetized patients recalled the entire surgical experience, including disparaging personal remarks made by OR personnel. As an advocate, the nurse never engages in this conversation and discourages others from doing so. Other advocacy activities include correcting for the clinical, dehumanizing aspects of being a surgical patient by making sure the patient is treated as a person, respecting cultural and spiritual values, providing physical privacy, and maintaining confidentiality.

MONITORING AND MANAGING POTENTIAL COMPLICATIONS

It is the responsibility of the surgeon and the anesthesiologist to monitor and manage complications. However, intraoperative nurses also play an important role. Being alert to and reporting changes in vital signs and symptoms of nausea and vomiting, anaphylaxis, hypoxia, hypothermia, malignant hyperthermia, or disseminated vascular coagulation and assisting with their management are important nursing functions (Dice, 2000; Fortunato-Phillips, 2000). Each of these complications was discussed earlier. Maintaining asepsis and preventing infection is the responsibility of all members of the surgical team.

Evaluation

EXPECTED PATIENT OUTCOMES

Expected patient outcomes may include:

1. Exhibits low level of anxiety
2. Remains free of perioperative positioning injury
3. Experiences no unexpected threats to safety
4. Has dignity preserved throughout OR experience
5. Is free of complications or experiences successful management of adverse effects of surgery and anesthesia

Critical Thinking Exercises

1. A patient in the holding area awaiting surgery indicates that he had not received instructions not to take his usual medications (antihypertensive agent, diuretic, digoxin, potassium chloride, and insulin injection); as a result, he took them a few hours ago. What implications does this have for the patient's care and well-being while awaiting surgery, during surgery, and in the immediate postoperative period?

2. What are the differences in responsibility of the operating room nurse for care of patients who receive general anesthesia, conscious sedation, spinal anesthesia, and regional anesthesia?

3. While she is being transferred from the stretcher to the operating table, a female patient says she is very anxious about her surgery because of previous negative experiences. What assessment and interventions are indicated at this time?

REFERENCES AND SELECTED READINGS

Books

American Society of Perianesthesia Nurses. (2000). *Standards of perianesthesia nursing practice.* Thorofare, NJ: ASPAN.

AORN Standards, Recommended Practice, and Guidelines (2002). Denver: AORN, Inc.

Canadian Anesthesiologists' Society. (2004). *Guidelines to the practice of anesthesia.* Toronto, ON: Author.

Canadian Standards Association. (2001). *Laser safety in health care facilities.* Toronto, ON: CSA International.

Dudek, S. G. (2001). *Nutrition essentials for nursing practice.* Philadelphia: Lippincott Williams & Wilkins.

Finkelmeier, B. (2000). *Cardiothoracic surgical nursing* (2d ed.). Philadelphia: Lippincott Williams & Wilkins.

Fortunato, N. (2000). *Berry and Kohn's operating room technique* (9th ed.). St. Louis: Mosby, Inc.

Joint Commission on Accreditation of Healthcare Organizations (JCAHO) (2001). *Revisions to anesthesia care standards for comprehensive accreditation manual for ambulatory care.* Philadelphia: Lippincott Williams & Wilkins.

Litwack, K. (Ed.). (1999). *Core curriculum for perianesthesia nursing practice.* Philadelphia: WB Saunders.

Operating Room Nurses Association of Canada (ORNAC). (2003). *Recommended standards, guidelines, and position statements for perioperative registered nursing practice.* Author.

Phippen, M., & Wells, M. (2000). *Patient care during operative and invasive procedures.* Philadelphia: WB Saunders.

Rothrock, J. C. (1999). *The RN first assistant: An expanded perioperative nursing role* (3rd ed.). Philadelphia: Lippincott.

Rothrock, J. C. (2003). *Alexander's care of the patient in surgery* (12th ed.). St. Louis: Mosby.

Schwartz, S., & Shires, G. T. (1999). *Principles of surgery.* New York: McGraw-Hill.

Townsend, C. (2002). *Pocket companion to Sabiston textbook of surgery* (16th ed.). Philadelphia: WB Saunders.

Journals

Asterisks indicate nursing research articles.

Aranda, M., & Hanson, W. (2000). Anesthetics, sedatives, and paralytics: Understanding their use in the intensive care unit. *Surgical Clinics of North America, 80*(3), 933–947.

Curet, M. (2000). Special problems in laparoscopic surgery: Previous abdominal surgery, obesity, and pregnancy. *Surgical Clinics of North America, 80*(4), 1093–1110.

Dice, R. (2000). Intraoperative disseminated intravascular coagulopathy. *Critical Care Nursing Clinics of North America, 12*(2), 175–180.

Fortunato-Phillips, N. (2000). Malignant hyperthermia: Update 2000. *Critical Care Nursing Clinics of North America, 12*(2), 199–210.

Friberg, B. (1998). Ultraclean laminar airflow ORs. *AORN Journal, 67*(4), 841–851.

Kassam, A., Carrau, R., Horowitz, M., Snyderman, C., Hirsch, B., & Welch, W. (2002). The role of fibrin sealants in cranial-based surgery. *Clinical Update, 1280,* 1–36.

*Larsen, E., Aiello, A., Heilman, J., Lyle, C., Cronquist, A., Stahl, J., & Dello-Latta, P. (2001). Comparison of different regimens for surgical hand preparation. *AORN Journal, 73*(2), 412–432.

Patterson, C. (2000*a*). New rules impact sedation and anesthesia care, Part 1. *Nursing Management, 31*(5), 22.

Patterson, C. (2000*b*). New rules impact sedation and anesthesia care, Part 2. *Nursing Management, 31*(6), 16–17.

Polanczyk, C., Marcantonio, E., Goldman, L., et al. (2001). Impact of age on perioperative complications and length of stay in patients undergoing noncardiac surgery. *Annals of Internal Medicine, 134*(8), 637–643.

Vargas, G., & Reger, T. (2000). An alternative to sutures. *MedSurg Nursing, 9*(2), 83–85.

Vermette, E. (1998). Emergency! Malignant hyperthermia. *American Journal of Nursing, 98*(4), 45.

Williams, H., & Reeves, F. (1998). Anesthetic techniques and positioning: Implications for perioperative nurses. *Seminars in Perioperative Nursing, 7*(1), 14–20.

Winslow, E., & Jacobson, A. (2000). Can a fashion statement harm the patients? *American Journal of Nursing, 100*(9), 63–65.

RESOURCES AND WEBSITES

American Society of Anesthesiologists, 520 N. Northwest Highway, Park Ridge, IL, 60068; (847) 825-2286; http://www.asahq.org/practice.

American Society of PeriAnesthesia Nurses, 10 Melrose Ave., Suite 110, Cherry Hill, NJ 08003-3696; 877-9696 (toll-free); fax (856) 616-9621; http://www.aspan.org.

Association of PeriOperative Registered Nurses, Inc., 2170 S. Parker Rd., Suite 300, Denver, CO 80231; (800) 755-2676; http://www.aorn.org.

Canadian Anesthesiologists' Society, 1 Eglinton Avenue East, Suite 208, Toronto, ON M4P 3A1; http://www.cas.ca.

Canadian Council on Health Services Accreditation, 1730 St. Laurent Boulevard, Suite 100, Ottawa, ON K1G 5L1; http://www.cchsa.ca.

Malignant Hyperthermia Association of Canada. 200 Elizabeth Street, Room ES3-403, Toronto, ON M5G 2C4; http://www.mhacanada.org/home.htm.

Operating Room Nurses Association of Canada (ORNAC), http://www.ornac.ca.

Public Health Agency of Canada. 130 Colonnade Road, A. L. 6501H, Ottawa, ON K1A 0K9; http://www.phac-aspc.gc.ca.

Postoperative Nursing Management

Adapted by Christy Raymond

On completion of this chapter, the learner will be able to:

1. Describe the responsibilities of the postanesthesia care unit nurse in the prevention of immediate postoperative complications.
2. Compare postoperative care of the ambulatory surgery patient and the hospitalized surgery patient.
3. Identify common postoperative problems and their management.
4. Describe the gerontologic considerations related to postoperative management of patients.
5. Describe variables that affect wound healing.
6. Demonstrate postoperative dressing techniques.
7. Identify assessment parameters appropriate for the early detection of postoperative complications.

*T*he postoperative period extends from the time the patient leaves the operating room until the last follow-up visit with the surgeon. This period may be as short as 1 week or as long as several months. During the postoperative period, nursing care focuses on reestablishing the patient's physiologic equilibrium, alleviating pain, preventing complications, and teaching the patient self-care. Careful assessment and immediate intervention assist the patient in returning to optimal function quickly, safely, and as comfortably as possible. Ongoing care in the community through home care, clinic visits, office visits, or telephone follow-up facilitates an uncomplicated recovery.

The Postanesthesia Care Unit

The **postanesthesia care unit (PACU)**, also called the postanesthesia recovery room, is located adjacent to the operating rooms. Patients still under anesthesia or recovering from anesthesia are placed in this unit for easy access to experienced, highly skilled nurses, anesthesiologists, surgeons, advanced hemodynamic and pulmonary monitoring and support, special equipment, and medications (Litwack, 1999; Rothrock, 2003).

The PACU is kept quiet, clean, and free of unnecessary equipment. This area is painted in soft, pleasing colours and has indirect lighting, a soundproof ceiling, equipment that controls or eliminates noise (eg, plastic emesis basins, rubber bumpers on beds and tables), and isolated but visible quarters for disruptive patients. The PACU should also be well ventilated. These features benefit the patient by helping to decrease anxiety and promote comfort. The PACU bed provides easy access to the patient, is safe and easily movable, can be readily placed in position to facilitate use of measures to counteract shock, and has features that facilitate care, such as intravenous (IV) poles, side rails, wheel brakes, and a chart storage rack.

PHASES OF POSTANESTHESIA CARE

Postanesthesia care in some hospitals and ambulatory surgical centres is divided into two phases (Litwack, 1999; Rothrock, 2003). In the **phase I PACU**, used during the immediate recovery phase, intensive nursing care is provided. The **phase II PACU** is reserved for patients who require less frequent observation and less nursing care. In the phase II unit, the patient is prepared for discharge. Recliners rather than stretchers or beds are standard in many phase II units, which may also be referred to as step-down, sit-up, or progressive care units. Patients may remain in a phase II PACU unit for as long as 4 to 6 hours, depending on the type of surgery and any preexisting conditions of the patient. In facilities without separate phase I and phase II units, the patient remains in the PACU and may be discharged home directly from this unit.

Both phase I and phase II PACU nurses have special skills. The phase I PACU nurse provides frequent (every 15 minutes) monitoring of the patient's pulse, electrocardiogram, respiratory rate, blood pressure, and pulse oximeter value (blood oxygen level). In some cases, end-tidal carbon dioxide ($ETCO_2$) levels are monitored as well. The patient's airway may become obstructed because of the latent effects of recent anesthesia, and the PACU nurse must be prepared to assist in reintubation and in handling other emergencies that may occur. The nurse in the phase II PACU must possess strong clinical assessment and patient teaching skills.

ADMITTING THE PATIENT TO THE PACU

Transferring the postoperative patient from the operating room to the PACU is the responsibility of the anesthesiologist. During transport from the operating room to the PACU, the anesthesia provider remains at the head of the stretcher (to maintain the airway), and a surgical team member remains at the opposite end. Transporting the patient involves special consideration of the incision site, potential vascular changes, and exposure. The surgical incision is considered every time the postoperative patient is moved; many wounds are closed under considerable tension, and every effort is made to prevent further strain on the incision. The patient is positioned so that he or she is not lying on and obstructing drains or drainage tubes. Serious orthostatic hypotension may occur when a patient is moved from one position to another (eg, from a lithotomy position to a horizontal position or from a lateral to a supine position), so the patient must be moved slowly and carefully. As soon as the patient is placed on the stretcher or bed, the soiled gown is removed and replaced with a dry gown. The patient is covered with lightweight blankets and warmed. The side rails are raised to guard against falls.

The nurse who admits the patient to the PACU reviews the following information with the anesthesiologist:

- Medical diagnosis and type of surgery performed
- Pertinent past medical history and allergies
- Patient's age and general condition, airway patency, vital signs
- Anesthetics and other medications used during the procedure (eg, opioids and other analgesic agents, muscle relaxants, antibiotic agents)

Glossary

dehiscence: partial or complete separation of wound edges

evisceration: protrusion of abdominal organs through the surgical incision

first-intention healing: method of healing in which wound edges are surgically approximated and integumentary continuity is restored without granulation

Phase I PACU: area designated for care of surgical patients immediately after surgery

and patients whose condition warrants close monitoring

Phase II PACU: area designated for care of surgical patients who have been transferred from a phase I PACU because their condition no longer requires the close monitoring provided in a phase I PACU

postanesthesia care unit (PACU): area where postoperative patients are monitored as they recover from anesthesia; for-

merly referred to as the recovery room or postanesthesia recovery room

second-intention healing: method of healing in which wound edges are not surgically approximated and integumentary continuity is restored by the process known as granulation

third-intention healing: method of healing in which surgical approximation of wound edges is delayed and integumentary continuity is restored by apposing areas of granulation

- Any problems that occurred in the operating room that might influence postoperative care (eg, extensive hemorrhage, shock, cardiac arrest)
- Pathology encountered (if malignancy is an issue during surgery, the nurse needs to know whether the patient and/or family have been informed)
- Fluid administered, estimated blood loss and replacement fluids
- Any tubing, drains, catheters, or other supportive aids
- Specific information about which the surgeon or anesthesiologist wishes to be notified (eg, blood pressure or heart rate below or above a specified level)

NURSING MANAGEMENT IN THE PACU

The nursing management objectives for the patient in the PACU are to provide care until the patient has recovered from the effects of anesthesia (eg, until resumption of motor and sensory functions), is oriented, has stable vital signs, and shows no evidence of hemorrhage or other complications.

Assessing the Patient

Frequent, skilled assessments of the blood oxygen saturation level, pulse rate and regularity, depth and nature of respirations, skin colour, level of consciousness, and ability to respond to commands are the cornerstones of nursing care in the PACU. The nurse performs a baseline assessment, then checks the surgical site for drainage or hemorrhage and makes sure that all drainage tubes and monitoring lines are connected and functioning.

After the initial assessment, vital signs are monitored and the patient's general physical status is assessed at least every 15 minutes. Patency of the airway and respiratory function are always evaluated first, followed by assessment of cardiovascular function, the condition of the surgical site, and function of the central nervous system. The nurse needs to be aware of any pertinent information from the patient's history that may be significant (eg, patient is hard of hearing, has a history of seizures, has diabetes, or is allergic to certain medications or to latex).

Maintaining a Patent Airway

The primary objective in the immediate postoperative period is to maintain pulmonary ventilation and thus prevent hypoxemia (reduced oxygen in the blood) and hypercapnia (excess carbon dioxide in the blood). Both can occur if the airway is obstructed and ventilation is reduced (hypoventilation). Besides checking the physician's orders for and administering supplemental oxygen, the nurse assesses respiratory rate and depth, ease of respirations, oxygen saturation, and breath sounds (Litwack, 1999; Rothrock, 2003).

Patients who have experienced prolonged anesthesia usually are unconscious, with all muscles relaxed. This relaxation extends to the muscles of the pharynx. When the patient lies on his or her back, the lower jaw and the tongue fall backward and the air passages become obstructed (Fig. 20-1*A*). This is called hypopharyngeal obstruction. Signs of occlusion include choking, noisy and irregular respirations, decreased oxygen saturation scores, and within minutes a blue, dusky colour (cyanosis) of the skin. Because movement of the thorax and the diaphragm does not necessarily indicate that the patient is breathing, the nurse needs to place the palm of the hand at the patient's nose and mouth to feel the exhaled breath.

> **! NURSING ALERT** The treatment of hypopharyngeal obstruction involves tilting the head back and pushing forward on the angle of the lower jaw, as if to push the lower teeth in front of the upper teeth (Figs. 20-1**B, C**). This manoeuvre pulls the tongue forward and opens the air passages.

The anesthesiologist may leave a hard rubber or plastic airway in the patient's mouth (Fig. 20-2) to maintain a patent airway. Such a device should not be removed until signs such as gagging indicate that reflex action is returning. Alternatively, the patient may enter the PACU with an endotracheal tube still in place and may require continued mechanical ventilation. The nurse assists in initiating the use of the ventilator and in the weaning and extubation processes. Some patients, particularly those who have had extensive or lengthy surgical procedures, may be transferred from the operating room directly to the intensive care unit or may be transferred from the PACU to the intensive care unit while still intubated and on mechanical ventilation.

Respiratory difficulty can also result from excessive secretion of mucus or aspiration of vomitus. Turning the patient to one side allows the collected fluid to escape from the side of the mouth. If the teeth are clenched, the mouth may be opened manually but cautiously with a padded tongue depressor. The head of the bed is elevated 15 to 30 degrees unless contraindicated, and the patient is closely observed to maintain the airway as well as to minimize the risk of aspiration. If vomiting occurs, the patient is turned to the side to prevent aspiration and the vomitus is collected in the emesis basin. Mucus or vomitus obstructing the pharynx or the trachea is suctioned with a pharyngeal suction tip or a nasal catheter introduced into the nasopharynx or oropharynx. The catheter can be passed into the nasopharynx or oropharynx safely to a distance of 15 to 20 cm. Caution is necessary in suctioning the throat of a patient who has had a tonsillectomy or other oral or laryngeal surgery because of risk for bleeding and discomfort.

Maintaining Cardiovascular Stability

To monitor cardiovascular stability, the nurse assesses the patient's mental status; vital signs; cardiac rhythm; skin temperature, colour, and moisture; and urine output. Central venous pressure, pulmonary artery pressure, and arterial lines are monitored if the patient's condition requires such assessment. The nurse also assesses the patency of all IV lines. The primary cardiovascular complications seen in the PACU include hypotension and shock, hemorrhage, hypertension, and dysrhythmias.

HYPOTENSION AND SHOCK
Hypotension can result from blood loss, hypoventilation, position changes, pooling of blood in the extremities, or side effects of medications and anesthetics; the most common cause is loss of circulating volume through blood and plasma loss. If the amount of blood loss exceeds 500 mL (especially if the loss is rapid), replacement is usually indicated.

Shock, one of the most serious postoperative complications, can result from hypovolemia. Shock may be described as inadequate cellular oxygenation accompanied by the inability to excrete waste products of metabolism. Hypovolemic shock is characterized by a fall in venous pressure, a rise in peripheral resistance, and tachycardia. Neurogenic shock, a less common cause of shock in the surgical patient, occurs as a result of decreased arterial resistance caused by spinal anesthesia. It is characterized by a fall in blood

FIGURE 20-1 (**A**) A hypopharyngeal obstruction occurs when neck flexion permits the chin to drop toward the chest; obstruction almost always occurs when the head is in the midposition. (**B**) Tilting the head back to stretch the anterior neck structure lifts the base of the tongue off the posterior pharyngeal wall. The direction of the arrows indicates the pressure of the hands. (**C**) Opening the mouth is necessary to correct valvelike obstruction of the nasal passage during expiration, which occurs in about 30% of unconscious patients. Open the patient's mouth (separate lips and teeth) and move the lower jaw forward so that the lower teeth are in front of the upper teeth. To regain backward tilt of the neck, lift with both hands at the ascending rami of the mandible.

FIGURE 20-2 Use of an airway to prevent respiratory difficulty after anesthesia. The airway passes over the base of the tongue and permits air to pass into the pharynx in the region of the epiglottis. Patients often leave the operating room with an airway in place. The airway should remain in place until the patient recovers sufficiently to breathe normally. As the patient regains consciousness, the airway usually causes irritation and should be removed.

pressure due to pooling of blood in dilated capacitance vessels (those with the ability to change volume capacity). Cardiogenic shock is unlikely in the surgical patient except if the patient has severe preexisting cardiac disease or experienced a myocardial infarction during surgery. See Chapter 15 for a detailed discussion of shock.

The classic signs of shock are:

- Pallor
- Cool, moist skin
- Rapid breathing
- Cyanosis of the lips, gums, and tongue
- Rapid, weak, thready pulse
- Decreasing pulse pressure
- Low blood pressure and concentrated urine

Hypovolemic shock can be avoided largely by the timely administration of IV fluids, blood, blood products, and medications that elevate blood pressure. Other factors may contribute to hemodynamic instability, and the PACU nurse implements multiple measures to manage these factors. Pain is controlled by making the patient as comfortable as possible and by using opioids judiciously. Exposure is avoided, and normothermia is maintained to prevent vasodilation.

Volume replacement is the primary intervention for shock. An infusion of lactated Ringer's solution or blood component therapy is initiated. Oxygen is administered by nasal cannula, facemask, or mechanical ventilation. Cardiotonic, vasodilator, and corticosteroid medications may be prescribed to improve cardiac function and reduce peripheral vascular resistance. The patient is kept warm while avoiding overheating to prevent cutaneous vessels from dilating and depriving vital organs of blood. The patient is placed flat in bed with the legs elevated. Respiratory and pulse rate, blood pressure, blood oxygen concentration, urinary output, level of consciousness, central venous pressure, pulmonary artery pressure, pulmonary capillary wedge pressure, and cardiac output are monitored to provide information on the patient's respiratory and cardiovascular status. Vital signs are monitored continuously until the patient's condition has stabilized.

HEMORRHAGE

Hemorrhage is an uncommon yet serious complication of surgery that can result in death (Finkelmeier, 2000). It can present insidiously or emergently at any time in the immediate postoperative period or up to several days after surgery (Table 20-1). When blood loss is extreme, the patient is apprehensive, restless, and thirsty; the skin is cold, moist, and pale. The pulse rate increases, the temperature falls, and respirations are rapid and deep, often of the gasping type spoken of as "air hunger." If hemorrhage progresses untreated, cardiac output decreases, arterial and venous blood pressure and hemoglobin level fall rapidly, the lips and the conjunctivae become pallid, spots appear before the eyes, a ringing is heard in the ears, and the patient grows weaker but remains conscious until near death.

Transfusing blood or blood products and determining the cause of hemorrhage are the initial therapeutic measures. The surgical site and incision should always be inspected for bleeding. If bleeding is evident, a sterile gauze pad and a pressure dressing are

applied, and the site of the bleeding is elevated to heart level if possible. The patient is placed in the shock position (flat on back; legs elevated at a 20-degree angle; knees kept straight). If the source of bleeding is concealed, the patient may be taken back to the operating room for emergency exploration of the surgical site.

 NURSING ALERT When IV fluids are given in cases of hemorrhage, it is important to remember that unless the hemorrhage has been well controlled, giving too large a quantity or administering the IV fluid too rapidly may raise the blood pressure enough to start the bleeding again.

Special considerations must be given to patients who decline blood transfusions, such as Jehovah's Witnesses and those who identify specific requests on their advance directives or living will.

HYPERTENSION AND DYSRHYTHMIAS

Hypertension is common in the immediate postoperative period secondary to sympathetic nervous system stimulation from pain, hypoxia, or bladder distention. Dysrhythmias are associated with electrolyte imbalance, altered respiratory function, pain, hypothermia, stress, and anesthetic medications. Both conditions are managed by treating the underlying causes.

Relieving Pain and Anxiety

Opioid analgesics are administered judiciously and often intravenously in the PACU (Rothrock, 2003). Intravenous opioids provide immediate relief and are short-acting, thus minimizing the potential for drug interactions or prolonged respiratory depression while anesthetics are still active in the patient's system. In addition to monitoring the patient's physiologic status and managing pain, the PACU nurse provides psychological support in an effort to relieve the patient's fears and concerns. The nurse checks the medical record for special needs and concerns of the patient. When the patient's condition permits, a close member of the family may visit in the PACU for a few moments. This often decreases the family's anxiety and makes the patient feel more secure.

Controlling Nausea and Vomiting

Nausea and vomiting are common problems in the PACU. The nurse should intervene at the patient's first report of nausea to control the problem rather than wait for it to progress to vomiting.

Many medications are available to control nausea and vomiting without oversedating the patient; they are commonly administered during surgery as well as in the PACU (Rothrock, 2003). Intravenous or intramuscular administration of droperidol (Inapsine) is common, especially in the ambulatory setting. Other medications such as metoclopramide (Reglan), prochlorperazine (Compazine), and promethazine (Phenergan) are commonly prescribed (Karch, 2002; Rothrock, 2003). Although it is costly, ondansetron (Zofran) is a frequently used, effective antiemetic with few side effects.

 NURSING ALERT At the slightest indication of nausea, the patient is turned completely to one side to promote mouth drainage and prevent aspiration of vomitus, which can cause asphyxiation and death.

Table 20-1 • **Classifications of Hemorrhage**

CLASSIFICATION	DEFINING CHARACTERISTIC
Time Frame	
Primary	Hemorrhage occurs at the time of surgery.
Intermediary	Hemorrhage occurs during the first few hours after surgery when the rise of blood pressure to its normal level dislodges insecure clots from untied vessels.
Secondary	Hemorrhage may occur some time after surgery if a ligature slips because a blood vessel was insecurely tied, became infected, or was eroded by a drainage tube.
Type of Vessel	
Capillary	Hemorrhage is characterized by a slow, general ooze.
Venous	Darkly coloured blood bubbles out quickly.
Arterial	Blood is bright red and appears in spurts with each heartbeat.
Visibility	
Evident	Hemorrhage is on the surface and can be seen.
Concealed	Hemorrhage is in a body cavity and cannot be seen.

Gerontologic Considerations

The elderly patient, like all other patients, is transferred from the operating room table to the bed or stretcher slowly and gently. The effects of this action on blood pressure and ventilation are monitored. Special attention is given to keeping the patient warm because the elderly are more susceptible to hypothermia. The patient's position is changed frequently to stimulate respirations and to promote circulation and comfort.

Immediate postoperative care for the elderly patient is the same as that for any surgical patient, but additional support is given if there is impaired cardiovascular, pulmonary, or renal function. With invasive monitoring, it is possible to detect cardiopulmonary deficits before signs and symptoms are apparent. The elderly patient has less physiologic reserve, and physiologic responses to stress are diminished or slowed. These changes reinforce the need for close monitoring and prompt treatment of hypotension, shock, and hemorrhage. Because of monitoring and improved individualized preoperative preparation, many older adults tolerate surgery well and have an uneventful recovery.

Postoperative confusion is common in older patients. The confusion is aggravated by social isolation, restraints, anesthetics and analgesics, and sensory deprivation. Reorienting the patient to the environment and using smaller amounts of sedatives, anesthetics, and analgesics may help prevent confusion. However, unrelieved pain, particularly pain at rest, may increase the risk for delirium and must be addressed (Lynch, Lazor, Gellis et al., 1998). Hypoxia can present as confusion and restlessness, as can blood loss and electrolyte imbalance. Excluding all other causes of confusion must precede the assumption that confusion is related to age, circumstances, and medications.

Determining Readiness for Discharge From the PACU

A patient remains in the PACU until he or she has fully recovered from the anesthetic agent (Rothrock, 2003). Indicators of recovery include stable blood pressure, adequate respiratory function, adequate oxygen saturation level compared with baseline, and spontaneous movement or movement on command. Usually the following measures are used to determine the patient's readiness for discharge from the PACU:

- Stable vital signs
- Orientation to person, place, events, and time
- Uncompromised pulmonary function
- Pulse oximetry readings indicating adequate blood oxygen saturation
- Urine output at least 30 mL/h
- Nausea and vomiting absent or under control
- Minimal pain

Many hospitals use a scoring system (eg, Aldrete score) to determine the patient's general condition and readiness for transfer from the PACU (Quinn, 1999). Throughout the recovery period, the patient's physical signs are observed and evaluated by means of a scoring system based on a set of objective criteria. This evaluation guide, a modification of the Apgar scoring system used for evaluating newborns, allows a more objective assessment of the patient's condition in the PACU (Fig. 20-3). The patient is assessed at regular intervals (eg, every 15 or 30 minutes), and the score is totalled on the assessment record. Patients with a score lower than 7 must remain in the PACU until their condition im-

proves or they are transferred to an intensive care area, depending on their preoperative baseline scores.

The patient is discharged from the phase I PACU by the anesthesiologist to the critical care unit, the medical-surgical unit, the phase II PACU, or home with a responsible family member (Quinn, 1999). Patients being discharged directly to home require verbal and written instructions and information about follow-up care.

Promoting Home and Community-Based Care

To ensure patient safety and recovery, expert patient teaching and discharge planning are necessary when a patient undergoes same-day or ambulatory surgery. Because anesthetics cloud memory for concurrent events, instructions should be given to both the patient and the adult who will be accompanying the patient home (Quinn, 1999).

TEACHING PATIENTS SELF-CARE
The patient and caregiver (eg, family member or friend) are informed about expected outcomes and immediate postoperative changes anticipated in the patient's capacity for self-care (Fox, 1998; Quinn, 1999). Written instructions about wound care, activity and dietary recommendations, medication, and follow-up visits to the same-day surgery unit or the surgeon are provided. Written instructions (designed to be copied and given to patients) about the postoperative care following many types of surgery are usually provided (Economou & Economou, 1999). The patient's caregiver at home is provided with verbal and written instructions about what to observe the patient for and about the actions to take if complications occur. Prescriptions are given to the patient. The nurse or surgeon's telephone number is provided, and the patient and caregiver are encouraged to call with questions and to schedule follow-up appointments (Chart 20-1).

Although recovery time varies depending on the type and extent of surgery and the patient's overall condition, instructions usually advise limited activity for 24 to 48 hours. During this time, the patient should not drive a vehicle, drink alcoholic beverages, or perform tasks that require energy or skill. Fluids may be consumed as desired, and smaller-than-normal amounts are eaten at mealtime. The patient is cautioned not to make important decisions at this time because the medications, anesthesia, and surgery may affect his or her decision-making ability.

CONTINUING CARE
Although most patients who undergo ambulatory surgery recover quickly and without complications, some patients require referral for home care. These may be elderly or frail patients, those who live alone, and patients with other health care problems that may interfere with self-care or resumption of usual activities. The home care nurse assesses the patient's physical status (eg, respiratory and cardiovascular status, adequacy of pain management, the surgical incision) and the patient's and family's ability to adhere to the recommendations given at the time of discharge. Previous teaching is reinforced as needed. The home care nurse may change surgical dressings, monitor the patency of a drainage system, or administer medications. The patient is assessed for any surgical complications. The patient and family are reminded about the importance of keeping follow-up appointments with the surgeon. Follow-up phone calls from the nurse or surgeon may also be used to assess the patient's progress and to answer any questions (Fox, 1998; Marley & Swanson, 2001).

Postanesthesia Care Unit:
MODIFIED ALDRETE SCORE

Patient: Final score:

Room: Surgeon:

Date: PACU nurse:

Area of Assessment	Point Score	Upon Admission	After		
			1 h	2 h	3 h
Muscle Activity:					
Moves spontaneously or on command:					
• Ability to move all extremities	2				
• Ability to move 2 extremities	1				
• Unable to control any extremity	0				
Respiration:					
• Ability to breathe deeply and cough	2				
• Limited respiratory effort (dyspnea or splinting)	1				
• No spontaneous effort	0				
Circulation:					
• BP ± 20% of preanesthetic level	2				
• BP ± 20%–49% of preanesthetic level	1				
• BP ± 50% of preanesthetic level	0				
Consciousness Level:					
• Fully awake	2				
• Arousable on calling	1				
• Not responding	0				
O_2 Saturation:					
• Able to maintain O_2 sat >92% on room air	2				
• Needs O_2 inhalation to maintain O_2 sat >90%	1				
• O_2 sat <90% even with O_2 supplement	0				
Totals:					

Required for discharge from Postanesthesia Care Unit: 7–8 points

_____   _____

Time of release   Signature of nurse

FIGURE 20-3 Postanesthesia care unit record; Modified Aldrete Score. (O_2 sat = oxygen saturation.)

The Hospitalized Postoperative Patient

The patient admitted to the clinical unit for postoperative care has multiple needs. Seriously ill patients or those who have undergone major cardiovascular, pulmonary, or neurologic surgery are admitted to specialized intensive care units for close monitoring and advanced interventions and support. The care required by these patients in the immediate postoperative period is discussed in specific chapters. Postoperative care for the surgical patient returning to the general medical-surgical unit is discussed below.

Chart 20-1
Home Care Checklist • Discharge From Surgery

At the completion of the home care instruction, the patient or caregiver will be able to:	Patient	Caregiver
• Name the procedure that was performed and identify any permanent changes in anatomic structure or function.	✓	✓
• Describe ongoing postoperative therapeutic regimen, including medications, diet, activities to perform (such as walking and breathing exercises) and to avoid (such as driving a car or contact sports), adjuvant therapies, dressing changes and wound care, and any other treatments.	✓	✓
• Describe signs and symptoms of complications.	✓	✓
• State time and date of follow-up appointments.	✓	✓
• Identify interventions and strategies to use in adapting to any permanent changes in structure or function.	✓	✓
• Relate how to reach health care provider with questions or complications.	✓	✓
• State understanding of community resources and referrals (if any).	✓	✓
• Describe pertinent health promotion activities (eg, weight reduction, smoking cessation, stress management).	✓	✓

RECEIVING THE PATIENT IN THE CLINICAL UNIT

The patient's room is readied by assembling the necessary equipment and supplies: IV pole, drainage receptacle holder, emesis basin, tissues, disposable pads (Chux), blankets, and postoperative charting forms. When the call comes to the unit about the patient's transfer from the PACU, the need for any additional items that may be needed is communicated. The PACU nurse reports the baseline data about the patient's condition to the receiving nurse. The report includes demographic data, medical diagnosis, procedure performed, comorbid conditions, allergies, unexpected intraoperative events, estimated blood loss, the type and amount of fluids received, medications administered for pain, whether the patient has voided, and information that the patient and family have received about the patient's condition. Usually the surgeon speaks to the family after surgery and relates the general condition of the patient. The receiving nurse reviews the postoperative orders, admits the patient to the unit, performs an initial assessment, and attends to the patient's immediate needs (Chart 20-2).

NURSING MANAGEMENT AFTER SURGERY

During the first 24 hours after surgery, nursing care of the hospitalized patient on the general medical-surgical unit involves continuing to help the patient recover from the effects of anesthesia, frequently assessing the patient's physiologic status, monitoring for complications, managing pain, and implementing measures designed to achieve the long-range goals of independence with self-care, successful management of the therapeutic regimen, discharge to home, and full recovery. In the initial hours after admission to the clinical unit, adequate ventilation, hemodynamic stability, incisional pain, surgical site integrity, nausea and vomiting, neurologic status, and spontaneous voiding are primary concerns. The pulse rate, blood pressure, and respiration rate are recorded at least every 15 minutes for the first hour and every 30 minutes for the next 2 hours. Thereafter, they are measured less frequently if they remain stable. The temperature is monitored every 4 hours for the first 24 hours.

Patients usually begin to feel better several hours after surgery or after waking up the next morning. Although pain may still be intense, many patients feel more alert, less nauseous, and less anxious. They have begun their breathing and leg exercises, and many will have dangled their legs over the edge of the bed, stood, and ambulated a few feet or been assisted out of bed to the chair at least once. Many will have tolerated a light meal and had IV fluids discontinued. The focus of care shifts from intense physiologic management and symptomatic relief of the adverse effects of anesthesia to regaining independence with self-care and preparing for discharge. Despite these gains, the postoperative patient is still at risk for complications. Atelectasis, pneumonia, deep vein thrombosis, pulmonary embolism, constipation, paralytic ileus, and wound infection are ongoing threats for the postoperative patient (Fig. 20-4).

Chart 20-2
Standard Postoperative Nursing Interventions

Once the patient leaves the PACU and is admitted to the unit, immediate nursing interventions include the following:

- Assess breathing and administer supplemental oxygen, if prescribed.
- Monitor vital signs and note skin warmth, moisture, and colour.
- Assess the surgical site and wound drainage systems.
- Assess level of consciousness, orientation, and ability to move extremities.
- Connect all drainage tubes to gravity or suction as indicated and monitor closed drainage systems.
- Assess pain level, pain characteristics (location, quality) and timing, type, and route of administration of last pain medication.
- Administer analgesics as prescribed and assess their effectiveness in relieving pain.
- Position patient to enhance comfort, safety, and lung expansion.
- Assess IV sites for patency and infusions for correct rate and solution.
- Assess urine output in closed drainage system or the patient's urge to void and bladder distention.
- Reinforce need to begin deep-breathing and leg exercises.
- Place call light, emesis basin, ice chips (if allowed), and bedpan or urinal within reach.
- Provide information to patient and family.

Neurologic
Delirium
Stroke

Respiratory
Atelectasis
Pneumonia
Pulmonary embolism
Aspiration

Cardiovascular
Shock
Thrombophlebitis

Urinary
Acute urine retention
Urinary tract infection

Gastrointestinal
Constipation
Paralytic ileus
Bowel obstruction

Wound
Infection
Dehiscence
Evisceration
Delayed healing
Hemorrhage
Hematoma

Functional
Weakness
Fatigue
Functional decline

FIGURE 20-4 The postoperative patient is subject to a number of potential complications.

NURSING PROCESS: THE HOSPITALIZED PATIENT RECOVERING FROM SURGERY

The ORNAC conceptual model for perioperative registered nursing practice is a helpful tool used by nurses in the postoperative phase of care (see Chap. 18, Fig. 18-1). Phenomena of concern to nurses on the clinical unit in the postoperative phase of care include nursing diagnoses, interventions, and outcomes for patients and their families. Additional areas of concern include collaborative problems and expected goals.

Assessment

Assessment of the hospitalized postoperative patient includes monitoring vital signs and completing a review of the systems upon arrival of the patient to the clinical unit and thereafter (see Chart 20-2).

Respiratory status is important because pulmonary complications are among the most frequent and serious problems encountered by the surgical patient. The nurse observes for airway patency and the quality of respirations, including depth, rate, and sound. Chest auscultation verifies that breath sounds are normal (or not normal) bilaterally, and the findings are documented as a baseline for later comparisons. Often, because of the effects of pain medications, respirations are slow. Shallow and rapid respirations may be due to pain, constricting dressings, gastric dilation, or obesity. Noisy breathing may be due to obstruction by secretions or the tongue.

The nurse assesses the patient's pain level using a verbal or visual analog scale and assesses the characteristics of the pain. The patient's appearance, pulse, respirations, blood pressure, skin colour (adequate or cyanotic), and skin temperature (cold and clammy, warm and moist, or warm and dry) are clues to cardiovascular function. When the patient arrives in the clinical unit, the surgical site is observed for bleeding, type and integrity of dressing, and drains.

Also assessed when the patient arrives on the clinical unit are the patient's mental status and level of consciousness, speech, and orientation in comparison with preoperative baseline measures. Although a change in mental status or postoperative restlessness may be related to anxiety, pain, or medications, it may also be a symptom of oxygen deficit or hemorrhage. These serious causes must be investigated and excluded before other causes are pursued.

General discomfort resulting from lying in one position on the operating table, the surgeon's handling of tissues, the body's reaction to anesthesia, and anxiety are also common causes of restlessness. These discomforts may be relieved by administering the prescribed analgesics, changing the patient's position frequently, and assessing and alleviating the cause of anxiety. If tight, drainage-soaked bandages are causing discomfort, reinforcing or changing the dressing completely makes the patient more comfortable. The bladder is palpated for distention because urinary retention can also cause restlessness.

Diagnosis

NURSING DIAGNOSES

Based on the assessment data, major nursing diagnoses may include the following:

- Risk for ineffective airway clearance related to depressed respiratory function, pain, and bed rest

- Acute pain related to surgical incision
- Decreased cardiac output related to shock or hemorrhage
- Activity intolerance related to generalized weakness secondary to surgery
- Impaired skin integrity related to surgical incision and drains
- Risk for imbalanced body temperature related to surgical environment and anesthetic agents
- Risk for imbalanced nutrition, less than body requirements related to decreased intake and increased need for nutrients secondary to surgery
- Risk for constipation related to effects of medications, surgery, dietary change, and immobility
- Risk for urinary retention related to anesthetic agents
- Risk for injury related to surgical procedure or anesthetic agents
- Anxiety related to surgical procedure
- Risk for ineffective management of therapeutic regimen related to insufficient knowledge about wound care, dietary restrictions, activity recommendations, medications, follow-up care, or signs and symptoms of complications

COLLABORATIVE PROBLEMS/ POTENTIAL COMPLICATIONS

Based on the assessment data, potential complications may include the following:

- Deep vein thrombosis
- Hematoma
- Infection
- Wound dehiscence or evisceration

Planning and Goals

The major goals for the patient include optimal respiratory function, relief of pain, optimal cardiovascular function, increased activity tolerance, unimpaired wound healing, maintenance of body temperature, and maintenance of nutritional balance. Further goals include resumption of usual pattern of bowel and bladder elimination, identification of any perioperative positioning injury, acquisition of sufficient knowledge to manage self-care after discharge, and absence of complications.

Nursing Interventions

PREVENTING RESPIRATORY COMPLICATIONS

Respiratory depressive effects of opioid medications, decreased lung expansion secondary to pain, and decreased mobility combine to put the patient at risk for common respiratory complications, particularly atelectasis (incomplete expansion of the lung), pneumonia, and hypoxemia (Finkelmeier, 2000; Rothrock, 2003). Atelectasis remains a risk for the patient who is not moving well or ambulating or who is not performing deep-breathing and coughing exercises or using an incentive spirometer. Signs and symptoms include decreased breath sounds over the affected area, crackles, and cough. Pneumonia is characterized by chills and fever, tachycardia, and tachypnea. Cough may or may not be present and may or may not be productive. Hypostatic pulmonary congestion, caused by a weakened cardiovascular system that permits stagnation of secretions at lung bases, may develop; it occurs most frequently in elderly patients who are not mobilized effectively. The symptoms are often vague, with perhaps a slight elevation of temperature, pulse, and respiratory rate and a

cough. Physical examination reveals dullness and crackles at the base of the lungs. If the condition progresses, the outcome may be fatal.

The types of hypoxemia that can affect postoperative patients are subacute and episodic. Subacute hypoxemia is a constant low level of oxygen saturation, although breathing appears normal. Episodic hypoxemia develops suddenly, and the patient may be at risk for cerebral dysfunction, myocardial ischemia, and cardiac arrest. Patients at risk for hypoxemia include those who have undergone major surgery (particularly abdominal), are obese, or have preexisting pulmonary problems. Hypoxemia can be detected by pulse oximetry, which measures blood oxygen saturation. Factors that may affect the accuracy of pulse oximetry readings include cold extremities, tremors, atrial fibrillation, acrylic nails, and black or blue nail polish (these colours interfere with the functioning of the pulse oximeter; other colours do not).

Preventive measures and timely recognition of signs and symptoms help avert pulmonary complications. Strategies to prevent respiratory complications include use of an incentive spirometer and deep-breathing and coughing exercises. Crackles indicate static pulmonary secretions that need to be mobilized by coughing and deep-breathing exercises. When a mucus plug obstructs one of the bronchi entirely, the pulmonary tissue beyond the plug collapses, and a massive atelectasis results.

To clear secretions and prevent pneumonia, the nurse encourages the patient to turn frequently and take deep breaths at least every 2 hours. Coughing is also encouraged to dislodge mucus plugs. These pulmonary exercises should begin as soon as the patient arrives on the clinical unit and continue until the patient is discharged. Even if he or she is not fully awake from anesthesia, the patient can be asked to take several deep breaths. This helps to expel residual anesthetic agents, mobilize secretions, and prevent alveolar collapse (atelectasis). Careful splinting of abdominal or thoracic incision sites helps the patient overcome the fear that the exertion of coughing might open the incision. Analgesic agents are administered to permit more effective coughing, and oxygen is administered as prescribed to prevent or relieve hypoxia. To encourage lung expansion, the patient is encouraged to yawn or take sustained maximal inspirations to create a negative intrathoracic pressure of −40 mm Hg and expand lung volume to total capacity. Chest physical therapy may be prescribed if indicated.

Coughing is contraindicated in patients who have head injuries or who have undergone intracranial surgery (because of the risk for increasing intracranial pressure), as well as in patients who have undergone eye surgery (risk for increasing intraocular pressure) or plastic surgery (risk for increasing tension on delicate tissues). In patients with an abdominal or thoracic incision, the nurse teaches the patient how to splint the incision while coughing.

Most postoperative patients, especially the elderly and those with an abdominal or thoracic incision, are given an incentive spirometer to use. In incentive spirometry, the patient performs sustained maximal inspirations and can see the results of these efforts as they register on the spirometer. Such feedback encourages the patient to continue to take deep breaths to maximize voluntary lung expansion. A target is established for each patient. The patient first exhales, then places the lips around the mouthpiece and slowly inhales, trying to drive the piston on the device to a marked goal. Using a spirometer has several advantages: it encourages the patient to participate actively in treatment; it ensures that the manoeuvre is physiologically appropriate and is repeated; and it is a cost-effective way of preventing complications. A common recommendation for use of the incentive spirometer is 10 deep breaths every hour while awake. Refer to Chapter 25 for additional discussion of incentive spirometry.

Early ambulation increases metabolism and pulmonary aeration and, in general, improves all body functions. The patient is encouraged to be out of bed as soon as possible (ie, on the day of surgery, or no later than the first postoperative day). This practice is especially valuable in preventing pulmonary complications in older patients.

RELIEVING PAIN

Most patients experience some pain after a surgical procedure (Rothrock, 2003). Many factors (motivational, affective, cognitive, and emotional) influence the pain experience. Research findings have led to a better understanding of how perception, learning, personality, ethnic and cultural factors, and environment can affect anxiety, depression, and pain response (Schafheutle, Cantrill & Noyce, 2001; Watt-Watson, Stevens, Garfinkel et al., 2001). The degree and severity of postoperative pain and the patient's tolerance for pain depend on the incision site, the nature of the surgical procedure, the extent of surgical trauma, the type of anesthetic agent, and how the agent was administered. The preoperative preparation received by the patient (including information about what to expect as well as reassurance and psychological support) is a significant factor in decreasing anxiety, apprehension, and even the amount of postoperative pain.

The reasons for controlling pain are compelling. There is a well-known correlation between frequency of complications and localization of pain (Moline, 2001). Intense pain stimulates the stress response, which adversely affects the cardiac and immune systems. When pain impulses are transmitted, muscle tension increases, as does local vasoconstriction. The ischemia in the affected area causes further stimulation of pain receptors. When these noxious impulses travel centrally, sympathetic activity is compounded, which increases myocardial demand and oxygen consumption. Research has shown that cardiovascular insufficiency occurs three times more frequently, and the incidence of infection is five times greater, in people with poor postoperative pain control (Moline, 2001; Schafheutle et al., 2001; Watt-Watson et al., 2001). The hypothalamic stress response is also responsible for an increase in blood viscosity and platelet aggregation. This can lead to phlebothrombosis and pulmonary embolism.

Often the physician has prescribed different medications or dosages to cover various levels of pain. The nurse should discuss these options with the patient to determine the best medication. Then the nurse should assess the effectiveness of the medication periodically, beginning 30 minutes after administration or sooner if the medication is being delivered by patient-controlled analgesia.

Opioid Analgesics

About one third of patients report severe pain, one third moderate pain, and one third little or no pain. These statistics do not mean that the patients in the last group have no pain; rather, they appear to activate psychodynamic mechanisms that impair the registering of pain ("gate closing" theory and nociceptive transmission). See Chapter 13 for a more detailed discussion of pain and the factors influencing the pain experience.

Opioid analgesics are commonly prescribed for pain and immediate postoperative restlessness. A preventive approach rather than an "as needed" (PRN) approach, is more effective in relieving pain. With a preventive approach, the medication is administered at prescribed intervals rather than when the pain becomes severe or unbearable. Many patients (and some health

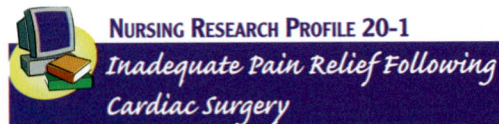

NURSING RESEARCH PROFILE 20-1
Inadequate Pain Relief Following Cardiac Surgery

Watt-Watson, J., Stevens, B., Garfinkel, P., Streiner, D., & Gallup, R. (2001). Relationships between nurses' pain knowledge and pain management outcomes for their postoperative cardiac patients. *Journal of Advanced Nursing, 36*(4), 535–545.

Purpose
Although studies have examined nurses' knowledge and perceived barriers to pain management, few studies have examined the relationship of nurses' knowledge and their actual implementation of pain management strategies. This Canadian study investigated the relationship between nursing pain knowledge and pain management outcomes for postoperative coronary artery bypass graft (CABG) patients.

Study Sample and Design
This was a descriptive, correlational, mixed between-within subjects design. A convenience sample of 94 nurses from four cardiovascular units in three university-affiliated hospitals were interviewed, along with 225 of their assigned patients. The nurses included 86 women and 8 men. The patients included 52 women and 173 men. Instruments used with the patients included the McGill Pain Questionnaire-Short Form (MPQ-SF), the present pain intensity (PPI) scale, and a visual analog scale (VAS); analgesic prescription and administration data were obtained by chart review. The Toronto Pain Management Inventory (TPMI) was used to measure pain knowledge in the nurses. The social desirability scale (SDS) was also used with the nurses.

Findings
The majority of patients reported moderate to severe pain during the previous 24 hours (86%) and at the time of interview while moving around (68%). The mean total score on the MPQ-SF, which has a range of possible scores from 0 to 45, was 11.8 ± 7. Chart review data indicated undermedication of patients for pain, with patients receiving only 47% of their prescribed analgesia. The nurses' scores on the TPMI indicated moderate pain knowledge, with the majority of nurses (53%) scoring 69% or less and only 15% scoring 75% or greater on the inventory. While hospital policy required documentation of pain as a fifth vital sign, charting of pain was minimal and high pain ratings did not result in an increase in analgesics administered.

Nursing Implications
Nurses caring for postoperative CABG patients need further education about pain management. Nurses also need to be aware that patients are undermedicated following CABG surgery and need to be more aware of patients' needs for medication, administer prescribed doses, and advocate for patients when pain medication is not prescribed.

care providers) are overly concerned with the risk of drug addiction in the postoperative patient. This risk, however, is negligible with the use of opioid medications for short-term pain control.

Patient-Controlled Analgesia

Given the negative impact of pain on recovery, nurses need to think "pain prevention" rather than sporadic pain control and should encourage the use of patient-controlled analgesia (PCA). Patients recover more quickly when adequate pain measures are used, and PCA permits patients to administer their own pain medication when needed (Quinn, 1999). The amount of medication delivered by the IV or epidural route and the time span during which the opioid medication is released are controlled by the PCA device. Self-administration promotes patient participation in care, eliminates delayed administration of pain medications, and maintains a therapeutic drug level.

Most patients are candidates for PCA. The two requirements for PCA are an understanding of the need to self-dose and the physical ability to self-dose. Upon sensing pain, the patient activates the medication-delivering pump with a hand-held button. PCA enables the patient to move, turn, cough, and take deep breaths with less pain, thus reducing postoperative pulmonary problems.

Epidural Infusions and Intrapleural Anesthesia

For thoracic, orthopedic, obstetric, and major abdominal surgery, certain opioid analgesics may be administered by epidural or intrathecal infusion. Epidural infusions produce a more profound analgesia. Epidural infusions are used with caution in chest procedures because the effect of the analgesic may ascend along the spinal cord and affect respiration. Intrapleural anesthesia involves the administration of local anesthetic by a catheter between the parietal and visceral pleura. It provides sensory anesthesia without affecting motor function to the intercostal muscles. This anesthesia allows more effective coughing and deep breathing in conditions such as cholecystectomy, renal surgery, and rib fractures in which pain in the thoracic region would interfere with these functions.

A local opioid or a combination anesthetic (opioid plus local anesthetic agent) is used in the epidural infusion. Other local anesthetic methods may be used to provide analgesia and anesthesia. Intrapleural anesthesia has fewer adverse effects than systemic or spinal opioids and a lower incidence of urinary retention, vomiting, and pruritus when compared with thoracic epidural opioids (Moline, 2001; Quinn, 1999).

Other Pain Relief Measures

For pain that is difficult to control, a subcutaneous pain management system may be used. This is a silicone catheter that is inserted at the affected area. The catheter is attached to a pump that delivers a continuous amount of local anesthetic at a specific amount determined and prescribed by the physician (Fig. 20-5).

Complete absence of pain in the area of the surgical incision may not occur for a few weeks, depending on the site and nature of surgery, but the intensity of postoperative pain gradually subsides on subsequent days. However, pain control continues to be an important concern for the patient and the nurse. Effective pain management allows the patient to participate in care, perform deep-breathing and leg exercises, and tolerate activity. As stated previously, poor pain control contributes to postoperative complications and increased length of stay. The nurse continues to assess the pain level, the effectiveness of pain medication, and factors that influence pain tolerance (eg, energy level, stress level, cultural background, meaning of pain to the patient). The nurse explains that taking pain medication before the pain becomes intense is more effective and offers pain medication at intervals rather than waiting for the patient to request medication. Nonpharmacologic pain relief measures, such as imagery, relaxation, massage, application of heat or cold (if prescribed), and distraction, can be used to supplement medications (Seers & Carroll, 1998). Changing the patient's position, using distraction, applying cool washcloths to the face, and rubbing the back with a soothing lotion may be useful in relieving general discomfort

FIGURE 20-5 Subcutaneous pain management system comprises a pump, filter, and catheter that delivers a specific amount of prescribed local anesthetic at a rate determined by the physician. With permission from I-Flow Corporation, Lake Forest, CA.

temporarily and rendering medication more effective when it is administered.

PROMOTING CARDIAC OUTPUT

If signs and symptoms of shock or hemorrhage occur, treatment and nursing care are implemented as described in the discussion of care in the PACU.

> **! NURSING ALERT** A systolic blood pressure of less than 90 mm Hg is usually considered reportable at once. However, the patient's preoperative or baseline blood pressure is used to make informed postoperative comparisons. A previously stable blood pressure that shows a downward trend of 5 mm Hg at each 15-minute reading should also be reported.

Although most patients do not hemorrhage or go into shock, changes in circulating volume, the stress of surgery, and the effects of medications and preoperative preparations all affect cardiovascular function. Intravenous fluid replacement is standard for up to 24 hours after surgery or until the patient is stable and tolerating oral fluids. Close monitoring is indicated to detect and correct conditions such as fluid volume deficit, altered tissue perfusion, and decreased cardiac output, all of which can increase the patient's discomfort, place him or her at risk for complications, and prolong the hospital stay. Some patients are at risk for fluid volume excess secondary to existing cardiovascular or renal disease, advanced age, or the release of adrenocorticotropic hormone and antidiuretic hormone as a result of the stress of surgery. Consequently, fluid replacement must be carefully managed, and intake and output records must be accurate.

Nursing management includes assessing the patency of the IV lines and ensuring that the appropriate fluids are administered at the prescribed rate. Intake and output, including emesis and output from wound drainage systems, are recorded separately and totalled to determine fluid balance. If the patient has an indwelling urinary catheter, hourly outputs are monitored and rates of less than 30 mL/h are reported; if the patient is voiding, an output of less than 240 mL per 8-hour shift is reported. Electrolyte levels and hemoglobin and hematocrit levels are monitored. Decreased hemoglobin and hematocrit levels can indicate blood loss or dilution of circulating volume by IV fluids. If dilution is contributing to the decreased levels, the hemoglobin and hematocrit rise as the stress response abates and fluids are mobilized and excreted.

Venous stasis from dehydration, immobility, and pressure on leg veins during surgery put the patient at risk for deep vein thrombosis. Leg exercises and frequent position changes are initiated early in the postoperative period to stimulate circulation. Patients should avoid positions that compromise venous return, such as raising the bed's knee gatch or placing a pillow under the knees, sitting for long periods, and dangling the legs with pressure at the back of the knees. Venous return is promoted by elastic compression stockings and early ambulation. Early ambulation has a significant effect on recovery and the prevention of complications and can begin, in many instances, the evening of surgery. Postoperative activity orders are checked before getting the patient out of bed. Sitting up at the edge of the bed for a few minutes may be all the patient can tolerate at first.

ENCOURAGING ACTIVITY

Most surgical patients are encouraged to be out of bed as soon as possible. Early ambulation reduces the incidence of postoperative complications, such as atelectasis, hypostatic pneumonia, gastrointestinal discomfort, and circulatory problems (Rothrock, 2003). Ambulation increases ventilation and reduces the stasis of bronchial secretions in the lung. It also reduces postoperative abdominal distention by increasing gastrointestinal tract and abdominal wall tone and stimulating peristalsis. Thrombophlebitis or phlebothrombosis occurs less frequently because early ambulation prevents stasis of blood by increasing the rate of circulation in the extremities. Pain is often decreased when early ambulation is possible, and the hospital stay is shorter and less costly, a further advantage to the patient and the hospital.

Despite the advantages of early ambulation, patients may be reluctant to get up the evening of surgery. Reminding them of the importance of early mobility in preventing complications may help them overcome their fears. One concern when the patient is to get out of bed for the first time is orthostatic hypotension, also called postural hypotension. Orthostatic hypotension is an abnormal drop in blood pressure that occurs as the patient changes from a supine to a standing position. It is common after surgery because of changes in circulating volume and bed rest. Signs and symptoms include a 20-mm Hg decrease in systolic blood pressure or a 10-mm Hg decrease in diastolic blood pressure, weakness, dizziness, and fainting. Older adults are at increased risk for

orthostatic hypotension secondary to age-related changes in vascular tone. To detect orthostatic hypotension, the nurse assesses the patient's feelings of dizziness and his or her blood pressure first in the supine position, after the patient sits up, again after the patient stands, and 2 to 3 minutes later. Gradual position change gives the circulatory system time to adjust. If the patient becomes dizzy, he or she should be returned to the supine position, and getting out of bed should be delayed for several hours.

To assist the postoperative patient in getting out of bed for the first time after surgery, the nurse performs the following actions:

1. Help the patient to move gradually from the lying position to the sitting position until dizziness passes. This can be achieved by raising the head of the bed.
2. Position the patient completely upright (sitting) and turned so that both legs are hanging over the edge of the bed.
3. Assist the patient to stand beside the bed.

When accustomed to the upright position, the patient may start to walk. The nurse should be at the patient's side to give physical support and encouragement. Care must be taken not to tire the patient; the extent of the first few periods of ambulation varies with the type of surgical procedure and the patient's physical condition and age.

Whether or not the patient can ambulate early in the postoperative period, bed exercises are encouraged to improve circulation. Bed exercises consist of the following:

- Arm exercises (full range of motion, with specific attention to abduction and external rotation of the shoulder)
- Hand and finger exercises
- Foot exercises to prevent deep vein thrombosis, foot drop, and toe deformities and to aid in maintaining good circulation
- Leg flexion and leg-lifting exercises to prepare the patient for ambulation
- Abdominal and gluteal contraction exercises

Hampered by pain, dressings, IV lines, or drains, many patients cannot engage in activity without assistance. Prolonged inactivity may lead to pressure ulcers, deep vein thrombosis, atelectasis, or hypostatic pneumonia. Helping the patient increase his or her activity level on the first postoperative day is an important nursing function. One way to increase the patient's activity is to have the patient perform as much routine hygiene care as possible. Setting up the patient to bathe with a bedside wash basin or, if possible, assisting the patient to the bathroom to sit in a chair at the sink not only gets the patient moving but helps restore a sense of self-control and prepares the patient for discharge.

To be safely discharged to home, patients need to be able to ambulate a functional distance (length of the house or apartment), get in and out of bed unassisted, and be independent with toileting. Patients can be asked to perform as much as they can and then to call for assistance. The patient and the nurse can collaborate on a schedule for progressive activity that includes ambulating in the room and hallway and sitting out of bed in the chair. Assessing the patient's vital signs before, during, and after a scheduled activity helps the nurse and patient determine the rate of progression. By providing physical support, the nurse maintains the patient's safety; by communicating a positive attitude about the patient's ability to perform the activity, the nurse promotes the patient's confidence. The nurse should make sure the patient continues to perform bed exercises, wears pneumatic compression or thigh-high elastic compression stockings when in bed, and rests as needed.

PROMOTING WOUND HEALING

Ongoing assessment of the surgical site involves inspection for approximation of wound edges, integrity of sutures or staples, redness, discolouration, warmth, swelling, unusual tenderness, or drainage. The area around the wound should also be inspected for reactions to tape or trauma from tight bandages.

Nursing interventions to promote wound healing also include management of surgical drains and dressings. Wound drains are tubes exiting the peri-incisional area into either a portable wound suction device (closed) or into the dressings (open). The principle involved is to allow the escape of blood and serous fluids that can otherwise serve as a culture medium for bacteria. In portable wound suction, the use of gentle, constant suction enhances drainage of these fluids and collapses the skin flaps against the underlying tissue, thus removing "dead space." Types of wound drains include the Penrose, Hemovac, and Jackson-Pratt drains (Fig. 20-6). Output from wound drainage systems and all new drainage is recorded. The amount of bloody drainage on the surgical dressing is assessed frequently. Spots of drainage on the dressings are outlined with a pen, and the date and time of the outline are recorded on the dressing so that increased drainage can be easily seen. A certain amount of bloody drainage in a wound drainage system or on the dressing is expected, but excessive amounts should be reported to the surgeon. Increasing amounts of fresh blood on the dressing should be reported immediately. Some wounds are irrigated heavily before closure in the operating room, and open drains exiting the wound may be embedded in the dressings. These wounds may drain large amounts of blood-tinged fluid that saturate the dressing. The dressing can be reinforced with sterile gauze bandages; the time that they were reinforced should be documented. If drainage continues, the surgeon should be notified so that the dressing can be changed. Multiple similar drains are numbered or otherwise labelled (eg, left lower quadrant, left upper quadrant) so that output measurements can be reliably and consistently recorded.

Surgical wound healing occurs in three phases: the inflammatory, proliferative, and maturation phases (Table 20-2). Wounds also heal by different mechanisms, depending on the condition of the wound. These mechanisms include first-, second-, or third-intention wound healing (Rothrock, 2003).

First-Intention Healing

Wounds made aseptically, with a minimum of tissue destruction, and properly closed heal with little tissue reaction by first intention (primary union) (Fig. 20-7). When wounds heal by **first-intention healing**, granulation tissue is not visible and scar formation is minimal. Postoperatively, many of these wounds are covered with a dry sterile dressing. If a cyanoacrylate tissue adhesive was used to close the incision without the use of sutures, a dressing is contraindicated (Vargas & Reger, 2000).

Second-Intention Healing

Second-intention healing (granulation) occurs in infected wounds (abscess) or in wounds in which the edges have not been approximated. When an abscess is incised, it collapses partly, but the dead and the dying cells forming its walls are still being released into the cavity. For this reason, drainage tubes or gauze packing are inserted into the abscess pocket to allow drainage to escape easily. Gradually, the necrotic material disintegrates and escapes, and the abscess cavity fills with a red, soft, sensitive tissue that bleeds easily. This tissue is composed of minute, thin-walled capillaries and buds that later form connective tissue. These buds, called granulations, enlarge until they fill the area left by the destroyed tissue (see Fig. 20-7). The cells surrounding the capillaries change their round shape to become long, thin, and intertwined to form a scar (cicatrix). Healing is complete when skin cells (epithelium) grow over these granulations. This method of repair is called healing by granulation, and it takes place whenever pus is formed or when loss of tissue has occurred for any reason. When the postoperative wound is allowed to heal by secondary intention, it is usually packed with saline-moistened sterile dressings and covered with a dry sterile dressing.

Third-Intention Healing

Third-intention healing (secondary suture) is used for deep wounds that have either not been sutured early or that break down and are resutured later, thus bringing together two apposing granulation surfaces. This results in a deeper and wider scar. These wounds are also packed postoperatively with moist gauze and covered with a dry sterile dressing.

Safety pin keeps drain from slipping into wound

A   Drain sponge   **B**   **C**

FIGURE 20-6 Types of surgical drains: (**A**) Penrose, (**B**) Jackson-Pratt, (**C**) Hemovac.

Table 20-2 • Phases of Wound Healing

PHASE	DURATION	EVENTS
Inflammatory (also called lag or exudative phase)	1–4 days	Blood clot forms Wound becomes edematous Debris of damaged tissue and blood clot are phagocytosed
Proliferative (also called fibroblastic or connective tissue phase)	5–20 days	Collagen produced Granulation tissue forms Wound tensile strength increases
Maturation (also called differentiation, resorptive, remodeling, or plateau phase)	21 days to months or even years	Fibroblasts leave wound Tensile strength increases Collagen fibres reorganize and tighten to reduce scar size

As a wound heals, many factors, such as adequate nutrition, cleanliness, rest, and position, determine how quickly healing occurs. These factors are influenced by nursing interventions. Specific nursing assessments and interventions that address these factors and help to promote wound healing are presented in Table 20-3. Other nursing interventions include assessment and care of the wound.

CHANGING THE DRESSING

While the first postoperative dressing is usually changed by a member of the surgical team, subsequent dressing changes in the immediate postoperative period are usually performed by the nurse. A dressing is applied to a wound for one or more of the following reasons: (1) to provide a proper environment for wound

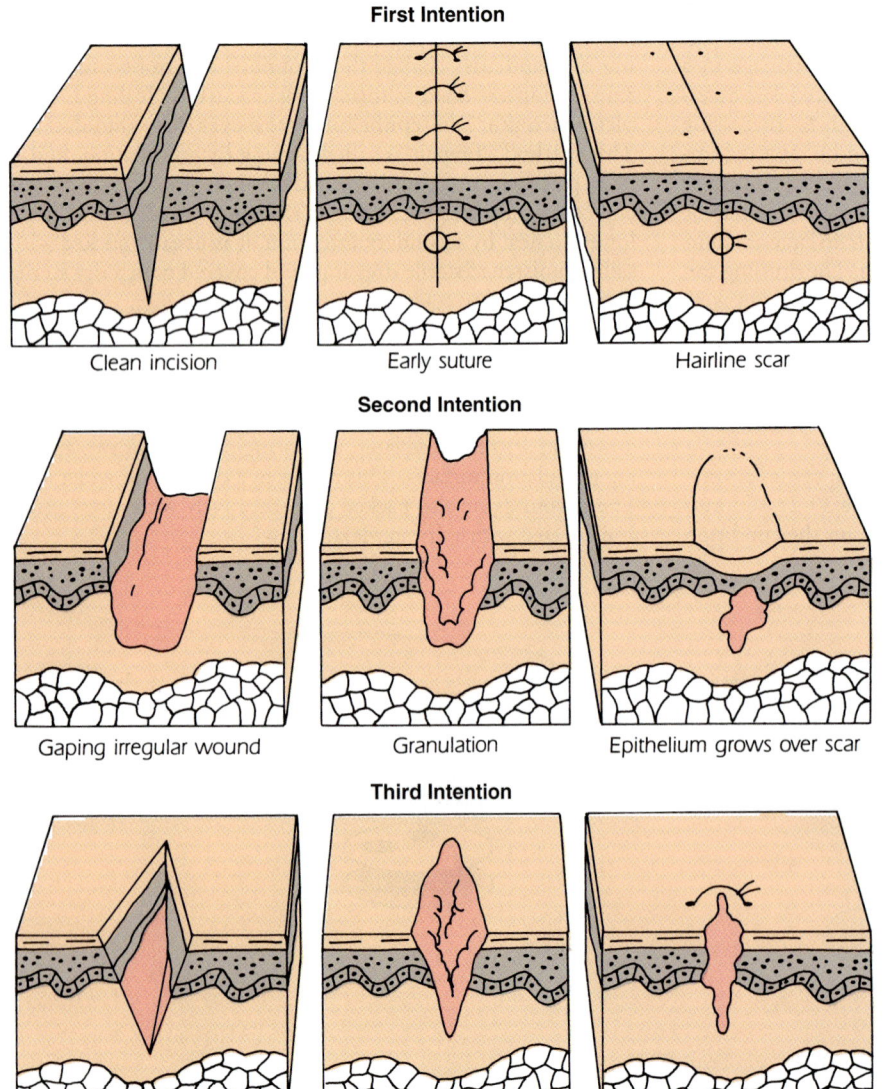

First Intention

Clean incision   Early suture   Hairline scar

Second Intention

Gaping irregular wound   Granulation   Epithelium grows over scar

Third Intention

Wound   Increased granulation   Late suturing with wide scar

FIGURE 20-7 Types of wound healing: first intention healing, second intention healing, and third intention healing.

Table 20-3 • Factors Affecting Wound Healing

FACTORS	RATIONALE	NURSING INTERVENTIONS
Age of patient	The older the patient, the less resilient the tissues.	Handle all tissues gently.
Handling of tissues	Rough handling causes injury and delayed healing.	Handle tissues carefully and evenly.
Hemorrhage	Accumulation of blood creates dead spaces as well as dead cells that must be removed. The area becomes a growth medium for organisms.	Monitor vital signs. Observe incision site for evidence of bleeding and infection.
Hypovolemia	Insufficient blood volume leads to vasoconstriction and reduced oxygen and nutrients available for wound healing.	Monitor for volume deficit (circulatory impairment). Correct by fluid replacement as prescribed.
Local factors		
Edema	Reduces blood supply by exerting increased interstitial pressure on vessels	Elevate part; apply cool compresses.
Inadequate dressing technique		
Too small	Permits bacterial invasion and contamination	Follow guidelines for proper dressing technique.
Too tight	Reduces blood supply carrying nutrients and oxygen	
Nutritional deficits	Protein-calorie depletion may occur. Insulin secretion may be inhibited, causing blood glucose to rise.	Correct deficits; this may require parenteral nutritional therapy. Monitor blood glucose levels. Administer vitamin supplements as prescribed.
Foreign bodies	Foreign bodies retard healing.	Keep wounds free of dressing threads, talcum, and powder from gloves.
Oxygen deficit (tissue oxygenation insufficient)	Insufficient oxygen may be due to inadequate lung and cardiovascular function as well as localized vasoconstriction.	Encourage deep breathing, turning, controlled coughing.
Drainage accumulation	Accumulated secretions hamper healing process.	Monitor closed drainage systems for proper functioning. Institute measures to remove accumulated secretions.
Medications		
Corticosteroids	May mask presence of infection by impairing normal inflammatory response	Be aware of action and effect of medications patient is receiving.
Anticoagulants	May cause hemorrhage	
Broad-spectrum and specific antibiotics	Effective if administered immediately before surgery for specific pathology or bacterial contamination. If administered after wound is closed, ineffective because of intravascular coagulation.	
Patient overactivity	Prevents approximation of wound edges. Resting favours healing.	Use measures to keep wound edges approximated: taping, bandaging, splints. Encourage rest.
Systemic disorders	These depress cell functions that directly affect wound healing.	Be familiar with the nature of the specific disorder. Administer prescribed treatment. Cultures may be indicated to determine appropriate antibiotic.
Hemorrhagic shock		
Acidosis		
Hypoxia		
Renal failure		
Hepatic disease		
Sepsis		
Immunosuppressed state	Patient is more vulnerable to bacterial and viral invasion; defense mechanisms are impaired.	Provide maximum protection to prevent infection. Restrict visitors with colds; institute mandatory hand hygiene by all staff.
Wound stressors	Produce tension on wounds, particularly of the torso.	Encourage frequent turning and ambulation and administer antiemetic medications as prescribed. Assist patient in splinting incision.
Vomiting		
Valsalva manoeuvre		
Heavy coughing		
Straining		

healing; (2) to absorb drainage; (3) to splint or immobilize the wound; (4) to protect the wound and new epithelial tissue from mechanical injury; (5) to protect the wound from bacterial contamination and from soiling by feces, vomitus, and urine; (6) to promote hemostasis, as in a pressure dressing; and (7) to provide mental and physical comfort for the patient.

The patient is told that the dressing is to be changed and that changing the dressing is a simple procedure associated with little discomfort. The dressing change is performed at a suitable time (eg, not at mealtimes or when visitors are present). Privacy is provided, and the patient is not unduly exposed. The nurse should avoid referring to the incision as a scar since the term may have negative connotations for the patient. Assurance is given that the incision will shrink as it heals and the redness will fade.

The nurse carries out hand hygiene before and after the dressing change and wears disposable gloves for the dressing change itself. The tape or adhesive portion of the dressing is removed by pulling it parallel with the skin surface and in the direction of hair growth, rather than at right angles. Alcohol wipes or nonirritating solvents aid in removing adhesive painlessly and quickly. The old dressing is removed and then deposited in a container designated for biomedical waste disposal. In accordance with standard precautions, dressings are never touched by ungloved hands because of the danger of transmitting pathogenic organisms.

If the patient is sensitive to adhesive tape, the dressing may be held in place with hypoallergenic tape. Many tapes are porous to permit ventilation and prevent skin maceration. The correct way to apply tape is to place the tape at the centre of the dressing and then press the tape down on both sides, applying tension evenly away from the midline. The wrong method of applying tape—fixing one end of the tape to the skin and pulling it tight over the dressing—often wrinkles and pulls the skin in the process. The resulting continuous and forceful traction produces a shearing effect, causing the epidermal layer to slip sideways and become separated from the deeper dermal layers. Some wounds become edematous after having been dressed, causing considerable tension on the tape. If the tape is not flexible, the stretching bandage will also cause a shear injury to the skin. This can result in denuded areas or large blisters. An elastic adhesive bandage (Elastoplast, Microfoam-3M) may be used to hold dressings in place over mobile areas, such as the neck or the extremities, or where pressure is required.

While changing the dressing, the nurse has an opportunity to teach the patient how to care for the incision and change the dressings at home. The nurse observes for indicators of the patient's readiness to learn, such as looking at the incision, expressing interest, or assisting in the dressing change. Information on self-care activities and possible signs of infection are summarized in Chart 20-3.

MAINTAINING NORMAL BODY TEMPERATURE

The patient is still at risk for malignant hyperthermia and hypothermia in the postoperative period (Fortunato-Phillips, 2000). Efforts are made to identify malignant hyperthermia and to treat it early and promptly (Redmond, 2001). (See the discussion of malignant hyperthermia in Chap. 19.)

Patients who have been anesthetized are susceptible to chills and drafts. Attention to hypothermia management, begun in the intraoperative period, extends into the postoperative period to prevent significant nitrogen loss and catabolism. Signs of hypothermia are reported to the physician. The room is maintained at a comfortable temperature, and blankets are provided to prevent chilling. Treatment includes oxygen administration, adequate

---

Chart 20-3 • PATIENT EDUCATION
Wound Care Instructions

Until Sutures Are Removed
1. Keep the wound dry and clean.
   - If there is no dressing, ask your nurse or physician if you can bathe or shower.
   - If a dressing or splint is in place, do not remove it unless it is wet or soiled.
   - If wet or soiled, change dressing yourself if you have been taught to do so; otherwise, call your nurse or physician for guidance.
   - If you have been taught, instruction might be as follows:
     Cleanse area *gently* with sterile normal saline once or twice daily.
     Cover with a sterile Telfa pad or gauze square large enough to cover wound.
     Apply hypoallergenic tape (Dermacel or paper). Adhesive is not recommended because it is difficult to remove without possible injury to the incisional site.
2. Immediately report any of these signs of infection:
   - Redness, marked swelling exceeding 2.5 cm from incision site; tenderness; or increased warmth around wound
   - Red streaks in skin near wound
   - Pus or discharge, foul odour
   - Chills or temperature higher than 37.7°C
3. If soreness or pain causes discomfort, apply a dry cool pack (containing ice or cold water) or take prescribed

acetaminophen tablets (2) every 4–6 hours. Avoid using aspirin without direction or instruction because bleeding can occur with its use.
4. Swelling after surgery is common. To help reduce swelling, elevate the affected part to the level of the heart.
   - Hand or arm
     Sleep—elevate arm on pillow at side
     Sitting—place arm on pillow on adjacent table
     Standing—rest affected hand on opposite shoulder; support elbow with unaffected hand
   - Leg or foot
     Sitting—place a pillow on a facing chair; provide support underneath the knee
     Lying—place a pillow under affected leg

After Sutures Are Removed
Although the wound appears to be healed when sutures are removed, it is still tender and will continue to heal and strengthen for several weeks.
1. Follow recommendations of physician or nurse regarding extent of activity.
2. Keep suture line clean; do not rub vigorously; pat dry. Wound edges may look red and may be slightly raised. This is normal.
3. If the site continues to be red, thick, and painful to pressure after 8 weeks, consult the health care provider. (This may be due to excessive collagen formation and should be checked.)

hydration, and proper nutrition. The patient is also monitored for cardiac dysrhythmias. The risk for hypothermia is greater in the elderly and in patients who were in the cool operating room environment for a prolonged period.

MANAGING GASTROINTESTINAL FUNCTION AND RESUMING NUTRITION

Gastrointestinal discomfort (nausea, vomiting, hiccups) and resumption of oral intake are issues for both the patient and the nurse. Nausea and vomiting are common after anesthesia (Litwack, 1999; Rothrock, 2003). They are more common in women, obese people (fat cells act as reservoirs for the anesthetic), patients prone to motion sickness, and patients who have undergone lengthy surgical procedures. Other causes of postoperative vomiting include an accumulation of fluid in the stomach, inflation of the stomach, and the ingestion of food and fluid before peristalsis resumes.

When vomiting is likely because of the nature of surgery, a nasogastric tube is inserted preoperatively and remains in place throughout the surgery and the immediate postoperative period. In addition, a nasogastric tube may be inserted when a patient who has food in the stomach requires emergency surgery.

Hiccups, produced by intermittent spasms of the diaphragm secondary to irritation of the phrenic nerve, can occur after surgery. The irritation may be direct, such as from stimulation of the nerve by a distended stomach, subdiaphragmatic abscess, or abdominal distention; indirect, such as from toxemia or uremia that stimulates the centre; or reflexive, such as irritation from a drainage tube or obstruction of the intestines. Usually these occurrences are mild, transitory attacks that cease spontaneously. When hiccups persist, they may produce considerable distress and serious effects such as vomiting, exhaustion, and wound dehiscence. The physician may prescribe phenothiazine medications for severe, persistent hiccups.

Once nausea and vomiting have subsided and the patient is fully awake and alert, the sooner he or she can tolerate a usual diet, the more quickly normal gastrointestinal function will resume. Taking food by mouth stimulates digestive juices and promotes gastric function and intestinal peristalsis. The return to normal dietary intake should proceed at the pace set by the patient. Of course, the nature of surgery and the type of anesthesia directly affect the rate at which normal gastric activity resumes. Liquids are typically the first substances desired and tolerated by the patient after surgery. Water, fruit juices, and tea may be given in increasing amounts. Cool fluids are tolerated more easily than those that are ice cold or hot. Soft foods (gelatin, custard, milk, and creamed soups) are added gradually after clear fluids have been tolerated. As soon as the patient tolerates soft foods well, solid food may be given.

Assessment and management of gastrointestinal function are important after surgery because the gastrointestinal tract is subject to uncomfortable or potentially life-threatening complications. Any postoperative patient may suffer from distention. Postoperative distention of the abdomen results from the accumulation of gas in the intestinal tract. Manipulation of the abdominal organs during surgery may produce a loss of normal peristalsis for 24 to 48 hours, depending on the type and extent of surgery. Even though nothing is given by mouth, swallowed air and gastrointestinal secretions enter the stomach and the intestines; if not propelled by peristalsis, they collect in the intestines, producing distention and causing the patient to complain of fullness or pain in the abdomen. Most often, the gas collects in the colon.

Abdominal distention is further increased by immobility, anesthetic agents, and the use of opioid medications.

After major abdominal surgery, distention may be avoided by having the patient turn frequently, exercise, and ambulate as early as possible. This also alleviates distention produced by swallowing air, which is common in anxious patients. When postoperative distention is anticipated, a nasogastric tube may be inserted before surgery. The tube may remain in place until full peristaltic activity (indicated by the passage of flatus) has resumed. The nurse can determine when peristaltic bowel sounds return by listening to the abdomen with a stethoscope. Bowel sounds are documented so that diet progression can occur.

Paralytic ileus and intestinal obstruction are potential postoperative complications that occur more frequently in patients undergoing intestinal or abdominal surgery. Refer to Chapter 37 for discussion of treatment.

PROMOTING BOWEL FUNCTION

Constipation is common after surgery and can range from a minor irritation to a serious complication (Fox, 1998). Decreased mobility, decreased oral intake, and opioid analgesics contribute to difficulty having a bowel movement. In addition, irritation and trauma to the bowel during surgery may inhibit intestinal movement for several days. The combined effect of early ambulation, improved dietary intake, and a stool softener (if prescribed) promotes bowel elimination. Until the patient reports return of normal bowel function, the nurse should assess the abdomen for distention and the presence and frequency of bowel sounds. If the abdomen is not distended and bowel sounds are normal, and if the patient does not have a bowel movement by the second or third postoperative day, the physician should be notified so that a laxative can be given that evening.

MANAGING VOIDING

Urinary retention after surgery can occur for various reasons. Anesthetics, anticholinergic agents, and opioids interfere with the perception of bladder fullness and the urge to void and inhibit the ability to initiate voiding and completely empty the bladder. Abdominal, pelvic, and hip surgery may increase the likelihood of retention secondary to pain. Additionally, some patients find it difficult to use the bedpan or urinal in the recumbent position.

Bladder distention and the urge to void should be assessed on the patient's arrival on the unit and frequently thereafter. The patient is expected to void within 8 hours of surgery (this includes time spent in the PACU). If the patient has an urge to void and cannot, or if the bladder is distended and no urge is felt or the patient cannot void, catheterization is not delayed solely on the basis of the 8-hour time frame. All methods to encourage the patient to void should be tried (eg, letting water run, applying heat to the perineum). The bedpan should be warm; a cold bedpan causes discomfort and automatic tightening of muscles (including the urethral sphincter). When the patient cannot void on a bedpan, it may be permissible to use a commode rather than resorting to catheterization. Male patients are often permitted to sit up or stand beside the bed to use the urinal, but safeguards should be taken to prevent the patient from falling or fainting due to loss of coordination from medications or orthostatic hypotension. If the patient cannot void in the specified time frame, the patient is catheterized and the catheter removed after the bladder has emptied. Straight intermittent catheterization is preferred over indwelling catheterization because the risk for infection is increased with an indwelling catheter.

Even if the patient voids, the bladder may not necessarily be empty. The nurse notes the amount of urine voided and palpates the suprapubic area for distention or tenderness. A portable ultrasound device may also be used to assess residual volume. Intermittent catheterization continues every 4 to 6 hours until the patient can void spontaneously and the postvoid residual is less than 100 mL.

MAINTAINING A SAFE ENVIRONMENT

During the immediate postoperative period, the patient recovering from anesthesia should have all side rails up, and the bed should be in the low position. The nurse assesses the patient's level of consciousness and orientation and determines if the patient needs his or her eyeglasses or hearing aid, because impaired vision, inability to hear postoperative instructions, or inability to communicate verbally place the patient at risk for injury. All objects the patient may need should be within reach, especially the call bell. Any immediate postoperative orders concerning special positioning, equipment, or interventions should be implemented as soon as possible. The patient is instructed to ask for assistance with any activity. Although they are occasionally necessary for the disoriented patient, restraints should not be used if at all possible.

Any surgical procedure has the potential for injury due to disrupted neurovascular integrity resulting from prolonged awkward positioning in the operating room, manipulation of tissues, inadvertent severing of nerves, or tight bandages. Any orthopedic surgery or surgery involving the extremities carries a risk for peripheral nerve damage. Vascular surgeries, such as replacing sections of diseased peripheral arteries or inserting an arteriovenous graft, put the patient at risk for thrombus formation at the surgical site and subsequent ischemia of tissues distal to the thrombus. Assessment includes having the patient move the hand or foot distal to the surgical site through a full range of motion, assessing that all surfaces have intact sensation, and assessing peripheral pulses.

PROVIDING EMOTIONAL SUPPORT TO THE PATIENT AND FAMILY

Although patients and families are undoubtedly relieved that surgery is over, anxiety levels may remain high in the immediate postoperative period. Many factors contribute to this anxiety: pain, being in an unfamiliar environment, feeling unable to control one's circumstances, fear of the long-term effects of surgery, fear of complications, loss of ability to care for self, fatigue, spiritual distress, altered role responsibilities, ineffective coping, and altered body image are all potential reactions to the surgical experience. The nurse helps the patient and family work through their anxieties by providing reassurance and information and by spending time listening to and addressing their concerns. The nurse describes hospital routines and what to expect in the ensuing hours and days until discharge and explains the purpose of nursing assessments and interventions. Informing patients when they will be able to drink fluids or eat, when they will be getting out of bed, and when tubes and drains will be removed helps them gain a sense of control and participation in recovery and engages them in the plan of care. Acknowledging family members' concerns and accepting and encouraging their participation in the patient's care assists them in feeling they are helping their loved one. The nurse can manipulate the environment to enhance rest and relaxation by providing privacy, reducing noise, adjusting the lighting, providing enough seating for family members, and performing any other measures that will produce a supportive atmosphere.

MANAGING POTENTIAL COMPLICATIONS

Deep Vein Thrombosis

Deep vein thrombosis and other complications, such as pulmonary embolism, are serious potential complications of surgery (Chart 20-4). The stress response that is initiated as a result of surgery inhibits the fibrinolytic system, resulting in blood hypercoagulability. Dehydration, low cardiac output, blood pooling in the extremities, and bed rest add to the risk of thrombosis formation. Although all postoperative patients are at some risk, certain surgeries and patient populations carry a greater risk. The first symptom of deep vein thrombosis may be a pain or cramp in the calf. Although not present in all cases, calf pain elicited on ankle dorsiflexion (Homans' sign) suggests thrombosis (Fig. 20-8). Initial pain and tenderness may be followed by a painful swelling of the entire leg, often accompanied by a fever, chills, and diaphoresis.

Prophylactic treatment for postoperative patients at risk is common practice. Low-dose heparin may be prescribed and administered subcutaneously until the patient is ambulatory. Low-molecular-weight heparin and low-dose warfarin are other anticoagulants that may be used. External pneumatic compression and thigh-high elastic compression stockings can be used alone or in combination with low-dose heparin.

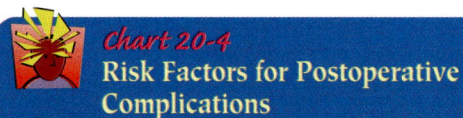

Chart 20-4
Risk Factors for Postoperative Complications

Patients at increased risk for postoperative complications (eg, deep vein thrombosis) and pulmonary problems include the following:

Deep Vein Thrombosis
- Orthopedic patients having hip surgery, knee reconstruction, and other lower extremity surgery
- Urologic patients having transurethral prostatectomy, and older patients having urologic surgery
- General surgical patients over 40 years of age, those who are obese, those with a malignancy, those who have had prior deep vein thrombosis or pulmonary embolism, or those undergoing extensive, complicated surgical procedures
- Gynecologic (and obstetric) patients over 40 years of age with added risk factors (varicose veins, previous venous thrombosis, infection, malignancy, obesity)
- Neurosurgical patients, similar to other surgical high-risk groups (in patients with stroke, for instance, the risk of deep vein thrombosis in the paralyzed leg is as high as 75%)

Pulmonary Complications
- Type of surgery—greater incidence after all forms of abdominal surgery when compared with peripheral surgery
- Location of incision—the closer the incision to the diaphragm, the higher the incidence of pulmonary complications
- Preoperative respiratory problems
- Age—greater risk after age 40 than before age 40
- Sepsis
- Obesity—weight greater than 110% of ideal body weight
- Prolonged bed rest
- Duration of surgical procedure—more than 3 hours
- Aspiration
- Dehydration
- Malnutrition
- Hypotension and shock
- Immunosuppression

FIGURE 20-8 Assessment of signs and symptoms of deep vein thrombosis. (**A**) With the knee flexed, the patient may complain of pain in the calf on dorsiflexion of the foot (Homans' sign). This is a sign of early and subclinical thrombosis, which may or may not be present. Gentle compression reveals tenderness of the calf muscles (note arrow). (**B**) The affected leg may swell; veins are more prominent and may be palpated easily.

The benefits of early ambulation and hourly leg exercises in preventing deep vein thrombosis cannot be overemphasized, and these activities are recommended for all patients, regardless of their risk. It is important to avoid the use of blanket rolls, pillow rolls, or any form of elevation that can constrict vessels under the knees. Even prolonged "dangling" (having the patient sit on the edge of the bed with legs hanging over the side) can be dangerous and is not recommended in susceptible patients because pressure under the knees can impede circulation. Adequate hydration is also encouraged; the patient can be offered juices and water throughout the day to avoid dehydration. Refer to Chapter 30 for a complete discussion of deep vein thrombosis and to Chapter 23 for discussion of pulmonary embolus.

Hematoma

At times, concealed bleeding occurs beneath the skin at the surgical site. This hemorrhage usually stops spontaneously but results in clot (hematoma) formation within the wound. If the clot is small, it will be absorbed and need not be treated. When the clot is large, the wound usually bulges somewhat, and healing will be delayed unless the clot is removed. After several sutures are removed by the physician, the clot is evacuated and the wound is packed lightly with gauze. Healing occurs usually by granulation, or a secondary closure may be performed.

Infection (Wound Sepsis)

The creation of a surgical wound disrupts the integrity of the skin and its protective function. Exposure of deep body tissues to pathogens in the environment places the patient at risk for infection of the surgical site, a potentially life-threatening complication. Surgical site infection increases hospital length of stay, costs of care, and risk for further complications. In postoperative patients, surgical site infection is the most common nosocomial infection, with 67% of these infections occurring within the incision and 33% occurring in an organ or space around the surgical site (CDC, 1999). Recent research suggests that the administration of supplemental oxygen during colorectal resection and for 2 hours postoperatively reduces the incidence of postoperative infection (Greif, Ozan, Horn et al., 2000).

Multiple factors place the patient at risk for wound infection. One risk factor is the wound classification. Surgical wounds are classified according to the degree of contamination. Table 20-4 defines the terms used to describe surgical wounds and gives the expected rate of wound infection per category. Other risk factors

Table 20-4 • Wound Classification and Associated Surgical Site Infection Risk

SURGICAL CATEGORY	DETERMINANTS OF CATEGORY	EXPECTED RISK OF POSTSURGICAL INFECTION (%)
Clean	Nontraumatic site Uninfected site No inflammation No break in aseptic technique No entry into respiratory, alimentary, genitourinary, or oropharyngeal tracts	1–3
Clean-contaminated	Entry into respiratory, alimentary, genitourinary or oropharyngeal tracts without unusual contamination Appendectomy Minor break in aseptic technique Mechanical drainage	3–7
Contaminated	Open, newly experienced traumatic wounds Gross spillage from gastrointestinal tract Major break in aseptic technique Entry into genitourinary or biliary tract when urine or bile is infected	7–16
Dirty	Traumatic wound with delayed repair, devitalized tissue, foreign bodies, or fecal contamination Acute inflammation and purulent drainage encountered during procedure	16–29

include both patient-related factors and those associated with the surgical procedure. Patient-related factors include age, nutritional status, diabetes, smoking, obesity, remote infections, endogenous mucosal microorganisms, altered immune response, length of preoperative stay, and severity of illness (Bryant, 2000). Factors related to the surgical procedure include the method of preoperative skin preparation, surgical attire of the team, method of sterile draping, duration of surgery, antimicrobial prophylaxis, aseptic technique, factors related to surgical technique, drains or foreign material, operating room ventilation, and exogenous microorganisms. Efforts to prevent wound infection are directed at reducing these risks. Preoperative and intraoperative risks and interventions are discussed in Chapters 18 and 19. Although the conditions for surgical site infection and serious contamination of the wound occur in the preoperative and intraoperative time frames, postoperative care of the wound centres on assessing the wound, preventing contamination and infection before wound edges have sealed, and enhancing healing.

Wound infection may not present until at least postoperative day 5. Most patients are discharged before that time, and more than half of wound infections are diagnosed after discharge, highlighting the importance of patient education regarding wound care. Risk factors for wound sepsis include wound contamination, foreign body, faulty suturing technique, devitalized tissue, hematoma, debilitation, dehydration, malnutrition, anemia, advanced age, extreme obesity, shock, length of preoperative hospitalization, duration of surgical procedure, and associated disorders (eg, diabetes mellitus, immunosuppression). Signs and symptoms of wound infection include pulse rate and temperature elevation; an elevated white blood cell count; wound swelling, warmth, tenderness, or discharge; and incisional pain. Local signs may be absent if the infection is deep. *Staphylococcus aureus* accounts for many postoperative wound infections. Other infections may result from *Escherichia coli, Proteus vulgaris, Aerobacter aerogenes, Pseudomonas aeruginosa,* and other organisms. Although rare, beta-hemolytic streptococcal or clostridial infections can be rapid and deadly. If wound infection due to beta-hemolytic streptococcus or clostridium occurs, extreme care is needed to prevent spread of infection to others. Intensive medical and nursing care is essential if the patient is to survive.

When a wound infection is diagnosed in a surgical incision, the surgeon may remove one or more sutures or staples and, using aseptic precautions, separate the wound edges with a pair of blunt scissors or a hemostat. Once the incision is opened, a drain is inserted. If the infection is deep, an incision and drainage procedure may be necessary. Antimicrobial therapy and a wound care regimen are also initiated (Byrant, 2000).

Wound Dehiscence and Evisceration

Wound **dehiscence** (disruption of surgical incision or wound) and **evisceration** (protrusion of wound contents) are serious surgical complications (Fig. 20-9). Dehiscence and evisceration are especially serious when they involve abdominal incisions or wounds. These complications result from sutures giving way, from infection, and, more frequently, after marked distention or strenuous cough. They may also occur because of increasing age, poor nutritional status, and pulmonary or cardiovascular disease in patients undergoing abdominal surgery.

When the wound edges separate slowly, the intestines may protrude gradually or not at all, and the earliest sign may be a gush of bloody (serosanguineous) peritoneal fluid from the wound. When a wound ruptures suddenly, coils of intestine may push out of the abdomen. The patient may report that "some-

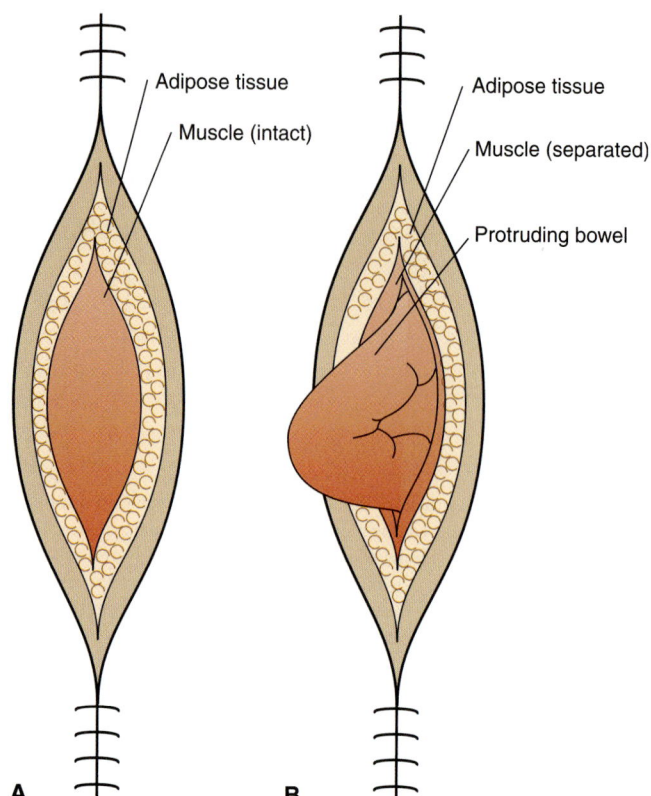

FIGURE 20-9   (**A**) Wound dehiscence; (**B**) wound evisceration.

thing gave way." The evisceration causes pain and can be associated with vomiting.

 NURSING ALERT   When disruption of a wound occurs, the patient is placed in low Fowler's position and instructed to lie quietly. These actions minimize protrusion of body tissues. The protruding coils of intestine are covered with sterile dressings moistened with sterile saline solution, and the surgeon is notified at once.

An abdominal binder, properly applied, is an excellent prophylactic measure against an evisceration and often is used along with the primary dressing, especially in patients with weak or pendulous abdominal walls or when rupture of a wound has occurred.

 ## Gerontologic Considerations

Older adults recover more slowly, have a longer hospital stay, and are at greater risk for developing postoperative complications (Polanczyk et al., 2001). Delirium, pneumonia, decline in functional ability, exacerbation of comorbid conditions, pressure ulcers, decreased oral intake, gastrointestinal disturbance, and falls are all threats to recovery in the older adult. Expert nursing care can help the older adult avoid these complications or minimize their effects.

Postoperative delirium, characterized by confusion, perceptual and cognitive deficits, altered attention levels, disturbed sleep patterns, and impaired psychomotor skills, is a significant problem for older adults. Causes of delirium are multifactorial (Chart 20-5).

Chart 20-5 Causes of Postoperative Delirium

- Fluid and electrolyte imbalance
- Dehydration
- Hypoxia
- Hypercarbia
- Acid–base disturbance
- Infection (urinary tract, wound, respiratory)
- Medications (anticholinergics, benzodiazepines, central nervous system depressants)
- Unrelieved pain
- Blood loss
- Decreased cardiac output
- Cerebral hypoxia
- Heart failure
- Acute myocardial infarction
- Hypothermia or hyperthermia
- Unfamiliar surroundings and sensory deprivation
- Emergent surgery
- Alcohol withdrawal
- Urinary retention
- Fecal impaction

Skilled and frequent assessment of mental status and of all physiologic factors influencing mental status helps the nurse plan care, because in the elderly patient delirium may be the initial or only early indicator of infection, fluid and electrolyte imbalance, or deterioration of respiratory or hemodynamic status. Factors that determine if the patient is at risk for delirium include age, history of alcohol abuse, preoperative cognitive function, physical function, serum chemistries, and type of surgery.

Recognizing postoperative delirium and identifying and treating its underlying cause are the goals of care. Postoperative delirium is sometimes mistaken for preexisting dementia or is attributed to age. In addition to monitoring and managing identifiable causes, nurses can implement supportive interventions. Keeping the patient in a well-lit room and close to the nurses' station can help with sensory deprivation. At the same time, distracting and unfamiliar noises should be minimized. Because pain can contribute to postoperative delirium, the nurse collaborates with the physician or geriatric nurse specialist and the patient to achieve pain relief without oversedation (Lynch, Lazor, Gellis et al., 1998). The patient is reoriented as often as necessary, and staff should introduce themselves each time they come in contact with the patient. Engaging the patient in conversation and care activities and placing a clock and calendar nearby may improve cognitive function. Physical activity should not be neglected while the patient is confused, because physical deterioration can worsen delirium and place the patient at increased risk for other complications. Restraints should be avoided because they can also worsen confusion. If possible, a family member or staff member is asked to sit with the patient instead. Haloperidol (Haldol) or lorazepam (Ativan) may be given during episodes of acute confusion, but these medications should be discontinued as soon as possible to avoid side effects.

Other problems confronting the older postoperative patient, such as pneumonia, altered bowel function, deep vein thrombosis, weakness, and functional decline, often can be prevented by early and progressive ambulation. Ambulation means walking, not just getting out of bed and sitting in a chair. Prolonged sitting positions that promote venous stasis in the lower extremities should be avoided. Assistance with ambulation may be required to keep the patient from bumping into objects and falling. A physical therapy referral may be indicated to promote safe, regular exercise for the older adult.

Urinary incontinence can be prevented by providing easy access to the call bell and the commode and by prompting voiding. Early ambulation and familiarity with the room help the patient to become self-sufficient sooner.

Optimal nutritional status is important for wound healing, return of normal bowel function, and fluid and electrolyte balance. The nurse and patient can consult with the dietitian to plan appealing, high-protein meals that provide sufficient fibre, calories, and vitamins. Nutritional supplements, such as Ensure or Sustacal, may be recommended. Multivitamins, iron, and vitamin C supplements aid in tissue healing, formation of new red blood cells, and overall nutritional status and are commonly prescribed postoperatively.

In addition to monitoring and managing the older adult's physiologic recovery, the nurse identifies and addresses psychosocial needs. The older adult may require more encouragement and support to resume activities, and the pace may be slower. Sensory deficits may require frequent repetition of instructions, and decreased physiologic reserve may necessitate frequent rest periods. The older adult may require extensive discharge planning to coordinate both professional and family care providers, and the nurse, social worker, or nurse case manager may institute the plan for continuing care.

PROMOTING HOME AND COMMUNITY-BASED CARE

Teaching Patients Self-Care

Patients have always required detailed discharge instructions to become proficient in special self-care needs after surgery; however, dramatically reduced hospital lengths of stay during the past decade have greatly increased the amount of information that should be provided while reducing the amount of time in which to provide it (Fox, 1998; Quinn, 1999). Although needs are specific to individual patients and the procedures they have undergone, general patient education needs for postoperative care have been identified (see Chart 20-1).

Continuing Care

Continuing care provided by community-based services is frequently necessary after surgery. Older patients, patients who live alone, patients without family support, and patients with preexisting disabilities are often in greatest need. Planning for discharge involves arranging for necessary services early in the acute care hospitalization. Wound care, drain management, catheter care, infusion therapy, and physical or occupational therapy are some of the needs addressed by community health care providers. The home care nurse coordinates these activities and services.

During home care visits, the nurse assesses the patient for postoperative complications; the nurse also assesses the surgical incision, respiratory and cardiovascular status, adequacy of pain management, fluid and nutritional status, and the patient's progress in returning to preoperative status. The nurse assesses the patient's and family's ability to manage dressing changes and drainage systems and other devices and to administer prescribed medications. The nurse may change dressings or catheters if needed. The nurse determines if any additional services are needed and assists the patient and family to arrange for them. Previous teaching is reinforced, and the patient is reminded to keep follow-up appointments. The patient and family are instructed about signs and symptoms to be reported to the surgeon. In addition, the nurse may provide information about how to obtain needed supplies and may suggest resources or support groups the patient may want to contact. In many settings, postoperative telephone calls are made to answer questions, assess recovery, and reassure patients and families.

Evaluation

EXPECTED PATIENT OUTCOMES

Expected patient outcomes may include:

1. Maintains optimal respiratory function
   a. Performs deep-breathing exercises
   b. Displays clear breath sounds
   c. Uses incentive spirometer as prescribed
   d. Splints incisional site when coughing to reduce pain
2. Indicates that pain is decreased in intensity
3. Exercises and ambulates as prescribed
   a. Alternates periods of rest and activity
   b. Progressively increases ambulation
   c. Resumes normal activities within prescribed time frame
   d. Performs activities related to self-care
4. Wound heals without complication
5. Maintains body temperature within normal limits
6. Resumes oral intake
   a. Reports absence of nausea and vomiting
   b. Takes at least 75% of usual diet
   c. Is free of abdominal distress and gas pains
   d. Exhibits normal bowel sounds
7. Reports resumption of usual bowel elimination pattern
8. Resumes usual voiding pattern
9. Is free of injury
10. Exhibits decreased anxiety
11. Acquires knowledge and skills necessary to manage therapeutic regimen
12. Experiences no complications

Critical Thinking Exercises

1. Your patient has a history of esophageal cancer and is HIV positive. After undergoing ambulatory surgery to insert a gastric feeding tube, he is to be discharged to home. Indicate which assessment findings would indicate his readiness for discharge. Describe a teaching plan for the patient and his family. How would you modify the plan if the patient lives alone?

2. A patient who has undergone abdominal surgery reports severe pain and as a result is unable to cough and deep breathe. When you listen to the patient's lungs you hear crackles in the bases. Analyze these findings and indicate the interventions you would implement in this situation. How would your care differ if the patient has a musculoskeletal disorder that makes turning and ambulation difficult?

3. You are visiting a 72-year-old woman who had emergency surgery for a broken hip 3 weeks ago and has returned to her home, where she is living alone. How would you direct your assessment to identify the factors that might affect her recovery? How would you modify your assessment and nursing care plan because of her age?

REFERENCES AND SELECTED READINGS

Books

American Pain Society. (1999). *Principles of analgesic use in the treatment of acute pain and cancer pain.* Glenview, IL: Author.

American Society of Anesthesiologists. (1995). *ASA standards for postanesthesia care.* Park Ridge, IL: Author.

American Society of PeriAnesthesia Nurses. (2000). *Standards of perianesthesia nursing practice.* Thorofare, NJ: ASPAN.

Byrant, R. (2000). *Acute and chronic wounds* (2d ed.). St. Louis: Mosby.

Economou, S. G., & Economou, T. S. (1999). *Instructions for surgery patients.* Philadelphia: WB Saunders.

Ethicon Endo-Surgery, Inc. (2000). *Nursing quick reference card: On-Q Soaker catheter 6.5 pain management system.* Cincinnati, OH: Author.

Finkelmeier, B. (2000). *Cardiothoracic surgical nursing* (2d ed.). Philadelphia: Lippincott Williams & Wilkins.

Karch, A. (Ed.). (2002). *Nursing drug guide.* Philadelphia: Lippincott Williams & Wilkins.

Litwack, K. (1999). *Core curriculum for perianesthesia nursing practice.* Philadelphia: WB Saunders.

Quinn, D. M. (Ed.). (1999). *Ambulatory surgical nursing core curriculum.* Philadelphia: WB Saunders.

Rothrock, J. C. (2003). *Alexander's care of the patient in surgery* (12th ed.). St. Louis: Mosby.

Schwartz, S., & Shires, G. T. (1999). *Principles of surgery.* New York: McGraw-Hill.

Journals

Asterisks indicate nursing research articles.

Anesthesia care: New guidelines on postanesthesia care (2002). *OR Manager, 18*(1), 21.

Aldreta, J. A. (1998). Modifications to the postanesthesia score for use in ambulatory surgery. *Journal of Perianesthesia Nursing, 12*(3), 148–155.

Aranda, M., & Hanson, W. (2000). Anesthetics, sedatives, and paralytics: Understanding their use in the intensive care unit. *Surgical Clinics of North America, 80*(3), 933–947.

Bennet, J., Haas, R., & Wren, K. R. (2001). Opioid use during the perianesthesia period: Nursing implications. *Journal of Perianesthesia Nursing, 16*(4), 255–258.

Buckle, J. (1999). Aromatherapy in perianesthesia nursing. *Journal of Perianesthesia Nursing, 14*(6), 336–344.

Centers for Disease Control and Prevention (1999). Guideline for prevention of surgical site infections. *Infection Control and Hospital Epidemiology, 20*(4), 247–280.

Fortunato-Phillips, N. (2000). Malignant hyperthermia: Update 2000. *Critical Care Nursing Clinics of North America, 12*(2), 199–210.

Fox, V. J. (1998). Postoperative education that works. *AORN Journal, 67*(5), 1010, 1012–1017.

Goodwin, S. A. (1998). A review of preemptive analgesia. *Journal of Perianesthesia Nursing, 13*(2), 109–114.

Gordon, D. B. (1999). Pain management in the elderly. *Journal of Perianesthesia Nursing, 14*(6), 367–372.

Greif, R., Ozan, A., Horn, E., et al. (2000). Supplemental perioperative oxygen to reduce the incidence of surgical wound infection. *New England Journal of Medicine, 342*(3), 161–167.

Hession, M. C. (1998). Factors influencing successful discharge after outpatient laparoscopic cholecystectomy. *Journal of Perianesthesia Nursing, 13*(1), 11–15.

Hilbig, J. I., & Manning, J. (1999) Accountability and responsibility underpins successful pain management. *Journal of Perianesthesia Nursing, 14*(6), 390–392.

Jeran, L. (2001). Patient temperature: An introduction to the clinical guideline for the prevention of unplanned perioperative hypothermia. *Journal of Perianesthesia Nursing, 16*(5), 303–314.

Lynch, E. P., Lazor, M. A., Gellis, J. E., et al. (1998). The impact of postoperative pain in the development of postoperative delirium. *Anesthesia and Analgesia, 86,* 761–785.

Mamaril, M., & Hooper, V. (1998). Fast tracking versus bypassing phase I: rapid PACU progression. *Breathline, 17*(7), 12.

Marley, R. A., & Swanson, J. (2001). Patient care after discharge from the ambulatory surgical center. *Journal of Perianesthesia Nursing, 16*(6), 399–419.

Moline, B. M. (2001). Pain management in the ambulatory surgical population. *Journal of Perianesthesia Nursing, 16*(6), 388–398.

Polanczyk, C., Marcantonio, E., Goldman, L., et al. (2001). Impact of age on perioperative complications and length of stay in patients undergoing noncardiac surgery. *Annals of Internal Medicine, 134*(8), 637–643.

Redmond, M. C. (2001). Malignant hyperthermia: Perianesthesia recognition, treatment, and care. *Journal of Perianesthesia Nursing, 16*(4), 259–270.

Scales, B. (2001). CAMPing in the PACU: Using complementary and alternative medical practices in the PACU. *Journal of Perianesthesia Nursing, 16*(5), 325–334.

Schroeter, K. (1999). Pain management: Ethical issues for the perianesthesia nurse. *Journal of Perianesthesia Nursing, 14*(6), 393–397.

Schafheutle, E., Cantrill, J. & Noyce, P. (2001). Why is pain management suboptimal on surgical wards? *Journal of Advanced Nursing, 33*(6), 728–737.

Schwartz, L. B. (1998). Conventional and alternative therapies for acute deep vein thrombosis. *Journal of Care Management, 4,* 9–12, 32.

Seers, K., & Carroll, D. (1998). Relaxation techniques for acute pain management. *Journal of Advanced Nursing, 27*(3), 466–476.

Vargas, G., & Reger, T. (2000). An alternative to sutures. *Medsurg Nursing, 9*(2), 83–85.

Watkins, A. C., & White, P. F. (2001). Fast-tracking after ambulatory surgery. *Journal of Perianesthesia Nursing, 16*(6), 379–387.

*Watt-Watson, J., Stevens, B., Garfinkel, P., et al. (2001). Relationships between nurses' pain knowledge and pain management outcomes for their postoperative cardiac patients. *Journal of Advanced Nursing, 36*(4), 535–545.

RESOURCES AND WEBSITES

American Academy of Ambulatory Care Nursing, East Holly Ave., Box 56, Pitman, NJ, 08071; (856) 256-2350; (800) AMB-NURS; http://www.aaacn.org.

American Society of PeriAnesthesia Nurses, 10 Melrose Ave., Suite 110, Cherry Hill, NJ 08003-3696; (856) 616-9600 or 9601; toll-free 1-877-737-9696; fax (856) 616-9621; http://www.aspan.org.

Association of PeriOperative Registered Nurses, Inc., 2170 S. Parker Road, Suite 300, Denver, CO 80231; (800) 755-2676, (303) 755-6304; http://www.aorn.org.

Canadian Anesthesiologists' Society. 1 Eglinton Avenue East, Suite 208, Toronto, ON M4P 3A1; http://www.cas.ca.

Malignant Hypothermia Association of Canada. 200 Elizabeth Street, Room ES3-403, Toronto, ON M5G 2C4; http://www.mhacanada.org/home.htm.

Operating Room Nurses Association of Canada (ORNAC), http://www.ornac.ca.

The Canadian Pain Society. 701 Rossland Road East, Suite 373, Whitby, ON L1N 9K3; http://www.canadianpainsociety.ca.

Gas Exchange and Respiratory Function

Applying Concepts from NANDA, NIC, and NOC

Mrs. Brant, age 73, is admitted to the hospital for LLL pneumonia. Her vital signs are: T: 38.11°C; HR: 90 and regular; RR: 28; BP: 142/74. She has a weak cough, diminished breath sounds over the lower left lung field, and coarse rhonchi over the mid-tracheal area. She can expectorate some sputum, which is thick and greyish-green. She has a history of stroke. Secondary to the stroke she has impaired gag and cough reflexes and mild weakness of her left side. She is allowed food and fluids because she can swallow safely if she uses the chin-tuck manoeuvre. The concept map illustrates the relationships that exist among the nursing diagnoses, interventions, and outcomes for one of Mrs. Brant's clinical problems.

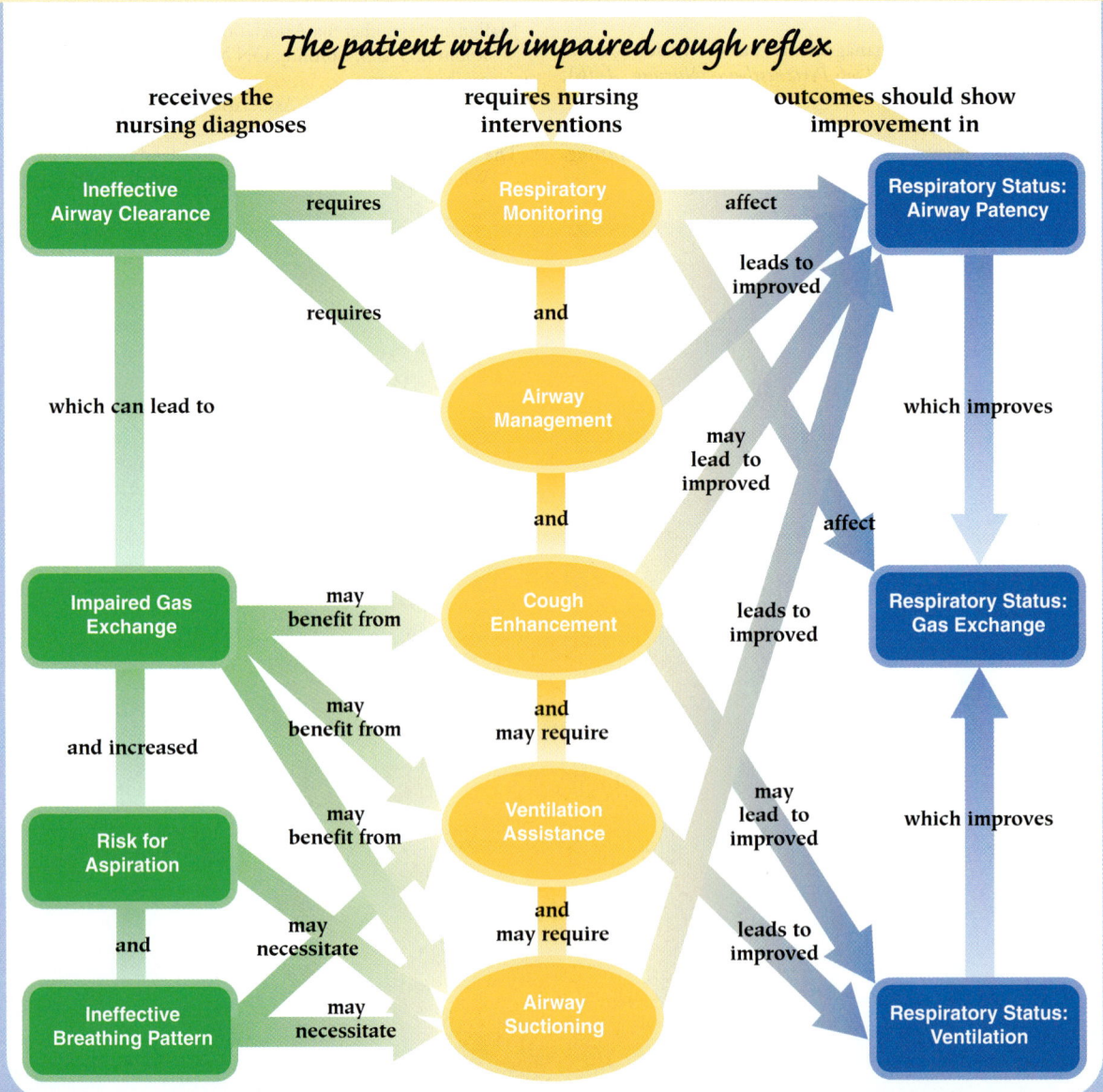

The patient with impaired cough reflex

receives the nursing diagnoses — requires nursing interventions — outcomes should show improvement in

Ineffective Airway Clearance — requires → Respiratory Monitoring — affect → Respiratory Status: Airway Patency

Ineffective Airway Clearance — requires → Airway Management

Ineffective Airway Clearance — which can lead to

Impaired Gas Exchange — may benefit from → Cough Enhancement

Impaired Gas Exchange — may benefit from → Ventilation Assistance

and increased

Risk for Aspiration — may benefit from → Ventilation Assistance

Risk for Aspiration — and → may necessitate → Airway Suctioning

Ineffective Breathing Pattern — may necessitate → Airway Suctioning

leads to improved — Respiratory Status: Airway Patency — which improves

may lead to improved

affect → Respiratory Status: Gas Exchange

leads to improved

may lead to improved — which improves

leads to improved

Respiratory Status: Ventilation

Nursing Classifications and Languages

NANDA
Nursing Diagnoses

Ineffective Airway Clearance— Inability to clear secretions or obstructions from the respiratory tract to maintain a clear airway

Impaired Gas Exchange—Excess or deficit in oxygenation and/or carbon dioxide elimination at the alveolar-capillary membrane

Risk for Aspiration—At risk for entry of gastrointestinal secretions, oropharyngeal secretions, solids or fluids into tracheobronchial passages

Ineffective Breathing Pattern— Inspiration and/or expiration that does not provide adequate ventilation

NIC
Nursing Interventions*

Respiratory Monitoring— Collection and analysis of patient data to ensure airway patency and adequate gas exchange

Airway Management—Facilitation of patency of air passages

Cough Enhancement—Promotion of deep inhalation by the patient with subsequent generation of high intrathoracic pressures and compression of underlying lung parenchyma for the forceful expulsion of air

Ventilation Assistance— Promotion of an optimal spontaneous breathing pattern that maximizes oxygen and carbon dioxide exchange in the lungs

Airway Suctioning—Removal of airway secretions by inserting a suction catheter into the patient's oral airway and/or trachea

NOC
Nursing Outcomes†

Return to functional baseline status, stabilization of, or improvement in

Respiratory Status: Airway Patency—Extent to which the tracheobronchial passages remain open; measured on a scale of extremely compromised to not compromised

Respiratory Status: Gas Exchange—The alveolar exchange of O_2 or CO_2 to maintain arterial blood gas concentrations; measured on a scale of extremely compromised to not compromised

Respiratory Status: Ventilation— Movement of air in and out of the lungs; measured on a scale of extremely compromised to not compromised

NANDA, North American Nursing Diagnosis Association; NIC, Nursing Interventions Classification; NOC, Nursing Outcomes Classification.

*Iowa Intervention Project © 2000. In McCloskey, J. C., & Bulechek, G. M. (2000). *Nursing interventions classification (NIC)* (3rd ed.). St. Louis: Mosby.

†Iowa Outcomes Project © 2000. In Johnson, M., Maas, M., & Moorhead, S. (2000). *Nursing outcomes classification (NOC)* (3rd ed.). St. Louis: Mosby.

Assessment of Respiratory Function

Adapted by Carolyn J. M. Ross

LEARNING OBJECTIVES

On completion of this chapter, the learner will be able to:

1. Describe the structures and functions of the upper and lower respiratory tracts.

2. Describe ventilation, perfusion, diffusion, shunting, and the relationship of pulmonary circulation to these processes.

3. Discriminate between normal and abnormal breath sounds.

4. Use assessment parameters appropriate for determining the characteristics and severity of the major symptoms of respiratory dysfunction.

5. Identify the nursing implications of the various procedures used for diagnostic evaluation of respiratory function.

*D*isorders of the respiratory system are common and are encountered by nurses in every setting from the community to the intensive care unit. To assess the respiratory system, the nurse must be skilled at differentiating normal assessment findings from abnormal ones. Good assessment skills must be developed and used when caring for patients with acute and chronic respiratory problems. In addition, an understanding of respiratory function and the significance of abnormal diagnostic test results is essential.

Anatomic and Physiologic Overview

The respiratory system is composed of the upper and lower respiratory tracts. Together, the two tracts are responsible for **ventilation** (movement of air in and out of the airways). The upper tract, known as the upper airway, warms and filters inspired air so that the lower respiratory tract (the lungs) can accomplish gas exchange. Gas exchange involves delivering oxygen to the tissues through the bloodstream and expelling waste gases, such as carbon dioxide, during expiration.

ANATOMY OF THE UPPER RESPIRATORY TRACT

Upper airway structures consist of the nose, sinuses and nasal passages, pharynx, tonsils and adenoids, larynx, and trachea.

Nose

The nose is composed of an external and an internal portion. The external portion protrudes from the face and is supported by the nasal bones and cartilage. The anterior nares (nostrils) are the external openings of the nasal cavities.

The internal portion of the nose is a hollow cavity separated into the right and left nasal cavities by a narrow vertical divider, the septum. Each nasal cavity is divided into three passageways by the projection of the turbinates (also called conchae) from the lateral walls. The nasal cavities are lined with highly vascular ciliated mucous membranes called the nasal mucosa. Mucus, secreted continuously by goblet cells, covers the surface of the nasal mucosa and is moved back to the nasopharynx by the action of the **cilia** (fine hairs).

The nose serves as a passageway for air to pass to and from the lungs. It filters impurities and humidifies and warms the air as it is inhaled. It is responsible for olfaction (smell) because the olfactory receptors are located in the nasal mucosa. This function diminishes with age.

Paranasal Sinuses

The paranasal sinuses include four pairs of bony cavities that are lined with nasal mucosa and ciliated pseudostratified columnar epithelium. These air spaces are connected by a series of ducts that drain into the nasal cavity. The sinuses are named by their location: frontal, ethmoidal, sphenoidal, and maxillary (Fig. 21-1). A prominent function of the sinuses is to serve as a resonating chamber in speech. The sinuses are a common site of infection.

Turbinate Bones (Conchae)

The turbinate bones are also called conchae (the name suggested by their shell-like appearance). Because of their curves, these bones increase the mucous membrane surface of the nasal passages and slightly obstruct the air flowing through them (Fig. 21-2).

Air entering the nostrils is deflected upward to the roof of the nose, and it follows a circuitous route before it reaches the nasopharynx. It comes into contact with a large surface of moist, warm mucous membrane that catches practically all the dust and organisms in the inhaled air. The air is moistened, warmed to body temperature, and brought into contact with sensitive nerves. Some of these nerves detect odours; others provoke sneezing to expel irritating dust.

Pharynx, Tonsils, and Adenoids

The pharynx, or throat, is a tubelike structure that connects the nasal and oral cavities to the larynx. It is divided into three regions: nasal, oral, and laryngeal. The nasopharynx is located posterior to the nose and above the soft palate. The oropharynx houses the faucial, or palatine, tonsils. The laryngopharynx extends from the hyoid bone to the cricoid cartilage. The epiglottis forms the entrance of the larynx.

The adenoids, or pharyngeal tonsils, are located in the roof of the nasopharynx. The tonsils, the adenoids, and other lymphoid tissue encircle the throat. These structures are important links in the chain of lymph nodes guarding the body from invasion by organisms entering the nose and the throat. The pharynx functions as a passageway for the respiratory and digestive tracts.

Larynx

The larynx, or voice organ, is a cartilaginous epithelium-lined structure that connects the pharynx and the trachea. The major function of the larynx is vocalization. It also protects the lower

Glossary

bronchoscopy: direct examination of larynx, trachea, and bronchi using an endoscope

cilia: short hairs that provide a constant whipping motion that serves to propel mucus and foreign substances away from the lung toward the larynx

crackles: soft, high-pitched, discontinuous popping sounds during inspiration caused by delayed reopening of the airways

diffusion: exchange of gas molecules from areas of high concentration to areas of low concentration

dyspnea: laboured breathing or shortness of breath

hemoptysis: expectoration of blood from the respiratory tract

hypoxemia: decrease in arterial oxygen tension in the blood

hypoxia: decrease in oxygen supply to the tissues and cells

orthopnea: inability to breathe easily except in an upright position

physiologic dead space: portion of the tracheobronchial tree that does not participate in gas exchange

pulmonary perfusion: blood flow through the pulmonary vasculature

respiration: gas exchange between atmospheric air and the blood and between the blood and cells of the body

ventilation: movement of air in and out of airways

wheezes: continuous musical sounds associated with airway narrowing or partial obstruction

Frontal
Ethmoid

Sphenoid
Maxillary

FIGURE 21-1 The paranasal sinuses.

airway from foreign substances and facilitates coughing. It is frequently referred to as the voice box and consists of the following:

- Epiglottis—a valve flap of cartilage that covers the opening to the larynx during swallowing
- Glottis—the opening between the vocal cords in the larynx
- Thyroid cartilage—the largest of the cartilage structures; part of it forms the Adam's apple
- Cricoid cartilage—the only complete cartilaginous ring in the larynx (located below the thyroid cartilage)
- Arytenoid cartilages—used in vocal cord movement with the thyroid cartilage

- Vocal cords—ligaments controlled by muscular movements that produce sounds; located in the lumen of the larynx

Trachea

The trachea, or windpipe, is composed of smooth muscle with C-shaped rings of cartilage at regular intervals. The cartilaginous rings are incomplete on the posterior surface and give firmness to the wall of the trachea, preventing it from collapsing. The trachea serves as the passage between the larynx and the bronchi.

ANATOMY OF THE LOWER RESPIRATORY TRACT: LUNGS

The lower respiratory tract consists of the lungs, which contain the bronchial and alveolar structures needed for gas exchange.

Lungs

The lungs are paired elastic structures enclosed in the thoracic cage, which is an airtight chamber with distensible walls (Fig. 21-3). Ventilation requires movement of the walls of the thoracic cage and of its floor, the diaphragm. The effect of these movements is alternately to increase and decrease the capacity of the chest. When the capacity of the chest is increased, air enters through the trachea (inspiration) because of the lowered pressure within and inflates the lungs. When the chest wall and diaphragm return to their previous positions (expiration), the lungs recoil and force the air out through the bronchi and trachea. The inspiratory phase of respiration normally requires energy; the expiratory phase is normally passive. Inspiration occurs during the first third of the respiratory cycle, expiration during the latter two thirds.

PLEURA

The lungs and wall of the thorax are lined with a serous membrane called the pleura. The visceral pleura covers the lungs; the parietal pleura lines the thorax. The visceral and parietal pleura and the small amount of pleural fluid between these two membranes serve to lubricate the thorax and lungs and permit smooth motion of the lungs within the thoracic cavity with each breath.

MEDIASTINUM

The mediastinum is in the middle of the thorax, between the pleural sacs that contain the two lungs. It extends from the sternum to the vertebral column and contains all the thoracic tissue outside the lungs.

Cribiform
plate
of ethmoid

Sphenoidal
sinus

Sella
turcica

Frontal
sinus

Superior
turbinate

Middle
turbinate

Inferior
turbinate

Hard
palate

Soft
palate

Orifice of auditory
(eustachian) tube

FIGURE 21-2 Cross-section of nasal cavity.

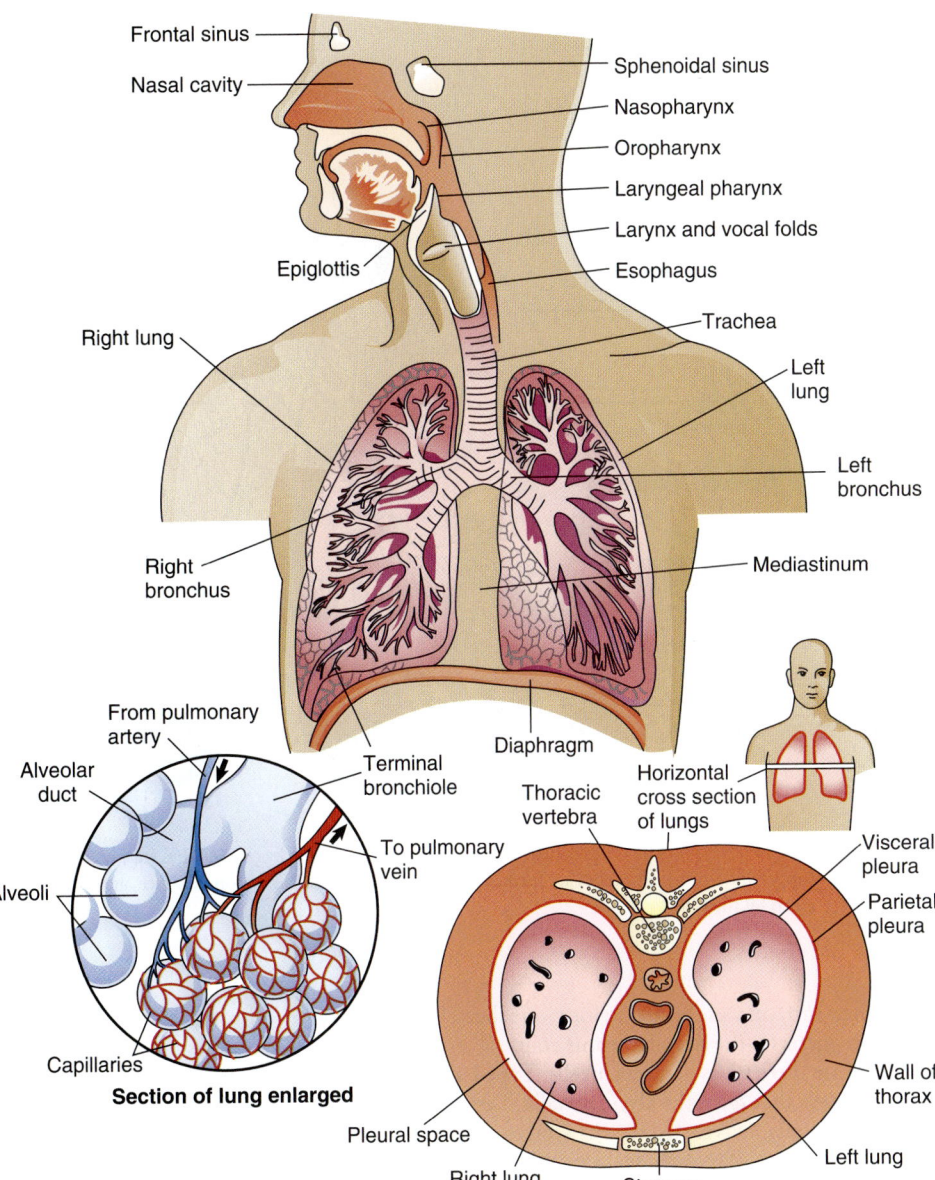

FIGURE 21-3 The respiratory system; upper respiratory structures and the structures of the thorax (*top*); alveoli and a horizontal cross section of the lungs (*bottom*).

LOBES
Each lung is divided into lobes. The left lung consists of an upper and lower lobe, whereas the right lung has an upper, middle, and lower lobe (Fig. 21-4). Each lobe is further subdivided into two to five segments separated by fissures, which are extensions of the pleura.

BRONCHI AND BRONCHIOLES
There are several divisions of the bronchi within each lobe of the lung. First are the lobar bronchi (three in the right lung and two in the left lung). Lobar bronchi divide into segmental bronchi (10 on the right and 8 on the left), which are the structures identified when choosing the most effective postural drainage position for a given patient. Segmental bronchi then divide into subsegmental bronchi. These bronchi are surrounded by connective tissue that contains arteries, lymphatics, and nerves.

The subsegmental bronchi then branch into bronchioles, which have no cartilage in their walls. Their patency depends entirely on the elastic recoil of the surrounding smooth muscle and

on the alveolar pressure. The bronchioles contain submucosal glands, which produce mucus that covers the inside lining of the airways. The bronchi and bronchioles are lined also with cells that have surfaces covered with cilia. These cilia create a constant whipping motion that propels mucus and foreign substances away from the lung toward the larynx.

The bronchioles then branch into terminal bronchioles, which do not have mucous glands or cilia. Terminal bronchioles then become respiratory bronchioles, which are considered to be the transitional passageways between the conducting airways and the gas exchange airways. Up to this point, the conducting airways contain about 150 mL of air in the tracheobronchial tree that does not participate in gas exchange. This is known as **physiologic dead space**. The respiratory bronchioles then lead into alveolar ducts and alveolar sacs and then alveoli. Oxygen and carbon dioxide exchange takes place in the alveoli.

ALVEOLI
The lung is made up of about 300 million alveoli, which are arranged in clusters of 15 to 20. These alveoli are so numerous

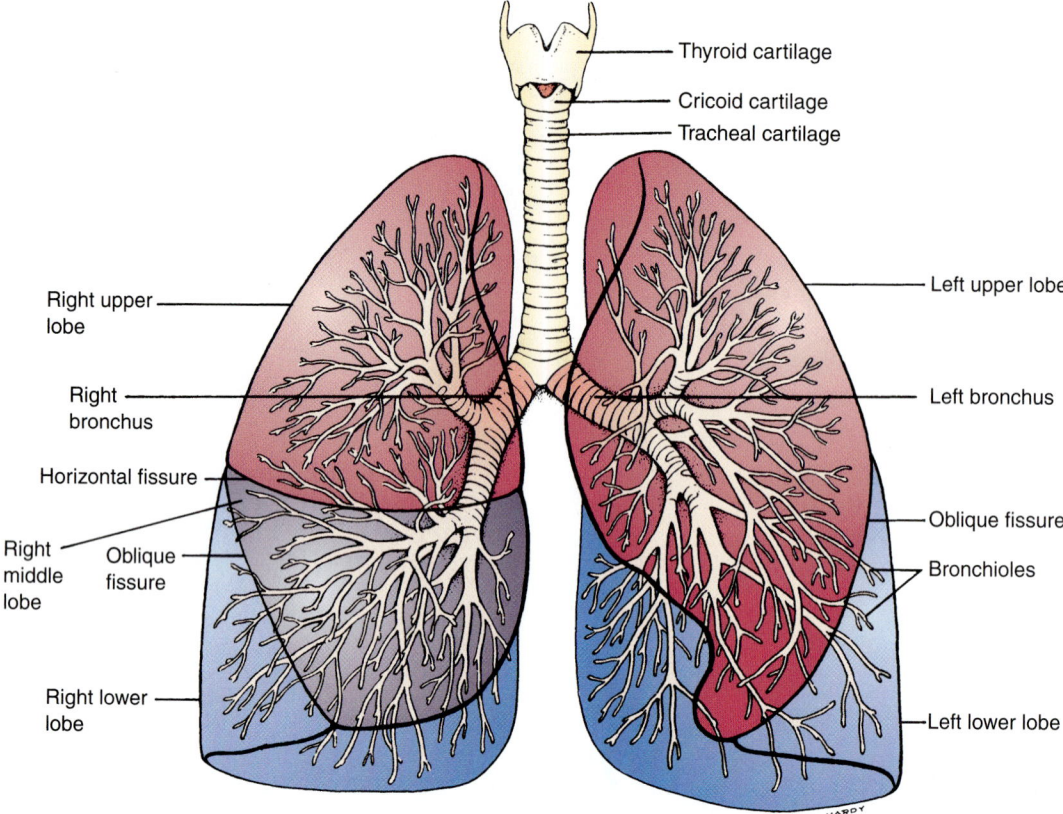

FIGURE 21-4   The lungs consist of five lobes. The right lung has three lobes (upper, middle, lower); the left has two (upper and lower). The lobes are further subdivided by fissures. The bronchial tree, another lung structure, inflates with air to fill the lobes.

that if their surfaces were united to form one sheet, it would cover 70 square meters—the size of a tennis court.

There are three types of alveolar cells. Type I alveolar cells are epithelial cells that form the alveolar walls. Type II alveolar cells are metabolically active. These cells secrete surfactant, a phospholipid that lines the inner surface and prevents alveolar collapse. Type III alveolar cell macrophages are large phagocytic cells that ingest foreign matter (eg, mucus, bacteria) and act as an important defense mechanism.

FUNCTION OF THE RESPIRATORY SYSTEM

The cells of the body derive the energy they need from the oxidation of carbohydrates, fats, and proteins. As with any type of combustion, this process requires oxygen. Certain vital tissues, such as those of the brain and the heart, cannot survive for long without a continuing supply of oxygen. However, as a result of oxidation in the body tissues, carbon dioxide is produced and must be removed from the cells to prevent the buildup of acid waste products. The respiratory system performs this function by facilitating life-sustaining processes such as oxygen transport, respiration and ventilation, and gas exchange.

Oxygen Transport

Oxygen is supplied to, and carbon dioxide is removed from, cells by way of the circulating blood. Cells are in close contact with capillaries, whose thin walls permit easy passage or exchange of oxygen and carbon dioxide. Oxygen diffuses from the capillary through the capillary wall to the interstitial fluid. At this point, it diffuses through the membrane of tissue cells, where it is used by mitochondria for cellular respiration. The movement of carbon dioxide occurs by diffusion in the opposite direction—from cell to blood.

Respiration

After these tissue capillary exchanges, blood enters the systemic veins (where it is called venous blood) and travels to the pulmonary circulation. The oxygen concentration in blood within the capillaries of the lungs is lower than in the lungs' air sacs (alveoli). Because of this concentration gradient, oxygen diffuses from the alveoli to the blood. Carbon dioxide, which has a higher concentration in the blood than in the alveoli, diffuses from the blood into the alveoli. Movement of air in and out of the airways (ventilation) continually replenishes the oxygen and removes the carbon dioxide from the airways in the lung. This whole process of gas exchange between the atmospheric air and the blood and between the blood and cells of the body is called **respiration**.

Ventilation

During inspiration, air flows from the environment into the trachea, bronchi, bronchioles, and alveoli. During expiration, alveolar gas travels the same route in reverse.

Physical factors that govern air flow in and out of the lungs are collectively referred to as the mechanics of ventilation and include air pressure variances, resistance to air flow, and lung compliance.

AIR PRESSURE VARIANCES

Air flows from a region of higher pressure to a region of lower pressure. During inspiration, movement of the diaphragm and other muscles of respiration enlarges the thoracic cavity and thereby lowers the pressure inside the thorax to a level below that of atmospheric pressure. As a result, air is drawn through the trachea and bronchi into the alveoli.

During normal expiration, the diaphragm relaxes and the lungs recoil, resulting in a decrease in the size of the thoracic cavity. The alveolar pressure then exceeds atmospheric pressure, and air flows from the lungs into the atmosphere.

AIRWAY RESISTANCE

Resistance is determined chiefly by the radius or size of the airway through which the air is flowing. Any process that changes the bronchial diameter or width affects airway resistance and alters the rate of air flow for a given pressure gradient during respiration (Chart 21-1). With increased resistance, greater-than-normal respiratory effort is required by the patient to achieve normal levels of ventilation.

COMPLIANCE

The pressure gradient between the thoracic cavity and the atmosphere causes air to flow in and out of the lungs. When pressure changes are applied in the normal lung, there is a proportional change in the lung volume. A measure of the elasticity, expandability, and distensibility of the lungs and thoracic structures is called compliance. Factors that determine lung compliance are the surface tension of the alveoli (normally low with the presence of surfactant) and the connective tissue (ie, collagen and elastin) of the lungs.

Compliance is determined by examining the volume–pressure relationship in the lungs and the thorax. In normal compliance (1.0 L/cm H_2O), the lungs and thorax easily stretch and distend when pressure is applied. High or increased compliance occurs when the lungs have lost their elasticity and the thorax is overdistended (ie, in emphysema). When the lungs and thorax are "stiff," there is low or decreased compliance. Conditions associated with this include pneumothorax, hemothorax, pleural effusion, pulmonary edema, atelectasis, pulmonary fibrosis, and acute respiratory distress syndrome (ARDS), all of which are discussed in later chapters in this unit. Measurement of compliance is one method used to assess the progression and improvement in ARDS. Lungs with decreased compliance require greater-than-normal energy expenditure to achieve normal levels of ventilation. Compliance is usually measured under static conditions.

Chart 21-1 Causes of Increased Airway Resistance

Common phenomena that may alter bronchial diameter, which affects airway resistance, include:
- Contraction of bronchial smooth muscle—as in asthma
- Thickening of bronchial mucosa—as in chronic bronchitis
- Obstruction of the airway—by mucus, a tumour, or a foreign body
- Loss of lung elasticity—as in emphysema, which is characterized by connective tissue encircling the airways, thereby keeping them open during both inspiration and expiration

Lung Volumes and Capacities

Lung function, which reflects the mechanics of ventilation, is viewed in terms of lung volumes and lung capacities. Lung volumes are categorized as tidal volume, inspiratory reserve volume, expiratory reserve volume, and residual volume. Lung capacity is evaluated in terms of vital capacity, inspiratory capacity, functional residual capacity, and total lung capacity. These terms are described in Table 21-1.

Diffusion and Perfusion

Diffusion is the process by which oxygen and carbon dioxide are exchanged at the air–blood interface. The alveolar–capillary membrane is ideal for diffusion because of its large surface area and thin membrane. In the normal healthy adult, oxygen and carbon dioxide travel across the alveolar–capillary membrane without difficulty as a result of differences in gas concentrations in the alveoli and capillaries.

Pulmonary perfusion is the actual blood flow through the pulmonary circulation. The blood is pumped into the lungs by the right ventricle through the pulmonary artery. The pulmonary artery divides into the right and left branches to supply both lungs. These two branches divide further to supply all parts of each lung. Normally about 2% of the blood pumped by the right ventricle does not perfuse the alveolar capillaries. This shunted blood drains into the left side of the heart without participating in alveolar gas exchange.

The pulmonary circulation is considered a low-pressure system because the systolic blood pressure in the pulmonary artery is 20 to 30 mm Hg and the diastolic pressure is 5 to 15 mm Hg. Because of these low pressures, the pulmonary vasculature normally can vary its capacity to accommodate the blood flow it receives. When a person is in an upright position, however, the pulmonary artery pressure is not great enough to supply blood to the apex of the lung against the force of gravity. Thus, when a person is upright, the lung may be considered to be divided into three sections: an upper part with poor blood supply, a lower part with maximal blood supply, and a section in between the two with an intermediate supply of blood. When a person lying down turns to one side, more blood passes to the dependent lung.

Perfusion also is influenced by alveolar pressure. The pulmonary capillaries are sandwiched between adjacent alveoli. If the alveolar pressure is sufficiently high, the capillaries will be squeezed. Depending on the pressure, some capillaries completely collapse, whereas others narrow.

Pulmonary artery pressure, gravity, and alveolar pressure determine the patterns of perfusion. In lung disease these factors vary, and the perfusion of the lung may become very abnormal.

Ventilation and Perfusion Balance and Imbalance

Ventilation is the flow of gas in and out of the lungs, and perfusion is the filling of the pulmonary capillaries with blood. Adequate gas exchange depends on an adequate ventilation–perfusion ratio. In different areas of the lung, the ratio varies.

Alterations in perfusion may occur with a change in the pulmonary artery pressure, alveolar pressure, and gravity. Airway blockages, local changes in compliance, and gravity may alter ventilation.

A ventilation–perfusion $\dot{V}/\dot{Q}$ imbalance occurs from inadequate ventilation, inadequate perfusion, or both. There are four possible $\dot{V}/\dot{Q}$ states in the lung: normal $\dot{V}/\dot{Q}$ ratio, low $\dot{V}/\dot{Q}$ ratio

Table 21-1 • **Lung Volumes and Lung Capacities**

TERM	SYMBOL	DESCRIPTION	NORMAL VALUE*	SIGNIFICANCE
Lung Volumes				
Tidal volume	V_T or TV	The volume of air inhaled and exhaled with each breath	500 mL or 5–10 mL/kg	The tidal volume may not vary, even with severe disease.
Inspiratory reserve volume	IRV	The maximum volume of air that can be inhaled after a normal inhalation	3,000 mL	
Expiratory reserve volume	ERV	The maximum volume of air that can be exhaled forcibly after a normal exhalation	1,100 mL	Expiratory reserve volume is decreased with restrictive conditions, such as obesity, ascites, pregnancy.
Residual volume	RV	The volume of air remaining in the lungs after a maximum exhalation	1,200 mL	Residual volume may be increased with obstructive disease.
Lung Capacities				
Vital capacity	VC	The maximum volume of air exhaled from the point of maximum inspiration VC = TV + IRV + ERV	4,600 mL	A decrease in vital capacity may be found in neuromuscular disease, generalized fatigue, atelectasis, pulmonary edema, and COPD.
Inspiratory capacity	IC	The maximum volume of air inhaled after normal expiration IC = TV + IRV	3,500 mL	A decrease in inspiratory capacity may indicate restrictive disease.
Functional residual capacity	FRC	The volume of air remaining in the lungs after a normal expiration FRV = ERV + RV	2,300 mL	Functional residual capacity may be increased with COPD and decreased in ARDS.
Total lung capacity	TLC	The volume of air in the lungs after a maximum inspiration TLC = TV + IRV + ERV + RV	5,800 mL	Total lung capacity may be decreased with restrictive disease (atelectasis, pneumonia) and increased in COPD.

*Values for healthy men; women are 20%–25% less.

(shunt), high $\dot{V}/\dot{Q}$ ratio (dead space), and absence of ventilation and perfusion (silent unit) (Chart 21-2).

Ventilation and perfusion imbalance causes shunting of blood, resulting in **hypoxia** (low cellular oxygen level). Shunting appears to be the main cause of hypoxia after thoracic or abdominal surgery and most types of respiratory failure. Severe hypoxia results when the amount of shunting exceeds 20%. Supplemental oxygen may eliminate hypoxia, depending on the type of $\dot{V}/\dot{Q}$ imbalance.

Gas Exchange

The air we breathe is a gaseous mixture consisting mainly of nitrogen (78.62%) and oxygen (20.84%), with traces of carbon dioxide (0.04%), water vapor (0.05%), helium, and argon. The atmospheric pressure at sea level is about 760 mm Hg. Partial pressure is the pressure exerted by each type of gas in a mixture of gases. The partial pressure of a gas is proportional to the concentration of that gas in the mixture. The total pressure exerted by the gaseous mixture is equal to the sum of the partial pressures.

PARTIAL PRESSURE OF GASES
Based on these facts, the partial pressures of nitrogen and oxygen can be calculated. The partial pressure of nitrogen is 79% of 760 (0.79 × 760), or 600 mm Hg; that of oxygen is 21% of 760 (0.21 × 760), or 160 mm Hg. Chart 21-3 spells out terms and abbreviations related to partial pressure of gases.

Once the air enters the trachea, it becomes fully saturated with water vapor, which displaces some of the gases so that the air pressure within the lung remains equal to the air pressure outside (760 mm Hg). Water vapor exerts a pressure of 47 mm Hg when

it fully saturates a mixture of gases at the body temperature of 37°C. Nitrogen and oxygen are responsible for the remaining 713 mm Hg (760 − 47) pressure. Once this mixture enters the alveoli, it is further diluted by carbon dioxide. In the alveoli, the water vapor continues to exert a pressure of 47 mm Hg. The remaining 713 mm Hg pressure is now exerted as follows: nitrogen, 569 mm Hg (74.9%); oxygen, 104 mm Hg (13.6%); and carbon dioxide, 40 mm Hg (5.3%).

PARTIAL PRESSURE IN GAS EXCHANGE
When a gas is exposed to a liquid, the gas dissolves in the liquid until an equilibrium is reached. The dissolved gas also exerts a partial pressure. At equilibrium, the partial pressure of the gas in the liquid is the same as the partial pressure of the gas in the gaseous mixture. Oxygenation of venous blood in the lung illustrates this point. In the lung, venous blood and alveolar oxygen are separated by a very thin alveolar membrane. Oxygen diffuses across this membrane to dissolve in the blood until the partial pressure of oxygen in the blood is the same as that in the alveoli (104 mm Hg). However, because carbon dioxide is a byproduct of oxidation in the cells, venous blood contains carbon dioxide at a higher partial pressure than that in the alveolar gas. In the lung, carbon dioxide diffuses out of venous blood into the alveolar gas. At equilibrium, the partial pressure of carbon dioxide in the blood and in alveolar gas is the same (40 mm Hg). The changes in partial pressure are shown in Figure 21-5.

EFFECTS OF PRESSURE ON OXYGEN TRANSPORT
Oxygen and carbon dioxide are transported simultaneously dissolved in blood or combined with some of the elements of blood. Oxygen is carried in the blood in two forms: first as physically dis-

Chart 21-2 Ventilation-Perfusion Ratios

Normal Ratio (A)
In the healthy lung, a given amount of blood passes an alveolus and is matched with an equal amount of gas (**A**). The ratio is 1:1 (ventilation matches perfusion).

Low Ventilation–Perfusion Ratio: Shunts (B)
Low ventilation–perfusion states may be called shunt-producing disorders. When perfusion exceeds ventilation, a shunt exists (**B**). Blood bypasses the alveoli without gas exchange occurring. This is seen with obstruction of the distal airways, such as with pneumonia, atelectasis, tumour, or a mucus plug.

High Ventilation–Perfusion Ratio: Dead Space (C)
When ventilation exceeds perfusion, dead space results (**C**). The alveoli do not have an adequate blood supply for gas exchange to occur. This is characteristic of a variety of disorders, including pulmonary emboli, pulmonary infarction, and cardiogenic shock.

Silent Unit (D)
In the absence of ventilation and perfusion or with limited ventilation and perfusion, a condition known as a silent unit occurs (**D**). This is seen with pneumothorax and severe acute respiratory distress syndrome.

solved oxygen in the plasma, and second in combination with the hemoglobin of the red blood cells. Each 100 mL of normal arterial blood carries 0.3 mL of oxygen physically dissolved in the plasma and 20 mL of oxygen in combination with hemoglobin. Large amounts of oxygen can be transported in the blood because it combines easily with hemoglobin to form oxyhemoglobin:

Chart 21-3 Partial Pressure Abbreviations

P = pressure
PO_2 = partial pressure of oxygen
PCO_2 = partial pressure of carbon dioxide
PAO_2 = partial pressure of alveolar oxygen
$PACO_2$ = partial pressure of alveolar carbon dioxide
PaO_2 = partial pressure of arterial oxygen
$PaCO_2$ = partial pressure of arterial carbon dioxide
$P\bar{v}O_2$ = partial pressure of venous oxygen
$P\bar{v}CO_2$ = partial pressure of venous carbon dioxide
P_{50} = partial pressure of oxygen when the hemoglobin is 50% saturated

$$O_2 + Hgb \leftrightarrow HgbO_2$$

The volume of oxygen physically dissolved in the plasma varies directly with the partial pressure of oxygen in the arteries (PaO_2). The higher the PaO_2, the greater the amount of oxygen dissolved. For example, at a PaO_2 of 10 mm Hg, 0.03 mL of oxygen is dissolved in 100 mL of plasma. At 20 mm Hg, twice this amount is dissolved in plasma, and at 100 mm Hg, 10 times this amount is dissolved. Therefore, the amount of dissolved oxygen is directly proportional to the partial pressure, regardless of how high the oxygen pressure rises.

The amount of oxygen that combines with hemoglobin also depends on PaO_2, but only up to a PaO_2 of about 150 mm Hg. When the PaO_2 is 150 mm Hg, hemoglobin is 100% saturated and will not combine with any additional oxygen. When hemoglobin is 100% saturated, 1 g of hemoglobin will combine with 1.34 mL of oxygen. Therefore, in a person with 140 g/L of hemoglobin, each 100 mL of blood will contain about 19 mL of oxygen associated with hemoglobin. If the PaO_2 is less than 150 mm Hg, the percentage of hemoglobin saturated with oxygen is lower. For example, at a PaO_2 of 100 mm Hg (normal value), saturation is 97%; at a PaO_2 of 40 mm Hg, saturation is 70%.

Abbreviation

A = alveolar
a = arterial
v̄ = venous
P = partial pressure
O_2 = oxygen
CO_2 = carbon dioxide
N_2 = nitrogen
H_2O = water vapor

PO_2 158 mm Hg
PCO_2 0.3 mm Hg
PN_2 596 mm Hg
PH_2O 5.7 mm Hg — Air from the lungs

PAO_2 100 mm Hg
$PACO_2$ 40 mm Hg
PAH_2O 47 mm Hg
PAN_2 573 mm Hg — Air in the alveolus

CO_2 O_2

$P\bar{v}O_2$ 40 mm Hg
$P\bar{v}CO_2$ 46 mm Hg

CO_2 Pulmonary Capillary O_2

PaO_2 97 mm Hg
$PaCO_2$ 40 mm Hg

Venous system blood
(Desaturated)

Arterial system blood
(Oxygenated)

FIGURE 21-5 Changes occur in the partial pressure of gases during respiration. These values vary as a result of the exchange of oxygen and carbon dioxide and the changes that occur in their partial pressures as venous blood flows through the lungs. Adapted from Willis, M. C. (1996). *Medical terminology: The language of healthcare.* Baltimore: Williams & Wilkins.

OXYHEMOGLOBIN DISSOCIATION CURVE

The oxyhemoglobin dissociation curve (Chart 21-4) shows the relationship between the partial pressure of oxygen (PaO_2) and the percentage of saturation of oxygen (SaO_2). The percentage of saturation can be affected by the following factors: carbon dioxide, hydrogen ion concentration, temperature, and 2,3-diphosphoglycerate. A rise in these factors shifts the curve to the right so that more oxygen is then released to the tissues at the same PaO_2. A reduction in these factors causes the curve to shift to the left, making the bond between oxygen and hemoglobin stronger, so that less oxygen is given up to the tissues at the same PaO_2. The unusual shape of the oxyhemoglobin dissociation curve is a distinct advantage to the patient for two reasons:

1. If the arterial PO_2 decreases from 100 to 80 mm Hg as a result of lung disease or heart disease, the hemoglobin of the arterial blood remains almost maximally saturated (94%) and the tissues will not suffer from hypoxia.
2. When the arterial blood passes into tissue capillaries and is exposed to the tissue tension of oxygen (about 40 mm Hg), hemoglobin gives up large quantities of oxygen for use by the tissues.

Clinical Significance. The normal value of PaO_2 is 80 to 100 mm Hg (95% to 98% saturation). With this level of oxygenation, there is a 15% margin of excess oxygen available to the tissues. With a normal hemoglobin level of 150 g/L and a PaO_2 level of 40 mm Hg (oxygen saturation 75%), there is adequate oxygen available for the tissues but no reserve for physiologic stresses that increase tissue oxygen demand. When a serious incident occurs (eg, bronchospasm, aspiration, hypotension, or cardiac dysrhythmias) that reduces the intake of oxygen from the lungs, tissue hypoxia will result.

An important consideration in the transport of oxygen is cardiac output, which determines the amount of oxygen delivered to the body and which affects lung and tissue perfusion. If the cardiac output is normal (5 L/min), the amount of oxygen delivered to the

Chart 21-4 **Oxyhemoglobin Dissociation Curve**

The oxyhemoglobin dissociation curve is marked to show three oxygen levels:
1. Normal levels—PaO_2 above 70 mm Hg
2. Relatively safe levels—PaO_2 45 to 70 mm Hg
3. Dangerous levels—PaO_2 below 40 mm Hg

The normal (middle) curve (N) shows that 75% saturation occurs at a PaO_2 of 40 mm Hg. If the curve shifts to the right (R), the same saturation (75%) occurs at a higher PaO_2. If the curve shifts to the left (L), 75% saturation occurs at a lower PaO_2.

body per minute is normal. If cardiac output falls, the amount of oxygen delivered to the tissues also falls. Under normal conditions, most of the oxygen delivered to the body is not used. In fact, only 250 mL of oxygen is used per minute. Under normal conditions, this is approximately 25% of available oxygen. The rest of the oxygen returns to the right side of the heart, and the PaO_2 of venous blood drops from 80 to 100 mm Hg to about 40 mm Hg.

Carbon Dioxide Transport

At the same time that oxygen diffuses from the blood into the tissues, carbon dioxide diffuses in the opposite direction (ie, from tissue cells to blood) and is transported to the lungs for excretion. The amount of carbon dioxide in transit is one of the major determinants of the acid–base balance of the body. Normally, only 6% of the venous carbon dioxide is removed, and enough remains in the arterial blood to exert a pressure of 40 mm Hg. Most of the carbon dioxide (90%) enters the red blood cells; the small portion (5%) that remains dissolved in the plasma (PCO_2) is the critical factor that determines carbon dioxide movement in or out of the blood.

In summary, the many processes involved in respiratory gas transport do not occur in intermittent stages; rather, they are rapid, simultaneous, and continuous.

Neurologic Control of Ventilation

Resting respiration is the result of cyclical excitation of the respiratory muscles by the phrenic nerve. The rhythm of breathing is controlled by respiratory centres in the brain. The inspiratory and expiratory centres in the medulla oblongata and pons control the rate and depth of ventilation to meet the body's metabolic demands.

The apneustic centre in the lower pons stimulates the inspiratory medullary centre to promote deep, prolonged inspirations. The pneumotaxic centre in the upper pons is thought to control the pattern of respirations.

Several groups of receptor sites assist in the brain's control of respiratory function. The central chemoreceptors are located in the medulla and respond to chemical changes in the cerebrospinal fluid, which result from chemical changes in the blood. These receptors respond to an increase or decrease in the pH and convey a message to the lungs to change the depth and then the rate of ventilation to correct the imbalance. The peripheral chemoreceptors are located in the aortic arch and the carotid arteries and respond first to changes in PaO_2, then to $PaCO_2$ and pH. The Hering–Breuer reflex is activated by stretch receptors in the alveoli. When the lungs are distended, inspiration is inhibited; as a result, the lungs do not become overdistended. In addition, proprioceptors in the muscles and joints respond to body movements, such as exercise, causing an increase in ventilation. Thus, range-of-motion exercises in an immobile patient stimulate breathing. Baroreceptors, also located in the aortic and carotid bodies, respond to an increase or decrease in arterial blood pressure and cause reflex hypoventilation or hyperventilation.

Gerontologic Considerations

A gradual decline in respiratory function begins in early to middle adulthood and affects the structure and function of the respiratory system. The vital capacity of the lungs and respiratory muscle strength peak between ages 20 and 25 and decrease thereafter. With aging (40 years and older), changes occur in the alveoli that reduce the surface area available for the exchange of oxygen and carbon dioxide. At approximately age 50, the alveoli begin to lose elasticity. A decrease in vital capacity occurs with loss of chest wall mobility, thus restricting the tidal flow of air. The amount of respiratory dead space increases with age. These changes result in a decreased diffusion capacity for oxygen with age, producing lower oxygen levels in the arterial circulation. Elderly people have a decreased ability to move air rapidly in and out of the lungs. Gerontologic changes in the respiratory system are summarized in Table 21-2. Despite these changes, in the absence of chronic pulmonary disease, elderly people are able to carry out activities of daily living, but they may have decreased tolerance for and require additional rest after prolonged or vigourous activity.

Assessment

HEALTH HISTORY

The health history focuses on the physical and functional problems of the patient and the effect of these problems on his or her life. The reason the patient is seeking health care often is related to one of the following: **dyspnea** (shortness of breath), pain, accumulation of mucus, wheezing, **hemoptysis** (blood spit up from the respiratory tract), edema of the ankles and feet, cough, and general fatigue and weakness.

In addition to identifying the chief reason why the patient is seeking health care, the nurse tries to determine when the health problem or symptom started, how long it lasted, if it was relieved at any time, and how relief was obtained. The nurse collects information about precipitating factors, duration, severity, and associated factors or symptoms and also assesses for risk factors and genetic factors that may contribute to the patient's lung condition (Chart 21-5).

The nurse assesses the impact of signs and symptoms on the patient's ability to perform activities of daily living and to participate in usual work and family activities. In addition, psychosocial factors that may affect the patient are explored (Chart 21-6). These factors include anxiety, role changes, family relationships, financial problems, employment status, and the strategies the patient uses to cope with them.

Many respiratory diseases are chronic and progressively debilitating. Therefore, ongoing assessment of the patient's physical abilities, psychosocial supports, and quality of life is needed to plan appropriate interventions. It is important for the patient with a respiratory disorder to understand the condition and to be familiar with necessary self-care interventions. The nurse evaluates these factors over time and provides education as needed.

Signs and Symptoms

The major signs and symptoms of respiratory disease are dyspnea, cough, sputum production, chest pain, wheezing, clubbing of the fingers, hemoptysis, and cyanosis. These clinical manifestations are related to the duration and severity of the disease.

DYSPNEA

Dyspnea (difficult or laboured breathing, shortness of breath) is a symptom common to many pulmonary and cardiac disorders, particularly when there is decreased lung compliance or increased airway resistance. The right ventricle of the heart will be affected ultimately by lung disease because it must pump blood through the lungs against greater resistance. It may also be associated with neurologic or neuromuscular disorders such as myasthenia gravis, Guillain-Barré syndrome, or muscular dystrophy.

Table 21-2 • Age-Related Changes of the Respiratory System

	STRUCTURAL CHANGES	FUNCTIONAL CHANGES	HISTORY AND PHYSICAL FINDINGS
Defense mechanisms (respiratory and nonrespiratory)	↓ Number of cilia and ↓ mucus ↓ Cough and gag reflex Loss of surface area of the capillary membrane Lack of a uniform or consistent ventilation and/or blood flow	↓ Protection against foreign particles ↓ Protection against aspiration ↓ Antibody response to antigens ↓ Response to hypoxia and hypercapnia (chemoreceptors)	↓ Cough reflex and mucus ↑ Infection rate History of respiratory infections, COPD, pneumonia. Risk factors: smoking, environmental exposure, TB exposure
Lung	↓ Size of airway ↑ Diameter of alveolar ducts ↑ Collagen of alveolar walls ↑ Thickness of alveolar membranes ↓ Elasticity of alveolar sacs	↑ Airway resistance ↑ Pulmonary compliance ↓ Expiratory flow rate ↓ Oxygen diffusion capacity ↑ Dead space Premature closure of airways ↑ Air trapping ↓ Expiratory flow rates Ventilation–perfusion mismatch ↓ Exercise capacity ↑ Anteroposterior (AP) diameter	Unchanged total lung capacity (TLC) ↑ Residual volume (RV) ↓ Inspiratory reserve volume (IRV) ↓ Expiratory reserve volume (ERV) ↓ Forced vital capacity (FVC) and vital capacity (VC) ↑ Functional residual capacity (FRC) ↓ PaO_2 ↑ CO_2
Chest wall and muscles	Calcification of intercostal cartilages Arthritis of costovertebral joints ↓ Continuity of diaphragm Osteoporotic changes ↓ Muscle mass Muscle atrophy	↑ Rigidity and stiffness of thoracic cage ↓ Respiratory muscle strength ↑ Work of breathing ↓ Capacity for exercise ↓ Peripheral chemosensitivity ↑ Risk for inspiratory muscle fatigue	Kyphosis, barrel chest Skeletal changes ↑ AP diameter Shortness of breath ↑ Abdominal and diaphragmatic breathing ↓ Maximum expiratory flow rates

Clinical Significance. In general, acute diseases of the lungs produce a more severe grade of dyspnea than do chronic diseases. Sudden dyspnea in a healthy person may indicate pneumothorax (air in the pleural cavity), acute respiratory obstruction, or ARDS. In immobilized patients, sudden dyspnea may denote pulmonary embolism. **Orthopnea** (inability to breathe easily except in an upright position) may be found in patients with heart disease and occasionally in patients with chronic obstructive pulmonary disease (COPD); dyspnea with an expiratory wheeze occurs with COPD. Noisy breathing may result from a narrowing of the airway or localized obstruction of a major bronchus by a tumour or foreign body. The presence of both inspiratory and expiratory wheezing usually signifies asthma if the patient does not have heart failure.

The circumstance that produces the dyspnea must be determined. Therefore, it is important to ask the patient the following questions:

- How much exertion triggers shortness of breath?
- Is there an associated cough?
- Is dyspnea related to other symptoms?
- Was the onset of shortness of breath sudden or gradual?

- At what time of day or night does the dyspnea occur?
- Is the shortness of breath worse when the patient is flat in bed?
- Does the shortness of breath occur at rest? With exercise? Running? Climbing stairs?
- Is the shortness of breath worse while walking? If so, when walking how far? How fast?

Relief Measures. The management of dyspnea is aimed at identifying and correcting its cause. Relief of the symptom sometimes is achieved by placing the patient at rest with the head elevated (high Fowler's position) and, in severe cases, by administering oxygen.

COUGH

Cough results from irritation of the mucous membranes anywhere in the respiratory tract. The stimulus producing a cough may arise from an infectious process or from an airborne irritant, such as smoke, smog, dust, or a gas. The cough is the patient's chief protection against the accumulation of secretions in the bronchi and bronchioles.

Clinical Significance. Cough may indicate serious pulmonary disease. The nurse needs to evaluate the character of the cough—is it dry, hacking, brassy, wheezing, loose, or severe? A dry, irritative cough is characteristic of an upper respiratory tract infection of viral origin or may be a side effect of angiotensin-converting enzyme (ACE) inhibitor therapy. Laryngotracheitis causes an irritative, high-pitched cough. Tracheal lesions produce a brassy cough. A severe or changing cough may indicate bronchogenic carcinoma. Pleuritic chest pain accompanying coughing may indicate pleural or chest wall (musculoskeletal) involvement.

Chart 21-5
Risk Factors for Respiratory Disease

Smoking (the single most important contributor to lung disease)
Personal or family history of lung disease
Occupation
Allergens and environmental pollutants
Recreational exposure

NURSING RESEARCH PROFILE 21-1
Dyspnea Self-Management

Nield, M. (2000). Dyspnea self-management in African Americans with chronic lung disease. *Heart & Lung, 29*(1), 50–55.

Purpose
The purpose of this qualitative analysis, part of a larger study of the relationship between dyspnea and respiratory muscle function in patients with chronic lung disease, was to explore dyspnea self-management in African Americans with COPD or chronic restrictive pulmonary disease resulting from sarcoidosis.

Study Sample and Design
A qualitative study approach was used with a convenience sample of 29 patients recruited from the pulmonary clinic at a large medical centre in the midwestern United States. Fifteen of the subjects had COPD and 14 had sarcoidosis. All routinely experienced dyspnea. A semistructured interview guide was used to obtain data. The taped interviews were transcribed and content analysis was performed using open coding methods.

Findings
The investigators identified the following self-management themes from the data:
- Traditional medical care (formal health care and prescription medications)
- Self-care wisdom (learned insight regarding the impact of dyspnea on quality of life)
- Self-care action (specific strategies for dyspnea relief included exercise, environmental control, cognitive strategies, and controlled breathing, which refers to patient-initiated position and breathing to manage dyspnea). Patients with sarcoidosis used inhalation-focused breathing only, while patients with COPD used both inhalation- and exhalation-focused breathing.
- Self-care resources (internal or external assets that could be used for sustenance of the self-care actions such as spiritual and social support)

Nursing Implications
These findings mirror previous research; however, this study extends previous knowledge as it focused on African Americans exclusively. When working with patients with chronic respiratory disorders, nurses should assess all four aspects of dyspnea self-management, which reflect a holistic approach to care. Self-care actions should be encouraged and taught, and self-care resources facilitated. The breathing techniques used by patients with COPD and those with sarcoidosis should be considered during patient and family education. Further research is warranted to determine if the differences in the breathing techniques used by these two populations of patients are also found in a research study with a larger sample size.

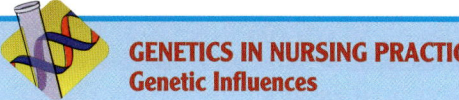

GENETICS IN NURSING PRACTICE— Genetic Influences

Various conditions that affect gas exchange and respiratory function are influenced by genetic factors, including:
- Asthma
- Chronic obstructive pulmonary disease
- Cystic fibrosis
- Alpha-1 antitrypsin deficiency

NURSING ASSESSMENTS
FAMILY HISTORY ASSESSMENT
- Assess family history for other family members with histories of respiratory impairment.
- Assess family history for individuals with early-onset chronic pulmonary disease, family history of hepatic disease in infants (clinical symptoms of alpha-1 antitrypsin deficiency).
- Inquire about family history of genetic cystic fibrosis.

MANAGEMENT ISSUES SPECIFIC TO GENETICS
- Inquire whether DNA mutation or other genetic testing has been performed on affected family members.
- Refer for further genetic counselling and evaluation so that family members can discuss inheritance, risk to other family members, availability of genetic testing and gene-based interventions.
- Offer appropriate genetics information and resources.
- Assess patient's understanding of genetics information.
- Provide support to families with newly diagnosed genetic-related respiratory disorders.
- Participate in management and coordination of care of patients with genetic conditions, individuals predisposed to develop or pass on a genetic condition.

GENETIC RESOURCES FOR NURSES AND THEIR PATIENTS ON THE WEB
Canadian Cystic Fibrosis Foundation http://www.ccff.ca.
Genetic Alliance http://www.geneticalliance.org—a directory of support groups for patients and families with genetic conditions
National Organization of Rare Disorders http://www.rarediseases.org—a directory of support groups and information for patients and families with rare genetic disorders
OMIM: Online Mendelian Inheritance in Man http://www.ncbi.nlm.nih.gov/omim/stats/html—a complete listing of inherited genetic conditions

---

The time of coughing is also noted. Coughing at night may herald the onset of left-sided heart failure or bronchial asthma. A cough in the morning with sputum production may indicate bronchitis. A cough that worsens when the patient is supine suggests postnasal drip (sinusitis). Coughing after food intake may indicate aspiration of material into the tracheobronchial tree. A cough of recent onset is usually from an acute infection.

SPUTUM PRODUCTION
A patient who coughs long enough almost invariably produces sputum. Violent coughing causes bronchial spasm, obstruction, and further irritation of the bronchi and may result in syncope (fainting). A severe, repeated, or uncontrolled cough that is nonproductive is exhausting and potentially harmful. Sputum pro-

duction is the reaction of the lungs to any constantly recurring irritant. It also may be associated with a nasal discharge.

Clinical Significance. A profuse amount of purulent sputum (thick and yellow, green, or rust-coloured) or a change in colour of the sputum probably indicates a bacterial infection. Thin, mucoid sputum frequently results from viral bronchitis. A gradual increase of sputum over time may indicate the presence of chronic bronchitis or bronchiectasis. Pink-tinged mucoid sputum suggests

Chart 21-6 • ASSESSMENT

Psychosocial Factors

Questions to consider when assessing psychosocial factors related to pulmonary disease and respiratory function include:

- What strategies does the patient use to cope with the signs and symptoms and challenges associated with pulmonary disease?
- Does the patient exhibit anxiety, anger, hostility, dependency, withdrawal, isolation, avoidance, noncompliance, acceptance, or denial?
- What support systems does the patient use to cope with the illness?
- Are resources (relatives, friends, or community groups) available? Do the patient and family use them effectively?

---

a lung tumour. Profuse, frothy, pink material, often welling up into the throat, may indicate pulmonary edema. Foul-smelling sputum and bad breath point to the presence of a lung abscess, bronchiectasis, or an infection caused by fusospirochetal or other anaerobic organisms.

Relief Measures. If the sputum is too thick for the patient to expectorate, it is necessary to decrease its viscosity by increasing its water content through adequate hydration (drinking water) and inhalation of aerosolized solutions, which may be delivered by any type of nebulizer. Strategies to assist the patient to cough productively are discussed later in this chapter.

Smoking is contraindicated with excessive sputum production because it interferes with ciliary action, increases bronchial secretions, causes inflammation and hyperplasia of the mucous membranes, and reduces production of surfactant. Thus, smoking impairs bronchial drainage. When the person stops smoking, sputum volume decreases and resistance to bronchial infections increases.

The patient's appetite may decrease because of the odour of the sputum or the taste it leaves in the mouth. The nurse encourages adequate oral hygiene and wise selection of food, measures that will stimulate appetite. In addition, the nurse encourages the patient and family to remove sputum cups, emesis basins, and soiled tissues before mealtime. Encouraging the patient to drink citrus juices at the beginning of the meal may increase the palatability of the rest of the meal because these juices cleanse the palate of the sputum taste.

CHEST PAIN

Chest pain or discomfort may be associated with pulmonary or cardiac disease. Chest pain associated with pulmonary conditions may be sharp, stabbing, and intermittent, or it may be dull, aching, and persistent. The pain usually is felt on the side where the pathologic process is located, but it may be referred elsewhere—for example, to the neck, back, or abdomen.

Clinical Significance. Chest pain may occur with pneumonia, pulmonary embolism with lung infarction, and pleurisy. It also may be a late symptom of bronchogenic carcinoma. In carcinoma the pain may be dull and persistent because the cancer has invaded the chest wall, mediastinum, or spine.

Lung disease does not always produce thoracic pain because the lungs and the visceral pleura lack sensory nerves and are insensitive to pain stimuli. However, the parietal pleura has a rich supply of sensory nerves that are stimulated by inflammation and stretching of the membrane. Pleuritic pain from irritation of the parietal pleura is sharp and seems to "catch" on inspiration; patients often describe

it as "like the stabbing of a knife." Patients are more comfortable when they lie on the affected side as this splints the chest wall, limits expansion and contraction of the lung, and reduces the friction between the injured or diseased pleurae on that side. Pain associated with cough may be reduced manually by splinting the rib cage.

The nurse assesses the quality, intensity, and radiation of pain and identifies and explores precipitating factors, along with their relationship to the patient's position. Also, it is important to assess the relationship of pain to the inspiratory and expiratory phases of respiration.

Relief Measures. Analgesic medications may be effective in relieving chest pain, but care must be taken not to depress the respiratory centre or a productive cough, if present. Nonsteroidal anti-inflammatory drugs (NSAIDs) achieve this goal and thus are used for pleuritic pain. A regional anesthetic block may be performed to relieve extreme pain.

WHEEZING

Wheezing is often the major finding in a patient with bronchoconstriction or airway narrowing. It is heard with or without a stethoscope, depending on its location. Wheezing is a high-pitched, musical sound heard mainly on expiration.

Relief Measures. Oral or inhalant bronchodilator medications reverse wheezing in most instances.

CLUBBING OF THE FINGERS

Clubbing of the fingers is a sign of lung disease found in patients with chronic hypoxic conditions, chronic lung infections, and malignancies of the lung. This finding may be manifested initially as sponginess of the nailbed and loss of the nailbed angle (Fig. 21-6).

HEMOPTYSIS

Hemoptysis (expectoration of blood from the respiratory tract) is a symptom of both pulmonary and cardiac disorders. The onset of hemoptysis is usually sudden, and it may be intermittent or continuous. Signs, which vary from blood-stained sputum to a large, sudden hemorrhage, always merit investigation. The most common causes are:

- Pulmonary infection
- Carcinoma of the lung

FIGURE 21-6 Clubbed finger. In clubbing, the distal phalanx of each finger is rounded and bulbous. The nail plate is more convex, and the angle between the plate and the proximal nail fold increases to 180 degrees or more. The proximal nail fold, when palpated, feels spongy or floating. Among the many causes are chronic hypoxia and lung cancer.

- Abnormalities of the heart or blood vessels
- Pulmonary artery or vein abnormalities
- Pulmonary emboli and infarction

Diagnostic evaluation to determine the cause includes several studies: chest x-ray, chest angiography, and bronchoscopy. A careful history and physical examination are necessary to diagnose the underlying disease, irrespective of whether the bleeding involved a very small amount of blood in the sputum or a massive hemorrhage. The amount of blood produced is not always proportional to the seriousness of the cause.

First, it is important to determine the source of the bleeding—the gums, nasopharynx, lungs, or stomach. The nurse may be the only witness to the episode. When documenting the bleeding episode, the nurse considers the following points:

- Bloody sputum from the nose or the nasopharynx is usually preceded by considerable sniffing, with blood possibly appearing in the nose.
- Blood from the lung is usually bright red, frothy, and mixed with sputum. Initial symptoms include a tickling sensation in the throat, a salty taste, a burning or bubbling sensation in the chest, and perhaps chest pain, in which case the patient tends to splint the bleeding side. The term "hemoptysis" is reserved for the coughing up of blood arising from a pulmonary hemorrhage. This blood has an alkaline pH (greater than 7.0).
- If the hemorrhage is in the stomach, the blood is vomited (hematemesis) rather than coughed up. Blood that has been in contact with gastric juice is sometimes so dark that it is referred to as "coffee grounds." This blood has an acid pH (less than 7.0).

CYANOSIS

Cyanosis, a bluish colouring of the skin, is a very late indicator of hypoxia. The presence or absence of cyanosis is determined by the amount of unoxygenated hemoglobin in the blood. Cyanosis appears when there is 50 g/L of unoxygenated hemoglobin. A patient with a hemoglobin level of 150 g/L will not demonstrate cyanosis until 50 g/L of that hemoglobin becomes unoxygenated, reducing the effective circulating hemoglobin to two thirds of the normal level. An anemic patient rarely manifests cyanosis, and a polycythemic patient may appear cyanotic even if adequately oxygenated. Therefore, cyanosis is *not* a reliable sign of hypoxia.

Assessment of cyanosis is affected by room lighting, the patient's skin colour, and the distance of the blood vessels from the surface of the skin. In the presence of a pulmonary condition, central cyanosis is assessed by observing the colour of the tongue and lips. This indicates a decrease in oxygen tension in the blood. Peripheral cyanosis results from decreased blood flow to a certain area of the body, as in vasoconstriction of the nailbeds or earlobes from exposure to cold, and does not necessarily indicate a central systemic problem.

PHYSICAL ASSESSMENT OF THE UPPER RESPIRATORY STRUCTURES

For a routine examination of the upper airway, only a simple light source, such as a penlight, is necessary. A more thorough examination requires the use of a nasal speculum.

Nose and Sinuses

The nurse inspects the external nose for lesions, asymmetry, or inflammation and then asks the patient to tilt the head backward.

Gently pushing the tip of the nose upward, the nurse examines the internal structures of the nose, inspecting the mucosa for colour, swelling, exudate, or bleeding. The nasal mucosa is normally redder than the oral mucosa, but it may appear swollen and hyperemic if the patient has a common cold. In allergic rhinitis, however, the mucosa appears pale and swollen.

Next the nurse inspects the septum for deviation, perforation, or bleeding. Most people have a slight degree of septal deviation, but actual displacement of the cartilage into either the right or left side of the nose may produce nasal obstruction. Such deviation usually causes no symptoms.

While the head is still tilted back, the nurse inspects the inferior and middle turbinates. In chronic rhinitis, nasal polyps may develop between the inferior and middle turbinates; they are distinguished by their grey appearance. Unlike the turbinates, they are gelatinous and freely movable.

Next the nurse may palpate the frontal and maxillary sinuses for tenderness (Fig. 21-7). Using the thumbs, the nurse applies gentle pressure in an upward fashion at the supraorbital ridges (frontal sinuses) and in the cheek area adjacent to the nose (maxillary sinuses). Tenderness in either area suggests inflammation. The frontal and maxillary sinuses can be inspected by transillumination (passing a strong light through a bony area, such as the sinuses, to inspect the cavity; Fig. 21-8). If the light fails to penetrate, the cavity may contain a tumour, fluid, or pus. Transillumination is controversial in adults. About 55% of patients with positive radiographic findings are likely to have abnormal transillumination of the maxillary and frontal sinuses (Low, Desrosiers, McSherry, Garber, Williams, Remmy et al., 1997)

Pharynx and Mouth

After the nasal inspection, the nurse may assess the mouth and pharynx, instructing the patient to open the mouth wide and take a deep breath. Usually this will flatten the posterior tongue and briefly allow a full view of the anterior and posterior pillars, tonsils, uvula, and posterior pharynx (Fig. 21-9). The nurse inspects these structures for colour, symmetry, and evidence of exudate, ulceration, or enlargement. If a tongue blade is needed to depress the tongue to visualize the pharynx, it is pressed firmly beyond the midpoint of the tongue to avoid a gagging response.

FIGURE 21-7 Technique for palpating the frontal sinuses at left and the maxillary sinuses at right. From Weber, J. & Kelley, J. (2003). *Health assessment in nursing* (2nd ed.). Philadelphia: Lippincott Williams & Wilkins.

FIGURE 21-8 At left, the nurse positions the light source for transillumination of the frontal sinus. At right, the nurse shields the patient's brow and shines the light. In normal conditions (a darkened room), the light should shine through the tissues and appear as a reddish glow (above the nurse's hand) over the sinus. From Weber, J. & Kelley, J. (2003). *Health assessment in nursing* (2nd ed.). Philadelphia: Lippincott Williams & Wilkins.

Trachea

Next the position and mobility of the trachea are usually noted by direct palpation. This is performed by placing the thumb and index finger of one hand on either side of the trachea just above the sternal notch. The trachea is highly sensitive, and palpating too firmly may trigger a coughing or gagging response. The trachea is normally in the midline as it enters the thoracic inlet behind the sternum, but it may be deviated by masses in the neck or mediastinum. Pleural or pulmonary disorders, such as a pneumothorax, may also displace the trachea.

PHYSICAL ASSESSMENT OF THE LOWER RESPIRATORY STRUCTURES AND BREATHING

Thorax

Inspection of the thorax provides information about the musculoskeletal structure, the patient's nutritional status, and the respiratory system. The nurse observes the skin over the thorax for colour and turgor and for evidence of loss of subcutaneous tissue. It is important to note asymmetry, if present. When findings are recorded or reported, anatomic landmarks are used as points of reference (Chart 21-7).

CHEST CONFIGURATION

Normally, the ratio of the anteroposterior diameter to the lateral diameter is 1:2. However, there are four main deformities of the chest associated with respiratory disease that alter this relationship: barrel chest, funnel chest (pectus excavatum), pigeon chest (pectus carinatum), and kyphoscoliosis.

Barrel Chest. Barrel chest occurs as a result of overinflation of the lungs. There is an increase in the anteroposterior diameter of the thorax. In a patient with emphysema, the ribs are more widely spaced and the intercostal spaces tend to bulge on expiration. The appearance of the patient with advanced emphysema is thus quite characteristic and often allows the observer to detect its presence easily, even from a distance.

Funnel Chest (Pectus Excavatum). Funnel chest occurs when there is a depression in the lower portion of the sternum. This may compress the heart and great vessels, resulting in murmurs. Funnel chest may occur with rickets or Marfan's syndrome.

Pigeon Chest (Pectus Carinatum). A pigeon chest occurs as a result of displacement of the sternum. There is an increase in the anteroposterior diameter. This may occur with rickets, Marfan's syndrome, or severe kyphoscoliosis.

Kyphoscoliosis. A kyphoscoliosis is characterized by elevation of the scapula and a corresponding S-shaped spine. This deformity limits lung expansion within the thorax. It may occur with osteoporosis and other skeletal disorders that affect the thorax.

BREATHING PATTERNS AND RESPIRATORY RATES

Observing the rate and depth of respiration is a simple but important aspect of assessment. The normal adult who is resting comfortably takes 12 to 18 breaths per minute. Except for occasional sighs, respirations are regular in depth and rhythm. This normal pattern is described as eupnea.

Bradypnea, also called slow breathing, is associated with increased intracranial pressure, brain injury, and drug overdose. Tachypnea, or rapid breathing, is commonly seen in patients with pneumonia, pulmonary edema, metabolic acidosis, septicemia,

Posterior pillar — Anterior pillar — Right tonsil

Hard palate — Soft palate — Uvula — Pharynx — Tongue

FIGURE 21-9 The pharynx and other oral structures—pillars, tonsils, uvula, hard and soft palates, posterior pharynx, and tongue—are easily seen when the mouth is open.

Chart 21-7 Locating Thoracic Landmarks

With respect to the thorax, location is defined both horizontally and vertically. With respect to the lungs, location is defined by lobe.

Horizontal Reference Points
Horizontally, thoracic locations are identified according to their proximity to the rib or the intercostal space under the examiner's fingers. On the anterior surface, identification of a specific rib is facilitated by first locating the angle of Louis. This is where the manubrium joins the body of the sternum in the midline. The second rib joins the sternum at this prominent landmark.

Other ribs may be identified by counting down from the second rib. The intercostal spaces are referred to in terms of the rib immediately above the intercostal space; for example, the fifth intercostal space is directly below the fifth rib.

Locating ribs on the posterior surface of the thorax is more difficult. The first step is to identify the spinous process. This is accomplished by finding the seventh cervical vertebra (*vertebra prominens*), which is the most prominent spinous process. When the neck is slightly flexed, the seventh cervical spinous process stands out. Other vertebrae are then identified by counting downward.

Vertical Reference Points
Several imaginary lines are used as vertical referents or landmarks to identify the location of thoracic findings. The *midsternal line* passes through the centre of the sternum. The *midclavicular line* is an imaginary line that descends from the middle of the clavicle. The *point of maximal impulse* of the heart normally lies along this line on the left thorax.

When the arm is abducted from the body at 90°, imaginary vertical lines may be drawn from the anterior axillary fold, from the middle of the axilla, and from the posterior axillary fold. These lines are called, respectively, the *anterior axillary line,* the *midaxillary line,* and the *posterior axillary line.* A line drawn vertically through the superior and inferior poles of the scapula is called the *scapular line,* and a line drawn down the centre of the vertebral column is called the *vertebral line.* Using these landmarks, for example, the examiner communicates findings by referring to an area of dullness extending from the vertebral to the scapular line between the seventh and tenth ribs on the right.

Lobes of the Lungs
The lobes of the lung may be mapped on the surface of the chest wall in the following manner. The line between the upper and lower lobes on the left begins at the fourth thoracic spinous process posteriorly, proceeds around to cross the fifth rib in the midaxillary line, and meets the sixth rib at the sternum. This line on the right divides the right middle lobe from the right lower lobe. The line dividing the right upper lobe from the middle lobe is an incomplete one that begins at the fifth rib in the midaxillary line, where it intersects the line between the upper and lower lobes and traverses horizontally to the sternum. Thus, the upper lobes are dominant on the anterior surface of the thorax and the lower lobes are dominant on the posterior surface. There is no presentation of the middle lobe on the posterior surface of the chest.

severe pain, and rib fracture. Shallow, irregular breathing is referred to as hypoventilation.

An increase in depth of respirations is called hyperpnea. An increase in both rate and depth that results in a lowered arterial PCO_2 level is referred to as hyperventilation. With rapid breathing, inspiration and expiration are nearly equal in duration. Hyperventilation that is marked by an increase in rate and depth, associated with severe acidosis of diabetic or renal origin, is called Kussmaul's respiration.

Apnea describes varying periods of cessation of breathing. If sustained, apnea is life-threatening.

Cheyne-Stokes respiration is characterized by alternating episodes of apnea (cessation of breathing) and periods of deep breathing. Deep respirations become increasingly shallow, followed by apnea that may last approximately 20 seconds. The cycle repeats after each apneic period. The duration of the period of apnea may vary and may progressively lengthen; therefore, it is timed and reported. Cheyne-Stokes respiration is usually associated with heart failure and damage to the respiratory centre (drug-induced, tumour, trauma).

Biot's respirations, or cluster breathing, are cycles of breaths that vary in depth and have varying periods of apnea. Biot's respirations are seen with some central nervous system disorders.

Certain patterns of respiration are characteristic of specific disease states. Respiratory rhythms and their deviation from normal are important observations that the nurse reports and documents. The rate and depth of different patterns of respiration are presented in Figure 21-10.

In thin people, it is quite normal to note a slight retraction of the intercostal spaces during quiet breathing. Bulging during expiration implies obstruction of expiratory airflow, as in emphysema. Marked retraction on inspiration, particularly if asymmetric, implies blockage of a branch of the respiratory tree. Asymmetric bulging of the intercostal spaces, on one side or the other, is created by an increase in pressure within the hemithorax. This may be a result of air trapped under pressure within the pleural cavity where it does not normally appear (pneumothorax) or the pressure of fluid within the pleural space (pleural effusion).

Thoracic Palpation

The nurse palpates the thorax for tenderness, masses, lesions, respiratory excursion, and vocal fremitus. If the patient has reported an area of pain or if lesions are apparent, the nurse performs direct palpation with the fingertips (for skin lesions and subcutaneous masses) or with the ball of the hand (for deeper masses or generalized flank or rib discomfort).

RESPIRATORY EXCURSION

Respiratory excursion is an estimation of thoracic expansion and may disclose significant information about thoracic movement during breathing. The nurse assesses the patient for range and symmetry of excursion. The patient is instructed to inhale deeply while the movement of the nurse's thumbs (placed along the costal margin on the anterior chest wall) during inspiration and expiration is observed. This movement is normally symmetric.

Posterior assessment is performed by placing the thumbs adjacent to the spinal column at the level of the tenth rib (Fig. 21-11). The hands lightly grasp the lateral rib cage. Sliding the thumbs medially about 2.5 cm raises a small skinfold between the thumbs. The patient is instructed to take a full inspiration and to exhale fully. The nurse observes for normal flattening of the skinfold and feels the symmetric movement of the thorax.

	Definition	Graphic Representation
Eupnea	Normal, breathing at 12-18 breaths/minute	
Bradypnea	Slower than normal rate (< 10 breaths/minute), with normal depth and regular rhythm	
Tachypnea	Rapid, shallow breathing > 24 breaths/minute	
Hypoventilation	Shallow, irregular breathing	
Hyperventilation	Increased rate and depth of breathing (called Kussmaul's respiration if caused by diabetic ketoacidosis)	
Apnea	Period of cessation of breathing. Time duration varies; apnea may occur briefly during other breathing disorders, such as with sleep apnea. Life threatening if sustained.	
Cheyne-Stokes	Regular cycle where the rate and depth of breathing increase, then decrease until apnea (usually about 20 seconds) occurs.	
Biot's respiration	Periods of normal breathing (3-4 breaths) followed by a varying period of apnea (usually 10 seconds to 1 minute).	

FIGURE 21-10 Graphic representation of different rates and depths of respiration.

true of consonant sounds. The detection of the resulting vibration on the chest wall by touch is called tactile fremitus.

Normal fremitus is widely varied. It is influenced by the thickness of the chest wall, especially if that thickness is muscular. However, the increase in subcutaneous tissue associated with obesity may also affect fremitus. Lower-pitched sounds travel better through the normal lung and produce greater vibration of the chest wall. Thus, fremitus is more pronounced in men than in women because of the deeper male voice. Normally, fremitus is most pronounced where the large bronchi are closest to the chest wall and least palpable over the distant lung fields. Therefore, it is most palpable in the upper thorax, anteriorly and posteriorly.

The patient is asked to repeat "ninety-nine" or "one, two, three," or "eee, eee, eee" as the nurse's hands move down the patient's thorax. The vibrations are detected with the palmar surfaces of the fingers and hands, or the ulnar aspect of the extended hands, on the thorax. The hand or hands are moved in sequence down the thorax. Corresponding areas of the thorax are compared (Fig. 21-12). Bony areas are not tested.

Air does not conduct sound well but a solid substance such as tissue does, provided that it has elasticity and is not compressed. Thus, an increase in solid tissue per unit volume of lung will enhance fremitus; an increase in air per unit volume of lung will impede sound. Patients with emphysema, which results in the rupture of alveoli and trapping of air, exhibit almost no tactile fremitus. A patient with consolidation of a lobe of the lung from pneumonia will have increased tactile fremitus over that lobe. Air in the pleural space will not conduct sound.

Thoracic Percussion

Percussion sets the chest wall and underlying structures in motion, producing audible and tactile vibrations. The nurse uses percussion to determine whether underlying tissues are filled with air, fluid, or solid material. Percussion also is used to estimate the size and location of certain structures within the thorax (eg, diaphragm, heart, liver).

FIGURE 21-11 Method for assessing posterior respiratory excursion. Place both hands posteriorly at the level of T9 or T10. Slide hands medially to pinch a small amount of skin between your thumbs. Observe for symmetry.

Decreased chest excursion may be due to chronic fibrotic disease. Asymmetric excursion may be due to splinting secondary to pleurisy, fractured ribs, trauma, or unilateral bronchial obstruction.

TACTILE FREMITUS
Sound generated by the larynx travels distally along the bronchial tree to set the chest wall in resonant motion. This is especially

FIGURE 21-12 When palpating for tactile fremitus (*left*), the nurse places the ball or ulnar surface of the hands on the chest area being assessed. The palpation sequence is at right. From Bickley L. S. (2003). *Bates' guide to physical examination and history taking* (8th ed.). Philadelphia: Lippincott Williams & Wilkins.

Percussion usually begins with the posterior thorax. Ideally, the patient is in a sitting position with the head flexed forward and the arms crossed on the lap. This position separates the scapulae widely and exposes more lung area for assessment. The nurse percusses across each shoulder top, locating the 5-cm width of resonance overlying the lung apices (Fig. 21-13). Then the nurse proceeds down the posterior thorax, percussing symmetric areas at 5- to 6-cm intervals. The middle finger is positioned parallel to the ribs in the intercostal space; the finger is placed firmly against the chest wall before striking it with the middle finger of the opposite hand. Bony structures (scapulae or ribs) are not percussed.

Percussion over the anterior chest is performed with the patient in an upright position with shoulders arched backward and arms at the side. The nurse begins in the supraclavicular area and proceeds downward, from one intercostal space to the next. In the female patient, it may be necessary to displace the breasts for an adequate examination. Dullness noted to the left of the sternum between the third and fifth intercostal spaces is a normal finding because it is the location of the heart. Similarly, there is a normal span of liver dullness in the right thorax from the fifth intercostal space to the right costal margin at the midclavicular line.

The anterior and lateral thorax is examined with the patient in a supine position. If the patient cannot sit up, percussion of the posterior thorax is performed with the patient positioned on the side.

Dullness over the lung occurs when air-filled lung tissue is replaced by fluid or solid tissue. Table 21-3 reviews percussion sounds and their characteristics.

DIAPHRAGMATIC EXCURSION

The normal resonance of the lung stops at the diaphragm. The position of the diaphragm is different during inspiration than during expiration.

FIGURE 21-13 Percussion of the posterior thorax. With the patient in a sitting position, symmetric areas of the lungs are percussed at 5-cm intervals. This progression starts at the apex of each lung and concludes with percussion of each lateral chest wall.

To assess the position and motion of the diaphragm, the nurse instructs the patient to take a deep breath and hold it while the maximal descent of the diaphragm is percussed. The point at which the percussion note at the midscapular line changes from resonance to dullness is marked with a pen. The patient is then instructed to exhale fully and hold it while the nurse again percusses downward to the dullness of the diaphragm. This point is also marked. The distance between the two markings indicates the range of motion of the diaphragm.

Maximal excursion of the diaphragm may be as much as 8 to 10 cm in healthy, tall young men, but for most people it is usually 5 to 7 cm. Normally, the diaphragm is about 2 cm higher on the right because of the position of the heart and the liver above and below the left and right segments of the diaphragm, respectively. Decreased diaphragmatic excursion may occur with pleural effusion and emphysema. An increase in intra-abdominal pressure, as in pregnancy or ascites, may account for a diaphragm that is positioned high in the thorax.

Thoracic Auscultation

Auscultation is useful in assessing the flow of air through the bronchial tree and in evaluating the presence of fluid or solid obstruction in the lung structures. The nurse auscultates for normal breath sounds, adventitious sounds, and voice sounds.

Examination includes auscultation of the anterior, posterior, and lateral thorax and is performed as follows. The nurse places the diaphragm of the stethoscope firmly against the chest wall as the patient breathes slowly and deeply through the mouth. Corresponding areas of the chest are auscultated in a systematic fashion from the apices to the bases and along midaxillary lines. The sequence of auscultation and the positioning of the patient are similar to those used for percussion. It often is necessary to listen to two full inspirations and expirations at each anatomic location for valid interpretation of the sound heard. Repeated deep breaths may result in symptoms of hyperventilation (eg, light-headedness); this is avoided by having the patient rest and breathe normally periodically during the examination.

BREATH SOUNDS

Normal breath sounds are distinguished by their location over a specific area of the lung and are identified as vesicular, bronchovesicular, and bronchial (tubular) breath sounds (Table 21-4).

The location, quality, and intensity of breath sounds are determined during auscultation. When airflow is decreased by bronchial obstruction (atelectasis) or when fluid (pleural effusion) or tissue (obesity) separates the air passages from the stethoscope, breath sounds are diminished or absent. For example, the breath sounds of the patient with emphysema are faint or often completely inaudible. When heard, the expiratory phase is prolonged. Bronchial and bronchovesicular sounds that are audible anywhere except over the main bronchus in the lungs signify pathology, usually indicating consolidation in the lung (eg, pneumonia, heart failure). This finding requires further evaluation.

ADVENTITIOUS SOUNDS

An abnormal condition that affects the bronchial tree and alveoli may produce adventitious (additional) sounds. Adventitious sounds are divided into two categories: discrete, noncontinuous sounds (crackles) and continuous musical sounds (wheezes). The duration of the sound is the important distinction to make in identifying the sound as noncontinuous or continuous. Pleural friction rubs are specific examples of crackles (Table 21-5).

Table 21-3 • Characteristics of Percussion Sounds

SOUND	RELATIVE INTENSITY	RELATIVE PITCH	RELATIVE DURATION	LOCATION EXAMPLE	EXAMPLES
Flatness	Soft	High	Short	Thigh	Large pleural effusion
Dullness	Medium	Medium	Medium	Liver	Lobar pneumonia
Resonance	Loud	Low	Long	Normal lung	Simple chronic bronchitis
Hyperresonance	Very loud	Lower	Longer	None normally	Emphysema, pneumothorax
Tympany	Loud	High*	*	Gastric air bubble or puffed-out cheek	Large pneumothorax

*Distinguished mainly by its musical timbre

Crackles (formerly referred to as rales) are discrete, noncontinuous sounds that result from delayed reopening of deflated airways. Crackles may or may not be cleared by coughing. Crackles reflect underlying inflammation or congestion and are often present in such conditions as pneumonia, bronchitis, heart failure, bronchiectasis, and pulmonary fibrosis.

Friction rubs result from inflammation of the pleural surfaces that induces a crackling, grating sound usually heard in inspiration and expiration. The sound can be enhanced by applying pressure to the chest wall with the diaphragm of the stethoscope. The sound is imitated by rubbing the thumb and index finger together near the ear. A friction rub is best heard over the lower lateral anterior surface of the thorax.

Wheezes are associated with bronchial wall oscillation and changes in airway diameter. Wheezes are commonly heard in patients with asthma, chronic bronchitis, and bronchiectasis.

VOICE SOUNDS

The sound heard through the stethoscope as the patient speaks is known as vocal resonance. The vibrations produced in the larynx are transmitted to the chest wall as they pass through the bronchi and alveolar tissue. During the process, the sounds are diminished in intensity and altered so that syllables are not distinguishable. Voice sounds are usually assessed by having the patient repeat "ninety-nine" or "eee" while the nurse listens with the stethoscope in corresponding areas of the chest from the apices to the bases.

Bronchophony describes vocal resonance that is more intense and clearer than normal. Egophony describes voice sounds that are distorted. It is best appreciated by having the patient repeat the letter E. The distortion produced by consolidation transforms the sound into a clearly heard A rather than E. Bronchophony and egophony have precisely the same significance as bronchial breathing with an increase in tactile fremitus. When an abnormality is detected, it should be evident using more than one assessment method. A change in tactile fremitus is more subtle and can be missed, but bronchial breathing and bronchophony can be noted loudly and clearly.

Whispered pectoriloquy is a very subtle finding, heard only in the presence of rather dense consolidation of the lungs. Transmission of high-frequency components of sound is so enhanced by the consolidated tissue that even whispered words are heard, a circumstance not noted in normal physiology. The significance is the same as that of bronchophony.

Table 21-4 • Breath Sounds

	DURATION OF SOUNDS	INTENSITY OF EXPIRATORY SOUND	PITCH OF EXPIRATORY SOUND	LOCATIONS WHERE HEARD NORMALLY
Vesicular*	Inspiratory sounds last longer than expiratory ones.	Soft	Relatively low	Entire lung field except over the upper sternum and between the scapulae
Broncho-vesicular	Inspiratory and expiratory sounds are about equal.	Intermediate	Intermediate	Often in the 1st and 2nd interspaces anteriorly and between the scapulae (over the main bronchus)
Bronchial	Expiratory sounds last longer than inspiratory ones.	Loud	Relatively high	Over the manubrium, if heard at all
Tracheal	Inspiratory and expiratory sounds are about equal.	Very loud	Relatively high	Over the trachea in the neck

*The thickness of the bars indicates intensity of breath sounds; the steeper their incline, the higher the pitch of the sounds.

BREATH SOUND	DESCRIPTION	ETIOLOGY
Crackles		
Crackles in general	Soft, high-pitched, discontinuous popping sounds that occur during inspiration	Secondary to fluid in the airways or alveoli or to opening of collapsed alveoli
Coarse crackles	Discontinuous popping sounds heard in early inspiration; harsh, moist sound originating in the large bronchi	Associated with obstructive pulmonary disease
Fine crackles	Discontinuous popping sounds heard in late inspiration; sounds like hair rubbing together; originates in the alveoli	Associated with interstitial pneumonia, restrictive pulmonary disease (eg, fibrosis). Fine crackles in early inspiration are associated with bronchitis or pneumonia.
Wheezes		
Sonorous wheezes (rhonchi)	Deep, low-pitched rumbling sounds heard primarily during expiration; caused by air moving through narrowed tracheobronchial passages	Secretions or tumour
Sibilant wheezes	Continuous, musical, high-pitched, whistle-like sounds heard during inspiration and expiration caused by air passing through narrowed or partially obstructed airways; may clear with coughing	Bronchospasm, asthma, and buildup of secretions
Friction rubs		
Pleural friction rub	Harsh, crackling sound, like two pieces of leather being rubbed together. Heard during inspiration alone or during both inspiration and expiration. May subside when patient holds breath. Coughing will not clear sound.	Secondary to inflammation and loss of lubricating pleural fluid

Table 21-5 • Abnormal (Adventitious) Breath Sounds

The physical findings for the most common respiratory diseases are summarized in Table 21-6.

PHYSICAL ASSESSMENT OF BREATHING ABILITY IN THE ACUTELY ILL PATIENT

Tests of the patient's breathing ability are easily performed at the bedside by measuring the respiratory rate (see the previous section "Breathing Patterns and Respiratory Rates"), tidal volume, minute ventilation, vital capacity, inspiratory force, and compliance. These tests are particularly important for patients at risk for developing pulmonary complications, including those who have undergone chest or abdominal surgery, have had prolonged anesthesia, have preexisting pulmonary disease, or are elderly. These tests are also used routinely for mechanically ventilated patients.

Patients whose chest expansion is limited by external restrictions such as obesity or abdominal distention and who cannot breathe deeply because of postoperative pain or sedation will inhale and exhale a low volume of air (referred to as low tidal volumes). Prolonged hypoventilation at low tidal volumes can produce alveolar collapse or atelectasis. The amount of air remaining in the lungs after a normal expiration (functional residual capacity) falls, the ability of the lungs to expand (compliance) is reduced, and the patient must breathe faster to maintain the same degree of tissue oxygenation. These events can be exaggerated in patients who have preexisting pulmonary diseases and in elderly patients whose airways are less compliant, because the small airways may collapse during expiration.

NURSING ALERT One should not rely only on visual inspection of the rate and depth of a patient's respiratory excursions to determine the adequacy of ventilation. Respiratory excursions may appear normal or exaggerated due to an increased work of breathing, but the patient may actually be moving only enough air to ventilate the dead space. If there is any question regarding adequacy of ventilation, auscultation and/or pulse oximetry should be used for additional assessment of respiratory status.

Tidal Volume

The volume of each breath is referred to as the tidal volume (see Table 21-1 to review lung capacities and volumes). A spirometer is an instrument that can be used at the bedside to measure volumes. If the patient is breathing through an endotracheal tube or tracheostomy, the spirometer is directly attached to it and the exhaled volume is obtained from the reading on the gauge. In other patients, the spirometer is attached to a facemask or a mouthpiece positioned so that it is airtight, and the exhaled volume is measured.

The tidal volume may vary from breath to breath. To make the measurement reliable, it is important to measure the volumes of several breaths and to note the range of tidal volumes, together with the average tidal volume.

Minute Ventilation

Respiratory rates and tidal volume alone are unreliable indicators of adequate ventilation because both can vary widely from breath to breath. Together, however, the tidal volume and respiratory

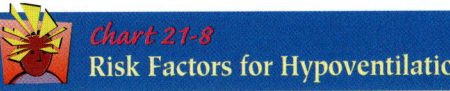

PROBLEM	TACTILE FREMITUS	PERCUSSION	AUSCULTATION
Consolidation (eg, pneumonia)	Increased	Dull	Bronchial breath sounds, crackles, bronchophony, egophony, whispered pectoriloquy
Bronchitis	Normal	Resonant	Normal to decreased breath sounds, wheezes
Emphysema	Decreased	Hyperresonant	Decreased intensity of breath sounds, usually with prolonged expiration
Asthma (severe attack)	Normal to decreased	Resonant to hyperresonant	Wheezes
Pulmonary edema	Normal	Resonant	Crackles at lung bases, possibly wheezes
Pleural effusion	Absent	Dull to flat	Decreased to absent breath sounds, bronchial breath sounds and bronchophony, egophony, and whispered pectoriloquy above the effusion over the area of compressed lung
Pneumothorax	Decreased	Hyperresonant	Absent breath sounds
Atelectasis	Absent	Flat	Decreased to absent breath sounds

Table 21-6 • **Assessment Findings in Common Respiratory Problems**

rate are important because the minute ventilation, which is useful in detecting respiratory failure, can be determined from them. Minute ventilation is the volume of air expired per minute. It is equal to the product of the tidal volume and the respiratory rate or frequency. In practice, the minute ventilation is not calculated but is measured directly using a spirometer.

Minute ventilation may be decreased by a variety of conditions that result in hypoventilation. When the minute ventilation falls, alveolar ventilation in the lungs also decreases, and the $PaCO_2$ increases. Risk factors for hypoventilation are listed in Chart 21-8.

Vital Capacity

Vital capacity is measured by having the patient take in a maximal breath and exhale fully through a spirometer. The normal value depends on the patient's age, gender, body build, and weight.

> **NURSING ALERT** Most patients can generate a vital capacity twice the volume they normally breathe in and out (tidal volume). If the vital capacity is less than 10 mL/kg, the patient will be unable to sustain spontaneous ventilation and will require respiratory assistance.

When the vital capacity is exhaled at a maximal flow rate, the forced vital capacity is measured. Most patients can exhale at least 80% of their vital capacity in 1 second (forced expiratory volume in 1 second, or FEV_1) and almost all of it in 3 seconds (FEV_3). A reduction in FEV_1 suggests abnormal pulmonary air flow. If the patient's FEV_1 and forced vital capacity are proportionately reduced, maximal lung expansion is restricted in some way. If the reduction in FEV_1 greatly exceeds the reduction in forced vital capacity, the patient may have some degree of airway obstruction.

Inspiratory Force

Inspiratory force evaluates the effort the patient is making during inspiration. It does not require patient cooperation and thus is

useful in the unconscious patient. The equipment needed for this measurement includes a manometer that measures negative pressure and adapters that are connected to an anesthesia mask or a cuffed endotracheal tube. The manometer is attached and the airway is completely occluded for 10 to 20 seconds while the inspiratory efforts of the patient are registered on the manometer. The normal inspiratory pressure is about 100 cm H_2O. If the negative pressure registered after 15 seconds of occluding the airway is less than about 25 cm H_2O, mechanical ventilation is usually required because the patient lacks sufficient muscle strength for deep breathing or effective coughing.

Diagnostic Evaluation

A wide range of diagnostic studies, described on the following pages, may be performed in patients with respiratory conditions.

PULMONARY FUNCTION TESTS

Pulmonary function tests (PFTs) are routinely used in patients with chronic respiratory disorders. They are performed to assess respiratory function and to determine the extent of dysfunction. Such tests include measurements of lung volumes, ventilatory

> *Chart 21-8*
> **Risk Factors for Hypoventilation**
>
> - Limited neurologic impulses transmitted from the brain to the respiratory muscles, as in spinal cord trauma, cerebrovascular accidents, tumours, myasthenia gravis, Guillain-Barré syndrome, polio, and drug overdose
> - Depressed respiratory centres in the medulla, as with anesthesia and drug overdose
> - Limited thoracic movement (kyphoscoliosis), limited lung movement (pleural effusion, pneumothorax), or reduced functional lung tissue (chronic pulmonary diseases, severe pulmonary edema)

function, and the mechanics of breathing, diffusion, and gas exchange (Table 21-7).

PFTs are useful in following the course of a patient with an established respiratory disease and assessing the response to therapy. They are useful as screening tests in potentially hazardous industries, such as coal mining and those that involve exposure to asbestos and other noxious fumes, dusts, or gases. They are useful for screening patients scheduled for thoracic and upper abdominal surgery, and symptomatic patients with a history suggesting high risk.

PFTs generally are performed by a technician using a spirometer that has a volume-collecting device attached to a recorder that demonstrates volume and time simultaneously. A number of tests are carried out because no single measurement provides a complete picture of pulmonary function. The most frequently used PFTs are described in Table 21-7. Technology is available that allows for more complex assessment of pulmonary function. Methods include exercise tidal flow-volume loops, negative expiratory pressure, nitric oxide, and forced oscillation. These assessment methods allow for detailed evaluation of expiratory flow limitations and airway inflammation (Johnson, Beck, Zeballos & Weisman, 1999).

PFT results are interpreted on the basis of the degree of deviation from normal, taking into consideration the patient's height, weight, age, and gender. Because there is a wide range of normal values, PFTs may not detect early localized changes. The patient with respiratory symptoms (dyspnea, wheezing, cough, sputum production) usually undergoes a complete diagnostic evaluation, even though the results of PFTs are "normal." Trends of results provide information about disease progression as well as the patient's response to therapy.

Patients with respiratory disorders may be taught how to measure their peak flow rate (reflects maximal expiratory flow) at home using a spirometer. This allows them to monitor the progress of therapy, to alter medications and other interventions as needed based on caregiver guidelines, or to notify the health care provider if there is inadequate response to their own interventions. Home care teaching instructions are described in Chapter 24, which discusses asthma.

ARTERIAL BLOOD GAS STUDIES

Measurements of blood pH and of arterial oxygen and carbon dioxide tensions are obtained when managing patients with respiratory problems and in adjusting oxygen therapy as needed. The arterial oxygen tension (PaO_2) indicates the degree of oxygenation of the blood, and the arterial carbon dioxide tension ($PaCO_2$) indicates the adequacy of alveolar ventilation. Arterial blood gas studies aid in assessing the ability of the lungs to provide adequate oxygen and remove carbon dioxide and the ability of the kidneys to reabsorb or excrete bicarbonate ions to maintain normal body pH. Serial blood gas analysis also is a sensitive indicator of whether the lung has been damaged after chest trauma. Arterial blood gas levels are obtained through an arterial puncture at the radial, brachial, or femoral artery or through an indwelling arterial catheter. Arterial blood gas levels are discussed in detail in Chapter 14.

PULSE OXIMETRY

Pulse oximetry is a noninvasive method of continuously monitoring the oxygen saturation of hemoglobin (SpO_2 or SaO_2). Although pulse oximetry does not replace arterial blood gas measurement, it is an effective tool to monitor for subtle or sudden changes in oxygen saturation. It is used in all settings where oxygen saturation monitoring is needed, such as the home, clinics, ambulatory surgical settings, and hospitals.

A probe or sensor is attached to the fingertip (Fig. 21-14), forehead, earlobe, or bridge of the nose. The sensor detects changes in oxygen saturation levels by monitoring light signals generated by the oximeter and reflected by blood pulsing through the tissue at the probe. Normal SpO_2 values are 95% to 100%. Values less than 85% indicate that the tissues are not receiving enough oxygen, and the patient needs further evaluation. SpO_2 values obtained by pulse oximetry are unreliable in cardiac arrest and shock, when dyes (ie, methylene blue) or vasoconstrictor medications have been used, or when the patient has severe anemia or a high carbon monoxide level.

Table 21-7 • Pulmonary Function Tests

TERM USED	SYMBOL	DESCRIPTION	REMARKS
Forced vital capacity	FVC	Vital capacity performed with a maximally forced expiratory effort	Forced vital capacity is often reduced in COPD because of air trapping.
Forced expiratory volume (qualified by subscript indicating the time intervals in seconds)	FEV_t, usually FEV_1	Volume of air exhaled in the specified time during the performance of forced vital capacity; FEV_1 is volume exhaled in 1 second	A valuable clue to the severity of the expiratory airway obstruction
Ratio of timed forced expiratory volume to forced vital capacity	$FEV_t/FVC\%$, usually $FEV_1/FVC\%$	FEV_t expressed as a percentage of the forced vital capacity	Another way of expressing the presence or absence of airway obstruction
Forced expiratory flow	$FEF_{200-1200}$	Mean forced expiratory flow between 200 and 1,200 mL of the FVC	An indicator of large airway obstruction
Forced midexpiratory flow	$FEF_{25\%-75\%}$	Mean forced expiratory flow during the middle half of the FVC	Slowed in small airway obstruction
Forced end expiratory flow	$FEF_{75\%-85\%}$	Mean forced expiratory flow during the terminal portion of the FVC	Slowed in obstruction of smallest airways
Maximal voluntary ventilation	MVV	Volume of air expired in a specified period (12 seconds) during repetitive maximal effort	An important factor in exercise tolerance

IMAGING STUDIES

Imaging studies, including x-rays, computed tomography (CT) scans, magnetic resonance imaging (MRI), contrast studies, and radioisotope diagnostic scans may be part of any diagnostic workup, ranging from a determination of the extent of infection in sinusitis to tumour growth in cancer.

Chest X-Ray

Normal pulmonary tissue is radiolucent; therefore, densities produced by fluid, tumours, foreign bodies, and other pathologic conditions can be detected by x-ray examination. A chest x-ray may reveal an extensive pathologic process in the lungs in the absence of symptoms. The routine chest x-ray consists of two views—the posteroanterior projection and the lateral projection. Chest x-rays are usually taken after full inspiration (a deep breath) because the lungs are best visualized when they are well aerated. Also, the diaphragm is at its lowest level and the largest expanse of lung is visible. If taken on expiration, x-ray films may accentuate an otherwise unnoticed pneumothorax or obstruction of a major artery.

Computed Tomography

CT is an imaging method in which the lungs are scanned in successive layers by a narrow-beam x-ray. The images produced provide a cross-sectional view of the chest. Whereas a chest x-ray shows major contrast between body densities, such as bones, soft tissues, and air, CT scans can distinguish fine tissue density. CT may be used to define pulmonary nodules and small tumours adjacent to pleural surfaces that are not visible on routine chest x-ray, and to demonstrate mediastinal abnormalities and hilar adenopathy, which are difficult to visualize with other techniques. Contrast agents are useful when evaluating the mediastinum and its contents.

Magnetic Resonance Imaging

MRIs are similar to CT scans except that magnetic fields and radiofrequency signals are used instead of a narrow-beam x-ray. MRIs yield a much more detailed diagnostic image than CT scans. MRI is used to characterize pulmonary nodules, stage bronchogenic carcinoma (assessment of chest wall invasion), and evaluate inflammatory activity in interstitial lung disease, acute pulmonary embolism, and chronic thrombolytic pulmonary hypertension (Kauczor & Kreitner, 2000).

Fluoroscopic Studies

Fluoroscopy is used to assist with invasive procedures, such as a chest needle biopsy or transbronchial biopsy, performed to identify lesions. It also may be used to study the movement of the chest wall, mediastinum, heart, and diaphragm, to detect diaphragm paralysis, and to locate lung masses.

Pulmonary Angiography

Pulmonary angiography is most commonly used to investigate thromboembolic disease of the lungs, such as pulmonary emboli and congenital abnormalities of the pulmonary vascular tree. It involves the rapid injection of a radiopaque agent into the vasculature of the lungs for radiographic study of the pulmonary vessels.

FIGURE 21-14 Measuring blood oxygenation with pulse oximetry reduces the need for invasive procedures, such as drawing blood for analysis of oxygen levels. After the pulse oximeter sensor slips easily over a patient's finger, the oxygen saturation level appears on the monitor. The oximeter is portable and ideal for home use. Courtesy Novametrix Medical Systems, Inc.

CULTURES

Throat cultures may be performed to identify organisms responsible for pharyngitis. Throat culture may also assist in identifying organisms responsible for infection of the lower respiratory tract. Nasal swabs also may be performed for the same purpose.

SPUTUM STUDIES

Sputum is obtained for analysis to identify pathogenic organisms and to determine whether malignant cells are present. It also may be used to assess for hypersensitivity states (in which there is an increase in eosinophils). Periodic sputum examinations may be necessary for patients receiving antibiotics, corticosteroids, and immunosuppressive medications for prolonged periods because these agents are associated with opportunistic infections. In general, sputum cultures are used in diagnosis, for drug sensitivity testing, and to guide treatment.

Expectoration is the usual method for collecting a sputum specimen. The patient is instructed to clear the nose and throat and rinse the mouth to decrease contamination of the sputum. After taking a few deep breaths, the patient coughs (rather than spits), using the diaphragm, and expectorates into a sterile container.

If the sputum cannot be raised spontaneously, the patient often can be induced to cough deeply by breathing an irritating aerosol of supersaturated saline, propylene glycol, or some other agent delivered with an ultrasonic nebulizer. Other methods of collecting sputum specimens include endotracheal aspiration, bronchoscopic removal, bronchial brushing, transtracheal aspiration, and gastric aspiration—usually for tuberculosis organisms (see Chap. 23). Generally, the deepest specimens (those from the base of the lungs) are obtained in the early morning after they have accumulated overnight.

The specimen is delivered to the laboratory within 2 hours by the patient or nurse. Allowing the specimen to stand for several hours in a warm room results in the overgrowth of contaminant organisms and may make it difficult to identify the organisms (especially *Mycobacterium tuberculosis*). The home care nurse may assist patients who need help obtaining the sample or who cannot deliver the specimen to the laboratory in a timely fashion.

FIGURE 21-15 Endoscopic bronchoscopy permits visualization of bronchial structures. The bronchoscope is advanced into bronchial structures orally. Bronchoscopy permits the clinician not only to diagnose but also to treat various lung problems.

piratory status and observes for hypoxia, hypotension, tachycardia, dysrhythmias, hemoptysis, and dyspnea. Any abnormality is reported promptly. The patient is not discharged from the recovery area until adequate cough reflex and respiratory status are present. The nurse instructs the patient and family caregivers to report any shortness of breath or bleeding immediately.

Thoracoscopy

Thoracoscopy is a diagnostic procedure in which the pleural cavity is examined with an endoscope (Fig. 21-16). Small incisions are made into the pleural cavity in an intercostal space; the location of the incision depends on the clinical and diagnostic findings. After any fluid present in the pleural cavity is aspirated, the fibreoptic mediastinoscope is inserted into the pleural cavity, and its surface is inspected through the instrument. After the procedure, a chest tube may be inserted, and the pleural cavity is drained by negative-pressure water-seal drainage.

Thoracoscopy is primarily indicated in the diagnostic evaluation of pleural effusions, pleural disease, and tumour staging. Biopsies of the lesions can be performed under visualization for diagnosis.

Thoracoscopic procedures have expanded with the availability of video monitoring, which permits improved visualization of the lung. Such procedures also have been used with the carbon dioxide laser in the removal of pulmonary blebs and bullae and in the treatment of spontaneous pneumothorax. Lasers have also

FIGURE 21-16 Endoscopic thoracoscopy. Like bronchoscopy, thoracoscopy uses fibreoptic instruments and video cameras for visualizing thoracic structures. Unlike bronchoscopy, thoracoscopy usually requires the surgeon to make a small incision before inserting the endoscope. A combined diagnostic–treatment procedure, thoracoscopy includes excising tissue for biopsy.

been used in the excision of peripheral pulmonary nodules. Although the laser does not replace the need for thoracotomy in the treatment of some lung cancers, its use continues to expand because it is less invasive.

NURSING INTERVENTIONS

Follow-up care in the health care facility and at home involves monitoring the patient for shortness of breath (which might indicate a pneumothorax), and minor activity restrictions, which vary depending on the intensity of the procedure. If a chest tube is in place, monitoring the chest drainage system and chest tube insertion site is essential (see Chap. 25).

THORACENTESIS

A thin layer of pleural fluid normally remains in the pleural space. An accumulation of pleural fluid may occur with some disorders. A sample of this fluid can be obtained by thoracentesis (aspiration of pleural fluid for diagnostic or therapeutic purposes). It is important to position the patient as shown in Chart 21-9.

A needle biopsy of the pleura may be performed at the same time. Studies of pleural fluid include Gram's stain culture and sensitivity, acid-fast staining and culture, differential cell count, cytology, pH, specific gravity, total protein, and lactic dehydrogenase.

BIOPSY

Biopsy, the excision of a small amount of tissue, may be performed to permit examination of cells from the pharynx, larynx, and nasal passages. Local, topical, or general anesthesia may be administered, depending on the site and the procedure (see also "Lung Biopsy Procedures" below).

Pleural Biopsy

Pleural biopsy is accomplished by needle biopsy of the pleura or by pleuroscopy, a visual exploration through a fibreoptic bronchoscope inserted into the pleural space. Pleural biopsy is performed when there is pleural exudate of undetermined origin and when there is a need to culture or stain the tissue to identify tuberculosis or fungi.

Lung Biopsy Procedures

When the chest x-ray findings are inconclusive or show pulmonary density (indicating an infiltrate or lesion), biopsy may be performed to obtain lung tissue for examination to identify the nature of the lesion. There are several nonsurgical lung biopsy techniques that are used because they yield accurate information with low morbidity: (1) transcatheter bronchial brushing, (2) transbronchial lung biopsy, or (3) percutaneous (through-the-skin) needle biopsy.

In transcatheter bronchial brushing, a fibreoptic bronchoscope is introduced into the bronchus under fluoroscopy. A small brush attached to the end of a flexible wire is inserted through the bronchoscope. Under direct visualization, the area under suspicion is brushed back and forth, causing cells to slough off and adhere to the brush. The catheter port of the bronchoscope may be used to irrigate the lung tissue with saline solution to secure material for additional studies. The brush is removed from the bronchoscope and a microscopic slide is made. The brush may be cut off and sent to the pathology laboratory for analysis.

This procedure is useful for cytologic evaluations of lung lesions and for the identification of pathogenic organisms (*Nocardia, Aspergillus, Pneumocystis carinii,* and other pathogens). It is especially useful in the immunologically compromised patient.

A transbronchial lung biopsy uses biting or cutting forceps introduced by a fibreoptic bronchoscope. A biopsy is indicated when a lung lesion is suspected and the results of routine sputum samples and bronchoscopic washings are negative.

Another method of bronchial brushing involves the introduction of the catheter through the transcricothyroid membrane by needle puncture. After this procedure, the patient is instructed to hold a finger or thumb over the puncture site while coughing to prevent air from leaking into the surrounding tissues.

Percutaneous needle biopsy may be accomplished with a cutting needle or by aspiration with a spinal-type needle that provides a tissue specimen for histologic study. Analgesia may be administered before the procedure. The skin over the biopsy site is cleansed and anesthetized and a small incision is made. The biopsy needle is inserted through the incision into the pleura with the patient holding the breath in mid-expiration. Using fluoroscopic monitoring, the surgeon guides the needle into the periphery of the lesion and obtains a tissue sample from the mass. Possible complications include pneumothorax, pulmonary hemorrhage, and empyema.

NURSING INTERVENTIONS

After the procedure, recovery and home care are similar to those for bronchoscopy and thoracoscopy. Nursing care involves monitoring the patient for shortness of breath, bleeding, and infection. In preparation for discharge, the patient and/or family is instructed to report pain, shortness of breath, visible bleeding, or redness of the biopsy site or pus to the health care provider immediately. Patients who have undergone biopsy are often anxious because of the need for the biopsy and the potential findings; the nurse must consider this in providing postbiopsy care and teaching.

Lymph Node Biopsy

The scalene lymph nodes are enmeshed in the deep cervical pad of fat overlying the scalenus anterior muscle. They drain the lungs and mediastinum and may show histologic changes from intrathoracic disease. When these nodes are palpable on physical examination, a scalene node biopsy may be performed. A biopsy of these nodes may be performed to detect lymph node spread of pulmonary disease and to establish a diagnosis or prognosis in such diseases as Hodgkin's disease, sarcoidosis, fungal disease, tuberculosis, and carcinoma.

Mediastinoscopy is the endoscopic examination of the mediastinum for exploration and biopsy of mediastinal lymph nodes that drain the lungs; this examination does not require a thoracotomy. Biopsy is usually performed through a suprasternal incision. Mediastinoscopy is carried out to detect mediastinal involvement of pulmonary malignancy and to obtain tissue for diagnostic studies of other conditions (eg, sarcoidosis).

An anterior mediastinotomy is thought to provide better exposure and diagnostic possibilities than a mediastinoscopy. An incision is made in the area of the second or third costal cartilage. The mediastinum is explored and biopsies are performed on any lymph nodes found. Chest tube drainage is required after the procedure. Mediastinotomy is particularly valuable to determine whether a pulmonary lesion is resectable.

Chart 21-9

GUIDELINES FOR Assisting the Patient Undergoing Thoracentesis

A thoracentesis (aspiration of fluid or air from the pleural space) is performed on patients with various clinical problems. A diagnostic or therapeutic procedure, thoracentesis may be used for:

- Removal of fluid and air from the pleural cavity
- Aspiration of pleural fluid for analysis
- Pleural biopsy
- Instillation of medication into the pleural space

The responsibilities of the nurse and rationale for the nursing actions are summarized below.

NURSING ACTIVITIES

1. Ascertain in advance that a chest x-ray has been ordered and completed and the consent form has been signed.

2. Assess the patient for allergy to the local anesthetic to be used. Administer sedation if prescribed.

3. Inform the patient about the nature of the procedure and:
   a. The importance of remaining immobile
   b. Pressure sensations to be experienced
   c. That minimal discomfort is anticipated after the procedure
4. Position the patient comfortably with adequate supports. If possible, place the patient upright or in one of the following positions:
   a. Sitting on the edge of the bed with the feet supported and arms and head on a padded over-the-bed table

RATIONALE

1. Posteroanterior and lateral chest x-ray films are used to localize fluid and air in the pleural cavity and to aid in determining the puncture site. When fluid is loculated (isolated in a pocket of pleural fluid), ultrasound scans are performed to help select the best site for needle aspiration.
2. If the patient is allergic to the initially prescribed anesthetic, assessment findings provide an opportunity to use a safer anesthetic.
3. An explanation helps to orient the patient to the procedure, assists the patient to mobilize resources, and provides an opportunity to ask questions and verbalize anxiety.

4. The upright position facilitates the removal of fluid that usually localizes at the base of the chest. A position of comfort helps the patient to relax.

Patient positioned for thoracentesis.

   b. Straddling a chair with arms and head resting on the back of the chair
   c. Lying on the unaffected side with the bed elevated 30 degrees to 45 degrees if unable to assume a sitting position
5. Support and reassure the patient during the procedure.
   a. Prepare the patient for the cold sensation of skin germicide solution and for a pressure sensation from infiltration of local anesthetic agent.
   b. Encourage the patient to refrain from coughing.

5. Sudden and unexpected movement, such as coughing, by the patient can traumatize the visceral pleura and lung.

(continued)

Chart 21-9

GUIDELINES FOR Assisting the Patient Undergoing Thoracentesis (Continued)

NURSING ACTIVITIES	RATIONALE
6. Expose the entire chest. The site for aspiration is visualized by chest x-ray film and percussion. If fluid is in the pleural cavity, the thoracentesis site is determined by the chest x-ray, ultrasound scanning, and physical findings, with attention to the site of maximal dullness on percussion.	6. If air is in the pleural cavity, the thoracentesis site is usually in the second or third intercostal space in the midclavicular line because air rises in the thorax.
7. The procedure is performed under aseptic conditions. After the skin is cleansed, the physician uses a small-calibre needle to inject a local anesthetic slowly into the intercostal space.	7. An intradermal wheal is raised slowly; rapid injection causes pain. The parietal pleura is very sensitive and should be well infiltrated with anesthetic before the physician passes the thoracentesis needle through it.
8. The physician advances the thoracentesis needle with the syringe attached. When the pleural space is reached, suction may be applied with the syringe.	
a. A 20-mL syringe with a three-way stopcock is attached to the needle (one end of the adapter is attached to the needle and the other to the tubing leading to a receptacle that receives the fluid being aspirated).	a. When a large quantity of fluid is withdrawn, a three-way stopcock serves to keep air from entering the pleural cavity.
b. If a considerable quantity of fluid is removed, the needle is held in place on the chest wall with a small hemostat.	b. The hemostat steadies the needle on the chest wall. Sudden pleuritic chest pain or shoulder pain may indicate that the needle point is irritating the visceral or the diaphragmatic pleura.
9. After the needle is withdrawn, pressure is applied over the puncture site and a small, sterile dressing is fixed in place.	9. Pressure helps to stop bleeding and the dressing protects the site.
10. Advise the patient that he or she will be on bed rest and a chest x-ray will be obtained after thoracentesis.	10. A chest x-ray verifies that there is no pneumothorax.
11. Record the total amount of fluid withdrawn from the procedure and document the nature of the fluid, its colour, and its viscosity. If indicated, prepare samples of fluid for laboratory evaluation. A specimen container with formalin may be needed for a pleural biopsy.	11. The fluid may be clear, serous, bloody, purulent, etc.
12. Monitor the patient at intervals for increasing respiratory rate; asymmetry in respiratory movement; faintness; vertigo; tightness in chest; uncontrollable cough; blood-tinged, frothy mucus; a rapid pulse; and signs of hypoxemia.	12. Pneumothorax, tension pneumothorax, subcutaneous emphysema, or pyrogenic infection are complications of a thoracentesis. Pulmonary edema or cardiac distress can occur after a sudden shift in mediastinal contents when large amounts of fluid are aspirated.

NURSING INTERVENTIONS

Postprocedure care focuses on providing adequate oxygenation, monitoring for bleeding, and providing pain relief. The patient may be discharged a few hours after the chest drainage system is removed. The nurse should instruct the patient and family about monitoring for changes in respiratory status, taking into consideration the impact of anxiety about the potential findings of the biopsy on their ability to remember those instructions.

Critical Thinking Exercises

1. After a transbronchial lung biopsy, your patient reports shortness of breath and appears anxious. He is coughing up blood-tinged sputum. Based on your knowledge of the risks associated with lung biopsy, how would you focus your assessment? What physical and psychological nursing interventions would be appropriate for the patient at this time?

2. Your patient is scheduled for a video-assisted thoracoscopy. Describe the postprocedure nursing care and teaching for a patient undergoing this procedure. Identify the specific assessment parameters that are indicated.

3. Your patient has had a thoracentesis to remove pleural fluid for laboratory analysis and to relieve shortness of breath. What assessment should be carried out following the procedure? What teaching is warranted for the patient and family if she is to be discharged an hour after the procedure? How would you modify your instructions to the patient if she lives alone?

4. Your frail, elderly patient has a diagnosis of long-standing cardiac disease and is scheduled for PFTs prior to surgery to repair her cardiac valves. What specific explanations about the tests would you provide to the patient? What problems would you monitor for following the PFT?

REFERENCES AND SELECTED READINGS

Books

Bickley, L. S. (2003). *Bates' guide to physical examination and history taking* (8th ed.). Philadelphia: Lippincott Williams & Wilkins.

Blair, K. A. (1999). The aging pulmonary system. In M. Stanley & P. G. Bear (Eds.), *Gerontological nursing* (2d ed.). Philadelphia: F. A. Davis.

Levitzky, M. G. (1999). *Pulmonary physiology* (4th ed.). New York: McGraw Hill.

Sole, M. L., & Byers, J. F. (2001). Ventilatory assistance. In M. L. Sole, J. C. Hartshorn, & M. L. Lamborn (Eds.), *Introduction to critical care nursing* (3rd ed.). Philadelphia: W. B. Saunders.

West, J. B. (2000). *Respiratory physiology: The essentials.* Philadelphia: Lippincott Williams & Wilkins.

West, J. B. (2001). *Pulmonary physiology and pathophysiology: An integrated, case-based approach.* Philadelphia: Lippincott Williams & Wilkins.

Wilkins, R. L., Sheldon, R. L., & Knider, S. J. (2000). *Clinical assessment in respiratory care* (4th ed.). St. Louis: Mosby-Year Book.

Journals

Asterisks indicate nursing research articles.

*Bailey, P. H. (2004). The dyspnea-anxiety-dyspnea cycle—COPD patients' stories of breathlessness: "It's scary when you can't breathe." *Qualitative Health Research, 14*(6), 760–778.

Boyle, A. H., & Waters, H. F. (2000). Issues in respiratory nursing: Focus on prevention: recommendations of the National Lung Health Education Program. *Heart & Lung, 29*(6), 446–449.

Camhi, S. L., & Enright, P. L. (2000). How to assess pulmonary function in older persons. *Journal of Respiratory Diseases, 21*(6), 395–399.

*Cicutto, L., Brooks, D., & Henderson, K. (2003). Self-care issues from the perspective of individuals with chronic obstructive pulmonary disease. *Patient Education and Counseling, 55*, 168–176.

Coleman, R. E. (1999). PET in lung cancer. *Journal of Nuclear Medicine, 40*(5), 814–820.

Graeber, G. M., Gupta, N. C., & Murray, G. F. (1999). Positron emission tomographic imaging with fluorodeoxyglucose is efficacious in evaluating malignant pulmonary disease. *Journal of Thoracic and Cardiovascular Surgery, 117*(4), 719–727.

Horne, C., & Derrico, D. (1999). Mastering ABGs. The art of arterial blood gas measurement. *American Journal of Nursing, 99*(8), 26–32.

Janssens, J. P., de Muralt, B., & Titelion, V. (2000). Management of dyspnea in severe chronic obstructive pulmonary disease. *Journal of Pain and Symptom Management, 19*(5), 378–392.

Johnson, B. D., Beck, K. C., Zeballos, R. J., & Weisman, I. M. (1999). Advances in pulmonary laboratory testing. *Chest, 116*(5), 1377–1387.

Kauczor, H. U., & Kreitner, K. E. (2000). Contrast-enhanced MRI of the lung. *European Journal of Radiology, 34*(3), 196–207.

Low, M., Desrosiers, J., McSherry, G., Garber, G., Williams, J. W., Remy, R. S. et al. (1997). A practical guide for the diagnosis and treatment of acute sinusitis. *Canadian Medical Association Journal, 156*(Suppl 6), S1–S14.

Lowe, V. J., Fletcher, J. W., Gobar, L., Lawson, M., et al. (1998). Prospective investigation of positron emission tomography in lung nodules. *Journal of Clinical Oncology, 16*(3), 1075–1084.

Martin, B., Llewellyn, J., Faut-Callahan, M., & Meyer, P. (2000). The use of telemetric oximetry in the clinical setting. *MedSurg Nursing, 9*(2), 71–76.

*Nield, M. (2000). Dyspnea self-management in African Americans with chronic lung disease. *Heart & Lung, 29*(1), 50–55.

Salzman, S. (1999). Pulmonary function testing: Tips on how to interpret the results. *Journal of Respiratory Diseases, 20*(12), 809–812.

Shortall, S. P., & Perkins, L. A. (1999). Interpreting the ins and outs of pulmonary function tests. *Nursing, 29*(12), 41–47.

Shuster, D. P. (1998). The evaluation of lung function with PET. *Seminars in Nuclear Medicine, 28*(4), 341–351.

Wong, F. W. H. (1999). A new approach to ABG interpretation. *American Journal of Nursing, 99*(8), 34–36.

RESOURCES AND WEBSITES

Canadian Lung Association, 3 Raymond Street, Suite 300, Ottawa, ON K1R 1A3; (613) 569-6411; 1-888-566-Lung (5864); http://www.lung.ca.

National Heart, Lung, and Blood Institute/National Institutes of Health, Rockville Pike, Bldg. 31, Bethesda, MD 20892; (301) 496-5166; http://www.nhlbi.nih.gov/nhlbi/index.htm.

National Lung Health Education Program: http://www.nlhep.org. Has easy-to-read teaching resources for patients.

Registered Nurses Association of Ontario, 111 Richmond Street West, Suite 1100, Toronto, ON M5H 2G4; www.rnao.org/bestpractice.

Management of Patients With Upper Respiratory Tract Disorders

Adapted By Carolyn J. M. Ross

LEARNING OBJECTIVES

On completion of this chapter, the learner will be able to:

1. Describe nursing management of patients with upper airway disorders.
2. Compare and contrast the upper respiratory tract infections with regard to cause, incidence, clinical manifestations, management, and the significance of preventive health care.
3. Use the nursing process as a framework for care of patients with upper airway infection.
4. Describe nursing management of the patient with epistaxis.
5. Use the nursing process as a framework for care of patients undergoing laryngectomy.

Many upper airway disorders are relatively minor, and their effects are limited to mild and temporary discomfort and inconvenience for the patient. However, other upper airway disorders are acute, severe, and life-threatening and may require permanent alterations in breathing and speaking. Thus, the nurse must have good assessment skills, an understanding of the wide variety of disorders that may affect the upper airway, and an awareness of the impact of these alterations on patients.

Because many of the disorders are treated outside the hospital or at home by patients themselves, patient teaching is an important aspect of nursing care. When caring for patients with acute, life-threatening disorders, the nurse needs highly developed assessment and clinical management skills, along with a focus on rehabilitation needs.

Upper Airway Infections

Upper airway infections are common conditions that affect most people on occasion. Some infections are acute, with symptoms that last several days; others are chronic, with symptoms that last a long time or recur. Patients with these conditions seldom require hospitalization. However, nurses working in community settings or long-term care facilities may encounter patients who have these infections. Thus, it is important for the nurse to recognize the signs and symptoms and to provide appropriate care.

RHINITIS

Rhinitis is a group of disorders characterized by inflammation and irritation of the mucous membranes of the nose. It may be classified as nonallergic or allergic. It is estimated that allergic rhinitis affects 10% to 25% of the North American population (Middleton et al., 1998). Rhinitis may be an acute or chronic condition.

Pathophysiology

Nonallergic rhinitis may be caused by a variety of factors, including environmental factors such as changes in temperature or humidity, odours, or foods; infection; age; systemic disease; drugs (cocaine) or prescribed medications; or the presence of a foreign body. Drug-induced rhinitis is associated with use of antihypertensive agents and oral contraceptives and chronic use of nasal decongestants. Rhinitis also may be a manifestation of an allergy (see Chap. 53), in which case it is referred to as allergic rhinitis. Figure 22-1 shows the pathological processes involved in rhinitis and sinusitis.

Clinical Manifestations

The signs and symptoms of rhinitis include **rhinorrhea** (excessive nasal drainage, runny nose), nasal congestion, nasal discharge (purulent with bacterial rhinitis), nasal itchiness, and sneezing. Headache may occur, particularly if sinusitis is also present.

Medical Management

The management of rhinitis depends on the cause, which may be identified in the history and physical examination. The examiner asks the patient about recent symptoms as well as possible exposure to allergens in the home, environment, or workplace. If viral rhinitis is the cause, medications are given to relieve the symptoms. In allergic rhinitis, tests may be performed to identify possible allergens. Depending on the severity of the allergy, desensitizing immunizations and corticosteroids may be required (see Chap. 53 for more details). If symptoms suggest a bacterial infection, an antimicrobial agent will be used (see "Medical Management of Sinusitis").

PHARMACOLOGIC THERAPY

Medication therapy for allergic and nonallergic rhinitis focuses on symptom relief. Antihistamines are administered for sneezing, itching, and rhinorrhea. Oral decongestant agents are used for nasal obstruction. In addition, intranasal corticosteroids may be used for severe congestion, and ophthalmic agents are used to relieve irritation, itching, and redness of the eyes.

Nursing Management

TEACHING PATIENTS SELF-CARE

The nurse instructs the patient with allergic rhinitis to avoid or reduce exposure to allergens and irritants, such as dusts, molds, animals, fumes, odours, powders, sprays, and tobacco smoke. The patient is instructed about the importance of controlling the environment at home and work. Saline nasal or aerosol sprays may be helpful in soothing mucous membranes, softening crusted secretions, and removing irritants. The nurse instructs the patient in the proper use of and technique for administrating nasal medications. To achieve maximal relief, the patient is instructed to blow the nose before applying any medication into the nasal cavity. In the case of infectious rhinitis, the nurse reviews with the patient hand hygiene technique as a measure to prevent transmission of organisms. The nurse teaches methods to treat symptoms of the viral rhinitis. In the elderly and other high-risk populations, the nurse reviews the value of receiving a vaccination

Glossary

alaryngeal communication: alternative modes of speaking that do not involve the normal larynx; used by patients whose larynx has been surgically removed

aphonia: impaired ability to use one's voice due to disease or injury to the larynx

apnea: cessation of breathing

dysphagia: difficulties in swallowing

epistaxis: hemorrhage from the nose due to rupture of tiny, distended vessels in the mucous membrane of any area of the nose

herpes simplex: cold sore (cutaneous viral infection with painful vesicles and erosions on the tongue, palate, gingival, buccal membranes, or lips)

laryngitis: inflammation of the larynx; may be due to voice abuse, exposure to irritants, or infectious organisms

laryngectomy: removal of all or part of the larynx and surrounding structures

pharyngitis: inflammation of the throat; usually viral or bacterial in origin

rhinitis: inflammation of the mucous membranes of the nose; may be infectious, allergic, or inflammatory in origin

rhinorrhea: drainage of a large amount of fluid from the nose

sinusitis: inflammation of the sinuses; may be acute or chronic; may be viral, bacterial, or fungal in origin

submucous resection: surgical procedure to correct nasal obstruction due to deviated septum; also called septoplasty

tonsillitis: inflammation of the tonsils, usually due to an acute infection

xerostomia: dryness of the mouth from a variety of causes

Physiology/Pathophysiology

A. Rhinitis

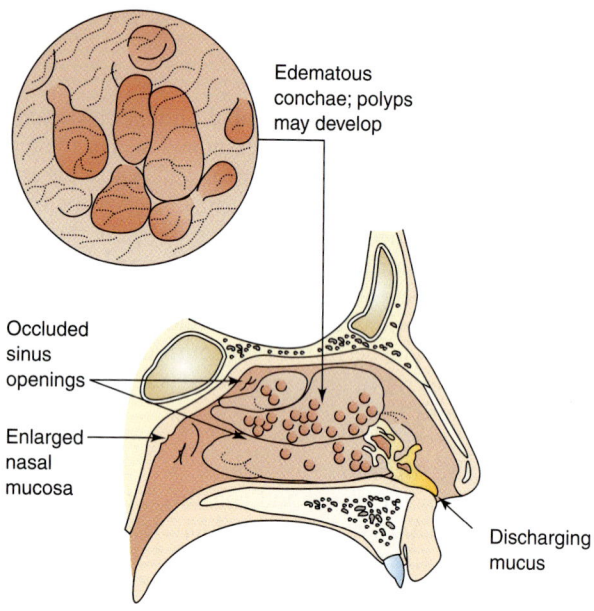

Edematous conchae; polyps may develop

Occluded sinus openings

Enlarged nasal mucosa

Discharging mucus

B. Sinusitis

Thick mucus occludes sinus cavity and prevents drainage

FIGURE 22-1 Pathophysiologic processes in rhinitis and sinusitis. Although pathophysiologic processes are similar in rhinitis and sinusitis, they affect different structures. In rhinitis (**A**), the mucous membranes lining the nasal passages become inflamed, congested, and edematous. The swollen nasal conchae block the sinus openings, and mucus is discharged from the nostrils. Sinusitis (**B**) is also marked by inflammation and congestion, with thickened mucous secretions filling the sinus cavities and occluding the openings.

in the fall in order to achieve immunity prior to the beginning of the "flu season."

VIRAL RHINITIS (COMMON COLD)

The term "common cold" often is used when referring to an upper respiratory tract infection that is self-limited and caused by a virus (viral rhinitis). Nasal congestion, rhinorrhea, sneezing, sore throat, and general malaise characterize it. Specifically, the term "cold" refers to an afebrile, infectious, acute inflammation

of the mucous membranes of the nasal cavity. More broadly, the term refers to an acute upper respiratory tract infection, whereas terms such as "rhinitis," "pharyngitis," and "laryngitis" distinguish the sites of the symptoms. It can also be used when the causative virus is influenza ("the flu"). Colds are highly contagious because virus is shed for about 2 days before the symptoms appear and during the first part of the symptomatic phase. It is estimated that adults in Canada have two to four colds per year. The common cold is the most common cause of absenteeism from work and school (Mandell, Bennett, & Dolin, 2000).

The six viruses known to produce the signs and symptoms of the viral rhinitis are rhinovirus, parainfluenza virus, coronavirus, respiratory syncytial virus (RSV), influenza virus, and adenovirus. Each virus may have multiple strains. For example, there are over 100 strains of rhinovirus, which accounts for 50% of all colds. The incidence of viral rhinitis follows a specific pattern during the year, depending on the causative agent (Fig. 22-2). Even though viral rhinitis can occur at any time of the year, three waves account for the epidemics in the United States:

- In September, just after the opening of school
- In late January
- Toward the end of April

Immunity after recovery is variable and depends on many factors, including a person's natural host resistance and the specific virus that caused the cold.

Clinical Manifestations

Signs and symptoms of viral rhinitis are nasal congestion, runny nose, sneezing, nasal discharge, nasal itchiness, tearing watery eyes, "scratchy" or sore throat, general malaise, low-grade fever, chills,

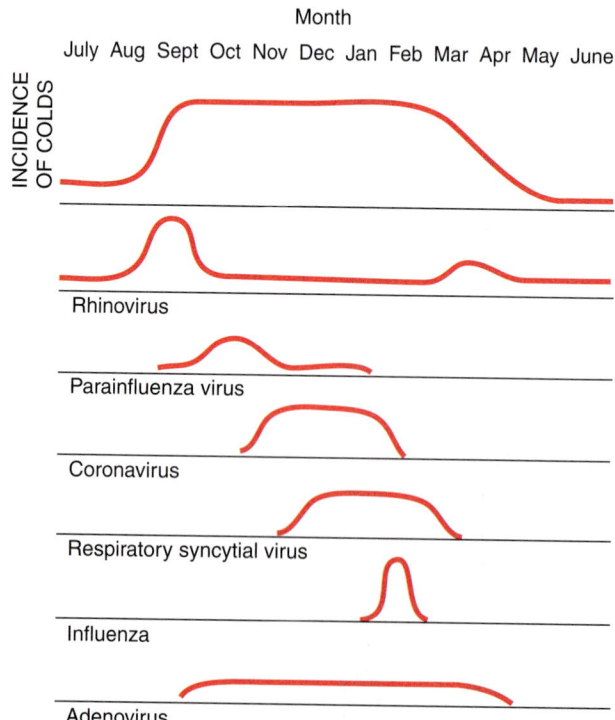

FIGURE 22-2 Schematic diagram incidence of viral rhinitis (common cold) in the United States and the frequency of the causative agents. Redrawn from Goldman, L. & Bennett, J. C. (eds.) (2000) *Cecil textbook of medicine* (21st ed., Vol. 2). Philadelphia: W. B. Saunders, p. 1791.

and often headache and muscle aches. As the illness progresses, cough usually appears. In some people, viral rhinitis exacerbates the **herpes simplex**, commonly called a cold sore (Chart 22-1).

The symptoms last from 1 to 2 weeks. If there is significant fever or more severe systemic respiratory symptoms, it is no longer viral rhinitis but one of the other acute upper respiratory tract infections. Allergic conditions can also affect the nose, mimicking the symptoms of a cold.

Medical Management

There is no specific treatment for the common cold or influenza. Management consists of symptomatic therapy. Some measures include providing adequate fluid intake, encouraging rest, preventing chilling, increasing intake of vitamin C, and using expectorants as needed. Warm salt-water gargles soothe the sore throat and nonsteroidal anti-inflammatory agents (NSAIDs) such as aspirin or ibuprofen relieve the aches, pains, and fever in adults. Antihistamines are used to relieve sneezing, rhinorrhea, and nasal congestion. Topical (nasal) decongestant agents may relieve nasal congestion; however, if they are overused they may create a rebound congestion that may be worse than the original symptoms. Some research suggests that zinc lozenges may reduce the duration of cold symptoms if taken within the first 24 hours of onset (Prasad, Fitzgerald, & Bao, 2000). Amantadine (Symmetrel) may be prescribed prophylactically to decrease the signs and symptoms as well. Antimicrobial agents (antibiotics) should not be used because they do not affect the virus or reduce the incidence of bacterial complications.

Nursing Management

TEACHING PATIENTS SELF-CARE

Most viruses can be transmitted in several ways: direct contact with infected secretions; inhalation of large particles that land on a mucosal surface from coughing or sneezing; or inhalation of small particles (aerosol) that may be suspended in the air for up to an hour. It is important to teach the patient how to break the chain of infection. Hand washing remains the most effective measure to prevent transmission of organisms. The nurse teaches methods to treat symptoms of the common cold and preventive measures (Chart 22-2).

ACUTE SINUSITIS

The sinuses, mucus-lined cavities filled with air that drain normally into the nose, are involved in a high proportion of upper respiratory tract infections. If their openings into the nasal passages are clear, the infections resolve promptly. However, if their drainage is obstructed by a deviated septum or by hypertrophied turbinates, spurs, or nasal polyps or tumours, sinus infection may persist as a smoldering secondary infection or progress to an acute suppurative process (causing purulent discharge). It is estimated that **sinusitis** affects over 14% of the population in Canada (Tierney, McPhee, & Papadakis, 2001). Some individuals are more prone to sinusitis because of their occupations. For example, continuous exposure to environmental hazards such as paint, sawdust, and chemicals may result in chronic inflammation of the nasal passages.

Pathophysiology

Acute sinusitis is an infection of the paranasal sinuses. It frequently develops as a result of an upper respiratory infection, such as an unresolved viral or bacterial infection, or an exacerbation of allergic rhinitis. Nasal congestion, caused by inflammation, edema, and transudation of fluid, leads to obstruction of the sinus cavities (see Fig. 22-1). This provides an excellent medium for bacterial growth. Bacterial organisms account for more than 60% of the cases of acute sinusitis, namely *Streptococcus pneumoniae*, *Haemophilus influenzae*, and *Moraxella catarrhalis* (Murray & Nadel, 2001). Dental infections also have been associated with acute sinusitis.

Clinical Manifestations

Symptoms of acute sinusitis may include facial pain or pressure over the affected sinus area, nasal obstruction, fatigue, purulent nasal discharge, fever, headache, ear pain and fullness, dental pain, cough, a decreased sense of smell, sore throat, eyelid edema, or facial congestion or fullness. Acute sinusitis can be difficult to differentiate from an upper respiratory infection or allergic rhinitis.

Chart 22-1 Colds and Cold Sores (Herpes Simplex Virus)

The herpes simplex virus (HSV-1) produces the familiar *herpes labialis,* commonly called a cold sore or fever blister. In the past, this painful blisterlike lip sore was thought to be caused by a cold or a fever. Even now that scientists recognize the origin of herpes labialis, the condition is still referred to as a cold sore. The herpes virus infection remains latent in cells of the lips or nose and is activated by stress, sunlight, and febrile illnesses from the common cold to streptococcal pneumonia, meningococcal meningitis, and even malaria.

The incubation period is 2 to 12 days. The virus is transmitted primarily by direct contact with infected secretions. The virus may also be transmitted from an asymptomatic person. Small vesicles, single or clustered, may erupt on the lips, inside the mouth, including the tongue, soft and hard palate, gums, buccal mucosa, and the pharynx. These soon rupture, forming sore shallow ulcers that increase in number. The gums may bleed and feel painful.

The herpes virus may subside spontaneously in 10 to 14 days. If it does not, acyclovir, an antiviral agent, may be administered orally or topically to minimize the symptoms and the duration or length of the flare-up. Analgesics, such as acetaminophen (Tylenol) with codeine or aspirin with codeine, are helpful in relieving pain and discomfort. Topical anesthetics, such as lidocaine (Xylocaine) or dyclonine (Dyclone), and over-the-counter preparations, such as Herpecin-L, may relieve oral pain. Applications of drying lotions or liquids may help to dry the lesions.

With permission from Goodheart, H. P. (1999). *Photoguide of common skin disorders: Diagnosis and management.* Baltimore: Lippincott Williams & Wilkins.

Chart 22-2
Home Care Checklist · Preventing and Managing Upper Respiratory Infections

At the completion of the home care instruction, the patient or caregiver will be able to:

	Patient	Caregiver
Prevention		
• Identify strategies to prevent infection and, if infected, to prevent spread of infection to others	✓	✓
Perform hand hygiene often		
Use disposable tissues		
Avoid crowds during the flu season		
Avoid individuals with colds or respiratory infections		
Obtain influenza vaccination, if recommended (especially if elderly or diagnosed with a chronic illness)		
• Practice good health habits	✓	✓
Eat a nutritious diet		
Get plenty of rest and sleep		
Avoid or reduce stress when possible		
Exercise appropriately		
Avoid smoking or second-hand smoke and excessive intake of alcohol		
Increase humidity in house, especially during winter		
Practice adequate oral hygiene		
• Avoid allergens, if allergies are associated with upper respiratory infections	✓	
Prevention and Management		
• Identify strategies to control the environment	✓	✓
Adequately humidify (avoid overhumidifying) living quarters		
Place a dehumidifier in the basement, if appropriate		
Provide central ventilation fans, air conditioning with microstatic air filters		
Reduce irritants (dust, chemical, tobacco smoke) when possible		
Limit exposure to animals and house pets, particularly in the bedroom		
Management		
• Describe strategies to relieve symptoms of upper respiratory infection	✓	✓
Gargle with salt water		
Increase fluid intake, particularly of hot liquids		
Provide warm, moist air by shower or humidifier to relieve swollen mucous membranes		
Avoid irritants (dust, chemicals, tobacco smoke) when possible		
• Recognize signs and symptoms of infection and state when to contact a health care provider	✓	✓
Upper respiratory infection symptoms persisting longer than 7 to 10 days		
Extreme red throat or white patches on the back of the throat		
Discoloured drainage or foul-smelling nasal discharge		
Prolonged fever of 38°C >2 days		
Shortness of breath, wheezing		
Swollen lymph nodes		
Severe pain or tenderness around the eyes or persistent pain in sinus areas		
Severe headache		

Assessment and Diagnostic Findings

A careful history and physical examination are performed. The head and neck, particularly the nose, ears, teeth, sinuses, pharynx, and chest, are examined. There may be tenderness to palpation over the infected sinus area. The sinuses are percussed using the index finger, tapping lightly to determine if the patient experiences pain. The affected area is also transilluminated; with sinusitis, there may be a decrease in the transmission of light (see Chap. 21, Fig. 21-8). Sinus x-rays may be performed to detect sinus opacity, mucosal thickening, bone destruction, and air–fluid levels. Computed tomography scanning of the sinuses is the most effective diagnostic tool. It is also used to rule out other local or systemic disorders, such as tumour, fistula, and allergy.

Complications

Acute sinusitis, if left untreated, may lead to severe and occasionally life-threatening complications such as meningitis, brain abscess, ischemic infarction, and osteomyelitis. Other complications of sinusitis, although uncommon, include severe orbital cellulitis, subperiosteal abscess, and cavernous sinus thrombosis.

Medical Management

The goals of treatment of acute sinusitis are to treat the infection, shrink the nasal mucosa, and relieve pain. There is a growing concern over the inappropriate use of antibiotics for viral upper respiratory infections; such overuse has resulted in antibiotics being less effective (more resistant) in treating bacterial infections such as sinusitis. As a result, careful consideration is given to the potential pathogen before antimicrobial agents are prescribed.

The antimicrobial agents of choice for a bacterial infection vary in clinical practice. First-line antibiotics include amoxicillin (Amoxil) or, if there is a β-lactam allergy, use TMP/SMX (cotrimoxazole). Second-line antibiotics include amoxicillin clavulanate (Augmentin) and cefuroxime axetil (Ceftin). Macrolides, such as azithromycin (Zithromax) and clarithromycin (Biaxin), and quinolones, such as levofloxacin (Levaquin), moxifloxacin, and gatifloxacin, should be reserved for patients with β-lactam allergy (Poole, 1999). The course of treatment is usually 10 days. A recent report found little difference in clinical outcomes between first-line and second-line antibiotics; however, costs were greater when newer second-line antibiotics were used (Piccirillo, Mager, Frisse et al., 2001).

Use of oral and topical decongestant agents may decrease mucosal swelling of nasal polyps, thereby improving drainage of the sinuses. Heated mist and saline irrigation also may be effective for opening blocked passages. Decongestant agents such as pseudoephedrine (Sudafed, Dimetapp) have proven effective because of their vasoconstrictive properties. Topical decongestant agents such as oxymetazoline (Afrin) may be used for up to 72 hours. It is important to administer them with the patient's head tilted back to promote maximal dispersion of the medication. Guaifenesin (Robitussin, Anti-Tuss), a mucolytic agent, may also be effective in reducing nasal congestion.

In 2000, the U.S. Food and Drug Administration issued a public health advisory concerning phenylpropanolamine, which previously had been commonly used in oral decongestants and diet pills. The voluntary recall of products containing this ingredient was based on a study linking its use with hemorrhagic stroke in women. Men may also be at risk (Kernan et al., 2000).

Antihistamines should be avoided in acute sinusitis because of their potential to aggravate sinusitis.

Nursing Management

TEACHING PATIENTS SELF-CARE

Patient teaching is an important aspect of nursing care for the patient with acute sinusitis. The nurse instructs the patient about methods to promote drainage such as inhaling steam (steam bath, hot shower, and facial sauna), increasing fluid intake, and applying local heat (hot wet packs). The nurse also informs the patient about the side effects of nasal sprays and about rebound congestion. In the case of rebound congestion, the body's receptors, which have become dependent on the decongestant sprays to keep the nasal passages open, close and congestion results after the spray is discontinued.

The nurse stresses the importance of following the recommended antibiotic regimen, because a consistent blood level of the medication is critical to treat the infection. The nurse teaches the patient the early signs of a sinus infection and recommends preventive measures such as following healthy practices and avoiding contact with people who have upper respiratory infections (see Chart 22-2).

The nurse should explain to the patient that fever, severe headache, and nuchal rigidity are signs of potential complications. If fever persists despite antibiotic therapy, the patient should seek additional care.

CHRONIC SINUSITIS

Chronic sinusitis is an inflammation of the sinuses that persists for more than 3 weeks in an adult and 2 weeks in a child. It is estimated that 32 million people a year develop chronic sinusitis.

Pathophysiology

A narrowing or obstruction in the ostia of the frontal, maxillary, and anterior ethmoid sinuses usually causes chronic sinusitis,

preventing adequate drainage to the nasal passages. This combined area is known as the osteomeatal complex. Blockage that persists for greater than 3 weeks in an adult may occur because of infection, allergy, or structural abnormalities. This results in stagnant secretions, an ideal medium for infection. The organisms that cause chronic sinusitis are the same as those implicated in acute sinusitis. Immunocompromised patients, however, are at increased risk for developing fungal sinusitis. *Aspergillus fumigatus* is the most common organism associated with fungal sinusitis.

Clinical Manifestations

Clinical manifestations of chronic sinusitis include impaired mucociliary clearance and ventilation, cough (because the thick discharge constantly drips backward into the nasopharynx), chronic hoarseness, chronic headaches in the periorbital area, and facial pain. These symptoms are generally most pronounced on awakening in the morning. Fatigue and nasal stuffiness are also common. In addition, some patients experience a decrease in smell and taste and a fullness in the ears.

Assessment and Diagnostic Findings

A careful history and diagnostic assessment, including a computed tomography scan of the sinuses or magnetic resonance imaging (if fungal sinusitis is suspected), are performed to rule out other local or systemic disorders, such as tumour, fistula, and allergy. Nasal endoscopy may be indicated to rule out underlying diseases such as tumours and sinus mycetomas (fungus balls). The fungus ball is usually a brown or greenish-black material with the consistency of peanut butter or cottage cheese.

Complications

Complications of chronic sinusitis, although uncommon, include severe orbital cellulitis, subperiosteal abscess, cavernous sinus thrombosis, meningitis, encephalitis, and ischemic infarction.

Medical Management

The goals of treatment of chronic sinusitis are to treat the infection, shrink the nasal mucosa, and relieve pain. The antimicrobial agents of choice include amoxicillin clavulanate (Augmentin) or clindamycin. The recommended course of treatment is 3 weeks, although longer periods may be required in exceptional circumstances. Topical nasal steroids, decongestant agents, saline sprays, and heated mist may also provide some symptom relief. Where a clear allergic component has been demonstrated antihistamines may be used. Decongestant agents, saline sprays, and heated mist may also provide some symptom relief.

SURGICAL MANAGEMENT

When standard medical therapy fails, surgery, usually endoscopic, may be indicated to correct structural deformities that obstruct the ostia (openings) of the sinus. Excising and cauterizing nasal polyps, correcting a deviated septum, incising and draining the sinuses, aerating the sinuses, and removing tumours are some of the specific procedures performed. When sinusitis is caused by a fungal infection, surgery is required to excise the fungus ball and necrotic tissue and drain the sinuses. Oral and topical corticosteroids are usually prescribed. Antimicrobial agents are administered before and after surgery. Some patients with severe chronic sinusitis obtain relief only by moving to a dry climate.

Nursing Management

Because the patient usually performs care measures for sinusitis at home, nursing management consists mainly of patient teaching.

TEACHING PATIENTS SELF-CARE

The nurse teaches the patient how to promote sinus drainage by increasing the environmental humidity (steam bath, hot shower, and facial sauna), increasing fluid intake, and applying local heat (hot wet packs). The nurse also instructs the patient about the importance of following the medication regimen. Instructions on the early signs of a sinus infection are provided and preventive measures are reviewed.

ACUTE PHARYNGITIS

Acute **pharyngitis** is an inflammation or infection in the throat, usually causing symptoms of a sore throat.

Pathophysiology

Most cases of acute pharyngitis are caused by viral infection. When group A beta-hemolytic streptococcus, the most common bacterial organism, causes acute pharyngitis, the condition is known as strep throat (Bisno, 2001). The body responds by triggering an inflammatory response in the pharynx. This results in pain, fever, vasodilation, edema, and tissue damage, manifested by redness and swelling in the tonsillar pillars, uvula, and soft palate. A creamy exudate may be present in the tonsillar pillars (Fig. 22-3).

Uncomplicated viral infections usually subside promptly, within 3 to 10 days after the onset. However, pharyngitis caused by more virulent bacteria such as group A beta-hemolytic streptococci is a more severe illness. If left untreated, the complications can be severe and life-threatening. Complications include sinusitis, otitis media, peritonsillar abscess, mastoiditis, and cervical adenitis. In rare cases the infection may lead to bacteremia, pneumonia, meningitis, rheumatic fever, or nephritis.

Clinical Manifestations

The signs and symptoms of acute pharyngitis include a fiery-red pharyngeal membrane and tonsils, lymphoid follicles that are swollen and flecked with white-purple exudate, and enlarged and tender cervical lymph nodes and no cough. Fever, malaise, and sore throat also may be present.

Assessment and Diagnostic Findings

Rapid screening tests for streptococcal antigens such as the latex agglutination (LA) antigen test and solid-phase enzyme immunoassays (ELISA), optical immunoassay (OIA), streptolysin titers, and throat cultures are used to determine the causative organism, after which appropriate therapy is prescribed. Nasal swabs and blood cultures may also be necessary to identify the organism (Corneli, 2001).

Medical Management

Viral pharyngitis is treated with supportive measures since antibiotics will have no effect on the organism. Bacterial pharyngitis is treated with a variety of antimicrobial agents.

PHARMACOLOGIC THERAPY

If a bacterial cause is suggested or demonstrated, penicillin is usually the treatment of choice. For patients who are allergic to penicillin or have organisms that are resistant to erythromycin (one fifth of group A beta-hemolytic streptococci and most *S. aureus* organisms are resistant to penicillin and erythromycin), clindamycin is a second-line alternative. Cephalosporins and macrolides (clarithromycin and azithromycin) are generally not recommended because of their broad spectrum and potential to increase resistance. Antibiotics are administered for at least 10 days to eradicate the infection from the oropharynx.

Severe sore throats can also be relieved by analgesic medications, as prescribed. For example, aspirin or acetaminophen (Tylenol) can be taken at 3- to 6-hour intervals; if required, acetaminophen with codeine can be taken three or four times daily. Antitussive medication, in the form of codeine, dextromethorphan (Robitussin DM), or hydrocodone bitartrate (Hycodan), may be required to control the persistent and painful cough that often accompanies acute pharyngitis.

NUTRITIONAL THERAPY

A liquid or soft diet is provided during the acute stage of the disease, depending on the patient's appetite and the degree of discomfort that occurs with swallowing. Occasionally, the throat is so sore that liquids cannot be taken in adequate amounts by mouth. In severe situations, fluids are administered intravenously. Otherwise, the patient is encouraged to drink as much fluid as possible (at least 2 to 3 L per day).

Nursing Management

The nurse instructs the patient to stay in bed during the febrile stage of illness and to rest frequently once up and about. Used tis-

FIGURE 22-3 Pharyngitis—inflammation without exudate. (**A**) Redness and vascularity of the pillars and uvula are mild to moderate. (**B**) Redness is diffuse and intense. Each patient would probably complain of a sore throat. From Bickley, L. S. (2003). *Bates' guide to physical examination and history taking* (8th ed.). Philadelphia: Lippincott Williams & Wilkins.

sues should be disposed of properly to prevent the spread of infection. It is important to examine the skin once or twice daily for possible rash, because acute pharyngitis may precede some other communicable diseases (ie, rubella).

Warm saline gargles or irrigations are used depending on the severity of the lesion and the degree of pain. The benefits of this treatment depend on the degree of heat that is applied. The nurse teaches the patient about the recommended temperature of the solution: high enough to be effective and as warm as the patient can tolerate, usually 40.6°C to 43.3°C. Irrigating the throat properly is an effective means of reducing spasm in the pharyngeal muscles and relieving soreness of the throat. Unless the purpose of the procedure and its technique are understood clearly by the patient and family, the results may be less than satisfactory.

An ice collar also can relieve severe sore throats. Mouth care may add greatly to the patient's comfort and prevent the development of fissures (cracking) of the lips and oral inflammation when bacterial infection is present. The nurse instructs the patient to resume activity gradually. A full course of antibiotic therapy is indicated in patients with group A beta-hemolytic streptococcal infection in view of the possible development of complications such as nephritis and rheumatic fever, which may have their onset 2 or 3 weeks after the pharyngitis has subsided. The nurse instructs the patient and family about the importance of taking the full course of therapy and informs them about the symptoms to watch for that may indicate complications.

CHRONIC PHARYNGITIS

Chronic pharyngitis is a persistent inflammation of the pharynx. It is common in adults who work or live in dusty surroundings, use their voice to excess, suffer from chronic cough, and habitually use alcohol and tobacco.

Three types of chronic pharyngitis are recognized:

- Hypertrophic: characterized by general thickening and congestion of the pharyngeal mucous membrane
- Atrophic: probably a late stage of the first type (the membrane is thin, whitish, glistening, and at times wrinkled)
- Chronic granular ("clergyman's sore throat"): characterized by numerous swollen lymph follicles on the pharyngeal wall

Clinical Manifestations

Patients with chronic pharyngitis complain of a constant sense of irritation or fullness in the throat, mucus that collects in the throat and can be expelled by coughing, and difficulty swallowing.

Medical Management

Treatment of chronic pharyngitis is based on relieving symptoms, avoiding exposure to irritants, and correcting any upper respiratory, pulmonary, or cardiac condition that might be responsible for a chronic cough.

Nasal congestion may be relieved by short-term use of nasal sprays or medications containing ephedrine sulfate (Kondon's Nasal) or phenylephrine hydrochloride (Neo-Synephrine). If there is a history of allergy, one of the antihistamine decongestant medications, such as Drixoral or Dimetapp, is taken orally every 4 to

6 hours. Aspirin or acetaminophen is recommended for its anti-inflammatory and analgesic properties.

Nursing Management

TEACHING PATIENTS SELF-CARE

To prevent the infection from spreading, the nurse instructs the patient to avoid contact with others until the fever subsides. Alcohol, tobacco, second-hand smoke, and exposure to cold are avoided, as are environmental or occupational pollutants if possible. The patient may minimize exposure to pollutants by wearing a disposable facemask. The nurse encourages the patient to drink plenty of fluids. Gargling with warm saline solutions may relieve throat discomfort. Lozenges will keep the throat moistened.

TONSILLITIS AND ADENOIDITIS

The tonsils are composed of lymphatic tissue and are situated on each side of the oropharynx. The faucial or palatine tonsils and lingual tonsils are located behind the pillars of fauces and tongue, respectively. They frequently serve as the site of acute infection (**tonsillitis**). Chronic tonsillitis is less common and may be mistaken for other disorders such as allergy, asthma, and sinusitis.

The adenoids or pharyngeal tonsils consist of lymphatic tissue near the centre of the posterior wall of the nasopharynx. Infection of the adenoids frequently accompanies acute tonsillitis. Group A beta-streptococcus is the most common organism associated with tonsillitis and adenoiditis.

Clinical Manifestations

The symptoms of tonsillitis include sore throat, fever, snoring, and difficulty swallowing. Enlarged adenoids may cause mouth-breathing, earache, draining ears, frequent head colds, bronchitis, foul-smelling breath, voice impairment, and noisy respiration. Unusually enlarged adenoids fill the space behind the posterior nares, making it difficult for the air to travel from the nose to the throat and resulting in a nasal obstruction. Infection can extend to the middle ears by way of the auditory (eustachian) tubes and may result in acute otitis media, which can lead to spontaneous rupture of the eardrums and further extension of the infection into the mastoid cells, causing acute mastoiditis. The infection also may reside in the middle ear as a chronic, low-grade, smoldering process that eventually may cause permanent deafness.

Assessment and Diagnostic Findings

A thorough physical examination is performed and a careful history is obtained to rule out related or systemic conditions. The tonsillar site is cultured to determine the presence of bacterial infection. In adenoiditis, if recurrent episodes of suppurative otitis media result in hearing loss, the patient should be given a comprehensive audiometric examination (see Chap. 59).

Medical Management

Tonsillectomy is usually performed for recurrent tonsillitis when medical treatment is unsuccessful and there is severe hypertrophy, asymmetry, or peritonsillar abscess that occludes the pharynx, making swallowing difficult and endangering the airway (particularly during sleep). Enlargement of the tonsils is rarely an indication for their removal; most children normally have large tonsils, which decrease in size with age.

Tonsillectomy or adenoidectomy is indicated only if the patient has had any of the following problems: repeated bouts of tonsillitis; hypertrophy of the tonsils and adenoids that could cause obstruction and obstructive sleep apnea; repeated attacks of purulent otitis media; suspected hearing loss due to serous otitis media that has occurred in association with enlarged tonsils and adenoids; and some other conditions, such as an exacerbation of asthma or rheumatic fever. Appropriate antibiotic therapy is initiated for patients undergoing tonsillectomy or adenoidectomy. The most common antimicrobial agent is oral penicillin, which is taken for 7 days. Amoxicillin and erythromycin are alternatives.

Nursing Management

PROVIDING POSTOPERATIVE CARE

Continuous nursing observation is required in the immediate postoperative and recovery period because of the significant risk of hemorrhage. In the immediate postoperative period, the most comfortable position is prone with the head turned to the side to allow drainage from the mouth and pharynx. The nurse must not remove the oral airway until the patient's gag and swallowing reflexes have returned. The nurse applies an ice collar to the neck, and a basin and tissues are provided for the expectoration of blood and mucus.

Bleeding may be bright red if the patient expectorates blood before swallowing it. Often, however, the patient swallows the blood, which immediately becomes brown because of the action of the acidic gastric juice.

Hemorrhage is a potential complication after a tonsillectomy and adenoidectomy. If the patient vomits large amounts of dark blood or bright-red blood at frequent intervals, or if the pulse rate and temperature rise and the patient is restless, the nurse notifies the surgeon immediately. The nurse should have the following items ready for examination of the surgical site for bleeding: a light, a mirror, gauze, curved hemostats, and a waste basin.

Occasionally, suture or ligation of the bleeding vessel is required. In such cases, the patient is taken to the operating room and given general anesthesia. After ligation, continuous nursing observation and postoperative care are required, as in the initial postoperative period.

If there is no bleeding, water and ice chips may be given to the patient as soon as desired. The patient is instructed to refrain from too much talking and coughing because these activities can produce throat pain.

TEACHING PATIENTS SELF-CARE

Tonsillectomy and adenoidectomy usually do not require hospitalization and are performed as outpatient surgery with a short length of stay. Because the patient will be sent home soon after surgery, the patient and family must understand the signs and symptoms of hemorrhage. Hemorrhage usually occurs in the first 12 to 24 hours. The patient is instructed to report frank red bleeding to the physician.

Alkaline mouthwashes and warm saline solutions are useful in coping with the thick mucus and halitosis that may be present after surgery. It is important to explain to the patient that a sore throat, stiff neck, and vomiting may occur in the first 24 hours. A liquid or semiliquid diet is given for several days. Sherbet and gelatin are acceptable foods. The patient should avoid spicy, hot, acidic, or rough foods. Milk and milk products (ice cream and yogurt) may be restricted because they may make removal of mucus more difficult.

The nurse explains to the patient that halitosis and some minor ear pain may occur for the first few days. The nurse instructs the patient to avoid vigorous tooth brushing or gargling, since these actions could cause bleeding.

PERITONSILLAR ABSCESS

A peritonsillar abscess is a collection of purulent exudate between the tonsillar capsule and the surrounding tissues, including the soft palate. It is believed to develop after an acute tonsillar infection, which progresses to a local cellulitis and abscess.

Clinical Manifestations

The usual symptoms of an infection are present, together with such local symptoms as a raspy voice, odynophagia (a severe sensation of burning, squeezing pain while swallowing), **dysphagia** (difficulty swallowing), otalgia (pain in the ear), and drooling. An examination shows marked swelling of the soft palate, often occluding almost half of the opening from the mouth into the pharynx, unilateral tonsillar hypertrophy, and dehydration.

Assessment and Diagnostic Findings

Aspiration of purulent material (pus) by needle aspiration is required to make the appropriate diagnosis. The aspirated material is sent for culture and Gram's stain. A CT scan is performed when it is not possible to aspirate the abscess.

Medical Management

Antibiotics (usually penicillin) are extremely effective in controlling the infection in peritonsillar abscess. If antibiotics are prescribed early in the course of the disease, the abscess may resolve without needing to be incised.

SURGICAL MANAGEMENT

If treatment is delayed, the abscess is evacuated as soon as possible. The mucous membrane over the swelling is first sprayed with a topical anesthetic and then injected with a local anesthetic. Single or repeated needle aspirations are performed to decompress the abscess. The abscess may also be incised and drained. These procedures are performed best with the patient in the sitting position to make it easier to expectorate the pus and blood that accumulate in the pharynx. Almost immediate relief is experienced. Approximately 30% of patients with peritonsillar abscess have indications for tonsillectomy (Tierney et al., 2001).

Nursing Management

Considerable relief may be obtained by the use of topical anesthetic agents and throat irrigations or the frequent use of mouthwashes or gargles, using saline or alkaline solutions at a temperature of 40.6°C to 43.3°C. The nurse instructs the patient to gargle at intervals of 1 or 2 hours for 24 to 36 hours. Liquids that are cool or at room temperature are usually well tolerated.

LARYNGITIS

Laryngitis, an inflammation of the larynx, often occurs as a result of voice abuse or exposure to dust, chemicals, smoke, and other pollutants, or as part of an upper respiratory tract infection.

It also may be caused by isolated infection involving only the vocal cords.

The cause of infection is almost always a virus. Bacterial invasion may be secondary. Laryngitis is usually associated with allergic rhinitis or pharyngitis. The onset of infection may be associated with exposure to sudden temperature changes, dietary deficiencies, malnutrition, and an immunosuppressed state. Laryngitis is common in the winter and is easily transmitted.

Clinical Manifestations

Signs of acute laryngitis include hoarseness or **aphonia** (complete loss of voice) and severe cough. Chronic laryngitis is marked by persistent hoarseness. Laryngitis may be a complication of upper respiratory infections.

Medical Management

Management of acute laryngitis includes resting the voice, avoiding smoking, resting, and inhaling cool steam or an aerosol. If the laryngitis is part of a more extensive respiratory infection due to a bacterial organism or if it is severe, appropriate antibacterial therapy is instituted. The majority of patients recover with conservative treatment; however, laryngitis tends to be more severe in elderly patients and may be complicated by pneumonia.

For chronic laryngitis, the treatment includes resting the voice, eliminating any primary respiratory tract infection, eliminating smoking, and avoiding second-hand smoke. Topical corticosteroids, such as beclomethasone dipropionate (Vanceril) inhalation, may also be used. These preparations have no systemic or long-lasting effects and may reduce local inflammatory reactions.

Nursing Management

The nurse instructs the patient to rest the voice and to maintain a well-humidified environment. If laryngeal secretions are present during acute episodes, expectorant agents are suggested, along with a daily fluid intake of 3 L to thin secretions.

NURSING PROCESS: THE PATIENT WITH UPPER AIRWAY INFECTION

Assessment

A health history may reveal signs and symptoms of headache, sore throat, pain around the eyes and on either side of the nose, difficulty in swallowing, cough, hoarseness, fever, stuffiness, and generalized discomfort and fatigue. Determining when the symptoms began, what precipitated them, what if anything relieves them, and what aggravates them is part of the assessment. It also is important to determine any history of allergy or the existence of a concomitant illness.

Inspection may reveal swelling, lesions, or asymmetry of the nose as well as bleeding or discharge. The nurse inspects the nasal mucosa for abnormal findings such as increased redness, swelling, or exudate, and nasal polyps, which may develop in chronic rhinitis.

The nurse palpates the frontal and maxillary sinuses for tenderness, which suggests inflammation, and then inspects the throat by having the patient open the mouth wide and take a deep breath. The tonsils and pharynx are inspected for abnormal findings such as redness, asymmetry, or evidence of drainage, ulceration, or enlargement.

Next the nurse palpates the trachea to determine the midline position in the neck and to detect any masses or deformities. The neck lymph nodes also are palpated for associated enlargement and tenderness.

Diagnosis

NURSING DIAGNOSES

Based on the assessment data, the patient's major nursing diagnoses may include the following:

- Ineffective airway clearance related to excessive mucus production secondary to retained secretions and inflammation
- Acute pain related to upper airway irritation secondary to an infection
- Impaired verbal communication related to physiologic changes and upper airway irritation secondary to infection or swelling
- Deficient fluid volume related to increased fluid loss secondary to diaphoresis associated with a fever
- Deficient knowledge regarding prevention of upper respiratory infections, treatment regimen, surgical procedure, or postoperative care

COLLABORATIVE PROBLEMS/ POTENTIAL COMPLICATIONS

Based on assessment data, potential complications may include:

- Sepsis
- Meningitis
- Peritonsillar abscess
- Otitis media
- Sinusitis

Planning and Goals

The major goals for the patient may include maintenance of a patent airway, relief of pain, maintenance of effective means of communication, normal hydration, knowledge of how to prevent upper airway infections, and absence of complications.

Nursing Interventions

MAINTAINING A PATENT AIRWAY

An accumulation of secretions can block the airway in patients with an upper airway infection. As a result, changes in the respiratory pattern occur, and the work of breathing required to get beyond the blockage increases. The nurse can implement several measures to loosen thick secretions or to keep the secretions moist so that they can be easily expectorated. Increasing fluid intake helps thin the mucus. Use of room vaporizers or steam inhalation also loosens secretions and reduces inflammation of the mucous membranes. To enhance drainage from the sinuses, the nurse instructs the patient about the best position to assume; this depends on the location of the infection or inflammation. For example, drainage for sinusitis or rhinitis is achieved in the upright position. In some conditions, topical or systemic medications, when prescribed, help to relieve nasal or throat congestion.

PROMOTING COMFORT

Upper respiratory tract infections usually produce localized discomfort. In sinusitis, pain may occur in the area of the sinuses or may produce a general headache. In pharyngitis, laryngitis, or tonsillitis, a sore throat occurs. The nurse encourages the patient to take analgesics, such as acetaminophen with codeine, as prescribed, which will help relieve this discomfort. Other helpful measures include topical anesthetic agents for symptomatic relief of herpes simplex blisters (see Chart 22-1) and sore throats, hot packs to relieve the congestion of sinusitis and promote drainage, and warm water gargles or irrigations to relieve the pain of a sore throat. The nurse encourages rest to relieve the generalized discomfort and fever that accompany many upper airway conditions (especially rhinitis, pharyngitis, and laryngitis). The nurse instructs the patient in general hygiene techniques to prevent the spread of infection. For postoperative care following tonsillectomy and adenoidectomy, an ice collar may reduce swelling and decrease bleeding.

PROMOTING COMMUNICATION

Upper airway infections may result in hoarseness or loss of speech. The nurse instructs the patient to refrain from speaking as much as possible and to communicate in writing instead, if possible. Additional strain on the vocal cords may delay full return of the voice.

ENCOURAGING FLUID INTAKE

In upper airway infections, the work of breathing and the respiratory rate increase as inflammation and secretions develop. This, in turn, may increase insensible fluid loss. Fever further increases the metabolic rate, diaphoresis, and fluid loss.

Sore throat, malaise, and fever may interfere with a patient's willingness to eat. The nurse encourages the patient to drink 2 to 3 L of fluid per day during the acute stage of airway infection, unless contraindicated, to thin secretions and promote drainage. Liquids (hot or cold) may be soothing, depending on the illness.

PROMOTING HOME AND COMMUNITY-BASED CARE

Teaching Patients Self-Care

Prevention of most upper airway infections is difficult because of the many potential causes. However, most upper respiratory infections are transmitted by hand-to-hand contact. Therefore, it is important to teach the patient and family how to minimize the spread of infection to others. Other preventive strategies are identified in Chart 22-2. The nurse advises the patient to avoid exposure to others at risk for serious illness if respiratory infection is transmitted. Those at risk include elderly adults, immunosuppressed people, and those with chronic health problems.

The nurse teaches patients and their families strategies to relieve symptoms of upper respiratory infections. These include increasing the humidity level, encouraging adequate fluid intake, getting adequate rest, using warm water gargles or irrigations and topical anesthetic agents to relieve sore throat, and applying hot packs to relieve congestion. The nurse reinforces the need to complete the treatment regimen, particularly when antibiotics are prescribed.

Continuing Care

Referral for home care is rare. However, it may be indicated for the person whose health status was compromised before the onset of the respiratory infection and for those who cannot manage self-care without assistance. In such circumstances, the home care nurse assesses the patient's respiratory status and progress in recovery. The nurse may advise elderly patients and those who would be at increased risk from a respiratory infection to consider an annual influenza vaccine. A follow-up appointment with the primary care provider may be indicated for patients with compromised health status to ensure that the respiratory infection has resolved.

MONITORING AND MANAGING POTENTIAL COMPLICATIONS

While major complications of upper respiratory infections are rare, the nurse must be aware of them and assess the patient for them. Because most patients with upper respiratory infections are managed at home, patients and their families must be instructed to monitor for signs and symptoms and to seek immediate medical care if the patient's condition does not improve or if the patient's physical status appears to be worsening.

Sepsis and meningitis may occur in patients with compromised immune status or in those with an overwhelming bacterial infection. The patient with an upper respiratory infection and family members are instructed to seek medical care if the patient's condition fails to improve within several days of the onset of symptoms, if unusual symptoms develop, or if the patient's condition deteriorates. They are instructed about signs and symptoms that require further attention: persistent or high fever, increasing shortness of breath, confusion, and increasing weakness and malaise. The patient with sepsis requires expert care to treat the infection, stabilize vital signs, and prevent or treat septicemia and shock. Deterioration of the patient's condition necessitates intensive care measures (eg, hemodynamic monitoring and administration of vasoactive medications, intravenous fluids, nutritional support, corticosteroids) to monitor the patient's status and to support the patient's vital signs. High doses of antibiotics may be administered to treat the causative organism. The nurse's role is to monitor the patient's vital signs, hemodynamic status, and laboratory values, administer needed treatment, alleviate the patient's physical discomfort, and provide explanations, teaching, and emotional support to the patient and family.

Peritonsillar abscess may develop following an acute infection of the tonsils. The patient requires treatment to drain the abscess and receives antibiotics for infection and topical anesthetic agents and throat irrigations to relieve pain and sore throat. Follow-up is necessary to ensure that the abscess resolves; tonsillectomy may be required. The nurse assists the patient in administering throat irrigations and instructs the patient and family about the importance of adhering to the prescribed treatment regimen and recommended follow-up appointments.

Otitis media and sinusitis may develop with upper respiratory infection. The patient and family are instructed about the signs and symptoms of otitis media and sinusitis and about the importance of follow-up with the primary health care practitioner to ensure adequate evaluation and treatment of these conditions.

Evaluation

EXPECTED PATIENT OUTCOMES

Expected patient outcomes may include:

1. Maintains a patent airway by managing secretions
   a. Reports decreased congestion
   b. Assumes best position to facilitate drainage of secretions
2. Reports feeling more comfortable
   a. Uses comfort measures: analgesics, hot packs, gargles, rest
   b. Demonstrates adequate oral hygiene
3. Demonstrates ability to communicate needs, wants, level of comfort

4. Maintains adequate fluid intake
5. Identifies strategies to prevent upper airway infections and allergic reactions
   a. Demonstrates hand hygiene technique
   b. Identifies the value of the influenza vaccine
6. Demonstrates an adequate level of knowledge and performs self-care adequately
7. Becomes free of signs and symptoms of infection
   a. Exhibits normal vital signs (temperature, pulse, respiratory rate)
   b. Absence of purulent drainage
   c. Free of pain in ears, sinuses, and throat

Obstruction and Trauma of the Upper Respiratory Airway

OBSTRUCTION DURING SLEEP

A variety of respiratory disorders are associated with sleep, the most common being sleep apnea syndrome. Sleep apnea syndrome is defined as cessation of breathing (**apnea**) during sleep.

Pathophysiology

Sleep apnea is classified into three types:

- Obstructive—lack of air flow due to pharyngeal occlusion
- Central—simultaneous cessation of both air flow and respiratory movements
- Mixed—a combination of central and obstructive apnea within one apneic episode

The most common type of sleep apnea syndrome, obstructive sleep apnea, will be presented here.

Clinical Manifestations

About 4% of men and 2% of women have obstructive sleep apnea. Obesity and cigarette smoking are risk factors. Obstructive sleep apnea is defined as frequent and loud snoring and breathing cessation for 10 seconds or more for five episodes per hour or more, followed by awakening abruptly with a loud snort as the blood oxygen level drops. Patients with sleep apnea may experience anywhere from five apneic episodes per hour to several hundred per night. Other symptoms include excessive daytime sleepiness, morning headache, sore throat, intellectual deterioration, personality changes, behavioural disorders, enuresis, impotence, obesity, and complaints by the partner that the patient snores loudly or is unusually restless during sleep (Chart 22-3).

The obstruction may be caused by mechanical factors such as a reduced diameter of the upper airway or dynamic changes in the upper airway during sleep. The activity of the tonic dilator muscles of the upper airway is reduced during sleep. These sleep-related changes may predispose the patient to increased upper airway collapse with the small amounts of negative pressure generated during inspiration. Obstructive sleep apnea may be associated with obesity and with other conditions that reduce pharyngeal muscle tone (eg, neuromuscular disease, sedative/hypnotic medications, acute ingestion of alcohol). The diagnosis of sleep apnea is made based on clinical features plus polysomnographic findings (sleep test), in which the cardiopulmonary status of the patient is monitored during an episode of sleep.

Chart 22-3 • ASSESSMENT

Obstructive Sleep Apnea

Clinical features of obstructive sleep apnea include:
   Excessive daytime sleepiness
   Frequent nocturnal awakening
   Insomnia
   Loud snoring
   Morning headaches
   Intellectual deterioration
   Personality changes, irritability
   Impotence
   Systemic hypertension
   Dysrhythmias
   Pulmonary hypertension, cor pulmonale
   Polycythemia
   Enuresis

The effects of obstructive sleep apnea can seriously tax the heart and lungs. Repetitive apneic events result in hypoxia and hypercapnia, which triggers a sympathetic response. As a consequence, patients have a high prevalence of hypertension and an increased risk of myocardial infarction and stroke. In patients with underlying cardiovascular disease, the nocturnal hypoxemia may predispose to dysrhythmias.

Medical Management

Patients usually seek medical treatment because their partners express concern or because they experience excessive sleeplessness at inappropriate times or settings (eg, while driving a car). A variety of treatments are used. In mild cases, the patient is advised to avoid alcohol and medications that depress the upper airway and to lose weight. In more severe cases involving hypoxemia with severe CO_2 retention (hypercapnia), the treatment includes continuous positive airway pressure or bilevel positive airway pressure therapy with supplemental oxygen via nasal cannula. These treatment methods are described in Chapter 25.

Surgical procedures (eg, uvulopalatopharyngoplasty) may be performed to correct the obstruction. As a last resort, a tracheostomy is performed to bypass the obstruction if the potential for respiratory failure or life-threatening dysrhythmias exists. The tracheostomy is unplugged only during sleep. Although this is an effective treatment, it is used in a limited number of patients because of its associated physical disfigurement (Murray & Nadel, 2001).

PHARMACOLOGIC THERAPY

Treatment of central sleep apnea also includes medication. Protriptyline (Triptil) given at bedtime is thought to increase the respiratory drive and improve upper airway muscle tone. Medroxyprogesterone acetate (Provera) and acetazolamide (Diamox) have been recommended for sleep apnea associated with chronic alveolar hypoventilation, but their benefits have not been well established. Administration of low-flow nasal oxygen at night can help relieve hypoxemia in some patients but has little effect on the frequency or severity of apnea.

Nursing Management

The patient with obstructive sleep apnea may not recognize the potential consequences of the disorder. Therefore, the nurse explains the disorder in language that is understandable to the patient and relates symptoms (daytime sleepiness) to the underlying disorder. The nurse also instructs the patient and family about treatments, including the correct and safe use of oxygen, if prescribed.

EPISTAXIS (NOSEBLEED)

A hemorrhage from the nose, referred to as **epistaxis**, is caused by the rupture of tiny, distended vessels in the mucous membrane of any area of the nose. Rarely does epistaxis originate in the densely vascular tissue over the turbinates. Most commonly, the site is the anterior septum, where three major blood vessels enter the nasal cavity: (1) the anterior ethmoidal artery on the forward part of the roof (Kesselbach's plexus), (2) the sphenopalatine artery in the posterosuperior region, and (3) the internal maxillary branches (the plexus of veins located at the back of the lateral wall under the inferior turbinate).

There are a variety of causes associated with epistaxis, including trauma, infection, inhalation of illicit drugs, cardiovascular diseases, blood dyscrasias, nasal tumours, low humidity, a foreign body in the nose, and a deviated nasal septum. Additionally, vigourous nose blowing and nose picking have been associated with epistaxis.

Medical Management

Management of epistaxis depends on the location of the bleeding site. A nasal speculum or headlight may be used to determine the site of bleeding in the nasal cavity. Most nosebleeds originate from the anterior portion of the nose. Initial treatment may include applying direct pressure. The patient sits upright with the head tilted forward to prevent swallowing and aspiration of blood and is directed to pinch the soft outer portion of the nose against the midline septum for 5 or 10 minutes continuously. If this measure is unsuccessful, additional treatment is indicated. In anterior nosebleeds, the area may be treated with a silver nitrate applicator and Gelfoam, or by electrocautery. Topical vasoconstrictors, such as adrenaline (1 : 1,000), cocaine (0.5%), and phenylephrine may be prescribed.

If bleeding is occurring from the posterior regions, cotton pledgets soaked in a vasoconstricting solution may be inserted into the nose to reduce the blood flow and improve the examiner's view of the bleeding site. Alternatively, a cotton tampon may be used to try to stop the bleeding. Suction may be used to remove excess blood and clots from the field of inspection. The search for the bleeding site should shift from the anteroinferior quadrant to the anterosuperior, then to the posterosuperior, and finally to the posteroinferior area. The field is kept clear by using suction and by shifting the cotton tampon. Only about 60% of the total nasal cavity can actually be seen, however.

When the origin of the bleeding cannot be identified, the nose may be packed with gauze impregnated with petrolatum jelly or antibiotic ointment; a topical anesthetic spray and decongestant agent may be used prior to inserting the gauze packing, or a balloon-inflated catheter may be used (Fig. 22-4). The packing may remain in place for 48 hours or up to 5 or 6 days if necessary to control bleeding. Antibiotics may be prescribed because of the risk of iatrogenic sinusitis and toxic shock syndrome.

Nursing Management

The nurse monitors the vital signs, assists in the control of bleeding, and provides tissues and an emesis basin to allow the patient to expectorate any excess blood. It is not uncommon for patients to be anxious in response to a nosebleed. Blood loss on clothing and handkerchiefs can be frightening, and the nasal examination and treatment are uncomfortable. Assuring the patient in a calm, efficient manner that bleeding can be controlled can help reduce anxiety.

TEACHING PATIENTS SELF-CARE
Discharge teaching includes reviewing ways to prevent epistaxis: avoiding forceful nose blowing, straining, high altitudes, and

FIGURE 22-4 Packing to control bleeding from the posterior nose. (**A**) Catheter is inserted and packing is attached. (**B**) Packing is drawn into position as the catheter is removed. (**C**) Strip is tied over a bolster to hold the packing in place with an anterior pack installed "accordion pleat" style. (**D**) Alternative method, using a balloon catheter instead of gauze packing.

nasal trauma (including nose picking). Adequate humidification may prevent drying of the nasal passages. The nurse instructs the patient how to apply direct pressure to the nose with the thumb and the index finger for 15 minutes in the case of a recurrent nosebleed. If recurrent bleeding cannot be stopped, the patient is instructed to seek additional medical attention.

NASAL OBSTRUCTION

The passage of air through the nostrils is frequently obstructed by a deviation of the nasal septum, hypertrophy of the turbinate bones, or the pressure of nasal polyps, which are grapelike swellings that arise from the mucous membrane of the sinuses, especially the ethmoids. This obstruction also may lead to a condition of chronic infection of the nose and result in frequent episodes of nasopharyngitis. Frequently, the infection extends to the sinuses of the nose. When sinusitis develops and the drainage from these cavities is obstructed by deformity or swelling within the nose, pain is experienced in the region of the affected sinus.

Medical Management

The treatment of nasal obstruction requires the removal of the obstruction, followed by measures to overcome whatever chronic infection exists. In many patients an underlying allergy requires treatment. At times endoscopic surgery is necessary to drain the nasal sinuses. The specific procedure performed depends on the type of nasal obstruction found. Usually, surgery is performed under local anesthesia.

If a deviation of the septum is the cause of the obstruction, the surgeon makes an incision into the mucous membrane and, after raising it from the bone, removes the deviated bone and cartilage with bone forceps. The mucosa then is allowed to fall back in place and is held there by tight packing. Generally, the packing is soaked in liquid petrolatum so that it can be removed easily in 24 to 36 hours. This operation is called a **submucous resection** or septoplasty.

Nasal polyps are removed by clipping them at their base with a wire snare. Hypertrophied turbinates may be treated by applying an astringent agent to shrink them.

Nursing Management

Most of these procedures are performed on an outpatient basis. If the patient is hospitalized, the nurse elevates the head of the bed to promote drainage and to help alleviate discomfort from edema. Frequent oral hygiene is encouraged to overcome dryness caused by breathing through the mouth.

FRACTURES OF THE NOSE

The location of the nose makes it susceptible to injury by a wide variety of causes. In fact, nasal fractures are more common than those of any other bone in the body. Fractures of the nose usually result from a direct assault. As a rule, no serious consequences result, but the deformity that may follow often gives rise to obstruction of the nasal air passages and to facial disfigurement.

Clinical Manifestations

The signs and symptoms of a nasal fracture are bleeding from the nose externally and internally into the pharynx, swelling of the soft tissues adjacent to the nose, and deformity.

Assessment and Diagnostic Findings

The nose is examined internally to rule out the possibility that the injury may be complicated by a fracture of the nasal septum and a submucosal septal hematoma. Because of the swelling and bleeding that occur with a nasal fracture, an accurate diagnosis can be made only after the swelling subsides.

Clear fluid draining from either nostril suggests a fracture of the cribriform plate with leakage of cerebrospinal fluid. Because cerebrospinal fluid contains glucose, it can readily be differentiated from nasal mucus by means of a dipstick (Dextrostix). Usually, careful inspection or palpation will disclose any deviations of the bone or disruptions of the nasal cartilages. An x-ray may reveal displacement of the fractured bones and may help rule out extension of the fracture into the skull.

Medical Management

As a rule, bleeding is controlled with the use of cold compresses. The nose is assessed for symmetry either before swelling has occurred or after it has subsided. The patient is referred to a specialist, usually 3 to 5 days after the injury, to evaluate the need to realign the bones. Nasal fractures are surgically reduced 7 to 10 days after the injury.

Nursing Management

The nurse instructs the patient to apply ice packs to the nose for 20 minutes four times each day to decrease swelling. The patient who experiences bleeding from the nose (epistaxis) because of injury or for unexplained reasons is usually frightened and anxious. The packing inserted to stop the bleeding may be uncomfortable and unpleasant, and obstruction of the nasal passages by the packing forces the patient to breathe through the mouth. This in turn causes the oral mucous membranes to become dry. Mouth rinses will help to moisten the mucous membranes and to reduce the odour and taste of dried blood in the oropharynx and nasopharynx.

LARYNGEAL OBSTRUCTION

Edema of the larynx is a serious, often fatal, condition. The larynx is a stiff box that will not stretch. It contains a narrow space between the vocal cords (glottis) through which air must pass. Swelling of the laryngeal mucous membranes, therefore, may close off the opening tightly, leading to suffocation. Edema of the glottis occurs rarely in patients with acute laryngitis, occasionally in patients with urticaria, and more frequently in patients with severe inflammations of the throat, as in scarlet fever. It is an occasional cause of death in severe anaphylaxis (angioneurotic edema).

Foreign bodies frequently are aspirated into the pharynx, the larynx, or the trachea and cause a twofold problem. First, they obstruct the air passages and cause difficulty in breathing, which may lead to asphyxia; later, they may be drawn farther down, entering the bronchi or a bronchial branch and causing symptoms of irritation, such as a croupy cough, expectoration of blood or mucus, or laboured breathing. The physical signs and x-ray findings confirm the diagnosis.

Medical Management

When the obstruction is caused by edema resulting from an allergic reaction, treatment includes administering subcutaneous epinephrine or a corticosteroid (see Chap. 53) and applying an ice pack to the neck. In emergencies caused by obstruction by a foreign body, when signs of asphyxia are apparent, immediate treatment is necessary. Frequently, if the foreign body has lodged in the pharynx and can be visualized, the finger can dislodge it.

If the obstruction is in the larynx or the trachea, the nurse or other rescuer tries the subdiaphragmatic abdominal thrust manoeuvre (Chart 22-4). If all efforts are unsuccessful, an immediate tracheotomy is necessary (see Chap. 25 for further discussion).

Cancer of the Larynx

Cancer of the larynx is a malignant tumour in the larynx (voice box). It is potentially curable if detected early. It represents less than 1% of all cancers and occurs about four times more frequently in men than in women, and most commonly in persons 50 to 70 years of age. The incidence of laryngeal cancer continues to decline, but the incidence in women versus men continues to increase. Each year in the United States, approximately 9,000 new cases are discovered, (American Cancer Society, 2002). Specific mortality rates for Canada are not available. However, based on data from the United States, about 40% of the new cases discovered each year will die (American Cancer Society, 2002).

Carcinogens that have been associated with the development of laryngeal cancer include tobacco (smoke, smokeless) and alcohol and their combined effects, exposure to asbestos, mustard gas, wood dust, cement dust, tar products, leather, and metals. Other contributing factors include straining the voice, chronic laryngitis, nutritional deficiencies (riboflavin), and family predisposition (Chart 22-5).

A malignant growth may occur in three different areas of the larynx: the glottic area (vocal cords), supraglottic area (area above the glottis or vocal cords, including epiglottis and false cords), and subglottis (area below the glottis or vocal cords to the cricoid). Two thirds of laryngeal cancers are in the glottic area. Supraglottic cancers account for approximately one third of the cases, subglottic tumours for less than 1%. Glottic tumours seldom spread if found early because of the limited lymph vessels found in the vocal cords (Lenhard, Osteen, & Gansler, 2001).

Chart 22-5
Risk Factors for Laryngeal Cancer

Carcinogens
Tobacco (smoke, smokeless)
Combined effects of alcohol and tobacco
Asbestos
Second-hand smoke
Paint fumes
Wood dust
Cement dust
Chemicals
Tar products
Mustard gas
Leather and metals

Other Factors
Straining the voice
Chronic laryngitis
Nutritional deficiencies (riboflavin)
History of alcohol abuse
Familial predisposition
Age (higher incidence after 60 years of age)
Gender (more common in men)
Race (more prevalent in African Americans)
Weakened immune system

Clinical Manifestations

Hoarseness of more than 2 weeks' duration is noted early in the patient with cancer in the glottic area because the tumour impedes the action of the vocal cords during speech. The voice may sound harsh, raspy, and lower in pitch. Affected voice sounds are not early signs of subglottic or supraglottic cancer. The patient may complain of a cough or sore throat that does not go away and pain and burning in the throat, especially when consuming hot liquids or citrus juices. A lump may be felt in the neck. Later symptoms include dysphagia, dyspnea (difficulty breathing), unilateral nasal

Chart 22-4 Performing the Abdominal Thrust Manoeuvre

To assist a patient or other person who is choking on a foreign object, the nurse performs the abdominal thrust manoeuvre (sometimes called the Heimlich manoeuvre) according to guidelines set forth by the American Heart Association. (*Note:* Hands crossed at the neck is the universal sign for choking.)

1. Stand behind the person who is choking.
2. Place both arms around the person's waist.
3. Make a fist with one hand with the thumb outside the fist.
4. Place thumb side of fist against the person's abdomen above the navel and below the xiphoid process.
5. Grasp fist with other hand.
6. Quickly and forcefully exert pressure against the person's diaphragm, pressing upward with quick, firm thrusts.
7. Apply thrusts 6 to 10 times until the obstruction is cleared.
8. The pressure from the thrusts should lift the diaphragm, force air into the lungs, and create an artificial cough powerful enough to expel the aspirated object.

obstruction or discharge, persistent hoarseness, persistent ulceration, and foul breath. Cervical lymph adenopathy, unplanned weight loss, a general debilitated state, and pain radiating to the ear may occur with metastasis.

Assessment and Diagnostic Findings

An initial assessment includes a complete history and physical examination of the head and neck. This will include assessment of risk factors, family history, and any underlying medical conditions. An indirect laryngoscopy, using a flexible endoscope, is initially performed in the otolaryngologist's office to visually evaluate the pharynx, larynx, and possible tumour. Mobility of the vocal cords is assessed; if normal movement is limited, the growth may affect muscle, other tissue, and even the airway. The lymph nodes of the neck and the thyroid gland are palpated to determine spread of the malignancy (Haskell, 2001).

If a tumour of the larynx is suspected on an initial examination, a direct laryngoscopic examination is scheduled. This examination is done under local or general anesthesia and allows evaluation of all areas of the larynx. Samples of the suspicious tissue are obtained for histologic evaluation. The tumour may involve any of the three areas of the larynx and may vary in appearance.

Squamous cell carcinoma accounts for over 90% of the cases of laryngeal carcinoma (Haskell, 2001). The staging of the tumour serves as a framework for the therapeutic regimen. The TNM classification system, developed by the American Joint Committee on Cancer (AJCC) (Chart 22-6), is the accepted method used to classify head and neck tumours. The classification of the tumour determines the suggested treatment modalities. Because many of

---

 Chart 22-6

Staging System for Cancer of Larynx: Tumour-Node-Metastasis (TNM) System

Primary Tumour (T)
TX: Primary tumour cannot be assessed
T0: No evidence of primary tumour
Tis: Carcinoma in situ

Supraglottis
T1: Tumour limited to one subsite of supraglottis with normal vocal cord mobility
T2: Tumour invades mucosa of more than one adjacent subsite of supraglottis or glottis or region outside the supraglottis (eg, mucosa of base of tongue, vallecula, medial wall of pyriform sinus) without fixation of the larynx
T3: Tumour limited to larynx with vocal cord fixation and/or invades any of the following: postcricoid area, pre-epiglottic tissues, paraglottic space, and/or minor thyroid cartilage erosion (eg, inner cortex)
T4a: Tumour invades through the thyroid cartilage, and/or invades tissues beyond the larynx (eg, trachea, soft tissues of neck including deep extrinsic muscle of the tongue, strap muscles, thyroid, or esophagus)
T4b: Tumour invades prevertebral space, encases carotid artery, or invades mediastinal structures

Glottis
T1: Tumour limited to vocal cord(s) (may involve anterior or posterior commissure) with normal mobility
T1a: Tumour limited to one vocal cord
T1b: Tumour involves both vocal cords
T2: Tumour extends to supraglottis and/or subglottis, and/or with impaired vocal cord mobility
T3: Tumour limited to the larynx with vocal cord fixation and/or invades paraglottic space, and or minor thyroid cartilage erosion (eg, inner cortex)
T4a: Tumour invades through the thyroid cartilage and/or invades tissues beyond the larynx (eg, trachea, soft tissues of neck including deep extrinsic muscle of the tongue, strap muscles, thyroid, or esophagus)
T4b: Tumour invades prevertebral space, encases carotid artery, or invades mediastinal structures

Subglottis
T1: Tumour limited to the subglottis
T2: Tumour extends to vocal cord(s) with normal or impaired mobility
T3: Tumour limited to larynx with vocal cord fixation

T4a: Tumour invades cricoid or thyroid cartilage and/or invades tissues beyond the larynx (eg, trachea, soft tissues of neck including deep extrinsic muscles of the tongue, strap muscles, thyroid, or esophagus)
T4b: Tumour invades prevertebral space, encases carotid artery, or invades mediastinal structures

Regional Lymph Nodes (N)
NX: Regional lymph nodes cannot be assessed
N0: No regional lymph node metastasis
N1: Metastasis in single ipsilateral lymph node, 3 cm or less in greatest dimension
N2: Metastasis in single ipsilateral lymph node, more than 3 cm but not more than 6 cm in greatest dimension, or in multiple ipsilateral lymph nodes, none more than 6 cm in greatest dimension, or in bilateral or contralateral lymph nodes, none more than 6 cm in greatest dimension
  N2a: Metastasis in a single ipsilateral lymph node more than 3 cm but not more than 6 cm in greatest dimension
  N2b: Metastasis in multiple ipsilateral lymph nodes, none more than 6 cm in greatest dimension
  N2c: Metastasis in bilateral or contralateral lymph nodes, none more than 6 cm in greatest dimension
N3: Metastasis in a lymph node more than 6 cm in greatest dimension

Distant Metastasis (M)
MX: Distant metastasis cannot be assessed
M0: No distant metastasis
M1: Distant metastasis

Stage Grouping

Stage	T	N	M
Stage 0	Tis	N0	M0
Stage I	T1	N0	M0
Stage II	T2	N0	M0
Stage III	T3	N0	M0
	T1	N1	M0
	T2	N1	M0
	T3	N1	M0
Stage IV A	T4a	N0	M0
	T4a	N1	M0
	Any T	N2	M0
Stage IV B	Any T	N3	M0
Stage IV C	Any T	Any N	M1

Used with the permission of the American Joint Committee on Cancer (AJCC), Chicago, Illinois. The original source for this material is the *AJCC Cancer Staging Manual, Sixth Edition* (2002) published by Springer-Verlag, New York, www.springer-ny.com.

these lesions are submucosal, biopsy may require that an incision be made using microlaryngeal techniques or using a CO_2 laser to transect the mucosa and reach the tumour.

Computed tomography and magnetic resonance imaging (MRI) are used to assess regional adenopathy and soft tissue and to help stage and determine the extent of a tumour. MRI is also helpful in post-treatment follow-up in order to detect a recurrence. Positron emission tomography (PET scan) may also be used to detect recurrence of a laryngeal tumour after treatment.

Medical Management

Treatment of laryngeal cancer depends on the staging of the tumour, which includes the location, size, and histology of the tumour and the presence and extent of cervical lymph node involvement. Treatment options include surgery, radiation therapy, and chemotherapy. The prognosis depends on a variety of factors: tumour stage, the patient's gender and age, and pathologic features of the tumour, including the grade and depth of infiltration. The treatment plan also depends on whether this is an initial diagnosis or a recurrence. Small glottic tumours, stage I and II, with no infiltration to the lymph nodes are associated with a 75% to 95% survival rate. Patients with stage III and IV or advanced tumours have a 50% to 60% survival rate and have a 50% chance of recurrence and a 30% chance of metastasis. The highest risk of laryngeal cancer recurrence is in the first 2 to 3 years. Recurrence after 5 years is rare and is usually due to a new primary malignancy (Lenhard et al., 2001) (Chart 22-7).

Surgery and radiation therapy are both effective methods in the early stages of cancer of the larynx. Chemotherapy traditionally has been used for recurrence or metastatic disease. It has also been used more recently in conjunction with either radiation therapy to avoid a total laryngectomy or preoperatively to shrink a tumour before surgery. A complete dental examination is performed to rule out any oral disease. Any dental problems are resolved, if possible, prior to surgery. If surgery is to be performed, a multidisciplinary team evaluates the needs of the patient and family to develop a successful plan of care (Forastiere et al., 2001).

SURGICAL MANAGEMENT

Recent advances in surgical techniques for treating laryngeal cancer may minimize the ensuing cosmetic and functional deficits. Depending on the location and staging of the tumour, four different types of **laryngectomy** (surgical removal of part or all of the larynx and surrounding structures) are considered:

- Partial laryngectomy
- Supraglottic laryngectomy
- Hemilaryngectomy
- Total laryngectomy

Some microlaryngeal surgery can be performed endoscopically. The CO_2 laser can be used for the treatment of many laryngeal tumours, with the exception of large vascular tumours.

Partial Laryngectomy. A partial laryngectomy (laryngofissure–thyrotomy) is recommended in the early stages of cancer in the glottic area when only one vocal cord is involved. The surgery is associated with a very high cure rate. It may also be performed for a recurrence when high-dose radiation has failed. A portion of the larynx is removed, along with one vocal cord and the tumour; all other structures remain. The airway remains intact and the patient is expected to have no difficulty swallowing. The voice quality may change or the patient may be hoarse.

Supraglottic Laryngectomy. A supraglottic laryngectomy is indicated in the management of early (stage I) supraglottic and stage II lesions. The hyoid bone, glottis, and false cords are removed. The true vocal cords, cricoid cartilage, and trachea remain intact. During surgery, a radical neck dissection is performed on the involved side. A tracheostomy tube (see Chap. 25) is left in the trachea until the glottic airway is established. It is usually removed after a few days and the stoma is allowed to close. Nutrition is provided through a nasogastric tube until there is healing, followed by a semisolid diet. Postoperatively, the patient may experience some difficulty swallowing for the first 2 weeks. Aspiration is a potential complication since the patient must learn a new method of swallowing (supraglottic swallowing). The chief advantage of this surgical procedure is that it preserves the voice, even though the quality of the voice may change. Speech therapy is required before and after surgery. The major problem is the high risk for recurrence of the cancer; therefore, patients are selected carefully.

Hemilaryngectomy. A hemilaryngectomy is performed when the tumour extends beyond the vocal cord but is less than 1 cm in size and is limited to the subglottic area. It may be used in stage I glottic lesions. In this procedure, the thyroid cartilage of the larynx is split in the midline of the neck and the portion of the vocal cord (one true cord and one false cord) is removed with the tumour. The arytenoid cartilage and half of the thyroid are removed. The patient will have a tracheostomy tube and nasogastric tube in place for 10 to 14 days following surgery. The patient is at risk for aspiration postoperatively. Some change may occur in the voice quality. The voice may be rough, raspy, and hoarse and have limited projection. The airway and swallowing remain intact.

Chart 22-7 • Ethics and Related Issues

Situation
A 68-year-old attorney was diagnosed with cancer of the larynx 8 years ago. He was treated successfully with radiation therapy, resulting in an altered voice quality. Recently, he has complained of shortness of breath and difficulty swallowing. In the past few months, he also has noticed a marked change in his voice and physical condition, which he attributed to "winter colds."

After a complete physical exam and an extensive diagnostic workup and biopsy, it is determined that the cancer has recurred at a new primary site. His health care provider recommends surgery (a total laryngectomy) and chemotherapy as the best options. The patient states that he is not willing to "lose my voice and my livelihood" but instead will "take my chances." He has also expressed concern about his quality of life after surgery. His family has approached you about trying to convince him to have surgery.

Dilemma
The patient's right to refuse treatment conflicts with the family's wishes and recommendation from his health care provider.

Discussion
1. Is the patient making a decision based upon all pertinent information concerning his health status, treatment, options, risk/benefits, and long-term prognosis?
2. What arguments can be made to support the patient's decision to forego treatment?
3. What arguments can be made to question the patient's decision to forego treatment?

Total Laryngectomy. A total laryngectomy is performed in the most advanced stage IV laryngeal cancer, when the tumour extends beyond the vocal cords, or for recurrent or persistent cancer following radiation therapy. In a total laryngectomy, the laryngeal structures are removed, including the hyoid bone, epiglottis, cricoid cartilage, and two or three rings of the trachea. The tongue, pharyngeal walls, and trachea are preserved. A total laryngectomy will result in permanent loss of the voice and a change in the airway.

Many surgeons recommend that a radical neck dissection be performed on the same side as the lesion even if no lymph nodes are palpable because metastasis to the cervical lymph nodes is common. Surgery is more difficult when the lesion involves the midline structures or both vocal cords. With or without neck dissection, a total laryngectomy requires a permanent tracheal stoma because the larynx that provides the protective sphincter is no longer present. The tracheal stoma prevents the aspiration of food and fluid into the lower respiratory tract. The patient will have no voice but will have normal swallowing. A total laryngectomy changes the manner in which airflow is used for breathing and speaking, as depicted in Figure 22-5. Complications that may occur include a salivary leak, wound infection from the development of a pharyngocutaneous fistula, stomal stenosis, and dysphagia secondary to pharyngeal and cervical esophageal stricture.

RADIATION THERAPY

The goal of radiation therapy is to eradicate the cancer and preserve the function of the larynx. The decision to use radiation therapy is based on several factors, including the staging of the tumour (usually used for stage I and stage II tumours as a standard treatment option) and the patient's overall health status, lifestyle (including occupation), and personal preference. Excellent results have been achieved with radiation therapy in patients with early-stage (I and II) glottic tumours when only one vocal cord is involved and there is normal mobility (ie, moves with phonation) and in small supraglottic lesions. One of the benefits of radiation therapy is that patients retain a near-normal voice. A few may develop chondritis (inflammation of the cartilage) or stenosis; a small number may later require laryngectomy.

Radiation therapy may also be used preoperatively to reduce the tumour size. Radiation therapy is combined with surgery in advanced (stages III and IV) laryngeal cancer as adjunctive therapy to surgery or chemotherapy, and as a palliative measure. A variety of clinical trials have combined chemotherapy and radiation therapy in the treatment of advanced laryngeal tumours. Early studies suggest that combined modality therapy may improve the tumour's response to radiation therapy. Radiation therapy combined with chemotherapy may be an alternative to a total laryngectomy.

The complications from radiation therapy are a result of external radiation to the head and neck area, which may also include the parotid gland responsible for mucus production. The symptoms may include acute mucositis, ulceration of the mucous membranes, pain, **xerostomia** (dry mouth), loss of taste, dysphasia, fatigue, and skin reactions. Later complications may include laryngeal necrosis, edema, and fibrosis.

SPEECH THERAPY

The loss or alteration of speech is discussed with the patient and family before surgery, and the speech therapist conducts a preoperative evaluation. During this time, the nurse should inform the patient and family about methods of communication that will be available in the immediate postoperative period. These include

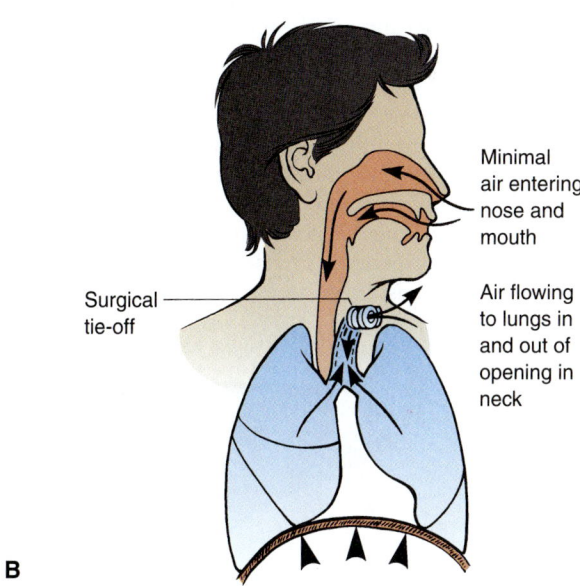

FIGURE 22-5 Total laryngectomy produces a change in airflow for breathing and speaking. (**A**) Normal airflow. (**B**) Airflow after total laryngectomy.

writing, lip speaking, and communication or word boards. A system of communication is established with the patient, family, nurse, and physician and implemented consistently after surgery.

A postoperative communication plan is also developed. The three most common techniques of **alaryngeal communication** are esophageal speech, artificial larynx (electrolarynx), and tracheoesophageal puncture. Training in these techniques begins once medical clearance is obtained from the physician.

Esophageal Speech. Esophageal speech was the primary method of alaryngeal speech taught to patients until the 1980s. The patient needs the ability to compress air into the esophagus and expel it, setting off a vibration of the pharyngeal esophageal segment. The technique can be taught once the patient begins oral feedings, approximately 1 week after surgery. First, the patient learns to belch and is reminded to do so an hour after eating. Then the technique is practiced repeatedly. Later, this conscious belching action is transformed into simple explosions of air from the esophagus for speech purposes. Thereafter, the speech therapist works with the patient in an attempt to make speech intelligible and as close to normal as possible. Because it takes a long time to become proficient, the success rate is low.

Electric Larynx. If esophageal speech is not successful, or until the patient masters the technique, an electric larynx may be used for communication. This battery-powered apparatus projects sound into the oral cavity. When the mouth forms words (articulated), the sounds from the electric larynx become audible words. The voice that is produced sounds mechanical, and some words may be difficult to distinguish. The advantage is that the patient is able to communicate with relative ease while working to become proficient at either esophageal or tracheoesophageal puncture speech.

Tracheoesophageal Puncture. The third technique of alaryngeal speech is tracheoesophageal puncture (Fig. 22-6). This technique is the most widely used because the speech associated with it most resembles normal speech (the sound produced is a combination of esophageal speech and voice), and it is easily learned. A valve is placed in the tracheal stoma to divert air into the esophagus and out of the mouth. Once the puncture is surgically created and has healed, a voice prosthesis (Blom–Singer) is fitted over the puncture site. To prevent airway obstruction, the prosthesis is removed and cleaned when mucus builds up. A speech therapist teaches the patient how to produce sounds. Moving the tongue and lips to form the sound into words produces speech as before. Tracheoesophageal speech is successful in 80% to 90% of patients (DeLisa & Gans, 1998).

Voice prosthesis

Tracheostoma valve

FIGURE 22-6 Schematic representation of tracheoesophageal puncture speech (TEP). Air travels from the lung through a puncture in the posterior wall of the trachea into the esophagus and out the mouth. A voice prosthesis is fitted over the puncture site.

NURSING PROCESS: THE PATIENT UNDERGOING LARYNGECTOMY

Assessment

The nurse assesses the patient for the following symptoms: hoarseness, sore throat, dyspnea, dysphagia, or pain and burning in the throat. The neck is palpated for swelling.

If treatment includes surgery, the nurse must know the nature of the surgery to plan appropriate care. If the patient is expected to have no voice, a preoperative evaluation by the speech therapist is indicated. The patient's ability to hear, see, read, and write is assessed. Visual impairment and functional illiteracy may create additional problems with communication and require creative approaches to ensure that the patient is able to communicate any needs.

In addition, the nurse determines the psychological readiness of the patient and family. The idea of cancer is terrifying to most people. Fear is compounded by the possibility of permanently losing one's voice and, in some cases, of having some degree of disfigurement. The nurse evaluates the patient's and family's coping methods to support them effectively both preoperatively and postoperatively.

Diagnosis

NURSING DIAGNOSES

Based on all the assessment data, major nursing diagnoses may include the following:

- Deficient knowledge about the surgical procedure and postoperative course
- Anxiety and depression related to the diagnosis of cancer and impending surgery
- Ineffective airway clearance related to excess mucus production secondary to surgical alterations in the airway
- Impaired verbal communication related to anatomic deficit secondary to removal of the larynx and to edema
- Imbalanced nutrition: less than body requirements, related to inability to ingest food secondary to swallowing difficulties
- Disturbed body image and low self-esteem secondary to major neck surgery, change in the structure and function of the larynx
- Self-care deficit related to pain, weakness, fatigue, musculoskeletal impairment related to surgical procedure and postoperative course

COLLABORATIVE PROBLEMS/ POTENTIAL COMPLICATIONS

Based on assessment data, potential complications that may develop include:

- Respiratory distress (hypoxia, airway obstruction, tracheal edema)
- Hemorrhage
- Infection
- Wound breakdown

Planning and Goals

The major goals for the patient may include attainment of an adequate level of knowledge, reduction in anxiety, maintenance of a patent airway (patient is able to handle own secretions), effective use of alternative means of communication, attainment of optimal levels of nutrition and hydration, improvement in body image and self-esteem, improved self-care management, and absence of complications.

Nursing Interventions

TEACHING THE PATIENT PREOPERATIVELY

The diagnosis of laryngeal cancer is associated with misconceptions and fears. Many people assume that loss of speech and disfigurement are inevitable with this condition. Once the physician explains the diagnosis to the patient, the nurse clarifies any misconceptions by identifying the location of the larynx, its function, the nature of the surgical procedure, and its effect on speech. Informational materials (written and audiovisual) about the surgery are given to the patient and family for review and reinforcement.

If a complete laryngectomy is planned, the patient should know that the natural voice will be lost, but that special training can provide a means for communicating. However, the ability to sing, laugh, or whistle will be lost. Until this training is initiated, the patient needs to know that communication will be possible by using the call light or special communication board and by writing. The nurse answers questions about the nature of the surgery and reinforces the physician's explanation that the patient will lose the ability to vocalize, but that a rehabilitation program is available. The multidisciplinary team conducts an initial assessment of the patient and family. The team might include the nurse, physician, respiratory therapist, speech therapist, clinical nurse specialist, social worker, dietitian, and home care nurse.

Next, the nurse reviews equipment and treatments for postoperative care with the patient and family, teaches important coughing and deep-breathing exercises, and assists the patient to perform a return demonstration. The nurse clarifies the patient's role in the postoperative and rehabilitation periods.

REDUCING ANXIETY AND DEPRESSION

Because surgery of the larynx is performed most commonly for a malignant tumour, the patient may have many questions: Will the surgeon be able to remove all of the tumour? Is it cancer? Will I die? Will I choke? Will I suffocate? Will I ever speak again? What will I look like? The psychological preparation of the patient is as important as the physical preparation.

Any patient undergoing surgery may have many fears. In laryngeal surgery, these fears may relate to the diagnosis of cancer and may be compounded by the possibility of permanent loss of the voice and disfigurement. The nurse provides the patient and family with opportunities to ask questions, verbalize feelings, and discuss perceptions. It is important to address any questions and misconceptions the patient and family have. During the preoperative or postoperative period, a visit from someone who has had a laryngectomy may reassure the patient that people are available to help and that rehabilitation is possible.

MAINTAINING A PATENT AIRWAY

The nurse promotes a patent airway by positioning the patient in the semi-Fowler's or Fowler's position after recovery from anesthesia. Observing the patient for restlessness, laboured breathing, apprehension, and increased pulse rate helps the nurse identify possible respiratory or circulatory problems. Medications that depress respiration, particularly opioids, should be used cautiously. As with other surgical patients, the nurse encourages the laryngectomy patient to turn, cough, and take deep breaths. If necessary, suctioning may be performed to remove secretions. The nurse also encourages and assists the patient with early ambulation to prevent atelectasis and pneumonia.

If a total laryngectomy was performed, a laryngectomy tube will most likely be in place. (In some instances a laryngectomy tube is not used; in others it is used temporarily, and in many it is used permanently.) The laryngectomy tube, which is shorter than a tracheostomy tube but has a larger diameter, is the patient's only airway. The care of this tube is the same as for a tracheostomy tube (see Chap. 25). The nurse cleans the stoma daily with saline solution or another prescribed solution. If a non–oil-based antibiotic ointment is prescribed, the nurse applies it around the stoma and suture line. If crusting appears around the stoma, the nurse removes the crusts with sterile tweezers and applies additional ointment.

Wound drains may be in place to assist in removal of fluid and air from the surgical site. Suction also may be used, but cautiously, to avoid trauma to the surgical site and incision. The nurse observes, measures, and records drainage. When drainage is less than 50 to 60 mL/day, the physician usually removes the drains.

Frequently, the patient coughs up large amounts of mucus through this opening. Because air passes directly into the trachea without being warmed and moistened by the upper respiratory mucosa, the tracheobronchial tree compensates by secreting excessive amounts of mucus. Therefore, the patient will have frequent coughing episodes and may develop a brassy-sounding, mucus-producing cough. The nurse should reassure the patient that these problems will diminish in time as the tracheobronchial mucosa adapts to the altered physiology.

After the patient coughs, the tracheostomy opening must be wiped clean and clear of mucus. A simple gauze dressing, washcloth, or even paper towel (because of its size and absorbency) worn below the tracheostomy may serve as a barrier to protect the clothing from the copious mucus that the patient may expel initially.

One of the most important factors in decreasing cough, mucus production, and crusting around the stoma is adequate humidification of the environment. Mechanical humidifiers and aerosol generators (nebulizers) increase the humidity and are important for the patient's comfort.

The laryngectomy tube may be removed when the stoma is well healed, within 3 to 6 weeks after surgery. The nurse can teach the patient how to clean and change the tube (see Chap. 25) and remove secretions.

PROMOTING ALTERNATIVE COMMUNICATION METHODS

Understanding the patient's postoperative needs is critical. Alternative means of communication are established and used consistently by all personnel who come in contact with the patient—for example, a call bell or hand bell may be placed within easy reach of the patient. Because a Magic Slate often is used for communication, the nurse should document which hand the patient uses for writing so that the opposite arm can be used for intravenous infusions. (The nurse should discard any old notes used for communication to ensure the patient's privacy.) If the patient cannot write, a picture-word-phrase board or hand signals can be used. Preoperatively, the nurse reviews the system of communication to be used postoperatively with the patient.

Because it is very time-consuming to have to write everything or communicate through gestures, the inability to speak can be very frustrating. The patient may become impatient and angry when not understood. In such cases, other staff members need to be alert to the problem and also recognize that the patient will be unable to use the intercom system.

The return of communication is generally the ultimate goal in the rehabilitation of the laryngectomy patient. The nurse works with the patient, speech therapist, and family to encourage use of alternative communication methods.

PROMOTING ADEQUATE NUTRITION

Postoperatively, the patient may not be permitted to eat or drink for 10 to 14 days. Alternative sources of nutrition and hydration include intravenous fluids, enteral feedings through a nasogastric tube, and parenteral nutrition.

Once the patient is ready to start oral feedings, the nurse explains that thick liquids will be used first because they are easy to swallow. The nurse instructs the patient to avoid sweet foods, which increase salivation and suppress the appetite. Solid foods are introduced as tolerated. The nurse instructs the patient to rinse the mouth with warm water or mouthwash and to brush the teeth frequently.

The patient can expect to have a diminished sense of taste and smell for a period of time after surgery. Inhaled air passes directly into the trachea, bypassing the nose and the olfactory end organs. Because taste and smell are so closely connected, taste sensations are altered. In time, however, the patient usually accommodates to this problem and olfactory sensation adapts, often with return of interest in eating. The nurse observes the patient for any difficulty swallowing, particularly when eating resumes, and reports its occurrence to the physician.

PROMOTING POSITIVE BODY IMAGE AND SELF-ESTEEM

Disfiguring surgery and an altered communication pattern are a threat to a patient's body image and self-esteem. The reaction of family members and friends is a major concern for the patient. The nurse encourages the patient to express any feelings about the changes brought about by surgery, particularly those related to fear, anger, depression, and isolation.

A positive approach is important when caring for the patient. Promoting self-care activities is part of this approach. It is important for the patient and family to begin participating in self-care activities as soon as possible. The nurse needs to be a good listener and a support to the family, especially when explaining the tubes, dressings, and drains that are in place postoperatively. Referral to a support group, such as Lost Chord or New Voice clubs (through the International Association of Laryngectomees) and I Can Cope (through the American Cancer Society), may help the patient and family deal with the changes in their lives. Groups such as Lost Chord and New Voice promote and support the rehabilitation of people who have had a laryngectomy by providing an opportunity for exchanging ideas and sharing information.

MONITORING AND MANAGING POTENTIAL COMPLICATIONS

The immediate potential complications after laryngectomy include respiratory distress and hypoxia, hemorrhage, infection, and wound breakdown.

Respiratory Distress and Hypoxia

The nurse monitors the patient for signs and symptoms of respiratory distress and hypoxia, particularly restlessness, irritation, agitation, confusion, tachypnea, use of accessory muscles, and decreased oxygen saturation on pulse oximetry (SpO_2). Any change in the respiratory status requires immediate intervention. Obstruction needs to be ruled out immediately by suctioning and having the patient cough and breathe deeply. Hypoxia and airway obstruction, if not immediately treated, are life-threatening.

The nurse contacts the physician immediately if nursing measures do not improve the patient's respiratory status.

Hemorrhage

Bleeding at the surgical site from the drains or with tracheal suctioning may signal the occurrence of hemorrhage. The nurse should notify the surgeon of any active bleeding immediately. Bleeding may occur at a variety of sites, including the surgical site, drains, or trachea. Rupture of the carotid artery is especially dangerous. Should this occur, the nurse should apply direct pressure over the artery, summon assistance, and provide emotional support to the patient until the vessel can be ligated. It is important to monitor vital signs for changes, particularly increased pulse rate, decreased blood pressure, and rapid deep respirations. Cold, clammy, pale skin may indicate active bleeding.

Infection

The nurse observes for postoperative infection. Early signs of infection include an increase in temperature and pulse, a change in the type of wound drainage, or increased areas of redness or tenderness at the surgical site. Other signs include purulent drainage, odour, and increased wound drainage. The nurse reports any significant change to the surgeon.

Wound Breakdown

Wound breakdown due to infection, poor wound healing, or development of a fistula or as a result of radiation therapy or tumour growth can create a life-threatening emergency. The carotid artery, which is close to the stoma, may rupture from erosion if the wound does not heal properly. The nurse observes the stoma area for wound breakdown, hematoma, and bleeding and reports any significant changes to the surgeon. If wound breakdown occurs, the patient must be monitored carefully and identified as being at high risk for carotid hemorrhage.

PROMOTING HOME AND COMMUNITY-BASED CARE

Teaching Patients Self-Care

The nurse has an important role in the recovery and rehabilitation of the laryngectomy patient. In an effort to facilitate the patient's ability to manage self-care, discharge instruction begins as soon as the patient is able to participate. Nursing care and patient teaching in the hospital, outpatient setting, and rehabilitation or long-term care facility must take into consideration the many emotions, physical changes, and lifestyle changes experienced by the patient. In preparing the patient to go home, the nurse assesses the patient's readiness to learn and the level of knowledge about self-care management. The nurse also reassures the patient and family that most self-care management strategies can be mastered. The patient will need to learn a variety of self-care behaviours, including tracheostomy and stoma care, wound care, and oral hygiene. In addition, the nurse instructs the patient about the need for safe hygiene and recreational activities.

Tracheostomy and Stoma Care. The nurse provides specific instructions to the patient and family about what to expect from the tracheostomy and its management. The nurse teaches the patient and family caregiver to perform suctioning and emergency measures and tracheostomy and stoma care. The nurse stresses the importance of humidification at home and instructs the family to set up a humidification system before the patient returns home. In addition, the nurse cautions the patient and family that air-conditioned air may be too cool or too dry, and thus too irritating, for the patient with a new laryngectomy. (See Chap. 25 for details about tracheostomy care.)

Hygiene and Safety Measures. The nurse instructs the patient and family about safety precautions needed because of the structural changes resulting from the surgery. Special precautions are needed in the shower to prevent water from entering the stoma. Wearing a loose-fitting plastic bib over the tracheostomy or simply holding the hand over the opening is effective. Swimming is not recommended, however, because people with a laryngectomy can drown without getting their face wet. Barbers and beauticians need to be alerted so that hair sprays, loose hair, and powder do not get near the stoma, because they can block or irritate the trachea and possibly cause infection. These self-care points are summarized in Chart 22-8.

Recreation and exercise are important, and all but very strenuous exercise can be enjoyed safely. Avoidance of strenuous exercise and fatigue is important because, when tired, the patient has more difficulty speaking, which can be discouraging. Additional safety points to address include the need for the patient to wear or carry medical identification, such as a bracelet or card, to alert medical personnel to the special requirements for resuscitation should this need arise. When resuscitation is needed, direct mouth-to-stoma ventilation should be performed. For home emergency situations, prerecorded emergency messages for police, the fire department, or other rescue services can be kept near the phone to be used quickly.

The nurse instructs and encourages the patient to perform oral care on a regular basis to prevent halitosis and infection. If the patient is receiving radiation therapy, there will be a decrease in saliva, and synthetic saliva may be required. The nurse instructs the patient to drink water or sugar-free liquids throughout the day and to use a humidifier at home. Brushing the teeth or dentures and rinsing the mouth several times a day will assist in maintaining proper oral hygiene.

Continuing Care

Referral for home care is an important aspect of postoperative care for the patient who has had a laryngectomy and will assist the patient and family in the transition to the home. The home care nurse assesses the patient's general health status and the ability of the patient and family to care for the stoma and tracheostomy.

The nurse assesses the surgical incisions, nutritional and respiratory status, and adequacy of pain management. The nurse assesses not only for signs and symptoms of complications but also for the patient's and family's knowledge of which signs and symptoms to report to the physician. During the home visit, the nurse identifies and addresses other learning needs of the patient and family, such as adaptation to physical, lifestyle, and functional changes. It is important to assess the patient's psychological status as well. The home care nurse reinforces previous teaching and provides reassurance and support to the patient and family as needed.

The nurse encourages the person who has had a laryngectomy to have regular physical examinations and to seek advice concerning any problems related to recovery and rehabilitation. The patient is also reminded to participate in health promotion activities and health screening and about the importance of keeping scheduled appointments with the physician, speech therapist, and other health care providers.

Evaluation

EXPECTED PATIENT OUTCOMES

Expected patient outcomes may include:

1. Acquires an adequate level of knowledge, verbalizing an understanding of the surgical procedure and performing self-care adequately
2. Demonstrates less anxiety and depression
   a. Expresses a sense of hope
   b. Is aware of available community organizations and agencies such as the Lost Chord or New Voice groups
   c. Participates in support group, such as I Can Cope
3. Maintains a clear airway and handles own secretions; also demonstrates practical, safe, and correct technique for cleaning and changing the laryngectomy tube
4. Acquires effective communication techniques
   a. Uses assistive devices and strategies for communication (Magic Slate, call bell, picture board, sign language, lip reading, computer aids)
   b. Follows the recommendations of the speech therapist

Chart 22-8

Home Care Checklist • The Patient With a Laryngectomy

At the completion of the home care instruction, the patient or caregiver will be able to:	Patient	Caregiver
• Demonstrate methods to clear the airway and handle secretions	✓	✓
• Explain the rationale for maintaining adequate humidification with a humidifier or nebulizer	✓	✓
• Demonstrate how to clean the skin around the stoma and how to use ointments and tweezers to remove encrustations	✓	✓
• State the rationale for wearing a loose-fitting protective cloth at the stoma	✓	✓
• Discuss the need to avoid cold air from air conditioning and the environment to prevent irritation of the airway	✓	✓
• Demonstrate safe technique in changing the laryngectomy tube	✓	✓
• Identify the signs and symptoms of wound infection and state what to do about them	✓	✓
• Describe safety or emergency measures to implement in case of breathing difficulty or bleeding	✓	✓
• State the rationale for wearing or carrying special medical identification and ways to obtain help in an emergency	✓	✓
• Explain the importance of covering the stoma when showering or bathing	✓	✓
• Identify fluid and caloric needs	✓	✓
• Describe mouth care and discuss its importance	✓	✓
• Demonstrate alternative communication methods	✓	✓
• Identify support groups and agency resources	✓	✓
• State the need for regular check-ups and reporting of any problems immediately	✓	✓

5. Maintains balanced nutrition and adequate fluid intake
6. Exhibits improved body image, self-esteem, and self-concept
   a. Expresses feelings and concerns
   b. Participates in self-care and decision making
   c. Accepts information about support group
7. Exhibits no complications
   a. Vital signs (blood pressure, temperature, pulse, respiratory rate) normal
   b. No redness, tenderness, or purulent drainage at surgical site
   c. Demonstrates a patent airway and appropriate respirations
   d. No bleeding from surgical site and minimal bleeding from drains
   e. No wound breakdown
8. Adheres to rehabilitation and home care program
   a. Practices recommended speech therapy
   b. Demonstrates proper methods for caring for stoma and laryngectomy tube (if present)
   c. Verbalizes understanding of symptoms that require medical attention
   d. States safety measures to take in emergencies
   e. Performs oral hygiene as prescribed

Critical Thinking Exercises

1. A 36-year-old teacher is diagnosed with acute sinusitis. She has been self-medicating with over-the-counter medications for the past 2 weeks with no relief. What assessment and treatment should the nurse anticipate? What teaching and management strategies would you discuss with the patient? What is the rationale for your approach?

2. Your 68-year-old patient is scheduled for total laryngectomy for treatment of laryngeal cancer. What information would you provide to the patient about managing changes in breathing and speech that are expected in the immediate postoperative period and in the long term? What information would you provide to the patient's family?

3. You are making the first home visit to a patient who has just been discharged from the hospital following treatment for pneumonia and a 27-kg weight loss. He had a laryngectomy 8 months ago to treat laryngeal cancer. What will be the focus of your initial home visit? What aspects of assessment and nursing management are key at this point in caring for this patient? How would you assist this patient and his family to plan his care for the next month? Next 6 months?

4. Your patient, age 36, has been admitted to the emergency department with profuse epistaxis following a car crash. He tells you that he has hemophilia and is HIV-positive as a result of repeated use of clotting factors. What are the initial measures you would use to stop the bleeding? What other options are available if the bleeding does not stop within a reasonable period? How will his HIV status and the diagnosis of hemophilia affect your plan of care for him?

REFERENCES AND SELECTED READINGS

Books

American Cancer Society. (2002). *Cancer facts and figures.* Atlanta: American Cancer Society Inc.

Bast, R. C., Kufe, D. W., Pollock, R. E., et al. (Eds.) (2000). *Holland & Frei cancer medicine* (5th ed.) Hamilton: B.C. Decker, Inc.

DeLisa, J. A., & Gans, B. M. (1998). *Rehabilitation medicine principles and practice* (3d ed.). Philadelphia: Lippincott-Raven.

Goldman, L., & Bennett, J. C. (Eds.) (2000). *Cecil textbook of medicine* (21st ed.). Philadelphia: W. B. Saunders.

Green, E., et al. (Eds.) (2002). *AJCC cancer staging manual* (6th ed.). New York: Springer-Verlag.

Haskell, C. M. (2001) *Cancer treatment* (5th ed.). Philadelphia: W. B. Saunders.

Lenhard, R. E., Osteen, R. T., & Gansler, T. (2001) *The American Cancer Society's clinical oncology* (1st ed.). Atlanta: American Cancer Society Inc.

Mandell, G. L., Bennett, J. E., & Dolin, R (Eds.) (2000). *Principles and practice of infectious diseases* (5th ed.). Philadelphia: Churchill Livingstone.

McKenry, L. M., & Salerno, E. (2001). *Mosby's principles in nursing* (21st ed.). St. Louis: Mosby.

Middleton, E., Ellis, E. F., Yuninger, J. W., et al. (1998). *Allergy: principles and practice* (Vol. II, 5th ed.). St. Louis: Mosby.

Murray, J. F., & Nadel, J. A. (2001). *Textbook of respiratory medicine* (Vols. 1 & 2, 3d ed.). Philadelphia: W. B. Saunders.

Peckenpaugh, N. J., & Poleman, C. M. (1999). *Nutrition essentials and diet therapy* (8th ed.). Philadelphia: W. B. Saunders.

Tierney, L. M., McPhee, S. J., & Papadakis, M. A. (2001). *Current medical diagnosis and treatment 2001* (40th ed.). New York: Lange Medical Books/McGraw Hill.

Tintinalli, J. E., Kelen, G. D., & Stapczynski, J. S. (2000). *Emergency medicine: A comprehensive study guide* (5th ed.). New York: McGraw-Hill.

Townsend, C. M. (Ed.) (2001). *Sabiston textbook of surgery* (16th ed.). Philadelphia: W. B. Saunders.

Yarbro, C. H., Goodman, M., Frogge, M. H., & Groenwald, S. L. I. (Eds.) (2000). *Cancer nursing: Principles and practice* (5th ed.). Boston: Jones & Bartlett.

Journals

Asterisks indicate nursing research articles.
General

Casale, T. B., Condemi, J., LaForce, C., et al. (2001). Effect of omalizumab on symptoms of seasonal allergic rhinitis: A randomized controlled trial. *Journal of the American Medical Association, 286*(23), 2956–2967.

Chan, E., & Welsh, C. H. (1998). Geriatric respiratory medicine. *Chest, 114*(6), 1704–1733.

Upper Respiratory Infections

Bisno, A. L. (2001) Primary care: Acute pharyngitis. *New England Journal of Medicine, 344*(3), 205–211.

Cifu, A., & Levinson, W. (2000) Influenza. *Journal of the American Medical Association, 284*(22), 2847–2849.

Cooper, R. J., Hoffman, J. R., Bartlett, J. G., et al. (June 2001). Centers for Disease Control and Prevention. Principles of appropriate antibiotic use for acute pharyngitis in adults: background. *Annals of Emergency Medicine. 37*(6), 711–719.

Corneli, H. (2001). Rapid strep tests in the emergency department: An evidence-based approach. *Pediatric Emergency Care, 17*(4), 272–278.

Ebell, M. H., Smith, M. A., Barry, H. C., Ives, K., & Carey, M. (2000). Does this patient have strep throat? *Journal of the American Medical Association, 284*(22), 2912–2918.

Hall, C. B. (2001). Respiratory syncytial virus and parainfluenza virus. *New England Journal of Medicine, 344*(25), 1917–1928.

Hickner, J. M. (2001). Acute rhinosinusitis: A diagnostic and therapeutic challenge. *Journal of Family Practice, 50*(1), 38–40.

Hickner, J. M., Bartlett, J. G., Besser, R. E., et al. (2001). American Academy of Family Physicians/American Society of Internal Medicine. Centers for Disease Control Infectious Diseases Society of America. Principles of appropriate antibiotic use for acute rhinosinusitis in adults: background. *Annals of Internal Medicine, 134*(6), 498–505.

Kearney, K. (2001). Emergency: Epiglottis. *American Journal of Nursing, 101*(8), 37–38.

Kernan, W. N., Viscoli, C. M., Brass, L. M., et al. (2000). Phenylpropanolamine and the risk of hemorrhagic stroke. *New England Journal of Medicine, 343*(25), 1826–1832.

Luna, B., Drew, R. H., & Perfect, J. R. (2000). Agents for the treatment of invasive fungal infections. *Otolaryngologic Clinics of North America, 33*(4), 277–299.

Mattila, P. (2001). Causes of tonsillar disease and frequency of tonsillectomy operations. *Archives of Otolaryngology—Head & Neck Surgery, 127*(1), 37–44.

Piccirillo, J. F., Mager, D. E., Frisse, M. E., Brophy, R. H. & Goggin, A. (2001). Impact of first-line vs. second-line antibiotics for the treatment of acute uncomplicated sinusitis. *Journal of the American Medical Association, 286*(15), 1849–1856.

Poole, M. (1999). A focus on acute sinusitis in adults: Changes in disease management. *American Journal of Medicine*, 106 (5A), 38S–47S.

Prasad, A. S., Fitzgerald, J. T., Bao, B., et al. (2000). Duration of symptoms and plasma cytokine levels in patients with the common cold treated with zinc acetate: A randomized, double-blind, placebo-controlled trial. *Annals of Internal Medicine, 133*(4), 245–252.

Sly, M. (1999). Changing prevalence of allergic rhinitis and asthma. *Annals of Allergy, Asthma, & Immunology, 82*(3), 233–252.

Snow, V., Mottur-Pilson, C., Hickner, J. M., et al. (2001). Principles of appropriate antibiotic use for acute sinusitis in adults. *Annals of Internal Medicine, 134*(6), 495–497.

Stephenson, K. (2000). Acute and chronic pharyngitis across the lifespan. *Lippincott's Primary Care Practice. Ear, Nose, and Throat Problems, 4*(5), 471–489.

Stone, S., Gonzales, R., Maselli, J., & Lowenstein, S. R. (2000). Antibiotic prescribing for patients with colds, upper respiratory tract infections, and bronchitis: A national study of hospital-based emergency departments. *Annals of Emergency Medicine. 36*(4), 320–327.

Youngs, R. (2000) Sinusitis in adults. *Current Opinion in Pulmonary Medicine, 6*(3), 217–220.

Obstruction and Trauma of the Airway

Boehlecke, B. A. (2000). Epidemiology and pathogenesis of sleep-disordered breathing. *Current Opinion in Pulmonary Medicine, 6*(6), 471–478.

Flemons, W. W. (2002). Clinical practice. Obstructive sleep apnea. *New England Journal of Medicine, 347*(7), 498–504.

Goldberg, R. (2000). Treatment of obstructive sleep apnea, other than with continuous positive airway pressure. *Current Opinion in Pulmonary Medicine, 6*(6), 496–500.

Harding, S. M. (2000). Complications and consequences of obstructive sleep apnea. *Current Opinion in Pulmonary Medicine, 6*(6), 485–489.

Krieger, A. C. & Redeker, N. S. (2002) Obstructive sleep apnea syndrome: its relationship with hypertension. *Journal of Cardiovascular Nursing, 17*(1), 1–11.

Krishna, P., & Lee, D. (2001). Post-tonsillectomy bleeding: A meta-analysis. *Laryngoscope, 111*(8), 1358–1361.

Liu, J., Anderson, K. E., Willging, J. P., et al. (2001). Post-tonsillectomy hemorrhage: What is it and what should be recorded? *Archives of Otolaryngology—Head & Neck Surgery, 127*(10), 1271–1275.

Marchiondo, K. (2000). Pickwickian syndrome: The challenge of severe sleep apnea. *MedSurg Nursing, 9*(4), 183–188.

Narkiewicz, K., Kato, M., Phillips, B. G., et al. (1999). Nocturnal continuous positive airway pressure decreases daytime sympathetic traffic in obstructive sleep apnea. *Circulation, 100*(23), 2332–2335.

National Institutes of Health. (2000). NHLBI study shows association between sleep apnea and hypertension (Press release, 4-11-00). http://www.nhlbi.nih.gov/about/ncsdr.

Nieto, F. J., Young, T. B., Lind, B. K., et al. (2000). Association of sleep-disordered breathing, sleep apnea, and hypertension in a large community-based study. Sleep Heart Health Study. *Journal of the American Medical Association, 283*(14), 1829–1836.

Parker, K. P. & Dunbar, S. B. (2002). Sleep and heart failure. *Journal of Cardiovascular Nursing, 17*(1), 12–29.

Peppard, P. E., Young, T., Palta, M., et al. (2000). Longitudinal study of moderate weight change and sleep-disordered breathing. *Journal of the American Medical Association, 284*(23), 3015–3021.

Redeker, N. S. (2002). Why is sleep relevant to cardiovascular disease? *Journal of Cardiovascular Nursing, 17*(1), v–ix.

Cancer of the Larynx

Bauer, A. M. (2001). Current trends in surgical management of head and neck carcinomas. *Nursing Clinics of North America, 36*(3), 501–506.

*Dropkin, M. J. (2001). Anxiety, coping strategies and coping behaviors in patients undergoing head and neck cancer surgery. *Cancer Nursing, 24*(2), 143–148.

Finizia, C., & Bergman, B. (2001). Health-related quality of life in patients with laryngeal cancer: A post-treatment comparison of different modes of communication. *Laryngoscope, 111*(5), 918–923.

Forastiere, A., Koch, W., Trotti, A., & Sidransky, D. (2001). Head and neck cancer. *New England Journal of Medicine, 345*(26), 1890–1900.

Friedman, M., Landsberg, R., Pryor, S., et al. (2001). The occurrence of sleep-disordered breathing among patients with head and neck cancer. *Laryngoscope, 111*(11), 1917–1919.

*Hemsley, B. (2001). Nursing the patient with severe communication impairment. *Journal of Advanced Nursing, 35*(6), 827–835.

Koch, W. (2001). A fail-safe technique for endoscopic tracheoesophageal puncture. *Laryngoscope, 111*(9), 1663–1665.

*Major, M. S., Bumpous, J. M., Flynn, M. B., & Schill, K. (2001). Quality of life after treatment for advanced laryngeal and hypopharyngeal cancer. *Laryngoscope, 111*(8), 1379–1382.

Owen, C., et al. (2001). The psychosocial impact of head and neck cancer. *Clinical Otolaryngology & Allied Sciences, 26*(5), 351–356.

Rose, P., & Yates, P. (2001). Quality of life experienced by patients receiving radiation treatment for cancers of the head and neck. *Cancer Nursing, 24*(4), 255–263.

Serra, A. (2000). Tracheostomy care. *Nursing Standard, 14*(42), 45–55.

Tamura, E. (2001). Clinical assessment of intralaryngeal ultrasonography. *Laryngoscope, 111*(10), 767–770.

Weinstein, G. S., El-Sawy, M. M., Ruiz, C., et al. (2001). Laryngeal preservation with supracricoid partial laryngectomy results in improved quality of life when compared with total laryngectomy. *Laryngoscope, 111*(12), 191–199.

RESOURCES AND WEBSITES

American Cancer Society, 1599 Clifton Rd., NE, Atlanta, GA 30329-4251; (404) 320-3333; (800) ACS-2345; http://www.cancer.org.

American Lung Association, 1740 Broadway, New York, NY 10019-4374; (212) 315-8700; http://www.lungusa.org.

American Sleep Apnea Association, 1424 K Street, NW, Suite 302, Washington, DC 20005; 202-293-3650; http://www.sleepapnea.org.

Canadian Cancer Society–British Columbian and Yukon Division, 565 West 10th Avenue, Vancouver, BC V5Z 4J4; 1-888-939-3333; http://www.cancer.ca.

Canadian Lung Association, 3 Raymond Street, Suite 300, Ottawa, ON K1R 1A3; 613-569-6411; 1-888-566-Lung (5864); http://www.lung.ca.

Canadian Medical Association; http://www.cma.ca.

Canadian Thoracic Society; http://www.lung.ca/cts.

Health Canada; http://www.hc-sc.gc.ca.

International Association of Laryngectomees, 7400 N. Shadeland Ave., Suite 100, Indianapolis, IN 46250; (317) 570-4568; http://www.larynxlink.com.

National Cancer Institute (NCI), Bldg. 31, 31 Center Drive, MSC 2580, Bethesda, MD 20892-2580; http://cancernet.nci.nih.gov.

National Institute of Allergy and Infectious Disease, Building 31, 31 Center Drive MSC 2520, Bethesda, MD 20892-2520; http://www.niaid.nih.gov.

National Heart, Lung, and Blood Institute (NHBLI), National Institutes of Health, Bldg. 31, Rm. 4A21, Bethesda, MD 20892; 301-592-8573 800-575-9355; http://www.nhlbi.nih.gov.

National Sleep Foundation, 1522 K Street NW, Suite 500, Washington, DC 20005; 202-437-3471; Fax: 202-347-3472; http://www.sleepfoundation.org.

Voice Center at Eastern Virginia Medical School, Norfolk, VA 23507; http://www.voice-center.com.

World Allergy Organization; http://www.worldallergy.org.

Management of Patients With Chest and Lower Respiratory Tract Disorders

Adapted by Carolyn J. M. Ross

LEARNING OBJECTIVES ●

On completion of this chapter, the learner will be able to:

1. Identify patients at risk for atelectasis and nursing interventions related to its prevention and management.
2. Compare the various pulmonary infections with regard to causes, clinical manifestations, nursing management, complications, and prevention.
3. Use the nursing process as a framework for care of the patient with pneumonia.
4. Relate pleurisy, pleural effusion, and empyema to pulmonary infection.
5. Describe smoking and air pollution as causes of pulmonary disease.
6. Relate the therapeutic management techniques of acute respiratory distress syndrome to the underlying pathophysiology of the syndrome.
7. Describe risk factors for and measures appropriate for prevention and management of pulmonary embolism.
8. Describe preventive measures appropriate for controlling and eliminating the problem of occupational lung disease.
9. Discuss the modes of therapy and related nursing management for patients with lung cancer.
10. Describe the complications of chest trauma and their clinical manifestations and nursing management.
11. Describe nursing measures to prevent aspiration.

*C*onditions affecting the lower respiratory tract range from acute problems to long-term chronic disorders. Many of these disorders are serious and often life-threatening. The patient with a lower respiratory tract disorder requires care from nurses with astute assessment and clinical management skills as well as an understanding of the impact of the disorder on the patient's quality of life and ability to carry out usual activities of daily living. Patient and family teaching is an important nursing intervention in the management of all lower respiratory tract disorders.

Atelectasis

Atelectasis refers to closure or collapse of alveoli and often is described in relation to x-ray findings and clinical signs and symptoms. Atelectasis may be acute or chronic and may cover a broad range of pathophysiologic changes, from microatelectasis (which is not detectable on chest x-ray) to macroatelectasis with loss of segmental, lobar, or overall lung volume. The most commonly described atelectasis is acute atelectasis, which occurs frequently in the postoperative setting or in people who are immobilized and have a shallow, monotonous breathing pattern. Excess secretions or mucus plugs may also cause obstruction of airflow and result in atelectasis in an area of the lung. Atelectasis also is observed in patients with a chronic airway obstruction that impedes or blocks air flow to an area of the lung (eg, obstructive atelectasis in the patient with lung cancer that is invading or compressing the airways). This type of atelectasis is more insidious and slower in onset.

Pathophysiology

Atelectasis may occur in the adult as a result of reduced alveolar ventilation or any type of blockage that impedes the passage of air to and from the alveoli that normally receive air through the bronchi and network of airways. The trapped alveolar air becomes absorbed into the bloodstream, but outside air cannot replace the absorbed air because of the blockage. As a result, the isolated portion of the lung becomes airless and the alveoli collapse. This may occur with altered breathing patterns, retained secretions, pain, alterations in small airway function, prolonged supine positioning, increased abdominal pressure, reduced lung volumes due to musculoskeletal or neurologic disorders, restrictive defects, and specific surgical procedures (eg, upper abdominal, thoracic, or open heart surgery). Persistent low lung volumes, secretions or a mass obstructing or impeding airflow, and compression of lung tissue may all cause collapse or obstruction of the airways, which leads to atelectasis.

The postoperative patient is at high risk for atelectasis because of the numerous respiratory changes that may occur. A monotonous low tidal breathing pattern may cause airway closure and alveolar collapse. This results from the effects of anesthesia or analgesic agents, supine positioning, splinting of the chest wall because of pain, and abdominal distention. The postoperative patient may also have secretion retention, airway obstruction, and an impaired cough reflex or may be reluctant to cough because of pain. Figure 23-1 shows the pathogenic mechanisms and consequences of acute atelectasis in the postoperative patient.

Atelectasis resulting from bronchial obstruction by secretions may occur in patients with impaired cough mechanisms (eg, postoperative, musculoskeletal or neurologic disorders) or in debilitated, bedridden patients. Atelectasis may also result from excessive pressure on the lung tissue, which restricts normal lung expansion on inspiration. Such pressure may be produced by fluid accumulating within the pleural space (**pleural effusion**), air in the pleural space (**pneumothorax**), or blood in the pleural space (**hemothorax**). The **pleural space** is the area between the parietal and the visceral pleurae. Pressure may also be produced

Glossary

acute respiratory distress syndrome (ARDS): nonspecific pulmonary response to a variety of pulmonary and non-pulmonary insults to the lung; characterized by interstitial infiltrates, alveolar hemorrhage, atelectasis, decreased compliance, and refractory hypoxemia

asbestosis: diffuse lung fibrosis resulting from exposure to asbestos fibres

atelectasis: collapse or airless condition of the alveoli caused by hypoventilation, obstruction to the airways, or compression

central cyanosis: bluish discolouration of the skin or mucous membranes due to hemoglobin carrying reduced amounts of oxygen

consolidation: lung tissue that has become more solid in nature due to collapse of alveoli or infectious process (pneumonia)

cor pulmonale: "heart of the lungs"; enlargement of the right ventricle from hypertrophy or dilation or as a secondary response to disorders that affect the lungs

empyema: accumulation of purulent material in the pleural space

fine-needle aspiration: insertion of a needle through the chest wall to obtain cells of a mass or tumour; usually performed under fluoroscopy or chest CT guidance

hemoptysis: the coughing up of blood from the lower respiratory tract

hemothorax: partial or complete collapse of the lung due to blood accumulating in the pleural space; may occur after surgery or trauma

induration: an abnormally hard lesion or reaction, as in a positive tuberculin skin test

nosocomial: pertaining to or originating from a hospitalization; not present at the time of hospital admission

open lung biopsy: biopsy of lung tissue performed through a limited thoracotomy incision

orthopnea: shortness of breath when reclining or in the supine position

pleural effusion: abnormal accumulation of fluid in the pleural space

pleural friction rub: localized grating or creaking sound caused by the rubbing together of inflamed parietal and visceral pleurae

pleural space: the area between the parietal and visceral pleurae; a potential space

pneumothorax: partial or complete collapse of the lung due to positive pressure in the pleural space

pulmonary edema: increase in the amount of extravascular fluid in the lung

pulmonary embolism: obstruction of the pulmonary vasculature with an embolus; embolus may be due to blood clot, air bubbles, or fat droplets

purulent: consisting of, containing, or discharging pus

restrictive lung disease: disease of the lung that causes a decrease in lung volumes

tension pneumothorax: pneumothorax characterized by increasing positive pressure in the pleural space with each breath; this is an emergency situation and the positive pressure needs to be decompressed or released immediately

thoracentesis: insertion of a needle into the pleural space to remove fluid that has accumulated and decrease pressure on the lung tissue; may also be used diagnostically to identify potential causes of a pleural effusion

transbronchial: through the bronchial wall, as in a transbronchial lung biopsy

ventilation–perfusion ratio: the ratio between ventilation and perfusion in the lung; matching of ventilation to perfusion optimizes gas exchange

Physiology/Pathophysiology

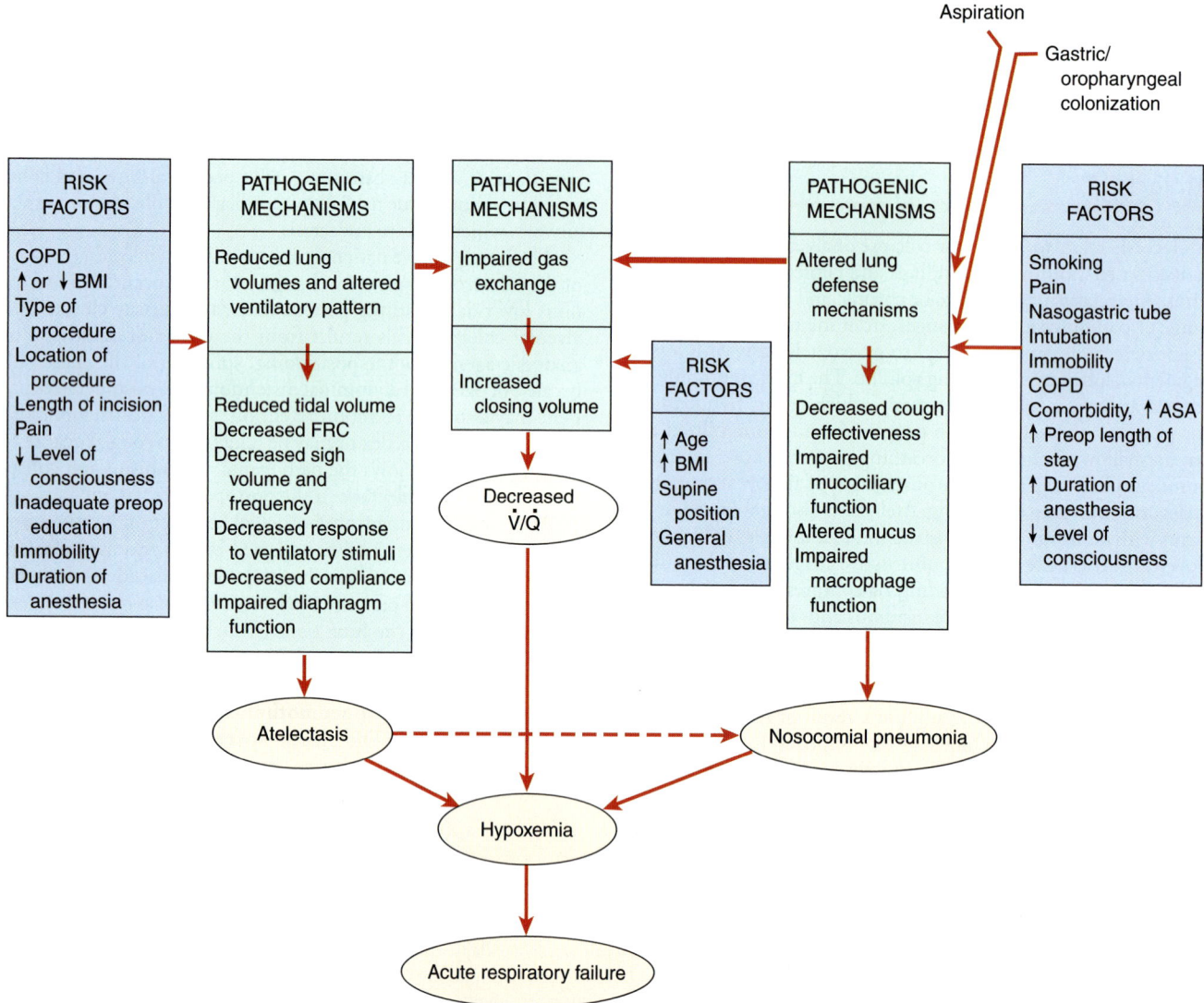

FIGURE 23-1   Relationship of risk factors, pathogenic mechanisms, and consequences of acute atelectasis in the postoperative patient. COPD, chronic obstructive pulmonary disease; BMI, body mass index; FRC, functional residual capacity; diaphragm fx, diaphragm function; ASA, American Society of Anesthesiology physical status; $\dot{V}/\dot{Q}$, ventilation-perfusion ratio. From the work of Jo Ann Brooks-Brunn, DNS, RN, FAAN, FCCP, Indiana University Medical Center, Indianapolis.

by a pericardium distended with fluid (pericardial effusion), tumour growth within the thorax, or an elevated diaphragm.

Clinical Manifestations

The development of atelectasis usually is insidious. Signs and symptoms include cough, sputum production, and low-grade fever. Fever is universally cited as a clinical sign of atelectasis, but there are few data to support this. Most likely the fever that accompanies atelectasis is due to infection or inflammation distal to the obstructed airway.

In acute atelectasis involving a large amount of lung tissue (lobar atelectasis), marked respiratory distress may be observed. In addition to the above signs and symptoms, dyspnea, tachycar-

dia, tachypnea, pleural pain, and **central cyanosis** (a bluish skin hue that is a late sign of hypoxemia) may be anticipated. The patient characteristically has difficulty breathing in the supine position and is anxious. Signs and symptoms of chronic atelectasis are similar to those of acute atelectasis. Because the alveolar collapse is chronic, infection may occur distal to the obstruction. Thus, the signs and symptoms of a pulmonary infection also may be present.

Assessment and Diagnostic Findings

Decreased breath sounds and crackles are heard over the affected area. In addition, chest x-ray findings may reveal patchy infiltrates or consolidated areas. In the patient who is confined to bed, atelectasis is usually diagnosed by chest x-ray or identified by physical assessment in the dependent, posterior, basilar areas of the lungs. Depending on the degree of hypoxemia, pulse oximetry (SpO_2) may demonstrate a low saturation of hemoglobin with oxygen (less than 90%) or a lower-than-normal partial pressure of arterial oxygen (PaO_2).

Prevention

Nursing measures to prevent atelectasis include frequent turning, early mobilization, and strategies to expand the lungs and to manage secretions. Deep-breathing manoeuvres (at least every 2 hours) assist in preventing and treating atelectasis. The performance of these manoeuvres requires a patient who is alert and cooperative. Patient education and reinforcement are key to the success of these interventions. The use of incentive spirometry or voluntary deep breathing enhances lung expansion, decreases the potential for airway closure, and may generate a cough. Secretion management techniques may include directed cough, suctioning, aerosol nebulizer treatments followed by chest physical therapy (postural drainage and chest percussion), or bronchoscopy. In some settings, a metered-dose inhaler (MDI) is used to dispense a bronchodilator rather than an aerosol nebulizer treatment. Chart 23-1 summarizes measures to prevent atelectasis.

Management

The goal in treating the patient with atelectasis is to improve ventilation and remove secretions. The strategies to prevent atelectasis, which include frequent turning, early ambulation, lung volume expansion manoeuvres (eg, deep-breathing exercises, incentive spirometry), and coughing also serve as the first-line measures to minimize or treat atelectasis by improving ventilation. In patients who do not respond to first-line measures or who cannot perform deep-breathing exercises, other treatments such as positive expiratory pressure or PEP therapy (a simple mask and one-way valve system that provides varying amounts of expiratory resistance [usually 5 to 15 cm H_2O]), continuous or intermittent positive pressure-breathing (IPPB), or bronchoscopy may be used. Although IPPB may be used in some settings, few data support its use in the postoperative setting (Duffy & Farley, 1993). Before initiating more complex, costly, and labour-intensive therapies, the nurse should ask several questions:

- Has the patient been given an adequate trial of deep-breathing exercises?

> **Chart 23-1**   **Preventing Atelectasis**

- Change patient's position frequently, especially from supine to upright position, to promote ventilation and prevent secretions from accumulating.
- Encourage early mobilization from bed to chair followed by early ambulation.
- Encourage appropriate deep breathing and coughing to mobilize secretions and prevent them from accumulating.
- Teach/reinforce appropriate technique for incentive spirometry.
- Administer prescribed opioids and sedatives judiciously to prevent respiratory depression.
- Perform postural drainage and chest percussion, if indicated.
- Institute suctioning to remove tracheobronchial secretions, if indicated.

- Has the patient received adequate education, supervision, and coaching to carry out the deep-breathing exercises?
- Have other factors been evaluated that may impair ventilation or prohibit a good patient effort (eg, lack of turning, mobilization; excessive pain; excessive sedation)?

If the cause of atelectasis is bronchial obstruction from secretions, the secretions must be removed by coughing or suctioning to permit air to re-enter that portion of the lung. Chest physical therapy (chest percussion and postural drainage) may also be used to mobilize secretions. Nebulizer treatments with a bronchodilator medication or sodium bicarbonate may be used to assist the patient in the expectoration of secretions. If respiratory care measures fail to remove the obstruction, a bronchoscopy is performed. Severe or massive atelectasis may lead to acute respiratory failure, especially in a patient with underlying lung disease. Endotracheal intubation and mechanical ventilation may be necessary. Prompt treatment reduces the risk for acute respiratory failure or pneumonia.

If atelectasis has resulted from compression of lung tissue, the goal is to decrease the compression. With a large pleural effusion that is compressing lung tissue and causing alveolar collapse, treatment may include **thoracentesis**, removal of the fluid by needle aspiration, or insertion of a chest tube. The measures to increase lung expansion described above also are used.

Management of chronic atelectasis focuses on removing the cause of the obstruction of the airways or the compression of the lung tissue. For example, bronchoscopy may be used to open an airway obstructed by lung cancer or a nonmalignant lesion, and the procedure may involve cryotherapy or laser therapy. The goal is to reopen the airways and provide ventilation to the collapsed area. In some cases, surgical management may be indicated.

Respiratory Infections

ACUTE TRACHEOBRONCHITIS

Acute tracheobronchitis, an acute inflammation of the mucous membranes of the trachea and the bronchial tree, often follows infection of the upper respiratory tract. A patient with a viral infection has decreased resistance and can readily develop a secondary bacterial infection. Thus, adequate treatment of upper respiratory tract infection is one of the major factors in the prevention of acute bronchitis. Aside from infection, inhalation of physical and chemical irritants, gases, and other air contaminants can also cause acute bronchial irritation.

Pathophysiology

In acute tracheobronchitis, the inflamed mucosa of the bronchi produces mucopurulent sputum, often in response to *Streptococcus pneumoniae, Haemophilus influenzae,* and *Mycoplasma pneumoniae.* In addition, a fungal infection (eg, *Aspergillus* tracheobronchitis) may also cause tracheobronchitis. A sputum culture is essential to identify the specific causative organism.

Clinical Manifestations

Initially, the patient has a dry, irritating cough and expectorates a scanty amount of mucoid sputum. The patient complains of sternal soreness from coughing and has fever or chills and night sweats, headache, and general malaise. As the infection progresses, the patient may be short of breath, have noisy inspiration and expiration (inspiratory stridor and expiratory wheeze), and produce **purulent** (pus-filled) sputum. With severe tracheobronchitis, blood-streaked secretions may be expectorated as a result of the irritation of the mucosa of the airways.

Medical Management

Antibiotic treatment may be indicated depending on the symptoms, sputum purulence, and results of the sputum culture. Antihistamines are usually not prescribed because they may cause excessive drying and make secretions more difficult to expectorate. Expectorants may be prescribed, although their efficacy is questionable. Fluid intake is increased to thin the viscous and tenacious secretions. Copious, purulent secretions that cannot be cleared by coughing place the patient at risk for increasing airway obstruction and the development of a more severe lower respiratory tract infection, such as pneumonia. Suctioning and bronchoscopy may be needed to remove secretions. Rarely, endotracheal intubation may be required in cases of acute tracheobronchitis leading to acute respiratory failure. This may be necessary for patients who are severely debilitated or who have coexisting diseases that also impair the respiratory system.

In most cases, treatment of tracheobronchitis is largely symptomatic. The patient is advised to rest. Increasing the vapor pressure (moisture content) in the air will reduce irritation. Cool vapor therapy or steam inhalations may help relieve laryngeal and tracheal irritation. Moist heat to the chest may relieve the soreness and pain. Mild analgesics or antipyretics may be indicated.

Nursing Management

Acute tracheobronchitis is frequently treated in the home setting. A primary nursing function is to encourage bronchial hygiene, such as increasing fluid intake and directed coughing to remove secretions. The nurse should encourage and assist the patient to sit up frequently to cough effectively and to prevent retention of mucopurulent sputum. If the patient is treated with antibiotics for an underlying infection, it is important to emphasize the need to complete the full course of antibiotics prescribed. Fatigue is a consequence of tracheobronchitis; therefore, the nurse must caution the patient against overexertion, which can induce a relapse or exacerbation of the infection.

PNEUMONIA

Pneumonia is an inflammation of the lung parenchyma that is caused by a microbial agent. "Pneumonitis" is a more general term that describes an inflammatory process in the lung tissue that may predispose a patient to or place a patient at risk for microbial invasion. Pneumonia is the leading cause of death from infection and the sixth leading cause of death overall in Canada (Health Canada, 2001). In persons 65 years of age and older, it is the fifth leading cause of death (National Center for Health Statistics, 2000; Minino & Smith, 2001). It is treated extensively on both an inpatient and outpatient basis.

Bacteria commonly enter the lower airway but do not cause pneumonia in the presence of an intact host defense mechanism. When pneumonia does occur, it is caused by various microorganisms, including bacteria, mycobacteria, chlamydiae, mycoplasma, fungi, parasites, and viruses. Several systems are used to classify pneumonias. Classically, pneumonia has been categorized into one of four categories: bacterial or typical, atypical, anaerobic/cavitary, and opportunistic. However, there is overlap in the microorganisms thought to be responsible for typical and atypical pneu-

monias. A more widely used classification scheme categorizes the major pneumonias as community-acquired pneumonia, hospital-acquired pneumonia, pneumonia in the immunocompromised host, and aspiration pneumonia (Table 23-1). There is overlap in how specific pneumonias are classified because they may occur in differing settings.

Community-acquired pneumonia (CAP) occurs either in the community setting or within the first 48 hours of hospitalization or institutionalization. The need for hospitalization for CAP depends on the severity of the pneumonia. The agents that most frequently cause CAP requiring hospitalization are *S. pneumoniae, H. influenzae, Legionella, Pseudomonas aeruginosa,* and other gram-negative rods. The specific etiologic agent of CAP is identified in about 50% of the cases. The absence of a responsible caregiver in the home may be another indication for hospitalization. In Canada it is estimated that each year community-acquired pneumonia accounts for 1 million doctor visits and 60,000 hospitalizations costing about $100 million (Helwig, 2000).

Pneumonia caused by *S. pneumoniae* (pneumococcus) is the most common CAP in people younger than 60 without comorbidity and in those older than 60 with comorbidity. It is most prevalent during the winter and spring, when upper respiratory tract infections are most frequent. *S. pneumoniae* is a gram-positive, capsulated, nonmotile coccus that resides naturally in the upper respiratory tract. The organism colonizes the upper respiratory tract and can cause the following types of illnesses: disseminated invasive infections, pneumonia and other lower respiratory tract infections, and upper respiratory tract infections, including otitis media and sinusitis (CDC, 1998). It may occur as a lobar or bronchopneumonic form in patients of any age and may follow a recent respiratory illness.

Mycoplasma pneumonia, another type of CAP, occurs most often in older children and young adults and is spread by infected respiratory droplets through person-to-person contact. Patients can be tested for mycoplasma antibodies. The inflammatory infiltrate is primarily interstitial rather than alveolar. It spreads throughout the entire respiratory tract, including the bronchioles, and has the characteristics of a bronchopneumonia. Earache and bullous myringitis are common. Impaired ventilation and diffusion may occur.

H. influenzae is another cause of CAP. It frequently affects elderly people or those with comorbid illnesses (eg, chronic obstructive pulmonary disease [COPD], alcoholism, diabetes mellitus). The presentation of this pneumonia is indistinguishable from that of other forms of bacterial CAP. The presentation may be subacute, with cough or low-grade fever for weeks before diagnosis. Chest x-rays may reveal multilobar, patchy bronchopneumonia or areas of **consolidation** (tissue that solidifies as a result of collapsed alveoli or pneumonia).

Viruses are the most common cause of pneumonia in infants and children but are relatively uncommon causes of CAP in adults. The chief causes of viral pneumonia in the immunocompetent adult are influenza viruses types A and B, adenovirus, parainfluenza virus, coronavirus, and varicella-zoster virus. In immunocompromised adults, cytomegalovirus is the most common viral pathogen, followed by herpes simplex virus, adenovirus, and respiratory syncytial virus. The acute stage of a viral respiratory infection occurs within the ciliated cells of the airways. This is followed by infiltration of the tracheobronchial tree. With pneumonia, the inflammatory process extends into the alveolar area, resulting in edema and exudation. The clinical signs and symptoms of a viral pneumonia are often difficult to distinguish from those of a bacterial pneumonia.

(text continues on page 528)

Table 23-1 • **Commonly Encountered Pneumonias**

TYPE	ORGANISM RESPONSIBLE	EPIDEMIOLOGY	CLINICAL FEATURES	TREATMENT	COMMENTS
Community-Acquired Pneumonia					
Streptococcal pneumonia (pneumococcal)	*Streptococcus pneumoniae*	Highest occurrence in winter months. Incidence greatest in the elderly and in patients with COPD, heart failure, alcoholism, asplenia, following influenza. Leading infectious cause of illness worldwide among young children, persons with underlying chronic health conditions, and the elderly. Death occurs in 14% of hospitalized adults with invasive disease.	Abrupt onset, toxic appearance, pleuritic chest pain. Usually involves one or more lobes. Lobar infiltrate common on chest x-ray or bronchopneumonia pattern. Bacteremia in 15% to 25% of all patients.	Penicillins Alternate antibiotic therapy, such as cefotaxime or ceftriaxone; antipseudomonal fluoroquinolones (levofloxacin, gatifloxacin, moxifloxacin).	Complications include shock, pleural effusion, superinfections, pericarditis, and otitis media.
Haemophilus influenzae	*Haemophilus influenzae*	Incidence greatest in alcoholics, the elderly, patients in chronic care facilities and nursing homes, patients with diabetes or COPD, and children <5 years old. Accounts for 5% to 20% of community-acquired pneumonias. Mortality rate: 30%.	Frequently insidious onset associated with upper respiratory tract infection 2 to 6 weeks before onset of illness. Fever, chills, productive cough. Usually involves one or more lobes. Bacteremia is common. Infiltrate, occasional bronchopneumonia pattern on chest x-ray.	Ampicillin, 3rd-generation cephalosporin, macrolides (azithromycin, clarithromycin), fluoroquinolones	Complications include lung abscess, pleural effusion, meningitis, arthritis, pericarditis, epiglottitis.
Legionnaires' disease	*Legionella pneumophila*	Highest occurrence in summer and fall. May cause disease sporadically or as part of an epidemic. Incidence greatest in middle-aged and older men, smokers, and patients with chronic diseases, those receiving immunosuppressive therapy, or those in close proximity to excavation sites. Accounts for 15% of community-acquired pneumonias. Mortality rate: 15% to 50%.	Flulike symptoms. High fevers, mental confusion, headache, pleuritic pain, myalgias, dyspnea, productive cough, hemoptysis, leukocytosis. Bronchopneumonia, unilateral or bilateral disease, lobar consolidation.	Erythromycin +/− rifampin (in severely compromised patient) or clarithromycin, or a macrolide (azithromycin), or a fluoroquinolone (ofloxacin, levofloxacin, sparfloxacin).	Complications include hypotension, shock, and acute renal failure.

(continued)

Table 23-1 • Commonly Encountered Pneumonias (Continued)

TYPE	ORGANISM RESPONSIBLE	EPIDEMIOLOGY	CLINICAL FEATURES	TREATMENT	COMMENTS
Mycoplasma pneumoniae	*Mycoplasma pneumoniae*	Increase in fall and winter. Responsible for epidemics of respiratory illness. Most common type of atypical pneumonia. Accounts for 20% of community-acquired pneumonias. More common in children and young adults. Mortality rate: <0.1%.	Onset is usually insidious. Patients not usually as ill as in other pneumonias. Sore throat, nasal congestion, ear pain, headache, low-grade fever, pleuritic pain, myalgias, diarrhea, erythematous rash, pharyngitis. Interstitial infiltrates on chest x-ray.	Erythromycin; macrolide, fluoroquinolone or tetracycline.	Complications include aseptic meningitis, meningo-encephalitis, transverse myelitis, cranial nerve palsies, pericarditis, myocarditis.
Viral pneumonia	Influenza viruses types A, B adenovirus, parainfluenza, cytomegalovirus, coronavirus	Incidence greatest in winter months. Epidemics occur every 2 to 3 years. Most common causative organisms in adults. Other organisms in children (eg, cytomegalovirus and respiratory syncytial virus). Accounts for 20% of community-acquired pneumonias.	Patchy infiltrate, small pleural effusion on chest x-ray. In majority of patients, influenza begins as an acute upper respiratory infection; others have bronchitis, pleurisy, etc., and still others develop gastrointestinal symptoms.	Amantadine; rimantadine; oseltamivir phosphate, ribavirin aerosol. Treated symptomatically. Does not respond to treatment with currently available antimicrobials.	Complications include a superimposed bacterial infection, bronchopneumonia.
Chlamydial pneumonia (TWAR agent)	*C. pneumoniae*	Reported mainly in college students, military recruits, and the elderly. May be a common cause of community-acquired pneumonia or observed in combination with other pathogens. Mortality rate is low as the majority of cases are relatively mild. The elderly with coexistent infections, comorbidities, and reinfections may require hospitalization.	Hoarseness, fever, chills, pharyngitis, rhinitis, nonproductive cough, myalgias, arthralgias. Single infiltrate on chest x-ray; pleural effusion possible.	Tetracycline, erythromycin, macrolide, quinolone.	Complications include reinfection and acute respiratory failure.

(continued)

Table 23-1 • Commonly Encountered Pneumonias (Continued)

TYPE	ORGANISM RESPONSIBLE	EPIDEMIOLOGY	CLINICAL FEATURES	TREATMENT	COMMENTS
Hospital-Acquired Pneumonia					
Pseudomonas pneumonia	*Pseudomonas aeruginosa*	Incidence greatest in those with pre-existing lung disease, cancer (particularly leukemia); those with homograft transplants, burns; debilitated persons; and patients receiving antimicrobial therapy and treatments such as tracheostomy, suctioning, and in postoperative settings. Almost always of nosocomial origin. Accounts for 15% of hospital-acquired pneumonias. Mortality rate: 40% to 60%.	Diffuse consolidation on chest x-ray. Toxic appearance: fever, chills, productive cough, relative bradycardia, leukocytosis.	Aminoglycoside and anti-pseudomonal agents (ticarcillin, piperacillin, mezlocillin, ceftazidine).	Complications include lung cavitation. Has capacity to invade blood vessels, causing hemorrhage and lung infarction. Usually requires hospitalization.
Staphylococcal pneumonia	*Staphylococcus aureus*	Incidence greatest in immunocompromised patients, IV drug users, and as a complication of epidemic influenza. Commonly nosocomial in origin. Accounts for 10% to 30% of hospital-acquired pneumonias. Mortality rate: 25% to 60%.	Severe hypoxemia, cyanosis, necrotizing infection. Bacteremia is common.	Nafcillin/oxacillin +/− rifampin or gentamicin; methicillin-resistant: vancomycin +/− rifampin or gentamicin.	Complications include pleural effusion/pneumothorax, lung abscess, empyema, meningitis, endocarditis. Frequently requires hospitalization. Treatment must be vigourous and prolonged because disease tends to destroy lung tissue.
Klebsiella pneumonia	*Klebsiella pneumoniae* (Friedlander's bacillus-encapsulated gram-negative aerobic bacillus)	Incidence greatest in the elderly; alcoholics; patients with chronic disease, such as diabetes, heart failure, COPD; patients in chronic care facilities and nursing homes. Accounts for 2% to 5% of community-acquired and 10% to 30% of hospital-acquired pneumonias. Mortality rate: 40% to 50%.	Tissue necrosis occurs rapidly. Toxic appearance: fever, cough, sputum production, bronchopneumonia, lung abscess. Lobar consolidation, bronchopneumonia pattern on chest x-ray.	Third-generation cephalosporins (cefotaxime, ceftriaxone) plus aminoglycoside, antipseudomonal penicillin, monobactam (aztreonam), or quinolone.	Complications include multiple lung abscesses with cyst formation, empyema, pericarditis, pleural effusion. May be fulminating, progressing to fatal outcome.

(continued)

Table 23-1 • **Commonly Encountered Pneumonias** (Continued)

TYPE	ORGANISM RESPONSIBLE	EPIDEMIOLOGY	CLINICAL FEATURES	TREATMENT	COMMENTS
Pneumonia in Immunocompromised Host					
Pneumocystis carinii pneumonia (PCP)	*Pneumocystis carinii*	Incidence greatest in patients with AIDS and patients receiving immunosuppressive therapy for cancer, organ transplants, and other disorders. Frequently seen with cytomegalovirus infection. Mortality rate 15% to 20% in hospitalized and fatal if not treated.	Pulmonary infiltrates on chest x-ray. Nonproductive cough, fever, dyspnea.	Trimethoprim/sulfamethoxazole (TMP-SMZ), dapsone-trimethoprim, pentamidine, primequine plus clindamycin.	Complications include respiratory failure.
Fungal pneumonia	*Aspergillus fumigatus*	Incidence greatest in immunocompromised and neutropenic patients. Mortality rate: 15% to 20%.	Cough, hemoptysis, infiltrates, fungus ball on chest x-ray.	Flucytosine with amphotericin B in non-neutropenic patients, amphotericin B, itraconazole, ketoconazole. Lobectomy for fungus ball.	Complications include dissemination to brain, myocardium, and/or thyroid gland.
Tuberculosis	*Mycobacterium tuberculosis*	Incidence increased in indigent, immigrant, and prison populations, people with AIDS, and the homeless. Mortality rate <1% (depending on comorbidity)	Weight loss, fever, night sweats, cough, sputum production, hemoptysis, nonspecific infiltrate (lower lobe), hilar node enlargement, pleural effusion on chest x-ray.	Rifampin, streptomycin, ethambutol, INH (isoniazid), pyrazinamide	Complications include reinfection and acute respiratory infection.

+/− = may add depending upon situation

Hospital-acquired pneumonia (HAP), also known as **nosocomial** pneumonia, is defined as the onset of pneumonia symptoms more than 48 hours after admission to the hospital. HAP accounts for approximately 15% of hospital-acquired infections but is the most lethal nosocomial infection. It is estimated to occur in 0.5% to 1% of all hospitalized patients and in 15% to 20% of intensive care patients. Ventilator-associated pneumonia can be considered a type of nosocomial pneumonia that is associated with endotracheal intubation and mechanical ventilation.

The common organisms responsible for HAP include the pathogens *Enterobacter* species, *Escherichia coli, Klebsiella* species, *Proteus, Serratia marcescens, P. aeruginosa,* and methicillin-sensitive or methicillin-resistant *Staphylococcus aureus.* These respiratory infections occur when at least one of three conditions exists: host defenses are impaired, an inoculum of organisms reaches the patient's lower respiratory tract and overwhelms the host's defenses, or a highly virulent organism is present. Certain illnesses may predispose a patient to HAP because of impaired host defenses. Examples include severe acute or chronic illness, a variety of comorbid conditions, coma, malnutrition, prolonged hospitalization, hypotension, and metabolic disorders. The hospitalized patient is also exposed to potential bacteria from other sources (eg, respiratory therapy devices and equipment, transmission of pathogens by the hands of health care personnel). Numerous intervention-related factors also may play a role in the development of HAP (eg, therapeutic agents leading to central nervous system depression with decreased ventilation, impaired removal of secretions, or potential aspiration; prolonged or complicated thoracoabdominal procedures, which may impair mucociliary function and cellular host defenses; endotracheal intubation; prolonged or inappropriate use of antibiotics; use of nasogastric tubes). In addition, immunocompromised patients are at particular risk. HAP is associated with a high mortality rate, in part because of the virulence of the organisms, their resistance to antibiotics, and the patient's underlying disorder.

Dominant pathogens for HAP are gram-negative bacilli (*P. aeruginosa* and *Enterobacteriaceae/Klebsiella* species, *Enterobacter, Proteus, Serratia*) and *S. aureus.* Pseudomonal pneumonia occurs in patients who are debilitated, those with altered mental status, and those with prolonged intubation or with tracheostomies. Staphylococcal pneumonia can occur through inhalation of the organism or spread through the hematogenous route. It is often accompanied by bacteremia and positive blood cultures. Although responsible for less than 10% of cases of CAP, staphylococcal pneumonia may be responsible for more than 30% of cases of HAP. Its mortality rate is high. Specific strains of staphylococci are resistant to all available antimicrobials except vancomycin. These strains of *S. aureus* are referred to as methicillin-resistant *S. aureus* (MRSA). Overuse and misuse of antimicrobial agents are major risk factors for the emergence of these resistant pathogens. Because MRSA is highly virulent, steps must be taken to prevent the spread of this organism. The patient with MRSA should be isolated in a private room, and contact precautions (gown, mask, glove, and antibacterial soap) are used. The number of people in contact with the patient should be minimized, and appropriate precautions must be taken when transporting the patient within or between facilities.

The usual presentation of an HAP is a new pulmonary infiltrate on chest x-ray combined with evidence of infection such as fever, respiratory symptoms, purulent sputum, and/or leukocytosis. Pneumonias from *Klebsiella* or other gram-negative organisms (*E. coli, Proteus, Serratia*) are characterized by destruction of lung structure and alveolar walls, consolidation, and bacteremia. Elderly patients and those with alcoholism, chronic lung disease, or diabetes are at particular risk. A sudden onset of cough is a common presentation, and blood-tinged sputum may be present. In the debilitated or dehydrated patient, sputum production may be minimal or absent. Pleural effusions, high fevers, and tachycardia are often observed. Even with treatment, the mortality rate remains high.

Pneumonia in the immunocompromised host is seen with greater frequency because immunocompromised hosts represent a growing portion of the patient population. Examples of pneumonia in the immunocompromised host are *Pneumocystis carinii* pneumonia (PCP), fungal pneumonias, and mycobacterium tuberculosis. These types of pneumonia may also occur in the immunocompetent person and in different settings, but these are less common. Immunocompromised states occur with the use of corticosteroids or other immunosuppressive agents, chemotherapy, nutritional depletion, use of broad-spectrum antimicrobial agents, AIDS, genetic immune disorders, and long-term advanced life-support technology (mechanical ventilation). Patients with compromised immune systems commonly acquire pneumonia from organisms of low virulence. In addition, increasing numbers of patients with impaired defenses develop HAP from gram-negative bacilli (*Klebsiella, Pseudomonas, E. coli, Enterobacteriaceae, Proteus, Serratia*).

Pneumonia in the compromised host may be caused by the organisms also observed in CAP or HAP (*S. pneumoniae, S. aureus, H. influenzae, P. aeruginosa, M. tuberculosis*). PCP is rarely observed in the immunocompetent host and is often an initial AIDS-defining complication. Whether the patient is immunocompromised or immunocompetent, the clinical presentation of pneumonia is similar. PCP has a subtle onset with progressive dyspnea, fever, and a nonproductive cough.

Aspiration pneumonia refers to the pulmonary consequences resulting from the entry of endogenous or exogenous substances into the lower airway. The most common form of aspiration pneumonia is bacterial infection from aspiration of bacteria that normally reside in the upper airways. Aspiration pneumonia may occur in the community or hospital setting; common pathogens are *S. pneumoniae, H. influenzae*, and *S. aureus*. Other substances may be aspirated into the lung, such as gastric contents, exogenous chemical contents, or irritating gases. This type of aspiration or ingestion may impair the lung defenses, cause inflammatory changes, and lead to bacterial growth and a resulting pneumonia. (Aspiration is described in more detail at the end of this chapter.)

Pathophysiology

Upper airway characteristics normally prevent potentially infectious particles from reaching the normally sterile lower respiratory tract. Thus, patients with pneumonia caused by infectious agents often have an acute or chronic underlying disease that impairs host defenses. Pneumonia arises from normally present flora in a patient whose resistance has been altered, or it results from aspiration of flora present in the oropharynx. It may also result from bloodborne organisms that enter the pulmonary circulation and are trapped in the pulmonary capillary bed, becoming a potential source of pneumonia.

Pneumonia often affects both ventilation and diffusion. An inflammatory reaction can occur in the alveoli, producing an exudate that interferes with the diffusion of oxygen and carbon dioxide. White blood cells, mostly neutrophils, also migrate into the alveoli and fill the normally air-containing spaces. Areas of the lung are not adequately ventilated because of secretions and mucosal edema that cause partial occlusion of the bronchi or alveoli, with a resultant decrease in alveolar oxygen tension. Bronchospasm may also occur in patients with reactive airway disease. Because of hypoventilation, a ventilation–perfusion mismatch occurs in the affected area of the lung. Venous blood entering the pulmonary circulation passes through the underventilated area and exits to the left side of the heart poorly oxygenated. The mixing of oxygenated and unoxygenated or poorly oxygenated blood eventually results in arterial hypoxemia.

If a substantial portion of one or more lobes is involved, the disease is referred to as "lobar pneumonia." The term "bronchopneumonia" is used to describe pneumonia that is distributed in a patchy fashion, having originated in one or more localized areas within the bronchi and extending to the adjacent surrounding lung parenchyma. Bronchopneumonia is more common than lobar pneumonia (Fig. 23-2).

Risk Factors

Being knowledgeable about the factors and circumstances that commonly predispose a person to pneumonia will aid in identifying patients at high risk for this disorder (Chart 23-2).

Physiology/Pathophysiology

Bronchopneumonia   Lobar pneumonia

FIGURE 23-2 Distribution of lung involvement in bronchial and lobar pneumonia. In bronchopneumonia (*left*), patchy areas of consolidation occur. In lobar pneumonia (*right*), an entire lobe is consolidated.

Chart 23-2
Risk Factors for Pneumonia

Risk Factor	Preventive Measure
Conditions that produce mucus or bronchial obstruction and interfere with normal lung drainage (eg, cancer, cigarette smoking, COPD)	Promote coughing and expectoration of secretions. Encourage smoking cessation.
Immunosuppressed patients and those with a low neutrophil count (neutropenic)	Initiate special precautions against infection.
Smoking; cigarette smoke disrupts both mucociliary and macrophage activity	Encourage smoking cessation.
Prolonged immobility and shallow breathing pattern	Reposition frequently and promote lung expansion exercises and coughing. Initiate suctioning and chest physical therapy if indicated.
Depressed cough reflex (due to medications, a debilitated state, or weak respiratory muscles); aspiration of foreign material into the lungs during a period of unconsciousness (head injury, anesthesia, depressed level of consciousness), or abnormal swallowing mechanism	Reposition frequently to prevent aspiration and administer medications judiciously, particularly those that increase risk for aspiration. Perform suctioning and chest physical therapy if indicated.
Nothing-by-mouth (NPO) status; placement of nasogastric, orogastric, or endotracheal tube	Promote frequent oral hygiene. Minimize risk for aspiration by checking placement of tube and proper positioning of patient.
Antibiotic therapy (in very ill people, the oropharynx is likely to be colonized by gram-negative bacteria)	
Alcohol intoxication (because alcohol suppresses the body's reflexes, may be associated with aspiration, and decreases white cell mobilization and tracheobronchial ciliary motion)	Encourage reduced or moderate alcohol intake (in case of alcohol stupor, position patient to prevent aspiration).
General anesthetic, sedative, or opioid preparations that promote respiratory depression, which causes a shallow breathing pattern and predisposes to the pooling of bronchial secretions and potential development of pneumonia	Observe the respiratory rate and depth during recovery from general anesthesia and before giving medications. If respiratory depression is apparent, withhold the medication and contact the physician.
Advanced age, because of possible depressed cough and glottic reflexes and nutritional depletion	Promote frequent turning, early ambulation and mobilization, effective coughing, breathing exercises, and nutritious diet.
Respiratory therapy with improperly cleaned equipment	Make sure that respiratory equipment is cleaned properly; participate in continuous quality improvement monitoring with the respiratory care department.

Increasing numbers of patients who have compromised defenses against infections are susceptible to pneumonia. Some types of pneumonia, such as those caused by viral infections, occur in previously healthy people and often follow a viral illness.

Pneumonia is common with certain underlying disorders such as heart failure, diabetes, alcoholism, COPD, and AIDS. Certain diseases also have been associated with specific pathogens. For example, staphylococcal pneumonia has been noted after epidemics of influenza, and patients with COPD are at increased risk for developing pneumonia caused by pneumococci or *H. influenzae*. In addition, cystic fibrosis is associated with respiratory infection caused by pseudomonal and staphylococcal organisms, and PCP has been associated with AIDS. Pneumonias occurring in hospitalized patients often involve organisms not usually found in CAP, including enteric gram-negative bacilli and *S. aureus*.

The CDC has identified three specific strategies for preventing HAP: (1) staff education and infection surveillance, (2) interruption of transmission of microorganisms through person-to-person transmission and equipment transmission, and (3) modification of host risk of infection (CDC, 1997). Providing anticipatory and preventive care is an important nursing measure.

To reduce or prevent serious complications of CAP in high-risk groups, vaccination against pneumococcal infection is advised for the following:

- People 65 years of age or older
- Immunocompetent people who are at increased risk for illness and death associated with pneumococcal disease because of chronic illness (eg, cardiovascular, pulmonary, diabetes mellitus, chronic liver disease)
- People with functional or anatomic asplenia
- People living in environments or social settings in which the risk of disease is high
- Immunocompromised people at high risk for infection (CDC, 1998)

The vaccine provides specific prevention against pneumococcal pneumonia and other infections caused by this organism (otitis media, other upper respiratory tract infections). Vaccines should be avoided in the first trimester of pregnancy.

Clinical Manifestations

Pneumonia varies in its signs and symptoms depending on the organism and the patient's underlying disease. However, regardless of the type of pneumonia (CAP, HAP, immunocompromised host, aspiration), a specific type of pneumonia cannot be diagnosed by clinical manifestations alone. For example, the patient with streptococcal (pneumococcal) pneumonia usually has a sudden onset of shaking chills, rapidly rising fever (38.5° to 40.5°C), and pleuritic chest pain that is aggravated by deep breathing and coughing. The patient is severely ill, with marked tachypnea (25 to 45 breaths/min), accompanied by other signs of respiratory distress (eg, shortness of breath, use of accessory muscles in respiration). The pulse is rapid and bounding, and it usually increases about 10 beats/min for every degree of temperature (Celsius) elevation. A relative bradycardia for the amount of fever may suggest viral infection, mycoplasma infection, or infection with a *Legionella* organism.

Some patients exhibit an upper respiratory tract infection (nasal congestion, sore throat), and the onset of symptoms of pneumonia is gradual and nonspecific. The predominant symptoms may be headache, low-grade fever, pleuritic pain, myalgia, rash, and pharyngitis. After a few days, mucoid or mucopurulent sputum is expectorated. In severe pneumonia, the cheeks are flushed and the lips and nailbeds demonstrate central cyanosis (a late sign of poor oxygenation [hypoxemia]).

Typically, the patient has **orthopnea** (shortness of breath when reclining); he or she prefers to be propped up in bed leaning forward (orthopneic position), trying to achieve adequate gas exchange without coughing or breathing deeply. Appetite is poor, and the patient is diaphoretic and tires easily. Sputum is often purulent; this is not a reliable indicator of the etiologic agent. Rusty, blood-tinged sputum may be expectorated with streptococcal (pneumococcal), staphylococcal, and *Klebsiella* pneumonia.

Signs and symptoms of pneumonia may also depend on underlying conditions. Differing signs occur in patients with other conditions, such as cancer, or in those who are undergoing treatment with immunosuppressants, which lower the resistance to infection. Such patients have fever, crackles, and physical findings that indicate consolidation of lung tissue, including increased tactile fremitus (vocal vibration detected on palpation), percussion dullness, bronchial breath sounds, egophony (when auscultated, the spoken "E" becomes a loud, nasal-sounding "A"), and whispered pectoriloquy (whispered sounds are easily auscultated through the chest wall). These changes occur because sound is transmitted better through solid or dense tissue (consolidation) than through normal air-filled tissue; these sounds are described in Chapter 21.

Purulent sputum or slight changes in respiratory symptoms may be the only sign of pneumonia in patients with COPD. It may be difficult to determine whether an increase in symptoms is an exacerbation of the underlying disease process or an additional infectious process.

Assessment and Diagnostic Findings

The diagnosis of pneumonia is made by history (particularly of a recent respiratory tract infection), physical examination, chest x-ray studies, blood culture (bloodstream invasion, called bacteremia, occurs frequently), and sputum examination. The sputum sample is obtained by having the patient: (1) rinse the mouth with water to minimize contamination by normal oral flora, (2) breathe deeply several times, (3) cough deeply, and (4) expectorate the raised sputum into a sterile container.

More invasive procedures may be used to collect specimens. Sputum may be obtained by nasotracheal or orotracheal suctioning with a sputum trap or by fibreoptic bronchoscopy (see Chap. 21). Bronchoscopy is often used in patients with acute severe infection, patients with chronic or refractory infection, or immunocompromised patients when a diagnosis cannot be made from an expectorated or induced specimen.

Medical Management

The treatment of pneumonia includes administration of the appropriate antibiotic as determined by the results of the Gram stain. However, an etiologic agent is not identified in 50% of CAP cases and empiric therapy must be initiated. Therapy for CAP is continuing to evolve. Guidelines exist to guide antibiotic choice; however, the resistance patterns, prevalence of etiologic agents, patient risk factors, and costs and availability of newer antibiotic agents must all be taken into consideration.

Several guidelines for the medical management of CAP have been published (American Thoracic Society, 2001; Bartlett et al., 2000; Blondel-Hill & Fryters, 2001; Canadian Infectious Disease Society [CIDS] & Canadian Thoracic Society [CTS], 2000). Recommendations are classified by existing risk factors, setting (inpatient vs. outpatient treatment), or specific pathogens. Examples of risk factors that may increase the risk of infection with certain types of pathogens appear in Chart 23-3.

Recommendations for treatment of outpatients with CAP who have no cardiopulmonary disease or other modifying factors include a macrolide (erythromycin, azithromycin [Zithromax], or clarithromycin [Biaxin]), doxycycline (Vibramycin), or a fluoroquinolone (eg, gatifloxacin [Tequin], levofloxacin [Levaquin]) with enhanced activity against *S. pneumoniae* (Bartlett et al., 2000; American Thoracic Society, 2001). Erythromycin should be avoided in areas where *H. influenzae* and *S. aureus* are more prevalent (Kenreigh & Wagner, 2000; Lynch, 2000). For those outpatients who have cardiopulmonary disease or other modifying factors, treatment should include a beta-lactam (oral cefpodoxime [Vantin], cefuroxime [Zinacef, Ceftin], high-dose amoxicillin or amoxicillin/clavulanate [Augmentin, Clavulin]) plus a macrolide or doxycycline. Also, a beta-lactam plus an antipneumococcal fluoroquinolone can be used (American Thoracic Society, 2001; CIDS & CTS, 2000). These are guidelines; treatment for individual patients may be modified.

For patients with CAP who are hospitalized and do not have cardiopulmonary disease or modifying factors, management consists of intravenous azithromycin (Zithromax) or monotherapy with an antipneumococcal fluoroquinolone. For inpatients with cardiopulmonary disease or modifying factors, the treatment involves an intravenous beta-lactam plus an intravenous or oral macrolide or doxycycline. An intravenous antipneumococcal fluoroquinolone may also be used alone (American Thoracic Society, 2001; CIDS & CTS, 2000). For acutely ill patients admitted to the intensive care unit, management includes an intravenous

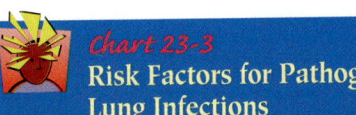

Chart 23-3

Risk Factors for Pathogenic Lung Infections

Risk Factors for Infection with Penicillin-Resistant and Drug-Resistant Pneumococci
- Age over 65 years
- Alcoholism
- Beta-lactam therapy (eg, cephalosporins) in past 3 months
- Immunosuppressive disorders
- Multiple medical comorbidities
- Exposure to a child in a day care facility

Risk Factors for Infection with Enteric Gram-Negative Bacteria
- Nursing home residency
- Underlying cardiopulmonary disease
- Multiple medical comorbidities
- Recent antibiotic therapy

Risk Factors for Infection with *Pseudomonas aeruginosa*
- Structural lung disease (eg, bronchiectasis)
- Corticosteroid therapy
- Broad-spectrum antibiotic therapy (more than 7 days in the past month)
- Malnutrition

(American Thoracic Society, 2001)

beta-lactam plus either an intravenous macrolide or fluoroquinolone. For patients at high risk for *P. aeruginosa,* more select antipseudomonal antibiotics are administered intravenously.

If specific pathogens have been identified for the CAP, more specific agents may be utilized. Mycoplasma pneumonia is treated with doxycycline or a macrolide. PCP responds best to pentamidine and trimethoprim–sulfamethoxazole (TMP-SMZ). Amantadine and rimantadine are effective with influenza A and have been shown to reduce the duration of fever and other systemic complications when administered within 24 to 48 hours of the onset of an uncomplicated influenza infection. These medications also reduce the duration and quantity of virus shedding in the respiratory secretions. They are most effective when used in combination with influenza vaccine. Ganciclovir is used to treat cytomegalovirus in the non-AIDS patient; cytomegalovirus immunoglobulin may also be used.

HAP has a different etiology from CAP. In suspected HAP or nosocomial pneumonia, empirical treatment is usually initiated with a broad-spectrum intravenous antibiotic and may be monotherapy or combination therapy. In patients who are mildly to moderately ill with a low risk of *Pseudomonas,* the following antibiotics may be used: second-generation cephalosporins (eg, cefuroxime [Ceftin, Zinacef] or cefamandole [Mandol]), nonpseudomonal third-generation cephalosporins (ceftriaxone [Rocephin], cefotaxime [Claforan], ampicillin-sulbactam [Unasyn]), or fluoroquinolones (eg, ciprofloxacin [Cipro], levofloxacin [Levaquin]). For combination therapy, any of the above may be used with an aminoglycoside.

For patients at high risk for *Pseudomonas* infection, an antipseudomonal penicillin plus an aminoglycoside (amikacin [Amikin], gentamicin) or beta-lactamase inhibitor (ampicillin/sulbactam [Unasyn], ticarcillin/clavulanate [Timentin]) may be used. Other types of combination therapy may also be used depending upon the individual characteristics of the patient.

Of concern is the rampant rise in respiratory pathogens that are resistant to available antibiotics. Examples include vancomycin-resistant enterococcus (VRE) and drug-resistant *S. pneumoniae* (McGeer & Low, 2000). There is a tendency for clinicians to aggressively use antibiotics inappropriately or to use broad-spectrum agents when narrow-spectrum agents are more appropriate. Mechanisms to monitor and minimize the inappropriate use of antibiotics are in place. Education of clinicians to use evidence-based guidelines in the treatment of respiratory infection is important. Monitoring and surveillance of susceptibility patterns for pathogens are also important.

Therapy with parenteral agents usually is changed to oral antimicrobial agents when there is evidence of a clinical response and the patient is able to tolerate oral medications. The recommended duration of treatment for pneumococcal pneumonia is 72 hours after the patient becomes afebrile. Most other forms of pneumonia caused by bacterial pathogens are treated for 1 to 2 weeks after the patient becomes afebrile. Atypical pneumonia is usually treated for 10 to 21 days (Bartlett, Dowell, Mandell et al., 2000).

Treatment of viral pneumonia is primarily supportive. Antibiotics are ineffective in viral upper respiratory infections and pneumonia and may be associated with adverse effects. Treatment of viral infections with antibiotics is a major reason for the overuse of these medications in Canada. Antibiotics are indicated with a viral respiratory infection *only* when a secondary bacterial pneumonia, bronchitis, or sinusitis is present. Hydration is a necessary part of therapy because fever and tachypnea may result in insensible fluid losses. Antipyretics may be used to treat headache and fever; antitussive medications may be used for the associated cough. Warm, moist inhalations are helpful in relieving bronchial

irritation. Antihistamines may provide benefit with reduced sneezing and rhinorrhea. Nasal decongestants may also be used to treat symptoms and improve sleep; however, excessive use may cause rebound nasal congestion. Treatment of viral pneumonia (with the exception of antimicrobial therapy) is the same as that for bacterial pneumonia. The patient is placed on bed rest until the infection shows signs of clearing. If hospitalized, the patient is observed carefully until the clinical condition improves.

If hypoxemia develops, oxygen is administered. Pulse oximetry or arterial blood gas analysis is performed to determine the need for oxygen and to evaluate the effectiveness of the therapy. A high concentration of oxygen is contraindicated in patients with COPD because it may worsen alveolar ventilation by decreasing the patient's ventilatory drive, leading to further respiratory decompensation. Respiratory support measures include high oxygen concentrations (fraction of inspired oxygen [FiO_2]), endotracheal intubation, and mechanical ventilation. Different modes of mechanical ventilation may be required; see Chapter 25.

Figure 23-3 provides an algorithm for patients with suspected CAP.

 ### Gerontologic Considerations

Pneumonia in the elderly patient may occur as a primary problem or as a complication of a chronic disease process. Pulmonary infections in the elderly frequently are difficult to treat and have a higher mortality rate than in younger patients. General deterioration, weakness, abdominal symptoms, anorexia, confusion, tachycardia, and tachypnea may signal the onset of pneumonia. The diagnosis of pneumonia may be missed because the classic symptoms of cough, chest pain, sputum production, and fever may be absent or masked in the elderly patient. Also, the presence of some signs may be misleading. Abnormal breath sounds, for example, may be due to microatelectasis that occurs in the aged as a result of decreased mobility, decreased lung volumes, and other respiratory function changes. Because chronic heart failure is often seen in the elderly, chest x-rays may be obtained to assist in differentiating it from pneumonia as the cause of clinical signs and symptoms.

Supportive treatment includes hydration (with caution and frequent assessment because of the risk of fluid overload in the elderly), supplemental oxygen therapy, assistance with deep breathing, coughing, frequent position changes, and early ambulation. All of these are particularly important in the care of the elderly patient with pneumonia. To reduce or prevent serious complications of pneumonia in the elderly, vaccination against pneumococcal and influenza infections is recommended.

Complications

SHOCK AND RESPIRATORY FAILURE

Severe complications of pneumonia include hypotension and shock and respiratory failure (especially with gram-negative bacterial disease in elderly patients). These complications are encountered chiefly in patients who have received no specific treatment or inadequate or delayed treatment. These complications are also encountered when the infecting organism is resistant to therapy and when a comorbid disease complicates the pneumonia.

If the patient is seriously ill, aggressive therapy may include hemodynamic and ventilatory support to combat peripheral collapse, maintain arterial blood pressure, and provide adequate oxygenation. A vasopressor agent may be administered intravenously by continuous infusion and at a rate adjusted in accordance with

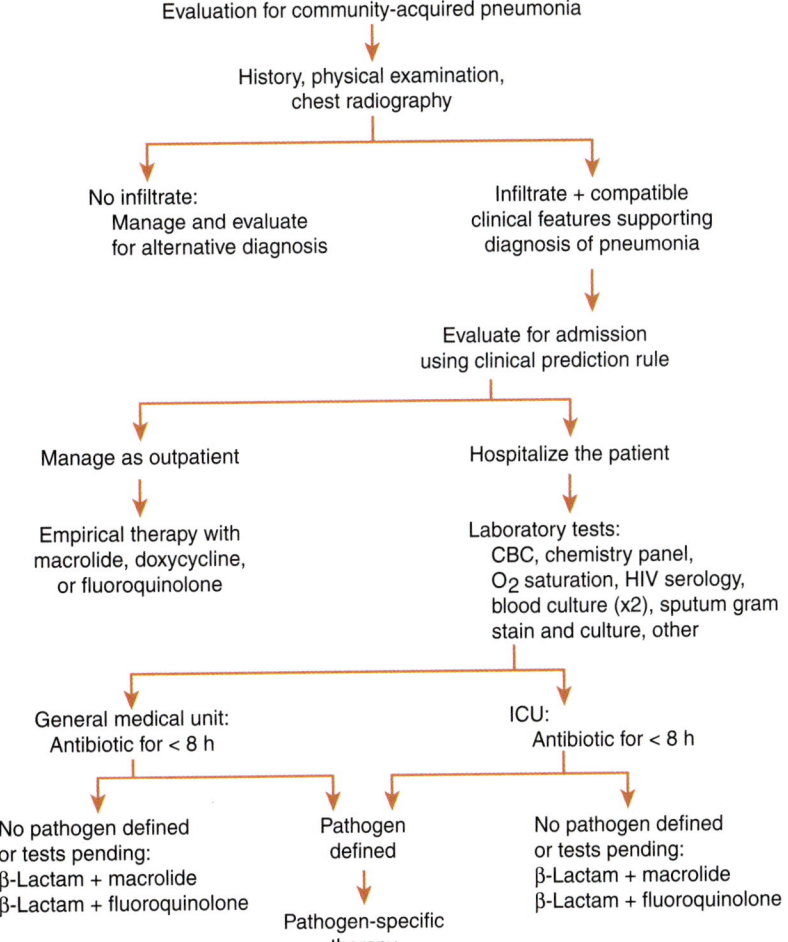

Evaluation for community-acquired pneumonia

History, physical examination, chest radiography

No infiltrate: Manage and evaluate for alternative diagnosis

Infiltrate + compatible clinical features supporting diagnosis of pneumonia

Evaluate for admission using clinical prediction rule

Manage as outpatient

Hospitalize the patient

Empirical therapy with macrolide, doxycycline, or fluoroquinolone

Laboratory tests: CBC, chemistry panel, O_2 saturation, HIV serology, blood culture (x2), sputum gram stain and culture, other

General medical unit: Antibiotic for < 8 h

ICU: Antibiotic for < 8 h

No pathogen defined or tests pending: β-Lactam + macrolide β-Lactam + fluoroquinolone

Pathogen defined

No pathogen defined or tests pending: β-Lactam + macrolide β-Lactam + fluoroquinolone

Pathogen-specific therapy

FIGURE 23-3 Treatment algorithm for patient with suspected CAP. From Bartlett, J. G. et al. (2000). Practice guidelines for the management of community-acquired pneumonia in adults. *Clinical Infectious Diseases, 31* (2), 347–382.

the pressure response. Corticosteroids may be administered parenterally to combat shock and toxicity in patients who are extremely ill with pneumonia and in apparent danger of dying of the infection. Patients may require endotracheal intubation and mechanical ventilation. Congestive heart failure, cardiac dysrhythmias, pericarditis, and myocarditis also are complications of pneumonia that may lead to shock.

ATELECTASIS AND PLEURAL EFFUSION

Atelectasis (from obstruction of a bronchus by accumulated secretions) may occur at any stage of acute pneumonia. Parapneumonic pleural effusions occur in at least 40% of bacterial pneumonias. A parapneumonic effusion is any pleural effusion associated with bacterial pneumonia, lung abscess, or bronchiectasis. After the pleural effusion is detected on a chest x-ray, a thoracentesis may be performed to remove the fluid. The fluid is sent to the laboratory for analysis. There are three stages of parapneumonic pleural effusions based on pathogenesis: uncomplicated, complicated, and thoracic empyema. An **empyema** occurs when thick, purulent fluid accumulates within the pleural space, often with fibrin development and a loculated (walled-off) area where the infection is located. (Empyema is discussed in greater detail in the section Pleural Conditions, below.) A chest tube may be inserted to treat pleural infection by establishing proper drainage of the empyema. Sterilization of the empyema cavity requires 4 to 6 weeks of antibiotics. Sometimes surgical management is required.

SUPERINFECTION

Superinfection may occur with the administration of very large doses of antibiotics, such as penicillin, or with combinations of antibiotics. Superinfection may also occur in the patient who has been receiving numerous courses and types of antibiotics. In such cases, bacteria may become resistant to the antibiotic therapy. If the patient improves and the fever diminishes after initial antibiotic therapy, but subsequently there is a rise in temperature with increasing cough and evidence that the pneumonia has spread, a superinfection is likely. Antibiotics are changed appropriately or discontinued entirely in some cases.

NURSING PROCESS: THE PATIENT WITH PNEUMONIA

Assessment

Nursing assessment is critical in detecting pneumonia. A fever, chills, or night sweats in a patient who also has respiratory symptoms should alert the nurse to the possibility of bacterial pneumonia. A respiratory assessment will further identify the clinical manifestations of pneumonia: pleuritic-type pain, fatigue, tachypnea, use of accessory muscles for breathing, bradycardia or relative bradycardia, coughing, and purulent sputum. It is important to identify the severity, location, and cause of the chest pain, along with any medications or procedures that provide relief. The nurse should monitor the following:

- Changes in temperature and pulse
- Amount, odour, and colour of secretions
- Frequency and severity of cough
- Degree of tachypnea or shortness of breath
- Changes in physical assessment findings (primarily assessed by inspecting and auscultating the chest)
- Changes in the chest x-ray findings

In addition, it is important to assess the elderly patient for unusual behaviour, altered mental status, dehydration, excessive fatigue, and concomitant heart failure.

Diagnosis

NURSING DIAGNOSES

Based on the assessment data, the patient's major nursing diagnoses may include:

- Ineffective airway clearance related to copious tracheobronchial secretions
- Activity intolerance related to impaired respiratory function
- Risk for deficient fluid volume related to fever and dyspnea
- Imbalanced nutrition: less than body requirements
- Deficient knowledge about the treatment regimen and preventive health measures

COLLABORATIVE PROBLEMS/POTENTIAL COMPLICATIONS

Based on the assessment data, collaborative problems or potential complications that may occur include:

- Continuing symptoms after initiation of therapy
- Shock
- Respiratory failure
- Atelectasis
- Pleural effusion
- Confusion
- Superinfection

Planning and Goals

The major goals for the patient may include improved airway patency, rest to conserve energy, maintenance of proper fluid volume, maintenance of adequate nutrition, an understanding of the treatment protocol and preventive measures, and absence of complications.

Nursing Interventions

IMPROVING AIRWAY PATENCY

Removing secretions is important because retained secretions interfere with gas exchange and may slow recovery. The nurse encourages hydration (2 to 3 L/day) because adequate hydration thins and loosens pulmonary secretions. Humidification may be used to loosen secretions and improve ventilation. A high-humidity facemask (using either compressed air or oxygen) delivers warm, humidified air to the tracheobronchial tree, helps to liquefy secretions, and relieves tracheobronchial irritation. Coughing can be initiated either voluntarily or by reflex. Lung expansion manoeuvres, such as deep breathing with an incentive spirometer, may induce a cough. A directed cough may be necessary to improve airway patency. The nurse encourages the patient to per-

form an effective, directed cough, which includes correct positioning, a deep inspiratory manoeuvre, glottic closure, contraction of the expiratory muscles against the closed glottis, sudden glottic opening, and an explosive expiration. In some cases, the nurse may assist the patient by placing both hands on the patient's lower rib cage (anteriorly or posteriorly) to focus the patient on a slow deep breath, and then manually assisting the patient by applying external pressure during the expiratory phase.

Chest physiotherapy (percussion and postural drainage) is important in loosening and mobilizing secretions (see Chap. 25). Indications for chest physiotherapy include sputum retention not responsive to spontaneous or directed cough, a history of pulmonary problems previously treated with chest physiotherapy, continued evidence of retained secretions (decreased or abnormal breath sounds, change in vital signs), abnormal chest x-ray findings consistent with atelectasis or infiltrates, or deterioration in oxygenation. The patient is placed in the proper position to drain the involved lung segments, and then the chest is percussed and vibrated either manually or with a mechanical percussor.

After each position change, the nurse encourages the patient to breathe deeply and cough. If the patient is too weak to cough effectively, the nurse may need to remove the mucus by nasotracheal suctioning (see Chap. 25). It may take time for secretions to mobilize and move into the central airways for expectoration. Thus, it is important for the nurse to monitor the patient for cough and sputum production after the completion of chest physiotherapy.

The nurse administers and titrates oxygen therapy as prescribed. The effectiveness of oxygen therapy is monitored by improvement in clinical signs and symptoms, and adequate oxygenation values measured by pulse oximetry or arterial blood gas analysis.

PROMOTING REST AND CONSERVING ENERGY

The nurse encourages the debilitated patient to rest and avoid overexertion and possible exacerbation of symptoms. The patient should assume a comfortable position to promote rest and breathing (eg, semi-Fowler's) and should change positions frequently to enhance secretion clearance and ventilation/perfusion in the lungs. It is important to instruct outpatients not to overexert themselves and to engage in only moderate activity during the initial phases of treatment.

PROMOTING FLUID INTAKE

The respiratory rate of a patient with pneumonia increases because of the increased workload imposed by laboured breathing and fever. An increased respiratory rate leads to an increase in insensible fluid loss during exhalation and can lead to dehydration. Therefore, it is important to encourage increased fluid intake (at least 2 L/day), unless contraindicated.

MAINTAINING NUTRITION

Patients with shortness of breath and fatigue often have a decreased appetite and will take only fluids. Fluids with electrolytes (commercially available drinks, such as Gatorade) may help provide fluid, calories, and electrolytes. Other nutritionally enriched drinks or shakes may be helpful. In addition, fluids and nutrients may be administered intravenously if necessary.

PROMOTING THE PATIENT'S KNOWLEDGE

The patient and family are instructed about the cause of pneumonia, management of symptoms of pneumonia, and the need for follow-up (discussed later). The patient also needs information about factors (both patient risk factors and external factors) that may have contributed to developing pneumonia and strategies to promote recovery and to prevent recurrence. If hospitalized for treatment, the patient is instructed about the purpose and importance of management strategies that have been implemented and about the importance of adhering to them during and after the hospital stay. Explanations need to be given simply and in language that the patient can understand. If possible, written instructions and information should be provided. Because of the severity of symptoms, the patient may require that instructions and explanations be repeated several times.

MONITORING AND MANAGING POTENTIAL COMPLICATIONS

Continuing Symptoms After Initiation of Therapy

Patients usually begin to respond to treatment within 24 to 48 hours after antibiotic therapy is initiated. The patient is observed for response to antibiotic therapy. The patient is monitored for changes in physical status (deterioration of condition or resolution of symptoms) and for persistent recurrent fever, which may be due to medication allergy (signaled possibly by a rash); medication resistance or slow response (greater than 48 hours) of the susceptible organism to therapy; superinfection; pleural effusion; or pneumonia caused by an unusual organism, such as *P. carinii* or *Aspergillus fumigatus*. Failure of the pneumonia to resolve or persistence of symptoms despite changes on the chest x-ray raises the suspicion of other underlying disorders, such as lung cancer. As described earlier, lung cancers may invade or compress airways, causing an obstructive atelectasis that may lead to a pneumonia.

In addition to monitoring for continuing symptoms of pneumonia, the nurse also monitors for other complications, such as shock and multisystem failure, atelectasis, pleural effusion, and superinfection, which may develop during the first few days of antibiotic treatment.

Shock and Respiratory Failure

The nurse assesses for signs and symptoms of shock and respiratory failure by evaluating the patient's vital signs, pulse oximetry values, and hemodynamic monitoring parameters. The nurse reports signs of deteriorating patient status and assists in administering intravenous fluids and medications prescribed to combat shock. Intubation and mechanical ventilation may be required if respiratory failure occurs. Shock is described in detail in Chapter 15, and care of the patient receiving mechanical ventilation is described in Chapter 25.

Atelectasis and Pleural Effusion

The patient is assessed for atelectasis, and preventive measures are initiated to prevent its development. If pleural effusion develops and thoracentesis is performed to remove fluid, the nurse assists in the procedure and explains it to the patient. After thoracentesis, the nurse monitors the patient for pneumothorax or recurrence of pleural effusion. If a chest tube needs to be inserted, the nurse monitors the patient's respiratory status (see Chap. 25 for more information on care of the patient with a chest tube).

Superinfection

The patient is monitored for manifestations of superinfection (ie, minimal improvement in signs and symptoms, rise in temperature with increasing cough, increasing fremitus and adventitious breath sounds on auscultation of the lungs). These signs are re-

ported, and the nurse assists in implementing therapy to treat superinfection.

Confusion

The patient with pneumonia is assessed for confusion and other more subtle changes in cognitive status. Confusion and changes in cognitive status resulting from pneumonia are poor prognostic signs. Confusion may be related to hypoxemia, fever, dehydration, sleep deprivation, or developing sepsis. The patient's underlying comorbid conditions may also play a part in the development of confusion. Addressing the underlying factors and ensuring the patient's safety are important nursing interventions.

PROMOTING HOME AND COMMUNITY-BASED CARE

Teaching Patients Self-Care

Depending on the severity of the pneumonia, treatment may occur in the hospital or in the outpatient setting. Patient education is crucial regardless of the setting, and the proper administration of antibiotics is important. In some instances, the patient may be initially treated with intravenous antibiotics as an inpatient and then be discharged to continue the intravenous antibiotics in the home setting. It is important that a seamless system of care be maintained for the patient from hospital to home; this includes communication between the nurses caring for this patient in both settings. In addition, if oral antibiotics are prescribed, it is important to teach the patient about their proper administration and potential side effects.

After the fever subsides, the patient may gradually increase activities. Fatigue and weakness may be prolonged after pneumonia, especially in the elderly. The nurse encourages breathing exercises to promote secretion clearance and volume expansion. It is important to instruct the patient to return to the clinic or caregiver's office for a follow-up chest x-ray and physical examination. Often improvement in chest x-ray findings lags behind improvement in clinical signs and symptoms.

The nurse encourages the patient to stop smoking. Smoking inhibits tracheobronchial ciliary action, which is the first line of defense of the lower respiratory tract. Smoking also irritates the mucous cells of the bronchi and inhibits the function of alveolar macrophage (scavenger) cells. The patient is instructed to avoid stress, fatigue, sudden changes in temperature, and excessive alcohol intake, all of which lower resistance to pneumonia. The nurse reviews with the patient the principles of adequate nutrition and rest, because one episode of pneumonia may make the patient susceptible to recurring respiratory tract infections.

Continuing Care

Patients who are severely debilitated or who cannot care for themselves may require referral for home care. During home visits, the nurse assesses the patient's physical status, monitors for complications, assesses the home environment, and reinforces previous teaching. The nurse evaluates the patient's adherence to the therapeutic regimen (ie, taking medications as prescribed, performing breathing exercises, consuming adequate fluid and dietary intake, and avoiding smoking, alcohol, and excessive activity). The nurse stresses to the patient and family the importance of monitoring for complications. The nurse encourages the patient to obtain an influenza vaccine at the prescribed times, because influenza increases susceptibility to secondary bacterial pneumonia, especially that caused by staphylococci, *H. influenzae*, and *S. pneumoniae*. The nurse also encourages the patient to seek medical advice about receiving the vaccine (Pneumovax) against *S. pneumoniae*.

NURSING RESEARCH PROFILE 23-1
Tobacco-Related Nursing Interventions

Sarna, L. P., Brown, J. K., Lillington, L., Rose, M., Wewers, M. E., & Brecht, M. (2000). Tobacco interventions by oncology nurses in clinical practice. *Cancer, 89*(4), 881–889.

Purpose

Smoking remains a major cause of death in all populations in the U.S. The purpose of this study was to describe the frequency of interventions related to the use of tobacco used by oncology nurses, using the Agency for Health Care Policy and Research (AHCPR) guidelines as a framework.

Study Sample and Design

This was a descriptive study; a self-report questionnaire was mailed to a random sample of 4,000 members of the Oncology Nursing Society. The response rate was 38%, with 1,508 completed questionnaires available for analysis. Subjects were asked to identify those interventions related to tobacco use that they used in their clinical practice.

Findings

The majority of respondents were female (98%), with an average age of 44 years. The educational background of respondents was varied, with 39% with baccalaureate preparation, 41% with associate or diploma education, and 20% with master's or doctoral level education. Sixty-two percent of the respondents reported their position as staff nurse. Overall, the sample was characterized as experienced nurses, with average number of years in nursing at 18 ± 9.4 years

and as an oncology nurse for 11.5 ± 5.5 years. Thirty percent of the sample were ex-smokers, while 7% were active smokers. The results demonstrated that most respondents (86%) encountered smokers in their clinical practice on a weekly basis, but only 10% had any knowledge of the AHCPR guidelines for smoking cessation. Sixty-four percent of the respondents assessed and documented smoking status in their clinical patients and 38% assessed readiness to quit. However, fewer nurses reported providing interventions for smoking cessation. The most frequent barriers cited included perceived lack of patient motivation (74%), time (52%), and skills to provide a cessation intervention (53%).

Nursing Implications

Nurses have frequent contacts with active smokers in the inpatient and outpatient setting and could have a tremendous impact on smoking prevention and cessation. Even in this sample of oncology nurses, few provided smoking cessation interventions on a regular basis. Nurses need a heightened awareness of the importance of smoking cessation and the potential impact they may have on this growing problem. It is imperative that students and practicing nurses receive improved education regarding smoking cessation techniques and use of evidence-based guidelines like those of the AHCPR.

Evaluation

EXPECTED PATIENT OUTCOMES

Expected patient outcomes may include:

1. Demonstrates improved airway patency, as evidenced by adequate oxygenation by pulse oximetry or arterial blood gas analysis, normal temperature, normal breath sounds, and effective coughing
2. Rests and conserves energy by limiting activities and remaining in bed while symptomatic and slowly increasing activities
3. Maintains adequate hydration, as evidenced by an adequate fluid intake and urine output and normal skin turgor
4. Consumes adequate dietary intake, as evidenced by maintenance or increase in body weight without excess fluid gain
5. States explanation for management strategies
6. Complies with management strategies
7. Exhibits no complications
    a. Has normal vital signs, pulse oximetry, and arterial blood gas measurements
    b. Reports productive cough that diminishes over time
    c. Has absence of signs or symptoms of shock, respiratory failure, or pleural effusion
    d. Remains oriented and aware of surroundings
    e. Maintains or increases weight
8. Complies with treatment protocol and prevention strategies

PULMONARY TUBERCULOSIS

Tuberculosis (TB) is an infectious disease that primarily affects the lung parenchyma. It also may be transmitted to other parts of

the body, including the meninges, kidneys, bones, and lymph nodes. The primary infectious agent, *Mycobacterium tuberculosis,* is an acid-fast aerobic rod that grows slowly and is sensitive to heat and ultraviolet light. *Mycobacterium bovis* and *Mycobacterium avium* have rarely been associated with the development of a TB infection.

TB is a worldwide public health problem, and the mortality and morbidity rates continue to rise. *M. tuberculosis* infects an estimated one third of the world's population and remains the leading cause of death from infectious disease in the world. It is the leading cause of death among HIV-positive people (World Health Organization, 2000). TB is closely associated with poverty, malnutrition, overcrowding, substandard housing, and inadequate health care.

The reported incidence of TB in Canada has been in significant decline since a peak in the early 1940s. It was thought that by the early part of the 21st century, TB might be eliminated in Canada. However, after decades of steady decline, the number of new cases per year has leveled off since 1987 (Health Canada, 2001). This change has been attributed to several factors, including increased immigration, the HIV epidemic, and the emergence of multidrug-resistant strains of TB.

Transmission and Risk Factors

TB spreads from person to person by airborne transmission. An infected person releases droplet nuclei (generally particles 1 to 5 micrometers in diameter) through talking, coughing, sneezing, laughing, or singing. Larger droplets settle; smaller droplets remain suspended in the air and are inhaled by the susceptible person. Risk factors for TB are listed in Chart 23-4. Chart 23-5 summarizes the CDC's recommendations for prevention of TB transmission in health care settings.

- Close contact with someone who has active TB. Inhalation of airborne nuclei from an infected person is proportional to the amount of time spent in the same air space, the proximity of the person, and the degree of ventilation.
- Immunocompromised status (eg, those with HIV infection, cancer, transplanted organs, and prolonged high-dose corticosteroid therapy)
- Substance abuse (IV or injection drug users and alcoholics)
- Any person without adequate health care (the homeless; impoverished; minorities, particularly children under age 15 years and young adults between ages 15 and 44 yrs)
- Preexisting medical conditions or special treatment (eg, diabetes, chronic renal failure, malnourishment, selected malignancies, hemodialysis, transplanted organ, gastrectomy, or jejunoileal bypass)
- Immigration from countries with a high prevalence of TB (southeastern Asia, Africa, Latin America, Caribbean)
- Institutionalization (eg, long-term care facilities, psychiatric institutions, prisons)
- Living in overcrowded, substandard housing
- Being a health care worker performing high-risk activities: administration of aerosolized pentamidine and other medications, sputum induction procedures, bronchoscopy, suctioning, coughing procedures, caring for the immunosuppressed patient, home care with the high-risk population, and administering anesthesia and related procedures (eg, intubation, suctioning)

Pathophysiology

A susceptible person inhales mycobacterium bacilli and becomes infected. The bacteria are transmitted through the airways to the alveoli, where they are deposited and begin to multiply. The bacilli also are transported via the lymph system and bloodstream to other parts of the body (kidneys, bones, cerebral cortex) and other areas of the lungs (upper lobes). The body's immune system responds by initiating an inflammatory reaction. Phagocytes (neutrophils and macrophages) engulf many of the bacteria, and TB-specific lymphocytes lyse (destroy) the bacilli and normal tissue. This tissue reaction results in the accumulation of exudate in the alveoli, causing bronchopneumonia. The initial infection usually occurs 2 to 10 weeks after exposure.

Granulomas, new tissue masses of live and dead bacilli, are surrounded by macrophages, which form a protective wall around the granulomas. Granulomas are then transformed to a fibrous tissue mass, the central portion of which is called a Ghon tubercle. The material (bacteria and macrophages) becomes necrotic, forming a cheesy mass. This mass may become calcified and form a collagenous scar. At this point, the bacteria become dormant, and there is no further progression of active disease.

After initial exposure and infection, the person may develop active disease because of a compromised or inadequate immune system response. Active disease also may occur with reinfection and activation of dormant bacteria. In this case, the Ghon tubercle ulcerates, releasing the cheesy material into the bronchi. The bacteria then become airborne, resulting in further spread of the disease. Then the ulcerated tubercle heals and forms scar tissue. This causes the infected lung to become more inflamed, resulting in further development of bronchopneumonia and tubercle formation.

Unless the process is arrested, it spreads slowly downward to the hilum of the lungs and later extends to adjacent lobes. The process may be prolonged and characterized by long remissions when the disease is arrested, only to be followed by periods of renewed activity. Approximately 10% of people who are initially infected develop active disease. Some people develop reactivation TB (also called adult-type TB). This type of TB results from a breakdown of the host defenses. It most commonly occurs within

CDC Recommendations for Preventing Transmission of Tuberculosis in Health Care Settings

1. Early identification and treatment of persons with active TB
   a. Maintain a high index of suspicion for TB to identify cases rapidly.
   b. Promptly initiate effective multidrug anti-TB therapy based on clinical and drug-resistance surveillance data.
2. Prevention of spread of infectious droplet nuclei by source control methods and by reduction of microbial contamination of indoor air
   a. Initiate acid-fast bacilli (AFB) isolation precautions immediately for all patients who are suspected or confirmed to have active TB and who may be infectious. AFB isolation precautions include use of a private room with negative pressure in relation to surrounding areas and a minimum of six air exchanges per hour. Air from the room should be exhausted directly to the outside. Use of ultraviolet lamps and/or high-efficiency particulate air filters to supplement ventilation may be considered.
   b. Persons entering the AFB isolation room should use disposable particulate respirators that fit snugly around the face.
   c. Continue AFB isolation precautions until there is clinical evidence of reduced infectiousness (ie, cough has substantially decreased, and the number of organisms on sequential sputum smears is decreasing). If drug resistance is suspected or confirmed, continue AFB precautions until the sputum smear is negative for AFB.
   d. Use special precautions during cough-inducing procedures.
3. Surveillance for TB transmission
   a. Maintain surveillance for TB infection among health care workers (HCWs) by routine, periodic tuberculin skin testing. Recommend appropriate preventive therapy for HCWs when indicated.
   b. Maintain surveillance for TB cases among patients and HCWs.
   c. Promptly initiate contact investigation procedures among HCWs, patients, and visitors exposed to an untreated, or ineffectively treated, infectious TB patient for whom appropriate AFB procedures are not in place. Recommend appropriate therapy or preventive therapy for contacts with disease or TB infection without current disease. Therapeutic regimens should be chosen based on the clinical history and local drug-resistance surveillance data.

the lungs, usually in the apical or posterior segments of the upper lobes, or the superior segments of the lower lobes.

Clinical Manifestations

The signs and symptoms of pulmonary TB are insidious. Most patients have a low-grade fever, cough, night sweats, fatigue, and weight loss. The cough may be nonproductive, or mucopurulent sputum may be expectorated. Hemoptysis also may occur. Both the systemic and pulmonary symptoms are usually chronic and may have been present for weeks to months. The elderly usually present with less pronounced symptoms than do younger patients. Nonrespiratory disease occurs in up to 25% of cases in Canada. In patients with AIDS, extrapulmonary disease is more prevalent and may occur in up to 70% of cases (Niederman & Sarosi, 2000; Small & Fujiwara, 2001).

Assessment and Diagnostic Findings

A complete history, physical examination, tuberculin skin test, chest x-ray, acid-fast bacillus smear, and sputum culture are used to diagnose TB. If the person is infected with TB, the chest x-ray usually reveals lesions in the upper lobes and the acid-fast bacillus smear contains mycobacterium.

TUBERCULIN SKIN TEST

The Mantoux test is used to determine if a person has been infected with the TB bacillus. The Mantoux test is a standardized procedure and should be performed only by those trained in its administration and reading. Tubercle bacillus extract (tuberculin), purified protein derivative (PPD), is injected into the intradermal layer of the inner aspect of the forearm, approximately 10 cm below the elbow (Fig. 23-4). Intermediate-strength (5 TU) PPD in a tuberculin syringe with a 1.3 cm 26- or 27-gauge needle is used. The needle, with the bevel facing up, is inserted beneath the skin. Then 0.1 mL of PPD is injected, creating an elevation in the skin, a wheal or bleb. The site, antigen name, strength, lot number, date, and time of the test are recorded. The test result is read 48 to 72 hours after injection. Tests read after 72 hours tend to underestimate the true size of **induration** (hardening). A delayed localized reaction indicates that the person is sensitive to tuberculin.

A reaction occurs when both induration and erythema (redness) are noted. After the area is inspected for induration, it is lightly palpated across the injection site, from the area of normal skin to the margins of the induration. The diameter of the induration (not erythema) is measured in millimetres at its widest part (see Fig. 23-4), and the size of the induration is documented. Erythema without induration is not considered significant.

Interpretation of Results. The size of the induration determines the significance of the reaction. A reaction of 0 to 4 mm is considered not significant; a reaction of 5 mm or greater may be significant in individuals who are considered at risk. An induration of 10 mm or greater is usually considered significant in individuals who have normal or mildly impaired immunity. A significant reaction indicates that a patient has been exposed to *M. tuberculosis* recently or in the past or has been vaccinated with bacille Calmette-Guérin (BCG) vaccine. The BCG vaccine is given to produce a greater resistance to developing TB. It is estimated to be effective in up to 80% of those who receive it. However, many countries, including Canada, limit the routine use of BCG to high risk groups (Health Canada, 2001).

A reaction of 5 mm or greater is defined as positive for patients who are HIV-positive or have HIV risk factors and are of unknown HIV status, those who are close contacts with an active case, and those who have chest x-ray results consistent with tuberculosis.

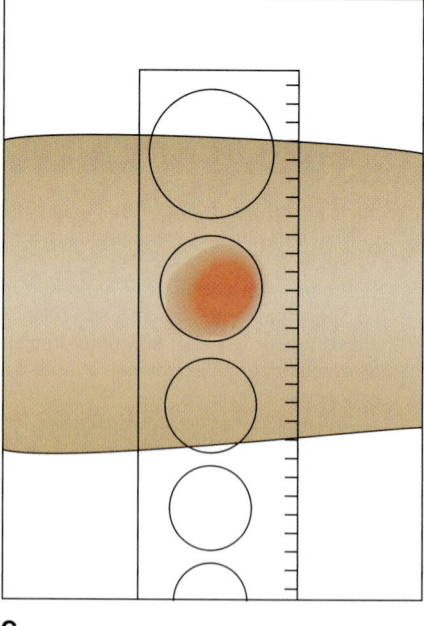

A   B   C

FIGURE 23-4 The Mantoux test for tuberculosis. (**A**) Correct technique for inserting the needle involves depositing the PPD subcutaneously with the needle bevel facing upward. (**B**) The reaction to the Mantoux test usually consists of a wheal, a hivelike, firm welt. (**C**) To determine the extent of the reaction, the wheal is measured using a commercially prepared gauge. A wheal measuring 5 mm or more is considered significant.

A significant (positive) reaction does not necessarily mean that active disease is present in the body. Most (more than 90%) people who are tuberculin-significant reactors do not develop clinical TB. However, all significant reactors are candidates for active TB. In general, the more intense the reaction, the greater the likelihood of an active infection.

A nonsignificant (negative) skin test does not exclude TB infection or disease because patients who are immunosuppressed cannot develop an immune response adequate to produce a positive skin test. This is referred to as anergy.

The accuracy of the skin test depends on the skill of the person interpreting the test reaction. One study (Kendig, Kirkpatrick, Carter et al., 1998) revealed that health care professionals tend to underestimate the size of induration: only 7% of a sample of 107 health care providers charted the correct size of induration.

CLASSIFICATION OF TB

Data from the history, physical examination, skin test, chest x-ray, and microbiologic studies are used to classify TB into one of five classes. A classification scheme provides public health officials with a systematic way to monitor epidemiology and treatment of the disease (American Thoracic Society, 2000).

- Class 0: no exposure; no infection
- Class 1: exposure; no evidence of infection
- Class 2: latent infection; no disease (eg, positive PPD reaction but no clinical evidence of active TB)
- Class 3: disease; clinically active
- Class 4: disease; not clinically active
- Class 5: suspected disease; diagnosis pending

 ## Gerontologic Considerations

TB may have atypical manifestations in elderly patients, whose symptoms may include unusual behaviour and altered mental status, fever, anorexia, and weight loss. Many elderly patients may have no reaction (loss of immunologic memory) or delayed reactivity for up to a week (recall phenomenon). A second skin test is performed in 1 to 2 weeks.

Medical Management

Pulmonary TB is treated primarily with chemotherapeutic agents (antituberculosis agents) for 6 to 12 months. A prolonged treatment duration is necessary to ensure eradication of the organisms and to prevent relapse. A worldwide concern and challenge in TB therapy is the continuing (since the 1950s) and increasing resistance of *M. tuberculosis* to TB medications. Several types of drug resistance must be considered when planning effective therapy:

- Primary drug resistance: resistance to one of the first-line antituberculosis agents in a person who has not had previous treatment
- Secondary or acquired drug resistance: resistance to one or more antituberculosis agents in a patient undergoing therapy
- Multidrug resistance: resistance to two agents, isoniazid (INH) and rifampin. The populations at highest risk for multidrug resistance are those who are HIV-positive, institutionalized, or homeless.

The increasing prevalence of drug resistance points out the need to begin TB treatment with four or more medications, to ensure completion of therapy, and to develop and evaluate new anti-TB medications.

PHARMACOLOGIC THERAPY

In current TB therapy, five first-line medications are used (Table 23-2): INH, rifampin, pyrazinamide, and either streptomycin or ethambutol.

Combination medications, such as INH and rifampin (Rifamate) or INH, pyrazinamide and rifampin and medications administered twice a week (eg, rifapentine) are available to help improve patient adherence. Capreomycin, ethionamide, para-aminosalicylate sodium, and cycloserine are second-line medications. Additional potentially effective medications include other aminoglycosides, quinolones, rifabutin, clofazimine, and combinations of medications.

Recommended Canadian treatment guidelines for newly diagnosed cases of pulmonary TB include two regimen options: (1) INH and rifampin, or (2) INH, rifampin, and pyrazinamide (Health Canada, 2000). In the former case, drugs are taken over a 9-month period using one of three dosing interval options. In the latter case, a combination of the drugs is taken over a 6-month period using one of two dosing interval options. Until drug susceptibility tests exclude the presence of resistance, ethambutol should be added. A person is considered noninfectious after 2 to 3 weeks of continuous medication therapy. Vitamin B (pyridoxine) is usually administered with INH to prevent INH-associated peripheral neuropathy (see Table 23-2).

INH also may be used as a prophylactic (preventive) measure for those at risk for significant disease, including:

- Household family members of patients with active disease
- HIV-infected patients with a PPD test reaction of 5 mm of induration or more
- Patients with fibrotic lesions detected on a chest x-ray, suggestive of old TB, and a PPD reaction of 5 mm of induration or more
- Patients whose current PPD test results show a change from former test results, suggesting recent exposure to TB and possible infection (also called skin test converters)
- Drug (intravenous or injectable) users with PPD test results of 10 mm of induration or more
- Patients with high-risk comorbid conditions with a PPD result of 10 mm of induration or more

Other candidates for preventive INH therapy are those age 35 years or younger with PPD test results of 10 mm of induration or more and one of the following criteria:

- Foreign-born individuals from countries with a high prevalence of TB
- High-risk, medically underserved populations
- Institutionalized patients

Prophylactic INH treatment involves taking daily doses for 6 to 12 months. Liver enzyme, blood urea nitrogen, and creatinine levels are monitored monthly. Sputum culture results are monitored for acid-fast bacillus to evaluate the effectiveness of treatment and the patient's compliance with therapy.

In 1998, the federal Advisory Council for the Elimination of Tuberculosis published recommendations for the development of TB vaccines. The recommendations include a focus on a "postinfection vaccine" to prevent people infected with TB from developing active disease (CDC, 1998). To date, this vaccine has

Table 23-2 • First-Line Antitubercular Medications

COMMONLY USED AGENTS	ADULT DAILY DOSAGE*	MOST COMMON SIDE EFFECTS	DRUG INTERACTIONS†	REMARKS*
isoniazid (INH)	5 mg/kg (300 mg maximum daily)	Peripheral neuritis, hepatic enzyme elevation, hepatitis, hypersensitivity	Phenytoin— synergistic Antabuse Alcohol	Bactericidal. Pyridoxine as prophylaxis for neuritis. Monitor AST (SGOT) and ALT (SGPT).
rifampin (Rifadin)	10 mg/kg (600 mg maximum daily)	Hepatitis, febrile reaction, purpura (rare), nausea, vomiting	Rifampin increases metabolism of oral contraceptives, quinidine, corticosteroids, coumarin derivatives and methadone, digoxin, oral hypoglycemics; PAS may interfere with absorption of rifampin.	Bactericidal. Orange urine and other body secretions. Discolouring of contact lenses. Monitor AST (SGOT) and ALT (SGPT).
rifabutin (Mycobutin)	5 mg/kg (300 mg maximum daily)			
streptomycin	15 mg/kg (1 g maximum daily)*	8th cranial nerve damage (may lead to deafness), nephrotoxicity	Neuromuscular blocking agents; may be potentiated to cause prolonged paralysis	Bactericidal in alkaline pH. Use with caution in elderly or in those with renal disease. Monitor vestibular function, audiograms, BUN and creatinine.
pyrazinamide	15 to 30 mg/kg (2.0 g maximum daily)*	Hyperuricemia, hepatotoxicity, skin rash, arthralgias, GI distress		Bactericidal. Monitor uric acid, AST (SGOT), ALT (SGPT).
ethambutol (Myambutol)	15 to 25 mg/kg (no maximum daily dose, but base on lean body wt)*	Optic neuritis (may lead to blindness; very rare at 15 mg/kg), skin rash		Bacteriostatic. Use with caution with renal disease or when eye testing is not feasible. Monitor visual acuity, colour discrimination.‡
Combinations: INH + rifampin (eg, Rifamate)	150-mg & 300-mg caps (2 caps daily)			

*Check product labelling for detailed information on dose, contraindications, drug interaction, adverse reactions, and monitoring.
†Refer to current literature, particularly on rifampin, because it increases hepatic microenzymes and therefore interacts with many drugs.
‡Initial examination should be performed at start of treatment.

not become clinically available. In 2000, recommendations were released regarding the treatment of latent TB infection (Health Canada, 2000). Isoniazid (INH) for 9 months is currently considered an optimal treatment for latent TB infection. Rifampin daily for 4 months is an option in persons infected with INH-resistant organisms and a high risk of tuberculous disease.

NURSING PROCESS: THE PATIENT WITH TUBERCULOSIS

Assessment

The nurse performs a complete history and physical examination. Clinical manifestations of fever, anorexia, weight loss, night sweats, fatigue, cough, and sputum production prompt a more thorough assessment of respiratory function—for example, as-

sessing the lungs for consolidation by evaluating breath sounds (diminished, bronchial sounds, crackles), fremitus, egophony, and dullness on percussion. Enlarged, painful lymph nodes may be palpated as well. The nurse also assesses the patient's living arrangements, perceptions and understanding of TB and its treatment, and readiness to learn.

Nursing Diagnoses

Based on the assessment data, the nursing diagnoses may include:

- Ineffective airway clearance related to copious tracheobronchial secretions
- Deficient knowledge about treatment regimen and preventive health measures and related ineffective individual management of the therapeutic regimen (noncompliance)

- Activity intolerance related to fatigue, altered nutritional status, and fever

Collaborative Problems/ Potential Complications

Based on the assessment data, collaborative problems or potential complications that may occur include:

- Malnutrition
- Adverse side effects of medication therapy: hepatitis, neurologic changes (deafness or neuritis), skin rash, gastrointestinal upset
- Multidrug resistance
- Spread of TB infection (miliary TB)

Planning and Goals

The major goals for the patient include maintenance of a patent airway, increased knowledge about the disease and treatment regimen and adherence to the medication regimen, increased activity tolerance, and absence of complications.

Nursing Interventions

PROMOTING AIRWAY CLEARANCE

Copious secretions obstruct the airways in many patients with TB and interfere with adequate gas exchange. Increasing fluid intake promotes systemic hydration and serves as an effective expectorant. The nurse instructs the patient about correct positioning to facilitate airway drainage (postural drainage); this is described in Chapter 25.

ADVOCATING ADHERENCE TO TREATMENT REGIMEN

The multiple-medication regimen that a patient must follow can be quite complex. Understanding the medications, schedule, and side effects is important. The patient must understand that TB is a communicable disease and that taking medications is the most effective means of preventing transmission. The major reason treatment fails is that patients do not take their medications regularly and for the prescribed duration. The nurse carefully instructs the patient about important hygiene measures, including mouth care, covering the mouth and nose when coughing and sneezing, proper disposal of tissues, and hand hygiene.

PROMOTING ACTIVITY AND ADEQUATE NUTRITION

Patients with TB are often debilitated from a prolonged chronic illness and impaired nutritional status. The nurse plans a progressive activity schedule that focuses on increasing activity tolerance and muscle strength. Anorexia, weight loss, and malnutrition are common in patients with TB. The patient's willingness to eat may be altered by fatigue from excessive coughing, sputum production, chest pain, generalized debilitated state, or cost, if the person has few resources. A nutritional plan that allows for small, frequent meals may be required. Liquid nutritional supplements may assist in meeting basic caloric requirements.

MONITORING AND MANAGING POTENTIAL COMPLICATIONS

Malnutrition

This may be a consequence of the patient's lifestyle, lack of knowledge about adequate nutrition and its role in health maintenance, lack of resources, fatigue, or lack of appetite because of coughing and mucus production. To counter the effects of these factors, the nurse collaborates with the dietitian, physician, social worker, family, and patient to identify strategies to ensure an adequate nutritional intake and availability of nutritious food. Identifying facilities (eg, shelters, soup kitchens, Meals on Wheels, and other community resources) that provide meals in the patient's neighbourhood may increase the likelihood that the patient with limited resources and energy will have access to a more nutritious intake. High-calorie nutritional supplements may be suggested as a strategy for increasing dietary intake using food products normally found in the home. Purchasing food supplements may be beyond the patient's budget, but a dietitian can help develop recipes to increase caloric intake despite minimal resources.

Side Effects of Medication Therapy

It is important to assess medication side effects because they are often a reason the patient fails to adhere to the prescribed medication regimen. Efforts are made to reduce the side effects to increase the patient's willingness to take the medications as prescribed.

The nurse instructs the patient to take the medication either on an empty stomach or at least 1 hour before meals, because food interferes with medication absorption (although taking medications on an empty stomach frequently results in gastrointestinal upset). Patients taking INH should avoid foods containing tyramine and histamine (tuna, aged cheese, red wine, soy sauce, yeast extracts). Eating these types of foods while taking INH may result in headache, flushing, hypotension, light-headedness, palpitations, and diaphoresis.

In addition, rifampin can increase the metabolism of other medications, making them less effective. These medications include beta-blockers, oral anticoagulants such as warfarin (Coumadin), digoxin, quinidine, corticosteroids, oral hypoglycemic agents, oral contraceptives, theophylline, and verapamil. This issue should be discussed with the physician and pharmacist so that medication dosages can be adjusted accordingly. The nurse informs the patient that rifampin may discolour contact lenses, so the patient may want to wear eyeglasses during treatment. The nurse monitors for other side effects of anti-TB medications, including hepatitis, neurologic changes (hearing loss, neuritis), and rash. Liver enzyme, blood urea nitrogen, and serum creatinine levels are monitored to detect medication-related changes in liver and kidney function. Sputum culture results are monitored for acid-fast bacillus to evaluate the effectiveness of the treatment regimen and adherence to therapy.

Multidrug Resistance

The nurse carefully monitors vital signs and observes for spikes in temperature or changes in the clinical status. The nurse reports any change in the patient's respiratory status to the primary health care provider. The nurse instructs the patient about the risk of drug resistance if the medication regimen is not strictly and continuously followed.

Spread of TB Infection

Spread of TB infection to nonpulmonary sites of the body is known as miliary TB. It is the result of invasion of the bloodstream by the tubercle bacillus (Ghon tubercle). Usually it results from late reactivation of a dormant infection in the lung or elsewhere. The origin of the bacilli that enter the bloodstream is either a chronic focus that has ulcerated into a blood vessel or multitudes of miliary tubercles lining the inner surface of the thoracic duct. The organisms migrate from these foci into the bloodstream, are carried throughout the body, and disseminate throughout all tissues, with tiny miliary tubercles developing in the lungs, spleen, liver, kidneys, meninges, and other organs.

The clinical course of miliary TB may vary from an acute, rapidly progressive infection with high fever to an indolent process with low-grade fever, anemia, and debilitation. At first, there may be no localizing signs except an enlarged spleen and a reduced number of leukocytes. Within a few weeks, however, the chest x-ray reveals small densities scattered diffusely throughout both lung fields; these are the miliary tubercles, which gradually grow.

The possibility of TB in nonpulmonary sites in the body requires careful monitoring for this very serious form of the infection. The nurse monitors vital signs and observes for spikes in temperature as well as changes in renal and cognitive function. Few physical signs may be elicited on physical examination of the chest, but at this stage the patient has a severe cough and dyspnea. Treatment of miliary TB is the same as for pulmonary TB.

PROMOTING HOME AND COMMUNITY-BASED CARE

Teaching Patients Self-Care

The nurse plays a vital role in caring for the patient with TB and the family, which includes assessing the patient's ability to continue therapy at home. The nurse instructs the patient and family about infection control procedures, such as proper disposal of tissues, covering the mouth during coughing, and hand hygiene. Assessment of the patient's adherence to the medication regimen is imperative because of the risk of developing resistant strains of TB if the regimen is not followed faithfully. In some cases, when the patient's ability to comply with the medication regimen is in question, referral to an outpatient clinic for daily medication administration may be required. This is referred to as directly observed therapy (DOT).

Continuing Care

The nurse evaluates the patient's environment, including home or workplace and social setting, to identify other people who may have been in contact with the patient during the infectious stage. It is important to arrange follow-up screening for any contacts of the infected person. Nurses who have contact with the patient in home, shelter, hospital, clinic, or work settings assess the patient's physical and psychological status and ability to adhere to the prescribed treatment. The nurse assesses the patient for adverse effects of medications and adherence to the therapeutic regimen (eg, taking medications as prescribed, practicing safe hygiene, consuming a nutritious and adequate diet, and participating in an appropriate level of activity). The nurse reinforces previous teaching and emphasizes the importance of keeping scheduled appointments with the primary health care provider. In addition, the patient is reminded of the importance

of other health promotion activities and recommended health screening.

Evaluation

EXPECTED PATIENT OUTCOMES

Expected patient outcomes may include:

1. Maintains a patent airway by managing secretions with hydration, humidification, coughing, and postural drainage
2. Demonstrates an adequate level of knowledge
   a. Lists medications by name and the correct schedule for taking them
   b. Names expected side effects of medications
   c. Identifies how and when to contact health care provider
3. Adheres to treatment regimen by taking medications as prescribed and reporting for follow-up screening
4. Participates in preventive measures
   a. Disposes of used tissues properly
   b. Encourages people who are close contacts to report for testing
   c. Adheres to hand hygiene recommendations
5. Maintains activity schedule
6. Exhibits no complications
   a. Maintains adequate weight or gains weight if indicated
   b. Exhibits normal results of tests of liver and kidney function
7. Takes steps to minimize side effects of medications
   a. Takes supplemental vitamins (vitamin B), as prescribed, to minimize peripheral neuropathy
   b. Avoids use of alcohol
   c. Avoids foods containing tyramine and histamine
   d. Has regular physical examinations and blood tests to evaluate liver and kidney function, neuropathy, hearing and visual acuity

LUNG ABSCESS

A lung abscess is a localized necrotic lesion of the lung parenchyma containing purulent material that collapses and forms a cavity. It is generally caused by aspiration of anaerobic bacteria. By definition, the chest x-ray will demonstrate a cavity of at least 2 cm. Patients who have impaired cough reflexes and cannot close the glottis, or those with swallowing difficulties, are at risk for aspirating foreign material and developing a lung abscess. Other at-risk patients include those with central nervous system disorders (seizure, stroke), drug addiction, alcoholism, esophageal disease, or compromised immune function, those without teeth, as well as patients receiving nasogastric tube feedings and those with an altered state of consciousness from anesthesia.

Pathophysiology

Most lung abscesses are a complication of bacterial pneumonia or are caused by aspiration of oral anaerobes into the lung. Abscesses also may occur secondary to mechanical or functional obstruction of the bronchi by a tumour, foreign body, or bronchial stenosis, or from necrotizing pneumonias, TB, pulmonary embolism, or chest trauma.

Most abscesses are found in areas of the lung that may be affected by aspiration. The site of the lung abscess is related to gravity and is determined by the patient's position. For patients who are confined to bed, the posterior segment of an upper lobe and the superior segment of the lower lobe are the most common areas in which lung abscess occurs. However, atypical presentations may occur, depending on the position of the patient when the aspiration occurred.

Initially, the cavity in the lung may or may not extend directly into a bronchus. Eventually the abscess becomes surrounded, or encapsulated, by a wall of fibrous tissue. The necrotic process may extend until it reaches the lumen of a bronchus or the pleural space and establishes communication with the respiratory tract, the pleural cavity, or both. If the bronchus is involved, the purulent contents are expectorated continuously in the form of sputum. If the pleura is involved, an empyema results. A communication or connection between the bronchus and pleura is known as a bronchopleural fistula.

The organisms frequently associated with lung abscesses are *S. aureus, Klebsiella,* and other gram-negative species. Anaerobic organisms, however, may also be present. The organism varies depending on the underlying predisposing factors.

Clinical Manifestations

The clinical manifestations of a lung abscess may vary from a mild productive cough to acute illness. Most patients have a fever and a productive cough with moderate to copious amounts of foul-smelling, often bloody, sputum. Leukocytosis may be present. Pleurisy or dull chest pain, dyspnea, weakness, anorexia, and weight loss are common. Fever and cough may develop insidiously and may have been present for several weeks before diagnosis.

Assessment and Diagnostic Findings

Physical examination of the chest may reveal dullness on percussion and decreased or absent breath sounds with an intermittent **pleural friction rub** (grating or rubbing sound) on auscultation. Crackles may be present. Confirmation of the diagnosis is made by chest x-ray, sputum culture, and in some cases fibreoptic bronchoscopy. The chest x-ray reveals an infiltrate with an air–fluid level. A computed tomography (CT) scan of the chest may be required to provide more detailed pictures of different cross-sectional areas of the lung.

Prevention

The following measures will reduce the risk of lung abscess:

- Appropriate antibiotic therapy before any dental procedures in patients who must have teeth extracted while their gums and teeth are infected
- Adequate dental and oral hygiene, because anaerobic bacteria play a role in the pathogenesis of lung abscess
- Appropriate antimicrobial therapy for patients with pneumonia

Medical Management

The findings of the history, physical examination, chest x-ray, and sputum culture indicate the type of organism and the treatment required. Adequate drainage of the lung abscess may be achieved through postural drainage and chest physiotherapy. The patient should be assessed for an adequate cough. A few patients need a percutaneous chest catheter placed for long-term drainage of the abscess. Therapeutic use of bronchoscopy to drain an abscess is uncommon. A diet high in protein and calories is necessary because

chronic infection is associated with a catabolic state, necessitating increased intake of calories and protein to facilitate healing. Surgical intervention is rare, but pulmonary resection (lobectomy) is performed when there is massive **hemoptysis** (coughing up of blood) or little or no response to medical management.

PHARMACOLOGIC THERAPY

Intravenous antimicrobial therapy depends on the results of the sputum culture and sensitivity and is administered for an extended period. Penicillin G or clindamycin (Cleocin) is the medication of choice, followed by penicillin with metronidazole. Large intravenous doses are generally required because the antibiotic must penetrate the necrotic tissue and the fluid in the abscess. The intravenous dose is continued until there is evidence of symptom improvement.

Long-term therapy with oral antibiotics replaces intravenous therapy after the patient shows signs of improvement (usually 3 to 5 days). Improvement is demonstrated by normal temperature, decreased white blood cell count, and improvement on the chest x-ray (resolution of surrounding infiltrate, reduction in cavity size, absence of fluid). Oral administration of antibiotic therapy is continued for an additional 4 to 8 weeks. If treatment stops too soon, a relapse may occur.

Nursing Management

The nurse administers antibiotics and intravenous therapies as prescribed and monitors for adverse effects. Chest physiotherapy is initiated as prescribed to facilitate drainage of the abscess. The nurse teaches the patient to perform deep-breathing and coughing exercises to help expand the lungs. To ensure proper nutritional intake, the nurse encourages a diet high in protein and calories. The nurse also offers emotional support because the abscess may take a long time to resolve.

PROMOTING HOME AND COMMUNITY-BASED CARE

Teaching Patients Self-Care. The patient who has had surgery may return home before the wound closes entirely or with a drain or tube in place. Thus, the patient or a caregiver needs instruction on how to change the dressings to prevent skin excoriation and odour, how to monitor for signs and symptoms of infection, and how to care for and maintain the drain or tube. The nurse instructs the patient to perform deep-breathing and coughing exercises every 2 hours during the day and shows a caregiver how to perform chest percussion and postural drainage to facilitate expectoration of lung secretions.

Continuing Care. Referral for home care may be required by some patients whose condition requires therapy at home. During visits to the patient at home, the nurse assesses the patient's physical condition, nutritional status, and home environment as well as the patient's and family's ability to carry out the therapeutic regimen. Patient teaching is reinforced during home visits, and nutrition counselling is provided with the goal of attaining and maintaining an optimal state of nutrition. To prevent a relapse, the nurse emphasizes the importance of completing the antibiotic regimen and of following the suggestions for rest and appropriate activity. If intravenous antibiotic therapy is to continue at home, the services of a home care nurse may be arranged to initiate intravenous therapy and to evaluate its administration by the patient or family. Although most outpatient intravenous therapy is administered in the home setting, a patient may visit a nearby clinic or physician's office for this treatment. In some cases the patient with lung abscess may have ignored his or her health. Therefore, it is important to use this opportunity to address health promotion strategies and health screening with the patient.

Pleural Conditions

Pleural conditions are disorders that involve the membranes covering the lungs (visceral pleura) and the surface of the chest wall (parietal pleura) or disorders affecting the pleural space.

PLEURISY

Pathophysiology

Pleurisy (pleuritis) refers to inflammation of both layers of the pleurae (parietal and visceral). Pleurisy may develop in conjunction with pneumonia or an upper respiratory tract infection, TB, or collagen disease; after trauma to the chest, pulmonary infarction, or pulmonary embolism; in patients with primary and metastatic cancer; and after thoracotomy. The parietal pleura has nerve endings; the visceral pleura does not. When the inflamed pleural membranes rub together during respiration (intensified on inspiration), the result is severe, sharp, knifelike pain.

Clinical Manifestations

The key characteristic of pleuritic pain is its relationship to respiratory movement. Taking a deep breath, coughing, or sneezing worsens the pain. Pleuritic pain is restricted in distribution rather than diffuse; it usually occurs only on one side. The pain may become minimal or absent when the breath is held, or it may be localized or radiate to the shoulder or abdomen. Later, as pleural fluid develops, the pain decreases.

Assessment and Diagnostic Findings

In the early period, when little fluid has accumulated, a pleural friction rub can be heard with the stethoscope, only to disappear later as more fluid accumulates and separates the inflamed pleural surfaces. Diagnostic tests may include chest x-rays, sputum examinations, thoracentesis to obtain a specimen of pleural fluid for examination, and less commonly a pleural biopsy.

Medical Management

The objectives of treatment are to discover the underlying condition causing the pleurisy and to relieve the pain. As the underlying disease (pneumonia, infection) is treated, the pleuritic inflammation usually resolves. At the same time, it is necessary to monitor for signs and symptoms of pleural effusion, such as shortness of breath, pain, assumption of a position that decreases pain, and decreased chest wall excursion.

Prescribed analgesics and topical applications of heat or cold provide symptomatic relief. Indomethacin, a nonsteroidal anti-inflammatory drug (NSAID), may provide pain relief while allowing the patient to take deep breaths and cough more effectively. If the pain is severe, an intercostal nerve block may be required.

Nursing Management

Because the patient has considerable pain on inspiration, the nurse can offer suggestions to enhance comfort, such as turning frequently onto the affected side to splint the chest wall and reduce the stretching of the pleurae. The nurse also can teach the patient to use the hands or a pillow to splint the rib cage while coughing.

PLEURAL EFFUSION

Pleural effusion, a collection of fluid in the pleural space, is rarely a primary disease process but is usually secondary to other diseases. Normally, the pleural space contains a small amount of fluid (5 to 15 mL), which acts as a lubricant that allows the pleural surfaces to move without friction (Fig. 23-5). Pleural effusion may be a complication of heart failure, TB, pneumonia, pulmonary infections (particularly viral infections), nephrotic syndrome, connective tissue disease, pulmonary embolism, and neoplastic tumours. Bronchogenic carcinoma is the most common malignancy associated with a pleural effusion.

Pathophysiology

In certain disorders, fluid may accumulate in the pleural space to a point where it becomes clinically evident. This almost always has pathologic significance. The effusion can be composed of a relatively clear fluid, or it can be bloody or purulent. An effusion

Physiology/Pathophysiology

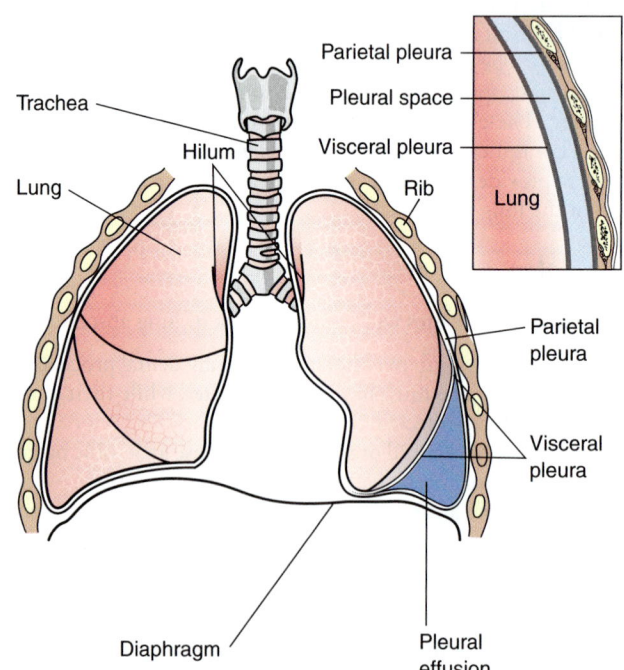

Trachea

Hilum

Lung

Parietal pleura

Pleural space

Visceral pleura

Rib

Lung

Parietal pleura

Visceral pleura

Diaphragm

Pleural effusion

FIGURE 23-5 In pleural effusion, an abnormal volume of fluid collects in the pleural space, causing pain and shortness of breath. Pleural effusion is usually secondary to other disease processes.

of clear fluid may be a transudate or an exudate. A transudate (filtrates of plasma that move across intact capillary walls) occurs when factors influencing the formation and reabsorption of pleural fluid are altered, usually by imbalances in hydrostatic or oncotic pressures. The finding of a transudative effusion generally implies that the pleural membranes are not diseased. The most common cause of a transudative effusion is heart failure. An exudate (extravasation of fluid into tissues or a cavity) usually results from inflammation by bacterial products or tumours involving the pleural surfaces.

Clinical Manifestations

Usually the clinical manifestations are those caused by the underlying disease. Pneumonia causes fever, chills, and pleuritic chest pain, whereas a malignant effusion may result in dyspnea and coughing. The size of the effusion and the patient's underlying lung disease determine the severity of symptoms. A large pleural effusion causes shortness of breath. When a small to moderate pleural effusion is present, dyspnea may be absent or only minimal. The severity of the symptoms assessed depends on the time course of the development of the pleural effusion and the patient's underlying disease.

Assessment and Diagnostic Findings

Assessment of the area of the pleural effusion reveals decreased or absent breath sounds, decreased fremitus, and a dull, flat sound when percussed. In an extremely large pleural effusion, the assessment reveals a patient in acute respiratory distress. Tracheal deviation away from the affected side may also be noted.

Physical examination, chest x-ray, chest CT scan, and thoracentesis confirm the presence of fluid. In some instances, a lateral decubitus x-ray is obtained. For this x-ray, the patient lies on the affected side in a side-lying position. A pleural effusion can be diagnosed because this position allows for the "layering out" of the fluid, and an air–fluid line is visible.

Pleural fluid is analyzed by bacterial culture, Gram stain, acid-fast bacillus stain (for TB), red and white blood cell counts, chemistry studies (glucose, amylase, lactic dehydrogenase, protein), cytologic analysis for malignant cells, and pH. A pleural biopsy also may be performed.

Medical Management

The objectives of treatment are to discover the underlying cause, to prevent reaccumulation of fluid, and to relieve discomfort, dyspnea, and respiratory compromise. Specific treatment is directed at the underlying cause (eg, heart failure, pneumonia, lung cancer, cirrhosis). If the pleural fluid is an exudate, more extensive diagnostic procedures are performed to determine the cause. Treatment for the primary cause is then instituted.

Thoracentesis is performed to remove fluid, to obtain a specimen for analysis, and to relieve dyspnea and respiratory compromise (see Chap. 21). Thoracentesis may be performed under ultrasound guidance. Depending on the size of the pleural effusion, the patient may be treated by removing the fluid during the thoracentesis procedure or by inserting a chest tube connected to a water-seal drainage system or suction to evacuate the pleural space and re-expand the lung.

If the underlying cause is a malignancy, however, the effusion tends to recur within a few days or weeks. Repeated thoracente-ses result in pain, depletion of protein and electrolytes, and sometimes pneumothorax. Once the pleural space is adequately drained, a chemical pleurodesis may be performed to obliterate the pleural space and prevent reaccumulation of fluid. Pleurodesis may be performed using a thoracoscopic approach or via a chest tube. Chemically irritating agents (eg., bleomycin or talc) are instilled in the pleural space. With the chest tube insertion approach, after the agent is instilled, the chest tube is clamped for 60 to 90 minutes and the patient is assisted to assume various positions to promote uniform distribution of the agent and to maximize its contact with the pleural surfaces. The tube is unclamped as prescribed, and chest drainage may be continued several days longer to prevent reaccumulation of fluid and to promote the formation of adhesions between the visceral and parietal pleurae.

Other treatments for malignant pleural effusions include surgical pleurectomy, insertion of a small catheter attached to a drainage bottle for outpatient management, or implantation of a pleuroperitoneal shunt. A pleuroperitoneal shunt consists of two catheters connected by a pump chamber containing two one-way valves. Fluid moves from the pleural space to the pump chamber and then to the peritoneal cavity. The patient manually pumps on the reservoir daily to move fluid from the pleural space to the peritoneal space (Taubert & Wright, 2000).

Nursing Management

The nurse's role in the care of the patient with a pleural effusion includes implementing the medical regimen. The nurse prepares and positions the patient for thoracentesis and offers support throughout the procedure. Pain management is a priority, and the nurse assists the patient to assume positions that are the least painful. However, frequent turning and ambulation are important to facilitate drainage. The nurse administers analgesics as prescribed and as needed.

If a chest tube drainage and water-seal system is used, the nurse is responsible for monitoring the system's function and recording the amount of drainage at prescribed intervals. Nursing care related to the underlying cause of the pleural effusion is specific to the underlying condition. Care of the patient with a chest tube is discussed in Chapter 25.

If the patient is to be managed as an outpatient with a pleural catheter for drainage, the nurse is responsible for educating the patient and family regarding management and care of the catheter and drainage system.

EMPYEMA

An empyema is an accumulation of thick, purulent fluid within the pleural space, often with fibrin development and a loculated (walled-off) area where infection is located. Most empyemas occur as complications of bacterial pneumonia or lung abscess. Other causes include penetrating chest trauma, hematogenous infection of the pleural space, nonbacterial infections, or iatrogenic causes (after thoracic surgery or thoracentesis).

Pathophysiology

At first the pleural fluid is thin, with a low leukocyte count, but it frequently progresses to a fibropurulent stage and, finally, to a stage where it encloses the lung within a thick exudative membrane (loculated empyema).

Clinical Manifestations

With an empyema, the patient is acutely ill and has signs and symptoms similar to those of an acute respiratory infection or pneumonia (fever, night sweats, pleural pain, cough, dyspnea, anorexia, weight loss). If the patient is immunocompromised, the symptoms may be more vague. If the patient has received antimicrobial therapy, the clinical manifestations may be less obvious.

Assessment and Diagnostic Findings

Chest auscultation demonstrates decreased or absent breath sounds over the affected area, and there is dullness on chest percussion as well as decreased fremitus. The diagnosis is established by a chest x-ray or chest CT scan. Usually a diagnostic thoracentesis is performed, often under ultrasound guidance.

Medical Management

The objectives of treatment are to drain the pleural cavity and to achieve full expansion of the lung. The fluid is drained and appropriate antibiotics, in large doses, are prescribed based on the causative organism. Sterilization of the empyema cavity requires 4 to 6 weeks of antibiotics. Drainage of the pleural fluid depends on the stage of the disease and is accomplished by one of the following methods:

- Needle aspiration (thoracentesis) with a thin percutaneous catheter, if the volume is small and the fluid not too purulent or thick
- Tube thoracostomy (chest drainage using a large-diameter intercostal tube attached to water-seal drainage [see Chap. 25]) with fibrinolytic agents instilled through the chest tube in patients with loculated or complicated pleural effusions
- Open chest drainage via thoracotomy, including potential rib resection, to remove the thickened pleura, pus, and debris and to remove the underlying diseased pulmonary tissue

With long-standing inflammation, an exudate can form over the lung, trapping it and interfering with its normal expansion. This exudate must be removed surgically (decortication). The drainage tube is left in place until the pus-filled space is obliterated completely. The complete obliteration of the pleural space is monitored by serial chest x-rays, and the patient should be informed that treatment may be long term. Patients are frequently discharged from the hospital with a chest tube in place, with instructions to monitor fluid drainage at home.

Nursing Management

Resolution of empyema is a prolonged process. The nurse helps the patient cope with the condition and instructs the patient in lung-expanding breathing exercises to restore normal respiratory function. The nurse also provides care specific to the method of drainage of the pleural fluid (eg, needle aspiration, closed chest drainage, or rib resection and drainage). When a patient is discharged to home with a drainage tube or system in place, the nurse instructs the patient and family on care of the drainage system and drain site, measurement and observation of drainage, signs and symptoms of infection, and how and when to contact the health care provider. (See Nursing Process: The Patient Undergoing Thoracic Surgery in Chapter 25.)

Pulmonary Edema

Pulmonary edema is defined as abnormal accumulation of fluid in the lung tissue and/or alveolar space. It is a severe, life-threatening condition.

Pathophysiology

Pulmonary edema most commonly occurs as a result of increased microvascular pressure from abnormal cardiac function. The backup of blood into the pulmonary vasculature resulting from inadequate left ventricular function causes an increased microvascular pressure, and fluid begins to leak into the interstitial space and the alveoli. Other causes of pulmonary edema are hypervolemia or a sudden increase in the intravascular pressure in the lung. One example of this is in the patient who has undergone pneumonectomy. When one lung has been removed, all the cardiac output then goes to the remaining lung. If the patient's fluid status is not monitored closely, pulmonary edema can quickly develop in the postoperative period as the patient's pulmonary vasculature attempts to adapt. This type of pulmonary edema is sometimes termed "flash" pulmonary edema. A second example is called re-expansion pulmonary edema. This may be due to a rapid reinflation of the lung after removal of air from a pneumothorax or evacuation of fluid from a large pleural effusion.

Clinical Manifestations

The patient has increasing respiratory distress, characterized by dyspnea, air hunger, and central cyanosis. The patient is usually very anxious and often agitated. As the fluid leaks into the alveoli and mixes with air, a foam or froth is formed. The patient coughs up or the nurse suctions out these foamy, frothy, and often blood-tinged secretions. The patient has acute respiratory distress and may become confused or stuporous.

Assessment and Diagnostic Findings

Auscultation reveals crackles in the lung bases (especially in the posterior bases) that rapidly progress toward the apices of the lungs. These crackles are due to the movement of air through the alveolar fluid. The chest x-ray reveals increased interstitial markings. The patient may be tachycardic, the pulse oximetry values begin to fall, and arterial blood gas analysis demonstrates increasing hypoxemia.

Medical Management

Management focuses on correcting the underlying disorder. If the pulmonary edema is cardiac in origin, then improvement in left ventricular function is the goal. Vasodilators, inotropic medications, afterload or preload agents, or contractility medications may be given. Additional cardiac measures (eg, intra-aortic balloon pump) may be indicated if the patient does not respond. If the problem is fluid overload, diuretics are given and the patient is placed on fluid restrictions. Oxygen is administered to correct the hypoxemia; in some circumstances, intubation and mechanical ventilation are necessary. The patient is extremely anxious, and morphine is administered to reduce anxiety and control pain.

Nursing Management

Nursing management of the patient with pulmonary edema includes assisting with administration of oxygen and intubation and mechanical ventilation if respiratory failure occurs. The nurse also administers medications (ie, morphine, vasodilators, inotropic medications, preload and afterload agents) as prescribed and monitors the patient's response. Nursing management in pulmonary edema is described in more detail in Chapter 30.

Acute Respiratory Failure

Respiratory failure is a sudden and life-threatening deterioration of the gas exchange function of the lung. It exists when the exchange of oxygen for carbon dioxide in the lungs cannot keep up with the rate of oxygen consumption and carbon dioxide production by the cells of the body.

Acute respiratory failure (ARF) is defined as a fall in arterial oxygen tension (PaO_2) to less than 50 mm Hg (hypoxemia) and a rise in arterial carbon dioxide tension ($PaCO_2$) to greater than 50 mm Hg (hypercapnia), with an arterial pH of less than 7.35. In ARF, the ventilation or perfusion mechanisms in the lung are impaired. Respiratory system mechanisms leading to ARF include:

- Alveolar hypoventilation
- Diffusion abnormalities
- Ventilation–perfusion mismatching
- Shunting

It is important to distinguish between ARF and chronic respiratory failure. Chronic respiratory failure is defined as a deterioration in the gas exchange function of the lung that has developed insidiously or has persisted for a long period after an episode of ARF. The absence of acute symptoms and the presence of a chronic respiratory acidosis suggest the chronicity of the respiratory failure. Two causes of chronic respiratory failure are COPD (discussed in Chap. 24) and neuromuscular diseases (discussed in Chap. 65). Patients with these disorders develop a tolerance to the gradually worsening hypoxemia and hypercapnia. However, a patient with chronic respiratory failure may develop ARF. This is seen in the COPD patient who develops an exacerbation or infection that causes additional deterioration of the gas exchange mechanism. The principles of management of acute versus chronic respiratory failure are different; the following discussion will be limited to ARF.

Pathophysiology

Common causes of ARF can be classified into four categories: decreased respiratory drive, dysfunction of the chest wall, dysfunction of the lung parenchyma, and other causes.

DECREASED RESPIRATORY DRIVE

Decreased respiratory drive may occur with severe brain injury, large lesions of the brain stem (multiple sclerosis), use of sedative medications, and metabolic disorders such as hypothyroidism. These disorders impair the normal response of chemoreceptors in the brain to normal respiratory stimulation.

DYSFUNCTION OF THE CHEST WALL

The impulses arising in the respiratory centre travel through nerves that extend from the brain stem down the spinal cord to receptors in the muscles of respiration. Thus, any disease or disorder of the nerves, spinal cord, muscles, or neuromuscular junc-

tion involved in respiration seriously affects ventilation and may ultimately lead to ARF. These include musculoskeletal disorders (muscular dystrophy, polymyositis), neuromuscular junction disorders (myasthenia gravis, poliomyelitis), some peripheral nerve disorders, and spinal cord disorders (amyotrophic lateral sclerosis, Guillain-Barré syndrome, and cervical spinal cord injuries).

DYSFUNCTION OF LUNG PARENCHYMA

Pleural effusion, hemothorax, pneumothorax, and upper airway obstruction are conditions that interfere with ventilation by preventing expansion of the lung. These conditions, which may cause respiratory failure, usually are produced by an underlying lung disease, pleural disease, or trauma and injury. Other diseases and conditions of the lung that lead to ARF include pneumonia, status asthmaticus, lobar atelectasis, pulmonary embolism, and pulmonary edema.

OTHER CAUSES

In the postoperative period, especially after major thoracic or abdominal surgery, inadequate ventilation and respiratory failure may occur because of several factors. During this period, for example, ARF may be caused by the effects of anesthetic agents, analgesics, and sedatives, which may depress respiration as described earlier or enhance the effects of opioids and lead to hypoventilation. Pain may interfere with deep breathing and coughing. A mismatch of ventilation to perfusion is the usual cause of respiratory failure after major abdominal, cardiac, or thoracic surgery.

Clinical Manifestations

Early signs are those associated with impaired oxygenation and may include restlessness, fatigue, headache, dyspnea, air hunger, tachycardia, and increased blood pressure. As the hypoxemia progresses, more obvious signs may be present, including confusion, lethargy, tachycardia, tachypnea, central cyanosis, diaphoresis, and finally respiratory arrest. Physical findings are those of acute respiratory distress, including use of accessory muscles, decreased breath sounds if the patient cannot adequately ventilate, and other findings related specifically to the underlying disease process and cause of ARF.

Medical Management

The objectives of treatment are to correct the underlying cause and to restore adequate gas exchange in the lung. Intubation and mechanical ventilation may be required to maintain adequate ventilation and oxygenation while the underlying cause is corrected.

Nursing Management

Nursing management of the patient with ARF includes assisting with intubation and maintaining mechanical ventilation (described in Chap. 25). The nurse assesses the patient's respiratory status by monitoring the patient's level of response, arterial blood gases, pulse oximetry, and vital signs and assessing the respiratory system. The nurse implements strategies (eg, turning schedule, mouth care, skin care, range of motion of extremities) to prevent complications. The nurse also assesses the patient's understanding of the management strategies that are used and initiates some form of communication to enable the patient to express his or her needs to the health care team. Nursing care also addresses the problems that led to ARF. As the patient's status improves, the nurse assesses the patient's knowledge of the underlying disorder and provides teaching as appropriate to address the underlying disorder.

Acute Respiratory Distress Syndrome

Acute respiratory distress syndrome (ARDS; previously called adult respiratory distress syndrome) is a clinical syndrome characterized by a sudden and progressive pulmonary edema, increasing bilateral infiltrates on chest x-ray, hypoxemia refractory to oxygen supplementation, and reduced lung compliance. These signs occur in the absence of left-sided heart failure. Patients with ARDS usually require mechanical ventilation with a higher-than-normal airway pressure. A wide range of factors are associated with the development of ARDS (Chart 23-6), including direct injury to the lungs (eg, smoke inhalation) or indirect insult to the lungs (eg, shock). ARDS has been associated with a mortality rate as high as 50% to 60%. The major cause of death in ARDS is nonpulmonary multiple-system organ failure, often with sepsis.

Pathophysiology

ARDS occurs as a result of an inflammatory trigger that initiates the release of cellular and chemical mediators, causing injury to the alveolar capillary membrane. This results in leakage of fluid into the alveolar interstitial spaces and alterations in the capillary bed.

Severe ventilation–perfusion mismatching occurs in ARDS. Alveoli collapse because of the inflammatory infiltrate, blood, fluid, and surfactant dysfunction. Small airways are narrowed because of interstitial fluid and bronchial obstruction. The lung compliance becomes markedly decreased (stiff lungs), and the result is a characteristic decrease in functional residual capacity and severe hypoxemia. The blood returning to the lung for gas exchange is pumped through the nonventilated, nonfunctioning areas of the lung, causing a shunt to develop. This means that blood is interfacing with nonfunctioning alveoli and gas exchange is markedly impaired, resulting in severe, refractory hypoxemia. Figure 23-6 shows the sequence of pathophysiologic events leading to ARDS.

Chart 23-6   Etiologic Factors Related to ARDS

Aspiration (gastric secretions, drowning, hydrocarbons)
Drug ingestion and overdose
Hematologic disorders (disseminated intravascular coagulopathy [DIC], massive transfusions, cardiopulmonary bypass)
Prolonged inhalation of high concentrations of oxygen, smoke, or corrosive substances
Localized infection (bacterial, fungal, viral pneumonia)
Metabolic disorders (pancreatitis, uremia)
Shock (any cause)
Trauma (pulmonary contusion, multiple fractures, head injury)
Major surgery
Fat or air embolism
Systemic sepsis

Clinical Manifestations

Clinically, the acute phase of ARDS is marked by a rapid onset of severe dyspnea that usually occurs 12 to 48 hours after the initiating event. A characteristic feature is arterial hypoxemia that does not respond to supplemental oxygen. On chest x-ray, the findings are similar to those seen with cardiogenic pulmonary edema and present as bilateral infiltrates that quickly worsen. The acute lung injury then progresses to fibrosing alveolitis with persistent, severe hypoxemia. The patient also has increased alveolar dead space (ventilation to alveoli, but poor perfusion) and decreased pulmonary compliance ("stiff lungs," which are difficult to ventilate). Clinically, a patient is thought to be in the recovery phase if the hypoxemia gradually resolves, the chest x-ray improves, and the lungs become more compliant (Ware & Matthay, 2000).

Assessment and Diagnostic Findings

Intercostal retractions and crackles, as the fluid begins to leak into the alveolar interstitial space, are evident on physical examination. A diagnosis of ARDS may be made based on the following crite-

 ## Physiology/Pathophysiology

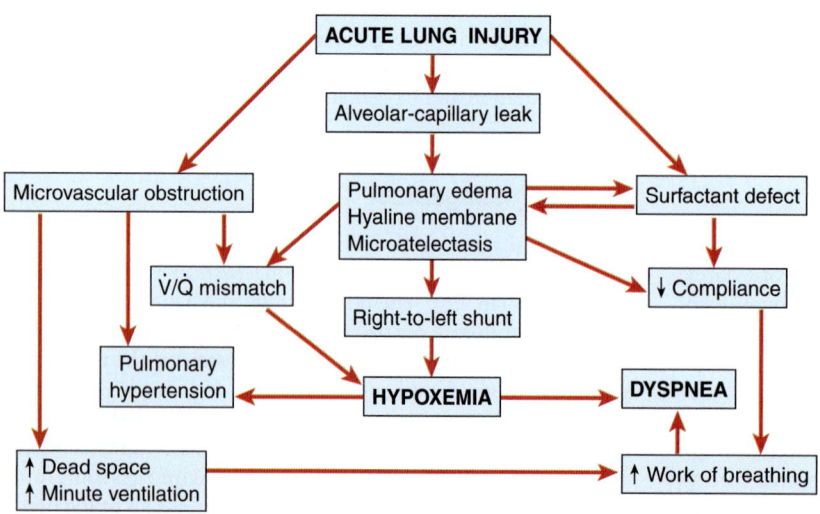

FIGURE 23-6 Pathogenesis and pathophysiology of acute respiratory distress syndrome. Adapted from Farzan, S. (1997). *A concise handbook of respiratory diseases* (4th ed.). Stamford, CT: Appleton & Lange.

ria: a history of systemic or pulmonary risk factors, acute onset of respiratory distress, bilateral pulmonary infiltrates, clinical absence of left-sided heart failure, and a ratio of partial pressure of oxygen of arterial blood to fraction of inspired oxygen (PaO_2/FiO_2) less than 200 mm Hg (severe refractory hypoxemia).

Medical Management

The primary focus in the management of ARDS includes identification and treatment of the underlying condition. Aggressive, supportive care must be provided to compensate for the severe respiratory dysfunction. This supportive therapy almost always includes intubation and mechanical ventilation. In addition, circulatory support, adequate fluid volume, and nutritional support are important. Supplemental oxygen is used as the patient begins the initial spiral of hypoxemia. As the hypoxemia progresses, intubation and mechanical ventilation are instituted. The concentration of oxygen and ventilator settings and modes are determined by the patient's status. This is monitored by arterial blood gas analysis, pulse oximetry, and bedside pulmonary function testing.

Positive end-expiratory pressure (PEEP) is a critical part of the treatment of ARDS. PEEP usually improves oxygenation, but it does not influence the natural history of the syndrome. Use of PEEP helps to increase functional residual capacity and reverse alveolar collapse by keeping the alveoli open, resulting in improved arterial oxygenation and a reduction in the severity of the ventilation–perfusion imbalance. By using PEEP, a lower FiO_2 may be required. The goal is a PaO_2 greater than 60 mm Hg or an oxygen saturation level of greater than 90% at the lowest possible FiO_2. PEEP and modes of mechanical ventilation are discussed in Chapter 25.

Systemic hypotension may occur in ARDS as a result of hypovolemia secondary to leakage of fluid into the interstitial spaces and depressed cardiac output from high levels of PEEP therapy. Hypovolemia must be carefully treated without causing further overload. Intravenous crystalloid solutions are administered, with careful monitoring of pulmonary status. Inotropic or vasopressor agents may be required. Pulmonary artery pressure catheters are used to monitor the patient's fluid status and the severe and progressive pulmonary hypertension sometimes observed in ARDS.

PHARMACOLOGIC THERAPY

Numerous pharmacologic treatments are under investigation to stop the cascade of events leading to ARDS. These include human recombinant interleukin-1 receptor antagonist, neutrophil inhibitors, pulmonary-specific vasodilators, surfactant replacement therapy, antisepsis agents, antioxidant therapy, and corticosteroids late in the course of ARDS (Ware & Matthay, 2000).

NUTRITIONAL THERAPY

Adequate nutritional support is vital in the treatment of ARDS. Patients with ARDS require 35 to 45 kcal/kg per day to meet caloric requirements. Enteral feeding is the first consideration; however, parenteral nutrition also may be required.

Nursing Management

GENERAL MEASURES

The patient with ARDS is critically ill and requires close monitoring because the condition could quickly change to a life-threatening situation. Most of the respiratory modalities discussed in Chapter 25 are used in this situation (oxygen administration, nebulizer therapy, chest physiotherapy, endotracheal intubation or tracheostomy, mechanical ventilation, suctioning, bronchoscopy). Frequent assessment of the patient's status is necessary to evaluate the effectiveness of treatment.

In addition to implementing the medical plan of care, the nurse considers other needs of the patient. Positioning is important. The nurse should turn the patient frequently to improve ventilation and perfusion in the lungs and enhance secretion drainage. However, the nurse must closely monitor the patient for deterioration in oxygenation with changes in position. Oxygenation in the ARDS patient is sometimes improved in the prone position and may be used in special circumstances; studies to assess the benefits and problems of such positioning are ongoing (Curley, 2000; Marion, 2001).

The patient is extremely anxious and agitated because of the increasing hypoxemia and dyspnea. The nurse should explain all procedures and provide care in a calm, reassuring manner. It is important to reduce the patient's anxiety because anxiety prevents rest and increases oxygen expenditure. Rest is essential to reduce oxygen consumption, thereby reducing oxygen needs.

VENTILATOR CONSIDERATIONS

If the patient is intubated and receiving mechanical ventilation with PEEP, several considerations must be addressed. PEEP, which causes increased end-expiratory pressure, is an unnatural pattern of breathing and feels strange to the patient. The patient may be anxious and "fight" the ventilator. Nursing assessment is important to assess for problems with ventilation that may be causing the anxiety reaction: tube blockage by kinking or retained secretions; other acute respiratory problems (eg, pneumothorax, pain); a sudden drop in the oxygen level; the patient's level of dyspnea; or ventilator malfunction. In some cases, sedation may be required to decrease the patient's oxygen consumption, allow the ventilator to provide full support of ventilation, and decrease the patient's anxiety. Possible sedatives are lorazepam (Ativan), midazolam (Versed), haloperidol (Haldol), propofol (Diprivan), and short-acting barbiturates.

If the PEEP level cannot be maintained despite the use of sedatives, neuromuscular blocking agents, such as pancuronium (Pavulon), vecuronium (Norcuron), atracurium (Tracrium), and rocuronium (Zemuron), may be given to paralyze the patient. This allows the patient to be ventilated more easily. With paralysis, the patient appears unconscious, loses motor function, and cannot breathe, talk, or blink independently. However, the patient retains sensation and is awake and able to hear. The nurse must reassure the patient that the paralysis is a result of the medication and is temporary. Paralysis should be used for the shortest possible time and never without adequate sedation.

Use of paralytic agents has many dangers and side effects. The nurse must be sure the patient does not become disconnected from the ventilator, because respiratory muscles are paralyzed and the patient will be apneic. Consequently, the nurse ensures that the patient is closely monitored at all times. All ventilator and patient alarms should be on at all times. Eye care is important as well because the patient cannot blink, increasing the risk of corneal abrasions. Neuromuscular blockers predispose patients to the development of deep venous thrombi, muscle atrophy, and skin breakdown. Nursing assessment is essential to minimize the complications related to neuromuscular blockade. The patient may have discomfort or pain but cannot communicate these sensations.

Analgesia is usually administered concurrently with neuromuscular blocking agents. The nurse must anticipate the patient's needs regarding pain and comfort. The nurse checks the patient's position to ensure it is comfortable and in normal alignment and talks to, and not about, the patient while in the patient's presence.

In addition, it is important for the nurse to describe the purpose and effects of the paralytic agents to the family. This experience can be very frightening to family members if they are unaware that these agents have been administered.

Pulmonary Hypertension

Pulmonary hypertension is a condition that is not clinically evident until late in its progression. Pulmonary hypertension exists when the systolic pulmonary artery pressure exceeds 30 mm Hg or the mean pulmonary artery pressure exceeds 25 mm Hg. These pressures cannot be measured indirectly as can systemic blood pressure; instead, they must be measured during right-sided heart catheterization. In the absence of these measurements, clinical recognition becomes the only indicator for the presence of pulmonary hypertension.

There are two forms of pulmonary hypertension: primary (or idiopathic) and secondary. Primary pulmonary hypertension is an uncommon disease in which the diagnosis is made by excluding all other possible causes. The exact cause is unknown, but there are several possible causes (Chart 23-7). The clinical presentation of primary pulmonary hypertension exists with no evidence of pulmonary and cardiac disease or pulmonary embolism. It occurs most often in women 20 to 40 years of age and is usually fatal within 5 years of diagnosis.

Chart 23-7

Causes of Pulmonary Hypertension

Primary or Idiopathic
  Altered immune mechanisms
  Silent pulmonary emboli
  Raynaud's phenomenon
  Oral contraceptive use
  Sickle cell disease
  Collagen diseases

Secondary
  Pulmonary vasoconstriction due to hypoxemia
    Chronic obstructive pulmonary disease
    Kyphoscoliosis
    Obesity
    Smoke inhalation
    High altitude
    Neuromuscular disorders
    Diffuse interstitial pneumonia
  Reduction of the pulmonary vascular bed (must impair 50% to 75% of the vascular bed)
    Pulmonary emboli
    Vasculitis
    Widespread interstitial lung disease (sarcoidosis, systemic sclerosis)
    Tumour emboli
  Primary cardiac disease
    Congenital (patent ductus arteriosus, atrial septal defect, ventricular septal defect)
    Acquired (rheumatic valvular disease, mitral stenosis, myxoma, left ventricular failure)

Secondary pulmonary hypertension is more common and results from existing cardiac or pulmonary disease. The prognosis depends on the severity of the underlying disorder and the changes in the pulmonary vascular bed. A common cause of secondary pulmonary hypertension is pulmonary artery constriction due to hypoxemia from COPD.

Pathophysiology

The underlying process of pulmonary hypertension varies, and multiple factors are often responsible. Normally, the pulmonary vascular bed can handle the blood volume delivered by the right ventricle. It has a low resistance to blood flow and compensates for increased blood volume by dilation of the vessels in the pulmonary circulation. However, if the pulmonary vascular bed is destroyed or obstructed, as in pulmonary hypertension, the ability to handle whatever flow or volume of blood it receives is impaired, and the increased blood flow then increases the pulmonary artery pressure. As the pulmonary arterial pressure increases, the pulmonary vascular resistance also increases. Both pulmonary artery constriction (as in hypoxemia or hypercapnia) and a reduction of the pulmonary vascular bed (which occurs with pulmonary emboli) result in an increase in pulmonary vascular resistance and pressure. This increased workload affects right ventricular function. The myocardium ultimately cannot meet the increasing demands imposed on it, leading to right ventricular hypertrophy (enlargement and dilation) and failure.

Clinical Manifestations

Dyspnea is the main symptom of pulmonary hypertension, occurring at first with exertion and eventually at rest. Substernal chest pain also is common, affecting 25% to 50% of patients. Other signs and symptoms include weakness, fatigue, syncope, occasional hemoptysis, and signs of right-sided heart failure (peripheral edema, ascites, distended neck veins, liver engorgement, crackles, heart murmur).

Assessment and Diagnostic Findings

A complete diagnostic evaluation includes a history, physical examination, chest x-ray, pulmonary function studies, electrocardiogram (ECG), echocardiogram, ventilation–perfusion scan, and cardiac catheterization. In some cases, a lung biopsy, performed by thoracotomy or thoracoscopy, may be needed to make a definite diagnosis. Cardiac catheterization of the right side of the heart reveals elevated pulmonary arterial pressure. An echocardiogram can assess the progression of the disease and rule out other conditions with similar signs and symptoms. The ECG reveals right ventricular hypertrophy, right axis deviation, and tall peaked P waves in inferior leads, tall anterior R waves, and ST-segment depression and/or T-wave inversion anteriorly. The PaO_2 also is decreased (hypoxemia). A ventilation–perfusion scan or pulmonary angiography detects defects in pulmonary vasculature, such as pulmonary emboli. Pulmonary function studies may be normal or show a slight decrease in vital capacity (VC) and lung compliance, with a mild decrease in the diffusing capacity.

Medical Management

The goal of treatment is to manage the underlying cardiac or pulmonary condition. Most patients with primary pulmonary hypertension do not have hypoxemia at rest but require supplemental oxygen with exercise. However, patients with severe ventricular failure, decreased cardiac output, and progressive disease may have resting hypoxemia and require continuous oxygen supplementation. Appropriate oxygen therapy (see Chap. 25) reverses the vasoconstriction and reduces the pulmonary hypertension in a relatively short time.

In the presence of cor pulmonale, which is discussed in the section that follows, treatment should include fluid restriction, diuretics to decrease fluid accumulation, cardiac glycosides (eg, digitalis) in an attempt to improve cardiac function, calcium channel blockers for vasodilation, and rest. In primary pulmonary hypertension, vasodilators have been administered with variable success (eg, calcium channel blockers, intravenous prostacyclin). Prostacyclin (PGX [Flolan]) is one of the prostaglandins produced by the pulmonary endothelium. Intravenous prostacyclin (epoprostenol) helps to decrease pulmonary hypertension by reducing pulmonary vascular resistance and pressures and increasing cardiac output. Anticoagulants such as warfarin (Coumadin) have been given to patients because of chronic pulmonary emboli. Heart–lung transplantation has been successful in select patients with primary hypertension who have not been responsive to other therapies.

Nursing Management

The major nursing goal is to identify patients at high risk for pulmonary hypertension, such as those with COPD, pulmonary emboli, congenital heart disease, and mitral valve disease. The nurse also must be alert for signs and symptoms, administer oxygen therapy appropriately, and instruct patients and their families about the use of home oxygen supplementation.

Pulmonary Heart Disease (Cor Pulmonale)

Cor pulmonale is a condition in which the right ventricle of the heart enlarges (with or without right-sided heart failure) as a result of diseases that affect the structure or function of the lung or its vasculature. Any disease affecting the lungs and accompanied by hypoxemia may result in cor pulmonale. The most frequent cause is severe COPD (see Chap. 24), in which changes in the airway and retained secretions reduce alveolar ventilation. Other causes are conditions that restrict or compromise ventilatory function, leading to hypoxemia or acidosis (deformities of the thoracic cage, massive obesity), or conditions that reduce the pulmonary vascular bed (primary idiopathic pulmonary arterial hypertension, pulmonary embolus). Certain disorders of the nervous system, respiratory muscles, chest wall, and pulmonary arterial tree also may be responsible for cor pulmonale.

Pathophysiology

Pulmonary disease can produce physiologic changes that in time affect the heart and cause the right ventricle to enlarge and eventually fail. Any condition that deprives the lungs of oxygen can cause hypoxemia and hypercapnia, resulting in ventilatory insufficiency. Hypoxemia and hypercapnia cause pulmonary arterial vasoconstriction and possibly reduction of the pulmonary vascular bed, as in emphysema or pulmonary emboli. The result is increased resistance in the pulmonary circulatory system, with a subsequent rise in pulmonary blood pressure (pulmonary hypertension). A mean pulmonary arterial pressure of 45 mm Hg or more may occur in cor pulmonale. Right ventricular hypertrophy

may result, followed by right ventricular failure. In short, cor pulmonale results from pulmonary hypertension, which causes the right side of the heart to enlarge because of the increased work required to pump blood against high resistance through the pulmonary vascular system.

Clinical Manifestations

Symptoms of cor pulmonale are usually related to the underlying lung disease, such as COPD. With right ventricular failure, the patient may develop increasing edema of the feet and legs, distended neck veins, an enlarged palpable liver, pleural effusion, ascites, and a heart murmur. Headache, confusion, and somnolence may occur as a result of increased levels of carbon dioxide (hypercapnia). Patients often complain of increasing shortness of breath, wheezing, cough, and fatigue.

Medical Management

The objectives of treatment are to improve the patient's ventilation and to treat both the underlying lung disease and the manifestations of heart disease. Supplemental oxygen is administered to improve gas exchange and to reduce pulmonary arterial pressure and pulmonary vascular resistance. Improved oxygen transport relieves the pulmonary hypertension that is causing the cor pulmonale.

Better survival rates and greater reduction in pulmonary vascular resistance have been reported with continuous, 24-hour oxygen therapy for patients with severe hypoxemia. Substantial improvement may require 4 to 6 weeks of oxygen therapy, usually in the home. Periodic assessment of pulse oximetry and arterial blood gases is necessary to determine the adequacy of alveolar ventilation and to monitor the effectiveness of oxygen therapy.

Ventilation is further improved with chest physical therapy and bronchial hygiene manoeuvres as indicated to remove accumulated secretions, and the administration of bronchodilators. Further measures depend on the patient's condition. If the patient is in respiratory failure, endotracheal intubation and mechanical ventilation may be necessary. If the patient is in heart failure, hypoxemia and hypercapnia must be relieved to improve cardiac function and output. Bed rest, sodium restriction, and diuretic therapy also are instituted judiciously to reduce peripheral edema (to lower pulmonary arterial pressure through a decrease in total blood volume) and the circulatory load on the right side of the heart. Digitalis may be prescribed to relieve pulmonary hypertension if the patient also has left ventricular failure, a supraventricular dysrhythmia, or right ventricular failure that does not respond to other therapy.

ECG monitoring may be indicated because of the high incidence of dysrhythmias in patients with cor pulmonale. Any pulmonary infection must be treated promptly to avoid further impaired gas exchange and exacerbations of hypoxemia and pulmonary heart disease. The prognosis depends on whether the pulmonary hypertension is reversible. (Management of acute respiratory failure was presented earlier in this chapter.)

Nursing Management

Nursing care of the patient with cor pulmonale addresses the underlying disorder leading to cor pulmonale as well as the problems related to pulmonary hyperventilation and right-sided cardiac failure. If intubation and mechanical ventilation are required to manage ARF, the nurse assists with the intubation procedure and maintains mechanical ventilation. The nurse assesses the patient's respiratory and cardiac status and administers medications as prescribed.

During the patient's hospital stay, the nurse instructs the patient about the importance of close monitoring (fluid retention, weight gain, edema) and adherence to the therapeutic regimen, especially the 24-hour use of oxygen. Factors that affect the patient's adherence to the treatment regimen are explored and addressed.

PROMOTING HOME AND COMMUNITY-BASED CARE

Teaching Patients Self-Care. Most of the care and monitoring of the patient with cor pulmonale is performed by the patient and family in the home because it is a chronic disorder. If supplemental oxygen is administered, the nurse instructs the patient and the family in its use. Nutrition counselling is warranted if the patient is on a sodium-restricted diet or is taking diuretics. The nurse teaches the family to monitor for signs and symptoms of right ventricular failure and about emergency interventions and when to call for assistance. Most importantly, the nurse urges the patient to stop smoking.

Continuing Care. A referral for home care may be warranted for the patient who cannot manage self-care or for the patient whose physical condition warrants close assessment. During the home visit, the home care nurse evaluates the patient's status and the patient's and family members' understanding of the therapeutic regimen and their adherence to it. If oxygen is used in the home, the nurse determines if it is being administered safely and as prescribed. It is important to assess the patient's progress in stopping smoking and to reinforce the importance of smoking cessation with the patient and family. The nurse identifies strategies to assist with smoking cessation and refers the patient and family to community support groups. In addition, the patient is reminded about the importance of other health promotion and screening practices.

Pulmonary Embolism

Pulmonary embolism (PE) refers to the obstruction of the pulmonary artery or one of its branches by a thrombus (or thrombi) that originates somewhere in the venous system or in the right side of the heart. Most commonly, PE is due to a blood clot or thrombus. However, there are other types of emboli: air, fat, amniotic fluid, and septic (from bacterial invasion of the thrombus). It is estimated that thromboembolism occurs for the first time in about 100 persons per 100,000 people each year. About 10% to 20% die within 48 hours following a major thromboembolic episode (White, 2003). PE is a common disorder and often is associated with trauma, surgery (orthopedic, major abdominal, pelvic, gynecologic), pregnancy, heart failure, age older than 50 years, hypercoagulable states, and prolonged immobility. It also may occur in an apparently healthy person. Risk factors for developing PE are identified in Chart 23-8.

Although most thrombi originate in the deep veins of the legs, other sites include the pelvic veins and the right atrium of the heart. A venous thrombosis can result from slowing of blood flow (stasis), secondary to damage to the blood vessel wall (particularly the endothelial lining) or changes in the blood coagulation mechanism. Atrial fibrillation is also a cause of pulmonary embolism. An enlarged right atrium in fibrillation causes blood to stagnate and form clots in this area. These clots are prone to travel into the pulmonary circulation.

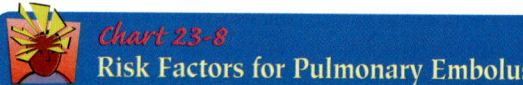

Chart 23-8
Risk Factors for Pulmonary Embolus

Venous Stasis (slowing of blood flow in veins)
Prolonged immobilization (especially postoperative)
Prolonged periods of sitting/traveling
Varicose veins
Spinal cord injury

Hypercoagulability (due to release of tissue thromboplastin after injury/surgery)
Injury
Tumour (pancreatic, GI, GU, breast, lung)
Increased platelet count (polycythemia, splenectomy)

Venous Endothelial Disease
Thrombophlebitis
Vascular disease
Foreign bodies (IV/central venous catheters)

Certain Disease States (combination of stasis, coagulation alterations, and venous injury)
Heart disease (especially heart failure)
Trauma (especially fracture of hip, pelvis, vertebra, lower extremities)
Postoperative state/postpartum period
Diabetes mellitus
Chronic obstructive pulmonary disease

Other Predisposing Conditions
Advanced age
Obesity
Pregnancy
Oral contraceptive use
History of previous thrombophlebitis, pulmonary embolism
Constrictive clothing

Pathophysiology

When a thrombus completely or partially obstructs a pulmonary artery or its branches, the alveolar dead space is increased. The area, although continuing to be ventilated, receives little or no blood flow. Thus, gas exchange is impaired or absent in this area. In addition, various substances are released from the clot and surrounding area, causing regional blood vessels and bronchioles to constrict. This causes an increase in pulmonary vascular resistance. This reaction compounds the ventilation–perfusion imbalance.

The hemodynamic consequences are increased pulmonary vascular resistance from the regional vasoconstriction and reduced size of the pulmonary vascular bed. This results in an increase in pulmonary arterial pressure and, in turn, an increase in right ventricular work to maintain pulmonary blood flow. When the work requirements of the right ventricle exceed its capacity, right ventricular failure occurs, leading to a decrease in cardiac output followed by a decrease in systemic blood pressure and the development of shock.

Clinical Manifestations

The symptoms of PE depend on the size of the thrombus and the area of the pulmonary artery occluded by the thrombus; they may be nonspecific. Dyspnea is the most frequent symptom; tachypnea (very rapid respiratory rate) is the most frequent sign (Goldhaber, 1998). The duration and intensity of the dyspnea depend on the extent of embolization. Chest pain is common and is usually sudden and pleuritic. It may be substernal and mimic angina pectoris or a myocardial infarction. Other symptoms include anxiety, fever, tachycardia, apprehension, cough, diaphoresis, hemoptysis, and syncope.

A massive embolism is best defined by the degree of hemodynamic instability rather than the percentage of pulmonary vasculature occlusion. It is described as an occlusion of the outflow tract of the main pulmonary artery or the bifurcation of the pulmonary arteries that produces pronounced dyspnea, sudden substernal pain, rapid and weak pulse, shock, syncope, and sudden death. Multiple small emboli can lodge in the terminal pulmonary arterioles, producing multiple small infarctions of the lungs. A pulmonary infarction causes ischemic necrosis of an area of the lung and occurs in less than 10% of cases of PE (Arroliga, Matthay & Matthay, 2000). The clinical picture may mimic that of bronchopneumonia or heart failure. In atypical instances, the disease causes few signs and symptoms, whereas in other instances it mimics various other cardiopulmonary disorders.

Assessment and Diagnostic Findings

Death from PE commonly occurs within 1 hour of symptoms; thus, early recognition and diagnosis are priorities. Because the symptoms of PE can vary from few to severe, a diagnostic workup is performed to rule out other diseases. Deep venous thrombosis is closely associated with the development of PE. Typically, patients report sudden onset of pain and/or swelling and warmth of the proximal or distal extremity, skin discolouration, and superficial vein distention. The pain is usually relieved with elevation. The diagnostic workup includes a ventilation–perfusion scan, pulmonary angiography, chest x-ray, ECG, peripheral vascular studies, impedance plethysmography, and arterial blood gas analysis.

The chest x-ray is usually normal but may show infiltrates, atelectasis, elevation of the diaphragm on the affected side, or a pleural effusion. The chest x-ray is most helpful in excluding other possible causes. The ECG usually shows sinus tachycardia, PR-interval depression, and nonspecific T-wave changes. Peripheral vascular studies may include impedance plethysmography, Doppler ultrasonography, or venography (see Chap. 31). Test results confirm or exclude the diagnosis of PE. Arterial blood gas analysis may show hypoxemia and hypocapnia (from tachypnea); however, arterial blood gas measurements are normal in up to 20% of patients with PE.

A ventilation–perfusion scan is the test of choice in patients with suspected PE. The perfusion portion of the scan may indicate areas of diminished or absent blood flow and is the most useful test to rule out clinically important PE. A ventilation scan may show whether there is also a ventilation abnormality present. A normal perfusion scan rules out the diagnosis of PE. If there is a ventilation–perfusion mismatch, the probability of PE is high. Spiral CT of the chest may also assist in the diagnosis.

If lung scan results are not definitive, pulmonary angiography, considered the gold standard for the diagnosis of PE, can be used. This test is invasive and is performed in the interventional radiology department. A contrast agent is injected into the pulmonary arterial system, allowing visualization of obstructions to blood flow and abnormalities.

Prevention

For those at risk, the most effective approach to preventing PE is to prevent deep venous thrombosis. Active leg exercises to avoid venous stasis, early ambulation, and use of elastic compression stockings are general preventive measures. Additional strategies for prevention are listed in the checklist in Chart 23-9.

Chart 23-9
Home Care Checklist • Prevention of Recurrent Pulmonary Embolism

At the completion of the home care instruction, the patient or caregiver will be able to:	Patient	Caregiver
• Describe the underlying process leading to pulmonary embolism.	✓	✓
• Describe the need for continued anticoagulant therapy after the initial embolism.	✓	✓
• Name the anticoagulant prescribed and identify dosage and schedule of administration.	✓	✓
• Describe potential side effects of coagulation such as bruising and bleeding and identify ways to prevent bleeding.	✓	✓
Avoid the use of sharps (razors, knives, etc.) to prevent cuts; shave with an electric shaver.		
Use a toothbrush with soft bristles to prevent gum injury.		
Do not take aspirin or antihistamines while taking warfarin sodium (Coumadin).		
Always check with health care provider before taking any medicine, including over-the-counter medications.		
Avoid laxatives, because they may affect vitamin K absorption.		
Report the occurrence of dark, tarry stools to the health care provider immediately.		
Wear an identification bracelet or carry a medicine card stating that you are taking anticoagulants.		
• Describe strategies to prevent recurrent deep venous thrombosis and pulmonary emboli:	✓	✓
Continue to wear elastic pressure stockings (compression hose) as long as directed.		
Avoid sitting with legs crossed or sitting for prolonged periods of time.		
When traveling, change position regularly, walk occasionally, and do active exercises of moving the legs and ankles while sitting.		
Drink fluids, especially while traveling and in warm weather, to avoid hemoconcentration due to fluid deficit.		
• Describe the signs and symptoms of lower extremity circulatory compromise and potential deep venous thrombosis: calf or leg pain, swelling, pedal edema.	✓	✓
• Describe the signs and symptoms of pulmonary compromise related to recurrent pulmonary embolism.	✓	✓
• Describe how and when to contact the health care provider if symptoms of circulatory compromise or pulmonary compromise are identified.	✓	✓

Patients who are older than 40, whose hemostasis is adequate, and who are undergoing major elective abdominal or thoracic surgery may receive anticoagulant therapy. Low doses of heparin may be given before surgery to reduce the risk of postoperative deep venous thrombus and PE. Heparin should be administered subcutaneously 2 hours before surgery and continued every 8 to 12 hours until the patient is discharged. Low-dose heparin is thought to enhance the activity of antithrombin III, a major plasma inhibitor of clotting factor X. This regimen is not recommended for patients with an active thrombotic process or for those undergoing major orthopedic surgery, open prostatectomy, or surgery on the eye or brain. Low-molecular-weight heparin (eg, enoxaparin [Lovenox]) is an alternative therapy. It has a longer half-life, enhanced subcutaneous absorption, a reduced incidence of thrombocytopenia, and reduced interaction with platelets as compared to unfractionated heparin (Ansell, Hickey, Kleinschmidt et al., 2000).

The intermittent pneumatic leg compression device is useful in preventing thromboembolism. The device inflates a bag that intermittently compresses the leg from the calf to the thigh, thereby improving venous return. It may be applied before surgery and continued until the patient is ambulatory. The device is particularly useful for patients who are not candidates for anticoagulant therapy (Clagett, Anderson, Geerts et al., 1998).

Medical Management

Because PE is often a medical emergency, emergency management is of primary concern. After emergency measures have been taken and the patient's condition stabilizes, the treatment goal is to dissolve (lyse) the existing emboli and prevent new ones from forming. The treatment of PE may include a variety of modalities:

- General measures to improve respiratory and vascular status
- Anticoagulation therapy
- Thrombolytic therapy
- Surgical intervention

EMERGENCY MANAGEMENT

Massive PE is a life-threatening emergency. The immediate objective is to stabilize the cardiopulmonary system. A sudden rise in pulmonary resistance increases the work of the right ventricle, which can cause acute right-sided heart failure with cardiogenic shock. Most patients who die of massive PE do so in the first 1 to 2 hours after the embolic event. Emergency management consists of the following:

- Nasal oxygen is administered immediately to relieve hypoxemia, respiratory distress, and central cyanosis.
- Intravenous infusion lines are started to establish routes for medications or fluids that will be needed.
- A perfusion scan, hemodynamic measurements, and arterial blood gas determinations are performed. Spiral (helical) CT or pulmonary angiography may be performed. Spiral CT is more advanced and quicker than routine tomography. With spiral CT, the patient continuously moves as the x-ray tube rotates. With this type of CT, images can be reconstructed at select levels and locations for diagnostic purposes.
- Hypotension is treated by a slow infusion of dobutamine (Dobutrex) (which has a dilating effect on the pulmonary vessels and bronchi) or dopamine (Intropin).

- The ECG is monitored continuously for dysrhythmias and right ventricular failure, which may occur suddenly.
- Digitalis glycosides, intravenous diuretics, and antiarrhythmic agents are administered when appropriate.
- Blood is drawn for serum electrolytes, complete blood count, and hematocrit.
- If clinical assessment and arterial blood gas analysis indicate the need, the patient is intubated and placed on a mechanical ventilator.
- If the patient has suffered massive embolism and is hypotensive, an indwelling urinary catheter is inserted to monitor urinary output.
- Small doses of intravenous morphine or sedatives are administered to relieve the patient's anxiety, to alleviate chest discomfort, to improve tolerance of the endotracheal tube, and to ease adaptation to the mechanical ventilator.

GENERAL MANAGEMENT

Measures are initiated to improve the patient's respiratory and vascular status. Oxygen therapy is administered to correct the hypoxemia, relieve the pulmonary vascular vasoconstriction, and reduce the pulmonary hypertension. Using elastic compression stockings or intermittent pneumatic leg compression devices reduces venous stasis. These measures compress the superficial veins and increase the velocity of blood in the deep veins by redirecting the blood through the deep veins. Elevating the leg (above the level of the heart) also increases venous flow.

PHARMACOLOGIC THERAPY

Anticoagulation Therapy. Anticoagulant therapy (heparin, warfarin sodium) has traditionally been the primary method for managing acute deep vein thrombosis and PE (Goldhaber, 1998). Heparin is used to prevent recurrence of emboli but has no effect on emboli that are already present. It is administered as an intravenous bolus of 5,000 to 10,000 units, followed by a continuous infusion initiated at a dose of 18 U/kg per hour, not to exceed 1,600 U/hour in otherwise healthy patients (Goldhaber, 1998). The rate is reduced in patients with a high risk of bleeding. The goal is to keep the partial thromboplastin time 1.5 to 2.5 times normal (or 46 to 70 seconds). Heparin is usually administered for 5 to 7 days. Low-molecular-weight heparin (eg, enoxaparin [Lovenox]) may also be used.

Warfarin sodium (Coumadin) administration is begun within 24 hours after the start of heparin therapy because its onset of action is 4 to 5 days. Warfarin is usually continued for 3 to 6 months. The prothrombin time is maintained at 1.5 to 2.5 times normal (or an INR [international normalized ratio] of 2.0 to 3.0). Anticoagulation therapy is contraindicated in patients who are at risk for bleeding (eg, those with gastrointestinal conditions or with postoperative or postpartum bleeding).

Thrombolytic Therapy. Thrombolytic therapy (urokinase, streptokinase, alteplase) also may be used in treating PE, particularly in patients who are severely compromised (eg, those who are hypotensive and have significant hypoxemia despite oxygen supplementation). Thrombolytic therapy resolves the thrombi or emboli more quickly and restores more normal hemodynamic functioning of the pulmonary circulation, thereby reducing pulmonary hypertension and improving perfusion, oxygenation, and cardiac output. Bleeding, however, is a significant side effect. Contraindications to thrombolytic therapy include a cerebrovascular accident within the past 2 months, other active intracranial processes, active bleeding, surgery within the past 10 days of the thrombotic event, recent labour and delivery, trauma, or severe hypertension. Consequently, thrombolytic agents are advocated only for PE affecting a significant area of blood flow to the lung and causing hemodynamic instability.

Before thrombolytic therapy is started, prothrombin time, partial thromboplastin time, hematocrit values, and platelet counts are obtained. Heparin is stopped prior to administration of a thrombolytic agent. During therapy, all but essential invasive procedures are avoided because of potential bleeding. If necessary, fresh whole blood, packed red cells, cryoprecipitate, or frozen plasma is administered to replace blood loss and reverse the bleeding tendency. After the thrombolytic infusion is completed (which varies in duration according to the agent used and the condition being treated), the patient is given anticoagulants.

SURGICAL MANAGEMENT

A surgical embolectomy is rarely performed but may be indicated if the patient has a massive PE or hemodynamic instability or if there are contraindications to thrombolytic therapy. Pulmonary embolectomy requires a thoracotomy with cardiopulmonary bypass technique. Transvenous catheter embolectomy is a technique in which a vacuum-cupped catheter is introduced transvenously into the affected pulmonary artery. Suction is applied to the end of the embolus and the embolus is aspirated into the cup. The surgeon maintains suction to hold the embolus within the cup, and the entire catheter is withdrawn through the right side of the heart and out the femoral vein. Catheters are available that pulverize the clot with high-velocity jets of normal saline solution (Goldhaber, 1998). An inferior caval filter is usually inserted at the time of surgery to protect against a recurrence.

Interrupting the inferior vena cava is another surgical technique used when PE recurs or when the patient is intolerant of anticoagulant therapy. This approach prevents dislodged thrombi from being swept into the lungs while allowing adequate blood flow. The preferred approach is the application of Teflon clips to the inferior vena cava to divide the lumen into small channels without occluding caval blood flow. Also, the use of transvenous devices that occlude or filter the blood through the inferior vena cava is a fairly safe way to prevent recurrent PE. One such technique involves inserting a filter (eg, Greenfield filter) through the internal jugular vein or common femoral vein (Fig. 23-7). This filter is advanced into the inferior vena cava, where it is opened. The perforated umbrella permits the passage of blood but prevents the passage of large thrombi. It is recommended that anticoagulation be continued in patients with a caval filter, if there are no contraindications to its use.

Nursing Management

MINIMIZING THE RISK OF PULMONARY EMBOLISM

A key role of the nurse is to identify patients at high risk for PE and to minimize the risk of PE in all patients. The nurse must have a high degree of suspicion for PE in any patient, but particularly in those with conditions predisposing to a slowing of venous return (see Chart 23-8).

FIGURE 23-7 An umbrella filter is in place in the inferior vena cava to prevent pulmonary embolism. The filter (compressed within an applicator catheter) is inserted through an incision in the right internal jugular vein. The applicator is withdrawn when the filter fixes itself to the wall of the inferior vena cava after ejection from the applicator.

PREVENTING THROMBUS FORMATION

Preventing thrombus formation is a major nursing responsibility. The nurse encourages ambulation and active and passive leg exercises to prevent venous stasis in patients on bed rest. The nurse instructs the patient to move the legs in a "pumping" exercise so that the leg muscles can help increase venous flow. The nurse also advises the patient not to sit or lie in bed for prolonged periods, not to cross the legs, and not to wear constricting clothing. Legs should not be dangled or feet placed in a dependent position while the patient sits on the edge of the bed; instead, the patient's feet should rest on the floor or on a chair. In addition, intravenous catheters (for parenteral therapy or measurements of central venous pressure) should not be left in place for prolonged periods.

ASSESSING POTENTIAL FOR PULMONARY EMBOLISM

The nurse examines patients who are at risk for developing PE for a positive Homans' sign, which may or may not indicate impending thrombosis of the leg veins (see Chap. 31). To test for Homans' sign, the patient assumes a supine position, lifts the leg, and dorsiflexes the foot. The nurse asks the patient to report whether calf pain occurs during this manoeuvre. The occurrence of pain—a positive Homans' sign—may indicate deep venous thrombosis.

MONITORING THROMBOLYTIC THERAPY

The nurse is responsible for monitoring thrombolytic and anticoagulant therapy. Thrombolytic therapy (streptokinase, urokinase, tissue plasminogen activator) causes lysis of deep vein thrombi and pulmonary emboli, which helps dissolve the clots. During thrombolytic infusion, the patient remains on bed rest, vital signs are assessed every 2 hours, and invasive procedures are limited. Tests to determine prothrombin time or partial thromboplastin time are performed 3 to 4 hours after the thrombolytic infusion is started to confirm that the fibrinolytic systems have been activated. Because of the prolonged clotting time, only essential arterial punctures or venipunctures are performed, and manual pressure is applied to any puncture site for at least 30 minutes. Pulse oximetry is used to monitor changes in oxygenation. The nurse immediately discontinues the infusion if uncontrolled bleeding occurs.

See Chapter 31 for nursing management for the patient receiving anticoagulant or thrombolytic therapy.

MANAGING PAIN

Chest pain, if present, is usually pleuritic rather than cardiac in origin. A semi-Fowler's position provides a more comfortable position for breathing. However, it is important to continue to turn the patient frequently and reposition the patient to improve the **ventilation–perfusion ratio** in the lung. The nurse administers opioid analgesics as prescribed for severe pain.

MANAGING OXYGEN THERAPY

Careful attention is given to the proper use of oxygen. It is important to ensure that the patient understands the need for continuous oxygen therapy. The nurse assesses the patient frequently for signs of hypoxemia and monitors the pulse oximetry values to evaluate the effectiveness of the oxygen therapy. Deep breathing and incentive spirometry are indicated for all patients to minimize or prevent atelectasis and improve ventilation. Nebulizer therapy or percussion and postural drainage may be used for management of secretions.

RELIEVING ANXIETY

The nurse encourages the stabilized patient to talk about any fears or concerns related to this frightening episode, answers the patient's and family's questions concisely and accurately, explains the therapy, and describes how to recognize untoward effects early.

MONITORING FOR COMPLICATIONS

When caring for a patient who has had PE, the nurse must be alert for the potential complication of cardiogenic shock or right ventricular failure subsequent to the effect of PE on the cardiovascular system. Nursing activities for managing shock are found in Chapter 15.

PROVIDING POSTOPERATIVE NURSING CARE

After surgery, the nurse measures the patient's pulmonary arterial pressure and urinary output. The nurse assesses the insertion site of the arterial catheter for hematoma formation and infection. It is important to maintain the blood pressure at a level that supports perfusion of vital organs. To prevent peripheral venous stasis and edema of the lower extremities, the nurse elevates the foot of the bed and encourages isometric exercises, use of elastic compression stockings, and walking when the patient is permitted out of bed. Sitting is discouraged because hip flexion compresses the large veins in the legs.

PROMOTING HOME AND COMMUNITY-BASED CARE

Teaching Patients Self-Care. Before hospital discharge and at follow-up visits to the clinic or during home visits, the nurse instructs the patient about how to prevent recurrence and what signs and symptoms to report immediately. Patient instructions, as presented in Chart 23-9, are intended to help prevent recurrences and side effects of treatment.

Sarcoidosis

Sarcoidosis is a multisystem, granulomatous disease of unknown etiology. It may involve almost any organ or tissue but most commonly involves the lungs, lymph nodes, liver, spleen, central nervous system, skin, eyes, fingers, and parotid glands. The disease is not gender-specific, but some manifestations are more common in women. Epidemiologic data are not currently available for Canada. Based on worldwide evidence available, sarcoidosis occurs primarily in adults aged 20 to 40 years. The peak incidence occurs in the third decade of life. The reported prevalence rates for sarcoidosis vary from 4 to 58 out of every 100,000 people (American Thoracic Society, 1999; Hosoda, Sasagawa, & Yasuda, 2002).

Pathophysiology

Sarcoidosis is thought to be a hypersensitivity response to one or more agents (bacteria, fungi, virus, chemicals) in people with an inherited or acquired predisposition to the disorder. The hypersensitivity response results in granuloma formation due to the release of cytokines and other substances that promote replication of fibroblasts. In the lung, granuloma infiltration and fibrosis may occur, resulting in low lung compliance, impaired diffusing capacity, and reduced lung volumes (American Thoracic Society, 1999).

Clinical Manifestations

A hallmark of this disease is its insidious onset and lack of prominent clinical signs or symptoms. The clinical picture depends on the systems involved. With pulmonary involvement, signs and symptoms may include dyspnea, cough, hemoptysis, and congestion. Generalized symptoms include anorexia, fatigue, and weight loss. Other signs include uveitis, joint pain, fever, and granulomatous lesions of the skin, liver, spleen, kidney, and central nervous system. The granulomas may disappear or gradually convert to fibrous tissue. With multisystem involvement, the patient has fatigue, fever, anorexia, weight loss, and joint pain.

Assessment and Diagnostic Findings

Chest x-rays and CT scans are used to assess pulmonary adenopathy. The chest x-ray may show hilar adenopathy and disseminated miliary and nodular lesions in the lungs. A mediastinoscopy or **transbronchial** biopsy (in which a tissue specimen is obtained through the bronchial wall) may be used to confirm the diagnosis. In rare cases, an **open lung biopsy** is performed. Diagnosis is confirmed by a biopsy that shows noncaseating granulomas. Pulmonary function test results are abnormal if there is restriction of lung function (reduction in total lung capacity). Arterial blood gas measurements may be normal or may show reduced oxygen levels (hypoxemia) and increased carbon dioxide levels (hypercapnia).

Medical Management

Many patients undergo remission without specific treatment. Corticosteroid therapy may benefit some patients because of its anti-inflammatory effect, which relieves symptoms and improves organ function. It is useful for patients with ocular and myocardial involvement, skin involvement, extensive pulmonary disease that compromises pulmonary function, hepatic involvement, and hypercalcemia. Other cytotoxic and immunosuppressive agents have been used, but without the benefit of controlled clinical trials. There is no single test that monitors the progression or recurrence of sarcoidosis. Multiple tests are used to monitor the involved systems.

Occupational Lung Diseases: Pneumoconioses

Diseases of the lungs occur in numerous occupations as a result of exposure to organic and inorganic (mineral) dusts and noxious gases (fumes and aerosols). The effects of inhaling these materials depend on the composition of the substance, its concentration, its ability to initiate an immune response, its irritating properties, the duration of exposure, and the individual's response or susceptibility to the irritant. Smoking may compound the problem and may increase the risk of lung cancers in people exposed to the mineral asbestos. Key aspects of any assessment of patients with a potential occupational respiratory history include job and job activities, exposure levels, general hygiene, time frame of exposure, amount of respiratory protection used, and direct versus indirect exposures.

Pneumoconiosis refers to a nonneoplastic alteration of the lung resulting from inhalation of mineral or inorganic dust (eg, "dusty lung"). The most common pneumoconioses are silicosis, asbestosis, and coal workers' pneumoconiosis.

SILICOSIS

Silicosis is a chronic fibrotic pulmonary disease caused by inhalation of silica dust (crystalline silicon dioxide particles). Exposure to silica and silicates occurs in almost all mining, quarrying, and tunneling operations. Glass manufacturing, stone-cutting, the manufacture of abrasives and pottery, and foundry work are other occupations with exposure hazards. Finely ground silica, such as that found in soaps, polishes and filters, is extremely dangerous.

Pathophysiology

When the silica particles, which have fibrogenic properties, are inhaled, nodular lesions are produced throughout the lungs. With the passage of time and further exposure, the nodules enlarge and coalesce. Dense masses form in the upper portion of the lungs, resulting in the loss of pulmonary volume. **Restrictive lung disease** (inability of the lungs to expand fully) and obstructive lung disease from secondary emphysema result. Cavities can form as a result of superimposed TB. Exposure of 15 to 20 years is usually required before the onset of the disease and shortness of breath are manifested. Fibrotic destruction of pulmonary tissue can lead to emphysema, pulmonary hypertension, and cor pulmonale.

Clinical Manifestations

Patients with acute silicosis present with dyspnea, fever, cough, and weight loss and have a rapid progression of the disease. Symptoms are more severe in patients whose disease is complicated by progressive massive fibrosis. More commonly, this disease is a chronic problem with a long latency period. The patient may have slowly progressive symptoms indicative of hypoxemia, severe air-flow obstruction, and right-sided heart failure. Edema may occur because of the cardiac failure.

Medical Management

There is no specific treatment for silicosis, because the fibrotic process in the lung is irreversible. Supportive therapy is directed at managing complications and preventing infection. Testing is performed to rule out other lung diseases, such as TB, lung cancer, and sarcoidosis. If TB is present, it is aggressively treated. Additional therapy might include oxygen, diuretics, inhaled beta-adrenergic agonists, anticholinergics, and bronchodilator therapy.

ASBESTOSIS

Asbestosis is a disease characterized by diffuse pulmonary fibrosis from the inhalation of asbestos dust. Current laws restrict the use of asbestos, but many industries used it in the past. Therefore, exposure occurred, and may still occur, in numerous occupations, including asbestos mining and manufacturing, shipbuilding, demolition of structures containing asbestos, and roofing. Materials such as shingles, cement, vinyl asbestos tile, fireproof paint and clothing, brake linings, and filters all contained asbestos at one time, and many of these materials are still in existence. Additional diseases related to asbestos exposure include lung cancer, mesothelioma, and asbestos pleural effusion.

Pathophysiology

Inhaled asbestos fibres enter the alveoli, where they are surrounded by fibrous tissue. The fibrous tissue eventually obliterates the alveoli. Fibrous changes also affect the pleura, which thickens and develops plaque. The result of these physiologic changes is a restrictive lung disease, with a decrease in lung volume, diminished exchange of oxygen and carbon dioxide, and hypoxemia.

Clinical Manifestations

The onset of the disease is insidious, and the patient has progressive dyspnea, persistent, dry cough, mild to moderate chest pain, anorexia, weight loss, and malaise. Early physical findings include bibasilar fine, end-inspiratory crackles and in more advanced cases clubbing of the fingers. Cor pulmonale and respiratory failure occur as the disease progresses. A high proportion of workers who have been exposed to asbestos dust die of lung cancer, especially those who smoke or have a history of smoking. Malignant mesotheliomas may also occur. These are rare cancers of the pleura or peritoneum that are strongly associated with asbestos exposure.

Medical Management

There is no effective treatment for asbestosis as the lung damage is permanent and often progressive. Management is directed at controlling infection and treating the lung disease. When oxygen–carbon dioxide exchange becomes severely impaired, continuous oxygen therapy may help improve activity tolerance. The patient must be instructed to avoid additional exposure to asbestos and to stop smoking. A significant contributing cause to mortality in this population is the high incidence of lung carcinoma.

COAL WORKERS' PNEUMOCONIOSIS

Coal workers' pneumoconiosis ("black lung disease") includes a variety of respiratory diseases found in coal workers who have inhaled coal dust over the years. Coal miners are exposed to dusts that are mixtures of coal, kaolin, mica, and silica.

Pathophysiology

When coal dust is deposited in the alveoli and respiratory bronchioles, macrophages engulf the particles (by phagocytosis) and transport them to the terminal bronchioles, where they are removed by mucociliary action. In time, the clearance mechanisms cannot handle the excessive dust load, and the macrophages aggregate in the respiratory bronchioles and alveoli. Fibroblasts appear and a network of reticulin is laid down surrounding the dust-laden macrophages. The bronchioles and the alveoli become clogged with coal dust, dying macrophages, and fibroblasts. This leads to the formation of the coal macule, the primary lesion of the disorder. Macules appear as blackish dots on the lungs. Fibrotic lesions develop and, as the macules enlarge, the weakening bronchioles dilate, with subsequent development of a localized emphysema. The disease begins in the upper lobes of the lungs but may progress to the lower lobes.

Clinical Manifestations

The first signs are a chronic cough and sputum production, similar to the signs encountered in chronic bronchitis. As the disease progresses, the patient develops dyspnea and coughs up large amounts of sputum with varying amounts of black fluid (melanoptysis), particularly if the individual is a smoker. Eventually, cor pulmonale and respiratory failure result. The diagnosis may first be made based on chest x-ray findings and a history of exposure.

Medical Management

Preventing this disease is key because there is no effective treatment. Instead, treatment focuses on early diagnosis and management of complications. (See Chap. 24 for discussion of emphysema.)

Nursing Management

TEACHING ABOUT PREVENTION

The occupational health nurse serves as an employee advocate, making every effort to promote measures to reduce the exposure of workers to industrial products. Laws require that the work environment be ventilated properly to remove any noxious agent. Dust control can prevent many of the pneumoconioses. Dust control includes ventilation, spraying an area with water to control dust, and effective and frequent floor cleaning. Air samples need to be monitored. Toxic substances should be enclosed and placed in restricted areas. Workers must wear or use protective devices (facemasks, hoods, industrial respirators) to provide a safe air supply when a toxic element is present. Employees who are at risk should be carefully screened and followed. There is a risk of developing serious smoking-related illness (cancer) in industries in which there are unsafe levels of certain gases, dusts, fumes, fluids, and other toxic substances. Additionally, there is the potential for second-hand exposure. Asbestos and toxic dusts and substances may be transferred to others through the handling of clothing or shoes that have been exposed. Ongoing educational programs should be designed to teach workers to take responsibility for their own health and to stop smoking and receive an influenza vaccination.

The Right to Know law stipulates that employees must be informed about all hazardous and toxic substances in the workplace. Specifically, they must be educated about any hazardous or toxic substances they work with, what effects these substances can have on their health, and the measures they can take to protect themselves. The responsibility for implementing these controls inevitably falls on the federal or state government.

Chest Tumours

Tumours of the lung may be benign or malignant. A malignant chest tumour can be primary, arising within the lung, chest wall, or mediastinum, or it can be a metastasis from a primary tumour site elsewhere in the body. Metastatic lung tumours occur fre-

quently because the bloodstream transports cancer cells from primary cancers elsewhere in the body to the lungs.

LUNG CANCER (BRONCHOGENIC CARCINOMA)

Lung cancer is the number-one cancer killer among men and women in Canada, accounting for 30% of cancer deaths in men and 20% in women (Health Canada, 2001). For men, the incidence of lung cancer has remained relatively constant, but in women it continues to rise. Lung cancer affects primarily those in the sixth or seventh decade of life; less than 5% of patients are under the age of 40. In approximately 70% of lung cancer patients, the disease has spread to regional lymphatics and other sites by the time of diagnosis. As a result, the long-term survival rate for lung cancer patients is low. Evidence indicates that carcinoma tends to arise at sites of previous scarring (TB, fibrosis) in the lung. More than 85% of lung cancers are caused by the inhalation of carcinogenic chemicals, most commonly cigarette smoke (Schottenfeld, 2000).

Pathophysiology

Lung cancers arise from a single transformed epithelial cell in the tracheobronchial airways. A carcinogen (cigarette smoke, radon gas, other occupational and environmental agents) binds to a cell's DNA and damages it. This damage results in cellular changes, abnormal cell growth, and eventually a malignant cell. As the damaged DNA is passed on to daughter cells, the DNA undergoes further changes and becomes unstable. With the accumulation of genetic changes, the pulmonary epithelium undergoes malignant transformation from normal epithelium to eventual invasive carcinoma.

Squamous cell carcinoma is more centrally located and arises more commonly in the segmental and subsegmental bronchi in response to repetitive carcinogenic exposures. Adenocarcinoma is the most prevalent carcinoma of the lung for both men and women; it presents more peripherally as peripheral masses or nodules and often metastasizes. Large cell carcinoma (also called undifferentiated carcinoma) is a fast-growing tumour that tends to arise peripherally. Bronchioalveolar cell cancer arises from the terminal bronchus and alveoli and is usually slower growing as compared to other bronchogenic carcinomas. Lastly, small cell carcinomas arise primarily as a proximal lesion or lesions but may arise in any part of the tracheobronchial tree.

Classification and Staging

Non-small cell carcinoma represents 70% to 75% of tumours; small cell carcinoma represents 15% to 20% of tumours. For non-small cell carcinoma, the cell types include squamous cell carcinoma (30%), large cell carcinoma (10% to 16%), and adenocarcinoma (31% to 34%), including bronchioalveolar carcinoma (3% to 4%). Most small cell carcinomas arise in the major bronchi and spread by infiltration along the bronchial wall. Small cell cancers account for 20% to 25% of all bronchogenic cancers (Matthay, Tanoue & Carter, 2000).

In addition to cell type, lung cancers also are staged. The stage of the tumour refers to the size of the tumour, its location, whether lymph nodes are involved, and whether the cancer has spread (American Joint Committee on Cancer, 2002). Non-small cell lung cancer is staged as I to IV. Stage I is the earliest stage with the highest cure rates, while stage IV designates metastatic spread.

Small cell lung cancers are classified as limited or extensive. Diagnostic tools and further information on staging are described in Chapter 16.

Risk Factors

Various factors have been associated with the development of lung cancer, including tobacco smoke, second-hand (passive) smoke, environmental and occupational exposures, gender, genetics, and dietary deficits. Other factors that have been associated with lung cancer include genetic predisposition and other underlying respiratory diseases, such as COPD and TB.

TOBACCO SMOKE

Tobacco is one of the leading causes of preventable illness and disability in Canada. Cigarette smoking is the predominate cause of lung cancer (Health Canada, 2001). It accounts for about 80% of all new cases of lung cancer in women and about 90% in men (Health Canada, 2001). Lung cancer is 10 times more common in cigarette smokers than nonsmokers. Risk is determined by the pack-year history (number of packs of cigarettes used each day, multiplied by the number of years smoked), the age of initiation of smoking, the depth of inhalation, and the tar and nicotine levels in the cigarettes smoked. The younger a person is when he or she starts smoking, the greater the risk of developing lung cancer. The risk of lung cancer decreases as the duration of smoking cessation increases.

SECOND-HAND SMOKE

Passive smoking has been identified as a possible cause of lung cancer in nonsmokers. In other words, people who are involuntarily exposed to tobacco smoke in a closed environment (home, car, building) are at increased risk for developing lung cancer as compared to unexposed nonsmokers. An average lifetime passive smoke exposure to a smoking spouse or partner increases a nonsmoker's risk of lung cancer by about 35% compared to the risk of 100% for a lifetime of active smoking (Matthay, Tanoue & Carter, 2000).

ENVIRONMENTAL AND OCCUPATIONAL EXPOSURE

Various carcinogens have been identified in the atmosphere, including motor vehicle emissions and pollutants from refineries and manufacturing plants. Evidence suggests that the incidence of lung cancer is greater in urban areas as a result of the buildup of pollutants and motor vehicle emissions.

Radon is a colourless, odourless gas found in soil and rocks. For many years it has been associated with uranium mines, but it is now known to seep into homes through ground rock. High levels of radon have been associated with the development of lung cancer, especially when combined with cigarette smoking. Homeowners are advised to have radon levels checked in their houses and to arrange for special venting if the levels are high.

Chronic exposure to industrial carcinogens, such as arsenic, asbestos, mustard gas, chromates, coke oven fumes, nickel, oil, and radiation, has been associated with the development of lung cancer. Laws have been passed to control exposure to such elements in the workplace.

GENETICS

Some familial predisposition to lung cancer seems apparent, because the incidence of lung cancer in close relatives of patients with lung cancer appears to be two to three times that of the general population regardless of smoking status.

DIETARY FACTORS

Prior research has demonstrated that smokers who eat a diet low in fruits and vegetables have an increased risk of developing lung cancer (Bast, Kufe, Pollock et al., 2000). The actual active agents in a diet rich in fruits and vegetables have yet to be determined. It has been hypothesized that carotenoids, particularly carotene or vitamin A, may be important. Several ongoing trials may help to determine if carotene supplementation has anticancer properties. Other nutrients, including vitamin E, selenium, vitamin C, fat, and retinoids, are also being evaluated regarding their protective role against lung cancer (Bast, Kufe, Pollock et al., 2000).

Clinical Manifestations

Often, lung cancer develops insidiously and is asymptomatic until late in its course. The signs and symptoms depend on the location and size of the tumour, the degree of obstruction, and the existence of metastases to regional or distant sites.

The most frequent symptom of lung cancer is cough or change in a chronic cough. People frequently ignore this symptom and attribute it to smoking or a respiratory infection. The cough starts as a dry, persistent cough, without sputum production. When obstruction of airways occurs, the cough may become productive due to infection.

 NURSING ALERT A cough that changes in character should arouse suspicion of lung cancer.

Wheezing is noted (occurs when a bronchus becomes partially obstructed by the tumour) in about 20% of patients with lung cancer. Patients also may report dyspnea. Hemoptysis or blood-tinged sputum may be expectorated. In some patients, a recurring fever occurs as an early symptom in response to a persistent infection in an area of pneumonitis distal to the tumour. In fact, cancer of the lung should be suspected in people with repeated unresolved upper respiratory tract infections. Chest or shoulder pain may indicate chest wall or pleural involvement by a tumour. Pain also is a late manifestation and may be related to metastasis to the bone.

If the tumour spreads to adjacent structures and regional lymph nodes, the patient may present with chest pain and tightness, hoarseness (involving the recurrent laryngeal nerve), dysphagia, head and neck edema, and symptoms of pleural or pericardial effusion. The most common sites of metastases are lymph nodes, bone, brain, contralateral lung, adrenal glands, and liver. Nonspecific symptoms of weakness, anorexia, and weight loss also may be diagnostic.

Assessment and Diagnostic Findings

If pulmonary symptoms occur in a heavy smoker, cancer of the lung is suspected. A chest x-ray is performed to search for pulmonary density, a solitary peripheral nodule (coin lesion), atelectasis, and infection. CT scans of the chest are used to identify small nodules not visualized on the chest x-ray and also to examine serially areas of the thoracic cage not clearly visible on the chest x-ray.

Sputum cytology is rarely used to make a diagnosis of lung cancer; however, fibreoptic bronchoscopy is more commonly used and provides a detailed study of the tracheobronchial tree and allows for brushings, washings, and biopsies of suspicious areas. For peripheral lesions not amenable to bronchoscopic biopsy, a transthoracic **fine-needle aspiration** may be performed under CT or fluoroscopic guidance to aspirate cells from a suspicious area. In some circumstances, an endoscopy with esophageal ultrasound (EUS) may be used to obtain a transesophageal biopsy of enlarged subcarinal lymph nodes that are not easily accessible by other means.

A variety of scans may be used to assess for metastasis of the cancer. These may include bone scans, abdominal scans, positron emission tomography (PET) scans, or liver ultrasound or scans. CT of the brain, magnetic resonance imaging (MRI), and other neurologic diagnostic procedures are used to detect central nervous system metastases. Mediastinoscopy or mediastinotomy may be used to obtain biopsy samples from lymph nodes in the mediastinum.

If surgery is a potential treatment, the patient is evaluated to determine whether the tumour is resectable and whether the physiologic impairment resulting from such surgery can be tolerated. Pulmonary function tests, arterial blood gas analysis, ventilation–perfusion scans, and exercise testing may all be used as part of the preoperative assessment (Knippel, 2001).

Medical Management

The objective of management is to provide a cure, if possible. Treatment depends on the cell type, the stage of the disease, and the physiologic status (particularly cardiac and pulmonary status) of the patient. In general, treatment may involve surgery, radiation therapy, or chemotherapy—or a combination of these. Newer and more specific therapies to modulate the immune system (gene therapy, therapy with defined tumour antigens) are under study and show promise in treating lung cancer.

SURGICAL MANAGEMENT

Surgical resection is the preferred method of treating patients with localized non-small cell tumours, no evidence of metastatic spread, and adequate cardiopulmonary function. If the patient's cardiovascular status, pulmonary function, and functional status are satisfactory, surgery is generally well tolerated. Coronary artery disease, pulmonary insufficiency, and other comorbidities, however, may contraindicate surgical intervention. The cure rate of surgical resection depends on the type and stage of the cancer. Surgery is primarily used for non-small cell carcinomas because small cell cancer of the lung grows rapidly and metastasizes early and extensively. Unfortunately, in many patients with bronchogenic cancer, the lesion is inoperable at the time of diagnosis.

Several different types of lung resections may be performed (Chart 23-10). The most common surgical procedure for a small, apparently curable tumour of the lung is lobectomy (removal of a lobe of the lung). In some cases, an entire lung may be removed (pneumonectomy) (see Chap. 25 for further details).

RADIATION THERAPY

Radiation therapy may cure a small percentage of patients. It is useful in controlling neoplasms that cannot be surgically resected but are responsive to radiation. Radiation also may be used to reduce the size of a tumour, to make an inoperable tumour operable, or to relieve the pressure of the tumour on vital structures. It can control symptoms of spinal cord metastasis and superior vena caval compression. Also, prophylactic brain irradiation is used in certain patients to treat microscopic metastases to the brain. Radiation may help relieve cough, chest pain, dyspnea, hemoptysis,

---

> **Chart 23-10** **Types of Lung Resections**
>
> - Lobectomy: a single lobe of lung is removed
> - Bilobectomy: two lobes of the lung are removed
> - Sleeve resection: cancerous lobe(s) is removed and a segment of the main bronchus is resected
> - Pneumonectomy: removal of entire lung
> - Segmentectomy: a segment of the lung is removed*
> - Wedge resection: removal of a small, pie-shaped area of the segment*
> - Chest wall resection with removal of cancerous lung tissue: for cancers that have invaded the chest wall
>
> ———————
> *Not recommended as curative resection for lung cancer.

---

and bone and liver pain. Relief of symptoms may last from a few weeks to many months and is important in improving the quality of the remaining period of life.

Radiation therapy usually is toxic to normal tissue within the radiation field, and this may lead to complications such as esophagitis, pneumonitis, and radiation lung fibrosis. These may impair ventilatory and diffusion capacity and significantly reduce pulmonary reserve. The patient's nutritional status, psychological outlook, fatigue level, and signs of anemia and infection are monitored throughout the treatment. See Chapter 16 for management of the patient receiving radiation therapy.

CHEMOTHERAPY

Chemotherapy is used to alter tumour growth patterns, to treat patients with distant metastases or small cell cancer of the lung, and as an adjunct to surgery or radiation therapy. Combinations of two or more medications may be more beneficial than single-dose regimens. A large number of medications are active against lung cancer. A variety of chemotherapeutic agents are used, including alkylating agents (ifosfamide), platinum analogues (cisplatin and carboplatin), taxanes (paclitaxel, docetaxel), vinca alkaloids (vinblastine and vindesine), doxorubicin, gemcitabine, vinorelbine, irinotecan (CPT-11), and etoposide (VP-16). The choice of agent depends on the growth of the tumour cell and the specific phase of the cell cycle that the medication affects. Numerous combinations of chemotherapy are undergoing investigation to identify the optimal regimen to treat differing types of lung cancer.

Chemotherapy may provide relief, especially of pain, but it does not usually cure the disease, nor does it often prolong life to any great degree. Chemotherapy is also accompanied by side effects. It is valuable in reducing pressure symptoms of lung cancer and in treating brain, spinal cord, and pericardial metastasis. See Chapter 16 for a discussion of chemotherapy for the patient with cancer.

PALLIATIVE THERAPY

Palliative therapy may include radiation therapy to shrink the tumour to provide pain relief, a variety of bronchoscopic interventions to open a narrowed bronchus or airway, and pain management and other comfort measures. Evaluation and referral for hospice care are important in planning for comfortable and dignified end-of-life care for the patient and family.

Treatment-Related Complications

A variety of complications may occur as a result of lung cancer treatments. Radiation therapy may result in diminished cardiopulmonary function and other complications, such as pulmonary fibrosis, pericarditis, myelitis, and cor pulmonale. Chemotherapy, particularly in combination with radiation therapy, can cause pneumonitis. Pulmonary toxicity is a potential side effect of chemotherapy. Surgical resection may result in respiratory failure, particularly when the cardiopulmonary system is compromised before surgery. Surgical complications and prolonged mechanical ventilation are potential outcomes.

Nursing Management

Nursing care of the patient with lung cancer is similar to that of other patients with cancer (see Chap. 16) and addresses the physiologic and psychological needs of the patient. The physiologic problems are primarily due to the respiratory manifestations of the disease. Nursing care includes strategies to ensure relief of pain and discomfort and to prevent complications.

MANAGING SYMPTOMS

The nurse instructs the patient and family about the potential side effects of the specific treatment and strategies to manage them. Strategies for managing such symptoms as dyspnea, fatigue, nausea and vomiting, and anorexia will assist the patient and family to cope with the therapeutic measures.

RELIEVING BREATHING PROBLEMS

Airway clearance techniques are key to maintaining airway patency through the removal of excess secretions. This may be accomplished through deep-breathing exercises, chest physiotherapy, directed cough, suctioning, and in some instances bronchoscopy. Bronchodilator medications may be prescribed to promote bronchial dilation. As the tumour enlarges or spreads, it may compress a bronchus or involve a large area of lung tissue, resulting in an impaired breathing pattern and poor gas exchange. At some stage of the disease, supplemental oxygen will probably be necessary.

Nursing measures focus on decreasing dyspnea by encouraging the patient to assume positions that promote lung expansion, breathing exercises for lung expansion and relaxation, and educating the patient on energy conservation and airway clearance techniques (Connolly & O'Neill, 1999). Many of the techniques used in pulmonary rehabilitation can be applied to the lung cancer patient. Depending on the severity of disease and the patient's wishes, a referral to a pulmonary rehabilitation program may be helpful in managing respiratory symptoms.

REDUCING FATIGUE

Fatigue is a devastating symptom that affects quality of life in the cancer patient. It is commonly experienced by the lung cancer patient and may be related to the disease itself, the cancer treatment and complications (eg, anemia), sleep disturbances, pain and discomfort, hypoxemia, poor nutrition, or the psychological ramifications of the disease (eg, anxiety, depression). The nurse is pivotal in thoroughly assessing the patient's level of fatigue, identifying potentially treatable causes, and validating with the patient that fatigue is indeed an important symptom. Educating the patient in energy conservation techniques or referring the patient to a physical therapy, occupational therapy, or pulmonary rehabilitation program may be helpful. In addition, guided exercise has been recently identified as a potential intervention for treating fatigue in cancer patients. This is an important area for research because few studies have been conducted, and only in select populations of cancer patients.

PROVIDING PSYCHOLOGICAL SUPPORT

Another important part of the nursing care of the patient with lung cancer is psychological support and identification of potential resources for the patient and family. Often, the nurse must help the patient and family deal with the poor prognosis and relatively rapid progression of this disease. The nurse must help the patient and family with informed decision making regarding the possible treatment options, methods to maintain the patient's quality of life during the course of this disease, and end-of-life treatment options.

TUMOURS OF THE MEDIASTINUM

Tumours of the mediastinum include neurogenic tumours, tumours of the thymus, lymphomas, germ cell, cysts, and mesenchymal tumours. These tumours may be malignant or benign. These tumours are usually described in relation to location: anterior, middle, or posterior masses or tumours.

Clinical Manifestations

Nearly all the symptoms of mediastinal tumours result from the pressure of the mass against important intrathoracic organs. Symptoms may include cough, wheezing, dyspnea, anterior chest or neck pain, bulging of the chest wall, heart palpitations, angina, other circulatory disturbances, central cyanosis, superior vena caval syndrome (ie, swelling of the face, neck, and upper extremities), marked distention of the veins of the neck and the chest wall (evidence of the obstruction of large veins of the mediastinum by extravascular compression or intravascular invasion), and dysphagia and weight loss from pressure or invasion into the esophagus.

Assessment and Diagnostic Findings

Chest x-rays are the major method used initially to diagnose mediastinal tumours and cysts. CT scans are the gold standard for assessment of the mediastinum and surrounding structures. MRI may be used in some circumstances, as well as PET scans.

Medical Management

If the tumour is malignant and has infiltrated surrounding tissue, radiation therapy and/or chemotherapy are the therapeutic modalities used when complete surgical removal (discussed below) is not feasible.

SURGICAL MANAGEMENT

Many mediastinal tumours are benign and operable. The location of the tumour (anterior, middle, or posterior compartments) in the mediastinum dictates the type of incision. The common incision used is a median sternotomy; however, a thoracotomy may be used, depending on the location of the tumour. Additional approaches may include a bilateral anterior thoracotomy (clamshell incision) or video-assisted thoracoscopic surgery (see Chap. 25). The care is the same as for any patient undergoing thoracic surgery. The major complications include hemorrhage, injury to the phrenic or recurrent laryngeal nerve, and infection.

Chest Trauma

Approximately 60% of all multisystem trauma victims have some type of chest or thoracic trauma (Owens, Chaudry, Eggerstedt & Smith, 2000). Chest trauma is classified as either blunt or penetrating. Blunt chest trauma results from sudden compression or positive pressure inflicted to the chest wall. Motor vehicle crashes (trauma due to steering wheel, seat belt), falls, and bicycle crashes (trauma due to handlebars) are the most common causes of blunt chest trauma. Penetrating trauma occurs when a foreign object penetrates the chest wall. The most common causes of penetrating chest trauma include gunshot wounds and stabbings.

BLUNT TRAUMA

Although blunt chest trauma is more common, it is often difficult to identify the extent of the damage because the symptoms may be generalized and vague. In addition, patients may not seek immediate medical attention, which may complicate the problem.

Pathophysiology

Injuries to the chest are often life-threatening and result in one or more of the following pathologic mechanisms:

- Hypoxemia from disruption of the airway; injury to the lung parenchyma, rib cage, and respiratory musculature; massive hemorrhage; collapsed lung; and pneumothorax
- Hypovolemia from massive fluid loss from the great vessels, cardiac rupture, or hemothorax
- Cardiac failure from cardiac tamponade, cardiac contusion, or increased intrathoracic pressure

These mechanisms frequently result in impaired ventilation and perfusion leading to ARF, hypovolemic shock, and death.

Assessment and Diagnostic Findings

Time is critical in treating chest trauma. Therefore, it is essential to assess the patient immediately to determine the following:

- When the injury occurred
- Mechanism of injury
- Level of responsiveness
- Specific injuries
- Estimated blood loss
- Recent drug or alcohol use
- Prehospital treatment

The initial assessment of thoracic injuries includes assessment of the patient for airway obstruction, tension pneumothorax, open pneumothorax, massive hemothorax, flail chest, and cardiac tamponade. These injuries are life-threatening and need immediate treatment. Secondary assessment would include simple pneumothorax, hemothorax, pulmonary contusion, traumatic aortic rupture, tracheobronchial disruption, esophageal perforation, traumatic diaphragmatic injury, and penetrating wounds to the mediastinum (Owens, Chaudry, Eggerstedt & Smith, 2000). Although listed as secondary, these injuries may be life-threatening as well depending upon the circumstances.

The physical examination includes inspection of the airway, thorax, neck veins, and breathing difficulty. Specifics include assessing the rate and depth of breathing for abnormalities, such as stridor, cyanosis, nasal flaring, use of accessory muscles, drooling, and overt trauma to the face, mouth, or neck. The chest should be assessed for symmetric movement, symmetry of breath sounds, open chest wounds, entrance or exit wounds, impaled objects, tracheal shift, distended neck veins, subcutaneous emphysema, and paradoxical chest wall motion. In addition, the chest wall should be assessed for bruising, petechiae, lacerations, and burns. The vital signs and skin colour are assessed for signs of shock. The thorax is palpated for tenderness and crepitus; the position of the trachea is also assessed.

The initial diagnostic workup includes a chest x-ray, CT scan, complete blood count, clotting studies, type and cross-match, electrolytes, oxygen saturation, arterial blood gas analysis, and ECG. The patient is completely undressed to avoid missing additional injuries that can complicate care. Many patients with injuries involving the chest have associated head and abdominal injuries that require attention. Ongoing assessment is essential to monitor the patient's response to treatment and to detect early signs of clinical deterioration.

Medical Management

The goals of treatment are to evaluate the patient's condition and to initiate aggressive resuscitation. An airway is immediately established with oxygen support and, in some cases, intubation and ventilatory support. Re-establishing fluid volume and negative intrapleural pressure and draining intrapleural fluid and blood are essential.

The potential for massive blood loss and exsanguination with blunt or penetrating chest injuries is high because of injury to the great blood vessels. Many patients die at the scene or are in shock by the time help arrives. Agitation and irrational and combative behaviour are signs of decreased oxygen delivery to the cerebral cortex. Strategies to restore and maintain cardiopulmonary function include ensuring an adequate airway and ventilation, stabilizing and re-establishing chest wall integrity, occluding any opening into the chest (open pneumothorax), and draining or removing any air or fluid from the thorax to relieve pneumothorax, hemothorax, or cardiac tamponade. Hypovolemia and low cardiac output must be corrected. Many of these treatment efforts, along with the control of hemorrhage, are usually carried out simultaneously at the scene of the injury or in the emergency department. Depending on the success of efforts to control the hemorrhage in the emergency department, the patient may be taken immediately to the operating room. Principles of management are essentially those pertaining to care of the postoperative thoracic patient (see Chap. 25).

Sternal and Rib Fractures

Sternal fractures are most common in motor vehicle crashes with a direct blow to the sternum via the steering wheel and are most common in women, patients over age 50, and those using shoulder restraints (Owens, Chaudry, Eggerstedt & Smith, 2000).

Rib fractures are the most common type of chest trauma, occurring in more than 60% of patients admitted with blunt chest injury. Most rib fractures are benign and are treated conservatively. Fractures of the first three ribs are rare but can result in a high mortality rate because they are associated with laceration of the subclavian artery or vein. The fifth through ninth ribs are the most common sites of fractures. Fractures of the lower ribs are associated with injury to the spleen and liver, which may be lacerated by fragmented sections of the rib.

CLINICAL MANIFESTATIONS

The patient with sternal fractures has anterior chest pain, overlying tenderness, ecchymosis, crepitus, swelling, and the potential of a chest wall deformity. For the patient with rib fractures, clinical manifestations are similar: severe pain, point tenderness, and muscle spasm over the area of the fracture, which is aggravated by coughing, deep breathing, and movement. The area around the fracture may be bruised. To reduce the pain, the patient splints the chest by breathing in a shallow manner and avoids sighs, deep breaths, coughing, and movement. This reluctance to move or breathe deeply results in diminished ventilation, collapse of unaerated alveoli (atelectasis), pneumonitis, and hypoxemia. Respiratory insufficiency and failure can be the outcomes of such a cycle.

ASSESSMENT AND DIAGNOSTIC FINDINGS

The patient with a sternal fracture must be closely evaluated for underlying cardiac injuries. A crackling, grating sound in the thorax (subcutaneous crepitus) may be detected with auscultation. The diagnostic workup may include a chest x-ray, rib films of a specific area, ECG, continuous pulse oximetry, and arterial blood gas analysis.

MEDICAL MANAGEMENT

Medical management of the patient with a sternal fracture is directed toward controlling pain, avoiding excessive activity, and treating any associated injuries. Surgical fixation is rarely necessary unless fragments are grossly displaced and pose a potential for further injury.

The goals of treatment for rib fractures are to control pain and to detect and treat the injury. Sedation is used to relieve pain and to allow deep breathing and coughing. Care must be taken to avoid oversedation and suppression of the respiratory drive. Alternative strategies to relieve pain include an intercostal nerve block and ice over the fracture site; a chest binder may decrease pain on movement. Usually the pain abates in 5 to 7 days, and discomfort can be controlled with epidural analgesia, patient-controlled analgesia, or nonopioid analgesia. Most rib fractures heal in 3 to 6 weeks. The patient is monitored closely for signs and symptoms of associated injuries.

Flail Chest

Flail chest is frequently a complication of blunt chest trauma from a steering wheel injury. It usually occurs when three or more adjacent ribs (multiple contiguous ribs) are fractured at two or more sites, resulting in free-floating rib segments. It may also result as a combination fracture of ribs and costal cartilages or sternum (Owens, Chaudry, Eggerstedt & Smith, 2000). As a result, the chest wall loses stability and there is subsequent respiratory impairment and usually severe respiratory distress.

PATHOPHYSIOLOGY

During inspiration, as the chest expands, the detached part of the rib segment (flail segment) moves in a paradoxical manner (pendelluft movement) in that it is pulled inward during inspiration, reducing the amount of air that can be drawn into the lungs. On expiration, because the intrathoracic pressure exceeds atmospheric pressure, the flail segment bulges outward, impairing the patient's ability to exhale. The mediastinum then shifts back to the affected side (Fig. 23-8). This paradoxical action results in increased dead space, a reduction in alveolar ventilation, and decreased compliance. Retained airway secretions and atelectasis frequently accompany flail chest. The patient has hypoxemia, and if gas exchange is greatly compromised, respiratory acidosis develops as a result of CO_2 retention. Hypotension, inadequate tissue perfusion, and metabolic acidosis often follow as the paradoxical motion of the mediastinum decreases cardiac output.

MEDICAL MANAGEMENT

As with rib fracture, treatment of flail chest is usually supportive. Management includes providing ventilatory support, clearing secretions from the lungs, and controlling pain. The specific management depends on the degree of respiratory dysfunction. If only a small segment of the chest is involved, the objectives are to clear the airway through positioning, coughing, deep breathing, and suctioning to aid in the expansion of the lung, and to relieve pain by intercostal nerve blocks, high thoracic epidural blocks, or cautious use of intravenous opioids.

For mild to moderate flail chest injuries, the underlying pulmonary contusion is treated by monitoring fluid intake and appropriate fluid replacement, while at the same time relieving chest pain. Pulmonary physiotherapy focusing on lung volume expansion and secretion management techniques are performed. The patient is closely monitored for further respiratory compromise.

When a severe flail chest injury is encountered, endotracheal intubation and mechanical ventilation are required to provide internal pneumatic stabilization of the flail chest and to correct abnormalities in gas exchange. This helps to treat the underlying

A Inspiration **B** Expiration

FIGURE 23-8 Flail chest is caused by a free-floating segment of rib cage resulting from multiple rib fractures. (**A**) Paradoxical movement on inspiration occurs when the flail rib segment is sucked inward and the mediastinal structures shift to the unaffected side. The amount of air drawn into the affected lung is reduced. (**B**) On expiration, the flail segment bulges outward and the mediastinal structures shift back to the affected side.

pulmonary contusion, serves to stabilize the thoracic cage to allow the fractures to heal, and improves alveolar ventilation and intrathoracic volume by decreasing the work of breathing. This treatment modality requires endotracheal intubation and ventilator support. Differing modes of ventilation are used depending on the patient's underlying disease and specific needs.

In rare circumstances, surgery may be required to more quickly stabilize the flail segment. This may be used in the patient who is difficult to ventilate or the high-risk patient with underlying lung disease who may be difficult to wean from mechanical ventilation.

Regardless of the type of treatment, the patient is carefully monitored by serial chest x-rays, arterial blood gas analysis, pulse oximetry, and bedside pulmonary function monitoring. Pain management is key to successful treatment. Patient-controlled analgesia, intercostal nerve blocks, epidural analgesia, and intrapleural administration of opioids may be used to control thoracic pain.

Pulmonary Contusion

Pulmonary contusion is observed in about 20% of adult patients with multiple traumatic injuries and in a higher percentage of children due to increased compliance of the chest wall. It is defined as damage to the lung tissues resulting in hemorrhage and localized edema. It is associated with chest trauma when there is rapid compression and decompression to the chest wall (ie, blunt trauma). It may not be evident initially on examination but will develop in the posttraumatic period.

PATHOPHYSIOLOGY

The primary pathologic defect is an abnormal accumulation of fluid in the interstitial and intra-alveolar spaces. It is thought that injury to the lung parenchyma and its capillary network results in a leakage of serum protein and plasma. The leaking serum protein exerts an osmotic pressure that enhances loss of fluid from the capillaries. Blood, edema, and cellular debris (from cellular response to injury) enter the lung and accumulate in the bronchioles and alveolar surface, where they interfere with gas exchange. An increase in pulmonary vascular resistance and pulmonary artery pressure occurs. The patient has hypoxemia and carbon dioxide retention. Occasionally, a contused lung occurs on the other side of the point of body impact; this is called a contrecoup contusion.

CLINICAL MANIFESTATIONS

Pulmonary contusion may be mild, moderate, or severe. The clinical manifestations vary from tachypnea, tachycardia, pleuritic chest pain, hypoxemia, and blood-tinged secretions to more severe tachypnea, tachycardia, crackles, frank bleeding, severe hypoxemia, and respiratory acidosis. Changes in sensorium, including increased agitation or combative irrational behaviour, may be signs of hypoxemia.

In addition, the patient with moderate pulmonary contusion has a large amount of mucus, serum, and frank blood in the tracheobronchial tree; the patient often has a constant cough but cannot clear the secretions. A patient with severe pulmonary contusion has the signs and symptoms of ARDS; these may include central cyanosis, agitation, combativeness, and productive cough with frothy, bloody secretions.

ASSESSMENT AND DIAGNOSTIC FINDINGS

The efficiency of gas exchange is determined by pulse oximetry and arterial blood gas measurements. Pulse oximetry is also used to measure oxygen saturation continuously. The chest x-ray may show pulmonary infiltration. The initial chest x-ray may show no changes; in fact, changes may not appear for 1 or 2 days after the injury.

MEDICAL MANAGEMENT

Treatment priorities include maintaining the airway, providing adequate oxygenation, and controlling pain. In mild pulmonary contusion, adequate hydration via intravenous fluids and oral intake is important to mobilize secretions. However, fluid intake must be closely monitored to avoid hypervolemia. Volume expansion techniques, postural drainage, physiotherapy including coughing, and endotracheal suctioning are used to remove the secretions. Pain is managed by intercostal nerve blocks or by opioids via patient-controlled analgesia or other methods. Usually, antimicrobial therapy is administered because the damaged lung is susceptible to infection. Supplemental oxygen is usually given by mask or cannula for 24 to 36 hours.

The patient with moderate pulmonary contusion may require bronchoscopy to remove secretions; intubation and mechanical ventilation with PEEP may also be necessary to maintain the pressure and keep the lungs inflated. Diuretics may be given to reduce edema. A nasogastric tube is inserted to relieve gastrointestinal distention.

The patient with severe contusion may develop respiratory failure and may require aggressive treatment with endotracheal intubation and ventilatory support, diuretics, and fluid restriction. Colloids and crystalloid solutions may be used to treat hypovolemia.

Antimicrobial medications may be prescribed for the treatment of pulmonary infection. This is a common complication of pulmonary contusion (especially pneumonia in the contused segment), because the fluid and blood that extravasates into the alveolar and interstitial spaces serve as an excellent culture medium.

PENETRATING TRAUMA: GUNSHOT AND STAB WOUNDS

Gunshot and stab wounds are the most common types of penetrating chest trauma. They are classified according to their velocity. Stab wounds are generally considered of low velocity because the weapon destroys a small area around the wound. Knives and switchblades cause most stab wounds. The appearance of the external wound may be very deceptive, because pneumothorax, hemothorax, lung contusion, and cardiac tamponade, along with severe and continuing hemorrhage, can occur from any small wound, even one caused by a small-diameter instrument such as an ice pick.

Gunshot wounds to the chest may be classified as of low, medium, or high velocity. The factors that determine the velocity and resulting extent of damage include the distance from which the gun was fired, the calibre of the gun, and construction and size of the bullet. A gunshot wound can produce a variety of pathophysiologic changes. A bullet can cause damage at the site of penetration and along its pathway. It also may ricochet off bony structures and damage the chest organs and great vessels. If the diaphragm is involved in either a gunshot wound or a stab wound, injury to the chest cavity must be considered.

Medical Management

The objective of immediate management is to restore and maintain cardiopulmonary function. After an adequate airway is ensured and ventilation is established, the patient is examined for shock and intrathoracic and intra-abdominal injuries. The patient is undressed completely so that additional injuries will not be missed. There is a high risk for associated intra-abdominal injuries with stab wounds below the level of the fifth anterior intercostal space. Death can result from exsanguinating hemorrhage or intra-abdominal sepsis.

After the status of the peripheral pulses is assessed, a large-bore intravenous line is inserted. The diagnostic workup includes a chest x-ray, chemistry profile, arterial blood gas analysis, pulse oximetry, and ECG. Blood typing and cross-matching are done in case blood transfusion is required. An indwelling catheter is inserted to monitor urinary output. A nasogastric tube is inserted to prevent aspiration, minimize leakage of abdominal contents, and decompress the gastrointestinal tract.

Shock is treated simultaneously with colloid solutions, crystalloids, or blood, as indicated by the patient's condition. Chest x-rays are obtained, and other diagnostic procedures are carried out as dictated by the needs of the patient (eg, CT scans of chest or abdomen, flat plate x-ray of the abdomen, abdominal tap to check for bleeding).

A chest tube is inserted into the pleural space in most patients with penetrating wounds of the chest to achieve rapid and continuing re-expansion of the lungs. The insertion of the chest tube frequently results in a complete evacuation of the blood and air. The chest tube also allows early recognition of continuing intrathoracic bleeding, which would make surgical exploration necessary. If the patient has a penetrating wound of the heart and great vessels, the esophagus, or the tracheobronchial tree, surgical intervention is required.

PNEUMOTHORAX

Pneumothorax occurs when the parietal or visceral pleura is breached and the pleural space is exposed to positive atmospheric pressure. Normally the pressure in the pleural space is negative or subatmospheric compared to atmospheric pressure; this negative pressure is required to maintain lung inflation. When either pleura is breached, air enters the pleural space, and the lung or a portion of it collapses. Types of pneumothorax include simple, traumatic, and tension pneumothorax.

Simple Pneumothorax

A simple, or spontaneous, pneumothorax occurs when air enters the pleural space through a breach of either the parietal or visceral pleura. Most commonly this occurs as air enters the pleural space through the rupture of a bleb or a bronchopleural fistula. A spontaneous pneumothorax may occur in an apparently healthy person in the absence of trauma due to rupture of an air-filled bleb, or blister, on the surface of the lung, allowing air from the airways to enter the pleural cavity. It may be associated with diffuse interstitial lung disease and severe emphysema.

Traumatic Pneumothorax

Traumatic pneumothorax occurs when air escapes from a laceration in the lung itself and enters the pleural space or enters the pleural space through a wound in the chest wall. It can occur with blunt trauma (eg, rib fractures) or penetrating chest trauma. It may also occur from abdominal trauma (eg, stab wounds or gunshot wounds to the abdomen) and from diaphragmatic tears. Traumatic pneumothorax may occur with invasive thoracic procedures (ie, thoracentesis, transbronchial lung biopsy, insertion

of a subclavian line) in which the pleura is inadvertently punctured, or with barotrauma from mechanical ventilation.

Traumatic pneumothorax resulting from major injury to the chest is often accompanied by hemothorax (collection of blood in the pleural space resulting from torn intercostal vessels, lacerations of the great vessels, and lacerations of the lungs). Often both blood and air are found in the chest cavity (hemopneumothorax) after major trauma. Chest surgery can cause what is classified as a traumatic pneumothorax as a result of the entry into the pleural space and the accumulation of air and fluid in the pleural space.

Open pneumothorax is one form of traumatic pneumothorax. It occurs when a wound in the chest wall is large enough to allow air to pass freely in and out of the thoracic cavity with each attempted respiration. Because the rush of air through the hole in the chest wall produces a sucking sound, such injuries are termed sucking chest wounds. In such patients, not only does the lung collapse, but the structures of the mediastinum (heart and great vessels) also shift toward the uninjured side with each inspiration and in the opposite direction with expiration. This is termed mediastinal flutter or swing, and it produces serious circulatory problems.

Clinical Manifestations

The signs and symptoms associated with pneumothorax depend on its size and cause. Pain is usually sudden and may be pleuritic. The patient may have only minimal respiratory distress with slight chest discomfort and tachypnea with a small simple or uncomplicated pneumothorax. If the pneumothorax is large and the lung collapses totally, acute respiratory distress occurs. The patient is anxious, has dyspnea and air hunger, has increased use of the accessory muscles, and may develop central cyanosis from severe hypoxemia. Severe chest pain may occur, accompanied by tachypnea, decreased movement of the affected side of the thorax, a tympanic sound on percussion of the chest wall, and decreased or absent breath sounds and tactile fremitus on the affected side.

Medical Management

Medical management of pneumothorax depends on its cause and severity. The goal of treatment is to evacuate the air or blood from the pleural space. A small chest tube (28 French) is inserted near the second intercostal space; this space is used because it is the thinnest part of the chest wall, minimizes the danger of contacting the thoracic nerve, and leaves a less visible scar. If the patient also has a hemothorax, a large-diameter chest tube (32 French or greater) is inserted, usually in the fourth or fifth intercostal space at the midaxillary line. The tube is directed posteriorly to drain the fluid and air. Once the chest tube or tubes are inserted and suction is applied (usually to 20 mm Hg suction), effective decompression of the pleural cavity (drainage of blood or air) occurs.

If an excessive amount of blood enters the chest tube in a relatively short period, an autotransfusion may be needed. This technique involves taking the patient's own blood that has been drained from the chest, filtering it, and then transfusing it back into the patient's vascular system.

> **! NURSING ALERT** Traumatic open pneumothorax calls for emergency interventions. Stopping the flow of air through the opening in the chest wall is a life-saving measure.

In such an emergency, anything may be used that is large enough to fill the chest wound—a towel, a handkerchief, or the heel of the hand. If conscious, the patient is instructed to inhale and strain against a closed glottis. This action assists in re-expanding the lung and ejecting the air from the thorax. In the hospital, the opening is plugged by sealing it with gauze impregnated with petrolatum. A pressure dressing is applied. Usually, a chest tube connected to water-seal drainage is inserted to permit air and fluid to drain. Antibiotics usually are prescribed to combat infection from contamination.

The severity of open pneumothorax depends on the amount and rate of thoracic bleeding and the amount of air in the pleural space. The pleural cavity can be decompressed by needle aspiration (thoracentesis) or chest tube drainage of the blood or air. The lung is then able to re-expand and resume the function of gas exchange. As a rule of thumb, the chest wall is opened surgically (thoracotomy) when more than 1,500 mL of blood is aspirated initially by thoracentesis (or is the initial chest tube output) or when chest tube output continues at greater than 200 mL/hour. The urgency with which the blood must be removed is determined by the respiratory compromise. An emergency thoracotomy may also be performed in the emergency department if there is suggested cardiovascular injury secondary to chest or penetrating trauma.

Tension Pneumothorax

A **tension pneumothorax** occurs when air is drawn into the pleural space from a lacerated lung or through a small hole in the chest wall. It may be a complication of other types of pneumothorax. In contrast to open pneumothorax, the air that enters the chest cavity with each inspiration is trapped; it cannot be expelled during expiration through the air passages or the hole in the chest wall. In effect, a one-way valve or ball valve mechanism occurs where air enters the pleural space but cannot escape. With each breath, tension (positive pressure) is increased within the affected pleural space. This causes the lung to collapse and the heart, the great vessels, and the trachea to shift toward the unaffected side of the chest (mediastinal shift). Both respiration and circulatory function are compromised because of the increased intrathoracic pressure. The increased intrathoracic pressure decreases venous return to the heart, causing decreased cardiac output and impairment of peripheral circulation. In extreme cases, the pulse may be undetectable—this is known as pulseless electrical activity.

CLINICAL MANIFESTATIONS
The clinical picture is one of air hunger, agitation, increasing hypoxemia, central cyanosis, hypotension, tachycardia, and profuse diaphoresis. A comparison of open and tension pneumothorax is shown in Figure 23-9.

 NURSING ALERT Relief of tension pneumothorax is considered an emergency measure.

MEDICAL MANAGEMENT
If a tension pneumothorax is suspected, the patient should immediately be given a high concentration of supplemental oxygen to treat the hypoxemia, and pulse oximetry should be used to monitor oxygen saturation.

In an emergency situation, a tension pneumothorax can be decompressed or quickly converted to a simple pneumothorax by inserting a large-bore needle (14-gauge) at the second intercostal

 Physiology/Pathophysiology

FIGURE 23-9 Open pneumothorax (*top*) and tension pneumothorax (*bottom*). In open pneumothorax, air enters the chest during inspiration and exits during expiration. A slight shift of the affected lung may occur because of a decrease in pressure as air moves out of the chest. In tension pneumothorax, air enters but cannot leave the chest. As the pressure increases, the heart and great vessels are compressed and the mediastinal structures are shifted toward the opposite side of the chest. The trachea is pushed from its normal midline position toward the opposite side of the chest, and the unaffected lung is compressed.

space, midclavicular line on the affected side. This relieves the pressure and vents the positive pressure to the external environment. A chest tube is then inserted and connected to suction to remove the remaining air and fluid, re-establish the negative pressure, and re-expand the lung. If the lung re-expands and air leakage from the lung parenchyma stops, further drainage may be unnecessary. If a prolonged air leak continues despite chest tube drainage to underwater seal, surgery may be necessary to close the leak.

CARDIAC TAMPONADE

Cardiac tamponade is the compression of the heart as a result of fluid within the pericardial sac. It usually is caused by blunt or penetrating trauma to the chest. A penetrating wound of the heart is associated with a high mortality rate. Cardiac tamponade also may follow diagnostic cardiac catheterization, angiographic procedures, and pacemaker insertion, which can produce perforations of the heart and great vessels. Pericardial effusion with fluid compressing the heart also may develop from metastases to the pericardium from malignant tumours of the breast, lung, and mediastinum and may occur with lymphomas and leukemias, renal failure, TB, and high-dose radiation to the chest. Cardiac tamponade is discussed in detail in Chapter 30.

SUBCUTANEOUS EMPHYSEMA

No matter what kind of chest trauma the patient has, when the lung or the air passages are injured, air may enter the tissue planes and pass for some distance under the skin (eg, neck, chest). The tissues give a crackling sensation when palpated, and the subcutaneous air produces an alarming appearance as the face, neck, body, and scrotum become misshapen by subcutaneous air. Fortunately, subcutaneous emphysema is of itself usually not a serious complication. The subcutaneous air is spontaneously absorbed if the underlying air leak is treated or stops spontaneously. In severe cases in which there is widespread subcutaneous emphysema, a tracheostomy is indicated if airway patency is threatened.

Aspiration

Aspiration of stomach contents into the lungs is a serious complication that may cause pneumonia and result in the following clinical picture: tachycardia, dyspnea, central cyanosis, hypertension, hypotension, and finally death. It can occur when the protective airway reflexes are decreased or absent from a variety of factors (Chart 23-11).

> **! NURSING ALERT** When a nonfunctioning nasogastric tube allows the gastric contents to accumulate in the stomach, a condition known as silent aspiration may result. Silent aspiration often occurs unobserved and may be more common than suspected. If untreated, massive inhalation of gastric contents develops in a period of several hours.

Pathophysiology

The primary factors responsible for death and complications after aspiration of gastric contents are the volume and character of the aspirated gastric contents. For example, a small, localized aspiration from regurgitation can cause pneumonia and acute respiratory distress; a massive aspiration is usually fatal.

A full stomach contains solid particles of food. If these are aspirated, the problem then becomes one of mechanical blockage of the airways and secondary infection. During periods of fasting, the stomach contains acidic gastric juice, which, if aspirated, may be very destructive to the alveoli and capillaries. Fecal contamination (more likely seen in intestinal obstruction) increases the

likelihood of death because the endotoxins produced by intestinal organisms may be absorbed systemically, or the thick proteinaceous material found in the intestinal contents may obstruct the airway, leading to atelectasis and secondary bacterial invasion.

Aspiration pneumonitis may develop from aspiration of substances with a pH of less than 2.5 and a volume of gastric aspirate greater than 0.3 mL per kilogram of body weight (20 to 25 mL in adults) (Marik, 2001). Aspiration of gastric contents causes a chemical burn of the tracheobronchial tree and pulmonary parenchyma (Marik, 2001). An inflammatory response occurs. This results in the destruction of alveolar–capillary endothelial cells, with a consequent outpouring of protein-rich fluids into the interstitial and intra-alveolar spaces. As a result, surfactant is lost, which in turn causes the airways to close and the alveoli to collapse. Finally, the impaired exchange of oxygen and carbon dioxide causes respiratory failure.

Aspiration pneumonia develops following inhalation of colonized oropharyngeal material. The pathologic process involves an acute inflammatory response to bacteria and bacterial products. Most commonly, the bacteriologic findings include gram-positive cocci, gram-negative rods, and occasionally anaerobic bacteria (Marik, 2001).

Prevention

Prevention is the primary goal when caring for patients at risk for aspiration.

COMPENSATING FOR ABSENT REFLEXES

Aspiration is likely to occur if the patient cannot adequately coordinate protective glottic, laryngeal, and cough reflexes. This hazard is increased if the patient has a distended abdomen, is in a supine position, has the upper extremities immobilized by intravenous infusions or hand restraints, receives local anesthetics to the oropharyngeal or laryngeal area for diagnostic procedures, has been sedated, or has had long-term intubation.

When vomiting, a person can normally protect the airway by sitting up or turning on the side and coordinating breathing, coughing, gag, and glottic reflexes. If these reflexes are active, an oral airway should not be inserted. If an airway is in place, it should be pulled out the moment the patient gags so as not to stimulate the pharyngeal gag reflex and promote vomiting and aspiration. Suctioning of oral secretions with a catheter should be performed with minimal pharyngeal stimulation.

ASSESSING FEEDING TUBE PLACEMENT

Even when the patient is intubated, aspiration may occur even with a nasogastric tube in place. This aspiration may result in nosocomial pneumonia. Assessment of tube placement is key to prevent aspiration. The best method for determining tube placement is via an x-ray. There are other nonradiologic methods that have been studied. Observation of the aspirate and testing of its pH are the most reliable. Gastric fluid may be grassy green, brown, clear, or colourless. An aspirate from the lungs may be off-white or tan mucus. Pleural fluid is watery and usually straw-coloured (Metheny & Titler, 2001). Gastric pH values are typically lower or more acidic that that of the intestinal or respiratory tract. Gastric pH is usually between 1 and 5, while intestinal or respiratory pH is 7 or higher (Metheny & Titler, 2001). There are differences in assessing tube placement with continuous versus intermittent feedings. For intermittent feedings with small-bore tubes, observation of aspirated contents and pH evaluation should be performed. For continuous feedings, the pH method

Chart 23-11
Risk Factors for Aspiration

Seizure activity
Decreased level of consciousness from trauma, drug or alcohol intoxication, excessive sedation, or general anesthesia
Nausea and vomiting in the patient with a decreased level of consciousness
Stroke
Swallowing disorders
Cardiac arrest
Silent aspiration

NURSING RESEARCH PROFILE 23-2
Pulmonary Aspiration

Elpern, E. H., Okonek, M. B., Bacon, M., Gerstung, C., & Skrzynski, M. (2000). Effect of the Passy-Muir tracheostomy speaking valve on pulmonary aspiration in adults. *Heart Lung, 29*(4), 287–293.

Purpose

The purpose of this study was to investigate the frequency of aspiration in adults with tracheostomies and to investigate the effect of the Passy-Muir speaking valve on aspiration occurrences.

Study Sample and Design

Fifteen subjects were included in this study. Inclusion criteria were that there was a tracheostomy in place and the patient was scheduled for a videofluoroscopic swallowing examination. During the swallowing examination, six presentations of thin liquids were recorded: three with and three without the Passy-Muir tracheostomy speaking valve applied.

Findings

Seven of the 15 subjects (47%) aspirated material on one or more presentations of the thin liquid. Five subjects aspirated without the valve and two subjects aspirated with and without the valve. No subjects aspirated only when the valve was applied. Aspiration occurred less frequently with the Passy-Muir tracheostomy speaking valve on than with it off.

Nursing Implications

Aspiration is a common problem that can lead to severe pulmonary complications. Potential complications of aspiration include obstruction, inflammation (pneumonitis), and infection (aspiration pneumonia). Nursing assessment and knowledge of risk factors are key in evaluating patients at risk for potential aspiration problems and preventing this complication.

is not clinically useful due to the infused formula (Metheny & Titler, 2001).

The patient who is receiving continuous or timed-interval tube feedings must be positioned properly. The patient receiving a continuous infusion is given small volumes under low pressure in an upright position, which helps to prevent aspiration. Patients receiving tube feedings at timed intervals are maintained in an upright position during the feeding and for a minimum of 30 minutes afterward to allow the stomach to empty partially. Tube feedings must be given only when it is certain that the feeding tube is positioned correctly in the stomach. Many patients today receive enteral feeding directly into the duodenum through a small-bore flexible feeding tube or surgically implanted tube. Feedings are given slowly and regulated by a feeding pump. Correct placement is confirmed by chest x-ray.

IDENTIFYING DELAYED STOMACH EMPTYING

A full stomach may cause aspiration because of increased intragastric or extragastric pressure. The following clinical situations cause a delayed emptying time of the stomach and may contribute to aspiration: intestinal obstruction; increased gastric secretions in gastroesophageal reflex disease; increased gastric secretions during anxiety, stress, or pain; or abdominal distention because of ileus, ascites, peritonitis, use of opioids and sedatives, severe illness, or vaginal delivery.

When a feeding tube is present, contents are aspirated, usually every 4 hours, to determine the amount of the last feeding left in the stomach (residual volume). If more than 50 mL is aspirated, there may be a problem with delayed emptying, and the next

feeding should be delayed or the continuous feeding stopped for a period of time.

MANAGING EFFECTS OF PROLONGED INTUBATION

Prolonged endotracheal intubation or tracheostomy can depress the laryngeal and glottic reflexes because of disuse. Patients with prolonged tracheostomies are encouraged to phonate and exercise their laryngeal muscles. For patients who have had long-term intubation or tracheostomies, it may be helpful to have a rehabilitation therapist experienced in speech and swallowing disorders work with the patient to assess the swallowing reflex.

Critical Thinking Exercises

1. Your patient, a 44-year-old unemployed man who lives with his 80-year-old mother, has recently been diagnosed with active TB. He has been started on treatment and given specific instructions about his medications. What strategies would you initiate to be sure that he takes his medications correctly? What strategies would you use to ensure that his mother is not infected? How would your care differ if the patient lived alone or were homeless?

2. You are working on a surgical unit. Your patient is a 67-year-old woman who has had surgery to repair a fractured hip that occurred following a fall associated with heavy alcohol use. She has been a heavy smoker for over 35 years and is reluctant to move in bed because of pain. What are the potential postoperative pulmonary complications? What assessment criteria would you use to assess her respiratory status? What interventions would you implement to prevent pulmonary complications in this patient? What changes, if any, would you implement if she had a history of deep vein thrombosis?

3. Your patient has experienced blunt chest trauma following a motor vehicle crash. A chest tube has been inserted to treat a pneumothorax. The chest drainage system has drained 400 mL of light-red fluid during the first 6 hours following the tube's insertion. The patient is unable to recall how he was injured or what has happened to him over the last 24 hours. The patient is experiencing pain requiring opioids and is asking that the chest tube be removed to enable him to walk to the bathroom. What additional information would you obtain through assessment and what actions would you take? How would you explain to the patient and his family the purpose of the chest tubes? How would you modify your explanation and teaching if he has little understanding of English?

REFERENCES AND SELECTED READINGS

Books

American Cancer Society. (2002). *Cancer facts and figures.* Atlanta: American Cancer Society.

American Joint Committee on Cancer (AJCC). (2002). *Cancer staging manual* (6th ed.). New York: Springer-Verlag.

Ansell, J. E., Hickey, A. D., Kleinschmidt, K. C., Merli, G. J., Tillman, D. J., & Yusen, R. D. (2000). *Advancing the treatment of deep venous thrombosis and pulmonary embolism.* Cincinnati: Sci-Health Communications.

Arroliga, A. C., Matthay, M. A., & Matthay, R. A. (2000). Pulmonary thromboembolism and other pulmonary vascular diseases. In R. George, R. Light, M. Matthay, & R. Matthay (eds.), *Chest medicine: Essentials of pulmonary and critical care medicine* (4th ed., pp 233–261). Philadelphia: Lippincott Williams & Wilkins.

Bartlett, J. G. (1999). *Management of respiratory tract infections* (2d ed). Philadelphia: Lippincott Williams & Wilkins.

Bast, R. C., Kufe, D. W., Pollock, R. E. et al. (eds.) (2000). *Cancer medicine* (5th ed.). Hamilton, Ontario: B. C. Decker, Inc.

Blondel-Hill, E., & Fryters, S. (2001). *Bugs and drugs antimicrobial pocket reference 2001.* Edmonton: Capital Health Authority.

Centers for Disease Control and Prevention (2000). *TB elimination: Now is the time.* National Center for HIV, STD and TB Prevention.

Cherniack, N. S., Homma, I., & Altose, M. (1999). *Rehabilitation of the patient with respiratory disease.* New York: McGraw-Hill.

Davis, G. S. (1999). *Medical management of pulmonary diseases.* New York: Marcel Dekker, Inc.

Duffy, S. Q., & Farley, D. E. (1993). *Intermittent positive pressure breathing: Old technologies rarely die* (AHCPR Publication No. 94-0001). Division of Provider Studies Research Note 18, Agency for Health Care Policy and Research, Rockville, MD: Public Health Service.

Farzan, S. (1997). *A concise handbook of respiratory diseases.* Stamford, CT: Appleton & Lange.

Health Canada. (2001). *Respiratory disease in Canada.* Ottawa: Author.

Health Canada. (2000). *Canadian tuberculosis standards* (5th ed.). Ottawa: Author.

Matthay, R. A., Tanoue, L. T., & Carter, D. C. (2000). Lung neoplasms. In R. George, R. Light, M. Matthay, & R. Matthay (eds.), *Chest medicine: essentials of pulmonary and critical care medicine* (4th ed., pp 346–376). Philadelphia: Lippincott Williams & Wilkins.

Niederman, M. S., & Sarosi, G. A. (2000). Respiratory tract infections. In R. George, R. Light, M. Matthay, & R. Matthay (eds.), *Chest medicine: Essentials of pulmonary and critical care medicine* (4th ed., pp 377–429). Philadelphia: Lippincott Williams & Wilkins.

Nield, M. J. (ed.). Committee on Regulating Occupational Exposure to Tuberculosis (2000). *Tuberculosis in the workplace.* Division of Health Promotion and Disease Prevention, National Academy of Sciences, Institute of Medicine.

Owens, M. W., Chaudry, M. S., Eggerstedt, J. M., & Smith, L. M. (2000). Thoracic trauma, surgery and perioperative management. In R. George, R. Light, M. Matthay, & R. Matthay (eds.), *Chest medicine: Essentials of pulmonary and critical care medicine* (4th ed., pp 592–619). Philadelphia: Lippincott Williams & Wilkins.

Respiratory Nursing Society and American Nurses Association. (1994). *Standards and scope of respiratory nursing practice/Joint Standards Task Force for Respiratory Nursing Practice.* Washington, DC: Author.

Schottenfeld, D. (2000). Etiology and epidemiology of lung cancer. In H. I. Pass, J. B. Mitchell, D. H. Johnson, & J. D. Minna (eds.) *Lung cancer: Principles and practice* (2d ed., pp 367–388). Philadelphia: Lippincott Williams & Wilkins.

Tanoue, L. T., & Elias, J. A. (1998). Systemic sarcoidosis. In G. L. Baum, J. D. Crapo, B. R. Celli, & J. B. Karlinsky (eds.), *Textbook of pulmonary disease* (pp 407–430). Philadelphia: Lippincott-Raven.

Velmahos, G. C., Kern, J., Chan, L., et al. (2000). *Prevention of venous thromboembolism after injury.* Evidence Report/Technology Assessment No. 22 (Prepared by Southern California Evidence-based Practice Center/RAND under Contract no. 290-97-0001). AHRQ Publication No. 01-E004. Rockville, MD: Agency for Healthcare Research and Quality.

Wilcox, W. (1998). *Public health sourcebook* (vol. 34, p 49). Detroit: Omnigraphics.

Winningham, M. L., & Barton-Burke, M. (2000). *Fatigue in cancer: A multidimensional approach.* Boston: Jones and Bartlett Publishers.

World Health Organization. (2000). *Global tuberculosis control: WHO report.* Geneva, Switzerland: Author.

Journals

Asterisks indicate nursing research articles.
General
American Thoracic Society. (1999). Statement on sarcoidosis. *American Journal of Respiratory and Critical Care Medicine, 160*(2), 736–755.

American Thoracic Society and European Respiratory Society. (2000). Idiopathic pulmonary fibrosis: diagnosis and treatment. International consensus statement. *American Journal of Respiratory and Critical Care Medicine, 161*(2), 646–664.

Bryce, J. C. (1995). Aspiration: causes, consequences, and prevention. *ORL Head and Neck Nursing, 13*(2), 14–19.

Centers for Disease Control and Prevention (1997). Premature deaths, monthly mortality and monthly physician contacts: United States. *MMWR Morbidity and Mortality Weekly Report, 46*(24), 556–561.

Clagett, G. P., Anderson, F. A. Jr., Geerts, W., et al. (1998). Prevention of venous thromboembolism. *Chest, 114*(5), 531S-560S.

Dalen, J. E., Hirsh, J., & Guyatt, G. H. (2001). Sixth ACCP consensus conference on antithrombotic therapy. *Chest, 119*(1), supplement, 1S-370S.

Elpern, E. H. (1997). Pulmonary aspiration in hospitalized adults. *Nutrition in Clinical Practice, 12*(1), 5–13.

*Elpern, E. H., Okonek, M. B., Bacon, M., et al. (2000). Effect of the Passy-Muir tracheostomy speaking valve on pulmonary aspiration in adults. *Heart Lung, 29*(4), 287–293.

Goldhaber, S. Z. (1998). Medical progress: Pulmonary embolism. *New England Journal of Medicine, 339*(2), 93–104.

Hosoda, Y., Sasagawa, S., & Yasuda, N. (2002). Epidemiology of sarcoidosis: New frontiers to explore. *Current Opinion in Pulmonary Medicine, 8*, 424–428.

Lomotan, J. R., George, S. S., & Brandsetter, R. D. (1997). Aspiration pneumonia: Strategies for early recognition and prevention. *Postgraduate Medicine, 102*(2), 225–231.

Marik, P. E. (2001). Aspiration pneumonitis and aspiration pneumonia. *New England Journal of Medicine, 344*(9), 665–671.

Metheny, N. A., & Titler, M. G. (2001). Assessing placement of feeding tubes. *American Journal of Nursing, 101*(5), 36–45.

Seijo, L. M., & Sterman, D. H. (2001). Interventional pulmonology. *New England Journal of Medicine, 344*(10), 740–749.

Taubert, J., & Wright, S. (2000). Malignant pleural effusion: nursing interventions using an indwelling pleural catheter with intermittent drainage. *Nursing Interventions in Oncology, 12*, 2–7.

White, R. H. (2003). Epidemiology of venous thromboembolism. *Circulation, 107*, I4–I8.

Acute Respiratory Failure and ARDS
Acute Respiratory Distress Syndrome Network. (2000). Ventilation with lower tidal volumes as compared with traditional tidal volumes for acute lung injury and the acute respiratory distress syndrome. *New England Journal of Medicine, 342*(18), 1301–1308.

Bernard, G. R., Artigas, A., Brigham, K. L., et al. (1994). Report of the American-European consensus conference on acute respiratory distress syndrome: Definitions, mechanisms, relevant outcomes, and clinical trial coordination. *American Journal of Critical Care Medicine, 9*(1), 72–81.

Brower, R. G., Ware, L. B., Berthiaume, Y., & Matthay, M. A. (2001). Treatment of ARDS. *Chest, 120*(4), 1347–1367.

Curley, M. A. (2000). Prone positioning of patients with acute respiratory distress syndrome: a systematic review. *American Journal of Critical Care, 9*(4), 295–296.

Davidson, T. A., Caldwell, E. S., Curtis, J. R., et al. (1999). Reduced quality of life in survivors of acute respiratory distress syndrome compared with critically ill control patients. *Journal of the American Medical Association, 281*(4), 354–360.

Marion, B. S. (2001). A turn for the better: 'Prone Positioning' of patients with ARDS. *American Journal of Nursing, 101*(5), 26–34.

Thompson, B. T., Hayden, D., Matthay, M. A., et al. (2001). Clinicians' approaches to mechanical ventilation in acute lung injury and ARDS. *Chest, 120*(5), 1622–1627.

Ware, L. B., & Matthay, M. A. (2000). The acute respiratory distress syndrome. *New England Journal of Medicine, 342*(18), 1334–1349.

Lung Cancer
Alpha-Tocopherol Beta-Carotene Cancer Prevention Study Group. (1994). The effect of vitamin E and beta-carotene on the incidence of lung cancer and other cancers in male smokers. *New England Journal of Medicine, 330*, 1029–1035.

American Thoracic Society. (2000). Management of malignant pleural effusions. *American Journal of Respiratory and Critical Care Medicine, 162*(5), 1987–2001.

*Brown, J. K., & Radke, K. J. (1998). Nutritional assessment, intervention, and evaluation of weight loss in patients with non-small-cell lung cancer. *Oncology Nursing Forum, 25*(3), 547–554.

*Connolly, M., & O'Neill, J. (1999). Teaching a research-based approach to the management of breathlessness in patients with lung cancer. *European Journal of Cancer Care, 8*(1), 30–36.

Greenlee, R. T., Hill-Harmon, M. B., Murray, T., & Thun, M. (2001). Cancer statistics 2001. *CA: A Cancer Journal for Clinicians, 51*(1), 15–36.

Hennekens, C., Buring, J., & Manson, J. (1996). Lack of effect of long-term supplementations with beta carotene on the incidence of malignant neoplasms and cardiovascular disease. *New England Journal of Medicine, 334,* 1145–1149.

Knippel, S. L. (2001). Surgical therapies for lung carcinomas. *Nursing Clinics of North America, 36*(3), 517–525.

Mountain, C. F. (1997). Revisions in the international system for staging lung cancer. *Chest, 111*(6), 1710–1717.

*Rice, V. H. (1999). Nursing intervention and smoking cessation: a meta-analysis. *Heart Lung, 28*(6), 438–454.

*Sarna, L. P., Brown, J. K., Lillington, L., et al. (2000). Tobacco interventions by oncology nurses in clinical practice. *Cancer, 89*(4), 881–889.

Taubert, J. (2001). Management of malignant pleural effusion. *Nursing Clinics of North America, 36*(4), 665–683.

Yeatman, T. J. (2000). Nutritional support for the surgical oncology patient. *Cancer Control, 7*(6), 563–565.

Pulmonary Infections

American Thoracic Society. (2001). Guidelines for the management of adults with community-acquired pneumonia. *American Journal of Respiratory and Critical Care Medicine, 163*(7), 1730–1754.

American Thoracic Society. (1995). Hospital-acquired pneumonia in adults: Diagnosis, assessment of severity, initial antimicrobial therapy, and preventive strategies. A consensus statement. *American Journal of Critical Care Medicine, 153*(5), 1711–1725.

Bartlett, J. G., Dowell, S. F., Mandell, L. A., File, T. M., Musher, D. M., & Fine, M. J. (2000). Practice guidelines for the management of community-acquired pneumonia in adults. *Clinical Infectious Diseases, 31*(2), 347–382.

*Brooks-Brunn, J. A. (1997). Predictors of postoperative pulmonary complications following abdominal surgery. *Chest, 111*(3), 564–571.

Brooks, J. A. (2001). Postoperative nosocomial pneumonia: nurse-sensitive interventions. *AACN Clinical Issues, 12*(2), 305–323.

Canadian Infectious Diseases Society and Canadian Thoracic Society. (2000). Canadian Guidelines for Initial Management of Community-Acquired Pneumonia: An evidence-based update by the Canadian Infectious Diseases Society and the Canadian Thoracic Society. *Clinical Infectious Diseases, 31,* 383–421.

Centers for Disease Control and Prevention. (1997). Guidelines for prevention of nosocomial pneumonia. *MMWR Morbidity and Mortality Weekly Report, 46:*RR1, 1–79.

Centers for Disease Control and Prevention. (1998). Influenza and pneumococcal vaccination levels among adults aged >65 years—United States. *MMWR Morbidity and Mortality Weekly Report, 47,* 797–802.

Centers for Disease Control and Prevention. (2000a). Prevention and control of influenza: recommendations of the Advisory Committee on Immunization Practices (ACIP). *MMWR Morbidity and Mortality Weekly Report, 49*(RR03), 1–38.

Centers for Disease Control and Prevention. (2000b). Influenza, pneumococcal, and tetanus toxoid vaccination of adults—United States, 1993–1997. *MMWR Morbidity and Mortality Weekly Report, 49*(SS09), 39–62.

Colice, G. L., Curtis, A., Deslauriers, J., et al. (2000). Medical and surgical treatment of parapneumonic effusions: an evidence-based guideline. *Chest, 18*(4), 1158–1171.

Fine, M. J., Auble, T. E., Yealy, D. M., et al. (1997). A prediction rule to identify low-risk patients with community-acquired pneumonia. *New England Journal of Medicine, 336*(4), 243–250.

Fine, M. J., Smith, M. A., Carson, C. A., et al. (1996). Prognosis and outcomes of patients with community-acquired pneumonia: a meta-analysis. *Journal of the American Medical Association, 75*(2), 134–141.

Goodwin, R. S. (1996). Prevention of aspiration pneumonia: A research-based protocol. *Dimensions of Critical Care Nursing, 15*(2), 58–74.

Gross, T. J., & Hunninghake, G. W. (2001). Idiopathic pulmonary fibrosis. *New England Journal of Medicine, 345*(7), 517–525.

Helwig, D. (2000). Major cost reductions reported in Canadian pneumonia study. *eCMAJ Today!* http://www.cma.cmaj/cmaj-today/2000/02_09.

Kenreigh, C. A., & Wagner, L. T. (2000). Treatment of CAP: optimizing formulary decisions. http://www.medscape.com.

Kollef, M. H. (1999). The prevention of ventilator-associated pneumonia. *New England Journal of Medicine, 340*(8), 627–634.

Lynch, J. P. (2000). Treating community-acquired pneumonia. *Journal of Respiratory Diseases, 23*(10), 602–608.

Marston, B. J., Plouffe, J. F., File, T. M., et al. (1997). Incidence of community-acquired pneumonia requiring hospitalizations: Results of a population-based active surveillance study in Ohio. *Archives of Internal Medicine, 157*(15), 1709–1718.

McGeer, A. J., & Low, D. E. (2000). Vancomycin-resistant enterococci. *Seminars in Respiratory Infections, 15*(4), 261–263.

McIntosh, K. (2002). Community-acquired pneumonia in children. *New England Journal of Medicine, 346*(6), 429–437.

Minino, A. M., & Smith, B. L. (2001). Deaths: preliminary data for 2000. *National Vital Statistics Reports, 49*(12), 1–40.

National Center for Health Statistics (2000). *United States Mortality Public Use Data Tape 1998,* Centers for Disease Control and Prevention.

Smith-Sims, K. (2001). Hospital-acquired pneumonia. *American Journal of Nursing, 101*(1), 24AA–24EE.

Tasota, F. J., Fisher, E. M., Coulson, C. F., & Hoffman, L. A. (1998). Protecting ICU patients from nosocomial infections: Practical measures for favorable outcomes. *Critical Care Nurse, 18*(1), 54–67.

Zimmer, J. G., & Hall, W. J. (1997). Nursing home-acquired pneumonia: Avoiding the hospital. *Journal of the American Geriatrics Society, 45*(3), 380–381.

Trauma

Collins, J. (2000). Chest wall trauma. *Journal of Thoracic Imaging, 15*(2), 112–119.

Flynn, M. B., & Bonini, S. (1999) Blunt chest trauma: Case report. *Critical Care Nurse, 19*(5), 68–77.

Karlet, M. C. (1997). Update for nurse anesthetists: Thoracic trauma. *American Association of Nurse Anesthetists Journal, 65*(1), 73–80.

Pape, H. C., Remmers, D., Rice, J., Ebisch, M., Krettek, C., & Tscherne, H. (2000). Appraisal of early evaluation of blunt chest trauma: Development of a standardized scoring system for initial clinical decision making. *Journal of Trauma-Injury Infection & Critical Care, 49*(3), 496–504.

Tuberculosis

American Thoracic Society. (2000). Diagnostic standards and classification of tuberculosis in adults and children. *American Journal of Respiratory and Critical Care Medicine, 161*(4), 1376–1395.

American Thoracic Society and Centers for Disease Control and Prevention. (2000). Targeted tuberculin testing and treatment of latent infection. *American Journal of Respiratory and Critical Care Medicine, 161*(4), S221–S247.

American Thoracic Society and Centers for Disease Control and Prevention. (2001). Fatal and severe liver injuries associated with rifampin and pyrazinamide for latent tuberculosis infection and revisions in American Thoracic Society/CDC Recommendations—United States 2001. *MMWR Morbidity Mortality Weekly Report, 50*(34), 733–735.

Centers for Disease Control and Prevention. (1995). Essential components of a tuberculosis prevention and control program: recommendations of the Advisory Council for the Elimination of Tuberculosis. *MMWR Morbidity and Mortality Weekly Report, 44*(RR-11), 1–16.

Centers for Disease Control and Prevention. (1995). Screening for tuberculosis and tuberculosis infection in high-risk populations: recommendations of the Advisory Council for the Elimination of Tuberculosis. *MMWR Morbidity and Mortality Weekly Report, 44*(RR-11), 18–34.

Centers for Disease Control and Prevention. (1998). Development of new vaccines for tuberculosis. *MMWR Morbidity and Mortality Weekly Report, 47*(RR13), 1–6.

Centers for Disease Control and Prevention. (1998). Tuberculosis morbidity, United States. *MMWR Morbidity and Mortality Weekly Report, 47*(13), 253–257.

Centers for Disease Control and Prevention. (2000). *Core curriculum on tuberculosis: What the clinician should know* (4th ed.). Atlanta: Author.

Corbett, E., Watt, C., Walker, N., Maher, D., Williams, B., Raviglione, C., et al. (2003). The growing burden of tuberculosis. *Archives of Internal Medicine, 163,* 1009–1021.

Fanning, A. E. (1998). Globalization of tuberculosis. *Canadian Medical Association Journal, 158*(5), 611–612.

Heywood, N., Kawa, B., Long, R., Howard, N., Panaro, L., et al. (2003). Guidelines for the investigation and follow-up of individuals under medical surveillance for tuberculosis after arriving in Canada: A summary. *Canadian Medical Association Journal, 168*(12), 1563–1565.

Horsburgh, C. R., Feldman, S., & Ridzon, R. (2000) Practice guidelines for the treatment of tuberculosis. *Clinical Infectious Diseases, 31*(3), 633–639.

Kendig, E. L., Kirkpatrick, B. V., Carter, W. H., Hill, F. A., Caldwell, K., & Entwistle, M. (1998). Underreading of the tuberculin skin test reaction. *Chest, 113*(5), 1175–1177.

Small, P. M., & Fujiwara, P. I. (2001). Management of tuberculosis in the United States. *New England Journal of Medicine, 345*(3), 189–200.

RESOURCES AND WEBSITES

Agency for Healthcare Quality and Research, 2101 E. Jefferson St., Suite 501, Rockville, MD 20852; 1-301-594-1364; http://www.ahrq.org.

American Association for Respiratory Care, 1720 Regal Row, Dallas, TX 75235; 1-214-630-3540; http://www.aarc.org.

American Cancer Society, 1599 Clifton Road NE, Atlanta, GA 30329; 1-888-ACS-5552; http://www.cancer.org.

American College of Chest Physicians, 3300 Dundee Road, Northbrook, IL 60062; 1-847-498-1400; http://www.chest.org.

American Lung Association, 1740 Broadway, New York, NY 10019-4374; 1-212-315-8700; http://www.lungusa.org.

American Thoracic Society, 1740 Broadway, New York, NY 10019; 1-212-315-8700; http://www.thoracic.org.

Canadian Cardiovascular Society; http://www.ccs.ca.

Canadian Council for Tobacco Control: National Clearinghouse on Tobacco and Health Program; http://www.ncth.ca/NCTHweb.nsf.

Canadian Lung Association, 3 Raymond Street, Suite 300, Ottawa, ON K1R 1A3; 613-569-6411; 1-888-566-Lung (5864); http://www.lung.ca.

Canadian Medical Association; http://www.cma.ca.

Canadian Thoracic Society; http://www.lung.ca/cts.

Centers for Disease Control and Prevention, 1600 Clifton Road, NE, Atlanta, GA 30333; http://www.cdc.gov.

Health Canada; http://www.hc-sc.gc.ca.

National Heart, Lung and Blood Institute, National Institutes of Health, 900 Rockville Pike, Bldg. 31, Bethesda, MD 20892; 1-301-496-5166; http://www.nhlbi.nih.gov.

National Cancer Institute, National Institutes of Health, 31 Center Drive MSC 2580, Bldg. 31, Room 10A16, Bethesda, MD 20892; 1-800-4-CANCER (Cancer Information Services); http://www.nci.nih.gov.

Respiratory Nursing Society, c/o NYSNA, 11 Cornell Road, Latham, NY 12110; 1-518-782-9400 × 286; http://www.respiratorynursingsociety.org.

U.S. Department of Labor, Occupational Safety and Health Administration (OSHA), Directorate of Technical Support, 200 Constitution Avenue, NW, Washington, DC 20210; 1-202-219-7047; http://www.osha.gov.

World Association of Sarcoidosis and Other Granulomatous Disorders; http://www.sarcoidosissharma.com.

Management of Patients With Chronic Obstructive Pulmonary Disease

Adapted by Carolyn J. M. Ross

LEARNING OBJECTIVES

On completion of this chapter, the learner will be able to:

1. Describe the pathophysiology of chronic obstructive pulmonary disease (COPD).
2. Discuss the major risk factors for developing COPD and nursing interventions to minimize or prevent these risk factors.
3. Use the nursing process as a framework for care of the patient with COPD.
4. Develop a teaching plan for patients with COPD.
5. Describe the pathophysiology of asthma.
6. Discuss the medications used in asthma management.
7. Describe asthma self-management strategies.
8. Describe the pathophysiology of cystic fibrosis.

Chronic obstructive pulmonary disease (COPD) is a leading cause of morbidity and mortality in Canada. Nurses are involved with COPD patients across the spectrum of care, from outpatient and home care to critical care and the hospice setting. Patients with COPD or asthma need care from nurses who not only have astute assessment and clinical management skills, but who also understand how these disorders can affect patients' quality of life. Patient and family teaching is an important nursing intervention to enhance self-management of COPD, asthma, and cystic fibrosis.

Chronic Obstructive Pulmonary Disease

Chronic obstructive pulmonary disease (COPD) is a disease state characterized by airflow limitation that is not fully reversible. This newest definition of COPD, provided by the Global Initiative for Chronic Obstructive Lung Disease, provides a broad description that better explains this disorder and its signs and symptoms (National Institutes of Health [NIH], 2001). While previous definitions have included emphysema and chronic bronchitis under the umbrella classification of COPD, this was often confusing because most patients with COPD present with overlapping signs and symptoms of these two distinct disease processes.

COPD may include diseases that cause airflow obstruction (eg, emphysema, chronic bronchitis) or a combination of these disorders. Other diseases such as cystic fibrosis, bronchiectasis, and asthma were previously classified as types of chronic obstructive lung disease. However, asthma is now considered a separate disorder and is classified as an abnormal airway condition characterized primarily by reversible inflammation. COPD can coexist with asthma. Both of these diseases have the same major symptoms; however, symptoms are generally more variable in asthma than in COPD. This chapter discusses COPD as a disease and briefly describes chronic bronchitis and emphysema as distinct disease states, providing a foundation for understanding the pathophysiology of COPD. Bronchiectasis, asthma, and cystic fibrosis are discussed separately.

COPD is the fifth leading cause of death in the United States for all ages and both genders; fifth for men and fourth for women (National Center for Health Statistics [NCHS], 2000). In 1998, more than 12,000 persons died of COPD. This represents a rise in the mortality rate for this disorder at a time when death rates from other serious illnesses, such as heart disease and cerebral vascular disease, were declining. In Canada, it is estimated that 3.8% of men and 4.8% of women over 34 years of age have COPD.

COPD was the fourth leading cause of death in men and the fifth in women (Health Canada, 2003). In 1999, 5,544 men and 3,974 women died of COPD. This represents a rise in the mortality rate for this disorder at a time when death rates from other serious illnesses, such as heart disease and cerebral vascular disease, were declining. Over 10% of individuals with COPD received home care services and over 30,000 individuals were hospitalized for COPD in 1998 (Health Canada, 2001). People with COPD commonly become symptomatic during the middle adult years, and the incidence of COPD increases with age. Although certain aspects of lung function normally decrease with age (eg, vital capacity and forced expiratory volume in 1 second [FEV_1]), COPD accentuates and accelerates these physiologic changes.

Pathophysiology

In COPD, the airflow limitation is both progressive and associated with an abnormal inflammatory response of the lungs to noxious particles or gases. The inflammatory response occurs throughout the airways, parenchyma, and pulmonary vasculature (Canadian Thoracic Society, 2003; NIH, 2001). Because of the chronic inflammation and the body's attempts to repair it, narrowing occurs in the small peripheral airways. Over time, this injury-and-repair process causes scar tissue formation and narrowing of the airway lumen. Airflow obstruction may also be due to parenchymal destruction as seen with emphysema, a disease of the alveoli or gas exchange units.

In addition to inflammation, processes relating to imbalances of proteinases and antiproteinases in the lung may be responsible for airflow limitation. When activated by chronic inflammation, proteinases and other substances may be released, damaging the parenchyma of the lung. The parenchymal changes may also be consequences of inflammation, environmental, or genetic factors (eg, alpha$_1$ antitrypsin deficiency).

Early in the course of COPD, the inflammatory response causes pulmonary vasculature changes that are characterized by thickening of the vessel wall. These changes may occur as a result of exposure to cigarette smoke or use of tobacco products or as a result of the release of inflammatory mediators (Canadian Thoracic Society, 2003; NIH, 2001).

Chronic Bronchitis

Chronic **bronchitis**, a disease of the airways, is defined as the presence of cough and sputum production for at least 3 months in each of 2 consecutive years. In many cases, smoke or other environ-

Glossary

air trapping: incomplete emptying of alveoli during expiration due to loss of lung tissue elasticity (emphysema), bronchospasm (asthma), or airway obstruction

alpha$_1$ antitrypsin deficiency: genetic disorder resulting from deficiency of alpha$_1$ antitrypsin, a protective agent for the lung; increases patient's risk for developing panacinar emphysema even in the absence of smoking

asthma: a disease with multiple precipitating mechanisms resulting in a common clinical outcome of reversible airflow obstruction; no longer considered a category of COPD

bronchiectasis: chronic dilation of a bronchus or bronchi; the dilated airways become saccular and are a medium for chronic infection. Is no longer considered a category of COPD.

bronchitis: a disease of the airways defined as the presence of cough and sputum production for at least a combined total of 3 months in each of 2 consecutive years; is a category of COPD

chronic obstructive pulmonary disease: disease state characterized by airflow limitation that is not fully reversible; sometimes referred to as chronic airway obstruction or chronic obstructive lung disease

emphysema: a disease of the airways characterized by destruction of the walls of overdistended alveoli; is a category of COPD

metered-dose inhaler (MDI): patient-activated medication canister that provides aerosolized medication that the patient inhales into the lungs

polycythemia: increase in the red blood cell concentration in the blood; in COPD, the body attempts to improve oxygen carrying capacity by producing increasing amounts of red blood cells

spirometry: pulmonary function tests that measure specific lung volumes (eg, FEV_1, FVC) and rates ($FEF_{25-75\%}$); may be measured before and after bronchodilator administration mental pollutants irritate the airways, resulting in hypersecretion of mucus and inflammation. This constant irritation causes the mucus-secreting glands and goblet cells to increase in number, ciliary function is reduced, and more mucus is produced. The bronchial walls become thickened, the bronchial lumen is narrowed, and mucus may plug the airway (Fig. 24-1). Alveoli adjacent to the bronchioles may become damaged and fibrosed, resulting in altered function of the alveolar macrophages. This is significant because the macrophages play an important role in destroying foreign particles, including bacteria. As a result, the patient becomes more susceptible to respiratory infection. A wide range of viral, bacterial, and mycoplasmal infections can produce acute episodes of bronchitis. Exacerbations of chronic bronchitis are most likely to occur during the winter.

Emphysema

In **emphysema**, impaired gas exchange (oxygen, carbon dioxide) results from destruction of the walls of overdistended alveoli. "Emphysema" is a pathological term that describes an abnormal distention of the air spaces beyond the terminal bronchioles, with destruction of the walls of the alveoli. It is the end stage of a process that has progressed slowly for many years. As the walls of the alveoli are destroyed (a process accelerated by recurrent infections), the alveolar surface area in direct contact with the pulmonary capillaries continually decreases, causing an increase in dead space (lung area where no gas exchange can occur) and impaired oxygen diffusion, which leads to hypoxemia. In the later stages of the disease, carbon dioxide elimination is impaired, resulting in increased carbon dioxide tension in arterial blood (hypercapnia) and causing respiratory acidosis. As the alveolar walls continue to break down, the pulmonary capillary bed is reduced. Consequently, pulmonary blood flow is increased, forcing the right ventricle to maintain a higher blood pressure in the pulmonary artery. Hypoxemia may further increase pulmonary artery pressure. Thus, right-sided heart failure (cor pulmonale) is one of the complications of emphysema. Congestion, dependent edema, distended neck veins, or pain in the region of the liver suggests the development of cardiac failure.

There are two main types of emphysema, based on the changes taking place in the lung: panlobular (panacinar) and centrilobular (centroacinar) (Fig. 24-2). Both types may occur in the same pa-

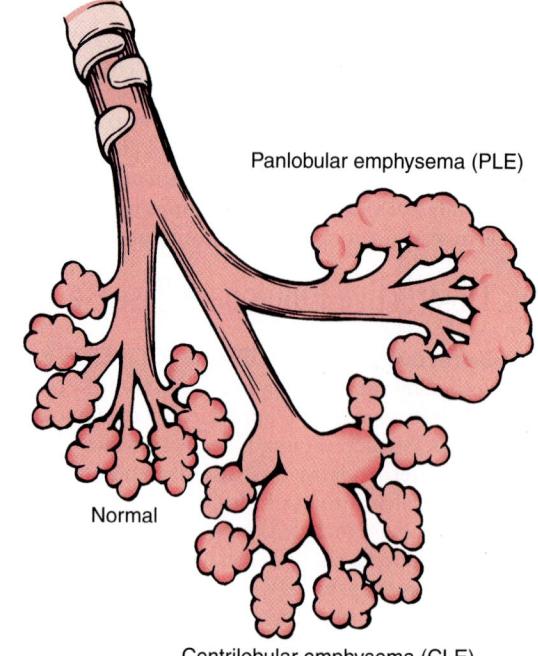

FIGURE 24-2 Changes in alveolar structure in centrilobular and panlobular emphysema. In panlobular emphysema, the bronchioles, alveolar ducts, and alveoli are destroyed and the air spaces within the lobule are enlarged. In centrilobular emphysema, the pathologic changes occur in the lobule, while the peripheral portions of the acinus are preserved.

tient. In the panlobular (panacinar) type, there is destruction of the respiratory bronchiole, alveolar duct, and alveoli. All air spaces within the lobule are essentially enlarged, but there is little inflammatory disease. The patient with this type of emphysema typically has a hyperinflated (hyperexpanded) chest (barrel chest on physical examination), marked dyspnea on exertion, and weight loss. To move air into and out of the lungs, negative pressure is required during inspiration, and an adequate level of positive pressure must be attained and maintained during expiration. The resting position is one of inflation. Instead of being an involuntary passive act, expiration becomes active and requires mus-

FIGURE 24-1 Pathophysiology of chronic bronchitis as compared to a normal bronchus. The bronchus in chronic bronchitis is narrowed and has impaired air flow due to multiple mechanisms: inflammation, excess mucus production, and potential smooth muscle constriction (bronchospasm).

cular effort. The patient becomes increasingly short of breath, the chest becomes rigid, and the ribs are fixed at their joints.

In the centrilobular (centroacinar) form, pathologic changes take place mainly in the centre of the secondary lobule, preserving the peripheral portions of the acinus. Frequently, there is a derangement of ventilation–perfusion ratios, producing chronic hypoxemia, hypercapnia (increased CO_2 in the arterial blood), **polycythemia,** and episodes of right-sided heart failure. This leads to central cyanosis, peripheral edema, and respiratory failure. The patient may receive diuretic therapy for edema.

Risk Factors

Risk factors for COPD include environmental exposures and host factors (Chart 24-1). The most important risk factor for COPD is cigarette smoking. Pipe, cigar, and other types of tobacco smoking are also risk factors. In addition, passive smoking contributes to respiratory symptoms and COPD (Health Canada, 2001; NIH, 2001). Smoking depresses the activity of scavenger cells and affects the respiratory tract's ciliary cleansing mechanism, which keeps breathing passages free of inhaled irritants, bacteria, and other foreign matter. When smoking damages this cleansing mechanism, airflow is obstructed and air becomes trapped behind the obstruction. The alveoli greatly distend, diminishing lung capacity. Smoking also irritates the goblet cells and mucus glands, causing an increased accumulation of mucus, which in turn produces more irritation, infection, and damage to the lung. In addition, carbon monoxide (a byproduct of smoking) combines with hemoglobin to form carboxyhemoglobin. Hemoglobin that is bound by carboxyhemoglobin cannot carry oxygen efficiently.

Smoking is not the only risk factor for COPD. Other factors include prolonged and intense exposure to occupational dusts and chemicals, indoor air pollution, and outdoor air pollution, which adds to the total burden of inhaled particles on the lung (NIH, 2001).

A host risk factor for COPD is a deficiency of alpha$_1$ antitrypsin, an enzyme inhibitor that protects the lung parenchyma from injury. This deficiency predisposes young patients to rapid development of lobular emphysema even in the absence of smoking. **Alpha$_1$ antitrypsin** deficiency is one of the most common genetically linked lethal diseases among Caucasians and affects approximately one in every 3,000 North Americans (George, San Pedro & Stoller, 2000). The genetically susceptible person is sensitive to environmental factors (smoking, air pollution, infectious agents, allergens) and in time develops chronic obstructive symptoms. Carriers of this genetic defect must be identified so that they can modify environmental risk factors to delay or prevent overt symptoms of disease. Genetic counselling should

also be offered. Alpha-protease inhibitor replacement therapy, which slows the progression of the disease, is available for patients with this genetic defect and for those with severe disease. This intermittent infusion therapy is costly and is required on an ongoing basis.

Clinical Manifestations

COPD is characterized by three primary symptoms: cough, sputum production, and dyspnea on exertion (Canadian Thoracic Society, 2001; NIH, 2001). These symptoms often worsen over time. Chronic cough and sputum production often precede the development of airflow limitation by many years. However, not all individuals with cough and sputum production will develop COPD. Dyspnea may be severe and often interferes with the patient's activities. Weight loss is common because dyspnea interferes with eating, and the work of breathing is energy-depleting. Often the patient cannot participate in even mild exercise because of dyspnea; as COPD progresses, dyspnea occurs even at rest. As the work of breathing increases over time, the accessory muscles are recruited in an effort to breathe. The patient with COPD is at risk for respiratory insufficiency and respiratory infections, which in turn increase the risk for acute and chronic respiratory failure.

In COPD patients with a primary emphysematous component, chronic hyperinflation leads to the "barrel chest" thorax configuration. This results from fixation of the ribs in the inspiratory position (due to hyperinflation) and from loss of lung elasticity (Fig. 24-3). Retraction of the supraclavicular fossae occurs on inspiration, causing the shoulders to heave upward (Fig. 24-4). In advanced emphysema, the abdominal muscles also contract on inspiration.

Assessment and Diagnostic Findings

The nurse should obtain a thorough health history for a patient with known or potential COPD. Chart 24-2 lists the key factors to assess. Pulmonary function studies are used to help confirm the diagnosis of COPD, determine disease severity, and follow disease progression. **Spirometry** is used to evaluate airflow obstruction, which is determined by the ratio of FEV_1 (volume of air that the patient can forcibly exhale in 1 second) to forced vital capacity (FVC). Spirometric results are expressed as an absolute volume and as percent-predicted using appropriate normal values for gender, age, and height. With obstruction, the patient either has difficulty exhaling or cannot forcibly exhale air from the lungs, reducing the FEV_1. Obstructive lung disease is defined as a FEV_1/FVC ratio of less than 70%.

In addition, bronchodilator reversibility testing may be performed to rule out the diagnosis of asthma and to guide initial treatment. With this type of testing, spirometry is first obtained, then the patient is given an inhaled bronchodilator per a protocol, and finally spirometry is repeated. The patient demonstrates a degree of reversibility if the pulmonary function values improve after administration of the bronchodilator.

Arterial blood gas measurements may also be obtained to assess baseline oxygenation and gas exchange. In addition, a chest x-ray may be obtained to exclude alternative diagnoses. Lastly, alpha$_1$ antitrypsin deficiency screening may be performed for patients under age 45 or for those with a strong family history of COPD.

The severity of COPD is classified into four stages (Table 24-1) (Canadian Thoracic Society, 2003). Factors that determine the clinical course and survival of patients with COPD include history

Chart 24-1
Risk Factors for COPD

Exposure to tobacco smoke accounts for an estimated 80% to 90% of COPD cases (Rennard, 1998)

Passive smoking

Occupational exposure

Ambient air pollution

Genetic abnormalities, including a deficiency of alpha$_1$-antitrypsin, an enzyme inhibitor that normally counteracts the destruction of lung tissue by certain other enzymes

NURSING RESEARCH PROFILE 24-1
Physical Activity in Patients With COPD

Belza, B., Steele, B. G., Hunziker, J., Lakshminaryan, S., Holt, L., & Buchner, D. M. (2001). Correlates of physical activity in chronic obstructive pulmonary disease. *Nursing Research, 50*(4), 195–202.

Purpose
For patients with chronic obstructive pulmonary disease (COPD), physical activity is an important part of their quality of life. Yet little is known about the contributions of psychological and physiologic variables to physical activity in this population. The purpose of this study was to determine the relationships among differing functional performance measures (physical activity, functional capacity, symptom experience, and health-related quality of life) in this population.

Study Sample and Design
This cross-sectional, descriptive study evaluated 63 outpatients with COPD prior to entry into a pulmonary rehabilitation program. The sample was predominantly male (60 men and 3 women) with a mean age of 65.4 ± 8.0 years. None of the participants had been hospitalized in the past 2 months for a respiratory problem, and none was engaged in a formalized exercise program. Functional performance was measured by physical activity (evaluated by an accelerometer and self-report). Functional capacity was measured by three measures of impairment (pulmonary function tests [FEV_1], 6-minute walk test, and

a self-efficacy questionnaire for walking). The symptom experiences of dyspnea and fatigue as well as health-related quality of life were measured by widely used reliable and valid questionnaires.

Findings
Sixty-nine subjects were initially enrolled in the study but six were withdrawn due to missing data. Daily physical activity as measured by the accelerometer was strongly associated with the maximal distance walked in the 6-minute walk test, the level of airway obstruction as measured by pulmonary function tests, walking self-efficacy, and physical health status. Physical activity was not correlated with the subjects' self-report of functional status. The 6-minute walk test was the only predictor of physical activity in this sample.

Nursing Implications
Functional performance status is an important multidimensional outcome measure for both nursing and medicine. This study demonstrates that the multiple measures of functional performance status, which are frequently used in clinical practice and research, may differ in their relationship to the actual physical activity level of the patient.

---

of cigarette smoking, passive smoking exposure, age, rate of decline of FEV_1, hypoxemia, pulmonary artery pressure, resting heart rate, weight loss, and reversibility of airflow obstruction (George, San Pedro & Stoller, 2000).

In diagnosing COPD, several differential diagnoses must be ruled out. The primary differential diagnosis is asthma. Key char-

acteristics of asthma include onset often early in life, variation in daily symptoms and day-to-day occurrence or timing of symptoms, family history of asthma, and a largely reversible airflow obstruction. It may be difficult to differentiate between a patient with COPD and one with chronic asthma. A key part of differentiation is the patient history, as well as the patient's respon-

A $$\frac{\text{A-P diameter}}{\text{Transverse diameter}} = \frac{1}{2}$$

B $$\frac{\text{A-P Diameter}}{\text{Transverse diameter}} = \frac{2}{1}$$

FIGURE 24-3 Characteristics of normal chest wall and chest wall in emphysema. The normal chest wall and its cross section are illustrated on the left (**A**). The barrel-shaped chest of emphysema and its cross section are illustrated on the right (**B**).

FIGURE 24-4 Typical posture of person with COPD—primarily emphysema. The person tends to lean forward and uses the accessory muscles of respiration to breathe, forcing the shoulder girdle upward and causing the supraclavicular fossae to retract on inspiration.

Table 24-1 • Chronic Obstructive Pulmonary Disease (COPD) Classification by Lung Function	
COPD STAGE	SPIROMETRY
At risk	Normal spirometry, chronic symptoms $FEV_1/FVC \geq 0.7$ and/or $FEV_1 \geq 80\%$ predicted
Mild	FEV_1 60% to 79% predicted, $FEV_1/FVC \leq 0.7$
Moderate	FEV_1 40% to 59% predicted, $FEV_1/FVC \leq 0.7$
Severe	$FEV_1 < 40\%$ predicted, $FEV_1/FVC \leq 70\%$

FEV_1 Forced expiratory volume in 1 second; FVC, forced vital capacity.
Canadian Thoracic Society. (2003). Executive summary: Canadian Thoracic Society recommendations for management of chronic obstructive pulmonary disease—2003. *Canadian Respiratory Journal, 10* (Suppl A), S4A-S65A.

siveness to bronchodilators. Other diseases that must be considered in the differential diagnosis include heart failure, bronchiectasis, and tuberculosis (Canadian Thoracic Society, 2003; NIH, 2001).

Complications

Respiratory insufficiency and failure are major life-threatening complications of COPD. The acuity of the onset and the severity of respiratory failure depend on the patient's baseline pulmonary function, pulse oximetry or arterial blood gas values,

comorbid conditions, and the severity of other complications of COPD. Respiratory insufficiency and failure may be chronic (with severe COPD) or acute (with severe bronchospasm or pneumonia in the patient with severe COPD). Acute respiratory insufficiency and failure may necessitate ventilatory support until other acute complications, such as infection, can be treated. Management of the patient requiring ventilatory support is discussed in Chapter 25. Other complications of COPD include pneumonia, atelectasis, pneumothorax, and cor pulmonale.

Medical Management

RISK REDUCTION

Smoking cessation is the single most effective intervention to prevent COPD or slow its progression (Canadian Thoracic Society, 2003; NIH, 2001). Recent surveys indicate that 25% of all Canadians aged 15 and over smoke cigarettes on a daily basis (Health Canada, 2001). Nurses play a key role in promoting smoking cessation and educating patients about ways to do so. Patients diagnosed with COPD who continue to smoke must be encouraged and assisted to quit. Factors associated with continued smoking vary among patients and may include the strength of nicotine addiction, continued exposure to smoking-associated stimuli (at work or in social settings), stress, depression, and habit. Continued smoking is also more prevalent among those with low incomes, a low level of education, and psychosocial problems (Pohl, 2000).

Because there are multiple factors associated with continued smoking, successful cessation often requires multiple strategies. The health care provider should promote cessation by explaining the risks of smoking and personalizing the "at-risk" message to the patient. After giving a strong warning about smoking, the health care provider should work with the patient to set a definite "quit date." Referral to a smoking cessation program may be helpful. Follow-up within 3 to 5 days after the quit date to review progress and to address any problems is associated with an increased rate of success; this should be repeated as needed. Continued reinforcement with telephone calls or clinic visits is extremely beneficial. Relapses should be analyzed, and the patient and health care provider should jointly identify possible solutions to prevent future backsliding. It is important to emphasize successes rather than failures. First-line pharmacotherapies that reliably

Chart 24-2 • ASSESSMENT

Key Factors to Assess in the COPD Patient's Health History

Exposure to risk factors—types, intensity, duration
Past medical history—respiratory diseases/problems, including asthma, allergy, sinusitis, nasal polyps, history of respiratory infections
Family history of COPD or other chronic respiratory diseases
Pattern of symptom development
History of exacerbations or previous hospitalizations for respiratory problems
Presence of comorbidities
Appropriateness of current medical treatments
Impact of the disease on quality of life
Available social and family support for patient
Potential for reducing risk factors (eg, smoking cessation)

increase long-term smoking abstinence rates are bupropion SR (Zyban, Wellbutrin), nicotine gum, nicotine inhaler, nicotine nasal spray, or nicotine patches. Second-line pharmacotherapies include clonidine (Catapres) and nortriptyline (Aventyl) (USPHS, 2000).

Smoking cessation can begin in a variety of health care settings—outpatient clinic, pulmonary rehabilitation, community, hospital, and the patient's home. Regardless of the setting, the nurse has the opportunity to teach the patient about the risks of smoking and the benefits of smoking cessation. A variety of materials, resources, and programs are available to assist with this effort (eg, Health Canada Tobacco Control Program, Canadian Lung Association, Canadian Council for Tobacco Control: National Clearinghouse on Tobacco and Health Program, Canadian Cancer Society).

PHARMACOLOGIC THERAPY

Bronchodilators. Bronchodilators relieve bronchospasm and reduce airway obstruction by allowing increased oxygen distribution throughout the lungs and improving alveolar ventilation. These medications, which are central in the management of COPD (Canadian Thoracic Society, 2003; NIH, 2001), are delivered through a metered-dose inhaler, by nebulization, or via the oral route in pill or liquid form. Bronchodilators are often administered regularly throughout the day as well as on an as-needed basis. They may also be used prophylactically to prevent breathlessness by having the patient use them before an activity, such as eating or walking.

A **metered-dose inhaler** (MDI) is a pressurized device containing an aerosolized powder of medication. A precise amount of medication is released with each activation of the canister (Dhand, 2000). Patients need to be instructed on the correct use of the device. A spacer (holding chamber) may also be used to enhance deposition of the medication in the lung and help the pa-

tient coordinate activation of the MDI with inspiration. Spacers come in several designs, but all are attached to the MDI and have a mouthpiece on the opposite end (Fig. 24-5). Once the canister is activated, the spacer holds the aerosol in the chamber until the patient inhales (Dhand, 2000). The patient should take a slow, 3- to 5-second inhalation immediately following activation of the MDI (Expert Panel Report II, 1997).

Several classes of bronchodilators are used: beta-adrenergic agonists, anticholinergic agents, and methylxanthines. These medications may be used in combination to optimize the bronchodilation effect. Some of these medications are short-acting; others are long-acting. Long-acting bronchodilators are more convenient for patient use. Examples of medications in these differing classes are shown in Table 24-2. Nebulized medications (nebulization of medication via an air compressor) may also be effective in patients who cannot use an MDI properly or who prefer this method of administration.

Corticosteroids. Inhaled and systemic corticosteroids (oral or intravenous) may also be used in COPD but are used more frequently in asthma. Although it has been shown that corticosteroids do not slow the decline in lung function, these medications may improve symptoms. A short trial course of oral corticosteroids may be prescribed for patients with moderate to severe COPD to see if pulmonary function improves and symptoms decrease. Inhaled corticosteroids via MDI may also be used. Examples of corticosteroids in the inhaled form are beclomethasone (Beclovent, Vanceril), budesonide (Pulmicort), flunisolide (AeroBid), fluticasone (Flovent), and triamcinolone (Azmacort).

Medication regimens used to manage COPD are based on disease severity. For mild COPD, a short-acting bronchodilator may be prescribed. For moderate COPD, one or more bronchodilators may be prescribed along with inhaled corticosteroids, if symptoms are significant. For severe COPD, medication therapy includes regular treatment with one or more bronchodilators

A   B

FIGURE 24-5 (**A**) Examples of metered dose inhalers and spacers. (**B**) A metered dose inhaler and spacer in use.

Table 24-2 • Types of Bronchodilator Medications

CLASS/DRUG	METHOD OF ADMINISTRATION			DURATION OF ACTION
	Metered-Dose Inhaler	Nebulizer	Oral	
Beta-Adrenergic Agonist Agents				
Albuterol (Proventil, Ventolin, Volmax)	X	X	X	Short
Bitolerol (Tornate)	X	X		Medium
Levalbuterol (Xopenax)		X		Medium
Metaproterenol (Alupent)	X	X	X	Short
Pirbuterol (Maxair)	X			Short
Salbutamol (Asmavent)	X	X	X	Short
Salmeterol (Serevent)	X			Long
Terbutaline (Brethaire)			X	Short
Anticholinergic Agents				
Ipratropium bromide (Atrovent)	X	X		Short
Oxitropium bromide (Oxivent)	X			Medium
Tiotropium (Spiriva)	X			Long
Methylxanthines				
Aminophylline (Phyllocontin)			X	Variable
Theophylline (Slo-bid, Theo-Dur)			X	Variable

Short-acting: 4–6 hours
Medium-acting: 6–9 hours
Long-acting: 12+ hours

and inhaled corticosteroids (Canadian Thoracic Society, 2003; NIH, 2001).

Other Medications. Patients should receive a yearly influenza vaccine and the pneumococcal vaccine every 5 to 7 years as preventive measures. In most healthy adults, pneumococcal vaccine titers persist for 5 or more years (George, San Pedro & Stoller, 2000). Other pharmacologic treatments that may be used in COPD include alpha$_1$ antitrypsin augmentation therapy, antibiotic agents, mucolytic agents, and antitussive agents.

MANAGEMENT OF EXACERBATION

An exacerbation of COPD is difficult to diagnose, but signs and symptoms may include increased dyspnea, increased sputum production and purulence, respiratory failure, changes in mental status, or worsening blood gas abnormalities. Primary causes for an acute exacerbation include tracheobronchial infection and air pollution (Canadian Thoracic Society, 2003; NIH, 2001). Secondary causes are pneumonia; pulmonary embolism; pneumothorax; rib fractures or chest trauma; inappropriate use of sedative, opioid, or beta-blocking agents; and right- or left-sided heart failure. First, the primary cause of the exacerbation is identified, and then specific treatment is administered. Optimization of bronchodilator medications is the first-line therapy and involves identifying the best medication or combinations of medications taken on a regular schedule for that patient. Depending on the signs and symptoms, corticosteroids, antibiotic agents, oxygen therapy, and intensive respiratory interventions may also be used. Indications for hospitalization of a patient with an acute exacerbation of COPD include severe dyspnea that does not respond adequately to initial therapy, confusion or lethargy, respiratory muscle fatigue, paradoxical chest wall movement, peripheral edema, worsening or new onset of central cyanosis, persistent or worsening hypoxemia, and/or need for non-invasive or invasive assisted mechanical ventilation (Canadian Thoracic Society, 2003; Celli, Snider, Heffner et al., 1995; NIH, 2001).

OXYGEN THERAPY

Oxygen therapy can be administered as long-term continuous therapy, during exercise, or to prevent acute dyspnea. Long-term oxygen therapy has been shown to improve the patient's quality of life and survival (Canadian Thoracic Society, 2003). For patients with an arterial oxygen pressure (PaO$_2$) of 55 mm Hg or less on room air, maintaining a constant and adequate oxygen saturation (>90%) is associated with significantly reduced mortality and improved quality of life. Indications for oxygen supplementation include a PaO$_2$ of 55 mm Hg or less or evidence of tissue hypoxia and organ damage such as cor pulmonale, secondary polycythemia, edema from right heart failure, or impaired mental status. In patients with exercise-induced hypoxemia, oxygen supplementation during exercise can improve performance. Patients who are hypoxemic while awake are likely to be so during sleep. Therefore, nighttime oxygen therapy is recommended as well, and the prescription for oxygen therapy is for continuous, 24-hour use. Intermittent oxygen therapy is indicated for those who desaturate only during exercise or sleep.

> **NURSING ALERT** Because hypoxemia stimulates respiration in the patient with severe COPD, increasing the oxygen flow to a high rate may greatly raise the patient's blood oxygen level. At the same time, this will suppress the respiratory drive, causing increased retention of carbon dioxide and CO$_2$ narcosis. The nurse should closely monitor the patient's respiratory response to oxygen administration via physical assessment, pulse oximetry, and/or arterial blood gases.

NURSING RESEARCH PROFILE 24-2

Oxygen Administration and Dyspnea Management in Patients With AAT Deficiency

Knebel, A. R., Bentz, E., & Barnes, P. (2000). Dyspnea management in alpha-1 antitrypsin deficiency: Effect of oxygen administration. *Nursing Research, 49*(6), 333–338.

Purpose

Limitations in activity due to dyspnea are common in persons with emphysema, including patients with alpha$_1$ antitrypsin (AAT) deficiency. The purpose of this study was to examine whether short-term oxygen administration decreased dyspnea and improved exercise tolerance in nonhypoxemic patients with emphysema caused by AAT deficiency.

Study Sample and Design

Thirty-one Caucasian subjects participated in a double-blind, crossover study. The subjects' mean age was 47 ± 7 years; 62% were male and 38% were female. Twenty-four percent had used oxygen supplementation at some point during their illness. Oxygen saturation, 6-minute walk distance, and end-of-walk dyspnea were measured during three practice walks and during walks with nasal cannula administration of oxygen (intervention) and compressed air (control).

Findings

Researchers found significant differences in subjects' oxygen saturation during walks with oxygen vs. walks with compressed air ($p = 0.0001$), with oxygen saturation higher with oxygen supplementation than with compressed air. There was no difference in subjects' walk distance and severity of self-reported dyspnea between oxygen and compressed air use. However, some gender differences were noted. Men showed no benefit from oxygen supplementation while walking, but women experienced less dyspnea, which corresponded with an increased walking distance.

Nursing Implications

The findings demonstrated that oxygen supplementation did not significantly improve the sensation of dyspnea or the distance walked in 6 minutes in the total sample of patients with AAT deficiency. However, there were trends in gender differences in relation to dyspnea levels and distance walked while receiving the intervention (oxygen supplementation). Future studies should examine subjects with differing levels of room air hypoxemia and explore potential gender differences in exercise performance with oxygen supplementation. Nurses should be aware that patients may respond differently to oxygen supplementation depending upon the underlying disease process, level of hypoxemia, and gender.

SURGICAL MANAGEMENT

Bullectomy. A bullectomy is a surgical option for select patients with bullous emphysema. Bullae are enlarged airspaces that do not contribute to ventilation but occupy space in the thorax; these areas may be surgically excised. Many times these bullae compress areas of the lung that do have adequate gas exchange. Bullectomy may help reduce dyspnea and improve lung function. It can be done thoracoscopically (with a video-assisted thoracoscope) or via a limited thoracotomy incision (see Chap. 25).

Lung Volume Reduction Surgery. Treatment options for patients with end-stage COPD with a primary emphysematous component are limited, although lung volume reduction surgery is an option for a specific subset of patients. This subset includes patients with homogenous disease or disease that is focused in one area and not widespread throughout the lungs. Lung volume reduction surgery involves the removal of a portion of the diseased lung parenchyma. This allows the functional tissue to expand, resulting in improved elastic recoil of the lung and improved chest wall and diaphragmatic mechanics. This type of surgery does not cure the disease, but it may decrease dyspnea, improve lung function, and improve the patient's overall quality of life. Careful selection of patients for this procedure is essential to decrease the morbidity and mortality. Delineation of the long-term benefits of lung volume reduction surgery awaits the results of several trials using larger sample sizes and longer duration follow-up: National Emphysema Treatment Trial, the Overholt Blue-Cross Emphysema Surgery Trial, and the Canadian Lung Volume Reduction Trial (Canadian Thoracic Society, 2003).

Lung Transplantation. Lung transplantation is a viable alternative for definitive surgical treatment of end-stage emphysema. It has been shown to improve quality of life and functional capacity (Canadian Thoracic Society, 2003; NIH, 2001). Specific criteria exist for referral for lung transplantation; however, organs are in short supply and many patients die while waiting for a transplant.

PULMONARY REHABILITATION

Pulmonary rehabilitation for patients with COPD is well established and widely accepted as a means to alleviate symptoms and optimize functional status. In both randomized and nonrandomized clinical trials, pulmonary rehabilitation has been shown to improve exercise tolerance, reduce dyspnea, and increase health-related quality of life (Rochester, 2000). The primary goal of rehabilitation is to restore patients to the highest level of independent function possible and to improve their quality of life. A successful rehabilitation program is individualized for each patient, is multidisciplinary, and attends to both the physiologic and emotional needs of the patient. Most pulmonary rehabilitation programs include educational, psychosocial, behavioural, and physical components. Breathing exercises and retraining and exercise programs are used to improve functional status, and the patient is taught methods to alleviate symptoms.

Pulmonary rehabilitation may be used therapeutically in other diseases besides COPD, including asthma, cystic fibrosis, lung cancer, interstitial lung disease, thoracic surgery, and lung transplantation. It may be conducted in the inpatient, outpatient, or home setting; the lengths of programs vary. Selection of a program depends upon the patient's physical, functional, and psychosocial status; insurance coverage; changing health care trends; availability of programs; and patient preference (Rochester, 2000).

Nursing Management

The nurse plays a key role in identifying potential candidates for pulmonary rehabilitation and in facilitating and reinforcing the material learned in the rehabilitation program. Not all patients have access to a formal rehabilitation program. However, the nurse can be instrumental in teaching the patient and family as well as facilitating specific services for the patient (eg, respiratory therapy education, physical therapy for exercise and breathing retraining, occupational therapy for conserving energy during activities of daily living, and nutritional counselling). In addition, numerous educational materials are available to assist the nurse in teaching patients with COPD. Potential resources include the American Thoracic Society, American Association of Cardiovascular and Pulmonary Rehabilitation, Canadian Lung Association, Canadian Thoracic Society, and Health Canada.

PATIENT EDUCATION

Patient education is a major component of pulmonary rehabilitation and includes a broad variety of topics. Depending on the length and setting of the program, topics may include normal anatomy and physiology of the lung, pathophysiology and changes with COPD, medications and home oxygen therapy, nutrition, respiratory therapy treatments, symptom alleviation, smoking cessation, sexuality and COPD, coping with chronic disease, communicating with the health care team, and planning for the future (advance directives, living wills, informed decision making about health care alternatives).

Breathing Exercises. The breathing pattern of most people with COPD is shallow, rapid, and inefficient; the more severe the disease, the more inefficient the breathing pattern. With practice, this type of upper chest breathing can be changed to diaphragmatic breathing, which reduces the respiratory rate, increases alveolar ventilation, and sometimes helps expel as much air as possible during expiration (see Chap. 25 for technique). Pursed-lip breathing helps to slow expiration, prevents collapse of small airways, and helps the patient to control the rate and depth of respiration. It also promotes relaxation, enabling the patient to gain control of dyspnea and reduce feelings of panic.

Inspiratory Muscle Training. Once the patient masters diaphragmatic breathing, a program of inspiratory muscle training may be prescribed to help strengthen the muscles used in breathing. This program requires that the patient breathe against resistance for 10 to 15 minutes every day. As the resistance is gradually increased, the muscles become better conditioned. Conditioning of the respiratory muscles takes time, and the patient is instructed to continue practicing at home (Larson, Covey, Wirtz et al., 1999; NIH, 2001).

Activity Pacing. A patient with COPD has decreased exercise tolerance during specific periods of the day. This is especially true on arising in the morning, because bronchial secretions collect in the lungs during the night while the person is lying down. The patient may have difficulty bathing or dressing. Activities requiring the arms to be supported above the level of the thorax may produce fatigue or respiratory distress but may be tolerated better after the patient has been up and moving around for an hour or more. Working with the nurse, the patient can reduce these limitations by planning self-care activities and determining the best time for bathing, dressing, and daily activities.

Self-Care Activities. As gas exchange, airway clearance, and the breathing pattern improve, the patient is encouraged to assume increasing participation in self-care activities. The patient is taught to coordinate diaphragmatic breathing with activities such as walking, bathing, bending, or climbing stairs. The patient should

bathe, dress, and take short walks, resting as needed to avoid fatigue and excessive dyspnea. Fluids should always be readily available, and the patient should begin to drink fluids without having to be reminded. If postural drainage is to be done at home, the nurse instructs and supervises the patient before discharge or in the outpatient setting.

Physical Conditioning. Physical conditioning techniques include breathing exercises and general exercises intended to conserve energy and increase pulmonary ventilation. There is a close relationship between physical fitness and respiratory fitness. Graded exercises and physical conditioning programs using treadmills, stationary bicycles, and measured level walks can improve symptoms and increase work capacity and exercise tolerance. Any physical activity that can be done regularly is helpful. Lightweight portable oxygen systems are available for ambulatory patients who require oxygen therapy during physical activity.

Oxygen Therapy. Oxygen supplied to the home comes in compressed gas, liquid, or concentrator systems. Portable oxygen systems allow the patient to exercise, work, and travel. To help the patient adhere to the oxygen prescription, the nurse explains the proper flow rate and required number of hours for oxygen use as well as the dangers of arbitrary changes in flow rates or duration of therapy. The nurse cautions the patient that smoking with or near oxygen is extremely dangerous. The nurse also reassures the patient that oxygen is not "addictive" and explains the need for regular evaluations of blood oxygenation by pulse oximetry or arterial blood gas analysis.

Nutritional Therapy. Nutritional assessment and counselling are important aspects in the rehabilitation process for the patient with COPD. Approximately 25% of patients with COPD are undernourished (NIH, 2001; Ferreira, Brooks, Lacasse & Goldstein, 2001). A thorough assessment of caloric needs and counselling about meal planning and supplementation are part of the rehabilitation process.

Coping Measures. Any factor that interferes with normal breathing quite naturally induces anxiety, depression, and changes in behaviour. Many patients find the slightest exertion exhausting. Constant shortness of breath and fatigue may make the patient irritable and apprehensive to the point of panic. Restricted activity (and reversal of family roles due to loss of employment), the frustration of having to work to breathe, and the realization that the disease is prolonged and unrelenting may cause the patient to react with anger, depression, and demanding behaviour. Sexual function may be compromised, which also diminishes self-esteem. In addition, the nurse needs to provide education and support to the spouse/significant other and family because the caregiver role in end-stage COPD can be difficult.

NURSING PROCESS: THE PATIENT WITH COPD

Assessment

Assessment involves obtaining information about current symptoms as well as previous disease manifestations. Chart 24-3 lists sample questions that may be used to obtain a clear history of the

Chart 24-3 • ASSESSMENT

Chronic Obstructive Pulmonary Disease

Health History
- How long has the patient had respiratory difficulty?
- Does exertion increase the dyspnea? What type of exertion?
- What are limits of the patient's tolerance for exercise?
- At what times during the day does the patient complain most of fatigue and shortness of breath?
- Which eating and sleeping habits have been affected?
- What does the patient know about the disease and his or her condition?
- What is the patient's smoking history (primary and secondary)?
- Is there occupational exposure to smoke or other pollutants?
- What are the triggering events (exertion, strong odours, dust, exposure to animals, etc.)?

Inspection and Examination Findings
- What position does the patient assume during the interview?
- What are the pulse and the respiratory rates?
- What is the character of respirations? Even and without effort? Other?
- Can the patient complete a sentence without having to take a breath?
- Does the patient contract the abdominal muscles during inspiration?
- Does the patient use accessory muscles of the shoulders and neck when breathing?
- Does the patient take a long time to exhale (prolonged expiration)?
- Is central cyanosis evident?
- Are the patient's neck veins engorged?
- Does the patient have peripheral edema?
- Is the patient coughing?
- What is the colour, amount, and consistency of the sputum?
- Is clubbing of the fingers present?
- What types of breath sounds (ie, clear, diminished or distant, crackles, wheezes) are heard? Describe and document findings and locations.
- What is the status of the patient's sensorium?
- Is there short-term or long-term memory impairment?
- Is there increasing stupor?
- Is the patient apprehensive?

---

disease process. In addition to the history, the nurse also reviews the results of available diagnostic tests.

Diagnosis

NURSING DIAGNOSES

Based on the assessment data, the patient's major nursing diagnoses may include the following:

- Impaired gas exchange and airway clearance due to chronic inhalation of toxins
- Impaired gas exchange related to ventilation–perfusion inequality
- Ineffective airway clearance related to bronchoconstriction, increased mucus production, ineffective cough, bronchopulmonary infection, and other complications
- Ineffective breathing pattern related to shortness of breath, mucus, bronchoconstriction, and airway irritants
- Activity intolerance due to fatigue, ineffective breathing patterns, and hypoxemia

- Deficient knowledge of self-care strategies to be performed at home.
- Ineffective coping related to reduced socialization, anxiety, depression, lower activity level, and the inability to work

COLLABORATIVE PROBLEMS/ POTENTIAL COMPLICATIONS

Based on the assessment data, potential complications that may develop include:

- Respiratory insufficiency or failure
- Atelectasis
- Pulmonary infection
- Pneumonia
- Pneumothorax
- Pulmonary hypertension

Planning and Goals

The major goals for the patient may include smoking cessation, improved gas exchange, airway clearance, improved breathing pattern, improved activity tolerance, maximal self-management, improved coping ability, adherence to the therapeutic program and home care, and absence of complications.

Nursing Interventions

PROMOTING SMOKING CESSATION

Because smoking has such a detrimental effect on the lungs, the nurse must discuss smoking cessation strategies with patients. Although patients may believe that it is too late to reverse the damage from years of smoking and that smoking cessation is futile, they should be informed that continuing to smoke impairs the mechanisms that clear the airways and keep them free of irritants. The nurse should educate the patient regarding the hazards of smoking and cessation strategies and provide resources regarding smoking cessation, counselling, and formalized programs available in the community.

IMPROVING GAS EXCHANGE

Bronchospasm, which occurs in many pulmonary diseases, reduces the calibre of the small bronchi and may cause dyspnea, static secretions, and infection. Bronchospasm can sometimes be detected when wheezing or diminished breath sounds are heard on auscultation with a stethoscope. Increased mucus production, along with decreased mucociliary action, contributes to further reduction in the calibre of the bronchi and results in decreased airflow and decreased gas exchange. This is further aggravated by the loss of lung elasticity that occurs with COPD (Canadian Thoracic Society, 2003; NIH, 2001).

These changes in the airway require that the nurse monitor the patient for dyspnea and hypoxemia. If bronchodilators or corticosteroids are prescribed, the nurse must administer the medications properly and be alert for potential side effects. The relief of bronchospasm is confirmed by measuring improvement in expiratory flow rates and volumes (the force of expiration, how long it takes to exhale, and the amount of air exhaled) and assessing whether the patient has less dyspnea.

ACHIEVING AIRWAY CLEARANCE

Diminishing the quantity and viscosity of sputum can clear the airway and improve pulmonary ventilation and gas exchange. All pulmonary irritants should be eliminated or reduced, particularly cigarette smoking, which is the most persistent source of pulmonary irritation. The nurse instructs the patient in directed or controlled coughing, which is more effective and reduces the fatigue associated with undirected forceful coughing. Directed coughing consists of a slow, maximal inspiration followed by breath-holding for several seconds and then two or three coughs. "Huff" coughing may also be effective. The technique consists of one or two forced exhalations ("huffs") from low to medium lung volumes with the glottis open.

Chest physiotherapy with postural drainage, intermittent positive-pressure breathing, increased fluid intake, and bland aerosol mists (with normal saline solution or water) may be useful for some patients with COPD. The use of these measures must be based on the patient's response and tolerance.

IMPROVING BREATHING PATTERNS

Ineffective breathing patterns and shortness of breath are due to the ineffective respiratory mechanics of the chest wall and lung resulting from **air trapping**, ineffective diaphragmatic movement, airway obstruction, the metabolic cost of breathing, and stress. Inspiratory muscle training and breathing retraining may help to improve breathing patterns. Training in diaphragmatic breathing reduces the respiratory rate, increases alveolar ventilation, and sometimes helps expel as much air as possible during expiration. Pursed-lip breathing helps to slow expiration, prevents collapse of small airways, and helps the patient to control the rate and depth of respiration. It also promotes relaxation, which enables the patient to gain control of dyspnea and reduce feelings of panic.

IMPROVING ACTIVITY TOLERANCE

Patients with COPD experience progressive activity and exercise intolerance. Education is focused on rehabilitative therapies to promote independence in executing activities of daily living. These may include pacing activities throughout the day or using supportive devices to decrease energy expenditure. The nurse evaluates the patient's activity tolerance and limitations and teaching strategies to promote independent activities of daily living. Also, the patient may be a candidate for exercise training to strengthen the muscles of the upper and lower extremities and improve exercise tolerance and endurance. Other health care professionals (rehabilitation therapy, occupational therapy, physical therapy) may be consulted as additional resources.

ENHANCING SELF-CARE STRATEGIES

In addition to a pulmonary rehabilitation program, the nurse helps the patient manage self-care by emphasizing the importance of setting realistic goals, avoiding temperature extremes, and modifying lifestyle (particularly stopping smoking) as applicable.

Setting Realistic Goals

A major area of teaching is the importance of setting and accepting realistic short-term and long-range goals. If the patient is severely disabled, the objectives of treatment are to preserve current pulmonary function and relieve symptoms as much as possible. If the disease is mild, the objectives are to increase exercise tolerance and prevent further loss of pulmonary function. It is important to plan and share the goals and expectations of treatment with the patient. The patient and those providing care need patience to achieve these goals.

Avoiding Temperature Extremes

The nurse instructs the patient to avoid extremes of heat and cold. Heat increases the body temperature, thereby raising oxygen requirements; cold tends to promote bronchospasm. Air pollutants such as fumes, smoke, dust, and even talcum, lint, and aerosol sprays may initiate bronchospasm. High altitudes aggravate hypoxemia.

Modifying Lifestyle

Patients with COPD should adopt a lifestyle of moderate activity, ideally in a climate with minimal shifts in temperature and humidity. As much as possible, the patient should avoid emotional disturbances and stressful situations that might trigger a coughing episode. The medication regimen for patients with COPD can be quite complex; patients receiving aerosol medications by an MDI may be particularly challenged. It is crucial to review this material and to have the patient perform a return demonstration before discharge, during follow-up visits to the caregiver's office or clinic, and during home visits (Chart 24-4).

Smoking cessation goes hand in hand with lifestyle changes, and reinforcement of the patient's efforts is a key nursing activity. Smoking cessation is the single most important therapeutic intervention for patients with COPD. There are many strategies, including prevention, cessation with or without oral or topical patch medications, and behaviour modification techniques.

ENHANCING INDIVIDUAL COPING STRATEGIES

COPD and its progression promote a cycle of physical, social, and psychological consequences, all which are interrelated. Patients experience depression, altered mood states, social isolation, and altered functional status. The nurse is key to identifying this cycle and promoting interventions for improved physical functioning, psychological and emotional stability, and social support. Following the initial assessment of the patient, the nurse may provide referrals to health care professionals in these specific areas.

MONITORING AND MANAGING POTENTIAL COMPLICATIONS

The nurse caring for the patient with COPD must assess for various complications, such as life-threatening respiratory insufficiency and failure and respiratory infection and atelectasis, which may increase the patient's risk for respiratory failure. The nurse also monitors for cognitive changes (personality and behavioural changes, memory impairment), increasing dyspnea, tachypnea, and tachycardia, which may indicate increasing hypoxemia and impending respiratory failure.

The nurse monitors pulse oximetry values to assess the patient's need for oxygen and administers supplemental oxygen as prescribed. The nurse also instructs the patient about signs and symptoms of respiratory infection that may worsen hypoxemia and reports changes in the patient's physical and cognitive status to the physician. Other activities require assisting with the management of developing complications, with possible intubation and mechanical ventilation (see Chap. 25).

Bronchopulmonary infections must be controlled to diminish inflammatory edema and to permit recovery of normal ciliary action. Minor respiratory infections that are of no consequence to the person with normal lungs can be life-threatening to the person with COPD. The cough associated with bronchial infection introduces a vicious cycle with further trauma and damage to the lungs, progression of symptoms, increased bronchospasm, and increased susceptibility to bronchial infection. Infection compromises lung function and is a common cause of respiratory failure in patients with COPD.

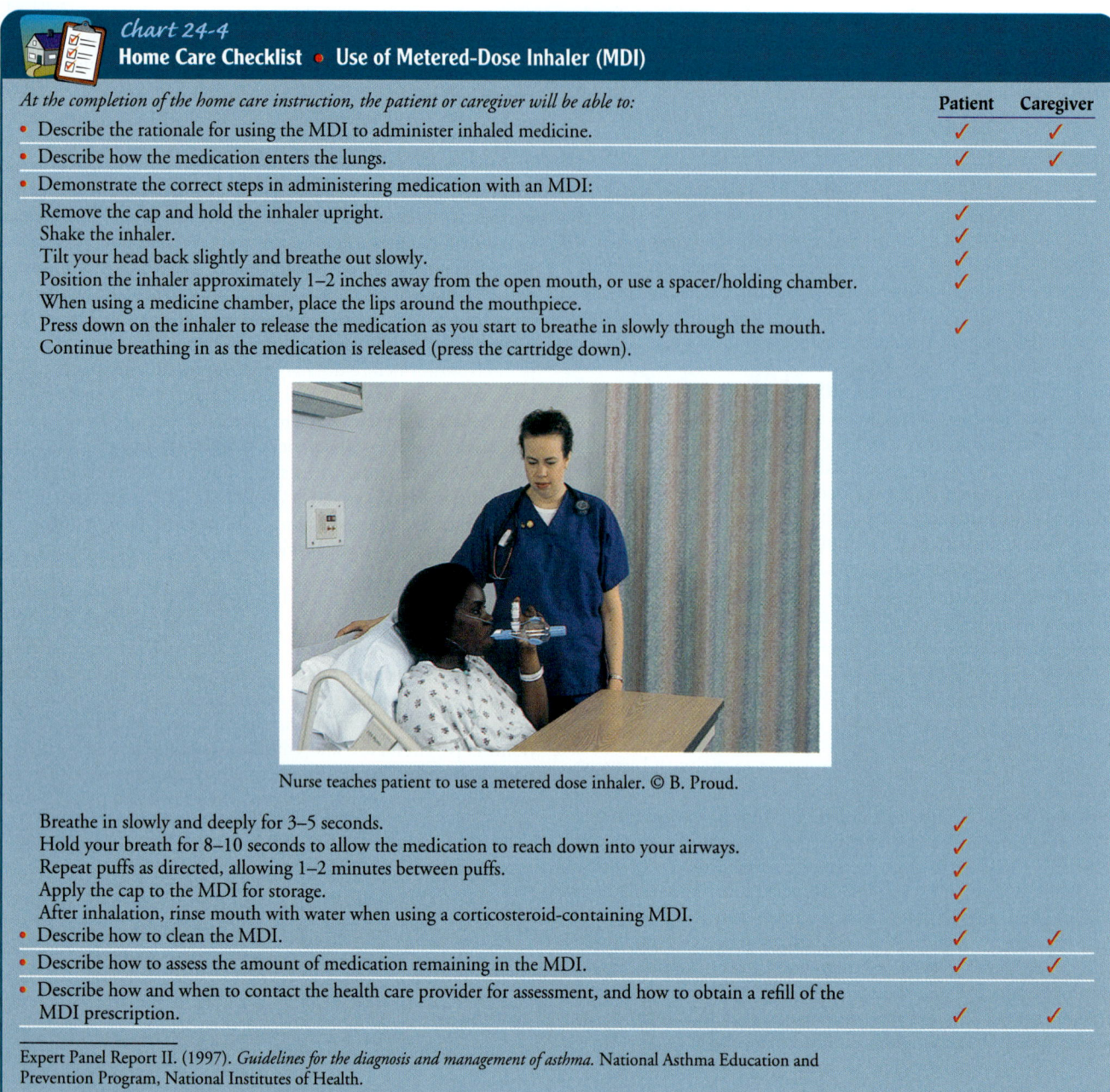

> ### Chart 24-4
> ### Home Care Checklist • Use of Metered-Dose Inhaler (MDI)
>
> *At the completion of the home care instruction, the patient or caregiver will be able to:*   **Patient**   **Caregiver**
>
> - Describe the rationale for using the MDI to administer inhaled medicine.   ✓   ✓
> - Describe how the medication enters the lungs.   ✓   ✓
> - Demonstrate the correct steps in administering medication with an MDI:
>   - Remove the cap and hold the inhaler upright.   ✓
>   - Shake the inhaler.   ✓
>   - Tilt your head back slightly and breathe out slowly.   ✓
>   - Position the inhaler approximately 1–2 inches away from the open mouth, or use a spacer/holding chamber.   ✓
>   - When using a medicine chamber, place the lips around the mouthpiece.
>   - Press down on the inhaler to release the medication as you start to breathe in slowly through the mouth.   ✓
>   - Continue breathing in as the medication is released (press the cartridge down).
>
> Nurse teaches patient to use a metered dose inhaler. © B. Proud.
>
>   - Breathe in slowly and deeply for 3–5 seconds.   ✓
>   - Hold your breath for 8–10 seconds to allow the medication to reach down into your airways.   ✓
>   - Repeat puffs as directed, allowing 1–2 minutes between puffs.   ✓
>   - Apply the cap to the MDI for storage.   ✓
>   - After inhalation, rinse mouth with water when using a corticosteroid-containing MDI.   ✓
> - Describe how to clean the MDI.   ✓   ✓
> - Describe how to assess the amount of medication remaining in the MDI.   ✓   ✓
> - Describe how and when to contact the health care provider for assessment, and how to obtain a refill of the MDI prescription.   ✓   ✓
>
> Expert Panel Report II. (1997). *Guidelines for the diagnosis and management of asthma.* National Asthma Education and Prevention Program, National Institutes of Health.

In COPD, infection may be accompanied by subtle changes. The nurse instructs the patient to report any signs of infection, such as a fever or change in sputum colour, character, consistency, or amount. Any worsening of symptoms (increased tightness of the chest, increased dyspnea and fatigue) also suggests infection and must be reported. Viral infections are hazardous to these patients because they are often followed by infections caused by bacterial organisms, such as *Streptococcus pneumoniae* and *Haemophilus influenzae.*

The nurse should encourage patients with COPD to be immunized against influenza and *S. pneumoniae* because these patients are prone to respiratory infection. It is important to caution patients to avoid going outdoors if the pollen count is high or if there is significant air pollution because of the risk of bronchospasm. The patient also should avoid exposure to high outdoor temperatures with high humidity.

Pneumothorax is a potential complication of COPD. Patients with severe emphysematous changes can develop large bullae, which may rupture and cause a pneumothorax. The development of a pneumothorax may be spontaneous or related to an activity such as severe coughing or large intrathoracic pressure changes. If the patient develops a rapid onset of shortness of breath, the nurse should quickly evaluate the patient for a potential pneumothorax by assessing the symmetry of chest movement, differences in breath sounds, and pulse oximetry. A pneumothorax is a life-threatening event in the patient with COPD who has minimal pulmonary reserve.

Over time, pulmonary hypertension may occur as a result of chronic hypoxemia. The pulmonary arteries respond to hypoxemia by constriction, thus leading to pulmonary hypertension. The complication may be prevented by maintaining adequate oxygenation through an adequate hemoglobin level, improved ventilation/perfusion of the lungs, or continuous administration of supplemental oxygen (if needed).

PROMOTING HOME AND COMMUNITY-BASED CARE

Teaching Patients Self-Care

Teaching is essential throughout the course of COPD and should be part of the nursing care given to every patient with COPD. Patients' and family members' knowledge and comfort level with their knowledge should be assessed and considered when providing instructions about self-management strategies. In addition to the aspects of patient education previously described, patients and family members must become familiar with the medications that are prescribed and knowledgeable about potential side effects. Patients and family members need to learn the early signs and symptoms of infection and other complications so that they seek appropriate health care promptly.

Continuing Care

Referral for home care is important to enable the nurse to assess the patient's home environment and physical and psychological status, to evaluate the patient's adherence to the prescribed regimen, and to assess the patient's ability to cope with changes in lifestyle and physical status. The nurse assesses the patient's and family's understanding of the complications and side effects of medications. The home care visit provides an opportunity to reinforce the information and activities learned in the inpatient or outpatient pulmonary rehabilitation program and to have the patient and family demonstrate correct administration of medications and oxygen, if indicated, and performance of exercises. If the patient does not have access to a formal pulmonary rehabilitation program, it is important for the nurse to provide the education and breathing retraining necessary to optimize the patient's functional status.

The nurse may direct patients to community resources such as pulmonary rehabilitation programs and smoking cessation programs to help improve their ability to cope with their chronic condition and the therapeutic regimen and to give them a sense of worth, hope, and well-being. In addition, the nurse reminds the patient and family about the importance of participating in general health promotion activities and health screening.

Evaluation

EXPECTED PATIENT OUTCOMES

Expected patient outcomes may include:

1. Demonstrates knowledge of hazards of smoking
   a. Verbalizes willingness/interest to quit smoking
   b. Verbalizes information about smoking, risks of continuing, benefits of quitting, and techniques to optimize cessation efforts
2. Demonstrates improved gas exchange
   a. Shows no signs of restlessness, confusion, or agitation
   b. Has stable pulse oximetry or arterial blood gas values (but not necessarily normal values due to chronic changes in the gas exchange ability of the lungs)
3. Achieves maximal airway clearance
   a. Stops smoking
   b. Avoids noxious substances and extremes of temperature
   c. Maintains adequate hydration
   d. If indicated, performs postural drainage correctly

e. Knows signs of early infection and is aware of how and when to report them if they occur
   f. Performs controlled coughing without experiencing excessive fatigue
4. Improves breathing pattern
   a. Practices and uses pursed-lip and diaphragmatic breathing
   b. Shows signs of decreased respiratory effort (decreased respiratory rate, less dyspnea)
5. Demonstrates knowledge of strategies to improve activity tolerance and maintain maximum level of self-care
   a. Performs self-care activities within tolerance range
   b. Paces self to avoid fatigue and dyspnea
   c. Uses controlled breathing while performing activities
   d. Uses devices to assist with activity tolerance and decrease energy expenditure
6. Demonstrates knowledge of self-care strategies
   a. Participates in determining the therapeutic program
   b. Understands the rationale for activities and medications
   c. Follows the medication plan
   d. Uses bronchodilators and oxygen therapy as prescribed
   e. Stops smoking
   f. Maintains acceptable activity level
7. Uses effective coping mechanisms for dealing with consequences of disease
   a. Uses self-care strategies to lessen stress associated with disease
   b. Verbalizes resources available to deal with psychological burden of disease
   c. Participates in pulmonary rehabilitation, if appropriate
8. Uses community resources and home-based care
   a. Verbalizes knowledge of community resources (eg, smoking cessation, hospital/community-based support groups)
   b. Participates in pulmonary rehabilitation, if appropriate
9. Avoids or reduces complications
   a. Has no evidence of respiratory failure or insufficiency
   b. Maintains adequate pulse oximetry and arterial blood gas values
   c. Shows no signs or symptoms of infection, pneumothorax, or pulmonary hypertension

For more information, see Plan of Nursing Care: Care of the Patient With COPD.

Bronchiectasis

Bronchiectasis is a chronic, irreversible dilation of the bronchi and bronchioles. Under the new definition of COPD, it is considered a separate disease process from COPD (Canadian Thoracic Society, 2003; NIH, 2001). Bronchiectasis may be caused by a variety of conditions, including:

- Airway obstruction
- Diffuse airway injury
- Pulmonary infections and obstruction of the bronchus or complications of long-term pulmonary infections
- Genetic disorders such as cystic fibrosis
- Abnormal host defense (eg, ciliary dyskinesia or humoural immunodeficiency)
- Idiopathic causes

(text continues on page 590)

Plan of Nursing Care
Care of the Patient With COPD

Nursing Interventions	Rationale	Expected Outcomes

Nursing Diagnosis: Impaired gas exchange and airway clearance due to chronic inhalation of toxins
Goal: Improvement in gas exchange

Nursing Interventions	Rationale	Expected Outcomes
1. Evaluate current smoking status, educate regarding smoking cessation, and facilitate efforts to quit. a. Evaluate current smoking habits of patient and family. b. Educate regarding hazards of smoking and relationship to COPD. c. Evaluate previous smoking cessation attempts. d. Provide educational materials. e. Refer to a smoking cessation program or resource. 2. Evaluate current exposure to occupational exposures and indoor/outdoor pollution. a. Evaluate current exposures to occupational toxins, indoor and outdoor air pollution (eg, smog, toxic fumes, chemicals). b. Emphasize primary prevention to occupational exposures. This is best achieved by elimination or reduction of exposures in the workplace. c. Educate regarding types of indoor and outdoor air pollution (eg, biomass fuel burned for cooking and heating in poorly ventilated buildings, outdoor air pollution). d. Advise patient to monitor public announcements regarding air quality.	1. Smoking causes permanent damage to the lung and diminishes the lungs' protective mechanisms. Airflow is obstructed, secretions are increased, and lung capacity is reduced. Continued smoking increases morbidity and mortality in COPD and is also a risk factor for lung cancer. 2. Chronic inhalation of both indoor and outdoor toxins causes damage to the airways and impairs gas exchange.	• Identifies the hazards of cigarette smoking • Enrolls in smoking cessation program • Reports success in stopping smoking • Identifies resources for smoking cessation • Verbalizes types of inhaled toxins • Minimizes or eliminates exposures • Monitors public announcements regarding air quality and minimizes or eliminates exposures during episodes of severe pollution

Nursing Diagnosis: Impaired gas exchange related to ventilation–perfusion inequality
Goal: Improvement in gas exchange

Nursing Interventions	Rationale	Expected Outcomes
1. Administer bronchodilators as prescribed: a. Inhalation is the preferred route. b. Observe for side effects: tachycardia, dysrhythmias, central nervous system excitation, nausea, and vomiting. c. Assess for correct technique of metered-dose inhaler (MDI) administration. 2. Evaluate effectiveness of nebulizer or MDI treatments. a. Assess for decreased shortness of breath, decreased wheezing or crackles, loosened secretions, decreased anxiety. b. Ensure that treatment is given before meals to avoid nausea and to reduce fatigue that accompanies eating. 3. Instruct and encourage patient in diaphragmatic breathing and effective coughing.	1. Bronchodilators dilate the airways. The medication dosage is carefully adjusted for each patient, in accordance with clinical response. 2. Combining medication with aerosolized bronchodilators is typically used to control bronchoconstriction in an acute exacerbation. Generally, however, the MDI with spacer is the preferred route (less cost and time to treatment). 3. These techniques improve ventilation by opening airways to facilitate clearing the airways of sputum. Gas exchange is improved and fatigue is minimized.	• Verbalizes need for bronchodilators and for taking as prescribed • Evidences minimal side effects; heart rate near normal, absence of dysrhythmias, normal mentation • Reports a decrease in dyspnea • Shows an improved expiratory flow rate • Uses and cleans respiratory therapy equipment as applicable • Demonstrates diaphragmatic breathing and coughing • Uses oxygen equipment appropriately when indicated • Evidences improved arterial blood gases or pulse oximetry • Demonstrates correct technique for use of MDI

(continued)

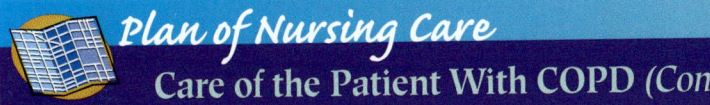

Plan of Nursing Care
Care of the Patient With COPD *(Continued)*

Nursing Interventions	Rationale	Expected Outcomes

4. Administer oxygen by the method prescribed.
  a. Explain rationale and importance to patient.
  b. Evaluate effectiveness; observe for signs of hypoxemia. Notify physician if restlessness, anxiety, somnolence, cyanosis, or tachycardia is present.
  c. Analyze arterial blood gases and compare with baseline values. When arterial puncture is performed and a blood sample is obtained, hold puncture site for 5 minutes to prevent arterial bleeding and development of ecchymoses.
  d. Initiate pulse oximetry to monitor oxygen saturation.
  e. Explain that no smoking is permitted by patient or visitors while oxygen is in use.
	4. Oxygen will correct the hypoxemia. Careful observation of the litre flow or the percentage administered and its effect on the patient is important. If the patient has chronic CO_2 retention, excessive oxygen could suppress the hypoxic drive and respirations. These patients generally need low-flow oxygen rates of 1 to 2 L/min. Periodic arterial blood gases and pulse oximetry help to evaluate adequacy of oxygenation. Smoking may render pulse oximetry inaccurate because the carbon monoxide from cigarette smoke also saturates hemoglobin.	

Nursing Diagnosis: Ineffective airway clearance related to bronchoconstriction, increased mucus production, ineffective cough, bronchopulmonary infection, and other complications

Goal: Achievement of airway clearance

1. Adequately hydrate the patient.	1. Systemic hydration keeps secretions moist and easier to expectorate. Fluids must be given with caution if right- or left-sided heart failure is present.	• Verbalizes need to drink fluids • Demonstrates diaphragmatic breathing and coughing • Performs postural drainage correctly • Coughing is minimized • Does not smoke • Verbalizes that pollens, fumes, gases, dusts, and extremes of temperature and humidity are irritants to be avoided • Identifies signs of early infection • Is free of infection (no fever, no change in sputum, lessening of dyspnea) • Verbalizes need to notify health care provider at the earliest sign of infection • Verbalizes need to stay away from crowds or people with colds in flu season • Discusses flu and pneumonia vaccines with clinician to help prevent infection
2. Teach and encourage the use of diaphragmatic breathing and coughing techniques.	2. These techniques help to improve ventilation and mobilize secretions without causing breathlessness and fatigue.	
3. Assist in administering nebulizer or MDI.	3. This ensures adequate delivery of medication to the airways.	
4. If indicated, perform postural drainage with percussion and vibration in the morning and at night as prescribed.	4. Uses gravity to help raise secretions so they can be more easily expectorated or suctioned.	
5. Instruct patient to avoid bronchial irritants such as cigarette smoke, aerosols, extremes of temperature, and fumes.	5. Bronchial irritants cause bronchoconstriction and increased mucus production, which then interferes with airway clearance.	

6. Teach early signs of infection that are to be reported to the clinician immediately:
  a. Increased sputum production
  b. Change in colour of sputum
  c. Increased thickness of sputum
  d. Increased shortness of breath, tightness in chest, or fatigue
  e. Increased coughing
  f. Fever or chills
	6. Minor respiratory infections that are of no consequence to the person with normal lungs can produce fatal disturbances in the lungs of the person with emphysema. Early recognition is crucial.	

7. Administer antibiotics as prescribed.	7. Antibiotics may be prescribed to prevent or treat infection.	
8. Encourage patient to be immunized against influenza and *Streptococcus pneumoniae*.	8. People with respiratory conditions are prone to respiratory infections and are encouraged to be immunized.	

(continued)

Plan of Nursing Care

Care of the Patient With COPD *(Continued)*

Nursing Interventions	Rationale	Expected Outcomes

Nursing Diagnosis: Ineffective breathing pattern related to shortness of breath, mucus, bronchoconstriction, and airway irritants

Goal: Improvement in breathing pattern

Nursing Interventions	Rationale	Expected Outcomes
1. Teach patient diaphragmatic and pursed-lip breathing.	1. Helps patient prolong expiration time and decreases air trapping. With these techniques, patient will breathe more efficiently and effectively.	• Practices pursed-lip and diaphragmatic breathing and uses them when short of breath and with activity
2. Encourage alternating activity with rest periods. Allow patient to make some decisions (bath, shaving) about care based on tolerance level.	2. Pacing activities permits patient to perform activities without excessive distress.	• Shows signs of decreased respiratory effort and paces activities • Uses inspiratory muscle trainer as prescribed
3. Encourage use of an inspiratory muscle trainer if prescribed.	3. Strengthens and conditions the respiratory muscles.	

Nursing Diagnosis: Self-care deficits related to fatigue secondary to increased work of breathing and insufficient ventilation and oxygenation

Goal: Independence in self-care activities

Nursing Interventions	Rationale	Expected Outcomes
1. Teach patient to coordinate diaphragmatic breathing with activity (eg, walking, bending).	1. This will allow the patient to be more active and to avoid excessive fatigue or dyspnea during activity.	• Uses controlled breathing while bathing, bending, and walking
2. Encourage patient to begin to bathe self, dress self, walk, and drink fluids. Discuss energy conservation measures.	2. As condition resolves, patient will be able to do more but needs to be encouraged to avoid increasing dependence.	• Paces activities of daily living to alternate with rest periods to reduce fatigue and dyspnea
3. Teach postural drainage if appropriate.	3. Encourages patient to become involved in own care. Prepares patient to manage at home.	• Describes energy conservation strategies • Performs same self-care activities as before • Performs postural drainage correctly

Nursing Diagnosis: Activity intolerance due to fatigue, hypoxemia, and ineffective breathing patterns

Goal: Improvement in activity tolerance

Nursing Interventions	Rationale	Expected Outcomes

1. Support patient in establishing a regular regimen of exercise using treadmill and exercycle, walking, or other appropriate exercises, such as mall walking.
  a. Assess the patient's current level of functioning and develop exercise plan based on baseline functional status.
  b. Suggest consultation with a physical therapist or pulmonary rehabilitation program to determine an exercise program specific to the patient's capability. Have portable oxygen unit available if oxygen is prescribed for exercise.
	1. Muscles that are deconditioned consume more oxygen and place an additional burden on the lungs. Through regular, graded exercise, these muscle groups become more conditioned, and the patient can do more without getting as short of breath. Graded exercise breaks the cycle of debilitation.	• Performs activities with less shortness of breath
		• Verbalizes need to exercise daily and demonstrates an exercise plan to be carried out at home
		• Walks and gradually increases walking time and distance to improve physical condition
		• Exercises both upper and lower body muscle groups

Nursing Diagnosis: Ineffective coping related to reduced socialization, anxiety, depression, lower activity level, and the inability to work

Goal: Attainment of an optimal level of coping

Nursing Interventions	Rationale	Expected Outcomes
1. Help the patient develop realistic goals.	1. Developing realistic goals will promote a sense of hope and accomplishment rather than defeat and hopelessness.	• Expresses interest in the future • Participates in the discharge plan • Discusses activities or methods that can be performed to ease shortness of breath
2. Encourage activity to level of symptom tolerance.	2. Activity reduces tension and decreases degree of dyspnea as patient becomes conditioned.	• Uses relaxation techniques appropriately • Expresses interest in a pulmonary rehabilitation program

(continued)

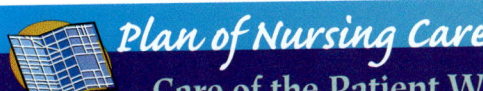

Plan of Nursing Care
Care of the Patient With COPD (Continued)

Nursing Interventions	Rationale	Expected Outcomes
3. Teach relaxation technique or provide a relaxation tape for patient.	3. Relaxation reduces stress, anxiety, and dyspnea and helps patient to cope with disability.	
4. Enroll patient in pulmonary rehabilitation program where available.	4. Pulmonary rehabilitation programs have been shown to promote a subjective improvement in a patient's status and self-esteem as well as increased exercise tolerance and decreased hospitalizations.	

Nursing Diagnosis: Deficient knowledge about self-management to be performed at home.
Goal: Adherence to therapeutic program and home care

1. Help patient understand short- and long-term goals.
  a. Teach the patient about disease, medications, procedures, and how and when to seek help.
  b. Refer patient to pulmonary rehabilitation.
2. Give strong message to stop smoking. Discuss smoking cessation strategies. Provide information about resource groups (eg, Canadian Cancer Society, Canadian Lung Association).
	1. Patient needs to be a partner in developing the plan of care and needs to know what to expect. Teaching about the condition is one of the most important aspects of care; it will prepare the patient to live and cope with the condition and improve quality of life.
	2. Smoking causes permanent damage to the lung and diminishes the lungs' protective mechanisms. Air flow is obstructed and lung capacity is reduced. Smoking increases morbidity and mortality and is also a risk factor for lung cancer.
		• Understands disease and what affects it
		• Verbalizes the need to preserve existing lung function by adhering to the prescribed program
		• Understands purposes and proper administration of medications
		• Stops smoking or enrolls in a smoking cessation program
		• Identifies when and whom to call for assistance

Collaborative Problem: Atelectasis
Goal: Absence of atelectasis on x-ray and physical examination

1. Monitor respiratory status, including rate and pattern of respirations, breath sounds, signs and symptoms of respiratory distress, and pulse oximetry. 2. Instruct in and encourage diaphragmatic breathing and effective coughing techniques. 3. Promote use of lung expansion techniques (eg, deep-breathing exercises, incentive spirometry) as prescribed.	1. A change in respiratory status, including tachypnea, dyspnea, and diminished or absent breath sounds, may indicate atelectasis. 2. These techniques improve ventilation and lung expansion and ideally improve gas exchange. 3. Deep-breathing exercises and incentive spirometry promote maximal lung expansion.	• Normal (baseline for patient) respiratory rate and pattern • Normal breath sounds for patient • Demonstrates diaphragmatic breathing and effective coughing • Performs deep-breathing exercises, incentive spirometry as prescribed • Pulse oximetry is ≥ 90%

Collaborative Problem: Pneumothorax
Goal: Absence of signs and symptoms of pneumothorax

1. Monitor respiratory status, including rate and pattern of respirations, symmetry of chest wall movement, breath sounds, signs and symptoms of respiratory distress, and pulse oximetry. 2. Assess pulse. 3. Assess for chest pain and precipitating factors. 4. Palpate for tracheal deviation/shift away from the affected side.	1. Dyspnea, tachypnea, tachycardia, acute pleuritic chest pain, tracheal deviation away from the affected side, absence of breath sounds on the affected side, and decreased tactile fremitus may indicate pneumothorax. 2. Tachycardia is associated with pneumothorax and anxiety. 3. Pain may accompany pneumothorax. 4. Early detection of pneumothorax and prompt intervention will prevent other serious complications.	• Normal respiratory rate and pattern for patient • Normal breath sounds bilaterally • Normal pulse for patient • Normal tactile fremitus • Absence of pain • Tracheal position is midline • Pulse oximetry ≥ 90% • Maintains normal oxygen saturation and arterial blood gas measurements for patient • Exhibits no hypoxemia and hypercapnia (or returns to baseline values)

(continued)

Plan of Nursing Care

Care of the Patient With COPD (Continued)

Nursing Interventions	Rationale	Expected Outcomes
5. Monitor pulse oximetry and if indicated arterial blood gases. 6. Administer supplemental oxygen therapy, as indicated. 7. Administer analgesics, as indicated, for chest pain. 8. Assist with chest tube insertion and use pleural drainage system, as prescribed.	5. Recognition of a deterioration in respiratory function will prevent serious complications. 6. Oxygen will correct hypoxemia; administer it with caution. 7. Pain interferes with deep breathing, resulting in a decrease in lung expansion. 8. Removal of air from the pleural space will reexpand the lung.	• Absence of pain • Symmetric chest wall movement • Lung is reexpanded on chest x-ray • Breath sounds are heard on the affected side

Collaborative Problem: Respiratory failure
Goal: Absence of signs and symptoms of respiratory failure; no evidence of respiratory failure on laboratory tests

1. Monitor respiratory status, including rate and pattern of respirations, breath sounds, and signs and symptoms of acute respiratory distress. 2. Monitor pulse oximetry and arterial blood gases. 3. Administer supplemental oxygen and initiate mechanisms for mechanical ventilation, as prescribed.	1. Early recognition of a deterioration in respiratory function will avert further complications, such as respiratory failure, severe hypoxemia, and hypercapnia. 2. Recognition of changes in oxygenation and acid–base balance will guide in correcting and preventing complications. 3. Acute respiratory failure is a medical emergency. Hypoxemia is a hallmark sign. Administration of oxygen therapy and mechanical ventilation (if indicated) are critical to survival.	• Normal respiratory rate and pattern for patient with no acute distress • Recognizes symptoms of hypoxemia and hypercapnia • Maintains normal arterial blood gases/pulse oximetry or returns to baseline values

Collaborative Problem: Pulmonary hypertension
Goal: Absence of evidence of pulmonary hypertension on physical examination or laboratory tests

1. Monitor respiratory status, including rate and pattern of respirations, breath sounds, pulse oximetry, and signs and symptoms of acute respiratory distress. 2. Assess for signs and symptoms of right-sided heart failure, including peripheral edema, ascites, distended neck veins, crackles, and heart murmur. 3. Administer oxygen therapy, as prescribed.	1. Dyspnea is the primary symptom of pulmonary hypertension. Other symptoms include fatigue, angina, near syncope, edema, and palpitations. 2. Right-sided heart failure is a common clinical manifestation of pulmonary hypertension due to increased right ventricular workload. 3. Continuous oxygen therapy is a major component of management of pulmonary hypertension by preventing hypoxemia and thereby reducing pulmonary vascular constriction (resistance) secondary to hypoxemia.	• Normal respiratory rate and pattern for patient • Exhibits no signs and symptoms of right-sided failure • Maintains baseline pulse oximetry values and arterial blood gases

A person may be predisposed to bronchiectasis as a result of recurrent respiratory infections in early childhood, measles, influenza, tuberculosis, and immunodeficiency disorders.

Pathophysiology

The inflammatory process associated with pulmonary infections damages the bronchial wall, causing a loss of its supporting structure and resulting in thick sputum that ultimately obstructs the bronchi. The walls become permanently distended and distorted, impairing mucociliary clearance. The inflammation and infection extend to the peribronchial tissues; in the case of saccular bronchiectasis, each dilated tube virtually amounts to a lung abscess, the exudate of which drains freely through the bronchus. Bronchiectasis is usually localized, affecting a segment or lobe of a lung, most frequently the lower lobes.

The retention of secretions and subsequent obstruction ultimately cause the alveoli distal to the obstruction to collapse (atelectasis). Inflammatory scarring or fibrosis replaces functioning lung tissue. In time the patient develops respiratory insufficiency with reduced vital capacity, decreased ventilation, and an increased ratio of residual volume to total lung capacity. There is impairment in the matching of ventilation to perfusion (ventilation–perfusion imbalance) and hypoxemia.

Clinical Manifestations

Characteristic symptoms of bronchiectasis include chronic cough and the production of purulent sputum in copious amounts. Many patients with this disease have hemoptysis. Clubbing of the fingers also is common because of respiratory insufficiency. The patient usually has repeated episodes of pulmonary infection. Even with modern treatment approaches, the average age at death is approximately 55 years.

Assessment and Diagnostic Findings

Bronchiectasis is not readily diagnosed because the symptoms can be mistaken for those of simple chronic bronchitis. A definite sign is offered by the prolonged history of productive cough, with sputum consistently negative for tubercle bacilli. The diagnosis is established by a computed tomography (CT) scan, which demonstrates either the presence or absence of bronchial dilation.

Medical Management

Treatment objectives are to promote bronchial drainage to clear excessive secretions from the affected portion of the lungs and to prevent or control infection. Postural drainage is part of all treatment plans because draining the bronchiectatic areas by gravity reduces the amount of secretions and the degree of infection. Sometimes mucopurulent sputum must be removed by bronchoscopy. Chest physiotherapy, including percussion and postural drainage, is important in secretion management.

Smoking cessation is important because smoking impairs bronchial drainage by paralyzing ciliary action, increasing bronchial secretions, and causing inflammation of the mucous membranes, resulting in hyperplasia of the mucous glands. Infection is controlled with antimicrobial therapy based on the results of sensitivity studies on organisms cultured from sputum. A year-round regimen of antibiotic agents may be prescribed, with different types of antibiotics at intervals. Some clinicians prescribe antibiotic agents throughout the winter or when acute upper respiratory tract infections occur. Patients should be vaccinated against influenza and pneumococcal pneumonia. Bronchodilators, which may be prescribed for patients who also have reactive airway disease, may also assist with secretion management.

Surgical intervention, although used infrequently, may be indicated for the patient who continues to expectorate large amounts of sputum and has repeated bouts of pneumonia and hemoptysis despite adhering to the treatment regimen. However, the disease must involve only one or two areas of the lung that can be removed without producing respiratory insufficiency. The goals of surgical treatment are to conserve normal pulmonary tissue and to avoid infectious complications. Diseased tissue is removed, provided that the postoperative lung function will be adequate. It may be necessary to remove a segment of a lobe (segmental resection), a lobe (lobectomy), or rarely an entire lung (pneumonectomy). (See Chart 25-16 for further information.) Segmental resection is the removal of an anatomic subdivision of a pulmonary lobe. The chief advantage is that only diseased tissue is removed and healthy lung tissue is conserved.

The surgery is preceded by a period of careful preparation. The objective is to obtain a dry (free of infection) tracheobronchial tree to prevent complications (atelectasis, pneumonia,

bronchopleural fistula, and empyema). This is accomplished by postural drainage or, depending on the location, by direct suction through a bronchoscope. A course of antibacterial therapy may be prescribed. After surgery, the care is the same as for any patient undergoing chest surgery (see Chap. 25).

Nursing Management

Nursing management of the patient with bronchiectasis focuses on alleviating symptoms and assisting the patient to clear pulmonary secretions. Smoking and other factors that increase the production of mucus and hamper its removal are targeted in patient teaching. The patient and family are taught to perform postural drainage and to avoid exposure to others with upper respiratory and other infections. If the patient experiences fatigue and dyspnea, strategies to conserve energy while maintaining as active a lifestyle as possible are discussed. The patient needs to become knowledgeable about early signs of respiratory infection and the progression of the disorder so that appropriate treatment can be implemented promptly. Because the presence of a large amount of mucus may decrease the patient's appetite and result in an inadequate dietary intake, the patient's nutritional status is assessed and strategies are implemented to ensure an adequate diet.

Asthma

Asthma is a chronic inflammatory disease of the airways that causes airway hyperresponsiveness, mucosal edema, and mucus production. This inflammation ultimately leads to recurrent episodes of asthma symptoms: cough, chest tightness, wheezing, and dyspnea (Fig. 24-6). About 2.5 million Canadians have asthma, and the mortality rate is 1.24 per 100,000 (Health Canada, 2001). It is estimated that 43% of individuals with asthma visit their doctors one to three times in a year. At least once each year, 18% of individuals with active asthma visit the emergency department and 5.3% require hospitalization (Health Canada, 2001).

Asthma differs from the other obstructive lung diseases in that it is largely reversible, either spontaneously or with treatment. Patients with asthma may experience symptom-free periods alternating with acute exacerbations, which last from minutes to hours or days. Asthma can occur at any age and is the most common chronic disease of childhood. Despite increased knowledge regarding the pathology of asthma and the development of better medications and management plans, the death rate from asthma continues to increase. For most patients it is a disruptive disease, affecting school and work attendance, occupational choices, physical activity, and general quality of life.

Allergy is the strongest predisposing factor for asthma. Chronic exposure to airway irritants or allergens also increases the risk for developing asthma. Common allergens can be seasonal (eg, grass, tree, and weed pollens) or perennial (eg, mold, dust, roaches, or animal dander). Common triggers for asthma symptoms and exacerbations in patients with asthma include airway irritants (eg, air pollutants, cold, heat, weather changes, strong odours or perfumes, smoke), exercise, stress or emotional upsets, sinusitis with postnasal drip, medications, viral respiratory tract infections, and gastroesophageal reflux. Most people who have asthma are sensitive to a variety of triggers. A patient's asthma condition will change depending upon the environment, activities, management practices, and other factors (Canadian Thoracic Society, 2003).

Physiology/Pathophysiology

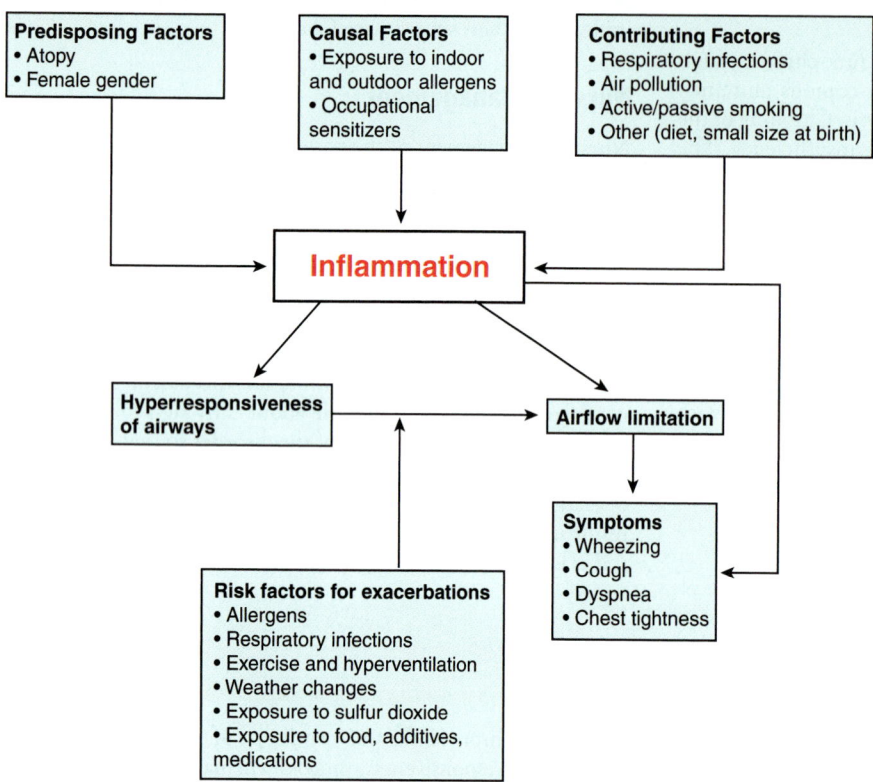

Predisposing Factors
• Atopy
• Female gender

Causal Factors
• Exposure to indoor and outdoor allergens
• Occupational sensitizers

Contributing Factors
• Respiratory infections
• Air pollution
• Active/passive smoking
• Other (diet, small size at birth)

Inflammation

Hyperresponsiveness of airways

Airflow limitation

Symptoms
• Wheezing
• Cough
• Dyspnea
• Chest tightness

Risk factors for exacerbations
• Allergens
• Respiratory infections
• Exercise and hyperventilation
• Weather changes
• Exposure to sulfur dioxide
• Exposure to food, additives, medications

FIGURE 24-6 Pathophysiology of asthma. Adapted from materials developed for the Global Initiative for Asthma (GINA): Global Strategy for Asthma Management and Prevention, National Institutes of Health–National Heart, Lung, and Blood Institute, revised 2002.

Pathophysiology

The underlying pathology in asthma is reversible and diffuse airway inflammation. The inflammation leads to obstruction from the following: swelling of the membranes that line the airways (mucosal edema), reducing the airway diameter; contraction of the bronchial smooth muscle that encircles the airways (bronchospasm), causing further narrowing; and increased mucus production, which diminishes airway size and may entirely plug the bronchi.

The bronchial muscles and mucus glands enlarge; thick, tenacious sputum is produced; and the alveoli hyperinflate. Some patients may have airway subbasement membrane fibrosis. This is called airway "remodeling" and occurs in response to chronic inflammation. The fibrotic changes in the airway lead to airway narrowing and potentially irreversible airflow limitation (NIH, 2001; NHLBI, 1998).

Cells that play a key role in the inflammation of asthma are mast cells, neutrophils, eosinophils, and lymphocytes. Mast cells, when activated, release several chemicals called mediators. These chemicals, which include histamine, bradykinin, prostaglandins, and leukotrienes, perpetuate the inflammatory response, causing increased blood flow, vasoconstriction, fluid leak from the vasculature, attraction of white blood cells to the area, and bronchoconstriction (NHLBI, 1998). Regulation of these chemicals is the aim of much of the current research regarding pharmacologic therapy for asthma.

Further, alpha- and beta$_2$-adrenergic receptors of the sympathetic nervous system are located in the bronchi. When the alpha-adrenergic receptors are stimulated, bronchoconstriction occurs; when the beta$_2$-adrenergic receptors are stimulated, bronchodilation results. The balance between alpha and beta$_2$ receptors is controlled primarily by cyclic adenosine monophosphate (cAMP).

Alpha-adrenergic receptor stimulation results in a decrease in cAMP, which leads to an increase of chemical mediators released by the mast cells and bronchoconstriction. Beta$_2$-receptor stimulation results in increased levels of cAMP, which inhibits the release of chemical mediators and causes bronchodilation (NHLBI, 1998).

Clinical Manifestations

The three most common symptoms of asthma are cough, dyspnea, and wheezing. In some instances, cough may be the only symptom. Asthma attacks often occur at night or early in the morning, possibly due to circadian variations that influence airway receptor thresholds.

An asthma exacerbation may begin abruptly but most frequently is preceded by increasing symptoms over the previous few days. There is cough, with or without mucus production. At times the mucus is so tightly wedged in the narrowed airway that the patient cannot cough it up. There may be generalized wheezing (the sound of airflow through narrowed airways), first on expiration and then possibly during inspiration as well. Generalized chest tightness and dyspnea occur. Expiration requires effort and becomes prolonged. As the exacerbation progresses, diaphoresis, tachycardia, and a widened pulse pressure may occur along with hypoxemia and central cyanosis (a late sign of poor oxygenation). Although life-threatening and severe hypoxemia can occur in asthma, it is relatively uncommon. The hypoxemia is secondary to a ventilation–perfusion mismatch and readily responds to supplemental oxygenation.

Symptoms of exercise-induced asthma include maximal symptoms during exercise, absence of nocturnal symptoms, and sometimes only a description of a "choking" sensation during exercise.

Asthma severity is likely to vary over time and optimal asthma management varies accordingly. A number of consensus guidelines describe categories of severity based on frequency and duration of respiratory symptoms, airflow limitation, and the medication required to maintain acceptable asthma control (Table 24-3) (Canadian Thoracic Society, 1999, 2003; Expert Panel Report II, 1997; Global Initiative for Asthma, 2004).

Assessment and Diagnostic Findings

A complete family, environmental, and occupational history is essential. To establish the diagnosis, the clinician must determine that periodic symptoms of airflow obstruction are present, airflow is at least partially reversible, and other etiologies have been excluded. A positive family history and environmental factors, including seasonal changes, high pollen counts, mold, climate changes (particularly cold air), and air pollution, are primarily associated with asthma. In addition, asthma is associated with a variety of occupation-related chemicals and compounds, including metal salts, wood and vegetable dust, medications (eg, aspirin, antibiotics, piperazine, cimetidine), industrial chemicals and plastics, biologic enzymes (eg, laundry detergents), animal and insect dusts, sera, and secretions. Comorbid conditions that may accompany asthma include gastroesophageal reflux, drug-induced asthma, and allergic bronchopulmonary aspergillosis. Other possible allergic reactions that may accompany asthma include eczema, rashes, and temporary edema.

During acute episodes, sputum and blood tests may disclose eosinophilia (elevated levels of eosinophils). Serum levels of immunoglobulin E may be elevated if allergy is present. Arterial blood gas analysis and pulse oximetry reveal hypoxemia during acute attacks. Initially, hypocapnia and respiratory alkalosis are present. As the condition worsens and the patient becomes more fatigued, the $PaCO_2$ may rise. A normal $PaCO_2$ value may be a signal of impending respiratory failure. Because CO_2 is 20 times more diffusible than oxygen, it is rare for $PaCO_2$ to be normal or elevated in a person who is breathing very rapidly. During an exacerbation, the FEV_1 and FVC are markedly decreased but improve with bronchodilator administration (demonstrating reversibility). Pulmonary function is usually normal between exacerbations.

The occurrence of a severe, continuous reaction is referred to as status asthmaticus and is considered life-threatening (see below).

Prevention

Patients with recurrent asthma should undergo tests to identify the substances that precipitate the symptoms. Possible causes are dust, dust mites, roaches, certain types of cloth, pets, horses, detergents, soaps, certain foods, molds, and pollens. If the attacks are seasonal, pollens can be strongly suspected. The patient is instructed to avoid the causative agents whenever possible.

Knowledge is the key to quality asthma care. Although national guidelines are available for the care of the asthma patient, unfortunately health care providers may not follow them. Failure to follow the guidelines in the following areas has been noted: lack of treatment of patients who have symptoms more than 2 days per week with a regular medication schedule, lack of patient-specific advice on improving the environment and an explanation about the importance of doing so, lack of encouragement for patients to monitor their peak flow measurements with a diary, and lack of written, up-to-date educational materials (Plaut, 2001).

A 1998 survey by a group called "Asthma in America" found that 11% of physicians were unaware of the national asthma guidelines. Only 35% of patients with asthma who were surveyed

reported having pulmonary function testing in the past year. While 83% of physicians reported prescribing peak flow meter monitoring, only 62% of patients had ever heard of a peak flow meter (Rickard & Stempel, 1999). All health care providers caring for asthma patients need to be aware of the national guidelines and use them (Expert Panel Report II, 1997).

Complications

Complications of asthma may include status asthmaticus, respiratory failure, pneumonia, and atelectasis. Airway obstruction, particularly during acute asthmatic episodes, often results in hypoxemia, requiring the administration of oxygen and the monitoring of pulse oximetry and arterial blood gases. Fluids are administered because people with asthma are frequently dehydrated from diaphoresis and insensible fluid loss with hyperventilation.

Medical Management

Immediate intervention is necessary because the continuing and progressive dyspnea leads to increased anxiety, aggravating the situation.

PHARMACOLOGIC THERAPY

Two general classes of asthma medications are long-acting medications to achieve and maintain control of persistent asthma and quick-relief medications for immediate treatment of asthma symptoms and exacerbations (Table 24-4). Because the underlying pathology of asthma is inflammation, control of persistent asthma is accomplished primarily with regular use of anti-inflammatory medications. These medications have systemic side effects when used long term. The route of choice for administration of these medications is the MDI because it allows for topical administration. Critical to the success of inhaled therapy is the proper use of the MDI (see Chart 24-4). If the patient has difficulty with this procedure, the use of a spacer device is indicated. Table 24-3 presents a stepwise approach for managing asthma (Expert Panel Report II, 1997). Information on use of the MDI and spacer device is given in the previous section on COPD.

Long-Acting Control Medications. Corticosteroids are the most potent and effective anti-inflammatory medications currently available. They are broadly effective in alleviating symptoms, improving airway function, and decreasing peak flow variability. Initially, the inhaled form is used. A spacer should be used with inhaled corticosteroids and the patient should rinse the mouth after administration to prevent thrush, a common complication of inhaled corticosteroid use. A systemic preparation may be used to gain rapid control of the disease; to manage severe, persistent asthma; to treat moderate to severe exacerbations; to accelerate recovery; and to prevent recurrence (Dhand, 2000).

Cromolyn sodium (Intal) and nedocromil (Tilade) are mild to moderate anti-inflammatory agents that are used more commonly in children. They also are effective on a prophylactic basis to prevent exercise-induced asthma or in unavoidable exposure to known triggers. These medications are contraindicated in acute asthma exacerbations.

Long-acting beta$_2$-adrenergic agonists are used with anti-inflammatory medications to control asthma symptoms, particularly those that occur during the night. These agents are also effective for preventing exercise-induced asthma. Long-acting beta$_2$-adrenergic agonists are not indicated for immediate relief of symptoms.

(text continues on page 596)

Table 24-3 • Stepwise Approach for Managing Asthma in Adults and Children Over 5 Years Old

Goals of Asthma Treatment
- Prevent chronic and troublesome symptoms (eg, coughing or breathlessness in the night, in the early morning, or after exertion)
- Maintain near-normal pulmonary function
- Maintain normal activity levels (including exercise and other physical activity)

- Prevent recurrent exacerbations of asthma and minimize the need for emergency department visits or hospitalizations
- Provide optimal pharmacotherapy with minimal or no adverse effects
- Meet patients' and families' expectation of and satisfaction with asthma care

	SYMPTOMS**	NIGHTTIME SYMPTOMS	LUNG FUNCTION	LONG-TERM CONTROL	QUICK RELIEF	EDUCATION
STEP 4 Severe Persistent*	• Continual symptoms • Limited physical activity • Frequent exacerbations	Frequent	• FEV_1 or PEF ≤60% predicted • PEF variability >30%	Daily medications: • Anti-inflammatory: inhaled corticosteroid (high dose) AND • Long-acting bronchodilator: either long-acting inhaled $beta_2$-agonist, sustained-release theophylline, or long-acting $beta_2$-agonist tablets AND • Corticosteroid tablets or syrup long term (2 mg/kg/day, generally do not exceed 60 mg per day).	• Short-acting bronchodilator: inhaled $beta_2$-agonists as needed for symptoms. • Intensity of treatment will depend on severity of exacerbation. • Use of short-acting inhaled $beta_2$-agonists on a daily basis, or increasing use, indicates the need for additional long-term control therapy.	Steps 2 and 3 actions plus: • Refer to individual education/counselling
STEP 3 Moderate Persistent	• Daily symptoms • Daily use of inhaled short-acting $beta_2$-agonist • Exacerbations affect activity • Exacerbations ≥2 times a week; may last days	>1 time a week	• FEV_1 or PEF 60% to 80% predicted • PEF variability >30%	Daily medication: • Either – Anti-inflammatory: inhaled corticosteroid (medium dose) OR – Inhaled corticosteroid (low–medium dose) and add a long-acting bronchodilator, especially for nighttime symptoms; either long-acting inhaled $beta_2$-agonist, sustained-release theophylline, or long-acting $beta_2$-agonist tablets. • If needed – Anti-inflammatory: inhaled corticosteroids (medium–high dose) AND – Long-acting bronchodilator, especially for nighttime symptoms; either long-acting inhaled $beta_2$-agonist, sustained-release theophylline, or long-acting $beta_2$-agonist tablets.	• Short-acting bronchodilator: inhaled $beta_2$-agonists as needed for symptoms. • Intensity of treatment will depend on severity of exacerbation. • Use of short-acting inhaled $beta_2$-agonists on a daily basis, or increasing use, indicates the need for additional long-term control therapy.	Step 1 actions plus: • Teach self-monitoring • Refer to group education if available • Review and update self-management plan
STEP 2 Mild Persistent	• Symptoms >2 times a week but <1 time a day • Exacerbations may affect activity	>2 times a month	• FEV_1 or PEF ≥80% predicted • PEF variability 20%–30%	Daily medication: • Anti-inflammatory: either inhaled corticosteroid (low doses) or cromolyn or nedocromil (children usually begin with a trial of cromolyn or nedocromil).	• Short-acting bronchodilator: inhaled $beta_2$-agonists as needed for symptoms. • Intensity of treatment will depend on severity of exacerbation.	Step 1 actions plus: • Teach self-monitoring • Refer to group education if available

Table 24-3 • Stepwise Approach for Managing Asthma in Adults and Children Over 5 Years Old (Continued)

	SYMPTOMS**	NIGHTTIME SYMPTOMS	LUNG FUNCTION	LONG-TERM CONTROL	QUICK RELIEF	EDUCATION
				• Sustained-release theophylline to serum concentration of 5–15 μg/mL is an alternative. Zafirlukast or zileuton may also be considered for patients ≥12 years of age, although their position in therapy is not fully established.	• Use of short-acting inhaled beta₂-agonists on a daily basis, or increasing use, indicates the need for additional long-term-control therapy.	• Review and update self-management plan
STEP 1 Mild Intermittent	• Symptoms ≤2 times a week • Asymptomatic and normal PEF between exacerbations • Exacerbations brief (from a few hours to a few days); intensity may vary	≤2 times a month	• FEV₁ or PEF ≥80% predicted • PEF variability <20%	• No daily medication needed.	• Short-acting bronchodilator: inhaled beta₂-agonists as needed for symptoms. • Intensity of treatment will depend on severity of exacerbation. • Use of short-acting inhaled beta₂-agonists more than 2 times a week may indicate the need to initiate long-term control therapy.	• Teach basic facts about asthma • Teach inhaler/spacer/holding chamber technique • Discuss roles of medications • Develop self-management plan • Develop action plan for when and how to take rescue actions • Discuss appropriate environmental control measures to avoid exposure to known allergens and irritants

↓*Step Down*
Review treatment every 1 to 6 months; a gradual stepwise reduction in treatment may be possible.

Notes:
• The stepwise approach presents general guidelines to assist clinical decision making; it is not intended to be a specific prescription. Asthma is highly variable; clinicians should tailor specific medication plans to the needs and circumstances of individual patients.
• Gain control as quickly as possible; then decrease treatment to the least medication necessary to maintain control. Gaining control may be accomplished either by starting treatment at the step most appropriate to the initial severity of the condition or by starting at a higher level of therapy (eg, a course of systemic corticosteroids or higher dose of inhaled corticosteroids).

↑ *Step Up*
If control is not maintained, consider step up. First, review patient medication technique, adherence, and environmental control (avoidance of allergens or other factors that contribute to asthma severity).
• A rescue course of systemic corticosteroid may be needed at any time and at any step.
• Some patients with intermittent asthma experience severe and life-threatening exacerbations separated by long periods of normal lung function and no symptoms. This may be especially common with exacerbations provoked by respiratory infections. A short course of systemic corticosteroids is recommended.
• At each step, patients should control their environment to avoid or control factors that make their asthma worse (eg, allergens, irritants); this requires specific diagnosis and education.

PEF, peak expiratory flow
*The presence of one of the features of severity is sufficient to place a patient in that category. An individual should be assigned to the most severe grade in which any feature occurs. The characteristics noted in this table are general and may overlap because asthma is highly variable. Furthermore, an individual's classification may change over time.
**Patients at any level of severity can have mild, moderate, or severe exacerbations. Some patients with intermittent asthma experience severe and life-threatening exacerbations separated by long periods of normal lung function and no symptoms.
Highlights of the Expert Panel Report 2. (1997). *Guidelines for the diagnosis and management of asthma.* National Institutes of Health, National Heart, Lung and Blood Institute, NIH Publication No 97-4051A, p. 29.

Table 24-4 • Classifications of Medications Used in Asthma

MEDICATION CLASS	DRUG (BRAND NAME)
Long-Acting Control Medications	
Corticosteroids	beclomethasone (Beclovent, Vanceril), budesonide (Pulmicort), flunisolide (AeroBid), fluticasone propionate (Flovent), triamcinolone acetonide (Azmacort), prednisone
Mast cell stabilizers	cromolyn sodium (Intal), nedocromil sodium (Tilade)
Long-acting beta$_2$-adrenergic agents	salmeterol (Serevent), albuterol (sustained release) (Volmax ER), formoterol fumarate (Foradil)
Xanthine derivatives	aminophylline, theophylline (Slo-bid, Theo-24, Theo-Dur)
Leukotriene modifiers (inhibitors)	zafirlukast (Accolate), zileuton (Zyflo), montelukast (Singulair)
Combination products	albuterol sulfate + ipratropium bromide (Combivent); fluticasone propionate + salmeterol inhalation powder (Advair Diskus)
Quick-Relief Medications	
Short-acting beta$_2$-adrenergic agents	Albuterol (Proventil), levalbuterol (Xopenex), pirbuterol (Maxair), bitolterol (Tornalate)
Anticholinergics	ipratropium bromide (Atrovent)

Expert Panel Report II. (1997). *Guidelines for the diagnosis and management of asthma.* National Asthma Education and Prevention Program, National Institutes of Health.

Methylxanthines (theophylline [Slo-bid, Theo-24, Theo-Dur]) are mild to moderate bronchodilators usually used in addition to inhaled corticosteroids, mainly for relief of nighttime asthma symptoms. There is some evidence that theophylline may have a mild anti-inflammatory effect (NHLBI, 1998).

Leukotriene modifiers (inhibitors) or antileukotrienes are a new class of medications. Leukotrienes are potent bronchoconstrictors that also dilate blood vessels and alter permeability. Leukotriene inhibitors act by either interfering with leukotriene synthesis or blocking the receptors where leukotrienes exert their action (Boushey, Fick, Lazarus & Martin, 2000). At this time, they may provide an alternative to inhaled corticosteroids for mild persistent asthma or may be added to a regimen of inhaled corticosteroids in more severe asthma to attain further control.

In addition, combination products are also available (eg, albuterol/ipratropium [Combivent]) and offer ease of use for the patient.

Quick-Relief Medications. Short-acting beta-adrenergic agonists are the medications of choice for relieving acute symptoms and preventing exercise-induced asthma. They have a rapid onset of action. Anticholinergics (eg, ipratropium bromide [Atrovent]) may bring added benefit in severe exacerbations, but they are used more frequently in COPD patients.

MANAGEMENT OF ASTHMA EXACERBATION

Asthma exacerbations are best managed by early treatment and education of the patient (Canadian Thoracic Society, 1999). Quick-acting beta-adrenergic medications are first used for prompt

relief of airflow obstruction. Systemic corticosteroids may be necessary to decrease airway inflammation in patients who fail to respond to inhaled beta-adrenergic medications. In some patients, oxygen supplementation may be required to relieve hypoxemia associated with a moderate to severe exacerbation (Canadian Thoracic Society, 1999). Also, response to treatment may be monitored by serial measurements of lung function.

A written action plan is the most useful tool for the patient (Fig. 24-7). This helps to guide the patient in self-management strategies regarding an exacerbation and also provides instructions regarding recognition of early warning signs of worsening asthma. Patient self-management and early recognition of problems lead to more efficient communication with health care providers regarding an asthma exacerbation (Canadian Thoracic Society, 1999; Expert Panel Report II, 1997).

PEAK FLOW MONITORING

Peak flow meters measure the highest airflow during a forced expiration (Fig. 24-8). Daily peak flow monitoring is recommended for all patients with moderate or severe asthma because it helps measure asthma severity and, when added to symptom monitoring, indicates the current degree of asthma control. The patient is instructed in the proper technique, particularly to give maximal effort. The "personal best" is determined after monitoring peak flows for 2 or 3 weeks after receiving optimal asthma therapy. The green (80% to 100% of personal best), yellow (60% to 80%), and red (less than 60%) zones are determined, and specific actions are delineated for each zone, enabling the patient to monitor and manipulate his or her own therapy after careful instruction (Expert Panel Report II, 1997). This reinforces compliance, independence, and self-efficacy (Reinke, 2000).

Nursing Management

The immediate nursing care of the patient with asthma depends on the severity of the symptoms. The patient may be treated successfully as an outpatient if asthma symptoms are relatively mild, or he or she may require hospitalization and intensive care for acute and severe asthma.

The patient and family are often frightened and anxious because of the patient's dyspnea. Thus, an important aspect of care is a calm approach. The nurse assesses the patient's respiratory status by monitoring the severity of symptoms, breath sounds, peak flow, pulse oximetry, and vital signs. The nurse obtains a history of allergic reactions to medications before administering medications and identifies the patient's current use of medications. The nurse administers medications as prescribed and monitors the patient's responses to those medications. Fluids may be administered if the patient is dehydrated, and antibiotic agents may be prescribed if the patient has an underlying respiratory infection. If the patient requires intubation because of acute respiratory failure, the nurse assists with the intubation procedure, continues close monitoring of the patient, and keeps the patient and family informed about procedures.

PROMOTING HOME AND COMMUNITY-BASED CARE

Teaching Patients Self-Care. A major challenge is to implement basic asthma management principles at the community level (Reinke, 2000). Key issues include education of health care providers, establishment of programs for asthma education (for patients and providers), use of outpatient follow-up care for patients, and a focus on chronic management versus acute episodic care. The nurse is pivotal to achieving all of these objectives.

ASTHMA ACTION PLAN FOR_____

Doctor's Name_____ Date_____

Doctor's Phone Number_____ Hospital/Emergency Room Phone Number_____

Take These Long-Term-Control Medicines Each Day (include an anti-inflammatory)

Medicine	How much to take	When to take it

GREEN ZONE: Doing Well
- No cough, wheeze, chest tightness, or shortness of breath during the day or night
- Can do usual activities

And, if a peak flow meter is used,
Peak flow: more than_____
(80% or more of my best peak flow)

My best peak flow is:_____

Before exercise ☐ ☐ 2 or ☐ 4 puffs 5 to 60 minutes before exercise

---

YELLOW ZONE: Asthma Is Getting Worse

FIRST → Add: Quick-Relief Medicine – and keep taking your GREEN ZONE medicine

- Cough, wheeze, chest tightness, or shortness of breath, or
- Waking at night due to asthma, or
- Can do some, but not all, usual activities

-Or-

Peak flow: _____ to _____
(50% - 80% of my best peak flow)

_____
(short-acting beta$_2$-agonist)

☐ 2 or ☐ 4 puffs, every 20 minutes for up to 1 hour
☐ Nebulizer, once

SECOND → If your symptoms (and peak flow, if used) return to GREEN ZONE after 1 hour of above treatment:
☐ Take the quick-relief medicine every 4 hours for 1 to 2 days.
☐ Double the dose of your inhaled steroid for _____ (7-10) days.

-Or-

If your symptoms (and peak flow, if used) do not return to GREEN ZONE after 1 hour of above treatment:

☐ Take: _____
(short-acting beta$_2$-agonist)
☐ 2 or ☐ 4 puffs or ☐ Nebulizer

☐ Add: _____ _____ mg. per day For _____ (3-10) days
(oral steroid)

☐ Call the doctor ☐ before/ ☐ within _____ hours after taking the oral steroid.

RED ZONE: Medical Alert!

Take this medicine:
- Very short of breath, or
- Quick-relief medicines have not helped, or
- Cannot do usual activities, or
- Symptoms are same or get worse after 24 hours in Yellow Zone

-Or-

Peak flow: less than_____
(50% of my best peak flow)

☐ _____
(short-acting beta$_2$-agonist)
☐ 4 or ☐ 6 puffs or ☐ Nebulizer

☐ _____ _____ mg.
(oral steroid)

Then call your doctor NOW. Go to the hospital or call for an ambulance if:
- You are still in the red zone after 15 minutes AND
- You have not reached your doctor.

DANGER SIGNS
- Trouble walking and talking due to shortness of breath
- Lips or fingernails are blue

→ ■ Take ☐ 4 or ☐ 6 puffs of your quick-relief medicine AND
■ Go to the hospital or call for an ambulance (_____) NOW!

FIGURE 24-7 Asthma action plan. From *Facts about controlling asthma,* National Asthma Education and Prevention Program, National Heart, Lung, and Blood Institute. NIH Publication No. 97-2339.

597

FIGURE 24-8 Peak flow meters measure the highest volume of air flow during a forced expiration (*left*). Volume is measured in colour-coded zones (*right*): the green zone signifies 80% to 100% of personal best; yellow, 60% to 80%; and red, less than 60%. If peak flow falls below the red zone, the patient should take the appropriate actions prescribed by his or her health care provider.

Patient teaching is a critical component of care for the patient with asthma (Plaut, 2001). Multiple inhalers, different types of inhalers, antiallergy therapy, antireflux medications, and avoidance measures are all integral for long-term control. This complex therapy requires a patient–provider partnership to determine the desired outcomes and to formulate a plan to achieve those outcomes. The patient then carries out daily therapy as part of self-care management, with input and guidance by the health care provider. Before a partnership can be established, the patient needs to understand the following:

- The nature of asthma as a chronic inflammatory disease
- The definition of inflammation and bronchoconstriction
- The purpose and action of each medication
- Triggers to avoid, and how to do so
- Proper inhalation technique
- How to perform peak flow monitoring (Chart 24-5)
- How to implement an action plan
- When to seek assistance, and how to do so

An assortment of excellent educational materials is available from the Expert Panel Report II (1997) and the National Heart,

Chart 24-5
Home Care Checklist • Use of Peak Flow Meter

At the completion of the home care instruction, the patient or caregiver will be able to:

	Patient	Caregiver
• Describe the rationale for using a peak flow meter in asthma management.	✓	✓
• Explain how peak flow monitoring is used along with symptoms to determine severity of asthma.	✓	✓
• Demonstrate steps for using the peak flow meter correctly:		
• Move the indicator to the bottom of the numbered scale.	✓	
• Stand up.	✓	
• Take a deep breath and fill the lungs completely.	✓	
• Place mouthpiece in mouth and close lips around mouthpiece (do not put tongue inside opening).	✓	
• Blow out hard and fast with a single blow.	✓	
• Record the number achieved on the indicator.	✓	
• Repeat steps 1–5 two more times and write the highest number in the asthma diary.	✓	
• Explain how to determine the "personal best" peak flow reading.	✓	✓
• Describe the significance of the colour zones for peak flow monitoring.	✓	✓
• Demonstrate how to clean the peak flow meter.	✓	✓
• Discuss how and when to contact the health care provider about changes or decreases in peak flow values.	✓	✓

Lung and Blood Institute. The nurse should obtain current educational materials for the patient based on the patient's diagnosis, causative factors, educational level, and cultural factors.

Continuing Care. The nurse who has contact with the patient in the hospital, clinic, school, or office uses the opportunity to assess the patient's respiratory status and ability to manage self-care to prevent serious exacerbations. The nurse emphasizes adherence to the prescribed therapy, preventive measures, and the need to keep follow-up appointments with the primary health care provider. A home visit to assess the home environment for allergens may be indicated for the patient with recurrent exacerbations. The nurse refers the patient to community support groups. In addition, the nurse reminds the patient and family about the importance of health promotion strategies and recommended health screening.

STATUS ASTHMATICUS

Status asthmaticus is severe and persistent asthma that does not respond to conventional therapy. The attacks can last longer than 24 hours. Infection, anxiety, nebulizer abuse, dehydration, increased adrenergic blockage, and nonspecific irritants may contribute to these episodes. An acute episode may be precipitated by hypersensitivity to aspirin.

Pathophysiology

The basic characteristics of asthma (constriction of the bronchiolar smooth muscle, swelling of the bronchial mucosa, and thickened secretions) decrease the diameter of the bronchi and are apparent in status asthmaticus. A ventilation–perfusion abnormality results in hypoxemia and respiratory alkalosis initially, followed by respiratory acidosis. There is a reduced PaO_2 and an initial respiratory alkalosis, with a decreased $PaCO_2$ and an increased pH. As status asthmaticus worsens, the $PaCO_2$ increases and the pH falls, reflecting respiratory acidosis.

Clinical Manifestations

The clinical manifestations are the same as those seen in severe asthma: laboured breathing, prolonged exhalation, engorged neck veins, and wheezing. However, the extent of wheezing does not indicate the severity of the attack. As the obstruction worsens, the wheezing may disappear, and this is frequently a sign of impending respiratory failure.

Assessment and Diagnostic Findings

Pulmonary function studies are the most accurate means of assessing acute airway obstruction. Arterial blood gas measurements are obtained if the patient cannot perform pulmonary function manoeuvres because of severe obstruction or fatigue, or if the patient does not respond to treatment. Respiratory alkalosis (low $PaCO_2$) is the most common finding in patients with asthma. A rising $PaCO_2$ (to normal levels or levels indicating respiratory acidosis) frequently is a danger sign of impending respiratory failure.

Medical Management

In the emergency setting, the patient is treated initially with a short-acting beta-adrenergic agonist and corticosteroids. The patient usually requires supplemental oxygen and intravenous fluids for hydration. Oxygen therapy is initiated to treat dyspnea, central cyanosis, and hypoxemia. Humidified oxygen by either Venturi mask or nasal catheter is administered. The flow is based on pulse oximetry or arterial blood gas values. The PaO_2 is maintained at 65 to 85 mm Hg. Sedative medications are contraindicated. If there is no response to repeated treatments, hospitalization is required. Other criteria indicating the need for hospitalization include poor pulmonary function test results and deteriorating blood gas levels (respiratory acidosis), which may indicate that the patient is tiring and will require mechanical ventilation. Although most patients do not need mechanical ventilation, it is used for patients in respiratory failure, for those who tire and are too fatigued by the attempt to breathe, or for those whose conditions do not respond to initial treatment.

Death from asthma is associated with several risk factors, including the following:

- Past history of sudden and severe exacerbations
- Prior endotracheal intubation for asthma
- Prior admission to the intensive care unit for an asthma exacerbation
- Two or more hospitalizations for asthma within the past year
- Three or more emergency care visits for asthma in the past year
- Excessive use of short-acting beta-adrenergic inhalers (more than two canisters per month)
- Recent withdrawal from systemic corticosteroids
- Comorbidity of cardiovascular disease or COPD
- Psychiatric disease
- Low socioeconomic status
- Urban residence (Expert Panel Report II, 1997)

Nursing Management

The nurse constantly monitors the patient for the first 12 to 24 hours, or until status asthmaticus is under control. The nurse also assesses the patient's skin turgor to identify signs of dehydration. Fluid intake is essential to combat dehydration, to loosen secretions, and to facilitate expectoration. The nurse administers intravenous fluids as prescribed, up to 3 to 4 L/day, unless contraindicated. The patient's energy needs to be conserved, and the room should be quiet and free of respiratory irritants, including flowers, tobacco smoke, perfumes, or odours of cleaning agents. A nonallergenic pillow should be used.

Cystic Fibrosis

Cystic fibrosis (CF) is the most common fatal autosomal recessive disease among the Caucasian population. An individual must inherit a defective copy of the CF gene (one from each parent) to have CF. About 1 in every 25 Canadians carries a defective version of the gene responsible for CF (Canadian Cystic Fibrosis Foundation, 2002). In Canada, it is estimated that 1 in every 2,500 children has cystic fibrosis. There are about 3,400 children, adolescents, and adults attending specialized CF clinics throughout Canada. Although CF was once considered a fatal childhood disease, in 2002, over 47% of Canadian CF patients were 18 years of age or older (Canadian Cystic Fibrosis Foundation, 2002, www.cysticfibrosis.ca). Cystic fibrosis is usually diagnosed in infancy or early childhood, but patients may be diagnosed later in life. For individuals diagnosed later in life, respiratory symptoms are frequently the major manifestation of the disease.

Pathophysiology

This disease is caused by mutations in the CF transmembrane conductance regulator protein, which is a chloride channel found in all exocrine tissues (Katkin, 2002). Chloride transport problems lead to thick, viscous secretions in the lungs, pancreas, liver, intestine, and reproductive tract as well as increased salt content in sweat gland secretions. In 1989, major breakthroughs were made in this disease with the identification of the CF gene. The ability to detect the common mutations of this gene allows for routine screening for this disease as well as the detection of carriers. Genetic counselling is an important part of health care for couples at risk.

Airflow obstruction is a key feature in the presentation of CF. This obstruction is due to bronchial plugging by purulent secretions, bronchial wall thickening due to inflammation, and, over time, airway destruction (Katkin, 2002). These chronic retained secretions in the airways set up an excellent reservoir for continued bronchial infections.

Clinical Manifestations

The pulmonary manifestations of this disease include a productive cough, wheezing, hyperinflation of the lung fields on chest x-ray, and pulmonary function test results consistent with obstructive airways disease (Katkin, 2002). Colonization of the airways with pathogenic bacteria usually occurs early in life. *Staphylococcus aureus* and *Haemophilus influenzae* are common organisms during early childhood. As the disease progresses, *Pseudomonas aeruginosa* is ultimately isolated from the sputum of most patients. Upper respiratory manifestations of the disease include sinusitis and nasal polyps.

Nonpulmonary clinical manifestations include gastrointestinal problems (eg, pancreatic insufficiency, recurrent abdominal pain, biliary cirrhosis, vitamin deficiencies, recurrent pancreatitis, weight loss), genitourinary problems (male and female infertility), and clubbing of the extremities. (See Chap. 40 for a discussion of pancreatitis.)

Assessment and Diagnostic Findings

Most of the time, the diagnosis of CF is made based on an elevated result of a sweat chloride concentration test, along with clinical signs and symptoms consistent with the disease. Repeated sweat chloride values of greater than 60 mmol/L distinguish most individuals with CF from those with other obstructive diseases. A molecular diagnosis may also be used in evaluating common genetic mutations of the CF gene.

Medical Management

Pulmonary problems remain the leading cause of morbidity and mortality in CF. Because chronic bacterial infection of the airways occurs in individuals with CF, control of infections is key in the treatment. Antibiotic medications are routinely prescribed for acute pulmonary exacerbations of the disease. Depending upon the severity of the exacerbation, aerosolized, oral, or intravenous antibiotic therapy may be used. Antibiotic agents are selected based upon the results of a sputum culture and sensitivity. Patients with CF have problems with bacteria that are resistant to multiple drugs and require multiple courses of antibiotic agents over long periods of time.

Bronchodilators are frequently administered to decrease airway obstruction. Differing pulmonary techniques are used to enhance secretion clearance. Examples include manual postural drainage and chest physical therapy, high-frequency chest wall oscillation, and other devices that assist in airway clearance (PEP masks [masks that generate positive expiratory pressure], "flutter devices" [devices that provide an oscillatory expiratory pressure pattern with positive expiratory pressure and assist with expectoration of secretions]).

Inhaled mucolytic agents such as dornase alfa (Pulmozyme) or N-acetylcysteine (Mucomyst) may also be used. These agents help to decrease the viscosity of the sputum and promote expectoration of secretions.

To decrease the inflammation and ongoing destruction of the airways, anti-inflammatory agents may also be used. These may include inhaled corticosteroids or systemic therapy. Other anti-inflammatory medications have also been studied in CF. Ibuprofen was studied in children with CF and some benefit was demonstrated, but there is little information on its use in young or older adults with CF (Katkin, 2002).

Supplemental oxygen is used to treat the progressive hypoxemia that occurs with CF. It helps to correct the hypoxemia and may minimize the complications seen with chronic hypoxemia (pulmonary hypertension).

Lung transplantation is an option for a small, select population of CF patients. A double lung transplant technique is used due to the chronically infected state of the lungs seen in end-stage CF. Because there is a long waiting list for lung transplant recipients, many patients die while awaiting a transplant.

Gene therapy is a promising approach to management, with many clinical trials underway. It is hoped that various methods of administering gene therapy will carry healthy genes to the damaged cells and correct defective CF cells. Efforts are underway to develop innovative methods of delivering therapy to the CF cells of the airways.

Nursing Management

Nursing care of the adult with CF includes assisting the patient to manage pulmonary symptoms and to prevent complications of CF. Specific nursing measures include strategies that promote removal of pulmonary secretions; chest physiotherapy, including postural drainage, chest percussion, and vibration, and breathing exercises are implemented and are taught to the patient and to the family when the patient is very young. The patient is reminded of the need to reduce risk factors associated with respiratory infections (eg, exposure to crowds and to persons with known infections). The patient is taught the early signs and symptoms of respiratory infection and disease progression that indicate the need to notify the primary health care provider.

The nurse emphasizes the importance of an adequate fluid and dietary intake to promote removal of secretions and to ensure an adequate nutritional status. Because CF is a life-long disorder, patients often have learned to modify their daily activities to accommodate their symptoms and treatment modalities. As the disease progresses, however, assessment of the home environment may be warranted to identify modifications required to address changes in the patient's needs, increasing dyspnea and fatigue, and nonpulmonary symptoms.

Although gene therapy and double lung transplantation are promising therapies for CF, they are limited in availability and largely experimental. As a result, the life expectancy of adults with CF is shortened. Therefore, end-of-life issues and concerns need to be addressed in patients when warranted. For the patient whose disease is progressing and who is developing increasing hypoxemia, preferences for end-of-life care should be discussed, documented, and honoured (see Chap. 17). Patients and family members need support as they face a shortened life span and an uncertain future.

Critical Thinking Exercises

1. A 75-year-old woman with end-stage COPD was recently admitted to your unit from the emergency room. She cannot lie flat in bed, she is extremely short of breath, and she has decreased breath sounds throughout the chest and crackles in the posterior basilar areas. What is the pathophysiology associated with these findings? What medical and nursing interventions might be used to decrease or alleviate these signs/symptoms?

2. Your patient at an outpatient asthma clinic is a 35-year-old inner-city Mexican-American mother with asthma. Use of an MDI on a regular daily schedule has been repeatedly prescribed for her, but she reports that she does not use the MDI except as needed when extremely short of breath. Describe teaching techniques you might use to assess the patient's knowledge of the medication and provide education about the action of the MDI, frequency of use, and correct administration of the medication. What methods would you use to monitor use of the MDI and reinforce education?

3. As a nurse in your hospital's community outreach clinic, you are responsible for providing group education and counselling to patients with asthma. What areas would you address regarding triggers for asthma? How might you have patients assess their home environments?

4. Your 64-year-old patient has a history of bronchiectasis and heart failure following two myocardial infarctions. To promote removal of pulmonary secretions, his physician has prescribed chest physiotherapy and postural drainage. The patient reports that he is able to breathe easily only in a sitting position. Describe how you would modify chest physiotherapy and postural drainage given his statement that he cannot breathe in a supine or prone position.

5. Your 22-year-old patient is a college student with a history of cystic fibrosis; he has been admitted to your unit for intravenous antibiotic therapy. Describe what pulmonary rehabilitation techniques would be appropriate for his disease process, which are age-specific and consistent with his activity level.

REFERENCES AND SELECTED READINGS

Books

American Association of Cardiovascular & Pulmonary Rehabilitation. (1998). *Guidelines for pulmonary rehabilitation programs* (2nd ed.). Champaign, IL: Human Kinetics.

Cystic Fibrosis Foundation (2002). What is CF? http://www.cff.org (accessed June 13, 2002).

Cherniack, N. S., Homma, I., & Altose, M. (Eds.). (1999). *Rehabilitation of the patient with respiratory disease.* New York: McGraw-Hill.

Expert Panel Report II. (1997). *Guidelines for the diagnosis and management of asthma.* National Asthma Education and Prevention Program, National Institutes of Health.

FitzGerald, J. M. (2001). *Evidence-based asthma management.* Hamilton, Ontario: B. C. Decker.

George, R. B., San Pedro, G. S., & Stoller, J. K. (2000). Chronic obstructive pulmonary disease, bronchiectasis, and cystic fibrosis. In R. B. George, R. W. Light, M. A. Matthay & R. A. Matthay (Eds.), *Chest medicine: Essentials of pulmonary and critical care medicine* (4th ed.). Philadelphia: Lippincott Williams & Wilkins.

Hall, J. B. (2000). *Acute asthma: Assessment and management.* New York: McGraw-Hill, Health Professions Division.

Health Canada. (2001). *Respiratory disease in Canada.* Ottawa: Author. Available at: http://www.hc-sc.gc.ca/pphb-dgspsp.

Katkin, J. P. (2002). *Clinical manifestations and diagnosis of cystic fibrosis.* UpToDate, Vol. 10(1), Wellesley, MA.

Kavuru, M. S., & Wiedemann, H. P. (2000). Asthma. In R. B. George, R. W. Light, M. A. Matthay & R. A. Matthay (Eds.), *Chest medicine: Essentials of pulmonary and critical care medicine* (4th ed., pp. 133–173). Philadelphia: Lippincott Williams & Wilkins.

Lieberman, P., & Anderson, J. A. (Eds.). (2000). *Allergic diseases: Diagnosis and treatment.* Totowa, NJ: Humana.

National Center for Health Statistics. (2000). *US mortality public use data tape 1998.* Centers for Disease Control and Prevention, Hyattsville, MD.

National Center for Health Statistics. (2001). *New asthma estimates: Tracking prevalence, health care, and mortality.* Fact sheet released Oct. 5, 2001, Hyattsville, MD.

National Heart, Lung and Blood Institute (1998). *Morbidity and mortality: 1998 chart book on cardiovascular, lung and blood diseases.*

National Heart, Lung and Blood Institute (2000). *Morbidity and mortality: 2000 chart book on cardiovascular, lung and blood diseases.*

National Institutes of Health. (2001) *Global initiative for chronic obstructive lung disease: Global strategy for the diagnosis, management, and prevention of chronic obstructive pulmonary disease.* U.S. Department of Health and Human Services, NIH Publication Number 2701B.

O'Byrne, P. M. (2001). *Manual of asthma management* (2d ed.). London: W. B. Saunders.

Journals

Asterisks indicate nursing research articles.

General

ACCP/AACVPR Pulmonary Rehabilitation Guidelines Panel. (1997). Pulmonary rehabilitation: Joint ACCP/AACVPR evidence-based guidelines. *Chest, 112*(5), 1363–1396.

Adatsi, G. (1999). Health going up in smoke: How can you prevent it? *American Journal of Nursing, 99*(3), 63–69.

American Thoracic Society. (1999). Statement on pulmonary rehabilitation. *American Journal of Respiratory and Critical Care Medicine, 159*(5), 1666–1682.

Lacasse, Y., Guyatt, G., & Goldstein, R. (1997). The components of a respiratory rehabilitation program: A systematic overview. *Chest, 111*(4), 1977–2088.

*McEntee, D. J., & Badenhop, D. T. (2000). Quality of life comparisons: Gender and population differences in cardiopulmonary rehabilitation. *Heart Lung, 29*(5), 340–347.

Rochester, C. L. (2000). Which pulmonary rehabilitation program is best for your patient? *Journal of Respiratory Diseases, 21*(9), 539–546.

Asthma

Boushey, H. A., Fick, R. B., Lazarus, S., & Martin, A. (2000). *Anti-IgE: A unique approach to asthma management.* Gardiner-Caldwell SynerMed, Califon, NJ, 2–24.

Busse, W. W., & Lemanske, R. F. Jr. (2001). Advances in immunology: Asthma. *New England Journal of Medicine, 344*(5), 350–362.

Caprioti, T. (1999). Leukotriene antagonists offer a new mechanism for asthma control. *MedSurg Nursing, 8*(5), 318–322.

Centers for Disease Control and Prevention. (1998). Forecasted state-specific estimates of self-reported asthma prevalence: United States, 1998. *MMWR Morbidity and Mortality Weekly Report, 47*(47), 1022–1025.

Centers for Disease Control and Prevention. (1999). Asthma Prevention Program of the National Center for Environmental Health, At-A-Glance, 1999, 1–6.

Dhand, R. (2000). Aerosol therapy in asthma. *Current Opinion in Pulmonary Medicine, 6*(1), 59–70.

Drazen, J. M., Israel, E., & O'Byrne, P. M. (1999). Treatment of asthma with drugs modifying the leukotriene pathway. *New England Journal of Medicine, 340*(3), 197–206.

Janson, S. (1998). National Asthma Education and Prevention Program, Expert Panel Report II: Overview and application for primary care. *Lippincott's Primary Care Practice, 2*(6), 578–588.

McGann, E. (1999). Medication compliance in adults with asthma. *American Journal of Nursing, 99*(3), 45–46.

National Heart, Lung and Blood Institute. (1998). Asthma diagnosis and management. A continuing education module. http://www.nhlbi.nih.gov.

Naureckas, E. T., & Solway, J. (2001). Mild asthma. *New England Journal of Medicine, 345*(17), 1257–1262.

Owen, C. L. (1999). New directions in asthma management. *American Journal of Nursing, 99*(3), 26–33.

Plaut, T. F. (2001). Lack of knowledge leads to poor asthma care. *Advance for Managers of Respiratory Care, 10*(3), 38, 40–41.

Reinke, L. F. (2000). Asthma education: Creating a partnership. *Heart Lung, 29*(3), 225–236.

Rickard, K. A., & Stempel, D. A. (1999). Asthma survey demonstrates that the goals of the NHLBI have not been accomplished [abstract]. *Journal of Allergy and Clinical Immunology, 103*(1 Pt 2), S171.

*Schott-Baer, D., & Christensen, M. (1999). A pilot program to increase self-care of adult asthma patients. *MedSurg Nursing, 8*(3), 178–183.

Togger, D. A., & Brenner, P. S. (2001). Metered dose inhalers. *American Journal of Nursing, 101*(10), 26–32.

COPD

Barnes, P. J. (2000). Medical progress: Chronic obstructive pulmonary disease. *New England Journal of Medicine, 343*(4), 269–280.

Barnes, P. J., & Stockley, R. A. (2005). COPD: Current therapeutic interventions and future approaches. *European Respiratory Journal, 25*(6), 1084–1106.

*Belza, B., Steele, B. G., Hunziker, J., Lakshminaryan, S., Holt, L., & Buchner, D. M. (2001). Correlates of physical activity in chronic obstructive pulmonary disease. *Nursing Research, 50*(4), 195–202.

Boyle, A. H., & Waters, H. F. (2000). COPD: Focus on prevention. Recommendations of the National Lung Health Education Program. *Heart Lung, 29*(6), 446–449.

Canadian Thoracic Society. (2003). Canadian Thoracic Society recommendations for management of chronic obstructive pulmonary disease-2003. *Canadian Respiratory Journal, 10*(Suppl A), S11A–S65A.

Canadian Thoracic Society and the Canadian Infectious Disease Society. (2003). Canadian guidelines for the management of acute exacerbations of chronic bronchitis. *Canadian Respiratory Journal, 10*(Suppl B), 3B–32B.

Canadian Thoracic Society. (2001). Alpha$_1$-antitirypsin deficiency: A position statement of the Canadian Thoracic Society. *Canadian Respiratory Journal, 8*, 81–88.

Celli, B. R., Snider, G. L, Heffner, J., et al. (1995). ATS standards for the diagnosis and care of patients with chronic obstructive pulmonary disease. *American Journal of Respiratory Critical Care Medicine, 152*(5), S77–S121.

*Cicutto, L., Brooks, D., & Henderson, K. (2004). Self-care issues from the perspective of individuals with chronic obstructive pulmonary disease. *Patient Education, 55*, 168–176.

Fein, A. (1998). Lung volume reduction surgery. *Chest, 113*(4), 277S–282S.

Ferreira, I., Brooks, D., Lacasse, Y., & Goldstein, R. (2001). Nutritional intervention in COPD: A systematic overview. *Chest, 119*(2), 353–363.

Fiel, S. B. (2000). Bronchiectasis: The changing clinical scenario. *Journal of Respiratory Disease, 21*(11), 666–681.

Garvey, C. (1998). COPD and exercise. *Lippincott's Primary Care Practice, 2*(6), 589–598.

*Knebel, A. R., Bentz, E., & Barnes, P. (2000). Dyspnea management in alpha-1 antitrypsin deficiency: Effect of oxygen administration. *Nursing Research, 49*(6), 333–338.

Lacasse, Y., Brooks, D., & Goldstein, R. S. (1998). Trends in the epidemiology of chronic obstructive pulmonary disease in Canada, 1980–1995. *Chest, 116*, 306–313.

Larson, J. L., Covey, M. K., Wirtz, S. E., et al. (1999). Cycle ergometer and inspiratory muscle training in chronic obstructive pulmonary disease. *American Journal of Respiratory and Critical Care Medicine, 160*(2), 500–507.

*Meek, P. M. (2000). Influence of attention and judgment on perception of breathlessness in healthy individuals and patient with chronic obstructive pulmonary disease. *Nursing Research, 49*(1), 11–19.

National Institutes of Health. (2001). *NHLBI-funded emphysema study finds certain patients at high risk for death following lung surgery.* NIH news release, Aug. 14, 2001.

National Institutes of Health. (2001). National emphysema treatment trial (NETT), evaluation of lung volume reduction surgery for emphysema. June 20, 2001. http://www.nhlbi.nih.gov/health/prof/lung/nett/lvrsweb.htm.

National Emphysema Treatment Trial Research Group (2001). Patients at high risk of death after lung-volume-reduction surgery. *New England Journal of Medicine, 345*(18), 1075–1083.

*Nield, M. (2000). Dyspnea self-management in African-Americans with chronic lung disease. *Heart Lung, 29*(1), 50–55.

Pohl, J. M. (2000). Smoking cessation and low-income women: Theory, research, and interventions. *Nurse Practice Forum, 11*(2), 101–108.

Rennard, S. I. (1998). COPD: Overview of definitions, epidemiology, and factors influencing its development. *Chest, 113*(4, Suppl.), 235S–241S.

*Skilbeck, J., Mott, L., Smith, D., Page, H., & Clark, D. (1997). Research and development. Nursing care for people dying from chronic obstructive airway disease. *International Journal of Palliative Nursing, 3*(2), 100–106.

Stoller, J. K. (2002). Acute exacerbations of chronic obstructive pulmonary medicine. *New England Journal of Medicine, 346*(13), 988–994.

*Trudeau, M. E., & Solano-McGuire, S. M. (1999). Evaluating the quality of COPD care. *American Journal of Nursing, 99*(3), 47–50.

Truesdell, S. (2000). Helping patients with COPD manage episodes of acute shortness of breath. *MedSurg Nursing, 9*(4), 178–182.

United States Public Health Service. (2000). Treating tobacco use and dependence. Summary, June 2000. http://www.surgeongeneral.gov/tobacco.smokesum.htm.

*Wu, C-Y., Lee, Y-Y., Baig, K., & Wichaikhum O. (2001). Coping behaviors of individuals with chronic obstructive pulmonary disease. *MedSurg Nursing, 10*(6), 315–320.

RESOURCES AND WEBSITES

Agency for Healthcare Research and Quality, 2101 E. Jefferson St., Suite 501, Rockville, MD 20852; (301) 594-1364; http://www.ahrq.org.

American Academy of Allergy, Asthma, and Immunology, 611 E. Wells St., Milwaukee, WI 53202; (414) 272-6071; http://www.aaaai.org.

American Association of Cardiovascular and Pulmonary Rehabilitation, 7611 Elmwood Ave., Suite 201, Middleton, WI 53562, (608) 831-5122; http://www.aacvpr.org.

American Association for Respiratory Care, 1720 Regal Row, Dallas, TX 75235; (214) 630-3540; http://www.aarc.org.

American Cancer Society, 1599 Clifton Road NE, Atlanta, GA 30329-4251; (800) ACS-2345; http://www.cancer.org.

American College of Chest Physicians, 3300 Dundee Road, Northbrook, IL 60062; (847) 498-1400; http://www.chest.org.

American Lung Association, 1740 Broadway, New York, NY 10019-4374; (212) 315-8700; http://www.lungusa.org.

American Thoracic Society, 1740 Broadway, New York, NY 10019; (212) 315-8700; http://www.thoracic.org.

Canadian COPD Alliance; http://www.lung.ca/cca.

Canadian Cystic Fibrosis Foundation (CCFF), 2221 Yonge Street, Suite 601, Toronto, ON, M4S 2B4; (416) 485-9149; (800) 378-2233; Fax (416) 485-0960; www.cysticfibrosis.ca.

Canadian Lung Association, 3 Raymond Street, Suite 300, Ottawa, ON K1R 1A3; (613) 569-6411; (888) 566-Lung (5864); http://www.lung.ca.

Canadian Network for Asthma Care, 16851 Mount Wolfe Road, Bolton, ON L7E 5R7; (905) 880-1092; www.cnac.net.

Centers for Disease Control and Prevention, 1600 Clifton Road, NE, Atlanta, GA 30333; http://www.cdc.gov.

Cystic Fibrosis Foundation, 6931 Arlington Road, Bethesda, MD 20814; (310) 951-4422 or (800) FIGHT CF; http://www.cff.org.

Global Initiative for Asthma (GINA); www.ginasthma.com.

Global Initiative for Chronic Obstructive Lung Disease; www.godcopd.com.

Health Canada, A.L. 0900C2 Ottawa, ON K1A 0K9; (613) 957-2991; (866) 225-0709; Fax: (613) 941-5366; www.hc-sc.gc.ca.

National Cancer Institute; (800) 4-Cancer or (301) 496-5585; http://www.cancer.gov or http://www.nci.nih.gov.

National Heart, Lung and Blood Institute, National Institutes of Health, 900 Rockville Pike, Bldg. 31, Bethesda, MD 20892; (301) 496-5166; http://www.nhlbi.nih.gov.

Physicians for a Smoke-Free Canada; 1226A Wellington Street, Ottawa, ON K1Y 3A1; 613-233-4878.

Respiratory Nursing Society, 11 Cornell Road, Latham, NY 12110; (518) 782-9400 x286l; e-mail: RNS@NYSNA.ORG.

U.S. Department of Health and Human Services, Department of Health and Human Services, 200 Independence Avenue, S.W., Washington DC 20201; (202) 619-0257; http://www.hhs.gov or http://www.healthfinder.gov.

World Allergy Organization; http://www.worldallergy.org.

Respiratory Care Modalities

Adapted by Carolyn J. M. Ross

LEARNING OBJECTIVES

On completion of this chapter, the learner will be able to:

1. Describe the nursing management for patients receiving oxygen therapy, intermittent positive-pressure breathing, mini-nebulizer therapy, incentive spirometry, chest physiotherapy, and breathing retraining.

2. Describe the patient education and home care considerations for patients receiving oxygen therapy.

3. Describe the nursing care for a patient with an endotracheal tube and for a patient with a tracheostomy.

4. Demonstrate the procedure of tracheal suctioning.

5. Use the nursing process as a framework for care of patients who are mechanically ventilated.

6. Describe the process of weaning the patient from mechanical ventilation.

7. Describe the significance of preoperative nursing assessment and patient teaching for the patient who is to have thoracic surgery.

8. Explain the principles of chest drainage and the nursing responsibilities related to the care of the patient with a chest drainage system.

9. Describe the patient education and home care considerations for patients who have had thoracic surgery.

Numerous treatment modalities are used when caring for patients with various respiratory conditions. The choice of modality is based on the oxygenation disorder and whether there is a problem with gas ventilation, diffusion, or both. Therapies range from simple and noninvasive modalities (oxygen and nebulizer therapy, chest physiotherapy, breathing retraining) to complex and highly invasive treatments (intubation, mechanical ventilation, surgery). Assessment and management of the patient with respiratory disorders are best accomplished when the approach is multidisciplinary and collaborative.

Noninvasive Respiratory Therapies

OXYGEN THERAPY

Oxygen therapy is the administration of oxygen at a concentration greater than that found in the environmental atmosphere. At sea level, the concentration of oxygen in room air is 21%. The goal of oxygen therapy is to provide adequate transport of oxygen in the blood while decreasing the work of breathing and reducing stress on the myocardium.

Oxygen transport to the tissues depends on factors such as cardiac output, arterial oxygen content, concentration of hemoglobin, and metabolic requirements. These factors must be kept in mind when oxygen therapy is considered. (Respiratory physiology and oxygen transport are discussed in Chap. 21.)

Indications

A change in the patient's respiratory rate or pattern may be one of the earliest indicators of the need for oxygen therapy. The change in respiratory rate or pattern may result from hypoxemia or hypoxia. **Hypoxemia** (a decrease in the arterial oxygen tension in the blood) is manifested by changes in mental status (progressing through impaired judgment, agitation, disorientation, confusion, lethargy, and coma), dyspnea, increase in blood pressure, changes in heart rate, dysrhythmias, central cyanosis (late sign), diaphoresis, and cool extremities. Hypoxemia usually leads to **hypoxia**, which is a decrease in oxygen supply to the tissues. Hypoxia, if severe enough, can be life-threatening.

The signs and symptoms signaling the need for oxygen may depend on how suddenly this need develops. With rapidly developing hypoxia, changes occur in the central nervous system because the higher neurologic centres are very sensitive to oxygen deprivation. The clinical picture may resemble that of alcohol intoxication, with the patient exhibiting lack of coordination and impaired judgment. Longstanding hypoxia (as seen in chronic obstructive pulmonary disease [COPD] and chronic heart failure) may produce fatigue, drowsiness, apathy, inattentiveness, and delayed reaction time. The need for oxygen is assessed by arterial blood gas analysis and pulse oximetry as well as by clinical evaluation. For more information about hypoxia, see Chart 25-1.

Cautions in Oxygen Therapy

As with other medications, the nurse administers oxygen with caution and carefully assesses its effects on each patient. Oxygen is a medication and except in emergency situations is administered only when prescribed by a physician.

In general, patients with respiratory conditions are given oxygen therapy only to raise the arterial oxygen pressure (PaO$_2$) back to the patient's normal baseline, which may vary from 60 to 95 mm Hg. In terms of the oxyhemoglobin dissociation curve (see Chap. 21),

Glossary

assist–control ventilation: mode of mechanical ventilation in which the patient's breathing pattern may trigger the ventilator to deliver a preset tidal volume; in the absence of spontaneous breathing, the machine delivers a controlled breath at a preset minimum rate and tidal volume

chest drainage system: use of a chest tube and closed drainage system to reexpand the lung and to remove excess air, fluid, and blood

chest percussion: manually cupping over the chest wall to mobilize secretions by mechanically dislodging viscous or adherent secretions in the lungs

chest physiotherapy (CPT): therapy used to remove bronchial secretions, improve ventilation, and increase the efficiency of the respiratory muscles. Types include postural drainage, chest percussion, and vibration.

controlled ventilation: mode of mechanical ventilation in which the ventilator completely controls the patient's ventilation according to preset tidal volumes and respiratory rate. Because of problems with synchrony, it is rarely used except in paralyzed or anesthetized patients.

endotracheal intubation: insertion of a breathing tube through the nose or mouth into the trachea

fraction of inspired oxygen (FiO$_2$): concentration of oxygen delivered (1.0 = 100% oxygen)

hypoxemia: decrease in arterial oxygen tension in the blood

hypoxia: decrease in oxygen supply to the tissues and cells

incentive spirometry: method of deep breathing that provides visual feedback to help the patient inhale deeply and slowly and achieve maximum lung inflation

mechanical ventilator: a positive- or negative-pressure breathing device that supports ventilation and oxygenation

pneumothorax: partial or complete collapse of the lung due to positive pressure in the pleural space

positive end-expiratory pressure (PEEP): positive pressure maintained by the ventilator at the end of exhalation (instead of a normal zero pressure) to increase functional residual capacity and open collapsed alveoli; improves oxygenation with lower FiO$_2$

postural drainage: positioning the patient to allow drainage from all the lobes of the lungs and airways

pressure support ventilation (PSV): mode of mechanical ventilation in which preset positive pressure is delivered with spontaneous breaths to decrease work of breathing

respiratory weaning: process of gradual, systematic withdrawal and/or removal of ventilator, breathing tube, and oxygen

synchronized intermittent mandatory ventilation (SIMV): mode of mechanical ventilation in which the ventilator allows the patient to breathe spontaneously while providing a preset number of breaths to ensure adequate ventilation; ventilated breaths are synchronized with spontaneous breathing

thoracotomy: surgical opening into the chest cavity

tracheotomy: surgical opening into the trachea

tracheostomy tube: indwelling tube inserted directly into the trachea to assist with ventilation

vibration: a type of massage administered by quickly tapping the chest with the fingertips or alternating the fingers in a rhythmic manner, or by using a mechanical device to assist in mobilizing lung secretions

---

Chart 25-1 — Types of Hypoxia

Hypoxia can occur from either severe pulmonary disease (inadequate oxygen supply) or from extrapulmonary disease (inadequate oxygen delivery) affecting gas exchange at the cellular level. The four general types of hypoxia are hypoxemic hypoxia, circulatory hypoxia, anemic hypoxia, and histotoxic hypoxia.

Hypoxemic Hypoxia
Hypoxemic hypoxia is a decreased oxygen level in the blood resulting in decreased oxygen diffusion into the tissues. It may be caused by hypoventilation, high altitudes, ventilation–perfusion mismatch (as in pulmonary embolism), shunts in which the alveoli are collapsed and cannot provide oxygen to the blood (commonly caused by atelectasis), and pulmonary diffusion defects. It is corrected by increasing alveolar ventilation or providing supplemental oxygen.

Circulatory Hypoxia
Circulatory hypoxia is hypoxia resulting from inadequate capillary circulation. It may be caused by decreased cardiac output, local vascular obstruction, low-flow states such as shock, or cardiac arrest. Although tissue partial pressure of oxygen (PO_2) is reduced, arterial oxygen (PaO_2) remains normal. Circulatory hypoxia is corrected by identifying and treating the underlying cause.

Anemic Hypoxia
Anemic hypoxia is a result of decreased effective hemoglobin concentration, which causes a decrease in the oxygen-carrying capacity of the blood. It is rarely accompanied by hypoxemia. Carbon monoxide poisoning, because it reduces the oxygen-carrying capacity of hemoglobin, produces similar effects but is not strictly anemic hypoxia because hemoglobin levels may be normal.

Histotoxic Hypoxia
Histotoxic hypoxia occurs when a toxic substance, such as cyanide, interferes with the ability of tissues to use available oxygen.

---

the blood at these levels is 80% to 98% saturated with oxygen; higher inspired oxygen flow (FiO_2) values add no further significant amounts of oxygen to the red blood cells or plasma. Instead of helping, increased amounts of oxygen may produce toxic effects on the lungs and central nervous system or may depress ventilation (see discussion below).

It is important to observe for subtle indicators of inadequate oxygenation when oxygen is administered by any method. Therefore, the nurse assesses the patient frequently for confusion, restlessness progressing to lethargy, diaphoresis, pallor, tachycardia, tachypnea, and hypertension. Intermittent or continuous pulse oximetry is used to monitor oxygen levels.

OXYGEN TOXICITY

Oxygen toxicity may occur when too high a concentration of oxygen (greater than 50%) is administered for an extended period (longer than 48 hours). It is caused by overproduction of oxygen free radicals, which are byproducts of cell metabolism. If oxygen toxicity is untreated, these radicals can severely damage or kill cells. Antioxidants such as vitamin E, vitamin C, and beta-carotene may help defend against oxygen free radicals (Scanlan, Wilkins & Stoller, 1999). The dietitian can adjust the patient's diet so that it is rich in antioxidants; supplements are also available for patients who have a decreased appetite or who are unable to eat.

Signs and symptoms of oxygen toxicity include substernal discomfort, paresthesias, dyspnea, restlessness, fatigue, malaise, progressive respiratory difficulty, and alveolar infiltrates evident on chest x-rays.

Prevention of oxygen toxicity is achieved by using oxygen only as prescribed. If high concentrations of oxygen are necessary, it is important to minimize the duration of administration and reduce its concentration as soon as possible. Often, **positive end-expiratory pressure** (PEEP) or continuous positive airway pressure (CPAP) is used with oxygen therapy to reverse or prevent microatelectasis, thus allowing a lower percentage of oxygen to be used. The level of PEEP that allows the best oxygenation without hemodynamic compromise is known as "best PEEP."

SUPPRESSION OF VENTILATION

In patients with COPD, the stimulus for respiration is a decrease in blood oxygen rather than an elevation in carbon dioxide levels. Thus, administration of a high concentration of oxygen removes the respiratory drive that has been created largely by the patient's chronic low oxygen tension. The resulting decrease in alveolar ventilation can cause a progressive increase in arterial carbon dioxide pressure ($PaCO_2$), ultimately leading to the patient's death from carbon dioxide narcosis and acidosis. Oxygen-induced hypoventilation is prevented by administering oxygen at low flow rates (1 to 2 L/min).

OTHER COMPLICATIONS

Because oxygen supports combustion, there is always a danger of fire when it is used. It is important to post "no smoking" signs when oxygen is in use. Oxygen therapy equipment is also a potential source of bacterial cross-infection; thus, the nurse changes the tubing according to infection control policy and the type of oxygen delivery equipment.

Methods of Oxygen Administration

Oxygen is dispensed from a cylinder or a piped-in system. A reduction gauge is necessary to reduce the pressure to a working level, and a flow meter regulates the flow of oxygen in litres per minute. When oxygen is used at high flow rates, it should be moistened by passing it through a humidification system to prevent it from drying the mucous membranes of the respiratory tract.

The use of oxygen concentrators is another means of providing varying amounts of oxygen, especially in the home setting. These devices are relatively portable, easy to operate, and cost-effective. However, they require more maintenance than tank or liquid systems and probably cannot deliver oxygen flows in excess of 4 L, which provides an FiO_2 of about 36%.

Many different oxygen devices are used, and all deliver oxygen if they are used as prescribed and maintained correctly (Table 25-1). The amount of oxygen delivered is expressed as a percentage concentration (eg, 70%). The appropriate form of oxygen therapy is best determined by arterial blood gas levels, which indicate the patient's oxygenation status.

Oxygen delivery systems are classified as low-flow or high-flow delivery systems. Low-flow systems contribute partially to the inspired gas the patient breathes. This means the patient breathes some room air along with the oxygen. These systems do not provide a constant or known concentration of inspired oxygen. The amount of inspired oxygen changes as the patient's breathing changes. Examples of low-flow systems include nasal cannula, oropharyngeal catheter, simple mask, and partial-rebreather and non-rebreather masks. High-flow systems provide the total amount of inspired air. A specific percentage of oxygen is delivered independent of the patient's breathing. High-flow systems are indicated for patients who require a constant and precise amount of oxygen. Examples of such systems include transtracheal catheters, Venturi

Table 25-1 • Oxygen Administration Devices

DEVICE	SUGGESTED FLOW RATE (L/MIN)	O_2 PERCENTAGE SETTING	ADVANTAGES	DISADVANTAGES
Low-Flow Systems				
Cannula	1–2	23–30	Lightweight, comfortable, inexpensive, continuous use with meals and activity	Nasal mucosal drying, variable FiO_2
	3–5	30–40		
	6	42		
Oropharyngeal catheter	1–6	23–42	Inexpensive, does not require a tracheostomy	Nasal mucosa irritation; catheter should be changed frequently to alternate nostril
Mask, simple	6–8	40–60	Simple to use, inexpensive	Poor fitting, variable FiO_2, must remove to eat
Mask, partial rebreather	8–11	50–75	Moderate O_2 concentration	Warm, poorly fitting, must remove to eat
Mask, non-rebreather	12	80–100	High O_2 concentration	Poorly fitting
High-Flow Systems				
Transtracheal catheter	¼–4	60–100	More comfortable, concealed by clothing, less oxygen litres per minute needed than nasal cannula	Requires frequent and regular cleaning, requires surgical intervention
Mask, Venturi	4–6	24, 26, 28	Provides low levels of supplemental O_2	Must remove to eat
	6–8	30, 35, 40	Precise FiO_2, additional humidity available	
Mask, aerosol	8–10	30–100	Good humidity, accurate FiO_2	Uncomfortable for some
Tracheostomy collar	8–10	30–100	Good humidity, comfortable, fairly accurate FiO_2	
T-piece	8–10	30–100	Same as tracheostomy collar	Heavy with tubing
Face tent	8–10	30–100	Good humidity, fairly accurate FiO_2	Bulky and cumbersome

masks, aerosol masks, tracheostomy collars, T-piece, and face tents (Cairo & Pilbeam, 1999; Scanlan, Wilkins & Stoller, 1999).

A nasal cannula is used when the patient requires a low to medium concentration of oxygen for which precise accuracy is not essential. This method is relatively simple and allows the patient to move about in bed, talk, cough, and eat without interrupting oxygen flow. Flow rates in excess of 6 to 8 L/min may lead to swallowing of air; this may cause irritation and drying of the nasal and pharyngeal mucosa.

The oropharyngeal catheter is rarely used but may be prescribed for short-term therapy to administer low to moderate concentrations of oxygen. The catheter should be changed every 8 hours, alternating nostrils to prevent infection and nasal irritation.

When oxygen is administered via cannula or catheter, the percentage of oxygen reaching the lungs varies with the depth and rate of respirations, particularly if the nasal mucosa is swollen or if the patient is a mouth breather.

Oxygen masks come in several forms. Each is used for different purposes (Fig. 25-1). *Simple masks* are used for low to moderate concentrations of oxygen. The body of the mask itself gathers and stores oxygen between breaths. The patient exhales directly through openings or ports in the body of the mask. If oxygen flow ceases, the patient can draw air in through these openings around the mask edges (Scanlan, Wilkins & Stoller, 1999). Although widely used, these masks cannot be used for controlled oxygen concentrations and must be adjusted for proper fit. They should not press too tightly against the skin, because this may cause a sense of claustrophobia and skin breakdown; adjustable elastic bands are provided to ensure comfort and security.

Partial-rebreathing masks have a reservoir bag that must remain inflated during both inspiration and expiration. The nurse should adjust the litre flow to ensure that the bag does not collapse during inhalation. A higher concentration of oxygen can be delivered because both the mask and bag serve as reservoirs for oxygen. Oxygen enters the mask through small-bore tubing that connects at the junction of the mask and bag. As the patient inhales, gas is drawn from the mask, the bag, and potentially from room air through the exhalation ports. As the patient exhales, the first third of the exhalation fills the reservoir bag. This is mainly dead space and does not participate in gas exchange in the lungs. Therefore, it has a high oxygen concentration. The remainder of the exhaled gas is vented through the exhalation ports. The actual percentage of oxygen delivered is influenced by the patient's ventilatory pattern (Cairo & Pilbeam, 1999).

Non-rebreathing masks are similar in design to partial-rebreathing masks except that they have two valves. The first valve is a one-way valve located between the reservoir bag and the base of the mask. The valve allows gas from the reservoir bag to enter the mask on inhalation and prevents gas in the mask from flowing back into the reservoir bag during exhalation. The second valve is a set of valves located at the exhalation ports. These one-way valves prevent room air from entering the mask during inhalation. They also allow the patient's exhaled gases to exit the mask on exhalation (Cairo & Pilbeam, 1999). As with the partial-rebreathing mask, it is important to adjust the litre flow so that the reservoir bag does not completely collapse on inspiration. In theory, if the non-rebreather mask fits the patient snugly and both side exhalation ports have one-way valves, it is possible for the patient to receive 100% oxygen, making the non-rebreather a high-flow oxygen system. However, because it is difficult to get an exact fit from the mask on every patient, and some non-rebreather masks have only one one-way exhalation valve, it is nearly impossible to ensure 100% oxygen delivery, making it a low-flow oxygen system.

Venturi mask

Nonrebreather mask

Partial rebreather mask

FIGURE 25-1 Types of oxygen masks used to deliver varying concentrations of oxygen. Photos © Ken Kaspar.

The *Venturi mask* is the most reliable and accurate method for delivering precise concentrations of oxygen through noninvasive means. The mask is constructed in a way that allows a constant flow of room air blended with a fixed flow of oxygen. It is used primarily for patients with COPD because it can provide low levels of supplemental oxygen, thus avoiding the risk of suppressing the hypoxic drive.

The Venturi mask employs the Bernoulli principle of air entrainment (trapping the air like a vacuum), which provides a high air flow with controlled oxygen enrichment. For each litre of oxygen that passes through a jet orifice, a fixed proportion of room air will be entrained. A precise volume of oxygen can be delivered by varying the size of the jet orifice and adjusting the flow of oxygen. Excess gas leaves the mask through the two exhalation ports, carrying with it the exhaled carbon dioxide. This method allows a constant oxygen concentration to be inhaled regardless of the depth or rate of respiration.

The mask should fit snugly enough to prevent oxygen from flowing into the patient's eyes. The nurse should check the patient's skin for irritation. It is necessary to remove the mask so that the patient can eat, drink, and take medications.

The *transtracheal oxygen catheter* is inserted directly into the trachea and is indicated for patients with chronic oxygen therapy needs. These catheters are more comfortable, less dependent on breathing patterns, and less obvious than other oxygen delivery methods. Because no oxygen is lost into the surrounding environment, the patient achieves adequate oxygenation at lower rates, making this method less expensive and more efficient.

The *T-piece* connects to the endotracheal tube and is useful in weaning patients from mechanical ventilation (Fig. 25-2).

Other oxygen devices include *aerosol masks, tracheostomy collars,* and *face tents,* all of which are used with aerosol devices (nebulizers) that can be adjusted for oxygen concentrations from 27% to 100% (0.27 to 1.00). If the gas mixture flow falls below patient demand, room air is pulled in, diluting the concentration. The aerosol mist must be available for the patient during the entire inspiratory phase.

Although most oxygen therapy is administered as continuous flow oxygen, new methods of oxygen conservation are coming into use. *Demand oxygen delivery systems* (DODS) interrupt the flow of oxygen during exhalation, when the oxygen flow is otherwise mostly wasted. Several versions of DODS are being researched for their effectiveness. Studies show that DODS models conserve oxygen and maintain oxygen saturations better than continuous-flow oxygen when the respiratory rate increases (Bliss, McCoy & Adams, 1999).

Hyperbaric oxygen therapy is the administration of oxygen at pressures greater than one atmosphere. As a result, the amount of oxygen dissolved in plasma is increased, which raises oxygen levels in the tissues. It is administered through a small (single patient use) or large (multiple patient use) cylinder chamber. During therapy, the patient is placed in the chamber. Hyperbaric oxygen therapy is used to treat conditions such as air embolism, carbon monoxide poisoning, gangrene, tissue necrosis, and hemorrhage. Other uses for this therapy include treatment for multiple sclerosis, diabetic foot ulcers, closed head trauma, and acute myocardial infarction. Research continues in the area of hyperbaric oxygen use because of potential side effects, including ear trauma, central nervous system disorders, and oxygen toxicity (Takezawa, 2000; Woodrow & Roe, 2000).

Gerontologic Considerations

The respiratory system changes throughout the aging process, and it is important for nurses to be aware of these changes when assessing patients who are receiving oxygen therapy. As the respiratory muscles weaken and the large bronchi and alveoli become enlarged, the available surface area of the lungs decreases, resulting in reduced ventilation and respiratory gas exchange. The number of functional cilia is also reduced, decreasing ciliary action and the cough reflex. As a result of osteoporosis and the calcification of the costal cartilages, chest wall compliance is decreased. Patients may display increased chest rigidity and respiratory rate and decreased PaO_2 and lung expansion. Nurses should be aware that the older adult is at risk for aspiration and infection related to these changes. In addition, patient education regarding adequate nutrition is essential, because appropriate dietary intake can help

FIGURE 25-2 T-pieces and tracheostomy collars are devices used when weaning patients from mechanical ventilation.

to diminish the excess build-up of carbon dioxide and to maintain optimal respiratory functioning (Abraham, Bottrell, Fulmer & Mezey, 1999; Eliopoulos, 2001).

Nursing Management

PROMOTING HOME AND COMMUNITY-BASED CARE

Teaching Patients Self-Care. At times oxygen must be administered to the patient at home. The nurse instructs the patient or family in the methods for administering oxygen and informs the patient and family that oxygen is available in gas, liquid, and concentrated forms. The gas and liquid forms come in portable de-

vices so that the patient can leave home while receiving oxygen therapy. Humidity must be provided while oxygen is used (except with portable devices) to counteract the dry, irritating effects of compressed oxygen on the airway (Chart 25-2).

Continuing Care. Home visits by a home health nurse or respiratory therapist may be arranged based on the patient's status and needs. It is important to assess the patient's home environment, the patient's physical and psychological status, and the need for further teaching. The nurse reinforces the teaching points on how to use oxygen safely and effectively, including fire safety tips because oxygen is flammable. To maintain a consistent quality of care and to maximize the patient's financial reimbursement for

Chart 25-2
Home Care Checklist • Oxygen Therapy

At the completion of the home care instruction, the patient or caregiver will be able to:	Patient	Caregiver
• State proper care of and administration of oxygen to patient		
State physician's prescription for oxygen and the manner in which it is to be used	✓	✓
Indicate when a humidifier should be used	✓	✓
Identify signs and symptoms indicating the need for change in oxygen therapy	✓	✓
Describe precautions and safety measures to be used when oxygen is in use	✓	✓
State how and when to place an order for more oxygen	✓	✓
Describe a diet that meets energy demands	✓	✓
• Maintain equipment properly		
Demonstrate correct adjustment of prescribed flow rate	✓	✓
Describe how to clean and when to replace oxygen tubing	✓	✓
Identify when a portable oxygen delivery device should be used	✓	✓
Demonstrate safe and appropriate use of portable oxygen delivery device	✓	✓
Identify causes of malfunction of equipment and when to call for replacement of equipment	✓	✓
Describe the importance of determining that all electrical outlets are working properly	✓	✓

home oxygen therapy, the nurse ensures that the physician's prescription includes the diagnosis, the prescribed oxygen flow, and conditions for use (eg, continuous use, nighttime use only). Because oxygen is a medication, the nurse reminds the patient receiving long-term oxygen therapy and family about the importance of keeping follow-up appointments with the physician. The patient is instructed to see the physician every 6 months or more often, if indicated. Blood gas measurements and laboratory tests are repeated annually, or more often if the patient's condition changes (Smith & Matti, 1999).

INTERMITTENT POSITIVE-PRESSURE BREATHING

Intermittent positive-pressure breathing (IPPB) is a form of assisted or controlled respiration produced by a ventilatory apparatus in which compressed gas is delivered under positive pressure into a person's airways until a preset pressure is reached. Passive exhalation is allowed through a valve. The specific pressure and volume amounts, along with the use of any nebulizing medications, are prescribed individually for patients. The nurse should encourage patients to relax and reassure them that the machine will automatically shut off airflow at the end of inspiration. The IPPB machine may be powered by electricity or gas and may be connected with a mouthpiece, mask, or tracheostomy adapter.

Indications

General indications for IPPB include difficulty in raising respiratory secretions, reduced vital capacity with ineffective deep breathing and coughing, or unsuccessful trials of simpler and less costly methods for loosening secretions, delivering aerosol, or expanding the lungs.

Complications

IPPB therapy is used rarely today because of its inherent hazards, which may include pneumothorax, mucosal drying, increased intracranial pressure, hemoptysis, gastric distention, vomiting with possible aspiration, psychological dependency (especially with long-term use, as in COPD patients), hyperventilation, excessive oxygen administration, and cardiovascular problems.

MINI-NEBULIZER THERAPY

The mini-nebulizer is a hand-held apparatus that disperses a moisturizing agent or medication, such as a bronchodilator or mucolytic agent, into microscopic particles and delivers it to the lungs as the patient inhales. The mini-nebulizer is usually air-driven by means of a compressor through connecting tubing. In some instances, the nebulizer is oxygen-driven rather than air-driven. To be effective, a visible mist must be available for the patient to inhale.

Indications

The indications for use of a mini-nebulizer are similar to the indications for IPPB, except that the patient must be able to generate a deep breath without the aid of the positive-pressure machine. Diaphragmatic breathing (Chart 25-3) is a helpful technique to prepare for proper use of the mini-nebulizer. Frequently,

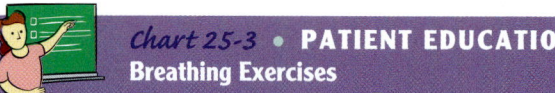

Chart 25-3 • PATIENT EDUCATION
Breathing Exercises

General Instructions

- Breathe slowly and rhythmically to exhale completely and empty the lungs completely.
- Inhale through the nose to filter, humidify, and warm the air before it enters the lungs.
- If you feel out of breath, breathe more slowly by prolonging the exhalation time.
- Keep the air moist with a humidifier.

Diaphragmatic Breathing

Goal: To use and strengthen the diaphragm during breathing

- Place one hand on the abdomen (just below the ribs) and the other hand on the middle of the chest to increase the awareness of the position of the diaphragm and its function in breathing.
- Breathe in slowly and deeply through the nose, letting the abdomen protrude as far as possible.
- Breathe out through pursed lips while tightening (contracting) the abdominal muscles.
- Press firmly inward and upward on the abdomen while breathing out.
- Repeat for 1 minute; follow with a rest period of 2 minutes.
- Gradually increase duration up to 5 minutes, several times a day (before meals and at bedtime).

Pursed-Lip Breathing

Goal: To prolong exhalation and increase airway pressure during expiration, thus reducing the amount of trapped air and the amount of airway resistance.

- Inhale through the nose while counting to 3—the amount of time needed to say "Smell a rose."
- Exhale slowly and evenly against pursed lips while tightening the abdominal muscles. (Pursing the lips increases intratracheal pressure; exhaling through the mouth offers less resistance to expired air.)
- Count to 7 while prolonging expiration through pursed lips—the length of time to say "Blow out the candle."
- While sitting in a chair:
  Fold arms over the abdomen.
  Inhale through the nose while counting to 3.
  Bend forward and exhale slowly through pursed lips while counting to 7.
- While walking:
  Inhale while walking two steps.
  Exhale through pursed lips while walking four or five steps.

mini-nebulizers are used for patients with COPD to dispense inhaled medications and are commonly used at home on a long-term basis.

Nursing Management

PROMOTING HOME AND COMMUNITY-BASED CARE

Teaching Patients Self-Care. The nurse instructs the patient to breathe through the mouth, taking slow, deep breaths, and then to hold the breath for a few seconds at the end of inspiration to increase intrapleural pressure and reopen collapsed alveoli, thereby increasing functional residual capacity. The nurse encourages the patient to cough and to monitor the effectiveness of the therapy. The nurse instructs the patient and family about the purpose of the treatment, equipment set-up, medication additive, and proper cleaning and storage of the equipment.

INCENTIVE SPIROMETRY (SUSTAINED MAXIMAL INSPIRATION)

Incentive spirometry is a method of deep breathing that provides visual feedback to help the patient inhale slowly and deeply to maximize lung inflation and prevent or reduce atelectasis. Ideally, the patient assumes a sitting or semi-Fowler's position to enhance diaphragmatic excursion (Chart 25-4). However, this procedure may be performed with the patient in any position.

Incentive spirometers may be one of two types: volume or flow. In the volume type, the tidal volume of the spirometer is set according to the manufacturer's instructions. The purpose of the device is to ensure that the volume of air inhaled is increased gradually as the patient takes deeper and deeper breaths. The patient takes a deep breath through the mouthpiece, pauses at peak lung inflation, and then relaxes and exhales. Taking several normal breaths before attempting another with the incentive spirometer helps avoid fatigue. The volume is periodically increased as tolerated.

A flow spirometer has the same purpose as a volume spirometer, but the volume is not preset. The spirometer contains a number of movable balls that are pushed up by the force of the breath and held suspended in the air while the patient inhales. The amount of air inhaled and the flow of the air are estimated by how long and how high the balls are suspended.

Indications

Incentive spirometry is used after surgery, especially thoracic and abdominal surgery, to promote the expansion of the alveoli and to prevent or treat atelectasis. As a preventive measure, incentive spirometry may be more effective than IPPB because it maximizes the amount of air inhaled while maintaining relatively low airway pressures.

Nursing Management

Nursing management of the patient using incentive spirometry includes placing the patient in the proper position, teaching the technique for using the incentive spirometer, setting realistic goals for the patient, and recording the results of the therapy.

CHEST PHYSIOTHERAPY

Chest physiotherapy (CPT) includes **postural drainage, chest percussion** and **vibration,** and breathing exercises/breathing retraining. In addition, teaching the patient effective coughing technique is an important part of chest physiotherapy. The goals of chest physiotherapy are to remove bronchial secretions, improve ventilation, and increase the efficiency of the respiratory muscles.

Postural Drainage (Segmented Bronchial Drainage)

Postural drainage uses specific positions that allow the force of gravity to assist in the removal of bronchial secretions. The secretions drain from the affected bronchioles into the bronchi and trachea and are removed by coughing or suctioning. Postural drainage is used to prevent or relieve bronchial obstruction caused by accumulation of secretions.

Because the patient usually sits in an upright position, secretions are likely to accumulate in the lower parts of the lungs. With postural drainage, different positions (Fig. 25-3) are used so that the force of gravity helps to move secretions from the smaller bronchial airways to the main bronchi and trachea. The secretions then are removed by coughing. The nurse should instruct the patient to inhale bronchodilators and mucolytic agents, if prescribed, before postural drainage because these medications improve bronchial tree drainage.

Chart 25-4 • PATIENT EDUCATION
Assisting the Patient to Perform Incentive Spirometry

- Explain the reason and objective for the therapy: the inspired air helps to inflate the lungs. The ball or weight in the spirometer will rise in response to the intensity of the intake of air. The higher the ball rises, the deeper the breath.
- Assess the patient's level of pain and administer pain medication if prescribed.
- Position the patient in semi-Fowler's position or in an upright position (although any position is acceptable).
- Demonstrate how to use diaphragmatic breathing.
- Instruct the patient to place the mouthpiece of the spirometer firmly in the mouth, to breathe air in (inspire), and to hold the breath at the end of inspiration for about 3 seconds. The patient then exhales slowly.
- Encourage approximately 10 breaths per hour with the spirometer during waking hours.
- Set a reasonable volume and repetition goal (to provide encouragement and give the patient a sense of accomplishment).
- Encourage coughing during and after each session.
- Assist the patient to splint the incision when coughing postoperatively.
- Place the spirometer within easy reach of the patient.
- For the postoperative patient, begin the therapy immediately. (If the patient begins to hypoventilate, atelectasis can start to occur within an hour.)

© B. Proud.

- Record how effectively the patient performs the therapy and the number of breaths achieved with the spirometer every 2 hours.

FIGURE 25-3 Postural drainage positions and the areas of lung drained by each position.

Postural drainage exercises can be directed at any of the segments of the lungs. The lower and middle lobe bronchi drain more effectively when the head is down; the upper lobe bronchi drain more effectively when the head is up. Frequently, five positions are used, one for drainage of each lobe: head down, prone, right and left lateral, and sitting upright.

Nursing Management

The nurse should be aware of the patient's diagnosis as well as the lung lobes or segments involved, the cardiac status, and any structural deformities of the chest wall and spine. Auscultating the chest before and after the procedure helps to identify the areas needing drainage and to assess the effectiveness of treatment. The nurse teaches family members who will be assisting the patient at home to evaluate breath sounds before and after treatment. The nurse explores strategies that will enable the patient to assume the indicated positions at home. This may require the creative use of objects readily available at home, such as pillows, cushions, or cardboard boxes.

Postural drainage is usually performed two to four times daily, before meals (to prevent nausea, vomiting, and aspiration) and at bedtime. Prescribed bronchodilators, water, or saline may be nebulized and inhaled before postural drainage to dilate the bronchioles, reduce bronchospasm, decrease the thickness of mucus and sputum, and combat edema of the bronchial walls. The recommended sequence of positioning is as follows: positions to drain the lower lobes first, then positions to drain the upper lobes.

The nurse makes the patient as comfortable as possible in each position and provides an emesis basin, sputum cup, and paper tissues. The nurse instructs the patient to remain in each position for 10 to 15 minutes and to breathe in slowly through the nose and then breathe out slowly through pursed lips to help keep the airways open so that secretions can drain while in each position. If a position cannot be tolerated, the nurse helps the patient to assume a modified position. When the patient changes position, the nurse explains how to cough and remove secretions (Chart 25-5).

If the patient cannot cough, the nurse may need to suction the secretions mechanically. It also may be necessary to use chest percussion and vibration to loosen bronchial secretions and mucus plugs that adhere to the bronchioles and bronchi and to propel sputum in the direction of gravity drainage (see "Chest Percussion and Vibration," below). If suctioning is required at home, the nurse instructs caregivers in safe suctioning technique and care of the suctioning equipment.

After the procedure, the nurse notes the amount, colour, viscosity, and character of the expelled sputum. It is important to evaluate the patient's skin colour and pulse the first few times the procedure is performed. It may be necessary to administer oxygen during postural drainage.

If the sputum is foul-smelling, it is important to perform postural drainage in a room away from other patients and/or family members and to use deodorizers unless contraindicated. Deodorizers delivered in aerosol sprays can cause bronchospasm and irritation to the patient with a respiratory disorder and should be used cautiously (Zang & Allender, 1999). After the procedure, the patient may find it refreshing to brush the teeth and use a mouthwash before resting.

Chest Percussion and Vibration

Thick secretions that are difficult to cough up may be loosened by tapping (percussing) and vibrating the chest. Chest percussion and vibration help to dislodge mucus adhering to the bronchioles and bronchi.

Percussion is carried out by cupping the hands and lightly striking the chest wall in a rhythmic fashion over the lung segment to be drained. The wrists are alternately flexed and extended so that the chest is cupped or clapped in a painless manner (Fig. 25-4). A soft cloth or towel may be placed over the segment of the chest that is being cupped to prevent skin irritation and redness from direct contact. Percussion, alternating with vibration, is performed for 3 to 5 minutes for each position. The patient uses diaphragmatic breathing during this procedure to promote relaxation (see "Breathing Retraining," below). As a precaution, percussion over chest drainage tubes, the sternum, spine, liver, kidneys, spleen, or breasts (in women) is avoided. Percussion is performed cautiously in the elderly because of their increased incidence of osteoporosis and risk of rib fracture.

Vibration is the technique of applying manual compression and tremor to the chest wall during the exhalation phase of respiration (see Fig. 25-4). This helps to increase the velocity of the air expired from the small airways, thus freeing the mucus. After three or four vibrations, the patient is encouraged to cough, using the abdominal muscles. (Contracting the abdominal muscles increases the effectiveness of the cough.)

A scheduled program of coughing and clearing sputum, together with hydration, reduces the amount of sputum in most patients. The number of times the percussion and vibration cycle is repeated depends on the patient's tolerance and clinical response. It is important to evaluate breath sounds before and after the procedures.

Nursing Management

When performing chest physiotherapy, the nurse ensures that the patient is comfortable, is not wearing restrictive clothing, and has not just eaten. The uppermost areas of the lung are treated first. The nurse gives medication for pain, as prescribed, before percussion and vibration and splints any incision and provides pillows for support as needed. The positions are varied, but focus is placed on the affected areas. On completion of the treatment, the nurse assists the patient to assume a comfortable position.

The nurse must stop treatment if any of the following occur: increased pain, increased shortness of breath, weakness, lightheadedness, or hemoptysis. Therapy is indicated until the patient has normal respirations, can mobilize secretions, and has normal breath sounds, and when the chest x-ray findings are normal.

Chart 25-5

Effective Coughing Technique

1. The patient assumes a sitting position and bends slightly forward. This upright position permits a stronger cough.
2. The patient's knees and hips are flexed to promote relaxation and reduce the strain on the abdominal muscles while coughing.
3. The patient inhales slowly through the nose and exhales through pursed lips several times.
4. The patient should cough twice during each exhalation while contracting (pulling in) the abdomen sharply with each cough.
5. The patient splints the incisional area, if any, with firm hand pressure or supports it with a pillow or rolled blanket while coughing (see Fig. 25-8). (The nurse can initially demonstrate this by using the patient's hands.)

FIGURE 25-4 Percussion and vibration. (**A**) Proper hand position for percussion. (**B**) Proper technique for vibration. The wrists and elbows remain stiff; the vibrating motion is produced by the shoulder muscles. (**C**) Proper hand position for vibration.

PROMOTING HOME AND COMMUNITY-BASED CARE

Teaching Patients Self-Care. Chest physiotherapy is frequently indicated at home for patients with COPD, bronchiectasis, and cystic fibrosis. The techniques are the same as described above, but gravity drainage is achieved by placing the hips over a box, a stack of magazines, or pillows (unless a hospital bed is available). The nurse instructs the patient and family in the positions and techniques of percussion and vibration so that therapy can be continued in the home. In addition, the nurse instructs the patient to maintain an adequate fluid intake and air humidity to prevent secretions from becoming thick and tenacious. It also is important to teach the patient to recognize early signs of infection, such as fever and a change in the colour or character of sputum. Resting 5 to 10 minutes in each postural drainage position before chest physiotherapy maximizes the amount of secretions obtained.

Continuing Care. Chest physical therapy may be carried out during visits by a home care nurse. The nurse also assesses the patient's physical status, understanding of the treatment plan, and compliance with recommended therapy, as well as the effectiveness of therapy. It is important to reinforce patient and family teaching during these visits. The nurse reports to the patient's physician any deterioration in the patient's physical status and inability to clear secretions.

Breathing Retraining

Breathing retraining consists of exercises and breathing practices designed to achieve more efficient and controlled ventilation and to decrease the work of breathing. Breathing retraining is especially indicated in patients with COPD and dyspnea. These exercises promote maximal alveolar inflation and muscle relaxation, relieve anxiety, eliminate ineffective, uncoordinated patterns of respiratory muscle activity, slow the respiratory rate, and decrease the work of breathing. Slow, relaxed, and rhythmic breathing also helps to control the anxiety that occurs with dyspnea. Specific breathing exercises include diaphragmatic and pursed-lip breathing (see Chart 25-3).

The goal of diaphragmatic breathing is to use and strengthen the diaphragm during breathing. Diaphragmatic breathing can become automatic with sufficient practice and concentration. Pursed-lip breathing, which improves oxygen transport, helps to

induce a slow, deep breathing pattern and assists the patient to control breathing, even during periods of stress. This type of breathing helps prevent airway collapse secondary to loss of lung elasticity in emphysema. The goal of pursed-lip breathing is to train the muscles of expiration to prolong exhalation and increase airway pressure during expiration, thus lessening the amount of airway trapping and resistance. The nurse instructs the patient in diaphragmatic breathing and pursed-lip breathing, as described earlier in Chart 25-3. Breathing exercises may be practiced in several positions because air distribution and pulmonary circulation vary with the position of the chest. Many patients require additional oxygen, using a low-flow method, while performing breathing exercises. Emphysema-like changes in the lung occur as part of the natural aging process of the lung; therefore, breathing exercises are appropriate for all elderly patients who are hospitalized and elderly patients in any setting who are sedentary, even without primary lung disease.

Nursing Management

PROMOTING HOME AND COMMUNITY-BASED CARE

Teaching Patients Self-Care. The nurse instructs the patient to breathe slowly and rhythmically in a relaxed manner and to exhale completely to empty the lungs. The patient is instructed always to inhale through the nose because this filters, humidifies, and warms the air. If short of breath, the patient should concentrate on breathing slowly and rhythmically. To avoid initiating a cycle of increasing shortness of breath and panic, it is often helpful to instruct the patient to concentrate on prolonging the length of exhalation rather than merely slowing the rate of breathing. Minimizing the amount of dust or particles in the air and providing adequate humidification may also make it easier for the patient to breathe. Strategies to decrease dust or particles in the air include removing drapes or upholstered furniture, using air filters, and washing floors and dusting and vacuuming frequently.

The nurse instructs the patient that an adequate dietary intake promotes gas exchange and increases energy levels. It is important to provide adequate nutrition without overfeeding patients. Nurses should teach patients to consume small, frequent meals and snacks. Having ready-prepared meals and favourite foods available helps encourage nutrient consumption. Gas-producing foods such as beans, legumes, broccoli, cabbage, and Brussels sprouts should be avoided to prevent gastric distress. Because many of these patients lack the energy to eat, they should be taught to rest before and after meals to conserve energy (Lutz & Przytulski, 2001).

Airway Management

Adequate ventilation is dependent on free movement of air through the upper and lower airways. In many disorders, the airway becomes narrowed or blocked as a result of disease, bronchoconstriction (narrowing of airway by contraction of muscle fibres), a foreign body, or secretions. Maintaining a patent (open) airway is achieved through meticulous airway management, whether in an emergency situation such as airway obstruction or in long-term management, as in caring for a patient with an endotracheal or a tracheostomy tube.

EMERGENCY MANAGEMENT OF UPPER AIRWAY OBSTRUCTION

Upper airway obstruction has a variety of causes. Acute upper airway obstruction may be caused by food particles, vomitus, blood clots, or any other particle that enters and obstructs the larynx or trachea. It also may occur from enlargement of tissue in the wall of the airway, as in epiglottitis, laryngeal edema, laryngeal carcinoma, or peritonsillar abscess, or from thick secretions. Pressure on the walls of the airway, as occurs in retrosternal goitre, enlarged mediastinal lymph nodes, hematoma around the upper airway, and thoracic aneurysm, also may result in upper airway obstruction.

The patient with an altered level of consciousness from any cause is at risk for upper airway obstruction because of loss of the protective reflexes (cough and swallowing) and the tone of the pharyngeal muscles, causing the tongue to fall back and block the airway.

The nurse makes the following rapid observations to assess for signs and symptoms of upper airway obstruction:

- Inspection—Is the patient conscious? Is there any inspiratory effort? Does the chest rise symmetrically? Is there use or retraction of accessory muscles? What is the skin colour? Are there any obvious signs of deformity or obstruction (trauma, food, teeth, vomitus)? Is the trachea midline?
- Palpation—Do both sides of the chest rise equally with inspiration? Are there any specific areas of tenderness, fracture, or subcutaneous emphysema (crepitus)?
- Auscultation—Is there any audible air movement, stridor (inspiratory sound), or wheezing (expiratory sound)? Are breath sounds present bilaterally in all lobes?

As soon as an upper airway obstruction is identified, the nurse takes emergency measures (Chart 25-6). (See "Guidelines for Managing a Foreign Body Airway Obstruction" in Chap. 71 for more details, or see Chap. 22.)

ENDOTRACHEAL INTUBATION

Endotracheal intubation involves passing an endotracheal tube through the mouth or nose into the trachea (Fig. 25-5). Intubation provides a patent airway when the patient is having respiratory distress that cannot be treated with simpler methods. It is the method of choice in emergency care. Endotracheal intubation is a means of providing an airway for patients who cannot maintain an adequate airway on their own (eg, comatose patients or pa-

tients with upper airway obstruction), for mechanical ventilation, and for suctioning secretions from the pulmonary tree.

An endotracheal tube usually is passed with the aid of a laryngoscope by specifically trained medical, nursing, or respiratory therapy personnel. (See "Guidelines for Inserting an Oropharyngeal Airway" in Chap. 71 for more details.) Once the tube is inserted, a cuff around the tube is inflated to prevent air from leaking around the outer part of the tube, to minimize the possibility of subsequent aspiration, and to prevent movement of the tube.

Nurses should be aware that complications could occur from pressure in the cuff on the tracheal wall. Cuff pressures should be checked with a calibrated aneroid manometer device every 8 to 12 hours to maintain cuff pressure between 20 and 25 mm Hg. High cuff pressure can cause tracheal bleeding, ischemia, and pressure necrosis, while low cuff pressure can increase the risk of aspiration pneumonia. Routine deflation of the cuff is not recommended due to the increased risk of aspiration and hypoxia. The cuff is deflated prior to removing the endotracheal tube (St. John, 1999b).

Tracheobronchial secretions are suctioned through the tube. Warmed, humidified oxygen should always be introduced through the tube, whether the patient is breathing spontaneously or is receiving ventilatory support. Endotracheal intubation may be used for no more than 3 weeks, by which time a tracheostomy must be considered to decrease irritation of and trauma to the tracheal lining, to reduce the incidence of vocal cord paralysis (secondary to laryngeal nerve damage), and to decrease the work of breathing. Chart 25-7 discusses the nursing care of the patient with an endotracheal tube.

There are several disadvantages of endotracheal and tracheostomy tubes. First, the tube causes discomfort. In addition, the cough reflex is depressed because closure of the glottis is hindered. Secretions tend to become thicker because the warming and humidifying effect of the upper respiratory tract has been bypassed. The swallowing reflexes, composed of the glottic, pharyngeal, and laryngeal reflexes, are depressed because of prolonged disuse and the mechanical trauma of the endotracheal or tracheostomy tube, which puts the patient at increased risk for aspiration. In addition, ulceration and stricture of the larynx or trachea may develop. Of great concern to the patient is the inability to talk and to communicate needs.

Unintentional or premature removal of the tube is a potentially life-threatening complication of endotracheal intubation. Removal of the tube is a frequent problem in intensive care units and occurs mainly during nursing care or by the patient. It is important for nurses to instruct patients and family members about the purpose of the tube and the dangers of removing it. Baseline and ongoing assessment of the patient and equipment ensures effective care. Providing comfort measures, including opioid analgesia and sedation, can improve the patient's tolerance of the endotracheal tube.

 NURSING ALERT Inadvertent removal of an endotracheal tube can cause laryngeal swelling, hypoxemia, bradycardia, hypotension, and even death. Measures must be taken to prevent premature or inadvertent removal.

To prevent tube removal by the patient, the nurse can use the following strategies: explain to the patient and family the purpose of the tube, distract the patient through one-to-one interaction with the nurse and family or with television, and maintain comfort measures. As a last resort, soft wrist restraints may be used, according to agency policy.

Chart 25-6   Clearing an Upper Airway Obstruction

Clearing the Airway

- Hyperextend the patient's neck by placing one hand on the forehead and placing the fingers of the other hand underneath the jaw and lifting upward and forward. This action pulls the tongue away from the back of the pharynx.

Opening the airway.

- Assess the patient by observing the chest and listening and feeling for the movement of air.
- Use a cross-finger technique to open the mouth and observe for obvious obstructions such as secretions, blood clots, or food particles.
- If no passage of air is detected, apply five quick sharp abdominal thrusts just below the xiphoid process to expel the obstruction (Heimlich maneuver). Repeat this procedure until the obstruction is expelled.
- After the obstruction is expelled, roll the patient as a unit onto the side for recovery.
- When the obstruction is relieved and the patient can breathe spontaneously but not cough, swallow, or gag, insert an oral or nasopharyngeal airway.

Abdominal thrust (Heimlich) maneuver administered to unconscious patient.

Bag and Mask Resuscitation

- Use a resuscitation bag and mask if assisted ventilation is required.
- Apply the mask to the patient's face and create a seal by pressing the thumb of the nondominant hand on the bridge of the nose and the index finger on the chin. Use the rest of the fingers on the hand and pull on the chin and the angle of the mandible to maintain the head in extension. Use the dominant hand to inflate the lungs by squeezing the bag to its full volume.

Resuscitation via bag and mask apparatus.

Studies have shown that the most effective way to prevent tube removal by the patient is through the use of soft wrist restraints (Happ, 2000). However, discretion and caution must always be used before applying any restraint. If the patient cannot move the arms and hands to the endotracheal tube, restraints would not be needed. If the patient is alert, oriented, able to follow directions, and cooperative to the point that it is highly unlikely that he or she will remove the endotracheal tube, restraints are not needed. On the other hand, if the nurse determines there is a risk that the patient may try to remove the tube, soft wrist restraints are appropriate with a physician's order (check agency policy). Close monitoring of the patient remains essential to ensure safety and prevent harm.

FIGURE 25-5 Endotracheal tube in place. Tube has been inserted using the oral route. The cuff has been inflated to maintain the tube's position and minimize the risk for aspiration.

TRACHEOSTOMY

A **tracheotomy** is a surgical procedure in which an opening is made into the trachea. The indwelling tube inserted into the trachea is called a **tracheostomy tube**. A tracheostomy may be either temporary or permanent.

A tracheostomy is used to bypass an upper airway obstruction, to allow removal of tracheobronchial secretions, to permit the long-term use of mechanical ventilation, to prevent aspiration of oral or gastric secretions in the unconscious or paralyzed patient (by closing off the trachea from the esophagus), and to replace an endotracheal tube. There are many disease processes and emergency conditions that make a tracheostomy necessary.

Procedure

The surgical procedure is usually performed in the operating room or in an intensive care unit, where the patient's ventilation can be well controlled and optimal aseptic technique can be maintained.

A surgical opening is made in the second and third tracheal rings. After the trachea is exposed, a cuffed tracheostomy tube of an appropriate size is inserted. The cuff is an inflatable attachment to the tracheostomy tube that is designed to occlude the space between the trachea walls and the tube to permit effective mechanical ventilation and to minimize the risk of aspiration.

The tracheostomy tube is held in place by tapes fastened around the patient's neck. Usually a square of sterile gauze is placed between the tube and the skin to absorb drainage and prevent infection.

Complications

Complications may occur early or late in the course of tracheostomy tube management. They may even occur years after the tube has been removed. Early complications include bleeding, pneumothorax, air embolism, aspiration, subcutaneous or mediastinal emphysema, recurrent laryngeal nerve damage, and posterior tracheal wall penetration. Long-term complications include airway obstruction from accumulation of secretions or protrusion of the cuff over the opening of the tube, infection, rupture of the innominate artery, dysphagia, tracheoesophageal fistula, tracheal dilation, and tracheal ischemia and necrosis. Tracheal stenosis may develop after the tube is removed. Chart 25-8 outlines measures nurses can take to prevent complications.

Postoperative Nursing Management

The patient requires continuous monitoring and assessment. The newly made opening must be kept patent by proper suctioning of secretions. After the vital signs are stable, the patient is placed in a semi-Fowler's position to facilitate ventilation, promote drainage, minimize edema, and prevent strain on the suture lines. Analgesia and sedative agents must be administered with caution because of the risk of suppressing the cough reflex.

Major objectives of nursing care are to alleviate the patient's apprehension and to provide an effective means of communica-

---

 Care of the Patient with an Endotracheal Tube

Immediately After Intubation
1. Check symmetry of chest expansion.
   - Auscultate breath sounds of anterior and lateral chest bilaterally.
   - Obtain order for chest x-ray to verify proper tube placement.
   - Check cuff pressure every 8–12 hours.
   - Monitor for signs and symptoms of aspiration.
2. Ensure high humidity; a visible mist should appear in the T-piece or ventilator tubing.
3. Administer oxygen concentration as prescribed by physician.
4. Secure the tube to the patient's face with tape, and mark the proximal end for position maintenance.
   - Cut proximal end of tube if it is longer than 7.5 cm to prevent kinking.
   - Insert an oral airway or mouth device to prevent the patient from biting and obstructing the tube.
5. Use sterile suction technique and airway care to prevent iatrogenic contamination and infection.
6. Continue to reposition patient every 2 hours and as needed to prevent atelectasis and to optimize lung expansion.
7. Provide oral hygiene and suction the oropharynx whenever necessary.

Extubation (Removal of Endotracheal Tube)
1. Explain procedure.
2. Have self-inflating bag and mask ready in case ventilatory assistance is required immediately after extubation.
3. Suction the tracheobronchial tree and oropharynx, remove tape, and then deflate the cuff.
4. Give oxygen for a few breaths, then insert a new, sterile suction catheter inside tube.
5. Have the patient inhale. At peak inspiration remove the tube, suctioning the airway through the tube as it is pulled out.
Note: In some hospitals this procedure can be performed by respiratory therapists; in others, by nurses. Check hospital policy.

Care of Patient Following Extubation
1. Give heated humidity and oxygen by face mask.
2. Monitor respiratory rate and quality of chest excursions. Note stridor, colour change, and change in mental alertness or behaviour.
3. Monitor the patient's oxygen level using a pulse oximeter.
4. Keep NPO or give only ice chips for next few hours.
5. Provide mouth care.
6. Teach patient how to perform coughing and deep-breathing exercises.

Preventing Complications Associated With Endotracheal and Tracheostomy Tubes

- Administer adequate warmed humidity.
- Maintain cuff around tube.
- Suction as needed per assessment findings.
- Maintain skin integrity. Change tape and dressing as needed or per protocol.
- Auscultate lung sounds.
- Monitor for signs and symptoms of infection, including temperature and white blood cell count.
- Administer prescribed oxygen and monitor oxygen saturation.
- Monitor for cyanosis.
- Maintain adequate hydration of the patient.
- Use sterile technique when suctioning and performing tracheostomy care.

---

tion. The nurse keeps paper and pencil or a Magic Slate and the call light within the patient's reach to ensure a means of communication. The care of the patient with a tracheostomy tube is summarized in Chart 25-9.

SUCTIONING THE TRACHEAL TUBE (TRACHEOSTOMY OR ENDOTRACHEAL TUBE)

When a tracheostomy or endotracheal tube is in place, it is usually necessary to suction the patient's secretions because of the decreased effectiveness of the cough mechanism. Tracheal suctioning is performed when adventitious breath sounds are detected or whenever secretions are obviously present. Unnecessary suctioning can initiate bronchospasm and cause mechanical trauma to the tracheal mucosa.

All equipment that comes into direct contact with the patient's lower airway must be sterile to prevent overwhelming pulmonary and systemic infections. The procedure for suctioning a tracheostomy is presented in Chart 25-10. In mechanically ventilated patients, an in-line suction catheter may be used to allow rapid suction when needed and to minimize cross-contamination of airborne pathogens. An in-line suction device allows the patient to be suctioned without being disconnected from the ventilator circuit.

MANAGING THE CUFF

As a general rule, the cuff on an endotracheal or tracheostomy tube should be inflated. The pressure within the cuff should be the lowest possible that allows delivery of adequate tidal volumes and prevents pulmonary aspiration. Usually the pressure is maintained at less than 25 cm H_2O to prevent injury and at more than 20 cm H_2O to prevent aspiration. Cuff pressure must be monitored at least every 8 hours by attaching a hand-held pressure gauge to the pilot balloon of the tube or by using the minimal leak volume or minimal occlusion volume technique. With long-term intubation, higher pressures may be needed to maintain an adequate seal.

PROMOTING HOME AND COMMUNITY-BASED CARE

Teaching Patients Self-Care. If the patient is at home with a tracheostomy, the nurse instructs the patient and family about its daily care as well as measures to take in an emergency. The nurse also makes sure the patient and family are aware of community contacts for education and support needs. It is important for the

nurse to teach the patient and family strategies to prevent infection when performing tracheostomy care (McConnell, 2000).

Mechanical Ventilation

Mechanical ventilation may be required for a variety of reasons, including the need to control the patient's respirations during surgery or during treatment of severe head injury, to oxygenate the blood when the patient's ventilatory efforts are inadequate, and to rest the respiratory muscles. Many patients placed on a ventilator can breathe spontaneously, but the effort needed to do so may be exhausting.

A mechanical ventilator is a positive- or negative-pressure breathing device that can maintain ventilation and oxygen delivery for a prolonged period. Caring for a patient on mechanical ventilation has become an integral part of nursing care in critical care or general medical-surgical units, extended care facilities, and the home. Nurses, physicians, and respiratory therapists must understand each patient's specific pulmonary needs and work together to set realistic goals. Positive patient outcomes depend on an understanding of the principles of mechanical ventilation and the patient's care needs as well as open communication among members of the health care team about the goals of therapy, weaning plans, and the patient's tolerance of changes in ventilator settings.

INDICATIONS FOR MECHANICAL VENTILATION

If a patient has a continuous decrease in oxygenation (PaO_2), an increase in arterial carbon dioxide levels ($PaCO_2$), and a persistent acidosis (decreased pH), mechanical ventilation may be necessary. Conditions such as thoracic or abdominal surgery, drug overdose, neuromuscular disorders, inhalation injury, COPD, multiple trauma, shock, multisystem failure, and coma all may lead to respiratory failure and the need for mechanical ventilation. The criteria for mechanical ventilation (Chart 25-11) guide the decision to place a patient on a ventilator. A patient with apnea that is not readily reversible also is a candidate for mechanical ventilation.

CLASSIFICATION OF VENTILATORS

Several types of mechanical ventilators exist; they are classified according to the manner in which they support ventilation. The two general categories are negative-pressure and positive-pressure ventilators. The most common category in use today is the positive-pressure ventilator.

Negative-Pressure Ventilators

Negative-pressure ventilators exert a negative pressure on the external chest. Decreasing the intrathoracic pressure during inspiration allows air to flow into the lung, filling its volume. Physiologically, this type of assisted ventilation is similar to spontaneous ventilation. It is used mainly in chronic respiratory failure associated with neuromuscular conditions, such as poliomyelitis, muscular dystrophy, amyotrophic lateral sclerosis, and myasthenia gravis. It is inappropriate for the unstable or complex patient or the patient whose condition requires frequent ventilatory changes. Negative-pressure ventilators are simple to use and do not require intubation of the airway; consequently, they are especially adaptable for home use.

Chart 25-9 Care of the Patient With a Tracheostomy Tube

Nursing Intervention	Rationale
1. Gather the needed equipment, including sterile gloves, hydrogen peroxide, normal saline solution or sterile water, cotton-tipped applicators, dressing and twill tape (and the type of tube prescribed, if the tube is to be changed).	Everything needed to care for a tracheostomy should be readily on hand for the most effective care.
A cuffed tube (air injected into cuff) is required during mechanical ventilation. A low-pressure cuff is most commonly used.	A cuffed tube prevents air from leaking during positive-pressure ventilation and also prevents tracheal aspiration of gastric contents. An adequate seal is indicated by the disappearance of any air leakage from the mouth or tracheostomy or by the disappearance of the harsh, gurgling sound of air coming from the throat.
Patients requiring long-term use of a tracheostomy tube and who can breathe spontaneously commonly use an uncuffed, metal tube.	Low-pressure cuffs exert minimal pressure on the tracheal mucosa and thus reduce the danger of tracheal ulceration and stricture.
2. Provide patient and family instruction on the key points for tracheostomy care, beginning with how to inspect the tracheostomy dressing for moisture or drainage.	The tracheostomy dressing is changed as needed to keep the skin clean and dry. To prevent potential breakdown, moist or soiled dressings should not remain on the skin.
3. Perform hand hygiene.	Hand hygiene reduces bacteria on hands.
4. Explain procedure to patient and family as appropriate.	A patient with a tracheostomy is apprehensive and requires ongoing assurance and support.
5. Put on clean gloves; remove and discard the soiled dressing in a biohazard container.	Observing body substance isolation reduces cross-contamination from soiled dressings.
6. Prepare sterile supplies, including hydrogen peroxide, normal saline solution or sterile water, cotton-tipped applicators, dressing, and tape.	Having necessary supplies and equipment readily available allows the procedure to be completed efficiently.
7. Put on sterile gloves. (Some physicians approve clean technique for long-term tracheostomy patients in the home.)	Sterile equipment minimizes transmission of surface flora to the sterile respiratory tract. Clean technique may be used in the home because of decreased exposure to potential pathogens.
8. Cleanse the wound and the plate of the tracheostomy tube with sterile cotton-tipped applicators moistened with hydrogen peroxide. Rinse with sterile saline solution.	Hydrogen peroxide is effective in loosening crusted secretions. Rinsing prevents skin residue.
9. Soak inner cannula in peroxide and rinse with saline solution or replace with a new disposable inner cannula.	Soaking loosens and removes secretions from the inner lumen of the tracheostomy tube.
10. Remove soiled twill tape with clean tape, after the new tape is in place. Place clean twill tape in position to secure the tracheostomy tube by inserting one end of the tape through the side opening of the outer cannula. Take the tape around the back of the patient's neck and thread it through the opposite opening of the outer cannula. Bring both ends around so that they meet on one side of the neck. Tighten the tape until only two fingers can be comfortably inserted under it. Secure with a knot. For a new tracheostomy, two people should assist with tape changes.	This taping technique provides a double thickness of tape around the neck, which is needed because the tracheostomy tube can be dislodged by movement or by a forceful cough if left unsecured. A dislodged tracheostomy tube is difficult to reinsert, and respiratory distress may occur. Dislodgement of a new tracheostomy is a medical emergency.
11. Remove old tapes and discard in a biohazard container.	Tapes with old secretions may harbour bacteria.
12. Although some long-term tracheostomies with healed stomas may not require a dressing, other tracheostomies do. In such cases, use a sterile tracheostomy dressing, fitting it securely under the twill tapes and flange of tracheostomy tube so that the incision is covered, as shown below.	Healed tracheostomies with minimal secretions do not need a dressing. Dressings that will shred are not used around a tracheostomy because of the risk that pieces of material, lint, or thread may get into the tube, and eventually into the trachea, causing obstruction or abscess formation. Special dressings that do not have a tendency to shred are used.

A   B   C

(A) The cuff of the tracheostomy tube fits smoothly and snugly in the trachea in a way that promotes circulation but seals off the escape of secretions and air surrounding the tube. **(B)** For a dressing change, a 4 × 4-inch gauze pad may be folded (cutting would promote shredding, placing the patient at risk for aspiration) around the tracheostomy tube and **(C)** stabilized by slipping the neck tape ties through the neck plate slots of the tracheostomy tube. The ties may be fastened to the side of the neck to eliminate the discomfort of lying on the knot.

Chart 25-10 Performing Tracheal Suction

Equipment
- Suction catheters
- Gloves
- Goggles for eye protection
- Basin for sterile normal saline solution for irrigation
- Manual resuscitation bag with supplemental oxygen
- Suction source

Procedure
1. Explain the procedure to the patient before beginning and offer reassurance during suctioning; the patient may be apprehensive about choking and about an inability to communicate.
2. Begin by carrying out hand hygiene.
3. Turn on suction source (pressure should not exceed 120 mm Hg).
4. Open suction catheter kit.
5. Fill basin with sterile normal saline solution.
6. Ventilate the patient with manual resuscitation bag and high-flow oxygen.
7. Put sterile glove on dominant hand.
8. Pick up suction catheter in gloved hand and connect to suction.
9. Hyperoxygenate the patient's lungs for several deep breaths. Instill normal saline solution into airway *only* if there are thick, tenacious secretions.
10. Insert suction catheter at least as far as the end of the tube without applying suction, just far enough to stimulate the cough reflex.
11. Apply suction while withdrawing and gently rotating the catheter 360° (no longer than 10 to 15 seconds, because hypoxia and dysrhythmias may develop, leading to cardiac arrest).
12. Reoxygenate and inflate the patient's lungs for several breaths.
13. Repeat previous three steps until the airway is clear.
14. Rinse catheter in basin with sterile normal saline solution between suction attempts if necessary.
15. Suction oropharyngeal cavity after completing tracheal suctioning.
16. Rinse suction tubing.
17. Discard catheter, gloves, and basin appropriately.

There are several types of negative-pressure ventilators: iron lung, body wrap, and chest cuirass.

IRON LUNG (DRINKER RESPIRATOR TANK)

The iron lung is a negative-pressure chamber used for ventilation. It was used extensively during polio epidemics in the past and currently is used by polio survivors and patients with other neuromuscular disorders.

BODY WRAP (PNEUMOWRAP) AND CHEST CUIRASS (TORTOISE SHELL)

Both of these portable devices require a rigid cage or shell to create a negative-pressure chamber around the thorax and abdomen.

Because of problems with proper fit and system leaks, these types of ventilators are used only with carefully selected patients.

Positive-Pressure Ventilators

Positive-pressure ventilators inflate the lungs by exerting positive pressure on the airway, similar to a bellows mechanism, forcing the alveoli to expand during inspiration. Expiration occurs passively. Endotracheal intubation or tracheostomy is necessary in most cases. These ventilators are widely used in the hospital setting and are increasingly used in the home for patients with primary lung disease. There are three types of positive-pressure ventilators, which are classified by the method of ending the inspiratory phase of respiration: pressure-cycled, time-cycled, and

---

NURSING RESEARCH PROFILE 25-1

The Effect of Normal Saline Instillation Before Suctioning on Oxygenation Status

Kinloch, D. (1999). Instillation of normal saline during endotracheal suctioning: Effects on mixed venous oxygen saturation. *American Journal of Critical Care, 8*(4), 231–240.

Purpose
Although it has been suggested that instilling normal saline into an endotracheal tube before suctioning facilitates the removal of secretions, few studies have addressed this issue using in vivo measures of patients' oxygenation status. The purpose of this study was to determine if instillation of normal saline before endotracheal suctioning improves patients' oxygenation status.

Study Sample and Design
A descriptive, observational study design was used to investigate the effect of normal saline instillation (NSI) before endotracheal suctioning on mixed venous oxygen saturations. Thirty-five patients recovering from coronary artery bypass grafting were included in the study. The decision to instill normal saline into the endotracheal tube was made by the clinician caring for the patient. Patients were divided into NSI (n = 15) and non-NSI groups (n = 20). Patients in the NSI group received 5 mL of normal saline before endotracheal suctioning, and patients in the non-NSI group did not. A standardized suctioning protocol was used; other than NSI, suctioning procedures for both groups were identical. Baseline levels of mixed venous oxygenated

blood saturation ($S\bar{v}O_2$) levels were obtained through the use of a pulmonary artery catheter at 1-minute intervals for 5 minutes before the start of suctioning; the mean of these levels was considered the patient's baseline value. After suctioning, $S\bar{v}O_2$ levels were measured at 1-minute intervals until they returned to baseline levels.

Findings
The mean post-suctioning $S\bar{v}O_2$ level of the NSI group was significantly lower ($p = .007$) than that of the non-NSI group. Further, the NSI group took an average of 3.8 minutes longer to return to baseline $S\bar{v}O_2$ than the non-NSI group; this difference was statistically significant ($p = .05$).

Nursing Implications
The current standard of practice for nurses is to instill normal saline before suctioning, especially if the secretions are thick and tenacious. Although the findings of this study suggest that this practice should no longer be used, the issue needs further study with a larger sample and with randomization of patients to groups. The findings of this study are relevant to nurses caring for patients requiring endotracheal suctioning.

Chart 25-11 Indications for Mechanical Ventilation

PaO_2 < 50 mm Hg with FiO_2 > 0.60
PaO_2 > 50 mm Hg with pH < 7.25
Vital capacity < 2 times tidal volume
Negative inspiratory force < 25 cm H_2O
Respiratory rate > 35/min

volume-cycled. Another type of positive-pressure ventilator used for selected patients is noninvasive positive-pressure ventilation.

PRESSURE-CYCLED VENTILATORS

The pressure-cycled ventilator ends inspiration when a preset pressure has been reached. In other words, the ventilator cycles on, delivers a flow of air until it reaches a predetermined pressure, then cycles off. Its major limitation is that the volume of air or oxygen can vary as the patient's airway resistance or compliance changes. As a result, the tidal volume delivered may be inconsistent, possibly compromising ventilation. Consequently, in adults, pressure-cycled ventilators are intended only for short-term use. The most common type is the IPPB machine (see previous discussion of IPPB).

TIME-CYCLED VENTILATORS

Time-cycled ventilators terminate or control inspiration after a preset time. The volume of air the patient receives is regulated by the length of inspiration and the flow rate of the air. Most ventilators have a rate control that determines the respiratory rate, but pure time-cycling is rarely used for adults. These ventilators are used in newborns and infants.

VOLUME-CYCLED VENTILATORS

Volume-cycled ventilators are by far the most commonly used positive-pressure ventilators today (Fig. 25-6). With this type of ventilator, the volume of air to be delivered with each inspiration is preset. Once this preset volume is delivered to the patient, the ventilator cycles off and exhalation occurs passively. From breath to breath, the volume of air delivered by the ventilator is relatively constant, ensuring consistent, adequate breaths despite varying airway pressures.

NONINVASIVE POSITIVE-PRESSURE VENTILATION

Positive-pressure ventilation can be given via facemasks that cover the nose and mouth, nasal masks, or other nasal devices. This eliminates the need for endotracheal intubation or tracheostomy and decreases the risk for nosocomial infections such as pneumonia. The most comfortable mode for the patient is pressure-controlled ventilation with pressure support. This eases the work of breathing and enhances gas exchange. The ventilator can be set with a minimum backup rate for patients with periods of apnea.

Patients are considered candidates for noninvasive ventilation if they have acute or chronic respiratory failure, acute pulmonary edema, COPD, or chronic heart failure with a sleep-related breathing disorder. The device also may be used at home to improve tissue oxygenation and to rest the respiratory muscles while the patient sleeps at night. It is contraindicated for those who have experienced respiratory arrest, serious dysrhythmias, cognitive impairment, or head or facial trauma. Noninvasive ventilation may also be used for patients at the end of life and those who do not want endotracheal intubation but may need short- or long-term ventilatory support (Scanlan, Wilkins & Stoller, 1999).

Bilevel positive airway pressure (bi-PAP) ventilation offers independent control of inspiratory and expiratory pressures while providing pressure support ventilation. It delivers two levels of

A

B

FIGURE 25-6 Control panels of positive pressure ventilators in current use illustrate functions made possible by technologic advances. (**A**) Bear 1000 ventilator. Courtesy Bear Medical Systems. (**B**) Servo Ventilator 300 with Automode allows weaning to begin with the patient still intubated. Courtesy Siemens Medical Systems, Inc.

positive airway pressure provided via a nasal or oral mask, nasal pillow, or mouthpiece with a tight seal and a portable ventilator. Each inspiration can be initiated either by the patient or by the machine if it is programmed with a backup rate. The backup rate ensures that the patient will receive a set number of breaths per minute (Perkins & Shortall, 2000). Bi-PAP is most often used for patients who require ventilatory assistance at night, such as those with severe COPD or sleep apnea. Tolerance is variable; bi-PAP is usually most successful with highly motivated patients.

ADJUSTING THE VENTILATOR

The ventilator is adjusted so that the patient is comfortable and breathes "in sync" with the machine. Minimal alteration of the normal cardiovascular and pulmonary dynamics is desired. Modes of mechanical ventilation are described in Figure 25-7. If the volume ventilator is adjusted appropriately, the patient's arterial blood gas values will be satisfactory and there will be little or no cardiovascular compromise. Chart 25-12 discusses how to achieve adequate mechanical ventilation for each patient.

ASSESSING THE EQUIPMENT

The ventilator needs to be assessed to make sure that it is functioning properly and that the settings are appropriate. Even though the nurse is not primarily responsible for adjusting the settings on the ventilator or measuring ventilator parameters (usually the responsibility of the respiratory therapist), the nurse is responsible for the patient and therefore needs to evaluate how the ventilator affects the patient's overall status.

In monitoring the ventilator, the nurse should note the following:

- Type of ventilator (such as volume-cycled, pressure-cycled, negative-pressure)
- Controlling mode (such as **controlled ventilation, assist–control ventilation, synchronized intermittent mandatory ventilation**)
- Tidal volume and rate settings (tidal volume is usually 10 to 15 mL/kg; rate is usually 12 to 16/min)
- FiO_2 (**fraction of inspired oxygen**) setting

A CONTROLLED VENTILATION

A Flow in the controlled ventilation mode. A preset volume of gas is delivered to the patient under positive pressure while spontaneous patient respiratory effort is "locked out."

B ASSIST/CONTROLLED VENTILATION (A/C)

B Gas flow in the assist/control ventilation mode. In this mode, a preset volume of gas is delivered to the patient at a preset rate, but the patient may trigger a ventilator breath with negative inspiratory effort.

C SYNCHRONIZED INTERMITTENT MANDATORY VENTILATION (SIMV)

C Gas flow in the synchronized intermittent mandatory ventilation (SIMV) mode. A preset minimum number of breaths are synchronously delivered to the patient but the patient may also take spontaneous breaths of varying volumes. Note how inspiratory and expiratory pressures differ between spontaneous and ventilator breaths.

D POSITIVE END EXPIRATORY PRESSURE (PEEP)

D Airway pressure with varying levels of positive end-expiratory pressure (PEEP). Note that at end expiration, the airway is not allowed to return to zero. (FRC: functional residual capacity.)

E CONTINUOUS POSITIVE AIRWAY PRESSURE (CPAP)

E Spontaneous ventilation with continuous positive airway pressure (CPAP). This ventilatory adjunct is used only with spontaneous ventilation; the patient breathes spontaneously through the ventilator at an elevated baseline pressure throughout the breathing cycle.

F PRESSURE SUPPORT (PS)

F Spontaneous ventilation with pressure support (PS). The patient breathes spontaneously with pressure assistance to each spontaneous inspiration.

☐ Inspiration ▮ Exhalation ◆ Patient-triggered breath

FIGURE 25-7 Modes of mechanical ventilation with air flow waveforms.

Chart 25-12 · Initial Ventilator Settings

The following guide is an example of the steps involved in operating a mechanical ventilator. The nurse, in collaboration with the respiratory therapist, always reviews the manufacturer's instructions, which vary according to the equipment, before beginning mechanical ventilation.

1. Set the machine to deliver the tidal volume required (10 to 15 mL/kg).
2. Adjust the machine to deliver the lowest concentration of oxygen to maintain normal PaO_2 (80 to 100 mm Hg). This setting may be high initially but will gradually be reduced based on arterial blood gas results.
3. Record peak inspiratory pressure.
4. Set mode (assist–control or synchronized intermittent mandatory ventilation) and rate according to physician order. (See the glossary for definitions of modes of mechanical ventilation.) Set PEEP and pressure support if ordered.
5. Adjust sensitivity so that the patient can trigger the ventilator with a minimal effort (usually 2 mm Hg negative inspiratory force).
6. Record minute volume and measure carbon dioxide partial pressure (PCO_2), pH, and PO_2 after 20 minutes of continuous mechanical ventilation.
7. Adjust setting (FiO_2 and rate) according to results of arterial blood gas analysis to provide normal values or those set by the physician.
8. If the patient suddenly becomes confused or agitated or begins bucking the ventilator for some unexplained reason, assess for hypoxia and manually ventilate on 100% oxygen with a resuscitation bag.

- Inspiratory pressure reached and pressure limit (normal is 15 to 20 cm H_2O; this increases if there is increased airway resistance or decreased compliance)
- Sensitivity (a 2-cm H_2O inspiratory force should trigger the ventilator)
- Inspiratory-to-expiratory ratio (usually 1 : 3 [1 second of inspiration to 3 seconds of expiration] or 1 : 2)
- Minute volume (tidal volume × respiratory rate, usually 6 to 8 L/min)
- Sigh settings (usually 1.5 times the tidal volume and ranging from 1 to 3 per hour), if applicable
- Water in the tubing, disconnection or kinking of the tubing
- Humidification (humidifier filled with water) and temperature
- Alarms (turned on and functioning properly)
- PEEP and/or pressure support level, if applicable. PEEP is usually 5 to 15 cm H_2O

NURSING ALERT If the ventilator system malfunctions and the problem cannot be identified and corrected immediately, the nurse must ventilate the patient with a manual resuscitation bag until the problem is resolved.

PROBLEMS WITH MECHANICAL VENTILATION

Because of the seriousness of the patient's condition and the highly complex and technical nature of mechanical ventilation, a number of problems or complications can occur. Such situations fall into two categories: ventilator problems and patient problems. In either case, the patient must be supported while the problem is identified and corrected. Ventilator complications include cardiovascular compromise, pneumothorax, and pulmonary infection. These problems, their probable causes, and solutions are listed in Table 25-2.

BUCKING THE VENTILATOR

The patient is "in sync" with the ventilator when thoracic expansion coincides with the inspiratory phase of the machine and exhalation occurs passively. The patient is said to fight or buck the ventilator when out of phase with the machine. This is manifested when the patient attempts to breathe out during the ventilator's mechanical inspiratory phase or when there is jerky and increased abdominal muscle effort. The following factors contribute to this problem: anxiety, hypoxia, increased secretions, hypercapnia, inadequate minute volume, and pulmonary edema. These problems must be corrected before resorting to the use of paralyzing agents to reduce bucking; otherwise, the underlying problem is simply masked and the patient's condition will continue to deteriorate.

Muscle relaxants, tranquilizers, analgesic agents, and paralyzing agents are sometimes administered to patients receiving mechanical ventilation. Their purpose is ultimately to increase the patient–machine synchrony by decreasing the patient's anxiety, hyperventilation, or excessive muscle activity. The selection and dose of the appropriate medication are determined carefully and are based on the patient's requirements and the cause of his or her restlessness. Paralyzing agents are always used as a last resort, and always in conjunction with a sedative medication.

Nursing Management

PROMOTING HOME AND COMMUNITY-BASED CARE

Increasingly, patients are being cared for in extended care facilities or at home while on mechanical ventilators, with tracheostomy tubes, or on oxygen therapy. Patients receiving home ventilator care usually have chronic neuromuscular conditions or COPD.

Teaching Patients Self-Care. Caring for the patient with mechanical ventilator support at home can be accomplished successfully, but the family must be emotionally, educationally, and physically able to assume the role of primary caregiver. A home care team consisting of the nurse, physician, respiratory therapist, social service or home care agency, and equipment supplier is needed. The home is evaluated to determine if the electrical equipment needed can be operated safely. A summary of the basic assessment criteria needed for successful home care is presented in Chart 25-13.

Once the decision is made to initiate mechanical ventilation at home, the nurse prepares the patient and family for home care. It is important to teach them about the ventilator, suctioning, tracheostomy care, signs of pulmonary infection, cuff inflation and deflation, and assessment of vital signs. Teaching often begins in the hospital and continues at home. Nursing responsibilities include evaluating the patient's and family's understanding of the information presented.

The nurse teaches the family cardiopulmonary resuscitation, including mouth-to-tracheostomy tube (instead of mouth-to-mouth) breathing. The nurse also explains how to handle a power failure, which usually involves converting the ventilator from an electrical power source to a battery power source. Conversion is

Table 25-2 • Troubleshooting Ventilator Problems

PROBLEM	CAUSE	SOLUTION
Ventilator		
Increase in peak airway pressure	Coughing or plugged airway tube	Suction airway for secretions, empty condensation fluid from circuit.
	Patient "bucking" ventilator	Adjust sensitivity.
	Decreasing lung compliance	Manually ventilate patient.
		Assess for hypoxia or bronchospasm.
		Check arterial blood gas values.
		Sedate only if necessary.
	Tubing kinked	Check tubing; reposition patient; insert oral airway if necessary.
	Pneumothorax	Manually ventilate patient; notify physician.
	Atelectasis or bronchospasm	Clear secretions.
Decrease in pressure or loss of volume	Increase in compliance	None
	Leak in ventilator or tubing; cuff on tube/ humidifier not tight	Check entire ventilator circuit for patency.
		Correct leak.
Patient		
Cardiovascular compromise	Decrease in venous return due to application of positive pressure to lungs	Assess for adequate volume status by measuring heart rate, blood pressure, central venous pressure, pulmonary capillary wedge pressure, and urine output. Notify physician if values are abnormal.
Barotrauma/pneumothorax	Application of positive pressure to lungs; high mean airway pressures lead to alveolar rupture	Notify physician. Prepare patient for chest tube insertion. Avoid high pressure settings for patients with COPD, ARDS, or history of pneumothorax.
Pulmonary infection	Bypass of normal defense mechanisms; frequent breaks in ventilator circuit; decreased mobility; impaired cough reflex	Use meticulous aseptic technique. Provide frequent mouth care. Optimize nutritional status.

Chart 25-13 • ASSESSMENT

Criteria for Successful Home Ventilator Care

The decision to proceed with home ventilation therapy is usually based on the following parameters.

Patient Criteria
• The patient has chronic underlying pulmonary abnormalities.
• The patient's clinical pulmonary status is stable.
• The patient is willing to go home on mechanical ventilation.

Home Criteria
• The home environment is conducive to care of the patient.
• The electrical facilities are adequate to operate all equipment safely.
• The home environment is controlled, without drafts in cold weather and with proper ventilation in warm weather.
• Space is available for cleaning and storing ventilator equipment.

Family Criteria
• Family members are competent, dependable, and willing to spend the time required for proper training with available professional support.
• Family members understand the diagnosis and prognosis.
• Family has sufficient financial and supportive resources.

automatic in most types of home ventilators and lasts approximately 1 hour. The nurse instructs the family on using a manual self-inflation bag should it be necessary. Some of the patient's and family's responsibilities are listed in Chart 25-14.

Continuing Care. A home care nurse monitors and evaluates how well the patient and family are adapting to providing care in the home. The nurse also assesses the adequacy of ventilation and oxygenation as well as airway patency. The nurse addresses any unique adaptation problems the patient may have and listens to the patient's and family's anxieties and frustrations, offering support and encouragement where possible. The home care nurse helps identify and contact community resources that may assist in home management of the patient with mechanical ventilation.

The technical aspects of the ventilator are managed by vendor follow-up. A respiratory therapist usually is assigned to the patient and makes frequent home visits to evaluate the patient and perform a maintenance check of the ventilator.

Transportation services are identified should the patient require transportation in an emergency. These arrangements must be made before an emergency arises.

Providing the opportunity for ventilator-dependent patients to return home to live with their families in familiar surroundings can be a positive experience. The ultimate goal of home ventilator therapy is to enhance the patient's quality of life, not simply to support or prolong life.

> **Chart 25-14**
> **Home Care Checklist** • **Ventilator Care**
>
> *At the completion of the home care instruction, the patient or caregiver will be able to:*
>
> | | Patient | Caregiver |
> |---|---|---|
> | • State proper care of patient on ventilator | | |
> | Observe physical signs such as colour, secretions, breathing pattern, and state of consciousness. | | ✓ |
> | Perform physical care such as suctioning, postural drainage, and ambulation. | | ✓ |
> | Observe the tidal volume and pressure manometer regularly. Intervene when they are abnormal (ie, suction if airway pressure increases). | | ✓ |
> | Provide a communication method for the patient (eg, pad and pencil, electric larynx, talking tracheostomy). | | ✓ |
> | Monitor vital signs as directed. | | ✓ |
> | Indicate when feeling short of breath or in distress by a predetermined signal. | ✓ | |
> | • Care for and maintain equipment properly | | |
> | Check the ventilator settings twice each day and whenever the patient is removed from the ventilator. | | ✓ |
> | Adjust the volume and pressure alarms if needed. | | ✓ |
> | Fill humidifier as needed and check its level three times a day. | | ✓ |
> | Empty water in tubing as needed. | ✓ | ✓ |
> | Use a clean humidifier when circuitry is changed. | | ✓ |
> | Keep exterior of ventilator clean and free of any objects. | | ✓ |
> | Change external circuitry once a week or more often as indicated. | ✓ | ✓ |
> | Report malfunction or strange noises immediately | ✓ | ✓ |

NURSING PROCESS:
THE PATIENT ON A VENTILATOR

Assessment

The nurse has a vital role in assessing the patient's status and the functioning of the ventilator.

In assessing the patient, the nurse evaluates the patient's physiologic status and how he or she is coping with mechanical ventilation. Physical assessment includes systematic assessment of all body systems, with an in-depth focus on the respiratory system. Respiratory assessment includes vital signs, respiratory rate and pattern, breath sounds, evaluation of spontaneous ventilatory effort, and potential evidence of hypoxia. Increased adventitious breath sounds may indicate a need for suctioning. The nurse also evaluates the settings and functioning of the mechanical ventilator, as described previously.

Assessment also addresses the patient's neurologic status and effectiveness of coping with the need for assisted ventilation and the changes that accompany it. The nurse should assess the patient's comfort level and ability to communicate as well. Finally, weaning from mechanical ventilation requires adequate nutrition. Therefore, it is important to assess the function of the gastrointestinal system and nutritional status.

Diagnosis

NURSING DIAGNOSES
Based on the assessment data, the patient's major nursing diagnoses may include:

- Impaired gas exchange related to underlying illness, or ventilator setting adjustment during stabilization or weaning.
- Ineffective airway clearance related to increased mucus production associated with continuous positive-pressure mechanical ventilation
- Risk for trauma and infection related to endotracheal intubation or tracheostomy
- Impaired physical mobility related to ventilator dependency

- Impaired verbal communication related to endotracheal tube and attachment to ventilator
- Defensive coping and powerlessness related to ventilator dependency

COLLABORATIVE PROBLEMS/
POTENTIAL COMPLICATIONS
Based on assessment data, potential complications may include:

- Alterations in cardiac function
- Barotrauma (trauma to the alveoli) and pneumothorax
- Pulmonary infection
- Sepsis

Planning and Goals

The major goals for the patient may include achievement of optimal gas exchange, maintenance of a patent airway, absence of trauma or infection, attainment of optimal mobility, adjustment to nonverbal methods of communication, acquisition of successful coping measures, and absence of complications.

Nursing Interventions

Nursing care of the mechanically ventilated patient requires expert technical and interpersonal skills. Nursing interventions are similar regardless of the setting; however, the frequency of interventions and the stability of the patient vary from setting to setting. Nursing interventions for the mechanically ventilated patient are not uniquely different from other pulmonary patients, but astute nursing assessment and a therapeutic nurse–patient relationship are critical. The specific interventions used by the nurse are determined by the underlying disease process and the patient's response.

Two general nursing interventions important in the care of the mechanically ventilated patient are pulmonary auscultation and interpretation of arterial blood gas measurements. The nurse is often the first to note changes in physical assessment findings or significant trends in blood gases that signal the development of a serious problem (eg, pneumothorax, tube displacement, pulmonary embolus).

ENHANCING GAS EXCHANGE

The purpose of mechanical ventilation is to optimize gas exchange by maintaining alveolar ventilation and oxygen delivery. The alteration in gas exchange may be due to the underlying illness or to mechanical factors related to the adjustment of the machine to the patient. The health care team, including the nurse, physician, and respiratory therapist, continually assesses the patient for adequate gas exchange, signs and symptoms of hypoxia, and response to treatment. Thus, the nursing diagnosis impaired gas exchange is, by its complex nature, multidisciplinary and collaborative. The team members must share goals and information freely. All other goals directly or indirectly relate to this primary goal.

Nursing interventions to promote optimal gas exchange include judicious administration of analgesic agents to relieve pain without suppressing the respiratory drive and frequent repositioning to diminish the pulmonary effects of immobility. The nurse also monitors for adequate fluid balance by assessing for the presence of peripheral edema, calculating daily intake and output, and monitoring daily weights. The nurse administers medications prescribed to control the primary disease and monitors for their side effects.

PROMOTING EFFECTIVE AIRWAY CLEARANCE

Continuous positive-pressure ventilation increases the production of secretions regardless of the patient's underlying condition. The nurse assesses for the presence of secretions by lung auscultation at least every 2 to 4 hours. Measures to clear the airway of secretions include suctioning, chest physiotherapy, frequent position changes, and increased mobility as soon as possible. Frequency of suctioning should be determined by patient assessment. If excessive secretions are identified by inspection or auscultation techniques, suctioning should be performed. Sputum is not produced continuously or every 1 to 2 hours but as a response to a pathologic condition. Therefore, there is no rationale for routine suctioning of all patients every 1 to 2 hours. Although suctioning is used to aid in the clearance of secretions, it can damage the airway mucosa and impair cilia action (Scanlan, Wilkins & Stoller, 1999).

The sigh mechanism on the ventilator may be adjusted to deliver at least one to three sighs per hour at 1.5 times the tidal volume if the patient is on assist–control. Because of the risk of hyperventilation and trauma to pulmonary tissue from excess ventilator pressure (barotrauma, pneumothorax), this feature is not being used as frequently today. If the patient is on the synchronized intermittent mandatory ventilation (SIMV) mode, the mandatory ventilations act as sighs because they are of greater volume than the patient's spontaneous breaths. Periodic sighing prevents atelectasis and the further retention of secretions.

Humidification of the airway via the ventilator is maintained to help liquefy secretions so they are more easily removed. Bronchodilators are administered to dilate the bronchioles and are classified as adrenergic or anticholinergic. Adrenergic bronchodilators are mostly inhaled and work by stimulating the beta-receptor sites, mimicking the effects of epinephrine in the body. The desired effect is smooth muscle relaxation, thus dilating the constricted bronchial tubes. Medications include albuterol (Proventil, Ventolin), isoetharine (Bronkosol), isoproterenol (Isuprel), metaproterenol (Alupent, Metaprel), pirbuterol acetate (Maxair), salmeterol (Serevent), and terbutaline (Brethine, Brethaire, Bricanyl). Tachycardia, heart palpitations, and tremors are side effects that have been reported with use of these medications (Zang & Allender, 1999). Anticholinergic bronchodilators

such as ipratropium (Atrovent) and ipratropium with albuterol (Combivent) produce airway relaxation by blocking cholinergic-induced bronchoconstriction. Patients receiving bronchodilator therapy of either type should be monitored for adverse effects including dizziness, nausea, decreased oxygen saturation, hypokalemia, increased heart rate, and urine retention. Mucolytic agents such as acetylcysteine (Mucomyst) are administered as prescribed to liquefy secretions so that they are more easily mobilized. Nursing management of patients receiving mucolytic therapy includes assessment for an adequate cough reflex, sputum characteristics, and improvement in incentive spirometry (McKenry & Salerno, 2001). Side effects include nausea, vomiting, bronchospasm, stomatitis (oral ulcers), urticaria, and runny nose (LeFever & Hayes, 2000).

PREVENTING TRAUMA AND INFECTION

Airway management must involve maintaining the endotracheal or tracheostomy tube. The nurse positions the ventilator tubing so that there is minimal pulling or distortion of the tube in the trachea; this reduces the risk of trauma to the trachea. Cuff pressure is monitored every 8 hours to maintain the pressure at less than 25 cm H_2O. The nurse evaluates for the presence of a cuff leak at the same time.

Patients with endotracheal intubation or a tracheostomy tube do not have the normal defenses of the upper airway. In addition, these patients frequently have multiple additional body system disturbances that lead to immunocompromise. Tracheostomy care is performed at least every 8 hours, and more frequently if needed, because of the increased risk of infection. The ventilator circuit and in-line suction tubing is replaced periodically, according to infection control guidelines, to decrease the risk of infection.

The nurse administers oral hygiene frequently because the oral cavity is a primary source of contamination of the lungs in the intubated and compromised patient. The presence of a nasogastric tube in the intubated patient can increase the risk for aspiration, leading to nosocomial pneumonia. The nurse positions the patient with the head elevated above the stomach as much as possible. Antiulcer medications such as sucralfate (Carafate) are given to maintain normal gastric pH; research has demonstrated a lower incidence of aspiration pneumonia when sucralfate is administered (Scanlan, Wilkins & Stoller, 1999).

PROMOTING OPTIMAL LEVEL OF MOBILITY

The patient's mobility is limited because he or she is connected to the ventilator. The nurse should assist a patient whose condition has become stable to get out of bed and to a chair as soon as possible. Mobility and muscle activity are beneficial because they stimulate respirations and improve morale. If the patient cannot get out of bed, the nurse encourages the patient to perform active range-of-motion exercises every 6 to 8 hours. If the patient cannot perform these exercises, the nurse performs passive range-of-motion exercises every 8 hours to prevent contractures and venous stasis.

PROMOTING OPTIMAL COMMUNICATION

It is important to develop alternative methods of communication for the patient on a ventilator. The nurse assesses the patient's communication abilities to evaluate for limitations. Questions to consider when assessing the ventilator-dependent patient's ability to communicate include the following:

- Is the patient conscious and able to communicate? Can the patient nod or shake the head?

- Is the patient's mouth unobstructed by the tube so that words can be mouthed?
- Is the patient's hand strong and available for writing? (For example, if the patient is right-handed, the intravenous line is placed in the left arm if possible so that the right hand is free.)

Once the patient's limitations are known, the nurse offers several appropriate communication approaches: lip reading (use single key words), pad and pencil or Magic Slate, communication board, gesturing, or electric larynx. Use of a "talking" or fenestrated tracheostomy tube may be suggested to the physician; this allows the patient to talk while on the ventilator. If indicated, the nurse should make sure that the patient's eyeglasses and hearing aid and a translator are available to enhance the patient's ability to communicate.

The patient must be assisted to find the most suitable communication method. Some methods may be frustrating to the patient, family, and nurse; these need to be identified and minimized. A speech therapist can assist in determining the most appropriate method.

PROMOTING COPING ABILITY

Dependence on a ventilator is frightening to both the patient and family and disrupts even the most stable families. Encouraging the family to verbalize their feelings about the ventilator, the patient's condition, and the environment in general is beneficial. Explaining procedures every time they are performed helps to reduce anxiety and familiarizes the patient with ventilator procedures. To restore a sense of control, the nurse encourages the patient to participate in decisions about care, schedules, and treatment when possible. The patient may become withdrawn or depressed while on mechanical ventilation, especially if its use is prolonged. To promote effective coping, the nurse informs the patient about progress when appropriate. It is important to provide diversions such as watching television, playing music, or taking a walk (if appropriate and possible). Stress reduction techniques (eg, a backrub, relaxation measures) help relieve tension and help the patient to deal with anxieties and fears about both the condition and the dependence on the ventilator.

MONITORING AND MANAGING POTENTIAL COMPLICATIONS

Alterations in Cardiac Function

Alterations in cardiac output may occur as a result of positive-pressure ventilation. The positive intrathoracic pressure during inspiration compresses the heart and great vessels, thereby reducing venous return and cardiac output. This is usually corrected during exhalation when the positive pressure is off. Patients may have decreased cardiac output and resultant decreased tissue perfusion and oxygenation.

To evaluate cardiac function, the nurse first looks for signs and symptoms of hypoxia (restlessness, apprehension, confusion, tachycardia, tachypnea, laboured breathing, pallor progressing to cyanosis, diaphoresis, transient hypertension, and decreased urine output). If a pulmonary artery catheter is in place, cardiac output, cardiac index, and other hemodynamic values can be used to assess the patient's status.

Barotrauma and Pneumothorax

Excessive positive pressure may cause barotrauma, which results in a spontaneous pneumothorax. This may quickly develop into a tension pneumothorax, further compromising venous return,

cardiac output, and blood pressure. The nurse should consider any sudden onset of changes in oxygen saturation or respiratory distress to be a life-threatening emergency requiring immediate action.

Pulmonary Infection

The patient is at high risk for infection, as described above. The nurse should report fever or a change in the colour or odour of sputum to the physician for follow-up.

Evaluation

EXPECTED PATIENT OUTCOMES

Expected patient outcomes may include:

1. Exhibits adequate gas exchange, as evidenced by normal breath sounds, acceptable arterial blood gas levels, and vital signs
2. Demonstrates adequate ventilation with minimal mucus accumulation
3. Is free of injury or infection, as evidenced by normal temperature and white blood count
4. Is mobile within limits of ability
   a. Gets out of bed to chair, bears weight, or ambulates as soon as possible
   b. Performs range-of-motion exercises every 6 to 8 hours
5. Communicates effectively through written messages, gestures, or other communication strategies
6. Copes effectively
   a. Verbalizes fears and concerns about condition and equipment
   b. Participates in decision making when possible
   c. Uses stress reduction techniques when necessary
7. Absence of complications
   a. Absence of cardiac compromise, as evidenced by stable vital signs and adequate urine output
   b. Absence of pneumothorax, as evidenced by bilateral chest excursion, normal chest x-ray, and adequate oxygenation
   c. Absence of pulmonary infection, as evidenced by normal temperature, clear pulmonary secretions, and negative sputum cultures

WEANING THE PATIENT FROM THE VENTILATOR

Respiratory weaning, the process of withdrawing the patient from dependence on the ventilator, takes place in three stages: the patient is gradually removed from the ventilator, then from the tube, and finally from oxygen. Weaning from mechanical ventilation is performed at the earliest possible time consistent with patient safety. The decision must be made from a physiologic rather than from a mechanical viewpoint. A thorough understanding of the patient's clinical status is required in making this decision. Weaning is started when the patient is recovering from the acute stage of medical and surgical problems and when the cause of respiratory failure is sufficiently reversed.

Successful weaning involves collaboration among the physician, respiratory therapist, and nurse. Each health care provider must understand the scope and function of other team members in relation to patient weaning to conserve the patient's strength, use resources efficiently, and maximize successful outcomes.

NURSING RESEARCH PROFILE 25-2
Early Versus Late Tracheostomy Decannulation

Clini, E., Vitacca, M., Bianchi, L., Porta, R., & Ambrosino, N. (1999). Long-term tracheostomy in severe COPD patients weaned from mechanical ventilation. *Respiratory Care, 44*(4), 241–244.

Purpose
Patients with chronic obstructive pulmonary disease (COPD) who require mechanical ventilation for management of acute respiratory failure are at risk for relapse. It is not known if patients with spontaneous respirations would benefit from retaining a tracheostomy after discharge from the intensive care unit. This study was conducted to determine the effects of maintaining a tracheal cannula in spontaneously breathing patients following discharge.

Study Sample and Design
Investigators studied 20 patients with severe COPD who were undergoing weaning from mechanical ventilation. The researchers used a prospective, randomized, and controlled design to measure tracheal cannula use in two groups of patients: 10 patients had the tracheal cannula removed, and 10 did not. Breathing pattern, forced lung volumes, respiratory muscle strength, and arterial blood gases were evaluated in patients at hospital discharge and at 1, 3, and 6 months after discharge. Investigators measured breathing patterns and forced lung volumes with a portable spirometer and assessed respiratory muscle strength by measuring maximal inspiratory pressure. They also recorded number of hospital days, mortality rate, and number of new exacerbations requiring antibiotics.

Results
No significant differences were found between the two groups with regard to breathing patterns, forced lung volumes, respiratory strength, or arterial blood gases. In both groups, 2 of the 10 patients (20%) died due to respiratory causes. During the follow-up period, exacerbations were significantly greater in the patients with tracheostomies than in those whose tracheostomies had been removed ($p < .005$).

Nursing Implications
The findings of this study suggest that retaining a chronic tracheostomy following weaning from mechanical ventilation in patients with COPD is associated with a higher frequency of adverse events, including exacerbations requiring treatment with antibiotics. Although there were no significant findings with regard to breathing pattern, forced lung volumes, respiratory muscle strength, and arterial blood gases, the patient population was small, thus necessitating further study. The results suggest that clinics should consider early decannulation in COPD patients weaned from mechanical ventilation.

Criteria for Weaning

Careful assessment is required to determine whether the patient is ready to be removed from mechanical ventilation. If the patient is stable and showing signs of improvement or reversal of the disease or condition that caused the need for mechanical ventilation, weaning indices should be assessed. These indices include:

- Vital capacity: the amount of air expired after maximum inspiration. Used to assess the patient's ability to take deep breaths. Vital capacity should be 10 to 15 mL/kg to meet the criteria for weaning.
- Maximum inspiratory pressure (MIP): used to assess the patient's respiratory muscle strength. It is also known as negative inspiratory pressure and should be at least −20 cm H_2O.
- Tidal volume: volume of air that is inhaled or exhaled from the lungs during an effortless breath. It is normally 7 to 9 mL/kg.
- Minute ventilation: equal to the respiratory rate multiplied by tidal volume. Normal is about 6 L/min.
- Rapid/shallow breathing index: used to assess the breathing pattern and is calculated by dividing the respiratory rate by tidal volume. Patients with indices below 100 breaths/min/L are more likely to be successful at weaning.

Other measurements used to assess readiness for weaning include a PaO_2 of greater than 60 mm Hg with an FiO_2 of less than 40%. Stable vital signs and arterial blood gases are also important predictors of successful weaning. Once readiness has been determined, the nurse records baseline measurements of weaning indices to monitor progress (Cull & Inwood, 1999).

Patient Preparation

To maximize the chances of success of weaning, the nurse must consider the patient as a whole, taking into account factors that impair the delivery of oxygen and elimination of carbon dioxide as well as those that increase oxygen demand (sepsis, seizures, thyroid imbalances) or decrease the patient's overall strength (nutrition, neuromuscular disease). Adequate psychological preparation is necessary before and during the weaning process. Patients need to know what is expected of them during the procedure. They are often frightened by having to breathe on their own again and need reassurance that they are improving and are well enough to handle spontaneous breathing. The nurse explains what will happen during weaning and what role the patient will play in the procedure. The nurse emphasizes that someone will be with or near the patient at all times, and answers any questions simply and concisely. Proper preparation of the patient can reduce the weaning time.

Methods of Weaning

Considerable effort has been devoted to finding the best method of weaning from mechanical ventilation, but research has not established which method is best (Tasota & Dobbin, 2000). Success depends on the combination of adequate patient preparation, available equipment, and an interdisciplinary approach to solving patient problems (Chart 25-15). The most common weaning methods in use today are described below.

Assist–control may be used as the resting mode for patients undergoing weaning trials. This mode provides full ventilatory support by delivering a preset tidal volume and respiratory rate; if the patient takes a breath, the ventilator delivers the preset volume. The cycle does not adapt to the patient's spontaneous efforts. The nurse assesses patients being weaned on this mode for the following signs of distress: rapid shallow breathing, use of accessory muscles, reduced level of consciousness, increase in carbon dioxide levels, decrease in oxygen saturations, and tachycardia.

The patient on intermittent mandatory ventilation (IMV) can increase the respiratory rate, but each spontaneous breath receives only the tidal volume the patient generates. Mechanical breaths

Chart 25-15

GUIDELINES FOR Care of the Patient Being Weaned From Mechanical Ventilation

NURSING INTERVENTIONS	RATIONALE

1. Assess patient for weaning criteria: Vital capacity—10 to 15 mL/kg
  Maximum inspiratory pressure (MIP) at least –20 cm H_2O
  Tidal volume—7 to 9 mL/kg
  Minute ventilation—6 L/min
  Rapid/shallow breathing index—below 100 breaths/minute/L
  PaO_2 greater than 60 mm Hg with FiO_2 less than 40%
	1. Careful assessment of multiple weaning indices helps to determine readiness for weaning. When the criteria have been met, the patient's likelihood of successful weaning increases.

2. Monitor activity level, assess dietary intake, and monitor results of laboratory tests of nutritional status.	2. Reestablishing independent spontaneous ventilation can be physically exhausting. It is crucial that the patient have enough energy reserves to succeed. Providing periods of rest and recommended nutritional intake can increase the likelihood of successful weaning.
3. Assess the patient's and family's understanding of the weaning process and address any concerns about the process. Explain that the patient may feel short of breath initially and provide encouragement as needed. Reassure the patient that he or she will be attended closely and that if the weaning attempt is not successful, it can be tried again later.	3. The weaning process can be psychologically tiring; emotional support can help promote a sense of security. Explaining that weaning will be attempted again later helps reduce the sense of failure if the first attempts are unsuccessful.
4. Implement the weaning method prescribed: A/C, IMV, SIMV, PSV, PAV, CPAP, or T-piece.	4. The prescribed weaning method should reflect the patient's individualized criteria for weaning and weaning history. By having different methods to choose from, the physician can select the one that best fits the patient.
5. Monitor vital signs, pulse oximetry, ECG, and respiratory pattern constantly for the first 20 to 30 minutes and every 5 minutes after that until weaning is complete.	5. Monitoring the patient closely provides ongoing indications of success or failure.
6. Maintain a patent airway; monitor arterial blood gas levels and pulmonary function tests. Suction the airway as needed.	6. These values can be compared to baseline measurements to evaluate weaning. Suctioning helps to reduce the risk of aspiration and maintain the airway.
7. In collaboration with the physician, terminate the weaning process if adverse reactions occur. These include a heart rate increase of 20 beats/min, systolic blood pressure increase of 20 mm Hg, a decrease in oxygen saturation to less than 90%, respiratory rate less than 8 or greater than 20 breaths/minute, ventricular dysrhythmias, fatigue, panic, cyanosis, erratic or laboured breathing, paradoxical chest movement.	7. These signs and symptoms indicate an unstable patient at risk for hypoxia and ventricular dysrhythmias. Continuing the weaning process can lead to cardiopulmonary arrest.
8. If the weaning process continues, measure tidal volume and minute ventilation every 20 to 30 minutes; compare with the patient's desired values, which have been determined in collaboration with the physician.	8. These values help to determine if weaning is successful and should be continued.
9. Assess for psychological dependence if the physiologic parameters indicate weaning is feasible and the patient still resists.	9. Psychological dependence is a common problem after mechanical ventilation. Possible causes include fear of dying and depression from chronic illness. It is important to address this issue before the next weaning attempt.

are delivered at preset intervals and a preselected tidal volume, regardless of the patient's efforts. IMV allows patients to use their own muscles of ventilation to help prevent muscle atrophy. IMV lowers mean airway pressure, which can assist in preventing barotrauma.

Synchronized intermittent mandatory ventilation (SIMV) delivers a preset tidal volume and number of breaths per minute. Between ventilator-delivered breaths, the patient can breathe spontaneously with no assistance from the ventilator on those extra breaths. As the patient's ability to breathe spontaneously increases, the preset number of ventilator breaths is decreased and the patient does more of the work of breathing. SIMV is indicated if the patient satisfies all the criteria for weaning but cannot sustain adequate spontaneous ventilation for long periods.

IMV and SIMV can be used to provide full or partial ventilatory support. Nursing interventions for both of these include

monitoring progress by recording respiratory rate, minute volume, spontaneous and machine-generated tidal volume, FiO_2, and arterial blood gas levels.

The **pressure support ventilation** (PSV) mode assists SIMV by applying a pressure plateau to the airway throughout the patient-triggered inspiration to decrease resistance by the tracheal tube and ventilator tubing. Pressure support is reduced gradually as the patient's strength increases. A SIMV backup rate may be added for extra support. The nurse must closely observe the patient's respiratory rate and tidal volumes on initiation of PSV. It may be necessary to adjust the pressure support to avoid tachypnea or large tidal volumes.

The proportional assist ventilation (PAV) mode of partial ventilatory support allows the ventilator to generate pressure in proportion to the patient's efforts. With every breath, the ventilator synchronizes with the patient's ventilatory efforts (Giannouli,

Webster, Roberts & Younes, 1999). Nursing assessment should include careful monitoring of the patient's respiratory rate, arterial blood gases, tidal volume, minute ventilation, and breathing pattern.

The continuous positive airway pressure (CPAP) mode allows the patient to breathe spontaneously, while applying positive pressure throughout the respiratory cycle to keep the alveoli open and promote oxygenation. Providing CPAP during spontaneous breathing also offers the advantage of an alarm system and may reduce patient anxiety if the patient has been taught that the machine is keeping track of breathing. It also maintains lung volumes and improves the patient's oxygenation status. CPAP is often used in conjunction with PSV. Nurses should carefully assess for tachypnea, tachycardia, reduced tidal volumes, decreasing oxygen saturations, and increasing carbon dioxide levels.

Weaning trials using a T-piece or tracheostomy mask (see Fig. 25-2) are normally conducted with the patient disconnected from the ventilator, receiving humidified oxygen only, and performing all work of breathing. Patients who do not have to overcome the resistance of the ventilator may find this mode more comfortable, or they may become anxious as they breathe with no support from the ventilator. During T-piece trials, the nurse monitors the patient closely and provides encouragement. This method of weaning is usually used when the patient is awake and alert, is breathing without difficulty, has good gag and cough reflexes, and is hemodynamically stable. During the weaning process, the patient is maintained on the same or a higher oxygen concentration than when on the ventilator. While on the T-piece, the patient should be observed for signs and symptoms of hypoxia, increasing respiratory muscle fatigue, or systemic fatigue. These include restlessness, increased respiratory rate greater than 35 breaths/min, use of accessory muscles, tachycardia with premature ventricular contractions, and paradoxical chest movement (asynchronous breathing, chest contraction during inspiration and expansion during expiration). Fatigue or exhaustion is initially manifested by an increased respiratory rate associated with a gradual reduction in tidal volume; later there is a slowing of the respiratory rate.

If the patient appears to be tolerating the T-piece trial, a second set of arterial blood gas measurements is drawn 20 minutes after the patient has been on spontaneous ventilation at a constant FiO_2 pressure support ventilation. (Alveolar–arterial equilibration takes 15 to 20 minutes to occur.)

Signs of exhaustion and hypoxia correlated with deterioration in the blood gas measurements indicate the need for ventilatory support. The patient is placed back on the ventilator each time signs of fatigue or deterioration develop.

If clinically stable, the patient usually can be extubated within 2 or 3 hours of weaning and allowed spontaneous ventilation by means of a mask with humidified oxygen. Patients who have had prolonged ventilatory assistance usually require more gradual weaning; it may take days or even weeks. They are weaned primarily during the day and placed back on the ventilator at night to rest.

Because patients respond in different manners to the various weaning methods, there is no definitive way to assess which method is best. With all of the methods, ongoing assessment of respiratory status is essential to monitor patient progress (Woodruff, 1999).

Successful weaning from the ventilator is supplemented by intensive pulmonary care. The following are continued:

- Oxygen therapy
- Arterial blood gas evaluation

- Pulse oximetry
- Bronchodilator therapy
- Chest physiotherapy
- Adequate nutrition, hydration, and humidification
- Incentive spirometry

These patients still have borderline pulmonary function and need vigorous supportive therapy before their respiratory status returns to a level that supports activities of daily living.

Weaning From the Tube

Weaning from the tube is considered when the patient can breathe spontaneously, maintain an adequate airway by effectively coughing up secretions, swallow, and move the jaw. If frequent suctioning is needed to clear secretions, tube weaning may be unsuccessful (Ecklund, 1999). Secretion clearance and aspiration risks are assessed to determine if active pharyngeal and laryngeal reflexes are intact.

Once the patient can clear secretions adequately, a trial period of mouth breathing or nose breathing is conducted. This can be accomplished by several methods. The first method requires changing to a smaller size tube to increase the resistance to airflow and simultaneously plugging the tracheostomy tube (deflating the cuff). The smaller tube is sometimes replaced by a cuffless tracheostomy tube, which allows the tube to be plugged at lengthening intervals to monitor patient progress. A second method involves changing to a fenestrated tube (a tube with an opening or window in its bend). This permits air to flow around and through the tube to the upper airway and enables talking. A third method involves switching to a smaller tracheostomy button (stoma button). A tracheostomy button is a plastic tube approximately 2.54 cm long that helps to keep the windpipe open after the larger tracheostomy tube has been removed. Finally, when the patient demonstrates the ability to maintain a patent airway without a tracheostomy tube, the tube can be removed. An occlusive dressing is placed over the stoma, which usually heals anywhere from several days to many weeks (Ecklund, 1999).

Weaning From Oxygen

The patient who has been successfully weaned from the ventilator, cuff, and tube and has adequate respiratory function is then weaned from oxygen. The FiO_2 is gradually reduced until the PaO_2 is in the range of 70 to 100 mm Hg while the patient is breathing room air. If the PaO_2 is less than 70 mm Hg on room air, supplemental oxygen is recommended. The Centers for Medicare and Medicaid Services, formerly the Health Care Financing Administration (HCFA), requires that the patient's PaO_2 on room air be less than 55 mm Hg for the patient to be eligible for financial reimbursement for in-home oxygen.

Nutrition

Success in weaning the long-term ventilator-dependent patient requires early and aggressive but judicious nutritional support. The respiratory muscles (diaphragm and especially intercostals) become weak or atrophied after just a few days of mechanical ventilation, especially if nutrition is inadequate. Fat kilocalories produce less carbon dioxide than carbohydrate kilocalories. For this reason, a high-fat diet may assist patients with respiratory failure who are being weaned from mechanical ventilation. Research is being conducted on the role of fatty acids in lung disease (Schwartz,

2000). A high-fat diet may provide as much as 50% of the total daily kilocalories. Adequate protein intake is important in increasing respiratory muscle strength. Protein intake should be approximately 25% of total daily kilocalories, or 1.2 to 1.5 g/kg/day. Because a high-carbohydrate diet can lead to increased carbon dioxide production and retention, total carbohydrate intake should not exceed 25% of total daily kilocalories, or 2 g/kg/day in patients being weaned from mechanical ventilation. Care must be taken not to overfeed patients because excessive intake can raise the demand for oxygen and the production of carbon dioxide. Total daily kilocalories should be closely monitored (Lutz & Przytulski, 2001).

Soon after the patient is admitted, a consultation with a dietitian or nutrition support team should be arranged to plan the best form of nutritional replacement. Adequate nutrition may decrease the duration of mechanical ventilation and prevent other complications, especially sepsis. Sepsis can occur if bacteria enter the bloodstream and release toxins that, in turn, cause vasodilation and hypotension, fever, tachycardia, increased respiratory rate, and coma. Aggressive treatment of sepsis is essential to reverse this threat to survival and to promote weaning from the ventilator when the patient's condition improves. Optimal nutritional intake is an essential part of the treatment of sepsis.

The Patient Undergoing Thoracic Surgery

Assessment and management are particularly important in the patient undergoing thoracic surgery. Frequently, patients undergoing such surgery also have obstructive pulmonary disease with compromised breathing. Preoperative preparation and careful postoperative management are crucial for successful patient outcomes because these patients may have a narrow range between their physical tolerance for certain activities and their limitations, which, if exceeded, can lead to distress. Various types of thoracic surgical procedures are performed to relieve disease conditions such as lung abscesses, lung cancer, cysts, and benign tumours (Chart 25-16). An exploratory **thoracotomy** (creation of a surgical opening into the thoracic cavity) may be performed to diagnose lung or chest disease. A biopsy may be performed in this procedure with a small amount of lung tissue removed for analysis; the chest incision is then closed.

The objectives of preoperative care for the patient undergoing thoracic surgery are to ascertain the patient's functional reserve to determine if the patient can survive the surgery and to ensure that the patient is in optimal condition for surgery.

PREOPERATIVE MANAGEMENT
Assessment and Diagnostic Findings

The nurse performs chest auscultation to assess breath sounds in the different regions of the lungs (see Chap. 21). It is important to note if breath sounds are normal, indicating a free flow of air in and out of the lungs. (In the patient with emphysema, the breath sounds may be markedly decreased or even absent on auscultation.) The nurse notes crackles and wheezes and assesses for hyperresonance and decreased diaphragmatic motion. Unilateral diminished breath sounds and rhonchi can be the result of occlusion of the bronchi by mucus plugs. The nurse assesses for retained secretions during auscultation by asking the patient to cough. It is important to note any signs of rhonchi or wheezing.

The patient history and assessment should include the following questions:

- What signs and symptoms are present (cough, sputum expectorated [amount and colour], hemoptysis, chest pain, dyspnea)?
- If there is a smoking history, how long has the patient smoked? Does the patient smoke currently? How many packs a day?
- What is the patient's cardiopulmonary tolerance while resting, eating, bathing, and walking?
- What is the patient's breathing pattern? How much exertion is required to produce dyspnea?
- Does the patient need to sleep in an upright position or with more than two pillows?
- What is the patient's physiologic status (eg, general appearance, mental alertness, behaviour, nutritional status)?
- What other medical conditions exist (eg, allergies, cardiac disorders, diabetes)?

A number of tests are performed to determine the patient's preoperative status and to assess the patient's physical assets and limitations. Many patients are seen by their surgeons in the office, and many tests and examinations are performed on an outpatient basis. The decision to perform any pulmonary resection is based on the patient's cardiovascular status and pulmonary reserve. Pulmonary function studies (especially lung volume and vital capacity) are performed to determine whether the planned resection will leave sufficient functioning lung tissue. Arterial blood gas values are assessed to provide a more complete picture of the functional capacity of the lung. Exercise tolerance tests are useful to determine if the patient who is a candidate for pneumonectomy can tolerate removal of one of the lungs.

Preoperative studies are performed to provide a baseline for comparison during the postoperative period and to detect any unsuspected abnormalities. These studies may include a bronchoscopic examination (a lighted scope is inserted into the airways to examine the bronchi), chest x-ray, electrocardiogram (for arteriosclerotic heart disease, conduction defects), nutritional assessment, determination of blood urea nitrogen and serum creatinine (renal function), glucose tolerance or blood glucose (diabetes), assessment of serum electrolytes and protein levels, blood volume determinations, and complete blood cell count.

PREOPERATIVE NURSING MANAGEMENT
Improving Airway Clearance

The underlying lung condition often is associated with increased respiratory secretions. Before surgery, the airway is cleared of secretions to reduce the possibility of postoperative atelectasis or infection. Risk factors for postoperative atelectasis and pneumonia are listed in Chart 25-17. Strategies to reduce the risk for atelectasis and infection include humidification, postural drainage, and chest percussion after bronchodilators are administered, if prescribed. The nurse estimates the volume of sputum if the patient expectorates large amounts of secretions. Such measurements are carried out to determine if and when the amount decreases. Antibiotics are administered as prescribed for infection, which may be causing the excessive secretions.

Chart 25-16 | Thoracic Surgeries and Procedures

Pneumonectomy

The removal of an entire lung (pneumonectomy) is performed chiefly for cancer when the lesion cannot be removed by a less extensive procedure. It also may be performed for lung abscesses, bronchiectasis, or extensive unilateral tuberculosis. The removal of the right lung is more dangerous than the removal of the left, because the right lung has a larger vascular bed and its removal imposes a greater physiologic burden.

A posterolateral or anterolateral thoracotomy incision is made, sometimes with resection of a rib. The pulmonary artery and the pulmonary veins are ligated and severed. The main bronchus is divided and the lung removed. The bronchial stump is stapled, and usually no drains are used because the accumulation of fluid in the empty hemithorax prevents mediastinal shift.

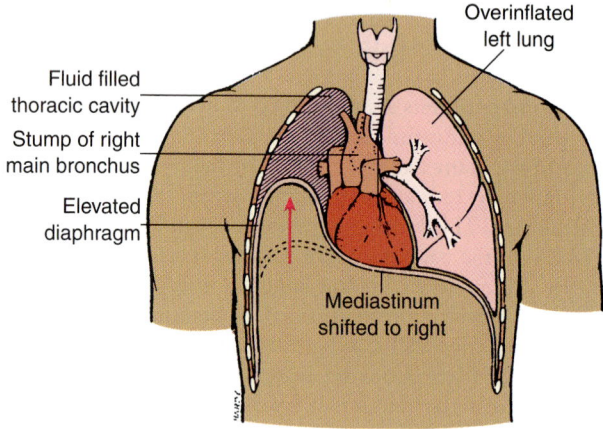

Pneumonectomy

Lobectomy

When the pathology is limited to one area of a lung, a lobectomy (removal of a lobe of a lung) is performed. Lobectomy, which is more common than pneumonectomy, may be carried out for bronchogenic carcinoma, giant emphysematous blebs or bullae, benign tumours, metastatic malignant tumours, bronchiectasis, and fungus infections.

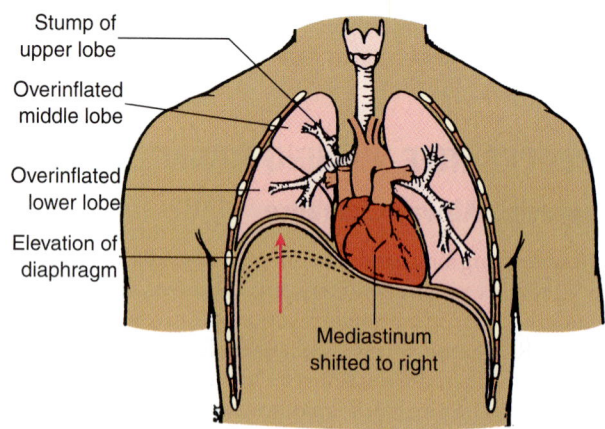

Lobectomy

The surgeon makes a thoracotomy incision: its exact location depends on the lobe to be resected. When the pleural space is entered, the involved lung collapses and the lobar vessels and the bronchus are ligated and divided. After the lobe is removed, the remaining lobes of the lung are reexpanded. Usually, two chest catheters are inserted for drainage. The upper tube is for air removal; the lower one is for fluid drainage. Sometimes, only one catheter is needed. The chest tube is connected to a chest drainage apparatus for several days.

Segmentectomy (Segmental Resection)

Some lesions are located in only one segment of the lung. Bronchopulmonary segments are subdivisions of the lung that function as individual units. They are held together by delicate connective tissue. Disease processes may be limited to a single segment. Care is used to preserve as much healthy and functional lung tissue as possible, especially in patients who already have limited cardiopulmonary reserve. Single segments can be removed from any lobe; the right middle lobe, which has only two small segments, invariably is removed entirely. On the left side, corresponding to a middle lobe, is a "lingular" segment of the upper lobe. This can be removed as a single segment or by lingulectomy. This segment frequently is involved in bronchiectasis.

Wedge Resection

A wedge resection of a small, well-circumscribed lesion may be performed without regard for the location of the intersegmental planes. The pleural cavity usually is drained because of the possibility of an air or blood leak. This procedure is performed for diagnostic lung biopsy and for the excision of small peripheral nodules.

Bronchoplastic or Sleeve Resection

Bronchoplastic resection is a procedure in which only one lobar bronchus, together with a part of the right or left bronchus, is excised. The distal bronchus is reanastomosed to the proximal bronchus or trachea.

Lung Volume Reduction

Lung volume reduction is a surgical procedure involving the removal of 20% to 30% of a patient's lung through a midsternal incision or video thoracoscopy. The diseased lung tissue is identified on a lung perfusion scan. Although some patients with chronic obstructive pulmonary disease have reported an improvement in the quality of their lives for at least 6 months to 1 year after the surgery, results have generally been disappointing. Research is ongoing to examine the benefits of lung volume reduction surgery using video thoracoscopy (Baker & Flynn, 1999; National Institutes of Health, 2001).

Video Thoracoscopy

A video thoracoscopy is an endoscopic procedure that allows the surgeon to look into the thorax without making a large incision. The procedure is performed to obtain specimens of tissue for biopsy, to treat recurrent spontaneous pneumothorax, and to diagnose either pleural effusions or pleural masses. Thoracoscopy has also been found to be an effective diagnostic and therapeutic alternative for the treatment of mediastinal disorders (Cirino et al., 2000). Some advantages of video thoracoscopy include rapid diagnosis and treatment of some conditions, a decrease in postoperative complications, and a shortened hospital stay (see Chap. 21).

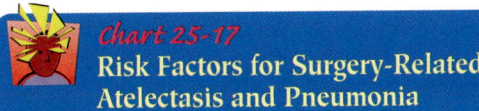

Chart 25-17
Risk Factors for Surgery-Related Atelectasis and Pneumonia

Preoperative Risk Factors
Increased age
Obesity
Poor nutritional status
Smoking history
Abnormal pulmonary function tests
Preexisting lung disease
Emergency surgery
History of aspiration
Comorbid states
Preexisting disability

Intraoperative Risk Factors
Thoracic incision
Prolonged anesthesia

Postoperative Risk Factors
Immobilization
Supine position
Decreased level of consciousness
Inadequate pain management
Prolonged intubation/mechanical ventilation
Presence of nasogastric tube
Inadequate preoperative education

Teaching the Patient

Increasingly, patients are admitted on the day of surgery, which does not provide much time for the acute care nurse to talk with the patient. Nurses in all settings must take an active role in educating the patient and relieving anxiety. The nurse informs the patient what to expect, from administration of anesthesia to thoracotomy and the likely use of chest tubes and a drainage system in the postoperative period. The patient is also informed about the usual postoperative administration of oxygen to facilitate breathing, and the possible use of a ventilator. It is essential to explain the importance of frequent turning to promote drainage of lung secretions. Instruction in the use of incentive spirometry begins before surgery to familiarize the patient with its correct use. The nurse should teach diaphragmatic and pursed-lip breathing, and the patient should begin practicing these techniques (see Chart 25-3, "Breathing Exercises," and Chart 25-4, "Assisting the Patient to Perform Incentive Spirometry").

Because a coughing schedule will be necessary in the postoperative period to promote the clearance or removal of secretions, the nurse instructs the patient in the technique of coughing and warns the patient that the coughing routine may be uncomfortable. The nurse teaches the patient to splint the incision with the hands, a pillow, or a folded towel (see Chart 25-5).

Another technique, "huffing," may be helpful for the patient with diminished expiratory flow rates or for the patient who refuses to cough because of severe pain. Huffing is the expulsion of air through an open glottis. This type of forced expiration technique (FET) stimulates pulmonary expansion and assists in alveolar inflation. The nurse instructs the patient as follows:

- Take a deep diaphragmatic breath and exhale forcefully against your hand in a quick, distinct pant, or huff.
- Practice doing small huffs and progress to one strong huff during exhalation.

Patients should be informed preoperatively that blood and other fluids may be administered, oxygen will be administered, and vital signs will be checked often for several hours after surgery. If a chest tube is needed, the patient should be informed that it will drain the fluid and air that normally accumulate after chest surgery. The patient and family are informed that the patient may be admitted to the intensive care unit for 1 to 2 days after surgery, that the patient may experience pain at the incision site, and that medication is available to relieve pain and discomfort (Finkelmeier, 2000).

Relieving Anxiety

The nurse listens to the patient to evaluate his or her feelings about the illness and proposed treatment. The nurse also determines the patient's motivation to return to normal or baseline function. The patient may reveal significant concerns: fear of hemorrhage because of bloody sputum, fear of discomfort from a chronic cough and chest pain, fear of ventilator dependence, or fear of death because of dyspnea and the underlying disease (eg, tumour).

The nurse helps the patient to overcome these fears and to cope with the stress of surgery by correcting any misconceptions, supporting the patient's decision to undergo surgery, reassuring the patient that the incision will "hold," and dealing honestly with questions about pain and discomfort and their treatment. The management and control of pain begin before surgery, when the nurse informs the patient that many postoperative problems can be overcome by following certain routines related to deep breathing, coughing, turning, and moving. If patient-controlled analgesia or epidural analgesia is to be used after surgery, the nurse instructs the patient in its use.

POSTOPERATIVE MANAGEMENT

After surgery the vital signs are checked frequently. Oxygen is administered by a mechanical ventilator, nasal cannula, or mask for as long as necessary. A reduction in lung capacity requires a period of physiologic adjustment, and fluids may be given at a low hourly rate to prevent fluid overload and pulmonary edema. When the patient is conscious and the vital signs have stabilized, the head of the bed may be elevated 30 to 45 degrees. Careful positioning of the patient is important. Following pneumonectomy, a patient is usually turned every hour from the back to the operative side and should not be completely turned to the unoperated side. This allows the fluid left in the space to consolidate and prevents the remaining lung and the heart from shifting (mediastinal shift) toward the operative side. The patient with a lobectomy may be turned to either side, and a patient with a segmental resection usually is not turned onto the operative side unless the surgeon prescribes this position (Finkelmeier, 2000).

Medication for pain is needed for several days after surgery. Because coughing can be painful, patients should be taught to splint the chest. Exercises are resumed early in the postoperative period to facilitate lung ventilation. The nurse assesses for signs of complications, including cyanosis, dyspnea, and acute chest pain. These may indicate atelectasis and should be reported immediately. Increased temperature or white blood cell count may indicate an infection, and pallor and increased pulse may indicate internal hemorrhage. Dressings should be assessed for fresh bleeding.

Mechanical Ventilation

Depending on the nature of the surgery, the patient's underlying condition, the intraoperative course, and the depth of anesthesia, the patient may require mechanical ventilation after surgery. The physician is responsible for determining the ventilator settings and modes, as well as determining the overall method and pace of weaning. However, the physician, nurse, and respiratory therapist work together closely to assess the patient's tolerance and weaning progress. Early extubation from mechanical ventilation can also lead to earlier removal of arterial lines (Zevola & Maier, 1999).

Chest Drainage

A crucial intervention for improving gas exchange and breathing in the postoperative period is the proper management of chest drainage and the **chest drainage system**. After thoracic surgery, chest tubes and a closed drainage system are used to re-expand the involved lung and to remove excess air, fluid, and blood. Chest

drainage systems also are used in treatment of spontaneous pneumothorax and trauma resulting in pneumothorax. Table 25-3 describes and compares the main features of these systems. Management of chest drainage systems is explained in Chart 25-18. Prevention of cardiopulmonary complications following thoracic surgery is discussed in Chart 25-19.

The normal breathing mechanism operates on the principle of negative pressure; that is, the pressure in the chest cavity normally is lower than the pressure of the atmosphere, causing air to move into the lungs during inspiration. Whenever the chest is opened, there is a loss of negative pressure, which can result in the collapse of the lung. The collection of air, fluid, or other substances in the chest can compromise cardiopulmonary function and can also cause the lung to collapse. Pathologic substances that collect in the pleural space include fibrin, or clotted blood; liquids (serous fluids, blood, pus, chyle); and gases (air from the lung, tracheobronchial tree, or esophagus).

Chest tubes may be inserted to drain fluid or air from any of the three compartments of the thorax (the right and left pleural spaces and the mediastinum). The pleural space, located between the visceral and parietal pleura, normally contains 20 mL or less of fluid, which helps to lubricate the visceral and parietal pleura. Surgical incision of the chest wall almost always causes some degree of pneumothorax (air accumulating in the pleural space) or hemothorax (build-up of serous fluid or blood in the pleural space). Air and fluid collect in the pleural space, restricting lung expansion and reducing gas exchange. Placement of a chest tube in the pleural space restores the negative intrathoracic pressure needed for lung re-expansion following surgery or trauma.

Table 25-3 • Comparison of Chest Drainage Systems

TYPES OF CHEST DRAINAGE SYSTEMS	DESCRIPTION	COMMENTS
Traditional Water Seal Also referred to as wet suction	Has 3 chambers: a collection chamber, water seal chamber (middle chamber), and wet suction control chamber	Requires that sterile fluid be instilled into water seal and suction chambers Has positive- and negative-pressure release valves Intermittent bubbling indicates that the system is functioning properly Additional suction can be added by connecting system to a suction source
Dry Suction Water Seal Also referred to as dry suction	Has 3 chambers: a collection chamber, water seal chamber (middle chamber), and wet suction control chamber	Requires that sterile fluid be instilled in water seal chamber at 2-cm level No need to fill suction chamber with fluid Suction pressure is set with a regulator Has positive- and negative-pressure release valves Has an indicator to signify that the suction pressure is adequate Quieter than traditional water seal systems
Dry Suction Also referred to as one-way valve system	Has a one-way mechanical valve that allows air to leave the chest and prevents air from moving back into the chest	No need to fill suction chamber with fluid; thus, can be set up quickly in an emergency Works even if knocked over, making it ideal for patients who are ambulatory

Chart 25-18

GUIDELINES FOR Managing Chest Drainage Systems

NURSING INTERVENTIONS

1. If using a chest drainage system with a water seal, fill the water seal chamber with sterile water to the level specified by the manufacturer.
2. When using suction in chest drainage systems with a water seal, fill the suction control chamber with sterile water to the 20-cm level or as prescribed. In systems without a water seal, set the regulator dial at the appropriate suction level.
3. Attach the drainage catheter exiting the thoracic cavity to the tubing coming from the collection chamber. Tape securely with adhesive tape.
4. If suction is used, connect the suction control chamber tubing to the suction unit. If using a wet suction system, turn on the suction unit and increase pressure until slow but steady bubbling appears in the suction control chamber. If using a chest drainage system with a dry suction control chamber, turn the regulator dial to 20 cm H_2O.

RATIONALE

Water seal drainage allows air and fluid to escape into a drainage chamber. The water acts as a seal and keeps the air from being drawn back into the pleural space.

The water level regulator dial setting determines the degree of suction applied.

In chest drainage units, the system is closed. The only connection is the one to the patient's catheter.

With a wet suction system, the degree of suction is determined by the amount of water in the suction control chamber and is not dependent on the rate of bubbling or the pressure gauge setting on the suction unit.

With a dry suction control chamber, the regulator dial replaces the water.

Example of a disposable chest drainage system.

5. Mark the drainage from the collection chamber with tape on the outside of the drainage unit. Mark hourly/daily increments (date and time) at the drainage level.

This marking shows the amount of fluid loss and how fast fluid is collecting in the drainage chamber. It serves as a basis for determining the need for blood replacement, if the fluid is blood. Visibly bloody drainage will appear in the chamber in the immediate postoperative period but should gradually becomes serous. If the patient is bleeding as heavily as 100 mL every 15 minutes, check the drainage every few minutes. A reoperation or autotransfusion may be needed. The transfusion of blood collected in the drainage chamber must be reinfused within 4 to 6 hours. Usually, however, drainage decreases progressively in the first 24 hours.

6. Ensure that the drainage tubing does not kink, loop, or interfere with the patient's movements.

Kinking, looping, or pressure on the drainage tubing can produce back-pressure, which may force fluid back into the pleural space or impede its drainage.

7. Encourage the patient to assume a comfortable position with good body alignment. With the lateral position, make sure that the patient's body does not compress the tubing. The patient should be turned and repositioned every 1.5 to 2 hours. Provide adequate analgesia.

Frequent position changes promote drainage, and good body alignment helps prevent postural deformities and contractures. Proper positioning also helps breathing and promotes better air exchange. Analgesics may be needed to promote comfort.

(continued)

Chart 25-18

GUIDELINES FOR Managing Chest Drainage Systems (Continued)

NURSING INTERVENTIONS	RATIONALE
8. Assist the patient with range-of-motion exercises for the affected arm and shoulder several times daily. Provide adequate analgesia.	Exercise helps to prevent ankylosis of the shoulder and to reduce postoperative pain and discomfort. Analgesics may be needed to relieve pain.
9. Gently "milk" the tubing in the direction of the drainage chamber as needed.	"Milking" prevents the tubing from becoming obstructed by clots and fibrin. Constant attention to maintaining the patency of the tube facilitates prompt expansion of the lung and minimizes complications.
10. Make sure there is fluctuation ("tidaling") of the fluid level in the water seal chamber (in wet systems), or check the air leak indicator for leaks (in dry systems with a one-way valve). *Note:* Fluid fluctuations in the water seal chamber or air leak indicator area will stop when: • The lung has reexpanded • The tubing is obstructed by blood clots, fibrin, or kinks • A loop of tubing hangs below the rest of the tubing • Suction motor or wall suction is not working properly	Fluctuation of the water level in the water seal shows effective connection between the pleural cavity and the drainage chamber and indicates that the drainage system remains patent. Fluctuation is also a gauge of intrapleural pressure in systems with a water seal (wet and dry, but not with the one-way valve). An air leak indicator shows changes in intrathoracic pressure in dry systems with a one-way valve. Bubbles will appear if a leak is present. The air leak indicator takes the place of fluid fluctuations in the water seal chamber.
11. With a dry system, assess for the presence of the indicator (bellows or float device) when setting the regulator dial to the desired level of suction.	The indicator shows that the vacuum is adequate to maintain the desired level of suction.
12. Observe for air leaks in the drainage system; they are indicated by constant bubbling in the water seal chamber, or by the air leak indicator in dry systems with a one-way valve. Also assess the chest tube system for correctable external leaks. Notify the physician immediately of excessive bubbling in the water seal chamber not due to external leaks.	Leaking and trapping of air in the pleural space can result in tension pneumothorax.
13. When turning down the dry suction, depress the manual high-negativity vent, and assess for a rise in the water level of the water seal chamber.	A rise in the water level of the water seal chamber indicates high negative pressure in the system that could lead to increased intrathoracic pressure.
14. Observe and immediately report rapid and shallow breathing, cyanosis, pressure in the chest, subcutaneous emphysema, symptoms of hemorrhage, or significant changes in vital signs.	Many clinical conditions can cause these signs and symptoms, including tension pneumothorax, mediastinal shift, hemorrhage, severe incisional pain, pulmonary embolus, and cardiac tamponade. Surgical intervention may be necessary.
15. Encourage the patient to breathe deeply and cough at frequent intervals. Provide adequate analgesia. If needed, request an order for patient-controlled analgesia. Also teach the patient how to perform incentive spirometry.	Deep breathing and coughing help to raise the intrapleural pressure, which promotes drainage of accumulated fluid in the pleural space. Deep breathing and coughing also promote removal of secretions from the tracheobronchial tree, which in turn promotes lung expansion and prevents atelectasis (alveolar collapse).
16. If the patient is lying on a stretcher and must be transported to another area, place the drainage system below the chest level. If the tubing disconnects, cut off the contaminated tips of the chest tube and tubing, insert a sterile connector in the cut ends, and reattach to the drainage system. Do *not* clamp the chest tube during transport.	The drainage apparatus must be kept at a level lower than the patient's chest to prevent fluid from flowing backward into the pleural space. Clamping can result in a tension pneumothorax.
17. When assisting in the chest tube's removal, instruct the patient to perform a gentle Valsalva manoeuvre or to breathe quietly. The chest tube is then clamped and quickly removed. Simultaneously, a small bandage is applied and made airtight with petrolatum gauze covered by a 4 × 4-inch gauze pad and thoroughly covered and sealed with nonporous tape.	The chest tube is removed as directed when the lung is reexpanded (usually 24 hours to several days), depending on the cause of the pneumothorax. During tube removal, the chief priorities are preventing air from entering the pleural cavity as the tube is withdrawn and preventing infection.

The mediastinal space is an extrapleural space that lies between the right and left thoracic cavities. Mediastinal chest tubes promote the removal of blood or other fluid from around the heart (Finkelmeier, 2000). Accumulating fluid can stop the heart from beating if it is not drained. A mediastinal tube can be inserted either anteriorly or posteriorly to the heart to drain blood after surgery or trauma. Without a tube, compression of the heart could occur, leading to death (Carroll, 2000).

There are two types of chest tubes: small-bore and large-bore catheters. Small-bore catheters (7F to 12F) have a one-way valve apparatus to prevent air from moving back into the patient. They can be inserted through a small skin incision. Large-bore catheters, which range in size up to 40F, are usually connected to a chest drainage system to collect any pleural fluid and monitor for air leaks (Scanlan, Wilkins & Stoller, 1999). After the chest tube is positioned, it is sutured to the skin and connected to a drainage apparatus to remove the residual air and fluid from the pleural or mediastinal space. This results in the re-expansion of remaining lung tissue.

CHEST DRAINAGE SYSTEMS

Chest drainage systems have a suction source, a collection chamber for pleural drainage, and a mechanism to prevent air from reentering the chest with inhalation. Various types of

Chart 25-19 Preventing Postoperative Cardiopulmonary Complications After Thoracic Surgery

Patient Management
- Auscultate lung sounds and assess for rate, rhythm, and depth.
- Monitor oxygenation with pulse oximetry.
- Monitor electrocardiogram for rate and rhythm changes.
- Assess capillary refill, skin colour, and status of the surgical dressing.
- Encourage and assist the patient to turn, cough, and take deep breaths.

Chest Drainage Management
- Verify that all connection tubes are patent and connected securely.
- Assess that the water seal is intact when using a wet suction system and assess the regulator dial in dry suction systems.
- Monitor characteristics of drainage including colour, amount, and consistency. Assess for significant increases or decreases in drainage output.
- Note fluctuations in the water seal chamber for wet suction systems and the air leak indicator for dry suction systems.
- Keep system below the patient's chest level.
- Assess suction control chamber for bubbling in wet suction systems.
- Keep suction at level ordered.
- Maintain appropriate fluid in water seal for wet suction systems.
- Keep air vent open when suction is off.

chest drainage systems are available for use in removal of air and fluid from the pleural space and re-expansion of the lungs. Chest drainage systems come with either wet (water seal) or dry suction control. In wet suction systems, the amount of suction is determined by the amount of water instilled in the suction chamber. The amount of bubbling in the suction chamber indicates how strong the suction is. Wet systems use a water seal to prevent air from moving back into the chest on inspiration. Dry systems use a one-way valve and a suction control dial in place of the water needed with wet or water seal system. Both systems can operate by gravity drainage, without a suction source.

Water Seal Chest Drainage Systems. The traditional water seal chest drainage system (or wet suction) has three chambers: a collection chamber, a water seal chamber, and a wet suction control chamber. The collection chamber acts as a reservoir for fluid draining from the chest tube. It is graduated to permit easy measurement of drainage. Suction may be added to create negative pressure and promote drainage of fluid and removal of air. The suction control chamber regulates the amount of negative pressure applied to the chest. The amount of suction is determined by the water level. It is generally set at 20-cm water; adding more fluid results in more suction. After the suction is turned on, bubbling appears in the suction chamber. A positive-pressure valve is located at the top of the suction chamber that automatically opens with increases in positive pressure within the system. Air will automatically be released through a positive-pressure relief valve if the suction tubing is inadvertently clamped or kinked.

The water seal chamber has a one-way valve or water seal that prevents air from moving back into the chest when the patient inhales. There will be an increase in the water level with inspiration and a return to the baseline level during exhalation; this is referred to as tidaling. Intermittent bubbling in the water seal chamber is normal, but continuous bubbling can indicate an air leak. Bubbling and tidaling do not occur when the tube is placed in the mediastinal space; however, fluid may pulsate with the patient's heartbeat. If the chest tube is connected to gravity drainage only, suction is not used. The pressure is equal to the water seal only. Two-chamber chest drainage systems (water seal chamber and collection chamber) are available for use with patients who need only gravity drainage.

The water level in the water seal chamber reflects the negative pressure present in the intrathoracic cavity. A rise in the water level indicates negative pressure in the pleural or mediastinal space. Excessive negative pressure can cause trauma to tissue (Bar-El, Ross, Kablawi & Egenburg, 2001). Most chest drainage systems have an automatic means to prevent excessive negative pressure. By pressing and holding a manual high-negativity vent (usually located on the top of the chest drainage system) until the water level in the water seal chamber returns to the 2-cm mark, excessive negative pressure is avoided, preventing damage to tissue.

> **! NURSING ALERT** When the wall vacuum is turned off, the drainage system must be open to the atmosphere so that intra-pleural air can escape from the system. This can be done by detaching the tubing from the suction port to provide a vent.

> **! NURSING ALERT** If the chest tube and drainage system become disconnected, air can enter the pleural space, producing a pneumothorax. To prevent pneumothorax if the chest tube is inadvertently disconnected from the drainage system, a temporary water seal can be established by immersing the chest tube's open end in a bottle of sterile water.

Dry Suction Water Seal Systems. Dry suction water seal systems, also referred to as dry suction, have a collection chamber for drainage, a water seal chamber, and a dry suction control chamber. The water seal chamber is filled with water to the 2-cm level. Bubbling in this area can indicate an air leak. The dry suction control chamber contains a regulator dial that conveniently regulates vacuum to the chest drain. Water is not needed for suction as it is in the wet system. Without the bubbling in the suction chamber, the machine is quieter.

Once the tube is connected to the suction source, the regulator dial allows the desired level of suction to be dialed in; the suction is increased until an indicator appears. The indicator has the same function as the bubbling in the traditional water seal system; that is, it indicates that the vacuum is adequate to maintain the desired level of suction. Some drainage systems use a bellows (a chamber that can be expanded or contracted) or an orange-coloured float device as an indicator of when the suction control regulator is set.

When the water in the water seal rises above the 2-cm level, intrathoracic pressure increases. Dry suction water seal systems have a manual high-negativity vent located on top of the drain. Pressing the manual high-negativity vent until the indicator appears (either a float device or bellows) and the water level in the water seal returns to the desired level, intrathoracic pressure is decreased.

> **! NURSING ALERT** The manual vent should not be used to lower the water level in the water seal when the patient is on gravity drainage (no suction) because intrathoracic pressure is equal to the pressure in the water seal.

Dry Suction with a One-Way Valve System. A third type of chest drainage system is dry suction with a one-way mechanical valve. This system has a collection chamber, a one-way mechanical valve, and a dry suction control chamber. The valve acts in the same way as a water seal and permits air to leave the chest but prevents it from moving back into the pleural space. This model lacks a water seal chamber and therefore has the advantage of a system that operates without water. For example, it can be set up quickly in emergency situations, and the dry control drain will still work even if it is knocked over. If the wet suction drain is knocked over, the water seal could be lost. This makes the dry suction systems useful for the patient who is ambulating or being transported. However, without the water seal chamber, there is no way to tell by inspection if the pressure in the chest has changed. An air leak indicator is present so that the system can be checked for air leaks. If an air leak is suspected, 30 mL of water are injected into the air leak indicator. Bubbles will appear if a leak is present (Carroll, 2000).

NURSING PROCESS: THE PATIENT UNDERGOING THORACIC SURGERY

Postoperative Assessment

The nurse monitors the heart rate and rhythm by auscultation and electrocardiography because episodes of major dysrhythmias are common after thoracic and cardiac surgery. In the immediate postoperative period, an arterial line may be maintained to allow frequent monitoring of arterial blood gases, serum electrolytes, hemoglobin and hematocrit values, and arterial pressure. Central venous pressure may be monitored to detect early signs of fluid volume disturbances. Central venous pressure monitoring devices are being used less frequently and for shorter periods of time than in the past. Early extubation from mechanical ventilation can also lead to earlier removal of arterial lines (Zevola & Maier, 1999). Another important component of postoperative assessment is to note the results of the preoperative evaluation of the patient's lung reserve by pulmonary function testing. A preoperative FEV_1 of more than 2 L or more than 70% of predicted value indicates a good lung reserve. Patients who have a postoperative predicted FEV_1 of less than 40% of predicted value have a higher incidence of morbidity and mortality (Scanlan, Wilkins & Stoller, 1999). This results in decreased tidal volumes, placing the patient at risk for respiratory failure.

Diagnosis

NURSING DIAGNOSES

Based on the assessment data, the patient's major postoperative nursing diagnoses may include:

- Impaired gas exchange related to lung impairment and surgery
- Ineffective airway clearance related to lung impairment, anesthesia, and pain
- Acute pain related to incision, drainage tubes, and the surgical procedure
- Impaired physical mobility of the upper extremities related to thoracic surgery
- Risk for imbalanced fluid volume related to the surgical procedure
- Imbalanced nutrition, less than body requirements related to dyspnea and anorexia
- Deficient knowledge about self-care procedures at home

COLLABORATIVE PROBLEMS/ POTENTIAL COMPLICATIONS

Based on assessment data, potential complications may include:

- Respiratory distress
- Dysrhythmias
- Atelectasis, pneumothorax, and bronchopleural fistula
- Blood loss and hemorrhage
- Pulmonary edema

Planning and Goals

The major goals for the patient may include improvement of gas exchange and breathing, improvement of airway clearance, relief of pain and discomfort, increased arm and shoulder mobility, maintenance of adequate fluid volume and nutritional status, understanding of self-care procedures, and absence of complications.

Nursing Interventions

IMPROVING GAS EXCHANGE AND BREATHING

Gas exchange is determined by evaluating oxygenation and ventilation. In the immediate postoperative period, this is achieved by measuring vital signs (blood pressure, pulse, and respirations) at least every 15 minutes for the first 1 to 2 hours, then less frequently as the patient's condition stabilizes.

Pulse oximetry is used for continuous monitoring of the adequacy of oxygenation. It is important to draw blood for arterial blood gas measurements early in the postoperative period to establish a baseline to assess the adequacy of oxygenation and ventilation and the possible retention of CO_2. The frequency with which postoperative arterial blood gases are measured depends on whether the patient is mechanically ventilated or exhibits signs of respiratory distress; these measurements can help determine appropriate therapy. It also is common practice for patients to have an arterial line in place to obtain blood for blood gas measurements and to monitor blood pressure closely. Hemodynamic monitoring may be used to assess hemodynamic stability.

Breathing techniques, such as diaphragmatic and pursed-lip breathing, that were taught before surgery should be performed by the patient every 2 hours to expand the alveoli and prevent atelectasis. Another technique to improve ventilation is sustained maximal inspiration therapy or incentive spirometry. This technique promotes lung inflation, improves the cough mechanism, and allows early assessment of acute pulmonary changes. (See Charts 25-3 and 25-4 for more information.)

Positioning also improves breathing. When the patient is oriented and blood pressure is stabilized, the head of the bed is elevated 30 to 40 degrees during the immediate postoperative period. This facilitates ventilation, promotes chest drainage from the lower chest tube, and helps residual air to rise in the upper portion of the pleural space, where it can be removed through the upper chest tube.

The nurse should consult with the surgeon about patient positioning. There is controversy regarding the best side-lying position. In general, the patient should be positioned from back to side frequently and moved from horizontal to semi-upright position as soon as tolerated. Most commonly, the patient is instructed to lie on the operative side. However, the patient with unilateral lung pathology may not be able to turn well onto that side because of pain. In addition, positioning the patient with the "good lung" (the nonoperated lung) down allows a better match of ventilation and perfusion and therefore may actually improve oxygenation. The patient's position is changed from horizontal to semi-upright as soon as possible, because remaining in one position tends to promote the retention of secretions in the dependent portion of the lungs. After a pneumonectomy, the operated side should be dependent so that fluid in the pleural space remains below the level of the bronchial stump, and the other lung can fully expand.

The procedure for turning the patient is as follows:

- Instruct the patient to bend the knees and use the feet to push.
- Have the patient shift hips and shoulders to the opposite side of the bed while pushing with the feet.
- Bring the patient's arm over the chest, pointing it in the direction toward which the patient is being turned. Have the patient grasp the side rail with the hand.
- Turn the patient in log-roll fashion to prevent twisting at the waist and pain from possible pulling on the incision.

IMPROVING AIRWAY CLEARANCE

Retained secretions are a threat to the thoracotomy patient after surgery. Trauma to the tracheobronchial tree during surgery, diminished lung ventilation, and diminished cough reflex all result in the accumulation of excessive secretions. If the secretions are retained, airway obstruction occurs. This, in turn, causes the air in the alveoli distal to the obstruction to become absorbed and the affected portion of the lung to collapse. Atelectasis, pneumonia, and respiratory failure may result.

Several techniques are used to maintain a patent airway. First, secretions are suctioned from the tracheobronchial tree before the endotracheal tube is discontinued. Secretions continue to be removed by suctioning until the patient can cough up secretions effectively. Nasotracheal suctioning may be needed to stimulate a deep cough and aspirate secretions that the patient cannot cough up. However, it should be used only after other methods to raise secretions have been unsuccessful (Chart 25-20).

Coughing technique is another measure used in maintaining a patent airway. The patient is encouraged to cough effectively; ineffective coughing results in exhaustion and retention of secretions (see Chart 25-5). To be effective, the cough must be low-pitched, deep, and controlled. Because it is difficult to cough in a supine position, the patient is helped to a sitting position on the edge of the bed, with the feet resting on a chair. The patient should cough at least every hour during the first 24 hours and when necessary thereafter. If audible crackles are present, it may be necessary to use chest percussion with the cough routine until the lungs are clear. Aerosol therapy is helpful in humidifying and mobilizing secretions so that they can easily be cleared with coughing. To minimize incisional pain during coughing, the nurse supports the incision or encourages the patient to do so (Fig. 25-8).

After helping the patient to cough, the nurse should listen to both lungs, anteriorly and posteriorly, to determine whether there are any changes in breath sounds. Diminished breath sounds may indicate collapsed or hypoventilated alveoli.

Chart 25-20 **Performing Nasotracheal Suction**

Sterile Technique to Be Used

1. Explain procedure to the patient.
2. Medicate patient for pain if necessary.
3. Place the patient in a sitting or semi-Fowler's position. Make sure the patient's head is not flexed forward. Remove excess pillows if necessary.
4. Oxygenate the patient several minutes before initiating the suctioning procedure. Have oxygen source ready nearby during procedure.
5. Put on sterile gloves.
6. Lubricate catheter with water-soluble gel.
7. Gently pass catheter through the patient's nose to the pharynx. If it is difficult to pass the catheter, and repeated suctioning is expected, a soft rubber nasal trumpet may be placed nasopharyngeally to provide easier catheter passage. Check the position of the tip of the catheter by asking the patient to open the mouth and inspecting it; the tip of the catheter should be in the lower pharynx.
8. Instruct the patient to take a deep breath or stick out the tongue. This action opens the epiglottis and promotes downward movement of the catheter.
9. Advance the catheter into the trachea only during inspiration. Listen for cough or for passage of air through the catheter.
10. Attach the catheter to suction apparatus. Apply intermittent suction while slowly withdrawing the catheter. Do not let suction exceed 120 mm Hg.
11. Do not suction for longer than 10 to 15 seconds, as dysrhythmias, bradycardia, or cardiac arrest may occur in patients with borderline oxygenation.
12. If additional suctioning is needed, withdraw the catheter to the back of the pharynx. Reassure patient and oxygenate for several minutes before resuming suctioning.

Chest physiotherapy is the final technique for maintaining a patent airway. If a patient is identified as being at high risk for developing postoperative pulmonary complications, then chest physiotherapy is started immediately (perhaps even before surgery). The techniques of postural drainage, vibration, and percussion help to loosen and mobilize the secretions so that they can be coughed up or suctioned.

RELIEVING PAIN AND DISCOMFORT

Pain after a thoracotomy may be severe, depending on the type of incision and the patient's reaction to and ability to cope with pain. Deep inspiration is very painful after thoracotomy. Pain can lead to postoperative complications if it reduces the patient's ability to breathe deeply and cough, and if it further limits chest excursions so that ventilation becomes ineffective.

Immediately after the surgical procedure and before the incision is closed, the surgeon may perform a nerve block with a long-acting local anesthetic such as bupivacaine (Marcaine, Sensorcaine). Bupivacaine is titrated to relieve postoperative pain while allowing the patient to cooperate in deep breathing, coughing, and mobilization. However, it is important to avoid depressing the respiratory system with excessive analgesia: the patient should not be so sedated as to be unable to cough. There is controversy about the effectiveness of injections of local anesthetic for pain relief after thoracotomy surgery. Research has shown that bupivacaine was no

A The nurse's hands should support the chest incision anteriorly and posteriorly. The patient is instructed to take several deep breaths, inhale, and then cough forcibly.

B With one hand, the nurse exerts downward pressure on the shoulder of the affected side while firmly supporting the area beneath the wound with the other hand. The patient is instructed to take several deep breaths, inhale, and then cough forcibly.

C The nurse can wrap a towel or sheet around the patient's chest and hold the ends together, pulling slightly as the patient coughs, and releasing during deep breaths.

D The patient can be taught to hold a pillow firmly against the incision while coughing. This can be done while lying down or sitting in an upright position.

FIGURE 25-8 Techniques for supporting incision while a patient recovering from thoracic surgery coughs.

more effective than saline injections in treating postoperative thoracotomy pain (Silomon et al., 2000).

Lidocaine and prilocaine are local anesthetic agents used to treat pain at the site of the chest tube insertion. These medications are administered as topical transdermal analgesics that penetrate the skin. Lidocaine and prilocaine have also been found to be effective when used together. EMLA cream, which is a mixture of the two medications, has been found to be effective in treating pain from chest tube removal, and recent studies found it to be more effective than intravenous morphine (Valenzuela & Rosen, 1999).

Because of the need to maximize patient comfort without depressing the respiratory drive, patient-controlled analgesia (PCA) is often used. Opioid analgesic agents such as morphine are commonly used. PCA, administered through an intravenous pump or an epidural catheter, allows the patient to control the frequency and total dosage. Preset limits on the pump avoid overdosage. With proper instruction, these methods are well tolerated and allow earlier mobilization and cooperation with the treatment regimen. (See Chap. 13 for a more extensive discussion of PCA and pain management.)

> **NURSING ALERT** It is important not to confuse the restlessness of hypoxia with the restlessness caused by pain. Dyspnea, restlessness, increasing respiratory rate, increasing blood pressure, and tachycardia are warning signs of impending respiratory insufficiency. Pulse oximetry is used to monitor oxygenation and to differentiate causes of restlessness.

PROMOTING MOBILITY AND SHOULDER EXERCISES

Because large shoulder girdle muscles are transected during a thoracotomy, the arm and shoulder must be mobilized by full range of motion of the shoulder. As soon as physiologically possible, usually within 8 to 12 hours, the patient is helped to get out of bed. Although this may be painful initially, the earlier the patient moves, the sooner the pain will subside. In addition to getting out of bed, the patient begins arm and shoulder exercises to restore movement and prevent painful stiffening of the affected arm and shoulder (Chart 25-21).

MAINTAINING FLUID VOLUME AND NUTRITION

Intravenous Therapy

During the surgical procedure or immediately after, the patient may receive a transfusion of blood products, followed by a continuous intravenous infusion. Because a reduction in lung capacity often occurs following thoracic surgery, a period of physiologic adjustment is needed. Fluids should be administered at a low hourly rate and titrated (as prescribed) to prevent overloading the vascular system and precipitating pulmonary edema. The nurse performs careful respiratory and cardiovascular assessments, as well as intake and output, vital signs, and assessment of jugular vein distention. The nurse should also monitor the infusion site for signs of infiltration, including swelling, tenderness, and redness.

Diet

It is not unusual for patients undergoing thoracotomy to have poor nutritional status before surgery because of dyspnea, sputum production, and poor appetite. Therefore, it is especially important

Chart 25-21 • **PATIENT EDUCATION**
Performing Arm and Shoulder Exercises

Arm and shoulder exercises are performed after thoracic surgery to restore movement, prevent painful stiffening of the shoulder, and improve muscle power.

(**A**) Hold hand of the affected side with the other hand, palms facing in. Raise the arms forward, upward, and then overhead, while taking a deep breath. Exhale while lowering the arms. Repeat five times. (**B**) Raise arm sideward, upward, and downward in a waving motion. (**C**) Place arm at side. Raise arm sideward, upward, and over the head. Repeat five times. These exercises can also be performed while lying in bed. (**D**) Extend the arm up and back, out to the side and back, down at the side and back. (**E**) Place hands in small of back. Push elbows as far back as possible. (**F**) Sit erect in an armchair; place the hands on the arms of the chair directly opposite the sides of the body. Press down on hands, consciously pulling the abdomen in and stretching up from the waist. Inhale while raising the body until the elbows are extended completely. Hold this position a moment, and begin exhaling while lowering the body slowly to the original position.

that adequate nutrition be provided. A liquid diet is provided as soon as bowel sounds return; the patient is progressed to a full diet as soon as possible. Small, frequent meals are better tolerated and are crucial to the recovery and maintenance of lung function.

MONITORING AND MANAGING POTENTIAL COMPLICATIONS

Complications after thoracic surgery are always a possibility and must be identified and managed early. In addition, the nurse monitors the patient at regular intervals for signs of respiratory distress or developing respiratory failure, dysrhythmias, bronchopleural fistula, hemorrhage and shock, atelectasis, and pulmonary infection.

Respiratory distress is treated by identifying and eliminating its cause while providing supplemental oxygen. If the patient progresses to respiratory failure, intubation and mechanical ventilation are necessary, eventually requiring weaning.

Dysrhythmias are often related to the effects of hypoxia or the surgical procedure. They are treated with antiarrhythmic medication and supportive therapy (see Chap. 27). Pulmonary infec-

tions or effusion, often preceded by atelectasis, may occur a few days into the postoperative course.

Pneumothorax may occur following thoracic surgery if there is an air leak from the surgical site to the pleural cavity or from the pleural cavity to the environment. Failure of the chest drainage system will prevent return of negative pressure in the pleural cavity and result in pneumothorax. In the postoperative patient pneumothorax is often accompanied by hemothorax. The nurse maintains the chest drainage system and monitors the patient for signs and symptoms of pneumothorax: increasing shortness of breath, tachycardia, increased respiratory rate, and increasing respiratory distress.

Bronchopleural fistula is a serious but rare complication preventing the return of negative intrathoracic pressure and lung re-expansion. Depending on its severity, it is treated with closed chest drainage, mechanical ventilation, and possibly talc pleurodesis (described in Chap. 23).

Hemorrhage and shock are managed by treating the underlying cause, whether by reoperation or by administration of blood products or fluids. Pulmonary edema from overinfusion of intravenous fluids is a significant danger. The early symptoms are dyspnea, crackles, bubbling sounds in the chest, tachycardia, and pink, frothy sputum. This constitutes an emergency and must be reported and treated immediately.

PROMOTING HOME AND COMMUNITY-BASED CARE

Teaching Patients Self-Care

The nurse instructs the patient and family about postoperative care that will be continued at home. The nurse explains signs and symptoms that should be reported to the physician. These include:

- Change in respiratory status: increasing shortness of breath, fever, increased restlessness or other changes in mental or cognitive status, increased respiratory rate, change in respiratory pattern, change in amount or colour of sputum
- Bleeding or other drainage from the surgical incision or chest tube exit sites
- Increased chest pain

In addition, respiratory care and other treatment modalities (oxygen, incentive spirometer, chest physiotherapy, and oral, inhaled, or intravenous medications) may be continued at home. Therefore, the nurse needs to instruct the patient and family in their correct and safe use.

The nurse emphasizes the importance of progressively increased activity. The nurse instructs the patient to ambulate within limits and explains that return of strength is likely to be very gradual. Another important aspect of patient teaching addresses shoulder exercises. It is important to instruct the patient to do these exercises five times daily. Additional patient teaching is described in Chart 25-22.

Continuing Care

Depending on the patient's physical status and the availability of family assistance, a home care referral may be indicated. The home care nurse assesses the patient's recovery from surgery, with special attention to respiratory status, the surgical incision, chest drainage, pain control, ambulation, and nutritional status. The patient's use of respiratory modalities should be assessed to ensure they are being used correctly and safely. In addition, the nurse assesses the patient's compliance with the postoperative treatment plan and identifies acute or late postoperative complications.

The recovery process may be longer than the patient had expected, and providing support to the patient is an important task for the home care nurse. Because of shorter hospital stays, attending follow-up physician appointments is essential. The nurse teaches the patient about the importance of keeping follow-up appointments and completing laboratory tests as prescribed to assist the physician in evaluating recovery. The home care nurse provides continuous encouragement and education to the patient and family during the process. As recovery progresses, the nurse also reminds the patient and family about the importance of participating in health promotion activities and recommended health screening.

Evaluation

EXPECTED PATIENT OUTCOMES

Expected patient outcomes may include:

1. Demonstrates improved gas exchange, as reflected in arterial blood gas measurements, breathing exercises, and use of incentive spirometry
2. Shows improved airway clearance, as evidenced by deep, controlled coughing and clear breath sounds or decreased presence of adventitious sounds
3. Has decreased pain and discomfort by splinting incision during coughing and increasing activity level
4. Shows improved mobility of shoulder and arm; demonstrates arm and shoulder exercises to relieve stiffening
5. Maintains adequate fluid intake and maintains nutrition for healing
6. Exhibits less anxiety by using appropriate coping skills, and demonstrates a basic understanding of technology used in care
7. Adheres to therapeutic program and home care
8. Is free of complications, as evidenced by normal vital signs and temperature, improved arterial blood gas measurements, clear lung sounds, and adequate respiratory function

For a detailed plan of nursing care for the patient who has had a thoracotomy, see the Plan of Nursing Care.

Chart 25-22
Home Care Checklist • The Patient With a Thoracotomy

At the completion of the home care instruction, the patient or caregiver will be able to:	Patient	Caregiver
• Use local heat and oral analgesia to relieve intercostal pain.	✓	✓
• Alternate walking and other activities with frequent rest periods, expecting weakness and fatigue for the first 3 weeks.	✓	✓
• Perform breathing exercises several times daily for the first few weeks at home.	✓	
• Avoid lifting more than 20 pounds until complete healing has taken place; the chest muscles and incision may be weaker than normal for 3 to 6 months after surgery.	✓	
• Walk at a moderate pace, gradually and persistently extending walking time and distance.	✓	
• Immediately stop any activity that causes undue fatigue, increased shortness of breath, or chest pain.	✓	
• Avoid bronchial irritants (smoke, fumes, air pollution, aerosol sprays).	✓	✓
• Avoid others with known colds or lung infections.	✓	✓
• Obtain an annual influenza vaccine and discuss vaccination against pneumonia with the physician.	✓	
• Report for follow-up care by the surgeon or clinic as necessary.	✓	✓
• Stop smoking, if applicable.	✓	✓

Plan of Nursing Care
Care of the Patient After Thoracotomy

Nursing Interventions	Rationale	Expected Patient Outcomes

Nursing Diagnosis: Impaired gas exchange related to lung impairment and surgery
Goal: Improvement of gas exchange and breathing

Nursing Interventions	Rationale	Expected Patient Outcomes

1. Monitor pulmonary status as directed and as needed:
  a. Auscultate breath sounds.
  b. Check rate, depth, and pattern of respirations.
  c. Assess blood gases for signs of hypoxemia or CO_2 retention.
  d. Evaluate patient's colour for cyanosis.
2. Monitor and record blood pressure, apical pulse, and temperature every 2–4 hours, central venous pressure (if indicated) every 2 hours.
3. Monitor continuous electrocardiogram for pattern and dysrhythmias.
 	
4. Elevate head of bed 30–40 degrees when patient is oriented and hemodynamic status is stable.
5. Encourage deep-breathing exercises (see section on Breathing Retraining) and effective use of incentive spirometer (sustained maximal inspiration).
6. Encourage and promote an effective cough routine to be performed every 1–2 hours during first 24 hours.
7. Assess and monitor the chest drainage system:*
  a. Assess for leaks and patency as needed.
  b. Monitor amount and character of drainage and document every 2 hours. Notify physician if drainage is 150 mL/h or greater.
  c. See Chart 25-18 for summary of nurse's role in management of chest drainage systems.
	1. Changes in pulmonary status indicate improvement or onset of complications.
	
	2. Aid in evaluating effect of surgery on cardiac status.
	
	3. Dysrhythmias (especially atrial fibrillation and atrial flutter) are more frequently seen after thoracic surgery. A patient with total pneumonectomy is especially prone to cardiac irregularity.
	4. Maximum lung excursion is achieved when patient is as close to upright as possible.
	5. Helps to achieve maximal lung inflation and to open closed airways.
	
	6. Coughing is necessary to remove retained secretions.
	
	7. System is used to eliminate any residual air or fluid after thoracotomy.
		• Lungs are clear on auscultation
		• Respiratory rate is within acceptable range with no episodes of dyspnea
		• Vital signs are stable
		• Dysrhythmias are not present or are under control
		• Demonstrates deep, controlled, effective breathing to allow maximal lung expansion
		• Uses incentive spirometer every 2 hours while awake
		• Demonstrates deep, effective coughing technique
		• Lungs are expanded to capacity (evidenced by chest x-ray)

Nursing Diagnosis: Ineffective airway clearance related to lung impairment, anesthesia, and pain
Goal: Improvement of airway clearance and achievement of a patent airway

Nursing Interventions	Rationale	Expected Patient Outcomes
1. Maintain an open airway. 2. Perform endotracheal suctioning until patient can raise secretions effectively. 3. Assess and medicate for pain. Encourage deep-breathing and coughing exercises. Help splint incision during coughing.	1. Provides for adequate ventilation and gas exchange 2. Endotracheal secretions are present in excessive amounts in post-thoracotomy patients due to trauma to the tracheobronchial tree during surgery, diminished lung ventilation, and cough reflex. 3. Helps to achieve maximal lung inflation and to open closed airways. Coughing is painful; incision needs to be supported.	• Airway is patent • Coughs effectively • Splints incision while coughing • Sputum is clear or colourless • Lungs are clear on auscultation

*A patient with a pneumonectomy usually does not have water seal chest drainage because it is desirable that the pleural space fill with an effusion, which eventually obliterates this space. Some surgeons do use a modified water seal system.

(continued)

Plan of Nursing Care

Care of the Patient After Thoracotomy (Continued)

Nursing Interventions	Rationale	Expected Patient Outcomes
4. Monitor amount, viscosity, colour, and odour of sputum. Notify physician if sputum is excessive or contains bright-red blood.	4. Changes in sputum suggest presence of infection or change in pulmonary status. Colourless sputum is not unusual; opacification or colouring of sputum may indicate dehydration or infection.	
5. Administer humidification and mini-nebulizer therapy as prescribed.	5. Secretions must be moistened and thinned if they are to be raised from the chest with the least amount of effort.	
6. Perform postural drainage, percussion, and vibration as prescribed. Do not percuss or vibrate directly over operative site.	6. Chest physiotherapy uses gravity to help remove secretions from the lung.	
7. Auscultate both sides of chest to determine changes in breath sounds.	7. Indications for tracheal suctioning are determined by chest auscultation.	

Nursing Diagnosis: Acute pain related to incision, drainage tubes, and the surgical procedure
Goal: Relief of pain and discomfort

1. Evaluate location, character, quality, and severity of pain. Administer analgesic medication as prescribed and as needed. Observe for respiratory effect of opioid. Is patient too somnolent to cough? Are respirations depressed?	1. Pain limits chest excursions and thereby decreases ventilation.	• Asks for pain medication, but verbalizes that he or she expects some discomfort while deep breathing and coughing • Verbalizes that he or she is comfortable and not in acute distress • No signs of incisional infection evident

2. Maintain care postoperatively in positioning the thoracotomy patient:
  a. Place patient in semi-Fowler's position.
  b. Patients with limited respiratory reserve may not be able to turn on unoperated side.
  c. Assist or turn patient every 2 hours.
	2. The patient who is comfortable and free of pain will be less likely to splint the chest while breathing. A semi-Fowler's position permits residual air in the pleural space to rise to upper portion of pleural space and be removed via the upper chest catheter.	

3. Assess incision area every 8 hours for redness, heat, induration, swelling, separation, and drainage.	3. These signs indicate possible infection.	
4. Request order for patient-controlled analgesia pump if appropriate for patient.	4. Allowing patient control over frequency and dose improves comfort and compliance with treatment regimen.	

Nursing Diagnosis: Anxiety related to outcomes of surgery, pain, technology
Goal: Reduction of anxiety to a manageable level

1. Explain all procedures in understandable language.	1. Explaining what can be expected in understandable terms decreases anxiety and increases cooperation.	• States that anxiety is at a manageable level • Participates with health care team in treatment regimen • Uses appropriate coping skills (verbalization, pain relief strategies, use of support systems such as family, clergy) • Demonstrates basic understanding of technology used in care
2. Assess for pain and medicate, especially before potentially painful procedures.	2. Premedication before painful procedures or activities improves comfort and minimizes undue anxiety.	
3. Silence all *unnecessary* alarms on technology (monitors, ventilators).	3. *Unnecessary* alarms increase the risk of sensory overload and may increase anxiety.	
4. Encourage and support patient while increasing activity level.	4. Positive reinforcement improves patient motivation and independence.	
5. Mobilize resources (family, clergy, social worker) to help patient cope with outcomes of surgery (diagnosis, change in functional abilities).	5. A multidisciplinary approach promotes the patient's strengths and coping mechanisms.	

(continued)

Nursing Interventions	Rationale	Expected Patient Outcomes

Nursing Diagnosis: Impaired physical mobility of the upper extremities related to thoracic surgery
Goal: Increased mobility of the affected shoulder and arm

1. Assist patient with normal range of motion and function of shoulder and trunk: a. Teach breathing exercises to mobilize thorax. b. Encourage skeletal exercises to promote abduction and mobilization of shoulder (see Chart 25-21). c. Assist out of bed to chair as soon as pulmonary and circulatory systems are stable (usually by evening of surgery). 2. Encourage progressive activities according to level of fatigue.	1. Necessary to regain normal mobility of arm and shoulder and to speed recovery and minimize discomfort 2. Increases patient's use of affected shoulder and arm	• Demonstrates arm and shoulder exercises and verbalizes intent to perform them on discharge • Regains previous range of motion in shoulder and arm

Nursing Diagnosis: Risk for imbalanced fluid volume related to the surgical procedure
Goal: Maintenance of adequate fluid volume

1. Monitor and record hourly intake and output. Urine output should be at least 30 mL/h after surgery. 2. Administer blood component therapy and parenteral fluids and/or diuretics as prescribed to restore and maintain fluid volume.	1. Fluid management may be altered before, during, and after surgery, and patient's response to and need for fluid management must be assessed. 2. Pulmonary edema due to transfusion or fluid overload is an ever-present threat; after pneumonectomy, the pulmonary vascular system has been greatly reduced.	• Patient is adequately hydrated, as evidenced by: • Urine output greater than 30 mL/h • Vital signs stable, heart rate, and central venous pressure approaching normal • No excessive peripheral edema

Nursing Diagnosis: Deficient knowledge of home care procedures
Goal: Increased ability to carry out care procedures at home

1. Encourage patient to practice arm and shoulder exercises five times daily at home. 2. Instruct patient to practice assuming a functionally erect position in front of a full-length mirror. 3. Instruct patient in following aspects of home care: a. Relieve intercostal pain by local heat or oral analgesia. b. Alternate activities with frequent rest periods. c. Practice breathing exercises at home. d. Avoid heavy lifting until complete healing has occurred. e. Avoid undue fatigue, increased shortness of breath, or chest pain. f. Avoid bronchial irritants. g. Prevent colds or lung infection. h. Get annual influenza vaccine. i. Keep follow-up appointment with physician. j. Stop smoking.	1. Exercise accelerates recovery of muscle function and reduces long-term pain and discomfort. 2. Practice will help restore normal posture. 3. Knowing what to expect facilitates recovery. a. Some soreness may persist for several weeks. b. Weakness and fatigue are common for the first 3 weeks or longer. c. Effective breathing is necessary to prevent splinting of affected side, which may lead to atelectasis. d. Chest muscles and incision may be weaker than normal for 3–6 months. e. Undue stress may prolong the healing process. f. The lung is more susceptible to irritants. g. The lung is more susceptible to infection during the recovery phase. h. Vaccination helps prevent flu. i. This allows timely follow-up assessment. j. Smoking will slow healing process by decreasing oxygen delivery to tissues and make lung susceptible to infection and other complications.	• Demonstrates arm and shoulder exercises • Verbalizes need to try to assume an erect posture • Verbalizes the importance of relieving discomfort, alternating walking and rest, performing breathing exercises, avoiding heavy lifting, avoiding undue fatigue, avoiding bronchial irritants, preventing colds or lung infections, getting flu vaccine, keeping follow-up visits, and stopping smoking

Critical Thinking Exercises

1. Oxygen therapy is required for the following patients: a 45-year-old patient who has undergone a right lower lobe lobectomy and needs short-term, low-flow oxygen; a 62-year-old patient with severe COPD admitted to the hospital for the fourth time in the past year; and a 74-year-old patient with dyspnea secondary to advanced lung cancer. Describe the explanations and safety precautions indicated for each of these patients and their families.

2. Your patient has just returned from the operating room after chest surgery with an endotracheal tube, a chest tube, and two intravenous lines and cardiac monitoring in place. Identify the priorities of assessment and interventions for this patient.

3. Your patient, who underwent a thoracotomy less than 24 hours ago, has a chest tube in place on the right side. Identify the actions that are indicated for each of the following situations and state the rationale for your actions:
    a. Output in chest drainage chamber of 500 mL of serous drainage in the last 8 hours
    b. Continuous bubbling in the water seal chamber
    c. Patient reports chest pain and dyspnea; absence of breath sounds on the right side of the thorax

4. A patient is being discharged home on oxygen therapy for the first time. The physician's prescription is for 2 L of oxygen via nasal cannula. Write a teaching plan for home oxygen therapy to be discussed with the patient before discharge from the hospital.

5. A patient who had a chest tube inserted 8 hours ago becomes confused and disconnects the chest tube from the drainage system. What immediate actions are indicated in this situation? What nursing assessments and interventions are needed once the immediate situation has been corrected?

REFERENCES AND SELECTED READINGS

Books

Abraham, I., Bottrell, M., Fulmer, T., & Mezey, M. (1999). *Geriatric nursing protocols for best practice.* New York: Springer.

Cairo, J., & Pilbeam, S. (1999). *Respiratory care equipment.* St. Louis: Mosby.

Clinical practice guidelines. (2000). Dallas, Texas: American Association for Respiratory Care.

Doenges, M. E., & Moorhouse, F. (2000). *Nurse's pocket guide. Diagnoses, interventions, and rationales.* Philadelphia: F. A. Davis.

Dudek, S. G. (2001). *Nutrition essentials for nursing practice.* Philadelphia: Lippincott.

Eliopoulos, C. (2001). *Gerontological nursing.* Philadelphia: Lippincott Williams & Wilkins.

Finkelmeier, B. (2000). *Cardiothoracic-surgical nursing.* Philadelphia: Lippincott Williams & Wilkins.

Hill, N. S. (2000). *Long-term mechanical ventilation.* New York: Marcel Dekker, Inc.

Hurford, W. E. (2000). *Airway management.* Philadelphia: Lippincott Williams & Wilkins.

Kacmarek, R. M. (2000). *Advanced respiratory care.* Philadelphia: Lippincott Williams & Wilkins.

LeFever, J., & Hayes, E. (2000). *Pharmacology: A nursing process approach.* Philadelphia: W. B. Saunders.

Lutz, C., & Przytulski, K. (2001). *Nutrition and diet therapy.* Philadelphia: F. A. Davis.

MacIntyre, N. R., & Branson, R. D. (2001). *Mechanical ventilation.* Philadelphia: W. B. Saunders.

McKenry, L., & Salerno, E. (2001). *Pharmacology in nursing.* St. Louis: Mosby.

Mishoe, S. C., & Welch, A. (2001). *Critical thinking in respiratory care: A problem-based learning approach.* New York: McGraw-Hill, Medical Publishing Division.

Ochroch, E. A., & Deutschman, C. S. (2000). *Managing the airway in the critically ill patient.* Philadelphia: W. B. Saunders.

Scanlan, C., Wilkins, R., & Stoller, J. (1999). *Fundamentals of respiratory care.* St. Louis: Mosby.

Wilkins, R. L., Krider, S. J., & Sheldon, R. L. (2000). *Clinical assessment in respiratory care.* St. Louis: Mosby.

Woodrow, P., & Roe, J. (2000). *Intensive care nursing: A framework for practice.* New York: Routledge.

Zang, S., & Allender, J. (1999). *Home care of the elderly.* Philadelphia: Lippincott Williams & Wilkins.

Journals

Asterisks indicate nursing research articles.

Avery, S. (2000). Insertion and management of chest drains. *Nursing Times, 96*(37), 1–6.

Baker, S., & Flynn, M. B. (1999). New hope for patients with emphysema: Lung volume reduction surgery. *Heart and Lung, 28*(6), 455–458.

Bar-El, Y., Ross, A., Kablawi, A., & Egenburg, S. (2001). Potentially dangerous negative intrapleural pressures generated by ordinary pleural drainage systems. *Chest, 119*(2), 511–514.

Blackwood, B. (1999). Normal saline instillation with endotracheal suctioning: Primum non nocere (first do no harm). *Journal of Advanced Nursing, 29*(4), 928–934.

Bliss, P., McCoy, R., & Adams, A. (1999). A bench study of comparison of demand oxygen delivery systems and continuous flow oxygen. *Respiratory Care, 44*(8), 925–929.

*Byers, J. F., & Sole, M. L. (2000). Analysis of factors related to the development of ventilator associated pneumonia: Use of existing databases. *American Journal of Critical Care, 9*(5), 344–351.

Carroll, P. (2000). Exploring chest drain options. *RN, 63*(10), 50–58.

Cirino, L., Campos, J., Fernandez, A., Samano, M., Fernandez, P., Filomeno, L. & Jatene, F. (2000). Diagnosis and treatment of mediastinal tumors by thoracoscopy. *Chest, 117*(6), 1787–1792.

Clini, E., Vitacca, M. D., Bianchi, L., Porta, R., & Ambrosino, N. (1999). Long-term tracheostomy in severe COPD patients weaned from mechanical ventilation. *Respiratory Care, 44*(4), 241–244.

Creechan, T. (2000). Combining mechanical ventilation with hospice care in the home: death with dignity. *Critical Care Nurse, 20*(3), 49–53.

Cull, C. (1999). Weaning patients from mechanical ventilation. *Professional Nurse, 14*(8), 535–538.

Cull, C., & Inwood, H. (1999). Extubation in ICU: Enhancing the nursing role. *Professional Nurse, 14*(9), 535–538.

Day, T. (2000). Tracheal suctioning: When, why, and how? *Nursing Times, 96*(20), 13–15.

Doherty, M. J., & Greenstone, M. A. (2000). Noninvasive ventilation in acute exacerbations of chronic obstructive pulmonary disease. *Care of the Critically Ill, 116*(4), 126–130.

Estaban, A., Anzueto, A., Frutos, F., et al. (2002). Characteristics and outcomes in adult patients receiving mechanical ventilation. A 28-day international study. *Journal of the American Medical Association, 287*(3), 345–355.

Ecklund, M. (1999). Successful outcomes for the ventilator-dependent patient. *Critical Care Nursing Clinics of North America, 11*(2), 249–260.

Ferreira, M. M., Brooks, D., Lacasse, Y., & Goldstein, R. S. (2000). Nutritional support for individuals with COPD: A meta-analysis. *Chest, 117*(3), 672–678.

Giannouli, E., Webster, K., Roberts, D., & Younes, M. (1999). Response of ventilator-dependent patients to different levels of pressure support and proportional assist. *American Journal of Respiratory and Critical Care Medicine, 159*(6), 1716–1725.

Goodfellow, L. T., & Jones, M. (2002). Bronchial hygiene therapy. *American Journal of Nursing, 102*(1), 37–43.

Hanneman, S. K. (1999). Protocols for practice: Applying research at the bedside. Weaning from short-term mechanical ventilation. *Critical Care Nurse, 19*(5), 86–89.

Hanneman, S. K. (1999). Weaning from short-term mechanical ventilation. *Critical Care Nurse, 19*(5), 86–89.

Happ, M. B. (2000). Preventing treatment interference: The nurse's role in maintaining technologic devices. *Heart & Lung, 29*(1), 60–69.

Kacmarek, R. M. (2000). Delivery systems for long-term oxygen therapy. State-of-the-art conference on long-term oxygen therapy. *Respiratory Care, 45*(1), 84–94.

*Kinloch, D. (1999). Instillation of normal saline during endotracheal suctioning: Effects on mixed venous oxygen saturation. *American Journal of Critical Care, 8*(4), 231–240.

Kruger, M., & Sandler, A. (1999). Post-thoracotomy pain control. *Current Opinion of Anaesthesiology, 12*(1), 55–58.

Manaligod, J. M., Bendel-Stenzel, E. M., Meyers, P. A., et al. (2000). Variations in end-expiratory pressure during partial liquid ventilation. *Chest, 117*(1), 184–190.

*Mazolewski, P., Turner, J., Baker, M., Kurtz, T., & Little, A. (1999). The impact of nutritional status on the outcome of lung volume reduction surgery. *Chest, 116*(3), 693–696.

McConnell, E. A. (2000). Do's and don'ts. Suctioning a tracheostomy. *Nursing, 30*(1), 79–80.

National Institutes of Health (2001). National emphysema treatment trial (NETT): Evaluation of lung volume reduction surgery for emphysema. June 20, 2001. http://www.nhlbi.nih.gov/health/prof/lung/nett/lvrsweb.htm

Perkins, L., & Shortall, S. P. (2000). Ventilation without intubation. *RN, 63*(1), 34–39.

*Powers, J., & Bennett, S. J. (1999). Measurement of dyspnea in patients treated with mechanical ventilation. *American Journal of Critical Care, 8*(4), 254–261.

Roviaro, G., Varoli, F., Nucca, O., Vergani, C., & Maciocco, M. (2000). Videothorascopic approach to primary mediastinal pathology. *Chest, 117*(4), 1179–1183.

Schwartz, J. (2000). Role of polyunsaturated fatty acids in lung disease. *American Journal of Clinical Nutrition, 71*(1), 393–396.

Sclafani, J. C. (1999). Clinical perspectives. Home oxygen for adults: selection of appropriate oxygen delivery system. *AARC Times, 23*(9), 51–54.

Seijo, L. M., & Sterman, D. H. (2001). Interventional pulmonology. *New England Journal of Medicine, 344*(10), 740–749.

Serra, A. (2000). Tracheostomy care. *Nursing Standard, 14*(42), 45–55.

Silomon, M., Claus, T., Hower, H., Biedler, A., Larsen, R., & Molter, G. (2000). Interpleural analgesia does not influence post-thoracotomy pain. *Anesthesia and Analgesia, 91*(1), 44–50.

Smith, L., & McDougall, C. (1999). Removal of chest drains. *Nursing Times, 95*(12), 24–30.

Smith, T., & Matti, A. M. (1999). Respiratory care. Air apparent long-term oxygen therapy. *Nursing Times, 95*(41), 34–38.

*Steuer, J. D., Stone, K. S., Nickel, J., & Steinfeld, Y. (2000). Methodologic issues associated with secretion weight as a dependent variable in research using closed-system suction catheters. *Nursing Research, 49*(5), 295–299.

St. John, R. E. (1999a). Advances in artificial airway management. *Critical Care Nursing Clinics of North America, 11*(1), 7–17.

St. John, R. E. (1999b). Protocols for practice: applying research at the bedside. Airway management. *Critical Care Nurse, 19*(4), 79–83.

Tasota, F. J., & Dobbin, K. (2000). Weaning your patient from mechanical ventilation. *Nursing, 30*(10), 41–47.

Takezawa, J. (2000). Hyperbaric oxygen therapy. *Critical Care Alert, 8*(8), 88–93.

Tamburri, L. M. (2000). Care of the patient with a tracheostomy. *Orthopaedic Nursing, 19*(2), 49–60.

Tobin, M. J. (2001). Advances in mechanical ventilation. *New England Journal of Medicine, 344*(26), 1986–1996.

Tonelli, M. R. (1999). Withdrawing mechanical ventilation: Conflicts and consensus. *Respiratory Care, 44*(11), 1383–1387.

Truesdell, S. (2000). Helping patients with COPD manage episodes of acute shortness of breath. *MedSurg Nursing, 9*(4), 178–182.

Valenzuela, R., & Rosen, D. (1999). Topical lidocaine-prilocaine cream (EMLA) for thoracostomy tube removal. *Anesthesia and Analgesia, 88*(1), 1107–1108.

Wilmoth, D. (1999). New strategies for mechanical ventilation: Lung protective ventilation. *Critical Care Nursing Clinics of North America, 11*(4), 447–454.

Woodruff, D. W. (1999). How to ward off complications of mechanical ventilation. *Nursing, 29*(11), 34–39.

Zevola, D. R., & Maier, B. (1999). Improving the care of cardiothoracic surgery patients through advanced nursing skills. *Critical Care Nurse, 19*(1), 34–36.

RESOURCES AND WEBSITES

American Association for Respiratory Care, 11030 Ables Lane, Dallas, TX 75229; (972) 243-2272; http://www.aarc.org.

American Lung Association, 1740 Broadway, New York, NY 10019; (212) 315-8700, (800) LUNG-USA; http://www.lungusa.org.

American Thoracic Society, 1740 Broadway, New York, NY 10019; (212) 315-8700; http://www.thoracic.org.

Canadian Lung Association, 3 Raymond Street, Suite 300, Ottawa, ON K1R 1A3; (613) 569-6411; (888) 566-LUNG (5864); http://www.lung.ca.

Health Canada, A.L. 0900C2, Ottawa, ON K1A 0K9; (613) 957-2991; (866) 225-0709; fax: (613) 941-5366; www.hc-sc.gc.ca.

National Heart, Lung and Blood Institute, National Institutes of Health, 9000 Rockville Pike, Bldg 31, Rm 5A52, Bethesda, MD 20892; (301) 496-5166 or (301) 496-4236; http://www.nhlbi.nih.gov.

Unit *6*

Cardiovascular, Circulatory, and Hematologic Function

Applying Concepts from NANDA, NIC, and NOC

Mr. Arno, age 57, has a history of peripheral arterial occlusive disease (2 years), hypertension, hypercholesterolemia, Type 2 diabetes, and smoking. He eats low-fat foods and cut back on smoking to half a pack a day. His home-monitored blood glucose levels range from 180 to 215 mg/dL. Because he has severe calf pain after walking, he now walks only two blocks a day: one block from home and one block back. He now receives medical treatment for a nonhealing ulcer on the plantar aspect of his left foot. The concept map illustrates the relationships that exist among the nursing diagnoses, interventions, and outcomes for one of Mr. Arno's clinical problems.

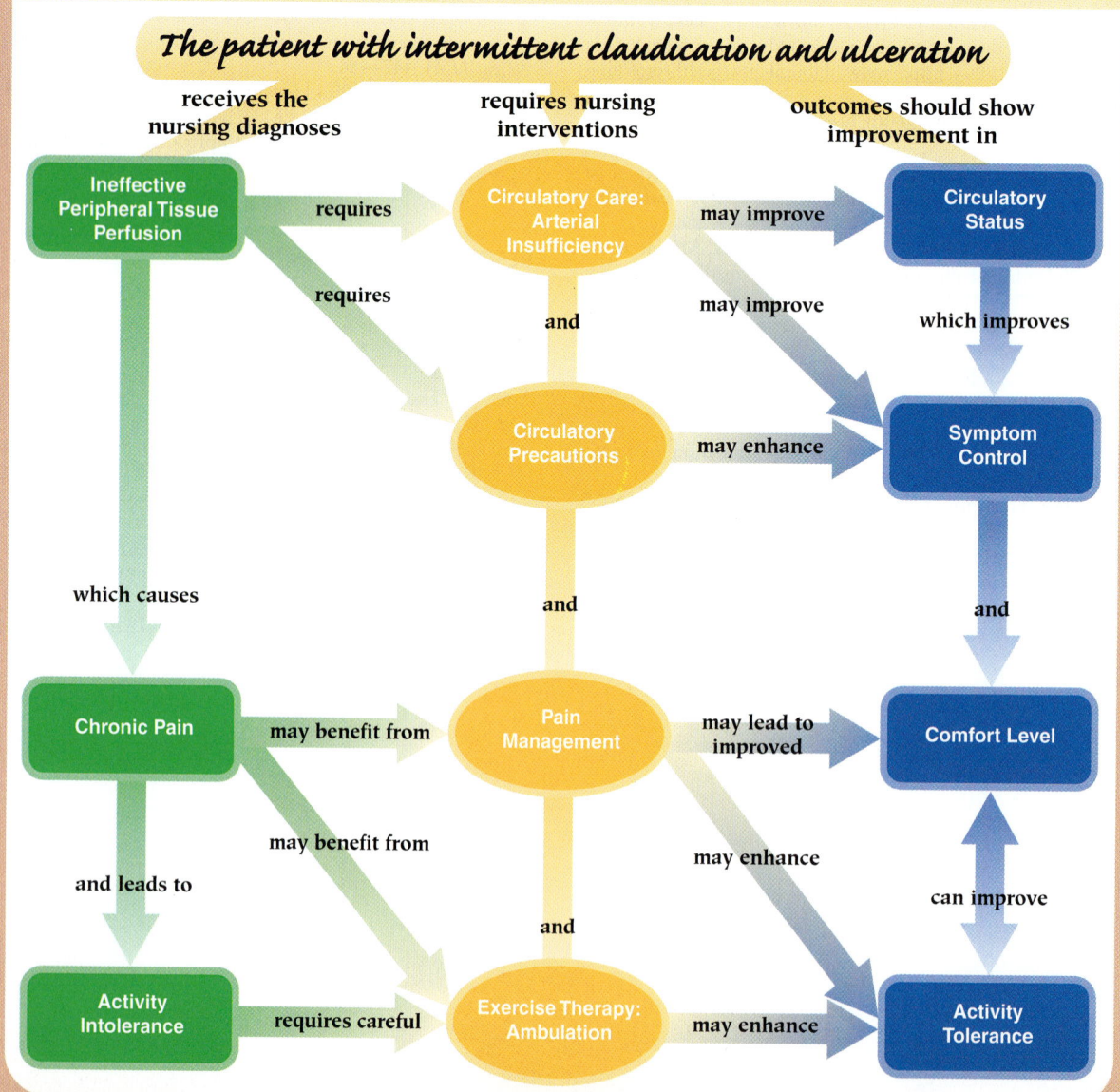

The patient with intermittent claudication and ulceration

| receives the nursing diagnoses | requires nursing interventions | outcomes should show improvement in |

Ineffective Peripheral Tissue Perfusion — requires → **Circulatory Care: Arterial Insufficiency** — may improve → **Circulatory Status**

requires → **Circulatory Precautions**

Circulatory Care: Arterial Insufficiency — may improve → **Symptom Control**

Circulatory Status — which improves → **Symptom Control**

Circulatory Precautions — may enhance → **Symptom Control**

Ineffective Peripheral Tissue Perfusion — which causes → **Chronic Pain**

Chronic Pain — may benefit from → **Pain Management**

Pain Management — may lead to improved → **Comfort Level**

Symptom Control — and → **Comfort Level**

Chronic Pain — and leads to → **Activity Intolerance**

Activity Intolerance — may benefit from → **Pain Management**

Activity Intolerance — requires careful → **Exercise Therapy: Ambulation**

Pain Management — and → **Exercise Therapy: Ambulation**

Exercise Therapy: Ambulation — may enhance → **Comfort Level**

Comfort Level — can improve → **Activity Tolerance**

Exercise Therapy: Ambulation — may enhance → **Activity Tolerance**

Nursing Classifications and Languages

NANDA
Nursing Diagnoses

Ineffective Tissue Perfusion—Decrease in oxygen resulting in the failure to nourish tissues at the capillary level

Chronic Pain—Unpleasant sensory and emotional experience arising from actual or potential tissue damage or described in terms of such damage; sudden or slow onset of any intensity from mild to severe, constant or recurring without an anticipated or predictable end and a duration of greater than 6 months

Activity Intolerance—Insufficient physiologic or psychological energy to endure or complete required or desired daily activities

NIC
Nursing Interventions*

Circulatory Care: Arterial Insufficiency—Promotion of arterial circulation

Circulatory Precautions—Protection of localized area with limited perfusion

Pain Management—Alleviation of pain or reduction in pain to a level of comfort that is acceptable to the patient

Exercise Therapy: Ambulation—Promotion and assistance with walking to maintain or restore autonomic and voluntary body functions during treatment and recovery from illness or injury

NOC
Nursing Outcomes†

Return to functional baseline status, stabilization of, or improvement in

Circulatory Status—Extent to which blood flows unobstructed, unidirectionally, and at an appropriate pressure through large vessels of the systemic and pulmonary circuits

Symptom Control—Personal actions to minimize perceived adverse changes in physical and emotional functioning

Comfort Level—Extent of physical and psychological ease

Activity Tolerance—Responses to energy-consuming body movements involved in required or desired daily activities

NANDA, North American Nursing Diagnosis Association; NIC, Nursing Interventions Classification; NOC, Nursing Outcomes Classification

*Iowa Intervention Project © 2000. In McCloskey, J. C., & Bulechek, G. M. (2000). *Nursing interventions classification (NIC)* (3rd ed.). St. Louis: Mosby.

†Iowa Outcomes Project © 2000. In Johnson, M., Maas, M., & Moorhead, S. (2000). *Nursing outcomes classification (NOC)* (3rd ed.). St. Louis: Mosby.

Assessment of Cardiovascular Function

Adapted by Alexander Clark and Colleen Norris

LEARNING OBJECTIVES

On completion of this chapter, the learner will be able to:

1. Explain cardiac physiology in relation to cardiac anatomy and the conduction system of the heart.

2. Incorporate assessment of functional health patterns and cardiac risk factors into the health history and physical assessment of the patient with cardiac conditions.

3. Identify the clinical significance and related nursing implications of the various tests and procedures used for diagnostic assessment of cardiac function.

4. Compare central venous pressure monitoring, pulmonary artery pressure monitoring, and systemic intra-arterial monitoring with regard to clinical usefulness and significance, possible complications, and nursing responsibilities.

Throughout the continuum of care, whether in a home, hospital, or rehabilitation setting, all patients with cardiovascular disease (disorders of the heart and major blood vessels; CVD) require similar assessments. Key components of the cardiovascular assessment include obtaining a health history, performing a physical assessment, and monitoring a variety of laboratory and diagnostic test results. An accurate and timely assessment of cardiovascular function provides the data necessary to identify nursing diagnoses, formulate a plan of care, and evaluate the response of the patient to the care provided. Essential to the development of these assessment skills is an understanding of the structure and function of the heart in health and in disease.

Anatomic and Physiologic Overview

The heart is a hollow, muscular organ located in the centre of the thorax, where it occupies the space between the lungs (mediastinum) and rests on the diaphragm. It weighs approximately 300 g, although heart weight and size are influenced by age, gender, body weight, extent of physical exercise and conditioning, and heart disease. The heart pumps blood to the tissues, supplying them with oxygen and other nutrients.

The pumping action of the heart is accomplished by the rhythmic contraction and relaxation of its muscular wall. During **systole** (contraction of the muscle), the chambers of the heart become smaller as the blood is ejected. During **diastole** (relaxation of the muscle), the heart chambers fill with blood in preparation for the subsequent ejection. A normal resting adult heart beats approximately 60 to 80 times per minute. Each ventricle ejects approximately 70 mL of blood per beat and has an output of approximately 5 L per minute.

ANATOMY OF THE HEART

The heart is composed of three layers (Fig. 26-1). The inner layer, or endocardium, consists of endothelial tissue and lines the inside of the heart and valves. The middle layer, or myocardium, is made up of muscle fibres and is responsible for the pumping action. The exterior layer of the heart is called the epicardium.

The heart is encased in a thin, fibrous sac called the pericardium, which is composed of two layers. Adhering to the epicardium is the visceral pericardium. Enveloping the visceral pericardium is the parietal pericardium, a tough fibrous tissue that attaches to the great vessels, diaphragm, sternum, and vertebral column and supports the heart in the mediastinum. The space between these two layers (pericardial space) is filled with about 30 mL of fluid, which lubricates the surface of the heart and reduces friction during systole.

Heart Chambers

The four chambers of the heart constitute the right- and left-sided pumping systems. The right side of the heart, made up of the right atrium and right ventricle, distributes venous blood (deoxygenated blood) to the lungs via the pulmonary artery (pulmonary circulation) for oxygenation. The right atrium receives blood returning from the superior vena cava (head, neck, and upper extremities), inferior vena cava (trunk and lower extremities), and coronary sinus (coronary circulation). The left

Glossary

afterload: the amount of resistance to ejection of blood from the ventricle

apical impulse (also called point of maximum impulse [PMI]): impulse normally palpated at the fifth intercostal space, left midclavicular line; caused by contraction of the left ventricle

baroreceptors: nerve fibres located in the aortic arch and carotid arteries that are responsible for reflex control of the blood pressure

cardiac catheterization: an invasive procedure used to measure cardiac chamber pressures and assess patency of the coronary arteries

cardiac conduction system: specialized heart cells strategically located throughout the heart that are responsible for methodically generating and coordinating the transmission of electrical impulses to the myocardial cells

cardiac output: amount of blood pumped by each ventricle in litres per minute; normal cardiac output is 5 L per minute in the resting adult heart

cardiac stress test: a test used to evaluate the functioning of the heart during a period of increased oxygen demand

contractility: ability of the cardiac muscle to shorten in response to an electrical impulse

depolarization: electrical activation of a cell caused by the influx of sodium into the cell while potassium exits the cell

diastole: period of ventricular relaxation resulting in ventricular filling

ejection fraction: percentage of the end-diastolic blood volume ejected from the ventricle with each heartbeat

hemodynamic monitoring: use of monitoring devices to measure cardiovascular function

hypertension: blood pressure greater than 140/90 mm Hg

hypotension: a decrease in blood pressure to less than 100/60 mm Hg

international normalized ratio (INR): a standard method for reporting prothrombin levels, eliminating the variation in test results from laboratory to laboratory

murmurs: sounds created by abnormal, turbulent flow of blood in the heart

myocardial ischemia: condition in which heart muscle cells receive less oxygen than needed

myocardium: muscle layer of the heart responsible for the pumping action of the heart

normal heart sounds: sounds produced when the valves close; normal heart sounds are S_1 (atrioventricular valves) and S_2 (semilunar valves)

postural (orthostatic) hypotension: a significant drop in blood pressure (usually 10 mm Hg systolic or more) after an upright posture is assumed

preload: degree of stretch of the cardiac muscle fibres at the end of diastole

pulmonary vascular resistance: resistance to right ventricle ejection of blood

radioisotopes: unstable atoms that emit small amounts of energy in the form of gamma rays; used in cardiac nuclear medicine studies

repolarization: return of the cell to resting state, caused by reentry of potassium into the cell while sodium exits the cell

sinoatrial (SA) node: primary pacemaker of the heart, located in the right atrium

stroke volume: amount of blood ejected from the ventricle per heartbeat; normal stroke volume is 70 mL in the resting heart

systemic vascular resistance: resistance to left ventricle ejection

systole: period of ventricular contraction resulting in ejection of blood from the ventricles into the pulmonary artery and aorta

telemetry: the process of continuous electrocardiographic monitoring by the transmission of radiowaves from a battery-operated transmitter worn by the patient

venodilating agent: medication causing dilation of veins

Physiology/Pathophysiology

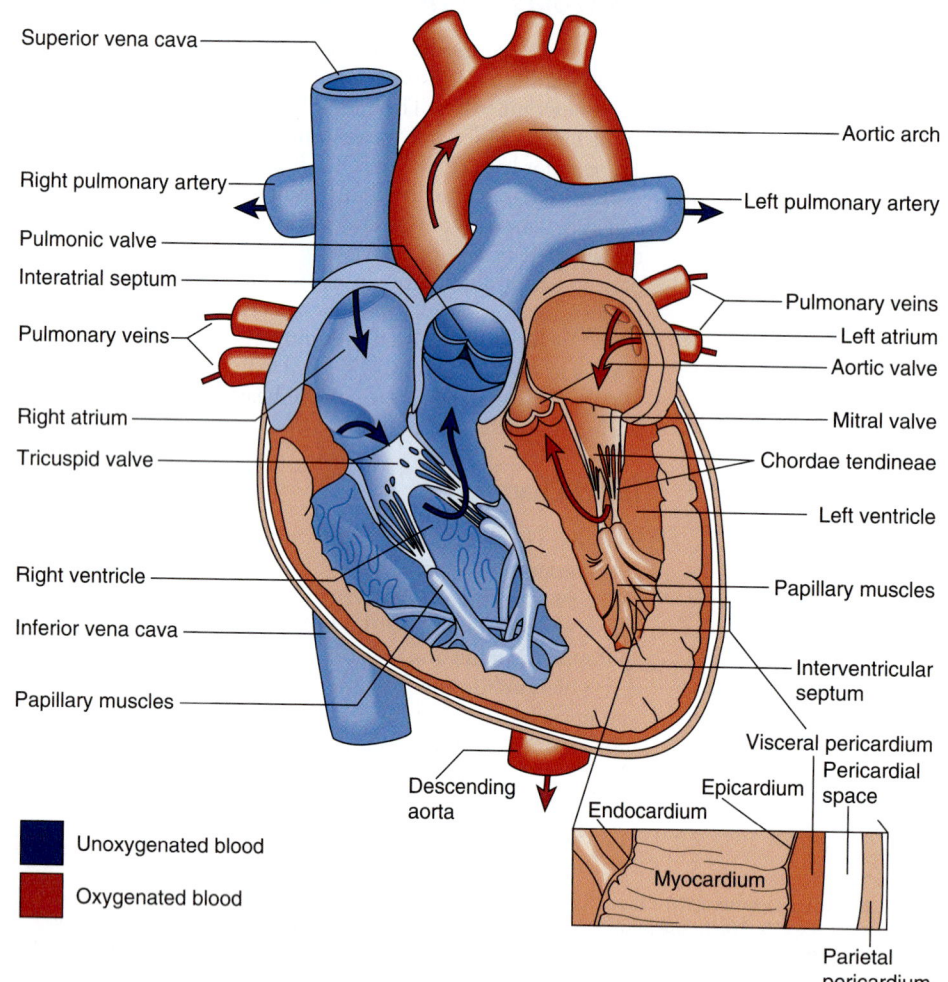

Superior vena cava

Right pulmonary artery

Pulmonic valve

Interatrial septum

Pulmonary veins

Right atrium

Tricuspid valve

Right ventricle

Inferior vena cava

Papillary muscles

Aortic arch

Left pulmonary artery

Pulmonary veins

Left atrium

Aortic valve

Mitral valve

Chordae tendineae

Left ventricle

Papillary muscles

Interventricular septum

Visceral pericardium

Pericardial space

Epicardium

Endocardium

Descending aorta

Myocardium

Parietal pericardium

Unoxygenated blood

Oxygenated blood

FIGURE 26-1 Structure of the heart. Arrows show course of blood flow through the heart chambers.

side of the heart, composed of the left atrium and left ventricle, distributes oxygenated blood to the remainder of the body via the aorta (systemic circulation). The left atrium receives oxygenated blood from the pulmonary circulation via the pulmonary veins. The relationships of the four heart chambers are shown in Figure 26-1.

The varying thicknesses of the atrial and ventricular walls relate to the workload required by each chamber. The atria are thin-walled because blood returning to these chambers generates low pressures. In contrast, the ventricular walls are thicker because they generate greater pressures during systole. The right ventricle contracts against low pulmonary vascular pressure and has thinner walls than the left ventricle. The left ventricle, with walls two-and-a-half times more muscular than those of the right ventricle, contracts against high systemic pressure.

Because the heart lies in a rotated position within the chest cavity, the right ventricle lies anteriorly (just beneath the sternum) and the left ventricle is situated posteriorly. The left ventricle is responsible for the apex beat or the point of maximum impulse (PMI), which is normally palpable in the left midclavicular line of the chest wall at the fifth intercostal space.

Heart Valves

The four valves in the heart permit blood to flow in only one direction. The valves, which are composed of thin leaflets of fibrous tissue, open and close in response to the movement of blood and pressure changes within the chambers. There are two types of valves: atrioventricular and semilunar.

ATRIOVENTRICULAR VALVES

The valves that separate the atria from the ventricles are termed atrioventricular valves. The tricuspid valve, so named because it is composed of three cusps or leaflets, separates the right atrium from the right ventricle. The mitral, or bicuspid (two cusps) valve, lies between the left atrium and the left ventricle (see Fig. 26-1).

Normally, when the ventricles contract, ventricular pressure rises, closing the atrioventricular valve leaflets. Two additional structures, the papillary muscles and the chordae tendineae, maintain valve closure. The papillary muscles, located on the sides of the ventricular walls, are connected to the valve leaflets by thin fibrous bands called chordae tendineae. During systole, contraction of the papillary muscles causes the chordae tendineae to become taut, keeping the valve leaflets approximated and closed.

SEMILUNAR VALVES

The two semilunar valves are composed of three half-moon-like leaflets. The valve between the right ventricle and the pulmonary artery is called the pulmonic valve; the valve between the left ventricle and the aorta is called the aortic valve.

Coronary Arteries

The left and right coronary arteries and their branches (Fig. 26-2) supply arterial blood to the heart. These arteries originate from the aorta just above the aortic valve leaflets. The heart has large metabolic requirements, extracting approximately 70% to 80% of the oxygen delivered (other organs consume, on average, 25%). Unlike other arteries, the coronary arteries are perfused during diastole. An increase in heart rate shortens diastole and can decrease myocardial perfusion. Patients, particularly those with coronary artery disease (CAD), can develop **myocardial ischemia** (inadequate oxygen supply) when the heart rate accelerates.

The left coronary artery has three branches. The artery from the point of origin to the first major branch is called the left main coronary artery. Two bifurcations arise off the left main coronary artery. These are the left anterior descending artery, which courses down the anterior wall of the heart, and the circumflex artery, which circles around to the lateral left wall of the heart.

The right side of the heart is supplied by the right coronary artery, which progresses around to the bottom or inferior wall of the heart. The posterior wall of the heart receives its blood supply by an additional branch from the right coronary artery called the posterior descending artery.

Superficial to the coronary arteries are the coronary veins. Venous blood from these veins returns to the heart primarily through the coronary sinus, which is located posteriorly in the right atrium.

Cardiac Muscle

The myocardium is composed of specialized muscle tissue. Microscopically, myocardial muscle resembles striated (skeletal) muscle, which is under conscious control. Functionally, however, myocardial muscle resembles smooth muscle because its contraction is involuntary. The myocardial muscle fibres are arranged in an interconnected manner (called a syncytium) that allows for coordinated myocardial contraction and relaxation. The sequential pattern of contraction and relaxation of individual muscle fibres ensures the rhythmic behaviour of the myocardium as a whole and enables it to function as an effective pump.

FUNCTION OF THE HEART: CONDUCTION SYSTEM

The specialized heart cells of the **cardiac conduction system** methodically generate and coordinate the transmission of electrical impulses to the myocardial cells. The result is sequential atrioventricular contraction, which provides for the most effective flow of blood, thereby optimizing cardiac output. Three physiologic characteristics of the cardiac conduction cells account for this coordination:

Automaticity: ability to initiate an electrical impulse
Excitability: ability to respond to an electrical impulse
Conductivity: ability to transmit an electrical impulse from one cell to another

The **sinoatrial (SA) node**, referred to as the primary pacemaker of the heart, is located at the junction of the superior vena cava and the right atrium (Fig. 26-3). The SA node in a normal resting heart has an inherent firing rate of 60 to 100 impulses per minute, but the rate can change in response to the metabolic demands of the body.

The electrical impulses initiated by the SA node are conducted along the myocardial cells of the atria via specialized tracts called internodal pathways. The impulses cause electrical stimulation

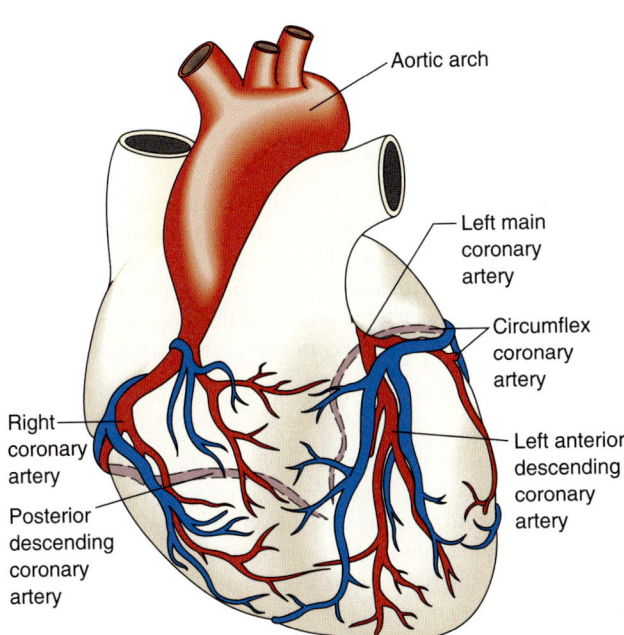

FIGURE 26-2 Coronary arteries (*red vessels*) arise from the aorta and encircle the heart. Coronary veins are shown in blue.

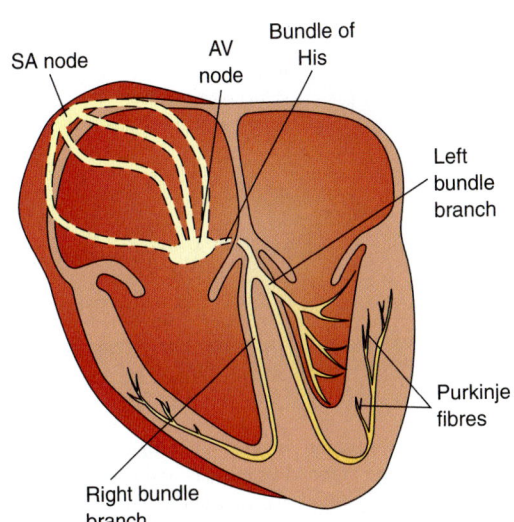

FIGURE 26-3 The cardiac conduction system. AV, atrioventricular; SA, sinoatrial.

and subsequent contraction of the atria. The impulses are then conducted to the atrioventricular (AV) node. The AV node (located in the right atrial wall near the tricuspid valve) consists of another group of specialized muscle cells similar to those of the SA node. The AV node coordinates the incoming electrical impulses from the atria and, after a slight delay (allowing the atria time to contract and complete ventricular filling), relays the impulse to the ventricles. This impulse is then conducted through a bundle of specialized conduction cells (bundle of His) that travel in the septum separating the left and right ventricles. The bundle of His divides into the right bundle branch (conducting impulses to the right ventricle) and the left bundle branch (conducting impulses to the left ventricle). To transmit impulses to the largest chamber of the heart, the left bundle branch bifurcates into the left anterior and left posterior bundle branches. Impulses travel through the bundle branches to reach the terminal point in the conduction system, called the Purkinje fibres. This is the point at which the myocardial cells are stimulated, causing ventricular contraction.

The heart rate is determined by the myocardial cells with the fastest inherent firing rate. Under normal circumstances, the SA node has the highest inherent rate, the AV node has the second-highest inherent rate (40 to 60 impulses per minute), and the ventricular pacemaker sites have the lowest inherent rate (30 to 40 impulses per minute). If the SA node malfunctions, the AV node generally takes over the pacemaker function of the heart at its inherently lower rate. Should both the SA and the AV nodes fail in their pacemaker function, a pacemaker site in the ventricle will fire at its inherent bradycardic rate of 30 to 40 impulses per minute.

Physiology of Cardiac Conduction

Cardiac electrical activity is the result of the movement of ions (charged particles such as sodium, potassium, and calcium) across the cell membrane. The electrical changes recorded within a single cell result in what is known as the cardiac action potential (Fig. 26-4).

In the resting state, cardiac muscle cells are polarized, which means an electrical difference exists between the negatively charged inside and the positively charged outside of the cell membrane.

As soon as an electrical impulse is initiated, cell membrane permeability changes and sodium moves rapidly into the cell, while potassium exits the cell. This ionic exchange begins **depolarization** (electrical activation of the cell), converting the internal charge of the cell to a positive one (see Fig. 26-4). Contraction of the myocardium follows depolarization. The interaction between changes in membrane voltage and muscle contraction is called electromechanical coupling. As one cardiac muscle cell is depolarized, it acts as a stimulus to its neighbouring cell, causing it to depolarize. Sufficient depolarization of a single specialized conduction system cell results in depolarization and contraction of the entire myocardium. **Repolarization** (return of the cell to its resting state) occurs as the cell returns to its baseline or resting state; this corresponds to relaxation of myocardial muscle.

After the rapid influx of sodium into the cell during depolarization, the permeability of the cell membrane to calcium is changed. Calcium enters the cell and is released from intracellular calcium stores. The increase in calcium, which occurs during the plateau phase of repolarization, is much slower than that of sodium and continues for a longer period.

Cardiac muscle, unlike skeletal or smooth muscle, has a prolonged refractory period during which it cannot be restimulated to contract. There are two phases of the refractory period, referred to as the absolute refractory period and the relative refractory period. The absolute refractory period is the time during which the heart cannot be restimulated to contract regardless of the strength of the electrical stimulus. This period corresponds with depolarization and the early part of repolarization. During the latter part of repolarization, however, if the electrical stimulus is stronger than normal, the myocardium can be stimulated to contract. This short period at the end of repolarization is called the relative refractory period.

Refractoriness protects the heart from sustained contraction (tetany), which would result in sudden cardiac death. Normal electromechanical coupling and contraction of the heart depend on the composition of the interstitial fluid surrounding the heart muscle cells. In turn, the composition of this fluid is influenced by the composition of the blood. A change in serum calcium concentration may alter the contraction of the heart muscle fibres. A change in serum potassium concentration is also important, because potassium affects the normal electrical voltage of the cell.

Cardiac Hemodynamics

An important determinant of blood flow in the cardiovascular system is the principle that fluid flows from a region of higher pressure to one of lower pressure. The pressures responsible for blood flow in the normal circulation are generated during systole and diastole. Figure 26-5 depicts the pressure differences in the great vessels and in the four chambers of the heart during systole and diastole.

CARDIAC CYCLE

Beginning with systole, the pressure inside the ventricles rapidly rises, forcing the atrioventricular valves to close. As a result, blood ceases to flow from the atria into the ventricles and regurgitation (backflow) of blood into the atria is prevented. The rapid rise of pressure inside the right and left ventricles forces the pulmonic and aortic valves to open, and blood is ejected into the pulmonary artery and aorta, respectively. The exit of blood is at first rapid;

FIGURE 26-4 Cardiac action potential. The arrows indicate the approximate time and direction of movement of each ion influencing membrane potential. Ca^{++} movement out of the cell is not well defined but is thought to occur during Phase 4.

Physiology/Pathophysiology

FIGURE 26-5 Great vessel and chamber pressures. Pressures are identified in millimeters of mercury (mm Hg) as mean pressure or systolic over diastolic pressure.

Labels in figure:
- Superior vena cava — 8–10
- Aortic arch — 110–130 / 70–80
- Right pulmonary artery
- Left pulmonary artery
- Pulmonic valve — 15–25 / 8–15
- Pulmonary veins
- Pulmonary veins
- Left atrium
- Right atrium — 0–8
- Aortic valve — 4–12
- Tricuspid valve
- Mitral valve
- Chordae tendineae
- Left ventricle — 110–130 / 4–12
- Right ventricle — 15–25 / 0–8
- Papillary muscles
- Inferior vena cava
- Interventricular septum
- Papillary muscles
- Descending aorta

then, as the pressure in each ventricle and its corresponding artery equalizes, the flow of blood gradually decreases. At the end of systole, pressure within the right and left ventricles rapidly decreases. This lowers pulmonary artery and aortic pressure, causing closure of the semilunar valves. These events mark the onset of diastole.

During diastole, when the ventricles are relaxed and the atrioventricular valves are open, blood returning from the veins flows into the atria and then into the ventricles. Toward the end of this diastolic period, the atrial muscles contract in response to an electrical impulse initiated by the SA node (atrial systole). The resultant contraction raises the pressure inside the atria, ejecting blood into the ventricles. Atrial systole augments ventricular blood volume by 15% to 25% and is sometimes referred to as the "atrial kick." At this point, ventricular systole begins in response to propagation of the electrical impulse that began in the SA node some milliseconds previously. The following section reviews the chamber pressures generated during systole and diastole.

Chamber Pressures. In the right side of the heart, the pressure generated during ventricular systole (15 to 25 mm Hg) exceeds the pulmonary artery diastolic pressure (8 to 15 mm Hg), and blood is ejected into the pulmonary circulation. During diastole, venous blood flows into the atrium because pressure in the superior and inferior vena cava (8 to 10 mm Hg) is higher than that in the atrium. Blood flows through the open tricuspid valve and

into the right ventricle until the two right chamber pressures equalize (0 to 8 mm Hg).

In the left side of the heart, similar events occur, although higher pressures are generated. As pressure mounts in the left ventricle during systole (110 to 130 mm Hg), resting aortic pressure (80 mm Hg) is exceeded and blood is ejected into the aorta. During left ventricular ejection, the resultant aortic pressure (110 to 130 mm Hg) forces blood progressively through the arteries. Forward blood flow into the aorta ceases as the ventricle relaxes and pressure drops. During diastole, oxygenated blood returning from the pulmonary circulation via the four pulmonary veins flows into the atrium, where pressure remains low. Blood readily flows into the left ventricle because ventricular pressure is also low. At the end of diastole, pressure in the atrium and ventricle equilibrates (4 to 12 mm Hg). Figure 26-5 depicts the systolic and diastolic pressures in the four chambers of the heart.

Pressure Measurement. Chamber pressures are measured with the use of special monitoring catheters and equipment. This technique is called hemodynamic monitoring. Nurses caring for critically ill patients must have a sophisticated working knowledge of normal chamber pressures and the hemodynamic changes that occur during serious illnesses. The data obtained from hemodynamic monitoring assist with the diagnosis and management of pathophysiologic conditions affecting critically ill patients. Hemodynamic monitoring is covered in more detail at the end of this chapter.

Cardiac Output

Cardiac output is the amount of blood pumped by each ventricle during a given period. The cardiac output in a resting adult is about 5 L per minute but varies greatly depending on the metabolic needs of the body. Cardiac output is computed by multiplying the stroke volume by the heart rate. **Stroke volume** is the amount of blood ejected per heartbeat. The average resting stroke volume is about 70 mL, and the heart rate is 60 to 80 beats per minute (bpm). Cardiac output can be affected by changes in either stroke volume or heart rate.

CONTROL OF HEART RATE

Cardiac output must be responsive to changes in the metabolic demands of the tissues. For example, during exercise the total cardiac output may increase fourfold, to 20 L per minute. This increase is normally accomplished by approximate doubling of both the heart rate and the stroke volume. Changes in heart rate are accomplished by reflex controls mediated by the autonomic nervous system, including its sympathetic and parasympathetic divisions. The parasympathetic impulses, which travel to the heart through the vagus nerve, can slow the cardiac rate, whereas sympathetic impulses increase it. These effects on heart rate result from action on the SA node, to either decrease or increase its inherent rate. The balance between these two reflex control systems normally determines the heart rate. The heart rate is stimulated also by an increased level of circulating catecholamines (secreted by the adrenal gland) and by excess thyroid hormone, which produces a catecholamine-like effect.

Heart rate is also affected by central nervous system and baroreceptor activity. **Baroreceptors** are specialized nerve cells located in the aortic arch and in both right and left internal carotid arteries (at the point of bifurcation from the common carotid arteries). The baroreceptors are sensitive to changes in blood pressure (BP). During elevations in BP (**hypertension**), these cells increase their rate of discharge, transmitting impulses to the medulla. This initiates parasympathetic activity and inhibits sympathetic response, lowering the heart rate and the BP. The opposite is true during **hypotension** (low BP). Hypotension results in less baroreceptor stimulation, which prompts a decrease in parasympathetic inhibitory activity in the SA node, allowing for enhanced sympathetic activity. The resultant vasoconstriction and increased heart rate elevate the BP.

CONTROL OF STROKE VOLUME

Stroke volume is primarily determined by three factors: preload, afterload, and contractility.

Preload is the term used to describe the degree of stretch of the cardiac muscle fibres at the end of diastole. The end of diastole is the period when filling volume in the ventricles is the highest and the degree of stretch on the muscle fibres is the greatest. The volume of blood within the ventricle at the end of diastole determines preload. Preload has a direct effect on stroke volume. As the volume of blood returning to the heart increases, muscle fibre stretch also increases (increased preload), resulting in stronger contraction and a greater stroke volume. This relationship, called the Frank-Starling law of the heart (or sometimes the Starling law of the heart), is maintained until the physiologic limit of the muscle is reached.

The Frank-Starling law is based on the fact that, within limits, the greater the initial length or stretch of the cardiac muscle cells (sarcomeres), the greater the degree of shortening that occurs. This result is caused by increased interaction between the thick and thin filaments within the cardiac muscle cells. Preload is decreased by a reduction in the volume of blood returning to the ventricles. Diuresis, **venodilating agents** (eg, nitrates), and loss of blood or body fluids from excessive diaphoresis, vomiting, or diarrhea reduce preload. Preload is increased by increasing the return of circulating blood volume to the ventricles. Controlling the loss of blood or body fluids and replacing fluids (ie, blood transfusions and intravenous fluid administration) are examples of ways to increase preload.

The second determinant of stroke volume is **afterload**, the amount of resistance to ejection of blood from the ventricle. The resistance of the systemic BP to left ventricular ejection is called **systemic vascular resistance**. The resistance of the pulmonary BP to right ventricular ejection is called **pulmonary vascular resistance**. There is an inverse relationship between afterload and stroke volume. For example, afterload is increased by arterial vasoconstriction, which leads to decreased stroke volume. The opposite is true with arterial vasodilation: afterload is reduced because there is less resistance to ejection, and stroke volume increases.

Contractility is a term used to denote the force generated by the contracting myocardium under any given condition. Contractility is enhanced by circulating catecholamines, sympathetic neuronal activity, and certain medications (eg, digoxin, intravenous dopamine or dobutamine). Increased contractility results in increased stroke volume. Contractility is depressed by hypoxemia, acidosis, and certain medications (eg, beta-adrenergic blocking agents such as atenolol [Tenormin]).

The heart can achieve a greatly increased stroke volume (eg, during exercise) by increasing preload (through increased venous return), increasing contractility (through sympathetic nervous system discharge), and decreasing afterload (through peripheral vasodilation with decreased aortic pressure).

The percentage of the end-diastolic volume that is ejected with each stroke is called the **ejection fraction**. With each stroke, about 42% (right ventricle) to 50% (left ventricle) or more of the end-diastolic volume is ejected by the normal heart. The ejection fraction can be used as an index of myocardial contractility: the ejection fraction decreases if contractility is depressed.

🍂 Gerontologic Considerations

Changes in cardiac structure and function are clearly observable in the older heart. To understand the changes specifically related to aging, it is helpful to distinguish the normal aging process from changes related to CVD. The anatomic and functional changes in the aging heart are listed in Table 26-1.

Studies show that the normal aging heart can produce adequate cardiac output under ordinary circumstances but may have a limited ability to respond to situations that cause physical or emotional stress. In an elderly person who is less active, the left ventricle may become smaller (atrophy) as a consequence of physical deconditioning. Aging also results in decreased elasticity and widening of the aorta, thickening and rigidity of the cardiac valves, and increased connective tissue in the SA and AV nodes and bundle branches.

These changes lead to decreased myocardial contractility, increased left ventricular ejection time (prolonged systole), and delayed conduction. Therefore, stressful physical and emotional conditions, especially those that occur suddenly, may have adverse effects on the aged person. The heart cannot respond to such conditions with an adequate rate increase and needs more time to return to a normal resting rate after even a minimal increase in heart rate. In some patients, the added stress may precipitate heart failure (HF).

Table 26-1 • Age-Related Changes of the Cardiac System

CARDIOVASCULAR SYSTEM	STRUCTURAL CHANGES	FUNCTIONAL CHANGES	HISTORY AND PHYSICAL FINDINGS
Atria	↑ Size of left atrium Thickening of the endocardium	↑ Atrial irritability	Irregular heart rhythm from atrial dysrhythmias
Left ventricle	Endocardial fibrosis Myocardial thickening (hypertrophy) Infiltration of fat into myocardium	Left ventricle stiff and less compliant Progressive decline in cardiac output ↑ Risk for ventricular dysrhythmias Prolonged systole	Fatigue ↓ Exercise tolerance Signs and symptoms of HF or ventricular dysrhythmias Point of maximal impulse palpated lateral to the midclavicular line ↓ Intensity S_1, S_2; split S_2 S_4 may be present
Valves	Thickening and rigidity of AV valves Calcification of aortic valve	Abnormal blood flow across valves during cardiac cycle	Murmurs may be present Thrill may be palpated if significant murmur is present
Conduction system	Connective tissue collects in SA node, AV node, and bundle branches ↓ Number SA node cells ↓ Number AV, bundle of His, right and left bundle branch cells	Slower SA node rate of impulse discharge Slowed conduction across AV node and ventricular conduction system	Bradycardia Heart block ECG changes consistent with slowed conduction (↑ PR interval, widened QRS complex)
Sympathetic nervous system	↓ Response to beta-adrenergic stimulation	↓ Adaptive response to exercise: contractility and heart rate slower to respond to exercise demands Heart rate takes more time to return to baseline	Fatigue Diminished exercise tolerance ↓ Ability to respond to stress
Aorta and arteries	Stiffening of vasculature ↓ Elasticity and widening of aorta Elongation of aorta, displacing the brachiocephalic artery upward	Left ventricular hypertrophy	Progressive increase in systolic BP; slight ↑ in diastolic BP Widening pulse pressure Pulsation visible above right clavicle
Baroreceptor response	↓ Sensitivity of baroreceptors in the carotid artery and aorta to transient episodes of hypertension and hypotension	Baroreceptors unable to regulate heart rate and vascular tone, causing slow response to postural changes in body position	Postural blood pressure changes and reports feeling dizzy, fainting when moving from lying to sitting or standing position

AV, atrioventricular; BP, blood pressure; CHF, congestive heart failure; ECG, electrocardiographic; SA, sinoatrial.

GENDER DIFFERENCES IN CARDIAC STRUCTURE AND FUNCTION

Compared with a man's heart, a woman's heart tends to be smaller. It weighs less and has smaller coronary arteries. These structural differences have significant implications. Because the coronary arteries of a woman are smaller, they occlude from atherosclerosis more easily, making procedures such as cardiac catheterization and angioplasty technically more difficult, with a higher incidence of postprocedure complications. In addition, the resting rate, stroke volume, and ejection fraction of a woman's heart are higher than those of a man's, and the conduction time of an electrical impulse coursing from the SA node through the AV node to the Purkinje fibres is briefer.

Another significant difference between the genders is the physiologic effects of estrogen on the cardiovascular system. Two important effects of estrogen, regulation of vasomotor tone and of response to vascular injury, may be the mechanisms that protect women against the development of atherosclerosis. An additional, potentially beneficial effect of estrogen is its action on the liver, which results in improved lipid profiles. On the other hand, less favourable effects of estrogen include an increase in coagulation proteins and a decrease in fibrinolytic protein, which enhance the risk of thrombus formation. Progesterone also has vascular effects, but its role in the development of CVD is unclear at this time. Beneficial effects of estrogen disappear after menopause, as evidenced by the increased incidence of CVD in this population. However, because of health risks associated with hormone replacement therapy, the American Heart Association does not recommend its use as a primary or secondary prevention intervention for CVD (Mosca et al., 2001; Roussouw et al., 2002).

Assessment

The severity of the patient's symptoms, the practice setting of the nurse, and the purpose of the assessment are factors that need to be considered when determining the frequency and extent of nursing assessment required. The assessment of the acutely ill cardiac patient will be different from that of a patient with stable or chronic cardiac conditions. For example, the assessment performed by an emergency department nurse caring for a patient who is experiencing an acute myocardial infarction (MI) must be very focused and must be performed rapidly. The nurse must assess the patient for complications associated with the MI, screen the patient for contraindications to coronary artery reperfusion strategies including thrombolytic therapy or primary percutaneous transluminal coronary angioplasty (PTCA), and evaluate the patient's response to medical and nursing interventions. For this patient, the health history, physical assessment, and important nursing interventions (eg, cardiac monitoring, administration of intravenous medications) are performed simultaneously.

HEALTH HISTORY AND CLINICAL MANIFESTATIONS

For the patient experiencing an acute MI, the nurse obtains the health history using a few specific questions about the onset and severity of chest discomfort, associated symptoms, current medications, and allergies. At the same time, the nurse observes the patient's general appearance and evaluates hemodynamic status (heart rate and rhythm, BP). Once the condition of the patient stabilizes, a more extensive history can be obtained.

With stable patients, a complete health history is obtained during the initial contact. Often, it is helpful to have the patient's spouse or partner available during the health history interview. Initially, demographic information regarding age, gender, and ethnic origin is obtained. The family history, as well as the physi-

cal examination, should include assessment for genetic abnormalities associated with cardiovascular disorders (see Genetics in Nursing Practice box). Height, current weight, and usual weight (if there has been a recent weight loss or gain) are established. During the interview, the nurse conveys sensitivity to the cultural background and religious practices of the patient. This removes barriers to communication that may result if the interview is based only on the nurse's personal frame of reference. Patients from different cultural and ethnic groups may have different ways of describing symptoms such as pain and may engage in different health practices before seeking formal medical attention.

The baseline information derived from the history assists in identifying pertinent issues related to the patient's condition and educational and self-care needs. Once these problems are clearly identified, a plan of care is instituted. During subsequent contacts or visits with the patient, a more focused health history is performed to determine whether goals have been met, whether the plan needs to be modified, and whether new problems have developed. During the interview, the nurse asks questions to evaluate cardiac symptoms and health status.

Cardiac Signs and Symptoms

Patients with cardiovascular disorders commonly have one or more of the following signs and symptoms:

- Chest pain or discomfort (angina pectoris, MI, valvular heart disease)

NURSING RESEARCH PROFILE 26-1

Women With Coronary Artery Disease Report Worse Health-Related Quality of Life Outcomes Compared to Men

Norris, C. M., Ghali W. A., Galbraith, P. D., Graham, M. M., Jensen L. A., Knudtson, M. L. for the APPROACH Investigators. (2004). *Health and Quality of Life Outcomes*, May 5(2), 21.

Purpose
Although there have been substantial medical advances that improve the outcomes following cardiac ischemic events, gender differences in the treatment and course of recovery for patients with coronary artery disease (CAD) continue to exist. There is a general paucity of data comparing the health-related quality of life (HRQOL) in men and women undergoing treatment for CAD. The purpose of this study was to compare HRQOL outcomes of men and women in Alberta, at 1 year following initial catheterization, after adjustment for known demographic, co-morbid, and disease severity predictors of outcome.

Study Sample and Design
The HRQOL outcome data were collected by means of a self-reported questionnaire mailed to patients on or near the 1-year anniversary of their initial cardiac catheterization. Using the Seattle Angina Questionnaire (SAQ), five dimensions of HRQOL were measured: exertional capacity, anginal stability, anginal frequency, quality of life, and treatment satisfaction. Data from the APPROACH registry were used to risk-adjust the SAQ scale scores. Two analytical strategies were used including general least-squares linear modeling, and proportional odds modeling sometimes referred to as the "ordinal logistic modeling."

Eligible subjects included all adult Alberta residents over the age of 18 years, undergoing their first cardiac catheterization with two or more coronary arteries having ≥ 50% occlusion (Duke Coronary Index between 3 and 13) registered in the Alberta Provincial Project for Outcome Assessment in Coronary Heart Disease (APPROACH) database. Patients were excluded if they did not consent to become part

of the APPROACH follow-up cohort. APPROACH is a province-wide inception cohort of all adult Alberta residents undergoing cardiac catheterization for ischemic heart disease. The APPROACH database contains detailed clinical and treatment information for adult patients with known or suspected CAD. The data provide a unique opportunity to study outcomes in an unselected patient population.

Findings
3392 (78.1%) patients responded to the follow-up survey. The adjusted proportional odds ratios for men relative to women (PORs >1 = better) indicated that men reported significantly better HRQOL on all five SAQ dimensions as compared to women. PORs: Exertional Capacity 3.38 (2.75–4.15), Anginal Stability 1.23 (1.03–1.47), Anginal Frequency 1.70 (1.43–2.01), Treatment Satisfaction 1.27 (1.07–1.50), and QOL 1.74 (1.48–2.04).

Nursing Implications
Women with CAD consistently reported worse HRQOL at 1-year follow-up compared to men. These findings underline the fact that conclusions based on research performed on men with CAD may not be valid for women and that more gender-related research is needed. Nurses can teach colleagues and the lay public that gender differences in psychosocial adjustment following treatment for CAD exist as adjustment for traditional clinical variables fails to explain sex differences in health-related quality of life outcomes and therefore needs further investigation.

GENETICS IN NURSING PRACTICE—Cardiovascular Disorders

Several cardiovascular disorders are associated with genetic abnormalities. Some examples are:

- Familial hypercholesterolemia
- Hypertrophic cardiomyopathy
- Long QT syndrome (LQTS)
- Hereditary hemochromatosis
- Elevated homocysteine levels

NURSING ASSESSMENTS

FAMILY HISTORY ASSESSMENT

- Assess all patients with cardiovascular symptoms for coronary artery disease, regardless of age (early-onset CAD occurs).
- Assess family history of sudden death in persons who may or may not have been diagnosed with coronary disease (especially of early onset).
- Ask about sudden death in a previously asymptomatic child, adolescent, or adult.
- Ask about other family members with biochemical or neuromuscular conditions (eg, hemochromatosis or muscular dystrophy).
- Assess whether DNA mutation or other genetic testing has been performed on an affected family member

ASSESSMENT

- Assess for signs and symptoms of hyperlipidemias (xanthomas, corneal arcus, abdominal pain of unexplained origin).
- Assess for muscular weakness.

MANAGEMENT ISSUES SPECIFIC TO GENETICS

- If indicated, refer for further genetic counselling and evaluation so that the family can discuss inheritance, risk to other family members, availability of genetic testing, and gene-based interventions
- Offer appropriate genetic information and resources (eg, Genetic Alliance website, American Heart Association, Muscular Dystrophy Association)
- Provide support to families newly diagnosed with genetic-related cardiovascular disease

GENETICS RESOURCES

Genetic Alliance—a directory of support groups for patients and families with genetic conditions; http://www.geneticalliance.org.

Gene Clinics—a listing of common genetic disorders with up-to-date clinical summaries, genetic counselling, and testing information; http://www.geneclinics.org.

National Organization of Rare Disorders—a directory of support groups and information for patients and families with rare genetic disorders; http://www.rarediseases.org.

OMIM: Online Mendelian Inheritance in Man—a complete listing of inherited genetic conditions; http://www.ncbi.nlm.nih.gov/omim/stats/html.

- Shortness of breath or dyspnea (MI, left ventricular failure, HF)
- Edema and weight gain (right ventricular failure, HF)
- Palpitations (dysrhythmias resulting from myocardial ischemia, valvular heart disease, ventricular aneurysm, stress, electrolyte imbalance)
- Fatigue (earliest symptom associated with several cardiovascular disorders)
- Dizziness and syncope or loss of consciousness (postural hypotension, dysrhythmias, vasovagal effect, cerebrovascular disorders)

Not all chest discomfort is related to myocardial ischemia. When a patient has chest discomfort, questions should focus on differentiating a serious, life-threatening condition such as MI from conditions that are less serious or that would be treated differently (see Table 26-2).

The following points should be remembered when assessing patients with cardiac symptoms:

- Women are more likely to present with atypical symptoms of MI than are men.
- There is little correlation between the severity of the chest discomfort and the gravity of its cause. Elderly people and those with diabetes may not have pain with angina or MI because of neuropathies. Fatigue and shortness of breath may be the predominant symptoms in these patients.

- There is poor correlation between the location of chest discomfort and its source.
- The patient may have more than one clinical condition occurring simultaneously.
- In a patient with a history of CAD, the chest discomfort should be assumed to be secondary to ischemia until proven otherwise.

NURSING ALERT People experiencing myocardial ischemia can have a variety of symptoms. The typical symptom is angina presenting as pressure, fullness, squeezing pain, or discomfort in the centre of the chest. This pain may radiate to the shoulders, neck, jaw, or arms. Angina can also have an atypical or uncommon presentation, referred to as anginal equivalent. It is characterized by shortness of breath, fatigue, weakness, or pain in other parts of the upper body, including the neck, shoulder, jaw, arm, back, or stomach. Angina patterns are usually predictable (eg, with activity). Rest or sublingual nitroglycerin relieves symptoms within a few minutes. A patient in the midst of an MI, however, can present with angina or its equivalent symptoms, which last longer than 15 minutes. Signs and symptoms associated with an MI include lightheadedness, fainting, diaphoresis, unexplained anxiety, nausea, and shortness of breath. Symptoms are unrelieved by rest or nitroglycerin.

HEALTH PERCEPTION AND MANAGEMENT

In an effort to determine how patients perceive their current health status. The nurse might ask some of the following questions:

Do you have any health problems? If so, what do you think caused them?

How has your health been recently? Have you noticed any changes from last year? from 5 years ago?

Do you have a cardiologist or primary health care provider? How often do you go for checkups?

Do you use tobacco or consume alcohol?

What are your risk factors for heart disease? What do you do to stay healthy and take care of your heart?

What prescription and over-the-counter medications are you taking? Do you take vitamins or herbal supplements?

Some patients may not be aware of their own medical diagnosis. For example, patients may not realize that their heart attack was caused by CAD. Patients who do not understand that their behaviours or diagnoses pose a threat to their health may be less motivated to make lifestyle changes or to manage their illness effectively. On the other hand, patients who perceive that their modifiable cardiovascular risk factors have contributed to their health conditions may be more likely to change these behaviours (Chart 26-1).

The patient's ability to recognize cardiac symptoms and to know what to do when they occur is essential for effective self-care management. All too often, patients' new symptoms or symptoms of progressing cardiac dysfunction go unrecognized. This results in prolonged delays in seeking life-saving treatment. Major barriers to seeking prompt medical care include lack of knowledge about symptoms to expect with heart disease, attribution of symptoms to a benign source, psychological factors such as denial of symptom significance, and social factors, specifically feeling embarrassed about having symptoms (Zerwic, 1999).

An additional issue to consider is the patient's medication history, dosages, and schedules. Is the patient independent in taking medications? Are the medications taken as prescribed? Does the patient understand why the medication regimen is important? Are doses ever forgotten or skipped, or does the patient ever decide to stop taking a medication? An aspirin a day is a common nonprescription medication that improves patient outcomes after an MI. However, if patients are not aware of this benefit, they may be inclined to stop taking aspirin if they think it is a trivial medication.

A careful medication history will often uncover common medication errors and causes for nonadherence to the medication regimen.

Table 26-2 summarizes the characteristics and patterns of the more common cardiac and noncardiac causes of chest pain. Table 26-3 identifies typical questions nurses use to assess cardiac signs and symptoms, as well as those used to determine the patient's ability to recognize and manage them. Some of the patient's responses may require further clarification and follow-up.

NUTRITION AND METABOLISM

Dietary modifications, exercise, weight loss, and careful monitoring are important strategies for managing three major cardiovascular risk factors: hyperlipidemia, hypertension, and hyperglycemia (diabetes mellitus). Diets that are restricted in sodium, fat, cholesterol, and/or calories are commonly prescribed. The nurse should obtain the following information:

- The patient's current height and weight (to determine body mass index), waist measurement (assessment for obesity), BP, and any laboratory test results such as blood glucose, glycosylated hemoglobin (diabetes), total blood cholesterol, high-density and low-density lipoprotein levels, and triglyceride levels (hyperlipidemia).
- How often the patient self-monitors BP, blood glucose, and weight as appropriate to the medical diagnoses.
- The patient's level of awareness regarding his or her target goals for each of the risk factors and any problems achieving or maintaining these goals.
- What the patient normally eats and drinks in a typical day and any food preferences (including cultural or ethnic preferences).
- Eating habits (canned or commercially prepared foods versus fresh foods, restaurant cooking versus home cooking, assessing for high sodium foods, dietary intake of fats).
- Who shops for groceries and prepares meals.

ELIMINATION

Typical bowel and bladder habits need to be identified. Nocturia (awakening at night to urinate) is common for patients with HF. Fluid collected in the dependent tissues (extremities) during the day redistributes into the circulatory system once the patient is recumbent at night. The increased circulatory volume is excreted by the kidneys (increased urine production). Patients need to be aware of their response to diuretic therapy and any changes in urination. This is vitally important for patients with HF. Patients may be taught to modify (titrate) their dose of diuretics based on urinary pattern, daily weight, and symptoms of dyspnea.

To avoid straining, patients who become easily constipated need to establish a regular bowel regimen. When straining, the patient tends to bear down (the Valsalva manoeuvre), which momentarily increases pressure on the baroreceptors. This triggers a vagal response, causing the heart rate to slow down and resulting in syncope in some patients. For the same reason, straining during urination should be avoided. Because many cardiac medications can cause gastrointestinal side effects or bleeding, the nurse asks about bloating, diarrhea, constipation, stomach upset, heartburn, loss of appetite, nausea, and vomiting. Patients taking platelet-inhibiting medications such as aspirin and clopidogrel (Plavix); intravenous GP IIb/IIIa platelet aggregation inhibitors such as abciximab (Reopro), eptifibatide (Integrilin), and tirofiban (Aggrastat); and anticoagulants such as low-molecular-weight heparin (ie, dalteparin [Fragmin]), enoxaparin (Lovenox), heparin, or warfarin (Coumadin) are screened for bloody urine or stools.

Chart 26-1

Risk Factors for Heart Disease

Nonmodifiable risk factors include the following:
Positive family history for premature coronary artery disease
Increasing age
Gender (men and postmenopausal women)
Race (higher incidence in African Americans than in Caucasians)

Modifiable risk factors include the following:
Hyperlipidemia
Hypertension
Cigarette smoking
Elevated blood glucose level (ie, diabetes mellitus)
Obesity
Physical inactivity
Type A personality characteristics, particularly hostility
Use of oral contraceptives

Table 26-2 • **Assessing Chest Pain**

	CHARACTER, LOCATION, AND RADIATION	DURATION	PRECIPITATING EVENTS	RELIEVING MEASURES
Angina Pectoris 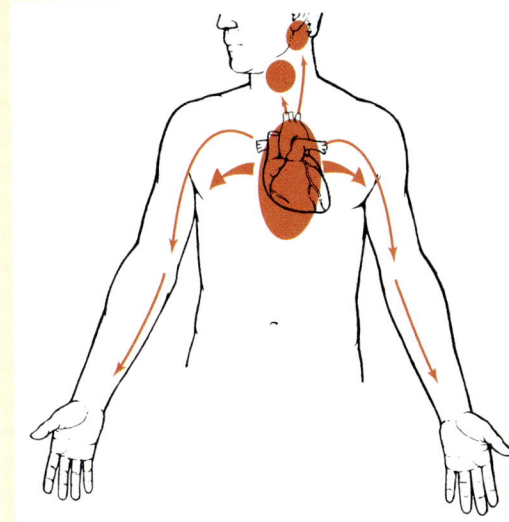	Substernal or retrosternal pain spreading across chest; may radiate to inside of arm, neck, or jaw	5–15 min	Usually related to exertion, emotion, eating, cold	Rest, nitroglycerin, oxygen
Myocardial Infarction 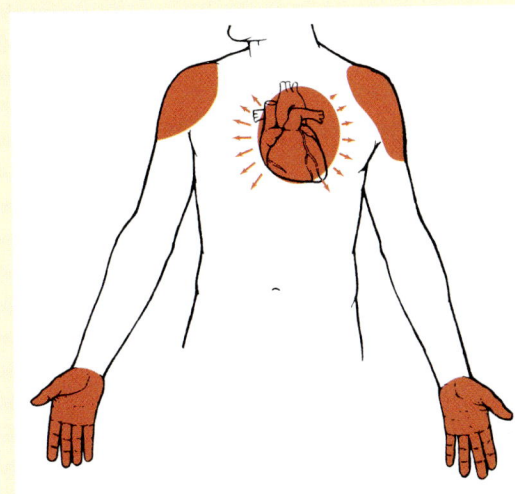	Substernal pain or pain over precordium; may spread widely throughout chest. Pain in shoulders and hands may be present.	>15 min	Occurs spontaneously but may be sequela to unstable angina	Morphine sulfate, successful reperfusion of blocked coronary artery
Pericarditis 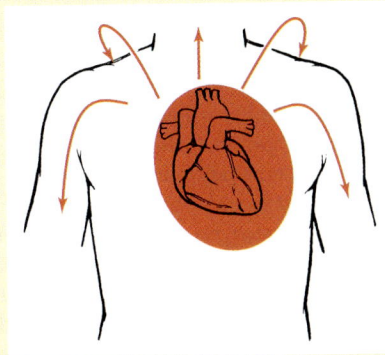	Sharp, severe substernal pain or pain to the left of sternum; may be felt in epigastrium and may be referred to neck, arms, and back	Intermittent	Sudden onset. Pain increases with inspiration, swallowing, coughing, and rotation of trunk.	Sitting upright, analgesia, anti-inflammatory medications

(continued)

Table 26-2 • **Assessing Chest Pain** (Continued)

	CHARACTER, LOCATION, AND RADIATION	DURATION	PRECIPITATING EVENTS	RELIEVING MEASURES
Pleuritic Pain	Pain arises from inferior portion of pleura; may be referred to costal margins or upper abdomen. Patient may be able to localize the pain.	30+ min	Often occurs spontaneously. Pain occurs or increases with inspiration.	Rest, time. Treatment of underlying cause, bronchodilators.
Esophageal Pain (Hiatal hernia, reflux esophagitis or spasm)	Substernal pain; may be projected around chest to shoulders.	5–60 min	Recumbency, cold liquids, exercise. May occur spontaneously.	Food, antacid. Nitroglycerin relieves spasm.
Anxiety	Pain over chest; may be variable. Does not radiate. Patient may complain of numbness and tingling of hands and mouth.	2–3 min	Stress, emotional tachypnea	Removal of stimulus, relaxation

ACTIVITY AND EXERCISE

As the nurse assesses the patient's activity and exercise history, it is important to note that decreases in activity tolerance are typically gradual and may go unnoticed by the patient. Therefore, the nurse needs to determine whether there has been a change in the activity pattern during the last 6 to 12 months. The patient's subjective response to activity is an essential assessment parameter. New symptoms or a change in the usual angina or angina equivalent during activity is a significant finding. Fatigue, associated with low ejection fraction and certain medications (eg, beta-blockers), can result in activity intolerance. Patients with fatigue may benefit from having their medications adjusted and learning energy conservation techniques.

Additional areas to ask about include possible architectural barriers and challenges in the home, and what the patient does for exercise. If the patient exercises, the nurse asks additional questions: What is the intensity, and how long and how often is exercise performed? Has the patient ever participated in a cardiac rehabilitation program? Functional levels are known to improve for almost all patients who participate in a cardiac rehabilitation program, and attendance is highly recommended (Smith et al., 2001). Patients with disabilities may require an individually tailored exercise program.

SLEEP AND REST

Clues to worsening cardiac disease, especially HF, can be revealed by sleep-related events. Determining where the patient sleeps or

Table 26-3 • **Asking Questions to Evaluate Cardiac Problems**

SYMPTOMS	ASSESSMENT QUESTIONS	ASSESSING PATIENT'S CAPACITY FOR SELF-MANAGEMENT
Chest pain, chest discomfort, angina pain	• Where is your pain (ask patient to point to location on chest) • What does the pain feel like? (pressure, heaviness, burning) • How severe is it on a scale of 0 to 10? • What causes the pain? (exertion, stress) • Does anything relieve it? (rest, nitroglycerin) • Does it spread to your arms, neck, jaw, shoulders, or back? • How long does the pain last? • Do you have any additional symptoms? (shortness of breath, palpitations, dizziness, sweating)	*Symptom Recognition* • If you have angina, what does it usually feel like? • If you have angina, how do your angina symptoms differ from the discomfort caused by your other medical conditions? (indigestion, GI disorders) • How do you think you would tell the difference between the symptoms of angina and a heart attack? • What were you doing when the pain started? *Symptom Management* • What did you do when the pain started? • How long did you wait before seeking medical attention (calling the doctor, coming to the emergency department, or calling the ambulance) *Use of Nitroglycerin* • Do you have a prescription for nitroglycerin (NTG) tablets or spray? • At the time of your chest pain, did you use your NTG? • How many tablets or sprays did you use and how frequently? • If you have NTG and did not take it with this angina episode, why do you think you did not take it? • When did you first open your NTG container? Where is it stored?
Shortness of breath, edema, weight gain	• When did you first notice feeling short of breath? • Do you have a cough? If yes, what do you cough up? • What makes you short of breath? Does anything make your breathing better or worse? • What activities are you no longer able to do because you are short of breath? • Do you ever wake up at night feeling short of breath? • What is your normal weight? • Have you had a recent weight gain? • Do you get up at night to urinate? Have you noticed an increase or decrease in the amount you usually urinate? • Have you noticed any weight gain or swelling in your feet, ankles, legs, or abdomen (sacrum if bedridden)? Do your shoes feel tight or clothes feel tight around your waist? • On how many pillows do you sleep, and has this changed recently? • Do you sleep in your bed, or do you breathe easier sleeping in a chair?	• Has anyone ever told you that you have heart failure? What does this mean to you? • Do you ever forget to take your diuretic medication (water pill) or other heart medicines or decide not to take them? If so, why do you think this happens? • What do you typically eat or drink? Who does the food shopping and meal preparation? • Are you on a sodium- or fluid-restricted diet? Have you been able to follow your special diet? • Do you have a scale to weigh yourself? How often do you weigh yourself? • What are important signs or symptoms to report to your doctor?
Palpitations	• Do you ever feel your heart racing, skipping beats, or pounding? • Do you ever feel lightheaded or dizzy? • Are there any other symptoms that occur at the same time? • How much caffeine do you consume? • Do you use tobacco (cigarettes, cigars, chew)? • Do you use any other stimulants, recreational drugs? • Do you use any nutritional supplements or herbs? • Have there been any changes in the amount of stress you experience?	• What did you do when your symptoms first occurred? • Is your primary health care provider aware of these symptoms? • Are you taking medication for this condition, and have you been taking it as directed?
Fatigue	• How would you describe your usual activity level? • What is your current activity level? • What were you able to do 1 month and 6 months ago? • What activities can you no longer do because of fatigue? • Do you feel rested when you wake up in the morning? • Can you rest during the day? • How often do you awaken at night, and for what reason?	• Have you spoken with your primary health care provider about decreases in your activity level? • Has anyone ever taught you energy conservation techniques? If so, are you able to use them?

(continued)

Table 26-3 • **Asking Questions to Evaluate Cardiac Problems** (Continued)

SYMPTOMS	ASSESSMENT QUESTIONS	ASSESSING PATIENT'S CAPACITY FOR SELF-MANAGEMENT
Dizziness, syncope (loss of consciousness)	• Do you ever feel dizzy or lightheaded? • Do you ever pass out or have fainting spells? • Does this happen when you move from a lying to a sitting or standing position? • Do you strain while having a bowel movement or when urinating? • Have you been urinating more than usual? • Have you decreased the amount of fluids you normally drink? • Do you have headaches?	• Have you ever been told you have high or low blood pressure? Has it been checked recently? • Are you taking any medications that can lower your blood pressure? • Before standing from a lying position, do you sit for a few minutes? Does that relieve the dizziness? • What are you using to prevent constipation?

rests is important. Recent changes, such as sleeping upright in a chair instead of in bed, increasing the number of pillows used, awakening short of breath at night (paroxysmal nocturnal dyspnea [PND]), or awakening with angina (nocturnal angina), are all indicative of worsening HF.

COGNITION AND PERCEPTION

Evaluating cognitive ability helps to determine whether the patient has the mental capacity to manage safe and effective self-care. Is the patient's short-term memory intact? Is there any history of dementia? Is there evidence of depression or anxiety? Can the patient read? Can the patient read English? What is the patient's reading level? What is the patient's preferred learning style? What information does the patient perceive as important?

Providing the patient with written information can be a valuable part of patient education, but only if the patient can read and comprehend the information. Related assessments include possible hearing or visual impairments. If vision is impaired, patients with HF may not be able to weigh themselves independently nor keep records of weight, BP, pulse, or other data requested by the health care team.

SELF-PERCEPTION AND SELF-CONCEPT

Personality factors are associated with the development of and recovery from CAD. Most commonly cited is "type A behaviour," which is characterized by competitive, hard-driving behaviours and a sense of time urgency. Although this behaviour is not an independent risk factor for CAD, anger and hostility (personality traits common in people with "type A behaviour") do affect the heart. People with these traits react to frustrating situations with an increase in BP, heart rate, and neuroendocrine responses. This physiologic activation, called cardiac reactivity, is thought to trigger acute cardiovascular events (Woods et al., 1999).

During the health history, the nurse discovers how patients feel about themselves by asking questions such as: How would you describe yourself? Have you changed the way you feel about yourself since your heart attack or surgery? Do you find that you are easily angered or hostile? How do you feel right now? What helps to manage these feelings? To fully evaluate this health pattern, assistance from a psychiatric clinical nurse specialist, psychologist, or psychiatrist may be necessary.

ROLES AND RELATIONSHIPS

Determining the patient's social support systems is vitally important in today's health care environment. Hospital stays for cardiac illnesses have shortened. Many invasive diagnostic cardiac procedures, such as cardiac catheterization and percutaneous

transluminal coronary angioplasty (PTCA) are performed as outpatient procedures. Patients are discharged back into the community with activity limitations, such as driving restrictions, and with greater nursing care and educational needs. These needs have significant implications for people who are independent under normal circumstances, and for people who are at higher risk for problems, such as older adults.

To assess support systems, the nurse needs to ask: Who is the primary caregiver? With whom does the patient live? Are there adequate services in place to provide a safe home environment? The nurse also assesses for any significant effects the cardiac illness has had on the patient's role in the family. Are there adequate finances and health insurance? The answers to these questions will assist the nurse in developing a plan to meet the patient's home care needs.

SEXUALITY AND REPRODUCTION

Although people recovering from cardiac illnesses or procedures are concerned about sexual activity, they are less likely to ask their nurse or other health care provider for information to help them resume their normal sex life. Lack of correct information and fear lead to reduced frequency and satisfaction with sexual activity. Therefore, nurses need to initiate this discussion with patients and not wait for them to bring it up in conversation. At first, inform the patient that it is common for people with similar heart problems to worry about resuming sexual activity. Then ask the patient to talk about his or her concerns.

The most commonly cited reasons for changes in sexual activity are fear of another heart attack or sudden death; untoward symptoms such as angina, dyspnea, or palpitations; and problems with impotence or depression. In men, impotence may develop as a side effect of cardiac medications (beta-adrenergic blocking agents) and may prompt patients to stop taking them. Other medications can be substituted, so patients should be encouraged to discuss this problem with their health care provider. Often, patients and their partners do not have adequate information about the physical demands related to sexual activity and ways in which these demands can be modified. The physiologic demands are greatest during orgasm, reaching 5 or 6 metabolic equivalents (METs). This level of activity is equivalent to walking 3 to 4 miles per hour on a treadmill. The METs expended before and after orgasm are considerably less, at 3.7 METs (Steinke, 2000). Having this information may make patients and their partners more comfortable with resuming sexual activity.

A reproductive history is necessary for women of childbearing age, particularly those with seriously compromised cardiac function. These women may be advised by their physicians not to become pregnant. The reproductive history includes information about previous pregnancies, plans for future pregnancies, oral contraceptive use (especially in women older than 35 years of age who are smokers), and use of hormone replacement therapy.

COPING AND STRESS TOLERANCE

It is important to determine the presence of psychosocial factors that adversely affect cardiac health. Anxiety, depression, and stress are known to influence both the development of and recovery from CAD. High levels of anxiety are associated with an increased incidence of CAD and increased in-hospital complication rates after MI. People with depression have an increased risk of MI- and heart disease–related death, compared to people without depression. It is postulated that people who are depressed feel hopeless and are less motivated to make lifestyle changes and follow treatment plans, explaining the association between mortality and depression (Buselli & Stuart, 1999).

Stress initiates a variety of physiologic responses, including increases in the circulation of catecholamines and cortisol, and has been strongly linked to cardiovascular events. Therefore, patients need to be assessed for presence of negative and positive emotions, as well as sources of stress. This is achieved by asking questions about recent or ongoing stressors, previous coping styles and effectiveness, and the patient's perception of his or her current mood and coping ability. To adequately evaluate this health pattern, consultation with a psychiatric clinical nurse specialist, psychologist, or psychiatrist may be indicated.

PREVENTION STRATEGIES

Additional features of the health history include identification of risk factors and measures taken by the patient to prevent disease. The nurse's questions need to focus on the patient's health promotion practices. Epidemiologic studies show that certain conditions or behaviours (ie, risk factors) are associated with a greater incidence of coronary artery, peripheral vascular, and cerebrovascular disease. Risk factors are classified by the extent to which they can be modified by changing one's lifestyle or modifying personal behaviours.

Once a patient's risk factors are determined, the nurse assesses whether the patient has a plan for making necessary behavioural changes and whether assistance is needed to support these lifestyle changes. For example, tobacco use is the most common avoidable cause of CAD. The first step in treating this health risk is to identify patients who use tobacco products and those who have recently quit. Because 70% of smokers visit a health care facility each year, nurses have ample opportunities to assess patients for tobacco use. For those who use tobacco, it is imperative to ask whether they are willing to quit. Provide cessation advice, motivation to quit, and relapse prevention strategies, as outlined in the Canadian Cardiovascular Society 1998 Consensus Conference on the Prevention of Cardiovascular Diseases: The Role of the Cardiovascular Specialist–Smoking (Canadian Cardiovascular Society, 1999). For patients who have obesity, hyperlipidemia, hypertension, and diabetes, the nurse determines any problems the patient may be having following the prescribed management plan (ie, diet, exercise, and medications). It may be necessary to clarify the patient's responsibilities, assist with finding additional resources, or make alternative plans for risk factor modification.

Comprehensive secondary prevention strategies (early diagnosis and prompt intervention to halt or slow the disease process and its consequences) aimed at reducing cardiovascular risk factors improve overall survival, improve quality of life, reduce the need for revascularization procedures (coronary artery bypass surgery and PTCA), and reduce the incidence of subsequent MIs. The overall benefits of secondary prevention also apply to other patient groups with atherosclerotic vascular disease, including patients with transient ischemic attacks, stroke, and peripheral vascular disease (the leading cause of disability and death in these patients being CAD). Despite these findings, only one third of eligible patients, over the long term, adhere to risk factor interventions. Patient compliance increases significantly with a team approach that includes long-term follow-up with office or clinic visits and telephone contact (Smith et al., 2001).

PHYSICAL ASSESSMENT

A physical examination is performed to confirm the data obtained in the health history. In addition to observing the patient's general appearance, a cardiac physical examination should include an evaluation of the following:

- Effectiveness of the heart as a pump
- Filling volumes and pressures
- Cardiac output
- Compensatory mechanisms

Indications that the heart is not contracting sufficiently or functioning effectively as a pump include reduced pulse pressure, cardiac enlargement, and murmurs and gallop rhythms (abnormal heart sounds).

The amount of blood filling the atria and ventricles and the resulting pressures (called filling volumes and pressures) are estimated by the degree of jugular vein distention and the presence or absence of congestion in the lungs, peripheral edema, and postural changes in BP that occur when the individual sits up or stands.

Cardiac output is reflected by cognition, heart rate, pulse pressure, colour and texture of the skin, and urine output. Examples of compensatory mechanisms that help maintain cardiac output are increased filling volumes and elevated heart rate. Note that the findings on the physical examination are correlated with data obtained from diagnostic procedures, such as hemodynamic monitoring (discussed later).

The examination, which proceeds logically from head to toe, can be performed in about 10 minutes with practice and covers the following areas: (1) general appearance, (2) cognition, (3) skin, (4) BP, (5) arterial pulses, (6) jugular venous pulsations and pressures, (7) heart, (8) extremities, (9) lungs, and (10) abdomen.

General Appearance and Cognition

The nurse observes the patient's level of distress, level of consciousness, and thought processes as an indication of the heart's ability to propel oxygen to the brain (cerebral perfusion). The nurse also observes for evidence of anxiety, along with any effects emotional factors may have on cardiovascular status. The nurse attempts to put the anxious patient at ease throughout the examination.

Inspection of the Skin

Examination of the skin begins during the evaluation of the general appearance of the patient and continues throughout the assessment. It includes all body surfaces, starting with the head and finishing with the lower extremities. Skin colour, temperature, and texture are assessed. The more common findings associated with cardiovascular disease are as follows.

- Pallor—a decrease in the colour of the skin—is caused by lack of oxyhemoglobin. It is a result of anemia or decreased arterial perfusion. Pallor is best observed around the fingernails, lips, and oral mucosa. In patients with dark skin, the nurse observes the palms of the hands and soles of the feet.
- Peripheral cyanosis—a bluish tinge, most often of the nails and skin of the nose, lips, earlobes, and extremities—suggests decreased flow rate of blood to a particular area, which allows more time for the hemoglobin molecule to become desaturated. This may occur normally in peripheral vasoconstriction associated with a cold environment, in patients with anxiety, or in disease states such as HF.
- Central cyanosis—a bluish tinge observed in the tongue and buccal mucosa—denotes serious cardiac disorders (pulmonary edema and congenital heart disease) in which venous blood passes through the pulmonary circulation without being oxygenated.
- Xanthelasma—yellowish, slightly raised plaques in the skin—may be observed along the nasal portion of one or both eyelids and may indicate elevated cholesterol levels (hypercholesterolemia).
- Reduced skin turgor occurs with dehydration and aging.
- Temperature and moistness are controlled by the autonomic nervous system. Normally the skin is warm and dry. Under stress, the hands may become cool and moist. In cardiogenic shock, sympathetic nervous system stimulation causes vasoconstriction, and the skin becomes cold and clammy. During an acute MI, diaphoresis is common.
- Ecchymosis (bruise)—a purplish-blue colour fading to green, yellow, or brown over time—is associated with blood outside of the blood vessels and is usually caused by trauma. Patients who are receiving anticoagulant therapy should be carefully observed for unexplained ecchymosis. In these patients, excessive bruising indicates prolonged clotting times (prothrombin or partial thromboplastin time) caused by an anticoagulant dosage that is too high.
- Wounds, scars, and tissue surrounding implanted devices should also be examined. Wounds are assessed for adequate healing, and any scars from previous surgeries are noted. The skin surrounding a pacemaker or implantable cardioverter defibrillator generator is examined for thinning, which could indicate erosion of the device through the skin.

Blood Pressure

Systemic arterial BP is the pressure exerted on the walls of the arteries during ventricular systole and diastole. It is affected by factors such as cardiac output, distention of the arteries, and the volume, velocity, and viscosity of the blood. BP usually is expressed as the ratio of the systolic pressure over the diastolic pressure, with normal adult values ranging from 100/60 to 140/90 mm Hg. The average normal BP usually cited is 120/80 mm Hg. An increase in BP above the upper normal range is called hypertension (see Chap. 32 for further definitions and management), whereas a decrease below the lower range is called hypotension.

BLOOD PRESSURE MEASUREMENT

BP can be measured with the use of invasive arterial monitoring systems (discussed later) or noninvasively by a sphygmomanometer and stethoscope or by an automated BP monitoring device. A detailed description of the procedure for obtaining BP can be found in nursing skills textbooks, and specific manufacturer's instructions review the proper use of the automated monitoring devices. Several important details must be observed to ensure that BP measurements are accurate; these are highlighted in Chart 26-2.

PULSE PRESSURE

The difference between the systolic and the diastolic pressures is called the pulse pressure. It is a reflection of stroke volume, ejection velocity, and systemic vascular resistance. Pulse pressure, which normally is 30 to 40 mm Hg, indicates how well the patient maintains cardiac output. The pulse pressure increases in conditions that elevate the stroke volume (anxiety, exercise, bradycardia), reduce systemic vascular resistance (fever), or reduce distensibility of the arteries (atherosclerosis, aging, hypertension). Decreased pulse pressure is an abnormal condition reflecting reduced stroke volume and ejection velocity (shock, HF, hypovolemia, mitral regurgitation) or obstruction to blood flow during systole (mitral or aortic stenosis). A pulse pressure of less than 30 mm Hg signifies a serious reduction in cardiac output and requires further cardiovascular assessment.

POSTURAL BLOOD PRESSURE CHANGES

Postural (orthostatic) hypotension occurs when the BP drops significantly after the patient assumes an upright posture. It is usually accompanied by dizziness, lightheadedness, or syncope.

Although there are many causes of postural hypotension, the three most common causes in patients with cardiac problems are a reduced volume of fluid or blood in the circulatory system (intravascular volume depletion, dehydration), inadequate vasoconstrictor mechanisms, and insufficient autonomic effect on vascular constriction. Postural changes in BP and an appropriate history help health care providers differentiate among these causes. The following recommendations are important when assessing postural BP changes:

Chart 26-2 — **Ensuring Accurate Blood Pressure Measurement**

- Cuff size must be appropriate for the patient. (The cuff size should have a bladder width at least 40% and length at least 80% of limb circumference.) The average adult cuff is 12 to 14 cm wide and 30 cm long. Using a cuff that is too small will give a high reading, whereas, too large a cuff results in a falsely low reading.
- Calibration of the sphygmomanometer should be performed routinely to ensure accuracy of blood pressure reading.
- Cuff is firmly wrapped around the arm, and cuff bladder is centred over the brachial artery.
- Patient's arm should be at heart level.
- Initial recordings are made on both arms, and subsequent measurements are taken on the arm with the higher pressure. Normally, in the absence of disease of the vasculature, there is a difference of no more than 5 mm Hg between arm pressures.
- Position of the patient and site of blood pressure measurement (eg, RA for right arm) are recorded.
- Palpation of the systolic pressure before auscultation helps to detect an auscultatory gap more readily.
- The patient is asked not to talk during blood pressure measurements. A significant increase in blood pressure and heart rate occurs when subjects are talking.

- Position the patient supine and flat (as symptoms permit) for 10 minutes before taking the initial BP and heart rate measurements.
- Check supine measurements before checking upright measurements.
- Do not remove the BP cuff between position changes, but check to see that it is still correctly placed.
- Assess postural BP changes with the patient sitting on the edge of the bed with feet dangling and, if appropriate, with the patient standing at the side of the bed.
- Wait 1 to 3 minutes after each postural change before measuring BP and heart rate.
- Be alert for any signs or symptoms of patient distress. If necessary, return the patient to a lying position before completing the test.
- Record both heart rate and BP and indicate the corresponding position (e.g., lying, sitting, standing) and any signs or symptoms that accompany the postural change.

Normal postural responses that occur when a person stands up or goes from a lying to a sitting position include (1) a heart rate increase of 5 to 20 bpm above the resting rate (to offset reduced stroke volume and maintain cardiac output); (2) an unchanged systolic pressure, or a slight decrease of up to 10 mm Hg; and (3) a slight increase of 5 mm Hg in diastolic pressure.

A decrease in the amount of blood or fluid in the circulatory system should be suspected after diuretic therapy or bleeding, when a postural change results in an increased heart rate and either a decrease in systolic pressure by 15 mm Hg or a drop in the diastolic pressure by 10 mm Hg. Vital signs alone do not differentiate between a decrease in intravascular volume and inadequate constriction of the blood vessels as a cause of postural hypotension. With intravascular volume depletion, the reflexes that maintain cardiac output (increased heart rate and peripheral vasoconstriction) function correctly; the heart rate increases, and the peripheral vessels constrict. However, because of lost volume, the BP falls. With inadequate vasoconstrictor mechanisms, the heart rate again responds appropriately, but because of diminished peripheral vasoconstriction the BP drops. The following is an example of a postural BP recording showing either intravascular volume depletion or inadequate vasoconstrictor mechanisms:

Lying down, BP 120/70, heart rate 70
Sitting, BP 100/55, heart rate 90
Standing, BP 98/52, heart rate 94

In autonomic insufficiency, the heart rate is unable to increase to completely compensate for the gravitational effects of an upright posture. Peripheral vasoconstriction may be absent or diminished. Autonomic insufficiency does not rule out a concurrent decrease in intravascular volume. The following is an example of autonomic insufficiency as demonstrated by postural BP changes:

Lying down, BP 150/90, heart rate 60
Sitting, BP 100/60, heart rate 60

Arterial Pulses

Factors to be evaluated in examining the pulse are rate, rhythm, quality, configuration of the pulse wave, and quality of the arterial vessel.

PULSE RATE

The normal pulse rate varies from a low of 50 bpm in healthy, athletic young adults to rates well in excess of 100 bpm after ex- ercise or during times of excitement. Anxiety frequently raises the pulse rate during the physical examination. If the rate is higher than expected, it is appropriate to reassess it near the end of the physical examination, when the patient may be more relaxed.

PULSE RHYTHM

The rhythm of the pulse is as important to assess as the rate. Minor variations in regularity of the pulse are normal. The pulse rate, particularly in young people, increases during inhalation and slows during exhalation. This is called sinus arrhythmia.

For the initial cardiac examination, or if the pulse rhythm is irregular, the heart rate should be counted by auscultating the apical pulse for a full minute while simultaneously palpating the radial pulse.

Any discrepancy between contractions heard and pulses felt is noted. Disturbances of rhythm (dysrhythmias) often result in a pulse deficit, a difference between the apical rate (the heart rate heard at the apex of the heart) and the peripheral rate. Pulse deficits commonly occur with atrial fibrillation, atrial flutter, premature ventricular contractions, and varying degrees of heart block. See Chapter 27 for a detailed discussion of these dysrhythmias.

To understand the complexity of dysrhythmias that may be encountered during the examination, the nurse needs to have a sophisticated knowledge of cardiac electrophysiology, obtained through advanced education and training.

PULSE QUALITY

The quality, or amplitude, of the pulse can be described as absent, diminished, normal, or bounding. It should be assessed bilaterally. Scales can be used to rate the strength of the pulse. The following is an example of a 0-to-4 scale:

0	pulse not palpable or absent
+1	weak, thready pulse; difficult to palpate; obliterated with pressure
+2	diminished pulse; cannot be obliterated
+3	easy to palpate, full pulse; cannot be obliterated
+4	strong, bounding pulse; may be abnormal

The numerical classification is quite subjective; therefore, when documenting the pulse quality, it helps to specify a scale range (eg, "left radial +3/+4").

PULSE CONFIGURATION

The configuration (contour) of the pulse conveys important information. In patients with stenosis of the aortic valve, the valve opening is narrowed, reducing the amount of blood ejected into the aorta. The pulse pressure is narrow, and the pulse feels feeble. In aortic insufficiency, the aortic valve does not close completely, allowing blood to flow back or leak from the aorta into the left ventricle. The rise of the pulse wave is abrupt and strong, and its fall is precipitous—a "collapsing" or "water hammer" pulse. The true configuration of the pulse is best appreciated by palpating over the carotid artery rather than the distal radial artery, because the dramatic characteristics of the pulse wave may be distorted when the pulse is transmitted to smaller vessels.

EFFECT OF VESSEL QUALITY ON PULSE

The condition of the vessel wall also influences the pulse and is of concern, especially in older patients. Once rate and rhythm have been determined, the nurse assesses the quality of the vessel by palpating along the radial artery and comparing it with normal vessels. Does the vessel wall appear to be thickened? Is it tortuous?

To assess peripheral circulation, the nurse locates and evaluates all arterial pulses. Arterial pulses are palpated at points where the arteries are near the skin surface and are easily compressed against bones or firm musculature. Pulses are detected over the temporal, carotid, brachial, radial, femoral, popliteal, dorsalis pedis, and posterior tibial arteries. A reliable assessment of the pulses of the lower extremities depends on accurate identification of the location of the artery and careful palpation of the area. Light palpation is essential; firm finger pressure can easily obliterate the dorsalis pedis and posterior tibial pulses and confuse the examiner. In approximately 10% of patients, the dorsalis pedis pulses are not palpable. In such circumstances, both are usually absent together, and the posterior tibial arteries alone provide adequate blood supply to the feet. Arteries in the extremities are often palpated simultaneously to facilitate comparison of quality.

 NURSING ALERT Do not palpate temporal or carotid arteries simultaneously, because it is possible to decrease the blood flow to the brain.

Jugular Venous Pulsations

An estimate of right-sided heart function can be made by observing the pulsations of the jugular veins of the neck. This provides a means of estimating central venous pressure, which reflects right atrial or right ventricular end-diastolic pressure (the pressure immediately preceding the contraction of the right ventricle).

Pulsations of the internal jugular veins are most commonly assessed. If they are difficult to see, pulsations of the external jugular veins may be noted. These veins are more superficial and are visible just above the clavicles, adjacent to the sternocleidomastoid muscles. The external jugular veins are frequently distended while the patient lies supine on the examining table or bed. As the patient's head is elevated, the distention of the veins disappears. The veins normally are not apparent if the head of the bed or examining table is elevated more than 30 degrees.

Obvious distention of the veins with the patient's head elevated 45 degrees to 90 degrees indicates an abnormal increase in the volume of the venous system. This is associated with right-sided HF, less commonly with obstruction of blood flow in the superior vena cava, and rarely with acute massive pulmonary embolism.

Heart Inspection and Palpation

The heart is examined indirectly by inspection, palpation, percussion, and auscultation of the chest wall. A systematic approach is the cornerstone of a thorough assessment. Examination of the chest wall is performed in the following six areas (Fig. 26-6):

1. *Aortic area*—second intercostal space to the right of the sternum. To determine the correct intercostal space, start at the angle of Louis by locating the bony ridge near the top of the sternum, at the junction of the body and the manubrium. From this angle, locate the second intercostal space by sliding one finger to the left or right of the sternum. Subsequent intercostal spaces are located from this reference point by palpating down the rib cage.
2. *Pulmonic area*—second intercostal space to the left of the sternum
3. *Erb's point*—third intercostal space to the left of the sternum

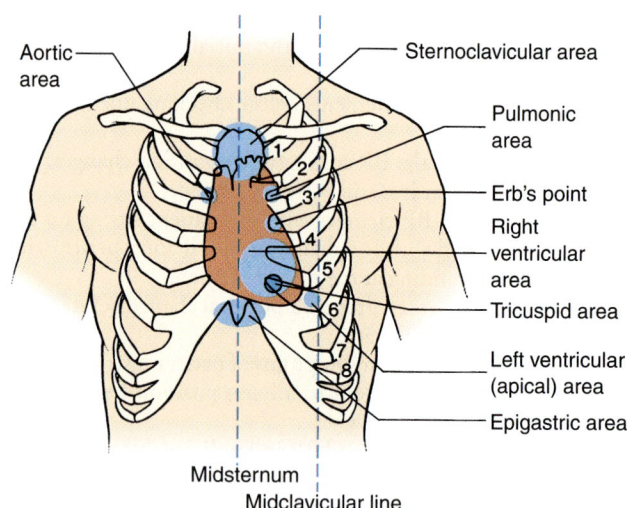

FIGURE 26-6 Areas of the precordium to be assessed when evaluating heart function. (Numerals identify ribs of adjacent intercostal spaces.)

4. *Right ventricular or tricuspid area*—fourth and fifth intercostal spaces to the left of the sternum
5. *Left ventricular or apical area*—the PMI, location on the chest where heart contractions can be palpated
6. *Epigastric area*—below the xiphoid process

For most of the examination, the patient lies supine, with the head slightly elevated. The right-handed examiner is positioned at the right side of the patient and the left-handed examiner at the left side.

In a systematic fashion, each area of the precordium is inspected and then palpated. Oblique lighting is used to assist the examiner in identifying subtle pulsation. A normal impulse that is distinct and located over the apex of the heart is called the **apical impulse** (PMI). It may be observed in young people and in older people who are thin. The apical impulse is normally located and auscultated in the left fifth intercostal space in the midclavicular line (Fig. 26-7).

In many cases, the apical impulse is palpable and is normally felt as a light pulsation, 1 to 2 cm in diameter. It is felt at the onset of the first heart sound and lasts for only half of systole. (See the next section for a discussion of heart sounds.) The nurse uses the palm of the hand to locate the apical impulse initially and the fingerpads to assess its size and quality. A broad and forceful apical impulse is known as a left ventricular heave or lift. It is so named because it appears to lift the hand from the chest wall during palpation.

An apical impulse below the fifth intercostal space or lateral to the midclavicular line usually denotes left ventricular enlargement from left ventricular failure. Normally, the apical impulse is palpable in only one intercostal space; palpability in two or more adjacent intercostal spaces indicates left ventricular enlargement. If the apical impulse can be palpated in two distinctly separate areas and the pulsation movements are paradoxical (not simultaneous), a ventricular aneurysm should be suspected.

Abnormal, turbulent blood flow within the heart may be palpated with the palm of the hand as a purring sensation. This phenomenon is called a thrill and is associated with a loud murmur. A thrill is always indicative of significant pathology within the heart. Thrills also may be palpated over vessels when blood flow is significantly and substantially obstructed and over the carotid arteries if aortic stenosis is present or if the aortic valve is narrowed.

FIGURE 26-7 Locating (**A**) and palpating (**B**) the apical impulse (also called the point of maximal impulse, PMI). The apical impulse normally is located at the fifth intercostal space to the left of the sternum at the mid-clavicular line. The nurse locates the impulse with the palm of the hand and palpates with the fingerpads. © B. Proud in Weber, J. W., & Kelley, J. (2003). *Health assessment in nursing* (2nd ed.). Philadelphia: Lippincott Williams & Wilkins.

Chest Percussion

Normally, only the left border of the heart can be detected by percussion. It extends from the sternum to the midclavicular line in the third to fifth intercostal spaces. The right border lies under the right margin of the sternum and is not detectable. Enlargement of the heart to either the left or right usually can be noted. In people with thick chests, obesity, or emphysema, the heart may lie so deep under the thoracic surface that not even its left border can be noted unless the heart is enlarged. In such cases, unless the nurse detects a displaced apical impulse and suspects cardiac enlargement, percussion is omitted.

Cardiac Auscultation

All areas identified in Figure 26-6, except the epigastric area, are auscultated. These include the aortic area, the pulmonary area, Erb's point, the tricuspid area, and the apical area. The actions of the four valves are uniquely reflected at specific locations on the chest wall. These locations do not correspond to the anatomic locations of the valves within the chest; rather, they reflect the patterns by which heart sounds radiate toward the chest wall. Sound in vessels through which blood is flowing is always reflected

downstream. For example, the actions of the mitral valve are usually heard best in the fifth intercostal space at the midclavicular line. This is called the mitral valve area.

HEART SOUNDS

The **normal heart sounds**, S_1 and S_2, are produced primarily by the closing of the heart valves. The time between S_1 and S_2 corresponds to systole (Fig. 26-8). This is normally shorter than the time between S_2 and S_1 (diastole). As the heart rate increases, diastole shortens.

In normal physiology, the periods of systole and diastole are silent. Ventricular disease, however, can give rise to transient sounds in systole and diastole that are called gallops, snaps, or clicks. Significant narrowing of the valve orifices at times when they should be open, or residual gapping of valves at times when they should be closed, gives rise to prolonged sounds called murmurs.

S_1—First Heart Sound. Closure of the mitral and tricuspid valves creates the first heart sound (S_1), although vibration of the myocardial wall also may contribute to this sound. Although S_1 is heard over the entire precordium, it is heard best at the apex of the heart (apical area). Its intensity increases when the valve leaflets are made rigid by calcium in rheumatic heart disease and in any circumstance in which ventricular contraction occurs at a time when the valve is caught wide open. The latter circumstance occurs, for example, when a premature ventricular contraction interrupts the normal cardiac cycle. S_1 varies in intensity from beat to beat when atrial contraction is not synchronous with ventricular contraction. This is because the valve may be fully or partially closed on one beat and open on the subsequent one as a function of irregular atrial activity. S_1 is easily identifiable and serves as the point of reference for the remainder of the cardiac cycle.

S_2—Second Heart Sound. Closing of the aortic and pulmonic valves produces the second heart sound (S_2). Although these two valves close almost simultaneously, the pulmonic valve usually lags slightly behind. Therefore, under certain circumstances, the two components of the second sound may be heard separately (split S_2). The splitting is more likely to be accentuated on inspiration and to disappear on exhalation. (More blood is ejected from the right ventricle during inspiration than during exhalation.)

S_2 is heard loudest at the base of the heart. The aortic component of S_2 is heard clearly in both the aortic and pulmonic areas, and less clearly at the apex. The pulmonic component of S_2, if present, may be heard only over the pulmonic area. Therefore, one may hear a "single" S_2 in the aortic area and a split S_2 in the pulmonic area.

Gallop Sounds. If the blood filling the ventricle is impeded during diastole, as occurs in certain disease states, then a tem-

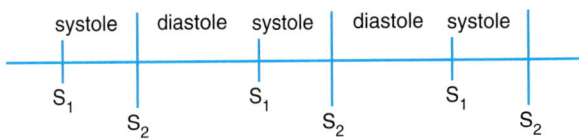

FIGURE 26-8 Normal heart sounds. The first heart sound (S_1) is produced by the closing of the mitral and tricuspid valves and is best heard at the apex of the heart (left ventricular or apical area). The second heart sound (S_2) is produced by the closing of the aortic and pulmonic valves and is loudest at the base of the heart. The time between S_1 and S_2 corresponds to systole. The time between S_2 and S_1 is diastole.

porary vibration may occur in diastole that is similar to, although usually softer than, S_1 and S_2. The heart sounds then come in triplets and have the acoustic effect of a galloping horse; they are called gallops. This may occur early in diastole, during the rapid-filling phase of the cardiac cycle, or later at the time of atrial contraction.

A gallop sound occurring during rapid ventricular filling is called a third heart sound (S_3); it represents a normal finding in children and young adults (Fig. 26-9A). Such a sound is heard in patients who have myocardial disease or in those who have HF and whose ventricles fail to eject all of their blood during systole. An S_3 gallop is heard best with the patient lying on the left side.

Gallop sounds heard during atrial contraction are called fourth heart sounds (S_4) (see Fig. 26-9B). An S_4 is often heard when the ventricle is enlarged or hypertrophied and therefore resistant to filling. Such a circumstance may be associated with CAD, hypertension, or stenosis of the aortic valve. On rare occasions, all four heart sounds are heard within a single cardiac cycle, giving rise to what is called a quadruple rhythm.

Gallop sounds are very low-frequency sounds and may be heard only with the bell of the stethoscope placed very lightly against the chest. They are heard best at the apex, although occasionally, when emanating from the right ventricle, they may be heard to the left of the sternum.

Snaps and Clicks. Stenosis of the mitral valve resulting from rheumatic heart disease gives rise to an unusual sound very early in diastole that is high-pitched and is best heard along the left sternal border. The sound is caused by high pressure in the left atrium with abrupt displacement of a rigid mitral valve. The sound is called an opening snap. It occurs too long after S_2 to be mistaken for a split S_2 and too early in diastole to be mistaken for a gallop. It almost always is associated with the murmur of mitral stenosis and is specific to this disorder.

In a similar manner, stenosis of the aortic valve gives rise to a short, high-pitched sound immediately after S_1 that is called an ejection click. This is caused by very high pressure within the ventricle, displacing a rigid and calcified aortic valve.

Murmurs. **Murmurs** are created by the turbulent flow of blood. The causes of the turbulence may be a critically narrowed valve, a malfunctioning valve that allows regurgitant blood flow, a congenital defect of the ventricular wall, a defect between the aorta and the pulmonary artery, or an increased flow of blood through a normal structure (eg, with fever, pregnancy, hyperthyroidism). Murmurs are characterized and consequently described by several characteristics, including timing in the cardiac cycle, location on the chest wall, intensity, pitch, quality, and pattern of radiation (Chart 26-3).

Friction Rub. In pericarditis, a harsh, grating sound that can be heard in both systole and diastole is called a friction rub. It is

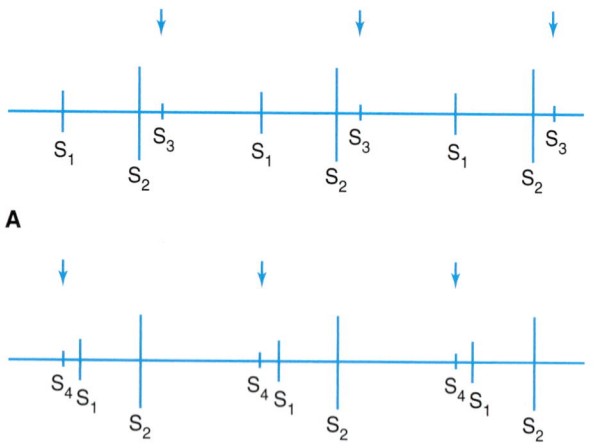

FIGURE 26-9 Gallops. (**A**) An S_3 gallop is heard immediately following the S_2 and occurs when the blood filling the ventricle is impeded during diastole, resulting in temporary vibrations. The heart sounds come in triplets and resemble the sound of a galloping horse. Myocardial disease and heart failure are associated with this sound. (**B**) An S_4 gallop is heard immediately preceding the S_1. The S_4 sound occurs during atrial contraction and is often heard when the ventricle is enlarged or hypertrophied. Associated conditions include coronary artery disease, hypertension, and stenosis of the aortic valve.

Chart 26-3   **Characteristics of Heart Murmurs**

Heart murmurs are described in terms of location, timing, intensity, pitch, quality, and radiation. These characteristics provide data about the location and nature of the cardiac abnormality.

Location
The location of the murmur (where it is detected on the chest wall) is crucial. Depending on the type of valvular disorder, a murmur can be heard only at the apex or more widely over the chest wall, or along the left sternal border between the third and fourth interspaces.

Timing
Timing of the murmur in the cardiac cycle is vital. The examiner first determines whether the murmur is occurring in systole or in diastole. Then, does it begin simultaneously with a heart sound, or is there some delay between the sound and the beginning of the murmur? Does the murmur continue to (or through) the second heart sound, or is there a delay between the end of the murmur and the second heart sound? Are diastolic murmurs (between the second and first heart sounds) continuous, or do they subside in mid- or late diastole?

Intensity
The intensity of murmurs is conventionally graded from I through VI. Sometimes, grade I murmurs are difficult to hear. However, a grade II cardiac murmur can be easily perceived by the experienced examiner. Murmurs of grades IV or louder are usually associated with thrills that may be palpated on the surface of the chest wall. A grade VI murmur can be heard with the stethoscope off the chest. A murmur may vary in intensity from its beginning to its conclusion. This is very characteristic of certain valvular disorders.

Pitch
The next important characteristic of a murmur is its pitch, which may be low, often heard only with the bell of the stethoscope placed lightly on the chest wall, or a very high-pitched murmur, heard best with the stethoscope's diaphragm. Other murmurs contain the full spectrum of sound frequency.

Quality
In addition to the intensity and pitch, the character of the sound. A murmur may be described as rumbling, blowing, whistling, harsh, or musical.

Radiation
The last feature of concern is radiation of the murmur. A murmur can radiate into the axilla, the carotid arteries in the neck, the left shoulder, or the back.

caused by abrasion of the pericardial surfaces during the cardiac cycle. Because a friction rub may be confused with a murmur, care should be taken to identify the sound and to distinguish it from murmurs that may be heard in both systole and diastole. A pericardial friction rub can be heard best using the diaphragm of the stethoscope, with the patient sitting up and leaning forward.

AUSCULTATION PROCEDURE

During auscultation, the patient remains supine and the examining room is as quiet as possible. A stethoscope with a diaphragm and a bell is necessary for accurate auscultation of the heart.

Using the diaphragm of the stethoscope, the examiner starts at the apical area and progresses upward along the left sternal border to the pulmonic and aortic areas. If desired, the examiner may choose to begin the examination at the aortic and pulmonic areas and progress downward to the apex of the heart. Initially, S_1 is identified and evaluated with respect to its intensity and splitting. Next, S_2 is identified, and its intensity and any splitting are noted. After concentrating on S_1 and S_2, the examiner listens for extra sounds in systole and then in diastole.

Sometimes it helps to ask the following questions: Do I hear snapping or clicking sounds? Do I hear any high-pitched blowing sounds? Is this sound in systole, or diastole, or both? The examiner again proceeds to move the stethoscope to all of the designated areas of the precordium, listening carefully for these sounds. Finally, the patient is turned on the left side and the stethoscope is placed on the apical area, where an S_3, an S_4, and a mitral murmur are more readily detected.

Once an abnormality is heard, the entire chest surface is re-examined to determine the exact location of the sound and its radiation. Also, the patient, who may be concerned about the prolonged examination, must be supported and reassured. The auscultatory findings, particularly murmurs, are documented by identifying the following characteristics:

- Location on chest wall.
- Timing of sound as either during systole or during diastole; described as early, middle, or late. (If heard throughout the systole, the sound is often referred to as pansystolic or holosystolic.)
- Intensity of the sound (I, very faint; II, quiet; III, moderately loud; IV, loud; V, very loud; or VI, heard with stethoscope removed from the chest).
- Pitch, described as high, medium, or low.
- Quality of the sound, commonly described as blowing, harsh, or musical.
- Location of radiation of the sound away from where it is heard the loudest.

INTERPRETATION OF CARDIAC SOUNDS

Interpreting cardiac sounds requires detailed knowledge of cardiac physiology and the pathophysiology of cardiac diseases. There are different levels of performance at which the nurse may be expected to function. The first level is simply recognizing that what one is hearing is not normal—such as a third heart sound, a murmur in systole or diastole, a pericardial friction rub over the midsternum, or a second heart sound that is widely split. These findings are reported to the physician and acted on accordingly. This level of function is useful in screening. It is the kind of activity involved in performing physical examinations in schools on normal children or in performing routine physical examinations or screening examinations.

The second level involves recognizing patterns. The nurse correctly observes the findings and can recognize the constellation of sounds and the diagnostic significance of common ones.

At its most sophisticated level, cardiac diagnosis can be interpretive. Highly skilled nurses can differentiate among dysrhythmias and respond accordingly. They can determine the significance of the appearance and disappearance of gallops during the treatment of patients who have had MIs or who have HF. This is the role that the coronary care nurse and the cardiovascular advanced practice nurse assume. They function with a team of other health care professionals who have highly tuned skills of cardiovascular assessment and diagnosis.

Inspection of the Extremities

The hands, arms, legs, and feet are observed for skin and vascular changes. The most noteworthy changes include the following:

- Decreased capillary refill time indicates a slower peripheral flow rate from sluggish reperfusion and is often observed in patients with hypotension or HF. Capillary refill time provides the basis for estimating the rate of peripheral blood flow. To test capillary refill, briefly compress the nailbed so that it blanches, and then release the pressure. Normally, reperfusion occurs within 3 seconds, as evidenced by the return of colour.
- Vascular changes from decreased arterial circulation include decrease in quality or loss of pulse, discomfort or pain, paresthesia, numbness, decrease in temperature, pallor, and loss of movement. During the first few hours after invasive cardiac procedures (eg, cardiac catheterization), affected extremities should be assessed for vascular changes frequently.
- Hematoma, or a localized collection of clotted blood in the tissue, may be observed in patients who have undergone invasive cardiac procedures such as cardiac catheterization, PTCA, or cardiac electrophysiology testing. Major blood vessels of the arms and legs are selected for catheter insertion. During these procedures, systemic anticoagulation with heparin is necessary, and minor or small hematomas may occur at the catheter puncture site. However, large hematomas are a serious complication that can compromise circulating blood volume and cardiac output, requiring blood transfusions. All patients who have undergone these procedures must have their puncture sites frequently observed until hemostasis is adequately achieved.
- Peripheral edema is fluid accumulation in dependent areas of the body (feet and legs, sacrum in the bedridden patient). Assess for pitting edema (a depression over an area of pressure) by pressing firmly for 5 seconds with the thumb over the dorsum of each foot, behind each medial malleolus, and over the shins. Pitting edema is graded as absent or as present on a scale from slight (1+ = 0 to 2 mm) to very marked (4+ = more than 8 mm). Peripheral edema is observed in patients with HF and in those with peripheral vascular diseases such as deep vein thrombosis or chronic venous insufficiency.
- Clubbing of the fingers and toes implies chronic hemoglobin desaturation, as in congenital heart disease.
- Lower extremity ulcers are observed in patients with arterial or venous insufficiency. Chapter 31 provides a complete description of differentiating characteristics.

Other Systems

LUNGS

The details of respiratory assessment are described in Chapter 21. Findings frequently exhibited by cardiac patients include the following:

Tachypnea: Rapid, shallow breathing may be noted in patients who have HF or pain, and in those who are extremely anxious.

Cheyne-Stokes respirations: Patients with severe left ventricular failure may exhibit Cheyne-Stokes breathing, a pattern of rapid respirations alternating with apnea. It is important to note the duration of the apnea.

Hemoptysis: Pink, frothy sputum is indicative of acute pulmonary edema.

Cough: A dry, hacking cough from irritation of small airways is common in patients with pulmonary congestion from HF.

Crackles: HF or atelectasis associated with bed rest, splinting from ischemic pain, or the effects of pain medications and sedatives often results in the development of crackles. Typically, crackles are first noted at the bases (because of gravity's effect on fluid accumulation and decreased ventilation of basilar tissue), but they may progress to all portions of the lung fields.

Wheezes: Compression of the small airways by interstitial pulmonary edema may cause wheezing. Beta-adrenergic blocking agents (beta-blockers), such as propranolol (Inderal), may precipitate airway narrowing, especially in patients with underlying pulmonary disease.

ABDOMEN

For the cardiac patient, two components of the abdominal examination are frequently performed.

Hepatojugular reflux: Liver engorgement occurs because of decreased venous return secondary to right ventricular failure. The liver is enlarged, firm, nontender, and smooth. The hepatojugular reflux may be demonstrated by pressing firmly over the right upper quadrant of the abdomen for 30 to 60 seconds and noting a rise of 1 cm or more in jugular venous pressure. This rise indicates an inability of the right side of the heart to accommodate increased volume.

Bladder distention: Urine output is an important indicator of cardiac function, especially when urine output is reduced. This may indicate inadequate renal perfusion or a less serious problem such as one caused by urinary retention. When the urine output is decreased, the patient needs to be assessed for a distended bladder or difficulty voiding. The bladder may be assessed with an ultrasound scanner or the suprapubic area palpated for an oval mass and percussed for dullness, indicative of a full bladder.

🍂 Gerontologic Considerations

When performing a cardiovascular examination on an elderly patient, the nurse may note such differences as more readily palpable peripheral pulses because of increased hardness of the arteries and a loss of adjacent connective tissue. Palpation of the precordium in the elderly is affected by the changes in the shape of the chest. For example, a cardiac impulse may not be palpable in patients with chronic obstructive pulmonary disease, because these patients usually have an increased anterior-posterior chest diameter. Kyphoscoliosis, a spinal deformity that occurs frequently in elderly patients, may dislocate the cardiac apex downward so that the diagnostic significance of palpating the apical impulse is obscured.

Systolic BP increases with age, but diastolic BP usually plateaus after 50 years. Medication therapy is usually initiated for high BP when consistent systolic readings of 160 mm Hg or diastolic readings of 95 mm Hg are observed. For the elderly patient, however, many factors are considered before initiating treatment. Orthostatic hypotension may reflect a decreasing sensitivity of postural reflexes, which must be considered when medication therapy is prescribed.

An S_4 is heard in about 90% of elderly patients; this is thought to be caused by decreased compliance of the left ventricle. The S_2 is usually split. At least 60% of elderly patients have murmurs, the most common being a soft systolic ejection murmur resulting from sclerotic changes of the aortic leaflets (see Table 26-1).

Diagnostic Evaluation

Diagnostic tests and procedures are used to confirm the data obtained by history and physical assessment. Some tests are easy to interpret, but others must be interpreted by expert clinicians. All tests should be explained to the patient. Some necessitate special preparation before they are performed and special monitoring by the nurse after the procedure.

LABORATORY TESTS

Laboratory tests may be performed for the following reasons:

- To assist in diagnosing an acute MI. (Angina pectoris, chest pain resulting from an insufficient supply of blood to the heart, cannot be confirmed by either blood or urine studies.)
- To identify abnormalities in the blood that affect the prognosis of a patient with a cardiac condition
- To assess the degree of inflammation
- To screen for risk factors associated with atherosclerotic coronary artery disease
- To determine baseline values before performing therapeutic interventions
- To monitor serum levels of medications
- To assess the effects of medications (e.g., the effects of diuretics on serum potassium levels)
- To screen generally for abnormalities

Because different laboratories use different equipment and different methods of measurements, normal test values may vary depending on the laboratory and the health care institution.

Cardiac Enzyme Analysis

Plasma cardiac enzyme analysis is part of a diagnostic profile that also includes the health history, symptoms, and electrocardiogram (ECG), associated with acute MI. Enzymes are released from injured cells when the cell membranes rupture. Most enzymes are nonspecific in relation to the particular organ that has been damaged. Certain isoenzymes, however, come only from myocardial cells and are released when the cells are damaged, such as by sustained hypoxia resulting in infarction or by trauma. The isoenzymes leak into the interstitial spaces of the myocardium and are carried into the general circulation by the lymphatic system and the coronary circulation, resulting in elevated serum enzyme concentrations.

Because different enzymes move into the blood at varying periods after MI, enzyme levels should be tested in relation to the time of onset of chest discomfort or other symptoms. Creatine kinase (CK) and its isoenzyme CK-MB are the most specific enzymes analyzed in acute MI, and they are the first enzyme levels to rise. Lactic dehydrogenase and its isoenzymes also are analyzed in patients who have delayed seeking medical attention, because these blood levels rise and peak in 2 to 3 days, much later than CK levels (see Table 28-5 in Chap. 28 for the time course of cardiac enzymes).

Myoglobin, an early marker of MI, is a heme protein with a small molecular weight. This allows it to be rapidly released from damaged myocardial tissue and accounts for its early rise, within 1 to 3 hours after the onset of an acute MI. Myoglobin peaks in 4 to 12 hours and returns to normal in 24 hours. Myoglobin is not used alone to diagnose MI, because elevations can also occur in patients with renal or musculoskeletal disease. However, negative results are helpful in ruling out an early diagnosis of MI.

Troponin I is measured in a laboratory test that has several advantages over traditional enzyme studies. Troponin I is a contractile protein found only in cardiac muscle. After myocardial injury, elevated serum troponin I concentrations can be detected within 3 to 4 hours; they peak in 4 to 24 hours and remain elevated for 1 to 3 weeks. These early and prolonged elevations make very early diagnosis of MI possible or allow for late diagnosis if the patient has delayed seeking treatment.

Blood Chemistry

LIPID PROFILE
Cholesterol, triglycerides, and lipoproteins are measured to evaluate a person's risk for developing atherosclerotic disease, especially if there is a family history of premature heart disease, or to diagnose a specific lipoprotein abnormality. Cholesterol and triglycerides are transported in the blood by combining with protein molecules to form lipoproteins. The lipoproteins are referred to as low-density lipoproteins (LDL) and high-density lipoproteins (HDL). The risk of CAD increases as the ratio of LDL to HDL or the ratio of total cholesterol (LDL + HDL) to HDL increases. Although cholesterol levels remain relatively constant over 24 hours, the blood specimen for the lipid profile should be obtained after a 12-hour fast.

CHOLESTEROL LEVELS
Cholesterol (normal level, less than 200 mg/dL) is a lipid required for hormone synthesis and cell membrane formation. It is found in large quantities in brain and nerve tissue. Two major sources of cholesterol are diet (animal products) and the liver, where cholesterol is synthesized. Elevated cholesterol levels are known to increase the risk for CAD. Factors that contribute to variations in cholesterol levels include age, gender, diet, exercise patterns, genetics, menopause, tobacco use, and stress levels.

LDLs (normal level, less than 130 mg/dL) are the primary transporters of cholesterol and triglycerides into the cell. One harmful effect of LDL is the deposition of these substances in the walls of arterial vessels. Elevated LDL levels are associated with a greater incidence of CAD. In people with known CAD or diabetes, the primary goal for lipid management is reduction of LDL levels to less than 100 mg/dL.

HDLs (normal range in men, 35 to 65 mg/dL; in women, 35 to 85 mg/dL) have a protective action. They transport cholesterol away from the tissue and cells of the arterial wall to the liver for excretion. Therefore, there is an inverse relationship between HDL levels and risk for CAD. Factors that lower HDL levels include smoking, diabetes, obesity, and physical inactivity. In patients with CAD, a secondary goal of lipid management is the increase of HDL levels to more than 40 mg/dL.

Triglycerides (normal range, 40 to 150 mg/dL), composed of free fatty acids and glycerol, are stored in the adipose tissue and are a source of energy. Triglyceride levels increase after meals and are affected by stress. Diabetes, alcohol use, and obesity can elevate triglyceride levels. These levels have a direct correlation with LDL and an inverse one with HDL.

SERUM ELECTROLYTE LEVELS
Sodium, potassium, and calcium are ions that are vital to cellular depolarization and repolarization. In addition, the serum sodium concentration reflects relative fluid balance. Generally, hyponatremia (low sodium level) indicates fluid excess, and hypernatremia (high sodium level) indicates fluid deficit.

Serum potassium is affected by renal function and may be decreased by diuretic agents that are used to treat HF. A decrease in potassium causes cardiac irritability and predisposes the patient receiving a digitalis preparation to digitalis toxicity and dysrhythmias. The effect of an elevated serum potassium concentration is myocardial depression and ventricular irritability. Both hypokalemia and hyperkalemia can lead to ventricular fibrillation or cardiac standstill. Calcium is necessary for blood coagulability and neuromuscular activity. Hypocalcemia and hypercalcemia can cause dysrhythmias.

Magnesium is integral to the absorption of calcium and the maintenance of potassium stores. It is required in the metabolism of adenosine triphosphate, playing a major role in protein synthesis, carbohydrate metabolism, and muscular contraction. Initial symptoms of hypermagnesemia are lethargy and decreased neuromuscular activity. On the ECG, hypomagnesemia lengthens the QT interval, predisposing the patient to life-threatening dysrhythmias.

BLOOD UREA NITROGEN LEVEL
Blood urea nitrogen (BUN) is an end product of protein metabolism and is excreted by the kidneys. In the patient with cardiac disease, an elevated BUN level may reflect reduced renal perfusion (from decreased cardiac output) or intravascular fluid volume deficit (from diuretic therapy or dehydration). The cause of elevated BUN is determined from the serum creatinine: high BUN and high creatinine reflect renal impairment, high BUN and normal creatinine reflect intravascular fluid volume deficit.

SERUM GLUCOSE LEVEL
The serum glucose level is important to monitor, because many patients with cardiac disease also have diabetes mellitus. In addition, the serum glucose level may be mildly elevated in stressful situations, when mobilization of endogenous epinephrine results in conversion of liver glycogen to glucose. Serum glucose levels are drawn in a fasting state. Glycosylated hemoglobin is an important measure to monitor in people with diabetes, because it reflects the blood glucose levels over 2 to 3 months. Hemoglobin A_{1C} is the common name for this test. The goal of diabetes management is to maintain the hemoglobin A_{1C} below 7% (normal range 4%–6%), reflecting consistent near-normal blood glucose

levels. This is particularly important for primary and secondary prevention of CVD (Brundy et al., 2002; Smith et al., 2001).

Coagulation Studies

The formation of a thrombus is initiated by injury to a vessel wall or to the tissue. These events activate the coagulation cascade, a complex series of interactions among phospholipids, calcium, and various clotting factors that converts prothrombin to thrombin. The coagulation cascade has two pathways, the intrinsic pathway and the extrinsic pathway. Coagulation studies are routinely performed before invasive procedures, such as cardiac catheterization, electrophysiology testing, and coronary or cardiac surgery.

Partial thromboplastin time (PTT) and activated partial thromboplastin time (aPTT) measure the activity of the intrinsic pathway. The values of PTT and aPTT are used to assess the effects of heparin therapy. Patients receiving heparin have their PTT or aPTT levels maintained at 1.5 to 2.5 times their baseline values (reference range, 25 to 38 seconds). Prothrombin time (PT) measures the extrinsic pathway activity and is used to monitor the effects of therapeutic anticoagulation with warfarin (Coumadin). Laboratory results of PT also include the **International Normalized Ratio (INR)**. The INR provides a standard method for reporting PT levels, eliminating the variation of PT results from laboratory to laboratory. The INR, rather than the PT alone, is used to monitor patients receiving warfarin therapy. The INR is maintained between 2.0 and 3.0 for patients with deep vein thrombosis, pulmonary embolism, valvular heart disease, or atrial fibrillation, and between 2.5 and 3.5 for patients with mechanical prosthetic heart valve replacements.

Hematologic Studies

The complete blood cell count (CBC) identifies the total number of white and red blood cells, the platelet count, and the hemoglobin and hematocrit. The CBC is carefully monitored in patients with CVD. White blood cell counts are monitored in immunocompromised patients, including patients with transplanted hearts, and in situations where there is concern for infection (eg, after invasive procedures or surgery). The red blood cells carry hemoglobin, which transports oxygen to the cells. The hematocrit is a measure of the relative proportion of red blood cells and plasma. Low hemoglobin and hematocrit levels have serious consequences for patients with CAD, such as more frequent angina episodes. Platelets are the first line of protection against bleeding. Once activated by blood vessel wall injury or rupture of atherosclerotic plaque, platelets undergo chemical changes that form a thrombus. Patients are prescribed medications to inhibit platelet function, including aspirin, clopidogrel (Plavix), and intravenous GP IIb/IIIa inhibitors (abciximab [Reopro], eptifibatide [Integrilin], tirofiban [Aggrastat]); therefore, it is essential to monitor for thrombocytopenia (low platelet counts). Chapter 33 provides an in-depth review of these laboratory tests and normal values.

CHEST X-RAY AND FLUOROSCOPY

A chest x-ray usually is obtained to determine the size, contour, and position of the heart. It reveals cardiac and pericardial calcifications and demonstrates physiologic alterations in the pulmonary circulation. It does not help diagnose acute MI but can help diagnose some complications (eg, HF). Correct placement of cardiac catheters, such as pacemakers and pulmonary artery catheters, is also confirmed by chest x-ray.

Fluoroscopy allows visualization of the heart on an x-ray screen. It shows cardiac and vascular pulsations and unusual cardiac contours. Fluoroscopy is useful for positioning intravenous pacing electrodes and for guiding catheter insertion during cardiac catheterization.

ELECTROCARDIOGRAPHY

The ECG is a diagnostic tool used in assessing the cardiovascular system. It is a graphic recording of the electrical activity of the heart; an ECG can be recorded with 12, 15, or 18 leads, showing the activity from those different reference points. The ECG is obtained by placing disposable electrodes in standard positions on the skin of the chest wall and extremities. The heart's electrical impulses are recorded as a tracing on special graph paper.

The standard 12-lead ECG is the most commonly used tool to diagnose dysrhythmias, conduction abnormalities, enlarged heart chambers, myocardial ischemia or infarction, high or low calcium and potassium levels, and effects of some medications. A 15-lead ECG adds 3 additional chest leads across the right precordium and is a valuable tool for the early diagnosis of right ventricular and posterior left ventricular infarction. The 18-lead ECG adds 3 posterior leads to the 15-lead ECG and is very useful for early detection of myocardial ischemia and injury (Wung & Drew, 1999). To enhance interpretation of the ECG, the patient's age, gender, BP, height, weight, symptoms, and medications (especially digitalis and antiarrhythmic agents) should be noted on the ECG requisition. The details of electrocardiography are covered in Chapter 27.

Continuous Electrocardiographic Monitoring

Continuous ECG monitoring is standard for patients who are at high risk for dysrhythmias. Two continuous ECG monitoring techniques are hardwire monitoring, found in critical care units and specialty step-down units, and telemetry, found in specialty step-down units and general nursing care units. Patients who are receiving continuous ECG monitoring need to be informed of its purpose and cautioned that this monitoring method will not detect symptoms such as dyspnea or chest pain. Therefore, patients need to be advised to report symptoms to the nurse whenever they occur.

HARDWIRE CARDIAC MONITORING

The patient's ECG can be continuously observed for dysrhythmias and conduction disorders on an oscilloscope at the bedside or at a central monitoring station by a hardwire monitoring system. This system is composed of three to five electrodes positioned on the patient's chest, a lead cable, and a bedside monitor. Hardwire monitoring systems vary in sophistication but in general can do the following:

- Monitor more than one lead simultaneously
- Monitor ST segments (ST-segment depression is a marker of myocardial ischemia; ST-segment elevation provides evidence of an evolving MI)
- Provide graded visual and audible alarms (based on priority, asystole would be highest)
- Computerize rhythm monitoring (dysrhythmias are interpreted and stored in memory)

- Print a rhythm strip
- Record a 12-lead ECG

Two leads commonly used for continuous monitoring are leads II and V1 or a modification of V1 (MCL1) (Fig. 26-10). Lead II provides the best visualization of atrial depolarization (represented by the P wave). Leads V1 and MCL1 best visualize the ventricle responsible for ectopic or abnormal ventricular beats.

TELEMETRY

In addition to hardwire monitoring systems, the ECG can be continuously observed by **telemetry**, the transmission of radio-waves from a battery-operated transmitter worn by the patient to a central bank of monitors. Although telemetry systems have the same capabilities as hardwire systems, they are wireless, allowing the patient to ambulate while being monitored. Following the guidelines for electrode placement will ensure good conduction and a clear picture of the patient's rhythm on the monitor:

- Clean the skin surface with soap and water and dry well (or as recommended by the manufacturer) before applying the electrodes. If the patient has much hair where the electrodes need to be placed, shave or clip the hair.
- Apply a small amount of benzoin to the skin if the patient is diaphoretic (sweaty) and the electrodes do not adhere well.
- Change the electrodes every 24 to 48 hours and examine the skin for irritation. Apply the electrodes to different locations each time they are changed.
- If the patient is sensitive to the electrodes, use hypoallergenic electrodes.

SIGNAL-AVERAGED ELECTROCARDIOGRAM

For some patients who are considered to be at high risk for sudden cardiac death, a signal-averaged ECG is performed. This high-resolution ECG assists in identifying the risk for life-threatening dysrhythmias and helps to determine the need for invasive diagnostic procedures. Signal averaging works by averaging about 150 to 300 QRS waveforms (QRS waveforms represent depolarization of the ventricle). The resulting averaged QRS complex is analyzed for certain characteristics that are likely to lead to lethal ventricular dysrhythmias. The recording is performed at the bedside and requires about 15 minutes.

CONTINUOUS AMBULATORY MONITORING

In ambulatory ECG monitoring, which may occur in the hospital but is more commonly prescribed for outpatients, one lead of the patient's ECG can be monitored by a Holter monitor. This monitor is a small tape recorder that continuously (for 10 to 24 hours) documents the heart's electrical activity on a magnetic tape. The tape recorder weighs approximately 2 pounds and can be carried over the shoulder or worn around the waist day and night to detect dysrhythmias or evidence of myocardial ischemia during activities of daily living. The patient keeps a diary of activity, noting the time of any symptoms, experiences, or unusual activities performed. The tape recording is then examined with a special scanner, analyzed, and interpreted. Evidence obtained in this way helps the physician diagnose dysrhythmias and myocardial ischemia and evaluate therapy, such as anti-arrhythmic and antianginal medications or pacemaker function.

TRANSTELEPHONIC MONITORING

Another method of evaluating the ECG of a patient at home is by transtelephonic monitoring. The patient attaches a specific lead system for transmitting the signals and places a telephone mouthpiece over the transmitter box; the ECG is recorded and evaluated at another location. This method is often used for diagnosing dysrhythmias and in follow-up evaluation of permanent cardiac pacemakers.

CARDIAC STRESS TESTING

Normally, the coronary arteries dilate to four times their usual diameter in response to increased metabolic demands for oxygen and nutrients. Coronary arteries with atherosclerosis, however, dilate much less, compromising blood flow to the myocardium and causing ischemia. Therefore, abnormalities in cardiovascular function are more likely to be detected during times of increased demand, or "stress." The **cardiac stress test** procedures—the exercise stress test, the pharmacologic stress test, and, more recently, the mental or emotional stress test—are noninvasive ways to evaluate the response of the cardiovascular system to stress. The stress test helps determine the following: (1) CAD, (2) cause of chest pain, (3) functional capacity of the heart after an MI or heart surgery, (4) effectiveness of antianginal or antiarrhythmic medications, (5) dysrhythmias that occur during physical exercise, and (6) specific goals for a physical fitness program. Contraindications

FIGURE 26-10 Two leads (views of the heart) commonly used for continuous monitoring. To monitor lead II, the negative electrode is placed on the right upper chest; the positive electrode is placed on the left lower chest. To monitor MCL1, the negative electrode is placed on the left upper chest; the positive electrode is placed in the V1 position. If three electrodes are used, the third electrode, which is the ground electrode, can be placed anywhere on the chest.

LEAD II   MCI₁

to stress testing include severe aortic stenosis, acute myocarditis or pericarditis, severe hypertension, suspected left main CAD, HF, and unstable angina. Because complications associated with stress testing can be life-threatening (MI, cardiac arrest, HF, and severe dysrhythmias), testing facilities must have staff and equipment ready to provide advanced cardiac life support.

Mental stress testing uses a mental arithmetic test or simulated public speech to determine whether an ischemic myocardial response occurs, similar to the response evoked by a conventional treadmill exercise test. Although its use for diagnostic purposes in patients with CAD is currently investigational, preliminary results indicate that the ischemic and hemodynamic measures obtained from mental stress testing may be useful in assessing the prognosis of patients with CHD who have had a positive exercise test (Krantz et al., 1999).

Stress testing is often combined with echocardiography or radionuclide imaging (discussed later). These techniques are performed during the resting state and immediately after stress.

Exercise Stress Testing

In an exercise stress test, the patient walks on a treadmill (most common) or pedals a stationary bicycle or arm crank. Exercise intensity progresses according to established protocols. The Bruce protocol, for example, is a common treadmill protocol in which the speed and grade of the treadmill are increased every 3 minutes. The goal of the test is to increase the heart rate to the "target heart rate." This is 80% to 90% of the maximum predicted heart rate and is based on the age and gender of the patient. During the test, the following are monitored: two or more ECG leads for heart rate, rhythm, and ischemic changes; BP; skin temperature; physical appearance; perceived exertion; and symptoms including chest pain, dyspnea, dizziness, leg cramping, and fatigue. The test is terminated when the target heart rate is achieved or when the patient experiences chest pain, extreme fatigue, a decrease in BP or pulse rate, serious dysrhythmias or ST segment changes on ECG, or other complications. When significant ECG abnormalities occur during the stress test (ST segment depressions), the test result is reported as positive and further diagnostic testing is required.

NURSING INTERVENTIONS

In preparation for the exercise stress test, the patient is instructed to fast for 4 hours before the test and to avoid stimulants such as tobacco and caffeine. Medications may be taken with sips of water. The physician may instruct patients not to take certain cardiac medications, such as beta-blockers, before the test. Clothes and sneakers or rubber-soled shoes suitable for exercising are to be worn. Women are advised to wear a bra that provides adequate support. The nurse describes the equipment used and the sensations and experiences that the patient may have during the test. The nurse explains the monitoring equipment used, the need to have an intravenous line placed, and the symptoms to report. The type of exercise is reviewed, and patients are asked to put forth their best exercise effort. If the test is to be performed with echocardiography or radionuclide imaging, this information is reviewed as well. After the test, patients are monitored for 10 to 15 minutes. Once stable, they may resume their usual activities.

Pharmacologic Stress Testing

Physically disabled or deconditioned patients will not be able to achieve their target heart rate by exercising on a treadmill or bi-

cycle. Two vasodilating agents, dipyridamole (Persantine) and adenosine (Adenocard), administered intravenously, are used to mimic the effects of exercise by maximally dilating the coronary arteries. The effects of dipyridamole last about 15 to 30 minutes. The side effects are related to its vasodilating action and include chest discomfort, dizziness, headache, flushing, and nausea. Adenosine has similar side effects, although patients report these symptoms as more severe. A unique property of adenosine is that it has an extremely short half-life (less than 10 seconds), so any severe effects rapidly subside. Dipyridamole and adenosine are the agents of choice used in conjunction with radionuclide imaging techniques. Theophylline and other xanthines, such as caffeine, block the effects of dipyridamole and adenosine and must be avoided before either of these pharmacologic stress tests.

Dobutamine (Dobutrex) is another medication that may be used for patients who cannot exercise. Dobutamine, a synthetic sympathomimetic, increases heart rate, myocardial contractility, and BP, thereby increasing the metabolic demands of the heart. It is the agent of choice when echocardiography is used because of its effects on altering myocardial wall motion (due to enhanced contractility). In addition, dobutamine is used for patients who have bronchospasm or pulmonary disease and cannot tolerate having doses of theophylline withheld.

NURSING INTERVENTIONS

In preparation for the pharmacologic stress test, patients are instructed not to eat or drink anything for at least 4 hours before the test. This includes chocolate, caffeine, caffeine-free coffee, tea, carbonated beverages, or medications with caffeine (eg, Anacin, Darvon). If caffeine is ingested before a dipyridamole or adenosine stress test, the test will have to be rescheduled. Patients taking aminophylline or theophylline are instructed to stop taking these medications for 24 to 48 hours before the test (if tolerated). Oral doses of dipyridamole are to be withheld as well. Patients are informed about the transient sensations they may experience during infusion of the vasodilating agent, such as flushing or nausea, which will disappear quickly. The patient is instructed to report any other symptoms occurring during the test to the cardiologist or nurse. An explanation of echocardiography or radionuclide imaging is also provided as necessary. The stress test may take about 1 hour, or up to 3 hours if imaging is performed.

ECHOCARDIOGRAPHY

Echocardiography is a noninvasive ultrasound test that is used to examine the size, shape, and motion of cardiac structures. It is a particularly useful tool for diagnosing pericardial effusions, determining the etiology of heart murmurs, evaluating the function of prosthetic heart valves, determining chamber size, and evaluating ventricular wall motion. It involves transmission of high-frequency sound waves into the heart through the chest wall and recording of the return signals. The ultrasound is generated by a hand-held transducer applied to the front of the chest. The transducer picks up the echoes, converts them to electrical impulses, and transmits them to the echocardiography machine for display on an oscilloscope and recording on a videotape. An ECG is recorded simultaneously to assist with interpreting the echocardiogram.

M-mode (motion), the unidimensional mode that was first introduced, provides information about the cardiac structures and their motion. Two-dimensional or cross-sectional echocardiography (Fig. 26-11), an enhancement of the technique, creates a sophisticated, spatially correct image of the heart. Other techniques, such as Doppler and colour flow imaging echocardiography, show the direction and velocity of the blood flow through the heart.

As previously mentioned, echocardiography may be performed with an exercise or pharmacologic stress test; resting and stress images are obtained. Myocardial ischemia from decreased perfusion during stress causes abnormalities in ventricular wall motion and is easily detected by echocardiography. A stress test using echocardiography is considered positive if abnormalities in ventricular wall motion are detected during stress but not during rest. These findings are highly suggestive of CAD and require further evaluation, such as a cardiac catheterization.

Transesophageal Echocardiography

A significant limitation of traditional echocardiography has been the poor quality of the images produced. Ultrasound loses its clarity as it passes through tissue, lung, and bone. Another echocardiographic technique involves threading a small transducer through the mouth and into the esophagus. This technique, called transesophageal echocardiography (TEE), provides clearer images because ultrasound waves are passing through less tissue. Pharmacologic stress testing using dobutamine and TEE can also be performed. The high-quality imaging obtained during TEE makes this technique an important adjunct to the technology available for detecting and evaluating the severity of CAD. Complications are uncommon during TEE, but if they do occur they are serious. These complications are caused by sedation and impaired swallowing from topical anesthesia (respiratory depression and aspiration) and by insertion and manipulation of the transducer into the esophagus and stomach (vasovagal response or esophageal perforation). The patient must be assessed before TEE for a history of dysphagia or radiation therapy to the chest that would increase the risk for complications.

NURSING INTERVENTIONS

Before traditional echocardiography, the nurse informs the patient about the test, explaining that it is painless. Echocardio-

graphic monitoring is performed while a transducer that emits the sound waves is moved about the chest. Gel applied to the skin helps transmit the sound waves. Periodically, the patient will have to turn onto the left side or hold a breath. The test takes about 30 to 45 minutes. If the patient is to undergo an exercise or pharmacologic stress test with echocardiography, information on stress testing is also reviewed.

In preparation for a TEE study, the following information is reviewed:

- The patient must fast for 6 hours before the study.
- An intravenous line is started for administering a sedative and any pharmacologic stress testing medications.
- The patient's throat is anesthetized before the probe is inserted.
- BP and the ECG are monitored throughout the study.
- The patient will be kept comfortable but not heavily sedated. The patient must be alert enough to follow instructions and to report symptoms such as chest pain.

After the study, monitoring continues for 30 to 60 minutes. The patient is to continue fasting for 4 hours. The patient may have a sore throat for the next 24 hours.

RADIONUCLIDE IMAGING

Radionuclide imaging studies involve the use of radioisotopes to evaluate coronary artery perfusion noninvasively, to detect myocardial ischemia and infarction, and to assess left ventricular function. **Radioisotopes** are atoms in an unstable form. Thallium 201 (Tl^{201}) and technetium 99m (Tc^{99m}) are two of the most common radioisotopes used in cardiac nuclear medicine studies. As they decay, they give off small amounts of energy in the form of gamma rays. When they are injected intravenously into the bloodstream, the energy emitted by the radioisotope can be detected by a gamma scintillation camera positioned over the body. Planar imaging, used with thallium, is a technique that provides a one-dimensional view of the heart from three locations. A relatively new technique called single photon emission computed tomography (SPECT) provides three-dimensional images. With SPECT, the patient is positioned supine with arms raised above the head, while the camera moves around the patient's chest in a 180- to 360-degree arc to identify the areas of decreased myocardial perfusion more precisely.

Myocardial Perfusion Imaging

The radioisotope Tl^{201} is used to assess myocardial perfusion. It resembles potassium and readily crosses into the cells of healthy myocardium. It is taken up more slowly and in smaller amounts by myocardial cells that are ischemic from decreased blood flow. However, thallium will not cross into the necrotic tissue that results from an MI.

Often, thallium is used with stress testing to assess changes in myocardial perfusion immediately after exercise (or after injection of one of the agents used in stress testing) and at rest. One or two minutes before the end of the stress test, a dose of Tl^{201} is injected into the intravenous line, allowing the radioisotope to be distributed into the myocardium. Images are taken immediately. Areas that do not show thallium uptake are noted as defects and indicate areas of either infarction or stress-induced myocardial ischemia. The resting images, taken 3 hours later, help to differentiate infarction

FIGURE 26-11 Two-dimensional echocardiogram, four-chamber view in a normal patient. The ventricles and atria are the dark areas outlined by the white. LA = left atrium, LV = left ventricle, RA = right atrium, RV = right ventricle. Courtesy of V. Bowles, RCS, CCT, Inova Alexandria Hospital, Alexandria, Virginia.

from ischemia. Infarcted tissue is unable to take up thallium regardless of when the scan is taken; the defect remains the same size. This is called a fixed defect, indicating that there is no perfusion in that area of the myocardium. Ischemic myocardium, on the other hand, recovers in a few hours. Once perfusion is restored, thallium crosses into the myocardial cells, and the area of defect on the resting images is either smaller or completely reversed. These reversible defects constitute positive stress test findings. Usually, cardiac catheterization is recommended after a positive test result to determine whether angioplasty or coronary artery bypass graft surgery is needed.

Another radioisotope used for cardiac imaging is Tc^{99m}. Technetium can be combined with various chemical compounds, giving it an affinity for different types of cells. For example, Tc^{99m} sestamibi (Cardiolite) is distributed to myocardial cells in proportion to their amount of perfusion, making this tracer excellent for assessing perfusion to the myocardium. The procedure for cardiac imaging using Tc^{99m} sestamibi with stress testing is similar to the one using thallium, with two differences. Patients receiving Tc^{99m} sestamibi can have their resting images recorded before or after the exercise images. Timing of the images is not important because the half-life of Tc^{99m} is short, and Tc^{99m} needs to be injected before each scan. Also, SPECT imaging with Tc^{99m} sestamibi provides high-quality images.

NURSING INTERVENTIONS

The patient undergoing nuclear imaging techniques with stress testing should be prepared for the type of stressor to be used (exercise or drug) and the type of imaging technique (planar or SPECT). The patient may be concerned about receiving a radioactive substance and needs to be reassured that these tracers are safe, the radiation exposure being similar to that of other diagnostic x-ray studies. No postprocedure radiation precautions are necessary.

When providing teaching for patients undergoing SPECT, the nurse should instruct them that their arms will need to be positioned over their head for about 20 to 30 minutes. If they are physically unable to do this, thallium with planar imaging can be used.

Test of Ventricular Function and Wall Motion

Equilibrium radionuclide angiocardiography (ERNA), also known as multiple-gated acquisition (MUGA) scanning, is a common noninvasive technique that uses a conventional scintillation camera interfaced with a computer to record images of the heart during several hundred heartbeats. The computer processes the data and allows for sequential viewing of the functioning heart. The sequential images are analyzed to evaluate left ventricular function, wall motion, and ejection fraction. MUGA scanning can also be used to assess the differences in left ventricular function during rest and exercise.

The patient is reassured that there is no known radiation danger and is instructed to remain motionless during the scan.

Computed Tomography

Computed tomography (CT), also called computerized axial tomographic (CAT) scanning or electron-beam computed tomography (EBCT), uses x-rays to provide cross-sectional images of the chest, including the heart and great vessels. These techniques are used to evaluate cardiac masses and diseases of the aorta and pericardium.

EBCT, also known as the Ultrafast CT, is an especially fast x-ray scanning technique that results in much faster image acquisition with a higher degree of resolution than traditional x-ray or CT scanning provides (Woods et al., 1999). It is used to evaluate bypass graft patency, congenital heart lesions, left and right ventricular muscle mass, chamber volumes, cardiac output, and ejection fraction. For people without previous MI, PTCA, or coronary artery bypass surgery, the EBCT is used to determine the amount of calcium deposits in the coronary arteries and underlying atherosclerosis. From this scan, a calcium score is derived that predicts the incidence of cardiac events, such as MI or the need for a revascularization procedure within the next 1 to 2 years.

The EBCT is not widely used, but it does show great promise for early detection of CAD that is not yet clinically significant and that would not be identified by traditional testing methods, such as the exercise stress test.

NURSING INTERVENTIONS

Patient preparation is the primary role of the nurse for these tests. The nurse should instruct the patient that he will be positioned on a table during the scan while the scanner rotates around him. The procedure is noninvasive and painless. However, to obtain adequate images, the patient must lie perfectly still during the scanning process. An intravenous access line is necessary if contrast enhancement is to be used.

Positron Emission Tomography

Positron emission tomography (PET) is a noninvasive scanning method that was used in the past primarily to study neurologic dysfunction. More recently, and with increasing frequency, PET has been used to diagnose cardiac dysfunction. PET provides more specific information about myocardial perfusion and viability than does TEE or thallium scanning. For cardiac patients, including those without symptoms, PET helps in planning treatment (eg, coronary artery bypass surgery, angioplasty). PET also helps evaluate the patency of native and previously grafted vessels and the collateral circulation.

During a PET scan, radioisotopes are administered by injection; one compound is used to determine blood flow in the myocardium, and another shows the metabolic function. The PET camera provides detailed three-dimensional images of the distributed compounds. The viability of the myocardium is determined by comparing the extent of glucose metabolism in the myocardium to the degree of blood flow. For example, ischemic but viable tissue would show decreased blood flow and elevated metabolism. For a patient with this finding, revascularization through surgery or angioplasty would be likely to improve heart function. Restrictions of food intake before the test vary among institutions, but, because PET evaluates glucose metabolism, the patient's blood glucose level should be in the normal range. Although PET equipment is costly, it is increasingly valued and available.

NURSING INTERVENTIONS

Nurses involved in PET and other scanning procedures may instruct the patient to refrain from using tobacco and ingesting caffeine for 4 hours before the procedure. They should also reassure the patient that radiation exposure is at safe and acceptable levels, similar to those of other diagnostic x-ray studies.

Magnetic Resonance Imaging

Magnetic resonance imaging (MRI) is a noninvasive, painless technique that is used to examine both the physiologic and anatomic properties of the heart. MRI uses a powerful magnetic field and computer-generated pictures to image the heart and great vessels. It is valuable in diagnosing diseases of the aorta, heart muscle, and pericardium, as well as congenital heart lesions. The application of this technique to the evaluation of coronary artery anatomy, cardiac blood flow, and myocardial viability in conjunction with pharmacologic stress testing is being investigated.

NURSING INTERVENTIONS

Because of the strong magnetic field used during MRI, diagnostic centres where these procedures are performed carefully screen patients for contraindications. Standardized questionnaires are commonly used to determine whether the patient has a pacemaker, metal plates, prosthetic joints, or other metallic implants that can become dislodged if exposed to MRI. During an MRI, the patient is positioned supine on a table that is placed into an enclosed imager or tube that contains the magnetic field. People who are claustrophobic may need to receive a mild sedative before undergoing an MRI. As the MRI is performed, there is an intermittent clanking or thumping sound from the magnetic coils that can be annoying to the patient, so patients are offered headsets to listen to music. The scanner is equipped with a microphone so that the patient can communicate with the staff. During the scanning, the patient is instructed to remain still and not move.

> **! NURSING ALERT** No metal can be in the MRI room because metal objects can become dangerous projectiles; this includes such items as clipboards, paperclips, oxygen tanks, and monitors.

CARDIAC CATHETERIZATION

Cardiac catheterization is an invasive diagnostic procedure in which radiopaque arterial and venous catheters are introduced into selected blood vessels of the right and left sides of the heart. Catheter advancement is guided by fluoroscopy. Most commonly, the catheters are inserted percutaneously through the blood vessels, or via a cutdown procedure if the patient has poor vascular access. Pressures and oxygen saturations in the four heart chambers are measured. Cardiac catheterization is used to diagnose CAD, assess coronary artery patency, and determine the extent of atherosclerosis based on the percentage of coronary artery obstruction. These results determine whether revascularization procedures including PTCA or coronary artery bypass surgery may be of benefit to the patient (see Chap. 28).

During cardiac catheterization, the patient has an intravenous line in place for the administration of sedatives, fluids, heparin, and other medications. Noninvasive hemodynamic monitoring that includes BP and multiple ECG tracings is necessary to continuously observe for dysrhythmias or hemodynamic instability. The myocardium can become ischemic and trigger dysrhythmias as catheters are positioned in the coronary arteries or during injection of contrast agents. Resuscitation equipment must be readily available during the procedure. Staff must be prepared to provide advanced cardiac life support measures as necessary.

Radiopaque contrast agents are used to visualize the coronary arteries; some contrast agents contain iodine. The patient is assessed before the procedure for previous reactions to contrast agents or allergies to iodine-containing substances (eg, seafood). If the patient has a suspected or known allergy to the substance, antihistamines or methylprednisolone (Solu-Medrol) may be administered before the procedure. In addition, the following blood tests are performed to identify abnormalities that may complicate recovery: BUN and creatinine levels, INR or PT, aPTT, hematocrit and hemoglobin values, platelet count, and electrolyte levels.

Diagnostic cardiac catheterizations are commonly performed on an outpatient basis and require 2 to 6 hours of bed rest before ambulation. For most patients, bed rest for 6 hours compared to 2 hours has no advantage with regard to groin bleeding complications (Logemann et al., 1999). However, variations in time to ambulation are most often related to the size of the catheter used during the procedure, the anticoagulation status of the patient, other patient variables (eg, advanced age, obesity, bleeding disorder), the method used for hemostasis of the arterial puncture site after the procedure, and institutional policies. The use of smaller (4 or 6 Fr) catheters, which are more amenable to shorter recovery times, is common in diagnostic cardiac catheterizations. There are several methods available to achieve arterial hemostasis after catheter removal, including manual pressure, mechanical compression devices such as the FemoStop (placed over puncture site for 30 minutes), and percutaneously deployed devices. The latter devices are positioned at the femoral arterial puncture site after completion of the procedure. They deploy collagen (VasoSeal), sutures (Perclose, Techstar), or a combination of both (Angio-Seal). Major benefits of these devices include reliable, immediate hemostasis and shorter time on bed rest without a significant increase in bleeding or other complications (Baim et al., 2000). A number of factors determine which hemostatic methods are used and are based on the physician's preference, the patient's condition, cost, and institutional availability of the equipment.

Patients hospitalized for angina or acute MI may also require cardiac catheterization. After the procedure, these patients usually return to their hospital rooms for recovery. In some cardiac catheterization laboratories, an angioplasty may be performed immediately after the catheterization if indicated.

ANGIOGRAPHY

Cardiac catheterization is usually performed with angiography, a technique of injecting a contrast agent into the vascular system to outline the heart and blood vessels. When a particular heart chamber or blood vessel is singled out for study, the procedure is known as selective angiography. Angiography makes use of cineangiograms, a series of rapidly changing films on an intensified fluoroscopic screen that record the passage of the contrast agent through the vascular site or sites. The recorded information allows for comparison of data over time. Common sites for selective angiography are the aorta, the coronary arteries, and the right and left sides of the heart.

Aortography

An aortogram is a form of angiography that outlines the lumen of the aorta and the major arteries arising from it. In thoracic aortography, a contrast agent is used to study the aortic arch and its major branches. The catheter may be introduced into the aorta using the translumbar or retrograde brachial or femoral artery approach.

Coronary Arteriography

In coronary arteriography, the catheter is introduced into the right or left brachial or femoral artery, then passed into the ascending aorta and manipulated into the appropriate coronary artery. Coronary arteriography is used to evaluate the degree of atherosclerosis and to guide the selection of treatment. It is also used to study suspected congenital anomalies of the coronary arteries.

Right Heart Catheterization

Right heart catheterization usually precedes left heart catheterization. It involves the passage of a catheter from an antecubital or femoral vein into the right atrium, right ventricle, pulmonary artery, and pulmonary arterioles. Pressures and oxygen saturations from each of these areas are obtained and recorded.

Although right heart catheterization is considered a relatively safe procedure, potential complications include cardiac dysrhythmias, venous spasm, infection of the insertion site, cardiac perforation, and, rarely, cardiac arrest.

Left Heart Catheterization

Left heart catheterization is performed to evaluate the patency of the coronary arteries and the function of the left ventricle and the mitral and aortic valves. Potential complications include dysrhythmias, MI, perforation of the heart or great vessels, and systemic embolization. Left heart catheterization is performed by retrograde catheterization of the left ventricle. In this approach, the physician usually inserts the catheter into the right brachial artery or a femoral artery and advances it into the aorta and left ventricle.

After the procedure, the catheter is carefully withdrawn and arterial hemostasis is achieved using manual pressure or other techniques previously described. If the physician performed an arterial or venous cutdown, the site is sutured and a sterile dressing is applied.

NURSING INTERVENTIONS
Nursing responsibilities before cardiac catheterization include the following:

- Instruct the patient to fast, usually for 8 to 12 hours, before the procedure. If catheterization is to be performed as an outpatient procedure, explain that a friend, family member, or other responsible person must transport the patient home.
- Prepare the patient for the expected duration of the procedure; indicate that it will involve lying on a hard table for less than 2 hours.
- Reassure the patient that mild sedatives or moderate sedation will be given intravenously.
- Prepare the patient to experience certain sensations during the catheterization. Knowing what to expect can help the patient cope with the experience. Explain that an occasional pounding sensation (palpitation) may be felt in the chest because of extrasystoles that almost always occur, particularly when the catheter tip touches the myocardium. The patient may be asked to cough and to breathe deeply, especially after the injection of contrast agent. Coughing may help to disrupt a dysrhythmia and to clear the contrast agent from the arteries. Breathing deeply and holding the breath helps to lower the diaphragm for better visualization of heart structures. The injection of a contrast agent into either side

of the heart may produce a flushed feeling throughout the body and a sensation similar to the need to void, which subsides in 1 minute or less.
- Encourage the patient to express fears and anxieties. Provide teaching and reassurance to reduce apprehension.

Nursing responsibilities after cardiac catheterization may include the following:

1. Observe the catheter access site for bleeding or hematoma formation, and assess the peripheral pulses in the affected extremity (dorsalis pedis and posterior tibial pulses in the lower extremity, radial pulse in the upper extremity) every 15 minutes for 1 hour, and then every 1 to 2 hours until the pulses are stable.
2. Evaluate temperature and colour of the affected extremity and any patient complaints of pain, numbness, or tingling sensations to determine signs of arterial insufficiency. Report changes promptly.
3. Monitor for dysrhythmias by observing the cardiac monitor or by assessing the apical and peripheral pulses for changes in rate and rhythm. A vasovagal reaction, consisting of bradycardia, hypotension, and nausea, can be precipitated by a distended bladder or by discomfort during removal of the arterial catheter, especially if a femoral site has been used. Prompt intervention is critical; this includes raising the feet and legs above the head, administering intravenous fluids, and administering intravenous atropine.
4. Inform the patient that if the procedure is performed percutaneously through the femoral artery (and without the use of devices such as VasoSeal, Perclose, or Angio-Seal), the patient will remain on bed rest for 2 to 6 hours with the affected leg straight and the head elevated to 30 degrees (Logemann et al., 1999). For comfort, the patient may be turned from side to side with the affected extremity straight. If the cardiologist uses deployed devices, check local nursing care standards, but anticipate that the patient will have less restrictions on elevation of the head of the bed and will be allowed to ambulate in 2 hours or less (Baim et al., 2000). Analgesic medication is administered as prescribed for discomfort.
5. Instruct the patient to report chest pain and bleeding or sudden discomfort from the catheter insertion sites immediately.
6. Encourage fluids to increase urinary output and flush out the dye.
7. Ensure safety by instructing the patient to ask for help when getting out of bed the first time after the procedure, because orthostatic hypotension may occur and the patient may feel dizzy and lightheaded.

For patients being discharged from the hospital on the same day as the procedure, additional instructions are provided. They appear in Chart 26-4.

ELECTROPHYSIOLOGIC TESTING

The electrophysiology study (EPS) is an invasive procedure that plays a major role in the diagnosis and management of serious dysrhythmias and is used (1) to distinguish atrial from ventricular tachycardias when the determination cannot be made from the 12-lead ECG, (2) to evaluate how readily a life-threatening dysrhythmia (eg, ventricular tachycardia, ventricular fibrillation)

Chart 26-4 • PATIENT EDUCATION
Self-Management After Cardiac Catheterization

After discharge from the hospital for cardiac catheterization, guidelines for self-care include the following:

- For the next 24 hours, do not bend at the waist (to lift anything), strain, or lift heavy objects.
- Avoid tub baths, but shower as desired.
- Talk with your physician about when you may return to work, drive, or resume strenuous activities.
- Call your physician if any of the following occur: bleeding, swelling, new bruising or pain from your procedure puncture site, temperature of 38.6°C or more.
- If test results show that you have coronary artery disease, talk with your physician about options for treatment, including cardiac rehabilitation programs in your community.
- Talk with your physician and nurse about lifestyle changes to reduce your risk for further or future heart problems, such as quitting smoking, lowering your cholesterol level, initiating dietary changes, beginning an exercise program, or losing weight.

can be induced, (3) to evaluate AV node function, (4) to evaluate the effectiveness of antiarrhythmic medications in suppressing the dysrhythmia, and (5) to determine the need for other therapeutic interventions, such as a pacemaker, implantable cardioverter defibrillator, or radiofrequency ablation (discussed in Chap. 27). EPS is indicated for patients with syncope and/or palpitations and for survivors of cardiac arrest from ventricular fibrillation (sudden cardiac death).

The initial study can take up to 4 hours. The patient receives moderate sedation. Catheters with recording and electrical stimulating (pacing) capabilities are inserted into the heart through the femoral and right subclavian veins to record electrical activity in the right and left atrium, bundle of His, and right ventricle. Fluoroscopy guides the positioning of these catheters. Baseline intracardiac recordings are obtained; programmed electrical stimulations of the atrium or ventricle are then administered in an attempt to induce the patient's dysrhythmia. If the dysrhythmia is induced, various antiarrhythmic medications are administered intravenously. The study is repeated after each medication to evaluate which medication or combination of medications is most effective in controlling the dysrhythmia.

After the study, the patient receives an equivalent oral antiarrhythmic agent, and subsequent studies may be necessary to evaluate the effectiveness of that medication. Results of the study may indicate the need for other therapeutic interventions, such as a pacemaker or implantable cardioverter defibrillator.

During EPS, lethal dysrhythmias may be induced; therefore, the procedure must be performed in a controlled environment with resuscitation equipment (eg, defibrillator) readily available. Possible complications include bleeding and hematoma from the catheter insertion sites, pneumothorax (air in the pleural cavity that may collapse portions of the lung), deep vein thrombosis, stroke, and sudden death.

Nursing Interventions

Patients receive nothing to eat or drink for 8 hours before the procedure. Antiarrhythmic medications are withheld for at least 24 hours before the initial study, and the patient's cardiac rate

and rhythm are carefully monitored for dysrhythmias. Other medications may be taken with sips of water.

Thorough preparation before EPS will help to minimize patient anxiety. Ensure that the patient understands the reason for the study and is able to describe the common sensations and experiences expected during and after the study. Often the EPS laboratory has relaxation interventions available for patients, such as headsets with music. Also, the patient needs to be aware that the nurses in the EPS laboratory will be monitoring carefully for signs of discomfort and will offer intravenous medications to reduce discomfort or anxiety. Patients should be reminded to request these medications if necessary. Postprocedure interventions include careful monitoring for complications. The nurse takes vital signs, reviews tracings of continuous ECG monitoring, assesses the apical pulse, auscultates for pericardial friction rub (which indicates bleeding into the pericardial sac), and inspects the catheter insertion sites for bleeding or hematoma formation.

In addition, the nurse assists the patient to maintain bed rest with the affected extremity kept straight and the head of the bed elevated to 30 degrees for 4 to 6 hours. The frequency of assessments and the duration of bed rest may vary based on institutional policy and physician preference.

HEMODYNAMIC MONITORING

Critically ill patients require continuous assessment of their cardiovascular system to diagnose and manage their complex medical conditions. This is most commonly achieved by the use of direct pressure monitoring systems, often referred to as **hemodynamic monitoring**. Central venous pressure (CVP), pulmonary artery pressure, and intra-arterial BP monitoring are common forms of hemodynamic monitoring. Patients requiring hemodynamic monitoring are cared for in specialty critical care units. Some critical care step-down units also admit stable patients with CVP or intra-arterial BP monitoring. Noninvasive hemodynamic monitoring is used in some facilities.

To perform invasive monitoring, specialized equipment is necessary and includes the following:

- A CVP, pulmonary artery, or arterial catheter, which is introduced into the appropriate blood vessel or heart chamber
- A flush system composed of intravenous solution (which may include heparin), tubing, stopcocks, and a flush device, which provides for continuous and manual flushing of the system
- A pressure bag placed around the flush solution that is maintained at 300 mm Hg of pressure; the pressurized flush system delivers 3 to 5 mL of solution per hour through the catheter to prevent clotting and backflow of blood into the pressure monitoring system
- A transducer to convert the pressure coming from the artery or heart chamber into an electrical signal
- An amplifier or monitor, which increases the size of the electrical signal for display on an oscilloscope

Central Venous Pressure Monitoring

The CVP, the pressure in the vena cava or right atrium, is used to assess right ventricular function and venous blood return to the right side of the heart. The CVP can be continuously measured by connecting either a catheter positioned in the vena cava or the proximal port of a pulmonary artery catheter to a pressure monitoring system. The pulmonary artery catheter, described in greater detail later, is used for critically ill patients. Patients in general medical-surgical units who require CVP monitoring may have a single-lumen or multilumen catheter placed into the superior vena cava. Intermittent measurement of the CVP can then be obtained with the use of a water manometer.

Because the pressures in the right atrium and right ventricle are equal at the end of diastole (0 to 8 mm Hg), the CVP is also an indirect method of determining right ventricular filling pressure (preload). This makes the CVP a useful hemodynamic parameter to observe when managing an unstable patient's fluid volume status. CVP monitoring is most valuable when pressures are monitored over time and are correlated with the patient's clinical status. A rising pressure may be caused by hypervolemia or by a condition, such as HF, that results in a decrease in myocardial contractility. Pulmonary artery monitoring is preferred for the patient with HF. Decreased CVP indicates reduced right ventricular preload, most often caused by hypovolemia. This diagnosis can be substantiated when a rapid intravenous infusion causes the CVP to rise. (CVP monitoring is not clinically useful in a patient with HF in whom left ventricular failure precedes right ventricular failure, because in these patients an elevated CVP is a very late sign of HF.)

Before insertion of a CVP catheter, the site is prepared by shaving if necessary and by cleansing with an antiseptic solution. A local anesthetic may be used. The physician threads a single-lumen or multilumen catheter through the external jugular, antecubital, or femoral vein into the vena cava just above or within the right atrium.

NURSING INTERVENTIONS

Once the CVP catheter is inserted, it is secured and a dry, sterile dressing is applied. Catheter placement is confirmed by a chest x-ray, and the site is inspected daily for signs of infection. The dressing and pressure monitoring system or water manometer are changed according to hospital policy. In general, the dressing is to be kept dry and air occlusive. Dressing changes are performed with the use of sterile technique. CVP catheters can be used for infusing intravenous fluids, administering intravenous medications, and drawing blood specimens in addition to monitoring pressure.

To measure the CVP, the transducer (when a pressure monitoring system is used) or the zero mark on the manometer (when a water manometer is used) must be placed at a standard reference point, called the phlebostatic axis (Fig. 26-12). After locating this position, the nurse may make an ink mark on the

FIGURE 26-12   The phlebostatic axis and the phlebostatic level. (**A**) The phlebostatic axis is the crossing of two reference lines: (1) a line from the fourth intercostal space at the point where it joins the sternum, drawn out to the side of the body beneath the axilla; and (2) a line midway between the anterior and posterior surfaces of the chest. (**B**) The phlebostatic level is a horizontal line through the phlebostatic axis. The air–fluid interface of the stopcock of the transducer, or the zero mark on the manometer, must be level with this axis for accurate measurements. When moving from the flat to erect positions, the patient moves the chest and therefore the reference level; the phlebostatic level stays horizontal through the same reference point. (**C**) Two methods for referencing the pressure system to the phlebostatic axis. The system can be referenced by placing the air–fluid interface of either the in-line stopcock or stopcock on top of the transducer at the phlebostatic level.

patient's chest to indicate the location. If the phlebostatic axis is used, CVP can be measured correctly with the patient supine at any backrest position up to 45 degrees. The range for a normal CVP is 0 to 8 mm Hg with a pressure monitoring system or 3 to 8 cm H_2O with a water manometer system. The most common complications of CVP monitoring are infection and air embolism.

Pulmonary Artery Pressure Monitoring

Pulmonary artery pressure monitoring is an important tool used in critical care for assessing left ventricular function, diagnosing the etiology of shock, and evaluating the patient's response to medical interventions (eg, fluid administration, vasoactive medications). Pulmonary artery pressure monitoring is achieved by using a pulmonary artery catheter and pressure monitoring system. Catheters vary in their number of lumens and their types of measurement (eg, cardiac output, oxygen saturation) or pacing capabilities. All types require that a balloon-tipped, flow-directed catheter be inserted into a large vein (usually the subclavian, jugular, or femoral vein); the catheter is then passed into the vena cava and right atrium. In the right atrium, the balloon tip is inflated, and the catheter is carried rapidly by the flow of blood through the tricuspid valve, into the right ventricle, through the pulmonic valve, and into a branch of the pulmonary artery. When the catheter reaches a small pulmonary artery, the balloon is deflated and the catheter is secured with sutures. Fluoroscopy may be used during insertion to visualize the progression of the catheter through the heart chambers to the pulmonary artery. This procedure can be performed in the operating room or cardiac catheterization laboratory or at the bedside in the critical care unit. During insertion of the pulmonary artery catheter, the bedside monitor is observed for waveform and ECG changes as the catheter is moved

through the heart chambers on the right side and into the pulmonary artery.

After the catheter is correctly positioned, the following pressures can be measured: CVP or right atrial pressure, pulmonary artery systolic and diastolic pressures, mean pulmonary artery pressure, and pulmonary artery wedge pressure (Fig. 26-13). If a thermodilution catheter is used, the cardiac output can be measured and systemic vascular resistance and pulmonary vascular resistance can be calculated.

Normal pulmonary artery pressure is 25/9 mm Hg, with a mean pressure of 15 mm Hg (see Fig. 26-5 for normal ranges). When the balloon tip is inflated, usually with 1 mL of air, the catheter floats farther out into the pulmonary artery until it becomes wedged. This is an occlusive manoeuvre that impedes blood flow through that segment of the pulmonary artery. A pressure measurement, called pulmonary artery wedge pressure, is taken within seconds after wedging of the pulmonary artery catheter; then the balloon is immediately deflated and blood flow is restored. The nurse who obtains the wedge reading ensures that the catheter has returned to its normal position in the pulmonary artery by evaluating the pulmonary artery pressure waveform. The pulmonary artery diastolic reading and the wedge pressure reflect the pressure in the ventricle at end-diastole and are particularly important to monitor in critically ill patients, because they are used to evaluate left ventricular filling pressures (preload). At end-diastole, when the mitral valve is open, the wedge pressure is the same as the pressure in the left atrium and the left ventricle, unless the patient has mitral valve disease or pulmonary hypertension. Pulmonary capillary wedge pressure is a mean pressure and is normally 4.5 to 13 mm Hg. Critically ill patients usually require higher left ventricular filling pressures to optimize cardiac output. These patients may need to have their wedge pressure maintained as high as 18 mm Hg.

FIGURE 26-13 Example of a pulmonary artery (PA) pressure monitoring system. PA catheter is inserted into the internal jugular vein and advanced into the pulmonary artery.

NURSING INTERVENTIONS

Catheter site care is essentially the same as for a CVP catheter. As in measuring CVP, the transducer must be positioned at the phlebostatic axis to ensure accurate readings (see Fig. 26-12). Complications of pulmonary artery pressure monitoring include infection, pulmonary artery rupture, pulmonary thromboembolism, pulmonary infarction, catheter kinking, dysrhythmias, and air embolism.

Intra-arterial Blood Pressure Monitoring

Intra-arterial BP monitoring is used to obtain direct and continuous BP measurements in critically ill patients who have severe hypertension or hypotension (Fig. 26-14). Arterial catheters are also useful when arterial blood gas measurements and blood samples need to be obtained frequently.

Once an arterial site is selected (radial, brachial, femoral, or dorsalis pedis), collateral circulation to the area must be confirmed before the catheter is placed. This is a safety precaution to prevent compromised arterial perfusion to the area distal to the arterial catheter insertion site. If no collateral circulation exists and the cannulated artery became occluded, ischemia and infarction of the area distal to that artery could occur. Collateral circulation to the hand can be checked by the Allen test to evaluate the radial and ulnar arteries or by an ultrasonic Doppler test for any of the arteries. With the Allen test, the nurse compresses the radial and ulnar arteries simultaneously and asks the patient to make a fist, causing the hand to blanch. After the patient opens the fist, the nurse releases the pressure on the ulnar artery while maintaining pressure on the radial artery. The patient's hand will turn pink if the ulnar artery is patent.

FIGURE 26-14 Example of an arterial pressure monitoring system. The arterial catheter is inserted into the radial artery. A three-way stopcock is used for drawing arterial blood samples.

NURSING INTERVENTIONS

Site preparation and care are the same as for CVP catheters. The catheter flush solution is the same as for pulmonary artery catheters. A transducer is attached, and pressures are measured in millimeters of mercury (mm Hg). Complications include local obstruction with distal ischemia, external hemorrhage, massive ecchymosis, dissection, air embolism, blood loss, pain, arteriospasm, and infection.

Critical Thinking Exercises

1. You are caring for an elderly man who has had three hospital admissions in 6 months for HF. To plan for his discharge you need to fully understand what is causing these recurrent HF episodes. What medical and nursing history, physical examination, and laboratory data will you need to collect to help you understand the recurrent episodes of HF? What types of information are necessary to help you formulate his plan for discharge? With what other team members might you consult before completing this plan?

2. While working in a primary care clinic, you notice that many of the patients use tobacco products including cigarettes and chewing tobacco. What are the health risks of tobacco use? The clinic does not have a smoking cessation protocol. You want to help people become tobacco free but have little experience in providing cessation advice. What information and resources will you need to obtain to devise and implement a smoking cessation protocol?

3. While making a home visit, your patient, a 54-year-old African American woman with a history of hypertension, diabetes, and tobacco use, tells you she has had overwhelming fatigue and right scapular and shoulder pain going down into her arm for the last 10 hours. Describe your rapid chest pain assessment and management plan for this patient. Discuss the factors that may be contributing to her delay in seeking care for symptoms of acute MI. Compare and contrast symptoms of acute MI and factors contributing to delay in seeking care.

REFERENCES AND SELECTED READINGS

Books

American Heart Association. (2003). *Heart and stroke facts: 2002 statistical supplement.* Dallas, TX: Author.

Apple, S., & Lindsey, J. (1999). *Principles and practices of interventional cardiology.* Philadelphia: Lippincott Williams & Wilkins.

Bickley, L. S., & Szilagyi, P. G. (2003). *Bates' guide to physical examination* (8th ed.). Philadelphia: Lippincott Williams & Wilkins.

Braunwald, E., Libby, P., & Zipes, D. P. (Eds.). (2001). *Heart disease: A textbook of cardiovascular medicine* (6th ed.). Philadelphia: W. B. Saunders.

Chernecky, C., & Berger, B. (2001). *Laboratory tests and diagnostic procedures* (3rd ed.). Philadelphia: W. B. Saunders.

Darvic, G. (2002). *Handbook of hemodynamic monitoring. Invasive and noninvasive clinical application* (3rd ed.). Philadelphia: W. B. Saunders.

Fuller, J., & Schaller-Ayers, J. (2000). *Health assessment: A nursing approach* (3rd ed.). Philadelphia: Lippincott Williams & Wilkins.

Huff, J. (2001). *ECG workout: Exercises in arrhythmia interpretation* (4th ed.). Philadelphia: Lippincott Williams & Wilkins.

Jairath, N. (1999). *Coronary heart disease and risk factor management: A nursing perspective.* Philadelphia: W. B. Saunders.

Kern, M. (2003). *The interventional cardiac catheterization handbook* (2nd ed.). St. Louis: C. V. Mosby.

Maas, M. L., Buckwalter, K. C., Hardy, M. D., Tripp-Reimer, T., Titler, M. G., Specht, J. P., et al. (2001). *Nursing care of older adults: Diagnoses, outcomes, and interventions.* St. Louis: C. V. Mosby.

Miller, C. (1999). *Nursing care of older adults: Theory and practice* (3rd ed.). Philadelphia: Lippincott Williams & Wilkins.

Pohost, G. M., O'Rourke, R. A., Berman, D. S., & Shah, P. M. (2000). *Imaging in cardiovascular disease.* Philadelphia: Lippincott Williams & Wilkins.

Weber, J., & Kelley, J. (2003). *Health assessment in nursing* (2nd ed.). Philadelphia: Lippincott Williams & Wilkins.

Woods, S. L., Froelicher, E. S. S., & Motzer, S. U. (1999). *Cardiac nursing* (4th ed.). Philadelphia: Lippincott Williams & Wilkins.

Journals

Asterisks indicate nursing research articles.

Attin, M. (2001). Electrophysiology study: A comprehensive review. *American Journal of Critical Care, 10*(4), 260–273.

*Baim, D., Knopf, W., Hinohara, T., Schwarten, D. E., Schatz, R. A., Pinkerton, C. A., et al. (2000). Suture-mediated closure of the femoral access site after cardiac catheterization: Results of the suture to ambulate and discharge (STAND I and STAND II) trials. *American Journal of Cardiology, 85*(7), 864–869.

Beattie, S. (1999). Cut the risks for cardiac cath patients. *RN, 62*(1), 50–55.

*Bosworth, H., Feaganes, J., Vitaliano, P., Mark, D. B., & Siegler, I. C. (2001). Personality and coping with a common stressor: Cardiac catheterization. *Journal of Behavioral Medicine, 24*(1), 17–31.

*Botti, M., Williamson, B., & Steen, K. (2001). Coronary angiographic observations: Evidence-based or ritualistic practice? *Heart & Lung, 30*(2), 138–145.

Buselli, E. F., & Stuart, E. M. (1999). Influence of psychosocial factors and biopsychosocial interventions on outcomes after myocardial infarction. *J Cardiovasc Nurs, 13*(3), 60–72.

Canadian Cardiovascular Society. (1999). 1998 Conference on the Prevention of Cardiovascular Diseases: The role of the cardiovascular specialist. *Canadian Journal of Cardiology, December 15* (Suppl. G) 1G–119G.

Chyun, D. (2001). Diabetes and coronary heart disease: A time for action. *Critical Care Nurse, 21*(1), 10–16.

Daleiden, A. M., & Schell, H. (2001). Setting a new gold standard: ST-segment monitoring provides early detection of myocardial ischemia. *American Journal of Nursing, 101,* (Suppl.), 4–8, 48–50.

Dracup, K., & Cannon, C. (1999). Combination treatment strategies for management of acute myocardial infarction: New directions with current therapies. *Critical Care Nurse, 19*(4), (Suppl.), 1–17.

Drew, B., & Krucoff, M. (1999). Multilead ST-segment monitoring in patients with acute coronary syndromes: A consensus statement for healthcare professionals. ST-segment monitoring practice guidelines international working group. *American Journal of Critical Care, 8*(6), 372–386.

Gibbar-Clements, T., Shirrell, D., Dooley, R., & Smiley, B. (2000). The challenge of warfarin therapy. *American Journal of Nursing, 100*(3), 38–40.

Grundy, S., Howard, B., Smith, S., Jr., Eckel, R., Redberg, R., & Bonow, R. O. (2002). Prevention Conference VI: Diabetes and cardiovascular disease executive summary: Conference proceeding for healthcare professionals from a special writing group of the American Heart Association. *Circulation, 105*(18), 2231–2239.

Hamel, W. (1999). Suppose a Perclose. *Progress in Cardiovascular Nursing, 14*(4), 136–142.

Hinkle, C., & Stegall, G. (2000). Ask the experts: Setting up 15 and 18 lead ECGs. *Critical Care Nurse, 20*(2), 125–126.

Jacobson, C. (2000). Optimum bedside cardiac monitoring. *Progress in Cardiovascular Nursing, 15*(4), 134–137.

*Krantz, D., Santiago, H., & Kop, W. (1999). Prognostic value of mental stress testing in coronary artery disease. *American Journal of Cardiology, 84*(11), 1292–1297.

*Logemann, T., Luetmer, P., Kaliebe, J., Olson, K., & Murdock, D. K. (1999). Two versus six hours of bed rest following left-sided cardiac catheterization and a meta-analysis of early ambulation trials. *American Journal of Cardiology, 84*(4), 486–488.

*Milner, K., Funk, M., Richards, S., Wilmes, R. M., Vaccarino, V., Krumholz, H. M., et al. (1999). Gender differences in symptom presentation associated with coronary heart disease. *American Journal of Cardiology, 84*(4), 396–399.

Mosca, L., Collins, P., Herrington, D., Mendelsohn, M. E., Pasternak, R. C., Robertson, R. M., et al. (2001). Hormone replacement therapy and cardiovascular disease: A statement for healthcare professionals from the American Heart Association. *Circulation, 104*(4), 499–503.

Mosca, L., Grungy, S. M., Judelson, D., King, K., Limacher, M., Oparil, S., et al. (1999). AHA/ACC scientific statement: Consensus panel statement. Guide to preventative cardiology for women. American Heart Association/American College of Cardiology. *Journal of the American College of Cardiology, 33*(6), 1751–1755.

*Mott, A. (1999). Psychologic preparation to decrease anxiety associated with cardiac catheterization. *Journal of Vascular Nursing, 17*(2), 41–49.

Pearson, T. A., Blair, S. W., Daniel, S. R., Eckel, R. H., Fair, J. M., Fortmann, S. P., et al. (2002). AHA guidelines for primary prevention of cardiovascular disease and stroke: 2002 update. Consensus panel guide to comprehensive risk reduction for adult patients without coronary or other atherosclerotic vascular diseases. *Circulation, 106*(3), 388–391.

*Richards, S., Funk, M., & Milner, K. (2000). Differences between blacks and whites with coronary heart disease in initial symptoms and delay in seeking care. *American Journal of Critical Care, 9*(4), 237–244.

Robertson, R. (2001). Women and cardiovascular disease: The risk of misperception and the need for action. *Circulation, 103*(19), 2318–2323.

*Roussouw, J. E., Anderson, G. L., Prentice, R. L., LaCroix, A. Z., Kooperberg, C., Stefanick, M. C., et al. (2002). Risk and benefits of estrogen plus progestin in healthy post menopausal women: Principle results from the Women's Health Initiative randomized controlled trial. *Journal of the American Medical Association, 288*(3), 321–333.

*Schickel, S., Adkisson, P., Miracle, V., Cronin, S. N. (1999). Achieving femoral artery hemostasis after cardiac catheterization: A comparison of methods. *American Journal of Critical Care, 8*(6), 406–415.

Siomko, A. J. (2000). Demystifying cardiac markers. *American Journal of Nursing, 100*(1), 36–41.

Smith, S. C. Jr., Blair, S. N., Bonow, R. O., Brass, L. M., Cerqueira, M. D., Dracup, K., et al. (2001). AHA/ACC guidelines for preventing heart attack and death in patients with atherosclerotic cardiovascular disease. *Circulation, 104*(13), 1577–1579.

Steinke, E. (2000). Sexual counseling: After myocardial infarction. *American Journal of Nursing, 100*(12), 38–44.

The Tobacco Use and Dependence Clinical Practice Guideline Update Panel, Staff, and Consortium Representatives. (2000). A clinical practice guideline for treating tobacco use and dependence: A U.S. Public Health Service Report. *Journal of the American Medical Association; 283*(24), 3244–3254.

*Then, K., Rankin, J., & Fofonoff, D. (2001). Atypical presentation of acute myocardial infarction in 3 age groups. *Heart & Lung, 30*(4), 285–293.

*Wung, S., & Drew, B. (1999). Comparison of 18-lead ECG and selected body surface potential mapping leads in determining maximally deviated ST lead and efficacy in detecting acute myocardial ischemia during coronary occlusion. *Journal of Electrophysiology, 32,* (Suppl.) 30–37.

Zerwic, J. (1999). Patient delay in seeking treatment for acute myocardial infarction symptoms. *Journal of Cardiovascular Nursing, 13*(3), 21–31.

RESOURCES AND WEBSITES

Canadian Council of Cardiovascular Nurses, 222 Queen Street, Suite 1402, Ottawa, ON K1P 5V9; 1-613-569-4361, ext 340; http://www.leverus.com/cccn/index2.cfm.

Heart and Stroke Foundation of Canada, 222 Queen Street, Suite 1402, Ottawa, ON K1P 5V9; 1-613-569-4361; http://ww1.heartandstroke.ca.

Management of Patients With Dysrhythmias and Conduction Problems

Adapted by Alexander Clark and Colleen Norris

LEARNING OBJECTIVES

On completion of this chapter, the learner will be able to:

1. Correlate the components of the normal ECG with physiologic events of the heart.
2. Define the ECG as a waveform that represents the cardiac electrical event in relation to the lead depicted (placement of electrodes).
3. Analyze elements of an ECG rhythm strip: ventricular and atrial rate, ventricular and atrial rhythm, QRS complex and shape, QRS duration, P wave and shape, PR interval, and P:QRS ratio.
4. Identify the ECG criteria, causes, and management of several dysrhythmias, including conduction disturbances.
5. Use the nursing process as a framework for care of patients with dysrhythmias.
6. Compare the different types of pacemakers, their uses, possible complications, and nursing implications.
7. Use the nursing process as a framework for care of patients with pacemakers.
8. Describe the key points of using a defibrillator.
9. Describe the purpose of an implantable cardioverter defibrillator (ICD), the types available, and the nursing implications.
10. Describe invasive methods to diagnose and treat recurrent dysrhythmias, and discuss the nursing implications.

Without a regular rate and rhythm, the heart may not perform efficiently as a pump to circulate oxygenated blood and other life-sustaining nutrients to all the body organs (including itself) and tissues. With an irregular or erratic rhythm, the heart is considered to be dysrhythmic (sometimes called arrhythmic). This has the potential to be a dangerous condition.

Dysrhythmias

Dysrhythmias are disorders of the formation or conduction (or both) of the electrical impulse within the heart. These disorders can cause disturbances of the heart rate, the heart rhythm, or both. Dysrhythmias may initially be evidenced by the hemodynamic effect they cause (eg, a change in conduction may change the pumping action of the heart and cause decreased blood pressure). Dysrhythmias are diagnosed by analyzing the electrocardiographic waveform. They are named according to the site of origin of the impulse and the mechanism of formation or conduction involved (Chart 27-1). For example, an impulse that originates in the sinoatrial (SA) node and that has a slow rate is called sinus bradycardia.

NORMAL ELECTRICAL CONDUCTION

The electrical impulse that stimulates and paces the cardiac muscle normally originates in the sinus node (SA node), an area located near the superior vena cava in the right atrium. Usually, the electrical impulse occurs at a rate ranging between 60 and 100 times a minute in the adult. The electrical impulse quickly travels from the sinus node through the atria to the atrioventricular (AV) node (Fig. 27-1). The electrical stimulation of the muscle cells of the atria causes them to contract. The structure of the AV node slows the electrical impulse, which allows time for the atria to contract and fill the ventricles with blood before the electrical impulse

travels very quickly through the bundle of His to the right and left bundle branches and the Purkinje fibres, located in the ventricular muscle. The electrical stimulation of the muscle cells of the ventricles, in turn, causes the mechanical contraction of the ventricles (systole). The cells repolarize and the ventricles then relax (diastole). The process from sinus node electrical impulse generation through ventricular repolarization completes the electromechanical circuit, and the cycle begins again.

Sinus rhythm promotes cardiovascular circulation. The electrical impulse causes (and, therefore, is followed by) the mechanical contraction of the heart muscle. The electrical stimulation is called **depolarization**; the mechanical contraction is called systole. Electrical relaxation is called **repolarization** and mechanical relaxation is called diastole. See Chapter 26 for a more complete explanation of cardiac function.

Chart 27-1

Identifying Dysrhythmias

Sites of Origin
Sinus (SA) node
Atria
Atrioventricular (AV) node or junction
Ventricles

Mechanisms of Formation or Conduction
Normal (idio) rhythm
Bradycardia
Tachycardia
Dysrhythmia
Flutter
Fibrillation
Premature complexes
Blocks

Glossary

ablation: purposeful destruction of heart muscle cells, usually in an attempt to control a dysrhythmia

antiarrhythmic: a medication that suppresses or prevents a dysrhythmia

automaticity: ability of the cardiac muscle to initiate an electrical impulse

cardioversion: electrical current administered in synchrony with the patient's own QRS to stop a dysrhythmia

conductivity: ability of the cardiac muscle to transmit electrical impulses

defibrillation: electrical current administered to stop a dysrhythmia, not synchronized with the patient's QRS complex

depolarization: process by which cardiac muscle cells change from a more negatively charged to a more positively charged intracellular state

dysrhythmia (also referred to as arrhythmia): disorder of the formation or conduction (or both) of the electrical impulse within the heart, altering the heart rate, heart rhythm, or both and potentially causing altered blood flow

implantable cardioverter defibrillator (ICD): a device implanted into the chest to treat dysrhythmias

inhibited: in reference to pacemakers, term used to describe the pacemaker withholding an impulse (not firing)

P wave: the part of an electrocardiogram (ECG) that reflects conduction of an electrical impulse through the atrium; atrial depolarization

paroxysmal: a dysrhythmia that has a sudden onset and/or termination and is usually of short duration

PR interval: the part of an ECG that reflects conduction of an electrical impulse from the sinoatrial (SA) node through the atrioventricular (AV) node

proarrhythmic: an agent (eg, a medication) that causes or exacerbates a dysrhythmia

QRS complex: the part of an ECG that reflects conduction of an electrical impulse through the ventricles; ventricular depolarization

QT interval: the part of an ECG that reflects the time from ventricular depolarization to repolarization

repolarization: process by which cardiac muscle cells return to a more negatively charged intracellular condition, their resting state

sinus rhythm: electrical activity of the heart initiated by the sinoatrial (SA) node

ST segment: the part of an ECG that reflects the end of ventricular depolarization (end of the QRS complex) through ventricular repolarization (end of the T wave)

supraventricular tachycardia (SVT): a rhythm that originates in the conduction system above the ventricles

T wave: the part of an ECG that reflects repolarization of the ventricles

triggered: in reference to pacemakers, term used to describe the release of an impulse in response to some stimulus

U wave: the part of an ECG that may reflect Purkinje fibre repolarization; usually seen when a patient's serum potassium level is low

ventricular tachycardia (VT): a rhythm that originates in the ventricles

FIGURE 27-1 Relationship of electrocardiogram (ECG) complex, lead system, and electrical impulse. The heart conducts electrical activity, which the ECG measures and shows. The configurations of electrical activity displayed on the ECG vary depending on the lead (or view) of the ECG and on the rhythm of the heart. Therefore, the configuration of a normal rhythm tracing from lead I will differ from the configuration of a normal rhythm tracing from lead II, lead II will differ from lead III, and so on. The same is true for abnormal rhythms and cardiac disorders. To make an accurate assessment of the heart's electrical activity or to identify where, when, and what abnormalities occur, the ECG needs to be evaluated from every lead, not just from lead II. Here the different areas of electrical activity are identified by colour.

Influences on Heart Rate and Contractility

The heart rate is influenced by the autonomic nervous system, which consists of sympathetic and parasympathetic fibres. Sympathetic nerve fibres (also referred to as adrenergic fibres) are attached to the heart and arteries as well as several other areas in the body. Stimulation of the sympathetic system increases heart rate (positive chronotropy), conduction through the AV node (positive dromotropy), and the force of myocardial contraction (positive inotropy). Sympathetic stimulation also constricts peripheral blood vessels, therefore increasing blood pressure. Parasympathetic nerve fibres are also attached to the heart and arteries. Parasympathetic stimulation reduces the heart rate (negative chronotropy), AV conduction (negative dromotropy), and the force of atrial myocardial contraction. The decreased sympathetic stimulation results in dilation of arteries, thereby lowering blood pressure.

Manipulation of the autonomic nervous system may increase or decrease the incidence of dysrhythmias. Increased sympathetic stimulation—caused, for example, by exercise, anxiety, fever, or administration of catecholamines (eg, dopamine [Intropin], aminophylline, dobutamine [Dobutrex])—may increase the incidence of dysrhythmias. Decreased sympathetic stimulation (eg, with rest, anxiety-reduction methods such as therapeutic communication or prayer, administration of beta-adrenergic blocking agents) may decrease the incidence of dysrhythmias.

INTERPRETATION OF THE ELECTROCARDIOGRAM

The electrical impulse that travels through the heart can be viewed by means of electrocardiography, the end product of which is an electrocardiogram (ECG). Each phase of the cardiac cycle is reflected by specific waveforms on the screen of a cardiac monitor or on a strip of ECG graph paper.

An ECG is obtained by slightly abrading the skin with a clean dry gauze pad and placing electrodes on the body at specific areas. Electrodes come in various shapes and sizes, but all have two components: (1) an adhesive substance that attaches to the skin to secure the electrode in place and (2) a substance that reduces the skin's electrical impedance and promotes detection of the electrical current.

The number and placement of the electrodes depend on the type of ECG needed. Most continuous monitors use two to five electrodes, usually placed on the limbs and the chest. These electrodes create an imaginary line, called a lead, that serves as a reference point from which the electrical activity is viewed. A lead is like an eye of a camera; it has a narrow peripheral field of vision, looking only at the electrical activity directly in front of it. Therefore, the ECG waveforms that appear on the paper or cardiac monitor represent the electrical current in relation to the lead (see Fig. 27-1). A change in the waveform can be caused by a change in the electrical current (where it originates or how it is conducted) or by a change in the lead.

Obtaining an Electrocardiogram

Electrodes are attached to cable wires, which are connected to one of the following:

- An ECG machine placed at the patient's side for an immediate recording (standard 12-lead ECG)
- A cardiac monitor at the patient's bedside for continuous reading; this kind of monitoring, usually called hardwire monitoring, is associated with intensive care units
- A small box that the patient carries and that continuously transmits the ECG information by radio waves to a central monitor located elsewhere (called telemetry)
- A small, lightweight tape recorder-like machine (called a Holter monitor) that the patient wears and that continuously records the ECG on a tape, which is later viewed and analyzed with a scanner

The placement of electrodes for continuous monitoring, telemetry, or Holter monitoring varies with the type of technology that is appropriate and available, the purpose of monitoring, and the standards of the institution. For a standard 12-lead ECG, 10 electrodes (six on the chest and four on the limbs) are placed on the body (Fig. 27-2). To prevent interference from the electrical activity of skeletal muscle, the limb electrodes are usually placed on areas that are not bony and that do not have significant movement. These limb electrodes provide the first six leads: leads I, II, III, aVR, aVL, and aVF. The six chest electrodes are attached to the chest at very specific areas. The chest electrodes provide the V or precordial leads, V_1 through V_6. To locate the fourth intercostal space and the placement of V_1, locate the sternal angle and then the sternal notch, which is about 1 or 2 inches below the sternal angle. When the fingers are moved to the patient's immediate right, the second rib can be palpated. The second intercostal space is the indentation felt just below the second rib.

Locating the specific intercostal space is critical for correct chest electrode placement. Errors in diagnosis can occur if electrodes are incorrectly placed. Sometimes, when the patient is in the hospital and needs to be monitored closely for ECG changes, the chest electrodes are left in place to ensure the same placement for follow-up ECGs.

A standard 12-lead ECG reflects the electrical activity primarily in the left ventricle. Placement of additional electrodes for

Supplemental right precordial leads

FIGURE 27-2 ECG electrode placement. The standard left precordial leads are V_1—4th intercostal space, right sternal border; V_2—4th intercostal space, left sternal border; V_3—diagonally between V_2 and V_4; V_4—5th intercostal space, left midclavicular line; V_5—same level as V_4, anterior axillary line; V_6 (not illustrated)—same level as V_4 and V_5, midaxillary line. The right precordial leads, placed across the right side of the chest, are the mirror opposite of the left leads. Adapted from Hosley, J. B., & Molle-Matthews, E. (1999). *Lippincott's pocket guide to medical assisting*. Philadelphia: Lippincott Williams & Wilkins.

other leads may be needed to obtain more complete information. For example, in patients with suspected right-sided heart damage, right-sided precordial leads are required to evaluate the right ventricle (see Fig. 27-2).

Analysis of the Electrocardiogram

The ECG waveform represents the function of the heart's conduction system, which normally initiates and conducts the electrical activity, in relation to the lead. When analyzed accurately, the ECG offers important information about the electrical activity of the heart. ECG waveforms are printed on graph paper that is divided by light and dark vertical and horizontal lines at standard intervals (Fig. 27-3). Time and rate are measured on the horizontal axis of the graph, and amplitude or voltage is measured on the vertical axis. When an ECG waveform moves toward the top of the paper, it is called a positive deflection. When it moves toward the bottom of the paper, it is called a negative deflection. When reviewing an ECG, each waveform should be examined and compared with the others.

WAVES, COMPLEXES, AND INTERVALS

The ECG is composed of waveforms (including the P wave, the QRS complex, the T wave, and possibly a U wave) and of segments or intervals (including the PR interval, the ST segment, and the QT interval) (see Fig. 27-3).

The **P wave** represents the electrical impulse starting in the sinus node and spreading through the atria. Therefore, the P wave represents atrial muscle depolarization. It is normally 2.5 mm or less in height and 0.11 second or less in duration.

The **QRS complex** represents ventricular muscle depolarization. Not all QRS complexes have all three waveforms. The first negative deflection after the P wave is the Q wave, which is normally less than 0.04 second in duration and less than 25% of the R wave amplitude; the first positive deflection after the P wave is the R wave; and the S wave is the first negative deflection after the R wave. When a wave is less than 5 mm in height, small letters (q, r, s) are used; when a wave is taller than 5 mm, capital letters (Q, R, S) are used. The QRS complex is normally less than 0.12 seconds in duration.

The **T wave** represents ventricular muscle repolarization (when the cells regain a negative charge; also called the resting state). It follows the QRS complex and is usually the same direction as the QRS complex.

The **U wave** is thought to represent repolarization of the Purkinje fibres, but it sometimes is seen in patients with hypokalemia (low potassium levels), hypertension, or heart disease. If present, the U wave follows the T wave and is usually smaller than the P wave. If tall, it may be mistaken for an extra P wave.

The **PR interval** is measured from the beginning of the P wave to the beginning of the QRS complex and represents the time needed for sinus node stimulation, atrial depolarization, and conduction through the AV node before ventricular depolarization. In adults, the PR interval normally ranges from 0.12 to 0.20 seconds in duration.

The **ST segment**, which represents early ventricular repolarization, lasts from the end of the QRS complex to the beginning of the T wave. The beginning of the ST segment is usually identified by a change in the thickness or angle of the terminal portion of the QRS complex. The end of the ST segment may be more difficult to identify because it merges into the T wave. The ST segment is normally isoelectric (see discussion of TP interval). It is analyzed to identify whether it is above or below the isoelectric line, which may be, among other signs and symptoms, a sign of cardiac ischemia (see Chap. 28).

The **QT interval**, which represents the total time for ventricular depolarization and repolarization, is measured from the beginning of the QRS complex to the end of the T wave. The QT interval varies with heart rate, gender, and age, and the measured interval needs to be corrected for these variables through a specific calculation. Several ECG interpretation books contain charts of these calculations. The QT interval is usually 0.32 to 0.40 seconds in duration if the heart rate is 65 to 95 beats per minute. If the QT interval becomes prolonged, the patient may be at risk for a lethal ventricular dysrhythmia called torsades de pointes.

The **TP interval** is measured from the end of the T wave to the beginning of the next P wave, an isoelectric period (see Fig 27-3).

FIGURE 27-3 ECG graph and commonly measured components. Each small box represents 0.04 seconds on the horizontal axis and 1 mm or 0.1 millivolt on the vertical axis. The PR interval is measured from the beginning of the P wave to the beginning of the QRS complex; the QRS complex is measured from the beginning of the Q wave to the end of the S wave; the QT interval is measured from the beginning of the Q wave to the end of the T wave; and the TP interval is measured from the end of the T wave to the beginning of the next P wave.

When no electrical activity is detected, the line on the graph remains flat; this is called the isoelectric line. The ST segment is compared with the TP interval to detect changes from the line on the graph during the isoelectric period.

The **PP interval** is measured from the beginning of one P wave to the beginning of the next. The PP interval is used to determine atrial rhythm and atrial rate. The RR interval is measured from one QRS complex to the next QRS complex. The RR interval is used to determine ventricular rate and rhythm (Fig. 27-4).

DETERMINING VENTRICULAR HEART RATE FROM THE ELECTROCARDIOGRAM

Heart rate can be obtained from the ECG strip by several methods. A 1-minute strip contains 300 large boxes and 1500 small boxes. Therefore, an easy and accurate method of determining heart rate with a regular rhythm is to count the number of small boxes within an RR interval and divide 1500 by that number. If, for example, there are 10 small boxes between two R waves, the heart rate is 1500 ÷ 10, or 150; if there are 25 small boxes, the heart rate is 1500 ÷ 25, or 60 (see Fig. 27-4A).

An alternative but less accurate method for estimating heart rate, which is usually used when the rhythm is irregular, is to count the number of RR intervals in 6 seconds and multiply that number by 10. The top of the ECG paper is usually marked at 3-second intervals, which is 15 large boxes horizontally (see Fig. 27-4B). The RR intervals are counted, rather than QRS complexes, because a computed heart rate based on the latter might be inaccurately high.

The same methods may be used for determining atrial rate, using the PP interval instead of the RR interval.

DETERMINING HEART RHYTHM FROM THE ELECTROCARDIOGRAM

The rhythm is often identified at the same time the rate is determined. The RR interval is used to determine ventricular rhythm and the PP interval to determine atrial rhythm. If the intervals are the same or nearly the same throughout the strip, the rhythm is called regular. If the intervals are different, the rhythm is called irregular.

ANALYZING THE ELECTROCARDIOGRAM RHYTHM STRIP

The ECG must be analyzed in a systematic manner to determine the patient's cardiac rhythm and to detect dysrhythmias and conduction disorders, as well as evidence of myocardial ischemia, injury, and infarction. Chart 27-2 is an example of a method that can be used to analyze the patient's rhythm.

Once the rhythm has been analyzed, the findings are compared with and matched to the ECG criteria for dysrhythmias to determine a diagnosis. It is important for the nurse to assess the patient to determine the physiologic effect of the dysrhythmia and to identify possible causes. Treatment of dysrhythmias is based on the etiology and the effect of the dysrhythmia, not on its presence alone.

Normal Sinus Rhythm

Normal sinus rhythm occurs when the electrical impulse starts at a regular rate and rhythm in the sinus node and travels through the normal conduction pathway. The following are the ECG criteria for normal sinus rhythm (Fig. 27-5):

Ventricular and atrial rate: 60 to 100 in the adult
Ventricular and atrial rhythm: Regular
QRS shape and duration: Usually normal, but may be regularly abnormal
P wave: Normal and consistent shape; always in front of the QRS
PR interval: Consistent interval between 0.12 and 0.20 seconds
P: QRS ratio: 1 : 1

Types of Dysrhythmias

Dysrhythmias include sinus node, atrial, junctional, and ventricular dysrhythmias and their various subcategories.

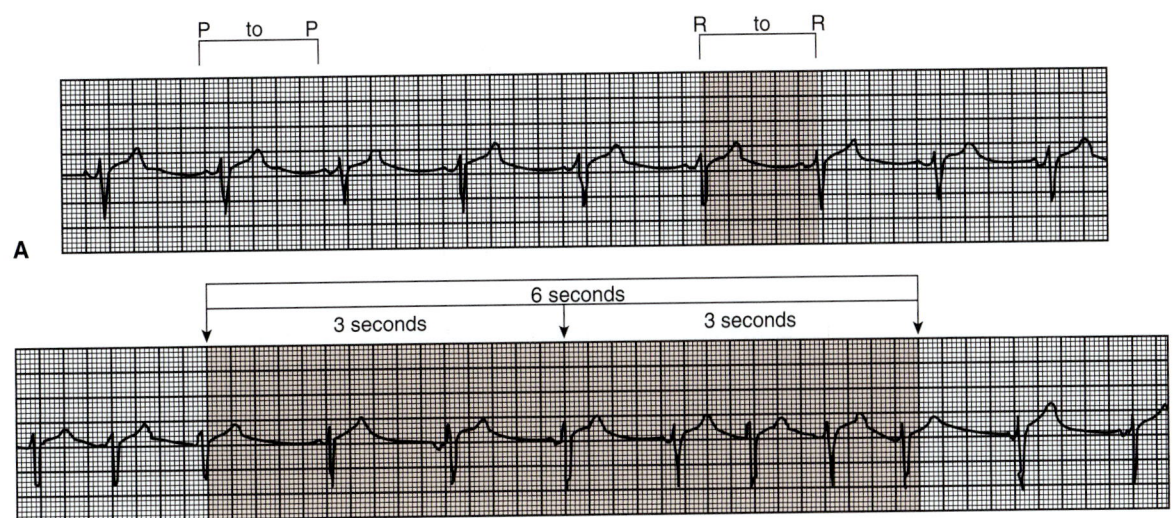

FIGURE 27-4 (**A**) Heart rate determination for a regular rhythm: 1500 divided by the number of small boxes between two R waves (there are 25 in this example) equals the ventricular heart rate. The heart rate in this example is 60. (**B**) Heart rate determination if the rhythm is irregular. There are approximately seven RR intervals in 6 seconds. Seven times 10 equals 70. The heart rate is 70.

Chart 27-2 Interpreting Dysrhythmias: Systematic Analysis of the Electrocardiogram

When examining an ECG rhythm strip to learn more about a patient's dysrhythmia, the nurse conducts the following assessment:

1. Determine the ventricular rate.
2. Determine the ventricular rhythm.
3. Determine QRS duration.
4. Determine whether the QRS duration is consistent throughout the strip. If not, identify other duration.
5. Identify QRS shape; if not consistent, then identify other shapes.
6. Identify P waves; is there a P in front of every QRS?
7. Identify P-wave shape; identify whether it is consistent or not.
8. Determine the atrial rate.
9. Determine the atrial rhythm.
10. Determine each PR interval.
11. Determine if the PR intervals are consistent, irregular but with a pattern to the irregularity, or just irregular.
12. Determine how many P waves for each QRS (P : QRS ratio).

In many cases, the nurse may use a checklist and document the findings next to the appropriate ECG criterion.

SINUS NODE DYSRHYTHMIAS

Sinus Bradycardia. Sinus bradycardia occurs when the sinus node creates an impulse at a slower-than-normal rate. Causes include lower metabolic needs (eg, sleep, athletic training, hypothermia, hypothyroidism), vagal stimulation (eg, from vomiting, suctioning, severe pain, extreme emotions), medications (eg, calcium channel blockers, amiodarone, beta-blockers), increased intracranial pressure, and myocardial infarction (MI), especially of the inferior wall. The following are characteristics of sinus bradycardia (Fig. 27-6):

Ventricular and atrial rate: Less than 60 in the adult
Ventricular and atrial rhythm: Regular
QRS shape and duration: Usually normal, but may be regularly abnormal
P wave: Normal and consistent shape; always in front of the QRS
PR interval: Consistent interval between 0.12 and 0.20 seconds
P : QRS ratio: 1 : 1

All characteristics of sinus bradycardia are the same as those of normal sinus rhythm, except for the rate. The patient is assessed to determine the hemodynamic effect and the possible cause of the dysrhythmia. If the decrease in heart rate results from stimulation of the vagus nerve, such as with bearing down during defecation or vomiting, attempts are made to prevent further vagal

stimulation. If the bradycardia is from a medication such as a beta-blocker, the medication may be withheld. If the slow heart rate causes significant hemodynamic changes, resulting in shortness of breath, decreased level of consciousness, angina, hypotension, ST-segment changes, or premature ventricular complexes, treatment is directed toward increasing the heart rate.

Atropine, 0.5 to 1.0 mg given rapidly as an intravenous (IV) bolus, is the medication of choice in treating sinus bradycardia. It blocks vagal stimulation, thus allowing a normal rate to occur. Rarely, catecholamines and emergency transcutaneous pacing also may be implemented.

Sinus Tachycardia. Sinus tachycardia occurs when the sinus node creates an impulse at a faster-than-normal rate. It may be caused by acute blood loss, anemia, shock, hypervolemia, hypovolemia, congestive heart failure, pain, hypermetabolic states, fever, exercise, anxiety, or sympathomimetic medications. The ECG criteria for sinus tachycardia follow (Fig. 27-7):

Ventricular and atrial rate: Greater than 100 in the adult
Ventricular and atrial rhythm: Regular
QRS shape and duration: Usually normal, but may be regularly abnormal
P wave: Normal and consistent shape; always in front of the QRS, but may be buried in the preceding T wave
PR interval: Consistent interval between 0.12 and 0.20 seconds
P : QRS ratio: 1 : 1

All aspects of sinus tachycardia are the same as those of normal sinus rhythm, except for the rate. As the heart rate increases, the diastolic filling time decreases, possibly resulting in reduced cardiac output and subsequent symptoms of syncope and low blood pressure. If the rapid rate persists and the heart cannot compensate for the decreased ventricular filling, the patient may develop acute pulmonary edema.

Treatment of sinus tachycardia is usually directed at abolishing its cause. Calcium channel blockers and beta-blockers (Table 27-1) may be used to reduce the heart rate quickly.

Sinus Arrhythmia. Sinus arrhythmia occurs when the sinus node creates an impulse at an irregular rhythm; the rate usually increases with inspiration and decreases with expiration. Nonrespiratory causes include heart disease and valvular disease, but these are rarely seen. The ECG criteria for sinus arrhythmia follow (Fig. 27-8):

Ventricular and atrial rate: 60 to 100 in the adult
Ventricular and atrial rhythm: Irregular
QRS shape and duration: Usually normal, but may be regularly abnormal

FIGURE 27-5 Normal sinus rhythm in lead II.

FIGURE 27-6   Sinus bradycardia in lead II.

P wave: Normal and consistent shape; always in front of the QRS
PR interval: Consistent interval between 0.12 and 0.20 seconds
P: QRS ratio: 1:1

Sinus arrhythmia does not cause any significant hemodynamic effect and usually is not treated.

ATRIAL DYSRHYTHMIAS

Premature Atrial Complex. A premature atrial complex (PAC) is a single ECG complex that occurs when an electrical impulse starts in the atrium before the next normal impulse of the sinus node. The PAC may be caused by caffeine, alcohol, nicotine, stretched atrial myocardium (as in hypervolemia), anxiety, hypokalemia (low potassium level), hypermetabolic states, or atrial ischemia, injury, or infarction. PACs are often seen with sinus tachycardia. PACs have the following characteristics (Fig. 27-9):

Ventricular and atrial rate: Depends on the underlying rhythm (eg, sinus tachycardia)
Ventricular and atrial rhythm: Irregular due to early P waves, creating a PP interval that is shorter than the others. This is sometimes followed by a longer-than-normal PP interval, but one that is less than twice the normal PP interval. This type of interval is called a noncompensatory pause.
QRS shape and duration: The QRS that follows the early P wave is usually normal, but it may be abnormal (aberrantly conducted PAC). It may even be absent (blocked PAC).
P wave: An early and different P wave may be seen or may be hidden in the T wave; other P waves in the strip are consistent.
PR interval: The early P wave has a shorter-than-normal PR interval, but still between 0.12 and 0.20 seconds.
P: QRS ratio: usually 1:1

PACs are common in normal hearts. The patient may say, "My heart skipped a beat." A pulse deficit (a difference between the apical and radial pulse rate) may exist.

If PACs are infrequent, no treatment is necessary. If they are frequent (more than 6 per minute), this may herald a worsening disease state or the onset of more serious dysrhythmias, such as atrial fibrillation. Treatment is directed toward the cause.

Atrial Flutter. Atrial flutter occurs in the atrium and creates impulses at an atrial rate between 250 and 400 times per minute. Because the atrial rate is faster than the AV node can conduct, not all atrial impulses are conducted into the ventricle, causing a therapeutic block at the AV node. This is an important feature of this dysrhythmia. If all atrial impulses were conducted to the ventricle, the ventricular rate would also be 250 to 400, which would result in ventricular fibrillation, a life-threatening dysrhythmia. Causes are similar to that of atrial fibrillation. Atrial flutter is characterized by the following (Fig. 27-10):

Ventricular and atrial rate: Atrial rate ranges between 250 and 400; ventricular rate usually ranges between 75 and 150.
Ventricular and atrial rhythm: The atrial rhythm is regular; the ventricular rhythm is usually regular but may be irregular because of a change in the AV conduction.
QRS shape and duration: Usually normal, but may be abnormal or may be absent
P wave: Saw-toothed shape. These waves are referred to as F waves.
PR interval: Multiple F waves may make it difficult to determine the PR interval.
P: QRS ratio: 2:1, 3:1, or 4:1

Atrial flutter can cause serious signs and symptoms, such as chest pain, shortness of breath, and low blood pressure. If the

FIGURE 27-7   Sinus tachycardia in lead II.

Table 27-1 • Summary of Antiarrhythmic Medications*

CLASS	ACTION	DRUGS: GENERIC (TRADE) NAMES	SIDE EFFECTS	NURSING INTERVENTIONS
1A	Moderate depression of depolarization; prolongs repolarization. Treats and prevents atrial and ventricular dysrhythmias	quinidine (Quinaglute, Quinalan, Quinora, Quinidex, Cardioquin) procainamide (Pronestyl) disopyramide (Norpace)	Decreased cardiac contractility Prolonged QRS, QT Proarrhythmic Hypotension with IV administration Lupus-like syndrome with Pronestyl Anticholinergic effects: dry mouth, decreased urine output	Observe for HF Monitor BP with IV administration Monitor QRS duration for increase >50% from baseline Monitor for prolonged QT Monitor N-acetyl procainamide (NAPA) laboratory values during procainamide therapy
1B	Minimal depression of depolarization; shortened repolarization. Treats ventricular dysrhythmias	lidocaine (Xylocaine) mexiletine (Mexitil) tocainide (Tonocard)	CNS changes (eg, confusion, lethargy)	Discuss with physician decreasing the dose in elderly patients and patients with cardiac/liver dysfunction
1C	Marked depression of depolarization; little effect on repolarization. Treats atrial and ventricular dysrhythmias	flecainide (Tambocor) propafenone (Rhythmol)	Proarrhythmic HF Bradycardia AV blocks	Discuss patient's left ventricular function with physician
II	Decreases automaticity and conduction. Treats atrial and ventricular dysrhythmias	acebutolol (Sectral) atenolol (Tenormin) esmolol (Brevibloc) labetalol (Normodyne) metoprolol (Lopressor, Toprol) nadolol (Corgard) propranolol (Betachron E-R, Inderal) sotalol (Betapace; also has class III actions)	Bradycardia, AV block Decreased contractility Bronchospasm Hypotension with IV administration Masks hypoglycemia and thyrotoxicosis CNS disturbances	Monitor heart rate, PR interval, signs and symptoms of HF Monitor blood glucose level in patients with type 2 diabetes mellitus
III	Prolongs repolarization. Primarily treats and prevents ventricular dysrhythmias; may also be used to treat atrial dysrhythmias	amiodarone (Cordarone, Pacerone) dofetilide (Tikosyn) ibutilide (Corvert)	Pulmonary toxicity (amiodarone) Corneal microdeposits (amiodarone) Photosensitivity (amiodarone) Hypotension with IV administration Polymorphic ventricular dysrhythmias Nausea and vomiting See beta-blockers (sotolol)	Make sure patient is sent for baseline pulmonary function tests (amiodarone) Closely monitor patient
IV	Blocks calcium channel. Treats atrial dysrhythmias	verapamil (Calan, Isoptin, Verlan) diltiazem (Cardizem, Dilacor, Tiazac)	Bradycardia, AV blocks Hypotension with IV administration HF, peripheral edema	Monitor heart rate, PR interval Monitor blood pressure closely with IV administration Monitor for signs and symptoms of HF

*Based on Vaughn-Williams classification.
AV, atrioventricular; BP, blood pressure; CNS, central nervous system; HF, heart failure; IV, intravenous.

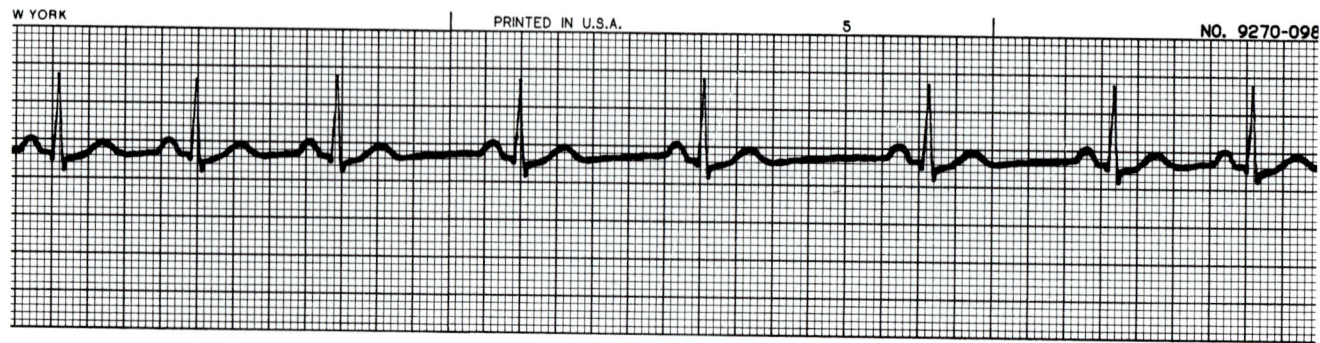

FIGURE 27-8 Sinus arrhythmia in lead II.

FIGURE 27-9 Premature atrial complexes (PACs) in lead II. Note pause following PAC that is longer than the normal PP interval, but shorter than twice the normal PP interval.

patient is unstable, electrical cardioversion (discussed later) is usually indicated. If the patient is stable, diltiazem (eg, Cardizem), verapamil (eg, Calan, Isoptin), beta-blockers, or digitalis may be administered intravenously to slow the ventricular rate. These medications can slow conduction through the AV node. Flecainide (Tambocor), ibutilide (Corvert), dofetilide (Tikosyn), quinidine (eg, Cardioquin, Quinaglute), disopyramide (Norpace), or amiodarone (Cordarone, Pacerone) may be given to promote conversion to sinus rhythm (see Table 27-1). If medication therapy is unsuccessful, electrical cardioversion is often successful. Once conversion has occurred, quinidine, disopyramide, flecainide, propafenone (Rhythmol), amiodarone, or sotalol (Betapace) may be given to maintain sinus rhythm (see Table 27-1).

Atrial Fibrillation. Atrial fibrillation causes a rapid, disorganized, and uncoordinated twitching of atrial musculature. It is the most common dysrhythmia that causes patients to seek medical attention. It may start and stop suddenly. Atrial fibrillation may occur for a very short time (**paroxysmal**), or it may be chronic. Atrial fibrillation is usually associated with advanced age, valvular heart disease, coronary artery disease, hypertension, cardiomyopathy, hyperthyroidism, pulmonary disease, acute moderate to heavy ingestion of alcohol ("holiday heart" syndrome), or the aftermath of open heart surgery. Sometimes it occurs in people without any underlying pathophysiology (termed lone atrial fibrillation). Atrial fibrillation is characterized by the following (Fig. 27-11):

Ventricular and atrial rate: Atrial rate is 300 to 600. Ventricular rate is usually 120 to 200 in untreated atrial fibrillation
Ventricular and atrial rhythm: Highly irregular
QRS shape and duration: Usually normal, but may be abnormal
P wave: No discernible P waves; irregular undulating waves are seen and are referred to as fibrillatory or f waves
PR interval: Cannot be measured
P: QRS ratio: many : 1

A rapid ventricular response reduces the time for ventricular filling, resulting in a smaller stroke volume. Because this rhythm causes the atria and ventricles to contract at different times, the atrial kick (the last part of diastole and ventricular filling, which accounts for 25% to 30% of the cardiac output) is also lost. This leads to symptoms of irregular palpitations, fatigue, and malaise. There is usually a pulse deficit, a numerical difference between apical and radial pulse rates. The shorter time in diastole reduces the time available for coronary artery perfusion, thereby increasing the risk for myocardial ischemia. The erratic atrial contraction promotes the formation of a thrombus within the atria, increasing the risk for an embolic event. There is a two- to five-fold increase in the risk of stroke (brain attack).

Treatment of atrial fibrillation depends on its cause and duration and the patient's symptoms, age, and comorbidities. In many patients, atrial fibrillation converts to sinus rhythm within 24 hours and without treatment. Both stable and unstable atrial fibrillation

FIGURE 27-10 Atrial flutter in lead II.

FIGURE 27-11 Atrial fibrillation in lead II.

of short duration are treated the same as stable and unstable atrial flutter. Cardioversion may be indicated for atrial fibrillation that has been present for less than 48 hours, a condition termed acute-onset atrial fibrillation. Cardioversion of atrial fibrillation that has lasted longer than 48 hours should be avoided unless the patient has received anticoagulants, due to the high risk for embolization of atrial thrombi.

For atrial fibrillation of acute onset, the medications quinidine, ibutilide, flecainide, dofetilide, propafenone, procainamide (Pronestyl), disopyramide, or amiodarone (see Table 27-1) may be given to achieve conversion to sinus rhythm (McNamara et al., 2001). Intravenous adenosine (Adenocard) has also been used for conversion, as well as to assist in the diagnosis. To prevent recurrence and to maintain sinus rhythm, quinidine, disopyramide, flecainide, propafenone, sotalol, or amiodarone may be prescribed. Calcium-channel blockers (diltiazem [Cardizem, Tiazac] and verapamil [Calan, Isoptin]) and beta blockers (see Table 27-1) are effective in controlling the ventricular rate in atrial fibrillation, especially during exercise (McNamara, et al., 2001). Use of digoxin is recommended to control the ventricular rate in those patients with poor cardiac function (ejection fraction less than 40%) (Hauptman & Kelly, 1999). In addition, warfarin is indicated if the patient is at higher risk for a stroke (ie, is elderly or has hypertension, heart failure, or a history of stroke). Aspirin may be substituted for warfarin for those with contraindications to warfarin and those who are at lower risk of stroke. The choice of antithrombotic medication can be guided by transesophageal echocardiography. Pacemaker implantation or surgery is sometimes indicated for patients who are unresponsive to medications.

JUNCTIONAL DYSRHYTHMIAS

Premature Junctional Complex. A premature junctional complex is an impulse that starts in the AV nodal area before the next normal sinus impulse reaches the AV node. Premature junctional complexes are less common than PACs. Causes of premature junctional complex include digitalis toxicity, congestive heart failure, and coronary artery disease. The ECG criteria for premature junctional complex are the same as for PACs, except for the P wave and the PR interval. The P wave may be absent, may follow the QRS, or may occur before the QRS but with a PR interval of less than 0.12 seconds. Premature junctional complexes rarely produce significant symptoms. Treatment for frequent premature junctional complexes is the same as for frequent PACs.

Junctional Rhythm. Junctional or idionodal rhythm occurs when the AV node, instead of the sinus node, becomes the pacemaker of the heart. When the sinus node slows (eg, from increased vagal tone) or when the impulse cannot be conducted through the AV node (eg, because of complete heart block), the AV node automatically discharges an impulse. The following are the ECG criteria for junctional rhythm not caused by complete heart block (Fig. 27-12):

Ventricular and atrial rate: Ventricular rate 40 to 60; atrial rate also 40 to 60 if P waves are discernible
Ventricular and atrial rhythm: Regular
QRS shape and duration: Usually normal, but may be abnormal
P wave: May be absent, after the QRS complex, or before the QRS; may be inverted, especially in lead II

FIGURE 27-12 Junctional rhythm in lead II; note short PR intervals.

FIGURE 27-13 AV nodal reentry tachycardia in lead II.

PR interval: If P wave is in front of the QRS, PR interval is less than 0.12 second.

P: QRS ratio: 1:1 or 0:1

Junctional rhythm may produce signs and symptoms of reduced cardiac output. If so, the treatment is the same as for sinus bradycardia. Emergency pacing may be needed.

Atrioventricular Nodal Reentry Tachycardia. AV nodal reentry tachycardia occurs when an impulse is conducted to an area in the AV node that causes the impulse to be rerouted back into the same area over and over again at a very fast rate. Each time the impulse is conducted through this area, it is also conducted down into the ventricles, causing a fast ventricular rate. AV nodal reentry tachycardia that has an abrupt onset and an abrupt cessation with a QRS of normal duration had been called paroxysmal atrial tachycardia (PAT). Factors associated with the development of AV nodal reentry tachycardia include caffeine, nicotine, hypoxemia, and stress. Underlying pathologies include coronary artery disease and cardiomyopathy. The ECG criteria are as follows (Fig. 27-13):

Ventricular and atrial rate: Atrial rate usually ranges between 150 to 250; ventricular rate usually ranges between 75 to 250
Ventricular and atrial rhythm: Regular; sudden onset and termination of the tachycardia
QRS shape and duration: Usually normal, but may be abnormal
P wave: Usually very difficult to discern
PR interval: If P wave is in front of the QRS, PR interval is less than 0.12 seconds
P: QRS ratio: 1:1, 2:1

The clinical symptoms vary with the rate and duration of the tachycardia and the patient's underlying condition. The tachycardia usually is of short duration, resulting only in palpitations. A fast rate may also reduce cardiac output, resulting in significant signs and symptoms such as restlessness, chest pain, shortness of breath, pallor, hypotension, and loss of consciousness.

Treatment is aimed at breaking the reentry of the impulse. Vagal manoeuvres, such as carotid sinus massage (Fig. 27-14), gag reflex, breath holding, and immersing the face in ice water, increase parasympathetic stimulation, causing slower conduction through the AV node and blocking the reentry of the rerouted impulse. Some patients have learned to use some of these methods to terminate the episode on their own. Because of the risk of a cerebral embolic event, carotid sinus massage is

contraindicated in patients with carotid bruits. If the vagal manoeuvres are ineffective, the patient may then receive a bolus of adenosine, verapamil, or diltiazem. Cardioversion is the treatment of choice if the patient is unstable or does not respond to the medications.

If P waves cannot be identified, the rhythm may be called **supraventricular tachycardia (SVT)**, which indicates only that it is not **ventricular tachycardia (VT)**. SVT could be atrial fibrillation, atrial flutter, or AV nodal reentry tachycardia, among others. Vagal manoeuvres and adenosine are used to slow conduction in the AV node to allow visualization of the P waves.

VENTRICULAR DYSRHYTHMIAS

Premature Ventricular Complex. Premature ventricular complex (PVC) is an impulse that starts in a ventricle and is conducted through the ventricles before the next normal sinus impulse. PVCs can occur in healthy people, especially with the use of caffeine, nicotine, or alcohol. They are also caused by cardiac ischemia or infarction, increased workload on the heart (eg, exercise, fever, hypervolemia, heart failure, tachycardia), digitalis toxicity, hypoxia, acidosis, or electrolyte imbalances, especially hypokalemia.

In the absence of disease, PVCs are not serious. In the patient with an acute MI, PVCs may indicate the need for more aggressive therapy. PVCs may indicate the possibility of ensuing VT. However, PVCs that are (1) more frequent than 6 per minute,

FIGURE 27-14 Carotid sinus massage.

(2) multifocal or polymorphic (having different shapes), (3) occur two in a row (pair), and (4) occur on the T wave (the vulnerable period of ventricular depolarization) have not been found to be precursors of VT (Cardiac Arrhythmia Suppression Trial Investigators, 1989). These PVCs are no longer considered as warning or complex PVCs.

In a rhythm called bigeminy, every other complex is a PVC. Trigeminy is a rhythm in which every third complex is a PVC, and quadrigeminy is a rhythm in which every fourth complex is a PVC. PVCs have the following characteristics on the ECG (Fig. 27-15):

Ventricular and atrial rate: Depends on the underlying rhythm (eg, sinus rhythm)
Ventricular and atrial rhythm: Irregular due to early QRS, creating one RR interval that is shorter than the others. PP interval may be regular, indicating that the PVC did not depolarize the sinus node.
QRS shape and duration: Duration is 0.12 seconds or longer; shape is bizarre and abnormal
P wave: Visibility of P wave depends on the timing of the PVC; may be absent (hidden in the QRS or T wave) or in front of the QRS. If the P wave follows the QRS, the shape of the P wave may be different.
PR interval: If the P wave is in front of the QRS, the PR interval is less than 0.12 seconds.
P: QRS ratio: 0:1; 1:1

The patient may feel nothing or may say that the heart "skipped a beat." The effect of a PVC depends on its timing in the cardiac cycle and how much blood was in the ventricles when they contracted. Initial treatment is aimed at correcting the cause, if possible. Lidocaine (Xylocaine) is the medication most commonly used for immediate, short-term therapy (see Table 27-1). Long-term pharmacotherapy for only PVCs is not indicated.

Ventricular Tachycardia. Ventricular tachycardia (VT) is defined as three or more PVCs in a row, occurring at a rate exceeding 100 beats per minute. The causes are similar to those for PVC. VT is usually associated with coronary artery disease and may precede ventricular fibrillation. VT is an emergency because the patient is usually (although not always) unresponsive and pulseless. VT has the following characteristics (Fig. 27-16):

Ventricular and atrial rate: Ventricular rate is 100 to 200 beats per minute; atrial rate depends on the underlying rhythm (eg, sinus rhythm)
Ventricular and atrial rhythm: Usually regular; atrial rhythm may also be regular.
QRS shape and duration: Duration is 0.12 seconds or more; bizarre, abnormal shape

P wave: Very difficult to detect, so atrial rate and rhythm may be indeterminable
PR interval: Very irregular, if P waves seen.
P: QRS ratio: Difficult to determine, but if P waves are apparent, there are usually more QRS complexes than P waves.

The patient's tolerance or lack of tolerance for this rapid rhythm depends on the ventricular rate and underlying disease. If the patient is stable, continuing the assessment, especially obtaining a 12-lead ECG, may be the only action necessary. Cardioversion may be the treatment of choice, especially if the patient is unstable. Several factors determine the initial medication used for treatment, including the following: identifying the rhythm as monomorphic (having a consistent QRS shape and rate) or polymorphic (having varying QRS shapes and rates); determining the existence of a prolonged QT interval before the initiation of VT; and ascertaining the patient's heart function (normal or decreased). VT in a patient who is unconscious and without a pulse is treated in the same manner as ventricular fibrillation: immediate **defibrillation** is the action of choice.

Ventricular Fibrillation. Ventricular fibrillation is a rapid but disorganized ventricular rhythm that causes ineffective quivering of the ventricles. There is no atrial activity seen on the ECG. Causes of ventricular fibrillation are the same as for VT; it may also result from untreated or unsuccessfully treated VT. Other causes include electrical shock and Brugada syndrome, in which the patient (frequently of Asian descent) has a structurally normal heart, few or no risk factors for coronary artery disease, and a family history of sudden cardiac death. Ventricular fibrillation has the following characteristics (Fig. 27-17):

Ventricular rate: Greater than 300 per minute
Ventricular rhythm: Extremely irregular, without specific pattern
QRS shape and duration: Irregular, undulating waves without recognizable QRS complexes

This dysrhythmia is always characterized by the absence of an audible heartbeat, a palpable pulse, and respirations. Because there is no coordinated cardiac activity, cardiac arrest and death are imminent if ventricular fibrillation is not corrected. Treatment of choice is immediate defibrillation and activation of emergency services. The importance of defibrillation is evident in one of the recent changes in basic life support (Introduction to the International Guidelines 2000 for CPR and ECC, 2000): placing a call for emergency assistance and calling for a defibrillator takes precedence over initiating cardiopulmonary resuscitation in the adult victim. Also, application of an automatic external defibrillator (AED) is included in basic life support classes. After defibrillation, eradicating causes and administering vasoactive and **antiarrhythmic** medications

FIGURE 27-15 Multifocal PVCs in quadrigeminy in lead V₁. Note regular PP interval.

FIGURE 27-16 Ventricular tachycardia in lead V₁.

alternating with defibrillation are treatments used to try to convert the rhythm to normal sinus rhythm.

Idioventricular Rhythm. Idioventricular rhythm, also called ventricular escape rhythm, occurs when the impulse starts in the conduction system below the AV node. When the sinus node fails to create an impulse (eg, from increased vagal tone), or when the impulse is created but cannot be conducted through the AV node (eg, due to complete AV block), the Purkinje fibres automatically discharge an impulse. The following are the ECG criteria when idioventricular rhythm is not caused by AV block (Fig. 27-18):

Ventricular rate: Ranges between 20 and 40; if the rate exceeds 40, the rhythm is known as accelerated idioventricular rhythm (AIVR).
Ventricular rhythm: Regular
QRS shape and duration: Bizarre, abnormal shape; duration is 0.12 seconds or more

Idioventricular rhythm commonly causes the patient to lose consciousness and experience other signs and symptoms of reduced cardiac output. In such cases, the treatment is the same as for pulseless electrical activity if the patient is in cardiac arrest or for bradycardia if the patient is not in cardiac arrest. Interventions may include identifying the underlying cause, administering intravenous atropine and vasopressor medications, and initiating emergency transcutaneous pacing. In some cases, idioventricular rhythm may cause no symptoms of reduced cardiac output. However, bed rest is prescribed so as not to increase the cardiac workload.

Ventricular Asystole. Commonly called flatline, ventricular asystole (Fig. 27-19) is characterized by absent QRS complexes, although P waves may be apparent for a short duration in two different leads. There is no heartbeat, no palpable pulse, and no respiration. Without immediate treatment, ventricular asystole is fatal. Cardiopulmonary resuscitation and emergency services are necessary to keep the patient alive. The guidelines for advanced cardiac life support (American Heart Association, 2000) state that the key to successful treatment is rapid assessment to identify a possible cause, which may be hypoxia, acidosis, severe electrolyte imbalance, drug overdose, or hypothermia. Intubation and establishment of intravenous access are the first recommended actions. Transcutaneous pacing may be attempted. A bolus of intravenous epinephrine should be administered and repeated at 3- to 5-minute intervals, followed by 1-mg boluses of atropine at 3- to 5-minute intervals. Because of the poor prognosis associated with asystole, if the patient does not respond to these actions and others aimed at correcting underlying causes, resuscitation efforts are usually ended ("the code is called") unless special circumstances (eg, hypothermia) exist.

CONDUCTION ABNORMALITIES

When assessing the rhythm strip, the nurse takes care first to identify the underlying rhythm (eg, sinus rhythm, sinus arrhythmia). Then the PR interval is assessed for the possibility of an AV block. AV blocks occur when the conduction of the impulse through the AV nodal area is decreased or stopped. These blocks can be caused by medications (eg, digitalis, calcium channel blockers, beta-blockers), myocardial ischemia and infarction, valvular disorders, or myocarditis. If the AV block is caused by increased vagal tone (eg, suctioning, pressure above the eyes or on large vessels, anal stimulation), it is commonly accompanied by sinus bradycardia.

The clinical signs and symptoms of a heart block vary with the resulting ventricular rate and the severity of any underlying dis-

FIGURE 27-17 Ventricular fibrillation in lead II.

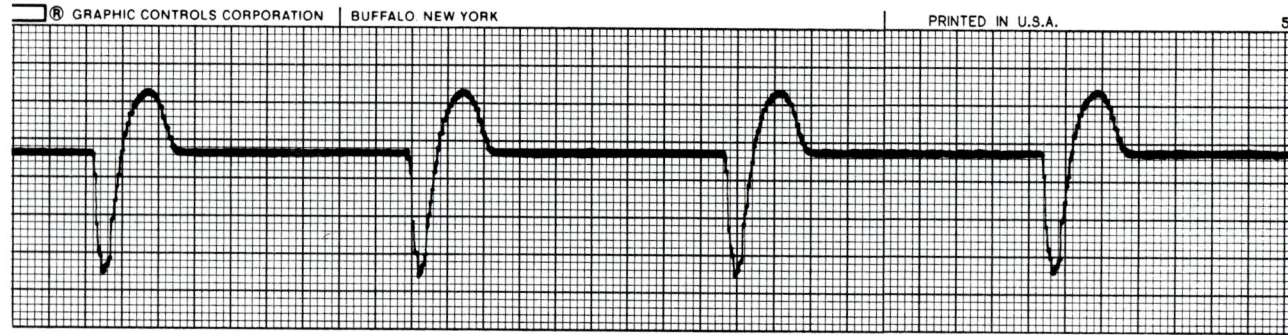

FIGURE 27-18 Idioventricular rhythm in lead V_1.

ease processes. Whereas first-degree AV block rarely causes any hemodynamic effect, the other blocks may result in decreased heart rate, causing a decrease in perfusion to vital organs, such as the brain, heart, kidneys, lungs, and skin. A patient with third-degree AV block caused by digitalis toxicity may be stable; another patient with the same rhythm caused by acute MI may be unstable. Health care providers must always keep in mind the need to treat the patient, not the rhythm. The treatment is based on the hemodynamic effect of the rhythm.

First-Degree Atrioventricular Block. First-degree heart block occurs when all the atrial impulses are conducted through the AV node into the ventricles at a rate slower than normal. This conduction disorder has the following characteristics (Fig. 27-20):

Ventricular and atrial rate: Depends on the underlying rhythm
Ventricular and atrial rhythm: Depends on the underlying rhythm
QRS shape and duration: Usually normal, but may be abnormal
P wave: In front of the QRS complex; shows sinus rhythm, regular shape
PR interval: Greater than 0.20 seconds; PR interval measurement is constant.
P: QRS ratio: 1:1

Second-Degree Atrioventricular Block, Type I. Second-degree, type I heart block occurs when all but one of the atrial impulses are conducted through the AV node into the ventricles. Each atrial impulse takes a longer time for conduction than the one before, until one impulse is fully blocked. Because the AV node is

not depolarized by the blocked atrial impulse, the AV node has time to fully repolarize, so that the next atrial impulse can be conducted within the shortest amount of time. Second-degree AV block, type I has the following characteristics (Fig. 27-21):

Ventricular and atrial rate: Depends on the underlying rhythm
Ventricular and atrial rhythm: The PP interval is regular if the patient has an underlying normal sinus rhythm; the RR interval characteristically reflects a pattern of change. Starting from the RR that is the longest, the RR interval gradually shortens until there is another long RR interval.
QRS shape and duration: Usually normal, but may be abnormal
P wave: In front of the QRS complex; shape depends on underlying rhythm
PR interval: PR interval becomes longer with each succeeding ECG complex until there is a P wave not followed by a QRS. The changes in the PR interval are repeated between each "dropped" QRS, creating a pattern in the irregular PR interval measurements.
P: QRS ratio: 3:2, 4:3, 5:4, and so forth

Second-Degree Atrioventricular Block, Type II. Second-degree, type II heart block occurs when only some of the atrial impulses are conducted through the AV node into the ventricles. Second-degree AV block, type II has the following characteristics (Fig. 27-22):

Ventricular and atrial rate: Depends on the underlying rhythm
Ventricular and atrial rhythm: The PP interval is regular if the patient has an underlying normal sinus rhythm. The RR

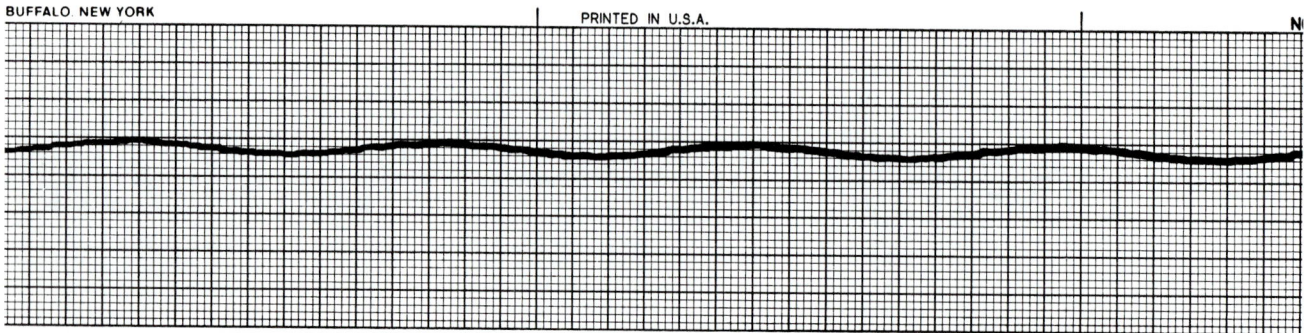

FIGURE 27-19 Asystole. (Always check two different leads to confirm rhythm.)

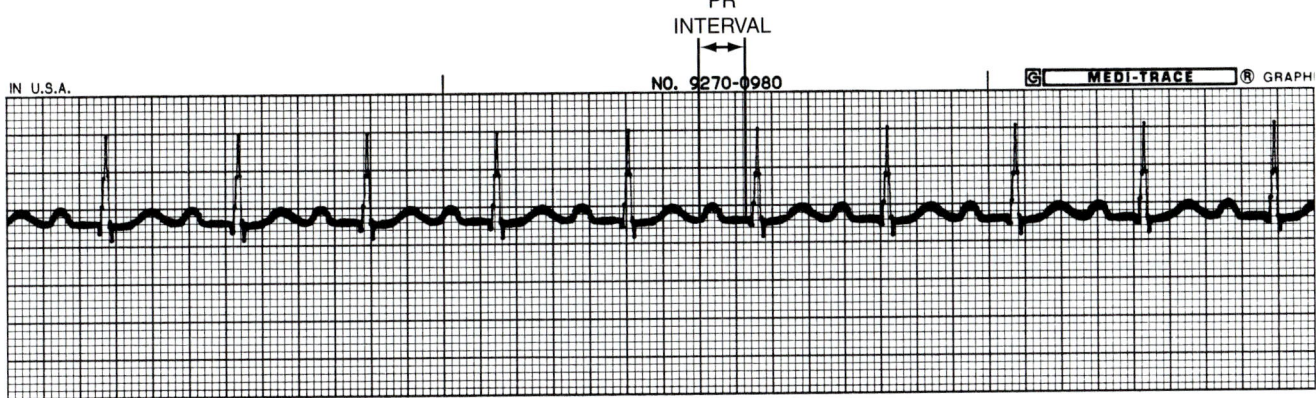

FIGURE 27-20 Sinus rhythm with first-degree AV block in lead II.

FIGURE 27-21 Sinus rhythm with second-degree AV block, type I in lead II. Note progressively longer PR durations until there is a nonconducted P wave, indicated by the asterisk (*).

★ = nonconducted P-waves

FIGURE 27-22 Sinus rhythm with second-degree AV block, type II in lead V_1; note constant PR interval.

interval is usually regular but may be irregular, depending on the P : QRS ratio.

QRS shape and duration: Usually abnormal, but may be normal
P wave: In front of the QRS complex; shape depends on underlying rhythm.
PR interval: PR interval is constant for those P waves just before QRS complexes.
P: QRS ratio: 2:1, 3:1, 4:1, 5:1, and so forth

Third-Degree Atrioventricular Block.
Third-degree heart block occurs when no atrial impulse is conducted through the AV node into the ventricles. In third-degree heart block, two impulses stimulate the heart: one stimulates the ventricles (eg, junctional or ventricular escape rhythm), represented by the QRS complex, and one stimulates the atria (eg, sinus rhythm, atrial fibrillation), represented by the P wave. P waves may be seen, but the atrial electrical activity is not conducted down into the ventricles to cause the QRS complex, the ventricular electrical activity. This is called AV dissociation. Complete block (third-degree AV block) has the following characteristics (Fig. 27-23):

Ventricular and atrial rate: Depends on the escape and underlying atrial rhythm
Ventricular and atrial rhythm: The PP interval is regular and the RR interval is regular; however, the PP interval is not equal to the RR interval.
QRS shape and duration: Depends on the escape rhythm; in junctional escape, QRS shape and duration are usually normal, and in ventricular escape, QRS shape and duration are usually abnormal.
P wave: Depends on underlying rhythm
PR interval: Very irregular
P: QRS ratio: More P waves than QRS complexes

Based on the cause of the AV block and the stability of the patient, treatment is directed toward increasing the heart rate to maintain a normal cardiac output. If the patient is stable and has no symptoms, no treatment is indicated other than decreasing or eradicating the cause (eg, withholding the medication or treatment). If the patient is short of breath, complains of chest pain or lightheadedness, or has low blood pressure, an intravenous bolus of atropine is the initial treatment of choice. If the patient does not respond to atropine or has an acute MI, transcutaneous pacing should be started. A permanent pacemaker may be necessary if the block persists.

NURSING PROCESS:
THE PATIENT WITH A DYSRHYTHMIA
Assessment

Major areas of assessment include possible causes of the dysrhythmia and the dysrhythmia's effect on the heart's ability to pump an adequate blood volume. When cardiac output is reduced, the amount of oxygen reaching the tissues and vital organs is diminished. This diminished oxygenation produces the signs and symptoms associated with dysrhythmias. If these signs and symptoms are severe or if they occur frequently, the patient may experience significant distress and disruption of daily life.

A health history is obtained to identify any previous occurrences of decreased cardiac output, such as syncope (fainting), lightheadedness, dizziness, fatigue, chest discomfort, and palpitations. Coexisting conditions that could be a possible cause of the dysrhythmia (eg, heart disease, chronic obstructive pulmonary disease) may also be identified. All medications, prescribed and over-the-counter (including herbs and nutritional supplements), are reviewed. Some medications (eg, digoxin) can cause dysrhythmias. A thorough psychosocial assessment is performed to identify the possible effects of the dysrhythmia and to determine whether anxiety is a significant contributing factor.

The nurse conducts a physical assessment to confirm the data obtained from the history and to observe for signs of diminished cardiac output during the dysrhythmic event, especially changes in level of consciousness. The nurse directs attention to the skin, which may be pale and cool. Signs of fluid retention, such as neck vein distention and crackles and wheezes auscultated in the lungs, may be detected. The rate and rhythm of apical and peripheral pulses are also assessed, and any pulse deficit is noted. The nurse auscultates for extra heart sounds (especially S_3 and S_4) and for heart murmurs, measures blood pressure, and determines pulse pressures. A declining pulse pressure indicates reduced cardiac output. Just one assessment may not disclose significant changes in cardiac output; therefore, the nurse compares multiple assessment findings over time, especially those that occur with and without the dysrhythmia.

Diagnosis

NURSING DIAGNOSES
Based on assessment data, major nursing diagnoses of the patient may include:

FIGURE 27-23   Sinus rhythm with third-degree AV block and idioventricular rhythm in lead V₁; note irregular PR intervals.

- Decreased cardiac output
- Anxiety related to fear of the unknown
- Deficient knowledge about the dysrhythmia and its treatment

COLLABORATIVE PROBLEMS/ POTENTIAL COMPLICATIONS

In addition to cardiac arrest, a potential complication that may develop over time is heart failure. Another potential complication, especially with atrial fibrillation, is a thromboembolic event. If the dysrhythmia necessitates treatment with medication, the beneficial and detrimental effects must be assessed.

Planning and Goals

The major goals for the patient may include eradicating or decreasing the incidence of the dysrhythmia (by decreasing contributory factors) to maintain cardiac output, minimizing anxiety, and acquiring knowledge about the dysrhythmia and its treatment.

Nursing Interventions

MONITORING AND MANAGING THE DYSRHYTHMIA

The nurse regularly evaluates blood pressure, pulse rate and rhythm, rate and depth of respirations, and breath sounds to determine the dysrhythmia's hemodynamic effect. The nurse also asks patients about episodes of lightheadedness, dizziness, or fainting as part of the ongoing assessment. If a patient with a dysrhythmia is hospitalized, the nurse may obtain a 12-lead ECG, continuously monitor the patient, and analyze rhythm strips to track the dysrhythmia.

Control of the incidence or the effect of the dysrhythmia, or both, is often achieved by the use of antiarrhythmic medications. The nurse assesses and observes for the beneficial and adverse effects of each of the medications. The nurse also manages medication administration carefully so that a constant serum blood level of the medication is maintained at all times.

In addition to medication, the nurse assesses for factors that contribute to the dysrhythmia (eg, caffeine, stress, nonadherence to the medication regimen) and assists the patient in developing a plan to make lifestyle changes that eliminate or reduce these factors.

MINIMIZING ANXIETY

When the patient experiences episodes of dysrhythmia, the nurse maintains a calm and reassuring attitude. This demeanor fosters a trusting relationship with the patient and assists in reducing anxiety (reducing the sympathetic response). Successes are emphasized with the patient to promote a sense of confidence in living with a dysrhythmia. For example, if a patient is experiencing episodes of dysrhythmia and a medication is administered that begins to reduce the incidence of the dysrhythmia, the nurse communicates that information to the patient. The nursing goal is to maximize the patient's control and to make the unknown less threatening.

PROMOTING HOME AND COMMUNITY-BASED CARE

Teaching Patients Self-Care

When teaching patients about dysrhythmias, the nurse presents the information in terms that are understandable and in a manner that is not frightening or threatening. The nurse explains the importance of maintaining therapeutic serum levels of anti-

arrhythmic medications so that the patient understands why medications should be taken regularly each day. In addition, the relationship between a dysrhythmia and cardiac output is explained so that the patient understands the rationale for the medical regimen. If the patient has a potentially lethal dysrhythmia, it is also important to establish with the patient and family a plan of action to take in case of an emergency. This allows the patient and family to feel in control and prepared for possible events.

A referral for home care usually is not necessary for the patient with a dysrhythmia unless the patient is hemodynamically unstable and has significant symptoms of decreased cardiac output. Home care is also warranted if the patient has significant comorbidities, socioeconomic issues, or limited self-management skills that could potentiate the risk for nonadherence to the therapeutic regimen.

Evaluation

EXPECTED PATIENT OUTCOMES

Expected patient outcomes may include:

1. Maintains cardiac output
   a. Demonstrates heart rate, blood pressure, respiratory rate, and level of consciousness within normal ranges
   b. Demonstrates no or decreased episodes of dysrhythmia
2. Experiences reduced anxiety
   a. Expresses a positive attitude about living with the dysrhythmia
   b. Expresses confidence in ability to take appropriate actions in an emergency
3. Expresses understanding of the dysrhythmia and its treatment
   a. Explains the dysrhythmia and its effects
   b. Describes the medication regimen and its rationale
   c. Explains the need for therapeutic serum level of the medication
   d. Describes a plan to eradicate or limit factors that contribute to the occurrence of the dysrhythmia
   e. States actions to take in the event of an emergency

Adjunctive Modalities and Management

Dysrhythmia treatments depend on whether the disorder is acute or chronic as well as on the cause of the dysrhythmia and its actual or potential hemodynamic effects.

Acute dysrhythmias may be treated with medications or with external electrical therapy. Many antiarrhythmic medications are used to treat atrial and ventricular tachydysrhythmias. These medications are summarized in Table 27-1. The choice of medication depends on the specific dysrhythmia, presence of cardiac failure and other diseases, and the patient's response to previous treatment. The nurse is responsible for monitoring and documenting the patient's responses to the medication and for making sure that the patient has the knowledge and ability to manage the medication regimen.

If medications alone are ineffective in eradicating or decreasing the dysrhythmia, certain adjunctive mechanical therapies are available. The most common are pacemakers for bradycardias and tachycardias, elective cardioversion and defibrillation for acute tachydysrhythmia, and implantable devices for chronic tachydysrhythmia. Surgical treatments, although less common, are also available.

PACEMAKER THERAPY

A pacemaker is an electronic device that provides electrical stimuli to the heart muscle. Pacemakers are usually used when a patient has a slower-than-normal impulse formation or a conduction disturbance that causes symptoms. They may also be used to control some tachydysrhythmias that do not respond to medication therapy. Biventricular (both ventricles) pacing may be used to treat advanced heart failure that does not respond to medication therapy.

Pacemakers can be permanent or temporary. Permanent pacemakers are used most commonly for irreversible complete heart block. Temporary pacemakers are used (eg, after MI, after open heart surgery) to support patients until they improve or receive a permanent pacemaker.

Pacemaker Design and Types

Pacemakers consist of two components: an electronic pulse generator and pacemaker electrodes, which are located on leads or wires. The generator contains the circuitry and batteries that generate the rate (measured in beats per minute) and the strength (measured in milliamperes [mA]) of the electrical stimulus delivered to the heart. The pacemaker electrodes convey the heart's electrical activity through a lead to the generator; the generator's electrical response to the information received is then transmitted to the heart.

Leads can be threaded through a major vein into the right ventricle (endocardial leads), or they can be lightly sutured onto the outside of the heart and brought through the chest wall during open heart surgery (epicardial wires). The epicardial wires are always temporary and are removed by a gentle tug within a few days after surgery. The endocardial leads may be temporarily placed with catheters through the femoral, antecubital, brachial, or jugular vein (transvenous wires), usually guided by fluoroscopy. The endocardial and epicardial wires are connected to a temporary generator, which is about the size of a small paperback book. The energy source for a temporary generator is a common household battery; monitoring for pacemaker malfunctioning and battery failure is a nursing responsibility. This type of pacemaker therapy necessitates hospitalization of the patient.

The endocardial leads also may be placed permanently, usually through the external jugular vein, and connected to a permanent generator, which is usually implanted underneath the skin in a subcutaneous pocket in the pectoral region or below the clavicle (Fig. 27-24). Sometimes an abdominal site is selected. This procedure is usually performed in a cardiac catheterization laboratory with the patient receiving a local anesthetic. Permanent pacemaker generators are insulated to protect against body moisture and warmth. There are several different energy sources for permanent generators: mercury-zinc batteries (which last 3 to 4 years), lithium cell units (up to 10 years), and nuclear-powered sources such as plutonium 238 (up to 20 years). Some of the batteries are rechargeable. If the battery is not rechargeable and failure is impending, the old generator is removed and the new one is connected to the existing leads and reimplanted in the already existing subcutaneous pocket. This procedure is usually performed with the patient receiving a local anesthetic. Hospitalization of the patient is needed for implantation or battery replacement.

If a patient suddenly develops a bradycardia, emergency pacing may be started with transcutaneous pacing, which most defibrillators are now equipped to perform. AEDs are not able to do transcutaneous pacing (see later discussion). Large pacing ECG electrodes (sometimes the same conductive pads that are used for

Pacemaker lead enters
external jugular vein

Pacemaker lead tunnelled
subcutaneously between
pacemaker and
external jugular
vein

Pacemaker placed
beneath skin in
pectoral region

Tip of lead (electrode)
lodged in apex of
right ventricle

FIGURE 27-24 Implanted transvenous pacing lead (with electrode) and pacemaker generator.

cardioversion and defibrillation) are placed on the patient's chest and back. The electrodes are connected to the defibrillator, which is the temporary pacemaker generator (Fig. 27-25). Because the impulse must travel through the patient's skin and tissue before reaching the heart, transcutaneous pacing can cause significant discomfort and is intended to be used only in emergencies. This type of pacing necessitates hospitalization. If the patient is alert, the use of sedation and analgesia should be discussed with the physician.

Pacemaker Generator Functions

Because of the sophistication and wide use of pacemakers, a universal code has been adopted to provide a means of safe communication about their function. The coding is referred to as the NASPE-BPEG code because it is sanctioned by the North American Society of Pacing and Electrophysiology and the British Pacing and Electrophysiology Group. The complete code consists of five letters, but only the first three are commonly used.

The first letter of the code identifies the chamber or chambers being paced—that is, the chamber containing a pacing electrode. The letter characters for this code are A (atrium), V (ventricle), or D (dual, meaning both A and V).

The second letter describes the chamber or chambers being sensed by the pacemaker generator. Information from the electrode within the chamber is sent to the generator for interpretation and action by the generator. The possible letter characters are A (atrium), V (ventricle), D (dual), and O (indicating that the sensing function is turned off).

The third letter of the code describes the type of response by the pacemaker to what is sensed. The possible letter characters used to describe this response are I (**inhibited**), T (**triggered**), D (dual, inhibited and triggered), and O (none). Inhibited response means that the response of the pacemaker is controlled by the activity of the patient's heart; that is, the pacemaker will not func-

FIGURE 27-25 Transcutaneous pacemaker with electrode pads connected to the anterior and posterior chest walls.

tion when the patient's heart beats but will pace if no beat is sensed. In contrast, triggered response means that the pacemaker will provide a response (pace the heart) when it senses intrinsic heart activity.

The fourth and fifth letters are used only with permanent pacemaker generators. The fourth letter of the code is related to a permanent generator's ability to be programmed or reset. The possible letters are O (none), P (simple programmability), M (multi-programmability; ability to change at least three factors, such as the rate at which pacing is initiated, the rate of pacing, and the amount of energy delivered), C (communicative or telemetry ability; information about the generator may be obtained [read or interrogated] with a hand-held device placed above the chest), and R (rate responsive capabilities; the ability of the pacemaker to change the rate from moment to moment based on parameters such as physical activity, acid-base changes, temperature, rate and depth of respirations, and oxygen saturation). A pacemaker with rate responsive ability will be capable of improving cardiac output during times of increased cardiac demand, such as with exercise.

The fifth letter of the code indicates that the permanent generator has antitachycardia and/or defibrillation capability. The possible letters are P (antitachycardia pacing), S (shock; defibrillation), D (dual—antitachycardia pacing and shock), and O (none). Antitachycardia pacing is used to terminate tachycardias caused by a conduction disturbance called reentry, which is repetitive restimulation of the heart by the same impulse. An impulse or series of impulses is delivered to the heart by the pacemaker at a fast rate to collide with and stop the heart's reentry conduction impulses, and therefore to stop the tachycardia.

An example of a NASPE-BPEG code is DVI:

D: Both the atrium and the ventricle have a pacing electrode in place.
V: The pacemaker is sensing the activity of the ventricle only.
I: The pacemaker's stimulating effect is inhibited by ventricular activity—in other words, it does not create an impulse when the patient's ventricle is active. The pacemaker paces the atrium and then the ventricle when no ventricular activity is sensed for a period of time (the time is individually programmed into the pacemaker for each patient).

The type of generator and its selected settings depend on the patient's dysrhythmia, underlying cardiac function, and age. A straight vertical line usually can be seen on the ECG when pacing is initiated. The line that represents pacing is called a pace-

maker spike. The appropriate ECG complex should immediately follow the pacing spike; therefore, a P wave should follow an atrial pacing spike and a QRS complex should follow a ventricular pacing spike. Because the impulse starts in a different place than the patient's normal rhythm, the QRS complex or P wave that responds to pacing looks different from the patient's normal ECG complex. *Capture* is a term used to denote that the appropriate complex followed the pacing spike.

Pacemakers are generally set to sense and respond to intrinsic activity, which is called on-demand pacing (Fig. 27-26). If the pacemaker is set to pace but not to sense, it is called a fixed or asynchronous pacemaker (Fig. 27-27); this is written in code as AOO or VOO. The pacemaker will pace at a constant rate, independent of the patient's intrinsic rhythm. Because AOO pacing stimulates only the atrium, it may be used in a patient who has undergone open heart surgery and develops sinus bradycardia. AOO pacing ensures synchrony between atrial stimulation and ventricular stimulation (and therefore contraction), as long as the patient has no conduction disturbances in the AV node. VOO is rare because of the risk that the pacemaker may deliver an impulse during the vulnerable repolarization phase, leading to VT.

Complications of Pacemaker Use

Complications associated with pacemakers relate to their presence within the body, and improper functioning. The following complications may arise from a pacemaker:

- Local infection at the entry site of the leads for temporary pacing, or at the subcutaneous site for permanent generator placement
- Bleeding and hematoma at the lead entry sites for temporary pacing, or at the subcutaneous site for permanent generator placement
- Hemothorax from puncture of the subclavian vein or internal mammary artery
- Ventricular ectopy and tachycardia from irritation of the ventricular wall by the endocardial electrode
- Movement or dislocation of the lead placed transvenously (perforation of the myocardium)
- Phrenic nerve, diaphragmatic (hiccuping may be a sign of this), or skeletal muscle stimulation if the lead is dislocated or if the delivered energy (mA) is set high
- Rarely, cardiac tamponade from bleeding resulting from removal of epicardial wires used for temporary pacing

FIGURE 27-26 Pacing with appropriate sensing (on-demand pacing) in lead V₁. Arrows denote pacing spike. Asterisk (*) denotes intrinsic (patient's own) beats, therefore no pacing. F denotes a fusion beat, which is a combination of an intrinsic beat and a paced beat occurring at the same time.

In the initial hours after a temporary or permanent pacemaker is inserted, the most common complication is dislodgment of the pacing electrode. Minimizing patient activity can help to prevent this complication. If a temporary electrode is in place, the extremity through which the catheter has been advanced is immobilized. With a permanent pacemaker, the patient is instructed initially to restrict activity on the side of the implantation.

The ECG is monitored very carefully to detect pacemaker malfunction. Improper pacemaker function, which can arise from failure in one or more components of the pacing system, is outlined in Table 27-2. The following data should be noted on the patient's record: model of pacemaker, type of generator, date and time of insertion, location of pulse generator, stimulation threshold, pacer settings (eg, rate, energy output [mA], and duration between atrial and ventricular impulses [AV delay]). This information is important for identifying normal pacemaker function and diagnosing pacemaker malfunction.

A patient experiencing pacemaker malfunction may develop signs and symptoms of decreased cardiac output. The degree to which these symptoms become apparent depends on the severity of the malfunction, the patient's level of dependency on the pacemaker, and the patient's underlying condition. Pacemaker malfunction is diagnosed by analyzing the ECG. Manipulating the electrodes, changing the generator's settings, or replacing the pacemaker generator or leads (or both) may be necessary.

Inhibition of permanent pacemakers can occur with exposure to strong electromagnetic fields (electromagnetic interference). However, recent pacemaker technology allows patients to safely use most household electronic appliances and devices (eg, microwave ovens, electric tools) as long as they are not held close to the pacemaker generator. Gas-powered engines should be turned off before working on them. Objects that contain magnets (eg, the earpiece of a standard phone; large stereo speakers; magnet therapy products such as mattresses, jewelry, and wraps) should not be near the generator for longer than a few seconds. Patients are advised to use digital cellular phones on the side opposite the pacemaker generator. Large electromagnetic fields, such as those produced by magnetic resonance imaging (MRI), radio and TV transmitter towers and lines, transmission power lines (these are different from the distribution lines that bring electricity into a home), and electrical substations may cause electromagnetic interference. Patients should be cautioned to avoid such situations or to simply move farther away from the area if they experience dizziness or a feeling of rapid or irregular heartbeats (palpitations). Welding and use of a chain saw should be avoided. If such tools are used, precautionary steps such as limiting the welding current to a 60- to 130-ampere range or using electric rather than gasoline-powered chain saws are advised.

The metal of the pacemaker generator may trigger some store and airport security alarms, but these alarm systems will not interfere with the pacemaker function. However, the handheld screening devices used in airports may interfere with the pacemaker. Patients should be advised to request a hand search instead of the handheld screening device. Patients also should be instructed to wear or carry medical identification to alert personnel to the presence of the pacemaker.

FIGURE 27-27 Fixed pacing or total loss of sensing pacing in lead V₁; arrows denote pacing spikes.

Table 27-2 • Assessing Pacemaker Malfunction

PROBLEM	POSSIBLE CAUSE	INTERVENTION
Loss of capture—complex does *not* follow pacing spike	Inadequate stimulus Catheter malposition Battery depletion Electronic insulation break	Check security of all connections; increase milliamperage. Reposition extremity; turn patient to left side. Change battery. Change generator.
Undersensing—pacing spike occurs at preset interval despite patient's intrinsic rhythm	Sensitivity too high Electrical interference (eg, by a magnet) Faulty generator	Decrease sensitivity. Eliminate interference. Replace generator.
Oversensing—loss of pacing artefact; pacing does *not* occur at preset interval despite lack of intrinsic rhythm	Sensitivity too low Electrical interference Battery depletion	Increase sensitivity. Eliminate interference. Change battery.
Loss of pacing—total absence of pacing spikes	Battery depletion Loose or disconnected wires Perforation	Change battery. Check security of all connections. Obtain 12-lead ECG and portable chest x-ray. Assess for murmur. Call physician.
Change in pacing QRS shape	Septal perforation	Obtain 12-lead ECG and portable chest x-ray. Assess for murmur. Call physician.
Rhythmic diaphragmatic or chest wall twitching or hiccuping	Output too high Myocardial wall perforation	Decrease milliamperage. Turn pacer off. Call physician at once. Monitor closely for decreased cardiac output.

Pacemaker Surveillance

Pacemaker clinics have been established to monitor patients and to test pulse generators for impending pacemaker battery failure. Several other factors, such as lead fracture, muscle inhibition, and insulation disruption, are assessed depending on the type of pacemaker and the equipment available. If indicated, the pacemaker is turned off for a few seconds, using a magnet or a programmer, while the ECG is recorded to assess the patient's underlying cardiac rhythm.

Another follow-up method is transtelephonic transmission of the generator's pulse rate. Special equipment is used to transmit information about the patient's pacemaker over the telephone to a receiving system at a pacemaker clinic. The information is converted into tones, which equipment at the clinic converts to an electronic signal and records on an ECG strip. The pacemaker rate and other data concerning pacemaker function are obtained and evaluated by a cardiologist. This simplifies the diagnosis of a failing generator, reassures the patient, and improves management when the patient is physically remote from pacemaker testing facilities.

NURSING PROCESS:
THE PATIENT WITH A PACEMAKER

Assessment

After a temporary or a permanent pacemaker is inserted, the patient's heart rate and rhythm are monitored by ECG. The pacemaker's settings are noted and compared with the ECG recordings to assess pacemaker function. Pacemaker malfunction is detected by examining the pacemaker spike and its relationship to the surrounding ECG complexes (Fig. 27-28). In addition, cardiac output and hemodynamic stability are assessed to identify the patient's response to pacing and the adequacy of pacing. The ap-

pearance or increasing frequency of dysrhythmia is observed and reported to the physician.

The incision site where the pulse generator was implanted (or the entry site for the pacing electrode, if the pacemaker is a temporary transvenous pacemaker) is observed for bleeding, hematoma formation, or infection, which may be evidenced by swelling, unusual tenderness, unusual drainage, and increased heat. The patient may complain of continuous throbbing or pain. These symptoms are reported to the physician.

The patient with a temporary pacemaker is also assessed for electrical interference and the development of microshock. The nurse observes for potential sources of electrical hazards. All electrical equipment used in the vicinity of the patient should be grounded. Improperly grounded equipment can generate leakage of current capable of producing ventricular fibrillation. Exposed wires must be carefully covered with nonconductive material to prevent accidental ventricular fibrillation from stray currents. The nurse, working with a biomedical engineer or electrician, should make certain that the patient is in an electrically safe environment.

Patients, especially those receiving a permanent pacemaker, should be assessed for anxiety. In addition, for those receiving permanent pacemakers, the level of knowledge and learning needs of the patient and the family and the history of adherence to the therapeutic regimen should be identified.

Diagnosis

NURSING DIAGNOSES

Based on assessment data, major nursing diagnoses of the patient may include the following:

- Risk for infection related to pacemaker lead or generator insertion
- Risk for ineffective coping
- Deficient knowledge regarding self-care program

FIGURE 27-28 (**A**) Ventricular pacing with intermittent loss of capture (a pacing spike not followed by a QRS complex). (**B**) Ventricular pacing with loss of sensing (a pacing spike occurring at an inappropriate time). *Key:* ↑ = pacing spike; * = loss of capture; P = pacemaker-induced QRS complex; I = patient's intrinsic QRS complex; F = fusion (a QRS complex formed by a merging of the patient's intrinsic QRS complex and the pacemaker-induced QRS complex). Both in lead V_1.

COLLABORATIVE PROBLEMS/ POTENTIAL COMPLICATIONS

Based on the assessment findings, potential complications that may develop include decreased cardiac output related to pacemaker malfunction.

Planning and Goals

The major goals for the patient may include absence of infection, adherence to a self-care program, effective coping, and maintenance of pacemaker function.

Nursing Interventions

PREVENTING INFECTION

The nurse changes the dressing regularly and inspects the insertion site for redness, swelling, soreness, or any unusual drainage. An increase in temperature should be reported to the physician. Changes in wound appearance are also reported to the physician.

PROMOTING EFFECTIVE COPING

The patient treated with a pacemaker experiences not only lifestyle and physical changes but also emotional changes. At different times during the healing process, the patient may feel angry, depressed, fearful, anxious, or a combination of these emotions. Although each patient uses individual coping strategies (eg, humour, prayer, communication with a significant other) to manage emotional distress, some strategies may work better than others. Signs that may indicate ineffective coping include social isolation, increased or prolonged irritability or depression, and difficulty in relationships.

To promote effective coping strategies, the nurse must recognize the patient's emotional state and assist the patient to explore his or her feelings. The nurse may help the patient to identify per-

ceived changes (eg, loss of ability to participate in contact sports), the emotional response to the change (eg, anger), and how the patient responded to that emotion (eg, quickly became angry when talking with spouse). The nurse reassures the patient that the responses are normal, then assists the patient to identify realistic goals (eg, develop interest in another activity) and to develop a plan to attain those goals. The nurse may also teach the patient easy-to-use stress reduction techniques (eg, deep-breathing exercises) to facilitate coping. Education (Chart 27-3) may assist a patient to cope with changes that occur with pacemaker treatment.

PROMOTING HOME AND COMMUNITY-BASED CARE

Teaching Patients Self-Care

After pacemaker insertion, the patient's hospital stay may be less than 1 day, and follow-up in an outpatient clinic or office is common. The patient's anxiety and feelings of vulnerability may interfere with the ability to learn information provided. Nurses often need to include home caregivers in the teaching and provide printed materials for use by the patient and caregiver. Priorities for learning are established with the patient and caregiver. Teaching may include the importance of periodic pacemaker monitoring, promoting safety, avoiding infection, and sources of electromagnetic interference (see Chart 27-3).

Evaluation

EXPECTED PATIENT OUTCOMES

Expected patient outcomes may include:

1. Remains free of infection
   a. Has normal temperature
   b. Has white blood cell count within normal range (5,000 to 10,000/mm³)

Chart 27-3
Home Care Checklist • The Patient With a Pacemaker

At the completion of the home care instruction, the patient or caregiver will be able to:	Patient	Caregiver
Monitor pacemaker function.		
• Describe the importance of reporting to physician or pacemaker clinic periodically as prescribed, so that the pacemaker's rate and function can be monitored. This is especially important during the first month after implantation.	✓	
• Adhere to monitoring schedule as instructed after implantation.	✓	
• Check pulse daily. Report *immediately* any sudden slowing or increasing of the pulse rate. This may indicate pacemaker malfunction.	✓	✓
• Resume more frequent monitoring when battery depletion is anticipated. (The time for reimplantation depends on the type of battery in use.)	✓	
Promote safety and avoid infection.		
• Wear loose-fitting clothing around the area of the pacemaker.	✓	
• State the reason for the slight bulge over the pacemaker implant.	✓	✓
• Notify physician if the pacemaker area becomes red or painful.	✓	✓
• Avoid trauma to the area of the pacemaker generator.	✓	
• Study the manufacturer's instructions and become familiar with the pacemaker.	✓	✓
• Recognize that physical activity does not usually have to be curtailed, with the exception of contact sports.	✓	
• Carry medical identification indicating physician's name, type and model number of pacemaker, manufacturer's name, pacemaker rate, and hospital where pacemaker was inserted.	✓	
Electromagnetic interference: Describe the importance of the following:		
• Avoid large magnetic fields such as those surrounding magnetic resonance imaging, large motors, arc welding, electrical substations. Magnetic fields can deactivate the pacemaker.	✓	
• Some electrical and small motor devices, as well as cellular phones, may interfere with pacemaker function if placed very close to the generator. Avoid leaning directly over devices, or ensure that contact is brief; place cellular phone on opposite side of generator.	✓	✓
• Household items, such as microwave ovens, should not cause any concern.	✓	✓
• When going through security gates (eg, at airports, government buildings) show identification card and request hand search.	✓	✓
• Hospitalization may be necessary periodically to change battery or replace pacemaker unit.	✓	✓

---

c. Exhibits no redness or swelling of pacemaker insertion site
2. Adheres to a self-care program
  a. Responds appropriately when queried about the signs and symptoms of infection
  b. Identifies when to seek medical attention (as demonstrated in responses to signs and symptoms)
  c. Adheres to monitoring schedule
  d. Describes appropriate methods to avoid electromagnetic interference
3. Maintains pacemaker function (see Chart 27-3)
  a. Measures and records pulse rate at regular intervals
  b. Experiences no abrupt changes in pulse rate or rhythm

CARDIOVERSION AND DEFIBRILLATION

Cardioversion and defibrillation are treatments for tachydysrhythmias. They are used to deliver an electrical current to depolarize a critical mass of myocardial cells. When the cells repolarize, the sinus node is usually able to recapture its role as the heart's pacemaker. One major difference between cardioversion and defibrillation has to do with the timing of the delivery of electrical current. Another major difference concerns the circumstance: defibrillation is usually performed as an emergency treatment, whereas cardioversion is usually, but not always, a planned procedure.

Electrical current may be delivered through paddles or conductor pads. Both paddles may be placed on the front of the chest (Fig. 27-29), which is the standard paddle placement, or one paddle may be placed on the front of the chest and the other connected to an adapter with a long handle and placed under the patient's back, which is called an anteroposterior placement (Fig. 27-30).

 NURSING ALERT When using paddles, apply the appropriate conductant between the paddles and the patient's skin. Do not substitute any other type of conductant, such as ultrasound gel.

FIGURE 27-29 Standard paddle placement for defibrillation.

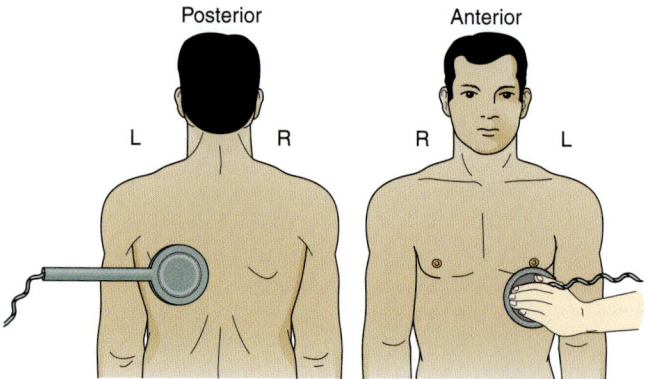

Posterior   Anterior

FIGURE 27-30 Anteroposterior paddle placement for defibrillation.

Instead of paddles, defibrillator multifunction conductor pads may be used (Fig. 27-31). The pads, which contain a conductive medium, are placed in the same position as the paddles. They are connected to the defibrillator and allow for hands-off defibrillation. This method reduces the risks of touching the patient during the procedure and increases electrical safety. AEDs use this type of delivery for the electrical current.

Whether using pads or paddles, the nurse must observe two safety measures. First, maintain good contact between the pads or paddles (with a conductive medium) and the patient's skin to prevent electrical current from leaking into the air (arcing) when the defibrillator is discharged. Second, ensure that no one is in contact with the patient or with anything that is touching the patient when the defibrillator is discharged, to minimize the chance that electrical current will be conducted to anyone other than the patient.

When performing defibrillation or cardioversion, the nurse should remember these key points:

- Use multifunction conductor pads or paddles with a conducting agent between the paddles and the skin (the conducting agent is available as a sheet, gel, or paste).
- Place paddles or pads so that they do not touch the patient's clothing or bed linen and are not near medication patches or direct oxygen flow.
- If cardioverting, ensure that the monitor leads are attached to the patient and that the defibrillator is in sync mode. If

defibrillating, ensure that the defibrillator is not in sync mode (most machines default to the "not-sync" mode).
- Do not charge the device until ready to shock; then keep thumbs and fingers off the discharge buttons until paddles or pads are on the chest and ready to deliver the electrical charge.
- Exert 20 to 25 pounds of pressure on the paddles to ensure good skin contact.
- Before pressing the discharge button, call "Clear!" three times: As "Clear" is called the first time, ensure that you are not touching the patient, bed or equipment; as "Clear" is called the second time, ensure that no one is touching the bed, the patient, or equipment, including the endotracheal tube or adjuncts; and as "Clear" is called the third time, perform a final visual check to ensure you and everyone else are clear of the patient and anything touching the patient.
- Record the delivered energy and the results (cardiac rhythm, pulse).
- After the event is complete, inspect the skin under the pads or paddles for burns; if any are detected, consult with the physician or a wound care nurse about treatment.

Cardioversion

Cardioversion involves the delivery of a "timed" electrical current to terminate a tachydysrhythmia. In cardioversion, the defibrillator is set to synchronize with the ECG on a cardiac monitor so that the electrical impulse discharges during ventricular depolarization (QRS complex). Because there may be a short delay until recognition of the QRS, the discharge buttons must be held down until the shock has been delivered. The synchronization prevents the discharge from occurring during the vulnerable period of repolarization (T wave), which could result in VT or ventricular fibrillation. When the synchronizer is on, no electrical current will be delivered if the defibrillator does not discern a QRS complex. Sometimes the lead and the electrodes must be changed for the monitor to recognize the patient's QRS complex.

If the cardioversion is elective, anticoagulation for a few weeks before cardioversion may be indicated. Digoxin is usually withheld for 48 hours before cardioversion to ensure the resumption of sinus rhythm with normal conduction. The patient is instructed not to eat or drink for at least 8 hours before the procedure. Gel-covered paddles or conductor pads are positioned front and back (anteroposteriorly) for cardioversion. Before cardio-

Back   Front

FIGURE 27-31 Multifunction pads for defibrillation.

version, the patient receives intravenous sedation as well as an analgesic medication or anesthesia. Respiration is then supported with supplemental oxygen delivered by a bag-mask-valve device with suction equipment readily available. Although patients rarely require intubation, equipment is nearby if it is needed. The amount of voltage used varies from 25 to 360 joules, depending on the defibrillator's technology and the type of dysrhythmia. If ventricular fibrillation occurs after cardioversion, the defibrillator is used to defibrillate the patient (sync mode is *not* used).

Indications of a successful response are conversion to sinus rhythm, adequate peripheral pulses, and adequate blood pressure. Because of the sedation, airway patency must be maintained and the patient's state of consciousness assessed. Vital signs and oxygen saturation are monitored and recorded until the patient is stable and recovered from sedation and the effects of analgesic medications or anesthesia. ECG monitoring is required during and after cardioversion.

Defibrillation

Defibrillation is used in emergency situations as the treatment of choice for ventricular fibrillation and pulseless VT. Defibrillation depolarizes a critical mass of myocardial cells at once; when they repolarize, the sinus node usually recaptures its role as the pacemaker. The electrical voltage required to defibrillate the heart is usually greater than that required for cardioversion. If three defibrillations of increasing voltage have been unsuccessful, cardiopulmonary resuscitation is initiated and advanced life support treatments are begun.

The use of epinephrine or vasopressin may make it easier to convert the dysrhythmia to a normal rhythm with defibrillation. These drugs may also increase cerebral and coronary artery blood flow. After the medication is administered and 1 minute of cardiopulmonary resuscitation is performed, defibrillation is again administered. Antiarrhythmic medications such as amiodarone (Cordarone), lidocaine (Xylocaine), magnesium, or procainamide (Pronestyl) are given if ventricular dysrhythmia persists (see Table 27-1). This treatment continues until a stable rhythm resumes or until it is determined that the patient cannot be revived.

IMPLANTABLE CARDIOVERTER DEFIBRILLATOR

The **implantable cardioverter defibrillator (ICD)** is a device that detects and terminates life-threatening episodes of VT or ventricular fibrillation in high-risk patients. Patients at high risk are those who have survived sudden cardiac death syndrome, usually caused by ventricular fibrillation, or have experienced symptomatic VT (syncope secondary to VT). In addition, an ICD may be indicated for patients who have survived an MI but are at high risk for cardiac arrest.

An ICD consists of a generator and at least one lead that can sense intrinsic electrical activity and deliver an electrical impulse. The device is usually implanted much like a pacemaker (Fig. 27-32). ICDs are designed to respond to two criteria: a rate that exceeds a predetermined level, and a change in the isoelectric line segments. When a dysrhythmia occurs, rate sensors take 5 to 10 seconds to sense the dysrhythmia. Then the device takes several seconds to charge and deliver the programmed charge through the lead to the heart. Battery life is about 5 years but varies depending on use of the ICD over time. The battery is checked during follow-up visits.

Antiarrhythmic medication usually is administered with this technology to minimize the occurrence of the tachydysrhythmia and to reduce the frequency of ICD discharge.

The first defibrillator, which was implanted in 1980 at Johns Hopkins University, simply defibrillated the heart. Today, however, several devices are available, and many are programmed for multiple treatments (Atlee & Bernstein, 2001). Each device offers a different delivery sequence, but all are capable of delivering high-energy (high-intensity) defibrillation to treat a tachycardia (atrial or ventricular). The device may deliver up to six shocks if necessary. Some ICDs can respond with antitachycardia pacing, in which the device delivers electrical impulses at a fast rate in an attempt to disrupt the tachycardia, by low-energy (low-intensity) cardioversion, by defibrillation, or all three (Atlee & Bernstein, 2001). Some also have pacemaker capability if the patient develops bradycardia, which sometimes occurs after treatment of the tachycardia. Usually the mode is VVI (V, paces the ventricle; V, senses ventricular activity; I, paces only if the ventricles do not depolarize) (Atlee & Bernstein, 2001). Some ICDs also deliver low-energy cardioversion, and some also treat atrial fibrillation (Bubien & Sanchez, 2001; Daoud et al., 2000). Which device is used and how it is programmed depends on the patient's dysrhythmia.

Complications are similar to those associated with pacemaker insertion. The primary complication associated with the ICD is surgery-related infection. There are a few complications associated with the technical aspects of the equipment, such as premature battery depletion and dislodged or fractured leads. Despite the possible complications, the consensus among clinicians is that the benefits of ICD therapy exceed the risks.

Nursing interventions for the patient with an ICD are provided throughout the preoperative, perioperative, and postoperative phases. In addition to providing the patient and family with explanations regarding implantation of the ICD in the preoperative phase, the nurse may need to manage acute episodes of life-threatening dysrhythmias. In the perioperative and postoperative phases, the nurse carefully observes the patient's responses to the ICD and provides the patient and family with further teaching as needed (White, 2000) (Chart 27-4). The nurse can also assist the patient and family in making lifestyle changes necessitated by the dysrhythmia and resulting ICD implantation (Dougherty, Benoliel, & Bellin, 2000).

FIGURE 27-32 The implantable cardioverter defibrillator (ICD) consists of a generator and a sensing/pacing/defibrillating electrode.

Chart 27-4
Home Care Checklist • The Patient With an ICD

At the completion of the home care instruction, the patient or caregiver will be able to:	Patient	Caregiver
Avoid infection at the ICD insertion site.		
• Observe incision site daily for redness, swelling, and heat.	✓	✓
• Take temperature; report any increase.	✓	✓
• Avoid tight restrictive clothing that may cause friction over the insertion site.	✓	✓
Adhere to activity restrictions.		
• Movement of arm may continue to be restricted until incision heals if the ICD was implanted in pectoral region.	✓	
• Avoid heavy lifting.	✓	
• Discuss safety of activities (eg, driving) with physician.	✓	✓
• Avoid contact sports.	✓	
Electromagnetic interference: Understand the importance of the following:		
• Avoid large magnetic fields such as those created by magnetic resonance imaging, large motors, arc welding, electrical substations, and so forth. Magnetic fields may deactivate the ICD, negating any effect on a dysrhythmia.	✓	
• At security gates at airports, government buildings, or other secured areas, show identification card and request a hand search.	✓	
• Some electrical and small motor devices, as well as cellular phones, may interfere with the functioning of the ICD if placed very close to the ICD. Avoid leaning directly over devices, or ensure contact is of brief duration; place cellular phone on opposite side of ICD.	✓	
• Household appliances (eg, microwave ovens) should not cause any concern.	✓	✓
Promote safety.		
• Describe what to do if symptoms occur and notify physician if any discharges seem unusual.	✓	✓
• Maintain a log that records discharges. Record events that precipitate the sensation of shock. This provides important data for the physician to use in readjusting the medical regimen.	✓	✓
• Encourage family members to attend a CPR class.		✓
• Call 911 for emergency assistance if feeling of dizziness occurs.	✓	✓
• Wear medical identification (eg, Medic-Alert) that includes physician information.	✓	
• Avoid frightening family or friends with unexpected shocks, which will not harm them. Inform family and friends that in the event they are in contact with the patient when a shock is delivered, they may also feel the shock. It is especially important to warn sexual partners that this may occur.	✓	✓
• Discuss psychological responses to the ICD implantation, such as changes in self-image, depression due to loss of mobility secondary to driving restrictions, fear of shocks, increased anxiety, concerns that sexual activity may trigger the ICD, and changes in partner relationship.	✓	✓
Follow-up care		
• Adhere to appointments that are scheduled to test electronic performance of ICD. Remember to take log of discharges to review with physician.	✓	✓
• Attend an ICD support group within the area.	✓	

ELECTROPHYSIOLOGIC STUDIES

An electrophysiology (EP) study is used to evaluate and treat various dysrhythmias that have caused cardiac arrest or significant symptoms. It also is indicated for patients with symptoms that suggest a dysrhythmia that has gone undetected and undiagnosed by other methods. An EP study is used to

- Identify the impulse formation and propagation through the cardiac electrical conduction system
- Assess the function or dysfunction of the SA and AV nodal areas
- Identify the location (called mapping) and mechanism dysrhythmogenic foci
- Assess the effectiveness of antiarrhythmic medications and devices for the patient with a dysrhythmia
- Treat certain dysrhythmias through the destruction of the causative cells (**ablation**)

An EP procedure is a type of cardiac catheterization that is performed in a specially equipped cardiac catheterization laboratory. The patient is awake but lightly sedated. Usually a catheter with multiple electrodes is inserted through the femoral vein, threaded through the inferior vena cava, and advanced into the heart. The electrodes are positioned within the heart at specific locations—for instance, in the right atrium near the sinus node, in the coronary sinus, near the tricuspid valve, and at the apex of the right ventricle. The number and placement of electrodes depend on the type of study being conducted. These electrodes allow the electrical signal to be recorded from within the heart (intracardiogram).

The electrodes also allow the clinician to introduce a pacing stimulus to the intracardiac area at a precisely timed interval and rate, thereby stimulating the area (programmed stimulation). An area of the heart may be paced at a rate much faster than the normal rate of **automaticity**, the rate at which impulses are spontaneously formed (eg, in the sinus node). This allows the pacemaker to become an artificial focus of automaticity and to assume control (overdrive suppression). Then the pacemaker is stopped suddenly, and the time it takes for the sinus node to resume control is assessed. A prolonged time indicates dysfunction of the sinus node.

One of the main purposes of programmed stimulation is to assess the ability of the area surrounding the electrode to cause a reentry dysrhythmia. One or a series of premature impulses is delivered to an area in an attempt to cause the tachydysrhythmia. Because the precise location of the suspected area and the specific timing of the pacing needed are unknown, the electrophysiologist uses several different techniques to cause the dysrhythmia during the study. If the dysrhythmia can be reproduced by programmed stimulation, it is called inducible. Once a dysrhythmia is induced, a treatment plan is determined and implemented. If, on the follow-up EP study, the tachydysrhythmia cannot be induced, then the treatment is determined to be effective. Different medications may be administered and combined with electrical devices (pacemaker, ICD) to determine the most effective treatment to suppress the dysrhythmia.

Complications of an EP study are the same as those that can occur with cardiac catheterization. Because an artery is not always used, there is a lower incidence of vascular complications than with other catheterization procedures. Cardiac arrest may occur, but the incidence is low (less than 1%).

Patients who are to undergo an EP study may be anxious about the procedure and about its outcome. A detailed discussion involving the patient, the family, and the electrophysiologist usually occurs to ensure that the patient is able to give informed consent and to reduce anxiety about the procedure. Before the procedure, patients should receive instructions about the procedure and its usual duration, the environment where the procedure is performed, and what to expect. Although an EP study is not painful, it does cause discomfort and can be tiring. It may also cause feelings that were experienced when the dysrhythmia occurred in the past. In addition, patients also are taught what will be expected of them (eg, lying very still during the procedure, reporting symptoms or concerns).

Patients need to know that the dysrhythmia may occur during the procedure, but under very controlled circumstances. It often stops on its own; if it does not, treatment is given to restore the patient's normal rhythm. During the procedure, patients benefit from a calm, reassuring approach.

Postprocedural care includes restriction of activity to promote hemostasis at the insertion site. To identify any complications and to ensure healing, the patient's vital signs and the appearance of the insertion site are assessed frequently.

CARDIAC CONDUCTION SURGERY

Atrial tachycardias and ventricular tachycardias that do not respond to medications and are not suitable for antitachycardia pacing may be treated by methods other than medications and devices. Such methods include endocardial isolation, endocardial resection, and ablation. An ICD may be used with these surgical interventions.

Endocardial Isolation

Endocardial isolation involves making an incision into the endocardium that separates the area where the dysrhythmia originates from the surrounding endocardium. The edges of the incision are then sutured together. The incision and its resulting scar tissue prevent the dysrhythmia from affecting the whole heart.

Endocardial Resection

In endocardial resection, the origin of the dysrhythmia is identified, and that area of the endocardium is peeled away. No reconstruction or repair is necessary.

Catheter Ablation Therapy

Catheter ablation destroys specific cells that are the cause or central conduction method of a tachydysrhythmia. It is performed with or after an EP study. Usual indications for ablation are AV nodal reentry tachycardia, atrial fibrillation, or VT unresponsive to previous therapy (or for which the therapy produced significant side effects).

Ablation is also indicated to eliminate accessory AV pathways or bypass tracts that exist in the hearts of patients with preexcitation syndromes such as Wolff-Parkinson-White (WPW) syndrome. During normal embryonic development, all connections between the atrium and ventricles disappear, except for that between the AV node and the bundle of His. In some people, embryonic connections of normal heart muscle between the atrium and ventricles remain, providing an accessory pathway or a tract through which the electrical impulse can bypass the AV node. These pathways can be located in several different areas. If the patient develops atrial fibrillation, the impulse may be conducted into the ventricle at a rate of 300 times per minute or more, which can lead to ventricular fibrillation and sudden cardiac death. Preexcitation syndromes are identified by specific ECG findings. For example, in WPW syndrome there is a shortened PR interval, slurring (called a delta wave) of the initial QRS deflection, and prolonged QRS duration (Fig. 27-33).

Ablation may be accomplished by three different methods: radiofrequency ablation, cryoablation, or electrical ablation. The most often used method is radiofrequency, which involves placing a special catheter at or near the origin of the dysrhythmia. High-frequency, low-energy sound waves are passed through the catheter, causing thermal injury and cellular changes that result in localized destruction and scarring. The tissue damage is more specific to the dysrhythmic tissue, with less trauma to the surrounding cardiac tissue than occurs with cryoablation or electrical ablation.

Cryoablation involves placing a special probe, cooled to a temperature of −60°C, on the endocardium at the site of the dysrhythmia's origin for 2 minutes. The tissue freezes and is later replaced by scar tissue, eliminating the origin of the dysrhythmia.

In electrical ablation, a catheter is placed at or near the origin of the dysrhythmia, and one to four shocks of 100 to 300 joules are administered through the catheter directly to the endocardium and surrounding tissue. The cardiac tissue burns and scars, thus eliminating the source of the dysrhythmia.

During the ablation procedure, defibrillation pads, an automatic blood pressure cuff, and a pulse oximeter are used on the patient, and an indwelling urinary catheter is inserted. The patient is given light sedation. An EP study is performed and attempts to induce the dysrhythmia are made. The ablation catheter is placed at the origin of the dysrhythmia, and the ablation procedure is performed. Multiple ablations may be necessary. Successful ablation is achieved when the dysrhythmia can no longer be induced. The patient is monitored for another 30 to 60 minutes and then retested to ensure that the dysrhythmia will not recur.

Postprocedural care is similar to that for an EP study, except that the patient is monitored more closely, depending on the time needed for recovery from sedation.

FIGURE 27-33 Wolff-Parkinson-White syndrome. (**A**) Sinus rhythm. Note the short PR interval, slurred initial upstroke of the QRS complex (delta wave, at the arrow), and prolonged QRS duration, upper lead II, lower lead V₁. (**B**) Rhythm strip of same patient following ablation, upper lead V₁, lower lead II. ECG strips courtesy of Linda Ardini and Catherine Berkmeyer, Inova Fairfax Hospital, Falls Church, VA.

Critical Thinking Exercises

1. You are caring for a 40-year-old male physician who had experienced a cardiac arrest at home, witnessed by his 9-year-old son and 15-year-old daughter. After having an ICD implanted, he appears sullen and withdrawn. On inquiry about how he feels, he replies, "I don't know if this device is a blessing or a punishment!" How would you respond? What other factors are important to assess? Discuss the impact that his children may have on his perception of the device. How would you alter your plan of care to address this patient's psychosocial concerns because he is a physician? How would the plan of care change if, instead of appearing sullen and withdrawn, he appeared irritable and confrontational?

2. Your patient is an active 80-year-old woman who has heart failure and chronic atrial fibrillation. She is taking an angiotensin-converting enzyme inhibitor, a beta-blocker, a diuretic, and digoxin. During your assessment, she tells you that she felt very dizzy this morning. How would you focus your assessment, and why? Identify some of the key assessment factors. What nursing interventions are needed? How would you modify your assessment and interventions if your patient also had chronic obstructive pulmonary disease and renal insufficiency?

REFERENCES AND SELECTED READINGS

Books and Pamphlets

Albert, J. S. (2001). *The AHA clinical cardiac consult.* Philadelphia: Lippincott Williams & Wilkins.

Braunwald, E., Zipes, D. P., & Libby, P. (2001). *Heart disease: A textbook of cardiovascular medicine* (6th ed.). Philadelphia: W. B. Saunders.

Conover, M. B. (1998). *Pocket guide to electrocardiology.* St. Louis: Mosby.

Ellenbogen, K. A., Kay, G. N, & Wilkoff, B. L. (Eds.). (2000). *Clinical cardiac pacing and defibrillation* (2nd ed.). Philadelphia: W. B. Saunders.

Fuster, V., Alexander R. W., & O'Rourke, R. A. (Eds.). (2001). *Hurst's the heart* (10th ed.). New York: McGraw-Hill.

Kinney, M., Brooks-Brunn, J. A., Molter, N., Dunbar, S. B., & Vitello-Ciccio, L. M. (Eds.). (1998). *AACN clinical reference for critical care nursing* (4th ed.). St. Louis: Mosby.

Management of new onset atrial fibrillation. Evidence Report/Technology Assessment: Number 12. AHRQ Publication No. 00-E007. (May 2000). Rockville, MD: Agency for Healthcare Research and Quality.

Marriott, H. J., & Conover, M. B. (1998). *Advanced concepts in arrhythmias.* St. Louis: Mosby.

McEvoy, G. K. (Ed.). (2001). *AHFS drug information 2001.* Bethesda, MD: American Society of Health System Pharmacists.

McNamara, R. L., Bass, E. B., Miller, M. R., Kim, N. L., Robinson, K. A., & Powe, N. R. (2001). *Management of new onset atrial fibrillation.* Evidence Report/Technology Assessment No. 12 (prepared by the Johns Hopkins University Evidence-Based Practice Center in Baltimore, MD, under Contract No. 290-97-0006). AHRQ Publication Number 01-E026. Rockville, MD: Agency for Healthcare Research and Quality.

Moses, H. W., Moulton, K. P., Miller, B. D., & Schneider, J. A. (2000). *A practical guide to cardiac pacing* (5th ed.). Philadelphia: Lippincott Williams & Wilkins.

Murphy, J. (Ed.). (2000). *Mayo Clinic cardiology review* (2nd ed.). Philadelphia: Lippincott Williams & Wilkins.

Singer, I. (2001). *Interventional electrophysiology*. Philadelphia: Lippincott.

Skidmore-Roth, L. (2002). *2002 Mosby's nursing drug reference*. St Louis: Mosby.

Wagner, G. S. (Ed.) (2001). *Marriott's practical electrocardiography* (10th ed.). Philadelphia: Lippincott Williams & Wilkins.

Journals

Asterisks indicate nursing research articles.

American College of Cardiology/American Heart Association Task Force on Practice Guidelines (Committee on Pacemaker Implantation). (1998). ACC/AHA Task Force Report. Guidelines for implantation of cardiac pacemakers and antiarrhythmia devices: Executive summary. *Circulation, 97*(13), 1325–1335.

American Heart Association, in collaboration with the International Liaison Committee on Resuscitation. (2000). Guidelines 2000 for cardiopulmonary resuscitation and emergency cardiovascular care: An international consensus on science. *Circulation, 102,* (8 Suppl.), I1–I384.

Aronow, W. S. (1999). Management of the older person with ventricular arrhythmias. *Journal of American Geriatrics Society, 47*(7), 886–895.

Asselin, M. E., & Cullen, H. A. (2001). What you need to know about the new ACLS guidelines: Find out about changes in algorithms and policies and how they'll affect your practice. *Nursing 2001, 31*(4), 48–50.

Atlee, J. L., & Bernstein, A. D. (2001). Cardiac rhythm management devices. Part I: Indications, device selection, and function. *Anesthesiology, 95*(5), 1265–1280.

Atkins, D. L., Dorian, P., Gonzalez, E. R., Gorgel, A. P., Kudenchuk, P. J., Luriek, K. G., Morley, P. T., Robertson, C., Samson, R. A., Silka, M. J., & Singh, B. N. (2001). Treatment of tachyarrhythmias: Proceedings of the International Guidelines 2000 Conference for Cardiopulmonary Resuscitation and Emergency Cardiovascular Care. *Annuals of Emergency Medicine, 37*(4), (Suppl.), S91–S109.

Bernstein, J. E. (1997). Recognizing when long QT intervals mean trouble. *Nursing 97, 27*(4), 32aa–32ff.

Boyle, J., & Rost, M. K. (2000). Present status of cardiac pacing: A nursing perspective. *Critical Care Nursing Quarterly, 23*(1), 1–19.

Brown, J., & Kellerman, A. L. (2000). The shocking truth about automated external defibrillators. *Journal of the American Medical Association, 284*(11), 1438–1441.

Bubien, R. S., & Sanchez, J. E. (2001). Atrial fibrillation: Treatment rationale and clinical utility of nonpharmacologic therapies. *AACN Clinical Issues: Advanced Practice Acute Critical Care 12*(1), 140–155.

The Cardiac Arrhythmia Suppression Trial Investigators. (1989). The Cardiac Arrhythmia Suppression Trial. *New England Journal of Medicine, 321*(25), 1754–1756.

Cannom, D. S. (2002). Implantable cardioverter defibrillator trials: What's new? *Current Opinion in Cardiology, 17*(1), 29–35.

Carroll, D. L., Hamilton, G. A., & McGovern, B. A. (1999). Changes in health status and quality of life and the impact of uncertainty in patients who survive life-threatening arrhythmia. *Heart & Lung, 28*(4), 251–260.

Daoud, E. G., Timmermans, C., Fellows, C., Hoyt, R., Lemery, R., Dawson, K., & Ayers, G. M. (2000). Initial clinical experience with ambulatory use of an implantable atrial defibrillator for conversion of atrial fibrillation. Metrix Investigators. *Circulation, 102*(12), 1407–1413.

Davis, D. R. & Tang, A. S. L. (2004). Implantable cardioverter defibrillator: Therapy against Canada's leading killer. *Canadian Medical Association Journal, 171*(9), 1053–1056.

Dickerson, S. S., Posluszny, M., & Kennedy, M. C. (2000). Help seeking in a support group for recipients of implantable cardioverter defibrillators and their support person. *Heart & Lung, 29*(2), 87–96.

Dougherty, C. M., Benoliel, J. Q., & Bellin, C. (2000). Domains of nursing intervention after sudden cardiac arrest and automatic internal cardioverter defibrillator implantation. *Heart & Lung, 29*(2), 79–86.

Drew, B. J., & Krucoff, M. W. (1999). Multilead ST-segment monitoring in patients with acute coronary syndromes: A consensus statement for healthcare professionals. *American Journal of Critical Care, 8*(6), 372–386.

Fenton, J. M. (2001). The clinician's approach to evaluating patients with dysrhythmias. *AACN Clinical Issues: Advanced Practice Acute Critical Care, 12*(1), 72–86.

Gilbert, C. J. (2001). Common supraventricular tachycardias: Mechanisms and management. *AACN Clinical Issues: Advanced Practice Acute Critical Care, 12*(1), 100–113, 170–172.

Gregoratos, G., Abrams, J., Epstein, A. E., Freedman, R. A., Hayes, D. L., Hlatky, M. A., Kerber, R. E., Naccarelli, G. V., Schoenfeld, M. H., Silka, M. J., Winters, S. L., Gibbons, R. J., Antman, E. M., Alpert, J. S., Gregoratos, G., Hiratzka, L. F., Faxon, D. P., Jacobs, A. K., Fuster, V., & Smith, S. C., Jr. ACC/AHA/NASPE 2002 guideline update for implantation of cardiac pacemakers and antiarrhythmia devices: Summary article. A report of the American College of Cardiology/American Heart Association Task Force on Practice Guidelines (ACC/AHA/NASPE Committee to Update the 1998 Pacemaker Guidelines). *Circulation, 106*(16), 2145–2161.

Hauptman, P. J., & Kelly, R. A. (1999). Digitalis. *Circulation, 99*(9), 1265–1270.

Introduction to the International Guidelines 2000 for CPR and ECC: A consensus on science. (2000). *Circulation, 102* (Suppl I), I-1–I-11.

Kellen, J. C., Ettinger, A., Todd, L., Brezsnyak, M. L., Campion, J., McBride, R., Thomas, S., Corum, J., & Schron, E. (1996). The cardiac arrhythmia suppression trial: Implications for nursing practice. *American Journal of Critical Care, 5*(1), 19–25.

*Malm, D., Karlsson, J., & Fridlund, B. (1998). Quality of life in pacemaker patients from a nursing perspective. *Coronary Health Care, 2*(1), 17–27.

Mirowski M., Mower M. M., & Reid, P. R. (1980). The automatic implantable defibrillator. *American Heart Journal, 100,* (6 Part II), 1089–1092.

Ocampo, C. M. (2000). Living with an implantable cardioverter defibrillator: Impact on the patient, family and society. *Nursing Clinics of North America, 35*(4), 1019–1030.

Reynolds, J., & Apple, S. (2001). A systematic approach to pacemaker assessment. *AACN Clinical Issues: Advanced Practice Acute Critical Care, 12*(1), 14–26.

Shaffer, R. S. (2002). ICD therapy: The patient's perspective. *American Journal of Nursing, 102*(2), 46–49.

Thomas, S. A., Friedmann, E., & Kelley, F. J. (2001). Living with an implantable cardioverter-defibrillator: A review of the current literature related to psychosocial factors. *AACN Clinical Issues: Advanced Practice Acute Critical Care, 12*(1), 156–163.

*Tyndall, A., Nystrom, K. V., & Funk, M. (1997). Nausea and vomiting in patients undergoing radiofrequency catheter ablation. *American Journal of Critical Care, 6*(6), 437–444.

Wallace, C. J. (2001). Diagnosing and treating pacemaker syndrome. *Critical Care Nurse, 21*(1), 24–31, 35–37.

White, E. (2000). Patients with implantable cardioverter defibrillators: Transition to home. *Journal of Cardiovascular Nursing, 14*(3), 42–52.

Yager, M., Benson, J., & Kamajian, M. (2001). Brugada syndrome: A case study of aborted sudden cardiac death manifesting as seizures. *Critical Care Nurse, 21*(1), 38, 40, 42–46.

Zipes, D. P., & Wellens, H. J. (2000). What have we learned about cardiac arrhythmias? *Circulation, 102,* (20 Suppl. 4), IV52–IV57.

RESOURCES AND WEBSITES

American Association of Critical Care Nurses, 101 Columbia, Aliso Viejo, CA 92656-4109; 800-899-2226; http://www.aacn.org.

American College of Cardiology, 911 Old Georgetown Road, Bethesda, MD 20814; 800-253-4636; http://www.acc.org.

American Heart Association, National Center, 7272 Greenville Ave., Dallas, TX 75231; 1-800-242-8721; http://www.americanheart.org.

National Heart, Lung, Blood Institute, Health Information Center, National Institutes of Health, PO Box 30105, Bethesda, MD 20824; 301-592-8573; http://www.nhlbi.nih.gov.

National Institute on Aging, Building 31, Room 5C27, 31 Center Drive, MSC 2292, Bethesda, MD 20892; 301-496-1752; http://www.nih.gov/nia.

North American Society of Pacing and Electrophysiology, Six Strathmore Road, Natick, MA 01760-2499; 508-647-0100; http://www.naspe.org.

Management of Patients With Coronary Vascular Disorders

Adapted by Alexander Clark and Colleen Norris

LEARNING OBJECTIVES

On completion of this chapter, the learner will be able to:

1. Describe the pathophysiology, clinical manifestations, and treatment of coronary atherosclerosis.
2. Describe the pathophysiology, clinical manifestations, and treatment of angina pectoris.
3. Use the nursing process as a framework for care of patients with angina pectoris.
4. Describe the pathophysiology, clinical manifestations, and treatment of myocardial infarction.
5. Use the nursing process as a framework for care of patients with myocardial infarction (acute coronary syndrome).
6. Describe the nursing care of a patient who has had an invasive interventional procedure for treatment of coronary artery disease.
7. Describe coronary artery revascularization procedures.
8. Describe the nursing care of the patient treated with cardiac surgery.

*I*n the past, identification and treatment of heart disease focused on white, middle-aged men. However, later studies showed that other segments of the population were also seriously affected by cardiac conditions. Cardiovascular disease affects over 5.7% of all Canadians and is the main cause of death for one in three Canadians (Heart and Stroke Foundation of Canada, 2003).

Coronary Artery Disease

Coronary artery disease (CAD) is the most prevalent type of cardiovascular disease. For this reason, it is important for nurses to become familiar with the various types of coronary artery conditions and the methods for assessing, preventing, and treating these disorders medically and surgically.

CORONARY ATHEROSCLEROSIS

The most common heart disease in the United States is **atherosclerosis**, which is an abnormal accumulation of lipid, or fatty, substances and fibrous tissue in the vessel wall. These substances create blockages or narrow the vessel in a way that reduces blood flow to the myocardium. Studies (Mehta et al., 1998) indicate that atherosclerosis involves a repetitious inflammatory response to artery wall injury and an alteration in the biophysical and biochemical properties of the arterial walls. An association between an infection (eg, gingivitis) and the later development of heart disease is being explored, as is the administration of antibiotics to prevent heart disease. Although authorities disagree about how atherosclerosis begins, they agree that atherosclerosis is a progressive disease that can be curtailed and, in some cases, reversed.

Pathophysiology

Atherosclerosis begins as fatty streaks, lipids that are deposited in the intima of the arterial wall. Although they are thought to be the precursors of atherosclerosis, fatty streaks are common, even in childhood. Moreover, not all develop into more advanced lesions. The reason why some fatty streaks continue to develop is unknown, although genetic and environmental factors are involved. The continued development of atherosclerosis involves an inflammatory response. T lymphocytes and monocytes (that become macrophages) infiltrate the area to ingest the lipids and then die; this causes smooth muscle cells within the vessel to proliferate and form a fibrous cap over the dead fatty core. These deposits, called **atheromas** or plaques, protrude into the lumen of the vessel, narrowing it and obstructing blood flow (Fig. 28-1). If the fibrous cap of the plaque is thick and the lipid pool remains relatively stable, it can resist the stress from blood flow and vessel movement. If the cap is thin, the lipid core may grow, causing it to rupture and hemorrhage into the plaque, allowing a thrombus to develop. The thrombus may obstruct blood flow, leading to sudden cardiac death or an acute **myocardial infarction (MI)**, which is the death of heart tissue.

The anatomic structure of the coronary arteries makes them particularly susceptible to the mechanisms of atherosclerosis. As Figure 28-2 shows, they twist and turn as they supply blood to the heart, creating sites susceptible to atheroma development. Although heart disease is most often caused by atherosclerosis of the coronary arteries, other phenomena decrease blood flow to the heart. Examples include vasospasm (sudden constriction or narrowing) of a coronary artery, myocardial trauma from internal or external forces, structural disease, congenital anomalies, decreased oxygen supply (eg, from acute blood loss, anemia, or low

Glossary

ACE inhibitor (ACE-I): abbreviation for medications that inhibit the angiotensin-converting enzyme

acute coronary syndrome (ACS): signs and symptoms that indicate unstable angina or acute myocardial infarction

angina pectoris: chest pain brought about by myocardial ischemia

atherosclerosis: abnormal accumulation of lipid deposits and fibrous tissue within arterial walls and lumen

atheroma: fibrous cap composed of smooth muscle cells that forms over lipid deposits within arterial vessels and that protrudes into the lumen of the vessel, narrowing the lumen and obstructing blood flow; also called plaque

collateral circulation: arteries that supply blood to tissue when the main arterial blood supply is partially or totally obstructed

contractility: ability of the cardiac muscle to shorten in response to an electrical impulse

coronary artery bypass graft (CABG): a surgical procedure in which a blood vessel from another part of the body is grafted onto the occluded coronary artery below the occlusion in such a way that blood flow bypasses the blockage

creatine kinase (CK): an enzyme found in human tissues; one of the three types of CK is specific to heart muscle and may be used as an indicator of heart muscle injury

high-density lipoprotein (HDL): a protein-bound lipid that transports cholesterol to the liver for excretion in the bile; composed of a higher proportion of protein to lipid than low-density lipoprotein; exerts a beneficial effect on the arterial wall

hormone replacement therapy (HRT): estrogen, progesterone, or both prescribed for postmenopausal or oophorectomized women

ischemia: insufficient tissue oxygenation

low-density lipoprotein (LDL): a protein-bound lipid that transports cholesterol to tissues in the body; composed of a lower proportion of protein to lipid than high-density lipoprotein; exerts a harmful effect on the arterial wall

myocardial infarction (MI): death of heart tissue caused by lack of oxygenated blood flow; if acute, abbreviated as AMI

percutaneous coronary intervention (PCI): an invasive procedure in which a catheter is placed in a coronary artery, and one of

several methods is employed to remove or reduce a blockage within the artery

percutaneous transluminal coronary angioplasty (PTCA): a type of percutaneous coronary intervention in which a balloon is inflated within a coronary artery to break an atheroma and open the vessel lumen, improving coronary artery blood flow

primary prevention: interventions taken to prevent the development of coronary artery disease

secondary prevention: interventions taken to prevent the advancement of existing coronary artery disease

streptokinase (SK): a thrombolytic agent

stent: a woven mesh that provides structural support to a coronary vessel, preventing its closure

sudden cardiac death: immediate cessation of effective heart activity

thrombolytic: an agent or process that breaks down blood clots

troponin: myocardial protein; measurement is used to indicate heart muscle injury

vasoconstrictor: an agent (usually a medication) that narrows the blood vessel lumen

vasodilator: an agent (usually a medication) that enlarges blood vessel lumen

Physiology/Pathophysiology

Adventitia
Media
Intima

Fibrous cap

Plaque

Thrombus

FIGURE 28-1 Atherosclerosis involves a normally patent artery (**A**) and an inflammatory response whereby smooth muscle cells proliferate within the blood vessel to form a fibrous cap (**B**). The proliferation results in deposits, called atheromas or plaques, which protrude into the lumen of the vessel, narrowing it and obstructing blood flow. If the cap ruptures and hemorrhages into the plaque (**C**), a thrombus (**D**) may develop and obstruct blood flow further.

blood pressure), and increased demand for oxygen (eg, from rapid heart rate, thyrotoxicosis, or ingestion of cocaine).

Clinical Manifestations

Coronary atherosclerosis produces symptoms and complications according to the location and degree of narrowing of the arterial lumen, thrombus formation, and obstruction of blood flow to the myocardium. This impediment to blood flow is usually progressive, causing an inadequate blood supply that deprives the muscle cells of oxygen needed for their survival. The condition is known as **ischemia**. **Angina pectoris** refers to chest pain that is brought about by myocardial ischemia. Angina pectoris usually is caused by significant coronary atherosclerosis. If the decrease in blood supply is great enough, of long enough duration, or both, irreversible damage and death of myocardial cells, or MI, may result. Over time, irreversibly damaged myocardium undergoes degener-

ation and is replaced by scar tissue, causing various degrees of myocardial dysfunction. Significant myocardial damage may cause inadequate cardiac output, and the heart cannot support the body's needs for blood, which is called heart failure (HF). A decrease in blood supply from CAD may even cause the heart to stop abruptly, an event that is called **sudden cardiac death**.

The most common manifestation of myocardial ischemia is acute onset of chest pain. However, an epidemiologic study of the people in Framingham, Massachusetts, showed that nearly 15% of men and women who had MIs were totally asymptomatic (Kannel, 1986). Another study found that 33% of those diagnosed with MI did not present to the emergency room with chest pain (Canto et al., 2000; Ishihara et al., 2000). Those without chest pain tend to be older or women, or to have diabetes or a history of heart failure. Women have been found to have more atypical symptoms of myocardial ischemia (eg, shortness of breath, nausea, unusual fatigue) than men (Meischke et al., 1999). The incidence of prodromal angina (ie, angina a few hours to days before the MI) was found to be significantly lower in patients older than 70 years of age (Ishihara et al., 2000). Other clinical manifestations of CAD may be abnormalities signaled by changes on the electrocardiogram (ECG), high levels of cardiac enzymes, dysrhythmias, and sudden death.

Risk Factors

Epidemiologic studies point to several factors that increase the probability that heart disease will develop. Major risk factors include use of tobacco, hypertension, elevated blood lipid levels, family history of premature cardiovascular disease (first-degree relative with cardiovascular disease at age 55 or younger for men and at age 65 or younger for women) and age (>45 years for men; >55 years for women). The Third Report of the Expert Panel on Detection, Evaluation, and Treatment of High Blood Cholesterol in Adults (Adult Treatment Panel III [ATP III]; 2001) represents the updated clinical guidelines for cholesterol testing and management. ATP III addresses **primary prevention** (preventing the occurrence of CAD) and **secondary prevention** (preventing the progression of CAD).

ATP III is the standard for cholesterol management. ATP III continues to identify elevated **low-density lipoprotein (LDL)**

FIGURE 28-2 Angles of the coronary arteries. The many angles and curves of the coronary arteries contribute to the vessels' susceptibility to atheromatous plaques. Arteries shown as dashed lines supply the posterior wall of the heart.

cholesterol as the primary target of cholesterol-lowering therapy. Those at highest risk for having a cardiac event within 10 years are those with existing CAD or those with diabetes, peripheral arterial disease, abdominal aortic aneurysm, or carotid artery disease. The latter diseases are called CAD risk equivalents, because patients with these diseases have the same risk for a cardiac event as patients with CAD (Chart 28-1). The possibility of having a cardiac event within 10 years is also determined by points given to several factors, such as age, level of total cholesterol, level of LDL, level of **high-density lipoprotein (HDL)**, systolic blood pressure, and tobacco use. If the total points add up to more than 15 for men or 23 for women, the person has a greater than 20% risk for a cardiac event within 10 years. A composite of lipid and nonlipid risk factors of metabolic origin, called *metabolic syndrome,* is another risk factor for CAD. Metabolic syndrome includes abdominal obesity, an elevated triglyceride level, low HDL level, elevated blood pressure, and impaired function of insulin.

Measurement of other emerging risk factors, such as elevations of Lipoprotein(a) [Lp(a)], remnant lipoproteins, small LDL, fibrinogen, homocysteine, and impaired fasting plasma glucose (110–125 mg/dL), is optional and is not routinely recommended (ATP III, 2001). For example, the Homocysteine Studies Collaboration (2002) found that lower levels of homocysteine, an amino acid, were modestly associated with reduced risk of ischemic heart disease and stroke. The results of these retrospective studies suggest that homocysteine may promote atherosclerosis. A meta-analysis of prospective studies was done that showed a significant association between homocysteine levels and ischemic heart disease as well as between homocysteine and stroke (Wald, Law, & Morris, 2002). The authors recommend a daily intake of approximately 0.8 mg of folic acid to decrease blood homocysteine levels and reduce the risk of ischemic heart disease and CVA (brain attack, stroke). The American Heart Association has stated that until the results of large-scale randomized trials become available, routine testing of homocysteine concentrations cannot be justified (Malinow, Bostom, & Krauss, 1999).

Prevention

Four modifiable risk factors—cholesterol abnormalities, cigarette smoking (tobacco use), hypertension, and diabetes mellitus—have been cited as major risk factors for CAD and its consequent complications. As a result, they receive much attention in health promotion programs (Chart 28-2).

 Chart 28-1

Coronary Artery Disease Risk Equivalents

Individuals at highest risk for a cardiac event within 10 years are those with existing coronary artery disease (CAD) and those with any of the following diseases, which are called CAD risk equivalents:

- Diabetes
- Peripheral arterial disease
- Abdominal aortic aneurysm
- Carotid artery disease

From Expert Panel on Detection, Evaluation, and Treatment of High Blood Cholesterol in Adults. (2001). Executive summary of the third report of the National Cholesterol Education Program (NCEP) Expert Panel on Detection, Evaluation, and Treatment of High Blood Cholesterol in Adults (Adult Treatment Panel III). *Journal of the American Medical Association, 285*(19), 2486–2497.

 Chart 28-2

Risk Factors for Coronary Artery Disease

A modifiable risk factor is one over which individuals may exercise control, such as by changing a lifestyle or personal habit or by using medication. A nonmodifiable risk factor is a circumstance over which individuals have no control, such as age or heredity. A risk factor may operate independently or in tandem with other risk factors. The more risk factors individuals have, the greater the likelihood of coronary artery disease. Those at risk are advised to seek regular medical examinations and to engage in "heart-healthy" behaviour (a deliberate effort to reduce the number and extent of risks).

Nonmodifiable Risk Factors
Family history of coronary heart disease
Increasing age
Gender (heart disease occurs three times more often in men than in premenopausal women)
Race (higher incidence of heart disease in African Americans than in Caucasians)

Modifiable Risk Factors
High blood cholesterol level
Cigarette smoking, tobacco use
Hypertension
Diabetes mellitus
Lack of estrogen in women
Physical inactivity
Obesity

CONTROLLING CHOLESTEROL ABNORMALITIES

The association of a high blood cholesterol level with heart disease is well established and accepted. The metabolism of fats is important in understanding the development of heart disease.

Fats, which are insoluble in water, are encased in water-soluble lipoproteins to allow them to be transported within a circulatory system that is water-based. Four elements of fat metabolism—total cholesterol, LDL, HDL, and triglycerides—are primary factors affecting the development of heart disease (Fig. 28-3). Cholesterol and the lipoproteins are synthesized by the liver or ingested as part of the diet. All adults 20 years of age or older should have a fasting lipid profile (total cholesterol, LDL, HDL, and triglyceride) performed at least once every 5 years and more often if the profile is abnormal. Patients who have had an acute event (MI), percutaneous coronary intervention (PCI), or **coronary artery bypass graft (CABG)** require assessment of the LDL-cholesterol level within 60 to 365 days after the event (LDL levels may be low immediately after the acute event). Subsequently, lipids should be monitored every 6 weeks until the desired level is achieved and then every 4 to 6 months (Expert Panel on Detection, Evaluation, and Treatment of High Blood Cholesterol in Adults, 2001).

LDL exerts a harmful effect on the arterial wall and accelerates atherosclerosis. In contrast, HDL promotes the use of total cholesterol by transporting LDL to the liver, where it is biodegraded and then excreted. The desired goal is to have low LDL values and high HDL values. The desired level of LDL depends on the patient:

- Less than 160 mg/dL for patients with one or no risk factors
- Less than 130 mg/dL for patients with two or more risk factors
- Less than 100 mg/dL for patients with CAD or a CAD risk equivalent

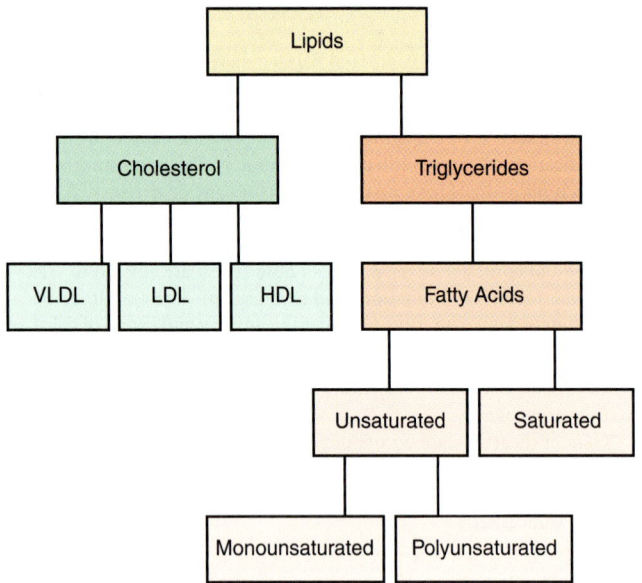

FIGURE 28-3 Types of lipids. Elevated levels of cholesterol, VLDL, LDL, and triglycerides, and low levels of HDL are risk factors for the development of atherosclerotic arterial disease, such as coronary artery disease. (VLDL, very low density lipoproteins; LDL, low density lipoproteins; HDL, high density lipoproteins.)

Serum cholesterol and LDL levels can usually be controlled by diet and physical activity. Depending on the patient's LDL level and risk of coronary heart disease, medication therapy may also be prescribed.

The level of HDL should exceed 40 mg/dL and should ideally be more than 60 mg/dL. A high HDL level is a strong negative risk factor (is protective) for heart disease.

Triglyceride is another fatty substance, made up of fatty acids, that is transported through the blood by a lipoprotein. Although an elevated triglyceride level (>200 mg/dL) may be genetic in origin, it also can be caused by obesity, physical inactiv-

ity, excessive alcohol intake, high-carbohydrate diets, diabetes mellitus, kidney disease, and certain medications, such as birth control pills, corticosteroids, and beta-adrenergic blockers when given in higher doses. Management of elevated triglyceride focuses on weight reduction and increased physical activity. Medications such as nicotinic acid and fibric acids (eg, fenofibrate [Tricor], clofibrate [Claripex]) may also be prescribed, especially if the triglyceride level is above 500 mg/dL (Expert Panel on Detection, Evaluation, and Treatment of High Blood Cholesterol in Adults, 2001).

Lipoprotein(a), or Lp(a), is a component of LDL and is attached to a special protein called apo(a). The level of Lp(a) is primarily determined by genetics. An elevated level of Lp(a) has been associated with a higher risk of CAD. However, clinical trials have not yet identified methods that lower the level of Lp(a) and have not demonstrated that lower levels of Lp(a) reduce the risk of CAD; therefore Lp(a) is not routinely monitored (Danesh, et al., 2000; Gibbons et al., 1999).

Dietary Measures. Table 28-1 provides recommendations of the Therapeutic Lifestyle Changes (TLC) diet (Expert Panel on Detection, Evaluation, and Treatment of High Blood Cholesterol in Adults, 2001). However, these recommendations may need to be adjusted to match the individual patient who has other nutritional needs, such as the requirements for pregnancy or diabetes. To assist in following the appropriate TLC diet, the patient should be referred to a registered dietitian. Other TLC recommendations are weight loss, cessation of tobacco use, and increased physical activity.

Soluble dietary fibre may also help lower cholesterol levels. Soluble fibres, which are found in fresh fruit, cereal grains, vegetables, and legumes, enhance the excretion of metabolized cholesterol. The ability of fibre to reduce serum cholesterol continues to be investigated. Intake of at least 20 to 30 grams of fibre each day is recommended (Expert Panel on Detection, Evaluation, and Treatment of High Blood Cholesterol in Adults, 2001).

Many resources are available to assist people who are attempting to control their cholesterol levels, including the Heart and Stroke Foundation of Canada, CAD support groups, and reliable

Table 28-1 • Nutrient Content of the Therapeutic Lifestyle Changes (TLC) Diet	
NUTRIENT	**RECOMMENDED INTAKE**
Total calories*	Balance intake and expenditure to maintain desirable weight
Total Fat	25%–35% of total calories
Saturated fat†	<7% of total calories
Polyunsaturated Fat	Up to 10% of total calories
Monounsaturated Fat	Up to 20% of total calories
Carbohydrate‡	50%–60% of total calories
Fibre	20–30 g/day
Protein	Approximately 15% of total calories
Cholesterol	<200 mg/day

*Daily energy expenditure should include at least moderate physical activity (contributing approximately 200 k/cal per day).
†Trans-fatty acids are formed from the processing (manufacturing, hydrogenation) of vegetable oils into a more solid form. The effects of trans-fatty acids are similar to saturated fats (ie, raising low-density lipoprotein and lowering high-density lipoprotein). Intake of trans-fatty acids should be kept low.
‡Carbohydrates should be derived predominately from foods rich in complex carbohydrates, including grains, especially whole grains, fruits, and vegetables.
From Expert Panel on Detection, Evaluation, and Treatment of High Blood Cholesterol in Adults. (2001). Executive summary of the third report of the National Cholesterol Education Program (NCEP) Expert Panel on Detection, Evaluation, and Treatment of High Blood Cholesterol in Adults (Adult Treatment Panel III). *Journal of the American Medical Association, 285*(19), 2486–2497.

Internet sources. Cookbooks and recipes that include the nutritional breakdown of foods can be included as resources for patients. Dietary control has been made easier because food manufacturers are required to provide comprehensive nutritional data on product labels. The label information of interest to a person attempting to eat a heart-healthy diet is as follows:

- Serving size, expressed in household measures
- Amount of total fat per serving
- Amount of saturated fat per serving
- Amount of cholesterol per serving
- Amount of fibre per serving

Physical Activity. Regular, moderate physical activity increases HDL levels and reduces triglyceride levels. The goal for the average person is a total of 30 minutes of exercise, three to four times per week. The nurse helps patients set realistic goals for physical activity. For example, the inactive patient should start with activity that lasts 3 minutes, such as parking farther from a building to increase the walking time. For sustained activity, patients should begin with a 5-minute warm-up period to stretch and prepare the body for the exercise. They should end the exercise with a 5-minute cool-down period in which they gradually reduce the intensity of the activity to prevent a sudden decrease in cardiac output. Patients should be instructed to engage in an activity or variety of activities that interest them, to maintain motivation. They should also be taught to exercise to an intensity that does not preclude their ability to talk; if they cannot have a conversation, they should slow down or switch to a less intensive activity. When the weather is hot and humid, the patient should be advised to exercise during the early morning or indoors and wear loose-fitting clothing. When the weather is cold, the patient should be instructed to layer clothing and to wear a hat. The nurse can also advise the patient to avoid adverse weather conditions by participating in local community programs, such as those held at shopping malls. The nurse should inform patients to stop any activity if they develop chest pain, unusual shortness of breath, dizziness, lightheadedness, or nausea.

Medications. Medications (Table 28-2) are used in some instances to control cholesterol levels. If diet alone cannot normalize serum cholesterol levels, several medications have a synergistic effect with the prescribed diet. Lipid-lowering medications can reduce CAD mortality in patients with elevated lipid levels and in those with normal lipid levels. The lipid-lowering agents affect the different lipid components and are usually grouped into four types:

- 3-Hydroxy-3-methylglutaryl coenzyme A (HMG-CoA) reductase inhibitors or statins (eg, lovastatin [Mevacor], pravastatin [Pravachol], simvastatin [Zocor]; see Table 28-2) block cholesterol synthesis, lower LDL and triglyceride levels, and increase HDL levels. These medications are frequently the initial medication therapy for significantly elevated cholesterol and LDL levels. Because of their effect on the liver, results of hepatic function tests are monitored.
- Nicotinic acids (niacin [Niaspan]; see Table 28-2) decrease lipoprotein synthesis, lower LDL and triglyceride levels, and increase HDL levels. The dose of niacin needs to be titrated weekly to achieve therapeutic dosage. Niacin is the medication most often used for minimally elevated cholesterol and LDL levels or as an adjunct to a statin when the lipid goal has not been achieved and the triglycerides are elevated. Side effects include gastrointestinal upset, gout, and flush-

ing. Because of its effect on the liver, hepatic function is monitored.
- Fibric acid or fibrates (eg, clofibrate [Abitrate], fenofibrate [Ticor]; see Table 28-2) decrease the synthesis of cholesterol, reduce triglyceride levels, and increase HDL levels. Because they have the potential to increase LDLs, fibrates are the medications of choice for patients with triglyceride levels above 400 mg/dL. Because of the risk of myopathy and acute renal failure, fibrates should be used with caution in patients who are also taking a statin.
- Bile acid sequestrants or resins (eg, cholestyramine [Questran]; see Table 28-2) bind cholesterol in the intestine, increase its breakdown, and lower LDL levels with minimal effect on HDLs and no effect (or minimal increase) on triglyceride levels. These medications are more often used as adjunct therapy when statins alone have not been effective in controlling lipid levels and the triglyceride levels are less than 200 mg/dL. Significant side effects, such as gastric distention and constipation, can occur from using these medications.

Medication therapy is reserved for at-risk patients and is not regarded as a substitute for dietary modification. All of these medications have been shown to reduce major coronary events (Expert Panel on Detection, Evaluation, and Treatment of High Blood Cholesterol in Adults, 2001). Some of these may be used in combination to achieve synergistic effects. For example, LDL cholesterol can be lowered more effectively by adding a low dose of resin to a dose of niacin or statins, or both, than a maximum dose of an individual agent.

Patients with elevated cholesterol levels should be monitored for adherence to the medical plan, the effect of cholesterol-lowering medications, and the development of side effects from cholesterol-lowering medications. Lipid levels are obtained and adjustments made to the diet and medication every 6 weeks until the lipid goal or maximum dose is achieved and then every 6 months thereafter.

PROMOTING CESSATION OF TOBACCO USE

Cigarette smoking contributes to the development and severity of CAD in three ways. First, the inhalation of smoke increases the blood carbon monoxide level, causing hemoglobin, the oxygen-carrying component of blood, to combine more readily with carbon monoxide than with oxygen. A decreased amount of available oxygen may decrease the heart's ability to pump.

Second, the nicotinic acid in tobacco triggers the release of catecholamines, which raise the heart rate and blood pressure. Nicotinic acid can also cause the coronary arteries to constrict. Smokers have a tenfold increase in risk for sudden cardiac death. The increase in catecholamines may be a factor in the increased incidence of sudden cardiac death.

Third, use of tobacco causes a detrimental vascular response and increases platelet adhesion, leading to a higher probability of thrombus formation. A person with increased risk for heart disease is encouraged to stop tobacco use through any means possible: counselling, consistent motivation and reinforcement messages, support groups, and medications. Some people have found complementary therapies (eg, acupuncture, guided imagery, hypnosis) to be helpful. People who stop smoking reduce their risk of heart disease by 30% to 50% within the first year, and the risk continues to decline as long as they refrain from smoking.

Exposure to other smokers' smoke (passive or second-hand smoke) is believed to cause heart disease in nonsmokers. Oral contraceptive use by women who smoke is inadvisable because

Table 28-2 • Medications Affecting Lipoprotein Metabolism

MEDICATION AND DAILY DOSAGE	LIPID/LIPOPROTEIN EFFECTS	SIDE EFFECTS	CONTRAINDICATIONS
HMG-CoA Reductase Inhibitors (statins)			
Lovastatin (Mevacor) 20–80 mg	LDL ↓ 18–55% HDL ↑ 5–15%	Myopathy, increased liver enzyme levels	Absolute: active or chronic liver disease Relative: concomitant use of certain drugs*
Pravastatin (Pravachol) 20–40 mg	TG ↓ 7–30%		
Simvastatin (Zocor) 20–80 mg			
Fluvastatin (Lescol) 20–80 mg			
Atorvastatin calcium (Lipitor) 10–80 mg			
Nicotinic Acid			
Niacin (Niaspan)			
Immediate-release nicotinic acid 1.5–3 g	LDL ↓ 5–25% HDL ↑ 15–35%	Flushing, hyperglycemia, hyperuricemia (or gout), upper gastrointestinal distress, hepatotoxicity	Absolute: chronic liver disease, severe gout Relative: diabetes, hyperuricemia, peptic ulcer disease
Extended-release nicotinic acid 1–2 g	TG ↓ 20–50%		
Sustained-release nicotinic acid 1–2 g			
Fibric Acids			
Fenofibrate (Tricor) 200 mg	LDL ↓ 5–20% (may be increased in patients with high TG)	Dyspepsia, gallstones, myopathy, unexplained non-CHD deaths in World Health Organization study	Absolute: severe renal disease, severe hepatic disease
Clofibrate (Abitrate) 1000 mg, b.i.d.	HDL ↑ 10–20% TG ↓ 20–50%		
Bile Acid Sequestrants			
Cholestryramine (Novo-Cholamine, PMS-Cholestyramine) 4–16 g	LDL ↓ 15–30% HDL ↑ 3–5% TG no change or increase	Gastrointestinal distress, constipation, decreased absorption of other drugs	Absolute: dysbetalipoproteinemia, TG >400 mg/dL Relative: TG >200 mg/dL
Colesevelam (Welchol) 2.6–3.8 g			
Colestipol HCl (Colestid) 5–20 g			

HMG-CoA, 3-hydroxy-3-methylglutaryl coenzyme A; LDL, low-density lipoprotein; HDL, high-density lipoprotein; TG, triglycerides; ↓ decrease, ↑ increase; CHD, coronary heart disease
*Cyclosporine (Neoral, Sandimmune, SangCya); macrolide antibiotics (azithromycin [Zithromax], clarithromycin [Biaxin]; dirithromycin [Dynabac]; erythromycin [Aknemycin, E-mycin, Ery-Tab]; various antifungal agents and cytochrome P-450 inhibitors; fibrates; and niacin should be used with appropriate caution).
From Expert Panel on Detection, Evaluation, and Treatment of High Blood Cholesterol in Adults. (2001). Executive summary of the third report of the National Cholesterol Education Program (NCEP) Expert Panel on Detection, Evaluation, and Treatment of High Blood Cholesterol in Adults (Adult Treatment Panel III). *Journal of the American Medical Association, 285*(19), 2486–2497.

these medications significantly increase the risk of CAD and sudden cardiac death.

Cessation of tobacco use results in a lower rate of cardiac events. Patients should be advised to participate in an educational class, support group, or behavioural program. Use of medications such as the nicotine patch (Nicotrol, Nicoderm CQ, Habitrol) or bupropion (Zyban) may assist with stopping use of tobacco, but do have the same systemic effects: catecholamine release (increasing heart rate and blood pressure) and increased platelet adhesion. These medications should be used for the shortest time and at the lowest effective doses.

MANAGING HYPERTENSION

Hypertension is defined as blood pressure measurements that repeatedly exceed 140/90 mm Hg. Long-standing elevated blood pressure may result in increased stiffness of the vessel walls, lead-ing to vessel injury and a resulting inflammatory response within the intima. Hypertension can also increase the work of the left ventricle, which must pump harder to eject blood into the arteries. Over time, the increased workload causes the heart to enlarge and thicken (ie, hypertrophy), a condition that may eventually lead to cardiac failure.

Early detection of high blood pressure and adherence to a therapeutic regimen can prevent the serious consequences associated with untreated elevated blood pressure. Hypertension is discussed in detail in Chapter 32.

CONTROLLING DIABETES MELLITUS

The relationship between diabetes mellitus and heart disease has been substantiated. For 65% to 75% of patients with diabetes, cardiovascular disease is listed as the cause of death (Braunwald et al., 2001; Grundy et al., 1999). Hyperglycemia fosters dyslipidemia, increased platelet aggregation, and altered red blood cell function, which can lead to thrombus formation. It has been suggested that these metabolic alterations impair endothelial cell–dependent vasodilation and smooth muscle function; treatment with insulin (eg, Humalog, Humulin, Novolin) and metformin (Glucophage) has demonstrated improvement in endothelial function: improved endothelial-dependent dilation (Gaenzer et al., 2002). Diabetes is considered equivalent to existing CAD in its risk of a cardiac event within 10 years (Expert Panel on Detection, Evaluation, and Treatment of High Blood Cholesterol in Adults, 2001). Diabetes is discussed in detail in Chapter 41.

Gender and Estrogen Level

Because heart disease had been considered to primarily affect white men, the disease was not as readily recognized and treated in women. However, in 1997 in Canada, rates of death for women from CAD were markedly higher (94 per 100,000 population) than for breast cancer (28 per 100,000 population) or lung cancer (33 per 100,000). (Statistics Canada, 2005). Women tend to have a higher incidence of complications from CAD (American Heart Association, 2002). African-American women have a mortality rate nearly twice that of Caucasian women (Office for Social Environment and Health Research at West Virginia University, 2001). Women tend not to recognize the symptoms as early as men and to wait longer to report their symptoms and seek medical assistance (Meischke et al., 1999; Penque et al., 1998). In the past, women were less likely than men to be referred for coronary artery diagnostic procedures, to receive medical therapy (eg, **thrombolytic** therapy to break down the blood clots that cause acute MI, or nitroglycerin), and to be treated with invasive interventions, eg, angioplasty (Sheifer et al., 2000). It is anticipated that with better education of the general public and health care professionals, gender and racial differences will have less influence on the diagnosis, treatment, and incidence of complications of heart disease in the future.

In women younger than age 55, the incidence of CAD is significantly lower than in men. However, after age 55, the incidence in women is approximately equal to that in men. The age difference of the incidence of CAD in women may be related to estrogen. Although **hormone replacement therapy (HRT)** for menopausal women had been promoted as prevention for CAD, research studies do not support HRT as an effective means of CAD prevention (Hulley et al., 1998; Mosca, 2000). HRT has decreased postmenopausal symptoms and the risk for osteoporosis-related bone fractures, but HRT also has been associated with an increased risk for CAD, breast cancer, deep vein thrombosis, cerebrovascular accident (CVA, brain attack, stroke), and pulmonary embolism. The Women's Health Initiative (Gebbie, 2002) demonstrated that long-term HRT may have more risks than benefits, and that HRT should not be initiated or continued for primary prevention of CAD.

Behaviour Patterns

Most clinicians believe that stress and certain behaviours contribute to the pathogenesis of CAD and a cardiac event, especially in women. Psychological and epidemiologic studies describe behaviours that characterize people who are prone to heart disease: excessive competitiveness, a sense of time urgency or impatience, aggressiveness, and hostility (Dembroski et al., 1989; Friedman & Rosenman, 1959; Krantz et al., 2000). A person with these behaviours is classified as type A coronary-prone.

The type A coronary-prone classification may not be as significant as was once thought; evidence of its precise role remains inconclusive (Rozanski et al., 1999). To be on the safer side, however, such a person may be wise to alter behaviours and responses to triggering events and to reduce other risk factors. Nurses can assist these people by teaching them cognitive restructuring and relaxation techniques. Because people who are depressed have worse outcomes, these patients should be assessed for signs and symptoms of depression and, if diagnosed, appropriately treated.

ANGINA PECTORIS

Angina pectoris is a clinical syndrome usually characterized by episodes or paroxysms of pain or pressure in the anterior chest. The cause is usually insufficient coronary blood flow. The insufficient flow results in a decreased oxygen supply to meet an increased myocardial demand for oxygen in response to physical exertion or emotional stress. In other words, the need for oxygen exceeds the supply. The severity of angina is based on the precipitating activity and its effect on the activities of daily living (Table 28-3).

Pathophysiology

Angina is usually caused by atherosclerotic disease. Almost invariably, angina is associated with a significant obstruction of a major coronary artery. The characteristics of the various types of angina are listed in Chart 28-3. Identifying angina requires obtaining a thorough history. Effective treatment begins with reducing the demands placed on the heart and teaching the patient about the condition. Several factors are associated with typical anginal pain:

- Physical exertion, which can precipitate an attack by increasing myocardial oxygen demand
- Exposure to cold, which can cause vasoconstriction and an elevated blood pressure, with increased oxygen demand
- Eating a heavy meal, which increases the blood flow to the mesenteric area for digestion, thereby reducing the blood supply available to the heart muscle (In a severely compromised heart, shunting of blood for digestion can be sufficient to induce anginal pain.)
- Stress or any emotion-provoking situation, causing the release of adrenaline and increasing blood pressure, which may accelerate the heart rate and increase the myocardial workload

Table 28-3 • **Canadian Cardiovascular Society Classification of Angina**		
CLASS	ACTIVITY EVOKING ANGINA	LIMITS TO ACTIVITY
I	Prolonged exertion	None
II	Walking >2 blocks	Slight
III	Walking <2 blocks	Marked
IV	Minimal or rest	Severe

Adapted from Campeau L. (1976). Grading of angina pectoris. *Circulation 54*, 522–523.

Chart 28-3 — Types of Angina

- **Stable angina:** predictable and consistent pain that occurs on exertion and is relieved by rest
- **Unstable angina** (also called preinfarction angina or crescendo angina): symptoms occur more frequently and last longer than stable angina. The threshold for pain is lower, and pain may occur at rest.
- **Intractable or refractory angina:** severe incapacitating chest pain
- **Variant angina** (also called Prinzmetal's angina): pain at rest with reversible ST-segment elevation; thought to be caused by coronary artery vasospasm
- **Silent ischemia:** objective evidence of ischemia (such as electrocardiographic changes with a stress test), but patient reports no symptoms

Atypical angina is not associated with the listed factors. It may occur at rest.

Clinical Manifestations

Ischemia of the heart muscle may produce pain or other symptoms, varying in severity from a feeling of indigestion to a choking or heavy sensation in the upper chest that ranges from discomfort to agonizing pain accompanied by severe apprehension and a feeling of impending death. The pain is often felt deep in the chest behind the upper or middle third of the sternum (retrosternal area). Typically, the pain or discomfort is poorly localized and may radiate to the neck, jaw, shoulders, and inner aspects of the upper arms, usually the left arm. The patient often feels tightness or a heavy, choking, or strangling sensation that has a vise-like, insistent quality. The patient with diabetes mellitus may not have severe pain with angina because the neuropathy that accompanies diabetes can interfere with neuroreceptors, dulling the patient's perception of pain.

A feeling of weakness or numbness in the arms, wrists, and hands may accompany the pain, as may shortness of breath, pallor, diaphoresis, dizziness or lightheadedness, and nausea and vomiting. These symptoms may also appear alone and still represent myocardial ischemia. When these symptoms appear alone, they are called angina-like symptoms. Anxiety may accompany angina. An important characteristic of angina is that it abates or subsides with rest or nitroglycerin.

Gerontologic Considerations

The elderly person with angina may not exhibit the typical pain profile because of the diminished responses of neurotransmitters that occur in the aging process. Often, the presenting symptom in the elderly is dyspnea. If they do have pain, it is atypical pain that radiates to both arms rather than just the left arm. Sometimes, there are no symptoms ("silent" CAD), making recognition and diagnosis a clinical challenge. Elderly patients should be encouraged to recognize their chest pain–like symptom (eg, weakness) as an indication that they should rest or take prescribed medications. Noninvasive stress testing used to diagnose CAD may not be as useful in elderly patients because of other conditions (eg,

peripheral vascular disease, arthritis, degenerative disk disease, physical disability, foot problems) that limit the patient's ability to exercise.

Assessment and Diagnostic Findings

The diagnosis of angina is often made by evaluating the clinical manifestations of ischemia and the patient's history. A 12-lead ECG and blood laboratory values help in making the diagnosis. The patient may undergo an exercise or pharmacologic stress test in which the heart is monitored by ECG, echocardiogram, or both. The patient may also be referred for an echocardiogram, nuclear scan, or invasive procedures (cardiac catheterization and coronary artery angiography).

CAD is believed to result from inflammation of the arterial endothelium. C-reactive protein (CRP) is a marker for inflammation of vascular endothelium. High blood levels of CRP have been associated with increased coronary artery calcification and risk of an acute cardiovascular event (eg, MI) in seemingly healthy individuals (Ridker et al., 2002; Wang et al., 2002). There is interest in using CRP blood levels as an additional risk factor for cardiovascular disease in clinical use and research, but the clinical value of CRP levels has not been fully established. The ability of CRP to predict cardiovascular disease when adjusted for other risk factors, how CRP levels can guide patient management, and if patient outcomes improve when using CRP levels must be established before CRP levels are used routinely for patient care (Mosca, 2002).

An elevated blood level of homocysteine, an amino acid, has also been proposed as an independent risk factor for cardiovascular disease. However, studies have not supported the relationship between mild to moderate elevations of homocysteine and atherosclerosis (Homocysteine Studies Collaboration, 2002). No study has yet shown that reducing homocysteine levels reduces the risk of CAD.

Medical Management

The objectives of the medical management of angina are to decrease the oxygen demand of the myocardium and to increase the oxygen supply. Medically, these objectives are met through pharmacologic therapy and control of risk factors.

Revascularization procedures to restore the blood supply to the myocardium include **percutaneous coronary interventional (PCI)** procedures (eg, **percutaneous transluminal coronary angioplasty [PTCA]**, intracoronary stents, and atherectomy), CABG, and percutaneous transluminal myocardial revascularization (PTMR).

PHARMACOLOGIC THERAPY

Among medications used to control angina are nitroglycerin, beta-adrenergic blocking agents, calcium channel blockers, and antiplatelet agents.

Nitroglycerin. Nitrates remain the mainstay for treatment of angina pectoris. A vasoactive agent, nitroglycerin (Nitrostat, Nitrol) is administered to reduce myocardial oxygen consumption, which decreases ischemia and relieves pain. Nitroglycerin dilates primarily the veins and, in higher doses, also dilates the arteries. It helps to increase coronary blood flow by preventing vasospasm and increasing perfusion through the collateral vessels.

Dilation of the veins causes venous pooling of blood throughout the body. As a result, less blood returns to the heart, and filling pressure (preload) is reduced. If the patient is hypovolemic (does not have adequate circulating blood volume), the decrease in filling pressure can cause a significant decrease in cardiac output and blood pressure.

Nitrates in higher doses also relax the systemic arteriolar bed and lower blood pressure (decreased afterload). Nitrates may increase blood flow to diseased coronary arteries and through collateral coronary arteries, arteries that have been underused until the body recognizes poorly perfused areas. These effects decrease myocardial oxygen requirements and increase oxygen supply, bringing about a more favourable balance between supply and demand.

Nitroglycerin may be given by several routes: sublingual tablet or spray, topical agent, and intravenous administration. Sublingual nitroglycerin is generally placed under the tongue or in the cheek (buccal pouch) and alleviates the pain of ischemia within 3 minutes. Topical nitroglycerin is also fast acting and is a convenient way to administer the medication. Both routes are suitable for patients who self-administer the medication. Chart 28-4 provides more information.

A continuous or intermittent intravenous infusion of nitroglycerin may be administered to the hospitalized patient with recurring signs and symptoms of ischemia or after a revascularization procedure. The amount of nitroglycerin administered is based on the patient's symptoms while avoiding side effects such as hypotension. It usually is not given if the systolic blood pressure is 90 mm Hg or less. Generally, after the patient is symptom free, the nitroglycerin may be switched to a topical preparation within 24 hours.

Beta-Adrenergic Blocking Agents. Beta-blockers such as propranolol (Inderal), metoprolol (Lopressor, Toprol-XL), and atenolol (Tenormin) appear to reduce myocardial oxygen consumption by blocking the beta-adrenergic sympathetic stimulation to the heart. The result is a reduction in heart rate, slowed conduction of an impulse through the heart, decreased blood pressure, and reduced myocardial **contractility** (force of contraction) that establishes a more favourable balance between myocardial oxygen needs (demands) and the amount of oxygen available (supply). This helps to control chest pain and delays the onset of ischemia during work or exercise. Beta-blockers reduce the incidence of recurrent angina, infarction, and cardiac mortality. The dose can be titrated to achieve a resting heart rate of 50 to 60 beats per minute.

Cardiac side effects and possible contraindications include hypotension, bradycardia, advanced atrioventricular block, and decompensated heart failure. If a beta-blocker is given intravenously for an acute cardiac event, the ECG, blood pressure, and heart rate are monitored closely after the medication has been administered. Because some beta-blockers also affect the beta-adrenergic receptors in the bronchioles, causing bronchoconstriction, they are contraindicated in patients with significant pulmonary constrictive diseases, such as asthma. Other side effects include worsening of hyperlipidemia, depression, fatigue, decreased libido, and masking of symptoms of hypoglycemia. Patients taking beta-blockers are cautioned not to stop taking them abruptly, because angina may worsen and MI may develop. Beta-blocker therapy needs to

Chart 28-4 • PHARMACOLOGY
Self-Administration of Nitroglycerin

Most patients with angina pectoris must self-administer nitroglycerin on an as-needed basis. A key nursing role in such cases is educating patients about the medication and how to take it. Sublingual nitroglycerin comes in tablet and spray forms.

Teaching About Sublingual Nitroglycerin
- Instruct the patient to make sure the mouth is moist, the tongue is still, and saliva is not swallowed until the nitroglycerin tablet dissolves. If the pain is severe, the patient can crush the tablet between the teeth to hasten sublingual absorption.
- Advise the patient to carry the medication at all times as a precaution. However, because nitroglycerin is very unstable, it should be carried securely in its original container (eg, capped dark glass bottle); tablets should never be removed and stored in metal or plastic pillboxes.
- Explain that nitroglycerin is volatile and is inactivated by heat, moisture, air, light, and time. Instruct the patient to renew the nitroglycerin supply every 6 months.
- Inform the patient that the medication should be taken in anticipation of any activity that may produce pain. Because nitroglycerin increases tolerance for exercise and stress when taken prophylactically (ie, before angina-producing activity, such as exercise, stair-climbing, or sexual intercourse), it is best taken before pain develops.
- Recommend that the patient note how long it takes for the nitroglycerin to relieve the discomfort. Advise the patient that if pain persists after taking three sublingual tablets at 5-minute intervals, emergency medical services should be called.

- Discuss possible side effects of nitroglycerin, including flushing, throbbing headache, hypotension, and tachycardia.

Teaching About Topical Nitroglycerin
Nitroglycerin is also available in a lanolin-petrolatum base that is applied to the skin as a paste or a patch. Patients who use topical nitroglycerin need additional instruction.
- Advise the patient to read the instructions that accompany the product, because instructions vary according to the preparation. Also remind the patient to rotate the site of application to avoid skin irritation.
- Explain that the area of application needs to be an area that is well perfused for absorption to occur. Therefore, the medication should not be applied to areas with extensive body hair or scar tissue.
- Recommend that the patient protect clothing from the oil base in the paste.
- Explain that a long-term equally spaced dosing schedule of application of topical nitroglycerin is generally avoided to prevent tolerance (when the body does not respond as well to the same amount of medication). Most physicians prescribe application of topical nitroglycerin paste three or four times daily or every 6 hours (excluding the mid-night dose), and application of the nitroglycerin patch every morning and removed at 10 PM. This dosing regimen allows for a 6- to 8-hour nitrate-free period to prevent the body's development of tolerance.

be decreased gradually over several days before discontinuing it. Patients with diabetes who take beta-blockers are instructed to assess their blood glucose levels more often and to observe for signs and symptoms of hypoglycemia.

Calcium Channel Blocking Agents.

Calcium channel blockers (calcium ion antagonists) have different effects. Some decrease sinoatrial node automaticity and atrioventricular node conduction, resulting in a slower heart rate and a decrease in the strength of the heart muscle contraction (negative inotropic effect). These effects decrease the workload of the heart. Calcium channel blockers also relax the blood vessels, causing a decrease in blood pressure and an increase in coronary artery perfusion. Calcium channel blockers increase myocardial oxygen supply by dilating the smooth muscle wall of the coronary arterioles; they decrease myocardial oxygen demand by reducing systemic arterial pressure and the workload of the left ventricle.

The calcium channel blockers most commonly used are amlodipine (Norvasc), verapamil (Calan, Isoptin, Verelan), and diltiazem (Cardizem, Dilacor, Tiazac). They may be used by patients who cannot take beta-blockers, who develop significant side effects from beta-blockers or nitrates, or who still have pain despite beta-blocker and nitroglycerin therapy. Calcium channel blockers are used to prevent and treat vasospasm, which commonly occurs after an invasive interventional procedure. Use of short-acting nifedipine (Procardia) was found to be poorly tolerated and to increase the risk of MI in patients with hypertension and the risk of death in patients with **acute coronary syndrome** (Braunwald et al., 2000; Furberg et al., 1996; Ryan et al., 1999).

First-generation calcium channel blockers should be avoided or used with great caution in people with heart failure, because they decrease myocardial contractility. Amlodipine (Norvasc) and felodipine (Plendil) are the calcium channel blockers of choice for patients with heart failure. Hypotension may occur after the intravenous administration of any of the calcium channel blockers. Other side effects that may occur include atrioventricular blocks, bradycardia, constipation, and gastric distress.

Antiplatelet and Anticoagulant Medications.

Antiplatelet medications are administered to prevent platelet aggregation, which impedes blood flow.

Aspirin.

Aspirin prevents platelet activation and reduces the incidence of MI and death in patients with CAD. A 160- to 325-mg dose of aspirin should be given to the patient with angina as soon as the diagnosis is made (eg, in the emergency room or physician's office) and then continued with 81 to 325 mg daily. Although it may be one of the most important medications in the treatment of CAD, aspirin may be overlooked because of its low cost and common use. Patients should be advised to continue aspirin even if concurrently taking nonsteroidal anti-inflammatory drugs (NSAIDs) or other analgesics. Because aspirin may cause gastrointestinal upset and bleeding, treatment of *Helicobacter pylori* and the use of H2-blockers (eg, cimetidine [Tagamet HB], famotidine [Mylanta AR, Pepcid], ranitidine [Zantac]) or misoprostol (Cytotec) should be considered to allow continued aspirin therapy.

Clopidogrel and Ticlopidine.

Clopidogrel (Plavix) or ticlopidine (Ticlid) is given to patients who are allergic to aspirin or given in addition to aspirin in patients at high risk for MI. Unlike aspirin, these medications take a few days to achieve their antiplatelet effect. They also cause gastrointestinal upset, including nausea, vomiting, and diarrhea, and they decrease the neutrophil level.

Heparin.

Unfractionated heparin prevents the formation of new blood clots. Use of heparin alone in treating patients with unstable angina reduces the occurrence of MI. If the patient's signs and symptoms indicate a significant risk for a cardiac event, the patient is hospitalized and may be given an intravenous bolus of heparin and started on a continuous infusion or given an intravenous bolus every 4 to 6 hours. The amount of heparin administered is based on the results of the activated partial thromboplastin time (aPTT). Heparin therapy is usually considered therapeutic when the aPTT is 1.5 to 2 times the normal aPTT value.

A subcutaneous injection of low-molecular-weight heparin (LMWH; enoxaparin [Lovenox] or dalteparin [Fragmin]) may be used instead of intravenous unfractionated heparin to treat patients with unstable angina or non–ST-segment elevation MIs. LMWH provides more effective and stable anticoagulation, potentially reducing the risk of rebound ischemic events, and it eliminates the need to monitor aPTT results (Cohen, 2001). LMWH may be beneficial before and during PCIs and for ST-segment elevation MIs.

Because unfractionated heparin and LMWH increase the risk of bleeding, the patient is monitored for signs and symptoms of external and internal bleeding, such as low blood pressure, an increased heart rate, and a decrease in serum hemoglobin and hematocrit values. The patient receiving heparin is placed on bleeding precautions, which include:

- Applying pressure to the site of any needle puncture for a longer time than usual
- Avoiding intramuscular injections
- Avoiding tissue injury and bruising from trauma or use of constrictive devices (eg, continuous use of an automatic blood pressure cuff)

A decrease in platelet count or skin lesions at heparin injection sites may indicate heparin-induced thrombocytopenia (HIT), an antibody-mediated reaction to heparin that may result in thrombosis (Hirsh et al., 2001). Patients who have received heparin within the past 3 months and those who have been receiving unfractionated heparin for 5 to 15 days are at high risk for HIT.

GPIIb/IIIa Agents.

Intravenous GPIIb/IIIa agents (abciximab [ReoPro], tirofiban [Aggrastat], eptifibatide [Integrelin]) are indicated for hospitalized patients with unstable angina and as adjunct therapy for PCI. These agents prevent platelet aggregation by blocking the GPIIb/IIIa receptors on the platelet, preventing adhesion of fibrinogen and other factors that crosslink platelets to each other and thereby allow platelets to form a thrombus (clot). As with heparin, bleeding is the major side effect, and bleeding precautions should be initiated.

Oxygen Administration.

Oxygen therapy is usually initiated at the onset of chest pain in an attempt to increase the amount of oxygen delivered to the myocardium and to decrease pain. Oxygen inhaled directly increases the amount of oxygen in the blood. The therapeutic effectiveness of oxygen is determined by observing the rate and rhythm of respirations. Blood oxygen saturation is monitored by pulse oximetry; the normal oxygen saturation (SpO_2) level is greater than 93%. Studies are being conducted to assess the use of oxygen in patients without respiratory distress and its effect on outcome.

ALTERNATIVE THERAPIES

Researchers have reported significant improvement in the exercise endurance of patients with angina who were treated with acupuncture as well as with an intravenous infusion of a combination of ginseng (*Panax quinquefolium*), astragalus (*Astragalus membranaceus*), and angelica (*Angelica sinensis*) (Ballegaard et al., 1991; Reichter et al., 1991). Coenzyme Q10 was advocated for preventing the occurrence and progression of heart failure (Khatta et al., 2000). However, there have not been large, randomized, placebo-controlled studies that identify the direct beneficial effect from these therapies.

NURSING PROCESS:
THE PATIENT WITH ANGINA PECTORIS

Assessment

The nurse gathers information about the patient's symptoms and activities, especially those that precede and precipitate attacks of angina pectoris. Appropriate questions are identified in Table 28-4, using a PQRST format. Other helpful questions may be asked. How long does the angina usually last? Does nitroglycerin relieve the angina? If so, how many tablets or sprays are needed to achieve relief? How long does it takes for relief to occur?

The answers to these questions form a basis for designing a logical program of treatment and prevention. In addition to assessing angina pectoris or its equivalent, the nurse also assesses the patient's risk factors for CAD, the patient's response to angina, the patient's and family's understanding of the diagnosis, and adherence to the current treatment plan.

Diagnosis

NURSING DIAGNOSES

Based on the assessment data, major nursing diagnoses for the patient may include:

- Ineffective myocardial tissue perfusion secondary to CAD, as evidenced by chest pain or equivalent symptoms
- Anxiety related to fear of death
- Deficient knowledge about the underlying disease and methods for avoiding complications
- Noncompliance, ineffective management of therapeutic regimen related to failure to accept necessary lifestyle changes

COLLABORATIVE PROBLEMS/
POTENTIAL COMPLICATIONS

Potential complications that may develop include the following, which are discussed in the chapters indicated:

- Acute pulmonary edema (see Chap. 30)
- Congestive heart failure (see Chap. 30)
- Cardiogenic shock (see Chap. 30)
- Dysrhythmias and cardiac arrest (see Chaps. 27 and 30)
- MI (described later in this chapter)
- Myocardial rupture (see Chap. 30)
- Pericardial effusion and cardiac tamponade (see Chap. 30)

Planning and Goals

The major patient goals include immediate and appropriate treatment when angina occurs, prevention of angina, reduction of anxiety, awareness of the disease process and understanding of the prescribed care, adherence to the self-care program, and absence of complications.

Nursing Interventions

TREATING ANGINA

If the patient reports pain (or the individual's equivalent to pain), the nurse takes immediate action. When a patient experiences angina, the nurse should direct the patient to stop all activities and sit or rest in bed in a semi-Fowler position to reduce the oxygen requirements of the ischemic myocardium. The nurse assesses the patient's angina, asking questions to determine whether the angina is the same as the patient typically experiences. A difference may indicate a worsening of the disease or a different cause. The nurse then continues to assess the patient, measuring vital signs and observing for signs of respiratory distress. If the patient is in the hospital, a 12-lead ECG is usually obtained and scrutinized for ST-segment and T-wave changes. If the patient has been placed on cardiac monitoring with continuous ST-segment monitoring, the ST segment is assessed for changes.

Nitroglycerin is administered sublingually, and the patient's response is assessed (relief of chest pain and effect on blood pressure and heart rate). If the chest pain is unchanged or is lessened but still present, nitroglycerin administration is repeated up to three doses.

Table 28-4 • Assessment of Angina

ACRONYM	FACTORS ABOUT PAIN THAT NEED TO BE ASSESSED	ASSESSMENT QUESTIONS
P	Position/Location	"Where is the pain? Can you point to it?"
	Provocation	"What were you doing when the pain began?"
Q	Quality	"How would you describe the pain?"
		"Is it like the pain you had before?"
	Quantity	"Has the pain been constant?"
R	Radiation	"Can you feel the pain anywhere else?"
	Relief	"Did anything make the pain better?"
S	Severity	"How would you rate the pain on a 0–10 scale with 0 being no pain and 10 being the most amount of pain?" (or use visual analog scale or adjective rating scale)
	Symptoms	"Did you notice any other symptoms with the pain?"
T	Timing	"How long ago did the pain start?"

From Casey, P. E., Morrissey, A., & Nolan, E. M. (1998). Ischemic heart disease. In M. R. Kinney, B. S. Dunbar, J. A. Brooks-Brunn, et al. (Eds.), *AACN clinical reference for critical care nursing* (4th ed.) St. Louis: Mosby.

Each time, blood pressure, heart rate, and the ST segment (if the patient is on a monitor with ST segment monitoring capability) are assessed. The nurse administers oxygen therapy if the patient's respiratory rate is increased or the oxygen saturation level is decreased. Although there is no documentation of its effect on outcome, oxygen is usually administered at 2 L/min by nasal cannula, even without evidence of respiratory distress. If the pain is significant and continues after these interventions, the patient is usually transferred to a higher-acuity nursing unit.

REDUCING ANXIETY

Patients with angina often fear loss of their roles within society and the family. They may also be fearful that the pain may lead to an MI or death. Exploring the implications that the diagnosis has for the patient and providing information about the illness, its treatment, and methods of preventing its progression are important nursing interventions. Various stress reduction methods should be explored with the patient. For example, music therapy, in which patients are given the opportunity to listen to selected music through headphones for a predetermined duration, has been shown to reduce anxiety in patients who are in a coronary care unit and may serve as an adjunct to therapeutic communication (Chlan & Tracy, 1999; Evans, 2002). Addressing the spiritual needs of the patient and family may also assist in allaying anxieties and fears.

PREVENTING PAIN

The nurse reviews the assessment findings, identifies the level of activity that causes the patient's pain, and plans the patient's activities accordingly. If the patient has pain frequently or with minimal activity, the nurse alternates the patient's activities with rest periods. Balance of activity and rest is an important aspect of the educational plan for the patient and family.

PROMOTING HOME AND COMMUNITY-BASED CARE

Teaching Patients Self-Care. Learning about the modifiable risk factors that contribute to the continued development of CAD and resulting angina is essential. Exploring with the patient and family what they see as their priority in managing the disease and developing a plan based on their priorities can assist with patient adherence to the therapeutic regimen. It is important to explore with the patient methods to avoid, modify, or adapt the triggers for anginal pain. The teaching program for the patient with angina is designed so that the patient and family can explain the illness, identify the symptoms of myocardial ischemia, state the actions to take when symptoms develop, and discuss methods to prevent chest pain and the advancement of CAD. The goals of the educational program are to reduce the frequency and severity of anginal attacks, to delay the progress of the underlying disease, if possible, and to prevent any complications. The factors outlined in the accompanying checklist Chart 28-5 are important in educating the patient with angina pectoris.

The self-care program is prepared in collaboration with the patient and family or friends. Activities should be planned to minimize the occurrence of angina episodes. The patient needs to understand that any pain unrelieved within 15 minutes by the usual methods (see Chart 28-4) should be treated at the closest emergency centre; the patient should call 911 for assistance.

Evaluation

EXPECTED PATIENT OUTCOMES

Expected patient outcomes may include:

1. Reports that pain is relieved promptly
   a. Recognizes symptoms
   b. Takes immediate action
   c. Seeks medical assistance if pain persists or changes in quality
2. Reports decreased anxiety
   a. Expresses acceptance of diagnosis
   b. Expresses control over choices within medical regimen
   c. Does not exhibit signs and symptoms that indicate a high level of anxiety
3. Understands ways to avoid complications and demonstrates freedom from complications
   a. Describes the process of angina

Chart 28-5

Home Care Checklist • Managing Angina Pectoris

At the completion of the home care instruction, the patient or caregiver will be able to:	Patient	Caregiver
• Reduce the probability of an episode of anginal pain by balancing rest with activity:		
– Participate in a regular daily program of activities that do not produce chest discomfort, shortness of breath, or undue fatigue.	✓	
– Avoid exercises requiring sudden bursts of activity; avoid isometric exercise.	✓	
– State that temperature extremes (particularly cold) may induce anginal pain; therefore, avoid exercise in temperature extremes.	✓	
– Alternate activity with periods of rest.	✓	
– Use appropriate resources for support during emotionally stressful times (eg, counselor, nurse, clergy, physician).	✓	✓
• Avoid using medications or any over-the-counter substances (eg, diet pills, nasal decongestants) that can increase the heart rate and blood pressure without first discussing with a health care provider.	✓	✓
• Stop smoking and other use of tobacco, and avoid second-hand smoke (because smoking increases the heart rate, blood pressure, and blood carbon monoxide levels).	✓	✓
• Eat a diet low in saturated fat, high in fibre, and if indicated, lower in calories.	✓	✓
• Achieve and maintain normal blood pressure.	✓	
• Achieve and maintain normal blood glucose levels.	✓	
• Take medications, especially aspirin and beta-blockers, as prescribed.	✓	
• Carry nitroglycerin at all times; state when and how to use it; identify its side effects.	✓	✓

b. Explains reasons for measures to prevent complications
c. Exhibits normal ECG and cardiac enzyme levels
d. Experiences no signs and symptoms of acute MI
4. Adheres to self-care program
   a. Takes medications as prescribed
   b. Keeps health care appointments
   c. Implements plan for reducing risk factors

MYOCARDIAL INFARCTION

Pathophysiology

MI refers to the process by which areas of myocardial cells in the heart are permanently destroyed. Like unstable angina, MI is usually caused by reduced blood flow in a coronary artery due to atherosclerosis and occlusion of an artery by an embolus or thrombus. Because unstable angina and acute MI are considered to be the same process but different points along a continuum, the term **acute coronary syndrome** (ACS) may be used for these diagnoses. Other causes of an MI include vasospasm (sudden constriction or narrowing) of a coronary artery; decreased oxygen supply (eg, from acute blood loss, anemia, or low blood pressure); and increased demand for oxygen (eg, from a rapid heart rate, thyrotoxicosis, or ingestion of cocaine). In each case, a profound imbalance exists between myocardial oxygen supply and demand.

Coronary occlusion, heart attack, and MI are terms used synonymously, but the preferred term is MI. The area of infarction takes time to develop. As the cells are deprived of oxygen, ischemia develops, cellular injury occurs, and over time, the lack of oxygen results in infarction, or the death of cells. The expression "time is muscle" reflects the urgency of appropriate treatment to improve patient outcomes. Each year in the United States, nearly 1 million people have acute MIs; one fourth of these people die of MI (American Heart Association, 2001; Ryan et al., 1999). One half of those who die never reach a hospital.

Various descriptions are used to further identify an MI: the location of the injury to the left ventricular wall (anterior, inferior, posterior, or lateral wall) or to the right ventricle and the point in time within the process of infarction (acute, evolving, or old).

The ECG usually identifies the location, and the ECG and patient history identify the timing. Regardless of the location of the infarction of cardiac muscle, the goal of medical therapy is to prevent or minimize myocardial tissue death and to prevent complications. The pathophysiology of heart disease and the risk factors involved are discussed earlier in this chapter.

Clinical Manifestations

Chest pain that occurs suddenly and continues despite rest and medication is the presenting symptom in most patients with an MI (Chart 28-6). One study showed that 2% of patients who eventually were diagnosed with an acute MI were incorrectly discharged and sent home from the emergency department (Pope et al., 2000). Most of these patients presented with atypical symptoms such as shortness of breath; they also tended to be female, younger than 55 years of age, of a minority group, and have normal ECGs. The Framingham Heart Study revealed that 50% of the men and 63% of the women who died suddenly of cardiovascular disease had no previous symptoms (Kannel, 1986). Patients may also be anxious and restless. They may have cool, pale, and moist skin. Their heart rate and respiratory rate may be faster than normal. These signs and symptoms, which are caused by stimulation of the sympathetic nervous system, may be present only for a short time or may not be present, or only some of them

Chart 28-6 • ASSESSMENT

Signs and Symptoms of an Acute Myocardial Infarction (MI) or Acute Coronary Syndrome (ACS)

Cardiovascular
Chest pain or discomfort, palpitations. Heart sounds may include S_3, S_4, and new onset of a murmur. Increased jugular venous distention may be seen if the MI has caused heart failure. Blood pressure may be elevated because of sympathetic stimulation or decreased because of decreased contractility, impending cardiogenic shock, or medications. Pulse deficit may indicate atrial fibrillation. In addition to ST-segment and T-wave changes, ECG may show tachycardia, bradycardia, and dysrhythmias.

Respiratory
Shortness of breath, dyspnea, tachypnea, and crackles if MI has caused pulmonary congestion. Pulmonary edema may be present.

Gastrointestinal
Nausea and vomiting.

Genitourinary
Decreased urinary output may indicate cardiogenic shock.

Skin
Cool, clammy, diaphoretic, and pale appearance due to sympathetic stimulation from loss of contractility may indicate cardiogenic shock. Dependent edema may also be present due to poor contractility.

Neurologic
Anxiety, restlessness, light-headedness may indicate increased sympathetic stimulation or a decrease in contractility and cerebral oxygenation. The same symptoms may also herald cardiogenic shock. Headache, visual disturbances, altered speech, altered motor function, and further changes in level of consciousness may indicate cerebral bleeding if patient is receiving thrombolytics.

Psychological
Fear with feeling of impending doom, or patient may deny that anything is wrong.

may occur. In many cases, the signs and symptoms of MI cannot be distinguished from those of unstable angina.

Assessment and Diagnostic Findings

Diagnosis of MI is generally based on the presenting symptoms, the ECG, and laboratory test results (eg, serial serum enzyme values). The prognosis depends on the severity of coronary artery obstruction and the extent of myocardial damage. Physical examination is always conducted, but the examination alone is insufficient to confirm the diagnosis.

PATIENT HISTORY

The patient history has two parts: the description of the presenting symptom (eg, pain) and the history of previous illnesses and family health history, particularly of heart disease. Previous history should also include information about the patient's risk factors for heart disease.

ELECTROCARDIOGRAM

The ECG provides information that assists in diagnosing acute MI. It should be obtained within 10 minutes from the time a patient reports pain or arrives in the emergency department. By monitoring the ECG over time, the location, evolution, and resolution of an MI can be identified and monitored.

The ECG changes that occur with an MI are seen in the leads that view the involved surface of the heart. The classic ECG changes are T-wave inversion, ST-segment elevation, and development of an abnormal Q wave (Fig. 28-4). Because infarction evolves over time, the ECG also changes over time. The first ECG signs of an acute MI are from myocardial ischemia and injury. Myocardial injury causes the T wave to become enlarged and symmetric. As the area of injury becomes ischemic, myocardial repolarization is altered and delayed, causing the T wave to invert. The ischemic region may remain depolarized while adjacent areas of the myocardium return to the resting state. Myocardial injury also causes ST-segment changes. The injured myocardial cells depolarize normally but repolarize more rapidly than normal cells, causing the ST segment to rise at least 1 mm above the isoelectric line (area between the T wave and the next P wave is used as the reference for the isoelectric line) when measured 0.08 seconds after the end of the QRS. If the myocardial injury is on the endocardial surface, the ST segment is depressed 1 mm or more for at least 0.08 seconds. The ST-segment depression is usually horizontal or has a downward slope (Wagner, 2001).

MI is classified as a Q-wave or non-Q-wave infarction. With Q-wave infarction, abnormal Q waves develop within 1 to 3 days because there is no depolarization current conducted from necrotic tissue (Wagner, 2001). The lead system then views the flow of current from other parts of the heart. An abnormal Q wave is 0.04 seconds or longer, 25% of the R-wave depth (provided the R wave exceeds a depth of 5 mm), or one that did not exist before the event (Wagner, 2001). An acute MI may cause a significant decrease in the height of the R wave. During an acute MI, injury and ischemic changes are also present. An abnormal Q wave may be present without ST-segment and T-wave changes, which indicates an old, not acute, MI. Patients with non-Q-wave MIs do not develop a Q wave on the ECG after the ST-segment and T-wave changes, but symptoms and cardiac enzyme analysis confirm the diagnosis of an MI.

During recovery from an MI, the ST segment often is the first to return to normal (1 to 6 weeks). The T wave becomes large and symmetric for 24 hours, and it then inverts within 1 to 3 days for 1 to 2 weeks. Q-wave alterations are usually permanent. An old Q-wave MI is usually indicated by an abnormal Q wave or decreased height of the R wave without ST-segment and T-wave changes.

ECHOCARDIOGRAM

The echocardiogram is used to evaluate ventricular function. It may be used to assist in diagnosing an MI, especially when the ECG is nondiagnostic. The echocardiogram can detect hypokinetic and akinetic wall motion and can determine the ejection fraction (see Chap. 26).

LABORATORY TESTS

Historically, laboratory tests used to diagnose an MI included **creatine kinase (CK)**, with evaluation of isoenzymes and lactic dehydrogenase (LDH) levels. Newer laboratory tests with faster results, resulting in earlier diagnosis, include myoglobin and troponin analysis. These tests are based on the release of cellular contents into the circulation when myocardial cells die. Table 28-5 shows the time courses of cardiac enzymes. An LDH test is now infrequently ordered because it is not useful in identifying cardiac events (Braunwald et al., 2000).

Creatine Kinase and Its Isoenzymes. There are three CK isoenzymes: CK-MM (skeletal muscle), CK-MB (heart muscle), and CK-BB (brain tissue). CK-MB is the cardiac-specific isoenzyme; CK-MB is found mainly in cardiac cells and therefore rises only when there has been damage to these cells. CK-MB assessed by mass assay is the most specific index for the diagnosis of acute MI (Braunwald et al., 2001). The level starts to increase within a few hours and peaks within 24 hours of an MI. If the area is reperfused (eg, due to thrombolytic therapy or PTCA), it peaks earlier.

Myoglobin. Myoglobin is a heme protein that helps to transport oxygen. Like CK-MB enzyme, myoglobin is found in cardiac and skeletal muscle. The myoglobin level starts to increase within 1 to 3 hours and peaks within 12 hours after the onset of symptoms.

Zone of ischemia

Zone of injury

Zone of infarction

Endocardium   Myocardium   Epicardium

FIGURE 28-4 Effects of ischemia, injury, and infarction on ECG recording. Ischemia causes inversion of T wave because of altered repolarization. Cardiac muscle injury causes elevation of the ST segment and tall, symmetrical T waves. With Q-wave infarction, Q or QS waves develop because of the absence of depolarization current from the necrotic tissue and opposing currents from other parts of the heart.

Table 28-5 • Serum Markers of Acute Myocardial Infarction

SERUM TEST		EARLIEST INCREASE (HR)	TEST RUNNING TIME (MIN)	PEAK (HR)	RETURN TO NORMAL
Total CK		3–6	30–60	24–36	3 days
CK-MB:	isoenzyme	4–8	30–60	12–24	3–4 days
	mass assay	2–3	30–60	10–18	3–4 days
Myoglobin		1–3	30–60	4–12	12 hr
Troponin T or I		3–4	30–60	4–24	1–3 wk

Resource assistance by June Price, Laboratory Manager, Kaiser Permanente.

The test takes only a few minutes to run. An increase in myoglobin is not very specific in indicating an acute cardiac event; however, negative results are an excellent parameter for ruling out an acute MI. If the first myoglobin test results are negative, the test may be repeated 3 hours later. Another negative test result confirms that the patient did not have an MI.

Troponin. **Troponin**, a protein found in the myocardium, regulates the myocardial contractile process. There are three isomers of troponin (C, I, and T). Because of the smaller size of this protein and the increased specificity of the troponins I and T for cardiac muscle, these tests are used more frequently to identify myocardial injury (unstable angina or acute MI). The increase in the level of troponin in the serum starts and peaks at approximately the same time as CK-MB. However, it remains elevated for a longer period, often up to 3 weeks, and it therefore cannot be used to identify subsequent extension or expansion of an MI.

Medical Management

The goal of medical management is to minimize myocardial damage, preserve myocardial function, and prevent complications. These goals are achieved by reperfusing the area with the emergency use of thrombolytic medications or PTCA. Minimizing myocardial damage is also accomplished by reducing myocardial oxygen demand and increasing oxygen supply with medications, oxygen administration, and bed rest. The resolution of pain and ECG changes are the primary clinical indicators that demand and supply are in equilibrium; they may also indicate reperfusion. Visualization of blood flow through an open vessel in the catheterization laboratory is evidence of reperfusion.

PHARMACOLOGIC THERAPY

The patient with an acute MI receives the same medications as the patient with unstable angina, with the possible additions of thrombolytics, analgesics, and angiotensin-converting enzyme (ACE) inhibitors. Patients should receive a beta-blocker initially, throughout the hospitalization, and a prescription to continue its use after hospital discharge.

Thrombolytics. Thrombolytics are medications that are usually administered intravenously, although some may also be given directly into the coronary artery in the cardiac catheterization laboratory (Chart 28-7). The purpose of thrombolytics is to dissolve and lyse the thrombus in a coronary artery (thrombolysis), allowing blood to flow through the coronary artery again (reperfusion), minimizing the size of the infarction, and preserving ventricular function. Even though thrombolytics may dissolve the thrombus, they do not affect the underlying atherosclerotic lesion. The patient may be referred for a cardiac catheterization and other invasive interventions.

Thrombolytics dissolve all clots, not just the one in the coronary artery. They should not be used if the patient has formed a protective clot, such as after major surgery or hemorrhagic stroke. Because thrombolytics reduce the patient's ability to form a stabilizing clot, the patient is at risk for bleeding. Thrombolytics should not be used if the patient is bleeding or has a bleeding disorder. All patients who receive thrombolytic therapy are placed on bleeding precautions to minimize the risk for bleeding. This means minimizing the number of punctures for inserting intravenous lines, avoiding intramuscular injections, preventing tissue trauma, and applying pressure for longer than usual after any puncture.

Chart 28-7 • Administration of Thrombolytic Therapy

Indications
- Chest pain for longer than 20 minutes, unrelieved by nitroglycerin
- ST-segment elevation in at least two leads that face the same area of the heart
- Less than 24 hours from onset of pain

Absolute Contraindications
- Active bleeding
- Known bleeding disorder
- History of hemorrhagic stroke
- History of intracranial vessel malformation
- Recent major surgery or trauma
- Uncontrolled hypertension
- Pregnancy

Nursing Considerations
- Minimize the number of times the patient's skin is punctured.
- Avoid intramuscular injections.
- Draw blood for laboratory tests when starting the IV line.
- Start IV lines before thrombolytic therapy; designate one line to use for blood draws.
- Avoid continual use of noninvasive blood pressure cuff.
- Monitor for acute dysrhythmias, hypotension, and allergic reaction.
- Monitor for reperfusion: resolution of angina or acute ST-segment changes.
- Check for signs and symptoms of bleeding: decrease in hematocrit and hemoglobin values, decrease in blood pressure, increase in heart rate, oozing or bulging at invasive procedure sites, back pain, muscle weakness, changes in level of consciousness, complaints of headache
- Treat major bleeding by discontinuing thrombolytic therapy and any anticoagulants; apply direct pressure and notify the physician immediately.
- Treat minor bleeding by applying direct pressure if accessible and appropriate; continue to monitor.

To be effective, thrombolytics must be administered as early as possible after the onset of symptoms that indicate an acute MI. They are not given to patients with unstable angina. Hospitals monitor their ability to administer these medications within 30 minutes from the time the patient arrives in the emergency department. This is called *door-to-needle time* (Ryan et al., 1999). The thrombolytic agents used most often are **streptokinase** (Kabikinase, Streptase), alteplase (Activase), and reteplase (r-PA, TNKase). Anistreplase (Eminase) is another thrombolytic agent that may be used.

Streptokinase increases the amount of plasminogen activator, which then increases the amount of circulating and clot-bound plasmin. Because streptokinase is made from a bacterium, its use also entails a risk of an allergic reaction. Vasculitis has occurred up to 9 days after administration. Streptokinase is not used if the patient has been exposed to a recent *Streptococcus* infection or has received streptokinase in the past 6 to 12 months.

Alteplase is a type of tissue plasminogen activator (t-PA). In contrast to streptokinase, alteplase activates the plasminogen on the clot more than the circulating plasminogen. Because it does not decrease the clotting factors as much as streptokinase, unfractionated or low molecular weight heparin is used with t-PA to prevent another clot from forming at the same lesion site. Because t-PA is a naturally occurring enzyme, allergic reactions are minimized, but t-PA costs considerably more than streptokinase.

Reteplase is structurally very similar to alteplase and has similar effects. Anistreplase is similar to streptokinase and has similar effects.

Analgesics. The analgesic of choice for acute MI is morphine sulfate (Duramorph, Astramorph) administered in intravenous boluses. Morphine reduces pain and anxiety. It reduces preload, which decreases the workload of the heart. Morphine also relaxes bronchioles to enhance oxygenation. The cardiovascular response to morphine is monitored carefully, particularly the blood pressure, which can be lowered, and the respiratory rate, which can be depressed. Because morphine decreases sensation of pain, ST-segment monitoring may be a better indicator of subsequent ischemia than assessment of pain.

Angiotensin-Converting Enzyme Inhibitors (ACE-I). Angiotensin I is formed when the kidneys release renin in response to decreased blood flow. Angiotensin I is converted to angiotensin II by ACE, a substance found in the lumen of all blood vessels, especially the pulmonary vasculature. Angiotensin II causes the blood vessels to constrict and the kidneys to retain sodium and fluid while excreting potassium. These actions increase circulating fluid and raise the pressure against which the heart must pump, resulting in significantly increased cardiac workload. **ACE inhibitors (ACE-I)** prevent the conversion of angiotensin from I to II. In the absence of angiotensin II, the blood pressure decreases and the kidneys excrete sodium and fluid (diuresis), decreasing the oxygen demand of the heart. Use of ACE inhibitors in patients after MI decreases the mortality rate and prevents the onset of heart failure. It is important to ensure that the patient is not hypotensive, hyponatremic, hypovolemic, or hyperkalemic before ACE-I administration. Blood pressure, urine output, and serum sodium, potassium, and creatinine levels need to be monitored closely.

EMERGENT PERCUTANEOUS CORONARY INTERVENTION (PCI)

The patient in whom an acute MI is suspected may be referred for an immediate PCI. PCI may be used to open the occluded coronary artery in an acute MI and promote reperfusion to the area that has been deprived of oxygen. PCI treats the underlying atherosclerotic lesion. Because the duration of oxygen deprivation is directly related to the number of cells that die, the time from the patient's arrival in the emergency department to the time PCI is performed should be less than 60 minutes (time is muscle). This is frequently referred to as *door-to-balloon time* (Smith et al., 2001). To perform an emergent PCI within this short time, a cardiac catheterization laboratory and staff must be available.

Cardiac Rehabilitation

After the MI patient is free of symptoms, an active rehabilitation program is initiated. Cardiac rehabilitation is a program that targets risk reduction by means of education, individual and group support, and physical activity. Most insurance programs, including Medicare, cover the cost of a cardiac rehabilitation program. However, some studies indicate that only 8% to 39% of patients who are candidates for cardiac rehabilitation services typically participate in these programs (Wenger et al., 1995; Williams et al., 2002).

The goals of rehabilitation for the patient with an MI are to extend and improve the quality of life. The immediate objectives are to limit the effects and progression of atherosclerosis, return the patient to work and a pre-illness lifestyle, enhance the psychosocial and vocational status of the patient, and prevent another cardiac event. These objectives are accomplished by encouraging physical activity and physical conditioning, educating patient and family, and providing counselling and behavioural interventions.

Throughout all phases of rehabilitation, the goals of activity and exercise tolerance are achieved through gradual physical conditioning, aimed at improving cardiac efficiency over time. Cardiac efficiency is achieved when work and activities of daily living can be performed at a lower heart rate and lower blood pressure, thereby reducing the heart's oxygen requirements and reducing cardiac workload.

Physical conditioning is achieved gradually over time. It is not unusual for patients to "overdo it" in an attempt to achieve their goals too rapidly. Patients are observed for chest pain, dyspnea, weakness, fatigue, and palpitations and are instructed to stop exercise if any of the symptoms develop. In a monitored program, they are also monitored for an increase in heart rate above the target heart rate, an increase in systolic or diastolic blood pressure more than 20 mm Hg, a decrease in systolic blood pressure, onset or worsening of dysrhythmias, or ST-segment changes on the ECG.

The target heart rate in phase I is an increase of less than 10% from the resting heart rate, or 120 beats per minute. In phase II, the target heart rate is based on the results of the patient's stress test (usually 60% to 85% of the heart rate at which symptoms occurred), medications, and underlying condition. Oxygen saturation may also be assessed to ensure that it remains higher than 93%. If signs or symptoms occur, the patient is instructed to slow down or stop exercising. If the patient is exercising in an unmonitored program, he or she is cautioned to cease activity immediately if signs or symptoms occur and to seek appropriate medical attention. Table 28-6 identifies conditions in which an unmonitored home exercise program is not recommended.

Patients who are able to walk at 3 to 4 miles per hour are usually able to resume sexual activities. The nurse recommends that the patient be well rested and in a familiar setting; wait at least 1 hour after eating or drinking alcohol; and use a comfortable position. The patient is cautioned against anal sex. Sexual dysfunction or cardiac symptoms should be reported to the health care provider.

PHASES OF CARDIAC REHABILITATION

Cardiac rehabilitation occurs along the continuum of the disease and is typically categorized in three phases. Phase I may begin with the diagnosis of atherosclerosis, which may occur when the

Table 28-6 • **Contraindications to Unsupervised Home Exercise**	
High-risk unstable angina (severe CAD)	Symptomatic severe aortic stenosis
Uncontrolled symptomatic dysrhythmia	Active pericarditis, myocarditis
Acute pulmonary embolism or infarction	High degree atrioventricular block
Acute aortic dissection	Resting diastolic BP > 110 mm Hg
Resting systolic BP > 200 mm Hg	Hypertrophic cardiomyopathy
Uncontrolled diabetes (BS > 400 mg/dL)	Active systemic illness or fever
Severe orthopedic problems	Orthostatic decrease in BP by ≥ 20 mm Hg
Uncompensated symptomatic HF	with symptoms

CAD, coronary artery disease; BS, blood sugar; BP, blood pressure; HF, heart failure; HR, heart rate.
Adapted from the American College of Cardiology Foundation and the American Heart Association (2002). *ACC/AHA 2002 Guideline Update for Exercise Testing: A report of the American College of Cardiology/American Heart Association Task Force on Practice Guidelines (Committee on Exercise Testing).* Available at: http://www.acc.org/clinical/guidelines/exercise. Accessed December 3, 2002.

patient is admitted to the hospital for ACS (unstable angina, acute MI). It consists of low-level activities and initial education for the patient and family. Because of the brief hospital stay, mobilization occurs earlier, and patient teaching is prioritized to the essentials of self-care, rather than instituting behavioural changes for risk reduction. Priorities for in-hospital education include the signs and symptoms that indicate the need to call 911 (seek emergency assistance), the medication regimen, rest-activity balance, and follow-up appointments with the physician. The nurse needs to reassure the patient that, although CAD is a lifelong disease and must be treated as such, most patients can resume a normal life after an MI. This positive approach while in the hospital helps to motivate and teach the patient to continue the education and lifestyle changes that are usually needed after discharge. The amount of activity recommended at discharge depends on the age of the patient, his or her condition before the cardiac event, the extent of the disease, the course of the hospital stay, and the development of any complications.

Phase II occurs after the patient has been discharged. It usually lasts for 4 to 6 weeks but may last up to 6 months. This outpatient program consists of supervised, often ECG-monitored, exercise training that is individualized based on the results of an exercise stress test. Support and guidance related to the treatment of the disease and education and counselling related to lifestyle modification for risk factor reduction are a significant part of this phase. Short-term and long-range goals are collaboratively determined based on the patient's needs. At each session, the patient is assessed for the effectiveness of and adherence to the current medical plan. To prevent complications and another hospitalization, the cardiac rehabilitation staff alerts the referring physician to any problems. Outpatient cardiac rehabilitation programs are designed to encourage patients and families to support each other. Many programs offer support sessions for spouses and significant others while the patients exercise. The programs involve group educational sessions for both patients and families that are given by cardiologists, exercise physiologists, dietitians, nurses, and other health care professionals. These sessions may take place outside a traditional classroom setting. For instance, a dietitian may take a group of patients and their families to a grocery store to examine labels and meat selections or to a restaurant to discuss menu offerings for a "heart-healthy" diet.

Phase III focuses on maintaining cardiovascular stability and long-term conditioning. The patient is usually self-directed during this phase and does not require a supervised program, although it may be offered. The goals of each phase build on the accomplishments of the previous phase.

NURSING PROCESS: THE PATIENT WITH MYOCARDIAL INFARCTION

Assessment

One of the most important aspects of care of the patient with an MI is the assessment. It establishes the baseline for the patient so that any deviations may be identified, systematically identifies the patient's needs, and helps determine the priority of those needs. Systematic assessment includes a careful history, particularly as it relates to symptoms: chest pain or discomfort, difficulty breathing (dyspnea), palpitations, unusual fatigue, faintness (syncope), or sweating (diaphoresis). Each symptom must be evaluated with regard to time, duration, the factors that precipitate the symptom and relieve it, and comparison with previous symptoms. A precise and complete physical assessment is critical to detect complications and any change in patient status. Chart 28-6 identifies important assessments and possible findings.

Intravenous sites are examined frequently. At least one and possibly two intravenous lines are placed for any patient with ACS to ensure that access is available for administering emergency medications. Medications are administered intravenously to achieve rapid onset and to allow for timely adjustment. Intramuscular medications are avoided because of unpredictable absorption, delayed effect, and the risk of causing elevated serum enzyme levels by injuring muscle cells with an injection. After the patient's condition stabilizes, the intravenous line may be changed into a saline lock to maintain intravenous access.

Diagnosis

NURSING DIAGNOSES

Based on the clinical manifestations, history, and diagnostic assessment data, the patient's major nursing diagnoses may include:

- Ineffective cardiopulmonary tissue perfusion related to reduced coronary blood flow from coronary thrombus and atherosclerotic plaque
- Potential impaired gas exchange related to fluid overload from left ventricular dysfunction
- Potential altered peripheral tissue perfusion related to decreased cardiac output from left ventricular dysfunction
- Anxiety related to fear of death
- Deficient knowledge about post-MI self-care

COLLABORATIVE PROBLEMS/ POTENTIAL COMPLICATIONS

Based on the assessment data, potential complications that may develop include the following:

- Acute pulmonary edema (see Chap. 30)
- Heart failure (see Chap. 30)
- Cardiogenic shock (see Chap. 30)
- Dysrhythmias and cardiac arrest (see Chaps. 27 and 30)
- Pericardial effusion and cardiac tamponade (see Chap. 30)
- Myocardial rupture (see Chap. 30)

Planning and Goals

The major goals of the patient include relief of pain or ischemic signs and symptoms (eg, ST-segment changes), prevention of further myocardial damage, absence of respiratory dysfunction, maintenance or attainment of adequate tissue perfusion by decreasing the heart's workload, reduced anxiety, adherence to the self-care program, and absence or early recognition of complications. Care of the patient with an uncomplicated MI is summarized in the Plan of Nursing Care on pages 735–737.

Nursing Interventions

RELIEVING PAIN AND OTHER SIGNS AND SYMPTOMS OF ISCHEMIA

Balancing the cardiac oxygen supply with its oxygen demand (eg, as evidenced by the relief of chest pain) is the top priority for the patient with an acute MI. Although medication therapy is required to accomplish this goal, nursing interventions are also important. Collaboration among the patient, nurse, and physician is critical in assessing the patient's response to therapy and in altering the interventions accordingly.

The accepted method for relieving symptoms associated with MI is revascularization with thrombolytic therapy or emergent PCI for patients who present to the health care facility immediately and who have no major contraindications. These therapies are important because, in addition to relieving symptoms, they aid in minimizing or avoiding permanent injury to the myocardium. With or without revascularization, administration of aspirin, intravenous beta-blocker, and nitroglycerin is indicated. Use of a GPIIb/IIIa agent or heparin may also be indicated. The nurse administers morphine for relief of pain and other symptoms, anxiety, and reduction of preload.

Oxygen should be administered along with medication therapy to assist with relief of symptoms. Administration of oxygen even in low doses raises the circulating level of oxygen to reduce pain associated with low levels of myocardial oxygen. The route of administration, usually by nasal cannula, and the oxygen flow rate are documented. A flow rate of 2 to 4 L/min is usually adequate to maintain oxygen saturation levels of 96% to 100% if no other disease is present.

Vital signs are assessed frequently as long as the patient is experiencing pain and other signs or symptoms of acute ischemia. Physical rest in bed with the backrest elevated or in a cardiac chair helps to decrease chest discomfort and dyspnea. Elevation of the head is beneficial for the following reasons:

- Tidal volume improves because of reduced pressure from abdominal contents on the diaphragm and better lung expansion and gas exchange.
- Drainage of the upper lung lobes improves.
- Venous return to the heart (preload) decreases, which reduces the work of the heart.

IMPROVING RESPIRATORY FUNCTION

Regular and careful assessment of respiratory function can help the nurse detect early signs of pulmonary complications. Scrupulous attention to fluid volume status prevents overloading the heart and lungs. Encouraging the patient to breathe deeply and change position frequently helps keep fluid from pooling in the bases of the lungs.

PROMOTING ADEQUATE TISSUE PERFUSION

Limiting the patient to bed or chair rest during the initial phase of treatment is particularly helpful in reducing myocardial oxygen consumption ($m\dot{V}O_2$). This limitation should remain until the patient is pain-free and hemodynamically stable. Checking skin temperature and peripheral pulses frequently is important to ensure adequate tissue perfusion. Oxygen may be administered to enrich the supply of circulating oxygen.

REDUCING ANXIETY

Alleviating anxiety and fears is an important nursing function to reduce the sympathetic stress response. Decreased sympathetic stimulation decreases the workload of the heart, which may relieve pain and other signs and symptoms of ischemia.

Developing a trusting and caring relationship with the patient is critical in reducing anxiety. Providing information to the patient and family in an honest and supportive manner invites the patient to be a partner in care and greatly assists in developing a positive relationship. Ensuring a quiet environment, preventing interruptions that disturb sleep, using a caring and appropriate touch, teaching the patient the relaxation response, using humour and assisting the patient to laugh, and providing the appropriate prayer book and assisting the patient to pray if consistent with the patient's beliefs are other nursing interventions that can be used to reduce anxiety. Frequent opportunities are provided for the patient to privately share concerns and fears. An atmosphere of acceptance helps the patient to know that these concerns and fears are both realistic and normal. Music therapy, in which the patient listens to selected music for a predetermined duration and at a set time, has been found to be an effective method for reducing anxiety and managing stress (Chlan & Tracy, 1999; Evans, 2002). Pet therapy, in which animals are brought to the patient, appears to provide emotional support and reduce anxiety. Administrative and infectious control practitioners are usually involved in developing standards for the animals, animal handlers, and patients who are eligible for pet therapy.

MONITORING AND MANAGING POTENTIAL COMPLICATIONS

Complications that can occur after acute MI are caused by the damage that occurs to the myocardium and to the conduction system as a result of the reduced coronary blood flow. Because these complications can be lethal, close monitoring for and early identification of the signs and symptoms is critical (see Plan of Nursing Care, pp. 735–737).

The nurse monitors the patient closely for changes in cardiac rate and rhythm, heart sounds, blood pressure, chest pain, respiratory status, urinary output, skin colour and temperature, sensorium, ECG changes, and laboratory values. Any changes in the patient's condition are reported promptly to the physician, and emergency measures are instituted when necessary.

PROMOTING HOME AND COMMUNITY-BASED CARE

Teaching Patients Self-Care

The most effective way to increase the probability the patient will implement a self-care regimen after discharge is to identify the

(text continues on page 737)

Plan of Nursing Care

Care of the Patient With an Uncomplicated Myocardial Infarction

Nursing Interventions	Rationale	Expected Outcomes

Nursing Diagnosis: Ineffective cardiopulmonary tissue perfusion related to reduced coronary blood flow
Goal: Relief of chest pain/discomfort

Nursing Interventions	Rationale	Expected Outcomes

1. Initially assess, document, and report to the physician the following:
 	
a. The patient's description of chest discomfort, including location, intensity, radiation, duration, and factors that affect it. Other symptoms such as nausea, diaphoresis, or complaints of unusual fatigue.
b. The effect of chest discomfort on cardiovascular perfusion—to the heart (eg, change in blood pressure, heart sounds), to the brain (eg, changes in LOC), to the kidneys (eg, decrease in urine output), and to the skin (eg, colour, temperature).
 	
2. Obtain a 12-lead ECG recording during the symptomatic event, as prescribed, to determine extension of infarction.
3. Administer oxygen as prescribed.
 	
4. Administer medication therapy as prescribed and evaluate the patient's response continuously.
 	
5. Ensure physical rest: use of the bedside commode with assistance; backrest elevated to promote comfort; diet as tolerated; arms supported during upper extremity activity; use of stool softener to prevent straining at stool. Provide a restful environment, and allay fears and anxiety by being supportive, calm, and competent. Individualized visitation, based on patient response.
	1. These data assist in determining the cause and effect of the chest discomfort and provide a baseline with which post-therapy symptoms can be compared.
	a. There are many conditions associated with chest discomfort. There are characteristic clinical findings of ischemic pain and symptoms.
	
	b. MI decreases myocardial contractility and ventricular compliance and may produce dysrhythmias. Cardiac output is reduced, resulting in reduced blood pressure and decreased organ perfusion. The heart rate may increase as a compensatory mechanism to maintain cardiac output.
	2. An ECG during symptoms may be useful in the diagnosis of an extension of MI.
	3. Oxygen therapy may increase the oxygen supply to the myocardium if actual oxygen saturation is less than normal.
	4. Medication therapy is the first line of defense in preserving myocardial tissue. The side effects of these medications can be hazardous and the patient's status must be assessed.
	5. Physical rest reduces myocardial oxygen consumption. Fear and anxiety precipitate the stress response; this results in increased levels of endogenous catecholamines, which increase myocardial oxygen consumption. Also, with increased epinephrine, the pain threshold is decreased, and pain increases myocardial oxygen consumption.
		• Reports beginning relief of chest discomfort and symptoms at once
		• Appears comfortable and pain or symptom free:
		  Is rested
		  Respiratory rate, cardiac rate, and blood pressure return to prediscomfort level
		  Skin warm and dry
		• Adequate cardiac output as evidenced by:
		  Heart rate and rhythm
		  Blood pressure
		  Mentation
		  Urine output
		  Serum BUN and creatinine
		  Skin colour, temperature, and moisture
		• Is pain and symptom free

Nursing Diagnosis: Potential ineffective air exchange related to fluid overload
Goal: Absence of respiratory difficulties

Nursing Interventions	Rationale	Expected Outcomes
1. Initially, every 4 hours, and with chest discomfort or symptoms, assess, document, and report to the physician abnormal heart sounds (particularly S_3 and S_4 gallops and the holosystolic murmur of left ventricular papillary muscle dysfunction), abnormal breath sounds (particularly crackles), and patient intolerance to specific activities.	1. These data are useful in diagnosing left ventricular failure. Diastolic filling sounds (S_3 and S_4 gallop) result from decreased left ventricular compliance associated with MI. Papillary muscle dysfunction (from infarction of the papillary muscle) can result in mitral regurgitation and a reduction in stroke volume, leading to left ventricular failure. The presence of crackles (usually at the lung bases) may indicate pulmonary	• No shortness of breath, dyspnea on exertion, orthopnea, or paroxysmal nocturnal dyspnea • Respiratory rate less than 20 breaths/min with physical activity and 16 breaths/min with rest • Skin colour normal • PaO_2 and $PaCO_2$ within normal range • Heart rate less than 100 beats/min and greater than 60 beats/min, with blood pressure within patient's normal limits

(continued)

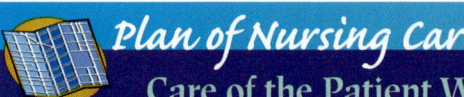

Plan of Nursing Care

Care of the Patient With an Uncomplicated Myocardial Infarction (*Continued*)

Nursing Interventions	Rationale	Expected Outcomes

	congestion from increased left heart pressures. The association of symptoms and activity can be used as a guide for activity prescription and a basis for patient teaching.	• Chest x-ray normal
		• Relief of chest discomfort
		• Appears comfortable:
		  Appears rested
		  Respiratory rate, cardiac rate, and blood
		    pressure return to prediscomfort level
		  Skin warm and dry

2. Teach patient:
  a. To adhere to the diet prescribed (for example, explain low-sodium, low-calorie diet)
 	
  b. To adhere to activity prescription
	2.
	
	  a. Low-sodium diet may reduce extracellular volume, thus reducing preload and afterload, and thus myocardial oxygen consumption. In the obese patient, weight reduction may decrease cardiac work and improve tidal volume.
	  b. The activity prescription is determined individually to maintain the heart rate and blood pressure within safe limits.	

Nursing Diagnosis: Potential ineffective peripheral tissue perfusion related to decreased cardiac output
Goal: Maintenance/attainment of adequate tissue perfusion

1. Initially, every 4 hours, and with chest discomfort, assess, document, and report to the physician the following:
  a. Hypotension
  b. Tachycardia and other dysrhythmia
  c. Activity intolerance
  d. Mentation changes (use family input)
  e. Reduced urine output (less than 200 mL per 8 hours)
  f. Cool, moist, cyanotic extremities
	1. These data are useful in determining a low cardiac output state. An ECG with pain may be useful in the diagnosis of an extension of myocardial ischemia, injury, and infarction, and of variant angina.	• Blood pressure within the patient's normal range
		• Ideally, normal sinus rhythm without dysrhythmia is maintained, or patient's baseline rhythm is maintained between 60 and 100 beats/min without further dysrhythmia.
		• No complaints of fatigue with prescribed activity
		• Remains fully alert and oriented and without cognitive or behavioural change
		• Appears comfortable
		  Appears rested
		    Respiratory rate, cardiac rate, and blood pressure return to prediscomfort level
		    Skin warm and dry
		• Urine output greater than 25 mL/hr
		• Extremities warm and dry with normal colour

Nursing Diagnosis: Anxiety related to fear of death, change in health status
Goal: Reduction of anxiety

1. Assess, document, and report to the physician the patient's and family's level of anxiety and coping mechanisms.	1. These data provide information about the psychological well-being and a baseline so that post-therapy symptoms can be compared. Causes of anxiety are variable and individual, and may include acute illness, hospitalization, pain, disruption of activities of daily living at home and at work, changes in role and self-image due to chronic illness, and lack of financial support. Because anxious family members can transmit anxiety to the patient, the nurse must also identify strategies to reduce the family's fear and anxiety.	• Reports less anxiety • Patient and family discuss their anxieties and fears about death • Patient and family appear less anxious • Appears restful, respiratory rate less than 16/min, heart rate less than 100/min without ectopic beats, blood pressure within patient's normal limits, skin warm and dry • Participates actively in a progressive rehabilitation program • Practices stress reduction techniques

(*continued*)

Plan of Nursing Care

Care of the Patient With an Uncomplicated Myocardial Infarction (*Continued*)

Nursing Interventions	Rationale	Expected Outcomes
2. Assess the need for spiritual counselling and refer as appropriate.	2. If a patient finds support in a religion, religious counselling may assist in reducing anxiety and fear.	
3. Allow patient (and family) to express anxiety and fear: a. By showing genuine interest and concern b. By facilitating communication (listening, reflecting, guiding) c. By answering questions	3. Unresolved anxiety (the stress response) increases myocardial oxygen consumption.	
4. Use of flexible visiting hours allows the presence of a supportive family to assist in reducing the patient's level of anxiety.	4. The presence of supportive family members may reduce both patient's and family's anxiety.	
5. Encourage active participation in a cardiac rehabilitation program.	5. Prescribed cardiac rehabilitation may help to eliminate fear of death, reduce anxiety, and enhance feelings of well-being.	
6. Teach stress reduction techniques.	6. Stress reduction may help to reduce myocardial oxygen consumption and may enhance feelings of well-being.	

Nursing Diagnosis: Deficient knowledge about post-MI self-care
Goal: Adheres to the home health care program
Chooses lifestyle consistent with heart-healthy recommendations.

(See Chart 28-8, Promoting Health After MI)

priorities as perceived by the patient, provide adequate education about heart-healthy living, and facilitate the patient's involvement in a cardiac rehabilitation program. Working with patients in developing plans to meet their specific needs further enhances the potential for an effective treatment plan (Chart 28-8).

Evaluation

EXPECTED PATIENT OUTCOMES

Expected patient outcomes may include the following:

1. Relief of angina
2. No signs of respiratory difficulties
3. Adequate tissue perfusion
4. Decreased anxiety
5. Adherence to a self-care program
6. Absence of complications

Invasive Coronary Artery Procedures

INVASIVE INTERVENTIONAL PROCEDURES

Angina pectoris may persist for many years in a stable form with brief attacks. However, unstable angina is a serious condition that can progress to MI or sudden cardiac death (ACS). Invasive interventional procedures to treat angina and CAD are PTCA, intracoronary stent implantation, atherectomy, brachytherapy, and transmyocardial laser revascularization. All of these procedures are classified as **percutaneous coronary interventions (PCIs)**.

Percutaneous Transluminal Coronary Angioplasty (PTCA)

PTCA may be used to treat patients who do not experience angina but are at high risk for a cardiac event as identified by non-invasive testing, with recurrent chest pain that is unresponsive to medical therapy, with a significant amount of myocardium at risk but are poor surgical candidates, or with an acute MI (as an alternate to thrombolysis and after thrombolysis) (Smith et al., 2001). The procedure is attempted when the cardiologist believes that PTCA can improve blood flow to the myocardium. PTCA alone is seldom attempted in the patient with occlusions of the left main coronary artery that do not demonstrate **collateral circulation** to the left anterior descending and circumflex arteries. The purpose of PTCA is to improve blood flow within a coronary artery by "cracking" the atheroma.

This invasive interventional procedure is carried out in the cardiac catheterization laboratory. The coronary arteries are examined by angiography, as they are during the diagnostic cardiac catheterization, and the location, extent, and calcification of the atheroma are verified. Hollow catheters, called sheaths, are inserted, usually in the femoral vein or artery (or both), providing a conduit for other catheters. After the presence of atheroma is verified, a balloon-tipped dilation catheter is passed through the sheath along a guide catheter and positioned over the lesion. The physician determines the catheter position by examining markers on the balloon that can be seen with fluoroscopy. When the catheter is properly positioned, the balloon is inflated with a radiopaque contrast agent (commonly called *dye*) to visualize the

---

Chart 28-8

Promoting Health After Myocardial Infarction and Other Acute Coronary Syndromes

To extend and improve the quality of life, a patient who has had an MI must learn to adjust his or her lifestyle to promote heart-healthy living. With this in mind, the nurse and patient develop a program to help the patient achieve desired outcomes.

Changing Lifestyle During Convalescence and Healing

Adaptation to a heart attack is an ongoing process and usually requires some modification of lifestyle. Some specific modifications include:

- Avoiding any activity that produces chest pain, extreme dyspnea, or undue fatigue
- Avoiding extremes of heat and cold and walking against the wind
- Losing weight, if indicated
- Stopping smoking and use of tobacco; avoiding second-hand smoke
- Using personal strengths to support lifestyle changes
- Developing heart-healthy eating patterns and avoiding large meals and hurrying while eating
- Modifying meals to align with the Therapeutic Lifestyle Changes (TLC) or the Dietary Approaches to Stopping Hypertension (DASH) diet
- Adhering to medical regimen, especially in taking medications
- Following recommendations that ensure blood pressure and blood glucose are in control
- Pursuing activities that relieve and reduce stress

Adopting an Activity Program

Additionally, the patient needs to undertake an *orderly* program of increasing activity and exercise for long-term rehabilitation as follows:

- Engaging in a regimen of physical conditioning with a gradual increase in activity duration and then a gradual increase in activity intensity
- Walking daily, increasing distance and time as prescribed
- Monitoring pulse rate during physical activity until the maximum level of activity is attained
- Avoiding activities that tense the muscles: isometric exercise, weight-lifting, any activity that requires sudden bursts of energy
- Avoiding physical exercise immediately after a meal
- Alternating activity with rest periods (some fatigue is normal and expected during convalescence)
- Participating in a daily program of exercise that develops into a program of regular exercise for a lifetime

Managing Symptoms

The patient must learn to recognize and take appropriate action for possible recurrences of symptoms as follows:

- Call 911 if chest pressure or pain (or anginal equivalent) is not relieved in 15 minutes by nitroglycerin
- Contacting the physician if any of the following occur: shortness of breath, fainting, slow or rapid heartbeat, swelling of feet and ankles

---

blood vessel and to provide a steady or oscillating pressure within the balloon. The balloon is inflated to a certain pressure for several seconds and then deflated. The pressure "cracks" and possibly compresses the atheroma (Fig. 28-5). The coronary artery's media and adventitia are also stretched.

Several inflations and several balloon sizes may be required to achieve the desired goal, usually defined as an improvement in blood flow and a residual stenosis of less than 20%. Other gauges of the success of a PTCA are an increase in the artery's lumen, a difference of less than 20 mm Hg in blood pressure from one side

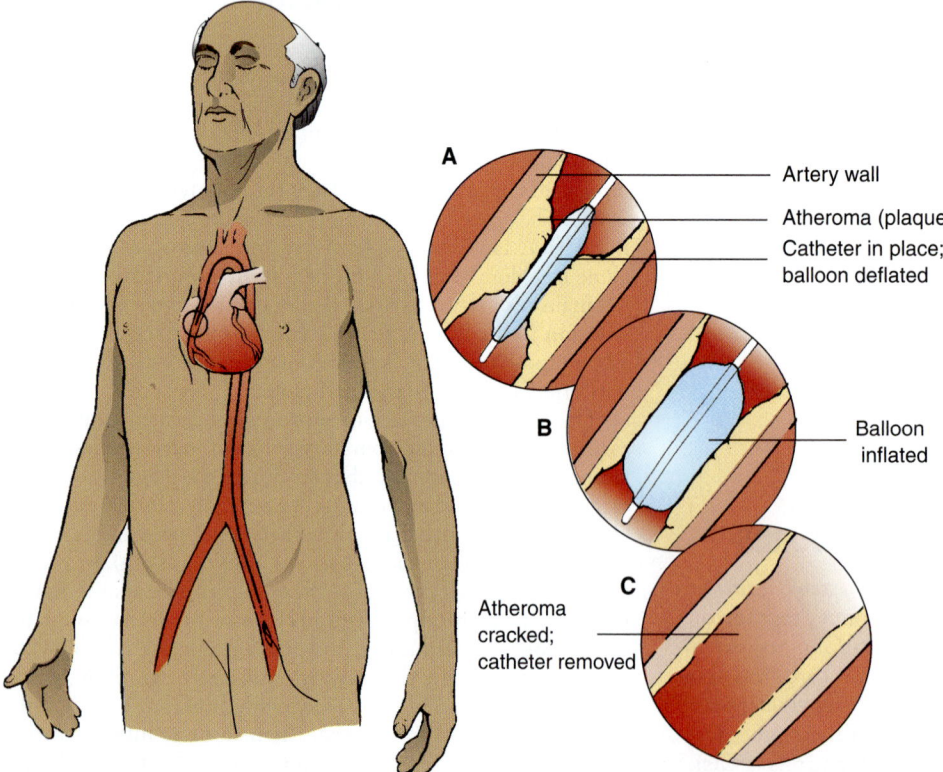

A — Artery wall
— Atheroma (plaque)
— Catheter in place; balloon deflated

B — Balloon inflated

C
Atheroma cracked; catheter removed

FIGURE 28-5 Percutaneous transluminal coronary angioplasty. (**A**) A balloon-tipped catheter is passed into the affected coronary artery and placed across the area of the atheroma (plaque). (**B**) The balloon is then rapidly inflated and deflated with controlled pressure. (**C**) After the atheroma is cracked, the catheter is removed, and blood flow improves.

of the lesion to the other, and no clinically obvious arterial trauma. Because the blood supply to the coronary artery decreases while the balloon is inflated, the patient may complain of chest pain (often called *stretch pain*), and the ECG may display significant ST-segment changes (Jeremias et al., 1998).

COMPLICATIONS

Possible complications during the PTCA procedure include dissection, perforation, abrupt closure, or vasospasm of the coronary artery, acute MI, acute dysrhythmias (eg, ventricular tachycardia), and cardiac arrest. These may require emergency surgical treatment. Complications after the procedure may include abrupt closure and vascular complications, such as bleeding at the insertion site, retroperitoneal bleeding, hematoma, pseudoaneurysm, arteriovenous fistula, or arterial thrombosis and distal embolization (Table 28-7).

POSTPROCEDURE CARE

Patient care is similar to that for a cardiac catheterization (see Chapter 26). Many patients are admitted to the hospital the day of the PTCA. Those with no complications go home the next day. During the PTCA, patients receive large amounts of heparin and are monitored closely for signs of bleeding. Most patients also receive intravenous nitroglycerin for a period after the procedure to prevent arterial spasm.

Hemostasis is usually achieved and sheaths are pulled immediately at the end of the procedure by using a vascular closure device (eg, Angio-Seal, VasoSeal, Duett, Syvek patch) or a device that sutures the vessels (Prostar, Perclose). Hemostasis after sheath removal may also be achieved by direct manual pressure, a mechanical compression device (eg, C-shaped clamp), or a pneumatic compression device (eg, FemStop).

The patient may return to the nursing unit with the large peripheral vascular access sheaths in place. The sheaths are removed after blood studies (eg, activated clotting time) indicate that the clotting time is within an acceptable range. This usually takes a few hours, depending on the amount of heparin given during the procedure. The patient must remain flat in bed and keep the affected leg straight until the sheaths are removed and then for a few hours after to maintain hemostasis. Because the immobility and bed rest usually cause the patient significant discomfort, treatment includes analgesics and sedation.

Several nursing interventions frequently used as part of the standard of care, such as applying a sandbag to the sheath insertion site, have not been shown to be effective in reducing the incidence of bleeding (Christensen et al., 1998; Juran et al., 1999). The method used to achieve hemostasis determines the length of time needed to achieve hemostasis, the duration of bed rest, and the risk of complications (Brachmann et al., 1998; Lehmann et al., 1999; Walker et al., 2001). Sheath removal and the application of pressure on the vessel insertion site may cause the heart rate to slow and the blood pressure to decrease (vasovagal response). An intravenous bolus of atropine is usually used to treat these side effects.

Some patients with unstable lesions and at high risk for abrupt vessel closure are restarted on heparin after sheath removal, or they receive an intravenous infusion of a GPIIb/IIIa inhibitor. These patients are monitored more closely and progressed more slowly.

After hemostasis is achieved, patients usually can be weaned from the intravenous medications, resume self-care, and ambulate unassisted within 1 to 12 hours of the procedure. The duration of immobilization depends on the size of the sheath inserted, the amount of anticoagulant administered, the method of hemostasis, the patient's underlying condition, and the physician's preference. The nurse teaches the patient to monitor the site for bleeding or development of a hard lump that is larger than a walnut. Most patients can return to their usual activities of daily living.

Table 28-7 • Complications After Percutaneous Transluminal Coronary Angioplasty (PTCA)

COMPLICATION	SIGNS AND SYMPTOMS	POSSIBLE CAUSES	NURSING ACTIONS
Bleeding or hematoma	Hard lump or bluish tinge at sheath insertion site	Coughing, vomiting, bending leg or hip, obesity, bladder distention, high blood pressure	Keep the head of the bed flat. Insert indwelling urinary catheter if needed. Apply manual pressure at site of sheath insertion. Outline extent of hematoma with a marking pen. If bleeding does not stop, notify physician or nurse practitioner.
Lost or weakened pulse distal to sheath insertion site	Extremity cool, cyanotic, pale, or painful	Arterial thrombus or embolus	Notify physician or nurse practitioner. Anticipate surgery and anticoagulation or thrombolytic therapy.
Pseudoaneurysm and arteriovenous fistula	Pulsatile mass felt or bruit heard near sheath insertion site	Vessel trauma during procedure	Notify physician or nurse practitioner. Anticipate ultrasound-guided compression. Prepare patient for surgery to close fistula.
Retroperitoneal bleeding	Back or flank pain, Low blood pressure, Tachycardia, Restlessness and agitation, Decreased hemoglobin, Decreased hematocrit	Arterial tear causing bleeding into flank area	Notify physician or nurse practitioner immediately. Stop any anticoagulation medication. Anticipate need for intravenous fluids and/or administration of blood.

Courtesy of Washington Adventist Hospital. Care of the interventional cardiology patient nursing protocol, based on communication from Amy Dukovic, Cardiac Interventional Nurse Practitioner.

Coronary Artery Stent

After PTCA, a portion of the plaque that was not removed may block the artery. The coronary artery may recoil (constrict) and the tissue remodels, increasing the risk for restenosis (Apple & Lindsay, 2000). A coronary artery stent is placed to overcome these risks. A **stent** is a woven mesh that provides structural support to a vessel at risk of acute closure. The stent is placed over the angioplasty balloon. When the balloon is inflated, the mesh expands and presses against the vessel wall, holding the artery open. The balloon is withdrawn, but the stent is left permanently in place within the artery (Fig. 28-6). Eventually, endothelium covers the stent and it is incorporated into the vessel wall. Because of the risk of thrombus formation in the stent, the patient receives antiplatelet medications (eg, clopidogrel [Plavix] therapy for 2 weeks and lifetime use of aspirin). Some stents have medication which may minimize the formation of thrombi or excessive scar tissue. It is estimated that 50% to 80% of all PCIs involve implanting at least one stent (Braunwald et al., 2001; Smith et al., 2001). Stents may be used in conjunction with PTCA or independently as a PCI. Use of stents without PTCA may decrease procedure time, use of the potentially nephrotoxic contrast agent, radiation exposure, and cost (Apple & Lindsay, 2000). Care of the patient after coronary artery stent placement is the same as for a patient after PTCA.

Atherectomy

Atherectomy is an invasive interventional procedure that involves the removal of the atheroma, or plaque, from a coronary artery (Smith et al., 2001). Directional (DCA) and transluminal extraction (TEC) coronary atherectomy procedures involve the use of a catheter that removes the lesion and its fragments. Rotational atherectomy uses a catheter with diamond chips impregnated on the tip (called a burr) that rotates like a dentist's drill at 130,000 to 180,000 rpm, pulverizing the lesion (Braunwald et al., 2001). Usually, several passes of these catheters are needed to achieve satisfactory results. Postprocedural patient care is the same as for a patient after PTCA.

Brachytherapy

PTCA and stent implantation cause a cellular reaction in the coronary artery that promotes proliferation of the intima of the artery, which also increases the possibility of arterial obstruction. Brachytherapy reduces the recurrence of obstruction, preventing vessel restenosis by inhibiting smooth muscle cell proliferation (Leon et al., 2001). Brachytherapy (from the Greek word, *brachys,* meaning *short*) involves the delivery of gamma or beta radiation by placing a radioisotope close to the lesion (Teirstein & Kuntz, 2001). The radioisotope may be delivered by a catheter or implanted with the stent. Long-term studies are needed to identify if the beneficial effects of radiation therapy are sustained and to determine the optimal dose and type of isotope to use for brachytherapy.

Transmyocardial Revascularization

Patients who have cardiac ischemia and who are not candidates for CABG may benefit from transmyocardial laser revascularization (TMR) (Burkhoff et al., 1999). The procedure may be performed percutaneously in the cardiac catheterization laboratory (percutaneous transmyocardial revascularization [PTMR]) or through a midsternal or thoracotomy incision in the operating room (Acorda et al., 2000). The tip of a fibreoptic catheter is held firmly against the ischemic area of the heart while a laser burns a channel into but not through the muscle. If the procedure is percutaneous, the catheter is positioned inside the ventricle. If the procedure is surgical, the catheter is positioned on the outer surface of the ventricle. Each procedure usually involves making 20 to 40 channels. It is thought that some blood flows into the channels, decreasing the ischemia directly. Within the next few days to months, the channels close as a result of the body's inflammatory process of healing a wound (Platek & Atzori, 1999). The long-term result is the formation of new blood vessels (angiogenesis) during the inflammatory process that follows the laser burns (Anderson, 2000; Braunwald et al., 2001; Fuster et al., 2001; Hayden, 1998; Platek, & Atzori, 1999). The new blood vessels provide enough blood to decrease the symptoms of cardiac ischemia. Nursing care before, during, and after the procedure depends on the approach: if the approach was percutaneous, the patient care is the same as following a PTCA; if the approach was surgical, the patient care is the same as following CABG.

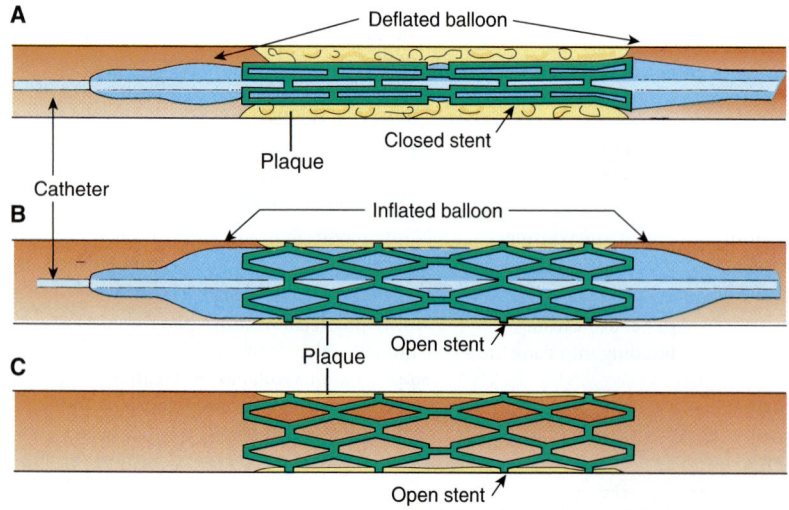

FIGURE 28-6 Intracoronary artery stent. (**A**) Stent closed, before balloon inflation. (**B**) Stent open, balloon inflated; stent will remain expanded after balloon is deflated and removed. (**C**) Stent open, balloon removed.

SURGICAL PROCEDURES

Coronary Artery Revascularization

Advances in diagnostics, medical management, surgical and anesthesia techniques, and cardiopulmonary bypass (CPB), as well as the care provided in critical care and surgical units, home care, and rehabilitation programs, have helped make surgery a viable treatment option for patients with cardiac disease. CAD has been treated by some form of myocardial revascularization since the 1960s; the most common CABG techniques have been performed for approximately 35 years. CABG is a surgical procedure in which a blood vessel from another part of the body is grafted to the occluded coronary artery so that blood can flow beyond the occlusion; it is also called a *bypass graft*.

Candidates for CABG are usually patients with the following conditions (Eagle et al., 1999):

- Angina that cannot be controlled by medical therapies
- Unstable angina
- A positive exercise tolerance test and lesions or blockage that cannot be treated by PCI
- A left main coronary artery lesion or blockage of more than 60%
- Blockage of two or three coronary arteries, one of which is the proximal left anterior descending artery
- Left ventricular dysfunction with blockages in two or more coronary arteries
- Complications from or unsuccessful PCIs

For a patient to be considered for CABG, the coronary arteries to be bypassed must have at least a 70% occlusion (60% if it is the left main coronary artery). If the lesion involves less than 70% of the artery, enough blood can flow through the blocked artery to prevent adequate blood flow through the bypass graft. As a result, the graft would clot, effectively negating the surgery.

The vessel most commonly used for CABG is the greater saphenous vein, followed by the lesser saphenous vein (Fig. 28-7). Cephalic and basilic veins are used also. The vein is removed from the leg (or arm) and grafted to the ascending aorta and to the coronary artery distal to the lesion. The saphenous veins are used in emergency CABG procedures because they can be obtained by one surgical team while another team performs the chest surgery. One side effect of using a large vein is edema, which may develop in the extremity from which it was taken. The degree of edema varies and may diminish over time. Approximately 5 to 10 years after CABG, symptomatic atherosclerotic changes develop in saphenous veins used for grafting. In arm veins, the same changes develop more quickly, approximately 3 to 6 years after the surgery.

The right and left internal mammary arteries and, occasionally, radial arteries are also used for CABG. Arterial grafts are preferred to vein grafts because they do not develop atherosclerotic changes as quickly and remain patent longer. In general, the surgeon leaves the proximal end of the mammary artery intact and detaches the distal end of the artery from the chest wall. This distal end of the artery is then grafted to the coronary artery distal to the occlusion. Disadvantages of using the internal mammary arteries are that they may not be long enough or wide enough for the bypass and ulnar nerve damage may result.

The gastroepiploic artery (located along the greater curvature of the stomach) may also be used, although it does not respond as well when used as a graft. It has a more extensive blood supply to its wall than the internal mammary arteries, making dissection from the stomach difficult and increasing the potential for injury

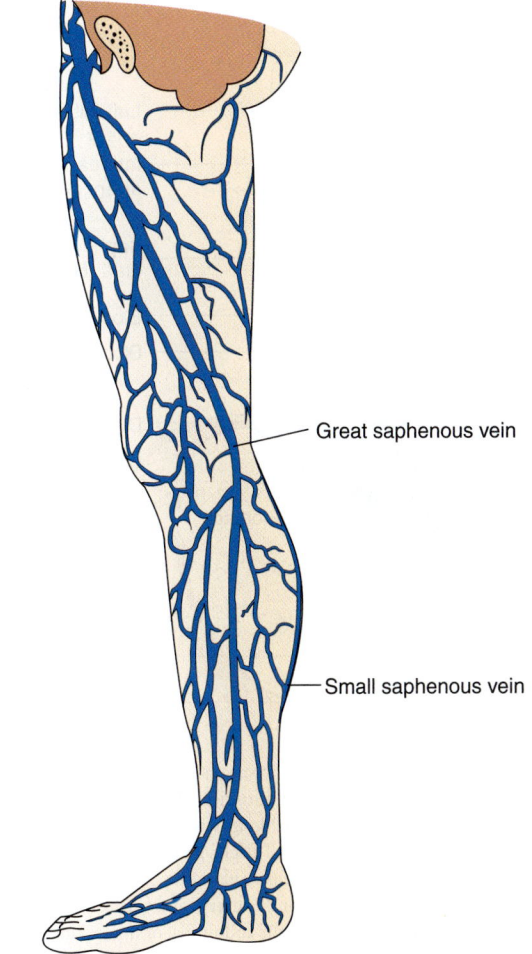

FIGURE 28-7 The greater and lesser saphenous veins are the vessels most commonly used in bypass graft procedures.

- Great saphenous vein
- Small saphenous vein

and ischemia of the graft. Use of the gastroepiploic artery requires the surgeon to extend the chest incision to the abdomen, thereby exposing the patient to the additional risks of an abdominal incision and infection at the surgical site from contamination by the gastrointestinal tract.

TRADITIONAL CORONARY ARTERY BYPASS GRAFT

The traditional CABG procedure is performed with the patient under general anesthesia. Usually, the surgeon makes a median sternotomy incision and connects the patient to the CPB machine. Next, a blood vessel from another part of the patient's body (eg, saphenous vein, left internal mammary artery) is grafted distal to the coronary artery lesion, bypassing the obstruction (Fig. 28-8). CPB is then discontinued and the incision is closed. The patient then is admitted to a critical care unit.

Cardiopulmonary Bypass (CPB). Many cardiac surgical procedures are possible because of CPB (ie, extracorporeal circulation). The procedure mechanically circulates and oxygenates blood for the body while bypassing the heart and lungs. CPB uses a heart-lung machine to maintain perfusion to other body organs and tissues while the surgeon works in a bloodless surgical field.

CPB, a common but complex technique, is accomplished by placing a cannula in the right atrium, vena cava, or femoral vein

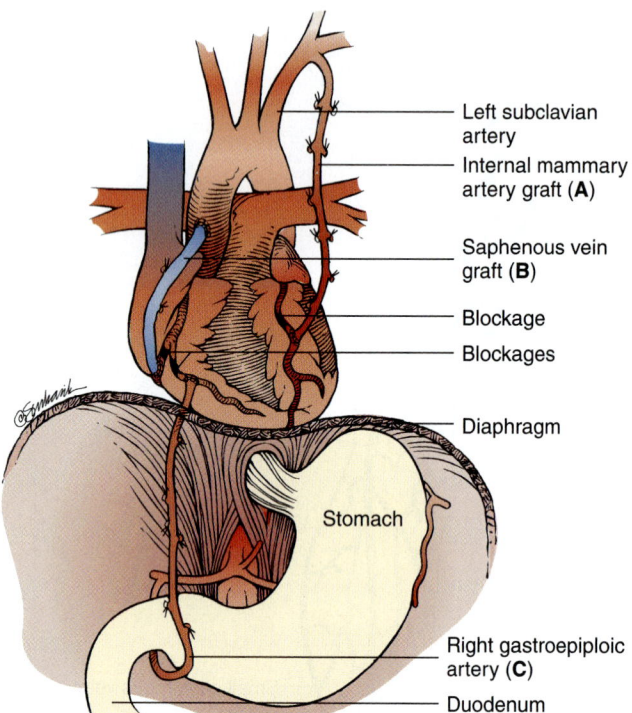

FIGURE 28-8 Three coronary artery bypass grafts. One or more procedures may be performed using various veins and arteries. (**A**) Left internal mammary artery, popular because of its functional longevity. (**B**) Saphenous vein, the most frequently constructed bypass. (**C**) Right gastroepiploic artery, rarely used because this artery has a more extensive blood supply to its wall (increasing the risk of bleeding and necrosis of the artery) and because of the risk of gastrointestinal tract contamination of the abdominal or mediastinal wound.

to withdraw blood from the body. The cannula is connected to tubing filled with an isotonic crystalloid solution (usually 5% dextrose in lactated Ringer's solution). Venous blood removed from the body by the cannula is filtered, oxygenated, cooled or warmed, and then returned to the body. The cannula used to return the oxygenated blood is usually inserted in the ascending aorta, but it may be inserted in the femoral artery (Fig. 28-9).

The patient receives heparin, an anticoagulant, to prevent thrombus formation and possible embolization that may occur when blood contacts the foreign surfaces of the CPB circuit and is pumped into the body by a mechanical pump (not the normal blood vessels and heart). After the patient is disconnected from the bypass machine, protamine sulfate is administered to reverse the effects of heparin.

During the procedure, hypothermia is maintained, usually 28°C to 32°C (82.4°F to 89.6°F). The blood is cooled during CPB and returned to the body. The cooled blood slows the body's basal metabolic rate, thereby decreasing its demand for oxygen. Cooled blood usually has a higher viscosity, but the crystalloid solution used to prime the bypass tubing dilutes the blood. When the surgical procedure is completed, the blood is rewarmed as it passes through the CPB circuit. Urine output, blood pressure, arterial blood gas measurements, electrolytes, coagulation studies, and the ECG are monitored to assess the patient's status during CPB.

MINIMALLY INVASIVE DIRECT CABG (MIDCAB)

For patients with single coronary artery blockages who cannot be treated by PTCA or with contraindications for CPB, an alternative to traditional CABG is minimally invasive direct CABG (MIDCAB). With the patient under general anesthesia, the surgeon makes one or more 2- to 4-inch (5- to 10-cm) incisions in

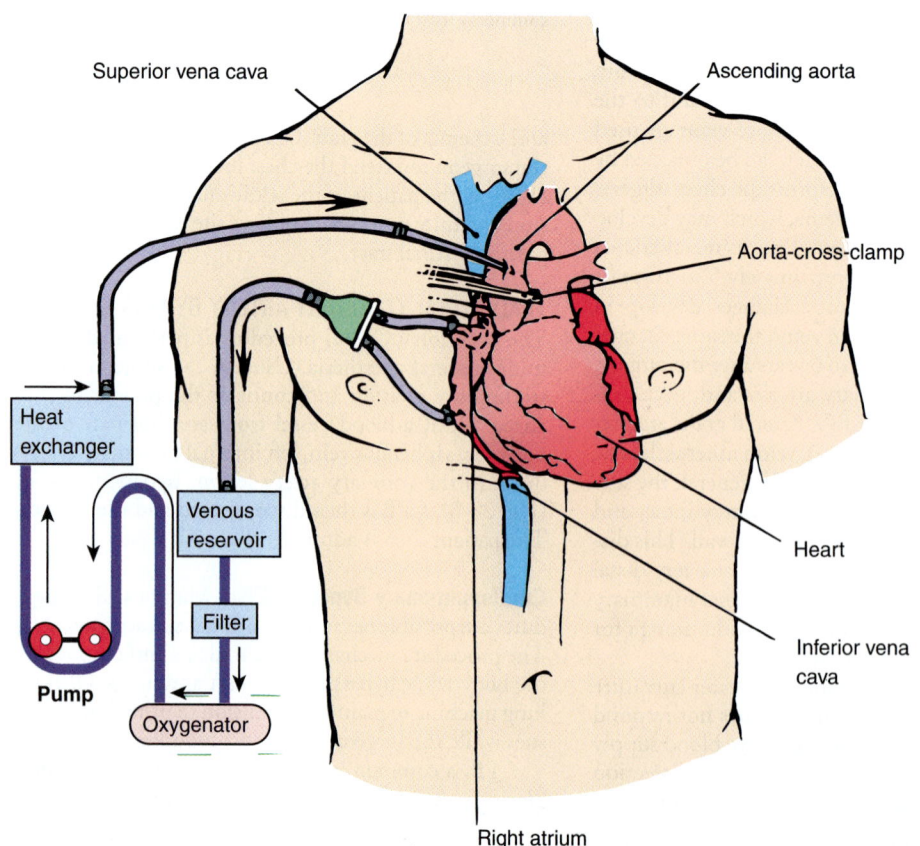

FIGURE 28-9 The cardiopulmonary bypass system, in which cannulae are placed through the right atrium into the superior and inferior vena cavae to divert blood from the body and into the bypass system. The pump system creates a vacuum, pulling blood into the venous reservoir. The blood is cleared of air bubbles, clots, and particulates by the filter, and then is passed through the oxygenator, releasing carbon dioxide and obtaining oxygen. Next, the blood is pulled to the pump and pushed out to the heat exchanger, where its temperature is regulated. The blood is then returned to the body via the ascending aorta.

the chest wall for a left or right anterior thoracotomy or for a midsternal or midline upper laparotomy. The graft is prepared for the bypass (see previous graft selection description). The surgeon identifies the location of the coronary artery for the CAB, and a special instrument, a myocardial stabilizer, is put around the site. The stabilizer holds the graft site still for the surgeon while the heart continues to beat. Other techniques to minimize movement of the beating heart are to temporarily collapse the lung on the side of the chest where the surgery is being performed, decrease the respiratory rate and the volume of each breath, and give medications to cause bradycardia or up to 20 seconds of asystole.

Patients treated with MIDCAB may recover from anesthesia in the postanesthesia care unit (PACU) and then be admitted to a telemetry unit for 1 to 3 days. Nursing care is often directed toward routine postoperative pulmonary interventions (especially if a lung was collapsed during the MIDCAB) and incisional pain management (especially if a thoracotomy incision was made).

PORT ACCESS CORONARY ARTERY BYPASS GRAFT

Port access CABG is another alternative to traditional CABG. With the patient under general anesthesia, the surgeon makes three or more incisions (ports) to perform the CABG. One 1.3- to 2.5-cm incision in the groin provides access to a femoral artery and vein. The femoral artery is used for a multipurpose catheter threaded retrograde through the aorta to the ascending aorta. The catheter is used to return blood from CPB to the patient, to occlude the aorta by inflating a balloon near the end of the catheter, to provide a cardioplegia solution to the coronary arteries, and to vent air from the aortic root during the surgical procedure. The femoral vein is used for a catheter threaded through the vena cava to the right atrium to drain blood from the patient for CPB. Another 1.3- to 2.5-cm incision in the neck provides access to the jugular vein for two catheters. One catheter is threaded into the pulmonary artery to remove air, fluid, and blood that may enter the right heart during surgery. The other catheter is threaded into the right atrium and the tip positioned in the coronary sinus for retrograde infusion of the cardioplegia solution. One or more thoracotomy incisions, usually 5 to 9 cm long, are made for insertion of the surgical instruments. One of the thoracotomy ports may be used for video-assisted imaging equipment.

CPB is begun when the equipment is in place through the groin, neck, and thoracotomy incisions. The balloon on the aortic catheter is inflated, and the cardioplegia solution is injected into the coronary arteries. Cardioplegia solution is a crystalloid and electrolyte liquid used to stop the heart and protect the myocardium during cardiac surgical procedures. One lung may be temporarily collapsed to assist with exposing the surgical site. The CABG is performed through a thoracotomy incision. When the CABG is complete, air is vented from the pulmonary artery and aorta. The balloon on the aortic catheter is deflated, and CPB is discontinued. The surgical instruments and the catheters are removed. The incisions are closed. The patient's postoperative care is similar to that after traditional CABG.

COMBINATION PERCUTANEOUS TRANSLUMINAL CORONARY ANGIOPLASTY AND CORONARY ARTERY BYPASS GRAFT

Patients who have blockages in the left anterior descending and at least one other coronary artery who are not candidates for traditional CABG or prefer less invasive procedures may be treated with both MIDCAB and PTCA. Because patients need their blood to be able to clot after MIDCAB, but require anticoagulation after PTCA, the sequence and timing of providing both treatments to the same patient are being investigated.

COMPLICATIONS

CABG may result in complications such as MI, dysrhythmias, and hemorrhage (see Table 28-2; these complications are discussed in depth in this chapter, in Chapter 27, and in Chapters 20 and 71). The patient's underlying heart disease remains, and angina, exercise intolerance, or other symptoms experienced before CABG may develop again. Medications required before surgery may need to be continued. Lifestyle modifications recommended before surgery remain important to treat the underlying CAD and for the continued viability of the newly implanted grafts (see Plan of Nursing Care, pp. 744–749).

NURSING PROCESS: THE PATIENT AWAITING CARDIAC SURGERY

The cardiac surgery patient has many of the same needs and requires the same perioperative care as other surgical patients (see Chaps. 18 through 20). The patient and family are experiencing a major life crisis. The association of the heart with life and death intensifies their emotional and psychological needs. Patients frequently are admitted the same day as the procedure. For these patients, the nurse must prioritize needs carefully; in the time allowed, the nurse focuses on the needs that have the highest priority.

Before surgery, physical and psychological assessments establish the baselines for future reference. The patient's understanding of the surgical procedure, informed consent, and adherence to treatment protocols are evaluated. Helping the patient to cope, understand the procedure, and maintain dignity are nursing responsibilities.

The preoperative phase of cardiac surgery begins before hospitalization. The nurse assesses the patient for other disorders, such as diabetes, hypertension, and respiratory, gastrointestinal, and hematologic diseases, and documents their treatment.

The nurse clarifies how the medication regimen is to be altered before surgery, such as tapering corticosteroids and digoxin, decreasing or discontinuing anticoagulants, and maintaining medications for treatment of blood pressure, angina, diabetes, and dysrhythmias. The nurse also clarifies the need to maintain activity patterns, a healthy diet, healthful sleep habits, and cessation of smoking to minimize the risks of surgery.

Assessment

Patients with nonacute heart disease may be admitted to the hospital the day of or the day before the surgery. Most of the preoperative evaluation is completed before the patient enters the hospital. Many surgeons' offices or hospitals mail an information packet to the patient's home.

A history and physical examination are performed by nursing and medical personnel. A chest x-ray, ECG, laboratory tests, blood typing and crossmatching, and autologous blood donation (patient's own blood) may also be performed. The health assessment focuses on obtaining baseline physiologic, psychological, and social information. The patient's and family's learning needs are identified and addressed as necessary. Of particular importance are the patient's usual functional level, coping mechanisms, and support systems. These are important because the support of the family or

(text continues on page 749)

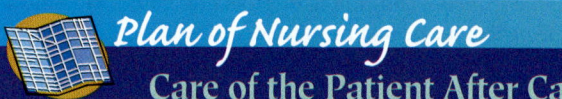

Plan of Nursing Care
Care of the Patient After Cardiac Surgery

Nursing Interventions	Rationale	Expected Outcomes

Nursing Diagnosis: Decreased cardiac output related to blood loss and compromised myocardial function
Goal: Restoration of cardiac output to maintain/attain desired lifestyle

Nursing Interventions	Rationale	Expected Outcomes
1. Monitor cardiovascular status. Serial readings of blood pressures (arterial, left atrial, pulmonary artery, pulmonary artery wedge pressure [PAWP], central venous pressure [CVP]), cardiac output/index, systemic and pulmonary vascular resistance, and cardiac rhythm and rate are obtained, recorded, and correlated with the patient's condition.	1. Effectiveness of cardiac output is determined by hemodynamic monitoring.	The following parameters are within the patient's normal ranges: • Arterial pressure • Left atrial pressures • PAWP • Pulmonary artery pressures • CVP • Heart sounds • Pulmonary and systemic vascular resistance • Cardiac output and cardiac index • Peripheral pulses • Cardiac rate and rhythm • Cardiac enzymes • Urine output • Skin and mucosal colour • Skin temperature
a. Assess arterial blood pressure every 15 minutes until stable; then arterial or cuff blood pressure every 1–4 hours × 24 hours; then every 8–12 hours until hospital discharge; then every visit.	a. Blood pressure is one of the most important physiologic parameters to follow; vasoconstriction after cardiopulmonary bypass may make auscultatory blood pressure unobtainable.	
b. Auscultate for heart sounds and rhythm.	b. Auscultation provides evidence of cardiac tamponade (muffled distant heart sounds), pericarditis (precordial rub), dysrhythmias.	
c. Assess peripheral pulses (pedal, tibial, radial, carotid).	c. Presence or absence and quality of pulses provide data about cardiac output as well as obstructive lesions.	
d. Measure left atrial pressure, pulmonary artery diastolic (PAD) pressure, and PAWP to determine left ventricular end-diastolic volume and to assess cardiac output.	d. Rising pressures may indicate congestive heart failure or pulmonary edema.	
e. Monitor PAWP, PAD, left atrial pressure, and CVP to assess blood volume, vascular tone, and pumping effectiveness of the heart. *Remember: Trends are more important than isolated readings.* Mechanical ventilation may elevate CVP.	e. High PAWP, PAD, left atrial pressure, or CVP may result from hypervolemia, heart failure, cardiac tamponade. If blood pressure drop is due to low blood volume, PAWP, PAD, left atrial pressure, and CVP will show corresponding drop.	
f. Monitor ECG pattern for cardiac dysrhythmias (see Chap. 27 for discussion of dysrhythmias).	f. Dysrhythmias may occur with coronary ischemia, hypoxia, alterations in serum potassium, edema, bleeding, acid-base or electrolyte disturbances, digitalis toxicity, cardiac failure. ST-segment changes may indicate myocardial ischemia or coronary artery spasm. Pacemaker capture and antiarrhythmic medication effects are used to maintain a heart rate and rhythm to support stable blood pressures.	
g. Assess cardiac enzyme test results when available.	g. Elevations may indicate myocardial infarction.	
h. Measure urine output every ½ hour to 1 hour at first, then with vital signs.	h. Urine output less than 25 mL/h indicates decreased renal perfusion and may reflect decreased cardiac output.	
i. Observe buccal mucosa, nailbeds, lips, earlobes, and extremities.	i. Duskiness and cyanosis may indicate decreased cardiac output.	
j. Assess skin; note temperature and colour.	j. Cool moist skin indicates vasoconstriction and decreased cardiac output.	

(continued)

Plan of Nursing Care
Care of the Patient After Cardiac Surgery (Continued)

Nursing Interventions	Rationale	Expected Outcomes
2. Observe for persistent bleeding: steady, continuous drainage of blood; hypotension; low CVP; tachycardia. Prepare to administer blood products, IV solutions.	2. Bleeding can result from cardiac incision, tissue fragility, trauma to tissues, clotting defects.	• Less than 200 mL/hr of drainage through chest tubes during first 4 to 6 hours • Vital signs stable • Chest tube drainage expected amount • CVP and left atrial pressures within normal limits • Urinary output within normal limits • Skin colour normal • Respirations unlaboured, clear breath sounds • Pain limited to incision • ECG and isoenzymes negative for ischemic changes
3. Observe for cardiac tamponade: hypotension; rising PAWP, PAD, left atrial pressure, or CVP; muffled heart sounds; weak, thready pulse; jugular vein distention; decreasing urinary output. Check for diminished amount of blood in chest drainage collection system. Prepare for pericardiocentesis. Assess for pulsus paradoxus.	3. Cardiac tamponade results from bleeding into the pericardial sac or accumulation of fluid in the sac, which compresses the heart and prevents adequate filling of the ventricles. Decrease in chest drainage may indicate fluid is accumulating in the pericardial sac.	
4. Observe for cardiac failure: hypotension, rising PAWP, PAD, CVP, and left atrial pressure, tachycardia, restlessness, agitation, cyanosis, venous distention, dyspnea, moist crackles, ascites. Prepare to administer diuretics and digoxin.	4. Cardiac failure results from decreased pumping action of the heart; can cause deficient blood perfusion to vital organs.	
5. Observe for myocardial infarction: ST-segment elevations, T-wave changes, decreased cardiac output in the presence of normal circulating volume and filling pressures. Obtain serial ECGs and isoenzymes. Differentiate myocardial pain from incisional pain.	5. Symptoms may be masked by the patient's level of consciousness and pain medication.	

Nursing Diagnosis: Impaired gas exchange related to trauma of extensive chest surgery
Goal: Adequate gas exchange

Nursing Interventions	Rationale	Expected Outcomes
1. Maintain mechanical ventilation until the patient is able to breathe independently.	1. Ventilatory support may be used to decrease work of the heart, to maintain effective ventilation, and to provide an airway in the event of cardiac arrest.	• Airway patent • ABGs within normal range • Endotracheal tube correctly placed, as evidenced by x-ray • Breath sounds clear • Ventilator synchronous with respirations • Breath sounds clear after suctioning/FET • Nailbeds and mucous membranes pink • Mental acuity consistent with amount of sedatives and analgesics received • Oriented to person; able to respond yes and no appropriately
2. Monitor arterial blood gases, tidal volumes, peak inspiratory pressures, and extubation parameters.	2. ABGs and tidal volume indicate effectiveness of ventilator and changes that need to be made to improve gas exchange.	
3. Auscultate chest for breath sounds.	3. Crackles indicate pulmonary congestion; decreased or absent breath sounds may indicate pneumothorax or hemothorax.	
4. Sedate patient adequately, as prescribed, and monitor respiratory rate and depth if ventilations are not "controlled."	4. Sedation helps the patient to tolerate the endotracheal tube and to cope with ventilatory sensations; sedatives can depress respiratory rate and depth.	
5. Promote deep breathing, forced expiratory technique (FET, coughing), and turning. Encourage use of the incentive spirometer and compliance with breathing treatments. Teach incisional splinting with a "cough pillow" to decrease discomfort during deep breathing and FET (coughing).	5. Aids in keeping airway patent, preventing atelectasis, and facilitating lung expansion.	
6. Suction tracheobronchial secretions as needed, using strict aseptic technique.	6. Retention of secretions leads to hypoxia and possible cardiac arrest; retained secretions promote infection.	
7. Assist in weaning and endotracheal tube removal.	7. Decreased risk of pulmonary infections and enhanced ability of patient to communicate without an endotracheal tube.	

(continued)

Plan of Nursing Care
Care of the Patient After Cardiac Surgery (Continued)

Nursing Interventions	Rationale	Expected Outcomes

Nursing Diagnosis: Risk for deficient fluid volume and electrolyte imbalance related to alterations in blood volume
Goal: Fluid and electrolyte balance

Nursing Interventions	Rationale	Expected Outcomes
1. Maintain fluid and electrolyte balance.	1. Adequate circulating blood volume is necessary for optimal cellular activity; metabolic acidosis and electrolyte imbalance can occur after use of cardiopulmonary bypass.	• Fluid intake and output balanced • Hemodynamic assessment parameters negative for fluid overload and dehydration • Normal blood pressure with position changes • Absence of dysrhythmia • Stable weight • Notify physician if weight gain of 2 lb or more in 1 day or 5 lb or more in 1 week. • Blood pH 7.35 to 7.45 • Serum potassium 3.5 to 5.0 mEq/L (3.5 to 5.0 mmol/L) • Serum magnesium 1.5 to 2.5 mEq/L (0.75 to 1.25 mmol/L) • Serum sodium 135 to 145 mEq/L (135 to 145 mmol/L) • Serum calcium 8.8 to 10.3 mg/100 mL (2.20 to 2.58 mmol/L)
a. Keep intake and output flow sheets; record urine volume every ½ hour to 4 hours while in critical care unit; then every 8 to 12 hours while hospitalized.	a. Provides a method to determine positive or negative fluid balance and fluid requirements.	
b. Assess the following parameters: pulmonary artery pressures, left atrial pressures, blood pressure, CVP, PAWP, weight, electrolyte levels, hematocrit, jugular venous pressure, tissue turgor, liver size, breath sounds, urinary output, and nasogastric tube drainage.	b. Provides information about state of hydration.	
c. Measure postoperative chest drainage (should not exceed 200 mL/hr for first 4 to 6 hours); cessation of drainage may indicate kinked or blocked chest tube. Ensure patency and integrity of the drainage system. Maintain autotransfusion system if in use.	c. Excessive blood loss from chest cavity can cause hypovolemia.	
d. Weigh daily once patient is ambulatory.	d. Indicator of fluid balance.	
2. Be alert to changes in serum electrolyte levels.	2. A specific concentration of electrolytes is necessary in both extracellular and intracellular body fluids to sustain life.	
a. Hypokalemia (low potassium) *Effects:* dysrhythmias, digitalis toxicity, metabolic alkalosis, weakened myocardium, cardiac arrest Observe for specific ECG changes. Administer IV potassium replacement as directed.	a. *Causes:* inadequate intake, diuretics, vomiting, excessive nasogastric drainage, stress from surgery	

b. Hyperkalemia (high potassium) *Effects:* mental confusion, restlessness, nausea, weakness, paresthesias of extremities
   Be prepared to administer an ion-exchange resin (sodium polystyrene sulfonate [Kayexalate]); IV sodium bicarbonate, or IV insulin and glucose.
	b. *Causes:* increased intake, hemolysis from cardiopulmonary bypass/mechanical assist devices, acidosis, renal insufficiency, tissue necrosis, adrenal cortical insufficiency.
	   The resin binds potassium and promotes intestinal excretion of it.
	   IV sodium bicarbonate drives potassium into the cells from extracellular fluid.
	   Insulin assists the cells with glucose absorption. The glucose provides the energy to activate the sodium–potassium pumps, which pull potassium into the cell while pumping sodium out.	

c. Hypomagnesemia (low magnesium) *Effects:* paresthesias, carpopedal spasm, muscle cramps, tetany, irritability, tremors, hyperexcitability, hyperreflexia, disorientation, depression, seizures, hypotension, dysrhythmias, prolonged PR and QT intervals, broad flat T waves.	c. *Causes:* decreased intake (chronic alcoholism, malnutrition, starvation), impaired absorption (malabsorption syndromes, excess intake of calcium) and increased excretion normal for 24 hours after major surgery, diuretic loss of intestinal fluids, diabetic ketoacidosis, primary aldosteronism, primary hyperparathyroidism.	

(continued)

Plan of Nursing Care

Care of the Patient After Cardiac Surgery *(Continued)*

Nursing Interventions	Rationale	Expected Outcomes
Be prepared to treat the cause. Magnesium supplements may be given (oral route preferred, extreme caution if IV).		
d. Hypermagnesemia (high magnesium) *Effects:* vasodilation, flushing, warm feeling, hypotension, loss of reflexes, slowing bowel function, drowsiness, respiratory depression, coma, apnea, cardiac arrest. Be prepared to treat cause; dialysis and calcium gluconate administration.	d. *Causes:* renal failure, excess intake of medications with magnesium (antacids, cathartics)	
e. Hyponatremia (low sodium) *Effects:* weakness, fatigue, confusion, seizures, coma Administer sodium or diuretics as prescribed.	e. *Causes:* reduction of total body sodium, or increased water intake causing dilution of sodium	
f. Hypocalcemia (low calcium) *Effects:* numbness and tingling in fingertips, toes, ears, nose; carpopedal spasm; muscle cramps; tetany Administer replacement therapy as prescribed.	f. *Causes:* alkalosis, multiple blood transfusions of citrated blood products	
g. Hypercalcemia (high calcium) *Effects:* dysrhythmias, digitalis toxicity, asystole Institute treatment as prescribed.	g. *Cause:* prolonged immobility	

Nursing Diagnosis: Disturbed sensory perception related to excessive environmental stimulation, sleep deprivation, electrolyte imbalance

Goal: Reduction of symptoms of sensory perceptual imbalance; prevention of postcardiotomy psychosis

1. Use measures to prevent postcardiotomy psychosis: a. Explain all procedures and the need for patient cooperation. b. Plan nursing care to provide for periods of uninterrupted sleep with patient's normal day–night pattern. c. Decrease sleep-preventing environmental stimuli as much as possible. d. Promote continuity of care from nurse to nurse. e. Orient to time and place frequently. Encourage family to visit at regular times. f. Assess for medications that may contribute to delirium. g. Teach relaxation techniques and diversions. h. Encourage self-care as much as tolerated to enhance self-control. Assess support systems and coping mechanisms 2. Observe for perceptual distortions, hallucinations, disorientation, and paranoid delusions.	1. Postcardiotomy psychosis may result from anxiety, sleep deprivation, increased sensory input, disorientation to night and day. Normally, sleep cycles are at least 50 min long. The first cycle may be as long as 90 to 120 min and then shorten during successive cycles. Sleep deprivation results when the sleep cycles are interrupted or there are not enough of them.	• Cooperates with procedures • Sleeps for long, uninterrupted intervals • Oriented to person, place, time • Experiences no perceptual distortions, hallucinations, disorientation, delusions

(continued)

Plan of Nursing Care
Care of the Patient After Cardiac Surgery *(Continued)*

Nursing Interventions	Rationale	Expected Outcomes
Nursing Diagnosis: Acute pain related to surgical trauma and pleural irritation caused by chest tubes and/or internal mammary artery dissection **Goal:** Relief of pain		
1. Record nature, type, location, intensity, and duration of pain. 2. Assist patient to differentiate between surgical pain and anginal pain. 3. Encourage routine pain medication dosing for the first 24 to 72 hours and observe for side effects of lethargy, hypotension, tachycardia, respiratory depression.	1. Pain and anxiety increase pulse rate, oxygen consumption, and cardiac workload. 2. Anginal pain requires immediate treatment. 3. Analgesia promotes rest, decreases oxygen consumption caused by pain, and aids patient in performing deep-breathing and FET (coughing) exercises; pain medications is more effective when taken before pain is severe.	• States pain is decreasing in severity • Reports absence of pain • Restlessness decreased • Vital signs stable • Participates in deep-breathing and forced expiratory technique (FET, coughing) exercises • Verbalizes fewer complaints of pain each day • Positions self; participates in care activities • Gradually increases activity
Nursing Diagnosis: Ineffective renal tissue perfusion related to decreased cardiac output, hemolysis, or vasopressor drug therapy **Goal:** Maintenance of adequate renal perfusion		

1. Assess renal function:
 	
  a. Measure urine output every ½ hour to 4 hours in critical care then every 8–12 hours until hospital discharge.
  b. Measure urine specific gravity.
 	
  c. Monitor and report lab results: BUN, serum creatinine, urine and serum electrolytes.
2. Prepare to administer rapid-acting diuretics or inotropic drugs (eg, dopamine, dobutamine).
3. Prepare patient for dialysis or continuous renal replacement therapy if indicated.
	1. Renal injury can be caused by deficient perfusion, hemolysis, low cardiac output, and use of vasopressor agents to increase blood pressure.
	  a. Less than 25 mL/h indicates decreased renal function.
	
	  b. Indicates kidneys' ability to concentrate urine in renal tubules.
	  c. Indicate kidneys' ability to excrete waste products.
	2. Promote renal function and increase cardiac output and renal blood flow.
	3. Patients have the right to know what care is prescribed; provides patient with the opportunity to ask questions and prepare for the procedure.
		• Urine output consistent with fluid intake; greater than 25 mL/hr
		• Urine specific gravity 1.015 to 1.025
		• BUN, creatinine, electrolytes within normal limits

Nursing Diagnosis: Ineffective thermoregulation related to infection or postpericardiotomy syndrome **Goal:** Maintenance of normal body temperature		
1. Assess temperature every hour. 2. Use aseptic technique when changing dressings, suctioning endotracheal tube; maintain closed systems for all intravenous and arterial lines and for indwelling urinary catheter. 3. Observe for symptoms of postpericardiotomy syndrome: fever, malaise, pericardial effusion, pericardial friction rub, arthralgia. 4. Administer anti-inflammatory agents as directed.	1. Fever can indicate infectious process or postpericardiotomy syndrome. 2. Decreases risk of infection. 3. Occurs in 10% to 40% of patients after cardiac surgery. 4. Relieve symptoms of inflammation (eg, warm or flushed sensation, swelling, fullness, stiffness or aching sensation, and fatigue).	• Normal body temperature • Incisions are free of infection and are healing • Absence of symptoms of postpericardiotomy syndrome

(continued)

Plan of Nursing Care

Care of the Patient After Cardiac Surgery (Continued)

Nursing Interventions	Rationale	Expected Outcomes
Nursing Diagnosis: Deficient knowledge about self-care activities **Goal:** Ability to perform self-care activities		
1. Develop teaching plan for patient and family. Provide specific instructions for the following: • Diet and daily weights • Activity progression • Exercise • Deep breathing, FET (coughing), lung expansion exercises • Temperature monitoring • Medication regimen • Pulse taking • CPR, if appropriate for the family to learn • Entry to the emergency medical system • Need for MedicAlert identification	1. Each patient will have unique learning needs.	• Patient and family members explain and comply with all therapeutic regimen • Patient and family members identify lifestyle changes necessitated by therapeutic regimen • Has copy of discharge instructions (in the patient's primary language) • Makes follow-up phone calls • Keeps follow-up appointments
2. Provide verbal and written instructions; provide several teaching sessions for reinforcement and answering questions.	2. Repetition promotes learning by allowing for clarification of misinformation. After cardiac surgery, patients have short-term memory difficulty; information written in the patient's primary language is essential because it can be used as a resource after discharge. The less familiar or greater the amount of the content the patient and family need to learn, the more time it will take to learn.	
3. Involve family in all teaching sessions.	3. Family member responsible for home care is usually anxious and requires adequate time for learning.	
4. Provide information regarding follow-up phone call to surgeon, cardiologist, or liaison nurse; follow-up visit with surgeon.	4. Arrangements for phone contacts with health care personnel help to allay anxieties.	
5. Make appropriate referrals: home care agency, cardiac rehabilitation program, community support groups, Mended Hearts Club.	5. Learning and lifestyle changes continue after discharge from the hospital.	

significant others will affect the patient's postoperative course and rehabilitation. Discharge plans are influenced by the lifestyle demands of the home situation and the physical environment of the home.

HEALTH HISTORY

The preoperative history and health assessment should be thorough and well documented because they provide a basis for postoperative comparison. A systematic assessment of all systems is performed, with emphasis on cardiovascular functioning.

Functional status of the cardiovascular system is determined by reviewing the patient's symptoms, including past and present experiences with chest pain, hypertension, palpitations, cyanosis, breathing difficulty (dyspnea), leg pain that occurs with walking (intermittent claudication), orthopnea, paroxysmal nocturnal dyspnea, and peripheral edema. Because alterations in cardiac output can affect renal, respiratory, gastrointestinal, integumentary, hematologic, and neurologic functioning, a history of

these systems is also reviewed. The patient's history of major illnesses, previous surgeries, medication therapies, and use of drugs, alcohol, and tobacco is also obtained.

PHYSICAL ASSESSMENT

A complete physical examination is performed, with special emphasis on the following:

- General appearance and behaviour
- Vital signs
- Nutritional and fluid status, weight, and height
- Inspection and palpation of the heart, noting the point of maximal impulse, abnormal pulsations, and thrills
- Auscultation of the heart, noting pulse rate, rhythm, and quality; S_3 and S_4, snaps, clicks, murmurs, and friction rub
- Jugular venous pressure
- Peripheral pulses
- Peripheral edema

PSYCHOSOCIAL ASSESSMENT

The psychosocial assessment and the assessment of the patient's and family's learning needs are as important as the physical examination. Anticipation of cardiac surgery is a source of great stress to the patient and family. They will be anxious and fearful and often have many unanswered questions. Their anxiety usually increases with the patient's admission to the hospital and the immediacy of surgery. An assessment of the level of anxiety is important. If it is low, it may indicate denial. If it is extremely high, it may interfere with the use of effective coping mechanisms and with preoperative teaching. Questions may be asked to obtain the following information:

- Meaning of the surgery to the patient and family
- Coping mechanisms that are being used
- Measures used in the past to deal with stress
- Anticipated changes in lifestyle
- Support systems in effect
- Fears regarding the present and the future
- Knowledge and understanding of the surgical procedure, postoperative course, and long-term rehabilitation

The nurse allows adequate time for the patient and family to express their fears. The fears most often expressed are fear of the unknown, fear of pain, fear of body image change, and fear of dying. During the assessment, the nurse determines how much the patient and family know about the impending surgery and the expected postoperative events. They are encouraged to ask questions and to indicate how much information they wish to receive. Some patients prefer not to have detailed information, whereas others want to know as much as possible. Patients are approached as unique individuals with their own specific learning needs, learning styles, and levels of understanding.

Patients requiring emergency heart surgery may have cardiac catheterization and surgery within several hours of admission. The nurse will have little opportunity to assess and meet their emotional and learning needs before surgery. As a result, patients will need extra help after surgery to adjust to the situation.

Diagnosis

NURSING DIAGNOSES

The nursing diagnoses for patients awaiting cardiac surgery vary according to each patient's cardiac disease and symptoms. Most patients have a nursing diagnosis of decreased cardiac output (see Cardiac Failure in Chap. 30). Preoperative nursing diagnoses for most patients may include:

- Fear related to the surgical procedure, its uncertain outcome, and the threat to well-being
- Deficient knowledge regarding the surgical procedure and the postoperative course

COLLABORATIVE PROBLEMS/POTENTIAL COMPLICATIONS

The stress of impending cardiac surgery may precipitate complications that require collaborative management with the physician. Based on the assessment data, potential complications that may develop include:

- Angina or anginal pain equivalent
- Severe anxiety requiring an anxiolytic (anxiety-reducing) medication
- Cardiac arrest

Planning and Goals

The major goals of the patient may include reducing fear, learning about the surgical procedure and postoperative course, and avoiding complications.

Nursing Interventions

During the preoperative phase of cardiac surgery, the nurse develops a plan of care that includes emotional support and teaching for the patient and family. Establishing rapport, answering questions, listening to fears and concerns, clarifying misconceptions, and providing information about what to expect are interventions the nurse uses to prepare the patient and family emotionally for the surgery and for the postoperative events.

REDUCING FEAR

The patient and family are provided time and opportunities to express their fears. If there is fear of the unknown, other surgical experiences that the patient has had can be compared with the impending surgery. It is often helpful to describe to the patient the sensations that are expected. If the patient has already had a cardiac catheterization, the similarities and differences between that procedure and the surgery may be compared. The patient is encouraged to talk about any concerns related to previous experiences.

A discussion of the patient's fears about pain is initiated. A comparison is made between the pain experienced with cardiac surgery and other pain experiences. The preoperative sedation, the anesthetic, and the postoperative pain medications are described. The nurse reassures the patient that the fear of pain is normal, that some pain will be experienced, that medication to relieve pain will be provided, and that the patient will be closely observed. The patient is encouraged to take pain medication before the pain becomes severe. Positioning and relaxation will make the pain more tolerable. Patients who have a fear of scarring from surgery are encouraged to discuss this concern, and misconceptions are corrected. It may be helpful to indicate that the health care team members will keep the patient informed about the healing process.

The patient and family are encouraged to talk about their fear of the patient dying. They should be reassured that this fear is normal. For those who only hint about this concern despite efforts to encourage them to talk about their fear, coaching may be helpful (eg, "Are you worrying about not making it through surgery? Most people who have heart surgery at least think about the possibility of dying."). After the fear is expressed, the patient and family can be helped to explore their feelings.

By alleviating undue anxiety and fear, preparing the patient emotionally for surgery decreases the chance of preoperative problems, promotes smooth anesthesia induction, and enhances the patient's involvement in care and recovery after surgery. Preparing the family for the events to come helps them to cope, be supportive to the patient, and participate in postoperative and rehabilitative care (Chart 28-9).

MONITORING AND MANAGING POTENTIAL COMPLICATIONS

Angina may occur because of increased stress and anxiety related to the forthcoming surgery. The patient who develops angina usually responds to normal angina therapy, most commonly nitroglycerin. Some patients require oxygen and intravenous nitroglycerin drips (see the Angina Pectoris section).

Chart 28-9 • Ethics and Related Issues

When Is Withholding or Withdrawing Life Support Discussed with Patients and Families?

Situation
Life support includes the use of intraaortic balloon pumps and ventricular assist devices, ventilators, vasoactive infusions, cardiopulmonary resuscitation, and antibiotics. Patients who receive these treatments include those who are acutely, chronically, and terminally ill. When dependent on life support, a patient may be unable to make decisions about his or her own care, and the patient's family may be asked to participate in decision making for the patient. At what point is the sensitive issue of withholding or withdrawing life support discussed?

Dilemma
A patient is unresponsive and utilizing life support in the critical care unit. The consulting cardiologist has written a progress note stating, "Patient is terminal. Further treatment is futile." The patient does not have a living will or a durable power of attorney for health care. The oldest child does not want the patient to suffer but states, "If there is any hope, I want everything done." The other child states that the patient "would not want to live like this."

Does the statement by the second child support the principle of autonomy? Does the statement by the oldest child provide precedence for the principles of sanctity of life, beneficence, or nonmaleficence? If you determined that the statement by the second child supported the principle of autonomy, should sanctity of life, beneficence, or nonmaleficence be used in decision making in this situation?

Discussion
What arguments would you offer to support the view that discussions about the extent of life-supporting treatments desired should occur before an individual experiences a life-threatening event?

What arguments would you offer to support the view that discussions about the extent of life-supporting treatment should occur only when certain circumstances arise?

For patients with extreme anxiety or fear and for whom emotional support and education are not successful, medication therapy may be helpful. The anxiolytic agents most commonly used before cardiac surgery are lorazepam (Ativan) and diazepam (Valium).

If cardiac arrest occurs in the preoperative period, advanced cardiac life support is provided (see Chap. 27).

PROMOTING HOME AND COMMUNITY-BASED CARE

Teaching Patients Self-Care
Patient and family teaching is based on assessed learning needs. Teaching usually includes information about hospitalization, surgery (eg, preoperative and postoperative care, length of surgery, pain and discomfort that can be expected, visiting hours, and procedures in the critical care unit), the recovery phase (eg, length of hospitalization, what to expect from home care and rehabilitation, when normal activities such as housework, shopping, and work can be resumed), and ongoing lifestyle habits. Any changes made in medical therapy and preoperative preparations need to be explained and reinforced.

The patient is informed that physical preparation usually involves several showers or scrubs with an antiseptic solution. A sedative may be prescribed the night before and the morning of

surgery. Most cardiac surgical teams use prophylactic antibiotic therapy, and the antibiotic therapy is initiated before surgery.

If no preadmission teaching has been done and the preoperative hospitalization period is very short, teaching the patient and family together may be most effective. Anxiety often increases with the admission process and impending surgery. Teaching the patient and family together capitalizes on their established support relationship. Teaching in this phase should be directed primarily by the patient's and family's questions. Too much detail may only increase anxiety.

The patient may be offered a tour of the critical care unit, the postanesthesia care unit, or both. (In some hospitals, the patient initially goes to the postanesthesia care unit.) The patient recovering from anesthesia may be reassured by having already seen the surroundings and having met someone from the unit. The patient and family are informed about the equipment, tubes, and lines that will be present after surgery and their purposes. They should know to expect monitors, several intravenous lines, chest tubes, and a urinary catheter. Explaining the purpose and the approximate time that these devices will be in place helps to reassure the patient. Most patients will remain intubated and on mechanical ventilation for 2 to 24 hours after surgery. They need to be aware that this prevents them from talking, and they should be reassured that the staff will be able to assist them with other means of communication.

The nurse takes care to answer the patient's questions about postoperative care and procedures. Deep breathing and huffing (or coughing), use of the incentive spirometer, and foot exercises are explained and practiced by the patient before surgery. The family's questions at this time usually focus on the length of the surgery, who will discuss the results of the procedure with them after surgery and when this may occur, where to wait during the surgery, the visiting procedures for the critical care unit, and how they can support the patient before surgery and in the critical care unit.

Evaluation

EXPECTED PATIENT OUTCOMES
Expected patient outcomes may include:
1. Demonstrates reduced fear
   a. Identifies fears
   b. Discusses fears with family
   c. Uses past experiences as a focus for comparison
   d. Expresses positive attitude about outcome of surgery
   e. Expresses confidence in measures to be used to relieve pain
2. Learns about the surgical procedure and postoperative course
   a. Identifies the purposes of the preoperative preparation procedure
   b. Tours the critical care unit, if desired
   c. Identifies limitations expected after surgery
   d. Discusses expected immediate postoperative environment (eg, tubes, machines, nursing surveillance)
   e. Demonstrates expected activities after surgery (eg, deep breathing, huffing [coughing], foot exercises)
3. Shows no evidence of complications
   a. Reports anginal pain is relieved with medications and rest
   b. Takes medications as prescribed

INTRAOPERATIVE NURSING MANAGEMENT

The perioperative nurse performs an assessment and prepares the patient for the operating room and recovery experience. Any changes in the patient's status and the need for changes in therapy are identified. Procedures are explained before they are performed, such as the application of electrodes and use of continuous monitoring, indwelling catheters, and an SpO_2 probe. Intravenous lines are inserted to administer fluids, medications, and blood products. The patient will receive general anesthesia, be intubated, and placed on mechanical ventilation. In addition to assisting with the surgical procedures, perioperative nurses are responsible for the comfort and safety of the patient. Some of the areas of intervention include positioning, skin care, wound care, and emotional support of the patient and family.

Before the chest incision is closed, chest tubes are positioned to evacuate air and drainage from the mediastinum and the thorax. Epicardial pacemaker electrodes are implanted on the surface of the right atrium and the right ventricle. These epicardial electrodes can be used to pace the heart and to monitor it for dysrhythmias through the atrial leads.

Possible intraoperative complications include dysrhythmias, hemorrhage, MI, CVA (stroke, brain attack), embolization, and organ failure from shock, embolus, or adverse drug reactions. Astute intraoperative patient assessment is critical in preventing these complications and for detecting symptoms and initiating prompt therapy.

NURSING PROCESS:
THE PATIENT WHO HAS HAD
CARDIAC SURGERY

Initial postoperative care focuses on achieving or maintaining hemodynamic stability and recovery from general anesthesia. Care may be provided in the postanesthesia care unit or intensive care unit. After hemodynamic stability and recovery from general anesthesia have been achieved, the patient is transferred to a surgical stepdown unit with telemetry. Care focuses on wound care, progressive activity, and nutrition. Education about medications and risk factor modification is emphasized (see Plan of Nursing Care: Care of the Patient After Cardiac Surgery). Discharge from the hospital usually occurs 3 to 5 days after CABG or 1 to 3 days after MIDCAB. Patients can expect fewer symptoms from CAD and an improved quality of life. CABG has been shown to increase the life span of high-risk patients—those with left main artery blockages, left ventricular dysfunction with multivessel blockages, three-vessel blockages with one being the left anterior descending artery, and diabetes (Eagle et al., 1999).

The immediate postoperative period for the patient who has undergone cardiac surgery presents many challenges to the health care team. All efforts are made to facilitate the transition from the operating room to the critical care unit or PACU with minimal risk. Specific information about the operation and important factors about postoperative management are communicated by the surgical team and anesthesia personnel to the critical care nurse, who then assumes responsibility for the patient's care. Figure 28-10 presents a graphic overview of the many aspects of postoperative care for the cardiac surgical patient.

Assessment

When the patient is admitted to the critical care unit or PACU and for at least every 12 hours thereafter, a complete assessment of all systems is performed to determine the postoperative status of the patient compared with the preoperative baseline and to identify anticipated changes since surgery. The following parameters are assessed:

Neurologic status: level of responsiveness, pupil size and reaction to light, reflexes, facial symmetry, movement of extremities, and hand grip strength

Cardiac status: heart rate and rhythm, heart sounds, arterial blood pressure, central venous pressure (CVP), pulmonary artery pressure, pulmonary artery wedge pressure (PAWP), left atrial pressure, waveforms from the invasive blood pressure lines, cardiac output or index, systemic and pulmonary vascular resistance, pulmonary artery oxygen saturation (SvO_2) if available, mediastinal chest tube drainage, and pacemaker status and function

Respiratory status: chest movement, breath sounds, ventilator settings (eg, rate, tidal volume, oxygen concentration, mode such as synchronized intermittent mandatory ventilation, positive end-expiratory pressure, pressure support), respiratory rate, ventilatory pressure, arterial oxygen saturation (SaO_2), percutaneous oxygen saturation (SpO_2), end-tidal CO_2, pleural chest tube drainage, arterial blood gases

Peripheral vascular status: peripheral pulses; colour of skin, nailbeds, mucosa, lips, and earlobes; skin temperature; edema; condition of dressings and invasive lines

Renal function: urinary output; urine specific gravity and osmolality may be assessed

Fluid and electrolyte status: intake, output from all drainage tubes, all cardiac output parameters, and the following indications of electrolyte imbalance:

- *Hypokalemia:* digitalis toxicity, dysrhythmias, ECG changes (U wave, atrioventricular block, flat or inverted T waves)
- *Hyperkalemia:* mental confusion, restlessness, nausea, weakness, paresthesias of extremities, dysrhythmias, ECG changes (tall, peaked T waves; increased amplitude, widening QRS complex; prolonged QT interval)
- *Hypomagnesemia:* paresthesias, carpopedal spasm, muscle cramps, tetany, irritability, tremors, hyperexcitability, hyperreflexia, cardiac dysrhythmias, ECG changes (prolonged PR and QT intervals; broad, flat T waves), disorientation, depression, hypotension, seizures
- *Hypermagnesemia:* vasodilation, hypotension, hyporeflexia, slow gastrointestinal motility (hypoactive bowel sounds), lethargy, respiratory depression, coma, apnea, cardiac arrest
- *Hyponatremia:* weakness, fatigue, confusion, seizures, coma
- *Hypocalcemia:* paresthesias, carpopedal spasm, muscle cramps, tetany
- *Hypercalcemia:* digitalis toxicity, asystole

Pain: nature, type, location, duration (incisional pain must be differentiated from anginal pain); apprehension; response to analgesics

Some patients who have had a MIDCAB using a midsternal incision or an internal mammary artery CABG experience ulnar nerve paresthesia on the same side of the body as the graft. The paresthesia may be temporary or permanent. Patients who have had CABG using the gastroepiploic artery may experience an ileus for a longer period after surgery and have abdominal pain at the site of the incision and pain at the site of the chest incision.

Assessment also includes observing all equipment and tubes to determine whether they are functioning properly: endotracheal tube, ventilator, end-tidal CO_2 monitor, SpO_2 monitor, pul-

Nasogastric tube to decompress stomach.

Endotracheal tube for providing ventilatory assistance, suctioning, and use of end-tidal CO_2 monitor.

Swan-Ganz catheter for monitoring central venous pressure, pulmonary artery and pulmonary artery wedge pressures, temperature, $S\bar{v}O_2$. Can be used for determining cardiac output, for venous and pulmonary artery blood sampling, and for medication administration. Venous lines can be used for fluid administration. Fluid intake is monitored.

ECG electrodes for monitoring heart rate and rhythm.

$S\bar{p}O_2$ monitor for measuring arterial oxygen saturation.

Assess peripheral pulses: radial, posterior tibial, dorsalis pedis.

Neurological assessment:
• Level of responsiveness
• Hand grasp
• Pupils
• Pain
• Movement

Assess skin colour and temperature, colour of lips, and colour and capillary refill of nail beds.

Epicardial pacing electrodes to temporarily pace the heart.

Mediastinal and pleural chest tubes attached to suction; drainage and wound healing are monitored.

Radial arterial line; used for monitoring arterial blood pressure and for blood sampling.

Indwelling catheter to closed drainage system for accurate measurement of urine output; a temperature probe may be part of the indwelling catheter.

FIGURE 28-10 Postoperative care of the cardiac surgical patient requires the nurse to be proficient in interpreting hemodynamics, correlating physical assessments with laboratory results, sequencing interventions, and evaluating progress toward desired outcomes.

monary artery catheter, $S\bar{v}O_2$ monitor, arterial and intravenous lines, intravenous infusion devices and tubing, cardiac monitor, pacemaker, chest tubes, and urinary drainage system.

As the patient regains consciousness and progresses through the postoperative period, the nurse expands the assessment to include parameters indicative of psychological and emotional status. The patient may exhibit behaviour that reflects denial or depression or may experience postcardiotomy psychosis. Characteristic signs of psychosis include transient perceptual illusions, visual and auditory hallucinations, disorientation, and paranoid delusions.

The family's needs also should be assessed. The nurse ascertains how they are coping with the situation; determines their psychological, emotional, and spiritual needs; and finds out whether they are receiving adequate information about the patient's condition.

ASSESSING FOR COMPLICATIONS

The patient is continuously assessed for indications of impending complications (Table 28-8). The nurse and the surgeon function collaboratively to identify early signs and symptoms of complications and to institute measures to reverse their progression.

(text continues on page 758)

Table 28-8 • **Potential Complications of Cardiac Surgery**

COMPLICATION	DESCRIPTION	ASSESSMENT AND MANAGEMENT
Cardiac Complications (The patient may require interventions for more than one complication at a time. Collaboration among nurses, physicians, pharmacists, respiratory therapists, and dietitians is necessary to achieve the desired patient outcomes.)		
Decreased Cardiac Output		
Preload Alterations (the amount of myocardial muscle fibre stretch at the end of diastole)		
Hypovolemia (most common cause of decreased cardiac output after cardiac surgery)	• Blood loss (although some blood may be replaced to provide sufficient hemoglobin to carry oxygen to the tissues) • Surgical hypothermia (As the reduced body temperature rises after surgery, blood vessels dilate, and more volume is needed to fill the vessels.) • Intravenous fluid loss to the interstitial spaces because cardiopulmonary bypass makes capillary beds more permeable • Arterial hypotension with low pulmonary artery wedge pressure (PAWP) and low central venous pressures (CVP) often are seen with an increased heart rate.	• Fluid replacement may be prescribed. Replacement fluids include: colloid (albumin or protein), starch (hetastarch), packed red blood cells, or crystalloid solution (normal saline, lactated Ringer's solution).
Persistent bleeding	• Cardiopulmonary bypass procedure, which may cause platelet malfunction (blood clots abnormally) and hypothermia, which alters clotting mechanisms • Surgical trauma causing tissues and blood vessels to ooze bloody drainage • Anticoagulant (heparin) therapy	• Accurate measurement of wound bleeding and drainage tube blood is essential. Bloody drainage should not exceed 200 mL/h for the first 4 to 6 hours. Drainage should decrease and stop within a few days, while progressing from sanguineous to serosanguineous and serous drainage. • Protamine sulfate may be administered to neutralize unfractionated heparin; vitamin K and blood products may be used to treat hematologic deficiencies. • If bleeding persists, the patient may return to the operating room for corrective surgery.
Cardiac tamponade (may decrease preload to the heart by preventing available blood from entering the heart)	• Fluid accumulates in the pericardial sac, which compresses the heart, preventing blood from filling the ventricles. • Signs and symptoms include arterial hypotension, tachycardia, muffled heart sounds, decreasing urine output and equalizing of the PAWP, CVP, and pulmonary artery diastolic pressures. Additional signs and symptoms: arterial and pulmonary artery pressure waveforms demonstrating a pulsus paradoxus (decrease of more than 10 mm Hg during inspiration) and decreased chest tube drainage (suggesting that the drainage is trapped or clotted in the mediastinum).	• Equipment is checked to eliminate possible kinks or obstructions in the tubing. • Drainage system patency may be reestablished by milking the tubing (taking care not to strip the tubing, creating massive negative pressure within the chest, which may harm the surgical repair or trigger a dysrhythmia). • Chest x-ray may show a widening mediastinum. • Emergency medical management is required; may include pericardiocentesis or return to surgery.
Fluid overload	• High PAWP, CVP, and pulmonary artery diastolic pressures as well as crackles indicate fluid overload.	• Diuretics are usually prescribed and the rate of IV fluid administration is reduced. • Fluid restriction may be prescribed. Alternative treatments include continuous renal replacement therapy, dialysis, and phlebotomy.
Afterload Alterations (The force that the ventricle must overcome to move blood forward. Vascular resistance may be calculated to assess afterload and the effects of any vasoactive treatments. Alteration in the patient's body temperature is the most common cause of alterations in afterload after cardiac surgery.)		
Hypothermia	• Blood vessel constriction, which increases afterload. (Blood vessel dilation from fever or other hyperthermic condition decreases afterload.)	• Patient is rewarmed gradually, although vasodilators may be required if the resistance is too great to wait for rewarming. The patient may require volume support or vasopressors during a fever or severe vasodilation.
Hypertension	• Various causes. Some patients have a history of this condition and the nurse can anticipate the need for treatment postoperatively. Other patients experience transient hypertension.	• Vasodilators (nitroglycerin [Nitro-Bid], nitroprusside [Nipride, Nitropress]) may be used to treat hypertension. If patient had hypertension before surgery, the preoperative management regimen resumes as soon as possible.

(continued)

Table 28-8 • Potential Complications of Cardiac Surgery (Continued)

COMPLICATION	DESCRIPTION	ASSESSMENT AND MANAGEMENT
Heart Rate Alterations Tachydysrhythmias	• May or may not result from preload or afterload alterations	• Rhythms are assessed to establish that they are not the result of preload or afterload alterations. • If a tachydysrhythmia is the primary symptom, the heart rhythm is assessed and medications (eg, adenosine [Adenocard], digoxin [Lanoxin], diltiazem [Cardizem], esmolol [Brevibloc], lidocaine [Xylocaine], procainamide [Pronestyl], propranolol [Inderal], quinidine [Cardioquin, Quinaglute, Quinidex], verapamil [Calan, Corvera, Isoptin]) are prescribed. (Patients may be prescribed antiarrhythmics before CABG to minimize the risk of postoperative tachydysrhythmias.) • Carotid massage may be performed by a physician to assist with diagnosing or treating the dysrhythmia. • Cardioversion and defibrillation are alternatives for symptomatic tachydysrhythmias.
Bradycardias	• Decreased heart rate	• Many postoperative patients will have temporary pacer wires that can be attached to a pulse generator (pacemaker) to stimulate the heart to beat faster. Less commonly, atropine, epinephrine or isoproterenol may be used to increase heart rate.
Dysrhythmias (may or may not affect cardiac output)	• Abnormal heart rates	• Treatment may include medication (Table 27-1), pacemakers (antibradycardiac, antitachycardiac), carotid massage, cardioversion, or defibrillation. Goal of treatment is to return the heart to a normal sinus rhythm. • For patients who cannot attain normal sinus rhythm, an alternate goal may be to establish a stable rhythm that produces a sufficient cardiac output.
Contractility Alterations Cardiac failure	• Possible when the heart fails as a pump and the chambers cannot adequately empty	• The nurse observes for and reports falling mean arterial pressure; rising PAWP, pulmonary artery diastolic pressure, and CVP; increasing tachycardia; restlessness and agitation; peripheral cyanosis; venous distention; laboured respirations; and edema. • Medical management includes diuretics and digoxin.
Myocardial infarction (may occur intraoperatively or post-operatively)	• Portion of the cardiac muscle dies, therefore contractility decreases. Until the infarcted area becomes edematous, the ventricular wall moves paradoxically during contractions, further decreasing cardiac output. Symptoms may be masked by the postoperative surgical discomfort or the anesthesia–analgesia regimen.	• Careful assessment to determine the type of pain the patient is experiencing; MI suspected if the mean blood pressure is low with normal preload. The systemic vascular resistance (afterload) and heart rate may be elevated to compensate for poor contractility. • Serial ECGs and cardiac enzymes assist in making the diagnosis (alterations may be due to the surgical intervention). Analgesics are prescribed in small amounts while the patient's blood pressure and respiratory rate are monitored (because vasodilation secondary to analgesics or decreasing pain may occur and compound the hypotension). • Activity progression depends on the patient's activity tolerance.
Pulmonary Complications Impaired gas exchange	• During and after anesthesia, patients require mechanical assistance to breathe. • Potential for postoperative atelectasis. • Endotracheal tubes stimulate production of mucus and chest incision pain may decrease the effectiveness of the forced expiratory technique (FET, cough).	• Pulmonary complications are often detected during assessment of breath sounds, oxygen saturation levels, and end-tidal CO_2 levels, and when monitoring peak pressure and exhaled tidal volumes on the ventilator. Arterial blood gas results and mixed venous saturations also are monitored when available.

(continued)

Table 28-8 • Potential Complications of Cardiac Surgery (Continued)

COMPLICATION	DESCRIPTION	ASSESSMENT AND MANAGEMENT
		• Extended periods of mechanical ventilation are often required while the complications are treated and until they are resolved. • In patients with hypoxia, ventricular stroke work index may be calculated to assist with assessment of contractility.
Fluid Volume Complications Hemorrhage	• Untoward and excessive bleeding may be life-threatening.	• Hemorrhage usually requires surgical intervention, and blood products are often administered. • Compression of a bleeding vessel is another treatment of hemorrhage. Lungs may be used to compress bleeding mediastinal blood vessels; lung volume and pressure are increased by adding PEEP to the ventilator settings of an intubated patient. The lungs slow or stop the bleeding by pushing in on the mediastinum and creating pressure on the bleeding vessels of the pericardium, coronary arteries, and bypass grafts.
Neurologic Complications Cerebrovascular accident (brain attack, stroke)	• Inability to follow simple command within 6 hours of recovery from anesthetic; different capabilities on right or left side of body	• Neurologically, most patients begin to recover from anesthesia in the operating room. • Patients who are elderly or who have renal or hepatic failure may take longer to recover. • Patient should be evaluated for CVA (brain attack, stroke) or air embolism.
Pain (see Chapter 13)		
Renal Failure and Electrolyte Imbalance Renal failure	• Usually acute and resolves within 3 months, but may become chronic and require ongoing dialysis	• May respond to diuretics or may require continuous renal replacement therapy (CRRT) or dialysis
Acute tubular necrosis	• Often results from hypoperfusion of the kidneys or from injury to the renal tubules by medications in the filtrate or from exacerbation of a pre-existing condition	• Fluids, electrolytes, and urine output are monitored frequently.
Hypokalemia (low potassium level; normal level is 3.5 to 5.0 mmol/L)	• May be caused by inadequate intake, diuretics, vomiting, diarrhea, excessive nasogastric drainage without potassium replacement, and stress due to surgery (increased aldosterone secretion produces decreased potassium and increased sodium retention). • Signs and symptoms: digitalis toxicity, dysrhythmias, metabolic alkalosis, a weakened myocardium, and cardiac arrest • One specific ECG change is a U wave (a positive deflection after the T wave) that is more than 1 mm high. Additional signs are atrioventricular block, flat or inverted T waves, and low voltage.	• Must be detected and treated immediately • Patient must be observed carefully when serum potassium rises or falls outside the normal level • Some cardiac surgeons strive to maintain potassium level at 4.0 mEq/L (4.0 mmol/L) or higher to avoid dysrhythmias in the postoperative period. • When necessary, IV potassium replacement is prescribed.
Hyperkalemia (high potassium level)	• Hyperkalemia may be caused by increased intake, red blood cell hemolysis caused by cardiopulmonary bypass or mechanical assist devices, acidosis, renal insufficiency, tissue necrosis, and adrenal cortical insufficiency. • Signs and symptoms: mental confusion, restlessness, nausea, weakness, and paresthesias of the extremities. • ECG changes specific for hyperkalemia are tall peaked T waves, increased amplitude and widening of the QRS complex, and a prolonged QT interval.	• An ion exchange resin, sodium polystyrene sulfonate (Kayexalate), may be prescribed to bind the potassium in the gastrointestinal tract and decrease serum potassium. • Alternative treatments include IV sodium bicarbonate, IV insulin, and glucose to temporarily drive the potassium back into the cells from the extracellular fluid. • Hemodialysis or peritoneal dialysis may be used to reduce the potassium level.

(continued)

Table 28-8 • Potential Complications of Cardiac Surgery (Continued)

COMPLICATION	DESCRIPTION	ASSESSMENT AND MANAGEMENT
Hypomagnesemia (low magnesium level, 0.75 mmol/L, although symptoms usually develop with <0.5 mmol/L). Normal magnesium level ranges from 0.75–1.25 mmol/L	• Can be caused by decreased intake, impaired absorption or increased excretion, and surgery, which causes the kidneys to excrete higher amounts of magnesium for 24 hours. Other causes may be decreased intake due to chronic alcoholism, malnutrition or starvation. Impaired absorption may be related to malabsorption syndromes (such as sprue, steatorrhea, or bowel resections) and excess intake of calcium. Increased excretion may result from diuretic use, loss of intestinal fluids (especially fistulas), diabetic ketoacidosis, primary aldosteronism, and primary hyperparathyroidism. Magnesium is important for the function of the neuromuscular system, so the signs and symptoms most often seen are neuromuscular. • Signs and symptoms: paresthesias, carpopedal spasm, muscle cramps, tetany, irritability, tremors, hyperexcitability, hyperreflexia, disorientation, depression, and seizures. Also, hypotension, dysrhythmias (atrial and ventricular), prolonged PR and QT intervals and broad flat T waves.	• Treatment is to correct the cause. If necessary, magnesium supplements may be given. The oral route is preferred to intramuscular injections, which are painful, and the IV route, which carries a significant risk for respiratory depression and hypotension. If the IV route is chosen for magnesium supplements, the nurse needs to assess the patient at least every 15 min for respiratory rate less than 16, hypotension, flushing, and diaphoresis. Loss of the patellar reflex may occur. If symptoms occur, the nurse slows or stops the infusion and notifies the physician.
Hypermagnesemia (high serum magnesium level, usually >1.5 mmol/L)	• Possibly caused by renal failure or intake of large amounts of medications with magnesium, such as some antacids and cathartics. • Signs and symptoms: vasodilation resulting in flushing, feeling warm, and hypotension. As the levels continue to rise, loss of reflexes, slowing bowel function, drowsiness, respiratory depression, coma, apnea and cardiac arrest may occur.	• Dialysis can be used to remove some magnesium but is not usually effective alone. Calcium gluconate is a temporary treatment until the cause can be identified and corrected.
Hypernatremia (high sodium level) and hyponatremia (low sodium level). Normal level is 135–145 mmol/L.	• Both may occur after cardiac surgery, but hyponatremia is more common. • Hyponatremia may result from reduced total body sodium or from increased water intake, which causes a dilution of body sodium. • Signs and symptoms of hyponatremia: weakness, fatigue, confusion, convulsions, and coma	• The patient must be observed for sodium values that vary from the normal ranges • When there is a true loss of sodium from the body, sodium replacement may be necessary. • Diuretics are prescribed when reduction in sodium is due to increased water intake.
Hypocalcemia (low calcium level). Normal level is 2.20–2.58 mmol/L.	• May result from alkalosis, which reduces the amount of calcium in the extracellular fluid, or from transfusions of large amounts of citrated blood products—packed red blood cells or whole blood. Citrate binds with calcium, reducing the amount of circulating ionized calcium. After 5–6 units of packed cells or whole blood from the blood bank, calcium binding may become a concern. • Signs and symptoms: numbness and tingling in the fingertips, toes, ears, and nose; carpopedal spasm; and muscle cramps and tetany	• Calcium level is monitored to determine if it is within normal limits. • Any symptoms of hypocalcemia are reported promptly so that calcium replacement can be instituted.
Hypercalcemia (high calcium level)	• Signs and symptoms: dysrhythmias that imitate those caused by digitalis toxicity (calcium can potentiate, or enhance, the action of digitalis)	• The nurse assesses the patient for signs of digitalis toxicity and reports these immediately so that the physician can institute treatment to prevent asystole and death.

(continued)

Table 28-8 • Potential Complications of Cardiac Surgery (Continued)

COMPLICATION	DESCRIPTION	ASSESSMENT AND MANAGEMENT
Other Complications		
Hepatic failure	• Most common in patients with cirrhosis, hepatitis, or prolonged right-sided heart failure	• Use of medications metabolized by the liver must be minimized. If hepatic failure cannot be reversed, death is inevitable. • Bilirubin, albumin, and amylase levels are monitored, and nutritional support must be provided.
Coagulopathies	• Result of hypothermia, blood component depletion, anticoagulation, or liver dysfunction	• Each patient must be carefully evaluated to determine the cause. Appropriate therapy is then provided.
Infection	• Cardiopulmonary bypass and anesthesia alter the patient's immune system. Many invasive devices are used to monitor and support the patient's recovery and may serve as a source of infection.	• The following must be monitored to detect signs of possible infection: body temperature, white blood cell counts and differential counts, incision and puncture sites, cardiac output and systemic vascular resistance, urine (clarity, colour, and odour), bilateral breath sounds, sputum (colour, odour, amount), as well as nasogastric secretions. • Antibiotic therapy may be expanded or modified as necessary. • Invasive devices must be discontinued as soon as they are no longer required. Institutional protocols for maintaining and replacing invasive lines and devices must be followed to minimize the patient's risk for infection.

Decreased Cardiac Output

A decrease in cardiac output is always a threat to the patient who has had cardiac surgery. It can have a variety of causes:

Preload alterations: too little or too much blood volume returning to the heart because of hypovolemia, persistent bleeding, cardiac tamponade, or fluid overload

Afterload alteration: hypertension and arterioles that are too constricted or too dilated because of alterations in body temperature or use of **vasoconstrictors** and **vasodilators**

Heart rate alterations: too fast, too slow, or dysrhythmias

Contractility alterations: cardiac failure, MI, electrolyte imbalances, hypoxia

Fluid Volume and Electrolyte Imbalance

The risk for fluid and electrolyte imbalance may occur after cardiac surgery. Nursing assessment for these complications includes monitoring of intake and output, weight, PAWP, left atrial pressure and CVP readings, hematocrit levels, distention of neck veins, edema, liver size, breath sounds (eg, fine crackles, wheezing), and electrolyte levels. Changes in serum electrolytes are reported promptly so that treatment can be instituted. Especially important are dangerously high or dangerously low levels of potassium, magnesium, sodium, and calcium.

Impaired Gas Exchange

Impaired gas exchange is another possible complication after cardiac surgery. All body tissues require an adequate supply of oxygen and nutrients for survival. To achieve this after surgery, an endotracheal tube with ventilator assistance may be used for 24 or more hours. The assisted ventilation is continued until the patient's blood gas measurements are acceptable and the patient demonstrates the ability to breathe independently. Patients who are stable after surgery may be extubated as early as 2 to 4 hours

after surgery, which reduces their anxiety regarding their limited ability to communicate.

The patient is continuously assessed for signs of impaired gas exchange: restlessness, anxiety, cyanosis of mucous membranes and peripheral tissues, tachycardia, and fighting the ventilator. Breath sounds are assessed often to detect fluid in the lungs and monitor lung expansion. Arterial blood gas values are monitored. Arterial blood gases, SpO_2, SaO_2, and end-tidal CO_2 are assessed for decreased oxygen and increased carbon dioxide.

Impaired Cerebral Circulation

Brain function depends on a continuous supply of oxygenated blood. The brain does not have the capacity to store oxygen and must rely on adequate continuous perfusion by the heart. It is important to observe the patient for any symptoms of hypoxia: restlessness, headache, confusion, dyspnea, hypotension, and cyanosis. An assessment of the patient's neurologic status includes level of consciousness, response to verbal commands and painful stimuli, pupil size and reaction to light, facial symmetry, movement of extremities, hand grip strength, presence of pedal and popliteal pulses, and temperature and colour of extremities. Any indication of a changing status is documented, and abnormal findings are reported to the surgeon because they may signal the beginning of a complication. Hypoperfusion or microemboli may produce central nervous system injury after cardiac surgery.

Diagnosis

NURSING DIAGNOSES

Based on the assessment data and the type of surgical procedure performed, major nursing diagnoses of the patient may include:

• Decreased cardiac output related to blood loss, compromised myocardial function, and dysrhythmias

- Impaired gas exchange related to trauma of extensive chest surgery
- Risk for deficient fluid volume (and electrolyte imbalance) related to alteration in circulating blood volume
- Disturbed sensory perception (visual or auditory) related to excessive environmental stimuli (critical care environment, surgical experience), insufficient sleep, psychological stress, altered sensory integration, and electrolyte imbalances
- Acute pain related to surgical trauma and pleural irritation caused by chest tubes
- Ineffective tissue perfusion (renal, cerebral, cardiopulmonary, gastrointestinal, peripheral) related to decreased cardiac output, hemolysis, vasopressor drug therapy, venous stasis, embolization, underlying atherosclerotic disease, effects of vasopressors, or coagulation problems
- Ineffective thermoregulation related to infection or post-pericardiotomy syndrome
- Deficient knowledge about self-care activities

COLLABORATIVE PROBLEMS/POTENTIAL COMPLICATIONS

Based on the assessment data, potential complications that may develop include:

- Cardiac complications: heart failure, MI, stunned myocardium, dysrhythmias, tamponade, cardiac arrest
- Pulmonary complications: pulmonary edema, pulmonary emboli, pleural effusions, pneumothorax or hemothorax, respiratory failure, acute respiratory distress syndrome
- Hemorrhage
- Neurologic complications: CVA (brain attack, stroke), air emboli
- Renal failure, acute or chronic
- Electrolyte imbalances
- Hepatic failure
- Coagulopathies
- Infection, sepsis

Planning and Goals

The major goals for the patient include restoration of cardiac output, adequate gas exchange, maintenance of fluid and electrolyte balance, reduction of symptoms of sensory-perception alterations, relief of pain, maintenance of adequate tissue perfusion, maintenance of normal body temperature, learning self-care activities, and absence of complications.

Nursing Interventions

RESTORING CARDIAC OUTPUT

Nursing management of the patient involves continuously observing the patient's cardiac status and notifying the surgeon of any changes that indicate decreased cardiac output. The nurse and the surgeon then work collaboratively to correct the problem.

In evaluating the patient's cardiac status, the nurse primarily determines the effectiveness of cardiac output through clinical observations and routine measurements: serial readings of blood pressure, heart rate, CVP, arterial pressure, and left atrial or pulmonary artery pressure.

Renal function is related to cardiac function, as blood pressure and heart rate drive glomerular filtration; therefore, urinary output is measured and recorded. Urine output of less than 25 mL/hr may indicate a decrease in cardiac output. Urine specific gravity may also be assessed (normal: 1.010 to 1.025), as may urine osmolality. Inadequate fluid volume may be manifested by low urinary output and high specific gravity, whereas overhydration is manifested by high urine output with low specific gravity.

The growth and function of body cells depend on adequate cardiac output to provide a continuous supply of oxygenated blood to meet the changing demands of the organs and body systems. Because the buccal mucosa, nailbeds, lips, and earlobes are sites with rich capillary beds, they should be observed for cyanosis or duskiness as possible signs of reduced heart action. Moist or dry skin may indicate vasodilation or vasoconstriction, respectively. Distention of the neck veins or of the dorsal surface of the hand raised to heart level may signal a changing demand or diminishing capacity of the heart. If cardiac output has fallen, the skin becomes cool, moist, and cyanotic or mottled.

Dysrhythmias, which may arise when poor perfusion of the heart exists, also serve as important indicators of cardiac function. The most common dysrhythmias encountered during the postoperative period are atrial fibrillation, bradycardias, tachycardias, and ectopic beats. Continuous observation of the cardiac monitor for various dysrhythmias is an essential part of patient care and management.

Any indications of decreased cardiac output are reported promptly to the physician. These assessment data and results of diagnostic tests are used by the physician to determine the cause of the problem. After a diagnosis has been made, the physician and the nurse work collaboratively to restore cardiac output and prevent further complications. When indicated, the physician prescribes blood components, fluids, digitalis or other antidysrhythmics, diuretics, vasodilators, or vasopressors. When additional surgery is necessary, the patient and family are prepared for the procedure.

PROMOTING ADEQUATE GAS EXCHANGE

To ensure adequate gas exchange, the nurse assesses and maintains the patency of the endotracheal tube. The patient is suctioned when wheezes, coarse crackles, or rhonchi are present. Suctioning may be performed with an in-line suction catheter; the nurse and respiratory therapist determine if the ventilator's fractional inspired oxygen (FiO_2) should be increased for three or more breaths before the patient is suctioned. Alternatively, 100% oxygen is delivered to the patient by a manual resuscitation bag (eg, Ambu-Bag) before and after suctioning to minimize the risk of hypoxia that can result from the suctioning procedure. Arterial blood gas determinations are compared with baseline data, and changes are reported to the physician promptly.

Because a patent airway is essential for oxygen and carbon dioxide exchange, the endotracheal tube must be secured to prevent it from slipping into the right mainstem bronchus and occluding the left bronchus. When the patient's condition stabilizes, body position is changed every 1 to 2 hours. Frequent changes of patient position provide for optimal pulmonary ventilation and perfusion by allowing the lungs to expand more fully. The nurse assesses breath sounds to detect crackles, wheezes, and fluid in the lungs.

The patient is usually weaned from the ventilator and extubated within 24 hours of CABG. Physical assessment and arterial blood gas results guide the process. Before being extubated, the patient should have cough and gag reflexes and stable vital signs; be able to lift the head off the bed or give firm hand grasps; have adequate vital capacity, negative inspiratory force, and minute volume appropriate for body size; and have acceptable arterial blood gas levels while breathing warmed humidified oxygen without the assistance of the ventilator.

Extubation has been performed within these parameters without any adverse effects on the patient's condition or prognosis.

During this time, the nurse assists with the weaning process and eventually with removal of the endotracheal tube. Deep breathing and forced expiration technique (FET, huffing) or coughing are encouraged at least every 1 to 2 hours after extubation to open the alveolar sacs and provide for increased perfusion. FET is the rapid exhalation of a deep breath using the diaphragm and abdominal muscles to force air out through an open mouth and glottis (the glottis is not held closed then suddenly opened, as in a cough). Patients may experience less pain with FET than coughing, which may increase the frequency with which a patient performs the exercises. The patient should be taught and assisted to splint the chest incision before and during FET or coughing to minimize discomfort.

MAINTAINING FLUID AND ELECTROLYTE BALANCE

To promote fluid and electrolyte balance, the nurse carefully assesses intake and output. Flow sheets are used to determine positive or negative fluid balance. All fluid intake is recorded, including intravenous, nasogastric tube, and oral fluids. All output is recorded, including urine, nasogastric drainage, and chest drainage.

Hemodynamic parameters (ie, blood pressure, pulmonary wedge and left atrial pressures, and CVP) are correlated with intake, output, and weight to determine the adequacy of hydration and cardiac output. Serum electrolytes are monitored, and the patient is observed for signs of potassium, magnesium, sodium, or calcium imbalance (ie, hypokalemia, hyperkalemia, hypomagnesemia, hyponatremia, or hypocalcemia).

Any indications of dehydration, fluid overload, or electrolyte imbalance are reported promptly, and the physician and nurse work collaboratively to restore fluid and electrolyte balance. The patient's response is monitored.

MINIMIZING SENSORY-PERCEPTION IMBALANCE

A large number of patients experience abnormal behaviours that occur with varying intensity and duration. In the early years of cardiac surgery, this phenomenon occurred more frequently than it does today. At that time, it was attributed to inadequate cerebral perfusion during surgery, microemboli, and the length of time that the patient remained on the CPB machine. Advances in surgical techniques have significantly decreased these factors. Today, when it occurs, it is thought to be caused by anxiety, sleep deprivation, increased sensory input, and disorientation to night and day when the patient loses track of time (Arrowsmith et al., 1999; Braunwald et al., 2001; Fuster et al., 2001). An important finding is that patients who do not or cannot express anxiety before surgery and those who are not able to sleep postoperatively are more prone to develop psychosis in the postoperative period. Psychosis may appear after a 2- to 5-day lucid interval.

Basic comfort measures used in conjunction with prescribed analgesics potentiate the effects of the analgesics and promote rest. The patient is assisted in changing positions every 1 to 2 hours and is positioned in such a way to avoid strain on incisions and chest tubes. Nursing care is scheduled as much as possible to provide undisturbed periods of rest. As the patient's condition stabilizes and the patient is disturbed less frequently for monitoring and therapeutic procedures, rest periods can be extended. As much uninterrupted sleep as possible is provided, especially during the patient's normal hours of sleep.

The nurse monitors the patient for signs of denial and provides an opportunity for emotional expression during the preoperative period. Careful explanations of all procedures and of the need for cooperation help to keep the patient oriented throughout the postoperative course. Continuity of care is desirable; a familiar face

and a nursing staff with a consistent approach promote the delivery of quality nursing care. A well-designed and individualized plan of nursing care can assist the nursing team in coordinating their efforts for the emotional well-being of the patient.

RELIEVING PAIN

Deep pain may not be reflected in the immediate area of injury but occur in a broader, more diffuse area. Patients who have had cardiac surgery experience pain caused by the interruption of intercostal nerves along the incision route and irritation of the pleura by the chest catheters. Incisional pain may also be experienced from peripheral vein or artery graft harvest sites.

It is essential to observe and listen to the patient for verbal and nonverbal clues about pain. The nurse accurately records the nature, type, location, and duration of the pain. (Chest incisional pain must be differentiated from anginal pain.) The patient is encouraged to use patient-controlled analgesia or accept medication as often as it is prescribed to reduce the amount of pain. Physical support of the incision during deep breathing and FET (or coughing) also helps to minimize pain. The patient should then be able to participate in respiratory exercises and to increase self-care progressively.

Pain produces tension, which may stimulate the central nervous system to release adrenaline, which results in constriction of the arterioles and increased heart rate. This can cause increased afterload and decreased cardiac output. Opioids alleviate anxiety and pain and induce sleep, which reduces the metabolic rate and oxygen demands. After the administration of opioids, any observations indicating relief of apprehension and pain are documented in the patient's record. The patient is observed for any respiratory depressant effects of the analgesic. If respiratory depression occurs, an opioid antagonist (eg, naloxone [Narcan]) is used to counteract the effect.

MAINTAINING ADEQUATE TISSUE PERFUSION

Peripheral pulses (eg, pedal, tibial, popliteal, femoral, radial, brachial) are routinely palpated to assess for arterial obstruction. If a pulse is absent in any extremity, the cause may be prior catheterization of that extremity. The newly identified absence of any pulse is immediately reported to the physician.

Thrombus formation and resulting embolus formation also can result from injury to the intima of the blood vessels, dislodging a clot from a damaged valve, loosening of mural thrombi, and coagulation problems. Air embolism may occur as a result of CPB or central venous cannulation. Symptoms of embolization vary according to site. The usual embolic sites are the lungs, coronary arteries, mesentery, spleen, extremities, kidneys, and brain. The patient is observed for:

- Chest pain and respiratory distress with pulmonary embolus or MI
- Midabdominal or midback pain
- Pain, cessation of pulses, blanching, numbness, or coldness in an extremity
- Decreased urine output
- One-sided weakness and pupillary changes, as occur in CVAs (brain attacks, strokes)

All such symptoms are promptly reported to the physician.

After surgery, the following measures are taken to prevent venous stasis, which can cause thrombus formation and subsequent embolization:

- Applying elastic compression stockings or elastic bandage wrap and pneumatic antiembolic stockings

- Discouraging crossing of legs
- Avoiding use of the knee gatch on the bed
- Omitting pillows in the popliteal space
- Instituting passive exercises followed by active exercises to promote circulation and prevent loss of muscle tone (patients need to ambulate as early as possible)

Inadequate renal perfusion can occur as a complication of cardiac surgery. One possible cause is low cardiac output. Trauma to blood cells during CPB can cause hemolysis of red blood cells, which then occlude the renal glomeruli. Use of vasopressor agents to increase blood pressure may constrict the renal arterioles and reduce blood flow to the kidneys.

Nursing management includes accurate measurement of urine output. An output of less than 25 mL/hr may indicate hypovolemia. Urine specific gravity can be monitored to determine the kidneys' ability to concentrate urine in the renal tubules. Rapid-acting diuretics or inotropic medications (eg, digoxin [Lanoxin], isoproterenol [Isuprel]) may be prescribed to increase cardiac output and renal blood flow. The nurse should be aware of the patient's blood urea nitrogen, serum creatinine, and urine and serum electrolyte levels. Abnormal levels are reported promptly because it may be necessary to adjust fluids and the dose or type of medication administered. If efforts to maintain renal perfusion are not effective, the patient may require dialysis or continuous renal replacement therapy (see Chap. 44).

MAINTAINING NORMAL BODY TEMPERATURE

Patients are usually hypothermic when admitted to the critical care unit from the cardiac surgical procedure. The patient must be gradually warmed to a normal temperature. This is accomplished partially by the patient's own basal metabolic processes and often with the assistance of warmed ventilator air, warm air or warm cotton blankets, or heat lamps. While the patient is hypothermic, the clotting process is less efficient, the heart is prone to dysrhythmias, and oxygen does not readily transfer from the hemoglobin to the tissues. Because anesthesia and hypothermia suppress the basal metabolism, oxygen supply usually meets the cellular demand.

After cardiac surgery, the patient is at risk for developing elevated body temperature caused by infection or postpericardiotomy syndrome. The resultant increase in metabolic rate increases tissue oxygen demands and increases cardiac workload. Measures are taken to prevent this sequence of events or to halt it as soon as it is recognized.

Sites of infection include the lungs, urinary tract, incisions, and intravascular catheters. Meticulous care is used to prevent contamination at the sites of catheter and tube insertions. Aseptic technique is used when changing dressings and when providing endotracheal tube and catheter care. Clearance of pulmonary secretions is accomplished by frequent repositioning of the patient, suctioning, and chest physical therapy, as well as teaching and encouraging the patient to breathe deeply and use FET (or cough). Closed systems are used to maintain all intravenous and arterial lines. All invasive equipment is discontinued as soon as possible after surgery.

Postpericardiotomy syndrome occurs in approximately 10% to 40% of patients who undergo cardiac surgery. Although the precise cause is unknown, a common factor appears to be trauma, with residual blood in the pericardial sac after surgery. The syndrome is characterized by fever, pericardial pain, pleural pain, dyspnea, pericardial effusion, pericardial friction rub, and arthralgia. There may be a combination of these signs and symptoms.

Leukocytosis occurs, along with elevation of the erythrocyte sedimentation rate. These symptoms frequently appear after the patient is discharged from the hospital.

The syndrome must be differentiated from other postoperative complications (eg, infection, incisional pain, MI, pulmonary embolus, bacterial endocarditis, pneumonia, atelectasis). Treatment depends on the severity of the symptoms. Bed rest and anti-inflammatory agents, such as salicylates and corticosteroids, produce a dramatic improvement in symptoms.

PROMOTING HOME AND COMMUNITY-BASED CARE

Teaching Patients Self-Care

Depending on the type of surgery and postoperative progress, the patient may be discharged from the hospital as early as 1 day after MIDCAB and 3 days after other surgery. Although the patient may be anxious to return home, the patient and family usually have apprehensions about this transition. The family members often express the fear that they are not capable of caring for the patient at home. They often are concerned that complications will occur that they are unprepared to handle.

The nurse helps the patient and family to set realistic, achievable goals. A teaching plan that meets the patient's individual needs is developed with the patient and family. This is done before admission and reviewed each shift through the hospitalization or with each home care and rehabilitation contact. Specific instructions are provided about incision care; signs and symptoms of infection; diet; activity progression and exercise; deep breathing, FET (or coughing), incentive spirometry; and smoking cessation; weight and temperature monitoring; the medication regimen; and follow-up visits with home care nurses, the rehabilitation personnel, the surgeon, and the cardiologist or internist.

Some patients may have difficulty learning and retaining information after cardiac surgery. Studies have documented that many patients have difficulties in cognitive function after cardiac surgery that do not occur after other types of major surgery (Arrowsmith et al., 1999; Roach et al., 1996). The patient may experience recent memory loss, short attention span, difficulty with simple math, poor handwriting, and visual disturbances. Patients with these difficulties often become frustrated when they try to resume normal activities and learn how to care for themselves at home. The patient and family are reassured that the difficulty is temporary and will subside, usually in 6 to 8 weeks. In the meantime, instructions are given to the patient at a much slower pace than normal, and a family member assumes responsibility for making sure that the prescribed regimen is followed. All information is provided in writing in the patient's primary language.

Continuing Care

Arrangements are made for a home care nurse to provide care when appropriate. Since the length of time that the patient remains in the hospital is relatively short, it is particularly important for the nurse to assess the patient's and family's ability to manage care in the home. The education plan is continued by the home care nurse. Vital signs and incisions are monitored, the patient is assessed for signs and symptoms of complications, and support for the patient and family is provided. Additional interventions may include dressing changes, intravenous antibiotic administration, diet counselling, and tobacco use cessation strategies. Patients and families need to know that cardiac surgery did not cure the patient's underlying heart disease. Lifestyle changes for risk factor reduction must be made, and medications taken preoperatively may be prescribed postoperatively.

NURSING RESEARCH PROFILE 28-1

Cardiac Surgery Patients' Transition From Hospital To Home

Weaver, L. A., & Doran, K. A. (2001). Telephone follow-up after cardiac surgery. *American Journal of Nursing*, 101(5), 24OO–24WW.

Purpose

Hospital length of stay (LOS) for patients after cardiac surgery may be 3 or 4 days. Formal patient/family education programs describing how to care for the patient at home are often provided during the hospitalization. These researchers identified that no health care professionals were contacting or seeing patients for 2 to 4 weeks after discharge from the hospital. The researchers implemented a telephone follow-up program. The purpose of the study was to evaluate the telephone follow-up program for patients who had undergone cardiac surgery.

Study Sample and Design

A convenience sample of heart surgery patients was selected, 46 of whom received usual care (control patients) and 44 of whom received usual care and postdischarge follow-up telephone calls (intervention patients). Patients in the intervention group were called by a cardiovascular stepdown unit registered nurse within 2 days after discharge, and then once a week for 1 month. At the end of this period, each participant was mailed a questionnaire to measure patient satisfaction, depression, recidivism, and complications. Patient satisfaction was measured with a modified four-question survey, the Continuity and Transition Dimensions, Picker Institute Survey. Depression was measured with a modified 15-question survey, the Geriatric Depression Scale. Recidivism was measured by the number of emergency department visits and hospital admissions during the 30 days after discharge from the hospital for cardiac surgery. Complications were self-reported by the participants.

Findings

Patient satisfaction in the intervention group was at least 10% higher than in the control group for three of four variables, but the results were not statistically significant. Twenty-two percent of the control group and 18% of the intervention group were readmitted or made emergency department visits during the first 30 days after discharge (recidivism); this difference in incidence was not statistically significant. There were no differences in the rate of depression or complications between the groups. The nurses who conducted the follow-up telephone program reported that they provided reassurance and support in each phone call. They provided reinforcement and clarification of postoperative education regarding leg swelling (31%), pain medication (23%), weight-taking and knowing when to call a health care provider (16%), and medication teaching (100%). The nurses also made referrals (to physicians, cardiac rehabilitation programs, dietitians, tobacco intervention programs [7%]) and coached patients with questions they wanted to ask their physicians (12%).

Nursing Implications

Telephone calls by step-down unit registered nurses to cardiac surgery patients after hospital discharge increase patient satisfaction (although not to statistical significance) and provide opportunities for reassurance and patient education. Development and use of scripts (algorithms, decision tree standards) may be helpful to the nurse making the telephone calls and facilitate consistency in the information provided to the patient. Script topics suggested by this study include incision care, leg swelling, fever, weight measurements and when to call a health care provider, pain management, medications (especially warfarin [Coumadin]), dysrhythmias, fluid status, constipation, nutrition, sleep, and depression.

Patient teaching does not end at the time of discharge from home health. The patient is encouraged to maintain telephone contact with the surgeon, cardiologist, and nurses. This provides the patient and family with reassurance that questions can be answered and problems can be resolved if they arise. Many hospitals provide family support sessions that help family members cope with their own stress related to the patient's home health care management. The patient is expected to have a follow-up visit with the surgeon.

Many patients and families benefit from supportive programs such as the postcardiac surgery rehabilitation programs offered by many medical centres. These programs provide exercise monitoring; instructions about diet and stress reduction; information about resuming exercise, work, driving, and sexual activity; assistance with tobacco use cessation; and support groups for patients and families. The Heart and Stroke Foundation of Canada provides a range of Internet resources to support families, share experiences, and provide care.

Evaluation

EXPECTED PATIENT OUTCOMES

Expected patient outcomes may include:

1. Maintains adequate cardiac output
2. Maintains adequate gas exchange
3. Maintains fluid (and electrolyte) balance
4. Experiences decreased symptoms of sensory-perception disturbances
5. Experiences relief of pain
6. Maintains adequate tissue perfusion
7. Maintains normal body temperature
8. Performs self-care activities

A typical plan of postoperative nursing care and more-detailed expected outcomes for the cardiac surgery patient are presented in the Plan of Nursing Care, on pages 744–749.

Critical Thinking Exercises

1. You are caring for a patient who has undergone a PTCA with stent placement. The patient suddenly develops chest discomfort. In addition to the characteristics of the chest discomfort, identify the key factors that need to be assessed. Describe the actions that you would take and state why.

2. You are caring for a patient who is scheduled to have MIDCAB surgery. He appears quite anxious and states that he is afraid he will need to have traditional CABG surgery as discussed in obtaining informed consent. He states he does not want to have his "whole sternum cut open." His wife tends to minimize the significance of his concerns, commenting that, as the surgeon explained it, the possibility of having a traditional CABG is very small. How would you respond to this patient and his wife? How might your response differ if the wife shares her husband's concerns?

3. You are caring for a patient who underwent traditional CABG surgery 2 days ago and is progressing well. After ambulating in the corridor with his daughter, he returns to his room and notices that the dressing on his saphenous vein site is stained with bright red blood. His daughter is visibly upset. Explain what your first action will be and why. If your initial actions do not achieve the desired outcome, how would you proceed? How would you explain the episode to the daughter to help her understand the bleeding?

4. You are caring for two patients, both of whom were hospitalized for acute MI. One patient lives in his home with a supportive family, the other patient is homeless and living on the street. How does your plan of care and patient teaching differ for these patients?

REFERENCES AND SELECTED READINGS

Books

Agency for Health Care Policy and Research. (1994). *Unstable angina: Diagnosis and management.* Clinical Practice Guideline Number 10. AHCPR Publication No. 94-0602. Rockville, MD: Public Health Service, U.S. Department of Health and Human Services.

Albert, J. S. (2001). *The AHA clinical cardiac consult.* Philadelphia: Lippincott Williams & Wilkins.

American Heart Association (2001). *2001 Heart and Stroke Statistical Update.* Dallas, TX: American Heart Association.

Apple, S., & Lindsay, J. (2000). *Principles and practices of interventional cardiology.* Philadelphia: Lippincott Williams & Wilkins.

Bickley, L. S., & Szilagyi, P. G. (2003). *Bates' guide to physical examination and history taking* (8th ed.). Philadelphia: Lippincott Williams & Wilkins.

Braunwald, E., Zipes, D. P., & Libby, P. (Eds.). (2001). *Heart disease: A textbook of cardiovascular medicine* (6th ed.). Philadelphia: W. B. Saunders.

Carpenito, L. J. (2004). *Nursing diagnosis: Application to clinical practice* (10th ed.). Philadelphia: Lippincott Williams & Wilkins.

Effron, D. M. (Ed.). (1998). *Cardiopulmonary resuscitation: CPR* (4th ed.). Tulsa, OK: CPR Publishers, Inc.

Fuster, V., Alexander, R. W., O'Rourke, R. A., Roberts, R., King, S. B., III, & Wellens, H. J. J. (Eds.). (2001). *Hurst's the heart* (10th ed.). New York: McGraw-Hill.

Hudak, C. M., Gallo, B. M., & Morton, P. G. (1998). *Critical care nursing: A holistic approach* (7th ed.). Philadelphia: Lippincott-Raven.

Kuhn, M. A. (1999). *Complementary therapies for healthcare providers.* Philadelphia: Lippincott Williams & Wilkins.

McHale, D. J., & Carlson, K. K. (2001). *AACN procedure manual for critical care* (4th ed.). Philadelphia: W. B. Saunders.

Murphy, J. (Ed.). (2000). *Mayo Clinic cardiology review* (2nd ed.). Philadelphia: Lippincott Williams & Wilkins.

National Heart, Lung, Blood Institute, National High Blood Pressure Education Program. (1997). *The sixth report of the Joint Committee on Prevention, Detection, and Treatment of High Blood Pressure.* NIH Publication No. 98-4080. Bethesda, MD: National Institutes of Health.

North American Nursing Diagnosis Association. (2001). *Nursing diagnoses: Definitions and classification 2001–2002.* Philadelphia: North American Nursing Diagnosis Association.

Office for Social Environment and Health Research at West Virginia University. (2001). *Women and heart disease: An atlas of racial and ethnic disparities in mortality* (2nd ed.). Washington, DC: National Center for Chronic Disease Prevention and Health Promotion Centers for Disease Control and Prevention, U.S. Department of Health & Human Services.

Wagner, G. S. (2001). *Marriott's practical electrocardiography* (10th ed.). Philadelphia: Lippincott Williams & Wilkins.

Wenger, N. K., Froelicher, E. S., Smith, L. K., Ades, P. A., Berra, K., Blumenthal, J. A., et al. (1995). *Cardiac rehabilitation.* Clinical Practice Guideline Number 17. AHCPR Publication No. 96-0672. Rockville, MD: Public Health Service, Agency for Health Care Policy and Research and the National Heart, Lung, and Blood Institute.

Journals

Asterisks indicate nursing research articles.

Acorda, R., Kraus, T., & Casey, P. E. (2000). Advances in the surgical treatment of coronary artery disease. *Nursing Clinics of North America, 35*(4), 911–932.

American College of Cardiology Foundation and American Heart Association. (2002). ACC/AHA 2002 guideline update for exercise testing: A report of the American College of Cardiology/American Heart Association Task Force on Practice Guidelines (Committee on Exercise Testing). Available at: http://www.acc.org/clinical/guidelines/exercise. Accessed December 3, 2002.

American Heart Association. (2002). Women, heart disease and stroke statistics. Available at: http://www.americanheart.org/presenter.jhtml?identifier=4787. Accessed March 12, 2002.

Anderson, J. J. (2000). Transmyocardial laser revascularization. *Progress on Cardiovascular Nursing, 15*(3), 76–81.

Arrowsmith, J. E., Grocott, H. P., & Newman, M. F. (1999). Neurologic risk assessment, monitoring and outcome in cardiac surgery. *Journal of Cardiothoracic Vascular Anesthesia, 13*(6), 736–743.

Ballegaard, S., Meyer, C. N., & Trojaborg, W. (1991). Acupuncture in angina pectoris: Does acupuncture have a specific effect? *Journal of Internal Medicine, 229*(4), 357–362.

*Bengtson, A., Karlsson, T., & Herlitz, J. (2000). Differences between men and women on the waiting list for coronary revascularization. *Journal of Advanced Nursing, 31*(6), 1361–1367.

Brachmann, J., Ansah, M., Kosinski, E. J., & Schuler, G. C. (1998). Improved clinical effectiveness with a collagen vascular hemostasis device for shortened immobilization time following diagnostic angiography and percutaneous transluminal coronary angioplasty. *American Journal of Cardiology, 81*(12), 1502–1505.

Braunwald, E., Antman, E. M., Beasley, J. W., Califf, R., Cheitlin, M. D., Hochman, J. S., Jones, R. H., Kereiakes, D., Kupersmith, J., Levin, T. N., Pepine, C. J., Schaeffer, J. W., Smith, E. E., 3rd, Steward, D. E., Theroux, P., Alpert, J. S., Eagle, K. A., Faxon, D. P., Fuster, V., Gardner, T. J., Gregoratos, G., Russell, R. O., & Smith, S. C., Jr. (2000). ACC/AHA guidelines for the management of patients with unstable angina and non-ST-segment elevation MI: Executive summary and recommendations. A report of the American College of Cardiology/American Heart Association Task Force on Practice Guidelines (Committee on the Management of Patients with Unstable Angina). *Circulation, 102*(10), 1193–1209.

Burkhoff, D., Schmidt, S., Schulman, S. P., Myers, J., Resar, J., Becker, L. C., Weiss, J., & Jones, J. W. (1999). Transmyocardial laser revascularization compared with continued medical therapy for treatment of refractory angina pectoris: A prospective randomized trial. ATLANTIC (Angina Treatments: Lasers and Normal Therapies in Comparison) Investigators. *Lancet, 354*(9182), 885–890.

Buselli, E. F., & Stuart, E. M. (1999). Influence of psychosocial factors and biopsychosocial interventions on outcomes after myocardial infarction. *Journal of Cardiovascular Nursing, 13*(3), 60–72.

Canto, J. G., Shlipak, M. G., Rogers, W. J., Malmgren, J. A., Fraterick, P. D., Lambrew, C. T., Ornato, J. P., Barron, H. V., & Kiefe, C. I. (2000). Prevalence, clinical characteristics, and mortality among patients with myocardial infarction presenting without chest pain. *Journal of the American Medical Association, 283*(24), 3223–3229.

Casey, K., Bedker, D. L., & Roussel-McElmeel, P. L. (1998). Myocardial infarction: Review of clinical trials and treatment strategies. *Critical Care Nurse, 18*(2), 39–54.

Chlan, L., & Tracy, M. F. (1999). Music therapy in critical care: Indications and guidelines for intervention. *Critical Care Nurse, 19*(3), 35–41.

*Christensen, B. V., Manion, R. V., Iacarella, C. L., Meyer, S. M., Cartland, J. L., Bruhn-Ding, B. J., & Wilson, R. F. (1998). Vascular complications after angiography with and without the use of sandbags. *Nursing Research, 47*(1), 51–53.

Cohen, M. (2001). The role of low-molecular-weight heparin in the management of acute coronary syndromes. *Current Opinion in Cardiology, 16*(6), 384–389.

*Corrêa, C. G., & da Cruz, D. A. L. M. (2000). Pain: Clinical validation with postoperative heart surgery patients. *Nursing Diagnosis, 11*(1), 5–14.

Creek, D. J., Granger, B. B., & Prinkley-Briggs, L. A. (Eds.). (2000). Issues in acute cardiology. Continuing care in adult cardiology: Living with a cardiac diagnosis. *Nursing Clinics of North America, 35*(4), 833–1046.

Cucinelli, C. (2000). Minimally invasive coronary artery bypass surgery. *Critical Care Nursing Quarterly, 23*(1), 54–65.

Danesh, J., Collins, R., & Peto, R. (2000). Lipoprotein(a) and coronary heart disease: Meta-analysis of prospective studies. *Circulation, 102*(10), 1082–1085.

*Davies, N. (2000). Patients' and carers' perceptions of factors influencing recovery after cardiac surgery. *Journal of Advanced Nursing, 32*(2), 318–326.

Dembroski, T. M., MacDougall, J. M., Costa, P. T., & Grandits, G. A. (1989). Components of hostility as predictors of sudden death and myocardial infarction in the Multiple Risk Factor Intervention Trial. *Psychosomatic Medicine, 51*(5), 514–522.

*Dixon, T., Lim, L. L. Y., Powell, H., & Fisher, J. D. (2000). Psychosocial experiences of cardiac patients in early recovery: A community-based study. *Journal of Advanced Nursing, 31*(6), 1368–1375.

Doering, L. V. (1999). Pathophysiology of acute coronary syndromes leading to acute myocardial infarction. *Journal of Cardiovascular Nursing, 13*(3), 1–20.

Eagle, K. A., Guyton, R. A., Davidoff, R., Ewy, G. A., Fonger, J., Gardner, T. J., Gott, J. P., Herrmann, H. C., Marlow, R. A., Nugent, W. C., O'Connor, G. T., Orszulak, T. A., Rieselbach, R. E., Winters, W. L., Yusuf, S., Gibbons, R. J., Alpert, J. S., Eagle, K. A., Garson, A., Jr., Gregoratos, G., Russell, R. O., Smith, S. C., Jr. (1999). ACC/AHA guidelines for coronary artery bypass surgery: A report of the American College of Cardiology/American Heart Association Task Force on Practice Guidelines (Committee to Revise the 1991 Guidelines for Coronary Artery Bypass Graft Surgery). *Journal of the American College of Cardiology, 34*(4), 1262–1347.

Edgar, W. F., Ebersole, N., & Mayfield, M. G. (1999). MIDCAB. *American Journal of Nursing, 99*(7), 40–46.

*Elliott, D. (1994). The effects of music and muscle relaxation on patient anxiety in a coronary care unit. *Heart & Lung, 23*(1), 27–35.

Evans, D. (2002). The effectiveness of music as an intervention for hospital patients: A systematic review. *Journal of Advanced Nursing, 37*(1), 8–18.

Expert Panel on Detection, Evaluation, and Treatment of High Blood Cholesterol in Adults. (2001). Executive summary of the third report of the National Cholesterol Education Program (NCEP) Expert Panel on Detection, Evaluation, and Treatment of High Blood Cholesterol in Adults (Adult Treatment Panel III). *Journal of the American Medical Association, 285*, 2486–2497.

Expert Panel on Detection, Evaluation, and Treatment of High Blood Cholesterol in Adults. (2001). Third report of the National Cholesterol Education Program (NCEP) Expert Panel on detection, evaluation, and treatment of high blood cholesterol in adults (Adult Treatment Panel III): Full report. Available at: http://www.nhlbi.nih.gov/guidelines/cholesterol/atp3_rpt.htm. Accessed June 30, 2002.

Fair, J., & Fletcher, B. J. (Eds.). (2000). Abnormal lipids. *Journal of Cardiovascular Nursing, 14*(2), 1–103.

Friedman, M., & Rosenman, R. H. (1959). Association of specific overt behavior patterns with blood and cardiovascular findings: Blood cholesterol level, blood clotting time, incidence of arcus senilis and clinical coronary artery disease. *Journal of the American Medical Association, 169*, 1286–1297.

Furberg, C. D., Psaty, B. M., & Meyer, J. V. (1996). Nifedipine: Dose-related increase in mortality in patients with coronary heart disease. *Circulation, 92*(5), 1326–1331.

Gaenzer, H., Neumayr, G., Marschang, P., Sturm, W., Lechleitner, M., Föger, B., Kirchmair, R., & Patsch, J. (2002). Effect of insulin therapy on endothelium-dependent dilation in type 2 diabetes mellitus. *American Journal of Cardiology, 89*(4), 431–434.

Gebbie, A. (2002). Risks and benefits of estrogen plus progestin in healthy postmenopausal women: Principal results from the Women's Health Initiative Randomized Controlled Trial. Writing Group for the Women's Health Initiative Number 10 Investigators. *Journal of the American Medical Association, 288*(3), 321–333.

Gibbons, R. J., Chatterjee, K., Daley, J., Douglas, J. S., Fihn, S. D., Gardin, J. M., Grunwald, M. A., Levy, D., Lytle, B. W., O'Rourke, R. A., Schafer, W. P., Williams, S. V., Ritchie, J. L., Cheitlin, M. D., Eagle, K. A., Gardner, T. J., Garson, A., Jr., Russell, R. O., Ryan, T. J., & Smith, S. C., Jr. (1999). ACC/AHA/ACP-ASIM guidelines for the management of patients with chronic stable angina: A report of the American College of Cardiology/American Heart Association Task Force on Practice Guidelines (Committee on Management of Patients with Chronic Stable Angina). *Journal of the American College of Cardiology, 33*(7), 2092–2197.

Giuliano, K. K., Bloniasz, E., & Bell, J. (1999). Implementation of a pet visitation program in critical care. *Critical Care Nurse, 19*(3), 43–50.

Grady, D., Herrington, D., Bittner, V., Blumenthal, R., Davidson, M., Hlatky, M., Hsia, J., Hulley, S., Herd, A., Khan, S., Newby, L. K., Waters, D., Vittinghoff, E., Wenger, N., & HERS Research Group. (2002). Cardiovascular disease outcomes during 6.8 years of hormone therapy: Heart and Estrogen/Progestin Replacement Study follow-up (HERS II). *Journal of the American Medical Association, 288*(1), 49–57.

Greeland, P., Smith, S. C., Jr., & Grundy, S. M. (2001). Improving coronary heart disease risk assessment in asymptomatic people: Role of traditional risk factors and noninvasive cardiovascular tests. *Circulation, 104*(15), 1863–1867.

Grundy, S. M., Benjamin, I. J., Burke, G. L., Chait, A., Eckel, R. H., Howard, B. V., Mitch, W., Smith, S. C., Jr., & Sowers, J. R. (1999). Diabetes and cardiovascular disease: A statement for healthcare professionals from the American Heart Association. *Circulation, 100*(10), 1134–1146.

Harrison, H. (1999). Troponin I. *American Journal of Nursing, 99*(5), 24TT–26TT.

Hayden, A. M. (1998). Transmyocardial revascularization surgery. *Critical Care Nursing Quarterly, 21*(1), 48–57.

Heart and Stroke Foundation of Canada. (2003). *The growing burden of heart disease and stroke.* Ottawa: Author.

Hirsh, J., Anand, S. S., Halperin, J. L., & Fuster, V. (2001). Guide to anticoagulant therapy: Heparin. A statement for healthcare professionals from the American Heart Association. *Circulation, 103*(24), 2994–3018.

Homocysteine Studies Collaboration. (2002). Homocysteine and risk of ischemic heart disease and stroke: A meta-analysis. *Journal of the American Medical Association, 288*(16), 2015–2022.

Hulley, S., Grady, D., Bush, T., Furberg, C., Herrington, D., Riggs, B., & Vittinghoff, E. (1998). Randomized trial of estrogen plus progestin for secondary prevention of coronary heart disease in postmenopausal women. *Journal of the American Medical Association, 280*(7), 605–613.

*Hussey, L. C., Hynan, L., & Leeper, B. (2001). Risk factors for sternal wound infection in men versus women. *American Journal of Critical Care, 10*(2), 112–116.

Ishihara, M., Sato, H., Tateishi, H., Kawagoe, T., Shimatani, Y., Ueda, K., Noma, K., Yumoto, A., & Nishioka, K. (2000). Beneficial effect of prodromal angina pectoris is lost in elderly patients with acute myocardial infarction. *American Heart Journal, 139*(5), 881–888.

The Israeli SPRINT Study Group. (1988). Secondary Prevention Reinfarction Israeli Nifedipine Trial (SPRINT): A randomized intervention trial of nifedipine in patients with acute myocardial infarction. *European Heart Journal, 9*(4), 354–364.

Jeremias, A., Kutscher, S., Haude, M., Heinen, D., Holtmann, G., Senf, W., & Erbel, R. (1998). Nonischemic chest pain induced by coronary intervention: A prospective study comparing coronary angioplasty and stent implantation. *Circulation, 98*(24), 2656–2658.

*Juran, N. B., Rouse, C. L., Smith, D. D., O'Brien, M. A., DeLuca, S. A., & Sigmon, K. (1999). Nursing interventions to decrease bleeding at the femoral site after percutaneous coronary intervention. SANDBAG Nursing Coordinators: Standards of Angioplasty Nursing techniques to Diminish Bleeding Around the Groin. *American Journal of Critical Care, 8*(5), 303–313.

Kannel, W. B. (1986). Silent myocardial ischemia and infarction: Insights from the Framingham study. *Cardiology Clinics, 4*(4), 583–591.

Khatta, M., Alexander, B. S., Krichten, C. M., Fisher, M. L., Freudenberger, R., Robinson, S. W., & Gottlieb, S. S. (2000). The effect of coenzyme Q10 in patients with congestive heart failure. *Annals of Internal Medicine, 132*(8), 636–640.

*Knoll, S. M., & Johnson, J. L. (2000). Uncertainty and expectations: Taking care of a cardiac surgery patient at home. *Journal of Cardiovascular Nursing, 14*(3), 64–75.

Krantz, D. S., Sheps, D. S., Carney, R. M., & Natelson, B. H. (2000). Effects of mental stress in patients with coronary artery disease. *Journal of the American Medical Association, 283*(14), 1800–1802.

Lehmann, K. G., Heath-Lange, S. J., & Ferris, S. T. (1999). Randomized comparison of hemostasis techniques after invasive cardiovascular procedures. *American Heart Journal, 138*, (6 Part 1), 1118–1125.

Leon, M. B., Teirstein, P. S., Moses, J. W., Tripuraneni, P., Lansky, A. J., Jani, S., Wong, S. C., Fish, D., Ellis, S., Holmes, D. R., Kerieakes, D., & Kuntz, R. E. (2001). Localized intracoronary gamma-radiation therapy to inhibit the recurrence of restenosis after stenting. *New England Journal of Medicine, 344*(4), 250–256.

Livorsi-Moore, J., Gulanick, M., & Rosko, P. N. (1999). Port access: Another advance in cardiovascular surgery. *American Journal of Nursing, 99*(7), 52–55.

Malinow, M. R., Bostom, A. G., & Krauss, R. M. (1999). Homocyste(e)ine, diet, and cardiovascular diseases: A statement for healthcare professionals from the Nutrition Committee, American Heart Association. *Circulation, 99*(1), 178–182.

McErlean, E. S. (Ed.). (2000). Unstable angina. *Journal of Cardiovascular Nursing, 15*(1), 1–79.

Mehta, R. H., & Eagle, K. A. (2000). Missed diagnoses of acute coronary syndromes in the emergency room: Continued challenges. *New England Journal of Medicine, 342*(16), 1207–1210.

Mehta, J. L., Saldeen, T. G., & Rand, K. (1998). Interactive role of infection, inflammation and traditional risk factors in atherosclerosis and coronary artery disease. *Journal of the American College of Cardiology, 31*(6), 1217–1225.

*Meischke, H., Yasui, Y., Kuniyuki, A., Bowen, D. J., Andersen, R. F., Urban, N. (1999). How women label and respond to symptoms of acute myocardial infarction: Responses to hypothetical symptom scenarios. *Heart & Lung, 28*(4), 261–269.

Miller, K., & Grindel, C. G. (1999). Coronary artery bypass surgery in women and men: Preoperative profile and postoperative outcomes. *MedSurg Nursing, 8*(3), 167–172.

Morse, J. M. (2000). On comfort and comforting. *American Journal of Nursing, 100*(9), 34–38.

Mortality from coronary heart disease and acute myocardial infarction–United States, 1998. (2001). *Morbidity and Mortality Weekly Report, 50*(06), 90–93.

Mosca, L. (2002). C-reactive protein: To screen or not to screen? *New England Journal of Medicine, 347*(20), 1615–1617.

Mosca, L. (2000). The role of hormone replacement therapy in the prevention of postmenopausal heart disease. *Archive of Internal Medicine, 160*(15), 2263–2272.

Mueller, X. M., Tinguely, F., Tevaearai, H. T., Revelly, J. P., Chioléro, R., & von Segesser, L. K. (2000). Pain location, distribution, and intensity after cardiac surgery. *Chest, 118*(2), 391–396.

O'Hanlon, J. V., Jr. (2000). Minimally invasive saphenous vein harvesting. *Critical Care Nursing Quarterly, 23*(1), 42–46.

O'Rourke, R. A., Hochman, J. S., Cohen, M. C., Lucore, C. L., Popma, J. J., & Cannon, C. P. (2001). New approaches to diagnosis and management of unstable angina and non-ST segment elevation myocardial infarction. *Annals of Internal Medicine, 161*(5), 674–682.

*Penque, S., Halm, M., Smith, M., Deutsch, J., Van Roekel, M., McLaughline, L., Dzubay, S., Doll, N., & Beahrs, M. (1998). Women and coronary disease: relationship between descriptors of signs and symptoms and diagnostic and treatment course. *American Journal of Critical Care, 7*(3), 175–182.

Pepys, M. B., & Berger, A. (2001). The renaissance of C-reactive protein: It may be a marker not only of acute illness but also of future cardiovascular disease. *British Medical Journal, 322*(7277), 4–5.

*Plach, S. K., & Heidrich, S. M. (2001). Women's perceptions of their social roles after heart surgery and coronary angioplasty. *Heart & Lung, 30*(2), 117–127.

Platek, Y. M., & Atzori, M. (1999). PTMR. *American Journal of Nursing, 99*(7), 64–66.

Pope, J. H., Aufderheide, T. P., Ruthazer, R., Woolard, R. H., Feldman, J. A., & Beshansky, J. R., et al. (2000). Missed diagnoses of acute cardiac ischemia in the emergency department. *New England Journal of Medicine, 342*(16), 1163–1170.

Reichter, A., Herlitz, J., & Hjalmarson, A. (1991). Effect of acupuncture in patients with angina pectoris. *European Heart Journal, 2*(2), 175–178.

Ridker, P. M., Rifai, N., Rose, L., Burning, J. E., Cook, N. R. (2002). Comparison of C-reactive protein and low-density lipoprotein cholesterol levels in the prediction of first cardiovascular events. *New England Journal of Medicine, 347*(20), 1557–1565.

Ridker, P. M., Stampfer, M. J., & Rifai, N. (2001). Novel risk factors for systemic atherosclerosis: A comparison of C-reactive protein, fibrinogen, homocysteine, lipoprotein(a), and standard cholesterol screening as predictors of peripheral arterial disease. *Journal of the American Medical Association, 285*(19), 2481–2485.

Roach, G. W., Kanchuger, M., Mangano, C. M., Newman, M., Nussmeier, N., Wolman, R., Aggarwal, A., Marschall, K., Graham, S. H., & Ley, C. (1996). Adverse cerebral outcomes after coronary bypass surgery: Multicenter study of Perioperative Ischemia Research Group and the Ischemia Research and Education Foundation investigators. *New England Journal of Medicine, 335*(25), 1857–1863.

Rozanski, A., Blumenthal, J. A., & Kaplan, J. (1999). Impact of psychological factors on the pathogenesis of cardiovascular disease and implications for therapy. *Circulation, 99*(16), 2192–2217.

Ryan, T. J., Antman, E. M., Brooks, N. H., Califf, R. M., Hillis, L. D., Hiratzka, L. F., Rapaport, E., Riegel, B., Russell, R. O., Smith, E. E., 3rd, Weaver, W. D., Gibbons, R. J., Alpert, J. S., Eagle, K. A., Gardner, T. J., Garson, A., Jr., Gregoratos, G., Ryan, T. J., & Smith, S. C., Jr. (1999). 1999 Update: ACC/AHA guidelines for the management of patients with acute myocardial infarction. A report of the American College of Cardiology/American Heart Association Task Force on Practice Guidelines (Committee on Management of Acute Myocardial Infarction). *Journal of the American College of Cardiology, 34*(3), 890–911.

Scanlon, P. J., Faxon, D. P., Audet, A. M., Carabello, B., Dehmer, G. J., Eagle, K. A., Legako, R. D., Leon, D. F., Murray, J. A., Nissen, S. E., Pepine, C. J., Watson, R. M., Ritchie, J. L., Gibbons, R. J., Cheitlin, M. D., Gardner, T. J., Garson, A., Jr., Russell, R. O., Jr., Ryan, T. J., & Smith, S. C., Jr. (1999). ACC/AHA guidelines for coronary angiography. A report of the American College of Cardiology/American Heart Association Task Force on Practice Guidelines (Committee on Coronary Angiography). *Journal of the American College of Cardiology, 33*(6), 1756–1824.

Schouchoff, B., & Belhumeur, J. (2000). Radial artery: An alternative revascularization conduit. *Critical Care Nursing Quarterly, 23*(1), 28–34.

Sheifer, S. E., Escarce, J. J., & Schulman, K. A. (2000). Race and sex differences in the management of coronary artery disease. *American Heart Journal, 139*(5), 848–857.

*Skaggs, B. G., & Chrisopherson, B. (1999). Quality of life comparisons after coronary angioplasty and coronary artery bypass graft surgery. *Heart & Lung, 28*(6), 409–417.

Smith, S. C., Dove, J. T., Jacobs, A. K., Kennedy, J. W., Kereiakes, D., Kern, M. J., Kuntz, R. E., Popma, J. J., Schaff, H. V., Williams, D. O., Gibbons, R. J., Alpert, J. P., Eagle, K. A., Faxon, D. P., Fuster, V., Gardner, T. J., Gregoratos, G., Russell, R. O., Smith, S. C., Jr., American College of Cardiology, American Heart Association Task Force on Practice Guidelines, Committee to Revise the 1993 Guidelines for Percutaneous Transluminal Coronary Angioplasty. (2001). ACC/AHA Guidelines for percutaneous coronary intervention (revision of the 1993 PTCA Guidelines): Executive summary. A report of the American College of Cardiology/American Heart Association Task Force on Practice Guidelines (Committee to Revise the 1993 Guidelines for Percutaneous Transluminal Coronary Angioplasty). *Journal of the American College of Cardiology, 37*(8), 2215–2238.

Statistics Canada. (2005). Age-standardized mortality rates by selected causes, by sex. Available at: http://www.statcan.ca/english?Pgdb/health30c.htm. Retrieved March 2005.

Steinke, E. E. (2000). Sexual counseling after myocardial infarction. *American Journal of Nursing, 100*(12), 38–44.

Strong, J. P. (1999). Prevalence and extent of atherosclerosis in adolescents and young adults. *Journal of the American Medical Association, 281*(8), 727–735.

Teirstein, P. S., & Kuntz, R. E. (2001). New frontiers in interventional cardiology: intravascular radiation to prevent restenosis. *Circulation, 104*(21), 2620–2626.

*Tooth, L. R., McKenna, K. T., & Maas, F. (1999). Prediction of functional and psychological status after transluminal coronary angioplasty. *Heart & Lung, 28*(4), 276–283.

Wald, D. S., Law, M., & Morris, J. K. (2002). Homocysteine and cardiovascular disease: Evidence on causality from a meta-analysis. *British Medical Journal, 325*(7374), 1202–1206.

*Walker, S. B., Cleary, S., & Higgins, M. (2001). Comparison of the FemoStop device and manual pressure in reducing groin puncture site complications following coronary angioplasty and coronary stent placement. *International Journal of Nursing Practice, 7*(6), 366–375.

Wang, T. J., Larson, M. G., Levy, D., Benjamin, E. J., Kupka, M. J., Manning, W. J., Clouse, M. E., D'Agostino, R. B., Wilson, P. W., & O'Donnell, C. J. (2002). C-reactive protein is associated with subclinical epicardial coronary calcification in men and women: The Framingham Heart Study. *Circulation, 106*(10), 1189–1191.

*Weaver, L. A., & Doran, K. A. (2001). Telephone follow-up after cardiac surgery. *American Journal of Nursing, 101*(5), 24OO–24WW.

Williams, M. A., Fleg, J. L., Ades, P. A., Chaitman, B. R., Miller, N. H., Mohiuddin, S. M., Ockene, I. S., Taylor, C. B., Wenger, N. K., & American Heart Association Council on Clinical Cardiology Subcommittee on Exercise, Cardiac Rehabilitation, and Prevention. (2002). Secondary prevention of coronary heart disease in the elderly (with emphasis on patients ≥75 years of age): An American Heart Association scientific statement from the Council on Clinical Cardiology Subcommittee on Exercise, Cardiac Rehabilitation, and Prevention. *Circulation, 105*(14), 1735–1743.

Zalenski, R. J., Selker, H. P., Cannon, C. P., Farin, H. M., Gibler, W. B., Goldberg, R. J., Lambrew, C. T., Ornato, J. P., Rydman, R. J., & Steele, P. (2000). National Heart Attack Alert Program position paper: Chest pain centers and programs for the evaluation of acute cardiac ischemia. *Annals of Emergency Medicine, 35*(5), 462–471.

RESOURCES AND WEBSITES

American Dietetic Association, 216 W Jackson Blvd., Chicago, IL 60606-6995; 1-800-366-1644; http://www.eatright.org.

American Heart Association, 7320 Greenville Ave., Dallas, TX 75231; 1-800-AHA-USA1 (1-800-242-8721); http://www.americanheart.org.

Healthy People 2010; managed by the Office of Disease Prevention and Health Promotion, U.S. Department of Health and Human Services, 200 Independence Ave., SW, Washington, DC 20201; 1-800-877-696-6775; http://www.health.gov/healthypeople.

Heart and Stroke Foundation of Canada, 222 Queen Street, Suite 1402, Ottawa, ON K1P 5V9; 1-613-569-4361; http://ww1.heartandstroke.ca.

Heartmates, P.O. Box 16202, Minneapolis, MN 55416; 952-929-3331; http://www.heartmates.com.

National Heart, Lung, and Blood Institute, National Institutes of Health, Building 31, Room 5A52, Bethesda, MD 20892; 301-592-8593; http://www.nhlbi.nih.gov.

National Institute on Aging, Building 31, Room 5C27, 31 Center Drive, MSC 2292, Bethesda, MD 20892; http://www.nih.gov/nia.

Management of Patients With Structural, Infectious, and Inflammatory Cardiac Disorders

Adapted by Alexander Clark and Colleen Norris

LEARNING OBJECTIVES

On completion of this chapter, the learner will be able to:

1. Define valvular disorders of the heart and describe the pathophysiology, clinical manifestations, and management of patients with mitral and aortic disorders.

2. Describe types of cardiac valve repair and replacement procedures used to treat valvular problems and the care needed by patients who undergo these procedures.

3. Describe the pathophysiology, clinical manifestations, and management of patients with cardiomyopathies.

4. Describe the pathophysiology, clinical manifestations, and management of patients with infections of the heart.

5. Describe the rationale for prophylactic antibiotic therapy for patients with mitral valve prolapse, valvular heart disease, rheumatic endocarditis, infective endocarditis, and myocarditis.

Structural disorders of the heart present many challenges for the patient, family, and health care team, as do the conduction and vascular disorders discussed in Chapters 27 and 28. Problems with the heart valves, holes in the intracardiac septum, cardiomyopathies, and infectious diseases of the heart muscle alter cardiac output. Treatments for these diagnoses may be noninvasive, such as medication therapy and activity and dietary modification. Invasive treatments, such as valve repair or replacement, septal repair, ventricular assist devices, total artificial hearts, cardiac transplantation, and other procedures may also be used. Nurses have an integral role in the care of patients with structural, infectious, and inflammatory cardiac conditions.

Acquired Valvular Disorders

The valves of the heart control the flow of blood through the heart into the pulmonary artery and aorta by opening and closing in response to the blood pressure changes as the heart contracts and relaxes through the cardiac cycle.

The atrioventricular valves separate the atria from the ventricles and include the **tricuspid valve**, which separates the right atrium from the right ventricle, and the **mitral valve**, which separates the left atrium from the left ventricle. The tricuspid valve has three leaflets; the mitral valve has two. Both valves have chordae tendineae that anchor the valve leaflets to the papillary muscles and ventricular wall.

The semilunar valves are located between the ventricles and their corresponding arteries. The **pulmonic valve** lies between the right ventricle and the pulmonary artery; the **aortic valve** lies between the left ventricle and the aorta. Figure 29-1 shows valves in the closed position.

When any of the heart valves do not close or open properly, blood flow is affected. When valves do not close completely, blood flows backward through the valve in a process called **regurgitation**. When valves do not open completely, a condition called **stenosis**, the flow of blood through the valve is reduced.

Disorders of the mitral valve fall into the following categories: mitral valve **prolapse** (ie, stretching of the valve leaflet into the atrium during systole), mitral regurgitation, and mitral stenosis. Disorders of the aortic valve are categorized as aortic regurgitation and aortic stenosis. These valvular disorders lead to various symptoms that, depending on their severity, may require surgical repair or replacement of the valve to correct the problem (Fig. 29-2). Tricuspid and pulmonic valve disorders also occur, usually with fewer symptoms and complications. Regurgitation and stenosis may occur at the same time in the same or different valves.

MITRAL VALVE PROLAPSE

Mitral valve prolapse, formerly known as mitral prolapse syndrome, is a deformity that usually produces no symptoms. Rarely, it progresses and can result in sudden death. Mitral valve prolapse occurs more frequently in women than in men. In recent years, this disorder has been diagnosed more frequently, probably as a result of improved diagnostic methods.

Pathophysiology

In mitral valve prolapse, a portion of a mitral valve leaflet balloons back into the atrium during systole. Rarely, the ballooning stretches the leaflet to the point that the valve does not remain closed during systole (ie, ventricular contraction). Blood then regurgitates from the left ventricle back into the left atrium (Braunwald et al., 2001).

Clinical Manifestations

Many people have a ballooned leaflet but no symptoms. Others have symptoms of fatigue, shortness of breath, light-headedness, dizziness, syncope, palpitations, chest pain, and anxiety (Braunwald et al., 2001; Freed et al., 1999; Fuster et al., 2001).

Fatigue may occur regardless of the person's activity level and amount of rest or sleep. Shortness of breath is not correlated with activity levels or pulmonary function. Atrial or ventricular dysrhythmias may produce the sensation of palpitations, but palpi-

Glossary

allograft: heart valve replacement made from a human heart valve (synonym: homograft)

annuloplasty: repair of a cardiac valve's outer ring

aortic valve: semilunar valve located between the left ventricle and the aorta

autograft: heart valve replacement made from the patient's own heart valve (ie, the pulmonic valve is excised and used as an aortic valve)

cardiomyopathy: disease of the heart muscle

chordoplasty: repair of the stringy, tendinous fibres that connect the free edges of the atrioventricular valve leaflets to the papillary muscles

commissurotomy: splitting or separating fused cardiac valve leaflets

heterograft: heart valve replacement made of tissue from an animal heart valve (synonym: xenograft)

heterotopic transplantation: procedure in which the recipient's heart remains in place and a donor heart is grafted to the right and anterior of it; the patient has two hearts

homograft: heart valve replacement made from a human heart valve (synonym: allograft)

leaflet repair: repair of a cardiac valve's movable "flaps" (leaflets)

mitral valve: atrioventricular valve located between the left atrium and left ventricle

orthotopic transplantation: the recipient's heart is removed, and a donor heart is grafted into the same site; the patient has one heart

prolapse (of a valve): stretching of an atrioventricular heart valve leaflet into the atrium during systole

pulmonic valve: semilunar valve located between the right ventricle and the pulmonary artery

regurgitation: backward flow of blood through a heart valve

stenosis: narrowing or obstruction of a cardiac valve's orifice

total artificial heart: mechanical device used to aid a failing heart, assisting the right and left ventricles

tricuspid valve: atrioventricular valve located between the right atrium and right ventricle

valve replacement: insertion of a device at the site of a malfunctioning heart valve to restore blood flow in one direction through the heart

valvuloplasty: repair of a stenosed or regurgitant cardiac valve by commissurotomy, annuloplasty, leaflet repair, or chordoplasty (or a combination of procedures)

ventricular assist device: mechanical device used to aid a failing right or left ventricle

xenograft: heart valve replacement made of tissue from an animal heart valve (synonym: heterograft)

FIGURE 29-1 The valves of the heart (aortic or semilunar, tricuspid, and mitral) in closed position.

Coronary arteries

Aortic (semilunar) valve   Tricuspid valve   Mitral valve

tations have been reported while the heart has been beating normally. Another puzzling symptom is chest pain, which is often localized to the chest and may last for days.

Anxiety may be a response to the symptoms experienced by the patient; however, some patients report anxiety as the only symptom. Some clinicians speculate that the symptoms may be explained by dysautonomia, a dysfunction of the autonomic nervous system, although no consensus exists about the cause of the symptoms experienced by some patients with mitral valve prolapse.

Physiology/Pathophysiology

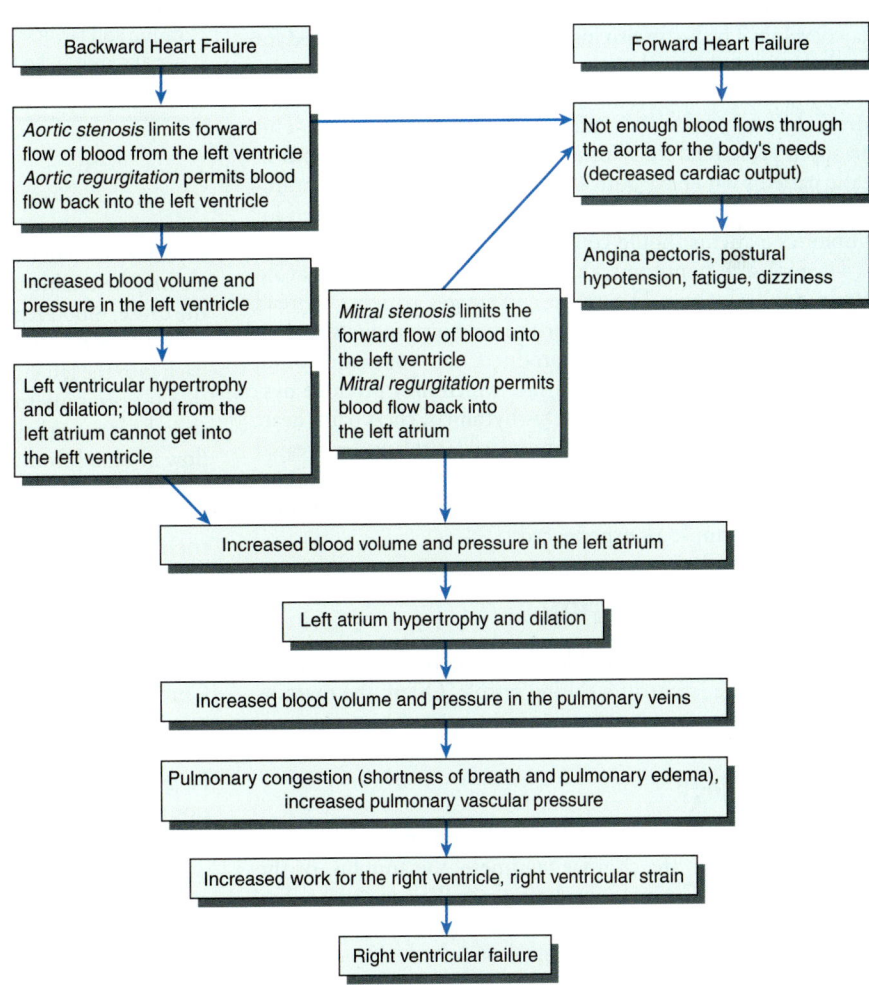

FIGURE 29-2 Pathophysiology: Left heart failure as a result of aortic and mitral valvular heart disease and the development of right ventricular failure.

Assessment and Diagnostic Findings

Often, the first and only sign of mitral valve prolapse is identified when a physical examination of the heart discloses an extra heart sound, referred to as a mitral click. The systolic click is an early sign that a valve leaflet is ballooning into the left atrium. In addition to the mitral click, a murmur of mitral regurgitation may be heard if progressive valve leaflet stretching and regurgitation have occurred. A small number of patients experience signs and symptoms of heart failure if mitral regurgitation exists.

Medical Management

Medical management is directed at controlling symptoms. If dysrhythmias are documented and cause symptoms, the patient is advised to eliminate caffeine and alcohol from the diet and to stop smoking; antiarrhythmic medications may be prescribed.

Chest pain that does not respond to nitrates may respond to calcium channel blockers or beta-blockers. Heart failure is treated the same as it would be for any other patient with heart failure (see Chap. 30). In advanced stages of disease, mitral valve repair or replacement may be necessary.

Nursing Management

The nurse educates patients about the diagnosis and the possibility that the condition is hereditary. Because most patients with mitral valve prolapse are asymptomatic, the nurse explains the need to inform the health care provider about any symptoms that may develop. The nurse also instructs patients about the need for prophylactic antibiotic therapy before undergoing invasive procedures (eg, dental work, genitourinary or gastrointestinal procedures) that may introduce infectious agents systemically. This therapy is prescribed for symptomatic patients and for asymptomatic patients who have both a systolic click and murmur or mitral regurgitation. If in doubt about risk factors and the need for antibiotics, patients should consult their physicians.

To minimize symptoms, the nurse teaches patients to avoid caffeine and alcohol. The nurse encourages patients to read product labels, particularly in over-the-counter products such as cough medicine, because these products may contain alcohol, caffeine, ephedrine, and epinephrine, which may produce dysrhythmias and other symptoms. Dysrhythmias, chest pain, heart failure, or other complications of mitral valve prolapse are treated as described in Chapter 30. The nurse also explores with patients possible diet, activity, sleep, and other lifestyle factors that may correlate with symptoms experienced.

MITRAL REGURGITATION

Mitral regurgitation involves blood flowing back from the left ventricle into the left atrium during systole. Often, the margins of the mitral valve cannot close during systole.

Pathophysiology

Mitral regurgitation may be caused by problems with one or more of the leaflets, the chordae tendineae, the annulus, or the papillary muscles. A mitral valve leaflet may shorten or tear. The chordae tendineae may elongate, shorten, or tear. The annulus may be stretched by heart enlargement or deformed by calcification. The papillary muscle may rupture, stretch, or be pulled out of position by changes in the ventricular wall (eg, scar from a

NURSING RESEARCH PROFILE 29-1

Mitral Valve Prolapse Support Group

Scordo, K. A. B. (2001). Factors associated with participating in a mitral valve prolapse support group. *Heart Lung, 30*(2), 128–137.

Purpose
The purpose of this study was to identify factors that influence a patient's attendance at mitral valve prolapse support groups.

Study Sample and Design
Questionnaires were used for this descriptive study of mitral valve support group leaders, current and former support group participants, and nonparticipants, all of whom had a diagnosis of mitral valve prolapse. A total of 376 questionnaires were analyzed.

Findings
People with mitral valve prolapse were more likely to participate in support groups if they were older than 50 years of age and participated in other self-help groups. The reason for attending was to obtain more information about mitral valve prolapse, information not usually available from family, friends, and physicians. No relationship was found between participation in a support group and patient gender, education level, marital status, age when first diagnosed, age when symptoms were first experienced, perceived social support, any symptoms experienced, or travel time or distance required to participate in the support group.

Nursing Implications
Nurses need to be aware that patients with mitral valve prolapse desire information about the condition, and not just at the time of diagnosis or development of symptoms. Nurses can provide education and facilitate support groups. Patients older than 50 years of age and those who participate in other self-help groups may be particularly interested in mitral valve prolapse support groups.

myocardial infarction or ventricular dilation). The papillary muscle may be unable to contract because of ischemia. Regardless of the cause, blood regurgitates back into the atrium during systole.

With each beat of the left ventricle, some of the blood is forced back into the left atrium. Because this blood is added to the blood that is beginning to flow in from the lungs, the left atrium must stretch. It eventually hypertrophies and dilates. The backward flow of blood from the ventricle diminishes the volume of blood flowing into the atrium from the lungs. As a result, the lungs become congested, eventually adding extra strain on the right ventricle. Mitral regurgitation ultimately involves the lungs and the right ventricle.

Clinical Manifestations

Chronic mitral regurgitation is often asymptomatic, but acute mitral regurgitation (eg, that resulting from a myocardial infarction) usually manifests as severe congestive heart failure. Dyspnea, fatigue, and weakness are the most common symptoms. Palpitations, shortness of breath on exertion, and cough from pulmonary congestion also occur.

Assessment and Diagnostic Findings

A systolic murmur is heard as a high-pitched, blowing sound at the apex. The pulse may be regular and of good volume, or it may be irregular as a result of extrasystolic beats or atrial fibrillation.

Echocardiography is used to diagnose and monitor the progression of mitral regurgitation.

Medical Management

Management of mitral regurgitation is the same as that for congestive heart failure. Surgical intervention consists of mitral valve replacement or valvuloplasty (ie, surgical repair of the heart valve).

MITRAL STENOSIS

Mitral stenosis is an obstruction of blood flowing from the left atrium into the left ventricle. It is most often caused by rheumatic endocarditis, which progressively thickens the mitral valve leaflets and chordae tendineae. The leaflets often fuse together. Eventually, the mitral valve orifice narrows and progressively obstructs blood flow into the ventricle.

Pathophysiology

Normally, the mitral valve opening is as wide as the diameter of three fingers. In cases of marked stenosis, the opening narrows to the width of a pencil. The left atrium has great difficulty moving blood into the ventricle because of the increased resistance of the narrowed orifice; it dilates (stretches) and hypertrophies (thickens) because of the increased blood volume it holds. Because there is no valve to protect the pulmonary veins from the backward flow of blood from the atrium, the pulmonary circulation becomes congested. As a result, the right ventricle must contract against an abnormally high pulmonary arterial pressure and is subjected to excessive strain. Eventually, the right ventricle fails.

Clinical Manifestations

The first symptom of mitral stenosis is often breathing difficulty (ie, dyspnea) on exertion as a result of pulmonary venous hypertension. Patients with mitral stenosis are likely to show progressive fatigue as a result of low cardiac output. They may expectorate blood (ie, hemoptysis), cough, and experience repeated respiratory infections.

Assessment and Diagnostic Findings

The pulse is weak and often irregular because of atrial fibrillation (caused by the strain on the atrium). A low-pitched, rumbling, diastolic murmur is heard at the apex. As a result of the increased blood volume and pressure, the atrium dilates, hypertrophies, and becomes electrically unstable, and the patient experiences atrial dysrhythmias. Echocardiography is used to diagnose mitral stenosis. Electrocardiography (ECG) and cardiac catheterization with angiography are used to determine the severity of the mitral stenosis.

Medical Management

Antibiotic prophylaxis therapy is instituted to prevent recurrence of infections. Congestive heart failure is treated as described in Chapter 30. Patients with mitral stenosis may benefit from anticoagulants to decrease the risk for developing atrial thrombus. They may also require treatment for anemia.

Surgical intervention consists of valvuloplasty, usually a commissurotomy to open or rupture the fused commissures of the mitral valve. Percutaneous transluminal valvuloplasty or mitral valve replacement may be performed.

AORTIC REGURGITATION

Aortic regurgitation is the flow of blood back into the left ventricle from the aorta during diastole. It may be caused by inflammatory lesions that deform the leaflets of the aortic valve, preventing them from completely closing the aortic valve orifice. This valvular defect also may result from endocarditis, congenital abnormalities, diseases such as syphilis, a dissecting aneurysm that causes dilation or tearing of the ascending aorta, or deterioration of an aortic valve replacement.

Pathophysiology

In aortic regurgitation, blood from the aorta returns to the left ventricle during diastole in addition to the blood normally delivered by the left atrium. The left ventricle dilates, trying to accommodate the increased volume of blood. It also hypertrophies, trying to increase muscle strength to expel more blood with above-normal force—raising systolic blood pressure. The arteries attempt to compensate for the higher pressures by reflex vasodilation; the peripheral arterioles relax, reducing peripheral resistance and diastolic blood pressure.

Clinical Manifestations

Aortic insufficiency develops without symptoms in most patients. Some patients are aware of a forceful heartbeat, especially in the head or neck. There may be marked arterial pulsations that are visible or palpable at the carotid or temporal arteries. This is a result of the increased force and volume of the blood ejected from the hypertrophied left ventricle. Exertional dyspnea and fatigue follow. Progressive signs and symptoms of left ventricular failure include breathing difficulties (eg, orthopnea, paroxysmal nocturnal dyspnea), especially at night.

Assessment and Diagnostic Findings

A diastolic murmur is heard as a high-pitched, blowing sound at the third or fourth intercostal space at the left sternal border. The pulse pressure (ie, difference between systolic and diastolic pressures) is considerably widened in patients with aortic regurgitation. One characteristic sign of the disease is the water-hammer pulse, in which the pulse strikes the palpating finger with a quick, sharp stroke and then suddenly collapses. Diagnosis may be confirmed by echocardiogram, radionuclide imaging, ECG, magnetic resonance imaging, and cardiac catheterization.

Medical Management

Before the patient undergoes invasive or dental procedures, antibiotic prophylaxis is needed to prevent endocarditis. Heart failure and dysrhythmias are treated as described in Chapters 27 and 30. Aortic valvuloplasty or valve replacement is the treatment of choice, preferably performed before left ventricular failure. Surgery is recommended for any patient with left ventricular hypertrophy, regardless of the presence or absence of symptoms.

AORTIC STENOSIS

Aortic valve stenosis is narrowing of the orifice between the left ventricle and the aorta. In adults, the stenosis may involve congenital leaflet malformations or an abnormal number of leaflets (ie, one or two rather than three), or it may result from rheumatic endocarditis or cusp calcification of unknown cause. The leaflets of the aortic valve may fuse.

Pathophysiology

There is progressive narrowing of the valve orifice, usually over a period of several years to several decades. The left ventricle overcomes the obstruction to circulation by contracting more slowly but with greater energy than normal, forcibly squeezing the blood through the very small orifice. The obstruction to left ventricular outflow increases pressure on the left ventricle, which results in thickening of the muscle wall. The heart muscle hypertrophies. When these compensatory mechanisms of the heart begin to fail, clinical signs and symptoms develop.

Clinical Manifestations

Many patients with aortic stenosis are asymptomatic. After symptoms develop, patients usually first have exertional dyspnea, caused by left ventricular failure. Other signs are dizziness and syncope because of reduced blood flow to the brain. Angina pectoris is a frequent symptom that results from the increased oxygen demands of the hypertrophied left ventricle, the decreased time in diastole for myocardial perfusion, and the decreased blood flow into the coronary arteries. Blood pressure can be low but is usually normal; there may be a low pulse pressure (30 mm Hg or less) because of diminished blood flow.

Assessment and Diagnostic Findings

On physical examination, a loud, rough systolic murmur may be heard over the aortic area. The sound to listen for is a systolic crescendo-decrescendo murmur, which may radiate into the carotid arteries and to the apex of the left ventricle. The murmur is low-pitched, rough, rasping, and vibrating. If the examiner rests a hand over the base of the heart, a vibration may be felt. The vibration is caused by turbulent blood flow across the narrowed valve orifice. Evidence of left ventricular hypertrophy may be seen on a 12-lead ECG and echocardiogram.

Echocardiography is used to diagnose and monitor the progression of aortic stenosis. After the stenosis progresses to the point that surgical intervention is considered, left-sided heart catheterization is necessary to measure the severity of the valvular abnormality and evaluate the coronary arteries. Pressure tracings are taken from the left ventricle and the base of the aorta. The systolic pressure in the left ventricle is considerably higher than that in the aorta during systole.

Medical Management

Antibiotic prophylaxis to prevent endocarditis is essential for anyone with aortic stenosis. After left ventricular failure or dysrhythmias occur, medications are prescribed. Definitive treatment for aortic stenosis is surgical replacement of the aortic valve. Patients who are symptomatic and are not surgical candidates may benefit from one- or two-balloon percutaneous valvuloplasty procedures.

VALVULAR HEART DISORDERS: NURSING MANAGEMENT

The nurse teaches all patients with valvular heart disease about the diagnosis, the progressive nature of valvular heart disease, and the treatment plan. The patient is taught to report any new symptoms or changes in symptoms to the health care provider. The nurse emphasizes the need for prophylactic antibiotic therapy before any invasive procedure (eg, dental work, genitourinary or gastrointestinal procedure) that may introduce infectious agents to the patient's bloodstream. The patient is taught that the infectious agent, usually a bacterium, is able to adhere to the diseased heart valve more readily than to a normal valve. Once attached to the valve, the infectious agent multiplies, resulting in endocarditis and further damage to the valve.

The patient's heart rate, blood pressure, and respiratory rate are measured and compared with previous data for any changes. Heart and lung sounds are auscultated and peripheral pulses palpated. The nurse assesses patients with valvular heart disease for signs and symptoms of heart failure: fatigue, dyspnea with exertion, an increase in coughing, hemoptysis, multiple respiratory infections, orthopnea, or paroxysmal nocturnal dyspnea (see Chap. 30). The nurse assesses for dysrhythmias by palpating the patient's pulse for strength and rhythm (ie, regular or irregular) and asks if the patient has experienced palpitations or felt forceful heartbeats (see Chap. 27). The nurse also assesses for dizziness, syncope, increased weakness, or angina pectoris (see Chap. 28).

The nurse collaborates with the patient to develop a medication schedule and teaches about the name, dosage, actions, side effects, and any drug-drug or drug-food interactions of the prescribed medications for heart failure, dysrhythmias, angina pectoris, or other symptoms. The nurse teaches the patient to weigh daily and report the gain of 2 pounds in 1 day or 5 pounds in 1 week to the health care provider. The nurse may assist the patient with planning activity and rest periods to achieve a lifestyle acceptable to the patient. If the patient is to have surgical valve replacement or valvuloplasty, the nurse teaches the patient about the procedure and anticipated recovery.

Valve Repair and Replacement Procedures

VALVULOPLASTY

The repair, rather than replacement, of a cardiac valve is referred to as **valvuloplasty**. The type of valvuloplasty depends on the cause and type of valve dysfunction. Repair may be made to the commissures between the leaflets in a procedure known as **commissurotomy**, to the annulus of the valve by annuloplasty, to the leaflets, or to the chordae by chordoplasty.

Most valvuloplasty procedures require general anesthesia and often require cardiopulmonary bypass. Some procedures, however, can be performed in the cardiac catheterization laboratory; these procedures do not always require general anesthesia or cardiopulmonary bypass. Percutaneous partial cardiopulmonary bypass is used in some cardiac catheterization laboratories. The cardiopulmonary bypass is achieved by inserting a large catheter (ie, cannula) into two peripheral blood vessels, usually a femoral vein and an artery. Blood is diverted from the body through the venous catheter to the cardiopulmonary bypass machine (see Chap. 28) and returned to the patient through the arterial catheter.

The patient is usually managed in a critical care unit for the first 24 to 72 hours after surgery. Care focuses on hemodynamic stabilization and recovery from anesthesia. Vital signs are assessed every 5 to 15 minutes and as needed until the patient recovers from anesthesia or sedation and then every 2 to 4 hours and as needed. Intravenous medications to increase or decrease blood pressure and to treat dysrhythmias or altered heart rates are administered, and their effects are monitored. The intravenous medications are gradually decreased until they are no longer required or the patient takes needed medication by another route (eg, oral, topical). Patient assessments are conducted every 1 to 4 hours and as needed, with particular attention to neurologic, respiratory, and cardiovascular assessments.

After the patient has recovered from anesthesia and sedation, is hemodynamically stable without intravenous medications, and assessments are stable, the patient is usually transferred to a telemetry or surgical unit for continued postsurgical care and teaching. The nurse provides wound care and patient teaching regarding diet, activity, medications, and self-care. Patients are discharged from the hospital in 1 to 7 days. In general, valves that have undergone valvuloplasty function longer than replacement valves, and the patients do not require continuous anticoagulation.

Commissurotomy

The most common valvuloplasty procedure is commissurotomy. Each valve has leaflets; the site where the leaflets meet is called the *commissure*. The leaflets may adhere to one another and close the commissure (ie, stenosis). Less commonly, the leaflets fuse in such a way that, in addition to stenosis, the leaflets are also prevented from closing completely, resulting in a backward flow of blood (ie, regurgitation). A commissurotomy is the procedure performed to separate the fused leaflets.

CLOSED COMMISSUROTOMY

Closed commissurotomies do not require cardiopulmonary bypass. The valve is not directly visualized. The patient receives a general anesthetic, a midsternal incision is made, a small hole is cut into the heart, and the surgeon's finger or a dilator is used to break open the commissure. This type of commissurotomy has been performed for mitral, aortic, tricuspid, and pulmonary valve disease.

Balloon Valvuloplasty. Balloon valvuloplasty (Fig. 29-3) is another type of closed commissurotomy beneficial for mitral valve stenosis in younger patients, for aortic valve stenosis in elderly patients, and for patients with complex medical conditions that place them at high risk for the complications of more extensive surgical procedures. Most commonly used for mitral and aortic valve stenosis, balloon valvuloplasty also has been used for tricuspid and pulmonic valve stenosis. The procedure is performed in the cardiac catheterization laboratory, and the patient may receive a local anesthetic. Patients remain in the hospital 24 to 48 hours after the procedure.

Mitral valvuloplasty is contraindicated for patients with left atrial or ventricular thrombus, severe aortic root dilation, significant mitral valve regurgitation, thoracolumbar scoliosis, rotation of the great vessels, and other cardiac conditions that require open heart surgery.

Mitral balloon valvuloplasty involves advancing one or two catheters into the right atrium, through the atrial septum into the left atrium, across the mitral valve into the left ventricle, and out into the aorta. A guide wire is placed through each catheter, and the original catheter is removed. A large balloon catheter is then placed over the guide wire and positioned with the balloon across the mitral valve. The balloon is then inflated with a dilute angiographic solution. When two balloons are used, they are inflated simultaneously. The advantage of two balloons is that they are each smaller than the one large balloon often used, making smaller atrial septal defects. As the balloons are inflated, they usually do not completely occlude the mitral valve, thereby permitting some forward flow of blood during the inflation period.

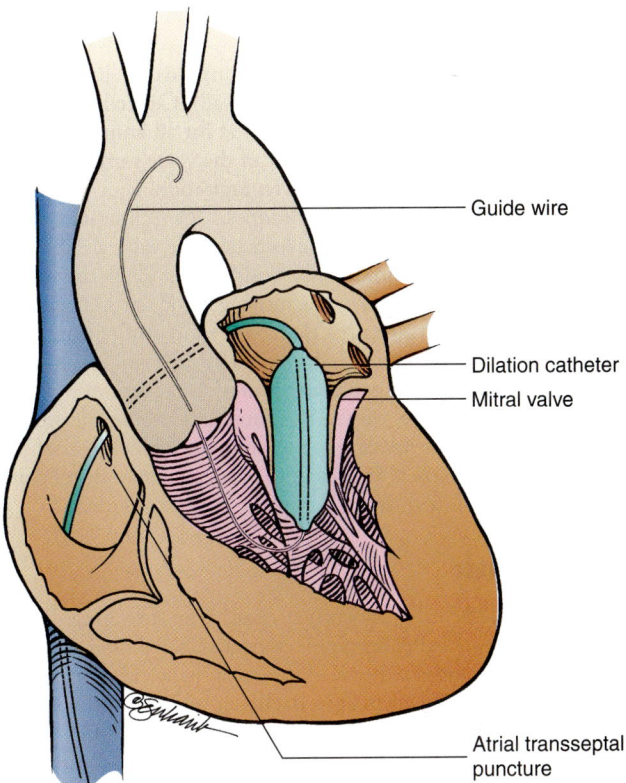

Guide wire

Dilation catheter
Mitral valve

Atrial transseptal puncture

FIGURE 29-3 Balloon valvuloplasty: cross-section of heart illustrating guide wire and dilation catheter placed through an atrial transseptal puncture and across the mitral valve. The guide wire is extended out from the aortic valve into the aorta for catheter support.

All patients have some degree of mitral regurgitation after the procedure. Other possible complications include bleeding from the catheter insertion sites, emboli resulting in complications such as strokes, and rarely, left-to-right atrial shunts through an atrial septal defect caused by the procedure.

Aortic balloon valvuloplasty also may be performed by passing the balloon or balloons through the atrial septum, but it is performed more commonly by introducing a catheter through the aorta, across the aortic valve, and into the left ventricle. The one-balloon or the two-balloon technique can be used for treating aortic stenosis. The aortic procedure is not as effective as the procedure for the mitral valve, and the rate of restenosis is nearly 50% in the first 12 to 15 months after the procedure (Braunwald et al., 2001). Possible complications include aortic regurgitation, emboli, ventricular perforation, rupture of the aortic valve annulus, ventricular dysrhythmias, mitral valve damage, and bleeding from the catheter insertion sites.

OPEN COMMISSUROTOMY

Open commissurotomies are performed with direct visualization of the valve. The patient is under general anesthesia, and a median sternotomy or left thoracic incision is made. Cardiopulmonary bypass is initiated, and an incision is made into the heart. A finger, scalpel, balloon, or dilator may be used to open the commissures. An added advantage of direct visualization of the valve is that thrombus may be identified and removed, calcifications can be seen, and if the valve has chordae or papillary muscles, they may be surgically repaired (chordoplasty is discussed later in this chapter).

Annuloplasty

Annuloplasty is the repair of the valve annulus (ie, junction of the valve leaflets and the muscular heart wall). General anesthesia and cardiopulmonary bypass are required for all annuloplasties. The procedure narrows the diameter of the valve's orifice and is useful for the treatment of valvular regurgitation.

There are two annuloplasty techniques. One technique uses an annuloplasty ring (Fig. 29-4). The leaflets of the valve are sutured to a ring, creating an annulus of the desired size. When the ring is in place, the tension created by the moving blood and contracting heart is borne by the ring rather than by the valve or a suture line, and progressive regurgitation is prevented by the repair. The other technique involves tacking the valve leaflets to the atrium with sutures or taking tucks to tighten the annulus. Because the valve's leaflets and the suture lines are subjected to the direct forces of the blood and heart muscle movement, the repair may degenerate more quickly than with the annuloplasty ring technique.

Leaflet Repair

Damage to cardiac valve leaflets may result from stretching, shortening, or tearing. **Leaflet repair** for elongated, ballooning, or other excess tissue leaflets is removal of the extra tissue. The elongated tissue may be folded over onto itself (ie, tucked) and sutured (ie, leaflet plication). A wedge of tissue may be cut from the middle of the leaflet and the gap sutured closed (ie., leaflet resection) (Fig. 29-5). Short leaflets are most often repaired by chordoplasty. After the short chordae are released, the leaflets often unfurl and can resume their normal function of closing the valve during systole. A piece of pericardium may also be sutured to extend the leaflet. A pericardial patch may be used to repair holes in the leaflets.

Chordoplasty

Chordoplasty is the repair of the chordae tendineae. The mitral valve is involved with chordoplasty (because it has the chordae tendineae); seldom is chordoplasty required for the tricuspid valve.

Regurgitation may be caused by stretched, torn, or shortened chordae tendineae. Stretched chordae tendineae can be shortened, torn ones can be reattached to the leaflet, and shortened ones can be elongated. Regurgitation may also be caused by stretched papillary muscles, which can be shortened.

VALVE REPLACEMENT

Prosthetic **valve replacement** began in the 1960s. When valvuloplasty or valve repair is not a viable alternative, such as when the annulus or leaflets of the valve are immobilized by calcifications, valve replacement is performed. General anesthesia and cardiopulmonary bypass are used for all valve replacements. Most procedures are performed through a median sternotomy (ie, incision through the sternum), although the mitral valve may be approached through a right thoracotomy incision.

After the valve is visualized, the leaflets and other valve structures, such as the chordae and papillary muscles, are removed. Some surgeons leave the posterior mitral valve leaflet, its chordae, and papillary muscles in place to help maintain the shape and function of the left ventricle after mitral valve replacement. Sutures are placed around the annulus and then into the valve prosthesis. The replacement valve is slid down the suture into position and tied into place (Fig. 29-6). The incision is closed, and the surgeon evaluates the function of the heart and the quality of the prosthetic repair. The patient is weaned from cardiopulmonary bypass, and surgery is completed.

Before surgery, the heart gradually adjusted to the pathology, but the surgery abruptly "corrects" the way blood flows through the heart. Complications unique to valve replacement are related to the sudden changes in intracardiac blood pressures. All prosthetic valve replacements create a degree of stenosis when they are implanted in the heart. Usually, the stenosis is mild and does not effect heart function. If valve replacement was for a stenotic valve, blood flow through the heart is often improved. The signs and symptoms of the backward heart failure resolve in a few hours or days. If valve replacement was for a regurgitant valve, it may take months for the chamber into which blood had been regurgitat-

FIGURE 29-4 Annuloplasty ring insertion. (**A**) Mitral valve regurgitation; leaflets do not close. (**B**) Insertion of an annuloplasty ring. (**C**) Completed valvuloplasty; leaflets close.

FIGURE 29-5 Valve leaflet resection and repair with a ring annuloplasty. (**A**) Mitral valve regurgitation; the section indicated by dashed lines is excised. (**B**) Approximation of edges and suturing. (**C**) Completed valvuloplasty, leaflet repair, and annuloplasty ring.

ing to achieve its optimal postoperative function. The signs and symptoms of heart failure resolve gradually as the heart function improves. The patient is at risk for many postoperative complications, such as bleeding, thromboembolism, infection, congestive heart failure, hypertension, dysrhythmias, hemolysis, and mechanical obstruction of the valve.

Types of Valve Prostheses

Two types of valve prostheses may be used: mechanical and tissue (ie, biologic) valves. Figure 29-7 shows mechanical and tissue valves.

MECHANICAL VALVES

The mechanical valves are of the ball-and-cage or disk design. Mechanical valves are thought to be more durable than tissue

prosthetic valves and often are used for younger patients. Mechanical valves are used if the patient has renal failure, hypercalcemia, endocarditis, or sepsis and requires valve replacement. The mechanical valves do not deteriorate or become infected as easily as the tissue valves used for patients with these conditions. Thromboemboli are significant complications associated with mechanical valves, and long-term anticoagulation with warfarin is required.

TISSUE OR BIOLOGIC VALVES

Tissue (ie, biologic) valves are of three types: xenografts, homografts, and autografts. Tissue valves are less likely to generate thromboemboli, and long-term anticoagulation is not required. Tissue valves are not as durable as mechanical valves and require replacement more frequently.

FIGURE 29-6 Valve replacement. (**A**) The native valve is excised and the prosthetic valve is sutured in place. (**B**) Once all sutures are placed through the ring, the surgeon slides the prosthetic valve down the sutures and into the natural orifice. The sutures are then tied off and trimmed.

FIGURE 29-7 Common mechanical and tissue valve replacements. (**A**) Caged ball valve (Starr-Edwards, mechanical). (**B**) Tilting-disk valve (Medtronic-Hall, mechanical). (**C**) Porcine heterograft valve (Carpenter-Edwards, tissue).

Xenografts. **Xenografts** are tissue valves (eg, bioprostheses, **heterografts**); most are from pigs (porcine), but valves from cows (bovine) may also be used. Their viability is 7 to 10 years. They do not generate thrombi, thereby eliminating the need for long-term anticoagulation. They are used for women of childbearing age because the potential complications of long-term anticoagulation associated with menses, placental transfer to a fetus, and delivery of a child do not exist. Xenografts also are used for patients older than 70 years of age, patients with a history of peptic ulcer disease, and others who cannot tolerate long-term anticoagulation. Xenografts are used for all tricuspid valve replacements.

Homografts. **Homografts**, or **allografts** (ie, human valves), are obtained from cadaver tissue donations. The aortic valve and a portion of the aorta or the pulmonic valve and a portion of the pulmonary artery are harvested and stored cryogenically. Homografts are not always available and are very expensive. Homografts last for about 10 to 15 years, somewhat longer than xenografts. Homografts are not thrombogenic and are resistant to subacute bacterial endocarditis. They are used for aortic and pulmonic valve replacement.

Autografts. Autografts (ie, autologous valves) are obtained by excising the patient's own pulmonic valve and a portion of the pulmonary artery for use as the aortic valve. Anticoagulation is unnecessary because the valve is the patient's own tissue and is not thrombogenic. The autograft is an alternative for children (it may grow as the child grows), women of childbearing age, young adults, patients with a history of peptic ulcer disease, and those who cannot tolerate anticoagulation. Aortic valve autografts have remained viable for more than 20 years.

Most aortic valve autograft procedures are double valve-replacement procedures, because a homograft also is performed for pulmonic valve replacement. If pulmonary vascular pressures are normal, some surgeons elect not to replace the pulmonic valve. The patient can recover without a valve between the right ventricle and the pulmonary artery.

VALVULOPLASTY AND REPLACEMENT: NURSING MANAGEMENT

Patients who have had valvuloplasty or valve replacements are admitted to the intensive care unit; care focuses on recovery from anesthesia and hemodynamic stability. Vital signs are assessed every 5 to 15 minutes and as needed until the patient recovers from anesthesia or sedation and then assessed every 2 to 4 hours and as needed. Intravenous medications to increase or decrease blood pressure and to treat dysrhythmias or altered heart rates are administered and their effects monitored. The intravenous medications are gradually decreased until they are no longer required or the patient takes needed medication by another route (eg, oral, topical). Patient assessments are conducted every 1 to 4 hours and as needed, with particular attention to neurologic, respiratory, and cardiovascular systems. (See Plan of Nursing Care 28-2: Care of the Patient After Cardiac Surgery, in Chap. 28).

After the patient has recovered from anesthesia and sedation, is hemodynamically stable without intravenous medications, and assessment values are stable, the patient is usually transferred to a telemetry unit, typically within 24 to 72 hours after surgery. Nursing care continues as for most postoperative patients, including wound care and patient teaching regarding diet, activity, medications, and self-care.

The nurse educates the patient about long-term anticoagulant therapy, explaining the need for frequent follow-up appointments and blood laboratory studies, and provides teaching about any prescribed medication: the name of the medication, dosage, its actions, prescribed schedule, potential side effects, and any drug-drug or drug-food interactions. Patients with a mechanical valve prosthesis require education to prevent bacterial endocarditis with antibiotic prophylaxis, which is prescribed before all dental and surgical interventions. Patients are discharged from the hospital in 3 to 7 days. Home care and office or clinic nurses reinforce all new information and self-care instructions with the patient and family for 4 to 8 weeks after the procedure.

Septal Repair

The atrial or ventricular septum may have an abnormal opening between the right and left sides of the heart (ie, septal defect). Although most septal defects are congenital and are repaired during infancy or childhood, adults may not have undergone early repair or may develop septal defects as a result of myocardial infarctions or diagnostic and treatment procedures.

Repair of septal defects requires general anesthesia and cardiopulmonary bypass. The heart is opened, and a pericardial or synthetic (usually polyester or Dacron) patch is used to close the opening. Atrial septal defect repairs have low morbidity and mortality rates. When the mitral or tricuspid valve is involved, however, the procedure is more complicated because valve repair or replacement may be required and the heart failure may be more severe. Generally, ventricular septal repairs are uncomplicated, but the proximity of the defect to the intraventricular conduction system and the valves may make this repair more complex. (See Chapter 28, Plan of Nursing Care: Care of the Patient After Cardiac Surgery.)

Cardiomyopathies

Cardiomyopathy is a heart muscle disease associated with cardiac dysfunction. It is classified according to the structural and functional abnormalities of the heart muscle: dilated cardiomyopathy

(DCM), hypertrophic cardiomyopathy (HCM), restrictive or constrictive cardiomyopathy, arrhythmogenic right ventricular cardiomyopathy (ARVC), and unclassified cardiomyopathy (Richardson et al., 1996). *Ischemic cardiomyopathy* is a term frequently used to describe an enlarged heart caused by coronary artery disease, which is usually accompanied by heart failure (see Chap. 30). Regardless of the category and the cause, cardiomyopathy may lead to severe heart failure, lethal dysrhythmias, and death. In 2002, there were 870 deaths in Canada due to cardiomyopathy (Statistics Canada, 2005). Cardiomyopathy is an important cause of sudden cardiac death in individuals under 30 years of age.

Pathophysiology

The pathophysiology of all cardiomyopathies is a series of progressive events that culminate in impaired cardiac output. Decreased stroke volume stimulates the sympathetic nervous system and the renin-angiotensin-aldosterone response, resulting in increased systemic vascular resistance and increased sodium and fluid retention, which places an increased workload on the heart. These alterations can lead to heart failure (see Chap. 30).

DILATED CARDIOMYOPATHY

DCM is the most common form of cardiomyopathy, with an incidence of 5 to 8 cases per 100,000 people per year and increasing (Braunwald et al., 2001). DCM occurs more often in men (Statistics Canada, 2005). DCM is distinguished by significant dilation of the ventricles (Fig. 29-8) without significant concomitant hypertrophy (ie, increased muscle wall thickness) and systolic dysfunction. DCM was formerly named *congestive cardiomyopathy,* but DCM may exist without signs and symptoms of congestion.

Microscopic examination of the muscle tissue shows diminished contractile elements of the muscle fibres and diffuse necrosis of myocardial cells. The result is poor systolic function. These structural changes decrease the amount of blood ejected from the ventricle with systole, increasing the amount of blood remaining in the ventricle after contraction. Less blood is then able to enter the ventricle during diastole, increasing end-diastolic pressure and eventually increasing pulmonary pressures. Altered valve function can result from the enlarged stretched ventricle, usually resulting in regurgitation. Embolic events caused by ventricular and atrial thrombi as a result of the poor blood flow through the ventricle may also occur. More than 75 conditions and diseases may cause DCM, including pregnancy, heavy alcohol intake, and viral infection (eg, influenza). When the causative factor cannot be identified, the term used is *idiopathic DCM.* Idiopathic DCM accounts for approximately 25% of all heart failure cases (Braunwald et al., 2001). Early diagnosis and treatment can prevent or delay significant symptoms and sudden death from DCM. Echocardiography and ECG are used to diagnose DCM and should be conducted for all first-degree relatives (eg, parents, siblings, children) of patients with DCM (Braunwald et al., 2001).

HYPERTROPHIC CARDIOMYOPATHY

In HCM, the heart muscle increases in size and mass, especially along the septum (see Fig. 29-8). The increased thickness of the heart muscle reduces the size of the ventricular cavities and causes the ventricles to take a longer time to relax, making it more difficult for the ventricles to fill with blood during the first part of diastole and making them more dependent on atrial contraction for

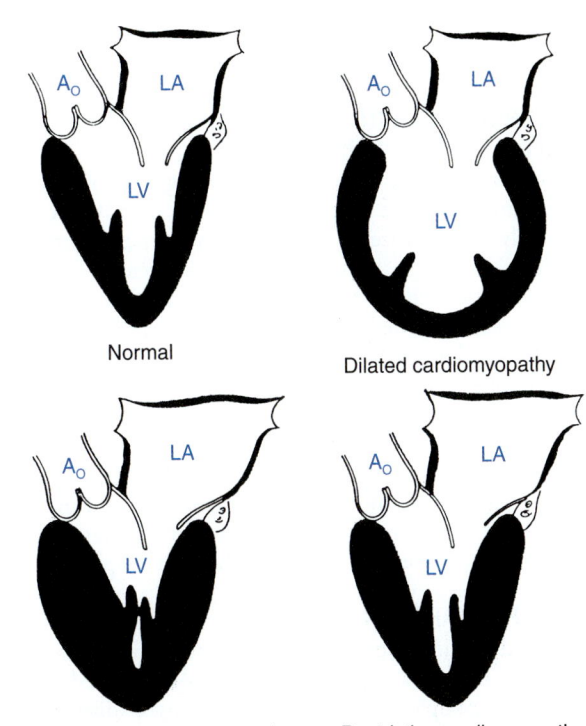

FIGURE 29-8 Cardiomyopathies that lead to congestive heart failure. A_O, aorta; LA, left atrium; LV, left ventricle. With permission from Braunwald, E., et al. (Eds.) (2001). *Heart disease: A textbook of cardiovascular medicine* (6th ed.). Philadelphia: W. B. Saunders.

filling. The increased septal size may misalign the papillary muscles so that the septum and mitral valve obstruct the flow of blood from the left ventricle into the aorta during ventricular contraction. Hence, HCM may be obstructive or nonobstructive. Because of the structural changes, HCM had also been called idiopathic hypertrophic subaortic stenosis (IHSS) or asymmetric septal hypertrophy (ASH). Structural changes may also result in a smaller than normal ventricular cavity and a higher velocity flow of blood out of the left ventricle into the aorta, which may be detected by echocardiography (Braunwald et al., 2001). HCM may cause significant diastolic dysfunction, but systolic function can be normal or high, resulting in a higher than normal ejection fraction.

Because HCM is a genetic disease, family members are observed closely for signs and symptoms indicating development of the disease (Fuster et al., 2001). HCM is rare, occurring in men, women, and children (often detected after puberty) (Oakley, 1997) with an estimated prevalence rate of 0.05% to 0.2% (Berul & Zevitz, 2002). It may also be idiopathic (ie, no cause can be found).

RESTRICTIVE CARDIOMYOPATHY

Restrictive cardiomyopathy (RCM) is characterized by diastolic dysfunction caused by rigid ventricular walls that impair ventricular stretch and diastolic filling (see Fig. 29-8). Systolic function is usually normal. Because RCM is the least common cardiomyopathy, representing approximately 5% of pediatric cardiomyopathies, its pathogenesis is the least understood (Shaddy, 2001). Restrictive cardiomyopathy can be associated with amyloidosis (in which amyloid, a protein substance, is deposited within the cells) and other such infiltrative diseases. However, the cause is unknown in most cases (ie, idiopathic).

ARRHYTHMOGENIC RIGHT VENTRICULAR CARDIOMYOPATHY

ARVC occurs when the myocardium of the right ventricle is progressively infiltrated and replaced by fibrous scar and adipose tissue. Initially, only localized areas of the right ventricle are affected, but as the disease progresses, the entire heart is affected. Eventually, the right ventricle dilates and develops poor contractility, right ventricular wall abnormalities, and dysrhythmias. The prevalence of ARVC is unknown because many cases are not recognized. ARVC should be suspected in patients with ventricular tachycardia originating in the right ventricle (ie, a left bundle branch block configuration on ECG) or sudden death, especially among previously symptom-free athletes (McRae et al., 2001). The disease may be genetic (ie, autosomal dominant) (Richardson et al., 1996). Family members should be screened for the disease with a 12-lead ECG, Holter monitor, and echocardiography.

UNCLASSIFIED CARDIOMYOPATHIES

Unclassified cardiomyopathies are different from or have characteristics of more than one of the previously described cardiomyopathies. Examples of unclassified cardiomyopathies include fibroelastosis, noncompacted myocardium, systolic dysfunction with minimal dilation, and mitochondrial involvement (Richardson et al., 1996).

Clinical Manifestations

The patient may have cardiomyopathy but remain stable and without symptoms for many years. As the disease progresses, so do symptoms. Frequently, dilated and restrictive cardiomyopathy are first diagnosed when the patient presents with signs and symptoms of heart failure (eg, dyspnea on exertion, fatigue). Patients with cardiomyopathy may also report paroxysmal nocturnal dyspnea, cough (especially with exertion), and orthopnea, which may lead to a misdiagnosis of bronchitis or pneumonia. Other symptoms include fluid retention, peripheral edema, and nausea, which is caused by poor perfusion of the gastrointestinal system. The patient may experience chest pain, palpitations, dizziness, nausea, and syncope with exertion. However, with HCM, cardiac arrest (ie, sudden cardiac death) may be the initial manifestation in young people, including athletes (Spirito et al., 2000).

Assessment and Diagnostic Findings

Physical examination in the early stage may reveal tachycardia and extra heart sounds. With disease progression, examination also reveals signs and symptoms of heart failure (eg, crackles on pulmonary auscultation, jugular vein distention, pitting edema of dependent body parts, enlarged liver).

Diagnosis is usually made from findings disclosed by the patient history and by ruling out other causes of heart failure, such as myocardial infarction. The echocardiogram is one of the most helpful diagnostic tools because the structure and function of the ventricles can be observed easily. ECG demonstrates dysrhythmias and changes consistent with left ventricular hypertrophy. The chest x-ray film reveals heart enlargement and possibly pulmonary congestion. Cardiac catheterization is sometimes used to rule out coronary artery disease as a causative factor. An endomyocardial biopsy may be performed to analyze myocardial tissue cells.

Medical Management

Medical management is directed toward determining and managing possible underlying or precipitating causes; correcting the heart failure with medications, a low-sodium diet, and an exercise-rest regimen (see Chap. 30); and controlling dysrhythmias with antiarrhythmic medications and possibly with an implanted electronic device, such as an implantable cardioverter-defibrillator (see Chap. 27). If patients exhibit signs and symptoms of congestion, their fluid intake may be limited to 2 litres each day. The person with HCM may also have to limit physical activity to avoid a life-threatening dysrhythmia. A pacemaker may be implanted to alter the electrical stimulation of the muscle and prevent the forceful hyperdynamic contractions that occur with HCM.

SURGICAL MANAGEMENT

When heart failure progresses and medical treatment is no longer effective, surgical intervention, including heart transplantation, is considered. However, because of the limited number of organ donors, many patients die waiting for transplantation. In some cases, a left ventricular assist device (LVAD) is implanted to support the failing heart until a suitable donor heart becomes available (mechanical assist devices and total artificial hearts are discussed later in this chapter).

Left Ventricular Outflow Tract Surgery. When a patient with HCM becomes symptomatic despite medical therapy and a difference in pressure of 50 mm Hg or more exists between the left ventricle and the aorta, surgery is considered. The most common procedure is a myectomy (sometimes referred to as a myotomy-myectomy), in which some of the heart tissue is excised. Septal tissue approximately 1 cm wide and deep is cut from the enlarged septum below the aortic valve. The length of septum removed depends on the degree of obstruction caused by the hypertrophied muscle.

Instead of a septal myectomy, the surgeon may open the left ventricular outflow tract to the aortic valve by removing the mitral valve, chordae, and papillary muscles. The mitral valve then is replaced with a low-profile disk valve. The space taken up by the mitral valve is substantially reduced by the prosthetic valve compared with the patient's own valve, chordae, and papillary muscles, allowing blood to move around the enlarged septum to the aortic valve in the area that the mitral valve once occupied. The primary complication of both procedures is dysrhythmia; additional complications are postoperative surgical complications such as pain, ineffective airway clearance, deep vein thrombosis, risk for infection, and delayed surgical recovery.

Heart Transplantation. The first human-to-human heart transplant was performed in 1967. Since then, transplant procedures, equipment, and medications have continued to improve. Since 1983, when cyclosporine became available, heart transplantation has become a therapeutic option for patients with end-stage heart disease. Cyclosporine (Neoral, Sandimmune, SangCya) is an immunosuppressant that greatly decreases the body's rejection of foreign proteins, such as transplanted organs. Unfortunately, cyclosporine also decreases the body's ability to resist infections, and a satisfactory balance must be achieved between suppressing rejection and avoiding infection.

Cardiomyopathy, ischemic heart disease, valvular disease, rejection of previously transplanted hearts, and congenital heart disease are the most common indications for transplantation (Becker & Petlin, 1999; Rourke et al., 1999). A typical candidate has severe symptoms uncontrolled by medical therapy, no other surgical options, and a prognosis of less than 12 months to live. A multidisciplinary team screens the candidate before recommending the transplantation procedure. The person's age, pulmonary status, other chronic health conditions, psychosocial status, family support, infections, history of other transplantations, compliance, and current health status are considered in the screening.

When a donor heart becomes available, a computer generates a list of potential recipients on the basis of ABO blood group compatibility, the sizes of the donor and the potential recipient, and the geographic locations of the donor and potential recipient; distance is a variable because postoperative function depends on the heart being implanted within 6 hours of harvest from the donor. Some patients are candidates for more than one organ transplant: heart-lung, heart-pancreas, heart-kidney, heart-liver.

Transplantation Techniques. **Orthotopic transplantation** is the most common surgical procedure for cardiac transplantation (Fig. 29-9). The recipient's heart is removed, and the donor heart is implanted at the vena cava and pulmonary veins. Some surgeons still prefer to remove the recipient's heart leaving a portion of the recipient's atria (with the vena cava and pulmonary veins) in place. The donor heart, which usually has been preserved in ice, is prepared for implant by cutting away a small section of the atria that corresponds with the sections of the recipient's heart that were left in place. The donor heart is implanted by suturing the donor atria to the residual atrial tissue of the recipient's heart. Both techniques then connect the recipient's pulmonary artery and aorta to those of the donor heart.

Heterotopic transplantation is less commonly performed (Fig. 29-10). The donor heart is placed to the right and slightly anterior to the recipient's heart; the recipient's heart is not removed. Initially, it was thought that the original heart might provide some protection for the patient in the event that the transplanted heart was rejected. Although the protective effect has not been proved, other reasons for retaining the original heart have been identified: a small donor heart or pulmonary hypertension (Becker & Petlin, 1999; Kadner et al., 2000).

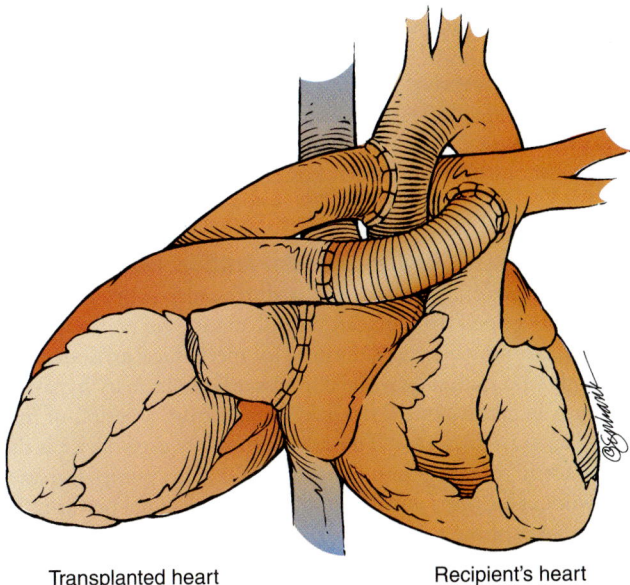

Transplanted heart   Recipient's heart

FIGURE 29-10 Heterotopic method of heart transplantation.

The transplanted heart has no nerve connections with the recipient's body (ie, denervated heart), and the sympathetic and vagus nerves do not affect the transplanted heart. The resting rate of the transplanted heart is approximately 70 to 90 beats per minute, but it increases gradually if catecholamines are in the circulation. Patients must gradually increase and decrease their exercise (ie, extended warm-up and cool-down periods), because 20 to 30 minutes may be required to achieve the desired heart rate. Atropine does not increase the heart rate of these patients.

Postoperative Course. Heart transplant patients are constantly balancing the risk of rejection with the risk of infection. They must comply with a complex regimen of diet, medications, activity, follow-up laboratory studies, biopsies (to diagnose rejection), and clinic visits. Most commonly, patients receive cyclosporine or tacrolimus (FK506, Prograf), azathioprine (Imuran) or mycophenolate mofetil (CellCept), and corticosteroids (ie, prednisone) to minimize rejection.

In addition to rejection and infection, complications may include accelerated atherosclerosis of the coronary arteries (ie, cardiac allograft vasculopathy [CAV] or accelerated graft atherosclerosis [AGA]). Although the cause is unknown, the disease is believed to be immunologically mediated (Augustine, 2000; Rourke et al., 1999). Hypertension may be experienced by patients taking cyclosporine or tacrolimus; the cause has not been identified. Osteoporosis frequently occurs as a side effect of the anti-rejection medications and pretransplantation dietary insufficiency and medications. Posttransplantation lymphoproliferative disease and cancer of the skin and lips are the most common malignancies after transplantation, possibly caused by immunosuppression. Weight gain, obesity, diabetes, dyslipidemias (eg, hypercholesterolemia), hypotension, renal failure, and central nervous system, respiratory, and gastrointestinal disturbances may be caused by the corticosteroids or other immunosuppressants. Other complications are immunosuppressant medication toxicities and responses to the psychosocial stresses imposed by organ transplantation. Patients may experience guilt that someone died for them to live, have anxiety about the new heart, experience depression or fear when rejection is identified, or have difficulty with family role changes before and after transplantation (Augustine, 2000; Becker &

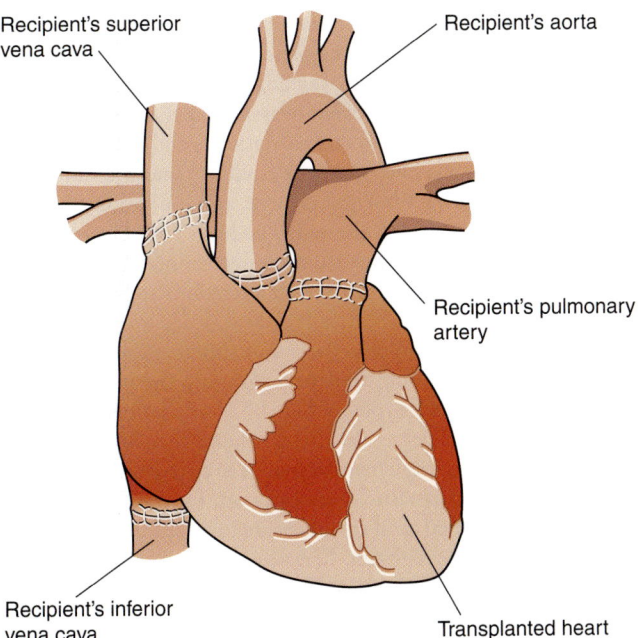

Recipient's superior vena cava

Recipient's aorta

Recipient's pulmonary artery

Recipient's inferior vena cava

Transplanted heart

FIGURE 29-9 Orthotopic method of heart transplantation.

Petlin, 1999; Braunwald et al., 2001; Fuster et al., 2001; Rourke et al., 1999).

The 1-year survival rate for patients with transplanted hearts is approximately 80% to 90%; the 5-year survival rate is approximately 60% to 70% (Augustine, 2000; Becker & Petlin, 1999; Braunwald et al., 2001; Fuster et al., 2001; Rourke et al., 1999).

Mechanical Assist Devices and Total Artificial Hearts. The use of cardiopulmonary bypass for cardiovascular surgery and the possibility of performing heart transplantation for end-stage cardiac disease have increased the need for mechanical assist devices. Patients who cannot be weaned from cardiopulmonary bypass or patients in cardiogenic shock may benefit from a period of mechanical heart assistance. The most commonly used device is the intra-aortic balloon pump (see Chap. 30). This pump decreases the work of the heart during contraction but does not perform the actual work of the heart.

Ventricular Assist Devices. More complex devices that actually perform some or all of the pumping function for the heart also are being used. These more sophisticated **ventricular assist devices** (VADs) (Fig. 29-11) can circulate as much blood per minute as the patient's heart, if not more. Each ventricular assist device is used to support one ventricle. Some ventricular assist devices can be combined with an oxygenator; the combination is called extracorporeal membrane oxygenation (ECMO). The oxygenator–ventricular assist device combination is used for the patient whose heart cannot pump adequate blood through the lungs or the body.

There are three basic types of devices: centrifugal, pneumatic, and electric or electromagnetic. Centrifugal VADs are external, nonpulsatile, cone-shaped devices with internal mechanisms that spin rapidly, creating a vortex (tornado-like action) that pulls blood from a large vein into the pump and then pushes it back into a large artery. Pneumatic VADs are external or implanted pulsatile devices with a flexible reservoir housed in a rigid exte-

rior. The reservoir usually fills with blood drained from the patient's atrium or ventricle. The VAD then forces pressurized air into the rigid housing, compressing the reservoir and returning the blood to the patient's circulation, usually into the aorta. Electric or electromagnetic VADs are similar to the pneumatic VADs, but instead of pressurized air, one or more flat metal plates are pushed against the reservoir to return the blood to the patient's circulation.

Total Artificial Hearts. **Total artificial hearts** are designed to replace both ventricles. Some require the removal of the patient's heart to implant the total artificial heart; others do not. All of these devices are experimental. Although there has been some short-term success, the long-term results have been disappointing. Researchers hope to develop a device that can be permanently implanted and that will eliminate the need for donated human heart transplantation for the treatment of end-stage cardiac disease (Braunwald et al., 2001; Chillcott et al., 1998; Fuster et al., 2001; Rose et al., 1999; Schakenbach, 2001).

Most VADs and total artificial hearts are temporary treatments while the patient's own heart recovers or until a donor heart becomes available for transplantation (ie, "bridge to transplant"). Some devices are being investigated for permanent use. Bleeding disorders, hemorrhage, thrombus, emboli, hemolysis, infection, renal failure, right heart failure, multisystem failure, and mechanical failure are some of the complications of VADs and total artificial hearts (Braunwald et al., 2001; Duke & Perna, 1999; Schakenbach, 2001; Scherr et al., 1999). The nursing care for these patients focuses on assessing for and minimizing these complications and involves providing emotional support and education about the mechanical assist device.

NURSING PROCESS:
THE PATIENT WITH CARDIOMYOPATHY

Assessment

Nursing assessment for the patient with cardiomyopathy begins with a detailed history of the presenting signs and symptoms. The nurse identifies possible etiologic factors, such as heavy alcohol intake, recent illness or pregnancy, or history of the disease in immediate family members. If the patient complains of chest pain, a thorough review of the pain, including its precipitating factors, should be performed. The review of systems includes the presence of orthopnea, paroxysmal nocturnal dyspnea, and syncope or dyspnea with exertion. The number of pillows that are needed to sleep, usual weight, any weight change, and limitation to activities of daily living also are assessed. The New York Heart Association Classification for heart failure is determined. The patient's usual diet is evaluated to determine if alterations are needed to reduce sodium intake.

Because of the chronicity of cardiomyopathy, the nurse compiles a careful psychosocial history exploring the impact of the disease on the patient's role within the family and community. Identification of all perceived stressors helps the patient and the health care team to implement activities to relieve anxiety related to changes in health status. Very early on, the patient's support systems are identified, and members are involved in the patient's care and therapeutic regimen. The assessment addresses the effect the diagnosis has had on the patient and members of his or her support system and the patient's emotional status. Depression is not uncommon in patients with cardiomyopathy who have developed heart failure.

FIGURE 29-11 Left ventricular assist device.

The physical assessment focuses on signs and symptoms of congestive heart failure. The baseline assessment includes such key components as:

- Vital signs
- Calculation of pulse pressure and identification of pulsus paradoxus
- Current weight; determination of weight gain or loss
- Detection by palpation of the point of maximal impulse, often shifted to the left
- Cardiac auscultation for a systolic murmur and third and fourth heart sounds
- Pulmonary auscultation for crackles
- Measurement of jugular vein distention
- Identification of presence and severity of edema

Diagnosis

NURSING DIAGNOSES

Based on the assessment data, major nursing diagnoses for the patient may include:

- Decreased cardiac output related to structural disorders caused by cardiomyopathy or to dysrhythmia from the disease process and medical treatments
- Ineffective cardiopulmonary, cerebral, peripheral, and renal tissue perfusion related to decreased peripheral blood flow (resulting from decreased cardiac output)
- Impaired gas exchange related to pulmonary congestion caused by myocardial failure (decreased cardiac output)
- Activity intolerance related to decreased cardiac output or excessive fluid volume, or both
- Anxiety related to the change in health status and in role functioning
- Powerlessness related to disease process
- Noncompliance with medication and diet therapies

COLLABORATIVE PROBLEMS/ POTENTIAL COMPLICATIONS

Based on the assessment data, potential complications include:

- Congestive heart failure
- Ventricular dysrhythmias
- Atrial dysrhythmias
- Cardiac conduction defects
- Pulmonary or cerebral embolism
- Valvular dysfunction

These complications are discussed earlier in this chapter and in Chapters 27 and 30.

Planning and Goals

The major goals for the patient include improved or maintained cardiac output, increased activity tolerance, reduction of anxiety, adherence to the self-care program, increased sense of power with decision making, and absence of complications.

Nursing Interventions

IMPROVING CARDIAC OUTPUT

During a symptomatic episode, rest is indicated. Many patients with DCM find that sitting up with their legs down is more comfortable than lying down in a bed. This position is helpful in pooling venous blood in the periphery and reducing preload. As-

sessing the patient's oxygen saturation at rest and during activity may assist with determining a need for supplemental oxygen. Oxygen is usually given through nasal cannula when indicated.

Ensuring that medications are taken as prescribed is important to preserving adequate cardiac output. It is important to ensure that patients with HCM avoid diuretics and that patients with DCM avoid verapamil (Calan, Isoptin) to maintain contractility. The nurse may assist the patient with planning a schedule for taking medications and identifying methods to remember to follow it, such as associating the time to take a medication with an activity (eg, eating a meal, brushing teeth). Ensuring that the patient receives or chooses food selections that are appropriate for the low-sodium diet is also important. Determining the patient's weight every day and identifying any significant change is one way to monitor the patient's response to treatment. Assessing if the patient experiences shortness of breath after more or less activity than before treatment is another indication of the effect of treatment. Patients with low cardiac output may need assistance keeping warm and frequently changing position to stimulate circulation and reduce the possibility of skin breakdown.

INCREASING ACTIVITY TOLERANCE

The nurse plans the patient's activities so that they occur in cycles, alternating rest with activity periods. This benefits the patient's physiologic status, and it helps to teach the patient about the need for planned cycles of rest and activity. For example, after taking a bath or shower, the patient should plan to sit and read the paper or pay bills. Suggesting that patients sit while chopping vegetables, drying their hair, or shaving helps them to identify methods to balance rest with activity. The nurse can also make sure that the patient recognizes the symptoms that indicate the need for rest and the actions to take when the symptoms occur. Patients with HCM need to avoid strenuous activity and sports.

REDUCING ANXIETY

Spiritual, psychological, and emotional support may be indicated for the patient, family, and significant others. Interventions are directed toward eradicating or alleviating perceived stressors. The patient is provided with appropriate information about cardiomyopathy and self-management activities. An atmosphere in which the patient feels free to verbalize concerns is provided, as is assurance that these concerns are legitimate. If the patient is facing death or awaiting transplantation, time must be provided to discuss these issues. Providing the patient with realistic hope helps to reduce anxiety while the patient awaits a donor heart. Nurses help the patient, family, and significant others with anticipatory grieving. Accomplishing a goal, no matter how small, also promotes the patient's sense of well-being.

DECREASING THE SENSE OF POWERLESSNESS

Patients need to recognize that they go through a grieving process when given a diagnosis of cardiomyopathy. They are assisted in identifying the things in their life that they have lost (eg, foods that they have enjoyed eating but are high in sodium, ability to engage in constant active lifestyle, ability to play sports, ability to lift grandchildren). They also are assisted in identifying their emotional responses to the loss (eg, anger, depression). The nurse then assists patients in identifying the amount of control that they have in their lives, such as making food choices, managing their medications, and working with their provider to achieve the best possible outcomes. The use of patient tools that track behaviours with the resulting symptoms may be helpful. For example, a diary in which the patient records his or her food selections and weight may assist the patient with understanding the relationship between sodium intake and weight gain. Some patients are able to manage a self-titrating diuretic regimen, in which the patient is able to adjust the dose of diuretic to his or her symptoms.

PROMOTING HOME AND COMMUNITY-BASED CARE

Teaching Patients Self-Care. Teaching patients about the medication regimen, symptom monitoring, and symptom management is a key part of the plan of nursing care. The nurse is integral to the learning process as patients learn to balance their lifestyle and work while accomplishing their therapeutic activities. Helping patients cope with their disease status assists them in adjusting their lifestyles and implementing a self-care program at home.

Continuing Care. The nurse reinforces previous teaching and performs ongoing assessment of the patient's symptoms and progress. The nurse also assists the patient and family to adjust to lifestyle changes. Teaching patients to read nutritional labels, to maintain a record of daily weights and symptoms, and to organize daily activities to increase activity tolerance can be helpful. The patient's responses to diet and fluid restrictions and to the medication regimen are assessed, and explanations about symptoms that should be reported to the physician are emphasized. Because of the risk of dysrhythmia, the patient's family may be taught cardiopulmonary resuscitation. Women are often advised to avoid pregnancy; each case is assessed individually. The nurse assesses the psychosocial needs of the patient and family on an ongoing basis. There may be concerns and fears about the prognosis, changes in lifestyle, effects of medications, and the possibility of others in the family having the same condition that increase the patient's anxiety and interfere with effective coping strategies. Establishing trust is vital to the relationship with these chronically ill patients and their families. This is particularly significant when the nurse is involved with the patient and family in discussions about end-of-life decisions. Patients who have significant symptoms of heart failure or other complications of cardiomyopathy may need a home care referral.

Evaluation

EXPECTED PATIENT OUTCOMES

Expected patient outcomes may include:

1. Maintains or improves cardiac function
   a. Exhibits heart and respiratory rates within normal limits
   b. Reports decreased dyspnea and increased comfort; maintains or improves gas exchange
   c. Reports no weight gain
   d. Maintains or improves peripheral blood flow
2. Maintains or increases activity tolerance
   a. Carries out activities of daily living (eg, brushes teeth, feeds self)
   b. Reports increased tolerance to activity
3. Is less anxious
   a. Discusses prognosis freely
   b. Verbalizes fears and concerns
   c. Participates in support groups if appropriate
4. Decreases sense of powerlessness
   a. Identifies emotional response to diagnosis
   b. Discusses the control he or she has in life
5. Adheres to the self-care program
   a. Takes medications according to prescribed schedule
   b. Modifies diet to accommodate sodium and fluid restrictions
   c. Modifies lifestyle to accommodate recommended activity and rest behaviours
   d. Identifies signs and symptoms to be reported to the health care professional

Cardiac Tumour and Trauma Surgery

TUMOUR EXCISION

Tumours of the heart are rare; most (75% to 88%) are benign (Braunwald et al., 2001; Kamiya et al., 2001). Primary tumours occur in less than 1% of the population; metastatic tumours have been reported in 1.5% to 35% of oncology patients (Braunwald et al., 2001; Reynan, 1996; Shapiro, 2001). Tumours may be sites for thrombus formation and therefore create a risk of embolism. Dysrhythmias may occur as the myocardium or conduction system is affected.

Surgical excision is performed to prevent obstruction of a chamber or valve. Cardiopulmonary bypass is used, except for epicardial tumours, which can be excised without entering the heart and without stopping the heart from beating. The tumour location may necessitate valve replacement, myocardial patching, or pacemaker implantation. The nursing care is the same as that for patients undergoing other forms of cardiac surgery (see Chap. 28).

TRAUMA REPAIR

Patients who have sustained nonpenetrating (ie, blunt force) injury or penetrating injury (eg, gunshot wound, stabbing) causing cardiac trauma often do not survive to treatment (Flynn & Bonini, 1999; Thourani et al., 1999). Patients who do survive to treatment often require surgical treatment (Thourani et al., 1999; Wall et al., 1997). The repairs are typically to the valves or septum in blunt force injuries and to the ventricular and atrial walls in penetrating injuries. The wound is débrided and closed surgically when possible, but valve repair and replacement or patch grafts of the septum and atrial or ventricular walls may be required. The surgery is usually an emergency procedure, and the risk of complications from the injury and surgery is high. The nursing care is the same as that for patients undergoing other forms of cardiac surgery (See Chap. 28).

Infectious Diseases of the Heart

Among the most common infections of the heart are infective endocarditis, myocarditis, and pericarditis. The ideal management is prevention.

RHEUMATIC ENDOCARDITIS

Acute rheumatic fever, which occurs most often in school-age children, follows 0.3% to 3% of cases of group A beta-hemolytic streptococcal pharyngitis (Chin, 2001). Prompt treatment of strep throat with antibiotics can prevent the development of rheumatic fever (Chart 29-1). The *Streptococcus* is spread by direct contact with oral or respiratory secretions. Although the bacteria are the causative agents, malnutrition, overcrowding, and lower socioeconomic status may predispose individuals to rheumatic fever (Beers et al., 1999). The incidence of rheumatic fever in Canada and other developed countries is believed to have steadily decreased, but the exact incidence is difficult to determine because the infection may

Chart 29-1 • ASSESSMENT

Recognizing and Preventing Rheumatic Fever

Rheumatic fever is a preventable disease. Eradicating rheumatic fever would eliminate rheumatic heart disease. Penicillin therapy in patients with streptococcal infections can prevent almost all primary attacks of rheumatic fever. A throat culture is the only method by which an accurate diagnosis can be determined.

The signs and symptoms of streptococcal pharyngitis are the following:

- Fever (38.9° to 40°C)
- Chills
- Sore throat (sudden in onset)
- Diffuse redness of throat with exudate on oropharynx (may not appear until after the first day)
- Enlarged and tender lymph nodes
- Abdominal pain (more common in children)
- Acute sinusitis and acute otitis media (if due to streptococci)

go unrecognized and patients may not seek treatment (Braunwald et al., 2001; Beers et al., 1999). As many as 39% of patients with rheumatic fever develop various degrees of rheumatic heart disease associated with valvular insufficiency, heart failure, and death (Chin, 2001). The disease also affects all bony joints, producing polyarthritis. Although it is difficult to determine the incidence in Canada since rheumatic fever is not a reportable disease, about 240 cases are expected per year (Templeton, Cooper, Human, et al., 2005). Acute rheumatic fever is still the most common cause of acquired heart disease in children worldwide. For chronic rheumatic heart disease, there was a significant trend of a decrease in death rate of about 0.22 per 100,000 population per year. These trends were observed for both men and women, although the death rates for women were consistently greater than those for men. (Rabkin & Chu-Chun-Lin, 1988.)

Pathophysiology

The heart damage and the joint lesions of rheumatic endocarditis are not infectious in the sense that these tissues are not invaded and directly damaged by destructive organisms; rather, they represent a sensitivity phenomenon or reaction occurring in response to hemolytic streptococci. Leukocytes accumulate in the affected tissues and form nodules, which eventually are replaced by scar tissue. The myocardium is certain to be involved in this inflammatory process; rheumatic myocarditis develops, which temporarily weakens the contractile power of the heart. The pericardium also is affected, and rheumatic pericarditis occurs during the acute illness. These myocardial and pericardial complications usually occur without serious sequelae. Rheumatic endocarditis, however, results in permanent and often crippling side effects.

Clinical Manifestations

Rheumatic endocarditis anatomically manifests first by tiny translucent vegetations or growths, which resemble pinhead-sized beads arranged in a row along the free margins of the valve flaps. These tiny beads look harmless enough and may disappear without injuring the valve leaflets. More often, however, they have serious effects. They are the starting point of a process that gradually

thickens the leaflets, rendering them shorter and thicker than normal and preventing them from closing completely. The result is leakage, a condition called *valvular regurgitation.* The most common site of valvular regurgitation is the mitral valve. In some patients, the inflamed margins of the valve leaflets become adherent, resulting in valvular stenosis, a narrowed or stenotic valvular orifice. Regurgitation and stenosis may occur in the same valve.

A few patients with rheumatic fever become critically ill with intractable heart failure, serious dysrhythmias, and pneumonia. These patients are treated in an intensive care unit. Most patients recover quickly. However, although the patient is free of symptoms, certain permanent residual effects remain that often lead to progressive valvular deformities. The extent of cardiac damage, or even its existence, might not have been apparent in clinical examinations during the acute phase of the disease. Eventually, however, the heart murmurs that are characteristic of valvular stenosis, regurgitation, or both become audible on auscultation and, in some patients, even detectable as thrills on palpation. Usually, the myocardium can compensate for these valvular defects very well for a time. As long as the myocardium can compensate, the patient remains in apparently good health. With continued valvular alterations, the myocardium is unable to compensate (see Fig. 29-2), as evidenced by signs and symptoms of heart failure, as described in Chapter 30.

Assessment and Diagnostic Findings

During assessment, the nurse should keep in mind that the symptoms depend on which side of the heart is involved. The mitral valve is most often affected, producing symptoms of left-sided heart failure: shortness of breath with crackles and wheezes in the lungs (see Chap. 30 for a discussion of left-sided versus right-sided failure). The severity of the symptoms depends on the size and location of the lesion. The systemic symptoms that are present are proportionate to the virulence of the invading organism. When a new murmur is detected in a patient with a systemic infection, infectious endocarditis should be suspected. The patient is also at risk for embolic phenomena of the lung (eg, recurrent pneumonia, pulmonary abscesses), kidney (eg, hematuria, renal failure), spleen (eg, left upper quadrant pain), heart (eg, myocardial infarction), brain (eg, stroke), or peripheral vessels.

Prevention

Rheumatic endocarditis is prevented through early and adequate treatment of streptococcal infections. A first-line approach in preventing initial attacks of rheumatic endocarditis is to recognize streptococcal infections, treat them adequately, and control epidemics in the community. Every nurse should be familiar with the signs and symptoms of streptococcal pharyngitis: high fever (38.9°C to 40°C), chills, sore throat, redness of the throat with exudate, enlarged lymph nodes, abdominal pain, and acute rhinitis.

NURSING ALERT A throat culture is the only method by which an accurate diagnosis of streptococcal infection of the throat can be made.

Medical Management

The objectives of medical management are to eradicate the causative organism and prevent additional complications, such as a thromboembolic event. Long-term antibiotic therapy is the recommended treatment, and penicillin administered parenterally remains the medication of choice.

The patient who has rheumatic endocarditis and whose valvular dysfunction is mild may require no further treatment. Nevertheless, the danger exists for recurrent attacks of acute rheumatic fever, bacterial endocarditis, embolism from vegetations or mural thrombi in the heart, and eventual cardiac failure.

Nursing Management

A key nursing role in rheumatic endocarditis is teaching patients about the disease, its treatment, and the preventive steps needed to avoid potential complications. After acute treatment with antibiotics, patients need to learn about the need to take prophylactic antibiotics before invasive procedures (see Prevention in the Infective Endocarditis section).

INFECTIVE ENDOCARDITIS

Infective endocarditis is an infection of the valves and endothelial surface of the heart. Endocarditis usually develops in people with cardiac structural defects (eg, valve disorders). Infective endocarditis is more common in older people, probably because of decreased immunologic response to infection and the metabolic alterations associated with aging. There is a high incidence of staphylococcal endocarditis among IV/injection drug users who most commonly have infections of the right heart valves (Bayer et al., 1998; Braunwald, 2001).

The incidence of infective endocarditis remained steady at about 4.2 cases per 100,000 patients in the years from 1950 to the mid-1980s (Braunwald et al., 2001). The incidence then increased, partially attributed to increased IV/injection drug abuse (Braunwald et al., 2001). In 2002, a total of 69 deaths in Canada were attributed to infective endocarditis (Statistics Canada, 2005). Invasive procedures, particularly those involving mucosal surfaces, can cause a bacteremia. The bacteremia rarely lasts for more than 15 minutes (Dajani et al., 1997). If a person has some anatomic cardiac defect, bacteremia can cause bacterial endocarditis (Dajani et al., 1997). The combination of the invasive procedure, the particular bacteria introduced into the bloodstream, and the cardiac defect may result in infective endocarditis.

Pathophysiology

Infective endocarditis is most often caused by direct invasion of the endocardium by a microbe (eg, streptococci, enterococci, pneumococci, staphylococci). The infection usually causes deformity of the valve leaflets, but it may affect other cardiac structures such as the chordae tendineae. Other causative microorganisms include fungi and rickettsiae. Patients at higher risk for infective endocarditis are those with prosthetic heart valves, a history of endocarditis, complex cyanotic congenital malformations, and systemic or pulmonary shunts or conduits that were surgically constructed (eg, saphenous vein grafts, internal mammary artery grafts). At high risk are patients with rheumatic heart disease or mitral valve prolapse and those who have prosthetic heart valves (Chart 29-2).

Hospital-acquired endocarditis occurs most often in patients with debilitating disease, those with indwelling catheters, and those receiving prolonged intravenous or antibiotic therapy. Patients receiving immunosuppressive medications or corticosteroids may develop fungal endocarditis.

Chart 29-2
Risk Factors for Infective Endocarditis

High Risk
Prosthetic cardiac valves
History of bacterial endocarditis (even without heart disease)
Complex cyanotic congenital malformations
Surgically constructed systemic or pulmonary shunts or conduits

Moderate Risk
Mitral valve prolapse with valvular regurgitation or thickened leaflets
Hypertrophic cardiomyopathy
Acquired valvular dysfunction
Most congenital cardiac malformations (other than those listed above and surgical repair of atrial and ventricular septal defect, or patent ductus arteriosus)

A diagnosis of acute infective endocarditis is made when the onset of infection and resulting valvular destruction is rapid, occurring within days to weeks. The onset of infection may take 2 weeks to months, diagnosed as subacute infective endocarditis (Braunwald et al., 2001).

Clinical Manifestations

Usually, the onset of infective endocarditis is insidious. The signs and symptoms develop from the toxic effect of the infection, from destruction of the heart valves, and from embolization of fragments of vegetative growths on the heart. The occurrence of peripheral emboli is not experienced by patients with right heart valve infective endocarditis (Bayer et al., 1998; Braunwald, 2001). The patient exhibits signs and symptoms similar to those described in rheumatic endocarditis (see previous discussion).

Assessment and Diagnostic Findings

The general manifestations, which may be mistaken for influenza, include vague complaints of malaise, anorexia, weight loss, cough, and back and joint pain. Fever is intermittent and may be absent in patients who are receiving antibiotics or corticosteroids or in those who are elderly or have heart failure or renal failure. Splinter hemorrhages (ie, reddish-brown lines and streaks) may be seen under the fingernails and toenails, and petechiae may appear in the conjunctiva and mucous membranes. Small, painful nodules (Osler's nodes) may be present in the pads of fingers or toes. Hemorrhages with pale centres (Roth's spots) that may be seen in the fundi of the eyes are caused by emboli in the nerve fibre layer of the eye.

The cardiac manifestations include heart murmurs, which may be absent initially. Progressive changes in murmurs over time may be encountered and indicate valvular damage from vegetations or perforation of the valve or the chordae tendineae. Enlargement of the heart or evidence of heart failure is also found.

The central nervous system manifestations include headache, temporary or transient cerebral ischemia, and strokes, which may be caused by emboli to the cerebral arteries. Embolization may be a presenting symptom; it may occur at any time and may involve other organ systems. Embolic phenomena may occur, as discussed in the previous section on rheumatic endocarditis.

Although the described characteristics may indicate infective endocarditis, the signs and symptoms may indicate other diseases as well. A definitive diagnosis is made when a microorganism is found in two separate blood cultures, in a vegetation, or in an abscess. Three sets of blood cultures (with each set including one aerobic and one anaerobic culture) should be obtained before administration of any antimicrobial agents. Negative blood cultures do not totally rule out the diagnosis of infective endocarditis. An echocardiogram may assist in the diagnosis by demonstrating a moving mass on the valve, prosthetic valve, or supporting structures and by identification of vegetations, abscesses, new prosthetic valve dehiscence, or new regurgitation (Braunwald et al., 2001). An echocardiogram may also demonstrate the development of heart failure.

Prevention

Although rare, bacterial endocarditis may be life-threatening. A key strategy is primary prevention in high-risk patients (ie, those with rheumatic heart disease, mitral valve prolapse, or prosthetic heart valves). Antibiotic prophylaxis is recommended for high-risk patients immediately before and sometimes after the following procedures:

- Dental procedures that induce gingival or mucosal bleeding, including professional cleaning and placement of orthodontic bands (not brackets)
- Tonsillectomy or adenoidectomy
- Surgical procedures that involve intestinal or respiratory mucosa
- Bronchoscopy with a rigid bronchoscope
- Sclerotherapy for esophageal varices
- Esophageal dilation
- Gallbladder surgery
- Cystoscopy
- Urethral dilation
- Urethral catheterization if urinary tract infection is present
- Urinary tract surgery if urinary tract infection is present
- Prostatic surgery
- Incision and drainage of infected tissue
- Vaginal hysterectomy
- Vaginal delivery

The type of antibiotic used for prophylaxis varies with the type of procedure and the degree of risk. The patient is usually instructed to take 2 g of amoxicillin (Amoxil) 1 hour before dental, oral, respiratory, or esophageal procedures. If the patient is allergic to penicillin (eg, ampicillin [Omnipen, Polycillin], carbenicillin [Geocillin], cloxacillin [Apo-Cloxi], methicillin [Staphcillin], nafcillin [Nallpen, Unipen], oxacillin [Prostaphlin, Bactocill], penicillin G [Bicillin]), clindamycin (Alti-Clindamyacin), cephalexin (Apo-Cephalex), cefadroxil (Duricef), azithromycin (Zithromax), or clarithromycin (Biaxin) may be used. Recommendations for gastrointestinal or genitourinary procedures are ampicillin and gentamicin (Garamycin) for high-risk patients, amoxicillin or ampicillin for moderate-risk patients, and substituting vancomycin (Vancocin) only for patients allergic to ampicillin or amoxicillin.

The severity of oral inflammation and infection is a significant factor in the incidence and degree of bacteremia. Poor dental hygiene can lead to bacteremia, particularly in the setting of a dental procedure. Regular personal and professional oral health care and rinsing with an antiseptic mouthwash for 30 seconds before dental procedures may assist in reducing the risk of bacteremia. Increased vigilance is also needed in patients with intravenous catheters. To minimize the risk of infection, nurses must ensure that meticulous hand hygiene, site preparation, and the use of

aseptic technique occur during the insertion and maintenance procedures (Schmid, 2000). All catheters are removed as soon as they are no longer needed or no longer function.

Complications

Even if the patient responds to the therapy, endocarditis can be destructive to the heart and other organs. Heart failure and cerebral vascular complications, such as stroke, may occur before, during, or after therapy. The development of heart failure, which may result from perforation of a valve leaflet, rupture of chordae, blood flow obstruction due to vegetations, or intracardiac shunts from dehiscence of prosthetic valves, indicates a poor prognosis with medical therapy alone and a higher surgical risk (Braunwald et al., 2001). Valvular stenosis or regurgitation, myocardial damage, and mycotic (fungal) aneurysms are potential heart complications. Many other organ complications can result from septic or nonseptic emboli, immunologic responses, abscess of the spleen, mycotic aneurysms, and hemodynamic deterioration.

Medical Management

The causative organism may be identified by serial blood cultures. The objective of treatment is to eradicate the invading organism through adequate doses of an appropriate antimicrobial agent.

PHARMACOLOGIC THERAPY

Antibiotic therapy is usually administered parenterally in a continuous intravenous infusion for 2 to 6 weeks. Parenteral therapy is administered in doses that achieve a high serum concentration and for a significant duration to ensure eradication of the dormant bacteria within the dense vegetations. This therapy is often delivered in the patient's home and is monitored by a home care nurse. Serum levels of the selected antibiotic are monitored. If the serum does not demonstrate bactericidal activity, increased dosages of the antibiotic are prescribed, or a different antibiotic is used. Numerous antimicrobial regimens are in use, but penicillin is usually the medication of choice. Blood cultures are taken periodically to monitor the effect of therapy. In fungal endocarditis, an antifungal agent, such as amphotericin B (Abelect, Amphocin, Fungizone), is the usual treatment.

The patient's temperature is monitored at regular intervals because the course of the fever is one indication of the effectiveness of treatment. However, febrile reactions also may occur as a result of medication. After adequate antimicrobial therapy is initiated, the infective organism usually disappears. The patient should begin to feel better, regain an appetite, and have less fatigue. During this time, patients require psychosocial support because, although they feel well, they may find themselves confined to the hospital or home with restrictive intravenous therapy.

SURGICAL MANAGEMENT

After the patient recovers from the infectious process, seriously damaged valves may need to be replaced. Surgical valve replacement greatly improves the prognosis for patients with severe symptoms from damaged heart valves. Aortic or mitral valve excision and replacement are required for patients who develop congestive heart failure despite adequate medical treatment, patients who have more than one serious systemic embolic episode, and patients with uncontrolled infection, recurrent infection, or fungal endocarditis. Many patients who have prosthetic valve endocarditis (ie, infected prostheses) require valve replacement.

Nursing Management

The nurse monitors the patient's temperature; the patient may have fever for weeks. Heart sounds are assessed; a new murmur may indicate involvement of the valve leaflets. The nurse monitors for signs and symptoms of systemic embolization, or for patients with right heart endocarditis, the nurse monitors for signs and symptoms of pulmonary infarction and infiltrates. The nurse assesses signs and symptoms of organ damage such as stroke (ie, cerebrovascular accident or brain attack), meningitis, heart failure, myocardial infarction, glomerulonephritis, and splenomegaly.

Patient care is directed toward management of infection. The patient is started on antibiotics as soon as blood cultures have been obtained. All invasive lines and wounds should be assessed daily for redness, tenderness, warmth, swelling, drainage, or other signs of infection. Patients and their families are instructed about any activity restrictions, medications, and signs and symptoms of infection. The nurse should instruct the patient and family about the need for prophylactic antibiotics before, and possibly after, dental, respiratory, gastrointestinal, or genitourinary procedures. Home care nurses supervise and monitor intravenous antibiotic therapy delivered in the home setting and educate the patient and family about prevention and health promotion. The nurse provides the patient and family with emotional support and facilitates coping strategies during the prolonged course of the infection and antibiotic treatment required. If the patient received surgical treatment, the nurse provides postoperative care and instruction.

MYOCARDITIS

Myocarditis is an inflammatory process involving the myocardium. Myocarditis can cause heart dilation, thrombi on the heart wall (mural thrombi), infiltration of circulating blood cells around the coronary vessels and between the muscle fibres, and degeneration of the muscle fibres themselves. In 2002, there were 46 deaths in Canada from myocarditis. The rate may be higher because the variety of clinical presentations may cause underreporting (Tang, 2001). Mortality varies with the severity of symptoms. Most patients with mild symptoms recover completely. Other patients may develop cardiomyopathy and heart failure. Patients with symptomatic heart failure and an ejection fraction of less than 45% had a 1-year mortality rate of 20% and a 4-year mortality rate of 56% (Tang, 2001).

Pathophysiology

Myocarditis usually results from a viral, bacterial, mycotic, parasitic, protozoal, or spirochetal infection. It also may occur in patients after acute systemic infections such as rheumatic fever, in those receiving immunosuppressive therapy, or in those with infective endocarditis. Myocarditis may result from an allergic reaction to pharmacologic agents used in the treatment of other diseases. It may begin in one small area and then spread throughout the myocardium. The degree of myocardial involvement determines the degree of hemodynamic effect and resulting signs and symptoms. It is theorized that dilated cardiomyopathy is a latent manifestation of myocarditis.

Clinical Manifestations

The symptoms of acute myocarditis depend on the type of infection, the degree of myocardial damage, and the capacity of the myocardium to recover. The patient may be asymptomatic, and the infection resolves on its own. The patient may develop mild to moderate symptoms and seek medical attention. The patient may also sustain sudden cardiac death or quickly develop severe congestive heart failure. The patient with mild to moderate symptoms often complains of fatigue and dyspnea, palpitations, and occasional discomfort in the chest and upper abdomen.

Assessment and Diagnostic Findings

Assessment of the patient may reveal no abnormalities; as a result, the entire illness goes unrecognized. The patient may complain of chest pain (with a subsequent cardiac catheterization demonstrating normal coronary arteries). The patient without any abnormal heart structure (at least initially) may suddenly develop dysrhythmias. If the patient has developed structural abnormalities (eg, systolic dysfunction), the clinical assessment may disclose cardiac enlargement, faint heart sounds, gallop rhythm, and a systolic murmur.

Prevention

Prevention of infectious diseases by means of appropriate immunizations (eg, influenza, hepatitis) and early treatment appears to be important in decreasing the incidence of myocarditis (Braunwald et al., 2001).

Medical Management

The patient receives specific treatment for the underlying cause if it is known (eg, penicillin for hemolytic streptococci) and is placed on bed rest to decrease the cardiac workload. Bed rest also helps to decrease myocardial damage and the complications of myocarditis. Activities, especially sports in young patients with myocarditis, should be limited for a 6-month period or at least until heart size and function have returned to normal. Physical activity is increased slowly, and the patient is instructed to report any symptoms that occur with increasing activity, such as a rapidly beating heart. The use of corticosteroids in treating myocarditis remains controversial (Braunwald et al., 2001). Nonsteroidal anti-inflammatory drugs (NSAIDs) such as aspirin and ibuprofen are not to be used during the acute phase or if the patient develops heart failure, because these medications can cause further myocardial damage. If the patient develops heart failure, management is essentially the same as for all causes of heart failure (see Chap. 30).

Nursing Management

The nurse assesses the patient's temperature to determine whether the disease is subsiding. The cardiovascular assessment focuses on signs and symptoms of heart failure and dysrhythmia. The patient experiencing dysrhythmias should receive continuous cardiac monitoring with personnel and equipment readily available to treat life-threatening dysrhythmias.

NURSING ALERT Patients with myocarditis are sensitive to digitalis. They must be closely monitored for digitalis toxicity, which is evidenced by dysrhythmia, anorexia, nausea, vomiting, headache, and malaise (see Chap. 30).

Elastic compression stockings and passive and active exercises should be used, because embolization from venous thrombosis and mural thrombi can occur.

PERICARDITIS

Pericarditis refers to an inflammation of the pericardium, the membranous sac enveloping the heart. It may be a primary illness, or it may develop in the course of a variety of medical and surgical disorders. The incidence of pericarditis varies with the cause. For example, pericarditis occurs after pericardectomy (opening of the pericardium) in 5% to 30% of patients after cardiac surgery (Beers et al., 1999). Pericarditis that occurs within 10 days to 2 months after acute myocardial infarction (Dressler's syndrome) causes 1% to 3% of all cases of pericarditis (Beers et al., 1999). Pericarditis may be acute or chronic. It may be classified by the layers of the pericardium becoming attached to each other (adhesive) or by what accumulates in the pericardial sac: serum (serous), pus (purulent), calcium deposits (calcific), clotting proteins (fibrinous), or blood (sanguinous).

Pathophysiology

The following are some of the causes underlying or associated with pericarditis:

- Idiopathic or nonspecific causes
- Infection: usually viral (eg, Coxsackie, influenza); rarely bacterial (eg, streptococci, staphylococci, meningococci, gonococci); and mycotic (fungal)
- Disorders of connective tissue: systemic lupus erythematosus, rheumatic fever, rheumatoid arthritis, polyarteritis
- Hypersensitivity states: immune reactions, medication reactions, serum sickness
- Disorders of adjacent structures: myocardial infarction, dissecting aneurysm, pleural and pulmonary disease (pneumonia)
- Neoplastic disease: caused by metastasis from lung cancer or breast cancer, leukemia, and primary (mesothelioma) neoplasms
- Radiation therapy
- Trauma: chest injury, cardiac surgery, cardiac catheterization, pacemaker implantation
- Renal failure and uremia
- Tuberculosis

Pericarditis can lead to an accumulation of fluid in the pericardial sac (pericardial effusion) and increased pressure on the heart, leading to cardiac tamponade (see Chap. 30). Frequent or prolonged episodes of pericarditis may also lead to thickening and decreased elasticity that restrict the heart's ability to fill properly with blood (constrictive pericarditis). The pericardium may become calcified, further restricting ventricular expansion during ventricular filling (diastole). With less filling, the ventricles pump out less blood, leading to decreased cardiac output and signs and symptoms of heart failure. Restricted diastolic filling may result in increased systemic venous pressure, causing peripheral edema and hepatic failure.

Clinical Manifestations

The most characteristic symptom of pericarditis is chest pain, although pain also may be located beneath the clavicle, in the neck, or in the left scapula region. The pain or discomfort usually remains fairly constant, but it may worsen with deep inspiration and when lying down or turning. It may be relieved with a forward-leaning or sitting position. The most characteristic sign of pericarditis is a friction rub. Other signs may include mild fever,

increased white blood cell count, and increased erythrocyte sedimentation rate (ESR). Dyspnea and other signs and symptoms of heart failure may occur as the result of pericardial compression due to constrictive pericarditis or cardiac tamponade.

Assessment and Diagnostic Findings

Diagnosis is most often made on the basis of the patient's history, signs, and symptoms. An echocardiogram may detect inflammation and fluid build-up, as well as indications of heart failure, and help to confirm the diagnosis. Because the pericardial sac surrounds the heart, a 12-lead ECG detects ST changes in many, if not all, leads.

Medical Management

The objectives of management are to determine the cause, administer therapy, and be alert for cardiac tamponade. When cardiac output is impaired, the patient is placed on bed rest until the fever, chest pain, and friction rub have subsided.

Analgesics and NSAIDs such as aspirin or ibuprofen may be prescribed for pain relief during the acute phase. They also hasten the reabsorption of fluid in the patient with rheumatic pericarditis. Corticosteroids (eg, prednisone) may be prescribed if the pericarditis is severe or if the patient does not respond to NSAIDs. Colchicine may also be used as an alternative medication.

Pericardiocentesis, a procedure in which some of the pericardial fluid is removed, may be performed to assist in the identification of the causative agent. It may also relieve symptoms, especially if there are signs and symptoms of heart failure. A pericardial window, a small opening made in the pericardium, may be performed to allow continuous drainage into the chest cavity. Surgical removal of the tough encasing pericardium (pericardiectomy) may be necessary to release both ventricles from the constrictive and restrictive inflammation.

Nursing Management

The nurse caring for the patient with pericarditis must be alert to the possibility of cardiac tamponade.

 NURSING ALERT Nursing assessment skills are key to anticipating and identifying the triad of symptoms of cardiac tamponade: falling arterial pressure, rising venous pressure, and distant heart sounds.

Patients with acute pericarditis require pain management with analgesics, positioning, and psychological support. Patients experiencing chest pain often benefit from education and reassurance that the pain is not a heart attack. To minimize complications, the nurse educates and assists the patient with activity restrictions until the pain and fever subside. As the patient's condition improves, the nurse encourages gradual increases of activity. If pain, fever, or friction rub reappear, however, activity restrictions must be resumed. The nurse educates the patient and family about a healthy lifestyle to enhance the patient's immune system.

The nurse monitors the patient for heart failure. A patient who is hemodynamically unstable or experiencing congestion is treated the same as a patient with acute heart failure (see Chap. 30).

NURSING PROCESS:
THE PATIENT WITH PERICARDITIS

Assessment

The primary symptom of the patient with pericarditis is pain, which is assessed by observing and evaluating the patient in various positions. While observing the patient, the nurse tries to discover whether the pain is influenced by respiratory movements, with or without the actual passage of air; by flexion, extension, or rotation of the spine, including the neck; by movements of the shoulders and arms; by coughing; or by swallowing. Recognizing the events that precipitate or intensify pain may help establish a diagnosis and differentiate the pain of pericarditis from the pain of myocardial infarction.

A pericardial friction rub occurs when the pericardial surfaces lose their lubricating fluid because of inflammation. The rub is audible on auscultation and is synchronous with the heartbeat. However, it may be elusive and difficult to detect.

> **! NURSING ALERT** A pericardial friction rub is diagnostic of pericarditis. The nurse should search diligently for the rub by placing the diaphragm of the stethoscope tightly against the thorax and auscultating the left sternal edge in the fourth intercostal space, the site where the pericardium comes into contact with the left chest wall. A pericardial friction rub has a scratching or leathery sound. The rub is louder at the end of exhalation and may be heard best with the patient sitting and leaning forward.

If there is difficulty in distinguishing a pericardial friction rub from a pleural friction rub, patients are asked to hold their breath; a pericardial friction rub will continue.

The patient's temperature is monitored frequently. Pericarditis may cause an abrupt onset of fever in a patient who has been afebrile.

Diagnosis

NURSING DIAGNOSES

Based on the assessment data, the major nursing diagnosis of the patient may include:

- Acute pain related to inflammation of the pericardium

COLLABORATIVE PROBLEMS/
POTENTIAL COMPLICATIONS

Based on the assessment data, potential complications that may develop include:

- Pericardial effusion
- Cardiac tamponade

Planning and Goals

The patient's major goals may include relief of pain and absence of complications.

Nursing Interventions

RELIEVING PAIN

Relief of pain is achieved by having the patient rest. Because sitting upright and leaning forward is the posture that tends to relieve pain, chair rest may be more comfortable. It is important to instruct the patient to restrict activity until the pain subsides. As the chest pain and friction rub abate, activities of daily living may

resume gradually. If the patient is receiving medications such as analgesics, antibiotics, or corticosteroids for the pericarditis, his or her responses are monitored and recorded. If chest pain and friction rub recur, bed or chair rest resumes.

MONITORING AND MANAGING
POTENTIAL COMPLICATIONS

Pericardial Effusion. If the patient does not respond to medical management, fluid may accumulate between the pericardial linings or in the sac. This condition is called *pericardial effusion* (see Chap. 30). Fluid in the pericardial sac can constrict the myocardium and interrupt its ability to pump. Cardiac output declines with each contraction. Failure to identify and treat this problem can lead to the development of cardiac tamponade and the possibility of sudden death.

Cardiac Tamponade. The signs and symptoms of cardiac tamponade begin with falling arterial pressure. Usually, the systolic pressure falls while the diastolic pressure remains stable; hence, the pulse pressure narrows. Heart sounds may progress from sounding distant to being imperceptible. Neck vein distention and other signs of rising central venous pressure are observed. These signs and symptoms occur because, as the fluid-filled pericardial sac compresses the myocardium, blood continues to return to the heart from the periphery but cannot flow into the heart to be pumped back into the circulation.

In such situations, the nurse notifies the physician immediately and prepares to assist with pericardiocentesis (see Chap. 30). The nurse stays with the patient and continues to assess and record signs and symptoms while intervening to decrease the patient's anxiety.

Evaluation

EXPECTED PATIENT OUTCOMES

Expected patient outcomes may include:

1. Is free of pain
   a. Performs activities of daily living without pain, fatigue, or shortness of breath
   b. Temperature returns to normal range
   c. Exhibits no pericardial friction rub
2. Absence of complications
   a. Sustains blood pressure in normal range
   b. Has heart sounds that are strong and can be auscultated
   c. Shows absence of neck vein distention

 Critical Thinking Exercises

1. One of your neighbours has been diagnosed with mitral regurgitation and does not understand why antibiotics need to be taken before undergoing any dental work, including routine checkups. How would you explain the rationale for these instructions?

2. Plans for discharge from the hospital are being made for a 26-year-old man with cardiomyopathy. His 24-year-old wife says she is prepared to care for him at home; she expects that he will be unable to participate extensively in his care. Based on your knowledge about developmental tasks of 24- to 26-year-olds, how would you explain the husband's emotional and physical needs to the wife and the ways she can address these needs, as well as her own? The cardiologist has requested a consult with the transplant services; how will your plan of care change?

3. A patient recovering from heart transplantation has a short attention span, has a poor short-term memory, and cannot sleep well. The family reports the patient is speaking more rapidly than usual and is excessively excited and happy. The surgeon states the high doses of steroids are most likely the reason and expects the symptoms to diminish as the steroids are tapered. Another patient who has undergone the same surgical procedure cries frequently and has reported being overwhelmed by the variety and schedule of medications. The family has not been in to visit the patient for 2 days. How would you explain the different reactions, and how would your teaching strategies for these two patients differ?

4. You are caring for a man with pericarditis. His systolic blood pressure begins to fall, and heart sounds cannot be heard. Describe the actions you would take and why.

REFERENCES AND SELECTED READINGS

Books and Pamphlets

American Heart Association. (2001). *Heart and stroke statistical update.* Dallas, TX: American Heart Association.

Beers, M. H., Berkow, R., & Burs, M. (1999). *The Merck manual of diagnosis and therapy* (17th ed.). Whitehouse Station, NJ: Merck & Co.

Bickley, L. S., & Szilagyi, P. G. (2003). *Bates's guide to physical examination and history taking* (8th ed.). Philadelphia: Lippincott Williams & Wilkins.

Braunwald, E., Zipes, D. P., & Libby, P. (Eds.). (2001). *Heart disease: A textbook of cardiovascular medicine* (6th ed.). Philadelphia: W. B. Saunders.

Fuster, V., Alexander, R. W., O'Rourke, R. A., Roberts, R., King, S. B., III, & Wellens, H. J. J. (Eds.). (2001). *Hurst's the heart* (10th ed.). New York: McGraw-Hill.

Hudak, C. M., Gallo, B. M., & Morton, P. G. (1998). *Critical care nursing: A holistic approach* (7th ed.). Philadelphia: Lippincott-Raven.

McHale, D. J., & Carlson, K. K. (2001). *AACN procedure manual for critical care* (4th ed.). Philadelphia: W. B. Saunders.

Schakenbach, L. H. (2001). Care of the patient with a ventricular assist device. In M. Chulay & S. Wingate (Eds.), *Care of the cardiovascular patient series.* Aliso Viejo, CA: American Association of Critical-Care Nurses.

Statistics Canada. (2005). *CANSIM Table 102-0529: Deaths, by cause, Chaper IX: Diseases of the circulatory system (100–199), age group and sex, Canada, annual (Number).* Available at: www.statcan.ca/english/freepub/84-208-X1E/2002/tables/table9.htm. Retrieved January 20, 2006.

Templeton, C. G., Cooper, A. R., Human, D. G., et al. (2005). *Acute rheumatic fever.* Available at: www.cps.ca/english/CPSP/Studies/rheumatic_fever.htm. Retrieved January 20, 2006.

Journals

Asterisks indicate nursing research articles.

Augustine, S. M. (2000). Heart transplantation. *Critical Care Nursing Clinics of North America, 12*(1), 69–77.

Baptiste, M. M. (2001). Aortic valve replacement. *RN, 64*(1), 58–64.

Bayer, A. S., Bolger, A. F., Taubert, K. A., Wilson, W., Stecklberg, J., Karchmer, A. W., et al. (1998). Diagnosis and management of infective endocarditis and its complications. *Circulation, 98*(25), 2936–2948.

Becker, C., & Petlin, A. (1999). Heart transplantation. *American Journal of Nursing, 99* (Suppl. 5), 5–14.

Berul, C., & Zevitz, M. E. (2002). Cardiomyopathy, hypertrophic. *eMedicine Journal, 3*(1). Available at: http://www.emedicine.com/ped/topic1102.htm. Accessed February 26, 2002.

Camp, D. (2000). The left ventricular assist device (LVAD). *Critical Care Nursing Clinics of North America, 12*(1), 61–68.

Canody, C. M., & Savage, L. (1999). The left ventricular assist device. *American Journal of Nursing, 99* (Suppl. 5), 15–20.

Chillcott, S. R., Atkins, P. J., & Adamson, R. M. (1998). Left ventricular assist as a viable alternative for cardiac transplantation. *Critical Care Nurse, 20*(4), 64–79.

Chin, T. K. (2001). Rheumatic heart disease. *eMedicine Journal, 2*(9). Available at: http://www.emedicine.com/ped/topic2007.htm. Accessed February 26, 2002.

Christensen, D. M. (2000). The ventricular assist device: An overview. *Nursing Clinics of North America, 35*(4), 945–959.

Dajani, A. S., Taubert, K. A., Wilson, W., Bolger, A. F., Bayer, A., Ferrieri, P., et al. (1997). Prevention of bacterial endocarditis. *Circulation, 96*(1), 358–366.

Duke, T., & Perna, J. (1999). The ventricular assist device as a bridge to cardiac transplantation. *AACN Clinical Issues, 10*(2), 217–228.

Flynn, M. B., & Bonini, S. (1999). Blunt chest trauma: Case report. *Critical Care Nurse, 19*(5), 68–77.

Fraund, S., Pethig, K., Franke, U., Wahlers, T., Harringer, W., Cremer, J., et al. (1999). Ten year survival after heart transplantation: Palliative procedure or successful long term treatment? *Heart, 82*(1), 47–51.

Freed, L. A., Levy, D., Levine, R. A., Larson, M. G., Evans, J. C., Fuller, D. L., et al. (1999). Prevalence and clinical outcome of mitral-valve prolapse. *New England Journal of Medicine, 34*(1), 1–7.

*Grady, K. L., Jalowiec, A., & White-Williams, C. (1999). Preoperative psychosocial predictors of hospital length of stay after heart transplantation. *Journal of Cardiovascular Nursing, 14*(1), 12–26.

Heijmeriks, J. A., Pourrier, S., Dassen, P., Prenger, K., & Wellens, H. J. J. (1999). Comparison of quality of life after coronary and/or valvular cardiac surgery in patients 75 years of age with younger patients. *American Journal of Cardiology, 83*(7), 1129–1132.

*Kaba, E., Thompson, D. R., & Burnard, P. (2000). Coping after heart transplantation: A descriptive study of heart transplant recipients' methods of coping. *Journal of Advanced Nursing, 32*(4), 930–936.

Kadner, A., Chen, R. H., & Adams, D. H. (2000). Heterotopic heart transplantation: Experiential development and clinical experience. *European Journal of Cardiothoracic Surgery, 7*(4), 474–481.

Kamiya, H., Yasuda, T., Nagamine, H., Sakakibara, N., Nishida, S., Kawasuji, M., et al. (2001). Surgical treatment of primary cardiac tumors: 28 years' experience in Kanazawa University Hospital. *Japan Circulation Journal, 65*(4), 315–319.

McRae, A. I., Chung, M. K., & Asher, C. R. (2001). Arrhythmogenic right ventricular cardiomyopathy: A cause of sudden death in young people. *Cleveland Clinic Journal of Medicine, 68*(5), 459–467.

Morse, C. J. (2001). Advance practice nursing in heart transplantation. *Progress in Cardiovascular Nursing, 16*(1), 21–24, 38.

Nagel, B. M., & O'Keefe, L. M. (1999). Closing in on mitral valve disease. *Nursing, 99* (Critical Care 4), 32cc1–2, 4–7.

Nauer, K. A., Schouchoff, B., & Demitras, K. (2000). Minimally invasive aortic valve surgery. *Critical Care in Nursing Quarterly, 23*(1), 66–71.

Oakley, C. (1997). Aetiology, diagnosis, investigation, and management of the cardiomyopathies. *British Medical Journal, 315*(7121), 1520–1524.

Rabkin, S. W., & Chu-Chun-Lin, S. F. (1988). Epidemiology of valvular heart disease in Canada. *Canadian Journal of Cardiology, 4*(8), 412–416.

Reynan, K. (1996). Frequency of primary tumor of the heart. *American Journal Cardiology, 77*(1), 107.

Richardson, P., McKenna, W., Bristow, M., Maisch, B., Mautner, B., O'Connell, J., et al. (1996). Report of the 1995 World Health Organization/International Society and Federation of Cardiology Task Force on the Definition and Classification of Cardiomyopathies. *Circulation, 93*(5), 841–842.

Rose, E. A., Moskowitz, A. J., Packer, M., Sollano, J. A., Williams, D. L., Tierney, A. R., et al. (1999). The REMATCH trial: Rationale, design, and endpoints. Randomized evaluation of mechanical assistance for the treatment of congestive heart failure. *Annals of Thoracic Surgery, 67*(3), 723–730.

Rosenhek, R., Binder, T., Porenta, G., Lang, I., Christ, G., Schemper, M., et al. (2000). Predictors of outcome in severe, asymptomatic aortic stenosis. *New England Journal of Medicine, 343*(9), 611–617.

Rourke, T. K., Droogan, M. T., & Ohler, L. (1999). Heart transplantation: State of the art. *AACN Clinical Issues, 10*(2), 185–201.

*Savage, L. S., & Canody, C. (1999). Life with a left ventricular assist device: The patient's perspective. *American Journal of Critical Care, 8*(5), 340–343.

Scherr, K., Jensen, L., & Koshal, A. (1999). Mechanical circulatory support as a bridge to cardiac transplantation: Toward the 21st century. *American Journal of Critical Care, 8*(5), 334–339.

Schmid, M. W. (2000). Risks and complications of peripherally and centrally inserted intravenous catheters. *Critical Care Nursing Clinics of North America, 12*(2), 165–174.

*Scordo, K. A. B. (2001). Factors associated with participating in a mitral valve prolapse support group. *Heart & Lung, 30*(2), 128–137.

Shaddy, R. E. (2001). Cardiomyopathy, restrictive. *eMedicine Journal, 2*(12). Accessed February 26, 2002 from http://www.emedicine.com/ped/topic2503.htm.

Shapiro, L. M. (2001). Cardiac tumors: Diagnosis and management. *Heart, 85*(2), 218–222.

Spirito, P., Bellone, P., Harris, K., Bernabo, P., Bruzzi, P., & Maron, B. (2000). Magnitude of left ventricular hypertrophy and risk of sudden death in hypertrophic cardiomyopathy. *New England Journal of Medicine, 42*(24), 1778–1785.

Sutaria, N., Elder, A. T., & Shaw, T. R. D. (2000). Mitral balloon valvotomy for the treatment of mitral stenosis in octogenarians. *Journal of the American Geriatrics Society, 48*(8), 971–974.

Tang, W. H. T., & Young, R. H. (2001). Myocarditis. *eMedicine Journal, 2*(11). Available at: http://www.emedicine.com/med/topic1569.htm. Accessed February 26, 2002.

Thourani, V. H., Feliciano, D. V., Cooper W. A., Brady, K. M., Adams, A. B., Rozycki, G. S., et al. (1999). Penetrating cardiac trauma in an urban trauma center: A 22-year experience. *American Surgeon, 65*(9), 811–818.

Wahi, S., Haluska, B., Pasquet, A., Case, C., Rimmerman, C. M., & Marwick, T. H. (2000). Exercise echocardiography predicts development of left ventricular dysfunction in medically and surgically treated patients with asymptomatic severe aortic regurgitation. *Heart, 84*(6), 606–614.

Wall, M. J., Jr., Mattox, K. C., Chen, C. D., & Baldwin, J. C. (1997). Acute management of complex cardiac injuries. *The Journal of Trauma, 42*(5), 905–912.

RESOURCES AND WEBSITES

Canadian Cardiovascular Society, 222 Queen Street, Suite 1403, Ottawa, ON K1P 5V9; 613-569-3407; toll-free: 877-569-3407; http://www.ccs.ca.

Heart and Stroke Foundation of Canada, 222 Queen Street, Suite 1402, Ottawa, ON K1P 5V9; 613-569-4361; http://ww1.heartandstroke.ca.

National Heart, Lung, and Blood Institute, Health Information Center, National Institutes of Health, P.O. Box 30105, Bethesda, MD 20824; 301-592-8573; http://www.nhlbi.nih.gov.

Management of Patients With Complications From Heart Disease

Adapted by Alexander Clark and Colleen Norris

LEARNING OBJECTIVES

On completion of this chapter, the learner will be able to:

1. Describe the management of patients with chronic heart failure.
2. Use the nursing process as a framework for care of patients with heart failure.
3. Describe the management of patients with acute heart failure.
4. Develop teaching plans for patients with heart failure.
5. Describe the management of patients with cardiogenic shock.
6. Describe the management of patients with thromboembolic episodes, pericardial effusion and cardiac tamponade, and myocardial rupture.
7. Demonstrate the techniques of cardiopulmonary resuscitation.

*T*oday, the patient with heart disease can be assisted to live longer and achieve a higher quality life than even a decade ago. Through advancements in diagnostic procedures that allow earlier and more accurate diagnoses, treatment can begin well before significant debilitation occurs. Newer treatments, technologies, and pharmacotherapies are being developed rapidly. However, heart disease remains a chronic condition, and complications may develop. This chapter presents the complications most often resulting from heart diseases and the treatments provided by the health care team for these complications.

Cardiac Hemodynamics

The basic function of the heart is to pump blood. The heart's ability to pump is measured by **cardiac output (CO)**, the amount of blood pumped in 1 minute. CO is determined by measuring the heart rate (HR) and multiplying it by the **stroke volume (SV)**, which is the amount of blood pumped out of the ventricle with each contraction. CO usually is calculated using the equation $CO = HR \times SV$.

One of the factors controlling HR is the autonomic nervous system. When SV falls, the nervous system is stimulated to increase HR and thereby maintain adequate CO. SV depends on three factors: preload, afterload, and contractility.

Preload is the amount of myocardial stretch just before systole caused by the pressure created by the volume of blood within the ventricle. Like a rubber band, the ventricular muscle fibres need to be stretched (by the blood) to produce optimal ejection of blood. Too little or too much muscle fibre stretch decreases the volume of blood ejected. The major factor that determines preload is venous return, the volume of blood that enters the ventricle during diastole. Another factor that determines preload is ventricular **compliance**, which is the elasticity or amount of "give" when blood enters the ventricle. Elasticity is decreased when the muscle thickens, as in hypertrophic cardiomyopathy (see Chap. 29) or when there is increased fibrotic tissue within the ventricle. Fibrotic tissue replaces dead cells, such as after a myocardial infarction (see Chap. 28). Fibrotic tissue has little compliance, making the ventricle stiff. Given the same volume of blood, a noncompliant ventricle has a higher intraventricular pressure than a compliant one. The higher pressure increases the workload of the heart and can lead to **heart failure (HF)**.

Afterload refers to the amount of resistance to the ejection of blood from the ventricle. To eject blood, the ventricle must overcome this resistance. Afterload is inversely related to SV. The major factors that determine afterload are the diameter and distensibility of the great vessels (aorta and pulmonary artery) and the opening and competence of the semilunar valves (pulmonic and aortic valves). The more open the valves, the lower the resistance. If the patient has significant vasoconstriction, hypertension, or a narrowed opening from a stenotic valve, resistance (afterload) increases. When afterload increases, the workload of the heart must increase to overcome the resistance and eject blood.

Contractility, which refers to the force of contraction, is related to the number and status of myocardial cells. Catecholamines, released by sympathetic stimulation such as exercise or from administration of positive inotropic medications, can increase contractility and stroke volume. MI causes necrosis of some myocardial cells, shifting the workload to the remaining cells. Significant loss of myocardial cells can decrease contractility and cause HF. Afterload must be reduced by stress reduction techniques or medications to match the lower contractility.

Glossary

afterload: the amount of resistance to ejection of blood from a ventricle
anuria: urine output of less than 50 mL per 24 hours
cardiac failure: heart failure
cardiac output (CO): the amount of blood pumped out of the heart in 1 minute
compliance: the elasticity or amount of "give" when blood enters the ventricle
congestive heart failure (CHF): a fluid overload condition (congestion) that may or may not be caused by HF; often an acute presentation of HF with increased amount of fluid in the blood vessels
contractility: the force of ventricular contraction; related to the number and state of myocardial cells
diastolic heart failure: the inability of the heart to pump sufficiently because of an alteration in the ability of the heart to fill; current term used to describe a type of HF
dyspnea on exertion (DOE): shortness of breath that occurs with exertion
ejection fraction (EF): percent of blood volume in the ventricles at the end of diastole that is ejected during systole; a measurement of contractility
heart failure (HF): the inability of the heart to pump sufficient blood to meet the needs

of the tissues for oxygen and nutrients; signs and symptoms of pulmonary and systemic congestion may or may not be present
left-sided heart failure (left ventricular failure): inability of the left ventricle to fill or pump (empty) sufficient blood to meet the needs of the tissues for oxygen and nutrients; traditional term used to describe patient's HF symptoms
oliguria: diminished urine output; less than 400 mL per 24 hours
orthopnea: shortness of breath when lying flat
paroxysmal nocturnal dyspnea (PND): shortness of breath that occurs suddenly during sleep
pericardiocentesis: procedure that involves surgically opening the pericardial sac
pericardiotomy: surgically created opening of the pericardium
preload: the amount of myocardial stretch just before systole caused by the pressure created by the volume of blood within a ventricle
pulmonary edema: abnormal accumulation of fluid occurring in the interstitial spaces or in the alveoli of the lungs
pulseless electrical activity (PEA): condition in which electrical activity is present

but there is not an adequate pulse or blood pressure because of ineffective cardiac contraction or circulating blood volume
pulsus paradoxus: systolic blood pressure that is more than 10 mm Hg higher during exhalation than during inspiration; difference is normally less than 10 mm Hg
right-sided heart failure (right ventricular failure): inability of the right ventricle to fill or pump (empty) sufficient blood to the pulmonary circulation
stroke volume (SV): amount of blood pumped out of the ventricle with each contraction
systolic heart failure: inability of the heart to pump sufficiently because of an alteration in the ability of the heart to contract; current term used to describe a type of HF
thermodilution: method of determining cardiac output that involves injecting fluid into the pulmonary artery catheter. A thermistor measures the difference between the temperature of the fluid and the temperature of the blood ejected from the ventricle. Cardiac output is calculated from the change in temperature.

NONINVASIVE ASSESSMENT OF CARDIAC HEMODYNAMICS

Several noninvasive assessment findings can indicate cardiac hemodynamic status, although the findings do not directly correlate to preload, afterload, or contractility. Right ventricular preload may be estimated by measuring jugular venous distention. Elevated left ventricular preload may be identified by a positive hepatojugular test. Mean arterial blood pressure is a rough indicator of left ventricular afterload. Activity tolerance may be used as an indicator of overall cardiac functioning. These assessments are described in more detail later in the chapter.

Impedance cardiography (ICG) is a noninvasive method for continuous calculation of SV, CO, systemic vascular resistance, ventricular contractility, and fluid status (Turner, 2000). Electrodes are placed on the patient's chest. The electrodes are connected to a device that transmits a very small amount of alternating electric current through the chest and measures the resistance (Z) to the flow (conduction) of the current. Because the current seeks the path of least resistance and fluid is an excellent conductor, the current flows through the blood. ICG measures the volume of blood flow.

The cardiac cycle produces normal changes in blood flow volume; for example, there is more blood flow volume during systole and less blood flow volume during diastole. The changes in blood flow volume change the resistance to flow of the current, which is called electrical impedance (dZ). During systole, the higher blood flow volume causes the red blood cells to be aligned in a more parallel pattern, which makes the flow of current faster and reduces impedance. During diastole, the lower blood flow volume causes the red blood cells to be more randomly arranged, which makes the flow of current slower and increases impedance. Stroke volume is determined by comparing dZ to the changes in time (dt) (Von Rueden & Turner, 1999). The preejection period (PEP) and ventricular ejection times (VET) can be measured, which further assists in understanding the hemodynamic status of the patient. For example, a dysfunctional left ventricle requires more time to generate pressure to overcome the resistance to ejection so that the aortic valve opens (increased PEP) and has less time during which blood is ejected into the aorta (decreased VET).

INVASIVE ASSESSMENT OF CARDIAC HEMODYNAMICS

An important method for evaluating the components of SV in a hemodynamically unstable patient is the pulmonary artery (PA) catheter, which is used to obtain the hemodynamic data essential for diagnosis and treatment (see Chap. 26). Connected to a computerized transducer apparatus, the PA catheter serves as a fluid-filled conduit for detecting pressure changes within the heart. The pulsatile changes in pressure are converted into electrical signals, which are displayed as waveforms on a monitor (Fig. 30-1; Chart 30-1).

CO is measured most often by the **thermodilution** method with the thermistor port of the catheter. The port is connected to a computer that calculates CO and other cardiac parameters. In thermodilution, a specific volume of fluid that is colder than the patient's blood is injected into the proximal port (right atrium). The fluid enters the right ventricle and is then ejected into the PA. The thermistor records the temperature before and after the ejection of fluid. The change in temperature is inversely related to CO; the greater the CO, the faster the blood and fluid moves, the less time the fluid has to mix with the blood to cause a change in temperature, and the less change in temperature detected by the thermistor.

Cardiac parameters for afterload and contractility are calculated at the same time as CO (Table 30-1). Measurements of the various pressures are made at intervals. Therapy, especially intravenous medication, is adjusted based on the assessment and diagnostic findings.

The patient with an invasive hemodynamic catheter is usually managed in an intensive care environment (see Chart 30-1) because of the need for frequent nursing assessments and interventions.

Heart Failure

HF, often referred to as **congestive heart failure (CHF)**, is the inability of the heart to pump sufficient blood to meet the needs of the tissues for oxygen and nutrients. However, the term CHF is misleading, because it indicates that patients must experience pulmonary or peripheral congestion to have HF, and it implies that patients with congestion have HF. The Agency for Health Care Policy and Research (AHCPR) HF guidelines panel (1994) defined HF as a clinical syndrome characterized by signs and symptoms of fluid overload or of inadequate tissue perfusion. These signs and symptoms result when the heart is unable to generate a CO sufficient to meet the body's demands. The HF guideline panel used the term *heart failure* because many patients with HF do not manifest pulmonary or systemic congestion. The term HF is preferred and indicates myocardial heart disease in which there is a problem with contraction of the heart (systolic dysfunction) or filling of the heart (diastolic dysfunction) and which may or may not cause pulmonary or systemic congestion. Some cases of HF are reversible, depending on the cause. Most often, HF is a life-long diagnosis that is managed with lifestyle changes and medications to prevent acute congestive episodes. CHF is usually an acute presentation of HF.

CHRONIC HEART FAILURE

As with coronary heart disease, the incidence of HF increases with age. However, the rate of coronary artery disease is decreasing and just the opposite is true for HF. Between 1% and 2% of all Canadians have HF; this rate is around 6% to 10% in those over 65 years of age (Heart and Stroke Foundation of Canada, 2003). The incidence and prevalence of CHF have increased so markedly that the condition is now considered to constitute an "epidemic" in most of the developed world (British Heart Foundation, 2002; McCullough, Philbin, Spertus, et al., 2002). As cardiovascular risk factors remain prevalent throughout young and middle-aged adults in Canada (Heart and Stroke Foundation of Canada, 2003), the prevalence of CHF is unlikely to decrease in the coming decades. Indeed, the absolute number of hospitalizations related to HF is projected to double in Canada over the next 25 years (Johansen, Strauss, et al., 2003). Rates of HF are higher in rural settings, in part because HF is more prevalent in older adults and the proportion of older adults in rural places is higher. While older adults account for 13% of Canada's population, this age group may represent up to 40% of the population in rural communities (Statistics Canada, 2002). Hospitalizations for HF are frequent, lengthy, and costly (Haldeman, Croft, et al., 1999). There were over 106,000 discharges for HF in Canada during 2000 (Tsuyuki, Shibata, et al., 2003). The total number of hospital days for HF is the second highest for any medical condition. Between 25% and 50% of HF patients in Canada are likely to be rehospitalized for CHF within 1 year of a previous hospitalization (Lee, Johansen, et al., 2004). Mean length of these stays is a costly 13 days (Tsuyuki, Shibata, et al., 2003). Many hospitalizations could be prevented by improved and appropriate outpatient care and home-based management.

FIGURE 30-1 The pulmonary artery (PA) catheter system serves as a fluid-filled conduit for detecting pressure changes within the heart. (**A**) The PA catheter is inserted through a sheath into the superior vena cava, usually via the right internal jugular or subclavian vein. It is connected to pressure tubing (**B**) which is then connected to a transducer (**C**). The transducer detects pulsatile changes in pressure and converts them into electrical signals. These signals are converted into waveforms, which are shown on a monitor (**D**). The transducer also contains a flush device (**E**) that automatically infuses a small amount of flush fluid through the catheter to help maintain its patency. Because of the pressure that the heart generates, pressure is applied to the flush fluid to ensure that the fluid flows into the catheter and into the bloodstream and that blood does not flow back into the catheter. The PA catheter contains several lumens (**F**) with openings located at various intervals. These lumens allow for the measurement of hemodynamic pressures at different points. The proximal port is usually in the right atrium and is used to measure central venous pressure (CVP). The distal tip of the catheter rests in the pulmonary artery and measures the pulmonary artery systolic and diastolic pressures. When the balloon is inflated (**G**), the tip floats into smaller branches of the pulmonary artery until it can no longer pass, that is, until it is "wedged" in the vessel. The distal tip then records the pressure in front of it, called pulmonary artery wedge pressure (PAWP). Cardiac output is measured most often by the thermodilution method with the thermistor port. The port is connected to a computer that calculates cardiac output and other cardiac parameters.

Chart 30-1

GUIDELINES FOR Hemodynamic Monitoring: Multilumen Pulmonary Artery Catheter

ACTIONS	RATIONALE/AMPLIFICATION
Preparatory Phase	
1. Explain the procedure to the patient, family, and significant others.	1. The information may assist in reducing the patient's anxiety, which may also help to limit the patient's movement during the procedure.
2. Check vital signs and apply ECG electrodes.	2. An initial assessment provides a baseline for comparison.
3. Position the patient to allow the physician access to the insertion site, decrease the risk of complications, and promote patient comfort. To ensure consistency, the angle of elevation should be documented if the patient cannot lie flat.	3. The patient is usually placed in a flat or Trendelenburg position to minimize the risk of air embolization and facilitate access.
4. Set up equipment according to manufacturer's directions.	4. Monitoring systems and setups vary according to manufacturer.
a. The pulmonary artery (PA) catheter requires pressure tubing, a transducer, a flush system, and a pressure amplifier connected to a monitoring–recording system. In addition, an IV pole and a transducer holder are usually needed.	a. The complexity of the setup requires an understanding of the equipment in use.
b. The pressure equipment is calibrated and flushed according to the manufacturer's directions.	b. Flushing the catheter system ensures patency and eliminates air bubbles.
c. The balloon is inflated with air to test for leakage.	c. Testing for leakage ensures that the balloon is intact.
5. Prepare the skin over the insertion site.	5. Decreases risk of infection at insertion site
Performance Phase (Physician Responsibility)	
1. The PA catheter is inserted through a sheath that has been placed in the internal jugular, subclavian, or any easily accessible, large-diameter vein by percutaneous puncture or venotomy. The sheath may be surrounded by a protective cover that maintains the sterility of the catheter.	1. The internal jugular vein insertion site has standard landmarks, establishes a straight route into the central venous system, and is associated with few complications. The subclavian insertion site allows the patient more mobility. It is also easier to secure the catheter from this site.
2. The catheter is advanced while observing the monitor for pressure waveforms, which indicate the placement of the tip of the catheter within the heart. Occasionally fluoroscopy is used to verify proper placement of the PA catheter.	2. Catheter placement is determined by characteristic waveforms and changes.
3. When the catheter is in the large vein, the balloon is inflated to its recommended volume.	3. The amount of air to be used is indicated on the catheter.
4. The patient's blood flow will gently pull the inflated balloon at the tip of the catheter through the right atrium and tricuspid valve into the right ventricle and into the main pulmonary artery. The monitoring equipment displays specific pressure waveforms as the catheter advances through the various chambers of the heart. These initial waveforms and pressures are recorded.	4. Watching the ECG monitor for signs of ventricular irritability as the catheter enters the right ventricle allows dysrhythmias to be reported to the physician promptly. Subsequent pressure readings are taken from this baseline.
5. The flowing blood will continue to direct the catheters more distally into the pulmonary arteries. When the catheter reaches a pulmonary vessel that is approximately the same size or slightly smaller in diameter than the inflated balloon, it will not advance any further. This is the wedge position from which pulmonary artery wedge pressure (PAWP) [pulmonary artery obstructive pressure (PAOP) or pulmonary capillary wedge pressure (PCWP)] is measured.	5. With the catheter in the wedge position, the balloon blocks the flow of blood from the right side of the heart toward the lungs. The resulting artery wedge pressure (PAWP) correlates with the mean left ventricular end-diastolic pressure.
6. The pressure is recorded with the balloon wedged in the pulmonary vascular bed. A mean capillary wedge pressure between 8 and 12 mm Hg indicates normal left ventricular function.	6. Wedge pressure is a valuable measure of cardiac function. Lower-than-normal pressure readings indicate hypovolemia. Higher-than-normal pressure readings indicate hypervolemia and/or left ventricular failure.
7. The balloon is then deflated, causing the catheter to retract spontaneously into a larger pulmonary artery. The change in the catheter tip position causes a reappearance of the pulmonary artery waveform. The pulmonary artery systolic, diastolic, and mean pressures are recorded.	7. The normal pulmonary artery systolic pressure is 15 to 30 mm Hg, and the diastolic pressure range is 10 to 15 mm Hg. The normal mean pulmonary artery pressure (average pressure in pulmonary artery throughout the entire cardiac cycle) ranges from 10 to 20 mm Hg. Elevated pulmonary pressures can indicate several clinical problems, such as pulmonary disease, mitral valve disease, and ventricular failure.

(continued)

ACTIONS	RATIONALE/AMPLIFICATION
8. The protective cover is attached to the introducer and secured to the catheter. The catheter is sutured in place and a dry dressing placed over the insertion site.	8. Maintaining catheter sterility in this manner allows for the advancement and repositioning of the catheter if needed. Apply sterile dressing.
9. A chest x-ray to confirm catheter position and to serve as a baseline for future reference is obtained after catheter insertion.	9. Accurate position will assure accurate readings and prevent complications.

To Obtain a Wedge Pressure Reading

1. Inflate the balloon slowly until the pulmonary artery pressure waveform changes (indicating a wedge pressure waveform) and an increase in resistance to injection is detected. Once these changes occur, no more air is introduced. (The amount of air to cause these changes should be less than 1.5 mL.) Most cardiac monitors allow for freezing the wedge pressure waveform and its immediate printing.	1. Do not allow the catheter to remain in the wedge position. The decrease in blood flow through the pulmonary artery that occurs when wedging the catheter may cause segmental pulmonary infarction.
2. As soon as the wedge pressure is obtained, allow passive deflation of the balloon by releasing pressure on the syringe. To make sure that the syringe cannot be inflated accidentally, remove it, push the plunger to the bottom of the barrel so that it is totally empty of air, reattach it to the PA catheter, and lock it closed.	2. These are standard safety measures.

Follow-up Phase

1. Inspect the insertion site daily. Observe for signs of infection, swelling, and bleeding.	1. Careful monitoring helps prevent complications. A foreign body (catheter) in the vascular system increases the risk of sepsis.
2. In accord with protocol, record date and time of dressing change and IV tubing change. If a peripheral vessel access site is used, assess the extremity for colour, temperature, capillary filling, and sensation.	2. Ischemia may occur from inadequate arterial flow.
3. Evaluate pulse.	3. Absence of a pulse may indicate occlusion of the vessel.
4. Assess for complications: pneumothorax, pulmonary ischemia or infarction (due to persistent balloon wedging from inflation or catheter migration), pulmonary artery rupture (due to overinflation of the balloon), dysrhythmias, heart block, damage to tricuspid valve, knotting of catheter within the heart or blood vessels, thromboembolus, infection, balloon rupture, hematoma at insertion site, and bleeding.	4. These are standard nursing practices.

For Removal of the Catheter

1. Explain the procedure to the patient, and make sure the balloon is not inflated.	1. An informed patient is less fearful; a deflated balloon is less likely to injure the patient's heart or blood vessels during catheter removal.
2. Place the patient in a supine position.	2. The supine position results in the least patient movement and is the best position for maintaining blood pressure and venous return.
3. Stop all IVs running through the PA catheter and turn stopcocks off.	3. This prevents fluid from infusing into tissues as the catheter is removed; it also prevents air from entering the catheter.
4. While the patient holds the breath or exhales, the catheter is withdrawn gently and continuously, without excessive force or traction; a sterile dressing is applied over the site.	4. Positive intrathoracic pressure minimizes the chance of air entering the chest and vasculature through or around the catheter. Continuous gentle traction minimizes the risk of the catheter becoming kinked, knotted, or tangled. A sterile dressing minimizes the risk of infection from the skin wound.

Medical management is based on the type, severity, and cause of HF. There are two types of HF, which are identified by assessment of left ventricular functioning: an alteration in ventricular filling (**diastolic heart failure**) and an alteration in ventricular contraction (**systolic heart failure**). An assessment of the **ejection fraction (EF)** is performed to assist in determining the type of HF. EF is the percentage of the end-diastolic blood volume in the ventricle minus the end-systolic blood volume in the ventricle divided by the end-diastolic blood volume in the ventricle—an indication of the amount of blood that was ejected and the contractile ability of the ventricle. The EF is normal in diastolic HF, whereas the EF is less than 40% in systolic HF. The severity of HF is frequently classified according to the patient's symptoms. The New York Heart Association classification is described in Table 30-2, and the causes are explained in subsequent sections of this chapter.

Pathophysiology

HF results from a variety of cardiovascular diseases but leads to some common heart abnormalities that result in decreased contraction (systole), decreased filling (diastole), or both. Significant myocardial dysfunction most often occurs before the patient experiences signs and symptoms of HF.

Systolic HF decreases the amount of blood ejected from the ventricle, which stimulates the sympathetic nervous system to release epinephrine and norepinephrine. The purpose of this initial

Table 30-1 • Hemodynamic Parameters

PARAMETER	RIGHT VENTRICLE	LEFT VENTRICLE
Preload		
Normal Values	CVP: 0–8 mm Hg	PAWP: 4–12 mm Hg
Afterload		
Normal Values	PVR: 20–120 dyne/sec/cm^{-5}	SVR: 800–1500 dyne/sec/cm^{-5}
Calculation	$\dfrac{\text{mean PAP} - \text{PAWP}}{\text{CO}} \times 80$	$\dfrac{\text{Mean arterial pressure} - \text{CVP}}{\text{CO}} \times 80$
Contractility		
Normal Values	Right ventricular stroke work index: 7–12 g/beat/m^2	Left ventricular stroke work index: 35–85 g/beat/m^2
Calculation	$\dfrac{(\text{PA systolic pressure} - \text{CVP}) \times \text{SV} \times 0.0136}{\text{Body Surface Area (height and weight)}}$	$\dfrac{(\text{Systolic BP} - \text{PAWP}) \times \text{SV} \times 0.0136}{\text{Body Surface Area (height and weight)}}$

BP, blood pressure; CO, cardiac output; CVP, central venous pressure; PA, pulmonary artery; PAP, pulmonary artery pressure; PAWP, pulmonary artery wedge pressure; PVR, pulmonary vascular resistance; SV, stroke volume; SVR, systemic vascular resistance.

response is to support the failing myocardium, but the continued response causes loss of beta$_1$-adrenergic receptor sites (downregulation) and further damage to the heart muscle cells. The sympathetic stimulation and the decrease in renal perfusion by the failing heart cause the release of renin by the kidney. Renin promotes the formation of angiotensin I, a benign, inactive substance. Angiotensin-converting enzyme (ACE) in the lumen of blood vessels converts angiotensin I to angiotensin II, a vasoconstrictor that also causes the release of aldosterone. Aldosterone promotes sodium and fluid retention and stimulates the thirst centre. Aldosterone causes additional detrimental effects to the myocardium and exacerbates myocardial fibrosis (Pitt et al., 1999; Weber, 2001). Angiotensin, aldosterone, and other neurohormones (eg, atrial natriuretic factor, endothelin, and prostacyclin) lead to an increase in preload and afterload, which increases stress on the ventricular wall, causing an increase in the workload of the heart.

Table 30-2 • New York Heart Association (NYHA) Classification of Heart Failure

CLASSIFICATION	SYMPTOMS	PROGNOSIS
I	Ordinary physical activity does not cause undue fatigue, dyspnea, palpitations, or chest pain No pulmonary congestion or peripheral hypotension Patient is considered asymptomatic Usually no limitations of activities of daily living (ADLs)	Good
II	Slight limitation on ADLs Patient reports no symptoms at rest but increased physical activity will cause symptoms Basilar crackles and S$_3$ murmur may be detected	Good
III	Marked limitation on ADL Patient feels comfortable at rest but less than ordinary activity will cause symptoms	Fair
IV	Symptoms of cardiac insufficiency at rest	Poor

As the heart's workload increases, contractility of the myofibrils decreases. Decreased contractility results in an increase in end-diastolic blood volume in the ventricle, stretching the myofibres and increasing the size of the ventricle (ventricular dilation). The increased size of the ventricle further increases the stress on the ventricular wall, adding to the workload of the heart. One way the heart compensates for the increased workload is to increase the thickness of the heart muscle (ventricular hypertrophy). However, the hypertrophy is not accompanied by an adequate increase in capillary blood supply, resulting in myocardial ischemia. The sympathetic-induced coronary artery vasoconstriction, increased ventricular wall stress, and decreased mitochondrial energy production also lead to myocardial ischemia. Eventually, the myocardial ischemia causes myofibril death, even in patients without coronary artery disease. The compensatory mechanisms of HF have been called the "vicious cycle of HF" because the heart does not pump sufficient blood to the body, which causes the body to stimulate the heart to work harder; the heart is unable to respond and failure becomes worse.

Diastolic HF develops because of continued increased workload on the heart, which responds by increasing the number and size of myocardial cells (ie, ventricular hypertrophy and altered myocellular functioning). These responses cause resistance to ventricular filling, which increases ventricular filling pressures despite a normal or reduced blood volume. Less blood in the ventricles causes decreased CO. The low CO and high ventricular filling pressures cause the same neurohormonal responses as described for systolic HF.

Etiology

Myocardial dysfunction is most often caused by coronary artery disease, cardiomyopathy, hypertension, or valvular disorders. Atherosclerosis of the coronary arteries is the primary cause of HF. Coronary artery disease is found in more than 60% of the patients with HF (Braunwald et al., 2001). Ischemia causes myocardial dysfunction because of resulting hypoxia and acidosis from the accumulation of lactic acid. Myocardial infarction causes focal heart muscle necrosis, the death of heart muscle cells, and a loss of contractility; the extent of the infarction correlates with the severity of HF. Revascularization of the coronary artery by a percutaneous coronary intervention or by coronary artery bypass surgery may correct the underlying cause so that HF is resolved.

Cardiomyopathy is a disease of the myocardium. There are three types: dilated, hypertrophic, and restrictive (see Chap. 29). Dilated cardiomyopathy, the most common type of cardio-myopathy, causes diffuse cellular necrosis, leading to decreased contractility (systolic failure). Dilated cardiomyopathy can be id-iopathic (unknown cause), or it can result from an inflammatory process, such as myocarditis, from pregnancy, or from a cytotoxic agent, such as alcohol or adriamycin. Hypertrophic cardiomy-opathy and restrictive cardiomyopathy lead to decreased disten-sibility and ventricular filling (diastolic failure). Usually, HF due to cardiomyopathy becomes chronic. However, cardiomyopathy and HF may resolve after the end of pregnancy or with the ces-sation of alcohol ingestion.

Systemic or pulmonary hypertension increases afterload (resis-tance to ejection), which increases the workload of the heart and leads to hypertrophy of myocardial muscle fibres; this can be con-sidered a compensatory mechanism because it increases contrac-tility. However, the hypertrophy may impair the heart's ability to fill properly during diastole.

Valvular heart disease is also a cause of HF. The valves ensure that blood flows in one direction. With valvular dysfunction, blood has increasing difficulty moving forward, increasing pres-sure within the heart and increasing cardiac workload, leading to diastolic HF. Chapter 29 discusses the effects of valvular heart disease.

Several systemic conditions contribute to the development and severity of HF, including increased metabolic rate (eg, fever, thyrotoxicosis), iron overload (eg, from hemochromatosis), hypoxia, and anemia (serum hematocrit less than 25%). All of these conditions require an increase in CO to satisfy the sys-temic oxygen demand. Hypoxia or anemia also may decrease the supply of oxygen to the myocardium. Cardiac dysrhythmias may cause HF, or they may be a result of HF; either way, the altered electrical stimulation impairs the myocardial contraction and de-creases the overall efficiency of myocardial function. Other factors, such as acidosis (respiratory or metabolic), electrolyte abnor-malities, and antiarrhythmic medications, can worsen the myo-cardial dysfunction.

Clinical Manifestations

The clinical manifestations produced by the different types of HF (systolic, diastolic, or both) are similar (Chart 30-2) and there-fore do not assist in differentiating the types of HF. The signs and symptoms of HF are most often described in terms of the effect on the ventricles. **Left-sided heart failure (left ventricular fail-ure)** causes different manifestations than **right-sided heart fail-ure (right ventricular failure)**. Chronic HF produces signs and symptoms of failure of both ventricles. Although dysrhythmias (especially tachycardias, ventricular ectopic beats, or atrioven-tricular [AV] and ventricular conduction defects) are common in HF, they may also be a result of treatments used in HF (eg, side effect of digitalis).

LEFT-SIDED HEART FAILURE

Pulmonary congestion occurs when the left ventricle cannot pump the blood out of the ventricle to the body. The increased left ven-tricular end-diastolic blood volume increases the left ventricular end-diastolic pressure, which decreases blood flow from the left atrium into the left ventricle during diastole. The blood volume and pressure in the left atrium increases, which decreases blood flow from the pulmonary vessels. Pulmonary venous blood vol-ume and pressure rise, forcing fluid from the pulmonary capillar-

Chart 30-2 • ASSESSMENT

Signs and Symptoms of Heart Failure

General
Pale, cyanotic skin (with decreased perfusion to extremities)
Dependent edema (with increased venous pressure)
Decreased activity tolerance

Cardiovascular
Apical impulse, enlarged and left lateral displacement (with cardiac enlargement)
Third heart sound (S_3)
Murmurs (with valvular dysfunction)
Tachycardia
Increased jugular venous distention (JVD)

Cerebrovascular
Lightheadness
Dizziness
Confusion

Gastrointestinal
Nausea and anorexia
Enlarged, pulsatile liver
Ascites
Hepatojugular test, increased (with increased right ventricular filling pressure)

Renal
Decreased urinary frequency during the day
Nocturia

Respiratory
Dyspnea on exertion
Orthopnea
Paroxysmal nocturnal dyspnea
Bilateral crackles that do not clear with cough

ies into the pulmonary tissues and alveoli, which impairs gas ex-change. These effects of left ventricular failure have been referred to as *backward failure*. The clinical manifestations of pulmonary venous congestion include dyspnea, cough, pulmonary crackles, and lower-than-normal oxygen saturation levels. An extra heart sound, S_3, may be detected on auscultation.

Dyspnea, or shortness of breath, may be precipitated by mini-mal to moderate activity (**dyspnea on exertion [DOE]**); dyspnea also can occur at rest. The patient may report **orthopnea**, difficulty in breathing when lying flat. Patients with orthopnea usually pre-fer not to lie flat. They may need pillows to prop themselves up in bed, or they may sit in a chair and even sleep sitting up. Some pa-tients have sudden attacks of orthopnea at night, a condition known as **paroxysmal nocturnal dyspnea (PND)**. Fluid that ac-cumulated in the dependent extremities during the day begins to be reabsorbed into the circulating blood volume when the person lies down. Because the impaired left ventricle cannot eject the in-creased circulating blood volume, the pressure in the pulmonary circulation increases, causing further shifting of fluid into the alve-oli. The fluid filled alveoli cannot exchange oxygen and carbon dioxide. Without sufficient oxygen, the patient experiences dys-pnea and has difficulty getting an adequate amount of sleep.

The cough associated with left ventricular failure is initially dry and nonproductive. Most often, patients complain of a dry hacking cough that may be mislabelled as asthma or chronic ob-structive pulmonary disease (COPD). The cough may become moist. Large quantities of frothy sputum, which is sometimes pink (blood tinged), may be produced, usually indicating severe pulmonary congestion (pulmonary edema).

Adventitious breath sounds may be heard in various lobes of the lungs. Usually, bi-basilar crackles that do not clear with coughing are detected in the early phase of left ventricular failure. As the failure worsens and pulmonary congestion increases, crackles may be auscultated throughout all lung fields. At this point, a decrease in oxygen saturation may occur.

In addition to increased pulmonary pressures that cause decreased oxygenation, the amount of blood ejected from the left ventricle may decrease, sometimes called *forward failure.* The dominant feature in HF is inadequate tissue perfusion. The diminished CO has widespread manifestations because not enough blood reaches all the tissues and organs (low perfusion) to provide the necessary oxygen. The decrease in SV can also lead to stimulation of the sympathetic nervous system, which further impedes perfusion to many organs.

Blood flow to the kidneys decreases, causing decreased perfusion and reduced urine output (**oliguria**). Renal perfusion pressure falls, which results in the release of renin from the kidney. Release of renin leads to aldosterone secretion. Aldosterone secretion causes sodium and fluid retention, which further increases intravascular volume. However, when the patient is sleeping, the cardiac workload is decreased, improving renal perfusion, which then leads to frequent urination at night (nocturia).

Decreased CO causes other symptoms. Decreased gastrointestinal perfusion causes altered digestion. Decreased brain perfusion causes dizziness, lightheadedness, confusion, restlessness, and anxiety due to decreased oxygenation and blood flow. As anxiety increases, so does dyspnea, enhancing anxiety and creating a vicious cycle. Stimulation of the sympathetic system also causes the peripheral blood vessels to constrict, so the skin appears pale or ashen and feels cool and clammy.

The decrease in the ejected ventricular volume causes the sympathetic nervous system to increase the heart rate (tachycardia), often causing the patient to complain of palpitations. The pulses become weak and thready. Without adequate CO, the body cannot respond to increased energy demands, and the patient is easily fatigued and has decreased activity tolerance. Fatigue also results from the increased energy expended in breathing and the insomnia that results from respiratory distress, coughing, and nocturia.

RIGHT-SIDED HEART FAILURE

When the right ventricle fails, congestion of the viscera and the peripheral tissues predominates. This occurs because the right side of the heart cannot eject blood and cannot accommodate all the blood that normally returns to it from the venous circulation. The increase in venous pressure leads to jugular vein distention (JVD).

The clinical manifestations that ensue include edema of the lower extremities (dependent edema), hepatomegaly (enlargement of the liver), distended jugular veins, ascites (accumulation of fluid in the peritoneal cavity), weakness, anorexia and nausea, and paradoxically, weight gain due to retention of fluid.

Edema usually affects the feet and ankles, worsening when the patient stands or dangles the legs. The swelling decreases when the patient elevates the legs. The edema can gradually progress up the legs and thighs and eventually into the external genitalia and lower trunk. Edema in the abdomen, as evidenced by increased abdominal girth, may be the only edema present. Sacral edema is not uncommon for patients who are on bed rest, because the sacral area is dependent. Pitting edema, in which

indentations in the skin remain after even slight compression with the fingertips (Fig. 30-2), is obvious only after retention of at least 4.5 kg (10 lb) of fluid (4.5 litres).

Hepatomegaly and tenderness in the right upper quadrant of the abdomen result from venous engorgement of the liver. The increased pressure may interfere with the liver's ability to perform (secondary liver dysfunction). As hepatic dysfunction progresses, pressure within the portal vessels may rise enough to force fluid into the abdominal cavity, a condition known as ascites. This collection of fluid in the abdominal cavity may increase pressure on the stomach and intestines and cause gastrointestinal distress. Hepatomegaly may also increase pressure on the diaphragm, causing respiratory distress.

Anorexia (loss of appetite) and nausea or abdominal pain results from the venous engorgement and venous stasis within the abdominal organs. The weakness that accompanies right-sided HF results from reduced CO, impaired circulation, and inadequate removal of catabolic waste products from the tissues.

Assessment and Diagnostic Findings

HF may go undetected until the patient presents with signs and symptoms of pulmonary and peripheral edema (congestion), which can lead the physician to make a preliminary diagnosis of CHF. However, the physical signs that suggest HF may also occur with other diseases, such as renal failure, liver failure, oncologic conditions, and COPD. If further assessment and evaluation are

FIGURE 30-2 Example of pitting edema. (**A**) The nurse applies finger pressure to an area near the ankle. (**B**) When the pressure is released, an indentation remains in the edematous tissue. Photographs © B. Proud.

not completed, these patients may be treated for HF inappropriately. The term *congestive heart failure* (CHF) means the patient has a fluid overload condition (congestion) that may or may not be caused by HF. CHF is caused by HF when ventricular dysfunction (systolic, diastolic, or both) has been identified. Assessment of ventricular function is an essential part of the initial diagnostic workup.

An echocardiogram is usually performed to confirm the diagnosis of HF, assist in the identification of the underlying cause, and determine the patient's ejection fraction, which assists in identification of the type and severity of HF. This information may also be obtained noninvasively by radionuclide ventriculography or invasively by ventriculogram as part of a cardiac catheterization procedure. A chest x-ray and an electrocardiogram (ECG) are obtained to assist in the diagnosis and to determine the underlying cause of HF. Laboratory studies usually completed in the initial workup include serum electrolytes, blood urea nitrogen (BUN), creatinine, B-type natriuretic peptide (BNP), thyroid-stimulating hormone (TSH), a complete blood cell count (CBC), and routine urinalysis. The results of these laboratory studies assist in determining the underlying cause and in establishing a baseline from which to measure effects of treatment. Exercise testing or cardiac catheterization may be performed to determine whether coronary artery disease and cardiac ischemia are causing the HF.

Ventricular function should be determined before discharge from a hospital of patients with acute myocardial infarction (MI) who are at risk for the development of HF. Patients who are at low risk for HF are those who meet all of the following criteria: no previous myocardial infarction, inferior myocardial infarction, small (less than two to four times normal) increase in cardiac enzymes, no Q waves on the ECG, and an uncomplicated clinical course (AHCPR, 1994). Evaluation of ventricular function may also be performed for patients whose initial assessment of HF suggested noncardiac causes but who failed to respond to treatment.

Medical Management

A critical step in the management of HF is early identification and documentation of the type of HF. Medical management, especially the pharmacologic therapy, varies with the type of HF. The basic objectives in treating patients with HF are the following:

- Eliminate or reduce any etiologic contributory factors, especially those that may be reversible, such as atrial fibrillation or excessive alcohol ingestion.
- Reduce the workload on the heart by reducing afterload and preload.

Managing the patient with HF includes providing general counselling and education about sodium restriction, monitoring daily weights and other signs of fluid retention, encouraging regular exercise, and recommending avoidance of excessive fluid intake, alcohol, and smoking. Medications are prescribed based on the patient's type and severity of HF. Oxygen therapy is based on the degree of pulmonary congestion and resulting hypoxia. Some patients may need supplemental oxygen therapy only during activity. Others may require hospitalization and endotracheal intubation. If the patient has underlying coronary artery disease, coronary artery revascularization with percutaneous transluminal coronary angioplasty (PTCA) or bypass surgery (see Chap. 28) may be considered. If the patient's condition is unresponsive to advanced aggressive medical therapy, innovative therapies, including mechanical assist devices and transplantation, may be considered.

Cardiac resynchronization, involving the use of left ventricular and biventricular pacing, is a treatment for HF with electrical conduction defects. Left bundle branch block (LBBB) is frequently found in patients with systolic dysfunction. LBBB occurs when the electrical impulse, which normally depolarizes the right and left bundle branches at the same time, depolarizes the right bundle branch but not the left bundle branch. The dyssynchronous electrical stimulation of the ventricles causes the right ventricle to contract before the left ventricle, which can lead to further decreased ejection fraction (Gerber et al., 2001). Use of a pacing device (eg, Medtronic InSync), with leads placed on the inner wall of the right atrium and right ventricle and on the outer wall of the left ventricle, provides synchronized electrical stimulation to the heart. In one study, 63% of the patients who had received these devices showed improvement in clinical status, including NYHA functional class and global assessment, compared with 38% of placebo patients (Abraham, 2002).

PHARMACOLOGIC THERAPY

Several medications are indicated for systolic HF. Medications for diastolic failure depend on the underlying condition, such as hypertension (see Chap. 32) or valvular dysfunction (see Chap. 29). If the patient is in mild systolic failure, an ACE inhibitor usually is prescribed. If the patient is unable to continue an ACE inhibitor (eg, because of development of renal impairment as evidenced by elevated serum creatinine or persistent serum potassium levels of 5.5 mEq/L or above), an angiotensin II receptor blocker (ARB) or hydralazine and isosorbide dinitrate are considered as part of the treatment plan. A diuretic is added if signs of fluid overload develop. Digitalis is added to ACE inhibitors if the symptoms continue. Although previously contraindicated in HF, specific beta-blockers decrease mortality and morbidity if added to the initial medications. Spironolactone, a weak diuretic, may also be added for persistent symptoms.

Angiotensin-Converting Enzyme Inhibitors. ACE inhibitors (ACE-Is) have a pivotal role in the management of HF due to systolic dysfunction. They have been found to relieve the signs and symptoms of HF and significantly decrease mortality and morbidity (when used to treat a symptomatic patient) by inhibiting neurohormonal activation (CONSENSUS Trial Study Group, 1987; SOLVD Investigators, 1992). Available as oral and intravenous medications, ACE-Is promote vasodilation and diuresis by decreasing afterload and preload. By doing so, they decrease the workload of the heart. Vasodilation reduces resistance to left ventricular ejection of blood, diminishing the heart's workload and improving ventricular emptying. In promoting diuresis, ACE-Is decrease the secretion of aldosterone, a hormone that causes the kidneys to retain sodium. ACE-Is stimulate the kidneys to excrete sodium and fluid (while retaining potassium), thereby reducing left ventricular filling pressure and decreasing pulmonary congestion. ACE-Is may be the first medication prescribed for patients in mild failure—patients with fatigue or dyspnea on exertion but without signs of fluid overload and pulmonary congestion.

Results from studies (Clement et al., 2000; NETWORK Investigators, 1998) to identify the specific dose to achieve this effect are equivocal, although one large study showed significant reductions in death and hospitalization with higher doses (Packer et al., 1999). However, it is recommended to start at a low dose and increase every 2 weeks until the optimal dose is achieved and the patient is hemodynamically stable. The final maintenance dose depends on the patient's blood pressure, fluid status, renal status, and degree of **cardiac failure**.

Patients receiving ACE-I therapy are monitored for hypotension, hypovolemia, hyponatremia, and alterations in renal function, especially if they are also receiving diuretics. When to observe for these effects and for how long depends on the onset, peak, and duration of the medication. Table 30-3 identifies several types of ACE-Is and their pharmacokinetics. Hypotension is most likely to develop from ACE-I therapy in patients older than age 75 and in those with a systolic blood pressure of 100 mm Hg or less, a serum sodium level of less than 135 mEq/L, or severe cardiac failure. Adjusting the dose or type of diuretic in response to the patient's blood pressure and renal function may allow for continued increases in the dosage of ACE-Is.

Because ACE-Is cause the kidneys to retain potassium, the patient who is also receiving a diuretic may not need to take oral potassium supplements. However, patients receiving potassium-sparing diuretics (which do not cause potassium loss with diuresis) must be carefully monitored for hyperkalemia, an increased level of potassium in the blood. Before the initiation of the ACE-I, hyperkalemic and hypovolemic states must be corrected. ACE-Is may be discontinued if the potassium remains above 5.0 mEq/L or if the serum creatinine is 3.0 mg/dL and continues to increase. Other side effects of ACE-Is include a dry, persistent cough that may not respond to cough suppressants. However, the cough could also indicate a worsening of ventricular function and failure. Rarely, the cough indicates angioedema. If angioedema affects the oropharyngeal area and impairs breathing, the ACE-I must be stopped immediately.

Angiotensin II Receptor Blockers (ARBs).

Although their action is different than that of ACE-Is, ARBs (eg, losartan [Cozaar]) have a similar hemodynamic effect as ACE-Is: lowered blood pressure and lowered systemic vascular resistance. Whereas ACE-Is block the conversion of angiotensin I to angiotensin II, ARBs block the effects of angiotensin II at the angiotensin II receptor. ACE-Is and ARBs also have similar side effects: hyperkalemia, hypotension, and renal dysfunction. ARBs are usually prescribed when patients are not able to tolerate ACE-Is.

Hydralazine and Isosorbide Dinitrate.

A combination of hydralazine (Apresoline) and isosorbide dinitrate (Apo-ISDN, Cedocard-SR, Coronex, NOVO-Sorbide, PMS-Isosorbide) may be another alternative for patients who cannot take ACE-Is. Nitrates (eg, iso-

sorbide dinitrate) cause venous dilation, which reduces the amount of blood return to the heart and lowers preload. Hydralazine lowers systemic vascular resistance and left ventricular afterload. It has also been shown to help avoid the development of nitrate tolerance. As with ARBs, this combination of medications is usually used when patients are not able to tolerate ACE-Is.

Beta-Blockers.

When used with ACE-Is, beta-blockers, such as carvedilol (Coreg), metoprolol (Lopressor, Toprol), or bisoprolol (Zebeta), have been found to reduce mortality and morbidity in NYHA class II or III HF patients by reducing the cytotoxic effects from the constant stimulation of the sympathetic nervous system (Beta-Blocker Evaluation of Survival Trial [BEST] Investigators, 2001; CIBIS-II Investigators and Committees, 1999; MERIT, 1999; Packer et al., 1996; Packer et al., 2001). These agents have also been recommended for patients with asymptomatic systolic dysfunction, such as after acute myocardial infarction or revascularization to prevent the onset of symptoms of HF. However, beta-blockers may also produce many side effects, including exacerbation of HF. The side effects are most common in the initial few weeks of treatment. The most frequent side effects are dizziness, hypotension, and bradycardia. To minimize these side effects, staggering the administration of the beta-blocker with the ACE-I is recommended. Because of the side effects, beta-blockers are initiated only after stabilizing the patient and ensuring a euvolemic (normal volume) state. They are titrated slowly (every 2 weeks), with close monitoring at each increase in dose. If the patient develops symptoms during the titration phase, treatment options include increasing the diuretic, reducing the dose of ACE-I, or decreasing the dose of the beta-blocker.

An important nursing role during titration is educating the patient about the potential worsening of symptoms during the early phase of treatment, and that improvement may take several weeks. It is very important that nurses provide support to patients going through this symptom-provoking phase of treatment. Because beta-blockade can cause bronchiole constriction, a beta$_1$-selective beta-blocker (ie, one that primarily blocks the beta-adrenergic receptor sites in the heart), such as metoprolol (Lopressor, Toprol), is recommended for patients with well-controlled, mild to moderate asthma. However, these patients need to be monitored closely for increased asthma symptoms. Any type of beta-blocker is contraindicated in patients with severe or uncontrolled asthma.

Table 30-3 • Angiotensin-Converting Enzyme (ACE) Inhibitors

ACE INHIBITOR	PHARMACOKINETICS			NURSING CONSIDERATIONS
	Onset	Peak (hr)	Duration (hr)	
benazepril (Lotensin)	within 1 hr	2–4	24	Monitor blood pressure, urine output, and electrolyte levels.
captopril (Capoten)	15–60 min	1–1.5	6–12*	Monitor serum creatinine and urine creatinine clearance.
enalapril (Vasotec)	1 hr	4–6	24	Monitor for development of cough that is resistant to cough
enalaprilat (Vasotec I.V.)	15 min	1–4	6	suppressants.
fosinopril (Monopril)	within 1 hr	2–6	24	Teach patient to change positions gradually and to report
lisinopril (Prinival, Zestril)	1 hr	6	24	signs of dizziness or lethargy.
quinapril (Accupril)	within 1 hr	2–4	up to 24*	
ramipril (Altace)	1–2 hr	4–6	24	
trandolapril (Mavik)	within 30 min	2–4	> 8 days	

*Duration of effect is related to the dose.

Diuretics. Diuretics are medications used to increase the rate of urine production and the removal of excess extracellular fluid from the body. Of the types of diuretics prescribed for patients with edema from HF, three are most common: thiazide, loop, and potassium-sparing diuretics. These medications are classified according to their site of action in the kidney and their effects on renal electrolyte excretion and reabsorption. Thiazide diuretics, such as metolazone (Mykrox, Zaroxolyn), inhibit sodium and chloride reabsorption mainly in the early distal tubules. They also increase potassium and bicarbonate excretion. Loop diuretics, such as furosemide (Lasix), inhibit sodium and chloride reabsorption mainly in the ascending loop of Henle. Patients with signs and symptoms of fluid overload should be started on a diuretic, a thiazide for those with mild symptoms or a loop diuretic for patients with more severe symptoms or with renal insufficiency (Brater, 1998). Both types of diuretics may be used for those in severe HF and unresponsive to a single diuretic. These medications may not be necessary if the patient responds to activity recommendations, avoidance of excessive fluid intake (<2 quarts/day), and a low-sodium diet (eg, <2 g/day).

Spironolactone (Aldactone) is a potassium-sparing diuretic that inhibits sodium reabsorption in the late distal tubule and collecting duct. It has been found to be effective in reducing mortality and morbidity in NYHA class III and IV HF patients when added to ACE-Is, loop diuretics, and digoxin. Serum creatinine and potassium levels are monitored frequently (eg, within the first week and then every 4 weeks) when this medication is first administered.

Side effects of diuretics include electrolyte imbalances, symptomatic hypotension (especially with overdiuresis), hyperuricemia (causing gout), and ototoxicity. Dosages depend on the indications, patient age, clinical signs and symptoms, and renal function. Table 30-4 lists commonly used diuretics, dosages, and pharmacokinetic properties. Careful patient monitoring and dose adjustments are necessary to balance the effectiveness with the side effects of therapy. Diuretics greatly improve the patient's symptoms, but they do not prolong life.

Table 30-4 • Diuretic Medications Used to Treat Heart Failure

DIURETIC	USUAL ADULT DOSE	ONSET (HR)	PEAK (HR)	DURATION (HR)
Thiazide Diuretics				
bendroflumethiazide (Naturetin)	2.5–20 mg in single or divided dose, once a day, once every other day, or once a day for 3–5 days per week	2	4	12–16
benzthiazide (Exna)	12.5–200 mg in single or divided dose	2	4–6	16–18
chlorothiazide (Diuril)	Oral: 0.25–2 g as single or divided dose; may be given on alternate days	2	4	16–18
	IV: 0.5–1 g in single or divided dose (note: avoid extravasation)	15 min	30 min	
chlorthalidone (Hygroton)	12.5–200 mg once a day, once every other day, or once a day for 3 days per week	2	2–6	24–72
hydrochlorothiazide (HydroDIURIL, Apo-Hydro, Diuchlor H)	12.5–200 mg as single or divided dose once a day, once every other day, or once a day for 3–5 days per week	2	4–6	12–16
hydroflumethiazide (Diucardin, Saluron)	25–200 mg as single or divided dose once a day, once every other day, or once a day for 3–5 days per week	2	4	12–16
methyclothiazide (Enduron)	2.5–10 mg once a day	2	6	24
metolazone (Zaroxolyn, Mykrox)	Zaroxolyn: 2.5–20 mg once a day Mykrox: 0.5–1 mg once a day	1	2	12–24
trichlormethiazide (Metahydrin, Naqua)	1–4 mg once or twice a day	2	6	24
Loop Diuretics				
bumetanide (Bumex)	0.5–2 mg once, twice or three times a day; may be given on alternate days or once every 3 days	30–60 min	1–2	4–6
	0.5–1 mg over 2 min; repeat every 2–3 h; a continuous infusion may be given at a rate of 1 mg/h.	5–10 min	15–30 min	½–1
ethacrynic acid (Edecrin)	50–400 mg as single or divided dose	<30 min	2	6–8
	0.5–1 mg/kg (max 100 mg) over several min; may be repeated within 2–6 h; repeat every hour in emergencies	<5 min	15–30 min	2
furosemide (Lasix)	20–600 mg as single daily dose, divided daily dose, as a dose given every other day or given once a day for 2–4 days per week	<1	1–2	6–8
	20–200 mg (max 6 mg/kg) given at a rate of 4 mg/min; after response obtained, given once or twice a day	<5 min	30 min	2
Potassium-Sparing Diuretics				
amiloride (Midamor)	5–20 mg daily as single dose	2	6–10	24
spironolactone (Aldactone)	25–400 mg as single dose or divided up to 4 doses	24–48	48–72	48–72
triamterene (Dyrenium)	50–300 mg as single dose	2–4	6–8	12–16

Digitalis. The most commonly prescribed form of digitalis for patients with HF is digoxin (Lanoxin). The medication increases the force of myocardial contraction and slows conduction through the AV node. It improves contractility, increasing left ventricular output. The medication also enhances diuresis, which removes fluid and relieves edema. The effect of a given dose of medication depends on the state of the myocardium, electrolyte and fluid balance, and renal and hepatic function. Although digitalis does not decrease the mortality rate, it is effective in decreasing the symptoms of systolic HF and in increasing the patient's ability to perform activities of daily living (Digitalis Investigation Group, 1997). It also has been shown to significantly decrease hospitalization rates and emergency room visits for NYHA class II and III HF patients (Uretsky et al., 1993).

A key concern associated with digitalis therapy is digitalis toxicity. Chart 30-3 summarizes the actions and uses of digitalis along with the nursing surveillance required when it is administered. The patient is observed for the effectiveness of digitalis therapy: lessening dyspnea and orthopnea, decrease in pulmonary crackles on auscultation, relief of peripheral edema, weight

---

Chart 30-3 • PHARMACOLOGY
Digoxin Use and Toxicity in Heart Failure

Digoxin, a cardiac glycoside derived from digitalis, is used for patients with systolic HF, atrial fibrillation, and atrial flutter. Digoxin improves cardiac function as follows:
- Increases the force of myocardial contraction
- Slows cardiac conduction through the AV node and therefore slows the ventricular rate in instances of supraventricular dysrhythmias
- Increases cardiac output by enhancing the force of ventricular contraction
- Promotes diuresis by increasing cardiac output

The therapeutic level is usually 0.5 to 2.0 ng/mL. Blood samples are usually obtained and analyzed to determine digitalis concentration at least 6 to 10 hours after the last dose. Toxicity may occur despite normal serum levels, and recommended dosages vary considerably.

Preparations
Digoxin
- Tablets: 0.125, 0.25, 0.5 mg (Lanoxin)
- Capsules: 0.05, 0.1, 0.2 mg (Lanoxicaps)
- Elixir: 0.05 mg/mL (Lanoxin Pediatric elixir)
- Injection: 0.25 mg/mL, 0.1 mg/mL (Lanoxin)

Digoxin Toxicity
A serious complication of digoxin therapy is toxicity. The incidence is high, and toxicity may occur even though the serum digoxin level remains within a normal range. Diagnosis of digoxin toxicity is based on the patient's clinical symptoms, which include the following:
- Fatigue, depression, malaise, anorexia, nausea, and vomiting (early effects of digitalis toxicity)
- Changes in heart rhythm: new onset of regular rhythm or new onset of irregular rhythm
- ECG changes indicating SA or AV block; new onset of irregular rhythm indicating ventricular dysrhythmias; and atrial tachycardia with block, junctional tachycardia, and ventricular tachycardia

Reversal of Toxicity
Digoxin toxicity is treated by holding the medication while monitoring the patient's symptoms and serum digoxin level. If the toxicity is severe, digoxin immune FAB (Digibind) may be prescribed. Digibind binds with digoxin and makes it unavailable for use. The Digibind dosage is based on the digoxin level and the patient's weight. Serum digoxin values are not accurate for several days after administration of Digibind because they do not differentiate between bound and unbound digoxin. Because Digibind quickly decreases the amount of available digoxin, an increase in ventricular rate due to atrial fibrillation and worsening of symptoms of HF may ensue shortly after its administration.

Nursing Considerations and Actions
1. Assess the patient's clinical response to digoxin therapy by evaluating relief of symptoms such as dyspnea, orthopnea, crackles, hepatomegaly, and peripheral edema.
2. Monitor serum potassium levels in patients receiving digoxin, especially those receiving both digoxin and diuretics. *An undetected, uncorrected potassium imbalance predisposes patients to digoxin toxicity and dysrhythmias.*
3. Assess for symptoms of electrolyte depletion: lassitude, apathy, mental confusion, anorexia, decreasing urinary output, azotemia.
4. Monitor the patient for factors that increase the risk of toxicity:
   - Oral antibiotics, quinidine, amiodarone, calcium channel blocker therapy (See Table 27-1).
   - Decreased potassium level (hypokalemia), which increases the action of digoxin and which may be caused by malnutrition, diarrhea, vomiting, or prolonged muscle wasting
   - Impaired renal function, particularly in patients age 65 and older with decreased renal clearance
5. Before administering digoxin, it is standard nursing practice to assess apical heart rate. When the patient's rhythm is atrial fibrillation and the heart rate is less than 60, or the rhythm becomes regular, the nurse may withhold the medication and notify the physician, because these signs indicate the development of AV conduction block. Although withholding digoxin is a common practice, the medication does not need to be withheld for a heart rate of less than 60 if the patient is in sinus rhythm because digoxin does not affect sinoatrial node automaticity. Measuring the PR interval for a patient with cardiac monitoring is more important than the apical pulse in determining whether digoxin should be held.
   Note: If monitoring discloses that the patient is in sinus rhythm, the nurse monitors the patient's PR interval instead of the patient's heart rate. If the patient is in atrial fibrillation, the nurse monitors for the development of regular R-R intervals, indicating AV block.
6. Monitor for gastrointestinal side effects: anorexia, nausea, vomiting, abdominal pain and distention.
7. Monitor for neurologic side effects: headache, malaise, nightmares, forgetfulness, social withdrawal, depression, agitation, confusion, paranoia, hallucinations, decreased visual acuity, yellow or green halo around objects (especially lights), or "snowy" vision.
8. Observe for and anticipate potential drug interactions when other medications are added to the patient's regimen. This is an important step in preventing toxicity. For example, antiarrhythmic and antibiotic medications may increase the amount of digoxin available to the patient. Diuretics may decrease the amount of potassium and increase the availability of digoxin. In addition, because digoxin is eliminated by the kidneys, renal function (serum creatinine and urine creatinine clearance) are monitored carefully.

loss, and increase in activity tolerance. The serum potassium level is measured at intervals because diuresis may have caused hypokalemia. The effect of digitalis is enhanced in the presence of hypokalemia, so digitalis toxicity may occur. Serum digoxin levels are obtained once each year or more frequently if there have been changes in the patient's medications, renal function, or symptoms.

Calcium Channel Blockers. First-generation calcium channel blockers, such as verapamil (Calan, Isoptin, Verelan), nifedipine (Adalat, Procardia), and diltiazem (Cardizem, Apo-Dilitiaz, Tiazac), are contraindicated in patients with systolic dysfunction, although they may be used in patients with diastolic dysfunction. Amlodipine (Norvasc) and felodipine (Plendil), dihydropyridine calcium channel blockers, cause vasodilation, reducing systemic vascular resistance. They may be used to improve symptoms especially in patients with nonischemic cardiomyopathy, although they have no effect on mortality.

Other Medications. Anticoagulants may be prescribed, especially if the patient has a history of an embolic event or atrial fibrillation or mural thrombus is present. Other medications such as antianginal medications may be given to treat the underlying cause of HF. Nonsteroidal anti-inflammatory drugs (NSAIDs), such as ibuprophen (Aleve, Advil, Motrin) should be avoided (Page & Henry, 2000). They can increase systemic vascular resistance and decrease renal perfusion, especially in the elderly. For similar reasons, use of decongestants should be avoided.

NUTRITIONAL THERAPY

A low-sodium (≤2 to 3 g/day) diet and avoidance of excessive amounts of fluid are usually recommended. Although it has not been shown to affect the mortality rate, this recommendation reduces fluid retention and the symptoms of peripheral and pulmonary congestion. The purpose of sodium restriction is to decrease the amount of circulating volume, which would decrease the need for the heart to pump that volume. A balance needs to be achieved between the ability of the patient to alter the diet and the amount of medications that are prescribed. Any change in diet needs to be done with consideration of good nutrition as well as the patient's likes, dislikes, and cultural food patterns.

> **! NURSING ALERT** The sources of sodium should be specified in describing the regimen, rather than simply saying "low-salt" or "salt-free," and the quantity should be indicated in milligrams. Salt is not 100% sodium; there are 393 mg of sodium in 1 g (1000 mg) of salt.

Nursing Management

The nurse is responsible for administering the medications and for assessing their beneficial and detrimental effects to the patient. It is the balance of these effects that determines the type and dosage of pharmacologic therapy. Nursing actions to evaluate therapeutic effectiveness include the following:

- Keeping an intake and output record to identify a negative balance (more output than input)
- Weighing the patient daily at the same time and on the same scale, usually in the morning after urination; monitoring for a 2- to 3-lb gain in a day or 5-lb gain in week
- Auscultating lung sounds at least daily to detect an increase or decrease in pulmonary crackles

- Determining the degree of JVD
- Identifying and evaluating the severity of dependent edema
- Monitoring pulse rate and blood pressure, as well as monitoring for postural hypotension and making sure that the patient does not become hypotensive from dehydration
- Examining skin turgor and mucous membranes for signs of dehydration
- Assessing symptoms of fluid overload (eg, orthopnea, paroxysmal nocturnal dyspnea, and dyspnea on exertion) and evaluating changes

MONITORING AND MANAGING POTENTIAL COMPLICATIONS

Profuse and repeated diuresis can lead to hypokalemia (ie, potassium depletion). Signs are weak pulse, faint heart sounds, hypotension, muscle flabbiness, diminished deep tendon reflexes, and generalized weakness. Hypokalemia poses new problems for the patient with HF because it markedly weakens cardiac contractions. In patients receiving digoxin, hypokalemia can lead to digitalis toxicity. Digitalis toxicity and hypokalemia increase the likelihood of dangerous dysrhythmias (see Chart 30-3). Low levels of potassium may also indicate a low level of magnesium, which can add to the risk for dysrhythmias. Hyperkalemia may also occur, especially with the use of ACE-Is or ARBs and spironolactone.

> **! NURSING ALERT** To reduce the risk for hypokalemia, the nurse advises patients to increase their dietary intake of potassium. Dried apricots, bananas, beets, figs, orange or tomato juice, peaches, and prunes (dried plums), potatoes, raisins, spinach, squash, and watermelon are good dietary sources of potassium. An oral potassium supplement (potassium chloride) may also be prescribed for patients receiving diuretic medications. If the patient is at risk for hyperkalemia, the nurse advises the patient to avoid the above products, including salt substitutes.

> **! NURSING ALERT** Grapefruit (fresh and juice) is a good dietary source of potassium but has serious drug–food interactions. Patients are advised to consult their physician or pharmacist before including grapefruit in their diet.

Prolonged diuretic therapy may also produce hyponatremia (deficiency of sodium in the blood), which results in apprehension, weakness, fatigue, malaise, muscle cramps and twitching, and a rapid, thready pulse.

> **! NURSING ALERT** Periodic assessment of the patient's electrolyte levels will alert health team members to hypokalemia, hypomagnesemia, and hyponatremia. Serum levels are assessed frequently when the patient starts diuretic therapy and then usually every 3 to 12 months. It is important to remember that serum potassium levels do not always indicate the total amount of potassium within the body.

Other problems associated with diuretic administration are hyperuricemia (excessive uric acid in the blood), volume depletion from excessive urination, and hyperglycemia.

Gerontologic Considerations

Several normal changes that occur with aging increase the frequency of diastolic HF: increased systolic blood pressure, increased ventricular wall thickness, increased atrial size, and increased myocardial fibrosis. Elderly people may present with atypical signs and symptoms: fatigue, weakness, and somnolence. Decreased renal function makes the elderly patient resistant to diuretics and more sensitive to changes in volume, especially with diastolic dysfunction. The administration of diuretics to elderly men requires nursing surveillance for bladder distention caused by urethral obstruction from an enlarged prostate gland. The bladder may be assessed with an ultrasound scanner, or the suprapubic area palpated for an oval mass and percussed for dullness, indicative of bladder fullness.

NURSING PROCESS:
THE PATIENT WITH HEART FAILURE

Assessment

The nursing assessment for the patient with HF focuses on observing for effectiveness of therapy and for the patient's ability to understand and implement self-management strategies. Signs and symptoms of pulmonary and systemic fluid overload are recorded and reported immediately so that adjustments can be made in therapy. The nurse also explores the patient's emotional response to the diagnosis of HF, a chronic illness.

HEALTH HISTORY

The nurse explores sleep disturbances, particularly sleep suddenly interrupted by shortness of breath. The nurse also asks about the number of pillows needed for sleep (an indication of orthopnea), activities of daily living, and the activities that cause shortness of breath. The nurse also explores the patient's understanding of HF, the self-management strategies, and the desire to adhere to those strategies. The nurse helps patients to identify things that they have lost because of the diagnosis, their emotional response to that loss, and successful coping skills that they have used previously. Family and significant others are often included in these discussions.

PHYSICAL EXAMINATION

The lungs are auscultated to detect crackles and wheezes or their absence. Crackles, which are produced by the sudden opening of small airways and alveoli that have adhered together by edema and exudate, may be heard at the end of inspiration and are not cleared with coughing. They may also sound like gurgling that may clear with coughing or suctioning. The rate and depth of respirations are also documented.

The heart is auscultated for an S_3 heart sound, a sign that the heart is beginning to fail and that increased blood volume remains in the ventricle with each beat. HR and rhythm are also documented. Rapid rates indicate that SV has decreased and that the ventricle has less time to fill, producing some blood stagnation in the atria and eventually in the pulmonary bed.

JVD is also assessed; distention greater than 3 cm above the sternal angle is considered abnormal. This is an estimate, not a precise measurement, of central venous pressure.

Sensorium and level of consciousness must be evaluated. As the volume of blood ejected by the heart decreases, so does the amount of oxygen transported to the brain.

The nurse makes sure that dependent parts of the patient's body are assessed for perfusion and edema. With significant decreases in SV, there is a decrease in perfusion to the periphery, causing the skin to feel cool and appear pale or cyanotic. If the patient is sitting upright, the feet and lower legs are examined for edema; if the patient is supine in bed, the sacrum and back are assessed for edema. Fingers and hands may also become edematous.

In extreme cases of HF, the patient may develop periorbital edema, in which the eyelids may swell shut.

The liver is assessed for hepatojugular reflux. The patient is asked to breathe normally while manual pressure is applied over the right upper quadrant of the abdomen for 30 to 60 seconds. If neck vein distention increases more than 1 cm, the test finding is positive for increased venous pressure.

If the patient is hospitalized, the nurse measures output carefully to establish a baseline against which to measure the effectiveness of diuretic therapy. Intake and output records are rigorously maintained. It is important to know whether the patient has ingested more fluid than he or she has excreted (positive fluid balance), which is then correlated with a gain in weight. The patient must be monitored for oliguria (diminished urine output, <400 mL/24 hours) or **anuria** (urine output <50 mL/24 hours).

The patient is weighed daily in the hospital or at home, at the same time of day, with the same type of clothing, and on the same scale. If there is a significant change in weight (ie, 2- to 3-lb increase in a day or 5-lb increase in a week), the patient is instructed to notify the physician or adjust the medications (eg, increase the diuretic dose).

Diagnosis

NURSING DIAGNOSES

Based on the assessment data, major nursing diagnoses for the patient with HF may include the following:

- Activity intolerance (or risk for activity intolerance) related to imbalance between oxygen supply and demand because of decreased CO
- Excess fluid volume related to excess fluid or sodium intake and retention of fluid because of HF and its medical therapy
- Anxiety related to breathlessness and restlessness from inadequate oxygenation
- Powerlessness related to inability to perform role responsibilities because of chronic illness and hospitalizations
- Noncompliance related to lack of knowledge

COLLABORATIVE PROBLEMS/
POTENTIAL COMPLICATIONS

Based on the assessment data, potential complications that may develop include the following:

- Cardiogenic shock (see also Chap. 15)
- Dysrhythmias (see Chap. 27)
- Thromboembolism (see Chap. 31)
- Pericardial effusion and cardiac tamponade (see also Chap. 29)

Planning and Goals

Major goals for the patient may include promoting activity and reducing fatigue, relieving fluid overload symptoms, decreasing the incidence of anxiety or increasing the patient's ability to manage anxiety, teaching the patient about the self-care program, and encouraging the patient to verbalize his or her ability to make decisions and influence outcomes.

Nursing Interventions

PROMOTING ACTIVITY TOLERANCE

Although prolonged bed rest and even short periods of recumbency promote diuresis by improving renal perfusion, they also promote decreased activity tolerance. Prolonged bed rest, which may be self-imposed, should be avoided because of the deconditioning effects and hazards, such as pressure ulcers (especially in edematous patients), phlebothrombosis, and pulmonary embolism. An acute event that causes severe symptoms or that requires hospitalization indicates the need for initial bed rest. Otherwise, a total of 30 minutes of physical activity three to five times each week should be encouraged (Georgiou et al., 2001). The nurse and patient can collaborate to develop a schedule that promotes pacing and prioritization of activities. The schedule should alternate activities with periods of rest and avoid having two significant energy-consuming activities occur on the same day or in immediate succession.

Before undertaking physical activity, the patient should be given the following safety guidelines:

- Begin with a few minutes of warm-up activities.
- Avoid performing physical activities outside in extreme hot, cold, or humid weather.
- Ensure that you are able to talk during the physical activity; if you are unable to do so, decrease the intensity of activity.
- Wait 2 hours after eating a meal before performing the physical activity.
- Stop the activity if severe shortness of breath, pain, or dizziness develops.
- End with cool-down activities and a cool-down period.

Because some patients may be severely debilitated, they may need to perform physical activities only 3 to 5 minutes at a time, one to four times per day. The patient then should be advised to increase the duration of the activity, then the frequency, before increasing the intensity of the activity (Meyer, 2001).

Barriers to performing an activity are identified, and methods of adjusting an activity to ensure pacing but still accomplish the task are discussed. For example, objects that need to be taken upstairs can be put in a basket at the bottom of the stairs throughout the day. At the end of the day, the person can carry the objects up the stairs all at once. Likewise, the person can carry cleaning supplies around in a basket or backpack rather than walk back and forth to obtain the items. Vegetables can be chopped or peeled while sitting at the kitchen table rather than standing at the kitchen counter. Small, frequent meals decrease the amount of energy needed for digestion while providing adequate nutrition. The nurse helps the patient to identify peak and low periods of energy and plan energy-consuming activities for peak periods. For example, the person may prepare the meals for the entire day in the morning. Pacing and prioritizing activities help maintain the patient's energy to allow participation in regular physical activity (see Chap. 28).

The patient's response to activities needs to be monitored. If the patient is hospitalized, vital signs and oxygen saturation level are monitored before, during, and immediately after an activity to identify whether they are within the desired range. Heart rate should return to baseline within 3 minutes. If the patient is at home, the degree of fatigue felt after the activity can be used as assessment of the response. If the patient tolerates the activity, short-term and long-term goals can be developed to gradually increase the intensity, duration, and frequency of activity. Referral to a cardiac rehabilitation program may be needed, especially for HF patients with recent myocardial infarction, recent open-heart surgery, or increased anxiety. A supervised program may also benefit those who need the structured environment, significant educational support, regular encouragement, and interpersonal contact.

MANAGING FLUID VOLUME

Patients with severe HF may receive intravenous diuretic therapy, but patients with less severe symptoms may receive oral diuretic medication (see Table 30-4 for a summary of common diuretics). Oral diuretics should be administered early in the morning so that diuresis does not interfere with the patient's nighttime rest. Discussing the timing of medication administration is especially important for patients, such as elderly people, who may have urinary urgency or incontinence. A single dose of a diuretic may cause the patient to excrete a large volume of fluid shortly after administration.

The nurse monitors the patient's fluid status closely—auscultating the lungs, monitoring daily body weights, and assisting the patient to adhere to a low-sodium diet by reading food labels and avoiding high-sodium foods such as canned, processed, and convenience foods (Chart 30-4). If the diet includes fluid restriction, the nurse can assist the patient to plan the fluid intake throughout the day while respecting the patient's dietary preferences. If the patient is receiving intravenous fluids, the

Chart 30-4 Facts About Dietary Sodium

Although the major source of sodium in the average Canadian diet is salt, many types of natural foods contain varying amounts of sodium. Even if no salt is added in cooking and if salty foods are avoided, the daily diet may still contain between 1000 and 2000 mg of sodium.

Additives in Food
Added food substances (additives), such as sodium alginate, which improves food texture; sodium benzoate, which acts as a preservative; and disodium phosphate, which improves cooking quality in certain foods, increase the sodium intake when included in the daily diet. Therefore, patients on low-sodium diets should be advised to check labels carefully for such words as "salt" or "sodium," especially on canned foods. For example, without looking at the sodium content per serving found on the nutrition labels, when given a choice between a serving of salt and vinegar potato chips and a cup of canned cream of mushroom soup, most would think that soup is lower in sodium. However, when the labels are examined, the lower sodium choice is found to be the chips. Although potato chips are *not* recommended in a low sodium diet, this example illustrates that it is important to read food labels to determine both sodium content and serving size.

Nonfood Sodium Sources
Sodium is also contained in toothpaste and local water supplies. Patients on sodium-restricted diets should be cautioned against using nonprescription medications such as antacids, cough syrups, laxatives, sedatives, or salt substitutes, because these products contain sodium or excessive amounts of potassium. Over-the-counter medications should not be used without first consulting the physician.

Promoting Dietary Adherence
If patients find food unpalatable because of the dietary sodium restrictions and/or the taste disturbances caused by the medications, they may refuse to eat or to comply with the dietary regimen. For this reason, severe sodium restrictions should be avoided and the amount of medication should be balanced with the patient's ability to restrict dietary sodium. A variety of flavourings, such as lemon juice, vinegar, and herbs, may be used to improve the taste of the food and increase acceptance of the diet. The patient's food preferences should be taken into account—diet counselling and educational handouts can be geared to individual and ethnic preferences. It is very important to involve the family in the dietary teaching.

amount of fluid needs to be monitored closely, and the physician or pharmacist can be consulted about the possibility of maximizing the amount of medication in the same amount of intravenous fluid (eg, double-concentrating to decrease the fluid volume administered).

The nurse positions the patient or teaches the patient how to assume a position that shifts fluid away from the heart. The number of pillows may be increased, the head of the bed may be elevated (20- to 30-cm blocks may be used), or the patient may sit in a comfortable armchair. In this position, the venous return to the heart (preload) is reduced, pulmonary congestion is alleviated, and impingement of the liver on the diaphragm is minimized. The lower arms are supported with pillows to eliminate the fatigue caused by the constant pull of their weight on the shoulder muscles.

The patient who can breathe only in the upright position may sit on the side of the bed with the feet supported on a chair, the head and arms resting on an overbed table, and the lumbosacral spine supported by a pillow. If pulmonary congestion is present, positioning the patient in an armchair is advantageous, because this position favours the shift of fluid away from the lungs.

Because decreased circulation in edematous areas increases the risk of skin injury, the nurse assesses for skin breakdown and institutes preventive measures. Frequent changes of position, positioning to avoid pressure, the use of elastic compression stockings, and leg exercises may help to prevent skin injury.

CONTROLLING ANXIETY

Because patients in HF have difficulty maintaining adequate oxygenation, they are likely to be restless and anxious and feel overwhelmed by breathlessness. These symptoms tend to intensify at night. Emotional stress stimulates the sympathetic nervous system, which causes vasoconstriction, elevated arterial pressure, and increased heart rate. This sympathetic response increases the amount of work that the heart has to do. By decreasing anxiety, the patient's cardiac work also is decreased. Oxygen may be administered during an acute event to diminish the work of breathing and to increase the patient's comfort.

When the patient exhibits anxiety, the nurse takes steps to promote physical comfort and psychological support. In many cases, a family member's presence provides reassurance. To help decrease the patient's anxiety, the nurse should speak in a slow, calm, and confident manner and maintain eye contact. When necessary, the nurse should also state specific, brief directions for an activity.

After the patient is comfortable, the nurse can begin teaching ways to control anxiety and to avoid anxiety-provoking situations. The nurse explains how to use relaxation techniques and assists the patient to identify factors that contribute to anxiety. Lack of sleep may increase anxiety, which may prevent adequate rest. Other contributing factors may include misinformation, lack of information, or poor nutritional status. Promoting physical comfort, providing accurate information, and teaching the patient to perform relaxation techniques and to avoid anxiety-triggering situations may relax the patient.

> **! NURSING ALERT** Cerebral hypoxia with superimposed carbon dioxide retention may be a problem in HF, causing the patient to react to sedative-hypnotic medications with confusion and increased anxiety. Hepatic congestion may slow the liver's metabolism of medication, leading to toxicity. Sedative-hypnotic medications must be administered with caution.

In cases of confusion and anxiety reactions that affect the patient's safety, the use of restraints should be avoided. Restraints are likely to be resisted, and resistance inevitably increases the cardiac workload. The patient who insists on getting out of bed at night can be seated comfortably in an armchair. As cerebral and systemic circulation improves, the degree of anxiety decreases, and the quality of sleep improves.

MINIMIZING POWERLESSNESS

Patients need to recognize that they are not helpless and that they can influence the direction of their lives and the outcomes of treatment. The nurse assesses for factors contributing to a sense of powerlessness and intervenes accordingly. Contributing factors may include lack of knowledge and lack of opportunities to make decisions, particularly if health care providers and family members behave in maternalistic or paternalistic ways. If the patient is hospitalized, hospital policies may promote standardization and limit the patient's ability to make decisions (eg, what time to have meals, take medications, prepare for bed).

Taking time to listen actively to patients often encourages them to express their concerns and ask questions. Other strategies include providing the patient with decision-making opportunities, such as when activities are to occur or where objects are to be placed, and increasing the frequency and significance of those opportunities over time; providing encouragement while identifying the patient's progress; and assisting the patient to differentiate between factors that can be controlled and those that cannot. In some cases, the nurse may want to review hospital policies and standards that tend to promote powerlessness and advocate for their elimination or change (eg, limited visiting hours, prohibition of food from home, required wearing of hospital gowns).

PROMOTING HOME AND COMMUNITY-BASED CARE

Teaching Patients Self-Care

The nurse provides patient education and involves the patient in implementing the therapeutic regimen to promote understanding and adherence to the plan. When the patient understands or believes that the diagnosis of HF can be successfully managed with lifestyle changes and medications, recurrences of acute HF lessen, unnecessary hospitalizations decrease, and life expectancy increases. Patients and their families need to be taught to follow the medication regimen as prescribed, maintain a low-sodium diet, perform and record daily weights, engage in routine physical activity, and recognize symptoms that indicate worsening HF. Although noncompliance is not well understood, interventions that may promote adherence include teaching to ensure accurate understanding. A summary of teaching points for the patient with HF is presented in Chart 30-5.

The patient and family members are supported and encouraged to ask questions so that information can be clarified and understanding enhanced. The nurse should be aware of cultural factors and adapt the teaching plan accordingly. Patients and their families need to be informed that the progression of the disease is influenced in part by choices made about health care and the decisions about following the treatment plan. They also need to be informed that health care providers are there to assist them in reaching their health care goals. Patients and family members need to make the decisions about the treatment plan, but they also need to understand the possible outcomes of those decisions. The treatment plan then will be based on what the patient wants, not just what the physician or other health care team members think is needed. Ultimately, the nurse needs to convey that monitoring symptoms and daily weights, restricting sodium intake, avoiding

Chart 30-5

Home Care Checklist • The Patient With Heart Failure

At the completion of the home care instruction, the patient or caregiver will be able to:	Patient	Caregiver
• Identify heart failure as a chronic disease that can be managed with medications and specific self-management behaviours.	✓	✓
• Take or administer medications daily, exactly as prescribed.	✓	✓
• Monitor effects of medication.	✓	✓
• Know signs and symptoms of orthostatic hypotension and how to prevent it.	✓	✓
• Weigh self daily. – Obtain weight at the same time each day (eg, every morning after urination). – Keep a record and report weight gain of ≥ 0.9–1.4 kg in 1 day or 2.3 kg in 1 week.	✓	
• Restrict sodium intake to 2–3 g daily: adapt diet by examining nutrition labels to check sodium content per serving; avoid canned or processed foods; eat fresh or frozen foods; consult the written diet plan and the list of permitted and restricted foods; avoid salt use; and avoid excesses in eating and drinking.	✓	✓
• Review activity program. – Participate in a daily exercise program. – Increase walking and other activities gradually, provided they do not cause unusual fatigue or dyspnea. – Conserve energies by balancing activity with rest periods. – Avoid activity in extremes of heat and cold, which increase the work of the heart. – Recognize that air conditioning may be essential in a hot, humid environment.	✓	
• Develop methods to manage stress.	✓	
• Keep regular appointments with physician or clinic.	✓	✓
• Be alert for symptoms that may indicate recurring heart failure. – Recall the symptoms experienced when illness began.	✓	✓
• Report immediately to the physician or clinic any of the following: – Gain in weight of ≥ 0.9–1.4 kg in 1 day, or 2.3 kg in 1 week – Loss of appetite – Unusual shortness of breath with activity – Swelling of ankles, feet, or abdomen – Persistent cough – Development of restless sleep; increase in number of pillows needed to sleep	✓	✓

excess fluids, preventing infection with influenza and pneumococcal immunizations, avoiding noxious agents (eg, alcohol, tobacco), and participating in regular exercise all aid in preventing exacerbations of HF.

Continuing Care

Depending on the patient's physical status and the availability of family assistance, a home care referral may be indicated for a patient who has been hospitalized. Elderly patients and those who have long-standing heart disease with compromised physical stamina often require assistance with the transition to home after hospitalization for an acute episode of HF. It is important for the home care nurse to assess the physical environment of the home. Suggestions for adapting the home environment to meet the patient's activity limitations are important. If stairs are the concern, the patient can plan the day's activities so that stair climbing is minimized; for some patients, a temporary bedroom may be set up on the main level of the home. The home care nurse collaborates with the patient and family to maximize the benefits of these changes.

The home care nurse also reinforces and clarifies information about dietary changes and fluid restrictions, the need to monitor symptoms and daily body weights, and the importance of obtaining follow-up health care. Assistance may be given in scheduling and keeping appointments as well. The patient is encouraged to gradually increase his or her self-care and responsibility for accomplishing the therapeutic regimen.

Evaluation

EXPECTED PATIENT OUTCOMES

Expected patient outcomes may include:

1. Demonstrates tolerance for increased activity
   a. Describes adaptive methods for usual activities
   b. Stops any activity that causes symptoms of intolerance
   c. Maintains vital signs (pulse, blood pressure, respiratory rate, and pulse oximetry) within the targeted range
   d. Identifies factors that contribute to activity intolerance and takes actions to avoid them
   e. Establishes priorities for activities
   f. Schedules activities to conserve energy and to reduce fatigue and dyspnea
2. Maintains fluid balance
   a. Exhibits decreased peripheral and sacral edema
   b. Demonstrates methods for preventing edema
3. Is less anxious
   a. Avoids situations that produce stress
   b. Sleeps comfortably at night
   c. Reports decreased stress and anxiety
4. Makes decisions regarding care and treatment
   a. States ability to influence outcomes
5. Adheres to self-care regimen
   a. Performs and records daily weights
   b. Ensures dietary intake includes no more than 2 to 3 g of sodium per day

c. Takes medications as prescribed
d. Reports any unusual symptoms or side effects

ACUTE HEART FAILURE (PULMONARY EDEMA)

Pulmonary edema is the abnormal accumulation of fluid in the lungs. The fluid may accumulate in the interstitial spaces or in the alveoli.

Pathophysiology

Pulmonary edema is an acute event that results from HF. It can occur acutely, such as with myocardial infarction, or it can occur as an exacerbation of chronic HF. Myocardial scarring as a result of ischemia can limit the ventricular distensibility and render it vulnerable to a sudden increase in workload. With increased resistance to left ventricular filling, the blood backs up into the pulmonary circulation. The patient quickly develops pulmonary edema, sometimes called flash pulmonary edema, from the blood volume overload in the lungs. Pulmonary edema can also be caused by noncardiac disorders, such as renal failure, liver failure, and oncologic conditions that cause the body to retain fluid. The left ventricle cannot handle the resulting hypervolemia, preventing blood from easily flowing from the left atrium into the left ventricle. This causes the pressure to increase in the left atrium. The increase in atrial pressure may result in an increase in pulmonary venous pressure, which produces an increase in hydrostatic pressure that forces fluid out of the pulmonary capillaries into the interstitial spaces and alveoli.

Impaired lymphatic drainage also contributes to the accumulation of fluid in the lung tissues. The fluid within the alveoli mixes with air, creating "bubbles" that are expelled from the mouth and nose, producing the classic symptom of pulmonary edema, frothy pink (blood-tinged) sputum. Because of the fluid within the alveoli, air cannot enter, and gas exchange is impaired. The result is hypoxemia, which is often severe. The onset may be preceded by premonitory symptoms of pulmonary congestion, but it also may develop quickly in the patient with a ventricle that has little reserve to meet increased oxygen needs.

In pulmonary edema, as well as in HF, preload, contractility, and afterload may be altered, thereby impairing CO. Technological advances (eg, impedance cardiography) have made it easier to implement effective pharmacologic therapy in treating acute pulmonary edema.

Clinical Manifestations

As a result of decreased cerebral oxygenation, the patient becomes increasingly restless and anxious. Along with a sudden onset of breathlessness and a sense of suffocation, the patient's hands become cold and moist, the nail beds become cyanotic (bluish), and the skin turns ashen (grey). The pulse is weak and rapid, and the neck veins are distended. Incessant coughing may occur, producing increasing quantities of mucoid sputum. As pulmonary edema progresses, the patient's anxiety and restlessness increase; the patient becomes confused, then stuporous. Breathing is rapid, noisy, and moist sounding. The patient's oxygen levels (saturation) are significantly decreased. The patient, nearly suffocated by the blood-tinged, frothy fluid filling the alveoli, is literally drowning in secretions. The situation demands immediate action.

Assessment and Diagnostic Findings

The diagnosis is made by evaluating the clinical manifestations resulting from pulmonary congestion. Most often, a chest x-ray is obtained to confirm that the pulmonary veins are engorged. Abrupt onset of signs and symptoms of left-sided HF (eg, crackles on auscultation of the lungs, flash pulmonary edema) without evidence of right-sided HF (eg, no JVD, no dependent edema) may indicate diastolic failure due to ischemia.

Prevention

Like most complications, pulmonary edema is easier to prevent than to treat. To recognize it in its early stages, the nurse auscultates the lung fields and heart sounds, measures JVD, and assesses the degree of peripheral edema and the severity of breathlessness. A dry, hacking cough; fatigue; weight gain; development or worsening of edema; and decreased activity tolerance may be early indicators of developing pulmonary edema.

In an early stage, the condition may be corrected by placing the patient in an upright position with the feet and legs dependent, eliminating overexertion, and minimizing emotional stress to reduce the left ventricular load. A re-examination of the patient's treatment regimen and the patient's understanding of and adherence to it are also needed. The long-range approach to preventing pulmonary edema must be directed at identifying its precipitating factors.

Medical Management

Clinical management of a patient with acute pulmonary edema due to HF is directed toward improving ventricular function and increasing respiratory exchange. These goals are accomplished through a combination of oxygen, medication therapies, and nursing support.

PHARMACOLOGIC THERAPY

Various treatments and medications are prescribed for pulmonary edema, among them oxygen, morphine, diuretics, and various intravenous medications.

Oxygen Therapy. Oxygen is administered in concentrations adequate to relieve hypoxemia and dyspnea. Usually, a face mask or non-rebreathing mask is initially used. If respiratory failure is severe or persists despite optimal management, endotracheal intubation and mechanical ventilation are required. The use of positive end-expiratory pressure (PEEP) is effective in reducing venous return, decreasing fluid movement from the pulmonary capillaries to the alveoli, and improving oxygenation. Oxygenation is monitored with pulse oximetry and by measurement of arterial blood gases.

Morphine. Morphine is administered intravenously in small doses (2 to 5 mg) to reduce peripheral resistance and venous return so that blood can be redistributed from the pulmonary circulation to other parts of the body. This action decreases pressure in the pulmonary capillaries and decreases seepage of fluid into the lung tissue. The effect of morphine in decreasing anxiety is also beneficial.

Diuretics. Diuretics promote the excretion of sodium and water by the kidneys. Furosemide (Lasix), for example, is administered intravenously to produce a rapid diuretic effect. Furosemide also causes vasodilation and pooling of blood in peripheral blood vessels, which reduces the amount of blood returned to the heart, even before the diuretic effect. Some physicians may prescribe bumetanide (Bumex) and metolazone (Mykrox, Zaroxolyn) in place of furosemide.

Dobutamine. Dobutamine (Dobutrex) is an intravenous medication given to patients with significant left ventricular dysfunction. A catecholamine, dobutamine stimulates the beta$_1$-adrenergic receptors. Its major action is to increase cardiac contractility. However, at higher amounts, it also increases the heart rate and the incidence of ectopic beats and tachydysrhythmias. Because it also increases AV conduction, care must be taken in patients who have underlying atrial fibrillation. A medication that protects the AV node, such as digitalis, a beta-blocker, or a calcium channel blocker, may be indicated before dobutamine therapy is initiated to prevent increased ventricular response rate.

Milrinone. Milrinone (Primacor) is a phosphodiesterase inhibitor that delays the release of calcium from intracellular reservoirs and prevents the uptake of extracellular calcium by the cells. This promotes vasodilation, decreasing preload and afterload, reducing the workload of the heart. Milrinone is administered intravenously, usually to patients who have not responded to other therapies. It is not usually used to treat patients with renal failure. The major side effects are hypotension (usually asymptomatic), gastrointestinal dysfunction, increased ventricular dysrhythmias, and decreased platelet counts. The patient's blood pressure is monitored closely.

Nesiritide. Nesiritide (Natrecor) is an intravenous medication that is indicated for acutely decompensated HF. Natriuretic peptides are produced by the myocardium as a compensatory response to increased ventricular end-diastolic pressure and myocardial wall stress and to the increased release of neurohormones (eg, norepinephrine, renin, aldosterone) that occur with HF. Nesiritide is a human B-type natriuretic peptide (BNP) made from *Escherichia coli* using recombinant technology. Human BNP binds to vascular smooth muscle and endothelial cells, causing dilation of arteries and veins and suppression of the neurohormones. The result is improved stroke volume and reduced preload and afterload (Colucci et al., 2000). This medication causes rapid improvement in the symptoms of HF and may be used with other HF medications (eg, beta-blockers, digoxin). The most common side effect is dose-related hypotension. This drug has been available in the United States since 2001 and may be more widely introduced in the future.

Nursing Management

POSITIONING THE PATIENT TO PROMOTE CIRCULATION
Proper positioning can help reduce venous return to the heart. The patient is positioned upright, preferably with the legs dangling over the side of the bed. This has the immediate effect of decreasing venous return, lowering the output of the right ventricle, and decreasing lung congestion. If the patient is unable to sit with the lower extremities dependent, the patient may be placed in an upright position in bed.

PROVIDING PSYCHOLOGICAL SUPPORT
As the ability to breathe decreases, the patient's sense of fear and anxiety rises proportionately, making the condition more severe. Reassuring the patient and providing skillful anticipatory nursing care are integral parts of the therapy. Because this patient feels a sense of impending doom and has an unstable condition, the nurse must remain with the patient. The nurse should give the pa-

tient simple, concise information in a reassuring voice about what is being done to treat the condition and the expected results. The nurse should also identify any anxiety-inducing factors (eg, a pet left alone at home, presence of an unwelcome family member at the bedside, a wallet full of money) and initiate strategies to eliminate the concern or reduce its effect.

MONITORING MEDICATIONS
The patient receiving morphine is observed for respiratory depression, hypotension, and vomiting; a morphine antagonist, such as naloxone hydrochloride (Narcan), is kept available and given to the patient who exhibits these side effects.

The patient receiving diuretic therapy may excrete a large volume of urine within minutes after a potent diuretic is administered. A bedside commode may be used to decrease the energy required by the patient and to reduce the resultant increase in cardiac workload induced by getting on and off a bedpan. If necessary, an indwelling urinary catheter may be inserted.

NURSING ALERT Because of the resulting diuresis, the patient's electrolyte levels, especially potassium and sodium, need to be monitored closely. Fluid balance in some patients is very brittle; they easily become hypovolemic or hypervolemic with small changes in the amount of circulating fluid. Falling blood pressure, increasing heart rate, and decreasing urine output indicate that the circulatory system is not tolerating diuresis and that measures must be taken to reverse the fluid imbalance that has occurred. Serum creatinine is monitored to assess renal function. Men with prostatic hyperplasia must be observed for signs of urinary retention. Additional monitoring activities are discussed in Chart 30-6.

Other Complications

CARDIOGENIC SHOCK
Cardiogenic shock occurs when the heart cannot pump enough blood to supply the amount of oxygen needed by the tissues. This may occur because of one significant or multiple smaller infarctions in which more than 40% of the myocardium becomes necrotic, because of a ruptured ventricle, significant valvular dysfunction, trauma to the heart resulting in myocardial contusion, or as the end stage of HF. It also can occur with cardiac tamponade, pulmonary embolism, cardiomyopathy, and dysrhythmias.

Pathophysiology
The signs and symptoms of cardiogenic shock reflect the circular nature of the pathophysiology of HF. The degree of shock is proportional to the extent of left ventricular dysfunction. The heart muscle loses its contractile power, resulting in a marked reduction in SV and CO, which is sometimes called forward failure. The damage to the myocardium results in a decrease in CO, which reduces arterial blood pressure and tissue perfusion in the vital organs (heart, brain, lung, kidneys). Flow to the coronary arteries is reduced, resulting in decreased oxygen supply to the myocardium, which increases ischemia and further reduces the heart's ability to pump. The inadequate emptying of the ventricle also leads to increased pulmonary pressures, pulmonary congestion, and pulmonary edema, exacerbating the hypoxia, causing ischemia of vital organs, and setting a vicious cycle in motion (Fig. 30-3).

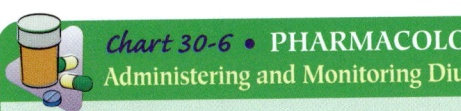

Chart 30-6 • PHARMACOLOGY
Administering and Monitoring Diuretic Therapy

When nursing care involves diuretic therapy for conditions such as pulmonary edema or heart failure, the nurse needs to administer the medication and monitor the patient's response carefully, as follows:

- Administer the diuretic at a time conducive to the patient's lifestyle; for example, early in the day to avoid nocturia.
- Give supplementary potassium with thiazide and loop diuretics as prescribed to replace potassium lost.
- Check laboratory results for electrolyte depletion, especially potassium, magnesium, and sodium; and for electrolyte elevation, especially potassium with potassium-sparing agents and calcium with thiazides.
- Monitor urine output or daily weights to identify appropriate response: intake and output balance, serum BUN and creatinine; notify the health care provider if renal impairment is suspected.
- Assess lung sounds, jugular vein distention, daily weight, and peripheral, abdominal, or sacral edema to identify need to adjust dose.
- Monitor for adverse reactions, such as nausea and gastrointestinal distress, vomiting, diarrhea, weakness, headache, fatigue, anxiety or agitation, and cardiac dysrhythmias.
- Assess for signs of volume depletion, such as postural hypotension, dizziness, imbalance, and reduced jugular venous distention (JVD).
- Monitor for glucose intolerance in patients with and without diabetes mellitus who are receiving thiazide diuretics.
- Monitor for potential ototoxicity in patients, especially those with renal failure, who are receiving a loop diuretic.
- Advise patients to avoid prolonged exposure to the sun because of the risk of photosensitivity.
- Monitor for elevated serum uric acid levels and the development of gout.
- Implement nursing actions to facilitate effect of medication, such as positioning patient upright with legs dangling.

Physiology/Pathophysiology

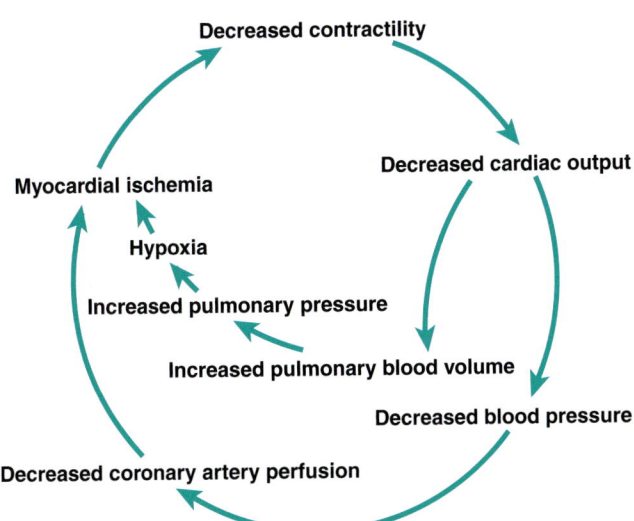

FIGURE 30-3 Pathophysiology of cardiogenic shock.

Clinical Manifestations

The classic signs of cardiogenic shock are tissue hypoperfusion manifested as cerebral hypoxia (restlessness, confusion, agitation), low blood pressure, rapid and weak pulse, cold and clammy skin, increased respiratory crackles, hypoactive bowel sounds, and decreased urinary output. Initially, arterial blood gas analysis may show respiratory alkalosis. Dysrhythmias are common and result from a decrease in oxygen to the myocardium.

Assessment and Diagnostic Findings

Use of a PA catheter to measure left ventricular pressures and CO is important in assessing the severity of the problem and planning management. The PA wedge pressure is elevated and the CO decreased as the left ventricle loses its ability to pump. The systemic vascular resistance is elevated because of the sympathetic nervous system stimulation that occurs as a compensatory response to the decrease in blood pressure. The decreased blood flow to the kidneys causes a hormonal response (ie, increased catecholamines and activation of the renin-angiotensin-aldosterone system) that causes fluid retention and further vasoconstriction. Increases in HR, circulating volume, and vasoconstriction occur to maintain circulation to the brain, heart, kidneys, and lungs, but at a cost: an increase in the workload of the heart.

The reduction in blood volume delivered to the tissues results in an increase in the amount of oxygen that is extracted from the blood that is delivered to the tissues (to try to meet the cellular demand for oxygen). The increased systemic oxygen extraction results in decreased venous (mixed and central) oxygen saturation. When the cellular oxygen needs cannot be met by the systemic oxygen delivery and the oxygen extraction, anaerobic metabolism and the resulting build up of lactic acid occur. Continuous central venous oximetry and measurement of blood lactic acid levels may assist in assessing the severity of the shock as well as the effectiveness of treatment.

Continued cellular hypoperfusion eventually results in organ failure. The patient becomes unresponsive, severe hypotension ensues, and the patient develops shallow respirations; cold, cyanotic or mottled skin; and absent bowel sounds. Arterial blood gas analysis shows metabolic acidosis, and all laboratory test results indicate organ dysfunction. Chapter 15 presents in more detail the pathophysiology and management of cardiogenic shock.

Medical Management

The major approach to treating cardiogenic shock is to correct the underlying problems, reduce any further demand on the heart, improve oxygenation, and restore tissue perfusion. For example, if the ventricular failure is the result of an acute myocardial infarction, emergency percutaneous coronary intervention may be indicated (Webb et al., 2001). Ventricular assist devices may be implanted to support the pumping action of the heart (Barron et al., 2001) (see Chap. 29). Major dysrhythmias are corrected because they may have caused or contributed to the shock. If the patient has hypervolemia, diuresis is indicated. Diuretics, vasodilators, and mechanical devices, such as filtration (continuous renal replacement therapy [CRRT]) and dialysis, have been used to reduce the circulating blood volume. If hypovolemia or low intravascular volume is suspected or detected through pressure readings, the patient is given intravenous volume expanders (eg, normal saline solution, lactated Ringer's solution, albumin) to increase the amount of circulating fluid. The patient is placed on strict bedrest to conserve energy. If the patient has hypoxemia, as detected by pulse oximetry or arterial blood gas analysis, oxygen administration is increased, often under positive pressure when regular flow is insufficient to meet tissue demands. Intubation and sedation may be necessary to maintain oxygenation. The settings for mechanical ventilation are adjusted according to the patient's oxygenation status and the need for conserving energy.

PHARMACOLOGIC THERAPY

Medication therapy is selected and guided according to CO, other cardiac parameters, and mean arterial blood pressure. Because of the decreased perfusion to the gastrointestinal system and the need to adjust the dosage quickly, most medications are administered intravenously.

Vasopressors, or pressor agents, are medications used to raise blood pressure and increase CO. Many pressor medications are catecholamines, such as norepinephrine (Levophed) and high-dose (>10 µg/kg per minute) dopamine (Intropin). Their purpose is to promote perfusion to the heart and brain, but they compromise circulation to other organs (eg, kidney). Because they also tend to increase the workload of the heart by increasing oxygen demand, they are not administered early in the cardiogenic shock process.

Diuretics and vasodilators may be administered carefully to reduce the workload of the heart as long as they do not cause worsening of the tissue hypoperfusion. Agents such as milrinone (Primacor), sodium nitroprusside (Nipride), and nitroglycerin (Nitrol) are effective vasoactive medications that lower the volume returning to the heart, decrease blood pressure, and decrease cardiac work. They cause the arteries and veins to dilate, thereby shunting much of the intravascular volume to the periphery and causing a reduction in preload and afterload.

Positive inotropic medications are given to increase myocardial contractility. Dopamine (Intropin, given at more than 2 µg/kg per minute), dobutamine (Dobutrex), and epinephrine (Adrenalin) are catecholamines that increase contractility. Each of these can cause tachydysrhythmias because they increase automaticity with increasing dosage. Monitoring baseline HR is therefore important. As the baseline HR increases, so does the risk of developing tachydysrhythmias.

OTHER TREATMENTS

Other therapeutic modalities for cardiogenic shock include use of circulatory assist devices. The most frequently used mechanical support device is the intra-aortic balloon pump (IABP). The IABP is a catheter with an inflatable balloon at the end. The catheter is usually inserted through the femoral artery, and the balloon is positioned in the descending thoracic aorta (Fig. 30-4). IABP uses internal counterpulsation through the regular inflation and deflation of the balloon to augment the pumping action of the heart. The device inflates during diastole, increasing the pressure in the aorta during diastole and therefore increasing blood flow through the coronary and peripheral arteries. It deflates just before systole, lessening the pressure within the aorta before left ventricular contraction, decreasing the amount of resistance the heart has to overcome to eject blood and therefore decreasing the amount of work the heart must put forth to eject blood. The device is connected to a console that synchronizes the inflation and deflation of the balloon with the ECG or the arterial pressure (as indicators for systole and diastole). Hemodynamic monitoring is essential to determine the patient's response to the IABP. Other ventricular assist devices are described in Chapter 29.

FIGURE 30-4 The intra-aortic balloon pump (IABP) inflates at the beginning of diastole, which results in increased perfusion of the coronary and peripheral arteries; it deflates just before systole, which results in a decrease in afterload (resistance to ejection) and in the left ventricular workload.

Nursing Management

The patient in cardiogenic shock requires constant monitoring and intensive care. The critical care (intensive care) nurse must carefully assess the patient, observe the cardiac rhythm, monitor hemodynamic parameters, and record fluid intake and urinary output. The patient must be closely assessed for responses to the medical interventions and for the development of complications, which must be corrected immediately.

Because of the frequency of nursing interventions and the technology required for effective medical management, the patient is always treated in an intensive care environment. Critical care nurses are responsible for the nursing management, which includes frequent assessments and timely adjustments to medications and therapies based on the assessment data. More information about nursing management of the patient in cardiogenic shock can be found in Chapter 15.

THROMBOEMBOLISM

The decreased mobility of the patient with cardiac disease and the impaired circulation that accompany these disorders contribute to the development of intracardiac and intravascular thrombosis. Intracardiac thrombus is especially common in patients with atrial fibrillation, because the atria do not contract forcefully and blood flow slows through the atrium, increasing thrombus formation. Intracardiac thrombus is detected by an echocardiogram and treated with anticoagulants, such as heparin and warfarin (Coumadin). A part of the thrombus may become detached (embolus) and may be carried to the brain, kidneys, intestines, or lungs. The most common problem is pulmonary embolism. The symptoms of pulmonary embolism include chest pain, cyanosis, shortness of breath, rapid respirations, and hemoptysis (bloody sputum).

The pulmonary embolus may block the circulation to a part of the lung, producing an area of pulmonary infarction. Usually, there is a significant decrease in oxygenation measured by arterial blood gas analysis or pulse oximetry. Pain experienced is usually pleuritic; it increases with respiration and may subside when the patient holds the breath. Cardiac pain is usually continuous and does not vary with respirations. However, it may be difficult to differentiate by symptoms alone. The patient usually undergoes a ventilation-perfusion scan or a pulmonary arteriogram for definitive diagnosis. The treatment and care for patients with pulmonary embolism are discussed in Chapter 23.

Systemic embolism may manifest as cerebral, mesenteric, or renal infarction; an embolism can also compromise the blood supply to an extremity, which is discussed in more detail in Chapter 31. The nurse must be aware of such possible complications and be prepared to identify and report signs and symptoms.

PERICARDIAL EFFUSION AND CARDIAC TAMPONADE

Pathophysiology

Pericardial effusion refers to the accumulation of fluid in the pericardial sac. This occurrence may accompany pericarditis (see Chap. 29), advanced HF, metastatic carcinoma, cardiac surgery, trauma, or nontraumatic hemorrhage.

Normally, the pericardial sac contains less than 50 mL of fluid, which is needed to decrease friction for the beating heart. An increase in pericardial fluid raises the pressure within the pericardial sac and compresses the heart. This has the following effects:

• Increased right and left ventricular end-diastolic pressures
• Decreased venous return
• Inability of the ventricles to distend adequately and to fill

Pericardial fluid may accumulate slowly without causing noticeable symptoms. A rapidly developing effusion, however, can stretch the pericardium to its maximum size and, because of increased pericardial pressure, reduce venous return to the heart and decrease CO. The result is cardiac tamponade (compression of the heart).

Clinical Manifestations

The patient may complain of a feeling of fullness within the chest or may have substantial or ill-defined pain. The feeling of pressure in the chest may result from stretching of the pericardial sac. Because of increased pressure within the pericardium, venous pressure tends to rise, as evidenced by engorged neck veins. Other signs include shortness of breath and a drop and fluctuation in blood pressure. Systolic blood pressure that is detected during exhalation but not heard with inhalation is called **pulsus paradoxus**. The difference in systolic pressure between the point that it is heard during exhalation and the point that it is heard during inhalation is measured. Pulsus paradoxus exceeding 10 mm Hg

is abnormal. The cardinal signs of cardiac tamponade are falling systolic blood pressure, narrowing pulse pressure, rising venous pressure (increased jugular venous distention), and distant (muffled) heart sounds (Chart 30-7).

 NURSING ALERT Cardiac tamponade is a life-threatening situation, demanding immediate intervention.

Assessment and Diagnostic Findings

Pericardial effusion is detected by percussing the chest and noticing an extension of flatness across the anterior aspect of the chest. An echocardiogram may be performed to confirm the diagnosis. The clinical signs and symptoms and chest x-ray findings are usually sufficient to diagnose pericardial effusion.

Medical Management

PERICARDIOCENTESIS

If cardiac function becomes seriously impaired, **pericardiocentesis** (puncture of the pericardial sac to aspirate pericardial fluid) is performed to remove fluid from the pericardial sac. The major

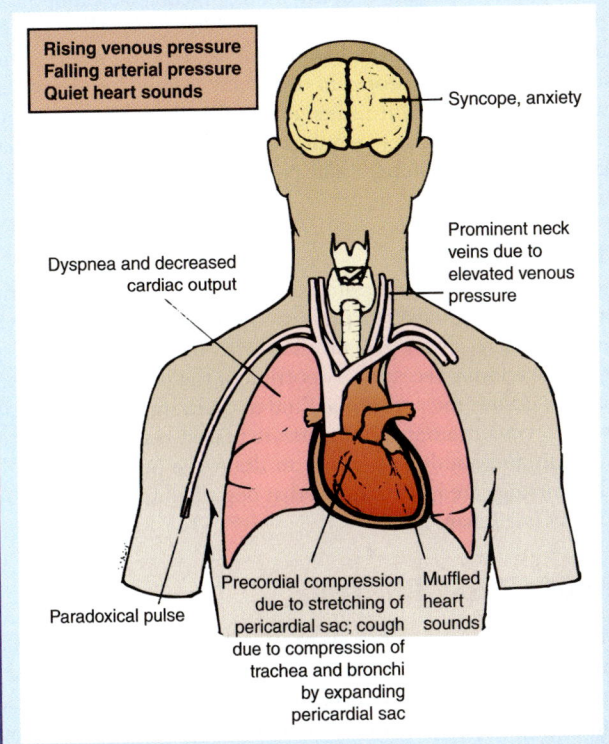

Chart 30-7 • ASSESSMENT

Signs and Symptoms of Cardiac Tamponade

Assessment findings in cardiac tamponade resulting from pericardial effusion include feelings of faintness, shortness of breath, anxiety, and pain from decreased cardiac output, cough from pressure created in the trachea from swelling of the pericardial sac, distended neck veins from rising venous pressure, paradoxical pulse, and muffled or distant heart sounds.

goal is to prevent cardiac tamponade, which restricts normal heart action.

During the procedure, the patient is monitored by ECG and hemodynamic pressure measurements. Emergency resuscitative equipment should be readily available. The head of the bed is elevated to 45 to 60 degrees, placing the heart in proximity to the chest wall so that the needle can be inserted into the pericardial sac more easily. If a peripheral intravenous device is not already in place, one is inserted, and a slow intravenous infusion is started in case it becomes necessary to administer emergency medications or blood products.

The pericardial aspiration needle is attached to a 50-mL syringe by a three-way stopcock. Several possible sites are used for pericardial aspiration. The needle may be inserted in the angle between the left costal margin and the xiphoid, near the cardiac apex; at the fifth or sixth intercostal space at the left sternal margin; or on the right sternal margin of the fourth intercostal space. The needle is advanced slowly until it has entered the epicardium and fluid is obtained. The ECG can help determine when the needle has contacted the epicardium. The cable of a precordial lead is attached to the aspirating needle with alligator clamps; contact with the epicardium is seen by ST segment elevation on the ECG. During the procedure, drainage fluid must be checked for clotting. Although not entirely accurate, the guideline is that pericardial blood does not clot readily, whereas blood obtained from inadvertent puncture of one of the heart chambers does clot.

A resulting fall in central venous pressure and an associated rise in blood pressure after withdrawal of pericardial fluid indicate that the cardiac tamponade has been relieved. The patient almost always feels immediate relief. If there is a substantial amount of pericardial fluid, a small catheter may be left in place to drain recurrent accumulation of blood or fluid. Pericardial fluid is sent to the laboratory for examination for tumour cells, bacterial culture, chemical and serologic analysis, and differential blood cell count.

Complications of pericardiocentesis include ventricular or coronary artery puncture, dysrhythmias, pleural laceration, gastric puncture, and myocardial trauma. After pericardiocentesis, the patient's heart rhythm, blood pressure, venous pressure, and heart sounds are monitored to detect any possible recurrence of cardiac tamponade. If it recurs, repeated aspiration is necessary. Cardiac tamponade may require treatment by open pericardial drainage (pericardiotomy). The patient is ideally in an intensive care unit.

PERICARDIOTOMY

Recurrent pericardial effusions, usually associated with neoplastic diseases, may be treated by a **pericardiotomy** (pericardial window). The patient receives a general anesthetic, but cardiopulmonary bypass is seldom necessary. A portion of the pericardium is excised to permit the pericardial fluid to drain into the lymphatic system. Uncommonly, catheters are placed between the pericardium and abdominal cavity to drain the pericardial fluid. The nursing care is the same as that described for other cardiac surgery (see Chap. 28).

MYOCARDIAL RUPTURE

Myocardial rupture is a rare event. However, it can occur when a myocardial infarction, infectious process, cardiac trauma, pericardial disease, or other myocardial dysfunction weakens the cardiac muscle (eg, ventricular aneurysm) substantially. Persistent elevation of the ST segment is an indication of ventricular aneurysm. In many cases, the result of myocardial rupture is immediate death, even if the patient undergoes immediate cardiac surgery.

CARDIAC ARREST

Cardiac arrest occurs when the heart ceases to produce an effective pulse and blood circulation. It may be caused by a cardiac electrical event, as when the HR is too fast (especially ventricular tachycardia or ventricular fibrillation) or too slow (bradycardia or AV block) or when there is no heart rate at all (asystole). Cardiac arrest may follow respiratory arrest; it may also occur when electrical activity is present but there is ineffective cardiac contraction or circulating volume, which is called **pulseless electrical activity (PEA)**. Formerly called electrical-mechanical dissociation (EMD), PEA can be caused by hypovolemia (eg, with excessive bleeding), cardiac tamponade, hypothermia, massive pulmonary embolism, medication overdoses (eg, tricyclic agents, digitalis, beta-blockers, calcium channel blockers), significant acidosis, and massive acute myocardial infarction.

Clinical Manifestations

Consciousness, pulse, and blood pressure are lost immediately. Ineffective respiratory gasping may occur. The pupils of the eyes begin dilating within 45 seconds. Seizures may or may not occur.

The risk of irreversible brain damage and death increases with every minute from the time that circulation ceases. The interval varies with the age and underlying condition of the patient. During this period, the diagnosis of cardiac arrest must be made, and measures must be taken immediately to restore circulation.

> **! NURSING ALERT** The most reliable sign of cardiac arrest is the absence of a pulse. In the adult and the child, the carotid pulse is assessed. In an infant, the brachial pulse is assessed. Valuable time should not be wasted taking the blood pressure, listening for the heartbeat, or checking proper contact of electrodes.

Emergency Management: Cardiopulmonary Resuscitation

The ABCDs of basic cardiopulmonary resuscitation (CPR) are *a*irway, *b*reathing, *c*irculation, and *d*efibrillation (Guidelines 2000 for Cardiopulmonary Resuscitation and Emergency Cardiovascular Care, 2000). Once loss of consciousness has been established, the resuscitation priority for the adult in most cases is placing a phone call to activate the code team or the emergency medical system (EMS). Exceptions to this include near drowning, drug or medication overdose, and respiratory arrest situations, for which 1 minute of CPR should be performed before activating the EMS. Because the underlying cause of arrest in an infant or child is usually respiratory, the priority is to begin CPR and then activate the EMS after 1 minute of CPR. Because the care of the pediatric patient is individualized, the following discussion on the care of a cardiac arrest patient applies only to adults.

Resuscitation consists of the following steps:

1. Airway: maintaining an open airway
2. Breathing: providing artificial ventilation by rescue breathing
3. Circulation: promoting artificial circulation by external cardiac compression
4. Defibrillation: restoring the heartbeat (see Chap. 27)

If the patient is monitored or is immediately placed on the monitor using the multifunction pads or the quick-look paddles (found on most defibrillators) and the ECG shows ventricular tachycardia or ventricular fibrillation, defibrillation rather than CPR is the treatment of choice. In this scenario, CPR is performed initially only if the defibrillator is not immediately available. The survival rate decreases by 10% for every minute that defibrillation is delayed (Guidelines, 2000). If the patient has not been defibrillated within 10 minutes, the chance of survival is close to zero. More information on defibrillation can be found in Chapter 27.

MAINTAINING AIRWAY AND BREATHING

The first step in CPR is to obtain an open airway. Any obvious material in the mouth or throat should be removed. The chin is directed up and back, or the jaw (mandible) is lifted forward. The rescuer "looks, listens, and feels" for air movement. An oropharyngeal airway is inserted if available. Two rescue ventilations over 3 to 4 seconds are provided using a bag-mask or mouth-mask device (Fig. 30-5). An obstructed airway should be suspected when the rescuer cannot give the initial ventilations, and the Heimlich manoeuvre or abdominal thrusts should be administered to relieve the obstruction.

If the first rescue ventilations enter easily, the patient is ventilated with 12 breaths per minute, and the open airway is maintained. Endotracheal intubation is frequently performed by a physician, nurse anesthetist, or respiratory therapist during a resuscitation procedure (also called a code) to ensure an adequate airway and ventilation. The resuscitation bag device is then connected directly to the endotracheal tube.

Because of the risk of unrecognized esophageal intubation or dislodgement of the endotracheal tube (ET), tracheal intubation must be confirmed by one technique from each of two different methods: a primary method (visualization of the ET through the vocal cords, auscultation of breath sounds in five areas on the chest, or bilateral chest expansion) and a secondary method (an esophageal detector device [such as Ambu TubeChek] or an end-tidal CO_2 detector). The end-tidal CO_2 detectors available give qualitative (yes/no) or quantitative (measurable; ie, capnometry) results. Because delivery of CO_2 is low in patients in cardiopulmonary arrest, the qualitative devices are not as accurate in detecting incorrect placement as are esophageal detector devices (EDDs). There are two main types of EDD: a bulb type and a syringe type.

The bulb is collapsed or the plunger of the syringe compressed before its attachment to the ET; each creates a suction force at the end of the ET. If the ET is in the trachea, the presence of air in the lungs and the rigid walls of the trachea allow re-inflation of the bulb or aspiration of the syringe. If the ET is in the esophagus, the suction pulls on the unsupported walls of the esophagus, causing them to collapse and preventing the bulb from re-inflating or the syringe to aspirate. A chest x-ray, which is frequently obtained after ET placement, is helpful in determining whether the ET is too high, too low, or in a main bronchus. However, a chest x-ray cannot confirm placement of an ET. The ET may be in the esophagus or the trachea and result in the same appearance on the x-ray (Guidelines, 2000). Arterial blood gas levels are measured to guide oxygen therapy.

RESTORING CIRCULATION

After performing ventilation, the carotid pulse is assessed and external cardiac compressions are provided when no pulse is detected. If a defibrillator is not yet available but a process has been put into place to obtain one, chest compressions are initiated. Compressions are performed with the patient on a firm surface, such as the floor, a cardiac board, or a meal tray. The rescuer (facing the patient's side) places the heel of one hand on the lower half of the sternum, two fingerwidths (3.8 cm) from the tip of the xiphoid and positions the other hand on top of the first hand (Fig. 30-6) (Guidelines, 2000). The fingers should not touch the chest wall.

Using the body weight while keeping the elbows straight, the rescuer presses quickly downward from the shoulder area to deliver a forceful compression to the victim's lower sternum about 3.8 to 5 cm toward the spine (Guidelines, 2000). The chest compression rate is 80 to 100 times per minute. If only one rescuer is available, the rate is two ventilations to every 15 cardiac compressions. When two rescuers are available, the first person performs the cardiac compressions, pausing after the fifth compression, when the second rescuer gives one ventilation over 1.5 to 2 seconds and at a tidal volume of less than 1 L.

FIGURE 30-6 Chest compressions in cardiopulmonary resuscitation (CPR) are performed by placing the heel of one hand on the lower half of the sternum and the other hand on top of the first hand. Elbows are kept straight and body weight is used to apply quick, forceful compressions to the lower sternum. For the most effective hand placement and outcome, the patient's chest should be bare.

FIGURE 30-5 The chin lift and bag-and-mask technique for ventilating patients who need cardiopulmonary resuscitation.

Table 30-5 • Medications Used in Cardiopulmonary Resuscitation

AGENT AND ACTION	INDICATIONS	NURSING CONSIDERATIONS
Oxygen—improves tissue oxygenation and corrects hypoxemia	Administered to all patients with acute cardiac ischemia or suspected hypoxemia, including those with COPD	• Use 100% FiO_2 during resuscitation. • Recognize that no lung damage occurs when used for less than 24 hours. • Monitor dose by end-tidal CO_2 or pulse oximeter.
Epinephrine (Adrenalin)—increases systemic vascular resistance and blood pressure; improves coronary and cerebral perfusion and myocardial contractility	Given to patients in cardiac arrest, especially caused by asystole or pulseless electrical activity; may be given if caused by ventricular tachycardia or ventricular fibrillation	• Administer by IV push (IVP) or through the endotracheal (ET) tube. • Avoid adding to IV lines that contain alkaline solution (eg, bicarbonate).
Atropine—blocks parasympathetic action; increases SA node automaticity and AV conduction	Given to patients with symptomatic bradycardia (hemodynamically unstable, frequent premature ventricular contractions and symptoms of ischemia)	• Give rapidly as 2.0 to 2.5 mg IVP or through the ET tube. • Be aware that less than 0.5 mg in the adult can cause the heart rate to decrease to a worse bradycardia. • Monitor patient for reflexive tachycardia.
Sodium bicarbonate ($NaHCO_3$)—corrects metabolic acidosis	Given to correct metabolic acidosis that is refractory to standard advanced cardiac life support interventions (cardiopulmonary resuscitation, intubation, and respiratory management)	• Administer initial dose of 1 mEq/kg IV; then administer the dose based on the base deficit calculated from arterial blood gas values. • Recognize that to prevent development of rebound metabolic alkalosis, complete correction of acidosis is not indicated
Magnesium—promotes adequate functioning of the cellular sodium–potassium pump	Given to patients with torsades de pointes	• May give diluted over 1–2 min or intravenous push. • Monitor for hypotension, asystole, bradycardia, respiratory paralysis.
Vasopressin (Pitressin)—increases inotropic action (contraction) of the heart	An alternative to epinephrine when cardiac arrest is caused by ventricular tachycardia or ventricular fibrillation	• Give 40 U IV one time only.

When the code team or emergency medical personnel arrive, the patient is quickly assessed to determine cardiac rhythm and respiratory status, as well as possible causes for the arrest. The specific subsequent advanced life support interventions depend on the assessment results. For example, after the patient is placed on a cardiac monitor and ventricular fibrillation is detected, the patient will be defibrillated up to three times, and then CPR will be resumed. However, if asystole is detected on the monitor, CPR is resumed immediately while trying to identify the underlying cause, such as hypovolemia, hypothermia, or hypoxia. CPR may be stopped when the patient responds and begins to breathe, the rescuers are too exhausted or at risk (eg, the building is at risk of collapsing) to continue CPR, or signs of death are obvious. If the patient does not respond to therapies given during the arrest, the resuscitation effort may be stopped or "called" by the physician. The decision to terminate resuscitation is based on medical considerations and takes into account the underlying condition of the patient and the chances for survival.

FOLLOW-UP MONITORING

Once successfully resuscitated, the patient is transferred to an intensive care unit for close monitoring. Continuous ECG monitoring and frequent blood pressure assessments are essential until hemodynamic stability is reestablished. Etiologic factors that precipitated the arrest, such as metabolic or rhythm abnormalities, must be identified and treated. Possible contributing factors, such as electrolyte or acid-base imbalances, need to be identified and corrected. Selected medications, as described in Table 30-5, may be used during and after resuscitation.

Critical Thinking Exercises

1. Your patient is a 55-year-old man who was diagnosed last year with systolic HF (due to coronary artery disease) and was stabilized with lisinopril, Lasix, and metoprolol. He follows a low-sodium diet, with only an occasional indiscretion. He is complaining of a nagging cough. What are some of the possible causes for the cough? What would be key assessment factors that would help identify the cause? What medical treatments and nursing interventions would be appropriate for each of the possible causes?

2. A 77-year-old female patient was readmitted for HF for the third time in 2 months. Identify the factors that possibly contribute to her readmission and that would need to be assessed. What interventions could be implemented to prevent another readmission? Describe the interaction (ie, behaviours, words, and communication techniques) that would demonstrate the concept of partnering with the patient.

REFERENCES AND SELECTED READINGS
Books

Agency for Health Care Policy and Research. (1994). *Heart failure: Evaluation and care of patients with left-ventricular systolic dysfunction.* Clinical Practice Guideline Number 11. AHCPR Publication

No. 94-0612. Rockville, MD: Public Health Service, U.S. Department of Health and Human Services.

American Heart Association. (2001). *2001 Heart and stroke statistical update.* Dallas, TX: American Heart Association.

Bickley, L. S., & Szilagyi, P. G. (2003). *Bates's guide to physical examination and history taking* (8th ed.). Philadelphia: Lippincott Williams & Wilkins.

British Heart Foundation. (2002). *Coronary heart disease statistics: Heart failure supplement.* London: Author.

Braunwald, E., Zipes, D. P., & Libby, P. (2001). *Heart disease: A textbook of cardiovascular medicine* (6th ed.). Philadelphia: W. B. Saunders.

Carpenito, L. J. (1997). *Nursing diagnosis: Application to clinical practice* (7th ed.). Philadelphia: Lippincott-Raven.

Fuster, V., Alexander, R. W., & O'Rourke, R. A. (Eds.). (2001). *Hurst's the heart* (10th ed.). New York: McGraw-Hill.

Heart and Stroke Foundation of Canada. (2003). *The growing burden of heart disease and stroke.* Ottawa: Author.

Kinney, M. R., Dunbar, S. B., Brooks-Brunn, J. A., Molter, N., & Vitello-Cicciu, J. M. (1998). *AACN clinical reference for critical care nursing* (4th ed.). St. Louis: Mosby.

Murphy, J. (Ed.). (2000). *Mayo Clinic cardiology review* (2nd ed.). Philadelphia: Lippincott Williams & Wilkins.

Journals

Asterisks indicate nursing research articles.

Abraham, W. T. (2002). Multicenter InSync Randomized Clinical Evaluation (MIRACLE). Available at: http://www.acc.org/education/online/trials/acc2001/miracle.html. Accessed January 22, 2002.

Ammon, S. (2001). Managing patients with heart failure. *American Journal of Nursing, 101*(12), 34–40.

Asselin, M. E., & Cullen, H. A. (2001). What you need to know about the new ACLS guidelines: Find out about changes in algorithms and policies and how they'll affect your practice. *Nursing 2001, 31*(4), 48–50.

Barron, H. V., Every, N. R., Parsons, L. S., Angeja, B., Goldberg, R. J., & Gore, J. M., Chou, T. M., & Investigators in the National Registry of Myocardial Infarction 2. (2001). The use of intra-aortic balloon counterpulsation in patients with cardiogenic shock complicating acute myocardial infarction: Data from the National Registry of Myocardial Infarction 2. *American Heart Journal, 141*(6), 933–939.

Beckett, J. L. (1999). Endothelial dysfunction and the promise of ACE inhibitors. *American Journal of Nursing, 99*(10), 44–50.

*Bennett, S. J., Huster, G. A., Baker, S. L., Milgrom, L. B., Kirchgassner, A., Birt, J., & Pressler, M. L. (1998). Characterization of the precipitants of hospitalization for heart failure decompensation. *American Journal of Critical Care, 7*(8), 168–174.

Beta-Blocker Evaluation of Survival Trial (BEST) Investigators. (2001). A trial of the beta-blocker bucindolol in patients with advanced chronic heart failure. *New England Journal of Medicine, 344*(22), 1659–1667.

Bither, C. J., & Apple, S. (2001). Home management of the failing heart. *American Journal of Nursing, 101*(12), 41–47.

Bixby, M. B., Konick-McMahon, J., & McKenna, C. G. (2000). Applying the transitional care model to elderly patients with heart failure. *Journal of Cardiovascular Nursing, 14*(3), 53–63.

Brater, D. C. (1998). Diuretic therapy. *New England Journal of Medicine, 339*(6), 387–395.

Carelock, J., & Clark, A. P. (2001). Heart failure: Pathophysiological mechanisms. *American Journal of Nursing, 101*, 26–33.

CIBIS-II Investigators and Committees. (1999). The Cardiac Insufficiency Bisoprolol Study II (CIBIS-II): A randomized trial. *Lancet, 353*(9146), 9–13.

Clement, D. L., De Buyzere, M., Tomas, M., & Vanavermaete, G. (2000). Long-term effects of clinical outcome with low and high dose captopril in the heart insufficient patients study (CHIPS). *Acta Cardiologica, 55*(1), 1–7.

Colucci, W. S., Elkayam, U., Horton, D. P., Abraham, W. T., Bourge, R. C., Johnson, A. D., Wagoner, L. E., Givertz, M. M., Liang, C. S., Neibaur, M., Haught, W. H., & LeJemtel, T. H. (2000). Intravenous nesiritide, a natriuretic peptide, in the treatment of decompensated heart failure. Nesiritide Study Group. *New England Journal of Medicine, 343*(4), 246–253.

The CONSENSUS Trial Study Group. (1987). Effects of enalapril on mortality in severe congestive heart failure: Results of the Cooperative North Scandinavian Enalapril Survival Study (CONSENSUS). *New England Journal of Medicine, 316*(23), 1429–1435.

Cook, D. M. (1993). The use of central nervous manifestations in the early detection of digitalis toxicity. *Heart & Lung, 22*(6), 477–480.

DeWald, T., Gaulden L., Beyler, M., Whellan, D., & Bowers, M. (2000). Current trends in the management of heart failure. *Nursing Clinics of North America, 35*(4), 855–875.

The Digitalis Investigation Group (DIG). (1997). The effect of digoxin on mortality and morbidity in patients with heart failure. *New England Journal of Medicine, 336*(8), 525–533.

Georgiou, D., Chen, Y., Appadoo, S., Belardinelli, R., Greene, R., Parides, M., & Glied, S. (2001). Cost-effectiveness analysis of long-term moderate exercise training in chronic heart failure. *American Journal of Cardiology, 87*(8), 984–988.

Gerber, T. C., Nishimura, R. A., Holmes, D. R., Jr., Lloyd, M. A., Zehr, K. J., Tajik, A. J., & Hayes, D. L. (2001). Left ventricular and biventricular pacing in congestive heart failure. *Mayo Clinic Proceedings, 76*(8), 803–812.

Guidelines 2000 for Cardiopulmonary Resuscitation and Emergency Cardiovascular Care: The American Heart Association in collaboration with the International Liaison Committee on Resuscitation. *Circulation, 102*(8)(Suppl. 8), I1–384.

Halm, M. A., & Penque, S. (1999). Heart disease in women. *American Journal of Nursing, 99*(4), 26–32.

*Happ, M. B., Naylor, M. D., & Roe-Prior, P. (1997). Factors contributing to rehospitalization of elderly patients with heart failure. *Journal of Cardiovascular Nursing, 11*(4), 75–84.

Haldeman, G. A., Croft, J. B., et al. (1999). Hospitalization of patients with heart failure: National Hospital Discharge Survey 1985 to 1995. *American Heart Journal 137*(2), 352–360.

Hunt, S. A., Baker, D. W., Chin, M. H., Cinquegrani, M. P., Feldman, A. M., Francis, G. S., Ganiats, T. G., Goldstein, S., Gregoratos, G., Jessup, M. L., Noble, R. J., Packer, M., Silver, M. A., Stevenson, L. W., Gibbons, R. J., Antman, E. M., Alpert, J. S., Faxon, D. P., Fuster, V., Gregoratos, G., Jacobs, A. K., Hiratzka, L. F., Russell, R. O., Smith, S. C., Jr., American College of Cardiology/American Heart Association Task Force on Practice Guidelines (Committee to Revise the 1995 Guidelines for the Evaluation and Management of Heart Failure), International Society for Heart and Lung Transplantation, & Heart Failure Society of America. (2001). ACC/AHA guidelines for the evaluation and management of chronic heart failure in the adult: A report of the American College of Cardiology/American Heart Association Task Force on Practice Guidelines (Committee to Revise the 1995 Guidelines for the Evaluation and Management of Heart Failure). *Journal of the American College of Cardiology, 38*(7), 2101–2113.

*Jaarsma, T., Halfens, R., Tan, F., Abu-Saad, H., Dracup, K., & Diederiks, J. (2000). Self-care and quality of life in patients with advanced heart failure: The effect of a supportive educational intervention. *Heart & Lung, 29*(5), 319–330.

Johansen, H., Strauss, B., et al. (2003). On the rise: The current and projected future burden of congestive heart failure hospitalization in Canada. *Canadian Journal of Cardiology, 19*(4), 430–435.

Lee, D., Johansen, H., et al. (2004). Canadian Cardiovascular Outcomes Research Team: Regional outcomes of heart failure in Canada. *Canadian Journal of Cardiology, 20*(6), 599–607.

Mancini, M. E., & Kaye, W. (1999). AEDs. Changing the way you respond to cardiac arrest. *American Journal of Nursing, 99*(5), 26–30.

McCullough, P. A., Philbin, E. F., Spertus, J. A., et al. (2002). Confirmation of a heart failure epidemic: Findings from the Resource Utilization Among Congestive Heart Failure (REACH) study. *Journal of the American College of Cardiology, 39*(1), 60–69.

MERIT-HF Study Group. (1999). Effect of metoprolol CR/XL in chronic heart failure: Metoprolol CR/XL randomized intervention trial in congestive heart failure (MERIT-HF). *Lancet, 353,* 2001–2007.

Meyer, K. (2001). Exercise training in heart failure: Recommendations based on current research. *Medicine and Science in Sports and Exercise, 33*(4), 525–531.

The NETWORK Investigators. (1998). Clinical outcome with enalapril in symptomatic chronic heart failure: A dose comparison. *European Heart Journal, 19*(3), 481–489.

Packer, M. (2000). *Carvedilol improves survival in patients with advanced heart failure: Results of the COPERNICUS study.* Presented at the 4th Scientific Meeting of the Heart Failure Society of America, Boca Raton, FL, September 10–13.

Packer, M., Bristow, M. R., Cohn, J. N., Colucci, W. S., Fowler, M. B., Gilbert, E. M., & Shusterman, N. H. (1996). The effect of carvedilol on morbidity and mortality in patients with chronic heart failure. U.S. Carvedilol Heart Failure Study Group. *New England Journal of Medicine, 334*(21), 1349–1355.

Packer, M., Coats, A. J. S., Fowler, M. B., Katus, H. A., Krum, H., Mohacsi, P., Rouleau, J. L., Tendera, M., Castaigne, A., Roecker, E. B., Schultz, M. K., DeMets, D. L., & Carvedilol Prospective Randomized Cumulative Survival Study Group. (2001). Effect of carvedilol on survival in severe chronic heart failure. *New England Journal of Medicine, 344* (22), 1651–1658.

Packer, M., Poole-Wilson, P. A., & Armstrong, P. W. (1999). Comparative effects of low and high doses of the angiotensin-converting enzyme inhibitor, lisinopril, on morbidity and mortality in chronic heart failure. ATLAS Study Group. *Circulation, 100*(23), 2312–2318.

Page, J., & Henry, D. (2000). Consumption of NSAIDs and the development of congestive heart failure in the elderly. *Archives of Internal Medicine, 160*(6), 777–784.

Pitt, B., Zannad, F., Remme, W. J., Cody, R., Castaigre, A., Perez, A., Palensky, J., & Wittes, J. (1999). The effect of spironolactone on morbidity and mortality in patients with severe heart failure. *New England Journal of Medicine, 341*(10), 709–717.

Rich, M. W., Beckham, V., Wittenberg, C., Leven, C. L., Freedland, K. E., Carney, R. M. (1995). A multidisciplinary intervention to prevent the readmission of elderly patients with congestive heart failure. *New England Journal of Medicine, 333*(18), 1190–1195.

*Riegle, B., Carlson, B., & Glaser, D. (2000). Developing and testing a clinical tool measuring self-management of heart failure. *Heart & Lung, 29*(1), 4–12.

Sanderson, J. E., Chan, S. K., Yip, G., Yeung, L. Y., Chan, K. W., Raymond, K., & Woo, K. S. (1999). Beta-blockade in heart failure: A comparison of carvedilol with metoprolol. *Journal of American College of Cardiology, 34*(5), 1522–1528.

Shamsham, F., & Mitchell, J. (2000). Essentials of the diagnosis of heart failure. *American Family Physician, 61*(5), 1319–1328.

The SOLVD Investigators. (1992). Effect of enalapril on mortality and the development of heart failure in asymptomatic patients with reduced left ventricular ejection fractions. *New England Journal of Medicine, 327*(10), 685–691.

Statistics Canada. (2002). Population by age group, CANSIM II, Table 051-001. Available at: http:www.statca.ca. Retrieved January 3, 2005.

*Ströberg, A., Broströ, A., Dahlström, U., & Fridlund, B. (1999). Factors influencing patient compliance with therapeutic regimens in chronic heart failure: A critical incident technique analysis. *Heart & Lung, 28*(5), 334–341.

*Stull, D., Starling, R., Hass, G., & Young, J. B. (1999). Becoming a patient with heart failure. *Heart & Lung, 28*(4), 284–292.

Tsuyuki, R. T., Shibata, M. S., et al. (2003). Burden of illness of congestive heart failure in Canada. *Canadian Journal of Cardiology, 19*(4), 436–438.

Turner, M. A. (2000). Impedance cardiography: A noninvasive way to monitor hemodynamics. *Dimensions in Critical Care Nursing, 19*(3), 2–12.

Uretsky, B. F., Young, J. B., Shahidi, F. E., Yellen, L. G., Harrison, M. C., & Jolly, M. K. (1993). Randomized study assessing the effect of digoxin withdrawal in patients with mild to moderate chronic congestive heart failure: Results of the PROVED trial. PROVED Investigative Group. *Journal of American College of Cardiology, 22*(4), 955–962.

Vasan, R. S., & Levy, K. (2000). Defining diastolic heart failure. *Circulation, 101*(17), 2118–2121.

Von Rueden, K. T., & Turner, M. (1999). Advances in continuous, noninvasive hemodynamic surveillance. *Critical Care Nursing Clinics of North America, 11*(1), 63–75.

Webb, J. G., Sanborn, T. A., Sleeper, L. A., Carere, R. G., Buller, C. E., Slater, J. N., Baran, K. W., Koller, P. T., Talley, J. D., Porway, M., Hochman, J. S., & SHOCK Investigators. (2001). Percutaneous coronary intervention for cardiogenic shock in the SHOCK Trial Registry. *American Heart Journal, 141*(6), 964–970.

Weber, K. T. (2001). Mechanisms of disease: Aldosterone in congestive heart failure. *New England Journal of Medicine, 345*(23), 1689–1697.

RESOURCES AND WEBSITES

Canadian Association of Cardiac Rehabilitation (CACR), 1390 Taylor Avenue, Winnipeg, MB R3M 3V8; 204-488-5854; http://www.cacr.ca.

Canadian Cardiovascular Society, 222 Queen Street, Suite 1403, Ottawa, ON K1P 5V9; 613-569-3407; http://www.ccs.ca.

Heart and Stroke Foundation of Canada, 222 Queen Street, Suite 1402, Ottawa, ON K1P 5V9; http://ww1.heartandstroke.ca.

Assessment and Management of Patients With Vascular Disorders and Problems of Peripheral Circulation

Adapted by Joe Noon

LEARNING OBJECTIVES ●

On completion of this chapter, the learner will be able to:

1. Identify anatomic and physiologic factors that affect peripheral blood flow and tissue oxygenation.
2. Use appropriate parameters for assessment of peripheral circulation.
3. Use the nursing process as a framework of care for patients with circulatory insufficiency of the extremities.
4. Compare the various diseases of the arteries, their causes, pathologic and physiologic changes, clinical manifestations, management, and prevention.
5. Describe the prevention and management of venous thrombosis.
6. Compare the preventive management of venous insufficiency, leg ulcers, and varicose veins.
7. Use the nursing process as a framework of care for patients with leg ulcers.
8. Describe the relationship between lymphangitis and lymphedema.

*A*dequate perfusion oxygenates and nourishes body tissues and depends in part on a properly functioning cardiovascular system. Adequate blood flow depends on the efficient pumping action of the heart, patent and responsive blood vessels, and adequate circulating blood volume. Nervous system activity, blood viscosity, and the metabolic needs of tissues influence the rate and adequacy of blood flow.

Anatomic and Physiologic Overview

The vascular system consists of two interdependent systems. The right side of the heart pumps blood through the lungs to the pulmonary circulation, and the left side of the heart pumps blood to all other body tissues through the systemic circulation. The blood vessels in both systems channel the blood from the heart to the tissues and back to the heart (Fig. 31-1). Contraction of the ventricles is the driving force that moves blood through the vascular systems.

Arteries distribute oxygenated blood from the left side of the heart to the tissues, whereas the veins carry deoxygenated blood from the tissues to the right side of the heart. Capillary vessels, located within the tissues, connect the arterial and venous systems and are the site of exchange of nutrients and metabolic wastes between the circulatory system and the tissues. Arterioles and venules immediately adjacent to the capillaries, together with the capillaries, make up the microcirculation.

The lymphatic system complements the function of the circulatory system. Lymphatic vessels transport lymph (a fluid similar to plasma), and tissue fluids (containing smaller proteins, cells, and cellular debris) from the interstitial space to systemic veins.

ANATOMY OF THE VASCULAR SYSTEM

Arteries and Arterioles

Arteries are thick-walled structures that carry blood from the heart to the tissues. The aorta, which has a diameter of approximately 25 mm, gives rise to numerous branches, which divide into smaller arteries that are about 4 mm in diameter by the time they reach the tissues. Within the tissues, the vessels divide

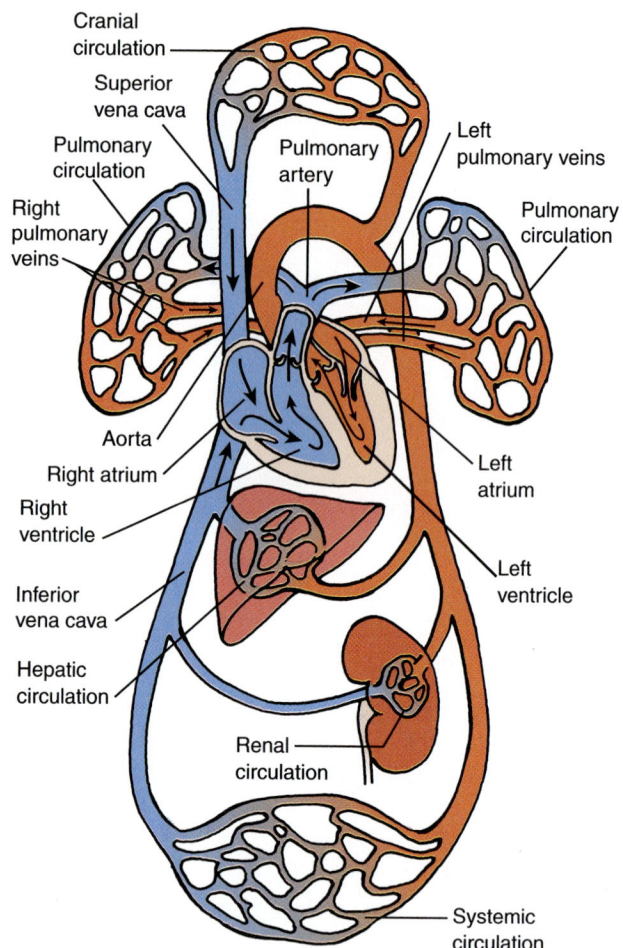

FIGURE 31-1 Systemic and pulmonary circulation. Oxygen-rich blood from the pulmonary circulation is pumped from the left heart into the aorta and the systemic arteries to the capillaries, where the exchange of nutrients and waste products takes place. The deoxygenated blood returns to the right heart by way of the systemic veins and is pumped into the pulmonary circulation. From *Stedman's Medical Dictionary* (27th ed.). (2000). Philadelphia: Lippincott Williams & Wilkins.

Glossary

anastomosis: surgical junction of two vessels

aneurysm: a localized sac or dilation of an artery formed at a weak point in the vessel wall

ankle-brachial index (ABI) or **ankle-arm index (AAI):** ratio of the ankle systolic pressure to the arm systolic pressure; an objective measurement of arterial disease that provides quantification of the degree of stenosis

angioplasty: an invasive procedure that uses a balloon-tipped catheter to dilate a stenotic area of a blood vessel

arteriosclerosis: diffuse process whereby the muscle fibres and the endothelial lining of the walls of small arteries and arterioles thicken

atherosclerosis: disease process involving the accumulation of lipids, calcium, blood components, carbohydrates, and fibrous tissue on the intimal layer of a large or medium-sized artery

bruit: sound produced by turbulent blood flow through an irregular, tortuous, stenotic, or dilated vessel

dissection: separation of the weakened elastic and fibromuscular elements in the medial layer of an artery

duplex ultrasonography: combines B-mode grey-scale imaging of tissue, organs, and blood vessels with capabilities of estimating velocity changes by use of a pulsed Doppler

intermittent claudication: a muscular, cramp-like pain in the extremities con-

sistently reproduced with the same degree of exercise or activity and relieved by rest

international normalized ratio (INR): method of measuring anticoagulation levels, such as warfarin (Coumadin); devised to bring a universal standard to monitoring of anticoagulation achieved by oral medications

ischemia: deficient blood supply

rest pain: persistent pain in the foot or digits when the patient is resting, indicating a severe degree of arterial insufficiency

rubor: reddish blue discolouration of the extremities; indicative of severe peripheral arterial damage in vessels that remain dilated and unable to constrict

stenosis: narrowing or constriction of a vessel

further, diminishing to approximately 30 μm in diameter; these vessels are called arterioles.

The walls of the arteries and arterioles are composed of three layers: the intima, an inner endothelial cell layer; the media, a middle layer of smooth elastic tissue; and the adventitia, an outer layer of connective tissue. The intima, a very thin layer, provides a smooth surface for contact with the flowing blood, and produces various compounds that locally cause vessels to constrict or dilate. The media makes up most of the vessel wall in the aorta and other large arteries of the body. This layer is composed chiefly of elastic and connective tissue fibres that give the vessels considerable strength and allow them to constrict and dilate to accommodate the blood ejected from the heart (stroke volume) and maintain an even, steady flow of blood. The adventitia is a layer of connective tissue that anchors the vessel to its surroundings. There is much less elastic tissue in the smaller arteries and arterioles, and the media in these vessels is composed primarily of smooth muscle.

Smooth muscle controls the diameter of the vessels by contracting and relaxing. Chemical, hormonal, and nervous system factors influence the activity of smooth muscle. Because arterioles can alter their diameter, thereby offering resistance to blood flow, they are often referred to as *resistance vessels*. Arterioles regulate the volume and pressure in the arterial system and the rate of blood flow to the capillaries. Because of the large amount of muscle, the walls of the arteries are relatively thick, accounting for approximately 25% of the total diameter of the artery. The walls of the arterioles account for approximately 67% of the total diameter of arterioles.

The intima and the inner third of the smooth muscle layer are in such close contact with the blood that the blood vessel receives its nourishment by direct diffusion. The adventitia and the outer media layers have a limited vascular system for nourishment and require their own blood supply to meet metabolic needs.

Capillaries

Capillary walls, which lack smooth muscle and adventitia, are composed of a single layer of endothelial cells. This thin-walled structure permits rapid and efficient transport of nutrients to the cells and removal of metabolic wastes. The diameter of capillaries ranges from 5 to 10 μm; this narrow channel requires red blood cells to alter their shape to pass through these vessels. Changes in a capillary's diameter are passive and are influenced by contractile changes in the blood vessels that carry blood to and from a capillary. The capillary's diameter also changes in response to chemical stimuli. In some tissues, a cuff of smooth muscle, called the precapillary sphincter, is located at the arteriolar end of the capillary and is responsible, along with the arteriole, for controlling capillary blood flow.

Some capillary beds, such as in the fingertips, contain arteriovenous anastomoses, through which blood passes directly from the arterial to the venous system. These vessels are believed to regulate heat exchange between the body and the external environment.

The distribution of capillaries varies with the type of tissue. For example, skeletal tissue, which is metabolically active, has a denser capillary network than does cartilage, which is less active.

Veins and Venules

Capillaries join to form larger vessels called venules, which join to form veins. The venous system is therefore structurally analogous to the arterial system; venules correspond to arterioles, veins to arteries, and the vena cava to the aorta. Analogous types of vessels in the arterial and venous systems have approximately the same diameters (see Fig. 31-1).

The walls of the veins, in contrast to those of the arteries, are thinner and considerably less muscular. The wall of the average vein amounts to only 10% of the vein diameter, in contrast to 25% in the artery. The walls of a vein, like those of arteries, are composed of three layers, although these layers are not as well defined.

The thin, less muscular structure of the vein wall allows these vessels to distend more than arteries. Greater distensibility and compliance permit large volumes of blood to be stored in the veins under low pressure. For this reason, veins are referred to as *capacitance vessels*. Approximately 75% of total blood volume is contained in the veins. The sympathetic nervous system, which innervates the vein musculature, can stimulate the veins to constrict (venoconstriction), thereby reducing venous volume and increasing the volume of blood in the general circulation. Contraction of skeletal muscles in the extremities creates the primary pumping action to facilitate venous blood flow back to the heart.

Some veins, unlike arteries, are equipped with valves. In general, veins that transport blood against the force of gravity, as in the lower extremities, have one-way bicuspid valves that interrupt the column of blood to prevent blood from seeping backward as it is propelled toward the heart. Valves are composed of endothelial leaflets, the competency of which depends on the integrity of the vein wall.

Lymphatic Vessels

The lymphatic vessels are a complex network of thin-walled vessels similar to the blood capillaries. This network collects lymphatic fluid from tissues and organs and transports the fluid to the venous circulation. The lymphatic vessels converge into two main structures: the thoracic duct and the right lymphatic duct. These ducts empty into the junction of the subclavian and the internal jugular veins. The right lymphatic duct conveys lymph primarily from the right side of the head, neck, thorax, and upper arms. The thoracic duct conveys lymph from the remainder of the body. Peripheral lymphatic vessels join larger lymph vessels and pass through regional lymph nodes before entering the venous circulation. The lymph nodes play an important role in filtering foreign particles.

The lymphatic vessels are permeable to large molecules and provide the only means by which interstitial proteins can return to the venous system. With muscular contraction, lymph vessels become distorted to create spaces between the endothelial cells, allowing protein and particles to enter. Muscular contraction of the lymphatic walls and surrounding tissues aids in propelling the lymph toward the venous drainage points.

FUNCTION OF THE VASCULAR SYSTEM
Circulatory Needs of Tissues

The amount of blood flow needed by body tissues constantly changes. The percentage of blood flow received by individual organs or tissues is determined by the rate of tissue metabolism, the availability of oxygen, and the function of the tissues (Table 31-1). When metabolic requirements increase, blood vessels dilate to increase the flow of oxygen and nutrients to the tissues. When metabolic needs decrease, vessels constrict, and blood flow to the tissues decreases. Metabolic demands of tissues increase with physical activity or exercise, local heat application, fever, and infection. Reduced metabolic requirements of tissues accompany rest or decreased physical activity, local cold application, and

Table 31-1 • Blood Flow and Oxygen Consumption for Selected Human Organs

Organ	Organ Weight (kg)	BLOOD FLOW DURING REST		OXYGEN USAGE DURING REST	
		Organ Blood Flow (mL/min)	% Total Cardiac Output	Organ O$_2$ Usage (mL/min)	% Total O$_2$ Usage
Brain	1.4	750	14	45	18
Heart	0.3	250	5	25	10
Liver	1.5	1300	23	75	30
GI tract	2.5	1000			
Kidneys	0.3	1200	22	15	6
Muscle	35.0	1000	18	50	20
Skin	2.0	200	4	5	2
Remainder (eg, skeleton, bone marrow, fat, connective tissue)	27.0	800	14	35	14
TOTAL	70	6500	100	250	100

Folkow B., & Neil E. *Circulation.* New York: Oxford University Press.

cooling of the body. If the blood vessels fail to dilate in response to the need for increased blood flow, tissue **ischemia** (ie, deficient blood supply to a body part) results. The mechanism by which blood vessels dilate and constrict to adjust for metabolic changes ensures that normal arterial pressure is maintained.

As blood passes through tissue capillaries, oxygen is removed, and carbon dioxide is added. The amount of oxygen extracted by each tissue differs. For example, the myocardium tends to extract about 50% of the oxygen from arterial blood in one pass through its capillary bed, whereas the kidneys extract only about 7% of the oxygen from the blood that passes through them. The average amount of oxygen removed collectively by all of the body tissues is about 25%. This means that the blood in the vena cavae contains about 25% less oxygen than aortic blood. This is known as the *systemic arteriovenous oxygen difference.* The value increases when the amount of oxygen delivered to the tissues is decreased relative to their metabolic needs (see Table 31-1).

Blood Flow

Blood flow through the cardiovascular system always proceeds in the same direction: left side of the heart to the aorta, arteries, arterioles, capillaries, venules, veins, vena cavae, and right side of the heart. This unidirectional flow is caused by a pressure difference that exists between the arterial and venous systems. Because arterial pressure (approximately 100 mm Hg) is greater than venous pressure (approximately 4 mm Hg) and fluid always flows from an area of high pressure to an area of lower pressure, blood flows from the arterial to the venous system.

The pressure difference (ΔP) between the two ends of the vessel provides the impetus for the forward propulsion of blood. Impediments to blood flow offer the opposing force, which is known as resistance (R). The rate of blood flow is determined by dividing the pressure difference by the resistance:

$$\text{Flow rate} = \Delta P/R$$

This equation clearly shows that, when resistance increases, a greater driving pressure is required to maintain the same degree of flow. In the body, an increase in driving pressure is accomplished by an increase in the force of contraction of the heart. If arterial resistance is chronically elevated, the myocardium of the left ventricle hypertrophies (enlarges) to sustain the greater contractile force.

In most long smooth blood vessels, flow is laminar or streamlined, with blood in the centre of the vessel moving slightly faster than the blood near the vessel walls. Laminar flow becomes turbulent when the blood flow rate increases, when blood viscosity increases, when the diameter of the vessel becomes greater than normal, or when segments of the vessel are narrowed or constricted. Turbulent blood flow creates a sound, called a **bruit**, that can be auscultated with a stethoscope.

Blood Pressure

Chapters 26 and 32 provide more information on the physiology and measurement of blood pressure.

Capillary Filtration and Reabsorption

Fluid exchange across the capillary wall is continuous. This fluid, which has the same composition as plasma without the proteins, forms the interstitial fluid. The equilibrium between hydrostatic and osmotic forces of the blood and interstitium, as well as capillary permeability, governs the amount and direction of fluid movement across the capillary. Hydrostatic force is a driving pressure that is generated by the blood pressure. Osmotic pressure is the pulling force created by plasma proteins. Normally, the hydrostatic pressure at the arterial end of the capillary is relatively high compared with that at the venous end. This high pressure at the arterial end of the capillaries tends to drive fluid out of the capillary and into the tissue space. Osmotic pressure tends to pull fluid back into the capillary from the tissue space, but this osmotic force cannot overcome the high hydrostatic pressure at the arterial end of the capillary. At the venous end of the capillary, however, the osmotic force predominates over the low hydrostatic pressure, and there is a net reabsorption of fluid from the tissue space back into the capillary.

Except for a very small amount, fluid that is filtered out at the arterial end of the capillary bed is reabsorbed at the venous end. The excess filtered fluid enters the lymphatic circulation. These processes of filtration, reabsorption, and lymph formation aid in maintaining tissue fluid volume and removing tissue waste and debris. Under normal conditions, capillary permeability remains constant.

Under certain abnormal conditions, the fluid filtered out of the capillaries may greatly exceed the amounts reabsorbed and carried away by the lymphatic vessels. This imbalance can result from damage to capillary walls and subsequent increased permeability, obstruction of lymphatic drainage, elevation of venous pressure, or decrease in plasma protein osmotic force. The accumulation of fluid that results from these processes is known as *edema*.

Hemodynamic Resistance

The most important factor that determines resistance in the vascular system is the vessel radius. Small changes in vessel radius lead to large changes in resistance. The predominant sites of change in the calibre or width of blood vessels, and therefore in resistance, are the arterioles and the precapillary sphincter. Peripheral vascular resistance is the opposition to blood flow provided by the blood vessels. Poiseuille's law provides the method by which resistance can be calculated:

$$R = 8\theta L/\pi r^4$$

where R = resistance, r = radius of the vessel, L = length of the vessel, θ = viscosity of the blood, and $8/\pi$ = a constant. This equation shows that the resistance is proportional to the viscosity or thickness of the blood and the length of the vessel but is inversely proportional to the fourth power of the vessel radius.

Under normal conditions, blood viscosity and vessel length do not change significantly, and these factors do not usually play an important role in blood flow. A large increase in hematocrit, however, may increase blood viscosity and reduce capillary blood flow.

Peripheral Vascular Regulating Mechanisms

Because the metabolic needs of body tissues, even at rest, are continuously changing, an integrated and coordinated regulatory system is necessary so that blood flow to individual areas is maintained in proportion to the needs of that area. As might be expected, this regulatory mechanism is complex and consists of central nervous system influences, circulating hormones and chemicals, and independent activity of the arterial wall itself.

Sympathetic (adrenergic) nervous system activity, mediated by the hypothalamus, is the most important factor in regulating the calibre and therefore the blood flow of peripheral blood vessels. All vessels are innervated by the sympathetic nervous system except the capillary and precapillary sphincters. Stimulation of the sympathetic nervous system causes vasoconstriction. The neurotransmitter responsible for sympathetic vasoconstriction is norepinephrine. Sympathetic activation occurs in response to physiologic and psychological stressors. Diminution of sympathetic activity by medications or sympathectomy results in vasodilation.

Other hormonal substances affect peripheral vascular resistance. Epinephrine, released from the adrenal medulla, acts like norepinephrine in constricting peripheral blood vessels in most tissue beds. In low concentrations, however, epinephrine causes vasodilation in skeletal muscles, the heart, and the brain. Angiotensin, a potent substance formed from the interaction of renin (synthesized by the kidney) and a circulating serum protein, stimulates arterial constriction. Although the amount of angiotensin concentrated in the blood is usually small, its profound vasoconstrictor effects are important in certain abnormal states, such as heart failure and hypovolemia.

Alterations in local blood flow are influenced by various circulating substances that have vasoactive properties. Potent vasodilators produced by the vascular endothelium include nitric oxide (NO), histamine, bradykinin, prostaglandin, and certain muscle metabolites. Potent vasoconstrictors produced by the vascular endothelium include endothelin (ET), angiotensin II, and vasoconstrictor prostaglandins. Nitric oxide also has anti-aggregatory effects on platelets, whereas endothelin causes them to aggregate. Thus, endothelial vasoactive agents have subluminal and intraluminal effects. A reduction in available oxygen and nutrients and changes in local pH also affect local blood flow. Serotonin, a substance liberated from platelets that aggregate at the site of vessel wall damage, constricts arterioles. The application of heat to parts of the body surface causes local vasodilation, whereas the application of cold causes vasoconstriction.

PATHOPHYSIOLOGY OF THE VASCULAR SYSTEM

Reduced blood flow through peripheral blood vessels characterizes all peripheral vascular diseases. The physiologic effects of altered blood flow depend on the extent to which tissue demands exceed the supply of oxygen and nutrients available. If tissue needs are high, even modestly reduced blood flow may be inadequate to maintain tissue integrity. Tissues then fall prey to ischemia (deficient blood supply), become malnourished, and ultimately die if adequate blood flow is not restored.

Pump Failure

Inadequate peripheral blood flow occurs when the heart's pumping action becomes inefficient. Left ventricular failure causes an accumulation of blood in the lungs and a reduction in forward flow or cardiac output, which results in inadequate arterial blood flow to the tissues. Right ventricular failure causes systemic venous congestion and a reduction in forward flow (see Chap. 30).

Alterations in Blood and Lymphatic Vessels

Intact, patent, and responsive blood vessels are necessary to deliver adequate amounts of oxygen to tissues and to remove metabolic wastes. Arteries can become obstructed by atherosclerotic plaque, a thrombus, or an embolus. They become less compliant ("stiffer") with age (see below), a process that is accelerated in cardiovascular diseases. Arteries can become damaged or obstructed as a result of chemical or mechanical trauma, infections or inflammatory processes, vasospastic disorders, and congenital malformations. A sudden arterial occlusion causes profound and often irreversible tissue ischemia and tissue death. When arterial occlusions develop gradually, there is less risk for sudden tissue death because collateral circulation has an opportunity to develop and the body adapts to the decreased blood flow.

Venous blood flow can be reduced by a thrombus obstructing the vein, by incompetent venous valves, or by a reduction in the effectiveness of the pumping action of surrounding muscles. Decreased venous blood flow results in increased venous pressure, a subsequent rise in capillary hydrostatic pressure, net filtration of fluid out of the capillaries into the interstitial space, and subsequent edema. Edematous tissues cannot receive adequate nutrition from the blood and consequently are more susceptible to breakdown, injury, and infection. Obstruction of lymphatic vessels also results in edema. Lymphatic vessels can become obstructed by tumour or by damage resulting from mechanical trauma or inflammatory processes.

🌾 Gerontologic Considerations

Aging produces changes in the walls of the blood vessels that affect the transport of oxygen and nutrients to the tissues. The intima thickens as a result of cellular proliferation and fibrosis. Elastin fibres of the media become calcified, thin, and fragmented, and collagen accumulates in the intima and the media. These changes cause the vessels to stiffen, which results in increased peripheral resistance, impaired blood flow, and increased left ventricular workload.

Circulatory Insufficiency of the Extremities

Although many types of peripheral vascular diseases exist, most result in ischemia and produce some of the same symptoms: pain, skin changes, diminished pulse, and possible edema. The type and severity of symptoms depend in part on the type, stage, and extent of the disease process and on the speed with which the disorder develops. Table 31-2 highlights the distinguishing features of arterial and venous insufficiency. In this chapter, peripheral vascular disease is categorized as arterial, venous, or lymphatic disorders.

Assessment

HEALTH HISTORY AND CLINICAL MANIFESTATIONS

A description of the pain and any precipitating factors, the skin colour and temperature, and the peripheral pulses are important for the diagnosis of arterial disorders.

Intermittent Claudication

A muscular, cramp-type pain in the extremities consistently reproduced with the same degree of exercise or activity and relieved by rest is experienced by patients with peripheral arterial insufficiency. Referred to as **intermittent claudication**, this pain is caused by the inability of the arterial system to provide adequate blood flow to the tissues in the face of increased demands for nutrients during exercise. As the tissues are forced to complete the energy cycle without the nutrients, muscle metabolites and lactic acid are produced. Pain is experienced as the metabolites aggravate the nerve endings of the surrounding tissue. Usually, about 50% of the arterial lumen or 75% of the cross-sectional area must be obstructed before intermittent claudication is experienced. When the patient rests and thereby decreases the metabolic needs of the muscles, the pain subsides. The progression of the arterial disease can be monitored by documenting the amount of exercise or the distance a patient can walk before pain is produced. Persistent pain in the forefoot when the patient is resting indicates a severe degree of arterial insufficiency and a critical state of ischemia. Known as **rest pain**, this discomfort is often worse at night and may interfere with sleep. This pain frequently requires that the extremity be lowered to a dependent position to improve perfusion pressure to the distal tissues.

The site of arterial disease can be deduced from the location of claudication, because pain occurs in muscle groups below the disease. As a general rule, the pain of intermittent claudication occurs one joint level below the disease process. Calf pain may accompany reduced blood flow through the superficial femoral or popliteal artery, whereas pain in the hip or buttock may result from reduced blood flow in the abdominal aorta or the common iliac or hypogastric arteries.

Changes in Skin Appearance and Temperature

Adequate blood flow warms the extremities and gives them a rosy colouring. Inadequate blood flow results in cool and pale extremities. Further reduction of blood flow to these tissues, which occurs when the extremity is elevated, for example, results in an even whiter or more blanched appearance (pallor). **Rubor**, a reddish blue discolouration of the extremities, may be observed within 20 seconds to 2 minutes after the extremity is dependent. Rubor suggests severe peripheral arterial damage in which vessels that cannot constrict remain dilated. Even with rubor, the extremity begins to turn pale with elevation. Cyanosis, a bluish tint on the skin, is manifested when the amount of oxygenated hemoglobin contained in the blood is reduced.

Additional changes resulting from a chronically reduced nutrient supply include loss of hair, brittle nails, dry or scaling skin, atrophy, and ulcerations. Edema may be apparent bilaterally or unilaterally and is related to the affected extremity's chronically dependent position because of severe rest pain. Gangrenous changes appear after prolonged, severe ischemia and represent tissue necrosis. In elderly patients who are inactive, gangrene may be the first sign of disease. These patients may have adjusted their lifestyle to accommodate the limitations imposed by the disease, and may not walk far enough to develop symptoms of claudication. Circulation is decreased, but this is not apparent to the patient until trauma occurs. At this point, gangrene develops when minimal arterial flow is impaired further by edema formation resulting from the traumatic event.

Table 31-2 • Characteristics of Arterial and Venous Insufficiency

CHARACTERISTIC	ARTERIAL	VENOUS
Pain	Intermittent claudication to sharp, unrelenting, constant	Aching, cramping
Pulses	Diminished or absent	Present, but may be difficult to palpate through edema
Skin characteristics	Dependent rubor—elevation pallor of foot, dry, shiny skin, cool-to-cold temperature, loss of hair over toes and dorsum of foot, nails thickened and ridged	Pigmentation in gaitor area (area of medial and lateral malleolus), skin thickened and tough, may be reddish blue, frequently with associated dermatitis
Ulcer characteristics		
Location	Tip of toes, toe webs, heel or other pressure areas if confined to bed	Medial malleolus; infrequently lateral malleolus or anterior tibial area
Pain	Very painful	Minimal pain if superficial or may be very painful
Depth of ulcer	Deep, often involving joint space	Superficial
Shape	Circular	Irregular border
Ulcer base	Pale to black and dry gangrene	Granulation tissue—beefy red to yellow fibrinous in chronic long-term ulcer
Leg edema	Minimal unless extremity kept in dependent position constantly to relieve pain	Moderate to severe

Pulses

Determining the presence or absence, as well as the quality, of peripheral pulses is important in assessing the status of peripheral arterial circulation (Fig. 31-2). Absence of a pulse may indicate that the site of **stenosis** (narrowing or constriction) is proximal to that location. Occlusive arterial disease impairs blood flow and can reduce or obliterate palpable pulsations in the extremities. Pulses should be palpated bilaterally and simultaneously, comparing both sides for symmetry in rate, rhythm, and quality.

Gerontologic Considerations

In elderly people, symptoms of peripheral arterial disease may be more pronounced than in younger people because of the condition's duration and coexisting chronic disease. Intermittent claudication may occur after walking only a few short blocks or after walking up a slight incline. Any prolonged pressure on the foot can cause pressure areas that become ulcerated, infected, and gangrenous. The outcomes of arterial insufficiency in the elderly person include reduced mobility and activity and a loss of independence.

Diagnostic Evaluation

In identifying and diagnosing the various abnormalities affecting the vascular structures (arteries, veins, and lymphatics), various tests may be performed.

DOPPLER ULTRASOUND FLOW STUDIES

Palpating pulses is subjective, and the examiner may mistake his or her own pulse for that of the patient. To prevent this, the examiner should use light touch and avoid using only the index finger for palpation, because this finger has the strongest arterial pulsation of all the fingers. The thumb should not be used for the same reason. When pulses cannot be reliably palpated, use of a microphone-like, hand-held Doppler ultrasound device, called a transducer or probe, may be helpful in detecting and assessing peripheral flow.

A continuous-wave (CW) Doppler ultrasound device may be used to hear (insonate) the blood flow in vessels when pulses cannot be palpated. This hand-held device emits a continuous signal through the patient's tissues. The signals are reflected by (echo off) the moving blood cells and are received by the device. The filtered-output Doppler signal is then transmitted to a loudspeaker or headphones, where it can be heard for interpretation. Because CW Doppler emits a continuous signal, all vascular structures in the path of the sound beam are insonated, and differentiating arterial from venous flow and detecting the site of a stenosis may be difficult. The depth at which blood flow can be detected by Doppler is determined by the frequency (in megahertz [MHz]) it generates. The lower the frequency, the deeper the tissue penetration; a 5- to 10-MHz probe may be used to evaluate the peripheral arteries.

To evaluate the lower extremities, the patient is placed in a supine position with the head of bed elevated 20 to 30 degrees; the legs are externally rotated, if possible, to permit adequate access to the medial malleolus. Acoustic gel is applied to the patient's skin

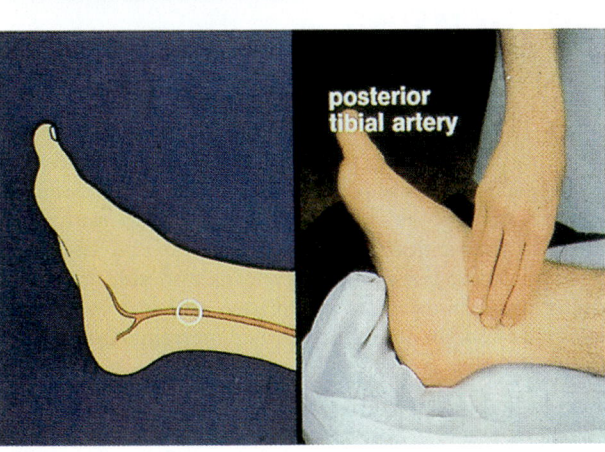

FIGURE 31-2 Assessing peripheral pulses. (*Left*) Popliteal pulse. (*Right*) Dorsalis pedis pulse. (*Bottom*) Posterior tibial pulse.

to permit uniform transmission of the ultrasound wave (electrocardiogram gel is not used because it contains sodium, which may dissolve the epoxy that covers the transducer's tip). The tip of the Doppler transducer is positioned at a 45- to 60-degree angle over the expected location of the artery and angled slowly to identify arterial blood flow. Excessive pressure is avoided because severely diseased arteries can collapse with even minimal pressure.

Because the equipment can detect blood flow in advanced arterial disease states, especially if collateral circulation has developed, identifying a signal documents only the presence of blood flow. However, it is clinically relevant to notify the primary care provider of the absence of a signal if one had been detected during a previous examination.

CW Doppler (Fig. 31-3) is more useful as a clinical tool when combined with ankle blood pressures, which are used to determine the **ankle-brachial index (ABI)**, also called the **ankle-arm index (AAI)**. The ABI is the ratio of the ankle systolic blood pressure to the arm systolic blood pressure. It is an objective indicator of arterial disease that allows the examiner to quantify the degree of stenosis. With increasing degrees of arterial narrowing, there is a progressive decrease in systolic pressure distal to the involved sites.

The first step in determining the ABI is to have the patient rest in a supine position (not seated) for at least 5 minutes. An appropriate-sized blood pressure cuff (typically, a 10-cm cuff) is applied to the patient's ankle above the malleolus. After identifying an arterial signal at the posterior tibial and dorsalis pedis arteries, the systolic ankle pressures are obtained in both feet. Diastolic pressures cannot be measured with a Doppler. If pressure in these arteries cannot be measured, pressure can be measured in the peroneal artery, which can also be assessed at the ankle (Fig. 31-4).

Doppler ultrasonography is used to measure brachial pressures in both arms. Both arms are evaluated because the patient may have an asymptomatic stenosis in the subclavian artery, causing brachial pressure on the affected side to be 20 mm Hg or more lower than systemic pressure. The abnormally low pressure should not be used for assessment.

To calculate ABI, the ankle systolic pressure for each foot is divided by the higher of the two brachial systolic pressures;

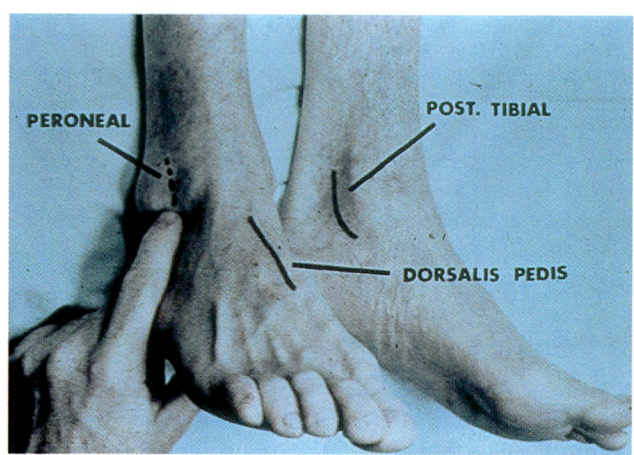

FIGURE 31-4 Location of peroneal artery; lateral malleolus. Photo reprinted with permission from Cantwell-Gab, K. (1996). Identifying chronic PAD. *American Journal of Nursing, 96*(7), 40–46.

Chart 31-1 offers more information. The ABI can be computed for a patient with the following systolic pressures:

Right brachial: 160 mm Hg
Left brachial: 120 mm Hg
Right posterior tibial: 80 mm Hg
Right dorsalis pedis: 60 mm Hg
Left posterior tibial: 100 mm Hg
Left dorsalis pedis: 120 mm Hg

The highest systolic pressure for each ankle (80 mm Hg for the right, 120 mm Hg for the left) would be divided by the highest brachial pressure (160 mm Hg).

Right: 80/160 mm Hg = 0.50 ABI
Left: 120/160 mm Hg = 0.75 ABI

In general, systolic pressure in the ankle of a healthy person is the same or slightly higher than the brachial systolic pressure, resulting in an ABI of about 1.0 (no arterial insufficiency). Patients with claudication usually have an ABI of 0.95 to 0.50 (mild to moderate insufficiency); patients with ischemic rest pain have an ABI of less than 0.50, and patients with severe ischemia or tissue loss have an ABI of 0.25 or less.

EXERCISE TESTING

Exercise testing is used to determine how long a patient can walk and to measure the ankle systolic blood pressure in response to walking. The patient walks on a treadmill at 1.5 mph with a 10% incline for a maximum of 5 minutes. Most patients can complete the test unless they have severe cardiac, pulmonary, or orthopedic problems or are physically disabled. A normal response to the test is little or no drop in ankle systolic pressure after exercise. In a patient with true claudication, however, ankle pressure drops. Combining this hemodynamic information with the walking time helps the physician determine whether intervention is necessary.

DUPLEX ULTRASONOGRAPHY

Duplex ultrasonography involves B-mode grey-scale imaging of the tissue, organs, and blood vessels (arterial and venous) and permits estimation of velocity changes by use of a pulsed Doppler

FIGURE 31-3 Continuous-wave (CW) Doppler ultrasound detects blood flow in peripheral vessels. Combined with computation of ankle or arm pressures, this diagnostic technique helps health care providers characterize the nature of peripheral vascular disease. Photo reprinted with permission from Cantwell-Gab, K. (1996). Identifying chronic PAD. *American Journal of Nursing, 96*(7), 40–46.

Chart 31-1 Avoiding Common Errors in Calculating Ankle-Brachial Index (ABI)

Take the following precautions to ensure an accurate ABI calculation:

- *Use the correctly sized blood pressure cuffs.* To obtain accurate blood pressure measurements, use a cuff with a bladder width at least 40% and length at least 80% of the limb circumference.
- *On the nursing plan of care, document the blood pressure cuff sizes used* (for example, "12-cm BP cuff used for brachial pressures; 10-cm BP cuff used for ankle pressures"). This minimizes the risk of shift-to-shift discrepancies in ABIs.
- *Use sufficient blood pressure cuff inflation.* To ensure complete closure of the artery and the most accurate measurements, inflate cuffs 20 to 30 mm Hg beyond the point at which the last arterial signal is detected.
- *Do not deflate blood pressure cuffs too rapidly.* Try to maintain a deflation rate of 2 to 4 mm Hg/second for patients without dysrhythmias and 2 mm Hg/second or slower for patients with dysrhythmias. Deflating the cuff more rapidly may miss the patient's highest pressure and result in recording an erroneous (low) blood pressure measurement.
- *Be suspicious of arterial pressures recorded at less than 40 mm Hg.* This may mean the venous signal has been mistaken for the arterial signal. If the arterial pressure, which is normally 120 mm Hg, is measured at less than 40 mm Hg, ask a colleague to double-check the findings before recording this as an arterial pressure.
- *Suspect medial calcific sclerosis anytime an ABI is 1.3 or greater or ankle pressure is more than 300 mm Hg.* Medial calcific sclerosis is associated with diabetes mellitus, chronic renal failure, and hyperparathyroidism. It produces falsely elevated ankle pressures by hardening the medra of the arteries; making the vessels noncompressible.

(From Cantwell-Gab, K. [1996]. Identifying chronic PAD. *American Journal of Nursing, 96*[1] 40–46, with permission.)

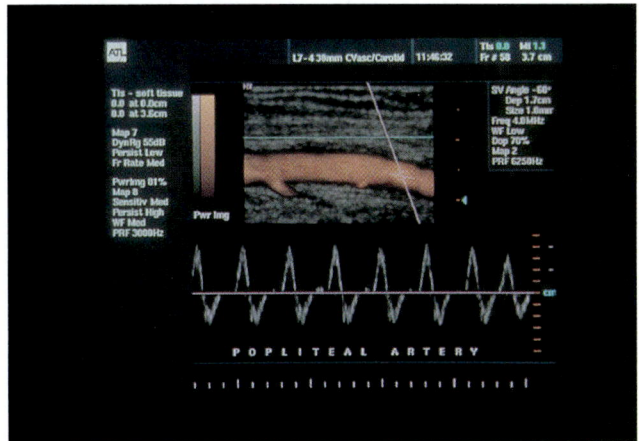

FIGURE 31-5 Colour flow duplex image of popliteal artery with normal triphasic Doppler flow.

(Fig. 31-5). Colour flow techniques, which can identify vessels, may be used to shorten the examination time. The procedure helps determine the level and extent of disease and is universally employed to evaluate the venous system. The technique makes it possible to image and assess blood flow, evaluate the runoff status of the distal vessels, locate the disease (stenosis versus occlusion), and determine anatomic morphology and the hemodynamic significance of plaque causing stenosis. Duplex ultrasound findings help in planning therapy and monitoring its outcomes. Moreover, the test is noninvasive and usually requires no patient preparation. The equipment is portable, making it useful anywhere for initial diagnosis or follow-up evaluations.

COMPUTED TOMOGRAPHY

Computed tomography (CT) provides cross-sectional images of soft tissue and can identify the area of volume changes to an extremity and the compartment where changes take place. CT of a lymphedematous arm or leg, for example, demonstrates a characteristic honeycomb pattern in the subcutaneous tissue.

In spiral (also called volumetric) CT, the scan head moves circumferentially around the patient as the patient passes through the scanner, creating a series of overlapping images that are connected to one another in a continuous spiral (Verta & Verta, 1998). Scan times are short; however, the patient is exposed to x-rays, and contrast agent usually must be injected to adequately visualize the blood vessels. Using computer software, the slicelike images are reconstructed into three-dimensional images that can be rotated and viewed from multiple angles.

COMPUTED TOMOGRAPHIC ANGIOGRAPHY

In computed tomographic angiography (CTA), a spiral CT scanner and rapid intravenous infusion of contrast agent are used to image very thin (1-mm) sections of the target area; the results are configured in three dimensions so that the image closely resembles a regular angiogram (Verta & Verta, 1998). CTA shows the aorta and main visceral arteries better than it shows smaller branch vessels. Scan times are usually between 20 and 30 seconds. The large volume of contrast agent required for CTA limits the usefulness of this study in patients with allergy to the contrast agent or with significantly impaired renal function.

MAGNETIC RESONANCE ANGIOGRAPHY

Magnetic resonance angiography is performed with a standard MRI scanner but with image-processing software specifically programmed to isolate the blood vessels. The images are reconstructed to resemble a standard angiogram, but because the images are reassembled in three dimensions, they can be rotated and viewed from multiple angles. Because no contrast agent is necessary, this study is useful in patients with poor renal function or allergy to contrast agent. Scan time is long, and motion artefacts are common, restricting the use of the test to relatively short segments of the vascular system (Verta & Verta, 1998).

ANGIOGRAPHY

An arteriogram produced by angiography may be used to confirm the diagnosis of occlusive arterial disease when considering surgery or other interventions. The procedure involves injecting a radiopaque contrast agent directly into the vascular system to visualize the vessels. The location of a vascular obstruction or an **aneurysm** (abnormal dilation of a blood vessel) and the collateral circulation can be demonstrated. Usually, patients experience a temporary sensation of warmth as the contrast agent is injected, and local irritation may occur at the injection site. Infrequently, a patient may have an immediate or delayed allergic reaction to the iodine contained in the contrast agent. Manifestations include dyspnea, nausea and vomiting, sweating, tachycardia, and numbness of the extremities. Any such reaction must be reported to the physician at once; treatment may include the administration of one or more of epinephrine (adrenaline), antihistamines, or corticosteroids. Additional risks include vessel injury, bleeding, and cerebrovascular accident (CVA; stroke).

AIR PLETHYSMOGRAPHY

Named for the standardized air chambers that fit around the lower leg and that are calibrated after being filled with a standard amount of air, air plethysmography quantifies venous reflux and calf muscle pump ejection. Changes in volume are measured with the patient's legs elevated, with the patient supine and standing, and after the patient performs toe-ups (patient extends ankle while standing; stands on tip-toes). Air plethysmography provides information about venous filling time, functional venous volume, ejected volume, and residual volume. It is useful in evaluating patients with suspected valvular incompetence or chronic venous insufficiency.

CONTRAST PHLEBOGRAPHY

Also known as venography, contrast phlebography involves injecting radiographic contrast media into the venous system through a dorsal foot vein. If a thrombus exists, the x-ray image discloses an unfilled segment of vein in an otherwise completely filled vein. Injection of the contrast agent may cause a brief but painful inflammation of the vein. The test is generally performed if the patient is to undergo thrombolytic therapy, but duplex ultrasonography is now accepted as the gold standard for diagnosing venous thrombosis.

LYMPHANGIOGRAPHY

Lymphangiography affords a means of detecting lymph node involvement that results from metastatic carcinoma, lymphoma, or infection in sites that are otherwise inaccessible to the examiner except by surgery. In this test, a lymphatic vessel in each foot (or hand) is injected with contrast agent. A series of x-rays are taken at the conclusion of the injection, 24 hours later, and periodically thereafter, as indicated. The failure to identify subcutaneous lymphatic collection of contrast agent and the persistence of contrast agent in the tissue for days afterward help to confirm a diagnosis of lymphedema.

LYMPHOSCINTIGRAPHY

Lymphoscintigraphy is a reliable alternative to lymphangiography. A radioactively labelled colloid is injected subcutaneously in the second interdigital space. The extremity is then exercised to facilitate the uptake of the colloid by the lymphatic system, and serial images are obtained at preset intervals. No adverse reactions have been reported.

Management of Arterial Disorders

ARTERIOSCLEROSIS AND ATHEROSCLEROSIS

Arteriosclerosis is the most common disease of the arteries; the term means *hardening of the arteries*. It is a diffuse process whereby the muscle fibres and the endothelial lining of the walls of small arteries and arterioles become thickened. **Atherosclerosis** involves a different process, affecting the intima of the large and medium-sized arteries. These changes consist of the accumulation of lipids, calcium, blood components, carbohydrates, and fibrous tissue that start by forming on the intimal layer of the artery but penetrate the medial (smooth muscle) layer as the disease progresses. These accumulations are referred to as atheromas or plaques.

Although the pathologic processes of arteriosclerosis and atherosclerosis differ, rarely does one occur without the other, and the terms are often used interchangeably. Because atherosclerosis is a generalized disease of the arteries, when it is present in the extremities, atherosclerosis is usually present elsewhere in the body.

Pathophysiology

The most common direct results of atherosclerosis in arteries include narrowing (stenosis) or complete occlusion of the lumen, obstruction by thrombosis, aneurysm, ulceration, and rupture. Its indirect results are malnutrition and the subsequent fibrosis of the organs that the sclerotic arteries supply with blood. All actively functioning tissue cells require an abundant supply of nutrients and oxygen and are sensitive to any reduction in the supply of these nutrients. If such reductions are severe and permanent, the cells undergo ischemic necrosis (death of cells due to deficient blood flow) and are replaced by fibrous tissue, which requires much less blood flow.

Atherosclerosis can develop at any point in the body, but certain sites are more vulnerable, typically bifurcation or branch areas. In the proximal lower extremity, these include the distal abdominal aorta, the common iliac arteries, the orifice of the superficial femoral and profunda femoris arteries, and the superficial femoral artery in the adductor canal. Distal to the knee, atherosclerosis occurs anywhere along the artery.

Atherosclerosis is an inflammatory disease. Numerous pathophysiologic observations in humans and animals led to the formulation of the response-to-injury hypothesis of atherosclerosis, which initially proposed that endothelial denudation was the first step in atherosclerosis (Ross & Glomset, 1973). The most recent version of this hypothesis emphasizes endothelial dysfunction rather than denudation (Ross, 1999 [see review]).

Morphologically, atherosclerotic lesions are of two types: fatty streaks and fibrous plaque. Fatty streaks are yellow and smooth, protrude slightly into the lumen of the artery, and are composed of lipids and elongated smooth muscle cells. These lesions have been found in the arteries of people of all age groups, including infants. It appears that fatty streaks are likely to lead to atherosclerotic plaque formation (Ross, 1999).

The fibrous plaque characteristic of atherosclerosis is composed of smooth muscle cells, collagen fibres, plasma components, and lipids. It is white to whitish yellow and protrudes in various degrees into the arterial lumen, sometimes completely obstructing it. These plaques are found predominantly in the abdominal aorta and the coronary, popliteal, and internal carotid arteries. This plaque is believed to be an irreversible lesion (Fig. 31-6). Gradual narrowing of the arterial lumen as the disease process progresses stimulates the development of collateral circulation (Fig. 31-7). Collateral circulation consists of preexisting vessels that enlarge to reroute blood flow in the presence of a hemodynamically significant stenosis or occlusion. Collateral flow allows continued perfusion to the tissues beyond the arterial obstruction,

FIGURE 31-6 Schematic concept of the progression of atherosclerosis. Fatty streaks constitute one of the earliest lesions of atherosclerosis. Many fatty streaks regress, whereas others progress to fibrous plaques and eventually to atheroma, which may be complicated by hemorrhage, ulceration, calcification, or thrombosis and may produce myocardial infarction, stroke, or gangrene.

but it is often inadequate to meet imposed metabolic demand, and ischemia results.

Risk Factors

Many risk factors are associated with atherosclerosis (Chart 31-2). There is ample evidence that modification of these risk factors

prevents the development of cardiovascular disease, evidence indicates that it may slow the disease process. Some risk factors, such as age or gender, cannot be modified. However, it is believed that genetic factors can be modified indirectly by altering other risk factors (Moore, 2002).

In peripheral vascular disease, tobacco use may be one of the strongest risk factors in the development of atherosclerotic lesions. Nicotine decreases blood flow to the extremities and increases heart rate and blood pressure by stimulating the sympathetic nervous system, causing vasoconstriction. It also increases the risk for clot formation by increasing the aggregation of platelets. Carbon monoxide, a toxin produced by burning tobacco, combines more readily with the hemoglobin than oxygen does, depriving the tissues of oxygen. The amount of tobacco use is directly related to the extent of the disease, and cessation of tobacco use reduces the risks. Major risk factors for cardiovascular disease include hypertension, hypercholesterolemia, and diabetes. Many other factors such as obesity, stress, and lack of exercise have been identified as contributing to the disease process.

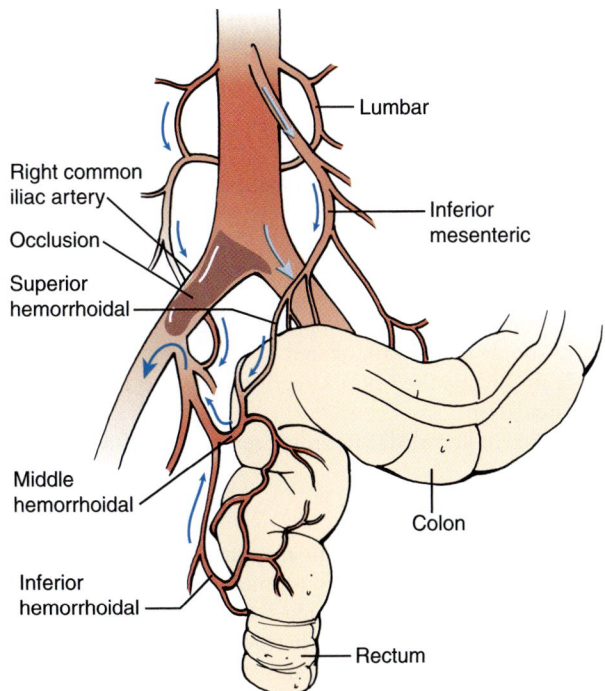

FIGURE 31-7 Development of channels for collateral blood flow in response to occlusion of the right common iliac artery and the terminal aortic bifurcation.

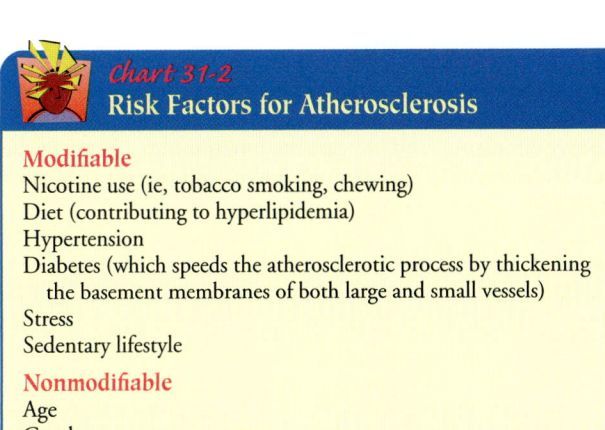

Chart 31-2
Risk Factors for Atherosclerosis

Modifiable
Nicotine use (ie, tobacco smoking, chewing)
Diet (contributing to hyperlipidemia)
Hypertension
Diabetes (which speeds the atherosclerotic process by thickening the basement membranes of both large and small vessels)
Stress
Sedentary lifestyle

Nonmodifiable
Age
Gender

Prevention

Intermittent claudication is a sign of generalized atherosclerosis and may be a marker of occult coronary artery disease. Because a high-fat diet is suspected of contributing to atherosclerosis, it is reasonable to measure serum cholesterol and to begin prevention efforts. The American Heart Association recommends reducing the amount of fat ingested in a healthy diet, substituting unsaturated fats for saturated fats, and decreasing cholesterol intake to no more than 300 mg daily to reduce the risk of cardiovascular disease (Krauss et al., 2000).

Certain medications combined with dietary modification and exercise are being used to reduce blood lipid levels. There is limited evidence that these medications can alter the course of peripheral arterial disease, but they may reduce the mortality rate from cardiovascular disease. Several classes of medication are used to prevent atherosclerosis by lowering lipids: statins (atorvastatin [Lipitor], lovastatin [Mevacor], pravastatin [Pravachol], simvastatin [Zocor]), bile acid sequestrants (cholestyramine [Questran] or colestipol [Colestid]), nicotinic acid (niacin, B_3, Niaspan), fibric acids (gemfibrozil [Lopid]), and lipophilic substances (probucol). Patients receiving long-term therapy with these medications require close medical supervision. Hypertension, which may accelerate the rate at which atherosclerotic lesions form in high-pressure vessels, can lead to cerebrovascular accident (CVA; brain attack; stroke), ischemic renal disease, severe peripheral arterial disease, or coronary artery disease. Results of large, randomized studies demonstrated dramatic reductions in myocardial infarction, stroke, and cardiovascular death when blood pressure was decreased to at least 140/90 mm Hg (Moser, 1999; McAlister et al., 2001).

It is clear that the greater the number of risk factors, the greater the likelihood of developing the disease. Reduction of all controllable risk factors, particularly hypertension, diabetes, and tobacco use, is strongly recommended.

Clinical Manifestations

The clinical signs and symptoms resulting from atherosclerosis depend on the organ or tissue affected. Coronary atherosclerosis (heart disease), angina, and acute myocardial infarction are discussed in Chapter 28. Cerebrovascular diseases, including transient cerebral ischemic attacks and stroke, are discussed in Chapter 62. Atherosclerosis of the aorta, including aneurysm, and atherosclerotic lesions of the extremities are discussed later in this chapter. Renovascular disease (renal artery stenosis and end-stage renal disease), including hypertension, is discussed in Chapter 45.

Medical Management

The traditional medical management of atherosclerosis involves modification of risk factors, a controlled exercise program to improve circulation and increase the functioning capacity of the circulation, medication, dietary control and interventional or surgical graft procedures.

SURGICAL MANAGEMENT

Vascular surgical procedures are divided into two groups: inflow procedures, which provide blood supply from the aorta into the femoral artery, and outflow procedures, which provide blood supply to vessels below the femoral artery. Inflow surgical procedures are discussed with diseases of the aorta and outflow procedures with peripheral arterial occlusive disease.

RADIOLOGIC INTERVENTIONS

Several interventional radiologic techniques are important adjunctive therapies to surgical procedures. If an isolated lesion or lesions are identified during the arteriogram, **angioplasty**, also called percutaneous transluminal angioplasty (PCTA), may be performed. After the patient receives a local anesthetic, a balloon-tipped catheter is manoeuvred across the area of stenosis. Exactly how PCTA works is controversial. Some theorize that it improves blood flow by overstretching (and thereby dilating) the elastic fibres of the nondiseased arterial segment, but most clinicians believe that the procedure widens the arterial lumen by cracking and flattening the plaque against the vessel wall (see Chap. 28). Complications from PCTA include hematoma formation, embolus, **dissection** (separation of the intima) of the vessel, and bleeding. To decrease the risk of reocclusion, stents (small, mesh tubes made of nitinol, titanium, or stainless steel) may be inserted to support the walls of blood vessels and prevent collapse immediately after balloon inflation (Fig. 31-8). A variety of covered wall stents and stent-grafts may be used for short-segment stenoses. Complications associated with stent or stent-graft use include distal embolization, intimal damage (dissection), and dislodgment. The advantage of angioplasty, stents, and stent-grafts is the decreased length of hospital stay required for the treatment; many of the procedures are performed on an outpatient basis.

NURSING PROCESS: THE PATIENT WHO HAS PERIPHERAL ARTERIAL INSUFFICIENCY OF THE EXTREMITIES

Assessment

The nursing assessment includes a complete health and medication history and identification of risk factors for peripheral artery disease. Signs and symptoms detected during the nursing assessment may include claudication pain; rest pain in the forefoot; pallor, rubor, or cyanosis; weak or absent peripheral pulses; and skin breakdown or ulcerations.

Nursing Diagnosis

Based on assessment data, major nursing diagnoses for the patient may include the following:

- Ineffective peripheral tissue perfusion related to compromised circulation
- Chronic pain related to impaired ability of peripheral vessels to supply tissues with oxygen
- Risk for impaired skin integrity related to compromised circulation
- Deficient knowledge regarding self-care activities

Planning and Goals

The major goals for the patient may include increased arterial blood supply to the extremities, promotion of vasodilation, prevention of vascular compression, relief of pain, attainment or maintenance of tissue integrity, and adherence to the self-care program.

Measures used by the patient and members of the health care team to accomplish a single goal must be evaluated in terms of the positive and the negative effects these measures may have on the simultaneous achievement of other goals. An overview of the

FIGURE 31-8 (**A**) Flexible stent. Courtesy of Medtronics, Peripheral Division, Santa Rosa, California. (**B**) Representation of a common iliac artery with a Wallstent (Boston Scientific).

care of a patient with peripheral arterial problems is provided in the Plan of Nursing Care: The Patient With Peripheral Vascular Problems.

Nursing Interventions

IMPROVING PERIPHERAL ARTERIAL CIRCULATION

Arterial blood supply to a body part can be enhanced by positioning the part below the level of the heart. For the lower extremities, this is accomplished by elevating the head of the patient's bed on 15-cm blocks or by having the patient use a reclining chair or sit with the feet resting on the floor.

The nurse can assist the patient with walking or other moderate or graded isometric exercises that may be prescribed to promote blood flow and encourage the development of collateral circulation. The nurse instructs the patient to walk to the point of pain, rest until pain subsides, and then resume walking so that endurance can be increased as collateral circulation develops. Pain can serve as a guide in determining the amount of exercise appropriate for an individual. The onset of pain indicates that the tissues are not receiving adequate oxygen, signaling the patient to rest before continuing activity. However, a regular exercise program can result in increased walking distance before the onset of claudication. The amount of exercise a patient can tolerate before the onset of pain is determined to provide a baseline for evaluation.

Not all patients with peripheral vascular disease should exercise. Before recommending any exercise program, the primary health care provider should be consulted. Conditions that worsen with activity include leg ulcers, cellulitis, gangrene, or acute thrombotic occlusions.

PROMOTING VASODILATION AND PREVENTING VASCULAR COMPRESSION

Arterial dilation promotes increased blood flow to the extremities and is therefore a desirable goal for patients with peripheral arterial disease. However, if the arteries are severely sclerosed, inelastic, or damaged, dilation is not possible. For this reason, measures to promote vasodilation, such as medications or surgery, may be only minimally effective.

Nursing interventions may involve applications of warmth to promote arterial flow and instructions to the patient to avoid exposure to cold temperatures, which causes vasoconstriction. Ad-

equate clothing and warm temperatures protect the patient from chilling. If chilling occurs, a warm bath or drink is helpful.

When heat is applied directly to ischemic extremities, the temperature of the heat source must not exceed body temperature. Even at lower temperatures, burn injuries can occur in ischemic extremities. Excess heat may increase the metabolic rate of the extremities and increase the need for oxygen beyond that provided by the reduced arterial flow through the diseased artery.

> **! NURSING ALERT** Patients are instructed to test the temperature of bath water and to avoid using hot-water bottles and heating pads on the extremities. Applying a heating pad to the abdomen can cause reflex vasodilation in the extremities and is safer than direct application of heat to affected extremities.

Nicotine causes vasospasm and can thereby dramatically reduce circulation to the extremities. Tobacco smoke also impairs transport and cellular use of oxygen and increases blood viscosity. Patients with arterial insufficiency who use tobacco (ie, smoke, chew) must be fully informed of the effects of nicotine on circulation and encouraged to stop using tobacco.

Emotional upsets stimulate the sympathetic nervous system, resulting in peripheral vasoconstriction. Although emotional stress is unavoidable, it can be minimized to some degree by avoiding stressful situations when possible or by consistently following a stress-management program. Counselling services or relaxation training may be indicated for people who cannot cope effectively with situational stressors.

Constrictive clothing and accessories such as tight socks, panty girdles, and shoelaces impede circulation to the extremities and promote venous stasis and therefore should be avoided. Crossing the legs should be discouraged because it compresses vessels in the legs.

RELIEVING PAIN

Frequently, the pain associated with peripheral arterial insufficiency is chronic and continuous. It limits activities, affects work and responsibilities, disturbs sleep, and alters patients' sense of well-being. Patients are often depressed, irritable, and unable to exert the energy necessary to execute prescribed therapies, making pain relief even more difficult. Analgesics such as oxycodone (OxyContin) plus acetylsalicylic acid (Aspirin) or oxycodone plus

Plan of Nursing Care
The Patient With Peripheral Vascular Problems

Nursing Interventions	Rationale	Expected Outcomes
Nursing Diagnosis: Ineffective peripheral tissue perfusion related to compromised circulation		
Goal: Increased arterial blood supply to extremities		
1. Lower the extremities below the level of the heart (if condition is arterial in nature). 2. Encourage moderate amount of walking or graded extremity exercises.	1. Dependency of lower extremities enhances arterial blood supply. 2. Muscular exercise promotes blood flow and the development of collateral circulation.	• Extremities warm to touch • Colour of extremities improved • Experiences decreased muscle pain with exercise
Goal: Decrease in venous congestion		
1. Elevate extremities above heart level (if condition is venous in nature). 2. Discourage standing still or sitting for prolonged periods. 3. Encourage walking.	1. Elevation of extremities counteracts gravitational pull, promotes venous return, and prevents venous stasis. 2. Prolonged standing still or sitting promotes venous stasis. 3. Walking promotes venous return by activating the "muscle pump."	• Elevates lower extremities as prescribed • Decreased edema of extremities • Avoids prolonged standing still or sitting • Gradually increases walking time daily
Goal: Promotion of vasodilation and prevention of vascular compression		
1. Maintain warm temperature and avoid chilling. 2. Discourage nicotine use. 3. Counsel in ways to avoid emotional upsets; stress management. 4. Encourage avoidance of constrictive clothing and accessories. 5. Encourage avoidance of leg crossing. 6. Administer vasodilator medications and adrenergic blocking agents as prescribed, with appropriate nursing considerations.	1. Warmth promotes arterial flow by preventing the vasoconstriction effects of chilling. 2. Nicotine causes vasospasm, which impedes peripheral circulation. 3. Emotional stress causes peripheral vasoconstriction by stimulating the sympathetic nervous system. 4. Constrictive clothing and accessories impede circulation and promote venous stasis. 5. Leg crossing causes compression of vessels with subsequent impediment of circulation, resulting in venous stasis. 6. Vasodilators relax smooth muscle; adrenergic blocking agents block the response to sympathetic nerve impulses or circulating catecholamines.	• Protects extremities from exposure to cold • Avoids nicotine • Uses stress-management program to minimize emotional upset • Avoids constricting clothing and accessories • Avoids leg crossing • Takes medication as prescribed
Nursing Diagnosis: Chronic pain related to impaired ability of peripheral vessels to supply tissues with oxygen		
Goal: Relief of pain		
1. Promote increased circulation. 2. Administer analgesics as prescribed, with appropriate nursing considerations.	1. Enhancement of peripheral circulation increases the oxygen supplied to the muscle and decreases the accumulation of metabolites that cause muscle spasms. 2. Analgesics help to reduce pain and allow the patient to participate in activities and exercises that promote circulation.	• Uses measures to increase arterial blood supply to extremities • Uses analgesics as prescribed
Nursing Diagnosis: Risk for impaired skin integrity related to compromised circulation		
Goal: Attainment/maintenance of tissue integrity		
1. Instruct in ways to avoid trauma to extremities.	1. Poorly nourished tissues are susceptible to trauma and bacterial invasion; healing of wounds is delayed or inhibited due to poor tissue perfusion.	• Inspects skin daily for evidence of injury or ulceration • Avoids trauma and irritation to skin

(continued)

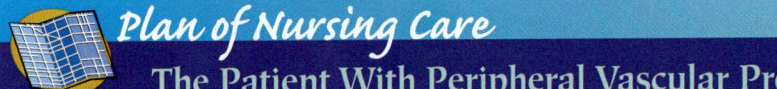

Plan of Nursing Care
The Patient With Peripheral Vascular Problems *(Continued)*

Nursing Interventions	Rationale	Expected Outcomes
2. Encourage wearing protective shoes and padding for pressure areas. 3. Encourage meticulous hygiene; bathing with neutral soaps, applying lotions, carefully trimming nails. 4. Caution to avoid scratching or vigourous rubbing. 5. Promote good nutrition; adequate intake of vitamins A and C, protein, and zinc; control of obesity.	2. Protective shoes and padding prevent foot injuries and blisters. 3. Neutral soaps and lotions prevent drying and cracking of skin. 4. Scratching and rubbing can cause skin abrasions and bacterial invasion. 5. Good nutrition promotes healing and prevents tissue breakdown.	• Wears protective shoes • Adheres to meticulous hygiene regimen • Eats a healthy diet that contains adequate protein and vitamins A and C

Nursing Diagnosis: Deficient knowledge regarding self-care activities
Goal: Adherence to the self-care program

1. Include family/significant others in teaching program. 2. Provide written instructions about foot care, leg care, and exercise program. 3. Assist to obtain properly fitting clothing, shoes, stockings. 4. Refer to self-help groups as indicated, such as smoking cessation clinics, stress management, weight management, and exercise program.	1. Adherence to the self-care program is enhanced when the patient receives support from family and from appropriate self-help groups and agencies. 2. Written instructions serve as reminder and reinforcement of information. 3. Constrictive clothing and accessories impede circulation and promote venous stasis. 4. Reducing risk factors may reduce symptoms or slow disease progression.	• Practices frequent position changes as prescribed • Practices postural exercises as prescribed • Takes medications as prescribed • Avoids vasoconstrictors • Uses measures to prevent trauma • Uses stress management program • Accepts condition as chronic but amenable to therapies that will decrease symptoms

acetaminophen (Tylenol) may be helpful in reducing pain to the point where the patient can participate in the therapies that can increase circulation and ultimately relieve pain more effectively.

MAINTAINING TISSUE INTEGRITY
Poorly nourished tissues are susceptible to damage and infection. When lesions develop, healing may be delayed or inhibited because of the poor blood supply to the area. Infected, nonhealing ulcerations of the extremities can be debilitating and may require prolonged and often expensive treatments. Amputation of an ischemic limb may eventually be necessary. Measures to prevent these complications must be a high priority and vigorously implemented.

Trauma to the extremities must be avoided. Advising the patient to wear sturdy, well-fitting shoes or slippers to prevent foot injury and blisters may be helpful, as may be recommending neutral soaps and body lotions to prevent drying and cracking of skin. Scratching and vigourous rubbing can abrade skin and create a site for bacterial invasion; therefore, feet should be patted dry. Stockings should be clean and dry. Fingernails and toenails should be carefully trimmed straight across and sharp corners filed to follow the contour of the nail. If nails are thick and brittle and cannot be trimmed safely, a podiatrist must be consulted. Corns and calluses need to be removed by a health care professional. Special shoe inserts may be needed to prevent calluses from recurring. All signs of blisters, ingrown toenails, infection, or other problems should be

reported to health care professionals for treatment and follow-up. Patients with diminished vision may require assistance in periodically examining the lower extremities for trauma.

Good nutrition promotes healing and prevents tissue breakdown and is therefore included in the overall therapeutic program for patients with peripheral vascular disease. Eating a well-balanced diet that contains adequate protein and vitamins is necessary for patients with arterial insufficiency. Key nutrients play specific roles in wound healing. Vitamin C is essential for collagen synthesis and capillary development. Vitamin A enhances epithelialization. Zinc is necessary for cell mitosis and cell proliferation. Obesity strains the heart, increases venous congestion, and reduces circulation; therefore, a weight-reduction plan may be necessary for some patients. A diet low in lipids may be indicated for patients with atherosclerosis.

PROMOTING HOME AND COMMUNITY-BASED CARE
The self-care program is planned with the patient so that activities that promote arterial and venous circulation, relieve pain, and promote tissue integrity are acceptable. The patient and family are helped to understand the reasons for each aspect of the program and the possible consequences of nonadherence. Long-term care of the feet and legs is of prime importance in the prevention of trauma, ulceration, and gangrene. The Plan of Nursing Care describes nursing care for patients with peripheral vascular disease. Chart 31-3 provides detailed patient instructions for foot and leg care.

Chart 31-3
Home Care Checklist • Foot and Leg Care in Peripheral Vascular Disease

At the completion of the home care instruction, the patient or caregiver will be able to:

	Patient	Caregiver
• Demonstrate daily foot bathing: Wash between toes with mild soap and lukewarm water, then rinse thoroughly and pat rather than rub dry.	✓	✓
• Recognize the dangers of thermal injury: – Wear clean, loose, soft cotton socks (they are comfortable, allow air to circulate, and will absorb moisture) – In cold weather, wear extra socks in extra-large shoes. – Avoid heating pads, whirlpools, and hot tubs. – Avoid sunburn.	✓	
• Identify safety concerns: – Inspect feet daily with a mirror for redness, dryness, cuts, blisters, etc. – Always wear soft shoes or slippers when out of bed. – Trim nails straight across after showering. – Consult podiatrist to trim nails if vision is decreased; also for care of corns, blisters, ingrown nails. – Clear pathways in house to prevent injury. – Avoid wearing thong sandals. – Use lamb's wool between toes if they overlap or rub each other.	✓	✓
• Demonstrate comfort measures: – Wear leather shoes with an extra-depth toebox. Synthetic shoes do not allow air to circulate. – If feet become dry and scaly, use cream with lanolin. Never put cream between toes. – If feet perspire, especially between toes, use powder daily and/or lamb's wool between toes to promote drying.	✓	
• Demonstrate ability to decrease risk of constricting blood vessels: – Avoid promoting circular compression around feet or knees—for example, by applying knee-high stockings or tight socks. – Do not cross legs at knees. – Stop using nicotine (ie, tobacco smoking or chewing) because nicotine causes vasoconstriction and vasospasm. – Avoid applying tight, constricting bandages. – Participate in a regular walking exercise program to stimulate circulation.	✓	
• Recognize when to seek medical attention: – Contact health care provider at the onset of skin breakdown such as abrasions, blisters, athlete's foot, or pain. – Do not use any medication on feet or legs unless prescribed. – Avoid using iodine, alcohol, corn/wart-removing compound, or adhesive products before checking with health care provider.	✓	✓

Evaluation
EXPECTED PATIENT OUTCOMES
Expected patient outcomes may include:

1. Demonstrates an increase in arterial blood supply to extremities
   a. Exhibits extremities warm to touch
   b. Has improved colour of extremities (ie, free of rubor or cyanosis)
   c. Experiences decreased muscle pain with exercise
   d. Demonstrates an increase in walking distance or duration
2. Promotes vasodilation; prevents vascular compression
   a. Protects extremities from exposure to cold
   b. Avoids use of tobacco
   c. Uses stress management strategies to minimize emotional upset
   d. Wears nonconstricting clothing
   e. Avoids leg crossing
   f. Takes medication as prescribed
3. Has decrease in severity and duration of pain
4. Attains or maintains tissue integrity
   a. Avoids trauma and irritation to skin
   b. Wears protective shoes
   c. Adheres to meticulous hygienic regimen
   d. Eats a healthy diet that contains adequate protein, vitamins A and C, and zinc
   e. Performs self-care activities

PERIPHERAL ARTERIAL OCCLUSIVE DISEASE

Arterial insufficiency of the extremities is usually found in individuals older than 50 years of age, most often in men. The legs are most frequently affected; however, the upper extremities may be involved. The age of onset and the severity are influenced by the type and number of atherosclerotic risk factors (Chart 31-4). In peripheral arterial disease, obstructive lesions are predominantly confined to segments of the arterial system extending from the aorta below the renal arteries to the popliteal artery (Fig. 31-9). However, distal occlusive disease is frequently seen in patients with diabetes mellitus and in elderly patients.

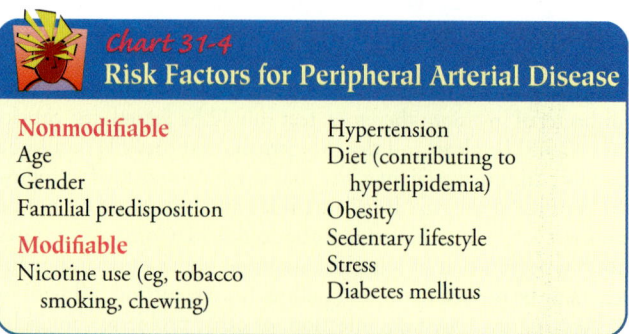

Chart 31-4
Risk Factors for Peripheral Arterial Disease

Nonmodifiable	Hypertension
Age	Diet (contributing to hyperlipidemia)
Gender	
Familial predisposition	Obesity
Modifiable	Sedentary lifestyle
Nicotine use (eg, tobacco smoking, chewing)	Stress Diabetes mellitus

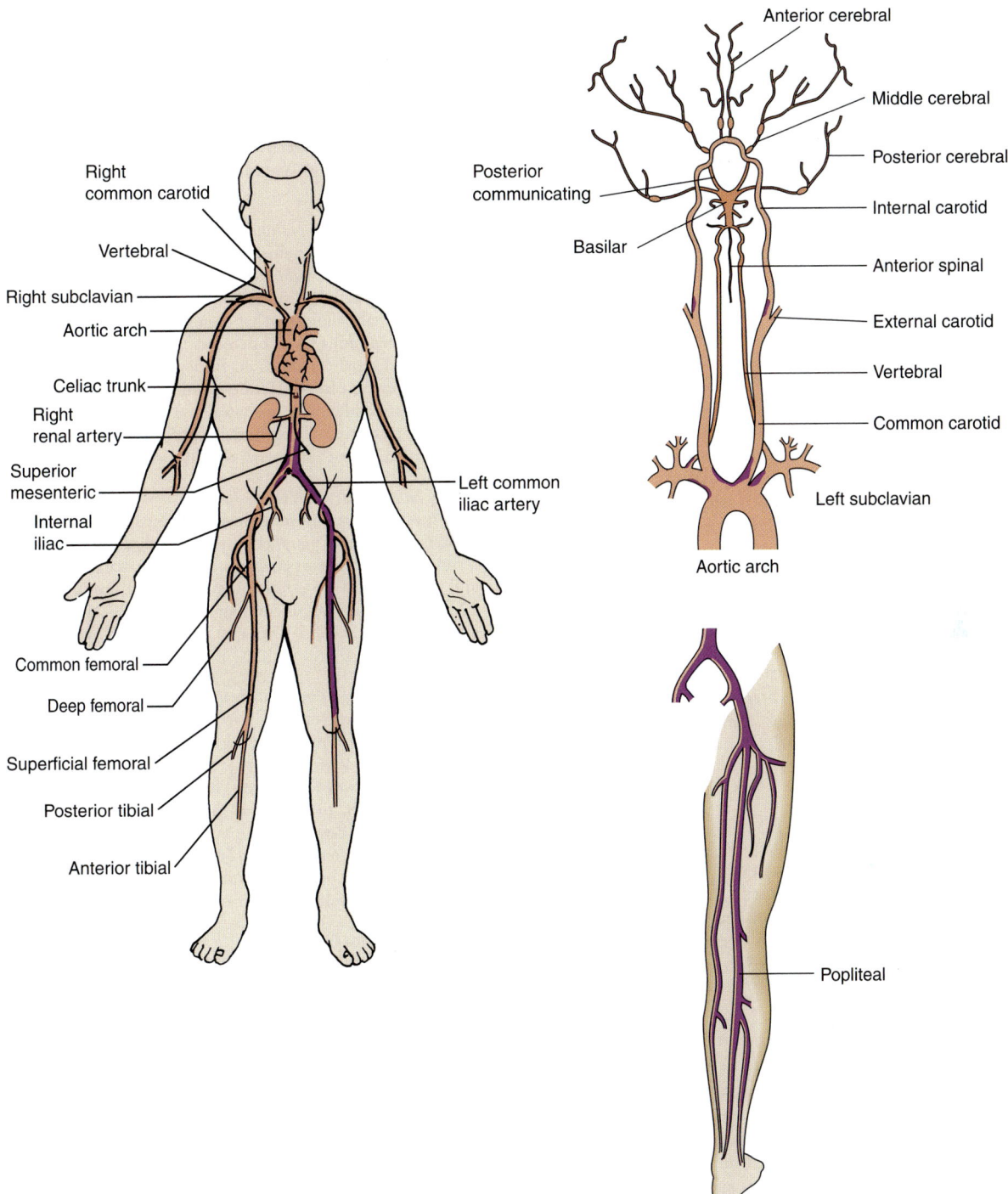

FIGURE 31-9   Common sites of atherosclerotic obstruction in major arteries.

Clinical Manifestations

The hallmark is intermittent claudication. This pain may be described as aching, cramping, fatigue, or weakness that is consistently reproduced with the same degree of exercise or activity and relieved with rest. The pain commonly occurs in muscle groups one joint level below the stenosis or occlusion. As the disease progresses, the patient may have a decreased ability to walk the same distance or may notice increased pain with ambulation. When the arterial insufficiency becomes severe, the patient begins to have rest pain. This pain is associated with critical ischemia of the distal extremity and is persistent, aching, or boring; it may be so excruciating that it is unrelieved by opioids. Ischemic rest pain is usually worse at night and often wakes the patient. Elevating the extremity or placing it in a horizontal position increases the pain, whereas placing the extremity in a dependent position reduces the pain. In bed, some patients sleep with the affected leg hanging over the side of the bed. Some patients sleep in a reclining chair in an attempt to relieve the pain.

Assessment and Diagnostic Findings

A sensation of coldness or numbness in the extremities may accompany intermittent claudication and is a result of the reduced arterial flow. When the extremity is examined, it may feel cool to the touch and look pale when elevated or ruddy and cyanotic when placed in a dependent position. Skin and nail changes, ulcerations, gangrene, and muscle atrophy may be evident. Bruits may be auscultated with a stethoscope; a bruit is the sound produced by turbulent blood flow through an irregular, tortuous, stenotic vessel or through a dilated segment of the vessel (aneurysm). Peripheral pulses may be diminished or absent.

Examining the peripheral pulses is an important part of assessing arterial occlusive disease. Unequal pulses between extremities or the absence of a normally palpable pulse is a sign of peripheral arterial disease. The femoral pulse in the groin and the posterior tibial pulse beside the medial malleolus are most easily palpated. The popliteal pulse is sometimes difficult to palpate; the location of the dorsalis pedis artery on the dorsum of the foot varies and is normally absent in about 7% of the population.

The presence, location, and extent of arterial occlusive disease are determined by a careful history of the symptoms and by physical examination. The colour and temperature of the extremity are noted and the pulses palpated. The nails may be thickened and opaque, and the skin may be shiny, atrophic, and dry, with sparse hair growth. The assessment includes comparison of the right and left extremities.

The diagnosis of peripheral arterial occlusive disease may be made using CW Doppler and ankle-brachial indices (ABIs), treadmill testing for claudication, duplex ultrasonography, or other imaging studies previously described.

Medical Management

Generally, patients feel better with some type of exercise program. If this program is combined with weight reduction and cessation of tobacco use, patients often can improve their activity tolerance. Patients should not be promised that their symptoms will be relieved if they stop tobacco use, because claudication may persist, and they may lose their motivation to stop using tobacco.

PHARMACOLOGIC THERAPY

Various medications are prescribed to treat the symptoms of peripheral arterial disease. Pentoxifylline (Trental) increases erythrocyte flexibility and reduces blood viscosity, and it is therefore thought to improve the supply of oxygenated blood to the muscle. Cilostazol (Pletal) works by inhibiting platelet aggregation, inhibiting smooth muscle cell proliferation, and increasing vasodilation. Antiplatelet aggregating agents such as aspirin, ticlopidine (Ticlid), and clopidogrel (Plavix) are thought to improve circulation throughout diseased arteries or prevent intimal hyperplasia leading to stenosis.

SURGICAL MANAGEMENT

In most patients, when intermittent claudication becomes severe and disabling or when the limb is at risk for amputation because of tissue loss, vascular grafting or endarterectomy is the treatment of choice. The choice of the surgical procedure depends on the degree and location of the stenosis or occlusion. Other important considerations are the overall health of the patient and the length of the procedure that can be tolerated. It is sometimes necessary to provide the palliative therapy of primary amputation rather than an arterial bypass. If endarterectomy is performed, an incision is made into the artery, and the atheromatous obstruction is

NURSING RESEARCH PROFILE 31-1
Does Exercise Relieve Pain of Peripheral Arterial Claudication?

Braun, C. M., Colucci, A. M., & Patterson, R. B. (1999). Components of an optimal exercise program for the treatment of patients with claudication. *Journal of Vascular Nursing, 17*(2), 32–36.

Purpose
Because patients with peripheral arterial claudication increasingly limit activity because of pain, they become physically deconditioned. The patients and their families report decreased quality of life (QOL) because of the activity limitations. Traditional treatment for peripheral arterial claudication has been surgical bypass. Exercise programs are beginning to be offered as treatment for patients with peripheral arterial claudication. Little is known about the effectiveness of exercise in the treatment of this patient population. This study evaluated whether a supervised exercise and education program increased pain-free walking distance and improved total fitness of patients with peripheral arterial claudication.

Study Sample and Design
This study was a retrospective review of 96 patients who had experienced symptoms of peripheral arterial claudication for longer than 3 months. Patients participated in a cardiovascular conditioning and muscle training exercise program with education classes for 12 weeks. Twenty-two patients were monitored for 2 years; data were collected at 1 year and 2 years after the original 12-week program.

Findings
Patients' walking distances increased threefold after participation in the 12-week program. The average maximum distance patients were able to walk at the beginning of the program was 190 meters. After the 12-week program the average distance was 580 m. The 22 patients followed for two years had an average maximum walking distance of 882 m 1 year after the 12-week program and 731 m 2 years after the 12-week program. The researchers concluded that patients were able to maintain and continue exercising after completion of the 12-week program. Families reported improvement in general health and psychosocial behaviour of the patients.

Nursing Implications
Patients with peripheral arterial claudication benefit from a supervised exercise program combined with education programs. Supervised exercise programs may enable patients with peripheral arterial claudication to increase the distance they can walk without symptoms, improve their quality of life, and avoid or delay surgical intervention.

removed. The artery is then sutured closed to restore vascular integrity (Fig. 31-10).

Bypass grafts are performed to reroute the blood flow around the stenosis or occlusion. Before bypass grafting, the surgeon determines where the distal **anastomosis** (site where the vessels are surgically joined) will be placed. The distal outflow vessel must be at least 50% patent for the graft to remain patent. A higher bypass graft patency rate is associated with keeping the length of the bypass as short as possible.

If the atherosclerotic occlusion is below the inguinal ligament in the superficial femoral artery, the surgical procedure of choice is the femoral-to-popliteal graft. This procedure is further classified as above-knee and below-knee grafts, referring to the location of the distal anastomosis.

Lower leg or ankle vessels with occlusions may also require grafts. Occasionally, the entire popliteal artery is occluded, and there is only collateral circulation. The distal anastomosis may be

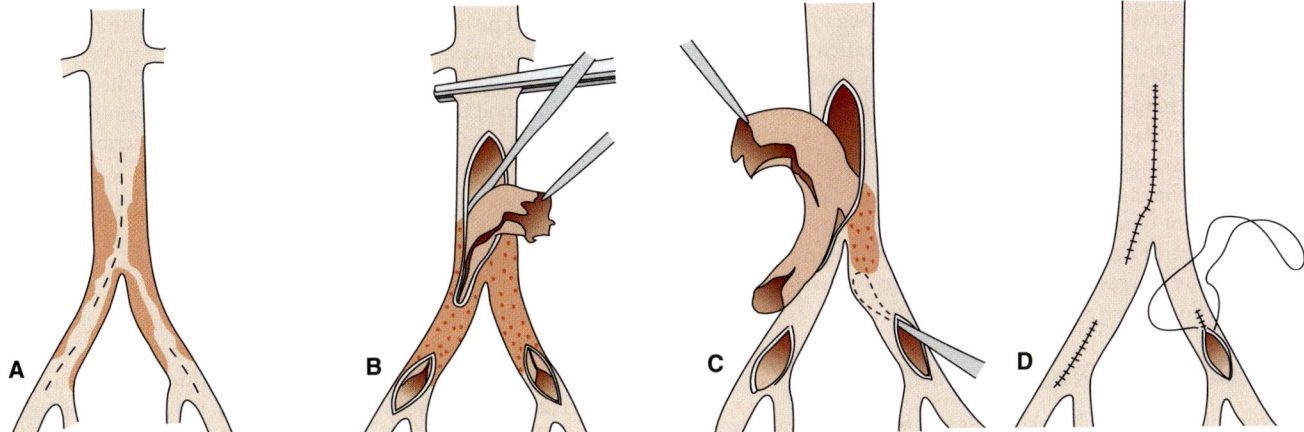

FIGURE 31-10 In an aortoiliac endarterectomy, the vascular surgeon (**A**) identifies the diseased area, (**B**) clamps off the blood supply to the vessel, (**C**) removes the plaque, and (**D**) sutures the vessel shut, after which blood flow is restored. Adapted with permission from Rutherford, R. B. (1999). *Vascular surgery: Vol. 1 and 2* (5th ed.). Philadelphia: W. B. Saunders.

made onto any of the tibial arteries (posterior tibial, anterior tibial, or peroneal arteries) or the dorsalis pedis or plantar artery. The distal anastomosis site is determined by the ease of exposure of the vessel in surgery and by which vessel provides the best flow to the distal limb. These grafts require the use of native vein to ensure patency. Native vein is autologous vein (the patient's own vein). The greater or lesser saphenous vein or a combination of one of the saphenous veins and an upper extremity vein such as the cephalic vein are used to meet the required length.

How long the graft remains patent is determined by several factors, including the size of the graft, graft location, and development of intimal hyperplasia at anastomosis sites. Bypass grafts may be synthetic or autologous vein. Several synthetic materials are available for use as a peripheral bypass graft: woven or knitted Dacron, expanded polytetrafluoroethylene (ePTFE, such as Gore-Tex or Impra), collagen-impregnated, and umbilical vein. Infection is a problem that threatens survival of the graft and almost always requires removal of the graft.

If a vein graft is the surgical choice, care must be taken in the operating room not to damage the vein after harvesting (removing the vein from the patient's body). The vein is occluded at one end and inflated with a heparinized solution to check for leakage and competency. When this is done, the graft is placed in a heparinized solution to keep it from becoming dry and brittle.

Nursing Management

MAINTAINING CIRCULATION
The primary objective in the postoperative management of patients who have undergone vascular procedures is to maintain adequate circulation through the arterial repair. Pulses, Doppler assessment, colour and temperature of the extremity, capillary refill, and sensory and motor function of the affected extremities are checked, compared with those of the other extremity, and recorded every hour for the first 8 hours and then every 2 hours for 24 hours. Doppler evaluation of the vessels distal to the bypass graft should be performed for all postoperative vascular patients, because it is more sensitive than palpation for pulses. The ABI is monitored at least once every 8 hours for the first 24 hours and then once each day until discharge (not usually assessed for pedal artery bypasses). An adequate circulating blood volume should be established and maintained. Disappearance of a pulse that was present may indicate thrombotic occlusion of the graft; the surgeon is immediately notified.

MONITORING AND MANAGING POTENTIAL COMPLICATIONS
Continuous monitoring of urine output (more than 30 mL/hour), central venous pressure, mental status, and pulse rate and volume permit early recognition and treatment of fluid imbalances. Bleeding can result from the heparin administered during surgery or from an anastomotic leak. A hematoma may form as well.

Leg crossing and prolonged extremity dependency are avoided to prevent thrombosis. Edema is a normal postoperative finding; however, elevating the extremities and encouraging the patient to exercise the extremities while in bed reduces edema. Elastic compression stockings may be prescribed for some patients, but care must be taken to avoid compressing distal vessel bypass grafts. Severe edema of the extremity, pain, and decreased sensation of toes or fingers can be an indication of compartment syndrome.

PROMOTING HOME AND COMMUNITY-BASED CARE
Discharge planning includes assessing the patient's ability to manage independently. The nurse determines if the patient has a network of family and friends to assist with activities of daily living. The patient may need to be encouraged to make the lifestyle changes necessary with a chronic disease, including pain management and modifications in diet, activity, and hygiene (skin care). The nurse ensures that the patient has the knowledge and ability to assess for any postoperative complications such as infection, occlusion of the artery or graft, and decreased blood flow. The nurse assists the patient in developing a plan to stop using tobacco. The Plan of Nursing Care describes nursing care for patients with peripheral vascular disease.

UPPER EXTREMITY ARTERIAL OCCLUSIVE DISEASE

Arterial occlusions occur less frequently in the upper extremities (arms) than in the legs and cause less severe symptoms because the collateral circulation is significantly better in the arms. The arms also have less muscle mass and are not subjected to the workload of the legs.

Clinical Manifestations

Stenosis and occlusions in the upper extremity result from atherosclerosis or trauma. The stenosis usually occurs at the origin of the vessel proximal to the vertebral artery, setting up the vertebral artery as the major contributor of flow. The patient may develop a "subclavian steal" syndrome characterized by reverse flow in the vertebral and basilar artery to provide blood flow to the arm. This syndrome may cause vertebrobasilar (cerebral) symptoms. Most patients are asymptomatic; however, some report vertigo, ataxia, syncope, or bilateral visual changes.

The patient typically complains of arm fatigue and pain with exercise (forearm claudication) and inability to hold or grasp objects (eg, painting, combing hair, placing objects on shelves above the head). Some even notice difficulties driving.

Assessment and Diagnostic Findings

Assessment findings include coolness and pallor of the affected extremity, decreased capillary refill, and a difference in arm blood pressures of more than 20 mm Hg. Noninvasive studies performed to evaluate for upper extremity arterial occlusions include upper and forearm blood pressure determinations and duplex ultrasonography to identify the anatomic location of the lesion and to evaluate the hemodynamics of the blood flow. Transcranial Doppler evaluation is performed to evaluate the intracranial circulation and to detect any siphoning of blood flow from the posterior circulation to provide blood flow to the affected arm. If a surgical or interventional procedure is planned, an arteriogram may be necessary.

Medical Management

If a short, focal lesion is identified in an upper extremity artery, a PCTA may be performed. If the lesion involves the subclavian artery with documented siphoning of blood flow from the intracranial circulation, several surgical procedures are available: carotid–to–subclavian artery bypass, axillary–to–axillary artery bypass, and autogenous reimplantation of the subclavian to the carotid artery.

Nursing Management

Nursing assessment involves bilateral comparison of upper arm blood pressures (obtained by stethoscope and Doppler); radial, ulnar, and brachial pulses; motor and sensory function; temperature; colour changes; and capillary refill every 2 hours. Disappearance of a pulse or Doppler flow that had been present may indicate an acute occlusion of the vessel, and the physician is notified immediately.

 NURSING ALERT Before and for 24 hours after surgery, the patient's arm is kept at heart level and protected from cold, venipunctures or arterial sticks, tape, and constrictive dressings.

After surgery, the arm is kept at heart level or elevated, with the fingers at the highest level. Pulses are monitored with Doppler assessment of the arterial flow every hour for 8 hours and then every 2 hours for 24 hours. Blood pressure (obtained by stethoscope and Doppler) is also assessed every hour for 8 hours and then every 2 hours for 24 hours. Motor and sensory function, warmth, colour, and capillary refill are monitored with each arterial flow (pulse) assessment.

Discharge planning includes assessing the patient's ability to manage independently. The nurse determines whether the patient has a network of family and friends to assist with activities of daily living. The patient may need to be encouraged to make the lifestyle changes necessary for a chronic disease, including pain management and modifications in diet, activity, and hygiene

(skin care). The nurse ensures that the patient has the knowledge and ability to assess for any postoperative complications such as infection, reocclusion of the artery or occlusion of the graft, and decreased blood flow. The patient is assisted in developing a plan to stop using tobacco. The Plan of Nursing Care describes nursing care for patients with peripheral vascular disease.

THROMBOANGIITIS OBLITERANS (BUERGER'S DISEASE)

Buerger's disease is characterized by recurring inflammation of the intermediate and small arteries and veins of the lower and (in rare cases) upper extremities. It results in thrombus formation and occlusion of the vessels. It is differentiated from other vessel diseases by its microscopic appearance. In contrast to atherosclerosis, Buerger's disease is believed to be an autoimmune disease that results in occlusion of distal vessels.

The cause of Buerger's disease is unknown, but it is believed to be an autoimmune vasculitis. It occurs most often in men between the ages of 20 and 35 years, and it has been reported in all races and in many areas of the world. There is considerable evidence that heavy smoking or chewing of tobacco is a causative or an aggravating factor (Frost-Rude et al., 2000). Generally, the lower extremities are affected, but arteries in the upper extremities or viscera can also be involved. Buerger's disease is generally bilateral and symmetric with focal lesions. Superficial thrombophlebitis may be present.

 ## Gerontologic Considerations

Although this condition is different from atherosclerosis, Buerger's disease in older patients may also be followed by atherosclerosis of the larger vessels after involvement of the smaller vessels. The patient's ability to walk may be severely limited. Patients are at higher risk for nonhealing wounds because of impaired circulation.

Clinical Manifestations

Pain is the outstanding symptom of Buerger's disease. The patient complains of foot cramps, especially of the arch (instep claudication), after exercise. The pain is relieved by rest; often, a burning pain is aggravated by emotional disturbances, nicotine, or chilling. Cold sensitivity of the Raynaud type is found in one half the patients and is frequently confined to the hands. Digital rest pain is constant, and the characteristics of the pain do not change between activity and rest.

Physical signs include intense rubor (reddish blue discolouration) of the foot and absence of the pedal pulse but with normal femoral and popliteal pulses. Radial and ulnar artery pulses are absent or diminished. Various types of paresthesia may develop.

As the disease progresses, definite redness or cyanosis of the part appears when the extremity is in a dependent position. Involvement is generally bilateral, but colour changes may affect only one extremity or only certain digits. Colour changes may progress to ulceration, and ulceration with gangrene eventually occurs.

Assessment and Diagnostic Findings

Segmental limb blood pressures are taken to demonstrate the distal location of the lesions or occlusions. Duplex ultrasonography is used to document patency of the proximal vessels and to visualize the extent of distal disease. Contrast angiography is performed to demonstrate the diseased portion of the anatomy.

Management

The treatment of Buerger's disease is essentially the same as that for atherosclerotic peripheral arterial disease. The main objectives are to improve circulation to the extremities, prevent the progression of the disease, and protect the extremities from trauma and infection. Treatment of ulceration and gangrene is directed toward minimizing infection and conservative débridement of necrotic tissue. Tobacco use is highly detrimental, and patients are strongly advised to stop using tobacco completely. Symptoms are often relieved by cessation of smoking and other uses of tobacco.

Vasodilators are rarely prescribed because these medications cause dilation of only healthy vessels; vasodilators may divert blood away from the partially occluded vessels, making the situation worse. A regional sympathetic block or ganglionectomy may be useful in some instances to produce vasodilation and increase blood flow.

SURGICAL MANAGEMENT OF COMPLICATIONS

If gangrene of a toe develops as a result of arterial occlusive disease in the leg, it is unlikely that toe amputation or even transmetatarsal amputation will be sufficient; usually, a below-knee amputation or, occasionally, an above-knee amputation is necessary. The indications for amputation are worsening gangrene, especially if the infected area is moist, severe rest pain, or fulminating sepsis.

NURSING MANAGEMENT OF COMPLICATIONS

If an amputation is performed, immediate postoperative care includes elevating the stump for the first 24 hours to promote venous return and minimize edema. The incision is monitored for signs of hematoma (unapproximated suture line, discolouration or ruddy colour changes of the skin along the suture line, tenderness with palpation, or oozing of dark blood from the suture line). The nurse assesses the fit of the elastic bandages and ensures the integrity of the wrap and continued ability to fit two fingers between layers of the wrap. Distal skin colour and warmth are assessed, if accessible, and recorded. Elastic bandages are removed and reapplied as prescribed by the surgeon (eg, every 6 hours using figure-of-eight turns).

The patient may experience grief, fear, or anxiety related to loss of the limb. The patient is encouraged to discuss his or her feelings. Spiritual advisors and other health care team members are consulted as appropriate. Recovery and rehabilitation require consultation among health care providers (eg, physicians, physical and occupational therapists, prosthetists, dietitians, nurses, discharge coordinators). The patient may decide to be fitted for and learn to use a prosthetic device. Rehabilitation facilities, home care, and outpatient therapy can assist the patient to adapt to the changes in lifestyle.

Discharge planning includes assessing the patient's ability to manage independently. The patient is assisted in developing a plan to stop using tobacco and to manage pain. The patient may need to be encouraged to make the lifestyle changes necessary with a chronic disease, including modifications in diet, activity, and hygiene (skin care). The nurse determines whether the patient has a network of family and friends to assist with activities of daily living. The nurse ensures that the patient has the knowledge and ability to assess for any postoperative complications such as infection and decreased blood flow. The Plan of Nursing Care describes nursing care for patients with peripheral vascular disease.

AORTITIS

The aorta, which is the main trunk of the arterial system, is divided into the ascending aorta (5 cm in diameter, contained in the pericardium), the aortic arch (extending upward, backward, and downward), and the descending aorta. The thoracic aorta is above the diaphragm; the abdominal aorta is below the diaphragm. The abdominal aorta is further designated as suprarenal (above renal artery level), perirenal level (at renal artery level), and infrarenal (below renal artery level).

Aortitis is inflammation of the aorta, particularly of the aortic arch. Two types are known to occur: Takayasu's disease and syphilitic aortitis. Takayasu's disease, or occlusive thromboaortopathy, is uncommon; today, syphilitic aortitis is rare.

Takayasu's disease, a chronic inflammatory disease of the aortic arch and its branches, primarily affects young or middle-aged women and is more common in those of Asian descent. It is nonatherosclerotic; the exact pathologic mechanism is unknown but thought to be immune complex mediated. It progresses from a systemic inflammation with localized arteritis to end-organ ischemia because of large vessel stenosis or obstruction. Magnetic resonance angiography, CT, duplex ultrasonography, or arteriography is used to diagnose and evaluate the lesions, which are typically long, smooth areas of narrowing with or without aneurysms. In the early stages, the disease may respond to corticosteroids, and patients may benefit from the addition of cytotoxic immunosuppressive agents (Strider et al., 1996). Selective PCTA and surgical revascularization may be performed after suppression of the systemic vascular inflammation.

AORTOILIAC DISEASE

If collateral circulation has developed, patients with a stenosis or occlusion of the aortoiliac segment may be asymptomatic, or they may complain of buttock or low back discomfort associated with walking. Men may experience impotence. These patients may have decreased or absent femoral pulses.

Medical Management

The treatment of aortoiliac disease is essentially the same as that for atherosclerotic peripheral arterial occlusive disease. The surgical procedure of choice is the aortobiiliac graft. If possible, the distal anastomosis is made to the iliac artery, and the entire surgical procedure can be performed within the abdomen. If the iliac vessels are diseased, the distal anastomosis is made to the femoral arteries (aortobifemoral graft). Bifurcated woven or knitted Dacron grafts are preferred for this surgical procedure.

Nursing Management

Preoperative assessment, in addition to the standard parameters (see Chap. 18), includes evaluating the brachial, radial, ulnar, femoral, posterior tibial, and dorsalis pedis pulses to establish a baseline for follow-up after arterial lines are placed and postoperatively. Patient teaching includes an overview of the procedure to be performed, the preparation for surgery, and the anticipated postoperative plan of care. Sights, sounds, and sensations that the patient may experience are discussed.

Postoperative care includes monitoring for signs of thrombosis in arteries distal to the surgical site. The nurse assesses colour and temperature of the extremity, capillary refill time, sensory and motor function, and pulses by palpation and Doppler every hour for the first 8 hours and then every 2 hours for the first

24 hours. Any dusky or bluish discolouration, coolness, capillary refill time greater than 3 seconds, decrease in sensory or motor function, or decrease in pulse quality are reported immediately to the physician.

Postoperative care also includes monitoring for urine output greater than or equal to 30 mL/hour. Renal function may be impaired as a result of hypoperfusion from hypotension, involvement of the renal arteries during the surgical procedure, hypovolemia, or embolization of the renal artery or renal parenchyma. Vital signs, pain, and intake and output are monitored with the pulse and extremity assessments. Results of laboratory tests are monitored and reported to the physician. Abdominal assessment for bowel sounds and paralytic ileus is performed at least every 8 hours. Bowel sounds may not return before the third postoperative day. The absence of bowel sounds, absence of flatus, and abdominal distention are indications of paralytic ileus. Manual manipulation of the bowel during surgery may have caused bruising, resulting in decreased peristalsis. Nasogastric suction may be necessary to decompress the bowel until peristalsis returns. A liquid bowel movement before the third postoperative day may indicate bowel ischemia, which may occur when the mesenteric blood supply (celiac, superior mesenteric, or inferior mesenteric arteries) is occluded. Ischemic bowel usually causes increased pain and an elevated white blood cell count (20,000 to 30,000 cells/mm^3).

AORTIC ANEURYSM

An aneurysm is a localized sac or dilation formed at a weak point in the wall of the aorta (Fig. 31-11). It may be classified by its shape or form. The most common forms of aneurysms are saccular or fusiform. A saccular aneurysm projects from one side of the vessel only. If an entire arterial segment becomes dilated, a fusiform aneurysm develops. Very small aneurysms due to localized infection are called mycotic aneurysms.

Historically, the cause of abdominal aortic aneurysm, the most common type of degenerative aneurysm, has been attributed to atherosclerotic changes in the aorta. Other causes of aneurysm formation are listed in Chart 31-5. Aneurysms are serious because they can rupture, leading to hemorrhage and death.

Chart 31-5 **Etiologic Classification of Arterial Aneurysms**

Congenital: Primary connective tissue disorders (Marfan's syndrome, Ehlers-Danlos syndrome) and other diseases (focal medial agenesis, tuberous sclerosis, Turner's syndrome, Menkes' syndrome)

Mechanical (hemodynamic): Poststenotic and arteriovenous fistula and amputation-related

Traumatic (pseudoaneurysms): Penetrating arterial injuries, blunt arterial injuries, pseudoaneurysms

Inflammatory (noninfectious): Associated with arteritis (Takayasu's disease, giant cell arteritis, systemic lupus erythematosus, Behçet's syndrome, Kawasaki's disease) and periarterial inflammation (ie, pancreatitis)

Infectious (mycotic): Bacterial, fungal, spirochetal infections

Pregnancy-related degenerative: Nonspecific, inflammatory variant

Anastomotic (postarteriotomy) and graft aneurysms: Infection, arterial wall failure, suture failure, graft failure

Adapted with permission from Rutherford, R. B. (1999). *Vascular surgery* (Vols. 1 and 2, 5th ed.). Philadelphia: W. B. Saunders.

THORACIC AORTIC ANEURYSM

Approximately 85% of all cases of thoracic aortic aneurysm are caused by atherosclerosis. They occur most frequently in men between the ages 40 and 70 years. The thoracic area is the most common site for a dissecting aneurysm. About one third of patients with thoracic aneurysms die of rupture of the aneurysm (Rutherford, 1999).

Clinical Manifestations

Symptoms are variable and depend on how rapidly the aneurysm dilates and how the pulsating mass affects surrounding intrathoracic structures. Some patients are asymptomatic. In most cases, pain is the most prominent symptom. The pain is usually constant and boring but may occur only when the person is supine.

FIGURE 31-11 Characteristics of arterial aneurysm. (**A**) Normal artery. (**B**) False aneurysm—actually a pulsating hematoma. The clot and connective tissue are outside the arterial wall. (**C**) True aneurysm. One, two, or all three layers of the artery may be involved. (**D**) Fusiform aneurysm—symmetric, spindle-shaped expansion of entire circumference of involved vessel. (**E**) Saccular aneurysm—a bulbous protrusion of one side of the arterial wall. (**F**) Dissecting aneurysm—this usually is a hematoma that splits the layers of the arterial wall.

Other conspicuous symptoms are dyspnea, the result of pressure of the sac against the trachea, a main bronchus, or the lung itself; cough, frequently paroxysmal and with a brassy quality; hoarseness, stridor, or weakness or complete loss of the voice (aphonia), resulting from pressure against the left recurrent laryngeal nerve; and dysphagia (difficulty in swallowing) due to impingement on the esophagus by the aneurysm.

Assessment and Diagnostic Findings

When large veins in the chest are compressed by the aneurysm, the superficial veins of the chest, neck, or arms become dilated, and edematous areas on the chest wall and cyanosis are often evident. Pressure against the cervical sympathetic chain can result in unequal pupils. Diagnosis of a thoracic aortic aneurysm is principally made by chest x-ray, transesophageal echocardiography, and CT.

Medical Management

In most cases, an aneurysm is treated by surgical repair. General measures such as controlling blood pressure and correcting risk factors may be helpful. It is important to control blood pressure in patients with dissecting aneurysms. Systolic pressure is maintained at about 100 to 120 mm Hg with antihypertensive medications (eg, hydralazine hydrochloride [Apresoline], esmolol hydrochloride [Brevibloc] or another beta-blocker such as atenolol [Tenormin] or timolol maleate [Timoptic]). Pulsatile flow is reduced by medications that reduce cardiac contractility (eg, propranolol [Inderal]). The goal of surgery is to repair the aneurysm and restore vascular continuity with a vascular graft (Fig. 31-12). Intensive monitoring is usually required after this type of surgery, and the patient is cared for in the critical care unit. Repair of thoracic aneurysms using endovascular grafts implanted (deployed) percutaneously in an interventional laboratory (eg, cardiac catheterization laboratory) may decrease postoperative recovery time and decrease complications compared with traditional surgical techniques.

ABDOMINAL AORTIC ANEURYSM

The most common cause of abdominal aortic aneurysm is atherosclerosis. The condition, which is more common among Caucasians, affects men four times more often than women and is most prevalent in elderly patients (Rutherford, 1999). Most of these aneurysms occur below the renal arteries (infrarenal aneurysms). Untreated, the eventual outcome may be rupture and death.

Pathophysiology

All aneurysms involve a damaged media layer of the vessel. This may be caused by congenital weakness, trauma, or disease. After an aneurysm develops, it tends to enlarge. Risk factors include genetic predisposition, smoking (or other tobacco use), and hypertension; more than one half of patients with aneurysms have hypertension.

FIGURE 31-12 Repair of an ascending aortic aneurysm and aortic valve replacement. (**A**) Incision into aortic aneurysm. (**B**) Aortic valve replacement with aortic graft implant to repair ascending aortic aneurysm. (**C**) Aortic aneurysm trimmed and closed over graft.

Clinical Manifestations

About two fifths of patients with abdominal aortic aneurysms have symptoms; the remainder do not. Some patients complain that they can feel their heart beating in their abdomen when lying down, or they may say they feel an abdominal mass or abdominal throbbing. If the abdominal aortic aneurysm is associated with thrombus, a major vessel may be occluded or smaller distal occlusions may result from emboli. A small cholesterol, platelet, or fibrin emboli may lodge in the interosseous or digital arteries, causing blue toes.

Assessment and Diagnostic Findings

The most important diagnostic indication of an abdominal aortic aneurysm is a pulsatile mass in the middle and upper abdomen. About 80% of these aneurysms can be palpated. A systolic bruit may be heard over the mass. Duplex ultrasonography or CT is used to determine the size, length, and location of the aneurysm (Fig. 31-13). When the aneurysm is small, ultrasonography is conducted at 6-month intervals until the aneurysm reaches a size at which surgery to prevent rupture is of more benefit than the possible complications of a surgical procedure. Some aneurysms remain stable over many years of observation.

Gerontologic Considerations

Most abdominal aneurysms occur in patients between the ages of 60 and 90 years. Rupture is likely with coexisting hypertension and with aneurysms wider than 6 cm. In most cases at this point, the chances of rupture are greater than the chance of death during surgical repair. If the elderly patient is considered at moderate risk for complications related to surgery or anesthesia, the aneurysm is not repaired until it is at least 5 cm (2 inches) wide.

Medical Management

An expanding or enlarging abdominal aneurysm is likely to rupture. Surgery is the treatment of choice for abdominal aneurysms wider than 5 cm (2 inches) wide or those that are enlarging.

SURGICAL MANAGEMENT

The standard treatment for abdominal aortic aneurysm repair has been open surgical repair of the aneurysm by resecting the vessel and sewing a bypass graft in place. The mortality rate associated with elective aneurysm repair, a major surgical procedure, is reported to be 1% to 4%. The prognosis for a patient with a ruptured aneurysm is poor, and surgery is performed immediately (Rutherford, 1999).

An alternative for treating an infrarenal abdominal aortic aneurysm is endovascular grafting. Endovascular grafting involves the transluminal placement and attachment of a sutureless aortic graft prosthesis across an aneurysm (Fig. 31-14). This procedure can be performed under local or regional anesthesia. Endovascular grafting of abdominal aortic aneurysms may be performed if the patient's abdominal aorta and iliac arteries are not extremely tortuous and if the aneurysm does not begin at the level of the renal arteries. Clinical trials are evaluating endograft treatment of abdominal aortic aneurysms at or above the level of the renal arteries and the thoracic aorta. Potential complications include bleeding, hematoma, or wound infection at the femoral insertion site; distal ischemia or embolization; dissection or perforation of the aorta; graft thrombosis; graft infection; break of the attachment system; graft migration; proximal or distal graft leaks; delayed rupture; and bowel ischemia.

Nursing Management

Before surgery, nursing assessment is guided by anticipating a rupture and by recognizing that the patient may have cardiovascular, cerebral, pulmonary, and renal impairment from atherosclerosis. The functional capacity of all organ systems should be assessed. Medical therapies designed to stabilize physiologic function should be promptly implemented.

Signs of impending rupture include severe back pain or abdominal pain, which may be persistent or intermittent and is often

FIGURE 31-13 Duplex ultrasonic image of abdominal aortic aneurysm at the perirenal level. Cross-sectional image documents the location of right and left renal arteries.

FIGURE 31-14 Ancure Endograft repair of an abdominal aortic aneurysm.

localized in the middle or lower abdomen to the left of the midline. Low back pain may also be present because of pressure of the aneurysm on the lumbar nerves. This is a serious symptom, usually indicating that the aneurysm is expanding rapidly and is about to rupture. Indications of a rupturing abdominal aortic aneurysm include constant, intense back pain; falling blood pressure; and decreasing hematocrit. Rupture into the peritoneal cavity is rapidly fatal. A retroperitoneal rupture of an aneurysm may result in hematomas in the scrotum, perineum, flank, or penis. Signs of heart failure or a loud bruit may suggest a rupture into the vena cava. Rupture into the vena cava results in the higher-pressure arterial blood entering the lower-pressure venous system and causing turbulence, which is heard as a bruit. The high blood pressure and increased blood volume returning to the right heart from the vena cava may cause the right heart to fail. The overall surgical mortality rate associated with a ruptured aneurysm is 50% to 75%.

Postoperative care requires intense monitoring of pulmonary, cardiovascular, renal, and neurologic status. Possible complications of surgery include arterial occlusion, hemorrhage, infection, ischemic bowel, renal failure, and impotence.

DISSECTING AORTA

Occasionally, in an aorta diseased by arteriosclerosis, a tear develops in the intima or the media degenerates, resulting in a dissection (see Fig. 31-11).

Pathophysiology

Arterial dissections (separations) are commonly associated with poorly controlled hypertension; they are three times more common in men than in women and occur most commonly in the 50- to 70-year-old age group (Rutherford, 1999). Dissection is caused by rupture in the intimal layer. A rupture may occur through adventitia or into the lumen through the intima, allowing blood to reenter the main channel and resulting in chronic dissection or occlusion of branches of the aorta.

As the separation progresses, the arteries branching from the involved area of the aorta shear and occlude. The tear occurs most commonly in the region of the aortic arch, with the highest mortality rate associated with ascending aortic dissection. The dissection of the aorta may progress backward in the direction of the heart, obstructing the openings to the coronary arteries or producing hemopericardium (effusion of blood into the pericardial sac) or aortic insufficiency, or it may extend in the opposite direction, causing occlusion of the arteries supplying the gastrointestinal tract, kidneys, spinal cord, and legs.

Clinical Manifestations

Onset of symptoms is usually sudden. Severe and persistent pain, described as tearing or ripping, may be reported. The pain is in the anterior chest or back and extends to shoulders, epigastric area, or abdomen. Aortic dissection may be mistaken for an acute myocardial infarction, which could confuse the clinical picture and initial treatment. Cardiovascular, neurologic, and gastrointestinal symptoms are responsible for other clinical manifestations, depending on the location and extent of the dissection. The patient may appear pale. Sweating and tachycardia may be detected. Blood pressure may be elevated or markedly different from one arm to the other if dissection involves the orifice of the subclavian artery on one side. Because of the variable clinical picture associated with this condition, early diagnosis is usually difficult.

Assessment and Diagnostic Findings

Arteriography, CT, transesophageal echocardiography, duplex ultrasonography, and magnetic resonance imaging aid in the diagnosis.

Medical Management

Medical or surgical treatment of a dissecting aneurysm depends on the type of dissection present and follows the general principles outlined for the treatment of thoracic aortic aneurysms.

Nursing Management

A patient with a dissecting aorta requires the same nursing care as a patient with an aortic aneurysm requiring surgical intervention, as described earlier in this chapter. Interventions described in the Plan of Nursing Care are also appropriate.

OTHER ANEURYSMS

Aneurysms may also arise in the peripheral vessels, most often as a result of atherosclerosis. These may involve such vessels as the subclavian artery, renal artery, femoral artery, or (most frequently) popliteal artery. Between 50% and 60% of popliteal aneurysms are bilateral and may be associated with abdominal aortic aneurysms.

The aneurysm produces a pulsating mass and disturbs peripheral circulation distal to it. Pain and swelling develop because of pressure on adjacent nerves and veins. Diagnosis is made by duplex ultrasonography and CT to determine the size, length, and extent of the aneurysm. Arteriography may be performed to evaluate the level of proximal and distal involvement.

Surgical repair is performed with replacement grafts or endovascular repair using a stent-graft or wall graft, which is a Dacron or PTFE (polytetrafluoroethylene) graft with external structures made from a variety of materials (nitinol, titanium, stainless steel) for additional support.

Nursing Management

The patient who has had an endovascular repair must lie supine for 6 hours; the head of the bed may be elevated up to 45 degrees after 2 hours. The patient needs to use a bedpan or urinal while on bed rest, or a Foley catheter may be used. Vital signs and Doppler assessment of peripheral pulses are performed every 15 minutes for four times, then every 30 minutes for four times, then every hour for four times, and then as directed by the physician or unit standards. The catheterization site is assessed when vital signs and pulses are monitored. The nurse assesses for bleeding, swelling, pain, and hematoma formation. Any changes in vital signs, pulse quality, bleeding, swelling, pain, or hematoma are reported to the physician. The physician is also notified of persistent coughing, sneezing, vomiting, or systolic blood pressure above 180 mm Hg because of the increased risk for hemorrhage. Most patients are able to resume their preprocedure diet and are encouraged to drink fluids. An intravenous infusion may be continued until the patient is able to drink normally. Fluids are important to maintain blood flow through the arterial repair site and to assist the kidneys with excreting intravenous contrast agent and other medications used during the procedure. Six hours after the procedure, the patient may be able to roll side to side and may be able to ambulate with assistance to the bathroom. After the patient is able to take adequate fluids orally, the intravenous infusion may be discontinued and the intravenous access converted to a saline lock.

ARTERIAL EMBOLISM AND ARTERIAL THROMBOSIS

Acute vascular occlusion may be caused by an embolus or acute thrombosis. Acute arterial occlusions may result from iatrogenic injury, which can occur during insertion of invasive catheters such as those used for arteriography, PCTA or stent placement, or an intra-aortic balloon pump. Other causes include trauma from a fracture, crush injury, and penetrating wounds that disrupt the arterial intima. The accurate diagnosis of an arterial occlusion as embolic or thrombotic in origin is necessary to initiate appropriate treatment.

Pathophysiology

Arterial emboli arise most commonly from thrombi that develop in the chambers of the heart as a result of atrial fibrillation, myocardial infarction, infective endocarditis, or chronic heart failure. These thrombi become detached and are carried from the left side of the heart into the arterial system, where they lodge in and obstruct an artery that is smaller than the embolus. Emboli may also develop in advanced aortic atherosclerosis because the atheromatous plaques ulcerate or become rough. Acute thrombosis frequently occurs in patients with preexisting ischemic symptoms.

Clinical Manifestations

The symptoms of arterial emboli depend primarily on the size of the embolus, the organ involved, and the state of the collateral vessels. The immediate effect is cessation of distal blood flow. The blockage can progress above and below the obstruction. Secondary vasospasm can contribute to the ischemia. The embolus can fragment or break apart, resulting in occlusion of distal vessels. Emboli tend to lodge at arterial bifurcations and areas narrowed by atherosclerosis. Cerebral, mesenteric, renal, and coronary arteries are often involved in addition to the large arteries of the extremities.

The symptoms of acute arterial embolism in extremities with poor collateral flow are acute, severe pain and a gradual loss of sensory and motor function. The six *P*s associated with acute arterial embolism are pain, pallor, pulselessness, paresthesia, poikilothermia (coldness), and paralysis. Eventually, superficial veins may collapse because of decreased blood flow to the extremity. The part of the extremity below the occlusion is markedly colder and paler than the part above the occlusion because of ischemia.

Arterial thrombosis can also acutely occlude an artery. A thrombosis is a slowly developing clot that usually occurs where the arterial wall has become damaged, generally as a result of atherosclerosis. Thrombi may also develop in an arterial aneurysm. The manifestations of an acute thrombotic arterial occlusion are similar to those described for embolic occlusion. However, treatment is more difficult with a thrombus because the arterial occlusion has occurred in a degenerated vessel and requires more extensive reconstructive surgery to restore flow than is required with an embolic event.

Assessment and Diagnostic Findings

An arterial embolus is usually diagnosed on the basis of the sudden nature of the onset of symptoms and an apparent source for the embolus. Two-dimensional echocardiography or transesophageal echocardiography, chest x-ray, and electrocardiography may reveal underlying cardiac disease. Noninvasive duplex and Doppler ultrasonography can determine the presence and extent of underlying atherosclerosis, and arteriography may be performed.

Medical Management

Management of arterial thrombosis depends on its cause. Management of acute embolic occlusion usually requires surgery because time is of the essence. Because the onset of the event is acute, collateral circulation has not developed, and the patient quickly moves through the list of six *P*s to paralysis, which is the most advanced stage. Heparin therapy is initiated immediately to prevent further development of emboli and to hamper the extension of existing thrombi. Typically, an initial bolus of 5,000 to 10,000 units is administered intravenously, followed by a continuous infusion of 1,000 units per hour until the patient is able to undergo surgery.

SURGICAL MANAGEMENT

Emergency embolectomy is the procedure of choice only if the involved extremity is viable (Fig. 31-15). Arterial emboli are usually treated by insertion of an embolectomy catheter. The catheter is passed through a groin incision into the affected artery and advanced past the occlusion. The balloon is inflated with sterile saline solution, and the thrombus is extracted as the catheter is withdrawn. This procedure involves incising the vessel and removing the clot.

PHARMACOLOGIC THERAPY

When the patient has collateral circulation, treatment may include intravenous anticoagulation with heparin, which can prevent the thrombus from spreading and reduce muscle necrosis. The use of intra-arterial thrombolytic medications helps to dissolve the embolus. Fibrin-specific thrombolytic medications (eg, tissue plasminogen activator [t-PA, alteplase, Activase] and single-chain urokinase-type plasminogen activator [scu-PA, pro-urokinase]) avoid systemic depletion of circulating fibrinogen and plasminogen, which prevents the development of systemic fibrinolysis.

FIGURE 31-15 Extraction of an embolus by balloon-tipped embolectomy catheter. The deflated balloon-tipped catheter is advanced past the embolus, inflated and then gently withdrawn, carrying the embolic material with it. Adapted with permission from Rutherford, R. B. (1999). *Vascular surgery: Vol. 1 and 2* (5th ed.). Philadelphia: W. B. Saunders.

Other thrombolytic medications are reteplase (r-PA, Retavase), tenecteplase (TNKase), and staphylokinase (Moore, 2002). Although these agents differ in their pharmacokinetics, they are administered in a similar manner. A catheter is advanced under x-ray visualization to the clot, and the thrombolytic agent is infused.

Thrombolytic therapy should not be used when there are known contraindications to therapy or when the extremity cannot tolerate the several additional hours of ischemia that it takes for the agent to lyse (disintegrate) the clot. Contraindications to thrombolytic therapy include active internal bleeding, CVA (brain attack, stroke), recent major surgery, uncontrolled hypertension, and pregnancy.

Nursing Management

Before surgery, the patient remains on bed rest with the extremity level or slightly dependent (15 degrees). The affected part is kept at room temperature and protected from trauma. Heating and cooling pads are contraindicated because ischemic extremities are easily traumatized by alterations in temperature. If possible, tape and electrocardiogram electrodes should not be used on the extremity; sheepskin and foot cradles are used to protect the leg from mechanical trauma.

If the patient is treated with thrombolytic therapy, she or he is accurately weighed in kilograms, and the dose of thrombolytic therapy is determined based on the patient's weight. The patient is admitted to a critical care unit for continuous monitoring. Vital signs are taken every 15 minutes for 2 hours, then every 30 minutes for the next 6 hours, and then every hour for 16 hours. Bleeding is the most common side effect of thrombolytic therapy, and the patient is closely monitored for any signs of bleeding. The nurse also minimizes the number of punctures for inserting intravenous lines, avoids intramuscular injections, prevents any possible tissue trauma, and applies pressure at least twice as long as usual after any puncture that is performed. If t-PA is used for the treatment, heparin is usually administered to prevent another thrombus from forming at the site of the lesion. The t-PA activates plasminogen on the thrombus more than circulating plasminogen, but it does not decrease the clotting factors as much as other thrombolytic therapies, so patients receiving t-PA are able to make new thrombi more easily than with some of the other thrombolytics.

During the postoperative period, the nurse collaborates with the surgeon about the patient's appropriate activity level based on the patient's condition. Generally, every effort is made to encourage the patient to move the leg to stimulate circulation and prevent stasis. Anticoagulant therapy may be continued after surgery to prevent thrombosis of the affected artery and to diminish the development of subsequent thrombi at the initiating site. The nurse assesses for evidence of local and systemic hemorrhage, including mental status changes, which can occur when anticoagulants are administered. Pulses, Doppler signals, ABI, and motor and sensory function are assessed every hour for the first 24 hours, because significant changes may indicate reocclusion. Metabolic abnormalities, renal failure, and compartment syndrome may be complications after an acute arterial occlusion.

RAYNAUD'S DISEASE

Raynaud's disease is a form of intermittent arteriolar vasoconstriction that results in coldness, pain, and pallor of the fingertips or toes. The cause is unknown, although many patients with the disease seem to have immunologic disorders. Symptoms may result from a defect in basal heat production that eventually decreases the ability of cutaneous vessels to dilate. Episodes may be triggered by emotional factors or by unusual sensitivity to cold. The disease is most common in women between 16 and 40 years of age, and it occurs more frequently in cold climates and during the winter.

The term *Raynaud's phenomenon* is used to refer to localized, intermittent episodes of vasoconstriction of small arteries of the feet and hands that cause colour and temperature changes. Generally unilateral and affecting only one or two digits, the phenomenon is always associated with underlying systemic disease. It may occur with scleroderma, systemic lupus erythematosus, rheumatoid arthritis, obstructive arterial disease, or trauma.

The prognosis for Raynaud's disease varies; some patients slowly improve, some become progressively worse, and others show no change. Ulceration and gangrene are rare; however, chronic disease may cause atrophy of the skin and muscles. With appropriate patient teaching and lifestyle modifications, the disorder is generally benign and self-limiting.

Clinical Manifestations

The classic clinical picture reveals pallor brought on by sudden vasoconstriction. The skin then becomes bluish (cyanotic) due to pooling of deoxygenated blood during vasospasm. As a result of exaggerated reflow (hyperemia) due to vasodilation, a red colour is produced (rubor) when oxygenated blood returns to the digits after the vasospasm stops. The characteristic sequence of colour change of Raynaud's phenomenon is described as white, blue, and red. Numbness, tingling, and burning pain occur as the colour changes. The involvement tends to be bilateral and symmetric.

Medical Management

Avoiding the particular stimuli (eg, cold, tobacco) that provoke vasoconstriction is a primary factor in controlling Raynaud's disease. Calcium channel blockers may be effective in relieving symptoms. Studies indicate that nifedipine (Procardia, Adalat) is an effective calcium channel blocker for treating an acute episode of vasospasm (Kaufman et al., 1996). Sympathectomy (interrupting the sympathetic nerves by removing the sympathetic ganglia or dividing their branches) may help some patients.

Nursing Management

The nurse teaches patients to avoid situations that may be stressful or unsafe. Stress management classes may be helpful. Exposure to cold must be minimized, and in areas where the fall and winter months are cold, the patient should remain indoors as much as possible and wear layers of clothing when outdoors. Hats and mittens or gloves should be worn at all times when outside. Fabrics specially designed for cold climates (eg, Thinsulate) are recommended. Patients should warm up their vehicles before getting in so that they can avoid touching a cold steering wheel or door handle, which could elicit an attack. During summer, a sweater should be available when entering air-conditioned rooms.

Concerns about serious complications, such as gangrene and amputation, are common among patients. However, these consequences are uncommon. Patients should avoid all forms of nicotine; the nicotine gum or patches used to help people quit smoking may induce attacks.

Patients should be careful about safety. Sharp objects should be handled carefully to avoid injuring the fingers. Patients should be informed about the postural hypotension that may result from medications, such as calcium channel blockers, used to treat Raynaud's disease. The nurse also discusses safety precautions related to alcohol, exercise, and hot weather.

Management of Venous Disorders

VENOUS THROMBOSIS, DEEP VEIN THROMBOSIS (DVT), THROMBOPHLEBITIS, AND PHLEBOTHROMBOSIS

Although the terms *venous thrombosis, deep vein thrombosis (DVT), thrombophlebitis,* and *phlebothrombosis* do not necessarily reflect identical disease processes, for clinical purposes, they are often used interchangeably.

Pathophysiology

Superficial veins, such as the greater saphenous, lesser saphenous, cephalic, basilic, and external jugular veins, are thick-walled muscular structures that lie just under the skin. Deep veins are thin walled and have less muscle in the media. They run parallel to arteries and bear the same names as the arteries. Deep and superficial veins have valves that permit unidirectional flow back to the heart. The valves lie at the base of a segment of the vein that is expanded into a sinus. This arrangement permits the valves to open without coming into contact with the wall of the vein, permitting rapid closure when the blood starts to flow backward. Other kinds of veins are known as perforating veins. These vessels have valves that allow one-way blood flow from the superficial system to the deep system.

Although the exact cause of venous thrombosis remains unclear, three factors, known as Virchow's triad, are believed to play a significant role in its development: stasis of blood (venous stasis), vessel wall injury, and altered blood coagulation (Chart 31-6). At least two of the factors seem to be necessary for thrombosis to occur. Venous stasis occurs when blood flow is reduced, as in heart failure or shock; when veins are dilated, as with some medication therapies; and when skeletal muscle contraction is reduced, as in immobility, paralysis of the extremities, or anesthesia. Moreover, bed rest reduces blood flow in the legs by at least 50%. Damage to the intimal lining of blood vessels creates a site for clot formation. Direct trauma to the vessels, as with fractures or dislocation, diseases of the veins, and chemical irritation of the vein from intravenous medications or solutions, can damage veins. Increased blood coagulability occurs most commonly in patients who have been abruptly withdrawn from anticoagulant medications. Oral contraceptive use and several blood dyscrasias (abnormalities) also can lead to hypercoagulability.

Formation of a thrombus frequently accompanies thrombophlebitis, which is an inflammation of the vein walls. When a thrombus develops initially in the veins as a result of stasis or hypercoagulability but without inflammation, the process is referred to as phlebothrombosis. Venous thrombosis can occur in any vein but occurs more in the veins of the lower extremities. The superficial and deep veins of the extremities may be affected.

Upper extremity venous thrombosis is not as common as lower extremity thrombosis. However, upper extremity venous thrombosis is more common in patients with intravenous catheters or in patients with an underlying disease that causes hypercoagulability. Internal trauma to the vessels may result from pacemaker leads, chemotherapy ports, dialysis catheters, or parenteral nutri-

Chart 31-6
Risk Factors for Deep Vein Thrombosis (DVT) and Pulmonary Embolism

Endothelial damage
  Trauma
  Surgery
  Pacing wires
  Central venous catheters
  Dialysis access catheters
  Local vein damage
  Repetitive motion injury
Venous stasis
  Bed rest or immobilization
  Obesity
  History of varicosities
  Spinal cord injury
  Age (>65 yr)
Coagulopathy
Cancer
Pregnancy
Oral contraceptive use
Presence of congenital proteins C and S
Presence of anticardiolipin antibody
Antithrombin III deficiency
Polycythemia
Septicemia

tion lines. The lumen of the vein may be decreased as a result of the catheter or from external compression, such as by neoplasms or an extra cervical rib. Effort thrombosis of the upper extremity is caused by repetitive motion, such as experienced by competitive swimmers, tennis players, and construction workers, that irritates the vessel wall, causing inflammation and subsequent thrombosis.

Venous thrombi are aggregates of platelets attached to the vein wall, along with a tail-like appendage containing fibrin, white blood cells, and many red blood cells. The "tail" can grow or can propagate in the direction of blood flow as successive layers of the thrombus form. A propagating venous thrombosis is dangerous because parts of the thrombus can break off and produce an embolic occlusion of the pulmonary blood vessels. Fragmentation of the thrombus can occur spontaneously as it dissolves naturally, or it can occur in association with an elevation in venous pressure, as occurs when a person stands suddenly or engages in muscular activity after prolonged inactivity. After an episode of acute deep vein thrombosis, recanalization of the lumen typically occurs. The time required for complete recanalization is an important determinant of venous valvular incompetence, which is one complication of venous thrombosis (Meissner et al., 2000). Other complications of venous thrombosis are listed in Chart 31-7.

Clinical Manifestations

A major problem associated with recognizing deep vein thrombosis is that the signs and symptoms are nonspecific. The exception is phlegmasia cerulea dolens (massive iliofemoral venous thrombosis), in which the entire extremity becomes massively swollen, tense, painful, and cool to the touch. Despite this variability, clinical signs should always be investigated.

DEEP VEINS

With obstruction of the deep veins comes edema and swelling of the extremity because the outflow of venous blood is inhibited.

<table>
</table>

| Chart 31-7 | **Complications of Vein Thrombosis** |

Chronic venous occlusion
Pulmonary emboli from dislodged thrombi
Valvular destruction
  Chronic venous insufficiency
  Increased venous pressure
  Varicosities
  Venous ulcers
Venous obstruction
  Increased distal pressure
  Fluid stasis
  Edema
  Venous gangrene

The amount of swelling can be determined by measuring the circumference of the affected extremity at various levels with a tape measure and comparing one extremity with the other at the same level to determine size differences. If both extremities are swollen, a size difference may be difficult to detect. The affected extremity may feel warmer than the unaffected extremity, and the superficial veins may appear more prominent.

Tenderness, which usually occurs later, is produced by inflammation of the vein wall and can be detected by gently palpating the affected extremity. Homans' sign (pain in the calf after the foot is sharply dorsiflexed) is not specific for deep vein thrombosis because it can be elicited in any painful condition of the calf. In some cases, signs of a pulmonary embolus are the first indication of deep vein thrombosis.

SUPERFICIAL VEINS

Thrombosis of superficial veins produces pain or tenderness, redness, and warmth in the involved area. The risk of the superficial venous thrombi becoming dislodged or fragmenting into emboli is very low because most of them dissolve spontaneously. This condition can be treated at home with bed rest, elevation of the leg, analgesics, and possibly anti-inflammatory medication.

Assessment and Diagnostic Findings

Careful assessment is invaluable in detecting early signs of venous disorders of the lower extremities. Patients with a history of varicose veins, hypercoagulation, neoplastic disease, cardiovascular disease, or recent major surgery or injury are at high risk. Other patients at high risk include those who are obese or elderly and women taking oral contraceptives.

When performing the nursing assessment, key concerns include limb pain, a feeling of heaviness, functional impairment, ankle engorgement, and edema; differences in leg circumference bilaterally from thigh to ankle; increase in the surface temperature of the leg, particularly the calf or ankle; and areas of tenderness or superficial thrombosis (ie, cordlike venous segment). Homans' sign (pain in the calf as the foot is sharply dorsiflexed) has been used historically to assess for DVT. It is not a reliable or valid sign for DVT and has no clinical value in the assessment of a patient for DVT.

Prevention

Venous thrombosis, thrombophlebitis, and DVT can be prevented, especially if patients who are considered at high risk are identified and preventive measures are instituted without delay.

Preventive measures include the application of elastic compression stockings, the use of intermittent pneumatic compression devices, and special body positioning and exercise (discussed later in the section on nursing management). A further method to prevent venous thrombosis in surgical patients is administration of subcutaneous unfractionated or low molecular weight heparin.

Medical Management

The objectives of treatment for deep vein thrombosis are to prevent the thrombus from growing and fragmenting (risking pulmonary embolism) and to prevent recurrent thromboemboli. Anticoagulant therapy (administration of a medication to delay the clotting time of blood, prevent the formation of a thrombus in postoperative patients, and forestall the extension of a thrombus after it has formed) can meet these objectives, although anticoagulants cannot dissolve a thrombus that has already formed.

ANTICOAGULATION THERAPY

Measures for preventing or reducing blood clotting within the vascular system are indicated in patients with thrombophlebitis, recurrent embolus formation, and persistent leg edema from heart failure. They are also indicated in elderly patients with a hip fracture that may result in lengthy immobilization.

Unfractionated Heparin. Unfractionated heparin (heparin) is administered subcutaneously to prevent development of deep vein thrombosis, or by intermittent intravenous infusion or continuous infusion for 5 to 7 days to prevent the extension of a thrombus and the development of new thrombi. Oral anticoagulants, such as warfarin (Coumadin), are administered with heparin therapy. Medication dosage is regulated by monitoring the activated partial thromboplastin time (aPTT), the **international normalized ratio** (INR), and the platelet count.

Low-Molecular-Weight Heparin. Subcutaneous low-molecular-weight heparin (LMWH) is an effective treatment for some cases of deep vein thrombosis. It has a longer half-life than unfractionated heparin, so doses can be given in one or two subcutaneous injections each day. Doses are adjusted according to weight. LMWH prevents the extension of a thrombus and development of new thrombi and is associated with fewer bleeding complications than unfractionated heparin. Because there are several preparations, the dosing schedule must be based on the product used and the protocol at each institution. The cost is higher than for unfractionated heparin; however, LMWH may be used safely in pregnant women, and the patients may be more mobile and have an improved quality of life.

Thrombolytic Therapy. Unlike the heparins, thrombolytic (fibrinolytic) therapy causes the thrombus to lyse and dissolve in 50% of patients. Thrombolytic therapy (eg, tissue plasminogen activator [t-PA, alteplase, Activase], reteplase [r-PA, Retavase], tenecteplase [TNKase], staphylokinase, urokinase, streptokinase) is given within the first 3 days after acute thrombosis. Therapy initiated beyond 5 days after the onset of symptoms is significantly less effective (Moore, 2002). The advantages of thrombolytic therapy include less long-term damage to the venous valves and a reduced incidence of postthrombotic syndrome and chronic venous insufficiency. However, thrombolytic therapy results in approximately a threefold greater incidence of bleeding than heparin. If bleeding occurs and cannot be stopped, the thrombolytic agent is discontinued.

SURGICAL MANAGEMENT

Surgery is necessary for deep vein thrombosis when anticoagulant or thrombolytic therapy is contraindicated (Chart 31-8), the danger of pulmonary embolism is extreme, or the venous drainage is so severely compromised that permanent damage to the extremity will probably result. A thrombectomy (removal of the thrombosis) is the procedure of choice. A vena cava filter may be placed at the time of the thrombectomy; this filter traps large emboli and prevents pulmonary emboli (see Chap. 23).

Nursing Management

If the patient is receiving anticoagulant therapy, the nurse must frequently monitor the activated partial thromboplastin time (aPTT), prothrombin time, hemoglobin and hematocrit values, platelet count, and fibrinogen level. Close observation is also required to detect bleeding; if bleeding occurs, it must be reported immediately and anticoagulant therapy discontinued.

ASSESSING AND MONITORING ANTICOAGULANT THERAPY

To prevent inadvertent infusion of large volumes of heparin, which could cause hemorrhage, continuous intravenous infusion by electronic infusion device is the preferred method of administering unfractionated heparin. Dosage calculations are based on the patient's weight, and any possible bleeding tendencies are detected by a pretreatment clotting profile. If renal insufficiency exists, lower doses of heparin are required. Periodic coagulation tests and hematocrit levels are obtained. Heparin is in the effective, or therapeutic, range when the aPTT is 1.5 times the control.

Intermittent intravenous injection is another means of administering heparin; a dilute solution of heparin is administered every 4 hours. Administration may be facilitated by using a heparin lock, an intravenous catheter or a small, butterfly-type scalp vein needle with an injection site at the end of the tubing.

Oral anticoagulants, such as warfarin, are monitored by the prothrombin time (PTT) or INR. Because their effect is delayed

for 3 to 5 days, they are usually administered with heparin until desired anticoagulation has been achieved (ie, when the prothrombin time is 1.5 to 2 times normal or the INR is 2.0 to 3.0).

MONITORING AND MANAGING POTENTIAL COMPLICATIONS

Bleeding. The principal complication of anticoagulant therapy is spontaneous bleeding anywhere in the body. Bleeding from the kidneys is detected by microscopic examination of the urine and is often the first sign of anticoagulant toxicity from excessive dosage. Bruises, nosebleeds, and bleeding gums are also early signs. To reverse the effects of heparin promptly, intravenous injections of protamine sulfate may be administered. Reversing the effects of warfarin, a coumarin derivative, is more difficult, but effective measures that may be prescribed include vitamin K and possibly transfusion of fresh frozen plasma.

Thrombocytopenia. Another complication of therapy may be heparin-induced thrombocytopenia (decrease in platelets), which may develop in patients who receive heparin for more than 5 days or on readministration after a brief interruption of heparin therapy. Beginning warfarin concomitantly with heparin can provide a stable INR or prothrombin time by day 5 of heparin treatment.

The use of LMWH is less frequently associated with heparin-induced thrombocytopenia. The thrombocytopenia is thought to result from an immunologic mechanism that causes aggregation of platelets. This serious complication results in thromboembolic manifestations, and the prognosis is extremely guarded.

Prevention of thrombocytopenia depends on regular monitoring of platelet counts. Early signs of thrombocytopenia are a falling platelet count to less than 100,000/mL, a decrease in platelet count exceeding 25% at one time, the need for increasing doses of heparin to maintain the therapeutic level, thromboembolic or hemorrhagic complications, and a history of heparin sensitivity (Stevens, 2000). If thrombocytopenia does occur, platelet aggregation studies are conducted, the heparin is discontinued, and protamine sulfate is administered to reverse heparin's effects.

Drug Interactions. Because oral anticoagulants interact with many other medications and herbal and nutritional supplements, close monitoring of the patient's medication schedule is necessary. Medications and supplements that potentiate oral anticoagulants include salicylates, anabolic steroids, chloral hydrate, glucagon, chloramphenicol, neomycin, quinidine, coenzyme Q10, dong quai, garlic, gingko, ginseng, green tea, and vitamin E; those that decrease the anticoagulant effect include phenytoin, barbiturates, diuretics, estrogen, and vitamin C. It is advisable to identify medication interactions for patients taking specific oral anticoagulants. Contraindications to anticoagulant therapy are summarized in Chart 31-8.

PROVIDING COMFORT

Bed rest, elevation of the affected extremity, elastic compression stockings, and analgesics for pain relief are adjuncts to therapy. They help to improve circulation and increase comfort. Depending on the extent and location of a venous thrombosis, bed rest may be required for 5 to 7 days after diagnosis. This is approximately the time necessary for the thrombus to adhere to the vein wall, preventing embolization.

Warm, moist packs applied to the affected extremity reduce the discomfort associated with deep vein thrombosis, as do mild analgesics prescribed for pain control. When the patient begins to ambulate, elastic compression stockings are used. Walking is

---

Chart 31-8 • PHARMACOLOGY
Contraindications to Anticoagulation Therapy

Lack of patient cooperation
Bleeding from the following systems:
  Gastrointestinal
  Genitourinary
  Respiratory
  Reproductive
Hemorrhagic blood dyscrasias
Aneurysms
Severe trauma
Alcoholism
Recent or impending surgery of:
  Eye
  Spinal cord
  Brain
Severe hepatic or renal disease
Recent cerebrovascular hemorrhage
Infections
Open ulcerative wounds
Occupations that involve a significant hazard for injury
Recent delivery of a baby

better than standing or sitting for long periods. Bed exercises, such as dorsiflexion of the foot, are also recommended.

APPLYING ELASTIC COMPRESSION STOCKINGS

Elastic compression stockings usually are prescribed for patients with venous insufficiency. These stockings exert a sustained, evenly distributed pressure over the entire surface of the calves, reducing the calibre of the superficial veins in the legs and resulting in increased flow in the deeper veins. The stockings may be knee-high, thigh-high, or panty hose. Thigh-high stockings are difficult for the patient to wear, because they have a tendency to roll down. The roll of the stocking further restricts blood flow rather than the stocking providing evenly distributed pressure over the thigh.

 NURSING ALERT Any type of stocking, including the elastic type, can inadvertently become a tourniquet if applied incorrectly (ie, rolled tightly at the top). In such instances, the stockings produce stasis rather than prevent it. For ambulatory patients, elastic compression stockings are removed at night and reapplied before the legs are lowered from the bed to the floor in the morning.

When the stockings are off, the skin is inspected for signs of irritation, and the calves are examined for possible tenderness. Any skin changes or signs of tenderness are reported. Stockings are contraindicated in patients with severe pitting edema because they can produce severe pitting at the knee.

Gerontologic Considerations

Because of decreased strength and manual dexterity, elderly patients may be unable to apply elastic compression stockings properly. If such is the case, a family member or friend should be taught to assist the patient to apply the stockings so that they do not cause undue pressure on any part of the feet or legs.

USING INTERMITTENT PNEUMATIC COMPRESSION DEVICES

These devices can be used with elastic compression stockings to prevent deep vein thrombosis. They consist of an electric controller that is attached by air hoses to plastic knee-high or thigh-high sleeves. The leg sleeves are divided into compartments, which sequentially fill to apply pressure to the ankle, calf, and thigh at 35 to 55 mm Hg of pressure. These devices can increase blood velocity beyond that produced by the stockings. Nursing measures include ensuring that prescribed pressures are not exceeded and assessing for patient comfort.

POSITIONING THE BODY AND ENCOURAGING EXERCISE

When the patient is on bed rest, the feet and lower legs should be elevated periodically above the level of the heart. This position allows the superficial and tibial veins to empty rapidly and to remain collapsed. Active and passive leg exercises, particularly those involving calf muscles, should be performed to increase venous flow. Early ambulation is most effective in preventing venous stasis. Deep-breathing exercises are beneficial because they produce increased negative pressure in the thorax, which assists in emptying the large veins. Once ambulatory, patients are instructed to avoid sitting for more than 2 hours at a time. The goal is to walk at least 10 minutes every 1 to 2 hours. Patients are also instructed to perform active and passive leg exercises when they are not able to ambulate as frequently as necessary, such as during long car, train, and plane trips.

PROMOTING HOME AND COMMUNITY-BASED CARE

In addition to teaching the patient how to apply elastic compression stockings and explaining the importance of elevating the legs and exercising adequately, the nurse teaches about the medication, its purpose, and the need to take the correct amount at the specific times prescribed (Chart 31-9). The patient should also be aware that blood tests are scheduled periodically to determine whether a change in medication or dosage is required. If the patient fails to adhere to the therapeutic regimen, continuation of the medication therapy should be questioned. A person who refuses to discontinue the use of alcohol should not receive anticoagulants because chronic alcohol use decreases their effectiveness. In patients with liver problems, the potential for bleeding may be exacerbated by anticoagulant therapy.

CHRONIC VENOUS INSUFFICIENCY

Venous insufficiency results from obstruction of the venous valves in the legs or a reflux of blood back through the valves. Superficial and deep leg veins can be involved. Resultant venous hypertension can occur whenever there has been a prolonged increase in venous pressure, such as occurs with deep venous thrombosis. Because the walls of veins are thinner and more elastic than

Chart 31-9 • PATIENT EDUCATION
Taking Anticoagulant Medications

- Take the anticoagulant at the same time each day, usually between 8:00 and 9:00 AM.
- Wear or carry identification indicating the anticoagulant being taken.
- Keep all appointments for blood tests.
- Because other medications affect the action of the anticoagulant, do not take any of the following medications or supplements without consulting with the primary health care provider: vitamins, cold medicines, antibiotics, aspirin, mineral oil, and anti-inflammatory agents, such as ibuprofen (Motrin) and similar medications or herbal or nutritional supplements. The primary health care provider should be contacted before taking any over-the-counter drugs.
- Avoid alcohol, because it may change the body's response to an anticoagulant.
- Avoid food fads, crash diets, or marked changes in eating habits.
- Do not take warfarin (Coumadin) unless directed.
- Do not stop taking Coumadin (when prescribed) unless directed.
- When seeking treatment from physician, a dentist, a podiatrist, or another health care provider, be sure to inform the caregiver that you are taking an anticoagulant.
- Contact your primary health care provider before having dental work or elective surgery.
- If any of the following signs appear, report them immediately to the primary health care provider:
  Faintness, dizziness, or increased weakness
  Severe headaches or abdominal pain
  Reddish or brownish urine
  Any bleeding—for example, cuts that do not stop bleeding
  Bruises that enlarge, nosebleeds, or unusual bleeding from any part of the body
  Red or black bowel movements
  Rash
- Avoid injury that can cause bleeding.
- For women: Notify the primary health care provider if you suspect pregnancy.

the walls of arteries, they distend readily when venous pressure is consistently elevated. In this state, leaflets of the venous valves are stretched and prevented from closing completely, allowing a backflow or reflux of blood in the veins. Duplex ultrasonography confirms the obstruction and identifies the level of valvular incompetence.

Clinical Manifestations

When the valves in the deep veins become incompetent after a thrombus has formed, postthrombotic syndrome may develop (Fig. 31-16). This disorder is characterized by chronic venous stasis, resulting in edema, altered pigmentation, pain, and stasis dermatitis. The patient may notice the symptoms less in the morning and more in the evening. Obstruction or poor calf muscle pumping in addition to valvular reflux must be present for the development of severe postthrombotic syndrome, which includes stasis ulceration (Caps et al., 1999). Superficial veins may be dilated. The disorder is long-standing, difficult to treat, and often disabling.

Stasis ulcers develop as a result of the rupture of small skin veins and subsequent ulcerations. When these vessels rupture, red blood cells escape into surrounding tissues and then degenerate, leaving a brownish discolouration of the tissues. The pigmentation and ulcerations usually occur in the lower part of the extremity, in the area of the medial malleolus of the ankle. The skin becomes dry, cracks, and itches; subcutaneous tissues fibrose and atrophy. The risk of injury and infection of the extremities is increased.

Complications

Venous ulceration is the most serious complication of chronic venous insufficiency and can be associated with other conditions affecting the circulation of the lower extremities. Cellulitis or dermatitis may complicate the care of chronic venous insufficiency and venous ulcerations.

Management

Management of the patient with venous insufficiency is directed at reducing venous stasis and preventing ulcerations. Measures that increase venous blood flow are antigravity activities, such as elevating the leg, and compression of superficial veins with elastic compression stockings.

FIGURE 31-16 Competent valves showing blood flow patterns when the valve is open (**A**) and closed (**B**), allowing blood to flow against gravity. (**C**) With faulty or incompetent valves, the blood is unable to move toward the heart.

Elevating the legs decreases edema, promotes venous return, and provides symptomatic relief. The legs should be elevated frequently throughout the day (at least 15 to 30 minutes every 2 hours). At night, the patient should sleep with the foot of the bed elevated about 15 cm. Prolonged sitting or standing still is detrimental; walking should be encouraged. When sitting, the patient should avoid placing pressure on the popliteal spaces, as occurs when crossing the legs or sitting with the legs dangling over the side of the bed. Constricting garments such as panty girdles or tight socks should be avoided.

Compression of the legs with elastic compression stockings reduces the pooling of venous blood and enhances venous return to the heart. Elastic compression stockings are recommended for people with venous insufficiency. The stocking should fit so that pressure is greater at the foot and ankle and then gradually declines to a lesser pressure at the knee or groin. If the top of the stocking is too tight or becomes twisted, a tourniquet effect is created, which worsens venous pooling. Stockings should be applied after the legs have been elevated for a period, when the amount of blood in the leg veins is at its lowest.

Extremities with venous insufficiency must be carefully protected from trauma; the skin is kept clean, dry, and soft. Signs of ulceration are immediately reported to the health care provider for treatment and follow-up.

LEG ULCERS

A leg ulcer is an excavation of the skin surface that occurs when inflamed necrotic tissue sloughs off. About 75% of all leg ulcers result from chronic venous insufficiency. Lesions due to arterial insufficiency account for approximately 20%; the remaining 5% are caused by burns, sickle cell anemia, and other factors (Gloviczki & Yao, 2001).

Pathophysiology

Inadequate exchange of oxygen and other nutrients in the tissue is the metabolic abnormality that underlies the development of leg ulcers. When cellular metabolism cannot maintain energy balance, cell death (necrosis) results. Alterations in blood vessels at the arterial, capillary, and venous levels may affect cellular processes and lead to the formation of ulcers.

Clinical Manifestations

The clinical appearance and associated characteristics of leg ulcers are determined by the cause of the ulcer. Most ulcers, especially in an elderly patient, have more than one cause. The symptoms depend on whether the problem is arterial or venous in origin (see Table 31-2). The severity of the symptoms depends on the extent and duration of the vascular insufficiency. The ulcer itself appears as an open, inflamed sore. The area may be draining or covered by eschar (dark, hard crust).

ARTERIAL ULCERS

Chronic arterial disease is characterized by intermittent claudication, which is pain caused by activity and relieved after a few minutes of rest. The patient may also complain of digital or forefoot pain at rest. If the onset of arterial occlusion is acute, ischemic pain is unrelenting and rarely relieved even with opioid analgesics. Typically, arterial ulcers are small, circular, deep ulcerations on the tips of toes or in the web spaces between toes. Ulcers often occur on the medial side of the hallux or lateral fifth toe and may be caused by a combination of ischemia and pressure (Fig. 31-17).

FIGURE 31-17 (**A**) Ulcers resulting from arterial emboli. (**B**) Gangrene of the toes resulting from severe arterial ischemia. (**C**) Ulcer from venous stasis.

Arterial insufficiency may result in gangrene of the toe (digital gangrene), which usually is caused by trauma. The toe is stubbed and then turns black (see Fig. 31-17). Usually, patients with this problem are elderly people without adequate circulation to provide revascularization. Débridement is contraindicated in these instances. Although the toe is gangrenous, it is dry. Managing dry gangrene is preferable to débriding the toe and causing an open wound that will not heal because of insufficient circulation. If the toe were to be amputated, the lack of adequate circulation would prevent healing and might make further amputation necessary—a below-knee or an above-knee amputation. A higher-level amputation in the elderly could result in a loss of independence and possibly institutional care. Dry gangrene of the toe in an elderly person with poor circulation is usually left undisturbed. The nurse keeps the toe clean and dry until it separates (without creating an open wound).

VENOUS ULCERS

Chronic venous insufficiency is characterized by pain described as aching or heaviness. The foot and ankle may be edematous. Ulcerations are in the area of the medial or lateral malleolus (gaiter area) and are typically large, superficial, and highly exudative. Venous hypertension causes extravasation of blood, which discolours the gaiter area (see Fig. 31-17). Patients with neuropathy frequently have ulcerations on the side of the foot over the metatarsal heads. These ulcers are painless and are described in further detail in Chapter 41.

Assessment and Diagnostic Findings

Because ulcers have many causes, the cause of each ulcer needs to be identified so appropriate therapy can be prescribed. The history of the condition is important in determining venous or arterial insufficiency. The pulses of the lower extremities (femoral, popliteal, posterior tibial, and dorsalis pedis) are carefully examined. More conclusive diagnostic aids are Doppler and duplex ultrasound studies, arteriography, and venography. Cultures of the ulcer bed may be necessary to determine whether the infecting agent is the primary cause of the ulcer.

Medical Management

Patients with ulcers can be effectively managed by advanced practice nurses or certified wound care nurses in collaboration with physicians. All ulcers have the potential to become infected.

PHARMACOLOGIC THERAPY

Antibiotic therapy is prescribed when the ulcer is infected; the specific antibiotic is selected on the basis of culture and sensitivity test results. Oral antibiotics usually are prescribed because topical antibiotics have not proven to be effective for leg ulcers.

DÉBRIDEMENT

To promote healing, the wound is kept clean of drainage and necrotic tissue. The usual method is to flush the area with normal saline solution. If this is unsuccessful, débridement may be necessary. Débridement is the removal of nonviable tissue from wounds. Removing the dead tissue is important, particularly in instances of infection. Débridement can be accomplished by several different methods:

- Sharp surgical débridement is the fastest method and can be performed by a physician, skilled advanced practice nurse, or certified wound care nurse in collaboration with the physician.
- Nonselective débridement can be accomplished by applying isotonic saline dressings of fine-mesh gauze to the ulcer. When the dressing dries, it is removed (dry), along with the debris adhering to the gauze. Pain management is usually necessary.
- Enzymatic débridement with the application of enzyme ointments may be prescribed to treat the ulcer. The ointment is applied to the lesion but not to normal surrounding skin. Most enzymatic ointments are covered with saline-soaked gauze that has been thoroughly wrung out. A dry gauze dressing and a loose bandage are then applied. The enzymatic ointment is discontinued when the necrotic tissue has been débrided and an appropriate wound dressing is applied.
- Débriding agents can be used. Dextranomer (Debrisan) beads are small, highly porous, spherical beads (0.1 to 0.3 mm in diameter) that can absorb wound secretions. Bacteria and the products of tissue necrosis and protein degradation are absorbed into the bead layer. When the beads are saturated, they take on a greyish yellow colour, at which point their cleansing action stops. They are then flushed from the wound with normal saline, and a fresh layer is applied.
- Calcium alginate dressings can also be used for débridement when absorption of exudate is needed. These dressings are changed when the exudate seeps through the cover dressing or at least every 7 days. The dressing can also be used on areas that are bleeding, because the material helps stop the bleeding. As the dry fibres absorb exudate, they become a gel that is painlessly removed from the ulcer bed. Calcium alginate dressings should not be used on dry or nonexudative wounds.

TOPICAL THERAPY

A variety of topical agents can be used in conjunction with cleansing and débridement therapies to promote healing of leg ulcers. The goals of treatment are to remove devitalized tissue and to keep the ulcer clean and moist while healing takes place. The treatment should not destroy developing tissue. For topical treatments to be successful, adequate nutritional therapy must be maintained.

WOUND DRESSING

After the circulatory status has been assessed and determined to be adequate for healing (ABI of more than 0.5), surgical dressings can be used to promote a moist environment. The simplest method is to use a wound contact material (eg, Tegapore) next to the wound bed and cover it with gauze. Tegapore maintains a moist environment, can be left in place for several days, and does not disrupt the capillary bed when removed for evaluation. Hydrocolloids (eg, Comfeel, DuoDerm CGF, Restore, Tegasorb) are also available options to promote granulation tissue and re-epithelialization. They also provide a barrier for protection because they adhere to the wound bed and surrounding tissue. However, deep wounds and infected wounds are often more appropriately treated with other dressings.

Knowledge deficit, frustration, fear, and depression can result in the patient's and family's decreased compliance with the prescribed therapy; therefore, patient and family education is necessary before beginning and throughout the wound care program.

STIMULATED HEALING

Tissue-engineered human skin equivalent along with therapeutic compression has been developed by Apligraf; it is a skin product cultured from human dermal fibroblasts and keratinocytes. When applied, it seems to react to factors in the wound and may interact with the patient's cells to stimulate the production of growth factors. Application is not difficult, no suturing is involved, and the procedure is painless.

NURSING PROCESS:
THE PATIENT WHO HAS LEG ULCERS

Assessment

A careful nursing history and assessment of symptoms are important. The extent and type of pain are carefully assessed, as are the appearance and temperature of the skin of both legs. The quality of all peripheral pulses is assessed, and comparisons are made of the pulses in both legs. The legs are checked for edema. If the extremity is edematous, the degree of edema is determined. Any limitation of mobility and activity that results from the vascular insufficiency is identified. The patient's nutritional status is assessed, and a history of diabetes, collagen disease, or varicose veins is obtained.

Diagnosis

NURSING DIAGNOSES

Based on the assessment data, major nursing diagnoses for the patient may include:

- Impaired skin integrity related to vascular insufficiency
- Impaired physical mobility related to activity restrictions of the therapeutic regimen and pain
- Imbalanced nutrition: less than body requirements, related to increased need for nutrients that promote wound healing

COLLABORATIVE PROBLEMS/POTENTIAL COMPLICATIONS

Based on the assessment data, potential complications that may develop include:

- Infection
- Gangrene

Planning and Goals

The major goals for the patient may include restoration of skin integrity, improved physical mobility, adequate nutrition, and absence of complications.

Nursing Interventions

The nursing challenge in caring for these patients is great, whether the patient is in the hospital, in a long-term care facility, or at home. The physical problem is often a long-term one that causes a substantial drain on the patient's physical, emotional, and economic resources.

RESTORING SKIN INTEGRITY

To promote wound healing, measures are used to keep the area clean. Cleansing requires very gentle handling, a mild soap, and lukewarm water. Positioning of the legs depends on whether the ulcer is of arterial or venous origin. If there is arterial insufficiency, the patient should be referred to be evaluated for vascular reconstruction. If there is venous insufficiency, dependent edema can be avoided by elevating the lower extremities. A decrease in edema promotes the exchange of cellular nutrients and waste products in the area of the ulcer, promoting healing.

Avoiding trauma to the lower extremities is imperative in promoting skin integrity. Protective boots may be used (eg, the Rooke Vascular boot, Lunax Boot, Bunny Boot); they are soft and provide warmth and protection from injury. If the patient is on bed rest, it is important to relieve pressure on the heels to prevent pressure ulcerations. When the patient is in bed, a bed cradle can be used to relieve pressure from bed linens and to prevent anything from touching the legs. When the patient is ambulatory, all obstacles are moved from the patient's path so that the patient's legs will not be bumped. Heating pads, hot-water bottles, or hot baths are avoided. Heat increases the oxygen demands and thus the blood flow demands of the tissue, which in this case are already compromised. The patient with diabetes mellitus suffers from neuropathy with decreased sensation, and heating pads may produce injury before the patient is aware of being burned.

IMPROVING PHYSICAL MOBILITY

Generally, physical activity is initially restricted to promote healing. When infection resolves and healing begins, ambulation should resume gradually and progressively. Activity promotes arterial flow and venous return and is encouraged after the acute phase of the ulcer process. Until full activity resumes, the patient is encouraged to move about when in bed, to turn from side to side frequently, and to exercise the upper extremities to maintain muscle tone and strength. Meanwhile, diversional activities that interest the patient are encouraged. Consultation with an occupational therapist may be helpful if a prolonged period of limited mobility and activity is anticipated.

If pain limits the patient's activity, analgesics may be prescribed by the physician. The pain of peripheral vascular disease, whether it is arterial or venous, is typically chronic. Analgesics may be taken before scheduled activities to help the patient participate more comfortably.

PROMOTING ADEQUATE NUTRITION

Nutritional deficiencies are determined from the patient's report of usual dietary intake. Alterations in the diet are made to remedy these deficiencies. A diet that is high in protein, vitamins C and A, iron, and zinc is encouraged in an attempt to promote healing.

Many patients with peripheral vascular disease are elderly. Their caloric intake may need to be adjusted because of their decreased metabolic rate and level of activity. Particular consideration should also be given to their iron intake, because many elderly people are anemic.

After a diet plan has been developed that meets the patient's nutritional needs and promotes healing, diet instruction is provided to the patient and family. The nurse and patient design the diet plan to be compatible with the lifestyle and preferences of the patient and family.

PROMOTING HOME AND COMMUNITY-BASED CARE

The self-care program is planned with the patient so that activities to promote arterial and venous circulation, relieve pain, and promote tissue integrity will be used. Reasons for each aspect of the program are explained to the patient and family. Leg ulcers are often chronic and difficult to heal; they frequently recur, even when patients rigorously follow the plan of care. Long-term care of the feet and legs to promote healing of wounds and prevent recurrence of ulcerations is the primary goal. Leg ulcers increase the patient's risk for infection, may be painful, and limit mobility, necessitating life-style changes. Participation of family members and home-health providers may be necessary for treatments such as dressing changes, reassessments, and evaluation of the plan of care. Regular follow-up with a primary health care provider is necessary.

Evaluation

EXPECTED PATIENT OUTCOMES

Expected patient outcomes may include:

1. Demonstrates restored skin integrity
   a. Exhibits absence of inflammation
   b. Exhibits absence of drainage; negative wound culture
   c. Avoids trauma to the legs
2. Increases physical mobility
   a. Progresses gradually to optimal level of activity
   b. Reports that pain does not impede activity
3. Attains adequate nutrition
   a. Selects foods high in protein, vitamins, iron, and zinc
   b. Discusses with family members dietary modifications that need to be made at home
   c. Plans, with the family, a diet that is nutritionally sound

VARICOSE VEINS

Varicose veins (varicosities) are abnormally dilated, tortuous, superficial veins caused by incompetent venous valves (see Fig. 31-16). Most commonly, this condition occurs in the lower extremities, the saphenous veins, or the lower trunk; however, it can occur elsewhere in the body, such as esophageal varices (see Chap. 39).

It is estimated that varicose veins occur in up to 15% of the adult population in Canada, with an increased incidence correlated with increased age. The condition is most common in women and in people whose occupations require prolonged standing, such as salespeople, hair stylists, teachers, nurses, ancillary medical personnel, and construction workers. A hereditary weakness of the vein wall may contribute to the development of varicosities, and it is not uncommon to see this condition occur in several members of the same family. Varicose veins are rare before puberty. Pregnancy may cause varicosities. The leg veins dilate during pregnancy because of hormonal effects related to distensibility, increased pressure by the gravid uterus, and increased blood volume which all contribute to the development of varicose veins (Johnson, 1997).

Pathophysiology

Varicose veins may be considered primary (without involvement of deep veins) or secondary (resulting from obstruction of deep veins). A reflux of venous blood in the veins results in venous stasis. If only the superficial veins are affected, the person may have no symptoms but may be troubled by the appearance of the dilated veins.

Clinical Manifestations

Symptoms, if present, may take the form of dull aches, muscle cramps, and increased muscle fatigue in the lower legs. Ankle edema and a feeling of heaviness of the legs may occur. Nocturnal cramps are common. When deep venous obstruction results in varicose veins, patients may develop the signs and symptoms of chronic venous insufficiency: edema, pain, pigmentation, and ulcerations. Susceptibility to injury and infection is increased.

Assessment and Diagnostic Findings

Diagnostic tests for varicose veins include the duplex scan, which documents the anatomic site of reflux and provides a quantitative measure of the severity of valvular reflux. Air plethysmography measures the changes in venous blood volume. Venography is not routinely performed to evaluate for valvular reflux. When it is used, however, it involves injecting an x-ray contrast agent into the leg veins so that the vein anatomy can be visualized by x-ray studies during various leg movements.

Prevention

The patient should avoid activities that cause venous stasis, such as wearing tight socks or a constricting panty girdle, crossing the legs at the thighs, and sitting or standing for long periods. Changing position frequently, elevating the legs when they are tired, and getting up to walk for several minutes of every hour promote circulation. The patient should be encouraged to walk 1.5 or 3 kilometres each day if there are no contraindications. Walking up the stairs rather than using the elevator or escalator is helpful in promoting circulation. Swimming is also good exercise for the legs.

Elastic compression stockings, especially knee-high stockings, are useful. Patients are more likely to use knee-high stockings than thigh-high stockings. The overweight patient should be encouraged to begin a weight-reduction plan.

Medical Management

Surgery for varicose veins requires that the deep veins be patent and functional. The saphenous vein is ligated and divided. The vein is ligated high in the groin, where the saphenous vein meets the femoral vein. Additionally, the vein may be removed (stripped). After the vein is ligated, an incision is made in the ankle, and a metal or plastic wire is passed the full length of the vein to the point of ligation. The wire is then withdrawn, pulling (removing, "stripping") the vein as it is removed (Fig. 31-18). Pressure and elevation keep bleeding at a minimum during surgery.

SCLEROTHERAPY

In sclerotherapy, a chemical is injected into the vein, irritating the venous endothelium and producing localized phlebitis and fibrosis, thereby obliterating the lumen of the vein. This treatment may be performed alone for small varicosities or may follow vein ligation or stripping. Sclerosing is palliative rather than curative. After the sclerosing agent is injected, elastic compression bandages are applied to the leg and are worn for approximately 5 days. The health care provider who performed sclerotherapy removes the first bandages. Elastic compression stockings are then worn for an additional 5 weeks.

After sclerotherapy, patients are encouraged to perform walking activities as prescribed to maintain blood flow in the leg. Walking enhances dilution of the sclerosing agent.

Nursing Management

Surgery can be performed in an outpatient setting, or patients can be admitted to the hospital on the day of surgery and discharged the next day, but nursing measures are the same as if the patient were hospitalized. Bed rest is maintained for 24 hours, after which the patient begins walking every 2 hours for 5 to 10 minutes. Elastic compression stockings are used to maintain compression of the leg. They are worn continuously for about 1 week after vein stripping. The nurse assists the patient to perform exercises and move the legs. The foot of the bed should be elevated. Standing still and sitting are discouraged.

PROMOTING COMFORT AND UNDERSTANDING

Analgesics are prescribed to help patients move affected extremities more comfortably. Dressings are inspected for bleeding, particularly at the groin, where the risk of bleeding is greatest. The nurse is alert for reported sensations of "pins and needles." Hyper-

sensitivity to touch in the involved extremity may indicate a temporary or permanent nerve injury resulting from surgery, because the saphenous vein and nerve are close to each other in the leg.

Usually, the patient may shower after the first 24 hours. The patient is instructed to dry the incisions well with a clean towel using a patting technique rather than rubbing. Application of skin lotion is to be avoided until the incisions are completely healed to decrease the chance of developing an infection.

If the patient underwent sclerotherapy, a burning sensation in the injected leg may be experienced for 1 or 2 days. The nurse may encourage the use of a mild analgesic (eg, propoxyphene napsylate and acetaminophen [Darvocet N], oxycodone and acetaminophen [Tylenol], oxycodone and acetylsalicylic acid [Asprin]) as prescribed by a physician or nurse practitioner and walking to provide relief.

PROMOTING HOME AND COMMUNITY-BASED CARE

Patients require long-term elastic support of the leg after discharge, and plans are made to obtain adequate supplies of elastic compression stockings or bandages as appropriate. Exercises of the legs are necessary; the development of an individualized plan requires consultation with the patient and the health care team.

Cellulitis

Pathophysiology and Clinical Manifestations

Cellulitis is the most common infectious cause of limb swelling. Cellulitis can occur as a single isolated event or a series of recurrent events. It is often misdiagnosed, usually as recurrent thrombophlebitis or chronic venous insufficiency. Cellulitis occurs when an entry point through normal skin barriers allows bacteria to enter and release their toxins in the subcutaneous tissues. The acute onset of swelling, localized redness, and pain is frequently associated with systemic signs of fever, chills, and sweating. The redness may not be uniform and often skips areas. Regional lymph nodes may also be tender and enlarged.

Femoral vein
Great saphenous vein
Alternate incision
Great saphenous vein

Small saphenous vein

FIGURE 31-18 Ligation and stripping of the great and the small saphenous veins. (**A**) The tributaries of the saphenous vein have been ligated at the saphenofemoral junction. (**B**) The vein stripper has been inserted from the ankle superiorly to the groin. The vein is removed ("stripped") from above downward. A number of alternate incisions may be needed to remove separate varicose masses. (**C**) The small saphenous vein is stripped from its junction with the popliteal vein to a point posterior to the lateral malleolus.

Medical Management

Mild cases of cellulitis can be treated on an outpatient basis with oral antibiotic therapy. If the cellulitis is severe, the patient is hospitalized and treated with intravenous antibiotics for at least 7 to 14 days. The key to preventing recurrent episodes of cellulitis lies in adequate antibiotic therapy for the initial event and in identifying the site of the bacterial entry. The most commonly overlooked areas are the cracks and fissures that occur in the skin between the toes. Other possible locations are drug use injection sites, contusions, abrasions, ulcerations, ingrown toenails, and hangnails.

Nursing Management

The patient is instructed to elevate the affected area above heart level and apply warm, moist packs to the site every 2 to 4 hours. Individuals with sensory and circulatory deficits, such as diabetes and paralysis, should use caution when applying warm packs because burns may occur; it is advisable to use a thermometer or have a caregiver ensure that the temperature is not more than lukewarm. Education should focus on preventing a recurrent episode. The patient with peripheral vascular disease or diabetes mellitus should receive education or re-education about skin and foot care.

Management of Lymphatic Disorders

The lymphatic system consists of a set of vessels that spread throughout most of the body. These vessels start as lymph capillaries that drain unabsorbed plasma from the interstitial spaces (spaces between the cells). The lymphatic capillaries unite to form the lymph vessels, which pass through the lymph nodes and then empty into the large thoracic duct that joins the jugular vein on the left side of the neck.

The fluid drained from the interstitial space by the lymphatic system is called lymph. The flow of lymph depends on the intrinsic contractions of the lymph vessels, the contraction of muscles, respiratory movements, and gravity. The lymphatic system of the abdominal cavity maintains a steady flow of digested fatty food (chyle) from the intestinal mucosa to the thoracic duct. In other parts of the body, the lymphatic system's function is regional; the lymphatic vessels of the head, for example, empty into clusters of lymph nodes located in the neck, and those of the extremities empty into nodes of the axillae and the groin.

LYMPHANGITIS AND LYMPHADENITIS

Lymphangitis is an acute inflammation of the lymphatic channels. It arises most commonly from a focus of infection in an extremity. Usually, the infectious organism is a hemolytic *Streptococcus*. The characteristic red streaks that extend up the arm or the leg from an infected wound outline the course of the lymphatic vessels as they drain.

The lymph nodes located along the course of the lymphatic channels also become enlarged, red, and tender (acute lymphadenitis). They can also become necrotic and form an abscess (suppurative lymphadenitis). The nodes involved most often are those in the groin, axilla, or cervical region.

Because these infections are nearly always caused by organisms that are sensitive to antibiotics, it is unusual to see abscess formation. Recurrent episodes of lymphangitis are often associated with progressive lymphedema. After acute attacks, an elastic compression stocking or sleeve should be worn on the affected extremity for several months to prevent long-term edema.

LYMPHEDEMA AND ELEPHANTIASIS

Lymphedemas are classified as primary (congenital malformations) or secondary (acquired obstructions). Tissue swelling occurs in the extremities because of an increased quantity of lymph that results from obstruction of lymphatic vessels. It is especially marked when the extremity is in a dependent position. Initially, the edema is soft, pitting, and relieved by treatment. As the condition progresses, the edema becomes firm, nonpitting, and unresponsive to treatment. The most common type is congenital lymphedema (lymphedema praecox), which is caused by hypoplasia of the lymphatic system of the lower extremity. This disorder is usually seen in women and first appears between ages 15 and 25.

The obstruction may be in the lymph nodes and the lymphatic vessels. Sometimes, it is seen in the arm after an axillary node dissection (eg, for breast cancer) and in the leg in association with varicose veins or chronic thrombophlebitis. In the latter case, the lymphatic obstruction usually is caused by chronic lymphangitis. Lymphatic obstruction caused by a parasite (filaria) is seen frequently in the tropics. When chronic swelling is present, there may be frequent bouts of acute infection characterized by high fever and chills and increased residual edema after the inflammation has resolved. These lead to chronic fibrosis, thickening of the subcutaneous tissues, and hypertrophy of the skin. This condition, in which chronic swelling of the extremity recedes only slightly with elevation, is referred to as elephantiasis.

Medical Management

The goal of therapy is to reduce and control the edema and prevent infection. Active and passive exercises assist in moving lymphatic fluid into the bloodstream. External compression devices milk the fluid proximally from the foot to the hip or from the hand to the axilla. When the patient is ambulatory, custom-fitted elastic compression stockings or sleeves are worn; those with the highest compression strength (exceeding 40 mm Hg) are required. When the leg is affected, strict bed rest with the leg elevated may aid in mobilizing the fluids.

PHARMACOLOGIC THERAPY

As initial therapy, the diuretic furosemide (Lasix) is prescribed as needed to prevent the fluid overload that can result from the mobilization of extracellular fluid. Diuretics have also been used palliatively for lymphedema in conjunction with elevating the leg and wearing elastic compression stockings or sleeves. However, the use of diuretics alone has little benefit because their main action is to limit capillary filtration by decreasing the circulating blood volume. If lymphangitis or cellulitis is present, antibiotic therapy is initiated. The patient is taught to inspect the skin for evidence of infection.

SURGICAL MANAGEMENT

Surgery is performed if the edema is severe and uncontrolled by medical therapy, if mobility is severely compromised, or if infection persists. One surgical approach involves the excision of the affected subcutaneous tissue and fascia, with skin grafting to cover the defect. Another procedure involves the surgical relocation of superficial lymphatic vessels into the deep lymphatic system by means of a buried dermal flap to provide a conduit for lymphatic drainage.

Nursing Management

After surgery, the management of skin grafts and flaps is the same as when these therapies are used for other conditions. Prophylactic antibiotics may be prescribed for 5 to 7 days. Constant elevation of the affected extremity and observations for complications are essential. Complications may include flap necrosis, hematoma or abscess under the flap, and cellulitis. The nurse instructs the patient or caregiver to inspect the dressing daily. Unusual drainage or any inflammation around the wound margin may suggest infection and should be reported to the physician. The patient is informed that there may be a loss of sensation in the skin graft area. The patient is also instructed to avoid the application of heating pads or exposure to sun to prevent burns or trauma to the area.

Critical Thinking Exercises

1. Your patient has been diagnosed with an enlarging abdominal aortic aneurysm (AAA). The physician gives the patient two surgical options: repair of the AAA using an endovascular graft or open surgical repair. What factors would you include in discussing the surgical options, postoperative care, continuing care, and home care? If the patient is taking warfarin (Coumadin) for atrial fibrillation and insulin for diabetes, how would you incorporate these factors into the plan of care?

2. Your 96-year-old patient presents with a 1-year history of experiencing symptoms of claudication after walking four or five blocks. The patient lives alone, six blocks from the local shopping area, and no longer drives a vehicle. The patient does not wish to undergo surgery at this time and wants to continue living at his current location. What options would you discuss with the patient? If this patient also had a nonhealing foot wound and had smoked two packs of cigarettes each day for the past 80 years, how would your plan of care change?

3. Your patient has been diagnosed with deep vein thrombosis of a calf. The physician gives the patient two treatment options: hospitalization with intravenous sodium heparin therapy or home treatment with LMWH. What factors would you include in discussing the treatment options with the patient?

REFERENCES AND SELECTED READINGS

Books

Bickley, L. S., & Szilagyi, P. G. (2003). *Bates' guide to physical examination and history taking* (8th ed.). Philadelphia: Lippincott Williams & Wilkins.

Bullock, B., & Henze R. (1999). *Focus on pathophysiology* (4th ed.). Philadelphia: Lippincott Williams & Wilkins.

Coleman, R. W., Hirsch, J., Marder, V. J., Clowes, A. W., George, J. N. (2000). *Hemostasis and thrombosis: Basic principles and clinical practice* (4th ed.). Philadelphia: Lippincott Williams & Wilkins.

Fahey, V. (1999). *Vascular nursing* (3rd ed.). Philadelphia: W. B. Saunders.

Gloviczki, P., & Yao, J. T. (2001). *Handbook of venous disorders—Guidelines of the American Venous Forum* (2nd ed.). New York: Oxford University Press.

Guyton, A., & Hall, J. (2000). *Textbook of medical physiology* (10th ed.). Philadelphia: W. B. Saunders.

Haimovici, H. (1996). *Vascular surgery principles and techniques* (4th ed.). Cambridge, MA: Blackwell Science.

Jarvis, C. (1999). *Physical examination and health assessment* (3rd ed.). Philadelphia: W. B. Saunders.

Moore, W. S. (2002). *Vascular surgery: A comprehensive review* (6th ed.). Philadelphia: W. B. Saunders.

Parodi, J. C., Veith, F. J., & Marin, M. (1999). *Endovascular grafting techniques.* Baltimore: Williams & Wilkins.

Rutherford, R. B. (1999). *Vascular surgery* (5th ed., Vols. I and II). Philadelphia: W. B. Saunders.

Strandness, D. E. (2002). *Duplex scanning in vascular disorders* (3rd ed.). Philadelphia: Lippincott Williams & Wilkins.

White, R. A., & Fogarty, T. J. (1999). *Peripheral endovascular interventions* (2nd ed.). New York: Singer-Verlag.

Yao, J. T. & Pearce, W. H. (1999). *Practical vascular surgery.* Stamford, CT: Appleton & Lange.

Journals

Beckey, N. P. (1999). Outpatient management of patients on warfarin. *Lippincott's Primary Care Practice, 3*(3), 280–289.

Berdejo, G. L., Lyon, R. T., Ohki, T., Sanchez, L. A., Wain, R. A., del Valle, W. N., et al. (1998). Color duplex ultrasound evaluation of transluminally placed endovascular grafts for aneurysm repair. *Journal of Vascular Technology, 22*(4), 201–207.

Bryant, J. L., & Turkoski, B. B. (1999). Relieving intermittent claudication: A nursing approach. *Journal of Vascular Nursing, 16*(4), 81–85.

Caps, M. T., Meissner, M. H., Tullis, M. J., Polissar, N. L., Manzo, R. A., Zierler, B. K., et al. (1999). Venous thrombus stability during acute phase of therapy. *Vascular Medicine, 4*(1), 9–14.

Finkelmeier, B. A. (1997). Dissection of the aorta: A clinical update. *Journal of Vascular Nursing, 15*(3), 88–93.

Frost-Rude, J. A., Nunnelee, J. D., & Spaner, S. (2000). Buerger's disease. *Journal of Vascular Nursing, 18*(4), 128–130.

Gramse, C. A., Hingorani, A., & Ascher, E. (2001). Postoperative anticoagulation in vascular surgery: Part 1. A retrospective comparison of clinical outcomes for unfractionated heparin versus low-molecular-weight heparin. *Journal of Vascular Nursing, 19*(2), 42–49.

Hirsch, A. T., Criqui, M. H., Treat-Jacobson, D., Regensteiner, J. G., Creager, M. A., Olin, J. W., et al. (2001). Peripheral arterial disease detection, awareness, and treatment in primary care. *Journal of the American Medical Association, 286*(11), 1317–1324.

Johnson, M. T. (1997). Treatment and prevention of varicose veins. *Journal of Vascular Nursing, 15*(3), 97–103.

Kaufman, M. W., & All, A. C. (1996). Raynaud's disease: Patient education as a primary nursing intervention. *Journal of Vascular Nursing, 14*(2), 34–39.

Kowallek, D. L., & DePalma, R. G. (1997). Venous ulceration: Active approaches to treatment. *Journal of Vascular Nursing, 15*(2), 50–57.

Krauss, R. M., Eckel, R. H., Howard, B., Appel, L. J., Daniels, S. R., Deckelbaum, R. J., et al. (2000). AHA dietary guidelines. Revision 2000: A statement for healthcare professionals from the Nutrition Committee of the American Heart Association. *Circulation, 102*(18), 2284–2299.

Lacey, K. O. (1996). Subclavian steal syndrome: A review. *Journal of Vascular Nursing, 14*(1), 1–7.

Lombardo, K. M. (1997). Endovascular grafting of abdominal aortic aneurysms. *Journal of Vascular Nursing, 15*(3), 83–87.

Mawhorter, S. D. (2000). Nonhealing cellulitis in a 54-year-old man with diabetes mellitus. *Cleveland Clinic Journal of Medicine, 67*(1), 21–24.

McAlister, F. A., Levine, M., Zarnke, K. B., Campbell, N., Lewanczuk, R., Leenen, F., et al. (2001). The 2000 Canadian recommendations for the management of hypertension: Part 1. Therapy. *Canadian Journal of Cardiology, 17*(5), 543–559.

Meissner, M. H., Caps, M. T., Zierler, B. F., Bergelin, R. O., Manzo, R. A., Stradnes, D. E., Jr. (2000). Deep venous thrombosis and superficial venous reflux. *Journal of Vascular Surgery, 32*(1), 48–56.

Moser, M. (1999). World Health Organization-International Society of Hypertension guidelines for the management of hypertension—Do these differ from the U.S. recommendations? Which guidelines should the practicing physician follow? *Journal of Clinical Hypertension, 1,* 48–54.

O'Connor, C. M. (2001). Raynaud's phenomenon. *Journal of Vascular Nursing, 19*(3), 87–92.

Phillips, L. (2000). Putting a damper on cellulitis. *Nursing, 30*(12), 52–53.

Ross, R. (1999). Atherosclerosis–an inflammatory disease. *New England Journal of Medicine, 340*(2), 115–126.

Ross, R., & Glomset, J. A. (1973). Atherosclerosis and the arterial smooth muscle cell: Proliferation of smooth muscle is a key event in the genesis of the lesions of atherosclerosis. *Science, 180,* 1332–1339.

Rudolph, D. (2001). Standards of care for venous leg ulcers: Compression therapy and moist wound healing. *Journal of Vascular Nursing, 19*(1), 20–27.

Stevens, S. L. (2000). Heparin-induced thrombocytopenia. *Journal of Vascular Nursing, 18*(2), 54–58.

Strider, D., Robinson, T., Guarini, J., Ivey, J. (1996). Challenges with Takayasu's arteritis: A case study. *Journal of Vascular Nursing, 14*(1), 12–17.

Verta, K. F., & Verta, M. J. (1998). Alternative imaging techniques in vascular surgery. *Journal of Vascular Nursing, 16*(4), 78–83.

Vogeley, C. L., & Coeling, H. (2000). Prevention of venous ulceration by use of compression after deep vein thrombosis. *Journal of Vascular Nursing, 18*(4), 123–127.

Zierler, R. E. (1999). Vascular surgery without arteriography: use of Duplex ultrasound. *Cardiovascular Surgery, 7*(1), 74–82.

RESOURCES AND WEBSITES

Canadian Healthcare Association: Guide to Canadian Healthcare Facilities, 17 York Street, Ottawa, ON K1N 9J6; 613-241-8005; www.cha.ca/publishing/guide.htm.

Canadian Society for Vascular Surgery, Sunnybrook and Women's College Health Science Centre, 2075 Bayview Avenue, H-185, Toronto, ON M4N 3M5; 416-480-4734; www.csvs.ca.

Centre for Chronic Disease Prevention and Control: Cardiovascular Disease, Public Health Agency of Canada, 130 Colonnade Road, AL 6501H Ottawa, ON K1A 0K9; 1-866-999-7612; http://www.phac-aspc.gc.ca/ccdpc-cpcmc/cvd-mcv/index_e.html.

National Heart, Lung, and Blood Institute, Health Information Center, P.O. Box 30105, Bethesda, MD 20824-0105; 301-592-8573; http://www.nhlbi.nih.gov.

Society for Vascular Surgery, 13 Elm Street, Manchester, MA 01944-1314; 978-526-8330; http://www.vascularweb.org.

Society of Vascular Nursing, 7794 Grow Drive, Pensacola, FL 32514; 888-536-4786; http://www.svnnet.org.

Assessment and Management of Patients With Hypertension

Adapted by Joe Noon

LEARNING OBJECTIVES

On completion of this chapter, the learner will be able to:

1. Define blood pressure and identify risk factors for hypertension.
2. Explain the difference between normal blood pressure and hypertension and discuss the significance of hypertension.
3. Describe the treatment approach for hypertension, including lifestyle changes and medication therapy.
4. Use the nursing process as a framework for care of the patient with hypertension.
5. Describe the necessity for immediate treatment of hypertensive crisis.

*B*lood pressure is the product of cardiac output multiplied by peripheral resistance. Cardiac output is the product of the heart rate multiplied by the stroke volume. In normal circulation, pressure is exerted by the flow of blood through the heart and blood vessels. High blood pressure, known as hypertension, can result from a change in cardiac output, a change in peripheral resistance, or both. The medications used for treating hypertension decrease peripheral resistance, blood volume, or the strength and rate of myocardial contraction.

Hypertension Defined

Hypertension is a systolic blood pressure greater than 140 mm Hg and a diastolic pressure greater than 90 mm Hg over a sustained period, based on the average of two or more blood pressure measurements taken in two or more contacts with the health care provider after an initial screening (Seventh Report of the Joint National Committee on Prevention, Detection, Evaluation, and Treatment of High Blood Pressure [**JNC VII**], 2003). Table 32-1 shows the categories of blood pressure established in 2003 by the JNC VII. The classification shows the direct relation between the risk of morbidity and mortality from hypertension and the level of systolic and diastolic blood pressures. The higher the systolic or diastolic pressure, the greater the risk.

Three stages (1, 2, and 3) of hypertension are defined by the JNC VII, which used these terms, similar to those used to describe cancer progression, so that the public and health care professionals would be aware that sustained elevations in blood pressure are associated with increased risks to health. Even within the normotensive range, three levels of blood pressure—optimal, normal, and high-normal—were specified to emphasize that the lower the blood pressure, the lower the risk. The JNC VII also developed recommendations for follow-up monitoring according to initial blood pressure readings at the time of diagnosis (Table 32-2).

Primary Hypertension

Twenty-two percent of Canadians aged 18–70 have hypertension, and 50% of Canadians over the age of 65 have hypertension. Of this population, between 90% and 95% have **primary hypertension**, meaning that the reason for the elevation in blood pressure cannot be identified. The remaining 5% to 10% of this group have high blood pressure related to specific causes, such as narrowing of the renal arteries, renal parenchymal disease, hyperal-

dosteronism (mineralocorticoid hypertension) certain medications, pregnancy, and coarctation of the aorta (Kaplan, 2001). **Secondary hypertension** is the term used to signify high blood pressure from an identified cause.

Hypertension is sometimes called "the silent killer" because people who have it are often symptom free. In a national survey (1991 to 1994), 32% of people who had pressures exceeding 140/90 mm Hg were unaware of their elevated blood pressure (Burt et al., 1995a). Once identified, elevated blood pressure should be monitored at regular intervals because hypertension is a lifelong condition.

Hypertension often accompanies risk factors for atherosclerotic heart disease, such as **dyslipidemia** (abnormal blood fat levels) and diabetes mellitus. Cigarette smoking does not cause high blood pressure; however, if a person with hypertension smokes, his or her risk of dying from heart disease or related disorders increases significantly.

High blood pressure can be viewed in three ways: as a sign, a risk factor for atherosclerotic cardiovascular disease, or a disease.

Table 32-1 • Classification of Blood Pressure for Adults Age 18 and Older*

CATEGORY	SYSTOLIC (mm Hg)		DIASTOLIC (mm Hg)
Optimal	<120	and	<80
Normal†	<130	and	<85
High-normal	130–139	or	85–89
Hypertension‡			
Stage 1	140–159	or	90–99
Stage 2	160–179	or	100–109
Stage 3	≥180	or	≥110

*Not taking antihypertensive drugs and not acutely ill. When systolic and diastolic blood pressures fall into different categories, the higher category should be selected to classify the individual's blood pressure status. For example, 160/92 mm Hg should be classified as stage 2 hypertension, and 174/120 mm Hg should be classified as stage 3 hypertension. Isolated systolic hypertension is defined as SBP of 140 mm Hg or greater and DBP below 90 mm Hg and staged appropriately (eg, 170/82 mm Hg is defined as stage 2 isolated systolic hypertension). In addition to classifying stages of hypertension on the basis of average blood pressure levels, clinicians should specify presence or absence of target organ disease and additional risk factors. This specificity is important for risk classification and treatment.
†Optimal blood pressure with respect to cardiovascular risk is below 120/80 mm Hg. However, unusually low readings should be evaluated for clinical significance.
‡Based on the average of two or more readings taken at each of two or more visits after an initial screening.
From the Seventh Report of the Joint National Committee on Prevention, Detection, Evaluation, and Treatment of High Blood Pressure. (2003). *Hypertension, 42*(6), 1206–1252.

Glossary

dyslipidemia: abnormally high or low blood lipid levels
hypertensive emergency: a situation in which blood pressure must be lowered immediately to prevent damage to target organs
hypertensive urgency: a situation in which blood pressure must be lowered within a few hours to prevent damage to target organs

JNC VII: Seventh Joint National Committee on the Prevention, Detection, Evaluation and Treatment of High Blood Pressure; committee established to study and make recommendations about hypertension in the United States. Findings and recommendations of JNC VII are contained in an extensive report published in 2003.
monotherapy: medication therapy with a single medication

primary hypertension: also called essential hypertension; denotes high blood pressure from an unidentified cause
rebound hypertension: pressure that is controlled with therapy and that becomes uncontrolled (abnormally high) with the discontinuation of therapy
secondary hypertension: high blood pressure from an identified cause, such as renal disease

Table 32-2 • Recommendations for Follow-up Based on Initial Blood Pressure Measurements for Adults

INITIAL BLOOD PRESSURE (mm Hg)*		FOLLOW-UP RECOMMENDED†
Systolic	Diastolic	
<130	<85	Recheck in 2 years
130–139	85–89	Recheck in 1 year‡
140–159	90–99	Confirm within 2 months
160–179	100–109	Evaluate or refer to source of care within 1 month
≥180	≥110	Evaluate or refer to source of care immediately or within 1 week depending on clinical situation

*If systolic and diastolic categories are different, follow recommendations for shorter follow-up time (eg, 160/86 mm Hg, evaluate or refer to source of care within 1 month).
†Modify the scheduling of follow-up according to reliable information about past blood pressure measurements, other cardiovascular risk factors, or target organ disease.
‡Provide advice about lifestyle modifications.
From the Seventh Report of the Joint National Committee on Prevention, Detection, Evaluation, and Treatment of High Blood Pressure. (2003). *Hypertension, 42*(6), 1206–1252.

As a sign, nurses and other health care professionals use blood pressure to monitor a patient's clinical status. Elevated pressure may indicate an excessive dose of vasoconstrictive medication or other problems. As a risk factor, hypertension contributes to the rate at which atherosclerotic plaque accumulates within arterial walls. As a disease, hypertension is a major contributor to death from cardiac, renal, and peripheral vascular disease.

Prolonged blood pressure elevation eventually damages blood vessels throughout the body, particularly in target organs such as the heart, kidneys, brain, and eyes. The usual consequences of prolonged, uncontrolled hypertension are myocardial infarction, heart failure, renal failure, strokes, and impaired vision. The left ventricle of the heart may become enlarged (left ventricular hypertrophy) as it works to pump blood against the elevated pressure. An echocardiogram is the recommended method of determining whether hypertrophy (enlargement) has occurred.

Pathophysiology

Although the precise cause for most cases of hypertension cannot be identified, it is understood that hypertension is a multifactorial condition. Because hypertension is a sign, it is most likely to have many causes, just as fever has many causes. For hypertension to occur, there must be a change in one or more factors affecting peripheral resistance or cardiac output (some of these factors are outlined in Fig. 32-1). In addition, there must also be a problem with the control systems that monitor or regulate pressure. Single gene mutations have been identified for a few rare types of hypertension, but most types of high blood pressure are thought to be polygenic (mutations in more than one gene) (Dominiczak et al., 2000).

Several hypotheses about the pathophysiologic bases of elevated blood pressure are associated with the concept of hypertension as a multifactorial condition. Given the overlap among these hypotheses, it is likely that aspects of all of them will eventually prove correct. Hypertension may be caused by one or more of the following:

- Increased sympathetic nervous system activity related to dysfunction of the autonomic nervous system

- Increased renal reabsorption of sodium, chloride, and water related to a genetic variation in the pathways by which the kidneys handle sodium
- Increased activity of the renin-angiotensin-aldosterone system, resulting in expansion of extracellular fluid volume and increased systemic vascular resistance
- Decreased vasodilation of the arterioles related to dysfunction of the vascular endothelium
- Resistance to insulin action, which may be a common factor linking hypertension, type 2 diabetes mellitus, hypertriglyceridemia, obesity, and glucose intolerance

 Gerontologic Considerations

Structural and functional changes in the heart and blood vessels contribute to increases in blood pressure that occur with age. The changes include accumulation of atherosclerotic plaque, fragmentation of arterial elastins, increased collagen deposits, and impaired vasodilation. The result of these changes is a decrease in the elasticity of the major blood vessels. Consequently, the aorta and large arteries are less able to accommodate the volume of blood pumped out by the heart (stroke volume), and the energy that would have stretched the vessels instead elevates the systolic blood pressure. Isolated systolic hypertension is more common in older adults.

Clinical Manifestations

Physical examination may reveal no abnormalities other than high blood pressure. Occasionally, retinal changes such as hemorrhages, exudates (fluid accumulation), arteriolar narrowing, and cotton-wool spots (small infarctions) occur. In severe hypertension, papilledema (swelling of the optic disc) may be seen. People with hypertension can be asymptomatic and remain so for many years. However, when specific signs and symptoms appear, they usually indicate vascular damage, with specific manifestations related to the organs served by the involved vessels. Coronary artery disease with angina or myocardial infarction is a common consequence of hypertension. Left ventricular hypertrophy occurs in response to the increased workload placed on the ventricle as it contracts against higher systemic pressure. When heart damage is extensive, heart failure ensues. Pathologic changes in the kidneys (indicated by increased blood urea nitrogen [BUN] and creatinine levels) may manifest as nocturia. Cerebrovascular involvement may lead to a stroke or transient ischemic attack (TIA), manifested by alterations in vision or speech, dizziness, weakness, a sudden fall, or temporary paralysis on one side (hemiplegia). Cerebral infarctions account for most of the strokes and TIAs in patients with hypertension.

Assessment and Diagnostic Evaluation

A thorough health history and physical examination are necessary. The retinas are examined, and laboratory studies are performed to assess possible target organ damage. Routine laboratory tests include urinalysis, blood chemistry (ie, analysis of sodium, potassium, creatinine, fasting glucose, and total and high-density lipoprotein [HDL] cholesterol levels), and a 12-lead electrocardiogram. Left ventricular hypertrophy can be assessed by echocardiography. Renal damage may be suggested by elevations in BUN and creatinine levels or by microalbuminuria or macroalbuminuria. Additional studies, such as creatinine clearance, renin level, urine tests, and 24-hour urine protein, may be performed.

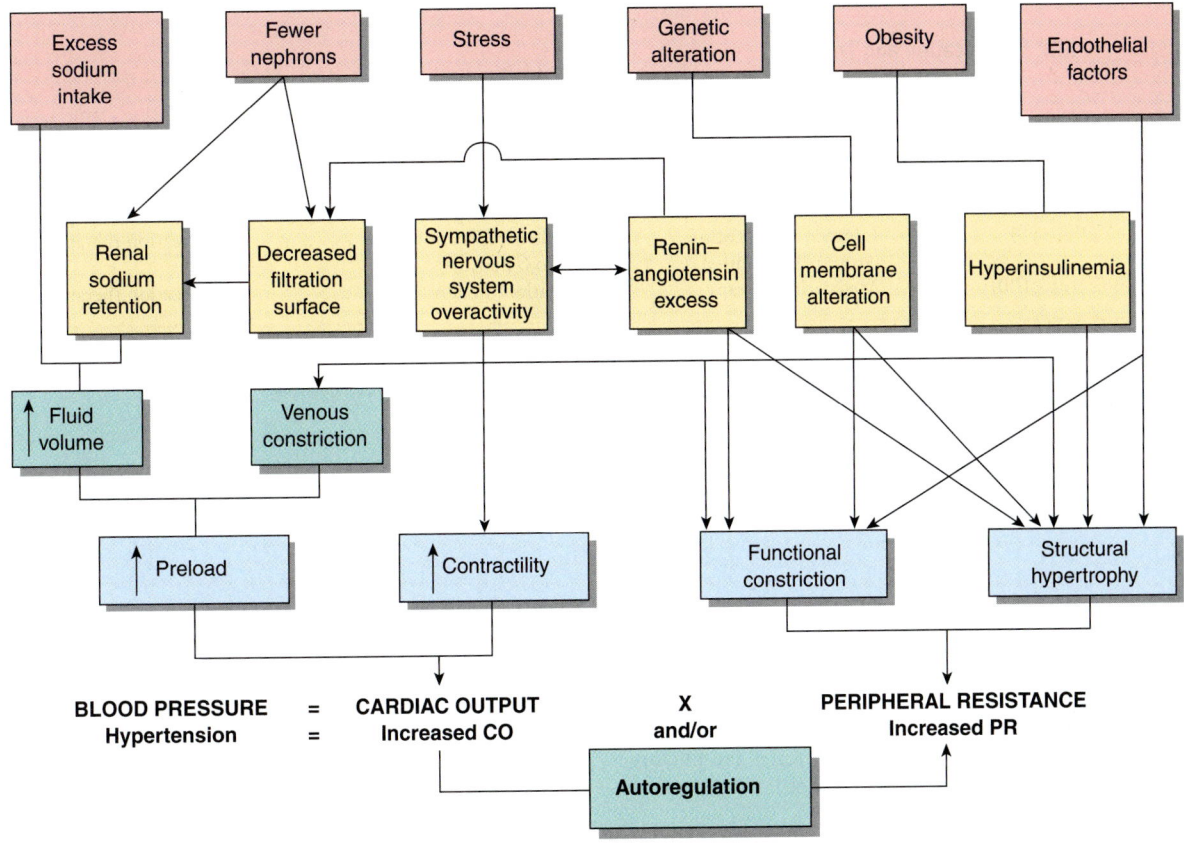

BLOOD PRESSURE = CARDIAC OUTPUT X PERIPHERAL RESISTANCE
Hypertension = Increased CO and/or Increased PR

Autoregulation

FIGURE 32-1 Factors involved in control of blood pressure, which is cardiac output multiplied by peripheral resistance. Adapted from Kaplan, N. M., Lieberman, E., & Neal, W. (2002). *Kaplan's clinical hypertension* (8th ed.). Philadelphia: Lippincott Williams & Wilkins.

A risk factor assessment, as advocated by the 2005 Canadian Hypertension Education Program Recommendations (CHEP), is needed to classify and guide treatment of hypertensive people at risk for cardiovascular damage. Risk factors and cardiovascular problems related to hypertension are presented in Chart 32-1 and Table 32-3.

Medical Management

The goal of hypertension treatment is to prevent death and complications by achieving and maintaining the arterial blood pressure at 140/90 mm Hg or lower. The CHEP specified a lower goal pressure of 130/85 mm Hg for people with diabetes mellitus or with proteinuria greater than 1 g per 24 hours. The optimal management plan is inexpensive, simple, and causes the least possible disruption in the patient's life.

The management options for hypertension are summarized in the treatment algorithm issued in the Seventh Report of the Joint National Committee on Prevention, Detection, Evaluation, and Treatment of High Blood Pressure (2003) (Fig. 32-2) and in Chart 32-2, which lists recommended lifestyle modifications. The clinician uses the algorithm in conjunction with the risk factor assessment data and the patient's blood pressure category to choose the initial and subsequent treatment plans for patients. Research findings demonstrate that weight loss, reduced alcohol and sodium intake, and regular physical activity are effective life-

Chart 32-1

Risk Factors for Cardiovascular Problems in Hypertensive Patients

Major Risk Factors (in Addition to Hypertension)
- Smoking
- Dyslipidemia
- Diabetes mellitus
- Age older than 60 years
- Gender (men and postmenopausal women)
- Family history of cardiovascular disease (in female relative younger than 65 years of age or male relative younger than 55 years)

Target Organ Damage/Clinical Cardiovascular Disease
- Heart disease (left ventricular hypertrophy, angina or previous myocardial infarction, previous coronary revascularization, heart failure)
- Stroke (cerebrovascular accident, brain attack) or TIA
- Nephropathy
- Peripheral arterial disease
- Retinopathy

Adapted from the 2005 Canadian Hypertension Education Program Recommendations. Canadian Stroke Network. www.canadianstrokenetwork.ca.

Table 32-3 • Risk Stratification and Treatment

BLOOD PRESSURE STAGES (mm HG)	RISK GROUP A (NO RISK FACTORS, NO TOD/CCD)	RISK GROUP B (AT LEAST 1 RISK FACTOR, NOT INCLUDING DIABETES; NO TOD/CCD)	RISK GROUP C (TOD/CCD AND/OR DIABETES, WITH OR WITHOUT OTHER RISK FACTORS)
High-normal (130–139/85–89)	Lifestyle modification	Lifestyle modification	Medication therapy†
Stage 1 (140–159/90–99)	Lifestyle modification (up to 12 months)	Lifestyle modification* (up to 6 months)	Medication therapy
Stages 2 and 3 (≥160/≥100)	Medication therapy	Medication therapy	Medication therapy

Example: A patient with diabetes and a blood pressure of 142/94 mm Hg plus left ventricular hypertrophy should be classified as having stage 1 hypertension with target organ disease (left ventricular hypertrophy) and with another major risk factor (diabetes). This patient would be categorized as Stage 1, Risk-Group C, and recommended for immediate initiation of pharmacologic treatment. Lifestyle modification should be adjunctive therapy for all patients recommended for pharmacologic therapy.
TOD/CCD, target organ disease/clinical cardiovascular disease (see Chart 32-1).
*For patients with multiple risk factors, clinicians should consider medications as initial therapy plus lifestyle modifications.
†For patients with heart failure, renal insufficiency, or diabetes.
From Seventh Report of the Joint National Committee on the Prevention, Detection, Evaluation, and Treatment of High Blood Pressure. (2003). *Hypertension, 42*(6), 1206–1252.

style adaptations to reduce blood pressure (Appel et al., 1997; Cushman et al., 1998; Hagberg et al., 2000; Sacks et al., 2001). Studies show that diets high in fruits, vegetables, and low-fat diary products can prevent the development of hypertension and can lower elevated pressures. Table 32-4 delineates the Dietary Approaches to Stop Hypertension (DASH) diet.

PHARMACOLOGIC THERAPY

For patients with uncomplicated hypertension and no specific indications for another medication, the recommended initial medications include diuretics, beta-blockers, or both. Patients are first given low doses of medication. If blood pressure does not fall to less than 140/90 mm Hg, the dose is increased gradually, and additional medications are included as necessary to achieve control. Table 32-5 describes the various pharmacologic agents used in treating hypertension. When the blood pressure has been less than 140/90 mm Hg for at least 1 year, gradual reduction of the types and doses of medication is recommended. To promote compliance, clinicians try to prescribe the simplest treatment schedule possible, ideally one pill once each day.

 Gerontologic Considerations

Hypertension, particularly elevated systolic blood pressure, increases the risk of death and complications in elderly patients. Treatment reduces this risk. Like younger patients, elderly patients should begin treatment with lifestyle modifications. If medications are needed to achieve the blood pressure goal of less than 140/90 mm Hg, the starting dose should be one-half that used in younger patients.

NURSING PROCESS: THE PATIENT WITH HYPERTENSION

Assessment

When hypertension is initially detected, nursing assessment involves carefully monitoring the blood pressure at frequent intervals and then, after diagnosis, at routinely scheduled intervals. The Canadian Heart Association, the Canadian Society of Hypertension, and the Heart and Stroke Foundation of Canada have defined the standards

for blood pressure measurement, including conditions required before measurements are made, equipment specifications, and techniques for measuring blood pressure to obtain accurate and reliable readings (Chart 32-3) (CHEP, 2005; Perloff et al., 1993). When the patient begins an antihypertensive treatment regimen, blood pressure assessments are needed to determine the effectiveness of medication therapy and to detect any changes in blood pressure that indicate the need for a change in the treatment plan.

A complete history is obtained to assess for symptoms that indicate target organ damage (whether other body systems have been affected by the elevated blood pressure). Such symptoms may include anginal pain; shortness of breath; alterations in speech, vision, or balance; nosebleeds; headaches; dizziness; or nocturia.

During the physical examination, the nurse must also pay specific attention to the rate, rhythm, and character of the apical and peripheral pulses to detect effects of hypertension on the heart and blood vessels. A thorough assessment can yield valuable information about the extent to which the hypertension has affected the body and about any other personal, social, or financial factors related to the condition.

Diagnosis

NURSING DIAGNOSES

Based on the assessment data, nursing diagnoses for the patient may include the following:

- Deficient knowledge regarding the relation between the treatment regimen and control of the disease process
- Noncompliance with therapeutic regimen related to side effects of prescribed therapy

COLLABORATIVE PROBLEMS/POTENTIAL COMPLICATIONS

Based on the assessment data, potential complications that may develop include the following:

- Left ventricular hypertrophy
- Myocardial infarction
- Heart failure
- TIAs
- Cerebrovascular accident (stroke or brain attack)

Lifestyle Modifications for Hypertension Prevention and Management

- Lose weight if overweight.
- Limit alcohol intake to no more than 30 mL ethanol (eg, 720 mL beer, 300 mL wine, or 60 mL 100-proof whiskey) per day or 15 mL ethanol per day for women and lighter weight people.
- Increase aerobic physical activity (30 to 45 minutes most days of the week).
- Reduce sodium intake to no more than 100 mmol per day (2.4 g sodium or 6 g sodium chloride).
- Maintain adequate intake of dietary potassium (approximately 90 mmol per day).
- Maintain adequate intake of dietary calcium and magnesium for general health.
- Stop smoking and reduce intake of dietary saturated fat and cholesterol for overall cardiovascular health.

From the 2005 Canadian Hypertension Education Program Recommendations. Canadian Stroke Network. www.canadianstrokenetwork.ca.

Nursing Interventions

The objective of nursing care for hypertensive patients focuses on lowering and controlling the blood pressure without adverse effects and without undue cost. To achieve these goals, the nurse must support and teach the patient to adhere to the treatment regimen by implementing necessary lifestyle changes, taking medications as prescribed, and scheduling regular follow-up appointments with the health care provider to monitor progress or identify and treat any complications of disease or therapy.

INCREASING KNOWLEDGE

The patient needs to understand the disease process and how lifestyle changes and medications can control hypertension. The nurse needs to emphasize the concept of controlling hypertension rather than curing it. The nurse can encourage the patient to consult a dietitian to help develop a plan for weight loss. The program usually consists of restricting sodium and fat intake, increasing intake of fruits and vegetables, and implementing regular physical activity. Explaining that it takes 2 to 3 months for the taste buds to adapt to changes in salt intake

(text continues on page 867)

* Unless contraindicated.
   ACE = angiotensin-converting enzyme; ISA, intrinsic sympathomimetic activity.
† Based on randomized controlled trials

FIGURE 32-2 Algorithm of hypertension treatment. Treatment begins with lifestyle modifications and continues with various medication regimens. From the Seventh Report of the Joint National Committee on Prevention, Detection, Evaluation, and Treatment of High Blood Pressure. (2003). *Hypertension, 42*(6), 1206–1252.

- Renal insufficiency and failure
- Retinal hemorrhage

Planning and Goals

The major goals for the patient include understanding of the disease process and its treatment, participation in a self-care program, and absence of complications.

Table 32-4 • **The DASH (Dietary Approaches to Stop Hypertension) Diet***	
FOOD GROUP	NO. SERVINGS PER DAY
Grains and grain products	7–8
Vegetables	4–5
Fruits	4–5
Lowfat or fat-free dairy foods	2–3
Meat, fish, and poultry	2 or fewer
Nuts, seeds, and dry beans	4–5 weekly

*Based on 2000 calories per day.
Source: www.nhlbi.nih.gov/health/public/heart/hbp/dash/new_dash.pdf

Table 32-5 • **Medication Therapy for Hypertension**

MEDICATIONS	MAJOR ACTION	ADVANTAGES AND CONTRAINDICATIONS	EFFECTS AND NURSING CONSIDERATIONS
Purpose: To maintain blood pressure within normal ranges by the simplest and safest means possible with the fewest side effects for each individual patient			
Diuretics and Related Drugs			
Thiazide Diuretics			
chlorthalidone (Hygroton) quinethazone (Hydromox) chlorothiazide (Diuril) hydrochlorothiazide (Esidrix; HydroDIURIL)	Decrease of blood volume, renal blood flow, and cardiac output Depletion of extracellular fluid Negative sodium balance (from natriuresis), mild hypokalemia Directly affect vascular smooth muscle	Effective orally Effective during long-term administration Mild side effects Enhance other antihypertensive medications Counter sodium retention effect of other antihypertensive medications *Contraindications:* Gout, known sensitivity to sulfonamide-derived medications, and severely impaired kidney function	Side effects include dry mouth, thirst, weakness, drowsiness, lethargy, muscle aches, muscular fatigue, tachycardia, GI disturbance. Postural hypotension may be potentiated by alcohol, barbiturates, opioids, or hot weather. Because thiazides cause loss of sodium, potassium, and magnesium, monitor for signs of electrolyte imbalance. Encourage intake of potassium-rich foods (eg, fruits). *Gerontological Considerations:* Risk of postural hypotension is significant because of volume depletion; measure blood pressure in three positions; caution patient to rise slowly.
Loop Diuretics			
furosemide (Lasix) bumetanide (Bumex)	Volume depletion Blocks reabsorption of sodium, chloride, and water in kidney	Action rapid Potent Used when thiazides fail or patient needs rapid diuresis *Contraindications:* Same as for thiazides	Volume depletion is rapid—profound diuresis can occur. Electrolyte depletion—replacement is required. Thirst, nausea, vomiting, skin rash, postural hypotension. Sweet taste noted; oral and gastric burning. *Gerontologic Considerations:* Same as for thiazides.
Potassium-Sparing Diuretics			
spironolactone (Aldactone) triamterene (Dyrenium)	Competitive inhibitor of aldosterone Acts on distal tubule independently of aldosterone	Spironolactone is effective in treating hypertension accompanying primary aldosteronism. Both spironolactone and triamterene cause retention of potassium. *Contraindications:* Renal disease, azotemia, severe hepatic disease, hyperkalemia	Drowsiness, lethargy, headache—decrease dosage. Monitor for hyperkalemia if given with ACE inhibitor. Diarrhea and other GI symptoms—administer medication after meals. Skin eruptions, urticaria Mental confusion, ataxia (with triamterene)—dosage may need to be reduced. Gynecomastia (not for triamterene)

(continued)

Table 32-5 • Medication Therapy for Hypertension (Continued)

MEDICATIONS	MAJOR ACTION	ADVANTAGES AND CONTRAINDICATIONS	EFFECTS AND NURSING CONSIDERATIONS
Adrenergic Agents *Peripheral Agents* reserpine (Serpasil)	Impairs synthesis and re-uptake of norepinephrine	Slows pulse, which counteracts tachycardia of hydralazine *Contraindications:* History of depression, psychosis, obesity, chronic sinusitis, peptic ulcer	May cause severe depression; report manifestations, as this may require that drug be omitted. Nasal stuffiness, which may require nasal vasoconstrictor. Increases appetite—therefore, weight control may be difficult. Recurrence of peptic ulcer—administer with meals or milk. *Gerontologic Considerations:* Depression and postural hypotension common in elderly
Central Alpha Agonists methyldopa (Aldomet)	Dopa-decarboxylase inhibitor; displaces norepinephrine from storage sites	Drug of choice for pregnant women with hypertension Useful in patients with renal failure Does not decrease cardiac output or renal blood flow Does not induce oliguria *Contraindications:* Liver disease	Drowsiness, dizziness Dry mouth; nasal stuffiness (troublesome at first but then tends to disappear) Hemolytic anemia (a hypersensitization reaction)—positive Coombs' test *Gerontologic Considerations:* May produce mental and behavioural changes in the elderly.
clonidine hydrochloride (Catapres)	Exact mode of action not understood, but acts through the central nervous system, apparently through centrally mediated alpha-adrenergic stimulation in the brain, producing blood pressure reduction	Little or no orthostatic effect. Moderately potent, and sometimes is effective when other medications fail to lower blood pressure. *Contraindications:* Severe coronary artery disease, pregnancy, children	Most common side effects are dry mouth, drowsiness, sedation, and occasional headaches and fatigue. Anorexia, malaise, and vomiting with mild disturbance of liver function have been reported. Rebound or withdrawal hypertension is relatively common; monitor blood pressure when stopping medication.
guanfacine (Tenex)	Stimulates central alpha-2 adrenergic receptors	Reduces heart rate and causes vasodilation. Serious adverse reactions are uncommon. Use with caution in persons with diminished liver function, recent myocardial infarction, or known cardiovascular disease.	Common side effects include dry mouth, dizziness, sleepiness, fatigue, headache, constipation, and impotence.
Beta-Blockers propranolol (Inderal) metoprolol (Lopressor) nadolol (Corgard)	Block the sympathetic nervous system (beta-adrenergic receptors), especially the sympathetics to the heart, producing a slower heart rate and lowered blood pressure	Reduce pulse rate in patients with tachycardia and blood pressure elevation and are useful as an adjunct with medications that act at the neuroeffector site of the blood vessel *Contraindications:* Bronchial asthma, allergic rhinitis, right ventricular failure from pulmonary hypertension, congestive heart failure, depression, diabetes mellitus, dyslipidemia, heart block, peripheral vascular disease, heart rate under 60 bpm	Mental depression manifested by insomnia, lassitude, weakness, and fatigue. Lightheadedness and occasional nausea, vomiting, and epigastric distress Check heart rate before giving. *Gerontologic Considerations:* Risk of toxicity is increased for elderly patients with decreased renal and liver function. Take blood pressure in three positions and observe for hypotension.

(continued)

Table 32-5 • Medication Therapy for Hypertension (Continued)

MEDICATIONS	MAJOR ACTION	ADVANTAGES AND CONTRAINDICATIONS	EFFECTS AND NURSING CONSIDERATIONS
Alpha Blocker prazosin hydrochloride (Minipress)	Peripheral vasodilator acting directly on the blood vessel; similar to hydralazine	Acts directly on the blood vessel and is an effective agent in patients with adverse reactions to hydralazine *Contraindications:* Angina pectoris and coronary artery disease. Induces tachycardia if not preceded by administration of propranolol and a diuretic.	Occasional vomiting and diarrhea, urinary frequency, and cardiovascular collapse, especially if given in addition to hydralazine without lowering the dose of the latter. Patients occasionally experience drowsiness, lack of energy, and weakness.
Combined Alpha and Beta Blocker labetalol hydrochloride (Normodyne, Trandate)	Blocks alpha- and beta-adrenergic receptors; causes peripheral dilation and decreases peripheral vascular resistance	Fast-acting No decrease in renal blood flow *Contraindications:* Asthma, cardiogenic shock, severe tachycardia, heart block	Orthostatic hypotension, tachycardia
Vasodilators fenoldopam mesylate	Stimulates dopamine and alpha-2 adrenergic receptors	Given intravenously for hypertensive emergencies. Use with caution in persons with glaucoma, recent stroke (brain attack), asthma, hypokalemia, or diminished liver function.	Headache, flushing, hypotension, sweating, tachycardia caused by vasodilation Observe for local reactions at the injection site.
hydralazine hydrochloride (Apresoline)	Decreases peripheral resistance but concurrently elevates cardiac output Acts directly on smooth muscle of blood vessels	Not used as initial therapy; used in combination with other medications. Used also in pregnancy-induced hypertension *Contraindications:* Angina or coronary disease, congestive heart failure, hypersensitivity	Headache, tachycardia, flushing, and dyspnea may occur—can be prevented by pretreating with reserpine. Peripheral edema may require diuretics. May produce lupus erythematosus-like syndrome
minoxidil	Direct vasodilating action on arteriolar vessels, causing decreased peripheral vascular resistance; reduces systolic and diastolic pressures	Hypotensive effect more pronounced than with hydralazine No effect on vasomotor reflexes so does not cause postural hypotension *Contraindications:* Pheochromocytoma	Tachycardia, angina pectoris, ECG changes, edema Take blood pressure and apical pulse before administration. Monitor intake and output and daily weights. Causes hirsutism
sodium nitroprusside (Nipride, Nitropress) nitroglycerin diazoxide (Hyperstat, NitroBid IV, Tridil)	Peripheral vasodilation by relaxation of smooth muscle	Fast-acting Used only in hypertensive emergencies *Contraindications:* Sepsis, azotemia, high intracranial pressure.	Dizziness, headache, nausea, edema, tachycardia, palpitations. Can cause thiocyanate and cyanide intoxication.
Angiotensin-Converting Enzyme Inhibitors benazepril (Lotensin) captopril (Capoten) enalaprilat (Vasotec IV) enalapril (Vasotec) lisinopril (Prinivil, Zestril) ramipril (Altace) trandolapril (Mavik)	Inhibit conversion of angiotensin I to angiotensin II Lower total peripheral resistance	Fewer cardiovascular side effects Can be used with thiazide diuretic and digitalis Hypotension can be reversed by fluid replacement. *Contraindications:* Renal impairment, pregnancy	*Gerontologic Considerations:* Require reduced dosages and the addition of loop diuretics when there is renal dysfunction
Angiotensin II Receptor Blockers candesartan (Atacand) losartan (Cozaar) valsartan (Diovan) irbesartan (Avapro)	Block the effects of angiotensin II at the receptor Reduce peripheral resistance	Minimal side effects *Contraindications:* Pregnancy, renovascular disease	Monitor for hypokalemia

(continued)

Table 32-5 • Medication Therapy for Hypertension (Continued)

MEDICATIONS	MAJOR ACTION	ADVANTAGES AND CONTRAINDICATIONS	EFFECTS AND NURSING CONSIDERATIONS
Calcium Antagonists			
Nondihydropyridines			
diltiazem hydrochloride (Cardizem SR, Cardizem CD, Dilacor XR, Tiazac)	Inhibits calcium ion influx Reduces cardiac afterload	Inhibits coronary artery spasm not controlled by beta-blockers or nitrates *Contraindications:* Sick sinus syndrome; AV block; hypotension; heart failure	Do not discontinue suddenly. Observe for hypotension. Report irregular heartbeat, dizziness, edema. Instruct on regular dental care because of potential gingivitis.
verapamil (Isoptin SR, Calan SR, Verelan, Covera HS)	Inhibits calcium ion influx Slows velocity of conduction of cardiac impulse	Effective antiarrhythmic Rapid IV onset Blocks SA and AV node channels *Contraindications:* Sinus or AV node disease; severe heart failure; severe hypotension	Administer on empty stomach or before meal. Do not discontinue suddenly. Depression may subside when medication is discontinued. To relieve headaches, reduce noise, monitor electrolytes. Decrease dose for patients with liver or renal failure.
Dihydropyridines			
nifedipine (Procardia, Adalat CC) amlodipine (Norvasc) felodipine (Plendil) nicardipine (Cardene) nisoldipine (Sular)	Inhibit calcium ion influx across membranes Vasodilating effects on coronary and peripheral arteriole Decrease cardiac work and energy consumption, increase delivery of oxygen to myocardium	Rapid action Effective by oral or sublingual route No tendency to slow SA nodal activity or prolong AV node conduction Isolated systolic hypertension *Contraindications:* None (except heart failure for nifedipine)	Administer on empty stomach. Use with caution in diabetic patients. Small frequent meals if nausea. Muscle cramps, joint stiffness, sexual difficulties may disappear when dose decreased. Report irregular heartbeat, constipation, shortness of breath, edema. May cause dizziness.

Chart 32-3 Measuring Blood Pressure

Instructions for Patient
- Avoid smoking cigarettes or drinking caffeine for 30 minutes before blood pressure is measured.
- Sit quietly for 5 minutes before the reading.
- Sit comfortably with the forearm supported at heart level on a firm surface, with both feet on the ground; avoid talking during measurement.

Equipment for Practitioner
- Mercury sphygmomanometer, recently calibrated aneroid manometer, or validated electronic device
- Choose from several cuffs of different size so that rubber bladder width is at least 40% and length at least 80% of the arm circumference

Equipment for Patient at Home
- Automatic or semiautomatic device with digital display of readings

Procedure
Assessment is based on the average of at least two readings. (If two readings differ by more than 5 mm Hg, additional readings are taken and an average reading is calculated from the results.)

Conclusion
Inform patient of the numeric blood pressure value and what it means. Emphasize the need for periodic reassessment, and encourage patients who measure blood pressure at home to keep a written record of readings.

may help the patient adjust to reduced salt intake. The patient should be advised to limit alcohol intake (see Chart 32-2 for specific recommendations), and tobacco should be avoided—not because smoking is related to hypertension, but because anyone with high blood pressure is already at increased risk for heart disease, and smoking amplifies this risk. Support groups for weight control, smoking cessation, and stress reduction may be beneficial for some patients; others can benefit from the support of family and friends. The nurse assists the patient to develop and adhere to an appropriate exercise regimen, because regular activity is a significant factor in weight reduction and a blood pressure–reducing intervention in the absence of any loss in weight (Seventh Report of the Joint National Committee on Prevention, Detection, Evaluation, and Treatment of High Blood Pressure, 2003).

PROMOTING HOME AND COMMUNITY-BASED CARE

If asked to participate in a blood pressure screening, the nurse should be sure that proper blood pressure measurement technique is being used (see Chart 32-3), that the manometers used are calibrated (Perloff et al., 1993), and that provision has been made to provide follow-up for any person identified as having an elevated blood pressure. Adequate time should also be allowed to teach people what the blood pressure numbers mean. Each person should be given a written record of his or her blood pressure at the screening.

Teaching Patients Self-Care

The therapeutic regimen is the responsibility of the patient in collaboration with the health care provider. Education about high blood pressure and how to manage it, including medications, lifestyle changes of diet, weight control, and exercise (see Table 32-2), setting goal blood pressures, and assistance with social support, can help the patient achieve blood pressure control. Involving family members in education programs enables them to support the patient's efforts to control hypertension. The Heart and Stroke Foundation of Canada provides printed and electronic patient education materials.

Written information about the expected effects and side effects of medications is important. When side effects occur, patients need to understand the importance of reporting them and to whom they should be reported. Patients need to be informed that **rebound hypertension** can occur if antihypertensive medications are suddenly stopped. Female and male patients should be informed that some medications, such as beta-blockers, may cause sexual dysfunction and that, if a problem with sexual function or satisfaction occurs, other medications are available. The nurse can encourage and teach patients to measure their blood pressure at home. This practice involves patients in their own care and emphasizes the fact that failing to take medications may result in an identifiable rise in blood pressure. Patients need to know that blood pressure varies continuously and that the range within which their pressure varies should be monitored.

Continuing Care

Regular follow-up care is imperative so that the disease process can be assessed and treated, depending on whether control or progression is found. A history and physical examination should be completed at each clinic visit. The history should include all data that pertain to any potential problem, specifically medication-related problems such as postural (orthostatic) hypotension (experienced as dizziness or lightheadedness).

Deviation from the therapeutic program is a significant problem for people with hypertension and other chronic conditions requiring lifetime management. It is estimated that 50% discontinue their medications within 1 year of beginning to take them. Blood pressure control is achieved by only 27% (JNC VII, 2003). However, when patients actively participate in self-care, including self-monitoring of blood pressure and diet, compliance increases—possibly because patients receive immediate feedback and have a greater sense of control.

Considerable effort is required by patients with hypertension to adhere to recommended lifestyle modifications and to take regularly prescribed medications. The effort needed to follow the therapeutic plan may seem unreasonable to some, particularly when they have no symptoms without medications but do have side effects with medications. The recommended lifestyle changes are listed in Chart 32-2. Continued education and encouragement are usually needed to enable patients to formulate an acceptable plan that helps them live with their hypertension and adhere to the treatment plan. Compromises may have to be made about some aspects of therapy to achieve success in higher-priority goals. The nurse can assist with behaviour change by supporting patients in making small changes with each visit that move them toward their goals. Another important factor is following up at each visit to see how the patient has progressed with the plans made at the prior visit. If the patient has had difficulty with a particular aspect of the plan, the patient and nurse can work together to develop an alternative or modification to the plan that the patient believes will be more successful.

MONITORING AND MANAGING POTENTIAL COMPLICATIONS

Symptoms suggesting that hypertension is progressing to the extent that target organ damage is occurring must be detected early so that appropriate treatment can be initiated accordingly. When the patient returns for follow-up care, all body systems must be assessed to detect any evidence of vascular damage. Examining the eyes with an ophthalmoscope is particularly important because retinal blood vessel damage indicates similar damage elsewhere in the vascular system. The patient is questioned about blurred vision, spots in front of the eyes, and diminished visual acuity. The heart, nervous system, and kidneys are also carefully assessed and examined. Any significant findings are promptly reported to determine whether additional diagnostic studies are required. Based on the findings, medications may be changed to improve blood pressure control.

 Gerontologic Considerations

Compliance with the therapeutic program may be more difficult for elderly people. The medication regimen can be difficult to remember, and the expense can be a problem. **Monotherapy** (treatment with a single agent), if appropriate, may simplify the medication regimen and make it less expensive. Special care must be taken to ensure that the elderly patient understands the regimen and can see and read instructions, open the medication container, and get the prescription refilled. The elderly person's family or caregivers should be included in the teaching program so that they can understand the patient's needs, encourage adherence to the treatment plan, and know when and whom to call if problems arise or information is needed.

> **NURSING ALERT** The patient and caregivers should be cautioned that antihypertensive medications can cause hypotension. Low blood pressure or postural hypotension should be reported immediately. Because elderly people have impaired cardiovascular reflexes, they are often more sensitive than younger people to the extracellular volume depletion caused by diuretic therapy and to the sympathetic inhibition caused by adrenergic antagonists. The nurse teaches patients to change positions slowly when moving from a lying or sitting position to a standing position. The nurse also counsels elderly patients to use supportive devices such as hand rails and walkers when necessary to prevent falls that could result from dizziness.

Evaluation

EXPECTED PATIENT OUTCOMES

Expected patient outcomes may include the following:

1. Maintains adequate tissue perfusion
   a. Maintains blood pressure at less than 140/90 mm Hg (or less than 130/85 mm Hg for persons with diabetes mellitus or proteinuria greater than 1 g per 24 hours) with lifestyle modifications, medications, or both
   b. Demonstrates no symptoms of angina, palpitations, or vision changes
   c. Has stable BUN and serum creatinine levels
   d. Has palpable peripheral pulses

2. Complies with the self-care program
   a. Adheres to the dietary regimen as prescribed: reduces calorie, sodium, and fat intake; increases fruit and vegetable intake
   b. Exercises regularly
   c. Takes medications as prescribed and reports any side effects
   d. Measures blood pressure routinely
   e. Abstains from tobacco and excessive alcohol intake
   f. Keeps follow-up appointments
3. Has no complications
   a. Reports no changes in vision
   b. Exhibits no retinal damage on vision testing
   c. Maintains pulse rate and rhythm and respiratory rate within normal ranges
   d. Reports no dyspnea or edema
   e. Maintains urine output consistent with intake
   f. Has renal function test results within normal range
   g. Demonstrates no motor, speech, or sensory deficits
   h. Reports no headaches, dizziness, weakness, changes in gait, or falls

Hypertensive Crises

There are two hypertensive crises that require nursing intervention: hypertensive emergency and hypertensive urgency. Hypertensive emergencies and urgencies may occur in patients whose hypertension has been poorly controlled or in those who have abruptly discontinued their medications. Once the hypertensive crisis has been managed, a complete evaluation is performed to review the patient's ongoing treatment plan and strategies to minimize the occurrence of subsequent hypertensive crises.

HYPERTENSIVE EMERGENCY

Hypertensive emergency is a situation in which blood pressure must be lowered immediately (not necessarily to less than 140/90 mm Hg) to halt or prevent damage to the target organs. Conditions associated with hypertensive emergency include acute myocardial infarction, dissecting aortic aneurysm, and intracranial hemorrhage. Hypertensive emergencies are acute, life-threatening blood pressure elevations that require prompt treatment in an intensive care setting because of the serious target organ damage that may occur. The medications of choice in hypertensive emergencies are those that have an immediate effect. Intravenous vasodilators, including sodium nitroprusside (Nipride), nicardipine hydrochloride (Cardene), fenoldopam mesylate (Corlopam), enalaprilat (Vasotec I.V.), and nitroglycerin (Nitro-Bid IV, Tridil), have an immediate action that is short lived (minutes to 4 hours), and they are therefore used as the initial treatment. Table 32-5 provides for more information about these medications.

HYPERTENSIVE URGENCY

Hypertensive urgency is a situation in which blood pressure must be lowered within a few hours. Severe perioperative hypertension is considered a hypertensive urgency. Hypertensive urgencies are managed with oral doses of fast-acting agents such as loop diuretics (bumetanide [Bumex], furosemide [Lasix]), beta-blockers propranolol (Inderal), metoprolol (Lopressor), nadolol

(Corgard), angiotensin-converting enzyme inhibitors (benazepril [Lotensin], captopril [Capoten], enalapril [Vasotec]), calcium antagonists (diltiazem [Cardizem], verapamil [Isoptin SR]), or alpha$_2$-agonists, such as clonidine (Catapres) and guanfacine (Tenex) (see Table 32-5).

Extremely close hemodynamic monitoring of the patient's blood pressure and cardiovascular status is required during treatment of hypertensive emergencies and urgencies. The exact frequency of monitoring is a matter of clinical judgment and varies with the patient's condition. The nurse may think that taking vital signs every 5 minutes is appropriate if the blood pressure is changing rapidly or may check vital signs at 15 or 30 minute intervals if the situation is more stable. A precipitous drop in blood pressure can occur, which would require immediate action to restore blood pressure to an acceptable level.

Critical Thinking Exercises

1. You are a nursing student assigned to a hypertension clinic. One of the patients is a 58-year-old telemarketer. During the physical assessment, the patient, who is 5 feet 6 inches tall and weighs 180 lb, asks you what he can do to reduce his blood pressure. How would you answer this patient's question? Identify what additional data you need to consider before you answer the patient's question. How would your assessment and plan change if the patient also had degenerative arthritis of his knees?

2. You are a home care nurse. One of your patients is an elderly man who lives alone and who has hypertension along with other health problems, including heart failure and atrial fibrillation. During a home visit, you learn that he has difficulty taking his medications as directed. What questions come to mind as you consider the situation? How will you direct your assessment to identify factors contributing to this problem? Using the factors identified, develop a sample follow-up home care teaching plan for this patient.

REFERENCES AND SELECTED READINGS

Books

Braunwald, E., Zipes, D. P., & Libby, P. (Eds.) (2001). *Heart disease: A textbook of cardiovascular medicine.* (6th ed.) Philadelphia: W. B. Saunders.

Kaplan, N. (2002). *Clinical hypertension* (8th ed.). Philadelphia: Lippincott Williams & Wilkins.

Journals

American Society of Hypertension. (1992). Recommendations for routine blood pressure measurement by indirect cuff sphygmomanometry. *American Journal of Hypertension, 5* (4, Pt. 1), 207–209.

Appel, L. J., Moore, T. J., Obarzanek, E., Vollmer, W. M., Svetkey, L. P., Sacks, F. M., et al. (1997). A clinical trial of the effects of dietary patterns on blood pressure. *New England Journal of Medicine, 336*(16), 1117–1124.

Burnier, M., & Brunner, H. R. (2000). Angiotensin II receptor antagonists. *Lancet, 355*(9204), 637–645.

Burt, V. L., Cutler, J. A., Higgins, M., Horan, M. J., Labarthe, D., Whelton, P., et al. (1995a). Trends in the prevalence, awareness, treatment, and control of hypertension in the adult US population. Data from the health examination surveys, 1960 to 1991. *Hypertension, 26*(1), 60–69.

Burt, V. L, Whelton, P., Roccella, E. J., Brown, C., Cutler, J. A., Higgins, M., et al. (1995b). Prevalence of hypertension in the US adult population: results from the Third National Health and Nutrition Examination Survey, 1988–1991. *Hypertension, 25,* 305–313.

Chase, S. L. (2000). Hypertensive crisis. *RN, 63*(6), 62–68.

Cushman, W. C., Cutler, J. A., Hanna, E., Bingham, S. F., Follmann, D., Harford, T., et al. (1998). Prevention and treatment of hypertension study (PATHS): Effects of an alcohol treatment program on blood pressure. *Archives of Internal Medicine, 158*(11), 1197–1207.

Dominiczak, A. F., Negrin, D. C., Clark, J. S., Brosnan, M. J., McBride, M. W., & Alexander, M. Y. (2000). Genes and hypertension: From gene mapping in experimental models to vascular gene transfer strategies. *Hypertension, 35* (1, Pt. 2), 164–172.

Gress, T. W., Nieto, F. J., Shahar, E., Wofford, M. R., & Brancati, F. L. (2000). Hypertension and antihypertensive therapy as risk factors for type 2 diabetes mellitus. *New England Journal of Medicine, 342*(13), 905–912.

Gus, M., Fuchs, F. D., Pimentel, M., Rosa, D., Melo, A. G., & Moreira, L. B. (2001). Behavior of ambulatory blood pressure surrounding episodes of headache in mildly hypertensive patients. *Archives of Internal Medicine, 161*(2), 252–255.

Hagberg, J. M., Park, J. J., & Brown, M. D. (2000). The role of exercise training in the treatment of hypertension: An update. *Sports Medicine, 30*(3), 193–206.

McAlister, F. A., & Straus, S. E. (2001). Evidence based treatment of hypertension. Measurement of blood pressure: An evidence based review. *British Medical Journal, 322*(7291), 908–911.

Miller, N. H., Hill, M., Kottke, T., & Ockene, I. S. (1997). The multilevel compliance challenge: Recommendations for a call to action. A statement for healthcare professionals. *Circulation, 95*(4), 1085–1090.

Neal, B., MacMahon, S., & Chapman, N. (2000). Effects of ACE inhibitors, calcium antagonists, and other blood-pressure-lowering drugs: Results of prospectively designed overviews of randomised trials. Blood Pressure Lowering Treatment Trialists' Collaboration. *Lancet, 356*(9246), 1955–1964.

Perloff, D., Grim, C., Flack, J., Frohlich, E. D., Hill, M., McDonald, M., et al. (1993). Human blood pressure determination by sphygmomanometry. *Circulation, 88,* (5, Pt. 1), 2460–2467.

Perry, H. M., Jr., Davis, B. R., Price, T. R., Applegate, W. B., Fields, W. S., Guralnik, J. M., et al. (2000). Effect of treating isolated systolic hypertension on the risk of developing various types and subtypes of stroke: The Systolic Hypertension in the Elderly Program (SHEP). *Journal of the American Medical Association, 284*(4), 465–471.

Pickering, T. G. (1999). Contempo 1999: Advances in the treatment of hypertension. *Journal of the American Medical Association, 281*(2), 114–116.

Sacks, F. M., Svetkey, L. P., Vollmer, W. M., Appel, L. J., Bray, G. A., Harsha, D., et al. (2001). Effects on blood pressure of reduced dietary sodium and the dietary approaches to stop hypertension (DASH) diet. *New England Journal of Medicine, 344*(1), 3–10.

Sixth Report of the Joint National Committee on Prevention, Detection, Evaluation, and Treatment of High Blood Pressure. (1997). *Archives of Internal Medicine, 157*(21), 2413–2446.

RESOURCES AND WEBSITES

Canadian Council of Cardiovascular Nurses, 222 Queen Street, Suite 1402, Ottawa, ON K1P 5V9; 1-613-569-4361, ext 340; http://www.leverus.com/cccn/index2.cfm.

Canadian Hypertension Society, CHS Secretariat, Dr. Venkat Gopal, Dept of Pharmacology, College of Medicine, University of Saskatchewan, 07 Wiggins Road, Saskatchewan, SK S7N 5ES; www.hypertension.ca.

Canadian Stroke Network. 2005 Canadian Hypertension Education Program Recommendations. www.canadianstrokenetwork.ca.

Centers for Disease Control and Prevention (CDC), 600 Clifton Rd., Atlanta, GA 30333; cardiovascular health program: 1-404-639-3534 or 1-800-311-3435; http://www.cdc.gov/nccdphp/cvd/.

Heart and Stroke Foundation of Canada, 222 Queen St., Suite 1402, Ottawa, ON K1P5V9, 1-613-569-4361; fax, 1-613-569-3278; http://www.heartandstroke.ca/.

World Health Organization (WHO), Avenue Appia 20, 1211 Geneva 27 Switzerland; cardiovascular diseases: http://www.who.int/ncd/cvd/index.htm.

Assessment and Management of Patients With Hematologic Disorders

Adapted by Joe Noon

LEARNING OBJECTIVES ●

On completion of this chapter, the learner will be able to:

1. Describe the process of hematopoiesis.
2. Describe the processes involved in maintaining hemostasis.
3. Differentiate between the hypoproliferative and the hemolytic anemias and compare and contrast the physiologic mechanisms, clinical manifestations, medical management, and nursing interventions for each.
4. Use the nursing process as a framework for care of patients with anemia.
5. Compare the leukemias, their incidence, physiologic alterations, clinical manifestations, management, and prognosis.
6. Use the nursing process as a framework for care of patients with acute leukemia.
7. Use the nursing process as a framework for care of patients with lymphoma or multiple myeloma.
8. Use the nursing process as a framework for care of patients with bleeding disorders.
9. Identify therapies for blood disorders, including the nursing implications for the administration of blood and blood components.

*U*nlike many other body systems, the hematologic system truly encompasses the entire human body. Patients with hematologic disorders can be quite challenging to nurses because they often have significant abnormalities in blood tests but few or no symptoms. It is therefore imperative that nurses have a good understanding of the pathophysiology of the patient's condition and can make a thorough assessment that relies heavily on the interpretation of laboratory tests. It is equally important for the nurse to anticipate potential patient needs and to target nursing interventions accordingly. Because it is so important to the understanding of most hematologic diseases, a basic appreciation of blood cells and bone marrow function is necessary.

Anatomic and Physiologic Overview

The hematologic system consists of the blood and the sites where blood is produced, including the bone marrow and the **reticuloendothelial system (RES).** Blood is a specialized organ that differs from other organs in that it exists in a fluid state. Blood is

Glossary

absolute neutrophil count (ANC): a mathematical calculation of the actual number of neutrophils in the circulation, derived from the total WBCs and the percentage of neutrophils counted in a microscope's visual field; provides a rough indication of infection risk

anemia: decreased RBC count

anergy: diminished reactivity to antigens (transient or complete)

angiogenesis: formation of new blood vessels, such as in a healing wound or in a malignant tumour

angular cheilosis: cracking sore at corner of mouth

aplasia: lack of cellular development (eg, of cells within the bone marrow)

apoptosis: complex process of programmed cell death

band cell: slightly immature neutrophil

blast cell: primitive WBC

cytokines: hormones produced by leukocytes that are vital to regulation of hematopoiesis, apoptosis, and immune responses

D-dimer: test that measures fibrin breakdown; considered to be more specific than fibrin degradation products in the diagnosis of disseminated intravascular coagulation (DIC)

differentiation: development of functions and characteristics that are different from those of the parent stem cell

dysplasia: abnormal development (eg, of blood cells); size, shape and appearance of cells are altered

ecchymosis: bruise

erythrocyte: see RBC

erythrocyte sedimentation rate (ESR): laboratory test that measures the rate of settling of RBCs; elevation is indicative of inflammation; also called the "sed rate"

erythroid cells: broad term used in reference to any cell that is or will become a mature RBC

erythropoiesis: process of formation of RBCs

erythropoietin: hormone produced primarily by the kidney; necessary for erythropoiesis

fibrin: filamentous protein; basis of thrombus and blood clot

fibrinogen: protein converted into fibrin to form thrombus and clot

granulocyte: granulated WBC (neutrophil, eosinophil, basophil); sometimes used synonymously with neutrophil

granulocytopenia: fewer than normal granulocytes

hematocrit: percentage of total blood volume consisting of RBCs

hematopoiesis: complex process of the formation and maturation of blood cells

hemoglobin: iron-containing protein of RBCs; delivers oxygen to tissues

hemolysis: destruction of RBCs; can occur within or outside of the vasculature

hemosiderin: iron-containing pigment derived from breakdown of hemoglobin

hemostasis: intricate balance between clot formation and clot dissolution

histiocytes: cells present in all loose connective tissue, capable of phagocytosis; part of the RES

hyperplasia: abnormally increased proliferation of normal cells

hypochromia: pallor within the RBC caused by decreased hemoglobin content

left shift, or **shift to the left:** increased release of immature forms of WBCs from the bone marrow in response to need

leukocyte: see WBC

leukemia: uncontrolled proliferation of WBCs, often immature

leukopenia: less than normal amount of WBCs in circulation

lymphoid: pertaining to lymphocytes

lymphocyte: form of WBC involved in immune functions

lysis: destruction of cells

macrocytosis: larger than normal RBCs

macrophage: cells of the RES that are capable of phagocytosis

mast cell: cells found in connective tissue involved in defense of the body and coagulation

microcytosis: smaller than normal RBCs

monocyte: large WBC that becomes a macrophage when it leaves the circulation and moves into body tissues

myeloid: pertaining to nonlymphoid blood cells that differentiate into RBCs, platelets, monocytes and macrophages, neutrophils, eosinophils, basophils, and mast cells

myelopoiesis: formation and maturation of cells derived from myeloid stem cell

neutropenia: lower than normal number of neutrophils

neutrophil: fully mature WBC capable of phagocytosis; primary defense against bacterial infection

normochromic: normal RBC colour, indicating normal amount of hemoglobin

normocytic: normal size of RBC

nucleated RBCs: immature form of RBC; portion of nucleus remains within the red cell; not normally seen in circulating blood

oxyhemoglobin: combined form of oxygen and hemoglobin; found in arterial blood

pancytopenia: abnormal decrease in WBCs, RBCs, and platelets

petechiae: tiny capillary hemorrhages

phagocytosis: process of ingestion and digestion of bacteria

plasma: liquid portion of blood

plasminogen: protein that is converted to plasmin to dissolve thrombi and clots

platelet: thrombocyte; a cellular component of blood involved in blood coagulation

poikilocytosis: variation in shape of RBCs

polycythemia: excess RBCs

RBC: red blood cell, erythrocyte; a cellular component of blood involved in the transport of oxygen and carbon dioxide

red blood cell: see RBC

reticulocytes: slightly immature RBCs, usually only 1% of total circulating RBCs

reticuloendothelial system (RES): complex system of cells throughout body capable of phagocytosis

serum: portion of blood remaining after coagulation occurs

stem cell: primitive cell, capable of self-replication and differentiation into myeloid or lymphoid stem cell

thrombin: enzyme necessary to convert fibrinogen into fibrin clot

thrombocyte: see platelet

thrombocytopenia: lower than normal platelet count

thrombocytosis: higher than normal platelet count

WBC: white blood cells, leukocytes; cellular components of blood involved in defense of the body; subtypes include neutrophils, eosinophils, basophils, monocytes, and lymphocytes

white blood cell: see WBC

composed of plasma and various types of cells. **Plasma** is the fluid portion of blood; it contains various proteins, such as albumin, globulin, **fibrinogen**, and other factors necessary for clotting, as well as electrolytes, waste products, and nutrients. About 55% of blood volume is plasma.

BLOOD

The cellular component of blood consists of three primary cell types (Table 33-1): **RBCs** (**red blood cells** or **erythrocytes**), **WBCs** (**white blood cells** or **leukocytes**), and **platelets** (**thrombocytes**). These cellular components of blood normally make up 40% to 45% of the blood volume. Because most blood cells have a short life span, the need for the body to replenish its supply of cells is continuous; this process is termed **hematopoiesis.** The primary site for hematopoiesis is the bone marrow. During embryonic development and in other conditions, the liver and spleen may also be involved.

Under normal conditions, the adult bone marrow produces about 175 billion RBCs, 70 billion **neutrophils** (mature form of a WBC), and 175 billion platelets each day. When the body needs more blood cells, as in infection (when WBCs are needed to fight the invading pathogen) or in bleeding (when more RBCs are required), the marrow increases its production of the cells required. Thus, under normal conditions, the marrow responds to increased demand and releases adequate numbers of cells into the circulation.

The volume of blood in humans is approximately 7% to 10% of the normal body weight and amounts to 5 to 6 L. Circulating through the vascular system and serving as a link between body organs, the blood carries oxygen absorbed from the lungs and nutri-

ents absorbed from the gastrointestinal tract to the body cells for cellular metabolism. Blood also carries waste products produced by cellular metabolism to the lungs, skin, liver, and kidneys, where they are transformed and eliminated from the body. Blood also carries hormones, antibodies, and other substances to their sites of action or use.

To function, blood must remain in its normally fluid state. Because blood is fluid, the danger always exists that trauma can lead to loss of blood from the vascular system. To prevent this, an intricate clotting mechanism is activated when necessary to seal any leak in the blood vessels. Excessive clotting is equally dangerous, because it can obstruct blood flow to vital tissues. To prevent this, the body has a fibrinolytic mechanism that eventually dissolves clots (thrombi) formed within blood vessels. The balance between these two systems, clot (thrombus) formation and clot (thrombus) dissolution or fibrinolysis, is called **hemostasis**.

BONE MARROW

The bone marrow is the site of hematopoiesis, or blood cell formation (Fig. 33-1). In a child all skeletal bones are involved, but as the child ages marrow activity decreases. By adulthood, marrow activity is usually limited to the pelvis, ribs, vertebrae, and sternum.

Marrow is one of the largest organs of the body, making up 4% to 5% of total body weight. It consists of islands of cellular components (red marrow) separated by fat (yellow marrow). As the adult ages, the proportion of active marrow is gradually replaced by fat; however, in the healthy person, the fat can again be replaced by active marrow when more blood cell production is required. In adults with disease that causes marrow destruction, fibrosis, or scarring, the liver and spleen can also resume production of blood cells by a process known as extramedullary hematopoiesis.

The marrow is highly vascular. Within it are primitive cells called **stem cells**. The stem cells have the ability to self-replicate, thereby ensuring a continuous supply of stem cells throughout the life cycle. When stimulated to do so, stem cells can begin a process of **differentiation** into either **myeloid** or **lymphoid** stem cells. These stem cells are committed to produce specific types of blood cells. Lymphoid stem cells produce either T or B **lymphocytes**. Myeloid stem cells differentiate into three broad cell types: RBCs, WBCs, and platelets. Thus, with the exception of lymphocytes, all blood cells are derived from the myeloid stem cell. A defect in the myeloid stem cell can cause problems not only with WBC production but also with RBC and platelet production. The entire process of hematopoiesis is highly complex. Research has identified many of the complex mechanisms involved, often at the molecular level. A thorough description of these processes is beyond the scope of this textbook; however, some mechanisms against which a specific treatment is targeted are briefly described in the relevant disease-specific sections of this chapter.

BLOOD CELLS

Red Blood Cells (RBCs)

The normal RBC is a biconcave disk that resembles a soft ball compressed between two fingers (Fig. 33-2). It has a diameter of about 8 μm and is so flexible that it can pass easily through capillaries that may be as small as 2.8 μm in diameter. The RBC membrane is so thin that gases, such as oxygen and carbon dioxide, can easily diffuse across it; the disk shape provides a large surface area that facilitates the absorption and release of oxygen molecules.

Table 33-1 • Blood Cells	
CELL TYPE	**MAJOR FUNCTION**
WBC (Leukocyte)	Fights infection
Neutrophil	Essential in preventing or limiting bacterial infection via phagocytosis; average life span is 2 to 4 h
Monocyte	Enters tissue as macrophage; highly phagocytic, especially against fungus; immune surveillance
Eosinophil	Involved in allergic reactions (neutralizes histamine); digests foreign proteins
Basophil	Contains histamine; integral part of hypersensitivity reactions
Lymphocyte	Integral component of immune system
T lymphocyte	Responsible for cell-mediated immunity; recognizes material as "foreign" (surveillance system)
B lymphocyte	Responsible for humoural immunity; many mature into plasma cells to form antibodies
Plasma cell	Secretes immunoglobulin (Ig, antibody); most mature form of B lymphocyte
RBC (Erythrocyte)	Carries hemoglobin to provide oxygen to tissues; average life span is 120 days
Platelet (Thrombocyte)	Fragment of megakaryocyte, not really a cell; provides basis for coagulation to occur; maintains hemostasis; average life span is 10 days

Physiology/Pathophysiology

Pluripotential stem cell

Myeloid stem cell

Lymphoid stem cell

BFU-E   CFU-Meg   CFU-GM   CFU-Eo   CFU-Ba   CFU-Mast   Pre-B cell   Pre-T cell

CFU-E   Megakaryocyte   CFU-G   CFU-M

Reticulocyte

Proplatelets

Monocyte

B Lymphocyte

Neutrophil

Eosinophil

Tissue mast cell

T Lymphocyte

Red blood cell
(RBC)

Macrophage
(in tissue)

Basophil

Plasma cell

Platelets

FIGURE 33-1 Hematopoiesis. Uncommitted (pluripotent) stem cells can differentiate into myeloid or lymphoid stem cells. These stem cells then undergo a complex process of differentiation and maturation into normal cells that are released into the circulation. The myeloid stem cell is responsible not only for all nonlymphoid white blood cells (WBCs) but also for the production of red blood cells (RBCs) and platelets. Each step of the differentiation process depends in part on the presence of specific growth factors for each cell type. When the stem cells are dysfunctional, they may respond inadequately to the need for more cells, or they may respond excessively, sometimes uncontrollably, as in leukemia. Adapted from Amgen, Inc., 1995, Thousand Oaks, CA.

FIGURE 33-2 Normal types of blood cells.

Mature RBCs consist primarily of **hemoglobin**, which contains iron and makes up 95% of the cell mass. RBCs have no nuclei, and they have many fewer metabolic enzymes than do most other cells. The presence of a large amount of hemoglobin enables the RBC to perform its principal function, the transport of oxygen between the lungs and tissues. Occasionally the marrow releases slightly immature forms of RBCs, called **reticulocytes**, into the circulation. This occurs as a normal response to an increased demand for RBCs (as in bleeding) or in some disease states.

The oxygen-carrying hemoglobin molecule is made up of four subunits, each containing a heme portion attached to a globin chain. Iron is present in the heme component of the molecule. An important property of heme is its ability to bind to oxygen loosely and reversibly. Oxygen readily binds to hemoglobin in the lungs and is carried as **oxyhemoglobin** in arterial blood. Oxyhemoglobin is a brighter red than hemoglobin that does not contain oxygen (reduced hemoglobin), which is why arterial blood is a brighter red than venous blood. The oxygen readily dissociates (detaches) from hemoglobin in the tissues, where the oxygen is needed for cellular metabolism. In venous blood, hemoglobin combines with hydrogen ions produced by cellular metabolism and thus buffers excessive acid. Whole blood normally contains about 15 g of hemoglobin per 100 mL of blood.

ERYTHROPOIESIS

Erythroblasts arise from the primitive myeloid stem cells in bone marrow. The erythroblast is a nucleated cell that, in the process of maturing within the bone marrow, accumulates hemoglobin and gradually loses its nucleus. At this stage, the cell is known as a reticulocyte. Further maturation into an RBC entails the loss of the dark-staining material and slight shrinkage. The mature RBC is then released into the circulation. Under conditions of rapid **erythropoiesis** (RBC production), reticulocytes and other immature cells (eg, **nucleated RBCs**) may be released prematurely into the circulation.

Differentiation of the primitive myeloid stem cell of the marrow into an erythroblast is stimulated by **erythropoietin**, a hormone produced primarily by the kidney. If the kidney detects low levels of oxygen (as would occur in **anemia**, in which fewer RBCs are available to bind oxygen, or in people living at high altitudes), the release of erythropoietin is increased. The increased erythropoietin then stimulates the marrow to increase production of RBCs. The entire process typically takes 5 days.

For normal RBC production, the bone marrow also requires iron, vitamin B_{12}, folic acid, pyridoxine (vitamin B_6), protein, and other factors. A deficiency of these factors during erythropoiesis can result in decreased RBC production and anemia.

Iron Stores and Metabolism. The average daily diet in Canada contains 10 to 15 mg of elemental iron; normally 0.5 to 1 mg of ingested iron is absorbed from the small intestine. The rate of iron absorption is regulated by the amount of iron already stored in the body and by the rate of RBC production. Additional amounts of iron, up to 2 mg daily, must be absorbed by women to replace blood lost during menstruation. Total body iron content in the average adult is approximately 3 g, most of which is present in hemoglobin or in one of its breakdown products. Iron is stored in the small intestine as ferritin and in reticuloendothelial cells. When required, the iron is released into the plasma, binds to transferrin, and is transported into the membranes of the normoblasts (RBC precursor cells) within the marrow, where it is incorporated into hemoglobin. Iron is lost in the feces, either in bile, blood, or mucosal cells from the intestine.

The concentration of iron in blood is normally about 75 to 175 µg/dL (13 to 31 µmol/L) for men and 65 to 165 µg/dL (11 to 29 µmol/L) for women. With iron deficiency, bone marrow iron stores are rapidly depleted; hemoglobin synthesis is depressed, and the RBCs produced by the marrow are small and low in hemoglobin. Iron deficiency in the adult generally indicates that blood has been lost from the body (eg, from bleeding in the gastrointestinal tract or heavy menstrual flow). In the adult, lack of dietary iron is rarely the sole cause of iron deficiency anemia. The source of iron deficiency should be investigated promptly, because iron deficiency in an adult may be a sign of bleeding in the gastrointestinal tract or colon cancer.

Vitamin B₁₂ and Folic Acid Metabolism. Vitamin B$_{12}$ and folic acid are required for the synthesis of DNA in many tissues, but deficiencies of either of these vitamins have the greatest effect on erythropoiesis. Both vitamin B$_{12}$ and folic acid are derived from the diet. Folic acid is absorbed in the proximal small intestine, but only small amounts are stored within the body. If the diet is deficient in folic acid, stores within the body quickly become depleted. Because vitamin B$_{12}$ is found only in foods of animal origin, strict vegetarians may ingest little B$_{12}$. Vitamin B$_{12}$ combines with intrinsic factor produced in the stomach. The vitamin B$_{12}$–intrinsic factor complex is absorbed in the distal ileum. People who have had a partial or total gastrectomy may have limited amounts of intrinsic factor, and therefore the absorption of B$_{12}$ may be diminished. The effects of either decreased absorption or decreased intake of B$_{12}$ are not apparent for 2 to 4 years.

Vitamin B$_{12}$ and folic acid deficiencies are characterized by the production of abnormally large RBCs called megaloblasts. Because these cells are abnormal, many are sequestered (trapped) while still in the bone marrow, and their rate of release is decreased. Some of these cells actually die in the marrow before they can be released into the circulation. This results in megaloblastic anemia.

RED BLOOD CELL DESTRUCTION

The average life span of a normal circulating RBC is 120 days. Aged RBCs lose their elasticity and become trapped in small blood vessels, particularly in the spleen. They are removed from the blood by the reticuloendothelial cells, particularly in the liver and the spleen. As the RBCs are destroyed, their hemoglobin is largely recycled. Some hemoglobin also breaks down to form bilirubin and is secreted in the bile. Most of the iron is recycled to form new hemoglobin molecules within the bone marrow; small amounts are lost daily in the feces and urine and monthly in menstrual flow.

White Blood Cells (WBCs)

Leukocytes are divided into two general categories: granulocytes and lymphocytes. In normal blood, the total leukocyte count is 5,000 to 10,000 cells per cubic millimeter. Of these, approximately 60% to 70% are granulocytes and 30% to 40% are lymphocytes. Primarily, WBCs protect the body against infection and tissue injury.

GRANULOCYTES

Granulocytes are defined by the presence of granules in the cytoplasm of the cell. Granulocytes are divided into three main subgroups, which are characterized by the staining properties of these granules (see Fig. 33-2). Eosinophils have bright-red granules in their cytoplasm, whereas the granules in basophils stain deep blue. The third and by far the most numerous cell in this class is the neutrophil, with granules that stain a pink to violet hue. Neutrophils are also called polymorphonuclear neutrophils (PMNs, or polys) or segmented neutrophils (segs).

The nucleus of the mature neutrophil has multiple lobes (usually two to five) that are connected by thin filaments of nuclear material, a "segmented" nucleus; it is usually twice the size of an RBC. The somewhat less mature granulocyte has a single-lobed, elongated nucleus and is called a **band cell**. Ordinarily, band cells account for only a small percentage of circulating granulocytes, although their percentage can increase greatly under conditions in which neutrophil production increases, such as infection. An increased number of band cells is sometimes called a "**left shift**" or "**shift to the left**." (Traditionally, the diagram of neutrophil maturation shows the stem cell on the left with progressive maturation stages toward the right, ending with a fully mature neutrophil on the right side. A shift to the left indicates that more immature cells are present in the blood than normally occurs.)

Granulocyte production from the myeloid stem cell pool results in the gradual differentiation of these cells from a myeloid **blast cell** into a fully mature neutrophil. The process, called **myelopoiesis**, is highly complex and depends on many factors. These factors, including specific **cytokines** such as growth factors, are normally present within the marrow itself. As the blast cell matures, the cytoplasm of the cell changes in colour (from blue to violet) and granules begin to form with the cytoplasm. The shape of the nucleus also changes. The entire process of maturation and differentiation takes about 10 days (see Fig. 33-1). Once the neutrophil is released into the circulation from the marrow, it stays there for only about 6 hours before it migrates into the body tissues to perform its function of **phagocytosis** (ingestion and digestion of bacteria and particles) (Fig. 33-3). Here, neutrophils last no more than 1 to 2 days before they die. The number of circulating granulocytes found in the healthy person is relatively constant, but in infection large numbers of these cells are rapidly released into the circulation.

MONONUCLEAR WHITE BLOOD CELLS (AGRANULOCYTES)

Monocytes. **Monocytes** (also called mononuclear leukocytes) are WBCs with a single-lobed nucleus and a granule-free cytoplasm—hence the term *agranulocyte*. In normal adult blood, monocytes account for approximately 5% of the total WBCs. Monocytes are the largest of the WBCs. Produced by the bone marrow, they remain in the circulation for a short time before entering the tissues and transforming into **macrophages**. Macrophages are particularly active in the spleen, liver, peritoneum, and the alveoli of the lungs.

Lymphocytes. Mature lymphocytes are small cells with scanty cytoplasm. Immature lymphocytes are produced in the marrow from the lymphoid stem cells. A second major source of production is the cortex of the thymus. Cells derived from the thymus are known as T lymphocytes (or T cells); those derived from the marrow can also be T cells but are more commonly B lymphocytes (or B cells). Lymphocytes complete their differentiation and maturation primarily in the lymph nodes and in the lymphoid tissue of the intestine and spleen after exposure to a specific antigen. Mature lymphocytes are antigen-specific cells.

Physiology/Pathophysiology

FIGURE 33-3 Phagocytosis. When foreign matter (such as bacteria or dead tissue) comes in contact with the cell membrane of the neutrophil, the membrane surrounds and pinches off the area, leaving the membrane intact. Thus, the engulfed material is left in a vacuole within the neutrophil, where enzymes within the cell destroy the foreign material.

FUNCTION OF WHITE BLOOD CELLS

WBCs protect the body from invasion by bacteria and other foreign entities. The major function of neutrophils is phagocytosis (see Fig. 33-3). Neutrophils arrive at the site within 1 hour after the onset of an inflammatory reaction and initiate phagocytosis, but they are short-lived. An influx of monocytes follows; these cells continue their phagocytic activities for long periods as macrophages. This process constitutes a second line of defense for the body against inflammation and infection. Although neutrophils can often work adequately against bacteria without the need for excessive involvement with macrophages, macrophages are particularly effective against fungi and viruses. Macrophages also digest senescent (aging or aged) blood cells, such as RBCs, primarily within the spleen.

The primary function of lymphocytes is to produce substances that aid in attacking foreign material. One group of lymphocytes (T lymphocytes) kills foreign cells directly or releases a variety of lymphokines, substances that enhance the activity of phagocytic cells. T lymphocytes are responsible for delayed allergic reactions, rejection of foreign tissue (eg, transplanted organs), and destruction of tumour cells. This process is known as *cellular immunity*. The other group of lymphocytes (B lymphocytes) is capable of differentiating into plasma cells. Plasma cells, in turn, produce immunoglobulin (Ig), or antibodies, which are protein molecules that destroy foreign material by several mechanisms. This process is known as *humoural immunity*.

Eosinophils and basophils function in hypersensitivity reactions. Eosinophils are important in the phagocytosis of parasites. The increase in eosinophil levels in allergic states indicates that these cells are involved in the hypersensitivity reaction; their function there is to neutralize histamine. Basophils produce and store histamine as well as other substances involved in hypersensitivity reactions. The release of these substances provokes allergic reactions.

Platelets (Thrombocytes)

Platelets, or thrombocytes, are not actually cells. Rather, they are granular fragments of giant cells in the bone marrow called megakaryocytes. Platelet production in the marrow is regulated in part by the hormone thrombopoietin, which stimulates the production and differentiation of megakaryocytes from the myeloid stem cell.

Platelets play an essential role in the control of bleeding. They circulate freely in the blood in an inactive state, where they nurture the endothelium of the blood vessels, maintaining the integrity of the vessel. When vascular injury does occur, platelets collect at the site and are activated. They adhere to the site of injury and to each other, forming a platelet plug that temporarily stops bleeding. Substances released from platelet granules activate coagulation factors in the blood plasma and initiate the formation of a stable clot composed of **fibrin**, a filamentous protein. Platelets have a normal life span of 7 to 10 days.

PLASMA AND PLASMA PROTEINS

After cellular elements are removed from blood, the remaining liquid portion is called plasma. More than 90% of plasma is water. The remainder consists primarily of plasma proteins, clotting factors (particularly fibrinogen), and small amounts of other substances such as nutrients, enzymes, waste products, and gases. If plasma is allowed to clot, the remaining fluid is called **serum**. Serum has essentially the same composition as plasma, except that fibrinogen and several clotting factors have been removed in the clotting process.

Plasma proteins consist primarily of albumin and globulins. The globulins can be separated into three main fractions—alpha, beta, and gamma—each of which consists of distinct proteins that have different functions. Important proteins in the alpha and beta fractions are the transport globulins and the clotting factors that are made in the liver. The transport globulins carry various substances in bound form around the circulation. For example, thyroid-binding globulin carries thyroxin, and transferrin carries iron. The clotting factors, including fibrinogen, remain in an inactive form in the blood plasma until activated by the clotting cascade. The gamma globulin fraction refers to the immunoglobulins, or antibodies. These proteins are produced by the well-differentiated lymphocytes and plasma cells. The actual fractionation of the globulins can be seen on a specific laboratory test (serum protein electrophoresis).

Albumin is particularly important for the maintenance of fluid balance within the vascular system. Capillary walls are impermeable to albumin, so its presence in the plasma creates an osmotic force that keeps fluid within the vascular space. Albumin, which is produced by the liver, has the capacity to bind to several substances that are transported in plasma (eg, certain medications, bilirubin, some hormones). People with poor hepatic function may have low concentrations of albumin, with a resultant decrease in osmotic pressure and the development of edema.

RETICULOENDOTHELIAL SYSTEM (RES)

The RES is composed of special tissue macrophages, which are derived from monocytes. When released from the marrow, monocytes spend a short time in the circulation (about 24 hours) and then enter the body tissues. Within the tissues, the monocytes continue to differentiate into cells called macrophages, which can survive for months. Macrophages have a variety of important functions. They defend the body against foreign invaders (ie, bacteria and other pathogens) via phagocytosis. They remove old or damaged cells from the circulation. They stimulate the inflammatory process and present antigen to the immune system (see Chapter 50). Macrophages give rise to tissue **histiocytes**, including Kupffer cells of the liver, peritoneal macrophages, alveolar macrophages, and other components of the RES. Thus, the RES is a component of many other organs within the body, particularly the spleen, lymph nodes, lung, and liver.

The spleen is the site of activity for most macrophages. Most of the spleen (75%) is made of red pulp; here the blood enters the venous sinuses through capillaries that are surrounded by macrophages. Within the red pulp are tiny aggregates of white pulp, consisting of B and T lymphocytes. The spleen sequesters newly released reticulocytes from the marrow, removing nuclear fragments and other materials (eg, denatured hemoglobin, iron) before the now fully mature RBC returns to the circulation. Although a minority of RBCs (less than 5%) is pooled in the spleen, a significant proportion of platelets (20%–40%) is pooled here. If the spleen is enlarged, a greater proportion of RBCs and platelets can be sequestered. The spleen is a major source of hematopoiesis in fetal life. It can resume hematopoiesis later in adulthood if necessary (eg, in bone marrow fibrosis). The spleen has important immunologic functions as well. It forms a substance that promotes the phagocytosis of neutrophils; it also forms the antibody IgM after exposure to antigen.

HEMOSTASIS

Hemostasis is the process of preventing blood loss from intact vessels and of stopping bleeding from a severed vessel. The prevention of blood loss from intact vessels requires adequate numbers of functional platelets. Platelets nurture the endothelium

and thereby maintain the structural integrity of the vessel wall. Two processes are involved in arresting bleeding: primary and secondary hemostasis.

In primary hemostasis, the severed blood vessel constricts. Circulating platelets aggregate at the site and adhere to the vessel and to one another. An unstable hemostatic plug is formed. For the coagulation process to be correctly activated, circulating inactive coagulation factors must be converted to active forms. This process occurs on the surface of the aggregated platelets at the site of vessel injury. The end result is the formation of fibrin, which reinforces the platelet plug and anchors it to the injury site. This process is termed secondary hemostasis (Fig. 33-4). The process of blood coagulation is highly complex. It can be activated by the intrinsic or the extrinsic pathway. Both pathways are needed for maintenance of normal hemostasis.

Many factors are involved in the reaction cascade that forms fibrin. When tissue is injured, the extrinsic pathway is activated by the release from the tissue of a substance called thromboplastin. As the result of a series of reactions, prothrombin is converted to **thrombin**, which in turn catalyzes the conversion of fibrinogen to fibrin. Clotting by the intrinsic pathway is activated when the collagen that lines blood vessels is exposed. Clotting factors are activated sequentially until, as with the extrinsic pathway, fibrin is ultimately formed. Although the intrinsic pathway is slower, this sequence is probably most often responsible for clotting in vivo.

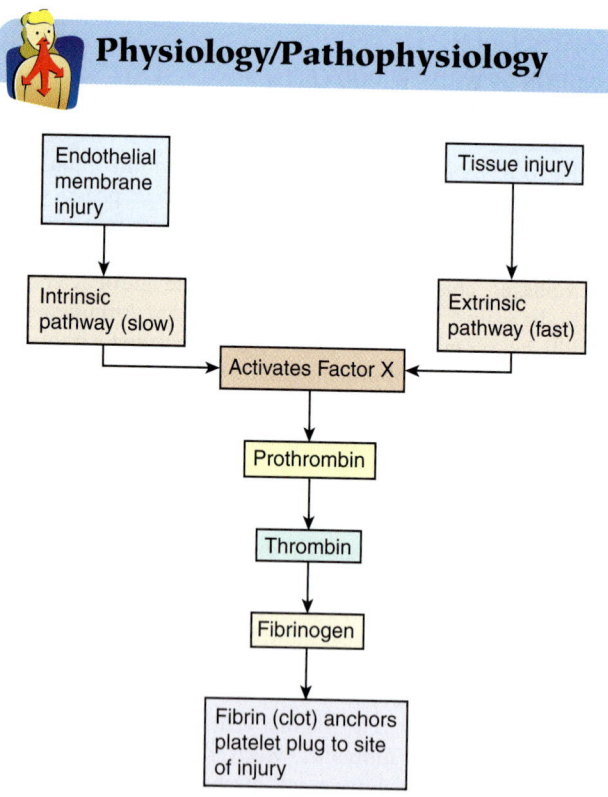

FIGURE 33-4 Secondary hemostasis. Based on the type of stimulus (injury to the endothelial membrane of a blood vessel or a tissue), one of two clotting pathways is initiated. The end result from either pathway is the conversion of prothrombin to thrombin. Thrombin is necessary for fibrinogen to be converted into fibrin, the stabilizing protein that anchors the fragile platelet plug to the site of injury to prevent further bleeding and permit the injured vessel or site to heal.

As the injured vessel is repaired and again covered with endothelial cells, the fibrin clot is no longer needed. The fibrin is digested via two systems: the plasma fibrinolytic system and the cellular fibrinolytic system. The substance **plasminogen** is required to lyse (break down) the fibrin. Plasminogen, which is present in all body fluids, circulates with fibrinogen and is therefore incorporated into the fibrin clot as it forms. When the clot is no longer needed (eg, after an injured blood vessel has healed), the plasminogen is activated to form plasmin. Plasmin digests the fibrinogen and fibrin. The breakdown particles of the clot (fibrin degradation products) are released into the circulation. Through this system, clots are dissolved as tissue is repaired, and the vascular system returns to its normal baseline state.

PATHOPHYSIOLOGY OF THE HEMATOLOGIC SYSTEM

Most hematologic diseases reflect a defect in the hematopoietic, hemostatic, or RES systems. The defect can be quantitative (eg, increased or decreased production of cells), qualitative (eg, the cells that are produced are defective in their normal functional capacity), or both.

 Gerontologic Considerations

In elderly patients, a common problem is decreased ability of the bone marrow to respond to the body's need for blood cells (RBCs, WBCs, and platelets). This inability is a result of many factors, including diminished production of the growth factors necessary for hematopoiesis by stromal cells within the marrow or a diminished response to the growth factors (in the case of erythropoietin). When an elderly person needs more blood cells (eg, WBCs in infection, RBCs in anemia), the bone marrow may not be able to increase production of these cells adequately. **Leukopenia** (a decreased number of circulating WBCs) or anemia can result. In the elderly, the bone marrow may be more susceptible to the myelosuppressive effects of medications.

Anemia is the most common hematologic condition affecting elderly patients; with each successive decade of life, the incidence of anemia increases. Anemia frequently results from iron deficiency (in the case of blood loss) or from a nutritional deficiency, particularly folate or B_{12} deficiency or protein-calorie malnutrition; it may also result from inflammation or chronic disease. Management of the disorder varies depending on the etiology. Therefore, it is important to identify the cause of the anemia rather than to consider it an inevitable consequence of aging. Elderly people with concurrent cardiac or pulmonary problems may not tolerate anemia very well, and a prompt, thorough evaluation is warranted.

Assessment and Diagnostic Findings

Many hematologic conditions cause few symptoms. Therefore, the use of extensive laboratory tests is often required to diagnose a hematologic disorder. For most hematologic conditions, continued monitoring via specific blood tests is required because it is very important to assess for changes in test results over time.

HEMATOLOGIC STUDIES

The most common tests used are the complete blood count (CBC) and the peripheral blood smear (Table 33-2). The CBC identifies the total number of blood cells (WBCs, RBCs, and platelets) as well as the hemoglobin, **hematocrit** (percentage of blood consisting of RBCs), and RBC indices. Because cellular morphology (shape and appearance of the cells) is particularly important in most hematologic disorders, the physician needs to examine the blood cells involved. This process is referred to as the manual examination of the peripheral smear, which may be part of the CBC. In this test, a drop of blood is spread on a glass slide, stained, and examined under a microscope. The shape and size of the RBCs and platelets as well as the actual appearance of the WBCs provides useful information in identifying hematologic conditions. Blood for the CBC is typically obtained by venipuncture.

BONE MARROW ASPIRATION AND BIOPSY

The bone marrow aspiration and biopsy are crucial when additional information is needed to assess how an individual's blood cells are being formed and to assess the quantity and quality of each type of cell produced within the marrow. These tests are also used to document infection or tumour within the marrow.

Normal bone marrow is in a semifluid state and can be aspirated through a special large needle. In adults, bone marrow is usually aspirated from the iliac crest and occasionally from the sternum. The aspirate provides only a sample of cells. Aspirate alone may be adequate for evaluating certain conditions, such as anemia. However, when more information is required, a biopsy is also performed. Biopsy samples are taken from the posterior iliac crest; occasionally, an anterior approach is required. A marrow biopsy shows the architecture of the bone marrow as well as its degree of cellularity.

Most patients need no more preparation than a careful explanation of the procedure, but for some very anxious patients, an antianxiety agent may be useful. It is always important for the physician or nurse to describe and explain to the patient the procedure and the sensations that will be experienced. The risks, benefits, and alternatives are also discussed. A signed informed consent is needed before the procedure is performed.

Before aspiration, the skin is cleansed as for any minor surgery, using aseptic technique. Then a small area is anesthetized with a local anesthetic through the skin and subcutaneous tissue to the periosteum of the bone. It is not possible to anesthetize the bone itself. The bone marrow needle is introduced with a stylet in place. When the needle is felt to go through the outer cortex of bone and enter the marrow cavity, the stylet is removed, a syringe is attached, and a small volume (0.5 mL) of blood and marrow is aspirated. Patients typically feel a pressure sensation as the needle is advanced into position. The actual aspiration always causes sharp but brief pain, resulting from the suction exerted as the marrow is aspirated into the syringe; the patient should be forewarned about this. Taking deep breaths or using relaxation techniques often helps ease the discomfort.

If a bone marrow biopsy is necessary, it is best performed after the aspiration and in a slightly different location, because the marrow structure may be altered after aspiration. A special biopsy needle is used. Because these needles are large, the skin is punctured first with a surgical blade to make a 3- or 4-mm incision. The biopsy needle is advanced well into the marrow cavity. When the needle is properly positioned, a portion of marrow is cored out, using a twisting or gentle rocking motion to free the sample and permit its removal within the biopsy needle. Patients feel a pressure sensation but should not feel actual pain. The nurse should instruct the patient to inform the physician if pain occurs so that additional anesthetic can be administered.

The major hazard of either bone marrow aspiration or biopsy is a slight risk of bleeding and infection. The bleeding risk is somewhat increased if the patient's platelet count is low or if the patient has been taking a medication (eg, aspirin) that alters platelet func-

Table 33-2 • Frequently Used Laboratory Tests in Hematology

TEST	NORMAL RANGE	DESCRIPTION	INDICATIONS/COMMENTS
Complete blood count (CBC)		General survey of bone marrow function; evaluates all three cell lines (WBCs, RBCs, platelets)	Important to note changes over time; many hematologic conditions show changes in CBC long before patient becomes symptomatic
Red blood cells (RBCs)	M: $4.7–6.1 \times 10^6$ F: $4.2–5.4 \times 10^6$	Carries hemoglobin; survival time, 120 days	
Hemoglobin (Hgb)	M: 13.5–17.5 g/dL F: 11.5–15.5 g/dL	Delivers O_2 through circulation to body tissues and returns CO_2 from tissues to lungs	Decreased in anemia; increased in polycythemia
Hematocrit (Hct)	M: 40–52% F: 36–48%	Indicates relative proportions of plasma and RBCs (volume of RBCs/L whole blood)	Usually three times the Hgb
Mean corpuscular volume (MCV)	81–96 μm³	Indicates size of RBCs; very useful in differentiating types of anemia	If <80, cells are microcytic; if >100, cells are macrocytic
Mean corpuscular hemoglobin concentration (MCHC)	33–36 g/dL	Average concentration of Hgb in RBCs; independent of cell size	
Red cell distribution width (RDW)	11–14.5%	Measures degree of variation in size of RBCs	
Reticulocyte count	0.5–1.5%	Measure of marrow production of erythrocytes; 1% of RBC mass is produced daily (to replace the 1% of old cells that die)	Indicates marrow's response to anemia (when anemia is present, reticulocyte level should rise)
White blood cells (WBCs)	4,500–11,000/mm³	Total WBC count	
Differential	Percentages of various types of WBCs	% of cell type × total WBC = absolute number of that cell type	Left shift: bone marrow ↑ production of WBCs; more immature forms released into the bloodstream
Neutrophils	40–75% (2,500–7,500/mm³)	Essential in preventing/limiting bacterial infection; average life span: 2–4 hr	If >8,000: infection, some inflammatory states, stress, steroids, other drugs, myeloproliferative disease. Absolute neutrophil count (ANC) <500: increased risk for infection; ANC <100: infection certain (if neutropenia persists)
Lymphocytes	20–50% (1,500–5,500/mm³)	Integral component of immune system	<1,500: lymphopenia; >4,000: lymphocytosis; increased in convalescent phase after bacterial or viral infection, lymphoproliferative disease
Monocytes	1–10% (100–800/mm³)	Enter tissue as macrophages; phagocytosis	Increased in acute and chronic infection, inflammation, some myeloproliferative disorders, chronic myelomonocytic leukemia (CMML)
Eosinophils	0–6% (0–440/mm³)	Involved in allergic reactions (neutralizes histamine); digest foreign proteins	Increased in allergic states, medications, parasites, chronic myeloid leukemia (CML), metastatic/necrotic tumours
Basophils	0–2% (0–200/mm³)	Contain histamine; integral part of hypersensitivity reactions	Increase is very rare (CML)
Platelets	150,000–400,000/mm³	Total number of platelets in circulation; average life span, 7–10 days	Thrombocytopenia: <20,000/mm³, serious; <10,000/mm³, potentially life-threatening

(continued)

Table 33-2 • Frequently Used Laboratory Tests in Hematology (Continued)

TEST	NORMAL RANGE	DESCRIPTION	INDICATIONS/COMMENTS
Prothrombin time (PT)	Varies (compare with control), 11–12.5 sec	Measure time elapsed until clot forms; measures extrinsic and common pathways	Increased in liver disease, disseminated intravascular coagulation (DIC), obstructive biliary disease, clotting factor depletion, warfarin (Coumadin) use
International normalized ratio (INR)	1.0 Standard warfarin (Coumadin) treatment, 2.0–3.0 INR; high-dose warfarin (Coumadin) treatment, 3.0–4.5 INR	A standard method of measuring PT independent of the thromboplastin reagent used in the test; calculated by dividing the PT result by the mean normal PT	Increased with anticoagulant excess and conditions that cause increased PT; decreased with insufficient anticoagulant and conditions that cause decreased PT
Partial thromboplastin time (PTT)	Varies (compare with control), 25–35 sec	Surface active agent added to plasma; measures time elapsed until clot forms; measures intrinsic and common pathways	Increased in clotting factor depletion, DIC, liver disease, biliary obstruction, circulating anticoagulants (heparin)
Thrombin time (TT)	Varies (compare with control), 8–11 sec	Tests conversion of fibrinogen to fibrin	Time to clot is inversely proportional to fibrinogen level
Fibrinogen	170–340 mg/100 mL	Measurement of fibrinogen concentration within plasma available for conversion to fibrin clot	Decreased in bleeding disorders, pregnancy, malignancy, inflammatory disease
D-dimer	0–0.5µg/mL	Measures the amount of fragments of fibrin when it is lysed (broken down); useful for distinguishing fibrinolysis from fibrinogenolysis	Increased with fibrinolytic activity, rheumatoid arthritis, ovarian cancer (with increased CA 125)
Fibrin degradation products (FDP)	<10 µg/mL	Byproduct of fibrinolysis	>40 µg/mL indicates DIC

tion. After the marrow sample is obtained, pressure is applied to the site for several minutes. The site is then covered with a sterile dressing. Most patients have no discomfort after a bone marrow aspiration, but the site of a biopsy may ache for 1 or 2 days. Warm tub baths and use of a mild analgesic (eg, acetaminophen) may be useful. Aspirin-containing analgesics should be avoided because they can aggravate or potentiate any bleeding that may occur.

Management of Hematologic Disorders

Commonly encountered blood disorders are anemia, polycythemia, leukopenia and **neutropenia**, leukocytosis, lymphoma, myeloma, **leukemia**, and various bleeding and coagulation disorders. Nursing management of patients with these disorders requires skillful assessment and monitoring as well as meticulous care and teaching to prevent deterioration and complications.

ANEMIA

Anemia, per se, is not a specific disease state but a sign of an underlying disorder. It is by far the most common hematologic condition. Anemia, a condition in which the hemoglobin concentration is lower than normal, reflects the presence of fewer than normal RBCs within the circulation. As a result, the amount of oxygen delivered to body tissues is also diminished.

There are many different kinds of anemia (Table 33-3), but all can be classified into three broad etiologic categories:

- Loss of RBCs—occurs with bleeding, potentially from any major source, such as the gastrointestinal tract, the uterus, the nose, or a wound
- Decreased production of RBCs—can be caused by a deficiency in cofactors (including folic acid, vitamin B_{12}, and iron) required for erythropoiesis; RBC production may also be reduced if the bone marrow is suppressed (eg, by tumour, medications, toxins) or is inadequately stimulated because of a lack of erythropoietin (as occurs in chronic renal disease).
- Increased destruction of RBCs—may occur because of an overactive RES (including hypersplenism) or because the bone marrow produces abnormal RBCs that are then destroyed by the RES (eg, sickle cell anemia).

A conclusion as to whether the anemia is caused by destruction or by inadequate production of RBCs usually can be reached on the basis of the following factors:

- The marrow's ability to respond to the decreased RBCs (as evidenced by an increased reticulocyte count in the circulating blood)
- The degree to which young RBCs proliferate in the bone marrow and the manner in which they mature (as observed on bone marrow biopsy)
- The presence or absence of end products of RBC destruction within the circulation (eg, increased bilirubin level, decreased haptoglobin level)

Table 33-3 • Classification of Anemias

TYPE OF ANEMIA	LABORATORY FINDINGS
Hypoproliferative (Resulting From Defective RBC Production)	
Iron deficiency	Decreased reticulocytes, iron, ferritin, iron saturation, MCV; increased TIBC
Vitamin B_{12} deficiency (megaloblastic)	Decreased vitamin B_{12} level; increased MCV
Folate deficiency	Decreased folate level; increased MCV
Decreased erythropoietin production (eg, from renal dysfunction)	Decreased erythropoietin level; normal MCV and MCH; increased creatinine level
Cancer/inflammation	Normal MCV, MCH, normal or decreased erythropoietin level; increased % of iron saturation, ferritin level; decreased iron; TIBC
Bleeding (Resulting From RBC Loss)	
Bleeding from gastro-intestinal tract, menorrhagia (excessive menstrual flow), epistaxis (nosebleed), trauma	Increased reticulocyte level; normal Hgb and Hct if measured soon after bleeding starts, but levels decrease thereafter; normal MCV initially but later decreases; decreased ferritin and iron levels (later)
Hemolytic (Resulting From RBC Destruction)	
Altered erythropoiesis (sickle cell anemia, thalassemia, other hemoglobinopathies)	Decreased MCV; fragmented RBCs; increased reticulocyte level
Hypersplenism (hemolysis)	Increased MCV
Drug-induced anemia	Increased spherocyte level
Autoimmune anemia	Increased spherocyte level
Mechanical heart valve–related anemia	Fragmented red cells

Hct, hematocrit; Hgb, hemoglobin concentration; MCH, mean corpuscular hemoglobin; MCV, mean corpuscular volume; RBCs, red blood cells; TIBC, total iron binding capacity.

Classification of Anemias

Anemia may be classified in several ways. The physiologic approach is to determine whether the deficiency in RBCs is caused by a defect in their production (hypoproliferative anemia), by their destruction (hemolytic anemia), or by their loss (bleeding).

In the hypoproliferative anemias, RBCs usually survive normally, but the marrow cannot produce adequate numbers of these cells. The decreased production is reflected in a low reticulocyte count. Inadequate production of RBCs may result from marrow damage due to medications or chemicals (eg, chloramphenicol, benzene) or from a lack of factors necessary for RBC formation (eg, iron, vitamin B_{12}, folic acid, erythropoietin).

Hemolytic anemias stem from premature destruction of RBCs, which results in a liberation of hemoglobin from the RBC into the plasma. The increased RBC destruction results in tissue hypoxia, which in turn stimulates erythropoietin production. This increased production is reflected in an increased reticulocyte count, as the bone marrow responds to the loss of RBCs. The released hemoglobin is converted in large part to bilirubin; therefore, the bilirubin concentration rises. **Hemolysis** can result from an abnormality within the RBC itself (eg, sickle cell anemia, glucose-6-phosphate

dehydrogenase [G-6-PD] deficiency) or within the plasma (eg, immune hemolytic anemias), or from direct injury to the RBC within the circulation (eg, hemolysis caused by mechanical heart valve). Chart 33-1 identifies the causes of hemolytic anemia.

Clinical Manifestations

Aside from the severity of the anemia itself, several factors influence the development of anemia-associated symptoms:

- The speed with which the anemia has developed
- The duration of the anemia (ie, its chronicity)
- The metabolic requirements of the individual
- Other concurrent disorders or disabilities (eg, cardiopulmonary disease)
- Special complications or concomitant features of the condition that produced the anemia

In general, the more rapidly an anemia develops, the more severe its symptoms. An otherwise healthy person can often tolerate as much as a 50% gradual reduction in hemoglobin without pronounced symptoms or significant incapacity, whereas the rapid loss of as little as 30% may precipitate profound vascular collapse in the same individual. A person who has been anemic for a very long time, with hemoglobin levels between 9 and 11 g/dL, usually has few or no symptoms other than slight tachycardia on exertion and fatigue.

Chart 33-1 **Causes of Hemolytic Anemias**

Inherited Hemolytic Anemia
Abnormal hemoglobin
   Sickle cell anemia*
   Thalassemia*
Red blood cell membrane abnormality
   Hereditary spherocytosis*
   Hereditary elliptocytosis
   Acanthocytosis
   Stomatocytosis
Enzyme deficiencies
   Glucose-6-phosphate dehydrogenase (G-6-PD) deficiency*

Acquired Hemolytic Anemia
Antibody-related
   Iso-antibody/transfusion reaction*
   Autoimmune hemolytic anemia (AIHA)*
   Cold agglutinin disease*
Not antibody-related
   Red blood cell membrane defects
   Paroxysmal nocturnal hemoglobinuria (PNH)
   Liver disease
   Uremia
   Trauma
   Mechanical heart valve
   Microangiopathic hemolytic anemia
   Infection
      Bacterial
      Parasitic
   Disseminated intravascular coagulation (DIC)*
   Toxins
   Hypersplenism*

*Discussed in text.

Patients who customarily are very active or who have significant demands on their lives (eg, a single, working mother of small children) are more likely to have symptoms, and those symptoms are more likely to be pronounced than in a more sedentary person. A patient with hypothyroidism with decreased oxygen needs may be completely asymptomatic, without tachycardia or increased cardiac output, at a hemoglobin level of 10 g/dL. Similarly, patients with coexistent cardiac, vascular, or pulmonary disease may develop more pronounced symptoms of anemia (eg, dyspnea, chest pain, muscle pain or cramping) at a higher hemoglobin level than those without these concurrent health problems.

Finally, some anemic disorders are complicated by various other abnormalities that do not result from the anemia but are inherently associated with these particular diseases. These abnormalities may give rise to symptoms that completely overshadow those of the anemia, as in the painful crises of sickle cell anemia.

Assessment and Diagnostic Findings

A variety of hematologic studies are performed to determine the type and cause of the anemia. In an initial evaluation, the hemoglobin, hematocrit, reticulocyte count, and RBC indices, particularly the mean corpuscular volume (MCV), are particularly useful. Iron studies (serum iron level, total iron-binding capacity [TIBC], percent saturation, and ferritin), as well as serum vitamin B_{12} and folate levels, are also frequently obtained. Other tests include haptoglobin and erythropoietin levels. The remaining CBC values are useful in determining whether the anemia is an isolated problem or part of another hematologic condition, such as leukemia or myelodysplastic syndrome (MDS). Bone marrow aspiration may be performed. In addition, other diagnostic studies may be performed to determine the presence of underlying chronic illness, such as malignancy, and the source of any blood loss, such as polyps or ulcers within the gastrointestinal tract.

Complications

General complications of severe anemia include heart failure, paresthesias, and confusion. At any given level of anemia, patients with underlying heart disease are far more likely to have angina or symptoms of heart failure than those without heart disease. Complications associated with specific types of anemia are included in the description of each type.

Medical Management

Management of anemia is directed toward correcting or controlling the cause of the anemia; if the anemia is severe, the RBCs that are lost or destroyed may be replaced with a transfusion of packed RBCs (PRBCs). The management of the various types of anemia is covered in the discussions that follow.

NURSING PROCESS: THE PATIENT WITH ANEMIA

Assessment

The health history and physical examination provide important data about the type of anemia involved, the extent and type of symptoms it produces, and the impact of those symptoms on the patient's life. Weakness, fatigue, and general malaise are common, as are pallor of the skin and mucous membranes (sclera, oral mucosa).

Jaundice may be present in patients with megaloblastic anemia or hemolytic anemia. The tongue may be smooth and red (in iron deficiency anemia) or beefy red and sore (in megaloblastic anemia); the corners of the mouth may be ulcerated (**angular cheilosis**) in both types of anemia. Individuals with iron deficiency anemia may crave ice, starch, or dirt (known as pica); their nails may be brittle, ridged, and concave.

The health history should include a medication history, because some medications can depress bone marrow activity or interfere with folate metabolism. An accurate history of alcohol intake, including the amount and duration, should be obtained. Family history is important, because certain anemias are inherited. Athletic endeavours should be assessed, because extreme exercise can decrease erythropoiesis and RBC survival in some athletes.

A nutritional assessment is important, because it may indicate deficiencies in essential nutrients such as iron, vitamin B_{12}, and folic acid. Children of indigent families may be at higher risk for anemia because of nutritional deficiencies. Strict vegetarians are also at risk for megaloblastic types of anemia if they do not supplement their diet with vitamin B_{12}.

Cardiac status should be carefully assessed. When the hemoglobin level is low, the heart attempts to compensate by pumping faster and harder in an effort to deliver more blood to hypoxic tissue. This increased cardiac workload can result in such symptoms as tachycardia, palpitations, dyspnea, dizziness, orthopnea, and exertional dyspnea. Heart failure may eventually develop, as evidenced by an enlarged heart (cardiomegaly) and liver (hepatomegaly) and by peripheral edema.

Assessment of the gastrointestinal system may disclose complaints of nausea, vomiting (with specific questions as to the appearance of any emesis [eg, looks like "coffee grounds"]), melena or dark stools, diarrhea, anorexia, and glossitis (inflammation of the tongue). Stools should be tested for occult blood. Women should be questioned about their menstrual periods (eg, excessive menstrual flow, other vaginal bleeding) and the use of iron supplements during pregnancy.

The neurologic examination is also important because of the effect of pernicious anemia on the central and peripheral nervous systems. Assessment should include the presence and extent of peripheral numbness and paresthesias, ataxia, poor coordination, and confusion. Finally, it is important to monitor relevant laboratory test results and to note any changes over time.

Diagnosis

NURSING DIAGNOSES
Based on the assessment data, major nursing diagnoses for the anemic patient may include:

- Activity intolerance related to weakness, fatigue, and general malaise
- Imbalanced nutrition, less than body requirements, related to inadequate intake of essential nutrients
- Ineffective tissue perfusion related to inadequate blood volume or hematocrit
- Noncompliance with prescribed therapy

COLLABORATIVE PROBLEMS/ POTENTIAL COMPLICATIONS
Based on the assessment data, potential complications that may develop include:

- Heart failure
- Paresthesias
- Confusion

Planning and Goals

The major goals for the patient may include increased tolerance of normal activity, attainment or maintenance of adequate nutrition, maintenance of adequate tissue perfusion, compliance with prescribed therapy, and absence of complications.

Nursing Interventions

MANAGING FATIGUE

The most frequent symptom and complication of anemia is fatigue. This distressing symptom is too often minimized by health care providers. Fatigue is often the symptom that has the greatest negative impact on the individual's level of functioning and consequent quality of life. Patients describe the fatigue from anemia as oppressive. Fatigue can be significant, yet the anemia may not be severe enough to warrant transfusion. Fatigue can interfere with an individual's ability to work, both inside and outside the home. It can harm relationships with family and friends. Patients often lose interest in hobbies and activities, including sexual activity. The distress from fatigue is often related to an individual's responsibilities and life demands as well as the amount of assistance and support received from others.

Nursing interventions can focus on assisting the patient to prioritize activities and to establish a balance between activity and rest that is realistic and feasible from the patient's perspective. Patients with chronic anemia need to maintain some physical activity and exercise to prevent the deconditioning that results from inactivity.

MAINTAINING ADEQUATE NUTRITION

Inadequate intake of essential nutrients, such as iron, vitamin B_{12}, folic acid, and protein can cause some anemias. The symptoms associated with anemia (eg, fatigue, anorexia) can in turn interfere with maintaining adequate nutrition. A healthy diet should be encouraged. Because alcohol interferes with the utilization of essential nutrients, the nurse should advise the patient to avoid alcoholic beverages or to limit their intake and should provide the rationale for this recommendation. Dietary teaching sessions should be individualized, including cultural aspects related to food preferences and food preparation. The involvement of family members enhances compliance with dietary recommendations. Dietary supplements (eg, vitamins, iron, folate, protein) may be prescribed as well.

Equally important, the patient and family must understand the role of nutritional supplements in the proper context, because many forms of anemia are not the result of a nutritional deficiency. In such cases, excessive intake of nutritional supplements will not improve the anemia. A potential problem in individuals with chronic transfusion requirements occurs with the indiscriminate use of iron. Unless an aggressive program of chelation therapy is implemented, these individuals are at risk for iron overload from their transfusions alone. The addition of an iron supplement only exacerbates the situation.

MAINTAINING ADEQUATE PERFUSION

Patients with acute blood loss or severe hemolysis may have decreased tissue perfusion from decreased blood volume or reduced circulating RBCs (decreased hematocrit). Lost volume is replaced with transfusions or intravenous fluids, based on the symptoms and the laboratory findings. Supplemental oxygen may be necessary, but it is rarely needed on a long-term basis unless there is underlying severe cardiac or pulmonary disease as well. The nurse monitors vital signs closely; other medications, such as antihypertensive agents, may need to be adjusted or withheld.

PROMOTING COMPLIANCE WITH PRESCRIBED THERAPY

For patients with anemia, medications or nutritional supplements are often prescribed to alleviate or correct the condition. These patients need to understand the purpose of the medication, how to take the medication and over what time period, and how to manage any side effects of therapy. To enhance compliance, the nurse can assist patients in developing ways to incorporate the therapeutic plan into their lives, rather than merely giving the patient a list of instructions. For example, many patients have difficulty taking iron supplements because of related gastrointestinal effects. Rather than seeking assistance from a health care provider in managing the problem, some of these patients simply stop taking the iron.

Abruptly stopping some medications can have serious consequences, as in the case of high-dose corticosteroids to manage hemolytic anemias. Some medications, such as growth factors, are extremely expensive. Patients receiving these medications may need assistance with obtaining needed insurance coverage or with exploring alternatives for obtaining these medications.

MONITORING AND MANAGING POTENTIAL COMPLICATIONS

A significant complication of anemia is heart failure from chronic diminished blood volume and the heart's compensatory effort to increase cardiac output. Patients with anemia should be assessed for signs and symptoms of heart failure. A serial record of body weights can be more useful than a record of dietary intake and output, because the intake and output measurements may not be accurate. In the case of fluid retention resulting from heart failure, diuretics may be required.

In megaloblastic forms of anemia, the significant potential complications are neurologic. A neurologic assessment should be performed for patients with known or suspected megaloblastic anemia. Patients may initially complain of paresthesias in their lower extremities. These paresthesias are usually manifested as numbness and tingling on the bottom of the foot, and they gradually progress. As the anemia progresses and damage to the spinal cord occurs, other signs become apparent. Position and vibration sense may be diminished; difficulty maintaining balance is not uncommon, and some patients have gait disturbances as well. Initially mild but gradually progressive confusion may develop.

Evaluation

EXPECTED PATIENT OUTCOMES

Expected patient outcomes may include:

1. Tolerates activity at a safe and acceptable level
   a. Follows a progressive plan of rest, activity, and exercise
   b. Prioritizes activities
   c. Paces activities according to energy level
2. Attains and maintains adequate nutrition
   a. Eats a healthy diet
   b. Develops meal plan that promotes optimal nutrition
   c. Maintains adequate amounts of iron, vitamins, and protein from diet or supplements
   d. Adheres to nutritional supplement therapy when prescribed
   e. Verbalizes understanding of rationale for using recommended nutritional supplements
   f. Verbalizes understanding of rationale for avoiding nonrecommended nutritional supplements
3. Maintains adequate perfusion
   a. Has vital signs within baseline for patient

b. Has pulse oximetry (arterial oxygenation) value within normal limits
4. Absence of complications
   a. Avoids or limits activities that cause dyspnea, palpitations, dizziness, or tachycardia
   b. Uses rest and comfort measures to alleviate dyspnea
   c. Has vital signs within baseline for patient
   d. Has no signs of increasing fluid retention (eg, peripheral edema, decreased urine output, neck vein distention)
   e. Remains oriented to time, place, and situation
   f. Ambulates safely, using assistive devices as necessary
   g. Remains free of injury
   h. Verbalizes understanding of importance of serial CBC measurements
   i. Maintains safe home environment; obtains assistance as necessary.

Hypoproliferative Anemias

IRON DEFICIENCY ANEMIA

Iron deficiency anemia typically results when the intake of dietary iron is inadequate for hemoglobin synthesis. The body can store about one fourth to one third of its iron, and it is not until those stores are depleted that iron deficiency anemia actually begins to develop. Iron deficiency anemia is the most common type of anemia in all age groups, and it is the most common anemia in the world. More than 500 million people are affected, more commonly in underdeveloped countries, where inadequate iron stores can result from inadequate intake of iron (seen with vegetarian diets) or from blood loss (eg, from intestinal hookworm). Iron deficiency is also common in the United States. In children, adolescents, and pregnant women, the cause is typically inadequate iron in the diet to keep up with increased growth. However, for most adults with iron deficiency anemia, the cause is blood loss. In fact, in adults, the cause of iron deficiency anemia should be considered to be bleeding until proven otherwise.

The most common cause of iron deficiency in men and postmenopausal women is bleeding (from ulcers, gastritis, inflammatory bowel disease, or gastrointestinal tumours). The most common cause of iron deficiency anemia in premenopausal women is menorrhagia (excessive menstrual bleeding) and pregnancy with inadequate iron supplementation. Patients with chronic alcoholism often have chronic blood loss from the gastrointestinal tract, which causes iron loss and eventual anemia. Other causes include iron malabsorption, as is seen after gastrectomy or with celiac disease.

Clinical Manifestations

Patients with iron deficiency primarily have the symptoms of anemia. If the deficiency is severe or prolonged, they may also have a smooth, sore tongue, brittle and ridged nails, and angular cheilosis (an ulceration of the corner of the mouth). These signs subside after iron-replacement therapy. The health history may be significant for multiple pregnancies, gastrointestinal bleeding, and pica (a craving for unusual substances, such as ice, clay, or laundry starch).

Assessment and Diagnostic Findings

The most definitive method of establishing the diagnosis of iron deficiency anemia is bone marrow aspiration. The aspirate is stained to detect iron, which is at a low level or even absent. However, few patients with suspected iron deficiency anemia undergo bone marrow aspiration. In many patients, the diagnosis can be established with other tests, particularly in patients with a history of conditions that predispose them to this type of anemia.

There is a strong correlation between laboratory values measuring iron stores and levels of hemoglobin. After the iron stores are depleted (as reflected by low serum ferritin levels), the hemoglobin level falls. The diminished iron stores cause small RBCs. Therefore, as the anemia progresses, the MCV, which measures the size of the RBC, also decreases. Hematocrit and RBC levels are also low in relation to the hemoglobin level. Other laboratory tests that measure iron stores are useful but are not as consistent indicators as a low ferritin level, which reflects low iron stores. Typically, patients with iron deficiency anemia have a low serum iron level and an elevated TIBC, which measures the transport protein supplying the marrow with iron as needed (also referred to as transferrin). However, other disease states, such as infection and inflammatory conditions, can also cause a low serum iron level and TIBC with an elevated ferritin level. Therefore, the most reliable laboratory findings in evaluating iron deficiency anemia are the ferritin and hemoglobin values.

Medical Management

Except in the case of pregnancy, the cause of iron deficiency should be investigated. Anemia may be a sign of a curable gastrointestinal cancer or of uterine fibroid tumours. Stool specimens should be tested for occult blood. People 50 years of age or older should have a colonoscopy, endoscopy, or x-ray examination of the gastrointestinal tract to detect ulcerations, gastritis, polyps, or cancer. Several oral iron preparations—ferrous sulfate, ferrous gluconate, and ferrous fumarate—are available for treating iron deficiency anemia. The hemoglobin level may increase in only a few weeks, and the anemia can be corrected in a few months. Iron store replenishment takes much longer, so it is important that the patient continue taking the iron for as long as 6 to 12 months.

In some cases, oral iron is poorly absorbed or poorly tolerated, or iron supplementation is needed in large amounts. In these situations, intravenous or intramuscular administration of iron dextran may be needed. Before parenteral administration of a full dose, a small test dose should be administered to avoid the risk of anaphylaxis with either intravenous or intramuscular injections. Emergency medications (eg, epinephrine) should be close at hand. If no signs of allergic reaction have occurred after 30 minutes, the remaining dose of iron may be administered. Several doses are required to replenish the patient's iron stores.

Nursing Management

Preventive education is important, because iron deficiency anemia is common in menstruating and pregnant women. Food sources high in iron include organ meats (beef or calf's liver, chicken liver), other meats, beans (black, pinto, and garbanzo), leafy green vegetables, raisins, and molasses. Taking iron-rich foods with a source of vitamin C enhances the absorption of iron.

The nurse helps the patient select a healthy diet. Nutritional counselling can be provided for those whose usual diet is inadequate. Patients with a history of eating fad diets or strict vegetarian diets are counselled that such diets often contain inadequate amounts of absorbable iron. The nurse encourages patients to continue iron therapy as long as it is prescribed, although they may no longer feel fatigued.

Because iron is best absorbed on an empty stomach, patients should be advised to take the supplement an hour before meals. Most patients can use the less expensive, more standard forms of ferrous sulfate. Tablets with enteric coating may be poorly

Chart 33-2 • PATIENT EDUCATION
Taking Iron Supplements

Iron supplementation is usually given in oral form, typically as ferrous sulfate, or $FeSO_4$. Many patients have difficulty tolerating iron supplements, primarily due to gastrointestinal toxicities (eg, nausea, abdominal discomfort, constipation). Here are some helpful guidelines for taking iron supplements:

- Take iron on an empty stomach (1 hour before or 2 hours after a meal). Iron absorption is reduced with food, especially dairy products.
- To prevent gastrointestinal distress, the following schedule may work better if more than one tablet a day is prescribed: Start with only one tablet per day for a few days, then increase to two tablets per day, then three tablets per day. This method permits the body to adjust gradually to the iron.
- Increase the intake of vitamin C (citrus fruits and juices, strawberries, tomatoes, broccoli), to enhance iron absorption.
- Eat foods high in fibre to minimize problems with constipation.
- Remember that stools will become dark in colour.

Polysaccharide iron complex forms are better tolerated but are more expensive. Liquid forms of iron supplementation may be better tolerated than solid forms, although they are more expensive. The liquid forms can discolour teeth. Use a straw or place the spoon at the back of the mouth to take the supplement; rinse mouth thoroughly afterward.

---

absorbed and should be avoided. Other patients have difficulty taking iron supplements because of gastrointestinal side effects (primarily constipation, but also cramping, nausea, and vomiting). Some iron formulations are designed to limit gastrointestinal side effects by the addition of a stool softener or use of sustained-release formulations to limit nausea or gastritis. Specific patient teaching aids, such as the accompanying patient education guide (Chart 33-2), can assist patients with the use of iron supplements.

If taking iron on an empty stomach causes gastric distress, the patient may need to take the iron supplement with meals. However, doing so diminishes iron absorption by as much as 50%, thus prolonging the time required to replenish iron stores. Antacids or dairy products should not be taken with iron, because they greatly diminish the absorption of iron. Polysaccharide iron complex forms that have less gastrointestinal toxicity are also available, but they are more expensive.

Liquid forms of iron that cause less gastrointestinal distress are available. However, they can stain the teeth; patients should be instructed to take this medication through a straw, to rinse the mouth with water, and to practice good oral hygiene after taking this medication. Finally, patients should be informed that iron salts may colour the stool dark green or black. However, iron replacement therapy does not cause a false-positive result on stool analyses for occult blood.

Intramuscular supplementation is used infrequently. The volume of iron required may be excessive. The intramuscular injection causes some local pain and can stain the skin. These side effects are minimized by using the Z-track technique for administering iron dextran deep into the gluteus maximus muscle (buttock). Avoid vigorously rubbing the injection site after the injection. Because of the problems with intramuscular administration, the intravenous route is preferred for administration of iron dextran.

ANEMIAS IN RENAL DISEASE

The degree of anemia in patients with end-stage renal disease varies greatly, but in general patients do not become significantly anemic until the serum creatinine level exceeds 3 mg/100 mL. The symptoms of anemia are often the most disturbing of the patient's symptoms. The hematocrit usually falls to between 20% and 30%, although in rare cases it may fall to less than 15%. The RBCs appear normal on the peripheral smear.

This anemia is caused by both a mild shortening of RBC life span and a deficiency of erythropoietin (necessary for erythro-

poiesis). As renal function decreases, erythropoietin, which is produced by the kidney, also decreases. Because erythropoietin is also produced outside the kidney, some erythropoiesis does continue, even in patients whose kidneys have been removed. However, the amount is small and the degree of erythropoiesis is inadequate.

Patients undergoing long-term hemodialysis lose blood into the dialyzer and therefore may become iron deficient. Folic acid deficiency develops because this vitamin passes into the dialysate. Therefore, patients who receive hemodialysis and who are anemic should be evaluated for iron and folate deficiency and treated appropriately.

The availability of recombinant erythropoietin (epoetin alfa [Eprex]) has dramatically altered the management of anemia in end-stage renal disease by decreasing the need for RBC transfusion, with its associated risks. Erythropoietin, in combination with oral iron supplements, can raise and maintain hematocrit levels to between 33% and 38%. This treatment has been successful with dialysis patients. Many patients report decreased fatigue, increased energy, increased feelings of well-being, improved exercise tolerance, better tolerance of dialysis treatments, and improved quality of life. Hypertension is the most serious side effect in this patient population when the hematocrit rapidly increases to a high level. Therefore, the hematocrit should be checked frequently when a patient with renal disease begins erythropoietin therapy. The dose of erythropoietin (epoetin alfa) should be titrated to the hematocrit. In some patients, the elevated hematocrit and associated hypertension may necessitate antihypertensive therapy.

ANEMIA OF CHRONIC DISEASE

The term "anemia of chronic disease" is a misnomer in that only the chronic diseases of inflammation, infection, and malignancy cause this type of anemia. Many chronic inflammatory diseases are associated with a **normochromic**, **normocytic** anemia (ie, the RBCs are normal in colour and size). These disorders include rheumatoid arthritis; severe, chronic infections; and many cancers. It is therefore imperative that the "chronic disease" be diagnosed when this form of anemia is identified so that it can be appropriately managed.

The anemia is usually mild to moderate and nonprogressive. It develops gradually over 6 to 8 weeks and then stabilizes at a hematocrit seldom less than 25%. The hemoglobin level rarely falls below 9 g/dL, and the bone marrow has normal cellularity with increased stores of iron as the iron is diverted from the serum (and thus is unavailable as a growth factor for invading pathogens). Erythropoietin levels are low, perhaps because of decreased production, and iron use is blocked by **erythroid cells** (cells that are or will become mature RBCs). A moderate shortening of RBC survival also occurs.

Most of these patients have few symptoms and do not require treatment for the anemia. With successful treatment of the underlying disorder, the bone marrow iron is used to make RBCs and the hemoglobin level rises.

APLASTIC ANEMIA

Aplastic anemia is a rather rare disease caused by a decrease in or damage to marrow stem cells, damage to the microenvironment within the marrow, and replacement of the marrow with fat. It results in bone marrow **aplasia** (markedly reduced hematopoiesis). Therefore, in addition to severe anemia, significant neutropenia and thrombocytopenia (a deficiency of platelets) are also seen.

Pathophysiology

Aplastic anemia can be congenital or acquired, but most cases are idiopathic (ie, without apparent cause). Infections and pregnancy can trigger it, or it may be caused by certain medications, chemicals, or radiation damage (Chart 33-3). Agents that regularly produce marrow aplasia include benzene and benzene derivatives (eg, airplane glue). Certain toxic materials, such as inorganic arsenic and several pesticides (including DDT, which is no longer used or available in Canada), have also been implicated as potential causes. Various medications have been associated with aplastic anemia.

Clinical Manifestations

The manifestations of aplastic anemia are often insidious. Complications resulting from bone marrow failure may occur before

---

Chart 33-3 **Substances Associated With Aplastic Anemia**

Analgesics
Antiseizure agents (mephenytoin, triethadione*)
Antihistamines
Antimicrobials*
Antineoplastic agents (alkylating agents, antitumour antibiotics, antimetabolites)
Antithyroid medications
Benzene*
Chloramphenicol*
Gold compounds*
Heavy metals
Hypoglycemic agents
Insecticides
Organic arsenicals*
Phenylbutazone*
Phenothiazines
Sulfonamides*
Sedatives

*Most common.

---

the diagnosis is established. Typical complications are infection and symptoms of anemia (eg, fatigue, pallor, dyspnea). Purpura (bruising) may develop later and should trigger a CBC and hematologic evaluation if these were not performed initially. If the patient has had repeated throat infections, cervical lymphadenopathy may be seen. Other lymphadenopathies and splenomegaly sometimes occur. Retinal hemorrhages are common.

Assessment and Diagnostic Findings

In many situations, aplastic anemia occurs when a medication or chemical is ingested in toxic amounts. However, in a few people, it develops after a medication has been taken at the recommended dosage. This may be considered an idiosyncratic reaction in those who are highly susceptible, possibly caused by a genetic defect in the medication biotransformation or elimination process. A bone marrow aspirate shows an extremely hypoplastic or even aplastic (very few to no cells) marrow replaced with fat.

Medical Management

It is presumed that the lymphocytes of patients with aplastic anemia destroy the stem cells and consequently impair the production of RBCs, WBCs, and platelets. Despite its severity, aplastic anemia can be successfully treated in most people. Potentially, those who are younger than 60 years of age, who are otherwise healthy, and who have a compatible donor can be cured of the disease by a bone marrow transplantation (BMT) or peripheral blood stem cell transplantation (PBSCT). In others, the disease can be managed with immunosuppressive therapy. A combination of antithymocyte globulin (Atgam) and cyclosporine (Neoral) is used most commonly. Immunosuppressants prevent the patient's lymphocytes from destroying the stem cells. If relapse occurs (ie, the patient becomes pancytopenic again), reinstitution of the same immunologic agents may induce another remission. Corticosteroids are not very useful as an immunosuppressive agent, because patients with aplastic anemia appear particularly susceptible to the development of bone complications from corticosteroids (ie, aseptic necrosis of the head of the femur).

Supportive therapy plays a major role in the management of aplastic anemia. Any offending agent is discontinued. The patient is supported with transfusions of RBCs and platelets as necessary. Death usually is caused by hemorrhage or infection.

Nursing Management

Patients with aplastic anemia are vulnerable to problems related to RBC, WBC, and platelet deficiencies. They should be assessed carefully for signs of infection and bleeding. Specific interventions are delineated in the sections on neutropenia and thrombocytopenia.

MEGALOBLASTIC ANEMIAS

In the anemias caused by deficiencies of vitamin B_{12} or folic acid, identical bone marrow and peripheral blood changes occur, because both vitamins are essential for normal DNA synthesis. In either anemia, the RBCs that are produced are abnormally large and are called megaloblastic RBCs. Other cells derived from the myeloid stem cell (nonlymphoid WBCs, platelets) are also abnormal. A bone marrow analysis reveals **hyperplasia** (abnormal increase in the number of cells), and the precursor erythroid and myeloid cells are large and bizarre in appearance. Many of these abnormal RBCs and myeloid cells are destroyed within the marrow, however, so the mature cells that do leave the marrow are actually fewer in number. Thus, **pancytopenia** (a decrease in all myeloid-derived cells) can develop. In an advanced situation, the hemoglobin value may be as low as 4 to 5 g/dL, the WBC count 2,000 to 3,000/mm^3, and the platelet count less than 50,000/mm^3. Those cells that are released into the circulation are often abnormally shaped. The neutrophils are hypersegmented. The platelets may be abnormally large. The RBCs are abnormally shaped, and the shapes may vary widely (**poikilocytosis**). Because the RBCs are very large, the MCV is very high, usually exceeding 110 µm^3.

Pathophysiology

FOLIC ACID DEFICIENCY

Folic acid, a vitamin that is necessary for normal RBC production, is stored as compounds referred to as folates. The folate stores in the body are much smaller than those of vitamin B$_{12}$, and they are quickly depleted when the dietary intake of folate is deficient (within 4 months). Folate is found in green vegetables and liver. Folate deficiency occurs in people who rarely eat uncooked vegetables. Alcohol increases folic acid requirements, and, at the same time, patients with alcoholism usually have a diet that is deficient in the vitamin. Folic acid requirements are also increased in patients with chronic hemolytic anemias and in women who are pregnant, because the need for RBC production is increased in these conditions. Some patients with malabsorptive diseases of the small bowel, such as sprue, may not absorb folic acid normally.

VITAMIN B$_{12}$ DEFICIENCY

A deficiency of vitamin B$_{12}$ can occur in several ways. Inadequate dietary intake is rare but can develop in strict vegetarians who consume no meat or dairy products. Faulty absorption from the gastrointestinal tract is more common. This occurs in conditions such as Crohn's disease, or after ileal resection or gastrectomy. Another cause is the absence of intrinsic factor, as in pernicious anemia. Intrinsic factor is normally secreted by cells within the gastric mucosa; normally it binds with the dietary vitamin B$_{12}$ and travels with it to the ileum, where the vitamin is absorbed. Without intrinsic factor, orally consumed vitamin B$_{12}$ cannot be absorbed, and RBC production is eventually diminished. Even if adequate vitamin B$_{12}$ and intrinsic factor are present, a deficiency may occur if disease involving the ileum or pancreas impairs absorption. Pernicious anemia, which tends to run in families, is primarily a disorder of adults, particularly the elderly. The abnormality is in the gastric mucosa: the stomach wall atrophies and fails to secrete intrinsic factor. Therefore, the absorption of vitamin B$_{12}$ is significantly impaired.

The body normally has large stores of vitamin B$_{12}$, so years may pass before the deficiency results in anemia. Because the body compensates so well, the anemia can be severe before the patient becomes symptomatic. For unknown reasons, patients with pernicious anemia have a higher incidence of gastric cancer than the general population; these patients should have endoscopies at regular intervals (every 1 to 2 years) to screen for early gastric cancer.

Clinical Manifestations

Symptoms of folic acid and vitamin B$_{12}$ deficiencies are similar, and the two anemias may coexist. However, the neurologic manifestations of vitamin B$_{12}$ deficiency do not occur with folic acid deficiency, and they persist if B$_{12}$ is not replaced. Therefore, careful distinction between the two anemias must be made. Serum levels of both vitamins can be measured. In the case of folic acid deficiency, even small amounts of folate will increase the serum folate level, sometimes to normal. Measuring the amount of folate within the RBC itself (red cell folate) is therefore a more sensitive test in determining true folate deficiency.

After the body stores of vitamin B$_{12}$ are depleted, patients may begin to show signs of the anemia. However, because the onset and progression of the anemia are so gradual, the body can compensate very well until the anemia is severe, so that the typical manifestations of anemia (weakness, listlessness, fatigue) may not be apparent initially. The hematologic effects of deficiency are accompanied by effects on other organ systems, particularly the gastrointestinal tract and nervous system. Patients with pernicious anemia develop a smooth, sore, red tongue and mild diarrhea. They are extremely pale, particularly in the mucous membranes. They may become confused; more often they have paresthesias in the extremities (particularly numbness and tingling in the feet and lower legs). They may have difficulty maintaining their balance because of damage to the spinal cord, and they also lose position sense (proprioception). These symptoms are progressive, although the course of illness may be marked by spontaneous partial remissions and exacerbations. Without treatment, patients can die after several years, usually from heart failure secondary to anemia.

Assessment and Diagnostic Findings

The classic method of determining the cause of vitamin B$_{12}$ deficiency is the Schilling test, in which the patient receives a small oral dose of radioactive vitamin B$_{12}$, followed in a few hours by a large, nonradioactive parenteral dose of vitamin B$_{12}$ (this aids in renal excretion of the radioactive dose). If the oral vitamin is absorbed, more than 8% will be excreted in the urine within 24 hours; therefore, if no radioactivity is present in the urine (ie, the radioactive vitamin B$_{12}$ stays within the gastrointestinal tract), the cause is gastrointestinal malabsorption of the vitamin B$_{12}$. Conversely, if the urine is radioactive, the cause of the deficiency is not ileal disease or pernicious anemia. Later, the same procedure is repeated, but this time intrinsic factor is added to the oral radioactive vitamin B$_{12}$. If radioactivity is now detected in the urine (ie, the B$_{12}$ was absorbed from the gastrointestinal tract in the presence of intrinsic factor), the diagnosis of pernicious anemia can be made. The Schilling test is useful only if the urine collections are complete; therefore, the nurse must promote the patient's understanding and ability to comply with this collection.

Another useful, easier test is the intrinsic factor antibody test. A positive test indicates the presence of antibodies that bind the vitamin B$_{12}$–intrinsic factor complex and prevent it from binding to receptors in the ileum, thus preventing its absorption. Unfortunately, this test is not specific for pernicious anemia alone, but it can aid in the diagnosis.

Medical Management

Folate deficiency is treated by increasing the amount of folic acid in the diet and administering 1 mg of folic acid daily. Folic acid is administered intramuscularly only for people with malabsorption problems. With the exception of the vitamins administered during pregnancy, most proprietary vitamin preparations do not contain folic acid, so it must be administered as a separate tablet. After the hemoglobin level returns to normal, the folic acid replacement can be stopped. However, patients with alcoholism should continue receiving folic acid as long as they continue alcohol consumption.

Vitamin B_{12} deficiency is treated by vitamin B_{12} replacement. Vegetarians can prevent or treat deficiency with oral supplements through vitamins or fortified soy milk. When, as is more common, the deficiency is due to defective absorption or absence of intrinsic factor, replacement is by monthly intramuscular injections of vitamin B_{12}, usually at a dose of 1000 µg. The reticulocyte count rises within 1 week, and in several weeks the blood counts are all normal. The tongue improves in several days. However, the neurologic manifestations require more time for recovery; if there is severe neuropathy, the patient may never recover fully. To prevent recurrence of pernicious anemia, vitamin B_{12} therapy must be continued for life.

> **NURSING ALERT** Even when the anemia is severe, RBC transfusions should not be used because the patient's body has compensated over time by expanding the total blood volume. Administration of blood transfusions to such patients, particularly those who are elderly or who have cardiac dysfunction, can precipitate pulmonary edema. If transfusions are required, the RBCs should be transfused slowly, with careful attention to signs and symptoms of fluid overload.

Nursing Management

Assessment of patients who have or are at risk for megaloblastic anemia includes inspection of the skin and mucous membranes. Mild jaundice may be apparent and is best seen in the sclera without using fluorescent lights. Vitiligo (patchy loss of skin pigmentation) and premature greying of the hair are often seen in patients with pernicious anemia. The tongue is smooth, red, and sore. Because of the neurologic complications associated with these anemias, a careful neurologic assessment is important, including tests of position and vibration sense.

PROMOTING HOME AND COMMUNITY-BASED CARE
The nurse needs to pay particular attention to ambulation and should assess the patient's gait and stability as well as the need for assistive devices (eg, canes, walkers) and for assistance in managing daily activities. Of particular concern is ensuring safety when position sense, coordination, and gait are affected. Physical and occupational therapy referrals may be needed.

If sensation is altered, patients need to be instructed to avoid excessive heat and cold.

Because mouth and tongue soreness may restrict nutritional intake, the nurse can advise patients and families to prepare bland, soft foods and to eat small amounts frequently. The nurse also may explain that other nutritional deficiencies, such as alcohol-induced anemia, can induce neurologic problems.

Patients must also be taught about the chronicity of their disorder and the necessity for monthly vitamin B_{12} injections even in the absence of symptoms. Many patients can be taught to self-administer their injections. The gastric atrophy associated with pernicious anemia increases the risk of gastric carcinoma, so these patients need to understand that ongoing medical follow-up and screening are important.

MYELODYSPLASTIC SYNDROMES (MDS)

The MDS are a group of disorders of the myeloid stem cell that cause **dysplasia** (abnormal development) in one or more types of cell lines. The most common feature of MDS—dysplasia of the RBCs—is manifested as a macrocytic anemia; however, the WBCs (myeloid cells, particularly neutrophils) and platelets can also be affected. Although the bone marrow is actually hypercellular, many of the cells within it die before being released into the circulation. Therefore, the number of affected cells in the circulation is typically lower than normal. In addition to the quantitative defect (ie, fewer cells than normal), there is also a qualitative defect: the cells are not as functional as normal. The neutrophils have diminished ability to destroy bacteria by phagocytosis; platelets are less able to aggregate and are less adhesive than usual. The result of these qualitative defects is an increased risk for infection and bleeding, even when the actual number of circulating cells may not be excessively low. A significant proportion of MDS cases evolve into acute myeloid leukemia (AML); this type of leukemia tends to be nonresponsive to standard therapy.

Primary MDS tends to be a disease of the elderly; more than 80% of patients with MDS are older than 60 years of age. Secondary MDS may occur at any age and results from prior toxic exposure to chemicals, including chemotherapeutic medications (particularly alkylating agents). Secondary MDS tends to have a poorer prognosis than does primary MDS.

Clinical Manifestations

The manifestations of MDS can vary widely. Many patients are asymptomatic, with the illness being discovered incidentally when a CBC is performed for other purposes. Other patients have profound symptoms and complications from the illness. Fatigue is often present, at varying levels. Neutrophil dysfunction renders the person at risk for infection; recurrent pneumonias are not uncommon. Because platelet function can also be altered, bleeding can occur. These problems may persist in a fairly steady state for months, even years. They may also progress over time; as the dysplasia evolves into a leukemic state, the complications increase in severity.

Assessment and Diagnostic Findings

The CBC typically reveals a macrocytic anemia; WBC and platelet counts may be diminished as well. Serum erythropoietin levels may be inappropriately low, as is the reticulocyte count. As the disease evolves into AML, more immature blast cells are noted on the CBC.

Medical Management

With the exception of allogeneic bone marrow transplantation (BMT), there is no known cure for MDS. Chemotherapy has been used, particularly in patients with more aggressive forms of the illness, typically with disappointing results (Deeg & Applebaum, 2000; Beran, 2000). However, patients with mild cytopenias (low blood counts) actually require no therapy. For most patients with MDS, transfusions of RBCs are required to control the anemia and its symptoms. These patients can develop significant problems with iron overload from the repeated transfusions; this problem can be diminished with prompt initiation of chelation therapy to remove the excess iron (see Nursing Management). In some patients, the use of erythropoietin can be successful in reducing the need for transfusions and their attendant complications. Some patients may also require ongoing platelet transfusions to prevent significant bleeding. Infections need to be managed aggressively and promptly. Administration of growth factors, particularly granulocyte colony-stimulating factor (G-CSF [Neupogen]), erythropoietin, or both, has been successful in increasing neutrophils and diminishing anemia in certain patients; however, these agents are expensive and the effect is lost if the medications are stopped. Because MDS tend to occur in elderly people, other chronic conditions may limit treatment options. Secondary MDS and MDS that evolve into AML tend to be much more refractory to conventional therapy for leukemia.

Nursing Management

Caring for patients with MDS can be challenging because the illness is unpredictable. As with other hematologic conditions, some patients (especially those with no symptoms) have difficulty perceiving that they have a serious illness that can place them at risk for life-threatening complications. At the other extreme, many patients have tremendous difficulty coping with the uncertain trajectory of the illness and fear that the illness will evolve into AML at a time when they are feeling very well physically.

Patients with MDS need extensive instruction about infection risk, measures to avoid it, signs and symptoms of developing infection, and appropriate actions to initiate should such symptoms occur. Instruction should also be given regarding the risk for bleeding. Patients with MDS who are hospitalized may require neutropenic precautions.

Laboratory values need to be monitored closely to anticipate the need for transfusion and to determine response to treatment with growth factors. Patients with chronic transfusion requirements usually benefit from a vascular access device for this purpose. Patients receiving growth factors or chelation therapy must be educated about these medications, their side effects, and administration techniques.

Chelation therapy is a process that is used to remove excess iron acquired from chronic transfusions. Iron is bound to a substance, the chelating agent, and then excreted in the urine. Oral forms of chelating agents have not been successful (due to either diminished efficacy or excessive toxicity). Chelation therapy is most effective as a subcutaneous infusion administered over 8 to 12 hours; most patients prefer to do this at night. Because chelation therapy removes only a small amount of iron with each treatment, patients with chronic transfusion requirements (and iron overload) need to continue chelation therapy as long as the iron overload exists, potentially for the rest of their lives. Patients who are embarking on chelation therapy must be highly motivated and need instruction in the subcutaneous infusion technique, infusion pump maintenance, and side effect management. Local erythema at the injection site is the most common reaction and typically requires no intervention. Patients should have baseline and annual auditory and eye examinations, because hearing loss and visual changes can occur with treatment.

Hemolytic Anemias

In hemolytic anemias, the RBCs have a shortened life span; thus, the number of RBCs in circulation is reduced. Fewer RBCs result in decreased available oxygen, causing hypoxia, which in turn stimulates an increase in erythropoietin release from the kidney. The erythropoietin stimulates the bone marrow to compensate by producing new RBCs and releasing some of them into the circulation somewhat prematurely as reticulocytes. If the RBC destruction persists, the hemoglobin is broken down excessively; about 80% of the heme is converted to bilirubin, conjugated in the liver, and excreted in the bile.

The mechanism of RBC destruction varies, but all types of hemolytic anemia share certain laboratory features: the reticulocyte count is elevated, the fraction of indirect (unconjugated) bilirubin is increased, and the supply of haptoglobin (a binding protein for free hemoglobin) is depleted as more hemoglobin is released. As a result, the plasma haptoglobin level is low. If the marrow cannot compensate to replace the RBCs (indicated by a decreased reticulocyte count), the anemia will progress.

Hemolytic anemia has various forms. Among the inherited forms are sickle cell anemia, thalassemia and thalassemia major, G-6-PD deficiency, and hereditary spherocytosis. Acquired forms include autoimmune hemolytic anemia, nonimmune-mediated paroxysmal nocturnal hemoglobinuria, microangiopathic hemolytic anemia, and heart valve hemolysis, as well as anemias associated with hypersplenism.

SICKLE CELL ANEMIA

Sickle cell anemia is a severe hemolytic anemia that results from inheritance of the sickle hemoglobin gene. This gene causes the hemoglobin molecule to be defective. The sickle hemoglobin (HbS) acquires a crystal-like formation when exposed to low oxygen tension. The oxygen level in venous blood can be low enough to cause this change; consequently, the RBC containing HbS loses its round, very pliable, biconcave disk shape and becomes deformed, rigid, and sickle-shaped (Fig. 33-5). These long, rigid RBCs can adhere to the endothelium of small vessels; when they pile up against each other, blood flow to a region or an organ may be reduced (Hoffman, et al., 2000). If ischemia or infarction results, the patient may have pain, swelling, and fever. The sickling process takes time; if the RBC is again exposed to adequate amounts of oxygen (eg, when it travels through the pulmonary circulation) before the membrane becomes too rigid, it can revert to a normal shape. For this reason, the "sickling crises" are intermittent. Cold can aggravate

FIGURE 33-5 A normal red blood cell (*upper left*) and a sickled red blood cell.

the sickling process, because vasoconstriction slows the blood flow. Oxygen delivery can also be impaired by an increased blood viscosity, with or without occlusion due to adhesion of sickled cells; in this situation, the effects are seen in larger vessels, such as arterioles.

The *HbS* gene is inherited in people of African descent and to a lesser extent in people from the Middle East, the Mediterranean area, and aboriginal tribes in India. Sickle cell anemia is the most severe form of sickle cell disease. Less severe forms include sickle cell hemoglobin C (SC) disease, sickle cell hemoglobin D (SD) disease, and sickle cell beta-thalassemia. The clinical manifestations and management are the same as for sickle cell anemia. The term *sickle cell trait* refers to the carrier state for SC diseases; it is the most benign type of SC disease, in that less than 50% of the hemoglobin within an RBC is HbS. However, in terms of genetic counselling, it is still an important condition. If two people with sickle cell trait have children, the children may inherit two abnormal genes. These children will produce only HbS and therefore will have sickle cell anemia.

Clinical Manifestations

Symptoms of sickle cell anemia vary and are only somewhat based on the amount of HbS. Symptoms and complications result from chronic hemolysis or thrombosis. The sickled RBCs have a shortened life span. Patients are always anemic, usually with hemoglobin values of 7 to 10 g/dL. Jaundice is characteristic and is usually obvious in the sclerae. The bone marrow expands in childhood in a compensatory effort to offset the anemia, sometimes leading to enlargement of the bones of the face and skull. The chronic anemia is associated with tachycardia, cardiac murmurs, and often an enlarged heart (cardiomegaly). Dysrhythmias and heart failure may occur in adults.

Virtually any organ may be affected by thrombosis, but the primary sites involve those areas with slowed circulation, such as the spleen, lungs, and central nervous system. All the tissues and organs are constantly vulnerable to microcirculatory interruptions by the sickling process and therefore are susceptible to hypoxic damage or true ischemic necrosis. Patients with sickle cell anemia are unusually susceptible to infection, particularly pneumonia and osteomyelitis. Complications of sickle cell anemia include infection, stroke, renal failure, impotence, heart failure, and pulmonary hypertension. Table 33-4 summarizes the complications resulting from sickle cell anemia.

SICKLE CELL CRISIS
There are three types of sickle cell crisis in the adult population. The most common is the very painful *sickle crisis,* which results from tissue hypoxia and necrosis due to inadequate blood flow to a specific region of tissue or organ. *Aplastic crisis* results from infection with the human parvovirus. The hemoglobin level falls rapidly and the marrow cannot compensate, as evidenced by an absence of reticulocytes. *Sequestration crisis* results when other organs pool the sickled cells. Although the spleen is the most common organ responsible for sequestration in children, by 10 years of age most children with sickle cell anemia have had a splenic infarction and the spleen is then no longer functional (autosplenectomy). In adults, the common organs involved in sequestration are the liver and, more seriously, the lungs.

ACUTE CHEST SYNDROME
Acute chest syndrome is manifested by a rapidly falling hemoglobin level, tachycardia, fever, and bilateral infiltrates seen on the chest x-ray. These signs often mimic infection; in fact, recent studies have identified infection as a major cause of acute chest syndrome (Vichinsky, et al., 2000). Another common cause is pulmonary fat embolism. Increased secretory phospholipase A_2

Table 33-4 • Summary of Complications in Sickle Cell Anemia*

ORGAN INVOLVED	MECHANISMS*	ASSESSMENT FINDINGS	SIGNS AND SYMPTOMS
Spleen	Primary site of sickling → infarctions → ↓ phagocytic function of macrophages	Autosplenectomy; ↑ infection (esp. pneumonia, osteomyelitis)	Abdominal pain; fever, signs of infection
Lungs	Infection	Pulmonary infiltrate	Chest pain; dyspnea
	Infarction → ↑ pulmonary pressure → pulmonary hypertension	↑ sPLA$_2$†	
Central Nervous System	Infarction	CVA (cerebral vascular accident, brain attack)	Weakness (if severe); learning difficulties (if mild)
Kidney	Sickling → damage to renal medulla	Hematuria; inability to concentrate urine; renal failure	Dehydration
Heart	Anemia	Tachycardia; cardiomegaly → heart failure	Weakness, fatigue, dyspnea
Bone	↑ Erythroid production	Widening of medullary spaces and cortical thinning	Ache
	Infarction of bone	Osteosclerosis → avascular necrosis	Bone pain, especially hips
Liver	Hemolysis	Jaundice and gallstone formation; hepatomegaly	Abdominal pain
Skin and peripheral vasculature	↑ Viscosity/stasis → infarction → skin ulcers	Skin ulcers; ↓ wound healing	Pain
Eye	Infarction	Scarring, hemorrhage, retinal detachment	↓ Vision; blindness
Penis	Sickling	Priapism → impotence	Pain, impotence

* Problems encountered in sickle cell anemia vary and are the result of a variety of mechanisms, as depicted in this table. Common physical findings and symptoms are also variable.
† sPLA$_2$: Secretory phospholipase A_2, a laboratory test that can predict impending acute chest syndrome (see text).

concentration has been identified as a predictor of impending acute chest syndrome; the increased amounts of free fatty acids can cause increased permeability of the pulmonary endothelium and leakage of the pulmonary capillaries. Although this syndrome is potentially lethal, prompt intervention can result in a favourable outcome.

Assessment and Diagnostic Findings

The patient with sickle cell trait usually has a normal hemoglobin level, a normal hematocrit, and a normal blood smear. In contrast, the patient with sickle cell anemia has a low hematocrit and sickled cells on the smear. The diagnosis is confirmed by hemoglobin electrophoresis.

Prognosis

Patients with sickle cell anemia are usually diagnosed in childhood, because they become anemic in infancy and begin to have sickle cell crises at 1 or 2 years of age. Some children die in the first years of life, typically from infection, but the use of antibiotics and parent teaching have greatly improved the outcomes for these children. However, with current management strategies, the average life expectancy is still suboptimal, at 42 years. Young adults are often forced to live with multiple, often severe, complications from their disease. In some patients, the symptoms and complications diminish by 30 years of age; these patients live into the sixth decade or longer. At this time, there is no way to predict which patients will fall into this subgroup.

Medical Management

Treatment for sickle cell anemia is the focus of continued research (Steinberg, 1999). Many trials of medications that have antisickling properties are being conducted, as is research using antiadhesion treatment for vasoocclusive crises. However, aside from the equally important aggressive management of symptoms and complications, currently there are only three primary treatment modalities for sickle cell diseases: BMT, hydroxyurea (Hydrea), and long-term RBC transfusion.

BMT offers the potential for cure for this disease. However, this treatment modality is available to only a small subset of the patient population, because of either the lack of a compatible donor or the severe organ (eg, renal, liver, lung) damage already present in the patient.

PHARMACOLOGIC THERAPY

Hydroxyurea (Hydrea), a chemotherapy agent, has been shown to be effective in increasing hemoglobin F levels in patients with sickle cell anemia, thereby decreasing the permanent formation of sickled cells. Patients who receive hydroxyurea appear to have fewer painful episodes of sickle cell crisis, a lower incidence of acute chest syndrome, and less need for transfusions (Ferster et al., 2001). However, whether hydroxyurea can prevent or reverse actual organ damage remains unknown. Side effects of hydroxyurea include chronic suppression of WBC formation, teratogenesis, and potential for later development of a malignancy. Patient response to the medication varies significantly. The incidence and severity of side effects are also highly variable within a dose range. Some patients have toxicity when receiving a very small dose (5 mg/kg per day), whereas others have little toxicity with a much higher dose (35 mg/kg per day). More research is needed to identify specific patient subgroups that are more likely to respond to this medication.

TRANSFUSION THERAPY

Chronic transfusions with RBCs have been shown to be highly effective in several situations: in an acute exacerbation of anemia (eg, aplastic crisis), in the prevention of severe complications from anesthesia and surgery, and in improving the response to infection (when it results in exacerbated anemia) (Ohene-Frempong, 2001). Chronic transfusions have also been shown to be effective in diminishing episodes of sickle cell crisis in pregnant women; however, these transfusions have not been shown to improve fetal survival. Transfusion therapy may be effective in preventing complications from sickle cell disease. Although controversial, some data support the use of chronic transfusions in patients with cerebral ischemic injury (as seen on magnetic resonance imaging [MRI] or Doppler studies) to prevent more severe injury (eg, CVA). More than 50% of asymptomatic patients have some cerebral ischemia documented by MRI. In a recent study (Adams, 2000), chronic transfusion with RBCs resulted in a 90% reduction of stroke in children at risk for this complication, as demonstrated by elevated blood viscosity on transcranial Doppler ultrasonography. Transfusions may also be useful in the management of severe cases of acute chest syndrome.

The risk of complications from transfusion is important to consider. These risks include iron overload, which necessitates chronic chelation therapy (see MDS Nursing Management); poor venous access, which necessitates a vascular access device (and its attendant risk for infection or thrombosis); infections (hepatitis, human immunodeficiency virus [HIV]); and alloimmunization from repeated transfusions. Another complication from transfusion is the increased viscosity of blood before the concentration of hemoglobin S is reduced. Exchange transfusion (in which the patient's own blood is removed and replaced via transfusion) may be performed to diminish the risk of increasing the viscosity excessively; the objective is to reduce the hematocrit to less than 30%, with transfusions supplying more than 80% of the patient's blood volume. Finally, it is important to consider the significant financial cost of an aggressive transfusion and chelation program.

Patients with sickle cell anemia require daily folic acid replacements to maintain the supply required for increased erythropoiesis from hemolysis. Infections must be treated promptly with appropriate antibiotics; infection remains a major cause of death in these patients.

Acute chest syndrome is managed by prompt initiation of antibiotic therapy. Incentive spirometry has been shown to decrease the incidence of pulmonary complications significantly. In severe cases, bronchoscopy may be required to identify the source of pulmonary disease. Fluid restriction may be more beneficial than aggressive hydration. Corticosteroids may also be useful. Transfusions reverse the hypoxia and decrease the level of secretory phospholipase A_2. Pulmonary function should be monitored regularly to detect pulmonary hypertension early, when therapy (hydroxyurea, transfusions, or transplantation) may have a positive impact.

Because repeated blood transfusions are necessary, patients may develop multiple autoantibodies, making cross-matching difficult. In this patient population, a hemolytic transfusion reaction (see later discussion) may mimic the signs and symptoms of a sickle cell crisis. The classic distinguishing factor is that, with a hemolytic transfusion reaction, the patient becomes more anemic after being transfused. These patients need very close observation. Further transfusion is avoided if possible until the hemolytic process abates. If possible, the patient is supported with corticosteroids (prednisone [Winpred]), intravenous immunoglobulin (Gammagard, Gamimune-N, Gamunex), and erythropoietin (Eprex).

SUPPORTIVE THERAPY

Supportive care is equally important. A significant issue is pain management. The incidence of painful sickle cell crises is highly variable; many patients have pain on a daily basis. The severity of the pain may not be enough to cause the patient to seek assistance from health care providers but severe enough to interfere with the ability to work and function within the family. Acute pain episodes tend to be self-limited, lasting hours to days. If the patient cannot manage the pain at home, intervention is frequently sought in the acute care setting, usually at an urgent care facility or emergency department. Adequate hydration is important during a painful sickling episode. Oral hydration is acceptable if the patient can maintain adequate amounts of fluids; intravenous hydration with dextrose 5% in water (D_5W) or dextrose 5% in 0.25 normal saline solution (3 L/m^2/24 hours) is usually required for sickle crisis. Supplemental oxygen may also be needed.

The use of medication to relieve pain is important (see Chap. 13 for a discussion of pain management). Aspirin is very useful in diminishing mild to moderate pain; it also diminishes inflammation and potential thrombosis (due to its ability to diminish platelet adhesion). Nonsteroidal anti-inflammatory drugs (NSAIDs) are useful for moderate pain or in combination with opioid analgesics. Although no tolerance develops with NSAIDs, a "ceiling effect" does develop whereby an increase in dosage does not increase analgesia. NSAID use must be carefully monitored, because these medications can precipitate renal dysfunction. When opioid analgesics are used, morphine is the medication of choice for acute pain. Patient-controlled analgesia is frequently used.

Chronic pain increases in incidence as the patient ages. Here, the pain is caused by complications from the sickling, such as avascular necrosis of the hip. With chronic pain management, the principal goal is to maximize functioning; pain may not be completely eliminated without sacrificing function. This concept may be difficult for patients to accept; they may need repeated explanations and support from nonjudgmental health care providers. Nonpharmacologic approaches to pain management are crucial in this setting. Examples include physical and occupational therapy, physiotherapy (including the use of heat, massage, and exercise), cognitive and behavioural intervention (including distraction, relaxation, and motivational therapy), and support groups.

Working with patients who have multiple episodes of severe pain can be challenging. It is important for health care providers to realize that patients with sickle cell disease must face a lifelong experience with severe and unpredictable pain. Such pain is disruptive to the person's level of functioning, including social functioning, and may result in a feeling of helplessness. Patients with inadequate social support systems may have more difficulty coping with chronic pain.

NURSING PROCESS: THE PATIENT WITH SICKLE CELL CRISIS

Patients in sickle cell crisis should be assessed for factors that could have precipitated the crisis, such as symptoms of infection or dehydration, or situations that promote fatigue or emotional stress.

Assessment

Patients are asked to recall factors that seemed to precipitate previous crises and measures they use to prevent and manage crises. Pain levels should always be monitored; a pain-rating scale, such as a 0-to-10 scale, best accomplishes this. The quality of the pain (eg, sharp, dull, burning), the frequency of the pain (constant versus intermittent), and factors that aggravate or alleviate the pain

are included in this assessment. If a sickle cell crisis is suspected, the nurse needs to determine whether the pain currently experienced is the same as or different than the pain typically encountered in crisis.

Because the sickling process can interrupt circulation in any tissue or organ, with resultant hypoxia and ischemia, a careful assessment of all body systems is necessary. Particular emphasis is placed on assessing for pain, swelling, and fever. All joint areas are carefully examined for pain and swelling. The abdomen is assessed for pain and tenderness because of the possibility of splenic infarction.

The respiratory system must be assessed carefully, including auscultation of breath sounds, measurement of oxygen saturation levels, and signs of cardiac failure, such as the presence and extent of dependent edema, an increased point of maximal impulse, and cardiomegaly (as seen on chest x-ray). The patient should be assessed for signs of dehydration by a history of fluid intake and careful examination of mucous membranes, skin turgor, urine output, and serum creatinine and blood urea nitrogen values.

A careful neurologic examination is important to elicit symptoms of cerebral hypoxia. However, ischemic findings on MRI or Doppler studies may significantly precede the findings on the physical examination. MRI and Doppler studies are used for early diagnosis and may be more beneficial to improve patient outcome, because therapy can be initiated more promptly.

Because patients with sickle cell anemia are so susceptible to infections, they are assessed for the presence of any infectious process. Particular attention is given to examination of the chest, long bones, and femoral head, because pneumonia and osteomyelitis are especially common. Leg ulcers, which may be infected and are slow to heal, are common.

The extent of anemia (as measured by the hemoglobin level and the hematocrit) and the ability of the marrow to replenish RBCs (as measured by the reticulocyte count) should be monitored and compared with the patient's baseline values. The patient's current and past history of medical management should also be assessed, particularly chronic transfusion therapy, hydroxyurea use, and prior treatment for infection.

Diagnosis

NURSING DIAGNOSES

Based on the assessment data, major nursing diagnoses for the patient with sickle cell crisis may include:

- Acute pain related to tissue hypoxia due to agglutination of sickled cells within blood vessels
- Risk for infection
- Risk for powerlessness related to illness-induced helplessness
- Deficient knowledge regarding sickle crisis prevention

COLLABORATIVE PROBLEMS/ POTENTIAL COMPLICATIONS

Based on the assessment data, potential complications may include:

- Hypoxia, ischemia, infection, and poor wound healing leading to skin breakdown and ulcers
- Dehydration
- Cerebrovascular accident (CVA, brain attack, stroke)
- Anemia
- Renal dysfunction
- Heart failure, pulmonary hypertension, and acute chest syndrome
- Impotence
- Poor compliance
- Substance abuse related to poorly managed chronic pain

Planning and Goals

The major goals for the patient are relief of pain, decreased incidence of crisis, enhanced sense of self-esteem and power, and absence of complications.

Nursing Interventions

MANAGING PAIN

Acute pain during a sickle cell crisis can be severe and unpredictable. The patient's subjective description and rating of pain on a pain scale must guide the use of analgesics, which are valuable in controlling the acute pain of a sickle crisis. Any joint that is acutely swollen should be supported and elevated until the swelling diminishes. Relaxation techniques, breathing exercises, and distraction are helpful for some patients. After the acute painful episode has diminished, aggressive measures should be implemented to preserve function. Physical therapy, whirlpool baths, and transcutaneous nerve stimulation are examples of such modalities.

PREVENTING AND MANAGING INFECTION

Nursing care focuses on monitoring the patient for signs and symptoms of infection. Prescribed antibiotics should be initiated promptly, and the patient should be assessed for signs of dehydration. If the patient is to take prescribed oral antibiotics at home, he or she must understand the need to complete the entire course of antibiotic therapy and must be able to identify a feasible administration schedule.

PROMOTING COPING SKILLS

This illness, because of its acute exacerbations that often result in chronic health problems, frequently leaves the patient feeling powerless and with decreased self-esteem. These feelings can be exacerbated by inadequate pain management. The patient's ability to use normal coping resources of physical strength, psychological stamina, and positive self-esteem is dramatically diminished. Enhancing pain management can be extremely useful in establishing a therapeutic relationship based on mutual trust. Nursing care that focuses on the patient's strengths rather than deficits can enhance effective coping skills. Providing the patient with opportunities to make decisions about daily care may increase the patient's feelings of control.

MINIMIZING DEFICIENT KNOWLEDGE

Patients with sickle cell anemia benefit from understanding what situations can precipitate a sickle cell crisis and the steps they can take to prevent or diminish such crises. Keeping warm and maintaining adequate hydration can be very effective in diminishing the occurrence and severity of attacks. Avoiding stressful situations is more challenging. Group education may be more effective if it is carried out by members of the community who are from the same ethnic group as those with the disease.

MONITORING AND MANAGING POTENTIAL COMPLICATIONS

Management measures for many of the potential complications were delineated in previous sections. Other measures follow.

Leg Ulcers

Leg ulcers require careful management and protection from trauma and contamination. Referral to a wound care specialist may facilitate healing and assist with prevention. If leg ulcers fail to heal, skin grafting may be necessary. Scrupulous aseptic technique is warranted to prevent nosocomial infections.

Priapism Leading to Impotence

Male patients may develop sudden, painful episodes of priapism (persistent penile erection). The patient is taught to empty his bladder at the onset of the attack, exercise, and take a warm bath. If an episode persists longer than 3 hours, medical attention is recommended. Repeated episodes may lead to extensive vascular thrombosis, resulting in impotence.

Chronic Pain and Substance Abuse

Many patients have considerable difficulty coping with chronic pain and repeated episodes of sickle crisis. Those who feel they have little control over their health and the physical complications that result from this illness may find it difficult to understand the importance of complying with a prescribed treatment plan. Being nonjudgmental and actively seeking involvement from the patient in establishing a treatment plan are useful strategies.

Some patients with sickle cell anemia develop problems with substance abuse. For many, this abuse results from inadequate management of acute pain during episodes of crisis. Some clinicians suggest that abuse may result from prescribing inadequate amounts of opioid analgesics for an inadequate time. The patient's pain may never be adequately relieved, promoting mistrust of the health care system and (from the patient's perspective) the need to seek care from a variety of sources when the pain is not severe. This cycle is best managed by prevention. Receiving care from a single provider over time is much more beneficial than receiving care from rotating physicians and staff in an emergency department. When crises do arise, the staff in the emergency department should be in contact with the patient's primary health care provider so that optimal management can be achieved. Once the pattern of substance abuse is established, it is very difficult to manage, but continuity of care and establishing written contracts with the patient can be useful management strategies.

PROMOTING HOME AND COMMUNITY-BASED CARE

Teaching Patients Self-Care

Because patients with sickle cell anemia are typically diagnosed as children, parents participate in the initial education. Based on the parents' education, literacy, socioeconomic level, and interest, teaching focuses on the disease process (including some pathophysiology), treatment, and the assessment and monitoring skills for potential complications. As the child ages, educational interventions prepare the child to assume more responsibility for self-care.

Vascular access device management and chelation therapy can be taught to most families. Follow-up and care for patients with vascular access devices may also need to be provided by nurses in an outpatient facility or by a home care agency.

Continuing Care

The illness trajectory of sickle cell anemia is highly varied, with unpredictable episodes of complications and crises. Care is often provided on an emergency basis, especially for some patients with pain management problems (see previous section). Nurses in all settings used by this patient population need to communicate regularly with each other. Patients need to learn which parameters are important for them to monitor and how to monitor them. Parameters should also be given as to when to seek urgent care.

Evaluation

EXPECTED PATIENT OUTCOMES

Expected patient outcomes may include:

1. Control of pain
   a. Acute pain is controlled with analgesics
   b. Uses relaxation techniques, breathing exercises, distraction to help relieve pain
2. Is free of infection
   a. Has normal temperature
   b. Shows WBC count within normal range (5,000 to 10,000/mm^3)
   c. Identifies importance of continuing antibiotics at home (if applicable)
3. Expresses improved sense of control
   a. Participates in goal setting and in planning and implementing daily activities
   b. Participates in decisions about care
4. Increases knowledge about disease process
   a. Identifies situations and factors that can precipitate sickle cell crisis
   b. Describes lifestyle changes needed to prevent crisis
   c. Describes the importance of warmth, adequate hydration, and prevention of infection in preventing crisis
5. Absence of complications

THALASSEMIA

The thalassemias are a group of hereditary disorders associated with defective hemoglobin-chain synthesis. These anemias occur worldwide, but the highest prevalence is found in people of Mediterranean, African, and Southeast Asian ancestry (Hoffman et al., 2000). Thalassemias are characterized by **hypochromia** (an abnormal decrease in the hemoglobin content of RBCs), extreme **microcytosis** (smaller-than-normal RBCs), destruction of blood elements (hemolysis), and variable degrees of anemia.

In thalassemia, the production of one or more globulin chains within the hemoglobin molecule is reduced. When this occurs, the imbalance in the configuration of the hemoglobin causes it to precipitate in the erythroid precursors or the RBCs themselves. This increases the rigidity of the RBCs and thus the premature destruction of these cells.

The thalassemias are classified into two major groups according to the globin chain diminished: alpha and beta. The alpha-thalassemias occur mainly in people from Asia and the Middle East; the beta-thalassemias are most prevalent in Mediterranean populations but also occur in people from the Middle East or Asia. The alpha-thalassemias are milder than the beta forms and often occur without symptoms. The RBCs are extremely microcytic, but the anemia, if present, is mild.

The severity of beta-thalassemia varies depending on the extent to which the hemoglobin chains are affected. Patients with mild forms have a microcytosis and mild anemia. If left untreated, severe beta-thalassemia (thalassemia major, or Cooley's anemia) can be fatal within the first few years of life. If it is treated with regular transfusion of RBCs, patients may survive into their 20s and 30s. Patient teaching during the reproductive years should include pre-conception counselling about the risk of congenital thalassemia major.

Thalassemia Major

Thalassemia major (Cooley's anemia) is characterized by severe anemia, marked hemolysis, and ineffective erythropoiesis (production of RBCs). With early regular transfusion therapy, growth and development through childhood are facilitated. Organ dysfunction due to iron overload results from the excessive amounts of iron obtained through the RBC transfusions. Regular chelation therapy (eg, via subcutaneous deferoxamine) has reduced the complications of iron overload and prolonged the life of these patients. This disease is potentially curable by BMT if the procedure can be performed before damage to the liver occurs (ie, during childhood).

GLUCOSE-6-PHOSPHATE DEHYDROGENASE DEFICIENCY

The abnormality in this disorder is in the G-6-PD gene; this gene produces an enzyme within the RBC that is essential for membrane stability. A few patients have inherited an enzyme so defective that they have a chronic hemolytic anemia; however, the most common type of defect results in hemolysis only when the RBCs are stressed by certain situations, such as fever or the use of certain medications. The disorder came to the attention of researchers during World War II, when some soldiers developed hemolysis while taking primaquine, an antimalarial agent. African Americans and people of Greek or Italian origin are those primarily affected by this disorder. The type of deficiency found in the Mediterranean population is more severe than that in the African Caribbean population, resulting in greater hemolysis and sometimes in life-threatening anemia. All types of G-6-PD deficiency are inherited as X-linked defects; therefore, many more men are at risk than women. In the United States, about 12% of African American males are affected. The deficiency is also common in those of Asian ancestry and in certain Jewish populations.

Medications that have hemolytic effects for people with G-6-PD deficiency are oxidant drugs. These medications include antimalarial agents (eg, chloroquine [Aralen]), sulfonamides (eg, trimethoprim and sulfamethoxazole [Septra]), nitrofurantoin (eg, Macrodantin), common coal tar analgesics (including aspirin in high doses), thiazide diuretics (eg, hydrochlorothiazide [Apo-Hydro, Novo-Hydrazide], chlorothiazide [Diuril]), oral hypoglycemic agents (eg, glyburide [Albert Glyburide, Englucon], metformin [Glucophage]), chloramphenicol (Chloromycetin), and vitamin K (phytonadione [Aqua-Mephyton]). In affected people, a severe hemolytic episode can result from ingestion of fava beans.

Clinical Manifestations

Patients are asymptomatic and have normal hemoglobin levels and reticulocyte counts most of the time. However, several days after exposure to an offending medication, they may develop pallor, jaundice, and hemoglobinuria (hemoglobin in the urine). The reticulocyte count rises, and symptoms of hemolysis develop. Special stains of the peripheral blood may then disclose Heinz bodies (degraded hemoglobin) within the RBCs. Hemolysis is often mild and self-limited. However, in the more severe Mediterranean type of G-6-PD deficiency, spontaneous recovery may not occur and transfusions may be necessary.

Assessment and Diagnostic Findings

The diagnosis is made by a screening test or by a quantitative assay of G-6-PD.

Medical Management

The treatment is to stop the offending medication. Transfusion is necessary only in the severe hemolytic state, which is more commonly seen in the Mediterranean variety of G-6-PD deficiency.

Nursing Management

The patient should be educated about the disease and given a list of medications to avoid. If hemolysis does develop, nursing interventions are the same as for hemolysis from other causes.

HEREDITARY SPHEROCYTOSIS

Hereditary spherocytosis is a relatively common (1 in 5,000 people) hemolytic anemia characterized by an abnormal permeability of the RBC membrane; this permits the cells to change into a spherical shape. These RBCs are destroyed prematurely in the spleen. The severity of this hemolytic anemia varies; jaundice can be intermittent, and splenomegaly (enlarged spleen) also can occur. Surgical removal of the spleen is the principal treatment for this disorder.

IMMUNE HEMOLYTIC ANEMIA

Hemolytic anemias can result from exposure of the RBC to antibodies. Alloantibodies (ie, antibodies against the host, or "self") result from the immunization of an individual with foreign antigens (eg, the immunization of an Rh-negative person with Rh-positive blood). Alloantibodies tend to be large (IgM type) and cause immediate destruction of the sensitized RBCs, either within the blood vessel (intravascular hemolysis) or within the liver. The most common type of alloimmune hemolytic anemia in adults results from a hemolytic transfusion reaction.

Autoantibodies are developed by an individual for varying reasons. In many instances, the person's immune system is dysfunctional, so that it falsely recognizes its own RBCs as foreign and produces antibodies against them. This mechanism is seen in people with chronic lymphocytic leukemia (CLL). Another mechanism is a deficiency in suppressor lymphocytes, which normally prevent antibody formation against a person's own antigens. Autoantibodies tend to be of the IgG type. The RBCs are sequestered in the spleen and destroyed by the macrophages outside the blood vessel (extravascular hemolysis).

Autoimmune hemolytic anemias can be classified based on the body temperature involved when the antibodies react with the RBC antigen. Warm-body antibodies bind to RBCs most actively in warm conditions (37°C); cold-body antibodies react in cold (0°C). Most autoimmune hemolytic anemias are the warm-body type. Autoimmune hemolytic anemia is associated with other disorders in most cases (eg, medication exposure, lymphoma, CLL, other malignancy, collagen vascular disease, autoimmune disease, infection). In idiopathic autoimmune hemolytic states, the reason why the immune system produces the antibodies is not known. All ages and both genders are equally vulnerable to this form, whereas the incidence of secondary forms is greater in people older than 45 years of age and in females.

Clinical Manifestations

Clinical manifestations can vary, and they usually reflect the degree of anemia. The hemolysis may be very mild, so that the patient's marrow compensates adequately and the patient is asymptomatic. At the other extreme, the hemolysis can be so severe that the resultant anemia is life-threatening. Most patients complain of fatigue and dizziness. Splenomegaly is the most common physical finding, occurring in more than 80% of patients; hepatomegaly, lymphadenopathy, and jaundice are also common.

Assessment and Diagnostic Findings

The laboratory tests show a low hemoglobin level and hematocrit, most often with an accompanying increase in the reticulocyte count. RBCs appear abnormal; spherocytes are common. The serum bilirubin level is elevated, and if the hemolysis is severe, the haptoglobin level is low or absent. The Coombs test (also referred to as the direct antiglobulin test [DAT]), which detects antibodies on the surface of RBCs, shows a positive result.

Medical Management

Any possibly offending medication should be immediately discontinued. The treatment consists of high doses of corticosteroids (1 mg/kg per day) until hemolysis decreases. Corticosteroids decrease the macrophage's ability to clear the antibody-coated RBCs. If the hemoglobin level returns toward normal, usually after several weeks, the corticosteroid dose can be lowered or, in some cases, tapered and discontinued. However, corticosteroids rarely produce a lasting remission. In severe cases, blood transfusions may be required. Because the antibody may react with all possible donor cells, careful blood typing is necessary, and the transfusion should be administered slowly and cautiously.

Splenectomy (removal of the spleen) removes the major site of RBC destruction; therefore, splenectomy may be performed if corticosteroids do not produce a remission. If neither corticosteroid therapy nor splenectomy is successful, immunosuppressive agents may be administered. The two immunosuppressive agents most frequently used are cyclophosphamide (Cytoxan, Procytox), which has a more rapid effect but more toxicity, or azathioprine (Imuran), which has a less rapid effect but less toxicity. The synthetic androgen danazol (eg, Cyclomen, Danocrine) can be useful in some patients, particularly in combination with corticosteroids. The mechanism for this success is unclear. If corticosteroids or immunosuppressive agents are used, the taper must be very gradual to prevent a rebound "hyperimmune" response and exacerbation of the hemolysis. Immunoglobulin administration is effective in about one third of patients, but the effect is transient and the medication is expensive. Transfusions may be necessary if the anemia is severe; it may be extremely difficult to cross-match samples of available units of RBCs with that of the patient.

For patients with cold-antibody hemolytic anemia, treatment may not be required, other than to advise the patient to keep warm; relocation to a warm climate may be necessary.

Nursing Management

Patients may have great difficulty understanding the pathologic mechanisms underlying the disease and need repeated explanations in terms they can understand. Patients who have had a splenectomy should be vaccinated against pneumococcal infections (Pneumovax) and informed that they are permanently at greater risk for infection. Patients receiving long-term corticosteroid therapy, particularly those with concurrent diabetes or hypertension, need careful monitoring. They must understand the need for this medication and the importance of never abruptly discontinuing it. A written explanation and a tapering schedule should be provided, and adjustments based on hemoglobin levels should be emphasized. Similar teaching should be provided when immunosuppressive agents are used. Corticosteroid therapy is not without significant risk, and patients need to be monitored closely for complications. The short- and long-term complications of corticosteroid therapy are presented in Chart 33-4 and in Chap. 42.

> **NURSING ALERT** It can be difficult to cross-match blood when antibodies are present. If imperfectly cross-matched RBCs must be transfused, the nurse begins the infusion very slowly (10 to 15 mL over 20 to 30 minutes) and monitors the patient very closely for signs and symptoms of a hemolytic transfusion reaction.

HEREDITARY HEMOCHROMATOSIS

Hemochromatosis is a genetic condition in which iron is abnormally (excessively) absorbed from the gastrointestinal tract. The excessive iron is deposited in various organs, particularly the liver, myocardium, testes, thyroid, and pancreas. Eventually, the affected organs become dysfunctional. The actual incidence of hemochromatosis is unknown; however, hereditary hemochromatosis is diagnosed in 0.5% of the population in Canada (ie, 1 million people). However, 1 in 250–300 Canadians is at risk of developing the full-blown disease (with two genes), and between 1 in 7 to 1 in 9 individuals is a carrier (with one gene). Recent data suggest that this defect may be a common cause of diabetes (Schechter, et al., 2000). Because of their natural loss of iron through menses, women are less affected than men.

Because the accumulation of iron in body organs occurs gradually, there often is no evidence of tissue injury until middle age. Symptoms of weakness, lethargy, arthralgia, weight loss, and loss of libido are common. The skin may be hyperpigmented with melanin deposits (occasionally **hemosiderin**, an iron-containing pigment) and appears bronze in colour. Cardiac dysrhythmias and cardiomyopathy can occur, with resulting dyspnea and edema. Endocrine dysfunction is manifested as hypothyroidism, diabetes mellitus, and hypogonadism (testicular atrophy, diminished libido, and impotence). A significant effect of hemochromatosis is the

---

Chart 33-4 • PHARMACOLOGY
Complications Associated with Corticosteroid Therapy

Whenever a patient begins a course of corticosteroid therapy, the potential for complications is great. Dosing regimens vary widely, depending on the underlying hematologic condition and the patient's response to the medication. For example, several chemotherapy protocols include high doses of corticosteroids for a period of several days. After that time, the medication is stopped abruptly without tapering the dosage. In other conditions, such as idiopathic thrombocytopenic purpura or hemolytic anemias, the corticosteroids are very carefully tapered to prevent a flare up of the underlying disease. With the exception of patients with preexisting conditions such as diabetes, hypertension, and osteoporosis, it is difficult to predict which complications will occur in a given patient. Patients who receive high doses of corticosteroids for longer than a few weeks should be screened for symptoms related to the potential complications listed here. If at all possible, patients who require long-term corticosteroid use should be switched to an alternate-day dosing schedule; this method may diminish the severity of complications that arise.

Short-Term Complications
Fluid and Electrolyte Complications
Fluid retention
Sodium retention
Potassium loss
Hypokalemic alkalosis
Hypertension

Endocrine Complications
Decreased carbohydrate tolerance
Diabetes mellitus
Uncontrolled glucose levels in diabetes mellitus

Neurologic Complications
Headache

Musculoskeletal Complications
Muscle weakness

Psychologic Complications
Depression
Euphoria
Mood swings
Insomnia
Psychosis

Long-Term Complications
Endocrine Complications
Decreased adrenocortical activity
Decreased ability to respond to stress
Decreased carbohydrate tolerance
Decreased growth rate (children)
Cushingoid state
Menstrual irregularities
Increased sweating

Metabolic Complications
Protein catabolism causing negative nitrogen balance

Gastrointestinal Complications
Gastritis
Ulcerative esophagitis
Peptic ulcer
Pancreatitis

Musculoskeletal Complications
Decreased muscle mass
Osteoporosis
Vertebral compression fracture
Pathologic fracture
Aseptic necrosis of femoral and humeral heads

Neurologic Complications
Vertigo
Increased intracranial pressure
Seizures

Ophthalmic Complications
Cataract formation
Glaucoma
Exophthalmos

Dermatologic Complications
Impaired wound healing
Ecchymoses
Increased skin fragility
Decreased skin thickness
Petechiae

Immunologic Complications
Decreased response to infection
Masked signs of early stages of infection
Suppressed reaction to skin tests
Increased risk for opportunistic infection (eg, *Pneumocystis*, herpes zoster)

development of hepatocellular carcinoma in one third of those affected. CBC values are typically normal. The most useful laboratory findings are an elevated serum iron level and high transferrin saturation (more than 60% in men, more than 50% in women). The definitive diagnostic test is a liver biopsy. Recently, a mutation in the *HFE* gene has been shown to occur in most patients with hereditary hemochromatosis (Gochee & Powell, 2001). Patients who are homozygous for the gene are at high risk for development of the disorder.

Medical Management

Therapy involves the removal of excess iron via therapeutic phlebotomy (removal of whole blood from a vein). Each unit of blood removed results in a decrease of 200–250 mg of iron. The objective typically is to reduce the serum ferritin to less than 50 μg/L and the transferrin saturation to 35% or less. To achieve this, a frequent phlebotomy schedule is required (1 to 2 units weekly), with a gradual reduction in frequency of phlebotomies over a 1- to 3-year period. After 1 to 3 years, the frequency of phlebotomy can be reduced to 1 unit of blood every several months to prevent reaccumulation of iron deposits. Removal of excess iron appears to diminish the severity of diabetes and skin hyperpigmentation; cardiac function also tends to improve.

Nursing Management

Patients with hemochromatosis often believe that it is important to limit their dietary intake of iron, although this management method has been shown to be very ineffective and need not be encouraged. However, it is important for these patients to avoid any additional insults to the liver, such as alcohol abuse. Serial screening tests for hepatoma are important; alpha-fetoprotein is used for this purpose. Other body systems should be monitored for signs of organ dysfunction, particularly the endocrine and cardiac systems. These systems should also be screened routinely for dysfunction so that appropriate management can be implemented quickly. Because patients with hemochromatosis require frequent phlebotomies, problems with venous access are common. Patients who are heterozygous for the *HFE* do not develop the disease but need to be counselled that they can transmit the gene to their children.

The Polycythemias

Polycythemia refers to an increased volume of RBCs. It is a term used when the hematocrit is elevated (to more than 55% in males, more than 50% in females). Dehydration (decreased volume of plasma) can cause an elevated hematocrit, but not typically to the level to be considered polycythemia. Polycythemia is classified as either primary or secondary.

POLYCYTHEMIA VERA

Polycythemia vera, or primary polycythemia, is a proliferative disorder in which the myeloid stem cells seem to have escaped normal control mechanisms. The bone marrow is hypercellular, and the RBC, WBC, and platelet counts in the peripheral blood are elevated. However, the RBC elevation is predominant; the hematocrit can exceed 60%. This phase can last for an extended period (10 years or longer). The spleen resumes its embryonic function of hematopoiesis and enlarges. Over time, the bone marrow may become fibrotic, with a resultant inability to produce as many cells

("burnt out" or spent phase). The disease evolves into myeloid metaplasia with myelofibrosis or AML in a significant proportion of patients; this form of AML is usually refractory to standard treatments (Hoffman, et al., 2000). The median survival time exceeds 15 years (Gruppo Italiano Studio Policitemia, 1995).

Clinical Manifestations

Patients typically have a ruddy complexion and splenomegaly (enlarged spleen). The symptoms result from the increased blood volume (headache, dizziness, tinnitus, fatigue, paresthesias, and blurred vision) or from increased blood viscosity (angina, claudication, dyspnea, and thrombophlebitis), particularly if the patient has atherosclerotic blood vessels. Another common and bothersome problem is generalized pruritus, which may be caused by histamine release due to the increased number of basophils. Erythromelalgia, a burning sensation in the fingers and toes, may be reported and is only partially relieved by cooling.

Assessment and Diagnostic Findings

Diagnosis is made by finding an elevated RBC mass (a nuclear medicine procedure), a normal oxygen saturation level, and an enlarged spleen. Other factors useful in establishing the diagnosis include elevated WBC and platelet counts. The erythropoietin level is not as low as would be expected with an elevated hematocrit; it is normal or only slightly low. Causes of secondary erythrocytosis should not be present (see later discussion).

Complications

Patients with polycythemia vera are at increased risk for thromboses resulting in a CVA (brain attack, stroke) or heart attack (MI); thrombotic complications are the most frequent cause of death. Bleeding is also a complication, possibly due to the fact that the platelets (often very large) are somewhat dysfunctional. The bleeding can be significant and can occur in the form of nosebleeds, ulcers, and frank gastrointestinal bleeding.

Medical Management

The objective of management is to reduce the high blood cell mass. Phlebotomy is an important part of therapy and can be performed repeatedly to keep the hematocrit within normal range. This is achieved by removing enough blood (initially 500 mL once or twice weekly) to deplete the patient's iron stores, thereby rendering the patient iron deficient and consequently unable to continue to manufacture RBCs excessively. Patients need to be instructed to avoid iron supplements, including those within multivitamin supplements. If the patient has an elevated uric acid concentration, allopurinol (Zyloprim) is used to prevent gouty attacks. Antihistamines are not particularly effective in controlling itching. If the patient develops ischemic symptoms, dipyridamole (eg, Persantine) is sometimes used. Radioactive phosphorus (^{32}P) or chemotherapeutic agents (eg, hydroxyurea [Hydrea]) can be used to suppress marrow function, but they may increase the risk for leukemia. Patients receiving hydroxyurea appear to have a lower incidence of thrombotic complications; this may result from a more controlled platelet count. The use of aspirin to prevent thrombotic complications is controversial. Low-dose aspirin is frequently used in patients with cardiovascular disease, but even this dose is often avoided in patients with prior bleeding, especially bleeding from the gastrointestinal tract. Aspirin is also useful in diminishing pain associated with erythromelalgia. Anagrelide (Agrylin) inhibits platelet aggregation and can also be useful in controlling the thrombocytosis associated with polycythemia vera. Interferon alfa-2b (Intron-A) has also been studied, but it may be difficult for patients to tolerate due to the frequent side effects experienced (Tefferi et al., 2000; Lengfelder, Berger, & Hehlmann, 2000).

Nursing Management

The nurse's role is primarily that of educator. Risk factors for thrombotic complications should be assessed, and patients should be instructed regarding the signs and symptoms of thrombosis. Patients with a history of bleeding are usually advised to avoid aspirin and aspirin-containing medications, because these medications alter platelet function. Minimizing alcohol intake should also be emphasized to further diminish any risk for bleeding. For pruritus, the nurse may recommend bathing in tepid or cool water, along with applications of cocoa butter–based lotions and bath products.

SECONDARY POLYCYTHEMIA

Secondary polycythemia is caused by excessive production of erythropoietin. This may occur in response to a reduced amount of oxygen, which acts as a hypoxic stimulus, as in cigarette smoking, chronic obstructive pulmonary disease, or cyanotic heart disease, or in nonpathologic conditions such as high altitude. It can also result from certain hemoglobinopathies in which the hemoglobin has an abnormally high affinity for oxygen (eg, hemoglobin Chesapeake). Secondary polycythemia can also occur from neoplasms (eg, renal cell carcinoma) that stimulate erythropoietin production.

Medical Management

Management of secondary polycythemia may not be necessary; when it is, it involves treating the primary conditions. If the cause cannot be corrected (eg, by treating the renal cell carcinoma or improving pulmonary function), therapeutic phlebotomy may be necessary in symptomatic patients to reduce blood viscosity and volume.

Leukopenia and Neutropenia

Leukopenia, a condition in which there are fewer WBCs than normal, results from neutropenia (diminished neutrophils) or lymphopenia (diminished lymphocytes). Even if other types of WBCs (eg, monocytes, basophils) are diminished, their numbers are too few to reduce the total WBC count significantly. Lymphopenia (lymphocytes less than 1,500/mm^3) can result from ionizing radiation, long-term use of corticosteroids, uremia, some neoplasms (eg, breast and lung cancers, advanced Hodgkin's disease), and some protein-losing enteropathies (in which the lymphocytes within the intestines are lost).

NEUTROPENIA

Neutropenia (neutrophils less than 2,000/mm^3) results from decreased production of neutrophils or increased destruction of these cells (Chart 33-5). Neutrophils are essential in preventing and limiting bacterial infection. A patient with neutropenia is at increased risk for infection, both exogenous and endogenous (the gastro-

Chart 33-5   Causes of Neutropenia

Decreased Production of Neutrophils
- Aplastic anemia, due to medications or toxins
- Metastatic cancer, lymphoma, leukemia
- Myelodysplastic syndromes
- Chemotherapy
- Radiation therapy

Ineffective Granulocytopoiesis
- Megaloblastic anemia

Increased Destruction of Neutrophils
- Hypersplenism
- Medication-induced*
- Immunologic disease (eg, systemic lupus erythematosus [SLE])
- Viral disease (eg, infectious hepatitis, mononucleosis)
- Bacterial infections

*Formation of antibody to medication, leading to a rapid decrease in neutrophils.

intestinal tract and skin are common endogenous sources). The risk for infection is based not only on the severity of the neutropenia (low neutrophil count), but also on the duration of the neutropenia. The actual number of neutrophils, known as the **absolute neutrophil count (ANC)**, is determined by a simple mathematical calculation using data obtained from the CBC and differential test (Chart 33-6). The risk of infection increases proportionately with the decrease in neutrophil count. The risk is significant when the ANC is less than 1000, is high when it is less than 500, and is almost certain when it is less than 100. The risk

Chart 33-6   Calculating the Absolute Neutrophil Count (ANC)

$$ANC = \frac{\text{Total WBC count} \times (\% \text{ neutrophils} + \% \text{ bands})}{100}$$

Normally, the neutrophil count is greater than 2000/mm^3. The actual (or absolute) neutrophil count (ANC) is calculated using the above formula.

For example, if the total white blood cell (WBC) count is 3000/mm^3 with 72% neutrophils and 3% bands, the ANC would be calculated as follows:

$$ANC = \frac{3000\,(72 + 3)}{100} = 2250$$

This result is not indicative of neutropenia, because the ANC is greater than 2000 despite the low total WBC count (3000/mm^3).

Conversely, in the following example, neutropenia is evident despite a normal WBC count (5500/mm^3) with 8% neutrophils and 0% bands:

$$ANC = \frac{5500\,(8 + 0)}{100} = 440$$

Here, the ANC is severely low (440) despite the normal total WBC count (5500/mm^3).

When evaluating neutropenia, it is important to calculate the ANC and not to rely solely on the total WBCs and percentage of neutrophils alone.

of developing infection increases with the length of time during which neutropenia persists, even if it is fairly mild. Conversely, even a severe neutropenia may not result in infection if the duration of the neutropenia is brief, as is often seen after chemotherapy (Chart 33-7).

Clinical Manifestations

There are no definite symptoms of neutropenia until the patient becomes infected. Routine CBC with differential tests, such as those obtained after chemotherapy treatment, can reveal neutropenia before the onset of infection.

Medical Management

Treatment of the neutropenia varies depending on its cause. If the neutropenia is medication induced, the offending agent needs to be stopped, if possible. Treatment of an underlying neoplasm can temporarily make the neutropenia worse, but with bone marrow recovery treatment may improve it. Corticosteroids may be used if the cause is an immunologic disorder. The use of growth factors such as G-CSF (Neupogen) or granulocyte/macrophage colony-stimulating factor (GM-CSF [Leukine]) can be effective in increasing neutrophil production when the cause of the neutropenia is decreased production. Withholding or reducing the dose of chemotherapy or radiation therapy may be required when the neutropenia is caused by these treatments; however, in the case of potentially curative therapy, administration of growth factor is considered to be preferable, so that the maximum antitumour effect can be achieved. Should the neutropenia be accompanied by fever, the patient is automatically considered to be infected and usually is admitted to the hospital. Cultures of blood, urine, and sputum should be obtained, as well as a chest x-ray. To ensure adequate therapy against the invading infectious organisms, broad-spectrum antibiotics are initiated as soon as the samples for culture are obtained, although the medications may be changed after culture and sensitivity results become available.

Nursing Management

Nurses in all settings have a crucial role in assessing the severity of neutropenia and in preventing and managing infectious complications. Patient teaching is equally important, particularly in the outpatient setting, so that the patient can implement appropriate self-care measures and know when and how to seek medical care (Chart 33-8). Patients at risk for neutropenia should have blood drawn for CBCs; the frequency is based on the suspected severity and duration of the neutropenia. Nurses need to be able to calculate the ANC (see Chart 33-6) and to assess the severity of neutropenia and the risk for infection. Chart 33-9 identifies nursing interventions related to neutropenia.

Leukocytosis and the Leukemias

The term *leukocytosis* refers to an increased level of WBCs in the circulation. Typically, only one specific cell type is increased. Usually, because the proportions of several types of WBCs are small (eg, eosinophils, basophils, monocytes), only an increase in neutrophils or lymphocytes can be great enough to elevate the total WBC count. Although leukocytosis can be a normal response to increased need (eg, in acute infection), the elevation in WBCs should decrease as the need decreases. A prolonged or progressively increasing elevation in WBCs is abnormal and should be evaluated. A significant cause for persistent leukocytosis is malignancy.

Hematopoiesis is characterized by a rapid, continuous turnover of cells. Normally, production of specific blood cells

---

Chart 33-7
Risk Factors for Development of Infection and Bleeding in Patients with Hematologic Disorders

Risk for Infection
Severity of neutropenia: Risk of infection is proportional to duration and severity of neutropenia

Duration of neutropenia: Increased duration leads to increased risk of infection

Nutritional status: Decreased protein stores lead to decreased immune response and anergy

Deconditioning: Decreased mobility leads to decreased respiratory effort, leading to increased pooling of secretions

Lymphocytopenia; disorders of lymphoid system (chronic lymphocytic leukemia [CLL], lymphoma, myeloma): Decreased cell-mediated and humoural immunity

Invasive procedures: Break in skin integrity leads to increased opportunity for organisms to enter blood system

Hypogammaglobulinemia: Decreased antibody formation

Poor hygiene: Increased organisms on skin, mucous membranes

Poor dentition; mucositis: Decreased endothelial integrity leads to increased opportunity for organisms to enter blood system

Antibiotic therapy: Increased risk for superinfection, often fungal

Certain medications: See text

Risk for Bleeding
Severity of thrombocytopenia: Risk increases when platelet count decreases; usually not a significant risk until platelet count is lower than 20,000/mm³; lower than 50,000/mm³ when invasive procedure performed

Duration of thrombocytopenia: Risk increases when duration increases (eg, risk is less when duration is transient after chemotherapy than when duration is permanent with poor marrow production)

Sepsis: Mechanism unknown; appears to cause increased platelet consumption

Increased intracranial pressure: Increased blood pressure leads to rupture of blood vessels

Liver dysfunction: Decreased synthesis of clotting factors

Renal dysfunction: Decreased platelet function

Dysproteinemia: Protein coats surface of platelet, leading to decreased platelet function; protein causes increased viscosity, which leads to increased stretching of capillaries and thus increased bleeding

Alcohol abuse: Suppressive effect on marrow leads to decreased platelet production, decreased platelet function; decreased liver function, resulting in decreased production of clotting factors

Splenomegaly: Increased platelet destruction; spleen traps circulating platelets

Concurrent medications: See text

Chart 33-8
Home Care Checklist • **The Patient at Risk for Infection**

At the completion of the home care instruction, the patient or caregiver will be able to:	Patient	Caregiver
• Describe consequences of alterations in neutrophils, lymphocytes, immunoglobulins, or their sources.	✓	✓
• Verbalize the rationale for being at risk for infection.	✓	✓
• Identify signs and symptoms of infection.	✓	✓
• Demonstrate how to monitor for signs of infection.	✓	✓
• Describe to whom, how, and when to report signs of infection.	✓	✓
• Identify appropriate behaviours to take to prevent infection:	✓	✓
– Maintain good hand hygiene technique, total body hygiene, and skin integrity.		
– Avoid fresh flowers, plants, garden work (soil), bird cages, and litter boxes.		
– Avoid fresh salads and unpeeled fruits or vegetables.		
– Maintain a high-calorie, high-protein diet, with fluid intake of 3,000 mL (unless fluids are restricted).		
– Avoid people with infections, crowds.		
– Perform deep breathing, use incentive spirometer every 4 hr while awake.		
– Provide adequate lubrication with gentle vaginal manipulation during sexual intercourse; avoid anal intercourse.		
• Describe appropriate actions to take should infection occur.	✓	✓

from their stem cell precursors is carefully regulated according to the body's needs. If the mechanisms that control the production of these cells are disrupted, the cells can proliferate to an excessive, potentially dangerous degree. Hematopoietic malignancies are often classified according to the cells involved. **Leukemia**, literally "white blood," is a neoplastic proliferation of one particular cell type (granulocytes, monocytes, lymphocytes, or megakaryocytes). The defect originates in the hematopoietic stem cell, the myeloid, or the lymphoid stem cell. The lymphomas are neoplasms of lymphoid tissue, usually derived from B lymphocytes. Multiple myeloma is a malignancy of the most mature form of B lymphocyte, the plasma cell.

The common feature of the leukemias is an unregulated proliferation of WBCs in the bone marrow. In acute forms (or late stages of chronic forms), the proliferation of leukemic cells leaves little room for normal cell production. There can also be a proliferation of cells in the liver and spleen (extramedullary hematopoiesis). With acute forms, there can be infiltration of other organs, such as the meninges, lymph nodes, gums, and skin. The cause of leukemia is not fully known, but there is some evidence that genetic influence and viral pathogenesis may be involved. Bone marrow damage from radiation exposure or from chemicals such as benzene and alkylating agents (eg, melphalan [Alkeran]) can cause leukemia.

The leukemias are commonly classified according to the stem cell line involved, either lymphoid or myeloid. They are also classified as either acute or chronic, based on the time it takes for symptoms to evolve and the phase of cell development that is halted (ie, with few WBCs differentiating beyond that phase).

In acute leukemia, the onset of symptoms is abrupt, often occurring within a few weeks. WBC development is halted at the blast phase, so that most WBCs are undifferentiated or are blasts. Acute leukemia progresses very rapidly; death occurs within weeks to months without aggressive treatment. In chronic leukemia, symptoms evolve over a period of months to years, and the majority of WBCs produced are mature. Chronic leukemia progresses more slowly; the disease trajectory can extend for years.

ACUTE MYELOID LEUKEMIA (AML)

AML results from a defect in the hematopoietic stem cell that differentiates into all myeloid cells: monocytes, granulocytes (neutrophils, basophils, eosinophils), erythrocytes, and platelets. All age groups are affected; the incidence rises with age, with a peak incidence at age 60 years. AML is the most common nonlymphocytic leukemia.

The prognosis is highly variable and is not consistently based on patient or disease variables. Patients with AML have a potentially curable disease. However, patients who are older or have a more undifferentiated form of AML tend to have a worse prognosis. Those who have preexisting MDS or who had previously received alkylating agents for cancer (secondary AML) have a much worse prognosis; the leukemia tends to be more resistant to treatment, resulting in a much shorter duration of remission. With treatment, these patients survive an average of less than 1 year, with death usually a result of infection or hemorrhage. Patients receiving supportive care also usually survive less than 1 year, dying from infection or bleeding.

Clinical Manifestations

Most of the signs and symptoms evolve from insufficient production of normal blood cells. Fever and infection result from neutropenia, weakness and fatigue from anemia, and bleeding tendencies from thrombocytopenia. The proliferation of leukemic cells within organs leads to a variety of additional symptoms: pain from an enlarged liver or spleen, hyperplasia of the gums, and bone pain from expansion of marrow.

Assessment and Diagnostic Findings

The disorder develops without warning, with symptoms occurring over a period of weeks to months. CBC results show a decrease in both erythrocytes and platelets. Although the total leukocyte count can be low, normal, or high, the percentage of normal cells is usually vastly decreased. A bone marrow analysis shows an ex-

Chart 33-9 · Neutropenia Precautions

Nursing Diagnosis
Risk for infection secondary to impaired immunoincompetence due to:
- Diminished neutrophil count (see below) secondary to bone marrow invasion or hypocellularity secondary to medications
- Dysfunctional neutrophils (eg, secondary to myelodysplastic syndrome [MDS])
- Dysfunctional or diminished lymphocytes
- Hypogammaglobulinemia
- Diminished immune response or anergy
- Malnutrition
- Surgery or invasive procedures
- Antibiotic therapy (increased risk for superimposed infection)
  - Neutropenic, infected patients often do *not* exhibit the classic signs of inflammation/infection (ie, redness, cloudiness of any drainage); the only initial sign may be fever (and it often occurs later in the infectious process with neutropenia).
  - Skin and mucous membranes are the body's first line of defense against infection; loss of endothelial cell integrity allows organisms to enter the blood and lymph systems.

Assessment
Patient
Assess the following areas thoroughly every shift or visit (with spot checks throughout shift if hospitalized) and notify physician of any signs of infection or worsening of status:
- *Skin:* Check for tenderness, edema, breaks in skin integrity, moisture, drainage, lesions (especially under breasts, axillae, groin, skin folds, bony prominences, perineum); check all puncture sites (eg, intravenous sites) for signs and symptoms of inflammation/infection.
- *Oral mucosa:* Check for moisture, lesions, colour (check palate, tongue, buccal mucosa, gums, lips, oropharynx).
- *Respiratory:* Check for presence of cough, sore throat; auscultate breath sounds.
- *Gastrointestinal:* Check for abdominal discomfort/distention, nausea, change in bowel pattern; auscultate bowel sounds.
- *Genitourinary:* Check for dysuria, urgency, frequency; check urine for colour, clarity, odour.
- *Neurologic:* Check for complaints of headache, neck stiffness, visual disturbances; assess level of consciousness, orientation, behaviour.
- *Temperature:* Check every 4 hr or every visit; call primary health care provider if temperature is >38°C, fever is unresponsive to acetaminophen, or patient shows a decline in hemodynamic status.

Diagnostic Studies
- Monitor complete blood count (CBC) and differential daily (especially absolute neutrophil count [ANC], lymphocyte count).
- Call physician if ANC is <1,000, significantly different from previous count, or whenever patient becomes symptomatic (eg, febrile).
- Monitor globulin, albumin, total protein levels.
- Monitor all culture and sensitivity reports.
- Monitor radiology reports.

Nursing Interventions
Environment and Staff
- **Thorough hand hygiene must be done by everyone before entering patient's room each and every time.**

- Allow no one with a cold or sore throat to care for the patient or to enter room, or come in contact with patient at home.
- Care for neutropenic patients before caring for other patients (as much as possible).
- Use private room for patient if ANC is <1,000.
- Allow no fresh flowers (stagnant water).
- Change water in containers every shift (include O_2 humidification systems every 24 hr).
- Ensure room is cleaned daily.

Dietary
- Provide low microbial diet.
- Eliminate fresh salads and unpeeled fresh fruits or vegetables.

Patient
- Avoid suppositories, enemas, rectal temperatures.
- Practice deep breathing (with incentive spirometer) every 4 hr while awake.
- Ambulate; wear high-efficiency particulate air (HEPA) filter mask if neutropenia is severe.
- Prevent skin dryness with water-soluble lubricants, especially in high-risk areas (eg, lips, corners of mouth, elbows, feet, bony prominences).

Hygiene
- Provide meticulous total body hygiene daily (preferably with antimicrobial solution), including perineal care after every bowel movement.
- Provide thorough oral hygiene after meals and every 4 hr while awake; warm saline, or salt and soda solution, is effective; avoid use of lemon-glycerine swabs, commercial mouthwashes, and hydrogen peroxide.

Intravenous (IV) Therapy
- Do not use plastic cannulas for peripheral IVs when ANC is <500 (if possible per agency); a central vascular access device is preferred for long-term or intensive IV therapy.
- Inspect IV sites every shift; monitor closely for any discomfort; erythema may not be present.
- Maintain meticulous IV site care.
- Cleanse skin with antimicrobial solution before venipuncture (unless patient is allergic).
- Moisture-vapor–permeable dressings are permissible with strict adherence to institutional protocol.
- Change IV tubing per institution policy, using aseptic technique.
- Administer antimicrobial agents on time.

Expected Patient Outcomes
- Patient demonstrates an absence of infection as evidenced by an absence of fever, chills, inflammation, drainage, cough, dyspnea, sore throat, dysuria, or urinary frequency.
- Patient demonstrates an absence of infection as evidenced by the presence of vital signs within normal limits, including intact neurologic status and intact skin.

Duration of Evaluation
Until patient is no longer neutropenic and any infection is resolved.

---

cess of immature blast cells (more than 30%). AML can be further classified into seven different subgroups, based on cytogenetics, histology, and morphology (appearance) of the blasts. The actual prognosis varies somewhat between subgroups, but the clinical course and treatment differ substantially with only one subtype, acute promyelocytic leukemia (APL, or AML-M3). Patients with this leukemia often have significantly more problems with bleed-

ing, in that they have underlying coagulopathy and a higher incidence of disseminated intravascular coagulation (DIC).

Complications

Complications of AML include bleeding and infection, the major causes of death. The risk of bleeding correlates with the level of platelet deficiency (thrombocytopenia). The low platelet count can result in **ecchymoses** (bruises) and **petechiae** (pinpoint red or purple hemorrhagic spots on the skin). Major hemorrhages also may develop when the platelet count drops to less than 10,000/mm³. The most common sites of bleeding are gastrointestinal, pulmonary, and intracranial. For undetermined reasons, fever and infection also increase the likelihood of bleeding.

Because of the lack of mature and normal granulocytes, patients with leukemia are always threatened by infection. The likelihood of infection increases with the degree and duration of neutropenia; neutrophil counts that persist at less than 100/mm³ make the chances of systemic infection extremely high. As the duration of severe neutropenia increases, the patient's risk for developing fungal infection also increases.

Medical Management

The overall objective of treatment is to achieve complete remission, in which there is no detectable evidence of residual leukemia remaining in the bone marrow. Attempts are made to achieve remission by the aggressive administration of chemotherapy, called induction therapy, which usually requires hospitalization for several weeks. Induction therapy typically involves high doses of cytarabine (Alkeron) and daunorubicin or mitoxantrone (Novantrone) or idarubicin (Idamycin); sometimes etoposide (VP-16, VePesid) is added to the regimen. The choice of agents is based on the patient's physical status and history of prior antineoplastic treatment.

The aim of induction therapy is to eradicate the leukemic cells, but this is often accompanied by the eradication of normal types of myeloid cells. Thus, the patient becomes severely neutropenic (an ANC of 0 is not uncommon), anemic, and thrombocytopenic (a platelet count of less than 10,000/mm³ is common). During this time, the patient is typically very ill, with bacterial, fungal, and occasionally viral infections, bleeding, and severe mucositis, which causes diarrhea and a marked decline in the ability to maintain adequate nutrition. Supportive care consists of administering blood products (RBCs and platelets) and promptly treating infections. The use of granulocytic growth factors, either G-CSF (filgrastim [Neupogen]) or GM-CSF (sargramostim [Leukine]), can shorten the period of significant neutropenia by stimulating the bone marrow to produce leukocytes more quickly; these agents do not appear to increase the risk of producing more leukemic cells.

When the patient has recovered from the induction therapy (ie, the WBC and platelet counts have returned to normal and any infection has resolved), the patient typically receives consolidation therapy (postremission therapy). The goal of consolidation therapy is to eliminate any residual leukemia cells that are not clinically detectable, thereby diminishing the chance for recurrence. Multiple treatment cycles of various agents are used, usually containing some form of cytarabine (eg, Alkeron). Frequently, the patient receives one cycle of treatment that is almost the same, if not identical, to the induction treatment but uses lower dosages (therefore resulting in less toxicity).

Despite the aggressive use of chemotherapy, the likelihood of remaining in remission for a prolonged period is not great. About 70% of patients with AML experience a relapse (Hiddemann & Buchner, 2001). A recent study of long-term survival of patients with AML found that only 11% survived 10 years or longer (Micallef et al., 2001).

Another aggressive treatment option is bone marrow transplantation (BMT) or peripheral blood stem cell transplantation (PBSCT). When a suitable tissue match can be obtained, the patient embarks on an even more aggressive regimen of chemotherapy (sometimes in combination with radiation therapy), with the treatment goal of destroying the hematopoietic function of the patient's bone marrow. The patient is then "rescued" with the infusion of the donor stem cells to reinitiate blood cell production. Patients who undergo PBSCT transplantation have a significant risk for problems with infection, potential graft-versus-host disease (in which the donor's lymphocytes [graft] recognize the patient's body as "foreign" and set up reactions to attack the "foreign" host), and other complications. PBSCT has been shown to cure AML in 25% to 50% of patients who are at high risk for relapse or who have relapsed (Radich & Sievers, 2000).

Recent advances in understanding of the molecular biology of myeloid blast cells have resulted in a new therapeutic option. After the uncommitted stem cell differentiates into a myeloid stem cell, it expresses a specific antigen on the cell surface, called CD33. It appears that 90% of blast cells found in AML express CD33; normal hematopoietic stem cells do not express this antigen (Radich & Sievers, 2000). Armed with that discovery, researchers developed a monoclonal antibody to target cells with the CD33 antigen. The anti-CD33 antibody is linked to a potent antitumour antibiotic, calicheamicin; this medication is called gemtuzumab ozogamicin (Mylotarg). When administered, the anti-CD33 antibody binds to cells with CD33 antigens, and the calicheamicin causes cell death. Normal myeloid and megakaryocyte precursors have the CD33 antigen, so the Mylotarg destroys them. Patients develop severe neutropenia and thrombocytopenia after receiving this medication. Nonetheless, Mylotarg shows promise as an effective agent against AML. In elderly patients, it appears to be somewhat less toxic than conventional induction therapy regimens.

Another important option for the patient to consider is supportive care alone. In fact, supportive care may be the only option if the patient has significant comorbidity, such as extremely poor cardiac, pulmonary, renal, or hepatic function. In such cases, aggressive antileukemia therapy is not used; occasionally, hydroxyurea (eg, Hydrea) may be used briefly to control the increase of blast cells. Patients are more commonly supported with antimicrobial therapy and transfusions as needed. This treatment approach provides the patient with some additional time at home; however, death frequently occurs within months, typically from infection or bleeding.

COMPLICATIONS OF TREATMENT

The massive leukemic cell destruction from chemotherapy results in release of electrolytes and fluids within the cell into the systemic circulation. Increases in uric acid levels, potassium, and phosphate are seen; this process is referred to as tumour **lysis** syndrome (see Chap. 16). The increased uric acid and phosphorus levels make patients vulnerable to renal stone formation and renal colic, which can progress to acute renal failure. Hyperkalemia and hypocalcemia can lead to cardiac dysrhythmias, hypotension, neuromuscular effects such as muscle cramps, weakness, spasm/tetany, confusion, and seizure. Patients require a high fluid intake, alkalization of the urine, and prophylaxis with allopurinol to prevent crystallization of uric acid and subsequent stone formation. Gastrointestinal problems may result from the infiltration of abnormal leukocytes into the abdominal organs and from the toxicity of the chemotherapeutic agents. Anorexia, nausea, vomiting, diarrhea, and severe mucositis are common. Because of the profound myelosuppressive effects of chemotherapy, significant neutropenia and thrombocytopenia typically result in serious infection and increased risk for bleeding.

Nursing Management

Nursing management of the patient with acute leukemia is discussed at the end of the leukemia section in this chapter.

CHRONIC MYELOID LEUKEMIA (CML)

Chronic myeloid leukemia (CML) arises from a mutation in the myeloid stem cell. Normal myeloid cells continue to be produced, but there is a preference for immature (blast) forms. Therefore, a wide spectrum of cell types exists within the blood, from blast forms through mature neutrophils. Because there is an uncontrolled proliferation of cells, the marrow expands into the cavities of long bones (eg, the femur), and cells are also formed in the liver and spleen (extramedullary hematopoiesis), resulting in enlargement of these organs that is sometimes painful. In 90% to 95% of patients with CML, a section of DNA is found to be missing from chromosome 22 (the Philadelphia chromosome [Ph1]); it is, in fact, translocated onto chromosome 9. The specific location of these changes is on the *BCR* gene of chromosome 22 and the *ABL* gene of chromosome 9. When these two genes fuse (*BCR-ABL* gene), they produce an abnormal protein (a tyrosine kinase protein) that causes WBCs to divide rapidly. This *BCR-ABL* gene is present in virtually all patients with this disease. CML is uncommon in people younger than 20 years of age, but the incidence increases with age (median age, 40 to 50 years).

Patients diagnosed with CML in the chronic phase have an overall median life expectancy of 3 to 5 years. During that time, they have very few symptoms and complications from the disease itself. Problems with infections and bleeding are rare. However, once the disease transforms to the acute phase (blast crisis), the overall survival time rarely exceeds several months.

Clinical Manifestations

The clinical picture of CML varies. Many patients are asymptomatic, and leukocytosis is detected by a CBC performed for some other reason. The WBC count commonly exceeds 100,000/mm³. Patients with extremely high WBC counts may be somewhat short of breath or slightly confused due to decreased capillary perfusion to the lungs and brain from leukostasis (the excessive amount of WBCs inhibits blood flow through the capillaries). Patients may complain of an enlarged, tender spleen. The liver may also be enlarged. Some patients have somewhat insidious symptoms, such as malaise, anorexia, and weight loss. Lymphadenopathy is rare. There are three stages in CML: chronic, transformation, and accelerated or blast crisis. Patients have more symptoms and complications as the disease progresses.

Medical Management

Advances in understanding of the pathology of CML at a molecular level have led to dramatic changes in its medical management. An oral formulation of a tyrosine kinase inhibitor, imatinib mesylate (Gleevec) works by blocking signals within the leukemia cells that express the *BCR-ABL* protein, thus preventing a series of chemical reactions that cause the cell to grow and divide (Tennant, 2001; Goldman & Melo, 2001). Gleevec appears to be more useful in the chronic phase of the illness. In clinical trials, it has been generally well tolerated. Antacids and grapefruit juice may limit drug absorption, and large doses of acetaminophen can cause hep-

atotoxicity. The long-term effects of Gleevec, its impact on survival, and the optimal length of treatment are being determined.

Conventional therapy depends on the stage of disease. In the chronic phase, the expected outcome is correction of the chromosomal abnormality (ie, conversion of the malignant stem cell population back to normal). Agents that have been used successfully for this purpose are interferon-alfa (Roferon-A) and cytosine (Cytosan), often in combination. These agents are administered daily as subcutaneous injections. This therapy is not benign; many patients cannot tolerate the profound fatigue, depression, anorexia, mucositis, and inability to concentrate. A less aggressive therapeutic approach focuses on reducing the WBC count to a more normal level, but does not alter cytogenetic changes. This goal can be achieved by using oral chemotherapeutic agents, typically hydroxyurea (eg, Hydrea) or busulfan (Myleran). In the case of an extreme leukocytosis at diagnosis (eg, WBC count higher than 300,000/mm³), a more emergent treatment may be required. In this instance, leukapheresis (in which the patient's blood is removed and separated, with the leukocytes withdrawn, and the remaining blood returned to the patient) can temporarily reduce the number of WBCs. An anthracycline chemotherapeutic agent (eg, daunomycin) may also be used to bring the WBC count down quickly to a safer level, where more conservative therapy can be instituted.

The transformation phase can be insidious, but it marks the process of evolution (or transformation) to the acute form of leukemia (blast crisis). In the transformation phase, the patient may complain of bone pain and may report fevers (without any obvious sign of infection) and weight loss. Even with chemotherapy, the spleen may continue to enlarge. The patient may become more anemic and thrombocytopenic; an increased basophil level is detected by the CBC. Despite its being a myeloid stem cell disease, CML will transform in up to 25% of patients to resemble not AML, but acute lymphoid leukemia (ALL), with lymphoid-appearing blasts (Derderian et al., 1993). Transformation into the acute phase can be gradual or rapid.

In the more acute form of leukemia (blast crisis), treatment may resemble induction therapy for acute leukemia, using the same medications as for AML or ALL. Patients whose disease evolves into a "lymphoid" blast crisis are more likely to be able to reenter a chronic phase after induction therapy. For those whose disease evolves into AML, therapy is largely ineffective in achieving a second chronic phase. Life-threatening infections and bleeding occur frequently in this phase. CML is a disease that can potentially be cured with BMT or PBSCT. Patients who receive such transplants while still in the chronic phase of the illness tend to have a greater chance for cure than those who receive them in the acute phase. The transplantation procedure may now be considered for otherwise healthy patients who are younger than 70 years of age.

ACUTE LYMPHOCYTIC LEUKEMIA (ALL)

ALL results from an uncontrolled proliferation of immature cells (lymphoblasts) derived from the lymphoid stem cell. The cell of origin is the precursor to the B lymphocyte in approximately 75% of ALL cases; T-lymphocyte ALL occurs in approximately 25% of ALL cases. The *BCR-ABL* translocation (see earlier discussion) is found in 20% of ALL blast cells. ALL is most common in young children, with boys affected more often than girls; the peak incidence is 4 years of age. After age 15 years, ALL is relatively uncommon. Increasing age appears to be associated with diminished survival (Nachman, 1999). Because of improvements in therapy for ALL, more than 80% of children survive at least

5 years. Even if relapse occurs, resumption of induction therapy can often achieve a second complete remission. Moreover, BMT may be successful even after a second relapse.

Clinical Manifestations

Immature lymphocytes proliferate in the marrow and crowd the development of normal myeloid cells. As a result, normal hematopoiesis is inhibited, resulting in reduced numbers of leukocytes, erythrocytes, and platelets. Leukocyte counts may be either low or high, but there is always a high proportion of immature cells. Manifestations of leukemic cell infiltration into other organs are more common with ALL than with other forms of leukemia and include pain from an enlarged liver or spleen, bone pain, and headache and vomiting (because of meningeal involvement).

Medical Management

The expected outcome of treatment is complete remission. Lymphoid blast cells are typically very sensitive to corticosteroids and to vinca alkaloids; therefore, these medications are an integral part of the initial induction therapy. Because ALL frequently invades the central nervous system, prophylaxis with cranial irradiation or intrathecal chemotherapy (eg, methotrexate [Folex]) or both is an integral part of the treatment plan.

Treatment protocols for ALL tend to be complex, using a wide variety of chemotherapeutic agents. They often include a maintenance phase, when lower doses of medications are given for up to 3 years. Despite the complexity, treatment can be provided in the outpatient setting in some circumstances until severe complications develop.

Infections are common, especially viral infections. The use of corticosteroids to treat ALL increases the patient's susceptibility to infection. Patients with ALL tend to have a better response to treatment than patients with AML do. BMT or PBSCT offers a chance for prolonged remission or even cure if the illness recurs after therapy.

Nursing Management

Nursing management of the patient with acute leukemia is discussed at the end of the leukemia section in this chapter.

CHRONIC LYMPHOCYTIC LEUKEMIA (CLL)

CLL is a common malignancy of older adults; two thirds of all patients are older than 60 years of age at diagnosis. It is the most common form of leukemia in the United States, Canada, and Europe, affecting more than 120,000 people, but is rarely seen in Asia. The average survival time for patients with CLL ranges from 14 years (early stage) to 2.5 years (late stage).

Pathophysiology

CLL typically derives from a malignant clone of B lymphocytes (T-lymphocyte CLL is rare). In contrast to the acute forms of leukemia, most of the leukemia cells in CLL are fully mature. It appears that these cells can escape **apoptosis** (programmed cell death), with the result being an excessive accumulation of the cells in the marrow and circulation. The antigen CD52 is prevalent on the surface of many of these leukemic B cells. The disease is classified into three or four stages (two classification systems are

in use). In the early stage, an elevated lymphocyte count is seen and can exceed 100,000/mm³. Because the lymphocytes are small, they can easily travel through the small capillaries within the circulation, and the pulmonary and cerebral complications of leukocytosis (as seen with myeloid leukemias) typically are not found in CLL.

Lymphadenopathy occurs as the lymphocytes are trapped within the lymph nodes. The nodes can become very large and are sometimes painful. Hepatomegaly and splenomegaly then develop.

In later stages, anemia and thrombocytopenia may develop. Treatment is typically initiated in the later stages; earlier treatment does not appear to increase survival. Autoimmune complications can also occur at any stage, as either autoimmune hemolytic anemia or idiopathic thrombocytopenic purpura (ITP). In the autoimmune process, the RES destroys the body's own RBCs or platelets.

Clinical Manifestations

Many patients are asymptomatic and are diagnosed incidentally during routine physical examinations or during the course of treatment for another disease. An increased lymphocyte count (lymphocytosis) is always present. The RBC and platelet counts may be normal or, in later stages of the illness, decreased. Enlargement of lymph nodes (lymphadenopathy) is common; it can be severe and sometimes painful. The spleen can also be enlarged (splenomegaly).

Patients with CLL can develop "B symptoms," a constellation of symptoms including fevers, drenching sweating (especially at night), and unintentional weight loss. These patients have defects in their humoural and cell-mediated immune systems; therefore, infections are common. The defect in cellular immunity is evidenced by an absent or decreased reaction to skin sensitivity tests (eg, *Candida*, mumps), which is known as **anergy**. Problems with life-threatening infections are common. Viral infections, such as herpes zoster, can become widely disseminated.

Medical Management

In early stages, CLL may require no treatment. When symptoms are severe (drenching night sweats, painful lymphadenopathy), or when the disease progresses to later stages (with resultant anemia and thrombocytopenia), chemotherapy with corticosteroids and chlorambucil (Leukeran) is often used. Other useful agents include cyclophosphamide (eg, Cytoxan), vincristine (Vincasar, PFS), and doxorubicin (Adriamycin). A significant number of patients who do not respond to these medications have achieved remission with fludarabine (Fludara), and this medication is increasingly being used as front-line therapy. The major side effect of fludarabine is prolonged bone marrow suppression, manifested by prolonged periods of neutropenia, lymphopenia, and thrombocytopenia. Patients are then at risk for such infections as *Pneumocystis carinii*, *Listeria*, mycobacteria, herpes viruses, and cytomegalovirus (CMV). The monoclonal antibody rituximab (Rituxan) also has efficacy in CLL therapy. It is often used in combination with other chemotherapeutic medications. Research has shown that the monoclonal antibody alemtuzumab (Campath) targets the CD52 antigen commonly found on CLL cells and that it is effective in clearing the marrow and circulation of these cells without affecting the stem cells. Because CD52 is present on both B and T lymphocytes, patients receiving alemtuzumab are at significant risk for infection; prophylactic use of antiviral agents and antibiotics (eg, trimethoprim and sulfamethoxazole [Septra]) is important and needs to continue for a minimum of 2 months after the patient stops treatment. Because bacterial infections are common in patients with CLL, intravenous treatment with immunoglobulin may be given to selected patients.

NURSING PROCESS:
THE PATIENT WITH ACUTE LEUKEMIA
Assessment

Although the clinical picture varies with the type of leukemia involved as well as the treatment implemented, the health history may reveal a range of subtle symptoms reported by the patient before the problem is manifested by findings on physical examination. Weakness and fatigue are common manifestations, not only of the leukemia but also of the resulting complications of anemia

and infection. If the patient is hospitalized, the assessments should be performed daily, or more frequently as warranted. Because the physical findings may be subtle initially, a thorough, systematic assessment incorporating all body systems is essential. For example, a dry cough, mild dyspnea, and diminished breath sounds may indicate a pulmonary infection. However, the infection may not be seen initially on the chest x-ray. The lack of neutrophils delays the inflammatory response against the pulmonary infection, and it is the inflammatory response that causes the x-ray changes. The platelet count can become dangerously low, leaving the patient at risk for significant bleeding. The specific body system assessments are delineated in the neutropenic precautions and bleeding precautions, found in Charts 33-9 and 33-10, respectively. When serial assessments are performed, current findings are compared with previous findings to evaluate improvement or worsening.

The nurse also must closely monitor the results of laboratory studies. Flow sheets and spreadsheets are particularly useful in

---

Chart 33-10 Bleeding Precautions

Nursing Diagnosis
Potential bleeding* and injury secondary to thrombocytopenia/altered coagulation due to:
- Malignant invasion in bone marrow
- Bone marrow suppression resulting from chemotherapy (particularly alkylators, antitumour antibiotics, antimetabolites) and radiation therapy
- Hypersplenism
- Disseminated intravascular coagulation (DIC)
- Altered coagulation

Assessment
Patient
Assess the following areas thoroughly every shift or visit (with spot checks throughout the shift if patient is hospitalized), and notify physician if there is new onset of the following and/or worsening of status:
- *Integument:* Petechiae (usually located on trunk, thighs), ecchymoses or hematomas, conjunctival hemorrhages, bleeding gums, bleeding at puncture sites (venipuncture, lumbar puncture, bone marrow)
- *Cardiovascular:* Hypotension, tachycardia, complaints of dizziness, epistaxis
- *Pulmonary:* Respiratory distress, tachypnea
- *Gastrointestinal:* Hemoptysis, abdominal distention, rectal bleeding
- *Genitourinary:* Vaginal or urethral bleeding
- *Neurologic:* Headache, blurred vision, mental status changes

Laboratory Tests
- Monitor complete blood count (CBC), platelets daily (at least); coagulation panel.
- Notify physician if platelet count is <10,000/mm³ or if count has changed significantly from previous count (including coagulation), or whenever patient becomes symptomatic.
- Ensure patient's blood was human leukocyte antigen (HLA) typed before transfusions or chemotherapy begins if admitted for induction therapy (eg, for acute leukemia).
- Obtain 1-hour posttransfusion platelet count if warranted.
- Test all urine, emesis, stools for occult blood.

Nursing Interventions
Prevent Complications
- Avoid aspirin and aspirin-containing medications or other medications known to inhibit platelet function, if possible.
- Do not give intramuscular injections.
- Do not insert indwelling catheters.
- Take no rectal temperatures; do not give suppositories, enemas.
- Use stool softeners, oral laxatives to prevent constipation.
- Use smallest possible needles when performing venipuncture.
- Apply pressure to venipuncture sites for 5 min or until bleeding has stopped.
- Permit no flossing of teeth and no commercial mouthwashes.
- Use only soft-bristled toothbrush for mouth care.
- Use only toothettes for mouth care if platelet count is <10,000/mm³, or if gums bleed.
- Lubricate lips with water-soluble lubricant every 2 hr while awake.
- Avoid suctioning if at all possible; if unavoidable, use only gentle suctioning.
- Discourage vigourous coughing or blowing of the nose.
- Use only electric razor for shaving.
- Pad side rails as needed.
- Prevent falls by ambulating with patient as necessary.

Control Bleeding
- Apply direct pressure.
- For epistaxis, position patient in high Fowler's position; apply ice pack to back of neck and direct pressure to nose.
- Notify physician for prolonged bleeding (eg, unable to stop within 10 min).
- Administer platelets, fresh frozen plasma, packed red blood cells, as prescribed.

Evaluation and Expected Patient Outcomes
- Patient demonstrates an absence of bleeding as evidenced by absence of spontaneous petechiae, ecchymoses, epistaxis, hemoptysis, bleeding gums, conjunctival hemorrhage, vaginal bleeding, hematuria, guaiac positive stool, blurred vision, orthostatic hypotension, and prolonged bleeding from puncture sites.
- Patient demonstrates an absence of bleeding as evidenced by the presence of vital signs within normal limits and intact neurologic status.

*Serious hemorrhage is unusual in mildly thrombocytopenic patients in absence of local lesions (peptic ulcer, bleeding from hemorrhoids, cystitis).

tracking the WBC count, ANC, hematocrit, platelet, and creatinine levels, hepatic function tests, and electrolyte levels. Culture results need to be reported immediately so that appropriate antimicrobial therapy can begin or be modified.

Diagnosis

NURSING DIAGNOSES

Based on the assessment data, major nursing diagnoses for the patient with acute leukemia may include:

- Risk for infection and bleeding
- Risk for impaired skin integrity related to toxic effects of chemotherapy, alteration in nutrition, and impaired mobility
- Impaired gas exchange
- Impaired mucous membranes due to changes in epithelial lining of the gastrointestinal tract from chemotherapy or prolonged use of antimicrobial medications
- Imbalanced nutrition, less than body requirements, related to hypermetabolic state, anorexia, mucositis, pain, and nausea
- Acute pain and discomfort related to mucositis, WBC infiltration of systemic tissues, fever, and infection
- Hyperthermia related to tumour lysis and infection
- Fatigue and activity intolerance related to anemia and infection
- Impaired physical mobility due to anemia and protective isolation
- Risk for excess fluid volume related to renal dysfunction, hypoproteinemia, need for multiple intravenous medications and blood products
- Diarrhea due to altered gastrointestinal flora, mucosal denudation
- Risk for deficient fluid volume related to potential for diarrhea, bleeding, infection, and increased metabolic rate
- Self-care deficit due to fatigue, malaise, and protective isolation
- Anxiety due to knowledge deficit and uncertain future
- Disturbed body image related to change in appearance, function, and roles
- Grieving related to anticipatory loss and altered role functioning
- Potential for spiritual distress
- Deficient knowledge about disease process, treatment, complication management, and self-care measures

COLLABORATIVE PROBLEMS/ POTENTIAL COMPLICATIONS

Based on the assessment data, potential complications that may develop include:

- Infection
- Bleeding
- Renal dysfunction
- Tumour lysis syndrome
- Nutritional depletion
- Mucositis

Planning and Goals

The major goals for the patient may include absence of complications and pain, attainment and maintenance of adequate

nutrition, activity tolerance, ability for self-care and to cope with the diagnosis and prognosis, positive body image, and an understanding of the disease process and its treatment.

Nursing Interventions

PREVENTING OR MANAGING INFECTION AND BLEEDING

The nursing interventions related to diminishing the risk for infection and for bleeding are delineated in Charts 33-9 and 33-10.

MANAGING MUCOSITIS

Although emphasis is placed on the oral mucosa, it is important to realize that the entire gastrointestinal mucosa can be altered, not only by the effects of chemotherapy but also from prolonged administration of antibiotics. Assessment of the oral mucosa must be thorough; therefore, dentures must be removed. Areas to assess include the palate, buccal mucosa, tongue, gums, lips, oropharynx, and the area under the tongue. In addition to identifying and describing lesions, the colour and moisture of the mucosa should be noted.

Oral hygiene is very important to diminish the bacteria within the mouth, maintain moisture, and provide comfort. Soft-bristled toothbrushes should be used until the neutrophil and platelet counts become very low; at that time, sponge-tipped applicators should be substituted. Lemon-glycerin swabs and commercial mouthwashes should never be used because the glycerin and alcohol within them are extremely drying to the tissues. Simple rinses with saline (or saline and baking soda) solutions are inexpensive but effective in cleaning and moistening the oral mucosa. Because the risk of yeast or fungal infection in the mouth is great, other medications are often prescribed, such as chlorhexidine rinses (eg, Peridex) or clotrimazole troches (eg, Mycelex). The nurse reminds the patient about the importance of these medications to enhance adherence to the therapeutic regimen. Chlorhexidine rinses may discolour the teeth.

To diminish perineal–rectal complications, it is important to cleanse the perineal–rectal area thoroughly after each bowel movement. Women are instructed to cleanse the perineum from front to back. Sitz baths are a comfortable method of cleansing; the perineal–anal region and buttocks must be carefully dried afterward to minimize the chance of excoriation. Stool softeners should be used to increase the moisture of bowel movements; however, the stool texture must be monitored so that the softeners can be decreased or stopped if the stool becomes too loose.

IMPROVING NUTRITIONAL INTAKE

The disease process can increase, and sepsis further increases, the patient's metabolic rate and nutritional requirements. Nutritional intake is often reduced because of pain and discomfort associated with stomatitis. Mouth care before and after meals and administration of analgesics before eating can help increase intake. If oral anesthetics are used, the patient must be warned to chew with extreme care to avoid inadvertently biting the tongue or buccal mucosa.

Nausea should not be a major contributing factor, because recent advances in antiemetic therapy are highly effective. However, nausea can result from antimicrobial therapy, so some antiemetic therapy may still be required after the chemotherapy has been completed.

Small, frequent feedings of foods that are soft in texture and moderate in temperature may be better tolerated. Low-microbial diets are typically prescribed (avoiding uncooked fruits or vegetables and those without a peelable skin). Nutritional supplements are frequently used. Daily body weights (as well as intake and output measurements) are useful in monitoring fluid status.

Calorie counts are useful, as are more formal nutritional assessments. Parenteral nutrition is often required to maintain adequate nutrition.

EASING PAIN AND DISCOMFORT

Recurrent fevers are common in acute leukemia; at times, they are accompanied by shaking chills, which can be severe (rigours). Myalgias and arthralgias can result. Acetaminophen is typically given to decrease fever, but it does so by increasing diaphoresis. Sponging with cool water may be useful, but cold water or ice packs should be avoided because the heat cannot dissipate from constricted blood vessels. Bedclothes need frequent changing as well. Gentle back and shoulder massage may provide comfort.

Stomatitis can also cause significant discomfort. In addition to oral hygiene practices, patient-controlled analgesia can be effective in controlling the pain (see Chap. 13).

Because patients with acute leukemia require hospitalization for extensive nursing care (either during induction or consolidation therapy or during resultant complications), sleep deprivation frequently results. Nurses need to implement creative strategies that permit uninterrupted sleep for at least a few hours while still administering necessary medications on time.

With the exception of severe mucositis, less pain is associated with acute leukemia than with many other forms of cancer. However, the amount of psychologic suffering that the patient must endure can be immense. Patients greatly benefit from active listening.

DECREASING FATIGUE AND DECONDITIONING

Fatigue is a common and oppressive problem. Nursing interventions should focus on assisting the patient to establish a balance between activity and rest. Patients with acute leukemia need to maintain some physical activity and exercise to prevent the deconditioning that results from inactivity. Use of a high-efficiency particulate air (HEPA) filter mask can permit the patient to ambulate outside the room despite severe neutropenia. Although many patients lack the motivation to use them, stationary bicycles within the room can also be used. At a minimum, patients should be encouraged to sit up in a chair while awake rather than staying in bed; even this simple activity can improve the patient's tidal volume and enhance circulation. Physical therapy can also be beneficial.

MAINTAINING FLUID AND ELECTROLYTE BALANCE

Febrile episodes, bleeding, and inadequate or overly aggressive fluid replacement can alter the patient's fluid status. Similarly, persistent diarrhea, vomiting, and long-term use of certain antimicrobial agents can cause significant deficits in electrolytes. Intake and output need to be measured accurately, and daily weights should also be monitored. The patient should be assessed for signs of dehydration as well as fluid overload, with particular attention to pulmonary status and the development of dependent edema. Laboratory test results, particularly electrolytes, blood urea nitrogen, creatinine, and hematocrit, should be monitored and compared with previous results. Replacement of electrolytes, particularly potassium and magnesium, is commonly required. Patients receiving amphotericin or certain antibiotics are at increased risk for electrolyte depletion.

IMPROVING SELF-CARE

Because hygiene measures are so important in this patient population, they must be performed by the nurse when the patient can-

not do so. However, the patient should be encouraged to do as much as possible, to preserve mobility and function as well as self-esteem. Patients may have negative feelings, even disgust that they can no longer care for themselves. Empathetic listening is helpful, as is realistic reassurance that these deficits are temporary. As the patient recovers, it is important to assist him or her to resume more self-care. Patients are usually discharged from the hospital with a central vascular access device (eg, Hickman catheter, PICC), and most patients can care for the catheter with adequate instruction and practice under observation.

MANAGING ANXIETY AND GRIEF

Being diagnosed with acute leukemia can be extremely frightening. In many instances, the need to begin treatment is emergent, and patients have little time to process the fact that they have the illness before making decisions about therapy. Providing emotional support and discussing the uncertain future are crucial. The nurse also needs to assess how much information patients want to have regarding the illness, its treatment, and potential complications. This desire should be reassessed at intervals, because needs and interest in information change throughout the course of the disease and treatment. Priorities must be identified so that procedures, assessments, and self-care expectations are adequately explained even to those who do not wish extensive information.

Many patients become depressed and begin to grieve for the losses they feel, such as normal family functioning, professional roles and responsibilities, and social roles, as well as physical functioning. Nurses can assist patients to identify the source of the grief and encourage them to allow time to adjust to the major life changes produced by the illness. Role restructuring, in both family and professional life, may be required. Again, when possible, permitting patients to identify options and to take time making significant decisions regarding such restructuring is helpful.

Discharge from the hospital can also provoke anxiety. Although most patients are extremely eager to go home, they may lack confidence in their ability to manage potential complications and to resume their normal activity. Close communication between nurses across care settings can reassure patients that they will not be abandoned.

ENCOURAGING SPIRITUAL WELL-BEING

Because acute leukemia is a serious, potentially life-threatening illness, the nurse may offer support to enhance the patient's spiritual well-being. The patient's spiritual and religious practices should be assessed and pastoral services offered. Throughout the patient's illness, it is important that the nurse assist the patient to maintain hope. However, that hope should be realistic and will certainly change over the course of the illness. For example, the patient may initially hope to be cured, but with repeated relapses and a change to terminal care the same patient may hope for a quiet, dignified death.

MONITORING AND MANAGING POTENTIAL COMPLICATIONS

Nursing interventions for potential complications were described previously.

PROMOTING HOME AND COMMUNITY-BASED CARE

Teaching Patients Self-Care

Most patients cope better when they have an understanding of what is happening to them. Based on their education, literacy level, and interest, teaching of patient and family should focus on the disease (including some pathophysiology), its treatment, and certainly the significant risk for infection and bleeding (Charts 33-8 and 33-11) that results.

Management of a vascular access device can be taught to most patients or family members. Follow-up and care for the devices may also need to be provided by nurses in an outpatient facility or by a home care agency or a health care provider.

Continuing Care. Shortened hospital stays and outpatient care have significantly altered care for patients with acute leukemia. In many instances, when the patient is clinically stable but still requires parenteral antibiotics or blood products, these procedures can be performed in an outpatient setting. Nurses in these various settings must communicate regularly. Patients need to learn which parameters are important for them to monitor, and how to monitor them. Specific instructions need to be given as to when the patient should seek care from the physician or a health care provider.

Patients and their families need to have a clear understanding of the disease and the prognosis. The nurse acts as an advocate to ensure that this information is provided. When patients no longer respond to therapy, it is important to respect their choices about treatment, including measures to prolong life and other end-of-life measures. Advance directives and living wills provide patients with some measure of control during terminal illness.

Many patients in this stage still choose to be cared for at home, and families often need support when considering this option. Coordination of home care services and instruction can help to alleviate anxiety about managing the patient's care in the home. As the patient becomes weaker, the caregivers must assume more of the patient's care. In addition, caregivers often need to be encouraged to take care of themselves, allowing time for rest and accepting emotional support. Hospice staff can assist in providing respite for family members as well as care for the patient. Patients and families also need assistance to cope with changes in their roles and responsibilities. Anticipatory grieving is an essential task during this time (see Chap. 17).

In patients with acute leukemia, death typically occurs from infection or bleeding. Family members need to have information about these complications and the measures to take should either occur. Many family members cannot cope with the care required when a patient begins to bleed actively. It is important to delineate alternatives to keeping the patient at home. Should another option be sought, family members who may feel guilty that they could not keep the patient at home will require support from the nurse.

Evaluation

EXPECTED PATIENT OUTCOMES

Expected patient outcomes may include:

1. Shows no evidence of infection
2. Experiences no bleeding
3. Has intact oral mucous membranes
   a. Participates in oral hygiene regimen
   b. Reports no discomfort in mouth
4. Attains optimal level of nutrition
   a. Maintains weight with increased food and fluid intake
   b. Maintains adequate protein stores (albumin)
5. Reports satisfaction with pain and discomfort levels
6. Has less fatigue and increased activity
7. Maintains fluid and electrolyte balance
8. Participates in self-care
9. Copes with anxiety and grief
   a. Discusses concerns and fears
   b. Uses stress management strategies appropriately
   c. Participates in decisions regarding end-of-life care
10. Absence of complications

AGNOGENIC MYELOID METAPLASIA (AMM)

Agnogenic myeloid metaplasia (AMM), also known as myelofibrosis, is a chronic myeloproliferative disorder that arises from neoplastic transformation of an early hematopoietic stem cell. The disease is characterized by marrow fibrosis or scarring, splenomegaly, extramedullary hematopoiesis (typically spleen, liver, or both), leukocytosis and thrombocytosis, and anemia. Some patients have suppressed WBC and platelet counts as well as anemia (pancytopenia). Patients with AMM have increased **angiogenesis** (formation of new blood vessels) within the marrow. Early forms of blood cells (including nucleated RBCs and megakaryocyte fragments) are frequently found in the circulation. AMM is a disease of the elderly, with a median age at diagnosis of 60 to 65 years. Survival time varies from as little as 1 year to more than 30 years; the average is 4 to 5 years (Anderson, Hamblin, & Traynor, 1999). Heart failure, complications of marrow failure, and transformation to AML are the common causes of death.

Chart 33-11
Home Care Checklist • The Patient at Risk for Bleeding

At the completion of the home care instruction, the patient or caregiver will be able to:	Patient	Caregiver
• Describe the source and function of platelets and clotting factors.	✓	✓
• Verbalize the rationale for being at risk for bleeding.	✓	✓
• Identify medications and other substances to avoid (eg, aspirin-containing medications, alcohol).	✓	✓
• Demonstrate how to monitor for signs of bleeding.	✓	✓
• Describe to whom, how, and when to report signs of bleeding.	✓	✓
• Notify health care professional before having dental work.	✓	
• Describe appropriate ways to prevent bleeding (avoid use of suppositories, enemas, tampons; avoid constipation, vigourous sexual intercourse, anal sex; use only electric razor for shaving and a soft-bristled toothbrush for teeth).	✓	✓
• Demonstrate appropriate actions to take should bleeding occur.	✓	✓

Medical Management

Medical management is directed toward palliation, reducing symptoms related to cytopenias, splenomegaly, and hypermetabolic state. Although one third of anemic patients respond to the combination of an androgen plus a corticosteroid, the primary treatment remains RBC transfusion. Because of the prolonged requirement for RBC transfusion, iron overload is a common problem. Iron chelation therapy should be initiated for those individuals in whom survival is expected to exceed a few years (Anderson, Hamblin, & Traynor, 1999). Hydroxyurea is often used to control high WBC and platelet counts and to reduce the size of the spleen. Splenic irradiation or splenectomy may also be used to control the massive splenomegaly that can develop. However, both modalities render the patient at significant risk for development of infection. BMT or PBSCT may be a useful treatment modality in younger, otherwise healthy individuals.

Nursing Management

The extent of splenomegaly can be profound in patients with AMM, with enlargement of the spleen that extends to the pelvic rim. This condition is extremely uncomfortable to the patient and can severely limit nutritional intake. Analgesics are often ineffective. Methods to reduce the spleen's size are usually more effective in controlling pain. Splenomegaly, coupled with a hypermetabolic state, results in weight loss (often severe) and muscle wasting. Patients benefit from very small, frequent meals of foods that are high in calories and protein. Weakness, fatigue, and altered body image are other significant problems. Energy conservation methods and active listening are important nursing interventions. Patients need to be educated about signs and symptoms of infection as well as appropriate interventions when an infection is suspected.

The Lymphomas

The lymphomas are neoplasms of cells of lymphoid origin. These tumours usually start in lymph nodes but can involve lymphoid tissue in the spleen, the gastrointestinal tract (eg, the wall of the stomach), the liver, or the bone marrow. They are often classified according to the degree of cell differentiation and the origin of the predominant malignant cell. Lymphomas can be broadly classified into two categories: Hodgkin's disease and non-Hodgkin's lymphoma (NHL).

HODGKIN'S DISEASE

Hodgkin's disease is a relatively rare malignancy that has an impressive cure rate. It is somewhat more common in men than women and has two peaks of incidence: one in the early 20s and the other after 50 years of age. Unlike other lymphomas, Hodgkin's disease is unicentric in origin in that it initiates in a single node. The disease spreads by contiguous extension along the lymphatic system. The cause of Hodgkin's disease is unknown, but a viral etiology is suspected. In fact, fragments of the Epstein-Barr virus have been found in 40% to 50% of patients; this occurs more commonly in the younger patient population (Weiss, 2000). There is a familial pattern associated with Hodgkin's disease: first-degree relatives have a higher-than-normal frequency of the disease. There is no increased incidence documented for non-blood relatives (eg, spouses).

The malignant cell of Hodgkin's disease is the Reed-Sternberg cell, a gigantic tumour cell that is morphologically unique and is thought to be of immature lymphoid origin. It is the pathologic hallmark and essential diagnostic criterion for Hodgkin's disease. However, the tumour is very heterogeneous and may actually contain few Reed-Sternberg cells. Repeated biopsies may be required to establish the diagnosis.

Hodgkin's disease is customarily classified into five subgroups based on pathologic analyses that reflect the natural history of the malignancy and suggest the prognosis. For example, when lymphocytes predominate, with few Reed-Sternberg cells and minimal involvement of the lymph nodes, the prognosis is much more favourable than when the lymphocyte count is low and the lymph nodes are virtually replaced by tumour cells of the most primitive type. The majority of patients with Hodgkin's disease have the types currently designated "nodular sclerosis" or "mixed cellularity." The nodular sclerosis type tends to occur more often in young women, at an earlier stage but with a worse prognosis than the mixed cellularity subgroup, which occurs more commonly in men and causes more constitutional symptoms but has a better prognosis.

Clinical Manifestations

Hodgkin's disease usually begins as a painless enlargement of one or more lymph nodes on one side of the neck. The individual nodes are painless and firm but not hard. The most common sites for lymphadenopathy are the cervical, supraclavicular, and mediastinal nodes; involvement of the iliac or inguinal nodes or spleen is much less common. A mediastinal mass may be seen on chest x-ray; occasionally, the mass is large enough to compress the trachea and cause dyspnea. Pruritus is common; it can be extremely distressing, and the cause is unknown. Approximately 20% of patients experience brief but severe pain after drinking alcohol (Cavalli, 1998). The pain is usually at the site of the Hodgkin's disease; again, the cause is unknown.

All organs are vulnerable to invasion by Hodgkin's disease. The symptoms result from compression of organs by the tumour, such as cough and pulmonary effusion (from pulmonary infiltrates), jaundice (from hepatic involvement or bile duct obstruction), abdominal pain (from splenomegaly or retroperitoneal adenopathy), or bone pain (from skeletal involvement). Herpes zoster infections are common. A cluster of constitutional symptoms has important prognostic implications. Referred to as "B symptoms," they include fever (without chills), drenching sweats (particularly at night), and unintentional weight loss of more than 10%. "B symptoms" are found in 40% of patients and are more common in advanced disease.

A mild anemia is the most common hematologic finding. The WBC count may be elevated or decreased. The platelet count is typically normal, unless the tumour has invaded the bone marrow, suppressing hematopoiesis. The **erythrocyte sedimentation rate (ESR)** and the serum copper level are used by some clinicians to assess disease activity. Patients with Hodgkin's disease have impaired cellular immunity, as evidenced by an absent or decreased reaction to skin sensitivity tests (eg, *Candida,* mumps).

Assessment and Diagnostic Findings

Because many manifestations are similar to those occurring with infection, diagnostic studies are performed to rule out an infectious origin for the disease. The diagnosis is made by means of an excisional lymph node biopsy and the finding of the Reed-Sternberg cell. Once the diagnosis is confirmed and the histologic type is established, it is necessary to assess the extent of the disease, a process referred to as staging.

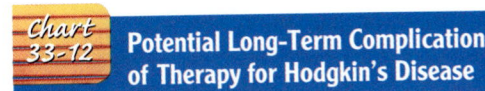

During the health history, the nurse should assess for any "B symptoms." Physical examination requires a careful, systematic evaluation of the lymph node chains, as well as the size of the spleen and liver. A chest x-ray and a CT scan of the chest, abdomen, and pelvis are crucial to identify the extent of lymphadenopathy within these regions. Laboratory tests include CBC, platelet count, ESR, and liver and renal function studies. A bone marrow biopsy is performed if there are signs of marrow involvement, and some physicians routinely perform bilateral biopsies. Bone scans may be performed to identify any involvement in these areas. A staging laparotomy and lymphangiography are no longer considered mandatory, primarily because of the accuracy of CT.

Medical Management

The general intent in treating Hodgkin's disease, regardless of stage, is cure. Treatment is determined primarily by the stage of the disease, not the histologic type; however, extensive research is ongoing to target treatment regimens to histologic subtypes or prognostic features. Traditionally, early Hodgkin's disease was treated by a staging laparotomy followed by radiation therapy. Recent data show improved results and decreased complications with a short course (2 to 4 months) of chemotherapy followed by radiation therapy in certain subsets of early-stage disease (IA and IIA); patients with early-stage disease and good prognostic features may receive radiation therapy alone (Hoppe et al., 2000). Combination chemotherapy, for example with doxorubicin (eg, Adriamycin), bleomycin (eg, Blenoxane), vinblastine (eg, Velban), and dacarbazine (eg, DTIC), referred to as ABVD, is now the standard treatment for more advanced disease (stages III and IV and all B stages).

Radiation therapy is still very useful for patients with extensive adenopathy (often termed bulky disease). In this group, residual disease often persists after the chemotherapy treatment is finished; radiation therapy to the areas of remaining adenopathy has been shown to improve survival.

Even when Hodgkin's disease does recur, the use of high doses of chemotherapeutic agents, followed by autologous BMT or stem cell transplantation (PBSCT), can be very effective in controlling the disease and extending survival time.

Long-Term Complications of Therapy

Much is now known about the long-term effects of chemotherapy and radiation therapy, primarily from the large numbers of people who were cured of Hodgkin's disease by these treatments. The various complications of treatment are listed in Chart 33-12. Risk factors for other cancers should be assessed, and long-term surveillance is crucial. The potential development of a second malignancy is obviously of concern to patients, and this potential should be addressed with the patient when treatment decisions are made. However, it is important to consider that Hodgkin's disease is curable. Revised treatment approaches are aimed at diminishing the risk for complications without sacrificing the potential for cure.

NON-HODGKIN'S LYMPHOMAS (NHLs)

The NHLs are a heterogeneous group of cancers that originate from the neoplastic growth of lymphoid tissue. As in CLL, the neoplastic cells are thought to arise from a single clone of lymphocytes; however, in NHL, the cells may vary morphologically. Most NHLs involve malignant B lymphocytes; only 5% involve T lymphocytes. In contrast to Hodgkin's disease, the lymphoid tissues involved are largely infiltrated with malignant cells. The spread of these ma-

> **Chart 33-12**
> ### Potential Long-Term Complications of Therapy for Hodgkin's Disease
>
> Immune dysfunction
> Herpes infections (zoster and varicella)
> Pneumococcal sepsis
> Acute myeloid leukemia (AML)
> Myelodysplastic syndromes (MDS)
> Non-Hodgkin's lymphoma
> Solid tumours
> Thyroid cancer
> Thymic hyperplasia
> Hypothyroidism
> Pericarditis (acute or chronic)
> Cardiomyopathy
> Pneumonitis (acute or chronic)
> Avascular necrosis
> Growth retardation
> Infertility
> Impotence
> Dental caries

lignant lymphoid cells occurs unpredictably, and true localized disease is uncommon. Lymph nodes from multiple sites may be infiltrated, as may sites outside the lymphoid system (extranodal tissue).

The incidence of NHL has increased dramatically over the past decade. This incidence in Canada is now 21 men and 14 women per 100,000, with 9 and 6 deaths per 100,000 (BC Cancer Agency, 2005). The incidence increases with each decade of life; the average age at diagnosis is 50 to 60 years. Although no common etiologic factor has been identified, there is an increased incidence of NHL in people with immunodeficiencies or autoimmune disorders, viral infections (including Epstein-Barr virus and HIV), or exposure to pesticides, solvents, or dyes. Prognosis varies greatly among the various types of NHL. Long-term survival (more than 10 years) is commonly achieved in low-grade, localized lymphomas. Even with aggressive disease forms, cure is possible in at least one third of patients who receive aggressive treatment.

Clinical Manifestations

Symptoms are highly variable, reflecting the diverse nature of these diseases. With early-stage disease, or with the types that are considered more indolent, symptoms may be virtually absent or very minor, and the illness typically is not diagnosed until it progresses to a later stage, when the patient is more symptomatic. At these stages (III or IV), lymphadenopathy is noticeable. One third of patients have "B symptoms" (recurrent fever, drenching night sweats, and unintentional weight loss of 10% or more).

Assessment and Diagnostic Findings

The actual diagnosis of NHL is categorized into a highly complex classification system based on histopathology, immunophenotyping, and cytogenetic analyses of the malignant cells. The specific histopathologic type of the disease has important prognostic implications. Treatment also varies and is based on these features. Indolent (less aggressive) types tend to have small cells and are distributed in a follicular pattern. Aggressive types tend to have large or immature cells distributed through the nodes in a diffuse pattern. Staging, also an important factor, is typically based on data obtained from CT scans, bone marrow biopsies, and occasionally cerebrospinal fluid analysis. The stage is based on the site of disease and its spread to other sites. For example, in stage I disease, only one area of involvement is detected; thus, stage I disease is highly localized and may respond well to localized therapy (eg, radiation therapy). In contrast, stage IV disease is detected in at least one extranodal site. Although low-grade lymphomas may not require treatment until the disease progresses to a later stage, historically they have also been relatively unresponsive to treatment in that most therapeutic modalities did not improve overall survival. More aggressive types of NHL (eg, lymphoblastic lymphoma, Burkitt's lymphoma) require prompt initiation of chemotherapy; however, these types tend to be more responsive to treatment.

Medical Management

Treatment is based on the actual classification of disease, the stage of disease, prior treatment (if any), and the patient's ability to tolerate therapy. If the disease is not an aggressive form and is truly localized, radiation alone may be the treatment of choice. With aggressive types of NHL, aggressive combinations of chemotherapeutic agents are given even in early stages. More intermediate forms are commonly treated with combination chemotherapy and radiation therapy for stage I and II disease. The biologic agent interferon has been approved for the treatment of follicular low-grade lymphomas, and an antibody to CD20, rituximab (Rituxan), has been effective in achieving partial responses in patients with recurrent low-grade lymphoma. Studies of this agent in combination with conventional chemotherapy have demonstrated an improvement in survival as well (Coiffier, 2002; Emmanouilides et al., 2000; Petryk & Grossbard, 2000). Central nervous system involvement is also common with some aggressive forms of NHL; in this situation, cranial radiation or intrathecal chemotherapy is used in addition to systemic chemotherapy. Treatment after relapse is controversial. BMT or PBSCT may be considered for patients younger than 60 years of age (See Chap. 16).

Nursing Management

Most of the care for patients with Hodgkin's disease or NHL is performed in the outpatient setting, unless complications occur (eg, infection, respiratory compromise due to mediastinal mass). For patients who require treatment, chemotherapy and radiation therapy are most commonly used. Chemotherapy causes systemic side effects (eg, myelosuppression, nausea, hair loss, risk for infection), whereas the side effects from radiation therapy are specific to the area being irradiated. For example, patients receiving abdominal radiation therapy may experience nausea and diarrhea but not hair loss. Regardless of the type of treatment, all patients may experience fatigue.

The risk of infection is significant for these patients, not only from treatment-related myelosuppression but also from the defective immune response that results from the disease itself. Patients need to be taught to minimize the risks for infection, to recognize signs of possible infection, and to contact the health care professional should such signs develop (see Chart 33-8).

Many lymphomas can be cured with current treatments. However, as survival rates increase, the incidence of second malignancies, particularly AML or MDS, also increases. Therefore, survivors should be screened regularly for the development of second malignancies.

Lymphoma is a highly complex constellation of diseases. When caring for the patient with lymphoma, it is extremely important to know the specific disease type, stage of disease, treatment history, and current treatment plan.

MULTIPLE MYELOMA

Multiple myeloma is a malignant disease of the most mature form of B lymphocyte, the plasma cell. It is not classified as a lymphoma. Plasma cells secrete immunoglobulins, proteins necessary for antibody production to fight infection.

Pathophysiology

In myeloma, the malignant plasma cells produce an increased amount of a specific immunoglobulin that is nonfunctional. Functional types of immunoglobulin are still produced by nonmalignant plasma cells, but in lower-than-normal quantity. The specific immunoglobulin secreted by the myeloma cells is detectable in the blood or urine and is referred to as the monoclonal protein, or M protein. This protein serves as a useful marker to monitor the extent of disease and the patient's response to therapy. It is measured by serum or urine protein electrophoresis. Moreover, the patient's total protein level is typically elevated, again due to the production of M protein. Malignant plasma cells also secrete certain substances to stimulate the creation of new blood vessels to enhance the growth of these clusters of plasma cells; this process is referred to as angiogenesis. Occasionally the plasma cells infiltrate other tissue, in which case they are referred to as plasmacytomas. Plasmacytomas can occur in the sinuses, spinal cord, and soft tissues. Median survival time is 3 to 5 years. Death usually results from infection.

Clinical Manifestations

The classic presenting symptom of multiple myeloma is bone pain, usually in the back or ribs. Bone pain is reported by two thirds of all patients at diagnosis. Unlike arthritic pain, the bone pain associated with myeloma increases with movement and decreases with rest; patients may report that they have less pain on awakening but the pain intensity increases during the day. In myeloma, a substance secreted by the plasma cells, osteoclast activating factor, as well as other substances (eg, interleukin-6 [IL-6]) are involved in stimulating osteoclasts. Both mechanisms appear to be involved in the process of bone breakdown. Thus, lytic lesions as well as osteoporosis may be seen on bone x-rays. (They are not well visualized on bone scans.) The bone destruction can be severe enough to cause fractures, including spinal fractures, which can impinge on the spinal cord and result in spinal cord compression. It is this bone destruction that causes significant pain.

 NURSING ALERT Any elderly patient whose chief complaint is back pain, and who has an elevated total protein level, should be evaluated for possible myeloma.

If the bone destruction is fairly extensive, excessive ionized calcium is lost from the bone and enters the serum; patients may therefore become hypercalcemic (frequently manifested by excessive thirst, dehydration, constipation, altered mental status, confusion, and perhaps coma). Renal failure may also be seen; the configuration of the circulating immunoglobulin molecule (particularly the shape of lambda light chains) can damage the renal tubules.

As more and more malignant plasma cells are produced, the marrow has less space for RBC production, and the patient can become anemic. This anemia is also caused to a great extent by a diminished production of erythropoietin (a glycoprotein necessary for RBC production) by the kidney. Patients may complain of fatigue and weakness due to the anemia. In the late stage of the disease, a reduced number of WBCs and platelets may also be seen because the bone marrow is infiltrated by malignant plasma cells.

When plasma cells secrete excessive amounts of immunoglobulin, particularly IgA, the serum viscosity can be elevated. Hyperviscosity may be manifested by bleeding from the nose or mouth, headache, blurred vision, paresthesias, or heart failure.

Assessment and Diagnostic Findings

Finding an elevated monoclonal protein spike in the serum (via serum protein electrophoresis) or urine (via urine protein electrophoresis) or light chain in the urine (sometimes referred to as Bence Jones protein) is considered to be a major criterion in the diagnosis of multiple myeloma. The presence of lytic bone lesions on x-ray aids in the diagnosis, as does the presence of anemia or hypercalcemia. The diagnosis of myeloma can be confirmed by bone marrow biopsy; the presence of sheets of plasma cells is the hallmark diagnostic criterion. Because the infiltration of the marrow by these malignant plasma cells is not uniform, the extent of plasma cells may not be increased in a given sample (a false-negative result).

Gerontologic Considerations

The incidence of multiple myeloma increases with age; the disease rarely occurs in patients younger than 40 years of age. Because of the increasing older population, more patients are seeking treatment for this disease. BMT or PBSCT is an option that can prolong remission and potentially cure some patients. However, it is unavailable to most because of age limitations. Back pain, which is often a presenting symptom in this disease, should be closely investigated in elderly patients.

Medical Management

There is no cure for multiple myeloma. Even BMT or PBSCT is considered by most authorities to extend remission rather than provide a cure. However, for many patients, it is possible to control the illness and maintain their level of functioning quite well for several years or longer. Chemotherapy is the primary treatment; corticosteroids, particularly dexamethasone (Decadron), are especially effective and are often combined with other agents (such as melphalan (Alkeran), cyclophosphamide (Cytoxan), doxorubicin (Adriamycin), vincristine (Vincasar, PFS), and BCNU (eg, Carmustine, BiCNU).

Radiation therapy is very useful in strengthening the bone at a specific lesion, particularly one at risk for bone fracture or spinal cord compression. It is also useful in relieving bone pain and reducing the size of plasma cell tumours that occur outside the skeletal system. However, because it is a nonsystemic form of treatment, it does not diminish the source of the bone conditions (ie, the production of malignant plasma cells). Therefore, radiation therapy is typically used with systemic treatment such as chemotherapy.

The biologic agent alpha-interferon has been used successfully to maintain remission in selected types of myeloma, particularly IgA type; however, its role in prolonging survival is controversial. Newer forms of bisphosphonates, such as pamidronate (Aredia) and zoledronic acid (Zometa), have been shown to strengthen bone

in this disease (by diminishing the secretion of osteoclast activating factor) (Berenson, 2001), controlling bone pain and potentially preventing bone fracture. They are also effective in managing and preventing hypercalcemia. Some evidence suggests that bisphosphonates may actually have activity against the myeloma cells themselves by inhibiting a growth factor necessary for myeloma cell survival (Berenson, 2001) (see later discussion).

When patients manifest signs and symptoms of hyperviscosity, plasmapheresis may be used to lower the immunoglobulin level. Symptoms may be more useful than serum viscosity levels in determining the need for this intervention.

Recent advances in the understanding of the process of angiogenesis have resulted in new therapeutic options. The sedative thalidomide (Thalomid), initially used as an antiemetic, has significant antimyeloma effects. It inhibits cytokines necessary for new vascular generation, such as vascular endothelial growth factor (VEGF), and for myeloma cell growth and survival, such as IL-6 and tumour necrosis factor (TNF), by boosting the body's immune response against the tumour and by creating favourable conditions for apoptosis (programmed cell death) of the myeloma cells. Thalidomide is effective in refractory myeloma and in "smoldering" disease states, and may prevent progression to a more active state. Thalidomide is not a typical chemotherapeutic agent and has a unique side effect profile. Fatigue, dizziness, constipation, rash, and peripheral neuropathy are commonly encountered; myelosuppression is not (Goldman, 2001). Thalidomide is contraindicated in pregnancy because of associated severe birth defects.

Nursing Management

Pain management is very important in this patient population. NSAIDs can be very useful for mild pain, or in combination with opioid analgesics. However, care needs to be taken, because NSAIDs can cause renal dysfunction. Patients need to be educated about activity restrictions (eg, lifting no more than 10 pounds, use of proper body mechanics). Braces are occasionally needed to provide support to the spinal column.

Patients also need to be instructed about the signs and symptoms of hypercalcemia. Maintaining mobility and hydration is important to diminish exacerbations of this complication; however, the primary cause is the disease itself. Renal function should also be monitored closely. Renal failure can become severe, and dialysis may be needed. Maintaining high urine output (3 L/day) can be very useful in preventing this complication.

Because antibody production is impaired, infections, particularly bacterial infections, are common and can be life-threatening. Patients need to be instructed in appropriate infection prevention measures (see Chart 33-8) and should be advised to contact their health care provider immediately if they have a fever or other signs and symptoms of infection. Patients should receive Pneumovax and flu vaccines. Prophylactic antibiotics are sometimes used. Intravenous immune globulin (IVIG) can be useful for patients with recurrent infections.

Bleeding Disorders

Normal hemostatic mechanisms can control bleeding from vessels and prevent spontaneous bleeding. The bleeding vessel constricts and platelets aggregate at the site, forming an unstable hemostatic plug. Circulating coagulation factors are activated on the surface of these aggregated platelets, forming fibrin, which anchors the platelet plug to the site of injury.

The failure of normal hemostatic mechanisms can result in bleeding, which is severe at times. This bleeding is commonly provoked by trauma, but in certain circumstances it can occur spontaneously. When the source is platelet or coagulation factor abnormalities, the site of spontaneous bleeding can be anywhere in the body. When the defect is caused by vascular abnormalities, the site of bleeding may be more localized. Some patients have defects in more than one hemostatic mechanism simultaneously.

In a variety of situations, the bone marrow may be stimulated to increase platelet production (thrombopoiesis). The increased production may be a reactive response, as in a compensatory response to significant bleeding, or a more general response to increase hematopoiesis, as in iron deficiency anemia. Sometimes, the increase in platelets does not result from increased production but from a loss in platelet pooling within the spleen. The spleen typically holds about one third of the circulating platelets at any time. If the spleen is lost (eg, splenectomy), the platelet reservoir is also lost, and an abnormally high amount of platelets enter the circulation. In time, the rate of thrombopoiesis slows to reestablish a more normal platelet level.

Clinical Manifestations

Signs and symptoms of bleeding disorders vary depending on the type of defect. A careful history and physical examination can be very useful in determining the source of the hemostatic defect. Abnormalities of the vascular system give rise to local bleeding, usually into the skin. Because platelets are primarily responsible for stopping bleeding from small vessels, patients with platelet defects develop petechiae, often in clusters; these are seen on the skin and mucous membranes but also occur throughout the body. Bleeding from platelet disorders can be severe. Unless the platelet disorder is severe, bleeding can often be stopped promptly when local pressure is applied; it does not typically recur when the pressure is released.

In contrast, coagulation factor defects do not tend to cause superficial bleeding, because the primary hemostatic mechanisms are still intact. Instead, bleeding occurs deeper within the body (eg, subcutaneous or intramuscular hematomas, hemorrhage into joint spaces). External bleeding diminishes very slowly when local pressure is applied; it often recurs several hours after pressure is removed. For example, severe bleeding may start several hours after a tooth extraction. Risk factors for bleeding are provided in Chart 33-7.

Medical Management

Management varies based on the underlying cause of the bleeding disorder. If bleeding is significant, transfusions of blood products are indicated. The specific blood product used is determined by the underlying defect. In specific situations in which fibrinolysis is excessive, hemostatic agents such as aminocaproic acid (Amicar) can be used to inhibit this process. This agent must be used with caution, because excessive inhibition of fibrinolysis can result in thrombosis.

Nursing Management

Patients who have bleeding disorders or who have the potential for development of such disorders as a result of disease or therapeutic agents must be taught to observe themselves carefully and frequently for bleeding. They need to understand the importance of avoiding activities that increase the risk of bleeding, such as

contact sports. The skin is observed for petechiae and ecchymoses (bruises) and the nose and gums for bleeding. Hospitalized patients may be monitored for bleeding by testing all drainage and excreta (feces, urine, emesis, and gastric drainage) for occult as well as obvious blood. Outpatients are often given fecal occult blood screening cards to detect occult blood in stools.

PRIMARY THROMBOCYTHEMIA

Primary thrombocythemia (also called essential thrombocythemia [ET]) is a stem cell disorder within the bone marrow. A marked increase in platelet production occurs, with the platelet count consistently greater than 600,000/mm³. Platelet size may be abnormal, but platelet survival is typically normal. Occasionally, the platelet increase is accompanied by an increase in RBCs or WBCs or both; however, these cells are not increased to the extent that they are in polycythemia vera, CML, or myelofibrosis. Although the exact cause is unknown, primary thrombocythemia is similar to other myeloproliferative disorders, particularly polycythemia vera. Unlike the other myeloproliferative disorders, however, it rarely evolves into acute leukemia.

Clinical Manifestations

Many patients with primary thrombocythemia are asymptomatic; the illness is diagnosed as the result of finding an elevated platelet count on a CBC. Symptoms, when they do occur, result primarily from hemorrhage or vasoocclusion in the microvasculature. Symptoms may occur more when the platelet count exceeds 1 million/mm³. However, symptoms do not always correlate with the extent to which the platelet count is elevated. Thrombosis is common and can be either arterial or venous; major thromboses occur in 15% to 40% of these patients (Jantunen et al., 2001). Because these platelets can be dysfunctional, minor or major hemorrhage can also occur. Bleeding from the mucous membranes of the nose and mouth is common, and significant gastrointestinal bleeding is also possible. Bleeding typically does not occur until the platelet count exceeds 1 million/mm³.

Vasoocclusive manifestations are most frequently seen in the form of erythromelalgia. The toxic effects of platelet substances include painful burning, warmth, and redness in a localized distal area of the extremities. Neurologic manifestations may also be seen, such as numbness, tingling, and visual disturbance; these occlusive manifestations can progress to stroke and seizure and, less commonly, to myocardial infarction. The spleen may be enlarged, but usually not to a significant extent.

Assessment and Diagnostic Findings

The diagnosis of primary thrombocythemia is made by ruling out other potential disorders. Iron deficiency should be excluded, because a reactive increase in the platelet count often accompanies this deficiency. The myeloproliferative disorders (CML, polycythemia vera) should also be excluded. Examination of the CBC shows markedly abnormal platelets. Analysis of the bone marrow (by aspiration and biopsy) shows a marked increase in megakaryocytes (platelet precursors) and is useful in excluding CML as a possible cause for the elevated platelet count. The disease, which affects men and women equally, tends to occur in late middle age. The median survival time exceeds 10 years.

No data reliably predict the development of complications. Risk factors for the development of thrombotic complications are age greater than 65 years, prior thrombotic events, and long duration of thrombocytosis. Major bleeding tends to occur when the platelet count is very high.

Medical Management

The management of primary thrombocythemia is highly controversial. The risk of significant thrombotic or hemorrhagic complications may not be increased until the platelet count exceeds 1 million/mm³ (Briere & Guilmin, 2001). A careful assessment of other risk factors, such as history of peripheral vascular disease, history of tobacco use, atherosclerosis, and prior thrombotic events, should be used in making the decision as to when to initiate therapy. In younger patients with no risk factors, low-dose aspirin therapy may be sufficient to prevent thrombotic complications; however, the use of aspirin can increase the risk for hemorrhagic complications and may be considered a contraindication in patients with a history of gastrointestinal bleeding. The neurologic symptoms (eg, headache and erythromelalgia) and visual symptoms of primary thrombocytopenia can be relieved by low-dose aspirin.

More aggressive measures may be required in older patients and in those with concurrent risk factors. Hydroxyurea (Hydrea), a chemotherapeutic medication, is effective in lowering the platelet count. It is taken orally and causes minimal side effects other than dose-related leukopenia. However, its potential for leukogenesis is in question. The medication anagrelide (Agrylin) is more specific in lowering the platelet count than is hydroxyurea, but it has more side effects. Severe headaches cause many patients to stop taking the medication. Tachycardia and chest pain may also occur, and anagrelide is contraindicated in patients with concurrent cardiac problems. Interferon-alfa-2b (eg, Intron-A) has been shown to lower platelet counts by an unknown mechanism. The medication is administered subcutaneously at varying frequency, commonly three times per week. Significant side effects, such as fatigue, weakness, memory defects, dizziness, anemia, and liver dysfunction, limit its usefulness.

Rarely, the occlusive symptoms are so great that the platelet count must be reduced immediately. Platelet pheresis (see later discussion) can reduce the amount of circulating platelets, but only transiently. The extent by which symptoms and complications (eg, thromboses) are reduced remains unclear.

Nursing Management

Patients with primary thrombocythemia need to be instructed about the accompanying risks of hemorrhage and thrombosis. Patients should be informed about signs and symptoms of thrombosis, particularly the neurologic manifestations, such as visual changes, numbness, tingling, and weakness. Risk factors for thrombosis should be assessed, and measures to diminish risk factors (particularly cessation of tobacco use) should be encouraged. Patients receiving aspirin therapy should be informed about the increased risk for bleeding. Patients who are at risk for bleeding should be instructed about medications that can alter platelet function, such as aspirin, NSAIDs, and alcohol. Patients receiving interferon therapy should be taught to self-administer the medication and manage side effects.

SECONDARY THROMBOCYTOSIS

Increased platelet production is the primary mechanism of secondary, or reactive, **thrombocytosis**. The platelet count is above

normal, but, in contrast to primary thrombocythemia, an increase above 1 million/mm³ is rare. Platelet function is normal; the platelet survival time is normal or decreased. Symptoms associated with hemorrhage or thrombosis are rare. Many disorders can cause a reactive increase in platelets, including chronic inflammatory disorders, iron deficiency, malignant disease, acute hemorrhage, and splenectomy (see previous discussion of primary thrombocythemia). Treatment is aimed at the underlying disorder. With successful management, the platelet count usually returns to normal.

THROMBOCYTOPENIA

Thrombocytopenia (low platelet level) can result from various factors: decreased production of platelets within the bone marrow, increased destruction of platelets, or increased consumption of platelets. Causes and treatments are summarized in Table 33-5.

Clinical Manifestations

Bleeding and petechiae usually do not occur with platelet counts greater than 50,000/mm³, although excessive bleeding can follow surgery or other trauma. When the platelet count drops below

Table 33-5 • Causes and Management of Thrombocytopenia

CAUSE	MANAGEMENT
Decreased Production	
Hematologic malignancy, especially acute leukemias	Treat leukemia; platelet transfusion
Myelodysplastic syndromes (MDS): metastatic involvement of bone marrow from solid tumours	Treat MDS; platelet transfusion Treat solid tumour
Aplastic anemia	Treat underlying condition
Megaloblastic anemia	Treat underlying anemia
Toxins	Remove toxin
Medications	Stop medication
Infection (esp. septicemia, viral infection, tuberculosis)	Treat infection
Alcohol	Refrain from alcohol consumption
Chemotherapy	Delay or decrease dose; growth factor; platelet transfusion
Increased Destruction	
Due to Antibodies Idiopathic thrombocytopenic purpura Lupus erythematosus Malignant lymphoma	Treat condition
Chronic lymphocytic leukemia (CLL)	Treat CLL and/or treat as ITP
Medications	Stop medication
Due to Infection Bacteremia Postviral infection	Treat infection
Sequestration of platelets in an enlarged spleen	If thrombocytopenia is severe, splenectomy may be needed
Increased Consumption	
Disseminated intravascular coagulation (DIC)	Treat underlying condition triggering DIC; administer heparin, EACA, blood products

20,000/mm^3, petechiae can appear, along with nose and gingival bleeding, excessive menstrual bleeding, and excessive bleeding after surgery or dental extractions. When the platelet count is less than 5000/mm^3, spontaneous, potentially fatal central nervous system or gastrointestinal hemorrhage can occur. If the platelets are dysfunctional due to disease (eg, MDS) or medications (eg, aspirin), the risk of bleeding may be much greater even when the actual platelet count is not significantly reduced.

Assessment and Diagnostic Findings

A platelet deficiency that results from decreased production (eg, leukemia, MDS) can usually be diagnosed by examining the bone marrow via aspiration and biopsy. When platelet destruction is the cause of thrombocytopenia, the marrow shows increased megakaryocytes (the cells from which the platelets originate) and normal or even increased platelet production as the body attempts to compensate for the decreased platelets in circulation. Another cause of thrombocytopenia is sequestration. Approximately one third of the circulating platelets are within the spleen, and a greatly enlarged spleen results in increased sequestration of platelets.

Medical Management

The management for secondary thrombocytopenia is usually treatment of the underlying disease. If platelet production is impaired, platelet transfusions may raise the platelet count and stop bleeding or prevent spontaneous hemorrhage. If excessive platelet destruction occurs, transfused platelets will also be destroyed, and the platelet count will not rise. The most common cause of excessive platelet destruction is ITP (see the following discussion). In some instances splenectomy can be a useful therapeutic intervention, but often it is not a therapeutic option, for example in patients in whom the enlarged spleen is due to portal hypertension related to excessive alcohol consumption.

Nursing Management

The interventions for a patient with thrombocytopenia are delineated in Chart 33-10.

IDIOPATHIC THROMBOCYTOPENIC PURPURA (ITP)

ITP is a disease that affects people of all ages, but it is more common among children and young women. There are two forms of ITP: acute and chronic. The acute form, which occurs predominantly in children, often appears 1 to 6 weeks after a viral illness. This form is self-limited; remission often occurs spontaneously within 6 months. Occasionally, corticosteroids are needed for a brief time. Chronic ITP is often diagnosed by exclusion of other causes of thrombocytopenia.

Pathophysiology

Although the precise cause remains unknown, viral infections sometimes precede ITP in children. Occasionally medications such as sulfa drugs can induce ITP. Other conditions, such as systemic lupus erythematosus (SLE) or pregnancy, can also induce ITP. Anti-platelet autoantibodies that bind to the patient's platelets are found in the blood of patients with ITP. When the platelets are bound by the antibodies, the RES or tissue macrophage system ingests the platelets, destroying them. The body attempts to compensate for this destruction by increasing platelet production within the marrow.

Clinical Manifestations

Many patients have no symptoms, and the low platelet count (often less than 20,000/mm^3, and less than 5000/mm^3 is not uncommon) is an incidental finding. Common physical manifestations are easy bruising, heavy menses, and petechiae on the extremities or trunk. Patients with simple bruising or petechiae ("dry purpura") tend to have fewer complications from bleeding than those with bleeding from mucosal surfaces, such as the gastrointestinal tract (including the mouth) and pulmonary system (eg, hemoptysis), which is termed "wet purpura." Patients with wet purpura have a greater risk for intracranial bleeding than do those with dry purpura. Despite low platelet counts, the platelets are young and very functional. They adhere to endothelial surfaces and to one another, so spontaneous bleeding does not always occur.

Assessment and Diagnostic Findings

Patients may have an isolated decrease in platelets (less than 20,000/mm^3 is common), but they may also have an increase in megakaryocytes (platelet precursors) within the marrow, as detected on bone marrow aspirate.

Medical Management

The primary goal of treatment is a safe platelet count. Because the risk of bleeding typically does not increase until the platelet count is lower than 10,000/mm^3, a patient whose count exceeds 30,000 to 50,000/mm^3 may be carefully observed without additional intervention. However, if the count is lower than 20,000/mm^3, or if bleeding occurs, the goal is to improve the patient's platelet count, rather than to cure the disease. Treatment for ITP usually requires several approaches. If the patient is taking a medication that is known to cause ITP (eg, quinine, sulfa-containing medications), that medication must be stopped immediately. The mainstay of short-term therapy is the use of immunosuppressive agents. The immunosuppressants block the binding receptors on macrophages so that the platelets are not destroyed. Prednisone is the agent typically used (at a dose of 1 mg/kg), and it is effective in about 75% of patients. Cyclophosphamide (Cytoxan) and azathioprine (Imuran) can also be used, and dexamethasone (Decadron) may be effective. Platelet counts rise within a few days after institution of corticosteroid therapy; this effect takes longer with azathioprine. Because of the associated side effects, patients cannot take high doses of corticosteroids indefinitely. It is not unusual for the platelet count to drop once the corticosteroid dose is tapered. Some patients can be successfully maintained on low doses of prednisone (eg, 2.5 to 10 mg every other day).

Intravenous immune globulin (IVIG) is also commonly used to treat ITP. It is effective in binding the receptors on the macrophages; however, high doses (1 g/kg for 2 days) are required, and the drug is very expensive. Splenectomy is an alternative treatment but results in a normal platelet count only 50% of the time; however, many patients can maintain a "safe" platelet count of more than 30,000/mm^3 after removal of the spleen. Even those who do respond to splenectomy may have recurrences of severe thrombocytopenia months or years later. Patients who have splenectomy are permanently at risk for sepsis; these patients should receive Pneumovax, *Haemophilus influenzae* B, and meningococcal vaccines, preferably 2 to 3 weeks before the splenectomy is performed. Pneumovax vaccine should be repeated at 5- to 10-year intervals.

Other options for management include use of the chemotherapy agent vincristine (Vincasar, PFS). Vincristine appears to work by blocking the receptors on the macrophages and therefore inhibiting platelet destruction; it may also stimulate thrombopoiesis. Some data support the efficacy of certain monoclonal antibodies (eg, rituximab) in increasing platelet counts, but more research is needed (Stasi, Pagano, Stipa, & Amadori, 2001; Saleh et al., 2000).

Another approach to the management of chronic ITP involves the use of anti-D (eg, WinRho) in patients who are Rh(D)-positive. The actual mechanism of action is unknown. One theory is that the anti-D binds to the patient's RBCs, which are in turn destroyed by the body's macrophages. While the macrophages destroy the anti-D/RBC complex, they are not able to destroy platelets. Anti-D produces a transient decreased hematocrit and increased platelet count in many, but not all, patients with ITP. Anti-D appears to be most effective in children with ITP and least effective in patients who have undergone splenectomy.

Despite the extremely low platelet count, platelet transfusions are usually avoided. Transfusions tend to be ineffective because the patient's anti-platelet antibodies bind with the transfused platelets, causing them to be destroyed. Platelet counts can actually drop after platelet transfusion. Occasionally, transfusion of platelets may protect against catastrophic bleeding in patients with severe wet purpura. Epsilon-aminocaproic acid (EACA; Amicar) may be useful for patients with significant mucosal bleeding refractory to other treatments.

Nursing Management

Nursing care for these patients should include an assessment of the patient's life style to determine the risk of bleeding from activity. A careful medication history should also be obtained, including use of over-the-counter medications, herbs, and nutritional supplements. The nurse must be alert for sulfa-containing medications and medications that alter platelet function (eg, medications that contain aspirin or other NSAIDs). The nurse should assess for any history of recent viral illness and reports of headache or visual disturbances (which could be initial symptoms of intracranial bleeding). Patients who are admitted to the hospital with wet purpura and low platelet counts should have a neurologic assessment incorporated into their routine vital sign measurements. No intramuscular injections or rectal medications should be administered, and rectal temperature measurements should not be performed, because they can stimulate bleeding.

Patient teaching should address signs of exacerbation of disease (petechiae, ecchymoses); how to contact appropriate health care personnel; the name and type of medication inducing ITP (if appropriate); current medical treatment (medications, tapering schedule if relevant, side effects); and the frequency of monitoring the platelet count. Patients should be instructed to avoid all agents that interfere with platelet function. The patient should avoid constipation, the Valsalva manoeuvre (eg, straining at stool), and flossing of the teeth. Electric razors should be used for shaving, and soft-bristled toothbrushes should replace stiff-bristled ones. Patients should also be counselled to refrain from vigourous sexual intercourse when the platelet count is less than 10,000/mm³. Patients who are receiving chronic corticosteroids are at risk for complications including osteoporosis, proximal muscle wasting,

cataract formation, and dental caries (see Chart 33-4). Bone mineral density should be monitored, and these patients may benefit from calcium and vitamin D supplementation and bisphosphonate therapy to prevent significant bone disease.

PLATELET DEFECTS

Quantitative platelet defects are relatively common (thrombocytopenia), but qualitative defects can also occur. With qualitative defects, the number of platelets may be normal, but the platelets do not function normally. Platelet function is most commonly evaluated by the bleeding time; however, this test is a crude measurement at best.

An important functional platelet disorder is that induced by aspirin. Even small amounts of aspirin reduce normal platelet aggregation, and the prolonged bleeding time lasts for several days after aspirin ingestion. Although this does not cause bleeding in most people, patients with a coagulation disorder (eg, hemophilia) or thrombocytopenia can have significant bleeding after taking aspirin, particularly if invasive procedures or trauma has occurred.

NSAIDs can also inhibit platelet function, but the effect is not as prolonged as with aspirin (about 5 days versus 7 to 10 days). Other causes of platelet dysfunction include end-stage renal disease, possibly from metabolic products affecting platelet function; MDS; multiple myeloma (due to abnormal protein interfering with platelet function); cardiopulmonary bypass; and other medications and substances (Chart 33-13).

Clinical Manifestations

Bleeding may be mild or severe. Its extent is not necessarily correlated with the platelet count or with tests that measure coagulation (prothrombin time [PT], activated partial thromboplastin time [aPTT]). Ecchymoses are common, particularly on the extremities. Patients with platelet dysfunction may be at risk for significant bleeding after trauma or invasive procedures (eg, biopsy, dental extraction).

Medical Management

If the platelet dysfunction is caused by medication, use of the offending medication should be stopped, if possible, particularly when bleeding occurs. If platelet dysfunction is marked, bleeding can often be prevented by transfusion of normal platelets before invasive procedures. Amniocaproic acid (Amicar) may be required to prevent significant bleeding after such procedures.

Nursing Management

Patients with significant platelet dysfunction need to be instructed to avoid agents that can diminish platelet function, such as certain over-the-counter medications, herbs, nutritional supplements, and alcohol. They also need to be assisted to serve as their own advocates and to inform their health care providers (including dentists) of the underlying condition before any invasive procedure is performed, so that appropriate steps can be initiated to diminish the risk of bleeding. Bleeding precautions should be initiated as appropriate (see Chart 33-10).

HEMOPHILIA

Two inherited bleeding disorders—hemophilia A and hemophilia B—are clinically indistinguishable, although they can be distinguished by laboratory tests. Hemophilia A is caused by a

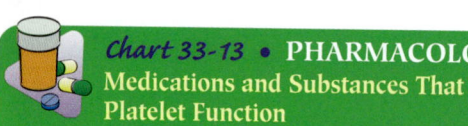

Chart 33-13 • PHARMACOLOGY
Medications and Substances That Impair Platelet Function

Anesthetic Agents
Local anesthetics
Halothane

Antibiotics
Beta-lactam antibiotics
  Penicillins
  Cephalosporins
Nitrofurantoin
Sulfonylureas

Anticoagulation Agents
Heparin
Fibrinolytic agents

Anti-inflammatory Agents (Nonsteroidal)
Aspirin
Ibuprofen
Naproxen

Antineoplastic Agents
BCNU
Daunorubicin
Mithramycin

Cardiovascular Drugs
Beta-blockers
Calcium channel blockers
Isosorbide
Nitroglycerine
Nitroprusside
Quinidine

Medications That Increase Platelet CAMP
Dipyridamole
Prostacycline
Theophylline

Food and Food Additives
Caffeine
Chinese black tree fungus
Clove
Cumin
Ethanol
Fish oils
Garlic
Onion extract
Turmeric

Plasma Expanders
Dextrans
Hydroxyethyl starch

Psychotropic Agents
Tricyclic antidepressants
Phenothiazines

Miscellaneous
Antihistamines
Clofibrate
Furosemide
Heroin
Contrast agents
Ticlopidine
Vitamin E

Herbal Supplements
Feverfew
Ginger
Gingko
Ginseng
Kava kava

---

genetic defect that results in deficient or defective factor VIII; hemophilia B (also called Christmas disease) stems from a genetic defect that causes deficient or defective factor IX. Hemophilia is a relatively rare disease; hemophilia A, which occurs in 1 of every 10,000 births, is three times more common than hemophilia B. Both types of hemophilia are inherited as X-linked traits, so almost all affected people are males; females can be carriers but are almost always asymptomatic. The disease is recognized in early childhood, usually in the toddler age group. However, patients with mild hemophilia may not be diagnosed until they experience severe trauma (eg, a high-school football injury) or surgery. Hemophilia occurs in all ethnic groups.

Clinical Manifestations

The disease, which can be severe, is manifested by hemorrhages into various parts of the body. Hemorrhage can occur even after minimal trauma. The frequency and severity of the bleeding depend on the degree of factor deficiency as well as the intensity of the precipitating trauma. For example, patients who have a mild factor VIII deficiency (ie, 6% to 50% of normal levels) rarely develop hemorrhage spontaneously; hemorrhage tends to occur

secondary to trauma. In contrast, spontaneous hemorrhages, particularly hemarthroses and hematomas, can frequently occur in patients with severe factor VIII deficiency (ie, less than 1% of normal levels). These patients require frequent factor replacement therapy.

About 75% of all bleeding in patients with hemophilia occurs into joints. The most commonly affected joints are the knees, elbows, ankles, shoulders, wrists, and hips. Patients often note pain in a joint before they are aware of swelling and limitation of motion. Recurrent joint hemorrhages can result in damage so severe that chronic pain or ankylosis (fixation) of the joint occurs. Many patients with severe factor deficiency are crippled by the joint damage before they become adults. Hematomas can be superficial or deep hemorrhages into muscle or subcutaneous tissue. With severe factor deficiency, they can occur without known trauma and progressively extend in all directions. When the hematomas occur within muscle, particularly in the extremities, peripheral nerves can be compressed. Over time, this compression results in decreased sensation, weakness, and atrophy of the area involved. Spontaneous hematuria and gastrointestinal bleeding can occur. Bleeding is also common in other mucous membranes, such as the nasal passages. The most dangerous site of hemorrhage is in the head (intracranial or extracranial). Any head trauma requires prompt evaluation and treatment. Surgical procedures typically result in excessive bleeding at the surgical site. Because clot formation is poor, wound healing is also poor. Such bleeding is most commonly associated with dental extraction.

Medical Management

In the past, the only treatment for hemophilia was infusion of fresh frozen plasma, which had to be administered in such large quantities that patients experienced fluid volume overload. Now factor VIII and factor IX concentrates are available to all blood banks. Recombinant forms of these factors have been made available and may diminish the use of factor concentrates. Patients are given concentrates when they are actively bleeding or as a preventive measure before traumatic procedures (eg, lumbar puncture, dental extraction, surgery). The patient and family are taught how to administer the concentrate intravenously at home at the first sign of bleeding. It is crucial to initiate treatment as soon as possible so that bleeding complications can be avoided. A few patients eventually develop antibodies to the concentrates, so their factor levels cannot be increased. Treatment of this problem is extremely difficult and often unsuccessful.

Aminocaproic acid (Amicar) is a fibrinolytic enzyme inhibitor that can slow the dissolution of blood clots that do form; it is very effective as an adjunctive measure after oral surgery. It is also useful in treating mucosal bleeding. Another agent, desmopressin (DDAVP), induces a transient rise in factor VIII levels; the mechanism for this response is unknown. In patients with mild forms of hemophilia A, desmopressin is extremely useful, significantly reducing the amount of blood products required. However, desmopressin is not effective in patients with severe factor VIII deficiency.

Nursing Management

Most patients with hemophilia are diagnosed as children. They often require assistance in coping with the condition because it is chronic, places restrictions on their lives, and is an inherited disorder that can be passed to future generations. From childhood, patients are helped to accept themselves and the disease and to identify the positive aspects of their lives. They are encouraged to be self-sufficient and to maintain independence by preventing unnecessary trauma that can cause acute bleeding episodes and temporarily interfere with normal activities. As they work through their feelings about the condition and progress to accepting it, they can assume more and more responsibility for maintaining optimal health.

Patients with mild factor deficiency may not be diagnosed until adulthood if they do not experience significant trauma or surgery as children. These patients need extensive teaching about activity restrictions and self-care measures to diminish the chance of hemorrhage and complications of bleeding. The nurse should emphasize safety at home and in the workplace.

Patients with hemophilia are instructed to avoid any agents that interfere with platelet aggregation, such as aspirin, NSAIDs, herbs, nutritional supplements, and alcohol. This restriction applies to over-the-counter medications such as cold remedies. Dental hygiene is very important as a preventive measure because dental extractions are so hazardous. Applying pressure may be sufficient to control bleeding resulting from minor trauma if the factor deficiency is not severe. Nasal packing should be avoided, because bleeding frequently resumes when the packing is removed. Splints and other orthopedic devices may be useful in patients with joint or muscle hemorrhages. All injections should be avoided; invasive procedures (eg, endoscopy, lumbar puncture) should be minimized or performed after administration of appropriate factor replacement. Patients with hemophilia should be encouraged to carry or wear medical identification.

During hemorrhagic episodes, the extent of bleeding must be assessed carefully. Patients who are at risk for significant compromise (eg, bleeding into the respiratory tract or brain) warrant close observation and systematic assessment for emergent complications (eg, respiratory distress, altered level of consciousness). If the patient has had recent surgery, the nurse frequently and carefully assesses the surgical site for bleeding. Frequent vital sign monitoring is needed until the nurse is certain that there is no excessive postoperative bleeding.

Analgesics are commonly required to alleviate the pain associated with hematomas and hemorrhage into joints. Many patients report that warm baths promote relaxation, improve mobility, and lessen pain. However, during bleeding episodes, heat, which can accentuate bleeding, is avoided; applications of cold are used instead.

Although recent technology (ie, the formulation of heat-solvent or detergent-treated factor concentrates) has rendered factor VIII and IX preparations free from viruses such as HIV and hepatitis, many patients have already been exposed to these infections. These patients and their families may need assistance in coping with the diagnosis and the consequences of these infections.

Between 15% and 50% of patients with hemophilia A and between 1% and 3% of patients with hemophilia B develop antibodies (inhibitors) to factor concentrates, complicating factor replacement management (Lusher, 2000; White, Greenwood, Escobar, & Frelinger, 2000). These patients may require plasmapheresis or concurrent immunosuppressive therapy, particularly in the setting of significant bleeding. Patients with severe factor deficiency should be screened for antibodies, particularly before major surgery.

VON WILLEBRAND'S DISEASE

Von Willebrand's disease, a common bleeding disorder affecting males and females equally, is usually inherited as a dominant trait. The disease is caused by a deficiency of von Willebrand factor (vWF), which is necessary for factor VIII activity. vWF is also nec-

essary for platelet adhesion at the site of vascular injury. Although synthesis of factor VIII is normal, its half-life is shortened; therefore, factor VIII levels commonly are mildly low (15% to 50% of normal).

Clinical Manifestations

Patients commonly have nosebleeds, excessively heavy menses, bleeding from cuts, and postoperative bleeding, although they do not suffer from massive soft tissue or joint hemorrhages. As the laboratory values fluctuate, so does the bleeding. For example, a careful history of prior bleeding may show little problem with postoperative bleeding on one occasion but significant bleeding from a dental extraction at another time.

Assessment and Diagnostic Findings

Laboratory test results show a normal platelet count but prolonged bleeding time and slightly prolonged aPTT. These defects are not static, and laboratory test results can vary widely within the same patient over time.

Medical Management

Both the factor deficiency and the platelet impairment can be corrected by administration of cryoprecipitate, which contains factor VIII, fibrinogen, and factor XIII (or fresh frozen plasma, if cryoprecipitate is unavailable). Replacement continues for several days to ensure correction of the factor VIII deficiency; up to 7 to 10 days of treatment may be necessary after major surgery. Desmopressin (DDAVP), a synthetic vasopressin analog, can be used to prevent bleeding associated with dental or surgical procedures or to manage mild bleeding after surgery. Desmopressin provides a transient increase in factor VIII coagulant activity and may also correct the bleeding time. It can be administered as an intravenous infusion or intranasally. With major surgery or invasive procedures, both desmopressin and cryoprecipitate may be needed to prevent hemorrhage.

Acquired Coagulation Disorders

LIVER DISEASE

With the exception of factor VIII, most blood coagulation factors are synthesized in the liver. Therefore, hepatic dysfunction (due to cirrhosis, tumour, or hepatitis; see Chap. 39) can result in diminished amounts of the factors needed to maintain coagulation and hemostasis. Prolongation of the PT, unless it is caused by vitamin K deficiency, may indicate severe hepatic dysfunction. Although minor bleeding is common (eg, ecchymoses), these patients are also at risk for significant bleeding, related especially to trauma or surgery. Transfusion of fresh frozen plasma may be required to replace clotting factors and to prevent or stop bleeding. Patients may also have life-threatening hemorrhage from peptic ulcers or esophageal varices. In these cases, replacement with fresh frozen plasma, PRBCs, and platelets is usually required.

VITAMIN K DEFICIENCY

The synthesis of many coagulation factors depends on vitamin K. Vitamin K deficiency is typical in malnourished patients, and some antibiotics decrease the intestinal flora that produce vitamin K, depleting vitamin K stores. Administration of vitamin K (phytonadione [eg, Mephyton], either orally or as a subcutaneous injection) can correct the deficiency quickly; adequate synthesis of coagulation factors is reflected by normalization of the PT.

COMPLICATIONS OF ANTICOAGULANT THERAPY

Anticoagulants are used in the treatment or prevention of thrombosis. These agents, particularly warfarin or heparin, can result in bleeding. If the PT or aPTT is longer than desired and bleeding has not occurred, the medication can be stopped or the dose decreased. Vitamin K is administered for warfarin toxicity. Protamine sulfate is rarely needed for heparin toxicity, because the half-life of heparin is very short. With significant bleeding, fresh frozen plasma replaces the vitamin K–dependent coagulation factors. Other complications of anticoagulant therapy are discussed in Chapter 31.

DISSEMINATED INTRAVASCULAR COAGULATION (DIC)

DIC is not a disease but a sign of an underlying condition. DIC may be triggered by sepsis, trauma, cancer, shock, abruptio placentae, toxins, or allergic reactions (Chart 33-14). It is potentially life-threatening.

Pathophysiology

In DIC, the normal hemostatic mechanisms are altered so that a massive amount of tiny clots forms in the microcirculation. Initially, the coagulation time is normal. However, as the platelets and clotting factors are consumed to form the microthrombi, coagulation fails. Thus, the paradoxical result of excessive clotting is bleeding. The clinical manifestations of DIC are reflected in the organs, which are affected either by excessive clot formation (with resultant ischemia to all or part of the organ) or by bleeding. The bleeding is characterized by low platelet and fibrinogen levels; prolonged PT, aPTT, and thrombin time; and elevated fibrin degradation products (**D-dimer**s) (Table 33-6).

The mortality rate can exceed 80% of patients who develop DIC. Identification of patients who are at risk for DIC and recognition of the early clinical manifestations of this syndrome can result in earlier medical intervention, which may improve the prognosis. However, the primary prognostic factor is the ability to treat the underlying condition that precipitated DIC.

Clinical Manifestations

Patients with DIC may bleed from mucous membranes, venipuncture sites, and the gastrointestinal and urinary tracts. The bleeding can range from minimal occult internal bleeding to profuse hemorrhage from all orifices. Patients may also develop organ dysfunction, such as renal failure and pulmonary and multifocal central nervous system infarctions as a result of microthromboses, macrothromboses, or hemorrhages.

During the initial process of DIC, the patient may have no new symptoms, the only manifestation being a progressive decrease in the platelet count. As the thrombosis becomes more extensive, the patient exhibits signs and symptoms of thrombosis in the organs involved. Then, as the clotting factors and platelets are consumed to form these thrombi, bleeding occurs. Initially the bleeding is subtle, but it can develop into frank hemorrhage. Signs and symptoms depend on the organs involved and are listed in Table 33-7.

Medical Management

The most important management issue is treating the underlying cause of the DIC. Until the cause is controlled, the mechanism for DIC will persist. A second goal is to correct the secondary effects of tissue ischemia by improving oxygenation, replacing fluids, correcting electrolyte imbalances, and administering vasopressor medications. If serious hemorrhage occurs, the depleted coagulation factors and platelets may be replaced to reestablish the potential for normal hemostasis and thereby diminish bleeding. Cryoprecipitate is given to replace fibrinogen and factors V and VII; fresh frozen plasma is administered to replace other coagulation factors.

A controversial method to interrupt the thrombosis process is the use of heparin infusion. Heparin may inhibit the formation of microthrombi and thus permit perfusion of the organs (skin, kidneys, or brain) to resume. Heparin is typically reserved for the patient in whom thrombotic manifestations predominate or in whom extensive blood component replacement fails to halt the hemorrhage or increase fibrinogen and other clotting levels. When heparin is administered, bleeding may actually worsen initially until the thrombotic process is interrupted. Consumed platelets and clotting factors need to be replaced. The effectiveness of heparin can best be determined by observing for normalization of the plasma fibrinogen concentration and diminishing signs of bleeding.

NURSING PROCESS: THE PATIENT WITH DISSEMINATED INTRAVASCULAR COAGULATION (DIC)

Assessment

Nurses need to be aware of patients who are at risk for DIC. Sepsis and acute promyelocytic leukemia are the most common causes of DIC. Patients need to be assessed thoroughly and frequently for signs and symptoms of thrombi and bleeding and monitored for any progression of these signs (see Table 33-7).

Diagnosis

NURSING DIAGNOSES

Based on the assessment data, major nursing diagnoses for the patient with DIC may include the following:

- Risk for deficient fluid volume related to bleeding
- Risk for impaired skin integrity related to ischemia or bleeding
- Potential for excess fluid volume related to excessive blood/factor component replacement
- Ineffective tissue perfusion related to microthrombi
- Anxiety and fear of the unknown and possible death

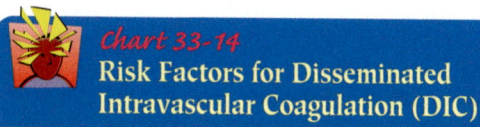

Chart 33-14
Risk Factors for Disseminated Intravascular Coagulation (DIC)

Sepsis
Obstetric complications
Acute hemolysis (eg, transfusion reaction)
Trauma
Shock
Cancer (especially prostate cancer and acute promyelocytic leukemia)
Allergic reactions

Table 33-6 • Laboratory Values Commonly Found in Disseminated Intravascular Coagulation (DIC)*

TEST	FUNCTION EVALUATED	NORMAL RANGE	CHANGES IN DIC
Platelet count	Platelet number	150,000–450,000/mm³	↓
Prothrombin time (PT)	Extrinsic pathway	11–12.5 sec	↑
Partial thromboplastin time (PTT)	Intrinsic pathway	23–35 sec	↑
Thrombin time (TT)	Clot formation	8–11 sec	↑
Fibrinogen	Amount available for coagulation	170–340 mg/dL	↓
D-dimer	Local fibrinolysis	0–250 ng/mL	↑
Fibrin degradation products (FDPs)	Fibrinolysis	0–5 µg/mL	↑
Euglobulin clot lysis	Fibrinolytic activity	≥2 hours	≤1 hour

*Because DIC is a dynamic condition, the laboratory values measured will change over time. Therefore, a progressive increase or decrease in a given laboratory value is likely to be more important than the actual value of a test at a single point in time.

COLLABORATIVE PROBLEMS/ POTENTIAL COMPLICATIONS

Collaborative problems include the clinical conditions that precipitated the DIC. Based on the assessment data, potential complications may include:

- Renal failure
- Gangrene
- Pulmonary embolism or hemorrhage
- Altered level of consciousness
- Acute respiratory distress syndrome
- Stroke

Planning and Goals

Major patient goals include maintenance of hemodynamic status, maintenance of intact skin and oral mucosa, maintenance of fluid balance, maintenance of tissue perfusion, enhanced coping, and absence of complications (see Plan of Nursing Care).

Nursing Interventions

See Plan of Nursing Care: The Patient with Disseminated Intravascular Coagulation.

MONITORING AND MANAGING POTENTIAL COMPLICATIONS

Despite aggressive measures, the lack of renal perfusion may result in acute renal failure, sometimes necessitating dialysis. Placement of a large-bore dialysis catheter is extremely hazardous in this patient population and should be accompanied by adequate platelet and plasma transfusions.

Table 33-7 • Recognizing Thrombosis and Bleeding in Disseminated Intravascular Coagulation (DIC)*

SYSTEM	SIGNS AND SYMPTOMS OF MICROVASCULAR THROMBOSIS	SIGNS AND SYMPTOMS OF MICROVASCULAR AND FRANK BLEEDING
Integumentary system (skin)	↓ Temperature, sensation; ↑ pain; cyanosis in extremities, nose, earlobes; focal ischemia, superficial gangrene	Petechiae, including periorbital and oral mucosa; bleeding: gums, oozing from wounds, previous injection sites, around catheters (IVs, tracheostomies); epistaxis; diffuse ecchymoses; subcutaneous hemorrhage; joint pain
Circulatory system	↓ Pulses; capillary filling time > 3 sec	Tachycardia
Respiratory system	Hypoxia (secondary to clot in lung); dyspnea; chest pain with deep inspiration; ↓ breath sounds over areas of large embolism	High-pitched bronchial breath sounds; tachypnea; ↑ consolidation; signs and symptoms of acute respiratory distress syndrome
Gastrointestinal system	Gastric pain; "heartburn"	Hematemesis (heme⊕† NG output) melana (heme⊕ stools → tarry stools → bright-red blood from rectum) retroperitoneal bleeding (abdomen firm and tender to palpation; distended; ↑ abdominal girth)
Renal system	↓ Urine output; ↑ creatinine, ↑ blood urea nitrogen	Hematuria
Neurologic system	↓ Alertness and orientation; ↓ pupillary reaction; ↓ response to commands; ↓ strength and movement ability	Anxiety; restlessness; ↓ mentation, altered level of consciousness; headache; visual disturbances; conjunctival hemorrhage

* *Note:* Signs of microvascular thrombosis are the result of an inappropriate activation of the coagulation system, causing thrombotic occlusion of small vessels within all body organs. As the clotting factors and platelets are consumed, signs of microvascular bleeding appear. This bleeding can quickly extend into frank hemorrhage. Treatment must be aimed at the disorder underlying the DIC; otherwise, the stimulus for the syndrome will persist.
†*heme⊕*, positive for hemoglobin

Nursing Interventions	Rationale	Expected Outcomes

Nursing Diagnosis: Potential for fluid volume deficit related to bleeding
Goals: Hemodynamic status maintained; urine output ≥30 mL/hr

Nursing Interventions	Rationale	Expected Outcomes
1. Avoid procedures/activities that can increase intracranial pressure (eg, coughing, straining to have a bowel movement).	1. Prevents intracranial bleeding.	• Level of consciousness (LOC) stable
2. Monitor vital signs closely, including neurologic checks: a. Monitor hemodynamics b. Monitor abdominal girth c. Monitor urine output	2. Identifies signs of hemorrhage/shock quickly.	• CVP 5–12 cm H$_2$O, systolic BP ≥70 mm Hg • Urine output ≥30 mL/hour • Decreased bleeding • Decreased oozing
3. Avoid medications that interfere with platelet function if possible (eg, ASA, NSAIDs, beta-lactam antibiotics).	3. Decreases problems with platelet aggregation and adhesion.	• Decreased ecchymoses • Amenorrhea • Absence of oral and bronchial bleeding
4. Avoid rectal probes, rectal medications.	4. Decreases chance for rectal bleeding.	• Oral mucosa clean, moist, intact
5. Avoid IM injections.	5. Decreases chance for intramuscular bleeding.	• Absence of bleeding
6. Monitor amount of external bleeding carefully a. Monitor number of dressings, % of dressing saturated; time to saturate a dressing is more objective than "dressing saturated a moderate amount." b. Monitor suction output, all excreta c. Monitor pad counts in menstruating females. d. Females may receive progesterone to prevent menses.	6. a. Provides accurate, objective assessment of extent of bleeding. b. Identifies presence of or quantifies extent of bleeding. c. Quantifies extent of bleeding d. Decreases chance for gynecologic source of hemorrhage.	
7. Use low pressure with any suctioning needed.	7. Prevents excessive trauma that could cause bleeding.	
8. Administer oral hygiene carefully. a. Avoid lemon-glycerine swabs, hydrogen peroxide, commercial mouthwashes. b. Use sponge-tipped swabs, salt/baking soda (bicarbonate of soda) mouth rinses.	8. Prevents excessive trauma that could cause bleeding. Glycerin and alcohol (in commercial mouthwashes) will dry mucosa, increasing risk for bleeding.	
9. Avoid dislodging any clots, including those around IV sites and injection sites.	9. Prevents excessive bleeding at sites.	

Nursing Diagnosis: Potential for impaired skin integrity secondary to ischemia or bleeding
Goals: Skin integrity remains intact; oral mucosa remains intact

Nursing Interventions	Rationale	Expected Outcomes
1. Assess skin, with particular attention to bony prominences, skin folds.	1. Prompt identification of any area at risk for skin breakdown or showing early signs of breakdown can facilitate prompt intervention and thus prevent complications.	• Skin integrity remains intact; skin is warm, and of normal colour • Oral mucosa is intact, pink, moist, without bleeding
2. Reposition carefully; use pressure-reducing mattress.	2–4. Meticulous skin care and use of measures to prevent pressure on bony prominences decrease the risk of skin trauma.	
3. Perform careful skin care every 2 hr, emphasizing dependent areas, all bony prominences, perineum.		
4. Use lamb's wool between digits, around ears, as needed.		
5. Use prolonged pressure after injection or procedure when such measures must be performed (at least 5 min)	5. Initial platelet plug is very unstable and easily dislodged, which can lead to increased bleeding.	
6. Administer oral hygiene carefully (see above).	6. Meticulous care to decreased trauma, bleeding, and risk of infection.	

(continued)

Plan of Nursing Care
The Patient With Disseminated Intravascular Coagulation (DIC) (Continued)

Nursing Interventions	Rationale	Expected Outcomes

Nursing Diagnosis: Potential for fluid volume excess
Goals: Absence of edema; absence of rales; intake not greater than output

1. Auscultate breath sounds every 2–4 hr.	1. Crackles can develop quickly.	• Breath sounds clear
2. Monitor extent of edema	2. Fluid may extend beyond intravascular system.	• Absence of edema
3. Monitor volume of IVs, blood products; decrease volume of IV medications if possible.	3. Helps prevent fluid overload.	• Intake does not exceed output
4. Administer diuretics as prescribed	4. Decreases fluid volume.	• Weight stable

Nursing Diagnosis: Potential for diminished tissue perfusion secondary to microthrombi
Goals: Neurologic status remains intact; absence of hypoxemia; peripheral pulses remain intact; skin integrity remains intact; urine output remains ≥30 mL/hr

1. Assess neurologic, pulmonary, integumentary systems.	1. Initial signs of thrombosis can be subtle.	• Arterial blood gases, O_2 saturation, pulse oximetry, LOC within normal limits.
2. Monitor response to heparin therapy.	2. Response to heparin is most accurately reflected in fibrinogen level.	• Breath sounds clear
3. Assess extent of bleeding.	3. Objective measurements of all sites of bleeding are crucial to accurately assess extent of blood loss.	• Absence of edema
4. Monitor fibrinogen levels.	4. Response to heparin is most accurately reflected in fibrinogen level.	• Intake does not exceed output
5. Stop ε-aminocaproic acid (EACA) if symptoms of thrombosis occur (see Table 33-7).	5. EACA should be used only in setting of extensive hemorrhage not responding to replacement therapy.	• Weight stable

Nursing Diagnosis: Potential for fear of unknown and possible death
Goals: Fears verbalized/identified; realistic hope maintained

1. Identify previous coping mechanisms, if possible: a. Encourage patient to use them as appropriate.	1. Identifying previous stressful situations can aid in recall of successful coping mechanisms.	• Previously used coping strategies identified and tried, to extent patient is able to do so
2. Explain all procedures and rationale for these in terms patient and family can understand.	2. Decreased knowledge and uncertainty can increase anxiety.	• Patient indicates understanding of procedures and situation as condition permits
3. Assist family in supporting patient.	3. Family can be useful in assisting patient to use coping strategies and to maintain hope.	
4. Use services from behavioural medicine, chaplain as needed.	4. Additional professional intervention may be necessary, particularly if previous coping mechanisms are maladaptive or ineffective. Spiritual dimension should be supported.	

Evaluation

See the Plan of Nursing Care for evaluation and expected outcomes for the patient with DIC.

THROMBOTIC DISORDERS

As in many bleeding disorders, several conditions can alter the balance within the normal hemostasis process and cause excessive thrombosis. Abnormalities that predispose a person to thrombotic events include decreased clotting inhibitors within the circulation (which enhances coagulation), altered hepatic function (which may decrease production of clotting factors or clearance of activated coagulation factors), lack of fibrinolytic enzymes, and tortuous vessels (which promote platelet aggregation). Thrombosis can be caused by more than one predisposing factor. Several conditions can result from thrombosis, such as myocardial infarction (see Chap. 28), cerebral vascular accident

(CVA, brain attack, or stroke; see Chap. 62), and peripheral arterial occlusion (see Chap. 31). Several inherited or acquired deficiency conditions, including hyperhomocystinemia, antithrombin III (AT III) deficiency, Protein C deficiency, activated Protein C resistance, factor V Leiden, and Protein S deficiency can predispose a patient to repeated episodes of thrombosis; they are referred to as hypercoagulable states or thrombophilia. Table 33-8 delineates these disorders, their abnormal laboratory values, and the need for family testing.

Thrombosis requires anticoagulation therapy. The duration of therapy varies with the location and extent of the thrombosis, precipitating events (eg, trauma, immobilization), and concurrent risk factors (eg, use of oral contraceptives, tortuous blood vessels, history of thrombotic events).

HYPERHOMOCYSTINEMIA

Increased plasma levels of homocystine are a significant risk factor not only for venous thrombosis (eg, deep venous thrombosis [DVT], pulmonary embolism) but also for arterial thrombosis (eg, stroke, myocardial infarction). This disorder can be heredi-

tary, or it can result from a nutritional deficiency of folic acid and, to a lesser extent, of vitamin B_{12} and B_6, because these vitamins are cofactors in homocystine metabolism. For unknown reasons, people who are elderly, have renal failure, or smoke tobacco may also have elevated levels of homocystine in the absence of nutritional deficiencies of these vitamins. Although a simple fasting measurement of plasma homocystine can serve as a useful screening test, people with heterozygous defects in this gene and those who are vitamin B_6 deficient may have normal or minimally elevated levels. A much more sensitive method involves obtaining a second measurement 4 hours after the patient consumes methionine; the prevalence of hyperhomocystinemia is twice as great when this method is used. In hyperhomocystinemia, the endothelial lining of the vessel walls is denuded; this can precipitate unnecessary thrombus formation. Recent studies have determined that this disorder is much more common than previously thought. In a long-term epidemiologic study on nurses' health (Rimm et al., 1998), women who used dietary supplements with folic acid and vitamin B_6 were found to have a lower incidence of thrombotic conditions such as DVT. Patients who are found to have hyperhomocystinemia should receive folic acid, B_6, and/or B_{12} supplements and should be instructed in the rationale for their use to enhance compliance.

ANTITHROMBIN III DEFICIENCY

Antithrombin is a protein that inhibits thrombin and certain coagulation factors. AT III deficiency is a common hereditary condition that can cause venous thrombosis, particularly when the level is less than 60% of normal. Patients with AT III deficiency can develop venous thrombosis as young adults; by 50 years of age, two thirds of patients with AT III deficiency have developed a venous thrombosis. The most common sites for thrombosis are the deep veins of the leg and the mesentery. Recurrent thrombosis often occurs. There is an increased resistance to heparin anticoagulation, so these patients may require greater amounts of heparin to achieve adequate anticoagulation. Patients with AT III deficiency should be encouraged to have their family members tested for the deficiency.

PROTEIN C DEFICIENCY

Protein C is an enzyme that, when activated, inhibits coagulation. When levels of Protein C are deficient, the risk of thrombosis increases, and thrombosis can often occur spontaneously. Protein C deficiency is at least as prevalent as AT III deficiency, and people who are Protein C–deficient can develop thrombosis early in life, as early as 15 years of age. Warfarin-induced skin necrosis is a rare but significant complication of anticoagulation management in patients with Protein C deficiency (Hoffman et al., 2000). This complication appears to result from progressive thrombosis in the capillaries within the skin; the extent of the necrosis can be extreme.

ACTIVATED PROTEIN C RESISTANCE AND FACTOR V LEIDEN MUTATION

Activated protein C resistance is a common condition that can occur with other hypercoagulable states. APC is an anticoagulant, and resistance to APC increases the risk for venous thrombosis. A molecular defect in the factor V gene has been identified in

Table 33-8 • Hypercoagulable States

DISORDER	ABNORMAL LABORATORY VALUE*
Inherited Disorders (Family Testing Necessary)	
Hyperhomocystinemia	Homocystine ↑ after methionine load
Antithrombin III (AT III) deficiency	AT III ↓
Protein C deficiency	Protein C activity ↓ (must be measured off warfarin [Coumadin])
Activated protein C (APC) resistance	Must be measured off anticoagulant; <2× prolongation of PTT when APC added. Patients with APC resistance have a smaller increase in clotting time than normal (ie, the prolongation of clotting time is less than normal).
Factor V Leiden	Positive
Protein S deficiency	Protein S activity ↓; must be measured off warfarin (Coumadin)
Dysfibrinogenemia	↑ thrombin time; ↑ reptilase time; ↓ functional fibrinogen; often requires special fibrinogen assays
Acquired Disorders (Family Testing Unnecessary)	
Anticardiolipin antibody Cancer	Positive
Lupus anticoagulant	Positive
Hyperhomocystinemia	Homocystine ↑ after methionine load
AT III Deficiency	AT III ↓
Paroxysmal nocturnal hemoglobinuria	+ Hamm's test; acid hemolysis
Myeloproliferative disorders	Varied, depending on disorder
Nephrotic syndrome	Varied, depending on disorder
Cancer chemotherapy	Varied, depending on disorder

* Protein C and Protein S are vitamin K–dependent proteins. Warfarin (Coumadin) interferes with the hepatic synthesis of vitamin K-dependent factors, which may decrease levels of Protein C or Protein S; therefore, Protein C and Protein S should be measured while the patient is off warfarin.

most (90%) of those with APC resistance; this defect is called factor V Leiden mutation. It has been identified as the most common cause of inherited hypercoagulability in Caucasians, but its incidence appears to be much lower in other ethnic groups. Factor V Leiden mutation synergistically increases the risk for thrombosis in patients with other risk factors (eg, use of oral contraceptives, hyperhomocystinemia, increased age). It does not appear that the use of postmenopausal hormone therapy in women increases the risk for thrombotic events as does the use of oral contraceptives; the dose of estrogen in the former situation is much lower than in the latter. People who are homozygous for the factor V Leiden mutation are at extremely high risk for thrombosis.

PROTEIN S DEFICIENCY

Protein S is another natural anticoagulant normally produced in the liver. APC requires Protein S to inactivate certain clotting factors. When the level of Protein S is deficient, this inactivation process is diminished, and the risk for thrombosis can be increased. Like patients with Protein C deficiency, those with Protein S deficiency have a greater risk for recurrent venous thrombosis at a young age, as young as 15 years.

ACQUIRED THROMBOPHILIA

Antibodies to phospholipids are common, acquired causes for thrombophilia (hypercoagulable states). The most common antibodies present against phospholipids are either lupus or anticardiolipin antibodies. Both of these antibodies can be transient, resulting from infection or certain medications. Most thrombotic events are venous, but arterial thrombosis can occur in up to one third of the cases. Patients who persistently test positive for either antibody and who have had a thrombotic event are at significant risk for recurrent thrombosis (greater than 50%). Recurrent thromboses tend to be of the same type—that is, venous thrombosis after an initial venous thrombosis, arterial thrombosis after an initial arterial thrombosis.

Another common acquired cause for thrombophilia is cancer. Specific types of stomach, pancreatic, lung, and ovarian cancers are most commonly associated with thrombophilia. The type of thrombosis that results is unusual. Rather than deep vein thrombosis or pulmonary embolism, the thrombosis occurs in unusual sites, such as the portal, hepatic, or renal vein or the inferior vena cava. Migratory superficial thrombophlebitis or nonbacterial thrombotic endocarditis can also occur. In these patients, anticoagulation can be difficult to manage in that the thrombosis can progress despite standard amounts of anticoagulation.

Medical Management

The primary method of treating thrombotic disorders is anticoagulation. However, in thrombophilic conditions, when to treat (prophylaxis or not) and how long to treat (lifelong or not) can be controversial. Anticoagulation therapy is not without risks; the most significant risk is bleeding. Risks of anticoagulation therapy are identified in Chapter 31. The most common anticoagulant medications are identified in the following section.

PHARMACOLOGIC THERAPY

Along with administering anticoagulant therapy, concerns include minimizing any risk factors that predispose a patient to

thrombosis. When risk factors (eg, immobility after surgery, pregnancy) cannot be avoided, prophylactic anticoagulation may be necessary.

Unfractionated Heparin Therapy. Heparin is a naturally occurring anticoagulant that enhances AT III and inhibits platelet function. To prevent thrombosis, heparin is typically given as a subcutaneous injection, two or three times daily. To treat thrombosis, heparin is usually administered intravenously. The therapeutic effect of heparin is monitored by serial measurements of the activated partial prothrombin time (aPTT); the dose is adjusted to maintain the range at 1.5 to 2.5 times the laboratory control. Oral forms are being evaluated, but their absorption remains variable (Money & York, 2001).

A significant potential complication of heparin-based therapy is heparin-induced thrombocytopenia (HIT). Antibodies are formed within the body against the heparin complex. The actual incidence of HIT is unknown, but it is thought to occur in as many as 5% of patients receiving heparin (Kelton, 1999). Whereas most patients remain asymptomatic, a significant proportion of those individuals with serologic HIT develop actual thrombocytopenia. A decline in platelet count typically develops after 5 to 8 days of heparin therapy, and the platelets can drop significantly, although in most instances the level stays higher than 50,000/mm^3. These patients are at increased risk for thrombosis, either venous or arterial, and the thrombosis can range from DVT to myocardial infarction, CVA (brain attack, stroke), and ischemic damage to an extremity necessitating amputation. The risk for development of HIT appears to be increased when heparin is used at higher concentrations (ie, therapeutic versus prophylactic dosage) and with preexisting comorbidity, such as underlying cardiac disease.

Low-Molecular-Weight Heparin Therapy. Low molecular-weight heparin (LMWH; eg, Dalteparin, Enoxaparin) is a special form of heparin that has a more selective effect on coagulation. Based on its biochemical properties, LMWH has a longer half-life and a less variable anticoagulant response than does standard heparin. These differences permit LMWH to be safely administered only once or twice daily, without the need for laboratory monitoring for dose adjustments. The incidence of HIT is much lower when LMWH is used. In certain conditions, the use of LMWH has allowed anticoagulation therapy to be moved entirely to the outpatient setting. Many cases of uncomplicated DVT are being managed outside the hospital setting. LMWH is also being increasingly used as "bridge therapy" when patients receiving anticoagulation therapy (warfarin) require an invasive procedure (eg, biopsy, surgery). In this situation, warfarin is stopped and LMWH is used in its place until the procedure is completed. After the procedure, warfarin therapy is resumed. LMWH is discontinued after a therapeutic level of warfarin is achieved.

Warfarin (Coumadin) Therapy. Coumarin anticoagulants (warfarin; eg, Coumadin) are antagonists of vitamin K and therefore interfere with the synthesis of vitamin K–dependent clotting factors. Coumarin anticoagulants bind to albumin, are metabolized in the liver, and have an extremely long half-life. Typically, a patient is initially treated with both heparin (either the unfractionated form or LMWH) and warfarin. When the international normalized ratio (INR) reaches the desired therapeutic range, the heparin is stopped. The dosage required to maintain the therapeutic range (typically using an INR of 2.0 to 3.0) varies widely among patients and even within the same patient. Frequent monitoring of the INR is extremely important so that the dosage of warfarin can be adjusted as needed. Warfarin is affected by many medications; consultation with a pharmacist is important to assess the extent to which concurrently administered medications, herbs, and nutritional supplements may interact with warfarin. It is also affected by many foods, so patients need dietary instruction and may benefit from consultation with a dietitian when receiving warfarin therapy. See Chart 33-15 for a listing of agents that interact with warfarin.

Nursing Management

Patients with thrombotic disorders should avoid activities that promote circulatory stasis (eg, immobility, crossing the legs). Exercise, especially ambulation, should be performed frequently throughout the day, particularly during long trips by car or plane.

Chart 33-15 • PHARMACOLOGY
Agents That Interact with Warfarin (Coumadin)

Although warfarin (Coumadin), an anticoagulant medication, is commonly used to treat and prevent thrombosis, many drug–drug and drug–food interactions are associated with its use. A careful medication history (including over-the-counter medications, herbs, and other substances, such as vitamins and minerals) is important when oral anticoagulation therapy is prescribed. Consultation with a pharmacist is recommended to assess the extent to which concurrent medications may affect the anticoagulant and for appropriate dosage adjustments. The following list contains a few examples of agents that interact with warfarin.

Agents That Inhibit Warfarin Function

Barbiturates	Glutethimide
Carbamazepine	Griseofulvin
Cholestyramine	Haloperidol
Corticosteroids	Oral contraceptives
Digitalis	Phenytoin
Estrogens	Rifampin
Ethanol	Spironolactone

Agents That Potentiate Warfarin Function

Acetaminophen	Vitamin C (in very large doses)
Allopurinol	Vitamin E (in very large doses)
Amiodarone	Isoniazid
Anabolic steroids	Mefenamic acid
Anti-inflammatory agents	Methotrexate
Antimalarial agents	Metronidazole
Aspirin	Oral hypoglycemic agents
Broad-spectrum antibiotics	Oxyphenbutazone
Chloral hydrate	Phenytoin
Chloramphenicol	Probenecid
Cimetidine	Propylthiouracil
Colchicine	Quinidine
Clofibrate	Quinine
Chlorpromazine	Salicylates
Danazol	Sulfinpyrazone
Disulfiram	Sulfonamides (long-acting)
Ethacrynic acid	Thyroxine
Feprazone	Triclofos
Herbal medicines:	Tricyclic antidepressants
feverfew, garlic, gingko,	
ginseng	

Medications that alter platelet aggregation, such as low-strength aspirin, may be prescribed. Some patients require life-long therapy with anticoagulants such as warfarin (eg, Coumadin).

Patients with thrombotic disorders, particularly those with thrombophilia, should be assessed for concurrent risk factors for thrombosis and should avoid concomitant risk factors if possible. For example, use of tobacco and nicotine products exacerbates the problem and should be avoided.

Just as for other conditions, patients with thrombotic disorders, particularly thrombophilia, should know the name of their specific condition and understand its significance. In many instances, younger patients with thrombophilia may not require prophylactic anticoagulation; however, with concomitant risk factors (eg, pregnancy), increasing age, or subsequent thrombotic events, prophylactic or lifelong anticoagulation therapy may be required. Being able to provide the health care provider with an accurate health history can be extremely useful and can help guide the selection of appropriate therapeutic interventions. Patients with hereditary disorders should be encouraged to have their siblings and children tested for the disorder.

When patients with thrombotic disorders are hospitalized, frequent assessments should be performed for signs and symptoms of beginning thrombus formation, particularly in the legs (DVT) and lungs (pulmonary embolism). Ambulation or range-of-motion exercises as well as the use of elastic compression stockings should be initiated promptly to decrease stasis. Prophylactic anticoagulants are commonly prescribed.

Therapies for Blood Disorders
SPLENECTOMY

The surgical removal of the spleen (splenectomy) is sometimes necessary after trauma to the abdomen. Because the spleen is very vascular, severe hemorrhage can result if the spleen is ruptured. Under such circumstances, splenectomy becomes an emergency procedure.

Splenectomy is also a possible treatment for other hematologic disorders. For example, an enlarged spleen may be the site of excessive destruction of blood cells. If the destruction is life-threatening, surgery may be lifesaving. This is the case in autoimmune hemolytic anemia or ITP when these disorders do not respond to more conservative measures, such as corticosteroid therapy. Some patients with severe anemia due to inherited RBC defects (eg, thalassemia) may also benefit from splenectomy.

In general, the mortality rate after splenectomy is low. Laparoscopic splenectomy can be used in selected patients, with a resultant decrease in the postoperative morbidity rate. Complications that may result from surgery are atelectasis, pneumonia, abdominal distention, and abscess formation. Although young children are at the highest risk after splenectomy, all age groups are vulnerable to overwhelming lethal infections and should receive Pneumovax before undergoing this surgical procedure, if possible.

Patients are instructed to seek prompt medical attention if even relatively minor symptoms of infection occur. Often, patients with high platelet counts have even higher counts after splenectomy—more than 1 million/mm³—which can predispose them to serious thrombotic or hemorrhagic problems. This increase is, however, transient.

THERAPEUTIC APHERESIS

Apheresis is a Greek word meaning separation. In therapeutic apheresis (or pheresis), blood is taken from the patient and passed through a centrifuge, where a specific component is separated from the blood and removed (Table 33-9). The remaining blood is then returned to the patient. The entire system is closed, so the risk of bacterial contamination is extremely low. When platelets or WBCs are removed, the decrease in these cells within the circulation is temporary. However, the temporary decrease provides a window of time until suppressive medications (eg, chemotherapy) can have therapeutic effects. Sometimes plasma is removed rather than blood cells—typically so that specific, abnormal proteins within the plasma will be transiently lowered until a long-term therapy can be initiated.

Apheresis is also used to obtain larger amounts of platelets from a donor than can be provided from a single unit of whole blood. A unit of platelets obtained in this way is equivalent to six to eight units of platelets obtained from six to eight separate donors via standard blood donation methods. Platelet donors can have their platelets apheresed as often as every 14 days. WBCs can be obtained similarly, typically after the donor has received growth factors (G-CSF, GM-CSF) to stimulate the formation of additional WBCs and thereby increase the WBC count. The use of these growth factors also stimulates the release of stem cells within the circulation. Apheresis is used to harvest these stem cells (typically over a period of several days) for use in PBSCT (peripheral blood stem cell transplant; see Chap. 16).

THERAPEUTIC PHLEBOTOMY

Therapeutic phlebotomy is the removal of a certain amount of blood under controlled conditions. Patients with elevated hematocrits (eg, those with polycythemia vera) or excessive iron absorption (eg, hemochromatosis) can usually be managed by periodically removing 1 unit (about 500 mL) of whole blood. Eventually this process can produce iron deficiency, leaving the patient unable to produce as many RBCs. The actual procedure for therapeutic phlebotomy is similar to that for blood donation (see later discussion).

BLOOD AND BLOOD COMPONENT THERAPY

A single unit of whole blood contains 450 mL of blood and 50 mL of an anticoagulant. A unit of whole blood can be processed and dispensed for administration. However, it is more appropriate, economical, and practical to separate that unit of whole blood into its primary components: RBCs, platelets, and plasma (WBCs are rarely used; see later discussion). Because the plasma is removed, a unit of RBCs (packed RBCs, PRBCs) is very concentrated (hematocrit, approximately 70%). Each component must be processed and stored differently to maximize the longevity of the viable cells and factors within it; each individual blood component has a different storage life. PRBCs are stored at 4°C. With special preservatives, they can be stored safely for up to 42 days before they must be discarded. In contrast, platelets must be stored at room temperature because they cannot withstand cold temperatures, and they last for only 5 days before they must be discarded. To prevent clumping, platelets are gently agitated while stored. Plasma is immediately frozen to maintain the activity of the clotting factors within; it lasts for 1 year if it remains frozen. Plasma can be further pooled and processed into blood derivatives, such as albumin, immune globulin, factor VIII, and factor IX. Table 33-10 describes each blood component and how it is commonly used.

SPECIAL PREPARATIONS

Factor VIII concentrate (antihemophilic factor) is a lyophilized, freeze-dried concentrate of pooled fractionated human plasma. It is used in treating hemophilia A. Factor IX concentrate (prothrombin complex) is similarly prepared and contains factors II,

---

Table 33-9 • Types of Apheresis*

PROCEDURE	PURPOSE	EXAMPLES OF CLINICAL USE
Platelet pheresis	Remove platelets	Extreme thrombocytosis, essential thrombocythemia (temporary measure); single-donor platelets transfusion
Leukapheresis	Remove WBCs (can be specific to neutrophils or lymphocytes)	Extreme leukocytosis (eg, AML, CML) (very temporary measure); harvest WBCs for transfusion
Erythrocytapheresis (RBC exchange)	Remove RBCs	RBC dyscrasias (eg, sickle cell disease); RBCs replaced via transfusion
Plasmapheresis (plasma exchange)	Remove plasma proteins	Hyperviscosity syndromes; treatment for some renal and neurologic diseases (eg, Goodpasture's syndrome, Guillain-Barré)
Stem cell harvest	Remove circulating stem cells	Transplantation (donor harvest or autologous)

*Therapeutic apheresis can be used to treat a wide variety of conditions. When it is used to treat a disease that causes an increase in a specific cell type with a short life in circulation (ie, WBCs, platelets), the reduction in those cells is temporary. However, this temporary reduction permits a margin of safety while waiting for a longer-lasting treatment modality (eg, chemotherapy) to take effect. Apheresis can also be used to obtain stem cells for transplantation, either from a matched donor (allogenic) or from the patient (autologous).
AML, acute myeloid leukemia; CML, chronic myeloid leukemia; RBC, red blood cell; WBC, white blood cell.

Table 33-10 • **Blood and Blood Components Commonly Used in Transfusion Therapy***

	COMPOSITION	INDICATIONS AND CONSIDERATIONS
Whole blood	Cells and plasma, hematocrit about 40%	Volume replacement and oxygen-carrying capacity; usually used only in significant bleeding (>25% blood volume lost)
Packed red blood cells (PRBCs)	RBCs with little plasma (hematocrit about 75%); some platelets and WBCs remain	↑ RBC mass Symptomatic anemia: platelets in the unit are not functional; WBCs in the unit may cause reaction and are not functional

Platelets—random	Platelets (5.5×10^{10} platelets/unit)
	Plasma; some RBCs, WBCs
		Bleeding due to severe ↓ platelets
		Prevent bleeding when platelets <5,000–10,000/mm³
		  Survival ↓ in presence of fever, chills, infection
		  Repeated treatment → ↓ survival due to alloimmunization

Platelets—single donor	Platelets (3×10^{11} platelets/unit) 1 unit is equivalent to 6–8 units of random platelets	Used for repeated treatment: ↓ alloimmunization risk by limiting exposure to multiple donors
Plasma (FFP)	Plasma; all coagulation factors Complement	Bleeding in patients with coagulation factor deficiencies; plasmapheresis
Granulocytes (pheresed)	Neutrophils (>1×10^{10}/unit); lymphocytes; some RBCs and platelets	Severe neutropenia in selected patients; controversial
Lymphocytes (WBCs) (apheresed)	Lymphocytes (number varies)	Stimulate graft-versus-disease effect
Cryoprecipitate	Fibrinogen ≥150 mg/bag, AHF (VIII:C) 80–110 units/bag, von Willebrand factor; fibronectin	von Willebrand's disease Hypofibrinoginemia Hemophilia A
Antihemophilic factor (AHF)	Factor VIII	Hemophilia A
Factor IX concentrate	Factor IX	Hemophilia B (Christmas disease)
Factor IX complex	Factor II, VII, IX, X	Hereditary factor VII, IX, X deficiency; Hemophilia A with factor VII inhibitors
Albumin	Albumin 5%, 25%	Hypoproteinemia; burns; volume expansion by 5% to ↑ blood volume; 25% → ↓ hematocrit
Intravenous gamma globulin	IgG antibodies	Hypogammaglobulinemia (in CLL, recurrent infections); ITP; primary immunodeficiency states
Antithrombin III concentrate (AT III)	AT III (trace amounts of other plasma proteins)	AT III deficiency with or at risk for thrombosis

* The composition of each type of blood component is described as well as the most common indications for using a given blood component. RBCs, platelets, and fresh frozen plasma are the blood products most commonly used. When transfusing these blood products, it is important to realize that the individual product is always "contaminated" with very small amounts of other blood products (eg, WBCs mixed in a unit of platelets). This contamination can cause some difficulties, particularly isosensitization, in certain patients.
AHF, antihemophilic factor; CLL, chronic lymphocytic leukemia; ITP, idiopathic thrombopenic purpura.

VII, IX, and X. It is used primarily for treatment of factor IX deficiency (hemophilia B). Factor IX concentrate is also useful in treating congenital factor VII and factor X deficiencies.

Plasma albumin is a large protein molecule that usually stays within vessels and is a major contributor to plasma oncotic pressure. This protein is used to expand the blood volume of patients in hypovolemic shock and, rarely, to increase the concentration of circulating albumin in patients with hypoalbuminemia.

Immune globulin is a concentrated solution of the antibody IgG; it contains very little IgA or IgM. It is prepared from large pools of plasma. The intravenous form (IVIG; Gammagard, Gamimune) is used in various clinical situations to replace inadequate amounts of IgG in patients who are at risk for recurrent bacterial infection (eg, those with CLL, those receiving BMT or PBSCT). IVIG, in contrast to all other fractions of human blood, cells, or plasma, are able to survive being subjected to heating at 60°C for 10 hours to free them of viral contaminants.

Procuring Blood and Blood Products

BLOOD DONATION

To protect both the donor and the recipients, all prospective donors are examined and interviewed before they are allowed to donate their blood. The intent of the interview is to assess the general health status of the donor and to identify risk factors that might harm a recipient of the donor's blood. Donors should be in good health and without any of the following:

- A history of viral hepatitis at any time in the past, or a history of close contact with a hepatitis or dialysis patient within 6 months
- A history of receiving a blood transfusion or an infusion of any blood derivative (other than serum albumin) within 6 months
- A history of untreated syphilis or malaria, because these diseases can be transmitted by transfusion even years later. A

person who has been free of symptoms and off therapy for 3 years after malaria may be a donor.

- A history or evidence of drug abuse in which substances were self-injected, because many intravenous/injection drug users are hepatitis carriers and because the risk for human immunodeficiency virus (HIV) is high in this group
- A history of possible exposure to HIV; the population at risk includes people who engage in anal sex, people with multiple sexual partners, intravenous/injection drug users, sexual partners of people at risk for HIV, and people with hemophilia
- A skin infection, because of the possibility of contaminating the phlebotomy needle, and subsequently the blood itself
- A history of recent asthma, urticaria, or allergy to medications, because hypersensitivity can be transferred passively to the recipient
- Pregnancy within 6 months, because of the nutritional demands of pregnancy on the mother
- A history of tooth extraction or oral surgery within 72 hours, because such procedures are frequently associated with transient bacteremia
- A history of exposure to infectious disease within the past 3 weeks, because of the risk of transmission to the recipient
- Recent immunizations, because of the risk of transmitting live organisms (2-week waiting period for live, attenuated organisms; 1 month for rubella; 1 year for rabies)
- A history of recent tattoo, because of the risk of blood-borne infections (eg, hepatitis, HIV)
- Cancer, because of the uncertainty about transmission of the disease
- A history of whole blood donation within the past 56 days

Potential donors should be asked whether they have consumed any aspirin or aspirin-containing medications within the past 3 days. Although aspirin use does not render the donor ineligible, the platelets obtained would be dysfunctional and therefore not useful. Aspirin does not affect the RBCs or plasma obtained from the donor.

All donors are expected to meet the following minimal requirements:

- Body weight should exceed 50 kg for a standard 450-mL donation. Donors weighing less than 50 kg donate proportionately less blood. People younger than 17 years of age are disqualified from donation.
- The oral temperature should not exceed 37.5°C.
- The pulse rate should be regular and between 50 and 100 beats per minute.
- The systolic arterial pressure should be 90 to 180 mm Hg, and the diastolic pressure should be 50 to 100 mm Hg.
- The hemoglobin level should be at least 12.5 g/dL for women and 13.5 g/dL for men.

Directed Donation

At times, friends and family of a patient wish to donate blood for that person. These blood donations are termed directed donations. These donations are not any safer than those provided by random donors, because directed donors may not be as willing to identify themselves as having a history of any of the risk factors that disqualify a person from donating blood.

Standard Donation

Phlebotomy consists of venipuncture and blood withdrawal. Standard precautions are used. Donors are placed in a semi-recumbent position. The skin over the antecubital fossa is carefully cleansed with an antiseptic preparation, a tourniquet is applied, and venipuncture is performed. Withdrawal of 450 mL of blood usually takes less than 15 minutes. After the needle is removed, donors are asked to hold the involved arm straight up, and firm pressure is applied with sterile gauze for 2 or 3 minutes or until bleeding stops. A firm bandage is then applied. Donors remain recumbent until they feel able to sit up, usually within a few minutes. Donors who experience weakness or faintness should rest for a longer period. Donors then receive food and fluids and are asked to remain another 15 minutes.

Donors are instructed to leave the dressing on and to avoid heavy lifting for several hours, to avoid smoking for 1 hour, to avoid drinking alcoholic beverages for 3 hours, to increase fluid intake for 2 days, and to eat healthy meals for 2 weeks. Specimens from this donated blood are tested to detect infections and to identify the specific blood type (see later discussion).

Autologous Donation

A patient's own blood may be collected for future transfusion; this method is useful for many elective surgeries where the potential need for transfusion is high (eg, orthopedic surgery). Preoperative donations are ideally collected 4 to 6 weeks before surgery. Iron supplements are prescribed during this period to prevent depletion of iron stores. Occasionally, erythropoietin (epoetin-alfa [eg, Epogen, Procrit]) is given to stimulate erythropoiesis to ensure that the donor's hematocrit remains high enough to be eligible for donation. Typically, 1 unit of blood is drawn each week; the number of units obtained varies with the type of surgical procedure to be performed (ie, the amount of blood anticipated to be transfused). Phlebotomies are not performed within 72 hours of surgery. Individual blood components can also be collected.

The primary advantage of autologous transfusions is the prevention of viral infections from another person's blood. Other advantages include safe transfusion for patients with a history of transfusion reactions, prevention of alloimmunization, and avoidance of complications in patients with alloantibodies. The policy of the Canadian Blood Services requires autologous blood to be transfused only to the donor. If the blood is not required, it can be frozen until the donor needs it in the future (for up to 10 years). The blood is never returned to the general donor supply of blood products to be used by someone else.

The disadvantage of autologous donation is that it may be performed even when the likelihood that the anticipated procedure will necessitate a transfusion is small. Needless autologous donation is expensive, takes time, and uses resources inappropriately. Moreover, in an emergency situation, the autologous units available may be inadequate, and the patient may still require additional units from the general donor supply.

Contraindications to donation of blood for autologous transfusion are acute infection, severely debilitating chronic disease, hemoglobin level less than 11 g/dL, hematocrit less than 33%, unstable angina, and acute cardiovascular or cerebrovascular disease. A history of poorly controlled epilepsy may be considered a contraindication in some centres. Patients with cancer may donate for themselves.

Intraoperative Blood Salvage

This transfusion method provides replacement for patients who are unable to donate before surgery and for those undergoing vascular, orthopedic, or thoracic surgery. During a surgical procedure, blood lost into a sterile cavity (eg, hip joint) is suctioned into a cell-saver machine. The RBCs are washed, often with saline solution, and then returned to the patient as an intravenous infusion. Salvaged blood cannot be stored, because bacteria cannot be completely removed from the blood.

Hemodilution

This transfusion method is initiated before or after induction of anesthesia. About 1 or 2 units of blood are removed from the patient through a venous or arterial line and simultaneously replaced with a colloid or crystalloid solution. The blood obtained is then reinfused after surgery (Kreimeier & Messmer, 2002). The advantage of this method is that the patient loses fewer RBCs during surgery, because the added intravenous solutions dilute the concentration of RBCs and lower the hematocrit. Patients who are at risk for myocardial injury, however, should not be further stressed by hemodilution.

COMPLICATIONS OF BLOOD DONATION

Excessive bleeding at the donor's venipuncture site is sometimes caused by a bleeding disorder in the donor but more often results from a technique error: laceration of the vein, excessive tourniquet pressure, or failure to apply enough pressure after the needle is withdrawn.

Fainting is common after blood donation and may be related to emotional factors, a vasovagal reaction, or prolonged fasting before donation. Because of the loss of blood volume, hypotension and syncope may occur when the donor assumes an erect position. A donor who appears pale or complains of faintness should immediately lie down or sit with head lowered below the knees; he or she should be observed for another 30 minutes.

Anginal chest pain may be precipitated in patients with unsuspected coronary artery disease. Seizures can occur in donors with epilepsy, although the incidence is very low. Both angina and seizures require further medical evaluation.

Many people have the misconception that donating blood can cause AIDS and other infections. Potential donors need to be educated that the equipment used in donation is sterile, a closed system, and not reusable; they are at no risk for acquiring such infections from donating blood.

BLOOD PROCESSING

Samples of the unit of blood are always taken immediately after donation so that the blood can be typed and tested. Each donation is tested for antibodies to HIV 1 and 2, hepatitis B core antibody (anti-HBc), hepatitis C virus (HCV), and human T-cell lymphotropic virus, type I (anti-HTLV-I/II). The blood is also tested for hepatitis B surface antigen (HbsAG) and for syphilis. Negative reactions are required for the blood to be used, and each unit of blood is labelled to certify the results. A new testing method, using nucleic acid amplification testing (NAT), has increased the ability to detect the presence of HCV and HIV infection, because it directly tests for genomic nucleic acids of the virus itself, rather than for the presence of antibodies to the virus (Korman, Leparc & Benson, 2001). This testing significantly shortens the "window" of inability to detect HIV and HCV from a donated unit, further ensuring the safety of the blood. Blood is also screened for CMV; if it tests positive for CMV, it can still be used, except in recipients who are negative for CMV and who are immunocompromised (eg, BMT or PBSCT recipients).

Equally important to viral testing is accurate determination of the blood type. More than 200 antigens have been identified on the surface of RBC membranes. Of these, the most important for safe transfusion are the ABO and Rh systems. The ABO system identifies which sugars are present on the membrane of an individual's RBCs: A, B, both A and B, or neither A nor B (type O). To prevent a significant reaction, the same type of RBCs should be transfused. Previously, it was thought that in an emergency situation in which the patient's blood type was not known, type O blood could be safely transfused. This practice is no longer advised by the American Red Cross.

The Rh antigen (also called D) is present on the surface of RBCs in 85% of the population (Rh-positive). Those who lack the D antigen are called Rh-negative. RBCs are routinely tested for the D antigen as well as ABO. Patients should receive PRBCs with a compatible Rh type.

TRANSFUSION

Administration of blood and blood components requires knowledge of correct administration techniques and possible complications. It is very important to be familiar with the agency's policies and procedures for transfusion therapy. Methods for transfusing blood components are presented in Charts 33-16 and 33-17. Potential complications of transfusion follow.

Setting

Although most blood transfusions are performed in the acute care setting, patients with chronic transfusion requirements often can receive transfusions in other settings. Free-standing infusion centres, ambulatory care clinics, a physician's office, and even the home may be appropriate settings for transfusion. Typically, patients who need chronic transfusions but are otherwise stable physically are appropriate candidates for outpatient therapy. Verification and administration of the blood product are performed much as in a hospital setting. Although most blood products can be transfused in the outpatient setting, the home is typically limited to transfusions of PRBCs and factor components (eg, factor VIII for patients with hemophilia).

Pretransfusion Assessment

PATIENT HISTORY

Patient history is an important component of the pretransfusion assessment to determine the history of previous transfusions as well as previous reactions to transfusion. The history should include the type of reaction, its manifestations, the interventions required, and whether any preventive interventions were used in subsequent transfusions. It is important to assess the number of pregnancies a woman has had, because a high number can increase her risk for reaction due to antibodies developed from exposure to fetal circulation. Other concurrent health problems should also be noted, with careful attention to cardiac, pulmonary, and vascular disease.

Chart 33-16
Transfusion of Packed Red Blood Cells (PRBCs)

Preprocedure
1. Confirm that the transfusion has been prescribed.
2. Check that patient's blood has been typed and cross-matched.
3. Verify that patient has signed a written consent form per institution policy.
4. Explain the procedure to the patient. Instruct patient in signs and symptoms of transfusion reaction (itching, hives, swelling, shortness of breath, fever, chills).
5. Take patient's temperature, pulse, respiration, and blood pressure to establish a baseline for comparing vital signs during transfusion.
6. Use hand hygiene and wear gloves in accordance with Standard Precautions.
7. Use a 20-gauge or larger needle for placement in a large vein. Use special tubing that contains a blood filter to screen out fibrin clots and other particulate matter. Do not vent the blood container.

Procedure
1. Obtain the PRBCs from the blood bank *after* the intravenous line is started. (Institution policy may limit release to only 1 unit at a time.)
2. Double-check the labels with another nurse or physician to make sure that the ABO group and Rh type agree with the compatibility record. Check to see that the number and type on the donor blood label and on the patient's chart are correct. Check the patient's identification by asking the patient's name and checking the identification wristband.
3. Check the blood for gas bubbles and any unusual colour or cloudiness. (Gas bubbles may indicate bacterial growth. Abnormal colour or cloudiness may be a sign of hemolysis.)

4. Make sure PRBC transfusion is initiated within 30 min after removal of the PRBCs from the blood bank refrigerator.
5. For first 15 minutes, run the transfusion slowly—no faster than 5 mL/min. Observe the patient carefully for adverse effects. If no adverse effects occur during the first 15 min, increase the flow rate unless the patient is at high risk for circulatory overload.
6. Monitor closely for 15–30 min to detect signs of reaction. Monitor vital signs at regular intervals per institution policy; compare results with baseline measurements. Increase frequency of measurements based on patient's condition. Observe the patient frequently throughout the transfusion for any signs of adverse reaction, including restlessness, hives, nausea, vomiting, torso or back pain, shortness of breath, flushing, hematuria, fever, or chills. Should any adverse reaction occur, stop infusion immediately, notify physician, and follow the agency's transfusion reaction standard.
7. Note that administration time does not exceed 4 hr because of the increased risk for bacterial proliferation.
8. Be alert for signs of adverse reactions: circulatory overload, sepsis, febrile reaction, allergic reaction, and acute hemolytic reaction.
9. Change blood tubing after every 2 units transfused, to decrease chance of bacterial contamination.

Postprocedure
1. Obtain vital signs and compare with baseline measurements.
2. Dispose of used materials properly.
3. Document procedure in patient's medical record, including patient assessment findings and tolerance to procedure.
4. Monitor patient for response to and effectiveness of the procedure.

Note: Never add medications to blood or blood products; if blood is too thick to run freely, normal saline may be added to the unit. If blood must be warmed, use an in-line blood warmer with a monitoring system.

Chart 33-17
Transfusion of Platelets or Fresh Frozen Plasma (FFP)

Preprocedure
1. Confirm that the transfusion has been prescribed.
2. Verify that patient has signed a written consent form per institution policy.
3. Explain the procedure to the patient. Instruct patient in signs and symptoms of transfusion reaction (itching, hives, swelling, shortness of breath, fever, chills).
4. Take patient's temperature, pulse, respiration, and blood pressure to establish a baseline for comparing vital signs during transfusion.
5. Use hand hygiene and wear gloves in accordance with Standard Precautions.
6. Use a 22-gauge or larger needle for placement in a large vein, if possible. Use appropriate tubing per institution policy (platelets often require different tubing from that used for other blood products).

Procedure
1. Obtain the platelets or FFP from the blood bank (only *after* the intravenous line is started.)
2. Double-check the labels with another nurse or physician to make sure that the ABO group matches the compatibility record (not usually necessary for platelets; here only if compatible platelets are ordered). Check to see that the number and type on the donor blood label and on the patient's chart are correct. Check the patient's identification by asking the patient's name and checking the identification wristband.
3. Check the blood product for any unusual colour or clumps (excessive redness indicates contamination with larger amounts of red blood cells).

4. Make sure platelets or FFP units are administered immediately after they are obtained.
5. Infuse each unit as fast as patient can tolerate to diminish platelet clumping during administration. Observe the patient carefully for adverse effects, including circulatory overload. Decrease rate of infusion if necessary.
6. Observe the patient closely throughout the transfusion for any signs of adverse reaction, including restlessness, hives, nausea, vomiting, torso or back pain, shortness of breath, flushing, hematuria, fever, or chills. Should any adverse reaction occur, stop infusion immediately, notify physician, and follow the agency's transfusion reaction standard.
7. Monitor vital signs at end of transfusion per institution policy; compare results with baseline measurements.
8. Flush line with saline after transfusion to remove blood component from tubing.

Postprocedure
1. Obtain vital signs and compare with baseline measurements.
2. Dispose of used materials properly.
3. Document procedure in patient's medical record, including patient assessment findings and tolerance to procedure.
4. Monitor patient for response to and effectiveness of procedure. A platelet count may be ordered 1 hr after platelet transfusion to facilitate this evaluation.

Note: FFP requires ABO but not Rh compatibility. Platelets are not typically cross-matched for ABO compatibility. Never add medications to blood or blood products.

PHYSICAL ASSESSMENT

A systematic physical assessment and measurement of baseline vital signs are important before transfusing any blood product. The respiratory system should be assessed, including careful auscultation of the lungs and for use of accessory muscles. Cardiac system assessment should include careful inspection for any edema as well as other signs of cardiac failure (eg, jugular venous distention). The skin should be observed for rashes, petechiae, and ecchymoses. The sclera should be examined for icterus. In the event of a possible transfusion reaction, a comparison of findings can help differentiate between types of reactions.

Patient Teaching

Reviewing the signs and symptoms of a potential transfusion reaction is crucial for patients who have not received a transfusion before. Even for those patients who have received prior transfusions, a brief review of signs and symptoms of potential transfusion reactions is advised. Signs and symptoms of a possible reaction include fever, chills, respiratory distress, low back pain, nausea, pain at the intravenous site, or anything "unusual." Although a thorough review is very important, it is also important to reassure the patient that the blood is carefully tested against the patient's own blood (cross-matched) to diminish the likelihood of any untoward reaction. Such assurance can be extremely beneficial in allaying anxiety. Similarly, it can be useful to mention again the very low possibility of contracting HIV from the transfusion; this fear persists among many people.

Transfusion Complications

Any patient who receives a blood transfusion may develop complications from that transfusion. When explaining the reasons for the transfusion, it is important to include the risks and benefits and what to expect during and after the transfusion. Patients must be informed that the supply of blood is not completely risk-free although it has been tested carefully. Nursing management is directed toward preventing complications, promptly recognizing complications if they develop, and promptly initiating measures to control any complications that occur. The following sections describe the most common or potentially severe transfusion-related complications.

FEBRILE, NONHEMOLYTIC REACTION

The nonhemolytic reaction, caused by antibodies to donor WBCs that are still present in the unit of blood or blood component, is the most common type of transfusion reaction, accounting for more than 90% of reactions. It occurs more frequently in patients who have had previous transfusions (exposure to multiple antigens from previous blood products) and in Rh-negative women who have borne Rh-positive children (exposure to an Rh-positive fetus raises antibody levels in the mother). These reactions occur in 1% of PRBC transfusions and 20% of platelet transfusions. More than 10% of patients with a chronic transfusion requirement develop this type of reaction.

NURSING RESEARCH PROFILE 33-1
Perspectives of Recipients of Blood Transfusions

Fitzgerald, M., Hodgkinson, B., & Thorp, D. (1999). Blood transfusion from the recipient's perspective. *Journal of Clinical Nursing 8(5)*, 593–600.

Purpose

The process of informed consent requires that information be provided to the patient before consent and implies that a dialogue between the patient and physicians and nurses occurs during this process. This study stemmed from previous studies examining transfusion practices in a large teaching hospital in Australia; the studies revealed that little is known about how much patients understood about the transfusion process. The purpose of this study was to more closely examine the meaning of patients' experiences with blood transfusions.

Study Sample and Design

The study design employed interpretive phenomenology, a qualitative analysis process that allowed researchers to identify meanings that may have been hidden in common actions. A convenience sample of 19 patients was interviewed; subjects were asked to discuss their experience of receiving a blood transfusion, beginning with the time they were told about it. Subjects received transfusions for a variety of clinical conditions, primarily surgery, cancer, and emergency situations. The interviews were tape recorded and transcribed verbatim. The data were analyzed and themes were identified.

Findings

Three broad themes were identified and more closely analyzed: information regarding the transfusion, reaction to receiving a transfusion, and care received during the transfusion. The focus of many of the interviews was on the information process. Physicians' explanations regarding the purpose of the transfusion were typically brief and were focused on providing factual information, particularly before the patient's signing of the consent for the procedure. Nurses' explanations continued as the procedure progressed but tended to focus only on potential reactions. Neither physicians nor nurses tended to encourage the patient to express his or her concerns, nor sought information from the patient. Few patients could actually recall any of the factual information presented to them. Fear of infection, particularly human immunodeficiency virus (HIV) infection, was present but was not excessive. Subjects verbalized understanding that the risk of acquiring HIV from their transfusion was very remote. Most subjects were told that the transfusion would make them feel better; in reality (and likely due to the severity of their illness/injury) such was not the case. Beyond the initial procedure by the nurse of double-checking the blood product for transfusion against the patient's identity and hanging the blood, patients did not notice any difference in the nursing care they received during the transfusion.

Nursing Implications

Findings from this study have important implications for nurses, particularly concerning the information process. Despite the focus of both physicians and nurses on providing information, patients demonstrated that they did not comprehend it well. Informational needs vary, as do learning styles. It is crucial that nurses assess their patients' level of understanding about the entire transfusion process. Not having the opportunity to deliberate on the information provided and to express concern was a common theme from the study subjects. Nurses need to make the time for patients to express their concerns and verbalize their feelings. This need exists not only for those receiving their first transfusion but also for those who have long-term transfusion requirements.

The diagnosis of a febrile, nonhemolytic reaction is made by excluding other potential causes, such as a hemolytic reaction or bacterial contamination of the blood product. The signs and symptoms of a febrile, nonhemolytic transfusion reaction are chills (absent to severe) followed by fever (more than 1°C elevation). The fever typically begins within 2 hours after the transfusion is begun. Although not life-threatening, the fever and particularly the chills and muscle stiffness can be frightening to the patient.

These reactions can be diminished, even prevented, by further depleting the blood component of donor WBCs; this is accomplished by a leukocyte reduction filter. The blood product may be filtered during processing, which achieves better results but is more expensive, or during the actual transfusion by adding the filter to the blood administration tubing. Antipyretics can be given to prevent fever, but routine premedication is not advised because it can mask the beginning of a more serious transfusion reaction.

ACUTE HEMOLYTIC REACTION

The most dangerous, and potentially life threatening, type of transfusion reaction occurs when the donor blood is incompatible with that of the recipient. Antibodies already present in the recipient's plasma rapidly combine with antigens on donor RBCs, and the RBCs are hemolyzed (destroyed) in the circulation (intravascular hemolysis). The most rapid hemolysis occurs in ABO incompatibility. This reaction can occur after transfusion of as little as 10 mL of RBCs. Rh incompatibility often causes a less severe reaction. The most common causes of acute hemolytic reaction are errors in blood component labelling and patient identification that result in the administration of an ABO-incompatible transfusion.

Symptoms consist of fever, chills, low back pain, nausea, chest tightness, dyspnea, and anxiety. As the RBCs are destroyed, the hemoglobin is released from the cells and excreted by the kidneys; therefore, hemoglobin is present in the urine (hemoglobinuria). Hypotension, bronchospasm, and vascular collapse may result. Diminished renal perfusion results in acute renal failure, and DIC may also occur.

The reaction must be recognized promptly and the transfusion discontinued immediately. Blood and urine specimens must be obtained and analyzed for evidence of hemolysis. Treatment goals include maintaining blood volume and renal perfusion and preventing and managing DIC.

Acute hemolytic transfusion reactions are preventable. Meticulous attention to detail in labelling blood samples and blood components and identifying the recipient cannot be overemphasized.

ALLERGIC REACTION

Some patients may develop urticaria (hives) or generalized itching during a transfusion. The cause of these reactions is thought to be a sensitivity reaction to a plasma protein within the blood component being transfused. Symptoms of an allergic reaction are urticaria, itching, and flushing. The reactions are usually mild and respond to antihistamines. If the symptoms resolve after administration of an antihistamine (eg, diphenhydramine [eg, Benadryl]), the transfusion may be resumed. Rarely, the allergic reaction is severe, with bronchospasm, laryngeal edema, and shock. These reactions are managed with epinephrine, corticosteroids, and pressor support, if necessary.

Giving the patient antihistamines before the transfusion may prevent future reactions. For severe reactions, future blood components are washed to remove any remaining plasma proteins. Leukocyte filters are not useful, because the offending plasma proteins can pass through the filter.

CIRCULATORY OVERLOAD

If too much blood infuses too quickly, hypervolemia can occur. This condition can be aggravated in patients who already have increased circulatory volume (eg, those with heart failure). PRBCs are safer to use than whole blood. If the administration rate is sufficiently slow, circulatory overload may be prevented. For patients who are at risk for, or already in, circulatory overload, diuretics are administered after the transfusion or between units of PRBCs. Patients receiving fresh frozen plasma or even platelets may also develop circulatory overload. The infusion rate of these blood components must also be titrated to the patient's tolerance.

Signs of circulatory overload include dyspnea, orthopnea, tachycardia, and sudden anxiety. Neck vein distention, crackles at the base of the lungs, and a rise in blood pressure can also occur. If the transfusion is continued, pulmonary edema can develop, as manifested by severe dyspnea and coughing of pink, frothy sputum.

If fluid overload is mild, the transfusion can often be continued after slowing the rate of infusion and administering diuretics. However, if the overload is severe, the patient is placed in an upright position with the feet in a dependent position, the transfusion is discontinued, and the physician is notified. The intravenous line is kept patent with a very slow infusion of normal saline solution or a saline or heparin lock device to maintain access to the vein in case intravenous medications are necessary. Oxygen and morphine may be needed for severe dyspnea.

BACTERIAL CONTAMINATION

The incidence of bacterial contamination of blood components is very low; however, administration of contaminated products puts the patient at great risk. Contamination can occur at any point during procurement or processing. Many bacteria cannot survive in the cold temperatures used to store PRBCs (platelets are at greater risk for contamination because they are stored at room temperature), but some organisms can survive cold temperatures.

Preventive measures include meticulous care in the procurement and processing of blood components. When PRBCs or whole blood is transfused, it should be administered within a 4-hour period, because warm room temperatures promote bacterial growth. A contaminated unit of blood product may appear normal, or it may have an abnormal colour.

The signs of bacterial contamination are fever, chills, and hypotension. These signs may not occur until the transfusion is complete, occasionally not until several hours after the transfusion. If the condition is not treated immediately with fluids and broad-spectrum antibiotics, shock can occur. Even with aggressive management, including vasopressor support, the mortality rate is high.

As soon as the reaction is recognized, any remaining transfusion is discontinued and the intravenous line is kept open with normal saline solution. The physician and the blood bank are notified, and the blood container is returned to the blood bank for testing and culture. Septicemia is treated with intravenous fluids and antibiotics; corticosteroids and vasopressors also may be necessary.

TRANSFUSION-RELATED ACUTE LUNG INJURY

This is a potentially fatal, idiosyncratic reaction that occurs in fewer than 1 in 5000 transfusions. Plasma antibodies (usually in the donor's plasma) that are present in the blood component stimulate the recipient's WBCs; aggregates of these WBCs form and occlude the microvasculature within the lungs. This lung injury is manifested as pulmonary edema; it can occur within 4 hours after the transfusion.

Signs and symptoms include fever, chills, acute respiratory distress (in the absence of other signs of left ventricular failure, such as elevated central venous pressure), and bilateral pulmonary infiltrates. Aggressive supportive therapy (oxygen, intubation, diuretics) may prevent death.

DELAYED HEMOLYTIC REACTION

Delayed hemolytic reactions usually occur within 14 days after transfusion, when the level of antibody has been increased to the extent that a reaction can occur. The hemolysis of the RBCs is extravascular, via the RES, and occurs gradually.

Signs and symptoms of a delayed hemolytic reaction are fever, anemia, increased bilirubin level, decreased or absent haptoglobin, and possibly jaundice. Rarely is there hemoglobinuria. Generally, these reactions are not dangerous, but it is useful to recognize them, because subsequent transfusions with blood products containing these antibodies may cause a more severe hemolytic reaction. However, recognition is also difficult, because the patient may not be in a health care setting to be tested for this reaction, and even if the patient is hospitalized, the reaction may be too mild to be recognized clinically. Because the amount of antibody present can be too low to detect, it is difficult to prevent delayed hemolytic reactions. The reaction is usually mild and requires no intervention.

DISEASES TRANSMITTED BY BLOOD TRANSFUSION

Despite the advances in donor screening and blood testing, certain diseases can still be transmitted by transfusion of blood components. The diseases in Chart 33-18 are examples of this phenomenon.

COMPLICATIONS OF LONG-TERM TRANSFUSION THERAPY

The complications that have been described represent a real risk for any patient any time a unit of blood is administered. However, patients with long-term transfusion therapy (eg, those with MDS, thalassemia, sickle cell anemia) are at greater risk for infection transmission and for becoming more sensitized to donor antigens, simply because they are exposed to more units of blood and, consequently, more donors. Iron overload is a complication unique to those individuals with long-term PRBC transfusions. A summary of complications associated with long-term transfusion therapy is depicted in Table 33-11.

Iron Overload. One unit of PRBCs contains 250 mg of iron. Patients with chronic transfusion requirements can quickly acquire more iron than they can use, leading to iron overload. Over time, the excess iron deposits in the tissues and can cause

Chart 33-18 — Diseases Transmitted by Blood Transfusion

Hepatitis (Viral Hepatitis B, C)
- Greater risk from pooled blood products and blood of paid donors than from volunteer donors
- Screening test detects most hepatitis B and C
- Transmittal risk estimated at 1:10,000

AIDS (HIV and HTLV)
- Donated blood screened for antibodies to HIV
- Transmittal risk estimated at 1:670,000
- People with high-risk behaviours (multiple sex partners, anal sex, intravenous/injection drug use) and people with signs and symptoms that suggest AIDS should not donate blood

Cytomegalovirus (CMV)
- Transmittal risk greater for premature newborns with CMV antibody-negative mothers and for immunocompromised recipients who are CMV-negative (eg, those with acute leukemia, organ or tissue transplant recipients).
- Blood products rendered "leukocyte-reduced" help reduce transmission of virus.

Graft-Versus-Host Disease (GVHD)
- Occurs only in severely immunocompromised recipients (eg, Hodgkin's disease, bone marrow transplantation).
- Transfused lymphocytes engraft in recipient and attack host lymphocytes or body tissues; signs and symptoms are fever, diffuse reddened skin rash, nausea, vomiting, diarrhea.
- Preventive measures include irradiating blood products to inactivate donor lymphocytes (no known radiation risks to transfusion recipient) and processing donor blood with leukocyte reduction filters.

Creutzfeldt-Jakob Disease (CJD)
- Rare, fatal disease causing irreversible brain damage
- No evidence of transmittal by transfusion, but hemophiliacs and others are concerned that transmittal is possible
- All blood donors must be screened for positive family history of CJD.
- Potential donors who spent 6 months or more in the United Kingdom (or Europe) from 1980 to 1996 cannot donate blood; blood products from a donor who develops CJD are recalled.

organ damage, particularly in the liver, heart, testes, and pancreas. Promptly initiating a program of iron chelation therapy (eg, with deferoxamine [Desferal]) can prevent end-organ damage from iron toxicity (Giardina & Grady, 1995).

NURSING MANAGEMENT FOR TRANSFUSION REACTIONS

If a transfusion reaction is suspected, the transfusion must be immediately stopped and the physician notified. A thorough patient assessment is crucial, because many complications have similar signs and symptoms. The following steps are taken to determine the type and severity of the reaction:

- Stop the transfusion. Maintain the intravenous line with normal saline solution through new intravenous tubing, administered at a slow rate.
- Assess the patient carefully. Compare the vital signs with those from the baseline assessment. Assess the patient's respiratory status carefully. Note the presence of adventitious breath sounds, use of accessory muscles, extent of dyspnea

Table 33-11 • Common Complications Resulting from Long-Term PRBC Transfusion Therapy*

	MANIFESTATION	MANAGEMENT
Infection	Hepatitis (B,C)	May immunize against hepatitis B; give alpha-interferon for hepatitis C; monitor hepatic function
	Cytomegalovirus (CMV)	WBC filters to protect against CMV
Iron overload	Heart failure	Prevent by chelation therapy
	Endocrine failure (diabetes, hypo-thyroidism, hypoparathyroidism, hypogonadism)	
Transfusion reaction	Sensitization	Diminish by RBC phenotyping, using WBC-filtered products
	Febrile reactions	Diminish by using WBC-filtered products

* Patients with long-term transfusion therapy requirements are at risk not only for the transfusion reactions discussed in the text but also for the complications noted above. In many cases, the use of WBC-filtered (eg, leukocyte-poor) blood products is standard for patients who receive long-term PRBC transfusion therapy. An aggressive chelation program initiated early in the course of therapy can prevent problems with iron overload.
PRBC, packed red blood cells; WBC, white blood cell; RBC, red blood cell.

(if any), and changes in mental status, including anxiety and confusion. Note any chills, diaphoresis, complaints of back pain, urticaria, and jugular vein distention.

- Notify the physician of the assessment findings, and implement any orders obtained. Continue to monitor the patient's vital signs and respiratory, cardiovascular, and renal status.
- Notify the blood bank that a suspected transfusion reaction has occurred.
- Send the blood container and tubing to the blood bank for repeat typing and culture. The identifying tags and numbers are verified.

If a hemolytic transfusion reaction or bacterial infection is suspected, the nurse should do the following:

- Obtain appropriate blood specimens from the patient.
- Collect a urine sample as soon as possible for a hemoglobin determination.
- Document the reaction, according to the institution's policy.

PHARMACOLOGIC ALTERNATIVES TO BLOOD TRANSFUSIONS

Pharmacologic agents to stimulate production of one or more types of blood cells by the marrow are commonly used. Chart 33-19 presents examples of such pharmacologic agents.

Researchers continue to seek a blood substitute that is practical and safe. Blood substitutes previously tried have not been successful. However, newer blood substitutes focus solely on oxygen delivery, as an RBC substitute (Rabinovici, 2001). Current blood substitutes in clinical trials have distinct advantages and disadvantages compared with human RBCs. They are manufactured hemoglobin solutions that can be sterilized without destroying the blood substitute. They require no refrigeration and appear to have a long shelf-life (possibly 1 year, versus little more than 1 month for PRBCs). Perhaps more importantly, they require no cross-matching, because there is no RBC membrane to interact with antibodies in the recipient's serum. The most significant disadvantage stems from the blood substitutes extremely short life within human circulation—approximately 1 day, instead of the 30-day life span of a conventionally trans-

fused RBC. Therefore, the use of these products would likely be limited to situations in which the need is short-term (eg, surgery, trauma). Finally, the blood substitutes are likely to be extremely expensive.

PERIPHERAL BLOOD STEM CELL TRANSPLANTATION (PBSCT) AND BONE MARROW TRANSPLANTATION (BMT)

PBSCT and BMT are therapeutic modalities that offer the possibility of cure for some patients with hematologic disorders such as severe aplastic anemia, some forms of leukemia, and thalassemia. Because most hematologic disease states arise from some form of bone marrow dysfunction, an autologous transplantation (receiving one's own stem cells) is not as common an option as is allogeneic transplantation. A patient receives intensive chemotherapy (sometimes with radiation therapy as well), with the goal being complete ablation of the patient's bone marrow. Stem cells from the donor (ideally, from a matched sibling), or actual marrow from the donor, is then infused into the patient using a process similar to an RBC transfusion. The stem cells travel to the marrow and slowly begin the process of resuming hematopoiesis. The advantage of autotransplantation is the reduced likelihood of complications and mortality; however, the risk of relapse is also higher.

A relatively new strategy is based on transplantation for adoptive cell therapy using certain immune mechanisms derived from the donor's lymphocytes (Slavin et al., 2001; Margolis, Borrello, & Flinn, 2000). In nonmyeloablative stem cell or marrow transplantation, also referred to as a "minitransplant," the conditioning regimen involves much less myelosuppression than in conventional regimens, rendering the patient immunosuppressed but for a shorter period of time. Consequently, the procedure is less toxic to the patient, and there is a significant decrease in morbidity.

After the deconditioning regimen (ie, during the time the patient is immunosuppressed), the allotransplantation is performed, using either marrow or stem cells. The goal is for the donor's lymphocytes to react against any residual malignant cells within the patient and destroy them. This process is typically augmented by

Chart 33-19 — Pharmacologic Alternatives to Blood Transfusions

Growth Factors

Recombinant technology has provided a means to produce hematopoietic growth factors necessary for the production of blood cells within the bone marrow. By increasing the body's production of blood cells, transfusions and complications resulting from diminished blood cells (eg, infection from neutropenia or transfusions) may be avoided. However, the successful use of growth factors requires functional bone marrow.

Erythropoietin

Erythropoietin (epoetin alpha [eg, Epogen, Procrit]) is an effective alternative treatment for patients with chronic anemia secondary to diminished levels of erythropoietin, as in chronic renal disease. This medication stimulates erythropoiesis. It also has been used for patients who are anemic from chemotherapy or zidovudine (AZT) therapy and for those who have diseases involving bone marrow suppression, such as myelodysplastic syndrome (MDS). The use of erythropoietin can also enable a patient to donate several units of blood for future use (eg, preoperative autologous donation). The medication can be administered intravenously or subcutaneously, although plasma levels are better sustained with the subcutaneous route. Side effects are rare, but erythropoietin can cause or exacerbate hypertension. If the anemia is corrected too quickly or is overcorrected, the elevated hematocrit can cause headache and, potentially, seizures. These adverse effects are rare except for patients with renal failure. Serial complete blood counts (CBCs) should be performed to evaluate the response to the medication. The dose and frequency of administration are titrated to the hematocrit.

Granulocyte-Colony Stimulating Factor (G-CSF)

G-CSF (filgrastim [Neupogen]) is a cytokine that stimulates the proliferation and differentiation of myeloid stem cells; a rapid increase in neutrophils is seen within the circulation. G-CSF is effective in improving transient but severe neutropenia after chemotherapy or in some forms of MDS. It is particularly useful in preventing bacterial infections that would be likely to occur with neutropenia. G-CSF is administered subcutaneously on a daily basis. The primary side effect is bone pain; this probably reflects the increase in hematopoiesis within the marrow. Serial CBCs should be performed to evaluate the response to the medication and to ensure that the rise in white blood cells is not excessive. The effect of G-CSF on myelopoiesis is short; the neutrophil count drops once the medication is stopped.

Granulocyte-Macrophage Colony Stimulating Factor (GM-CSF)

GM-CSF (sargramostim [Leukine]) is a cytokine that is naturally produced by a variety of cells, including monocytes and endothelial cells. It works either directly or synergistically with other growth factors to stimulate myelopoiesis. GM-CSF is not as specific to neutrophils as is G-CSF; thus, an increase in erythroid (RBC) and megakaryocytic (platelet) production may also be seen. GM-CSF serves the same purpose as G-CSF. However, it may have a greater effect on macrophage function and therefore may be more useful against fungal infections, whereas G-CSF may be better used to fight bacterial infections. GM-CSF is also administered subcutaneously. Side effects include bone pain, fevers, and myalgias.

Thrombopoietin

Thrombopoietin (TPO) is a cytokine that is necessary for the proliferation of megakaryocytes and subsequent platelet formation. Clinical studies have demonstrated efficacy of TPO in the setting of chemotherapy-induced thrombocytopenia with few side effects (Vadhan-Raj, 2000). Further studies are ongoing to assess the efficacy of TPO in other, more chronic conditions associated with thrombocytopenia (Kuter, 2000).

infusion of the donor's lymphocytes as well (referred to as donor lymphocyte infusion, or DLI). If relapse occurs, repeated DLI has been effective in reestablishing remission in many patients. This approach has great promise, particularly in the setting of hematologic malignancy, and may provide a mechanism to increase the utility of transplantation for more patients than is possible with conventional methods.

Success of transplantation depends on tissue compatibility and the patient's tolerance of the immunosuppression that results from the ablative therapy. Patients require intensive nursing care that is directed toward preventing infection and assessing for early signs and symptoms of complications. One common complication involves the formation of lymphocytes that respond to their new host (ie, the patient) as foreign and mount a reaction against the body. This process, known as graft-versus-host disease (GVHD), can involve the skin, gastrointestinal tract, and liver and can be life-threatening. In hematologic malignancies, some GVHD is actually desirable in that the donor lymphocytes can also mount a reaction against any lingering tumour cells; this process is referred to as graft-versus-malignancy. GVHD is a significant complication in nonmyeloablative transplantation therapy, as well as in conventional allotransplantation. Late complications (occurring more than 100 days after transplantation) are frequent; these patients, particularly those who receive an allogeneic transplant, require careful follow-up for years after transplantation. (See Chap. 16 for further information on GVHD.)

Critical Thinking Exercises

1. You are working in a hematology-oncology clinic. The laboratory reports a critical study result for one of your patients with CLL: the reticulocyte count is 25%. What other laboratory results would be important to review or consider? The patient is profoundly anemic; does this support your original thinking and problem solving? What medical treatment orders would you anticipate? What nursing interventions would be appropriate?

2. You are caring for a young adult patient who has had repeated hospitalizations for sickle cell crisis. What factors should be assessed to determine the patient's education, coping, and pain management needs? What is important for the patient's discharge plan?

3. You are caring for a patient diagnosed with leukemia. The family members are very concerned about the patient's risk for infection at home. What assessments will assist you to determine the patient's risk of developing an infection at home? What instructions should you give about decreasing the risks for infection? How would you alter your interventions if the family members are not fluent in English?

4. You are caring for a patient who is septic and is now receiving a transfusion of 2 units of PRBCs. The patient's temperature spikes to 38.5°C after half of the second unit has been transfused. What are the possible causes of the fever? What are the appropriate nursing interventions?

REFERENCES AND SELECTED READINGS

Books

Abrams, A. C. (2001). *Clinical drug therapy: Rationales for nursing practice.* Philadelphia: Lippincott Williams & Wilkins.

American Association of Blood Banks. (2002). *Blood transfusion therapy: A physician's handbook* (7th ed.). Bethesda, MD: Author.

Anderson, K. C., & Ness, P. M. (Eds.). (2000). *Scientific basis of transfusion medicine: Implications for clinical practice.* Philadelphia: W. B. Saunders.

Blumenthal, M., Goldberg, A., & Brinkman, J. (Eds.). (2000). *Herbal medicine.* Newton, MA: Integrative Medicine Communications.

Hoffman, R., Benz, E. J., Shattil, S. J., Furie, B., Cohen, H. J., Silberstein, L. E., et al. (Eds.). (2000). *Hematology: Basic principles and practice* (3rd ed.). New York: Churchill Livingstone.

Lee, G., Foerster, J., Lukens, J., Paraskevas, F., Rogers, G. (1999). *Wintrobe's clinical hematology* (10th ed.). Baltimore: Williams & Wilkins.

Mintz, P. D. (Ed.). (1999). *Transfusion therapy: Clinical principles and practice.* Bethesda, MD: American Association of Blood Banks Press.

Rieger, P. T. (Ed.). (2001). *Biotherapy: A comprehensive overview* (2nd ed.). Boston: Jones and Bartlett.

Schechter, G., Berliner, N., & Telen, M. J. (Eds.). (2000). *Hematology 2000.* [Monograph]. San Francisco: American Society of Hematology Educational Program Book.

Schechter, G., Hoffman, R., & Schrier, S. (Eds.). (1999). *Hematology.* [Monograph]. New Orleans: American Society of Hematology Educational Program Book.

Skeel, R. (Ed.). (1999). *Handbook of cancer chemotherapy* (5th ed.). Philadelphia: Lippincott Williams & Wilkins.

Westphal, R. G. (1996). *Handbook of transfusion medicine* (3rd ed.). Washington, DC: American Red Cross Blood Services.

Wilkes, G. M., Ingwersen, K., & Barton-Burke, M. (2000). *2000 Oncology nursing drug handbook.* Boston: Jones and Bartlett.

Winningham, M. L., & Barton-Burke, M. (Eds.). (2000). *Fatigue in cancer: A multidimensional approach.* Boston: Jones and Bartlett.

Journals

Asterisks indicate nursing research articles.

Aaronson, L. S., Teel, C. S., Cassmeyer, V., Neuberger, G. B., Pallikkathayil, L., Pierce, J., Press, A. N., Williams, P. D., & Wingate, A. (1999). Defining and measuring fatigue. *Image: The Journal of Nursing Scholarship, 31*(1), 45–50.

Adams, R. J. (2000). Lessons from the Stroke Prevention Trial in Sickle Cell Anemia (STOP) study. *Journal of Child Neurology, 15*(5), 344–349.

Alcoser, P. W., & Burchetts, S. (1999). Bone marrow transplantation: Immune system suppression and reconstitution. *American Journal of Nursing, 99*(6), 26–30.

Anderson, K., Hamblin, T. J., & Traynor, A. (1999). Management of multiple myeloma today. *Seminars in Hematology, 36,* (1 Suppl. 3), 3–8.

Andrews, N. C. (1999). Disorders of iron metabolism. *New England Journal of Medicine, 341*(26), 1986–1995.

Applebaum, F. R., Baer, M. R., Carabisi, M. H., Coutre, S. E., Erba, H. P., Estey, E., Glenn, M. J., Kraut, E. H., Maslak, P., Millenson, M., Miller, C. B., Saba, H. I., Stone, R., & Tallman, M. S.; National Comprehensive Cancer Network. (2000). NCCN practice guidelines for acute myelogenous leukemia. *Oncology, 14*(11A), 53–61.

*Baker, F., Zabora, J., Pollard, A., & Wingard, J. (1999). Reintegration after bone marrow transplantation. *Cancer Practice, 7*(4), 190–197.

Barbui, T., & Finazzi, G. (1999). Clinical parameters for determining when and when not to treat essential thrombocytopenia. *Seminars in Hematology, 36* (1, Suppl. 2), 14–18.

BC Cancer Agency. (2005). Types of cancer and sequelae: Non-Hodgkins lymphoma. Available at: http://www.bccancer.bc.ca/PPI/TypesofCancer/NonHodgkinsLymphoma/default.htm.

Bensinger, W., Martin, P. J., Storer, B., Clift, R., Forman, S. J., Negrin, R., Kashyap, A., Flowers, M. E., Lilleby, K., Chauncey, T. R., Storb, R., & Appelbaum, F. R. (2001). Transplantation of bone marrow as compared with peripheral-blood cells from HLA-identical relatives in patients with hematologic cancers. *New England Journal of Medicine, 344*(3), 175–181.

Beran, M. (2000). Intensive chemotherapy for patients with high-risk myelodysplastic syndrome. *International Journal of Hematology, 72*(2), 139–150.

Berman, E., Clift, R. A., Copelan, E. A., Emanuel, P. D., Erba, H. P., Glenn, M. J., Greenberg, P. L., Jones, R. J., O'Brien, S., Saba, H. I., Schilder, R., Snyder, D. S., Soiffer, R. J., Tallman, M. S., Wetzler, M., Ravansi-Kashani, F., Kantarjian, H., & Talpaz, M. (2000). NCCN practice guidelines for chronic myelogenous leukemia. *Oncology, 14*(11A), 229–240.

Berenson, J. (2001). New advances in the biology and treatment of myeloma bone disease. *Seminars in Hematology, 38*(2, Suppl. 3), 15–20.

Bick, R. L. (1999). Low molecular weight heparins in the outpatient management of venous thromboembolism. *Seminars in Thrombosis and Hemostasis, 25* (Suppl. 3), 97–99.

Bradbury, M., & Cruickshank, J. P. (2000). Blood transfusion: Crucial steps in maintaining safe practice. *British Journal of Nursing, 9*(3), 134–138.

Briere, J., & Guilmin, F. (2001). Management of patients with essential thrombocythemia: Current concepts and perspectives. *Pathologie-biologie, 49*(2), 178–183.

Brown, P. (2001). Transfusion medicine and spongiform encephalopathy. *Transfusion, 41*(4), 433–436.

Burney, K. (2000). Tips for timely management of febrile neutropenia. *Oncology Nursing Forum, 27*(4), 617–618.

Carella, A. M., Cavaliere, M., Lerma, E., Ferrara, R., Tedeschi, L., Romanelli, A., Vinci, M., Pinotti, G., Lambelet, P., Loni, C., Verdiani, S., De Stefano, F., Valbonesi, M., & Corsetti, M. T. (2000). Autografting followed by nonmyeloablative immunosuppressive chemotherapy and allogeneic peripheral-blood hematopoietic stem-cell transplantation as treatment of resistant Hodgkin's disease and non-Hodgkin's lymphoma. *Journal of Clinical Oncology, 18*(23), 3918–3924.

Carella, A. M., Giralt, S., & Slavin, S. (2000). Low intensity regimens with allogeneic hematopoietic stem cell transplantation as treatment of hematologic neoplasia. *Haematologica, 85*(3), 304–313.

Cassileth, P. A., Harrington, D. P., Appelbaum, F., Lazarus, H. M., Rowe, J. M., Paietta, E., Willman, C., Hurd, D. D., Bennett, J. M., Blume, K. G., Head, D. R., & Wiernik, P. H. (1998). Chemotherapy compared with autologous or allogeneic bone marrow transplantation in the management of acute myeloid leukemia in first remission. *New England Journal of Medicine, 339*(23), 1649–1656.

Cavalli, F. (1998). Rare syndromes in Hodgkin's disease. *Annals of Oncology, 9* (Suppl. 5), S109–S113.

Cervantes, F. (2001). Prognostic factors and current practice in treatment of myelofibrosis with myeloid metaplasia: An update anno 2000. *Pathologie-biologie, 49*(2), 148–152.

Champlin, R., Khouri, I., Komblau, S., Molidrem, J., & Giralt, S. (1999). Reinventing bone marrow transplantation: Nonmyeloablative preparative regimens and induction of graft vs malignancy effect. *Oncology, 13*(5), 621–628.

Cheson, B., Horning, S., Coiffier, B., Shipp, M., Fisher, R., Conners, J., Lister, T., Vose, J., Grillo-Lopez, A., Hagenbeek, A., Cabanillas, F., Klippensten, D., Hiddemann, W., Castellino, R., Harris, N., Armitage, J., Carter, W., Hoppe, R., & Canellos, G. (1999). Report of an international workshop to standardize response criteria for non-Hodgkin's lymphomas. *Journal of Clinical Oncology, 17*(4), 1244–1253.

Coiffer, B. (2002). Rituximab in the treatment of diffuse large B-cell lymphomas. *Seminars in Oncology, 29*(1, Suppl. 2), 30–35.

Corwin, E. J. (2000). Understanding cytokines. Part I: Physiology and mechanisms of action. *Biologic Research for Nursing, 2*(1), 30–40.

Corwin, E. J. (2000). Understanding cytokines. Part II: Implications for nursing research and practice. *Biologic Research for Nursing, 2*(1), 41–48.

Creteur, J., Sibbald, W., & Vincent, J. L. (2000). Hemoglobin solutions: Not just red blood cell substitutes. *Critical Care Medicine, 28*(8), 3025–3034.

Derderian, P. M., Kantarjian, H. M., Talpaz, M., O'Brien, S., Cork, A., Estey, E., Pierce, S., & Keating, M. (1993). Chronic myelogenous leukemia in the lymphoid blastic phase: Characteristics, treatment response, and prognosis. *American Journal of Medicine, 94*(1), 69–74.

Deagle, J., & Kelaher, N. (1999). Deep-vein thrombosis: The shift to outpatient care. *Nursing Times, 95*(46), 48–49.

*de Carvalho, E. C., Goncalves, P. G., Bontempo, A. M., & Sloer, V. (2000). Interpersonal needs expressed by patients during bone marrow transplantation. *Cancer Nursing, 23*(6), 462–467.

Deeg, H. J., & Applebaum, F. R. (2000). Hematopoietic stem cell transplantation in patients with myelodysplastic syndrome. *Leukemia Research, 24*(8), 653–663.

Delmore, B. A., Hansen, D., Mooney, K. A., Paplanus, L. M., & Sutton, P. R. (2000). An anticoagulation pathway for quality management. *Applied Nursing Research, 13*(2), 105–110.

Druker, B., Talpaz, M., Resta, D., Peng, B., Buchdinger, E., Ford., J., Lydon, N., Kantargian, H., Capdeville, R., Ohno-Jones, S., & Sawyers, C. L. (2001). Efficacy and safety of a specific inhibitor of the BCR-ABL tyrosine kinase in chronic myeloid leukemia. *New England Journal of Medicine, 344*(14), 1031–1037.

*Duquette-Petersen, L., Francis, M., Dohnalek, L., Skinner, R., & Dudas, P. (1999). The role of protective clothing in infection prevention in patients undergoing autologous bone marrow transplantation. *Oncology Nursing Forum, 26*(8), 1319–1324.

Elalamy, I., Lecrubier, C., Horellou, M. H., Conard, J., & Samama, M. M. (2000). Heparin-induced thrombocytopenia: Laboratory diagnosis and management. *Annals of Medicine, 32*, (Suppl. 1), 60–67.

Ely, E. W., & Bernard, G. R. (1999). Transfusions in critically ill patients. *New England Journal of Medicine, 340*(6), 467–468.

Emmanouilides, C., Rosen, P., Telatar, M., Malone, R., Bosserman, L., Menco, H., Patel, R., Barstis, J., & Grody, W. (2000). Excellent tolerance of rituximab when given after mitoxantrone/cyclophosphamide: An effective and safe combination for indolent non-Hodgkin's lymphoma. *Clinical Lymphoma, 1*(2), 146–151.

Engstrom, C. A., & Sarkodee-Adoo, C. (1998). The molecular biology of lymphoma. *Seminars in Oncology Nursing, 14*(4), 256–261.

Fareed, J., Hoppensteadt, D. A., & Bick, R. L. (2000). An update on heparins at the beginning of the new millennium. *Seminars in Thrombosis and Hemostasis, 26* (Suppl. 1), 5–21.

Ferster, A., Tahriri, P., Vermylen, C., Sturbois, G., Corazza, F., Fondu, P., Devalck, C., Dresse, M., Feremans, W., Hunninck, K., Toppet, M., Philippet, P., Van Geet, C., & Sariban, E. (2001). Five years of experience with hydroxyurea in children and young adults with sickle cell disease. *Blood, 97*(11), 3628–3632.

*Fitzgerald, M., Hodgkinson, B., & Thorp, D. (1999). Blood transfusion from the recipient's perspective. *Journal of Clinical Nursing, 8*(5), 593–600.

George, J. N., Kojouri, K., Perdue, J. J., & Vesely, S. K. (2000). Management of patients with chronic, refractory idiopathic thrombocytopenic purpura. *Seminars in Hematology, 37*(3), 290–298.

Giardina, P. J., & Grady, R. W. (1995). Chelation therapy in beta-thalassemia: The benefits and limitations of desferrioxamine. *Seminars in Hematology, 32*(4), 304–312.

Gilbert, H. S. (1999). Historical perspective on the treatment of essential thrombocythemia and polycythemia vera. *Seminars in Hematology, 36* (1, Suppl. 2), 19–22.

Gobel, B. H. (1999). Disseminated intravascular coagulation. *Seminars in Oncology Nursing, 15*(3), 174–182.

Gochee, P. A., & Powell, L. W. (2001). What's new in hemochromatosis. *Current Opinion in Hematology, 8*(2), 98–104.

Goldman, D. A. (2001). Thalidomide use: Past history and current implications for practice. *Oncology Nursing Forum, 28*(3), 471–477.

Goldman, J., & Melo, J. (2001). Targeting the BCR-ABL tyrosine kinase in chronic myeloid leukemia. *New England Journal of Medicine, 344*(14), 1084–1086.

Gorman, K. (1999). Sickle cell disease. *American Journal of Nursing, 99*(3), 38–43.

Greenberg, P., Baer, M., Bennett, J., Bloomfield, C., Deeg, H., J., Erba, H. P., et al. (2000). NCCN practice guidelines for myelodysplastic syndromes, Version 2000. In *The Complete Library of NCCN Guidelines* [CD-ROM]. Rockledge, PA. National Comprehensive Cancer Network.

Greenlee, R. T., Hill-Harmon, M., Murray, T., & Thun, M. (2001). Cancer statistics, 2001. *CA: A Cancer Journal for Clinicians, 51*(1), 15–36.

Gruppo Italiano Studio Policitemia (GISP). (1995). Polycythemia vera: The natural history of 1213 patients followed over 20 years. *Annals of Internal Medicine, 123*(9), 656–664.

Hainsworth, J., Burris, H., Morrissey, L., Litchy, S., Scullin, D., Bearden, J., Richards, P., & Greco, F. (2000). Rituximab monoclonal antibody as initial systemic therapy for patients with low-grade non-Hodgkin lymphoma. *Blood, 95*(10), 3052–3056.

Hays, K., & McCartney, S. (1998). Nursing care of the patient with chronic lymphocytic leukemia. *Seminars in Oncology, 25*(1), 75–79.

Heaney, M. L., & Golde, D. W. (1999). Myelodysplasia. *New England Journal of Medicine, 340*(21), 1649–1660.

Hiddemann, W., & Buchner, T. (2001). Current status and perspectives of therapy for acute myeloid leukemia. *Seminars in Hematology, 38* (3, Suppl. 6), 3–9.

Hoelzer, D., & Gokbuget, N. (2000). New approaches to acute lymphoblastic leukemia in adults: Where do we go? *Seminars in Oncology, 27*(5), 540–559.

Hu, K., & Yahalom, J. (2000). Radiotherapy in the management of plasma cell tumors. *Oncology, 14*(1), 101–108.

Huffstutler, S. Y. (2000). Adult anemia. *Advance for Nurse Practitioners, 8*(3), 89–91.

Jantunen, R., Juvonen, E., Ikkala, E., Okansen, K., Antilla, P., & Ruutu, T. (2001). The predictive value of vascular risk factors and gender for the development of thrombotic complications in essential thrombocythemia. *Annals of Hematology, 80*(2), 74–78.

Josting, A., & Diehl, V. (2001). Early-stage Hodgkin's disease. *Current Oncology Reports, 3*(3), 279–284.

Kanis, J. A., & McCloskey, E. V. (2000). Bisphosphonates in multiple myeloma. *Cancer, 88* (12, Suppl.), 3022–3032.

Kelton, J. G. (1999). The clinical management of heparin-induced thrombocytopenia. *Seminars in Hematology, 36*, (1 Suppl. 1), 17–21.

Kelton, J. G., & Bussel, J. B. (2000). Idiopathic immune thrombocytopenic purpura: An update. *Seminars in Hematology, 37*(3), 219–221.

Korman, M. T., Leparc, G., & Benson, K. (2001). Nucleic acid amplification testing: The new infectious disease testing method for donor blood. Available at: http://www.moffitt.usf.edu/pubs/ccj/v6n5/dept5.htm. Accessed June 28, 2001.

Kornblith, A. B., Herndon, J. E. II, Silverman, L. R., Demakos, E. P., Holland, J. F., et al. (1998). The impact of 5-azacytidine on the quality of life of patients with myelodysplastic syndrome (MDS) treated in a randomized phase III trial of the cancer and leukemia group B (CALGB). *Proceedings of the American Society of Clinical Oncology, 17*, Abstract 189.

Kosits, C., & Callaghan M. (2000). Rituximab: A new monoclonal antibody therapy for non-Hodgkin's lymphoma. *Oncology Nursing Forum, 27*(1), 51–59.

Kreimeier, U., & Messmer, K. (2002). Perioperative hemodilution. *Transfusions and Apheresis Science, 27*(1), 59–72.

Kuter, D. J. (2000) Future directions with platelet growth factors. *Seminars in Hematology, 37*(2, Suppl. 4), 41–49.

Lengfelder, E., Berger, U., & Hehlmann, R. (2002). Interferon alpha in the treatment of polycythemia vera. *Annals of Hematology, 79*(3), 103–109.

Loney, M., & Chernecky, C. (2000). Anemia. *Oncology Nursing Forum, 27*(6), 951–962.

Lusher, J. M. (2000). Inhibitor antibodies to factor VIII and factor IX: Management. *Seminars in Thrombosis and Hemostasis, 26*(2), 179–188.

Major, P., Lortholary, A., Hon, J., Abdi, E., Mills, G., Menssen, H. D., Yunus, F., Bell, R., Body, J., Quebe-Fehling, E., & Seaman, J. (2001). Zolendronic acid is superior to pamidronate in the treatment of tumor-induced hypercalcemia: A pooled analysis of two randomized, controlled clinical trials. *Journal of Clinical Oncology, 19*(2), 558–567.

Marcaccio, M. J. (2000). Laparoscopic splenectomy in chronic idiopathic thrombocytopenic purpura. *Seminars in Hematology, 37*(3), 267–274.

Margolis, J., Borrello, I., & Flynn, I. W. (2000). New approaches to treating malignancies with stem cell transplantation. *Seminars in Oncology, 27*(5), 524–530.

McCullough, J. (2000). Current issues with platelet transfusion in patients with cancer. *Seminars in Hematology, 37* (2, Suppl. 4), 3–10.

Micallef, I. N., Rohatiner, A. Z., Carter, M., Boyle, M., Slater, S., Amess, J. A., & Lister, T. A. (2001). Long-term outcome of patients surviving for more than ten years following treatment for acute leukemia. *British Journal of Haematology, 113*(2), 443–445.

Michiels, J. J., Barbui, T., Finazzi, G., Fuchtman, S. M., Kutti, J., Rain, J. D., et al. (2000). Diagnosis and treatment of polycythemia vera and possible future study designs of the PVSG. *Leukemia and Lymphoma, 36*(3–4), 239–253.

Mitka, M. (2001). FDA wants more restrictions on donated blood. *Journal of the American Medical Association, 286*(4), 408.

Money, S. R., & York, J. W. (2001). Development of oral heparin therapy for prophylaxis and treatment of deep venous thrombosis. *Cardiovascular Surgery, 9*(3), 211–218.

Murphy, S. (1999). Diagnostic criteria and prognosis in polycythemia vera and essential thrombocythemia. *Seminars in Hematology, 36* (1, Suppl. 2), 9–13.

NCCN practice guidelines for Hodgkin's disease. National Comprehensive Cancer Network. *Oncology, 13*(5A), 78–110.

Ohene-Frempong, K. (2001). Indications for red cell transfusion in sickle cell disease. *Seminars in Hematology, 38* (1, Suppl. 1), 5–13.

O'Rourke, M. E., & High, K. (2000). Diagnosing graft versus host disease. *Clinical Journal of Oncology Nursing, 4*(1), 47–48.

Osterbor, A. (2000). The role of recombinant human erythropoietin in the management of anaemic cancer patients: Focus on haematological malignancies. *Medical Oncology, 17* (Suppl 1), S17–S22.

Patt, J., & Morrison, S. (2001). National Cancer Institute resources for patients and their caregivers. *Cancer Practice, 9*(5), 257–261.

*Pederson, C., & Parren, L. (1999). Pain in adult recipients of blood or marrow transplant. *Cancer Nursing, 22*(6), 397–407.

Petrykk, M., & Grossbard, M. L. (2000). Rituximab therapy of B-cell neoplasms. *Clinical Lymphoma, 1*(3), 186–194.

Rabinovici, R. (2001). The status of hemoglobin-based red cell substitutes. *Israel Medical Association Journal, 3*(9), 691–697.

Radich, J., & Sievers, E. (2000). New developments in the treatment of acute myeloid leukemia. *Oncology, 14*(11A), 125–131.

Reed, W., Walker, P., Haddix, T., & Perkins, H. A. (2000). Acute anemic events in sickle cell disease. *Transfusion, 40*(3), 267–273.

Rimm, E. B., Willett, W. C., Hu, F. B., Sampson, L., Colditz, G. A., Manson, J. E., Hennekens, C., & Stampfer, M. J. (1998). Folate and vitamin B6 from diet and supplements in relation to risk of coronary heart disease among women. *Journal of the American Medical Association, 279*(5), 359–364.

Rust, D., Simpson, J., & Lister, J. (2000). Nutritional issues in patients with severe neutropenia. *Seminars in Oncology Nursing, 16*(16), 152–162.

Saleh, M. N., Gutheil, J., Moore, M., Bunch, P. W., Butler, J., Kunkel, L., Grillo-Lopez, A. J., & LoBuglio, A. F. (2000). A pilot study of the anti-CD20 monoclonal antibody rituximab in patients with refractory immune thrombocytopenia. *Seminars in Oncology, 27* (6, Suppl. 12), 99–103.

Scaradavou, A. (2000). Splenectomy-sparing, long-term maintenance with anti-D for chronic immune (idiopathic) thrombocytopenic purpura: The New York Hospital experience. *Seminars in Hematology, 37* (1, Suppl. 1), 42–44.

Seligsohn, U., & Lubetsky, A. (2001). Genetic susceptibility to venous thrombosis. *New England Journal of Medicine, 344*(16), 1222–1231.

Shapiro, A. D. (2000). Platelet function disorders. *Haemophilia, 6* (Suppl. 1), 120–127.

Shelton, B. K. (1999). Sepsis. *Seminars in Oncology Nursing, 15*(3), 209–221.

Sievers, E., Appelbaum, F., Speilberger, R. T., Forman, S., Flowers, D., Smith, F., Shannon-Dorcy, K., Berger, M. S., & Bernstein, I. D. (1999). Selective ablation of acute myeloid leukemia using antibody-targeted chemotherapy: A phase I study of anti-CD33 calicheamicin immunoconjugate. *Blood, 93*(11), 3678–3684.

Silverstein, M. R., & Tefferi, A. (1999). Treatment of essential thrombocythemia with anagrelide. *Seminars in Hematology, 36* (1, Suppl. 2), 23–25.

Singhal, S., Mehta, J., Desikan, R., Ayers, D., Roberson, P., Eddlemon, P., Munshi, N., Anaissie, E., Wilson, C., Dhodapkar, M., Zeddis, J., & Barlogie, B. (1999). Antitumor activity of thalidomide in refractory multiple myeloma. *New England Journal of Medicine, 341*(21), 1565–1571.

Slavin, S., Or, R., Aker, M., Shapira, M. Y., Panigrahi, S., Symeonidis, A., Cividalli, G., & Nagler, A. (2001). Nonmyeloablative stem cell transplantation for the treatment of cancer and life-threatening nonmalignant disorders: Past accomplishments and future goals. *Cancer Chemotherapy and Pharmacology, 48* (Suppl. 1), S79–S84.

*Smith, L. H., & Besser, S. G. (2000). Dietary restrictions for patients with neutropenia: A survey of institutional practices. *Oncology Nursing Forum, 27*(3), 515–520.

Stampfer, M. J., Hu, F. B., Manson, J. E., Rimm, E. B., & Willett, W. C. (2000). Primary prevention of coronary heart disease in women through diet and lifestyle. *New England Journal of Medicine, 343*(1), 16–22.

Stasi, R., Pagano, A., Stipa, E., & Amadori, S. (2001). Rituximab chimeric anti-CD20 monoclonal antibody treatment for adults with chronic idiopathic thrombocytopenic purpura. *Blood, 98*(4), 952–957.

Steinberg, M. H. (1999). Management of sickle cell disease. *New England Journal of Medicine, 340*(13), 1021–1030.

Tefferi, A., Fonseca, R., Pereira, D. L., & Hoagland, H. C. (2001). A long-term retrospective study of young women with essential thrombocythemia. *Mayo Clinic Proceedings, 76*(1), 22–28.

Tefferi, A., Solberg, L. A., & Silverstein, M. N. (2000). A clinical update in polycythemia vera and essential thrombocythemia. *American Journal of Medicine, 109*(2), 141–149.

Tennant, L. (2001). Chronic myelogenous leukemia: An overview. *Clinical Journal of Oncology Nursing, 5*(5), 218–219.

Terpos, E., Palermos, J., Tsinos, K., Anargyrou, K., Viniou, N., Papassavas, P., Meletis, J., & Yataganas, X. (2000). Effect of pamidronate administration on markers of bone turnover and disease activity in multiple myeloma. *European Journal of Haematology, 65*(5), 331–336.

Tesch, H., Sieber, M., & Diehl, V. (2001). Treatment of advanced stage Hodgkin's disease. *Oncology, 60*(2), 101–109.

Thomas, M. L. (1998). Anemia and quality of life in cancer patients: Impact of transfusion and erythropoietin. *Medical Oncology, 15* (Suppl. 1), S13–S18.

Thomas, M. L. (1998). Quality of life and psychsocial adjustment in patients with myelodysplastic syndromes. *Leukemia Research, 22* (Suppl. 1), S41–S47.

Traynor, A. E., & Noga, S. J. (2001). NCCN: multiple myeloma. *Cancer Control, 8* (6, Suppl. 2), 78–87.

Vadhan-Raj, S. (2000). Clinical experience with recombinant human thrombopoietin in chemotherapy-induced thrombocytopenia. *Seminars in Hematology, 37* (2, Suppl. 4), 28–34.

Viale, P. H. (1999). Management of thromboembolism in patients with cancer. *Oncology Nursing Forum, 26*(10), 1625–1632.

Vichinsky, E. P., Neumayr, L. D., Earles, A. N., Williams, R., Lennett, E. T., Dean, D. D., Nickerson, B., Orringer, E., McKie, V., Bellevue, R., Daeschner, C., & Manci, E. A. (2000). Causes and outcomes of the acute chest syndrome in sickle cell disease. National Acute Chest Syndrome Study Group. *New England Journal of Medicine, 342*(25), 1855–1865.

Wazny, L. D., & Ariano, R. E. (2000). Evaluation and management of drug-induced thrombocytopenia in the acutely ill patient. *Pharmacotherapy, 20*(3), 292–307.

Weiss, L. M. (2000). Epstein-Barr virus and Hodgkin's disease. *Current Oncology Reports 2*(2), 199–204.

White, G. C., Greenwood, R., Escobar, M., & Frelinger, J. A. (2000). Hemophilia factor VIII therapy: Immunological tolerance. *Haematologica, 85* (10, Suppl.), 113–116.

Young, N. S. (2000). Hematopoietic cell destruction by immune mechanisms in acquired aplastic anemia. *Seminars in Hematology, 37*(1), 3–14.

Young, N. S. (1999). Acquired aplastic anemia. *Journal of the American Medical Association, 282*(3), 271–278.

Zaidi, A. A., & Vesole, D. H. (2001). Multiple myeloma: An old disease with new hope for the future. *CA: A Cancer Journal for Clinicians, 51*(5), 273–285.

Zelenetz, A., & Hoppe, R. T. (2001). NCCN: Non-Hodgkin's lymphomas. *Cancer Control, 8*(6, Suppl. 2), 102–113.

RESOURCES AND WEBSITES

American Pain Society, 4700 W. Lake Ave., Glenview, IL 60025 USA; 1-847-375-4715; http://www.ampainsoc.org.

BC Cancer Agency, Provincial Health Services Authority (PHSA), 700-1380 Burrard Street, Vancouver, BC V6Z 2H3; 604-675-7400; www.bcccancer.bc.ca.

Blood and Marrow Transplant Newsletter, 1985 Spruce Ave., Highland Park, IL 60036.

Canadian Blood Services, 1800 Alta Vista Drive, Ottawa, ON K1G 4J5; 613-739-2300; www.bloodservices.ca.

Canadian Cancer Society, Suite 200, 10 Alcorn Ave., Toronto ON M4B 3V1; 416-961-7223; http://www.cancer.ca

Canadian Hemochromatosis Society, 272-7000 Minoru Blvd, Richmond, BC V6Y 3Z5; 1-877-BAD-IRON (223-4766); http://www.cdnhemochromatosis.ca.

Canadian Hemophilia Society, 625 President Kennedy Ave., Suite 1210, Montreal, PQ, H3A 1K2; 514-848-0503; http://www.hemophilia.ca.

Canadian Oncology Societies; http://www.cos.ca/en/index.asp.

Canadian Pain Society, 701 Rossland Road East, Suite 373, Whitby, ON L1N 9K3; 905-668-9545; http://www.canadianpainsociety.ca.

Illness: Health Care Information Resources: Sickle Cell Disorder links; http://www-hsl.mcmaster.ca/tomflem/sickle.html.

International Myeloma Foundation, 12650 Riverside Drive, Suite 206, North Hollywood, CA 91607 USA; 1-800-452-2873; http://www.myeloma.org.

Leukemia and Lymphoma Society of Canada, 936 The East Mall, Toronto, ON M9B 6J9; 1-877-668-8326; http://leukemia.ca.

Neutropenia Support Association, PO Box 243, 971 Corydon, Winnipeg, MN R3M 3S7; 1-800-6-NEUTRO or 1-204-489-8454; http://www.neutropenia.ca/research/mds.html.

Digestive and Gastrointestinal Function

Applying Concepts from NANDA, NIC, and NOC

Mr. Sullivan is a 32-year-old man who has had several episodes of bloody diarrhea with severe cramping, nausea, and vomiting after attending a party 12 hours earlier where he drank eggnog and ate foods from a buffet table. His temperature is 39.44°C, heart rate 108, respiratory rate 20, and BP 118/80. Because he is a kidney transplant recipient and is on immunosuppressive medications, he is admitted to the hospital; his diagnosis is salmonellosis. The concept map illustrates the relationships that exist among the nursing diagnoses, interventions, and outcomes for one of Mr. Sullivan's clinical problems.

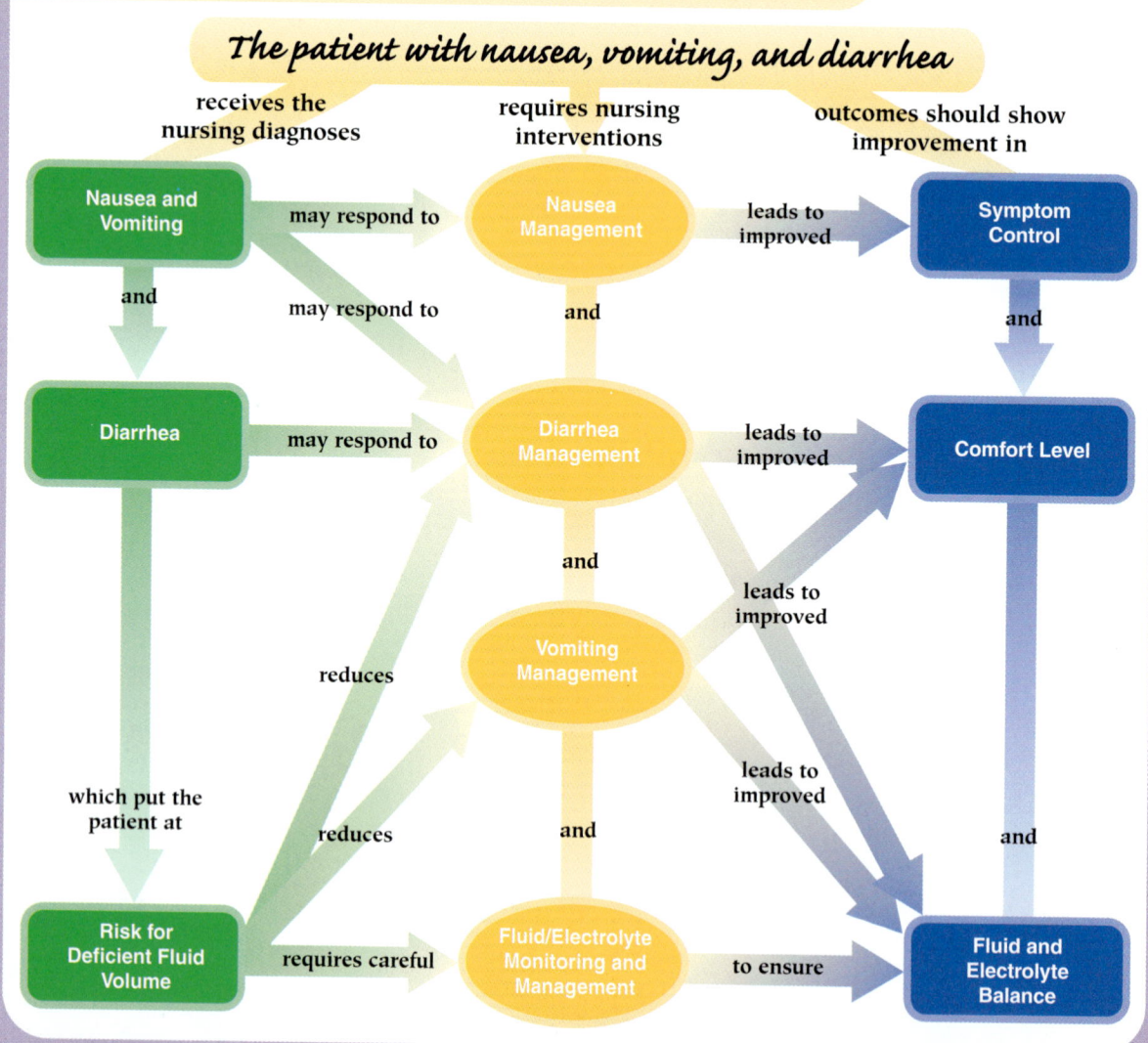

The patient with nausea, vomiting, and diarrhea

receives the nursing diagnoses — requires nursing interventions — outcomes should show improvement in

Nausea and Vomiting — may respond to → Nausea Management — leads to improved → Symptom Control

and — may respond to

Diarrhea — may respond to → Diarrhea Management — leads to improved → Comfort Level

and → Vomiting Management — leads to improved

reduces

which put the patient at — reduces — and — leads to improved

Risk for Deficient Fluid Volume — requires careful → Fluid/Electrolyte Monitoring and Management — to ensure → Fluid and Electrolyte Balance

Nursing Classifications and Languages

NANDA
Nursing Diagnoses

Nausea—Unpleasant wavelike sensation in the back of the throat, epigastrium, or throughout the abdomen that may or may not lead to vomiting

Diarrhea—Passage of loose, unformed stools

Risk for Deficient Fluid Volume—Risk for decreased intravascular, interstitial, and/or intracellular fluid. This refers to dehydration, water loss alone, without change in sodium.

NIC
Nursing Interventions*

Nausea Management—Prevention and alleviation of nausea

Diarrhea Management—Management and alleviation of diarrhea

Vomiting Management—Prevention and alleviation of vomiting

Fluid/Electrolyte Monitoring and Management—Collection and analysis of patient data to regulate fluid balance, and regulation and prevention of complications from altered fluid and/or electrolyte levels

NOC
Nursing Outcomes†

Return to functional baseline status, stabilization of, or improvement in

Symptom Control—Personal actions to minimize perceived adverse changes in physical functioning

Comfort Level—Extent of physical and psychological ease

Fluid/Electrolyte Balance—Balance of water and electrolytes in the intracellular and extracellular compartments of the body

NANDA, North American Nursing Diagnosis Association; NIC, Nursing Interventions Classification; NOC, Nursing Outcomes Classification

*Iowa Intervention Project © 2000. In McCloskey, J. C., & Bulechek, G. M. (2000). *Nursing interventions classification (NIC)* (3rd ed.). St. Louis: Mosby.

†Iowa Outcomes Project © 2000. In Johnson, M., Maas, M., & Moorhead, S. (2000). *Nursing outcomes classification (NOC)* (3rd ed.). St. Louis: Mosby.

Assessment of Digestive and Gastrointestinal Function

Adapted by Christy Raymond

LEARNING OBJECTIVES

On completion of this chapter, the learner will be able to:

1. Describe the structure and function of the organs of the gastrointestinal tract.

2. Describe the mechanical and chemical processes involved in digesting and absorbing foods and eliminating waste products.

3. Use assessment parameters appropriate for determining the status of gastrointestinal function.

4. Describe the appropriate preparation, teaching, and follow-up care for patients who are undergoing diagnostic testing of the gastrointestinal tract.

Anatomic and Physiologic Overview

ANATOMY OF THE GASTROINTESTINAL TRACT

The GI tract is a 5.76- to 6.5-m long pathway that extends from the **mouth** through the esophagus, stomach, and intestines to the anus (Fig. 34-1). The **esophagus** is located in the mediastinum in the thoracic cavity, anterior to the spine and posterior to the trachea and heart. This collapsible tube, which is about 25 cm (10 inches) in length, becomes distended when food passes through it. It passes through the diaphragm at an opening called the diaphragmatic hiatus.

The remaining portion of the GI tract is located within the peritoneal cavity. The **stomach** is situated in the upper portion of the abdomen to the left of the midline, just under the left diaphragm. It is a distensible pouch with a capacity of approximately 1500 mL. The inlet to the stomach is called the esophagogastric junction; it is surrounded by a ring of smooth muscle called the lower esophageal sphincter (or cardiac sphincter), which, on contraction, closes off the stomach from the esophagus. The stomach can be divided into four anatomic regions: the cardia (entrance), fundus, body, and pylorus (outlet). Circular smooth muscle in the wall of the pylorus forms the pyloric sphincter and controls the opening between the stomach and the small intestine.

The **small intestine** is the longest segment of the GI tract, accounting for about two thirds of the total length. It folds back and forth on itself, providing approximately 7000 cm of surface area for secretion and **absorption,** the process by which nutrients enter the bloodstream through the intestinal walls. The small intestine is divided into three anatomic parts: the upper part, called the duodenum; the middle part, called the jejunum; and the lower part, called the ileum. The common bile duct, which allows for the passage of both bile and pancreatic secretions, empties into the duodenum at the ampulla of Vater. The junction between the small and large intestine, the cecum, is located in the right lower portion of the abdomen. The ileocecal valve is located at this junction. It controls the passage of intestinal contents into the large intestine and prevents reflux of bacteria into the small intestine. The vermiform appendix is located near this junction.

The **large intestine** consists of an ascending segment on the right side of the abdomen, a transverse segment that extends from right to left in the upper abdomen, and a descending segment on the left side of the abdomen. The terminal portion of the large intestine consists of two parts: the sigmoid colon and the rectum. The rectum is continuous with the **anus**. A network of striated muscle that forms both the internal and the external anal sphincters regulates the anal outlet.

The GI tract receives blood from arteries that originate along the entire length of the thoracic and abdominal aorta. Of particular importance are the gastric artery and the superior and inferior mesenteric arteries. Oxygen and nutrients are supplied to the stomach by the gastric artery and to the intestine by the mesenteric arteries (Fig. 34-2). Blood is drained from these organs by veins that merge with others in the abdomen to form a large vessel called the portal vein. Nutrient-rich blood is then carried to the liver. The blood flow to the GI tract is about 20% of the total cardiac output and increases significantly after eating.

Both the sympathetic and parasympathetic portions of the autonomic nervous system innervate the GI tract. In general, sympathetic nerves exert an inhibitory effect on the GI tract, decreasing gastric secretion and motility and causing the sphincters and blood vessels to constrict. Parasympathetic nerve stimulation causes peristalsis and increases secretory activities. The sphincters relax under the influence of parasympathetic stimulation. The only portions of the tract that are under voluntary control are the upper esophagus and the external anal sphincter.

FUNCTION OF THE DIGESTIVE SYSTEM

All cells of the body require nutrients. These nutrients are derived from the intake of food that contains proteins, fats, carbohydrates, vitamins and minerals, and cellulose fibres and other vegetable matter of no nutritional value. The primary digestive functions of the GI tract are the following:

- To break down food particles into the molecular form for digestion

Glossary

absorption: phase of the digestive process that occurs when small molecules, vitamins, and minerals pass through the walls of the small and large intestine and into the bloodstream

amylase: an enzyme that aids in the digestion of starch

anus: last section of the GI tract; outlet for waste products from the system

chyme: mixture of food with saliva, salivary enzymes, and gastric secretions that is produced as the food passes through the mouth, esophagus, and stomach

digestion: phase of the digestive process that occurs when digestive enzymes and secretions mix with ingested food and when proteins, fats, and sugars are broken down into their component smaller molecules

elimination: phase of digestive process that occurs after digestion and absorption, when waste products are evacuated from the body

esophagus: collapsible tube connecting the mouth to the stomach, through which food passes as it is ingested

fibroscopy (gastrointestinal): intubation of a part of the GI system with a flexible, lighted tube to assist in diagnosis and treatment of diseases of that area

hydrochloric acid: acid secreted by the glands in the stomach; mixes with chyme to break it down into absorbable molecules and to aid in the destruction of bacteria

ingestion: phase of the digestive process that occurs when food is taken into the GI tract via the mouth and esophagus

intrinsic factor: a gastric secretion that combines with vitamin B_{12} so that the vitamin can be absorbed

large intestine: the portion of the GI tract into which waste material from the small intestine passes as absorption continues and elimination begins; consists of several parts—ascending segment, transverse segment, descending segment, sigmoid colon, and rectum

lipase: an enzyme that aids in the digestion of fats

mouth: first portion of the GI tract, through which food is ingested

pepsin: a gastric enzyme that is important in protein digestion

small intestine: longest portion of the GI tract, consisting of three parts—duodenum, jejunum, and ileum—through which food mixed with all secretions and enzymes passes as it continues to be digested and begins to be absorbed into the bloodstream

stomach: distensible pouch into which the food bolus passes to be digested by gastric enzymes

trypsin: enzyme that aids in the digestion of protein

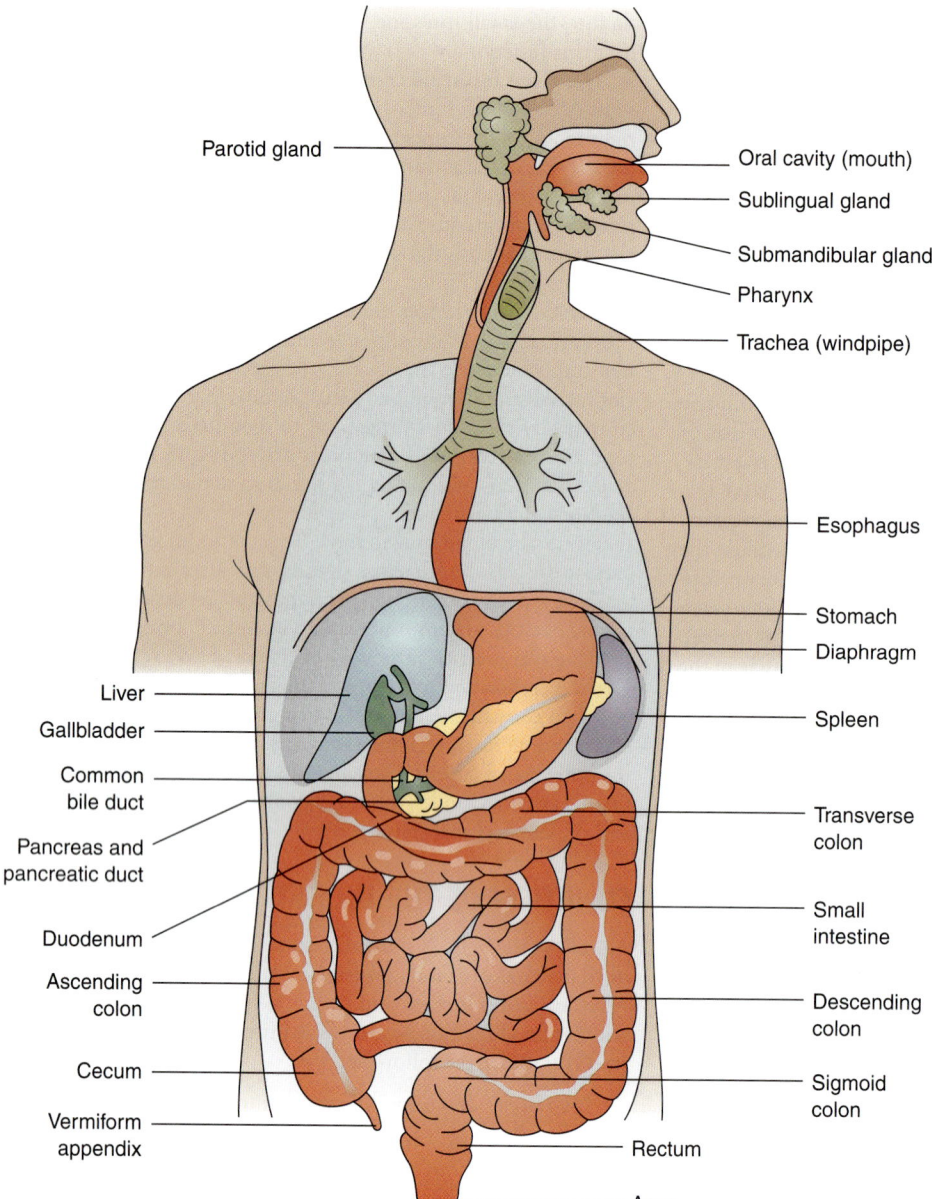

Parotid gland

Oral cavity (mouth)

Sublingual gland

Submandibular gland

Pharynx

Trachea (windpipe)

Esophagus

Stomach

Diaphragm

Liver

Gallbladder

Spleen

Common
bile duct

Pancreas and
pancreatic duct

Transverse
colon

Duodenum

Small
intestine

Ascending
colon

Descending
colon

Cecum

Sigmoid
colon

Vermiform
appendix

Rectum

Anus

FIGURE 34-1 Organs of the digestive system and associated structures.

- To absorb into the bloodstream the small molecules produced by **digestion**
- To eliminate undigested and unabsorbed foodstuffs and other waste products from the body

After food is ingested, it is propelled through the GI tract, coming into contact with a wide variety of secretions that aid in its digestion, absorption, or **elimination** from the GI tract.

Chewing and Swallowing

The process of digestion begins with the act of chewing, in which food is broken down into small particles that can be swallowed and mixed with digestive enzymes. Eating—or even the sight, smell, or taste of food—can cause reflex salivation. Saliva is secreted from three pairs of glands: the parotid, the submaxillary, and the sublingual glands. Approximately 1.5 L of saliva is se-

creted daily. Saliva is the first secretion that comes in contact with food. Saliva contains the enzyme ptyalin, or salivary amylase, which begins the digestion of starches (Table 34-1). Saliva also contains mucus and water, which help to lubricate the food as it is chewed, thereby facilitating swallowing.

Swallowing begins as a voluntary act that is regulated by a swallowing centre in the medulla oblongata of the central nervous system. As food is swallowed, the epiglottis moves to cover the tracheal opening and prevent aspiration of food into the lungs. Swallowing, which propels the bolus of food into the upper esophagus, thus ends as a reflex action. The smooth muscle in the wall of the esophagus contracts in a rhythmic sequence from the upper esophagus toward the stomach to propel the bolus of food along the tract. During this process of esophageal peristalsis, the lower esophageal sphincter relaxes and permits the bolus of food to enter the stomach. Subsequently, the lower esophageal sphincter closes tightly to prevent reflux of stomach contents into the esophagus.

glands of the stomach. The function of this gastric secretion is two-fold: to break down food into more absorbable components and to aid in the destruction of most ingested bacteria. The stomach can produce about 2.4 L per day of these gastric secretions. Gastric secretions also contain the enzyme **pepsin**, which is important for initiating protein digestion. **Intrinsic factor** is also secreted by the gastric mucosa. This compound combines with dietary vitamin B_{12} so that the vitamin can be absorbed in the ileum. In the absence of intrinsic factor, vitamin B_{12} cannot be absorbed and pernicious anemia results (see Chapter 33).

Peristaltic contractions in the stomach propel its contents toward the pylorus. Because large food particles cannot pass through the pyloric sphincter, they are churned back into the body of the stomach. In this way, food in the stomach is agitated mechanically and broken down into smaller particles. Food remains in the stomach for a variable length of time, from a half-hour to several hours, depending on the size of food particles, the composition of the meal, and other factors. Peristalsis in the stomach and contractions of the pyloric sphincter allow the partially digested food to enter the small intestine at a rate that permits efficient absorption of nutrients. This food mixed with gastric secretions is called **chyme**. Hormones, neuroregulators, and local regulators found in the gastric secretions control the rate of gastric secretions and influence gastric motility (Table 34-2).

Small Intestine Function

The digestive process continues in the duodenum. Secretions in the duodenum come from the accessory digestive organs—the pancreas, liver, and gallbladder—and the glands in the wall of the intestine itself. These secretions contain digestive enzymes and bile. Pancreatic secretions have an alkaline pH because of high concentrations of bicarbonate. This neutralizes the acid entering the duodenum from the stomach. The pancreas also secretes digestive enzymes, including **trypsin**, which aids in digesting protein; **amylase**, which aids in digesting starch; and **lipase**, which

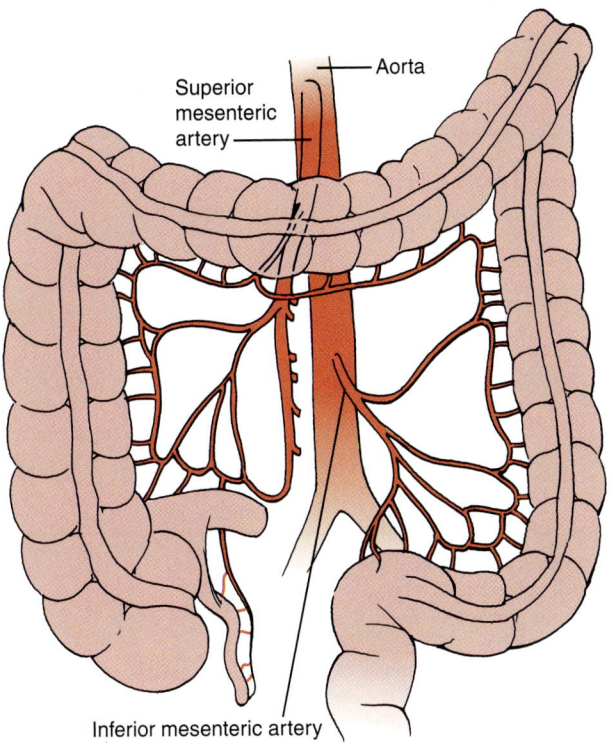

FIGURE 34-2 Anatomy and blood supply of the large intestine.

Gastric Function

The stomach stores and mixes the food with secretions. It secretes a highly acidic fluid in response to the presence or anticipated **ingestion** of food. This fluid, which may have a pH as low as 1, derives its acidity from the **hydrochloric acid** (HCl) secreted by the

Table 34-1 • The Major Digestive Enzymes and Secretions

ENZYME/SECRETION	ENZYME SOURCE	DIGESTIVE ACTION
Action of Enzymes That Digest Carbohydrates		
Ptyalin (salivary amylase)	Salivary glands	Starch→dextrin, maltose, glucose
Amylase	Pancreas and intestinal mucosa	Starch→dextrin, maltose, glucose
		Dextrin→maltose, glucose
Maltase	Intestinal mucosa	Maltose→glucose
Sucrase	Intestinal mucosa	Sucrose→glucose, fructose
Lactase	Intestinal mucosa	Lactose→glucose, galactose
Action of Enzymes/Secretions That Digest Protein		
Pepsin	Gastric mucosa	Protein→polypeptides
Trypsin	Pancreas	Proteins and polypeptides→polypeptides, dipeptides, amino acids
Aminopeptidase	Intestinal mucosa	Polypeptides→dipeptides, amino acids
Dipeptidase	Intestinal mucosa	Dipeptides→amino acids
Hydrochloric acid	Gastric mucosa	Protein→polypeptides, amino acids
Action of Enzymes That Digest Fat (Triglyceride)		
Pharyngeal lipase	Pharynx mucosa	Triglycerides→fatty acids, diglycerides, monoglycerides
Steapsin	Gastric mucosa	Triglycerides→fatty acids, diglycerides, monoglycerides
Pancreatic lipase	Pancreas	Triglycerides→fatty acids, diglycerides, monoglycerides
Bile	Liver and gallbladder	Fat emulsification

Table 34-2 • The Major Gastrointestinal Regulatory Substances

SUBSTANCE	STIMULUS FOR PRODUCTION	TARGET TISSUE	EFFECT ON SECRETIONS	EFFECT ON MOTILITY
Neuroregulators				
Acetylcholine	Sight, smell, chewing food, stomach distention	Gastric glands, other secretory glands, gastric and intestinal muscle	Increased gastric acid	Generally increased; decreased sphincter tone
Norepinephrine	Stress, other various stimuli	Secretory glands, gastric and intestinal muscle	Generally inhibitory	Generally decreased; increased sphincter tone
Hormonal Regulators				
Gastrin	Stomach distention with food	Gastric glands	Increased secretion of gastric juice, which is rich in HCl	Increased motility of stomach, decreased time required for gastric emptying Relaxation of ileocecal sphincter Excitation of colon Constriction of gastro-esophageal sphincter
Cholecystokinin	Fat in duodenum	Gallbladder Pancreas Stomach	Release of bile into duodenum Increased production of enzyme-rich pancreatic secretions Inhibits gastric secretion somewhat	
Secretin	pH of chyme in duodenum below 4–5	Stomach Pancreas	Inhibits gastric secretion somewhat Increased production of bicarbonate-rich pancreatic juice	Inhibits stomach contractions
Local Regulator				
Histamine	Unclear; substances in food	Gastric glands	Increased gastric acid production	

aids in digesting fats. Bile (secreted by the liver and stored in the gallbladder) aids in emulsifying ingested fats, making them easier to digest and absorb.

The intestinal glands secrete mucus, hormones, electrolytes, and enzymes. The mucus coats the cells and protects the mucosa from injury by HCl. Hormones, neuroregulators, and local regulators found in these intestinal secretions control the rate of intestinal secretions and also influence GI motility. Intestinal secretions total approximately 1 L/day of pancreatic juice, 0.5 L/day of bile, and 3 L/day of secretions from the glands of the small intestine. Tables 34-1 and 34-2 summarize the actions of digestive enzymes and GI regulatory substances.

Two types of contractions occur regularly in the small intestine: segmentation contractions and intestinal peristalsis. *Segmentation contractions* produce mixing waves that move the intestinal contents back and forth in a churning motion. *Intestinal peristalsis* propels the contents of the small intestine toward the colon. Both movements are stimulated by the presence of chyme.

Food, initially ingested in the form of fats, proteins, and carbohydrates, is broken down into absorbable particles (constituent nutrients) by the process of digestion. Carbohydrates are broken down into disaccharides (eg, sucrose, maltose, galactose) and monosaccharides (eg, glucose, fructose). Glucose is the major carbohydrate that the tissue cells use as fuel. Proteins are broken down into amino acids and peptides. Ingested fats are emulsified into monoglycerides and fatty acids. These smaller molecules are then ready to be absorbed. Chyme stays in the small intestine for 3 to 6 hours, allowing for continued breakdown and absorption of nutrients.

Small, finger-like projections called villi are present throughout the entire intestine and function to produce digestive enzymes as well as to absorb nutrients. Absorption is the primary function of the small intestine. Vitamins and minerals are not digested but rather absorbed essentially unchanged. Absorption begins in the jejunum and is accomplished by both active transport and diffusion across the intestinal wall into the circulation. Absorption of different nutrients takes place at different locations in the small intestine. Iron and calcium absorption takes place in the duodenum. Fats, proteins, carbohydrates, sodium, and chloride are absorbed in the jejunum. Vitamin B_{12} and bile salts are absorbed in the ileum. Magnesium, phosphate, and potassium are absorbed throughout the small intestine (Society of Gastroenterologic Nursing and Associates, 1998).

Colonic Function

Within 4 hours after eating, residual waste material passes into the terminal ileum and passes slowly into the proximal portion of the colon through the ileocecal valve. This valve, which is normally closed, helps prevent colonic contents from refluxing into the small intestine. With each peristaltic wave of the small intestine, the valve opens briefly and permits some of the contents to pass into the colon.

Bacteria make up a major component of the contents of the large intestine. They assist in completing the breakdown of waste material, especially of undigested or unabsorbed proteins and bile salts. Two types of colonic secretions are added to the residual material: an electrolyte solution and mucus. The electrolyte solution is chiefly a bicarbonate solution that acts to neutralize the end products formed by the colonic bacterial action. The mucus protects the colonic mucosa from the interluminal contents and also provides adherence for the fecal mass.

Slow, weak peristaltic activity moves the colonic contents slowly along the tract. This slow transport allows efficient reabsorption of water and electrolytes, which is the primary purpose of the colon. Intermittent strong peristaltic waves propel the contents for considerable distances. This generally occurs after another meal is eaten, when intestine-stimulating hormones are released. The waste materials from a meal eventually reach and distend the rectum, usually in about 12 hours. As much as one fourth of the waste materials from a meal may still be in the rectum 3 days after the meal was ingested.

Waste Products of Digestion

Feces consist of undigested foodstuffs, inorganic materials, water, and bacteria. Fecal matter is about 75% fluid and 25% solid material. The composition is relatively unaffected by alterations in diet, because a large portion of the fecal mass is of nondietary origin, derived from the secretions of the GI tract. The brown colour of the feces results from the breakdown of bile by the intestinal bacteria. Chemicals formed by intestinal bacteria (especially indole and skatole) are responsible in large part for the fecal odour. Gases formed contain methane, hydrogen sulfide, and ammonia, among others. The GI tract normally contains approximately 150 mL of these gases, which are either absorbed into the portal circulation and detoxified by the liver or expelled from the rectum as flatus.

Elimination of stool begins with distention of the rectum, which reflexively initiates contractions of the rectal musculature and relaxes the normally closed internal anal sphincter. The internal sphincter is controlled by the autonomic nervous system; the external sphincter is under the conscious control of the cerebral cortex. During defecation, the external anal sphincter voluntarily relaxes to allow colonic contents to be expelled. Normally, the external anal sphincter is maintained in a state of tonic contraction. Thus, defecation is seen to be a spinal reflex (involving the parasympathetic nerve fibres) that can be inhibited voluntarily by keeping the external anal sphincter closed. Contracting the abdominal muscles (straining) facilitates emptying of the colon. The average frequency of defecation in humans is once daily, but the frequency varies among individuals.

Assessment

HEALTH HISTORY AND CLINICAL MANIFESTATIONS

The nurse begins by taking a complete history, focusing on symptoms common to GI dysfunction. These symptoms include pain, indigestion, intestinal gas, nausea and vomiting, hematemesis, and changes in bowel habits and stool characteristics. Information about any previous GI disease is important. The nurse notes past and current medication use and any previous treatment or surgery. Information pertaining to medications is of particular interest because medications are a frequent cause of GI symptoms. The nurse takes a dietary history to assess nutritional status. Questioning about the use of tobacco and alcohol includes details about type and amount. The nurse and patient discuss changes in appetite or eating patterns and any examples of unexplained weight gain or loss over the past year. The nurse also assesses the stool characteristics. The nurse records all abnormal findings and reports them to the physician. It is important to include in the history questions about psychosocial, spiritual, or cultural factors that may be affecting the patient.

Pain

Pain can be a major symptom of GI disease. The character, duration, pattern, frequency, location, distribution of referred pain (Fig. 34-3), and time of the pain vary greatly depending on the underlying cause. Other factors, such as meals, rest, defecation, and vascular disorders, may directly affect this pain.

Indigestion

Upper abdominal discomfort or distress associated with eating (commonly called *indigestion*) is the most common symptom of patients with GI dysfunction. The basis for this abdominal distress may be the patient's own gastric peristaltic movements. Bowel movements may or may not relieve the pain. Indigestion can result from disturbed nervous system control of the stomach

FIGURE 34-3 Common sites of referred abdominal pain.

or from a disorder in the GI tract or elsewhere in the body. Fatty foods tend to cause the most discomfort, because they remain in the stomach longer than proteins or carbohydrates do. Coarse vegetables and highly seasoned foods can also cause considerable distress.

Intestinal Gas

The accumulation of gas in the GI tract may result in belching (the expulsion of gas from the stomach through the mouth) or flatulence (the expulsion of gas from the rectum). It is through belching that swallowed air is expelled quickly when it reaches the stomach. Usually, gases in the small intestine pass into the colon and are released as flatus. Patients often complain of bloating, distention, or being "full of gas." Excessive flatulence may be a symptom of gallbladder disease or food intolerance.

Nausea and Vomiting

Vomiting is another major symptom of GI disease. Vomiting is usually preceded by nausea, which can be triggered by odours, activity, or food intake. The emesis, or vomitus, may vary in colour and content. It may contain undigested food particles or blood (hematemesis). When vomiting occurs soon after hemorrhage, the emesis is bright red. If blood has been retained in the stomach, it takes on a coffee-ground appearance because of the action of the digestive enzymes.

Change in Bowel Habits and Stool Characteristics

Changes in bowel habits may signal colon disease. Diarrhea (an abnormal increase in the frequency and liquidity of the stool or in daily stool weight or volume) commonly occurs when the contents move so rapidly through the intestine and colon that there is inadequate time for the GI secretions to be absorbed. Diarrhea is sometimes associated with abdominal pain or cramping and nausea or vomiting. Constipation (a decrease in the frequency of stool, or stools that are hard, dry, and of smaller volume than normal) may be associated with anal discomfort and rectal bleeding. See Chapter 38 for further discussion of diarrhea and constipation.

The characteristics of the stool can vary greatly. Stool is normally light to dark brown. However, many circumstances, including the ingestion of certain foods and medications, can change the appearance of stool (Table 34-3). Blood in the stool can present in various ways and must be investigated. If blood is shed in sufficient quantities into the upper GI tract, it produces a tarry-black colour

(melena). Blood entering the lower portion of the GI tract or passing rapidly through it will appear bright or dark red. Lower rectal or anal bleeding is suspected if there is streaking of blood on the surface of the stool or if blood is noted on toilet tissue. Other common abnormalities in stool characteristics that the patient may describe during the health history include the following:

- Bulky, greasy, foamy stools that are foul in odour; stool colour is grey, with a silvery sheen
- Light grey or clay-coloured stool, caused by the absence of urobilin
- Stool with mucus threads or pus that may be visible on gross inspection of the stool
- Small, dry, rock-hard masses called scybala; sometimes streaked with blood from rectal trauma as they pass through the rectum
- Loose, watery stool that may or may not be streaked with blood

PHYSICAL ASSESSMENT

The physical examination includes assessment of the mouth, abdomen, and rectum. The mouth, tongue, buccal mucosa, teeth, and gums are inspected, and ulcers, nodules, swelling, discolouration, and inflammation are noted. People with dentures should remove them during this part of the examination to allow good visualization.

The patient lies supine with knees flexed slightly for inspection, auscultation, palpation, and percussion of the abdomen (Fig. 34-4). The nurse performs inspection first, noting skin changes and scars from previous surgery. It also is important to note the contour and symmetry of the abdomen, to identify any localized bulging, distention, or peristaltic waves.

The nurse performs auscultation before percussion and palpation (which can increase intestinal motility and thereby change bowel sounds) and notes the character, location, and frequency of bowel sounds. The nurse assesses bowel sounds in all four quadrants using the diaphragm of the stethoscope; the high-pitched and gurgling sounds can be heard best in this manner. It is important to document the frequency of the sounds, using the terms *normal* (sounds heard about every 5 to 20 seconds), *hypoactive* (one or two sounds in 2 minutes), *hyperactive* (5 to 6 sounds heard in less than 30 seconds), or *absent* (no sounds in 3 to 5 minutes).

The nurse notes tympany or dullness during percussion. Use of light palpation is appropriate for identifying areas of tenderness or swelling; the nurse may use deep palpation to identify masses in any of the four quadrants. If the patient identifies any area of discomfort, the nurse can assess for rebound tenderness. To elicit rebound tenderness, the nurse exerts pressure over the area and then releases it quickly. It is important to note any pain experienced on withdrawal of the pressure. The nurse notes any abnormal finding in relation to the surface landmarks (xiphoid process, costal margins, anterior iliac spine, and symphysis pubis) or in relation to the four quadrants commonly used to describe the abdomen (right upper quadrant, RUQ; right lower quadrant, RLQ; left upper quadrant, LUQ; and left lower quadrant, LLQ) (Bickley & Hoekelman, 1999).

The final part of the examination is inspection of the anal and perineal area. The nurse should inspect and palpate areas of excoriation or rash, fissures or fistula openings, or external hemorrhoids. A digital rectal examination can be performed to note any areas of tenderness or mass.

Table 34-3 • Foods and Medications That Alter Stool Colour	
ALTERING SUBSTANCE	COLOUR
Meat protein	Dark brown
Spinach	Green
Carrots and beets	Red
Cocoa	Dark red or brown
Senna	Yellow
Bismuth, iron, licorice, and charcoal	Black
Barium	Milky white

Inspecting the abdomen

Auscultating the abdomen

Palpating the abdomen

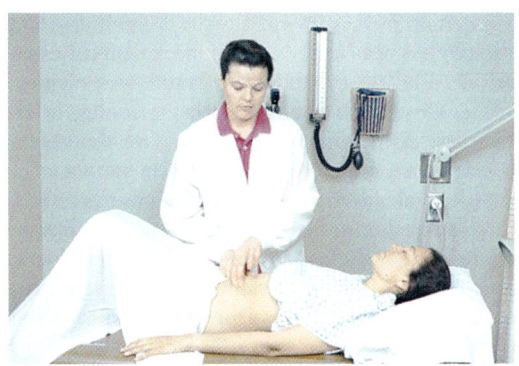

Percussing the abdomen

FIGURE 34-4 Examination of the abdomen includes inspection, auscultation, palpation, and percussion.

Diagnostic Evaluation

Blood tests are ordered initially. Common blood tests include complete blood count (CBC), liver function tests, serum cholesterol, and triglycerides. The carcinoembryonic antigen (CEA) is not routinely used as a screening tool but may be used as one diagnostic test. Serum CEA assays may also be used as one measure to guide physician's clinical management of a specific disorder (Gold & Goldenberg, 1997). Test findings may reveal alterations in basal metabolic function and may indicate the severity of a disorder.

Many other modalities are available for diagnostic assessment of the GI tract. The majority of these tests and procedures are performed on an outpatient basis in special units designed for this purpose (eg, endoscopy or GI laboratory). The nurse supports and educates patients who are undergoing diagnostic evaluation, whether in an inpatient or an outpatient setting. Patients who require such tests frequently are anxious, elderly, or debilitated. The preparation for many of these studies includes fasting, the use of laxatives or enemas, and ingestion or injection of a contrast agent or a radiopaque dye. These preparatory measures are poorly tolerated by weak and many elderly patients and have the potential to cause fluid and electrolyte imbalances. If further assessment or treatment is needed after any outpatient procedure, the patient may be admitted to the hospital.

Specific nursing interventions for each test are provided later in this chapter. General nursing interventions for the patient who is having GI diagnostic assessment include the following:

- Providing general information about a healthy diet and the nutritional factors that can cause GI disturbances; after a diagnosis has been confirmed, the nurse provides informa-

tion about specific nutrients that should be included in the diet
- Providing needed information about the test and the activities required of the patient
- Providing instructions about postprocedure care and activity restrictions
- Alleviating anxiety
- Helping the patient cope with discomfort
- Encouraging family members or others to offer emotional support to the patient during the diagnostic testing
- Assessing for adequate hydration before, during, and immediately after the procedure, and providing education about maintenance of hydration

STOOL TESTS

Basic examination of the stool includes inspecting the specimen for consistency and colour and testing for occult (not visible) blood. Special tests, including tests for fecal urobilinogen, fat, nitrogen, parasites, pathogens, food residues, and other substances, require that the specimen be sent to the laboratory.

Stool samples are usually collected on a random basis unless a quantitative study (eg, fecal fat, urobilinogen) is to be performed. Random specimens should be sent promptly to the laboratory for analysis. The quantitative 24- to 72-hour collections must be kept refrigerated until they are taken to the laboratory. Some stool collections require the patient to follow a special diet or to refrain from taking certain medications before the collection. It is important to follow test guidelines closely for accurate results.

Fecal occult blood testing is one of the most commonly performed stool tests. It can be useful in initial screening for several disorders. It tests only for the presence of blood, so other follow-up testing is required. It is most frequently used in cancer screening programs and for early cancer detection (Chart 34-1). The test can be performed at the bedside, in the laboratory, or at home. It tests for heme, the iron-containing portion of the hemoglobin molecule that is altered during transit through the intestines.

Probably the most widely used occult blood test is the Hemoccult test. It is inexpensive and noninvasive, and it carries no risk to the patient. It should not, however, be performed when there is hemorrhoidal bleeding. The test can be performed at home as well as in the doctor's office. The patient provides a stool specimen, and the physician smears it on a dry, guaiac-impregnated paper slide. If the test is done at home, the patient takes the sample to a laboratory location. The stool specimen is then examined for occult blood. Serial 3- to 6-day testing is recommended. The test is not perfect, because certain factors interfere with its sensitivity and specificity. False-positive results may occur if the patient has eaten rare meat, liver, poultry, turnips, broccoli, cauliflower, melons, salmon, sardines, or horseradish within 7 days before testing. Medications that can cause gastric irritation, such as aspirin, ibuprofen, indomethacin, colchicine, corticosteroids, cancer chemotherapeutic agents, and anticoagulants, may also cause false-positive results. Extensive research has demonstrated that therapeutic doses of iron preparations do not cause false-positive results. Ingestion of vitamin C from supplements or foods can cause false-negative results. Therefore, a careful assessment of the patient's diet and medication regimen is essential to reduce incorrect interpretation of results (Ahmed, 2000).

Other occult blood tests may yield more specific and more sensitive readings. Immunologic tests are more specific to human hemoglobin and decrease the problem of dietary interference. Hemoporphyrin assays detect the broadest range of blood derivatives, but a strict dietary protocol is essential. Immunochemical tests using anti-human antibodies that are extremely sensitive to human hemoglobin are also available.

BREATH TESTS

The *hydrogen breath test* was developed to evaluate carbohydrate absorption. It also is used to aid in the diagnosis of bacterial overgrowth in the intestine and short bowel syndrome. This test determines the amount of hydrogen expelled in the breath after it has been produced in the colon (on contact of galactose with fermenting bacteria) and absorbed into the blood.

Urea breath tests detect the presence of *Helicobacter pylori,* the bacteria that can live in the mucosal lining of the stomach and cause peptic ulcer disease. The patient takes a capsule of carbon-labelled urea and then provides a breath sample 10 to 20 minutes later. Because *H. pylori* metabolizes urea rapidly, the labelled carbon is absorbed quickly; it can then be measured as carbon dioxide in the expired breath to determine whether *H. pylori* is present. The patient is instructed to avoid antibiotics or loperamide (Pepto-Bismol) for 1 month before the test; sucralfate (Sulcrate) and omeprazole (Losec) for 1 week before the test; and cimetidine (Novo-Cimetidine), famotidine (Pepcid), ranitidine (Zantac), and nizatidine (Axid) for 24 hours before urea breath testing. *H. pylori* also can be detected by assessing serum antibody levels.

ABDOMINAL ULTRASONOGRAPHY

Ultrasonography is a noninvasive diagnostic technique in which high-frequency sound waves are passed into internal body structures and the ultrasonic echoes are recorded on an oscilloscope as they strike tissues of different densities. During abdominal ultrasonography, an image of the abdominal organs and structures is produced on the oscilloscope. This procedure is generally used to indicate the size and configuration of abdominal structures. It is particularly useful in the detection of cholelithiasis, cholecystitis, and appendicitis. Most recently this technique has proven useful in diagnosing acute colonic diverticulitis.

Advantages of abdominal ultrasonography are that it requires no ionizing radiation, there are no noticeable side effects, and it is relatively inexpensive. One disadvantage is that it cannot be used to examine structures that lie behind bony tissue, because bone prevents sound waves from passing to deeper structures. Gas and fluid in the abdomen or air in the lungs also prevent transmission of ultrasound.

Nursing Interventions

The patient fasts for 8 to 12 hours before the test to decrease the amount of gas in the bowel. If gallbladder studies are being performed, the patient should eat a fat-free meal the evening before the test. If barium studies are to be performed, the nurse should make sure they are scheduled after this test; otherwise, the barium will interfere with the transmission of the sound waves.

DNA TESTING

Researchers have refined methods for genetic risk assessment, preclinical diagnosis, and prenatal diagnosis to identify persons who are at risk for certain GI disorders (eg, gastric cancer, lactose deficiency, inflammatory bowel disease, colon cancer). In some cases, DNA testing allows practitioners to prevent (or minimize) disease, by intervening before its onset, and to improve therapy. Persons who are identified as at risk for certain GI disorders may choose to undergo genetic counselling to learn about the disease; to understand options for preventing and treating the disease; and to receive support in coping with the situation (Yamada, 1999).

Chart 34-1
Guidelines for Colon Cancer Screening

Those older than age 50 with no affected family member(s):
Are encouraged to have regular screening including FOBT, x-ray, endoscopy, or a combination.

Those younger than age 60 with a first-degree relative with colon cancer or polyps:
Are encouraged to have colonoscopy every 5 years at age 40 or 10 years younger than diagnosis of polyps or colon cancer in affected individual.

Those older than age 60 or having two or more first-degree relatives with colon cancer:
Are encouraged to have regular screening starting at age 40.

Those with one second- or third-degree relative affected with polyps or colon cancer:
Are encouraged to have regular screening beginning at age 50.

Definitions
FOBT–fecal occult blood test
First-degree relative–parent, child, or sibling
Second-degree relative–grandparent, aunt/uncle, nephew/niece
Third-degree relative–cousin, great grandparent, great grandchild

Source: Colon Cancer Screening Guidelines, Colorectal Cancer Screening Initiative Foundation, Canadian Association of Gastroenterology, and Canadian Digestive Health Foundation.

Persons at risk for colon cancer often are targeted for DNA testing because it can provide a head start on this preventable cancer.

IMAGING STUDIES

Imaging studies include x-ray and contrast studies, computed tomography (CT) scans, magnetic resonance imaging (MRI), and scintigraphy (radionuclide imaging).

Upper Gastrointestinal Tract Study

X-rays can delineate the entire GI tract after the introduction of a contrast agent. A radiopaque liquid (eg, barium sulfate) is commonly used. The patient ingests this tasteless, odourless, nongranular, and completely insoluble (hence, not absorbable) powder in the form of a thick or thin aqueous suspension for the purpose of studying the upper GI tract (upper GI series or barium swallow).

The upper GI series enables the examiner to detect or exclude anatomic or functional derangement of the upper GI organs or sphincters. It also aids in the diagnosis of ulcers, varices, tumours, regional enteritis, and malabsorption syndromes. The procedure may be extended to examine the duodenum and small bowel (small bowel follow-through).

The patient swallows barium under direct fluoroscopic examination. As the barium descends into the stomach, the position, patency, and calibre of the esophagus are visualized, enabling the examiner to detect or exclude any anatomic or functional derangement of that organ. Fluoroscopic examination next extends to the stomach as its lumen fills with barium, allowing observation of stomach motility, thickness of the gastric wall, the mucosal pattern, patency of the pyloric valve, and the anatomy of the duodenum. Multiple x-ray films are obtained during the procedure, and additional images may be taken at intervals for up to

---

GENETICS IN NURSING PRACTICE—Digestive and Gastrointestinal Disorders

SELECTED DIGESTIVE AND GASTROINTESTINAL DISORDERS INFLUENCED BY GENETIC FACTORS
- Cleft lip and/or palate
- Familial adenomatous polyposis
- Hereditary nonpolyposis colorectal cancer (HNPCC)
- Hirschsprung disease (aganglionic megacolon)
- Inflammatory bowel disease (eg, Crohn's disease)
- Pyloric stenosis

NURSING ASSESSMENTS
FAMILY HISTORY ASSESSMENT
- Careful family history assessment for other family members with a similar condition (eg, cleft lip/palate, pyloric stenosis)
- Assess for other family members in several generations with early-onset colorectal cancer
- Inquire about other family members with inflammatory bowel disease
- Assess family history for other cancers (eg, endometrial, ovarian, renal)

PHYSICAL ASSESSMENT
Assess for presence of other clinical symptoms:
- With clefting—congenital heart defect, mental retardation, other birth defects suggestive of a genetic syndrome
- With familial adenomatous polyposis—congenital hypertrophy of retinal pigment epithelium (CHRPE)

MANAGEMENT ISSUES SPECIFIC TO GENETICS
- Inquire whether any affected family member has had DNA mutation testing
- If indicated, refer for further genetic counselling and evaluation so that family members can discuss inheritance, risk to other family members, availability of genetic testing, and gene-based interventions
- Offer appropriate genetics information and resources
- Assess patients' understanding of genetics information
- Provide support to families with newly diagnosed genetics-related digestive disorders

- Participate in management and coordination of care for patients with genetic conditions and for those who are predisposed to develop or pass on a genetic condition

GENETIC RESOURCES
CANADA
Canadian Association of Genetic Counsellors—the purpose of the CAGC is to establish minimum standards of practice, encourage professional growth, and gain recognition of the genetic counselling profession in Canada; www.cagc-accg.ca.

Canadian Directory of Genetic Support Groups—a resource guide for families and professionals seeking information on genetic support groups in Canada; www.lhsc.on.ca/programs/medgenet.

Canadian Genetic Diseases Network—advancing Canada's scientific and commercial competitiveness in genetic research, and the application of genetic discoveries to prevent, diagnose, and treat disease; www.cgdn.ca.

Canadian Organization for Rare Disorders—an educational and informational support network for the enhancement of the lives of all persons affected by rare disorders; www.cord.ca.

UNITED STATES
Genetic Alliance—a directory of support groups for patients and families with genetic conditions; http://www.geneticalliance.org.

American Cancer Society—offers general information about cancer and support resources for families; http://www.cancer.org.

Gene Clinics—a listing of common genetic disorders with up-to-date clinical summaries, genetic counselling and testing information; http://www.geneclinics.org.

National Organization of Rare Disorders—a directory of support groups and information for patients and families with rare genetic disorders; http://www.rarediseases.org.

National Cancer Institute—current information about cancer research, treatment, resources for health providers, individuals, and families; http://www.nci.nih.gov.

Online Mendelian Inheritance in Man (OMIM)—a complete listing of inherited genetic conditions; http://www.ncbi.nlm.nih.gov/omim/stats/html.

24 hours to evaluate the rate of gastric emptying. Small bowel x-rays taken while the barium is passing through that area allow for observation of the motility of the small bowel. Obstructions, ileitis, and diverticula can be detected if present.

Variations of the upper GI study include double-contrast studies and enteroclysis. The double-contrast method of examining the upper GI tract involves administration of a thick barium suspension to outline the stomach and esophageal wall, after which tablets that release carbon dioxide in the presence of water are given. This technique has the advantage of showing the esophagus and stomach in finer detail, permitting signs of early superficial neoplasms to be noted.

Enteroclysis is a very detailed, double-contrast study of the entire small intestine that involves the continuous infusion, through a duodenal tube, of 500 to 1000 mL of a thin barium sulfate suspension. Methylcellulose is then infused into the small intestine through the tube. The barium and methylcellulose fill the intestinal loops and are observed continuously by fluoroscopy and viewed at frequent intervals as they progress through the jejunum and the ileum. This process (even with normal motility) can take up to 6 hours. The procedure aids in the diagnosis of partial small-bowel obstructions or diverticula.

NURSING INTERVENTIONS

The patient may need to maintain a low-residue diet for several days before the test. He or she should receive nothing by mouth after midnight before the test. The physician may prescribe a laxative to clean out the intestinal tract. Because smoking can stimulate gastric motility, the nurse discourages the patient from smoking on the morning before the examination. In addition, the nurse withholds all medications.

Follow-up care is needed after any of the upper GI procedures to ensure that the patient has completely eliminated the ingested barium. Fluids must be increased to facilitate evacuation of stool and barium. The nurse monitors the patient's stools until they return to their normal colour (the barium will look like clay). A laxative or enema may be needed.

Lower Gastrointestinal Tract Study

When barium is instilled rectally to visualize the lower GI tract, the procedure is called a barium enema. The purpose of a barium enema is to detect the presence of polyps, tumours, and other lesions of the large intestine and to demonstrate any abnormal anatomy or malfunction of the bowel.

The radiopaque substance is instilled rectally in the radiology department during fluoroscopy. If the patient has been prepared adequately and the colon has been evacuated completely, the contour of the entire colon, including the cecum and appendix (if patent), is clearly visible and the motility of each portion may be observed readily. The procedure usually takes about 15 to 30 minutes, during which time x-ray images are taken.

Other means for visualizing the colon include double-contrast studies and a water-soluble contrast study. A double-contrast or air-contrast barium enema involves the instillation of a thicker barium solution, followed by the instillation of air. The patient may feel some cramping or discomfort with this process. This test provides a contrast between the air-filled lumen and the barium-coated mucosa, allowing easier detection of smaller lesions.

If active inflammatory disease, fistulas, or perforation of the colon is suspected, a water-soluble iodinated contrast agent (eg, Gastrografin) can be used. The procedure is the same as for a barium enema; however, the patient must be assessed for allergy to iodine or contrast agent. The contrast agent is eliminated readily after the procedure, so there is no need for postprocedure laxatives. Some diarrhea may occur in a few patients until the contrast agent has been totally eliminated.

NURSING INTERVENTIONS

Preparing the patient includes emptying and cleansing the lower bowel. This often necessitates a low-residue diet 1 to 2 days before the test (the preparation required by different radiology departments may vary); a clear liquid diet and a laxative the evening before; nothing by mouth after midnight; and cleansing enemas until returns are clear the following morning. The nurse should make sure that barium enemas are scheduled before any upper GI studies. If the patient has active inflammatory disease of the colon, enemas are contraindicated. Barium enema also is contraindicated in patients with signs of perforation or obstruction; instead, a water-soluble contrast study may be performed in these situations. Active GI bleeding may prohibit the use of laxatives and enemas.

The nurse administers an enema or laxative after these tests to facilitate barium removal. Increasing fluid intake also will assist in eliminating the barium. As with any barium study, the nurse monitors the patient for complete elimination of the barium.

Computed Tomography

CT provides cross-sectional images of abdominal organs and structures. Multiple x-ray images are taken from many different angles, digitized in the computer, reconstructed, and then viewed on a computer monitor. Indications for abdominal CT scanning are diseases of the liver, spleen, kidney, pancreas, and pelvic organs. CT is a valuable tool for detecting and localizing many inflammatory conditions in the colon, such as appendicitis, diverticulitis, regional enteritis, and ulcerative colitis. Because the adequacy of detail in the test depends on the presence of fat, this diagnostic tool is not useful for very thin, cachectic patients. The procedure is completely painless, but radiation doses are considerable. Because a scanning time of 5 seconds is required, motion artefacts produced by heartbeat and respiration cannot be avoided, resulting in pictures that are less than clear.

New, continuous-motion (helical or spiral), three-dimensional CT scans have been developed that provide very detailed pictures of the GI organs and vasculature (Yamada, 1999). Colonography can be completed in minutes. It involves inserting a thin, straw-like tube into the colon and inflating the bowel with air to generate a computer image of the intestine. There is little discomfort, and sedation is not needed.

NURSING INTERVENTIONS

The patient should not eat or drink for 6 to 8 hours before the test. The practitioner may prescribe an intravenous or oral contrast agent. Therefore, the nurse should question the patient about contrast dye allergies. If barium studies are to be performed, it is important to schedule them after CT scanning, so as not to interfere with imaging.

Magnetic Resonance Imaging

MRI is used in gastroenterology to supplement ultrasonography and CT scanning. It is a noninvasive technique that uses magnetic fields and radio waves to produce an image of the area being studied. The use of oral contrast agents to enhance the image has increased the application of this technique for the diagnosis of GI diseases. It is useful in evaluating abdominal soft tissues as well as blood vessels, abscesses, fistulas, neoplasms, and other sources of bleeding.

The physiologic artefacts of heartbeat, respiration, and peristalsis may create a less-than-clear image. Newer, fast-imaging MRI techniques help to eliminate these physiologic motion artefacts. MRI is contraindicated for patients with permanent pacemakers, artificial heart valves and defibrillators, implanted insulin pumps, or implanted transcutaneous electrical nerve stimulation devices, because the magnetic field could cause malfunction. MRI is also contraindicated for patients with internal metal devices (eg, aneurysm clips) or intraocular metallic fragments.

NURSING INTERVENTIONS

The patient should not eat or drink for 6 to 8 hours before the test. Before the test, the patient must remove all jewelry and other metals. The patient lies in a machine that constructs an image based on the magnetic field created between the machine and the structures scanned. The entire procedure takes 30 to 90 minutes.

It is important to warn patients that the close-fitting scanners used in many MRI facilities may induce feelings of claustrophobia and that the machine will make a knocking sound during the procedure. Open MRIs that are less close-fitting eliminate the claustrophobia that many patients experience.

Scintigraphy

Scintigraphy is the diagnostic testing procedure where radionuclides are administered to examine specific tissues and organs (Lippincott Williams & Wilkins, 2005). Scintigraphy (radionuclide testing) relies on the use of radioactive isotopes (ie, technetium, iodine, and indium) to reveal displaced anatomic structures, changes in organ size, and the presence of neoplasms or other focal lesions, such as cysts or abscesses.

Scintigraphic scanning is also used to measure the uptake of tagged red blood cells and leukocytes. Tagging of red blood cells and leukocytes by injection of a radionuclide is performed to define areas of inflammation, abscess, blood loss, or neoplasm. A sample of blood is removed, mixed with a radioactive substance, and reinjected into the patient. Abnormal concentrations of blood cells are then detected at 24- and 48-hour intervals.

Gastrointestinal Motility Studies

Radionuclide testing also is used to assess gastric emptying and colonic transit time. For gastric emptying studies, the liquid and solid components of a meal are tagged with radionuclide markers. After the patient ingests the meal, the patient is positioned under a scintiscanner, which measures the rate of passage of the radioactive substance out of the stomach. This is useful in diagnosing disorders of gastric motility. Radionuclide evaluation of gastric emptying is now preferred over intubation methods because it gives more defined results (Phillips & Wingate, 1998). This procedure is helpful for evaluating any functional cause of gastric emptying, but its most common clinical uses at this time are in the evaluation of diabetic gastroparesis and of the rapid emptying process in the dumping syndrome.

Colonic transit studies are used to evaluate colonic motility instances of chronic constipation and obstructive defecation syndromes. This is usually an outpatient study. The patient is given a capsule containing 20 radionuclide markers and instructions to follow a regular diet and normal daily activities. Abdominal x-rays are taken every 24 hours until all markers are passed. This process usually takes 4 to 5 days, but in the presence of severe constipation it may take as long as 10 days. People with chronic diarrhea may be evaluated at 8-hour intervals. The amount of time it takes for the radioactive material to move through the colon indicates colonic motility.

ENDOSCOPIC PROCEDURES

Endoscopic procedures used in GI tract assessment include fibroscopy/esophagogastroduodenoscopy, anoscopy, proctoscopy, sigmoidoscopy, colonoscopy, small-bowel enteroscopy, and endoscopy through ostomy.

Upper Gastrointestinal Fibroscopy/ Esophagogastroduodenoscopy

Fibrescopes are flexible scopes equipped with fibreoptic lenses. **Fibroscopy** of the upper GI tract allows direct visualization of the esophageal, gastric, and duodenal mucosa through a lighted endoscope (gastroscope) (Fig. 34-5). This procedure,

FIGURE 34-5 Patient undergoing gastroscopy.

called esophagogastroduodenoscopy (EGD), is especially valuable when esophageal, gastric, or duodenal abnormalities or inflammatory, neoplastic, or infectious processes are suspected. This procedure also can be used to evaluate esophageal and gastric motility and to collect secretions and tissue specimens for further analysis.

The gastroenterologist views the GI tract through a viewing lens and can take still or video photographs through the scope to document findings. Electronic video endoscopes also are available that attach directly to a video processor, converting the electronic signals into pictures on a television screen. This allows larger and continuous viewing capabilities, as well as the simultaneous recording of the procedure.

Side-viewing flexible scopes are used to visualize the common bile duct and the pancreatic and hepatic ducts through the ampulla of Vater in the duodenum. This procedure, called endoscopic retrograde cholangiopancreatography (ERCP), uses the endoscope in combination with radiographic techniques to view the ductal structures of the biliary tract. ERCP is helpful in evaluating jaundice, pancreatitis, pancreatic tumours, common duct stones, and biliary tract disease. ERCP is described further in Chapter 40.

Upper GI fibroscopy also can be a therapeutic procedure when it is combined with other procedures. Therapeutic endoscopy can be used to remove common bile duct stones, dilate strictures, and treat gastric bleeding and esophageal varices. Laser-compatible scopes can be used to provide laser therapy for upper GI neoplasms. Sclerosing solutions can be injected through the scope in an attempt to control upper GI bleeding.

After the patient is sedated, the endoscope is lubricated with a water-soluble lubricant and passed smoothly and slowly along the back of the mouth and down into the esophagus. The gastroenterologist views the gastric wall and the sphincters, and then advances the endoscope into the duodenum for further examination. Biopsy forceps to obtain tissue specimens or cytology brushes to obtain cells for microscopic study can be passed through the scope. The procedure usually takes about 30 minutes.

The patient may experience nausea, gagging, or choking. Use of topical anesthetics and moderate sedation makes it important to monitor and maintain the oral airway during and after the procedure. Finger or ear oximeters are used to monitor oxygen saturation, and supplemental oxygen may be used if needed. Emergency equipment must be readily available. Precautions must be taken to protect the scope, because the fibreoptic bundles can be broken if the scope is bent at an acute angle. The patient wears a mouth guard to keep from biting the scope.

NURSING INTERVENTIONS

The patient should not eat or drink for 6 to 12 hours before the examination. Patient preparation includes helping the patient spray or gargle with a local anesthetic, and administering midazolam (Versed) intravenously just before the scope is introduced. Midazolam is a sedative that provides moderate sedation and relieves anxiety during the procedure. The nurse also may administer atropine to reduce secretions, and may give glucagon, if needed and prescribed, to relax smooth muscle. The nurse positions the patient on the left side to facilitate saliva drainage and to provide easy access for the endoscope. After the procedure, the nurse instructs the patient not to eat or drink until the gag reflex returns (in 1 to 2 hours), to prevent aspiration of food or fluids into the lungs. The nurse places the patient in the Sims' position until he or she is awake and then places the patient in the semi-Fowler's position until ready for discharge. After gastroscopy, as-

sessment by the nurse includes observing for signs of perforation, such as pain, bleeding, unusual difficulty swallowing, and an elevated temperature. The nurse monitors the pulse and blood pressure for changes that can occur with sedation. The nurse can test the gag reflex by placing a tongue blade onto the back of the throat to see whether gagging occurs. After the patient's gag reflex has returned, the nurse can offer lozenges, saline gargle, and oral analgesics to relieve minor throat discomfort. Patients who were sedated for the procedure must stay on bed rest until fully alert. After moderate sedation, the patient must be accompanied and transported home if the procedure was performed on an outpatient basis. The nurse instructs the patient not to drive for 10 to 12 hours if sedation was used.

Anoscopy, Proctoscopy, and Sigmoidoscopy

The lower portion of the colon also can be viewed directly to evaluate rectal bleeding, acute or chronic diarrhea, or change in bowel patterns and to observe for ulceration, fissures, abscesses, tumours, polyps, or other pathologic processes. Rigid or flexible fibreoptic scopes can be used. The anoscope is a rigid scope that is used to examine the anus and lower rectum. Proctoscopes and sigmoidoscopes are rigid scopes that are used to inspect the rectum and the sigmoid colon.

Flexible scopes have largely replaced the rigid scopes for routine examinations. The flexible fibreoptic sigmoidoscope (Fig. 34-6) permits the colon to be examined up to 40 to 50 cm (16 to 20 inches) from the anus, much more than the 25 cm (10 inches) that can be visualized with the rigid sigmoidoscope. The flexible scope has many of the same capabilities as the scopes used for the upper GI study, including the use of still or video images to document findings.

For rigid scope procedures, the patient assumes the knee-chest position at the edge of the bed or the examining table. With the back inclined at about a 45-degree angle, the patient is properly positioned for the introduction of an anoscope, proctoscope, or

FIGURE 34-6 Flexible fibreoptic sigmoidoscopy. The flexible scope is advanced past the proximal sigmoid and then into the descending colon.

sigmoidoscope. During the examination, it is important to keep the patient informed about the progress of the examination and to explain that the pressure exerted by the instrument will create the urge to have a bowel movement.

For flexible scope procedures, the patient assumes a comfortable position on the left side with the right leg bent and placed anteriorly. Again, it is important to keep the patient informed throughout the examination and to explain the sensations associated with the examination. Biopsies and polypectomies can be performed during this procedure. Biopsy is performed with small biting forceps introduced through the endoscope; one or more small pieces of tissue may be removed. If rectal or sigmoid polyps are present, they may be removed with a wire snare, which is used to grasp the pedicle, or stalk. An electrocoagulating current is then used to sever the polyp and prevent bleeding. It is extremely important that all excised tissue be placed immediately in moist gauze or in an appropriate receptacle, labelled correctly, and delivered without delay to the pathology laboratory for examination.

NURSING INTERVENTIONS

These examinations require only limited bowel preparation, including a warm tap water or Fleet's enema until returns are clear. Dietary restrictions usually are not necessary, and sedation usually is not required. During the procedure, the nurse monitors vital signs, skin colour and temperature, pain tolerance, and vagal response (Society of Gastroenterologic Nursing and Associates, 2003). After the procedure, the nurse monitors the patient for rectal bleeding and signs of intestinal perforation (ie, fever, rectal drainage, abdominal distention, and pain). On completion of the examination, the patient can resume regular activities and dietary practices.

Fibreoptic Colonoscopy

Direct visual inspection of the colon to the cecum is possible by means of a flexible fibreoptic colonoscope (Fig. 34-7). These scopes have the same capabilities as those used for esophagogastro-

duodenoscopy; however, they are larger in diameter and longer. Still and video recordings can be used to document the procedure and findings.

This procedure is used commonly as a diagnostic aid and screening device. It is most frequently used for cancer screening (see Chart 34-1) and for surveillance in patients with previous colon cancer or polyps. In addition, tissue biopsies can be obtained as needed, and polyps can be removed and evaluated. Other uses of colonoscopy include the evaluation of patients with diarrhea of unknown cause, occult bleeding, or anemia; further study of abnormalities detected on barium enema; and diagnosis, clarification, and determination of the extent of inflammatory or other bowel disease.

Therapeutically, the procedure can be used to remove all visible polyps with a special snare and cautery through the colonoscope. Many colon cancers begin with adenomatous polyps of the colon; therefore, one goal of colonoscopic polypectomy is early detection and prevention of colorectal cancer. This procedure also can be used to treat areas of bleeding or stricture. Use of bipolar and unipolar coagulators, use of heater probes, and injections of sclerosing agents or vasoconstrictors are all possible during this procedure. Laser-compatible scopes provide laser therapy for bleeding lesions or colonic neoplasms. Bowel decompression can also be completed during the procedure.

Colonoscopy is performed while the patient is lying on the left side with the legs drawn up toward the chest. The patient's position may be changed during the test to facilitate advancement of the scope. The procedure usually takes about 1 hour. Discomfort may result from instillation of air to expand the colon or from insertion and moving of the scope. Biopsy forceps or a cytology brush may be passed through the scope to obtain specimens for histology and cytology examinations. Potential complications of colonoscopy include cardiac dysrhythmias and respiratory depression resulting from the medications administered, vasovagal reactions, and circulatory overload or hypotension resulting from overhydration or underhydration during bowel preparation. Therefore, it is important to monitor the patient's cardiac and respiratory function continuously. Oxygen saturation is monitored with a

FIGURE 34-7 Colonoscopy. The flexible scope is passed through the rectum and sigmoid colon into the descending, transverse, and ascending colon.

finger or ear oximeter. Supplemental oxygen should be used as necessary.

NURSING INTERVENTIONS

The success of the procedure depends on how well the colon is prepared. Adequate colon cleansing provides optimal visualization and decreases the time needed for the procedure. First, the patient should limit the intake of liquids for 24 to 72 hours before the examination. Then, cleansing of the colon can be accomplished in various ways. The physician may prescribe a laxative for two nights before the examination and a Fleet's or saline enema until the return runs clear the morning of the test. More frequently, however, polyethylene glycol electrolyte and magnesium citrate lavage solutions are used as intestinal lavages for effective cleansing of the bowel. The patient maintains a clear liquid diet starting at noon the day before the procedure. Then the patient ingests lavage solutions orally at intervals over 3 to 4 hours. If necessary, the nurse can give this solution through a feeding tube if the patient is unable to swallow. Patients with a colostomy can receive this same bowel preparation. With the use of lavage solutions, bowel cleansing is fast (rectal effluent is clear in about 4 hours) and is tolerated fairly well by most patients. Side effects of the electrolyte solutions include nausea, bloating, cramps or abdominal fullness, fluid and electrolyte imbalance, and hypothermia (patients are often told to drink the preparation as cold as possible to make it more palatable). The side effects are especially problematic for elderly patients, and sometimes they have difficulty ingesting the required volume of solution. The use of lavage solutions is contraindicated in patients with intestinal obstruction or inflammatory bowel disease.

Additional nursing actions include the following:

- Instructing the patient not to take routine medications when the lavage solution is ingested; the medications will not be digested and therefore will be ineffective
- Advising the diabetic patient to consult with his or her physician about medication adjustment to prevent hyperglycemia or hypoglycemia resulting from dietary modifications required in preparation for the test
- Instructing all patients, especially the elderly, to maintain adequate fluid, electrolyte, and caloric intake while undergoing bowel cleansing

Special precautions must be taken for some patients. Implantable defibrillators and pacemakers are at high risk for malfunction if electrosurgical procedures (ie, polypectomy) are performed in conjunction with colonoscopy. A cardiologist should be consulted before the test is performed, and the defibrillator should be turned off. These patients require careful cardiac monitoring during the procedure. Colonoscopy cannot be performed if there is a suspected or documented colon perforation, acute severe diverticulitis, or fulminant colitis. Therapeutic colonoscopy may be contraindicated in patients with coagulopathies and in those receiving anticoagulation therapy, because of the high risk for excessive bleeding during and after the procedure. Nonsteroidal anti-inflammatory agents (NSAIDs), aspirin, ticlopidine, and pentoxifylline must be discontinued before the test and for 2 weeks after the procedure. Patients taking coumadin or heparin must consult the physician for specific instructions. Those with prosthetic heart valves or a history of endocarditis require prophylactic antibiotics before the procedure.

Informed consent is obtained before the test. The patient receives nothing by mouth (NPO) after midnight before the test,

but most medications can be taken with a small amount of water; the physician should be consulted about medication use. Before the examination, the nurse may administer intravenously an opioid analgesic or a sedative (eg, midazolam) to provide moderate sedation and relieve anxiety during the procedure. Glucagon may be used, if needed, to relax the colonic musculature and to reduce spasm during the test. Elderly or debilitated patients may require a reduced dosage of these medications to decrease the risks of oversedation and cardiopulmonary complications.

During the procedure, the nurse monitors for changes in oxygen saturation, vital signs, colour and temperature of the skin, level of consciousness, abdominal distention, vagal response, and pain intensity. After the procedure, patients who were sedated are maintained on bed rest until fully alert. Some will have abdominal cramps caused by increased peristalsis stimulated by the air insufflated into the bowel during the procedure. Immediately after the test, the nurse observes the patient for signs and symptoms of bowel perforation (eg, rectal bleeding, abdominal pain or distention, fever, focal peritoneal signs). If midazolam was used, the nurse explains its amnesic effects. It is important to provide written instructions, because the patient may be unable to recall verbal information. If the procedure is performed on an outpatient basis, someone must accompany and transport the patient home. After a therapeutic procedure, the nurse instructs the patient to report any bleeding to the physician.

Small-Bowel Enteroscopy

Technology for the use of the small-calibre transnasal endoscope to allow direct inspection of the wall of the small intestine continues to be developed. Two methods are being used at this time: the "push" and the "pull" endoscope methods. The "pull" endoscope is very long and flexible and has a balloon at its tip. When inflated, the balloon tip advances the scope by peristalsis through the small intestine. Reglan may be administered intravenously to assist passage. This procedure takes up to 10 hours to complete. The patient may be kept in the recovery area or sent home during this period. Once the scope has entered the distal ileum, the balloon is deflated and the tube is retracted slowly while the endoscopist examines the intestinal wall. "Push" endoscopes have been designed to be smaller in calibre and longer in length, while still allowing the use of biopsy forceps and probes (Lightdale, 2000). These two methods are especially useful in the evaluation of patients who have continued bleeding even after extensive diagnostic testing has identified no other problem area. They can also be used when biopsy of the small bowel is needed to diagnose malabsorption syndromes.

Endoscopy Through Ostomy

Endoscopy using a flexible endoscope through an ostomy stoma is useful for visualizing a segment of the small or large intestine. It may be indicated to evaluate an anastomosis, to screen for recurrent disease, or to visualize and treat bleeding in a segment of the bowel. Nursing interventions are similar to those for other endoscopic procedures.

MANOMETRY

Manometry studies are methods for evaluating patients with GI motility disorders. The manometry test measures changes in intraluminal pressures and the coordination of muscle activity in the GI tract. The pressures can be recorded manually, on a physiograph, or on a computer.

Esophageal manometry is used to detect motility disorders of the esophagus and the lower esophageal sphincter. Patients must refrain from eating or drinking for 8 to 12 hours before the test. Medications that could have a direct effect on motility (eg, calcium channel blockers, anticholinergic agents, sedatives) are withheld for 24 to 48 hours. A pressure-sensitive catheter is inserted through the nose and is connected to a transducer and a video recorder. The patient then swallows small amounts of water while the resultant pressure changes are recorded.

Gastroduodenal, small-intestine, and colonic manometry are used to evaluate delayed gastric emptying and gastric and intestinal motility disorders such as irritable bowel syndrome or atonic colon. This is often an ambulatory outpatient procedure lasting 24 to 72 hours. Anorectal manometry measures the resting tone of the internal anal sphincter and the contractibility of the external anal sphincter. It is helpful in evaluating patients with chronic constipation or fecal incontinence and is useful in biofeedback for the treatment of fecal incontinence. It can be performed in conjunction with rectal sensory functioning tests. Phospho-Soda or a saline cleansing enema is administered 1 hour before the test. Positioning for the test is either the prone or the lateral position.

A rectal sensory function test is used to evaluate rectal sensory function and neuropathy. A catheter and balloon are passed into the rectum, and the balloon is inflated until the patient feels distention. Then the tone and pressure of the rectum and anal sphincter are measured. The results are especially helpful in the evaluation of patients with chronic constipation, diarrhea, or incontinence.

Defecography

Defecography measures anorectal function. Very thick barium paste is instilled into the rectum, and then fluoroscopy is performed to assess the function of the rectum and anal sphincter while the patient attempts to expel the barium. The test requires no preparation. The use of scintigraphic techniques to measure rectal emptying of radioisotope-labelled artificial stool can provide more quantitative information.

Electromyographic studies can supplement anorectal manometry to measure the integrity and function of the anal sphincters in an effort to treat functional bowel incontinence and constipation.

GASTRIC ANALYSIS, GASTRIC ACID STIMULATION TEST, AND pH MONITORING

Analysis of the gastric juice yields information about the secretory activity of the gastric mucosa and the presence or degree of gastric retention in patients thought to have pyloric or duodenal obstruction. It is also useful for diagnosing diseases such as Zollinger-Ellison syndrome.

The patient is kept NPO for 8 to 12 hours before the procedure. Any medications that affect gastric secretions are withheld for 24 to 48 hours before the test. Smoking is not allowed on the morning before the test, because it increases gastric secretions. A small nasogastric tube with a catheter tip marked at various points is inserted through the nose. When the tube is at a point slightly less than 50 cm (21 inches) distant, it should be within the stomach, lying along the greater curvature. Once in place, the tube is secured to the patient's cheek and the patient is placed in a semi-reclining position. The entire stomach contents are aspirated by gentle suction into a syringe, and gastric samples are collected every 15 minutes for the next hour.

The gastric acid stimulation test usually is performed in conjunction with gastric analysis. Histamine or pentagastrin is administered subcutaneously to stimulate gastric secretions. It is important to inform the patient that this injection may produce a flushed feeling. The nurse monitors blood pressure and pulse frequently to detect hypotension. Gastric specimens are collected after the injection every 15 minutes for 1 hour and are labelled to indicate the time of specimen collection after histamine injection. The volume and pH of the specimen are measured. In certain instances, cytologic study by the Papanicolaou technique may be used to determine the presence or absence of malignant cells. Enzyme analysis of the gastric juice may be indicated.

Important diagnostic information to be gained from gastric analysis includes the ability of the mucosa to secrete HCl. This ability is altered in various disease states, including

- Pernicious anemia—patients with this disease secrete no acid under basal conditions or after stimulation
- Severe chronic atrophic gastritis or gastric cancer—patients with these diseases secrete little or no acid
- Peptic ulcer—patients with peptic ulcers secrete some acid
- Duodenal ulcers—patients with duodenal ulcers usually secrete an excess amount of acid

Esophageal reflux of gastric acid may be diagnosed by ambulatory pH monitoring. The patient is NPO for 6 hours before the test, and all medications affecting gastric secretions are withheld for 24 to 36 hours before the test. A probe that measures pH is placed through the nose and into position about 5 inches above the lower esophageal sphincter. It is connected to an external recording device and is worn for 24 hours while the patient continues his or her normal daily activities. The end result is a computer analysis and graphic display of the results. This test allows for the direct correlation between chest pain and reflux episodes (Wolfe, 2000).

A Bernstein test may be performed to evaluate complaints of acid-related chest or epigastric pain. HCl is instilled through a small feeding tube positioned in the esophagus. This is done to try to elicit reported chest pain. Resultant signs and symptoms are compared with the usual symptoms the patient reports. However, since the advent of ambulatory pH monitoring, this previously popular evaluation tool is used infrequently (Wolfe, 2000).

LAPAROSCOPY (PERITONEOSCOPY)

Laparoscopy can be used for the diagnosis of GI disease. This procedure is performed through a small incision in the abdominal wall. Special fibreoptic laparoscopes allow direct visualization of the organs and structures within the abdomen, permitting visualization and identification of any growths, anomalies, and inflammatory processes. In addition, biopsy samples can be taken from the structures and organs as necessary. This procedure can be used to evaluate peritoneal disease, chronic abdominal pain, abdominal masses, and gallbladder and liver disease. However, laparoscopy has not become an important diagnostic modality in patients with acute abdominal pain, because less invasive tools (ie, CT and MRI) are readily available (Wolfe, 2000). Laparoscopy usually requires general anesthesia and sometimes requires that the stomach and bowel be decompressed. Gas (usually carbon dioxide) is insufflated into the peritoneal cavity to create a working space for visualization. One of the most positive benefits of this procedure is that after visualization of a problem, excision (eg, removal of the gallbladder) can then be performed at the same time, if appropriate.

Pathophysiologic and Psychological Considerations

Abnormalities of the GI tract are numerous and represent every type of major pathology that can affect other organ systems, including bleeding, perforation, obstruction, inflammation, and cancer. Congenital, inflammatory, infectious, traumatic, and neoplastic lesions have been encountered in every portion, and at every site, along the length of the GI tract. As with all other organ systems, the GI tract is subject to circulatory disturbances, faulty nervous system control, and aging.

Apart from the many organic diseases to which the GI tract is susceptible, there are many extrinsic factors that can interfere with its normal function and produce symptoms. Stress and anxiety, for example, often find their chief expression in indigestion, anorexia, or motor disturbances of the intestines, sometimes producing constipation or diarrhea. In addition to the state of mental health, physical factors such as fatigue and an inadequate or abruptly changed dietary intake can markedly affect the GI tract. When assessing and instructing the patient, the nurse should consider the variety of mental and physical factors that affect the function of the GI tract.

 Gerontologic Considerations

Normal physiologic changes of the GI system that occur with aging are identified in the accompanying Gerontologic Considerations box. The nurse should carefully assess and monitor signs and symptoms related to these changes. Age-related changes in the mouth include loss of teeth, diminished number of taste buds, decreased production of saliva, and atrophy of gingival tissue. These changes cause difficulty in chewing and swallowing. Changes in the esophagus include decreased muscle tone and weakness in the lower esophageal sphincter, leading to reflux and heartburn.

Decreased gastric motility leads to delayed gastric emptying. Atrophy of the mucosa causes a decrease in HCl production, and this can lead to food intolerances, malabsorption, or decrease in vitamin B_{12} absorption. Changes in the small and large intestine are evidenced largely by decreased motility and decreased transit time, which lead to complaints of indigestion and constipation. Other changes lead to decreased absorption of nutrients (dextrose, fats, calcium, and iron) in the large intestine. The nerve supply to the anal sphincter is sometimes impaired, causing fecal incontinence (Luekenotte, 2000).

Gerontologic Considerations
Age-Related Changes of the Gastrointestinal System

Oral Cavity and Pharynx
- Injury/loss or decay of teeth
- Atrophy of taste buds
- Decreased saliva production
- Reduced ptyalin and amylase in saliva

Esophagus
- Decreased motility and emptying
- Weakened gag reflex
- Decreased resting pressure of lower esophageal sphincter

Stomach
- Degeneration and atrophy of gastric mucosal surfaces with decreased production of HCl
- Decreased secretion of gastric acids and most digestive enzymes
- Decreased motility and emptying

Small Intestine
- Atrophy of muscle and mucosal surfaces
- Thinning of villi and epithelial cells

Large Intestine
- Decrease in mucus secretion
- Decrease in elasticity of rectal wall
- Decreased tone of internal anal sphincter
- Slower and duller nerve impulses in rectal area

Critical Thinking Exercises

1. You are caring for a 24-year-old male patient who was admitted for acute abdominal pain. He has just arrived from the emergency room and is being scheduled for tests this afternoon. What laboratory tests would you expect to be ordered? He is scheduled for a CT and ultrasound in 2 hours. What preparation is needed for these tests? What preprocedure education is needed?

2. A 58-year-old patient assigned to you this morning has just left to go to the Endoscopy Suite, where she will undergo a colonoscopy. You know that your patient will receive moderate sedation during the procedure and that she will be returned to your care once she is fully alert. What should you anticipate in the course of recovery for your patient after the colonoscopy? What medications might be used for the moderate sedation, and what effects of those medications would you expect to see during the recovery period? Describe the potential complications that could occur and what you will monitor. What are the goals for care during this period?

REFERENCES AND SELECTED READINGS
Books

Bickley, L. S., & Szilagyi, P. G. (2003). *Bates' guide to physical examination and history taking* (8th ed.). Philadelphia: Lippincott Williams & Wilkins.

Castell, D. (1999). *The esophagus* (3rd ed.). Philadelphia: Lippincott Williams & Wilkins.

Grendell, J., et al. (Eds.). (1996). *Current diagnosis and treatment in gastroenterology.* Stamford, CT: Appleton & Lange.

Heuther, S. E., & McCance, K. L. (2004). *Understanding pathophysiology* (3rd ed.). St. Louis: Mosby.

Keeffe, E. (Ed.). (1998). *Atlas of gastrointestinal endoscopy.* New York: McGraw-Hill Professional.

Kirsner, J. (Ed.). (2000). *Inflammatory bowel disease* (5th ed.). Philadelphia: W. B. Saunders.

Levine, M. (Ed.). (2000). *Double contrast gastrointestinal radiology.* Philadelphia: W. B. Saunders.

Lippincott Williams & Wilkins. (2005). *Stedman's medical dictionary for the health professional and nursing* (5th ed.). Baltimore, MD: Lippincott Williams & Wilkins.

Luekenotte, A. (2000). *Gerontologic nursing* (2nd ed.). St. Louis: Mosby.

Phillips, S., & Wingate, D. (1998). Functional disorders of the gut. New York: Churchill-Livingstone.

Rosenthal, M. (1999). *The gastrointestinal sourcebook.* Los Angeles: Lowell House.

Society of Gastroenterologic Nursing and Associates. (2003). *Core curriculum* (2nd ed.). St. Louis: Mosby.

Wilson, B. A., Shannon, M. T., & Stang, C. L. (2004). *Nurses' drug guide 2004.* Upper Saddle River, NJ: Pearson Education.

Wolfe, M. (Ed). (2000). *Therapy of digestive disorders.* Philadelphia: W. B. Saunders.

Yamada, T. (1998). *Atlas of gastroenterology* (2nd ed.). Philadelphia: Lippincott-Raven.

Yamada, T. (Ed.). (1999). *Textbook of gastroenterology* (3rd ed.). Philadelphia: Lippincott Williams & Wilkins.

Journals

Ahmed, D. (2000). Hidden factors in occult blood testing. *American Journal of Nursing, 100*(2), 25.

Anonymous. (2000). SGNA guideline for nursing care of patients during sedation and analgesia in the GI endoscopy setting. *Gastroenterology Nursing, 23*(3), 125–129.

Forsberg, F. (1999). Advances in ultrasound contrast techniques. *Applied Radiology (Supplement), 16,* 5–10.

Gavaghan, M. (1999). Anatomy and physiology of the esophagus. *AORN J, 69*(2), 370, 372, 374.

Glaser, Y. (2001). Colorectal cancer screening: New directions, evolving guidelines. *Patient Care, 35*(4), 24–30, 33–34.

Gold, P., & Goldenberg, N. A. (1997). The carcinoembryonic antigen (CEA): Past, present, and future. *McGill Journal of Medicine, 3,* 46–66.

Heflin, M. (2001). Cancer screening in the elderly. *Hospital Practice, 36*(3), 61–69.

Lightdale, C. (2000). Small bowel endoscopy. *Gastrointestinal Endoscopy, 9*(1), 101–108.

Lessick, M. (2001). Advances in genetic testing for cancer risk. *MedSurg Nursing, 10*(3), 123–127.

O'Hanlon-Nichols, T. (1998). Basic assessment series: Gastrointestinal system. *American Journal of Nursing, 98*(4), 48–53.

Pontieri-Lewis, V. (2000). Colorectal cancer. *MedSurg Nursing, 9*(1), 9–15, 20.

Staff, D., & Shaker, R. (2001). Aging and the gastrointestinal tract. *Disease a Month, 47*(3), 69–104.

RESOURCES AND WEBSITES

Canadian Association of Gastroenterology (CAG); www.cag-acg.org.

Canadian Cancer Society, 10 Alcorn Avenue, Suite 200, Toronto, ON M4V 3B1; www.cancer.ca.

Canadian Digestive Health Foundation; www.CDHF.ca.

Canadian Society of Gastroenterology Nurses and Associates; www.csgna.com.

National Cancer Institute of Canada; www.ncic.cancer.ca.

The Colorectal Cancer Screening Initiative Foundation; www.screencolons.ca.

Management of Patients With Oral and Esophageal Disorders

Adapted by Christy Raymond

LEARNING OBJECTIVES

On completion of this chapter, the learner will be able to:

1. Use the nursing process as a framework for care of patients with conditions of the oral cavity.
2. Describe the relationship of dental hygiene and dental problems to nutrition.
3. Describe the nursing management of patients with abnormalities of the lips, gums, teeth, mouth, and salivary glands.
4. Use the nursing process as a framework for care of patients with cancer of the oral cavity.
5. Identify the physical and psychosocial long-term needs of patients with oral cancer.
6. Use the nursing process as a framework for care of patients undergoing neck dissection.
7. Use the nursing process as a framework for care of patients with conditions of the esophagus.
8. Describe the various conditions of the esophagus and their clinical manifestations and management.

Because digestion normally begins in the mouth, adequate nutrition is related to good dental health and the general condition of the mouth. Any discomfort or adverse condition in the oral cavity can affect a person's nutritional status. Changes in the oral cavity may influence the type and amount of food ingested as well as the degree to which food particles are properly mixed with salivary enzymes. Disease of the mouth or tongue can interfere with speech and thus affect communication and self-image. Esophageal problems related to swallowing can also adversely affect food and fluid intake, thereby jeopardizing general health and well-being. Given the close relationship between adequate nutritional intake and the structures of the upper gastrointestinal tract (lips, mouth, teeth, pharynx, esophagus), health teaching can help prevent disorders associated with these structures.

The oral cavity, which includes the lips, mouth, and gums, is subject to many disorders and diseases. Table 35-1 reviews common abnormalities, their possible causes, and nursing management. In 2000/2001, over 25 million individuals are reported to have had contact with dental professionals in Canada (Statistics Canada, 2005).

Disorders of the Teeth

DENTAL PLAQUE AND CARIES

Tooth decay is an erosive process that begins with the action of bacteria on fermentable carbohydrates in the mouth, which produces acids that dissolve tooth enamel. The extent of damage to the teeth depends on the following:

- The presence of dental plaque
- The strength of the acids and the ability of the saliva to neutralize them
- The length of time the acids are in contact with the teeth
- The susceptibility of the teeth to decay

Dental plaque is a gluey, gelatin-like substance that adheres to the teeth. The initial action that causes damage to a tooth occurs under dental plaque.

Dental decay begins with a small hole, usually in a fissure (a break in the tooth's enamel) or in an area that is hard to clean. Left unchecked, the affected area penetrates the enamel into the dentin. Because dentin is not as hard as enamel, decay progresses more rapidly and in time reaches the pulp. When the blood, lymph vessels, and nerves are exposed, they become infected and an abscess may form, either within the tooth or at the tip of the root. Soreness and pain usually occur with an abscess. As the infection continues, the patient's face may swell, and there may be

pulsating pain. The dentist can determine by x-ray studies the extent of damage and the type of treatment needed. Treatment for dental caries includes fillings, dental implants, and extractions. If treatment is not successful, the tooth may need to be extracted. In general, dental decay is associated with young people, but older adults are subject to decay as well, particularly from drug-induced or age-related oral dryness (see the accompanying Gerontologic Considerations box).

Prevention

Measures used to prevent and control dental caries include practicing effective mouth care, reducing the intake of starches and sugars (refined carbohydrates), applying fluoride to the teeth or drinking fluoridated water, refraining from smoking, controlling diabetes, and using pit and fissure sealants (Chart 35-1).

MOUTH CARE

Healthy teeth must be conscientiously and effectively cleaned on a daily basis. Brushing and flossing are particularly effective in mechanically breaking up the bacterial plaque that collects around teeth.

Normal mastication (chewing) and the normal flow of saliva also aid greatly in keeping the teeth clean. Because many ill patients do not eat adequate amounts of food, they produce less saliva, which in turn reduces this natural tooth cleaning process. The nurse may need to assume the responsibility for brushing the patient's teeth. In any case, merely wiping the patient's mouth and teeth with a swab is ineffective. The most effective method is mechanical cleansing (brushing). If brushing is impossible, it is better to wipe the teeth with a gauze pad, then have the patient swish an antiseptic mouthwash several times before expectorating into an emesis basin. A soft-bristled toothbrush is more effective than a sponge or foam stick. The lips may be coated with a water-soluble gel to prevent drying.

DIET

Dental caries may be prevented by decreasing the amount of sugar and starch in the diet. Patients who snack should be encouraged to choose less cariogenic alternatives, such as fruits, vegetables, nuts, cheeses, or plain yogurt.

FLUORIDATION

Fluoridation of public water supplies has been found to decrease dental caries. Some areas of the country have natural fluoridation; other communities have added fluoride to public water supplies. Fluoridation may be achieved also by having a dentist apply a concentrated gel or solution to the teeth, adding fluoride to home

Glossary

achalasia: absent or ineffective peristalsis (wavelike contraction) of the distal esophagus accompanied by failure of the esophageal sphincter to relax in response to swallowing
dysphagia: difficulty swallowing
gastroesophageal reflux: back-flow of gastric or duodenal contents into the esophagus

hernia: protrusion of an organ or part of an organ through the wall of the cavity that normally contains it
lithotripsy: use of shock waves to break up or disintegrate stones
odynophagia: pain on swallowing
parotitis: inflammation of the parotid gland
pyrosis: heartburn
periapical abscess: abscessed tooth

sialadenitis: inflammation of the salivary glands
stomatitis: inflammation of the oral mucosa
temporomandibular disorders: a group of conditions that cause pain or dysfunction of the temporomandibular joint (TMJ) and surrounding structures
xerostomia: dry mouth

Table 35-1 • Disorders of the Lips, Mouth, and Gums

CONDITION	SIGNS AND SYMPTOMS	POSSIBLE CAUSES AND SEQUELAE	NURSING CONSIDERATIONS
Abnormalities of the Lips			
Actinic cheilitis	Irritation of lips associated with scaling, crusty, fissure; white overgrowth of horny layer of epidermis (hyperkeratosis) Considered a premalignant squamous cell skin cancer	Exposure to sun; more common in fair-skinned people and in those whose occupations involve sun exposure, such as farmers May lead to squamous cell cancer	Teach patient importance of protecting lips from the sun by using protective ointment such as sun block Instruct patient to have a periodic checkup by physician
Herpes simplex 1 (cold sore or fever blister)	Symptoms may be delayed up to 20 days after exposure; singular or clustered painful vesicles that may rupture	An opportunistic infection; frequently seen in immunosuppressed patients; very contagious May recur with menstruation, fever, or sun exposure	Use acyclovir or zovirax ointment or systemic medications as prescribed Administer analgesics as prescribed Instruct patient to avoid irritating foods
Chancre	Reddened circumscribed lesion that ulcerates and becomes crusted	Primary lesion of syphilis; very contagious	Comfort measures: cold soaks to lip, mouth care Administer antibiotics as prescribed Instruct patient regarding contagion
Contact dermatitis	Red area or rash; itching	Allergic reaction to lipstick, cosmetic ointments, or toothpaste	Instruct patient to avoid possible causes Administer corticosteroids as prescribed
Abnormalities of the Mouth			
Leukoplakia	White patches; may be hyperkeratotic; usually in buccal mucosa; usually painless	Fewer than 2% are malignant, but may progress to cancer Common among tobacco users	Instruct patient to see a physician if leukoplakia persists longer than 2 weeks Eliminate risk factors, such as tobacco
Hairy leukoplakia	White patches with rough hair-like projections; typically found on lateral border of the tongue	Possibly viral; smoking and use of tobacco Often seen in people who are HIV positive	Instruct patient to see a physician if condition persists longer than 2 weeks
Lichen planus	White papules at the intersection of a network of interlacing lesions; usually ulcerated and painful	Recurrences are common May lead to a malignant process Unknown cause	Apply topical corticosteroids such as fluocinolone acetonide oral base gel Avoid foods that irritate Administer corticosteroids systemically or intralesionally as prescribed Instruct the patient of need for follow-up if condition is chronic
Candidiasis (moniliasis/thrush)	Cheesy white plaque that looks like milk curds; when rubbed off, it leaves an erythematous and often bleeding base	*Candida albicans* fungus; predisposing factors include diabetes, antibiotic therapy, and immunosuppression	Antifungal medications such as nystatin (Mycostatin), Amphotericin B, clotrimazole, or ketoconazole may be prescribed; these may be taken in pill form or as a suspension; when used as a suspension, instruct the patient to swish vigourously for at least 1 minute and then swallow
Aphthous stomatitis (canker sore)	Shallow ulcer with a white or yellow centre and red border; seen on the inner side of the lip and cheek or on the tongue; it begins with a burning or tingling sensation and slight swelling; painful; usually lasts 7–10 days and heals without a scar	Associated with emotional or mental stress, fatigue, hormonal factors, minor trauma (such as biting), allergies, acidic foods and juices, and dietary deficiencies Associated with HIV infection May recur	Instruct the patient in comfort measures, such as saline rinses, and a soft or bland diet Antibiotics or corticosteroids may be prescribed
Nicotine stomatitis (smoker's patch)	Two stages—begins as a red stomatitis; over time the tongue and mouth become covered with a creamy, thick, white mucous membrane, which may slough, leaving a beefy red base	Chronic irritation by tobacco	Cessation of tobacco use; if condition exists for longer than 2 weeks a physician should be consulted and a biopsy may be needed

(continued)

Table 35-1 • **Disorders of the Lips, Mouth, and Gums** (Continued)

CONDITION	SIGNS AND SYMPTOMS	POSSIBLE CAUSES AND SEQUELAE	NURSING CONSIDERATIONS
Krythoplakia	Red patch on the oral mucous membrane	Nonspecific inflammation; more frequently seen in the elderly	
Kaposi's sarcoma	Appears first on the oral mucosa as a red, purple, or blue lesion; may be singular or multiple; may be flat or raised	HIV infection	Instruct patient regarding side effects of planned treatment
Abnormalities of the Gums			
Gingivitis	Painful, inflamed, swollen gums; usually the gums bleed in response to light contact	Poor oral hygiene: food debris, bacterial plaque, and calculus (tartar) accumulate; the gums may also swell in response to normal processes such as puberty and pregnancy	Teach patient proper oral hygiene; see Preventive Oral Hygiene chart
Necrotizing gingivitis (trench mouth)	Grey-white pseudomembranous ulcerations affecting the edges of the gums, mucosa of the mouth, tonsils, and pharynx; foul breath; painful, bleeding gums; swallowing and talking are painful	Poor oral hygiene; bacterial infection, inadequate rest, overwork, emotional stress, smoking, and poor nutrition may contribute to development	Teach patient proper oral hygiene; see Preventive Oral Hygiene chart Irrigate with 2% to 3% hydrogen peroxide or normal saline solution Avoid irritants such as smoking and spicy foods
Herpetic gingivostomatitis	Burning sensation with the appearance of small vesicles 24–48 hours later; vesicles may rupture, forming sore, shallow ulcers covered with a grey membrane	Herpes simplex virus; occurs most frequently in people who are immunosuppressed; may occur in other infectious processes such as streptococcal pneumonia, meningococcal meningitis, and malaria	Apply topical anesthetics as prescribed; may need opioids if pain is severe Saline or 2% to 3% hydrogen peroxide irrigations Antiviral agents such as acyclovir may be prescribed
Periodontitis	Little discomfort at onset; may have bleeding, infection, gum recession, and loosening of teeth; later in the disease tooth loss may occur	May result from untreated gingivitis Poor or inadequate dental hygiene and inadequate diet contribute to development	Instruct patient in proper oral hygiene Instruct patient to consult a dentist

water supplies, using fluoridated toothpaste or mouth rinse, or using sodium fluoride tablets, drops, or lozenges.

PIT AND FISSURE SEALANTS

The occlusal surfaces of the teeth have pits and fissures, areas that are prone to caries. Some dentists apply a special coating to fill and seal these areas from potential exposure to cariogenic processes. These sealants last up to 7 years.

DENTOALVEOLAR ABSCESS OR PERIAPICAL ABSCESS

Periapical abscess, more commonly referred to as an abscessed tooth, involves the collection of pus in the apical dental periosteum (fibrous membrane supporting the tooth structure) and

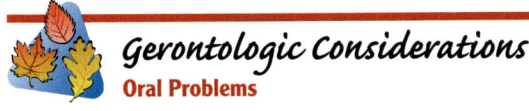

Gerontologic Considerations
Oral Problems

Many medications taken by the elderly cause dry mouth, which is uncomfortable, impairs communication, and increases the risk of oral infection. These medications include the following:
- Diuretics
- Antihypertensive medications
- Anti-inflammatory agents
- Antidepressant medications

Poor dentition can exacerbate problems of aging, such as
- Decreased food intake
- Loss of appetite
- Social isolation
- Increased susceptibility to systemic infection (from periodontal disease)
- Trauma to the oral cavity secondary to thinner, less vascular oral mucous membranes

Chart 35-1 • PATIENT EDUCATION
Preventive Oral Hygiene

- Brush teeth using a soft toothbrush at least two times daily. Hold toothbrush at a 45-degree angle between the brush and the gums and teeth. A small brush is better than a large brush. Gums and tongue surface should be brushed.
- Floss at least once daily.
- Use an antiplaque mouth rinse.
- Visit a dentist at least every 6 months, or when you have a chipped tooth, a lost filling, an oral sore that persists longer than 2 weeks, or a toothache.
- Avoid alcohol and tobacco products, including smokeless tobacco.
- Maintain adequate nutrition and avoid sweets.
- Replace toothbrush at first signs of wear, usually every 2 months.

the tissue surrounding the apex of the tooth (where it is suspended in the jaw bone). The abscess has two forms: acute and chronic. Acute periapical abscess is usually secondary to a suppurative pulpitis (a pus-producing inflammation of the dental pulp) that arises from an infection extending from dental caries. The infection of the dental pulp extends through the apical foramen of the tooth to form an abscess around the apex.

Chronic dentoalveolar abscess is a slowly progressive infectious process. It differs from the acute form in that the process may progress to a fully formed abscess without the patient's knowing it. The infection eventually leads to a "blind dental abscess," which is really a periapical granuloma. It may enlarge to as much as 1 cm in diameter. It is often discovered on x-ray films and is treated by extraction or root canal therapy, often with apicectomy (excision of the apex of the tooth root).

Clinical Manifestations

The abscess produces a dull, gnawing, continuous pain, often with a surrounding cellulitis and edema of the adjacent facial structures, and mobility of the involved tooth. The gum opposite the apex of the tooth is usually swollen on the cheek side. Swelling and cellulitis of the facial structures may make it difficult for the patient to open the mouth. In well-developed abscesses, there may be a systemic reaction, fever, and malaise.

Management

In the early stages of an infection, a dentist or dental surgeon may perform a needle aspiration or drill an opening into the pulp chamber to relieve tension and pain and to provide drainage. Usually, the infection will have progressed to a periapical abscess. Drainage is provided by an incision through the gingiva down to the jawbone. Pus (purulent material) escapes under pressure. This procedure is commonly performed in the dentist's office, but it may be performed in an outpatient surgery centre or a same-day surgery department. After the inflammatory reaction has subsided, the tooth may be extracted or root canal therapy performed. Antibiotics may be prescribed.

Nursing Management

The nurse assesses the patient for bleeding after treatment and instructs the patient to use a warm saline or warm water mouth rinse to keep the area clean. The patient is also instructed to take antibiotics and analgesics as prescribed, to advance from a liquid diet to a soft diet as tolerated, and to keep follow-up appointments.

MALOCCLUSION

Malocclusion is a misalignment of the teeth of the upper and lower dental arcs when the jaws are closed. Malocclusion can be inherited or acquired (from thumb-sucking, trauma, or some medical conditions). Malocclusion makes the teeth difficult to clean and can lead to decay, gum disease, and excess wear on supporting bone and gum tissues. About 50% of the population has some form of malocclusion. Correction of malocclusion requires an orthodontist with special training, a patient who is motivated and cooperative, and adequate time. Most treatments begin when the patient has shed the last primary tooth and the last permanent successor has erupted, usually at about 12 or 13 years of age, but treatment may occur in adulthood. Preventive orthodontics may be started at age 5 years if malocclusion is diagnosed early. The need for teeth straightening in adolescence is reduced if preventive orthodontics is started with the primary teeth.

Management

People with malocclusion have an obviously misaligned bite or crooked, crowded, widely spaced, or protruding teeth. To realign the teeth, the orthodontist gradually forces the teeth into a new location by using wires or plastic bands (braces). These devices may be unattractive, but this psychological burden must be overcome if good results are to be achieved. In the final phase of treatment, a retaining device is worn for several hours each day to support the tissues as they adjust to the new alignment of the teeth.

Nursing Management

The patient must practice meticulous oral hygiene, and the nurse encourages the patient to persist in this important part of the treatment. An adolescent undergoing orthodontic correction who is admitted to the hospital for some other problem may have to be reminded to continue wearing the retainer (if it does not interfere with the problem requiring hospitalization).

Disorders of the Jaw

Abnormal conditions affecting the mandible (jaw) and of the temporomandibular joint (which connects the mandible to the temporal bone at the side of the head in front of the ear) include congenital malformation, fracture, chronic dislocation, cancer, and syndromes characterized by pain and limited motion. Temporomandibular disorders and jaw surgery (a treatment common in many structural abnormalities or cancer of the jaw) are presented in this section.

TEMPOROMANDIBULAR DISORDERS

Temporomandibular disorders are categorized as follows (National Oral Health Information Clearinghouse, 2000):

- Myofascial pain—a discomfort in the muscles controlling jaw function and in neck and shoulder muscles
- Internal derangement of the joint—a dislocated jaw, a displaced disc, or an injured condyle
- Degenerative joint disease—rheumatoid arthritis or osteoarthritis in the jaw joint

Diagnosis and treatment of temporomandibular disorders remain somewhat ambiguous, but the condition is thought to affect about 10 million people in the United States. Misalignment of the joints in the jaw and other problems associated with the ligaments and muscles of mastication are thought to result in tissue damage and muscle tenderness. Suggested causes include arthritis of the jaw, head injury, trauma or injury to the jaw or joint, stress, and malocclusion (although research does not support malocclusion as a cause).

Clinical Manifestations

Patients have pain ranging from a dull ache to throbbing, debilitating pain that can radiate to the ears, teeth, neck muscles, and facial sinuses. They often have restricted jaw motion and locking of the jaw. They may hear clicking and grating noises, and chewing and swallowing may be difficult. Depression may occur in response to these symptoms.

Assessment and Diagnostic Findings

Diagnosis is based on the patient's subjective symptoms of pain, limitations in range of motion, dysphagia, difficulty chewing, difficulty with speech, or hearing difficulties. Magnetic resonance imaging, x-ray studies, and an arthrogram may be performed.

Management

Although some practitioners think the role of stress in temporomandibular joint (TMJ) disorders is overrated, patient education in stress management may be helpful (to reduce grinding and clenching of teeth). Patients may also benefit from range-of-motion exercises. Pain management measures may include nonsteroidal anti-inflammatory drugs (NSAIDs), with the possible addition of opioids, muscle relaxants, or mild antidepressants. Occasionally, a bite plate or splint (plastic guard worn over the upper and lower teeth) may be worn to protect teeth from grinding; however, this is a short-term therapy. Conservative and reversible treatment is recommended. If irreversible surgical options are recommended, the patient is encouraged to seek a second opinion.

SURGICAL MANAGEMENT

Correction of mandibular structural abnormalities may require surgery involving repositioning or reconstruction of the jaw. Simple fractures of the mandible without displacement, resulting from a blow on the chin, and planned surgical interventions, as in the correction of long or short jaw syndrome, may require treatment by these means. Jaw reconstruction may be necessary in the aftermath of trauma from a severe injury or cancer, both of which can cause tissue and bone loss.

Mandibular fractures are usually closed fractures. Rigid plate fixation (insertion of metal plates and screws into the bone to approximate and stabilize the bone) is the current treatment of choice in many cases of mandibular fracture and in some mandibular reconstructive surgery procedures. Bone grafting may be performed to replace structural defects using bones from the patient's own ilium, ribs, or cranial sites. Rib tissue may also be harvested from cadaver donors.

Nursing Management

The patient who has had rigid fixation should be instructed not to chew food in the first 1 to 4 weeks after surgery. A liquid diet is recommended, and dietary counselling should be obtained to ensure optimal caloric and protein intake.

PROMOTING HOME AND COMMUNITY-BASED CARE

The patient needs specific guidelines for mouth care and feeding. Any irritated areas in the mouth should be reported to the physician. The importance of keeping scheduled appointments for assessing the stability of the fixation appliance is emphasized.

Consultation with a dietitian may be indicated so that the patient and family can learn about foods that are high in essential nutrients and ways in which these foods can be prepared so that they can be consumed through a straw or spoon, while remaining palatable. Nutritional supplements may be recommended.

Disorders of the Salivary Glands

The salivary glands consist of the parotid glands, one on each side of the face below the ear; the submandibular and sublingual glands, both in the floor of the mouth; and the buccal gland, beneath the lips. About 1200 mL of saliva are produced daily. The glands' primary functions are lubrication, protection against harmful bacteria, and digestion.

PAROTITIS

Parotitis (inflammation of the parotid gland) is the most common inflammatory condition of the salivary glands, although inflammation can occur in the other salivary glands as well. Mumps (epidemic parotitis), a communicable disease caused by viral infection and most commonly affecting children, is an inflammation of a salivary gland, usually the parotid.

Elderly, acutely ill, or debilitated people with decreased salivary flow from general dehydration or medications are at high risk for parotitis. The infecting organisms travel from the mouth through the salivary duct. The organism is usually *Staphylococcus aureus* (except in mumps). The onset of this complication is sudden, with an exacerbation of both the fever and the symptoms of the primary condition. The gland swells and becomes tense and tender. The patient feels pain in the ear, and swollen glands interfere with swallowing. The swelling increases rapidly, and the overlying skin soon becomes red and shiny.

Preventive measures are essential and include advising the patient to have necessary dental work performed before surgery. In addition, maintaining adequate nutritional and fluid intake, good oral hygiene, and discontinuing medications (eg, tranquilizers, diuretics) that can diminish salivation may help prevent the condition. If parotitis occurs, antibiotic therapy is necessary. Analgesics may also be prescribed to control pain. If antibiotic therapy is not effective, the gland may need to be drained by a surgical procedure known as parotidectomy. This procedure may be necessary to treat chronic parotitis.

SIALADENITIS

Sialadenitis (inflammation of the salivary glands) may be caused by dehydration, radiation therapy, stress, malnutrition, salivary gland calculi (stones), or improper oral hygiene. The inflammation is associated with infection by *S. aureus, Streptococcus viridans,* or pneumococcus. In hospitalized or institutionalized patients the infecting organism may be methicillin-resistant *S. aureus* (MRSA) (McQuone, 1999). In Canada, the incidence of MRSA infections and colonizations is approximately 5 of every 1000 admissions (Public Health Agency of Canada, 2005). Symptoms include pain, swelling, and purulent discharge. Antibiotics are used to treat infections. Massage, hydration, and corticosteroids frequently cure the problem. Chronic sialadenitis with uncontrolled pain is treated by surgical drainage of the gland or excision of the gland and its duct.

SALIVARY CALCULUS (SIALOLITHIASIS)

Sialolithiasis, or salivary calculi (stones), usually occurs in the submandibular gland. Salivary gland ultrasonography or sialography (x-ray studies filmed after the injection of a radiopaque substance into the duct) may be required to demonstrate obstruction of the duct by stenosis. Salivary calculi are formed mainly from calcium phosphate. If located within the gland, the calculi are irregular and vary in diameter from 3 to 30 mm. Calculi in the duct are small and oval.

Calculi within the salivary gland itself cause no symptoms unless infection arises; however, a calculus that obstructs the gland's duct causes sudden, local, and often colicky pain, which is abruptly relieved by a gush of saliva. This characteristic symptom is often disclosed in the patient's health history. On physical assessment, the gland is swollen and quite tender, the stone itself can be palpable, and its shadow may be seen on x-ray films.

The calculus can be extracted fairly easily from the duct in the mouth. Sometimes, enlargement of the ductal orifice permits the stone to pass spontaneously. Occasionally **lithotripsy**, a procedure that uses shock waves to disintegrate the stone, may be used instead of surgical extraction for parotid stones and smaller submandibular stones. Lithotripsy requires no anesthesia, sedation, or analgesia. Side effects can include local hemorrhage and swelling. Surgery may be necessary to remove the gland if symptoms and calculi recur repeatedly.

NEOPLASMS

Although they are uncommon, neoplasms (tumours or growths) of almost any type may develop in the salivary gland. Tumours occur more often in the parotid gland. The incidence of salivary gland tumours is similar in men and women. Risk factors include prior exposure to radiation to the head and neck. Diagnosis is based on the health history and physical examination and the results of fine needle aspiration biopsy.

Management of salivary gland tumours evokes controversy, but the common procedure involves partial excision of the gland, along with all of the tumour and a wide margin of surrounding tissue. Dissection is carefully performed to preserve the seventh cranial nerve (facial nerve), although it may not be possible to preserve the nerve if the tumour is extensive. If the tumour is malignant, radiation therapy may follow surgery. Radiation therapy alone may be a treatment choice for tumours that are thought to be contained or if there is risk of facial nerve damage from surgical intervention. Chemotherapy is usually used for palliative purposes. Local recurrences are common, and the recurrent growth usually is more aggressive than the original. It has also been observed that patients with salivary gland tumours have an increased incidence of second primary cancers (Bull, 2001).

Cancer of the Oral Cavity

Cancers of the oral cavity, which can occur in any part of the mouth or throat, are curable if discovered early. These cancers are associated with the use of alcohol and tobacco. The combination of alcohol and tobacco seems to have a synergistic carcinogenic effect. In Canada, approximately 3000 new cases of oral cancer are discovered each year (Canadian Dental Association, 1999; Canadian Cancer Society, 2005). Most cases occur among older individuals with a history of tobacco use and excessive alcohol consumption (Hawkins, Wang, & Leake, 1999).

Cancer of the oral cavity accounts for approximately 1.5% of all new cases of cancer and 1.1% of related deaths in Canadian women. Men are afflicted with oral cancer more often than women and represent 2.8% of established new cases of cancer. Men experience 1.9% of cancer deaths from oral cancer (Canadian Cancer Society, 2005). The 5-year survival rate for cancer of the oral cavity and pharynx is 55% for whites and 33% for African Americans. Of the 7400 annual deaths from oral cancer, the distribution by site is estimated as follows: tongue, 1700; mouth, 2000; pharynx, 2100; other, 1600 (American Cancer Society, Cancer Facts and Figures, 2002).

Chronic irritation by a warm pipestem or prolonged exposure to the sun and wind may predispose a person to lip cancer. Predisposing factors for other oral cancers are exposure to tobacco (including smokeless tobacco), ingestion of alcohol, dietary deficiency, and ingestion of smoked meats.

Pathophysiology

Malignancies of the oral cavity are usually squamous cell cancers. Any area of the oropharynx can be a site for malignant growths, but the lips, the lateral aspects of the tongue, and the floor of the mouth are most commonly affected.

Clinical Manifestations

Many oral cancers produce few or no symptoms in the early stages. Later, the most frequent symptom is a painless sore or mass that will not heal. A typical lesion in oral cancer is a painless indurated (hardened) ulcer with raised edges. Tissue from any ulcer of the oral cavity that does not heal in 2 weeks should be examined through biopsy. As the cancer progresses, the patient may complain of tenderness; difficulty in chewing, swallowing, or speaking; coughing of blood-tinged sputum; or enlarged cervical lymph nodes.

Assessment and Diagnostic Findings

Diagnostic evaluation consists of an oral examination as well as an assessment of the cervical lymph nodes to detect possible metastases. Biopsies are performed on suspicious lesions (those that have not healed in 2 weeks). High-risk areas include the buccal mucosa and gingiva for people who use snuff or smoke cigars or pipes. For those who smoke cigarettes and drink alcohol, high-risk areas include the floor of the mouth, the ventrolateral tongue, and the soft palate complex (soft palate, anterior and posterior tonsillar area, uvula, and the area behind the molar and tongue junction).

Medical Management

Management varies with the nature of the lesion, the preference of the physician, and patient choice. Surgical resection, radiation therapy, chemotherapy, or a combination of these therapies may be effective.

In cancer of the lip, small lesions are usually excised liberally; larger lesions involving more than one third of the lip may be more appropriately treated by radiation therapy because of superior cosmetic results. The choice depends on the extent of the lesion and what is necessary to cure the patient while preserving the best appearance. Tumours larger than 4 cm often recur.

Cancer of the tongue may be treated with radiation therapy and chemotherapy to preserve organ function and maintain quality of life. A combination of radioactive interstitial implants (surgical implantation of a radioactive source into the tissue adjacent to or at the tumour site) and external beam radiation may be used. If the cancer has spread to the lymph nodes, the surgeon may perform a neck dissection. Surgical treatments leave a less functional tongue; surgical procedures include hemiglossectomy (surgical removal of half of the tongue) and total glossectomy (removal of the tongue).

Often cancer of the oral cavity has metastasized through the extensive lymphatic channel in the neck region (Fig. 35-1), requiring a neck dissection and reconstructive surgery of the oral

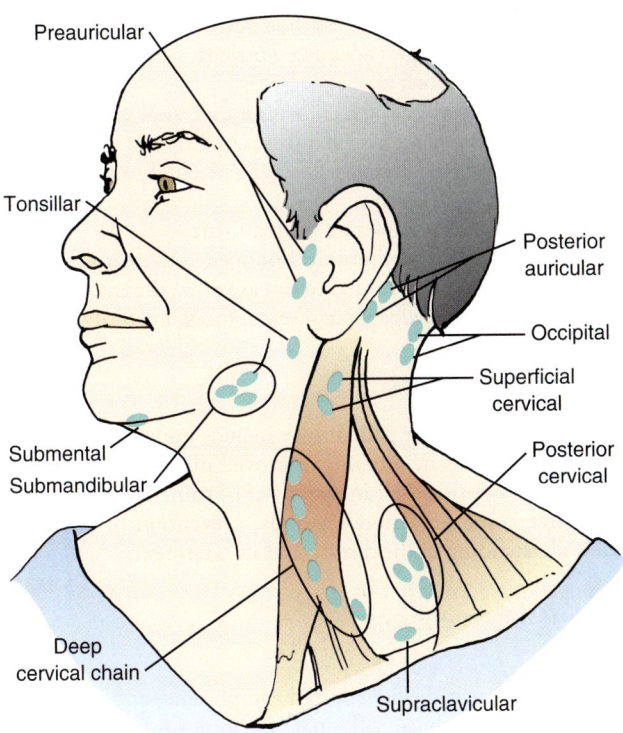

FIGURE 35-1 Lymphatic drainage of the head and neck.

Labels: Preauricular, Tonsillar, Submental, Submandibular, Deep cervical chain, Posterior auricular, Occipital, Superficial cervical, Posterior cervical, Supraclavicular

cavity. A common reconstructive technique involves use of a radial forearm free flap (a thin layer of skin from the forearm along with the radial artery).

Nursing Management

The nurse assesses the patient's nutritional status preoperatively, and a dietary consultation may be necessary. The patient may require enteral (through the intestine) or parenteral (intravenous) feedings before and after surgery to maintain adequate nutrition. If a radial graft is to be performed, an Allen test on the donor arm must be performed to ensure that the ulnar artery is patent and can provide blood flow to the hand after removal of the radial artery. The Allen test is performed by asking the patient to make a fist and then manually compressing the ulnar artery. The patient is then asked to open the hand into a relaxed, slightly flexed position. The palm will be pale. Pressure on the ulnar artery is released. If the ulnar artery is patent, the palm will flush within about 3 to 5 seconds.

Postoperatively, the nurse assesses for a patent airway. The patient may be unable to manage oral secretions, making suctioning necessary. If grafting was included in the surgery, suctioning must be performed with care to prevent damage to the graft. The graft is assessed postoperatively for viability. Although colour should be assessed (white may indicate arterial occlusion, and blue mottling may indicate venous congestion), it can be difficult to assess the graft by looking into the mouth. A Doppler ultrasound device may be used to locate the radial pulse at the graft site and to assess graft perfusion.

NURSING PROCESS: THE PATIENT WITH CONDITIONS OF THE ORAL CAVITY

Assessment

Obtaining a health history allows the nurse to determine the patient's learning needs concerning preventive oral hygiene and to identify symptoms requiring medical evaluation. The history includes questions about the patient's normal brushing and flossing routine; frequency of dental visits; awareness of any lesions or irritated areas in the mouth, tongue, or throat; recent history of sore throat or bloody sputum; discomfort caused by certain foods; daily food intake; use of alcohol and tobacco, including smokeless chewing tobacco; and the need to wear dentures or a partial plate. For more information about dentures, see the accompanying Gerontologic Considerations box.

A careful physical assessment follows the health history. Both the internal and the external structures of the mouth and throat are inspected and palpated. Dentures and partial plates are removed to ensure a thorough inspection of the mouth. In general, the examination can be accomplished by using a bright light source (penlight) and a tongue depressor. Gloves are worn to palpate the tongue and any abnormalities.

LIPS

The examination begins with inspection of the lips for moisture, hydration, colour, texture, symmetry, and the presence of ulcerations or fissures. The lips should be moist, pink, smooth, and symmetric. The patient is instructed to open the mouth wide; a tongue blade is then inserted to expose the buccal mucosa for an assessment of colour and lesions. Stensen's duct of each parotid gland is visible as a small red dot in the buccal mucosa next to the upper molars.

GUMS

The gums are inspected for inflammation, bleeding, retraction, and discolouration. The odour of the breath is also noted. The hard palate is examined for colour and shape.

TONGUE

The dorsum (back) of the tongue is inspected for texture, colour, and lesions. A thin white coat and large, vallate papillae in a "V" formation on the distal portion of the dorsum of the tongue are

Gerontologic Considerations
Denture Care

Many older adults wear dentures. Mouth care and regular checkups remain part of the denture-wearing older adult's health promotion activities.
- Brush dentures twice a day.
- Remove dentures at night and soak them in water or a denture product. (Never put dentures in hot water, because they may warp.)
- Rinse mouth with warm salt water in the morning, after meals, and at bedtime.
- Clean well under partial dentures, where food particles tend to get caught.
- Consume nonsticky foods that have been cut into small pieces; chew slowly.
- See dentist regularly to assess and readjust fit.

normal findings. The patient is instructed to protrude the tongue and move it laterally. This provides the examiner with an opportunity to estimate the tongue's size as well as its symmetry and strength (to assess the integrity of the 12th cranial nerve [hypoglossal]).

Further inspection of the ventral surface of the tongue and the floor of the mouth is accomplished by asking the patient to touch the roof of the mouth with the tip of the tongue. Any lesions of the mucosa or any abnormalities involving the frenulum or superficial veins on the undersurface of the tongue are assessed for location, size, colour, and pain. This is a common area for oral cancer, which presents as a white or red plaque, an indurated ulcer, or a warty growth.

A tongue blade is used to depress the tongue for adequate visualization of the pharynx. It is pressed firmly beyond the midpoint of the tongue; proper placement avoids a gagging response. The patient is told to tip the head back, open the mouth wide, take a deep breath, and say "ah." Often this flattens the posterior tongue and briefly allows a full view of the tonsils, uvula, and posterior pharynx (Fig. 35-2). These structures are inspected for colour, symmetry, and evidence of exudate, ulceration, or enlargement. Normally, the uvula and soft palate rise symmetrically with a deep inspiration or "ah"; this indicates an intact vagus nerve (10th cranial nerve).

A complete assessment of the oral cavity is essential because many disorders, such as cancer, diabetes, and immunosuppressive conditions resulting from medication therapy or AIDS, may be manifested by changes in the oral cavity. The neck is examined for enlarged lymph nodes (adenopathy).

Nursing Diagnoses

Based on all the assessment data, major nursing diagnoses may include the following:

- Impaired oral mucous membrane related to a pathologic condition, infection, or chemical or mechanical trauma (eg, medications, ill-fitting dentures)

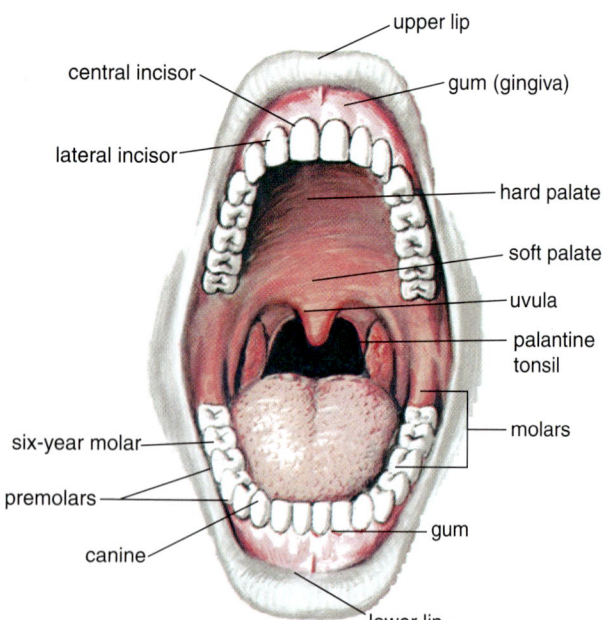

FIGURE 35-2 Structures of the mouth, including the tongue and palate.

- Imbalanced nutrition, less than body requirements, related to inability to ingest adequate nutrients secondary to oral or dental conditions
- Disturbed body image related to a physical change in appearance resulting from a disease condition or its treatment
- Fear of pain and social isolation related to disease or change in physical appearance
- Pain related to oral lesion or treatment
- Impaired verbal communication related to treatment
- Risk for infection related to disease or treatment
- Deficient knowledge about disease process and treatment plan

Planning and Goals

The major goals for the patient may include improved condition of the oral mucous membrane, improved nutritional intake, attainment of a positive self-image, relief of pain, identification of alternative communication methods, prevention of infection, and understanding of the disease and its treatment.

Nursing Interventions

PROMOTING MOUTH CARE

The nurse instructs the patient in the importance and techniques of preventive mouth care. If a patient cannot tolerate brushing or flossing, an irrigating solution of 1 teaspoon of baking soda to 8 ounces of warm water, half-strength hydrogen peroxide, or normal saline solution is recommended. The nurse reinforces the need to perform oral care and provides such care to patients who are unable to provide it for themselves.

If a bacterial or fungal infection is present, the nurse administers the appropriate medications and instructs the patient in how to administer the medications at home. The nurse monitors the patient's physical and psychological response to treatment.

Xerostomia, dryness of the mouth, is a frequent sequela of oral cancer, particularly when the salivary glands have been exposed to radiation or major surgery. It is also seen in patients who are receiving psychopharmacologic agents, patients with HIV infection, and patients who cannot close the mouth and as a result become mouth-breathers. To minimize this problem, the patient is advised to avoid dry, bulky, and irritating foods and fluids, as well as alcohol and tobacco. The patient is also encouraged to increase intake of fluids (when not contraindicated) and to use a humidifier during sleep. The use of synthetic saliva, a moisturizing antibacterial gel such as Oral Balance, or a saliva production stimulant such as Salagen may be helpful.

Stomatitis, or mucositis, which involves inflammation and breakdown of the oral mucosa, is often a side effect of chemotherapy or radiation therapy. Prophylactic mouth care is started when the patient begins receiving treatment; however, mucositis may become so severe that a break in treatment is necessary. If a patient receiving radiation therapy has poor dentition, extraction of the teeth before radiation treatment in the oral cavity is often initiated to prevent infection. Many radiation therapy centres recommend the use of fluoride treatments for patients receiving radiation to the head and neck.

ENSURING ADEQUATE FOOD AND FLUID INTAKE

The patient's weight, age, and level of activity are recorded to determine whether nutritional intake is adequate. A daily calorie count may be necessary to determine the exact quantity of food and fluid ingested. The frequency and pattern of eating are recorded to determine whether any psychosocial or physiologic factors are

At the completion of the home care instruction, the patient or caregiver will be able to:	Patient	Caregiver
• Demonstrate use of suction equipment if indicated.	✓	✓
• State rationale for humidification.	✓	✓
• State foods necessary to meet caloric needs and dietary needs (ie, change in consistency, seasoning limitations, supplements).	✓	✓
• Demonstrate oral hygiene.	✓	✓
• Demonstrate care of incision.	✓	✓
• State when next medical/dental follow-up appointment will be scheduled.	✓	✓

affecting ingestion. The nurse recommends changes in the consistency of foods and the frequency of eating, based on the disorder and the patient's preferences. Consultation with a dietitian can be helpful. The goal is to help the patient attain and maintain desirable body weight and level of energy, as well as to promote the healing of tissue.

SUPPORTING A POSITIVE SELF-IMAGE

A patient who has a disfiguring oral condition or has undergone disfiguring surgery may experience an alteration in self-image. The patient is encouraged to verbalize the perceived change in body appearance and to realistically discuss actual changes or losses. The nurse offers support while the patient verbalizes fears and negative feelings (withdrawal, depression, anger). The nurse listens attentively and determines whether the patient's needs are primarily psychosocial or cognitive-perceptual. This determination will help the nurse to individualize a plan of care. The patient's strengths, achievements, and positive attributes are reinforced.

The nurse should determine the patient's anxieties concerning relationships with others. Referral to support groups, a psychiatric liaison nurse, a social worker, or a spiritual advisor may be useful in helping the patient to cope with anxieties and fears. Emphasizing that the patient's worth is not diminished by a physical change in a body part can be a helpful approach. The patient's progress toward development of positive self-esteem is documented. The nurse should be alert to signs of grieving and should record emotional changes. By providing acceptance and support, the nurse encourages the patient to verbalize feelings.

MINIMIZING PAIN AND DISCOMFORT

Oral lesions can be painful. Strategies to reduce pain and discomfort include avoiding foods that are spicy, hot, or hard (eg, pretzels, nuts). The patient is instructed about mouth care. It may be necessary to provide the patient with an analgesic such as viscous lidocaine (Xylocaine Viscous 2%) or opioids, as prescribed. The nurse can reduce the patient's fear of pain by providing information about pain control methods.

PROMOTING EFFECTIVE COMMUNICATION

Verbal communication may be impaired by radical surgery for oral cancer. It is therefore vital to assess the patient's ability to communicate in writing before surgery. Pen and paper are provided postoperatively to patients who can use them to communicate. A communication board with commonly used words or pictures is obtained preoperatively and given after surgery to patients who cannot write so that they may point to needed items. A speech therapist is also consulted postoperatively.

PREVENTING INFECTION

Leukopenia (a decrease in white blood cells) may result from radiation, chemotherapy, AIDS, and some medications used to treat HIV infection. Leukopenia reduces defense mechanisms, increasing the risk for infections. Malnutrition, which is also common among these patients, may further decrease resistance to infection. If the patient has diabetes, the risk of infection is further increased.

Laboratory results should be evaluated frequently and the patient's temperature checked every 4 to 8 hours for an elevation that may indicate infection. Visitors who might transmit microorganisms are prohibited because the patient's immunologic system is depressed. Sensitive skin tissues are protected from trauma to maintain skin integrity and prevent infection. Aseptic technique is necessary when changing dressings. Desquamation (shedding of the epidermis) is a reaction to radiation therapy that causes dryness and itching and can lead to a break in skin integrity and subsequent infection.

As described earlier, adequate nutrition is helpful in preventing infection. Signs of wound infection (redness, swelling, drainage, tenderness) are reported to the physician. Antibiotics may be prescribed prophylactically.

PROMOTING HOME AND COMMUNITY-BASED CARE

Teaching Patients Self-Care

The patient who is recovering from treatment of an oral condition is instructed about mouth care, nutrition, prevention of infection, and signs and symptoms of complications (Chart 35-2). Methods of preparing nutritious foods that are seasoned according to the patient's preference and at the preferred temperature are explained. For some patients, it may be more convenient to use commercial baby foods than to prepare liquid and soft diets. The patient who cannot take foods orally may receive enteral or parenteral nutrition; the administration of these feedings is explained and demonstrated to the patient and the care provider.

For patients with cancer, instructions are provided in the use and care of any prostheses. The importance of keeping dressings clean is emphasized, as is the need for conscientious oral hygiene.

Continuing Care

The need for ongoing care in the home depends on the patient's condition. The patient, the family members or others responsible for home care, the nurse, and other health care professionals (eg, speech therapist, nutritionist, psychologist) work together to prepare an individual plan of care.

If suctioning of the mouth or tracheostomy tube is required, the necessary equipment is obtained and the patient and care providers are taught how to use it. Considerations include the control of odours and humidification of the home to keep secretions moist. The patient and the care providers are taught how to assess for obstruction, hemorrhage, and infection and what actions to take if they occur. The home care nurse may provide physical care, monitor for changes in the patient's physical status (eg, skin integrity, nutritional status, respiratory function), and assess the adequacy of pain control measures. The nurse also assesses the patient's and family's ability to manage incisions, drains, and feeding tubes and the use of recommended strategies for communication. The ability of the patient and family to accept physical, psychological, and role changes is assessed and addressed.

Follow-up visits to the physician are important to monitor the patient's condition and to determine the need for modifications in treatment and general care. The nurse reinforces instructions in an effort to promote the patient's self-care and comfort.

Because patients and their family members and health care providers tend to focus on the most obvious needs and issues, the nurse reminds the patient and family about the importance of continuing health promotion and screening practices. Those patients who have not been involved in these practices in the past are educated about their importance and are referred to appropriate health care providers.

Evaluation

EXPECTED PATIENT OUTCOMES

Expected patient outcomes may include:

1. Shows evidence of intact oral mucous membranes
   a. Is free of pain and discomfort in the oral cavity
   b. Has no visible alteration in membrane integrity
   c. Identifies and avoids foods that are irritating (eg, nuts, pretzels, spicy foods)
   d. Describes measures that are necessary for preventive mouth care
   e. Complies with medication regimen
   f. Limits or avoids use of alcohol and tobacco (including smokeless tobacco)
2. Attains and maintains desirable body weight
3. Has a positive self-image
   a. Verbalizes anxieties
   b. Is able to accept change in appearance and modify self-concept accordingly
4. Attains an acceptable level of comfort
   a. Verbalizes that pain is absent or under control
   b. Avoids foods and liquids that cause discomfort
   c. Adheres to medication regimen
5. Has decreased fears related to pain, isolation, and the inability to cope
   a. Accepts that pain will be managed if not eliminated
   b. Freely expresses fears and concerns
6. Is free of infection
   a. Exhibits normal laboratory values
   b. Is afebrile
   c. Performs oral hygiene after every meal and at bedtime
7. Acquires information about disease process and course of treatment

Neck Dissection

Malignancies of the head and neck include those of the oral cavity, oropharynx, hypopharynx, nasopharynx, nasal cavity, paranasal sinus, and larynx (Fig. 35-3). (Laryngeal cancer is

FIGURE 35-3 Anatomy of the head and neck.

presented in Chapter 22.) These cancers account for fewer than 5% of all cancers. Depending on the location and stage, treatment may consist of radiation therapy, chemotherapy, surgery, or a combination of these modalities. Deaths from malignancies of the head and neck are primarily attributable not to recurrence at the primary site but to local-regional metastasis to the cervical lymph nodes in the neck. This often occurs by way of the lymphatics before the primary lesion has been treated. This local-regional metastasis is not amenable to surgical resection and responds poorly to chemotherapy and radiation therapy.

A radical neck dissection involves removal of all cervical lymph nodes from the mandible to the clavicle and removal of the sternocleidomastoid muscle, internal jugular vein, and spinal accessory muscle on one side of the neck. The associated morbidities include shoulder drop and poor cosmesis (visible neck depression). Modified radical neck dissection, which preserves one or more of the nonlymphatic structures, is used more often. A selective neck dissection (in comparison to a radical dissection) preserves one or more of the lymph node groups, the internal jugular vein, the sternocleidomastoid muscle, and the spinal accessory nerve (Fig. 35-4).

Reconstructive techniques may be performed with a variety of grafts. A cutaneous flap (skin and subcutaneous tissue), such as the deltopectoral flap, may be used. A more frequently used graft for head and neck reconstruction is a myocutaneous flap (subcutaneous tissue, muscle and skin). The pectoralis major muscle is usually used. A microvascular free flap may be used for large defects. This involves the transfer of muscle, skin, or bone with an artery and vein to the area of reconstruction, using microinstrumentation. Areas used for a free flap include the scapula, the radial area of the forearm, or the fibula. The fibula, which provides a larger bone area, may be used if mandibular reconstruction is involved.

FIGURE 35-4 (**A**) A classic radical neck dissection in which the sternocleidomastoid and smaller muscles are removed. All tissue is removed, from the ramus of the jaw to the clavicle. The jugular vein has also been removed. The selective neck dissection (**B**) is similar but preserves the sternocleidomastoid muscle, internal jugular vein, and spinal accessory nerve. The wound is closed (**C**), and portable suction drainage tubes are in place.

NURSING PROCESS: THE PATIENT UNDERGOING A NECK DISSECTION

Assessment

Preoperatively, the patient's physical and psychological preparation for major surgery is assessed, along with his or her knowledge of the preoperative and postoperative procedures. Postoperatively, the patient is assessed for complications such as altered respiratory status, wound infection, and hemorrhage. As healing occurs, neck range of motion is assessed to determine whether there has been a decrease in range of motion due to nerve or muscle damage.

Diagnosis

NURSING DIAGNOSES

Based on all the assessment data, major nursing diagnoses may include the following:

- Deficient knowledge about preoperative and postoperative procedures
- Ineffective airway clearance related to obstruction by mucus, hemorrhage, or edema
- Acute pain related to surgical incision
- Risk for infection related to surgical intervention secondary to decreased nutritional status, or immunosuppression from chemotherapy or radiation therapy
- Impaired tissue integrity secondary to surgery and grafting
- Imbalanced nutrition, less than body requirements, related to disease process or treatment
- Situational low self-esteem related to diagnosis or prognosis
- Impaired verbal communication secondary to surgical resection
- Impaired physical mobility secondary to nerve injury

COLLABORATIVE PROBLEMS/ POTENTIAL COMPLICATIONS

Potential postoperative complications that may develop include the following:

- Hemorrhage
- Chyle fistula
- Nerve injury

Planning and Goals

The major goals for the patient include participation in the treatment plan, maintenance of respiratory status, absence of infection, viability of the graft, maintenance of adequate intake of food and fluids, effective coping strategies, attainment of comfort, effective communication, and absence of complications.

Nursing Interventions

PROVIDING PREOPERATIVE PATIENT EDUCATION

Before surgery, the patient should be informed about the nature and extent of the surgery, and what the postoperative period will be like. The patient is encouraged to ask questions and to express concerns about the upcoming surgery and the expected results. During this exchange, the nurse has an opportunity to assess the patient's coping abilities, answer questions, and develop a plan for offering assistance. A sense of mutual understanding and rapport will make the postoperative experience less traumatic for the patient. The patient's expressions of concern, anxieties, and fears can guide the nurse in providing support postoperatively.

PROVIDING GENERAL POSTOPERATIVE CARE

The general postoperative nursing interventions are similar to those presented in Chapter 20. For the patient who has had extensive neck surgery, specific postoperative interventions include maintenance of a patent airway and continuous assessment of respiratory status, wound care and oral hygiene, maintenance of adequate nutrition, and observation for hemorrhage or nerve injury.

MAINTAINING THE AIRWAY

After the endotracheal tube or airway has been removed and the effects of the anesthesia have worn off, the patient may be placed in Fowler's position to facilitate breathing and promote comfort. This position also increases lymphatic and venous drainage, facilitates swallowing, and decreases venous pressure on the skin flaps.

In the immediate postoperative period, the nurse assesses for stridor (coarse, high-pitched sound on inspiration) by listening frequently over the trachea with a stethoscope. This finding must be reported immediately because it indicates obstruction of the airway. Signs of respiratory distress, such as dyspnea, cyanosis, changes in mental status, and changes in vital signs, are assessed because they may suggest edema, hemorrhage, inadequate oxygenation, or inadequate drainage.

Pneumonia may occur in the postoperative phase if pulmonary secretions are not removed. Coughing and deep breathing are encouraged to aid in the removal of secretions. The patient should assume a sitting position, with the nurse supporting the neck so that the patient can bring up excessive secretions. If this is ineffective, the patient's respiratory tract may have to be suctioned. Care is taken to protect the suture lines during suctioning. If a tracheostomy tube is in place, suctioning is performed through the tube. The patient may also be instructed on use of Yankauer suction (tonsil tip suction) to remove oral secretions. Temperature should not be taken orally.

RELIEVING PAIN

Pain and the patient's fear of pain are assessed and managed. Patients with head and neck cancer often report less pain than patients with other types of cancer; however, the nurse needs to be aware that each person's pain experience is individual. The nurse administers analgesics as prescribed and assesses their effectiveness.

PROVIDING WOUND CARE

Wound drainage tubes are usually inserted during surgery to prevent the collection of fluid subcutaneously. The drainage tubes are connected to portable suction device (eg, Jackson-Pratt), and the container is emptied periodically. Between 80 and 120 mL of serosanguineous secretions may drain over the first 24 hours. Excessive drainage may be indicative of a chyle fistula or hemorrhage (see later discussion). If dressings are present, they may need to be reinforced from time to time. Dressings are observed for evidence of hemorrhage and constriction, which impairs respiration and perfusion of the graft. The graft is assessed for colour and temperature, and for the presence of a pulse if applicable, to determine viability. The graft should be pale pink and warm to the touch. The surgical incisions are also assessed for infection, which is reported immediately. Prophylactic antibiotics may be prescribed.

MAINTAINING ADEQUATE NUTRITION

Nutritional status is assessed preoperatively; early intervention to correct nutritional imbalances may decrease the risk of postoperative complications. Frequently, nutrition is less than optimal because of inadequate intake, and the patient often requires enteral or parenteral supplements preoperatively to attain a positive nitrogen balance. This therapy may need to be continued postoperatively if the patient cannot take enough nutrients by mouth. Supplements (eg, Ensure, Sustacal) that are nutritionally dense may help reestablish a positive nitrogen balance. They may be taken enterally by mouth, by nasogastric feeding tube, or by gastrostomy feeding tube. (See the Plan of Nursing Care for further discussion.)

The patient who is able to chew may take food by mouth; the level of the patient's chewing ability will determine whether some diet modification (eg, soft, pureed, or liquid foods) is necessary. Food preferences should also be discussed with the patient. Oral care before eating may enhance the patient's appetite, and oral care after eating is important to prevent infection and dental caries. Most patients are able to maintain and gain weight.

SUPPORTING COPING MEASURES

Preoperatively, information about the planned surgery is given to the patient and family. The psychological postoperative nursing intervention is aimed at supporting the patient who has had a change in body image or who has major concerns regarding the prognosis. The patient may have difficulty communicating and may be concerned about his or her ability to breathe and swallow normally. The nurse enlists the support of family or friends in encouraging and reassuring the patient that adjusting to the results of this surgery will take time.

The person who has had extensive neck surgery often is sensitive about his or her appearance. This can occur when the operative area is covered by bulky dressings, when the incision line is visible, or later after healing has occurred but the appearance of the neck and possibly the lower face has been significantly altered. If the nurse accepts the patient's appearance and expresses a positive, optimistic attitude, the patient is more likely to be encouraged. The patient also needs an opportunity to express concerns regarding the success of the surgery and the prognosis. The Canadian Cancer Society may be a resource to provide a volunteer to meet with the patient either preoperatively or postoperatively.

People with cancer of the head and neck frequently have used alcohol or tobacco before surgery; postoperatively, the patient is encouraged to abstain from these substances. Alternative methods of coping need to be explored. A referral to Alcoholics Anonymous may be appropriate.

PROMOTING EFFECTIVE COMMUNICATION

If a laryngectomy was performed, the nurse explores other methods of communicating with the patient and obtains a consultation with a speech/language therapist. Alternatives to verbal communication may include use of a pencil and paper or pointing to needed items on a picture pad. Alternative speech techniques, such as an electrolarynx (a mechanical device held against the neck) or esophageal speech, may be taught by a speech/language therapist.

MAINTAINING PHYSICAL MOBILITY

Excision of muscles and nerves results in weakness at the shoulder that can cause shoulder drop, a forward curvature of the shoulder. Many problems can be avoided with a conscientious exercise program. These exercises are usually begun after the drains have been removed and the neck incision is sufficiently healed. The purpose of the exercises depicted in Figure 35-5 is to promote maximal shoulder function and neck motion after surgery. Physical therapists and occupational therapists can assist patients in performing these exercises.

MONITORING AND MANAGING POTENTIAL COMPLICATIONS

Hemorrhage

Hemorrhage may occur from carotid artery rupture as a result of necrosis of the graft or damage to the artery itself from tumour or infection. The following measures are indicated:

- Vital signs are assessed. Tachycardia, tachypnea, and hypotension may indicate hemorrhage and impending hypovolemic shock.
- The patient is instructed to avoid the Valsalva manoeuvre to prevent stress on the graft and carotid artery.
- Signs of impending rupture, such as high epigastric pain or discomfort, are reported.

Exercise 1

Gently turn head to each side and look as far as possible. Gently tip right ear toward right shoulder as far as possible. Repeat on left side. Move chin to chest and then lift head up and back.

Exercise 2

Place hands in front with elbows at right angles away from body.

Rotate shoulders back, bringing elbows to side. Then relax whole body.

Lean or hold onto low table or chair with hand on the unaffected side. Bend body slightly at waist and swing shoulder and arm from left to right.

Exercise 3

Swing shoulder and arm from front to back.

Swing shoulder and arm in a wide circle, gradually bringing arm above head.

FIGURE 35-5 Three rehabilitation exercises after head and neck surgery. The objective is to regain maximum shoulder function and neck motion after neck surgery. From *Exercise for Radical Neck Surgery Patients.* Head and Neck Service, Department of Surgery, Memorial Hospital, New York, NY.

- Dressings and wound drainage are observed for excessive bleeding.
- If hemorrhage occurs, assistance is summoned immediately.
- Hemorrhage requires the continuous application of pressure to the bleeding site or major associated vessel.
- Although some advocate placing the patient in modified Trendelenburg position to maintain blood pressure, others recommend that the head of the patient's bed be elevated to maintain airway patency and prevent aspiration.
- A controlled, calm manner will allay the patient's anxiety.
- The surgeon is notified immediately, because a vascular or ligature tear requires surgical intervention.

Chyle Fistula

A chyle fistula (milk-like drainage from the thoracic duct into the thoracic cavity) may develop as a result of damage to the thoracic duct during surgery. The diagnosis is made if there is excess drainage which has a 3% fat content and a specific gravity of 1.012 or greater. Treatment of a small leak (500 mL or less) includes application of a pressure dressing and a diet of medium-chain fatty acids or parenteral nutrition. Surgical intervention to repair the damaged duct is necessary for larger leaks.

Nerve Injury

Nerve injury can occur if the cervical plexus or spinal accessory nerves are severed during surgery. Because lower facial paralysis may occur as a result of injury to the facial nerve, this complication is observed for and reported. Likewise, if the superior laryngeal nerve is damaged, the patient may have difficulty swallowing liquids and food because of the partial lack of sensation of the glottis. Speech therapy may be indicated to assist with the problems related to nerve injury.

PROMOTING HOME AND COMMUNITY-BASED CARE

Teaching Patients Self-Care

The patient and care provider will require instructions about management of the wound, the dressing, and any drains that remain in place. Patients who require oral suctioning or who have a tracheostomy may be very anxious about their care at home; the transition to home can be eased if the care provider is given several opportunities to demonstrate the ability to meet the patient's needs (Chart 35-3).

If the patient cannot take food by mouth, detailed instructions and demonstration of enteral or parenteral feedings will be required. Education in techniques of effective oral hygiene is also important.

Chart 35-3
Home Care Checklist • Recovering From Neck Surgery

At the completion of the home care instruction, the patient or caregiver will be able to:	Patient	Caregiver
• Demonstrate use of suction equipment.	✓	✓
• State rationale for humidification.	✓	✓
• State dietary modifications needed to meet caloric needs.	✓	✓
• Demonstrate enteral or parenteral feeding techniques.	✓	✓
• Demonstrate care of incision and drains.	✓	✓
• State when next checkup is needed.	✓	✓
• Demonstrate exercises.	✓	
• Identify available support groups.	✓	✓

Continuing Care

A referral for home care nursing may be necessary in the early period after discharge. The nurse will assess healing, ensure that feedings are being administered properly, and detect any complications. The home care nurse assesses the patient's adjustment to changes in physical appearance and status, ability to communicate, and ability to eat normally. Physical and speech therapy also may be continued at home.

The patient is given information regarding local support groups, if indicated. The local chapter of the Canadian Cancer Society may be contacted for information and equipment needed for the patient.

Evaluation

EXPECTED PATIENT OUTCOMES

Expected patient outcomes may include:

1. Discusses expected course of treatment
2. Demonstrates good respiratory exchange
   a. Lungs are clear to auscultation
   b. Breathes easily with no shortness of breath
   c. Demonstrates ability to use suction effectively
3. Remains free of infection
   a. Maintains normal laboratory values
   b. Is afebrile
4. Graft is pink and warm to touch
5. Maintains adequate intake of foods and fluids
   a. Accepts altered route of feeding
   b. Is well hydrated
   c. Maintains or gains weight
6. Demonstrates ability to cope
   a. Discusses emotional responses to the diagnosis
   b. Attends support group meetings
7. Verbalizes comfort
8. Attains maximal mobility
   a. Adheres to physical therapy exercises
   b. Attains maximal range of motion

The Plan of Nursing Care presents an overview of the care of a patient undergoing a neck dissection.

Disorders of the Esophagus

The esophagus is a mucus-lined, muscular tube that carries food from the mouth to the stomach. It begins at the base of the pharynx and ends about 4 cm below the diaphragm. Its ability to transport food and fluid is facilitated by two sphincters. The upper esophageal sphincter, also called the hypopharyngeal sphincter, is located at the junction of the pharynx and the esophagus. The lower esophageal sphincter, also called the gastroesophageal sphincter, is located at the junction of the esophagus and the stomach. An incompetent lower esophageal sphincter allows reflux (backward flow) of gastric contents. There is no serosal layer of the esophagus; therefore, if surgery is necessary, it is more difficult to perform suturing or anastomosis.

DYSPHAGIA

Dysphagia (difficulty swallowing) is the most common symptom of esophageal disease. This symptom may vary from an uncomfortable feeling that a bolus of food is caught in the upper esophagus (before it eventually passes into the stomach) to acute pain on swallowing (**odynophagia**). Obstruction of food (solid and soft) and even liquids may occur anywhere along the esophagus. Often the patient can indicate that the problem is located in the upper, middle, or lower third of the esophagus.

There are many pathologic conditions of the esophagus, including motility disorders (achalasia, diffuse spasm), gastroesophageal reflux, hiatal hernias, diverticula, perforation, foreign bodies, chemical burns, benign tumours, and carcinoma.

ACHALASIA

Achalasia is absent or ineffective peristalsis of the distal esophagus, accompanied by failure of the esophageal sphincter to relax in response to swallowing. Narrowing of the esophagus just above the stomach results in a gradually increasing dilation of the esophagus in the upper chest. Achalasia may progress slowly and occurs most often in people 40 years of age or older.

Clinical Manifestations

The primary symptom of achalasia is difficulty in swallowing both liquids and solids. The patient has a sensation of food sticking in the lower portion of the esophagus. As the condition progresses, food is commonly regurgitated, either spontaneously or intentionally by the patient to relieve the discomfort produced by prolonged distention of the esophagus by food that will not pass into the stomach. The patient may also complain of chest pain and heartburn (**pyrosis**). Pain may or may not be associated with eating. There may be secondary pulmonary complications from aspiration of gastric contents.

Assessment and Diagnostic Findings

X-ray studies show esophageal dilation above the narrowing at the gastroesophageal junction. Barium swallow, computed tomography

(text continues on page 979)

Plan of Nursing Care
The Patient Who Has Undergone Neck Dissection

Nursing Interventions	Rationale	Expected Outcomes

Nursing Diagnosis: Ineffective airway clearance related to obstruction secondary to edema, hemorrhage, or inadequate wound drainage

Goal: Maintenance of normal respiratory function

Nursing Interventions	Rationale	Expected Outcomes
1. Place the patient in Fowler's position.	1. Fowler's position facilitates expansion of the lungs because the diaphragm is pulled downward and the abdominal viscera are pulled away from the lungs. Breathing is promoted. This position also increases lymphatic and venous drainage, decreases swallowing, and decreases venous pressure on the graft. Regurgitation and aspiration of stomach contents are prevented postoperatively.	• Achieves a normal respiratory rate • Breathes comfortably • Avoids use of accessory muscles of respiration • Maintains vital signs within normal range • Shows evidence of normal breath sounds • Coughs effectively • Maintains a patent airway • Does not develop a mucus plug
2. Monitor vital signs according to postoperative routine.	2. Edema, hemorrhage, or inadequate drainage will alter heart rate and respirations. Tachypnea and restlessness may indicate respiratory distress.	
3. Auscultate breath sounds as needed. In the immediate postoperative period, place the stethoscope over the trachea to assess for stridor.	3. Abnormal breath sounds may indicate ineffective ventilation, decreased perfusion, and fluid accumulation. Stridor, a harsh, high-pitched sound primarily heard on inspiration, indicates airway obstruction.	
4. Encourage deep breathing and coughing. Place the patient in a sitting position and support the neck area with both hands.	4. Deep breathing before coughing promotes expansion of the airways and a more forceful cough. The coughing mechanism assists airway cilia with removal of secretions. Splinting the incision during coughing reduces strain and promotes the expulsion of secretions by allowing deeper inspirations.	
5. Suction the airway as needed using sterile technique and a soft catheter.	5. Suctioning assists in removal of secretions that the patient may be unable to cough up, thereby assisting with maintaining a patent airway.	
6. Provide humidified air or oxygen if the patient has a tracheostomy.	6. Keeps secretions thin.	

Nursing Diagnosis: Risk for infection

Goal: Absence of infection

Nursing Interventions	Rationale	Expected Outcomes
1. Instruct the patient in preoperative and postoperative oral hygiene using slightly alkaline solutions such as 8 oz of water mixed with 1 teaspoon of baking soda, or normal saline solution, every 4 hours.	1. Oral care decreases oral bacteria, thereby decreasing the risk of bacterial infection postoperatively. Hydrogen peroxide should not be used, because it may break down fresh granulation tissue.	• Patient performs oral hygiene preoperatively and postoperatively every 4 hours • Mouth remains clean • Wound drains less than 200 mL of serosanguineous drainage on the first postoperative day • No hematoma at skin graft • Serosanguineous drainage is within normal limits • Dressing remains intact with no constriction of airway or blood flow • Wound and surrounding skin remain clean and free of infection • Patient is afebrile with normal respirations and a normal heart rate • Patient is alert and aware of surroundings
2. Monitor wound suction drainage.	2. Suction drainage negates the need for pressure dressings because the skin flaps are pulled down tightly. Drainage should be 80–120 mL of serosanguineous secretions for the first 24 hours; then the secretions should decrease daily. Continuous bloody drainage indicates small vessel oozing.	

(continued)

Plan of Nursing Care

The Patient Who Has Undergone Neck Dissection (Continued)

Nursing Interventions	Rationale	Expected Outcomes
3. Note drainage quantity and odour.	3. Purulent, malodourous drainage indicates an infection. Drainage greater than 300 mL in the first 24 hours is considered abnormal.	
4. Assess condition of dressing and reinforce pressure dressings as needed. Assess for any possible constrictions that would affect respirations or decrease blood flow to graft.	4. If portable wound suction is not used, pressure dressings may be applied to obliterate dead spaces and provide immobilization. These dressings are reinforced, not changed, as needed.	
5. Use aseptic technique to cleanse skin around the drains; change the dressings as ordered by surgeon (usually the second through fifth postoperative days).	5. Aseptic technique prevents wound contamination. Sterile saline effectively cleans the skin around the drains.	
6. Monitor vital signs. Assess for symptoms of infection: chills, diaphoresis, altered level of consciousness.	6. An elevated temperature, tachypnea, and tachycardia may indicate an infection.	

Nursing Diagnosis: Impaired skin integrity

Goal: Maintenance of intact skin and viability of graft

1. Assess condition of graft for viability.	1. Cyanotic, cool graft indicates possible necrosis. (Pale graft indicates arterial thrombosis; purple graft indicates venous congestion.)	• Graft is pale pink in colour and warm to touch • Tissue blanches to gentle touch • Graft has pulse via Doppler ultrasound
2. Assess wound for signs and symptoms of infection.	2. Infected wound interferes with healing and threatens the viability of the graft.	• Patient does not have wound infection

Nursing Diagnosis: Imbalanced nutrition, less than body requirements, related to anorexia and dysphagia

Goal: Attainment/maintenance of adequate nutrition

1. Assess nutritional status preoperatively, consult with dietitian.	1. Poor nutritional status preoperatively impairs wound healing and increases potential for infection.	• Does not have weight loss greater than 10% of body weight. (If weight loss is greater than 10%, supplements are given to maintain/increase weight and obtain positive nitrogen balance.)
2. Administer tube feedings as prescribed. Keep head of bed elevated during feeding to prevent aspiration. Monitor for signs of tracheoesophageal fistula (feeding in tracheal secretions).	2. A nasogastric tube may be in place for several days to administer enteral feedings.	• Tolerates tube feedings • No signs of aspiration • No sign of fistula
3. Provide oral hygiene before and after meals.	3. Oral hygiene enhances appetite.	• Expresses a desire for food
4. Assist with oral intake: a. Offer easily chewed foods; mash or blenderize if necessary. b. Suggest that the head be tilted to the unaffected side when swallowing. c. Inquire whether privacy is desired when eating. d. Provide altered eating utensils as needed.	4. Soft-textured foods facilitate swallowing. Passage of food may be tolerated better when the head is tilted to the unaffected side. Self-feeding difficulties may cause embarrassment and interfere with intake quantity.	• Swallows food easily • Is comfortable eating alone or with others

(continued)

Plan of Nursing Care
The Patient Who Has Undergone Neck Dissection *(Continued)*

Nursing Interventions	Rationale	Expected Outcomes

Nursing Diagnosis: Situational low self-esteem and body image related to changes in appearance and alterations in communication

Goal: Attainment of positive self-image

Nursing Interventions	Rationale	Expected Outcomes
1. Assist the patient to communicate effectively: a. Provide materials for writing messages. b. Make certain that the call bell is readily accessible. c. Develop nonverbal ways to communicate (eg, finger-tapping, sign language, sign board). d. Consult speech/language therapist.	1. Temporary hoarseness is common after neck surgery. A tracheostomy may be performed, and verbal communication may not be possible. Communication with head movement may be impossible because of incisional pain and need to maintain position of neck for graft. A speech/language therapist may assist with other forms of communication, such as esophageal speech or electrolarynx.	• Recognizes that hoarseness is temporary • Develops alternative forms of communication • Willingly conveys fears and concerns • Accepts prognosis with realistic limitations • Accepts support as offered • Absence of facial paralysis • Absence of drooling and dysphagia • Maintains normal shoulder function • Verbalizes methods to enhance physical appearance
2. Encourage verbalization of fears: a. Provide time to listen. b. Project a positive, optimistic attitude. c. Reinforce reality. d. Collaborate with family members to elicit their support and encouragement. e. Consult support groups such as New Voice Club through the American Cancer Society.	2. Listening conveys acceptance and encourages further verbalization. An optimistic approach conveys interest and hope. Honesty will promote a trusting relationship. This includes confirming cosmetic and functional limitations. Family members or significant others can provide valuable support to the patient.	
3. Observe for facial paralysis.	3. Injury to facial nerve will cause lower facial paralysis.	
4. Observe for excessive drooling.	4. Damage to the hypoglossal nerve will result in excessive drooling and decreased ability to swallow.	
5. Check for normal shoulder position and function.	5. Damage to the spinal accessory nerve will result in drooping of the shoulder. Rehabilitation exercises are begun after the incision is healed.	
6. Provide information on clothing/cosmetics to deemphasize physical defects (offer information on "Look Good, Feel Better" program through American Cancer Society).	6. Physical appearance may be enhanced through use of cosmetics or clothing.	

(CT) of the esophagus, and endoscopy may be used for diagnosis; however, the diagnosis is confirmed by manometry, a process in which the esophageal pressure is measured by a radiologist or gastroenterologist.

Management

The patient should be instructed to eat slowly and to drink fluids with meals. As a temporary measure, calcium channel blockers and nitrates have been used to decrease esophageal pressure and improve swallowing. Injection of botulinum toxin (Botox) to quadrants of the esophagus via endoscopy has been helpful because it inhibits the contraction of smooth muscle. Periodic injections are required to maintain remission. If these methods are unsuccessful, pneumatic (forceful) dilation or surgical separation of the muscle fibres may be recommended (Streeter, 1999; Annese et al., 2000).

Achalasia may be treated conservatively by pneumatic dilation to stretch the narrowed area of the esophagus (Fig. 35-6). Pneumatic dilation has a high success rate. Although perforation is a

potential complication, its incidence is low. The procedure can be painful; therefore, moderate sedation in the form of an analgesic or tranquilizer, or both, is administered for the treatment. The patient is monitored for perforation. Complaints of abdominal tenderness and fever may be indications of perforation (see later discussion).

Achalasia may be treated surgically by esophagomyotomy (Fig. 35-7). The procedure usually is performed laparoscopically, either with a complete lower esophageal sphincter myotomy and an antireflux procedure (see later discussion of fundoplasty), or without an antireflux procedure. The esophageal muscle fibres are separated to relieve the lower esophageal stricture. Although patients with a history of achalasia have a slightly higher incidence of esophageal cancer, long-term follow-up with esophagoscopy for early detection has not proved beneficial.

DIFFUSE SPASM

Diffuse spasm is a motor disorder of the esophagus. The cause is unknown, but stressful situations can produce contractions of the

FIGURE 35-6 Treatment of achalasia by the conservative approach. (**A–C**) The dilator is passed, guided by a previously inserted guidewire. (**D**) When the balloon is in proper position, it is distended by pressure sufficient to dilate the narrowed area of the esophagus.

Catheter passed through narrowed end of esophagus

Fully inflated balloon

esophagus. It is more common in women and usually manifests in middle age.

Clinical Manifestations

Diffuse spasm is characterized by difficulty or pain on swallowing (dysphagia, odynophagia) and by chest pain similar to that of coronary artery spasm.

Assessment and Diagnostic Findings

Esophageal manometry, which measures the motility of the esophagus and the pressure within the esophagus, indicates that simultaneous contractions of the esophagus occur irregularly. Diagnostic x-ray studies after ingestion of barium show separate areas of spasm.

Management

Conservative therapy includes administration of sedatives and long-acting nitrates to relieve pain. Calcium channel blockers have also been used to manage diffuse spasm. Small, frequent feedings and a soft diet are usually recommended to decrease the esophageal pressure and irritation that lead to spasm. Dilation performed by bougienage (use of progressively sized flexible dilators), pneumatic dilation, or esophagomyotomy may be necessary if the pain becomes intolerable.

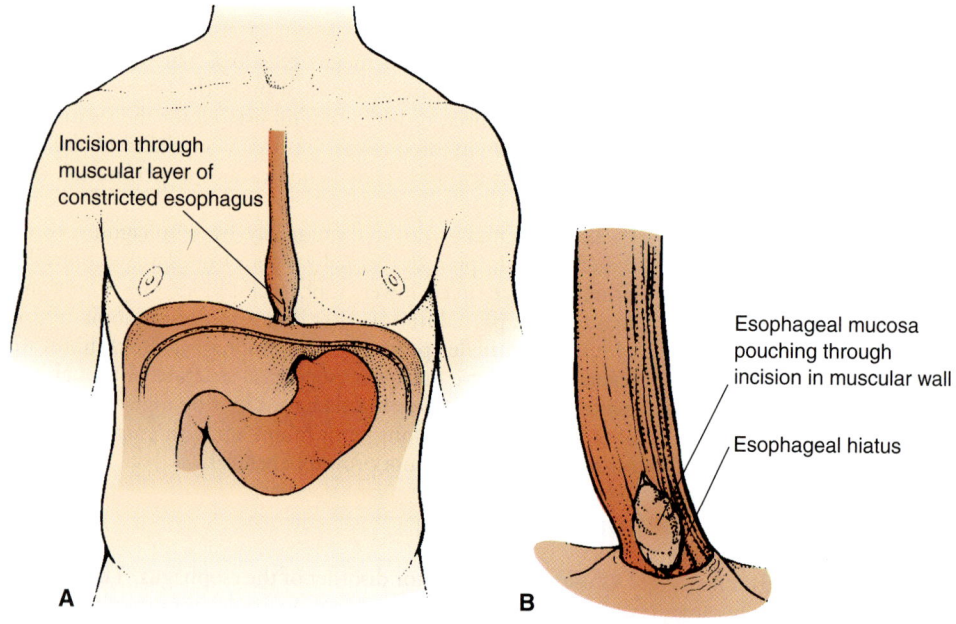

Incision through muscular layer of constricted esophagus

Esophageal mucosa pouching through incision in muscular wall

Esophageal hiatus

FIGURE 35-7 Treatment of achalasia: esophagomyotomy. (**A**) The esophagus is approached via thoracotomy from the front, on the left side. An incision is made through the muscularis of the esophagus extending about 1 cm into the gastric area. (**B**) The incision is large enough to allow a pouching of the esophageal mucosa. Separation of the muscular fibres relieves the narrowing at the lower end of the esophagus and permits the patient to swallow normally again.

HIATAL HERNIA

The esophagus enters the abdomen through an opening in the diaphragm and empties at its lower end into the upper part of the stomach. Normally, the opening in the diaphragm encircles the esophagus tightly, and the stomach lies completely within the abdomen. In a condition known as hiatus (or hiatal) **hernia**, the opening in the diaphragm through which the esophagus passes becomes enlarged, and part of the upper stomach tends to move up into the lower portion of the thorax. Hiatal hernia occurs more often in women than men. There are two types of hiatal hernias: sliding and paraesophageal. Sliding, or type I, hiatal hernia occurs when the upper stomach and the gastroesophageal junction (GEJ) are displaced upward and slide in and out of the thorax (Fig. 35-8A). About 90% of patients with esophageal hiatal hernia have a sliding hernia. A paraesophageal hernia occurs when all or part of the stomach pushes through the diaphragm beside the esophagus (see Fig. 35-8B). Paraesophageal hernias may be further classified as types II, III, or IV, depending on the extent of herniation, with type IV having the greatest herniation.

Clinical Manifestations

The patient with a sliding hernia may have heartburn, regurgitation, and dysphagia, but at least 50% of patients are asymptomatic. Sliding hiatal hernia is often implicated in reflux. The patient with a paraesophageal hernia usually feels a sense of fullness after eating or may be asymptomatic. Reflux usually does not occur, because the gastroesophageal sphincter is intact. The complications of hemorrhage, obstruction, and strangulation can occur with any type of hernia.

Assessment and Diagnostic Findings

Diagnosis is confirmed by x-ray studies, barium swallow, and fluoroscopy.

Management

Management for an axial hernia includes frequent, small feedings that can pass easily through the esophagus. The patient is advised not to recline for 1 hour after eating, to prevent reflux or movement of the hernia, and to elevate the head of the bed on 10- to 20-cm blocks to prevent the hernia from sliding upward. Surgery is indicated in about 15% of patients. Medical and surgical management of a paraesophageal hernia is similar to that for gastroesophageal reflux; however, paraesophageal hernias may require emergency surgery to correct torsion (twisting) of the stomach or other body organ that leads to restriction of blood flow to that area.

DIVERTICULUM

A diverticulum is an outpouching of mucosa and submucosa that protrudes through a weak portion of the musculature. Diverticula may occur in one of the three areas of the esophagus—the pharyngoesophageal or upper area of the esophagus, the midesophageal area, or the epiphrenic or lower area of the esophagus—or they may occur along the border of the esophagus intramurally.

The most common type of diverticulum, which is found three times more frequently in men than in women, is Zenker's diverticulum (also known as pharyngoesophageal pulsion diverticulum or a pharyngeal pouch). It occurs posteriorly through the cricopharyngeal muscle in the midline of the neck. It is usually seen in people older than 60 years of age. Other types of diverticula include midesophageal, epiphrenic, and intramural diverticula.

Midesophageal diverticula are uncommon. Symptoms are less acute, and usually the condition does not require surgery. Epiphrenic diverticula are usually larger diverticula in the lower esophagus just above the diaphragm. They are thought to be related to the improper functioning of the lower esophageal sphincter or to motor disorders of the esophagus. Intramural diverticulosis is the occurrence of numerous small diverticula associated with a stricture in the upper esophagus.

Clinical Manifestations

Symptoms experienced by the patient with a pharyngoesophageal pulsion diverticulum include difficulty swallowing, fullness in the neck, belching, regurgitation of undigested food, and gurgling

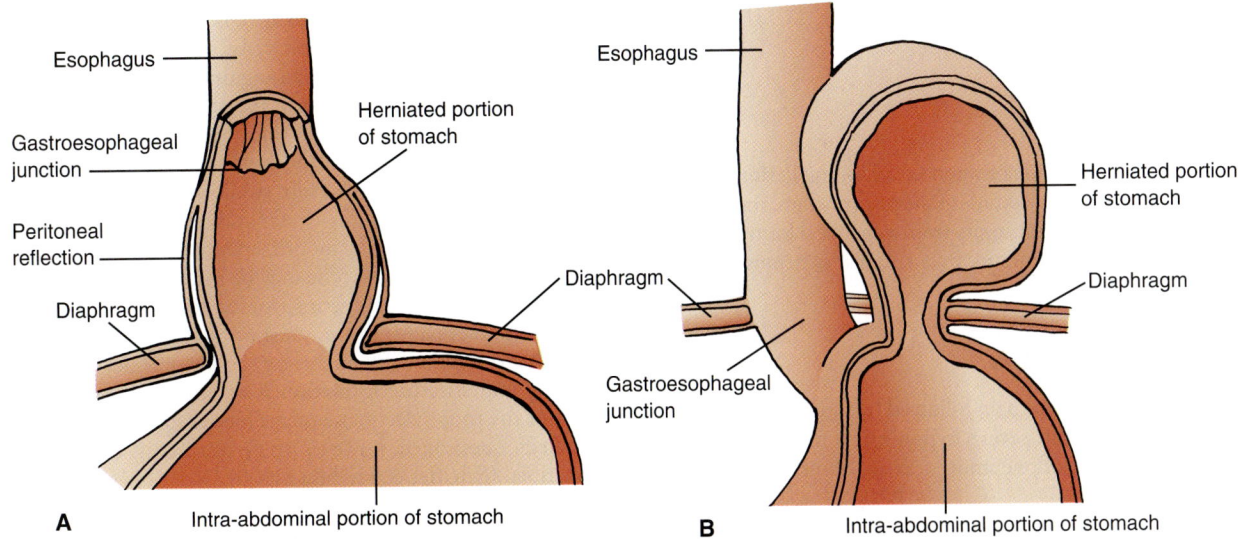

FIGURE 35-8 Sliding esophageal and paraesophageal hernias. (**A**) Sliding esophageal hernia. The upper stomach and cardioesophageal junction have moved upward and slide in and out of the thorax. (**B**) Paraesophageal hernia. All or part of the stomach pushes through the diaphragm next to the gastroesophageal junction.

noises after eating. The diverticulum, or pouch, becomes filled with food or liquid. When the patient assumes a recumbent position, undigested food is regurgitated, and coughing may be caused by irritation of the trachea. Halitosis and a sour taste in the mouth are also common because of the decomposition of food retained in the diverticulum.

Symptoms produced by midesophageal diverticula are less acute. One third of patients with epiphrenic diverticula are asymptomatic, and the remaining two thirds complain of dysphagia and chest pain. Dysphagia is the most common complaint of patients with intramural diverticulosis.

Assessment and Diagnostic Findings

A barium swallow may be performed to determine the exact nature and location of a diverticulum. Manometric studies are often performed for patients with epiphrenic diverticula to rule out a motor disorder. Esophagoscopy usually is contraindicated because of the danger of perforation of the diverticulum, with resulting mediastinitis (inflammation of the organs and tissues that separate the lungs). Blind insertion of a nasogastric tube should be avoided.

Management

Because pharyngoesophageal pulsion diverticulum is progressive, the only means of cure is surgical removal of the diverticulum. During surgery, care is taken to avoid trauma to the common carotid artery and internal jugular veins. The sac is dissected free and amputated flush with the esophageal wall. In addition to a diverticulectomy, a myotomy of the cricopharyngeal muscle is often performed to relieve spasticity of the musculature, which otherwise seems to contribute to a continuation of the previous symptoms. Postoperatively, the patient may have a nasogastric tube inserted at the time of surgery. The surgical incision must be observed for evidence of leakage from the esophagus and a developing fistula. Food and fluids are withheld until x-ray studies show no leakage at the surgical site. The diet begins with liquids and progresses as tolerated.

Surgery is indicated for epiphrenic and midesophageal diverticula only if the symptoms are troublesome and becoming worse. Treatment consists of a diverticulectomy and long myotomy. Intramural diverticula usually regress after the esophageal stricture is dilated.

PERFORATION

The esophagus is not an uncommon site of injury. Perforation may result from stab or bullet wounds of the neck or chest, trauma from motor vehicle crash, caustic injury from a chemical burn (described later), or inadvertent puncture by a surgical instrument during examination or dilation.

Clinical Manifestations

The patient has persistent pain followed by dysphagia. Infection, fever, leukocytosis, and severe hypotension may be noted. In some instances, signs of pneumothorax are observed.

Assessment and Diagnostic Findings

Diagnostic x-ray studies and fluoroscopy are used to identify the site of the injury.

Management

Because of the high risk of infection, broad-spectrum antibiotic therapy is initiated. A nasogastric tube is inserted to provide suction and to reduce the amount of gastric juice that can reflux into the esophagus and mediastinum. Nothing is given by mouth; nutritional needs are met by parenteral nutrition. Parenteral nutrition is preferred to gastrostomy because the latter might cause reflux into the esophagus.

Surgery may be necessary to close the wound, and postoperative nutritional support then becomes a primary concern. Depending on the incision site and the nature of surgery, the postoperative nursing management is similar to that for patients who have had thoracic or abdominal surgery.

FOREIGN BODIES

Many swallowed foreign bodies pass through the gastrointestinal tract without the need for medical intervention. However, some swallowed foreign bodies (eg, dentures, fish bones, pins, small batteries, items containing mercury or lead) may injure the esophagus or obstruct its lumen and must be removed. Pain and dysphagia may be present, and dyspnea may occur as a result of pressure on the trachea. The foreign body may be identified by x-ray film. Perforation may have occurred (see earlier discussion).

Glucagon, because of its relaxing effect on the esophageal muscle, may be injected intramuscularly. An endoscope (with a covered hood or overtube) may be used to remove the impacting food or object from the esophagus. A mixture consisting of sodium bicarbonate and tartaric acid may be used to increase intraluminal pressure by the formation of a gas. Caution must be used with this treatment because there is risk of perforation.

CHEMICAL BURNS

Chemical burns of the esophagus may be caused by undissolved medications in the esophagus. This occurs more frequently in the elderly than it does among the general adult population. A chemical burn may also occur after swallowing of a battery, which may release caustic alkaline. Chemical burns of the esophagus occur most often when a patient, either intentionally or unintentionally, swallows a strong acid or base (eg, lye). This patient is emotionally distraught as well as in acute physical pain. An acute chemical burn of the esophagus may be accompanied by severe burns of the lips, mouth, and pharynx, with pain on swallowing. There may be difficulty in breathing due to either edema of the throat or a collection of mucus in the pharynx.

The patient, who may be profoundly toxic, febrile, and in shock, is treated immediately for shock, pain, and respiratory distress. Esophagoscopy and barium swallow are performed as soon as possible to determine the extent and severity of damage. The patient is given nothing by mouth, and intravenous fluids are administered. A nasogastric tube may be inserted by the physician. Vomiting and gastric lavage are avoided to prevent further exposure of the esophagus to the caustic agent. The use of corticosteroids to reduce inflammation and minimize subsequent scarring and stricture formation is of questionable value. The value of the prophylactic use of antibiotics for these patients has also been questioned; however, these treatments continue to be prescribed (Schaffer & Herbert, 2000).

After the acute phase has subsided, the patient may need nutritional support via enteral or parenteral feedings. The patient may require further treatment to prevent or manage strictures of the esophagus. For strictures that do not respond to dilation, surgical management is necessary. Reconstruction may be accomplished by esophagectomy and colon interposition to replace the portion of esophagus removed.

GASTROESOPHAGEAL REFLUX DISEASE

Some degree of **gastroesophageal reflux** (back-flow of gastric or duodenal contents into the esophagus) is normal in both adults and children. Excessive reflux may occur because of an incompetent lower esophageal sphincter, pyloric stenosis, or a motility disorder. The incidence of reflux seems to increase with aging. In Canada, approximately 17% of individuals have reported experiencing heartburn in the last 3 months (Armstrong, Marshall, Chiba, et al., 2004).

Clinical Manifestations

Symptoms of gastroesophageal reflux disease (GERD) may include pyrosis (burning sensation in the esophagus), dyspepsia (indigestion), regurgitation, dysphagia or odynophagia (difficulty swallowing, pain on swallowing), hypersalivation, and esophagitis. The symptoms may mimic those of a heart attack. The patient's history aids in obtaining an accurate diagnosis.

Assessment and Diagnostic Findings

Diagnostic testing may include an endoscopy or barium swallow to evaluate damage to the esophageal mucosa. Ambulatory 12- to 36-hour esophageal pH monitoring is used to evaluate the degree of acid reflux. Bilirubin monitoring (Bilitec) is used to measure bile reflux patterns. Exposure to bile can cause mucosal damage (Aronson, 2000; Stein et al., 1999).

Management

Management begins with teaching the patient to avoid situations that decrease lower esophageal sphincter pressure or cause esophageal irritation. The patient is instructed to eat a low-fat diet; to avoid caffeine, tobacco, beer, milk, foods containing peppermint or spearmint, and carbonated beverages; to avoid eating or drinking 2 hours before bedtime; to maintain normal body weight; to avoid tight-fitting clothes; to elevate the head of the bed on 6- to 8-inch (15- to 20-cm) blocks; and to elevate the upper body on pillows. If reflux persists, the patient may be given medications such as antacids or histamine receptor blockers. Proton pump inhibitors (medications that decrease the release of gastric acid, such as lansoprazole [Prevacid] or rabeprazole [Aciphex]) may be used; however, there is concern that these products may increase intragastric bacterial growth and the risk for infection. In addition, the patient may receive prokinetic agents, which accelerate gastric emptying. These agents include bethanechol (Urecholine), domperidone (Motilium), and metoclopramide (Maxeran). Metoclopramide has central nervous system complications with long-term use.

If medical management is unsuccessful, surgical intervention may be necessary. Surgical management involves a fundoplication (wrapping of a portion of the gastric fundus around the sphincter area of the esophagus). Fundoplication may be performed by laparoscopy.

BARRETT'S ESOPHAGUS

It is believed that long-standing untreated GERD may result in a condition known as Barrett's esophagus. This has been identified as a precancerous condition that, if left untreated, can result in adenocarcinoma of the esophagus, which has a poor prognosis. It is more common among middle-aged white men.

Clinical Manifestations

The patient complains of symptoms of GERD, notably frequent heartburn. The heartburn is a result of reflux, which eventually causes changes in the cells lining the lower esophagus. The patient may also complain of symptoms related to peptic ulcers or esophageal stricture, or both.

Assessment and Diagnostic Findings

An esophagogastroduodenoscopy (EGD) is performed. This usually reveals an esophageal lining that is red rather than pink. Biopsies are taken, and the cells resemble those of the intestine.

Management

Monitoring varies depending on the amount of cell changes. Some physicians may recommend a repeat endoscopy in 6 to 12 months if there are minor cell changes. Medical and surgical management is similar to that for GERD. Because this is a condition that is increasing in incidence, research is underway to determine the best monitoring and surgical interventions (Mueller et al., 2000; Stein et al., 1999).

BENIGN TUMOURS OF THE ESOPHAGUS

Benign tumours can arise anywhere along the esophagus. The most common lesion is a leiomyoma (tumour of the smooth muscle), which can occlude the lumen of the esophagus. Most benign tumours are asymptomatic and are distinguished from cancerous lesions by a biopsy. Small lesions are excised during esophagoscopy; lesions that occur within the wall of the esophagus may require treatment via a thoracotomy.

CANCER OF THE ESOPHAGUS

In Canada, carcinoma of the esophagus occurs more than three times as often in men compared to women. Canadian cancer statistics show that over 1050 new cases are discovered in men and approximately 400 new cases in women yearly (Canadian Cancer Society, 2005). This represents 1.3 % of all new cases of cancer for males and 0.5% of all new cases of cancer for females. There are 1200 deaths related to oral cancer in the male population, compared with 420 oral cancer deaths in females yearly (Canadian Cancer Society, 2005).

Chronic irritation is a risk factor for esophageal cancer. In the United States, cancer of the esophagus has been associated with ingestion of alcohol and with the use of tobacco. There seems to be an association between GERD and adenocarcinoma of the esophagus. People with Barrett's esophagus (which is caused by chronic irritation of mucous membranes due to reflux of gastric and duodenal contents) have a higher incidence of esophageal cancer (Stein, 1999).

Pathophysiology

Esophageal cancer is usually of the squamous cell epidermoid type; however, the incidence of adenocarcinoma of the esophagus is increasing in the United States. Tumour cells may spread beneath the esophageal mucosa or directly into, through, and beyond the muscle layers into the lymphatics. In the latter stages, obstruction of the esophagus is noted, with possible perforation into the mediastinum and erosion into the great vessels.

Clinical Manifestations

Many patients have an advanced ulcerated lesion of the esophagus before symptoms are manifested. Symptoms include dysphagia, initially with solid foods and eventually with liquids; a sensation of a mass in the throat; painful swallowing; substernal pain or fullness; and, later, regurgitation of undigested food with foul breath and hiccups. The patient first becomes aware of intermittent and increasing difficulty in swallowing. As the tumour progresses and the obstruction becomes more complete, even liquids cannot pass into the stomach. Regurgitation of food and saliva occurs, hemorrhage may take place, and progressive loss of weight and strength occurs from starvation. Later symptoms include substernal pain, persistent hiccup, respiratory difficulty, and foul breath. The delay between the onset of early symptoms and the time when the patient seeks medical advice is often 12 to 18 months. Anyone with swallowing difficulties should be encouraged to consult a physician immediately.

Assessment and Diagnostic Findings

Although new endoscopic techniques are being studied for screening and diagnosis of esophageal cancer, currently diagnosis is confirmed most often by endoscopy with biopsy and brushings. Bronchoscopy usually is performed, especially in tumours of the middle and the upper third of the esophagus, to determine whether the trachea has been affected and to help determine whether the lesion can be removed. Endoscopic ultrasound or mediastinoscopy is used to determine whether the cancer has spread to the nodes and other mediastinal structures. Cancer of the lower end of the esophagus may be caused by adenocarcinoma of the stomach that extends upward into the esophagus.

Medical Management

If esophageal cancer is found at an early stage, treatment goals may be directed toward cure; however, it is often found in late stages, making relief of symptoms the only reasonable goal of therapy. Treatment may include surgery, radiation, chemotherapy, or a combination of these modalities, depending on the extent of the disease.

Standard surgical management includes a total resection of the esophagus (esophagectomy) with removal of the tumour plus a wide tumour-free margin of the esophagus and the lymph nodes in the area. The surgical approach may be through the thorax or the abdomen, depending on the location of the tumour. When tumours occur in the cervical or upper thoracic area, esophageal continuity may be maintained by free jejunal graft transfer, in which the tumour is removed and the area is replaced with a portion of the jejunum (Fig. 35-9). A segment of the colon may be used, or the stomach can be elevated into the chest and the proximal section of the esophagus anastomosed to the stomach.

Tumours of the lower thoracic esophagus are more amenable to surgery than are tumours located higher in the esophagus, and gastrointestinal tract integrity is maintained by anastomosing the lower esophagus to the stomach.

Surgical resection of the esophagus has a relatively high mortality rate because of infection, pulmonary complications, or leakage through the anastomosis. Postoperatively, the patient will have a nasogastric tube in place that should not be manipulated. The patient is given nothing by mouth until x-ray studies confirm that the anastomosis is secure and not leaking.

FIGURE 35-9 Esophageal reconstruction with free jejunal transfer. A portion of the jejunum is grafted between the esophagus and pharynx to replace the abnormal portion of the esophagus. The vascular structures are also anastomosed. A portion of the graft may be externalized through the neck wound to evaluate graft viability.

Preoperative radiation therapy or chemotherapy, or both, may be used; however, treatment is based on type of cell, tumour spread, and patient condition.

Palliative treatment may be necessary to keep the esophagus open, to assist with nutrition, and to control saliva. Palliation may be accomplished with dilation of the esophagus, laser therapy, placement of an endoprosthesis (stent), radiation, or chemotherapy. Because the ideal method of treating esophageal cancer has not yet been found, treatment is individually determined.

Nursing Management

Intervention is directed toward improving the patient's nutritional and physical condition in preparation for surgery, radiation therapy, or chemotherapy. A program to promote weight gain based on a high-calorie and high-protein diet, in liquid or soft form, is provided if adequate food can be taken by mouth. If this is not possible, parenteral or enteral nutrition is initiated. Nutritional status is monitored throughout treatment. The patient is informed about the nature of the postoperative equipment that will be used, including that required for closed chest drainage, nasogastric suction, parenteral fluid therapy, and gastric intubation. Immediate postoperative care is similar to that provided for patients undergoing thoracic surgery. After recovering from the effects of anesthesia, the patient is placed in a low Fowler's position, and later in a Fowler's position, to assist in preventing reflux of gastric secretions. The patient is observed carefully for regurgitation and dyspnea. A common postoperative complication is aspiration pneumonia. The patient's temperature is monitored to detect any elevation that may indicate aspiration or seepage of fluid through the operative site into the mediastinum.

If jejunal grafting has been performed, the nurse checks for graft viability hourly for at least the first 12 hours. To make the graft visible, the surgeon usually brings a portion of the jejunum to the exterior neck by way of a small incision. Moist gauze covers the external portion of the graft. The gauze is removed briefly to assess the graft for colour and to assess for the presence of a pulse by means of Doppler ultrasonography.

If an endoprosthesis has been placed or an anastomosis has been performed, a functioning continuum will exist between the throat and the stomach. Immediately after surgery, the nasogastric tube should be marked for position, and the physician is notified if displacement occurs. The nurse does not attempt to reinsert a displaced nasogastric tube, because damage to the anastomosis may occur. The nasogastric tube is removed 5 to 7 days after surgery, and a barium swallow is performed to assess for any anastomotic leak before the patient is allowed to eat.

Once feeding begins, the nurse encourages the patient to swallow small sips of water and, later, small amounts of pureed food. When the patient is able to increase food intake to an adequate amount, parenteral fluids are discontinued. If an endoprosthesis is used, it may easily become obstructed if food is not chewed sufficiently. After each meal, the patient remains upright for at least 2 hours to allow the food to move through the gastrointestinal tract. It is a challenge to encourage the patient to eat, because appetite is usually poor. Family involvement and home-cooked favourite foods may help the patient to eat. Antacids may help those with gastric distress.

If radiation is part of the therapy, the patient's appetite is further depressed and esophagitis may occur, causing pain when food is eaten. Liquid supplements may be more easily tolerated.

Often, in either the preoperative or the postoperative period, an obstructed or nearly obstructed esophagus causes difficulty with excess saliva, so that drooling becomes a problem. Oral suction may be used if the patient is unable to handle oral secretions, or a wick-type gauze may be placed at the corner of the mouth to direct secretions to a dressing or emesis basin. The possibility that the patient may aspirate saliva into the tracheobronchial tree and develop pneumonia is of great concern.

When the patient is ready to go home, the family is instructed about how to promote nutrition, what observations to make, what measures to take if complications occur, how to keep the patient comfortable, and how to obtain needed physical and emotional support.

NURSING PROCESS:
THE PATIENT WITH A CONDITION
OF THE ESOPHAGUS

Assessment

Emergency conditions of the esophagus (perforation, chemical burns) usually occur in the home or away from medical help and require emergency medical care. The patient is treated for shock and respiratory distress and transported as quickly as possible to a medical facility. Foreign bodies in the esophagus do not pose an immediate threat to life unless pressure is exerted on the trachea, resulting in dyspnea or interfering with respiration, or unless there is leakage of caustic alkali from a battery. Educating the public to prevent inadvertent swallowing of foreign bodies or corrosive agents is a major health issue.

For nonemergency symptoms, a complete health history may reveal the nature of the esophageal disorder. The nurse asks about the patient's appetite. Has it remained the same, increased, or decreased? Is there any discomfort with swallowing? If so, does it occur only with certain foods? Is it associated with pain? Does a change in position affect the discomfort? The patient is asked to describe the pain. Does anything aggravate it? Are there any other symptoms that occur regularly, such as regurgitation, nocturnal regurgitation, eructation (belching), heartburn, substernal pressure, a sensation that food is sticking in the throat, a feeling of becoming full after eating a small amount of food, nausea, vom-

iting, or weight loss? Are the symptoms aggravated by emotional upset? If the patient reports any of these symptoms, the nurse asks about the time of their occurrence, their relationship to eating, and factors that relieve or aggravate them (eg, position change, belching, antacids, vomiting).

This history also includes questions about past or present causative factors, such as infections and chemical, mechanical, or physical irritants; the degree to which alcohol and tobacco are used; and the amount of daily food intake. The nurse determines whether the patient appears emaciated and auscultates the patient's chest to determine whether pulmonary complications exist.

Nursing Diagnosis

Based on the assessment data, the nursing diagnoses may include the following:

- Imbalanced nutrition, less than body requirements, related to difficulty swallowing
- Risk for aspiration related to difficulty swallowing or to tube feeding
- Acute pain related to difficulty swallowing, ingestion of an abrasive agent, tumour, or frequent episodes of gastric reflux
- Deficient knowledge about the esophageal disorder, diagnostic studies, medical management, surgical intervention, and rehabilitation

Planning and Goals

The major goals for the patient may include attainment of adequate nutritional intake, avoidance of respiratory compromise from aspiration, relief of pain, and increased knowledge level.

Nursing Interventions

ENCOURAGING ADEQUATE NUTRITIONAL INTAKE
The patient is encouraged to eat slowly and to chew all food thoroughly so that it can pass easily into the stomach. Small, frequent feedings of nonirritating foods are recommended to promote digestion and to prevent tissue irritation. Sometimes liquid swallowed with food helps the food pass through the esophagus. Food should be prepared in an appealing manner to help stimulate the appetite. Irritants such as tobacco and alcohol should be avoided. A baseline weight is obtained, and daily weights are recorded. The patient's intake of nutrients is assessed.

DECREASING RISK OF ASPIRATION
The patient who has difficulty swallowing or difficulty handling secretions should be kept in at least a semi-Fowler's position to decrease the risk of aspiration. The patient can be instructed in the use of oral suction to decrease the risk of aspiration further.

RELIEVING PAIN
Small, frequent feedings are recommended, because large quantities of food overload the stomach and promote gastric reflux. The patient is advised to avoid any activities that increase pain, and to remain upright for 1 to 4 hours after each meal to prevent reflux. The head of the bed should be placed on 10- to 20-cm blocks. Eating before bedtime is discouraged.

The patient is advised that excessive use of over-the-counter antacids can cause rebound acidity. Antacid use should be directed by the primary care provider, who can recommend the daily, safe dose needed to neutralize gastric juices and prevent esophageal

Chart 35-4
Home Care Checklist • The Patient With an Esophageal Condition

At the completion of the home care instruction, the patient or caregiver will be able to:	Patient	Caregiver
• Demonstrate use of suction equipment.	✓	✓
• State dietary modifications needed to meet caloric needs.	✓	✓
• Demonstrate enteral or parenteral feeding techniques.	✓	✓
• Demonstrate care of incision if indicated.	✓	✓
• State when next checkup is needed.	✓	✓
• Identify available support groups.	✓	✓

irritation. Histamine$_2$ antagonists are administered as prescribed to decrease gastric acid irritation.

PROVIDING PATIENT EDUCATION

The patient is prepared physically and psychologically for diagnostic tests, treatments, and possible surgical intervention. The principal nursing interventions include reassuring the patient and discussing the procedures and their purposes. Some disorders of the esophagus evolve over time, whereas others are the result of trauma (eg, chemical burns, perforation). In instances of trauma, the emotional and physical preparation for treatment is more difficult because of the short time available and the circumstances of the injury. Treatment interventions must be evaluated continually; the patient is given sufficient information to participate in care and diagnostic tests. If endoscopic diagnostic methods are used, the patient is instructed regarding the moderate sedation that will be used during the procedure. If procedures are being performed on an outpatient basis with the use of moderate sedation, the patient is instructed to have someone available to drive him or her home after the procedure. If surgery is required, immediate and long-term evaluation is similar to that for a patient undergoing thoracic surgery.

PROMOTING HOME AND COMMUNITY-BASED CARE

Teaching Patients Self-Care

The self-care required of the patient depends on the nature of the disorder and on the surgery or treatment measures used (eg, diet, positioning, medications). If an ongoing condition exists, the nurse helps the patient plan for needed physical and psychological adjustments and for follow-up care (Chart 35-4).

Special equipment, such as suction or enteral or parenteral feeding devices, may be required. The patient may need assistance in planning meals, using medications as prescribed, and resuming activities. Education about nutritional requirements and how to measure the adequacy of nutrition is important. Elderly and debilitated patients in particular often need assistance and education in ways to adjust to their limitations and to resume activities that are important to them.

Continuing Care

Patients with chronic esophageal conditions require an individualized approach to their management at home. Foods may need to be prepared in a special way (blenderized foods, soft foods), and the patient may need to eat more frequently (eg, four to six small servings per day). The medication schedule is adjusted to the patient's daily activities as much as possible. Analgesic medications and antacids can usually be taken as needed every 3 to 4 hours.

Postoperative home health care focuses on nutritional support, management of pain, and respiratory function. Some patients are discharged from the hospital with enteral feeding by means of a gastrostomy or jejunostomy tube or parenteral nutrition. The patient and care provider need specific instructions regarding management of the equipment and treatments. Home care visits by a nurse may be necessary to assess the patient's care and the care provider's ability to provide the necessary care. (See Chapter 36 for more information about parenteral nutrition and management of the patient with a gastrostomy.) For some patients, a multidisciplinary team comprising a dietitian, a social worker, and family members is helpful. Hospice care is appropriate for some patients.

Evaluation

EXPECTED PATIENT OUTCOMES

Expected patient outcomes may include:

1. Achieves an adequate nutritional intake
   a. Eats small, frequent meals
   b. Drinks water with small servings of food
   c. Avoids irritants (alcohol, tobacco, very hot beverages)
   d. Maintains desired weight
2. Does not aspirate or develop pneumonia
   a. Maintains upright position during feeding
   b. Uses oral suction equipment effectively
3. Is free of pain or able to control pain within a tolerable level
   a. Avoids large meals and irritating foods
   b. Takes medications as prescribed and with adequate fluids (at least 4 ounces), and remains upright for at least 10 minutes after taking medications
   c. Maintains an upright position after meals for 1 to 4 hours
   d. Reports that there is less eructation and chest pain
4. Increases knowledge level of esophageal condition, treatment, and prognosis
   a. States cause of condition
   b. Discusses rationale for medical or surgical management and diet or medication regimen
   c. Describes treatment program
   d. Practices preventive measures so injuries are avoided

Critical Thinking Exercises

1. You are interviewing a patient in the medical clinic. The patient is complaining of difficulty swallowing as well as indigestion. Describe how you would continue to assess this patient to obtain the additional information that is needed. Identify the various factors that may be causing this patient's symptoms.

2. You are caring for two postoperative patients. One patient is being treated for cancer of the mouth, the other for cancer of the esophagus. How will the nutritional care of these two patients differ? Describe the communication needs and psychosocial needs of these patients.

REFERENCES AND SELECTED READINGS

Books

Bickley, L. S., & Szilagyi, P. G. (2003). *Bates' guide to physical examination and history taking* (8th ed.). Philadelphia: Lippincott Williams & Wilkins.

Brandt, L. J. (Ed.). (1999). *Clinical practice of gastroenterology* (Vols. I & II). Philadelphia: Churchill-Livingstone.

Castell, D. O., & Richter, J. E. (1999). *The esophagus* (3rd ed.). Philadelphia: Lippincott Williams & Wilkins.

DeVita, V. T., Hellman, S., & Rosenberg, S. A. (Eds.). (2001). *Cancer: Principles and practice of oncology* (6th ed.). Philadelphia: Lippincott Williams & Wilkins.

Fonseca, R. J. (Ed.). (2000). *Oral and maxillofacial surgery*. Philadelphia: W. B. Saunders.

Garber, T. M. (Ed.). (2000). *Orthodontics: Current principles and techniques*. St. Louis: Mosby.

Harris, N. O., & Garcia-Godoy, F. (1999). *Primary preventive dentistry* (5th ed.). Norwalk, CT: Appleton & Lange.

Harrison, L. B., et al. (1999). *Head and neck cancer: A multidisciplinary approach*. Philadelphia: Lippincott Williams & Wilkins.

McEvoy, G. R. (Ed.). (2000). *American Hospital Formulary Service*. Bethesda, MD: American Society of Health-System Pharmacists.

Murray, J. (1999). *Manual of dysphagia assessment in adults*. San Diego: Singular Publishing.

Pappas, T. N., et al. (1999). *Atlas of laparoscopic surgery* (2nd ed.). Norwalk, CT: Appleton & Lange.

Proffit, W. R. (2000). *Contemporary orthodontics*. St. Louis: Mosby.

U.S. Department of Health and Human Services. (2000). *Oral health in America: A report of the surgeon general. Executive summary*. Rockville, MD: National Institutes of Dental and Craniofacial Research, National Institutes of Health.

Yamada, T. (Ed.). (1999). *Textbook of gastroenterology* (3rd ed., Vols. I & II). Philadelphia: Lippincott Williams & Wilkins.

Journals

Conditions and Cancer of the Oral Cavity

Armstrong, D. A., Marshall, J. K., Chiba, N., et al., for the Canadian Association of Gastroenterology Consensus Group. (2004). Canadian consensus conference on the management of gastroesophageal reflux disease in adults. *Canadian Journal of Gastroenterology, 19*(1), 15–35.

Armstrong, R. (2005). Access and care: Towards a national oral health strategy. A report of the symposium. *Journal of the Canadian Dental Association, 71*(1), 19–22.

Baldota, K. K., & Leake, J. (2004). A macroeconomic review of dentistry in Canada in the 1990's. *Journal of the Canadian Dental Association, 70*(9), 604–609.

Bull, P. D. (2001). Salivary gland stones: Diagnosis and treatment. *Hospital Medicine, 62*(7), 396–399.

Canadian Cancer Society. (2005). Specific cancers. Available at: www.cancer.ca.

Greenlee, R. T. (2001). Cancer statistics, 2001. *CA Cancer Journal for Clinicians, 51*(1), 15–36.

Hawkins, R. J., Wang, E. E., & Leake, J. C. (1999). Preventative health care update: Prevention of oral cancer mortality. *Journal of the Canadian Dental Association, 65*(11), 617–628.

Kimata, Y., et al. (2000). Postoperative complications and functional results after total glossectomy with microvascular reconstruction. *Plastic Reconstructive Surgery, 106*(5), 1028–1035.

Lingstrom, P., et al. (2000). Food starches and dental caries. *Critical Reviews in Oral Biology and Medicine, 11*(3), 366–380.

McQuone, S. J. (1999). Acute viral and bacterial infections of the salivary glands. *Otolaryngology Clinics of North America, 32*(5), 793–811.

Public Health Agency of Canada. (2005). *Surveillance for methicillin-resistant staphylococcus aureus in Canadian hospitals: A report update from the Canadian nosocomial infection surveillance program*. Available at: http://www.phac-aspc.gc.ca. Retrieved May 9, 2005.

Reimers, M., et al. (2000). Results after shock wave lithotripsy for salivary gland stones. *Schweizerische Medizinische Wochenschrift, 125*, 122s–126s.

Rethman, J. (2000). Trends in preventive care: Caries risk assessment and indications for sealants. *Journal of the American Dental Association, 131*, (Suppl.), 8S–12S.

Rice, D. H. (1999a). Chronic inflammatory disorders of the salivary glands. *Otolaryngology Clinics of North America, 32*(5), 813–818.

Rice, D. H. (1999b). Noninflammatory, non-neoplastic disorders of the salivary gland. *Otolaryngology Clinics of North America, 32*(5), 835–843.

Sessons, D. G., et al. (2000). Analysis of treatment results for floor-of-mouth cancer. *Laryngoscope, 110*(10 Pt. 1), 1764–1772.

Statistics Canada. (2005). Health indicators. Volume 2004, No. 1: Contact with dental professionals. Report No. 82-221-XIE. Available at: http://www.statcan.ca/english/freepub/82-221-XIE/00604/tables/html/4295.htm. Retrieved March 15, 2005.

Villarrel, P. M., et al. (2000). Study of mandibular repair using quantitative radiodensitometry: A comparison between maxillomandibular and rigid internal fixation. *Journal of Oral and Maxillofacial Surgery, 58*, 776–781.

Williamson, M., & Maze, B. (2004). *A Canadian oral health strategy*. Ottawa: Federal, provincial, and territorial dental directors.

Wright, E. F. (2000). Referred craniofacial pain patterns in patients with temporomandibular disorder. *Journal of the American Dental Association, 131*(9), 1307–1315.

Conditions and Treatment of the Esophagus

Annese, V., et al. (2000). A multicenter randomized study of intrasphincteric botulism toxin in patients with oesophageal achalasia. *Gut, 46*, 597–600.

Aronson, B. S. (2000). Applying clinical practice guidelines to a patient with complicated gastroesophageal reflux disease. *Gastroenterology Nursing, 23*(4), 143–147.

Bowrey, D. J. (2000). Laparoscopic esophageal surgery. *Surgical Clinics of North America, 80*(4), 1213–1242.

Frenken, M. (2001). Best palliation in esophageal cancer: Surgery, stenting, radiation therapy. *Diseases of the Esophagus, 14*(2), 120–123.

Heath, E. I., et al. (2000). Adenocarcinoma of the esophagus: Risk factors and prevention. *Oncology, 14*(2), 507–514.

Hirano, I. (1999). Pathophysiology of achalasia. *Current Gastroenterology Report, 1*(3), 198–202.

Mueller, J., et al. (2000). Malignant progression in Barrett's esophagus: Pathology and biology. *Recent Results in Cancer Research, 155*, 29–41.

Nguyen, N. T., et al. (2000). Laparoscopy or thoracoscopy for achalasia. *Seminars in Thoracic and Cardiovascular Surgery, 12*(3), 201–205.

Para, M. Epidemiology of esophageal cancer, especially adenocarcinoma of the esophagus and esophagogastric junction. *Recent Results in Cancer Research, 155*, 1–14.

Schaffer, S. B., & Herbert, A. F. (2000). Caustic ingestion. *Journal of the Louisiana State Medical Society, 152*(12), 590–596.

Stein, H. J., et al. (2000). Malignant degeneration of Barrett's esophagus: Clinical point options. *Recent Results in Cancer Research, 155*, 42–53.

Stein, H. J., et al. (1999). Bile acids as components of the duodenogastric refluate: Detection, relationship to bilirubin, mechanism of injury, and clinical relevance. *Hepatogastroenterology, 46*, 66–73.

Streeter, B. L. (1999). Botulinum toxin: A case study. *Gastroenterology Nursing, 22*(2), 59–61.

Vaezi, M. F., & Shay, S. S. (2001). New techniques in measuring nonacidic esophageal reflux. *Seminars in Thoracic Cardiovascular Surgery, 13*(3), 255–264.

Conditions and Treatment of the Head and Neck

Ferlito, A. (2001), Evolution in the philosophy of neck dissection. *Acta Otolaryngol, 121,* 963–966.

Richards, B. L., & Spiro, J. D. (2000). Controlling advanced neck disease: Efficacy of neck dissection and radiotherapy. *Laryngoscope, 110*(7), 1124–1127.

Talmi, Y. P., et al. (2000). Pain in the neck after neck dissection. *Otolaryngology Head and Neck Surgery, 123*(3), 302–306.

Weymuller, E. A. (2000). Quality of life in patient with head and neck cancer: Lessons learned from 549 prospectively evaluated patients. *Archives of Otolaryngology Head and Neck Surgery, 126*(3), 329–335.

RESOURCES AND WEBSITES

Canadian Cancer Society; www.cancer.ca.

Canadian Dental Association; www.cda-adc.ca.

Health Canada; www.hc-sc.gc.ca.

Statistics Canada; www.statscan.ca.

American Cancer Society, 1599 Clifton Rd. NE, Atlanta, GA 30329; 1-800-ACS-2345; http://www.cancer.org.

American Dental Association, 211 E. Chicago Ave., Chicago, IL 60611; 312-440-2806; http://www.ada.org.

Centers for Disease Control and Prevention, 1600 Clifton Rd., Atlanta, GA 30333; 404-639-7000; http://www.cdc.gov/health.

National Institute of Dental and Craniofacial Research, National Institutes of Health, 900 Rockville Pike, Bethesda, MD 20892; 301-496-4261; http://www.nidr.nih.gov.

National Oral Health Information Clearinghouse, 1 NOHIC Way, Bethesda, MD 20892-3500; 1-301-402-7364; http://www.nohic.nider.nih.gov.

Gastrointestinal Intubation and Special Nutritional Modalities

Adapted by Christy Raymond

LEARNING OBJECTIVES

On completion of this chapter, the learner will be able to:

1. Describe the purposes and types of GI intubation.
2. Discuss nursing management of the patient who has a nasogastric or nasoenteric tube.
3. Use the nursing process as a framework for care of the patient receiving an enteral feeding.
4. Explain the preoperative and postoperative care of the patient with a gastrostomy.
5. Use the nursing process as a framework for care of the patient with a gastrostomy.
6. Identify the purposes and uses of parenteral nutrition.
7. Use the nursing process as a framework for care of the patient receiving parenteral nutrition.
8. Describe the nursing measures used to prevent complications from parenteral nutrition.

*T*his chapter presents several topics related to gastrointestinal (GI) intubation. Nursing management topics relate to managing the care of patients with nasogastric (NG) and nasoenteric tubes and gastrostomies, providing tube feedings, and teaching points related to home health care and nutritional therapy. In addition, parenteral nutrition is presented, including general indications for this nutritional modality and nursing care of patients receiving these support measures.

Gastrointestinal Intubation

GI intubation is the insertion of a rubber or plastic tube into the stomach, the **duodenum** (first section of the small intestine), or the intestine. The tube may be inserted through the mouth, the nose, or the abdominal wall. The tubes can be short, medium, or long, depending on their intended use; **nasogastric (NG) tubes** are short, **nasoduodenal tubes** are of medium length, and nasoenteric tubes are long. GI intubation may be performed for the following reasons:

- To decompress the stomach and remove gas and fluid
- To lavage the stomach and remove ingested toxins
- To diagnose disorders of GI motility and other disorders
- To administer medications and feedings
- To treat an obstruction
- To compress a bleeding site
- To aspirate gastric contents for analysis

A variety of tubes are used for decompression, aspiration, and lavage. The Sengstaken-Blakemore tube is a type of NG tube used to treat bleeding esophageal varices (see Chapter 39). Orogastric tubes are large-bore tubes with wide proximal outlets for removal of particles of ingested substances (eg, pills); they are primarily used in emergency departments. Various other tubes are used to administer feedings and medications. The tubes are made of various materials (rubber, polyurethane, silicone), and they vary in length

(90 cm to 3 m), in size (6 to 18 French [Fr]), in purpose, and in placement in the GI tract (stomach, duodenum, jejunum) (Table 36-1). Any solution administered through a tube is either poured through a syringe or delivered by a drip mechanism regulated by gravity or by an electric pump. **Aspiration** (suctioning) to remove gas and fluids is accomplished with the use of a syringe, an electric suction machine, or a wall suction outlet.

SHORT TUBES

An NG tube or short tube is introduced through the nose into the stomach, often before or during esophageal or stomach surgery. Commonly used short tubes include the Levin tube and the gastric sump tube. Short tubes are used in adults primarily to remove fluid and gas from the upper GI tract or to obtain a specimen of gastric contents for laboratory studies. They are occasionally used for the short-term (3 to 4 weeks) administration of medications or feedings.

Levin Tube

The Levin tube has a single lumen (the hollow part of the tube), ranges from 14 to 18 Fr in size, and is made of plastic or rubber with openings near its tip. It is 125 cm long. Circular markings at specific points on the tube serve as guides for insertion. A marking is made on the tube to indicate the midpoint. The tube is advanced cautiously until this marking reaches the patient's nostril, suggesting that the tube is in the stomach. Placement is checked by observing the characteristics of the aspirate and by testing the **pH** (which varies according to the source of the aspirate). Seeing the tube on an x-ray study is the only sure way to verify its location. The Levin tube can be connected to low intermittent suction (30 to 40 mm Hg) versus constant suction. Intermittent suction is used to avoid erosion or tearing of the stomach lining, which can result from constant adherence of the tube's lumen to the mucosal lining of the stomach.

Glossary

antireflux valve: valve that prevents return or backward flow of fluid

aspiration: breathing of fluids or foods into the trachea and lungs; removal of substance by suction

bolus: a feeding administered into the stomach in large amounts and at designated intervals

central venous access device (CVAD): a device designed and used for long-term administration of medications and fluids into central veins

cyclic feeding: periodic feeding/infusion given over a short period (8 to 12 hours)

decompression (intestinal): removal of intestinal contents to prevent gas and fluid from distending the coils of the intestine

dumping syndrome: rapid emptying of the stomach contents into the small intestine; characterized by sweating and weakness

duodenum: the first part of the small intestine, which connects with the pylorus of the stomach and extends to the jejunum

feeding tube: tube through which nutritional products, water, and other fluids can be introduced into the GI tract

gastrostomy: surgical creation of an opening into the stomach for the purpose of administering foods and fluids

irrigation: flushing of the tube with water or other fluids to clear it

jejunum: second portion of the small intestine, extending from the duodenum to the ileum

low-profile gastrostomy device (LPGD, G-button): an enteral feeding access device that is flush with the skin and is used for long-term feeding

nasoduodenal tube: tube inserted through the nose into the beginning of the small intestine (duodenum)

nasogastric (NG) tube: tube inserted through the nose into the stomach

nasojejunal tube: tube inserted through the nose into the second portion of the small intestine (jejunum)

osmolality: ionic concentration of fluid

osmosis: passage of solvent through a semipermeable membrane; the solvent, usually water, passes through the membrane from a region of low concentration of solute to that of a higher concentration of solute

parenteral nutrition: method of supplying nutrients to the body by an intravenous route

percutaneous endoscopic gastrostomy (PEG): an endoscopic procedure for placing a permanent feeding tube into the stomach

peristalsis: wavelike movement that occurs involuntarily in the alimentary canal

pH: the degree of acidity or alkalinity of a substance or solution

peripherally inserted central catheter (PICC): a device used for intermediate-term intravenous therapy

stoma: artificially created opening between a body cavity (eg, intestine) and the body surface

total nutrient admixture: an admixture of lipid emulsions, proteins, carbohydrates, electrolytes, vitamins, trace minerals, and water

Table 36-1 • Nasogastric, Nasoenteric, and Feeding Tubes

TUBE TYPE	LENGTH (CM)	SIZE (FRENCH)	LUMEN	OTHER CHARACTERISTICS
Nasogastric Tubes				
Levin (plastic or rubber)	125	14–18	Single	Circular markings at intervals along the tube serve as guidelines for insertion
Gastric sump or Salem (plastic)	120	12–18	Double	Smaller lumen acts as a vent
Moss	90	12–16	Triple	Contains both a gastric decompression lumen and a duodenal lumen for postoperative feedings
Sengstaken-Blakemore (rubber)			Triple	Two lumens are used to inflate the gastric and esophageal balloons
Nasoenteric Decompression Tubes				
Miller-Abbott (rubber)	300	12–18	Double	One lumen uses mercury, water, saline, or air for balloon inflation
Harris	180	14, 16	Single	Mercury-weighted tip (or may use water as a weight)
Cantor (rubber)	300	16	Single	Mercury-weighted bag (or may use water as a weight)
Baker (plastic)	270	16	Double	One lumen is used for balloon inflation
Nasoenteric Feeding Tubes				
Dobbhoff or EnteraFlo (polyurethane or silicone rubber)	160–175	8–12	Single	Tungsten-weighted tip, radiopaque, stylet
Kaofeed or Corpak	56–140	5–12	Single	Available with or without stylets, tungsten tip and radiopaque

Gastric Sump

The gastric sump (Salem) tube is a radiopaque, clear plastic, double-lumen NG tube used to decompress the stomach and keep it empty. It is 120 cm long and is passed into the stomach in the same way as the Levin tube. The inner, smaller tube vents the larger suction-drainage tube to the atmosphere by means of an opening at the distal end of the tube. The sump tube can protect gastric suture lines because, when used properly, it maintains the force of suction at the drainage openings, or outlets, at less than 25 mm Hg, the level of capillary fragility. The small vent tube (known as the blue pigtail) controls this action. These tubes are connected to low continuous suction. The suction lumen is irrigated as prescribed to maintain patency.

To prevent reflux of gastric contents through the vent lumen (blue pigtail), the vent lumen is kept above the patient's waist; otherwise it will act as a siphon. A one-way **antireflux valve** seated in the blue pigtail prevents the reflux of gastric contents out the vent lumen (Fig. 36-1). The valve is removed after irrigation of the suction lumen, and 20 mL of air is injected to reestablish a buffer of air between the gastric contents and the valve.

MEDIUM TUBES

Medium-length nasoenteric tubes are used for feeding. Feeding tubes placed in the duodenum are 160 cm long; feeding tubes placed in the **jejunum** (portion of the small intestine adjacent to the duodenum) are 175 cm long. They can be inserted at the time of surgery or before surgery, by interventional radiologists assisted by fluoroscopy or at the bedside. If the tube is inserted at the bedside, placement is verified by radiography. After insertion, the tip of the tube will initially be in the stomach; it usually takes 24 hours for the tube to pass through the stomach and into the

intestines. Some tubes remain situated in the stomach and are up to 140 cm long.

 NURSING ALERT Having the patient lie on the right side facilitates passage, because gravity and peristaltic motion will move the weighted tube into the duodenum.

Polyurethane or silicone rubber feeding tubes have narrow diameters (6 to 12 Fr) and tungsten tips (rather than mercury-filled bags); some have a water-activated lubricant that makes it easier to insert the tube. The tubing may kink when a stylet is not used, particularly if the patient is uncooperative or unable to swallow. Feeding tubes with a stylet are inserted with caution in patients who are predisposed to esophageal puncture, such as elderly and frail patients with thin tissues. These tubes are advanced in the same way as an NG tube; that is, with the patient in Fowler's position. If this is not feasible, the patient is placed on the right side.

LONG TUBES

Nasoenteric decompression tubes are not commonly used due to the potential for mercury leakage. When used, a long nasoenteric tube is introduced through the nose and passed through the esophagus and stomach into the intestinal tract. It is used to aspirate intestinal contents so that gas and fluid do not distend the intestine; this is called **decompression**. Three major nasoenteric tubes used for aspiration and decompression are the Miller-Abbott tube, the Harris tube, and the Cantor tube. These tubes are used to relieve obstruction of the small intestine. They are also used prophylactically; they may be inserted the night before GI surgery to prevent postoperative obstruction. The use of these tubes is not

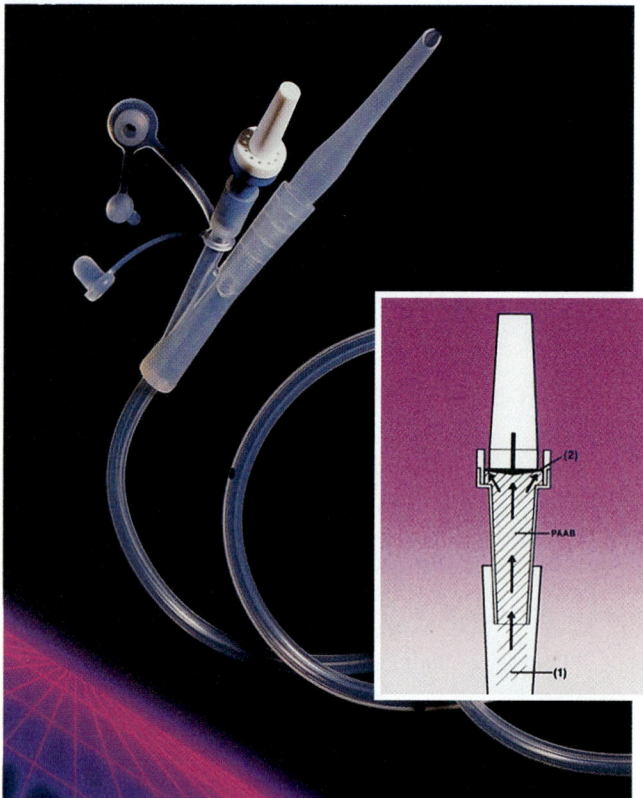

FIGURE 36-1 Gastric sump tube (Salem) equipped with a one-way anti-reflux valve that allows air to enter and prevents gastric contents from escaping. The antireflux valve is designed with a pressure activated air buffer (PAAB). The buffer is activated (1) and the valve closes (2) when pressure from gastric contents enters the tubing. Argyle Silicone Salem Sump Tube with preattached Argyle Salem Sump Anti-Reflux Valve courtesy of Sherwood Medical, St. Louis, Missouri.

commonly seen in Canada. In some care areas, the Salem sump or Levin tube is more commonly used for gastric decompression.

Because **peristalsis** is either stopped or slowed for 24 to 48 hours after surgery as a result of anesthesia and visceral manipulation, NG or nasoenteric suction is used to evacuate fluids and flatus so that vomiting is prevented, tension is reduced along the incision line, and obstruction is prevented. Usually, the tube remains in place until peristalsis returns, as evidenced by the resumption of bowel sounds and the passage of flatus.

Miller-Abbott Tube

The Miller-Abbott tube is a double-lumen rubber tube that is 300 cm long and 12, 14, 16, or 18 Fr in size. One lumen is used to introduce mercury, water, or saline into the balloon at the end of the tube for weighting of the tube; the other lumen is used for aspiration. Before the tube is inserted, the balloon should be tested and its capacity measured; then it should be deflated completely. The tube should be lubricated sparingly and chilled well (chilling causes the tube to become stiff and facilitates its passage) before the tip is inserted through the patient's nose. Markings on the tube indicate the distance it has been passed. Before removal, the balloon at the end of the lumen must be completely deflated.

Harris Tube

The Harris tube is a single-lumen (14 Fr), mercury-weighted tube of about 180 cm. This tube has a metal tip that is lubri-

cated and introduced through the nose. The mercury-weighted bag follows. The weight of the mercury promotes the passage of the bag by gravity. This tube is used solely for suction and **irrigation**. Usually, a Y-tube is attached to the end of the Harris tube. The suction is applied to one side of the Y and the other side is clamped, except when irrigation of the tube is being performed.

Cantor Tube

The Cantor tube is 300 cm long and has a 16-Fr lumen. Its distinguishing feature is that it is larger than the other long tubes. It has a 4- or 5-mL bag at the extreme end of the rubber tubing; mercury, water or saline is introduced into this bag to weight the tube. Before the tube is inserted, the bag is wrapped around the tube. After the tube is lubricated, it is advanced through the nose and into the esophagus. The patient assumes a sitting position and may be offered sips of water to facilitate passage of the tube. Fluoroscopy helps to verify that the tube has passed into the duodenum.

NURSING MANAGEMENT OF PATIENTS UNDERGOING NASOGASTRIC OR NASOENTERIC INTUBATION

Nursing interventions include the following:

- Instructing the patient about the purpose of the tube and the procedure required for inserting and advancing it
- Describing the sensations to be expected during tube insertion
- Inserting the NG tube and assisting with insertion of the nasoenteric tube
- Confirming the placement of the NG tube
- Advancing the nasoenteric tube
- Monitoring the patient and maintaining tube function
- Providing oral and nasal hygiene and care
- Monitoring for potential complications
- Removing the tube

Providing Instruction

Before the patient is intubated, the nurse explains the purpose of the tube; this information may assist the patient to be cooperative and tolerant of what is often an unpleasant procedure. The general activities related to inserting the tube are then reviewed, including the fact that the patient may have to breathe through the mouth and that the procedure may cause gagging until the tube has passed the area of the gag reflex.

Inserting the Tube

Before inserting the tube, the clinician determines how much tubing will be needed to reach the stomach or the small intestine. A mark is made on the tube to indicate the desired length. This length is determined by measuring the distance from the tip of the nose to the earlobe, and from the earlobe to the xiphoid process (Fig. 36-2).

While the tube is being inserted, the patient usually sits upright with a towel spread bib-fashion over the chest. Tissue wipes are made available. Privacy and adequate light are provided. The physician may swab the nostril and spray the oropharynx with Tetracaine or benzocaine can be ordered and applied to numb the nasal passage and suppress the gag reflex. This makes the entire

Measuring distance from nostril to tip of earlobe.

Measuring distance from earlobe to tip of xiphoid process.

Traditional Measurement Method

1. Have the patient sit supine in either the semi-Fowler's or high Fowler's position with the neck in a neutral position.
2. Place the distal tip of the tubing at the tip of the patient's nose and mark this location on the tubing.
3. Extend the tubing from the point of the last measurement to the tragus (tip) of the ear and mark this location on the tubing.
4. Extend the tubing from the point of the last measurement to the tip of the patient's xyphoid process and mark the point on the tubing.

FIGURE 36-2 Measuring length of nasogastric tube for placement into stomach.

procedure more tolerable. Having the patient gargle with a liquid anesthetic or hold ice chips in the mouth for a few minutes can have the same effect. Encouraging the patient to breathe through the mouth or to pant often helps, as does swallowing water, if permitted.

A polyurethane tube may need to be warmed to make it more pliable. To make the tube easier to insert, it should be lubricated with a water-soluble substance (K-Y jelly) unless it has a dry coating called hydromer, which, when moistened, provides its own lubrication. The nurse wears gloves during the procedure.

The patient is placed in Fowler's position, and the nostrils are inspected for any obstruction. The more patent nostril is selected for use. The tip of the patient's nose is tilted, and the tube is aligned to enter the nostril. When the tube reaches the nasopharynx, the patient is instructed to lower the head slightly and to begin to swallow as the tube is advanced. The patient may also sip water through a straw to facilitate advancement of the tube. The oropharynx is inspected to ensure that the tube has not coiled in the pharynx or mouth.

Confirming Placement

To ensure patient safety, it is essential to confirm that the tube has been placed correctly, particularly because tubes may be accidentally inserted in the lungs, which may be undetected in high-risk patients. Examples of high-risk patients are those with a decreased level of consciousness, confused mental state, poor or absent cough and gag reflexes, or agitation during insertion. Presence of an endotracheal tube and recent removal of an endotracheal tube also increase the risk for inadvertent placement of the tube in the lung (Metheny, 1998). Initially, an x-ray study should confirm tube placement. However, each time liq-

uids or medications are administered, and once a shift for continuous feedings, the tube must be checked to ensure that it remains properly placed. The traditional recommendation has been to inject air through the tube while auscultating the epigastric area with a stethoscope to detect air insufflations. However, studies indicate that this auscultatory method is not accurate in determining whether the tube has been inserted into the stomach, intestines, or respiratory tract (Lord, 2001; Metheny et al., 1999). Instead of the auscultation method, a combination of three methods is recommended:

- Measurement of tube length
- Visual assessment of aspirate
- pH measurement of aspirate

After the tube is inserted, the exposed portion of the tube is measured and the length is documented. The nurse measures the exposed tube length every shift and compares it with the original measurement. An increase in the length of exposed tube may indicate dislodgement, or a leaking or ruptured balloon if the tube has a balloon.

Visual assessment of the colour of the aspirate may help identify tube placement. Metheny et al. (1994) found that gastric aspirate is most frequently cloudy and green, tan or off-white, or bloody or brown. Intestinal aspirate is primarily clear and yellow to bile-coloured. Pleural fluid is usually pale yellow and serous, and tracheobronchial secretions are usually tan or off-white mucus. Researchers suggest that the appearance of the aspirate may be helpful in distinguishing between gastric and intestinal placement but is of little value in ruling out respiratory placement. This method is less helpful when the patient is receiving continuous feedings, because aspirate often looks like the formula that is used for the feeding (Metheny & Titler, 2001).

Determining the pH of the tube aspirate is a more accurate method of confirming tube placement. The pH method can also be used to monitor the advancement of the tube into the small intestines. The pH of gastric aspirate is acidic (1 to 5). The pH of intestinal aspirate is approximately 6 or greater, and the pH of respiratory aspirate is more alkaline (7 or greater). pH testing is best suited for distinguishing between gastric and intestinal placement. A pH sensor enteral tube is available which does not require fluid aspirate to obtain pH values; it can be useful in distinguishing gastric from small bowel placement of the tube. The pH method is less helpful with continuous feedings, because tube feedings have a pH value of 6.6 and neutralize the GI pH (Metheny & Titler, 2001). For more information, see Nursing Research Profile 36-1.

Using gastric aspiration as a means of verifying that the NG tube has been placed correctly may be a problem because of the characteristic properties and diameter of the tubes. Studies suggest that aspiration may be performed more easily with polyurethane tubes and tubes with a size 10 Fr diameter. Metheny et al. (1993) recommended the following steps if problems occur with aspiration of fluid from small-bore feeding tubes:

1. Insufflate 20 mL of air through the tube with a large syringe (30 to 60 mL).
2. Pull back on the plunger.
3. If step 2 is ineffective, insufflate another 20 mL of air and replace the large syringe with a smaller one (12 mL); attempt to aspirate.
4. If the measure is still ineffective, repeat step 3.
5. Change the patient's position and attempt to aspirate.

Securing the Tube

After the correct position of the tip has been confirmed, the NG tube is secured to the nose (Fig. 36-3). A liquid skin barrier should be applied to the skin where the NG tube will be secured. The prepared area is covered with a strip of hypoallergenic tape or Op-site; the tube is then placed over the tape and secured with a second piece of tape. The nasoenteric tube can be secured by taping it to the forehead (see Fig. 36-3). This keeps the tube from dislodging when the patient moves but still allows it to pass into the intestine. Instead of tape, a feeding tube attachment device (Hollister) can be used to secure the tube. This device adheres to the nose and uses an adjustable clip to hold the tube in place (Fig. 36-4). The nurse should ensure thorough skin care and proper skin preparation is completed prior to applying the feeding tube attachment device. After the nasoenteric tube has progressed into the intestine (after approximately 24 hours), the tube may be taped in place.

Advancing the Nasoenteric Decompression Tube

After the tube has passed through the pyloric sphincter, it may be advanced 5 to 7.5 cm every hour. To enable gravity and peristalsis to assist in the passage of the tube, the patient is generally asked to lie in the following positions in this order: on the right side for 2 hours, on the back for 2 hours, and then on the left side for 2 hours. Ambulation, if possible, also helps advance the tube. If the tube is advanced too rapidly, it will curl and kink in the stomach. The tube is irrigated with normal saline

---

NURSING RESEARCH PROFILE 36-1

Assessment of Feeding Tube Location

Metheny, N. A., Smith, L., & Stewart, B. J. (2000). Development of a reliable and valid bedside test for bilirubin and its utility for improving prediction of feeding tube location. *Nursing Research, 49,* 302–309.

Purpose

Although a wide variety of methods have been used to assess feeding tube location at the bedside, pH testing of aspirate has been found to be the most reliable in differentiating between gastric and respiratory placement of the tube and between gastric and intestinal placement of the tube. However, it is not reliable in distinguishing intestinal from respiratory fluids, because both of these fluids are alkaline. One new method that is being studied to distinguish these fluids is testing the tube aspirate for bilirubin, which is normally found in intestinal fluids but not in respiratory fluids.

The purposes of this study were (1) to assess the validity of a visual bilirubin teststrip used with a colourimetric visual bilirubin (VBIL) scale to predict laboratory bilirubin values, (2) to evaluate the interrater reliability of staff nurses using the visual bilirubin test strip and VBIL scale, and (3) to evaluate the ability of the visual bilirubin test strip and VBIL scale in combination with pH testing to predict feeding tube placement in the respiratory tract, stomach, or intestine.

Study Sample and Design

Concurrent pH and bilirubin testing was conducted on 631 GI specimens obtained from adult, acutely ill patients with newly inserted feeding tubes; the testing was done within 5 minutes of x-ray studies obtained to confirm tube placement. Also, 225 respiratory specimens were tested. A teststrip and VBIL scale as well as laboratory assay were used to measure bilirubin. A pH meter and pH teststrips were used to measure pH. Results were read by research assistants and staff nurses, who were blinded to (unaware of) the source or type of specimens. These readings were compared with the x-ray results.

Findings

There was a high correlation (0.93) between the readings made from the VBIL scale and the laboratory bilirubin assay. A pH reading greater than 5 and a bilirubin reading lower than 5 mg/dL accurately identified 100% of the respiratory specimens. A pH of 5 or less and a bilirubin concentration lower than 5 mg/dL accurately identified 98% of the gastric specimens. Approximately 88% of the specimens with a pH greater than 5 and a bilirubin value of 5 mg/dL or higher were intestinal specimens.

Nursing Implications

Use of the VBIL scale and bilirubin test strip has the potential for greatly improving the accuracy of determining feeding tube placement at the bedside. However, before its approval by the U.S. Food and Drug Administration for this purpose, further refinements are required to make sure that the most accurate readings can be made. Until such approval, nurses must rely on the auscultatory method, pH measurements, and observations of the patient's physical status to determine tube placement. Any question about correct tube placement should be investigated, and placement should be confirmed by x-ray studies whenever indicated.

A

B

FIGURE 36-3 Securing NG and naso-enteric tubes. (**A**) The NG tube is secured to the nose with tape to prevent injury to the nasopharyngeal passages. (**B**) Tape is placed on the forehead and the nasoenteric tube is taped to it, thereby allowing the tube to be advanced until desired placement is achieved. (**C, D**) Secure tubing to the patient's gown with either an elastic band or tape attached to a safety pin to prevent tension on the line during movement of the patient.

C

D

solution every 6 to 8 hours to prevent blockage. Again, this type of tube placement is not commonly seen.

Monitoring the Patient and Maintaining Tube Function

If the NG tube is used for decompression, it is attached to intermittent low suction. If it is used for enteral nutrition, the end of the tube is plugged between feedings. The nurse confirms tube placement before any fluids or medications are instilled and once a shift for continuous feedings. Displacement of the tube may be caused by tension on the tube (when the patient moves around in the bed or room), coughing, tracheal or nasotracheal suctioning, or airway intubation. If the NG tube is removed inadvertently in a patient who has undergone esophageal or gastric surgery, it is replaced by the physician, usually under fluoroscopy to avoid trauma to the suture line.

It is important to keep an accurate record of all fluid intake, feedings, and irrigation. To maintain patency, the tube is irrigated every 4 to 6 hours with normal saline to avoid electrolyte loss through gastric drainage. If an automatic flush enteral pump is used, the flushing schedule may be altered. The nurse records the amount, colour, and type of all drainage every 8 hours.

When double- or triple-lumen tubes are used, each lumen is labelled according to its intended use: aspiration, feeding, or balloon inflation. To avoid tension on the tube, the portion of the tube from the nose to the drainage unit is fixed in position, either with a safety pin or with adhesive tape loops that are pinned to the patient's pajamas or gown. The tube must be looped loosely to prevent tension and dislodgement (see Fig. 36-3).

FIGURE 36-4 Feeding tube attachment device. Courtesy of Hollister, Incorporated.

Providing Oral and Nasal Hygiene

Regular and conscientious oral and nasal hygiene is a vital part of patient care, because the tube causes discomfort and pressure and may be in place for several days. Moistened cotton-tipped swabs can be used to clean the nose, followed by cleansing with a water-soluble lubricant. Frequent mouth care is comforting for the patient. The nasal tape is changed every 2 to 3 days, and the nose is inspected for skin irritation. If the nasal and pharyngeal mucosa are excessively dry, steam or cool vapor inhalations may be beneficial. Throat lozenges, an ice collar, chewing gum, or sucking on hard candies (if permitted), and frequent movement also assist in relieving patient discomfort. These activities keep the mucous membranes moist and help prevent inflammation of the parotid glands.

Monitoring and Managing Potential Complications

Patients with NG or nasoenteric intubation are susceptible to a variety of problems, including fluid volume deficit, pulmonary complications, and tube-related irritations. These potential complications require careful ongoing assessment.

Symptoms of fluid volume deficit include dry skin and mucous membranes, decreased urinary output, lethargy, and decreased body temperature. Assessment of fluid volume deficit involves maintaining an accurate record of intake and output. This includes measuring NG drainage, fluid instilled by irrigation of the NG tube, water taken by mouth, vomitus, water administered with tube feedings, and intravenous (IV) fluids. Laboratory values, particularly blood urea nitrogen and creatinine, are monitored. The nurse assesses 24-hour fluid balance and reports negative fluid balance, increased NG output, interruption of IV therapy, or any other disturbance in fluid intake or output.

Pulmonary complications from NG intubation occur because coughing and clearing of the pharynx are impaired, because gas buildup can irritate the phrenic nerve, and because tubes may become dislodged, retracting the distal end above the esophagogastric sphincter. Medications (antacids, simethicone, and metoclopramide) are administered to decrease potential problems. Signs and symptoms of complications include coughing during the administration of foods or medications, difficulty clearing the airway, tachypnea, and fever. Assessment includes regular auscultation of lung sounds and routine assessment of vital signs. It is important to encourage the patient to cough and to take deep breaths regularly. The nurse also carefully confirms the proper placement of the tube before instilling any fluids or medications.

Irritation of the mucous membranes is a common complication of NG intubation. The nostrils, oral mucosa, esophagus, and trachea are susceptible to irritation and necrosis. Visible areas are inspected frequently, and the adequacy of hydration is assessed. When providing oral hygiene, the nurse carefully inspects the mucous membranes for signs of irritation or excessive dryness. The nurse palpates the area around the parotid glands to detect any tenderness or enlarged nodes, indicating parotitis, and observes for any skin or mucous membrane irritation or necrosis. In addition, it is important to assess the patient for esophagitis and tracheitis; symptoms include sore throat and hoarseness.

Removing the Tube

Before removing a tube, the nurse may have orders to intermittently clamp and unclamp the NG tube for a trial period of 24 hours to ensure that the patient does not experience nausea, vomiting, or distention. Before the tube is removed, it is flushed with 10 mL of normal saline to ensure that it is free of debris and away from the gastric lining; then the balloon (if present) is deflated. Gloves are worn to remove the tube. The tube is withdrawn gently and slowly for 15 to 20 cm until the tip reaches the esophagus; the remainder is withdrawn rapidly from the nostril. A nasointestinal tube is withdrawn at intervals of 10 minutes until the end reaches the esophagus. If the tube does not come out easily, force should

not be used, and the problem should be reported to the physician. As the tube is withdrawn, it is concealed in a towel, because the sight of it may be unpleasant to the patient. After the tube is removed, the nurse provides oral hygiene.

Tube Feedings With Nasogastric and Nasoenteric Devices

Tube feedings are given to meet nutritional requirements when oral intake is inadequate or not possible and the GI tract is functioning normally. Tube feedings have several advantages over parenteral nutrition: they are low in cost, safe, well tolerated by the patient, and easy to use both in extended care facilities and in the patient's home. Tube feedings have other advantages:

- They preserve GI integrity by delivery of nutrients and medications (antacids, simethicone, and metoclopramide) intraluminally
- They preserve the normal sequence of intestinal and hepatic metabolism
- They maintain fat metabolism and lipoprotein synthesis
- They maintain normal insulin/glucagon ratios

Tube feedings are delivered to the stomach (in the case of NG intubation or gastrostomy) or to the distal duodenum or proximal jejunum (in the case of nasoduodenal or **nasojejunal tube** feeding). Nasoduodenal or nasojejunal feeding is indicated when the esophagus and stomach need to be bypassed or when the patient is at risk for **aspiration** (breathing fluids or foods into the trachea and lungs). For long-term feedings (longer than 4 weeks), nasoduodenal, gastrostomy, or jejunostomy tubes are preferred for administration of medications or food. The numerous conditions requiring enteral nutrition are summarized in Table 36-2.

OSMOSIS AND OSMOLALITY

Osmolality is an important consideration for patients receiving tube feedings through the duodenum or jejunum, because feeding formulas with a high osmolality may lead to undesirable effects, such as dumping syndrome (described below).

Fluid balance is maintained by **osmosis**, the process by which water moves through membranes from a dilute solution of lower **osmolality** (ionic concentration) to a more concentrated solution of higher osmolality until both solutions are of nearly equal osmolality. The osmolality of normal body fluids is approximately 300 mOsm/kg. The body attempts to keep the osmolality of the contents of the stomach and intestines at approximately this level.

Highly concentrated solutions and certain foods can upset the normal fluid balance in the body. Individual amino acids and carbohydrates are small particles that have great osmotic effect. Proteins are extremely large particles and therefore have less osmotic effect. Fats are not water-soluble and do not enter into a solution in water; thus, they have no osmotic effect. Electrolytes, such as sodium and potassium, are comparatively small particles; they have a great effect on osmolality and consequently on the patient's ability to tolerate a given solution.

When a concentrated solution of high osmolality is taken in large amounts, water will move to the stomach and intestines from fluid surrounding the organs and the vascular compartment. The patient has a feeling of fullness, nausea, and diarrhea; this causes

Table 36-2 • Conditions Requiring Enteral Therapy

CONDITION OR NEED	EXAMPLES
Preoperative bowel preparation	—
Gastrointestinal problems	Fistula, short-bowel syndrome, mild pancreatitis, Crohn's disease, ulcerative colitis, nonspecific maldigestion or malabsorption
Cancer therapy	Radiation, chemotherapy
Convalescent care	Surgery, injury, severe illness
Coma, semiconsciousness*	Stroke, head injury, neurologic disorder, neoplasm
Hypermetabolic conditions	Burns, trauma, multiple fractures, sepsis, AIDS, organ transplantation
Alcoholism, chronic depression, anorexia nervosa*	Chronic illness, psychiatric or neurologic disorder
Debilitation*	Disease or injury
Maxillofacial or cervical surgery	Disease or injury
Oropharyngeal or esophageal paralysis*	Disease or injury, neoplasm, inflammation, trauma, respiratory failure

*Because some of these patients are at risk for regurgitating or vomiting and aspirating administered formula, each condition must be considered individually.

dehydration, hypotension, and tachycardia, collectively termed the **dumping syndrome**. Starting with a more dilute solution and increasing the concentration over several days can generally alleviate this problem. Patients vary in the degree to which they tolerate the effects of high osmolality; usually debilitated patients are more sensitive. The nurse needs to be knowledgeable about the osmolality of the patient's formula and needs to observe for and take steps to prevent undesired effects.

TUBE FEEDING FORMULAS

The choice of formula to be delivered by tube feeding is influenced by the status of the GI tract and the nutritional needs of the patient. The formula characteristics evaluated include chemical composition of the nutrient source (protein, carbohydrates, fat), caloric density, osmolality, residue, bacteriologic safety, vitamins, minerals, and cost.

Various major formula types for tube feedings are available commercially. Blenderized formulas can be made by the patient's family or obtained in a ready-to-use form that is carefully prepared according to directions. Commercially prepared polymeric formulas (formulas with high molecular weight) are composed of protein, carbohydrates, and fats in a high-molecular-weight form (Boost Plus, TwoCal HN, Isosource). Chemically defined formulas contain predigested and easy-to-absorb nutrients (Osmolite HN). Modular products contain only one major nutrient, such as protein (Promote). Disease-specific formulas are available for various conditions, such as renal failure (Nepro), severe chronic obstructive pulmonary disease (Pulmocare). Nepro is high in calories and low in electrolytes. It is ideal for patients who require electrolyte and fluid restriction. Pulmocare is high in fat and low in carbohydrates. Its high density (1.5 calories/mL) is ideal for patients who require fluid restriction, and it is also designed to reduce carbon dioxide production. Fibre has also been added to formulas (Jevity) in an attempt to decrease the occurrence of diarrhea. Some feedings are given as supplements, and others are designed to meet the patient's total nutritional needs. Dietitians collaborate with physicians and nurses in determining the best formula for the individual patient.

NURSING ALERT Commercial formulas frequently present problems because the composition is fixed and some patients are not able to tolerate certain ingredients, such as sodium, protein, or potassium. Modular products may be substituted, and the critical constituents of sodium, potassium, and fat can be added. Attention is given to including all essential minerals and vitamins. Total intake of calories, nutrients, and fluids must be assessed when there is a reduction in total intake or excessive dilution of feedings.

TUBE FEEDING ADMINISTRATION METHODS

Many patients do not tolerate NG and nasoenteric tube feedings well. Often a medium- or fine-bore Silastic nasoenteric tube is tolerated better than a plastic or rubber tube. The finer-bore tube requires a finely dispersed formula to ensure that the patency of the tube is maintained. For long-term tube feeding therapy, a gastrostomy or jejunostomy tube is used (see later discussion).

The tube feeding method chosen depends on the location of the tube, patient tolerance, convenience, and cost. Intermittent bolus feedings are administered into the stomach (usually by gastrostomy tube) in large amounts at designated intervals and may be given 4 to 8 times per day. The intermittent gravity drip is another method for administering tube feedings into the stomach and is commonly used when the patient is at home. In this instance, the tube feeding is administered over 30 minutes at designated intervals. Both of these tube-feeding methods are practical and inexpensive. However, the feedings delivered at variable rates may be poorly tolerated and time-consuming.

The continuous infusion method is used when feedings are administered into the small intestine. This method is preferred for patients who are at risk for aspiration or who tolerate the tube feedings poorly. The feedings are given continuously at a constant rate by means of a pump. The continuous tube feeding method, which requires a pump device, decreases abdominal distention, gastric residuals, and the risk of aspiration. However, pumps are expensive, and they permit the patient less flexibility than intermittent feedings do.

An alternative to the continuous infusion method is **cyclic feeding**. The infusion is given at a faster rate over a shorter time (usually 8 to 12 hours). Feeding may be infused at night to avoid interrupting the patient's lifestyle. Cyclic continuous infusions may be appropriate for patients who are being weaned from tube feedings to an oral diet, as a supplement for a patient who cannot eat enough, and for patients at home who need daytime hours free from the pump.

Tube feeding solutions vary in terms of required preparation, consistency, and the number of calories and supplemental vitamins they contain. The choice of solution depends on the size and location of the tube, the patient's nutrient needs, the type of nutritional supplement, the method of delivery, and the convenience for the patient at home. A wide variety of containers, feeding tubes and catheters, delivery systems, and pumps are available for use with tube feedings.

NURSING PROCESS: THE PATIENT RECEIVING A TUBE FEEDING

Assessment

A preliminary assessment of the patient who requires a tube feeding includes several considerations, as well as the family's need for information:

- What is the patient's nutritional status, as judged by current physical appearance, dietary history, and recent weight loss?
- Are there any existing chronic illnesses or factors that will increase metabolic demands on the body (eg, surgical stress, fever)?
- What is the patient's hydration status? What are the electrolyte levels?
- Is the patient's digestive tract functioning?
- Are the kidneys functioning normally?
- Are fluid requirements (ie, 30 to 40 mL/kg body weight) being met?
- What medications and other therapies is the patient receiving that may affect digestive intake and function of the digestive system?
- Does the dietary prescription fulfill the patient's needs?

In addition, a more elaborate assessment is performed for patients who require extensive nutritional therapy. A team that includes the nurse, physician, and dietitian conducts this assessment. In addition to the history and physical examination (which includes anthropometric measurements), nutritional assessment consists of recording any weight change; determining albumin, prealbumin, and transferrin levels and total lymphocyte count; testing for the delayed hypersensitivity reaction; and evaluating muscle function. (See Chapter 5 for a detailed description of nutritional assessment.)

Diagnosis

NURSING DIAGNOSES

Based on the assessment data, the major nursing diagnoses may include the following:

- Imbalanced nutrition, less than body requirements, related to inadequate intake of nutrients
- Risk for diarrhea related to the dumping syndrome or to tube feeding intolerance
- Risk for ineffective airway clearance related to aspiration of tube feeding
- Risk for deficient fluid volume related to hypertonic dehydration
- Risk for ineffective coping related to discomfort imposed by the presence of the NG or nasoenteric tube
- Risk for ineffective therapeutic regimen management
- Deficient knowledge about home tube feeding regimen

COLLABORATIVE PROBLEMS/ POTENTIAL COMPLICATIONS

Complications of NG and nasoenteric tube feeding therapy are classified into three types—GI, mechanical, and metabolic. Table 36-3 lists complications, possible causes, and appropriate interventions.

Planning and Goals

The major goals for the patient may include nutritional balance, normal bowel elimination pattern, reduced risk of aspiration, adequate hydration, individual coping, knowledge and skill in self-care, and prevention of complications.

Nursing Interventions

MAINTAINING FEEDING EQUIPMENT AND NUTRITIONAL BALANCE

The temperature and volume of the feeding, the flow rate, and the total fluid intake are important factors to be considered when tube feedings are administered. The schedule of tube feedings, including the correct quantity and frequency, is maintained. The nurse must carefully monitor the drip rate and avoid administering fluids too rapidly.

Feedings are administered by gravity (drip), bolus, or continuous controlled pump (mL/hour or drops/hour). Gravity feedings are placed above the level of the stomach, with the speed of administration determined by gravity. **Bolus** feedings are given in large volumes (300 to 400 mL every 4 to 6 hours). Continuous feeding is the preferred method; delivery of the feeding in small amounts over long periods reduces the incidence of aspiration, distention, nausea, vomiting, and diarrhea. Continuous administration rates of about 100 to 150 mL/hour (2400 to 3600 calories/day) are effective in inducing positive nitrogen balance and progressive weight gain without producing abdominal cramps and diarrhea. If the feeding is intermittent, 200 to 350 mL is given in 10 to 15 minutes. Enteral pumps are mechanical devices that control the delivery rate of feeding formula (Fig. 36-5). Pumps allow for a constant flow rate and can infuse a viscous formula through a small-diameter feeding tube. These pumps are relatively heavy and must be attached to an IV pole. For home use, there are portable lightweight enteral pumps available that weigh about 1.75 kilograms and are easy to handle. An enteral pump is available with an automatic water flush system. In addition to administering the feeding formula, these pumps provide hourly water flushes that are designed to prevent clogged feeding tubes (Petnicki, 1998).

Residual gastric content is measured before each intermittent feeding and every 4 to 8 hours during continuous feedings. (This aspirated fluid is readministered to the patient.) The research findings of McClave et al. (1992) indicated that, if the amount of aspirated gastric content is greater than or equal to 200 mL for

Table 36-3 • Complications of Enteral Therapy

COMPLICATIONS	CAUSES	SELECTED NURSING INTERVENTIONS
Gastrointestinal		
Diarrhea (most common)	Hyperosmolar feedings Rapid infusion/bolus feedings Bacteria-contaminated feedings Lactase deficiency Medications/antibiotic therapy Decreased serum osmolality level Food allergies Cold formula	Assess fluid balance and electrolyte levels; report findings Assess rate of infusion and temperature of formula Implement changes in tube feeding formula or rate Replace formula every 4 hours; change tube feeding container and tubing daily
Nausea/vomiting	Change in rate Hyperosmolar formula Inadequate gastric emptying	Check residuals; if ≥ 200 mL for NG or >100 mL for gastrostomy, continue feeding and recheck; report if residual is still high Review medications
Gas/bloating/cramping	Air in tube	Keep tubing free of air
Dumping syndrome	Bolus feedings/rapid rate Cold formula	Check fibre and water content; report findings Check rate and temperature of formula
Constipation	High milk (lactose) content Lack of fibre Inadequate fluid intake/dehydration	Check fibre and water content; report findings
Mechanical		
Aspiration pneumonia	Improper tube placement Vomiting and aspirated tube feeding Flat in bed Use of large tube	Implement reliable method for checking small-bore enteral tube placement (ie, measuring length of exposed tube) Keep head of bed elevated 30 degrees continuously
Tube displacement	Excessive coughing/vomitus Tension on the tube or unsecured tube Tracheal suctioning Airway intubation	Check tube placement before administering feeding
Tube obstruction	Inadequate flushing/formula rate	Follow policy for flushing of tube and for crushing medications
Residue	Inadequate crushing of medications and flushing after administration	Obtain liquid medications when possible Flush feeding tube before and after medication administration
Nasopharyngeal irritation	Tube position/improper taping Use of large tubes	Tape tube to prevent pressure on nares Assess nasopharyngeal mucous membranes every 4 hours
Metabolic		
Hyperglycemia	Glucose intolerance High carbohydrate content of the feeding	Check blood glucose levels periodically
Dehydration and azotemia (excessive urea in the blood)	Hyperosmolar feedings with insufficient fluid intake	Report signs and symptoms of dehydration Implement changes in tube feeding formula, rate, or ratio to water
Tube feeding syndrome	Excessive urea from high-protein mix- ture and formulas lacking fat Dehydration	Implement changes in tube feeding formula, rate, or ratio to water

NG tubes or if residual volumes are greater than or equal to 100 mL for gastrostomy tubes, tube feeding intolerance should be considered. Tube feedings may be continued with close monitoring of gastric residual volume, radiographic studies, and the patient's physical status. If excessive residual volumes occur twice, the nurse notifies the physician.

Maintaining tube function is an ongoing responsibility of the nurse, patient, or primary caregiver. To ensure patency and to decrease the chance of bacterial growth, crusting, or occlusion of the tube, 20 to 30 mL of water is administered in each of the following instances:

- Before and after each dose of medication and each tube feeding
- After checking for gastric residuals and gastric pH

- Every 4 to 6 hours with continuous feedings
- If the tube feeding is discontinued for any reason

PROVIDING MEDICATIONS BY TUBE

When different types of medications are administered, each type is given separately, using a bolus method that is compatible with the medication's preparation (Table 36-4). The tube is flushed with 20 to 30 mL of water after each dose. If a liquid form of a medication is not available and the medication can be crushed, it must first be reduced to a fine powder or the tube will become clogged. Devices are available (eg, Handicrush Irrigation Syringe by Nestle) that crush and dissolve tablets with water (Fig. 36-6). Medications are not mixed with each other or with the feeding formula. When small-bore feeding tubes for continuous infusion

Enteral feeding container

Enteral feeding pump

8 Fr. feeding tube

Flexible weighted tip

FIGURE 36-5 Nasoenteric tube feeding by continuous controlled pump.

are irrigated after medication administration, a 30-mL or larger syringe is used, because the pressure generated by smaller syringes could rupture the tube.

MAINTAINING FEEDING REGIMENS AND DELIVERY SYSTEMS

Tube feeding formula is delivered to patients by either an open or a closed system. The open system comes in cans or as a powder and may be mixed with water. The feeding container (which is hung on a pole) and the tubing used with the open system are changed—usually every 24 to 72 hours. To avoid bacterial contamination, the amount of feeding formula in the bag should never exceed what is expected to be infused in 4 hours.

Closed delivery systems use a prefilled, sterile container that is spiked with enteral tubing. The bag holding the feeding formula for the closed system can be hung safely for 24 to 48 hours.

The tube-feeding regimen must be assessed frequently to evaluate its effectiveness and avoid complications (Chart 36-1).

MAINTAINING NORMAL BOWEL ELIMINATION PATTERN

Patients receiving NG or nasoenteric tube feedings commonly have diarrhea (watery stools occurring three or more times in 24 hours). Pasty, unformed stool is expected with enteral therapy, because many formulas have little or no residue. The dumping syndrome also leads to diarrhea, but to confirm dumping syndrome as the cause of diarrhea other possible causes must be ruled out, among them the following:

- Zinc deficiency—Adding 15 mg of zinc to the tube feeding every 24 hours is recommended to maintain a normal serum level of 7.65 to 22.95 fmol/L
- Contaminated formula

Table 36-4 • Preparing Medication for Delivery by Feeding Tube

MEDICATION FORM	PREPARATION
Liquid	None
Simple compressed tablets	Crush and dissolve in water
Buccal or sublingual tablets	Administer as prescribed
Soft gelatin capsules filled with liquid	Make an opening in capsule and squeeze out contents
Enteric-coated tablets	Do not crush; change in form is required
Timed-release tablets	Do not crush tablets because doing so may release too much drug too quickly (overdose); check with pharmacist for alternative formulation
Timed-release capsules or sustained-release capsules	Some can be opened and contents added to tube-feeding formula; *always* check with pharmacist before doing this

FIGURE 36-6 The Pill Crusher™ Syringe (from Welcon, Inc.) crushes medications to a fine powder and then allows them to be administered to persons with feeding tubes. The Pill Crusher™ is also used to irrigate the feeding tube and assists in hydrating the patient. Courtesy of Welcon, Inc., Fort Worth, TX (www.welcon.com).

- Malnutrition—A decrease in the intestinal absorptive area resulting from malnutrition can cause diarrhea
- Medication therapy—Antibiotics, such as clindamycin (Dalacin) and lincomycin (Lincocin); antiarrhythmics, such as quinidine and propranolol (Apo-Propranolol, Novopranolol); and aminophylline, theophylline, and digitalis have been found to increase the frequency of diarrhea in some patients

The dumping syndrome results from rapid distention of the jejunum when hypertonic solutions are administered quickly (over 10 to 20 minutes). Foods high in carbohydrates and electrolytes draw extracellular fluid from the vascular system into the jejunum so that dilution and absorption can occur. Measures for managing the GI symptoms (diarrhea, nausea) associated with the dumping syndrome are presented in Chart 36-2.

REDUCING THE RISK OF ASPIRATION

Aspiration pneumonia occurs when stomach contents or enteral feedings are regurgitated and aspirated, or when an NG tube is improperly positioned and feedings are instilled into the pharynx or the trachea. Nasoenteric tubes, especially those that provide for gastric and esophageal or duodenal decompression, have helped decrease the frequency of regurgitation and aspiration.

To prevent aspiration, the nurse must establish the correct tube feeding placement before every feeding, each time medications are administered, and once every shift if the tube feeding is continuous. Feedings and medications should always be given with the patient in the proper position to prevent regurgitation. To reduce the risk of reflux and pulmonary aspiration, the semi-Fowler's position is necessary for an NG feeding, with the patient's head elevated at least 30 to 45 degrees. This position is maintained at least 1 hour after completion of an intermittent tube feeding and is maintained at all times for patients receiving continuous tube feedings. Another prevention strategy is to monitor residual volumes (Edwards & Metheny, 2000).

If aspiration is suspected, the feeding is stopped immediately, the pharynx and trachea are suctioned, and the patient is placed on the right side with the head of the bed down. The physician is notified immediately.

MAINTAINING ADEQUATE HYDRATION

The nurse carefully monitors hydration because, in many cases, the patient cannot communicate the need for water. Water (at least 2 L/day) is given every 4 to 6 hours and after feedings to prevent hypertonic dehydration. At the beginning of administration, the feeding is diluted to at least half-strength and not more than 50 to 100 mL is given at a time, or 40 to 60 mL/hour is given in continuous drip administration. This gradual administration helps the patient to develop tolerance, especially for hyperosmo-

---

Chart 36-1 • ASSESSMENT

Measures for Assessing Tube Feeding Regimens

The following nursing measures may be implemented when assessing the effectiveness and safety of tube feeding:

1. Assess tube placement, patient's position (head of bed elevated 30 to 45 degrees), and formula flow rate.
2. Determine the patient's ability to tolerate the formula. Observe for fullness, bloating, distention, urticaria, nausea, vomiting, and stool pattern and character.
3. Check clinical responses, as noted in laboratory findings (blood urea nitrogen, serum protein, prealbumin, electrolytes, renal function, hemoglobin, hematocrit).
4. Observe for signs of dehydration (dry mucous membranes, thirst, decreased urine output).
5. Record the amount of formula actually taken in by the patient.
6. Report an elevated blood glucose level, decreased urinary output, sudden weight gain, and periorbital or dependent edema.
7. Replace any formula administered by an open system every 4 hours with fresh formula. Formula should be at room temperature or cool (not cold).
8. Change tube feeding container and tubing every 24 to 72 hours.
9. Assess residual volume before each feeding or, in the case of continuous feedings, every 4 hours. Return the aspirate to the stomach.
10. Monitor intake and output.
11. Weigh the patient twice weekly.
12. Consult the dietitian regularly.

Chart 36-2 **Preventing Symptoms of Dumping Syndrome**

The following strategies may help prevent some of the uncomfortable symptoms of dumping syndrome related to tube feeding:

- Slow the formula instillation rate to provide time for carbohydrates and electrolytes to be diluted.
- Administer feedings at room temperature, because temperature extremes stimulate peristalsis.
- Administer feeding by continuous drip (if tolerated) rather than by bolus, to prevent sudden distention of the intestine.
- Advise the patient to remain in semi-Fowler's position for 1 hour after the feeding; this position prolongs intestinal transit time by decreasing the effect of gravity.
- Instill the minimal amount of water needed to flush the tubing before and after a feeding, because fluid given with a feeding increases intestinal transit time.

lar solutions. Key nursing interventions include observing for signs of dehydration (dry mucous membranes, thirst, decreased urine output); administering water routinely and as needed; and monitoring intake, output, and fluid balance (24-hour intake versus output).

PROMOTING COPING ABILITY

The psychosocial goal of nursing care is to support and encourage the patient to accept physical changes and to convey hope that daily progressive improvement is possible. If the patient is having difficulty adjusting to the treatment, the nurse intervenes by encouraging self-care (eg, recording daily weight and intake and output), within the parameters of the patient's activity level. In addition, the nurse reinforces an optimistic approach by identifying signs and symptoms that indicate progress (daily weight gain, electrolyte balance, absence of nausea and diarrhea).

PROMOTING HOME AND COMMUNITY-BASED CARE

Teaching Patients Self-Care

Patients who require long-term tube feedings in the home care setting have conditions such as obstruction of the upper GI tract, malabsorption syndrome, surgery of the GI tract or of the head or neck region, or decreased level of consciousness. For a patient to be considered for tube feeding at home, the following criteria must be met: The patient must be medically stable and must have successfully completed a tube feeding trial (tolerated 70% of feeding). In addition, the patient must be capable of self-care or have a caregiver who is willing to assume the responsibility, and the patient or caregiver must have access to supplies and interest in learning how to administer tube feedings at home.

Preparation of the patient for home administration of enteral feedings begins while the patient is still hospitalized. Ideally, the nurse teaches while administering the feedings so that the patient can observe the mechanics of the procedure, participate in the procedure, ask questions, and express any concerns. Before discharge, the nurse provides information about the equipment needed, formula purchase and storage, and administration of the feedings (frequency, quantity, rate of instillation).

Family members who will be active in the patient's home care are encouraged to participate in all teaching sessions. Available printed information about the equipment, the formula, and the procedure is reviewed. The nurse encourages the patient and caregiver to learn to use the equipment with the supervision of the nurse. Arrangements are made for the caregiver to obtain the equipment and formula and have it ready for use before the patient's discharge.

Continuing Care

Referral to a home care agency is important so that a nurse can arrange to be present to supervise and provide support during the first feeding at home. Further visits will depend on the skill and comfort of the patient or caregiver in administering the feedings. During all visits, the nurse monitors the patient's physical status (weight, vital signs, activity level) and the ability of the patient and family to administer the tube feedings correctly. In addition, the nurse assesses for any complications (dumping syndrome, nausea or vomiting, weight loss, lethargy, confusion, excessive thirst). The patient or caregiver is encouraged to keep a diary to record times and amounts of feedings and any symptoms that occur. The nurse reviews the diary with the patient and caregiver during home visits.

Evaluation

EXPECTED PATIENT OUTCOMES

Expected patient outcomes may include the following:

1. Attains or maintains nutritional balance
   a. Has a positive nitrogen balance
   b. Maintains laboratory values within normal limits (ie, blood urea nitrogen, hemoglobin, hematocrit, prealbumin, serum protein)
   c. Attains or maintains hydration of body tissue
   d. Attains or maintains desired body weight
2. Is free of episodes of diarrhea
   a. Has fewer than three watery stools a day
   b. Does not have a bowel movement after a bolus feeding
   c. States that there is no intestinal cramping
   d. Has normal bowel sounds
3. Avoids aspiration
   a. Lungs are clear to auscultation
   b. Exhibits normal heart rate and respirations
4. Attains or maintains hydration of body tissue
   a. Has a balanced intake and output every 24 hours
   b. Does not have dry skin or dry mucous membranes
5. Copes effectively with tube feeding regimen
6. Demonstrates skill in managing tube feeding regimen
7. Experiences no complications
   a. Has no GI disturbances
   b. Tube remains intact and patent for duration of therapy
   c. Maintains metabolic balance within normal limits

Gastrostomy

A **gastrostomy** is a surgical procedure in which an opening is created into the stomach for the purpose of administering foods and fluids. In some instances, a gastrostomy is preferred for prolonged nutrition (greater then 3 to 4 weeks)—for example, in the elderly or debilitated patient. Gastrostomy is also preferred over NG feedings in the comatose patient because the gastroesophageal sphincter remains intact. Regurgitation and aspiration are less likely to occur with a gastrostomy than with NG feedings.

Different types of feeding gastrostomies may be used, including the Stamm (temporary and permanent), Janeway (permanent), and percutaneous endoscopic gastrostomy (temporary) systems. The Stamm and Janeway gastrostomies require either an upper abdominal midline incision or a left upper quadrant transverse incision. The Stamm procedure requires the use of concentric purse-string sutures to secure the tube to the anterior gastric wall. To create the gastrostomy, an exit wound is created in the left upper abdomen. The Janeway procedure necessitates the creation of a tunnel (called a gastric tube) that is brought out through the abdomen to form a permanent **stoma**.

A **percutaneous endoscopic gastrostomy (PEG)** is a procedure that requires the services of two physicians (or a physician and a nurse with specialty skills). After administering a local anesthetic, one physician inserts a cannula into the stomach through an abdominal incision and then threads a nonabsorbable suture through the cannula; the second physician looks through an endoscope that has been passed into the upper GI tract and uses the endoscopic snare to grasp the end of the suture and guide it up through the patient's mouth. The suture is knotted to the dilator tip at the end of the PEG tube. The endoscopist then advances the dilator tip through the patient's mouth while the first physician pulls the suture through the cannula site. The attached PEG tube is guided down the esophagus, into the stomach, and out through the abdominal incision (Fig. 36-7A). The mushroom catheter tip and internal crossbar secure the tube against the stomach wall. An external crossbar or bumper keeps the catheter in place. A tubing adaptor is in place between feedings, and a clamp or plug is used to close or open the tubing. If an endoscope is unable to pass through the esophagus, then the gastrostomy can be performed under x-ray guidance through the abdominal wall. This procedure is known as fluoroscopically guided percutaneous gastrostomy, or FGPG (Johnson, 1997).

The initial PEG device can be removed and replaced once the tract is well established (10 to 14 days after insertion). Replacement of the PEG device is indicated to provide long-term nutritional support, to replace a clotted or migrated tube, or to enhance patient comfort. The PEG replacement device should be fitted securely to the stoma to prevent leakage of gastric acid and is maintained in place through traction between the internal and anchoring devices.

An alternative to the PEG device is a **low-profile gastrostomy device (LPGD)** (see Fig. 36-7B). The LPGD may be inserted 3 to 6 months after initial gastrostomy tube placement. These devices are inserted flush with the skin; they eliminate the possibility of tube migration and obstruction and have antireflux valves to prevent gastric reflux. Two types of devices may be used—obturated or nonobturated. The obturated devices (G-button) have a dome tip that acts as an internal stabilizer. A major drawback is the need for a physician to obturate (insert a tube that is larger than the actual stoma). The nonobturated device (MIC-KEY) has an external skin disk and is inserted into the stoma without force; a balloon is inflated to secure placement. A nurse in the home setting can insert these devices easily. The drawbacks of both types of LPGDs are the inability to check residual volumes (one-way valve) and the need for a special adaptor to connect the device to the feeding container.

Patients with severe gastroesophageal reflux are at risk for aspiration pneumonia and therefore are not candidates for a gastrostomy. A jejunostomy is preferred, or jejunal feeding through a nasojejunal tube may be recommended.

NURSING PROCESS:
THE PATIENT WITH A GASTROSTOMY
Assessment

The focus of the preoperative assessment is to determine the patient's ability both to understand and to cope with the impending surgical experience. The nurse evaluates the patient's ability to adjust to a change in body image and to participate in self-care, along with the patient's and the family's psychological status.

The purpose of the operative procedure is explained so that the patient will have a better understanding of the expected postoperative course. The patient needs to know that the result of this surgery is to bypass the mouth and esophagus so that liquid feedings can be administered directly into the stomach by means of a rubber or plastic tube or a prosthesis. If the prosthesis is to be permanent, the patient should be made aware of this. Psychologically, this is often difficult for the patient to accept. If the procedure is being performed to relieve discomfort, prolonged vomiting, debilitation, or an inability to eat, the patient may find it more acceptable.

The nurse evaluates the patient's skin condition and determines whether a delay in healing may be anticipated because of a systemic disorder (eg, diabetes mellitus, cancer).

In a Canadian-based article, preoperative nutritional assessments and patient teaching, occurring at least 1 week preoperatively, was implemented (Watt & Lewis, 2001). Watt and Lewis (2001) described the potential benefits of this patient-focused approach, including reduced hospital stays.

In the postoperative period, the patient's fluid and nutritional needs are assessed to ensure proper intake of food and fluids. The nurse inspects the tube for proper maintenance and the incision for signs of infection. At the same time, the nurse evaluates the patient's response to the change in body image and the patient's understanding of the feeding methods. Interventions are identified to help the patient cope with the tube and learn self-care measures.

Diagnosis
NURSING DIAGNOSES
Based on the assessment data, the major nursing diagnoses in the postoperative period may include the following:

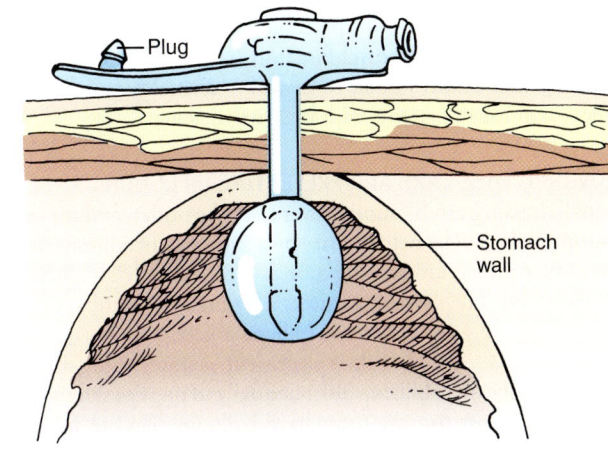

FIGURE 36-7 (**A**) A detail of the abdomen and the PEG tube, showing catheter fixation. (**B**) A detail of the abdomen and the nonobturated LPGD, showing balloon fixation.

- Imbalanced nutrition, less than body requirements, related to enteral feeding problems
- Risk for infection related to presence of wound and tube
- Risk for impaired skin integrity at tube site
- Ineffective coping related to inability to eat normally
- Disturbed body image related to presence of tube
- Risk for ineffective therapeutic regimen management related to knowledge deficit about home care and the feeding procedure

COLLABORATIVE PROBLEMS/ POTENTIAL COMPLICATIONS

Potential complications that may develop include the following:

- Wound infection, cellulitis, and abdominal wall abscess
- GI bleeding
- Premature removal of the tube

Planning and Goals

The major goals for the patient may include attaining an optimal level of nutrition, preventing infection, maintaining skin integrity, enhancing coping, adjusting to changes in body image, acquiring knowledge of and skill in self-care, and preventing complications.

Nursing Interventions

MEETING NUTRITIONAL NEEDS

The first fluid nourishment is administered soon after surgery and usually consists of tap water and 10% glucose. At first, only 30 to 60 mL is given at one time, but the amount is increased gradually. By the second day, 180 to 240 mL may be given at one time, provided it is tolerated and no leakage of fluid occurs around the tube. Water and milk can be instilled after 24 hours for a permanent gastrostomy. High-calorie liquids are added gradually. In some settings, during the early postoperative period the nurse aspirates gastric secretions and reinstills them after adding enough feeding solution to bring the volume to the desired total. By this method, gastric dilation is avoided.

Blenderized foods are added gradually to clear liquids until a full diet is achieved. Powdered feedings that are easily liquefied are commercially available. The patient who receives blenderized tube feedings typically is not forced to give up usual dietary patterns, which may prove to be psychologically more acceptable. In addition, near-normal bowel function is promoted because the fibre and residue are similar to that of a normal diet. Intake of milk is avoided in patients with lactase deficiency.

PROVIDING TUBE CARE AND PREVENTING INFECTION

A small dressing can be applied over the tube outlet, and the gastrostomy tube can be held in place by a thin strip of adhesive tape that is first placed around the tube and then firmly attached to the abdomen. The dressing protects the skin around the incision from seepage of gastric acid and spillage of feedings.

The nurse verifies the tube's placement, assesses residuals, and rotates the tube or stabilizing disk once daily to prevent skin breakdown. Some gastrostomy tubes have balloons that are inflated with water to anchor the tube in the stomach. The adequacy of balloon inflation is checked weekly by deflating the balloon using a Luer-tip syringe.

PROVIDING SKIN CARE

The skin surrounding a gastrostomy requires special care because it may become irritated from the enzymatic action of gastric juices that leak around the tube. Left untreated, the skin becomes macerated, red, raw, and painful. The nurse washes the area around the tube with soap and water daily, removes any encrustation with saline solution, rinses the area well with water, and pats it dry. Once the stoma heals and drainage ceases, a dressing is not required. A long-term gastrostomy may require a special dressing or stabilization device to protect the skin around the tube from gastric secretions and to help secure the tube in place (Fig. 36-8).

Skin at the exit site is evaluated daily for signs of breakdown, irritation, excoriation, and the presence of drainage or gastric leakage. The nurse encourages the patient and family members to participate in this inspection and in hygiene activities. If skin problems do occur, an enterostomal therapist or wound care specialist can be of assistance.

ENHANCING BODY IMAGE

The patient with a gastrostomy has experienced a major assault to body image. Eating, a physiologic and social function, can no longer be taken for granted. The patient is also aware that gastrostomy as a therapeutic intervention is performed only in the presence of a major, chronic, or perhaps terminal illness.

Calm discussion of the purposes and routines of gastrostomy feeding can help keep the patient from feeling overwhelmed. Talking with a person who has had a gastrostomy can also help the patient to accept the expected changes. Adjusting to a change in body image takes time and requires family support and acceptance. Evaluating the existing family support system is necessary. One family member may emerge as the primary support person.

MONITORING AND MANAGING POTENTIAL COMPLICATIONS

During the postoperative course, the nurse monitors the patient for potential complications. The most common complications are wound infection and other wound problems, including cellulitis at the wound site and abscesses in the abdominal wall. Because many patients who receive tube feedings are debilitated and have compromised nutritional status, any signs of infections are promptly

FIGURE 36-8 Protection at the gastrostomy site. A PEG tube may be protected by a dressing that allows access to the tube but covers the exit site. Typically the tube is stabilized with tape over the dressing. From Craven, R., & Hirnle, C. (2002). *Fundamentals of nursing: Human health and function* (4th ed.). Philadelphia: Lippincott Williams & Wilkins.

reported to the physician so that appropriate antibiotic therapy can be instituted.

Bleeding from the insertion site in the stomach may also occur. The nurse closely monitors the patient's vital signs and observes all drainage from the operative site, vomitus, and stool for evidence of bleeding. Any signs of bleeding are reported promptly.

Premature removal of the tube, whether it is done inadvertently by the patient or by the caregiver, is another complication. If the tube is removed prematurely, the skin is cleansed and a sterile dressing is applied; the nurse immediately notifies the physician. The tract will close within 4 to 6 hours if the tube is not replaced promptly. Some Canadian institutions and care settings request that a sterile Foley catheter be inserted into the stoma tract until a physician can assess the patient.

PROMOTING HOME AND COMMUNITY-BASED CARE

Teaching Patients Self-Care

The patient who is to receive gastrostomy tube feedings in the home setting must be capable of, and responsible for, administering the tube feedings or have a caregiver who is able to do so. There must also be the physical, financial, and social resources to maintain care.

The nurse assesses the patient's level of knowledge, interest in learning about the tube feeding, and ability to understand and apply the information before providing detailed instructions about how to prepare the formula and manage the tube feeding. Written materials for patients and caregivers are designed to outline the care instructions. To facilitate self-care, the nurse encourages the patient to participate in the tube feedings during hospitalization and to establish as normal a routine as possible.

Demonstration of the tube feeding begins by showing the patient how to check for residual gastric contents before the feeding. The patient then learns how to check and maintain the patency of the tube by administering room-temperature water before and after the feeding. This will establish patency before the feeding and then clear the tube of food particles, which could decompose if allowed to remain in the tube. All feedings are given at room temperature or near body temperature.

For a bolus feeding, the nurse shows the patient how to introduce the liquid into the catheter by using a funnel or the barrel of a syringe. The receptacle is tilted to allow air to escape while the liquid is being instilled initially. As the funnel or syringe fills with liquid, the feeding is allowed to flow into the stomach by gravity by holding the barrel or syringe perpendicular to the abdomen (Fig. 36-9). Raising or lowering the receptacle to no higher than 45 cm above the abdominal wall regulates the rate of flow.

A bolus feeding of 300 to 500 mL usually is given for each meal and requires 10 to 15 minutes to complete. The amount is often determined by the patient's reaction. If the patient feels full, it may be desirable to give smaller amounts more frequently.

The patient and caregiver must understand that keeping the head of the bed elevated for at least 1 hour after feeding facilitates digestion and decreases the risk for aspiration. Any obstruction requires that the feeding be stopped and the physician notified.

The patient or caregiver is instructed to flush the tube with 30 mL of water after each bolus or medication administration, and otherwise to flush the tube daily to keep it patent. Adaptors are available that can be secured to the end of the tube to create a "Y" site for ease of flushing or medication delivery. The flushing

FIGURE 36-9 Bolus gastrostomy feeding by gravity. **(A)** Feeding is instilled at an angle so that air does not enter the stomach. **(B)** Syringe is raised perpendicular to the abdomen so that feeding can enter by gravity.

equipment is cleaned with warm, soapy water and rinsed after each use.

The patient and caregiver are made aware that the tube is marked at skin level to provide the patient a baseline for later comparison. They are advised to monitor the tube's length and to notify the physician or home care nurse if the segment of the tube outside the body becomes shorter or longer.

If the patient is to use an intermittent or continuous-pressure feeding pump at home, instruction in the use of the particular type of pump is essential. Most feeding pumps have built-in alarms that signal when the bag is empty, when the battery is low, or when an occlusion is present. The patient and caregiver need to be aware of these alarms and how to troubleshoot the pump.

Continuing Care

Referral to a home care agency is important to ensure initial supervision and support for the patient and caregiver. The home care nurse assesses the patient's status and progress and evaluates the techniques that are used in administering the tube feeding. Further instruction and supervision in the home setting may be required to help the patient and caregiver adapt to a physical environment and equipment that are different from the hospital setting. The nurse also reviews with the patient and caregiver information about complications to report (eg, dumping syndrome, nausea and vomiting, infection of the skin at the insertion site of the tube).

The home care nurse assists the patient and family in establishing as normal a routine as possible. Some patients will want to experience a sensation of normal eating and are advised that they can try smelling, tasting, and chewing small amounts of food before taking their tube feedings. This stimulates the flow of salivary and gastric secretions and may give some sensation of a normal meal. The chewed food can then be deposited by the patient into a funnel or syringe attached to the gastrostomy tube for administration into the stomach. The patient or caregiver is encouraged to keep a diary to record the times and amounts of feedings and any symptoms that occur. The nurse reviews the diary during home visits. When the tube is to be replaced, the patient or caregiver must be taught how to do this.

Evaluation

EXPECTED PATIENT OUTCOMES

Expected patient outcomes may include the following:

1. Achieves an adequate intake of nutrients
   a. Tolerates quantity and frequency of tube feedings
   b. Has 50 mL or less of residual gastric content before each feeding
   c. Has no diarrhea
   d. Maintains or gains weight
   e. Has normal electrolyte values
2. Is free from infection and skin breakdown
   a. Is afebrile
   b. Has no drainage from the incision
   c. Demonstrates intact skin surrounding the exit site
   d. Inspects exit site twice a day
3. Adjusts to change in body image
   a. Is able to discuss expected changes
   b. Verbalizes concerns
   c. Asks to speak with someone who has experienced this procedure
4. Demonstrates skill in managing feeding regimen
   a. Helps prepare prescribed formula or blenderized food
   b. Handles equipment competently
   c. Helps administer the feeding or does so independently
   d. Demonstrates how to maintain tube patency
   e. Cleans tubing as needed
   f. Keeps an accurate record of intake
   g. Can remove and reinsert the tube as appropriate and needed for feedings
5. Avoids complications
   a. Exhibits adequate wound healing
   b. Has no abnormal bleeding from puncture site
   c. Tube remains intact for the duration of therapy

Parenteral Nutrition

Parenteral nutrition (PN) is a method of providing nutrients to the body by an IV route. It is a very complex admixture of individual chemicals combined in a single container. The components of a PN admixture are proteins, carbohydrates, fats, electrolytes, vitamins, trace minerals, and sterile water. The goals of PN are to improve nutritional status, establish a positive nitrogen balance, maintain muscle mass, promote weight gain, and enhance the healing process.

ESTABLISHING POSITIVE NITROGEN BALANCE

When a patient's intake of protein and nutrients is significantly less than that required by the body to meet energy expenditures, a state of negative nitrogen balance results. In response, the body begins to convert the protein found in muscles into carbohydrates to be used to meet energy needs. The result is muscle wasting, weight loss, fatigue, and, if left uncorrected, death.

The average postoperative adult patient requires approximately 1500 calories per day to keep the body from using its own store of protein. Traditional IV fluids do not provide sufficient calories or nitrogen to meet the body's daily requirements. PN solutions, which supply nutrients such as dextrose, amino acids, electrolytes, vitamins, minerals, and fat emulsions, provide enough calories and nitrogen to meet the patient's daily nutritional needs. In general, PN can provide 30 to 35 kcal/kg of body weight and 1.0 to 1.5 g of protein/kg of body weight (Rombeau & Rolandelli, 2000).

The patient with fever, trauma, burns, major surgery, or hypermetabolic disease may require up to 10,000 additional calories daily. The volume of fluid necessary to provide these calories would surpass fluid tolerance and lead to pulmonary edema or heart failure. To provide the required calories in small volume, it is necessary to increase the concentration of nutrients and use a route of administration (ie, a large, high-flow vein [subclavian vein]) that will rapidly dilute incoming nutrients to the proper levels of body tolerance.

When highly concentrated glucose is administered, caloric requirements are satisfied and the body uses amino acids for protein synthesis rather than for energy. Additional potassium is added to the solution to maintain proper electrolyte balance and to transport glucose and amino acids across cell membranes. To prevent deficiencies and fulfill requirements for tissue synthesis, other elements, such as calcium, phosphorus, magnesium, and sodium chloride, are added (Rombeau & Rolandelli, 2000).

CLINICAL INDICATIONS

The indications for PN include a 10% deficit in body weight (compared with preillness weight), an inability to take oral food or fluids within 7 days after surgery, and hypercatabolic situations such as major infection with fever. In both the home and hospital setting, PN is indicated in the following situations:

- The patient's intake is insufficient to maintain an anabolic state (eg, severe burns, malnutrition, short bowel syndrome, AIDS, sepsis, cancer).
- The patient's ability to ingest food orally or by tube is impaired (eg, paralytic ileus, Crohn's disease with obstruction, postradiation enteritis, severe hyperemesis gravidarum in pregnancy).
- The patient is not interested in or is unwilling to ingest adequate nutrients (eg, anorexia nervosa, postoperative elderly patients).
- The underlying medical condition precludes being fed orally or by tube (eg, acute pancreatitis, high enterocutaneous fistula).
- Preoperative and postoperative nutritional needs are prolonged (eg, extensive bowel surgery).

FORMULAS

A total of 2 to 3 L of solution is administered over a 24-hour period using a filter (1.2-micron particulate filter). Before administration, the PN infusion must be inspected for clarity and any precipitate. The label is compared with the physician's order, noting the expiration date. Fat emulsions (Intralipid) may be infused simultaneously with PN through a Y-connector close to the infusion site. Fat emulsions should not be filtered. Before administration, the fat emulsion solution is inspected for frothiness, separation, or oily appearance. Usually 500 mL of a 10% emulsion is administered over 4 to 6 hours, one to three times a week. Fat emulsions can provide up to 30% of the total daily calorie intake.

INITIATING THERAPY

PN solutions are initiated slowly and advanced gradually each day to the desired rate, as the patient's fluid and glucose tolerance permits. The patient's laboratory test results and response to PN therapy are monitored on an ongoing basis by the nutritional support team. Standing orders are initiated for weighing the patient; monitoring intake, output, and blood glucose; and baseline and periodic monitoring of complete blood count, platelet count, and chemistry panel, including serum carbon dioxide, magnesium, phosphorus, triglycerides, and prealbumin. A 24-hour urine nitrogen determination may be performed for analysis of nitrogen balance. In most hospitals, the physician prescribes PN solutions on a daily standard PN order form. The formulation of the PN solutions is calculated carefully each day to meet the complete nutritional needs of the individual patient.

ADMINISTRATION METHODS

Various vascular access devices are used to administer PN solutions in clinical practice. PN may be administered by either peripheral or central IV lines, depending on the patient's condition and the anticipated length of therapy.

Peripheral Method

To supplement oral intake when complete bowel rest is not indicated and NG or nasoenteric suction is not required, a peripheral parenteral nutrition (PPN) formula may be prescribed. PPN is administered through a peripheral vein; this is possible because the solution is less hypertonic than PN solution. PPN formulas are not nutritionally complete. Protein and dextrose are limited. Dextrose concentrations of more than 10% should not be administered through peripheral veins because they irritate the intima (innermost walls) of small veins, causing chemical phlebitis. Lipids are administered simultaneously to buffer the PPN and to protect the peripheral vein from irritation. The usual length of therapy using PPN is 5 to 7 days (Hamilton, 2000).

Central Method

Because PN solutions have five or six times the solute concentration of blood (and exert an osmotic pressure of about 2000 mOsm/L), they are injurious to the intima of peripheral veins. Therefore, to prevent phlebitis and other venous complications, these solutions are administered into the vascular system through a catheter inserted into a high-flow, large blood vessel (the subclavian vein). Concentrated solutions are then very rapidly diluted to isotonic levels by the blood in this vessel.

Four types of **central venous access devices (CVAD)** are available—nontunnelled (or percutaneous) central catheters, peripherally inserted central catheters, tunnelled catheters, and implanted ports. Whenever one of these catheters is inserted, catheter tip placement should be confirmed by x-ray studies before PN therapy is initiated. The optimal position is the midproximal third of the superior vena cava.

NONTUNNELLED CENTRAL CATHETERS

Nontunnelled central catheters are used for short-term (less than 30 days) IV therapy in the acute care, long-term care, and home care settings. The physician inserts these catheters. Examples of nontunnelled central catheters are Vas Cath, Percutaneous Subclavian, and Hohn catheters. The subclavian vein is the most common vessel used, because the subclavian area provides a stable insertion site to which the catheter can be anchored, allows the patient freedom of movement, and provides easy access to the dressing site. The jugular or femoral vein also may be used. Single-, double-, and triple-lumen central catheters are available for central lines. To ensure accessibility, a triple-lumen subclavian catheter should be used, because it offers three ports for various uses (Fig. 36-10). The 16-gauge distal lumen can be used to infuse blood or other viscous fluids. The 18-gauge middle lumen is reserved for PN infusion.

FIGURE 36-10 Subclavian triple-lumen catheter used for parenteral nutrition and other adjunctive therapy. (**A**) The catheter is threaded through the subclavian vein into the vena cava. (**B**) Each lumen is an avenue for solution administration. The lumens are secured with threaded needleless adapters or Luer-Lok caps when the device is not in use.

A   B

The 18-gauge proximal port can be used for administration of blood or medications. A port not being used for fluid administration can be used for obtaining blood specimens if indicated.

If a single-lumen central catheter is used for administering PN, various restrictions apply. Blood cannot be drawn from the catheter and medications cannot be administered through it, because the medication may be incompatible with the components of the nutritional solution (insulin is an exception). If medications must be given, they must be infused through a separate peripheral IV line, not by piggyback into the PN line. Transfusions of blood products also cannot be given through the main line, because red cells may possibly coat the lumen of the catheter, thereby reducing the flow of the nutritional solution.

PERIPHERALLY INSERTED CENTRAL CATHETERS

Peripherally inserted central catheters (PICC) are used for intermediate-term (3 to 12 months) IV therapy in the hospital, long-term care, or home setting. These catheters may be inserted at the bedside or in the outpatient setting by a specially trained nurse. The basilic or cephalic vein is accessed through the antecubital space, and the catheter is threaded to a designated location, depending on the type of solution to be infused (superior vena cava for PN). Taking of blood pressure and blood specimens from the extremity with the PICC is avoided (see Chapter 14).

TUNNELLED CENTRAL CATHETERS

Tunnelled central catheters are for long-term use and may remain in place for many years. These catheters are cuffed and can have single or double lumens; examples are the Hickman, Groshong, and Permacath. These catheters are inserted surgically. They are threaded under the skin (reducing the risk of ascending infection) to the subclavian vein, and the distal end of the catheter is advanced into the superior vena cava 2 to 3 cm above the junction with the right atrium (see Chapter 16).

IMPLANTED PORTS

Implanted ports are also used for long-term home IV therapy; examples include the Port-A-Cath, Mediport, Hickman Port, and P.A.S. Port. Instead of exiting from the skin, as do the Hickman and Groshong catheters, the end of the catheter is attached to a small chamber that is placed in a subcutaneous pocket, either on the anterior chest wall or on the forearm. The subcutaneous port requires minimal care and allows the patient complete freedom of activity. Implanted ports are more expensive than the external catheters, and access requires passing a special needle (Huber-tipped) through the skin into the chamber to initiate IV therapy (see Chapter 16). Taking of blood pressure and blood specimens from the extremity with the port system is avoided.

NONTUNNELLED CENTRAL CATHETER INSERTION

The procedure is explained so that the patient understands the importance of not touching the catheter insertion site and is aware of what to expect during the insertion procedure. To insert the catheter, the patient is placed supine, in head-low position (to produce dilation of neck and shoulder vessels, which makes entry easier and prevents air embolus). The area is shaved if necessary, and the skin is prepared with acetone and alcohol to remove surface oils. Final skin preparation includes cleaning with tincture of 2% iodine or chlorhexidine. To afford maximal accuracy in the placement of the catheter, the patient is instructed to turn the head away from the site of venipuncture and to remain motionless while the catheter is inserted and the wound is dressed.

The preferred insertion route is the subclavian vein, which leads into the superior vena cava. The external jugular route can be used, but usually only in emergency situations. Because a nontunnelled central catheter is always a potential source of serious infection, the site should be changed every 4 weeks or as recommended by the Centers for Disease Control and Prevention.

Sterile drapes are applied to the upper chest. The patient may be asked to wear a facemask to prevent the spread of microorganisms. Procaine or lidocaine is injected to anesthetize the skin and underlying tissues. The target area is the inferior border at the midpoint of the clavicle. A large-bore needle on a syringe is inserted and moved parallel to and beneath the clavicle until it enters the vein. The syringe is then detached and a radiopaque catheter is inserted through the needle into the vein.

When the catheter is positioned, the needle is withdrawn and the hub of the catheter is attached to the IV tubing. Until the syringe is detached from the needle and the catheter is inserted, the patient may be asked to perform the Valsalva manoeuvre. (To do this, the patient is instructed to take a deep breath, hold it, and bear down with mouth closed. Compression of the abdomen may also accomplish the manoeuvre.) The Valsalva manoeuvre is performed to produce a positive phase in central venous pressure, to lessen the possibility of air being drawn into the circulatory system (air embolism). The physician sutures the catheter to the skin to avoid inadvertent removal.

The catheter insertion site is swabbed with either tincture of 2% iodine or a chlorhexidine solution. A gauze or transparent dressing is applied using strict sterile technique. An isotonic IV solution, such as dextrose 5% in water (D_5W), is administered to keep the vein patent.

The position of the tip of the catheter is checked with fluoroscopy to confirm its location in the superior vena cava and to rule out a pneumothorax resulting from puncture of the pleura. Once the catheter position is confirmed, the prescribed PN solution is started. The initial rate of infusion is usually 50 mL/hour, and the rate is gradually increased to the maintenance rate or predetermined dose (eg, 100 to 125 mL/hour). An infusion pump is always used for administration of PN or PPN.

An injection site cap is attached to the end of each central catheter lumen, creating a closed system. IV infusion tubing is connected to the insertion site cap of the central catheter with a threaded needleless adapter or Luer-Lok device. Each lumen is labelled according to location (proximal, middle, distal). To ensure patency, all lumens are flushed with a diluted heparin flush initially, daily when not in use, after each intermittent infusion, after blood drawing, and whenever an infusion is disconnected. Force is never used to flush the catheter. If resistance is met, aspiration may be effective in cleansing the lumen; if this is not effective, the physician is notified. Low-dose t-PA (alteplase) may be prescribed to dissolve a clot or fibrin sheath. If attempts to clear the lumen are ineffective, the lumen is labelled as "clotted off."

DISCONTINUING PARENTERAL NUTRITION

The PN solution is discontinued gradually to allow the patient to adjust to decreased levels of glucose. After administration of the PN solution is terminated, isotonic glucose is administered for several hours to protect against rebound hypoglycemia. Providing oral carbohydrates will shorten the tapering time. Specific symptoms of rebound hypoglycemia include weakness, faintness, sweating, shakiness, feeling cold, confusion, and increased heart rate. Once all IV therapy is completed, the nurse (with a physician's order) removes the nontunnelled central venous catheter or PICC and applies an occlusive dressing to the exit site. Tunnelled catheters and implanted ports are removed by the physician.

In cases of serious illness when death is imminent, some patients or families may request that PN be discontinued. This difficult issue poses many ethical questions, some of which are discussed in Chart 36-3.

NURSING PROCESS: THE PATIENT RECEIVING PARENTERAL NUTRITION

Assessment

The nurse assists in identifying patients who may be candidates for PN. Indicators include any significant weight loss (10% or more of usual weight), a decrease in oral food intake for more than 1 week, any significant sign of protein loss (serum albumin levels less than 32 g/L, muscle wasting, decreased tissue healing, or abnormal urea nitrogen excretion), and persistent vomiting and diarrhea. The nurse carefully monitors the patient's hydration, electrolyte levels, and calorie intake.

Chart 36-3 • Ethics and Related Issues

Is It Ethical to Withhold or Withdraw Nutrition and Hydration?

Situation
It is generally agreed that patients (or their designated decision makers) can refuse life-saving treatment, particularly if the means of treatment are extraordinary (eg, ventilators, dialysis machines, extracorporeal oxygenators). Extraordinary means include medications, treatments, and procedures that can be obtained only at excessive cost, pain, or inconvenience and offer no reasonable hope of benefit. Nutrition and hydration therapy, however, are perceived as ordinary means by many.

Ordinary means are those medications, treatments, and procedures that offer a reasonable hope of benefit and can be obtained without excessive expense, pain, or inconvenience. Additionally, withdrawing or withholding nutrition and hydration can in and of itself cause death. Thus, some have argued that nutrition and hydration should always be provided to every patient, regardless of the patient's preference or condition.

Dilemma
The patient's desire to have nutrition or hydration withdrawn or withheld may conflict with the reluctance of others to harm the patient by withdrawing the food and water needed for survival (autonomy versus nonmaleficence).

Discussion
- What arguments would you offer against the withholding and withdrawing of nutrition and hydration?
- What arguments would you offer in favour of withholding and withdrawing of nutrition and hydration?
- Are foods and fluids always "ordinary means," or are there instances in which they might be considered "extraordinary"? Support your answer.

Answer the above questions using as an example a patient in a persistent vegetative state (ie, unable to express his or her wishes).

Diagnosis

NURSING DIAGNOSES

Based on the assessment data, the major nursing diagnoses may include the following:

- Imbalanced nutrition, less than body requirements, related to inadequate oral intake of nutrients
- Risk for infection related to contamination of the central catheter site or infusion line
- Risk for excess or deficient fluid volume related to altered infusion rate
- Risk for immobility related to fear that the catheter will become dislodged or occluded
- Risk for ineffective therapeutic regimen management related to knowledge deficit about home PN therapy

COLLABORATIVE PROBLEMS/ POTENTIAL COMPLICATIONS

The most common complications are pneumothorax, air embolism, a clotted or displaced catheter, sepsis, hyperglycemia, rebound hypoglycemia, and fluid overload. These problems and the associated collaborative interventions are described in Table 36-5.

Planning and Goals

The major goals for the patient may include optimal level of nutrition, absence of infection, adequate fluid volume, optimal level of activity (within individual limitations), knowledge of and skill in self-care, and prevention of complications.

Nursing Interventions

MAINTAINING OPTIMAL NUTRITION

A continuous, uniform infusion of PN solution over a 24-hour period is desired. In some cases, however (eg, home care patients), cyclic PN may be appropriate. With cyclic PN, there is a set time during a 24-hour period when PN is infused and a set time when it is not. The time periods for infusion are sufficient to meet the patient's nutritional and pharmacologic needs. Ideally, cyclic PN is infused over an 8- to 10-hour period during the night.

The patient is weighed daily (this may be decreased to two or three times per week), at the same time of the day under the same conditions for accurate comparison. Under the PN regimen (without additional energy expenditure), a satisfactory weight gain is usually achieved. It is important to keep accurate intake and output records and calculations of fluid balance. A calorie count is kept of any oral nutrients. Trace elements (copper, zinc, chromium, manganese, and selenium) are included in PN solutions and are individualized for each patient. The PN solutions are prescribed daily by the physician on a standard PN order form based on laboratory values and patient tolerance.

PREVENTING INFECTION

The high glucose content of PN solutions makes these solutions ideal culture media for bacterial and fungal growth, and CVADs provide a port of entry. *Candida albicans* is the most common infectious organism. Other infectious organisms include *Staphylococcus aureus, Staphylococcus epidermidis,* and *Klebsiella pneumoniae.* Meticulous technique is essential to prevent infection.

Table 36-5 • Complications of Parenteral Nutrition

COMPLICATION	CAUSE	NURSING ACTIONS AND COLLABORATIVE INTERVENTIONS
Pneumothorax	Improper catheter placement and inadvertent puncture of the pleura	Place patient in Fowler's position. Offer reassurance. Monitor vital signs. Prepare for thoracentesis or chest tube insertion.
Air embolism	Disconnected tubing	Tape all tubing connection sites securely. Replace tubing immediately and notify physician.
	Cap missing from port	Replace cap and notify physician.
	Blocked segment of vascular system	Turn patient on left side and place in the head-low position. Notify physician.
Clotted catheter line	Inadequate/infrequent heparin flushes Disruption of infusion	Administer heparin flush in unused lines twice a day. Monitor infusion rate hourly and inspect the integrity of the line. On *rare* occasions, flush with urokinase as prescribed.
Catheter displacement and contamination	Excessive movement, possibly with a nonsecured catheter	Stop the infusion and notify the physician.
	Separation of tubing and contamination	Tape all tubing connection sites. Avoid interrupting the main line or piggybacking other lines.
Sepsis	Separation of dressings	Reinforce or change dressing quickly using aseptic technique.
	Contaminated solution	Discard. Notify pharmacist.
	Infection at insertion site of catheter	Notify physician. Monitor vital signs every 4 hours. Catheter site is changed every 4 weeks.
Hyperglycemia	Glucose intolerance	Monitor glucose levels (blood and urine). Monitor urine output. Observe for stupor, confusion, lethargy. Notify physician; the addition of insulin to the PN solution may be prescribed.
Fluid overload	Fluid infusing rapidly	Decrease infusion rate, use infusion pump. Monitor vital signs. Notify physician. Treat respiratory distress by sitting patient upright and administering oxygen as needed, if prescribed.
Rebound hypoglycemia	Feedings stopped too abruptly	Monitor for symptoms (weakness, tremors, diaphoresis, headache, hunger, and apprehension); notify physician. Gradually wean patient from PN.

The primary sources of microorganisms for catheter-related infections are the skin and the catheter hub. The catheter site is covered with an occlusive gauze dressing that is usually changed every other day. Alternatively, a transparent dressing may be used and changed weekly. The Centers for Disease Control and Prevention recommends changing dressings for CVADs only if they are damp, bloody, loose, or soiled. The dressings are changed using sterile technique. The nurse and patient wear masks during dressing changes to reduce the possibility of airborne contamination. The area is checked for leakage, bloody drainage, a kinked catheter, and skin reactions such as inflammation, redness, swelling, tenderness, or purulent drainage. The nurse puts on sterile gloves and cleanses the area with tincture of 2% iodine or a chlorhexidine solution on a sterile gauze. The site is cleaned thoroughly using circular motion from the site outward approximately 7.5 cm. This is repeated two times. This is followed with the same cleaning procedure using 2 × 2-inch gauze pads moistened with sterile water or saline solution (alcohol is used to remove iodine). Next the catheter lumens are cleaned from the exit site to the distal end with an alcohol wipe. The insertion site is covered with an occlusive gauze pad or transparent dressing centred over the area.

The advantages of using a transparent dressing over the gauze pad are that it allows frequent examination of the catheter site without changing the dressing, it adheres well, and it is more comfortable for the patient. When an extension set is used with a central catheter, it is considered an extension of the catheter itself. It is not routinely changed with dressing or tubing changes. The connection (hub) between the catheter and extension tubing is secured with adhesive tape to prevent separation and exposure to air. Main-line IV tubing and filters are changed every 72 to 96 hours, and all connections are taped securely to avoid breaks in the integrity of the system. The dressing and tubing are labelled with the date, time of insertion, time of dressing change, and initials of the person who carried out the procedure; this information is also documented in the medical record.

The catheter is another major source of colonization and infection. Antiseptic-impregnated central venous catheters are new devices that reduce catheter colonization by coating of the catheter surfaces with antimicrobial agents. Two types are available, one coated with chlorhexidine/silver sulfadiazine and the other with minocycline/rifampin (Hanna et al., 2001).

MAINTAINING FLUID BALANCE

An infusion pump is necessary for PN to maintain an accurate rate of administration. A designated rate is set in millilitres per hour, and the rate checked every 30 to 60 minutes. An alarm signals a problem. The infusion rate should not be increased or decreased to compensate for fluids that have infused too quickly or too slowly. If the solution runs out, 10% dextrose and water is infused until the next PN solution is available from the pharmacy.

If the rate is too rapid, hyperosmolar diuresis occurs (excess sugar will be excreted), which, if severe enough, can cause intractable seizures, coma, and death. Symptoms of rapid hypertonic fluid intake include headache, nausea, fever, chills, and increasing lethargy.

If the flow rate is too slow, the patient does not get the maximal benefit of calories and nitrogen. Intake and output are recorded every 8 hours so that fluid imbalance can be readily detected. The patient is weighed two or three times a week; in ideal situations, the patient will show neither weight loss nor significant weight gain. The nurse assesses for signs of dehydration (eg, thirst, decreased skin turgor, decreased central venous pressure) and reports these findings to the physician immediately. It is essential to monitor blood glucose levels, because hyperglycemia can cause diuresis and excessive fluid loss.

ENCOURAGING ACTIVITY

Activities and ambulation are encouraged when the patient is physically capable. With a catheter in the subclavian vein, the patient is free to move the extremities and should be encouraged to maintain good muscle tone. If applicable, the teaching and exercise program initiated in the occupational and physical therapy departments should be reinforced.

PROMOTING HOME AND COMMUNITY-BASED CARE

Teaching Patients Self-Care

Successful home PN requires teaching the patient and family specialized skills using an intensive training program and follow-up supervision in the home. This is accomplished through a team effort. The financial costs of such programs, although high, are less than those incurred in a hospital. Initiation of a home program may be the only way the patient can be discharged from the hospital.

Ideal candidates for home PN are those patients who have a reasonable life expectancy after return home, have only a limited number of medical illnesses other than the one that has resulted in the need for PN, and are highly motivated and fairly self-sufficient. In addition, ability to learn, availability of family interest and support, adequate finances, and the physical plan of the home are factors that must be assessed when the decision for home PN is made.

Home health care agencies sponsoring home PN programs have developed teaching brochures for every aspect of the treatment, including catheter and dressing care, use of an infusion pump, administration of fat emulsions, and instillation of heparin flushes. Teaching begins in the hospital and continues in the home or in an ambulatory infusion centre.

Continuing Care

The home care nurse should be aware that the average patient needs about 2 weeks of instruction and reinforcement. For more information about home patient education, see Charts 36-4 and 36-5.

Evaluation

EXPECTED PATIENT OUTCOMES

Expected patient outcomes may include the following:

1. Attains or maintains nutritional balance
2. Is free of infection at the catheter site
    a. Is afebrile
    b. Has no purulent drainage from the catheter insertion site
    c. Has intact IV line

Chart 36-4 • PATIENT EDUCATION
Teaching Patients About Home Parenteral Nutrition

An effective home care teaching program prepares the patient to manage the appropriate form of PN: how to store solutions, set up the infusion, flush the line with heparin, change the dressings, and troubleshoot for problems. The most common complication is sepsis. Strict aseptic technique is taught for hand hygiene, handling equipment, changing the dressing, and preparing the solution.

Troubleshooting Mechanical Difficulties

Mechanical problems usually arise from technical complications in the infusion pump or catheter site. The patient needs to know how to measure the length of the external portion of the catheter; this measurement is used as a comparison if the line is pulled or if dislodgement is suspected. The patient also needs to know how to recognize catheter problems (eg, leakage, loose cap, blood clot, dislodgement) and should receive a list of instructions explaining what to do for each problem.

Recognizing Metabolic Complications

The patient is given a list of symptoms that indicate metabolic complications (neuropathies, mentation changes, diarrhea, nausea, skin changes, decreased urine output) and directions on how to contact the home health care nurse or physician if any of these complications occurs. The patient is instructed to have weekly serum chemistry and hematology tests as well.

Obtaining Psychosocial Support

The psychosocial aspects of home PN are as important as the physiologic and technical concerns. Patients must cope with the loss of eating and with changes in lifestyle brought on by sleep disturbances (frequent urination during infusions, usually two or three times during the night).

Major psychosocial reactions include depression, anger, withdrawal, anxiety, and impaired self-image. A successful home parenteral nutrition program depends on the patient's and family's motivation, emotional stability, and technical competence. Patients and families need to know which support groups are available in the community to help them cope with the transition and to minimize disruption of lifestyle.

> **Chart 36-5**
> **Home Care Checklist • The Patient Receiving Parenteral Nutrition**
>
> | At the completion of the home care instruction, the patient or caregiver will be able to: | Patient | Caregiver |
> | --- | :---: | :---: |
> | • Discuss goal and purpose of PN therapy | ✓ | ✓ |
> | • Discuss basic components of PN solution. | ✓ | ✓ |
> | • List emergency phone numbers. | ✓ | ✓ |
> | • Demonstrate how to handle PN solutions and medications correctly. | ✓ | ✓ |
> | • Demonstrate how to operate infusion pump. | ✓ | ✓ |
> | • Demonstrate how to prime tubing and filter. | ✓ | ✓ |
> | • Demonstrate how to connect and disconnect PN infusion. | ✓ | ✓ |
> | • Demonstrate how to perform catheter dressing changes. | ✓ | ✓ |
> | • Demonstrate how to heparinize central line. | ✓ | ✓ |
> | • Identify possible PN complications and interventions. | ✓ | ✓ |

3. Is hydrated, as evidenced by good skin turgor
4. Achieves an optimal level of activity, within limitations
5. Demonstrates skill in managing PN regimen
6. Prevents complications
   a. Maintains proper catheter and equipment function
   b. Has no symptoms of sepsis
   c. Maintains metabolic balance within normal limits
   d. Shows improved and stabilized nutritional status

Critical Thinking Exercises

1. You are caring for a patient with an NG feeding tube. Before administering the patient's tube feeding, you explain to the patient that you will be checking to make sure the tube is placed correctly. The patient responds that she is accustomed to this and that the other nurses "check the tube by placing the end of it in a cup of water;" the patient also states that the nurses then "put air in the tube and use a stethoscope to listen for bubbles in my stomach." How would you respond to the patient? What research findings guide your actions in confirming the placement of the tube? What follow-up actions would you take to ensure that there is consistency among the nursing staff in the procedure used for confirmation of tube placement?

2. A patient who is receiving gastrostomy tube feedings is to be discharged from the hospital to return home within the next few days. Several family members are to be taught how to administer the tube feedings. What are the learning priorities that should be accomplished before the patient is discharged? What assessment parameters should be used to determine whether the family has the necessary resources for providing care for the patient at home?

3. A patient who had major abdominal surgery 1 week ago and who has developed a paralytic ileus is to begin receiving PN. What explanation would you give to this patient about the benefits of PN and the procedure for its administration? How would you alter your plan of care to include assessment for complications of PN? What assessment would you conduct to determine whether the patient is a candidate for home PN therapy?

REFERENCES AND SELECTED READINGS

Books

Brandt, L. J., & Daum, F. (Eds.). (1999). *Clinical practice of gastroenterology.* New York: Churchill-Livingstone.

Domkowski, K. (Ed.). (1998). *Gastroenterology nursing: A core curriculum* (2nd ed.). St. Louis: Mosby–Year Book.

Guenter, P., & Silkroski, M. (2001). *Tube Feeding: Practical guidelines and nursing protocols.* Gaithersburg, MD: Aspen.

Hamilton, H. (2000). *Total parenteral nutrition: A practical guide for nurses.* New York: Churchill-Livingstone.

Hankins, J., Lonsway, R. A. W., Hedrick, C., et al. (Eds.). (2001). *Infusion therapy in clinical practice* (2nd ed.). Philadelphia: W. B. Saunders.

Rombeau, J. L., & Rolandelli, R. (Eds.). (2000). *Clinical nutrition: Parenteral nutrition* (3rd ed.). Philadelphia: W. B. Saunders.

Ross-Kerr, J.C., & Wood, M.J. (2001). *Potter and Perry Canadian fundamentals of nursing* (2nd ed.). Toronto, ON: Harcourt Canada.

Yamada, T., Alpers, D. H., & Laine, L. (Eds.). (1999). *Textbook of gastroenterology.* Philadelphia: Lippincott Williams & Wilkins.

Weinstein, S. (Ed.). (2001). *Plumer's principles & practice of intravenous therapy.* Philadelphia: Lippincott Williams & Wilkins.

Wilson, B.A., Shannon, M.T., & Stang, C.L. (2005). *Prentice Hall nurse's drug guide 2005.* Upper Saddle River, NJ: Pearson Education.

Journals

Asterisks indicate nursing research articles.

Gastrostomies

Bowers, S. (1996). Tubes: A nurse's guide to enteral feeding devices. *MedSurg Nursing, 5*(5), 313–325.

Johnson, M. S. (1997). Radiologic placement of gastrostomy tubes. *Nutrition in Clinical Practice, 12*(1), S20–S22.

O'Brien, B., Davis, S., & Erwin-Toth, P. (1999). G-tube site care: A practical guide. *RN, 62*(2), 52–56.

*Smarszez, R. M. (2000). Microbial contamination of low-profile balloon gastrostomy extension tubes and three cleaning methods. *Nutrition in Clinical Practice, 15*(3), 138–142.

Thompson, L. (1995). Percutaneous endoscopic gastrostomy. *Nursing '95, 25*(4), 62–63.

Nasogastric and Nasoenteric Intubation and Feeding

Bowers, S. (1999). Nutrition support for malnourished, acutely ill adults. *MedSurg Nursing, 8*(3), 145–166.

Case, K. O., Cuddy, P. G., & McGurk, E. P. D. (2000). Nutrition support in the critically ill patient. *Critical Care Nursing Quarterly, 22*(4), 75–89.

Edwards, S. J., & Metheny, N. A. (2000). Measurement of gastric residual volume: State of the science. *MedSurg, 9*(1), 125–128.

Fellows, L. S., Miller, R. H., Frederickson, M., et al. (2000). Evidence-based practice for enteral feedings: Aspiration prevention strategies, bedside detection, and practice change. *MedSurg, 9*(1), 27–31.

Livingston, A., Seamons, C., & Dalton, T. (2000). If the gut works use it. *Nursing Management, 7*(2), 39–42.

Lord, L. (2001). Photo guide: How to insert a large-bore nasogastric tube. *Nursing2001, 31*(9), 46–48.

*McClave, S. A., Snider, H. L., & Lowen, C. C., et al. (1992). Use of residual volume as a marker for enteral feeding intolerance: Prospective blinded comparison with physical examination and radiographic findings. *Journal of Parenteral and Enteral Nutrition, 16*(2), 99–105.

Metheny, N. A. (1998). Detection of improperly positioned feeding tubes. *Journal of Health Care Risk Management, 18*(3), 37–45.

*Metheny, N. A., Dettenmeier, P., Hampton, K., et al. (1990a). Detection of inadvertent respiratory placement of small-bore feeding tubes: A report of 10 cases. *Heart and Lung, 19*(6), 631–638.

*Metheny, N. A., McSweeney, M., Wehrle, M. A., et al. (1990b). Effectiveness of the auscultatory method in predicting feeding tube location. *Nursing Research, 39*(5), 262–267.

*Metheny, N. A., Reed, L., Berglund, B., et al. (1994). Visual characteristics of aspirates from feeding tubes as a method for predicting tube location. *Nursing Research, 43*(5), 282–287.

*Metheny, N. A., Reed, L., Worseck, M., et al. (1993). How to aspirate fluid from small-bore feeding tubes. *American Journal of Nursing, 93*(5), 86–88.

*Metheny, N. A., Smith, L., & Stewart, B. J., et al. (2000). Development of a reliable and valid bedside test for bilirubin and its utility for improving prediction of feeding tube location. *Nursing Research, 49*(6), 302–309.

*Metheny, N. A., Stewart, B. J., Smith, L, et al. (1999). pH and concentration of bilirubin in feeding tube aspirates as predictors of tube placement. *Nursing Research, 48*(3), 189–197.

*Metheny, N. A., & Titler, M. G. (2001). Assessing placement of feeding tubes. *American Journal of Nursing, 101*(5), 36–46.

*Metheny, N. A., Webrle, M. A., Wiersema, L., et al. (1998). Testing feeding tube placement: Auscultation vs. pH method. *American Journal of Nursing, 98*(5), 37–43.

Mitchell, J. F. (2000). Oral dosage forms that should not be crushed: 2000 update. *Hospital Pharmacy, 35*(5), 553–567.

Noble, K. A. (2003). Name that tube. *Nursing2003, 33*(3), 56–62.

Petnicki, P. J. (1998). Cost savings and improved patient care with the use of a flush enteral feeding pump. Proceedings of the Third Annual Ross Enteral Device Conference, Winston-Salem, NC, September 19–21, 1997. *Nutrition in Clinical Practice, 13,* (3 Suppl. l), s39–s41, s50–s51.

Trujillo, E. B., Robinson, M. K., & Jacobs, D. O. (2001). Nutrition: Feeding critically ill patients. Current concepts. *Critical Care Nurse, 21*(4), 60–71.

Watt, R., & Lewis, R. (2001). Improving care for patients with gastrostomy tubes. *Canadian Nurse, 97*(10), 30–33.

Parenteral Nutrition

*Collin, G. R. (1999). Decreasing catheter colonization through the use of an antiseptic-impregnated catheter. *Clinical Investigations in Critical Care, 111*(6), 1632–1639.

Driscoll, M., Buckenmyer, C., Spirk, M., et al. (1997). Inserting and maintaining peripherally inserted central catheters. *MedSurg Nursing, 6*(6), 350–358.

Griffiths, V. R., & Philpot, P. (2002). Peripherally inserted central catheters (PICCs): Do they have a role in the care of the critically ill patient? *Intensive and Critical Care Nursing 18*(1), 37–47.

Hanna, H., Darouicher, R., & Raad, I. (2001). New approaches for prevention of intravascular catheter-related infections. *Infections in Medicine, 18*(9), 38–48.

Masoorli, S., & Angeles, T. (2002). Getting a line on CVAD: Central vascular access devices. *Nursing 02, 32*(4), 36–45.

McConnell, E. A. (2001). Clinical do's and don'ts: Administering total parenteral nutrition. *Nursing 01, 31*(7), 17.

Moureau, N. (2001). Preventing complications with vascular access devices. *Nursing 01, 31*(7), 52–54.

*Norwood, S. (2000). The safety of prolonging the use of central catheters: A prospective analysis of the effects of using antiseptic-bonded catheters with daily site care. *Critical Care Medicine, 28*(5), 1376–1382.

RESOURCES AND WEBSITES

American Cancer Society, 1599 Clifton Rd. N.E., Atlanta, GA 30329; 1-404-320-3333; http://www.cancer.org.

American Society for Clinical Nutrition, 9650 Rockville Pike, Bethesda, MD 20814-3998; http://www.faseb.org/assn.

American Society for Gastrointestinal Endoscopy, 13 Elm St., Manchester, MA 01944; http://www.asge.org.

American Society of Parenteral and Enteral Nutrition (ASPEN), 8630 Fenton St., #412, Silver Spring, MD 20910-3805; http://www.nutritioncare.org.

Canadian Parenteral-Enteral Nutrition Association; www.cpena.ca.

Canadian Society for Clinical Nutrition, 2175 Sheppard Ave East, Suite 310, Toronto, ON M2J 1W8; www.cscn-scnc.ca.

Oley Foundation for Home Parenteral and Enteral Nutrition, 214 Hun Memorial, A-23, New Scotland Ave., Albany, NY 12208; http://www.wizvax.net/oleyfdn.

Ross.com: enteral nutrition product information; www.ross.com.

Society of Gastroenterology Nurses & Associates, Inc., 140 North Michigan Ave., Chicago, IL 60611-4267; 800-245-7462; in Illinois, 312-321-5165; http://www.sgna.org.

VIASYS Healthcare Inc., 100 Chaddick Drive, Wheeling, IL 60090, USA; www.corpakmedsystems.com/eneteral.html.

Management of Patients With Gastric and Duodenal Disorders

Adapted by Christy Raymond

On completion of this chapter, the learner will be able to:

1. Compare the etiology, clinical manifestations, and management of acute gastritis, chronic gastritis, and peptic ulcer.

2. Use the nursing process as a framework for care of patients with gastritis.

3. Use the nursing process as a framework for care of patients with peptic ulcer.

4. Describe the dietary, pharmacologic, and surgical treatment of peptic ulcer.

5. Describe the nursing management of patients who undergo surgical procedures to treat obesity.

6. Use the nursing process as a framework for care of patients with gastric cancer.

7. Use the nursing process as a framework for care of patients undergoing gastric surgery.

8. Identify the complications of gastric surgery and their prevention and management.

9. Describe the home health care needs of the patient who has had gastric surgery.

*A*n individual's nutritional status depends not only on the type and amount of intake but also on the functioning of the gastric and intestinal portions of the gastrointestinal (GI) system. This chapter describes disorders of the stomach and duodenum and their treatment.

Gastritis

Gastritis (inflammation of the **gastric** or stomach mucosa) is a common GI problem. Gastritis may be acute, lasting several hours to a few days, or chronic, resulting from repeated exposure to irritating agents or recurring episodes of acute gastritis.

Acute gastritis is often caused by dietary indiscretion—the person eats food that is contaminated with disease-causing microorganisms or that is irritating or too highly seasoned. Other causes of acute gastritis include overuse of aspirin and other nonsteroidal anti-inflammatory drugs (NSAIDs), excessive alcohol intake, bile reflux, and radiation therapy. A more severe form of acute gastritis is caused by the ingestion of strong acid or alkali, which may cause the mucosa to become gangrenous or to perforate. Scarring can occur, resulting in pyloric obstruction. Gastritis also may be the first sign of an acute systemic infection.

Chronic gastritis and prolonged inflammation of the stomach may be caused by either benign or malignant ulcers of the stomach or by the bacteria *Helicobacter pylori.* Chronic gastritis is sometimes associated with autoimmune diseases such as pernicious anemia; dietary factors such as caffeine; the use of medications, especially NSAIDs; alcohol; smoking; or reflux of intestinal contents into the stomach.

Pathophysiology

In gastritis, the gastric mucous membrane becomes edematous and hyperemic (congested with fluid and blood) and undergoes superficial erosion (Fig. 37-1). It secretes a scanty amount of gastric juice, containing very little acid but much mucus. Superficial ulceration may occur and can lead to hemorrhage.

Clinical Manifestations

The patient with acute gastritis may have abdominal discomfort, headache, lassitude, nausea, anorexia, vomiting, and hiccuping. Some patients, however, have no symptoms. The patient with chronic gastritis may complain of anorexia, heartburn after eating, belching, a sour taste in the mouth, or nausea and vomiting. Patients with chronic gastritis from vitamin deficiency usually have evidence of malabsorption of vitamin B_{12} caused by antibodies against intrinsic factor.

Assessment and Diagnostic Findings

Gastritis is sometimes associated with achlorhydria or hypochlorhydria (absence or low levels of hydrochloric acid [HCl]) or with hyperchlorhydria (high levels of HCl). Diagnosis can be determined by endoscopy, upper GI radiographic studies, and histologic examination of a tissue specimen obtained by biopsy. In addition to biopsy, other diagnostic measures for detecting *H. pylori* include serologic testing for antibodies against the *H. pylori* antigen, a 1-minute ultrarapid urease test, and a breath test. *H. pylori* is said to be present in approximately 20% to 40% of all individual Canadians (Fallone, Veldhuyzen van Zuten, & Chiba, 2000).

Medical Management

The gastric mucosa is capable of repairing itself after a bout of gastritis. As a rule, the patient recovers in about 1 day, although the appetite may be diminished for an additional 2 or 3 days. Acute gastritis is also managed by instructing the patient to refrain from alcohol and food until symptoms subside. After the patient can take nourishment by mouth, a nonirritating diet is recommended. If the symptoms persist, fluids may need to be administered parenterally. If bleeding is present, management is similar to the procedures used for upper GI tract hemorrhage (discussed later in this chapter).

If gastritis is caused by ingestion of strong acids or alkalis, treatment consists of diluting and neutralizing the offending agent. To neutralize acids, common antacids (eg, aluminum hydroxide) are used; to neutralize an alkali, diluted lemon juice or diluted vinegar is used. If corrosion is extensive or severe, emetics and lavage are avoided because of the danger of perforation and damage to the esophagus.

Therapy is supportive and may include nasogastric (NG) intubation, analgesic agents and sedatives, antacids, and intravenous (IV) fluids. Fibreoptic endoscopy may be necessary. In extreme cases, emergency surgery may be required to remove gangrenous or perforated tissue. Gastrojejunostomy or gastric resection may be necessary to treat pyloric obstruction, a narrowing of the pyloric orifice.

Chronic gastritis is managed by modifying the patient's diet, promoting rest, reducing stress, and initiating pharmacotherapy. *H. pylori* may be treated with antibiotics (eg, tetracycline or amoxicillin, combined with clarithromycin) and a proton pump inhibitor (eg, lansoprazole [Prevacid]), and possibly bismuth salts (Pepto-Bismol) (Table 37-1). Research is being conducted to develop a vaccine against *H. pylori* (Alsahli et al., 2001).

NURSING PROCESS: THE PATIENT WITH GASTRITIS

Assessment

When obtaining the history, the nurse asks about the patient's presenting signs and symptoms. Does the patient have heartburn,

Glossary

antrectomy: removal of the pyloric (antrum) portion of the stomach with anastomosis (surgical connection) to the duodenum (gastroduodenostomy or Billroth I) or anastomosis to the jejunum (gastrojejunostomy or Billroth II)

dumping syndrome: physiologic response to rapid emptying of gastric contents into the jejunum, manifested by nausea, weakness, sweating, palpitations, syncope, and possibly diarrhea; occurs in patients who have had partial gastrectomy and gastrojejunostomy

duodenum: first portion of the small intestine, between the stomach and the jejunum

gastric: refers to the stomach

gastritis: inflammation of the stomach

hematemesis: vomiting of blood

melena: tarry or black stools; indicative of blood in stools

morbid obesity: 45 kg or more over ideal body weight

pyloroplasty: surgical procedure to increase the opening of the pyloric orifice

pylorus: opening between the stomach and the duodenum

pyrosis: heartburn

FIGURE 37-1 Endoscopic view of erosive gastritis (*left*). Damage from irritants (*right*) results in increased intracellular pH, impaired enzyme function, disrupted cellular structures, ischemia, vascular stasis, and tissue death. From Porth, C. (2002). *Pathophysiology: Concepts of altered health states* (6th ed.). Philadelphia: Lippincott Williams & Wilkins.

indigestion, nausea, or vomiting? Do the symptoms occur at any specific time of the day, before or after meals, after ingesting spicy or irritating foods, or after the ingestion of certain drugs or alcohol? Has there been recent weight gain or loss? Are the symptoms related to anxiety, stress, allergies, eating or drinking too much, or eating too quickly? How are the symptoms relieved? Is there a history of previous gastric disease or surgery? A diet history plus a 72-hour dietary recall (a list of everything the patient ate and drank in the last 72 hours) may be helpful.

A thorough history is important because it helps the nurse to identify whether known dietary excesses or other indiscretions are associated with the current symptoms, whether others in the patient's environment have similar symptoms, whether the patient is vomiting blood, and whether any known caustic element has been ingested. The nurse also identifies the duration of the current symptoms, any methods used by the patient to treat these symptoms, and whether the methods are effective. Signs to note during the physical examination include abdominal tenderness, dehydration, and evidence of any systemic disorder that might be responsible for the symptoms of gastritis.

Nursing Diagnoses

Based on the assessment data, the patient's major nursing diagnoses may include the following:

- Anxiety related to treatment
- Imbalanced nutrition, less than body requirements, related to inadequate intake of nutrients
- Risk for imbalanced fluid volume related to insufficient fluid intake and excessive fluid loss subsequent to vomiting
- Deficient knowledge about dietary management and disease process
- Acute pain related to irritated stomach mucosa

Planning and Goals

The major goals for the patient may include reduced anxiety, avoidance of irritating foods, adequate intake of nutrients, maintenance of fluid balance, increased awareness of dietary management, and relief of pain.

Nursing Interventions

REDUCING ANXIETY

If the patient has ingested acids or alkalis, emergency measures may be needed. The nurse offers supportive therapy to the patient and family during treatment and after the ingested acid or alkali has been neutralized or diluted. In some cases, the nurse may need to prepare the patient for additional diagnostic studies (endoscopy) or surgery. The patient usually feels anxious about the pain and the treatment modalities. The nurse uses a calm approach to assess the patient and to answer all questions as completely as possible. It is important to explain all procedures and treatments according to the patient's level of understanding.

PROMOTING OPTIMAL NUTRITION

For acute gastritis, the nurse provides physical and emotional support and helps the patient manage the symptoms, which may include nausea, vomiting, heartburn, and fatigue. The patient should take no foods or fluids by mouth—possibly for days—until the acute symptoms subside, thus allowing the gastric mucosa to heal. If IV therapy is necessary, the nurse monitors it regularly, along with serum electrolyte values. After the symptoms subside, the nurse can offer the patient ice chips followed by clear liquids. Introducing solid food as soon as possible will provide oral nutrition, decrease the need for IV therapy, and minimize irritation to the gastric mucosa. As food is introduced, the nurse evaluates and reports any symptoms that suggest a repeat episode of gastritis.

Table 37-1 • Pharmacologic Therapy for Peptic Ulcer Disease and Gastritis

PHARMACOLOGIC AGENT	MAJOR ACTION	NURSING CONSIDERATIONS
Antibiotics and Bismuth Salts		
Tetracycline (Novotetra) (plus metronidazole, proton pump inhibitor, and bismuth salts)	Exerts bacteriostatic effects to eradicate *Helicobacter pylori* bacteria in the gastric mucosa	May cause photosensitivity reaction; warn patient to use sunscreen. Use with caution in patients with renal or hepatic impairment. Milk or dairy products may reduce medication effectiveness.
Amoxicillin (Apo-Amoxi) (plus clarithromycin and proton pump inhibitor such as omeprazole [Losec])	A bactericidal antibiotic that assists with eradicating *H. pylori* bacteria in the gastric mucosa	May cause diarrhea. Do not use in patients allergic to penicillin.
Metronidazole (Flagyl); use with clarithromycin and proton pump inhibitor	An amebocide that assists with eradicating *H. pylori* bacteria in the gastric mucosa	Administer with meals to decrease GI distress. Administer with other antibiotics and proton pump inhibitors.
Clarithromycin (Biaxin); use with proton pump inhibitor and amoxicillin	Exerts bactericidal effects to eradicate *H. pylori* bacteria in the gastric mucosa	May cause GI upset.
Bismuth subsalicylate (Pepto-Bismol); use with antibiotics	Suppresses *H. pylori* bacteria in the gastric mucosa and assists with healing of mucosal lesions	Given concurrently with antibiotics to cure *H. pylori* infection. Should be taken on an empty stomach.
Histamine 2 (H$_2$) Receptor Antagonists		
Cimetidine (Peptol)	Inhibits acid secretion by blocking the action of histamine on the histamine receptors of the parietal cells in the stomach	Least expensive of the H$_2$ receptor antagonists. May cause confusion, agitation, or coma in the elderly or those with renal or hepatic insufficiency. Long-term use may cause gynecomastia, impotence, and diarrhea.
Ranitidine (Zantac)	Inhibits acid secretion by blocking the action of the histamine on the histamine receptors of the parietal cells in the stomach	Prolonged drug half-life in patients with renal and hepatic insufficiency. Causes fewer side effects than cimetidine. Rarely causes constipation, diarrhea, dizziness, and depression.
Famotidine (Pepcid)	Inhibits acid secretion by blocking the action of histamine on the histamine receptors on the parietal cells in the stomach	Best choice for critically ill patient because it is known to have least risk of interaction with other medications. (It is unclear whether other H$_2$ receptor antagonists are as safe as famotidine.) Does not alter medication metabolism in the liver. Prolonged half-life in patients with renal insufficiency. Short-term relief for gastroesophageal reflux. Dilute before IV injection. Rarely causes constipation or diarrhea.
Nizantidine (Axid)	Inhibits acid secretion by blocking the action of histamine on the histamine receptors on the parietal cells in the stomach	Used for duodenal ulcers. Prolonged half-life in patients with renal insufficiency. Rarely causes sweating, increased liver enzymes, nausea, urticaria.
Proton (Gastric Acid) Pump Inhibitor		
Omeprazole (Losec)	Decreases gastric acid secretion by slowing the hydrogen-potassium adenosine triphosphatase (H+, K+-ATPase) pump on the surface of the parietal cells	Long-term use may cause gastric tumours and bacterial invasion. May cause diarrhea, additional pain, and nausea.
Lansoprazole (Prevacid)	Decreases gastric acid secretion by slowing the H+, K+-ATPase pump on the surface of the parietal cells.	A delayed-release capsule that is to be swallowed whole and taken before meals.
Rabeprazole (Aciphex)	Decreases gastric acid secretion by slowing the H+, K+-ATPase pump on the surface of the parietal cells	A delayed-release tablet; swallow whole.

(continued)

Table 37-1 • Pharmacologic Therapy for Peptic Ulcer Disease and Gastritis (Continued)

PHARMACOLOGIC AGENT	MAJOR ACTION	NURSING CONSIDERATIONS
Cytoprotective Medications		
Misoprostol (Cytotec)	A synthetic prostaglandin; protects the gastric mucosa from ulcerogenic agents; also increases mucus production and bicarbonate levels	Used as a preventive medication (to prevent ulceration in patients using NSAIDs). Administer with food. May cause diarrhea and cramping (including uterine cramping).
Sucralfate (Sulcrate)	In the presence of gastric acid, sucralfate creates a viscous substance that forms a protective layer at the site of the ulcer and prevents digestion by pepsin	May cause constipation or nausea. Approved for duodenal—*not gastric*—ulcers.

The nurse discourages the intake of caffeinated beverages, because caffeine is a central nervous system stimulant that increases gastric activity and pepsin secretion. It also is important to discourage alcohol use. Discouraging cigarette smoking is important because nicotine reduces the secretion of pancreatic bicarbonate and thus inhibits the neutralization of gastric acid in the duodenum (Eastwood, 1997). When appropriate, the nurse refers the patient for alcohol counselling and smoking cessation programs.

PROMOTING FLUID BALANCE

Daily fluid intake and output are monitored to detect early signs of dehydration (minimal urine output of 30 mL/hour, minimal intake of 1.5 L/day). If food and fluids are withheld, IV fluids (3 L/day) usually are prescribed and a record of fluid intake plus caloric value (1 L of 5% dextrose in water = 170 calories of carbohydrate) needs to be maintained. Electrolyte values (sodium, potassium, chloride) are assessed every 24 hours to detect imbalance.

The nurse must always be alert for any indicators of hemorrhagic gastritis, which include **hematemesis** (vomiting of blood), tachycardia, and hypotension. If these occur, the physician is notified and the patient's vital signs are monitored as the patient's condition warrants. Guidelines for managing upper GI tract bleeding are discussed later in this chapter.

RELIEVING PAIN

Measures to help relieve pain include instructing the patient to avoid foods and beverages that may be irritating to the gastric mucosa (described earlier) and instructing the patient about using medications to relieve chronic gastritis. To follow up, the nurse assesses the patient's level of pain and the extent of comfort attained from the use of medications and avoidance of irritating substances.

PROMOTING HOME AND COMMUNITY-BASED CARE

Teaching Patients Self-Care

The nurse evaluates the patient's knowledge about gastritis and develops an individualized teaching plan that includes information about stress management, diet, and medications (Chart 37-1). Dietary instructions take into account the patient's daily caloric needs, food preferences, and pattern of eating. The nurse and patient review foods and other substances to be avoided (eg, spicy, irritating, or highly seasoned foods; caffeine; nicotine; alcohol). Consultation with a dietitian may be recommended.

Providing information about prescribed antibiotics, bismuth salts, medications to decrease gastric secretion, and medications to protect mucosal cells from gastric secretions can help the patient recover and prevent recurrence. Patients with pernicious anemia need information about long-term vitamin B_{12} injections; the nurse may instruct a family member about administering these injections or make arrangements for the patient to receive the injections from a health care provider. Finally, the nurse emphasizes the importance of keeping follow-up appointments with health care providers.

Evaluation

EXPECTED PATIENT OUTCOMES

Expected patient outcomes may include the following:

1. Exhibits less anxiety
2. Avoids eating irritating foods or drinking caffeinated beverages or alcohol
3. Maintains fluid balance
   a. Has intake of at least 1.5 L daily
   b. Drinks six to eight glasses of water daily

Chart 37-1
Home Care Checklist • The Patient With Gastritis

At the completion of the home care instruction, the patient or caregiver will be able to:	Patient	Caregiver
• Identify foods and other substances that may cause gastritis.	✓	✓
• Describe medication regimen to follow.	✓	✓
• State need for vitamin B_{12} injections if patient has pernicious anemia.	✓	✓

c. Has a urinary output of about 1 L daily
d. Displays adequate skin turgor
4. Adheres to medical regimen
  a. Selects nonirritating foods and beverages
  b. Takes medications as prescribed
5. Maintains appropriate weight
6. Reports less pain

Gastric and Duodenal Ulcers

A peptic ulcer is an excavation (hollowed-out area) that forms in the mucosal wall of the stomach, in the **pylorus** (opening between stomach and duodenum), in the **duodenum** (first part of small intestine), or in the esophagus. A peptic ulcer is frequently referred to as a gastric, duodenal, or esophageal ulcer, depending on its location, or as peptic ulcer disease. Erosion of a circumscribed area of mucous membrane is the cause (Fig. 37-2). This erosion may extend as deeply as the muscle layers or through the muscle to the peritoneum. Peptic ulcers are more likely to be in the duodenum than in the stomach. As a rule they occur alone, but they may occur in multiples. Chronic gastric ulcers tend to occur in the lesser curvature of the stomach, near the pylorus. Table 37-2 compares the features of gastric and duodenal ulcers.

Peptic ulcer disease occurs with the greatest frequency in people between the ages of 40 and 60 years. It is relatively uncommon in women of childbearing age, but it has been observed in children and even in infants. After menopause, the incidence of peptic ulcers in women is almost equal to that in men. Peptic ulcers in the body of the stomach can occur without excessive acid secretion.

Table 37-2 • Comparing Duodenal and Gastric Ulcers	
DUODENAL ULCER	**GASTRIC ULCER**
Incidence	
Age 30–60	Usually 50 and over
Male: female = 2–3:1	Male: female = 1:1
80% of peptic ulcers are duodenal	15% of peptic ulcers are gastric
Signs, Symptoms, and Clinical Findings	
Hypersecretion of stomach acid (HCl)	Normal—hyposecretion of stomach acid (HCl)
May have weight gain	Weight loss may occur
Pain occurs 2–3 hours after a meal; often awakened between 1–2 AM; ingestion of food relieves pain	Pain occurs ½ to 1 hour after a meal; rarely occurs at night; may be relieved by vomiting; ingestion of food does not help, sometimes increases pain
Vomiting uncommon	Vomiting common
Hemorrhage less likely than with gastric ulcer, but if present melena more common than hematemesis	Hemorrhage more likely to occur than with duodenal ulcer; hematemesis more common than melena
More likely to perforate than gastric ulcers	
Malignancy Possibility	
Rare	Occasionally
Risk Factors	
H. pylori, alcohol, smoking, cirrhosis, stress	*H. pylori,* gastritis, alcohol, smoking, use of NSAIDs, stress

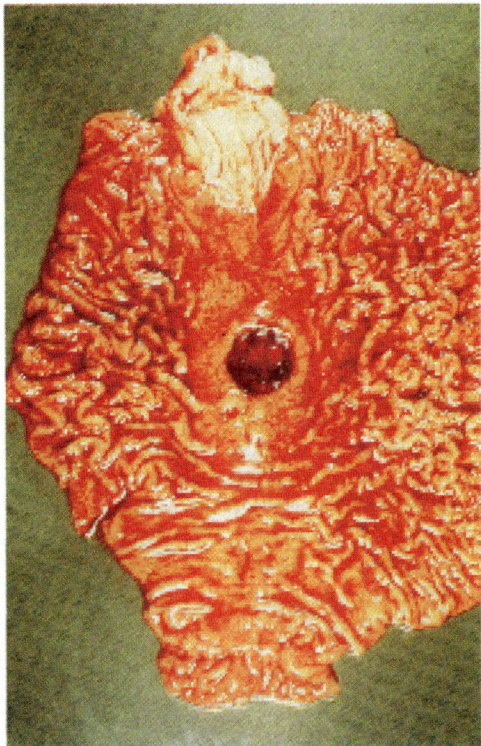

FIGURE 37-2 Deep peptic ulcer. From Porth, C. (2002). *Pathophysiology: Concepts of altered health states* (6th ed). Philadelphia: Lippincott Williams & Wilkins.

In the past, stress and anxiety were thought to be causes of ulcers. Research has identified that peptic ulcers result from infection with the gram-negative bacteria *H. pylori* (Tytgat, 2000). However, ulcers do seem to develop more commonly in people who are tense; whether this is a contributing factor to the condition is uncertain. In addition, excessive secretion of HCl in the stomach may contribute to the formation of gastric ulcers, and stress may be associated with its increased secretion. The ingestion of milk and caffeinated beverages, smoking, and alcohol also may increase HCl secretion.

Familial tendency may be a significant predisposing factor. A further genetic link is noted in the finding that people with blood type O are more susceptible to peptic ulcers than are those with blood type A, B, or AB. There also is an association between duodenal ulcers and chronic pulmonary disease or chronic renal disease. Other predisposing factors associated with peptic ulcer include chronic use of NSAIDs, alcohol ingestion, and excessive smoking.

Rarely, ulcers are caused by excessive amounts of the hormone gastrin, produced by tumours. This Zollinger-Ellison syndrome (ZES) consists of severe peptic ulcers, extreme gastric hyperacidity, and gastrin-secreting benign or malignant tumours of the pancreas. Stress ulcers, which are clinically different from peptic ulcers, are ulcerations in the mucosa that can occur in the gastroduodenal area. Stress ulcers may occur in patients who are exposed to stressful conditions. Esophageal ulcers occur as a result of the backward flow of HCl from the stomach into the esophagus (gastroesophageal reflux disease [GERD]).

Pathophysiology

Peptic ulcers occur mainly in the gastroduodenal mucosa because this tissue cannot withstand the digestive action of gastric acid (HCl) and pepsin. The erosion is caused by the increased concentration or activity of acid-pepsin, or by decreased resistance of the mucosa. A damaged mucosa cannot secrete enough mucus to act as a barrier against HCl. The use of NSAIDs inhibits the secretion of mucus that protects the mucosa. Patients with duodenal ulcer disease secrete more acid than normal, whereas patients with gastric ulcer tend to secrete normal or decreased levels of acid.

ZES is suspected when a patient has several peptic ulcers or an ulcer that is resistant to standard medical therapy. It is identified by the following findings: hypersecretion of gastric juice, duodenal ulcers, and gastrinomas (islet cell tumours) in the pancreas. Ninety percent of tumours are found in the "gastric triangle," which encompasses the cystic and common bile ducts, the second and third portions of the duodenum, and the neck and body of the pancreas. Approximately one third of gastrinomas are malignant. Diarrhea and steatorrhea (unabsorbed fat in the stool) may be evident. The patient may have coexisting parathyroid adenomas or hyperplasia and may therefore exhibit signs of hypercalcemia. The most common complaint is epigastric pain. *H. pylori* is not a risk factor for ZES.

Stress ulcer is the term given to the acute mucosal ulceration of the duodenal or gastric area that occurs after physiologically stressful events, such as burns, shock, severe sepsis, and multiple organ traumas. These ulcers are most common in ventilator-dependent patients after trauma or surgery. Fibreoptic endoscopy within 24 hours after injury reveals shallow erosions of the stomach wall; by 72 hours, multiple gastric erosions are observed. As the stressful condition continues, the ulcers spread. When the patient recovers, the lesions are reversed. This pattern is typical of stress ulceration.

Differences of opinion exist as to the actual cause of mucosal ulceration in stress ulcers. Usually, it is preceded by shock; this leads to decreased gastric mucosal blood flow and to reflux of duodenal contents into the stomach. In addition, large quantities of pepsin are released. The combination of ischemia, acid, and pepsin creates an ideal climate for ulceration.

Stress ulcers should be distinguished from Cushing's ulcers and Curling's ulcers, two other types of gastric ulcers. Cushing's ulcers are common in patients with trauma to the brain. They may occur in the esophagus, stomach, or duodenum and are usually deeper and more penetrating than stress ulcers. Curling's ulcer is frequently observed about 72 hours after extensive burns and involves the antrum of the stomach or the duodenum.

Clinical Manifestations

Symptoms of an ulcer may last for a few days, weeks, or months and may disappear only to reappear, often without an identifiable cause. Many people have symptomless ulcers, and in 20% to 30% perforation or hemorrhage may occur without any preceding manifestations.

As a rule, the patient with an ulcer complains of dull, gnawing pain or a burning sensation in the midepigastrium or in the back. It is believed that the pain occurs when the increased acid content of the stomach and duodenum erodes the lesion and stimulates the exposed nerve endings. Another theory suggests that contact of the lesion with acid stimulates a local reflex mechanism that initiates contraction of the adjacent smooth muscle. Pain is usually relieved by eating, because food neutralizes the acid, or by taking alkali; however, once the stomach has emptied or the alkali's effect has decreased, the pain returns. Sharply localized tenderness can be elicited by applying gentle pressure to the epigastrium at or slightly to the right of the midline.

Other symptoms include **pyrosis** (heartburn), vomiting, constipation or diarrhea, and bleeding. Pyrosis is a burning sensation in the esophagus and stomach that moves up to the mouth. Heartburn is often accompanied by sour eructation, or burping, which is common when the patient's stomach is empty.

Although vomiting is rare in uncomplicated duodenal ulcer, it may be a symptom of a peptic ulcer complication. It results from obstruction of the pyloric orifice, caused by either muscular spasm of the pylorus or mechanical obstruction from scarring or acute swelling of the inflamed mucous membrane adjacent to the ulcer. Vomiting may or may not be preceded by nausea; usually it follows a bout of severe pain and bloating, which is relieved by ejection of the gastric contents. Emesis often contains undigested food eaten many hours earlier. Constipation or diarrhea can occur, probably as a result of diet and medications.

Fifteen percent of patients with gastric ulcers experience bleeding. Patients may present with GI bleeding as evidenced by the passage of tarry stools. A small portion of patients who bleed from an acute ulcer have had no previous digestive complaints, but they develop symptoms thereafter (Yamada, 1999).

Assessment and Diagnostic Findings

A physical examination may reveal pain, epigastric tenderness, or abdominal distention. A barium study of the upper GI tract may show an ulcer; however, endoscopy is the preferred diagnostic procedure because it allows direct visualization of inflammatory changes, ulcers, and lesions. Through endoscopy, a biopsy of the gastric mucosa and of any suspicious lesions can be obtained. Endoscopy may reveal lesions that are not evident on x-ray studies because of their size or location.

Stools may be tested periodically until they are negative for occult blood. Gastric secretory studies are of value in diagnosing achlorhydria and ZES. *H. pylori* infection may be determined by biopsy and histology with culture. There is also a breath test that detects *H. pylori,* as well as a serologic test for antibodies to the *H. pylori* antigen. Pain that is relieved by ingesting food or antacids and absence of pain on arising are also highly suggestive of an ulcer.

Medical Management

Once the diagnosis is established, the patient is informed that the problem can be controlled. Recurrence may develop; however, peptic ulcers treated with antibiotics to eradicate *H. pylori* have a lower recurrence rate than those not treated with antibiotics. The goals are to eradicate *H. pylori* and to manage gastric acidity. Methods used include medications, lifestyle changes, and surgical intervention.

PHARMACOLOGIC THERAPY

Currently, the most commonly used therapy in the treatment of ulcers is a combination of antibiotics, proton pump inhibitors, and bismuth salts that suppresses or eradicates *H. pylori;* histamine 2 (H_2) receptor antagonists and proton pump inhibitors are used to treat NSAID-induced and other ulcers not associated with *H. pylori* ulcers. Table 37-1 provides details about pharmacologic treatment.

The patient is advised to adhere to the medication regimen to ensure complete healing of the ulcer. Because most patients become symptom-free within a week, it becomes a nursing responsibility to stress the importance of following the prescribed regimen so that the healing process can continue uninterrupted and the return of chronic ulcer symptoms can be prevented. Rest, sedatives, and tranquilizers may add to the patient's comfort and are prescribed as needed. Maintenance dosages of H$_2$ receptor antagonists are usually recommended for 1 year.

For patients with ZES, hypersecretion of acid may be controlled with high doses of H$_2$ receptor antagonists. These patients may require twice the normal dose, and dosages usually need to be increased with prolonged use. Octreotide (Sandostatin), a medication that suppresses gastrin levels, also may be prescribed.

Patients at risk for stress ulcers may be treated prophylactically with IV H$_2$ receptor antagonists and cytoprotective agents (e.g., misoprostol, sucralfate) because of the risk for upper GI tract hemorrhage. Frequent gastric aspiration is performed to allow monitoring of gastric secretion pH.

STRESS REDUCTION AND REST

Reducing environmental stress requires physical and psychological modifications on the patient's part as well as the aid and cooperation of family members and significant others. The patient may need help in identifying situations that are stressful or exhausting. A rushed lifestyle and an irregular schedule may aggravate symptoms and interfere with regular meals taken in relaxed settings and with the regular administration of medications. The patient may benefit from regular rest periods during the day, at least during the acute phase of the disease. Biofeedback, hypnosis, or behaviour modification may be helpful.

SMOKING CESSATION

Studies have shown that smoking decreases the secretion of bicarbonate from the pancreas into the duodenum, resulting in increased acidity of the duodenum. Research indicates that continuing to smoke cigarettes may significantly inhibit ulcer repair. Therefore, the patient is strongly encouraged to stop smoking. Smoking cessation support groups and other smoking cessation approaches are helpful for many patients (Eastwood, 1997).

DIETARY MODIFICATION

The intent of dietary modification for patients with peptic ulcers is to avoid oversecretion of acid and hypermotility in the GI tract. These can be minimized by avoiding extremes of temperature and overstimulation from consumption of meat extracts, alcohol, coffee (including decaffeinated coffee, which also stimulates acid secretion) and other caffeinated beverages, and diets rich in milk and cream (which stimulate acid secretion). In addition, an effort is made to neutralize acid by eating three regular meals a day. Small, frequent feedings are not necessary as long as an antacid or a histamine blocker is taken. Diet compatibility becomes an individual matter: the patient eats foods that can be tolerated and avoids those that produce pain.

SURGICAL MANAGEMENT

The introduction of antibiotics to eradicate *H. pylori* and of H$_2$ receptor antagonists as treatment for ulcers has greatly reduced the need for surgical interventions. However, surgery is usually recommended for patients with intractable ulcers (those that fail to heal after 12 to 16 weeks of medical treatment), life-threatening hemorrhage, perforation, or obstruction, and for those with ZES not responding to medications (Yamada, 1999). Surgical procedures include vagotomy, with or without pyloroplasty, and the Billroth I and Billroth II procedures (Table 37-3; see also the section on gastric surgery later in this chapter). Patients who need ulcer surgery may have had a long illness. They may be discouraged and have had interruptions in their work role and pressures in their family life.

FOLLOW-UP CARE

Recurrence within 1 year may be prevented with the prophylactic use of H$_2$ receptor antagonists given at a reduced dose. Not all patients require maintenance therapy; it may be prescribed only for those with two or three recurrences per year, those who have had a complication such as bleeding or outlet obstruction, or those who are candidates for gastric surgery but are at too high a risk for surgery. The likelihood of recurrence is reduced if the patient avoids smoking, coffee (including decaffeinated coffee) and other caffeinated beverages, alcohol, and ulcerogenic medications (eg, NSAIDs).

NURSING PROCESS: THE PATIENT WITH ULCER DISEASE

Assessment

The nurse asks the patient to describe the pain and the methods used to relieve it (e.g., food, antacids). The patient usually describes peptic ulcer pain as burning or gnawing; it occurs about 2 hours after a meal and frequently awakens the patient between midnight and 3 AM. Taking antacids, eating, or vomiting often relieves the pain. If the patient reports a recent history of vomiting, the nurse determines how often emesis has occurred and notes important characteristics of the vomitus: Is it bright red, does it resemble coffee grounds, or is there undigested food from previous meals? Has the patient noted any bloody or tarry stools?

The nurse also asks the patient to list his or her usual food intake for a 72-hour period and to describe food habits (e.g., speed of eating, regularity of meals, preference for spicy foods, use of seasonings, use of caffeinated beverages and decaffeinated coffee). Lifestyle and habits are a concern as well. Does the patient use irritating substances? For example, does he or she smoke cigarettes? If yes, how many? Does the patient ingest alcohol? If yes, how much and how often? Are NSAIDs used? The nurse inquires about the patient's level of anxiety and his or her perception of current stressors. How does the patient express anger or cope with stressful situations? Is the patient experiencing occupational stress or problems within the family? Is there a family history of ulcer disease?

The nurse assesses vital signs and reports tachycardia and hypotension, which may indicate anemia from GI bleeding. The stool is tested for occult blood, and a physical examination, including palpation of the abdomen for localized tenderness, is performed as well.

Diagnosis

NURSING DIAGNOSES

Based on the assessment data, the patient's nursing diagnoses may include the following:

- Acute pain related to the effect of gastric acid secretion on damaged tissue
- Anxiety related to coping with an acute disease
- Imbalanced nutrition related to changes in diet
- Deficient knowledge about prevention of symptoms and management of the condition

Table 37-3 • Surgical Procedures for Peptic Ulcer Disease

OPERATION	DESCRIPTION	COMMENTS
Vagotomy 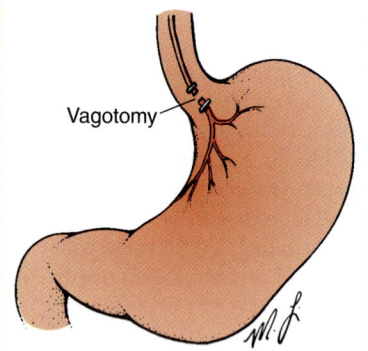	Severing of the vagus nerve. Decreases gastric acid by diminishing cholinergic stimulation to the parietal cells, making them less responsive to gastrin. May be done via open surgical approach, laparoscopy, or thoracoscopy	May be performed to reduce gastric acid secretion. A drainage type of procedure (see pyloroplasty) is usually performed to assist with gastric emptying (because there is total denervation of the stomach). Some patients experience problems with feeling of fullness, dumping syndrome, diarrhea, and gastritis.
Truncal vagotomy	Severs the right and left vagus nerves as they enter the stomach at the distal part of the esophagus.	This type of vagotomy is most commonly used to decrease acid secretions and reduce gastric and intestinal motility. Recurrence rate of ulcer is 10%–15%.
Selective vagotomy	Severs vagal innervation to the stomach but maintains innervation to the rest of the abdominal organs.	
Proximal (parietal cell) gastric vagotomy without drainage	Denervates acid-secreting parietal cells but preserves vagal innervation to the gastric antrum and pylorus.	No dumping syndrome. No need for drainage procedure. Recurrence rate of ulcer is 10%–15%.
Pyloroplasty 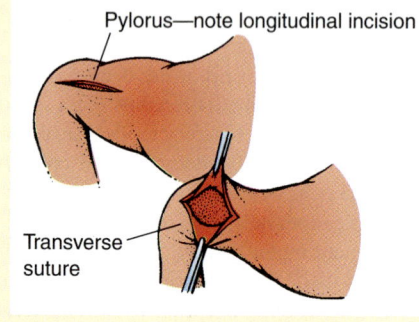	A surgical procedure in which a longitudinal incision is made into the pylorus and transversely sutured closed to enlarge the outlet and relax the muscle	Usually accompanies truncal and selective vagotomies, which produce delayed gastric emptying due to decreased innervation.
Antrectomy Billroth I (Gastroduodenostomy) 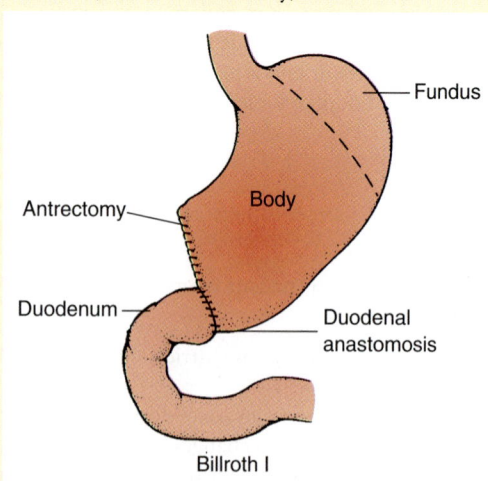	Removal of the lower portion of the antrum of the stomach (which contains the cells that secrete gastrin) as well as a small portion of the duodenum and pylorus. The remaining segment is anastomosed to the duodenum (Billroth I) or to the jejunum (Billroth II)	May be performed in conjunction with a truncal vagotomy. The patient may have problems with feeling of fullness, dumping syndrome, and diarrhea. Recurrence rate of ulcer is <1%.

Image labels:

Vagotomy

Pylorus—note longitudinal incision

Transverse suture

Fundus

Antrectomy

Body

Duodenum

Duodenal anastomosis

Billroth I

(continued)

Table 37-3 • Surgical Procedures for Peptic Ulcer Disease (Continued)

OPERATION	DESCRIPTION	COMMENTS
Billroth II (Gastrojejunostomy) 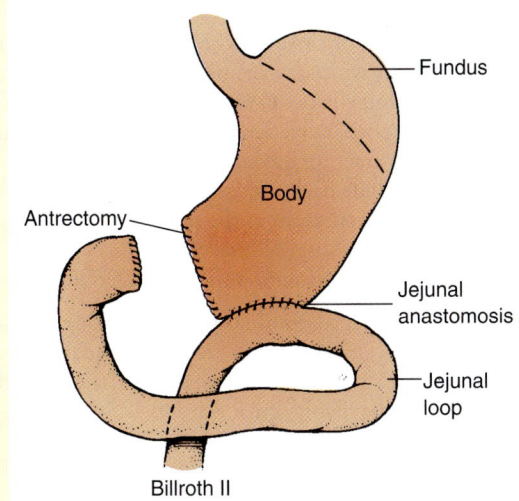		
Subtotal gastrectomy with Billroth I or II anastomosis	Removal of distal third of stomach; anastomosis with duodenum or jejunum. Removes gastrin-producing cells in the antrum and part of the parietal cells.	Dumping syndrome, anemia, malabsorption, weight loss. Recurrence rate of ulcer is 10%–15%.

COLLABORATIVE PROBLEMS/ POTENTIAL COMPLICATIONS

Potential complications may include the following:

- Hemorrhage
- Perforation
- Penetration
- Pyloric obstruction (gastric outlet obstruction)

Planning and Goals

The goals for the patient may include relief of pain, reduced anxiety, maintenance of nutritional requirements, knowledge about the management and prevention of ulcer recurrence, and absence of complications.

Nursing Interventions

RELIEVING PAIN

Pain relief can be achieved with prescribed medications. The patient should avoid aspirin, foods and beverages that contain caffeine, and decaffeinated coffee, and meals should be eaten at regularly paced intervals in a relaxed setting. Some patients benefit from learning relaxation techniques to help manage stress and pain and to enhance smoking cessation efforts.

REDUCING ANXIETY

The nurse assesses the patient's level of anxiety. Patients with peptic ulcers are usually anxious, but their anxiety is not always obvious. Appropriate information is provided at the patient's level of understanding, all questions are answered, and the patient is encouraged to express fears openly. Explaining diagnostic tests and administering medications on schedule also help to reduce anxiety. The nurse interacts with the patient in a relaxed manner, helps identify stressors, and explains various coping techniques

and relaxation methods, such as biofeedback, hypnosis, or behaviour modification. The patient's family is also encouraged to participate in care and to provide emotional support.

MAINTAINING OPTIMAL NUTRITIONAL STATUS

The nurse assesses the patient for malnutrition and weight loss. After recovery from an acute phase of peptic ulcer disease, the patient is advised about the importance of complying with the medication regimen and dietary restrictions.

MONITORING AND MANAGING POTENTIAL COMPLICATIONS

Hemorrhage

Gastritis and hemorrhage from peptic ulcer are the two most common causes of upper GI tract bleeding (which may also occur with esophageal varices, as discussed in Chapter 39). Hemorrhage, the most common complication, occurs in about 15% of patients with peptic ulcers (Yamada, 1999). The site of bleeding is usually the distal portion of the duodenum. Bleeding may be manifested by hematemesis or **melena** (tarry stools). The vomited blood can be bright red, or it can have a "coffee grounds" appearance (which is dark) from the oxidation of hemoglobin to methemoglobin. When the hemorrhage is large (2000 to 3000 mL), most of the blood is vomited. Because large quantities of blood may be lost quickly, immediate correction of blood loss may be required to prevent hemorrhagic shock. When the hemorrhage is small, much or all of the blood is passed in the stools, which will appear tarry black because of the digested hemoglobin. Management depends on the amount of blood lost and the rate of bleeding.

The nurse assesses the patient for faintness or dizziness and nausea, which may precede or accompany bleeding. It is important to monitor vital signs frequently and to evaluate the patient for tachycardia, hypotension, and tachypnea. Other nursing interventions include monitoring the hemoglobin and hematocrit, testing the stool for gross or occult blood, and recording hourly urinary output to detect anuria or oliguria (absence or decreased urine production).

Many times the bleeding from a peptic ulcer stops spontaneously; however, the incidence of recurrent bleeding is high. Because bleeding can be fatal, the cause and severity of the hemorrhage must be identified quickly and the blood loss treated to prevent hemorrhagic shock. Management of upper GI tract bleeding consists of quickly determining the amount of blood lost and the rate of bleeding, rapidly replacing the blood that has been lost, stopping the bleeding, stabilizing the patient, and diagnosing and treating the cause. Related nursing and collaborative interventions include the following:

- Inserting a peripheral IV line for the infusion of saline or lactated Ringer's solution and blood products. The nurse may need to assist with the placement of a pulmonary artery catheter for hemodynamic monitoring. Blood component therapy is initiated if there are signs of shock (eg, tachycardia, sweating, coldness of the extremities).
- Monitoring the hemoglobin and hematocrit to assist in evaluating blood loss
- Inserting an NG tube to distinguish fresh blood from "coffee grounds" material, to aid in the removal of clots and acid, to prevent nausea and vomiting, and to provide a means of monitoring further bleeding
- Administering a room-temperature lavage of saline solution or water. This is controversial; some authorities recommend using ice lavage (Yamada, 1999).
- Inserting an indwelling urinary catheter and monitoring urinary output
- Monitoring vital signs and oxygen saturation and administering oxygen therapy
- Placing the patient in the recumbent position with the legs elevated to prevent hypotension; or, to prevent aspiration from vomiting, placing the patient on the left side
- Treating hemorrhagic shock (described in Chapter 15)

If bleeding cannot be managed by the measures described, other treatment modalities may be used. Transendoscopic coagulation by laser, heat probe, medication, a sclerosing agent, or a combination of these therapies can halt bleeding and make surgical intervention unnecessary. There is much debate regarding how soon endoscopy should be performed. Some believe that endoscopy should be performed in the first 24 hours after hemorrhage has been stabilized. Others believe that endoscopy may be performed during acute bleeding, as long as the esophageal or gastric area can be visualized (blood may decrease visibility) (Yamada, 1999).

For those who are unable to undergo surgery, selective embolization may be used. This procedure involves forcing emboli of autologous blood clots with or without Gelfoam (absorbable gelatin sponge) through a catheter in the artery to a point above the bleeding lesion. A radiologist performs this procedure.

Rebleeding may occur and often warrants surgical intervention. The nurse monitors the patient carefully so that bleeding can be detected quickly. Signs of bleeding include tachycardia, tachypnea, hypotension, mental confusion, thirst, and oliguria. If bleeding recurs within 48 hours after medical therapy has begun, or if more than 6 to 10 units of blood are required within 24 hours to maintain blood volume, the patient is likely to require surgery. Some physicians recommend surgical intervention if a patient hemorrhages three times. Other criteria for surgery are the patient's age (massive hemorrhaging is three times more likely to be fatal in those older than 60 years of age); a history of chronic duodenal ulcer; and

a coincidental gastric ulcer (Yamada, 1999). The area of the ulcer is removed or the bleeding vessels are ligated. Many patients also undergo procedures (eg, vagotomy and pyloroplasty, gastrectomy) aimed at controlling the underlying cause of the ulcers (see Table 37-3).

Perforation and Penetration

Perforation is the erosion of the ulcer through the gastric serosa into the peritoneal cavity without warning. It is an abdominal catastrophe and requires immediate surgery. Penetration is erosion of the ulcer through the gastric serosa into adjacent structures such as the pancreas, biliary tract, or gastrohepatic omentum. Symptoms of penetration include back and epigastric pain not relieved by medications that were effective in the past. Like perforation, penetration usually requires surgical intervention.

Signs and symptoms of perforation include the following:

- Sudden, severe upper abdominal pain (persisting and increasing in intensity); pain may be referred to the shoulders, especially the right shoulder, because of irritation of the phrenic nerve in the diaphragm.
- Vomiting and collapse (fainting)
- Extremely tender and rigid (boardlike) abdomen
- Hypotension and tachycardia, indicating shock

Because chemical peritonitis develops within a few hours after perforation and is followed by bacterial peritonitis, the perforation must be closed as quickly as possible. In a few patients, it may be deemed safe and advisable to perform surgery for the ulcer disease in addition to suturing the perforation.

Postoperatively, the stomach contents are drained by means of an NG tube. The nurse monitors fluid and electrolyte balance and assesses the patient for peritonitis or localized infection (increased temperature, abdominal pain, paralytic ileus, increased or absent bowel sounds, abdominal distention). Antibiotic therapy is administered parenterally as prescribed.

Pyloric Obstruction

Pyloric obstruction, also called gastric outlet obstruction (GOO), occurs when the area distal to the pyloric sphincter becomes scarred and stenosed from spasm or edema or from scar tissue that forms when an ulcer alternately heals and breaks down. The patient has nausea and vomiting, constipation, epigastric fullness, anorexia, and, later, weight loss.

In treating the patient with pyloric obstruction, the first consideration is to insert an NG tube to decompress the stomach. Confirmation that obstruction is the cause of the discomfort is accomplished by assessing the amount of fluid aspirated from the NG tube. A residual of more than 400 mL strongly suggests obstruction. Usually an upper GI study or endoscopy is performed to confirm gastric outlet obstruction. Decompression of the stomach and management of extracellular fluid volume and electrolyte balances may improve the patient's condition and avert the need for surgical intervention. A balloon dilatation of the pylorus via endoscopy may be beneficial. If the obstruction is unrelieved by medical management, surgery (in the form of a vagotomy and **antrectomy** or gastrojejunostomy and vagotomy) may be required.

PROMOTING HOME AND COMMUNITY-BASED CARE

Teaching Patients Self-Care

To manage ulcer disease successfully, the patient is instructed about the factors that will help or aggravate the condition (Chart 37-2). The nurse reviews information about medications to be taken at

---

Chart 37-2
Home Care Checklist • The Patient With Peptic Ulcer Disease

At the completion of the home care instruction, the patient or caregiver will be able to:	Patient	Caregiver
• State the medication regimen and importance of complying with medication schedule.	✓	✓
• State dietary restrictions and foods that may exacerbate condition (caffeine products, milk).	✓	✓
• Identify smoking cessation groups.	✓	
• Identify methods to reduce stress.	✓	✓

• State signs and symptoms of complications:
    Hemorrhage—cool skin, confusion, increased heart rate, laboured breathing, blood in stool
    Penetration and perforation—severe abdominal pain, rigid and tender abdomen, vomiting, elevated temperature, increased heart rate
    Pyloric obstruction—nausea and vomiting, distended abdomen, abdominal pain
	✓	✓

• State need for follow-up medical care.	✓	✓

---

home, including name, dosage, frequency, and possible side effects, stressing the importance of continuing to take medications even after signs and symptoms have decreased or subsided. Then the patient is instructed to avoid certain medications and foods that exacerbate symptoms as well as substances that have acid-producing potential (eg, alcohol; caffeinated beverages such as coffee, tea, and colas). It is important to counsel the patient to eat meals at regular times and in a relaxed setting, and to avoid overeating. If relevant, the nurse also informs the patient about the irritant effects of smoking on the ulcer and provides information about smoking cessation programs.

> **NURSING ALERT** The nurse reviews with the patient and family the signs and symptoms of complications to be reported. They include hemorrhage (cool skin, confusion, increased heart rate, laboured breathing, and blood in the stool); penetration and perforation (severe abdominal pain, rigid and tender abdomen, vomiting, elevated temperature, and increased heart rate); and pyloric obstruction (nausea, vomiting, distended abdomen, and abdominal pain).

The nurse reinforces the importance of follow-up care for approximately 1 year, the need to report recurrence of symptoms, and the need for treating possible problems that occur after surgery, such as intolerance to dairy products and sweet foods.

Evaluation

EXPECTED PATIENT OUTCOMES
Expected patient outcomes may include the following:

1. Reports freedom from pain between meals
2. Feels less anxiety by avoiding stress
3. Complies with therapeutic regimen
   a. Avoids irritating foods and beverages
   b. Eats regularly scheduled meals
   c. Takes prescribed medications as scheduled
   d. Uses coping mechanisms to deal with stress
4. Maintains weight
5. Is free of complications

Morbid Obesity

In Canada, approximately 25% of children and close to 50% of adults are overweight (Canadian Institutes of Health Research, 2004). Close to 2.8 million Canadians are obese (Government of

Alberta, 2004). **Morbid obesity** is the term applied to people who are more than two times their ideal body weight or whose body mass index (BMI) exceeds 30 kg/m². (See Chapter 5.)

Another definition of morbid obesity is body weight that is more than 45 kg greater than the ideal body weight (Monteforte & Turkelson, 2000). Patients with morbid obesity are at higher risk for health complications, such as cardiovascular disease, arthritis, asthma, bronchitis, and diabetes. They frequently suffer from low self-esteem, impaired body image, and depression.

Medical Management

Conservative management consists of placing the person on a weight loss diet in conjunction with behavioural modification and exercise; however, diet therapy is usually unsuccessful. There is a belief that depression may be a contributing factor to weight gain, and treatment of the depression with bupropion hydrochloride (Wellbutrin) may be helpful (Wangsness, 2000). Some physicians recommend acupuncture and hypnosis before recommending surgery.

PHARMACOLOGIC MANAGEMENT
Several medications have recently been approved for obesity. They include sibutramine HCl (Meridia) and orlistat (Xenical). By inhibiting the reuptake of serotonin and norepinephrine, sibutramine decreases appetite. Orlistat reduces caloric intake by binding to gastric and pancreatic lipase to prevent digestion of fats. Both medications require a physician's prescription. Sibutramine may increase blood pressure and should not be taken by people with a history of coronary artery disease, angina pectoris, dysrhythmias, or kidney disease; by those taking antidepressants or monoamine oxidase inhibitors; or by pregnant or nursing women. Side effects may include dry mouth, insomnia, headache, increased sweating, and increased heart rate. Side effects of orlistat may include increased bowel movements, gas with oily discharge, decreased food absorption, decreased bile flow, and decreased absorption of some vitamins. A multivitamin is usually recommended for patients taking orlistat. Women who are pregnant or nursing should not take orlistat (Hussar, 2000, Wilson, Shannon, & Stang 2005).

SURGICAL MANAGEMENT
Bariatric surgery, or surgery for morbid obesity, is performed only after other nonsurgical attempts at weight control have failed. The first surgical procedure to treat morbid obesity was the jejunoileal bypass. This procedure, which resulted in significant

complications, has been largely replaced by gastric restriction procedures. Gastric bypass and vertical banded gastroplasty are the current operations of choice. These procedures may be performed laparoscopically or by an open surgical technique.

In gastric bypass surgery, the proximal segment of the stomach is transected to form a small pouch with a small gastroenterostomy stoma. The Roux-en-Y gastric bypass is the recommended procedure for long-term weight loss. In this procedure, a horizontal row of staples creates a stomach pouch with a 1-cm stoma that is anastomosed with a portion of distal jejunum, creating a gastroenterostomy. The transected proximal portion of the jejunum is anastomosed to the distal jejunum (Fig. 37-3A).

In vertical banded gastroplasty, a double row of staples is applied vertically along the lesser curvature of the stomach, beginning at the angle of His. A small stoma is created at the end of the staples by adding a circle of staples or a band of polypropylene mesh or silicone tubing (see Fig. 37-3B).

After weight loss, the patient may need surgical intervention for body contouring. This may include lipoplasty to remove fat deposits or a panniculectomy to remove excess abdominal skinfolds.

Nursing Management

Nursing management focuses on care of the patient after surgery. General postoperative nursing care is similar to that for a patient recovering from a gastric resection, but with attention given to the risks of complications associated with morbid obesity. Complications that may occur in the immediate postoperative period include peritonitis, stomal obstruction, stomal ulcers, atelectasis and pneumonia, thromboembolism, and metabolic imbalances resulting from prolonged vomiting and diarrhea. After bowel sounds have returned and oral intake is resumed, the nurse provides six

small feedings consisting of a total of 600 to 800 calories per day and encourages fluid intake to prevent dehydration.

Patients are usually discharged in 4 to 5 days with detailed dietary instructions. The nurse instructs patients to report excessive thirst or concentrated urine, both of which are indications of dehydration. Psychosocial interventions are also essential for these patients. Efforts are directed toward helping them modify their eating behaviours and cope with changes in body image. The nurse explains that noncompliance by eating too much or too fast or eating high-calorie liquid and soft foods results in vomiting and painful esophageal distention. The nurse discusses dietary instructions before discharge and schedules monthly outpatient visits. Long-term side effects may include increased risk of gallstones, nutritional deficiencies, and potential to regain weight.

Gastric Cancer

In Canada, there are an estimated 2800 new cases of stomach cancer reported yearly (Canadian Cancer Society, 2005). Most of these deaths occur in people older than 40 years of age, but they occasionally occur in younger people. Men have a higher incidence of gastric cancers than women do. The incidence of gastric cancer is much greater in Japan, which has instituted mass screening programs for earlier diagnosis. Diet appears to be a significant factor. A diet high in smoked foods and low in fruits and vegetables may increase the risk of gastric cancer. Other factors related to the incidence of gastric cancer include chronic inflammation of the stomach, pernicious anemia, achlorhydria, gastric ulcers, *H. pylori* infection, and genetics. The prognosis is poor, because most patients have metastases at the time of diagnosis (Greenlee, 2001).

FIGURE 37-3 Surgical procedures for morbid obesity. (**A**) Gastric bypass with roux-en-Y. A horizontal row of staples creates a pouch with a capacity of 50 mL or less. The proximal jejunum is transected and the distal end anastomosed to the new pouch. The proximal segment is anastomosed to the jejunum. (**B**) Vertical banded gastroplasty. A vertical row of staples along the lesser curvature of the stomach creates a new, smaller stomach pouch of 10 to 15 mL.

Pathophysiology

Most gastric cancers are adenocarcinomas and can occur in any portion of the stomach. The tumour infiltrates the surrounding mucosa, penetrating the wall of the stomach and adjacent organs and structures. The liver, pancreas, esophagus, and duodenum are often affected at the time of diagnosis. Metastasis through lymph to the peritoneal cavity occurs later in the disease.

Clinical Manifestations

In the early stages of gastric cancer, symptoms may be absent. Early symptoms are seldom definitive because most gastric tumours begin on the lesser curvature, where they cause little disturbance of gastric functions. Some studies show that early symptoms, such as pain relieved with antacids, resemble those of benign ulcers. Symptoms of progressive disease may include anorexia, dyspepsia (indigestion), weight loss, abdominal pain, constipation, anemia, and nausea and vomiting.

Assessment and Diagnostic Findings

Usually the physical examination is not helpful in detecting cancer because most gastric tumours are not palpable. Ascites may be apparent if the cancer cells have metastasized to the liver. Endoscopy for biopsy and cytologic washings is the usual diagnostic study, and a barium x-ray examination of the upper GI tract may also be performed. Because metastasis often occurs before warning signs develop, a computed tomography (CT) scan, bone scan, and liver scan are valuable in determining the extent of metastasis. A complete x-ray examination of the GI tract should be performed when any person older than 40 years of age has had indigestion (dyspepsia) of more than 4 weeks' duration.

Medical Management

There is no successful treatment for gastric carcinoma except removal of the tumour. If the tumour can be removed while it is still localized to the stomach, the patient can be cured. If the tumour has spread beyond the area that can be excised, cure is impossible. Palliative rather than radical surgery is performed if there is metastasis to other vital organs, such as the liver. In many of these patients, effective palliation to prevent discomfort caused by obstruction or dysphagia may be obtained by resection of the tumour (see Gastric Surgery).

If a radical subtotal gastrectomy is performed, the stump of the stomach is anastomosed to the jejunum, as in the gastrectomy for ulcer. When a total gastrectomy is performed, GI continuity is restored by means of an anastomosis between the ends of the esophagus and the jejunum.

If surgical treatment does not offer cure, treatment with chemotherapy may offer further control of the disease or palliation. Commonly used chemotherapeutic medications include cisplatin, irinotecan, or a combination of 5-fluorouracil, doxorubicin (Adriamycin), and mitomycin-C. Some studies are being conducted on the use of chemotherapy before surgery. Radiation therapy also may be used for palliation. Assessment of tumour markers (blood analysis for antigens indicative of colon cancer) such as carcinoembryonic antigen, CA 19-9, and CA 50 may help determine the effectiveness of treatment. If these values were elevated before treatment, they should decrease if the tumour is responding to the treatment (Bobbio-Pallavicini et al., 2001; Kerby & Heslin, 1999).

NURSING PROCESS: THE PATIENT WITH GASTRIC CANCER

Assessment

The nurse elicits a dietary history from the patient, focusing on recent nutritional intake and status. Has the patient lost weight? If so, how much and over what period of time? Can the patient tolerate a full diet? If not, what foods can he or she eat? What other changes in eating habits have occurred? Does the patient have an appetite? Is the patient in pain? Do foods, antacids, or medications relieve the pain, make no difference, or worsen the pain? Is there a history of infection with *H. pylori* bacteria? Other health information to obtain includes the patient's smoking and alcohol history and the family history (any first- or second-degree relatives with gastric or other cancer). A psychosocial assessment, including questions about social support, individual and family coping skills, and financial resources, will help the nurse plan for care in acute and community settings.

After the interview, the nurse performs a complete physical examination, carefully assesses the patient's abdomen for tenderness or masses, and also palpates and percusses to detect ascites.

Nursing Diagnosis

Based on the assessment data, the patient's major nursing diagnoses may include the following:

- Anxiety related to the disease and anticipated treatment
- Imbalanced nutrition, less than body requirements, related to anorexia
- Pain related to tumour mass
- Anticipatory grieving related to the diagnosis of cancer
- Deficient knowledge regarding self-care activities

Planning and Goals

The major goals for the patient may include reduced anxiety, optimal nutrition, relief of pain, and adjustment to the diagnosis and anticipated lifestyle changes.

Nursing Interventions

REDUCING ANXIETY

A relaxed, nonthreatening atmosphere is provided so that patient can express fears, concerns, and possibly anger about the diagnosis and prognosis. The nurse encourages the family in their efforts to support the patient, offering reassurance and supporting positive coping measures. The nurse advises the patient about any procedures and treatments so that the patient knows what to expect. The nurse also may suggest talking with a support person (eg, spiritual advisor), if the patient desires.

PROMOTING OPTIMAL NUTRITION

The nurse encourages the patient to eat small, frequent portions of nonirritating foods to decrease gastric irritation. Food supplements should be high in calories, as well as vitamins A and C and iron, to enhance tissue repair. If the patient is unable to eat adequately to meet nutritional requirements, parenteral nutrition may be necessary. Because the patient may develop dumping syndrome when enteral feeding resumes after gastric resection, the nurse explains ways to prevent and manage it (six small feedings daily that are low in carbohydrates and sugar; fluids between meals rather than with meals) and informs the patient that symptoms often resolve after several months. If a total gastrectomy is performed, parenteral vitamin B_{12} will be required indefinitely, because dietary vitamin B_{12} is absorbed in the stomach. The nurse monitors the IV therapy and nutritional status and records intake, output, and daily weights to ensure that the patient is maintaining or gaining weight. The nurse assesses for signs of dehydration (thirst, dry mucous membranes, poor skin turgor, tachycardia, decreased urine output) and reviews the results of daily laboratory studies to note any metabolic abnormalities (sodium, potassium, glucose, blood urea nitrogen). Antiemetics are administered as prescribed.

RELIEVING PAIN

The nurse administers analgesics as prescribed. A continuous infusion of an opioid may be necessary for severe pain. The nurse assesses the frequency, intensity, and duration of the pain to determine the effectiveness of the analgesic being administered. The nurse works with the patient to manage pain by suggesting nonpharmacologic methods for pain relief, such as position changes, imagery, distraction, relaxation exercises (using relaxation audiotapes), backrubs, massage, and periods of rest and relaxation.

PROVIDING PSYCHOSOCIAL SUPPORT

The nurse helps the patient express fears, concerns, and grief about the diagnosis. It is important to answer the patient's questions honestly and to encourage the patient to participate in treatment decisions. Some patients mourn the loss of a body part and perceive their surgery as a type of mutilation. Some express disbelief and need time and support to accept the diagnosis.

The nurse offers emotional support and involves family members and significant others whenever possible. This includes recognizing mood swings and defense mechanisms (eg, denial, rationalization, displacement, regression) and reassuring the patient and family members that emotional responses are normal and expected. The services of clergy, psychiatric clinical nurse specialists, psychologists, social workers, and psychiatrists are made available, if needed. The nurse projects an empathetic attitude and spends time with the patient. Most patients will begin to participate in self-care activities after they have acknowledged their loss.

PROMOTING HOME AND COMMUNITY-BASED CARE

Teaching Patients Self-Care

Self-care activities will depend on the mode of treatment used—surgery, chemotherapy, radiation, or palliative care. Patient and family teaching will include information about diet and nutrition, treatment regimens, activity and lifestyle changes, pain management, and possible complications (Chart 37-3). Consul-

tation with a dietitian is essential to determine how the patient's nutritional needs can best be met at home. The nurse teaches the patient or care provider about administration of enteral or parenteral nutrition. If chemotherapy or radiation is prescribed, the nurse provides explanations to the patient and family about what to expect, including the length of treatments, the expected side effects (eg, nausea, vomiting, anorexia, fatigue, neutropenia), and the need for transportation to appointments for treatment. Psychological counselling may also be helpful.

Continuing Care

The need for ongoing care in the home will depend on the patient's condition and treatment. The home care nurse reinforces nutritional counselling and supervises the administration of any enteral or parenteral feedings; the patient or family member must become skillful in administering the feedings and in detecting and preventing untoward effects or complications related to the feedings (see Chapter 36 to review management of enteral and parenteral feedings). The nurse teaches the patient or a family member to record the patient's daily intake, output, and weight and explains strategies to manage pain, nausea, vomiting, or other symptoms. The nurse also teaches the patient or caregiver to recognize and report signs and symptoms of complications that require medical attention, such as bleeding, obstruction, perforation, or any symptoms that become progressively worse. It is important to explain the chemotherapy or radiation therapy regimen. The patient and family need to know about the care that will be needed during and after treatments (see Chapter 16). Because the prognosis for gastric cancer is so poor, the nurse may need to assist the patient and family with decisions regarding end-of-life care. Referral to hospice may be warranted.

Evaluation

EXPECTED PATIENT OUTCOMES

Expected patient outcomes may include the following:

1. Reports less anxiety
   a. Expresses fears and concerns about surgery
   b. Seeks emotional support
2. Attains optimal nutrition
   a. Eats small, frequent meals high in calories, iron, and vitamins A and C
   b. Complies with enteral or parenteral nutrition as needed
3. Has less pain
4. Performs self-care activities and adjusts to lifestyle changes
   a. Resumes normal activities within 3 months
   b. Alternates periods of rest and activity
   c. Manages tube feedings

Chart 37-3
Home Care Checklist • The Patient With Gastric Cancer

At the completion of the home care instruction, the patient or caregiver will be able to:	Patient	Caregiver
• Demonstrate safe management of enteral or parenteral feedings, if applicable.	✓	✓
• Describes dietary restrictions.	✓	✓
• Identifies potential side effects of chemotherapy or radiation therapy, if applicable	✓	✓
• Identifies signs and symptoms of wound infection.	✓	✓
• State signs and symptoms of obstruction or perforation.	✓	✓
• Describes follow-up needs.	✓	✓

Gastric Surgery

Gastric surgery may be performed on patients with peptic ulcers who have life-threatening hemorrhage, obstruction, perforation, or penetration or whose condition does not respond to medication. It also may be indicated for patients with gastric cancer or trauma. Surgical procedures include a vagotomy and **pyloroplasty** (disconnecting nerves that stimulate acid secretion and opening the pylorus), a partial gastrectomy, and a total gastrectomy (removal of the stomach) with either an end-to-end or an end-to-side esophagojejunal anastomosis (see Table 37-3).

NURSING PROCESS: THE PATIENT UNDERGOING GASTRIC SURGERY

Assessment

Before surgery, the nurse assesses the patient's and family's knowledge of preoperative and postoperative surgical routines and the rationale for surgery. The nurse also assesses the patient's nutritional status: Has the patient lost weight? How much? Over how much time? Does the patient have nausea and vomiting? Has the patient had hematemesis? The nurse assesses for the presence of bowel sounds and palpates the abdomen to detect masses or tenderness.

After surgery, the nurse assesses the patient for complications secondary to the surgical intervention, such as hemorrhage, infection, abdominal distention, or decreased nutritional status. (See Chapters 20 and 25.)

Diagnosis

NURSING DIAGNOSES

Based on the assessment data, the patient's major nursing diagnoses may include the following:

- Anxiety related to surgical intervention
- Acute pain related to surgical incision
- Deficient knowledge about surgical procedures and postoperative course
- Imbalanced nutrition, less than body requirements, related to poor nutrition before surgery and altered GI system after surgery

COLLABORATIVE PROBLEMS/POTENTIAL COMPLICATIONS

In addition to the complications to which all postoperative patients are subject, the patient undergoing gastric surgery is at increased risk for:

- Hemorrhage
- Dietary deficiencies
- Bile reflux
- Dumping syndrome

Planning and Goals

The major goals for the patient undergoing gastric surgery may include reduced anxiety, increased knowledge and understanding about the surgical procedure and postoperative course, optimal nutrition and management of the complications that can interfere with nutrition, relief of pain, avoidance of hemorrhage and steatorrhea, and enhanced self-care skills at home. General postoperative care for the patient who has received general anesthesia, as discussed in Chapter 20, should be followed.

Nursing Interventions

REDUCING ANXIETY

An important part of the preoperative nursing care involves allaying the patient's fears and anxieties about the impending surgery and its implications. The nurse encourages the patient to express feelings and answers the patient's and family's questions. If the patient has an acute obstruction, a perforated bowel, or an active GI hemorrhage, adequate psychological preparation may not be possible. In this event, the nurse caring for the patient after surgery should anticipate the concerns, fears, and questions that are likely to surface and should be available for support and further explanations.

RELIEVING PAIN

After surgery, analgesics may be administered as prescribed to relieve pain and discomfort. It is important to avoid sedating the patient so as not to impair his or her ability to perform pulmonary care activities (deep breathing and coughing) and to ambulate. The nurse assesses the effectiveness of analgesic intervention. Positioning the patient in a Fowler's position promotes comfort and allows emptying of the stomach after a partial gastrectomy.

The nurse maintains functioning of the NG tube to prevent distention and resultant pain and damage to the suture line. Normally, the amount of NG drainage after a total gastrectomy is small.

INCREASING KNOWLEDGE

The nurse explains routine preoperative and postoperative activities to the patient, which include preoperative medications, NG intubation, IV fluids, abdominal dressings, and pulmonary care. These explanations need to be reinforced after surgery, especially if the patient had emergency surgery.

RESUMING ENTERAL INTAKE

The patient's nutritional status is evaluated before surgery, because many patients with gastric cancer are malnourished and may require preoperative enteral or, more often, parenteral nutrition (see Chapter 36). After surgery, parenteral nutrition may be continued to meet caloric needs, to replace fluids lost through drainage and vomitus, and to support the patient metabolically until oral intake is adequate.

After the return of bowel sounds and removal of the NG tube, the nurse may give fluids, followed by food in small portions. The nurse adds foods gradually until the patient is able to eat six small meals a day and drink 120 mL of fluid between meals. The key to increasing the dietary content is to offer food and fluids gradually as tolerated and to recognize that each patient's tolerance is different.

RECOGNIZING OBSTACLES TO ADEQUATE NUTRITION

Dysphagia and Gastric Retention

Dysphagia may occur in patients who have had truncal vagotomy, a surgical procedure that can result in trauma to the lower esophagus. Gastric retention may be evidenced by abdominal distention, nausea, and vomiting. Regurgitation may also occur if the patient has eaten too much or too quickly. It also may indicate that edema along the suture line is preventing fluids and food from moving into the intestinal tract. If gastric retention occurs, it may be necessary to reinstate NG suction; pressure must be low to avoid disrupting the suture line.

Bile Reflux

Bile reflux gastritis and esophagitis may occur with the removal of the pylorus, which acts as a barrier to the reflux of duodenal contents. Burning epigastric pain and vomiting of bilious material manifest this condition. Eating or vomiting does not relieve the situation. Agents that bind with bile acid, such as cholestyramine (Questran), may be helpful. Aluminum hydroxide gel (an antacid) and metoclopramide hydrochloride (Reglan) have been used with some success.

Dumping Syndrome

The term **dumping syndrome** refers to an unpleasant set of vasomotor and GI symptoms that sometimes occur in patients who have had gastric surgery or a form of vagotomy. It may be the mechanical result of surgery in which a small gastric remnant is connected to the jejunum through a large opening. Foods high in carbohydrates and electrolytes must be diluted in the jejunum before absorption can take place, but the passage of food from the stomach remnant into the jejunum is too rapid to allow this to happen. The symptoms that occur are probably a result of rapid distention of the jejunal loop anastomosed to the stomach. The hypertonic intestinal contents draw extracellular fluid from the circulating blood volume into the jejunum to dilute the high concentration of electrolytes and sugars. The ingestion of fluid at mealtime is another factor that causes the stomach contents to empty rapidly into the jejunum.

Early symptoms include a sensation of fullness, weakness, faintness, dizziness, palpitations, diaphoresis, cramping pains, and diarrhea. Later, there is a rapid elevation of blood glucose, followed by increased insulin secretion. This results in a reactive hypoglycemia, which also is unpleasant for the patient. Vasomotor symptoms that occur 10 to 90 minutes after eating are pallor, perspiration, palpitations, headache, and feelings of warmth, dizziness, and even drowsiness. Anorexia may also be a result of the dumping syndrome.

Steatorrhea also may occur in the patient with gastric surgery. It is partially the result of rapid gastric emptying, which prevents adequate mixing with pancreatic and biliary secretions. In mild cases, reducing the intake of fat and administering an antimotility medication can control steatorrhea.

Vitamin and Mineral Deficiencies

Other dietary deficiencies the nurse should be aware of include malabsorption of organic iron, which may require supplementation with oral or parenteral iron, and a low serum level of vitamin B_{12}, which may require supplementation by the intramuscular route. Total gastrectomy results in lack of intrinsic factor, a gastric secretion required for the absorption of vitamin B_{12} from the GI tract. Unless this vitamin is supplied by parenteral injection after gastrectomy, the patient inevitably will suffer vitamin B_{12} deficiency, which eventually leads to a condition identical to pernicious anemia. All manifestations of pernicious anemia, including macrocytic anemia and combined system disease, may be expected to develop within a period of 5 years or less; they progress in severity thereafter and, in the absence of therapy, are fatal. This complication is avoided by the regular monthly intramuscular injection of 100 to 1000 μg (usual dose is 300 μg) of vitamin B_{12}.

This regimen should be started without delay after gastrectomy. Weight loss is a common long-term problem because the patient experiences early fullness, which suppresses the appetite.

TEACHING DIETARY SELF-MANAGEMENT

Because the patient may experience any of the described conditions affecting nutrition, nursing intervention includes proper dietary instruction. The following teaching points are emphasized:

- To delay stomach emptying, the patient should assume a low Fowler's position during mealtime, and after the meal the patient should lie down for 20 to 30 minutes.
- Antispasmodics, as prescribed, also may aid in delaying the emptying of the stomach.
- Fluid intake with meals is discouraged; instead, fluids may be consumed up to 1 hour before or 1 hour after mealtime.
- Meals should contain more dry items than liquid items.
- The patient can eat fat as tolerated but should keep carbohydrate intake low and avoid concentrated sources of carbohydrates.
- The patient should eat smaller but more frequent meals.
- Dietary supplements of vitamins and medium-chain triglycerides and injections of vitamin B_{12} and iron may be prescribed.

The nurse also gives instructions regarding enteral or parenteral supplementation if it is needed.

MONITORING AND MANAGING POTENTIAL COMPLICATIONS

Occasionally hemorrhage complicates gastric surgery. The patient has the usual signs of rapid blood loss and shock (see Chapter 15) and may vomit considerable amounts of bright red blood. The nurse assesses NG drainage for type and amount; some bloody drainage for the first 12 hours is expected, but excessive bleeding should be reported. The nurse also assesses the abdominal dressing for bleeding. Because this situation is upsetting to the patient and family, the nurse should remain calm. The nurse performs emergency measures, such as NG lavage and administration of blood and blood products.

PROMOTING HOME AND COMMUNITY-BASED CARE

Teaching Patients Self-Care

Nurse-patient teaching stems from the assessment of the patient's physical and psychological readiness to participate in self-care. The nurse provides information about nutrition, enteral or parenteral nutrition if required, nutritional supplements, pain management, and the symptoms of dumping syndrome and measures to use to prevent or minimize these symptoms (Chart 37-4). It is important to emphasize the continued need for vitamin B_{12} injections.

Chart 37-4
Home Care Checklist • The Patient With Gastric Resection

At the completion of the home care instruction, the patient or caregiver will be able to:

	Patient	Caregiver
• Demonstrate enteral or parenteral feedings as applicable.	✓	✓
• State necessary dietary changes.	✓	✓
• Identify available support groups.	✓	✓
• Explain medication regimen.	✓	✓
• Identify signs and symptoms of complications	✓	✓

Continuing Care

Both the patient and the family can benefit from a team approach to discharge planning. The team members include the home care nurse, physician, dietitian, social worker, patient and family; written instructions about meals, activities, medications, and follow-up care are helpful. The home care nurse supervises the administration of any enteral or parenteral feedings, emphasizing information about detection and prevention of untoward effects or complications related to the feedings. Information about community support groups is provided to the patient and family.

Evaluation

EXPECTED PATIENT OUTCOMES

Expected patient outcomes may include:

1. Reports decreased anxiety; expresses fears and concerns about surgery
2. Demonstrates knowledge regarding postoperative course by discussing the surgical procedure and postoperative course
3. Attains optimal nutrition
   a. Maintains a reasonable weight
   b. Does not have excessive diarrhea
   c. Tolerates 6 small meals a day
   d. Does not experience dysphagia, gastric retention, bile reflux, dumping syndrome, or vitamin and mineral deficiencies
4. Attains optimal level of comfort
5. Has no evidence of hemorrhage

Critical Thinking Exercises

1. You are working in the office of a gastroenterologist. You have a patient coming in today with symptoms of a peptic ulcer. What questions will you ask the patient, and what types of teaching regimen do you anticipate you will need to review with this patient?

2. You are caring for a patient who is to have a gastrectomy to treat gastric cancer. What nutritional needs do you anticipate for this patient preoperatively, immediately postoperatively, and after discharge from the hospital?

3. Your 45-year-old patient who weighs 170.1 kg has had gastric bypass to treat morbid obesity. Describe the preoperative interventions for this patient. How would you modify your interventions if the patient had diabetes? If he had angina?

REFERENCES AND SELECTED READINGS

Books

Brandt, L. J. (Ed.). (1999). *Clinical practice of gastroenterology* (Vols. I & II). Philadelphia: Churchill-Livingstone.

DeVita, V. T., Hellman, S., & Rosenberg, S. A. (Eds.). (1997). *Cancer: Principles and practice of oncology* (5th ed.). Philadelphia: Lippincott-Raven.

McEvoy, G. R. (Ed.). (2000). *American hospital formulary service.* Bethesda, MD: American Society of Health-System Pharmacists.

Pappas, T. N., et al. (1999). *Atlas of laparoscopic surgery* (2nd ed.). Norwalk, CT: Appleton & Lange.

Porth, C. (2002). *Pathophysiology: Concepts of altered health states* (6th ed.). Philadelphia: Lippincott Williams & Wilkins.

Townsend, C. M. Jr. (Ed.). (2001). *Textbook of surgery* (7th ed.). Philadelphia: W. B. Saunders.

U.S. Department of Health and Human Services. (2001). *The surgeon general's call to action to prevent and decrease overweight and obesity.* Rockville, MD: Author.

Wilson, B. A., Shannon, M. T., & Stang, C. L. (2005). *Prentice Hall nurse's drug guide 2005.* Upper Saddle River, NJ: Pearson Education.

Wolfe, M. M. (2000). *Therapy of digestive disorders.* Philadelphia: W. B. Saunders.

Yamada, T. (1999). *Textbook of gastroenterology* (3rd ed., Vols. I & II). Philadelphia: Lippincott Williams & Wilkins.

Journals

Gastric Cancer

Bobbio-Pallavicini, E., et al. (2001). Cisplatin, mitomycin-C, 5-fluorouracil and leucovorin combination chemotherapy (L-FCM) in locally advanced unresectable or metastatic gastric carcinoma: A phase-II study. *Oncology Reports, 8*(1), 167–171.

Canadian Cancer Society. (2005). Canadian cancer encyclopedia. Available at: www.cancer.ca.

Greenlee, R. T. (2001). Cancer statistics, 2001. *CA: A Cancer Journal for Clinicians, 5*(1), 15–16.

Hanazaki, K., et al. (2000). Postoperative chemotherapy in elderly patients with advanced cancer. *Hepatogastroenterology, 47*(36), 1761–1764.

Kerby, J. D., & Heslin, M. J. (1999). Gastric cancer. *Current Treatment Options in Gastroenterology, 2*(3), 163–170.

La Veccha, J. C., & Franceschi, S. (2000). Nutrition and gastric cancer. *Canadian Journal of Gastroenterology, 14,* (Suppl D), 51D–54D.

Stucky-Marshall, L. S. (1999). New agents in gastrointestinal malignancies. Part 1: Irinotecan in clinical practice. *Cancer Nursing, 22*(3), 212–219.

Morbid Obesity

Canadian Institute for Health Research. (2004). *Obesity.* Available at: www.cihr-irsc.gc.ca. Retrieved May 10, 2005.

Canadian Institute for Health Research. (2004). *Obesity research in Canada: Backgrounder.* Available at: www.cihr-irsc.gc.ca. Retrieved May 9, 2005.

Davila-Cervantes, A, et al. (2000). Open vs laparoscopic vertical banded gastroplasty: A case control study with a 1-year follow-up. *Obesity Surgery 2000, 10*(5), 409–412.

Government of Alberta: Agriculture, Food and Rural Development. (2004). *Canadian consumer trends in obesity and food consumption.* Available at: www.agric.gov.ab.ca. Retrieved May 8, 2005.

Hussar, D. A. (1999). New drugs 1999: Part II. *Nursing 99, 29*(2), 45–51.

Hussar, D. A. (2000). New drugs 2000: Part I. *Nursing 00, 30*(1), 50–62.

Monteforte M. J., & Turkelson, C. M. (2000). Bariatric surgery for morbid obesity. *Obesity Surgery, 10*(5), 391–401.

Schirmer, B. D. (2000). Laparoscopic bariatric surgery. *Surgical Clinics of North America, 80*(4), 1253–1267.

Wangsness, M. (2000). Pharmacological treatment of obesity: Past, present and future. *Minnesota Medicine, 83*(11), 21–26.

Weiss, D. (2000). How to help your patients lose weight: Current therapy for obesity. *Cleveland Clinic Journal of Medicine, 67*(10), 739, 743–746, 749–754.

Peptic Ulcers and Gastritis

Alsahli, M., et al. (2001). Vaccines: An ongoing promise? *Digestive Diseases, 19*(2), 148–157.

Axon, A. T. (2000). Treatment of *Helicobacter pylori:* An overview. *Alimentary Pharmacology and Therapeutics, 14* (Suppl. 3), 1–6.

Beehrie, D. M., & Evans, D. (1999). A review of NSAID complications: Gastrointestinal and more. *Primary Care Practice, 3*(3), 305–315.

Eastwood, G. L. (1997). Is smoking still important in the pathogenesis of peptic ulcer disease? *Journal of Clinical Gastroenterology, 25* (Suppl. 1), S1–S7.

Fallone, C. A., Veldhuyzen van Zanten, S. J., & Chiba, N. (2000). Does the urea breath test tell us what we need to know? *Canadian Medical Association Journal, 162*(10), 1401–1402. Available at: www.cmaj.ca.

Fallone, C. A., Veldhuyzen van Zanten, S. J., & Chiba, N. (2000). The urea breath test for *Helicobacter pylori* infection. *Canadian Medical Association Journal, 162*(3), 371–372. Available at: www.cmaj.ca.

McManus, T. J. (2000). *Helicobacter pylori:* An emerging infectious disease. *Nurse Practitioner, 25*(8), 40–50.

Tytgat, G. (2000). *Helicobacter pylori:* Past, present and future. *Journal of Gastroenterology and Hepatology, 15* (Suppl.) G30–G33.

Weart, C. W. (2000). Peptic ulcer disease: Let's help cure it. *Journal of the American Pharmaceutical Association, 40*(4), 560–561.

RESOURCES AND WEBSITES

American Cancer Society, 1599 Clifton Rd., N.E., Atlanta, GA 30329; 1-800-ACS-2345; http://www.cancer.org.
American Gastroenterological Association, 7910 Woodmont Ave., Seventh Floor, Bethesda, MD 20814; http://www.gastro.org.
Canadian Cancer Society; www.cancer.ca.

Management of Patients With Intestinal and Rectal Disorders

Adapted by Christy Raymond

LEARNING OBJECTIVES

On completion of this chapter, the learner will be able to:

1. Identify the health care teaching needs of patients with constipation or diarrhea.
2. Compare the conditions of malabsorption with regard to their pathophysiology, clinical manifestations, and management.
3. Use the nursing process as a framework for care of patients with diverticulitis.
4. Compare regional enteritis and ulcerative colitis with regard to their pathophysiology, clinical manifestations, diagnostic evaluation, and medical, surgical, and nursing management.
5. Use the nursing process as a framework for care of the patient with an inflammatory bowel disease.
6. Describe the responsibilities of the nurse in meeting the needs of the patient with an ileostomy.
7. Describe the various types of intestinal obstructions and their management.
8. Use the nursing process as a framework for care of the patient with cancer of the colon or rectum.
9. Use the nursing process as a framework for care of the patient with an anorectal condition.

From 2000 to 2001, diseases of the gastrointestinal tract accounted for approximately 12.5% of all hospitalizations for men in Canada. The percentage of all hospitalizations for women related to gastrointestinal disease for the same time period was 10% (Canadian Institutes for Health Information, 2002).

In all age groups, a fast-paced lifestyle, high levels of stress, irregular eating habits, insufficient intake of fibre and water, and lack of daily exercise contribute to GI problems. Nurses can have an impact on these chronic problems by identifying behaviour patterns that put patients at risk, by educating the public about prevention and management, and by helping those affected to improve their condition and prevent complications.

Abnormalities of Fecal Elimination

Changes in patterns of fecal elimination are symptoms of functional disorders or disease of the GI tract. The most common changes seen are constipation, diarrhea, and fecal incontinence. The nurse should be aware of the possible causes and therapeutic management of these problems and of nursing management techniques. Education is important for patients with these abnormalities.

CONSTIPATION

Constipation is a term used to describe an abnormal infrequency or irregularity of defecation, abnormal hardening of stools that makes their passage difficult and sometimes painful, a decrease in stool volume, or retention of stool in the rectum for a prolonged period. Any variation from normal habits may be considered a problem. Constipation is common in North America, with approximately 63 million people experiencing it. Prevalence increases with age and it is more predominant in women (Higgins & Johanson, 2004).

Constipation can be caused by certain medications (ie, tranquilizers, anticholinergics, antidepressants, antihypertensives, opioids, antacids with aluminum, and iron); rectal or anal disorders (eg, hemorrhoids, fissures); obstruction (eg, cancer of the bowel); metabolic, neurologic, and neuromuscular conditions (eg, diabetes mellitus, Hirschsprung's disease, Parkinson's disease, multiple sclerosis); endocrine disorders (eg, hypothyroidism, pheochromocytoma); lead poisoning; and connective tissue disorders (eg, scleroderma, lupus erythematosus). Constipation is a major problem for patients taking opioids for chronic pain. Diseases of the colon commonly associated with constipa-tion are irritable bowel syndrome (IBS) and diverticular disease. Constipation can also occur with an acute disease process in the abdomen (eg, appendicitis).

Other causes include weakness, immobility, debility, fatigue, and an inability to increase intra-abdominal pressure to facilitate the passage of stools, as occurs with emphysema. Many people develop constipation because they do not take the time to defecate or they ignore the urge to defecate. In the United States, constipation is also a result of dietary habits (ie, low consumption of fibre and inadequate fluid intake), lack of regular exercise, and a stress-filled life.

Perceived constipation can also be a problem. This subjective problem occurs when an individual's bowel elimination pattern is not consistent with what he or she perceives as normal. Chronic laxative use is attributed to this problem and is a major health concern, especially among the elderly population.

Pathophysiology

The pathophysiology of constipation is poorly understood, but it is thought to include interference with one of three major functions of the colon: mucosal transport (ie, mucosal secretions facilitate the movement of colon contents), myoelectric activity (ie, mixing of the rectal mass and propulsive actions), or the processes of defecation. Any of the causative factors previously identified can interfere with any of these three processes.

The urge to defecate is stimulated normally by rectal distention, which initiates a series of four actions: stimulation of the inhibitory rectoanal reflex, relaxation of the internal sphincter muscle, relaxation of the external sphincter muscle and muscles in the pelvic region, and increased intra-abdominal pressure. Interference with any of these processes can lead to constipation.

If all organic causes are eliminated, idiopathic constipation is diagnosed. If the urge to defecate is ignored, the rectal mucous membrane and musculature become insensitive to the presence of fecal masses, and consequently, a stronger stimulus is required to produce the necessary peristaltic rush for defecation. The initial effect of fecal retention is to produce irritability of the colon, which at this stage frequently goes into spasm, especially after meals, giving rise to colicky midabdominal or low abdominal pains. After several years of this process, the colon loses muscular tone and becomes essentially unresponsive to normal stimuli. Atony or decreased muscle tone occurs with aging. This also leads to constipation because the stool is retained for longer periods.

Glossary

appendicitis: infectious and inflammatory process of the appendix creating acute abdominal pain and nausea

azotorrhea: excess of nitrogenous matter in the feces or urine

colostomy: surgical opening into the colon by means of a stoma to allow drainage of bowel contents; one type of fecal diversion

diverticulitis: inflammation of a diverticulum from obstruction (by fecal matter), resulting in abscess formation

diverticulosis: presence of a number of diverticula in the intestine; common in middle age

diverticulum: saclike outpouching of the lining of the bowel protruding through the muscle of the intestinal wall, usually caused by high intraluminal pressure

hemorrhoids: dilated portions of the anal veins; can occur internal or external to the anal sphincter

ileostomy: surgical opening into the ileum by means of a stoma to allow drainage of bowel contents; one type of fecal diversion

inflammatory bowel disease: group of chronic disorders (most common are ulcerative colitis and regional enteritis [Crohn's disease]) that result in inflamma-tion or ulceration (or both) of the bowel lining, associated with abdominal pain, diarrhea, fever, and weight loss

irritable bowel syndrome: functional disorder that affects frequency of defecation and consistency of stool; associated with crampy abdominal pain and bloating

malabsorption: impaired transport across the mucosa

peritonitis: inflammation of the lining of the abdominal cavity, usually as a result of a bacterial infection of an area in the GI tract with leakage of contents into the abdominal cavity

Clinical Manifestations

Clinical manifestations include abdominal distention, borborygmus (ie, gurgling or rumbling sound caused by passage of gas through the intestine), pain and pressure, decreased appetite, headache, fatigue, indigestion, a sensation of incomplete emptying, straining at stool, and the elimination of small-volume, hard, dry stools.

Assessment and Diagnostic Findings

Chronic constipation is usually considered idiopathic, but secondary causes should be excluded. In patients with severe, intractable constipation, further diagnostic testing is needed (Wong, 1999). The diagnosis of constipation is based on results of the patient's history, physical examination, possibly a barium enema or sigmoidoscopy, and stool testing for occult blood. These tests are completed to determine whether this symptom results from spasm or narrowing of the bowel. Anorectal manometry (ie, pressure studies) may be performed to determine malfunction of the muscle and sphincter. Defecography and bowel transit studies can also assist in the diagnosis (see Chap. 34).

Complications

Complications of constipation include hypertension, fecal impaction, hemorrhoids and fissures, and megacolon. Increased arterial pressure can occur with defecation. Straining at stool, which results in the Valsalva manoeuvre (ie, forcibly exhaling with the glottis closed), has a striking effect on arterial blood pressure. During active straining, the flow of venous blood in the chest is temporarily impeded because of increased intrathoracic pressure. This pressure tends to collapse the large veins in the chest. The atria and the ventricles receive less blood, and consequently less is delivered by the systolic contractions of the left ventricle. The cardiac output is decreased, and there is a transient drop in arterial pressure. Almost immediately after this period of hypotension, a rise in arterial pressure occurs; the pressure is elevated momentarily to a point far exceeding the original level (ie, rebound phenomenon). In patients with hypertension, this compensatory reaction may be exaggerated greatly, and the peaks of pressure attained may be dangerously high—sufficient to rupture a major artery in the brain or elsewhere.

Fecal impaction occurs when an accumulated mass of dry feces cannot be expelled. The mass may be palpable on digital examination, may produce pressure on the colonic mucosa that results in ulcer formation, and frequently may cause seepage of liquid stools.

Hemorrhoids and anal fissures can develop as a result of constipation. **Hemorrhoids** develop as a result of perianal vascular congestion caused by straining. Anal fissures may result from the passage of the hard stool through the anus, tearing the lining of the anal canal.

Megacolon is a dilated and atonic colon caused by a fecal mass that obstructs the passage of colon contents. Symptoms include constipation, liquid fecal incontinence, and abdominal distention. Megacolon can lead to perforation of the bowel.

Gerontologic Considerations

Physician visits for constipation are more frequent by individuals 65 years of age or older (Yamada et al., 1999). Elderly people report problems with constipation five times more frequently than younger people. A number of factors contribute to this increased frequency. People who have loose-fitting dentures or have lost their teeth have difficulty chewing and frequently choose soft, processed foods that are low in fibre. Convenience foods, also low

in fibre, are widely used by those who have lost interest in eating. Some older people reduce their fluid intake if they are not eating regular meals. Lack of exercise and prolonged bed rest also contribute to constipation by decreasing abdominal muscle tone and intestinal motility as well as anal sphincter tone. Nerve impulses are dulled, and there is decreased sensation to defecate. Many older people who overuse laxatives in an attempt to have a daily bowel movement become dependent on them.

Medical Management

Treatment is aimed at the underlying cause of constipation and includes education, bowel habit training, increased fibre and fluid intake, and judicious use of laxatives. Management may also include discontinuing laxative abuse. Routine exercise to strengthen abdominal muscles is encouraged. Biofeedback is a technique that can be used to help patients learn to relax the sphincter mechanism to expel stool. Daily addition to the diet of 6 to 12 teaspoonfuls of unprocessed bran is recommended, especially for the treatment of constipation in the elderly. If laxative use is necessary, one of the following may be prescribed: bulk-forming agents, saline and osmotic agents, lubricants, stimulants, or fecal softeners. The physiologic action and patient education information related to these laxatives are identified in Table 38-1. Enemas and rectal suppositories are generally not recommended for constipation and should be reserved for the treatment of impaction or for preparing the bowel for surgery or diagnostic procedures. If long-term laxative use is necessary, a bulk-forming agent may be prescribed in combination with an osmotic laxative.

Doctors prescribe the use of specific medications to enhance colonic transit by increasing propulsive motor activity. Further studies are being carried out on cholinergic agents (eg, bethanechol), cholinesterase inhibitors (eg, neostigmine), and prokinetic agents (eg, metoclopramide) to determine the role these agents can play in treating constipation (Yamada et al., 1999).

Nursing Management

The nurse elicits information about the onset and duration of constipation, current and past elimination patterns, the patient's expectation of normal bowel elimination, and lifestyle information (eg, exercise and activity level, occupation, food and fluid intake, and stress level) during the health history interview. Past medical and surgical history, current medications, and laxative and enema use are important, as is information about the sensation of rectal pressure or fullness, abdominal pain, excessive straining at defecation, and flatulence.

Patient education and health promotion are important functions of the nurse (Chart 38-1). After the health history is obtained, the nurse sets specific goals for teaching. Goals for the patient include restoring or maintaining a regular pattern of elimination, ensuring adequate intake of fluids and high-fibre foods, learning about methods to avoid constipation, relieving anxiety about bowel elimination patterns, and avoiding complications.

DIARRHEA

Diarrhea is increased frequency of bowel movements (more than three per day), increased amount of stool (more than 200 g per day), and altered consistency (ie, looseness) of stool. It is usually associated with urgency, perianal discomfort, incontinence, or a combination of these factors. Any condition that causes increased intestinal secretions, decreased mucosal absorption, or altered

Table 38-1 • Laxatives: Classification, Agent, Action, and Patient Education

CLASSIFICATION	SAMPLE AGENT	ACTION	PATIENT EDUCATION
Bulk forming	Psyllium hydrophilic (Metamucil, Karasil, mucilloid)	Polysaccharides and cellulose derivatives mix with intestinal fluids, swell, and stimulate peristalsis.	Take with 8 oz water and follow with 8 oz water; do not take dry. Report abdominal distention or unusual amount of flatulence.
Saline agent	Magnesium hydroxide (Milk of Magnesia)	Nonabsorbable magnesium ions alter stool consistency by drawing water into the intestines by osmosis; peristalsis is stimulated. Action occurs within 2 h.	The liquid preparation is more effective than the tablet form. Only short-term use is recommended because of toxicity (CNS or neuromuscular depression, electrolyte imbalance). Magnesium laxatives should not be taken by patients with renal insufficiency.
Lubricant	Mineral oil	Nonabsorbable hydrocarbons soften fecal matter by lubricating the intestinal mucosa; the passage of stool is facilitated. Action occurs within 6–8 h.	Do not take with meals, because mineral oils can impair the absorption of fat-soluble vitamins and delay gastric emptying. Swallow carefully, because drops of oil that gain access to the pharynx can produce a lipid pneumonia.
Stimulant	Bisacodyl (Bisco-lax, Dulcolax)	Irritates the colon epithelium by stimulating sensory nerve endings and increasing mucosal secretions. Action occurs within 6–8 h.	Catharsis may cause fluid and electrolyte imbalance, especially in the elderly. Tablets should be swallowed, not crushed or chewed. Avoid milk or antacids within 1 hour of taking the medication, because the enteric coating may dissolve prematurely.
Fecal softener	Dioctyl sodium sulfosuccinate (Colace)	Hydrates the stool by its surfactant action on the colonic epithelium (increases the wetting efficiency of intestinal water); aqueous and fatty substances are mixed. Does not exert a laxative action.	Can be used safely by patients who should avoid straining (cardiac patients, patients with anorectal disorders).
Osmotic agent	Polyethylene glycol and electrolytes (Colyte)	Cleanses colon rapidly and induces diarrhea.	This is a large-volume product. It takes time to consume it safely. It can cause considerable nausea and bloating.

motility can produce diarrhea. Irritable bowel syndrome (IBS), inflammatory bowel disease (IBD), and lactose intolerance are frequently the underlying disease processes that cause diarrhea (Stone et al., 1999).

Diarrhea can be acute or chronic. Acute diarrhea is most often associated with infection and is usually self-limiting; chronic diarrhea persists for a longer period and may return sporadically. Diarrhea can be caused by certain medications (eg, thyroid hormone replacement, stool softeners and laxatives, antibiotics, chemotherapy, antacids), certain tube feeding formulas, metabolic and endocrine disorders (eg, diabetes, Addison's disease, thyrotoxicosis), and viral or bacterial infectious processes (eg, dysentery, shigellosis, food poisoning). Other disease processes associated with diarrhea are nutritional and malabsorptive disorders (eg, celiac disease), anal sphincter defect, Zollinger-Ellison syndrome, paralytic ileus, intestinal obstruction, and acquired immunodeficiency syndrome (AIDS).

Pathophysiology

Types of diarrhea include secretory, osmotic, and mixed diarrhea. Secretory diarrhea is usually high-volume diarrhea and is caused by increased production and secretion of water and electrolytes by the intestinal mucosa into the intestinal lumen. Osmotic diarrhea occurs when water is pulled into the intestines by the osmotic pressure of unabsorbed particles, slowing the reabsorption of water. Mixed diarrhea is caused by increased peristalsis (usually from IBD) and a combination of increased secretion and decreased absorption in the bowel. The physiology of diarrhea related to infection is discussed in Chapter 70.

Clinical Manifestations

In addition to the increased frequency and fluid content of stools, the patient usually has abdominal cramps, distention, intestinal rumbling (ie, borborygmus), anorexia, and thirst. Painful spasmodic

Chart 38-1
Health Promotion: Preventing Constipation

- Describe the physiology of defecation.
- Emphasize the importance of heeding the urge to defecate.
- Discuss normal variations in patterns of defecation.
- Teach how to establish a bowel routine, and explain that having a regular time for defecation (eg, best time is after breakfast) may aid in initiating the reflex.
- Provide dietary information; suggest eating high-residue, high-fibre foods, adding bran daily (must be introduced gradually), and increasing fluid intake (unless contraindicated).
- Explain how an exercise regimen, increased ambulation, and abdominal muscle toning will increase muscle strength and help propel colon contents.
- Describe abdominal toning exercises (contracting abdominal muscles 4 times daily and leg-to-chest lifts 10 to 20 times each day).
- Explain that the normal position (semisquatting) maximizes use of abdominal muscles and force of gravity.

contractions of the anus and ineffectual straining (ie, tenesmus) may occur with defecation. Other symptoms depend on the cause and severity of the diarrhea but are related to dehydration and to fluid and electrolyte imbalances.

Watery stools are characteristic of small bowel disease, whereas loose, semisolid stools are associated more often with disorders of the colon. Voluminous, greasy stools suggest intestinal malabsorption, and the presence of mucus and pus in the stools suggests inflammatory enteritis or colitis. Oil droplets on the toilet water are almost always diagnostic of pancreatic insufficiency. Nocturnal diarrhea may be a manifestation of diabetic neuropathy.

Assessment and Diagnostic Findings

When the cause of the diarrhea is not obvious, the following diagnostic tests may be performed: complete blood cell count, chemical profile, urinalysis, routine stool examination, and stool examinations for infectious or parasitic organisms, bacterial toxins, blood, fat, and electrolytes. Endoscopy or barium enema may assist in identifying the cause.

Complications

Complications of diarrhea include the potential for cardiac dysrhythmias because of significant fluid and electrolyte loss (especially loss of potassium). Urinary output of less than 30 mL per hour for 2 to 3 consecutive hours, muscle weakness, paresthesia, hypotension, anorexia, and drowsiness with a potassium level of less than 3.0 mEq/L (3 mmol/L) must be reported. Decreased potassium levels cause cardiac dysrhythmias (ie, atrial and ventricular tachycardia, ventricular fibrillation, and premature ventricular contractions) that can lead to death.

Medical Management

Primary management is directed at controlling symptoms, preventing complications, and eliminating or treating the underlying disease. Certain medications (eg, antibiotics, anti-inflammatory agents) may reduce the severity of the diarrhea and treat the underlying disease.

Nursing Management

The nurse's role includes assessing and monitoring the characteristics and pattern of diarrhea. A health history addresses the patient's medication therapy, medical and surgical history, and dietary patterns and intake. Reports of recent exposure to an acute illness or recent travel to another geographic area are important. Assessment includes abdominal auscultation and palpation for abdominal tenderness. Inspection of the abdomen and mucous membranes and skin is important to determine hydration status. Stool samples are obtained for testing.

During an episode of acute diarrhea, the nurse encourages bed rest and intake of liquids and foods low in bulk until the acute attack subsides. When food intake is tolerated, the nurse recommends a bland diet of semisolid and solid foods. The patient should avoid caffeine, carbonated beverages, and very hot and very cold foods, because they stimulate intestinal motility. It may be necessary to restrict milk products, fat, whole-grain products, fresh fruits, and vegetables for several days. The nurse administers antidiarrheal medications such as diphenoxylate (Lomotil) and loperamide (Imodium) as prescribed. Intravenous fluid therapy may be necessary for rapid rehydration, especially for the el-

derly and those with preexisting GI conditions (eg, IBD). It is important to closely monitor serum electrolyte levels. The nurse immediately reports evidence of dysrhythmias or a change in the level of consciousness.

NURSING ALERT Elderly persons can become dehydrated quickly and develop low potassium levels (ie, hypokalemia) as a result of diarrhea. The older person taking digitalis must be aware of how quickly dehydration and hypokalemia can occur with diarrhea. The nurse instructs this person to recognize the signs of hypokalemia, because low levels of potassium intensify the action of digitalis, which can lead to digitalis toxicity.

The perianal area may become excoriated because diarrheal stool contains digestive enzymes that can irritate the skin. The patient should follow a perianal skin care routine to decrease irritation and excoriation. It is important to use skin sealants and moisture barriers as needed. The older person's skin is very sensitive because of decreased turgor and reduced subcutaneous fat layers.

FECAL INCONTINENCE

The term *fecal incontinence* describes the involuntary passage of stool from the rectum. Several factors influence fecal continence—the ability of the rectum to sense and accommodate stool, the amount and consistency of stool, the integrity of the anal sphincters and musculature, and rectal motility.

Pathophysiology

Fecal incontinence can result from trauma (eg, after surgical procedures involving the rectum), a neurologic disorder (eg, stroke, multiple sclerosis, diabetic neuropathy, dementia), inflammation, infection, radiation treatment, fecal impaction, pelvic floor relaxation, laxative abuse, medications, or advancing age (ie, weakness or loss of anal or rectal muscle tone). It is an embarrassing and socially incapacitating problem that requires a many-tiered approach to treatment and much adaptation on the patient's part.

Clinical Manifestations

Patients may have minor soiling, occasional urgency and loss of control, or complete incontinence. Patients may also experience poor control of flatus, diarrhea, or constipation.

Assessment and Diagnostic Findings

Diagnostic studies are necessary because the treatment of fecal incontinence depends on the cause. A rectal examination and other endoscopic examinations such as a flexible sigmoidoscopy are performed to rule out tumours, inflammation, or fissures. X-ray studies such as barium enema, computed tomography (CT) scans, anorectal manometry, and transit studies may be helpful in identifying alterations in intestinal mucosa and muscle tone or in detecting other structural or functional problems.

Medical Management

Although there is no known cause or cure for fecal incontinence, specific management techniques can help the patient achieve a better quality of life. If fecal incontinence is related to diarrhea, the incontinence may disappear when diarrhea is successfully treated. Fecal incontinence is frequently a symptom of a fecal impaction. After the impaction is removed and the rectum is cleansed, normal functioning of the anorectal area can resume. If the fecal incontinence is related to a more permanent condition, other treatments are initiated. Biofeedback therapy can be of assistance if the problem is decreased sensory awareness or sphincter control. Bowel training programs can also be effective. Surgical procedures include surgical reconstruction, sphincter repair, or fecal diversion.

Nursing Management

The nurse takes a thorough health history, including information about previous surgical procedures, chronic illnesses, bowel habits and problems, and current medication regimen. The nurse also completes an examination of the rectal area.

The nurse initiates a bowel-training program that involves setting a schedule to establish bowel regularity. The goal is to assist the patient to achieve fecal continence. If this is not possible, the goal should be to manage the problem so the person can have predictable, planned elimination (Stone et al., 1999). Sometimes, it is necessary to use suppositories to stimulate the anal reflex. After the patient has achieved a regular schedule, the suppository can be discontinued. Biofeedback can be used in conjunction with these therapies to help the patient improve sphincter contractility and rectal sensitivity.

Fecal incontinence can also cause problems with perineal skin integrity. Maintaining skin integrity is a priority, especially in the debilitated or elderly patient. Incontinence briefs, although helpful in containing the fecal material, allow for increased skin contact with the feces and may cause excoriation of the skin. The nurse encourages and teaches meticulous skin hygiene.

Continence sometimes cannot be achieved, and the nurse assists the patient and family to accept and cope with this chronic situation. The patient can use fecal incontinence devices, which include external collection devices and internal drainage systems. External devices are special pouches that are drainable. They are attached to a synthetic adhesive skin barrier specially designed to conform to the buttocks. Internal drainage systems can be used to eliminate fecal skin contact and are especially useful when there is extensive excoriation or skin breakdown. A large catheter is inserted into the rectum and is connected to a drainage system.

IRRITABLE BOWEL SYNDROME

IBS is one of the most common GI problems. Approximately one in six otherwise healthy persons report classic symptoms of IBS (Wolfe, 2000). It occurs more commonly in women than in men, and the cause is still unknown. Although no anatomic or biochemical abnormalities have been found that explain the common symptoms, various factors are associated with the syndrome: heredity, psychological stress or conditions such as depression and anxiety, a diet high in fat and stimulating or irritating foods, alcohol consumption, and smoking. The small intestine has become a focus of investigation as an additional site of dysmotility in IBS, and cluster contractions in the jejunum and ileum are being studied (Wolfe, 2000). The diagnosis is made only after tests have been completed that prove the absence of structural or other disorders.

Pathophysiology

IBS results from a functional disorder of intestinal motility. The change in motility may be related to the neurologic regulatory system, infection or irritation, or a vascular or metabolic disturbance. The peristaltic waves are affected at specific segments of the intestine and in the intensity with which they propel the fecal matter forward. There is no evidence of inflammation or tissue changes in the intestinal mucosa.

Clinical Manifestations

There is a wide variability in symptom presentation. Symptoms range in intensity and duration from mild and infrequent to severe and continuous. The primary symptom is an alteration in bowel patterns—constipation, diarrhea, or a combination of both. Pain, bloating, and abdominal distention often accompany this change in bowel pattern. The abdominal pain is sometimes precipitated by eating and is frequently relieved by defecation.

Assessment and Diagnostic Findings

A definite diagnosis of IBS requires tests that prove the absence of structural or other disorders. Stool studies, contrast x-ray studies, and proctoscopy may be performed to rule out other colon diseases. Barium enema and colonoscopy may reveal spasm, distention, or mucus accumulation in the intestine (Fig. 38-1). Manometry and electromyography are used to study intraluminal pressure changes generated by spasticity.

Medical Management

The goals of treatment are aimed at relieving abdominal pain, controlling the diarrhea or constipation, and reducing stress. Restriction and then gradual reintroduction of foods that are possibly irritating may help determine what types of food are acting as irritants (eg, beans, caffeinated products, fried foods, alcohol, spicy foods). A healthy, high-fibre diet is prescribed to help control the diarrhea and constipation. Exercise can assist in reducing anxiety and increasing intestinal motility. Patients often find it helpful to participate in a stress reduction or behaviour-modification program.

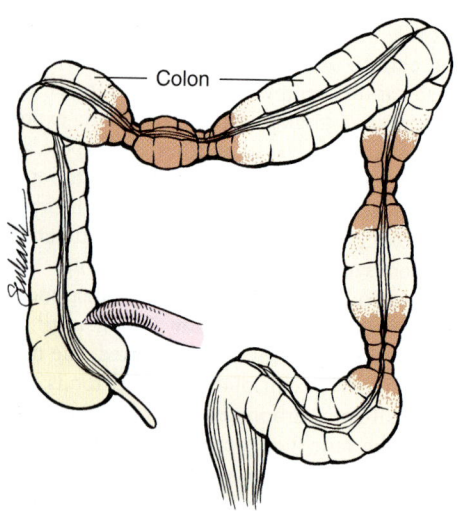

Colon

FIGURE 38-1 In IBS, the spastic contractions of the bowel can be seen in x-ray contrast studies.

Hydrophilic colloids (ie, bulk) and antidiarrheal agents (eg, loperamide) may be given to control the diarrhea and fecal urgency. Antidepressants can assist in treating underlying anxiety and depression. Anticholinergics and calcium channel blockers decrease smooth muscle spasm, decreasing cramping and constipation.

Nursing Management

The nurse's role is to provide patient and family education. The nurse emphasizes teaching and reinforces good dietary habits. The patient is encouraged to eat at regular times and to chew food slowly and thoroughly. The patient should understand that, although adequate fluid intake is necessary, fluid should not be taken with meals because this results in abdominal distention. Alcohol use and cigarette smoking are discouraged.

CONDITIONS OF MALABSORPTION

Malabsorption is the inability of the digestive system to absorb one or more of the major vitamins (especially vitamin B$_{12}$), minerals (ie, iron and calcium), and nutrients (ie, carbohydrates, fats, and proteins). Interruptions in the complex digestive process may occur anywhere in the digestive system and cause decreased absorption. Diseases of the small intestine are the most common cause of malabsorption.

Pathophysiology

The conditions that cause malabsorption can be grouped into the following categories:

- Mucosal (transport) disorders causing generalized malabsorption (eg, celiac sprue, regional enteritis, radiation enteritis)
- Infectious diseases causing generalized malabsorption (eg, small bowel bacterial overgrowth, tropical sprue, Whipple's disease)
- Luminal problems causing malabsorption (eg, bile acid deficiency, Zollinger-Ellison syndrome, pancreatic insufficiency)
- Postoperative malabsorption (eg, after gastric or intestinal resection)
- Disorders that cause malabsorption of specific nutrients (eg, disaccharidase deficiency leading to lactose intolerance)

Table 38-2 lists the clinical and pathologic aspects of malabsorptive diseases.

Clinical Manifestations

The hallmarks of malabsorption syndrome from any cause are diarrhea or frequent, loose, bulky, foul-smelling stools that have increased fat content and are often greyish. Patients often have associated abdominal distention, pain, increased flatus, weakness, weight loss, and a decreased sense of well-being. The chief result of malabsorption is malnutrition, manifested by weight loss and other signs of vitamin and mineral deficiency (eg, easy bruising, osteoporosis, anemia). Patients with a malabsorption syndrome, if untreated, become weak and emaciated because of starvation and dehydration. Failure to absorb the fat-soluble vitamins A, D, and K causes a corresponding avitaminosis.

Assessment and Diagnostic Findings

Several diagnostic tests may be prescribed, including stool studies for quantitative and qualitative fat analysis, lactose tolerance tests, D-xylose absorption tests, and Schilling tests. The hydrogen breath test that is used to evaluate carbohydrate absorption (see Chap. 34) is performed if carbohydrate malabsorption is suspected. Endoscopy with biopsy of the mucosa is the best diagnostic tool. Biopsy of the small intestine is performed to assay enzyme activity or to identify infection or destruction of mucosa. Ultrasound studies, CT scans, and x-ray findings can reveal pancreatic or intestinal tumours that may be the cause. A complete blood cell count is used to detect anemia. Pancreatic function tests can assist in the diagnosis of specific disorders.

Medical Management

Intervention is aimed at avoiding dietary substances that aggravate malabsorption and at supplementing nutrients that have been lost. Common supplements are water-soluble vitamins (eg, B$_{12}$, folic acid), fat-soluble vitamins (ie, A, D, and K), and minerals (eg, calcium, iron). Primary disease states may be managed surgically or nonsurgically. Dietary therapy is aimed at reducing gluten intake in patients with celiac sprue. Folic acid supplements are prescribed for patients with tropical sprue. Antibiotics (eg, tetracycline, ampicillin) are sometimes needed in the treatment of tropical sprue and bacterial overgrowth syndromes. Antidiarrheal agents may be used to decrease intestinal spasms. Parenteral fluids may be necessary to treat dehydration.

Nursing Management

The nurse provides patient and family education regarding diet and the use of nutritional supplements (Chart 38-2). It is important to monitor patients with diarrhea for fluid and electrolyte imbalances. The nurse conducts ongoing assessments to determine if the clinical manifestations related to the nutritional deficits have abated. Patient education includes information about the risk of osteoporosis related to malabsorption of calcium.

Acute Inflammatory Intestinal Disorders

Any part of the lower GI tract is susceptible to acute inflammation caused by bacterial, viral, or fungal infection. Two such situations are appendicitis and diverticulitis. These two conditions can lead to **peritonitis**, an inflammatory process within the abdomen.

APPENDICITIS

The appendix is a small, finger-like appendage about 10 cm long that is attached to the cecum just below the ileocecal valve. The appendix fills with food and empties regularly into the cecum. Because it empties inefficiently and its lumen is small, the appendix is prone to obstruction and is particularly vulnerable to infection (ie, appendicitis).

Appendicitis is the most common cause of acute abdomen and the most common reason for emergency abdominal surgery. About 7% of the population will have appendicitis at some time in their lives; males are affected more than females, and teenagers more than adults. Although it can occur at any age, it occurs most frequently between the ages of 10 and 30 years (Yamada et al., 1999). In Canada, appendicitis is the leading digestive disease resulting in hospitalization (Canadian Institute of Health Information, 2002).

Pathophysiology

The appendix becomes inflamed and edematous as a result of either becoming kinked or occluded by a fecalith (ie, hardened mass of stool), tumour, or foreign body. The inflammatory pro-

Table 38-2 • **Characteristics of Diseases of Malabsorption**

DISEASES/DISORDERS	PHYSIOLOGIC PATHOLOGY	CLINICAL FEATURES
Gastric resection with gastrojejunostomy	Decreased pancreatic stimulation because of duodenal bypass; poor mixing of food, bile, pancreatic enzymes; decreased intrinsic factor	Weight loss, moderate steatorrhea, anemia (combination of iron deficiency, vitamin B_{12} malabsorption, folate deficiency)
Pancreatic insufficiency (chronic pancreatitis, pancreatic carcinoma, pancreatic resection, cystic fibrosis)	Reduced intraluminal pancreatic enzyme activity, with maldigestion of lipids and proteins	History of abdominal pain followed by weight loss; marked steatorrhea, **azotorrhea** (excess of nitrogenous matter in the feces or urine); also frequent glucose intolerance (70% in pancreatic insufficiency)
Ileal dysfunction (resection or disease)	Loss of ileal absorbing surface leads to reduced bile-salt pool size and reduced vitamin B_{12} absorption; bile in colon inhibits fluid absorption	Diarrhea, weight loss with steatorrhea, especially when greater than 100 cm resection, decreased vitamin B_{12} absorption
Stasis syndromes (surgical strictures, blind loops, enteric fistulas, multiple jejunal diverticula, scleroderma)	Overgrowth of intraluminal intestinal bacteria, especially anaerobic organisms, to greater than 10^6/mL results in deconjugation of bile salts, leading to decreased effective bile-salt pool size, also bacterial utilization of vitamin B_{12}	Weight loss, steatorrhea; low vitamin B_{12} absorption; may have low D-xylose absorption
Zollinger-Ellison syndrome	Hyperacidity in duodenum inactivates pancreatic enzymes	Ulcer diathesis, steatorrhea
Lactose intolerance	Deficiency of intestinal lactase results in high concentration of intraluminal lactose with osmotic diarrhea	Varied degrees of diarrhea and cramps after ingestion of lactose-containing foods; positive lactose intolerance test, decreased intestinal lactase
Celiac disease (gluten enteropathy)	Toxic response to a gluten fraction by surface epithelium results in destruction of absorbing surface	Weight loss, diarrhea, bloating, anemia (low iron, folate), osteomalacia, steatorrhea, azotorrhea, low D-xylose absorption; folate and iron malabsorption
Tropical sprue	Unknown toxic factor results in mucosal inflammation, partial villous atrophy	Weight loss, diarrhea, anemia (low folate, vitamin B_{12}); steatorrhea; low D-xylose absorption, low vitamin B_{12} absorption
Whipple's disease	Bacterial invasion of intestinal mucosa	Arthritis, hyperpigmentation, lymphadenopathy, serous effusions, fever, weight loss; steatorrhea, azotorrhea
Certain parasitic diseases (giardiasis, strongyloidiasis, coccidiosis, capillariasis)	Damage to or invasion of surface mucosa	Diarrhea, weight loss; steatorrhea; organism may be seen on jejunal biopsy or recovered in stool
Immunoglobulinopathy	Decreased local intestinal defenses, lymphoid hyperplasia, lymphopenia	Frequent association with *Giardia:* hypogammaglobulinemia or isolated IgA deficiency

cess increases intraluminal pressure, initiating a progressively severe, generalized or upper abdominal pain that becomes localized in the right lower quadrant of the abdomen within a few hours. Eventually, the inflamed appendix fills with pus.

Clinical Manifestations

Vague epigastric or periumbilical pain progresses to right lower quadrant pain and is usually accompanied by a low-grade fever and nausea and sometimes by vomiting. Loss of appetite is common. Local tenderness is elicited at McBurney's point when pressure is applied (Fig. 38-2). Rebound tenderness (ie, production or intensification of pain when pressure is released) may be present. The extent of tenderness and muscle spasm and the existence of constipation or diarrhea depend not so much on the severity of the appendiceal infection as on the location of the appendix. If the appendix curls around behind the cecum, pain and tenderness may be felt in the lumbar region. If its tip is in the pelvis, these signs may be elicited only on rectal examination. Pain on

defecation suggests that the tip of the appendix is resting against the rectum; pain on urination suggests that the tip is near the bladder or impinges on the ureter. Some rigidity of the lower portion of the right rectus muscle may occur. Rovsing's sign may be elicited by palpating the left lower quadrant; this paradoxically causes pain to be felt in the right lower quadrant (see Fig. 38-2). If the appendix has ruptured, the pain becomes more diffuse; abdominal distention develops as a result of paralytic ileus, and the patient's condition worsens.

Constipation can also occur with an acute process such as appendicitis. Laxatives administered in this instance may produce perforation of the inflamed appendix. In general, a laxative or cathartic should never be given while the person has fever, nausea, or pain.

Assessment and Diagnostic Findings

Diagnosis is based on results of a complete physical examination and on laboratory and x-ray findings. The complete blood cell count demonstrates an elevated white blood cell count. The leukocyte

Chart 38-2 • PATIENT EDUCATION
Managing Lactose Intolerance

The following information may be helpful for patients who cannot tolerate lactose:

- Deficiency of lactase, a digestive enzyme essential for the absorption of lactose from the intestines, results in an intolerance to milk.
- Elimination of milk and milk substances can abolish symptoms.
- Many processed foods have fillers, such as dried milk, added to them.
- Pretreatment of foods with lactase preparations (eg, LactAid drops) before ingestion can reduce symptoms.
- Most people can tolerate 1 to 2 cups of milk or milk products daily without major problems; they are best tolerated if ingested in small amounts during the day.
- Lactase activity of yogurt with "active cultures" helps the digestion of lactose within the intestine better than lactase preparations do.
- Milk and milk products are rich sources of calcium and vitamin D; elimination of milk from the diet may result in calcium and vitamin D deficiencies; decreased intake without supplements can lead to osteoporosis.

count may exceed 10,000 cells/mm³, and the neutrophil count may exceed 75%. Abdominal x-ray films, ultrasound studies, and CT scans may reveal a right lower quadrant density or localized distention of the bowel.

Complications

The major complication of appendicitis is perforation of the appendix, which can lead to peritonitis or an abscess. The incidence of perforation is 10% to 32%. The incidence is higher in young children and the elderly. Perforation generally occurs 24 hours after the onset of pain. Symptoms include a fever of 37.7°C or higher, a toxic appearance, and continued abdominal pain or tenderness.

Gerontologic Considerations

Acute appendicitis does not occur frequently in the elderly population. Classic signs and symptoms are altered and may vary greatly. Pain may be absent or minimal. Symptoms may be vague, suggesting bowel obstruction or another process. Fever and leukocytosis may not be present. As a result, diagnosis and prompt treatment may be delayed, causing potential complications and mortality. The patient may have no symptoms until the appendix ruptures. The incidence of perforated appendix is higher in the elderly population because many of these patients do not seek health care as quickly as younger patients.

Medical Management

Surgery is indicated if appendicitis is diagnosed. To correct or prevent fluid and electrolyte imbalance and dehydration, antibiotics and intravenous fluids are administered until surgery is performed. Analgesics can be administered after the diagnosis is made. Appendectomy (ie, surgical removal of the appendix) is performed as soon as possible to decrease the risk of perforation. It may be performed under a general or spinal anesthetic with a low abdominal incision or by laparoscopy.

Nursing Management

Goals include relieving pain, preventing fluid volume deficit, reducing anxiety, eliminating infection from the potential or actual disruption of the GI tract, maintaining skin integrity, and attaining optimal nutrition.

The nurse prepares the patient for surgery, which includes an intravenous infusion to replace fluid loss and promote adequate renal function and antibiotic therapy to prevent infection. If there is evidence or likelihood of paralytic ileus, a nasogastric tube is inserted. An enema is not administered because it can lead to perforation.

After surgery, the nurse places the patient in a semi-Fowler position. This position reduces the tension on the incision and abdominal organs, helping to reduce pain. An opioid, usually morphine sulfate, is prescribed to relieve pain. When tolerated, oral fluids are administered. Any patient who was dehydrated before surgery receives intravenous fluids. Food is provided as desired and tolerated on the day of surgery.

The patient may be discharged on the day of surgery if the temperature is within normal limits, there is no undue discomfort in the operative area, and the appendectomy was uncomplicated. Discharge teaching for the patient and family is imperative. The nurse instructs the patient to make an appointment to have the surgeon remove the sutures between the fifth and seventh days after surgery. Incision care and activity guidelines are discussed; normal activity can usually be resumed within 2 to 4 weeks.

If there is a possibility of peritonitis, a drain is left in place at the area of the incision. Patients at risk for this complication may be kept in the hospital for several days and are monitored carefully for signs of intestinal obstruction or secondary hemorrhage. Secondary abscesses may form in the pelvis, under the diaphragm, or

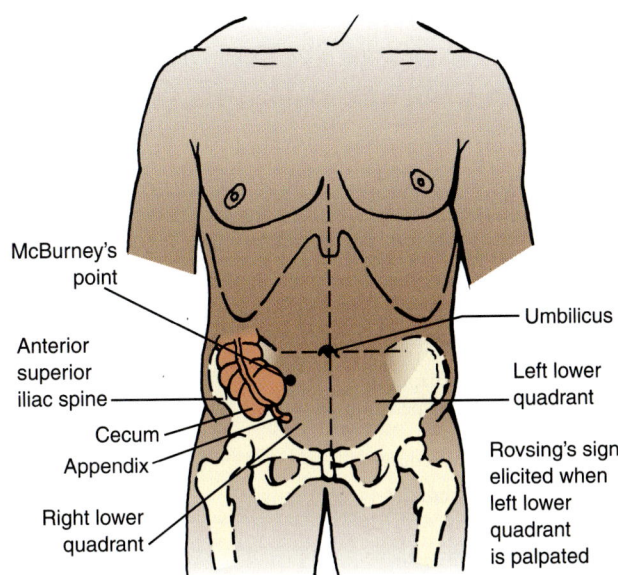

FIGURE 38-2 When the appendix is inflamed, tenderness can be noted in the right lower quadrant at McBurney's point, which is between the umbilicus and the anterior superior iliac spine. Rovsing's sign is pain felt in the right lower quadrant after the left lower quadrant has been palpated.

in the liver, elevating the temperature and pulse rate and increasing the leukocyte count.

When the patient is ready for discharge, the nurse teaches the patient and family to care for the incision and perform dressing changes and irrigations as prescribed. A home care nurse may be needed to assist with this care and to monitor the patient for complications and wound healing. Other potential complications of appendectomy are listed in Table 38-3.

DIVERTICULAR DISEASE

A **diverticulum** is a saclike outpouching of the lining of the bowel that extends through a defect in the muscle layer. Diverticula may occur anywhere along the GI tract. **Diverticulosis** exists when multiple diverticula are present without inflammation or symptoms. Diverticular disease of the colon is very common in developed countries, and its prevalence increases with age. More than 35% of Americans older than 60 years of age have diverticulosis. The incidence increases to 50% among those in the ninth decade of life (Keighley, 1999). **Diverticulitis** results when food and bacteria retained in a diverticulum produce infection and inflammation that can impede drainage and lead to perforation or abscess formation. Diverticulitis is most common (95%) in the sigmoid colon. Approximately 20% of patients with diverticulosis have diverticulitis at some point. A congenital predisposition is suspected when the disorder occurs in those younger than 40 years of age. A low intake of dietary fibre is considered a predisposing factor, but the exact cause is unknown. Diverticulitis may occur in acute attacks or may persist as a continuing, smoldering infection. Most patients remain entirely asymptomatic. The symptoms manifested generally result from its potential complications—abscesses, fistulas, obstruction, and hemorrhage.

Pathophysiology

A diverticulum forms when the mucosa and submucosal layers of the colon herniate through the muscular wall because of high intraluminal pressure, low volume in the colon (ie, fibre-deficient contents), and decreased muscle strength in the colon wall (ie, muscular hypertrophy from hardened fecal masses). Bowel contents can accumulate in the diverticulum and decompose, causing inflammation and infection. A diverticulum can become obstructed and then inflamed if the obstruction continues. The inflammation tends to spread to the surrounding bowel wall, giving rise to irritability and spasticity of the colon (ie, diverticulitis). Abscesses develop and may eventually perforate, leading to peritonitis and erosion of the blood vessels (arterial) with bleeding.

Clinical Manifestations

Chronic constipation often precedes the development of diverticulosis by many years. Frequently, no problematic symptoms occur with diverticulosis. Signs of acute diverticulosis are bowel irregularity and intervals of diarrhea, abrupt onset of crampy pain in the left lower quadrant of the abdomen, and a low-grade fever. The patient may have nausea and anorexia, and some bloating or abdominal distention may occur. With repeated local inflammation of the diverticula, the large bowel may narrow with fibrotic strictures, leading to cramps, narrow stools, and increased constipation. Weakness, fatigue, and anorexia are common symptoms. With acute diverticulosis, the patient reports mild to severe pain in the lower left quadrant. The condition, if untreated, can lead to septicemia.

Assessment and Diagnostic Findings

A CT scan is the procedure of choice and can reveal abscesses. Abdominal x-ray findings may demonstrate free air under the diaphragm if a perforation has occurred from the diverticulitis. Diverticulosis may be diagnosed using barium enema, which shows narrowing of the colon and thickened muscle layers. If there are symptoms of peritoneal irritation and when the diagnosis is diverticulitis, barium enema is contraindicated because of the potential for perforation.

A colonoscopy may be performed if there is no acute diverticulitis or after resolution of an acute episode to visualize the colon, determine the extent of the disease, and rule out other conditions. Laboratory tests that assist in diagnosis include a complete blood cell count, revealing an elevated leukocyte count, and elevated sedimentation rate.

COMPLICATION	NURSING INTERVENTIONS
Peritonitis	Observe for abdominal tenderness, fever, vomiting, abdominal rigidity, and tachycardia.
	Employ constant nasogastric suction.
	Correct dehydration as prescribed.
	Administer antibiotic agents as prescribed.
Pelvic abscess	Evaluate for anorexia, chills, fever, and diaphoresis.
	Observe for diarrhea, which may indicate pelvic abscess.
	Prepare patient for rectal examination.
	Prepare patient for surgical drainage procedure.
Subphrenic abscess (abscess under the diaphragm)	Assess patient for chills, fever, and diaphoresis.
	Prepare for x-ray examination.
	Prepare for surgical drainage of abscess.
Ileus (paralytic and mechanical)	Assess for bowel sounds.
	Employ nasogastric intubation and suction.
	Replace fluids and electrolytes by intravenous route as prescribed.
	Prepare for surgery, if diagnosis of mechanical ileus is established.

Table 38-3 • **Potential Complications and Nursing Interventions After Appendectomy**

Complications

Complications of diverticulitis include peritonitis, abscess formation, and bleeding. If an abscess develops, the associated findings are tenderness, a palpable mass, fever, and leukocytosis. An inflamed diverticulum that perforates results in abdominal pain localized over the involved segment, usually the sigmoid; local abscess or peritonitis follows. Abdominal pain, a rigid boardlike abdomen, loss of bowel sounds, and signs and symptoms of shock occur with peritonitis. Noninflamed or slightly inflamed diverticula may erode areas adjacent to arterial branches, causing massive rectal bleeding.

Gerontologic Considerations

The incidence of diverticular disease increases with age because of degeneration and structural changes in the circular muscle layers of the colon and because of cellular hypertrophy. The symptoms are less pronounced in the elderly than in other adults. The elderly may not have abdominal pain until infection occurs. They may delay reporting symptoms because they fear surgery or are afraid that they may have cancer. Blood in the stool is overlooked frequently, especially in the elderly, because of a failure to examine the stool or the inability to see changes because of diminished vision.

Medical Management

DIETARY AND MEDICATION MANAGEMENT

Diverticulitis can usually be treated on an outpatient basis with diet and medicine therapy. When symptoms occur, rest, analgesics, and antispasmodics are recommended. Initially, the diet is clear liquid until the inflammation subsides; then, a high-fibre, low-fat diet is recommended. This type of diet helps to increase stool volume, decrease colonic transit time, and reduce intraluminal pressure. Antibiotics are prescribed for 7 to 10 days. A bulk-forming laxative also is prescribed.

In acute cases of diverticulitis with significant symptoms, hospitalization is required. Hospitalization is often indicated for those who are elderly, immunocompromised, or taking corticosteroids. Withholding oral intake, administering intravenous fluids, and instituting nasogastric suctioning if vomiting or distention occurs rests the bowel. Broad-spectrum antibiotics are prescribed for 7 to 10 days. An opioid is prescribed for pain relief; morphine is not used because it increases segmentation and intraluminal pressures. Oral intake is increased as symptoms subside. A low-fibre diet may be necessary until signs of infection decrease.

Antispasmodics such as propantheline bromide (Pro-Banthine) and oxyphencyclimine (Daricon) may be prescribed. Normal stools can be achieved by using bulk preparations (Metamucil) or stool softeners (Colace), by instilling warm oil into the rectum, or by inserting an evacuant suppository (Dulcolax). Such a prophylactic plan can reduce the bacterial flora of the bowel, diminish the bulk of the stool, and soften the fecal mass so that it moves more easily through the area of inflammatory obstruction.

SURGICAL MANAGEMENT

Although acute diverticulitis usually subsides with medical management, immediate surgical intervention is necessary if complications (eg, perforation, peritonitis, abscess formation, hemorrhage, obstruction) occur. Alternatively, when the acute episode of diverticulitis resolves, surgery may be recommended to prevent repeated episodes. Two types of surgery are considered:

- One-stage resection in which the inflamed area is removed and a primary end-to-end anastomosis is completed
- Multiple-staged procedures for complications such as obstruction or perforation (Fig. 38-3)

The type of surgery performed depends on the extent of complications found during surgery. When possible, the area of diverticulitis is resected and the remaining bowel is joined end to end (ie, primary resection and end-to-end anastomosis). This is performed through traditional surgical or laparoscopically assisted colectomy. A two-stage resection may be performed in which the diseased colon is resected (as in a one-stage procedure) but no anastomosis is performed; both ends of the bowel are brought out onto the abdomen as stomas. This "double-barrel" colostomy is then reanastomosed in a later procedure. Fecal diversion procedures are discussed later in this chapter.

NURSING PROCESS: THE PATIENT WITH DIVERTICULITIS

Assessment

During the health history, the nurse asks the patient about the onset and duration of pain and about past and present elimination patterns. The nurse reviews dietary habits to determine fibre intake and asks the patient about straining at stool, history of constipation with periods of diarrhea, tenesmus (ie, spasms of the anal sphincter with pain and persistent urge to defecate), abdominal bloating, and distention.

Assessment includes auscultation for the presence and character of bowel sounds and palpation for lower left quadrant pain, tenderness, or firm mass. The stool is inspected for pus, mucus, or blood. It is important to monitor temperature, pulse, and blood pressure for abnormal variations.

Diagnosis

NURSING DIAGNOSES

Based on the assessment data, the nursing diagnoses may include the following:

- Constipation related to narrowing of the colon from thickened muscular segments and strictures
- Acute pain related to inflammation and infection

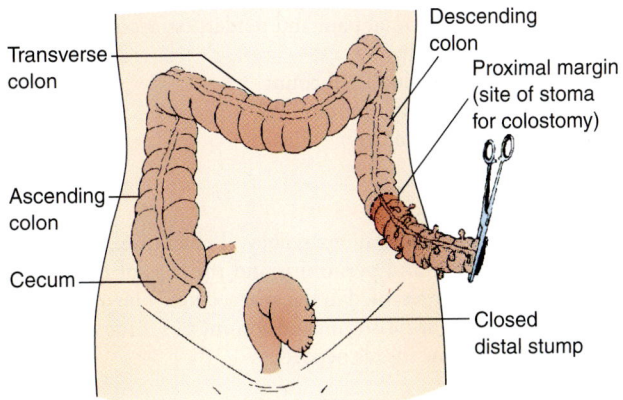

FIGURE 38-3 The Hartmann procedure for diverticulitis: primary resection for diverticulitis of the colon. The affected segment (*clamp attached*) has been divided at its distal end. In a primary anastomosis, the proximal margin (*dotted line*) is transected and the bowel attached end-to-end. In a two-stage procedure, a colostomy is constructed at the proximal margin with the distal stump oversewn (Hartmann procedure, as shown) or brought to the outer surface as a mucous fistula. The second stage consists of colostomy takedown and anastomosis.

COLLABORATIVE PROBLEMS/ POTENTIAL COMPLICATIONS

Potential complications that may develop include the following:

- Peritonitis
- Abscess formation
- Bleeding

Planning and Goals

The major goals for the patient may include attainment and maintenance of normal elimination patterns, pain relief, and absence of complications.

Nursing Interventions

MAINTAINING NORMAL ELIMINATION PATTERNS

The nurse recommends a fluid intake of 2 L per day (within limits of the patient's cardiac and renal reserve) and suggests foods that are soft but have increased fibre to increase the bulk of the stool and facilitate peristalsis, thereby promoting defecation. An individualized exercise program is encouraged to improve abdominal muscle tone. It is important to review the patient's daily routine to establish a schedule for meals and a set time for defecation and to assist in identifying habits that may have suppressed the urge to defecate. The nurse encourages daily intake of bulk laxatives such as Metamucil, which helps to propel feces through the colon. Stool softeners are administered as prescribed to decrease straining at stool, which decreases intestinal pressure. Oil retention enemas may be prescribed to soften the stool, making it easier to pass.

RELIEVING PAIN

Analgesics (eg, meperidine) to relieve the pain of diverticulitis and antispasmodic agents to decrease intestinal spasm are administered as prescribed. The nurse records the intensity, duration, and location of pain to determine if the inflammatory process worsens or subsides.

MONITORING AND MANAGING POTENTIAL COMPLICATIONS

The major nursing focus is to prevent complications by identifying patients at risk and managing their symptoms as needed. The nurse assesses for the following signs of perforation:

- Increased abdominal pain and tenderness accompanied by abdominal rigidity
- Elevated white blood cell count
- Elevated sedimentation rate
- Increased temperature
- Tachycardia
- Hypotension

Perforation is a surgical emergency. The clinical manifestations of perforation and peritonitis and the care of the patient with peritonitis are presented in the next section. The nurse monitors vital signs and urine output and administers intravenous fluids to replace volume loss as needed.

HOME AND COMMUNITY-BASED CARE

Because patients and their family members and health care providers tend to focus on the most obvious needs and issues, the nurse reminds the patient and family about the importance of continuing health promotion and screening practices. The nurse educates patients who have not been involved in these practices in the past about their importance and refers the patients to appropriate health care providers.

Evaluation

EXPECTED PATIENT OUTCOMES

Expected patient outcomes may include the following:

1. Attains a normal pattern of elimination
   a. Reports less abdominal cramping and pain
   b. Reports the passage of soft, formed stool without pain
   c. Adds unprocessed bran to foods
   d. Drinks at least 10 glasses of fluid each day (if fluid intake is tolerated)
   e. Exercises daily
2. Reports decreased pain
   a. Requests analgesics as needed
   b. Adheres to a low-fibre diet during acute episodes
3. Recovers without complications
   a. Is afebrile
   b. Has normal blood pressure
   c. Has a soft, nontender abdomen with normal bowel sounds
   d. Maintains adequate urine output
   e. Has no blood in the stool

PERITONITIS

Peritonitis is inflammation of the peritoneum, the serous membrane lining the abdominal cavity and covering the viscera. Usually, it is a result of bacterial infection; the organisms come from diseases of the GI tract or, in women, from the internal reproductive organs. Peritonitis can also result from external sources such as injury or trauma (eg, gunshot wound, stab wound) or an inflammation that extends from an organ outside the peritoneal area, such as the kidney. The most common bacteria implicated are *Escherichia coli, Klebsiella, Proteus,* and *Pseudomonas.* Inflammation and paralytic ileus are the direct effects of the infection. Other common causes of peritonitis are appendicitis, perforated ulcer, diverticulitis, and bowel perforation (Fig. 38-4). Peritonitis may also be associated with abdominal surgical procedures and peritoneal dialysis.

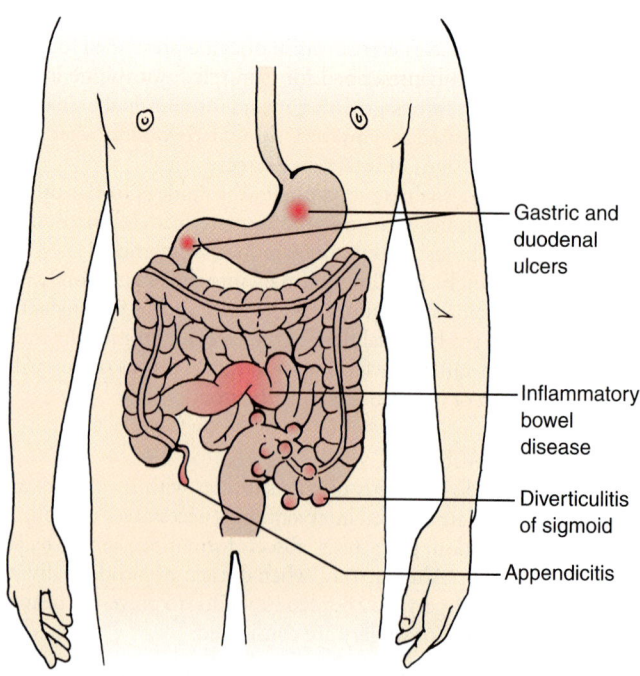

FIGURE 38-4 Common gastrointestinal causes of peritonitis.

Pathophysiology

Peritonitis is caused by leakage of contents from abdominal organs into the abdominal cavity, usually as a result of inflammation, infection, ischemia, trauma, or tumour perforation. Bacterial proliferation occurs. Edema of the tissues results, and exudation of fluid develops in a short time. Fluid in the peritoneal cavity becomes turbid with increasing amounts of protein, white blood cells, cellular debris, and blood. The immediate response of the intestinal tract is hypermotility, soon followed by paralytic ileus with an accumulation of air and fluid in the bowel.

Clinical Manifestations

Symptoms depend on the location and extent of the inflammation. The early clinical manifestations of peritonitis frequently are the symptoms of the disorder causing the condition. At first, a diffuse type of pain is felt. The pain tends to become constant, localized, and more intense near the site of the inflammation. Movement usually aggravates it. The affected area of the abdomen becomes extremely tender and distended, and the muscles become rigid. Rebound tenderness and paralytic ileus may be present. Usually, nausea and vomiting occur and peristalsis is diminished. The temperature and pulse rate increase, and there is almost always an elevation of the leukocyte count.

Assessment and Diagnostic Findings

The leukocyte count is elevated. The hemoglobin and hematocrit levels may be low if blood loss has occurred. Serum electrolyte studies may reveal altered levels of potassium, sodium, and chloride.

An abdominal x-ray is obtained, and findings may show air and fluid levels as well as distended bowel loops. A CT scan of the abdomen may show abscess formation. Peritoneal aspiration and culture and sensitivity studies of the aspirated fluid may reveal infection and identify the causative organisms.

Complications

Frequently, the inflammation is not localized and the whole abdominal cavity becomes involved in a generalized sepsis. Sepsis is the major cause of death from peritonitis. Shock may result from septicemia or hypovolemia. The inflammatory process may cause intestinal obstruction, primarily from the development of bowel adhesions.

The two most common postoperative complications are wound evisceration and abscess formation. Any suggestion from the patient that an area of the abdomen is tender or painful or "feels as if something just gave way" must be reported. The sudden occurrence of serosanguineous wound drainage strongly suggests wound dehiscence (see Chap. 20).

Medical Management

Fluid, colloid, and electrolyte replacement is the major focus of medical management. The administration of several litres of an isotonic solution is prescribed. Hypovolemia occurs because massive amounts of fluid and electrolytes move from the intestinal lumen into the peritoneal cavity and deplete the fluid in the vascular space.

Analgesics are prescribed for pain. Antiemetics are administered as prescribed for nausea and vomiting. Intestinal intubation and suction assist in relieving abdominal distention and in promoting intestinal function. Fluid in the abdominal cavity can cause pressure that restricts expansion of the lungs and causes respiratory distress. Oxygen therapy by nasal cannula or mask can promote adequate oxygenation, but airway intubation and ventilatory assistance occasionally are required.

Massive antibiotic therapy is usually initiated early in the treatment of peritonitis. Large doses of a broad-spectrum antibiotic are administered intravenously until the specific organism causing the infection is identified and the appropriate antibiotic therapy can be initiated.

Surgical objectives include removing the infected material and correcting the cause. Surgical treatment is directed toward excision (ie, appendix), resection with or without anastomosis (ie, intestine), repair (ie, perforation), and drainage (ie, abscess). With extensive sepsis, a fecal diversion may need to be created.

Nursing Management

Ongoing assessment of pain, vital signs, GI function, and fluid and electrolyte balance is important. The nurse reports the nature of the pain, its location in the abdomen, and any shifts in location. Administering analgesic medication and positioning the patient for comfort are helpful in decreasing pain. The patient is placed on the side with knees flexed; this position decreases tension on the abdominal organs. Accurate recording of all intake and output and central venous pressure assists in calculating fluid replacement. The nurse administers and monitors closely intravenous fluids.

Signs that indicate that peritonitis is subsiding include a decrease in temperature and pulse rate, softening of the abdomen, return of peristaltic sounds, passing of flatus, and bowel movements. The nurse increases fluid and food intake gradually and reduces parenteral fluids as prescribed. A worsening clinical condition may indicate a complication, and the nurse must prepare the patient for emergency surgery.

Drains are frequently inserted during the surgical procedure, and the nurse must observe and record the character of the drainage postoperatively. Care must be taken when moving and turning the patient to prevent the drains from being dislodged. It is also important for the nurse to prepare the patient and family for discharge by teaching the patient to care for the incision and drains if the patient will be sent home with the drains still in place.

Inflammatory Bowel Disease

The term **inflammatory bowel disease** refers to two chronic inflammatory GI disorders: regional enteritis (ie, Crohn's disease or granulomatous colitis) and ulcerative colitis. Both disorders have striking similarities but also several differences. Table 38-4 compares regional enteritis and ulcerative colitis.

There is an increasing number of annually diagnosed cases of inflammatory bowel disease in Canada. Approximately 10,000 new cases are reported each year (Canadian Society of Intestinal Research, 2005).

Despite vast amounts of research, the cause of IBD is still unknown. Researchers think it is triggered by environmental agents such as pesticides, food additives, tobacco, and radiation (Kirsner & Shorter, 2000). Nonsteroidal anti-inflammatory drugs have been found to exacerbate IBD. Allergies and immune disorders have also been suggested as causes. Abnormal response to dietary

Table 38-4 • Comparison of Regional Enteritis and Ulcerative Colitis

FACTOR	REGIONAL ENTERITIS	ULCERATIVE COLITIS
Course	Prolonged, variable	Exacerbations, remissions
Pathology		
Early	Transmural thickening	Mucosal ulceration
Late	Deep, penetrating granulomas	Mucosal minute ulceration
Clinical Manifestations		
Location	Ileum, right colon (usually)	Rectum, left colon
Bleeding	Usually not, but may occur	Common—severe
Perianal involvement	Common	Rare—mild
Fistulas	Common	Rare
Rectal involvement	About 20%	Almost 100%
Diarrhea	Less severe	Severe
Diagnostic Study Findings		
Radiography	Regional, discontinuous lesions	Diffuse involvement
	Narrowing of colon	No narrowing of colon
	Thickening of bowel wall	No mucosal edema
	Mucosal edema	Stenosis rare
	Stenosis, fistulas	Shortening of colon
Sigmoidoscopy	May be unremarkable unless accompanied by perianal fistulas	Abnormal inflamed mucosa
Colonoscopy	Distinct ulcerations separated by relatively normal mucosa in right colon	Friable mucosa with pseudopolyps or ulcers in left colon
Therapeutic Management	Corticosteroids, sulfonamides (sulfasalazine [Salazopyrine, SAS Enteric 500])	Corticosteroids, sulfonamides; sulfasalazine useful in preventing recurrence
	Antibiotics	Bulk hydrophilic agents
	Parenteral nutrition	Antibiotics
	Partial or complete colectomy, with ileostomy or anastomosis	Proctocolectomy, with ileostomy
	Rectum can be preserved in some patients	Rectum can be preserved in only a few patients "cured" by colectomy
	Recurrence common	
Systemic Complications	Small bowel obstruction	Toxic megacolon
	Right-sided hydronephrosis	Perforation
	Nephrolithiasis	Hemorrhage
	Cholelithiasis	Malignant neoplasms
	Arthritis	Pyelonephritis
	Retinitis, iritis	Nephrolithiasis
	Erythema nodosum	Cholangiocarcinoma
		Arthritis
		Retinitis, iritis
		Erythema nodosum

or bacterial antigens has been studied extensively, and genetic factors also are being studied. There is a high prevalence of coexistent IBS, which complicates the overall symptom presentation.

REGIONAL ENTERITIS (CROHN'S DISEASE)

Regional enteritis commonly occurs in adolescents or young adults but can appear at any time of life. It is more common in women, and it occurs frequently in the older population (between the ages of 50 and 80). It can occur anywhere along the GI tract, but the most common areas are the distal ileum and colon. The incidence of Crohn's disease has risen over the past 30 years. Crohn's disease is seen two times more often in patients who smoke than in nonsmokers (Rose, 1998).

Pathophysiology

Regional enteritis is a subacute and chronic inflammation that extends through all layers (ie, transmural lesion) of the bowel wall from the intestinal mucosa. It is characterized by periods of remissions and exacerbations. The disease process begins with edema and thickening of the mucosa. Ulcers begin to appear on the inflamed mucosa. These lesions are not in continuous contact with one another and are separated by normal tissue. Fistulas, fissures, and abscesses form as the inflammation extends into the peritoneum. Granulomas occur in one half of patients. In advanced cases, the intestinal mucosa has a cobblestone appearance. As the disease advances, the bowel wall thickens and becomes fibrotic, and the intestinal lumen narrows. Diseased bowel loops sometimes adhere to other loops surrounding them.

Clinical Manifestations

In regional enteritis, the onset of symptoms is usually insidious, with prominent lower right quadrant abdominal pain and diarrhea unrelieved by defecation. Scar tissue and the formation of granulomas interfere with the ability of the intestine to transport products of the upper intestinal digestion through the constricted lumen, resulting in crampy abdominal pains. There is abdominal tenderness and spasm. Because eating stimulates intestinal peristalsis, the crampy pains occur after meals. To avoid these bouts of crampy pain, the patient tends to limit food intake, reducing the amounts and types of food to such a degree that normal nutritional requirements are not met. The result is weight loss, malnutrition, and secondary anemia. Ulcers in the membranous lining of the intestine and other inflammatory changes result in a weeping, swollen intestine that continually empties an irritating discharge into the colon. Disrupted absorption causes chronic diarrhea and nutritional deficits. The result is a person who is thin and emaciated from inadequate food intake and constant fluid loss. In some patients, the inflamed intestine may perforate, leading to intra-abdominal and anal abscesses. Fever and leukocytosis occur. Chronic symptoms include diarrhea, abdominal pain, steatorrhea, anorexia, weight loss, and nutritional deficiencies.

Abscesses, fistulas, and fissures are common. Symptoms extend beyond the GI tract and commonly include joint involvement (eg, arthritis), skin lesions (eg, erythema nodosum), ocular disorders (eg, conjunctivitis), and oral ulcers. The clinical course and symptoms can vary; in some patients, periods of remission and exacerbation occur, but in others, the disease follows a fulminating course.

Assessment and Diagnostic Findings

A proctosigmoidoscopic examination is usually performed initially to determine whether the rectosigmoid area is inflamed. A stool examination is also performed; the result may be positive for occult blood and steatorrhea (ie, excessive fat in the feces). The most conclusive diagnostic aid for regional enteritis is a barium study of the upper GI tract that shows the classic "string sign" on an x-ray film of the terminal ileum, indicating the constriction of a segment of intestine. Endoscopy and intestinal biopsy may be used for confirmation of the diagnosis. A barium enema may show ulcerations (the cobblestone appearance described earlier), fissures, and fistulas. A CT scan may show bowel wall thickening and fistula tracts.

A complete blood cell count is performed to assess hematocrit and hemoglobin levels (usually decreased) and the white blood cell count (may be elevated). The sedimentation rate is usually elevated. Albumin and protein levels may be decreased, indicating malnutrition.

Complications

Complications of regional enteritis include intestinal obstruction or stricture formation, perianal disease, fluid and electrolyte imbalances, malnutrition from malabsorption, and fistula and abscess formation. A fistula is an abnormal communication between two body structures, either internal (ie, between two structures) or external (ie, between an internal structure and the outside surface of the body). The most common type of small bowel fistula that results from regional enteritis is the enterocutaneous fistula (ie, between the small bowel and the skin). Abscesses can be the result of an internal fistula tract into an area that results in fluid accumulation and infection. Patients with regional enteritis are also at increased risk for colon cancer.

ULCERATIVE COLITIS

Ulcerative colitis is a recurrent ulcerative and inflammatory disease of the mucosal and submucosal layers of the colon and rectum. The incidence of ulcerative colitis is highest in Caucasians and people of Jewish heritage (Yamada et al., 1999). The peak incidence is between 30 and 50 years of age. It is a serious disease, accompanied by systemic complications and a high mortality rate. Eventually, 10% to 15% of the patients develop carcinoma of the colon.

Pathophysiology

Ulcerative colitis affects the superficial mucosa of the colon and is characterized by multiple ulcerations, diffuse inflammations, and desquamation or shedding of the colonic epithelium. Bleeding occurs as a result of the ulcerations. The mucosa becomes edematous and inflamed. The lesions are contiguous, occurring one after the other. Abscesses form, and infiltrate is seen in the mucosa and submucosa with clumps of neutrophils in the crypt lumens (ie, crypt abscesses). The disease process usually begins in the rectum and spreads proximally to involve the entire colon. Eventually, the bowel narrows, shortens, and thickens because of muscular hypertrophy and fat deposits.

Clinical Manifestations

The clinical course is usually one of exacerbations and remissions. The predominant symptoms of ulcerative colitis are diarrhea, lower left quadrant abdominal pain, intermittent tenesmus, and rectal bleeding. The bleeding may be mild or severe, and pallor results. The patient may have anorexia, weight loss, fever, vomiting, and dehydration, as well as cramping, the feeling of an urgent need to defecate, and the passage of 10 to 20 liquid stools each day. The disease is classified as mild, severe, or fulminant, depending on the severity of the symptoms. Hypocalcemia and anemia frequently develop. Rebound tenderness may occur in the right lower quadrant. Extraintestinal symptoms include skin lesions (eg, erythema nodosum), eye lesions (eg, uveitis), joint abnormalities (eg, arthritis), and liver disease.

Assessment and Diagnostic Findings

The patient should be assessed for tachycardia, hypotension, tachypnea, fever, and pallor. Other assessments include the level of hydration and nutritional status. The abdomen should be examined for characteristics of bowel sounds, distention, and tenderness. These findings assist in determining the severity of the disease.

The stool is positive for blood, and laboratory test results reveal a low hematocrit and hemoglobin concentration in addition to an elevated white blood cell count, low albumin levels, and an electrolyte imbalance. Abdominal x-ray studies are useful for determining the cause of symptoms. Free air in the peritoneum and bowel dilation or obstruction should be excluded as a source of the presenting symptoms. Sigmoidoscopy or colonoscopy and barium enema are valuable in distinguishing this condition from other diseases of the colon with similar symptoms. A barium enema may show mucosal irregularities, focal strictures or fistulas, shortening of the colon, and dilation of bowel loops. Endoscopy may reveal friable, inflamed mucosa with exudate and ulcerations. This procedure assists in defining the extent and severity of the disease. CT scanning, magnetic resonance imaging, and ultrasound can identify abscesses and perirectal involvement. Leukocyte scanning (see Chap. 34) is useful when severe colitis prohibits the use of endoscopy to determine the extent of inflammation.

> **! NURSING ALERT** In acute ulcerative colitis, cathartics are contraindicated when the patient is being prepared for barium enema or endoscopy because they may exacerbate the condition, which can lead to megacolon (ie, excessive dilation of the colon), perforation, and death. If the patient needs to have these diagnostic tests, a liquid diet for a few days before radiography and a gentle tap-water enema on the day of the examination may be prescribed. Colonoscopy is contraindicated in severe disease because of the risk of perforation.

Careful stool examination for parasites and other microbes is performed to rule out dysentery caused by common intestinal organisms, especially *Entamoeba histolytica* and *Clostridium difficile*.

Complications

Complications of ulcerative colitis include toxic megacolon, perforation, and bleeding as a result of ulceration, vascular engorgement, and highly vascular granulation tissue. In toxic megacolon, the inflammatory process extends into the muscularis, inhibiting its ability to contract and resulting in colonic distention. Symptoms include fever, abdominal pain and distention, vomiting, and fatigue. Colonic perforation from toxic megacolon is associated with a high mortality rate (15% to 50%) (Grendell et al., 1998). If the patient with toxic megacolon does not respond within 24 to 48 hours to medical management with nasogastric suction, intravenous fluids with electrolytes, corticosteroids, and antibiotics, surgery is required. Total colectomy is indicated. For many patients, surgery becomes necessary to relieve the effects of the disease and to treat these serious complications; an ileostomy usually is performed. The surgical procedures involved and the care of patients with this type of fecal diversion are discussed later in this chapter.

Patients with IBD also have a significantly increased risk of osteoporotic fractures due to decreased bone mineral density. Corticosteroid therapy may also contribute to the diminished bone mass.

Medical Management of Chronic Inflammatory Bowel Disease

Medical treatment for regional enteritis and ulcerative colitis is aimed at reducing inflammation, suppressing inappropriate immune responses, providing rest for a diseased bowel so that healing may take place, improving quality of life, and preventing or minimizing complications.

Most patients maintain long-term well-being interspersed with short intervals of illness (Hanauer, 2001). Management depends on the disease location, severity, and complications.

NUTRITIONAL THERAPY

Oral fluids and a low-residue, high-protein, high-calorie diet with supplemental vitamin therapy and iron replacement are prescribed to meet nutritional needs, reduce inflammation, and control pain and diarrhea. Fluid and electrolyte imbalances from dehydration caused by diarrhea are corrected by intravenous therapy as necessary if the patient is hospitalized or by oral supplementation if the patient can be managed at home. Any foods that exacerbate diarrhea are avoided. Milk may contribute to diarrhea in those with lactose intolerance. Cold foods and smoking are avoided because

both increase intestinal motility. Parenteral nutrition may be indicated.

PHARMACOLOGIC THERAPY

Sedatives and antidiarrheal and antiperistaltic medications are used to minimize peristalsis to rest the inflamed bowel. They are continued until the patient's stools approach normal frequency and consistency.

Aminosalicylate formulations such as sulfasalazine (Azulfidine) are often effective for mild or moderate inflammation and are used to prevent or reduce recurrences in long-term maintenance regimens. Newer sulfa-free aminosalicylates (eg, mesalamine [Asacol, Pentasa]) have been developed and shown effective in preventing and treating recurrence of inflammation (Wolfe, 2000). Antibiotics are used for secondary infections, particularly for purulent complications such as abscesses, perforation, and peritonitis.

Corticosteroids are used to treat severe and fulminant disease. These corticosteroids (eg, prednisone) can be administered orally in outpatient treatment or parenterally in hospitalized patients. Topical (ie, rectal administration) corticosteroids are also widely used in the treatment of distal colon disease. When the dosage of corticosteroids is reduced or stopped, the symptoms of disease may return. If corticosteroids are continued, adverse sequelae such as hypertension, fluid retention, cataracts, hirsutism (ie, abnormal hair growth), adrenal suppression, and loss of bone density may develop.

Immunomodulators (eg, azathioprene [Imuran], 6-mercaptopurine, methotrexate, cyclosporin) have been used to alter the immune response (Wolfe, 2000). The exact mechanism of action of these medications in treating IBD is unknown. They are used for patients with severe disease who have failed other therapies. These medications are useful in maintenance regimens to prevent relapses. Newer biologic therapies are being studied, and it is hoped that they will lead to improvement in the treatment of patients with chronically active disease (Yamada et al., 1999).

SURGICAL MANAGEMENT

When nonsurgical measures fail to relieve the severe symptoms of IBD, surgery may be recommended. The most common indications for surgery are medically intractable disease, poor quality of life, or complications from the disease or medical therapy (Wolfe, 2000).

More than one half of all patients with regional enteritis require surgery at some point. Recurrence of inflammation and disease after surgery in regional enteritis is inevitable. The rate of recurrence after surgery is 20% to 40% in the first 5 years. Patients younger than 25 years of age have the highest recurrence rate. Surgery for regional enteritis is indicated for refractory disease or complications (Wolfe, 2000). The procedure of choice is a total colectomy and ileostomy.

A newer surgical procedure developed for patients with severe regional enteritis is intestinal transplant. This technique is now available to children and to young and middle-age adults who have lost intestinal function from disease. Although not a cure, this procedure may eventually provide improvement in quality of life for some who are terminally ill. The technical and immunologic problems with this procedure remain formidable, and the costs and mortality rates remain high (Wolfe, 2000).

Approximately 15% to 20% of patients with ulcerative colitis require surgical intervention (Tierney et al., 2000). Indications for surgery include lack of improvement and continued deterioration, profuse bleeding, perforation, stricture formation, and cancer. Surgical excision usually improves quality of life.

Proctocolectomy with ileostomy (ie, complete excision of colon, rectum, and anus) is recommended when the rectum is severely involved.

One type of surgical technique that can be helpful is strictureplasty, in which the blocked or narrowed section of the bowel is widened, leaving the bowel intact. If a lesion can be delineated in regional enteritis or if a complication has occurred, the lesion is resected, and the remaining portions of the bowel are anastomosed. Surgical removal of up to 50% of the small bowel usually can be tolerated. Other types of surgical procedures, known as fecal diversions, are discussed later in this chapter.

Total Colectomy With Ileostomy. An **ileostomy**, the surgical creation of an opening into the ileum or small intestine (usually by means of an ileal stoma on the abdominal wall), is commonly performed after a total colectomy (ie, excision of the entire colon). It allows for drainage of fecal matter (ie, effluent) from the ileum to the outside of the body. The drainage is very mushy and occurs at frequent intervals. Nursing management of the patient with an ileostomy is discussed in a later section of this chapter.

Total Colectomy With Continent Ileostomy. Another procedure involves the removal of the entire colon and creation of the continent ileal reservoir (ie, Kock pouch). This procedure eliminates the need for an external fecal collection bag. Approximately 30 cm of the distal ileum is reconstructed to form a reservoir with a nipple valve that is created by pulling a portion of the terminal ileal loop back into the ileum. GI effluent can accumulate in the pouch for several hours and then be removed by means of a catheter inserted through the nipple valve. The major problem with the Kock pouch is malfunction of the nipple valve, which occurs in about 20% of the patients (Yamada et al., 1999).

Total Colectomy With Ileoanal Anastomosis. A total colectomy with ileoanal anastomosis is another surgical procedure that eliminates the need for a permanent ileostomy. It establishes an ileal reservoir, and anal sphincter control of elimination is retained. The procedure involves connecting a portion of the ileum to the anus (ie, ileoanal anastomosis) in conjunction with removal of the colon and the rectal mucosa (ie, total abdominal colectomy and mucosal proctectomy) (Fig. 38-5). A temporary diverting loop ileostomy is constructed at the time of surgery and closed about 3 months later.

With ileoanal anastomosis, the diseased colon and rectum are removed, voluntary defecation is maintained, and anal continence is preserved. The ileal reservoir decreases the number of bowel movements by 50%, from approximately 14 to 20 per day to 7 to 10 per day. Nighttime elimination is gradually reduced to one bowel movement. Complications of ileoanal anastomosis include irritation of the perianal skin from leakage of fecal contents, stricture formation at the anastomosis site, and small bowel obstruction.

Nursing Management

Nursing management of patients with IBD may be medical, surgical, or both. Patients in the community setting or those recently diagnosed may primarily require education about diet and medications and referral to support groups. Hospitalized patients with long-standing or severe disease also require careful monitoring, parenteral nutrition, fluid replacement, and possibly emergent surgery. The surgical procedures may involve a fecal diversion, with attendant needs for physical care, emotional support, and extensive teaching about management of the ostomy.

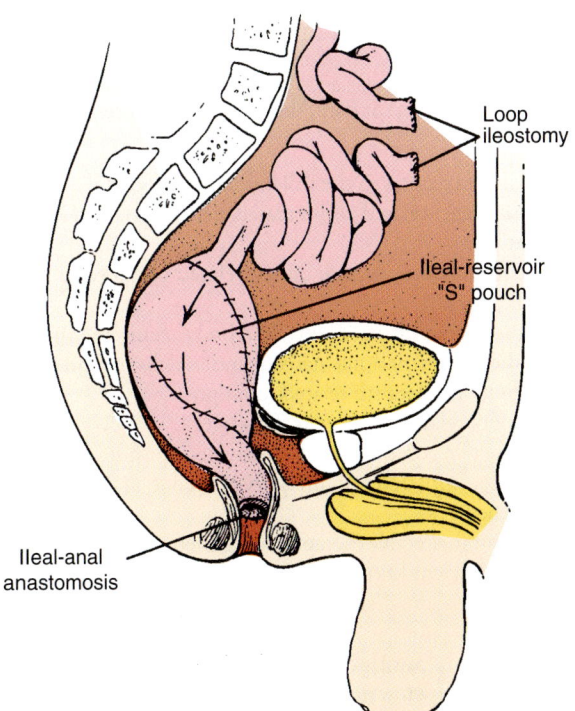

FIGURE 38-5 A mucosal proctectomy precedes anastomosis of the ileal reservoir. A temporary loop ileostomy diverts effluent for several months.

NURSING PROCESS: MANAGEMENT OF THE PATIENT WITH INFLAMMATORY BOWEL DISEASE

Assessment

The nurse takes a health history to identify the onset, duration, and characteristics of abdominal pain; the presence of diarrhea or fecal urgency, straining at stool (tenesmus), nausea, anorexia, or weight loss; and family history of IBD. It is important to discuss dietary patterns, including the amounts of alcohol, caffeine, and nicotine containing products used daily and weekly. The nurse asks about patterns of bowel elimination, including character, frequency, and presence of blood, pus, fat, or mucus. It is important to note allergies and food intolerance, especially milk (lactose) intolerance. The patient may identify sleep disturbances if diarrhea or pain occurs at night.

Assessment includes auscultating the abdomen for bowel sounds and their characteristics; palpating the abdomen for distention, tenderness, or pain; and inspecting the skin for evidence of fistula tracts or symptoms of dehydration. The stool is inspected for blood and mucus.

With regional enteritis, pain is usually localized in the right lower quadrant, where hyperactive bowel sounds can be heard because of borborygmus and increased peristalsis. Abdominal tenderness is noticed on palpation. The most prominent symptom is intermittent pain that occurs with diarrhea but does not decrease after defecation. Pain in the periumbilical region usually indicates involvement of the terminal ileum. With ulcerative colitis, the abdomen may be distended, and rebound tenderness may be present. Rectal bleeding is a significant sign.

Diagnosis

NURSING DIAGNOSES

Based on the assessment data, the nursing diagnoses may include the following:

- Diarrhea related to the inflammatory process
- Acute pain related to increased peristalsis and GI inflammation
- Deficient fluid volume deficit related to anorexia, nausea, and diarrhea
- Imbalanced nutrition, less than body requirements, related to dietary restrictions, nausea, and malabsorption
- Activity intolerance related to fatigue
- Anxiety related to impending surgery
- Ineffective coping related to repeated episodes of diarrhea
- Risk for impaired skin integrity related to malnutrition and diarrhea
- Risk for ineffective therapeutic regimen management related to insufficient knowledge concerning the process and management of the disease

COLLABORATIVE PROBLEMS/POTENTIAL COMPLICATIONS

Potential complications that may develop include the following:

- Electrolyte imbalance
- Cardiac dysrhythmia related to electrolyte depletion
- GI bleeding with fluid volume loss
- Perforation of the bowel

Planning and Goals

The major goals for the patient include attainment of normal bowel elimination patterns, relief of abdominal pain and cramping, prevention of fluid volume deficit, maintenance of optimal nutrition and weight, avoidance of fatigue, reducing anxiety, promoting effective coping, absence of skin breakdown, learning about the disease process and therapeutic regimen, and avoidance of complications.

Nursing Interventions

MAINTAINING NORMAL ELIMINATION PATTERNS

The nurse determines if there is a relationship between diarrhea and certain foods, activity, or emotional stress. Identifying precipitating factors, the frequency of bowel movements, and the character, consistency, and amount of stool passed is important. The nurse provides ready access to a bathroom, commode, or bedpan and keeps the environment clean and odour free. It is important to administer antidiarrheal medications as prescribed, to record the frequency and consistency of stools after therapy is initiated, and to encourage bed rest to decrease peristalsis.

RELIEVING PAIN

The character of the pain is described as dull, burning, or crampy. Asking about its onset is relevant. Does it occur before or after meals, during the night, or before elimination? Is the pattern constant or intermittent? Is it relieved with medications? The nurse administers anticholinergic medications as prescribed 30 minutes before a meal to decrease intestinal motility and administers analgesics as prescribed for pain. Position changes, local application of heat (as prescribed), diversional activities, and the prevention of fatigue also are helpful for reducing pain.

MAINTAINING FLUID INTAKE

To detect fluid volume deficit, the nurse keeps an accurate record of oral and intravenous fluids and maintains a record of output (ie, urine, liquid stool, vomitus, and wound or fistula drainage). The nurse monitors daily weights for fluid gains or losses and assesses the patient for signs of fluid volume deficit (ie, dry skin and mucous membranes, decreased skin turgor, oliguria, exhaustion, decreased temperature, increased hematocrit, elevated urine specific gravity, and hypotension). It is important to encourage oral intake of fluids and to monitor the intravenous flow rate. The nurse initiates measures to decrease diarrhea (eg, dietary restrictions, stress reduction, antidiarrheal agents).

MAINTAINING OPTIMAL NUTRITION

Parenteral nutrition (PN) is used when the symptoms of IBD are severe. With PN, the nurse maintains an accurate record of fluid intake and output as well as the patient's daily weight. The patient should gain 0.5 kg daily during PN therapy. Because PN is very high in glucose and can cause hyperglycemia, blood glucose levels are monitored every 6 hours. Elemental feedings high in protein and low in fat and residue are instituted after PN therapy because they are digested primarily in the jejunum, do not stimulate intestinal secretions, and allow the bowel to rest. The nurse notes intolerance if the patient exhibits nausea, vomiting, diarrhea, or abdominal distention.

If oral foods are tolerated, small, frequent, low-residue feedings are given to avoid overdistending the stomach and stimulating peristalsis. It is important for the patient to restrict activity to conserve energy, reduce peristalsis, and reduce calorie requirements.

PROMOTING REST

The nurse recommends intermittent rest periods during the day and schedules or restricts activities to conserve energy and reduce the metabolic rate. It is important to encourage activity within the limits of the patient's capacity. The nurse suggests bed rest for a patient who is febrile, has frequent diarrheal stools, or is bleeding. The patient on bed rest should perform active exercises to maintain muscle tone and prevent thromboembolic complications. If the patient is unable to perform these active exercises, the nurse performs passive exercises and joint range of motion. Activity restrictions are modified as needed on a day-to-day basis.

REDUCING ANXIETY

Rapport can be established by being attentive and displaying a calm, confident manner. The nurse allows time for the patient to ask questions and express feelings. Careful listening and sensitivity to nonverbal indicators of anxiety (eg, restlessness, tense facial expressions) are helpful. The patient may be emotionally labile because of the consequences of the disease; the nurse tailors information about possible impending surgery to the patient's level of understanding and desire for detail. If surgery is planned, pictures and illustrations help to explain the surgical procedure and help the patient to visualize what a stoma looks like.

ENHANCING COPING MEASURES

Because the patient may feel isolated, helpless, and out of control, understanding and emotional support are essential. The patient may respond to stress in a variety of ways that may alienate others, including anger, denial, and social self-isolation.

The nurse needs to recognize that the patient's behaviour may be affected by a number of factors unrelated to inherent emotional characteristics. Any patient suffering the discomforts of frequent bowel movements and rectal soreness is anxious, discouraged, and depressed. It is important to develop a relationship with the patient that supports all attempts to cope with these stresses. It is also important to communicate that the patient's feelings are understood by encouraging the patient to talk and express his or her feelings and to discuss any concerns. Stress reduction measures that may be used include relaxation techniques, visualization, breathing exercises, and biofeedback. Professional counselling may be needed to help the patient and family manage issues associated with chronic illness.

PREVENTING SKIN BREAKDOWN

The nurse examines the patient's skin frequently, especially the perianal skin. Perianal care, including the use of a skin barrier, is important after each bowel movement. The nurse gives immediate attention to reddened or irritated areas over a bony prominence and uses pressure-relieving devices to prevent skin breakdown. Consultation with a wound care specialist or enterostomal therapist is often helpful.

MONITORING AND MANAGING POTENTIAL COMPLICATIONS

Serum electrolyte levels are monitored daily, and electrolyte replacements are administered as prescribed. It is important to report evidence of dysrhythmias or change in level of consciousness immediately.

The nurse closely monitors rectal bleeding and administers blood component therapy and volume expanders as prescribed to prevent hypovolemia. It is important to monitor the blood pressure for hypotension and to obtain coagulation and hematocrit and hemoglobin profiles frequently. Vitamin K may be prescribed to increase clotting factors.

The nurse closely monitors the patient for indications of perforation (ie, acute increase in abdominal pain, rigid abdomen, vomiting, or hypotension) and obstruction and toxic megacolon (ie, abdominal distention, decreased or absent bowel sounds, change in mental status, fever, tachycardia, hypotension, dehydration, and electrolyte imbalances).

PROMOTING HOME AND COMMUNITY-BASED CARE

Teaching Patients Self-Care

The nurse assesses the patient's understanding of the disease process and his or her need for additional information about medical management (eg, medications, diet) and surgical interventions. The nurse provides information about nutritional management; a bland, low-residue, high-protein, high-calorie, and high-vitamin diet relieves symptoms and decreases diarrhea. It is important to provide the rationale for the use of corticosteroids and anti-inflammatory, antibacterial, antidiarrheal, and antispasmodic medications. The nurse emphasizes the importance of taking medications as prescribed and not abruptly discontinuing them (especially corticosteroids) to avoid development of serious medical problems (Chart 38-3). The nurse reviews ileostomy care as necessary (see Nursing Management of the Patient with an Ileostomy). Patient education information can be obtained from the National Foundation for Ileitis and Colitis.

Continuing Care

Patients with chronic inflammatory disease are managed at home with follow-up care by their physician or through an outpatient clinic. Those whose nutritional status is compromised and who are receiving PN need home care nursing to ensure that their nutritional requirements are being met and that they or their caregivers can follow through with the instructions for PN. Patients who are medically managed need to understand that their disease can be controlled and that they can lead a healthy life between exacerbations. Control implies management based on an understanding of the disease and its treatment. Patients in the home setting need information about their medications (ie, name, dose, side effects, and frequency of administration) and need to take medications on schedule. Medication reminders such as containers that separate pills according to day and time or daily checklists are helpful.

During a flare-up, the nurse encourages patients to rest as needed and to modify activities according to their energy levels. Patients should limit tasks that impose strain on the lower abdominal muscles. They should sleep in a room close to the bathroom because of the frequent diarrhea (10 to 20 times per day); quick access to a toilet helps alleviate the worry of embarrassment if an accident occurs. Room deodourizers help control odours.

Dietary modifications can control but not cure the disease; the nurse recommends a low-residue, high-protein, high-calorie diet, especially during an acute phase. It is important to encourage patients to keep a record of the foods that irritate the bowel and to eliminate them from the diet and to remind patients to drink at least eight glasses of water each day.

Chart 38-3
Home Care Checklist • Managing Inflammatory Bowel Disease

At the completion of the home care instruction, the patient or caregiver will be able to:	Patient	Caregiver
• Verbalize an understanding of the disease process.	✓	✓
• Discuss nutritional management: bland, low-residue, high-protein, high-vitamin diet; identify foods to include and foods to be avoided.	✓	✓
• Describe medication regimen; identify medications by name, use, route, and frequency.	✓	✓
• Identify measures to be used to treat exacerbation of symptoms, to include rest, dietary modifications, medications.	✓	✓
• Identify measures to be used to promote fluid and electrolyte balance during acute exacerbations	✓	✓
• Demonstrate management of PN therapy, if applicable; identifies possible complications and interventions	✓	✓
• Incorporate stress reduction measures into life-style	✓	

The prolonged nature of the disease has an impact on the patient and often strains his or her family life and financial resources as well. Family support is vital; however, some family members may be resentful, guilty, and tired and feel unable to continue coping with the emotional demands of the illness and the physical demands of caring for another. Some patients with IBD do not socialize for fear of being embarrassed. Many prefer to eat alone. Because they have lost control over elimination, they may fear losing control over other aspects of their lives. They need time to express their fears and frustrations. Individual and family counselling may be helpful.

Evaluation

EXPECTED PATIENT OUTCOMES

Expected patient outcomes may include the following:

1. Reports a decrease in the frequency of diarrhea stools
   a. Complies with dietary restrictions; maintains bed rest
   b. Takes medications as prescribed
2. Has reduced pain
3. Maintains fluid volume balance
   a. Drinks 1 to 2 L of oral fluids daily
   b. Has a normal body temperature
   c. Displays adequate skin turgor and moist mucous membranes
4. Attains optimal nutrition; tolerates small, frequent feedings without diarrhea
5. Avoids fatigue
   a. Rests periodically during the day
   b. Adheres to activity restrictions
6. Is less anxious
7. Copes successfully with diagnosis
   a. Expresses feelings freely
   b. Uses appropriate stress reduction behaviours
8. Maintains skin integrity
   a. Cleans perianal skin after defecation
   b. Uses lotion or ointment as skin barrier
9. Acquires an understanding of the disease process
   a. Modifies diet appropriately to decrease diarrhea
   b. Adheres to medication regimen
10. Recovers without complications
    a. Maintains electrolytes within normal ranges
    b. Maintains normal sinus or baseline cardiac rhythm
    c. Maintains fluid balance
    d. Experiences no perforation or rectal bleeding

NURSING MANAGEMENT OF THE PATIENT REQUIRING AN ILEOSTOMY

Some patients with IBD eventually require permanent fecal diversion with creation of an ileostomy to manage symptoms and to treat or prevent complications. The Plan of Nursing Care 38-1 summarizes care for the patient requiring an ostomy.

Providing Preoperative Care

A period of preparation with intensive replacement of fluid, blood, and protein is necessary before surgery is performed. Antibiotics may be prescribed. If the patient has been taking corticosteroids, they will be continued during the surgical phase to prevent steroid-induced adrenal insufficiency. Usually, the patient is given a low-residue diet, provided in frequent, small feedings. All other preoperative measures are similar to those for general

abdominal surgery. The abdomen is marked for the proper placement of the stoma by the surgeon or the enterostomal therapist. Care is taken to ensure that the ostomy stoma is conveniently placed–usually in the right lower quadrant about 2 inches below the waist, in an area away from previous scars, bony prominence, skin folds, or fistulas.

The patient must have a thorough understanding of the surgery to be performed and what to expect after surgery. Information about an ileostomy is presented to the patient by means of written materials, models, and discussion. Preoperative teaching includes management of drainage from the stoma, the nature of drainage, and the need for nasogastric intubation, parenteral fluids, and possibly perineal packing.

Providing Postoperative Care

General abdominal surgery wound care is required. The nurse observes the stoma for colour and size. It should be pink to bright red and shiny. For the traditional ileostomy, a temporary plastic bag with adhesive facing is placed over the ileostomy and firmly pressed onto surrounding skin. The nurse monitors the ileostomy for fecal drainage, which should begin about 72 hours after surgery. The drainage is a continuous liquid from the small intestine because the stoma does not have a controlling sphincter. The contents drain into the plastic bag and are thus kept from coming into contact with the skin. They are collected and measured when the bag becomes full. If a continent ileal reservoir was created, as described for the Kock pouch, continuous drainage is provided by an indwelling reservoir catheter for 2 to 3 weeks after surgery. This allows the suture lines to heal.

As with other patients undergoing abdominal surgery, the nurse encourages those with an ileostomy to engage in early ambulation. It is important to administer prescribed pain medications as required.

Because these patients lose much fluid in the early postoperative period, an accurate record of fluid intake, urinary output, and fecal discharge is necessary to help gauge the fluid needs of the patient. There may be 1000 to 2000 mL of fluid lost each day in addition to expected fluid loss through urine, perspiration, respiration, and other sources. With this loss, sodium and potassium are depleted. The nurse monitors laboratory values and administers electrolyte replacements as prescribed. Intravenous fluids are administered to replace fluid losses for 4 to 5 days.

Nasogastric suction is also a part of immediate postoperative care, with the tube requiring frequent irrigation, as prescribed. The purpose of nasogastric suction is to prevent a buildup of gastric contents. After the tube is removed, the nurse offers sips of clear liquids and gradually progresses the diet. It is important to immediately report nausea and abdominal distention, which may indicate obstruction.

By the end of the first week, rectal packing is removed. Because this procedure may be uncomfortable, the nurse may administer an analgesic an hour before it is performed. After the packing is removed, the perineum is irrigated two or three times daily until full healing takes place.

PROVIDING EMOTIONAL SUPPORT

The patient understandably may think that everyone is aware of the ileostomy and may view the stoma as a mutilation compared with other abdominal incisions that heal and are hidden. Because

(text continues on page 1055)

Plan of Nursing Care
The Patient Undergoing Ostomy Surgery

Nursing Interventions	Rationale	Expected Outcomes

Nursing Diagnosis: Deficient knowledge about the surgical procedure and preoperative preparation
Goal: Understands the surgical process and the necessary preoperative preparations

Preoperative Care

1. Ascertain whether the patient has had a previous surgical experience and ask for recollections of positive and negative impressions.

2. Determine what information the surgeon gave the patient and family and whether it was understood. Clarify and elaborate as necessary. Determine whether the stoma is permanent or temporary. Be aware of the patient's prognosis if carcinoma exists.

3. Use pictures or drawings to illustrate the location and appearance of the surgical wounds (abdominal, perineal) and the stoma if the patient is receptive.

4. Explain that oral/parenteral antimicrobials will be administered to cleanse the bowel preoperatively. Mechanical cleansing may also be required.

5. Assist the patient during nasogastric/nasoenteric intubation. Measure drainage from the tube.

1. Fear of a repeated negative experience increases anxiety. Talking about the experience with a nurse helps clarify misconceptions and helps the patient ventilate any repressed emotions. Positive experiences are reinforced.

2. Clarification prevents misunderstandings and alleviates anxiety. A positive affect may be more difficult to project if the ostomy is permanent or the prognosis poor.

3. Knowledge, for some, alleviates anxiety because fear of the unknown is decreased. Others choose not to know because it makes them more anxious.

4. Antimicrobials and mechanical cleansing reduce intestinal bacterial flora.

5. Nasoenteral intubation is used for decompression and drainage of gastrointestinal contents before surgery.

- Expresses anxieties and fears about the surgical process
- Projects a positive attitude toward the surgical procedure
- Repeats in own words information given by the surgeon
- Identifies normal anatomy and physiology of gastrointestinal tract and how it will be altered; can point to expected location of abdominal wound and stoma; describes stoma appearance and size
- Adheres to "bowel prep" regimen of antimicrobials or mechanical cleansing
- Tolerates the presence of nasogastric/nasoenteric tube

Nursing Diagnosis: Disturbed body image
Goal: Attainment of a positive self-concept

1. Encourage the patient to verbalize feelings about the stoma. Offer to be present when the stoma is first viewed and touched.

2. Suggest that the spouse or significant other view the stoma.

3. Offer counselling, if desired.

4. Arrange for a visit with an ostomate.

1. Free expression of feelings allows the patient the opportunity to verbalize and identify concerns. Expressed concerns can be therapeutically addressed by health care team members.

2. Helps patient to overcome fears about partner's response.

3. Provides opportunity for additional support.

4. Ostomates can offer support and share mutual feelings and experiences.

- Freely expresses concerns
- Accepts support
- Seeks help as needed
- States is willing to talk with an ostomate

Nursing Diagnosis: Anxiety related to the loss of bowel control
Goal: Reduction of anxiety

Postoperative Care

1. Provide information about expected bowel function:
   a. Characteristics of effluent
   b. Frequency of discharge

2. Teach the patient how to prepare the appliance for an adequate fit.

1. Emotional adjustment is facilitated if adequate information is provided at the level of the learner.

2. Adequate fit is necessary for successful use of the appliance.

- Expresses interest in learning about altered bowel function
- Handles equipment correctly
- Changes the appliance unassisted
- Irrigates colostomy successfully
- Progresses toward a regular schedule of elimination

(continued)

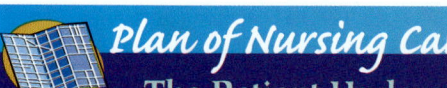

Plan of Nursing Care

The Patient Undergoing Ostomy Surgery (Continued)

Nursing Interventions	Rationale	Expected Outcomes
a. Choose the drainage appliance that will provide a secure fit around the stoma. Measure the stoma size with a measuring guide provided by the ostomy manufacturer and compare with the opening on the pouch. About 3-mm clearance should be provided around the stoma.	a. The appliance opening should be larger than the stoma for an adequate fit. Available brands come in different sizes to fit the stoma. Adjustments are made as necessary.	
b. Remove any plastic covering that protects the appliance adhesive. *Note:* The pouch is applied by pressing the adhesive for 30 s to the skin or skin barrier.	b. The appliance is ready to apply directly to the skin or skin protector.	
3. Demonstrate how to change the appliance before leakage occurs. Be aware that the elderly person may have diminished vision and difficulty handling equipment.	3. Manipulation of the appliance is a learned motor skill that requires practice and positive reinforcement.	
4. When appropriate, demonstrate how to irrigate the colostomy (usually on the 4th–5th day). Recommend that irrigation be performed at a consistent time, depending on the type of colostomy.	4. Colostomy irrigation is used to regulate the passage of fecal material; alternatively the bowel can be allowed to evacuate naturally.	

Nursing Diagnosis: Risk for impaired skin integrity related to irritation of the peristomal skin by the effluent
Goal: Maintenance of skin integrity

1. Provide information about signs and symptoms of irritated or inflamed skin. Use pictures if possible.	1. Peristomal skin should be slightly pink without abrasions and similar to that of the entire abdomen.	• Describes appearance of healthy skin
2. Teach patient how to cleanse the peristomal skin gently.	2. Mild friction with warm water and a gentle soap cleanses the skin and minimizes irritation and possible abrasions. Patting the skin dry prevents tissue trauma.	• Correctly cleanses the skin • Successfully applies a skin barrier • Gently removes the drainage appliance without skin damage • Demonstrates intact skin around the colostomy stoma
3. Demonstrate how to apply a skin barrier (powder, gel, paste, wafer).	3. Skin barriers protect the peristomal skin from enzymes and bacteria.	
4. Demonstrate how to remove the pouch.	4. Gently separate adhesive from the skin to avoid irritation. Never pull!	

Nursing Diagnosis: Potential imbalanced nutrition, less than body requirements, related to avoidance of foods that may cause GI discomfort
Goal: Achievement of an optimal nutritional intake

1. Conduct a complete nutritional assessment to identify any foods that may increase peristalsis by irritating the bowel.	1. Patients react differently to certain foods because of individual sensitivity.	• Modifies diet to avoid offensive foods yet maintains adequate nutritional intake
2. Advise the patient to avoid food products with a cellulose or hemicellulose base (nuts, seeds).	2. Cellulose food products are the nondigestible residue of plant foods. They hold water, provide bulk, and stimulate elimination.	• Avoids foods such as peanuts • Modifies intake of certain fruits
3. Recommend moderation in intake of certain irritating fruits such as prunes, grapes, and bananas.	3. These fruits tend to increase the quantity of effluent.	

(continued)

Plan of Nursing Care
The Patient Undergoing Ostomy Surgery (Continued)

Nursing Interventions	Rationale	Expected Outcomes
Nursing Diagnosis: Sexual dysfunction related to altered body image **Goal:** Attainment of satisfactory sexual performance		
1. Encourage the patient to verbalize concerns and fears. The sexual partner is welcomed to participate in the discussion.	1. Expressed needs help the therapist develop a plan of care.	• Expresses fears and concerns
2. Recommend alternative sexual positions.	2. Avoid patient embarrassment with the visual appearance of the stoma. Avoid peristomal skin irritation secondary to friction.	• Discusses alternative sexual positions
3. Seek assistance from a sexual therapist, enterostomal therapist, or advanced practice nurse.	3. Some patients need professional sexual counselling.	• Accepts services of a professional counselor
Nursing Diagnosis: Risk for deficient fluid volume related to anorexia and vomiting and increased loss of fluids and electrolytes from GI tract **Goal:** Attainment of fluid balance		
1. Estimate fluid intake and output: a. Strict intake and output b. Daily weights	1. Provides indication of fluid balance. a. An early indicator of fluid imbalance is a daily, significant difference between intake and output. The average person ingests (food, fluids) and loses (urine, feces, lungs) about 2 L of fluid every 24 h. b. A gain/loss of 1 L of fluid is reflected in a body weight change of 1 kg.	• Maintains fluid balance
2. Assess serum and urinary values of sodium and potassium.	2. Sodium is the major electrolyte regulating water balance. Vomiting results in decreased urinary and serum sodium levels. Urinary sodium values, in contrast to serum values, reflect early, sensitive changes in sodium balance. Sodium works in conjunction with potassium, which is also decreased with vomiting. A significant deficiency in potassium is associated with a decrease in intracellular potassium bicarbonate, which leads to acidosis and compensatory hyperventilation.	• Maintains normal serum and urinary values for sodium and potassium
3. Observe and record skin turgor and the appearance of the tongue.	3. Adequate hydration is reflected by the skin's ability to return to its normal shape after being grasped between the fingers. *Note:* In the older person, it is normal for the return to be delayed. Changes in the mucous membrane covering the tongue are accurate and early indicators of hydration status.	• Normal skin turgor • Surface of tongue is pink, with a moist mucous membrane

there is loss of a body part and a major change in anatomy, the patient often goes through the various phases of grieving—shock, disbelief, denial, rejection, anger, and restitution. Nursing support through these phases is important, and understanding of the patient's emotional outlook in each instance should determine the approach taken. For example, teaching may be ineffective until the patient is ready to learn. Concern about body image may

lead to questions related to family relationships, sexual function, and for women, the ability to become pregnant and to deliver a baby normally. Patients need to know that someone understands and cares about them. A calm, nonjudgmental attitude exhibited by the nurse aids in gaining the patient's confidence. It is important to recognize the dependency needs of these patients. Their prolonged illness can make them irritable, anxious, and depressed. The nurse can coordinate patient care through meetings attended by consultants such as the physician, psychologist, psychiatrist, social worker, enterostomal therapist, and dietitian. The team approach is important in facilitating the often complex care of this patient.

Conversely, a surgical procedure to create an ileostomy can produce dramatic positive changes in patients who have suffered from IBD for several years. After the continuous discomfort of the disease has decreased and patients learn how to take care of the ileostomy, they often develop a more positive outlook. Until they progress to this phase, an empathetic and tolerant approach by the nurse plays an important part in recovery. The sooner the patient masters the physical care of the ileostomy, the sooner he or she will psychologically accept it.

The support of other ostomates is also helpful. The United Ostomy Association is dedicated to the rehabilitation of ostomates. This organization gives patients useful information about living with an ostomy through an educational program of literature, lectures, and exhibits. Local associations offer visiting services by qualified members who provide hope and rehabilitation services to new ostomy patients. Hospitals and other health care agencies may have an enterostomal therapy nurse on staff who can serve as a valuable resource person for the ileostomy patient.

MANAGING SKIN AND STOMA CARE

The patient with a traditional ileostomy cannot establish regular bowel habits because the contents of the ileum are fluid and are discharged continuously. The patient must wear a pouch at all times. Stomal size and pouch size vary initially; the stoma should be rechecked 3 weeks after surgery, when the edema has subsided. The final size and type of appliance is selected in 3 months, after the patient's weight has stabilized, and the stoma shrinks to a stable shape.

The location and length of the stoma are significant in the management of the ileostomy by the patient. The surgeon positions the stoma as close to the midline as possible and at a location where even an obese patient with a protruding abdomen can care for it easily. Usually, the ileostomy stoma is about 2.5 cm long, which makes it convenient for the attachment of an appliance.

Skin excoriation around the stoma can be a persistent problem. Peristomal skin integrity may be compromised by several factors, such as an allergic reaction to the ostomy appliance, skin barrier, or paste; chemical irritation from the effluent; mechanical injury from the removal of the appliance; and possible infection. If irritation and yeast growth occur, nystatin powder (Mycostatin) is dusted lightly on the peristomal skin.

CHANGING AN APPLIANCE

A regular schedule for changing the pouch before leakage occurs must be established for those with a traditional ileostomy. The patient can be taught to change the pouch in a manner similar to that described in Chart 38-4.

The amount of time a person can keep the appliance sealed to the body surface depends on the location of the stoma and on body structure. The usual wearing time is 5 to 7 days. The appliance is emptied every 4 to 6 hours or at the same time the patient empties the bladder. An emptying spout at the bottom of the appliance is closed with a special clip made for this purpose.

Most pouches are disposable and odour-proof. Foods such as spinach and parsley act as deodourizers in the intestinal tract; foods that cause odours include cabbage, onions, and fish. Bismuth subcarbonate tablets, which may be prescribed and taken by mouth three or four times each day, are effective in reducing odour. A stool thickener, such as diphenoxylate (Lomotil), can also be prescribed and taken orally to assist in odour control.

IRRIGATING A CONTINENT ILEOSTOMY

For a continent ileostomy (ie, Kock pouch), the nurse teaches the patient to drain the pouch, as described in Chart 38-5. A catheter is inserted into the reservoir to drain the fluid. The length of time between drainage periods is gradually increased until the reservoir needs to be drained only every 4 to 6 hours and irrigated once each day. A pouch is not necessary; instead, most patients wear a small dressing over the opening.

When the fecal discharge is thick, water can be injected through the catheter to loosen and soften it. The consistency of the effluent is affected by food intake. At first, drainage is only 60 to 80 mL, but as time goes on, the amount increases significantly. The internal Kock pouch stretches, eventually accommodating 500 to 1000 mL. The patient learns to use the sensation of pressure in the pouch as a gauge to determine how often the pouch should be drained.

MANAGING DIETARY AND FLUID NEEDS

A low-residue diet is followed for the first 6 to 8 weeks. Strained fruits and vegetables are given. These foods are important sources of vitamins A and C. Later, there are few dietary restrictions, except for avoiding foods that are high in fibre or hard-to-digest kernels, such as celery, popcorn, corn, poppy seeds, caraway seeds, and coconut. Foods are reintroduced one at a time. The nurse assesses the patient's tolerance for these foods and reminds him or her to chew food thoroughly.

Fluids may be a problem during the summer, when fluid lost through perspiration adds to the fluid loss through the ileostomy. Fluids such as Gatorade are helpful in maintaining the electrolyte balance. If the fecal discharge is too watery, fibrous foods (eg, whole-grain cereals, fresh fruit skins, beans, corn, nuts) are restricted. If the effluent is excessively dry, salt intake is increased. Increased intake of water or fluid does not increase the effluent, because excess water is excreted in the urine.

PREVENTING COMPLICATIONS

Monitoring for complications is an ongoing activity for the patient with an ileostomy. Minor complications occur in about 40% of patients who have an ileostomy; less than 20% of the complications require surgical intervention (Kirsner & Shorter, 2000).

Common complications include skin irritation, diarrhea, stomal stenosis, urinary calculi, and cholelithiasis. Peristomal skin irritation, the most common complication of an ileostomy, results from leakage of effluent. A pouch that does not fit well is often the cause. The nurse or an enterostomal therapist adjusts the pouch and skin barriers are applied. Diarrhea, manifested by very irritating effluent that rapidly fills the pouch (every hour or sooner), can quickly lead to dehydration and electrolyte losses. Supplemental water, sodium, and potassium are administered to prevent hypovolemia and hypokalemia. Antidiarrheal agents are administered. Stenosis is caused by circular scar tissue that forms at the stoma site. The scar tissue must be surgically released. Urinary calculi occur in about 10% of ileostomy patients because of dehydration from decreased fluid intake. Intense lower abdominal pain that radiates to the legs, hematuria, and signs of dehydration indicate that the urine should be strained. Fluid intake is encouraged. Sometimes, small stones are passed during urination; otherwise, treatment is necessary to crush or remove the calculi (see Chap. 45).

Cholelithiasis (ie, gallstones) occurs three times more commonly in patients with an ileostomy than in the general population

Chart 38-4

GUIDELINES FOR Changing an Ostomy Appliance

Changing an ileostomy appliance is necessary to prevent leakage (the bag is usually changed every 5 to 7 days), to allow for examination of the skin around the stoma, and to assist in controlling odour if this becomes a problem. The appliance should be changed at any time that the patient complains of burning or itching under the disk or pain in the area of the stoma; routine changes should be performed early in the morning before breakfast or 2 to 4 hours after a meal, when the bowel is least active.

NURSING ACTION

1. Promote patient comfort and involvement in the procedure.
   a. Have the patient assume a relaxed position.
   b. Provide privacy.
   c. Explain details of the procedure.
   d. Expose the ileostomy area; remove the ileostomy belt (if worn).
2. Remove the appliance.
   a. Have the patient sit on the toilet or on a chair facing the toilet. A patient who prefers to stand should face the toilet.
   b. The appliance (pouch) can be removed by gently pushing the skin away from the adhesive.

RATIONALE

1. Providing a relaxed atmosphere and adequate explanations help the patient to become an active participant in the procedure.

2. These positions facilitate disposal or drainage.

Selected Ostomy Pouches and Accessories

One-piece drainable pouch

One-piece drainable pouch

One-piece nondrainable pouch

Two-piece drainable pouch

Wafer

Clip

Wire closure

Clamp

Narrow valve

Skin barriers

(continued)

Chart 38-4

GUIDELINES FOR Changing an Ostomy Appliance (Continued)

NURSING ACTION	RATIONALE

3. Cleanse the skin:
  a. Wash the skin gently with a soft cloth moistened with tepid water and mild soap; the patient may prefer to bathe before putting on a clean appliance.
  b. Rinse and dry the skin thoroughly after cleansing.
4. Apply appliance (when there is *no* skin irritation):
  a. An appropriate skin barrier is applied to the peristomal skin before the appliance is applied.
  b. Remove cover from adherent surface of disk of disposable plastic appliance and apply directly to the skin.
  c. Press firmly in place for 30 s to ensure adherence.
	3. The patient may shower with or without the pouch.
	  a. Micropore or waterproof tape applied to the sides of the face-plate will keep it secure during bathing.
	
	  b. Moisture or soap residue will interfere with appliance adhesion.
	4. Many appliances have a built-in skin barrier. The skin should be thoroughly dried before applying the appliance.

Pressing the appliance into place. Courtesy of Convatec, a Squibb Company.

5. Apply appliance (when there is skin irritation):
  a. Cleanse the skin thoroughly but gently; pat dry.
  b. Apply Kenalog spray; blot excess moisture with a cotton pledget and dust lightly with nystatin (Mycostatin) powder.
 	
 OR
  Apply as an alternative a wafer of Stomahesive (Squibb), which is commercially available. The stomal opening should be cut the same size as the stoma; use a cutting guide (supplied with Stomahesive). The wafer is applied directly to the skin.
  c. Another alternative is to moisten a karaya gum washer and apply when it is tacky. If the skin is moist, karaya powder may be applied first and any excess dusted off gently.
  d. The pouch is then applied to the treated skin.
6. Check the pouch bottom for closure; use the rubber band or clip provided.
	5.
	  a. To remove debris.
	  b. The corticosteroid preparation (Kenalog) helps to decrease inflammation. The antifungal agent (nystatin) treats those types of infections that are common around stomas. A prescription is required for either medication.
	
	  Stomahesive is a substance that facilitates healing of excoriated skin. It adheres well even to moist, irritated skin.
	
	  c. Karaya also facilitates skin healing. Tackiness promotes adherence.
	
	  d. This will allow skin to heal while the appliance is in place.
	6. Proper closure controls leakage.

because of changes in the absorption of bile acids that occur postoperatively. Spasm of the gallbladder causes severe upper right abdominal pain that can radiate to the back and right shoulder (see Chap. 40).

PROMOTING HOME AND COMMUNITY-BASED CARE

Teaching Patients Self-Care

The spouse and family should be familiar with the adjustment that will be necessary when the patient returns home. They need to know why it is necessary for the patient to occupy the bathroom for 10 minutes or more at certain times of the day and why certain equipment is needed. Their understanding is necessary to re-

duce tension; a relaxed patient tends to have fewer problems. Visits from an enterostomal therapy nurse may be arranged to ensure that the patient is progressing as expected and to provide additional guidance and teaching as needed.

The patient needs to know the commercial name of the pouch to be used so that he or she can obtain a ready supply and should have information about obtaining other supplies. The names and contact information of the local enterostomal therapy nurse and local self-help groups are often helpful. Any special restrictions on driving or working also need to be reviewed. The nurse teaches the patient about common postoperative complications and how to recognize and report them (Chart 38-6).

Chart 38-5
GUIDELINES FOR Draining a Continent Ileostomy (Kock Pouch)

A continent ileostomy is the surgical creation of a pouch of small intestine that can serve as an internal receptacle for fecal discharge; a nipple valve is constructed at the outlet. Postoperatively, a catheter extends from the stoma and is attached to a closed drainage suction system. To ensure patency of the catheter, usually every 3 hours 10 to 20 mL of normal saline is instilled gently into the pouch; return flow is not aspirated but is allowed to drain by gravity.

After approximately 2 weeks, when the healing process has progressed to the point at which the catheter is removed from the stoma, the patient is taught to drain the pouch. The equipment required includes a catheter, tissues, water-soluble lubricant, gauze squares, a syringe, irrigating solution in a bowl, and an emesis or receiving basin.

The following procedure is used to drain the pouch; the patient is helped to participate in this procedure to learn to perform it unassisted.

NURSING ACTION	RATIONALE
1. Lubricate the catheter and gently insert it about 5 cm, at which point some resistance may be felt at the valve or nipple.	1. When gentle pressure is used, the catheter usually will enter the pouch.
2. If there is much resistance, fill a syringe with 20 mL of air or water and inject it through the catheter, while still exerting some pressure on the catheter.	2. This will permit the catheter to enter the pouch.
3. Place the other end of the catheter in a drainage basin held below the level of the stoma. Later this process can be carried out at the toilet with drainage delivered into the toilet bowl.	3. Gravity facilitates drainage. Drainage may include flatus as well as effluent.
4. After drainage, the catheter is removed and the area around the stoma is gently washed with warm water. Pat dry and apply an absorbent pad over the stoma. Fasten the pad with hypoallergenic tape.	4. The entire procedure requires about 5 to 10 min; at first it is performed every 3 h. The time between procedures is gradually lengthened to three times daily.

Intestinal Obstruction

Intestinal obstruction exists when blockage prevents the normal flow of intestinal contents through the intestinal tract. Two types of processes can impede this flow.

- *Mechanical obstruction:* An intraluminal obstruction or a mural obstruction from pressure on the intestinal walls occurs. Examples are intussusception, polypoid tumours and neoplasms, stenosis, strictures, adhesions, hernias, and abscesses, diverticulitis, and gallstones.
- *Functional obstruction:* The intestinal musculature cannot propel the contents along the bowel. Examples are amyloidosis, muscular dystrophy, electrolyte imbalance (hypokalemia), myocardial infarction, endocrine disorders such as diabetes mellitus, or neurologic disorders such as Parkinson's disease.

The blockage also can be temporary and the result of the manipulation of the bowel during surgery (paralytic ileus).

The obstruction can be partial or complete. Its severity depends on the region of bowel affected, the degree to which the lumen is occluded, and especially the degree to which the vascular supply to the bowel wall is disturbed.

Most bowel obstructions occur in the small intestine. Adhesions are the most common cause of small bowel obstruction, followed by hernias and neoplasms. Other causes include intussusception, volvulus (ie, twisting of the bowel), and paralytic ileus. About 15% of intestinal obstructions occur in the large bowel; most of these are found in the sigmoid colon (Wolfe, 2000). The most common causes are carcinoma, diverticulitis, inflammatory bowel disorders, and benign tumours. Table 38-5 and Figure 38-6 list mechanical causes of obstruction and describe how they occur.

Chart 38-6
Home Care Checklist • Managing Ostomy Care

At the completion of the home care instruction, the patient or caregiver will be able to:	Patient	Caregiver
• Demonstrate ostomy care, including wound cleansing, irrigation, and appliance changing.	✓	✓
• Describe the importance of maintaining peristomal skin integrity.	✓	✓
• Identify sources for obtaining additional dressing and appliance supplies.	✓	✓
• Identify dietary restrictions (foods that can cause diarrhea and constipation).	✓	✓
• Identify measures to be used to promote fluid and electrolyte balance	✓	✓
• Describe medication regimen: identify medications by name, use, route, and frequency.	✓	✓
• Describe potential complications and necessary actions to be taken if complications occur.	✓	✓
• Identify how to contact enterostomal therapist or home health nurse.	✓	✓

Table 38-5 • **Mechanical Causes of Intestinal Obstruction**

CAUSE	COURSE OF EVENTS	RESULT
Adhesions	Loops of intestine become adherent to areas that heal slowly or scar after abdominal surgery.	After surgery, adhesions produce a kinking of an intestinal loop.
Intussusception	One part of the intestine slips into another part located below it (like a telescope shortening).	The intestinal lumen becomes narrowed.
Volvulus	Bowel twists and turns on itself.	Intestinal lumen becomes obstructed. Gas and fluid accumulate in the trapped bowel.
Hernia	Protrusion of intestine through a weakened area in the abdominal muscle or wall.	Intestinal flow may be completely obstructed. Blood flow to the area may be obstructed as well.
Tumour	A tumour that exists within the wall of the intestine extends into the intestinal lumen, or a tumour outside the intestine causes pressure on the wall of the intestine.	Intestinal lumen becomes partially obstructed; if the tumour is not removed, complete obstruction results.

SMALL BOWEL OBSTRUCTION

Pathophysiology

Intestinal contents, fluid, and gas accumulate above the intestinal obstruction. The abdominal distention and retention of fluid reduce the absorption of fluids and stimulate more gastric secretion. With increasing distention, pressure within the intestinal lumen increases, causing a decrease in venous and arteriolar capillary pressure. This causes edema, congestion, necrosis, and eventual rupture or perforation of the intestinal wall, with resultant peritonitis.

Reflux vomiting may be caused by abdominal distention. Vomiting results in a loss of hydrogen ions and potassium from the stomach, leading to a reduction of chlorides and potassium in the blood and to metabolic alkalosis. Dehydration and acidosis develop from loss of water and sodium. With acute fluid losses, hypovolemic shock may occur.

Clinical Manifestations

The initial symptom is usually crampy pain that is wavelike and colicky. The patient may pass blood and mucus, but no fecal matter and no flatus. Vomiting occurs. If the obstruction is complete, the peristaltic waves initially become extremely vigourous and eventually assume a reverse direction, with the intestinal contents propelled toward the mouth instead of toward the rectum. If the

Small intestine
Peritoneum
Hernial sac
Testicle

FIGURE 38-6 Three causes of intestinal obstruction. (**A**) Intussusception invagination or shortening of the colon caused by the movement of one segment of bowel into another. (**B**) Volvulus of the sigmoid colon; the twist is counterclockwise in most cases. Note the edematous bowel. (**C**) Hernia (inguinal). The sac of the hernia is a continuation of the peritoneum of the abdomen. The hernial contents are intestine, omentum, or other abdominal contents that pass through the hernial opening into the hernial sac.

obstruction is in the ileum, fecal vomiting takes place. First, the patient vomits the stomach contents, then the bile-stained contents of the duodenum and the jejunum, and finally, with each paroxysm of pain, the darker, fecal-like contents of the ileum. The unmistakable signs of dehydration become evident: intense thirst, drowsiness, generalized malaise, aching, and a parched tongue and mucous membranes. The abdomen becomes distended. The lower the obstruction is in the GI tract, the more marked the abdominal distention. If the obstruction continues uncorrected, hypovolemic shock occurs from dehydration and loss of plasma volume.

Assessment and Diagnostic Findings

Diagnosis is based on the symptoms described previously and on x-ray findings. Abdominal x-ray studies show abnormal quantities of gas, fluid, or both in the bowel. Laboratory studies (ie, electrolyte studies and a complete blood cell count) reveal a picture of dehydration, loss of plasma volume, and possible infection.

Medical Management

Decompression of the bowel through a nasogastric or small bowel tube (see Chap. 36) is successful in most cases. When the bowel is completely obstructed, the possibility of strangulation warrants surgical intervention. Before surgery, intravenous therapy is necessary to replace the depleted water, sodium, chloride, and potassium.

The surgical treatment of intestinal obstruction depends largely on the cause of the obstruction. In the most common causes of obstruction, such as hernia and adhesions, the surgical procedure involves repairing the hernia or dividing the adhesion to which the intestine is attached. In some instances, the portion of affected bowel may be removed and an anastomosis performed. The complexity of the surgical procedure for intestinal obstruction depends on the duration of the obstruction and the condition of the intestine.

Nursing Management

Nursing management of the nonsurgical patient with a small bowel obstruction includes maintaining the function of the nasogastric tube, assessing and measuring the nasogastric output, assessing for fluid and electrolyte imbalance, monitoring nutritional status, and assessing improvement (eg, return of normal bowel sounds, decreased abdominal distention, subjective improvement in abdominal pain and tenderness, passage of flatus or stool). The nurse reports discrepancies in intake and output, worsening of pain or abdominal distention, and increased nasogastric output. If the patient's condition does not improve, the nurse prepares him or her for surgery. The exact nature of the surgery depends on the cause of the obstruction. Nursing care of the patient after surgical repair of a small bowel obstruction is similar to that for other abdominal surgeries (see Chap. 20).

LARGE BOWEL OBSTRUCTION

Pathophysiology

As in small bowel obstruction, large bowel obstruction results in an accumulation of intestinal contents, fluid, and gas proximal to the obstruction. Obstruction in the large bowel can lead to severe distention and perforation unless some gas and fluid can flow back through the ileal valve. Large bowel obstruction, even if complete, may be undramatic if the blood supply to the colon is not disturbed. If the blood supply is cut off, however, intestinal strangulation and necrosis (ie, tissue death) occur; this condition is life threatening. In

the large intestine, dehydration occurs more slowly than in the small intestine because the colon can absorb its fluid contents and can distend to a size considerably beyond its normal full capacity.

Clinical Manifestations

Large bowel obstruction differs clinically from small bowel obstruction in that the symptoms develop and progress relatively slowly. In patients with obstruction in the sigmoid colon or the rectum, constipation may be the only symptom for days. Eventually, the abdomen becomes markedly distended, loops of large bowel become visibly outlined through the abdominal wall, and the patient has crampy lower abdominal pain. Finally, fecal vomiting develops. Symptoms of shock may occur.

Assessment and Diagnostic Findings

Diagnosis is based on symptoms and on x-ray studies. Abdominal x-ray studies (flat and upright) show a distended colon. Barium studies are contraindicated.

Medical Management

A colonoscopy may be performed to untwist and decompress the bowel. A cecostomy, in which a surgical opening is made into the cecum, may be performed for patients who are poor surgical risks and urgently need relief from the obstruction. The procedure provides an outlet for releasing gas and a small amount of drainage. A rectal tube may be used to decompress an area that is lower in the bowel. The usual treatment, however, is surgical resection to remove the obstructing lesion. A temporary or permanent colostomy may be necessary. An ileoanal anastomosis may be performed if it is necessary to remove the entire large colon.

Nursing Management

The nurse's role is to monitor the patient for symptoms that indicate that the intestinal obstruction is worsening and to provide emotional support and comfort. The nurse administers intravenous fluids and electrolytes as prescribed. The nurse performs assessments related to vital sign monitoring, signs of potential shock, pain evaluation, fluid input/output, and effectiveness of the nasogastric tube. The nurse also can provide comfort measures, such as having the patient elevate the head to relieve some of the discomfort associated with abdominal pressure (McConnell, 2001). If the patient's condition does not respond to nonsurgical treatment, the nurse prepares the patient for surgery. This preparation includes preoperative teaching as the patient's condition indicates. After surgery, general abdominal wound care and routine postoperative nursing care are provided.

COLORECTAL CANCER

Tumours of the colon and rectum are relatively common; the colorectal area (the colon and rectum combined) is now the third most common site of new cancer cases and deaths in Canada. There are approximately 17,600 new cases reported yearly, two thirds of which are in the large intestine and one third in the rectum (Canadian Cancer Society, 2005).

The incidence increases with age (the incidence is highest for people older than 85 years of age) and is higher for people with a family history of colon cancer and those with IBD or polyps. The exact cause of colon and rectal cancer is still unknown, but risk factors have been identified (Chart 38-7).

Chart 38-7
Risk Factors for Colorectal Cancer

Increasing age
Family history of colon cancer or polyps
Previous colon cancer or adenomatous polyps
History of inflammatory bowel disease
High-fat, high-protein (with high intake of beef), low-fibre diet
Genital cancer or breast cancer (in women)
Lifestyle habits (tobacco, alcohol)

The distribution of cancer sites throughout the colon is shown in Figure 38-7 (Goldman, & Bennett, 2000). Changes in this distribution have occurred in recent years. The incidence of cancer in the sigmoid and rectal areas has decreased, whereas the incidence of cancer in the cecum, ascending, and descending colon has increased.

Improved screening strategies have helped to reduce the number of deaths in recent years. Of the more than 148,000 people diagnosed each year, fewer than half that number die annually (Beyers et al., 2001). Early diagnosis and prompt treatment could save almost three of every four people with colorectal cancer. If the disease is detected and treated at an early stage, the 5-year survival rate is 90%, but only 34% of colorectal cancers are found at an early stage. Survival rates after late diagnosis are very low. Most people are asymptomatic for long periods and seek health care only when they notice a change in bowel habits or rectal bleeding. Prevention and early screening are key to detection and reduction of mortality rates.

Pathophysiology

Cancer of the colon and rectum is predominantly (95%) adenocarcinoma (ie, arising from the epithelial lining of the intestine). It may start as a benign polyp but may become malignant, invade and destroy normal tissues, and extend into surrounding structures. Cancer cells may break away from the primary tumour and spread to other parts of the body (most often to the liver).

Clinical Manifestations

The symptoms are greatly determined by the location of the cancer, the stage of the disease, and the function of the intestinal segment in which it is located. The most common presenting symptom is a change in bowel habits. The passage of blood in the stools is the second most common symptom. Symptoms may also include unexplained anemia, anorexia, weight loss, and fatigue.

The symptoms most commonly associated with right-sided lesions are dull abdominal pain and melena (ie, black, tarry stools). The symptoms most commonly associated with left-sided lesions are those associated with obstruction (ie, abdominal pain and cramping, narrowing stools, constipation, and distention), as well as bright red blood in the stool. Symptoms associated with rectal lesions are tenesmus (ie, ineffective, painful straining at stool), rectal pain, the feeling of incomplete evacuation after a bowel movement, alternating constipation and diarrhea, and bloody stool.

Assessment and Diagnostic Findings

Along with an abdominal and rectal examination, the most important diagnostic procedures for cancer of the colon are fecal occult blood testing, barium enema, proctosigmoidoscopy, and colonoscopy (see Chap. 34). As many as 60% of colorectal cancer cases can be identified by sigmoidoscopy with biopsy or cytology smears (Yamada et al., 1999).

Carcinoembryonic antigen (CEA) studies may also be performed. Although CEA may not be a highly reliable indicator in diagnosing colon cancer because not all lesions secrete CEA, studies show that CEA levels are reliable in predicting prognosis. With complete excision of the tumour, the elevated levels of CEA should return to normal within 48 hours. Elevations of CEA at a later date suggest recurrence (Yamada et al., 1999).

Complications

Tumour growth may cause partial or complete bowel obstruction. Extension of the tumour and ulceration into the surrounding blood vessels results in hemorrhage. Perforation, abscess formation, peritonitis, sepsis, and shock may occur.

 Gerontologic Considerations

The incidence of carcinoma of the colon and rectum increases with age. These cancers are considered common malignancies in advanced age. Only prostate cancer and lung cancer in men exceed colorectal cancer. Among women, only breast cancer exceeds the incidence of colorectal cancer (Lueckenotte, 2000). Symptoms are often insidious. Cancer patients usually report fatigue, which is caused primarily by iron-deficiency anemia. In early stages, minor changes in bowel patterns and occasional bleeding may occur. The later symptoms most commonly reported by the elderly are abdominal pain, obstruction, tenesmus, and rectal bleeding.

Colon cancer in the elderly has been closely associated with dietary carcinogens. Lack of fibre is a major causative factor because the passage of feces through the intestinal tract is prolonged, which extends exposure to possible carcinogens. Excess fat is believed to alter bacterial flora and convert steroids into compounds that have carcinogenic properties.

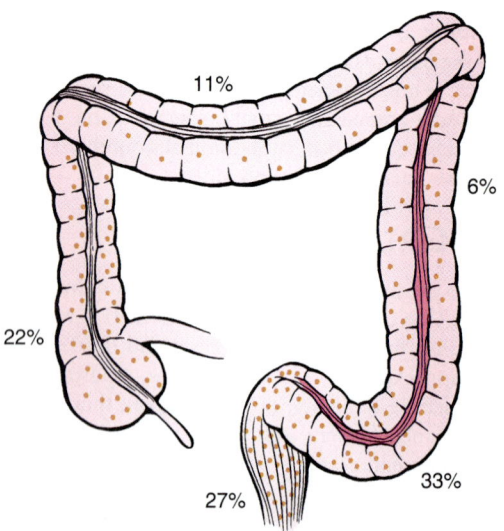

11%

6%

22%

27%

33%

FIGURE 38-7 Percentage distribution of cancer sites in the colon and rectum.

Medical Management

The patient with symptoms of intestinal obstruction is treated with intravenous fluids and nasogastric suction. If there has been significant bleeding, blood component therapy may be required.

Treatment for colorectal cancer depends on the stage of the disease (Chart 38-8) and consists of surgery to remove the tumour, supportive therapy, and adjuvant therapy. Data demonstrate delays in tumour recurrence and increases in survival time for patients who receive some form of adjuvant therapy—chemotherapy, radiation therapy, immunotherapy, or multimodality therapy.

ADJUVANT THERAPY

The standard adjuvant therapy administered to patients with Dukes' class C colon cancer is the 5-fluorouracil plus levamisole regimen (Wolfe, 2000). Patients with Dukes' class B or C rectal cancer are given 5-fluorouracil and high doses of pelvic irradiation. Mitomycin is also used. Radiation therapy is used before, during, and after surgery to shrink the tumour, to achieve better results from surgery, and to reduce the risk of recurrence. For inoperative or unresectable tumours, irradiation is used to provide significant relief from symptoms. Intracavity and implantable devices are used to deliver radiation to the site. The response to adjuvant therapy varies.

SURGICAL MANAGEMENT

Surgery is the primary treatment for most colon and rectal cancers. It may be curative or palliative. Advances in surgical techniques can enable the patient with cancer to have sphincter-saving devices that restore continuity of the GI tract (Tierney et al., 2000). The type of surgery recommended depends on the location and size of the tumour. Cancers limited to one site can be removed through the colonoscope. Laparoscopic colotomy with polypectomy minimizes the extent of surgery needed in some cases. A laparoscope is used as a guide in making an incision into the colon; the tumour mass is then excised. Use of the neodymium/yttrium-aluminum-garnet (Nd:YAG) laser has proved effective with some lesions as well. Bowel resection is indicated for most class A lesions and all class B and C lesions. Surgery is sometimes recommended for class D colon cancer, but the goal of surgery in this instance is

palliative; if the tumour has spread and involves surrounding vital structures, it is considered nonresectable.

Surgical procedures include the following:

- Segmental resection with anastomosis (ie, removal of the tumour and portions of the bowel on either side of the growth, as well as the blood vessels and lymphatic nodes) (Fig. 38-8).
- Abdominoperineal resection with permanent sigmoid colostomy (ie, removal of the tumour and a portion of the sigmoid and all of the rectum and anal sphincter) (Fig. 38-9).
- Temporary colostomy followed by segmental resection and anastomosis and subsequent reanastomosis of the colostomy, allowing initial bowel decompression and bowel preparation before resection
- Permanent colostomy or ileostomy for palliation of unresectable obstructing lesions
- Construction of a coloanal reservoir called a colonic J pouch is performed in two steps. A temporary loop ileostomy is constructed to divert intestinal flow, and the newly constructed J pouch (made from 6 to 10 cm of colon) is reattached to the anal stump. About 3 months after the initial stage, the ileostomy is reversed, and intestinal continuity is restored. The anal sphincter and therefore continence are preserved.

A **colostomy** is the surgical creation of an opening (ie, stoma) into the colon. It can be created as a temporary or permanent fecal diversion. It allows the drainage or evacuation of colon contents to the outside of the body. The consistency of the drainage is related to the placement of the colostomy, which is dictated by the location of the tumour and the extent of invasion into surrounding tissues (Fig. 38-10). With improved surgical techniques, colostomies are performed on fewer than one third of patients with colorectal cancer.

 Gerontologic Considerations

The elderly are at increased risk for complications after surgery and may have difficulty managing colostomy care. They may have decreased vision, impaired hearing, and difficulty with fine motor coordination. It may be helpful for the patient to handle ostomy equipment and simulate cleaning the peristomal skin and irrigating the stoma before surgery. Skin care is a major concern in the elderly ostomate because of the skin changes that occur with aging—the epithelial and subcutaneous fatty layers become thin, and the skin is irritated easily. To prevent skin breakdown, special attention is paid to skin cleansing and the proper fit of an appliance. Arteriosclerosis causes decreased blood flow to the wound and stoma site. As a result, transport of nutrients is delayed, and healing time may be prolonged. Some patients have delayed elimination after irrigation because of decreased peristalsis and mucus production. Most patients require 6 months before they feel comfortable with their ostomy care.

NURSING PROCESS:
THE PATIENT WITH COLORECTAL CANCER

Assessment

The nurse completes a health history to obtain information about fatigue, abdominal or rectal pain (eg, location, frequency, duration, association with eating or defecation), past and present elimination patterns, and characteristics of stool (eg, colour, odour,

---

Chart 38-8	**Staging of Colorectal Cancer: Dukes' Classification–Modified Staging System**

Class A: Tumour limited to muscular mucosa and submucosa
Class B₁: Tumour extends into mucosa
Class B₂: Tumour extends through entire bowel wall into serosa or pericolic fat, no nodal involvement
Class C₁: Positive nodes, tumour is limited to bowel wall
Class C₂: Positive nodes, tumour extends through entire bowel wall
Class D: Advanced and metastasis to liver, lung, or bone

Another staging system, the TNM (tumour, nodal involvement, metastasis) classification, may be used to describe the anatomic extent of the primary tumour, depending on

- Size, invasion depth and surface spread
- Extent of nodal involvement
- Presence or absence of metastasis

Rudy, D. R., & Zdon, M. J. (2000). Update on colorectal cancer. *American Family Physician, 61* (6), 1759–1770, 1773–1774.

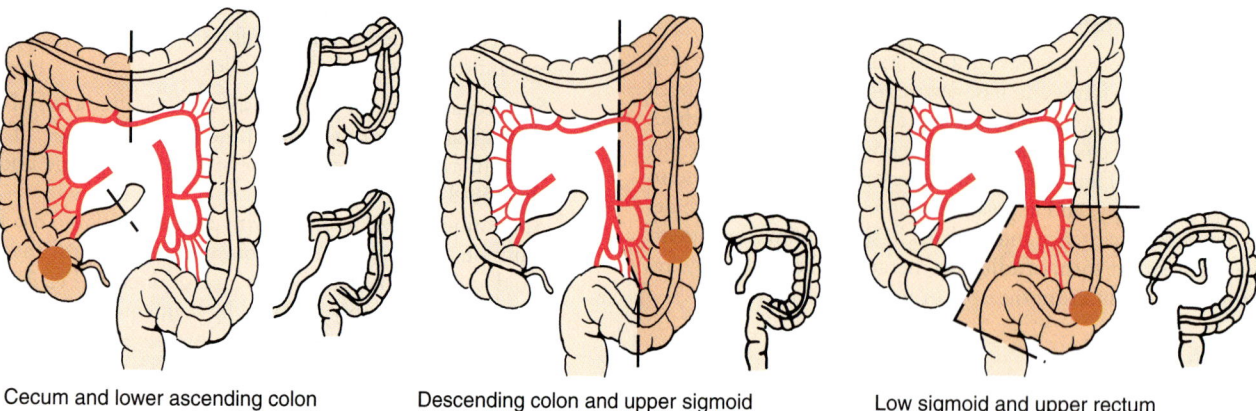

Cecum and lower ascending colon

Descending colon and upper sigmoid

Low sigmoid and upper rectum

Rectal sigmoid resection

FIGURE 38-8 Examples of areas where cancer can occur, the area that is removed, and how the anastomosis is performed (*small diagrams*).

consistency, presence of blood or mucus). Additional information includes a history of IBD or colorectal polyps, a family history of colorectal disease, and current medication therapy. The nurse identifies dietary habits, including fat and fibre intake, as well as amounts of alcohol consumed. The nurse describes and documents a history of weight loss.

Assessment includes auscultating the abdomen for bowel sounds and palpating the abdomen for areas of tenderness, distention, and solid masses. Stool specimens are inspected for character and presence of blood.

Diagnosis

NURSING DIAGNOSES

Based on the assessment data, the major nursing diagnoses may include the following:

- Imbalanced nutrition, less than body requirements, related to nausea and anorexia
- Risk for deficient fluid volume related to vomiting and dehydration
- Anxiety related to impending surgery and the diagnosis of cancer
- Risk for ineffective therapeutic regimen management related to knowledge deficit concerning the diagnosis, the surgical procedure, and self-care after discharge
- Impaired skin integrity related to the surgical incisions (abdominal and perianal), the formation of a stoma, and frequent fecal contamination of peristomal skin
- Disturbed body image related to colostomy

- Ineffective sexuality patterns related to presence of ostomy and changes in body image and self-concept

COLLABORATIVE PROBLEMS/ POTENTIAL COMPLICATIONS

Potential complications that may develop include the following:

- Intraperitoneal infection
- Complete large bowel obstruction
- GI bleeding
- Bowel perforation
- Peritonitis, abscess, and sepsis

Planning and Goals

The major goals for the patient may include attainment of optimal level of nutrition; maintenance of fluid and electrolyte balance; reduction of anxiety; learning about the diagnosis, surgical procedure, and self-care after discharge; maintenance of optimal tissue healing; protection of peristomal skin; learning how to irrigate the colostomy and change the appliance; expressing feelings and concerns about the colostomy and the impact on himself or herself; and avoidance of complications.

PREPARING THE PATIENT FOR SURGERY

The patient anticipating surgery for colorectal cancer has many concerns, needs, and fears. He or she may be physically debilitated and emotionally distraught with concern about lifestyle changes after surgery, prognosis, ability to perform in established roles, and finances. Priorities for nursing care include preparing

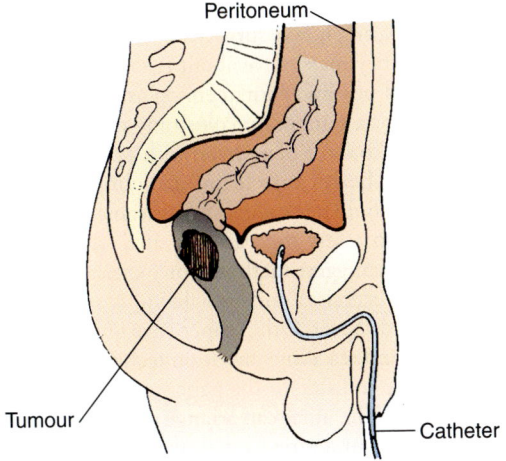

1. Prior to surgery. Note tumour in rectum.

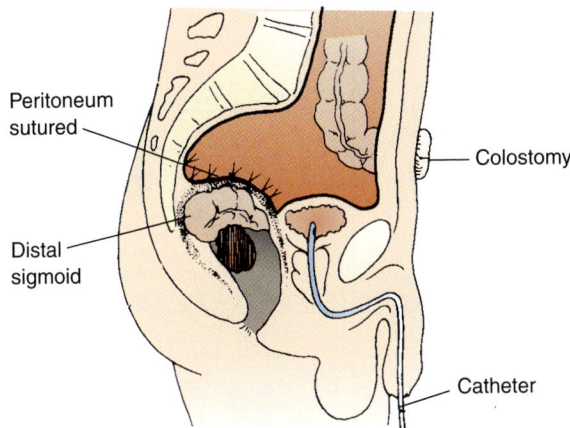

2. During surgery, the sigmoid is removed and colostomy established. The distal bowel has been dissected free to a point below the pelvic peritoneum, which is sutured over the closed end of the distal sigmoid and rectum.

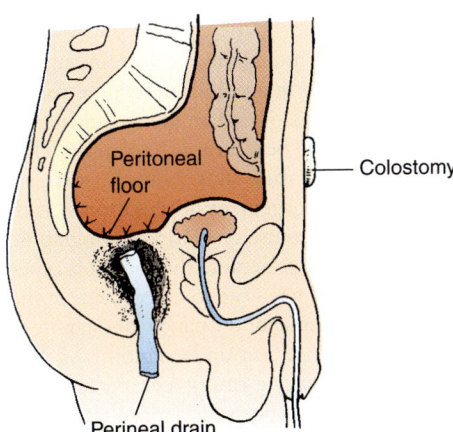

3. Perineal resection includes removal of the rectum and free portion of the sigmoid from below. A perineal drain is inserted.

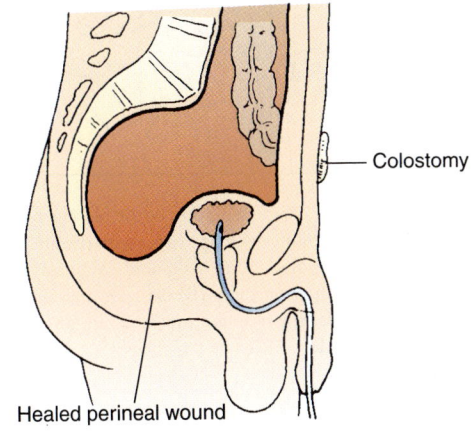

4. The final result after healing. Note healed perineal wound and the permanent colostomy.

FIGURE 38-9 Abdominoperineal resection for carcinoma of the rectum.

the patient physically for surgery, providing information about postoperative care, including stoma care if a colostomy is to be created, and supporting the patient and family emotionally.

Physical preparation for surgery involves building the patient's stamina in the days preceding surgery and cleansing and sterilizing the bowel the day before surgery. If the patient's condition permits, the nurse recommends a diet high in calories, protein, and carbohydrates and low in residue for several days before surgery to provide adequate nutrition and minimize cramping by decreasing excessive peristalsis. A full-liquid diet may be prescribed 24 to 48 hours before surgery to decrease bulk. If the patient is hospitalized in the days preceding surgery, PN may be required to replace depleted nutrients, vitamins, and minerals. In some instances, PN may be given at home before surgery. Antibiotics such as sulfonamides, neomycin, and cephalexin are administered the day before surgery to reduce intestinal bacteria. The bowel is cleansed with laxatives, enemas, or colonic irrigations the evening before and the morning of surgery.

For the patient who is very ill and hospitalized, the nurse measures and records intake and output, including vomitus, to provide an accurate record of fluid balance. The patient's intake of oral food and fluids may be restricted to prevent vomiting. The

nurse administers antiemetics as prescribed. Full or clear liquids may be tolerated, or the patient may be allowed nothing by mouth. A nasogastric tube may be inserted to drain accumulated fluids and prevent abdominal distention. The nurse monitors the abdomen for increasing distention, loss of bowel sounds, and pain or rigidity, which may indicate obstruction or perforation. It also is important to monitor intravenous fluids and electrolytes. Monitoring serum electrolyte levels can detect the hypokalemia and hyponatremia that occur with GI fluid loss. The nurse observes for signs of hypovolemia (eg, tachycardia, hypotension, decreased pulse volume), assesses hydration status, and reports decreased skin turgor, dry mucous membranes, and concentrated urine.

The nurse assesses the patient's knowledge about the diagnosis, prognosis, surgical procedure, and expected level of functioning after surgery. It is important to include information about the physical preparation for surgery, the expected appearance and care of the wound, the technique of ostomy care (if applicable), dietary restrictions, pain control, and medication management in the teaching plan (see Plan of Nursing Care 38-1). If the patient will be admitted the day of surgery, the physician's office may arrange for the patient to be seen by an enterostomal therapist in the days preceding surgery. The ther-

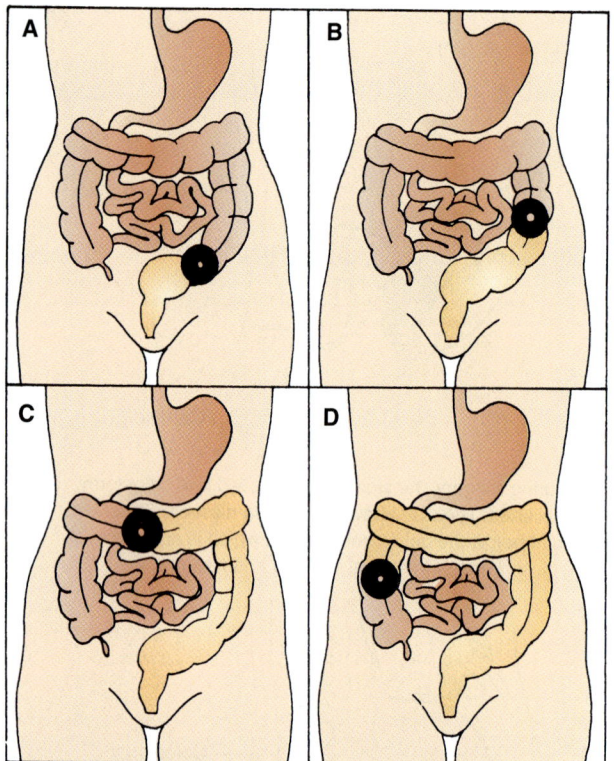

FIGURE 38-10 A diagrammatic representation of the placement of permanent colostomies. The nature of the discharge varies with the site. Shaded areas show sections of bowel removed. With a sigmoid colostomy (**A**) the feces are solid. With a descending colostomy (**B**) the feces are semimushy. With a transverse colostomy (**C**) the feces are mushy. With an ascending colostomy (**D**) the feces are fluid.

apist helps determine the optimal site for the stoma and provides teaching about care. If the patient is hospitalized before the day of surgery, the staff enterostomal therapist is involved in the preoperative teaching. All procedures are explained in language the patient understands.

PROVIDING EMOTIONAL SUPPORT

Patients anticipating bowel surgery for colorectal cancer may be very anxious. They may grieve about the diagnosis, the impending surgery, and possible permanent colostomy. Patients undergoing surgery for a temporary colostomy may express fears and concerns similar to those of a person with a permanent stoma. All members of the health care team, including the enterostomal therapy nurse, should be available for assistance and support. The nurse's role is to assess the patient's anxiety level and coping mechanisms and suggest methods for reducing anxiety such as deep-breathing exercises and visualizing a successful recovery from surgery and cancer. Other supportive measures include providing privacy and teaching relaxation techniques to the patient. Time is set aside to listen to the patient who wishes to talk, cry, or ask questions. The nurse can arrange a meeting with a spiritual advisor if the patient desires or with the physicians if the patient wishes to discuss the treatment or prognosis. To promote patient comfort, the nurse projects a relaxed, professional, and empathetic attitude. See Nursing Research Profile 38-1 about the importance of spiritual well-being for patients with colorectal cancer.

The patient undergoing a colostomy may find the anticipated changes in body image and lifestyle profoundly disturbing. Because the stoma is located on the abdomen, the patient may think that everyone will be aware of the ostomy. The nurse helps reduce this fear by presenting facts about the surgical procedure and the creation and management of the ostomy. If the patient is receptive, the nurse can use diagrams, photographs, and appliances to explain and clarify. Because the patient is experiencing emotional stress, the nurse may need to repeat some of the information. The nurse provides time for the patient and family to ask questions; the nurse's acceptance and understanding of the patient's concerns and feelings convey a caring, competent attitude that promotes confidence and cooperation. Consultation with an enterostomal therapist during the preoperative period can be extremely helpful, as can speaking with a person who is successfully managing a colostomy. The United Ostomy Association provides useful information about living with an ostomy through literature, lectures, and exhibits. Visiting services by qualified members and rehabilitation services for new ostomy patients are provided.

NURSING RESEARCH PROFILE 38-1

Spiritual Needs of Patients with Colorectal Cancer

Fernsler, J., Klemm, P., & Miller, M. (1999). Spiritual well-being and demands of illness in people with colorectal cancer. *Cancer Nursing, 22*(2), 134–140.

Purpose
Patients with colorectal cancer must be assisted in coping with the demands of the illness and its treatment. Using the Demands of Illness Inventory (DOI) and the Spiritual Well-Being Scale (SWBS), the authors of this descriptive study looked closely at the events that individuals experience in response to a cancer diagnosis and attempted to determine whether those events relate to spiritual well-being. The purpose of the study was to identify the demands of the illness and determine their relationship to spiritual well-being.

Study Sample and Findings
The sample for this study consisted of 121 respondents to questionnaires who were at least 21 years old and had been treated for colon, rectal, or anal cancer. Two thirds of the respondents reported a Christian affiliation. Results showed that the illness exerted the greatest demands (highest DOI scores) on those in the youngest age group

(21–45 years) and on those with terminal illness. These respondents also reported lower levels of spiritual well-being.

Subjects who reported significantly lower ($p < .05$) DOI levels related to their physical symptoms, monitoring symptoms, and treatment issues also reported higher levels of spiritual well-being.

Nursing Implications
Nurses who care for cancer patients must be aware of the intense illness-related demands placed on their patients, especially on those in the younger age range and those with a terminal diagnosis. Nurses should explore interventions to assist patients in coping with these demands, especially interventions to enhance the patients' spiritual resources.

This study had several limitations. All responses were self-reported, and measures were taken at only one point in time. Other studies need to be conducted to determine whether the findings can be generalized.

PROVIDING POSTOPERATIVE CARE

Postoperative nursing care for patients undergoing colon resection or colostomy is similar to nursing care for any abdominal surgery patient (see Chap. 20), including pain management during the immediate postoperative period. The nurse also monitors the patient for complications such as leakage from the site of the anastomosis, prolapse of the stoma, perforation, stoma retraction, fecal impaction, skin irritation, and pulmonary complications associated with abdominal surgery. The nurse assesses the abdomen for returning peristalsis and assesses the initial stool characteristics. It is important to help patients with a colostomy out of bed on the first postoperative day and encourage them to begin participating in managing the colostomy.

MAINTAINING OPTIMAL NUTRITION

The nurse teaches all patients undergoing surgery for colorectal cancer about the health benefits to be derived from consuming a healthy diet. The diet is individualized as long as it is well balanced and does not cause diarrhea or constipation. The return to normal diet is rapid.

A complete nutritional assessment is important for patients with a colostomy. The patient avoids foods that cause excessive odour and gas, including foods in the cabbage family, eggs, fish, beans, and high-cellulose products such as peanuts. It is important to determine whether the elimination of specific foods is causing any nutritional deficiency. Nonirritating foods are substituted for those that are restricted so that deficiencies are corrected. The nurse advises the patient to experiment with an irritating food several times before restricting it, because an initial sensitivity may decrease with time. The nurse can help the patient identify any foods or fluids that may be causing diarrhea, such as fruits, high-fibre foods, soda, coffee, tea, or carbonated beverages. Paregoric, bismuth subgallate, bismuth subcarbonate, or diphenoxylate with atropine (Lomotil) help control the diarrhea. For constipation, prune or apple juice or a mild laxative is effective. The nurse suggests fluid intake of at least 2 L of fluid per day.

PROVIDING WOUND CARE

The nurse frequently examines the abdominal dressing during the first 24 hours after surgery to detect signs of hemorrhage. It is important to help the patient splint the abdominal incision during coughing and deep breathing to lessen tension on the edges of the incision. The nurse monitors temperature, pulse, and respiratory rate for elevations, which may indicate an infectious process. If the patient has a colostomy, the stoma is examined for swelling (slight edema from surgical manipulation is normal), colour (a healthy stoma is pink or red), discharge (a small amount of oozing is normal), and bleeding (an abnormal sign).

If the malignancy has been removed using the perineal route, the perineal wound is observed for signs of hemorrhage. This wound may contain a drain or packing, which is removed gradually. Bits of tissue may slough off for a week. This process is hastened by mechanical irrigation of the wound or with sitz baths performed two or three times each day initially. The condition of the perineal wound and any bleeding, infection, or necrosis are documented.

MONITORING AND MANAGING COMPLICATIONS

The patient is observed for signs and symptoms of complications. It is important to frequently assess the abdomen, including decreasing or changing bowel sounds and increasing abdominal girth, to detect bowel obstruction. The nurse monitors vital signs for increased temperature, pulse, and respirations and for decreased blood pressure, which may indicate an intra-abdominal infectious process. It is important to report rectal bleeding immediately because it indicates hemorrhage. The nurse monitors hematocrit and hemoglobin levels and administers blood component therapy as prescribed. Any abrupt change in abdominal pain is reported promptly. Elevated white blood cell counts and temperature or symptoms of shock are reported because they may indicate sepsis. The nurse administers antibiotics as prescribed.

Pulmonary complications are always a concern with abdominal surgery; patients older than 50 years of age are at risk, especially if they are or have been receiving sedatives or are being maintained on bed rest for a prolonged period. Two primary pulmonary complications are pneumonia and atelectasis. Frequent activity (eg, turning the patient from side to side every 2 hours), deep breathing, coughing, and early ambulation can reduce the risks for these complications. Table 38-6 lists possible postoperative complications.

The incidence of complications related to the colostomy is about one half that seen with an ileostomy. Some common complications are prolapse of the stoma (usually from obesity), perforation (from improper stoma irrigation), stoma retraction, fecal impaction, and skin irritation. Leakage from an anastomotic site can occur if the remaining bowel segments are diseased or weakened. Leakage from an intestinal anastomosis causes abdominal distention and rigidity, temperature elevation, and signs of shock. Surgical repair is necessary.

REMOVING AND APPLYING THE COLOSTOMY APPLIANCE

The colostomy begins to function 3 to 6 days after surgery. The nurse manages the colostomy and teaches the patient about its care until the patient can take over. The nurse teaches skin care and how to apply and remove the drainage pouch. Care of the peristomal skin is an ongoing concern because excoriation or ulceration can develop quickly. The presence of such irritation makes adhering the ostomy appliance difficult, and adhering the ostomy appliance to irritated skin can worsen the skin condition. The effluent discharge and the degree to which it is irritating vary with the type of ostomy. With a transverse colostomy, the stool is soft and mushy and irritating to the skin. With a descending or sigmoid colostomy, the stool is fairly solid and less irritating to the skin. Other skin problems include yeast infections and allergic dermatitis.

If the patient wants to bathe or shower before putting on the clean appliance, micropore tape applied to the sides of the pouch will keep it secure during bathing. To remove the appliance, the patient assumes a comfortable sitting or standing position and gently pushes the skin down from the faceplate while pulling the pouch up and away from the stoma. Gentle pressure prevents the skin from being traumatized and any liquid fecal contents from spilling out. The nurse advises the patient to protect the peristomal skin by then washing the area gently with a moist, soft cloth and a mild soap. Soap acts as a mild abrasive agent to remove enzyme residue from fecal spillage. The patient should remove any excess skin barrier. While the skin is being cleansed, a gauze dressing can cover the stoma, or a vaginal tampon can be inserted gently to absorb excess drainage. After cleansing, the patient pats the skin completely dry with a gauze pad, taking care not to rub the area. The patient can lightly dust nystatin (Mycostatin) powder on the peristomal skin if irritation or yeast growth is present.

Smoothly applying the drainage appliance for a secure fit requires practice and a well-fitting appliance. Patients can choose from a wide variety of appliances, depending on their individual

---

Table 38-6 • **Potential Complications and Nursing Interventions After Intestinal Surgery**

COMPLICATION	NURSING INTERVENTIONS
Paralytic ileus	Initiate or continue nasogastric intubation as prescribed. Prepare patient for x-ray study. Ensure adequate fluid and electrolyte replacement. Administer prescribed antibiotics if patient has symptoms of peritonitis.
Mechanical obstruction	Assess patient for intermittent colicky pain, nausea, and vomiting.
Intra-abdominal Septic Conditions	
Peritonitis	Evaluate patient for nausea, hiccups, chills, spiking fever, tachycardia. Administer antibiotics as prescribed. Prepare patient for drainage procedure. Administer parenteral fluid and electrolyte therapy as prescribed. Prepare patient for surgery if condition deteriorates.
Abscess formation	Administer antibiotics as prescribed. Apply warm compresses as prescribed. Prepare for surgical drainage.
Surgical Wound Complications	
Infection	Monitor temperature; report temperature elevation. Observe for redness, tenderness, and pain around wound. Assist in establishing local drainage. Obtain specimen of drainage material for culture and sensitivity studies.
Wound disruption	Observe for sudden appearance of profuse serous drainage from wound. Cover wound area with sterile towels held in place with binder. Prepare patient immediately for surgery.
Intraperitoneal infection and abdominal wound infection	Monitor for evidence of constant or generalized abdominal pain, rapid pulse, and elevation of temperature. Prepare for tube decompression of bowel. Administer fluids and electrolytes by IV route as prescribed. Administer antibiotics as prescribed.
Anastomotic Complications	
Dehiscence of anastomosis	Prepare patient for surgery.
Fistulas	Assist in bowel decompression. Administer parenteral fluids as prescribed to correct fluid and electrolyte deficits.

---

needs. The stoma is measured to determine the correct size for the pouch; the pouch opening should be about 0.3 cm larger than the stoma. After the skin is cleansed according to the previously described procedure, the patient applies the peristomal skin barrier (ie, wafer, paste, or powder). Mild skin irritation may require dusting the skin with karaya or Stomahesive powder before attaching the pouch. The patient removes the backing from the adherent surface of the appliance, and places the bag down over the stoma for 30 seconds. The patient empties or changes the drainage appliance when it is one-third to one-fourth full so that the weight of its contents does not cause the appliance to separate from the adhesive disk and spill the contents. Most appliances are disposable and odour resistant; commercially prepared deodourizers are available.

For some patients, colostomy appliances are not always necessary. As soon as the patient has learned a routine for evacuation, bags may be dispensed with, and a closed ostomy appliance or a simple dressing of disposable tissue (often covered with plastic wrap) is used, held in place by an elastic belt. Except for gas and a slight amount of mucus, nothing escapes from the colostomy opening between irrigations. Colostomy plugs that expand on insertion to prevent passage of flatus and feces are available.

IRRIGATING THE COLOSTOMY

The purpose of irrigating a colostomy is to empty the colon of gas, mucus, and feces so that the patient can go about social and business activities without fear of fecal drainage. A stoma does not have voluntary muscular control and may empty at irregular intervals. Regulating the passage of fecal material is achieved by irrigating the colostomy or allowing the bowel to evacuate naturally without irrigations. The choice often depends on the individual and the type of the colostomy. By irrigating the stoma at a regular time, there is less gas and retention of the irrigant. The time for irrigating the colostomy should be consistent with the schedule the person will follow after leaving the hospital. Chart 38-9 delineates the irrigating procedure.

SUPPORTING A POSITIVE BODY IMAGE

The patient is encouraged to verbalize feelings and concerns about altered body image and to discuss the surgery and the stoma (if one was created). A supportive environment and a supportive attitude on the nurse's part are crucial in promoting the patient's adaptation to the changes brought about by the surgery. If applicable, the patient must learn colostomy care and begin to plan for incorporating stoma care into daily life. The nurse helps the patient overcome aversion to the stoma or fear

Chart 38-9

GUIDELINES FOR Irrigating a Colostomy

A colostomy is irrigated to empty the colon of feces, gas, or mucus, cleanse the lower intestinal tract, and establish a regular pattern of evacuation so that normal life activities may be pursued. A suitable time for the irrigation is selected that is compatible with the patient's posthospital pattern of activity (preferably after a meal). Irrigation should be performed at the same time each day.

Before the procedure, the patient sits on a chair in front of the toilet or on the toilet itself. An irrigating reservoir containing 500 to 1500 mL of lukewarm tapwater is hung 45 to 50 cm above the stoma (shoulder height when the patient is seated). The dressing or pouch is removed. The following procedure is used; the patient is helped to participate in the procedure to learn to perform it unassisted.

NURSING ACTION	RATIONALE
1. Apply an irrigating sleeve or sheath to the stoma. Place the end in the commode.	1. This helps to control odour and splashing and allows feces and water to flow directly into the commode.

Colostomy irrigation. (**A**) Irrigating catheter has a cone attachment to prevent injury to stomal tissue. (**B**) Irrigating fluid is instilled with sleeve in place. Drainage contents empty into toilet. (**C**) The bulb syringe method can be used to stimulate fecal drainage. Note that a portion of the hard nozzle is removed and a catheter attached to minimize stomal irritation.

NURSING ACTION	RATIONALE
2. Allow some of the solution to flow through the tubing and catheter/cone.	2. Air bubbles in the setup are released so that air is not introduced into the colon, which would cause crampy pain.
3. Lubricate the catheter/cone and gently insert it into the stoma. Insert the catheter no more than 8 cm. Hold the shield/cone gently, but firmly, against the stoma to prevent backflow of water.	3. Lubrication permits ease of insertion of the catheter/cone.
4. If the catheter does not advance easily, allow water to flow slowly while advancing catheter. *Never force the catheter!*	4. A slow rate of flow helps to relax the bowel and facilitates passage of the catheter.
5. Allow tepid fluid to enter the colon slowly. If cramping occurs, clamp off the tubing and allow the patient to rest before progressing. Water should flow in over a 5- to 10-minute period.	5. Painful cramps usually are caused by too rapid a flow or by too much solution; 300 mL of fluid may be all that is needed to stimulate evacuation. Volume may be increased with subsequent irrigations to 500, 1000, or 1500 mL as needed by the patient for effective results.
6. Hold the shield/cone in place 10 seconds after the water has been instilled; then gently remove it.	
7. Allow 10 to 15 minutes for most of the return; then dry the bottom of the sleeve/sheath and attach it to the top, or apply the appropriate clamp to the bottom of the sleeve.	7. Most of the water, feces, and flatus will be expelled in 10 to 15 minutes.
8. Leave the sleeve/sheath in place for 30 to 45 minutes while the patient gets up and moves around.	8. Ambulation stimulates peristalsis and completion of the irrigation return.
9. Cleanse the area with a mild soap and water; pat the area dry.	9. Cleanliness and dryness will provide the patient with hours of comfort.
10. Replace the colostomy dressing or appliance.	10. The patient should use an appliance until the colostomy is sufficiently controlled. A dressing may be all that is needed.

of self-injury by providing care and teaching in an open, accepting manner and by encouraging the patient to talk about his or her feelings about the stoma.

DISCUSSING SEXUALITY ISSUES

The nurse encourages the patient to discuss feelings about sexuality and sexual function. Some patients may initiate questions about sexual activity directly or give indirect clues about their fears. Some may view the surgery as mutilating and a threat to their sexuality; some fear impotence. Others may express worry about odour or leakage from the pouch during sexual activity. Although the appliance presents no deterrent to sexual activity, some patients wear silk or cotton covers and smaller pouches during sex. Alternative sexual positions are recommended, as well as alternative methods of stimulation to satisfy sexual drives. The nurse assesses the patient's needs and attempts to identify specific concerns. If the nurse is uncomfortable with this or if the patient's concerns seem complex, it is appropriate for the nurse to seek assistance from an enterostomal therapy nurse, sex counselor or therapist, or advanced practice nurse.

PROMOTING HOME AND COMMUNITY-BASED CARE

Teaching Patients Self-Care

Patient education and discharge planning require the combined efforts of the physician, nurse, enterostomal therapist, social worker, and dietitian. Patients are given specific information, individualized to their needs, about ostomy care and signs and symptoms of potential complications. Dietary instructions are essential to help patients identify and eliminate irritating foods that can cause diarrhea or constipation. It is important to teach patients about their prescribed medications (ie, action, purpose, and possible side effects).

The nurse reviews treatments (eg, irrigations, wound cleansing) and dressing changes and encourages the family to participate. Because the hospital stay is short, the patient may not be able to become proficient in stoma care techniques before discharge. Many patients need referral to a home care agency and the telephone number of the provincial or territorial division of the Canadian Cancer Society. The home care nurse goes to the home to provide further care and teaching and to assess how well the patient and family are adjusting to the colostomy. The home environment is assessed for adequacy of resources that allow the patient to accomplish self-care. A family member may assume responsibility for purchasing the equipment and supplies needed at home.

Patients need very specific directions about when to call the physician. They need to know which complications require prompt attention (ie, bleeding, abdominal distention and rigidity, diarrhea, fever, wound drainage, and disruption of suture line). If radiation therapy is planned, the possible side effects (ie, anorexia, vomiting, diarrhea, and exhaustion) are reviewed.

Continuing Care

Ongoing care of the patient with cancer and a colostomy often extends well beyond the initial hospital stay. Home care nurses manage ostomy follow-up care, manage the assessment and care of the debilitated patient, and coordinate adjuvant therapy. The home care visits also provide the nurse with opportunities to assess the patient's physical and emotional status and the patient's and family's ability to carry out recommended management strategies. Visits from an enterostomal therapy nurse are available to the patient and family as they learn to care for the ostomy and work through their feelings about it, the diagnosis of cancer, and the

future. Some patients are interested in and can benefit from involvement in an ostomy support group.

Evaluation

EXPECTED PATIENT OUTCOMES

Expected patient outcomes may include the following:

1. Consumes a healthy diet
   a. Avoids foods and fluids that cause diarrhea
   b. Substitutes nonirritating foods and fluids for those that are restricted
2. Maintains fluid balance
   a. Experiences no vomiting or diarrhea
   b. Experiences no signs or symptoms of dehydration
3. Feels less anxious
   a. Expresses concerns and fears freely
   b. Uses coping measures to manage stress
4. Acquires information about diagnosis, surgical procedure, preoperative preparation, and self-care after discharge
   a. Discusses the diagnosis, surgical procedure, and postoperative self-care
   b. Demonstrates techniques of ostomy care
5. Maintains clean incision, stoma, and perineal wound
6. Expresses feelings and concerns about self
   a. Gradually increases participation in stoma and peristomal skin care
   b. Discusses feelings related to changed appearance
7. Discusses sexuality in relation to ostomy and to changes in body image
8. Recovers without complications
   a. Is afebrile
   b. Regains normal bowel activity
   c. Exhibits no signs and symptoms of perforation or bleeding

POLYPS OF THE COLON AND RECTUM

A polyp is a mass of tissue that protrudes into the lumen of the bowel. Polyps can occur anywhere in the intestinal tract and rectum. They can be classified as neoplastic (ie, adenomas and carcinomas) or non-neoplastic (ie, mucosal and hyperplastic). Non-neoplastic polyps, which are benign epithelial growths, are common in the Western world. They occur more commonly in the large intestine than in the small intestine. Although most polyps do not develop into invasive neoplasms, they must be identified and followed closely. Adenomatous polyps are more common in men. The proportion of these polyps arising in the proximal part of the colon increases with age (after 40 years of age). Prevalence rates vary from 25% to 60%, depending on age. Non-neoplastic polyps occur in 80% of the population, and their frequency increases with age (Wolfe, 2000).

Clinical manifestations depend on the size of the polyp and the amount of pressure it exerts on intestinal tissue. The most common symptom is rectal bleeding. Lower abdominal pain may also occur. If the polyp is large enough, symptoms of obstruction occur. The diagnosis is based on history and digital rectal examination, barium enema studies, sigmoidoscopy, or colonoscopy.

After a polyp is identified, it should be removed. There are several methods: colonoscopy with the use of special equipment (ie, biopsy forceps and snares), laparoscopy, or colonoscopic excision with laparoscopic visualization. The latter technique enables immediate detection of potential problems and allows laparoscopic resection and repair of the major complications of perforation and bleeding that may occur with polypectomy. Microscopic examination of the polyp then identifies the type of polyp and indicates what further surgery is required.

Diseases of the Anorectum

Anorectal disorders are common, and more than one half of the population will experience one at some time during their lives (Yamada et al., 1999). Patients with anorectal disorders seek medical care primarily because of pain, rectal bleeding, or change in bowel habits. Other common complaints are protrusion of hemorrhoids, anal discharge, perianal itching, swelling, anal tenderness, stenosis, and ulceration. Constipation results from delaying defecation because of anorectal pain.

There has been a steady increase in the frequency of sexually transmitted diseases in recent decades, leading to the identification of new anorectal syndromes. The prevalence of these conditions is increasing. These syndromes include venereal infections such as syphilis, gonorrhea, herpes, chlamydia, and candidiasis, and they are most commonly seen in male homosexuals who practice anorectal intercourse (Wolfe, 2000).

ANORECTAL ABSCESS

An anorectal abscess is caused by obstruction of an anal gland, resulting in retrograde infection. People with regional enteritis or immunosuppressive conditions such as AIDS are particularly susceptible to these infections. Many of these abscesses result in fistulas.

An abscess may occur in a variety of spaces in and around the rectum. It often contains a quantity of foul-smelling pus and is painful. If the abscess is superficial, swelling, redness, and tenderness are observed. A deeper abscess may result in toxic symptoms, lower abdominal pain, and fever.

Palliative therapy consists of sitz baths and analgesics. However, prompt surgical treatment to incise and drain the abscess is the treatment of choice. When a deeper infection exists with the possibility of a fistula, the fistulous tract must be excised. If possible, the fistula is excised when the abscess is incised and drained, or a second procedure to do so may be necessary. The wound may be packed with gauze and allowed to heal by granulation.

ANAL FISTULA

An anal fistula is a tiny, tubular, fibrous tract that extends into the anal canal from an opening located beside the anus (Fig. 38-11A). Fistulas usually result from an infection. They may also develop from trauma, fissures, or regional enteritis. Pus or stool may leak constantly from the cutaneous opening. Other symptoms may be the passage of flatus or feces from the vagina or bladder, depending on the fistula tract. Untreated fistulas may cause systemic infection with related symptoms.

Surgery is always recommended, because few fistulas heal spontaneously. A fistulectomy (ie, excision of the fistulous tract) is the recommended surgical procedure. The lower bowel is evacuated thoroughly with several prescribed enemas. During surgery, the sinus tract is identified by inserting a probe into it or by injecting the tract with methylene blue solution. The fistula is dissected out or laid open by an incision from its rectal opening to its outlet. The wound is packed with gauze.

ANAL FISSURE

An anal fissure is a longitudinal tear or ulceration in the lining of the anal canal (see Fig. 38-11B). Fissures are usually caused by the trauma of passing a large, firm stool or from persistent tightening of the anal canal because of stress and anxiety (leading to constipation). Other causes include childbirth, trauma, and overuse of laxatives.

Extremely painful defecation, burning, and bleeding characterize fissures. Most of these fissures heal if treated by conservative measures, which include stool softeners and bulk agents, an increase in water intake, sitz baths, and emollient suppositories. A suppository combining an anesthetic with a corticosteroid helps relieve the discomfort. Anal dilation under anesthesia may be required.

If fissures do not respond to conservative treatment, surgery is indicated. The procedure considered by most surgeons to be the procedure of choice is the lateral internal sphincterotomy with excision of the fissure; the success rate is 90% to 95% (Keighley & Williams, 1999).

HEMORRHOIDS

Hemorrhoids are dilated portions of veins in the anal canal. They are very common. By the age of 50, about 50% of people have hemorrhoids to some extent (Corman, 1998). Shearing of the

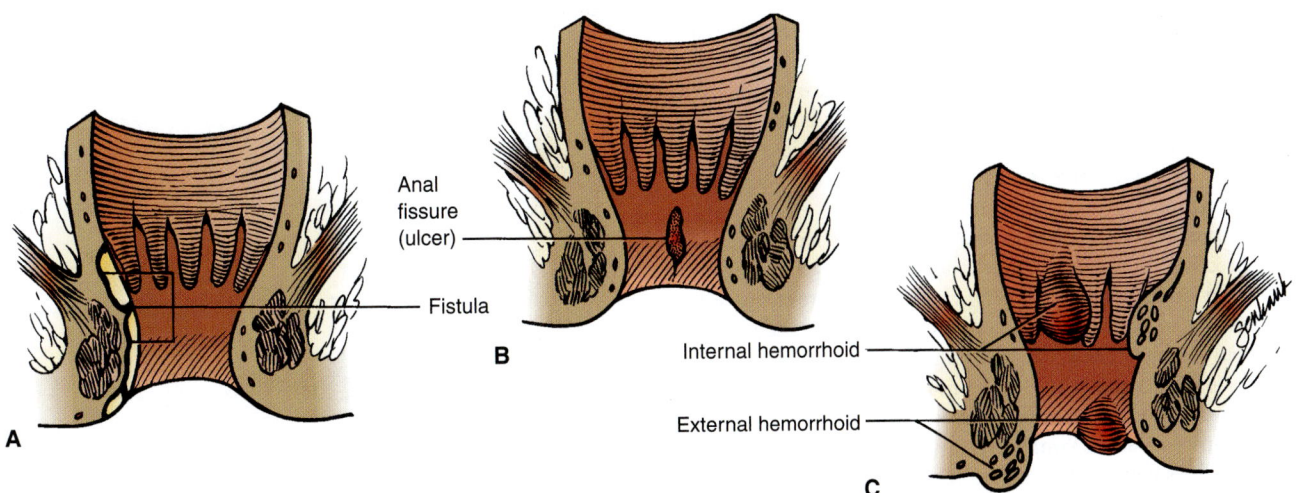

FIGURE 38-11 Various types of anal lesions. (**A**) Fistula. (**B**) Fissure. (**C**) External and internal hemorrhoids.

mucosa during defecation results in the sliding of the structures in the wall of the anal canal, including the hemorrhoidal and vascular tissues. Increased pressure in the hemorrhoidal tissue due to pregnancy may initiate hemorrhoids or aggravate existing ones. Hemorrhoids are classified as one of two types. Those above the internal sphincter are called internal hemorrhoids, and those appearing outside the external sphincter are called external hemorrhoids (see Fig. 38-11C).

Hemorrhoids cause itching and pain and are the most common cause of bright red bleeding with defecation. External hemorrhoids are associated with severe pain from the inflammation and edema caused by thrombosis (ie, clotting of blood within the hemorrhoid). This may lead to ischemia of the area and eventual necrosis. Internal hemorrhoids are not usually painful until they bleed or prolapse when they become enlarged.

Hemorrhoid symptoms and discomfort can be relieved by good personal hygiene and by avoiding excessive straining during defecation. A high-residue diet that contains fruit and bran along with an increased fluid intake may be all the treatment that is necessary to promote the passage of soft, bulky stools to prevent straining. If this treatment is not successful, the addition of hydrophilic bulk-forming agents such as psyllium and mucilloid may help. Warm compresses, sitz baths, analgesic ointments and suppositories, astringents (eg, witch hazel), and bed rest allow the engorgement to subside.

There are several types of nonsurgical treatments for hemorrhoids. Infrared photocoagulation, bipolar diathermy, and laser therapy are newer techniques that are used to affix the mucosa to the underlying muscle. Injecting sclerosing solutions is also effective for small, bleeding hemorrhoids. These procedures help prevent prolapse.

A conservative surgical treatment of internal hemorrhoids is the rubber-band ligation procedure. The hemorrhoid is visualized through the anoscope, and its proximal portion above the mucocutaneous lines is grasped with an instrument. A small rubber band is then slipped over the hemorrhoid. Tissue distal to the rubber band becomes necrotic after several days and sloughs off. Fibrosis occurs; the result is that the lower anal mucosa is drawn up and adheres to the underlying muscle. Although this treatment has been satisfactory for some patients, it has proven painful for others and may cause secondary hemorrhage. It has been known to cause perianal infection.

Cryosurgical hemorrhoidectomy, another method for removing hemorrhoids, involves freezing the hemorrhoid for a sufficient time to cause necrosis. Although it is relatively painless, this procedure is not widely used because the discharge is very foul smelling and wound healing is prolonged. The Nd:YAG laser is useful in excising hemorrhoids, particularly external hemorrhoidal tags. The treatment is quick and relatively painless. Hemorrhage and abscess are rare postoperative complications.

The previously described methods of treating hemorrhoids are not effective for advanced thrombosed veins, which must be treated by more extensive surgery. Hemorrhoidectomy, or surgical excision, can be performed to remove all the redundant tissue involved in the process. During surgery, the rectal sphincter is usually dilated digitally and the hemorrhoids are removed with a clamp and cautery or are ligated and then excised. After the operative procedures are completed, a small tube may be inserted through the sphincter to permit the escape of flatus and blood; pieces of Gelfoam or Oxycel gauze may be placed over the anal wounds.

SEXUALLY TRANSMITTED ANORECTAL DISEASES

Three infectious syndromes that are related to sexually transmitted diseases have been identified. Proctitis involves the rectum. It is commonly associated with recent anal-receptive intercourse with an infected partner. Symptoms include a mucopurulent discharge or bleeding, pain in the area, and diarrhea. The pathogens most frequently involved are *Neisseria gonorrheae* (53%), *Chlamydia* (20%), herpes simplex virus (18%), and *Treponema pallidum* (9%) (Yamada et al., 1999). Proctocolitis involves the rectum and lowest portion of the descending colon. Symptoms are similar to proctitis but may also include watery or bloody diarrhea, cramps, pain, and bloating. Enteritis involves more of the descending colon, and symptoms include watery, bloody diarrhea; abdominal pain; and weight loss. The most common pathogens causing enteritis are *E. histolytica, Giardia lamblia, Shigella,* and *Campylobacter* (Wolfe, 2000).

Sigmoidoscopy is performed to identify portions of the anorectum involved. Samples are taken with rectal swabs, and cultures are obtained to identify the pathogens involved. The treatment of choice for bacterial infections is antibiotics (ie, cefixime, doxycycline, and penicillin). Acyclovir is given to those with viral infections. Infections from *E. histolytica* and *G. lamblia* are treated with antiamebic therapy (ie, metronidazole). Ciprofloxacin is an effective treatment for *Shigella*. Antibiotics of choice for *Campylobacter* infection are erythromycin and ciprofloxacin.

PILONIDAL SINUS OR CYST

A pilonidal sinus or cyst is found in the intergluteal cleft on the posterior surface of the lower sacrum (Fig. 38-12). Current theories suggest that it results from local trauma that causes the pen-

A Pilonidal sinus   Intergluteal cleft

Posterior surface of lower sacrum

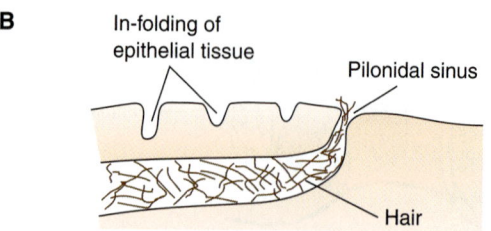

B In-folding of epithelial tissue

Pilonidal sinus

Hair

FIGURE 38-12 (**A**) Pilonidal sinus on lower sacrum about 5 cm above the anus in the intergluteal cleft. (**B**) Note: Hair particles emerge from the sinus tract and localized indentations (pits) can appear on the skin near the sinus openings.

etration of hairs into the epithelium and subcutaneous tissue (Yamada et al., 1999). It may also be formed congenitally by an infolding of epithelial tissue beneath the skin, which may communicate with the skin surface through one or several small sinus openings. Hair frequently is seen protruding from these openings, and this gives the cyst its name, *pilonidal* (ie, a nest of hair). The cysts rarely cause symptoms until adolescence or early adult life, when infection produces an irritating drainage or an abscess. Perspiration and friction easily irritate this area.

In the early stages of the inflammation, the infection may be controlled by antibiotic therapy, but after an abscess has formed, surgery is indicated. The abscess is incised and drained under local anesthesia. After the acute process resolves, further surgery is performed to excise the cyst and the secondary sinus tracts. The wound is allowed to heal by granulation. Gauze dressings are placed in the wound to keep its edges separated while healing occurs.

NURSING PROCESS: THE PATIENT WITH AN ANORECTAL CONDITION

Assessment

The nurse takes a health history to determine the presence and characteristics of itching, burning, or pain. Does it occur during bowel movements? How long does it last? Is any abdominal pain associated with it? Does any bleeding occur from the rectum? How much? How frequently? Is it bright red? Is there any other discharge, such as mucus or pus? Other questions relate to elimination patterns and laxative use, diet history (including fibre intake), the amount of exercise, activity levels, and occupation (especially one that involves prolonged sitting or standing). Assessment also includes inspection of the stool for blood or mucus and the perianal area for hemorrhoids, fissures, irritation, or pus.

Diagnosis

NURSING DIAGNOSES
Based on the assessment data, the major nursing diagnoses may include the following:

- Constipation related to ignoring the urge to defecate because of pain during elimination
- Anxiety related to impending surgery and embarrassment
- Acute pain related to irritation, pressure, and sensitivity in the anorectal area from anorectal disease and sphincter spasms after surgery
- Urinary retention related to postoperative reflex spasm and fear of pain
- Risk for ineffective therapeutic regimen management

COLLABORATIVE PROBLEMS/ POTENTIAL COMPLICATIONS

- Hemorrhage

Planning and Goals

The major goals for the patient may include adequate elimination patterns, reduction of anxiety, pain relief, promotion of urinary elimination, managing the therapeutic regimen, and absence of complications.

Nursing Interventions

RELIEVING CONSTIPATION
The nurse encourages intake of at least 2 L of water daily to provide adequate hydration and recommends high-fibre foods to promote bulk in the stool and to make it easier to pass fecal matter through the rectum. Bulk laxatives such as Metamucil and stool softeners are administered as prescribed. The patient is advised to set aside a time for moving the bowels and to heed the urge to defecate as promptly as possible. It may be helpful to have the patient perform relaxation exercises before defecating to relax the abdominal and perineal muscles, which may be constricted or in spasm. Administering an analgesic before a bowel movement is beneficial.

REDUCING ANXIETY
Patients facing rectal surgery may be upset and irritable because of discomfort, pain, and embarrassment. The nurse identifies specific psychosocial needs and individualizes the plan of care. The nurse maintains the patient's privacy while providing care and by limiting visitors, if the patient desires. Soiled dressings are removed from the room promptly to prevent unpleasant odours; room deodourizers may be needed if dressings are foul smelling.

RELIEVING PAIN
During the first 24 hours after rectal surgery, painful spasms of the sphincter and perineal muscles may occur. Control of pain is a prime consideration. The patient is encouraged to assume a comfortable position. Flotation pads under the buttocks when sitting help to decrease the pain, as may ice and analgesic ointments. Warm compresses may promote circulation and soothe irritated tissues. Sitz baths taken three or four times each day can relieve soreness and pain by relaxing sphincter spasm. Twenty-four hours after surgery, topical anesthetic agents may be beneficial in relieving local irritation and soreness. Medications may include topical anesthetics (ie, suppositories), astringents, antiseptics, tranquilizers, and antiemetics. Patients are more compliant and less apprehensive if they are free of pain.

Wet dressings saturated with equal parts of cold water and witch hazel help relieve edema. When wet compresses are being used continuously, the petrolatum is applied around the anal area to prevent skin maceration. The patient is instructed to assume a prone position at intervals because this position promotes dependent drainage of edematous fluid.

PROMOTING URINARY ELIMINATION
Voiding may be a problem after surgery because of a reflex spasm of the sphincter at the outlet of the bladder and a certain amount of muscle guarding from apprehension and pain. The nurse tries all methods to encourage voluntary voiding (ie, increasing fluid intake, listening to running water, and dripping water over the urinary meatus) before resorting to catheterization. After rectal surgery, urinary output is closely monitored.

MONITORING AND MANAGING COMPLICATIONS
The operative site is examined frequently for rectal bleeding. The nurse assesses the patient for systemic indicators of excessive bleeding (ie, tachycardia, hypotension, restlessness, and thirst). After hemorrhoidectomy, hemorrhage may occur from the veins that were cut. If a tube has been inserted through the sphincter after surgery, evidence of bleeding may be visible on the dressings. If bleeding is obvious, direct pressure is applied to the area, and the physician is notified. It is important to avoid using moist heat because it encourages vessel dilation and bleeding.

PROMOTING HOME AND COMMUNITY-BASED CARE

Teaching Patients Self-Care

Most patients with anorectal conditions are not hospitalized. Those who have surgical procedures to correct the condition often are discharged directly from the outpatient surgical centre. If they are hospitalized, it is for a short time, usually only 24 hours. Patient teaching is essential to facilitate recovery at home.

The nurse instructs the patient to keep the perianal area as clean as possible by gently cleansing with warm water and then drying with absorbent cotton wipes. The patient avoids rubbing the area with toilet tissue. Instructions are provided about how to take a sitz bath and how to test the temperature of the water. Sitz baths may be given in the bathtub or plastic sitz bath unit three or four times each day. Sitz baths should follow each bowel movement for 1 to 2 weeks after surgery. The nurse encourages the patient to respond quickly to the urge to defecate to prevent constipation. The diet is modified to increase fluids and fibre. Moderate exercise is encouraged, and the patient is taught about the prescribed diet, the significance of proper eating habits and exercise, and the laxatives that can be taken safely.

Evaluation

EXPECTED PATIENT OUTCOMES

Expected patient outcomes may include the following:

1. Attains a normal pattern of elimination
   a. Sets aside a time for defecation, usually after a meal or at bedtime
   b. Responds to the urge to defecate and takes the time to sit on the toilet and try to defecate
   c. Uses relaxation exercises as needed
   d. Increases fluid intake to 2 L per day
   e. Adds high-fibre foods to diet
   f. Reports passage of soft, formed stools
   g. Reports decreased abdominal discomfort
2. Is less anxious
3. Has less pain
   a. Modifies body position and activities to minimize pain and discomfort
   b. Applies warmth or cold to anorectal area
   c. Takes sitz baths four times each day
4. Voids without difficulty
5. Adheres to the therapeutic regimen
   a. Keeps perianal area dry
   b. Eats bulk-forming foods
   c. Has a soft, formed stool on a regular basis
6. Exhibits no evidence of complications
   a. Has a clean incision
   b. Has normal vital signs
   c. Shows no signs of hemorrhage

 Critical Thinking Exercises

1. You are caring for an elderly man who was just admitted to the hospital. He complains that he has had pain throughout his abdomen for the past 2 days. He states that his bowel patterns have changed recently and that he has not had a bowel movement in 4 days. He has not eaten since yesterday. He states he has no appetite and that he is concerned because he has type 2 diabetes mellitus. When you complete your initial nursing assessment, you notice that his abdomen is distended and rigid and that bowel sounds are absent throughout all fields. Analyze these findings, indicate what you think the possible causes may be, and explain the actions you would take and why. Explain how this man's diagnosis of diabetes mellitus affects his plan of nursing care and his medical management.

2. During a conversation with a neighbour, you learn that she has recently seen her doctor and that she has been diagnosed with IBS. She asks you to help her understand this process and to explain the reason for the dietary restrictions her doctor has given her. Her doctor also prescribed a laxative and an antidepressant. She explains the amount of stress she has been under at work. Identify the facts that you know about this process and how the actions of the doctor would help in this situation. What will you tell your neighbour?

3. You are caring for a patient who has been diagnosed with colon cancer. He recently underwent a colonoscopy where the growth was detected in the lower portion of the descending colon. The patient is scheduled for a colon resection. You know that he will return from surgery with a sigmoid colostomy. What will you need to do during the preoperative period to prepare your patient for this surgery? What will be the nursing diagnoses and related interventions that are a priority during the immediate postoperative period? Explain how you would meet the postoperative emotional and health education needs of the patient with a colostomy.

4. You are assigned to a general medical clinic. Two patients with inflammatory bowel disease arrive for their appointments. One of the patients, a 52-year-old woman, has recently been diagnosed with Crohn's disease. The other patient, a 21-year-old woman, was diagnosed with ulcerative colitis at 15 years of age and has had an ileostomy since the age of 19 years. Compare the two disease processes in terms of their pathophysiology, clinical manifestations, course of the illness, and therapeutic management. What similarities and differences would you expect to find in the nutritional and pharmacologic therapies for these two patients? What assessment parameters would you use to identify the psychosocial needs of each of these patients?

REFERENCES AND SELECTED READINGS

Books

Brandt, L., & Daum, F. (1999). *Clinical practice of gastroenterology.* New York: Churchill-Livingstone.

Bruce, F. (1997). *Nursing in gastroenterology.* Philadelphia: W. B. Saunders.

Corman, M. (1998). *Colon and rectal surgery* (4th ed.). Philadelphia: Lippincott-Raven.

Eliopoulos, C. (1999). *Manual of gerontological nursing* (2nd ed.). St. Louis: Mosby.

Goldman, L., & Bennett, J. C. (2000). *Cecil textbook of medicine* (21st ed.). Philadelphia: W. B. Saunders.

Greene, F. L., Page, D. L., Fleming, I. D., et al. (2002). *AJCC Cancer Staging Manual.* New York: Springer-Verlag.

Grendell, J., et al. (Eds.). (1998). *Current diagnosis and treatment in gastroenterology.* Stamford, CT: Appleton & Lange.

Kirsner, J., & Shorter, R. (2000). *Inflammatory bowel disease* (5th ed.), Philadelphia: W. B. Saunders.

Keighley, M., & Willaims, N. S. (1999). *Surgery of the anus, rectum and colon* (2nd ed.). Philadelphia: W. B. Saunders.

Lipsky, M. S. (2000). *Gastrointestinal problems.* Philadelphia: Lippincott Williams & Wilkins.

Lueckenotte, A. (2000). *Gerontologic nursing.* St. Louis: Mosby.

Ming, S. (Ed.). (1998). *Pathology of the gastrointestinal tract* (2nd ed.). Baltimore: Williams & Wilkins.

Phillips, S. (1998). *Functional disorders of the gut.* London: Churchill-Livingstone.

Rose, S. (1998). *Gastrointestinal and hepatobiliary physiology.* Madison, WI: Fena Creek Publishers.

Society of Gastroenterology Nurses and Associates. (1998). *Gastroenterology nursing: A core curriculum* (2nd ed.). St. Louis: Mosby.

Stone, J., et al. (1999). *Clinical gerontological nursing* (2nd ed.). Philadelphia: W. B. Saunders.

Tierney, L., et al. (Eds.). (2000). *Current medical diagnosis and treatment.* New York: Lange Medical Books.

Williams, N. (Ed.). (1996). *Colorectal cancer.* New York: Churchill-Livingstone.

Wilson, B. A., Shannon, M. T., & Stang, C. L. (2005). *Prentice Hall nurse's drug guide 2005.* Upper Saddle River, NJ: Pearson Education.

Wolfe, M. (Ed.). (2000). *Therapy of digestive disorders.* Philadelphia: W. B. Saunders.

Yamada, T., Alpers, D. H., Owyang, C., Powell, D. W., Silverstein, F., Hasler, W. L., & Traber, P. G. (Eds.). (1998). *Handbook of gastroenterology.* Philadelphia: Lippincott Williams & Wilkins.

Yamada, T., Alpers, D. H., Laine, L., Owyang, C., & Powell, D. W. (Eds.). (1999). *Textbook of gastroenterology* (3rd ed.). Philadelphia: Lippincott Williams & Wilkins.

Journals

General

Andersson, R. E., Olaison, G., Tysk, C., & Ekbom, A. (2001). Appendectomy and protection against ulcerative colitis. *New England Journal of Medicine, 344*(11), 808–814.

Canadian Institute for Health Information (CIHI). (2002). *Rate of hospitalizations continues to decline: News brief.* Available at: www.cihi.ca. Retrieved May 8, 2005.

Creason, N., & Sparks, D. (2000). Fecal impaction: A review. *Nursing Diagnosis, 11*(1), 15–23.

Cox, J. A., Rogers, M. A., & Cox, S. D. (2001). Treating benign colon disorders using laparoscopic colectomy. *AORN Journal, 73*(2), 377–382, 384–389, 391.

Ebert, E. (2001). Maldigestion and malabsorption. *Disease of the Month, 4*(2), 45–68.

Gauf, C. L. (2000). Diagnosing appendicitis across the life span. *Journal of the American Academy of Nurse Practitioners, 12*(4), 129–133.

Higgins, P. D., & Johanson, J. F. (2004). Epistemology of constipation in North America: A systematic review. *American Journal of Gastroenterology* (in press).

Hyde, C. (2000). Diverticular disease. *Nursing Standard, 14*(51), 38–42.

Madick, S. S. (2001). Perioperative care of the patient with Zenker's diverticulum. *AORN Journal, 73*(5), 904–913.

McConnell, E. A., (1999). Myths and facts about lactose intolerance. *Nursing, 29*(3), 71.

McConnell, E. A. (2001). What is behind intestinal obstruction? *Nursing2001, 31*(10), 58–63.

Murphy-Ende, K. (2000). Bowel obstruction. *Clinical Journal of Oncology Nursing, 4*(6), 291–293.

Murphy-Ende, K. (2001). Palliation of gastrointestinal obstructive disorders. *Nursing Clinics of North America, 36*(4) 761–768.

Posarra, V. H. (1999). Recognizing the various presentations of appendicitis. *Nurse Practitioner, 24*(8), 42, 44, 49, 52–53.

Scheidler, M. & Giannella, R. (2001). Practical management of acute diarrhea. *Hospital Practice, 36*(2), 49–56.

Waldman, A. R. (2001). Bowel obstruction. *Clinical Journal of Oncology Nursing, 5*(6), 281–281, 286.

Whitehead, W. E., Wald, A., Norton, N. J. (2001). Treatment options for fecal incontinence. *Diseases of the Colon and Rectum, 44*(1), 131–142.

Wong, P. W. (1999). How to deal with chronic constipation. *Postgraduate Medicine, 106*(6), 199–200, 203–204, 207–210.

Cancer of the Colon and Rectum

Anderson, J. (2000). Review of recommendations for colorectal screening. *Geriatrics, 55*(2), 67–73.

Baker, D. (2001). Current surgical management of colorectal cancer. *Nursing Clinic of North America, 36*(3), 579–592.

Beyers, T. (2001). Colorectal cancer screening: New directions, evolving guidelines. *Patient Care, 35*(4), 24–34.

Burrer, C. V., & Bauer, S. M. (2000). Insights into genetic testing for colon cancer: The nurse practitioner role. *Clinical Excellence for Nurse Practitioners, 4*(6), 349–355.

Canadian Cancer Society. (2005). Canadian cancer encyclopedia. Available at: www.cancer.ca.

Dest, V. M. (2000). Colorectal cancer. *RN, 63*(3), 54–59.

Greenberg, M. J. (2001). Screening for colorectal cancer. *New England Journal of Medicine, 345*(25), 1851–1852.

Longo, W. E. & Johnson, F. E. (2002). The preoperative assessment and postoperative surveillance of patients with colon and rectal cancer. *Surgical Clinic of North America, 8*(5) 1091–1098.

Olsen, S. J. & Zawacki, K. (2000). Hereditary colorectal cancer. *Nursing Clinics of North America, 35*(3), 671–685.

Pontieri-Lewis, V. (2000). Colorectal cancer: Prevention and screening. *Medsurg Nursing, 9*(1) 9–15.

Rothenberger, D. (2000). Colorectal cancer. *Surgical Oncology Clinics of North America, 9*(4), 665–730.

Rudy, D. & Zdon, M. (2000). Update on colorectal cancer. *American Family Physician, 61*(6), 1759–1770, 1773–1774.

Sarna, L. & Chang, B. I. (2000). Colon cancer screening among older women caregivers. *Cancer Nursing, 23*(2), 109–116.

Stefanik, D. (2000). Colon cancer. *American Journal of Nursing 100*(Suppl. 4), 36–40.

Young, M. (2000) Caring for patients with coloanal reservoirs for rectal cancer. *Medsurg Nursing, 9*(4), 193–197.

Inflammatory Bowel Disease

Alpers, D. (2001). Is irritable bowel syndrome more than just a gastrointestinal problem? *American Journal of Gastroenterology, 96*(6), 943–949.

Blackington, E. (2000). Irritable bowel syndrome; an update on treatment options. *Advanced Nurse Practitioner, 8*(10), 41–70.

Brown, M. (1999). Inflammatory bowel disease. *Primary Care, 26*(1), 41–70.

Canadian Society of Intestinal Research. (2005). Inflammatory bowel disease. Available at: www.badgut.com.

Colwell, J. C. & Gray, M. (2001). What functional outcomes and complications should be taught to the patient with ulcerative colitis or familial adenomatous polyposis who undergoes ileal pouch anal anastomosis? *Journal of Wound Ostomy Continence Nursing, 28*(4), 184–189.

Dudley-Brown, S. (2002). Prevention of psychological distress in persons with inflammatory bowel disease. *Issues in Mental Health Nursing, 23*(4), 403–422.

Hanauer, S. (2001). Management of Crohn's disease in adults. *American Journal of Gastroenterology, 96*(3), 635–644.

Heitkemper, M. (2001). Irritable bowel syndrome. *American Journal of Nursing, 101*(1), 26–34.

Joachim, G. (2000). Responses of people with inflammatory bowel disease to foods consumed. *Gastroenterology Nursing, 23*(4), 160–167.

*Joachim, G. (2002). An assessment of social support in people with inflammatory bowel disease. *Gastroenterology Nursing, 25*(6), 246–252.

Kefalides, P. T. & Hanauer, S. B. (2002). Ulcerative colitis: diagnosis and management. *Hospital Physician, 38*(6), 53–63.

Klonowski, E. (1999). The patient with Crohn's disease. *RN, 62*(3), 32–37.

Licht, H. (2000). Irritable bowel syndrome: Diagnostic criteria. *Postgraduate Nursing, 107*(3), 203–207.

Lombardi, D. A., Feller, E. R., & Shah, S. A. (2002). Medical management of inflammatory bowel disease in the new millennium. *Comprehensive Therapy, 28*(1), 39–49.

*Mukherjee, S., Sloper, P., & Turnbull, A. (2002). An insight into the experiences of parents with inflammatory bowel disease. *Journal of Advanced Nursing, 37*(4), 355–363.

Parascandolo, M. E. (2001). Multiple ostomy complications in a patient with Crohn's disease: A case study. *Journal of Wound Ostomy Continence Nursing, 28*(5), 236–241.

Rayhorn, N. (1999). Understanding inflammatory bowel disease. *Nursing, 29*(12), 57–61.

Rayhorn, N. & Rayhorn, D. J. (2002). An in-depth look at inflammatory bowel disease. *Nursing, 32*(7), 36–45.

Rayhorn, N. & Rayhorn, D. J. (2002). Inflammatory bowel disease: Symptoms in the bowel and beyond. *Nurse Practitioner, 27*(11), 13–27.

*Smith, G. D., Watson, R., & Palmer, K. R. (2002). Inflammatory bowel disease: Developing a short disease specific scale to measure health related quality of life. *International Journal of Nursing Studies, 39*(6), 583–590.

Smith, G. D., Watson, R., Roger, D., McRorie, E., et. al. (2002). Impact of a nurse-led counselling service on quality of life in patients with inflammatory bowel disease. *Journal of Advanced Nursing, 38*(2), 152–160.

Tung, J. K. & Warner, A. S. (2002). Colonic inflammatory bowel disease. Medical therapies for colonic Crohn's disease and ulcerative colitis. *Postgraduate Medicine, 112*(5), 45–48.

Ostomy

Ball, E. M. (2000). Ostomy guide. Part one. A practical ostomy guide. *RN, 63*(11), 61–66.

Ball, E. M. (2000). Ostomy guide. Part two. A teaching guide for continent ileostomy. *RN, 63*(12), 35–38, 40.

Bryant, D. (2000). Photo guide: Changing an ostomy appliance. *Nursing, 30*(11), 51–53.

Floruta, C. V. (2001). Dietary choices of people with ostomies. *Journal of Wound Ostomy Continence Nursing, 28*(1), 28–31.

Haugen, V. & Loehner, D. (2001). *Journal of Wound Ostomy Continence Nursing, 28*(4), 219–222.

Hocevar, B. J. & Remzi, F. (2001). The ileal pouch anal anastomosis: Past, present, and future. *Journal of Wound Ostomy Continence Nursing, 28*(1), 32–36.

Schultz, J. M. (2002). Preparing the patient for colostomy care: A lesson well learned. *Ostomy Wound Management, 48*(10), 22–25.

Taylor, P. (2001). Choosing the right stoma appliance for an ileostomy. *Community Nurse, 6*(12), 33–4.

RESOURCES AND WEBSITES

American Cancer Society, 1599 Clifton Rd., N.E., Atlanta, GA 30329; 1-800-277-2345; http://www.cancer.org.

Canadian Digestive Health Foundation; www.CDHF.ca.

Colon Cancer Alliance, 175 Ninth Ave., New York, NY 10011; 1-212-627-7451; http://www.ccalliance.org.

Crohn's & Colitis Foundation of America, 386 Park Avenue South, New York, NY 10016-8804; 1-800-932-2423; http://www.ccfa.org.

Crohn's and Colitis Foundation of Canada; www.ccfc.ca.

Health Canada; www.hc-sc.gc.ca.

International Foundation for Functional Gastrointestinal Disorders, P.O. Box 17864, Milwaukee, WI 17864; 1-888-964-2001; http://www.iffgd.org.

Intestinal Disease Foundation, Inc., 1323 Forbes Ave., Suite 200, Pittsburgh, PA 15219; 1-412-261-5888; Ischorr@aol.com.

National Association for Continence, P.O. Box 544, Union, SC 29379; 1-803-585-8789; http://www.nafc.org/site2/index.html.

National Cancer Institute of Canada; www.ncic.cancer.ca.

National Foundation for Ileitis and Colitis, 295 Madison Ave., New York, NY 10017; 1-212-685-3440.

STOP Colon/Rectal Cancer Foundation, P.O. Box 1616, Barrington, IL 60010; 1-312-782-4828; http://www.coloncancerprevention.org.

The Canadian Association for Enterostomal Therapy; www.caet.ca.

The Colorectal Cancer Screening Initiative Foundation; www.screencolons.ca.

United Ostomy Association, 19772 MacArthur Blvd., Suite 200, Irvine, CA 92612-2405; 1-800-826-0826; http://www.uoa.org.

United Ostomy Association of Canada; www.ostomycanada.ca.

Metabolic and Endocrine Function

Applying Concepts from NANDA, NIC, and NOC

Mr. Lee is a 52-year-old man with Type 2 diabetes, peripheral vascular disease, hyperlipidemia, and peripheral neuropathy. He is also 50 pounds over his ideal body weight. He takes an oral antidiabetic agent twice daily and lovastatin for elevated cholesterol levels. Mr. Lee comes to the clinic for treatment of an unrelated respiratory infection. While there, he tells the nurse that he cannot feel his feet well and has burning pain in his legs if he stands for long periods of time. The nurse inspects his feet and notes an ulcer on his left great toe where his shoes have been pinching. The nurse asks Mr. Lee when he first noticed the ulcer on his toe, and he replies that he had no idea there was an ulcer on his toe. He states he has not seen his doctor for over 1 year and only comes to the clinic if he feels sick. The concept map illustrates the relationships that exist among selected nursing diagnoses, interventions, and outcomes for one of Mr. Lee's clinical problems.

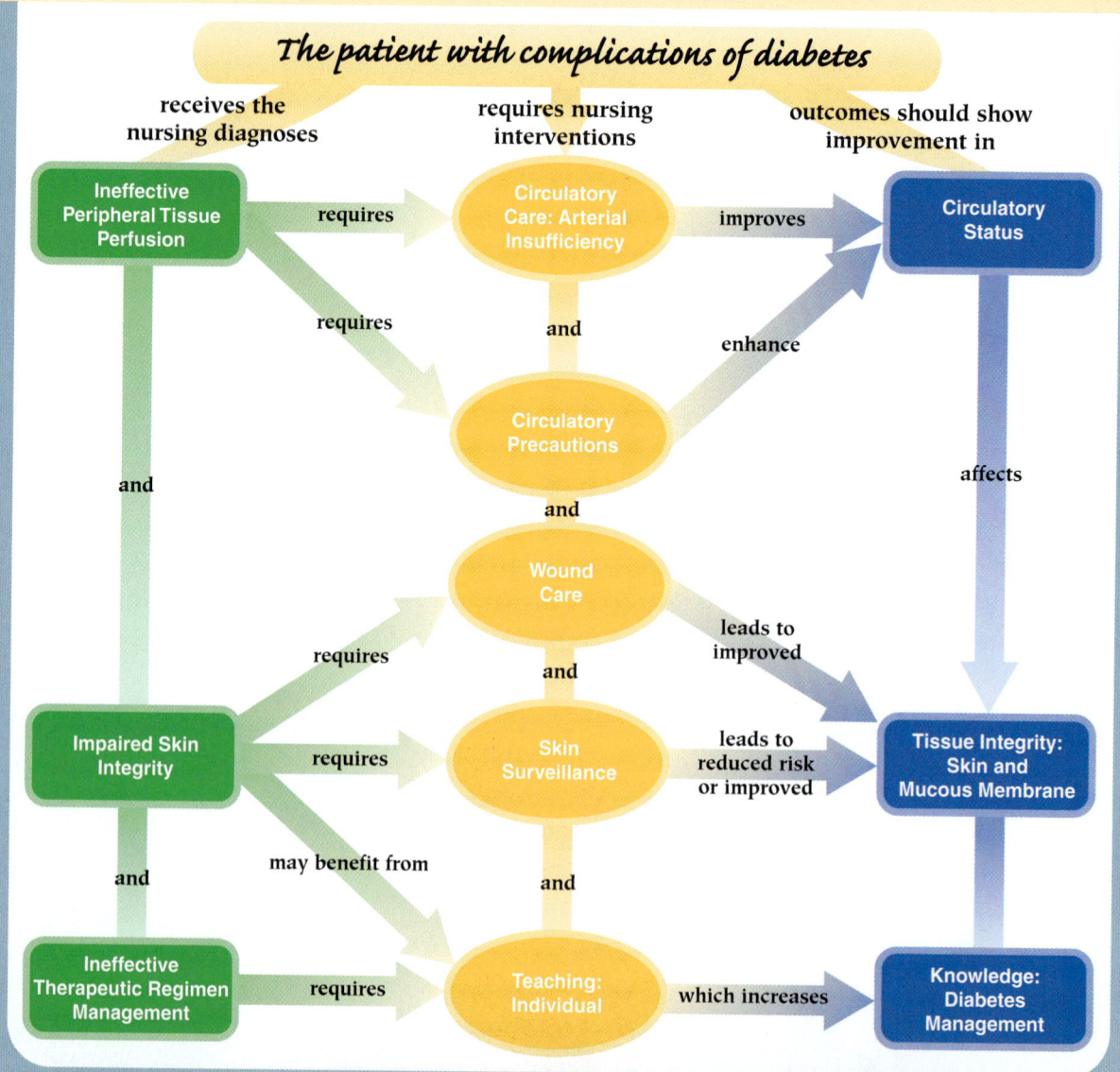

The patient with complications of diabetes

receives the nursing diagnoses — requires nursing interventions — outcomes should show improvement in

Ineffective Peripheral Tissue Perfusion — requires → Circulatory Care: Arterial Insufficiency — improves → Circulatory Status

and

Circulatory Care: Arterial Insufficiency — and — Circulatory Precautions — enhance → Circulatory Status

Ineffective Peripheral Tissue Perfusion — requires → Circulatory Precautions

Circulatory Precautions — and — Wound Care

Wound Care — leads to improved → Tissue Integrity: Skin and Mucous Membrane

Circulatory Status — affects → Tissue Integrity: Skin and Mucous Membrane

Impaired Skin Integrity — requires → Wound Care

Impaired Skin Integrity — requires → Skin Surveillance

Skin Surveillance — leads to reduced risk or improved → Tissue Integrity: Skin and Mucous Membrane

Wound Care — and — Skin Surveillance

Impaired Skin Integrity — may benefit from → Teaching: Individual

Skin Surveillance — and — Teaching: Individual

Ineffective Therapeutic Regimen Management — requires → Teaching: Individual — which increases → Knowledge: Diabetes Management

Nursing Classifications and Languages

NANDA
Nursing Diagnoses

Ineffective Tissue Perfusion (all types)—At risk for decrease in oxygen resulting in the failure to nourish tissues at the capillary level

Impaired Skin Integrity—Altered epidermis and/or dermis

Ineffective Therapeutic Regimen Management—Pattern of regulating and integrating into daily living a program for treatment of illness and the sequelae of illness that is unsatisfactory for meeting specific health goals

NIC
Nursing Interventions*

Circulatory Care: Arterial Insufficiency—Promotion of arterial circulation

Circulatory Precautions—Protection of localized area with limited perfusion

Wound Care—Prevention of wound complications and promotion of wound healing

Skin Surveillance—Collection and analysis of patient data to maintain skin and mucous membrane integrity

Teaching: Individual—Planning, implementation, and evaluation of a teaching program designed to address a patient's particular needs

NOC
Nursing Outcomes†

Return to functional baseline status, stabilization of, or improvement in

Circulation Status—Extent to which blood flows unobstructed, unidirectionally, and at an appropriate pressure through large vessels of the systemic and pulmonary circuits

Tissue Integrity: Skin and Mucous Membranes—Structural intactness and normal physiological function of skin and mucous membranes

Knowledge: Diabetes Management—Extent of understanding conveyed about diabetes mellitus and its control

NANDA, North American Nursing Diagnosis Association; NIC, Nursing Interventions Classification; NOC, Nursing Outcomes Classification.

*Iowa Intervention Project © 2000. In McCloskey, J. C., & Bulechek, G. M. (2000). *Nursing interventions classification (NIC)* (3rd ed.). St. Louis: Mosby.

†Iowa Outcomes Project © 2000. In Johnson, M., Maas, M., & Moorhead, S. (2000). *Nursing outcomes classification (NOC)* (3rd ed.). St. Louis: Mosby.

Assessment and Management of Patients With Hepatic Disorders

Adapted by Bev Williams and Bernadette Dodd

LEARNING OBJECTIVES

On completion of this chapter, the learner will be able to:

1. Identify the metabolic functions of the liver and the alterations in these functions that occur with liver disease.
2. Explain liver function tests and the clinical manifestations of liver dysfunction in relation to pathophysiologic alterations of the liver.
3. Relate jaundice, portal hypertension, ascites, varices, nutritional deficiencies, and hepatic coma to pathophysiologic alterations of the liver.
4. Describe the medical, surgical, and nursing management of patients with esophageal varices.
5. Compare the various types of hepatitis and their causes, prevention, clinical manifestations, management, prognosis, and home health care needs.
6. Use the nursing process as a framework for care of the patient with cirrhosis of the liver.
7. Compare the nonsurgical and surgical management of patients with cancer of the liver.
8. Describe the postoperative nursing care of the patient undergoing liver transplantation.

Liver disorders are common and may result from a virus or exposure to toxic substances such as alcohol. Another liver disorder is cancer: hepatocellular carcinoma is a highly malignant tumour that is difficult to treat and often fatal. In Canada, hepatocellular cancer accounts for less than 1% of all cancers, but in other parts of the world, it accounts for up to 50% of cancer cases. The difference is thought to be due to the percentage of the population who are carriers of the hepatitis B virus, which predisposes individuals to hepatocellular cancer. Liver cancer can originate in the liver or can metastasize to the liver from other sites.

Liver function is complex, and liver dysfunction affects all body systems. For this reason, the nurse must understand how the liver functions and must have expert assessment and clinical management skills to care for patients undergoing complex diagnostic and treatment procedures. The nurse also must understand technological advances in the management of liver disorders.

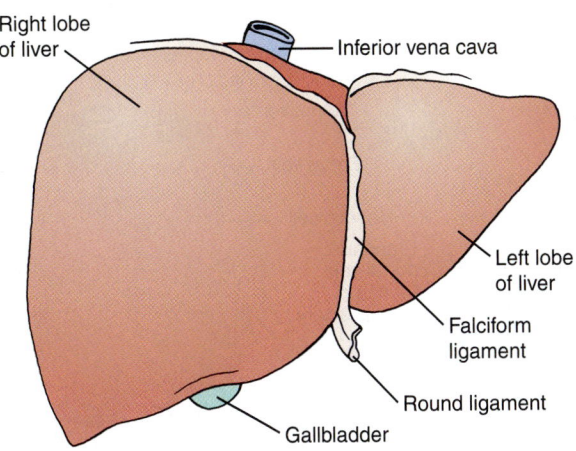

FIGURE 39-1 The liver and biliary system.

Anatomic and Physiologic Overview

The liver, the largest gland of the body, can be considered a chemical factory that manufactures, stores, alters, and excretes a large number of substances involved in metabolism. The location of the liver is essential in this function, because it receives nutrient-rich blood directly from the gastrointestinal (GI) tract and then either stores or transforms these nutrients into chemicals that are used elsewhere in the body for metabolic needs. The liver is especially important in the regulation of glucose and protein metabolism. The liver manufactures and secretes bile, which has a major role in the digestion and absorption of fats in the GI tract. It removes waste products from the bloodstream and secretes them into the bile. The bile produced by the liver is stored temporarily in the gallbladder until it is needed for digestion, at which time the gallbladder empties and bile enters the intestine (Fig. 39-1).

ANATOMY OF THE LIVER

The liver is located behind the ribs in the upper right portion of the abdominal cavity. It weighs about 1,500 g and is divided into four lobes. A thin layer of connective tissue surrounds each lobe,

extending into the lobe itself and dividing the liver mass into small units called lobules (O'Grady, Lake & Howdle, 2000).

The circulation of the blood into and out of the liver is of major importance in its function. The blood that perfuses the liver comes from two sources. Approximately 75% of the blood supply comes from the portal vein, which drains the GI tract and is rich in nutrients. The remainder of the blood supply enters by way of the hepatic artery and is rich in oxygen. Terminal branches of these two blood supplies join to form common capillary beds, which constitute the sinusoids of the liver (Fig. 39-2). Thus, a mixture of venous and arterial blood bathes the liver cells (hepatocytes). The sinusoids empty into a venule that occupies the centre of each liver lobule and is called the central vein. The central veins join to form the hepatic vein, which constitutes the venous drainage from the liver and empties into the inferior vena cava, close to the diaphragm. Thus, there are two sources of blood flowing into the liver and only one exit pathway (O'Grady et al., 2000).

In addition to hepatocytes, phagocytic cells belonging to the reticuloendothelial system are present in the liver. Other organs that contain reticuloendothelial cells are the spleen, bone marrow,

Glossary

asterixis: involuntary flapping movements of the hands associated with metabolic liver dysfunction

balloon tamponade: use of balloons placed within the esophagus and proximal portion of the stomach and inflated to compress bleeding vessels (esophageal and gastric varices)

Budd-Chiari syndrome: hepatic vein thrombosis resulting in noncirrhotic portal hypertension

cirrhosis: a chronic liver disease characterized by fibrotic changes and the formation of dense connective tissue within the liver, subsequent degenerative changes, and loss of functioning cells

constructional apraxia: inability to draw figures in two or three dimensions

cryoablation: method of treating malignant hepatic lesions that involves exposing the

tumour to temperatures below −20°C and subsequent thawing. This surgical intervention is performed via a probe through which liquid nitrogen flows.

hepatic encephalopathy: central nervous system dysfunction resulting from liver disease; frequently associated with elevated ammonia levels that produce changes in mental status, altered level of consciousness, and coma

fetor hepaticus: sweet, slightly fecal odour to the breath, presumed to be of intestinal origin; prevalent with the extensive collateral portal circulation in chronic liver disease

fulminant hepatic failure: sudden, severe onset of acute liver failure that occurs within 8 weeks of the first symptoms of jaundice

orthotopic liver transplantation (OLT): grafting of a donor liver into the normal

anatomic location, with removal of the diseased native liver

portal hypertension: elevated pressure in the portal circulation resulting from obstruction of venous flow into and through the liver

sclerotherapy: the injection of substances into or around esophagogastric varices to cause constriction, thickening, and hardening of the vessel and thus to stop bleeding

variceal banding: procedure that involves the endoscopic placement of a rubber band-like device over esophageal varices to ligate the area and stop bleeding

xenograft: transplantation of organs from one species to another

Cross section of liver lobule

Schematic diagram of section of liver lobule

To hepatic veins

FIGURE 39-2 A section of liver lobule showing the location of hepatic veins, hepatic cells, liver sinusoids, and branches of the portal vein and hepatic artery.

lymph nodes, and lungs. In the liver, these cells are called Kupffer cells. Their main function is to engulf particulate matter (such as bacteria) that enters the liver through the portal blood.

The smallest bile ducts, called canaliculi, are located between the lobules of the liver. The canaliculi receive secretions from the hepatocytes and carry them to larger bile ducts, which eventually form the hepatic duct. The hepatic duct from the liver and the cystic duct from the gallbladder join to form the common bile duct, which empties into the small intestine. The sphincter of Oddi, located at the junction where the common bile duct enters the duodenum, controls the flow of bile into the intestine. Disorders of the gallbladder are described in Chapter 40.

FUNCTIONS OF THE LIVER

Glucose Metabolism

The liver plays a major role in the metabolism of glucose and the regulation of blood glucose concentration. After a meal, glucose is taken up from the portal venous blood by the liver and converted into glycogen, which is stored in the hepatocytes. Subsequently, the glycogen is converted back to glucose and released as needed into the bloodstream to maintain normal levels of blood glucose. Additional glucose can be synthesized by the liver through a process called gluconeogenesis. For this process, the liver uses amino acids from protein breakdown or lactate produced by exercising muscles (Bacon & Di Bisceglie, 2000).

Ammonia Conversion

Use of amino acids from protein for gluconeogenesis results in the formation of ammonia as a byproduct. The liver converts this metabolically generated ammonia into urea. Ammonia produced by bacteria in the intestines is also removed from portal blood for

urea synthesis. In this way, the liver converts ammonia, a potential toxin, into urea, a compound that can be excreted in the urine.

Protein Metabolism

The liver also plays an important role in protein metabolism. It synthesizes almost all of the plasma proteins (except gamma globulin), including albumin, alpha and beta globulins, blood clotting factors, specific transport proteins, and most of the plasma lipoproteins. Vitamin K is required by the liver for synthesis of prothrombin and some of the other clotting factors. Amino acids serve as the building blocks for protein synthesis.

Fat Metabolism

The liver is also active in fat metabolism. Fatty acids can be broken down for the production of energy and the production of ketone bodies (acetoacetic acid, beta-hydroxybutyric acid, and acetone). Ketone bodies are small compounds that can enter the bloodstream and provide a source of energy for muscles and other tissues. Breakdown of fatty acids into ketone bodies occurs primarily when the availability of glucose for metabolism is limited, as during starvation or in uncontrolled diabetes. Fatty acids and their metabolic products are also used for the synthesis of cholesterol, lecithin, lipoproteins, and other complex lipids. Under some conditions, lipids may accumulate in the hepatocytes, resulting in the abnormal condition called fatty liver.

Vitamin and Iron Storage

Vitamins A, B, and D and several of the B-complex vitamins are stored in large amounts in the liver. Certain substances, such as iron and copper, are also stored in the liver. Because the liver is rich in these substances, liver extracts have been used for therapy for a wide range of nutritional disorders.

Drug Metabolism

The liver metabolizes many medications, such as barbiturates, opioids, sedative agents, anesthetics, and amphetamines. Metabolism generally results in loss of activity of the medication, although in some cases activation of the medication may occur. One of the important pathways for medication metabolism involves conjugation (binding) of the medication with a variety of compounds, such as glucuronic or acetic acid, to form more soluble substances. The conjugated products may be excreted in the feces or urine, similar to bilirubin excretion. If an oral medication (absorbed from the GI tract) is metabolized by the liver to a great extent before it reaches the systemic circulation (first-pass effect), the amount of medication actually reaching the systemic circulation (oral bioavailability) will be decreased. Bioavailability is the fraction of the administered drug that reaches the systemic circulation. Some medications have such a large first-pass effect that their use is essentially limited to the parenteral route, or oral doses must be substantially larger than parenteral doses to achieve the same effect.

Bile Formation

Bile is continuously formed by the hepatocytes and collected in the canaliculi and bile ducts. It is composed mainly of water and electrolytes such as sodium, potassium, calcium, chloride, and bicarbonate, and it also contains significant amounts of lecithin, fatty acids, cholesterol, bilirubin, and bile salts. Bile is collected and stored in the gallbladder and is emptied into the intestine when needed for digestion. The functions of bile are excretory, as in the excretion of bilirubin; bile also serves as an aid to digestion through the emulsification of fats by bile salts.

Bile salts are synthesized by the hepatocytes from cholesterol. After conjugation or binding with amino acids (taurine and glycine), they are excreted into the bile. The bile salts, together with cholesterol and lecithin, are required for emulsification of fats in the intestine, which is necessary for efficient digestion and absorption. Bile salts are then reabsorbed, primarily in the distal ileum, into portal blood for return to the liver and are again excreted into the bile. This pathway from hepatocytes to bile to intestine and back to the hepatocytes is called the enterohepatic circulation. Because of the enterohepatic circulation, only a small fraction of the bile salts that enter the intestine are excreted in the feces. This decreases the need for active synthesis of bile salts by the liver cells.

Bilirubin Excretion

Bilirubin is a pigment derived from the breakdown of hemoglobin by cells of the reticuloendothelial system, including the Kupffer cells of the liver. Hepatocytes remove bilirubin from the blood and chemically modify it through conjugation to glucuronic acid, which makes the bilirubin more soluble in aqueous solutions. The conjugated bilirubin is secreted by the hepatocytes into the adjacent bile canaliculi and is eventually carried in the bile into the duodenum.

In the small intestine, bilirubin is converted into urobilinogen, which is in part excreted in the feces and in part absorbed through the intestinal mucosa into the portal blood. Much of this reabsorbed urobilinogen is removed by the hepatocytes and is secreted into the bile once again (enterohepatic circulation). Some of the urobilinogen enters the systemic circulation and is excreted by the kidneys in the urine. Elimination of bilirubin in the bile represents the major route of excretion for this compound.

The bilirubin concentration in the blood may be increased in the presence of liver disease, when the flow of bile is impeded (ie, with gallstones in the bile ducts), or with excessive destruction of red blood cells. With bile duct obstruction, bilirubin does not enter the intestine; as a consequence, urobilinogen is absent from the urine and decreased in the stool. Biliary tract disorders are discussed in Chapter 40.

Gerontologic Considerations

The Gerontologic Considerations Box outlines age-related changes in the liver. The most common change in the liver in the elderly is a decrease in its size and weight, accompanied by a decrease in total hepatic blood flow. In general, however, these decreases are proportional to the decreases in body size and weight seen in normal aging. Results of liver function tests do not normally change in the elderly; abnormal results in an elderly patient indicate abnormal liver function and are not the result of the aging process itself.

The immune system is altered in the aged, and a less responsive immune system may be responsible for the increased incidence and severity of hepatitis B in the elderly and the increased incidence of liver abscesses secondary to decreased phagocytosis by the Kupffer cells. With the advent of hepatitis B vaccine as the standard for prevention, the incidence of hepatic diseases may decrease in the future.

Metabolism of medications by the liver appears to decrease in the elderly, but such changes are usually accompanied by changes

Gerontologic Considerations
Age-Related Changes of the Hepatobiliary System

- Steady decrease in size and weight of the liver, particularly in women
- Decrease in blood flow
- Decrease in replacement/repair of liver cells after injury
- Reduced drug metabolism
- Slow clearance of hepatitis B surface antigen
- Decline in drug clearance capability
- Increased prevalence of gallstones due to the increase in cholesterol secretion in bile
- Decreased gallbladder contraction after a meal
- Atypical clinical presentation of biliary disease
- More severe complications of biliary tract disease

in intestinal absorption, renal excretion, and altered body distribution of some medications secondary to changes in fat deposition. These alterations necessitate careful medication administration and monitoring; if appropriate, reduced dosages may be needed to prevent medication toxicity.

Assessment

HEALTH HISTORY

If liver function test results are abnormal, the patient may need to be evaluated for liver disease. In such cases, the health history will focus on exposure of the patient to hepatotoxic substances or infectious agents. The patient's occupational, recreational, and travel history may assist in identifying exposure to hepatotoxins (eg, industrial chemicals, other toxins) responsible for illness. The patient's history of alcohol and drug use, including but not limited to the use of injectable drugs, provides additional information about exposure to toxins and infectious agents. Many medications (including acetaminophen, ketoconazole, and valproic acid) are responsible for hepatic dysfunction and disease. A careful medication history to assess hepatic dysfunction should address all prescribed and over-the counter medications, herbal remedies, and dietary supplements used by the patient currently and in the past.

Lifestyle behaviours that increase the risk for exposure to infectious agents are identified. Injectable drug use, illegal street tattooing, sexual practices, and a history of foreign travel are all potential risk factors for liver disease. The amount and type of alcohol consumption are identified using screening tools (questionnaires) that have been developed for this purpose (see Chap. 5).

The history also includes an evaluation of the patient's past medical history to identify risk factors for the development of liver disease. Current and past medical conditions, including those of a psychological or psychiatric nature, are identified. The family history includes questions about familial liver disorders that may have their etiology in alcohol abuse or gallstone disease, as well as other familial or genetic diseases, such as hemochromatosis, Wilson's disease, or alpha-1 antitrypsin disease (see "Genetics in Nursing Practice" in Chap. 42).

The history also includes reviewing symptoms that suggest liver disease. Symptoms that may have their etiology in liver disease but are not specific to hepatic dysfunction include jaundice, malaise, weakness, fatigue, pruritus, abdominal pain, fever, anorexia, weight gain, edema, increasing abdominal girth, hematemesis, melena, hematochezia (passage of bloody stools), easy bruising, decreased libido in men and secondary amenorrhea in women, changes in mental acuity, personality changes, and sleep disturbances.

PHYSICAL EXAMINATION

The nurse assesses the patient for physical signs that may occur with liver dysfunction, including pallor of chronic illness and jaundice. The skin, mucosa, and sclerae are inspected for jaundice, and the extremities are assessed for muscle atrophy, edema, and skin excoriation secondary to scratching. The nurse observes the skin for petechiae or ecchymotic areas (bruises), spider angiomas, and palmar erythema. The male patient is assessed for unilateral or bilateral gynecomastia and testicular atrophy due to endocrine changes. The patient's cognitive status (recall, memory, abstract thinking) and neurologic status are assessed. The nurse observes for general tremor, asterixis, weakness, and slurred speech. These symptoms are discussed later.

The nurse assesses the abdomen for dilated abdominal wall veins, ascites, and a fluid wave (discussed later). The abdomen is palpated to assess liver size and to detect any tenderness over the liver. The liver may be palpable in the right upper quadrant. A palpable liver presents as a firm, sharp ridge with a smooth surface (Fig. 39-3). The nurse estimates liver size by percussing its upper and lower borders. When the liver is not palpable but tenderness is suspected, tapping the lower right thorax briskly may elicit tenderness. For comparison, the nurse then performs a similar manoeuvre on the left lower thorax.

If the liver is palpable, the examiner notes and records its size and consistency, whether it is tender, and whether its outline is regular or irregular. If the liver is enlarged, the degree to which it descends below the right costal margin is recorded to provide some indication of its size. The examiner determines whether the liver's edge is sharp and smooth or blunt, and whether the enlarged liver is nodular or smooth. The liver of a patient with cir-

rhosis is small and hard, whereas the liver of a patient with acute hepatitis is soft, and the hand easily moves the edge.

Tenderness of the liver implies recent acute enlargement with consequent stretching of the liver capsule. The absence of tenderness may imply that the enlargement is of long-standing duration. The liver of a patient with viral hepatitis is tender, whereas that of a patient with alcoholic hepatitis is not. Enlargement of the liver is an abnormal finding requiring evaluation.

Diagnostic Evaluation

LIVER FUNCTION TESTS

More than 70% of the parenchyma of the liver may be damaged before liver function test results become abnormal. Function is generally measured in terms of serum enzyme activity (ie, alkaline phosphatase, lactic dehydrogenase, serum aminotransferases) and serum concentrations of proteins (albumin and globulins), bilirubin, ammonia, clotting factors, and lipids. Several of these tests may be helpful for assessing patients with liver disease. However, the nature and extent of hepatic dysfunction cannot be determined by these tests alone, as many other disorders can affect their results.

Serum aminotransferases (also called transaminases) are sensitive indicators of injury to the liver cells and are useful in detecting acute liver disease such as hepatitis. Alanine aminotransferase (ALT) (formerly called serum glutamic-pyruvic transaminase [SGPT]), aspartate aminotransferase (AST) (formerly called serum glutamic-oxaloacetic transaminase [SGOT]), and gamma glutamyl transferase (GGT) (also called G-glutamyl transpeptidase) are the most frequently used tests of liver damage. ALT levels increase primarily in liver disorders and may be used to monitor the course of hepatitis or cirrhosis or the effects of treatments that may be toxic to the liver. AST is present in tissues that have high metabolic activity; thus, the level may be increased if there is damage to or death of tissues of organs such as the heart, liver, skeletal muscle, and kidney. Although not specific to liver disease, levels of AST may be increased in cirrhosis, hepatitis, and liver cancer. Increased GGT levels are associated with cholestasis but can also be due to alcoholic liver disease. Although the kidney has the highest level of the enzyme, the liver is considered the source of normal serum activity. The test determines liver cell dysfunction and is a sensitive indicator of cholestasis. Its main value in liver disease is confirming the hepatic origin of an elevated alkaline phosphatase level. Common liver function tests are listed in Table 39-1.

LIVER BIOPSY

Liver biopsy is the removal of a small amount of liver tissue, usually through needle aspiration. It permits examination of liver cells. The most common indication is to evaluate diffuse disorders of the parenchyma and to diagnose space-occupying lesions. Liver biopsy is especially useful when clinical findings and laboratory tests are not diagnostic. Bleeding and bile peritonitis after liver biopsy are the major complications; therefore, coagulation studies are obtained, their values are noted, and abnormal results are treated before liver biopsy is performed. Other techniques for liver biopsy are preferred if ascites or coagulation abnormalities exist. A liver biopsy can be performed percutaneously under ultrasound guidance or transvenously through the right internal jugular vein to right hepatic vein under fluoroscopic control. Liver biopsy can also be performed laparoscopically. Nursing responsibilities related to percutaneous liver biopsy are summarized in Chart 39-1.

FIGURE 39-3 Technique for palpating the liver. The examiner places one hand under the right lower rib cage and presses downward with light pressure with the other hand.

Table 39-1 • Liver Function Studies

TEST	NORMAL	CLINICAL FUNCTIONS
Pigment Studies		
Serum bilirubin, direct	0–5.1 μmol/L	These studies measure the ability of the liver to con-
Serum bilirubin, total	1.7–20.5 μmol/L	jugate and excrete bilirubin. Results are abnormal
Urine bilirubin	0	in liver and biliary tract disease and are associated
Urine urobilinogen	0.09–4.23 μmol/24 h	with jaundice clinically.
Fecal urobilinogen (infrequently used)	0.068–0.34 mmol/24 h	
Protein Studies		
Total serum protein	70–75 g/L	Proteins are manufactured by the liver. Their levels
Serum albumin	40–55 g/L	may be affected in a variety of liver impairments.
Serum globulin	17–33 g/L	Albumin: Cirrhosis
Serum protein electrophoresis		Chronic hepatitis
Albumin	40–55 g/L	Edema, ascites
α_1-Globulin	1.5–2.5 g/L	Globulin: Cirrhosis
α_2-Globulin	4.3–7.5 g/L	Liver disease
β-Globulin	5–10 g/L	Chronic obstructive jaundice
γ-Globulin	6–13 g/L	Viral hepatitis
Albumin/globulin (A/G) ratio	A > G or 1.5:1–2.5:1	A/G ratio is reversed in chronic liver disease (decreased albumin and increased globulin).
Prothrombin Time	100% or 12–16 seconds	Prothrombin time may be prolonged in liver disease. It will not return to normal with vitamin K in severe liver cell damage.
Serum Alkaline Phosphatase	Varies with method: 2–5 Bodansky units 17–142 U/L at 30°C (20–90 U/L at 30°C)	Serum alkaline phosphatase is manufactured in bones, liver, kidneys, and intestine and excreted through biliary tract. In absence of bone disease, it is a sensitive measure of biliary tract obstruction.
Serum Aminotransferase or Transaminase Studies		
AST (SGOT)	4.8–19 U/L	The studies are based on release of enzymes from
ALT (SGPT)	2.4–17 U/L	damaged liver cells. These enzymes are elevated in liver cell damage.
GGT, GGTP	10–48 U/L	Elevated in alcohol abuse. Marker for biliary
LDH	100–225 U/L	cholestasis.
Serum Ammonia	11.1–67.0 μmol/L 3.90–6.50 mmol/L	Liver converts ammonia to urea. Ammonia level rises in liver failure.
Cholesterol		
Ester	fraction of total cholesterol: 0.60	Cholesterol levels are elevated in biliary obstruction
HDL (high-density lipoprotein)	HDL Male: 0.91–1.81 mmol/L, Female: 0.91–2.20 mmol/L	and decreased in parenchymal liver disease.
LDL (low-density lipoprotein)	LDL < 3.40 mmol/L	

ADDITIONAL STUDIES	CLINICAL FUNCTIONS
Barium study of esophagus	For varices, which indicate increased portal blood pressure
Abdominal x-ray	To determine gross liver size
Liver scan with radiotagged iodinated rose bengal, gold, technetium, or gallium	To show size and shape of liver; to show replacement of liver tissue with scars, cysts, or tumour
Cholecystogram and cholangiogram	For gallbladder and bile duct visualization
Celiac axis arteriography	For liver and pancreas visualization
Splenoportogram (splenic portal venography)	To determine adequacy of portal blood flow
Laparoscopy	Direct visualization of anterior surface of liver, gallbladder, and mesentery through a trocar
Liver biopsy (percutaneous or transjugular)	To determine anatomic changes in liver tissue
Measurement of portal pressure	Elevated in cirrhosis of the liver
Esophagoscopy/endoscopy	To search for esophageal varices and other abnormalities
Electroencephalogram	Abnormal in hepatic coma and impending hepatic coma
Ultrasonography	To show size of abdominal organs and presence of masses
Computed tomography (CT scan)	To detect hepatic neoplasms; diagnose cysts, abscesses, and hematomas; and distinguish between obstructive and nonobstructive jaundice. Detects cerebral atrophy in hepatic encephalopathy.
Angiography	Visualizes hepatic circulation and detects presence and nature of hepatic masses
Magnetic resonance imaging (MRI)	To detect hepatic neoplasms; diagnose cysts, abscesses, and hematomas. Detects cerebral atrophy in encephalopathy.
Endoscopic retrograde cholangiopancreatography (ERCP)	Visualizes biliary structures via endoscopy

Chart 39-1

GUIDELINES FOR Assisting With Percutaneous Liver Biopsy

NURSING ACTIVITIES	RATIONALE
PREPROCEDURE	

1. Ascertain that results of coagulation tests (prothrombin time, partial thromboplastin time, and platelet count) are available and that compatible donor blood is available.

   Many patients with liver disease have clotting defects and are at risk for bleeding.

2. Check for signed consent; confirm that informed consent has been provided.

3. Measure and record the patient's pulse, respirations, and blood pressure immediately before biopsy.

   Prebiopsy values provide a basis on which to compare the patient's vital signs and evaluate status after the procedure.

4. Describe to the patient in advance: steps of the procedure; sensations expected; after-effects anticipated; restrictions of activity and monitoring procedures to follow.

   Explanations allay fears and ensure cooperation.

DURING PROCEDURE

5. Support the patient during the procedure.

   Encouragement and support of the nurse enhance comfort and promote a sense of security.

6. Expose the right side of the patient's upper abdomen (right hypochondriac).

   The skin at the site of penetration will be cleansed and a local anesthetic will be infiltrated.

7. Instruct the patient to inhale and exhale deeply several times, finally to exhale, and to hold breath at the end of expiration. The physician promptly introduces the biopsy needle by way of the transthoracic (intercostal) or transabdominal (subcostal) route, penetrates the liver, aspirates, and withdraws.

   Holding the breath immobilizes the chest wall and the diaphragm; penetration of the diaphragm thereby is avoided, and the risk of lacerating the liver is minimized.

8. Instruct the patient to resume breathing.

POSTPROCEDURE

9. Immediately after the biopsy, assist the patient to turn onto the right side; place a pillow under the costal margin, and caution the patient to remain in this position, recumbent and immobile, for several hours. Instruct the patient to avoid coughing or straining.

   In this position, the liver capsule at the site of penetration is compressed against the chest wall, and the escape of blood or bile through the perforation is prevented.

10. Measure and record the patient's pulse, respiratory rate, and blood pressure at 10- to 15-minute intervals for the first hour, then every 30 minutes for the next 1 to 2 hours or until the patient's condition stabilizes.

    Changes in vital signs may indicate bleeding, severe hemorrhage, or bile peritonitis, the most frequent complications of liver biopsy.

11. If the patient is discharged after the procedure, instruct the patient to avoid heavy lifting and strenuous activity for 1 week.

    Activity restriction reduces the risk of bleeding at the biopsy puncture site.

OTHER DIAGNOSTIC TESTS

Ultrasonography, computed tomography (CT), and magnetic resonance imaging (MRI) are used to identify normal structures and abnormalities of the liver and biliary tree. A radioisotope liver scan may be performed to assess liver size and hepatic blood flow and obstruction.

Laparoscopy (insertion of a fibre-optic endoscope through a small abdominal incision) is used to examine the liver and other pelvic structures. It is also used to perform guided liver biopsy, to determine the etiology of ascites, and to diagnose and stage tumours of the liver and other abdominal organs.

Hepatic Dysfunction

Hepatic dysfunction results from damage to the liver's parenchymal cells, either directly from primary liver diseases or indirectly from obstruction of bile flow or derangements of hepatic circulation. Liver dysfunction may be acute or chronic; chronic dysfunction is far more common than acute.

The impact of liver disease on the Canadian health care system may be greater than previously thought. Statistics Canada (2005) reports chronic liver disease and **cirrhosis** as the 13th most common cause of death among Canadians. This includes only the 40.2% of deaths associated with liver disease as viral hepatitis and neoplasms of the liver are reported separately (Desai & Peltekian, 2004). Hepatitis C is now the leading cause of liver disease in Canada (Public Health Agency of Canada, 2004). The rate of liver disease for men is almost twice that for women and is more common among Aboriginal than Caucasian Canadians.

Disease processes that lead to hepatocellular dysfunction may be caused by infectious agents such as bacteria and viruses and by anoxia, metabolic disorders, toxins and medications, nutritional deficiencies, and hypersensitivity states. The most common cause of parenchymal damage is malnutrition, especially that related to alcoholism.

The parenchymal cells respond to most noxious agents by replacing glycogen with lipids, producing fatty infiltration with or without cell death or necrosis. This is commonly associated with inflammatory cell infiltration and growth of fibrous tissue. Cell regeneration can occur if the disease process is not too toxic to the cells. The result of chronic parenchymal disease is the shrunken, fibrotic liver seen in cirrhosis.

The consequences of liver disease are numerous and varied. Their ultimate effects are often incapacitating or life-threatening, and their presence is ominous. Treatment often is difficult. Among the most common and significant symptoms of liver disease are the following:

- Jaundice, resulting from increased bilirubin concentration in the blood
- Portal hypertension, ascites, and varices, resulting from circulatory changes within the diseased liver and producing severe GI hemorrhages and marked sodium and fluid retention
- Nutritional deficiencies, which result from the inability of the damaged liver cells to metabolize certain vitamins; responsible for impaired functioning of the central and peripheral nervous systems and for abnormal bleeding tendencies
- Hepatic encephalopathy or coma, reflecting accumulation of ammonia in the serum due to impaired protein metabolism by the diseased liver

JAUNDICE

When the bilirubin concentration in the blood is abnormally elevated, all the body tissues, including the sclerae and the skin, become yellow-tinged or greenish-yellow, a condition called jaundice. Jaundice becomes clinically evident when the serum bilirubin level exceeds 43 µmol/L. Increased serum bilirubin levels and jaundice may result from impairment of hepatic uptake, conjugation of bilirubin, or excretion of bilirubin into the biliary system. There are several types of jaundice: hemolytic, hepatocellular, obstructive, or jaundice due to hereditary hyperbilirubinemia. Hepatocellular and obstructive jaundice are the two types commonly associated with liver disease.

Hemolytic Jaundice

Hemolytic jaundice is the result of an increased destruction of the red blood cells, the effect of which is to flood the plasma with bilirubin so rapidly that the liver, although functioning normally, cannot excrete the bilirubin as quickly as it is formed. This type of jaundice is encountered in patients with hemolytic transfusion reactions and other hemolytic disorders. The bilirubin in the blood of these patients is predominantly of the unconjugated, or free, type. Fecal and urine urobilinogen levels are increased, but the urine is free of bilirubin. Patients with this type of jaundice, unless their hyperbilirubinemia is extreme, do not experience symptoms or complications as a result of the jaundice per se. Prolonged jaundice, however, even if mild, predisposes to the formation of pigment stones in the gallbladder, and extremely severe jaundice (levels of free bilirubin exceeding 300 to 400 µmol/L) poses a risk for brain stem damage.

Hepatocellular Jaundice

Hepatocellular jaundice is caused by the inability of damaged liver cells to clear normal amounts of bilirubin from the blood. The cellular damage may be from infection, such as in viral hepatitis (eg, hepatitis A, B, C, D, or E) or other viruses that affect the liver (eg, yellow fever virus, Epstein-Barr virus), from medication or chemical toxicity (eg, carbon tetrachloride, chloroform, phosphorus, arsenicals, certain medications), or from alcohol. Cirrhosis of the liver is a form of hepatocellular disease that may produce jaundice. It is usually associated with excessive alcohol intake, but it may also be a late result of liver cell necrosis caused by viral infection. In prolonged obstructive jaundice, cell damage eventually develops, so that both types appear together.

Patients with hepatocellular jaundice may be mildly or severely ill, with lack of appetite, nausea, malaise, fatigue, weakness, and possible weight loss. In some cases of hepatocellular disease, jaundice may not be obvious. The serum bilirubin concentration and urine urobilinogen level may be elevated. In addition, AST and ALT levels may be increased, indicating cellular necrosis. The patient may report headache, chills, and fever if the cause is infectious. Depending on the cause and extent of the liver cell damage, hepatocellular jaundice may or may not be completely reversible.

Obstructive Jaundice

Obstructive jaundice of the extrahepatic type may be caused by occlusion of the bile duct by a gallstone, an inflammatory process, a tumour, or pressure from an enlarged organ. The obstruction may also involve the small bile ducts within the liver (ie, intrahepatic obstruction), caused, for example, by pressure on these channels from inflammatory swelling of the liver or by an inflammatory exudate within the ducts themselves. Intrahepatic obstruction resulting from stasis and inspissation (thickening) of bile within the canaliculi may occur after the ingestion of certain medications, which are referred to as cholestatic agents. These include phenothiazines, antithyroid medications, sulfonylureas, tricyclic antidepressant agents, nitrofurantoin, androgens, and estrogens.

Whether the obstruction is intrahepatic or extrahepatic, and whatever its cause may be, bile cannot flow normally into the intestine but is backed up into the liver substance. It is then reabsorbed into the blood and carried throughout the entire body, staining the skin, mucous membranes, and sclerae. It is excreted in the urine, which becomes deep orange and foamy. Because of the decreased amount of bile in the intestinal tract, the stools become light or clay-coloured. The skin may itch intensely, requiring repeated soothing baths. Dyspepsia and intolerance to fatty foods may develop because of impaired fat digestion in the absence of intestinal bile. AST, ALT, and GGT levels generally rise only moderately, but bilirubin and alkaline phosphatase levels are elevated.

Hereditary Hyperbilirubinemia

Increased serum bilirubin levels (hyperbilirubinemia) resulting from several inherited disorders can also produce jaundice. Gilbert's syndrome is a familial disorder characterized by an increased level of unconjugated bilirubin that causes jaundice. Although serum bilirubin levels are increased, liver histology and liver function test results are normal, and there is no hemolysis. This syndrome affects 3% to 7% of the population.

Other conditions that are probably caused by inborn errors of biliary metabolism include Dubin–Johnson syndrome (chronic idiopathic jaundice, with pigment in the liver) and Rotor's syndrome (chronic familial conjugated hyperbilirubinemia without pigment in the liver); "benign" cholestatic jaundice of pregnancy, with retention of conjugated bilirubin, probably secondary to unusual sensitivity to the hormones of pregnancy; and probably also benign recurrent intrahepatic cholestasis.

PORTAL HYPERTENSION

Obstructed blood flow through the damaged liver results in increased blood pressure (**portal hypertension**) throughout the portal venous system. Although portal hypertension is commonly associated with hepatic cirrhosis, it can also occur with noncirrhotic liver disease. While splenomegaly (enlarged spleen) with possible hypersplenism is a common manifestation of portal hypertension, two major consequences of portal hypertension are ascites and varices.

In ascites, fluid accumulates in the abdominal cavity. Although ascites is often a result of liver damage, it may also occur with disorders such as cancer, kidney disease, and heart failure. Varices are varicosities that develop from elevated pressures transmitted to all of the veins that drain into the portal system. They are prone to rupture and often are the source of massive hemorrhages from the upper GI tract and the rectum. In addition, blood clotting abnormalities, often seen in patients with severe liver disease, increase the likelihood of bleeding.

ASCITES

Pathophysiology

The mechanisms responsible for the development of ascites are not completely understood. Portal hypertension and the resulting increase in capillary pressure and obstruction of venous blood flow through the damaged liver are contributing factors. The failure of the liver to metabolize aldosterone increases sodium and

water retention by the kidney. Sodium and water retention, increased intravascular fluid volume, and decreased synthesis of albumin by the damaged liver all contribute to fluid moving from the vascular system into the peritoneal space. Loss of fluid into the peritoneal space causes further sodium and water retention by the kidney in an effort to maintain the vascular fluid volume, and the process becomes self-perpetuating.

As a result of liver damage, large amounts of albumin-rich fluid, 15 L or more, may accumulate in the peritoneal cavity as ascites. With the movement of albumin from the serum to the peritoneal cavity, the osmotic pressure of the serum decreases. This, combined with increased portal pressure, results in movement of fluid into the peritoneal cavity (Fig. 39-4).

Clinical Manifestations

Increased abdominal girth and rapid weight gain are common presenting symptoms of ascites. The patient may be short of breath and uncomfortable from the enlarged abdomen, and striae and distended veins may be visible over the abdominal wall. Fluid and electrolyte imbalances are common.

Assessment and Diagnostic Evaluation

The presence and extent of ascites are assessed by percussion of the abdomen. When fluid has accumulated in the peritoneal cavity, the flanks bulge when the patient assumes a supine position. The presence of fluid can be confirmed either by percussing for shifting dullness or by detecting a fluid wave (Fig. 39-5). A fluid wave

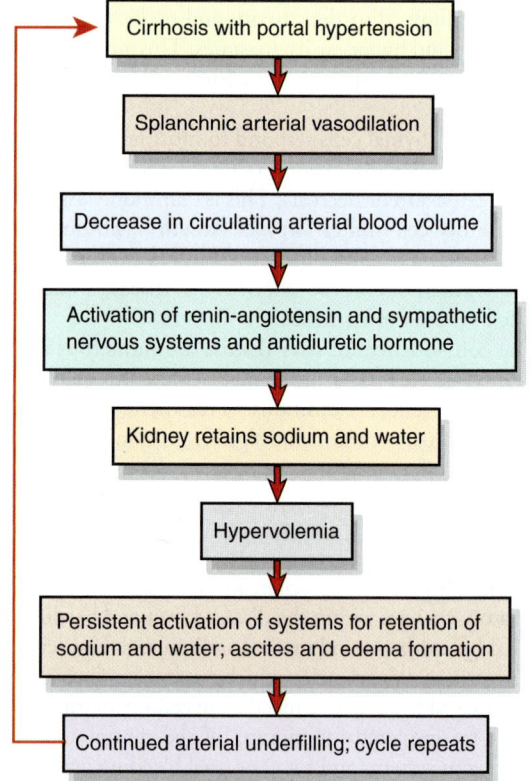

FIGURE 39-4 Pathogenesis of ascites (arterial vasodilation theory).

FIGURE 39-5 Assessing for abdominal fluid wave. The examiner places the hands along the side of the patient's flank, then strikes one flank sharply, detecting any fluid wave with the other hand. An assistant's hand is placed (ulnar side down) along the patient's midline to prevent the fluid wave from being transmitted through the tissues of the abdominal wall.

is likely to be found only when a large amount of fluid is present. Daily measurement and recording of abdominal girth and body weight are essential to assess the progression of ascites and its response to treatment.

Medical Management

DIETARY MODIFICATION

The goal of treatment for the patient with ascites is a negative sodium balance to reduce fluid retention. Table salt, salty foods, salted butter and margarine, and all ordinary canned and frozen foods (foods that are not specifically prepared for low-sodium diets) should be avoided. It may take 2 to 3 months for the patient's taste buds to adjust to unsalted foods. In the meantime, the taste of unsalted foods can be improved by using salt substitutes such as lemon juice, oregano, and thyme. Commercial salt substitutes need to be approved by the physician because those containing ammonia could precipitate hepatic coma. Most salt substitutes contain potassium and should be avoided if the patient has impaired renal function. The patient should make liberal use of powdered, low-sodium milk and milk products. If fluid accumulation is not controlled with this regimen, the daily sodium allowance may be reduced further to 500 mg, and diuretics may be administered.

Dietary control of ascites via strict sodium restriction is difficult to achieve at home. The likelihood that the patient will follow even a 2-g sodium diet increases if the patient and the person preparing meals understand the rationale for the diet and receive periodic guidance about selecting and preparing appropriate foods. Approximately 10% of patients with ascites respond to these measures alone. Nonresponders and those who find sodium restriction difficult require diuretic therapy.

DIURETICS

Use of diuretics along with sodium restriction is successful in 90% of patients with ascites. Spironolactone (Aldactone), an aldosterone-blocking agent, is most often the first-line therapy in patients with ascites from cirrhosis. When used with other diuretics, spironolactone helps prevent potassium loss. Oral diuretics such as furosemide (Lasix) may be added but should be used cautiously because with long-term use they may also induce severe sodium depletion (hyponatremia).

Ammonium chloride and acetazolamide (Diamox) are contraindicated because of the possibility of precipitating hepatic coma. Daily weight loss should not exceed 1 to 2 kg in patients with ascites and peripheral edema or 0.5 to 0.75 kg in patients without edema. Fluid restriction is not attempted unless the serum sodium concentration is very low.

Possible complications of diuretic therapy include fluid and electrolyte disturbances (including hypovolemia, hypokalemia, hyponatremia, and hypochloremic alkalosis) and encephalopathy. Encephalopathy may be precipitated by dehydration and hypovolemia. Also, when potassium stores are depleted, the amount of ammonia in the systemic circulation increases, which may cause impaired cerebral functioning and encephalopathy.

BED REST

In patients with ascites, an upright posture is associated with activation of the renin-angiotensin-aldosterone system and sympathetic nervous system (Porth, 2002). This results in reduced renal glomerular filtration and sodium excretion and a decreased response to loop diuretics. Bed rest may be a useful therapy, especially for patients whose condition is refractory to diuretics.

PARACENTESIS

Paracentesis is the removal of fluid (ascites) from the peritoneal cavity through a small surgical incision or puncture made through the abdominal wall under sterile conditions. Ultrasound guidance may be indicated in some patients at high risk for bleeding because of an abnormal coagulation profile or in those who have had previous abdominal surgery and who may have adhesions. Paracentesis was once considered a routine form of treatment for ascites but is now performed primarily for diagnostic examination of ascitic fluid, for treatment of massive ascites that is resistant to nutritional and diuretic therapy and that is causing severe problems to the patient, and as a prelude to diagnostic imaging studies, peritoneal dialysis, or surgery. A sample of the ascitic fluid may be sent to the laboratory for analysis. Cell count, albumin and total protein levels, culture, and occasionally other tests are performed.

Use of large-volume (5 to 6 litres) paracentesis has been shown to be a safe method for treating patients with severe ascites. This technique, in combination with the intravenous infusion of salt-poor albumin or other colloid, has become the standard treatment for refractory, massive ascites (Krige & Beckingham, 2001; Menon & Kamath, 2000). The salt-poor albumin helps reduce edema by causing the ascitic fluid to be drawn back into the bloodstream and ultimately eliminated by the kidneys. The procedure provides only temporary removal of fluid; it rapidly recurs, necessitating repeated removal. Nursing care of the patient undergoing paracentesis is presented in Chart 39-2.

OTHER METHODS OF TREATMENT

Insertion of a peritoneovenous shunt to redirect ascitic fluid from the peritoneal cavity into the systemic circulation is a treatment modality for ascites, but this procedure is seldom used because of the high complication rate and high incidence of shunt failure. The shunt is reserved for those who are resistant to diuretic therapy, are not candidates for liver transplantation, have abdominal adhesions, or are ineligible for other procedures because of severe medical conditions, such as cardiac disease.

Chart 39-2 Assisting With a Paracentesis

Preprocedure

1. Prepare the patient by providing the necessary information and instructions about the procedure and by offering reassurance.
2. Instruct the patient to void.
3. Gather appropriate sterile equipment and collection receptacles.
4. Place patient in upright position on edge of bed with feet supported on stool, or place in chair. Fowler's position should be used for the patient confined to bed.
5. Place sphygmomanometer cuff around patient's arm to allow monitoring of blood pressure during the procedure.

Procedure

1. The physician, using aseptic technique, inserts the trocar through a puncture wound below the umbilicus. The fluid drains from the abdomen through a drainage tube into a container.
2. Help the patient maintain position throughout procedure.
3. Measure and record blood pressure at frequent intervals from the beginning of the procedure.
4. Monitor the patient closely for signs of vascular collapse: pallor, increased pulse rate, or decreased blood pressure.

Postprocedure

1. Return patient to bed or to a comfortable sitting position.
2. Measure, describe, and record the fluid collected.
3. Label samples of fluid and send to laboratory.
4. Continue to monitor vital signs every 15 minutes for 1 hour, every 30 minutes over 2 hours, then every hour over 2 hours and then every 4 hours. Monitor temperature after procedure and every 4 hours.
5. Assess for hypovolemia, electrolyte loss, changes in mental status, and encephalopathy.
6. Check puncture site when taking vital signs for bleeding and leakage.
7. Provide patient education (especially if patient is discharged after procedure) regarding monitoring for bleeding or excess drainage from puncture site, avoiding heavy lifting or straining, changing position slowly, and monitoring for fever.

Figure on *left* shows possible sites for insertion of trocar.

Nursing Management

If a patient with ascites from liver dysfunction is hospitalized, nursing measures include assessment and documentation of intake and output, abdominal girth, and daily weight to assess fluid status. The nurse monitors serum ammonia and electrolyte levels to assess electrolyte balance, response to therapy, and indicators of encephalopathy.

PROMOTING HOME AND COMMUNITY-BASED CARE

Teaching Patients Self-Care. The patient treated for ascites is likely to be discharged with some ascites still present. Before hospital discharge, the nurse teaches the patient and family about the treatment plan, including the need to avoid all alcohol intake, adhere to a low-sodium diet, take medications as prescribed, and check with the physician before taking any new medications (Chart 39-3). Additional patient and family teaching addresses skin care and the need to weigh the patient daily and to watch for and report signs and symptoms of complications.

Continuing Care. A referral for home care may be warranted, especially if the patient lives alone or cannot provide self-care. The home visit enables the nurse to assess changes in the patient's condition and weight, abdominal girth, skin, and cognitive and emotional status. The home care nurse assesses the home environment and the availability of resources needed to adhere to the treatment plan (eg, a scale to obtain daily weights, facilities to prepare and store appropriate foods, resources to purchase needed medications). It is important to assess the patient's adherence to the treatment plan and the ability to buy, prepare, and eat

Chart 39-3
Home Care Checklist • Management of Ascites

At the completion of the home care instruction, the patient or caregiver will be able to: | **Patient** | **Caregiver**

- Make appropriate dietary choices consistent with dietary prescription and recommendations. ✓ ✓
- State the importance of weighing self daily and keeping a daily record of weight. ✓ ✓
- Maintain record of weight daily and identify daily weight-loss goals. ✓ ✓
- List weight changes (loss or gain) that should be reported to the primary health care provider. ✓ ✓
- Explain the rationale for monitoring and recording daily intake and output. ✓ ✓
- Identify changes in output that should be reported to primary health care provider (decreasing urine output). ✓ ✓
- Identify rationale for fluid restrictions (if needed), and comply with fluid restriction. ✓ ✓
- Discuss importance of avoiding nonsteroidal anti-inflammatory agents, medications (eg, cough mixtures) containing alcohol, antibiotics or antacids containing salt. ✓ ✓
- Describe effects, side effects, and monitoring parameters for diuretic therapy. ✓ ✓
- Identify need to stop all alcohol intake as critical to well-being. ✓ ✓
- Explain how to contact Alcoholics Anonymous or alcohol counselors in related organizations. ✓ ✓
- Demonstrate how to care for skin, alleviate pressure over bony prominences by turning when in bed or chair, and decrease edema by position changes. ✓ ✓
- Identify early signs and symptoms of complications (encephalopathy, spontaneous bacterial peritonitis, dehydration, electrolyte abnormalities, azotemia). ✓ ✓

appropriate foods. The nurse reinforces previous teaching and emphasizes the need for regular follow-up and the importance of keeping scheduled health care appointments.

ESOPHAGEAL VARICES

Bleeding or hemorrhage from esophageal varices occurs in approximately one third of patients with cirrhosis and varices. The mortality rate resulting from the first bleeding episode is 45% to 50%; it is one of the major causes of death in patients with cirrhosis (Pomier-Layrargues, Villeneuve, Deschenes et al., 2001). The mortality rate increases with each subsequent bleeding episode.

Pathophysiology

Esophageal varices are dilated, tortuous veins usually found in the submucosa of the lower esophagus, but they may develop higher in the esophagus or extend into the stomach. This condition nearly always is caused by portal hypertension, which in turn is due to obstruction of the portal venous circulation within the damaged liver.

Because of increased obstruction of the portal vein, venous blood from the intestinal tract and spleen seeks an outlet through collateral circulation (new pathways of return to the right atrium). The effect is increased pressure, particularly in the vessels in the submucosal layer of the lower esophagus and upper part of the stomach. These collateral vessels are not very elastic but rather are tortuous and fragile and bleed easily (Fig. 39-6). Less common causes of varices are abnormalities of the circulation in the splenic vein or superior vena cava and hepatic venothrombosis.

Bleeding esophageal varices are life-threatening and can result in hemorrhagic shock, producing decreased cerebral, hepatic, and renal perfusion. In turn, there is an increased nitrogen load from bleeding into the GI tract and an increased serum ammonia level, increasing the risk for encephalopathy. Usually the dilated veins cause no symptoms unless the portal pressure increases sharply and the mucosa or supporting structures become thin. Then massive hemorrhage takes place.

Factors that contribute to hemorrhage are muscular exertion from lifting heavy objects; straining at stool; sneezing, coughing, or

vomiting; esophagitis; irritation of vessels by poorly chewed foods or irritating fluids; or reflux of stomach contents (especially alcohol). Salicylates and any medication that erodes the esophageal mucosa or interferes with cell replication also may contribute to bleeding.

Clinical Manifestations

The patient with bleeding esophageal varices may present with hematemesis, melena, or general deterioration in mental or physical status and often has a history of alcohol abuse. Signs and

Physiology/Pathophysiology

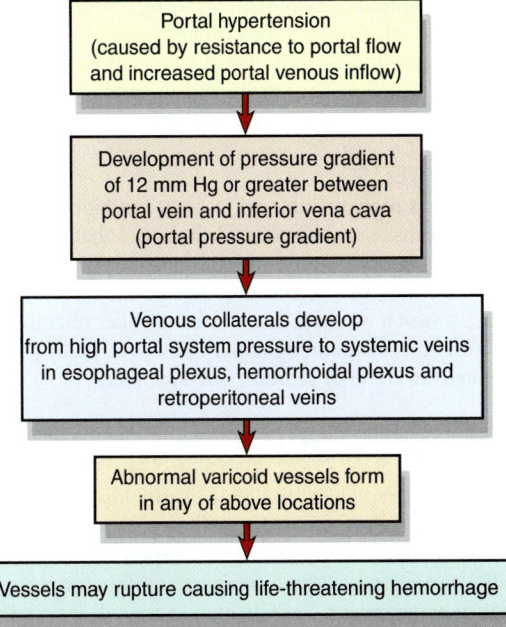

FIGURE 39-6 Pathogenesis of bleeding esophageal varices.

symptoms of shock (cool clammy skin, hypotension, tachycardia) may be present.

Assessment and Diagnostic Findings

Endoscopy is used to identify the bleeding site, along with barium swallow, ultrasonography, CT, and angiography.

ENDOSCOPY

Immediate endoscopy (see Chap. 34) is indicated to identify the cause and the site of bleeding; at least 30% of patients suspected of bleeding from esophageal varices bleed from other sources (gastritis, ulcers). Nursing support can be effective in relieving anxiety during this often-stressful experience. Careful monitoring can detect early signs of cardiac dysrhythmias, perforation, and hemorrhage.

After the examination, fluids are not given until the gag reflex returns. Lozenges and gargles may be used to relieve throat discomfort if the patient's physical condition and mental status permit. If the patient is actively bleeding, oral intake will not be permitted and the patient will be prepared for further diagnostic and therapeutic procedures.

PORTAL HYPERTENSION MEASUREMENTS

Portal hypertension may be suspected if dilated abdominal veins and hemorrhoids are detected. A palpable enlarged spleen (splenomegaly) and ascites may also be present. Portal venous pressure can be measured directly or indirectly. Indirect measurement of the hepatic vein pressure gradient is the most common procedure; it requires insertion of a fluid-filled balloon catheter into the antecubital or femoral vein. The catheter is advanced under fluoroscopy to a hepatic vein. A "wedged" pressure (similar to pulmonary artery wedge pressure) is obtained by occluding the blood flow in the blood vessel; pressure in the unoccluded vessel is also measured. Although the values obtained may underestimate portal pressure, this measurement may be obtained several times to evaluate the results of therapy.

Direct measurement of portal vein pressure can be obtained by several methods. During laparotomy, a needle may be introduced into the spleen; a manometer reading of more than 20 mL saline is abnormal. Another direct measurement requires insertion of a catheter into the portal vein or one of its branches. Endoscopic measurement of pressure within varices is used only in conjunction with endoscopic sclerotherapy.

LABORATORY TESTS

Laboratory tests may include various liver function tests, such as serum aminotransferase, bilirubin, alkaline phosphatase, and serum proteins. Splenoportography, which involves serial or segmental x-rays, is used to detect extensive collateral circulation in esophageal vessels, which would indicate varices. Other tests are hepatoportography and celiac angiography. These are usually performed in the operating room or radiology department.

Medical Management

Bleeding from esophageal varices can quickly lead to hemorrhagic shock and is an emergency. This patient is critically ill, requiring aggressive medical care and expert nursing care, and is usually transferred to the intensive care unit for close monitoring and management. See Chapter 15 for a discussion of care of the patient in shock.

The extent of bleeding is evaluated and vital signs are monitored continuously when hematemesis and melena are present. Signs of potential hypovolemia are noted, such as cold clammy skin, tachycardia, a drop in blood pressure, decreased urine output, restlessness, and weak peripheral pulses. Blood volume is monitored by a central venous pressure or arterial catheter. Oxygen is administered to prevent hypoxia and to maintain adequate blood oxygenation.

Because patients with bleeding esophageal varices have intravascular volume depletion and are subject to electrolyte imbalance, intravenous fluids with electrolytes and volume expanders are provided to restore fluid volume and replace electrolytes. Transfusion of blood components also may be required. An indwelling urinary catheter is usually inserted to permit frequent monitoring of urine output.

A variety of pharmacologic, endoscopic, and surgical approaches are used to treat bleeding esophageal varices, but none is ideal and most are associated with considerable risk to the patient. Nonsurgical treatment of bleeding esophageal varices is preferable because of the high mortality rate of emergency surgery for control of bleeding esophageal varices and because of the poor physical condition of the patient with severe liver dysfunction.

PHARMACOLOGIC THERAPY

In an actively bleeding patient, medications are administered initially because they can be obtained and administered quickly; other therapies take longer to initiate. Vasopressin (Pitressin) may be the initial mode of therapy because it produces constriction of the splanchnic arterial bed and a resulting decrease in portal pressure. It may be administered intravenously or by intra-arterial infusion (Menon & Kamath, 2000). Either method requires close monitoring by the nurse. Vital signs and the presence or absence of blood in the gastric aspirate indicate the effectiveness of vasopressin. Monitoring of fluid intake and output and electrolyte levels is necessary because hyponatremia may occur and vasopressin may have an antidiuretic effect. Coronary artery disease is a contraindication to the use of vasopressin, because coronary vasoconstriction is a side effect that may precipitate myocardial infarction.

The combination of vasopressin and nitroglycerin (administered by the intravenous, sublingual, or transdermal route) has been effective in reducing or preventing the side effects (constriction of coronary vessels and angina) caused by vasopressin alone.

Somatostatin and octreotide (Sandostatin) have been reported to be more effective than vasopressin in decreasing bleeding from esophageal varices without the vasoconstrictive effects of vasopressin. These medications cause selective splanchnic vasoconstriction. Propranolol (Inderal) and nadolol (Corgard), beta-blocking agents that decrease portal pressure, have been shown to prevent bleeding from esophageal varices in some patients; however, it is recommended that they be used only in combination with other treatment modalities such as sclerotherapy, variceal banding, or balloon tamponade. Nitrates such as isosorbide (Isordil) lower portal pressure by venodilation and decreased cardiac output. Further studies of these and other medications are necessary to evaluate their use in the treatment and prevention of bleeding episodes.

BALLOON TAMPONADE

To control hemorrhage in certain patients, **balloon tamponade** may be used. In this procedure, pressure is exerted on the cardia (upper orifice of the stomach) and against the bleeding varices by a double-balloon tamponade (Sengstaken-Blakemore tube) (Fig. 39-7). The tube has four openings, each with a specific purpose: gastric aspiration, esophageal aspiration, inflation of the gastric balloon, and inflation of the esophageal balloon.

The balloon in the stomach is inflated with 100 to 200 mL of air. An x-ray confirms proper positioning of the gastric balloon. Then the tube is pulled gently to exert a force against the gastric

FIGURE 39-7 Esophageal balloon tamponade to treat esophageal varices. (**A**) Dilated, bleeding esophageal veins (varices) of the lower esophagus. (**B**) A four-lumen esophageal tamponade tube with balloons (uninflated) in place. (**C**) Compression of bleeding esophageal varices by inflated esophageal and gastric balloons. The gastric and esophageal outlets permit the nurse to aspirate secretions.

cardia. Traction may be applied with weights or by attachment to a football helmet. Irrigation of the tubing is performed to detect bleeding; if returns are clear, the esophageal balloon is not inflated. If bleeding continues, the esophageal balloon is inflated. The desired pressure in the esophageal and gastric balloons is 25 to 40 mm Hg, as measured by the manometer. There is a possibility of injury or rupture of the esophagus with inflation of the esophageal balloon, so constant nursing surveillance is necessary.

Gastric suction is provided by connecting the gastric catheter outlet to suction. The tubing is irrigated hourly, and drainage will indicate whether bleeding has been controlled. Room-temperature lavage or irrigation may be used in the gastric balloon. The pressure within the esophageal balloon is measured and recorded every 2 to 4 hours via the manometer to detect underinflation or overinflation with potential for esophageal injury. When it appears that bleeding has stopped, the balloons are carefully and sequentially deflated. The esophageal balloon is deflated first and the patient is monitored for recurrent bleeding. After several hours without bleeding, the gastric balloon may be deflated safely. If there is still no bleeding, the tamponade tube is removed. The therapy is used for as short a time as possible to control bleeding while emergency treatment is completed and definitive therapies are instituted (no longer than 24 hours).

Although balloon tamponade has been fairly successful, there are some inherent dangers. Displacement of the tube and the inflated balloon into the oropharynx can cause life-threatening obstruction of the airway and asphyxiation. This may occur if a patient pulls on the tube because of confusion or discomfort. It may also result from rupture of the gastric balloon, allowing the esophageal balloon to move into the oropharynx. Sudden rupture of the balloon causes airway obstruction and aspiration of gastric contents into the lungs. The tube is tested before insertion to minimize this risk. Aspiration of blood and secretions into the lungs is frequently associated with balloon tamponade, especially in the stuporous or comatose patient. Endotracheal intubation before insertion of the tube protects the airway and minimizes the risk of aspiration. Ulceration and necrosis of the nose, the mucosa of the stomach, or the esophagus may occur if the tube is left in place or inflated too long or at too high a pressure.

> **NURSING ALERT** The patient being treated with balloon tamponade must never be left alone because of the risk for serious complications. The patient must be monitored closely and continuously. Precautions must be taken to ensure that the patient does not pull on or inadvertently displace the tube.

These potential complications necessitate intensive and expert care. A confused or restless patient with this tube in place and balloons inflated requires close monitoring to prevent its displacement. Nursing measures include frequent mouth and nasal care. For secretions that accumulate in the mouth, tissues should be within easy reach of the patient. Oral suction may be necessary to remove oral secretions. Because of the many potential complications, balloon tamponade tubes are used only as a temporary measure.

The patient with esophageal hemorrhage is usually extremely anxious and frightened. Knowing that the nurse is nearby and will respond immediately can help alleviate some of this anxiety. Tube insertion is uncomfortable and never pleasant. Explanations during the procedure and while the tube is in place may be reassuring to the patient.

Although the use of balloon tamponade stops the bleeding in 90% of patients, bleeding recurs in 60% to 70%, necessitating other treatment modalities (eg, sclerotherapy or banding) (Menon & Kamath, 2000). Once the balloons are deflated or the tube is removed, the patient must be assessed frequently because of the high risk for recurrent bleeding.

ENDOSCOPIC SCLEROTHERAPY

In endoscopic **sclerotherapy** (Fig. 39-8) (also referred to as injection sclerotherapy), a sclerosing agent is injected through a fibreoptic endoscope into the bleeding esophageal varices to promote thrombosis and eventual sclerosis. The procedure has been used successfully to treat acute GI hemorrhage (Menon & Kamath, 2000; O'Grady et al., 2000). Endoscopic variceal sclerotherapy has been used in the primary prophylaxis of variceal bleeding, but the results are poorer than those of pharmacotherapy (Sarin, Lamba, Kumar et al., 1999).

After treatment, the patient must be observed for bleeding, perforation of the esophagus, aspiration pneumonia, and esophageal stricture. Antacids may be administered after the procedure to counteract the effects of peptic reflux.

ESOPHAGEAL BANDING THERAPY (VARICEAL BAND LIGATION)

In **variceal banding** (Fig. 39-9), a modified endoscope loaded with an elastic rubber band is passed through an overtube directly onto the varix (or varices) to be banded. After suctioning the bleeding varix into the tip of the endoscope, the rubber band is slipped over the tissue, causing necrosis, ulceration, and eventual sloughing of the varix.

FIGURE 39-8 Endoscopic or injection sclerotherapy. Injection of sclerosing agent into esophageal varices through an endoscope promotes thrombosis and eventual sclerosis, thereby obliterating the varices.

Pre-emptive variceal banding is superior to endoscopic sclerotherapy in the effective prevention of bleeding. Compared with sclerotherapy, variceal banding also significantly reduces rebleeding rates, mortality, procedure-related complications, and the number of sessions needed to eradicate varices (de Franchis & Primighani, 1999). Complications include superficial ulceration and dysphagia, transient chest discomfort, and rarely esophageal strictures (Menon & Kamath, 2000). Recently, endoscopic variceal band ligation has been shown to be safe and more effective than propranolol for preventing a first bleeding episode (Sarin et al., 1999). Scolerotherapy and banding are equivalent in the emergency setting.

TRANSJUGULAR INTRAHEPATIC PORTOSYSTEMIC SHUNTING

Transjugular intrahepatic portosystemic shunting (TIPS) is a method of treating esophageal varices in which a cannula is threaded into the portal vein by the transjugular route. An expandable stent is inserted and serves as an intrahepatic shunt between the portal circulation and the hepatic vein (Fig. 39-10), reducing portal hypertension.

Creation of a TIPS is indicated for the treatment of recurrent variceal bleeding refractory to pharmacologic or endoscopic therapy. It has also been indicated for the control of refractory ascites. This technique is also used as a bridge to liver transplantation. Complications may include bleeding, sepsis, heart failure, organ perforation, shunt thrombosis, and progressive liver failure (Pomier-Layrargues et al., 2001).

SURGICAL MANAGEMENT

Several surgical procedures have been developed to treat esophageal varices and to minimize rebleeding, but they are often accompanied by significant risk. Procedures that may be used for esophageal varices are direct surgical ligation of varices; splenorenal, mesocaval, and portacaval venous shunts to relieve portal pressure; and esophageal transection with devascularization. Use of these procedures is controversial, and studies regarding their effectiveness and outcomes are ongoing (Bacon & Di Bisceglie, 2000).

Surgical Bypass Procedures. Surgical decompression of the portal circulation can prevent variceal bleeding if the shunt remains patent (Bacon & Di Bisceglie, 2000). One of the various surgical shunting procedures (Fig. 39-11) is the distal splenorenal shunt made between the splenic vein and the left renal vein after splenectomy. A mesocaval shunt is created by anastomosing the superior mesenteric vein to the proximal end of the vena cava or to the side of the vena cava using grafting material. The goal of distal splenorenal and mesocaval shunts is to drain only a portion of venous blood from the portal bed to decrease portal pressure; thus, they are considered selective shunts. The liver continues to receive some portal flow, and the incidence of encephalopathy may be reduced. Portacaval shunts divert all portal flow to the vena cava via end-to-side or side-to-side approaches, so they are considered nonselective shunts.

These procedures are extensive and are not always successful because of secondary thrombosis in the veins used for the shunt as well as complications (eg, encephalopathy, accelerated liver failure). The efficacy of these procedures has been studied extensively. The most recent studies have found that all shunts are equally effective in preventing recurrent variceal bleeding but may cause further impairment of liver function and encephalopathy. Partial portacaval shunts with interposition grafts are as effective as other shunts but are associated with a lower rate of encephalopathy (de Franchis, 2000; Krige & Beckingham, 2001; Orozco & Mercado, 2000). The severity of the disease (by Child's classification) and the

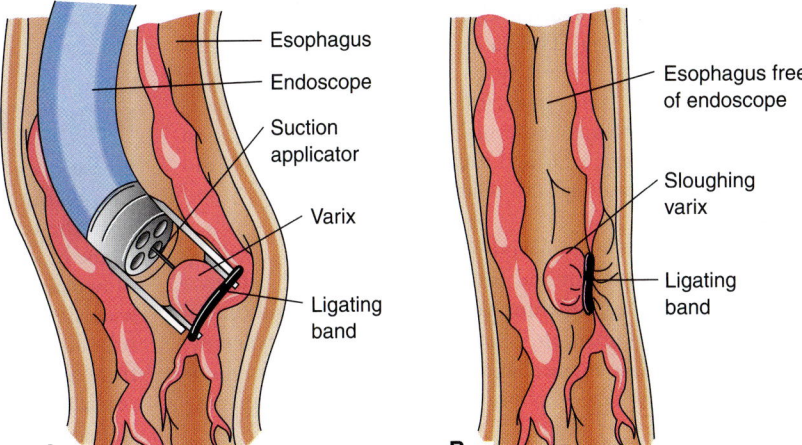

FIGURE 39-9 Esophageal banding. (**A**) A rubber band–like ligature is slipped over an esophageal varix via an endoscope. (**B**) Necrosis results and the varix eventually sloughs off.

potential for future liver transplantation guide the physician's choice of intervention. If the cause of portal hypertension is the rare **Budd-Chiari syndrome** or other venous obstructive disease, a portacaval or a mesoatrial shunt may be performed (see Fig. 39-11). The mesoatrial shunt is required when the infrahepatic vena cava is thrombosed and must be bypassed.

Devascularization and Transection. Devascularization and staple-gun transection procedures to separate the bleeding site from the high-pressure portal system have been used in the emergency management of variceal bleeding. The lower end of the esophagus is reached through a small gastrostomy incision; a staple gun permits anastomosis of the transected ends of the esophagus. Rebleeding is a risk, and the outcomes of these procedures vary among patient populations.

> **NURSING ALERT** Postoperative care is similar to that for any abdominal surgery, but the risk for complications (hypovolemic or hemorrhagic shock, hepatic encephalopathy, electrolyte imbalance, metabolic and respiratory alkalosis, alcohol withdrawal syndrome, and seizures) is high. The surgical procedures do not alter the course of the progressive liver disease, and bleeding may recur as new collateral vessels develop.

Nursing Management

Overall nursing assessment includes monitoring the patient's physical condition and evaluating emotional responses and cognitive status. The nurse monitors and records vital signs and assesses the patient's nutritional and neurologic status. This assessment will assist in identifying hepatic encephalopathy resulting from the breakdown of blood in the GI tract and a rising serum ammonia level. Manifestations range from drowsiness to encephalopathy and coma.

Complete rest of the esophagus may be indicated with bleeding, so parenteral nutrition is initiated. Gastric suction usually is

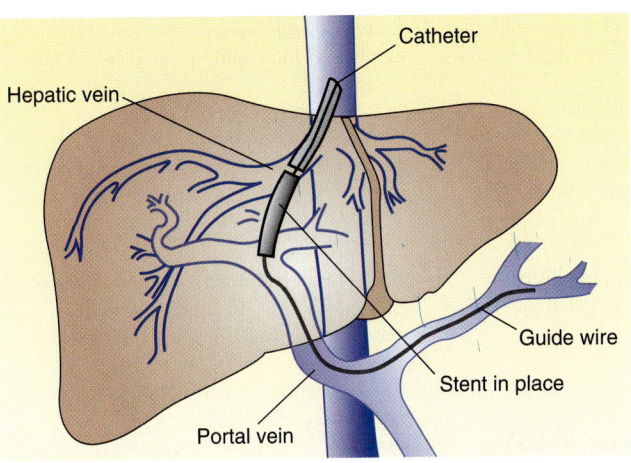

FIGURE 39-10 Transjugular intrahepatic portosystemic shunt (TIPS). A stent is inserted via catheter to the portal vein to divert blood flow and reduce portal hypertension.

FIGURE 39-11 Portal systemic shunts. Normal portal system is shown in (**A**); examples of portal shunts to reduce portal pressure are shown in (**B**) to (**D**).

initiated to keep the stomach as empty as possible and to prevent straining and vomiting. The patient often complains of severe thirst, which may be relieved by frequent oral hygiene and moist sponges to the lips. The nurse closely monitors the blood pressure. Vitamin K therapy and multiple blood transfusions often are indicated because of blood loss. A quiet environment and calm reassurance may help to relieve the patient's anxiety and reduce agitation.

Bleeding anywhere in the body is anxiety-provoking, resulting in a crisis for the patient and family. If the patient has been a heavy user of alcohol, delirium secondary to alcohol withdrawal can complicate the situation. The nurse provides support and explanations regarding medical and nursing interventions. Monitoring the patient closely will help in detecting and managing complications.

Management modalities and nursing care of the patient with bleeding esophageal varices are summarized in Table 39-2.

HEPATIC ENCEPHALOPATHY AND COMA

Hepatic encephalopathy, a life-threatening complication of liver disease, occurs with profound liver failure and may result from the accumulation of ammonia and other toxic metabolites in the blood. Hepatic coma represents the most advanced stage of hepatic encephalopathy. Some researchers describe a false or weak neurotransmitter as a cause, but the exact mechanism is not fully understood. These false neurotransmitters may be generated from an intestinal source and result in the precipitation of encephalopathy. Many other theories exist about the causes of encephalopathy, including excess tryptophan and its metabolites,

---

Table 39-2 • **Management Modalities and Nursing Care for the Patient With Bleeding Esophageal Varices**

TREATMENT MODALITY*	ACTION	NURSING PRIORITIES
Nonsurgical Modalities		
Pharmacologic agents		
Vasopressin (Pitressin)	Reduces portal pressure by constricting splanchnic arteries	Observe response to therapy. Monitor for side effects: *vasopressin*—angina; nitroglycerin may be prescribed to prevent or treat angina.
Propranolol (Inderal)/nadolol (Corgard)	Reduces portal pressure by β-adrenergic blocking action	*propranolol and nadolol*—decreased pulse pressure, impaired cardiovascular response to hemorrhage.
Somatostatin/octreotide (Sandostatin)	Reduces portal pressure by selective vasodilation of portal system	Support patient during treatment.
Balloon tamponade	Exerts pressure directly to bleeding sites in esophagus and stomach	Explain procedure to patient briefly to obtain cooperation with insertion and maintenance of esophageal tamponade tube and reduce patient's fear of the procedure. Monitor closely to prevent inadvertent removal or displacement of tube, subsequent airway obstruction, and aspiration. Provide frequent oral hygiene.
Room-temperature saline lavage	Clears blood and secretions before endoscopy and other procedures	Ensure patency of the nasogastric tube to prevent aspiration. Observe gastric aspirate for blood and cessation of bleeding.
Injection sclerotherapy	Promotes thrombosis and sclerosing of bleeding sites by injection of sclerosing agent into the esophageal varices	Observe for aspiration, perforation of the esophagus, and recurrence of bleeding after treatment.
Variceal banding	Provides thrombosis and mucosal necrosis of bleeding sites by band ligation	Observe for recurrence of bleeding, esophageal perforation.
Transjugular intrahepatic portosystemic shunting (TIPS)	Reduces portal pressure by creating a shunt within the liver between the portal and systemic venous system.	Observe for rebleeding and signs of infection.
Surgical Modalities		
Portal-systemic shunting	Reduces portal hypertension by diverting blood flow away from obstructed portal system	Observe for development of portal-systemic encephalopathy (altered mental status, neurologic dysfunction), hepatic failure, and rebleeding. Requires intensive, expert nursing care for prolonged period.
Surgical ligation of varices	Ties off blood vessels at the site of bleeding	Observe for rebleeding.
Esophageal transection and devascularization	Separates bleeding site from portal system	Observe for rebleeding. Provide postthoracotomy care.

*Several modalities may be used concurrently or in sequence.

and endogenous benzodiazepines or opiates. Benzodiazepine-like chemicals (compounds) have been detected in the plasma and cerebrospinal fluid of patients with hepatic encephalopathy due to cirrhosis (Bacon & Di Bisceglie, 2000).

Portal-systemic encephalopathy, the most common type of hepatic encephalopathy, occurs primarily in patients with cirrhosis with portal hypertension and portal-systemic shunting.

Pathophysiology

Ammonia accumulates because damaged liver cells fail to detoxify and convert to urea the ammonia that is constantly entering the bloodstream. Ammonia enters the bloodstream as a result of its absorption from the GI tract and its liberation from kidney and muscle cells. The increased ammonia concentration in the blood causes brain dysfunction and damage, resulting in hepatic encephalopathy.

Circumstances that increase serum ammonia levels tend to aggravate or precipitate hepatic encephalopathy. The largest source of ammonia is the enzymatic and bacterial digestion of dietary and blood proteins in the GI tract. Ammonia from these sources is increased as a result of GI bleeding (ie, bleeding esophageal varices or chronic GI bleeding), a high-protein diet, bacterial infections, and uremia. The ingestion of ammonium salts also increases the blood ammonia level. In the presence of alkalosis or hypokalemia, increased amounts of ammonia are absorbed from the GI tract and from the renal tubular fluid. Conversely, serum ammonia is decreased by elimination of protein from the diet and by the administration of antibiotic agents, such as neomycin sulfate, that reduce the number of intestinal bacteria capable of converting urea to ammonia (Dudek, 2001).

Other factors unrelated to increased serum ammonia levels that may cause hepatic encephalopathy in susceptible patients include excessive diuresis, dehydration, infections, surgery, fever, and some medications (sedative agents, tranquilizers, analgesic agents, and diuretic medications that cause potassium loss). Table 39-3 presents the stages of hepatic encephalopathy, common signs and symptoms, and potential nursing diagnoses for each stage.

Clinical Manifestations

The earliest symptoms of hepatic encephalopathy include minor mental changes and motor disturbances. The patient appears slightly confused, has alterations in mood, becomes unkempt, and has altered sleep patterns. The patient tends to sleep during the day and have restlessness and insomnia at night. As hepatic encephalopathy progresses, the patient may be difficult to awaken.

Asterixis (flapping tremor of the hands) may occur (Fig. 39-12). Simple tasks, such as handwriting, become difficult. A handwriting or drawing sample (eg, star figure), taken daily, may provide graphic evidence of progression or reversal of hepatic encephalopathy. Inability to reproduce a simple figure (Fig. 39-13) is referred to as **constructional apraxia**. In the early stages of hepatic encephalopathy, the deep tendon reflexes are hyperactive; with worsening of hepatic encephalopathy, these reflexes disappear and the extremities may become flaccid.

Assessment and Diagnostic Findings

The electroencephalogram (EEG) shows generalized slowing, an increase in the amplitude of brain waves, and characteristic triphasic waves. Occasionally, **fetor hepaticus**, a sweet, slightly fecal odour to the breath presumed to be of intestinal origin may be noticed. The odour has also been described as similar to that of freshly mowed grass, acetone, or old wine. Fetor hepaticus is prevalent with extensive collateral portal circulation in chronic liver disease. In a more advanced stage, there are gross disturbances of consciousness and the patient is completely disoriented with respect to time and place. With further progression of the disorder, the patient lapses into frank coma and may have seizures. Approximately 35% of all patients with cirrhosis of the liver die in hepatic coma.

Medical Management

Lactulose (Cephulac) is administered to reduce serum ammonia levels. It acts by several mechanisms that promote the excretion of ammonia in the stool: (1) ammonia is kept in the ionized state, resulting in a fall in colon pH, reversing the normal passage of ammonia from the colon to the blood; (2) evacuation of the bowel takes place, which decreases the ammonia

---

Table 39-3 • Stages of Hepatic Encephalopathy and Possible Nursing Diagnoses*

STAGE	CLINICAL SYMPTOMS	CLINICAL SIGNS AND EEG CHANGES	SELECTED POTENTIAL NURSING DIAGNOSES
1	Normal level of consciousness with periods of lethargy and euphoria; reversal of day–night sleep patterns	Asterixis; impaired writing and ability to draw line figures. Normal EEG.	Activity intolerance Self-care deficit Disturbed sleep pattern
2	Increased drowsiness; disorientation; inappropriate behaviour; mood swings; agitation	Asterixis; fetor hepaticus. Abnormal EEG with generalized slowing.	Impaired social interaction Ineffective role performance Risk for injury
3	Stuporous; difficult to rouse; sleeps most of time; marked confusion; incoherent speech	Asterixis; increased deep tendon reflexes; rigidity of extremities. EEG markedly abnormal.	Imbalanced nutrition Impaired mobility Impaired verbal communication
4	Comatose; may not respond to painful stimuli	Absence of asterixis; absence of deep tendon reflexes; flaccidity of extremities. EEG markedly abnormal.	Risk for aspiration Impaired gas exchange Impaired tissue integrity Disturbed sensory perception

*Nursing diagnoses are likely to progress, so that most nursing diagnoses present at earlier stages will occur during later stages as well.

FIGURE 39-12 Asterixis or "liver flap" may occur in hepatic encephalopathy. The patient is asked to hold the arm out with the hand held upward (dorsiflexed). Within a few seconds, the hand falls forward involuntarily and then quickly returns to the dorsiflexed position.

absorbed from the colon; and (3) the fecal flora are changed to organisms that do not produce ammonia from urea. Two or three soft stools per day are desirable; this indicates that lactulose is performing as intended.

 NURSING ALERT The patient receiving lactulose is monitored closely for the development of watery diarrheal stools, because they indicate a medication overdose.

Possible side effects include intestinal bloating and cramps, which usually disappear within a week. To mask the sweet taste,

FIGURE 39-13 Effects of constructional apraxia. Deterioration of handwriting and inability to draw a simple star figure occurs with progressive hepatic encephalopathy. With permission from Sherlock S. & Dooley, J. (1997). *Diseases of the liver and biliary system* (10th ed). Olney Mead, Blackwell Scientific Ltd.

to which some patients object, lactulose can be diluted with fruit juice. The patient is closely monitored for hypokalemia and dehydration. Other laxatives are not prescribed during lactulose administration because their effects would disturb dosage regulation. Lactulose can be administered by nasogastric tube or enema for patients who are comatose or in whom oral administration is contraindicated or impossible.

Other aspects of management include intravenous administration of glucose to minimize protein breakdown, administration of vitamins to correct deficiencies, and correction of electrolyte imbalances (especially potassium). Additional principles of management of hepatic encephalopathy include the following:

- Therapy is directed toward treating or removing the cause.
- Neurologic status is assessed frequently. A daily record is kept of handwriting and performance in arithmetic to monitor mental status.
- Fluid intake and output and body weight are recorded each day.
- Vital signs are measured and recorded every 4 hours.
- Potential sites of infection (peritoneum, lungs) are assessed frequently, and abnormal findings are reported promptly.
- Serum ammonia level is monitored daily.
- Protein intake is restricted in patients who are comatose or who have encephalopathy that is refractory to lactulose and antibiotic therapy (Chart 39-4).
- Reduction in the absorption of ammonia from the GI tract is accomplished by the use of gastric suction, enemas, or oral antibiotics.
- Electrolyte status is monitored and corrected if abnormal.
- Sedatives, tranquilizers, and analgesic medications are discontinued.
- Benzodiazepine antagonists (flumazenil [Romazicon]) may be administered to improve encephalopathy whether or not the patient has previously taken benzodiazepines.

Nursing Management

The nurse is responsible for maintaining a safe environment to prevent injury, bleeding, and infection. The nurse administers the prescribed treatments and monitors the patient for the many potential complications. The nurse also communicates with the pa-

> **Chart 39-4**
>
> ### Nutritional Management of Hepatic Encephalopathy
>
> - Prevent the formation and absorption of toxins, principally ammonia, from the intestine.
> - Keep daily protein intake between 1.0 and 1.5 g/kg, depending on the degree of decompensation.
> - Avoid protein restriction if possible, even in those with encephalopathy. If necessary, implement temporary restriction of 0.5 g/kg.
> - For patients who are truly protein-intolerant, provide additional nitrogen in the form of an amino acid supplement. Use of branched-chain amino acids is still controversial.
> - Provide small, frequent meals and an evening snack of complex carbohydrates to avoid protein loading.
> - Substitute vegetable protein for animal protein in as high a percentage as possible.

tient's family to keep them informed about the patient's status, and supports them by explaining the procedures and treatments that are part of the patient's care. If the patient recovers from hepatic encephalopathy and coma, rehabilitation is likely to be prolonged. Thus, the patient and family will require assistance to understand the causes of this severe complication and to recognize that it may recur.

PROMOTING HOME AND COMMUNITY-BASED CARE

Teaching Patients Self-Care. If the patient has recovered from hepatic encephalopathy and is to be discharged home, the nurse instructs the family to watch for subtle signs of recurrent encephalopathy. In the acute phase of hepatic encephalopathy, dietary protein may be reduced to 0.8 to 1.0 g/kg per day. During recovery, and in the home situation, it is important to instruct the patient in maintenance of a low-protein, high-calorie diet. Protein may then be added in 10-g increments every 3 to 5 days. Any relapse is treated by a return to the previous level. The limits of tolerance are usually 1.0 to 1.5 g/kg per day. Continued use of lactulose in the home environment is not uncommon, and the patient and family should monitor its efficacy and side effects closely. Use of vegetable rather than animal protein may be indicated in patients whose total daily protein tolerance is less than 1 g/kg. Vegetable protein intake may result in improved nitrogen balance without precipitating or advancing hepatic encephalopathy (Menon & Kamath, 2000; Seymour & Whelan, 1999).

Continuing Care. Referral for home care is warranted for the patient who returns home after recovery from hepatic encephalopathy. The home care nurse assesses the patient's physical and mental status and collaborates closely with the physician. The home visit also provides an opportunity for the nurse to assess the home environment and the ability of the patient and family to monitor signs and symptoms and to follow the treatment regimen. Home care visits are particularly important if the patient lives alone, because encephalopathy may affect the patient's ability to remember or follow the treatment regimen. The nurse reinforces previous teaching and reminds the patient and family about the importance of dietary restrictions, close monitoring, and follow-up.

OTHER MANIFESTATIONS OF LIVER DYSFUNCTION

Edema and Bleeding

Many patients with liver dysfunction develop generalized edema from hypoalbuminemia that results from decreased hepatic production of albumin. The production of blood clotting factors by the liver is also reduced, leading to an increased incidence of bruising, epistaxis, bleeding from wounds, and, as described above, GI bleeding.

Vitamin Deficiency

Decreased production of several clotting factors may be due, in part, to deficient absorption of vitamin K from the GI tract. This probably is caused by the inability of liver cells to use vitamin K to make prothrombin. Absorption of the other fat-soluble vitamins (vitamins A, D, and E) as well as dietary fats may also be impaired because of decreased secretion of bile salts into the intestine.

Another group of problems common to patients with severe chronic liver dysfunction results from inadequate intake of sufficient vitamins. Among the specific deficiency states that occur on this basis are:

- Vitamin A deficiency, resulting in night blindness and eye and skin changes
- Thiamine deficiency, leading to beriberi, polyneuritis, and Wernicke-Korsakoff psychosis
- Riboflavin deficiency, resulting in characteristic skin and mucous membrane lesions
- Pyridoxine deficiency, resulting in skin and mucous membrane lesions and neurologic changes
- Vitamin C deficiency, resulting in the hemorrhagic lesions of scurvy
- Vitamin K deficiency, resulting in hypoprothrombinemia, characterized by spontaneous bleeding and ecchymoses
- Folic acid deficiency, resulting in macrocytic anemia

The threat of these avitaminoses provides the rationale for supplementing the diet of every patient with chronic liver disease (especially if alcohol-related) with ample quantities of vitamins A, B complex, C, and K and folic acid.

Metabolic Abnormalities

Abnormalities of glucose metabolism also occur; the blood glucose level may be abnormally high shortly after a meal (a diabetic-type glucose tolerance test result), but hypoglycemia may occur during fasting because of decreased hepatic glycogen reserves and decreased gluconeogenesis. Because the ability to metabolize medications is decreased, medications must be used cautiously and usual medication dosages must be reduced for the patient with liver failure.

Many endocrine abnormalities also occur with liver dysfunction because the liver cannot metabolize hormones normally, including androgens or sex hormones. Gynecomastia, amenorrhea, testicular atrophy, loss of pubic hair in the male, and menstrual irregularities in the female and other disturbances of sexual function and sex characteristics are thought to result from failure of the damaged liver to inactivate estrogens normally.

Pruritus and Other Skin Changes

Patients with liver dysfunction resulting from biliary obstruction commonly develop severe itching (pruritus) due to retention of bile salts. Patients may develop vascular (or arterial) spider angiomas (Fig. 39-14) on the skin, generally above the waistline. These are numerous small vessels resembling a spider's legs. These are most frequently associated with cirrhosis, especially in alcoholic liver disease. Patients may also develop reddened palms ("liver palms" or palmar erythema).

Management of Patients With Viral Hepatic Disorders

VIRAL HEPATITIS

Viral hepatitis is a systemic, viral infection in which necrosis and inflammation of liver cells produce a characteristic cluster of clinical, biochemical, and cellular changes. To date, five definitive

Table 39-4 • Comparison of Major Forms of Viral Hepatitis

	HEPATITIS A	HEPATITIS B	HEPATITIS C	HEPATITIS D	HEPATITIS E
Previous names	Infectious hepatitis	Serum hepatitis	Non-A, non-B hepatitis		
Epidemiology					
Cause	Hepatitis A virus (HAV)	Hepatitis B virus (HBV)	Hepatitis C virus (HCV)	Hepatitis D virus (HDV)	Hepatitis E virus (HEV)
Mode of transmission	Fecal–oral route; poor sanitation. Person-to-person contact. Water-borne; foodborne. Transmission possible with oral–anal contact during sex.	Parenterally; by intimate contact with carriers or those with acute disease; sexual and oral–oral contact. Perinatal transmission from mothers to infants. An important occupational hazard for health care personnel.	Transfusion of blood and blood products; exposure to contaminated blood through equipment or drug paraphernalia. Transmission possible with sex with infected partner; risk increased with STD.	Same as HBV. HBV surface antigen necessary for replication; pattern similar to that of hepatitis B.	Fecal–oral route; person to person contact may be possible, although risk appears low
Incubation (days) *Immunity*	15–50 days Average: 30 days Homologous	28–160 days Average: 70–80 days Homologous	15–160 days Average: 50 days Second attack may indicate weak immunity or infection with another agent.	21–140 days Average: 35 days Homologous	15–65 days Average: 42 days Unknown
Nature of Illness					
Signs and symptoms	May occur with or without symptoms; flulike illness *Preicteric phase:* Headache, malaise, fatigue, anorexia, fever *Icteric phase:* Dark urine, jaundice of sclera and skin, tender liver	May occur without symptoms May develop arthralgias, rash	Similar to HBV; less severe and anicteric	Similar to HBV	Similar to HAV. Very severe in pregnant women.
Outcome	Usually mild with recovery. Fatality rate: <1%. No carrier state or increased risk of chronic hepatitis, cirrhosis, or hepatic cancer.	May be severe. Fatality rate: 1%–10%. Carrier state possible. Increased risk of chronic hepatitis, cirrhosis, and hepatic cancer.	Frequent occurrence of chronic carrier state and chronic liver disease. Increased risk of hepatic cancer.	Similar to HBV but greater likelihood of carrier state, chronic active hepatitis, and cirrhosis	Similar to HAV except very severe in pregnant women

oral–anal contact, anal intercourse, and a greater number of sex partners (CDC, 2002).

The incubation period is estimated to be 15 to 50 days, with an average of 30 days (O'Grady et al., 2000). The illness may be prolonged, lasting 4 to 8 weeks. It generally lasts longer and is more severe in those older than 40 years of age. Recovery is the rule; hepatitis A rarely progresses to acute liver necrosis or fulminant hepatitis, terminating in cirrhosis of the liver or death. Hepatitis A confers immunity against itself, but the person may contract other forms of hepatitis. The mortality rate of hepatitis A is approximately 0.5% for those under 40 years of age and increases to 1% to 2% for those over 40. No carrier state exists, and no chronic hepatitis is associated with hepatitis A. The virus is present only briefly in the serum; by the time jaun-dice occurs, the patient is likely to be noninfectious (O'Grady et al., 2000).

Clinical Manifestations

Many patients are anicteric (without jaundice) and symptomless. When symptoms appear, they are of a mild, flu-like upper respiratory tract infection, with low-grade fever. Anorexia, an early symptom, is often severe. It is thought to result from release of a toxin by the damaged liver or by failure of the damaged liver cells to detoxify an abnormal product. Later, jaundice and dark urine may become apparent. Indigestion is present in varying degrees, marked by vague epigastric distress, nausea, heartburn, and flatulence. The patient may also develop a strong aversion to the taste of cigarettes or the presence of cigarette smoke and other strong odours. These symptoms tend to clear as soon as the jaundice reaches its peak, perhaps 10 days after its initial appearance. Symptoms may be mild in children; in adults, the symptoms may be more severe and the course of the disease prolonged.

Assessment and Diagnostic Findings

The liver and spleen are often moderately enlarged for a few days after onset; otherwise, apart from jaundice, there are few physical signs. Hepatitis A antigen may be found in the stool a week to 10 days before illness and for 2 to 3 weeks after symptoms appear. HAV antibodies are detectable in the serum, but usually not until symptoms appear. Analysis of subclasses of immunoglobulins can help determine whether the antibody represents acute or past infection.

Prevention

A number of strategies exist to prevent transmission of HAV. Patients and their families need to be made aware of these and encouraged to consider them if recommended by their primary health care provider.

Effective and safe HAV vaccines include Havrix and Vagta (Koff, 2001). It is recommended that the two-dose vaccine be given to adults 18 years of age or older, with the second dose 6 to 12 months after the first. Protection against hepatitis A develops within several weeks after the first dose of the vaccine. Children and adolescents 2 to 18 years of age receive three doses, with the second dose 1 month after the first and the third dose 6 to 12 months later. It is estimated that protection against hepatitis A may last for at least 20 years (CDC, 1999). No country has as yet recommended universal vaccination against hepatitis A. Hepatitis A vaccine is recommended for travelers to locations where sanitation and hygiene are unsatisfactory. Vaccination is also recommended for those from other high-risk groups (homosexual men, injection/intravenous drug users, staff of day care centres, and health care personnel) (CDC, 2002). The vaccine has also been used to interrupt community-wide outbreaks. As with other vaccinations, precautions must be taken to ensure prevention, detection, and treatment of hypersensitivity reactions to the vaccine.

Type A hepatitis can be prevented in those not previously vaccinated by the intramuscular administration of globulin during the incubation period, if given within 2 weeks of exposure. This bolsters the person's antibody production and provides 6 to 8 weeks of passive immunity. Immune globulin may suppress overt symptoms of the disease; the resulting subclinical case of hepatitis A would produce active immunity to subsequent episodes of the virus.

Immune globulin is also recommended for household members and sexual contacts of people with hepatitis A. Susceptible people in the same household as the patient are usually also infected by the time the diagnosis is made and should receive immune globulin. Day care centre and restaurant workers with exposure to or infected with hepatitis A should also receive immune globulin to provide passive immunity (CDC, 1999). Although rare, systemic reactions to immune globulin may occur. Caution is required when anyone who has previously had angioedema, hives, or other allergic reactions is treated with any human immune globulin. Epinephrine should be available in case a systemic, anaphylactic reaction occurs.

Chart 39-6 Community Prevention of Hepatitis A

- Proper community and home sanitation
- Conscientious individual hygiene
- Safe practices for preparing and dispensing food
- Effective health supervision of schools, dormitories, extended care facilities, barracks, and camps
- Community health education programs
- Mandatory reporting of viral hepatitis to local health departments
- Vaccination for travelers to developing countries, illegal drug users (injection and noninjection drug users), men who have sex with men, and persons with chronic liver disease
- Vaccination to interrupt community-wide outbreaks

Preexposure prophylaxis is recommended for those traveling to developing countries and settings with poor or uncertain sanitation conditions but who do not have sufficient time to acquire protection by administration of hepatitis A vaccine (CDC, 1999). Community interventions for preventing hepatitis A are outlined in Chart 39-6.

Medical Management

Bed rest during the acute stage and a diet that is both acceptable to the patient and nutritious are part of the treatment and nursing care. During the period of anorexia, the patient should receive frequent small feedings, supplemented, if necessary, by IV fluids with glucose. Because this patient often has an aversion to food, gentle persistence and creativity may be required to stimulate the appetite. Optimal food and fluid levels are necessary to counteract weight loss and slow recovery. Even before the icteric phase, however, many patients recover their appetites (Chart 39-7).

The patient's sense of well-being as well as laboratory test results are generally appropriate guides to bed rest and restriction of physical activity. Gradual but progressive ambulation seems to hasten recovery, provided the patient rests after activity and does not participate in activities to the point of fatigue.

Nursing Management

The patient is usually managed at home unless symptoms are severe. Therefore, the nurse assists the patient and family in coping with the temporary disability and fatigue that are common in hepatitis and instructs them to seek additional health care if the

Chart 39-7 Dietary Management of Viral or Drug-Related Hepatitis

- Recommend small, frequent meals.
- Provide intake of 8,000 to 12,000 KJ/day (2,000 to 3,000 kcal/day) during acute illness.
- Although early studies indicate that a high-protein, high-calorie diet may be beneficial, advise patient not to force food and to restrict fat intake.
- Carefully monitor fluid balance.
- If anorexia and nausea and vomiting persist, enteral feedings may be necessary.
- Instruct patient to abstain from alcohol during acute illness and for 6 months after recovery.
- Advise patient to avoid substances (medication, herbs, illicit drugs, and toxins) that may affect liver function.

symptoms persist or worsen. The patient and family also need specific guidelines about diet, rest, follow-up blood work, and the importance of avoiding alcohol, as well as sanitation and hygiene measures (particularly hand washing) to prevent spread of the disease to other family members.

Specific teaching to patients and families about reducing the risk of contracting hepatitis A includes good personal hygiene, stressing careful hand washing (after bowel movements and before eating), and environmental sanitation (safe food and water supply, as well as effective sewage disposal).

> **! NURSING ALERT** Since 1997 the National Advisory Committee on Immunization recommends a combined hepatitis A and B vaccine (Twinrix) for vaccination of persons 18 years of age and older with indications for both hepatitis A and B vaccination. Vaccination consists of three doses, on the same schedule as that used for single-antigen hepatitis B vaccine.

HEPATITIS B VIRUS (HBV)

Unlike hepatitis A, which is transmitted primarily by the fecal–oral route, hepatitis B is transmitted primarily through blood (percutaneous and permucosal routes). HBV has been found in blood, saliva, semen, and vaginal secretions and can be transmitted through mucous membranes and breaks in the skin. HBV is also transferred from carrier mothers to their babies, especially in areas with a high incidence (ie, Africa and Southeast Asia). The infection is usually not via the umbilical vein, but from the mother at the time of birth and during close contact afterward.

HBV has a long incubation period. It replicates in the liver and remains in the serum for relatively long periods, allowing transmission of the virus. Those at risk for developing hepatitis B include surgeons, clinical laboratory workers, dentists, nurses, and respiratory therapists. Staff and patients in hemodialysis and oncology units and sexually active homosexual and bisexual men and injection drug users are also at increased risk. Screening of blood donors has greatly reduced the occurrence of hepatitis B after blood transfusion.

Most people (>90%) who contract hepatitis B infections will develop antibodies and recover spontaneously in 6 months. The mortality rate from hepatitis B has been reported to be as high as 10%. Another 10% of patients who have hepatitis B progress to a carrier state or develop chronic hepatitis with persistent HBV infection and hepatocellular injury and inflammation. It remains a major cause of cirrhosis and hepatocellular carcinoma worldwide (Chart 39-8).

> ### Chart 39-8
> ### Risk Factors for Hepatitis B
>
> - Frequent exposure to blood, blood products, or other body fluids
> - Health care workers: hemodialysis staff, oncology and chemotherapy nurses, personnel at risk for needlesticks, operating room staff, respiratory therapists, surgeons, dentists
> - Hemodialysis
> - Male homosexual and bisexual activity
> - IV/injection drug use
> - Close contact with carrier of HBV
> - Travel to or residence in area with uncertain sanitary conditions
> - Multiple sexual partners
> - Recent history of sexually transmitted disease
> - Receipt of blood or blood products (eg, clotting factor concentrate)

Clinical Manifestations

Clinically, the disease closely resembles hepatitis A, but the incubation period is much longer (1 to 6 months). Signs and symptoms of hepatitis B may be insidious and variable. Fever and respiratory symptoms are rare; some patients have arthralgias and rashes. The patient may have loss of appetite, dyspepsia, abdominal pain, generalized aching, malaise, and weakness. Jaundice may or may not be evident. If jaundice occurs, light-coloured stools and dark urine accompany it. The liver may be tender and enlarged to 12 to 14 cm vertically. The spleen is enlarged and palpable in a few patients; the posterior cervical lymph nodes may also be enlarged. Subclinical episodes also occur frequently.

Assessment and Diagnostic Findings

HBV is a DNA virus composed of the following antigenic particles:

- HBcAg—hepatitis B core antigen (antigenic material in an inner core)
- HBsAg—hepatitis B surface antigen (antigenic material on surface of HBV)
- HBeAg—an independent protein circulating in the blood
- HBxAg—gene product of X gene of HBV/DNA

Each antigen elicits its specific antibody and is a marker for different stages of the disease process:

- anti-HBc—antibody to core antigen or HBV; persists during the acute phase of illness; may indicate continuing HBV in the liver
- anti-HBs—antibody to surface determinants on HBV; detected during late convalescence; usually indicates recovery and development of immunity
- anti-HBe—antibody to hepatitis B e-antigen; usually signifies reduced infectivity
- anti-HBxAg—antibody to the hepatitis B x-antigen; may indicate ongoing replication of HBV

HBsAg appears in the circulation in 80% to 90% of infected patients 1 to 10 weeks after exposure to HBV and 2 to 8 weeks before the onset of symptoms or an increase in transferase (transaminase) levels. Patients with HBsAg that persists for 6 or more months after acute infection are considered HBsAg carriers (Befeler & Di Bisceglie, 2000). HBeAg is the next antigen of HBV to appear in the serum. It usually appears within a week of the appearance of HBsAg and before changes in aminotransferase levels, disappearing from the serum within 2 weeks. HBV DNA, detected by polymerase chain reaction testing, appears in the serum at about the same time as HBeAg. HBcAg is not always detected in the serum in HBV infection.

An average of 2868 new cases of hepatitis B are reported annually in Canada, with the highest rate in young adults aged 20 to 39. Forty percent of all reported cases are from British Columbia.

Prevention

The goals of prevention are to interrupt the chain of transmission, to protect people at high risk with active immunization through the use of hepatitis B vaccine, and to use passive immunization for unprotected people exposed to HBV.

PREVENTING TRANSMISSION

Continued screening of blood donors for the presence of hepatitis B antigens will further decrease the risk of transmission by blood transfusion. The use of disposable syringes, needles, and lancets and the introduction of needleless IV administration systems reduce the risk of spreading this infection from one patient to another or to health care personnel during the collection of blood samples or the administration of parenteral therapy. Good personal hygiene is fundamental to infection control. In the clinical laboratory, work areas should be disinfected daily. Gloves are worn when handling all blood and body fluids as well as HBAg-positive specimens, or when there is potential exposure to blood (blood drawing) or to patients' secretions. Eating and smoking are prohibited in the laboratory and in other areas exposed to secretions, blood, or blood products. Patient education regarding the nature of the disease, its infectiousness, and prognosis is a critical factor in preventing transmission and protecting contacts.

ACTIVE IMMUNIZATION: HEPATITIS B VACCINE

Active immunization is recommended for individuals at high risk for hepatitis B (eg, health care personnel and hemodialysis patients). In addition, individuals with hepatitis C and other chronic liver diseases should receive the vaccine (CDC, 1999). A yeast-recombinant hepatitis B vaccine (Recombivax HB) is used to provide active immunity. Long-term studies of healthy adults and children indicate that immunologic memory remains intact for at least 5 to 10 years, although antibody levels may become low or undetectable. Measurable levels of antibodies may not be essential for protection. In those with normal immune systems, booster doses are not generally required. The CDC (2002) does not recommend booster doses at this time except for hemodialysis patients. The need for booster doses may be revisited if reports of hepatitis B increase or an increased prevalence of the carrier state develops, indicating that protection is declining.

A hepatitis B vaccine prepared from plasma of humans chronically infected with HBV is used only rarely and in patients who are immunodeficient or allergic to recombinant yeast-derived vaccines.

Both forms of the hepatitis B vaccine are administered intramuscularly in three doses, the second and third doses 1 and 6 months after the first dose. The third dose is very important in producing prolonged immunity. Hepatitis B vaccination should be administered to adults in the deltoid muscle. Antibody response may be measured by anti-HBs levels 1 to 3 months after completing the basic course of vaccine, but this testing is not routine and not currently recommended. Individuals who fail to respond may benefit from one to three additional doses (Koff, 2001).

People at high risk, including nurses and other health care personnel exposed to blood or blood products, should receive active immunization. Health care workers who have had frequent contact with blood are screened for anti-HBs to determine whether immunity is already present from previous exposure. The vaccine produces active immunity to HBV in 90% of healthy people (Koff, 2001). It does not provide protection to those already exposed to HBV and provides no protection against other types of viral hepatitis. Side effects of immunization are infrequent; soreness and redness at the injection site are the most common complaints.

Because hepatitis B infection is frequently transmitted sexually, hepatitis B vaccination is recommended for all unvaccinated persons being evaluated for a sexually transmitted disease (STD). It is also recommended for those with a history of an STD, persons with multiple sex partners, those who have sex with injection drug users, and sexually active men who have sex with other men (CDC, 2002).

Universal childhood vaccination for hepatitis B prevention has been instituted in all provinces and territories of Canada. The age at vaccination differs across regions, but vaccination com-

monly occurs in grade four. Although the efficacy of the vaccine in childhood is 98%, the response to the vaccine generally declines with age. Studies (Chang, 2000; Wu et al., 1999) show that universal vaccination of all newborns in endemic areas has dramatically reduced the carrier rate among children and the incidence of childhood hepatocellular carcinoma. In the United States, studies regarding the effectiveness of the vaccine are ongoing, but it is known that clinical infection is rarely observed during long-term follow-up of known responders (ie, health care workers) who seroconverted within 3 months of the third dose of vaccine (Bircher et al., 1999). Development of chronic carrier states has not been reported in adult responders to the vaccine.

PASSIVE IMMUNITY: HEPATITIS B IMMUNE GLOBULIN

Hepatitis B immune globulin (HBIG) provides passive immunity to hepatitis B and is indicated for people exposed to HBV who have never had hepatitis B and have never received hepatitis B vaccine. Specific indications for postexposure vaccine with HBIG include: (1) inadvertent exposure to HBAg-positive blood through percutaneous (needlestick) or transmucosal (splashes in contact with mucous membrane) routes, (2) sexual contact with people positive for HBAg, and (3) perinatal exposure (babies born to HBV-infected mothers should receive HBIG within 12 hours of delivery). HBIG, which provides passive immunity, is prepared from plasma selected for high titers of anti-HBs. Prompt immunization with HBIG (within hours to a few days after exposure to hepatitis B) increases the likelihood of protection. Both active and passive immunization are recommended for people exposed to hepatitis B through sexual contact or through percutaneous or transmucosal routes. If HBIG and hepatitis B vaccine are administered at the same time, separate sites and separate syringes should be used. Prophylaxis with high doses of HBIG started at the time of liver transplantation and continued indefinitely improves survival by thwarting recurrence of hepatitis B (Bacon & Di Bisceglie, 2000). There has been no evidence that HIV infection can be transmitted by HBIG.

 Gerontologic Considerations

The elderly patient who contracts hepatitis B has a serious risk of severe liver cell necrosis or fulminant hepatic failure, particularly if other illnesses are present. The patient is seriously ill and the prognosis is poor, so efforts should be undertaken to eliminate other factors (eg, medications, alcohol) that may affect liver function.

Medical Management

The goals of treatment are to minimize infectivity, normalize liver inflammation, and decrease symptoms. In 1998 an antiviral agent oral nucleoside analogue (lamivudine) that was developed in Canada became the first oral agent for use in the management of hepatitis B (Ko, Lennon & Roy, 1998). Prior to the availability of antiviral oral nucleoside analogues (lamivudine, adefovir dipivoxil, entecavir, and famciclovir), treatment of hepatitis B was limited to injectable interferon. Interferon has significant side effects including fever, chills, anorexia, nausea, myalgias, and fatigue. Late, and perhaps more serious, side effects include bone marrow suppression, thyroid dysfunction, alopecia, and bacterial infections, which often lead to dosage reduction or discontinuation of the medication. The oral antiviral agents are well tolerated and work by interfering with the replication of the hepatitis B virus. They reduce hepatitis-associated inflammation in the liver, halt the progression of fibrosis to cirrhosis, and are used to prevent recurrent infection following liver transplant. These actions contribute to liver transplantation success. Viral resistance is an issue with antiviral agents and lamivudine-resistant YMDD mutants are common. However, adefovir has been effective against this mutant (Farrell, 2000). Recently combination treatments of oral agents and interferon have been investigated (Yurdaydin, Bozkaya, Cetinkaya, Sahin, Karaoguz, Toruner, et al.). Although lamivudine alone was as effective in treating hepatitis B as a combination of lamivudine and interferon, the group treated with combination therapy exhibited fewer mutant strains. Combination therapy may indeed be a benefit to patients but needs to be further studied in relation to its costs and side effects.

Bed rest may be recommended, regardless of other treatment, until the symptoms of hepatitis have subsided. Activities are restricted until the hepatic enlargement and elevated levels of serum bilirubin and liver enzymes have disappeared. Gradually increased activity is then allowed.

Adequate nutrition should be maintained; proteins are restricted when the liver's ability to metabolize protein byproducts is impaired, as demonstrated by symptoms. Measures to control the dyspeptic symptoms and general malaise include the use of antacids and antiemetics, but all medications should be avoided if vomiting occurs. If vomiting persists, the patient may require hospitalization and fluid therapy. Because of the mode of transmission, the patient is evaluated for other bloodborne diseases (eg, +HCV and HIV infection).

Nursing Management

Convalescence may be prolonged, with complete symptomatic recovery sometimes requiring 3 to 4 months or longer. During this stage, gradual resumption of physical activity is encouraged after the jaundice has resolved.

The nurse identifies psychosocial issues and concerns, particularly the effects of separation from family and friends if the patient is hospitalized during the acute and infective stages. Even if not hospitalized, the patient will be unable to work and must avoid sexual contact. Planning is required to minimize alterations in sensory perception. Planning that includes the family helps to decrease their fears and anxieties about the spread of the disease.

PROMOTING HOME AND COMMUNITY-BASED CARE

Teaching Patients Self-Care. Because of the prolonged period of convalescence, the patient and family must be prepared for home care. Provision for adequate rest and nutrition must be ensured. The nurse informs family members and friends who have had intimate contact with the patient about the risks of contracting hepatitis B and makes arrangements for them to receive hepatitis B vaccine or hepatitis B immune globulin as prescribed. Those at risk must be aware of the early signs of hepatitis B and of ways to reduce risk to themselves by avoiding all modes of transmission. Patients with all forms of hepatitis should avoid drinking alcohol. Patients should also be aware that disruptions in medication schedules can increase the probability of viral mutation.

Continuing Care. Follow-up visits by a home care nurse may be needed to assess the patient's progress and answer family members' questions about disease transmission. A home visit also permits assessment of the patient's physical and psychological status and the patient and family's understanding of the importance of adequate rest and nutrition. The nurse also reinforces previous instructions. Because of the risk of transmission through sexual intercourse, strategies to prevent exchange of body fluids are advised, such as abstinence or the use of condoms. The nurse emphasizes the importance of keeping follow-up appointments and participating in other health promotion activities and recommended health screenings.

HEPATITIS C VIRUS (HCV)

Although hepatitis C was first identified in 1989, a diagnostic test to detect its presence was not available until 1990. Prior to this, the disease was referred to as non-A, non-B hepatitis. Since 1990, all blood donors in Canada have been screened for the hepatitis C virus. While blood transfusions and transplanted organs once accounted for the majority of hepatitis C incidences in Canada, injection drug use now accounts for 57.4 % of new infections. Hemodialysis (20%), sexual exposure (1 to 10%), household exposure (1 to 10%), and occupational exposure (1 to 2%) account for the remaining incidence (Bowker, Soskolne, Houston, Newman, & Jhangri, 2004). There are approximately 5000 new cases of hepatitis C in Canada each year. Between 210,000 and 275,000 persons have been infected with HCV in Canada, of whom only 30% are aware they carry the disease. HCV is the most common cause of liver cirrhosis and the leading indication for liver transplantation (Public Health Agency of Canada, 2004).

Individuals at special risk for hepatitis C include IV/injection drug users, sexually active people with multiple partners, patients receiving frequent transfusions or those who require large volumes of blood, and health care personnel. The incubation period is variable and may range from 15 to 160 days. The clinical course of acute hepatitis C is similar to that of hepatitis B; symptoms are usually mild. A chronic carrier state occurs frequently, however, and there is an increased risk of chronic liver disease, including cirrhosis or liver cancer, after hepatitis C. Small amounts of alcohol taken regularly appear to encourage progression of the disease. Therefore, alcohol and medications that may affect the liver should be avoided (Chart 39-9).

There is no benefit from rest, diet, or vitamin supplements. Recent studies have demonstrated that a combination of interferon (Intron-A) and ribavirin (Rebetol), two antiviral agents, is effective in producing improvement in patients with hepatitis C and in treating relapses. Some patients experience complete remission with combination therapy, which is the treatment of choice according to the FDA (Cheney, Chopra & Graham, 2000). Hemolytic anemia, the most frequent side effect, may be severe enough to require discontinuation of treatment. Ribavirin must be used with caution in women of childbearing age. A molecule (polyethylene glycol moiety [PEG]) added to the interferon keeps it in the body longer without reducing its efficacy and extends the dosing interval to once a week. Pegylated interferon (Pegasys) is now available (Lauer & Walker, 2001; Sheffield et al., 2001).

Screening of blood has reduced the incidence of hepatitis associated with blood transfusions, and public health programs are helping to reduce the number of cases associated with shared needles in illicit drug use.

Chart 39-9
Risk Factors for Hepatitis C

- Recipient of blood products or organ transplant prior to 1989 or clotting factor concentrates before 1987
- Health care and public safety workers after needlestick injuries or mucosal exposure to blood
- Children born to women infected with hepatitis C virus
- Past/current illicit IV/injection drug use
- Past treatment with chronic hemodialysis
- Sex with infected partner, having multiple sex partners, history of STD, unprotected sex

HEPATITIS D VIRUS (HDV)

Hepatitis D (delta agent) occurs in some cases of hepatitis B. Because the virus requires hepatitis B surface antigen for its replication, only individuals with hepatitis B are at risk for hepatitis D. Anti-delta antibodies in the presence of HBAg on testing confirm the diagnosis. It is also common among IV/injection drug users, hemodialysis patients, and recipients of multiple blood transfusions. Sexual contact with those with hepatitis B is considered to be an important mode of transmission of hepatitis B and D. The incubation period varies between 21 and 140 days (Bacon & Di Bisceglie, 2000).

The symptoms of hepatitis D are similar to those of hepatitis B, except that patients are more likely to develop fulminant hepatitis and to progress to chronic active hepatitis and cirrhosis. Treatment is similar to that of other forms of hepatitis; interferon as a specific treatment for hepatitis D is under investigation.

HEPATITIS E VIRUS (HEV)

Hepatitis E is believed to be transmitted by the fecal–oral route, principally through contaminated water in areas with poor sanitation. The incubation period is variable, estimated to range between 15 and 65 days. In general, hepatitis E resembles hepatitis A. It has a self-limiting course with an abrupt onset. Jaundice is nearly always present. Chronic forms do not develop.

Avoiding contact with the virus through good hygiene, including hand washing, is the major method of prevention of hepatitis E. The effectiveness of immune globulin in protecting against hepatitis E virus is uncertain.

HEPATITIS G (HGV) AND GB VIRUS-C

It has long been believed that there is another non-A, non-E agent causing hepatitis in humans. The incubation period for post-transfusion hepatitis is 14 to 145 days, too long for hepatitis B or C. Thus, a new form of hepatitis (hepatitis G or GBV-C) has been described. They are two different isolates of the same virus. Autoantibodies are absent. HGV has no clinical significance as an agent of liver disease. Researchers continue to look for causes of non-A, non-E hepatitis (Yoshida, 2002).

Management of Patients With Nonviral Hepatic Disorders

Certain chemicals have toxic effects on the liver and when taken by mouth, inhaled, or injected parenterally produce acute liver cell necrosis, or toxic hepatitis. The chemicals most commonly implicated in this disease are carbon tetrachloride, phosphorus, chloroform, and gold compounds. These substances are true hepatotoxins. Many medications may induce hepatitis but are sensitizing rather than toxic. The result, drug-induced hepatitis, is similar to acute viral hepatitis, but parenchymal destruction tends to be more extensive. Some medications that can lead to hepatitis are isoniazid, halothane, acetaminophen, and certain antibiotics, antimetabolites, and anesthetic agents.

TOXIC HEPATITIS

Toxic hepatitis resembles viral hepatitis in onset. Obtaining a history of exposure to hepatotoxic chemicals, medications, or other agents assists in early treatment and removal of the offending agent. Anorexia, nausea, and vomiting are the usual symptoms; jaundice and hepatomegaly are noted on physical assessment. Symptoms are more intense for the more severely toxic patient.

Recovery from acute toxic hepatitis is rapid if the hepatotoxin is identified early and removed or if exposure to the agent has been limited. Recovery is unlikely if there is a prolonged period between exposure and onset of symptoms. There are no effective antidotes. The fever rises; the patient becomes toxic and prostrated. Vomiting may be persistent, with the emesis containing blood. Clotting abnormalities may be severe, and hemorrhages may appear under the skin. The severe GI symptoms may lead to vascular collapse. Delirium, coma, and seizures develop, and within a few days the patient may die of fulminant hepatic failure (discussed below) unless he or she receives a liver transplant.

Short of liver transplantation, few treatment options are available. Therapy is directed toward restoring and maintaining fluid and electrolyte balance, blood replacement, and comfort and supportive measures. A few patients recover from acute toxic hepatitis only to develop chronic liver disease. If the liver heals, there may be scarring, followed by postnecrotic cirrhosis.

DRUG-INDUCED HEPATITIS

Manifestations of sensitivity to a medication may occur on the first day of its use or not until several months later, depending on the medication. Usually the onset is abrupt, with chills, fever, rash, pruritus, arthralgia, anorexia, and nausea. Later, there may be jaundice and dark urine and an enlarged and tender liver. When the offending medication is withdrawn, symptoms may gradually subside. However, reactions may be severe and even fatal, even though the medication is stopped. If fever, rash, or pruritus occurs from any medication, its use should be stopped immediately.

Although any medication can affect liver function, use of acetaminophen (found in many over-the counter medications used to treat fever and pain) has been identified as the leading cause of acute liver failure (Ostapowicz, Fontana, Schiodt, et al., 2002). Others commonly associated with liver injury include but are not limited to anesthetic agents, medications used to treat rheumatic and musculoskeletal disease, antidepressants, psychotropic medications, anticonvulsants, and anti-tuberculosis agents.

Inhalational agents of the halothane family (halokanes) are metabolized by the liver and excreted in bile. These volatile anesthetics may also decrease hepatic blood flow. Halothane hepatitis is a dreaded but rare complication of halothane administration. Sevoflurane and desflurane may have less hepatotoxic effects than halokanes. Nitrous oxide, an adjunct to halokanes, is not hepatotoxic. Because it undergoes little hepatic metabolism, isoflurane is considered the anesthetic agent of choice in patients with liver disease (Bacon & Di Bisceglie, 2000).

Although its efficacy is uncertain, a short course of high-dose corticosteroids may be used in patients with severe hypersensitivity. Liver transplantation is an option for drug-induced hepatitis, but outcomes may not be as successful as with other causes of liver failure.

FULMINANT HEPATIC FAILURE

Fulminant hepatic failure is the clinical syndrome of sudden and severely impaired liver function in a previously healthy person. According to the original and generally accepted definition, fulminant hepatic failure develops within 8 weeks of the first symptoms of jaundice (Maddrey et al., 2001). Patterns of the progression from jaundice to encephalopathy have been identified and have led to proposals of time-based classifications, but no agreement as to these classifications has been reached. However, three categories are frequently cited: hyperacute, acute, and subacute liver failure. In hyperacute liver failure, the duration of jaundice before the onset of encephalopathy is 0 to 7 days; in acute liver failure, it is 8 to 28 days; and in subacute liver failure, it is 28 to 72 days. The prognosis for fulminant hepatic failure is much worse than for chronic liver failure. However, in fulminant failure, the hepatic lesion is potentially reversible, with survival rates of approximately 50% to 85% (survival rates depend greatly on the etiology of liver failure). Those who do not survive die of massive hepatocellular injury and necrosis (Maddrey et al., 2001).

Viral hepatitis is a common cause of fulminant hepatic failure; other causes include toxic medications (eg, acetaminophen) and chemicals (eg, carbon tetrachloride), metabolic disturbances (Wilson's disease, a hereditary syndrome with deposition of copper in the liver), and structural changes (Budd-Chiari syndrome, an obstruction to outflow in major hepatic veins).

Jaundice and profound anorexia may be the initial reasons the patient seeks health care. Fulminant hepatic failure is often accompanied by coagulation defects, renal failure and electrolyte disturbances, infection, hypoglycemia, encephalopathy, and cerebral edema.

Management

The key to optimizing treatment is rapid recognition of acute liver failure and institution of intensive interventions. Supportive measures include monitoring for and treating hypoglycemia, infection, coagulopathy, and encephalopathy. Hypoglycemia is seen in 45% of patients who present in fulminant liver failure. In the case of hypoglycemia, immediate glucose replacement therapy is required. Broad-spectrum antibiotics are recommended to minimize the infection risks that are associated with a high incidence of mortality. Extreme coagulopathy and progressive hepatic encephalopathy occur with the onset of fulminant hepatic failure and are also associated with significant mortality. Coagulopathy should be corrected with fresh frozen plasma, but only when there is evidence of overt bleeding. Otherwise, the INR is used to monitor the progression of liver failure. There is some debate in the literature regarding the treatment of encephalopathy in liver disease. Traditionally lactulose was used; however, nonabsorbable disaccharides, dopaminergic agonists, and benzodiazepine receptor antagonists have recently been studied as possible treatment options for encephalopathy (Als-Nielsen, Gluud, & Gluud, 2005a, 2005b, 2005c). Intubation may be necessary to protect the airway as encephalopathy progresses.

There is a high risk for cerebral edema, a life-threatening complication, in patients with fulminant liver failure with stage 4 encephalopathy. The cause is not fully understood, although disruption of the blood–brain barrier and plasma leaking into the cerebrospinal fluid has been proposed as one theory (Sherlock & Dooley, 2002). These patients require intracranial pressure monitoring. Measures to promote adequate cerebral perfusion include careful fluid balance and hemodynamic assessments, a quiet environment, and diuresis with mannitol, an osmotic diuretic.

To prevent surges in intracranial pressure related to agitation, barbiturate anesthesia or pharmacologic paralysis and sedation are indicated. Other support measures include monitoring for and treating hypoglycemia, coagulopathies, and infection. Despite these treatment modalities, the mortality rate remains high. Consequently, liver transplantation (discussed later in this chapter) has become the treatment of choice for fulminant hepatic failure.

Management may also be determined based on the etiology of liver failure. For example, *N*-acetylcysteine is the treatment of choice for acetaminophen overdose (Marrero, Martinez & Hyzy, 2003). Over the last decade, a number of treatment modalities have been suggested to support those in acute failure as a bridge to recovery or to transplantation, but to date, none of these has made a significant difference in outcomes. Liver dialysis or liver assist systems have been shown to reduce mortality in chronic liver failure but have no affect on acute liver failure outcomes (Liu, Gluud, Als-Nielsen, & Gluud, 2005). Further studies are recommended before these systems can be used routinely.

HEPATIC CIRRHOSIS

Cirrhosis is a chronic disease characterized by replacement of normal liver tissue with diffuse scarring that disrupts the structure and function of the liver. There are three main categories of cirrhosis based on etiology:

- Hepatocellular disease that is the result of HCV, HBV, alcohol, nonalcoholic fatty liver disease (NAFLD), autoimmune and cryptogenic causes. The scarring begins in the hepatocytes that surround the portal areas. Biopsies taken of cirrhotic livers caused by alcoholic hepatitis and nonalcoholic steatosis hepatitis contain fatty infiltrates and are indistinguishable from each other. Hepatocellular carcinoma is a concern in these populations.
- Metabolic liver disease is generally the result of metabolic diseases such as Wilson's disease, hemachromatosis, and alpha1-antitrypsin deficiency. Glycogen storage disorders may also cause cirrhosis.
- Cholestatic disease is usually the result of chronic biliary obstruction or infection (cholangitis) and involves scarring around the bile ducts. It is much less common than the other two types. The areas become sites of inflammation, and the bile ducts become occluded with thickened bile and purulent matter. The liver attempts to form new bile channels with subsequent overgrowth of tissue. Cholangiocarcinoma can be a problem for this group of people.

Clinical manifestations include intermittent jaundice, fever, anorexia, muscle wasting, diarrhea, depleted platelet count, and fatigue. Further deterioration is evidenced by the development of ascites, varices, and encephalopathy. Initially, the liver is enlarged, hard, and irregular, but as it atrophies, it decreases in size.

Pathophysiology

Fibrosis is the healing response of the liver to injury, but over time, fibrosis can progress to cirrhosis. Cirrhosis is the permanent scarring of the liver and is considered the end-stage of liver disease. There are over 100 recognized forms of liver disease that may lead to cirrhosis. Hepatitis C is the leading cause of liver disease in Canada, followed by alcoholic cirrhosis. Recently, NAFLD, which is indistinguishable histologically from alcoholic fatty liver disease, has become an increasing concern in North America. The incidence of NAFLD is increasing as obesity and the incidence of type 2 diabetes becomes more common. Chemical exposure is another factor that influences the development of cirrhosis. Twice as many men as women are affected, and most patients are between 40 and 60 years of age. Each year, more than 2000 people in Canada die of chronic liver disease and cirrhosis (Statistics Canada, 2005). The goal of treatment for fibrosis and cirrhosis is to minimize the effects of the underlying cause of liver disease. It is anticipated that antifibrotic research will revolutionize hepatology (Iredale, 2003).

The prognosis of different forms of cirrhosis caused by various liver diseases has been investigated in several studies. Of the many prognostic indicators, the Child's classification seems most useful in predicting the outcome of patients with liver disease (Table 39-5). It is also used in choosing management approaches.

Clinical Manifestations

Signs and symptoms of cirrhosis increase in severity as the disease progresses. The severity of the manifestations helps to categorize the disorder into two main presentations (Chart 39-10).

Compensated cirrhosis, with its less severe, often vague symptoms, may be discovered secondarily at a routine physical examination. The hallmarks of decompensated cirrhosis result from failure of the liver to synthesize proteins, clotting factors, and other substances and manifestations of portal hypertension (see the "Hepatic Dysfunction" section of this chapter for clinical manifestations and management of portal hypertension, ascites, varices, and hepatic encephalopathy).

LIVER ENLARGEMENT
Early in the course of cirrhosis, the liver tends to be large and its cells loaded with fat. The liver is firm and has a sharp edge noticeable on palpation. Abdominal pain may be present because of recent, rapid enlargement of the liver, producing tension on the fibrous covering of the liver (Glisson's capsule). Later in the disease, the liver decreases in size as scar tissue contracts the liver tissue. The liver edge, if palpable, is nodular.

PORTAL OBSTRUCTION AND ASCITES
These late manifestations are due partly to chronic failure of liver function and partly to obstruction of the portal circulation. Practically all the blood from the digestive organs is collected in the portal veins and carried to the liver. Because a cirrhotic liver does not allow the blood free passage, it backs up into the spleen and the GI tract and these organs become the seat of chronic passive congestion; that is, they are stagnant with blood and thus cannot function properly. Indigestion and altered bowel function result. Fluid rich in protein may accumulate in the peritoneal cavity, producing ascites. This can be demonstrated through percussion for shifting dullness or a fluid wave (see Fig. 39-5).

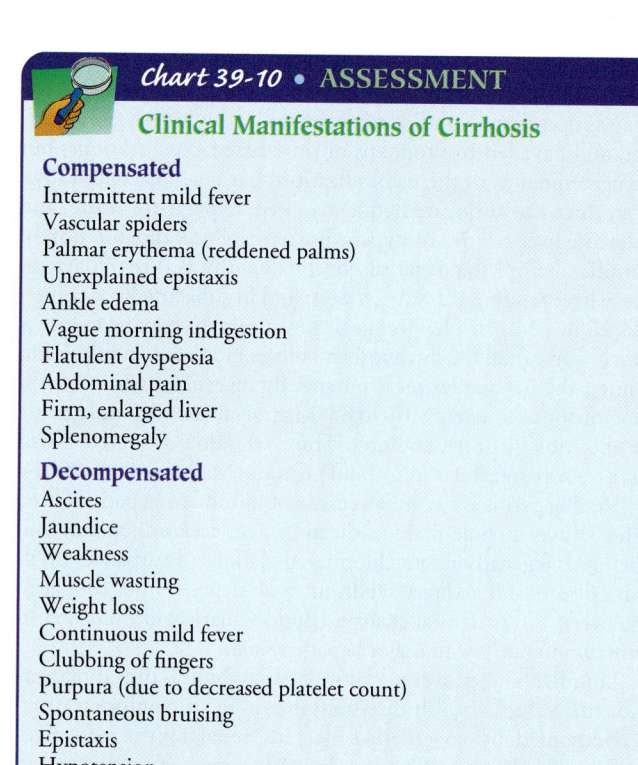

Chart 39-10 • ASSESSMENT

Clinical Manifestations of Cirrhosis

Compensated
Intermittent mild fever
Vascular spiders
Palmar erythema (reddened palms)
Unexplained epistaxis
Ankle edema
Vague morning indigestion
Flatulent dyspepsia
Abdominal pain
Firm, enlarged liver
Splenomegaly

Decompensated
Ascites
Jaundice
Weakness
Muscle wasting
Weight loss
Continuous mild fever
Clubbing of fingers
Purpura (due to decreased platelet count)
Spontaneous bruising
Epistaxis
Hypotension
Sparse body hair
White nails
Gonadal atrophy

INFECTION AND PERITONITIS
Bacterial peritonitis may develop in cirrhotic patients with ascites in the absence of an intra-abdominal source of infection or an abscess. This condition is referred to as spontaneous bacterial peritonitis (SBP). Bacteremia is believed to be the most likely route of infection. Clinical signs may be absent; paracentesis may be necessary for diagnosis. Antibiotic therapy is effective in the treatment and prevention of recurrent episodes of spontaneous bacterial peritonitis. Undiagnosed SBP often results in life-threatening episodes of sepsis.

GASTROINTESTINAL VARICES
The obstruction to blood flow through the liver resulting from the fibrotic changes also results in the formation of collateral blood vessels in the GI system and shunting of blood from the portal vessels into blood vessels with lower pressures. As a result, the patient with cirrhosis often has prominent, distended abdominal blood vessels, which are visible on abdominal inspection (caput medusae), and

Table 39-5 • Child's Classification of Hepatocellular Dysfunction in Cirrhosis

GROUP DESIGNATION	A (LEAST SEVERE)	B	C (MOST SEVERE)
Serum bilirubin (μmol/L)	Below 30	30–50	Over 50
Serum albumin (g/L)	Over 35	30–35	Under 30
Ascites	None	Easily controlled	Poorly controlled
Neurologic disorder (degree of encephalopathy)	None	Minimal	Advanced coma
Nutrition	Excellent	Good	Poor with "wasting"

From Sherlock, S., & Dooley, J. (2002). *Diseases of the liver and biliary system* (11th ed.). Oxford: Blackwell, p. 171.

distended blood vessels throughout the GI tract. The esophagus, stomach, and lower rectum are common sites of collateral blood vessels. These distended blood vessels form varices or hemorrhoids, depending on their location (see Fig. 39-6).

Because these vessels were not intended to carry the high pressure and volume of blood imposed by cirrhosis, they may rupture and bleed. Therefore, assessment must include observation for occult and frank bleeding from the GI tract. Approximately 25% of patients develop minor hematemesis; others have profuse hemorrhage from gastric and esophageal varices (Bacon & Di Bisceglie, 2000).

EDEMA

Another late symptom of cirrhosis is edema, which is attributed to chronic liver failure. A reduced plasma albumin concentration predisposes the patient to the formation of edema. Edema is generalized but often affects lower extremities, upper extremities, and the presacral area. Facial edema is not typical. Overproduction of aldosterone occurs, causing sodium and water retention and potassium excretion.

VITAMIN DEFICIENCY AND ANEMIA

Because of inadequate formation, use, and storage of certain vitamins (notably vitamins A, C, and K), signs of their deficiency are common, particularly hemorrhagic phenomena associated with vitamin K deficiency. Chronic gastritis and impaired GI function, together with inadequate dietary intake and impaired liver function, account for the anemia often associated with cirrhosis. The anemia and the patient's poor nutritional status and poor state of health result in severe fatigue, which interferes with the ability to carry out routine daily activities.

MENTAL DETERIORATION

Additional clinical manifestations include deterioration of mental function with impending hepatic encephalopathy and hepatic coma. Neurologic assessment is indicated and includes the patient's general behaviour, cognitive abilities, orientation to time and place, and speech patterns.

Assessment and Diagnostic Findings

The extent of liver disease and the type of treatment are determined after reviewing the laboratory findings. Because the functions of the liver are complex, there are many diagnostic tests that may provide information about liver function (see Table 39-1). The patient needs to know why these tests are being performed and ways to cooperate.

In severe parenchymal liver dysfunction, the serum albumin level tends to decrease and the serum globulin level rises. Enzyme tests indicate liver cell damage: serum alkaline phosphatase, AST, ALT, and GGT levels increase, and the serum cholinesterase level may decrease. Bilirubin tests are performed to measure bile excretion or bile retention; elevated levels can occur with cirrhosis and other liver disorders. Prothrombin time is prolonged.

Ultrasound scanning is used to measure the difference in density of parenchymal cells and scar tissue. CT, MRI, and radioisotope liver scans give information about liver size and hepatic blood flow and obstruction. Arterial blood gas analysis may reveal a ventilation–perfusion imbalance and hypoxia.

Medical Management

The management of the patient with cirrhosis is usually based on the presenting symptoms. For example, antacids are prescribed to decrease gastric distress and minimize the possibility of GI bleeding. Vitamins and nutritional supplements promote healing of damaged liver cells and improve the general nutritional status. Potassium-sparing diuretics (spironolactone [Aldactone], triamterene [Dyrenium]) may be indicated to decrease ascites, if present; these diuretics are preferable to other diuretic agents because they minimize the fluid and electrolyte changes common with other agents. An adequate diet and avoidance of alcohol are essential. Although the fibrosis of the cirrhotic liver cannot be reversed, its progression may be halted or slowed by such measures.

Preliminary studies indicate that colchicine, an anti-inflammatory agent used to treat the symptoms of gout, may increase the length of survival in patients with mild to moderate cirrhosis. Improved survival has been observed in patients with alcoholic cirrhosis. Colchicine is believed to reverse the fibrotic processes in cirrhosis, and this has improved survival (Bacon & Di Bisceglie, 2000).

NURSING PROCESS: THE PATIENT WITH HEPATIC CIRRHOSIS

Assessment

Nursing assessment focuses on the onset of symptoms and the history of precipitating factors, particularly long-term alcohol abuse, as well as dietary intake and changes in the patient's physical and mental status. The patient's past and current patterns of alcohol use (duration and amount) are assessed and documented. It is also important to document any exposure to toxic agents encountered in the workplace or during recreational activities. The nurse documents and reports exposure to potentially hepatotoxic substances (medications, illicit IV/injection drugs, inhalants) or general anesthetic agents. The patient's surgical history, transfusion history, tattoos, and body piercings should be listed, along with dates and locations.

The nurse assesses the patient's mental status through the interview and other interactions with the patient; orientation to person, place, and time is noted. The patient's ability to carry out a job or household activities provides some information about physical and mental status. The patient's relationships with family, friends, and coworkers may give some indication about incapacitation secondary to alcohol abuse and cirrhosis. Abdominal distention and bloating, GI bleeding, bruising, and weight changes are noted.

The nurse assesses nutritional status, which is of major importance in cirrhosis, by daily weights and monitoring of plasma proteins, transferrin, and creatinine levels.

Diagnosis

NURSING DIAGNOSES

Based on all the assessment data, the patient's major nursing diagnoses may include the following:

- Activity intolerance related to fatigue, general debility, muscle wasting, and discomfort
- Imbalanced nutrition, less than body requirements, related to chronic gastritis, decreased GI motility, and anorexia
- Impaired skin integrity related to compromised immunologic status, edema, and poor nutrition

- Risk for injury and bleeding related to altered clotting mechanisms

COLLABORATIVE PROBLEMS/ POTENTIAL COMPLICATIONS

Based on assessment data, potential complications may include:

- Bleeding and hemorrhage
- Hepatic encephalopathy
- Fluid volume excess

Planning and Goals

The goals for the patient may include increased participation in activities, improvement of nutritional status, improvement of skin integrity, decreased potential for injury, improvement of mental status, and absence of complications.

Nursing Interventions

PROMOTING REST

The patient with active liver disease requires rest and other supportive measures to permit the liver to reestablish its functional ability. If the patient is hospitalized, weight and fluid intake and output are measured and recorded daily. The nurse adjusts the patient's position in bed for maximal respiratory efficiency, which is especially important if ascites is marked because it interferes with adequate thoracic excursion. Oxygen therapy may be required in liver failure to oxygenate the damaged cells and prevent further cell destruction.

Rest reduces the demands on the liver and increases the liver's blood supply. Because the patient is susceptible to the hazards of immobility, efforts to prevent respiratory, circulatory, and vascular disturbances are initiated. These measures may help prevent such problems as pneumonia, thrombophlebitis, and pressure ulcers. When nutritional status improves and strength increases, the nurse encourages the patient to increase activity gradually. Activity and mild exercise, as well as rest, are planned.

IMPROVING NUTRITIONAL STATUS

The patient with cirrhosis who has no ascites or edema and exhibits no signs of impending hepatic coma should receive a nutritious, high-protein diet if tolerated, supplemented by vitamins of the B complex and others as indicated (including vitamins A, C, K and folic acid). Because proper nutrition is so important, the nurse makes every effort to encourage the patient to eat. This is as important as any medication. Often small, frequent meals are tolerated better than three large meals because of the abdominal pressure exerted by ascites. Protein supplements may also be indicated.

Patient preferences are considered. Patients with prolonged or severe anorexia, or those who are vomiting or eating poorly for any reason, may receive nutrients enterally or parenteral nutrition.

Patients with fatty stools (steatorrhea) should receive water-soluble forms of fat-soluble vitamins—A, D, and E (Aquasol A, D, and E). Folic acid and iron are prescribed to prevent anemia. If the patient shows signs of impending or advancing coma, the amount of protein in the diet is decreased temporarily. In the absence of hepatic encephalopathy, a moderate-protein, high-calorie intake is provided, with protein foods of high biologic value. A diet containing 1 to 1.5 g of protein per kilogram of body weight per day is required unless the patient is malnourished. Protein is restricted if encephalopathy develops. Incorporating vegetable protein to meet protein needs may decrease the risk of encephalopathy. Sodium restriction is also indicated to prevent ascites.

A high-calorie intake should be maintained, and supplemental vitamins and minerals should be provided (eg, oral potassium if the serum potassium level is normal or low and if renal function is normal).

PROVIDING SKIN CARE

Providing careful skin care is important because of subcutaneous edema, the patient's immobility, jaundice, and increased susceptibility to skin breakdown and infection. Frequent position changes are necessary to prevent pressure ulcers. It is important to avoid irritating soaps and the use of adhesive tape to prevent trauma to the skin. Lotion may be soothing to irritated skin; the nurse takes measures to minimize scratching by the patient.

REDUCING RISK OF INJURY

The nurse protects the patient with cirrhosis from falls and other injuries. The side rails should be in place and padded with blankets in case the patient becomes agitated or restless. To minimize agitation, the nurse orients the patient to time and place and explains all procedures. The nurse instructs the patient to ask for assistance to get out of bed. The nurse carefully evaluates any injury because of the possibility of internal bleeding.

Because of the risk for bleeding from abnormal clotting, the patient should use an electric rather than a safety razor. A soft-bristled toothbrush will help to minimize bleeding gums, and pressure applied to all venipuncture sites will help to minimize bleeding.

MONITORING AND MANAGING POTENTIAL COMPLICATIONS

Bleeding and Hemorrhage

The patient is at increased risk for bleeding and hemorrhage because of decreased production of prothrombin and decreased ability of the diseased liver to synthesize the substances necessary for blood coagulation. Precautionary measures include protecting the patient with padded side rails, applying pressure to injection sites, and avoiding injury from sharp objects. The nurse observes for melena and assesses stools for blood (signs of possible internal bleeding). Vital signs are monitored regularly. Precautions are taken to minimize rupture of esophageal varices by avoiding further increases in portal pressure (discussed previously). Dietary modification and appropriate use of stool softeners may help prevent straining during defecation. The nurse closely monitors the patient for GI bleeding and keeps readily available equipment (Sengstaken–Blakemore tube), IV fluids, and medications needed to treat hemorrhage from esophageal and gastric varices.

If hemorrhage occurs, the nurse assists the physician in initiating measures to halt the bleeding, administering fluid and blood component therapy and medications. The patient with massive hemorrhage from bleeding esophageal or gastric varices may be transferred to the intensive care unit and may require emergency surgery or other treatment modalities. The patient and family require explanations about the event and the necessary treatment.

Hepatic Encephalopathy

Hepatic encephalopathy and coma, possible complications of cirrhosis, may present as deteriorating mental status and dementia as well as physical signs such as abnormal voluntary and involuntary movements. Hepatic encephalopathy is mainly caused by the accumulation of ammonia in the blood and its effect on cerebral metabolism. Many factors predispose the patient with cirrhosis to hepatic encephalopathy; therefore, the patient may require extensive diagnostic testing to identify hidden sources of bleeding, ammonia and infection (SBP).

Treatment may include the use of lactulose and nonabsorbable intestinal tract antibiotics to decrease ammonia levels, modification in medications to eliminate those that may precipitate or worsen hepatic encephalopathy, and bed rest to minimize energy expenditure.

Monitoring is an essential nursing function to identify early deterioration in mental status. The nurse monitors the patient's mental status closely and reports changes so that treatment of encephalopathy can be initiated promptly. Because electrolyte disturbances can contribute to encephalopathy, serum electrolyte levels are carefully monitored and corrected if abnormal. Oxygen is administered if oxygen desaturation occurs. The nurse monitors for fever or abdominal pain, which may signal the onset of bacterial peritonitis or other infection (see the discussion of hepatic encephalopathy in the "Hepatic Dysfunction" section of this Chapter).

Fluid Volume Excess

Patients with advanced chronic liver disease develop cardiovascular abnormalities. These occur due to an increased cardiac output and decreased peripheral vascular resistance, possibly resulting from the release of vasodilators. A hyperdynamic circulatory state develops in patients with cirrhosis, and plasma volume increases. This increase in circulating plasma volume may be due in part to splanchnic venous congestion (Bircher et al., 1999). The greater the degree of hepatic decompensation, the more severe the hyperdynamic state. Close assessment of the cardiovascular and respiratory status is key for the nurse caring for patients with this disorder. Pulmonary compromise is always a potential complication of end-stage liver disease due to plasma volume excess, making prevention of pulmonary complications an important role for the nurse. Administering diuretics, implementing fluid restrictions, and enhancing patient positioning can optimize pulmonary function. Fluid retention may be noted in the development of ascites and lower extremity swelling and dyspnea. Monitoring intake and output, daily weight changes, changes in abdominal girth, and edema formation is part of nursing assessment in the hospital or in the home setting. Patients are also monitored for nocturia and, later, oliguria as these states indicate increasing severity of liver function (Bacon & Di Bisceglie, 2000).

PROMOTING HOME AND COMMUNITY-BASED CARE

Teaching Patients Self-Care

During the patient's hospital stay, the nurse and other health care providers prepare the patient with cirrhosis for discharge, focusing on dietary instruction. Of greatest importance is the exclusion of alcohol from the diet. The patient may need referral to Alcoholics Anonymous, psychiatric care, or counselling or may benefit from support from a spiritual advisor.

Sodium restriction will continue for a considerable time, if not permanently. The patient will require written instructions, teaching, reinforcement, and support from the staff as well as the family members.

The success of treatment depends on convincing the patient of the need to adhere completely to the therapeutic plan. This includes rest, lifestyle changes, adequate dietary intake, and the elimination of alcohol. The nurse also instructs the patient and family about the symptoms of impending encephalopathy, possible bleeding tendencies, and susceptibility to infection.

Recovery is neither rapid nor easy; there are frequent setbacks and apparent lack of improvement. Many patients find it difficult to refrain from using alcohol for comfort or escape. The nurse has a significant role in offering support and encouragement to this patient.

Continuing Care

Referral of the patient for home care may assist the patient in dealing with the transition from hospital to home, where the use of alcohol may have been an important part of normal home and social life. The home care nurse assesses the patient's progress at home and the manner in which the patient and family cope with the elimination of alcohol and the dietary restrictions. The nurse also reinforces previous teaching and answers questions that may not have occurred to the patient or family until the patient is back home and trying to establish new patterns of eating, drinking, and lifestyle. For an overall view of the nursing management of the patient with impaired liver function, refer to the Plan of Nursing Care.

Evaluation

EXPECTED PATIENT OUTCOMES

Expected patient outcomes may include:

1. Participates in activities
   a. Plans activities and exercises to allow alternating periods of rest and activity
   b. Reports increased strength and well-being
   c. Participates in hygiene care
2. Increases nutritional intake
   a. Demonstrates intake of appropriate nutrients and avoidance of alcohol as reflected by diet log
   b. Gains weight without increased edema and ascites formation
   c. Reports decrease in GI disturbances and anorexia
   d. Identifies foods and fluids that are nutritious and allowed on diet or restricted from diet
   e. Adheres to vitamin therapy regimen
   f. Describes the rationale for small, frequent meals
3. Exhibits improved skin integrity
   a. Has intact skin without evidence of breakdown, infection, or trauma
   b. Demonstrates normal turgor of skin of extremities and trunk, without edema
   c. Changes position frequently and inspects bony prominences daily
   d. Uses lotions to decrease pruritus
4. Avoids injury
   a. Is free of ecchymotic areas or hematoma formation
   b. States rationale for side rails and asks for assistance to get out of bed
   c. Uses measures to prevent trauma (eg, uses electric razor and soft toothbrush, blows nose gently, arranges furniture to prevent bumps and falls, avoids straining during defecation)
5. Is free of complications
   a. Reports absence of frank bleeding from GI tract (ie, absence of melena and hematemesis)
   b. Is oriented to time, place, and person and demonstrates normal attention span
   c. Has serum ammonia level within normal limits
   d. Identifies early, reportable signs of impaired thought processes

(text continues on page 1119)

Plan of Nursing Care
The Patient With Impaired Liver Function

Nursing Interventions	Rationale	Expected Outcomes

Nursing Diagnosis: Activity intolerance related to fatigue, lethargy, and malaise

Goal: Patient reports decrease in fatigue and reports increased ability to participate in activities

Nursing Interventions	Rationale	Expected Outcomes
1. Assess level of activity tolerance and degree of fatigue, lethargy, and malaise when performing routine ADLs.	1. Provides baseline for further assessment and criteria for assessment of effectiveness of interventions	• Exhibits increased interest in activities and events
2. Assist with activities and hygiene when fatigued.	2. Promotes exercise and hygiene within patient's level of tolerance	• Participates in activities and gradually increases exercise within physical limits
3. Encourage rest when fatigued or when abdominal pain or discomfort occurs.	3. Conserves energy and protects the liver	• Reports increased strength and well-being
4. Assist with selection and pacing of desired activities and exercise.	4. Stimulates patient's interest in selected activities	• Reports absence of abdominal pain and discomfort
5. Provide diet high in carbohydrates with protein intake consistent with liver function.	5. Provides calories for energy and protein for healing	• Plans activities to allow ample periods of rest
6. Administer supplemental vitamins (A, B complex, C, and K).	6. Provides additional nutrients	• Takes vitamins as prescribed

Nursing Diagnosis: Imbalanced nutrition: less than body requirements, related to abdominal distention and discomfort and anorexia

Goal: Positive nitrogen balance, no further loss of muscle mass; meets nutritional requirements

Nursing Interventions	Rationale	Expected Outcomes
1. Assess dietary intake and nutritional status through diet history and diary, daily weight measurements and laboratory data.	1. Identifies deficits in nutritional intake and adequacy of nutritional state	• Exhibits improved nutritional status by increased weight (without fluid retention) and improved laboratory data.
2. Provide diet high in carbohydrates with protein intake consistent with liver function.	2. Provides calories for energy, sparing protein for healing	• States rationale for dietary modifications
3. Assist patient in identifying low-sodium foods.	3. Reduces edema and ascites formation	• Identifies foods high in carbohydrates and within protein requirements (moderate to high protein in cirrhosis and hepatitis, low protein in hepatic failure)
4. Elevate the head of the bed during meals.	4. Reduces discomfort from abdominal distention and decreases sense of fullness produced by pressure of abdominal contents and ascites on the stomach	• Reports improved appetite
5. Provide oral hygiene before meals and pleasant environment for meals at meal time.	5. Promotes positive environment and increased appetite; reduces unpleasant taste	• Participates in oral hygiene measures
6. Offer smaller, more frequent meals (6 per day).	6. Decreases feeling of fullness, bloating	• Reports increased appetite; identifies rationale for smaller, frequent meals
7. Encourage patient to eat meals and supplementary feedings.	7. Encouragement is essential for the patient with anorexia and gastrointestinal discomfort.	• Demonstrates intake of high-calorie diet; adheres to protein restriction
8. Provide attractive meals and an aesthetically pleasing setting at meal time.	8. Promotes appetite and sense of well-being	• Identifies foods and fluids that are nutritious and permitted on diet
9. Eliminate alcohol.	9. Eliminates "empty calories" and further damage from alcohol	• Gains weight without increased edema or ascites formation
10. Apply an ice collar for nausea.	10. May reduce incidence of nausea	• Reports increased appetite and well-being
11. Administer medications prescribed for nausea, vomiting, diarrhea, or constipation.	11. Reduces gastrointestinal symptoms and discomforts that decrease the appetite and interest in food	• Excludes alcohol from diet
12. Encourage increased fluid intake and exercise if the patient reports constipation.	12. Promotes normal bowel pattern and reduces abdominal discomfort and distention	• Takes medications for gastrointestinal disorders as prescribed
		• Reports normal gastrointestinal function with regular bowel function

(continued)

Plan of Nursing Care
The Patient With Impaired Liver Function (Continued)

Nursing Interventions	Rationale	Expected Outcomes

Nursing Diagnosis: Impaired skin integrity related to pruritus from jaundice and edema
Goal: Decrease potential for pressure ulcer development; breaks in skin integrity

1. Assess degree of discomfort related to pruritus and edema.	1. Assists in determining appropriate interventions	• Exhibits intact skin without redness, excoriation, or breakdown
2. Note and record degree of jaundice and extent of edema.	2. Provides baseline for detecting changes and evaluating effectiveness of interventions	• Reports relief from pruritus • Exhibits no skin excoriation from scratching
3. Keep patient's fingernails short and smooth.	3. Prevents skin excoriation and infection from scratching	• Uses nondrying soaps and lotions. States rationale for use of nondrying soaps and lotions.
4. Provide frequent skin care; avoid use of soaps and alcohol-based lotions.	4. Removes waste products on skin while preventing dryness of skin	• Turns self periodically. Exhibits reduced edema of dependent parts of the body.
5. Massage every 2 hours with emollients; turn every 2 hours	5. Promotes mobilization of edema	• Exhibits no areas of skin breakdown • Exhibits decreased edema; normal skin turgor
6. Initiate use of alternating-pressure mattress or low air loss bed.	6. Minimizes prolonged pressure on bony prominences susceptible to breakdown	
7. Recommend avoiding use of harsh detergents.	7. May decrease skin irritation and need for scratching	
8. Assess skin integrity every 4–8 hours. Instruct patient and family in this activity.	8. Edematous skin and tissue has compromised nutrient supply and is vulnerable to pressure and trauma	
9. Restrict sodium as prescribed.	9. Minimizes edema formation	
10. Perform range of motion exercises every 4 hours; elevate edematous extremities whenever possible.	10. Promotes mobilization of edema	

Nursing Diagnosis: High risk for injury related to altered clotting mechanisms and altered level of consciousness
Goal: Reduced risk of injury

1. Assess level of consciousness and cognitive level.	1. Assists in determining patient's ability to protect self and comply with required self-protective actions; may detect deterioration of hepatic function	• Is oriented to time, place, and person • Exhibits no hallucinations, and demonstrates no efforts to get up unassisted or to leave hospital
2. Provide safe environment (pad side rails, remove obstacles in room, prevent falls).	2. Minimizes falls and injury if falls occur	• Exhibits no ecchymoses (bruises), cuts, or hematoma
3. Provide frequent surveillance to orient patient and avoid use of restraints.	3. Protects patient from harm while stimulating and orienting patient; use of restraints may disturb patient further	• Uses electric razor rather than sharp-edged razor
4. Replace sharp objects (razors) with safer items.	4. Avoids cuts and bleeding	• Exhibits absence of frank bleeding from gastrointestinal tract
5. Observe each stool for colour, consistency, and amount.	5. Permits detection of bleeding in gastrointestinal tract	• Exhibits absence of restlessness, epigastric fullness, and other indicators of hemorrhage and shock
6. Be alert for symptoms of anxiety, epigastric fullness, weakness, and restlessness.	6. May indicate early signs of bleeding and shock	• Exhibits negative results of test for occult gastrointestinal bleeding
7. Test each stool and emesis for occult blood.	7. Detects early evidence of bleeding	• Is free of ecchymotic areas or hematoma formation
8. Observe for hemorrhagic manifestations: ecchymosis, epistaxis, petechiae, and bleeding gums.	8. Indicates altered clotting mechanisms	• Exhibits normal vital signs • Maintains rest and remains quiet if active bleeding occurs
9. Record vital signs at frequent intervals, depending on patient acuity (every 1–4 hours).	9. Provides baseline and evidence of hypovolemia, and hemorrhagic shock	• Identifies rationale for blood transfusions and measures to treat bleeding
10. Keep patient quiet and limit activity.	10. Minimizes risk of bleeding and straining	• Uses measures to prevent trauma (eg, uses soft toothbrush, blows nose gently, avoids bumps and falls, avoids straining during defecation)
11. Assist physician in passage of tube for esophageal balloon tamponade, if its insertion is indicated.	11. Promotes nontraumatic insertion of tube in anxious and combative patient for immediate treatment of bleeding	• Experiences no side effects of medications • Takes all medications as prescribed

(continued)

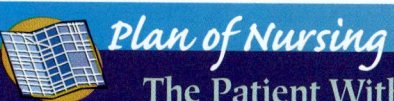

Plan of Nursing Care

The Patient With Impaired Liver Function *(Continued)*

Nursing Interventions	Rationale	Expected Outcomes
12. Observe during blood transfusions.	12. Permits detection of transfusion reactions (risk is increased with multiple blood transfusions needed for active bleeding from esophageal varices)	• Identifies rationale for precautions with use of all medications • Cooperates with treatment modalities
13. Measure and record nature, time, and amount of vomitus.	13. Assists in evaluating extent of bleeding and blood loss	
14. Maintain patient in fasting state, if indicated.	14. Reduces risk of aspiration of gastric contents and minimizes risk of further trauma to esophagus and stomach by preventing vomiting	
15. Administer vitamin K as prescribed.	15. Promotes clotting by providing fat-soluble vitamin necessary for clotting.	
16. Remain with patient during episodes of bleeding.	16. Reassures anxious patient and permits monitoring and detection of further needs of the patient	
17. Offer cold liquids by mouth when bleeding stops (if prescribed).	17. Minimizes risk of further bleeding by promoting vasoconstriction of esophageal and gastric blood vessels	

18. Institute measures to prevent trauma:
  a. Maintain safe environment.
 	
  b. Encourage *gentle* blowing of nose.
 	
  c. Provide soft toothbrush and avoid use of toothpicks.
  d. Encourage intake of foods with high content of vitamin C.
  e. Apply cold compresses where indicated.
  f. Record location of bleeding sites.
 	
  g. Use small-gauge needles for injections.
	18. Promotes safety of patient
	  a. Minimizes risk of trauma and bleeding by avoiding falls and cuts, etc.
	  b. Reduces risk of nosebleed (epistaxis) secondary to trauma and decreased clotting
	  c. Prevents trauma to oral mucosa while promoting good oral hygiene
	  d. Promotes healing
	
	  e. Minimizes bleeding into tissues by promoting local vasoconstriction
	  f. Permits detection of new bleeding sites and monitoring of previous sites of bleeding
	  g. Minimizes oozing and blood loss from repeated injections	

19. Administer medications carefully; monitor for side effects.	19. Reduces risk of side effects secondary to damaged liver's inability to detoxify (metabolize) medications normally	

Nursing Diagnosis: Disturbed body image related to changes in appearance, sexual dysfunction, and role function
Goal: Patient verbalizes feelings consistent with improvement of body image and self-esteem

1. Assess changes in appearance and the meaning these changes have for patient and family.	1. Provides information for assessing impact of changes in appearance, sexual function, and role on the patient and family	• Verbalizes concerns related to changes in appearance, life, and lifestyle • Shares concerns with significant others • Identifies past coping strategies that have been effective • Uses past effective coping strategies to deal with changes in appearance, life, and lifestyle • Maintains good grooming and hygiene • Identifies short-term goals and strategies to achieve them • Exercises an active role in decision making about self and care
2. Encourage patient to verbalize reactions and feelings about these changes.	2. Enables patient to identify and express concerns; encourages patient and significant others to share these concerns	
3. Assess patient's and family's previous coping strategies.	3. Permits encouragement of those coping strategies that are familiar to patient and have been effective in the past	
4. Assist and encourage patient to maximize appearance and explore alternatives to previous sexual and role functions.	4. Encourages patient to continue safe roles and functions while encouraging exploration of alternatives	

(continued)

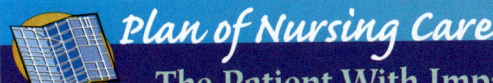

Plan of Nursing Care

The Patient With Impaired Liver Function (Continued)

Nursing Interventions	Rationale	Expected Outcomes
5. Assist patient in identifying short-term goals. 6. Encourage and assist patient in decision making about care. 7. Identify with patient resources to provide additional support (counselor, spiritual advisor). 8. Assist patient in identifying previous practices that may have been harmful to self (alcohol and drug abuse).	5. Accomplishing these goals serves as positive reinforcement and increases self-esteem. 6. Promotes patient's control of life and improves sense of well-being and self-esteem 7. Assists patient in identifying resources and accepting assistance from others when indicated 8. Recognition and acknowledgment of the harmful effects of these practices are necessary for identifying a healthier lifestyle.	• Identifies resources that are not harmful • Verbalizes that some of previous lifestyle practices have been harmful • Uses healthy expressions of frustration, anger, anxiety

Nursing Diagnosis: Chronic pain and discomfort related to enlarged tender liver and ascites
Goal: Increased level of comfort

1. Maintain bed rest when patient experiences abdominal discomfort. 2. Administer antispasmodic and sedative agents as prescribed. 3. Observe, record, and report presence and character of pain and discomfort. 4. Reduce sodium and fluid intake if prescribed. 5. Prepare patient and assist with paracentesis.	1. Reduces metabolic demands and protects the liver 2. Reduces irritability of the gastrointestinal tract and decreases abdominal pain and discomfort 3. Provides baseline to detect further deterioration of status and to evaluate interventions 4. Minimizes further formation of ascites 5. Removal of ascites fluid may decrease abdominal discomfort	• Reports pain and discomfort if present • Maintains bed rest and decreases activity in presence of pain • Takes antispasmodic and sedatives as indicated and as prescribed • Reports decreased pain and abdominal discomfort • Reduces sodium and fluid intake to prescribed levels if indicated to treat ascites • Exhibits decreased abdominal girth and appropriate weight changes • Reports decreased discomfort after paracentesis

Nursing Diagnosis: Fluid volume excess related to ascites and edema formation
Goal: Restoration of normal fluid volume

1. Restrict sodium and fluid intake if prescribed. 2. Administer diuretics, potassium, and protein supplements as prescribed. 3. Record intake and output every 1 to 8 hours depending on response to interventions and on patient acuity. 4. Measure and record abdominal girth and weight daily. 5. Explain rationale for sodium and fluid restriction. 6. Prepare patient and assist with paracentesis.	1. Minimizes formation of ascites and edema 2. Promotes excretion of fluid through the kidneys and maintenance of normal fluid and electrolyte balance 3. Indicates effectiveness of treatment and adequacy of fluid intake 4. Monitors changes in ascites formation and fluid accumulation 5. Promotes patient's understanding of restriction and cooperation with it 6. Paracentesis will temporarily decrease amount of ascites present.	• Consumes diet low in sodium and within prescribed fluid restriction • Takes diuretics, potassium, and protein supplements as indicated without experiencing side effects • Exhibits increased urine output • Exhibits decreasing abdominal girth • Exhibits no rapid increase in weight • Identifies rationale for sodium and fluid restriction • Shows a decrease in ascites with decreased weight

(continued)

Plan of Nursing Care

The Patient With Impaired Liver Function (Continued)

Nursing Interventions	Rationale	Expected Outcomes

Nursing Diagnosis: Disturbed thought processes related to deterioration of liver function and increased serum ammonia level

Goal: Improved mental status; safety maintained

Nursing Interventions	Rationale	Expected Outcomes
1. Restrict dietary protein as prescribed.	1. Reduces source of ammonia (protein foods)	• Adheres to protein restriction
2. Give frequent, small feedings of carbohydrates.	2. Promotes consumption of adequate carbohydrates for energy requirements and spares protein from breakdown for energy	• Demonstrates an interest in events and activities in environment
3. Protect from infection.	3. Minimizes risk for further increase in metabolic requirements	• Demonstrates normal attention span
4. Keep environment warm and draft-free.	4. Minimizes shivering, which would increase metabolic requirements	• Follows and participates in conversation appropriately
5. Pad the side rails of the bed.	5. Provides protection for the patient should hepatic coma and seizure activity occur	• Is oriented to person, place, and time
6. Limit visitors.	6. Minimizes patient's activity and metabolic requirements	• Remains in bed when indicated
7. Provide careful nursing surveillance to ensure patient's safety.	7. Provides close monitoring of new symptoms and minimizes trauma to the confused patient	• Reports no urinary or fecal incontinence
8. Avoid opioids and barbiturates.	8. Prevents masking of symptoms of hepatic coma and prevents drug overdose secondary to reduced ability of the damaged liver to metabolize opioids and barbiturates	• Experiences no seizures
9. Awaken at intervals (every 2–4 hours) to assess cognitive status.	9. Provides stimulation to the patient and opportunity for observing the patient's level of consciousness	

Nursing Diagnosis: Risk for imbalanced body temperature: hyperthermia related to inflammatory process of cirrhosis or hepatitis

Goal: Maintenance of normal body temperature, free from infection

Nursing Interventions	Rationale	Expected Outcomes
1. Record temperature regularly (every 4 hours).	1. Provides baseline to detect fever and to evaluate interventions	• Exhibits normal temperature and reports absence of chills or sweating
2. Encourage fluid intake.	2. Corrects fluid loss from perspiration and fever and increases patient's level of comfort	• Demonstrates adequate intake of fluids
3. Apply cool sponges or icebag for elevated temperature.	3. Promotes reduction of fever and increases patient's comfort	• Exhibits no evidence of local or systemic infection
4. Administer antibiotics as prescribed.	4. Ensures appropriate serum concentration of antibiotics to treat infection	
5. Avoid exposure to infections.	5. Minimizes risk of further infection and further increases in body temperature and metabolic rate	
6. Keep patient at rest while temperature is elevated.	6. Reduces metabolic rate	
7. Assess for abdominal pain, tenderness.	7. May occur with bacterial peritonitis	

(continued)

Plan of Nursing Care
The Patient With Impaired Liver Function *(Continued)*

Nursing Interventions	Rationale	Expected Outcomes

Nursing Diagnosis: Ineffective breathing pattern related to ascites and restriction of thoracic excursion secondary to ascites, abdominal distention, and fluid in the thoracic cavity

Goal: Improved respiratory status

Nursing Interventions	Rationale	Expected Outcomes
1. Elevate head of bed to at least 30 degrees.	1. Reduces abdominal pressure on the diaphragm and permits fuller thoracic excursion and lung expansion	• Experiences improved respiratory status • Reports decreased shortness of breath • Reports increased strength and sense of well-being
2. Conserve patient's strength by providing rest periods and assisting with activities.	2. Reduces metabolic and oxygen requirements	• Exhibits normal respiratory rate (12–18/min) with no adventitious sounds
3. Change position every 2 hours.	3. Promotes expansion and oxygenation of all areas of the lungs	• Exhibits full thoracic excursion without shallow respirations
4. Assist with paracentesis or thoracentesis.	4. Paracentesis and thoracentesis (performed to remove fluid from the abdominal and thoracic cavities, respectively) may be frightening to the patient.	• Exhibits normal arterial blood gases • Exhibits adequate oxygen saturation by pulse oximetry • Experiences absence of confusion or cyanosis
a. Explain procedure and its purpose to patient.	a. Helps obtain patient's cooperation with procedures	
b. Have patient void before paracentesis.	b. Prevents inadvertent bladder injury	
c. Support and maintain position during procedure.	c. Prevents inadvertent organ or tissue injury	
d. Record both the amount and the character of fluid aspirated.	d. Provides record of fluid removed and indication of severity of limitation of lung expansion by fluid	
e. Observe for evidence of coughing, increasing dyspnea, or pulse rate.	e. Indicates irritation of the pleural space and evidence of pneumothorax or hemothorax.	

Collaborative Problem: Gastrointestinal bleeding and hemorrhage

Goal: The patient will develop no episodes of gastrointestinal bleeding and hemorrhage

Nursing Interventions	Rationale	Expected Outcomes

1. Assess patient for evidence of gastrointestinal bleeding or hemorrhage. If bleeding does occur:
  a. Monitor vital signs (blood pressure, pulse, respiratory rate) every 4 hours or more frequently, depending on acuity.
  b. Assess skin temperature, level of consciousness every 4 hours or more frequently, depending on acuity.
  c. Monitor gastrointestinal secretions and output (emesis, stool for occult or obvious bleeding). Test emesis for blood once per shift and with any change. Hematest each stool.
  d. Monitor hematocrit and hemoglobin for trends and changes.
	1. Allows early detection of signs and symptoms of bleeding and hemorrhage	• Experiences no episodes of bleeding and hemorrhage
		• Vital signs are within acceptable range for patient
		• No evidence of bleeding from gastrointestinal tract
		• Hematocrit and hemoglobin levels within acceptable limits
		• Turns and moves without straining and increasing intra-abdominal pressure
		• No straining with bowel movements
		• No further bleeding episodes if aggressive treatment of bleeding and hemorrhage was needed
		• Patient and family state rationale for treatments
		• Patient and family identify supports available to them
		• Patient and family describe signs and symptoms of a recurrent bleeding episode and identify needed action

2. Avoid activities that increase intra-abdominal pressure (straining, turning).
  a. Avoid coughing/sneezing.
  b. Assist patient to turn.
  c. Keep all needed items within easy reach.
  d. Use measures to prevent constipation such as adequate fluid intake; stool softeners.
  e. Ensure small meals.
	2. Minimizes increases in intra-abdominal pressure that could lead to rupture and bleeding of esophageal or gastric varices	

(continued)

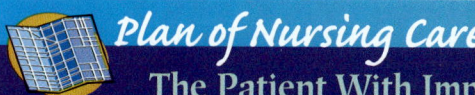

Nursing Interventions	Rationale	Expected Outcomes
3. Have equipment (Blakemore tube, medications, intravenous fluids) available if indicated.	3. Equipment, medications, and supplies will be readily available if patient experiences bleeding from ruptured esophageal or gastric varices.	
4. Assist with procedures and therapy needed to treat gastrointestinal bleeding and hemorrhage.	4. Gastrointestinal bleeding and hemorrhage require emergency measures (eg, insertion of Blakemore tube, administration of fluids and medications).	
5. Monitor respiratory status every hour and minimize risk of respiratory complications if esophageal tamponade is needed.	5. The patient is at high risk for respiratory complications, including asphyxiation if gastric balloon of Blakemore tube ruptures or migrates upward.	
6. Prepare patient physically and psychologically for other treatment modalities if needed.	6. The patient who experiences hemorrhage is very anxious and fearful; minimizing anxiety assists in control of hemorrhage.	
7. Monitor patient for recurrence of bleeding and hemorrhage.	7. Risk of rebleeding is high with all treatment modalities used to halt gastrointestinal bleeding.	
8. Keep family informed of patient's status.	8. Family members are likely to be anxious about the patient's status; providing information will reduce their anxiety level and promote more effective coping.	
9. Once recovered from bleeding episode, provide patient and family with information regarding signs and symptoms of gastrointestinal bleeding.	9. Risk of rebleeding is high. Subtle signs may be more quickly identified.	

Collaborative Problem: Hepatic encephalopathy
Goal: Patient will be maintained safely and without injury

Nursing Interventions	Rationale	Expected Outcomes
1. Assess cognitive status every 4–8 hours: a. Assess patient's orientation to person, place, and time. b. Monitor patient's level of activity, restlessness, and agitation. Assess for presence of flapping hand tremors (asterixis). c. Obtain and record daily sample of patient's handwriting or ability to construct a simple figure (eg, star). d. Assess neurologic signs (deep tendon reflexes, ability to follow instructions).	1. Data will provide baseline of patient's cognitive status and enable detection of changes.	• Remains awake, alert, and aware of surroundings • Is oriented to time, place, and person • Exhibits no restlessness or agitation • Record of handwriting demonstrates no deterioration in cognitive function • States rationale for treatment used to prevent or treat hepatic encephalopathy • Demonstrates stable serum ammonia level within acceptable limits • Consumes adequate caloric intake and adheres to protein restriction • Takes medications as prescribed • Breath sounds are normal without adventitious sounds • Skin and tissue intact without evidence of pressure or breaks in integrity
2. Monitor medications to prevent administration of those that may precipitate hepatic encephalopathy (sedatives, hypnotics, analgesics).	2. Medications are a common precipitating factor in development of hepatic encephalopathy in patients at risk.	
3. Monitor laboratory data, especially serum ammonia level.	3. Increases in serum ammonia level are associated with hepatic encephalopathy and coma.	
4. Notify physician of even subtle changes in patient's neurologic status and cognitive function.	4. Allows early initiation of treatment of hepatic encephalopathy and prevention of hepatic coma	
5. Limit sources of protein from diet if indicated.	5. Reduces breakdown and conversion of protein to ammonia	
6. Administer medications prescribed to reduce serum ammonia level (eg, lactulose, antibiotics, glucose, benzodiazepine antagonist [flumazenil] if indicated).	6. Reduces serum ammonia level	
7. Assess respiratory status and initiate measures to prevent complications.	7. The patient who develops hepatic coma is at risk for respiratory complications (ie, pneumonia, atelectasis, infection).	
8. Protect patient's skin and tissue from pressure and breakdown.	8. The patient in coma is at risk for skin breakdown and pressure ulcer formation.	

Cancer of the Liver

Hepatic tumours may be malignant or benign. Benign liver tumours were uncommon until the widespread use of oral contraceptives. With the use of oral contraceptives, benign tumours of the liver occur most frequently in women in their reproductive years.

PRIMARY LIVER TUMOURS

Few cancers originate in the liver. Primary liver tumours usually are associated with chronic liver disease, hepatitis B and C infections, and cirrhosis. Hepatocellular carcinoma (HCC) is by far the most common type of primary liver cancer, but it is rare in Canada (Bacon & Di Bisceglie, 2000). HCC is usually nonresectable because of rapid growth and metastasis. Other types of primary liver cancer include cholangiocellular carcinoma and combined hepatocellular and cholangiocellular carcinoma. If found early, resection may be possible, but early detection is unlikely. Cirrhosis, chronic infection with hepatitis B and C, and exposure to certain chemical toxins (eg, vinyl chloride, arsenic) have been implicated as causes of HCC. Cigarette smoking has also been identified as a risk factor, especially when combined with alcohol use. Some evidence suggests that aflatoxin, a metabolite of the fungus *Aspergillus flavus,* may be a risk factor for HCC. This is especially true in areas where HCC is endemic (ie, Asia and Africa). Aflatoxin and other similar toxic molds can contaminate food such as ground nuts and grains and may act as a co-carcinogen with hepatitis B. The risk of contamination is greatest when these foods are stored unrefrigerated in tropical or subtropical climates.

LIVER METASTASES

Metastases from other primary sites are found in the liver in about half of all advanced cancer cases (Bacon & Di Bisceglie, 2000). Malignant tumours are likely to reach the liver eventually, by way of the portal system or lymphatic channels, or by direct extension from an abdominal tumour. Moreover, the liver apparently is an ideal place for these malignant cells to thrive. Often the first evidence of cancer in an abdominal organ is the appearance of liver metastases; unless exploratory surgery or an autopsy is performed, the primary tumour may never be identified.

Clinical Manifestations

The early manifestations of malignancy of the liver include pain, a continuous dull ache in the right upper quadrant, epigastrium, or back. Weight loss, loss of strength, anorexia, and anemia may also occur. The liver may be enlarged and irregular on palpation. Jaundice is present only if the larger bile ducts are occluded by the pressure of malignant nodules in the hilum of the liver. Ascites develops if such nodules obstruct the portal veins or if tumour tissue is seeded in the peritoneal cavity.

Assessment and Diagnostic Findings

The liver cancer diagnosis is based on clinical signs and symptoms, the history and physical examination, and the results of laboratory and x-ray studies. Increased serum levels of bilirubin, alkaline phosphatase, AST, GGT, and lactic dehydrogenase may occur. Leukocytosis (increased white blood cells), erythrocytosis (increased red blood cells), hypercalcemia, hypoglycemia, and hypocholesterolemia may also be seen on laboratory assessment.

The serum level of alpha-fetoprotein (AFP), which serves as a tumour marker, is elevated in 30% to 40% of patients with primary liver cancer. Levels of carcinoembryonic antigen (CEA), a marker of advanced cancer of the digestive tract, may be elevated. These two markers together are useful to distinguish between metastatic liver disease and primary liver cancer.

Many patients have metastases from the primary liver tumour to other sites by the time diagnosis is made; metastases occur primarily to the lung but may also occur to regional lymph nodes, adrenals, bone, kidneys, heart, pancreas, and stomach.

X-rays, liver scans, CT scans, ultrasound studies, MRI, arteriography, and laparoscopy may be part of the diagnostic workup and may be performed to determine the extent of the cancer. Positive emission tomograms (PET scans) are used to evaluate a wide range of metastatic tumours of the liver.

Confirmation of a tumour's histology can be made by biopsy under imaging guidance (CT scan or ultrasound) or laparoscopically. Local or systemic dissemination of the tumour by needle biopsy or fine-needle biopsy can occur but is rare. Some clinicians believe that these procedures should not be performed if the tumour is thought to be resectable; rather, for primary HCC diagnosis should be confirmed by frozen section at the time of laparotomy.

Medical Management

Although surgical resection of the liver tumour is possible in some patients, the underlying cirrhosis, so prevalent in cancer of the liver, increases the risks associated with surgery. Radiation therapy and chemotherapy have been used in treating cancer of the liver with varying degrees of success. Although these therapies may prolong survival and improve quality of life by reducing pain and discomfort, their major effect is palliative.

RADIATION THERAPY

The use of external beam radiation for the treatment of liver tumours has been limited by the radiosensitivity of normal hepatocytes. Doses over 2,500 to 3,000 cGy may result in radiation hepatitis (O'Grady et al., 2000). More effective methods of delivering radiation to tumours of the liver include (1) intravenous or intra-arterial injection of antibodies that are tagged with radioactive isotopes and specifically attack tumour-associated antigens and (2) percutaneous placement of a high-intensity source for interstitial radiation therapy (delivering radiation directly to the tumour cells).

CHEMOTHERAPY

Chemotherapy has been used to improve quality of life and prolong survival; it also may be used as adjuvant therapy after surgical resection of hepatic tumours. Systemic chemotherapy and regional infusion chemotherapy are two methods used to administer antineoplastic agents to patients with primary and metastatic hepatic tumours (O'Grady et al., 2000).

An implantable pump has been used to deliver a high concentration of chemotherapy to the liver through the hepatic artery. This method provides a reliable, controlled, and continuous infusion of medication that can be carried out in the patient's home. Recent studies have begun to show some effective palliation and modestly improved survival rates (Bacon & Di Bisceglie, 2000).

PERCUTANEOUS BILIARY DRAINAGE

Percutaneous biliary or transhepatic drainage is used to bypass biliary ducts obstructed by liver, pancreatic, or bile duct tumours in patients with inoperable tumours or in those considered poor surgical risks. Under fluoroscopy, a catheter is inserted through the abdominal wall and past the obstruction into the duodenum. Such procedures are used to reestablish biliary drainage, relieve pressure and pain from the buildup of bile behind the obstruction, and decrease pruritus and jaundice. As a result, the patient is made more comfortable and quality of life and survival are improved.

For several days after its insertion, the catheter is opened to external drainage. The bile is observed closely for amount, colour, and presence of blood and debris. Complications of percutaneous biliary drainage include sepsis, leakage of bile, hemorrhage, and reobstruction of the biliary system by debris in the catheter or from encroaching tumour. Therefore, the patient is observed for fever and chills, bile drainage around the catheter, changes in vital signs, and evidence of biliary obstruction, including increased pain or pressure, pruritus, and recurrence of jaundice.

OTHER NONSURGICAL TREATMENTS

Laser hyperthermia has been used to treat hepatic metastases. Heat has been directed to tumours through several methods to cause necrosis of the tumour cells while sparing normal tissue. In radiofrequency thermal ablation, a needle electrode is inserted into the liver tumour under imaging guidance. Radiofrequency energy passes through to the noninsulated needle tip, causing heat and tumour cell death from coagulation necrosis.

Immunotherapy is another treatment modality under investigation. In this therapy, lymphocytes with antitumour reactivity are administered to the patient with hepatic cancer. Regression of the tumour, the desired outcome, has been demonstrated in patients with metastatic cancer in whom standard treatment has failed.

Transcatheter arterial embolization interrupts the arterial blood flow to small tumours by injecting small particulate embolic or chemotherapeutic agents into the artery supplying the tumour. Ischemia and necrosis of the tumour occur as a result.

For multiple small lesions, ultrasound-guided injection of alcohol promotes dehydration of tumour cells and tumour necrosis (Habib, 2000; O'Grady et al., 2000).

SURGICAL MANAGEMENT

Surgical resection is the treatment of choice when HCC is confined to one lobe of the liver and the function of the remaining liver is considered adequate for postoperative recovery. In the case of metastasis, hepatic resection can be performed when the primary site can be completely excised and the metastasis is limited. Metastases to the liver, however, are rarely limited or solitary. Capitalizing on the regenerative capacity of the liver cells, some surgeons have successfully removed 90% of the liver. However, the presence of cirrhosis limits the ability of the liver to regenerate. Staging of liver tumours aids in predicting the likelihood of surgical cure. A staging system for liver tumours is summarized in Chart 39-11.

In preparation for surgery, the patient's nutritional, fluid, and general physical status is assessed and efforts are undertaken to ensure the best physical condition possible. Support, explanation, and encouragement are provided to help the patient prepare psychologically for the surgery.

Extensive diagnostic studies may be performed. Specific studies may include liver scan, liver biopsy, cholangiography, selective hepatic angiography, percutaneous needle biopsy, peritoneoscopy, laparoscopy, ultrasound, CT scans, MRI, and blood tests, particularly determinations of serum alkaline phosphatase, AST, and GGT and its isoenzymes.

Chart 39-11

TNM Staging for Liver Tumours

Primary Tumour (T)

TX	Primary tumour cannot be assessed
T0	No evidence of primary tumour
T1	Solitary tumour without vascular invasion
T2	Solitary tumour with vascular invasion or multiple tumours none more than 5 cm
T3	Multiple tumours more than 5 cm or tumour involving a major branch of the portal or hepatic vein(s)
T4	Tumour(s) with direct invasion of adjacent organs other than the gallbladder or with perforation of visceral peritoneum.

Regional Lymph Nodes (N)

NX	Regional lymph nodes cannot be assessed
N0	No regional lymph node metastasis
N1	Regional lymph node metastasis

Distant Metastasis (M)

MX	Distant metastasis cannot be assessed
M0	No distant metastasis
M1	Distant metastasis

Stage Grouping			
Stage I	T1	N0	M0
Stage II	T2	N0	M0
Stage IIIA	T3	N0	M0
IIIB	T4	N0	M0
IIIC	Any T	N1	M0
Stage IV	Any T	Any N	M1

Used with the permission of the American Joint Committee on Cancer (AJCC), Chicago, Illinois. The original source for this material is the *AJCC Cancer Staging Manual, Sixth Edition* (2002) published by Springer-Verlag New York, www.springer-ny.com.

Lobectomy. Removal of a lobe of the liver is the most common surgical procedure for excising a liver tumour. If it is necessary to restrict blood flow from the hepatic artery and portal vein beyond 15 minutes, it is likely that hypothermia will be used. For a right-liver lobectomy or an extended right lobectomy (including the medial left lobe), a thoracoabdominal incision is used. An extensive abdominal incision is made for a left lobectomy.

Cryosurgery. In cryosurgery (**cryoablation**), tumours are destroyed by liquid nitrogen at −196° C. To destroy the diseased tissue, two or three freeze-and-thaw cycles are administered via probes during open laparotomy. This technique has been used alone or as an adjunct to hepatic resection in HCC and colorectal metastases not amenable to radical surgical excision. The efficacy of cryosurgery is still being evaluated; indications and outcomes require further investigation.

Liver Transplantation. Removing the liver and replacing it with a healthy donor organ is another way to treat liver cancer. Recurrence of the primary liver malignancy after transplantation, however, has been reported to occur in 70% to 85% of cases, and the survival time after recurrence is brief. Metastasis and recurrence may be enhanced by the immunosuppressive therapy needed to prevent rejection. The patient with small tumours may have a good prognosis after transplantation, but recurrence is common with tumours greater than 8 cm in diameter or those that are multifocal or have vascular invasion (Bacon & Di Bisceglie, 2000). See the discussion of liver transplantation that follows.

Nursing Management

If the patient has had surgery to treat liver cancer, potential problems related to cardiopulmonary involvement include vascular complications and respiratory and liver dysfunction. Metabolic abnormalities require careful attention. A constant infusion of 10% glucose may be required in the first 48 hours to prevent a precipitous fall in the blood glucose level resulting from decreased gluconeogenesis. Because extensive blood loss may occur as well, the patient will receive infusions of blood and IV fluids. The patient requires constant, close monitoring and care for the first 2 or 3 days, similar to postsurgical abdominal and thoracic nursing care.

The patient undergoing cryosurgery is monitored closely for hypothermia, hemorrhage, or bile leak; myoglobinuria can occur as a result of tissue necrosis and is minimized by hydration, diuresis, and at times medications (allopurinol) to bind to and aid in the excretion of toxic products.

If the patient will receive chemotherapy or radiation therapy in an effort to relieve symptoms, he or she may be discharged home while still receiving one or both of these therapies. The patient may also go home with a biliary drainage system in place. The need for teaching is great because of the need for the patient to participate in care and the family's role in care at home.

PROMOTING HOME AND COMMUNITY-BASED CARE

Teaching Patients Self-Care. The nurse instructs the patient to recognize and report the complications and side effects of the chemotherapy that may occur and the actions and desired and undesirable effects of the specific chemotherapy regimen. The nurse also emphasizes the importance of follow-up visits to assess the patient and the tumour's response to chemotherapy and radiation therapy.

If the patient is receiving chemotherapy on an outpatient basis, the nurse explains the patient's and family's role in managing the chemotherapy infusion and in assessing the infusion/insertion site. The nurse encourages the patient to resume routine activities as soon as possible, while cautioning him or her to avoid activities that may damage the infusion pump or site.

The family and the patient at home with a biliary drainage system in place typically fear that the catheter will be dislodged. They need reassurance and instruction to reduce their fear that the catheter will fall out easily. The patient and family also require instruction on catheter care. They need to learn how to keep the catheter site clean and dry and how to assess the catheter and its insertion site. Irrigation of the catheter with sterile normal saline solution or water may be prescribed to keep the catheter patent and free of debris. The patient and caregivers are taught proper technique to avoid introducing bacteria into the biliary system or catheter during irrigation. They are instructed not to aspirate or draw back on the syringe during irrigation to prevent entry of irritating duodenal contents into the biliary tree or catheter. The patient and caregivers are also instructed about the signs of complications and are encouraged to notify the nurse or physician if problems or questions arise.

Continuing Care. In many cases, referral for home care enables the patient with liver cancer to be at home in a familiar environment with family and friends. Because of the poor prognosis associated with liver cancer, the home care nurse serves a vital role in assisting the patient and family to cope with the symptoms that may occur and the prognosis. The home care nurse assesses the patient's physical and psychological status, the adequacy of pain relief, nutritional status, and the presence of symptoms indicating complications of treatment or progression of disease. During home visits, the nurse assesses the function of the chemotherapy pump, the infusion site, and the biliary drainage system, if indicated. The nurse collaborates with the other members of the health care team, the patient, and the family to ensure effective pain management and to manage other problems that may occur: weakness, pruritus, inadequate dietary intake, jaundice, and symptoms associated with metastasis to other sites. The home care nurse also assists the patient and family in making decisions about hospice care and assists with initiation of referrals. The patient is encouraged to discuss preferences for end-of-life care with family members and health care providers (see Chap. 17).

Liver Transplantation

Liver transplantation is used to treat life-threatening, end-stage liver disease for which no other form of treatment is available. The transplantation procedure involves total removal of the diseased liver and its replacement with a healthy liver in the same anatomic location (**orthotopic liver transplantation** [OLT]). Removal of the liver leaves a space for the new liver and permits anatomic reconstruction of the hepatic vasculature and biliary tract as close to normal as possible. Today, 1-year graft and patient survival rates are as high as 90%. (Cohen, 2002).

The success of liver transplantation depends on successful immunosuppression, which prevents rejection. Immunosuppressant medications generally fall into four categories. The first category includes the calcineurin inhibitors (cyclosporine, tacrolimus). Cyclosporine (Neoral) was introduced to the market in 1980 and revolutionized transplantation. The 1990 discovery that tacrolimus (Prograf) was significantly more potent than cyclosporine had a similar effect on the field of transplantation (Cohen, 2002). Both medications have similar side effect profiles, but tacrolimus does not cause the hirsutism and gingival hyperplasia that many recipients experienced when taking cyclosporine. The second category is comprised of the antimetabolite and antiproliferative medications. These include azathioprine (Imuran), mycophenolate mofetil (CellCept), and sirolimus (Rapamune). Azathioprine is rarely used in current practice, but recipients who received their transplant several years ago may still be taking this medication. There is some controversy regarding the use of sirolimus in liver transplant recipients, so mycophenolate mofetil is currently the antimetabolite of choice. Corticosteroids are the third category of immunosuppressants. Although corticosteroids once formed the first line of defense against rejection, they are only occasionally used today because of their lengthy side effects profile (Reding, Gras, Sokal, Otte, & Davies, 2003). Antibodies are the last category of immunosuppressants. These include OKT3 (muromonab-CD30), antithymocyte globulin (equine and rabbit), anti-CD25 and anti-IL2 receptor antibodies (daclizumab, basiliximab), anti-tumour necrosis factor-alpha (infliximab), and anti-CD20 (rituximab). The antibodies have been used to induce tolerance and treat steroid resistance, chronic rejection, and post-transplant lymphoproliferative disease. The goals of ongoing research are to find the most effective combinations of immunosuppressive agents and to identify new agents with fewer side effects.

Despite the success of immunosuppression in reducing the incidence of rejection of transplanted organs, liver transplantation is not a routine procedure and may be accompanied by complications related to the lengthy surgical procedure, immunosuppressive therapy, infection, and the technical difficulties encountered in reconstructing the blood vessels and biliary tract. Long-standing systemic problems resulting from the primary liver disease may complicate the preoperative and postoperative course. Previous surgery of the abdomen, including procedures to treat complications of advanced liver disease (ie, shunt procedures used to treat portal hypertension and esophageal varices) increase the complexity of the transplantation procedure.

The indications for liver transplantation are not as limited today as they were when the procedure was first introduced, due to advances in immunosuppressive therapy, improvements in biliary tract reconstruction, and in some cases the use of venovenous bypass. General indications for liver transplantation include irreversible advanced chronic liver disease, fulminant hepatic failure, metabolic liver diseases, and some hepatic malignancies. Examples of disorders that are indications for liver transplantation include hepatocellular liver disease (eg, viral hepatitis, drug- and alcohol-induced liver disease, and Wilson's disease) and cholestatic diseases (primary biliary cirrhosis, sclerosing cholangitis, and biliary atresia).

The patient being considered for liver transplantation frequently has many systemic problems that influence preoperative and postoperative care. Because transplantation is more difficult when the patient has developed severe GI bleeding and hepatic coma, efforts are made to perform the procedure before this stage.

Liver transplantation is now recognized as an established therapeutic modality rather than an experimental procedure to treat these disorders. As a result, the number of centres where liver transplantation is performed is increasing. There are seven sites across Canada where liver transplantation is performed. Patients requiring transplantation are often referred from distant hospitals to these sites. To prepare the patient and family for liver transplantation, nurses in all settings must understand the processes and procedures of liver transplantation.

SURGICAL PROCEDURE

The donor liver is freed from other structures, the bile is flushed from the gallbladder to prevent damage to the walls of the biliary tract, and the liver is perfused with a preservative and cooled. Before the donor liver is placed in the recipient, it is flushed with cold lactated Ringer's solution to remove potassium and air bubbles.

Anastomoses (connections) of the blood vessels and bile duct are performed between the donor liver and the recipient liver. Biliary reconstruction is performed with an end-to-end anastomosis of the donor and recipient common bile ducts; a stented T-tube is rarely inserted for external drainage of bile. If an end-to-end anastomosis is not possible because of diseased or absent bile ducts, an end-to-side anastomosis is made between the common bile duct of the graft and a loop (Roux-en-Y portion) of jejunum (Fig. 39-15*A*); in this case, bile drainage will be internal and a T-tube will not be inserted (Maddrey et al., 2001). Figure 39-15*B* and *C* illustrates the final appearance of the grafted liver and final closure and drain placement.

Liver transplantation is a long surgical procedure, partly because the patient with liver failure often has portal hypertension and subsequently many venous collateral vessels that must be ligated. Blood loss during the surgical procedure may be extensive. If the patient has adhesions from previous abdominal surgery, lysis of adhesions is often necessary. If a shunt procedure was performed previously, it must be surgically reversed to permit adequate portal venous blood supply to the new liver. During the lengthy surgery, providing regular updates to the family about the progress of the operation and the patient's status is helpful.

COMPLICATIONS

The postoperative complication rate is high, primarily because of technical complications or infection. Immediate postoperative complications may include bleeding, infection, and rejection. Disruption, infection, or obstruction of the biliary anastomosis and impaired biliary drainage may occur. Vascular thrombosis and stenosis are other potential complications.

Bleeding

Bleeding is common in the postoperative period and may result from coagulopathy, portal hypertension, and fibrinolysis caused by ischemic injury to the donor liver. Hypotension may occur in this phase secondary to blood loss. Administration of platelets, fresh-frozen plasma, and other blood products may be necessary. Hypertension is more common, but its cause is uncertain. Blood pressure elevation that is significant or sustained is treated.

Infection

Infection is the leading cause of death after liver transplantation. Pulmonary and fungal infections are common; susceptibility to infection is increased by the immunosuppression needed to prevent rejection (Maddrey et al., 2001). Therefore, precautions must be taken to prevent nosocomial infections by strict asepsis when manipulating arterial lines and urine, bile, and other drainage systems; obtaining specimens; and changing dressings. Meticulous hand hygiene is crucial.

Rejection

Rejection is a key concern. A transplanted liver is perceived by the immune system as a foreign antigen. This triggers an immune response, leading to the activation of T lymphocytes that attack and destroy the transplanted liver. Immunosuppressive agents are used long term to prevent this response and rejection of the transplanted liver. These agents inhibit the activation of immunocompetent T lymphocytes to prevent the production of effector T cells.

Although the 1- and 5-year survival rates have increased dramatically with the use of new immunosuppressive therapies, these advances are not without major side effects. A major side effect of calcineurin inhibitors (cyclosporine, tacrolimus), which are widely used in transplantation, is nephrotoxicity; this problem seems to be dose-related, and renal dysfunction may be reversed if the dose is appropriately decreased or if its use is not initiated immediately. Cyclosporine-related side effects have caused many centres to use tacrolimus as first-line therapy because of its efficacy and lower side effect profile.

Corticosteroids, azathioprine, mycophenolate mofetil, rapamycin, antithymocyte globulin, OKT3, and the new IL-Z receptor antagonists are also elements of the various regimens of immunosuppression and may be used as the initial therapy to prevent re-

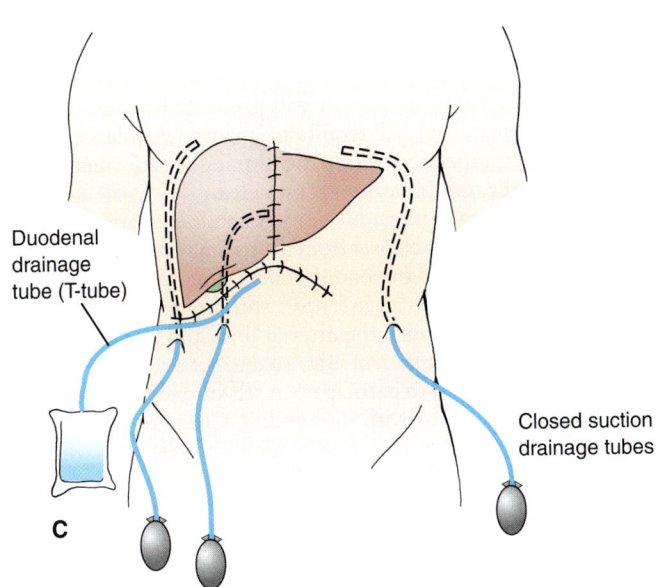

FIGURE 39-15A–C (**A**) Roux-en-Y hepatojejunostomy. (**B**) Final appearance of implanted liver graft. (**C**) Final closure and drain placement after liver transplant.

jection, or later to treat rejection. The trend is to use steroids and polyclonal antibodies because of their longer side effect profiles. Liver biopsy and ultrasound are required to evaluate suspected episodes of rejection.

Retransplantation is usually attempted if the transplanted liver fails, but the success rate of retransplantation does not approach that of initial transplantation.

Nursing Management

The patient considering transplantation and the family have difficult decisions to make about treatment, use of financial resources, and relocation to another area to be closer to the medical centre. They also must cope with the patient's long-standing health prob-

lems and perhaps social and family problems associated with behaviours that may be responsible for the patient's liver failure. Therefore, the time during which the patient and family are considering liver transplantation and awaiting the news that a liver is available is often stressful. The nurse must be aware of these issues and attuned to the emotional and psychological status of the patient and family. Referral of the patient and family to a psychiatric liaison nurse, psychologist, psychiatrist, or spiritual advisor may be helpful to them as they deal with the stressors associated with end-stage liver disease and liver transplantation.

PREOPERATIVE NURSING INTERVENTIONS

If irreversible, severe liver dysfunction has been diagnosed, the patient may be a candidate for transplantation. An extensive diagnostic evaluation will be carried out to determine whether the patient is a candidate. The nurse and other health care team members provide the patient and family with full explanations about the procedure, the chances of success, and the risks, including the side effects of long-term immunosuppression. The need for close follow-up and lifelong compliance with the therapeutic regimen, including immunosuppression, is explained to the patient and family.

Once accepted as a candidate, the patient is placed on a waiting list at the transplant centre and patient information is shared with the local Organ Procurement Organization (OPD) so that candidates may be matched with appropriate organs as they become available.

Unless the patient is having a living donor liver transplantation (Chart 39-12), a liver becomes available for transplantation only with the nerological determination of death of another individual, who is usually healthy except for severe brain injury. Thus, the patient and family undergo a stressful waiting period, and the nurse is often the major source of support. The patient must be accessible at all times in case an appropriate liver becomes available. During this time, liver function may deteriorate further and the patient may experience other complications from the primary liver disease. Because of the current shortage of donor organs, many patients die awaiting transplantation.

Malnutrition, massive ascites, and fluid and electrolyte disturbances are treated before surgery to increase the chance of a successful outcome. If the patient's liver dysfunction has a very rapid onset, as in fulminant hepatic failure, there is little time or opportunity for the patient to consider and weigh options and their consequences; often this patient is in a coma, and the decision to proceed with transplantation is made by the family.

The nurse coordinator is an integral member of the transplant team and plays an important role in preparing the patient for liver transplantation. The nurse serves as a patient and family advocate and assumes the important role of link between the patient and the other members of the transplant team. The nurse also serves as a resource to other nurses and health care team members involved in evaluating and caring for the patient.

POSTOPERATIVE NURSING INTERVENTIONS

The patient is maintained in an environment as free from bacteria, viruses, and fungi as possible, because immunosuppressive medications reduce the body's natural defenses. In the immediate postoperative period, cardiovascular, pulmonary, renal, neurologic, and metabolic functions are monitored continuously. Mean arterial and pulmonary artery pressures are monitored continuously. Cardiac output, central venous pressure, pulmonary capillary wedge pressure, arterial and mixed venous blood gases, oxygen saturation, oxygen demand and delivery, urine output, heart rate, and blood pressure are used to evaluate the patient's hemodynamic status and intravascular fluid volume. Liver function tests, electrolyte levels, the coagulation profile, chest x-ray, electrocardiogram, and fluid output, including urine and drainage from Jackson-Pratt tubes, are monitored closely. Because the liver is responsible for the storage of glycogen and the synthesis of protein and clotting factors, these substances need to be monitored and replaced in the immediate postoperative period.

Because of the likelihood of atelectasis and an altered ventilation–perfusion ratio as a result of the insult to the diaphragm during the surgical procedure, prolonged anesthesia, immobility, and postoperative pain, the patient will probably have an endotracheal tube in place and will require mechanical ventilation during the initial postoperative period. Suctioning is performed as required and sterile humidification is provided.

As the vital signs and condition stabilize, efforts are made to assist the patient to recover from the trauma of this complex surgery. After removal of the endotracheal tube, the nurse encourages the patient to use an incentive spirometer to decrease the risk for atelectasis. Once the arterial lines and the urinary catheter are removed, the patient is assisted to get out of bed, to ambulate as tolerated, and to participate in self-care to prevent the complications associated with immobility. Close monitoring for signs and symptoms of liver dysfunction and rejection will continue throughout the hospital stay. Plans will be made for close follow-up after discharge as well. Teaching, initiated during the preoperative period, continues after surgery.

PROMOTING HOME AND COMMUNITY-BASED CARE

Teaching Patients Self-Care. Teaching the patient and family about long-term measures to promote health is crucial for success of the transplant and represents an important role of the nurse. The patient and family must understand why they should adhere continuously to the therapeutic regimen, with special emphasis on the methods of administration, rationale, and side effects of the prescribed immunosuppressive agents. The nurse provides written as well as verbal instructions about how and when to take the medications. To avoid running out of medication or skipping a dose, the patient must make sure that an adequate supply of medication is available. Instructions are also provided about the signs and symptoms that indicate problems that require consultation with the transplant team. The patient with a T-tube in place must be taught how to manage the tube.

Continuing Care. The nurse emphasizes the importance of follow-up blood tests and visits to the transplant team. Trough blood levels of immunosuppressive agents are obtained, along with other blood tests that assess the function of the liver and kidneys. During the first months, the patient is likely to require blood tests two or three times a week. As the patient's condition

---

Chart 39-12 **Innovative Strategies in Liver Transplantation**

Living donor liver transplantation in adults using part of the liver of a living donor is a relatively new technique (Bacon & Di Bisceglie, 2000) that is becoming the norm in an era of cadaveric donor shortfall. Many ethical and medical questions remain.

Issues Related to Donation

There are two key issues in donor selection:
- The living donor of the liver segment must be a volunteer, without coercion and without financial incentives.
- The potential donor must be assessed for medical conditions that would increase his or her risk, since liver resection poses serious risks to the donor (Maddrey et al., 2001).

Other issues concern risks, benefits, and education of the donor and recipient. An acceptable level of risk and benefits must exist for the potential recipient. In addition, a satisfactory process for educating both the donor and recipient and the family (or families in the case of unrelated parties) should be in place. Informed consent for the donor must also be ensured (Maddrey et al., 2001).

Nurse's Role

During the period of evaluation and planning for the elective procedure, nurses are involved in supporting and educating both parties. Addressing the concerns each may have for the other's welfare requires a multidisciplinary approach of all transplant team members.

NURSING RESEARCH PROFILE 39-1
The Experience of Liver Failure and Liver Transplantation

Robertson, G. (1999). Individuals' perception of their quality of life following a liver transplant: An exploratory study. *Journal of Advanced Nursing, 30*(2), 497–505.

Purpose

Although advances in liver transplantation have increased the survival of persons who undergo the procedure, little is known about their quality of life. This study explored individuals' perceptions of the effect a liver transplant had on their quality of life and focused on the progression from dependence to independence physically, socially, and psychologically.

Study Sample and Design

A phenomenologic approach was used; patients were interviewed in the outpatient clinic. Interviews were audiotaped and transcribed. Cluster analysis was used to identify groups of shared issues. The sample included five patients who had undergone liver transplantation for chronic liver disease at least 1 year before the study. Participants were asked about their quality of life before and after transplantation, the meaning of a good quality of life, and the transition from being dependent before transplantation to independent.

Findings

Physical problems present before transplantation prevented the subjects from fulfilling personal goals and participating in their usual activities. Their physical problems kept them from achieving a good quality of life. Following transplant, the subjects identified their interest in social integration and their desire to be treated normally. The return to independence was identified as the key factor in their quality of life. However, their family and friends restricted their return to independence by overprotecting them. The study participants identified the importance of support from liver transplant unit staff and other patients in their transition during the first 3 months following transplantation.

Nursing Implications

It is important to recognize the issues shared by liver transplant patients and to devise strategies to assist them in achieving independence after surgery. Patient and family education regarding factors such as overprotectiveness versus using good judgment in social situations can be explored before the transplant. Educating the patient's family and friends about the need for independence is important in helping to improve the patient's quality of life after liver transplantation.

---

stabilizes, blood studies and visits to the transplant team are less frequent. The importance of routine ophthalmologic examinations is emphasized because of the increased incidence of cataracts and glaucoma with the long-term corticosteroid therapy used with transplantation. Regular oral hygiene and follow-up dental care, with administration of prophylactic antibiotics before dental treatments, are recommended because of the immunosuppression.

The nurse reminds the patient that although a successful transplantation will not return him or her to normal, it does increase the chances for survival and a more normal life than before transplantation if rejection and infection can be prevented. Many patients have lived successful and productive lives after receiving a liver transplant. In fact, pregnancy can be considered 1 year after transplantation, depending on the medication regimen. Successful outcomes have been reported, but these pregnancies are considered high risk for mother and infant (Sherlock & Dooley, 2002).

Liver Abscesses

Two categories of liver abscess have been identified: amebic and pyogenic. Amebic liver abscesses are most commonly caused by *Entamoeba histolytica*. Most amebic liver abscesses occur in the developing countries of the tropics and subtropics because of poor sanitation and hygiene. Pyogenic liver abscesses are much less common but are more common in developed countries than the amebic type.

Pathophysiology

Whenever an infection develops anywhere along the biliary or GI tract, infecting organisms may reach the liver through the biliary system, portal venous system, or hepatic arterial or lymphatic system. Most bacteria are destroyed promptly, but occasionally some gain a foothold. The bacterial toxins destroy the neighboring liver cells, and the resulting necrotic tissue serves as a protective wall for the organisms.

Meanwhile, leukocytes migrate into the infected area. The result is an abscess cavity full of a liquid containing living and dead leukocytes, liquefied liver cells, and bacteria. Pyogenic abscesses of this type may be either single or multiple and small. Examples of causes of pyogenic liver abscess include cholangitis and abdominal trauma.

Clinical Manifestations

The clinical picture is one of sepsis with few or no localizing signs. Fever with chills and diaphoresis, malaise, anorexia, nausea, vomiting, and weight loss may occur. The patient may complain of dull abdominal pain and tenderness in the right upper quadrant of the abdomen. Hepatomegaly, jaundice, anemia, and pleural effusion may develop. Sepsis and shock may be severe and life-threatening. In the past, the mortality rate was 100% because of the vague clinical symptoms, inadequate diagnostic tools, and inadequate surgical drainage of the abscess. With the aid of ultrasound, CT and MRI scans, and liver scans, early diagnosis and surgical drainage of the abscess have greatly reduced the mortality rate.

Assessment and Diagnostic Findings

Blood cultures are obtained but may not identify the organism. Aspiration of the liver abscess, guided by ultrasound, CT, or MRI, may be performed to assist in diagnosis and to obtain cultures of the organism. Percutaneous drainage of pyogenic abscesses is carried out to evacuate the abscess material and promote healing. A catheter may be left in place for continuous drainage; the patient must be instructed about its management.

Medical Management

Treatment includes IV antibiotic therapy; the specific antibiotic used in treatment depends on the organism identified. Continuous supportive care is indicated because of the serious condition of the patient. Open surgical drainage may be required if antibiotic therapy and percutaneous drainage are ineffective.

Nursing Management

Although the manifestations of liver abscess vary with the type of abscess, most patients appear acutely ill. Others appear to be chronically ill and debilitated. The nursing management depends on the patient's physical status and the medical management that is indicated. For patients who undergo evacuation and drainage of the abscess, monitoring of the drainage and skin care are imperative. Strategies must be implemented to contain the drainage and to protect the patient from other sources of infection. Vital signs are monitored to detect changes in the patient's physical status. Deterioration in vital signs or the onset of new symptoms such as increasing pain, which may indicate rupture or extension of the abscess, is reported promptly. The nurse administers IV antibiotic therapy as prescribed. The white blood cell count and other laboratory test results are monitored closely for changes consistent with worsening infection. The nurse prepares the patient for discharge by providing instruction about symptom management, signs and symptoms that should be reported to the physician, management of drainage, and the importance of taking antibiotics as prescribed.

Critical Thinking Exercises

1. A 54-year-old man is admitted to the hospital with end-stage liver disease due to postnecrotic cirrhosis from hepatitis C, which developed following a blood transfusion in 1986. He is on the waiting list for a liver transplant due to incapacitating ascites and until now has been managed at home with diuretics, low sodium intake, daily weights, and fluid restriction. He also requires a weekly ultrasound-guided paracentesis. He has become unresponsive to oral diuretics, and his ascites is quickly reaccumulating after the paracentesis. His serum blood urea nitrogen (BUN) and creatinine levels are also rising. He is admitted to the hospital to receive intravenous diuretics and for closer monitoring as his renal function worsens. His worsening condition has placed him high on the waiting list for a liver transplant. As his nurse, what nursing interventions would you anticipate? What are the educational needs of the patient and his family?

2. A 59-year-old white woman received an orthotopic liver transplant 6 months ago. She did well postoperatively and was discharged on immunosuppressive therapy. She now presents with a low-grade fever (38.2° C), 2-kg weight gain, tenderness over her transplanted liver, and mild jaundice. She also reports that her urine has become dark and has decreased in amount over the past 2 weeks. Her liver function test results are abnormal. Additional laboratory test results reveal that the serum level of tacrolimus (one of her immunosuppressant medications) is subtherapeutic. Describe the relationship of each of her current symptoms to liver dysfunction. What treatment would you anticipate, and what are the nursing measures for her at this time? What explanation would you give to her for her symptoms?

3. A 20-year-old college student has been diagnosed with hepatitis B. What teaching is warranted for this patient to prevent transmission to others and to reduce the risk of complications? What symptomatic treatment would you an-

ticipate, and what are the nursing implications associated with treatment? How would patient teaching, treatment, and nursing implications differ if the patient's diagnosis were hepatitis A? What instructions about hepatitis B or hepatitis A would you give to the patient's family or roommates?

4. A 66-year-old man is admitted to the hospital with a tentative diagnosis of bleeding esophageal varices. Describe the monitoring you would initiate. Describe the possible management strategies to prevent bleeding and to treat active bleeding of the esophageal varices. Identify the nursing implications for each of these strategies. How would medical management and nursing care be modified if the patient had chronic obstructive pulmonary disease in addition to esophageal varices?

REFERENCES AND SELECTED READINGS

Books

American Cancer Society. (2002). *Cancer facts and figures.* Atlanta: American Cancer Society.

Bacon, B. R., & Di Bisceglie, A. M. (Eds). (2000). *Liver disease.* New York: Churchill Livingstone.

Blumgart, L. H., & Fong, Y. (Eds). (2000). *Surgery of the liver and biliary tract* (3d ed.). London: WB Saunders.

Clavien, P. A. (Ed.) (1999). *Malignant liver tumors.* Malden, MA: Blackwell Science.

Dudek, S. G. (2001). *Nutrition essentials for nursing practice* (4th ed.). Philadelphia: Lippincott Williams & Wilkins.

Evans, S. R. T., & Ascher, S. M. (Eds.) (1998). *Hepatobiliary and pancreatic surgery.* New York: Wiley-Liss.

Ginns, L. C., Cosimi, A. B., & Morris, P. J. (Eds.) (1999). *Transplantation.* Malden, MA: Blackwell Science.

Greene, F. L., Page, D. L., Fleming, I. D. et al. (Eds.) (2002). *AJCC cancer staging manual* (6th ed.). New York: Springer-Verlag.

Habib, N. A. (Ed.) (2000). *Hepatocellular carcinoma: Methods and protocols.* Totowa, NJ: Humana Press.

Maddrey, W. C., Schiff, E. R., & Sorrell, M. F. (Eds.) (2001). *Transplantation of the liver* (3d ed.). Philadelphia: Lippincott Williams & Wilkins.

National Digestive Diseases Information Clearinghouse (NIDDK) (2000). *Cirrhosis of the liver.* NIH Publication No. 00-1134, Bethesda, MD.

National Institutes of Health. National Institute on Alcohol Abuse and Alcoholism. (1999). *Alcohol research and health: The journal of the national institution on alcohol and alcoholism.* Alexandria, VA: U.S. Department of Health and Human Services.

O'Grady, J. G., Lake, J. R., & Howdle, P. D. (Eds.) (2000). *Comprehensive clinical hepatology.* London: Mosby.

Porth, C. M. (2002). *Pathophysiology: Concepts of altered health states* (6th ed.). Philadelphia: Lippincott Williams & Wilkins.

Schiff, E. R., Sorrell, M. F., & Maddrey, W. C. (1999). *Schiff's diseases of the liver* (8th ed.). Philadelphia: Lippincott-Raven.

Sherlock, S., & Dooley, J. (2002). *Diseases of the liver and biliary system.* Osney Mead, Oxford: Blackwell Science.

Wolfe, M. M. (2000). *Therapy of digestive disorders.* Philadelphia: WB Saunders.

Zimmerman, H. J. (1999). *Hepatotoxicity: The adverse effects of drugs and other chemicals on the liver* (2d ed.). Philadelphia: Lippincott Williams & Wilkins.

Journals

Asterisks indicate nursing research articles.
General
Als-Nielsen, B., Gluud, L.L., & Gluud, C., (2005a). Benzodiazepine receptor antagonists for hepatic encephalopathy. The Cochrane Library, (2) ID #CD002798. Available at: http://www.cochrane.org/cochrane/revabstr/AB002798.htm. Retrieved June 13, 2005.

Als-Nielsen, B., Gluud, L.L., & Gluud, C., (2005b). Dopaminergic agonists for hepatic encephalopathy. *The Cochrane Library*, (2) ID #CD003047. Available at: http://www.cochrane.org/cochrane/revabstr/AB003047.htm. Retrieved June 13, 2005.

Als-Nielsen, B., Gluud, L.L., & Gluud, C., (2005c). Nonabsorbable disaccharides for hepatic encephalopathy. *The Cochrane Library*, (2) ID #CD003044. Available at: http://www.cochrane.org/cochrane/revabstr/AB003047.htm. Retrieved June 13, 2005.

Angulo, P. (2002). Nonalcoholic fatty liver disease. *New England Journal of Medicine, 346*(16), 1221–1231.

Blow, F. C., Walton, M. A., Barry, K. L., et al. (2000). The relationship between alcohol problems and health functioning of older adults in primary care settings. *Journal of American Geriatrics Society, 48*(7), 856–908.

Bravo, A. A., Sheth, S. G., & Chopra, S. (2001). Liver biopsy. *New England Journal of Medicine, 344*(7), 495–500.

Chikritzhs, T. N., Jonas, H. A., Stockwell, T. R., et al. (2001). Mortality and life years lost due to alcohol: A comparison of acute and chronic causes. *Medical Journal of Australia, 174*(6), 281–284.

Desai, S., & Peltekian, K. M. (2004). Canadian mortality rates for liver disease: Taking a closer look at ICD coding. *Canadian Journal of Public Health, 95*(3), 198–200.

de Franchis, R., & Primighani, M. (1999). Endoscopic treatment of portal hypertension. *Seminars in Liver Disease, 19*, 439–455.

Fingerhood, M. (2000). Substance abuse in older people. *Journal of the American Geriatrics Society, 48*(8), 86–99.

Garcia, N., Jr. & Sanyal, A. J. (2001). Portal hypertension. *Clinics in Liver Disease, 5*(2), 509–540.

Hussain, H., Lapin, S., & Cappell, M. S. (2000). Clinical scoring systems for determining the prognosis of gastrointestinal bleeding. *Gastroenterology Clinics, 29*(2), 46–59.

Kaptanoglu, L., & Blei, A. T. (2000). Current status of liver support systems. *Clinics in Liver Disease, 4*(3), 711–729.

Jonsen, P. L. (2002). Liver disease in the elderly. *Best Practice and Research in Clinical Gastroenterology, 16*(1), 149–158.

Lake, J. R. (2000). The role of transjugular portosystemic shunting in patients with ascites. *New England Journal of Medicine, 342*(23), 1745–1747.

Liu, J.P., Gluud, L.L., Als-Nielsen, B., & Gluud, C. (2005). Artificial and bioartificial support systems for liver failure. *The Cochrane Library*, (2) ID #CD003628. Available at: http://www.cochrane.org/cochrane/revabstr/AB003628.htm. Retrieved June 9, 2005.

Maddrey, W. C. (2000). Alcohol-induced liver disease. *Clinics in Liver Disease, 4*(1), 115–131.

Pastorelli, R., Bardozzi, G., Saieva, C., et al. (2001). Genetic determinants of alcohol addiction and metabolism: A survey in Italy. *Alcoholism: Clinical and Experimental Research, 25*(2), 221–227.

Pratt, D. S., & Kaplan, M. M. (2000). Primary care: Evaluation of abnormal liver-enzyme results in asymptomatic patients. *New England Journal of Medicine, 342*(17), 1266–1271.

Public Health Agency of Canada. (2004). Sex differences in injecting practices and hepatitis C: A systematic review of the literature. Canada Communicable Disease Report, 30(14). Available at: www.hc-sc.gc.ca/pphb-dgspsp/publicat/ccdr.rmtc. Retrieved June 4, 2005.

Reynolds, T. B. (2000). Ascites. *Clinics in Liver Disease, 4*(1), 151–168.

Schiff, E. R. (2000). Update in hepatology. *Annals of Internal Medicine, 132*(6), 460–466.

Yu, A. S., & Hu, K. Q. (2001). Management of ascites. *Clinics in Liver Disease, 5*(2), 541–568.

Zimmerman, H. J. (2000). Drug-induced liver disease. *Clinics in Liver Disease, 4*(1), 73–96.

Cirrhosis and Esophageal Varices

Chalasani, N., & Imperiale, T. F. (2001). Screening for varices in patients with cirrhosis: Where do we stand? *American Journal of Gastroenterology, 96*(3), 623–624.

de Franchis, R. (2000). Updating consensus: Portal hypertension: Report of the Bavena III Consensus Workshop on definitions, methodology, and therapeutic strategies in portal hypertension. *Journal of Hepatology, 33*(5), 846–852.

Inadomi, J. M., Kapur, S., Kinkhabwala, M., & Cello, J. P. (2001). The laparoscopic evaluation of ascites. *Gastrointestinal Endoscopy Clinics of North America, 11*(1), 79–91.

Iredale, J. P. (2003). Cirrhosis: New research provides a basis for rational and targeted treatments. *British Medical Journal, 346*, 143–147.

Krige, J. J., & Beckingham, I. J. (2001). Portal hypertension. *British Medical Journal, 322*(7283), 348–351, 416–418.

Medical consequences of alcohol abuse. (2002). *Alcohol Research and Health: The Journal of the National Institute on Alcohol Abuse & Alcoholism, 24*(1), 27–31.

Menon, K. V., & Kamath, P. S. (2000). Managing the complications of cirrhosis. *Mayo Clinic Proceedings, 75*(5), 501–509.

Orozco, H., & Mercado, M. A. (2000). The evolution of portal hypertension: Lessons from 1,000 operations and 50 years' experience. *Archives of Surgery, 135*(12), 1389–1393.

Pomier-Layrargues, G., Villeneuve, J. P., Deschenes, M., et al. (2001). Transjugular intrahepatic portosystemic shunts (TIPS) versus endoscopic variceal ligation in the prevention of variceal rebleeding in patients with cirrhosis: A randomized trial. *Gut, 48*(3), 390–396.

Sarin, S. K., Lamba, G. S., Kumar, M., et al. (1999). Comparison of endoscopic ligation and propanolol for the primary prevention of variceal bleeding. *New England Journal of Medicine, 340*(13), 988–993.

Seymour, C. A., & Whelan, K. (1999). Dietary management of hepatic encephalopathy: Too many myths persist. *British Medical Journal, 318*(7195), 1364–1365.

Sharara, A. I., & Rockey, D. C. (2001). Medical progress: Gastroesophageal variceal hemorrhage. *New England Journal of Medicine, 345*(9), 669–681.

Statistics Canada, Health Sciences Division. (2005). Available at: http://www.40.statsca/101/cstoi/health36.htm.

Hepatitis

Al-Saden, P. C., McPartlin, F., Daly-Gawenda, D., et al. (1999). Hepatitis C: An emerging dilemma. *AAOHN Journal, 47*(5), 217–222.

Befeler, A. S., & Di Bisceglie, A. M. (2000). Hepatitis B. *Infectious Disease Clinics of North America, 14*(3), 617–632.

Birkel, A., Caldwell, L., Stafford-Fox, V., et al. (2000). Combination interferon alfa-2b/ribavirin therapy for the treatment of hepatitis C: Nursing implications. *Gastroenterology Nursing, 23*(2), 55–62.

Bockhold, K. M. (2000). Who's afraid of hepatitis C? *American Journal of Nursing, 100*(5), 26–32.

Bowker, S., Soskolne, C., Houston, S. Newman, S., & Jhangri, G. (2004). Human immunodeficiency virus (HIV) and Hepatitis C virus (HCV) in a northern Alberta population. *Canadian Journal of Public Health, 95*(3), 188–192.

Centers for Disease Control and Prevention (CDC). (2002). Sexually transmitted diseases treatment guidelines 2002. *MMWR: Morbidity and Mortality Weekly Report, 51*(RR-6), 1–84.

Centers for Disease Control and Prevention (CDC). (2001). FDA approval for a combined hepatitis A and B vaccine. *MWWR: Morbidity and Mortality Weekly Report, 50*(37), 806–807.

Centers for Disease Control and Prevention (CDC). (1999). Prevention of hepatitis A through active or passive immunizations: Recommendations of the Advisory Committee on Immunization Practice (ACIP). *MMWR: Morbidity and Mortality Weekly Report, 48*(RR-12), 1–37.

Chang, M. H. (2000). Hepatitis B vaccination and control of hepatitis B-related liver disease. *Journal of Pediatric Gastroenterology and Nutrition, 31*(2), 112–117.

Chang, M. H., Shau, W. Y., & Chen, C. J. (2000). Hepatitis B vaccination and hepatocellular carcinoma rates in boys and girls. *Journal of the American Medical Association, 284*(23), 3040–3042.

Cheney, C. P., Chopra, S., & Graham, C. (2000). Hepatitis C. *Infectious Disease Clinics of North America, 14*(3), 633–659.

Di Bisceglie, A. M., Thompson, J., et al. (2001). Combination of interferon and ribavirin in chronic hepatitis C: Re-treatment of non-responders to interferon. *Hepatology, 33*(3), 704–707.

Dougherty, A. S., & Dreher, H. M. (2001). Hepatitis C: Current treatment strategies for an emerging epidemic. *MedSurg Nursing, 10*(1), 9–15.

Farrell, G. C. (2000). Clinical potential of emerging new agents in hepatitis B. *Drugs. 60*(4), 701–710.

Fried, M. W. (2001). Advances in therapy for chronic hepatitis C. *Clinics in Liver Disease, 5*(4), 1009–1023.

Kenny-Walsh, E. (2001). The natural history of hepatitis C virus infection. *Clinics in Liver Disease, 5*(4), 969–977.

Ko, J., Lennon, C., & Roy, M. (1998). Canadian discovery for the treatment of chronic hepatitis B is approved in Canada…offers real hope to thousands of infected Canadians. *The Aboriginal Nurse, 13*(3), 4.

Koff, R. S. (2001). Hepatitis vaccines. *Infectious Disease Clinics of North America, 15*(1), 83–93.

Lauer, G. M., & Walker, B. D. (2001). Hepatitis C virus infection. *New England Journal of Medicine, 345*(1), 41–52.

Lin, O. S., & Keeffe, E. B. (2001). Current treatment strategies for chronic hepatitis B and C. *Annual Review of Medicine, 52,* 29–49.

Marrero, J., Martinez, F. J., & Hyzy, R. (2003). *Advances in Critical Care Hepatology, 168*(12), 1421–1426.

National Advisory Committee on Immunization: Supplementary Statement on Hepatitis Prevention. (1997). *Canadian Communicable Disease Report, 23* (ACS–4), 1–6.

National Institutes of Health (1997). Management of hepatitis C. *NIH Consensus Statement Online, 15*(3), 1–41.

Ostapowicz, G., Fontana, R. J., Schiodt, F. V., et al. (2002). Results of a prospective study of acute liver failure at 17 tertiary care centers in the United States. *Annals of Internal Medicine, 137*(12), 947–954.

Public Health Agency of Canada Immunization and Respiratory Infections Division. (2002). Vaccine preventable diseases: Hepatitis B. Available at: http://www.phac-aspc.gc.ca/dird-dimr/vpd-mev/hepatitis-b_e.html. Retrieved June 7, 2005.

Public Health Agency of Canada Immunization and Respiratory Infections Division. (2002). Vaccine preventable diseases: Hepatitis B. Available at: http://www.phac-aspc.gc.ca/dird-dimr/vpd-mev/hepatitis-b_e.html. Retrieved June 7, 2005.

Public Health Agency of Canada. (2004). Sex differences in injecting practices and hepatitis C: A systematic review of the literature. Canada Communicable Disease Report, 30(14). Available at: www.hc-sc.gc.ca/pphb-dgspsp/publicat/ccdr.rmtc. Retrieved June 4, 2005.

Regev, A., & Schiff, E. R. (2000). Viral hepatitis A, B, and C. *Clinics in Liver Disease, 4*(1), 47–71.

Riordan, S. M., & Williams, R. (2000). Fulminant liver failure. *Clinics in Liver Disease, 4*(1), 25–45.

Ryder, S. D., & Beckingham, I. J. (2001). Acute hepatitis: Clinical review: ABC of diseases of liver, pancreas, and biliary system. *British Medical Journal, 322*(7279), 151–153.

Sheffield, J. V., Larson, E. B., Gillock, M. R., et al. (2001). Update in general internal medicine. *Annals of Internal Medicine, 135*(4), 269–278.

Shovein, J. T., Damazo, R. J., & Hyams, I. (2000). Hepatitis A: How benign is it? *American Journal of Nursing, 100*(3), 43–47.

Thomas, D. L., Astemborski, J., Rai, R. M., et al. (2000). The natural history of hepatitis C virus infection: Host, viral and environmental factors. *Journal of the American Medical Association, 284*(4), 450–456.

Wong, J. B., McQuillan, G. M., McHutchinson, J. G., & Poynard, T. (2000). Estimating future hepatitis C morbidity, mortality and costs in the United States. *American Journal of Public Health, 90*(10), 1562–1569.

Wu, J. S., Hwang, L. Y., Goodman, K. J., et al. (1999). Hepatitis B vaccination in high-risk infants: 10-year follow-up. *Journal of Infectious Diseases, 179*(6), 1319–1325.

Yashida, H., Arakawa, Y., Sata, M., et al. (2002). Interferon therapy prolonged life expectancy among chronic hepatitis C patients. *Gastroenterology, 123*(2), 483–491.

Yoshida, E. M. (2002). Is there an association between SEN virus and liver disease? Reviewing the evidence. *Canadian Communicable Disease Report, 28*(7). Available at: www.phac-aspc.gc. Retrieved June, 2005.

Yurdaydin, C., Bozkaya, H., Cetinkaya, H., Sahin, T., Karaoguz, D., Toruner, M., et al. (2005). Lamivudine vs lamivudine and interferon combination treatment of HbeAg-Negative chronic hepatitis B. *Journal of Viral Hepatology, 12*(3), 262–268.

Wu, J., Zou, S., & Giulivi, A. (2001). Hepatitis A and its control. Canadian Communicable Disease Report (Vol. 2753). Available at: www.phac-aspc.gc/publicat/ccdr-rmtc/01vol27/2753/2753d-e.html. Retrieved June, 2005.

Liver Cancer

Aguayo, A., & Patt, Y. Z. (2001). Liver cancer. *Clinics in Liver Disease, 5*(2), 479–507.

Gonzalez, K. B. & Woodall, M. (2001). Hepatocellular carcinoma: Surgical treatment options. *Nursing Clinics of North America, 36*(3), 593–602.

Nagasue, N., Ond, T., Yamanoi, A., et al. (2001). Prognostic factors and survival after hepatic resection for hepatocellular carcinoma without cirrhosis. *British Journal of Surgery, 88*(4), 515–522.

Tsao, J. I., DeSanctis, J., Rossi, R. L., & Oberfield, R. A. (2000). Hepatic malignancies. *Surgical Clinics of North America, 80*(2), 18–32.

Liver Transplantation

Cohen, S. M. (2002). Current immunosuppression in liver transplantation. *American Journal of Therapeutics, 9*(2), 119–25.

Dabbs, A. D., Dauber, J. H., & Hoffman, L. A. (2000). Rejection after organ transplantation: A historical review. *American Journal of Critical Care, 9*(6), 419–429.

*Forsberg, A., Backman, L., & Moller, A. (2000). Experiencing liver transplantation: A phenomenological approach. *Journal of Advanced Nursing, 32*(2), 327–334.

Gomez-Manero, N., Herrero, J. I., Quiroga, J., et al. (2001). Prognostic model for early acute rejection after liver transplant. *Liver Transplantation, 7*(3), 246–254.

Gopal, D. V., Rabkin, J. M., Berk, B. S., et al. (2001). Treatment of progressive hepatitis C recurrence after liver transplantation with combination interferon plus ribavirin. *Liver Transplantation, 7*(3), 181–190.

Hebert, M. F., Ascher, M. L., Lake, J. R., et al. (1999). Four-year follow-up of mycophenolate mofetil for grant rescue in liver allograft recipients. *Transplantation, 67*(5), 707–712.

Niklason, L. E., & Langer, R. (2001). Prospects for organ and tissue replacement. *Journal of the American Medical Association, 285*(5), 573–576.

Reding, R., Gras, J., Sokal, E., Otte, J., & Davies, H.F.S. (2003). Steroid-free liver transplantation in children. *Lancet, 362*(9401), 2068–2070.

*Robertson, G. (1999). Individuals' perception of their quality of life following a liver transplant: An exploratory study. *Journal of Advanced Nursing, 30*(2), 497–505.

Surman, O. S. (2002). The ethics of partial-liver donation. *New England Journal of Medicine, 346*(14), 1038.

Trotter, J. F., Wachs, M., Everson, G. T., & Kam, I. (2002). Adult-to-adult transplantation of the right hepatic lobe from a living donor. *New England Journal of Medicine, 346*(14), 1074–1082.

Watson, C. J., Friend, P. J., Jamieson, N. V., et al. (1999). Sirolimus: A potent new immunosuppressant for liver transplantation. *Transplantation, 67*(4), 505–509.

RESOURCES AND WEBSITES

Alcoholics Anonymous World Services, 475 Riverside Drive, 11th Floor, New York, NY 10115; (212) 870-3400; http://aa.org.

Al-Anon Family Group Headquarters, 1600 Corporate Landing Parkway, Virginia Beach, VA 23454-5617; for meetings, (800) 344-2666 (8 a.m. to 6 p.m., Monday through Friday); for information, (800) 356-9996 (7 days a week, 24 hours); http://www.al-anon.alateen.org.

Canadian Association of Transplantation; http://www.transplant.ca.

Canadian Liver Foundation, Suite 1500, 2235 Sheppherd Ave East, Toronto, ON M2J 5B5; http://liver.ca.

Hepatitis Foundation International, 30 Sunrise Terrace, Cedar Grove, NJ 07009; (800) 891-0707; http://www.hepfi.org.

National Council on Alcoholism and Drug Dependence, 12 W. 21st St., New York, NY 10010; (800) NCA-CALL; http://www.ncadd.org.

National Digestive Diseases Information Clearing House, 2 Information Way, Bethesda, MD 20892-3570; (301) 654-3810; http://www.niddk.nih.gov.

National Institute on Alcohol Abuse and Alcoholism, Scientific Communications Branch, 6000 Executive Boulevard, Suite 409, Bethesda, MD 20892-7003; (301) 443-3860; http://www.niaaa.nih.gov.

Assessment and Management of Patients With Biliary Disorders

Adapted by Bev Williams

LEARNING OBJECTIVES

On completion of this chapter, the learner will be able to:

1. Compare approaches to management of cholelithiasis.
2. Use the nursing process as a framework for care of patients with cholelithiasis and those undergoing laparoscopic or open cholecystectomy.
3. Differentiate between acute and chronic pancreatitis.
4. Use the nursing process as a framework for care of patients with acute pancreatitis.
5. Describe the nutritional and metabolic effects of surgical treatment of tumours of the pancreas.

*D*isorders of the biliary tract and pancreas are common and include gallbladder stones and pancreatic dysfunction. An understanding of the structure and function of the biliary tract and pancreas is essential, along with an understanding of the close link of biliary tract disorders with liver disease. Patients with acute or chronic biliary tract or pancreatic disease require care from nurses knowledgeable about the diagnostic procedures and interventions that are used in the management of gallbladder and pancreatic disorders.

Anatomic and Physiologic Overview

ANATOMY OF THE GALLBLADDER

The gallbladder, a pear-shaped, hollow, saclike organ, 7.5 to 10 cm long, lies in a shallow depression on the inferior surface of the liver, to which it is attached by loose connective tissue. The capacity of the gallbladder is 30 to 50 mL of bile. Its wall is composed largely of smooth muscle. The gallbladder is connected to the common bile duct by the cystic duct (Fig. 40-1).

FUNCTION OF THE GALLBLADDER

The gallbladder functions as a storage depot for bile. Between meals, when the sphincter of Oddi is closed, bile produced by the hepatocytes enters the gallbladder. During storage, a large portion of the water in bile is absorbed through the walls of the gallbladder, so that gallbladder bile is five to ten times more concentrated than that originally secreted by the liver. When food enters the duodenum, the gallbladder contracts and the sphincter of Oddi (located at the junction where the common bile duct enters the duodenum) relaxes. Relaxation of the sphincter of Oddi allows the bile to enter the intestine. This response is mediated by secretion of the hormone **cholecystokinin–pancreozymin (CCK-PZ)** from the intestinal wall. Bile is composed of water and electrolytes (sodium, potassium, calcium, chloride, and bicarbonate) and significant amounts of lecithin, fatty acids, cholesterol, bilirubin, and bile salts. The bile salts, together with cholesterol, assist in emulsification of fats in the distal ileum. They then are reabsorbed into the portal blood for return to the liver and again excreted into the bile. This pathway from hepa-

tocytes to bile to intestine and back to the hepatocytes is called the enterohepatic circulation. Because of the enterohepatic circulation, only a small fraction of the bile salts that enter the intestine are excreted in the feces. This decreases the need for active synthesis of bile salts by the liver cells.

If the flow of bile is impeded (ie, with gallstones in the bile ducts), bilirubin, a pigment derived from the breakdown of red blood cells, does not enter the intestine. As a result, bilirubin levels in the blood increase. This results, in turn, in increased renal excretion of urobilinogen, which results from conversion of bilirubin in the small intestine, and decreased excretion in the stool. These changes produce many of the signs and symptoms seen in gallbladder disorders.

THE PANCREAS

The pancreas, located in the upper abdomen, has **endocrine** as well as **exocrine** functions (see Fig. 40-1). The secretion of pancreatic enzymes into the gastrointestinal tract through the pancreatic duct represents its exocrine function. The secretion of insulin, glucagon, and somatostatin directly into the bloodstream represents its endocrine function.

Exocrine Pancreas

The secretions of the exocrine portion of the pancreas are collected in the pancreatic duct, which joins the common bile duct and enters the duodenum at the ampulla of Vater. Surrounding the ampulla is the sphincter of Oddi, which partially controls the rate at which secretions from the pancreas and the gallbladder enter the duodenum.

The secretions of the exocrine pancreas are digestive enzymes high in protein content and an electrolyte-rich fluid. The secretions are very alkaline because of their high concentration of sodium bicarbonate and are capable of neutralizing the highly acid gastric juice that enters the duodenum. The enzyme secretions include **amylase**, which aids in the digestion of carbohydrates; **trypsin**, which aids in the digestion of proteins; and **lipase**, which aids in the digestion of fats. Other enzymes that promote the breakdown of more complex foodstuffs are also secreted.

Glossary

amylase: pancreatic enzyme; aids in the digestion of carbohydrates
cholecystitis: inflammation of the gallbladder
cholecystokinin-pancreozymin (CCK-PZ): hormone; major stimulus for digestive enzyme secretion; stimulates contraction of the gallbladder
cholecystectomy: removal of the gallbladder
cholecystojejunostomy: anastomosis of the jejunum to the gallbladder to divert bile flow
cholecystostomy: opening and drainage of the gallbladder
choledocholithiasis: stones in the common duct
choledochostomy: opening into the common duct
cholelithiasis: calculi in the gallbladder

dissolution therapy: use of medications to break up/dissolve gallstones
endocrine: secreting internally; hormonal secretion of a ductless gland
endoscopic retrograde cholangiopancreatography (ERCP): an endoscopic procedure using fibreoptic technology to visualize the biliary system
exocrine: secreting externally; hormonal secretion from excretory ducts
laparoscopic cholecystectomy: removal of gallbladder through endoscopic procedure
lipase: pancreatic enzyme; aids in the digestion of fats
lithotripsy: disintegration of gallstones by shock waves
pancreaticojejunostomy: joining of the pancreatic duct to the jejunum by side-to-

side anastomosis; allows drainage of the pancreatic secretions into the jejunum
pancreatitis: inflammation of the pancreas; may be acute or chronic
secretin: hormone responsible for stimulating secretion of pancreatic juice; also used as an aid in diagnosing pancreatic exocrine disease and in obtaining desquamated pancreatic cells for cytologic examination
steatorrhea: frothy, foul-smelling stools with a high fat content; results from impaired digestion of proteins and fats due to a lack of pancreatic juice in the intestine
trypsin: pancreatic enzyme; aids in digestion of proteins
Zollinger-Ellison tumour: hypersecretion of gastric acid that produces peptic ulcers as a result of a non-beta cell tumour of the pancreatic islets

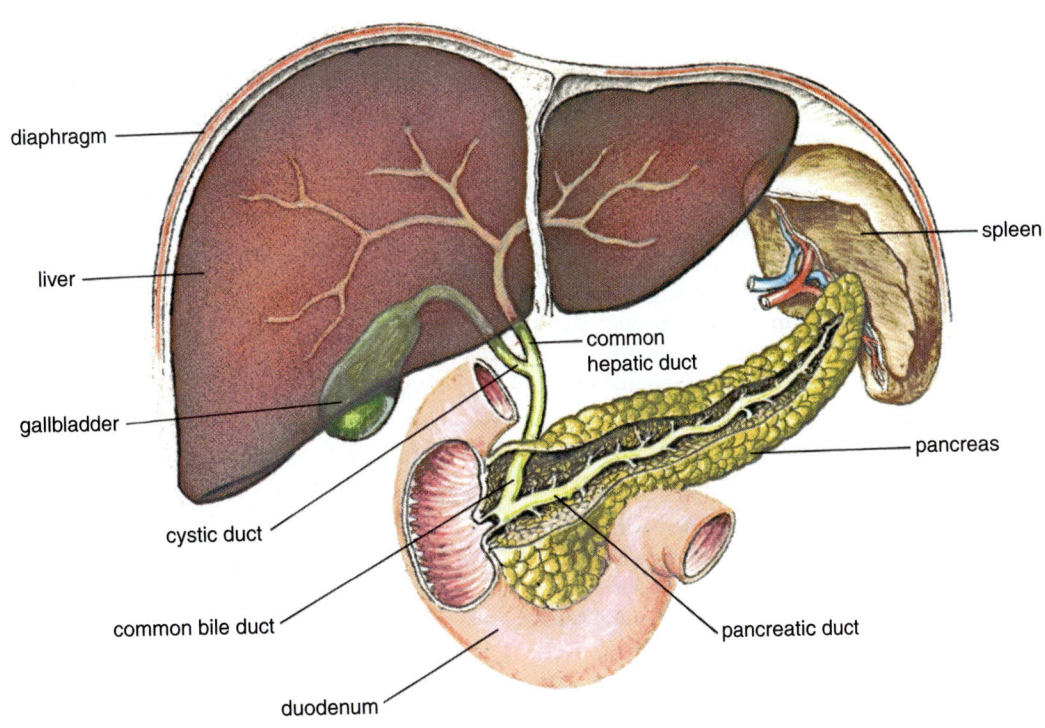

FIGURE 40-1 The liver, biliary system, and pancreas.

Hormones originating in the gastrointestinal tract stimulate the secretion of these exocrine pancreatic juices. **Secretin** is the major stimulus for increased bicarbonate secretion from the pancreas, and the major stimulus for digestive enzyme secretion is the hormone CCK-PZ. The vagus nerve also influences exocrine pancreatic secretion.

Endocrine Pancreas

The islets of Langerhans, the endocrine part of the pancreas, are collections of cells embedded in the pancreatic tissue. They are composed of alpha, beta, and delta cells. The hormone produced by the beta cells is called insulin; the alpha cells secrete glucagon and the delta cells secrete somatostatin.

INSULIN

A major action of insulin is to lower blood glucose by permitting entry of the glucose into the cells of the liver, muscle, and other tissues, where it is either stored as glycogen or used for energy. Insulin also promotes the storage of fat in adipose tissue and the synthesis of proteins in various body tissues. In the absence of insulin, glucose cannot enter the cells and is excreted in the urine. This condition, called diabetes mellitus, can be diagnosed by high levels of glucose in the blood. In diabetes mellitus, stored fats and protein are used for energy instead of glucose, with consequent loss of body mass. (Diabetes mellitus is discussed in detail in Chap. 41.) The level of glucose in the blood normally regulates the rate of insulin secretion from the pancreas.

GLUCAGON

The effect of glucagon (opposite to that of insulin) is chiefly to raise the blood glucose by converting glycogen to glucose in the liver. Glucagon is secreted by the pancreas in response to a decrease in the level of blood glucose.

SOMATOSTATIN

Somatostatin exerts a hypoglycemic effect by interfering with release of growth hormone from the pituitary and glucagon from the pancreas, both of which tend to raise blood glucose levels.

Endocrine Control of Carbohydrate Metabolism

Glucose for body energy needs is derived by metabolism of ingested carbohydrates and also from proteins by the process of gluconeogenesis. Glucose can be stored temporarily in the liver, muscles, and other tissues in the form of glycogen. The endocrine system controls the level of blood glucose by regulating the rate at which glucose is synthesized, stored, and moved to and from the bloodstream. Through the action of hormones, blood glucose is normally maintained at about 5.5 mmol/L. Insulin is the primary hormone that lowers the blood glucose level. Hormones that raise the blood glucose level are glucagon, epinephrine, adrenocorticosteroids, growth hormone, and thyroid hormone.

The endocrine and exocrine functions of the pancreas are interrelated. The major exocrine function is to facilitate digestion through secretion of enzymes into the proximal duodenum. Secretin and CCK-PZ are hormones from the gastrointestinal tract that aid in the digestion of food substances by controlling the secretions of the pancreas. Neural factors also influence pancreatic enzyme secretion. Considerable dysfunction of the pancreas must occur before enzyme secretion decreases and protein and fat digestion becomes impaired. Pancreatic enzyme secretion is normally 1,500 to 2,500 mL/day.

Gerontologic Considerations

There is little change in the size of the pancreas with age. There is, however, an increase in fibrous material and some fatty deposition in the normal pancreas in patients older than 70 years of age. Some localized arteriosclerotic changes occur with age. There is also a decreased rate of pancreatic secretion (decreased lipase, amylase, and trypsin) and bicarbonate output in older patients. Some impairment of normal fat absorption occurs with increasing age, possibly because of delayed gastric emptying and pancreatic insufficiency. Decreased calcium absorption may also occur. These changes require care in interpreting diagnostic tests in the normal elderly person and in providing dietary counselling.

Disorders of the Gallbladder

Several disorders affect the biliary system and interfere with normal drainage of bile into the duodenum. These disorders include inflammation of the biliary system and carcinoma that obstructs the biliary tree. Gallbladder disease with gallstones is the most common disorder of the biliary system. Although not all occurrences of gallbladder inflammation (**cholecystitis**) are related to gallstones (**cholelithiasis**), more than 90% of patients with acute cholecystitis have gallstones. Most of the one in ten Canadians with gallstones have no pain, however, and are unaware of the presence of stones. For a guide to the terminology associated with biliary disorders and procedures, see Chart 40-1.

CHOLECYSTITIS

Acute inflammation (cholecystitis) of the gallbladder causes pain, tenderness, and rigidity of the upper right abdomen that may radiate to the midsternal area or right shoulder and is associated with nausea, vomiting, and the usual signs of an acute inflammation. An empyema of the gallbladder develops if the gallbladder becomes filled with purulent fluid.

Calculous cholecystitis is the cause of more than 90% of cases of acute cholecystitis (Ahmed, Cheung & Keefe, 2000). In calculous cholecystitis, a gallbladder stone obstructs bile outflow.

Bile remaining in the gallbladder initiates a chemical reaction; autolysis and edema occur; and the blood vessels in the gallbladder are compressed, compromising its vascular supply. Gangrene of the gallbladder with perforation may result. Bacteria play a minor role in acute cholecystitis; however, secondary infection of bile with *Escherichia coli*, *Klebsiella* species, and other enteric organisms occurs in about 60% of patients (Schwartz, 1999).

Acalculous cholecystitis describes acute gallbladder inflammation in the absence of obstruction by gallstones. Acalculous cholecystitis occurs after major surgical procedures, severe trauma, or burns. Other factors associated with this type of cholecystitis include torsion, cystic duct obstruction, primary bacterial infections of the gallbladder, and multiple blood transfusions. It is speculated that acalculous cholecystitis results from alterations in fluids and electrolytes and in regional blood flow in the visceral circulation. Bile stasis (lack of gallbladder contraction) and increased viscosity of the bile are also thought to play a role. The occurrence of acalculous cholecystitis with major surgical procedures or trauma makes its diagnosis difficult.

CHOLELITHIASIS

Calculi, or gallstones, usually form in the gallbladder from the solid constituents of bile; they vary greatly in size, shape, and composition (Fig. 40-2). They are uncommon in children and young adults but become increasingly prevalent after 40 years of age. The incidence of cholelithiasis increases thereafter to such an extent that up to 50% of those over the age of 70 and over 50% of those over 80 will develop stones in the bile tract (Borzellino, deManzoni & Ricci, 1999). Chart 40-2 identifies common risk factors.

Pathophysiology

There are two major types of gallstones: those composed predominantly of pigment and those composed primarily of cholesterol. Pigment stones probably form when unconjugated pigments in the bile precipitate to form stones; these stones account for about one third of all cases (Donovan, 1999). The risk of developing such stones is increased in patients with cirrhosis, hemolysis, and infections of the biliary tract. Pigment stones cannot be dissolved and must be removed surgically.

Cholesterol stones account for most of the remaining cases of gallbladder disease in Canada. Cholesterol, a normal constituent of bile, is insoluble in water. Its solubility depends on bile acids and lecithin (phospholipids) in bile. In gallstone-prone patients, there is decreased bile acid synthesis and increased cholesterol synthesis in the liver, resulting in bile supersaturated with cholesterol, which precipitates out of the bile to form stones. The cholesterol-saturated bile predisposes to the formation of gallstones and acts as an irritant, producing inflammatory changes in the gallbladder.

Four times more women than men develop cholesterol stones and gallbladder disease; the women are usually older than 40, multiparous, and obese. The incidence of stone formation rises in users of oral contraceptives, estrogens, and clofibrate; these substances are known to increase biliary cholesterol saturation. The incidence of stone formation increases with age as a result of increased hepatic secretion of cholesterol and decreased bile acid synthesis. In addition, there is an increased risk because of malabsorption of bile salts in patients with gastrointestinal disease or

---

Chart 40-1

Definition of Terms: Biliary

Cholecystitis: inflammation of the gallbladder
Cholelithiasis: the presence of calculi in the gallbladder
Cholecystectomy: removal of the gallbladder
Cholecystostomy: opening and drainage of the gallbladder
Choledochotomy: opening into the common duct
Choledocholithiasis: stones in the common duct
Choledocholithotomy: incision of common bile duct for removal of stones
Choledochoduodenostomy: anastomosis of common duct to duodenum
Choledochojejunostomy: anastomosis of common duct to jejunum
Lithotripsy: disintegration of gallstones by shock waves
Laparoscopic cholecystectomy: removal of gallbladder through endoscopic procedure
Laser cholecystectomy: removal of gallbladder using laser rather than scalpel and traditional surgical instruments

FIGURE 40-2 Examples of cholesterol gallstones (*left*) made up of a coalescence of multiple small stones (*left*) and pigment gallstones (*right*) composed of calcium bilirubinate. Rubin, E., & Farber, J. L. (1999). *Pathology* (3rd ed.). Philadelphia: Lippincott Williams & Wilkins.

T-tube fistula or in those who have had ileal resection or bypass. The incidence also increases in people with diabetes.

Clinical Manifestations

Gallstones may be silent, producing no pain and only mild gastrointestinal symptoms. Such stones may be detected incidentally during surgery or evaluation for unrelated problems.

The patient with gallbladder disease from gallstones may develop two types of symptoms: those due to disease of the gallbladder itself and those due to obstruction of the bile passages by a gallstone. The symptoms may be acute or chronic. Epigastric distress, such as fullness, abdominal distention, and vague pain in the right upper quadrant of the abdomen, may occur. This distress may follow a meal rich in fried or fatty foods.

Chart 40-2
Risk Factors for Cholelithiasis

- Obesity
- Women, especially those who have had multiple pregnancies or who are of Aboriginal ethnicity
- Frequent changes in weight
- Rapid weight loss (leads to rapid development of gallstones and high risk of symptomatic disease)
- Treatment with high-dose estrogen (ie, in prostate cancer)
- Low-dose estrogen therapy—a small increase in the risk of gallstones
- Ileal resection or disease
- Cystic fibrosis
- Diabetes mellitus

PAIN AND BILIARY COLIC

If a gallstone obstructs the cystic duct, the gallbladder becomes distended, inflamed, and eventually infected (acute cholecystitis). The patient develops a fever and may have a palpable abdominal mass. The patient may have biliary colic with excruciating upper right abdominal pain that radiates to the back or right shoulder, is usually associated with nausea and vomiting, and is noticeable several hours after a heavy meal. The patient moves about restlessly, unable to find a comfortable position. In some patients the pain is constant rather than colicky.

Such a bout of biliary colic is caused by contraction of the gallbladder, which cannot release bile because of obstruction by the stone. When distended, the fundus of the gallbladder comes in contact with the abdominal wall in the region of the right ninth and tenth costal cartilages. This produces marked tenderness in the right upper quadrant on deep inspiration and prevents full inspiratory excursion.

The pain of acute cholecystitis may be so severe that analgesics are required. Morphine is thought to increase spasm of the sphincter of Oddi and may be avoided in many cases in favour of meperidine (Porth, 2002). This is controversial because morphine is the preferred analgesic agent for management of acute pain, and meperidine has metabolites toxic to the CNS.

If the gallstone is dislodged and no longer obstructs the cystic duct, the gallbladder drains and the inflammatory process subsides after a relatively short time. If the gallstone continues to obstruct the duct, abscess, necrosis, and perforation with generalized peritonitis may result.

JAUNDICE

Jaundice occurs in a few patients with gallbladder disease and usually occurs with obstruction of the common bile duct. The bile, which is no longer carried to the duodenum, is absorbed by the blood and gives the skin and mucous membrane a yellow colour. This is frequently accompanied by marked itching of the skin.

CHANGES IN URINE AND STOOL COLOUR

The excretion of the bile pigments by the kidneys gives the urine a very dark colour. The feces, no longer coloured with bile pigments, are greyish, like putty, and usually described as clay-coloured.

VITAMIN DEFICIENCY

Obstruction of bile flow also interferes with absorption of the fat-soluble vitamins A, D, E, and K. Therefore, the patient may exhibit deficiencies (eg, bleeding caused by vitamin K deficiency, which interferes with normal blood clotting) of these vitamins if biliary obstruction has been prolonged.

Assessment and Diagnostic Findings

ABDOMINAL X-RAY

An abdominal x-ray may be obtained if gallbladder disease is suggested to exclude other causes of symptoms. However, only 15% to 20% of gallstones are calcified sufficiently to be visible on such x-ray studies.

ULTRASONOGRAPHY

Ultrasonography has replaced oral cholecystography as the diagnostic procedure of choice because it is rapid and accurate and can be used in patients with liver dysfunction and jaundice. It does not expose patients to ionizing radiation. The procedure is most accurate if the patient fasts overnight so that the gallbladder is distended. The use of ultrasound is based on reflected sound waves. Ultrasonography can detect calculi in the gallbladder or a dilated common bile duct. It is reported to detect gallstones with 95% accuracy.

RADIONUCLIDE IMAGING OR CHOLESCINTIGRAPHY

Cholescintigraphy is used successfully in the diagnosis of acute cholecystitis. In this procedure, a radioactive agent is administered intravenously. It is taken up by the hepatocytes and excreted rapidly through the biliary tract. The biliary tract is then scanned, and images of the gallbladder and biliary tract are obtained. This test is more expensive than ultrasonography, takes longer to perform, exposes the patient to radiation, and cannot detect gallstones. Its use may be limited to cases in which ultrasonography is not conclusive.

CHOLECYSTOGRAPHY

Although it has been replaced by ultrasonography as the test of choice, cholecystography is still used if ultrasound equipment is not available or if the ultrasound results are inconclusive. Oral cholangiography may be performed to detect gallstones and to assess the ability of the gallbladder to fill, concentrate its contents, contract, and empty. An iodide-containing contrast agent excreted by the liver and concentrated in the gallbladder is administered to the patient. The normal gallbladder fills with this radiopaque substance. If gallstones are present, they appear as shadows on the x-ray film.

Contrast agents include iopanoic acid (Telepaque), iodipamide meglumine (Cholografin), and sodium ipodate (Oragrafin). These agents are administered orally 10 to 12 hours before the x-ray study. To prevent contraction and emptying of the gallbladder, the patient is permitted nothing by mouth after the contrast agent is administered.

The patient is asked about allergies to iodine or seafood. If no allergy is identified, the patient receives the oral form of the contrast agent the evening before the x-rays are obtained. An x-ray of the right upper abdomen is obtained. If the gallbladder is found to fill and empty normally and to contain no stones, gallbladder disease is ruled out. If gallbladder disease is present, the gallbladder may not be visualized because of obstruction by gallstones. A repeat of the oral cholecystogram with a second dose of the contrast agent may be necessary if the gallbladder is not visualized on the first attempt.

Cholecystography in the obviously jaundiced patient is not useful because the liver cannot excrete the radiopaque dye into the gallbladder in the presence of jaundice. Oral cholecystography is likely to continue to be used as part of the evaluation of the few patients who have been treated with gallstone **dissolution therapy** or lithotripsy.

ENDOSCOPIC RETROGRADE CHOLANGIOPANCREATOGRAPHY

Endoscopic retrograde cholangiopancreatography (ERCP) permits direct visualization of structures that could once be seen only during laparotomy. The examination of the hepatobiliary system is carried out via a side-viewing flexible fibreoptic endoscope inserted into the esophagus to the descending duodenum (Fig. 40-3). Multiple position changes are required during the procedure, beginning in the left semiprone position to pass the endoscope.

Fluoroscopy and multiple x-rays are used during ERCP to evaluate the presence and location of ductal stones. Careful insertion of a catheter through the endoscope into the common bile duct is the most important step in sphincterotomy (division of the muscles of the biliary sphincter) for gallstone extraction via this technique. This is described later in the chapter.

Nursing Implications. The procedure requires a cooperative patient to permit insertion of the endoscope without damage to the gastrointestinal tract structures, including the biliary tree. Before

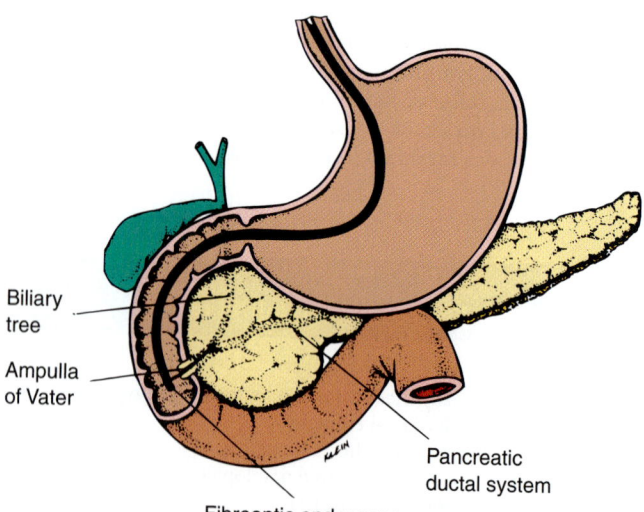

FIGURE 40-3 Endoscopic retrograde cholangiopancreatography (ERCP). A fibreoptic duodenoscope, with side-viewing apparatus, is inserted into the duodenum. The ampulla of Vater is catheterized and the biliary tree injected with contrast agent. The pancreatic ductal system is also assessed, if indicated. This procedure is of special value in visualizing neoplasms of the ampulla area and extracting a biopsy specimen.

the procedure, the patient is given an explanation of the procedure and his or her role in it. The patient takes nothing by mouth for several hours before the procedure. Moderate sedation is used with this procedure, so the sedated patient must be monitored closely. Most endoscopists use a combination of an opioid and a benzodiazepine. Medications such as glucagon or anticholinergics may also be necessary to eliminate duodenal peristalsis to make cannulation easier. The nurse observes closely for signs of respiratory and central nervous system depression, hypotension, oversedation, and vomiting (if glucagon is given). During ERCP, the nurse monitors intravenous fluids, administers medications, and positions the patient.

After the procedure, the nurse monitors the patient's condition, observing vital signs and monitoring for signs of perforation or infection. The nurse also monitors the patient for side effects of any medications received during the procedure and for return of the gag and cough reflexes after the use of local anesthetics.

PERCUTANEOUS TRANSHEPATIC CHOLANGIOGRAPHY

Percutaneous transhepatic cholangiography involves the injection of dye directly into the biliary tract. Because of the relatively large concentration of dye that is introduced into the biliary system, all components of the system, including the hepatic ducts within the liver, the entire length of the common bile duct, the cystic duct, and the gallbladder, are outlined clearly.

This procedure can be carried out even in the presence of liver dysfunction and jaundice. It is useful for distinguishing jaundice caused by liver disease (hepatocellular jaundice) from that caused by biliary obstruction, for investigating the gastrointestinal symptoms of a patient whose gallbladder has been removed, for locating stones within the bile ducts, and for diagnosing cancer involving the biliary system.

This sterile procedure is performed under moderate sedation on a patient who has been fasting; the patient receives local anesthesia and intravenous sedation. Coagulation parameters and platelet count should be normal to minimize the risk for bleeding. Broad-spectrum antibiotics are administered during the procedure due to the high prevalence of bacterial colonization from obstructed biliary systems. After infiltration with a local anesthetic agent, a flexible needle is inserted into the liver from the right side in the midclavicular line immediately beneath the right costal margin. Successful entry of a duct is noted when bile is aspirated or upon the injection of a contrast agent. Ultrasound guidance can be used for duct puncture. Bile is aspirated and samples are sent for bacteriology and cytology. A water-soluble contrast agent is injected to fill the biliary system. The fluoroscopy table is tilted and the patient repositioned to allow x-rays to be taken in multiple projections. Delayed x-ray views can identify abnormalities of more distant ducts and determine the length of a stricture or multiple strictures. Before the needle is removed, as much dye and bile as possible are aspirated to forestall subsequent leakage into the needle tract and eventually into the peritoneal cavity, thus minimizing the risk of bile peritonitis.

Table 40-1 identifies various procedures and their diagnostic uses.

> **NURSING ALERT** Although the complication rate after this procedure is low, the nurse must closely observe the patient for symptoms of bleeding, peritonitis, and septicemia. The nurse should immediately report pain and indicators of these complications. Antibiotic agents are often prescribed to minimize the risk of sepsis and septic shock.

Medical Management

The major objectives of medical therapy are to reduce the incidence of acute episodes of gallbladder pain and cholecystitis by supportive and dietary management and, if possible, to remove the cause of cholecystitis by pharmacologic therapy, endoscopic procedures, or surgical intervention.

Although nonsurgical approaches have the advantage of eliminating risks associated with surgery, they are associated with persistent symptoms or recurrent stone formation. Most of the nonsurgical approaches, including lithotripsy and dissolution of gallstones, provide only temporary solutions to the problems associated with gallstones. They are therefore rarely used in Canada. In some instances, other treatment approaches may be indicated; these are described below.

Table 40-1 • Studies Used in the Diagnosis of Biliary Tract and Pancreatic Disease

STUDIES	DIAGNOSTIC USES
Cholecystogram, cholangiogram	To visualize gallbladder and bile duct
Celiac axis arteriography	To visualize liver and pancreas
Laparoscopy	To visualize anterior surface of liver, gallbladder, and mesentery through a trocar
Ultrasonography	To show size of abdominal organs and presence of masses
Magnetic resonance imaging (MRI)	To detect neoplasms; diagnose cysts, abscess, and hematomas
Endoscopic retrograde cholangiopancreatography (ERCP)	To visualize biliary structures and pancreas via endoscopy
Serum alkaline phosphatase	In absence of bone disease, to measure of biliary tract obstruction
GGT, GGTP, LDH	Markers for biliary stasis; also elevated in alcohol abuse
Cholesterol levels	Elevated in biliary obstruction; decreased in parenchymal liver disease

Removal of the gallbladder (**cholecystectomy**) through traditional surgical approaches was considered the standard approach to management for more than 100 years. However, dramatic changes have occurred in the surgical management of gallbladder disease. There is now widespread use of **laparoscopic cholecystectomy** (removal of the gallbladder through a small incision through the umbilicus). As a result, surgical risks have decreased, along with the length of hospital stay and the long recovery period associated with the standard surgical cholecystectomy.

NUTRITIONAL AND SUPPORTIVE THERAPY

Approximately 80% of the patients with acute gallbladder inflammation achieve remission with rest, intravenous fluids, nasogastric suction, analgesia, and antibiotic agents. Unless the patient's condition deteriorates, surgical intervention is delayed until the acute symptoms subside and a complete evaluation can be carried out.

The diet immediately after an episode is usually limited to low-fat liquids. The patient can stir powdered supplements high in protein and carbohydrate into skim milk. Cooked fruits, rice or tapioca, lean meats, mashed potatoes, non–gas-forming vegetables, bread, coffee, or tea may be added as tolerated. The patient should avoid eggs, cream, pork, fried foods, cheese and rich dressings, gas-forming vegetables, and alcohol. It is important to remind the patient that fatty foods may bring on an episode. Dietary management may be the major mode of therapy in patients who have had only dietary intolerance to fatty foods and vague gastrointestinal symptoms (Dudek, 2001).

PHARMACOLOGIC THERAPY

Ursodeoxycholic acid (UDCA) and chenodeoxycholic acid (chenodiol or CDCA) have been used to dissolve small, radiolucent gallstones composed primarily of cholesterol. UDCA has fewer side effects than chenodiol and can be administered in smaller doses to achieve the same effect. It acts by inhibiting the synthesis and secretion of cholesterol, thereby desaturating bile. Existing stones can be reduced in size, small ones dissolved, and new stones prevented from forming. Six to 12 months of therapy are required in many patients to dissolve stones, and monitoring of the patient is required during this time. The effective dose of medication depends on body weight. This method of treatment is generally indicated for patients who refuse surgery or for whom surgery is considered too risky.

Patients with significant, frequent symptoms, cystic duct occlusion, or pigment stones are not candidates for this therapy. Symptomatic patients with acceptable operative risk are more appropriate for laparoscopic or open cholecystectomy.

NONSURGICAL REMOVAL OF GALLSTONES

Dissolving Gallstones. Several methods have been used to dissolve gallstones by infusion of a solvent (mono-octanoin or methyl tertiary butyl ether [MTBE]) into the gallbladder. The solvent can be infused through the following routes: a tube or catheter inserted percutaneously directly into the gallbladder; a tube or drain inserted through a T-tube tract to dissolve stones not removed at the time of surgery; an ERCP endoscope; or a transnasal biliary catheter.

In the last procedure, the catheter is introduced through the mouth and inserted into the common bile duct. The upper end of the tube is then rerouted from the mouth to the nose and left in place. This enables the patient to eat and drink normally while passage of stones is monitored or chemical solvents are infused to dissolve the stones. This method of dissolution of stones is not widely used in patients with gallstone disease.

Stone Removal by Instrumentation. Several nonsurgical methods are used to remove stones that were not removed at the time of cholecystectomy or have become lodged in the common bile duct (Fig. 40-4*A, B*). A catheter and instrument with a basket attached are threaded through the T-tube tract or fistula formed at the time of T-tube insertion; the basket is used to retrieve and remove the stones lodged in the common bile duct.

A second procedure involves the use of the ERCP endoscope (see Fig. 40-4*C*). After the endoscope is inserted, a cutting instrument is passed through the endoscope into the ampulla of Vater of the common bile duct. It may be used to cut the submucosal fibres, or papilla, of the sphincter of Oddi, enlarging the opening, which may allow the lodged stones to pass spontaneously into the duodenum. Another instrument with a small basket or balloon at its tip may be inserted through the endoscope to retrieve the stones (see Fig. 40-4*D–F*). Although complications after this procedure are rare, the patient must be observed closely for bleeding, perforation, and the development of pancreatitis or sepsis.

The ERCP procedure is particularly useful in the diagnosis and treatment of patients who have symptoms after biliary tract surgery, for patients with intact gallbladders, and for patients in whom surgery is particularly hazardous.

Extracorporeal Shock-Wave Lithotripsy. Extracorporeal shock-wave therapy (lithotripsy or ESWL) has been used for nonsurgical fragmentation of gallstones. The word **lithotripsy** is derived from *lithos,* meaning stone, and *tripsis,* meaning rubbing or friction. This noninvasive procedure uses repeated shock waves directed at the gallstones in the gallbladder or common bile duct to fragment the stones. The energy is transmitted to the body through a fluid-filled bag, or it may be transmitted while the patient is immersed in a water bath. The converging shock waves are directed to the stones to be fragmented.

After the stones are gradually broken up, the stone fragments pass from the gallbladder or common bile duct spontaneously, are removed by endoscopy, or are dissolved with oral bile acid or solvents. Because the procedure requires no incision and no hospitalization, patients are usually treated as outpatients, but several sessions are generally necessary.

The advent of laparoscopic cholecystectomy has reduced the use of this method to treat gallbladder stones. It is used in some centres for a small percentage of suitable patients (those with common bile duct stones who may not be surgical candidates), sometimes in combination with dissolution therapy.

Intracorporeal Lithotripsy. Stones in the gallbladder or common bile duct may be fragmented by means of laser pulse technology. A laser pulse is directed under fluoroscopic guidance with the use of devices that can distinguish between stones and tissue. The laser pulse produces rapid expansion and disintegration of plasma on the stone surface, resulting in a mechanical shock wave. Electrohydraulic lithotripsy uses a probe with two electrodes that deliver electric sparks in rapid pulses, creating expansion of the liquid environment surrounding the gallstones. This results in pressure waves that cause stones to fragment. This technique can be employed percutaneously with the use of a basket or balloon catheter system or by direct visualization through an endoscope. Repeated procedures may be necessary due to stone size, local anatomy, bleeding, or technical difficulty. A nasobiliary tube can be inserted to allow for biliary decompression and prevent stone impaction in the common bile duct. This approach allows time for improvement in the patient's clinical condition until gallstones are cleared endoscopically, percutaneously, or surgically.

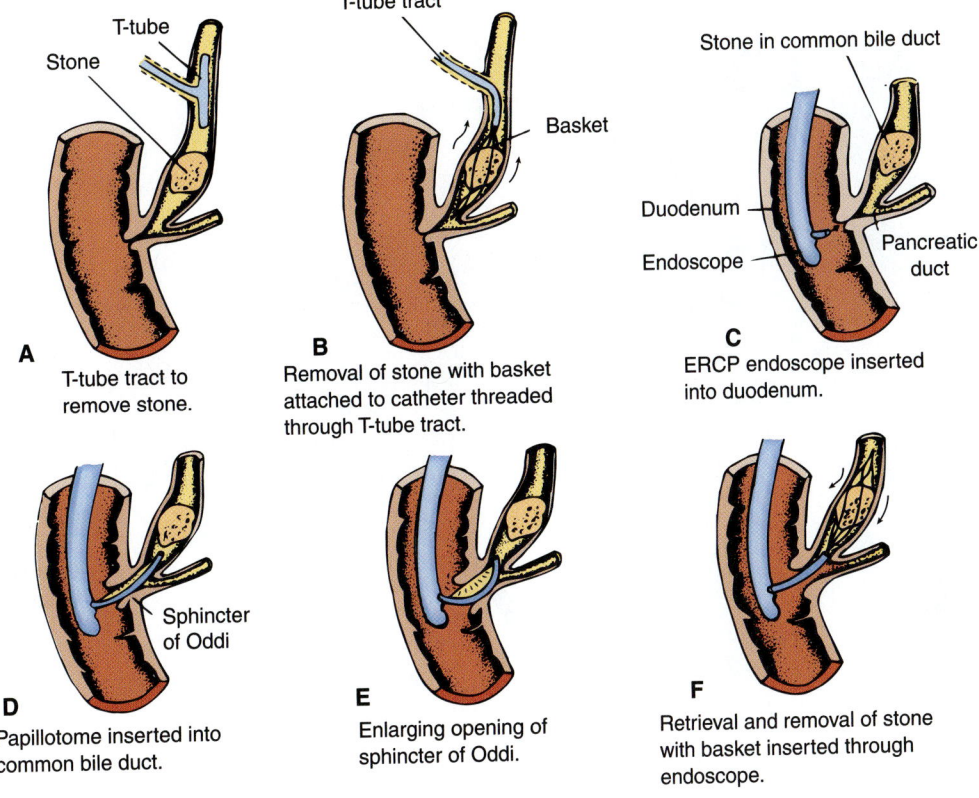

A — T-tube tract to remove stone.

B — Removal of stone with basket attached to catheter threaded through T-tube tract.

C — ERCP endoscope inserted into duodenum.

D — Papillotome inserted into common bile duct.

E — Enlarging opening of sphincter of Oddi.

F — Retrieval and removal of stone with basket inserted through endoscope.

FIGURE 40-4 Nonsurgical techniques for removing gallstones.

SURGICAL MANAGEMENT

Surgical treatment of gallbladder disease and gallstones is carried out to relieve persistent symptoms, to remove the cause of biliary colic, and to treat acute cholecystitis. Surgery may be delayed until the patient's symptoms have subsided or may be performed as an emergency procedure if the patient's condition necessitates it.

Preoperative Measures. A chest x-ray, electrocardiogram, and liver function tests may be performed in addition to x-ray studies of the gallbladder. Vitamin K may be administered if the prothrombin level is low. Blood component therapy may be administered before surgery. Nutritional requirements are considered; if the nutritional status is suboptimal, it may be necessary to provide intravenous glucose with protein hydrolysate supplements to aid wound healing and help prevent liver damage.

Preparation for gallbladder surgery is similar to that for any upper abdominal laparotomy or laparoscopy. Instructions and explanations are given before surgery with regard to turning and deep breathing. Pneumonia and atelectasis are possible postoperative complications that can be avoided by deep-breathing exercises and frequent turning. The patient should be informed that drainage tubes and a nasogastric tube and suction may be required during the immediate postoperative period if an open cholecystectomy is performed.

Laparoscopic Cholecystectomy. Laparoscopic cholecystectomy (Fig. 40-5) has dramatically changed the approach to the management of cholecystitis. It has become the new standard for therapy of symptomatic gallstones. The majority of people who require surgery each year for removal of the gallbladder are candidates for laparoscopic cholecystectomy (Bornman & Beckingham, 2001).

If the common bile duct is thought to be obstructed by a gallstone, an ERCP with sphincterotomy may be performed to explore the duct before laparoscopy.

Before the procedure, the patient is informed that an open abdominal procedure may be necessary, and general anesthesia is administered. Laparoscopic cholecystectomy is performed through a small incision or puncture made through the abdominal wall in the umbilicus. The abdominal cavity is insufflated with carbon dioxide (pneumoperitoneum) to assist in inserting the laparoscope and to aid the surgeon in visualizing the abdominal structures. The fibreoptic scope is inserted through the small umbilical incision. Several additional punctures or small incisions are made in the abdominal wall to introduce other surgical instruments into the operative field. The surgeon visualizes the biliary system through the laparoscope; a camera attached to the scope permits a view of the intra-abdominal field to be transmitted to a television monitor. After the cystic duct is dissected, the common bile duct is imaged by ultrasound or cholangiography to evaluate the anatomy and identify stones. The cystic artery is dissected free and clipped. The gallbladder is separated away from the hepatic bed and dissected. The gallbladder is then removed from the abdominal cavity after bile and small stones are aspirated. Stone forceps also can be used to remove or crush larger stones.

The advantage of the laparoscopic procedure is that the patient does not experience the paralytic ileus that occurs with open abdominal surgery and has less postoperative abdominal pain. The patient is often discharged from the hospital on the day of surgery or within a day or two and can resume full activity and employment within a week of the surgery.

Conversion to a traditional abdominal surgical procedure may be necessary if problems are encountered during the laparoscopic procedure; this occurs in 2% to 8% of reported surgical cases.

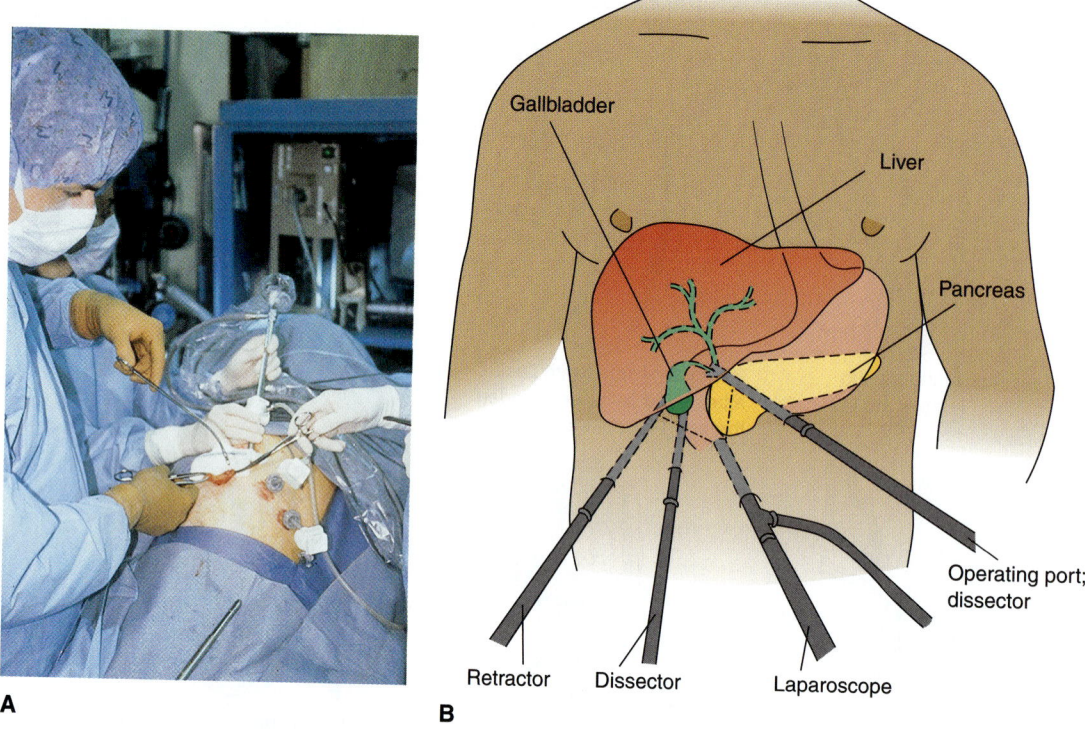

A   **B**

FIGURE 40-5 In (**A**) laparoscopic cholecystectomy, (**B**) the surgeon makes four small incisions (less than 1.12 cm each) in the abdomen and inserts a laparoscope with a miniature camera through the umbilical incision. The camera apparatus displays the gallbladder and adjacent tissues on a screen, allowing the surgeon to visualize the sections of the organ for removal.

Conversion is required more often, approximately 20% of the time, in those with acute cholecystitis (Lai et al., 1998). Careful screening of patients and identification of those at low risk for complications limits the frequency of conversion to an open abdominal procedure. With wider use of laparoscopic procedures, however, there may be an increase in the number of such conversions. The most serious complication after laparoscopic cholecystectomy is a bile duct injury.

Because of the short hospital stay, it is important to provide written as well as verbal instructions about managing postoperative pain and reporting signs and symptoms of intra-abdominal complications, including loss of appetite, vomiting, pain, distention of the abdomen, and temperature elevation. Although recovery from laparoscopic cholecystectomy is rapid, patients are drowsy afterward. The nurse must ensure that the patient has assistance at home during the first 24 to 48 hours. If pain occurs in the right shoulder or scapular area (from migration of the CO_2 used to insufflate the abdominal cavity during the procedure), the nurse may recommend use of a heating pad for 15 to 20 minutes hourly, walking, and sitting up when in bed.

Cholecystectomy. In this procedure, the gallbladder is removed through an abdominal incision (usually right subcostal) after the cystic duct and artery are ligated. The procedure is performed for acute and chronic cholecystitis. In some patients a drain may be placed close to the gallbladder bed and brought out through a puncture wound if there is a bile leak. The drain type is chosen based on the physician's preference. A small leak should close spontaneously in a few days with the drain preventing accumulation of bile. Usually only a small amount of serosanguineous fluid will drain in the initial 24 hours after surgery, and then the drain will be removed.

The drain is usually maintained if there is excess oozing or bile leakage. Use of a T-tube inserted into the common bile duct during the open procedure is now uncommon; it is used only in the setting of a complication (ie, retained common bile duct stone). Bile duct injury is a serious complication of this procedure but occurs less frequently than with the laparoscopic approach. Once one of the most common surgical procedures in Canada, this procedure has largely been replaced by laparoscopic cholecystectomy.

Mini-cholecystectomy. Mini-cholecystectomy is a surgical procedure in which the gallbladder is removed through a small incision. If needed, the surgical incision is extended to remove large gallbladder stones. Drains may or may not be used. The cost savings resulting from the shorter hospital stay have been identified as a major reason for pursuing this type of procedure. Debate exists about this procedure because it limits exposure to all the involved biliary structures.

Choledochostomy. Choledochostomy involves an incision into the common duct, usually for removal of stones. After the stones have been evacuated, a tube usually is inserted into the duct for drainage of bile until edema subsides. This tube is connected to gravity drainage tubing. The gallbladder also contains stones, and as a rule a cholecystectomy is performed at the same time.

Surgical Cholecystostomy. Cholecystostomy is performed when the patient's condition prevents more extensive surgery or when an acute inflammatory reaction is severe. The gallbladder is surgically opened, the stones and the bile or the purulent drainage are removed, and a drainage tube is secured with a purse-string suture. The drainage tube is connected to a drainage system to prevent bile from leaking around the tube or escaping into the peritoneal cavity. After recovery from the acute episode, the patient may return for cholecystectomy. Despite its lower risk, surgical cholecystostomy has a high mortality rate (reported as high as 20% to 30%) because of the underlying disease process.

Percutaneous Cholecystostomy. Percutaneous cholecystostomy has been used in the treatment and diagnosis of acute cholecystitis in patients who are poor risks for any surgical procedure or for general anesthesia. These may include patients with sepsis or severe cardiac, renal, pulmonary, or liver failure. Under local anesthesia, a fine needle is inserted through the abdominal wall and liver edge into the gallbladder under the guidance of ultrasound or computed tomography. Bile is aspirated to ensure adequate placement of the needle, and a catheter is inserted into the gallbladder to decompress the biliary tract. Almost immediate relief of pain and resolution of signs and symptoms of sepsis and cholecystitis have been reported with this procedure. Antibiotic agents are administered before, during, and after the procedure.

 Gerontologic Considerations

Surgical intervention for disease of the biliary tract is the most common operative procedure performed in the elderly. Cholesterol saturation of bile increases with age due to increased hepatic secretion of cholesterol and decreased bile acid synthesis.

Although the incidence of gallstones increases with age, the elderly patient may not exhibit the typical picture of fever, pain, chills, and jaundice. Symptoms of biliary tract disease in the elderly may be accompanied or preceded by those of septic shock, which include oliguria, hypotension, changes in mental status, tachycardia, and tachypnea.

Although surgery in the elderly presents a risk because of preexisting associated diseases, the mortality rate from serious complications from biliary tract disease itself is also high. The risk of death and complications is increased in the elderly patient who undergoes emergency surgery for life-threatening disease of the biliary tract. Despite chronic illness in many elderly patients, elective cholecystectomy is usually well tolerated and can be carried out with low risk if expert assessment and care are provided before, during, and after the surgical procedure.

Because of recent changes in the health care system, there has been a decrease in the number of elective surgical procedures performed, including cholecystectomies. As a result, patients requiring the procedure are seen in the later stages of disease. Simultaneously, patients undergoing surgery are increasingly older than 60 years of age and have complicated acute cholecystitis. The higher risk of complications and shorter hospital stays make it essential that older patients and their family members receive specific information about signs and symptoms of complications and measures to prevent them.

NURSING PROCESS: THE PATIENT UNDERGOING SURGERY FOR GALLBLADDER DISEASE

Assessment

The patient who is to undergo surgical treatment of gallbladder disease is often admitted to the hospital or same-day surgery unit on the morning of surgery. Preadmission testing is often completed a week or more before admission; at that time, the nurse instructs the patient about the need to avoid smoking to enhance pulmonary recovery postoperatively and to avoid respiratory complications. It also is important to instruct the patient to avoid the use of aspirin and other agents (over-the-counter medications and herbal remedies) that can alter coagulation and other biochemical processes.

Assessment should focus on the patient's respiratory status. If a traditional surgical approach is planned, the high abdominal incision required during surgery may interfere with full respiratory excursion. The nurse notes a history of smoking, previous respiratory problems, shallow respirations, a persistent or ineffective cough, and the presence of adventitious breath sounds. Nutritional status is evaluated through a dietary history and general examination performed at the time of preadmission testing. The nurse also reviews previously obtained laboratory results to obtain information about the patient's nutritional status.

Diagnosis
NURSING DIAGNOSES
Based on all the assessment data, the major postoperative nursing diagnoses for the patient undergoing surgery for gallbladder disease may include the following:

- Acute pain and discomfort related to surgical incision
- Impaired gas exchange related to the high abdominal surgical incision (if traditional surgical cholecystectomy is performed)
- Impaired skin integrity related to altered biliary drainage after surgical intervention (if a T-tube is inserted because of retained stones in the common bile duct or another drainage device is employed)
- Imbalanced nutrition, less than body requirements, related to inadequate bile secretion
- Deficient knowledge about self-care activities related to incision care, dietary modifications (if needed), medications, reportable signs or symptoms (eg, fever, bleeding, vomiting)

COLLABORATIVE PROBLEMS/ POTENTIAL COMPLICATIONS
Based on assessment data, potential complications may include:

- Bleeding
- Gastrointestinal symptoms (may be related to biliary leak)

Planning and Goals

The goals for the patient include relief of pain, adequate ventilation, intact skin and improved biliary drainage, optimal nutritional intake, absence of complications, and understanding of self-care routines.

Postoperative Nursing Interventions

After recovery from anesthesia, the nurse places the patient in the low Fowler's position. Intravenous fluids may be given, and nasogastric suction (a nasogastric tube was probably inserted immediately before surgery for a nonlaparoscopic procedure) may be instituted to relieve abdominal distention. Water and other fluids are given in about 24 hours, and a soft diet is started when bowel sounds return.

RELIEVING PAIN
The location of the subcostal incision in nonlaparoscopic gallbladder surgery is likely to cause the patient to avoid turning and moving, to splint the affected site, and to take shallow breaths to prevent pain. Because full aeration of the lungs and gradually increased activity are necessary to prevent postoperative complica-

tions, the nurse should administer analgesic agents as prescribed to relieve the pain and to promote well-being in addition to helping the patient turn, cough, breathe deeply, and ambulate as indicated. Use of a pillow or binder over the incision may reduce pain during these manoeuvres.

IMPROVING RESPIRATORY STATUS

Patients undergoing biliary tract surgery are especially prone to pulmonary complications, as are all patients with upper abdominal incisions. Thus, the nurse reminds patients to take deep breaths and cough every hour to expand the lungs fully and prevent atelectasis. The early and consistent use of incentive spirometry also helps improve respiratory function. Early ambulation prevents pulmonary complications as well as other complications, such as thrombophlebitis. Pulmonary complications are more likely to occur in the elderly and in obese patients.

PROMOTING SKIN CARE AND BILIARY DRAINAGE

In patients who have undergone a cholecystostomy or choledochostomy, the drainage tubes must be connected immediately to a drainage receptacle. The nurse should fasten tubing to the dressings or to the patient's gown, with enough leeway for the patient to move without dislodging or kinking it. Because a drainage system remains attached when the patient is ambulating, the drainage bag may be placed in a bathrobe pocket or fastened so that it is below the waist or common duct level. If a Penrose drain is used, the nurse changes the dressings as required.

After these surgical procedures, the patient is observed for indications of infection, leakage of bile into the peritoneal cavity, and obstruction of bile drainage. If bile is not draining properly, an obstruction is probably causing bile to be forced back into the liver and bloodstream. Because jaundice may result, the nurse should be particularly observant of the colour of the sclerae. The nurse should also note and report right upper quadrant abdominal pain, nausea and vomiting, bile drainage around any drainage tube, clay-coloured stools, and a change in vital signs.

Bile may continue to drain from the drainage tract in considerable quantities for a time, necessitating frequent changes of the outer dressings and protection of the skin from irritation because bile is corrosive to the skin.

To prevent total loss of bile, the physician may want the drainage tube or collection receptacle elevated above the level of the abdomen so that the bile drains externally only if pressure develops in the duct system. Every 24 hours, the nurse measures the bile collected and records the amount, colour, and character of the drainage. After several days of drainage, the tube may be clamped for an hour before and after each meal to deliver bile to the duodenum to aid in digestion. Within 7 to 14 days, the drainage tube is removed. The patient who goes home with a drainage tube in place requires instruction and reassurance about its function and care of the tube.

In all patients with biliary drainage, the nurse observes the stools daily and notes their colour. Specimens of both urine and stool may be sent to the laboratory for examination for bile pigments. In this way, it is possible to determine whether the bile pigment is disappearing from the blood and is draining again into the duodenum. Maintaining a careful record of fluid intake and output is important.

IMPROVING NUTRITIONAL STATUS

The nurse encourages the patient to eat a diet low in fats and high in carbohydrates and proteins immediately after surgery. At the time of hospital discharge, there are usually no special dietary instructions other than to maintain a nutritious diet and avoid excessive fats. Fat restriction usually is lifted in 4 to 6 weeks when

the biliary ducts dilate to accommodate the volume of bile once held by the gallbladder and when the ampulla of Vater again functions effectively. After this, when the patient eats fat, adequate bile will be released into the digestive tract to emulsify the fats and allow their digestion. This is in contrast to before surgery, when fats may not be digested completely or adequately, and flatulence may occur. However, one purpose of gallbladder surgery is to allow a normal diet.

MONITORING AND MANAGING POTENTIAL COMPLICATIONS

Bleeding may occur as a result of inadvertent puncture or nicking of a major blood vessel. Postoperatively, the nurse closely monitors vital signs and inspects the surgical incisions and drains, if in place, for evidence of bleeding. The nurse also periodically assesses the patient for increased tenderness and rigidity of the abdomen. If these signs and symptoms occur, they are reported to the surgeon. The nurse instructs the patient and family to report to the surgeon any change in the colour of stools because this may indicate complications. Gastrointestinal symptoms, although not common, may occur with manipulation of the intestines during surgery.

After laparoscopic cholecystectomy, the nurse assesses the patient for loss of appetite, vomiting, pain, distention of the abdomen, and temperature elevation. These may indicate infection or disruption of the gastrointestinal tract and should be reported to the surgeon promptly. Because the patient is discharged soon after laparoscopic surgery, the patient and family are instructed verbally and in writing about the importance of reporting these symptoms promptly.

PROMOTING HOME AND COMMUNITY-BASED CARE

Teaching Patients Self-Care

The nurse instructs the patient about the medications that are prescribed (vitamins, anticholinergics, and antispasmodics) and their actions. It also is important to inform the patient and family about symptoms that should be reported to the physician, including jaundice, dark urine, pale-coloured stools, pruritus, or signs of inflammation and infection, such as pain or fever.

Some patients report one to three bowel movements a day. This is the result of a continual trickle of bile through the choledochoduodenal junction after cholecystectomy. Usually, such frequency diminishes over a period of a few weeks to several months.

If a patient is discharged from the hospital with a drainage tube still in place, the patient and family may need instructions about its management. The nurse instructs them in proper care of the drainage tube and the importance of reporting to the physician promptly any changes in the amount or characteristics of drainage. Assistance in securing the appropriate dressings will reduce the patient's anxiety about going home with the drain or tube still in place. (See Chart 40-3 for more details.)

Continuing Care

With sufficient support at home, most patients recover quickly from cholecystectomy. However, elderly or frail patients and those who live alone may require a referral for home care. During home visits, the nurse assesses the patient's physical status, especially wound healing, and progress toward recovery. Assessing the patient for adequacy of pain relief and pulmonary exercises also is important. If the patient has a drainage system in place, the nurse assesses it for patency and appropriate management by the patient and family. Assessing for signs of infection and teaching the patient about the signs and symptoms of infection are also important nursing interventions. The patient's understanding of the therapeutic regimen (medications, gradual return to normal activities) is assessed, and previous teaching is reinforced. The nurse emphasizes the importance of keeping follow-up appointments and reminds the patient and family of the importance of participating in health promotion activities and recommended health screening.

Evaluation

EXPECTED PATIENT OUTCOMES

Expected patient outcomes may include:

1. Reports decrease in pain
   a. Splints abdominal incision to decrease pain
   b. Avoids foods that cause pain
   c. Uses postoperative analgesia as prescribed
2. Demonstrates appropriate respiratory function
   a. Achieves full respiratory excursion, with deep inspiration and expiration
   b. Coughs effectively, using pillow to splint abdominal incision
   c. Uses postoperative analgesia as prescribed
   d. Exercises as prescribed (eg, turns, ambulates)
3. Exhibits normal skin integrity around biliary drainage site (if applicable)
   a. Is free of fever, abdominal pain, change in vital signs, or bile, foul-smelling drainage, or pus around drainage tube
   b. Demonstrates proper management of drainage tube (if applicable)
   c. Identifies signs and symptoms of biliary obstruction to be noted and reported
   d. Has serum bilirubin level within normal range
4. Obtains relief of dietary intolerance
   a. Maintains adequate dietary intake and avoids foods that cause gastrointestinal symptoms
   b. Reports decreased or absent nausea, vomiting, diarrhea, flatulence, and abdominal discomfort
5. Absence of complications
   a. Has normal vital signs (blood pressure, pulse, respiratory rate and pattern, and temperature)

b. Reports absence of bleeding from gastrointestinal tract, biliary drainage tube/catheter (if present) and no evidence of bleeding in stool
c. Reports return of appetite and no evidence of vomiting, abdominal distention, and pain
d. Lists symptoms that should be reported to surgeon promptly and demonstrates an understanding of self-care, including wound care

Disorders of the Pancreas

Pancreatitis (inflammation of the pancreas) is a serious disorder. The most basic classification system used to describe or categorize the various stages and forms of pancreatitis divides the disorder into acute or chronic forms. Acute pancreatitis can be a medical emergency associated with a high risk for life-threatening complications and mortality, whereas chronic pancreatitis often goes undetected until 80% to 90% of the exocrine and endocrine tissue is destroyed. Acute pancreatitis does not usually lead to chronic pancreatitis unless complications develop. However, chronic pancreatitis can be characterized by acute episodes. Typically, patients are men 40 to 45 years of age with a history of alcoholism or women 50 to 55 years of age with a history of biliary disease (Hale et al., 2000).

Although the mechanisms causing pancreatic inflammation are unknown, pancreatitis is commonly described as autodigestion of the pancreas. Generally, it is believed that the pancreatic duct becomes obstructed, accompanied by hypersecretion of the exocrine enzymes of the pancreas. These enzymes enter the bile duct, where they are activated and, together with bile, back up (reflux) into the pancreatic duct, causing pancreatitis.

ACUTE PANCREATITIS

Acute pancreatitis ranges from a mild, self-limiting disorder to a severe, rapidly fatal disease that does not respond to any treatment. Mild acute pancreatitis is characterized by edema and inflammation confined to the pancreas. Minimal organ dysfunction is present, and return to normal usually occurs within 6 months. Although this is considered the milder form of pancreatitis, the patient is acutely ill and at risk for hypovolemic shock, fluid and electrolyte disturbances, and sepsis. A more widespread and complete enzymatic digestion of the gland characterizes severe acute pancreatitis. The tissue becomes necrotic, and the damage extends into the retroperitoneal tissues. Local complications consist of pancreatic cysts or abscesses and acute fluid collections in or near the pancreas. Systemic complications, such as acute respiratory distress syndrome, shock, disseminated intravascular coagulopathy, and pleural effusion, can increase the mortality rate to 50% or higher (Aronson, 1999).

Gerontologic Considerations

Acute pancreatitis affects people of all ages, but the mortality rate associated with acute pancreatitis increases with advancing age. In addition, the pattern of complications changes with age. Younger patients tend to develop local complications; the incidence of multiple organ failure increases with age, possibly as a result of progressive decreases in physiologic function of major organs with increasing age. Close monitoring of major organ function (ie, lungs, kidneys) is essential, and aggressive treatment is necessary to reduce mortality from acute pancreatitis in the elderly.

Pathophysiology

Self-digestion of the pancreas by its own proteolytic enzymes, principally trypsin, causes acute pancreatitis. Eighty percent of patients with acute pancreatitis have biliary tract disease; however, only 5% of patients with gallstones develop pancreatitis. Gallstones enter the common bile duct and lodge at the ampulla of Vater, obstructing the flow of pancreatic juice or causing a reflux of bile from the common bile duct into the pancreatic duct, thus activating the powerful enzymes within the pancreas. Normally, these remain in an inactive form until the pancreatic secretions reach the lumen of the duodenum. Activation of the enzymes can lead to vasodilation, increased vascular permeability, necrosis, erosion, and hemorrhage (Quillen, 2001).

Long-term use of alcohol is commonly associated with acute episodes of pancreatitis, but the patient usually has had undiagnosed chronic pancreatitis before the first episode of acute pancreatitis occurs. Other less common causes of pancreatitis include bacterial or viral infection, with pancreatitis a complication of mumps virus. Spasm and edema of the ampulla of Vater, resulting from duodenitis, can probably produce pancreatitis. Blunt abdominal trauma, peptic ulcer disease, ischemic vascular disease, hyperlipidemia, hypercalcemia, and the use of corticosteroids, thiazide diuretics, and oral contraceptives also have been associated with an increased incidence of pancreatitis. Acute pancreatitis may follow surgery on or near the pancreas or after instrumentation of the pancreatic duct. Acute idiopathic pancreatitis accounts for up to 20% of the cases of acute pancreatitis (Hale, Moseley & Warner, 2000). In addition, there is a small incidence of hereditary pancreatitis.

The mortality rate of patients with acute pancreatitis is high (10%) because of shock, anoxia, hypotension, or fluid and electrolyte imbalances. Attacks of acute pancreatitis may result in complete recovery, may recur without permanent damage, or may progress to chronic pancreatitis. The patient admitted to the hospital with a diagnosis of pancreatitis is acutely ill and needs expert nursing and medical care.

Severity and mortality predictions of acute alcoholic pancreatitis are generally assessed using Ranson's criteria (Tierney,

McPhee & Papadakis, 2001). The Acute Physiology and Chronic Health Evaluation (APACHE) grading system may also be used. Predictors of the severity of pancreatitis and its prognosis are listed in Chart 40-4.

Clinical Manifestations

Severe abdominal pain is the major symptom of pancreatitis that causes the patient to seek medical care. Abdominal pain and tenderness and back pain result from irritation and edema of the inflamed pancreas that stimulate the nerve endings. Increased tension on the pancreatic capsule and obstruction of the pancreatic ducts also contribute to the pain. Typically, the pain occurs in the midepigastrium. Pain is frequently acute in onset, occurring 24 to 48 hours after a very heavy meal or alcohol ingestion, and it may be diffuse and difficult to localize. It is generally more severe after meals and is unrelieved by antacids. Pain may be accompanied by abdominal distention; a poorly defined, palpable abdominal mass; and decreased peristalsis. Pain caused by pancreatitis is accompanied frequently by vomiting that does not relieve the pain or nausea.

The patient appears acutely ill. Abdominal guarding is present. A rigid or board-like abdomen may develop and is generally an ominous sign; the abdomen may remain soft in the absence of peritonitis. Ecchymosis (bruising) in the flank or around the umbilicus may indicate severe pancreatitis. Nausea and vomiting are common in acute pancreatitis. The emesis is usually gastric in origin but may also be bile-stained. Fever, jaundice, mental confusion, and agitation also may occur.

Hypotension is typical and reflects hypovolemia and shock caused by the loss of large amounts of protein-rich fluid into the tissues and peritoneal cavity. The patient may develop tachycardia, cyanosis, and cold, clammy skin in addition to hypotension. Acute renal failure is common.

Respiratory distress and hypoxia are common, and the patient may develop diffuse pulmonary infiltrates, dyspnea, tachypnea, and abnormal blood gas values. Myocardial depression, hypocalcemia, hyperglycemia, and disseminated intravascular coagulopathy (DIC) may also occur with acute pancreatitis.

Chart 40-4 — Criteria for Predicting Severity of Pancreatitis*

Criteria on Admission to Hospital

Age >55 years
WBC >16 × 10⁹/L
Serum glucose >11.1 mmol/L
Serum LDH >350 U/L
AST >120 U/L

Criteria Within 48 Hours of Hospital Admission

Fall in hematocrit >0.10
BUN increase >1.7 mmol/L
Serum calcium <2.0 mmol/L
Base deficit >4 mmol/L
Fluid retention or sequestration >6 L
PO₂ <60 mm Hg

Two or fewer signs: 1% mortality; 3 or 4 signs: 15% mortality; 5 or 6 signs: 40% mortality; >6 signs: 100% mortality.
*Note: The more risk factors a patient has, the greater the severity and the greater the likelihood of a complicated course or death.

Assessment and Diagnostic Findings

The diagnosis of acute pancreatitis is based on a history of abdominal pain, the presence of known risk factors, physical examination findings, and diagnostic findings. Serum amylase and lipase levels are used in making the diagnosis of acute pancreatitis. In 90% of the cases, serum amylase and lipase levels usually rise in excess of three times their normal upper limit within 24 hours (Tierney, McPhee & Papadakis, 2001). Serum amylase usually returns to normal within 48 to 72 hours. Serum lipase levels may remain elevated for 7 to 14 days (Braunwald et al., 2001). Urinary amylase levels also become elevated and remain elevated longer than serum amylase levels. The white blood cell count is usually elevated; hypocalcemia is present in many patients and correlates well with the severity of pancreatitis. Transient hyperglycemia and glucosuria and elevated serum bilirubin levels occur in some patients with acute pancreatitis.

X-ray studies of the abdomen and chest may be obtained to differentiate pancreatitis from other disorders that may cause similar symptoms and to detect pleural effusions. Ultrasound and contrast-enhanced computed tomography scans are used to identify an increase in the diameter of the pancreas and to detect pancreatic cysts, abscesses, or pseudocysts.

Hematocrit and hemoglobin levels are used to monitor the patient for bleeding. Peritoneal fluid, obtained through paracentesis or peritoneal lavage, may contain increased levels of pancreatic enzymes. The stools of patients with pancreatic disease are often bulky, pale, and foul-smelling. Fat content of stools varies between 50% and 90% in pancreatic disease; normally, the fat content is 20%. ERCP is rarely used in the diagnostic evaluation of acute pancreatitis because the patient is acutely ill; however, it may be valuable in the treatment of gallstone pancreatitis.

Medical Management

Management of the patient with acute pancreatitis is directed toward relieving symptoms and preventing or treating complications. All oral intake is withheld to inhibit pancreatic stimulation and secretion of pancreatic enzymes. Parenteral nutrition is usually an important part of therapy, particularly in debilitated patients, because of the extreme metabolic stress associated with acute pancreatitis (Dejong, Greve & Soeters, 2001). Nasogastric suction may be used to relieve nausea and vomiting, to decrease painful abdominal distention and paralytic ileus, and to remove hydrochloric acid so that it does not enter the duodenum and stimulate the pancreas. Histamine-2 (H_2) antagonists (eg, cimetidine [Tagamet] and ranitidine [Zantac]) may be prescribed to decrease pancreatic activity by inhibiting HCl secretion.

PAIN MANAGEMENT

Adequate pain medication is essential during the course of acute pancreatitis to provide sufficient pain relief and minimize restlessness, which may stimulate pancreatic secretion further. Morphine and morphine derivatives are often avoided because it has been thought that they cause spasm of the sphincter of Oddi; meperidine (Demerol) is often prescribed because it is less likely to cause spasm of the sphincter (Porth, 2002). Antiemetic agents may be prescribed to prevent vomiting.

INTENSIVE CARE

Correction of fluid and blood loss and low albumin levels is necessary to maintain fluid volume and prevent renal failure. The patient is usually acutely ill and is monitored in the intensive care unit, where hemodynamic monitoring and arterial blood gas monitoring are initiated. Antibiotic agents may be prescribed if infection is present; insulin may be required if significant hyperglycemia occurs.

RESPIRATORY CARE

Aggressive respiratory care is indicated because of the high risk for elevation of the diaphragm, pulmonary infiltrates and effusion, and atelectasis. Hypoxemia occurs in a significant number of patients with acute pancreatitis even with normal x-ray findings. Respiratory care may range from close monitoring of arterial blood gases to use of humidified oxygen to intubation and mechanical ventilation (see Chap. 25 for further discussion).

BILIARY DRAINAGE

Placement of biliary drains (for external drainage) and stents (indwelling tubes) in the pancreatic duct through endoscopy has been performed to reestablish drainage of the pancreas. This has resulted in decreased pain and increased weight gain.

SURGICAL INTERVENTION

Although often risky because the acutely ill patient is a poor surgical risk, surgery may be performed to assist in the diagnosis of pancreatitis (diagnostic laparotomy), to establish pancreatic drainage, or to resect or débride a necrotic pancreas. The patient who undergoes pancreatic surgery may have multiple drains in place postoperatively as well as a surgical incision that is left open for irrigation and repacking every 2 to 3 days to remove necrotic debris (Fig. 40-6).

FIGURE 40-6 Multiple sump tubes are used after pancreatic surgery. Triple-lumen tubes consist of ports that provide tubing for irrigation, air venting, and drainage.

POSTACUTE MANAGEMENT

Antacids may be used when acute pancreatitis begins to resolve. Oral feedings low in fat and protein are initiated gradually. Caffeine and alcohol are eliminated from the diet. If the episode of pancreatitis occurred during treatment with thiazide diuretics, corticosteroids, or oral contraceptives, these medications are discontinued. Follow-up of the patient may include ultrasound, x-ray studies, or ERCP to determine whether the pancreatitis is resolving and to assess for abscesses and pseudocysts. ERCP may also be used to identify the cause of acute pancreatitis if it is in question and for endoscopic sphincterotomy and removal of gallstones from the common bile duct.

NURSING PROCESS:
THE PATIENT WITH ACUTE PANCREATITIS

Assessment

The health history focuses on the presence and character of the abdominal pain and discomfort. The nurse assesses the presence of pain, its location, its relationship to eating and to alcohol consumption, and the effectiveness of pain relief measures. It also is important to assess the patient's nutritional and fluid status and history of gallbladder attacks and alcohol use. A history of gastrointestinal problems, including nausea, vomiting, diarrhea, and passage of fatty stools, is elicited. The nurse assesses the abdomen for pain, tenderness, guarding, and bowel sounds, noting the presence of a board-like or soft abdomen. It also is important to assess respiratory status, respiratory rate and pattern, and breath sounds. Normal and adventitious breath sounds and abnormal findings on chest percussion, including dullness at the bases of the lungs and abnormal tactile fremitus, are documented. The nurse assesses the emotional and psychological status of the patient and family and their coping, because they are often anxious about the severity of the symptoms and the acuity of illness.

Diagnosis

NURSING DIAGNOSES

Based on all the assessment data, the major nursing diagnoses of the patient with acute pancreatitis include the following:

- Acute pain related to inflammation, edema, distention of the pancreas, and peritoneal irritation
- Ineffective breathing pattern related to severe pain, pulmonary infiltrates, pleural effusion, atelectasis, and elevated diaphragm
- Imbalanced nutrition, less than body requirements, related to reduced food intake and increased metabolic demands
- Impaired skin integrity related to poor nutritional status, bed rest, and multiple drains and surgical wound

COLLABORATIVE PROBLEMS/
POTENTIAL COMPLICATIONS

Based on assessment data, potential complications that may occur include the following:

- Fluid and electrolyte disturbances
- Necrosis of the pancreas
- Shock and multiple organ dysfunction

Planning and Goals

The major goals for the patient include relief of pain and discomfort, improved respiratory function, improved nutritional status, maintenance of skin integrity, and absence of complications.

Nursing Interventions

RELIEVING PAIN AND DISCOMFORT

Because the pathologic process responsible for pain is autodigestion of the pancreas, the objectives of therapy are to relieve pain and decrease secretion of the enzymes of the pancreas. The pain of acute pancreatitis is often very severe, necessitating the liberal use of analgesic agents. Meperidine (Demerol) is the medication of choice; morphine sulfate is avoided because it causes spasm of the sphincter of Oddi (Porth, 2002). Oral feedings are withheld to decrease the formation and secretion of secretin. The patient is maintained on parenteral fluids and electrolytes to restore and maintain fluid balance. Nasogastric suction is used to remove gastric secretions and to relieve abdominal distention. The nurse provides frequent oral hygiene and care to decrease discomfort from the nasogastric tube and relieve dryness of the mouth.

The acutely ill patient is maintained on bed rest to decrease the metabolic rate and reduce the secretion of pancreatic and gastric enzymes. If the patient experiences increasing severity of pain, the nurse reports this to the physician because the patient may be experiencing hemorrhage of the pancreas, or the dose of analgesic may be inadequate.

The patient with acute pancreatitis often has a clouded sensorium because of severe pain, fluid and electrolyte disturbances, and hypoxia. Therefore, the nurse provides frequent and repeated but simple explanations about the need for withholding fluid intake and about maintenance of gastric suction and bed rest.

IMPROVING BREATHING PATTERN

The nurse maintains the patient in a semi-Fowler's position to decrease pressure on the diaphragm by a distended abdomen and to increase respiratory expansion. Frequent changes of position are necessary to prevent atelectasis and pooling of respiratory secretions. Pulmonary assessment and monitoring of pulse oximetry or arterial blood gases are essential to detect changes in respiratory status so that early treatment can be initiated. The nurse instructs the patient in techniques of coughing and deep breathing to improve respiratory function and encourages and assists the patient to cough and deep breathe every 2 hours.

IMPROVING NUTRITIONAL STATUS

The patient with acute pancreatitis is not permitted food and oral fluid intake; however, it is important to assess the patient's nutritional status and to note factors that alter the patient's nutritional requirements (eg, temperature elevation, surgery, drainage). Laboratory test results and daily weights are useful in monitoring the nutritional status.

Parenteral nutrition may be prescribed. In addition to administering parenteral nutrition, the nurse monitors serum glucose levels every 4 to 6 hours. As the acute symptoms subside, the nurse gradually reintroduces oral feedings. Between acute attacks, the patient receives a diet high in carbohydrates and low in fat and proteins. The patient should avoid heavy meals and alcoholic beverages.

IMPROVING SKIN INTEGRITY

The patient is at risk for skin breakdown because of poor nutritional status, enforced bed rest, and restlessness, which may result in pressure ulcers and breaks in tissue integrity. In addition, the patient who has undergone surgery, has had multiple drains inserted, or has an open surgical incision is at risk for skin breakdown and infection. The nurse carefully assesses the wound, drainage sites, and skin for signs of infection, inflammation, and breakdown. The nurse carries out wound care as prescribed and takes precautions to protect intact skin from contact with drainage. Consultation with an enterostomal therapist is often helpful in identifying appropriate skin care devices and protocols. It is important to turn the patient every 2 hours; use of specialty beds may be indicated to prevent skin breakdown.

MONITORING AND MANAGING POTENTIAL COMPLICATIONS

Fluid and electrolyte disturbances are common complications because of nausea, vomiting, movement of fluid from the vascular compartment to the peritoneal cavity, diaphoresis, fever, and the use of gastric suction. The nurse assesses the patient's fluid and electrolyte status by noting skin turgor and moistness of mucous membranes. The nurse weighs the patient daily and carefully measures fluid intake and output, including urine output, nasogastric secretions, and diarrhea. In addition, it is important to assess the patient for other factors that may affect fluid and electrolyte status, including increased body temperature and wound drainage. The nurse assesses the patient for ascites and measures abdominal girth daily if ascites is suspected.

Intravenous fluids are administered and may be accompanied by infusion of blood, blood products, and albumin to maintain the blood volume and to prevent or treat hypovolemic shock. It is important to keep emergency medications readily available because of the risk of circulatory collapse and shock. The nurse promptly reports decreased blood pressure and reduced urine output because they may indicate hypovolemia and shock or renal failure. Low serum calcium and magnesium levels may occur and require prompt treatment.

Pancreatic necrosis is a major cause of morbidity and mortality in patients with acute pancreatitis. The patient who develops necrosis is at risk for hemorrhage, septic shock, and multiple organ failure. The patient may undergo diagnostic procedures to confirm pancreatic necrosis; surgical débridement or insertion of multiple drains may be performed. The patient with pancreatic necrosis is usually critically ill and requires expert medical and nursing management, including hemodynamic monitoring in the intensive care unit.

In addition to carefully monitoring vital signs and other signs and symptoms, the nurse is responsible for administering prescribed fluids, medications, and blood products; assisting with supportive management, such as use of a ventilator; preventing additional complications; and attending to the patient's physical and psychological care.

Shock and multiple organ failure may occur with acute pancreatitis. Hypovolemic shock may occur as a result of hypovolemia and sequestering of fluid in the peritoneal cavity. Hemorrhagic shock may occur with hemorrhagic pancreatitis. Septic shock may occur with bacterial infection of the pancreas. Cardiac dysfunction may occur as a result of fluid and electrolyte disturbances, acid–base imbalances, and release of toxic substances into the circulation.

The nurse closely monitors the patient for early signs of neurologic, cardiovascular, renal, and respiratory dysfunction. The nurse must be prepared to respond quickly to rapid changes in the patient's status, treatments, and therapies. In addition, it is important to inform the family about the status and progress of the patient and allow them to spend time with the patient. (Management of the patient in shock is discussed in detail in Chap. 15.)

PROMOTING HOME AND COMMUNITY-BASED CARE

Teaching Patients Self-Care

The patient who has survived an episode of acute pancreatitis has been acutely ill. A prolonged period is needed to regain strength and return to previous level of activity. The patient is often still weak and debilitated weeks or months after an acute episode of pancreatitis. Because of the severity of the acute illness, the patient may not recall many of the explanations and instructions given during the acute phase, so these often need to be repeated and reinforced. The nurse instructs the patient about the factors implicated in the onset of acute pancreatitis and about the need to avoid high-fat foods, heavy meals, and alcohol. It is important to give the patient and family verbal and written instructions about signs and symptoms of acute pancreatitis and possible complications that should be reported promptly to the physician.

If acute pancreatitis is a result of biliary tract disease, such as gallstones and gallbladder disease, additional explanations are needed about required dietary modifications. If the pancreatitis is a result of alcohol abuse, the nurse reminds the patient of the importance of eliminating all alcohol.

Continuing Care

A referral for home care often is indicated; this enables the nurse to assess the patient's physical and psychological status and adherence to the therapeutic regimen. The nurse also assesses the home situation and reinforces instructions about fluid and nutrition intake and avoidance of alcohol.

When the acute attack has subsided, some patients may be inclined to return to their previous drinking habits. The nurse provides specific information about resources and support groups that may be of assistance in avoiding alcohol in the future. Referral to Alcoholics Anonymous or other appropriate support groups is essential. A summary of nursing management of the patient with acute pancreatitis is provided in the Plan of Nursing Care.

Evaluation

EXPECTED PATIENT OUTCOMES

Expected patient outcomes may include:

1. Reports relief of pain and discomfort
   a. Uses analgesics and anticholinergics as prescribed, without overuse
   b. Maintains bed rest as prescribed
   c. Avoids alcohol to decrease abdominal pain
2. Experiences improved respiratory function
   a. Changes position in bed frequently
   b. Coughs and takes deep breaths at least every hour
   c. Demonstrates normal respiratory rate and pattern, full lung expansion, normal breath sounds
   d. Demonstrates normal body temperature and absence of respiratory infection
3. Achieves nutritional and fluid and electrolyte balance
   a. Reports decrease in number of episodes of diarrhea
   b. Identifies and consumes high-carbohydrate, low-protein foods
   c. Explains rationale for eliminating alcohol intake
   d. Maintains adequate fluid intake within prescribed guidelines
   e. Exhibits adequate urine output

(text continues on page 1148)

Plan of Nursing Care
Care of the Patient With Acute Pancreatitis

Nursing Interventions	Rationale	Expected Outcomes

Nursing Diagnosis: Acute pain and discomfort related to edema, distention of the pancreas, and peritoneal irritation

Goal: Relief of pain and discomfort

Nursing Interventions	Rationale	Expected Outcomes
1. Administer meperidine (Demerol) frequently, as prescribed, to achieve level of pain acceptable to patient based on patient's level of pain and discomfort.	1. Meperidine acts by depressing the central nervous system and thereby increasing the patient's pain threshold. Morphine is avoided because it produces spasm of the sphincter of Oddi.	• Reports relief of pain • Moves and turns without increasing pain and discomfort • Rests comfortably and sleeps for increasing periods • Reports less frequent episodes of pain, discomfort, and cramping • Experiences enhanced pain relief • Reports increased feelings of well-being and security with the health care team
2. Using a pain scale, assess pain level before and after administration of analgesic.	2. Assessment and control of pain are important because restlessness increases body metabolism, which stimulates the secretion of pancreatic and gastric enzymes.	
3. Report unrelieved pain or increasing intensity of pain.	3. Pain may increase pancreatic enzymes and may also indicate pancreatic hemorrhage.	
4. Assist the patient to assume positions of comfort; turn and reposition every 2 hours.	4. Frequent turning relieves pressure and assists in preventing pulmonary and vascular complications.	
5. Use nonpharmacologic interventions for relieving pain (eg, relaxation, focused breathing, diversion).	5. Use of nonpharmacologic methods will enhance the effects of analgesics. Gate control theory states that cutaneous stimulation closes the pain pathways.	
6. Listen to patient's expression of pain experience.	6. Demonstration of caring can help to decrease anxiety.	

Goal: Relief of pain related to stimulation of the pancreas

Nursing Interventions	Rationale	Expected Outcomes
1. Administer anticholinergic medications as prescribed.	1. Anticholinergic medications reduce gastric and pancreatic secretion.	• Reports relief of pain, discomfort, and abdominal cramping • Consumes no fluid and food during acute phase • Maintains bed rest • Identifies rationale for fluid and dietary restrictions and use of nasogastric drainage • Cooperates with insertion of nasogastric tube and suction
2. Withhold oral intake.	2. Pancreatic secretion is increased by food and fluid intake.	
3. Maintain the patient on bed rest.	3. Bed rest decreases body metabolism and thus reduces pancreatic and gastric secretions.	
4. Maintain continuous nasogastric drainage. a. Measure gastric secretions at specified intervals. b. Observe and record colour and viscosity of gastric secretions. c. Ensure that the nasogastric tube is patent to permit free drainage.	4. Nasogastric suction removes gastric contents and prevents gastric secretions from entering the duodenum and stimulating the secretin mechanism. Decompression of the intestines (if intestinal intubation is used) also assists in relieving respiratory distress.	

Nursing Diagnosis: Discomfort related to nasogastric tube

Goal: Relief of discomfort associated with nasogastric intubation

Nursing Interventions	Rationale	Expected Outcomes
1. Use water-soluble lubricant around external nares.	1. Prevents irritation of nares	• Exhibits intact skin and tissue of nares at site of nasogastric tube insertion • Reports no pain or irritation of nares or oropharynx • Exhibits moist, clean mucous membranes of mouth and nasopharynx • States that thirst is relieved by oral hygiene • Identifies rationale for nasogastric tube and suction
2. Turn patient at intervals; avoid pressure or tension on nasogastric tube	2. Relieves pressure of tube on esophageal and gastric mucosa	
3. Provide oral hygiene and gargling solutions without alcohol.	3. Relieves dryness and irritation of oropharynx	
4. Explain rationale for use of nasogastric drainage.	4. Assists patient to cooperate with the drainage, nasogastric tube, and suction.	

(continued)

Plan of Nursing Care
Care of the Patient With Acute Pancreatitis (Continued)

Nursing Interventions	Rationale	Expected Outcomes

Nursing Diagnosis: Imbalanced nutrition: less than body requirements related to inadequate dietary intake, impaired pancreatic secretions, increased nutritional needs secondary to acute illness, and increased body temperature

Goal: Improvement in nutritional status

Nursing Interventions	Rationale	Expected Outcomes
1. Assess current nutritional status and increased metabolic requirements.	1. Alteration in pancreatic secretions interferes with normal digestive processes. Acute illness, infection, and fever increase metabolic needs.	• Maintains normal body weight • Demonstrates no additional weight loss • Maintains normal serum glucose levels • Reports decreasing episodes of vomiting and diarrhea
2. Monitor serum glucose levels and administer insulin as prescribed.	2. Impairment of endocrine function of the pancreas leads to increased serum glucose levels.	• Reports return of normal stool characteristics and bowel pattern • Consumes foods high in carbohydrate, low in fat and protein
3. Administer intravenous fluid and electrolytes and parenteral nutrition as prescribed.	3. Parenteral administration of fluids, electrolytes, and nutrients is essential to provide fluids, calories, electrolytes, and nutrients when oral intake is prohibited.	• Explains rationale for high-carbohydrate, low-fat, low-protein diet • Eliminates alcohol from diet
4. Provide high-carbohydrate, low-protein, low-fat diet when tolerated.	4. These foods increase caloric intake without stimulating pancreatic secretions beyond the ability of the pancreas to respond.	• Explains rationale for limiting coffee intake and avoiding spicy foods • Participates in Alcoholics Anonymous or other counselling approach • Returns to and maintains desirable weight
5. Instruct patient to eliminate alcohol and refer to Alcoholics Anonymous if indicated. 6. Counsel patient to avoid excessive use of coffee and spicy foods. 7. Monitor daily weights.	5. Alcohol intake produces further damage to pancreas and precipitates attacks of acute pancreatitis. 6. Coffee and spicy foods increase pancreatic and gastric secretions. 7. This provides a baseline and a means to measure desirable weight.	

Nursing Diagnosis: Ineffective breathing pattern related to splinting from severe pain, pulmonary infiltrates, pleural effusion, and atelectasis

Goal: Improvement in respiratory function

Nursing Interventions	Rationale	Expected Outcomes
1. Assess respiratory status (rate, pattern, breath sounds), pulse oximetry, and arterial blood gases.	1. Acute pancreatitis produces retroperitoneal edema, elevation of the diaphragm, pleural effusion, and inadequate lung ventilation. Intra-abdominal infection and laboured breathing increase the body's metabolic demands, which further decreases pulmonary reserve and leads to respiratory failure.	• Demonstrates normal respiratory rate and pattern and full lung expansion • Demonstrates normal breath sounds and absence of adventitious breath sounds • Demonstrates normal arterial blood gases and pulse oximetry • Maintains semi-Fowler's position when in bed
2. Maintain semi-Fowler's position. 3. Instruct and encourage patient to take deep breaths and to cough every hour. 4. Assist patient to turn and change position every 2 hours.	2. Decreases pressure on diaphragm and allows greater lung expansion. 3. Taking deep breaths and coughing will clear the airways and reduce atelectasis. 4. Changing position frequently assists aeration and drainage of all lobes of the lungs.	• Changes position in bed frequently • Coughs and takes deep breaths at least every hour • Demonstrates normal body temperature • Exhibits no signs or symptoms of respiratory infection or impairment • Is alert and responsive to environment
5. Reduce the excessive metabolism of the body. a. Administer antibiotics as prescribed. b. Place patient in an air-conditioned room. c. Administer nasal oxygen as required for hypoxia. d. Use a hypothermia blanket if necessary.	5. Pancreatitis produces a severe peritoneal and retroperitoneal reaction that causes fever, tachycardia, and accelerated respirations. Placing the patient in an air-conditioned room and supporting the patient with oxygen therapy decrease the workload of the respiratory system and the tissue utilization of oxygen. Reduction of fever and pulse rate decreases the metabolic demands on the body.	

(continued)

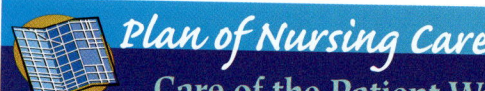

Plan of Nursing Care
Care of the Patient With Acute Pancreatitis *(Continued)*

Nursing Interventions	Rationale	Expected Outcomes
Collaborative Problem: Fluid and electrolyte disturbances, hypovolemia, shock		
Goal: Improvement in fluid and electrolyte status, prevention of hypovolemia and shock		
1. Assess fluid and electrolyte status (skin turgor, mucous membranes, urine output, vital signs, hemodynamic parameters).	1. The amount and type of fluid and electrolyte replacement are determined by the status of the blood pressure, the laboratory evaluations of serum electrolyte and blood urea nitrogen levels, the urinary volume, and the assessment of the patient's condition.	• Exhibits moist mucous membranes and normal skin turgor • Exhibits normal blood pressure without evidence of postural (orthostatic) hypotension • Excretes adequate urine volume • Exhibits normal, not excessive, thirst • Maintains normal pulse and respiratory rate • Remains alert and responsive • Exhibits normal arterial pressures and blood gases • Exhibits normal electrolyte levels • Exhibits no signs or symptoms of calcium deficit (eg, tetany, carpopedal spasm) • Exhibits no additional losses of fluids and electrolytes through vomiting, diarrhea, or diaphoresis • Reports stabilization of weight • Demonstrates no increase in abdominal girth • Demonstrates no fluid wave on palpation of the abdomen • Demonstrates stable organ function without manifestations of failure
2. Assess sources of fluid and electrolyte loss (vomiting, diarrhea, nasogastric drainage, excessive diaphoresis).	2. Electrolyte losses occur from nasogastric suctioning, severe diaphoresis, emesis, and as a result of the patient's being in a fasting state.	

3. Combat shock if present.
  a. Administer corticosteroids as prescribed if patient does not respond to conventional treatment.
  b. Evaluate the amount of urinary output. Attempt to maintain this at 50 mL/h.
	3. Extensive acute pancreatitis may cause peripheral vascular collapse and shock. Blood and plasma may be lost into the abdominal cavity, and, therefore, there is a decreased blood and plasma volume. The toxins from the bacteria of a necrotic pancreas may cause shock.	

4. Administer blood products, fluids, and electrolytes (sodium, potassium, chloride) as prescribed.	4. Patients with hemorrhagic pancreatitis lose large amounts of blood and plasma, which decreases effective circulation and blood volume.	
5. Administer plasma, albumin, and blood products as prescribed.	5. Replacement with blood, plasma or albumin assists in ensuring effective circulating blood volume.	
6. Keep a supply of intravenous calcium gluconate readily available.	6. Calcium may be prescribed to prevent or treat tetany.	

7. Assess abdomen for ascites formation:
  a. Measure abdominal girth daily.
  b. Weigh patient daily.
  c. Palpate abdomen for fluid wave.
	7. During acute pancreatitis, plasma may be lost into the abdominal cavity, which diminishes the blood volume.	

8. Monitor for manifestations of multiple organ failure: neurologic, cardiovascular, renal, and respiratory dysfunction.	8. All body systems may fail if pancreatitis is severe and treatment is ineffective.	

4. Exhibits intact skin
   a. Skin is without breakdown or infection
   b. Drainage is contained adequately
5. Absence of complications
   a. Demonstrates normal skin turgor, moist mucous membranes, normal serum electrolyte levels
   b. Exhibits stabilization of weight, with no increase in abdominal girth
   c. Exhibits normal neurologic, cardiovascular, renal, and respiratory function

CHRONIC PANCREATITIS

Chronic pancreatitis is an inflammatory disorder characterized by progressive anatomic and functional destruction of the pancreas. As cells are replaced by fibrous tissue with repeated attacks of pancreatitis, pressure within the pancreas increases. The end result is mechanical obstruction of the pancreatic and common bile ducts and the duodenum. Additionally, there is atrophy of the epithelium of the ducts, inflammation, and destruction of the secreting cells of the pancreas.

Alcohol consumption in Western societies and malnutrition worldwide are the major causes of chronic pancreatitis. Excessive and prolonged consumption of alcohol accounts for approximately 70% of the cases (Clain & Pearson, 1999). The incidence of pancreatitis is 50 times greater in alcoholics than in the nondrinking population. Long-term alcohol consumption causes hypersecretion of protein in pancreatic secretions, resulting in protein plugs and calculi within the pancreatic ducts. Alcohol also has a direct toxic effect on the cells of the pancreas. Damage to these cells is more likely to occur and to be more severe in patients whose diets are poor in protein content and either very high or very low in fat.

Clinical Manifestations

Chronic pancreatitis is characterized by recurring attacks of severe upper abdominal and back pain, accompanied by vomiting. Attacks are often so painful that opioids, even in large doses, do not provide relief. As the disease progresses, recurring attacks of pain are more severe, more frequent, and of longer duration. Some patients experience continuous severe pain; others have a dull, nagging constant pain. The risk of dependence on opioids is increased in pancreatitis because of the chronic nature and severity of the pain.

Weight loss is a major problem in chronic pancreatitis: more than 75% of patients experience significant weight loss, usually caused by decreased dietary intake secondary to anorexia or fear that eating will precipitate another attack. Malabsorption occurs late in the disease, when as little as 10% of pancreatic function remains. As a result, digestion, especially of proteins and fats, is impaired. The stools become frequent, frothy, and foul-smelling because of impaired fat digestion, which results in stools with a high fat content. This is referred to as **steatorrhea**. As the disease progresses, calcification of the gland may occur, and calcium stones may form within the ducts.

Assessment and Diagnostic Findings

ERCP is the most useful study in the diagnosis of chronic pancreatitis. It provides detail about the anatomy of the pancreas and the pancreatic and biliary ducts. It is also helpful in obtaining tissue for analysis and differentiating pancreatitis from other conditions, such as carcinoma. Various imaging procedures, including magnetic resonance imaging, computed tomography, and ultrasound, have been useful in the diagnostic evaluation of patients with suspected pancreatic disorders. Computed tomography scanning or ultrasound is helpful to detect pancreatic cysts.

A glucose tolerance test evaluates pancreatic islet cell function, information necessary for making decisions about surgical resection of the pancreas. An abnormal glucose tolerance test indicative of diabetes may be present. In contrast to the patient with acute pancreatitis, serum amylase levels and the white blood cell count may not be elevated significantly.

Medical Management

The management of chronic pancreatitis depends on its probable cause in each patient. Treatment is directed toward preventing and managing acute attacks, relieving pain and discomfort, and managing exocrine and endocrine insufficiency of pancreatitis.

NONSURGICAL MANAGEMENT

Nonsurgical approaches may be indicated for the patient who refuses surgery, who is a poor surgical risk, or whose disease and symptoms do not warrant surgical intervention. Endoscopy to remove pancreatic duct stones and stent strictures may be effective in selected patients to manage pain and relieve obstruction. However, such therapy is available only in special centres and is suitable for few patients (Bornman & Beckingham, 2001).

Management of abdominal pain and discomfort is similar to that of acute pancreatitis; however, the focus is usually on the use of nonopioid methods to manage pain. Persistent, unrelieved pain is often the most difficult aspect of management (Bornman & Beckingham, 2001). The physician, nurse, and dietitian emphasize to the patient and family the importance of avoiding alcohol and other foods that the patient has found tend to produce abdominal pain and discomfort. The fact that no other treatment is likely to relieve pain if the patient continues to consume alcohol is stressed to the patient.

Diabetes mellitus resulting from dysfunction of the pancreatic islet cells is treated with diet, insulin, or oral antidiabetic agents.

The hazard of severe hypoglycemia with alcohol use is stressed to the patient and family. Pancreatic enzyme replacement is indicated in the patient with malabsorption and steatorrhea (Trolli, Conwell & Zuccaro, 2001).

SURGICAL MANAGEMENT

Surgery is generally carried out to relieve abdominal pain and discomfort, restore drainage of pancreatic secretions, and reduce the frequency of acute attacks of pancreatitis. The surgery performed depends on the anatomic and functional abnormalities of the pancreas, including the location of disease within the pancreas, diabetes, exocrine insufficiency, biliary stenosis, and pseudocysts of the pancreas. Other factors taken into consideration in determining whether surgery is to be performed and what procedure is indicated include the patient's continued use of alcohol and the likelihood that the patient will be able to manage the endocrine or exocrine changes that are expected after surgery.

Pancreaticojejunostomy (also referred to as Roux-en-Y) with a side-to-side anastomosis or joining of the pancreatic duct to the jejunum allows drainage of the pancreatic secretions into the jejunum. Pain relief occurs by 6 months in more than 80% of the patients who undergo this procedure, but pain returns in a substantial number of patients as the disease itself progresses (Tierney et al., 2001).

Other surgical procedures may be performed for different degrees and types of disease, ranging from revision of the sphincter of the ampulla of Vater, to internal drainage of a pancreatic cyst into the stomach (see Pancreatic Cyst discussion), to insertion of a stent, to wide resection or removal of the pancreas. A Whipple resection (pancreaticoduodenectomy) has been carried out to relieve the pain of chronic pancreatitis.

Autotransplantation or implantation of the patient's pancreatic islet cells has been attempted to preserve the endocrine function of the pancreas in patients who have undergone total pancreatectomy. Testing and refinement of this procedure continue in an effort to improve outcomes.

When chronic pancreatitis develops as a result of gallbladder disease, the obstruction is treated by surgery to explore the common duct and remove the stones; usually, the gallbladder is removed at the same time. In addition, an attempt is made to improve the drainage of the common bile duct and the pancreatic duct by dividing the sphincter of Oddi, a muscle that is located at the ampulla of Vater (this surgical procedure is known as a sphincterotomy). A T-tube usually is placed in the common bile duct, requiring a drainage system to collect the bile postoperatively. Nursing care after such surgery is similar to that indicated after other biliary tract surgery.

Patients who undergo surgery for chronic pancreatitis may experience weight gain and improved nutritional status; this may result from reduction in pain associated with eating rather than from correction of malabsorption. However, morbidity and mortality after these surgical procedures are high because of the poor physical condition of the patient before surgery and the concomitant occurrence of cirrhosis. Even after undergoing these surgical procedures, the patient is likely to continue to have pain and impaired digestion secondary to pancreatitis unless alcohol is avoided completely.

PANCREATIC CYSTS

As a result of the local necrosis that occurs at the time of acute pancreatitis, collections of fluid may form in the vicinity of the pancreas. These become walled off by fibrous tissue and are called pancreatic pseudocysts. They are the most common type of pancreatic cysts. Less common cysts occur as a result of congenital anomalies or are secondary to chronic pancreatitis or trauma to the pancreas.

Diagnosis of pancreatic cysts and pseudocysts is made by ultrasound, computed tomography, and ERCP. ERCP may be used to define the anatomy of the pancreas and evaluate the patency of pancreatic drainage. Pancreatic pseudocysts may be of considerable size. Because of their location behind the posterior peritoneum, when they enlarge they impinge on and displace the stomach or the colon, which are adjacent. Eventually, through pressure or secondary infection, they produce symptoms and require drainage.

Drainage into the gastrointestinal tract or through the skin and abdominal wall may be established. In the latter instance, the drainage is likely to be profuse and destructive to tissue because of the enzyme contents. Hence, steps must be taken to protect the skin near the drainage site from excoriation. Ointments protect the skin if they are applied before excoriation takes place. Another method involves the constant aspiration of digestive secretions from the drainage tract by means of a suction apparatus, so that skin contact with the digestive enzymes is avoided. This method requires expert nursing attention to ensure that the suction tube does not become dislodged and suction is not interrupted. Consultation with an enterostomal therapist is indicated to identify appropriate strategies to maintain drainage and protect the skin.

CANCER OF THE PANCREAS

The incidence of pancreatic cancer has decreased slightly over the past 25 years in non-Caucasian men. It accounts for approximately 3300 deaths annually in Canada and occurs most frequently in the fifth to seventh decades of life (Canadian Cancer Society, 2005). Cigarette smoking, exposure to industrial chemicals or toxins in the environment, and a diet high in fat, meat, or both are associated with pancreatic cancer, although their role is not completely clear. The risk for pancreatic cancer increases as the extent of cigarette smoking increases. Diabetes mellitus, chronic pancreatitis, and hereditary pancreatitis are also associated with pancreatic cancer. The pancreas can also be the site of metastasis from other tumours.

Cancer may arise in any portion of the pancreas (in the head, the body, or the tail); clinical manifestations vary depending on the location of the lesion and whether functioning, insulin-secreting pancreatic islet cells are involved. Approximately 75% of pancreatic cancers originate in the head of the pancreas and give rise to a distinctive clinical picture. Functioning islet cell tumours, whether benign (adenoma) or malignant (carcinoma), are responsible for the syndrome of hyperinsulinism. With these exceptions, the symptoms are nonspecific, and patients usually do not seek medical attention until late in the disease; 80% to 85% of patients have advanced, unresectable tumour when first detected. In fact, pancreatic carcinoma has only a 2% to 5% survival rate at 5 years regardless of the stage of disease at diagnosis or treatment (Tierney et al., 2001).

Clinical Manifestations

Pain, jaundice, or both are present in more than 90% of patients and, along with weight loss, are considered classic signs of pancreatic carcinoma. However, they often do not appear until the disease is far advanced. Other signs include rapid, profound, and progressive weight loss as well as vague upper or midabdominal pain or discomfort that is unrelated to any gastrointestinal function and is often difficult to describe. Such discomfort radiates as a boring pain in the midback and is unrelated to posture or activity. It is often progressive and severe, requiring the use of opioids. It is often more severe at night. Relief may be obtained by sitting up and leaning forward, or accentuated when lying supine.

Malignant cells from pancreatic cancer are often shed into the peritoneal cavity, increasing the likelihood of metastasis. The formation of ascites is common. An important sign, when present, is the onset of symptoms of insulin deficiency: glucosuria, hyperglycemia, and abnormal glucose tolerance. Thus, diabetes may be an early sign of carcinoma of the pancreas. Meals often aggravate epigastric pain, which usually occurs before the appearance of jaundice and pruritus.

Assessment and Diagnostic Findings

Magnetic resonance imaging and computed tomography are used to identify the presence of pancreatic tumours. ERCP is also used in the diagnosis of pancreatic carcinoma. Cells obtained during ERCP are sent to the laboratory for examination. Gastrointestinal x-ray findings may demonstrate deformities in adjacent viscera caused by the impinging pancreatic mass.

Percutaneous fine-needle aspiration biopsy of the pancreas is used to diagnose pancreatic tumours and confirm the diagnosis in patients whose tumours are not resectable, eliminating the stress and postoperative pain of ineffective surgery. In this procedure, a needle is inserted through the anterior abdominal wall into the pancreatic mass, guided by computed tomography, ultrasound, ERCP, or other imaging techniques. The aspirated material is examined for malignant cells. Although percutaneous biopsy is a valuable diagnostic tool, it has some potential drawbacks: a false-negative result if small tumours are missed and seeding of cancer cells along the needle track. Low-dose radiation to the site may be used before the biopsy to reduce the risk of seeding.

Percutaneous transhepatic cholangiography is another procedure that may be performed to identify obstructions of the biliary tract by a pancreatic tumour. Several tumour markers (eg, CA 19-9, CEA, DU-PAN-2) may be used in the diagnostic workup, but they are nonspecific for pancreatic carcinoma. These tumour markers are useful as indicators of disease progression.

Angiography, computed tomography, and laparoscopy may be performed to determine whether the tumour can be removed surgically. Intraoperative ultrasonography has been used to determine if there is metastatic disease to other organs.

Medical Management

If the tumour is resectable and localized (typically tumours in the head of the pancreas), the surgical procedure to remove it is usually extensive (see Medical Management in Tumours of the Head of the Pancreas). However, definitive surgical treatment (ie, total excision of the lesion) is often not possible because of the extensive growth when the tumour is finally diagnosed and because of the probable widespread metastases (especially to the liver, lungs, and bones). More often, treatment is limited to palliative measures.

Although pancreatic tumours may be resistant to standard radiation therapy, the patient may be treated with radiation and chemotherapy (fluorouracil and gemcitabine). If the patient undergoes surgery, intraoperative radiation therapy (IORT) may be used to deliver a high dose of radiation to the tumour with minimal injury to other tissues. IORT may also be helpful in relief of pain. Interstitial implantation of radioactive sources has also been used, although the rate of complications is high. A large biliary stent inserted percutaneously or by endoscopy may be used to relieve jaundice.

Nursing Management

Pain management and attention to nutritional requirements are important nursing measures to improve the level of comfort. Skin care and nursing measures are directed toward relief of pain and discomfort associated with jaundice, anorexia, and profound weight loss. Specialty mattresses are beneficial and protect bony prominences from pressure. Pain associated with pancreatic cancer may be severe and may require liberal use of opioids; patient-controlled analgesia should be considered for the patient with severe, escalating pain.

Because of the poor prognosis and likelihood of short survival, end-of-life preferences are discussed and honoured. If appropriate, the nurse refers the patient to hospice care. (See Chaps. 16 and 17, respectively, for discussion of care of the patient with cancer and end-of-life care.)

PROMOTING HOME AND COMMUNITY-BASED CARE

Teaching Patients Self-Care. The specific patient and family teaching indicated varies with the stage of disease and the treatment choices made by the patient. If the patient elects to receive chemotherapy, the nurse focuses teaching on prevention of side effects and complications of the agents used. If surgery is performed to relieve obstruction and establish biliary drainage, teaching addresses management of the drainage system and monitoring for complications. The nurse instructs the family about changes in the patient's status that should be reported to the physician.

Continuing Care. A referral for home care is indicated to help the patient and family deal with the physical problems and discomforts associated with pancreatic cancer and the psychological impact of the disease. The home care nurse assesses the patient's physical status, fluid and nutritional status, and skin integrity and the adequacy of pain management. The nurse teaches the patient and family strategies to prevent skin breakdown and relieve pain, pruritus, and anorexia. It is important to discuss and arrange palliative care (hospice services) in an effort to relieve patient discomfort, assist with care, and comply with the patient's end-of-life decisions and wishes.

TUMOURS OF THE HEAD OF THE PANCREAS

Sixty to eighty percent of pancreatic tumours occur in the head of the pancreas. Tumours in this region of the pancreas obstruct the common bile duct where the duct passes through the head of the pancreas to join the pancreatic duct and empty at the ampulla of Vater into the duodenum. The tumours producing the obstruction may arise from the pancreas, the common bile duct, or the ampulla of Vater.

Clinical Manifestations

The obstructed flow of bile produces jaundice, clay-coloured stools, and dark urine. Malabsorption of nutrients and fat-soluble vitamins may result from obstruction by the tumour to entry of bile in the gastrointestinal tract. Abdominal discomfort or pain

and pruritus may be noted, along with anorexia, weight loss, and malaise. If these signs and symptoms are present, cancer of the head of the pancreas is suspected.

The jaundice of this disease must be differentiated from that due to a biliary obstruction caused by a gallstone in the common duct, which is usually intermittent and appears typically in obese patients, most often women, who have had previous symptoms of gallbladder disease.

Assessment and Diagnostic Findings

Diagnostic studies may include duodenography, angiography by hepatic or celiac artery catheterization, pancreatic scanning, percutaneous transhepatic cholangiography, ERCP, and percutaneous needle biopsy of the pancreas. Results of a biopsy of the pancreas may aid in the diagnosis.

Medical Management

Before extensive surgery can be performed, a fairly long period of preparation is often necessary because the patient's nutritional and physical condition is often quite compromised. Various liver and pancreatic function studies are performed. A diet high in protein along with pancreatic enzymes is often prescribed. Preoperative preparation includes adequate hydration, correction of prothrombin deficiency with vitamin K, and treatment of anemia to minimize postoperative complications. Parenteral nutrition and blood component therapy are frequently required.

A biliary-enteric shunt may be performed to relieve the jaundice and, perhaps, to provide time for a thorough diagnostic evaluation. Total pancreatectomy (removal of the pancreas) may be performed if there is no evidence of direct extension of the tumour to adjacent tissues or regional lymph nodes. A pancreaticoduodenectomy (Whipple's procedure or resection) is used for potentially resectable cancer of the head of the pancreas (Fig. 40-7). This procedure involves removal of the gallbladder, distal portion of the stomach, duodenum, head of the pancreas, and common bile duct and anastomosis of the remaining pancreas and stomach to the jejunum (Stanford, 2001). The result is removal of the tumour, allowing flow of bile into the jejunum. When the tumour cannot be excised, the jaundice may be relieved by diverting the bile flow into the jejunum by anastomosing the jejunum to the gallbladder, a procedure known as **cholecystojejunostomy**.

The postoperative management of patients who have undergone a pancreatectomy or a pancreaticoduodenectomy is similar to the management of patients after extensive gastrointestinal and biliary surgery. The patient's physical status is often less than optimal, increasing the risk for postoperative complications. Hemorrhage, vascular collapse, and hepatorenal failure remain the major complications of these extensive surgical procedures. The mortality rate after these procedures has improved because of advances in nutritional support and improved surgical techniques. A nasogastric tube and suction and parenteral nutrition allow the gastrointestinal tract to rest while promoting adequate nutrition.

Nursing Management

Preoperatively and postoperatively, nursing care is directed toward promoting patient comfort, preventing complications, and assisting the patient to return to and maintain as normal and comfortable a life as possible. The nurse closely monitors the patient in the intensive care unit after surgery; the patient will have

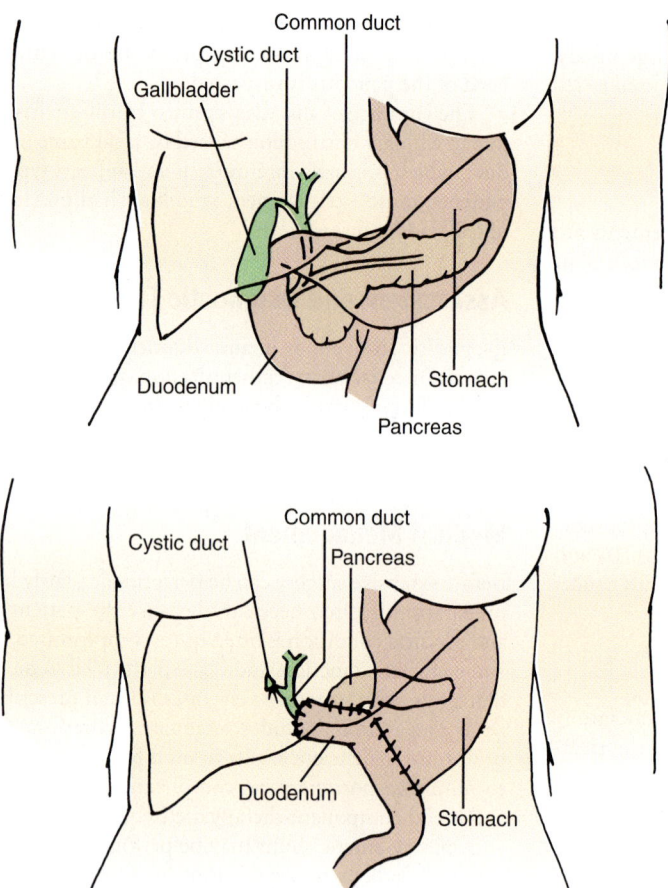

Common duct
Cystic duct
Gallbladder
Duodenum
Stomach
Pancreas

Cystic duct
Common duct
Pancreas
Duodenum
Stomach

FIGURE 40-7 Pancreatoduodenectomy (Whipple's procedure or resection). End result of the resection of the carcinoma of the head of the pancreas or the ampulla of Vater. The common duct is sutured to the end of the jejunum, and the remaining portion of the pancreas and the end of the stomach are sutured to the side of the jejunum.

multiple intravenous and arterial lines in place for fluid and blood replacement as well as for monitoring arterial pressures, and is on a mechanical ventilator in the immediate postoperative period. It is important to give careful attention to changes in vital signs, arterial blood gases and pressures, pulse oximetry, laboratory values, and urine output. The nurse must also consider the patient's compromised nutritional status and risk for bleeding. Depending on the type of surgical procedure performed, malabsorption syndrome and diabetes mellitus are likely; the nurse must address these issues during acute and long-term patient care.

Although the patient's physiologic status is the focus of the health care team in the immediate postoperative period, the patient's psychological and emotional state must be considered, along with that of the family. The patient has undergone major and risky surgery and is critically ill; thus, anxiety and depression may affect recovery. The immediate and long-term outcome of this extensive surgical resection is uncertain, and the patient and family require emotional support and understanding in the critical and stressful preoperative and postoperative periods.

PROMOTING HOME AND COMMUNITY-BASED CARE

Teaching Patients Self-Care. The patient who has undergone this extensive surgery requires careful and thorough preparation for self-care at home. The nurse instructs the patient and family about the need for modifications in the diet because of malabsorption and hyperglycemia resulting from the surgery. It is important to instruct them about the continuing need for pancreatic enzyme replacement, a low-fat diet, and vitamin supplementation.

The nurse teaches the patient and family strategies to relieve pain and discomfort, along with strategies to manage drains, if present, and to care for the surgical incision. The patient and family members may require instruction about use of patient-controlled analgesia, parenteral nutrition, wound care, skin care, and management of drainage. It is important to describe, verbally and in writing, the signs and symptoms of complications, and to teach the patient and family about indicators of complications that should be reported promptly.

Discharge of the patient to a long-term care setting may be warranted after surgery as extensive as pancreatectomy or pancreaticoduodenectomy, particularly if the patient's preoperative status was not optimal. Efforts are made to communicate to the long-term care staff about the teaching that has been provided so that instructions can be clarified and reinforced. During the recovery or long-term phase of care, the patient and family receive further instructions about care that they will carry out at home.

Continuing Care. A referral for home care may be indicated when the patient returns home. The home care nurse assesses the patient's physical and psychological status and the ability of the patient and family to manage needed care. The home care nurse provides needed physical care and monitors the adequacy of pain management. In addition, it is important to assess the patient's nutritional status and monitor the use of parenteral nutrition. The nurse discusses the use of hospice services with the patient and family and makes a referral if indicated.

PANCREATIC ISLET TUMOURS

The pancreas contains the islets (islands) of Langerhans, small nests of cells that secrete directly into the bloodstream and therefore are part of the endocrine system. The hormone insulin is essential for the metabolism of glucose. Diabetes mellitus (see Chap. 41) is the result of deficient secretion of insulin.

At least two types of tumours of the pancreatic islet cells are known: those that secrete insulin (insulinoma) and those in which insulin secretion is not increased ("nonfunctioning" islet cell cancer). Insulinomas produce hypersecretion of insulin and cause an excessive rate of glucose metabolism. The resulting hypoglycemia may produce symptoms of weakness, mental confusion, and seizures. These symptoms may be relieved almost immediately by oral or intravenous administration of glucose. The 5-hour glucose tolerance test is helpful in diagnosing insulinoma and in distinguishing it from other causes of hypoglycemia.

Surgical Management

When a tumour of the islet cells has been diagnosed, surgical treatment with removal of the tumour usually is recommended. The tumours may be benign adenomas or they may be malignant. Complete removal usually results in almost immediate relief of symptoms. In some patients, symptoms may be produced by simple hypertrophy of this tissue rather than a tumour of the islet cells. In such cases, a partial pancreatectomy (removal of the tail and part of the body of the pancreas) is performed.

Nursing Management

In preparing the patient for surgery, the nurse must be alert for symptoms of hypoglycemia and be ready to administer glucose as prescribed if symptoms occur. Postoperatively, the nursing management is the same as that after other upper abdominal surgical procedures, with special emphasis on monitoring serum glucose levels. Patient teaching is determined by the extent of surgery and the alterations in pancreatic function that result.

HYPERINSULINISM

Hyperinsulinism results from overproduction of insulin by the pancreatic islets. Symptoms resemble those of excessive doses of insulin and are attributable to the same mechanism, an abnormal reduction in blood glucose levels. Clinically, it is characterized by episodes during which the patient experiences unusual hunger, nervousness, sweating, headache, and faintness; in severe cases, seizures and episodes of unconsciousness may occur. The findings at the time of surgery or at autopsy may indicate hyperplasia (overgrowth) of the islets of Langerhans or a benign or malignant tumour involving the islets and capable of producing large amounts of insulin (see preceding discussion). Occasionally, tumours of nonpancreatic origin produce an insulin-like material that can cause severe hypoglycemia that may be responsible for seizures coinciding with blood glucose levels too low to sustain normal brain function (ie, below 1.6 mmol/L).

All the symptoms that accompany spontaneous hypoglycemia are relieved by the oral or parenteral administration of glucose. Surgical removal of the hyperplastic or neoplastic tissue from the pancreas is the only successful method of treatment. About 15% of patients with spontaneous or functional hypoglycemia eventually develop diabetes mellitus.

ULCEROGENIC TUMOURS

Some tumours of the islets of Langerhans are associated with hypersecretion of gastric acid that produces ulcers in the stomach, duodenum, and jejunum. The result is referred to as **Zollinger-Ellison syndrome**. The hypersecretion is so great that even after partial gastric resection, enough acid is produced to cause further ulceration. When a marked tendency to develop gastric and duodenal ulcers is noted, an ulcerogenic tumour of the islets of Langerhans is considered.

These tumours, which may be benign or malignant, are treated, when possible, by excision. Frequently, however, because of extension beyond the pancreas, removal is not possible. In many patients, a total gastrectomy may be necessary to reduce the secretion of gastric acid sufficiently to prevent further ulceration.

Critical Thinking Exercises

1. A 48-year-old woman is scheduled for a laparoscopic cholecystectomy. What postoperative care is indicated for this patient? What factors would you consider in preparing her for discharge? How would your care differ if she lived alone? How would you modify teaching for her if she understood little English?

2. A 73-year-old man presents to the emergency department with an oral temperature of 38° C, nausea, vomiting of bile, and abdominal distention. He reports mild upper abdominal pain but is not a good historian due to a new onset of mild confusion and lethargy. His sclerae are slightly icteric, blood pressure is 88/50, and heart rate 116 per minute and regular. His primary physician reports fluctuating mild abnormalities in liver function studies over the past 6 months. Considering gerontologic changes in the hepatobiliary system, what diagnostic tests and medical and nursing interventions do you anticipate?

3. A 57-year-old man has a history of alcoholism and cirrhosis. He is admitted to your unit with a diagnosis of acute pancreatitis. He is complaining of severe epigastric pain, vomiting, and diarrhea. What medications and laboratory tests would you expect to see prescribed for this patient? What physical assessment findings will you see? Describe nursing care for this patient, and compare and contrast care with and without the diagnosis of cirrhosis.

4. A 69-year-old woman is being discharged to home with a diagnosis of advanced cancer of the pancreas. She has had a biliary drain inserted to relieve obstruction. What teaching about management of the drainage system is needed for the patient and her family? How would you modify your discharge plans for her if she lives alone and has no family support available?

REFERENCES AND SELECTED READINGS

Books

Canadian Cancer Society/National Cancer Institute of Canada. (2005). *Canadian cancer statistics 2005*. Toronto: Canada.

Blumgart, L. H., & Fong, Y. (Eds). (2000). *Surgery of the liver and biliary tract* (3rd ed.). London: W. B. Saunders Co. Ltd.

Braunwald, E., Fauci, A. S., Kasper, D. L., et al. (Eds.). (2001). *Harrison's principles of internal medicine* (15th ed.). New York: McGraw-Hill.

Dudek, S. (2001) *Nutrition essentials for nursing practice.* Philadelphia: Lippincott Williams & Wilkins.

Evans, S. R. T., & Ascher, S. M. (Eds.) (1998). *Hepatobiliary and pancreatic surgery.* New York: Wiley-Liss.

Feldman, M., Friedman, L. S., & Sleisenger, M. H. (Eds.). (2002). *Sleisenger & Fordtran's gastrointestinal and liver disease: pathophysiology, diagnosis, and management.* Philadelphia: W. B. Saunders.

Grenvik, A., Ayres, S. M., Holbrook, P. R., & Shoemaker, W. C. (Eds.). (2000). *Textbook of critical care* (4th ed.). Philadelphia: W. B. Saunders.

Kacsoh, B. (2000). *Endocrine physiology.* New York: McGraw-Hill.

Porth, C. M. (2002). *Pathophysiology: Concepts of altered health states* (6th ed.). Philadelphia: Lippincott Williams & Wilkins.

Rakel, R. E., & Bope, E. T. (Eds.). (2001). *Conn's current therapy.* Philadelphia: W. B. Saunders.

Schiff, E. R., Sorrell, M. F., & Maddrey, W. C. (1999). *Schiff's diseases of the liver* (8th ed.). Philadelphia: Lippincott-Raven.

Schwartz, S. I. (Ed.) (1999). *Principles of surgery* (7th ed.). New York: McGraw-Hill.

Tierney, L. M., McPhee, S. J., & Papadakis, M. A. (Eds.). (2001). *Current medical diagnosis and treatment.* New York: Lange Medical Books/McGraw-Hill.

Van Leeuwen, D. J., Reeders, W. A. J., & Ariyama, J. (Eds.). (2000). *Imaging in hepatobiliary and pancreatic disease.* London: W. B. Saunders Co. Ltd.

Wolfe, M. M. (2000). *Therapy of digestive disorders.* Philadelphia: W. B. Saunders.

Wu, G. Y., & Israel, J. (Eds.). (1998). *Diseases of the liver and bile ducts.* Totowa, NJ: Humana Press.

Journals

Asterisks indicate nursing research articles.

General

Barish, M. A., Yucel, E. K., & Ferrucci, J. T. (1999). Magnetic resonance cholangiopancreatography. *New England Journal of Medicine, 341*(4), 258–264.

Kalloo, A. N., & Kantsevoy, S. V. (2001). Gallstones and biliary diseases. *Primary Care Clinics in Office Practice, 28*(3), 591–606.

Gallbladder Disease

Ahmed, A., Cheung, R. C., & Keefe, E. B. (2000). Management of gallstones and their complications. *American Family Physician, 61*(6), 1673–1688.

Borzellino, G., deManzoni, G., & Ricci, F., et al. (1999). Emergency cholecystostomy and subsequent cholecystectomy for acute gallstone cholecystitis in the elderly. *British Journal of Surgery, 86*(12), 1521–1525.

Bowser, L., & Schutz, S. M. (2000). The role of surveillance ERCP in preventing episodic cholangitis in patients with recurrent bile duct stones. *Gastrointestinal Endoscopy, 51*(2), 118–121.

De Groen, P. C., Gores, G. J., LaRusso, N. F., et al. (1999). Biliary tract cancers. *New England Journal of Medicine, 341*(18), 1368–1378.

Donovan, J. M. (1999). Physical and metabolic factors in gallstone pathogenesis. *Gastroenterology Clinics of North America, 28*(1), 75–97.

Farrar, J. A. (2001). Acute cholecystitis. *American Journal of Nursing, 101*(1), 35–36.

Kowdley, K. V. (2000). Ursodeoxycholic acid therapy in hepatobiliary disease. *American Journal of Medicine, 108*(6), 481–486.

Lai, P. B. S., Kwong, K. H., & Leung, K. L., et al. (1998). Randomized trial of early versus delayed laparoscopic cholecystectomy for acute cholecystitis. *British Journal of Surgery, 85*(6), 764–767.

Lauter, D. M., & Froines, E. J. (2000). Laparoscopic common duct exploration in the management of choledocholithiasis. *American Journal of Surgery, 179*(5), 372–374.

Lee, L., & Yee, J. (2000). Diagnostic dilemma. *American Journal of Medicine, 108*(6), 503, 511.

Memon, M., Hassaballa, H., & Memon, M. (2000). Laparoscopic common bile duct exploration: The past, the present, and the future. *American Journal of Surgery, 179*(4), 309–315.

Shaffer, E. A. (2000). Morphine and biliary pain revisited. *Gut, 46*(6), 750–751.

Siddiqui, M. N. (1999). Laparoscopic management of complicated gallstone disease. *British Journal of Surgery, 86*(11), 1481–1482.

Strasberg, S. M. (1999). Laparoscopic biliary surgery. *Gastroenterology Clinics of North America, 28*(1), 117–132.

Pancreatic Disorders

Aronson, B. S. (1999). Update on acute pancreatitis. *MedSurg Nursing, 8*(1), 9–16.

Berger, H. G., & Isenmann, R. (1999). Surgical management of necrotizing pancreatitis. *Surgical Clinics of North America, 79*(4), 783–799.

Bornman, P. C., & Beckingham, I. J. (2001). ABC of diseases of liver, pancreas, and biliary system. Chronic pancreatitis. *British Medical Journal, 322*(7287), 660–663.

Clain, J. E., & Pearson, R. K. (1999). Diagnosis of chronic pancreatitis. *Surgical Clinics of North America, 79*(4), 829–843.

Dejong, C. H., Greve, J. W. & Soeters, P. B. (2001). Nutrition in patients with acute pancreatitis. *Current Opinion in Critical Care, 7*(4), 251–256.

Hale, A. S., Moseley, M. J., & Warner, S. C. (2000). Treating pancreatitis in the acute care setting. *Dimensions of Critical Care Nursing, 19*(4), 16–21.

Johnson, F. M. G. (2001). Alterations in taste sensation: A case presentation of a patient with end-stage pancreatic cancer. *Cancer Nursing, 24*(2), 149–155.

Lankish, P. G. (1999). Progression from acute to chronic pancreatitis: A physician's view. *Surgical Clinics of North America, 79*(4), 815–824.

Munoz, A., & Katerndahl, D. A. (2000). Diagnosis and management of acute pancreatitis. *American Family Physician, 62*(1), 164–174, 39–42, 244.

Pennachio, D. L. (2002). The latest approaches to pancreatic disease. *Patient Care for the Nurse Practitioner, 4*(9), 41–44, 47–48.

Quillen, S. M. (2001). Identification of pancreatitis in the ambulatory setting. *Gastroenterology Nursing, 24*(1), 20–22.

Sakorafas, G. H., Farnell, M. B., Nagorney, D. M., & Sarr, M. G. (2001). Surgical management of chronic pancreatitis at the Mayo Clinic. *Surgical Clinics of North America, 81*(2), 457–465.

Schlapman, N. (2001). Spotting acute pancreatitis. *RN, 64*(11), 55–58.

Stanford, P. (2001). Surgical approaches to pancreatic cancer. *Nursing Clinics of North America, 36*(3), 567–577.

*Trolli, P. A., Conwell, D. L., & Zuccaro, G. Jr. (2001). Pancreatic enzyme therapy and nutritional status of outpatients with chronic pancreatitis. *Gastroenterology Nursing, 24*(2), 84–87.

RESOURCES AND WEBSITES

Canadian Cancer Society/Société Canadienne du Cancer, National Office, Suite 200, 10 Alcorn Avenue, Toronto, ON M4V 3B1; (416) 961-7223; fax: (416) 961-4189; www.cancer.ca.

Canadian Digestive Health Foundation; http://cdhf.ca.

Canadian Gastroenterological Association; http://www.cag-acg.org.

National Cancer Institute of Canada/Institut National du Cancer du Canada, Suite 200, 10 Alcorn Avenue, Toronto, ON M4V 3B1; (416) 961-7223; fax: (416) 961-4189; www.ncic.cancer.ca.

National Digestive Diseases Information Clearing House, 2 Information Way, Bethesda, MD 20892-3570; (301) 654-3810; http://www.niddk.nih.gov.

National Endocrine Society, 4350 East West Highway, Suite 500, Bethesda, MD 20814; (301) 941-0200; http://www.endo-society.org.

National Pancreas Foundation, P.O. Box 15333, Boston, MA 02215; http://www.pancreasfoundation.org.

Assessment and Management of Patients With Diabetes Mellitus

Adapted by Lorraine Watson

On completion of this chapter, the learner will be able to:

1. Differentiate between type 1 and type 2 diabetes.
2. Describe etiologic factors associated with diabetes.
3. Relate the clinical manifestations of diabetes to the associated pathophysiologic alterations.
4. Identify the diagnostic and clinical significance of blood glucose tests.
5. Explain the dietary modifications used for management of people with diabetes.
6. Describe the relationship between diet, exercise, and medication (ie, insulin or oral hypoglycemic agents) for people with diabetes.
7. Develop a plan for teaching insulin self-administration.
8. Identify the role of oral antidiabetic agents in diabetic therapy.
9. Differentiate between hypoglycemia and diabetic ketoacidosis, and hyperosmolar nonketotic syndrome.
10. Describe management strategies for a person with diabetes to use during "sick days."
11. Describe the major macrovascular, microvascular, and neuropathic complications of diabetes and the self-care behaviours important in their prevention.
12. Identify the teaching aids and community support groups available for people with diabetes.
13. Use the nursing process as a framework for care of the patient with diabetes.

Diabetes is a condition in which the body either cannot produce insulin or cannot effectively use the insulin it produces (Canadian Diabetes Association, 2003). **Diabetes mellitus** is a group of metabolic diseases characterized by elevated levels of glucose in the blood (**hyperglycemia**) (American Diabetes Association [ADA], Expert Committee on the Diagnosis and Classification of Diabetes Mellitus, 2003). Normally a certain amount of glucose circulates in the blood. The major sources of this glucose are absorption of ingested food in the gastrointestinal (GI) tract and formation of glucose by the liver from food substances.

Insulin, a hormone produced by the pancreas, controls the level of glucose in the blood by regulating the production and storage of glucose. In the diabetic state, the cells may stop responding to insulin or the pancreas may stop producing insulin entirely. This leads to hyperglycemia, which may result in acute metabolic complications such as **diabetic ketoacidosis** (DKA) and **hyperglycemic hyperosmolar nonketotic syndrome** (HHNS). Long-term effects of hyperglycemia contribute to macrovascular complications (coronary artery disease, cerebrovascular disease, and peripheral vascular disease), chronic microvascular complications (kidney and eye disease), and neuropathic complications (diseases of the nerves).

More than 2 million Canadians have been diagnosed with some type of diabetes mellitus. It is suspected that about 2.7% of the general adult population may have undiagnosed type 2 diabetes. By the end of this decade it is estimated that the number of individuals diagnosed with diabetes will reach 3 million. Approximately 10% of the population who have been diagnosed with diabetes have type 1; the remaining 90% have type 2. A third classification, gestational diabetes mellitus, occurs in approximately 3.5% to 3.8% of non-Aboriginal populations and 8.0% to 18.0% of Aboriginal populations for all pregnancies. Aboriginal people are three to five times more likely to develop type 2 diabetes than the general population. Canadians who are of Hispanic, Asian, South Asian, or African descent have a greater risk of developing type 2 diabetes. There is an increase in the incidence of type 2 diabetes occurring in children from high-risk groups; risk factors include ethnicity or the presence of obesity (Canadian Diabetes Association, 2003). Chart 41-1 summarizes other risk factors of diabetes mellitus.

The far-reaching and devastating physical, social, and economic consequences of diabetes are as follows:

- Diabetes is a leading cause of nontraumatic amputations, blindness among working-age adults, and end-stage renal disease.
- There is a high rate of cardiovascular disease (myocardial infarction, stroke, and peripheral vascular disease) among people with diabetes.
- In Canada, diabetes is the seventh leading cause of death with a rate of 17/100,000 (Statistics Canada, 1997)

Glossary

alpha glucosidase inhibitor: a category of oral agents used to treat type 2 diabetes that delay the absorption of carbohydrate, resulting in lower postprandial blood glucose levels

continuous subcutaneous insulin infusion: a small device that delivers insulin on a 24-hour basis as basal insulin; it is also programmed by the patient to deliver a bolus dose before eating a meal in an attempt to mimic normal pancreatic function

diabetes mellitus: a group of metabolic diseases characterized by hyperglycemia resulting from defects in insulin secretion, insulin action, or both

diabetic ketoacidosis (DKA): a metabolic derangement in type 1 diabetes that results from a deficiency of insulin. Highly acidic ketone bodies are formed, resulting in acidosis; usually requires hospitalization for treatment and is usually caused by nonadherence to the insulin regimen, concurrent illness, or infection.

fasting plasma glucose (FPG): blood glucose determination obtained in the laboratory after fasting for more than 8 hours. Although plasma levels are specified in diagnostic criteria, blood glucose levels, which are slightly higher than plasma levels, are more commonly used.

glycosylated hemoglobin (hemoglobin A$_{1c}$): a long-term measure of glucose control that is a result of glucose attaching to hemoglobin for the life of the red blood cell (120 days). The goal of diabetes therapy is a normal to near-normal level of glycosy-lated hemoglobin (referred to as HgbA$_{1C}$ or A1C), the same as in the nondiabetic population.

hyperglycemia: elevated blood glucose level—fasting level greater than 6.1 mmol/L; 2-hour postprandial level greater than 7.8 mmol/L

hyperglycemic hyperosmolar nonketotic syndrome (HHNS): a metabolic disorder of type 2 diabetes resulting from a relative insulin deficiency initiated by an intercurrent illness that raises the demand for insulin; associated with polyuria and severe dehydration

hypoglycemia: low blood glucose level less than 2.7 mmol/L

insulin: a hormone secreted by the beta cells of the islets of Langerhans of the pancreas that is necessary for the metabolism of carbohydrates, proteins, and fats; a deficiency of insulin results in diabetes mellitus

impaired fasting glucose (IFG), impaired glucose tolerance (IGT): a metabolic stage intermediate between normal glucose homeostasis and diabetes; not clinical entities in their own right but risk factors for future diabetes and cardiovascular disease

islet cell transplant: an investigational procedure in which purified islet cells from cadaver donors are injected into the portal vein of the liver, with the goal of having these cells secrete insulin and cure type 1 diabetes.

ketone: a highly acidic substance formed when the liver breaks down free fatty acids in the absence of insulin. The result is diabetic ketoacidosis.

nephropathy: a long-term complication of diabetes in which the kidney cells are damaged; characterized by microalbuminuria in early stages and progressing to end-stage renal disease

neuropathy: a long-term complication of diabetes resulting from damage to the nerve cell.

retinopathy: a long-term complication of diabetes in which the microvascular system of the eye is damaged

self-monitoring of blood glucose (SMBG): a method of capillary blood glucose testing in which the patient pricks his/her finger and applies a drop of blood to a test strip that is read by a meter

sulfonylurea: a classification of oral anti-diabetic medication for treating type 2 diabetes; enhances insulin secretion and insulin action

thiazolidinedione: a class of oral anti-diabetic medications that reduce insulin resistance in target tissues, enhancing insulin action without directly stimulating insulin secretion

type 1 diabetes: a metabolic disorder characterized by an absence of insulin production and secretion from autoimmune destruction of the beta cells of the islets of Langerhans in the pancreas. Formerly called insulin-dependent, juvenile or type I diabetes.

type 2 diabetes: a metabolic disorder characterized by the relative deficiency of insulin production and a decreased insulin action and increased insulin resistance. Formerly called non-insulin-dependent, adult-onset, or type II diabetes.

Chart 41-1
Risk Factors for Diabetes Mellitus

Family history (ie, parents or siblings with diabetes)
Membership in a high-risk group (Aboriginal, Hispanic, Asian, South Asian, or African descent)
Excess weight, especially around the waist
Hypertension
Elevated lipid or cholesterol levels
Gestational diabetes – gave birth to a baby over 4 kilograms at birth
Polycystic ovary syndrome, acanthosis nigricans, schizophrenia
Age over 40 years
Impaired glucose tolerance or fasting glucose levels
Presence of heart disease, kidney disease, eye disease, impotence, or nerve damage
Poor or slow wound healing

(Canadian Diabetes Association, 2003)

• Hospitalization rates for people with diabetes are 2.4 times greater for adults and 5.3 times greater for children than for the general population.
• Canadian data indicate that diabetes can shorten life span by an average of 13 years (Manuel & Schultz, 2003).

The economic cost of diabetes continues to rise because of increasing health care costs and an aging population. Half of all people who have diabetes and who are older than 65 are hospitalized each year, and severe and life-threatening complications often contribute to the increased rates of hospitalization. Costs related to diabetes are estimated to be almost $13.2 billion annually, including direct medical care expenses and indirect costs attributable to disability and premature death (Canadian Diabetes Association, 2005).

The primary goals of treatment for patients with diabetes include maintaining blood glucose levels within normal range and preventing acute and long-term complications. Thus, the nurse who cares for diabetic patients must work with them to develop self-care management skills.

Classification of Diabetes

There are several different types of diabetes mellitus; they may differ in cause, clinical course, and treatment. The major classifications of diabetes are:

• **Type 1 diabetes**—marked by immune-mediated destruction of pancreatic beta cells; insulin dependent
• **Type 2 diabetes**—may range from predominantly insulin resistance with some insulin deficiency to a predominantly insulin secretory defect with insulin resistance; may be preventable
• Gestational diabetes mellitus—glucose intolerance with first onset or recognition occurring during pregnancy
• Diabetes associated with other conditions or syndromes

(Canadian Diabetes Association, 2005)

OVERVIEW

The terms "insulin-dependent diabetes" and "non-insulin-dependent diabetes" and their acronyms (IDDM and NIDDM, respectively) are no longer used because they have resulted in classification of patients on the basis of the treatment of their diabetes rather than the underlying etiology. Use of Roman numerals (type I and type II) to distinguish between the two types has been changed to type 1 and type 2 to reduce confusion (ADA, Expert Committee on the Diagnosis and Classification of Diabetes Mellitus, 2003).

Approximately 10% of people with diabetes have type 1 diabetes, in which the insulin-producing pancreatic beta cells are destroyed by an autoimmune process. As a result, they produce little or no insulin and require insulin injections to control their blood glucose levels. Type 1 diabetes is characterized by an acute onset, usually before age 30 (Canadian Diabetes Association, 2005).

Approximately 90% of people with diabetes have type 2 diabetes (Canadian Diabetes Association, 2005), which results from decreased sensitivity to insulin (called insulin resistance) and impaired beta cell functioning resulting in decreased insulin production. Type 2 diabetes is first treated with diet and exercise. If elevated glucose levels persist, diet and exercise are supplemented with oral hypoglycemic agents. In some individuals with type 2 diabetes, oral agents do not control hyperglycemia, and insulin injections are required. In addition, some individuals whose type 2 diabetes can usually be controlled with diet, exercise, and oral agents may require insulin injections during periods of acute physiologic stress (eg, illness or surgery). The development of type 2 diabetes is insidious and it usually develops in people older than 30 years who have increased amounts of visceral fat.

Diabetes complications may develop in any person with type 1 or type 2 diabetes, not only in patients who take insulin. Some patients with type 2 diabetes who are treated with oral medications may have the impression that they do not *really* have diabetes or that they simply have "borderline" diabetes. They may believe that, compared with diabetic patients who require insulin injections, their diabetes is not a serious problem. It is important for the nurse to emphasize to these individuals that they *do* have diabetes and not a borderline problem with sugar (glucose). Borderline diabetes is classified as **impaired glucose tolerance (IGT)** or **impaired fasting glucose (IFG)** and refers to a condition in which blood glucose levels fall between normal levels and levels considered diagnostic for diabetes.

Table 41-1 summarizes the major classifications of diabetes, current terminology, old labels, and major clinical characteristics. This classification system is dynamic in two ways. First, research findings suggest many differences among individuals within each category. Second, except for those with type 1 diabetes, patients may move from one category to another. For example, a woman with gestational diabetes may, after delivery, move into the type 2 category. These types also differ in their etiology, clinical course, and management.

PHYSIOLOGY AND PATHOPHYSIOLOGY OF DIABETES

Insulin is secreted by beta cells, which are one of four types of cells in the islets of Langerhans in the pancreas. Insulin is an anabolic, or storage, hormone. When a person eats a meal, insulin secretion increases and moves glucose from the blood into muscle, liver, and fat cells. In those cells, insulin:

• Transports and metabolizes glucose for energy
• Stimulates storage of glucose in the liver and muscle (in the form of glycogen)
• Signals the liver to stop the release of glucose
• Enhances storage of dietary fat in adipose tissue
• Accelerates transport of amino acids (derived from dietary protein) into cells

Table 41-1 • Classification of Diabetes Mellitus and Related Glucose Intolerances

CURRENT CLASSIFICATION	PREVIOUS CLASSIFICATIONS	CLINICAL CHARACTERISTICS AND CLINICAL IMPLICATIONS
Type 1 (10% of all diabetes)	Juvenile diabetes Juvenile-onset diabetes Ketosis-prone diabetes Brittle diabetes Insulin-dependent diabetes mellitus (IDDM)	Onset any age, but usually young (<30 yrs) Usually thin at diagnosis because of recent weight loss Etiology includes genetic, immunologic, or environmental factors (eg, virus). Often have islet cell antibodies Often have antibodies to insulin even before insulin treatment Little or no endogenous insulin Need insulin to preserve life Ketosis-prone when insulin absent Acute complication of hyperglycemia: diabetic ketoacidosis
Type 2 (90% of all diabetes: obese—80% of type 2; nonobese—20% of type 2)	Adult-onset diabetes Maturity-onset diabetes Ketosis-resistant diabetes Stable diabetes Non–insulin-dependent diabetes (NIDDM)	Onset any age, usually over 30 years Usually abdominal obesity present at diagnosis Causes include presence of visceral fat, heredity, or lifestyle factors. No islet cell antibodies Decrease in endogenous insulin, or increased with insulin resistance Most patients can control blood glucose levels through proper eating, physical activity, and weight loss (if obese). Oral antidiabetic agents may improve blood glucose levels if dietary modification and exercise are unsuccessful. May need insulin on a short- or long-term basis to prevent hyperglycemia Ketosis rare, except in stress or infection Acute complication: hyperglycemic hyperosmolar nonketotic syndrome
Diabetes mellitus associated with other conditions or syndromes	Secondary diabetes	Accompanied by conditions known or suspected to cause the disease: pancreatic diseases, hormonal abnormalities, medications such as corticosteroids and estrogen-containing preparations. Depending on the ability of the pancreas to produce insulin, the patient may require treatment with oral antidiabetic agents or insulin.
Gestational diabetes	Gestational diabetes	Onset during pregnancy, usually in the second or third trimester Due to hormones secreted by the placenta, which inhibit the action of insulin Above-normal risk for perinatal complications, especially macrosomia (abnormally large babies) Treated with diet and, if needed, insulin to strictly maintain normal blood glucose levels Occurs in about 3.5%–3.8% of all pregnancies Glucose intolerance transitory but may recur: • In subsequent pregnancies • 30%–40% will develop overt diabetes (usually type 2) within 10 years (especially if abdominal obesity is present) Risk factors include obesity, age older than 30 years, family history of diabetes, previous large babies (over 4 kg). Screening tests (glucose challenge test) should be performed on all pregnant women between 24 and 28 weeks' gestation.
Impaired glucose tolerance	Borderline diabetes Latent diabetes Chemical diabetes Subclinical diabetes Asymptomatic diabetes	Fasting blood glucose > 7.0 mmol/L Random blood glucose > 11.1 mmol/L A person with abnormally high readings, even just on the very high end of normal, but may not have any overt symptoms associated with diabetes. 29% eventually develop diabetes. Above-normal susceptibility to atherosclerotic disease Renal and retinal complications usually not significant May be obese or nonobese; obese should reduce weight Should be screened for diabetes periodically
Prediabetes	Previous abnormality of glucose tolerance (PrevAGT)	Current normal glucose metabolism Previous history of hyperglycemia (eg, during pregnancy or illness) Periodic blood glucose screening after age 40 if there is a family history of diabetes or if symptomatic Encourage ideal body weight, even a weight loss of 5%–10% of body weight may improve glycemic control for a person who is overweight or obese.
Prediabetes	Potential abnormality of glucose tolerance (PotAGT)	No history of glucose intolerance Increased risk of diabetes if: • Positive family history • Visceral obesity • Mother of babies over 4 kg at birth • Member of high-risk populations Screening and weight advice as in PrevAGT

Insulin also inhibits the breakdown of stored glucose, protein, and fat.

During fasting periods (between meals and overnight), the pancreas continuously releases a small amount of insulin (basal insulin); another pancreatic hormone called glucagon (secreted by the alpha cells of the islets of Langerhans) is released when blood glucose levels decrease and stimulate the liver to release stored glucose. The insulin and the glucagon together maintain a constant level of glucose in the blood by stimulating the release of glucose from the liver.

Initially, the liver produces glucose through the breakdown of glycogen (glycogenolysis). After 8 to 12 hours without food, the liver forms glucose from the breakdown of noncarbohydrate substances, including amino acids (gluconeogenesis).

TYPE 1 DIABETES

Type 1 diabetes is characterized by destruction of the pancreatic beta cells. It is thought that combined genetic, immunologic, and possibly environmental (eg, viral) factors contribute to beta cell destruction. Although the events that lead to beta cell destruction are not fully understood, it is generally accepted that a genetic susceptibility is a common underlying factor in the development of type 1 diabetes. People do not inherit type 1 diabetes itself; rather, they inherit a genetic predisposition, or tendency, toward developing type 1 diabetes. This genetic tendency has been found in people with certain HLA (human leukocyte antigen) types. HLA refers to a cluster of genes responsible for transplantation antigens and other immune processes. About 95% of Caucasians with type 1 diabetes exhibit specific HLA types (DR3 or DR4). The risk of developing type 1 diabetes is increased three to five times in people who have one of these two HLA types. The risk increases 10 to 20 times in people who have both DR3 and DR4 HLA types (as compared with the general population). Immune-mediated diabetes commonly develops during childhood and adolescence, but it can occur at any age (ADA, Expert Committee on the Diagnosis and Classification of Diabetes Mellitus, 2003).

There is also evidence of an autoimmune response in type 1 diabetes. This is an abnormal response in which antibodies are directed against normal tissues of the body, responding to these tissues as if they are foreign. Autoantibodies against islet cells and against endogenous (internal) insulin have been detected in people at the time of diagnosis and even several years before the development of clinical signs of type 1 diabetes. In addition to genetic and immunologic components, environmental factors, such as viruses or toxins, that may initiate destruction of the beta cell are being investigated.

Regardless of the specific etiology, the destruction of the beta cells results in decreased insulin production, unchecked glucose production by the liver, and fasting hyperglycemia. In addition, glucose derived from food cannot be stored in the liver but instead remains in the bloodstream and contributes to postprandial (after meals) hyperglycemia. If the concentration of glucose in the blood exceeds the renal threshold for glucose, usually 9.9 to 11.1 mmol/L, the kidneys may not reabsorb all of the filtered glucose; the glucose then appears in the urine (glucosuria). When excess glucose is excreted in the urine, it is accompanied by excessive loss of fluids and electrolytes. This is called osmotic diuresis.

Because insulin normally inhibits glycogenolysis (breakdown of stored glucose) and gluconeogenesis (production of new glucose from amino acids and other substrates), in people with insulin deficiency, these processes occur in an unrestrained fashion

> **NURSING ALERT** Ketone bodies are acids that disturb the acid–base balance of the body when they accumulate in excessive amounts. The resulting DKA may cause signs and symptoms such as abdominal pain, nausea, vomiting, hyperventilation, a fruity breath odour, and, if left untreated, altered level of consciousness, coma, and death. Initiation of insulin treatment, along with fluid and electrolytes as needed, is essential to treat hyperglycemia and DKA and rapidly improves the metabolic abnormalities.

and contribute further to hyperglycemia. In addition, when there is a deficiency in the presence of insulin, the stored fat is broken down to provide a source of energy, resulting in the production of **ketone** bodies, which can lead to the development of ketosis.

TYPE 2 DIABETES

Type 2 diabetes differs from type 1 diabetes in many different ways. The onset of type 1 diabetes is more abrupt, whereas the development of hyperglycemia in type 2 may take years before the person experiences symptoms. There is no autoimmune destruction of the islet cells of the pancreas for type 2 diabetes, so the production of insulin continues. As the disease progresses over time, however, there is loss of function of the pancreatic B cells. Although there is a strong genetic predisposition to type 2 diabetes, it is not linked to HLA markers on the sixth chromosome. Genetic predisposition coupled with environmental factors, such as the presence of visceral/abdominal obesity and a sedentary lifestyle, seem to be the major contributors to the development of insulin resistance, the most salient characteristic of type 2 diabetes. The pathogenesis of insulin resistance is complex. There are numerous coexisting signs that are associated with the development of insulin resistance. They are hypertension (blood pressure of 130/85 mm Hg or greater), fasting blood glucose of 6.1 mmol/L or higher, triglycerides of 1.7 mmol/L or higher, HDL (high density lipids) of less than 1.0 mmol/L for men or 1.3 mmol/L for women, and the presence of visceral or abdominal obesity (defined as a waist circumference of 102 cm or greater for men and 88 cm or greater for women) (Canadian Diabetes Association, 2003; Health Canada, 1997).

This constellation of abnormal signs is often referred to as metabolic syndrome or syndrome X. Other concomitant illness such as Cushing's syndrome or polycystic ovarian syndrome (PCOS) may also lead to the development of type 2 diabetes. Another major difference between type 1 and 2 diabetes is the fact that those with type 2 diabetes are not as prone to developing the complication of diabetic ketoacidosis (DKA). Because fat is not broken down for use as an alternative energy source in type 2 diabetes, there is no production of ketone bodies. This can change, however, if the person with type 2 diabetes must take insulin to normalize glucose levels.

The symptoms experienced with type 2 diabetes are frequently mild and may include fatigue, irritability, polyuria, polydipsia, skin wounds that heal poorly, vaginal infections, or blurred vision (if glucose levels are very high).

For most patients (approximately 75%), type 2 diabetes is detected incidentally (eg, when routine laboratory tests or ophthalmoscopic examinations are performed). One consequence of undetected diabetes is that long-term diabetes complications (eg, eye disease, peripheral neuropathy, peripheral vascular disease) may have developed before the actual diagnosis of diabetes is made (ADA, Expert Committee on the Diagnosis and Classification of Diabetes Mellitus, 2003).

Because insulin resistance is associated with abdominal obesity, the primary treatment of type 2 diabetes is weight loss. Exercise is also important in enhancing the effectiveness of insulin. Oral antidiabetic agents may be added if diet and exercise are not successful in controlling blood glucose levels. If maximum doses of a single category of oral agents fail to reduce glucose levels to satisfactory levels, additional oral agents may be used. Insulin may be added to oral agent therapy, or patients may move to insulin therapy entirely. Some patients require insulin on an ongoing basis, and others may require insulin on a temporary basis during periods of acute physiologic stress, such as illness or surgery.

A recent report has demonstrated that type 2 diabetes can be prevented or delayed in persons at high risk for the disease through weight reduction and increased participation in moderate exercise (Diabetes Prevention Program Research Group, 2002). Metformin, one of the antidiabetic agents, also prevented or delayed the onset of type 2 diabetes, but to a lesser degree. The findings of this study support the role that weight reduction and exercise have in the prevention of type 2 diabetes (Chart 41-2).

GESTATIONAL DIABETES

Gestational diabetes is any degree of glucose intolerance with its onset during pregnancy. Hyperglycemia develops during pregnancy because of the secretion of placental hormones, which causes insulin resistance. For women who meet one or more of the following criteria, selective screening for diabetes during pregnancy is now being recommended between the 24th and 28th weeks of gestation: age 25 years or older; presence of obesity; family history of diabetes in first-degree relatives or gestational diabetes in a previous pregnancy; or member of an ethnic/racial group with a high prevalence of diabetes (eg, Hispanic, Aboriginal or African Canadian).

Gestational diabetes occurs in up to 3.5%–3.8% of pregnant women and increases their risk for hypertensive disorders during pregnancy. Initial management includes dietary modification and blood glucose monitoring. If hyperglycemia persists, insulin is prescribed. Oral antidiabetic agents should not be used during pregnancy. Goals for blood glucose levels during pregnancy are 5.3 mmol/L (fasting) or less; 7.8 mmol/L (one hour after meal) or less; or 6.7 mmol/L (2 hours after meal) or less.

After delivery of the infant, blood glucose levels in the woman with gestational diabetes return to normal. However, many women who have had gestational diabetes develop type 2 diabetes later in life. Therefore, all women who have had gestational diabetes should be counselled to maintain their ideal body weight and to exercise regularly to reduce their risk for type 2 diabetes (Canadian Diabetes Association, 2003).

CLINICAL MANIFESTATIONS

Classic clinical manifestations of all types of diabetes include the "three Ps": polyuria, polydipsia, and polyphagia. Polyuria (increased urination) and polydipsia (increased thirst) occur as a result of the excess loss of fluid associated with osmotic diuresis. The patient also experiences polyphagia (increased appetite) resulting from the catabolic state induced by insulin deficiency. Other symptoms include fatigue and weakness, sudden vision changes, tingling or numbness in hands or feet, dry skin, skin lesions or wounds that are slow to heal, and recurrent infections. The onset of type 1 diabetes may also be associated with sudden weight loss or nausea, vomiting, or abdominal pains, if DKA has developed.

ASSESSMENT AND DIAGNOSTIC FINDINGS

An abnormally high blood glucose level is the basic criterion for the diabetes diagnosis. Levels of 7.1 mmol/L or more or random plasma glucose levels exceeding 11.1 mmol/L on more than one occasion are diagnostic of diabetes. See Chart 41-3 for the diagnostic criteria for diabetes mellitus.

Plasma glucose values may be 10% to 15% higher than whole blood values, which are obtained with finger sticks (Porth, 2002). In addition to the assessment and diagnostic evaluation performed to diagnose diabetes, ongoing specialized assessment of

---

Chart 41-2   **Prevention of Type 2 Diabetes**

In 2002, the Diabetes Prevention Program Research Group reported that type 2 diabetes can be prevented with appropriate changes in lifestyle. Persons at high risk for type 2 diabetes (with a BMI ≥ 24 and fasting and postprandial plasma glucose levels elevated but not to levels diagnostic of diabetes) received either standard lifestyle recommendations plus metformin, standard lifestyle recommendations plus placebo, or an intensive program of lifestyle modifications. The 16-lesson curriculum of the intensive program of lifestyle modifications focused on weight reduction of >7% of initial body weight and physical activity of moderate intensity. It also included behaviour modification strategies designed to help patients achieve the goals of weight reduction and participation in exercise. The lifestyle intervention group had a 58% lower incidence of diabetes and the metformin group had a 31% lower incidence of diabetes compared to the placebo group. These findings were found in both genders and all racial and ethnic groups. These findings demonstrate that type 2 diabetes can be prevented or delayed in persons at high risk for the disease.

Diabetes Prevention Program Research Group (2002). Reduction in the incidence of type 2 diabetes with lifestyle intervention or metformin. *New England Journal of Medicine, 346*(6), 393–403.

Chart 41-3   **Criteria for the Diagnosis of Diabetes Mellitus**

FPG ≥ 7.0 mmol/L (fasting means no caloric intake for at least 8 hours)

OR

Casual PG ≥ 11.1 mmol/L + symptoms of diabetes (casual means any time of day, without regard to the interval since the last meal; classic symptoms of diabetes include polyuria, polydipsia, and unexplained weight loss)

OR

2hPG in a 75-g OGTT ≥ 11.1 mmol/L

A confirmatory laboratory glucose test (a FPG, casual PG, or 2h PG in a 75-g OGTT) must be done in all cases on another day in the absence of unequivocal hyperglycemia accompanied by acute metabolic decompensation.

2hPG = 2-hour plasma glucose
FPG = fasting plasma glucose
OGTT = oral glucose tolerance test
PG = plasma glucose

(Canadian Diabetes Association, 2003, p. 57)

patients with known diabetes and evaluation for complications in patients with newly diagnosed diabetes are important components of care. Parameters that should be regularly assessed are discussed in Chart 41-4.

Gerontologic Considerations

Elevated blood glucose levels appear to be age-related and occur in both men and women throughout the world. Elevated blood glucose levels commonly appear in the fifth decade of life and increase in frequency with advancing age. When elderly people with overt diabetes are excluded from the statistics, approximately 10% to 30% of elderly people have age-related hyperglycemia. What causes age-related changes in carbohydrate metabolism is unresolved. Possibilities include poor diet, physical inactivity, a decrease in the lean body mass in which ingested carbohydrate may be stored, altered insulin secretion, and increase in fat tissue, which increases insulin resistance.

Diabetes Management

The main goal of diabetes treatment is to normalize insulin activity and blood glucose levels to reduce the development of vascular and neuropathic complications. The importance of tight blood glucose control was demonstrated by the Diabetes Control and Complications Trial (DCCT), a 10-year prospective clinical trial conducted from 1983 to 1993. The trial investigated the impact of intensive glucose control on the development and progression of complications such as **retinopathy**, **nephropathy**, and **neuropathy**. A cohort of 1,441 people with type 1 diabetes were randomly assigned to conventional treatment (one or two insulin injections per day) or intensive treatment (three or four insulin injections per day or insulin pump therapy plus frequent blood glucose monitoring and weekly contacts with diabetes educators). Results demonstrated that the risk for developing retinopathy, neuropathy, and early signs of nephropathy (microalbuminuria and albuminuria) was dramatically reduced. The reduction was attributed to control of blood glucose levels to normal or near-normal levels. The ADA now recommends that all patients with diabetes strive for glucose control to reduce their risks for complications (ADA, Implications of the Diabetes Control and Complications Trial, 2003).

The major adverse effect of intensive therapy was a threefold increase in the incidence of severe **hypoglycemia** (severe enough to require assistance from another person), coma, or seizure. Because of these adverse effects, intensive therapy must be initiated with caution and must be accompanied by thorough education of the patient and family and by responsible behaviour of the patient. Careful screening of patients is a key step in initiating intensive therapy. (For situations that preclude the initiation of very tight blood glucose control, see the discussion of insulin in this chapter.)

A study conducted in the United Kingdom and reported in 1998 supported the results of the DCCT in type 2 diabetes and demonstrated a decrease in complications in patients with type 2 diabetes receiving intensive therapy compared to those receiving conventional therapy (United Kingdom Prospective Diabetes Study Group [UKPDS], 1998; ADA, Implications of the United Kingdom Prospective Diabetes Study, 2003).

Therefore, the therapeutic goal for diabetes management is to achieve normal blood glucose levels (euglycemia) without hypoglycemia and without seriously disrupting the patient's usual lifestyle and activity. There are five components of diabetes management (Fig. 41-1):

- Nutritional management
- Exercise
- Monitoring

Chart 41-4 • ASSESSMENT

The Patient With Diabetes

History
Symptoms related to the diagnosis of diabetes:
  Symptoms of hyperglycemia
  Symptoms of hypoglycemia
    Frequency, timing, severity, and resolution
Results of blood glucose monitoring
Status, symptoms, and management of chronic complications of diabetes
  Eye; kidney; nerve; genitourinary and sexual, bladder, and gastrointestinal
  Cardiac; peripheral vascular; foot complications associated with diabetes
Compliance with prescribed dietary management plan
Adherence to prescribed exercise regimen
Compliance with prescribed pharmacologic treatment (insulin or oral antidiabetic agents)
Use of tobacco, alcohol, and prescribed and over-the-counter medications/drugs
Lifestyle, cultural, psychosocial, and economic factors that may affect diabetes treatment

Physical Examination
Blood pressure (sitting and standing to detect orthostatic changes)

Waist circumference
Body mass index (height and weight)
Fundoscopic examination
Foot examination (lesions, signs of infection, pulses)
Skin examination (lesions and insulin-injection sites)
Neurologic examination
  Vibratory and sensory examination using monofilament
  Deep tendon reflexes
Oral examination

Laboratory Examination
HgbA$_{1C}$ (A1C)
Fasting lipid profile
Test for microalbuminuria
Serum creatinine level
Urinalysis
Electrocardiogram

Need for Referrals
Ophthalmology
Podiatry
Dietitian
Diabetes educator
Others if indicated

FIGURE 41-1 The five components of diabetes management.

- Pharmacologic therapy
- Education

Treatment varies because of changes in lifestyle and physical and emotional status as well as advances in treatment methods. Therefore, diabetes management involves constant assessment and modification of the treatment plan by health professionals and daily adjustments in therapy by the patient. Although the health care team directs the treatment, it is the patient who must manage the complex therapeutic regimen. For this reason, patient and family education is an essential component of diabetes treatment and is as important as all other components of the regimen.

NUTRITIONAL MANAGEMENT

Nutrition, diet, and weight control, along with exercise, are the foundation of diabetes management. The most important objective in the dietary and nutritional management of diabetes is control of total caloric intake to attain or maintain a reasonable body weight and control of blood glucose levels. Success of this alone is often associated with reversal of hyperglycemia in type 2 diabetes. However, achieving this goal is not always easy. Because nutritional management of diabetes is so complex, a registered dietitian who understands diabetes management has the major responsibility for this aspect of the therapeutic plan. However, the nurse and all other members of the health care team need to be knowledgeable about nutritional therapy and supportive of the patient who needs to implement dietary and lifestyle changes (ADA, Expert Committee on the Diagnosis and Classification of Diabetes Mellitus, 2003). Nutritional management of the patient with diabetes includes the following goals (ADA, Evidence-Based Nutrition Principles and Recommendations for the Treatment and Prevention of Diabetes and Related Complications, 2003):

- Providing all the essential food constituents (eg, vitamins, minerals) necessary for optimal nutrition
- Meeting energy needs
- Achieving and maintaining a reasonable weight

- Preventing wide daily fluctuations in blood glucose levels, with blood glucose levels as close to normal as is safe and practical to prevent or reduce the risk for complications
- Decreasing serum lipid levels, if elevated, to reduce the risk for macrovascular disease

For patients who require insulin to help control blood glucose levels, maintaining as much consistency as possible in the amount of calories and carbohydrates ingested at different meal times is essential. In addition, consistency in the approximate time intervals between meals, with the addition of snacks if necessary, helps in preventing hypoglycemic reactions and in maintaining overall blood glucose control.

For overweight or obese patients with diabetes (especially those with type 2 diabetes), weight loss is a key to treatment. (It is also a major factor in preventing type 2 diabetes.) In general, overweight is considered to be a Body Mass Index (BMI) of 25.0 to 29.9 and obesity is a BMI of 30.0 or greater (Canadian Diabetes Association, 2003).

Because the location of the adipose tissue is of critical importance in the development of type 2 diabetes, it is also important to consider the waist circumference of the individual. A waist circumference of more than 102 cm for men and 88 cm for women is indicative of visceral or abdominal obesity (Canadian Diabetes Association, 2003). Calculation of BMI is discussed in Chapter 5. Obesity is associated with an increased resistance to insulin; it is also a main factor in type 2 diabetes. Some obese patients who have type 2 diabetes and who require insulin or oral agents to control blood glucose levels may be able to reduce or eliminate the need for medication through weight loss. A weight loss as small as 5%–10% of total weight may significantly improve blood glucose levels, insulin sensitivity, hypertension, and dyslipidemia. For diabetic patients who do not take insulin, consistent meal content or timing is not as critical. Rather, decreasing the overall caloric intake assumes more importance for the overweight or obese diabetic. However, meals should not be skipped. Pacing food intake throughout the day places more manageable demands on the pancreas.

Long-term adherence to the meal plan is one of the most challenging aspects of diabetes management. For overweight or obese patients, it may be more realistic to restrict calories only moderately. For those who have lost weight, maintaining the weight loss may be difficult. To help these patients incorporate new dietary habits into their lifestyles, diet education, behavioural therapy, group support, and ongoing nutrition counselling are encouraged.

Meal Planning and Related Teaching

Because of limited evidence to support one dietary prescription over another, meal planning for all patients with diabetes must consider the patient's food preferences, lifestyle, usual eating times, ethnic and cultural background, and readiness to change (Canadian Diabetes Association, 2003). For patients using intensive insulin therapy, there may be greater flexibility in the timing and content of meals by allowing adjustments in insulin dosage for changes in eating and exercise habits. Advances in insulin management (new insulin analogs, insulin algorithms, insulin pumps) permit greater flexibility of schedules than previously possible. This is in contrast to the older concept of maintaining a constant dose of insulin and requiring the patient to adjust his or her schedule to the actions and duration of the insulin.

The first step in preparing a meal plan is a thorough review of the patient's diet history to identify his or her eating habits and

NURSING RESEARCH PROFILE 41-1
Diabetes Mismanagement in Adolescents and Young Adults

Hanna, K., & Guthrie, D. (2001). The health-compromising behavior and diabetes mismanagement among adolescents and young adults with diabetes. *Diabetes Educator, 27*(2), 223–228.

Purpose

Adolescence and young adulthood are periods often associated with health-compromising behaviours. This study was conducted to determine the relationship between health-compromising behaviour, age, gender, and diabetes mismanagement in adolescents and young adults.

Study Sample and Design

A correlational study was conducted; the sample included 107 adolescents and young adults with type 1 diabetes. Health-compromising behaviour was measured by a 10-item Problem Behaviour Survey that assessed subjects' involvement with hard drugs, marijuana, alcohol, smoking/chewing tobacco, physical violence, fighting, carrying weapons, riding with a drinking driver, driving while drinking, and having sexual intercourse. Higher scores indicate higher levels of health-compromising behaviour. Diabetes mismanagement was measured using a 6-item questionnaire that addressed glucose monitoring, diet, and insulin administration for the previous 10 days. Higher scores indicate higher levels of diabetes mismanagement. $HgbA_{1c}$ levels were used as indicators of metabolic control. The mean age of the sample was 17.4 (SD ± 3.2); their ages ranged from 12 to 24 years. It was largely a Caucasian sample. Age since diagnosis of diabetes was 7 years and 5 months. Subjects reported a mean daily insulin dose of 1.0 units per kilogram of body weight. The mean $HgbA_{1c}$ of the sample was 8.9%. $HgbA_{1c}$ values ranged from 5.1% to 16.6%; the normal range of $HgbA_{1c}$ was 3.4% to 6.2%.

Findings

The mean scores on the diabetes mismanagement scale and the health-compromising scale were below the medians and indicated relatively low levels of diabetes mismanagement and health-compromising behaviours, respectively. Participants were categorized into two groups by scores on the health-compromising scale: those involved in health-compromising behaviour and those not involved in such behaviour. On multiple regression analysis, correlations were found of diabetes mismanagement with age ($r = 0.23$, $p = 0.05$), female gender ($r = 0.24$, p = 0.05), and participation in health-compromising behaviours ($r = 0.32$, $p = 0.001$). Additionally, there was a significant relationship ($r = 0.66$, $p = 0.001$) between age and health-compromising behaviour. Further analyses revealed that being female and having greater health-compromising behaviour contributed to diabetes mismanagement; female subjects were found to have poorer metabolic control than males.

Nursing Implications

The results of this study reveal some issues important to nurses involved in the care of adolescents and young adults with type 1 diabetes. Participation in health-compromising behaviour and gender are two of the many factors that affect diabetes management and metabolic control. Assessment of health-compromising behaviour and diabetes mismanagement should be considered in nurses' assessment of adolescents and young adults with diabetes. Differentiating those adolescents and young adults who are involved in health-compromising behaviours and those who are not involved in those behaviours may provide information about those at risk for difficulty associated with management of diabetes. It is important to maintain open communication to determine if health-compromising behaviours are being practiced and to discuss these behaviours in a nonjudgmental way to decrease the risk for diabetes mismanagement.

---

lifestyle. A thorough assessment of the patient's need for weight loss, gain, or maintenance is also undertaken. In most instances, the person with type 2 diabetes requires weight reduction.

In teaching about meal planning, the clinical dietitian uses various educational tools, materials, and approaches. Initial education addresses the importance of consistent eating habits, the relationship of food and insulin, and the provision of an individualized meal plan. In-depth follow-up education then focuses on management skills, such as eating at restaurants, reading food labels, and adjusting the meal plan for exercise, illness, and special occasions. The nurse plays an important role in communicating pertinent information to the dietitian and reinforcing the patient's understanding.

For some patients, certain aspects of meal planning may be difficult to learn. This may be related to limitations in the patient's intellectual level or to emotional issues, such as difficulty accepting the diagnosis of diabetes or feelings of deprivation and undue restriction in eating. In any case, it helps to emphasize that using Canada's Guidelines for Healthy Eating (Health Canada, 1997)(or any food classification system) provides a way of thinking about food. It is also important to simplify information as much as possible and to provide opportunities for the patient to practice and repeat activities and information.

CALORIC REQUIREMENTS

Calorie-controlled diets are planned by first calculating the individual's energy needs and caloric requirements based on the patient's age, gender, height, and weight. An activity element is then factored in to provide the actual number of calories required for weight maintenance. To promote a .5–1.0 kilogram weight loss per week, 500 to 1,000 calories are subtracted from the daily total.

The priority for a young patient with type 1 diabetes, for example, should be a diet with enough calories to maintain normal growth and development. Some patients may be underweight at the onset of type 1 diabetes because of rapid weight loss from severe hyperglycemia. The goal with these patients initially may be to provide a higher-calorie diet to regain lost weight. The calories are distributed into carbohydrates, proteins, and fats, and a meal plan is then developed.

CALORIC DISTRIBUTION

A diabetic meal plan also focuses on the percentage of calories to come from carbohydrates, proteins, and fats. In general, carbohydrate foods have the greatest effect on blood glucose levels because they are more quickly digested than other foods and are converted into glucose rapidly.

Carbohydrates. The caloric distribution currently recommended is higher in carbohydrates than in fats and protein. Carbohydrates consist of sugars and starches, which are essential to provide fuel for our bodies. There is much debate about the amount, source, and type of carbohydrates a person with diabetes should consume. The Canadian Diabetes Association Clinical Practice

Guidelines, Nutrition Therapy (2003) recommend that people with diabetes choose carbohydrates that have the lowest postprandial response (a low glycemic index) to optimise blood glucose control. Also, counting the number of carbohydrates the person consumes at each meal is recommended.

Carbohydrate counting is a nutritional tool used for blood glucose management because carbohydrates are the main nutrients in food that influence blood glucose levels. This method provides flexibility in food choices, can be less complicated to understand than the diabetic food exchange list, and allows more accurate management with multiple daily injections (insulin before each meal). However, if carbohydrate counting is not used with other meal-planning techniques, weight gain can result. A variety of methods are used to count carbohydrates. When developing a diabetic meal plan using carbohydrate counting, all food sources should be considered. Once digested, 100% of carbohydrates are converted to glucose. However, approximately 50% of protein foods (meat, fish, and poultry) are also converted to glucose.

One method of carbohydrate counting includes counting grams of carbohydrates. If target goals are not reached by counting carbohydrates alone, protein will be factored into the calculations. This is especially true if the meal consists of only meat, fish, and non-starchy vegetables.

An alternative to counting grams of carbohydrate is measuring servings or choices. This method is used more often by people with type 2 diabetes. It emphasizes portion control of total servings of carbohydrate at meals and snacks. One carbohydrate serving is equivalent to 15 g of carbohydrate. Examples of one serving are an apple 5 centimeters in diameter and one slice of bread. Vegetables and meat are counted as one third of a carbohydrate serving.

Although carbohydrate counting is now commonly used for blood glucose management with type 1 and type 2 diabetes, it is not a perfect system. All carbohydrates, to some extent, affect the blood glucose to different degrees, regardless of equivalent serving size.

Fats. The recommendations regarding fat content of the diabetic diet include both reducing the total percentage of calories from fat sources to less than 30% of the total calories and limiting the amount of saturated fats and transfatty acids to 10% of total calories. Meal plans should favour foods rich in omega-3 fatty acids and plant oils. This approach may help to reduce risk factors such as elevated serum cholesterol levels, which are associated with the development of coronary artery disease, the leading cause of death and disability among people with diabetes.

The meal plan may include the use of some nonanimal sources of protein (eg, legumes and whole grains) to help reduce saturated fat and cholesterol intake. In addition, the amount of protein intake may be reduced in patients with early signs of renal disease.

Fibre. The use of fibre in diabetic diets has received increased attention as researchers study the effects on diabetes of a high-carbohydrate, high-fibre diet. This type of diet plays a role in lowering total cholesterol and low-density lipoprotein cholesterol in the blood. Increasing fibre in the diet may also improve blood glucose levels and decrease the need for exogenous insulin.

There are two types of dietary fibres: soluble and insoluble. Soluble fibre—in foods such as legumes, oats, and some fruits—plays more of a role in lowering blood glucose and lipid levels than does insoluble fibre, although the clinical significance of this effect is probably small (ADA, Expert Committee on the Diagnosis and Classification of Diabetes Mellitus, 2003). Soluble fibre is thought to be related to the formation of a gel in the GI tract.

This gel slows stomach emptying and the movement of food through the upper digestive tract. The potential glucose-lowering effect of fibre may be caused by the slower rate of glucose absorption from foods that contain soluble fibre. Insoluble fibre is found in whole-grain breads and cereals and in some vegetables. This type of fibre plays more of a role in increasing stool bulk and preventing constipation. Both insoluble and soluble fibres increase satiety, which is helpful for weight loss.

One risk involved in suddenly increasing fibre intake is that it may require adjusting the dosage of insulin or oral agents to prevent hypoglycemia. Other problems may include abdominal fullness, nausea, diarrhea, increased flatulence, and constipation if fluid intake is inadequate. If fibre is added to or increased in the meal plan, it should be done gradually and in consultation with a dietitian.

FOOD CLASSIFICATION SYSTEMS

To teach diet principles and to help patients in meal planning, several systems have been developed in which foods are organized into groups with common characteristics, such as number of calories, composition of foods (ie, amount of protein, fat, or carbohydrate in the food), or effect on blood glucose levels.

Canada's Guidelines for Healthy Eating. The dietary goal for patients diagnosed with diabetes is to maintain their blood glucose levels within normal limits to reduce or prevent the occurrence of complications. They must therefore learn to balance the carbohydrates, protein, and fats they ingest to control the amount of glucose that enters their bloodstream. Improvement in glycemic control can be monitored through regular readings of the diabetic individual's glycosylated hemoglobin (AIC). To achieve sustained metabolic control through lifestyle and behavioural changes, the nutritional therapy must be based upon the individual's needs and preferences and should be regularly re-evaluated and reinforced.

Generally, individuals with diabetes should follow Canada's Food Guide to Healthy Eating (Health Canada, 1997) (see Chapter 5). These guidelines encourage the selection of a variety of foods from four food groups: grain products, fruits and vegetables, milk products, and meat or alternatives. Using these guidelines, the individual should plan his or her total daily caloric or energy intake to reflect the following: 50% to 55% of their total caloric intake comes from carbohydrates, 15% to 20% of their energy intake comes from protein sources, 30% of their energy intake comes from fats (<10% from polyunsaturated fat, <10% from saturated fats or trans fatty acids; select foods that contain monounsaturated fats or are rich in omega-3 fatty acids).

Canadian Diabetes Association Food Choice System. Individuals with diabetes can use the Canadian Diabetes Association Food Choice System (www.diabetes.ca/) which has been developed to help people make choices that will promote blood glucose control. This system is based on two concepts: 1) food portions should be measured, and 2) foods within the seven food groupings can be interchanged. The seven food groups in the Food Choice System are starch foods, fruits and vegetables, milk, sugars, protein foods, fats and oils, and extras. Health Canada has introduced new labelling regulations that appear on food packages to assist consumers with making healthier food choices. For more information on these nutrition labels, go to www.healthyeatingisinstore.ca.

Glycemic Index. One of the main goals of diet therapy in diabetes is to avoid sharp, rapid increases in blood glucose levels after food is eaten. The term "glycemic index (GI)" is used to describe how much a given food raises the blood glucose level compared with an equivalent amount of glucose (Canadian Diabetes Association, 2005). However, because knowing the effect a food item has on the person's blood glucose level is not exact, there is debate about the utility of the GI. Although more research is necessary, the following guidelines can be helpful when making dietary recommendations:

- Combining starchy foods with protein- and fat-containing foods tends to slow their absorption and lower the glycemic response.
- In general, eating foods that are raw and whole results in a lower glycemic response than eating chopped, puréed, or cooked foods.
- Eating whole fruit instead of drinking juice decreases the glycemic response because fibre in the fruit slows absorption.
- Adding foods with sugars to the diet may produce a lower glycemic response if these foods are eaten with foods that are more slowly absorbed.

Patients can create their own glycemic index by monitoring their blood glucose level after ingesting a particular food. This can help patients improve blood glucose levels through individualized manipulation of the diet. Many patients who use frequent monitoring of blood glucose levels can use this information to adjust their insulin doses for variations in food intake.

Other Dietary Concerns

ALCOHOL CONSUMPTION

Patients with diabetes do not need to give up alcoholic beverages entirely, but patients and health care professionals need to be aware of the potential adverse effects of alcohol specific to diabetes. In general, the same precautions regarding the use of alcohol by people without diabetes should be applied to patients with diabetes. Moderation is recommended. The main danger of alcohol consumption by a diabetic patient is hypoglycemia, especially for patients who take insulin. Alcohol may decrease the normal physiologic reactions in the body that produce glucose (gluconeogenesis). Thus, if a diabetic patient takes alcohol on an empty stomach, there is an increased likelihood that hypoglycemia will develop. In addition, excessive alcohol intake may impair the patient's ability to recognize and treat hypoglycemia and to follow a prescribed meal plan to prevent hypoglycemia.

For the person with type 2 diabetes treated with the sulfonylurea agent chlorpropamide (Diabinese), a potential side effect of alcohol consumption is a disulfiram (Antabuse) type of reaction, which involves facial flushing, warmth, headache, nausea, vomiting, sweating, or thirst within minutes of consuming alcohol. The intensity of the reaction depends on the amount of alcohol consumed; the reaction seems to be less common with other sulfonylureas.

Alcohol consumption may lead to excessive weight gain (from the high caloric content of alcohol), hyperlipidemia, and elevated glucose levels (especially with mixed drinks and liqueurs).

Patient teaching regarding alcohol intake must emphasize moderation in the amount of alcohol consumed. Lower-calorie or less sweet drinks, such as light beer or dry wine, and food intake along with alcohol consumption are advised. For patients with type 2 diabetes especially, incorporating the calories from alcohol into the overall meal plan is important for weight control.

SWEETENERS

Using sweeteners is acceptable for patients with diabetes, especially if it assists in overall dietary adherence. Moderation in the amount of sweetener used is encouraged to avoid potential adverse effects. There are two main types of sweeteners: nutritive and non-nutritive. The nutritive sweeteners contain calories, and the non-nutritive sweeteners have few or no calories in the amounts normally used.

Nutritive sweeteners include fructose (fruit sugar), sorbitol, and xylitol. They are not calorie-free; they provide calories in amounts similar to those in sucrose (table sugar). They cause less elevation in blood sugar levels than sucrose and are often used in "sugar-free" foods. Sweeteners containing sorbitol may have a laxative effect.

Non-nutritive sweeteners have minimal or no calories. They are used in food products and are also available for table use. They produce minimal or no elevation in blood glucose levels and have been approved by Health Canada as safe for people with diabetes. Saccharin contains no calories. Aspartame (NutraSweet) is packaged with dextrose; it contains 4 calories per packet and loses sweetness with heat. Acesulfame-K (Ace-K) is also packaged with dextrose; it contains 1 calorie per packet. Sucralose (Splenda) is a newer nonnutritive, high-intensity sweetener that is about 600 times sweeter than sugar. It has been approved for use in baked goods, nonalcoholic beverages, chewing gum, coffee, confections, frostings, and frozen dairy products.

MISLEADING FOOD LABELS

Foods labelled "sugarless" or "sugar-free" may still provide calories equal to those of the equivalent sugar-containing products if they are made with nutritive sweeteners. Thus, for weight loss, these products may not always be useful. In addition, patients must not consider them "free" foods to be eaten in unlimited quantity, because they may elevate blood glucose levels.

Foods labelled "dietetic" are not necessarily reduced-calorie foods. They may be lower in sodium or have other special dietary uses. Patients are advised that foods labelled "dietetic" may still contain significant amounts of sugar or fat.

It is also important to read the labels of "health foods"—especially snacks—because they often contain carbohydrates such as honey, brown sugar, and corn syrup. In addition, these supposedly healthy snacks frequently contain saturated vegetable fats (eg, coconut or palm oil), hydrogenated vegetable fats, or animal fats, which may be contraindicated in patients with elevated blood lipid levels.

EXERCISE

Benefits

Exercise is extremely important in managing diabetes because of its effects on lowering blood glucose and reducing cardiovascular risk factors. Exercise lowers the blood glucose level by increasing the uptake of glucose by body muscles and by improving insulin utilization. It also improves circulation and muscle tone. Resistance (strength) training, such as weight lifting, can increase lean muscle mass, thereby increasing the resting metabolic rate. These effects are useful in diabetes in relation to losing weight, easing stress, and maintaining a feeling of well-being. Exercise also alters blood lipid levels, increasing levels of high-density lipoproteins and decreasing total cholesterol and triglyceride levels. This is especially important to the person with diabetes because of the increased risk of cardiovascular disease (Creviston & Quinn, 2001). General guidelines for exercise in diabetes are presented in Chart 41-5.

General Precautions for Exercise in Diabetics

- Use proper footwear and, if appropriate, other protective equipment.
- Avoid exercise in extreme heat or cold.
- Inspect feet daily after exercise.
- Avoid exercise during periods of poor metabolic control.

Exercise Precautions

Patients who have blood glucose levels exceeding 14 mmol/L and who have ketones in their urine should not begin exercising until the urine tests negative for ketones and the blood glucose level is closer to normal. Exercising with elevated blood glucose levels increases the secretion of glucagon, growth hormone, and catecholamines. The liver then releases more glucose, and the result is an increase in the blood glucose level (ADA, Physical Activity/ Exercise and Diabetes Mellitus, 2003).

The physiologic decrease in circulating insulin that normally occurs with exercise cannot occur in patients treated with insulin. Initially, the patient who requires insulin should be taught to eat a 15-g carbohydrate snack (a fruit choice) or a snack of complex carbohydrate with a protein before engaging in moderate exercise, to prevent unexpected hypoglycemia. The exact amount of food needed varies from person to person and should be determined by blood glucose monitoring. Some patients find that they do not require a pre-exercise snack if they exercise within 1 to 2 hours after a meal. Other patients may require extra food regardless of when they exercise. If extra food is required, it need not be deducted from the regular meal plan.

Another potential problem for patients who take insulin is hypoglycemia that occurs many hours after exercise. To avoid postexercise hypoglycemia, especially after strenuous or prolonged exercise, the patient may need to eat a snack at the end of the exercise session and at bedtime and monitor the blood glucose level more frequently. In addition, it may be necessary to have the patient reduce the dosage of insulin that peaks at the time of exercise. Patients who are capable, knowledgeable, and responsible can learn to adjust their own insulin doses. Others need specific instructions on what to do when they exercise.

Patients participating in extended periods of exercise should test their blood glucose levels before, during, and after the exercise period, and they should snack on carbohydrates as needed to maintain blood glucose levels (Canadian Diabetes Association, 2003). Other participants or observers should be aware that the person exercising has diabetes, and they should know what assistance to give if severe hypoglycemia occurs.

In obese people with type 2 diabetes, exercise in addition to dietary management both improves glucose metabolism and enhances loss of body fat. Exercise coupled with weight loss improves insulin sensitivity and may decrease the need for insulin or oral agents. Eventually, the patient's glucose tolerance may return to normal. The patient with type 2 diabetes who is not taking insulin or an oral agent may not need extra food before exercise.

Exercise Recommendations

People with diabetes should exercise at the same time (preferably when blood glucose levels are at their peak) and in the same amount each day. Regular daily exercise, rather than sporadic exercise,

should be encouraged. Exercise recommendations must be altered as necessary for patients with diabetic complications such as retinopathy, autonomic neuropathy, sensorimotor neuropathy, and cardiovascular disease (ADA, Physical Activity/Exercise and Diabetes Mellitus, 2003). Increased blood pressure associated with exercise may aggravate diabetic retinopathy and increase the risk of a hemorrhage into the vitreous or retina. Patients with ischemic heart disease risk triggering angina or a myocardial infarction, which may be silent. Avoiding trauma to the lower extremities is especially important in the patient with numbness related to neuropathy.

In general, a slow, gradual increase in the exercise period is encouraged. For many patients, walking is a safe and beneficial form of exercise that requires no special equipment (except for proper shoes) and can be performed anywhere. People with diabetes should discuss an exercise program with their physician and undergo a careful medical evaluation with appropriate diagnostic studies before beginning an exercise program (ADA, Physical Activity/Exercise and Diabetes Mellitus, 2003; Creviston & Quinn, 2001; Flood & Constance, 2002).

For patients who are older than 30 years and who have two or more risk factors for heart disease, an exercise stress test is recommended. Risk factors for heart disease include hypertension, obesity, high cholesterol levels, abnormal resting electrocardiogram, sedentary lifestyle, smoking, male gender, and a family history of heart disease.

Gerontologic Considerations

Physical activity that is consistent and realistic is beneficial to the elderly person with diabetes. Physical fitness in the elderly population with diabetes may lead to less chronic vascular disease and an improved quality of life (ADA, Physical Activity/Exercise and Diabetes Mellitus, 2003). Advantages of exercise in this population include a decrease in hyperglycemia, a general sense of well-being, and the use of ingested calories, resulting in weight reduction. Because there is an increased incidence of cardiovascular problems in the elderly, a pattern of gradual, consistent exercise should be planned that does not exceed the patient's physical capacity. Physical impairment from other chronic diseases must also be considered. In some cases a physical therapy evaluation may be warranted with the goal of determining exercises specific to the patient's needs and abilities. Tools such as the "Armchair Fitness" video may be helpful. For more information about age-related changes that affect diabetes management see Chart 41-6.

MONITORING GLUCOSE LEVELS AND KETONES

Blood glucose monitoring is a cornerstone of diabetes management, and **self-monitoring of blood glucose (SMBG)** levels by patients has dramatically altered diabetes care. Frequent SMBG enables people with diabetes to adjust the treatment regimen to obtain optimal blood glucose control. This allows for detection and prevention of hypoglycemia and hyperglycemia and plays a crucial role in normalizing blood glucose levels, which in turn may reduce the risk of long-term diabetic complications.

Various SMBG methods are available. Most involve obtaining a drop of blood from the fingertip, applying the blood to a special reagent strip, and allowing the blood to stay on the strip for the amount of time specified by the manufacturer (usually 5 to 30 seconds). The meter gives a digital readout of the blood glucose value.

Chart 41-6 Age-Related Changes That May Affect Diabetes and Its Management

Sensory changes
Decreased vision
Decreased smell
Taste changes
Decreased proprioception
Diminished thirst

Gastrointestinal changes
Dental problems
Appetite changes
Delayed gastric emptying
Decreased bowel motility

Activity/exercise pattern changes
More sedentary

Renal function changes
Decreased function
Decreased drug clearance

Affective/cognitive changes
Medications/meals omitted or taken erratically

Socioeconomic factors
Fad diets
Loneliness/living alone
Lack of money/lack of support system

Chronic diseases
Hypertension
Arthritis
Neoplasms
Acute/chronic infections

Potential drug interactions
Use of another person's medications
Consulting multiple physicians for different illnesses
Alcohol use/abuse

The meters available for SMBG offer different features and benefits. Newer monitors have eliminated the step of blood removal from the strip. The strip is placed in the meter first, before blood is applied to it. Once the blood is placed on the strip, it remains there for the duration of the test. The meter automatically displays the blood glucose level after a short time (less than 1 minute). Some meters are biosensors that use blood obtained from alternate test sites, such as the forearm. They have a special lancing device that is useful for patients who have painful fingertips or pain with finger sticks.

Some meters can be used by patients with visual impairments. They have audio components that assist the patient in performing the test and obtaining the result. In addition, meters are available to check both blood glucose and blood ketone levels by those who are particularly susceptible to development of DKA.

Advantages and Disadvantages of SMBG Systems

The monitoring method used by the patient must match his or her skill level. Factors affecting SMBG performance include visual acuity, fine motor coordination, cognitive ability, comfort with technology, willingness, and cost.

Visual methods are the least expensive and require less equipment. However, they require the ability to distinguish colours and

---

to be exact in timing the procedures. Further, they involve subjective interpretation of results. Monitoring blood glucose using meters is recommended because meters have become much less expensive and less technique-dependent, making the results more accurate. Referral to a social worker may be warranted to assist individuals without the financial means to purchase a meter.

Older meters that required removal of blood from the reagent strip are generally obsolete. These procedures have more steps that must be performed in an exact sequence. The newer meters that do not require removal of blood from the strip generally are easier to use. However, most do not provide a backup method for visually assessing the meter results. Figure 41-2 illustrates a system for glucose monitoring.

A potential hazard of all SMBG methods is that the patient may obtain and report erroneous blood glucose values as a result of using incorrect techniques. Some common sources of error include:

- Improper application of blood (eg, drop too small)
- Improper meter cleaning and maintenance (eg, allowing dust or blood to accumulate on the optic window). This is not an issue in the biosensor type of meter.
- Damage to the reagent strips by heat or humidity; use of outdated strips

The nurse plays an important role in providing initial teaching about SMBG techniques. Equally important is evaluating the techniques of patients who are experienced in self-monitoring. Patients should be discouraged from purchasing SMBG products from stores or catalogues that do not provide direct education. Every 6 to 12 months, patients should conduct a comparison of their meter with a simultaneous laboratory-measured blood glucose level in their physician's office. The accuracy of the meter and strips should also be assessed with control solutions specific to that meter whenever a new vial of strips is used or whenever the validity of the reading is in doubt.

Candidates for SMBG

For everyone with diabetes, SMBG is useful for managing self-care. It is a key component of treatment for any intensive insulin therapy regimen (including two to four injections per day or insulin pumps) and for diabetes management during pregnancy. It is also recommended for patients with:

- Unstable diabetes
- A tendency for severe ketosis or hypoglycemia
- Hypoglycemia without warning symptoms

FIGURE 41-2 Example of blood glucose monitors.

For patients not taking insulin, SMBG is helpful for monitoring the effectiveness of exercise, diet, and oral antidiabetic agents. It can also help motivate patients to continue with treatment. For patients with type 2 diabetes, SMBG is recommended during periods of suspected hyperglycemia (eg, illness) or hypoglycemia (eg, unusual increased activity levels) (Canadian Diabetes Association, 2003).

Frequency of SMBG

For most patients who require insulin, SMBG is recommended two to four times daily (usually before meals and at bedtime). For patients who take insulin before each meal, SMBG is required at least three times daily before meals to determine each dose (Canadian Diabetes Association, 2003). Patients not receiving insulin may be instructed to assess their blood glucose levels at least two or three times per week, including a 2-hour postprandial test. For all patients, testing is recommended whenever hypoglycemia or hyperglycemia is suspected. The patient should increase the frequency of SMBG with changes in medications, activity, or diet and with stress or illness.

Responding to SMBG Results

Patients are instructed to keep a record or logbook of blood glucose levels so that they can detect patterns. Testing is done at the peak action time of the medication to evaluate the need for dosage adjustments. To evaluate basal insulin and determine bolus insulin doses, testing is performed before meals. To titrate bolus insulin doses, regular or lispro, testing is done 2 hours after meals. Patients with type 2 diabetes are encouraged to test before and 2 hours after the largest meal of the day. Patients who take insulin at bedtime or who are on an insulin infusion pump must also test at 3 a.m. once a week to document that the blood glucose level is not decreasing during the night. If a patient is unwilling or cannot afford to test frequently, then once or twice a day may be sufficient if the patient varies the time of day to test (eg, before breakfast one day, before lunch the next day).

A tendency to discontinue SMBG is more likely to occur when patients do not receive instruction about using the results to alter their treatment regimen. Instructions vary according to the patient's understanding and the physician's philosophy of diabetes management. At the very least, patients should be given parameters for calling the physician. Patients using intensive insulin therapy regimens may be instructed in the use of algorithms (rules or decision trees) for changing the insulin doses based on patterns of values greater or less than the target range and the amount of carbohydrate to be consumed. Baseline patterns should be established by SMBG for 1 to 2 weeks.

Glycosylated Hemoglobin

Glycosylated hemoglobin (referred to as $HgbA_{1C}$ or A1C) is a blood test that reflects average blood glucose levels over a period of approximately 2 to 3 months (Canadian Diabetes Association, 2003). When blood glucose levels are elevated, glucose molecules attach to hemoglobin in the red blood cell. The longer the amount of glucose in the blood remains above normal, the more glucose binds to the red blood cell and the higher the glycosylated hemoglobin level. This complex (the hemoglobin attached to the glucose) is permanent and lasts for the life of the red blood cell, approxi-

mately 120 days. If near-normal blood glucose levels are maintained, with only occasional increases in blood glucose, the overall value will not be greatly elevated. However, if the blood glucose values are consistently high, then the test result will also be elevated. If patients report mostly normal SMBG results but the glycosylated hemoglobin is high, there may be errors in the methods used for glucose monitoring, errors in recording results, or frequent elevations in glucose levels at times during the day when the patient is not usually monitoring the blood.

Recommended blood glucose targets for people with diabetes are A1C levels ≤ 7% (Canadian Diabetes Association, 2003).

Urine Testing for Glucose

Before SMBG methods were available, urine glucose testing was the only way to monitor diabetes on a daily basis. Today its use is limited to patients who cannot or will not perform SMBG. The advantages of urine glucose testing are that it is less expensive than SMBG and it is not invasive. The general procedure involves applying urine to a reagent strip or tablet and matching colours on the strip with a colour chart at the end of a specified period.

Disadvantages of urine testing include the following:

- Results do not accurately reflect the blood glucose level at the time of the test.
- The renal threshold for glucose is 9.9 to 11.1 mmol/L, far above target blood glucose levels.
- Hypoglycemia cannot be detected because a "negative" urine glucose result may occur when the blood glucose level is 9.9 mmol/L or higher.
- Patients may have a false sense of being in good control when results are always negative.
- Various medications (eg, aspirin, vitamin C, some antibiotics) may interfere with test results.
- In elderly patients and patients with kidney disease, the renal threshold (the level of blood glucose at which glucose starts to appear in the urine) is raised; thus, false-negative readings may occur at dangerously elevated glucose levels.

Testing for Ketones

Ketones (or ketone bodies) in the urine signal that control of type 1 diabetes is deteriorating, and the risk of DKA is high. When there is almost no effective insulin available, the body starts to break down stored fat for energy. Ketone bodies are byproducts of this fat breakdown, and they accumulate in the blood and urine. Urine testing is the most common method used for self-testing of ketone bodies by patients. A meter that enables testing of blood for ketones is available but not widely used.

Most commonly, patients use a urine dipstick (Ketostix or Chemstrip uK) to detect ketonuria. The reagent pad on the strip turns purplish when ketones are present. (One of the ketone bodies is called acetone, and this term is frequently used interchangeably with the term "ketones.") Other strips are available for measuring both urine glucose and ketones (Keto-Diastix or Chemstrip uGK). Large amounts of ketones may depress the colour response of the glucose test area.

Urine ketone testing should be performed whenever patients with type 1 diabetes have glucosuria or persistently elevated blood glucose levels (more than 13.2 mmol/L for two testing periods in a row) and during illness, in pregnancy with pre-existing diabetes, and in gestational diabetes (Canadian Diabetes Association, 2003).

PHARMACOLOGIC THERAPY

As stated earlier, insulin is secreted by the beta cells of the islets of Langerhans and works to lower the blood glucose level after meals by facilitating the uptake and utilization of glucose by muscle, fat, and liver cells. In the absence of adequate insulin, pharmacologic therapy is essential.

Insulin Therapy and Insulin Preparations

Because the body loses the ability to produce insulin in type 1 diabetes, exogenous insulin must be administered for life. In type 2 diabetes, insulin may be necessary on a long-term basis to control glucose levels if diet and oral agents fail. In addition, some patients in whom type 2 diabetes is usually controlled by diet alone or by diet and an oral agent may require insulin temporarily during illness, infection, pregnancy, surgery, or some other stressful event. In many cases, insulin injections are administered two or more times daily to control the blood glucose level. Because the insulin dose required by the individual patient is determined by the level of glucose in the blood, accurate monitoring of blood glucose levels is essential; thus, SMBG has become a cornerstone of insulin therapy. A number of insulin preparations are available. They vary according to three main characteristics: time course of action, species (source), and manufacturer.

TIME COURSE OF ACTION

Insulins may be grouped into several categories based on the onset, peak, and duration of action (Table 41-2). Human insulin preparations have a shorter duration of action than insulin from animal sources because the presence of animal proteins triggers an immune response that results in the binding of animal insulin, which slows its availability.

Rapid-acting analogue (clear) insulins such as insulin lispro (Humalog) and insulin aspart (NovoRapid) are blood glucose-lowering agents that produce a more rapid effect that is of shorter duration than regular insulin. These insulins have an onset of 10 to 15 minutes, a peak action of 60 to 90 minutes after injection, and a duration of 4 to 5 hours. Because of their rapid onset, patients should be instructed to eat no more than 10 to 15 minutes after injection. Because of the short duration of action of these insulin analogues, patients with type 1 diabetes and some patients with type 2 or gestational diabetes also require a long-acting insulin to maintain glucose control. Basal insulin is necessary to maintain blood glucose levels irrespective of meals. A constant level of insulin is required at all times. Intermediate-acting insulins function as basal insulins but may have to be split into two injections to achieve 24-hour coverage.

Fast-acting (clear) insulins have an onset of 30 minutes to 1 hour; peak, 2 to 4 hours; and duration, 5 to 8 hours. They are usually administered 20 to 30 minutes before a meal, either alone or in combination with a longer-acting insulin. Humulin R and Novolin ge Toronto are examples of this type of insulin.

Intermediate-acting (cloudy) insulins, called NPH insulin (neutral protamine Hagedorn), have an onset of 1 to 3 hours; peak, 5 to 8 hours; and duration, 18 hours. Intermediate-acting insulins, which are similar in their time course of action, appear white and cloudy. If NPH insulin is taken alone, it is not crucial that it be taken 30 minutes before the meal. It is important, however, for the patient to eat some food around the time of the onset and peak of these insulins. Humulin N, Novolin ge NPH, and Humulin L are examples of these insulins.

Long-acting (cloudy) human insulins have an onset of 3 to 4 hours; peak, 8 to 15 hours; and duration, 22 to 26 hours. Humulin-U is an example.

"Peakless" basal insulin, insulin glargine (Lantus), is approved for use as a basal insulin—that is, the insulin is absorbed very slowly over 24 hours and can be given once a day. Because the insulin is in a suspension with a pH of 4, it cannot be mixed with other insulins because this would cause precipitation. It is given once a day at bedtime. This insulin has been approved, but is not yet available in Canada (Canadian Diabetes Association, 2003).

> **! NURSING ALERT** When administering insulin, it is very important to read the label carefully and to be sure that the correct type of insulin is administered.

In the future, "inhaled insulin" may be approved for use. This type of insulin is in the form of a very fine powder, which is in-

---

 Table 41-2 • **Categories of Insulin**

TIME COURSE	AGENT	ONSET	PEAK	DURATION	INDICATIONS
Rapid-acting analogue	Humalog (insulin lispro) NovoRapid (insulin aspart)	10–15 min	60–70 min	4–5 h	Used for rapid reduction of glucose level, to treat postprandial hyperglycemia, and/or to prevent nocturnal hypoglycemia
Fast-acting	Humalog R, Novolin ge Toronto	½–1 h	2–4 h	5–8 h	Usually administered 20–30 minutes before a meal; may be taken alone or in combination with longer-acting insulin
Intermediate-acting	Humulin L, Humulin N, Novolin ge NPH	1–3 h	5–8 h	up to 18	Usually taken after food
Long-acting	Humulin U	3–4 h	8–15 h	22–26 h	Used primarily to control fasting glucose level
Extended long-acting analogue	Lantus (insulin glargine)	90 min	Continuous (no peak)	24 h	Used for basal dose

haled through a device similar to that used to administer asthma medications. The patient's program would consist of a "basal" rate of insulin such as glargine supplemented by an inhaled dose before each meal.

The nurse may find that different sources list differing numbers of hours for the onset, peak, and duration of action of the main types of insulin, and patients' responses may vary (ie, larger doses prolong onset, duration, and peak). The nurse should focus on which meals—and snacks—are being "covered" by which insulin doses. In general, the rapid- and short-acting insulins are expected to cover the rise in glucose levels after meals, immediately after the injection; the intermediate-acting insulins are expected to cover subsequent meals; and the long-acting insulins provide a relatively constant level of insulin and act as a basal insulin.

SPECIES (SOURCE)

In the past, all insulins were obtained from beef (cow) and pork (pig) pancreases. "Human insulins" are now widely available. They are produced by recombinant DNA technology and have largely replaced insulin from animal sources (Canadian Diabetes Association, 2003).

Insulin Regimens

Insulin regimens vary from one to four injections per day. Usually there is a combination of a short-acting insulin and a longer-acting insulin. The normally functioning pancreas continuously secretes small amounts of insulin during the day and night. In addition, whenever blood glucose rises after ingestion of food, there is a rapid burst of insulin secretion in proportion to the glucose-raising effect of the food. The goal of all but the simplest, one-injection insulin regimens is to mimic this normal pattern of insulin secretion in response to food intake and activity patterns. Table 41-3 depicts several insulin regimens and the advantages and disadvantages of each.

Patients can learn to use SMBG results and carbohydrate counting to vary the insulin doses. This allows patients more flexibility in the timing and content of meals and exercise periods. However, complex insulin regimens require a strong level of commitment, intensive education, and close follow-up by the health care team. In addition, patients aiming for normal blood glucose levels run the risk of more hypoglycemic reactions.

The type of regimen used by any particular patient varies. For example, patient knowledge, willingness, goals, health status, and finances all may affect decisions regarding insulin treatment. In addition, the physician's philosophy about blood glucose control and the availability of equipment and support staff may influence decisions regarding insulin therapy. There are two general approaches to insulin therapy: conventional and intensive.

CONVENTIONAL REGIMEN

One approach is to simplify the insulin regimen as much as possible, with the aim of avoiding the acute complications of diabetes (hypoglycemia and symptomatic hyperglycemia). With this type of simplified regimen (eg, one or more injections of a mixture of short- and intermediate-acting insulins per day), patients may frequently have blood glucose levels well above normal. The exception is the patient who never varies meal patterns and activity levels. This approach would be appropriate for the terminally ill, the frail elderly with limited self-care abilities, or any patient who is completely unwilling or unable to engage in the self-management activities that are part of a more complex insulin regimen.

INTENSIVE REGIMEN

The second approach is to use a more complex insulin regimen to achieve as much control over blood glucose levels as is safe and practical. The results of the landmark DCCT study (1993) and the UKPDS study (1998) have demonstrated that maintaining blood glucose levels as close to normal as possible prevents or slows the progression of long-term diabetic complications. Another reason for using a more complex insulin regimen is to allow patients more flexibility to change their insulin doses from day to day in accordance with changes in their eating and activity patterns, with stress and illness, and as needed for variations in the prevailing glucose level.

Although the DCCT found that intensive treatment (three or four injections of insulin per day) reduced the risk of complications, not all people with diabetes are candidates for very tight control of blood glucose. The risk for severe hypoglycemia was increased threefold in patients receiving intensive treatment in the DCCT (ADA, Implications of the Diabetes Control and Complications Trial, 2003). Those who may not be candidates include patients with:

- Nervous system disorders rendering them unaware of hypoglycemic episodes (eg, those with autonomic neuropathy)
- Recurring severe hypoglycemia
- Irreversible diabetic complications, such as blindness or end-stage renal disease
- Cerebrovascular and/or cardiovascular disease
- Ineffective self-care skills

An exception is the patient who has received a kidney transplant because of nephropathy and chronic renal failure; this patient should be on an intensive regimen to preserve function of the new kidney.

The patient needs to be involved in the decision regarding which insulin regimen to use. Patients need to compare the potential benefits of different regimens with the potential costs (eg, time involved, number of injections or finger sticks for glucose testing, amount of record-keeping). There are no set guidelines as to which insulin regimen should be used for which patients. It must not be assumed that an elderly patient or a patient with visual impairment should automatically be given a simplified regimen. Likewise, it must not be assumed that all people will want to be involved in a complex treatment regimen. Nurses play an important role in educating patients about the different approaches to insulin therapy. Nurses should refer patients to diabetes specialists or diabetes education centres, when available, for further training and education in the various insulin treatment regimens.

Complications of Insulin Therapy

LOCAL ALLERGIC REACTIONS

A local allergic reaction (redness, swelling, tenderness, and induration or a 2- to 4-cm wheal) may appear at the injection site 1 to 2 hours after the insulin administration. These reactions, which usually occur during the beginning stages of therapy and disappear with continued use of insulin, are becoming rare because of the increased use of human insulins. The physician may prescribe an antihistamine to be taken 1 hour before the injection if such a local reaction occurs.

SYSTEMIC ALLERGIC REACTIONS

Systemic allergic reactions to insulin are rare. When they do occur, there is an immediate local skin reaction that gradually

Table 41-3 • Insulin Regimens

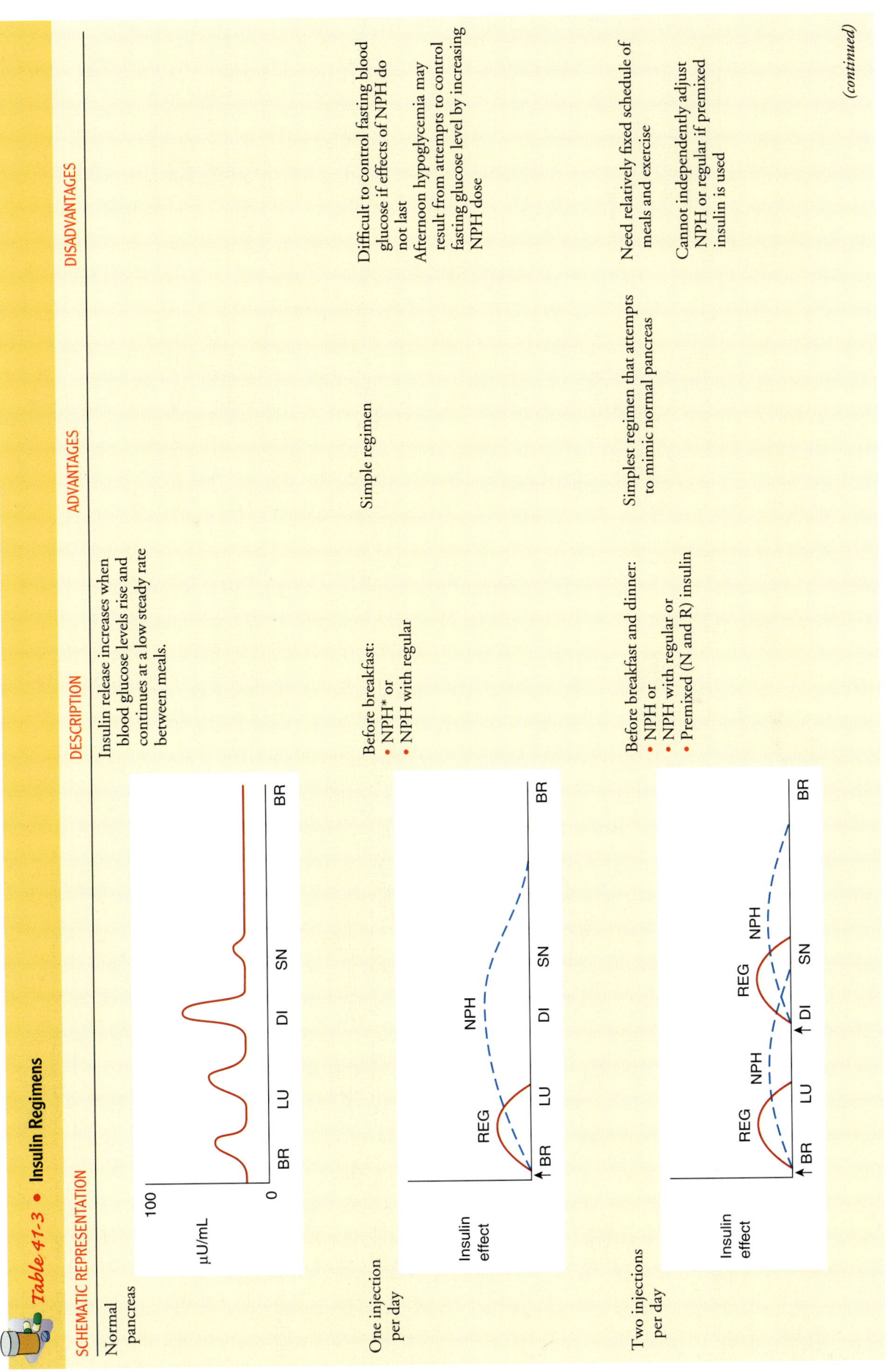

SCHEMATIC REPRESENTATION	DESCRIPTION	ADVANTAGES	DISADVANTAGES
Normal pancreas	Insulin release increases when blood glucose levels rise and continues at a low steady rate between meals.		
One injection per day	Before breakfast: • NPH* or • NPH with regular	Simple regimen	Difficult to control fasting blood glucose if effects of NPH do not last Afternoon hypoglycemia may result from attempts to control fasting glucose level by increasing NPH dose
Two injections per day	Before breakfast and dinner: • NPH or • NPH with regular or • Premixed (N and R) insulin	Simplest regimen that attempts to mimic normal pancreas	Need relatively fixed schedule of meals and exercise Cannot independently adjust NPH or regular if premixed insulin is used

(continued)

Table 41-3 • Insulin Regimens (Continued)

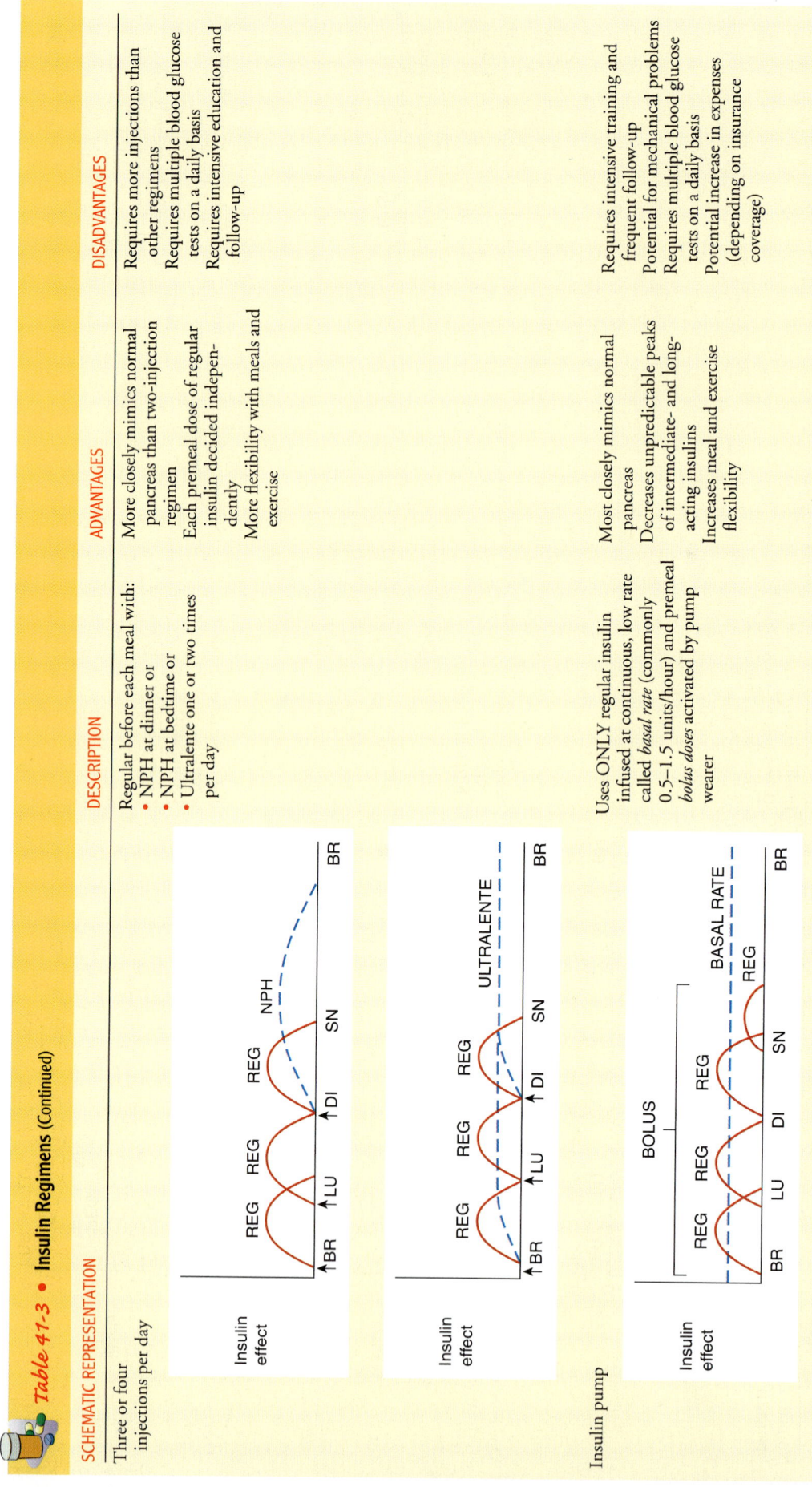

SCHEMATIC REPRESENTATION	DESCRIPTION	ADVANTAGES	DISADVANTAGES
Three or four injections per day	Regular before each meal with: • NPH at dinner or • NPH at bedtime or • Ultralente one or two times per day	More closely mimics normal pancreas than two-injection regimen Each premeal dose of regular insulin decided independently More flexibility with meals and exercise	Requires more injections than other regimens Requires multiple blood glucose tests on a daily basis Requires intensive education and follow-up
Insulin pump	Uses ONLY regular insulin infused at continuous, low rate called *basal rate* (commonly 0.5–1.5 units/hour) and premeal *bolus doses* activated by pump wearer	Most closely mimics normal pancreas Decreases unpredictable peaks of intermediate- and long-acting insulins Increases meal and exercise flexibility	Requires intensive training and frequent follow-up Potential for mechanical problems Requires multiple blood glucose tests on a daily basis Potential increase in expenses (depending on insurance coverage)

BR, breakfast; LU, lunch; DI, dinner; SN, snack; REG, regular; ↑ indicates insulin injections.

spreads into generalized urticaria (hives). The treatment is desensitization, with small doses of insulin administered in gradually increasing amounts using a desensitization kit. These rare reactions are occasionally associated with generalized edema or anaphylaxis.

INSULIN LIPODYSTROPHY

Lipodystrophy refers to a localized reaction, in the form of either lipoatrophy or lipohypertrophy, occurring at the site of insulin injections. Lipoatrophy is loss of subcutaneous fat and appears as slight dimpling or more serious pitting of subcutaneous fat. The use of human insulin has almost eliminated this disfiguring complication.

Lipohypertrophy, the development of fibrofatty masses at the injection site, is caused by the repeated use of an injection site. If insulin is injected into scarred areas, absorption may be delayed. This is one reason that rotation of injection sites is so important. The patient should avoid injecting insulin into these areas until the hypertrophy disappears.

INSULIN RESISTANCE

Most patients at one time or another have some degree of insulin resistance. This may occur for various reasons, the most common being obesity, which can be overcome by weight loss. Clinical insulin resistance has been defined as a daily insulin requirement of 200 units or more. In most diabetic patients taking insulin, immune antibodies develop and bind the insulin, thereby decreasing the insulin available for use. All animal insulins, as well as human insulins to a lesser degree, cause antibody production in humans.

Very few resistant patients develop high levels of antibodies. Many of these patients have a history of insulin therapy interrupted for several months or more. Treatment consists of administering a more concentrated insulin preparation, such as U-500, which is available by special order. Occasionally, prednisone is needed to block the production of antibodies. This may be followed by a gradual reduction in insulin requirement. Therefore, patients need to monitor themselves for hypoglycemia.

Table 41-4 • Causes of Morning Hyperglycemia

CHARACTERISTIC	TREATMENT
Insulin Waning Progressive rise in blood glucose from bedtime to morning	Increase evening (predinner or bedtime) dose of intermediate- or long-acting insulin, or institute a dose of insulin before the evening meal if one is not already in use.
Dawn Phenomenon Relatively normal blood glucose until about 3 AM, when the level begins to rise	Change time of injection of evening intermediate-acting insulin from dinnertime to bedtime.
Somogyi Effect Normal or elevated blood glucose at bedtime, a decrease at 2–3 AM to hypoglycemic levels, and a subsequent increase caused by the production of counterregulatory hormones	Decrease evening (predinner or bedtime) dose of intermediate-acting insulin, or increase bedtime snack.

MORNING HYPERGLYCEMIA

An elevated blood glucose level upon arising in the morning may be caused by an insufficient level of insulin due to several causes: the dawn phenomenon, the Somogyi effect, or insulin waning. The dawn phenomenon is characterized by a relatively normal blood glucose level until approximately 3 a.m., when blood glucose levels begin to rise. The phenomenon is thought to result from nocturnal surges in growth hormone secretion that create a greater need for insulin in the early morning hours in patients with type 1 diabetes. It must be distinguished from insulin waning (the progressive increase in blood glucose from bedtime to morning) or the Somogyi effect (nocturnal hypoglycemia followed by rebound hyperglycemia). Insulin waning is frequently seen if the evening NPH dose is administered before dinner and is prevented by moving the evening dose of NPH insulin to bedtime.

It may be difficult to tell from the patient's history which of these causes is responsible for morning hyperglycemia. To determine the cause, the patient must be awakened once or twice during the night to test blood glucose levels. Testing the blood glucose level at bedtime, at 3 a.m., and on awakening provides information that can be used in making adjustments in insulin to avoid morning hyperglycemia caused by the dawn phenomenon. Table 41-4 provides a summary of the differences among insulin waning, the dawn phenomenon, and the Somogyi effect.

Alternative Methods of Insulin Delivery

INSULIN PENS

These devices use small (150- to 300-unit) prefilled insulin cartridges that are loaded into a penlike holder. A disposable needle is attached to the device for insulin injection. Insulin is delivered by dialing in a dose or pushing a button for every 1- or 2-unit increment administered. People using these devices still need to insert the needle for each injection; however, they do not need to carry insulin bottles or to draw up insulin before each injection. These devices are most useful for patients who need to inject only one type of insulin at a time (eg, premeal regular insulin three times a day and bedtime NPH insulin) or who can use the premixed insulins. These pens are convenient for those who administer insulin before dinner if eating out or traveling. They are also useful for patients with impaired manual dexterity, vision, or cognitive function that makes the use of traditional syringes difficult.

JET INJECTORS

As an alternative to needle injections, jet injection devices deliver insulin through the skin under pressure in an extremely fine stream. These devices are more expensive than other alternative devices mentioned above and require thorough training and supervision when first used. In addition, patients should be cautioned that absorption rates, peak insulin activity, and insulin levels may be different when changing to a jet injector. (Insulin administered by jet injector is usually absorbed faster.) Bruising has occurred in some patients with use of the jet injector.

INSULIN PUMPS

Continuous subcutaneous insulin infusion involves the use of small, externally worn devices that closely mimic the functioning of the normal pancreas (ADA, Continuous Subcutaneous Insulin Infusion, 2003). Insulin pumps contain a 3-mL syringe attached to a long, thin, narrow-lumen tube with a needle or Teflon catheter attached to the end (Figs. 41-3 and 41-4). The patient inserts the

FIGURE 41-3 (**A**) Diagram of an insulin pump showing syringe in place inside pump and connection of pump via tubing to needle site. (**B–E**) Actual insertion site before, during, and after the needle and catheter have been inserted.

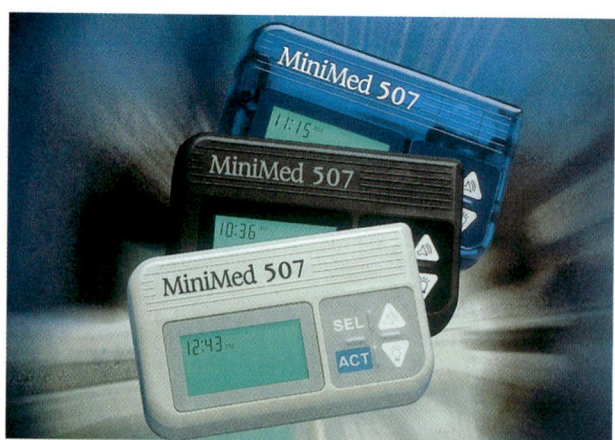

FIGURE 41-4 MiniMed insulin pump.

needle or catheter into the subcutaneous tissue (usually on the abdomen) and secures it with tape or a transparent dressing. The needle or catheter is changed at least every 3 days. The pump is then worn either on a belt or in a pocket. Some women keep the pump tucked into the front or side of the bra or wear it on a garter belt on the thigh.

The rapid-acting lispro insulin is used in the insulin pump and is delivered at a basal rate and as a bolus with meals. A continuous basal rate of insulin is typically 0.5 to 2.0 units/hour, depending on the patient's needs. A bolus dose of insulin is delivered before each meal when the patient activates the pump (by pushing buttons). The patient determines the amount of insulin to infuse based on blood glucose levels and anticipated food intake and activity level. Advantages of insulin pumps include increased flexibility in lifestyle (in terms of timing and amount of meals, exercise, and travel) and, for many patients, improved blood glucose control.

A disadvantage of insulin pumps is that unexpected disruptions in the flow of insulin from the pump may occur if the tubing or needle becomes occluded, if the supply of insulin runs out, or if the battery is depleted, increasing the risk of DKA. Effective teaching and a knowledgeable patient can minimize this risk. Another disadvantage is the potential for infection at needle insertion sites. Hypoglycemia may occur with insulin pump therapy; however, this is usually related to the lowered blood glucose levels many patients achieve rather than to a specific problem with the pump itself. The tight diabetic control associated with using an insulin pump may increase the incidence of hypoglycemia unawareness because of the very gradual decline in serum glucose level from levels greater than 3.9 mmol/L to those less than 3.3 mmol/L.

Some patients find that wearing the pump for 24 hours each day is an inconvenience. However, the pump can easily be disconnected, per patient preference, for limited periods (eg, for showering, exercise, or sexual activity).

Insulin pump candidates must be willing to assess blood glucose levels multiple times daily while on pump therapy. In addition, they must be psychologically stable and open about having diabetes, because the insulin pump is often a visible sign to others and a constant reminder to the patient that he or she has diabetes. Most important, patients using insulin pumps must have extensive education in the use of the insulin pump and in self-management of blood glucose and insulin doses. They must work closely with a team of health care professionals who are experienced in insulin pump therapy—specifically, a diabetologist/endocrinologist, a dietitian, and a certified diabetes educator.

IMPLANTABLE AND INHALANT INSULIN DELIVERY

Research into mechanical delivery of insulin has involved implantable insulin pumps that can be externally programmed according to blood glucose test results. Clinical trials with these devices are continuing. In addition, there is research into the development of implantable devices that both measure the blood glucose level and deliver insulin as needed. Methods of administering insulin by the oral route (oral spray or capsule), skin patch, and inhalation are undergoing intensive study.

TRANSPLANTATION OF PANCREATIC CELLS

Transplantation of the whole pancreas or a segment of the pancreas is being performed on a limited population (mostly diabetic patients receiving kidney transplantations simultaneously). One main issue regarding pancreatic transplantation is weighing the risks of antirejection medications against the advantages of pancreas transplantation. Another approach under investigation is the implantation of insulin-producing pancreatic islet cells (Canadian Diabetes Association, 2003). This latter approach involves a less extensive surgical procedure and a potentially lower incidence of immunogenic problems. However, thus far, independence from exogenous insulin has been limited to 2 years after transplantation of islet cells. A recent study of patients with **islet cell transplants** using less toxic antirejection drugs has shown promise (Edmonton Protocol) (Shapiro et al., 2000).

Oral Antihyperglycemic Agents

Oral antihyperglycemic agents may be effective for patients who have type 2 diabetes that cannot be treated by diet and exercise alone; however, they cannot be used during pregnancy. In Canada, oral antihyperglycemic agents include the sulfonylureas, biguanides, alpha glucosidase inhibitors, thiazolidinediones, and meglitinides. Sulfonylureas and meglitinides are considered insulin secretagogues because their action increases the secretion of insulin by the pancreatic beta cells.

SULFONYLUREAS

The **sulfonylureas** exert their primary action by directly stimulating the pancreas to secrete insulin. Therefore, a functioning pancreas is necessary for these agents to be effective, and they cannot be used in patients with type 1 diabetes. These agents improve insulin action at the cellular level and may also directly decrease glucose production by the liver. The sulfonylureas can be divided into first- and second-generation categories.

The most common side effects of these medications are GI symptoms and dermatologic reactions. Hypoglycemia may occur when an excessive dose of a sulfonylurea is used or when the patient omits or delays meals, reduces food intake, or increases activity. Because of the prolonged hypoglycemic effects of these agents (especially chlorpropamide), some patients need to be hospitalized for treatment of oral agent-induced hypoglycemia. Another side effect of chlorpropamide is a disulfiram (Antabuse) type of reaction when alcohol is ingested (see section on alcohol consumption for more information). Some medications may directly interact with sulfonylureas, potentiating their hypoglycemic effects (eg, sulfonamides, chloramphenicol, clofibrate, phenylbutazone, and bishydroxycoumarin). In addition, certain medications may independently affect blood glucose levels, thereby indirectly interfering with these agents. Medications that may increase glucose levels include potassium-losing diuretics, corticosteroids, estrogen compounds, and diphenylhydantoin (Dilantin). Medications that may cause hypoglycemia include salicylates, propranolol, monoamine oxidase inhibitors, and pentamidine.

Second-generation sulfonylureas have the advantage of a shorter half-life and excretion by both the kidney and the liver. This makes these medications safer to use in the elderly, in whom accumulation of the medication can cause recurring hypoglycemia.

BIGUANIDES

The biguanides are other kinds of oral antidiabetic agents. Metformin (Glucophage) produces its antidiabetic effects by facilitating insulin's action on peripheral receptor sites. Therefore, it can be used only in the presence of insulin. Biguanides have no effect on pancreatic beta cells. Biguanides used with a sulfonylurea may enhance the glucose-lowering effect more than either medication used alone. Lactic acidosis is a potential and serious complication of biguanide therapy; the patient must be monitored closely when therapy is initiated or when dosage changes. Medications that may interact with biguanides include anticoagulants, corticosteroids, diuretics, and oral contraceptives. Metformin is contraindicated in patients with renal impairment (serum creatinine level more than 1.4) or those at risk for renal dysfunction (eg, those with acute myocardial infarction). Renal function studies should be performed periodically to ensure that function is not impaired. Metformin should not be administered for 2 days before any diagnostic testing that may require use of a contrast agent. These situations increase the risk for lactic acidosis.

An extended-release form and a combination form (Glucovance) combines metformin with a sulfonylurea, such as glyburide. The combination provides two mechanisms of action and improved patient compliance. Hypoglycemia is a risk.

ALPHA GLUCOSIDASE INHIBITORS

Acarbose (Prandase) is an oral **alpha glucosidase inhibitor** used in type 2 diabetes management. It works by delaying the absorption of glucose in the intestinal system, resulting in a lower postprandial blood glucose level. As a consequence of plasma glucose reduction, hemoglobin A_{1C} levels drop. In contrast to the sulfonylureas, acarbose and miglitol do not enhance insulin secretion. It can be used alone with dietary treatment as monotherapy or in combination with sulfonylureas, thiazolidinediones, or meglitinides. When this medication is used in combination with sulfonylureas or meglitinides, hypoglycemia may occur. The patient must be advised that if hypoglycemia occurs, sucrose absorption will be blocked and treatment for hypoglycemia should be in the form of glucose, such as glucose tablets. The advantage of an oral alpha glucosidase inhibitor is that it is not systemically absorbed and is safe to use. The side effects are diarrhea and flatulence. These effects may be minimized by starting at a very low dose and increasing the dose gradually. Because acarbose and miglitol affect food absorption, they must be taken immediately before a meal, making therapeutic adherence a potential problem.

THIAZOLIDINEDIONES (TZDs)

Rosiglitazone (Avandia) and pioglitazone (Actos) are oral diabetes medications categorized as **thiazolidinediones.** They are indicated for patients with type 2 diabetes who take insulin injections and whose blood glucose control is inadequate (hemoglobin A_{1C} level greater than 8.5%). They have also been approved as first-line agents to treat type 2 diabetes, in combination with diet. Thiazolidinediones enhance insulin action at the receptor site without increasing insulin secretion from the beta cells of the pancreas. These medications may affect liver function; therefore, liver function studies must be performed at baseline and at frequent intervals (monthly for the first 12 months of treatment, and quarterly thereafter). Women should be informed that thiazolidinediones can cause resumption of ovulation in perimenopausal anovulatory women, making pregnancy a possibility.

MEGLITINIDES

Repaglinide (GlucoNorm), an oral glucose-lowering agent of the class of oral agents called meglitinides, lowers the blood glucose level by stimulating insulin release from the pancreatic beta cells. Its effectiveness depends on the presence of functioning beta cells. Therefore, repaglinide is contraindicated in patients with type 1 diabetes. Repaglinide has a fast action and a short duration. It should be taken before each meal to stimulate the release of insulin in response to that meal. It is also indicated for use in combination with metformin in patients whose hyperglycemia cannot be controlled by exercise, diet, and either metformin or repaglinide alone. The principal side effect of repaglinide is hypoglycemia; however, this side effect is less severe and frequent than for a sulfonylurea because repaglinide has a short half-life (approximately 1 hour). Patients must be taught the signs and symptoms of hypoglycemia and should understand that the medication should not be taken unless the patient eats a meal. Repaglinide is supplied in 0.5-, 1-, and 2-mg tablets.

Naglitinide (Starlix), another meglitinide, has a very rapid onset and short duration. It should be taken with meals and not taken if the meal is skipped. Hypoglycemia risk is low if taken correctly.

General Considerations for Oral Agents

Patients need to understand that oral agents are prescribed as an addition to (not as a substitute for) other treatment modalities, such as diet and exercise. Use of oral antidiabetic medications may need to be halted temporarily and insulin prescribed if hyperglycemia develops that is attributable to infection, trauma, or surgery.

In time, oral antidiabetic agents may no longer be effective in controlling the patient's diabetes. In such cases, the patient is treated with insulin. Approximately half of all patients who initially use oral antidiabetic agents eventually require insulin. This is referred to as a secondary failure. Primary failure occurs when the blood glucose level remains high a month after initial medication use.

Because the mechanisms of action vary (Fig. 41-5), the effect may be enhanced using multidose, multiple medications (Inzucchi et al., 1998). Use of multiple medications with different mechanisms of action is very common today (Quinn, 2001b). Using a combination of oral agents with insulin has been proposed as a treatment for some patients with type 2 diabetes. However, the effectiveness of this approach has not yet been demonstrated.

Nursing Management

Nursing management of the patient with diabetes can involve treatment of a wide variety of physiologic disorders, depending on the patient's health status and whether the patient is newly diagnosed or seeks care for an unrelated health problem. Nursing management of the newly diagnosed patient and the patient with diabetes as a secondary diagnosis is presented in subsequent sections of this chapter. Because all diabetic patients must master the concepts and skills necessary for long-term management of diabetes and its potential complications, a solid educational foundation is necessary for competent self-care and is an ongoing focus of nursing care.

EDUCATION

Diabetes mellitus is a chronic illness requiring a lifetime of special self-management behaviours. Because diet, physical activity, and physical and emotional stress affect diabetic control, patients must learn to balance a multitude of factors. They must learn daily self-care skills to prevent acute fluctuations in blood glucose, and they must also incorporate into their lifestyle many preventive behaviours for avoidance of long-term diabetic complications. Diabetic patients must become knowledgeable about nutrition, medication effects and side effects, exercise, disease progression, prevention strategies, blood glucose monitoring techniques, and medication adjustment. In addition, they must learn the skills associated with monitoring and managing diabetes and must incorporate many new activities into their daily routines. An appreciation for the knowledge and skills that diabetic patients must acquire can help the nurse in providing effective patient education and counselling (Beebe & O'Donnell, 2001).

DEVELOPING A DIABETIC TEACHING PLAN

Changes in the health care delivery system as a whole have had a major impact on diabetes education and training. Patients with new-onset type 1 diabetes have much shorter hospital stays or may be managed completely on an outpatient basis; patients with new-onset type 2 diabetes are rarely hospitalized for initial care. There has been a proliferation of outpatient diabetes education and training programs, with increasing support of third-party reimbursement. For some patients, however, exposure to diabetes education during hospitalization may be the only op-

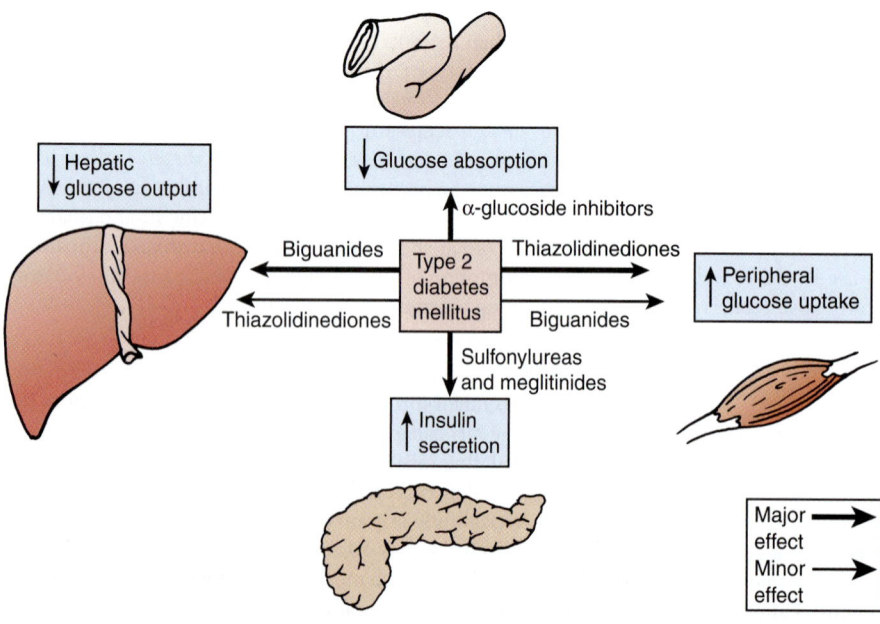

FIGURE 41-5 Sites of action of oral antidiabetic medications.

portunity for learning self-management skills and preventing complications.

Many hospitals employ nurses who specialize in diabetes education and management. However, because of the large number of patients with diabetes who are admitted to every unit of a hospital for reasons other than diabetes or its complications, the staff nurse plays a vital role in identifying diabetic patients, assessing self-care skills, providing basic education, reinforcing the teaching provided by the specialist, and referring patients for follow-up care after discharge.

Organizing Information

There are various strategies for organizing and prioritizing the vast amount of information that must be taught to diabetic patients. In addition, many hospitals and outpatient diabetes centres have devised written guidelines, care plans, and documentation forms (often based on guidelines from the CDA) that may be used to document and evaluate teaching. A general approach is to organize information and skills into two main types: basic, initial, or "survival" skills and information, and in-depth (advanced) or continuing education.

TEACHING SURVIVAL SKILLS

This information must be taught to any patient with newly diagnosed type 1 or type 2 diabetes and any patient receiving insulin for the first time. This basic information is literally what the patient must know to survive—that is, to avoid severe hypoglycemic or acute hyperglycemic complications after discharge. An outline of survival information includes:

1. Simple pathophysiology
   a. Basic definition of diabetes (having a high blood glucose level)
   b. Normal blood glucose ranges and target blood glucose levels
   c. Effect of insulin and exercise (decrease glucose)
   d. Effect of food and stress, including illness and infections (increase glucose)
   e. Basic treatment approaches
2. Treatment modalities
   a. Administration of insulin and oral antidiabetes medications
   b. Diet information (food groups, timing of meals)
   c. Monitoring of blood glucose and ketones
3. Recognition, treatment, and prevention of acute complications
   a. Hypoglycemia
   b. Hyperglycemia
4. Pragmatic information
   a. Where to buy and store insulin, syringes, and glucose monitoring supplies
   b. When and how to reach the physician

For patients with newly diagnosed type 2 diabetes, emphasis is initially placed on diet. Patients starting to take oral sulfonylureas or meglitinides need to know about detecting, preventing, and treating hypoglycemia. If diabetes has gone undetected for many years, the patient may already be experiencing some chronic diabetic complications. Thus, for some patients with newly diagnosed type 2 diabetes, the basic diabetes teaching must include information on preventive skills, such as foot care and eye care—for example, planning yearly or more frequent complete (dilated eye) examinations by the ophthalmologist and under-

standing that retinopathy is largely asymptomatic until the advanced stages.

Patients also need to realize that once they master the basic skills and information, further diabetes education must be pursued. Acquiring in-depth and advanced diabetes knowledge occurs throughout the patient's lifetime, both formally through programs of continuing education and informally through experience and sharing of information with other people with diabetes.

PLANNING IN-DEPTH AND CONTINUING EDUCATION

This involves teaching more detailed information related to survival skills (eg, learning to vary diet and insulin and preparing for travel) as well as learning preventive measures for avoiding long-term diabetic complications. Preventive measures include:

- Foot care
- Eye care
- General hygiene (eg, skin care, oral hygiene)
- Risk factor management (eg, control of blood pressure and blood lipid levels, and normalizing blood glucose levels)

More advanced continuing education may include alternative methods for insulin delivery, such as the insulin pump, and algorithms or rules for evaluating and adjusting insulin doses. For example, patients can be taught to increase or decrease insulin doses based on a several-day pattern of blood glucose levels. The degree of advanced diabetes education to be provided depends on the patient's interest and ability. However, learning preventive measures (especially foot care and eye care) is mandatory for reducing the occurrence of amputations and blindness in diabetic patients.

Assessing Readiness to Learn

Before initiating diabetes education, the nurse assesses the patient's (and family's) readiness to learn (Beebe & O'Donnell, 2001). When patients are first diagnosed with diabetes (or first told of their need for insulin), they often go through various stages of the grieving process. These stages may include shock and denial, anger, depression, negotiation, and acceptance. The amount of time it takes for patients and family members to work through the grieving process varies from patient to patient. They may experience helplessness, guilt, altered body image, loss of self-esteem, and concern about the future. The nurse must assess the patient's coping strategies and reassure patients and families that feelings of depression and shock are normal.

Asking the patient and family about their major concerns or fears is an important way to learn about any misinformation that may be contributing to anxiety. Some common misconceptions regarding diabetes and its treatment are listed in Table 41-5. Simple, direct information should be provided to dispel misconceptions. More information can be provided once the patient masters survival skills.

After dispelling misconceptions or answering questions that concern the patient the most, the nurse focuses attention on concrete survival skills. Because of the immediate need for multiple new skills, teaching is initiated as soon as possible after diagnosis. Nurses whose patients are in the hospital rarely have the luxury of waiting until the patient feels ready to learn; short hospital stays necessitate initiation of survival skill education as early as possible. This gives the patient the opportunity to practice skills with supervision by the nurse before discharge. Follow-up by home health nurses is often necessary for reinforcement of survival skills.

Table 41-5 • Misconceptions Related to Insulin Treatment

MISCONCEPTION	RESPONSE
Once insulin injections are started (for treatment of type 2 diabetes), they can never be discontinued.	During periods of acute stress (eg, illness, infection, or surgery) or when receiving certain medications that cause elevations in blood glucose, some patients with type 2 diabetes require insulin. If the diabetes had previously been well controlled with diet alone or diet with oral antidiabetic agents, the patient should be able to resume previous methods for control of diabetes when the stress is resolved. In addition, insulin is sometimes used to control blood glucose levels in obese type 2 diabetic patients who have been unsuccessful at weight loss. If the patient can lose weight after insulin therapy is initiated, the insulin doses may be tapered and the patient may be able to switch to diet and exercise alone or with oral antidiabetic agents for control of blood glucose. (For patients with type 1 diabetes, insulin is needed on an ongoing basis. For thin patients with type 2 diabetes, once insulin has to be started, it is usually required permanently).
If increasing doses of insulin are needed to control the blood glucose, the diabetes must be getting "worse."	Explain to the patient that unlike other medications that are given in standard doses, there is not a standard dose of insulin that is effective for all patients. Rather, the dose must be adjusted according to blood glucose test results. If the initial insulin dose prescribed for the patient does not adequately decrease the glucose level, the patient may assume that he or she has a "bad" case of diabetes or that the diabetes is getting worse. It is important to instruct patients that many different factors may affect the ability of insulin to lower the glucose, including obesity, puberty, pregnancy, illness, and certain medications. In addition, to avoid hypoglycemia, physicians frequently initiate insulin therapy with smaller dosages than will eventually be needed. The doses are then increased in small increments until blood glucose levels are in the desired range.
Insulin causes blindness (or other diabetic complications).	When patients have a diabetic acquaintance in whom the initiation of insulin therapy happened to coincide with the onset of diabetic complications, the patient may view insulin as the cause of complications such as blindness or amputation. In these situations, the acquaintance probably had type 2 diabetes that was no longer controllable with diet and oral hypoglycemic agents. It must be explained to the patient that factors such as elevated blood glucose (and not insulin therapy) contribute to some of the diabetic complications. Further, emphasize that insulin is a natural hormone that is present in every person's body, helps control blood glucose levels, and definitely does *not* cause long-term complications of diabetes.
Insulin must be injected directly into the vein.	When patients first learn that one area used for insulin injections is on the arm, they may envision inserting the needle directly into a vein in the antecubital area, as in blood withdrawal. The patient must be reassured that insulin is injected into the fat tissue on the *back* of the arm (or on the abdomen, thigh, or hip) and that the needle is much shorter than that used for venipuncture.
There is extreme danger in injecting insulin if there are any air bubbles in the syringe.	Patients may have a fear of dying if air bubbles are injected with a syringe. (This may be related to the misconception that insulin is injected directly into the vein.) Reassure patients that the main danger in having air bubbles in the insulin syringe is that the amount of insulin being injected is less than the required dose. It is often difficult to remove every small "champagne" bubble from the syringe. Thus, patients should be reassured that injection of insulin when these bubbles are present does not cause any harm.
Insulin always causes people to have bad (hypoglycemic) reactions.	First, make sure that patients are aware that low blood sugar reactions are often related to an imbalance with the insulin, food, and activity and can often be avoided. Thus, before starting on insulin, patients should discuss their usual schedule of meals and activities as well as the content of meals with the health care team. Make sure that patients are aware that various different insulins and insulin schedules can be used to try to allow patients to maintain some of their usual lifestyle habits. Reassure patients that avoiding hypoglycemic reactions is a high priority for the diabetes team. In addition, tell patients of the importance of reporting any hypoglycemic reactions to the health care team immediately so that early adjustments can be made in the insulin dosage. Focus early insulin education on treatment and prevention of hypoglycemia.
People who take insulin must travel only where there is a refrigerator to store the insulin.	Insulin bottles in use may be kept at room temperature. Therefore, for most business trips or vacations, keeping the insulin in a purse or briefcase (or special diabetes supply case) is acceptable. If a prolonged trip is planned (more than 2 to 3 months), patients may want to consult the pharmacist or insulin manufacturer for suggestions. Most importantly, emphasize with patients that taking insulin should never deter them from pursuing activities they enjoy.

Pearce, M. A., Rosenberg, C. S., & Davidson, M. B. (1998). Patient education. In M. B. Davidson (Ed.), *Diabetes mellitus: Diagnosis and treatment* (4th ed.). New York: Churchill Livingstone. Reprinted with permission from Elsevier Science.

A major goal of patient teaching is an educated consumer, a patient who is informed about the wide variations in the prices of medications and supplies and about the importance of comparing prices.

Determining Teaching Methods

Maintaining flexibility in teaching approaches is important. Teaching skills and information in a logical sequence is not always the most helpful for patients. For example, many patients fear the injection. Before they learn how to draw up, purchase, store, and mix insulins, they should be taught to insert the needle and inject insulin (or practice with saline solution). Numerous demonstrations by the nurse or practice injections before the patient (or family) gives the first injection may actually increase the patient's anxiety and fear of self-injection. Once patients have actually performed the injection, most are more prepared to hear and to comprehend other information. (If they then want to practice further using a pillow or an orange, that would be appropriate.) Thus, having patients self-inject first or having patients perform a fingerstick for glucose monitoring first may enhance learning to draw up the insulin or to operate the glucose meter. Ample opportunity should be provided for the patient and family to practice skills under supervision (including self-injection, self-testing, meal selection, verbalization of symptoms, and treatment of hypoglycemia). Once skills have been mastered, participation in ongoing support groups may assist patients in incorporating new habits and maintaining adherence to the treatment regimen.

Various tools can be used to complement teaching. Many of the companies that manufacture products for diabetes self-care also provide booklets and videotapes to assist in patient teaching. It is important to use a variety of written handouts that match the patient's learning needs (including different languages, low-literacy information, large print). Patients can continue learning about diabetes care by participating in activities sponsored by local hospitals and diabetes organizations. In addition, magazines with information on all aspects of diabetes management are available for people with diabetes.

IMPLEMENTING THE PLAN

Teaching Experienced Patients with Diabetes

The nurse should continue to assess the skills of patients who have had diabetes for many years, because it is estimated that up to 50% of patients may make errors in self-care. Assessment of these patients must include direct observation of skills, not just their self-report of self-care behaviours. In addition, these patients must be fully aware of preventive measures related to foot care, eye care, and risk factor management. If patients are experiencing long-term diabetic complications for the first time, they may go through the grieving process again. Some of these patients may have a renewed interest in diabetes self-care in the hope of delaying further complications. Other patients may be overwhelmed by feelings of guilt and depression. The patient is encouraged to discuss feelings and fears related to complications; the nurse meanwhile provides appropriate information regarding diabetic complications.

Teaching Patients to Self-Administer Insulin

Insulin injections are administered into the subcutaneous tissue with the use of special insulin syringes. A variety of syringes and injection-aid devices are available. Chart 41-7 provides important information to include and evaluate when teaching patients about insulin. Basic information includes explanation of the equipment, insulins, syringes, and mixing insulin.

STORING INSULIN

Cloudy insulins should be thoroughly mixed by gently inverting the vial or rolling it between the hands before drawing the solution into a syringe or a pen.

Whether insulin is the short- or long-acting preparation, the vials not in use should be refrigerated and extremes of temperature should be avoided; insulin should not be allowed to freeze and should not be kept in direct sunlight or in a hot car. The insulin vial in use should be kept at room temperature to reduce local irritation at the injection site, which may occur when cold insulin is injected. If a vial of insulin will be used up in 1 month, it may be kept at room temperature. Patients should be instructed to always have a spare vial of the type or types of insulin they use. Spare vials should be refrigerated.

Insulin bottles should also be inspected for flocculation, which is a frosted, whitish coating inside the bottle of intermediate- or long-acting insulins. This occurs most commonly with human insulins that are not refrigerated. If a frosted, adherent coating is present, some of the insulin is bound and should not be used.

SELECTING SYRINGES

Syringes must be matched with the insulin concentration (eg, U-100). Currently, three sizes of U-100 insulin syringes are available:

- 1-mL (cc) syringes that hold 100 units
- 0.5-mL syringes that hold 50 units
- 0.3-mL syringes that hold 30 units

The concentration of insulin used in Canada is U-100; that is, there are 100 units per millilitre (or cubic centimeter). Syringe size varies. Small syringes allow patients who require small amounts of insulin to measure and draw up the amount of insulin accurately. Patients who require large amounts of insulin would use larger syringes. Although there is a U-500 (500 units/mL) concentration of insulin available by special order for patients who have severe insulin resistance and require massive doses of insulin, it is rarely used.

Most insulin syringes have a disposable 27- to 29-gauge needle that is approximately 13 mm long. The smaller syringes are marked in 1-unit increments and may be easier to use for patients with visual deficits or patients taking very small doses of insulin. The 1-mL syringes are marked in 2-unit increments. A small disposable insulin needle (29- to 30-gauge, 8 mm long) is available for very thin patients and children.

PREPARING THE INJECTION: MIXING INSULINS

When rapid- or short-acting insulins are to be given simultaneously with longer-acting insulins, they are usually mixed together in the same syringe; the longer-acting insulins must be mixed thoroughly before use. There is some question as to whether the two insulins are stable if the mixture is kept in the syringe for more than 5 to 15 minutes. This may depend on the ratio of the insulins as well as the time between mixing and injecting. When regular insulin is mixed with long-acting insulin, there is a binding reaction that slows the action of the regular insulin. This may also occur to a greater degree when mixing regular insulin with one of the Lente insulins. Patients are advised to consult their

Chart 41-7 • PATIENT EDUCATION
Self-Injection of Insulin

1. With one hand, stabilize the skin by spreading it or pinching up a large area.

Pinching the skin

2. Pick up syringe with the other hand and hold it as you would a pencil. Insert needle straight into the skin.*

Inserting the needle into the skin

3. To inject the insulin, push the plunger all the way in.

Injecting the insulin

4. Pull needle straight out of skin. Press cotton ball over injection site for several seconds.

Removing the needle and holding cotton ball over site

5. Use disposable syringe *only once* and discard into hard plastic container (with a tight-fitting top) such as an empty bleach or detergent container.† Follow provincial regulations for disposal of syringes and needles.

Disposing of syringe

---

*Some patients may be taught to insert the needle at a 45-degree angle.
†Although some studies suggest that reusing disposable syringes may be safe, it is recommended that this be done only in the absence of poor personal hygiene, an acute concurrent illness, open wounds on the hands, or decreased resistance to infection.

---

health care provider for advice on this matter. The most important issue is that patients be consistent in how they prepare their insulin injections from day to day.

While there are varying opinions regarding which type of insulin (short- or longer-acting) should be drawn up into the syringe first when they are going to be mixed, the Canadian Diabetes Association recommends that the regular insulin be drawn up first. The most important issues are, again, that patients be consistent in technique so as not to draw up the wrong dose accidentally or the wrong type of insulin, and that patients not inject one type of insulin into the bottle containing a different type of insulin.

For patients who have difficulty mixing insulins, two options are available: they may use a premixed insulin, or they may have prefilled syringes prepared. For patients who can inject insulin but who have difficulty drawing up a single or mixed dose, syringes can be prefilled with the help of home care nurses or fam-

ily and friends. A 3-week supply of insulin syringes may be prepared and kept in the refrigerator. The prefilled syringes should be stored with the needle in an upright position to avoid clogging of the needle.

WITHDRAWING INSULIN
Most (if not all) of the printed materials available on insulin dose preparation instruct patients to inject air into the bottle of insulin equivalent to the number of units of insulin to be withdrawn. The rationale for this is to prevent the formation of a vacuum inside the bottle, which would make it difficult to withdraw the proper amount of insulin. Some nurses who specialize in diabetes report that some patients (who have been taking insulin for many years) have stopped injecting air before withdrawing the insulin. These patients found that the extra step was not necessary for accurately drawing up the insulin dose. Most patients find it easier

to withdraw the insulin by eliminating the step and report no difficulty in preparing the proper insulin dose.

Eliminating this step (or alternating it by, for instance, injecting a syringe full of air into the vial once per week) facilitates the teaching process for some patients learning to draw up insulin for the first time. Some patients become confused with the sequence of steps involved in injecting air into two separate bottles in two different amounts before drawing up a mixed dose. For many individuals, including elderly ones, simplifying the procedure for preparing insulin injections may help them maintain independence in daily living.

As with other variations in insulin injection technique, the most important factors are that the patient maintain consistency in the procedure and that the nurse be flexible when teaching new patients or assessing the skills of experienced patients.

SELECTING AND ROTATING THE INJECTION SITE

The four main areas for injection are the abdomen, arms (posterior surface), thighs (anterior surface), and hips (Fig. 41-6). Insulin is absorbed faster in some areas of the body than others. The speed of absorption is greatest in the abdomen and decreases progressively in the arm, thigh, and hip.

Systematic rotation of injection sites within an anatomic area is recommended to prevent localized changes in fatty tissue (lipodystrophy). In addition, to promote consistency in insulin absorption, patients should be encouraged to use all available injection sites within one area rather than randomly rotating sites from area to area (Canadian Diabetes Association, 2003). For example, some patients almost exclusively use the abdominal area, administering each injection 1–2 cm away from the previous injection. Another approach to rotation is always to use the same area at the same time of day. For example, patients may inject

morning doses into the abdomen and evening doses into the arms or legs.

A few general principles apply to all rotation patterns. First, patients should try not to use the same site more than once in 2 to 3 weeks. In addition, if the patient is planning to exercise, insulin should not be injected into the limb that will be exercised, because it will be absorbed faster, and this may result in hypoglycemia.

In the past, patients were taught to rotate injections from one area to the next (eg, injecting once in the right arm, then once in the right abdomen, then once in the right thigh). Patients who still use this system must be taught to avoid repeated injections into the same site within an area. However, as previously stated, it is preferable for the patient to use the same anatomic area at the same time of day consistently; this reduces day-to-day variation in blood glucose levels because of different absorption rates.

PREPARING THE SKIN

Use of alcohol to cleanse the skin is not recommended, but patients who have learned this technique often continue to use it. They should be cautioned to allow the skin to dry after cleansing with alcohol. If the skin is not allowed to dry before the injection, the alcohol may be carried into the tissues, resulting in a localized reddened area.

INSERTING THE NEEDLE

There are varying approaches to inserting the needle for insulin injections. The correct technique is based on the need for the insulin to be injected into the subcutaneous tissue. Injection that is too deep (eg, intramuscular) or too shallow may affect the rate of absorption of the insulin. Aspiration (inserting the needle and then pulling back on the plunger to assess for blood being drawn into the syringe) is generally not recommended with self-injection of insulin. Many patients who have been using insulin for an extended period have eliminated this step from their insulin injection routine with no apparent adverse effects.

PROMOTING HOME AND COMMUNITY-BASED CARE

Teaching Patients Self-Care. Adherence to the therapeutic plan is the most important goal of self-care the patient must master. Patients who are having difficulty adhering to the diabetes treatment plan must be approached with care and understanding. Using scare tactics (such as threats of blindness or amputation if the patient does not adhere to the treatment plan) or making the patient feel guilty is not productive and may interfere with establishing a trusting relationship with the patient. Judgmental actions, such as asking the patient if he or she has "cheated" on the diet, only promote feelings of guilt and low self-esteem.

If problems exist with glucose control or with the development of preventable complications, it is important to distinguish among nonadherence, knowledge deficit, and self-care deficit. It should not be assumed that problems with diabetes management are related to nonadherence. The patient may simply have forgotten or never learned certain information. The problem may be correctable simply through providing complete information and ensuring that the patient comprehends the information. Chart 41-8 details how to evaluate the effectiveness of self-injection of insulin.

If knowledge deficit is not the problem, certain physical or emotional factors may be impairing the patient's ability to perform self-care skills. For example, decreased visual acuity may impair the patient's ability to administer insulin accurately, measure the blood

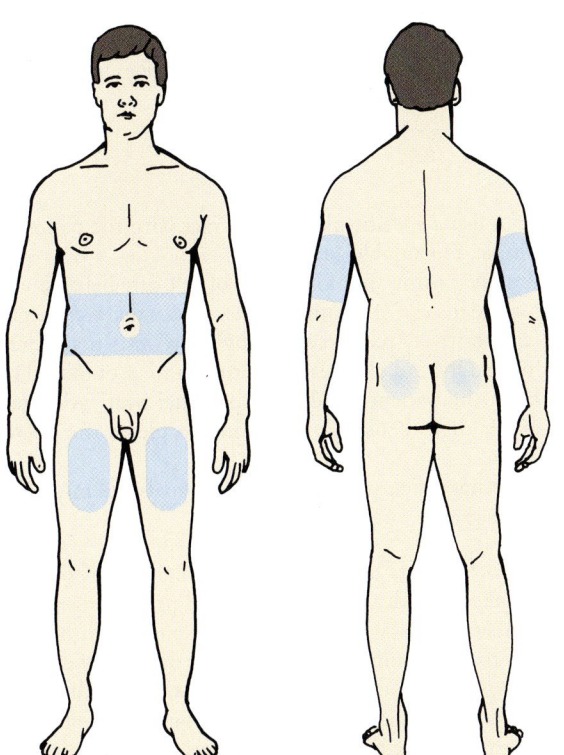

FIGURE 41-6 Suggested areas for insulin injection.

Chart 41-8   **Outcome Criteria for Determining Effectiveness of Self-Injection of Insulin Education**

Equipment

Insulin

1. Identifies information on label of insulin bottle:
   - Type (eg, NPH, regular, 70/30)
   - Species (human, biosynthetic, pork)
   - Concentration (eg, U-100)
   - Expiration date
2. Checks appearance of insulin:
   - Clear or milky white
   - Checks for flocculation (clumping, frosted appearance)
3. Identifies where to purchase and store insulin:
   - Indicates approximately how long bottle will last (1,000 units per bottle U-100 insulin)
   - Indicates how long opened bottles can be used

Syringes

1. Identifies concentration (U-100) marking on syringe
2. Identifies size of syringe (eg, 100-unit, 50-unit, 30-unit)
3. Describes appropriate disposal of used syringe

Preparation and Administration of Insulin Injection

1. Draws up correct amount and type of insulin
2. Properly mixes two insulins if necessary
3. Inserts needle and injects insulin
4. Describes site rotation:
   - Demonstrates injection with all anatomic areas to be used
   - Describes pattern for rotation, such as using abdomen only or using certain areas at the same time of day
   - Describes system for remembering site locations, such as horizontal pattern across the abdomen as if drawing a dotted line

Knowledge of Insulin Action

1. Lists prescription:
   - Type and dosage of insulin
   - Timing of insulin injections
2. Describes approximate time course of insulin action:
   - Identifies long- and short-acting insulins by name
   - States approximate time delay until onset of insulin action
   - Identifies need to delay food until 15 to 30 minutes after injection of rapid-acting insulin (lispro, aspart).

- Knows that longer time delays are safe when blood glucose level is high, and time delays may need to be shortened when blood glucose level is low

Incorporation of Insulin Injections Into Daily Schedule

1. Recites proper order of premeal diabetes activities:
   - May use mnemonic device such as the word "tie," which helps the patient remember the order of activities ("t" = test [blood glucose], "i" = insulin injection, "e" = eat)
   - Describes daily schedule, such as test, insulin, eat, before breakfast and dinner; test and eat, before lunch and bedtime
2. Describes information regarding hypoglycemia:
   - Symptoms: shakiness, sweating, nervousness, hunger, weakness
   - Causes: too much insulin, too much exercise, not enough food
   - Treatment: 15 g concentrated carbohydrate, such as two or three glucose tablets, 1 tube glucose gel, 0.5 cup (125 mL) of juice
   - After initial treatment, follow with snack including starch and protein, such as cheese and crackers, milk and crackers, half sandwich.
3. Describes information regarding prevention of hypoglycemia:
   - Avoid delays in meal timing.
   - Eat a meal or snack approximately every 4 to 5 hours (while awake).
   - Do not skip meals.
   - Increase food intake before exercise if blood glucose level is < 5 mmol/L
   - Check blood glucose regularly.
   - Change insulin doses only with medical supervision.
   - Carry a form of fast-acting sugar at all times.
   - Wear a medical identification bracelet.
   - Teach family, friends, coworkers about signs and treatment of hypoglycemia.
   - Have family, roommates, traveling companions learn to use injectable glucagon for severe hypoglycemic reactions.
4. Maintains regular follow-up for evaluation of diabetes control:
   - Keeps written record of blood glucose, insulin doses, hypoglycemic reactions, variations in diet
   - Keeps all appointments with health professionals
   - Sees physician regularly (usually two to four times per year)
   - States how to contact physician in case of emergency
   - States when to call physician to report variations in blood glucose levels

---

glucose level, or inspect the skin and feet. In addition, decreased joint mobility (especially in the elderly) impairs the ability to inspect the bottom of the feet. Emotional factors such as denial of the diagnosis or depression may impair the patient's ability to carry out multiple daily self-care measures. In other circumstances, family, personal, or work problems may be of higher priority to the patient. The patient facing competing demands for time and attention may benefit from assistance in establishing priorities. It is also important to assess the patient for infection or emotional stress that may lead to elevated blood glucose levels despite adherence to the treatment regimen.

The following approaches by the nurse are helpful for promoting self-care management skills:

- Address any underlying factors (eg, knowledge deficit, self-care deficit, illness) that may affect diabetic control.
- Simplify the treatment regimen if it is too difficult for the patient to follow.
- Adjust the treatment regimen to meet patient requests (eg, adjust diet or insulin schedule to allow increased flexibility in meal content or timing).

- Establish a specific plan or contract with the patient with simple, measurable goals.
- Provide positive reinforcement of self-care behaviours performed instead of focusing on behaviours that were neglected (eg, positively reinforce blood glucose tests that were performed instead of focusing on the number of missed tests).
- Help the patient to identify personal motivating factors rather than focusing on wanting to please the doctor or nurse.
- Encourage the patient to pursue life goals and interests; discourage an undue focus on diabetes.

Continuing Care. As discussed, continuing care of the patient with diabetes is critical in managing and preventing complications. The degree to which the client interacts with health care providers to obtain ongoing care depends on many factors. Age, socioeconomic level, existing complications, type of diabetes, and comorbid conditions all may dictate the frequency of follow-up visits. Many patients with diabetes may be seen by home health nurses for diabetic education, wound care, insulin preparation, or assistance with glucose monitoring. Even patients who achieve excellent glucose control and have no complications can expect to see their primary health care provider at least twice a year for ongoing evaluation.

In addition to follow-up care with health professionals, participation in support groups is encouraged for those who have had diabetes for many years as well as those who are newly diagnosed. Such participation may assist the patient and family in coping with changes in lifestyle that occur with the onset of diabetes and with its complications. Those who participate in support groups often have an opportunity to share valuable information and experiences and to learn from others. Support groups provide an opportunity for discussion of strategies to deal with diabetes and its management and to clarify and verify information with the nurse or other health care professionals. Participation in support groups may help patients and their families to become more knowledgeable about diabetes and its management and may promote adherence to the management plan. Another very important role of the nurse is to remind the patient about the importance of participating in other health promotion activities and recommended health screening.

Acute Complications of Diabetes

There are three major acute complications of diabetes related to short-term imbalances in blood glucose levels: hypoglycemia, DKA, and HHNS, which is also called hyperglycemic hyperosmolar nonketotic coma or hyperglycemic hyperosmolar syndrome.

HYPOGLYCEMIA (INSULIN REACTIONS)

Hypoglycemia (abnormally low blood glucose level) occurs when the blood glucose falls to less than 2.7 to 3.3 mmol/L. It can be caused by too much insulin or oral hypoglycemic agents, too little food, or excessive physical activity. Hypoglycemia may occur at any time of the day or night. It often occurs before meals, especially if meals are delayed or snacks are omitted. For example, midmorning hypoglycemia may occur when the morning regular insulin is peaking, whereas hypoglycemia that occurs in the late afternoon coincides with the peak of the morning NPH or Lente insulin. Middle-of-the-night hypoglycemia may occur because of peaking evening or predinner NPH or Lente insulins, especially in patients who have not eaten a bedtime snack.

Clinical Manifestations

The clinical manifestations of hypoglycemia may be grouped into two categories: adrenergic symptoms and central nervous system (CNS) symptoms. In mild hypoglycemia, as the blood glucose level falls, the sympathetic nervous system is stimulated, resulting in a surge of epinephrine and norepinephrine. This causes symptoms such as sweating, tremor, tachycardia, palpitation, nervousness, and hunger.

In moderate hypoglycemia, the fall in blood glucose level deprives the brain cells of needed fuel for functioning. Signs of impaired function of the CNS may include inability to concentrate, headache, lightheadedness, confusion, memory lapses, numbness of the lips and tongue, slurred speech, impaired coordination, emotional changes, irrational or combative behaviour, double vision, and drowsiness. Any combination of these symptoms (in addition to adrenergic symptoms) may occur with moderate hypoglycemia.

In severe hypoglycemia, CNS function is so impaired that the patient needs the assistance of another person for treatment of hypoglycemia. Symptoms may include disoriented behaviour, seizures, difficulty arousing from sleep, or loss of consciousness

Assessment and Diagnostic Findings

Hypoglycemic symptoms can occur suddenly and unexpectedly. The combination of symptoms varies considerably from person to person. To some degree, this may be related to the actual level to which the blood glucose drops or to the rate at which it is dropping. For example, patients who usually have a blood glucose level in the hyperglycemic range (eg, 10.5 mmol/L or greater) may feel hypoglycemic (adrenergic) symptoms when their blood glucose quickly drops to 6.6 mmol/L or less. Conversely, patients who frequently have a glucose level in the low range of normal may be asymptomatic when the blood glucose slowly falls to less than 2.7 mmol/L.

Another factor contributing to altered hypoglycemic symptoms is a decreased hormonal (adrenergic) response to hypoglycemia. This occurs in some patients who have had diabetes for many years. It may be related to one of the chronic diabetic complications, autonomic neuropathy (see the section in this chapter on hypoglycemic unawareness). As the blood glucose level falls, the normal surge in adrenalin does not occur. The patient does not feel the usual adrenergic symptoms, such as sweating and shakiness. The hypoglycemia may not be detected until moderate or severe CNS impairment occurs. These patients must perform SMBG on a frequent regular basis, especially before driving or engaging in other potentially dangerous activities.

Gerontologic Considerations

In the elderly diabetic patient, hypoglycemia is a particular concern for many reasons:

- Elderly people frequently live alone and may not recognize the symptoms of hypoglycemia.
- With decreasing renal function, it takes longer for oral hypoglycemic agents to be excreted by the kidneys.
- Skipping meals may occur because of decreased appetite or financial limitations.
- Decreased visual acuity may lead to errors in insulin administration.

Management

Immediate treatment must be given when hypoglycemia occurs. The usual recommendation is for 15 g of a fast-acting concentrated source of carbohydrate such as the following, given orally:

- Three or four commercially prepared glucose tablets
- 120–180 mL of fruit juice or regular soft drink
- 6 to 10 Life Savers or other hard candies
- 2 to 3 teaspoons of sugar or honey

It is not necessary to add sugar to juice, even if it is labelled as unsweetened juice: the fruit sugar in juice contains enough carbohydrate to raise the blood glucose level. Adding table sugar to juice may cause a sharp increase in the blood glucose level, and the patient may experience hyperglycemia for hours after treatment.

The blood glucose level should be retested in 15 minutes and retreated if it is less than 3.8 to 4 mmol/L. If the symptoms persist more than 10 to 15 minutes after initial treatment, the treatment is repeated even if blood glucose testing is not possible. Once the symptoms resolve, a snack containing protein and starch (eg, milk or cheese and crackers) is recommended unless the patient plans to eat a regular meal or snack within 30 to 60 minutes.

TEACHING PATIENTS

It is important for patients with diabetes, especially those receiving insulin, to learn that they must carry some form of simple sugar with them at all times (Canadian Diabetes Association, 2003). There are many different commercially prepared glucose tablets and gels that patients may find convenient to carry. If the patient has a hypoglycemic reaction and does not have any of the recommended emergency foods available, any available food (preferably a carbohydrate food) should be eaten.

Patients are advised to refrain from eating high-calorie, high-fat dessert foods (eg, cookies, cakes, doughnuts, ice cream) to treat hypoglycemia. The high fat content of these foods may slow the absorption of the glucose, and the hypoglycemic symptoms may not resolve as quickly as they would with the intake of carbohydrates. The patient may subsequently eat more of the foods when symptoms do not resolve rapidly. This in turn may cause very high blood glucose levels for several hours after the reaction and may also contribute to weight gain.

Patients who feel unduly restricted by their meal plan may view hypoglycemic episodes as a time to reward themselves with desserts. It may be more prudent to teach these patients to incorporate occasional desserts into the meal plan. This may make it easier for them to limit their treatment of hypoglycemic episodes to simple (low-calorie) carbohydrates such as juice or glucose tablets.

INITIATING EMERGENCY MEASURES

For patients who are unconscious and cannot swallow, an injection of glucagon 1 mg can be administered either subcutaneously or intramuscularly. Glucagon is a hormone produced by the alpha cells of the pancreas that stimulates the liver to release glucose (through the breakdown of glycogen, the stored glucose). Injectable glucagon is packaged as a powder in 1-mg vials and must be mixed with a diluent before being injected. After injection of glucagon, it may take up to 20 minutes for the patient to regain consciousness. A concentrated source of carbohydrate followed by a snack should be given to the patient on awakening to prevent recurrence of hypoglycemia (because the duration of the action of 1 mg of glucagon is brief [its onset is 8 to 10 minutes and its action lasts 12 to 27 minutes]) and to replenish liver stores of glucose. Some patients experience nausea after the administration of glucagon; if this occurs, the patient should be turned to the side to prevent aspiration. The patient should be instructed to notify the physician after severe hypoglycemia has occurred.

Glucagon is sold by prescription only and should be part of the emergency supplies kept available by patients with diabetes who require insulin. Family members, neighbours, or coworkers should be instructed in the use of glucagon. This is especially true for patients who receive little or no warning of hypoglycemic episodes.

In the hospital or emergency department, patients who are unconscious or cannot swallow may be treated with 25 to 50 mL 50% dextrose in water ($D_{50}W$) administered intravenously. The effect is usually seen within minutes. Patients may complain of a headache and of pain at the injection site. Assuring patency of the intravenous (IV) line used for injection of 50% dextrose is essential because hypertonic solutions such as 50% dextrose are very irritating to the vein.

PROMOTING HOME AND COMMUNITY-BASED CARE

Teaching Patients Self-Care. Hypoglycemia is prevented by a consistent pattern of eating, administering insulin, and exercising. Between-meal and bedtime snacks may be needed to counteract the maximum insulin effect. In general, the patient should cover the time of peak activity of insulin by eating a snack and by taking additional food when physical activity is increased. Routine blood glucose tests are performed so that changing insulin requirements may be anticipated and the dosage adjusted. Because unexpected hypoglycemia may occur, all patients treated with insulin should wear an identification bracelet or tag stating that they have diabetes.

Patients and family members must be instructed about the symptoms of hypoglycemia. Family members in particular must be made aware that any subtle (but unusual) change in behaviour may be an indication of hypoglycemia. They should be taught to encourage and even insist that the person with diabetes assess blood glucose levels if hypoglycemia is suspected. Some patients (when hypoglycemic) become very resistant to testing or eating and become angry at family members trying to treat the hypoglycemia. Family members must be taught to persevere and to understand that the hypoglycemia can cause irrational behaviour.

Some patients with autonomic neuropathy or those taking beta blockers such as propranolol to treat hypertension or cardiac dysrhythmias may not experience the typical symptoms of hypoglycemia. It is very important for these patients to perform blood glucose tests on a frequent and regular basis. Patients who have type 2 diabetes and who take oral sulfonylurea agents may also develop hypoglycemia (especially those taking chlorpropamide, a long-lasting oral hypoglycemic agent).

DIABETIC KETOACIDOSIS

DKA is caused by an absence or markedly inadequate amount of insulin. This deficit in available insulin results in disorders in the metabolism of carbohydrate, protein, and fat. The three main clinical features of DKA are:

- Hyperglycemia
- Dehydration and electrolyte loss
- Acidosis

Pathophysiology

Without insulin, the amount of glucose entering the cells is reduced and the liver increases glucose production. Both factors lead to hyperglycemia. In an attempt to rid the body of the excess glucose, the kidneys excrete the glucose along with water and electrolytes (eg, sodium and potassium). This osmotic diuresis, which is characterized by excessive urination (polyuria), leads to dehydration and marked electrolyte loss. Patients with severe DKA may lose up to 6.5 litres of water and up to 400 to 500 mmol/L each of sodium, potassium, and chloride over a 24-hour period.

Another effect of insulin deficiency or deficit is the breakdown of fat (lipolysis) into free fatty acids and glycerol. The free fatty acids are converted into ketone bodies by the liver. In DKA there is excessive production of ketone bodies because of the lack of insulin that would normally prevent this from occurring. Ketone bodies are acids; their accumulation in the circulation leads to metabolic acidosis.

Three main causes of DKA are decreased or missed dose of insulin, illness or infection, and undiagnosed and untreated diabetes (DKA may be the initial manifestation of diabetes). An insulin deficit may result from an insufficient dosage of insulin prescribed or from insufficient insulin being administered by the patient. Errors in insulin dosage may be made by patients who are ill and who assume that if they are eating less or if they are vomiting, they must decrease their insulin doses. (Because illness, especially infections, may cause increased blood glucose levels, patients do not need to decrease their insulin doses to compensate for decreased food intake when ill and may even need to increase the insulin dose.)

Other potential causes of decreased insulin include patient error in drawing up or injecting insulin (especially in patients with visual impairments), intentional skipping of insulin doses (especially in adolescents with diabetes who are having difficulty coping with diabetes or other aspects of their lives), or equipment problems (eg, occlusion of insulin pump tubing).

Illness and infections are associated with insulin resistance. In response to physical (and emotional) stressors, there is an increase in the level of "stress" hormones—glucagon, epinephrine, norepinephrine, cortisol, and growth hormone. These hormones promote glucose production by the liver and interfere with glucose utilization by muscle and fat tissue, counteracting the effect of insulin. If insulin levels are not increased during times of illness and infection, hyperglycemia may progress to DKA (Quinn, 2001c).

Clinical Manifestations

The signs and symptoms of DKA are listed in Figure 41-7. The hyperglycemia of DKA leads to polyuria and polydipsia (increased thirst). In addition, patients may experience blurred vision, weakness, and headache. Patients with marked intravascular volume depletion may have orthostatic hypotension (drop in systolic blood pressure of 20 mm Hg or more on standing). Volume depletion may also lead to frank hypotension with a weak, rapid pulse.

The ketosis and acidosis of DKA lead to GI symptoms such as anorexia, nausea, vomiting, and abdominal pain. The abdominal pain and physical findings on examination can be so severe that they resemble an acute abdominal disorder that requires surgery. Patients may have acetone breath (a fruity odour), which occurs with elevated ketone levels. In addition, hyperventilation (with very deep, but not laboured, respirations) may occur. These Kussmaul respirations represent the body's attempt to decrease the acidosis, counteracting the effect of the ketone buildup. In addition, mental status changes in DKA vary widely from patient to patient. Patients may be alert, lethargic, or comatose, most likely depending on the plasma osmolarity (concentration of osmotically active particles).

Assessment and Diagnostic Findings

Blood glucose levels may vary from 16.6 to 44.4 mmol/L. Some patients have lower glucose values, and others have values of 55.5 mmol/L or more (usually depending on the degree of dehydration). The severity of DKA is not necessarily related to the blood glucose level. Some patients may have severe acidosis with modestly elevated blood glucose levels, whereas others may have no evidence of DKA despite blood glucose levels of 22.2 to 27.7 mmol/L (Quinn, 2001c).

Evidence of ketoacidosis is reflected in low serum bicarbonate (0 to 15 mmol/L) and low pH (6.8 to 7.3) values. A low PCO_2 level (10 to 30 mm Hg) reflects respiratory compensation (Kussmaul respirations) for the metabolic acidosis. Accumulation of ketone bodies (which precipitates the acidosis) is reflected in blood and urine ketone measurements.

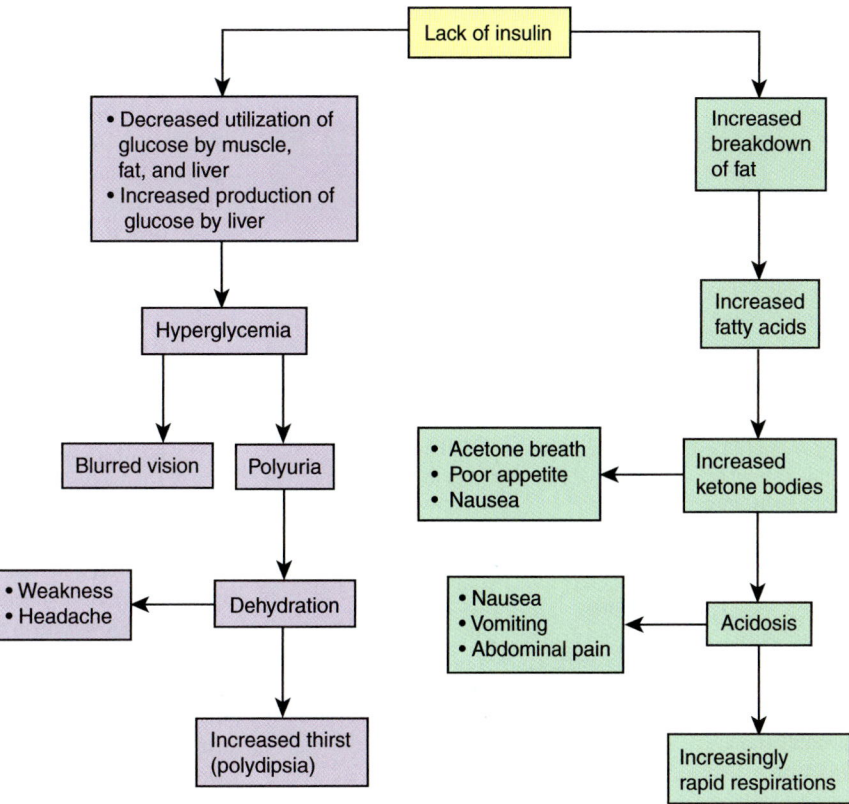

FIGURE 41-7 Abnormal metabolism that causes signs and symptoms of diabetic ketoacidosis. Pearce, M. A., Rosenberg, C. S., & Davidson, M. D. (1998). Patient education. In M. B. Davidson (Ed.). *Diabetes mellitus: Diagnosis and treatment.* New York: Churchill Livingstone.

Sodium and potassium levels may be low, normal, or high, depending on the amount of water loss (dehydration). Despite the plasma concentration, there has been a marked total body depletion of these (and other) electrolytes. Ultimately, these electrolytes will need to be replaced.

Elevated levels of creatinine, blood urea nitrogen (BUN), hemoglobin, and hematocrit may also be seen with dehydration. After rehydration, continued elevation in the serum creatinine and BUN levels will be present in the patient with underlying renal insufficiency.

Prevention

For prevention of DKA related to illness, patients must be taught "sick day" rules for managing their diabetes when ill (Chart 41-9). The most important issue to teach patients is not to eliminate insulin doses when nausea and vomiting occur. Rather, they should take their usual insulin dose (or previously prescribed special "sick day" doses) and then attempt to consume frequent small portions of carbohydrates (including foods usually avoided, such as juices, regular sodas, and gelatin). Drinking fluids every hour is important to prevent dehydration. Blood glucose and urine ketones must be assessed every 3 to 4 hours.

If the patient cannot take fluids without vomiting, or if elevated glucose or ketone levels persist, the physician must be contacted. Patients are taught to have available foods for use on sick days. In addition, a supply of urine test strips (for ketone testing) and blood glucose test strips should be available. Patients must know how to contact their physician 24 hours a day.

Diabetes self-management skills (including insulin administration and blood glucose testing) should be assessed to ensure that an error in insulin administration or blood glucose testing did not occur. Psychological counselling is recommended for patients and family members if an intentional alteration in insulin dosing was the cause of the DKA.

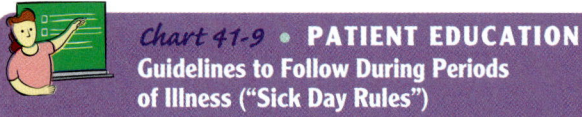

Chart 41-9 • PATIENT EDUCATION
Guidelines to Follow During Periods of Illness ("Sick Day Rules")

- Take insulin or oral antihyperglycemic agents as usual.
- Test blood glucose and test urine ketones every 3 to 4 hours.
- Report elevated glucose levels (greater than 16.6 mmol/L or as otherwise specified) or urine ketones to the physician.
- Insulin-requiring patients may need supplemental doses of regular insulin every 3 to 4 hours.
- If usual meal plan cannot be followed, substitute soft foods (eg, ⅓ cup [80 mL] regular gelatin, 1 cup [250 mL] cream soup, ½ cup [125 mL] custard, 3 squares of graham crackers) six to eight times per day.
- If vomiting, diarrhea, or fever persists, take liquids (eg, ½ cup [125 mL] regular cola or orange juice, ½ cup [125 mL] broth, 1 cup [250 mL] Gatorade) every ½ to 1 hour to prevent dehydration and to provide calories.
- Report nausea, vomiting, and diarrhea to the physician, because extreme fluid loss may be dangerous.
- For patients with type 1 diabetes, inability to retain oral fluids, may warrant hospitalization to avoid diabetic ketoacidosis and possibly coma.

Medical Management

In addition to treating hyperglycemia, management of DKA is aimed at correcting dehydration, electrolyte loss, and acidosis (Quinn, 2001c).

REHYDRATION

In dehydrated patients, rehydration is important for maintaining tissue perfusion. In addition, fluid replacement enhances the excretion of excessive glucose by the kidneys. Patients may need up to 6 to 10 litres of IV fluid to replace fluid losses caused by polyuria, hyperventilation, diarrhea, and vomiting.

Initially, 0.9% sodium chloride (normal saline) solution is administered at a rapid rate, usually 0.5 to 1 L per hour for 2 to 3 hours. Half-strength normal saline (0.45%) solution (also known as hypotonic saline solution) may be used for patients with hypertension or hypernatremia or those at risk for heart failure. After the first few hours, half-normal saline solution is the fluid of choice for continued rehydration, if the blood pressure is stable and the sodium level is not low. Moderate to high rates of infusion (200 to 500 mL per hour) may continue for several more hours. When the blood glucose level reaches 16.6 mmol/L or less, the IV fluid may be changed to dextrose 5% in water (D_5W) to prevent a precipitous decline in the blood glucose level (ADA, Hyperglycemic Crisis in Patients with Diabetes Mellitus, 2003).

Monitoring fluid volume status involves frequent measurements of vital signs (including monitoring for orthostatic changes in blood pressure and heart rate), lung assessment, and monitoring intake and output. Initial urine output will lag behind IV fluid intake as dehydration is corrected. Plasma expanders may be necessary to correct severe hypotension that does not respond to IV fluid treatment. Monitoring for signs of fluid overload is especially important for older patients, those with renal impairment, or those at risk for heart failure.

RESTORING ELECTROLYTES

The major electrolyte of concern during treatment of DKA is potassium. Although the initial plasma concentration of potassium may be low, normal, or even high, there is a major loss of potassium from body stores and an intracellular to extracellular shift of potassium. Further, the serum level of potassium drops during the course of treatment of DKA as potassium re-enters the cells; therefore, it must be monitored frequently. Some of the factors related to treating DKA that reduce the serum potassium concentration include:

- Rehydration, which leads to increased plasma volume and subsequent decreases in the concentration of serum potassium. Rehydration also leads to increased urinary excretion of potassium.
- Insulin administration, which enhances the movement of potassium from the extracellular fluid into the cells.

Cautious but timely potassium replacement is vital to avoid dysrhythmias that may occur with hypokalemia. Up to 40 mmol/L per hour may be needed for several hours. Because extracellular potassium levels drop during DKA treatment, potassium must be infused even if the plasma potassium level is normal.

Frequent (every 2 to 4 hours initially) electrocardiograms and laboratory measurements of potassium are necessary during the first 8 hours of treatment. Potassium replacement is withheld only if hyperkalemia is present or if the patient is not urinating.

NURSING ALERT Because the patient's serum potassium level may drop quickly due to rehydration and insulin treatment, potassium replacement must begin once potassium levels drop to normal.

REVERSING ACIDOSIS

Ketone bodies (acids) accumulate as a result of fat breakdown. The acidosis that occurs in DKA is reversed with insulin, which inhibits fat breakdown, thereby stopping acid buildup. Insulin is usually infused intravenously at a slow, continuous rate (eg, 5 units per hour). Hourly blood glucose values must be measured. IV fluid solutions with higher concentrations of glucose, such as normal saline (NS) solution (eg, D_5NS or $D_{50}.45NS$), are administered when blood glucose levels reach 13.8 to 16.6 mmol/L to avoid too rapid a drop in the blood glucose level.

Various IV mixtures of regular insulin may be used. The nurse must convert hourly rates of insulin infusion (frequently prescribed as "units per hour") to IV drip rates. For example, if 100 units of regular insulin are mixed in 500 mL 0.9% NS, then 1 unit of insulin equals 5 mL. Thus, an initial insulin infusion rate of 5 units per hour would equal 25 mL per hour. The insulin is often infused separately from the rehydration solutions to allow frequent changes in the rate and content of rehydration solutions.

 NURSING ALERT When mixing the insulin drip, it is important to flush the insulin solution through the entire IV infusion set and to discard the first 50 mL of fluid. Insulin molecules adhere to the inner surface of IV infusion sets; thus, the initial fluid may contain a decreased concentration of insulin.

Insulin must be infused continuously until subcutaneous administration of insulin resumes. Any interruption in administration may result in the reaccumulation of ketone bodies and worsening acidosis. Even if blood glucose levels are dropping to normal, the insulin drip must not be stopped; rather, the rate or concentration of the dextrose infusion should be increased. Blood glucose levels are usually corrected before the acidosis is corrected. Thus, IV insulin may be continued for 12 to 24 hours until the serum bicarbonate level improves (to at least 15 to 18 mmol/L) and until the patient can eat. In general, bicarbonate infusion to correct severe acidosis is avoided during treatment of DKA because it precipitates further, sudden (and potentially fatal) decreases in serum potassium levels. Continuous insulin infusion is usually sufficient for reversing DKA.

Nursing Management

Nursing care of the patient with DKA focuses on monitoring fluid and electrolyte status as well as blood glucose levels; administering fluids, insulin, and other medications; and preventing other complications such as fluid overload. Urine output is monitored to ensure adequate renal function before potassium is administered to prevent hyperkalemia. The electrocardiogram is monitored for dysrhythmias indicating abnormal potassium levels. Vital signs, arterial blood gases, and other clinical findings are recorded on a flow sheet. The nurse documents the patient's laboratory values and the frequent changes in fluids and medications that are prescribed and monitors the patient's responses. As DKA resolves and the potassium replacement rate is decreased, the nurse makes sure that:

- There are no signs of hyperkalemia on the electrocardiogram (tall, peaked [or tented] T waves).
- The laboratory values of potassium are normal or low.
- The patient is urinating (ie, no renal shutdown).

As the patient recovers, the nurse reassesses the factors that may have led to DKA and teaches the patient and family about strategies to prevent its recurrence (Quinn, 2001c). If indicated, the nurse initiates a referral for home care to ensure the patient's continued recovery.

HYPERGLYCEMIC HYPEROSMOLAR NONKETOTIC SYNDROME

HHNS is a serious condition in which hyperosmolarity and hyperglycemia predominate, with alterations of the sensorium (sense of awareness). At the same time, ketosis is minimal or absent. The basic biochemical defect is lack of effective insulin (ie, insulin resistance). The patient's persistent hyperglycemia causes osmotic diuresis, resulting in losses of water and electrolytes. To maintain osmotic equilibrium, water shifts from the intracellular fluid space to the extracellular fluid space. With glucosuria and dehydration, hypernatremia and increased osmolarity occur. Table 41-6 compares DKA and HHNS.

This condition occurs most often in older people (ages 50 to 70) with no known history of diabetes or with mild type 2 diabetes. HHNS can be traced to a precipitating event such as an acute illness (eg, pneumonia or stroke), medications that exacerbate hyperglycemia (thiazides), or treatments, such as dialysis. The history includes days to weeks of polyuria with adequate fluid intake. What distinguishes HHNS from DKA is that ketosis and acidosis do not occur in HHNS partly because of differences in insulin levels. In DKA no insulin is present, and this promotes the breakdown of stored glucose, protein, and fat, which leads to the production of ketone bodies and ketoacidosis. In HHNS the insulin level is too low to prevent hyperglycemia (and subsequent osmotic diuresis), but it is high enough to prevent fat breakdown. Patients with HHNS do not have the ketosis-related GI symptoms that lead them to seek medical attention. Instead, they may tolerate polyuria and polydipsia until neurologic changes or an underlying illness (or family members or others) prompts them to seek treatment. Because of possible delays in therapy, hyperglycemia, dehydration, and hyperosmolarity may be more severe in HHNS (Quinn, 2001c).

Clinical Manifestations

The clinical picture of HHNS is one of hypotension, profound dehydration (dry mucous membranes, poor skin turgor), tachycardia, and variable neurologic signs (eg, alteration of sensorium, seizures, hemiparesis). The mortality rate ranges from 10% to 40%, usually related to an underlying illness.

Assessment and Diagnostic Findings

Diagnostic assessment includes a range of laboratory tests, including blood glucose, electrolytes, BUN, complete blood count, serum osmolality, and arterial blood gas analysis. The blood glucose level, and the osmolality are exceptionally high. Electrolyte and BUN levels are consistent with the clinical picture of severe dehydration. Mental status changes, focal neurologic deficits, and hallucinations

Table 41-6 • Comparison of Diabetic Ketoacidosis (DKA) and Hyperglycemic Hyperosmolar Nonketotic Syndrome (HHNS)

CHARACTERISTICS	DKA	HHNS
Patients most commonly affected	Can occur in type 1 or type 2 diabetes; more common in type 1	Can occur in type 1 or type 2 patients; more common in type 2 diabetes, especially elderly patients with type 2 diabetes
Precipitating event	Omission of insulin; physiologic stress (infection, surgery, CVA, MI)	Physiologic stress (infection, surgery, CVA, MI)
Onset	Rapid (<24 hrs)	Slower (over several days)
Blood glucose levels	Usually >13.9 mmol/L	Usually >33.3 mmol/L
Arterial pH level	<7.3	Normal
Serum and urine ketones	Present	Absent
Serum bicarbonate level	Decreased	Normal
BUN and creatinine levels	Elevated	Elevated
Mortality rate	<5%	10%–40%

are common secondary to the cerebral dehydration that results from extreme hyperosmolality. Postural hypotension accompanies the dehydration (ADA, Hyperglycemic Crises in Patients With Diabetes Mellitus, 2003).

Medical Management

The overall approach to the treatment of HHNS is similar to that of DKA: fluid replacement, correction of electrolyte imbalances, and insulin administration. Because of the older age of the typical patient with HHNS, close monitoring of volume and electrolyte status is important for prevention of fluid overload, heart failure, and cardiac dysrhythmias. Fluid treatment is started with 0.9% or 0.45% NS, depending on the patient's sodium level and the severity of volume depletion. Central venous or arterial pressure monitoring guides fluid replacement. Potassium is added to IV fluids when urinary output is adequate and is guided by continuous electrocardiographic monitoring and frequent laboratory determinations of potassium.

Extremely elevated blood glucose levels drop as the patient is rehydrated. Insulin plays a less important role in the treatment of HHNS because it is not needed for reversal of acidosis, as in DKA. Nonetheless, insulin is usually administered at a continuous low rate to treat hyperglycemia, and replacement IV fluids with dextrose are administered (as in DKA) when the glucose level is decreased to the range of 13.8 to 16.6 mmol/L (ADA, Hyperglycemic Crises in Patients With Diabetes Mellitus, 2003).

Other therapeutic modalities are determined by the underlying illness of the patient and the results of continuing clinical and laboratory evaluation. Treatment is continued until metabolic abnormalities are corrected and neurologic symptoms clear. It may take 3 to 5 days for neurologic symptoms to resolve; thus, treatment of HHNS usually continues well beyond the time when metabolic abnormalities are resolved.

After recovery from HHNS, many patients can control their diabetes with diet alone or with diet and oral antidiabetic agents. Insulin may not be needed once the acute hyperglycemic complication is resolved.

Nursing Management

Nursing care of the patient with HHNS includes close monitoring of vital signs, fluid status, and laboratory values. In addition, strategies are implemented to maintain safety and prevent injury related to changes in the patient's sensorium secondary to HHNS. Fluid status and urine output are closely monitored because of the high risk for renal failure secondary to severe dehydration. In addition, the nurse must direct nursing care to the condition that may have precipitated the onset of HHNS. Because HHNS tends to occur in older patients, the physiologic changes that occur with aging make careful assessment of cardiovascular, pulmonary, and renal function important throughout the acute and recovery phases of HHNS (Quinn, 2001c).

NURSING PROCESS: THE PATIENT NEWLY DIAGNOSED WITH DIABETES MELLITUS

Assessment

The history and physical assessment focus on the signs and symptoms of prolonged hyperglycemia and on physical, social, and emotional factors that may affect the patient's ability to learn and perform diabetes self-care activities. The patient is asked to describe symptoms that preceded the diagnosis of diabetes, such as polyuria, polydipsia, polyphagia, skin dryness, blurred vision, weight loss, vaginal itching, and nonhealing ulcers. The blood glucose and, for patients with type 1 diabetes, urine ketone levels are measured.

Patients with type 1 diabetes are assessed for signs of DKA, including ketonuria, Kussmaul respirations, orthostatic hypotension, and lethargy. The patient is questioned about symptoms of DKA, such as nausea, vomiting, and abdominal pain. Laboratory values are monitored for metabolic acidosis (ie, decreased pH and decreased bicarbonate level) and for electrolyte imbalance. Patients with type 2 diabetes are assessed for signs of HHNS, including hypotension, altered sensorium, seizures, and decreased skin turgor. Laboratory values are monitored for hyperosmolality and electrolyte imbalance.

If the patient exhibits signs and symptoms of DKA or HHNS, nursing care first focuses on treatment of these acute complications, as outlined in previous sections. Once these complications are resolving, nursing care then focuses on long-term management of diabetes, as discussed in this section.

Then the patient is assessed for physical factors that may impair his or her ability to learn or perform self-care skills, such as:

- Visual deficits (the patient is asked to read numbers or words on the insulin syringe, menu, newspaper, or written teaching materials)
- Deficits in motor coordination (the patient is observed eating or performing other tasks or handling a syringe or finger-lancing device)
- Neurologic deficits (eg, due to stroke, other neurologic disorders; other disabling conditions) (from history in chart; the patient is assessed for aphasia or decreased ability to follow simple commands)

The nurse evaluates the patient's social situation for factors that may influence the diabetes treatment and education plan, such as:

- Low literacy level (may be evaluated while assessing for visual deficits by the patient read from teaching materials)
- Limited financial resources
- Presence or absence of family support
- Typical daily schedule (patient is asked about timing and number of usual daily meals, work and exercise schedule, plans for travel)

The patient's emotional status is assessed by observing general demeanor (eg, withdrawn, anxious) and body language (eg, avoids eye contact). The patient is asked about major concerns and fears about diabetes; this allows the nurse to assess for any misconceptions or misinformation regarding diabetes. Coping skills are assessed by asking how the patient has dealt with difficult situations in the past.

Diagnosis

NURSING DIAGNOSES
Based on the assessment data, the patient's major nursing diagnoses may include the following:

- Risk for fluid volume deficit related to polyuria and dehydration
- Imbalanced nutrition related to imbalance of insulin, food, and physical activity
- Deficient knowledge about diabetes self-care skills/information
- Potential self-care deficit related to physical impairments or social factors
- Anxiety related to loss of control, fear of inability to manage diabetes, misinformation related to diabetes, fear of diabetes complications

COLLABORATIVE PROBLEMS/POTENTIAL COMPLICATIONS
Based on assessment data, potential complications may include:

- Fluid overload, pulmonary edema, heart failure
- Hypokalemia
- Hyperglycemia and ketoacidosis

- Hypoglycemia
- Cerebral edema

Planning and Goals

The major goals for the patient may include maintenance of fluid and electrolyte balance, optimal control of blood glucose levels, reversal of weight loss, ability to perform survival diabetes skills and self-care activities, decreased anxiety, and absence of complications.

Nursing Interventions

MAINTAINING FLUID AND ELECTROLYTE BALANCE
Intake and output are measured. IV fluids and electrolytes are administered as prescribed, and oral fluid intake is encouraged when it is permitted. Laboratory values of serum electrolytes (especially sodium and potassium) are monitored. Vital signs are monitored for signs of dehydration (tachycardia, orthostatic hypotension).

IMPROVING NUTRITIONAL INTAKE
The diet is planned with the control of glucose as the primary goal. It must take into consideration the patient's lifestyle, cultural background, activity level, and food preferences. An appropriate caloric intake allows the patient to achieve and maintain the desired body weight. The patient is encouraged to eat full meals and snacks as prescribed per the diabetic diet. Arrangements are made with the dietitian for extra snacks before increased physical activity. It is important for the nurse to ensure that insulin orders are altered as needed for delays in eating because of diagnostic and other procedures.

REDUCING ANXIETY
The nurse provides emotional support and sets aside time to talk with the patient who wishes to express feelings, cry, or ask questions about this new diagnosis. Any misconceptions the patient or family may have regarding diabetes are dispelled (see Table 41-5). The patient and family are assisted to focus on learning self-care behaviours. The patient is encouraged to perform the skills that are feared most and must be reassured that once a skill such as self-injection or lancing a finger for glucose monitoring is performed for the first time, anxiety will decrease. Positive reinforcement is given for the self-care behaviours attempted, even if the technique is not yet completely mastered.

IMPROVING SELF-CARE
Patient teaching (discussed earlier in the Nursing Management section and below) is the major strategy used to prepare the patient for self-care. Special equipment may be needed for instruction on diabetes survival skills, such as a magnifying glass for insulin preparation or an injection-aid device for insulin injection. Low-literacy information and literature in other languages can be obtained from the ADA. The family is also taught so that they can assist in diabetes management by, for instance, prefilling syringes or monitoring the blood glucose level. The diabetes specialist is consulted regarding various blood glucose monitors and other equipment for use by patients with physical impairments. The patient is assisted in identifying community resources for education and supplies as needed. Other members of the health care team are informed about variations in the timing of meals and the work schedule (eg, if the patient works at night or

in the evenings and sleeps during the day) so that the diabetes treatment regimen can be adjusted accordingly.

MONITORING AND MANAGING POTENTIAL COMPLICATIONS

Fluid Overload

Fluid overload can occur because of the administration of a large volume of fluid at a rapid rate that is often required to treat the patient with DKA or HHNS. This risk is increased in elderly patients and in those with preexisting cardiac disease. To avoid fluid overload and resulting congestive heart failure and pulmonary edema, the nurse monitors the patient closely during treatment by measuring vital signs at frequent intervals. Central venous pressure monitoring and hemodynamic monitoring may be initiated to provide additional measures of the fluid status. Physical examination focuses on assessment of cardiac rate and rhythm, breath sounds, venous distention, skin turgor, and urine output. The nurse monitors fluid intake and keeps careful records of IV and other fluid intake, along with urine output measurements.

Hypokalemia

As previously described, hypokalemia is a potential complication during the treatment of DKA as potassium is lost from body stores. Low serum potassium levels may result from rehydration, increased urinary excretion of potassium, and movement of potassium from the extracellular fluid into the cells with insulin administration. Prevention of hypokalemia includes cautious replacement of potassium; before its administration, however, it is important to ensure that the patient's kidneys are functioning. Because of the adverse effects of hypokalemia on cardiac function, monitoring of the cardiac rate, cardiac rhythm, electrocardiogram, and serum potassium levels is essential.

Hyperglycemia and Ketoacidosis

Although the hyperglycemia and ketoacidosis that may have led to the new diagnosis of diabetes may be resolved, the patient is at risk for their subsequent recurrence. Therefore, blood glucose levels and urine ketones are monitored, and medications (insulin, oral antidiabetic agents) are administered as prescribed. The patient is monitored for signs and symptoms of impending hyperglycemia and ketoacidosis; if they occur, insulin and IV fluids are administered.

Hypoglycemia

Hypoglycemia may occur if the patient skips or delays meals or does not follow the prescribed diet or greatly increases the amount of exercise without modifying diet and insulin. Also, the hospitalized patient or outpatient who fasts in preparation for diagnostic testing is at risk for hypoglycemia. Juice or glucose tablets are used for treatment of hypoglycemia. The patient is encouraged to eat full meals and snacks as prescribed per the diabetic diet. If hypoglycemia is a recurrent problem, the total therapeutic regimen should be re-evaluated.

Because of the risk of hypoglycemia, especially with intensive insulin regimens, it is important for the nurse to review with the patient its signs and symptoms, possible causes, and measures to prevent and treat it. The nurse stresses to the patient and family the importance of having information on diabetes at home for reference.

Cerebral Edema

Although the cause of cerebral edema is unknown, it is thought to be caused by rapid correction of hyperglycemia, resulting in fluid shifts. Cerebral edema can be prevented by gradual reduction in the blood glucose level (ADA, Hyperglycemic Crises in Patients With Diabetes Mellitus, 2003). An hourly flow sheet is used to enable close monitoring of the blood glucose level, serum electrolyte levels, urine output, mental status, and neurologic signs. Precautions are taken to minimize activities that could increase intracranial pressure.

PROMOTING HOME AND COMMUNITY-BASED CARE

Teaching Patients Self-Care

The patient is taught survival skills, including simple pathophysiology; treatment modalities (insulin administration, monitoring of blood glucose, and, for type 1 diabetes, urine ketones, and diet); recognition, treatment, and prevention of acute complications (hypoglycemia and hyperglycemia); and practical information (where to obtain supplies, when to call the physician). If the patient has signs of long-term diabetes complications at the time of diagnosis of diabetes, teaching about appropriate preventive behaviours (eg, foot care or eye care) should be included at this time (Chart 41-10).

Continuing Care

Follow-up education is arranged with a home care nurse or an outpatient diabetes education centre. This is particularly important for the patient who has had difficulty coping with the diagnosis, the patient who has limitations that may affect his or her ability to learn or to carry out the management plan, or the patient without any family or social supports. Referral to social services and community resources (eg, centres for the visually impaired) may be needed, depending on the patient's financial circumstances and physical limitations. The importance of self-monitoring and of monitoring and follow-up by primary health care providers is reinforced, and the patient is reminded about the importance of keeping follow-up appointments. The patient who is newly diagnosed with diabetes is also reminded about the importance of participating in other health promotion activities and health screening. Chart 41-11 is a checklist of home care skills.

Evaluation

EXPECTED PATIENT OUTCOMES

Expected patient outcomes may include:

1. Achieves fluid and electrolyte balance
   a. Demonstrates intake and output balance
   b. Exhibits electrolyte values within normal limits
   c. Exhibits vital signs that remain stable with resolution of orthostatic hypotension and tachycardia
2. Achieves metabolic balance
   a. Avoids extremes of glucose levels (hypoglycemia or hyperglycemia)
   b. Demonstrates rapid resolution of hypoglycemic episodes
   c. Avoids further weight loss (if applicable) and begins to approach desired weight
3. Demonstrates/verbalizes diabetes survival skills
   a. Defines diabetes as a condition in which high blood glucose levels are present

Chart 41-10 • PATIENT EDUCATION
Foot Care Tips

1. Take care of your diabetes.
   - Work with your health care team to keep your blood glucose level within a normal range.
2. Inspect your feet every day.
   - Look at your bare feet every day for cuts, blisters, red spots, and swelling.
   - Use a mirror to check the bottoms of your feet or ask a family member for help if you have trouble seeing.
   - Check for changes in temperature.
3. Wash your feet every day.
   - Wash your feet in warm, not hot, water.
   - Dry your feet well. Be sure to dry between the toes.
   - Do not soak your feet.
   - Do not check water temperature with your feet; use a thermometer or elbow.
4. Keep the skin soft and smooth.
   - Rub a thin coat of skin lotion over the tops and bottoms of your feet, but not between your toes.
5. Smooth corns and calluses gently.
   - Use a pumice stone to smooth corns and calluses.
6. Trim your toenails each week or when needed.
   - Trim your toenails straight across and file the edges with an emery board or nail file.
7. Wear shoes and socks at all times.
   - Never walk barefoot.
   - Wear comfortable shoes that fit well and protect your feet.
   - Feel inside your shoes before putting them on each time to make sure the lining is smooth and there are no objects inside.
8. Protect your feet from hot and cold.
   - Wear shoes at the beach or on hot pavement.
   - Wear socks at night if your feet get cold.
9. Keep the blood flowing to your feet.
   - Put your feet up when sitting.
   - Wiggle your toes and move your ankles up and down for 5 minutes, 2 or 3 times a day.
   - Do not cross your legs for long periods of time.
   - Do not smoke.
10. Check with your doctor.
    - Have your doctor check your bare feet and find out whether you are likely to have serious foot problems. Remember that you may not feel the pain of an injury.
    - Call your doctor right away if a cut, sore, blister, or bruise on your foot does not begin to heal after one day.
    - Follow your doctor's advice about foot care.
    - Do not self-medicate or use home remedies or over-the-counter agents to treat foot problems.

h. Verbalizes plan for rotating insulin injection sites
i. States dose, timing, peak action, and duration of prescribed oral agents
j. Verbalizes understanding of food group classifications (depending on system used)
k. Verbalizes appropriate schedule for eating snacks and meals; orders appropriate foods on menus; identifies foods that may be substituted for one another on the meal plan
l. Demonstrates proper technique for monitoring blood glucose, including using finger-lancing device; obtaining a drop of blood; applying blood properly to strip; obtaining value of blood glucose; and recording blood glucose value. Also, is able to calibrate and clean meter, change batteries, identify alarms and warnings on meter, and use control solutions to validate strips.
m. Demonstrates proper technique for disposing of lancets and needles used for blood glucose monitoring and insulin injections (discarding them into hard plastic container such as empty bleach or detergent container or medical waste containers)
n. Demonstrates proper technique for urine ketone testing (for patients with type 1 diabetes) and verbalizes appropriate times to assess for ketones (when ill or when blood glucose test results are repeatedly and inexplicably more than 13.8 to 16.6 mmol/L)
o. Identifies community, outpatient resources for obtaining further diabetes education
p. Identifies acute complications (hypoglycemia and hyperglycemia)
q. Verbalizes symptoms of hypoglycemia (shakiness, sweating, headache, hunger, numbness or tingling of lips or fingers, weakness, fatigue, difficulty concentrating, change of mood) and dangers of untreated hypoglycemia (seizures and coma)
r. Identifies appropriate treatment of hypoglycemia, including 15 g simple carbohydrate (eg, two to four glucose tablets, 120 to 180 mL juice or soft drinks, 2 to 3 teaspoons sugar, or 6 to 10 hard candies) followed by a snack of protein and carbohydrate (eg, cheese and crackers or milk) or by a regularly scheduled meal
s. States potential causes of hypoglycemia (too much insulin, delayed or decreased food intake, increased physical activity) and verbalizes preventive behaviours, such as frequent monitoring of blood glucose when daily schedule is changed and eating a snack before exercise
t. Verbalizes importance of wearing medical identification and carrying a source of simple carbohydrate at all times
v. Verbalizes symptoms of prolonged hyperglycemia (increased thirst and urination)
w. Verbalizes rules for sick day management
x. Describes where to purchase and store insulin, syringes, and glucose monitoring supplies
y. Identifies appropriate circumstances for calling the physician (when ill, when glucose levels repeatedly exceed a certain level [per physician guidelines], or when skin wounds fail to heal) and also identifies name of physician (or other health care team member) and 24-hour phone number

4. Absence of complications
   a. Exhibits normal cardiac rate and rhythm and normal breath sounds
   b. Exhibits jugular venous pressure and distention within normal limits

b. States normal and target blood glucose ranges
c. Identifies factors that cause the blood glucose level to fall (insulin, exercise, some oral anti-diabetes medications)
d. Identifies factors that cause the blood glucose level to rise (food, illness, stress, and infections)
e. Describes the major treatment modalities: diet, exercise, monitoring, medication, education
f. Demonstrates proper technique for drawing up and injecting insulin (including mixing two types of insulin if necessary)
g. States dose and timing of injections, peak action, duration, and adverse effects of insulin

---

Chart 41-11

Home Care Checklist • The Person With Newly Diagnosed Diabetes

At the completion of the home care instruction, the patient or caregiver will be able to:	Patient	Caregiver
• State the importance of diabetes survival skills.	✓	✓
• Explain underlying pathology of diabetes.	✓	✓
• State normal range of blood glucose.	✓	✓
• Identify factors that cause hyper- and hypoglycemia.	✓	✓
• Describe the major modalities used to control diabetes (diet, exercise, monitoring, medication, education).	✓	✓
• Demonstrate proper technique for drawing up and injecting insulin (including mixing two types of insulin if necessary).	✓	✓
• State dose and timing of injections, peak action and duration of insulin.	✓	✓
• Explain insulin injection rotation plan and its rationale.	✓	✓
• State dose, timing, peak action and duration of prescribed oral agents.	✓	✓
• Describe where to purchase and store insulin, syringes, and glucose monitoring supplies.	✓	✓
• Identify classification of food groups (depending on system used).	✓	✓
• State appropriate schedule for eating snacks and meals.	✓	✓
• Select appropriate foods on menus and identify foods that may be substituted for one another on the meal plan.	✓	
• Demonstrate proper technique for monitoring blood glucose.	✓	
• Describe strategies to be used to treat hypoglycemic episodes.	✓	✓
• Use proper technique for disposing of lancets used for blood glucose monitoring and equipment used for insulin injections.	✓	
• Demonstrate proper technique for urine ketone testing (for patients with type 1 diabetes), and verbalize appropriate times to assess for ketones.	✓	✓
• Identify community, outpatient resources for obtaining further diabetes education.	✓	✓
• Identify signs and symptoms of hypoglycemia.	✓	✓
• Describe appropriate treatment of hypoglycemia.	✓	✓
• Identify factors that may cause hypoglycemia.	✓	✓
• State strategies that minimize risk for hypoglycemia.	✓	✓
• State rationale for wearing medical identification and carrying a source of simple carbohydrate at all times.	✓	
• Identify signs and symptoms of hyperglycemia.	✓	✓
• Describe appropriate treatment of hyperglycemia.	✓	✓
• Identify factors that may cause hyperglycemia.	✓	✓
• Identify rules for sick-day management.	✓	✓
• Identify appropriate circumstances for contacting physician.	✓	✓

---

c. Exhibits blood glucose and urine ketone levels within normal limits

d. Exhibits no manifestations of hypoglycemia or hyperglycemia

e. Shows improved mental status without signs of cerebral edema

f. States measures to prevent complications

Long-Term Complications of Diabetes

There has been a steady decline in the number of deaths of diabetic patients attributable to ketoacidosis and infection, but an alarming rise in the number of deaths from cardiovascular and renal complications. Long-term complications are becoming more common as more people live longer with diabetes. The long-term complications of diabetes can affect almost every organ system of the body. In Canada, hospitalization rates are more than double (18% compared to 8% admitted each year) among adults who have diabetes compared with adults who do not have diabetes (Millar & Young, 2003). The general categories of chronic diabetic complications are macrovascular disease, microvascular disease, and neuropathy.

The specific causes and pathogenesis of each type of complication are still being investigated. It appears, however, that increased levels of blood glucose may play a role in neuropathic disease, microvascular complications, and risk factors contributing to macrovascular complications. Hypertension may also be a major contributing factor, especially in macrovascular and microvascular diseases.

Long-term complications are seen in both type 1 and type 2 diabetes but usually do not occur within the first 5 to 10 years of the diagnosis. However, evidence of these complications may be present at the time of diagnosis of type 2 diabetes, as the patient may have had undiagnosed diabetes for many years. Renal (microvascular) disease is more prevalent among patients with type 1 diabetes, and cardiovascular (macrovascular) complications are more prevalent among older patients with type 2 diabetes.

MACROVASCULAR COMPLICATIONS

Diabetic macrovascular complications result from changes in the medium to large blood vessels. Blood vessel walls thicken, sclerose, and become occluded by plaque that adheres to the vessel walls. Eventually, blood flow is blocked. These atherosclerotic changes are indistinguishable from atherosclerotic changes in people without diabetes, but they tend to occur more often and at an earlier age in diabetes. Coronary artery disease, cerebrovascular disease, and peripheral vascular disease are the three main types of macrovascular complications that occur more frequently in the diabetic population.

Myocardial infarction is twice as common in diabetic men and three times as common in diabetic women. There is also an increased risk for complications resulting from myocardial infarction and an increased likelihood of a second myocardial infarction. Coronary artery disease may account for 50% to 60% of all deaths in patients with diabetes. One unique feature of coronary artery disease in patients with diabetes is that the typical ischemic symptoms may be absent. Thus, patients may not experience the early warning signs of decreased coronary blood flow and may have "silent" myocardial infarctions. These silent myocardial infarctions may be discovered only as changes on the electrocardiogram. This lack of ischemic symptoms may be secondary to autonomic neuropathy (see below).

Cerebral blood vessels are similarly affected by accelerated atherosclerosis. Occlusive changes or the formation of an embolus elsewhere in the vasculature that lodges in a cerebral blood vessel can lead to transient ischemic attacks and strokes. People with diabetes have twice the risk of developing cerebrovascular disease, and studies suggest there may be a greater likelihood of death from cerebrovascular disease in patients with diabetes. In addition, recovery from a stroke may be impaired in patients who have elevated blood glucose levels at the time of and immediately after a stroke. Because symptoms of cerebrovascular disease may be similar to symptoms of acute diabetic complications (HHNS or hypoglycemia), it is very important to rapidly assess the blood glucose level (and treat abnormal levels) in patients reporting these symptoms so that testing and treatment of cerebrovascular disease (stroke) can be initiated if indicated.

Atherosclerotic changes in the large blood vessels of the lower extremities are responsible for the increased incidence (two to three times higher than in nondiabetic people) of occlusive peripheral arterial disease in patients with diabetes. Signs and symptoms of peripheral vascular disease include diminished peripheral pulses and intermittent claudication (pain in the buttock, thigh, or calf during walking). The severe form of arterial occlusive disease in the lower extremities is largely responsible for the increased incidence of gangrene and subsequent amputation in diabetic patients. Neuropathy and impairments in wound healing also play a role in diabetic foot disease (see below).

Role of Diabetes in Macrovascular Diseases

Diabetes researchers continue to investigate the relation between diabetes and macrovascular diseases. The main feature unique to diabetes is an elevated blood glucose level; however, a direct link has not been found between hyperglycemia and atherosclerosis. Although it may be tempting to attribute the increased prevalence of macrovascular diseases to the increased prevalence of certain risk factors (eg, obesity, increased triglyceride levels, hypertension) among patients with diabetes, there is a higher-than-expected rate of macrovascular diseases among patients with diabetes when compared with nondiabetic patients with the same risk factors (ADA, Management of Dyslipidemia in Adults With Diabetes, 2003). Thus, diabetes itself is seen as an independent risk factor for the development of accelerated atherosclerosis. Other potential factors that may play a role in diabetes-related atherosclerosis include platelet and clotting factor abnormalities,

decreased flexibility of red blood cells, decreased oxygen release, changes in the arterial wall related to hyperglycemia, and possibly hyperinsulinemia.

Management

Management of macrovascular complications involves prevention and treatment of the commonly accepted risk factors for atherosclerosis. Diet and exercise are important in managing obesity, hypertension, and hyperlipidemia. In addition, the use of medications to control hypertension and hyperlipidemia may be indicated. Smoking cessation is essential. Control of blood glucose levels may reduce triglyceride levels and can significantly reduce the incidence of complications.

When macrovascular complications do occur, treatment is the same as with nondiabetic patients. In addition, patients may require increased amounts of insulin or may need to switch from oral antidiabetic agents to insulin during illnesses.

MICROVASCULAR COMPLICATIONS AND DIABETIC RETINOPATHY

Although macrovascular atherosclerotic changes are seen in both diabetic and nondiabetic patients, the microvascular changes are unique to diabetes. Diabetic microvascular disease (or microangiopathy) is characterized by capillary basement membrane thickening. The basement membrane surrounds the endothelial cells of the capillary. Researchers believe that increased blood glucose levels react through a series of biochemical responses to thicken the basement membrane to several times its normal thickness. Two areas affected by these changes are the retina and the kidneys. Diabetic retinopathy is the leading cause of legal blindness in people between 20 and 70 years of age in North America; it occurs in both type 1 (86%) and type 2 (33%) diabetes (Public Health Agency of Canada, 2000). Between 1996 and 1999, the Canadian National Institute for the Blind (CNIB), the major vision rehabilitation agency in Canada, reported that diabetic retinopathy was the second leading cause of vision loss in people of all ages (Public Health Agency of Canada, 2000). Similarly, about one in every four individuals starting dialysis has diabetic nephropathy.

People with diabetes are subject to multiple visual complications (Table 41-7). The eye pathology referred to as diabetic retinopathy is caused by changes in the small blood vessels in the retina, the area of the eye that receives images and sends information about the images to the brain (Fig. 41-8). It is richly supplied with blood vessels of all kinds: small arteries and veins, arterioles, venules, and capillaries. There are three main stages of retinopathy: nonproliferative (background) retinopathy, preproliferative retinopathy, and proliferative retinopathy.

Nearly all patients with type 1 diabetes and more than 60% of patients with type 2 diabetes have some degree of retinopathy after 20 years (ADA, Diabetic Retinopathy, 2003). Changes in the microvasculature include microaneurysms, intraretinal hemorrhage, hard exudates, and focal capillary closure. Although most patients do not develop visual impairment, it can be devastating if it occurs. A complication of nonproliferative retinopathy, macular edema, occurs in approximately 10% of people with type 1 and type 2 diabetes and may lead to visual distortion and loss of central vision.

An advanced form of background retinopathy, preproliferative retinopathy, is considered a precursor to the more serious proliferative retinopathy. In preproliferative retinopathy, there

EYE DISORDER	CHARACTERISTICS
Retinopathy	Deterioration of the small blood vessels that nourish the retina
Background	Early stage, asymptomatic retinopathy. Blood vessels within the retina develop micro-aneurysms that leak fluid, causing swelling and forming deposits (exudates). In some cases, macular edema causes distorted vision.
Preproliferative	Represents increased destruction of retinal blood vessels
Proliferative	Abnormal growth of new blood vessels on the retina. New vessels rupture, bleeding into the vitreous and blocking light. Ruptured blood vessels in the vitreous form scar tissue, which can pull on and detach the retina.
Cataracts	Opacity of the lens of the eye; cataracts occur at an earlier age in patients with diabetes.
Lens changes	The lens of the eye can swell when blood glucose levels are elevated. For some patients, visual changes related to lens swelling may be the first symptoms of diabetes. It may take up to 2 months of improved blood glucose control before hyperglycemic swelling subsides and vision stabilizes. Therefore, patients are advised not to change eyeglass prescriptions during the 2 months after discovery of hyperglycemia.
Extraocular muscle palsy	This may occur as a result of diabetic neuropathy. The involvement of various cranial nerves responsible for ocular movements may lead to double vision. This usually resolves spontaneously.
Glaucoma	Results from occlusion of the outflow channels by new blood vessels. Glaucoma may occur with slightly higher frequency in the diabetic population.

Table 41-7 • Ocular Complications of Diabetes

are more widespread vascular changes and loss of nerve fibres. Epidemiologic evidence suggests that 10% to 50% of patients with preproliferative retinopathy will develop proliferative retinopathy within a short time (possibly as little as 1 year). As with background retinopathy, if visual changes occur during the preproliferative stage, they are usually caused by macular edema.

Proliferative retinopathy represents the greatest threat to vision. Proliferative retinopathy is characterized by the proliferation of new blood vessels growing from the retina into the vitreous. These new vessels are prone to bleeding. The visual loss associated with proliferative retinopathy is caused by this vitreous hemorrhage and/or retinal detachment. The vitreous is normally clear, allowing light to be transmitted to the retina. When there is a hemorrhage, the vitreous becomes clouded and cannot transmit light, resulting in loss of vision. Another consequence of vitreous hemorrhage is that resorption of the blood in the vitreous leads to the formation of fibrous scar tissue. This scar tissue may place traction on the retina, resulting in retinal detachment and subsequent visual loss.

Clinical Manifestations

Retinopathy is a painless process. In nonproliferative and preproliferative retinopathy, blurry vision secondary to macular edema occurs in some patients, although many patients are asymptomatic. Even patients with a significant degree of proliferative retinopathy and some hemorrhaging may not experience major visual changes. However, symptoms indicative of hemorrhaging include floaters or cobwebs in the visual field, or sudden visual changes including spotty or hazy vision, or complete loss of vision.

Assessment and Diagnostic Findings

Diagnosis is by direct visualization with an ophthalmoscope or with a technique known as fluorescein angiography. Fluorescein angiography can document the type and activity of the retinopathy. Dye is injected into an arm vein and is carried to various parts of the body through the blood, but especially through the vessels of the retina of the eye. This technique allows the ophthalmologist, using special instruments, to see the retinal vessels in bright detail and gives useful information that cannot be obtained with just an ophthalmoscope.

Side effects of this diagnostic procedure may include nausea during the dye injection; yellowish, fluorescent discolouration of the skin and urine lasting 12 to 24 hours; and occasional allergic reactions, usually manifested by hives or itching. Generally, however, it is a safe diagnostic procedure. Patient preparation includes explaining:

- The steps of the procedure
- The fact that the procedure is painless

FIGURE 41-8 Diabetic retinopathy. **(A)** In the fundus photograph of a normal eye, the light circular area over which a number of blood vessels converge is the optic disc, where the optic nerve meets the back of the eye. **(B)** The fundus photograph of a patient with diabetic retinopathy shows characteristic waxy-looking retinal lesions, microaneurysms of the vessels, and hemorrhages. Courtesy of American Optometric Association.

- The potential side effects
- The type of information the technique can provide
- That the flash of the camera may be slightly uncomfortable for a short time

Medical Management

The first focus of management is on primary and secondary prevention. The results of the DCCT study demonstrated that maintenance of blood glucose to a normal or near-normal level in type 1 diabetes through intensive insulin therapy and patient education decreased the risk for development of retinopathy by 76% when compared with conventional therapy in patients without preexisting retinopathy. The progression of retinopathy was decreased by 54% in patients with very mild to moderate nonproliferative retinopathy at the time of initiation of treatment. Similarly, the UKPDS study demonstrated a reduced risk of retinopathy in type 2 diabetes with better control of blood glucose levels (Canadian Diabetes Association, 2003).

For advanced cases, the main treatment of diabetic retinopathy is argon laser photocoagulation. The laser treatment destroys leaking blood vessels and areas of neovascularization. For patients at increased risk for hemorrhaging, panretinal photocoagulation may significantly reduce the rate of progression to blindness. Panretinal photocoagulation involves the systematic application of multiple (more than 1,000) laser burns throughout the retina (except in the macular region). This stops the widespread growth of new vessels and hemorrhaging of damaged vessels. The role of "mild" panretinal photocoagulation (with only a third to a half as many laser burns) in the early stages of proliferative retinopathy or in patients with preproliferative changes is being investigated. For macular edema, focal photocoagulation is used to apply smaller laser burns to specific areas of microaneurysms in the macular region. This may reduce the rate of visual loss from macular edema by 50% (ADA, Diabetic Retinopathy, 2003).

Photocoagulation treatments are usually performed on an outpatient basis, and most patients can return to their usual activities by the next day. For some patients, limitations may be placed on activities involving weight bearing or bearing down. For most patients, the treatment does not cause intense pain, although they may report varying degrees of discomfort. Usually an anesthetic eye drop is all that is needed during the treatment. A few patients may experience slight visual loss, loss of peripheral vision, or impairments in adaptation to the dark. For most patients, however, the risk of slight visual changes from the laser treatment itself is much less than the potential for loss of vision from progression of retinopathy.

When a major hemorrhage into the vitreous occurs, the vitreous fluid becomes mixed with blood and prevents light from passing through the eye; this can cause blindness. A vitrectomy is a surgical procedure in which vitreous humour filled with blood or fibrous tissue is removed with a special drill-like instrument and replaced with saline or another liquid. A vitrectomy is performed on patients who already have visual loss and in whom the vitreous hemorrhage has not cleared on its own after 6 months. The purpose is to restore useful vision; recovery to near-normal vision is not usually expected. Other strategies that may slow the progression of diabetic retinopathy include:

- Control of hypertension
- Control of blood glucose
- Cessation of smoking

Nursing Management

Nursing management of patients with diabetic retinopathy or other eye disorders involves implementing the individual plan of care and providing patient education. Education focuses on prevention through regular ophthalmologic examinations and blood glucose control and self-management of eye care regimens. The effectiveness of early diagnosis and prompt treatment is emphasized in teaching the patient and family. If vision loss occurs, nursing care must also address the patient's adjustment to impaired vision and use of adaptive devices for diabetes self-care as well as activities of daily living. Nursing care for the patient with low vision or loss of vision is discussed in detail in Chapter 58.

PROMOTING HOME AND COMMUNITY-BASED CARE

Teaching Patients Self-Care. In all forms of therapy for retinopathy, something is destroyed in the process of saving vision, and the facts must be presented to the patient and family as honestly as possible. The course of the retinopathy may be long and stressful. In teaching and counselling the patient, it is important to stress the following:

- Retinopathy may appear after many years of diabetes, and its appearance does not necessarily mean that the diabetes is on a downhill course.
- The odds for maintaining vision are in the patient's favour, especially with adequate control of glucose levels and blood pressure.
- Frequent eye examinations are the best way to preserve vision, because they allow for the detection of any retinopathy.

Some additional points to keep in mind when the patient with diabetes has some type of visual impairment include the following:

- Visual impairment can be a shock. The person's response to vision loss depends on personality, self-concept, and coping mechanisms.
- As in any loss, acceptance of blindness by the patient occurs in stages; some patients may learn to accept blindness in a rather short period, and others may never do so.
- Although retinopathy occurs bilaterally, the severity may differ in the two eyes.
- Many of the chronic complications of diabetes occur simultaneously. For example, a patient who is blind due to diabetic retinopathy may also have peripheral neuropathy and may experience impairment of manual dexterity and tactile sensation.

Continuing Care. Continuing care for the patient with impaired vision due to diabetic changes depends on the severity of the impairment and the effectiveness of the patient's coping in response to the impairment. The importance of careful diabetes management is emphasized as one means of slowing the progression of visual changes. The patient is reminded of the need to see the ophthalmologist regularly. If eye changes are progressive and unrelenting, the patient needs to be prepared for inevitable blindness. Therefore, consideration is given to making referrals for teaching the patient Braille and for training with a guide dog. Referral to provincial/territorial agencies should be made to ensure that the patient receives services for the blind. Family members are also taught how to assist the patient to remain as independent as possible despite decreasing visual acuity.

Referral for home care may be indicated for some patients, particularly those who live alone, those not coping well, and those who have other health problems or complications of diabetes that may interfere with their ability to perform self-care. During home visits, the nurse can assess the patient's home environment and ability to manage diabetes despite visual impairments. Medical management and nursing care of patients with visual disturbances are discussed in detail in Chapter 58.

NEPHROPATHY

Nephropathy, or renal disease secondary to diabetic microvascular changes in the kidney, is a common complication of diabetes. People with diabetes account for nearly half of new cases of end-stage renal disease (ESRD) each year and about a quarter of those requiring dialysis or transplantation each year in the United States. About 28% of Canadians with type 1 or type 2 diabetes have kidney failure (3300 Canadians in 1996 were being treated, mainly by dialysis) (Public Health Agency of Canada, 2000).

Patients with type 1 diabetes frequently show initial signs of renal disease after 10 to 15 years, whereas patients with type 2 diabetes develop renal disease within 10 years of the diagnosis of diabetes. Many patients with type 2 diabetes have had diabetes for many years before it was diagnosed and treated. Therefore, they have evidence of nephropathy at the time of diagnosis.

There is no reliable method to predict whether a person will develop renal disease. The DCCT results showed that intensive treatment of diabetes with a goal of achieving a hemoglobin A_{1C} level as close to the nondiabetic range as possible reduced the occurrence of early signs of nephropathy, such as microalbuminuria by 39%, and albuminuria by 54%. Similarly, the UKPDS study demonstrated a reduced incidence of overt nephropathy in type 2 diabetes with control of blood glucose levels (ADA, Diabetic Nephropathy, 2003).

Soon after the onset of diabetes, and especially if the blood glucose levels are elevated, the kidney's filtration mechanism is stressed, allowing blood proteins to leak into the urine. As a result, the pressure in the blood vessels of the kidney increases. It is thought that the elevated pressure serves as the stimulus for the development of nephropathy. Various medications and diets are being tested to prevent these complications.

Clinical Manifestations

Most of the signs and symptoms of renal dysfunction in the patient with diabetes are similar to those seen in patients without diabetes. (See Chap. 45 for the management of patients with renal disorders.) Also, as renal failure progresses, the catabolism (breakdown) of both exogenous and endogenous insulin decreases, and frequent hypoglycemic episodes may result. Insulin needs change as a result of changes in the catabolism of insulin, and also as a result of changes in diet related to the treatment of nephropathy. The stress of renal disease affects self-esteem, family relationships, marital relations, and virtually all aspects of daily life. As renal function decreases, the patient commonly has multiple-system failure (eg, declining visual acuity, impotence, foot ulcerations, heart failure, and nocturnal diarrhea).

Assessment and Diagnostic Findings

One of the most important blood proteins that leaks into the urine is albumin. Small amounts may leak undetected for years. Of patients with microalbuminuria, clinical nephropathy eventually

develops in more than 85%. However, if microalbuminuria is not present, nephropathy develops in fewer than 5%. Early microalbuminuria can be discovered by testing a random urine sample for the albumin to creatinine ratio (ACR) along with a urine dipstick test to rule out nondiabetic renal disease. If the urinary albumin is 30 to 300 mg/day (ACR is 2.0 to 20.0 mg/mmol in men and 2.8 to 28.0 mg/mmol in women) two more random urine tests are required between 1 week and 2 months apart. Nephropathy is diagnosed if two of the three urine specimens show an ACR greater than 2.0 mg/mmol (men) or greater than 2.8 mg/mmol (women) (Canadian Diabetes Association, 2003).

When a urine dipstick test reads consistently positive for significant amounts of albumin, serum creatinine and BUN levels are obtained. At this point in the development of renal disease, diagnostic testing for cardiac or other systemic problems may also be required. Some of the tests involve injection of special dyes that are not easily cleared by the damaged kidney, so the value of the diagnostic test must be weighed against the potential risks.

Hypertension often develops in patients (both diabetic and nondiabetic) who are in the early stages of renal disease. However, essential hypertension occurs in up to 50% of all individuals with diabetes (for unknown reasons). Thus, it should not be assumed that someone with diabetes who has hypertension also has renal disease; other diagnostic criteria must also be present.

Medical Management

In addition to achieving and maintaining near-normal blood glucose levels, management for all patients with diabetes should include careful attention to the following:

- Control of hypertension (the use of angiotensin-converting enzyme [ACE] inhibitors, such as captopril, because control of hypertension may also decrease or delay the onset of early proteinuria)
- Prevention or vigourous treatment of urinary tract infections
- Avoidance of nephrotoxic substances
- Adjustment of medications as renal function changes
- Low-sodium diet
- Low-protein diet

If the patient has already developed microalbuminuria and its level exceeds 30 mg/24 hours on two consecutive tests, an ACE inhibitor should be prescribed. ACE inhibitors lower blood pressure and reduce microalbuminuria and therefore protect the kidney. Alternatively, angiotensin-receptor blocking (ARB) agents may be prescribed. This preventive strategy should be part of the standard of care for the person with diabetes. Carefully designed low-protein diets also appear to reverse early leakage of small amounts of protein from the kidney (ADA, Clinical Practice Recommendations, 2003; ADA, Diabetic Nephropathy, 2003).

In chronic or end-stage renal failure, two types of treatment are available: dialysis (hemodialysis or peritoneal dialysis) and transplantation from a relative or a cadaver. Hemodialysis for the patient with diabetes is similar to that for patients without the disease (see Chap. 44). Because hemodialysis creates additional stress on patients with cardiovascular disease, it may not be appropriate for certain patients. In addition, it is extremely intrusive into a patient's life.

Continuous ambulatory peritoneal dialysis is being used by an increasing number of patients with diabetes, mainly because of the independence it allows patients. In addition, insulin can be mixed into the dialysate, which may result in better blood glucose control and end the need for insulin injections. However, these patients may require more insulin because the dialysate contains glucose. Major risks of peritoneal dialysis are infection and peritonitis. The mortality rate for diabetic patients undergoing dialysis is higher than that in patients without diabetes undergoing dialysis and is closely related to the severity of cardiovascular problems.

Renal disease is frequently accompanied by advancing retinopathy that may require laser treatments and surgery. Severe hypertension also worsens eye disease because of the additional stress it places on the blood vessels. Patients being treated with hemodialysis who require eye surgery may be changed to peritoneal dialysis and have their hypertension aggressively controlled for several weeks before surgery. The rationale for this change is that hemodialysis requires anticoagulants that can increase the risk of bleeding after the surgery, and peritoneal dialysis minimizes pressure changes in the eyes.

The success rate for kidney transplantation in patients with diabetes has improved. In medical centres performing large numbers of transplants, the chances are 75% to 80% that the transplanted kidney will continue to function in the patient with diabetes for at least 5 years. Like the original kidneys, transplanted kidneys in patients with diabetes can eventually be damaged if blood glucose levels are consistently high after the transplantation. Therefore, monitoring blood glucose levels frequently and adjusting insulin levels in diabetic patients with transplanted kidneys are essential for long-term success. Pancreas transplants are sometimes attempted when a kidney transplant is performed. Pancreatic transplants have not been successful enough to be performed alone because of the risks associated with immunosuppression.

DIABETIC NEUROPATHIES

Diabetic neuropathy refers to a group of diseases that affect all types of nerves, including peripheral (sensorimotor), autonomic, and spinal nerves. The disorders appear to be clinically diverse and depend on the location of the affected nerve cells. The prevalence increases with the age of the patient and the duration of the disease and may be as high as 40%–50% in patients who have had diabetes for 10 years. For people with type 1 diabetes, neuropathy rarely occurs within the first 5 years from onset. However, for those with type 2 diabetes, neuropathy may be present very soon after onset (Canadian Diabetes Association, 2003).

Elevated blood glucose levels over a period of years have been implicated in the etiology of neuropathy. The pathogenesis of neuropathy may be attributed to either a vascular or a metabolic mechanism or both, but their relative contributions have yet to be determined. Capillary basement membrane thickening and capillary closure may be present. In addition, there may be demyelinization of the nerves, which is thought to be related to hyperglycemia. Nerve conduction is disrupted when there are aberrations of the myelin sheaths. Control of blood glucose levels to normal or near-normal levels was shown in the DCCT study to decrease the incidence of neuropathy by 60%.

The two most common types of diabetic neuropathy are sensorimotor polyneuropathy and autonomic neuropathy. Cranial mononeuropathies, for example, those affecting the oculomotor nerve, also occur in diabetes, especially among the elderly.

Sensorimotor polyneuropathy is a diabetic neuropathy also called peripheral neuropathy. It most commonly affects the distal portions of the nerves, especially the nerves of the lower extremities. It affects both sides of the body symmetrically and may spread in a proximal direction.

Peripheral Neuropathy

CLINICAL MANIFESTATIONS

Initial symptoms include paresthesias (prickling, tingling, or heightened sensation) and burning sensations (especially at night). As the neuropathy progresses, the feet become numb. In addition, a decrease in proprioception (awareness of posture and movement of the body and of position and weight of objects in relation to the body) and a decreased sensation of light touch may lead to an unsteady gait. Decreased sensations of pain and temperature place patients with neuropathy at increased risk for injury and undetected foot infections. Deformities of the foot may also occur, with neuropathy-related joint changes producing Charcot joints. These joint deformities result from the abnormal weight distribution on joints due to lack of proprioception.

On physical examination, a decrease in deep tendon reflexes and vibratory sensation is found. For patients who have few or no symptoms of neuropathy, these physical findings may be the only indication of neuropathic changes. For patients with signs or symptoms of neuropathy, it is important to rule out other possible neuropathies, including alcohol-induced or vitamin-deficiency neuropathies.

MANAGEMENT

The results of the DCCT study demonstrate that intensive insulin therapy and control of blood glucose levels delay the onset and slow the progression of neuropathy. Pain, particularly of the lower extremities, is a disturbing symptom in some people with neuropathy secondary to diabetes. For some patients, neuropathic pain spontaneously resolves within 6 months. For other patients, pain persists for many years. Various approaches to pain management can be tried. These include analgesics (preferably nonopioid); tricyclic antidepressants; phenytoin, carbamazepine, or gabapentin (antiseizure medications); mexiletine (an antiarrhythmic); or transcutaneous electrical nerve stimulation (TENS).

The use of aldose reductase inhibitors is under study to determine whether they block the damaging effects of hyperglycemia. The topical medication capsaicin (Axscain) also has been shown in preliminary reports to decrease lower-extremity neuropathic pain. Studies of the role of this topical medication in neuropathy continue.

Autonomic Neuropathies

Neuropathy of the autonomic nervous system results in a broad range of dysfunctions affecting almost every organ system of the body. Three manifestations of autonomic neuropathy are related to the cardiac, GI, and renal systems Cardiovascular symptoms range from fixed, slightly tachycardic heart rate; orthostatic hypotension; and silent, or painless, myocardial ischemia and infarction. Delayed gastric emptying may occur with the typical symptoms of early satiety, bloating, nausea, and vomiting. In addition, there may be unexplained wide swings in blood glucose levels related to inconsistent absorption of the glucose from ingested foods secondary to the inconsistent gastric emptying. "Diabetic" constipation or diarrhea (especially nocturnal diarrhea) may occur as a result.

Urinary retention, a decreased sensation of bladder fullness, and other urinary symptoms of neurogenic bladder result from autonomic neuropathy. Patients with a neurogenic bladder are predisposed to developing urinary tract infections due to inability to completely empty the bladder. This is especially true in patients with poorly controlled diabetes, because hyperglycemia impairs resistance to infection

HYPOGLYCEMIC UNAWARENESS

Autonomic neuropathy of the adrenal medulla is responsible for diminished or absent adrenergic symptoms of hypoglycemia. Patients may report that they no longer feel the typical shakiness, sweating, nervousness, and palpitations associated with hypoglycemia. Strict blood glucose monitoring, including frequent SMBG, is recommended for these patients. Their inability to detect and treat these warning signs of hypoglycemia puts them at risk for developing dangerously low blood glucose levels. Therefore, their goals for blood glucose levels may need to be adjusted to reduce the risk for hypoglycemia. The patient and family need to be taught to recognize subtle signs and symptoms of hypoglycemia (Tkacs, 2002).

SUDOMOTOR NEUROPATHY

This neuropathic condition refers to a decrease or absence of sweating (anhidrosis) of the extremities, with a compensatory increase in upper body sweating. Dryness of the feet increases the risk for the development of foot ulcers.

SEXUAL DYSFUNCTION

Sexual dysfunction, especially impotence in men, is a complication of diabetes. The effects of autonomic neuropathy on female sexual functioning are not well documented. Reduced vaginal lubrication has been mentioned as a possible neuropathic effect; other possible changes in sexual function in women with diabetes include decreased libido and lack of orgasm. Vaginal infection, increased in incidence in women with diabetes, may be associated with decreased lubrication and vaginal itching and tenderness. Urinary tract infections and vaginitis may also affect sexual function (Tilton, 1997).

Impotence (inability of the penis to become rigid and sustain an erection adequate for penetration) occurs with greater frequency in diabetic men than in nondiabetic men of the same age. However, diabetic neuropathy is not the only cause of impotence in men with diabetes. Medications such as antihypertensive agents, psychological factors, and other medical conditions (eg, vascular insufficiency) that may affect nondiabetic men also play a role in impotence in diabetic men.

Some men with autonomic neuropathy have normal erectile function and can experience orgasm but do not ejaculate. Retrograde ejaculation occurs: seminal fluid is propelled backward through the posterior urethra and into the urinary bladder. Examination of the urine confirms the diagnosis because of the large number of active sperm present. Fertility counselling is necessary for couples attempting conception.

MANAGEMENT

Management strategies depend on the symptoms. There is no treatment for painless cardiac ischemia, and the prognosis is poor. Detection, however, is important so that education about avoiding strenuous exercise can be provided. Orthostatic hypotension may respond to a diet high in sodium, the discontinuation of medications that impede autonomic nervous system responses, the use of sympathomimetics and other agents (eg, caffeine) that stimulate an autonomic response, and the use of lower-body elastic garments that maximize venous return and prevent pooling of blood in the extremities.

Treatment of delayed gastric emptying includes a low-fat diet, frequent small meals, close blood glucose control, and use of agents that increase gastric motility (eg, metoclopramide, bethanechol). Treatment of diabetic diarrhea may include bulk-forming laxatives or antidiarrheal agents. Constipation is treated with a high-fibre diet and adequate hydration; medications, laxatives, and enemas may be necessary when constipation is severe. Management of the patient with a neurogenic bladder is discussed in Chapter 44.

Treatment of sudomotor dysfunction focuses on education about skin care and heat intolerance. Erectile dysfunction is discussed in Chapter 49.

FOOT AND LEG PROBLEMS

From 50% to 75% of lower extremity amputations are performed on people with diabetes. More than 50% of these amputations are thought to be preventable, provided patients are taught foot care measures and practice them on a daily basis (ADA, Preventive Foot Care in People With Diabetes, 2003). Complications of diabetes that contribute to the increased risk of foot infections include:

- Neuropathy: Sensory neuropathy leads to loss of pain and pressure sensation, and autonomic neuropathy leads to increased dryness and fissuring of the skin (secondary to decreased sweating). Motor neuropathy results in muscular atrophy, which may lead to changes in the shape of the foot.
- Peripheral vascular disease: Poor circulation of the lower extremities contributes to poor wound healing and the development of gangrene.
- Immunocompromise: Hyperglycemia impairs the ability of specialized leukocytes to destroy bacteria. Thus, in poorly controlled diabetes, there is a lowered resistance to certain infections.

The typical sequence of events in the development of a diabetic foot ulcer begins with a soft tissue injury of the foot, formation of a fissure between the toes or in an area of dry skin, or formation of a callus (Fig. 41-9). Injuries are not felt by the patient with an insensitive foot and may be thermal (eg, from using

FIGURE 41-9 Neuropathic ulcers occur on pressure points in areas with diminished sensation in diabetic polyneuropathy. Pain is absent (and therefore the ulcer may go unnoticed).

heating pads, walking barefoot on hot concrete, or testing bath water with the foot), chemical (eg, burning the foot while using caustic agents on calluses, corns, or bunions), or traumatic (eg, injuring skin while cutting nails, walking with an undetected foreign object in the shoe, or wearing ill-fitting shoes and socks).

If the patient is not in the habit of thoroughly inspecting both feet on a daily basis, the injury or fissure may go unnoticed until a serious infection has developed. Drainage, swelling, redness (from cellulitis) of the leg, or gangrene may be the first sign of foot problems that the patient notices. Treatment of foot ulcers involves bed rest, antibiotics, and débridement. In addition, controlling glucose levels, which tend to increase when infections occur, is important for promoting wound healing. In patients with peripheral vascular disease, foot ulcers may not heal because of the decreased ability of oxygen, nutrients, and antibiotics to reach the injured tissue. Amputation may be necessary to prevent the spread of infection.

Foot assessment and foot care instructions are most important when caring for patients who are at high risk for developing foot infections. Some of the high-risk characteristics include:

- Duration of diabetes more than 10 years
- Age older than 40 years
- History of smoking
- Decreased peripheral pulses
- Decreased sensation
- Anatomic deformities or pressure areas (eg, bunions, calluses, hammer toes)
- History of previous foot ulcers or amputation

Management

Teaching patients proper foot care is a nursing intervention that can prevent costly, painful, and debilitating complications. Preventive foot care begins with careful daily assessment of the feet. The feet must be inspected on a daily basis for any redness, blisters, fissures, calluses, ulcerations, changes in skin temperature, and the development of foot deformities (ie, hammer toes, bunions).

For patients with visual impairment or decreased joint mobility (especially the elderly), use of a mirror to inspect the bottom of the feet or the help of a family member in foot inspection may be necessary. The interior surfaces of shoes should be inspected for any rough spots or foreign objects.

In addition to the daily visual and manual inspection of the feet, the feet should be examined during every health care visit or at least once per year (more often if there is an increase in the patient's risk) by a podiatrist, physician, or nurse (Fritschi, 2001). Patients with neuropathy should also undergo evaluation of neurologic status using a monofilament device by an experienced examiner (Fig. 41-10). Patients with pressure areas, such as calluses, or thick toenails should see the podiatrist routinely for treatment of calluses and trimming of nails.

Additional aspects of preventive foot care that are taught to the patient and family include the following:

- Properly bathing, drying, and lubricating the feet, taking care not to allow moisture (water or lotion) to accumulate between the toes
- Wearing closed-toe shoes that fit well. Podiatrists can provide patients with inserts (orthotics) to remove pressure from pressure points on the foot. New shoes should be broken in slowly (ie, worn for 1 to 2 hours initially, with gradual increases in the length of time worn) to avoid blister formation. Patients with bony deformities may need extra-wide shoes or extra-depth shoes. High-risk behaviours should be avoided, such as walking barefoot, using heating pads on the feet, wearing open-toed shoes, soaking the feet, and shaving calluses.
- Trimming toenails straight across and filing sharp corners to follow the contour of the toe (American Association of Diabetes Educators, 1998). If patients have visual deficits or thickened toenails, a podiatrist should cut the nails.
- Reducing risk factors, such as smoking and elevated blood lipids, that contribute to peripheral vascular disease
- Avoiding home remedies or over-the-counter agents or self-medicating to treat foot problems (Fritschi, 2001)

FIGURE 41-10 The monofilament test is used to assess the sensory threshold in patients with diabetes. The test instrument—a monofilament—is gently applied to about five pressure points on the foot (as shown in image on left). (**A**) This is an example of a monofilament used for advanced quantitative assessment; (**B**) Sennes-Weinstein monofilament used by clinicians; (**C**) disposable monofilament used by patients. The examiner applies the monofilament to the test area to determine if the patient feels the device. Adapted with permission from Cameron, B. L. (2002). Making diabetes management routine. *American Journal of Nursing, 102* (2); 26–32.

Blood glucose control is important for avoiding decreased resistance to infections and for preventing diabetic neuropathy. The patient may be referred by the physician to a wound care centre for managing persistent wounds of the feet or legs. Many wound care centres provide diabetes education; however, the patient needs to discuss recommendations for treating wounds with his or her own physician, as well as raising any questions about diabetes management.

Special Issues in Diabetes Care

THE PATIENT WITH DIABETES UNDERGOING SURGERY

During periods of physiologic stress such as surgery, blood glucose levels tend to rise as a result of an increase in the level of stress hormones (epinephrine, norepinephrine, glucagon, cortisol, and growth hormone). If hyperglycemia is not controlled during surgery, the resulting osmotic diuresis may lead to excessive loss of fluids and electrolytes. Patients with type 1 diabetes also risk developing ketoacidosis during periods of stress.

Hypoglycemia is also a concern in diabetic patients undergoing surgery. This is especially a concern during the preoperative period if surgery is delayed beyond the morning in a patient who received a morning injection of intermediate-acting insulin.

There are various approaches to managing glucose control during the perioperative period. Frequent capillary glucose monitoring is essential throughout the preoperative and postoperative periods, regardless of the method used for glucose control. Examples of these approaches are as follows, although the use of IV insulin and dextrose has become widespread with the increased availability of meters for intraoperative glucose monitoring:

- The morning of surgery, all subcutaneous insulin doses are withheld (unless the blood glucose level is elevated—for example, more than 11.1 mmol/L, in which case a small dose of subcutaneous regular insulin may be prescribed). The blood glucose level is controlled during surgery with the IV infusion of regular insulin, which is balanced by an infusion of dextrose. The insulin and dextrose infusion rates are adjusted according to frequent (hourly) capillary glucose determinations. After surgery, the insulin infusion may be continued until the patient can eat. If IV insulin is discontinued, subcutaneous regular insulin may be administered at set intervals (every 4 to 6 hours), or intermediate-acting insulin may be administered every 12 hours with supplemental regular insulin as necessary until the patient is eating and the usual pattern of insulin dosing is resumed. The nurse caring for a patient with diabetes who is receiving IV insulin must carefully monitor the insulin infusion rate and blood glucose levels. IV insulin has a much shorter duration of action than subcutaneous insulin. Thus, if the infusion is interrupted or discontinued, hyperglycemia will develop rapidly (within 1 hour in type 1 diabetes and within a few hours in type 2 diabetes). The nurse must ensure that subcutaneous insulin is administered 30 minutes before discontinuing the IV insulin infusion.
- One half to two thirds of the patient's usual morning dose of insulin (either intermediate-acting insulin alone or both short- and intermediate-acting insulins) is administered subcutaneously in the morning before surgery. The remainder is then administered after surgery.

- The patient's usual daily dose of subcutaneous insulin is divided into four equal doses of regular insulin. These are then administered at 6-hour intervals. The last two approaches do not provide the control achieved by IV administration of insulin and dextrose.
- Patients with type 2 diabetes who do not usually take insulin may require insulin during the perioperative period to control blood glucose elevations. Patients who are taking chlorpropamide, a long-acting oral antidiabetic agent, may be instructed to discontinue the oral agent 24 to 48 hours before surgery. Some of these patients may resume their usual regimen of diet and oral agent during the recovery period. Other patients (whose diabetes is probably not well controlled with diet and an oral antidiabetic agent before surgery) need to continue with insulin injections after discharge.
- For patients with type 2 diabetes who are undergoing minor surgery but who do not normally take insulin, glucose levels may remain stable provided no dextrose is infused during the surgery. After surgery, they may require small doses of regular insulin until the usual diet and oral agent are resumed.

During the postoperative period, diabetic patients must also be closely monitored for cardiovascular complications because of the increased prevalence of atherosclerosis in patients with diabetes, wound infections, and skin breakdown (especially in the patient with decreased pain sensation in the extremities due to neuropathy). Maintaining adequate nutrition and blood glucose control promotes wound healing.

MANAGEMENT OF HOSPITALIZED DIABETIC PATIENTS

At any one time, 10% to 20% of general medical-surgical patients in the hospital have diabetes. This number will increase as elderly patients make up a greater proportion of the population. Although some hospitals may have a specialized diabetic/metabolic unit, typically patients with diabetes are admitted throughout the hospital.

Often diabetes is not the primary medical diagnosis, yet problems with the control of diabetes frequently result from changes in the patient's normal routine or from surgery or illness. Some of the main issues pertinent to nursing care of the hospitalized diabetic patient are presented in the following section.

Self-Care Issues

All patients admitted to the hospital must relinquish control of some aspects of their daily care to the hospital staff. For the patient with diabetes who is actively involved in diabetes self-management (especially insulin dose adjustment), relinquishing control over meal timing, insulin timing, and insulin dosage may be particularly difficult. The patient may fear hypoglycemia and express much concern over possible delays in receiving attention from the nurse if hypoglycemic symptoms occur.

It is important for the nurse to acknowledge the patient's concerns and to involve the patient as much as possible in the plan of care. If the patient disagrees with certain aspects of the nursing or medical care related to diabetes, the nurse must communicate this to other members of the health care team and, where appropriate, make changes in the plan to meet the patient's needs. The nurse and other health care providers need to pay particular attention to patients who are successful in managing self-care, assess their self-care management skills, and encourage them to continue their self-care management if correct and appropriate.

Hyperglycemia During Hospitalization

Hyperglycemia may occur in the hospitalized patient as a result of the original illness that led to the need for hospitalization. In addition, a number of other factors may contribute to hyperglycemia, such as:

- Changes in the usual treatment regimen (eg, increased food, decreased insulin, decreased activity)
- Medications (eg, glucocorticoids such as prednisone, which are used in the treatment of a variety of inflammatory disorders)
- IV dextrose, which may be part of the maintenance fluids or may be used for the administration of antibiotics and other medications
- Overly vigourous treatment of hypoglycemia
- Mismatched timing of meals and insulin (eg, postmeal hyperglycemia may occur if short-acting insulin is administered immediately before or even after meals)

Nursing actions to correct some of these factors are important for avoiding hyperglycemia. Assessment of the patient's usual home routine is important. The nurse should try to approximate as much as possible the home schedule of insulin, meals, and activities. Monitoring blood glucose levels has been identified by the ADA as an additional "vital sign" essential in assessing the patient's status (ADA, Bedside Blood Glucose Monitoring in Hospitals, 2003). The results of blood glucose monitoring provide information needed to obtain orders for extra doses of insulin (at times when insulin is usually taken by the patient), an important nursing function. The insulin doses must not be withheld when blood glucose levels are normal.

Short-acting insulin is usually needed to avoid postprandial hyperglycemia (even in the patient with normal premeal glucose levels), and NPH insulin does not peak until many hours after the dose is given. IV antibiotics should be mixed in normal saline (if possible) to avoid excess infusion of dextrose (especially in the patient who is eating). It is important to avoid overly vigourous treatment of hypoglycemia, which may lead to hyperglycemia. Treatment of hypoglycemia should be based on the established hospital protocol (usually 15 g carbohydrate in the form of juice, glucose tablets, or, if necessary, 0.5 to 1 ampule of 50% dextrose administered intravenously). Extra sugar should not be added to the juice. If the initial treatment does not increase the glucose level adequately, the same treatment may be repeated.

Hypoglycemia During Hospitalization

Hypoglycemia in a hospitalized patient is usually the result of too much insulin or delays in eating. Specific examples include:

- Overuse of "sliding scale" regular insulin, particularly as a supplement to regularly scheduled, twice-daily short- and intermediate-acting insulins
- Lack of dosage change when dietary intake is changed (eg, in the patient taking nothing by mouth)
- Overly vigourous treatment of hyperglycemia (eg, giving too-frequent successive doses of regular insulin before the time of peak insulin activity is reached) so that there is an accumulated effect

- Delayed meal after administration of lispro or aspart insulin (patient should eat within 15 minutes of administration)

Nurses must assess the pattern of glucose values and avoid giving doses of insulin that repeatedly lead to hypoglycemia. Successive doses of subcutaneous regular insulin should be administered no more frequently than every 3 to 4 hours. For patients receiving intermediate insulin before breakfast and dinner, the nurse must use caution in administering supplemental doses of regular insulin at lunch and bedtime. Hypoglycemia may occur when two insulins peak at similar times (eg, morning NPH peaks with lunchtime regular insulin and may lead to late-afternoon hypoglycemia, and dinnertime NPH peaks with bedtime regular insulin and may lead to nocturnal hypoglycemia). To avoid hypoglycemic reactions caused by delayed food intake, the nurse should arrange for a snack to be given to the patient if meals are going to be delayed because of procedures, physical therapy, or other activities.

Common Alterations in Diet

Dietary modifications common during hospitalization require special consideration when the patient has diabetes.

NPO (NOTHING BY MOUTH)

For the patient who must have nothing by mouth in preparation for diagnostic or surgical procedures, the nurse must ensure that the usual insulin dosage has been changed. These changes may include eliminating the regular insulin and giving a decreased amount (eg, half the usual dose) of intermediate-acting insulin. Another approach is to use frequent (every 3 to 4 hours) dosing of regular insulin only. IV dextrose may be administered to provide calories and to avoid hypoglycemia.

Even when no food is taken, glucose levels may rise as a result of hepatic glucose production, especially in patients with type 1 diabetes and lean patients with type 2 diabetes. Further, in type 1 diabetes, elimination of the insulin dose may lead to the development of DKA. Thus, administering insulin to the patient with type 1 diabetes who is NPO is an important nursing action.

For patients with type 2 diabetes who are taking insulin, DKA does not develop when insulin doses are eliminated because the patient's pancreas produces some insulin. Thus, skipping the insulin dose altogether when the patient has type 2 diabetes (and is receiving IV dextrose) may be safe; however, close monitoring is essential.

For patients who are NPO for extended periods, glucose testing and insulin administration should be performed at regular intervals, usually two to four times per day. Insulin regimens for the patient who is NPO for an extended period may include NPH insulin every 12 hours (with regular insulin added to the NPH, depending on the results of glucose testing) or regular insulin only every 4 to 6 hours. These patients should receive dextrose infusions to provide some calories and limit ketosis.

To prevent these problems resulting from the need to withhold food, diagnostic tests and procedures and surgery should be scheduled early in the morning if possible.

CLEAR LIQUID DIET

When the diet is advanced to include clear liquids, the diabetic patient will be receiving more simple carbohydrate foods, such as juice and gelatin desserts, than are usually included in the diabetic diet. It is important for hospitalized patients to maintain their nutritional status as much as possible to promote healing. Thus, the use of reduced-calorie substitutes such as diet soft drinks or diet gelatin desserts would not be appropriate when the only source of calories is clear liquids. Simple carbohydrates, when eaten alone, cause a rapid rise in blood glucose levels; thus, it is important to try to match peak times of insulin with peaks in glucose. If a patient was receiving insulin at regular intervals while NPO, the scheduled times for glucose tests and insulin injections must be changed to match meal times.

ENTERAL TUBE FEEDINGS

Tube feeding formulas contain more simple carbohydrates and less protein and fat than the typical diabetic diet. This results in increased levels of glucose in the diabetic patient receiving tube feedings. It is important that insulin doses be administered at regular intervals (eg, NPH every 12 hours or regular insulin every 4 to 6 hours) when tube feedings are administered at a continuous rate. If insulin is administered at routine (prebreakfast and predinner) times, hypoglycemia during the day may result from patients receiving more insulin without more calories, and hyperglycemia may occur during the night when feedings continue but insulin action decreases.

A common cause of hypoglycemia in patients receiving continuous tube feedings and insulin is inadvertent or purposeful discontinuation of the feeding. The nurse must discuss with the medical team any plans for temporarily discontinuing the tube feeding (eg, when the patient is away from the unit). Planning ahead may allow alterations to be made in the insulin dose, or it may allow for IV dextrose to be administered. In addition, if problems with the tube feeding develop unexpectedly (eg, the patient pulls out the tube, the tube clogs, or the feeding is discontinued when residual gastric contents are found), the nurse must notify the physician, assess blood glucose levels more frequently, and administer IV dextrose if indicated.

PARENTERAL NUTRITION

The patient with diabetes receiving parenteral nutrition may receive both IV insulin (added to the parenteral nutrition container) and subcutaneous intermediate- or short-acting insulins. If the patient is receiving continuous parenteral nutrition, the blood glucose level should be monitored and insulin administered at regular intervals. If the parenteral nutrition is infused over a limited number of hours, subcutaneous insulin should be administered so that peak times of insulin action coincide with times of parenteral nutrition infusion.

Hygiene

The nurse caring for a hospitalized diabetic patient must focus attention on oral hygiene and skin care. Because diabetic patients are at increased risk for periodontal disease, it is important for the nurse to assist patients with daily dental care. The patient may also require assistance in keeping the skin clean and dry, especially in areas of contact between two skin surfaces (eg, groin, axilla, and, in obese women, under the breasts), where chafing and fungal infections tend to occur.

For the bedridden diabetic patient, nursing care must emphasize the prevention of skin breakdown at pressure points. The heels are particularly susceptible to breakdown because of loss of sensation of pain and pressure associated with sensory neuropathy.

Feet should be cleaned, dried, lubricated with lotion (but not between the toes), and inspected frequently. If the patient is in the supine position, pressure on the heels can be alleviated by elevating the lower legs on a pillow, with the heels positioned over the edge of the pillow. When the patient is seated in a chair, the feet should be positioned so that pressure is not placed on the heels. If the patient has a foot ulcer, it is important to provide preventive foot care to the unaffected foot as well as to carry out special care of the affected foot.

As always, every opportunity should be taken to teach the patient about diabetes self-management, including daily oral, skin, and foot care. Female diabetic patients should also be instructed about measures for the avoidance of vaginal infections, which occur more frequently when blood glucose levels are elevated. Patients often take their cues from the nurse and realize the importance of daily personal hygiene if this is emphasized during their hospitalization.

Stress

As mentioned earlier, physiologic stress, such as infections and surgery, contributes to hyperglycemia and may precipitate DKA or HHNS. Emotional stress may have a negative impact on diabetic control as well. An increase in stress hormones leads to an increase in glucose levels, especially when the intake of food and insulin remains unchanged. In addition, during periods of emotional stress, the person with diabetes may alter the usual pattern of meals, exercise, and medication. This contributes to hyperglycemia or even hypoglycemia (eg, in the patient taking insulin or oral antidiabetic agents who stops eating in response to stress).

People who have diabetes must be made aware of the potential deterioration in diabetic control that can accompany emotional stress. They must be encouraged to try to adhere to the diabetes treatment plan as much as possible during times of stress. In addition, learning strategies for minimizing stress and coping with stress when it does occur are important aspects of diabetes education.

Gerontologic Considerations

People with diabetes are living longer; therefore, both type 1 and type 2 diabetes are seen more frequently in the elderly population. Regardless of the type or duration of diabetes, the goals of diabetes treatment may need to be altered when caring for the elderly. The focus is on quality of life issues, such as maintaining independent functioning and promoting general well-being. Although striving for strict blood glucose control may not be safe or appropriate, prolonged symptomatic hyperglycemia should be avoided.

Some elderly patients cannot manage a detailed diabetes treatment plan, but the nurse must not assume that all patients older than a certain age can adhere only to the simplest regimen. Although the goal may be simply to avoid hypoglycemia and symptomatic hyperglycemia, certain patients may prefer more complex regimens that allow more flexibility in meals and daily schedule. As with all people with diabetes, individualization of the treatment plan with frequent follow-up by the health care team is important.

Some of the barriers to learning and self-care that may be seen in the elderly include decreased vision, hearing loss, memory deficits, decreased mobility and fine motor coordination, increased tremors, depression and loneliness, decreased financial resources, and limitations related to other medical illnesses. Assessing patients for these barriers as well as discussing any misconceptions or folk beliefs regarding the cause and treatment of diabetes is important in setting up a diabetes treatment plan and educational activities. Presenting brief, simplified instructions with ample opportunity for practice of skills is important. The use of special devices such as a magnifier for the insulin syringe, an insulin pen, or a mirror for foot inspection is helpful. If necessary, family members and other community resources are called on to assist with diabetes survival skills. It is preferable to teach patients or family members to test blood glucose at home; the choice of meter should be tailored to the patient's visual and cognitive status and dexterity. Frequent evaluation of self-care skills (insulin administration, blood glucose monitoring, foot care, diet planning) is essential, especially in patients with deteriorating vision and memory.

Dietary adherence is difficult for some elderly patients because of decreased appetite, poor dentition, and decreased physical and financial ability to prepare meals. In addition, patients may be unwilling to change long-standing dietary habits. Altering the meal plan to incorporate these eating habits or other limitations may be necessary.

> **NURSING ALERT** Careful monitoring for diabetes complications must not be neglected in elderly patients. Hypoglycemia is especially dangerous because it may go undetected and result in falls. Dehydration is a concern in patients who have chronically elevated blood glucose levels. Assessment for long-term complications, especially eye and foot problems, is important. Avoiding blindness and amputation through early detection and treatment of retinopathy and foot ulcers may mean the difference between institutionalization and continued independent living for the elderly person with diabetes.

NURSING PROCESS: THE PATIENT WITH DIABETES AS A SECONDARY DIAGNOSIS

People with diabetes frequently seek medical attention for problems not directly related to blood glucose control. However, during the course of treatment for the primary medical diagnosis, blood glucose control may worsen. In addition, the only opportunity for some patients with diabetes to update their knowledge about diabetes self-care and prevention of complications is during hospitalization. Therefore, it is important for the nurse caring for the patient with diabetes to focus attention on diabetes, regardless of the primary problem. Further, control of blood glucose levels is important because hyperglycemia impairs resistance to certain infections and impedes wound healing.

Assessment

Assessment of the patient with diabetes with a primary problem such as cardiac disease, renal disease, cerebrovascular disease, peripheral vascular disease, surgery, or any other type of illness is the same as that for a nondiabetic patient and is described in other chapters. In addition to nursing assessment for the primary problem, assessment of the patient with diabetes must also focus on hypoglycemia and hyperglycemia, skin breakdown, and diabetes self-care skills, including survival skills and measures for prevention of long-term complications. In addition, the patient is asked about use of alternative or complementary therapies; studies have demonstrated that patients with diabetes are twice as

likely as other patients to use these therapies, and some may be harmful (Egede et al., 2002).

The patient is assessed for hypoglycemia and hyperglycemia with frequent blood glucose monitoring (usually prescribed before meals and at bedtime) and with monitoring for signs and symptoms of hypoglycemia or prolonged hyperglycemia (including DKA or HHNS), as described in previous sections.

Careful assessment of the skin, especially at pressure points and on the lower extremities, is important. The skin is assessed for dryness, cracks, skin breakdown, and redness. The patient is asked about symptoms of neuropathy, such as tingling and pain or numbness of the feet. Deep tendon reflexes are assessed.

Assessment of diabetes self-care skills is performed as early as possible to determine whether the patient requires further diabetes teaching. The nurse observes the patient preparing and injecting the insulin, monitoring blood glucose, and performing foot care. (Simply questioning the patient about these skills without actually observing performance of the skills is not sufficient.) Knowledge about diet can be assessed with the help of the dietitian through direct questioning and review of patient choices on the menu. The patient is questioned regarding signs, treatment, and prevention of hypoglycemia and hyperglycemia. The patient's knowledge of risk factors for macrovascular disease, including hypertension, increased lipids, and smoking, is assessed. The patient is asked the date of the last eye examination (including dilation of the pupil). It is also important to assess the patient's use of preventive health measures: annual influenza vaccination (flu shot), date of last pneumonia vaccine (ADA, Immunization and the Prevention of Influenza and Pneumococcal Disease in People With Diabetes, 2003), daily dose of aspirin (unless contraindicated) (ADA, Aspirin Therapy in Diabetes, 2003), and smoking cessation (ADA, Smoking and Diabetes, 2003).

Diagnosis

NURSING DIAGNOSES

Based on the assessment data, the patient's major nursing diagnoses may include:

- Imbalanced nutrition related to increase in stress hormones (caused by primary medical problem) and imbalances in insulin, food, and physical activity
- Risk for impaired skin integrity related to immobility and lack of sensation (caused by neuropathy)
- Deficient knowledge about diabetes self-care skills (caused by lack of basic diabetes education or lack of continuing in-depth diabetes education)

COLLABORATIVE PROBLEMS/ POTENTIAL COMPLICATIONS

Based on the assessment data, potential complications may include:

- Inadequate control of blood glucose levels (hyperglycemia, hypoglycemia)
- DKA and HNNS

Planning and Goals

The major goals for the patient may include improved nutritional status, maintenance of skin integrity, ability to perform basic diabetes self-care skills as well as preventive care for the avoidance of chronic diabetes complications, and absence of complications.

Nursing Interventions

IMPROVING NUTRITIONAL STATUS

The patient's diet is planned with the primary goal of glucose control; however, the dietary prescription must also consider the patient's primary health problem in addition to lifestyle, cultural background, activity level, and food preferences. If alterations are needed in the patient's diet because of the primary health problem (eg, GI problems), alternative strategies to ensure adequate nutritional intake must be implemented. The patient's nutritional intake is monitored carefully along with blood glucose, urine ketones, and daily weight. Blood glucose records are assessed for patterns of hypoglycemia and hyperglycemia at the same time of day, and findings are reported to the physician for alteration in insulin orders. In the patient with elevated blood glucose levels that are prolonged, laboratory values and the patient's physical condition are monitored for signs of DKA or HHNS.

MAINTAINING SKIN CARE

The skin is assessed daily for dryness or breaks. The feet are cleaned with warm water and soap. Excessive soaking of the feet is avoided. The feet are dried thoroughly, especially between the toes, and lotion is applied to the entire foot except between the toes. For bedridden patients (especially those with a history of neuropathy), the heels are elevated off the bed with a pillow placed under the lower legs and the heels resting over the edge of the pillow. Dermal ulcers are treated as indicated and prescribed. The nurse promotes optimal blood glucose control in patients with skin breakdown.

ADDRESSING KNOWLEDGE DEFICITS

Hospital admission of the patient with diabetes provides an ideal opportunity for the nurse to assess the patient's level of knowledge about diabetes and its management. The nurse uses this opportunity to assess the patient's understanding of diabetes management, including blood glucose monitoring, administration of medications (ie, insulin, oral agents), dietary requirements, exercise, and strategies to prevent long- and short-term complications of diabetes. The nurse also assesses the adjustment of the patient and family to diabetes and its management and identifies any misconceptions they have.

MONITORING AND MANAGING POTENTIAL COMPLICATIONS

Inadequate control of blood glucose levels may hinder recovery from the immediate health problem. Blood glucose levels are monitored, and insulin is administered as prescribed. It is important for the nurse to ensure that insulin prescribed is modified as needed to compensate for changes in the patient's schedule or eating pattern. Treatment is given for hypoglycemia (with oral glucose) or hyperglycemia (with supplemental regular insulin no more often than every 3 to 4 hours). Blood glucose records are assessed for patterns of hypoglycemia and hyperglycemia at the same time of day, and findings are reported to the physician for modification in insulin orders. In the patient with elevated blood glucose levels that are prolonged, laboratory values and the patient's physical condition are monitored for signs of DKA or HHNS.

Development of acute complications of diabetes secondary to inadequate control of blood glucose levels may be associated with other health care problems because of changes in activity level and diet and physiologic alterations related to the primary health prob-

lem itself. Therefore, the patient must be monitored for acute complications (hyperglycemia, hypoglycemia) and measures must be implemented for their prevention and early treatment.

PROMOTING HOME AND COMMUNITY-BASED CARE

Teaching Patients Self-Care

Even if the patient has had diabetes for many years, it is important to assess his or her knowledge and adherence to the plan of care. It may be necessary to plan and implement a teaching plan that includes basic information about diabetes, its cause and symptoms, and acute and chronic complications and their treatment. The nurse asks the patient to give repeated return demonstrations of skills that were not performed correctly during the initial assessment. The patient is taught self-care activities for the prevention of long-term complications, including foot care, eye care, and risk factor management. The nurse also reminds the patient and family about the importance of health promotion activities and recommended health screening.

Continuing Care

The patient who is hospitalized for another health problem may require referral for home care for that problem or if gaps in knowledge about self-care are uncovered. In either case, the home care nurse can use this opportunity to assess the patient's knowledge about diabetes management and the patient's and family's ability to carry out that management. Teaching provided in the hospital, clinic, office, or diabetes education centre is reinforced by the nurse. The home care environment is assessed to determine its adequacy for self-care and safety.

During home care visits, the nurse assesses the patient for signs and symptoms of long-term complications and assesses the patient's and family's techniques in blood glucose monitoring, insulin administration, and food selection. In addition, the patient and family are reminded of the importance of participating in health promotion activities as well as recommended health screening.

Evaluation

EXPECTED PATIENT OUTCOMES

Expected patient outcomes may include:

1. Achieves optimal control of blood glucose
   a. Avoids extremes of hypoglycemia and hyperglycemia
   b. Takes steps to resolve rapidly any hypoglycemic episodes
2. Maintains skin integrity
   a. Demonstrates intact skin without dryness and cracking
   b. Avoids ulcers caused by pressure and neuropathy
3. Demonstrates/verbalizes diabetes survival skills and preventive care
4. Understands treatment modalities
   a. Demonstrates proper technique for administering insulin or oral antidiabetic medications and assessing blood glucose
   b. Demonstrates appropriate knowledge of diet through proper menu selections and identification of pattern used for selecting foods at home
   c. Verbalizes signs, appropriate treatment, and prevention of hypoglycemia and hyperglycemia
5. Demonstrate proper foot care
   a. Inspects feet (using mirror if necessary to see bottom of foot), including inspection for cracks or fungal infections between toes

b. Washes feet with warm water and soap; dries feet thoroughly
c. Applies lotion to entire foot except between toes
d. Verbalizes behaviours that decrease the risk of foot ulcers, including wearing shoes at all times; using hand or elbow, not foot, to test temperature of bath water; avoiding use of heating pad on feet; avoiding constrictive shoes; wearing new shoes for brief periods; avoiding home remedies for treatment of corns and calluses; having feet examined at every appointment with the physician; and consulting a podiatrist for regular nail care if necessary

6. Takes steps to prevent eye disease
   a. Verbalizes need for yearly or more frequent thorough dilated eye examinations by an ophthalmologist (starting at 5 years after diagnosis for type 1 diabetes or the year of diagnosis for type 2 diabetes)
   b. Verbalizes that retinopathy usually does not cause change in vision until serious damage to the retina has occurred
   c. States that early laser treatment along with good control of blood glucose and blood pressure may prevent visual loss from retinopathy
   d. Identifies hypoglycemia and hyperglycemia as two causes of temporary blurred vision

7. States measures to control macrovascular risk factors
   a. Smoking cessation
   b. Limitation of fats and cholesterol
   c. Control of hypertension
   d. Exercise
   e. Regular monitoring of renal function

8. Reports absence of acute complications
   a. Maintains blood glucose and urine ketones within normal limits
   b. Experiences no signs or symptoms of hypoglycemia or hyperglycemia
   c. Identifies signs and symptoms of hypoglycemia or hyperglycemia
   d. Reports appearance of symptoms so that treatment can be initiated

Critical Thinking Exercises

1. A patient is newly diagnosed with type 1 diabetes. Identify the major nursing assessment issues and nursing interventions in each of the following situations: (1) the patient is in the first trimester of pregnancy, (2) the patient refuses to use insulin, and (3) the patient is developmentally disabled and able to understand only simple instructions.

2. A patient with type 2 diabetes is scheduled for major abdominal surgery. What modifications in nursing assessment and care before, during, and after surgery are indicated because of the diagnosis of type 2 diabetes? How would these differ if the patient had type 1 diabetes?

3. A 57-year-old patient is brought to the emergency department by his daughter because he has become drowsy and has developed slurred speech over the last hour. His daughter, who lives out of town, tells you that he has re-

cently been diagnosed with diabetes and has been depressed ever since. She does not know how the diabetes is being managed. What assessment data would you initially obtain? What diagnostic tests and treatments would you anticipate? Provide the rationale for those tests and treatments.

4. A 48-year-old patient with three children has had diabetes for 5 years and has not adhered to the prescribed treatment regimen. He says, "My father and grandfather both died from diabetes. I don't see any point in modifying my life if I'm going to die from diabetes anyway." How would you approach this patient? What resources would you use? How would you alter your approach if your first efforts to convince him of the benefits of treatment were unsuccessful?

5. Your patient has diabetes, and blood glucose monitoring is recommended. Develop a plan for teaching blood glucose monitoring to him. Explain how the results of monitoring are used in the management of type 1 and type 2 diabetes. How would you modify your teaching plan if the patient is blind? If he understands little English?

REFERENCES AND SELECTED READINGS

Books

Centers for Disease Control and Prevention. (2002). *National diabetes fact sheet: National estimates and general information and national estimates on diabetes in the United States, 2000.* Atlanta, GA: U.S. Department of Health and Human Services, Centers for Disease Control and Prevention.

Health Canada. Office of Nutrition Policy and Promotion. Health Products and Food Branch. (1997). *Canada's food guide to healthy eating.* Ottawa: Author.

National Institutes of Health, National Heart, Lung and Blood Institute, North American Association for the Study of Obesity. (2000). *The practical guide: Identification, evaluation and treatment of overweight and obesity in adults.* NIH Publication Number 00-4084. Bethesda, MD.

Porth, C. M. (2002). *Pathophysiology: Concepts of altered health states* (6th ed.). Philadelphia: Lippincott Williams & Wilkins.

Tilton, M. C. (1997). Diabetes and amputation. In M. L. Sipski & C. J. Alexander (Eds.), *Sexual function in people with disability and chronic illness: A health professional's guide.* Gaithersburg, MD: Aspen Publishers.

Journals

Asterisks indicate nursing research articles.

General

ADA. (2003). Screening for type 2 diabetes. *Diabetes Care, 26*(1), 21–24.

ADA. (2003). Implications of the Diabetes Control and Complications Trial. (Position Statement). *Diabetes Care, 26*(1), 25–27.

ADA. (2003). Implications of the United Kingdom Prospective Diabetes Study. (Position Statement). *Diabetes Care, 26*(1), 28–32.

ADA. (1998). Economic consequences of diabetes mellitus in the U.S. in 1997. *Diabetes Care, 21*(2), 296–309.

ADA. (2003). Immunization and the prevention of influenza and pneumococcal disease in people with diabetes. (Position Statement) *Diabetes Care, 26*(1), 126–128.

ADA. (2003). Prevention of type 1 diabetes mellitus. (Position Statement). *Diabetes Care, 26*(1), 140.

Anderson-Loftin, W., & Moneyham, L., (2000). Long-term disease management needs of southern African Americans with diabetes. *Diabetes Educator, 26*(5), 821–832.

Bohannon, N. J. (1999). Coronary artery disease and diabetes. *Postgraduate Medicine, 105*(2), 66–80.

Canadian Diabetes Association. (2005). *About diabetes.* Available at: www.diabetes.ca/section_about/index.asp. Retrieved December 15, 2005.

Canadian Diabetes Association. (2003). Clinical practice guidelines for the prevention and management of diabetes in Canada. [Special issue]. *Canadian Journal of Diabetes, 27*(Suppl. 2).

CDC Diabetes Cost-Effectiveness Study Group. (1998). The cost-effectiveness of screening for type 2 diabetes. *Journal of the American Medical Association, 280,* 1757–1763.

Dewey, C. M., & Riley, W. J. (1999). Have diabetes, will travel. *Post-graduate Medicine, 105*(2), 111–126.

Diabetes Prevention Program Research Group (2002). Reduction in the incidence of type 2 diabetes with lifestyle intervention or metformin. *New England Journal of Medicine, 346*(6), 393–403.

Dyck, B. (1998). Clinical update. Diabetes update with a cardiac perspective. *Progress in Cardiovascular Nursing, 13*(2), 28–36.

Egede, L. E., Ye, X., Zheng, D., & Silverstein, M. D. (20002). The prevalence and pattern of complementary and alternative medicine use in individuals with diabetes. *Diabetes Care, 25*(2), 324–329.

Funnell, M. M. (1999). Care of the nursing-home resident with diabetes. *Clinics in Geriatric Medicine, 15*(2), 413–422.

Funnell, M. M., Arnold, M. S., Fogler, J., Merritt, J. H., & Anderson, I. A. (1998). Participation in a diabetes education and care program: Experience from the Diabetes Care for Older Adults project. *Diabetes Educator, 24*(2), 163–167.

Goldstein, I., et al. (1998). Oral sildenafil in the treatment of erectile dysfunction. *New England Journal of Medicine, 338*(20), 1397–1404.

Guay, A. T. (1998). Treatment of erectile dysfunction in men with diabetes. *Diabetes Spectrum, 11*(2), 101–111.

Martin, W. (1999). Oral health and the older diabetic. *Clinics in Geriatric Medicine, 15*(2), 339–350.

Mensing, C., Boucher, J., Cypress, M., et al. (2003). National standards for diabetes self-management education. (Position Statement). *Diabetes Care, 26*(1), 149–156.

Mokdad, A., Ford, E. S., Bowman, B. A., et al. (2000). Diabetes trends in the U.S.: 1990–1998. *Diabetes Care, 23*(9), 1278–1283.

Quinn, L., (2001a). Type 2 diabetes. Epidemiology, pathophysiology, and diagnosis. *Nursing Clinics of North America, 36*(2), 175–192.

Rendell, M. S., et al. (1999). Sildenafil for treatment of erectile dysfunction in men with diabetes. *Journal of the American Medical Association, 281*(5), 421–426.

Statistics Canada, Health Statistics Division. (1997). *Selected leading causes of death, by sex.* Available at: www.40.statcan.ca/101/cst01/health36.htm. Retrieved December 15, 2005.

Weiss, R. (1999). Communication strategies. Diabetics learn while they shop in disease-management program. *Health Progress, 80*(1), 68.

Complications

Aljahlan, M., Lee, K. C., & Toth, E. (1999). Limited joint mobility in diabetes. *Postgraduate Medicine, 105*(2), 99–106.

ADA. (2003). Diabetic retinopathy. (Position Statement). *Diabetes Care, 26*(1), 99–102.

ADA. (2003). Hyperglycemic crisis in patients with diabetes mellitus. (Position Statement). *Diabetes Care, 26*(1), 109–117.

Beckwith, S. (1999). Complications in diabetes: Measures to reduce the risks. *Community Nurse, 4*(12), 24–26.

DCCT Research Group. (1993). The effect of intensive treatment of diabetes on the development and progression of long-term complications in insulin-dependent diabetes mellitus. *New England Journal of Medicine, 329*(14), 977–986.

Fritschi, C. (2001). Preventive care of the diabetic foot. *Nursing Clinics of North America, 36*(2), 303–320.

Grinslade, S., & Buck, E. A. (1999). Diabetic ketoacidosis: Implications for the medical-surgical nurse. *MedSurg Nursing, 8*(1), 37–45.

Halpin-Landry, J. E., & Goldsmith, S. (1999). Feet first: Diabetes care. *American Journal of Nursing, 99*(2), 26–34.

Harman, K. (1999). Focus on feet to reduce risk from diabetes. *Practice Nurse, 17*(2), 91–96.

*Hathaway, D. K., Cashion, A. K., Wicks, M. N., Milstead, E. J., & Gaber, A. O. (1998). Cardiovascular dysautonomia of patients with end-stage renal disease and type 1 or type 2 diabetes. *Nursing Research, 47*(3), 171–179.

Hernandes, D. (1998). Hospitalization can exacerbate devastating complications of type II diabetes, including retinopathy, neuropathy, and nephropathy. *American Journal of Nursing, 98*(6), 27–31.

Magee, M. F., & Bhatt, B. A. (2001). Management of decompensated diabetes. Diabetic ketoacidosis and hyperglycemic hyperosmolar syndrome. *Critical Care Clinics, 17*(1), 75–106.

Millar, W. J., & Young, T. K. (2003). Tracking diabetes: Prevalence, incidence and risk factors. *Health Reports, 14*(3), 35–47.

Pudner, R. (2002). Assessing diabetic patients at risk for foot ulceration. *Journal of Community Nursing, 16*(1), 18–22.

Quinn, L., (2001c). Diabetic emergencies in the patient with type 2 diabetes. *Nursing Clinics of North America, 36*(2), 341–360.

Ramsey, S. D., Newton, K., Blough, D., et al. (1999). Incidence, outcomes, and cost of foot ulcers in patients with diabetes. *Diabetes Care, 22*(3), 382–387.

Rendell, M. S., Rajfer, J., Wicker, P. A., & Smith, M. D. (1999). Sildenafil for treatment of erectile dysfunction in men with diabetes: A randomized controlled trial. Sildenafil Diabetes Study Group. *Journal of American Medical Association, 281*(5), 421–426.

Setter, S. M., Baker, D. E., Campbell, R. K., & Johnson, S. B. (1999). Sildenafil (Viagra) for the treatment of erectile dysfunction in men with diabetes. *Diabetes Educator, 25*(1), 79–87.

Tkacs, N. C. (2002). Hypoglycemia unawareness: Your patients with diabetes won't always know when their blood sugar is low. *American Journal of Nursing, 102*(2), 34–40.

Management

ADA. (2003). Standards of medical care for patients with diabetes mellitus. (Position Statement). *Diabetes Care, 26*(1), 33–50.

ADA. (2003). Hospital admission guidelines for diabetes mellitus. (Position Statement). *Diabetes Care, 26*(1), 118.

ADA. (2003). Bedside blood glucose monitoring in hospitals. (Position Statement). *Diabetes Care, 26*(1), 119.

ADA. (2003). Continuous subcutaneous insulin infusion. (Position Statement). *Diabetes Care, 26*(1), 125.

ADA. (2003). Evidence-based nutrition principles and recommendations for the treatment and prevention of diabetes and related complications. (Position Statement). *Diabetes Care, 26*(1), 51–61.

ADA. (2003). Translation of the diabetes nutrition recommendations for health care institutions. (Position Statement). *Diabetes Care, 26*(1), 70–72.

ADA. (2003). Preventive foot care in adults with diabetes. (Position Statement). *Diabetes Care, 26*(1), 78–79.

ADA. (2003). Treatment of hypertension in adults with diabetes. (Position Statement). *Diabetes Care, 26*(1), 80–82.

ADA. (2003). Management of dyslipidemia in adults with diabetes. (Position Statement). *Diabetes Care, 26*(1), 83–86.

ADA. (2003). Aspirin therapy in diabetes. (Position Statement). *Diabetes Care, 26*(1), 87–88.

ADA. (2003). Smoking and diabetes. (Position Statement). *Diabetes Care, 26*(1), 89–91.

American Dietetic Association. (1999). Position of the American Dietetic Association: Medical nutrition therapy and pharmacotherapy. *Journal of the American Dietetic Association, 99*(2), 227–230.

Beebe, C., & O'Donnell, M. (2001). Educating patients with type 2 diabetes. *Nursing Clinics of North America, 36*(2), 375–386.

Braun, L. T. (2001). Lipid disorders in type 2 diabetes. *Nursing Clinics of North America, 36*(2), 291–302.

Colwell, L., & Quinn, L. (2001). Glycemic control and heart disease. *Nursing Clinics of North America, 36*(2), 321–331.

Conlon, P. C. (2001). A practical approach to type 2 diabetes. *Nursing Clinics of North America, 36*(2), 193–202.

Cooper, J. W. (1998). Oral agent treatment of diabetes mellitus in older adults. *Annals of Long Term Care, 6*(3), 414–422.

Creviston, T., & Quinn, L. (2001). Exercise and physical activity in the treatment of type 2 diabetes. *Nursing Clinics of North America, 36*(2), 243–272.

Cunningham, M. A. (2001). Glucose monitoring in type 2 diabetes. *Nursing Clinics of North America, 36*(2), 361–374.

Emilien, G., Maloteaux, J. M., & Ponchon, M. (1999). Pharmacological management of diabetes: Recent progress and future perspective in daily drug treatment. *Pharmacology and Therapeutics, 81*(1), 37–51.

Fleming, D. R. (1999). Challenging traditional insulin injection practices. *American Journal of Nursing, 99*(2), 72–74.

Flood, L., & Constance, A. (2002). Diabetes and exercise safety. *American Journal of Nursing, 102*(6), 47–55.

Inzucchi, S. E., et al. (1998). Efficacy and metabolic effects of metformin and troglitazone in type II diabetes mellitus. *New England Journal of Medicine, 338*(13), 867–872.

Jacobson, A. F. (1999). Saving limbs with Semmes-Weinstein monofilament. *American Journal of Nursing, 99*(2), 76.

O'Neill, S. (1999). How to achieve effective diabetes management. *Nursing Times, 95*(1), 53–54.

Quinn, L. (2001*b*). Pharmacologic management of the patient with Type 2 Diabetes. *Nursing Clinics of North America, 36*(2), 217–242.

Reed, R. L., & Mooradian, A. D. (1998). Management of diabetes mellitus in the nursing home. *Annals of Long Term Care, 6*(3), 100–107.

Schlater, A. L. (1998). Diabetes in older persons: Special considerations. *Western Journal of Medicine, 168*(6), 532–533.

Sengewald, J. M. (1999). Update on diabetes medications. *Journal of Emergency Nursing, 25*(1), 28–30.

Shapiro, A. M., Ryan, E. A., & Lakey, J. R. (2001). Pancreatic islet transplantation in the treatment of diabetes mellitus. *Best Practices Research in Clinical Endocrinology and Metabolism, 15*(2), 241–264.

Swenson, K., & Brackenridge, B. (1998). Lispro insulin for improved glucose control in obese patients with Type 2 diabetes. *Diabetes Spectrum, 11*(1), 13–15.

United Kingdom Prospective Diabetes Study Group. (1998). Intensive blood glucose control with sulfonylureas or insulin compared with conventional treatment and risk of complications with type 2 diabetes. *Lancet, 352,* 837–853.

Pregnancy and Gestational Diabetes

ADA. (2003). Preconception care of women with diabetes. (Position Statement). *Diabetes Care, 26*(1), 91–93.

ADA. (2003). Gestational diabetes mellitus. (Position Statement). *Diabetes Care, 26*(1), 103–105.

RESOURCES AND WEBSITES

Agencies

American Association of Diabetes Educators, 444 N. Michigan Ave., Suite 1240, Chicago, IL 60611; (800) 832-6874; http://www.diabetesnet.com/aade.html.

American Diabetes Association (ADA), 1660 Duke St., Alexandria, VA 22314; (800) 232-3472; http://www.diabetes.org.

American Dietetic Association, 216 W. Jackson Boulevard, Chicago, IL 60606; (800) 366-1655; http://www.eatright.org.

American Foundation for the Blind, 15 W. 16th St., New York, NY 10011; (800) 232-5463; http://www.afb.org.

Centers for Disease Control and Prevention, 1600 Clifton Rd., Atlanta, GA 30333; (404) 639-3311, http://www.cdc.gov/diabetes//pubs/factsheet.htm.

Canadian Diabetes Association, National Life Building, 400-522 University Avenue, Toronto, ON M5G 2R5; 416-363-0177; toll free: 1-800 BANTING (1-800-226-8464); fax: 416-408-7117; email: info@diabetes.ca; http://www.diabetes.ca.

Dietitians of Canada, 480 University Avenue, Suite 604, Toronto, ON M5G 1V2; 416-596-0857; fax: 416-596-0603; http://www.dietitians.ca.

Juvenile Diabetes Foundation International, 120 Wall St., 19th Floor, New York, NY 10005; (800) JDF-CURE, (800) 223-1138; http://www.jdfcure.com.

MedicAlert Foundation International, 2323 Colorado St., Turlock, CA 95381-1009; (209) 668-3333; http://www.medicalert.org.

National Library Services for the Blind and Physically Handicapped (NLSBPH), Library of Congress, 1291 Taylor St., NW, Washington DC 20542; (202) 287-5100; (800) 424-8567; http://www.lcweb.loc.gov/nls.

National Diabetes Information Clearinghouse, 1 Information Way, Bethesda, MD 20892; (800) GETWELL, (301) 654-3327; http://www.niddk.nih.gov.

Nutrition Labelling Education Centre; http://www.healthyeatingisinstore.ca.

Sources for Patients

Blumer, I. & Rubin, A. L. (2004). *Diabetes for Canadians for dummies.* Etobicoke, ON: John Wiley & Sons Canada, Ltd.

Canadian Diabetes Association: Beyond the Basics: Meal Planning for Healthy Eating, Diabetes Prevention and Management; http://www.diabetes.ca/Section_Professionals/btb.asp. More nutrition pages; http://www.diabetes.ca/Section_Professionals/ng_index.asp.

Health Canada: Canada's Food Guide to Healthy Eating; http://www.hc-sc.gc.ca/hpfb-dgpsa/onpp-bppn/food_guide_rainbow_e.html.

Rosenthal, M. S. (2002). *The Canadian type 2 diabetes sourcebook.* Toronto, ON: Macmillan.

Assessment and Management of Patients With Endocrine Disorders

Adapted by Bev Williams

LEARNING OBJECTIVES

On completion of this chapter, the learner will be able to:

1. Describe the functions of each of the endocrine glands and their hormones.
2. Identify the diagnostic tests used to determine alterations in function of each of the endocrine glands.
3. Compare hypothyroidism and hyperthyroidism: their causes, clinical manifestations, management, and nursing interventions.
4. Develop a plan of nursing care for the patient undergoing thyroidectomy.
5. Compare hyperparathyroidism and hypoparathyroidism: their causes, clinical manifestations, management, and nursing interventions.
6. Compare Addison's disease with Cushing's syndrome: their causes, clinical manifestations, management, and nursing interventions.
7. Use the nursing process as a framework for care of patients with adrenal insufficiency.
8. Use the nursing process as a framework for care of patients with Cushing's syndrome.
9. Identify the teaching needs of patients requiring corticosteroid therapy.

*T*he nervous system and the interconnected network of glands known as the endocrine system control body systems. Disorders of the endocrine system are common and have the potential to affect the function of every organ system in the body. Understanding the function of each of the endocrine glands, and the consequences of hypofunction and hyperfunction of each gland, enables the nurse to anticipate physiologic changes and to plan interventions to address them. Nursing interventions that are essential in managing endocrine disorders are carried out in every setting from the intensive care unit to the outpatient setting and the home.

Anatomic and Physiologic Overview

The endocrine system has far-reaching effects in the human body because of its links with the nervous system and the immune system. The hormones secreted by the endocrine system are affected in large part by structures in the central nervous system, such as the hypothalamus. Other structures located in the brain, such as the pituitary gland, are endocrine glands that influence the function of a large number of other endocrine glands. The effects of hormones secreted by the endocrine system affect the nervous system and are, in turn, mediated by the nervous system. The adrenal medulla, for example, secretes a number of substances (eg, norepinephrine and epinephrine) that act as neurotransmitters. The immune system also interacts closely with the endocrine system. It responds to the introduction of foreign agents by means of chemicals (eg, interleukins, interferons) and is regulated by hormones secreted by the adrenal cortex.

In addition to the hormones secreted by the major endocrine glands, other tissues produce hormones that are secreted into body fluids and act on nearby cells and tissues. The gastrointestinal mucosa produces hormones (eg, gastrin, enterogastrone, secretin, and cholecystokinin) that are important in the digestive process. The kidneys produce erythropoietin, a hormone that stimulates the bone marrow to produce red blood cells. The white blood cells produce cytokines that actively participate in inflammatory and immune responses.

Hormones are important in regulation of the internal environment of the body and affect every aspect of life. Some hormones target specific tissues; for example, **adrenocorticotropic hormone (ACTH)**, or corticotrophin, is secreted by the anterior pituitary gland and targets the adrenal cortex to increase the secretion of the hormones of the adrenal cortex (ie, glucocorticoids, mineralocorticoids, and androgens). Other hormones affect a wide variety of cells and tissues of the body. Thyroid hormone is one example; it affects metabolic activity of cells throughout the body.

GLANDS OF THE ENDOCRINE SYSTEM

The **endocrine** glands include the pituitary, thyroid, parathyroids, adrenals, pancreatic islets, ovaries, and testes (Fig. 42-1). Endocrine glands secrete their products directly into the bloodstream, which differentiates them from **exocrine** glands, such as sweat glands, which secrete their products through ducts onto epithelial surfaces or into the gastrointestinal tract. The hypothalamus is the link between the nervous system and the endocrine system. (Because of the unique endocrine and exocrine functions of the pancreas, pancreatic function and disorders are discussed

Glossary

acromegaly: disease process resulting from excessive secretion of somatotropin causing progressive enlargement of peripheral body parts, commonly the face, head, hands, and feet

Addison's disease: chronic adrenocortical insufficiency secondary to destruction of the adrenal glands

addisonian crisis: acute adrenocortical insufficiency; characterized by acute hypotension, cyanosis, fever, nausea and vomiting, and the classic signs of shock; precipitated by stress or abrupt withdrawal of therapeutic glucocorticoids

adrenalectomy: surgical removal of one or both adrenal glands.

adrenocorticotropic hormone (ACTH): hormone secreted by the anterior pituitary, essential for growth and development

androgens: hormones secreted by the adrenal cortex; stimulate activity of accessory male sex organs and development of male sex characteristics

adrenogenital syndrome: masculinization in women, feminization in men, or premature sexual development in children; result of abnormal secretion of adrenocortical hormones, especially androgen

basal metabolic rate: chemical reactions occurring when the body is at rest

calcitonin: hormone secreted by the parafollicular cells of the thyroid gland; participates in calcium regulation

Chvostek's sign: spasm of the facial muscles produced by sharply tapping over the facial nerve in front of the parotid gland and anterior to the ear; causes spasm or twitching of the mouth, nose, and eye; suggestive of latent tetany in patients with hypocalcemia

corticosteroids: hormones produced by the adrenal cortex or their synthetic equivalents; also referred to as adrenal-cortical hormone and adrenocorticosteroid; consist of glucocorticoids, mineralocorticoids, and androgens

cretinism: stunted body growth and mental development appearing during the first year of life as a result of congenital hypothyroidism

Cushing's syndrome: group of symptoms produced by an excess of free circulating cortisol from the adrenal cortex; characterized by truncal obesity, "moon face," acne, abdominal striae, and hypertension

diabetes insipidus: condition in which abnormally large volumes of dilute urine are

excreted as a result of deficient production of vasopressin

dilutional hyponatremia: sodium deficiency developed as a result of fluid retention; associated with excessive ADH secretion in patients with SIADH

dwarfism: generalized limited growth; condition caused by insufficient secretion of growth hormone during childhood

endocrine: secreting internally; hormonal secretion of a ductless gland

euthyroid: state of normal thyroid hormone production

exocrine: secreting externally; hormonal secretion from excretory ducts

exophthalmos: abnormal protrusion of one or both eyeballs; produces a startled expression; usually due to hyperthyroidism

glucocorticoids: steroid hormones (ie, cortisol, cortisone, and corticosterone) secreted by the adrenal cortex in response to ACTH; produce a rise of liver glycogen and blood glucose

Graves' disease: a form of hyperthyroidism; characterized by a diffuse goitre, exophthalmos

goitre: enlargement of the thyroid gland; usually caused by an iodine-deficient diet

Hashimoto's disease: thyroiditis characterized by high levels of antimicrosomal antibodies; most common cause of hypothyroidism in the United States; also known as chronic lymphocytic thyroiditis or autoimmune thyroiditis

hormones: chemical transmitter substances produced in one organ or part of the body and carried by the bloodstream to other cells or organs on which they have a specific regulatory effect; produced mainly by endocrine glands (eg, pituitary, thyroid, gonads)

hypophysectomy: surgical removal or destruction of all or part of the pituitary gland

mineralocorticoid: steroid of the adrenal cortex; influences sodium and potassium

myxedema: severe form of hypothyroidism characterized by an accumulation of mucopolysaccharides in subcutaneous and other interstitial tissues; masklike expression, puffy eyelids, hair loss in the eyebrows, thick lips, and a broad tongue

negative feedback: regulating mechanism in which an increase or decrease in the level of a substance decreases or increases the function of the organ producing the substance

oxytocin: hormone secreted by the posterior pituitary; causes myometrial contraction at term and milk release during lactation

pheochromocytoma: chromaffin cell tumour, usually benign, located in the adrenal medulla; characterized by secretion of catecholamines resulting in hypertension, severe headache, profuse sweating, visual blurring, anxiety, and nausea

radioimmunoassay: measurement of hormone or other substance using radioisotope-labelled antigen

syndrome of inappropriate antidiuretic hormone (SIADH) secretion: excessive secretion of antidiuretic hormone (ADH) from the pituitary gland despite subnormal serum osmolality; occurs with oat cell carcinoma of the lung and other malignant tumours that produce ADH

thyroid-stimulating hormone (TSH): released from the pituitary gland; causes stimulation of the thyroid gland, resulting in release of T_3 and T_4

thyroid storm: severe life-threatening form of hyperthyroidism precipitated by stress; usually of abrupt onset; characterized by high fever, extreme tachycardia, and altered mental state

thyroidectomy: surgical removal of all or part of the thyroid gland

thyroiditis: inflammation of the thyroid gland; may lead to chronic hypothyroidism or resolve spontaneously

thyrotoxicosis: condition produced by excessive endogenous or exogenous thyroid hormone

thyroxine (T_4) thyroid hormone: active iodine compound formed and stored in the thyroid; deiodinated in peripheral tissues to form triiodothyronine (T_3); maintains body metabolism in a steady state

triiodothyronine (T_3): thyroid hormone; formed and stored in the thyroid; released in smaller quantities, biologically more active and faster onset of action than thyroxine (T_4); widespread effect on cellular metabolism, influences every major organ system

Trousseau's sign: carpopedal spasm induced when blood flow to the arm is occluded using a blood pressure cuff or tourniquet, causing ischemia to the distal nerves; suggestive sign for latent tetany in hypocalcemia

vasopressin: antidiuretic hormone secreted by the posterior pituitary; causes contraction of smooth muscle, particularly blood vessels

in Chaps. 40 and 41; reproductive structures, such as the ovaries and testes, are discussed in Chaps. 47 and 49.)

FUNCTION AND REGULATION OF HORMONES

The chemical substances secreted by the endocrine glands are called **hormones**. Hormones help to regulate organ function in concert with the nervous system. This dual regulatory system, in which rapid action by the nervous system is balanced by slower hormonal action, permits precise control of organ functions in response to varied changes within and outside the body. Table 42-1 lists the major hormones, their target tissue, and some of their properties.

The endocrine glands are composed of secretory cells arranged in minute clusters known as acini. No ducts are present, but the glands have a rich blood supply so that the hormones they produce enter the bloodstream rapidly. In the healthy physiologic state, hormone concentration in the bloodstream is maintained at a relatively constant level. When the hormone concentration rises, further production of that hormone is inhibited. When the hormone concentration falls, the rate of production of that hormone increases. This mechanism for regulating hormone concentration in the bloodstream is called **negative feedback**, which is important in the regulation of many biologic processes.

CLASSIFICATION AND ACTION OF HORMONES

Hormones are classified as steroid hormones (such as hydrocortisone), peptide or protein hormones (such as insulin), and amine hormones (such as epinephrine). These different classes of hormones act on the target tissues by different mechanisms. Hormones can alter the function of the target tissue by interacting with chemical receptors located either on the cell membrane or in the interior of the cell.

Peptide and protein hormones interact with receptor sites on the cell surface, which results in the stimulation of the intracellular enzyme adenyl cyclase. This results in increased production of cyclic 3′, 5′-adenosine monophosphate (cyclic AMP). The cyclic AMP inside the cell alters enzyme activity. Thus, cyclic AMP is the "second messenger" that links the peptide hormone at the cell surface to a change in the intracellular environment. Some of the protein and peptide hormones may also act by changing membrane permeability. These hormones act within seconds or minutes. The mechanism of action for amine hormones is similar to that for peptide hormones.

Steroid hormones, because of their smaller size and higher lipid solubility, penetrate the cell membranes and interact with intracellular receptors. This steroid–receptor complex modifies cell metabolism and formation of messenger ribonucleic acid (RNA) from deoxyribonucleic acid (DNA). The messenger RNA then stimulates protein synthesis within the cell. Steroid hormones require several hours to exert their effects because they exert their action by the modification of protein synthesis.

Assessment

HEALTH HISTORY AND CLINICAL MANIFESTATIONS

Because of the widespread effects of the endocrine system on the body, a wide variety of signs and symptoms may occur with endocrine disorders. Although specific endocrine disorders are

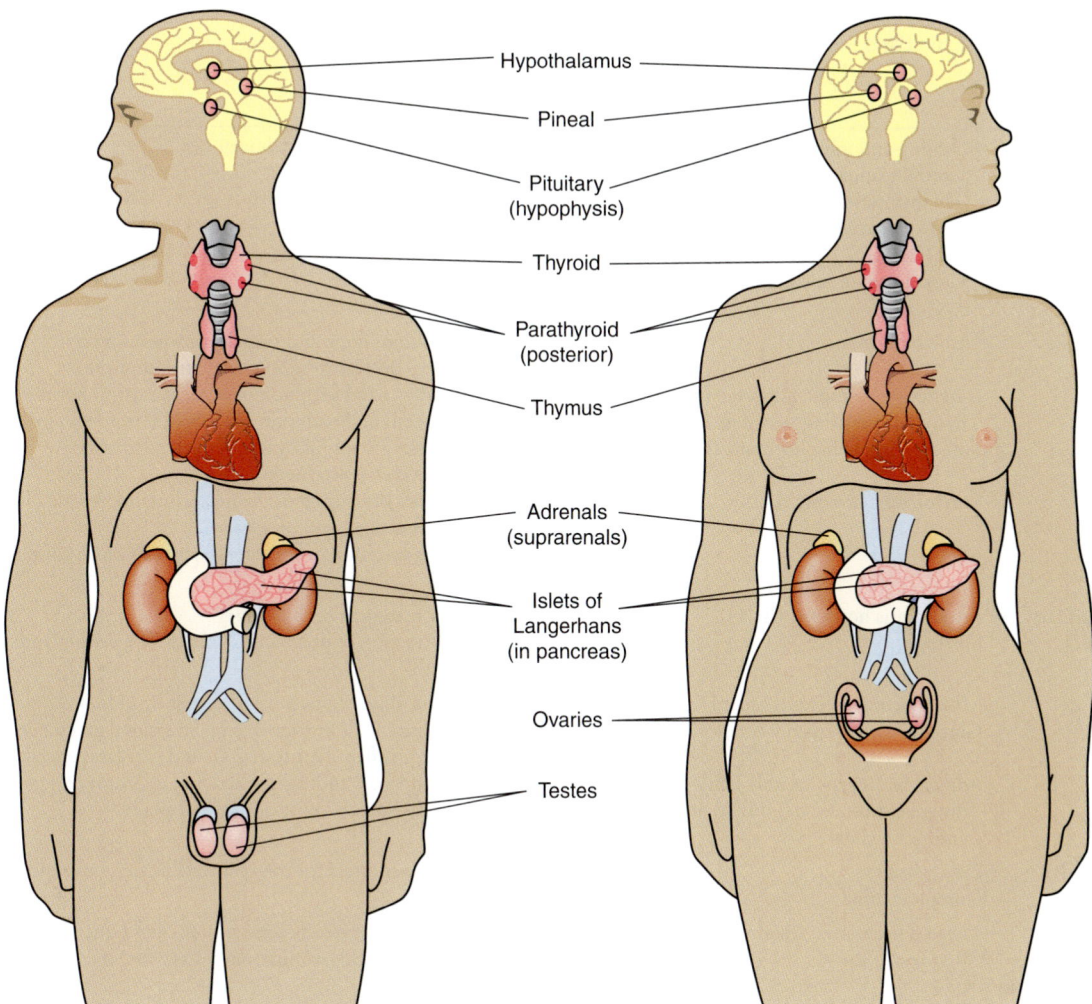

FIGURE 42-1 Major hormone-secreting glands of the endocrine system.

often accompanied by specific clinical symptoms, more general manifestations may occur with a number of endocrine disorders. Changes in energy level and fatigue are common to many endocrine imbalances. During the health history, the nurse asks the patient about fatigue and changes in usual energy levels and about how the changes affect the patient's ability to carry out activities of daily life. The nurse also asks about changes in heat and cold tolerance as well as recent changes in weight: increases or decreases may occur with changes in adrenal and thyroid disorders and may be a result of changes in fat distribution or fluid loss or retention.

Changes in sexual function and secondary sex characteristics may occur with any number of endocrine disorders and are assessed by obtaining a sexual history. Asking the patient or family about changes in mood, memory, and ability to concentrate and altered sleep patterns is important because these changes are common in endocrine disorders. Other specific symptoms that occur with specific endocrine disorders are discussed with each of those disorders.

PHYSICAL ASSESSMENT

The patient is observed for obvious changes in appearance that may indicate endocrine dysfunction. Changes in the skin texture are common with both hypofunction and hyperfunction of the thyroid gland. Eye changes, such as exophthalmos, may occur with hyperthyroidism and Graves' disease. Changes in physical appearance (eg, appearance of facial hair in women, "moon face," "buffalo hump," thinning of the skin, obesity of the trunk and thinness of the extremities, increased size of the feet and hands, edema) may signify disorders of the thyroid, adrenal cortex, or pituitary gland.

Vital signs are measured and compared with previous values if known. Elevated blood pressure may occur with hyperfunction of the adrenal cortex or tumour of the adrenal medulla. Decreased blood pressure may occur with hypofunction of the adrenal cortex. Other specific physical assessment findings are discussed with each endocrine disorder.

Diagnostic Evaluation

Although a wide variety of diagnostic tests can be used in the diagnostic workup, three major categories of diagnostic tests are common: blood tests, urine tests, and stimulation and suppression tests. Specific blood tests, urine tests, and stimulation and suppression tests are discussed with the specific endocrine disorders that follow in this chapter.

Table 42-1 • **Major Action and Source of Selected Hormones**

SOURCE	HORMONE	MAJOR ACTION

Hypothalamus	Releasing and inhibiting hormones
	  Corticotropin-releasing hormone (CRH)
	  Thyrotropin-releasing hormone (TRH)
	  Growth hormone-releasing hormone
	    (GHRH)
	  Gonadotropin-releasing hormone
	    (GnRH)
		Controls the release of pituitary hormones

Anterior pituitary	Growth hormone (GH)	Stimulates growth of bone and muscle, promotes protein synthesis and fat metabolism, decreases carbohydrate metabolism
	Adrenocorticotropic hormone (ACTH)	Stimulates synthesis and secretion of adrenal cortical hormones
	Thyroid-stimulating hormone (TSH)	Stimulates synthesis and secretion of thyroid hormone
	Follicle-stimulating hormone (FSH)	Female: stimulates growth of ovarian follicle, ovulation Male: stimulates sperm production
	Luteinizing hormone (LH)	Female: stimulates development of corpus luteum, release of oocyte, production of estrogen and progesterone Male: stimulates secretion of testosterone, development of interstitial tissue of testes
Posterior pituitary	Antidiuretic hormone (ADH)	Increases water reabsorption by kidney
	Oxytocin	Stimulates contraction of pregnant uterus, milk ejection from breasts after childbirth
Adrenal cortex	Mineralocorticosteroids, mainly aldosterone	Increases sodium absorption, potassium loss by kidney
	Glucocorticoids, mainly cortisol	Affects metabolism of all nutrients; regulates blood glucose levels, affects growth, has anti-inflammatory action, and decreases effects of stress
	Adrenal androgens, mainly dehydroepiandrosterone (DHEA) and androstenedione	Have minimal intrinsic androgenic activity; they are converted to testosterone and dihydrotestosterone in the periphery
Adrenal medulla	Epinephrine Norepinephrine	Serve as neurotransmitters for the sympathetic nervous system
Thyroid (follicular cells)	Thyroid hormones: triiodothyronine (T$_3$), thyroxine (T$_4$)	Increase the metabolic rate; increase protein and bone turnover; increase responsiveness to catecholamines; necessary for fetal and infant growth and development
Thyroid C cells	Calcitonin	Lowers blood calcium and phosphate levels
Parathyroid glands	Parathyroid hormone	Regulates serum calcium
Pancreatic islet cells	Insulin	Lowers blood glucose by facilitating glucose transport across cell membranes of muscle, liver, and adipose tissue
	Glucagon	Increases blood glucose concentration by stimulation of glycogenolysis and glyconeogenesis
	Somatostatin	Delays intestinal absorption of glucose
Gastrointestinal tract	Gastrin	Stimulates release of hydrochloric acid in stomach
	Cholecystokinin	Stimulates release of pancreatic secretions
	Secretin	Stimulates release of pancreatic enzymes, gallbladder contraction
Kidney	1,25-Dihydroxyvitamin D	Stimulates calcium absorption from the intestine
	Renin	Activates renin-angiotensin-aldosterone system
	Erythropoietin	Increases red blood cell production
Heart	Atrial natriuretic peptide (ANP)	Produces natriuresis
Ovaries	Estrogen	Affects development of female sex organs and secondary sex characteristics
	Progesterone	Influences menstrual cycle; stimulates growth of uterine wall; maintains pregnancy
	Inhibin	Inhibits FSH secretion by anterior pituitary
Testes	Androgens, mainly testosterone	Affect development of male sex organs and secondary sex characteristics; aid in sperm production
	Inhibin	Inhibits FSH secretion by anterior pituitary
Placenta	Human chorionic gonadotropin	Maintains pregnancy
Adipose cells	Leptin	Decreases appetite and food intake, increases sympathetic activity and metabolic rate, decreases insulin secretion to reduce fat storage
	Resistin	Suppresses insulin's ability to stimulate glucose uptake by adipose cells

Reproduced with permission from Porth, C. (2002). *Pathophysiology: Concepts of altered health states* (6th ed.). Philadelphia: Lippincott Williams & Wilkins.

Blood tests may be used to determine hormone blood levels. For example, in a patient thought to have a thyroid disorder, serum levels of **thyroid-stimulating hormone** (TSH) and thyroid hormone provide information about the nature (hypofunction or hyperfunction) and site (the thyroid gland, the pituitary, or the hypothalamus) of the disorder. Other blood tests are used to detect antibodies or assess the effect of the hormone on other substances (eg, the effect of insulin on blood glucose levels). **Radioimmunoassays**, which are radioisotope-labelled antigen tests used to measure hormones or other substances, may be performed.

Urine tests may be used to measure the amount of hormone or the end products of hormones excreted by the kidneys. One-time specimens may be obtained, or in some disorders 24-hour urine specimens are collected to measure hormones or their metabolites. For example, urinary levels of free catecholamines (norepinephrine, epinephrine, and dopamine) may be measured in patients with suspected tumours of the adrenal medulla (**pheochromocytoma**).

Stimulation and suppression tests may be used to diagnose endocrine disorders. Stimulation tests can determine how an endocrine gland responds to the administration of stimulating hormones that are normally produced or released by the hypothalamus or pituitary gland. If the endocrine gland responds to this stimulation, the specific disorder may be in the hypothalamus or pituitary. Failure of the endocrine gland to respond to this stimulation helps to identify the problem as being in the endocrine gland itself. Suppression tests may be used to determine whether negative feedback mechanisms that normally control secretion of hormones from the hypothalamus or pituitary gland are intact.

Management of Patients With Pituitary Disorders

The pituitary gland, or the hypophysis, is a round structure about 1.27 cm in diameter located on the inferior aspect of the brain. It is divided into the anterior, intermediate, and posterior lobes.

PITUITARY FUNCTION AND DYSFUNCTION

Commonly referred to as the master gland, the pituitary secretes hormones that control the secretion of hormones by other endocrine glands (Fig. 42-2). The pituitary itself is controlled by the hypothalamus, an adjacent area of the brain connected to the pituitary by the pituitary stalk.

Posterior Pituitary

The important hormones secreted by the posterior lobe of the pituitary gland are **vasopressin** (antidiuretic hormone [ADH]) and **oxytocin**. These hormones are synthesized in the hypothalamus and travel from the hypothalamus to the posterior pituitary gland for storage. Vasopressin controls the excretion of water by the kidney; its secretion is stimulated by an increase in the osmolality of the blood or by a decrease in blood pressure. Oxytocin facilitates milk ejection during lactation and increases the force of uterine contractions during labour and delivery. Oxytocin secretion is stimulated during pregnancy and at childbirth.

Anterior Pituitary

The major hormones of the anterior pituitary gland are follicle-stimulating hormone (FSH), luteinizing hormone (LH), prolactin, ACTH, thyroid-stimulating hormone (TSH), and growth hormone (also referred to as somatotropin). The secretion of these major hormones is controlled by releasing factors secreted by the hypothalamus. These releasing factors reach the anterior pituitary by way of the bloodstream in a special circulation called the pituitary portal blood system. Other hormones include melanocyte-stimulating hormone and beta-lipotropin; the function of lipotropin is poorly understood.

The hormones released by the anterior pituitary enter the general circulation and are transported to their target organs. The main function of TSH, ACTH, FSH, and LH is the release of hormones from other endocrine glands. Prolactin acts on the breast to stimulate milk production. Growth hormone has widespread effects on many target tissues and is discussed later. Hormones that stimulate other organs and tissues are discussed in conjunction with their target organs.

Growth hormone is a protein hormone that increases protein synthesis in many tissues, increases the breakdown of fatty acids in adipose tissue, and increases the glucose level in the blood. These actions of growth hormone are essential for normal growth, although other hormones, such as thyroid hormone and insulin, are required as well. Stress, exercise, and low blood glucose levels increase the secretion of growth hormone. The half-life of growth hormone activity in the blood is 20 to 30 minutes; the hormone is largely inactivated in the liver.

Pathophysiology

Abnormalities of pituitary function are caused by oversecretion or undersecretion of any of the hormones produced or released by the gland. Abnormalities of the anterior and posterior portions of the gland may occur independently. Oversecretion (hypersecretion) most commonly involves ACTH or growth hormone and results in **Cushing's syndrome** or **acromegaly**, respectively. Acromegaly, an excess of growth hormone in adults, results in bone and soft tissue deformities and enlargement of the viscera without an increase in height. In children, oversecretion of growth hormone results in gigantism, with a person reaching 210 or even 240 cm tall. Conversely, insufficient secretion of growth hormone during childhood results in generalized limited growth and **dwarfism**.

Undersecretion (hyposecretion) commonly involves all of the anterior pituitary hormones and is termed *panhypopituitarism*. In this condition, the thyroid gland, the adrenal cortex, and the gonads atrophy (shrink) because of loss of the trophic-stimulating hormones.

The most common disorder related to posterior lobe dysfunction is **diabetes insipidus**, a condition in which abnormally large volumes of dilute urine are excreted as a result of deficient production of vasopressin.

HYPOPITUITARISM

Hypofunction of the pituitary gland (hypopituitarism) can result from disease of the pituitary gland itself or of the hypothalamus, but the result is essentially the same. Hypopituitarism may result from destruction of the anterior lobe of the pituitary gland. Panhypopituitarism (Simmonds' disease) is total absence of all pituitary secretions and is rare. Postpartum pituitary necrosis (Sheehan's syndrome) is another uncommon cause of failure of the anterior pituitary. It is more likely to occur in women with severe blood loss, hypovolemia, and hypotension at the time of delivery.

Internal and external stimuli
Neurotransmitters
Hypothalamus

ADH and oxytocin
Nerve tracts
Posterior pituitary

Releasing hormones
Portal system
Anterior pituitary

Antidiuretic hormone
(ADH, vasopressin)

Oxytocin

Prolactin

Kidney

Breast

Uterus

Breast

FSH and LH (ICSH)

FSH and LH

GH

ACTH

TSH

Corpus luteum

Ovary

Testes

Bone and soft tissues

Adrenal gland

Thyroid gland

Progesterone

Adrenocorticosteroids

Thyroid hormones

Testosterone

Estrogen

Blood levels exert regulatory influences upon the anterior pituitary gland and the hypothalamus

FIGURE 42-2 The pituitary gland, the relationship of the brain to pituitary action, and the hormones secreted by the anterior pituitary and the posterior pituitary.

Hypopituitarism is also a complication of radiation therapy to the head and neck area. The total destruction of the pituitary gland by trauma, tumour, or vascular lesion removes all stimuli that are normally received by the thyroid, the gonads, and the adrenal glands. The result is extreme weight loss, emaciation, atrophy of all endocrine glands and organs, hair loss, impotence, amenorrhea, hypometabolism, and hypoglycemia. Coma and death occur if the missing hormones are not replaced.

PITUITARY TUMOURS

Pituitary tumours are usually benign, although their location and effects on hormone production by target organs can cause life-threatening effects. Three principal types of pituitary tumours rep-

resent an overgrowth of (1) eosinophilic cells, (2) basophilic cells, or (3) chromophobic cells (ie, cells with no affinity for either eosinophilic or basophilic stains).

Clinical Manifestations

Eosinophilic tumours that develop early in life result in gigantism. The affected person may be more than 210 cm tall and large in all proportions, yet so weak and lethargic that he or she can hardly stand. If the disorder begins during adult life, the excessive skeletal growth occurs only in the feet, the hands, the superciliary ridge, the molar eminences, the nose, and the chin, giving rise to the clinical picture called acromegaly. Enlargement, however, involves all tissues and organs of the body. Many of these patients suffer from severe headaches and visual disturbances because the tumours exert pressure on the optic nerves (Sachse, 2001). Assessment of central vision and visual fields may indicate loss of colour discrimination, diplopia (double vision), or blindness of a portion of a field of vision. Decalcification of the skeleton, muscular weakness, and endocrine disturbances, similar to those occurring in patients with hyperthyroidism, also are associated with this type of tumour.

Basophilic tumours give rise to Cushing's syndrome with features largely attributable to hyperadrenalism, including masculinization and amenorrhea in females, truncal obesity, hypertension, osteoporosis, and polycythemia.

Chromophobic tumours represent 90% of pituitary tumours. These tumours usually produce no hormones but destroy the rest of the pituitary gland, causing hypopituitarism. People with this disease are often obese and somnolent and exhibit fine, scanty hair, dry, soft skin, a pasty complexion, and small bones. They also experience headaches, loss of libido, and visual defects progressing to blindness. Other signs and symptoms include polyuria, polyphagia, a lowering of the **basal metabolic rate**, and a subnormal body temperature.

Assessment and Diagnostic Findings

Diagnostic evaluation requires a careful history and physical examination, including assessment of visual acuity and visual fields. Computed tomography (CT) and magnetic resonance imaging (MRI) are used to diagnose the presence and extent of pituitary tumours. Serum levels of pituitary hormones may be obtained along with measurements of hormones of target organs (eg, thyroid, adrenal) to assist in diagnosis if other information is inconclusive.

Medical Management

Surgical removal of the pituitary tumour through a transsphenoidal approach is the usual treatment. Stereotactic radiation therapy, which requires use of a neurosurgery-type stereotactic frame, may be used to deliver external-beam radiation therapy precisely to the pituitary tumour with minimal effect on normal tissue (see Chap. 16). Other treatments include conventional radiation therapy, bromocriptine (dopamine antagonist), and octreotide (synthetic analog of growth hormone). These medications inhibit the production or release of growth hormone and may bring about marked improvement of symptoms. Octreotide (Sandostatin) may also be used preoperatively to improve the patient's clinical condition and to shrink the tumour.

SURGICAL MANAGEMENT: HYPOPHYSECTOMY

Hypophysectomy, or removal of the pituitary gland, may be performed to treat primary pituitary gland tumours. It is the treatment of choice in patients with Cushing's syndrome due to excessive production of ACTH by a tumour of the pituitary gland. Hypophysectomy may also be performed on occasion as a palliative measure to relieve bone pain secondary to metastasis of malignant lesions of the breast and prostate.

Several approaches are used to remove or destroy the pituitary gland: surgical removal by transfrontal, subcranial, or oronasal–transsphenoidal approaches or irradiation or cryosurgery. (See Chap. 61 for the transsphenoidal approach to the removal of a pituitary tumour and for the nursing management of a patient undergoing cranial surgery.) Even if surgery succeeds at removing the tumour, many of the features or symptoms of acromegaly will be unaffected (Sachse, 2001).

The absence of the pituitary gland alters the function of many body systems. Menstruation ceases and infertility occurs after total or near-total ablation of the pituitary gland. Replacement therapy with corticosteroids and thyroid hormone is necessary; therefore, patient teaching is imperative and is discussed later in this chapter.

DIABETES INSIPIDUS

Diabetes insipidus is a disorder of the posterior lobe of the pituitary gland characterized by a deficiency of antidiuretic hormone (ADH), or vasopressin. Great thirst (polydipsia) and large volumes of dilute urine characterize the disorder. It may be secondary to head trauma, brain tumour, or surgical ablation or irradiation of the pituitary gland. It may also occur with infections of the central nervous system (meningitis, encephalitis, tuberculosis) or tumours (eg, metastatic disease, lymphoma of the breast or lung). Another cause of diabetes insipidus is failure of the renal tubules to respond to ADH; this nephrogenic form may be related to hypokalemia, hypercalcemia, and a variety of medications (eg, lithium, demeclocycline [Declomycin]).

Clinical Manifestations

Without the action of ADH on the distal nephron of the kidney, an enormous daily output of very dilute, water-like urine with a specific gravity of 1.001 to 1.005 occurs. The urine contains no abnormal substances such as glucose and albumin. Because of the intense thirst, the patient tends to drink 2 to 20 litres of fluid daily and craves cold water. In the hereditary form of diabetes insipidus, the primary symptoms may begin at birth. In adults, the onset of diabetes insipidus may be abrupt or insidious.

The disease cannot be controlled by limiting fluid intake because the high-volume loss of urine continues even without fluid replacement. Attempts to restrict fluids cause the patient to experience an insatiable craving for fluid and to develop hypernatremia and severe dehydration.

Assessment and Diagnostic Findings

The fluid deprivation test is carried out by withholding fluids for 8 to 12 hours or until 3% to 5% of the body weight is lost. The patient is weighed frequently during the test. Plasma and urine osmolality studies are performed at the beginning and end of the test. The inability to increase the specific gravity and osmolality of the urine is characteristic of diabetes insipidus. The patient continues to excrete large volumes of urine with low specific gravity and experiences weight loss, rising serum osmolality, and elevated serum sodium levels. The patient's condition needs to be monitored frequently during the test, and the test is terminated if tachycardia, excessive weight loss, or hypotension develops.

Other diagnostic procedures include concurrent measurements of plasma levels of ADH (vasopressin) and plasma and urine osmolality, a trial of desmopressin (synthetic vasopressin) therapy and intravenous infusion of hypertonic saline solution. When the diagnosis is confirmed and the cause is not obvious (eg, head injury), the patient is carefully assessed for tumours that may be causing the disorder.

Medical Management

The objectives of therapy are (1) to replace ADH (which is usually a long-term therapeutic program), (2) to ensure adequate fluid replacement, and (3) to identify and correct the underlying intracranial pathology. Nephrogenic causes require different management approaches.

PHARMACOLOGIC THERAPY

Desmopressin (DDAVP), a synthetic vasopressin without the vascular effects of natural ADH, is particularly valuable because it has a longer duration of action and fewer adverse effects than other preparations previously used to treat the disease. It is administered intranasally; the patient sprays the solution into the nose through a flexible calibrated plastic tube. One or two administrations daily or every 12 to 24 hours usually control the symptoms (Tierney, McPhee, & Papadakis, 2001).

Another form of therapy is the intramuscular administration of ADH, or vasopressin tannate in oil, which is used when the intranasal route is not possible. It is administered every 24 to 96 hours. The vial of medication should be warmed or shaken vigorously before administration. The injection is administered in the evening so that maximum results are obtained during sleep. Abdominal cramps are a side effect of this medication. Rotation of injection sites is necessary to prevent lipodystrophy.

Clofibrate, a hypolipidemic agent, has been found to have an antidiuretic effect on patients with diabetes insipidus who have some residual hypothalamic vasopressin. Chlorpropamide (Diabinese) and thiazide diuretics are also used in mild forms of the disease because they potentiate the action of vasopressin. The patient receiving chlorpropamide should be warned of the possibility of hypoglycemic reactions.

If the diabetes insipidus is renal in origin, the previously described treatments are ineffective. Thiazide diuretics, mild salt depletion, and prostaglandin inhibitors (ibuprofen, indomethacin, and aspirin) are used to treat the nephrogenic form of diabetes insipidus.

Nursing Management

The patient with possible diabetes insipidus needs encouragement and support while undergoing studies for a possible cranial lesion. The nurse needs to inform the patient and family about follow-up care and emergency measures. The nurse also needs to provide specific verbal and written instructions, show the patient how to administer the medications, and observe return demonstrations as appropriate. The nurse also advises the patient to wear a medical identification bracelet and to carry medication and information about this disorder at all times. Vasopressin must be administered with caution if the patient has coronary artery disease because the medication causes vasoconstriction.

SYNDROME OF INAPPROPRIATE ANTIDIURETIC HORMONE SECRETION

The **syndrome of inappropriate antidiuretic hormone (SIADH) secretion** includes excessive growth hormone (ADH) secretion from the pituitary gland even in the face of subnormal serum osmolality. Patients with this disorder cannot excrete a dilute urine. They retain fluids and develop a sodium deficiency known as **dilutional hyponatremia**. SIADH is often of nonendocrine origin; for instance, the syndrome may occur in patients with bronchogenic carcinoma in which malignant lung cells synthesize and release ADH. SIADH has also occurred with severe pneumonia, pneumothorax, and other disorders of the lungs, in addition to malignant tumours that affect other organs (Terpstra & Terpstra, 2000).

Disorders of the central nervous system, such as head injury, brain surgery or tumour, and infection, are thought to produce SIADH by direct stimulation of the pituitary gland. Some medications (vincristine, phenothiazines, tricyclic antidepressants, thiazide diuretics, and others) and nicotine have been implicated in SIADH; they either directly stimulate the pituitary gland or increase the sensitivity of renal tubules to circulating ADH.

Eliminating the underlying cause, if possible, and restricting fluid intake are typical interventions for managing this syndrome. Because retained water is excreted slowly through the kidneys, the extracellular fluid volume contracts and the serum sodium concentration gradually increases toward normal. Diuretics (eg, furosemide [Lasix]) may be used along with fluid restriction if severe hyponatremia is present.

Close monitoring of fluid intake and output, daily weight, urine and blood chemistries, and neurologic status is indicated for the patient at risk for SIADH. Supportive measures and explanations of procedures and treatments assist the patient to deal with this disorder (Terpstra & Terpstra, 2000).

Management of Patients With Thyroid Disorders

The thyroid gland is a butterfly-shaped organ located in the lower neck anterior to the trachea (Fig. 42-3). It consists of two lateral lobes connected by an isthmus. The gland is about 5 cm long and 3 cm wide and weighs about 30 g. The blood flow to the thyroid is very high (about 5 mL/min per gram of thyroid tissue), about five times the blood flow to the liver. This reflects the high metabolic activity of the thyroid gland. The thyroid gland produces three hormones: **thyroxine** (T_4), **triiodothyronine** (T_3), and **calcitonin**. Thyroxine and triiodothyronine are referred to collectively as thyroid hormone.

THYROID FUNCTION AND DYSFUNCTION

Various hormones and chemicals are responsible for normal thyroid function. Key among them are thyroid hormone, calcitonin, and iodine.

Thyroid Hormone

The two separate hormones, thyroxine (T_4) and triiodothyronine (T_3), that are produced by the thyroid gland and that make up thyroid hormone, are amino acids that have the unique property of

FIGURE 42-3 The thyroid gland and surrounding structures. From Weber, J. W. & Kelley, J. (2003). *Health assessment in nursing* (2nd ed.). Philadelphia: Lippincott Williams & Wilkins.

containing iodine molecules bound to the amino acid structure. T_4 contains four iodine atoms in each molecule, and T_3 contains only three. These hormones are synthesized and stored bound to proteins in the cells of the thyroid gland until needed for release into the bloodstream. About 75% of bound thyroid hormone is bound to thyroxine-binding globulin (TBG); the remaining bound thyroid hormone is bound to thyroid-binding prealbumin and albumin.

ROLE OF IODINE

Iodine is essential to the thyroid gland for synthesis of its hormones. In fact, the major use of iodine in the body is by the thyroid, and the major derangement in iodine deficiency is alteration of thyroid function. Iodide is ingested in the diet and absorbed into the blood in the gastrointestinal tract. The thyroid gland is extremely efficient in taking up iodide from the blood and concentrating it within the cells, where iodide ions are converted to iodine molecules, which react with tyrosine (an amino acid) to form the thyroid hormones.

REGULATION OF THYROID HORMONE

The secretion of T_3 and T_4 by the thyroid gland is controlled by thyroid-stimulating hormone (TSH, or thyrotropin) from the anterior pituitary gland. TSH controls the rate of thyroid hormone release. In turn, the level of thyroid hormone in the blood determines the release of TSH. If thyroid hormone concentration in the blood decreases, the release of TSH increases, which causes increased output of T_3 and T_4. This is an example of negative feedback.

Thyrotropin-releasing hormone (TRH), secreted by the hypothalamus, exerts a modulating influence on the release of TSH from the pituitary. Environmental factors, such as a decrease in temperature, may lead to increased secretion of TRH, resulting in elevated secretion of thyroid hormones. Figure 42-4 shows the hypothalamic-pituitary-thyroid axis, which regulates thyroid hormone production.

FUNCTION OF THYROXINE AND TRIIODOTHYRONINE

The primary function of the thyroid hormone is to control the cellular metabolic activity. T_4, a relatively weak hormone, maintains body metabolism in a steady state. T_3 is about five times as potent as T_4 and has a more rapid metabolic action. These hormones accelerate metabolic processes by increasing the level of specific enzymes that contribute to oxygen consumption and altering the responsiveness of tissues to other hormones. The thyroid hormones influence cell replication and are important in brain development. Thyroid hormone is also necessary for normal growth. The thyroid hormones, through their widespread effects on cellular metabolism, influence every major organ system.

Calcitonin

Calcitonin, or thyrocalcitonin, is another important hormone secreted by the thyroid gland. It is secreted in response to high plasma levels of calcium, and it reduces the plasma level of calcium by increasing its deposition in bone.

Assessment and Diagnostic Findings

The thyroid gland is inspected and palpated routinely on all patients. Inspection begins with identification of landmarks. The lower neck region between the sternocleidomastoid muscles is inspected for swelling or asymmetry. The patient is instructed to extend the neck slightly and swallow. Thyroid tissue rises normally with swallowing. The thyroid is then palpated for size, shape, consistency, symmetry, and the presence of tenderness.

Physiology/Pathophysiology

FIGURE 42-4 The hypothalamic-pituitary-thyroid axis. Thyroid-releasing hormone (TRH) from the hypothalamus stimulates the pituitary gland to secrete thyroid-stimulating hormone (TSH). TSH stimulates the thyroid to produce thyroid hormone (T_3 and T_4). High circulating levels of T_3 and T_4 inhibit further TSH secretion and thyroid hormone production through a negative feedback mechanism (*dashed lines*).

The examiner may examine the thyroid from an anterior or posterior position. In the posterior position, both hands encircle the patient's neck. The thumbs rest on the nape of the neck, while the index and middle fingers palpate for the thyroid isthmus and the anterior surfaces of the lateral lobes. When palpable, the isthmus is perceived as firm and of a rubber-band consistency.

The left lobe is examined by positioning the patient so that the neck flexes slightly forward and to the left. The thyroid cartilage is then displaced to the left with the fingers of the right hand. This manoeuvre displaces the left lobe deep into the sternocleidomastoid muscle, where it can be more easily palpated. The left lobe is then palpated by placing the left thumb deep into the posterior area of the sternocleidomastoid muscle, while the index and middle fingers exert opposite pressure in the anterior portion of the muscle. Having the patient swallow during the manoeuvre may assist the examiner to locate the thyroid as it ascends in the neck. The procedure is reversed to examine the right lobe. The isthmus is the only portion of the thyroid that is normally palpable. If a patient has a very thin neck, two thin, smooth, nontender lobes may also be palpable.

If palpation discloses an enlarged thyroid gland, both lobes are auscultated using the diaphragm of the stethoscope. Auscultation identifies the localized audible vibration of a bruit. This abnormal finding indicates increased blood flow through the thyroid gland and necessitates referral to a physician. Tenderness, enlargement, and nodularity within the thyroid also require referral for additional evaluation (Table 42-2).

THYROID FUNCTION TESTS

Assessment measures in addition to palpation and auscultation include thyroid function tests, such as laboratory measurement of thyroid hormones, thyroid scanning, biopsy, and ultrasonography. The most widely used tests are serum immunoassay for TSH and free thyroxine (FT_4). Measurement of TSH has a sensitivity and specificity of greater than 95% (Larson, Anderson & Koslawy, 2000). FT_4 levels correlate with metabolic status and are elevated in hyperthyroidism and decreased in hypothyroidism.

THYROID-STIMULATING HORMONE

Measurement of the serum TSH concentration is the single best screening test of thyroid function in outpatients because of its high sensitivity. The ability to detect minute changes in serum TSH makes it possible to distinguish subclinical thyroid disease from euthyroid states in patients with low or high normal values. Values above the normal range of 0.4 to 4.2 mμ/L indicate primary hypothyroidism, and low values indicate hyperthyroidism. When the TSH is normal, there is a 98% chance that the FT_4 is also normal. Measurement of TSH is also used for monitoring thyroid hormone replacement therapy and for differentiating between disorders of the thyroid gland itself and disorders of the pituitary or hypothalamus. Current recommendations suggest TSH screening for all adults beginning at age 35, and every 5 years thereafter (Ladenson, Singer, Ain, et al., 2000).

SERUM FREE THYROXINE

The test most commonly used to confirm an abnormal TSH is FT_4. FT_4 is a direct measurement of free (unbound) thyroxine, the only metabolically active fraction of T_4. The range of FT_4 in serum is normally 10.3 to 35 pmol/L. When measured by the dialysis method, FT_4 is not affected by variations in protein binding and is the procedure of choice for following the changes in T_4 secretion during treatment of hyperthyroidism. Measurement of FT_4 by the immunoassay technique is less reliable because it may be affected by medication, illness, or changes in protein binding. An estimate (or index) of FT_4 can also be calculated by multiplying total T_4 by T_3 resin uptake.

SERUM T_3 AND T_4

Measurement of total T_3 or T_4 includes protein-bound and free hormone levels that occur in response to TSH secretion. T_4 is 80% bound to thyroxine-binding globulin (TBG); T_3 is bound less firmly. Only 0.03% of T_4 and 0.3% of T_3 is unbound. Any factor that alters binding proteins also changes the T_3 and T_4 levels. Serious systemic illnesses, medications (eg, oral contraceptives, corticosteroids, phenytoin, salicylates), and protein wasting as a result of nephrosis and use of androgens may interfere with accurate test results. Normal range for T_4 is 65 to 138 nmol/L. Although serum T_3 and T_4 levels generally increase or decrease together, the T_3 level appears to be a more accurate indicator of hyperthyroidism, which causes a greater rise in T_3 than T_4 levels. The normal range for serum T_3 is 1.08 to 3.14 nmol/L.

T_3 RESIN UPTAKE TEST

The T_3 resin uptake test is an indirect measure of unsaturated TBG. Its purpose is to determine the amount of thyroid hormone bound to TBG and the number of available binding sites. This provides an index of the amount of thyroid hormone already present in the circulation. Normally, TBG is not fully saturated with thyroid hormone, and additional binding sites are available to combine with radioiodine-labelled T_3 added to the blood specimen. The normal T_3 relative uptake fraction is 0.24 to 0.34, which indicates that about one third of the available sites of TBG are occupied by thyroid hormone. If the number of free or unoccupied binding sites is low, as in hyperthyroidism, the T_3 uptake is greater than 0.35. If the number of available sites is high, as occurs in hypothyroidism, the test results are less than 0.25.

T_3 uptake is useful in the evaluation of thyroid hormone levels in patients who have received diagnostic or therapeutic doses of

Table 42-2 • Summary of Findings on Physical Examination of the Thyroid Gland

PHYSICAL FINDING	DIFFERENTIAL DIAGNOSIS	SPECIAL FEATURES
Single nodule	Autonomously functioning adenoma	Opposite lobe not palpable
	Adenoma or adenomatous nodule	Rubbery, firm; tenderness suggests recent hemorrhage or infarction
	Cancer	Usually hard; may have associated lymph node enlargement or vocal cord palsy
	Hyperplasia secondary to unilobar agenesis	Opposite lobe not palpable
Multiple nodules	Multinodular goitre	Firm lobes or irregular surface may be misinterpreted as multiple nodules
	Hashimoto's thyroditis	
Diffuse goitre	Graves' disease	Bruit or thrill; pyramidal lobe
	Hashimoto's thyroiditis	Irregular surface; pyramidal lobe; rubbery or firm; occasionally tender; fibrous variant may be hard
	Thyroid lymphoma	Rapidly growing goitre, particularly in setting of preexisting Hashimoto's thyroiditis
	Multinodular goitre	Nodules may be hidden within gland and may become apparent with thyroid hormone suppression
Tenderness	Subacute thyroiditis	Unilateral or bilateral; tenderness often severe
	Hemorrhagic or infarcted adenoma	Discrete nodule with tenderness
	Hashimoto's thyroiditis	Mild tenderness
	Cancer	Irregular, firm thyroid nodule with chronic tenderness

iodine. The test results may be altered by the use of estrogens, androgens, salicylates, phenytoin, anticoagulants, or corticosteroids.

THYROID ANTIBODIES

Autoimmune thyroid diseases include both hypothyroid and hyperthyroid conditions. Results of testing by immunoassay techniques for antithyroid antibodies, specifically antimicrosomal antibodies, are positive in chronic autoimmune thyroid disease (90%), Hashimoto's thyroiditis (100%), Graves' disease (80%), and other organ-specific autoimmune disease, such as lupus erythematosus and rheumatoid arthritis. Antithyroid antibody titers are normally present in 5% to 10% of the population and increase with age.

RADIOACTIVE IODINE UPTAKE

The radioactive iodine uptake test measures the rate of iodine uptake by the thyroid gland. The patient is administered a tracer dose of iodine-123 (^{123}I) or another radionuclide, and a count is made over the thyroid gland with use of a scintillation counter, which detects and counts the gamma rays released from the breakdown of ^{123}I in the thyroid. It measures the proportion of the administered dose present in the thyroid gland at a specific time after its administration. It is a simple test and provides reliable results. It is affected by the patient's intake of iodide or thyroid hormone; therefore, a careful preliminary clinical history is essential in evaluating results. Normal values vary from one geographic region to another and with the intake of iodine. Patients with hyperthyroidism exhibit a high uptake of the ^{123}I (in some patients, up to 90%), whereas patients with hypothyroidism exhibit a very low uptake. This test is also used to determine what dose of ^{123}I should be administered to treat a patient with hyperthyroidism.

FINE-NEEDLE ASPIRATION BIOPSY

Using a small-gauge needle to sample the thyroid tissue for biopsy is a safe and accurate method of detecting malignancy. It is often the initial test for evaluation of thyroid masses. Results are reported as (1) negative (benign), (2) positive (malignant), (3) indeterminate (suspicious), and (4) inadequate (nondiagnostic).

THYROID SCAN, RADIOSCAN, OR SCINTISCAN

In a thyroid scan, a scintillation detector or gamma camera moves back and forth across the area to be studied in a series of parallel tracks, and a visual image is made of the distribution of radioactivity in the area being scanned. Although ^{123}I has been the most commonly used isotope, several other radioactive isotopes, including technetium-99m (^{99m}Tc) pertechnetate, thallium, and americium, are also used.

Scans are helpful in determining the location, size, shape, and anatomic function of the thyroid gland, particularly when thyroid tissue is substernal or large. Identifying areas of increased function ("hot" areas) or decreased function ("cold" areas) can assist in diagnosis. Although most areas of decreased function do not represent malignancies, lack of function increases the likelihood of malignancy, particularly if only one nonfunctioning area is present. Scanning of the entire body, to obtain the total body profile, may be carried out in a search for a functioning thyroid metastasis.

OTHER DIAGNOSTIC TESTS

Ultrasound, CT scans, and MRI may be used to clarify or confirm the results of other diagnostic studies. Thyroglobulin (Tg), a precursor for T_3 and T_4, can be measured reliably in the serum by radioimmunoassay. Clinically, it is used to detect persistence or recurrence of thyroid carcinoma.

NURSING IMPLICATIONS

When thyroid tests are scheduled, it is necessary to determine whether the patient has taken medications or agents that contain iodine because these may alter the test results. Iodine-containing medications include contrast agents and those used to treat thyroid disorders. Less obvious sources of iodine are topical antiseptics, multivitamin preparations, and food supplements frequently found in health food stores; cough syrups; and amiodarone, an antiarrhythmic agent. Other medications that may affect test results are estrogens, salicylates, amphetamines, chemotherapeutic agents, antibiotics, corticosteroids, and mercurial diuretics. The nurse asks the patient about the use of these medications and notes their use on the laboratory requisition. Chart 42-1 gives a partial list of agents that may interfere with accurate testing of thyroid gland function.

ABNORMAL THYROID FUNCTION

Inadequate secretion of thyroid hormone during fetal and neonatal development results in stunted physical and mental growth (**cretinism**) because of general depression of metabolic activity. In adults, hypothyroidism manifests as lethargy, slow mentation, and generalized slowing of body functions.

Oversecretion of thyroid hormones (hyperthyroidism) is manifested by a greatly increased metabolic rate. Many of the other characteristics of hyperthyroidism result from the increased response to circulating catecholamines (epinephrine and norepinephrine). Hypothyroidism and hyperthyroidism are discussed in detail in the following sections of this chapter.

Oversecretion of thyroid hormones is usually associated with an enlarged thyroid gland (**goitre**). Goitre also commonly occurs with iodine deficiency. In this latter condition, lack of iodine results in low levels of circulating thyroid hormones, which causes increased release of TSH; the elevated TSH causes overproduction of thyroglobulin and hypertrophy of the thyroid gland. The term **euthyroid** refers to thyroid hormone production that is within normal limits.

HYPOTHYROIDISM

Hypothyroidism results from suboptimal levels of thyroid hormone. Thyroid deficiency can affect all body functions and can range from mild, subclinical forms to **myxedema**, an advanced form. The most common cause of hypothyroidism in adults is autoimmune thyroiditis (**Hashimoto's disease**), in which the immune system attacks the thyroid gland. Symptoms of hyper-

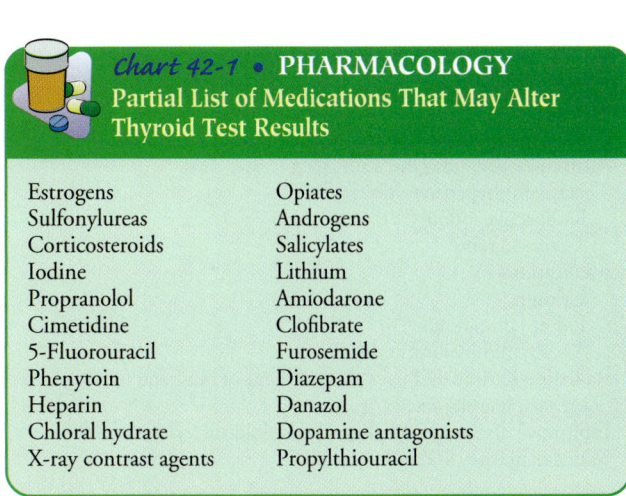

Chart 42-1 • PHARMACOLOGY
Partial List of Medications That May Alter Thyroid Test Results

Estrogens	Opiates
Sulfonylureas	Androgens
Corticosteroids	Salicylates
Iodine	Lithium
Propranolol	Amiodarone
Cimetidine	Clofibrate
5-Fluorouracil	Furosemide
Phenytoin	Diazepam
Heparin	Danazol
Chloral hydrate	Dopamine antagonists
X-ray contrast agents	Propylthiouracil

thyroidism may later be followed by those of hypothyroidism and myxedema. Hypothyroidism also commonly occurs in patients with previous hyperthyroidism who have been treated with radioiodine or antithyroid medications or who have had surgery. It occurs most frequently in older women. Radiation therapy for head and neck cancer can also cause hypothyroidism in older men; therefore, testing of thyroid function is recommended for all patients who receive such treatment. Other causes of hypothyroidism are presented in Chart 42-2.

Pathophysiology

More than 95% of patients with hypothyroidism have primary or thyroidal hypothyroidism, which refers to dysfunction of the thyroid gland itself. When thyroid dysfunction is caused by failure of the pituitary gland, the hypothalamus, or both, it is known as central hypothyroidism. It may be referred to as pituitary or secondary hypothyroidism if it is caused entirely by a pituitary disorder, and hypothalamic or tertiary hypothyroidism if it is attributable to a disorder of the hypothalamus resulting in inadequate secretion of TSH because of decreased stimulation by TRH. When thyroid deficiency is present at birth, the condition is known as cretinism. In such instances, the mother may also suffer from thyroid deficiency.

The term myxedema refers to the accumulation of mucopolysaccharides in subcutaneous and other interstitial tissues. Although myxedema occurs in long-standing hypothyroidism, the term is used appropriately only to describe the extreme symptoms of severe hypothyroidism.

Clinical Manifestations

Early symptoms of hypothyroidism are nonspecific, but extreme fatigue makes it difficult for the person to complete a full day's work or participate in usual activities. Reports of hair loss, brittle nails, and dry skin are common, and numbness and tingling of the fingers may occur. On occasion, the voice may become husky, and the patient may complain of hoarseness. Menstrual disturbances such as menorrhagia or amenorrhea occur, in addition to loss of libido. Hypothyroidism affects women five times more frequently than men and occurs most often between 30 and 60 years of age.

Severe hypothyroidism results in a subnormal temperature and pulse rate. The patient usually begins to gain weight even without an increase in food intake, although severely hypothyroid patients may be cachectic. The skin becomes thickened because of an ac-

cumulation of mucopolysaccharides in the subcutaneous tissues (the origin of the term myxedema). The hair thins and falls out; the face becomes expressionless and masklike. The patient often complains of being cold even in a warm environment.

At first, the patient may be irritable and may complain of fatigue, but as the condition progresses, the emotional responses are subdued. The mental processes become dulled, and the patient appears apathetic. Speech is slow, the tongue enlarges, and hands and feet increase in size. The patient frequently complains of constipation. Deafness may also occur.

Advanced hypothyroidism may produce personality and cognitive changes characteristic of dementia. Inadequate ventilation and sleep apnea can occur with severe hypothyroidism. Pleural effusion, pericardial effusion, and respiratory muscle weakness may also occur.

Severe hypothyroidism is associated with an elevated serum cholesterol level, atherosclerosis, coronary artery disease, and poor left ventricular function. The patient with advanced hypothyroidism is hypothermic and abnormally sensitive to sedatives, opioids, and anesthetic agents. Therefore, these medications are administered only with extreme caution.

Patients with unrecognized hypothyroidism who are undergoing surgery are at increased risk for intraoperative hypotension and postoperative heart failure and altered mental status.

Myxedema coma describes the most extreme, severe stage of hypothyroidism, in which the patient is hypothermic and unconscious. Myxedema coma may follow increasing lethargy, progressing to stupor and then coma. Undiagnosed hypothyroidism may be precipitated by infection or other systemic disease or by use of sedatives or opioid analgesic agents. The patient's respiratory drive is depressed, resulting in alveolar hypoventilation, progressive CO_2 retention, narcosis, and coma. These symptoms, along with cardiovascular collapse and shock, require aggressive and intensive therapy if the patient is to survive. Even with early vigourous therapy, however, mortality is high.

 ## Gerontologic Considerations

Most patients with primary hypothyroidism are 40 to 70 years of age and present with long-standing mild to moderate hypothyroidism. Subclinical disease is common among older women and can be asymptomatic or mistaken for other medical conditions. Subtle symptoms of hypothyroidism, such as fatigue, muscle aches, and mental confusion, may be attributed to the normal aging process by the patient, family, and health care provider. The higher prevalence of hypothyroidism in elderly people may be related to alterations in immune function with age. Regular screening of TSH levels is recommended for people older than 60 because they are at high risk for hypothyroidism (Ladenson et al., 2000).

The signs and symptoms of hypothyroidism are often atypical in elderly people; the elderly patient may have few or no symptoms until the dysfunction is severe. Depression, apathy, or decreased mobility or activity may be the major initial symptom. The major symptoms of hypothyroidism may be depression and apathy, and may be accompanied by significant weight loss. One fourth of affected elderly patients experience constipation.

Chart 42-2	**Causes of Hypothyroidism**

Chronic lymphocytic thyroiditis (Hashimoto's thyroiditis)
Atrophy of thyroid gland with aging
Therapy for hyperthyroidism
    Radioactive iodine (^{131}I)
    Thyroidectomy
Medications
    Lithium
    Iodine compounds
    Antithyroid medications
Radiation to head and neck for treatment of head and neck
    cancers, lymphoma
Infiltrative diseases of the thyroid (amyloidosis, scleroderma)
Iodine deficiency and iodine excess

 NURSING ALERT In all patients with hypothyroidism, the effects of analgesic agents, sedatives, and anesthetic agents are prolonged; particular caution is necessary in administering these agents to elderly patients because of concurrent changes in liver and renal function.

Medical Management

The primary objective in the management of hypothyroidism is to restore a normal metabolic state by replacing the missing hormone.

PHARMACOLOGIC THERAPY

Synthetic levothyroxine (Synthroid or Levothroid) is the preferred preparation for treating hypothyroidism and suppressing nontoxic goitres. The dosage for hormone replacement is based on the patient's serum TSH concentration. Desiccated thyroid is used less frequently because it often results in transient elevated serum concentrations of T_3, with occasional symptoms of hyperthyroidism. If replacement therapy is adequate, the symptoms of myxedema disappear and normal metabolic activity is resumed.

Prevention of Cardiac Dysfunction. Any patient who has had hypothyroidism for a long period is almost certain to have elevated serum cholesterol levels, atherosclerosis, and coronary artery disease. As long as metabolism is subnormal and the tissues, including the myocardium, require relatively little oxygen, a reduction in blood supply is tolerated without overt symptoms of coronary artery disease. When thyroid hormone is administered, however, the oxygen demand increases, but oxygen delivery cannot be increased unless, or until, the atherosclerosis improves. This occurs very slowly, if at all. The occurrence of angina is the signal that the oxygen needs of the myocardium exceed its blood supply. Angina or dysrhythmias may occur when thyroid replacement is initiated because thyroid hormones enhance the cardiovascular effects of catecholamines.

 NURSING ALERT The nurse must monitor for myocardial ischemia or infarction, which may occur in response to therapy in patients with severe, long-standing hypothyroidism or myxedema coma. The nurse must also be alert for signs of angina, especially during the early phase of treatment; if detected, it must be reported and treated at once to avoid a fatal myocardial infarction.

Obviously, if angina or dysrhythmias occur, thyroid hormone administration must be discontinued immediately. Later, when it can be resumed safely, thyroid hormone replacement should be prescribed cautiously at a lower dosage and under the close observation of the physician and the nurse.

Prevention of Medication Interactions. Precautions must be taken during the course of therapy because of the interaction of thyroid hormones with other medications. Thyroid hormones may increase blood glucose levels, which may necessitate adjustment in the dosage of insulin or oral antidiabetic agents in patients with diabetes. The effects of thyroid hormone may be increased by phenytoin (Dilantin) and tricyclic antidepressant agents. Thyroid hormones may also increase the pharmacologic effects of digitalis glycosides, anticoagulant agents, and indomethacin, requiring careful observation and assessment by the nurse for side effects. Bone loss and osteoporosis may also occur with thyroid therapy.

 NURSING ALERT Severe untreated hypothyroidism is characterized by an increased susceptibility to the effects of all hypnotic and sedative agents.

Even in small doses, hypnotic and sedative agents may induce profound somnolence, lasting far longer than anticipated. More-over, they are likely to cause respiratory depression, which can easily be fatal because of decreased respiratory reserve and alveolar hypoventilation. If their use is necessary, the dose is one-half or one-third that ordinarily prescribed in patients of similar age and weight with normal thyroid function. If these medications must be used, the patient must be monitored closely for signs of impending narcosis (stupor-like condition) or respiratory failure.

 Gerontologic Considerations

In the elderly patient with mild to moderate hypothyroidism, thyroid hormone replacement must be started with low dosages and increased gradually to prevent serious cardiovascular and neurologic side effects. Angina, for example, may occur with rapid thyroid replacement in the presence of coronary artery disease secondary to the hypothyroid state. Heart failure and tachydysrhythmias may worsen during the transition from the hypothyroid state to the normal metabolic state. Dementia may become more apparent during early thyroid hormone replacement in the elderly patient.

Elderly patients with severe hypothyroidism and atherosclerosis may also become confused and agitated if their metabolic rates are raised too quickly. Marked clinical improvement follows the administration of hormone replacement; such medication must be continued for life, even though signs of hypothyroidism disappear within 3 to 12 weeks.

Myxedema and myxedema coma generally occur exclusively in patients older than 50 years. The high mortality rate of myxedema coma mandates immediate intravenous administration of high doses of thyroid hormone as well as supportive care.

SUPPORTIVE THERAPY

In severe hypothyroidism and myxedema coma, management includes maintaining vital functions. Arterial blood gases may be measured to determine CO_2 retention and to guide the use of assisted ventilation to combat hypoventilation. Pulse oximetry may also be helpful in monitoring oxygen saturation levels. Fluids are administered cautiously because of the danger of water intoxication. Application of external heat (eg, heating pads) is avoided because it increases oxygen requirements and may lead to vascular collapse. If hypoglycemia is evident, concentrated glucose may be prescribed to provide glucose without precipitating fluid overload. Thyroid hormone (usually Synthroid) is administered intravenously until consciousness is restored if myxedema has progressed to myxedema coma. The patient is then continued on oral thyroid hormone therapy. Because of an associated adrenocortical insufficiency, corticosteroid therapy may be necessary.

Nursing Management

Nursing care of the patient with hypothyroidism and myxedema is summarized in the Plan of Nursing Care.

MODIFYING ACTIVITY

The patient with hypothyroidism experiences decreased energy and moderate to severe lethargy. As a result, the risk for complications from immobility increases. The patient's ability to exercise and participate in activities is further limited by the changes in cardiovascular and pulmonary status secondary to hypothyroidism. A major role of the nurse is assisting with care and hygiene while encouraging the patient to participate in activities within established tolerance levels to prevent the complications of immobility.

(text continues on page 1124)

Plan of Nursing Care
Care of the Patient With Hypothyroidism

Nursing Interventions	Rationale	Expected Outcomes

Nursing Diagnosis: Activity intolerance related to fatigue and depressed cognitive process
Goal: Increased participation in activities and increased independence

Nursing Interventions	Rationale	Expected Outcomes

1. Promote independence in self-care activities.
  a. Space activities to promote rest and exercise as tolerated.
  b. Assist with self-care activities when patient is fatigued.
  c. Provide stimulation through conversation and nonstressful activities.
  d. Monitor patient's response to increasing activities.
	1. Encouragement needed in fatigued, often depressed patient
	  a. Encourages activities while allowing time for adequate rest
	  b. Permits patient to participate to the extent possible in self-care activities
	  c. Promotes interest without overly stressing the patient
	  d. Guards against over- and under-exertion by the patient
		• Participates in self-care activities
		• Reports decreased level of fatigue
		• Displays interest and awareness in environment
		• Participates in activities and events in environment
		• Participates in family events and activities
		• Reports no chest pain, increased fatigue, or breathlessness with increased level of activity

Nursing Diagnosis: Risk for imbalanced body temperature
Goal: Maintenance of normal body temperature

Nursing Interventions	Rationale	Expected Outcomes
1. Provide extra layer of clothing or extra blanket. 2. Avoid and discourage use of external heat source (eg, heating pads, electric or warming blankets). 3. Monitor patient's body temperature and report decreases from patient's baseline value. 4. Protect from exposure to cold and drafts.	1. Minimizes heat loss 2. Reduces risk of peripheral vasodilation and vascular collapse 3. Detects decreased body temperature and onset of myxedema coma 4. Increases patient's level of comfort and decreases further heat loss	• Experiences relief of discomfort and cold intolerance • Maintains baseline body temperature • Reports adequate feeling of warmth and lack of chilling • Uses extra layer of clothing or extra blanket • Explains rationale for avoiding external heat source

Nursing Diagnosis: Constipation related to depressed gastrointestinal function
Goal: Return of normal bowel function

Nursing Interventions	Rationale	Expected Outcomes
1. Encourage increased fluid intake within limits of fluid restriction. 2. Provide foods high in fibre. 3. Instruct patient about foods with high water content. 4. Monitor bowel function. 5. Encourage increased mobility within patient's exercise tolerance. 6. Encourage patient to use laxatives and enemas sparingly.	1. Promotes passage of soft stools 2. Increases bulk of stools and more frequent bowel movements 3. Provides rationale for patient to increase fluid intake 4. Permits detection of constipation and return to normal bowel pattern 5. Promotes evacuation of the bowel 6. Minimizes patient's dependence on laxatives and enemas and encourages normal pattern of bowel evacuation	• Reports normal bowel function • Identifies and consumes foods high in fibre • Drinks recommended amount of fluid each day • Participates in gradually increasing exercises • Uses laxatives as prescribed and avoids excessive dependence on laxatives and enemas

Nursing Diagnosis: Deficient knowledge about the therapeutic regimen for lifelong thyroid replacement therapy
Goal: Knowledge and acceptance of the prescribed therapeutic regimen

Nursing Interventions	Rationale	Expected Outcomes
1. Explain rationale for thyroid hormone replacement. 2. Describe desired effects of medication to patient. 3. Assist patient to develop schedule and checklist to ensure self-administration of thyroid replacement.	1. Provides rationale for patient to use thyroid hormone replacement as prescribed 2. Provides encouragement to patient by identifying improved physical status and well-being that will occur with thyroid hormone therapy and return to a euthyroid state 3. Increases chances that medication will be taken as prescribed	• Describes therapeutic regimen correctly • Explains rationale for thyroid hormone replacement • Identifies positive outcomes of thyroid hormone replacement • Administers medication to self as prescribed

(continued)

Plan of Nursing Care
Care of the Patient With Hypothyroidism (Continued)

Nursing Interventions	Rationale	Expected Outcomes
4. Describe signs and symptoms of over- and underdose of medication. 5. Explain the necessity for long-term follow-up to patient and family.	4. Serves as check for patient to determine if therapeutic goals are met 5. Increases likelihood that hypo- or hyperthyroidism will be detected and treated	• Identifies adverse side effects that should be reported promptly to physician: recurrence of symptoms of hypothyroidism and occurrence of symptoms of hyperthyroidism • Restates need for periodic/long-term follow-up visits to physician

Nursing Diagnosis: Ineffective breathing pattern related to depressed ventilation
Goal: Improved respiratory status and maintenance of normal breathing pattern

1. Monitor respiratory rate, depth, pattern, pulse oximetry, and arterial blood gases. 2. Encourage deep breathing, coughing, and use of incentive spirometry. 3. Administer medications (hypnotics and sedatives) with caution. 4. Maintain patent airway through suction and ventilatory support if indicated (see Chap. 25 for care of patients requiring mechanical ventilation).	1. Identifies patient's baseline to monitor further changes and evaluate effectiveness of interventions 2. Prevents atelectasis and promotes adequate ventilation 3. Patients with hypothyroidism are *very* susceptible to respiratory depression with use of hypnotics and sedatives. 4. Use of an artificial airway and ventilatory support may be necessary with respiratory depression.	• Shows improved respiratory status and maintenance of normal breathing pattern • Demonstrates normal respiratory rate, depth, and pattern • Takes deep breaths, coughs, and uses incentive spirometry when encouraged • Demonstrates normal breath sounds without adventitious sounds on auscultation • Explains rationale for cautious use of medications • Cooperates with suction procedure and ventilator when necessary

Nursing Diagnosis: Disturbed thought processes related to depressed metabolism and altered cardiovascular and respiratory status
Goal: Improved thought processes

1. Orient patient to time, place, date, and events around him or her. 2. Provide stimulation through conversation and nonthreatening activities. 3. Explain to patient and family that change in cognitive and mental functioning is a result of disease process. 4. Monitor cognitive and mental processes and response of these to medication and other therapy.	1. Provides reality orientation to patient 2. Provides stimulation within patient's level of tolerance for stress 3. Reassures patient and family about the cause of the cognitive changes and that a positive outcome is possible with appropriate treatment 4. Permits evaluation of the effectiveness of treatment	• Shows improved cognitive functioning • Identifies time, place, date, and events correctly • Responds when stimulated • Responds spontaneously as treatment becomes effective • Interacts spontaneously with family and environment • Explains that change in mental and cognitive processes is a result of disease processes • Takes medications as prescribed to prevent decrease in cognitive processes

Collaborative Problem: Myxedema and myxedema coma
Goal: Absence of complications

1. Monitor patient for increasing severity of signs and symptoms of hypothyroidism:
  a. Decreased level of consciousness; dementia
  b. Decreased vital signs (blood pressure, respiratory rate, temperature, pulse rate)
  c. Increasing difficulty in awakening or arousing patient
	1. Extreme hypothyroidism may lead to myxedema, myxedema coma, and slowing of all body systems if untreated	• Exhibits reversal of myxedema and myxedema coma
		• Responds appropriately to questions and surroundings
		• Vital signs return to normal or near-normal ranges
		• Respiratory status improves with adequate spontaneous ventilatory effort
		• Reports no episodes of angina or other indicators of cardiac insufficiency

(continued)

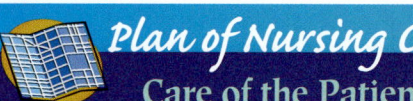

Plan of Nursing Care
Care of the Patient With Hypothyroidism *(Continued)*

Nursing Interventions	Rationale	Expected Outcomes
2. Assist in ventilatory support if respiratory depression and failure occur.	2. Ventilatory support is necessary to maintain adequate oxygenation and maintenance of an airway	• Experiences minimal or no complications caused by immobility
3. Administer prescribed medications (eg, thyroxine) with extreme caution.	3. The slow metabolism and atherosclerosis of myxedema may result in angina with administration of thyroxine	
4. Turn and reposition patient at intervals.	4. Minimizes risks associated with immobility	
5. Avoid use of hypnotic, sedative, and analgesic agents.	5. Altered metabolism of these agents greatly increases the risks of their use in myxedema	

MONITORING PHYSICAL STATUS

The nurse closely monitors the patient's vital signs and cognitive level to detect the following:

- Deterioration of physical and mental status
- Signs and symptoms indicating that treatment has resulted in the metabolic rate exceeding the ability of the cardiovascular and pulmonary systems to respond
- Continued limitations or complications of myxedema

 NURSING ALERT Medications are administered to the patient with hypothyroidism with extreme caution because of the potential for altered metabolism and excretion and depressed metabolic rate and respiratory status.

PROMOTING PHYSICAL COMFORT

The patient often experiences chilling and extreme intolerance to cold, even if the room feels comfortable or hot to others. Extra clothing and blankets are provided, and the patient is protected from drafts. Use of heating pads and electric blankets is avoided because of the risk of peripheral vasodilation, further loss of body heat, and vascular collapse. Additionally, the patient could be burned by these items without being aware of it because of delayed responses and decreased mental status.

PROVIDING EMOTIONAL SUPPORT

The patient with moderate to severe hypothyroidism may experience severe emotional reactions to changes in appearance and body image and the frequent delay in diagnosis. The nonspecific, early symptoms may produce negative reactions by family members and friends, and the family and friends may have labelled the patient mentally unstable, uncooperative, or unwilling to participate in self-care activities.

As hypothyroidism is treated successfully and symptoms subside, the patient may experience depression and guilt as a result of the progression and severity of symptoms that occurred. The nurse informs the patient and family that the symptoms and inability to recognize them are common and part of the disorder itself. The patient and family may require assistance and counselling to deal with the emotional concerns and reactions that result.

PROMOTING HOME AND COMMUNITY-BASED CARE

Teaching Patients Self-Care. Because most hypothyroidism treatment takes place at home, the patient and family require information and instruction that will enable them to monitor the patient's condition and response to therapy. The nurse instructs the patient about the desired actions and side effects of medications and about how and when to take prescribed medications. The importance of continuing to take medications as prescribed even after symptoms improve is stressed to the patient. Because of the slowed mental processes that occur with hypothyroidism, it is important that a family member also be informed and instructed about treatment goals, medication schedules, and side effects to be reported to the physician. The nurse provides written instructions and guidelines for the patient and family.

Dietary instruction is provided to promote weight loss once medication has been initiated and to promote return of normal bowel patterns. The patient and family are often very concerned about the changes they have observed as a result of the hypothyroid state. It is often reassuring to the patient and family to be informed that many of the symptoms will disappear with effective treatment (Chart 42-3).

Continuing Care. The patient with hypothyroidism and myxedema coma needs considerable follow-up and health care. Before hospital discharge, arrangements are made to ensure that the patient returns to an environment that will promote adherence to the prescribed treatment plan. Assistance in devising a schedule or record ensures accurate and complete administration of medications. The nurse reinforces the importance of continued thyroid hormone replacement and periodic follow-up testing and instructs the patient and family members about the signs of overmedication and undermedication.

If indicated, a referral is made for home care. The home care nurse assesses the patient's progress toward recovery and ability to cope with the recent changes, along with the patient's physical and cognitive status and the patient's and family's understanding of the importance of prescribed long-term medication therapy and compliance with the medication schedule and recommended follow-up tests and appointments. The nurse documents, and reports to the patient's primary health care provider, subtle signs and symptoms that may indicate either inadequate or excessive thyroxine hormone.

> ### Chart 42-3
> ### Home Care Checklist • The Patient With Hypothyroidism (Myxedema)
>
> | *At the completion of the home care instruction, the patient or caregiver will be able to:* | Patient | Caregiver |
> | --- | :---: | :---: |
> | • State present and potential effects of hypothyroidism on the body | ✓ | ✓ |
> | • State precipitating factors and interventions for complications (hyperthyroidism, myxedema coma) | ✓ | ✓ |
> | • Explain the purpose, dose, route, schedule, side effects, and precautions of prescribed medication (synthetic thyroid hormone) | ✓ | ✓ |
> | • State that compliance with medical regimen is lifelong | ✓ | ✓ |
> | • State the need to avoid extreme cold temperature until condition is stable | ✓ | ✓ |
> | • State importance of regular follow-up visits with health care provider | ✓ | ✓ |
> | • Identify dietary strategies to promote weight reduction and prevent constipation (high fibre, low calorie, adequate fluid intake) | ✓ | ✓ |
> | • State potential for menstrual irregularities and potential for pregnancy for women | ✓ | ✓ |
> | • State the importance of avoiding infection | ✓ | ✓ |
> | • Identify changes in personality as related to hypothyroidism | ✓ | ✓ |
> | • Identify areas of activity limitations and impact on lifestyle | ✓ | ✓ |

Gerontologic Considerations

The elderly patient requires periodic follow-up monitoring of serum TSH levels because poor compliance with therapy may occur or the patient may take the medications erratically. A careful history may identify the need for further teaching about the importance of the medication. Because of the prevalence of hypothyroidism, testing of serum TSH levels in elderly people every 5 years has been recommended (Smallridge, 2000). In addition, the patient is reminded of the importance of participating in general health promotion activities and recommended health screening.

HYPERTHYROIDISM

Hyperthyroidism is the second most prevalent endocrine disorder, after diabetes mellitus. **Graves' disease**, the most common type of hyperthyroidism, results from an excessive output of thyroid hormones caused by abnormal stimulation of the thyroid gland by circulating immunoglobulins. It affects women eight times more frequently than men, with onset usually between the second and fourth decades (Tierney et al., 2001). It may appear after an emotional shock, stress, or an infection, but the exact significance of these relationships is not understood. Other common causes of hyperthyroidism include thyroiditis and excessive ingestion of thyroid hormone.

Clinical Manifestations

Patients with well-developed hyperthyroidism exhibit a characteristic group of signs and symptoms (sometimes referred to as **thyrotoxicosis**). The presenting symptom is often nervousness. These patients are often emotionally hyperexcitable, irritable, and apprehensive; they cannot sit quietly; they suffer from palpitations; and their pulse is abnormally rapid at rest as well as on exertion. They tolerate heat poorly and perspire unusually freely. The skin is flushed continuously, with a characteristic salmon colour, and is likely to be warm, soft, and moist. Elderly patients, however, may report dry skin and diffuse pruritus. A fine tremor of the hands may be observed. Patients may exhibit **exophthalmos** (bulging eyes), which produces a startled facial expression.

Other manifestations include an increased appetite and dietary intake, progressive weight loss, abnormal muscular fatigability and weakness (difficulty in climbing stairs and rising from a chair), amenorrhea, and changes in bowel function. The pulse rate ranges constantly between 90 and 160 beats/min; the systolic, but characteristically not the diastolic, blood pressure is elevated; atrial fibrillation may occur; and cardiac decompensation in the form of heart failure is common, especially in elderly patients. Osteoporosis and fracture are also associated with hyperthyroidism.

Cardiac effects may include sinus tachycardia or dysrhythmias, increased pulse pressure, and palpitations; it has been suggested that these changes may be related to increased sensitivity to catecholamines or to changes in neurotransmitter turnover. Myocardial hypertrophy and heart failure may occur if the hyperthyroidism is severe and untreated.

The course of the disease may be mild, characterized by remissions and exacerbations and terminating with spontaneous recovery in a few months or years. Conversely, it may progress relentlessly, with the untreated person becoming emaciated, intensely nervous, delirious, and even disoriented; eventually, the heart fails.

Symptoms of hyperthyroidism may occur with the release of excessive amounts of thyroid hormone as a result of inflammation after irradiation of the thyroid or destruction of thyroid tissue by tumour. Such symptoms may also occur with excessive administration of thyroid hormone for treatment of hypothyroidism. Long-standing use of thyroid hormone in the absence of close monitoring may be a cause of symptoms of hyperthyroidism. It is also likely to result in premature osteoporosis, particularly in women.

Assessment and Diagnostic Findings

The thyroid gland invariably is enlarged to some extent. It is soft and may pulsate; a thrill often can be palpated, and a bruit is heard over the thyroid arteries. These are signs of greatly increased blood flow through the thyroid gland. In advanced cases, the diagnosis is made on the basis of the symptoms and an increase in serum T_4 and an increased ^{123}I or ^{125}I uptake by the thyroid in excess of 50%.

Gerontologic Considerations

Although hyperthyroidism is much less common in elderly people than hypothyroidism, patients older than 60 years account for 10% to 15% of the cases of thyrotoxicosis. Although some older patients develop typical signs and symptoms of thyrotoxicosis, in most an atypical picture is present, which is often subclinical (Toft, 2001).

Elderly patients commonly present with vague and nonspecific signs and symptoms, making disorders hard to detect. Symptoms such as tachycardia, fatigue, mental confusion, weight loss, change in bowel habits, and depression can be attributed to age and other illnesses common to elderly people. In addition, the patient may report cardiovascular symptoms and difficulty climbing stairs or rising from a chair because of muscle weakness. New or worsening heart failure or angina is more likely to occur in elderly than in younger patients. The elderly patient may experience a single manifestation, such as atrial fibrillation, anorexia, or weight loss. These signs and symptoms may mask the underlying thyroid disease.

Spontaneous remission of hyperthyroidism is rare in elderly patients. Measurement of TSH is indicated in elderly patients with unexplained physical or mental deterioration.

Medical Management

Treatment of hyperthyroidism is directed toward reducing thyroid hyperactivity to relieve symptoms and remove the cause of important complications. Treatment depends on the cause of the hyperthyroidism and may require a combination of therapeutic approaches.

PHARMACOLOGIC THERAPY

Two forms of pharmacotherapy are available for treating hyperthyroidism and controlling excessive thyroid activity: (1) use of irradiation by administration of the radioisotope ^{123}I or ^{131}I for destructive effects on the thyroid gland and (2) antithyroid medications that interfere with the synthesis of thyroid hormones and other agents that control manifestations of hyperthyroidism. Surgical removal of most of the thyroid gland is a nonpharmacologic alternative.

Radioactive Iodine Therapy. The goal of radioactive iodine therapy (^{123}I or ^{131}I) is to destroy the overactive thyroid cells. Use of radioactive iodine is the most common treatment in elderly patients. Almost all the iodine that enters and is retained in the body becomes concentrated in the thyroid gland. Therefore, the radioactive isotope of iodine is concentrated in the thyroid gland, where it destroys thyroid cells without jeopardizing other radiosensitive tissues. Over a period of several weeks, thyroid cells exposed to the radioactive iodine are destroyed, resulting in reduction of the hyperthyroid state and inevitably hypothyroidism.

The patient is instructed about what to expect with this tasteless, colourless radioiodine, which may be administered by the radiologist. A single oral dose of the agent is administered, based on 80 to 160 µCi/g estimated thyroid weight. About 70% to 85% of patients are cured by one dose of radioactive iodine. An additional 10% to 20% require two doses; rarely is a third dose necessary. Use of an ablative dose of radioactive iodine initially causes an acute release of thyroid hormone from the thyroid gland and may cause an increase of symptoms. The patient is observed for signs of **thyroid storm**; propranolol is useful in controlling these symptoms.

After treatment with radioactive iodine, the patient is followed closely until the euthyroid state is reached. In 3 to 4 weeks, symptoms of hyperthyroidism subside. Because the incidence of hypothyroidism after this form of treatment is very high (ie, more than 90% at 10 years), close follow-up is required to evaluate thyroid function. Thyroid hormone replacement is necessary; small doses are usually prescribed, with the dose gradually increased over a period of months (up to about 1 year) until the FT$_4$ and TSH levels stabilize within normal ranges.

Radioactive iodine has been used to treat toxic adenomas and multinodular goitre and most varieties of thyrotoxicosis (rarely permanently successful); it is preferred for treating patients beyond the childbearing years with diffuse toxic goitre. It is contraindicated in pregnancy and in nursing mothers because radioiodine crosses the placenta and is secreted in breast milk. A major advantage of treatment with radioactive iodine is that it avoids many of the side effects associated with antithyroid medications. However, many patients and their families fear medications that are radioactive. Because of this fear, many patients elect to take antithyroid medications rather than radioactive iodine.

 Gerontologic Considerations

The use of radioactive iodine is generally recommended for treatment of thyrotoxicosis in elderly patients unless an enlarged thyroid gland is pressing on the airway. The hypermetabolic state of thyrotoxicosis must be controlled by antithyroid medications before radioactive iodine is administered because radiation may precipitate thyroid storm by increasing the release of hormone from the thyroid gland. Thyroid storm, if it occurs, has a mortality rate of 10% in elderly patients (Chart 42-4).

Antithyroid Medications. The objective of pharmacotherapy is to inhibit one or more stages in thyroid hormone synthesis or hormone release; another goal may be to reduce the amount of thyroid tissue, with resulting decreased thyroid hormone production.

Antithyroid agents block the utilization of iodine by interfering with the iodination of thyrosine and the coupling of iodothyrosines in the synthesis of thyroid hormones. This prevents the synthesis of thyroid hormone. The most commonly used medications are propylthiouracil (Propacil, PTU) or methimazole (Tapazole) until the patient is euthyroid (ie, neither hyperthyroid nor hypothyroid). These medications block extrathyroidal conversion of T$_4$ to T$_3$. Because antithyroid medications do not interfere with release or activity of previously formed thyroid hormones, it may take several weeks for relief of symptoms. At this time the maintenance dose is established, followed by a gradual withdrawal of the medication over the next several months.

Therapy is determined on the basis of clinical criteria, including changes in pulse rate, pulse pressure, body weight, size of the goitre, and results of laboratory studies of thyroid function.

Toxic complications of antithyroid medications are relatively uncommon; nevertheless, the importance of periodic follow-up is emphasized because medication sensitization, fever, rash, urticaria, or even agranulocytosis and thrombocytopenia (decrease in granulocytes and platelets) may develop. With any sign of infection, especially pharyngitis and fever or the occurrence of mouth ulcers, the patient is advised to stop the medication, notify the physician immediately, and undergo hematologic studies. Rash, arthralgias, and fever occur in 5% of patients. Agranulocytosis, the most serious toxic side effect, occurs in 1 of every 200 patients. Its incidence is higher in patients older than 40 years. It generally occurs within the first 3 months of therapy but may occur up to 1 year after it is started.

Thyroid Storm (Thyrotoxic Crisis, Thyrotoxicosis)

Thyroid storm (thyrotoxic crisis) is a form of severe hyperthyroidism, usually of abrupt onset. Untreated it is almost always fatal, but with proper treatment the mortality rate is reduced substantially. The patient with thyroid storm or crisis is critically ill and requires astute observation and aggressive and supportive nursing care during and after the acute stage of illness.

Clinical Manifestations
Thyroid storm is characterized by:
- High fever (hyperpyrexia) above 38.5°C
- Extreme tachycardia (more than 130 beats/min)
- Exaggerated symptoms of hyperthyroidism with disturbances of a major system—for example, GI (weight loss, diarrhea, abdominal pain), or cardiovascular (edema, chest pain, dyspnea, palpitations)
- Altered neurologic or mental state, which frequently appears as delirium psychosis, somnolence, or coma

Life-threatening thyroid storm is usually precipitated by stress, such as injury, infection, thyroid and nonthyroid surgery, tooth extraction, insulin reaction, diabetic acidosis, pregnancy, digitalis intoxication, abrupt withdrawal of antithyroid medications, extreme emotional stress, or vigourous palpation of the thyroid. These factors can precipitate thyroid storm in the partially controlled or completely untreated patient with hyperthyroidism. Current methods of diagnosis and treatment for hyperthyroidism have greatly decreased the incidence of thyroid storm, making it uncommon today.

Management
Immediate objectives are reduction of body temperature and heart rate and prevention of vascular collapse. Measures to accomplish these objectives include:
- A hypothermia mattress or blanket, ice packs, a cool environment, hydrocortisone, and acetaminophen (Tylenol). Salicylates (eg, aspirin) are not used because they displace thyroid hormone from binding proteins and worsen the hypermetabolism.
- Humidified oxygen is administered to improve tissue oxygenation and meet the high metabolic demands. Arterial blood gas levels or pulse oximetry may be used to monitor respiratory status.
- Intravenous fluids containing dextrose are administered to replace liver glycogen stores that have been decreased in the hyperthyroid patient.
- PTU or methimazole is administered to impede formation of thyroid hormone and block conversion of T_4 to T_3, the more active form of thyroid hormone.
- Hydrocortisone is prescribed to treat shock or adrenal insufficiency.
- Iodine is administered to decrease output of T_4 from the thyroid gland. For cardiac problems such as atrial fibrillation, dysrhythmias, and heart failure, sympatholytic agents may be administered. Propranolol, combined with digitalis, has been effective in reducing severe cardiac symptoms.

Patients taking antithyroid medications are instructed not to use decongestants for nasal stuffiness because they are poorly tolerated. Antithyroid medications are contraindicated in late pregnancy because they may produce goitre and cretinism in the fetus.

Thyroid hormone is occasionally administered with antithyroid medications to put the thyroid gland at rest. In this approach, hypothyroidism from excess antithyroid medication is avoided, as is stimulation of the thyroid gland by TSH. Thyroid hormone is available as thyroglobulin (Proloid) and levothyroxine sodium (Synthroid). These slow-acting preparations take about 10 days to achieve their full effect. Liothyronine sodium (Cytomel) has a more rapid onset, and its action is of short duration.

Gerontologic Considerations

If antithyroid agents are used in elderly patients, the patient must be monitored closely because elderly patients are more likely to develop granulocytopenia. The dosage of other medications to treat other chronic illnesses in elderly patients may need to be modified because of the altered rate of metabolism in hyperthyroidism.

Adjunctive Therapy. Iodine or iodide compounds, once the only therapy available for patients with hyperthyroidism, are no longer used as the sole method of treatment. Such compounds decrease the release of thyroid hormones from the thyroid gland and reduce the vascularity and size of the thyroid. Compounds such as potassium iodide (KI), Lugol's solution, and saturated solution of potassium iodide (SSKI) may be used in combination with antithyroid agents or beta-adrenergic blockers to prepare the patient with hyperthyroidism for surgery. These agents reduce the activity of the thyroid hormone and the vascularity of the thyroid gland, making the surgical procedure safer. Solutions of iodine and iodide compounds are more palatable in milk or fruit juice and are administered through a straw to prevent staining of the teeth. These compounds

reduce the metabolic rate more rapidly than antithyroid medications, but their action does not last as long.

NURSING ALERT Patients receiving these medications should be observed for the development of goitre and should be cautioned against use of over-the-counter medications that contain iodides and can increase the response to iodide therapy. Cough medications, expectorants, bronchodilators, and salt substitutes may contain iodide and should be avoided by the patient receiving iodide therapy.

Beta-adrenergic blocking agents are important in controlling the sympathetic nervous system effects of hyperthyroidism. For example, propranolol (Inderal) is used to control nervousness, tachycardia, tremor, anxiety, and heat intolerance. The patient continues taking propranolol until the FT_4 is within the normal range and the TSH level approaches normal.

Gerontologic Considerations

Use of beta-adrenergic blocking agents (eg, propranolol [Inderal]) may be indicated to decrease the cardiovascular and neurologic signs and symptoms of thyrotoxicosis. These agents must be used with extreme caution in elderly patients to minimize adverse effects on cardiac function that may produce heart failure.

SURGICAL MANAGEMENT
Surgery to remove thyroid tissue was once the primary method of treating hyperthyroidism; today, surgery is reserved for special circumstances—for example, in pregnant women allergic to antithyroid medications, patients with large goitres, or patients unable to take antithyroid agents. Surgery for treatment of hyperthyroidism is performed soon after the thyroid function has returned to normal (4 to 6 weeks).

The surgical removal of about five sixths of the thyroid tissue (subtotal thyroidectomy) practically ensures a prolonged remission in most patients with exophthalmic goitre. Its use today is reserved for large goitres, presence of obstructive symptoms, pregnant women, or when there is a need for rapid normalization of thyroid function (Argueta & Whitaker, 2000; Fatourechi, 2000). Before surgery, propylthiouracil is administered until signs of hyperthyroidism have disappeared. A beta-adrenergic blocking agent (propranolol) may be used to reduce the heart rate and other signs and symptoms of hyperthyroidism; however, this does not create a euthyroid state. Iodine (Lugol's solution or potassium iodide) may be prescribed in an effort to reduce blood loss; however, the effectiveness of this is unknown. Patients receiving iodine medication must be monitored for evidence of iodine toxicity (iodism), which requires immediate withdrawal of the medication. Symptoms of iodism include swelling of the buccal mucosa, excessive salivation, coryza, and skin eruptions.

Recurrent Hyperthyroidism

No treatment for thyrotoxicosis is without side effects, and all three treatments (radioactive iodine therapy, antithyroid medications, and surgery) share the same complications: relapse or recurrent hyperthyroidism and permanent hypothyroidism. The rate of relapse increases in patients who had very severe disease, a long history of dysfunction, ocular and cardiac symptoms, large goitre, and relapse after previous treatment. The relapse rate after radioactive iodine therapy depends on the dose used in treatment. Patients receiving a lower dose of radioactive iodine are more likely to require subsequent treatment than those being treated with a higher dose. Hypothyroidism occurs in almost 80% of patients at 1 year and in 90% to 100% by 5 years for both the multiple low-dose and single high-dose methods.

Although rates of relapse and the occurrence of hypothyroidism vary, relapse with antithyroid medications is about 45% by 1 year after completion of therapy and almost 75% by 5 years later (Larson et al., 2000). Discontinuation of antithyroid medications before therapy is complete usually results in relapse within 6 months in most patients. The incidence of relapse with subtotal thyroidectomy is 19% at 18 months; an incidence of hypothyroidism of 25% has been reported at 18 months after surgery. The risk for these complications illustrates the importance of long-term follow-up of patients treated for hyperthyroidism.

NURSING PROCESS:
THE PATIENT WITH HYPERTHYROIDISM
Assessment

The health history and examination focus on symptoms related to accelerated or exaggerated metabolism. These include the patient's and family's report of irritability and increased emotional reaction and the impact these changes have had on the patient's interaction with family, friends, and coworkers. The history includes other stressors and the patient's ability to cope with stress.

The nurse assesses the patient's nutritional status and the presence of symptoms. Symptoms related to excessive nervous system output and changes in vision and appearance of the eyes are noted. The nurse periodically assesses and monitors the patient's cardiac status, including heart rate, blood pressure, heart sounds, and peripheral pulses.

Because emotional changes are associated with hyperthyroidism, the patient's emotional state and psychological status are evaluated, as are such symptoms as irritability, anxiety, sleep disturbances, apathy, and lethargy, all of which may occur with hyperthyroidism. The family may also provide information about recent changes in the patient's emotional status.

Diagnosis
NURSING DIAGNOSES

Based on all the assessment data, the major nursing diagnoses of the patient with hyperthyroidism include the following:

- Imbalanced nutrition, less than body requirements, related to exaggerated metabolic rate, excessive appetite, and increased gastrointestinal activity
- Ineffective coping related to irritability, hyperexcitability, apprehension, and emotional instability
- Low self-esteem related to changes in appearance, excessive appetite, and weight loss
- Altered body temperature

COLLABORATIVE PROBLEMS/ POTENTIAL COMPLICATIONS

Based on assessment data, potential complications may include the following:

- Thyrotoxicosis or thyroid storm
- Hypothyroidism

Planning and Goals

The goals for the patient may be improved nutritional status, improved coping ability, improved self-esteem, maintenance of normal body temperature, and absence of complications.

Nursing Interventions
IMPROVING NUTRITIONAL STATUS

Hyperthyroidism affects all body systems, including the gastrointestinal system. The appetite is increased but may be satisfied by several well-balanced meals of small size, even up to six meals a day. Foods and fluids are selected to replace fluid lost through diarrhea and diaphoresis and to control the diarrhea that results from increased peristalsis. Rapid movement of food through the gastrointestinal tract may result in nutritional imbalance and further weight loss. To reduce diarrhea, highly seasoned foods and stimulants such as coffee, tea, cola, and alcohol are discouraged. High-calorie, high-protein foods are encouraged. A quiet atmosphere during mealtime may aid digestion. Weight and dietary intake are recorded to monitor nutritional status.

ENHANCING COPING MEASURES

The patient with hyperthyroidism needs reassurance that the emotional reactions being experienced are a result of the disorder and that with effective treatment those symptoms will be controlled. Because of the negative effect these symptoms have on family and friends, they too need reassurance that these symptoms are expected to disappear with treatment.

It is important to use a calm, unhurried approach with the patient. Stressful experiences are minimized; therefore, if hospitalized, the patient is not placed in a room with very ill or talkative patients. The environment is kept quiet and uncluttered. Noises, such as loud music, conversation, and equipment alarms, are minimized. The nurse encourages relaxing activities if they do not overstimulate the patient.

If thyroidectomy is planned, the patient needs to know that pharmacologic therapy is necessary to prepare the thyroid gland for surgical treatment. The nurse instructs and reminds the patient to take the medications as prescribed. Because of hyperexcitability and shortened attention span, the patient may require repetition of this information and written instructions.

IMPROVING SELF-ESTEEM

The hyperthyroid patient is likely to experience changes in appearance, appetite, and weight. These factors, along with the patient's inability to cope well with family and the illness, may result in loss of self-esteem. The nurse conveys an understanding of the patient's concern about these problems and assists the patient to develop effective coping strategies. The patient and family need to know that these changes are a result of the thyroid dysfunction and are, in fact, out of the patient's control.

If changes in appearance are very disturbing to the patient, mirrors may be covered or removed. In addition, the nurse reminds family members and personnel to avoid bringing these changes to the patient's attention. The nurse explains to the patient and family that most of these changes are expected to disappear with effective treatment.

If the patient experiences eye changes secondary to hyperthyroidism, eye care and protection may become necessary. The patient may need instructions about instillation of eye drops or ointment prescribed to soothe the eyes and protect the exposed cornea.

The patient may be embarrassed by the need to eat large meals. Therefore, the nurse arranges for the patient to eat alone if desired and avoids commenting on the patient's large dietary intake while making sure that the patient receives sufficient food.

MAINTAINING NORMAL BODY TEMPERATURE

The patient with hyperthyroidism frequently finds a normal room temperature too warm because of an exaggerated metabolic rate and increased heat production. The nurse maintains the environment at a cool, comfortable temperature and changes bedding and clothing as needed. Cool baths and cool or cold fluids may provide relief. The reason for the patient's discomfort and the importance of providing a cool environment are explained to the family and staff.

MONITORING AND MANAGING POTENTIAL COMPLICATIONS

The nurse closely monitors the patient with hyperthyroidism for signs and symptoms that may be indicative of thyroid storm. Cardiac and respiratory function are assessed by measuring vital signs and cardiac output, ECG monitoring, arterial blood gases, and pulse oximetry. Assessment continues when treatment is initiated because of the potential side effects on cardiac function. Oxygen is administered to prevent hypoxia, to improve tissue oxygenation, and to meet the high metabolic demands. Intravenous fluids may be necessary to maintain blood glucose levels and to replace lost fluids. Antithyroid medications (PTU or methimazole) may be prescribed to reduce thyroid hormone levels. In addition, propranolol and digitalis may be prescribed to treat cardiac symptoms. If shock develops, treatment strategies must be implemented (see Chap. 15).

Hypothyroidism is likely to occur with any of the treatments used to treat hyperthyroidism. Therefore, the nurse periodically monitors the patient. Most patients report a greatly improved sense of well-being after treatment of hyperthyroidism, and some fail to continue to take prescribed thyroid replacement therapy. Therefore, part of patient and family teaching is instruction about the importance of continuing therapy indefinitely after discharge and a discussion of the consequences of failing to take medication.

PROMOTING HOME AND COMMUNITY-BASED CARE

Teaching Patients Self-Care

The nurse teaches the patient with hyperthyroidism how and when to take prescribed medication, and provides instruction about the essential role of the medication in the broader therapeutic plan. Because of the hyperexcitability and decreased attention span associated with hyperthyroidism, the nurse provides a written plan for the patient to use at home. The type and amount of information given depend on the patient's stress and anxiety levels. The patient and family members receive verbal and written information about the actions and possible side effects of the medications. The nurse identifies adverse effects that should be reported if they occur (Chart 42-5).

If a total or subtotal thyroidectomy is anticipated, the patient needs information about what to expect. This information is repeated as the time of surgery approaches. The nurse also advises

---

Chart 42-5
Home Care Checklist • The Patient With Hyperthyroidism

At the completion of the home care instruction, the patient or caregiver will be able to:	Patient	Caregiver
• State present and potential effects of hyperthyroidism on the body	✓	✓
• State precipitating factors and interventions for complications (hypothyroidism, thyroid storm)	✓	✓
• State the purpose, dose, route, schedule, side effects, and precautions of prescribed medications (propylthiouracil, radioactive iodine)	✓	✓
• State the need to contact health care provider before taking over-the-counter medications	✓	✓
• State need for regular follow-up visits with health care provider	✓	✓
• Identify the need for planned rest periods and methods to improve sleep patterns	✓	✓
• Identify the need for increased dietary intake until weight stabilizes	✓	✓
• Identify areas of physical and emotional stress	✓	✓
• State that emotional lability is part of disease process	✓	✓
• Describe the potential benefits and risks of surgical intervention or radioactive iodine therapy	✓	✓
• Identify potential for menstrual irregularities, increased risk for osteoporosis, and potential for pregnancy for women	✓	✓
• State need to wear medical identification and carry medical information card	✓	✓

the patient to avoid stressful situations that may precipitate thyroid storm.

Continuing Care

Referral for home care, if indicated, allows the home care nurse to assess the home and family environment and the patient's and family's understanding of the importance of adhering to the therapeutic regimen and the recommended follow-up monitoring. The nurse reinforces to the patient and family the importance of long-term follow-up because of the risk for hypothyroidism after thyroidectomy or treatment with antithyroid medications or radioactive iodine. The nurse also assesses the patient for changes indicating return to normal thyroid function and signs and symptoms of hyperthyroidism and hypothyroidism. Further, the nurse reminds the patient and family about the importance of health promotion activities and recommended health screening.

Evaluation

EXPECTED PATIENT OUTCOMES

Expected patient outcomes may include:

1. Improves nutritional status
   a. Reports adequate dietary intake and decreased hunger
   b. Identifies high-calorie, high-protein foods; identifies foods to be avoided
   c. Avoids use of alcohol and other stimulants
   d. Reports decreased episodes of diarrhea
2. Demonstrates effective coping methods in dealing with family, friends, and coworkers
   a. Explains reasons for irritability and emotional instability
   b. Avoids stressful situations, events, and people
   c. Participates in relaxing, nonstressful activities
3. Achieves increased self-esteem
   a. Verbalizes feelings about self and illness
   b. Describes feelings of frustration and loss of control to others
   c. Describes reasons for increased appetite
4. Maintains normal body temperature
5. Absence of complications
   a. Serum thyroid hormone and TSH levels are within normal limits
   b. Identifies signs and symptoms of thyroid storm and hypothyroidism
   c. Vital signs and results of ECG, arterial blood gases, and pulse oximetry are within normal limits
   d. States importance of regular follow-up and lifelong maintenance of prescribed therapy

THYROIDITIS

Thyroiditis, inflammation of the thyroid gland, can be acute, subacute, or chronic. Each type of thyroiditis is characterized by inflammation, fibrosis, or lymphocytic infiltration of the thyroid gland.

ACUTE THYROIDITIS

Acute thyroiditis is a rare disorder caused by infection of the thyroid gland by bacteria, fungi, mycobacteria, or parasites. *Staphylococcus aureus* and other staphylococci are the most common causes. Infection typically causes anterior neck pain and swelling, fever, dysphagia, and dysphonia. Pharyngitis or pharyngeal pain is often present. Examination may reveal warmth, erythema (redness), and tenderness of the thyroid gland. Treatment of acute thyroiditis includes antimicrobial agents and fluid replacement. Surgical incision and drainage may be needed if an abscess is present.

SUBACUTE THYROIDITIS

Subacute thyroiditis may be subacute granulomatous thyroiditis (deQuervain's thyroiditis) or painless thyroiditis (silent thyroiditis or subacute lymphocytic thyroiditis). Subacute granulomatous thyroiditis is an inflammatory disorder of the thyroid gland that predominantly affects women between 40 and 50 years old (Smallridge, 2000). The condition presents as a painful swelling in the anterior neck that lasts 1 to 2 months and then disappears spontaneously without residual effect. It often follows a respiratory infection. The thyroid enlarges symmetrically and may be painful. The overlying skin is often reddened and warm. Swallowing may be difficult and uncomfortable. Irritability, nervousness, insomnia, and weight loss—manifestations of hyperthyroidism—are common, and many patients experience chills and fever as well.

Treatment aims to control the inflammation. In general, nonsteroidal anti-inflammatory drugs (NSAIDs) are used to relieve neck pain. Acetylsalicylic acid (aspirin) is avoided if symptoms of hyperthyroidism occur because aspirin displaces thyroid hormone from its binding sites and increases the amount of circulating hormone. Beta-blocking agents (eg, propranolol [Inderal]) may be used to control symptoms of hyperthyroidism. Antithyroid agents, which block the synthesis of T_3 and T_4, are not effective in thyroiditis because the associated thyrotoxicosis results from the release of stored thyroid hormones rather than from their increased synthesis. In more severe cases, oral corticosteroids may be prescribed to reduce swelling and relieve pain; however, they do not usually affect the underlying cause. In some cases, temporary hypothyroidism may develop and may necessitate thyroid hormone therapy. Follow-up monitoring is necessary to document the patient's return to a euthyroid state.

Painless thyroiditis (subacute lymphocytic thyroiditis) often occurs in the postpartum period and is thought to be an autoimmune process. Symptoms of hyperthyroidism or hypothyroidism are possible. Treatment is directed at symptoms, and yearly follow-up is recommended to determine the patient's need for treatment of subsequent hypothyroidism.

CHRONIC THYROIDITIS (HASHIMOTO'S DISEASE)

Chronic thyroiditis, which occurs most frequently in women between 30 and 50 years old, has been termed Hashimoto's disease, or chronic lymphocytic thyroiditis; its diagnosis is based on the histologic appearance of the inflamed gland. In contrast to acute thyroiditis, the chronic forms are usually not accompanied by pain, pressure symptoms, or fever, and thyroid activity is usually normal or low rather than increased. Cell-mediated immunity may play a significant role in the pathogenesis of chronic thyroiditis, and there may be a genetic predisposition to it. If untreated, the disease runs a slow, progressive course, leading eventually to hypothyroidism.

The objective of treatment is to reduce the size of the thyroid gland and prevent hypothyroidism. Thyroid hormone therapy is prescribed to reduce thyroid activity and the production of thyroglobulin. If hypothyroid symptoms are present, thyroid hormone therapy is prescribed. Surgery may be required if pressure symptoms persist.

THYROID TUMOURS

Tumours of the thyroid gland are classified on the basis of being benign or malignant, the presence or absence of associated thyrotoxicosis, and the diffuse or irregular quality of the glandular enlargement. If the enlargement is sufficient to cause a visible swelling in the neck, the tumour is referred to as a goitre.

GENETICS IN NURSING PRACTICE—Metabolic Disorders

Some examples of metabolic and endocrine disorders influenced by genetic factors include the following:

- Alpha-1 antitrypsin deficiency
- Cystic fibrosis
- Diabetes mellitus type 1 and type 2
- Hereditary hemochromatosis
- Multiple endocrine neoplasia (MEN) type I and type II
- Von Hippel-Lindau syndrome
- Possibly, the chronic thyroiditis known as Hashimoto's disease

NURSING ASSESSMENTS

FAMILY HISTORY ASSESSMENT

- Assess family history for relatives with early-onset hepatic, pancreatic, endocrine disease.
- Inquire about family members with diabetes and their ages at onset.
- Assess family history of other related genetic conditions such as cystic fibrosis, alpha-1 antitrypsin deficiency, hereditary hemochromatosis.

PHYSICAL ASSESSMENT

- Assess for physical symptoms such as mucosal neuromas, hypertrophied lips, skeletal abnormalities, and marfanoid appearance.
- Assess for signs of arthritis, bronze pigmentation of the skin (hereditary hemochromatosis).

MANAGEMENT ISSUES SPECIFIC TO GENETICS

- Inquire whether DNA mutation testing has been performed on any affected family member.
- If indicated, refer for further genetic counselling and evaluation so that family members can discuss inheritance, risk to other family members, availability of genetic testing and gene-based interventions.
- Offer appropriate genetics information and resources.
- Assess patient's understanding of genetics information.

- Provide support to families with newly diagnosed genetic-related metabolic and endocrine conditions.
- Participate in management and coordination of care of patients with genetic conditions, individuals predisposed to develop or pass on a genetic condition.

GENETICS RESOURCES FOR NURSES AND THEIR PATIENTS ON THE WEB

Canadian Association of Genetic Counsellors (CAGC): www.cagc-accg.ca—provides a listing of genetic centres across Canada.

Canadian Cancer Society: www.cancer.ca—information on the genetic factors/risk and genetic testing.

Canadian Directory of Genetic Support Groups: www.lhsc.on.ca/programs/medgenet—a resource guide for families and professionals.

Canadian Genetic Disease Network: www.cgdn.ca—its stated mission is to be the primary catalyst in advancing Canada's scientific and commercial competitiveness in genetic research and the application of genetic discoveries to the prevention, diagnosis, and treatment of human disease.

Canadian Organization for Rare Disorders (CORD): www.cord.ca—information on over 6000 rare disorders and links individuals/families together with the same rare disorder.

Genetic Alliance: www.geneticalliance.org—increases the capacity of genetic advocacy groups to achieve their missions and leverages the voices of millions of individuals and families living with genetic conditions.

The Genetics Society of Canada (GSC): http://life.biology.mcmaster.ca/GSC—promotes research and communicates the results and implications of genetics to the public.

GeneTests: www.genetests.org—a publicly funded medical genetics information resource developed for physicians, other health care providers, and researchers.

OMIM Online Mendelian Inheritance in Man: www.ncbi.nlm.nih.gov/entrez/query.fcgi?db=OMIM—a catalogue of human genes and genetic disorders.

All grades of goitre are encountered, from those that are barely visible to those producing disfigurement. Some are symmetric and diffuse; others are nodular. Some are accompanied by hyperthyroidism, in which case they are described as toxic; others are associated with a euthyroid state and are called nontoxic goitres.

ENDEMIC (IODINE-DEFICIENT) GOITRE

The most common type of goitre, encountered chiefly in geographic regions where the natural supply of iodine is deficient (eg, the Great Lakes areas of Canada), is the so-called simple or colloid goitre. In addition to being caused by an iodine deficiency, simple goitre may be caused by an intake of large quantities of goitrogenic substances in patients with unusually susceptible glands. These substances include excessive amounts of iodine or lithium, which is used in treating bipolar disorders.

Simple goitre represents a compensatory hypertrophy of the thyroid gland, caused by stimulation by the pituitary gland. The pituitary gland produces thyrotropin or TSH, a hormone that controls the release of thyroid hormone from the thyroid gland. Its pro-

duction increases if there is subnormal thyroid activity, as when insufficient iodine is available for production of the thyroid hormone. Such goitres usually cause no symptoms, except for the swelling in the neck, which may result in tracheal compression when excessive.

Many goitres of this type recede after iodine imbalance is corrected. Supplementary iodine, such as SSKI, is prescribed to suppress the pituitary's thyroid-stimulating activity. When surgery is recommended, the risk for postoperative complications is minimized by ensuring a preoperative euthyroid state by treatment with antithyroid medications and iodide to reduce the size and vascularity of the goitre.

Providing children in iodine-poor regions with iodine compounds can prevent simple or endemic goitre. If the mean iodine intake is less than 40 µg/day, the thyroid gland hypertrophies. The World Health Organization recommends that salt be iodized to a concentration of 1 part in 100,000, which is adequate for the prevention of endemic goitre. In the United States, salt is iodized to 1 part in 10,000. The introduction of iodized salt has been the single most effective means of preventing goitre in at-risk populations.

NODULAR GOITRE

Some thyroid glands are nodular because of areas of hyperplasia (overgrowth). No symptoms may arise as a result of this condition, but not uncommonly these nodules slowly increase in size, with some descending into the thorax, where they cause local pressure symptoms. Some nodules become malignant, and some are associated with a hyperthyroid state. Thus, the patient with many thyroid nodules may eventually require surgery.

THYROID CANCER

Cancer of the thyroid is much less prevalent than other forms of cancer; however, it accounts for 90% of endocrine malignancies. According to the Canadian Cancer Society (2005), about 3100 new cases of thyroid cancer are diagnosed each year. Women account for 2400 of the new cases and men 710. About 100 women and 65 men die annually from this malignancy. There are several types of cancer of the thyroid gland; the type determines the course and prognosis (Table 42-3).

External radiation of the head, neck, or chest in infancy and childhood increases the risk of thyroid carcinoma. Between 1940 and 1960, radiation therapy was occasionally used to shrink enlarged tonsillar and adenoid tissue, to treat acne, or to reduce an enlarged thymus. For people exposed to external radiation in childhood, there appears to be an increased incidence of thyroid cancer 5 to 40 years after irradiation. Consequently, people who underwent such treatment should consult a physician, request an isotope thyroid scan as part of the evaluation, follow recommended treatment of abnormalities of the gland, and continue with annual checkups (Chart 42-6).

Assessment and Diagnostic Findings

Lesions that are single, hard, and fixed on palpation or associated with cervical lymphadenopathy suggest malignancy. Thyroid function tests may be helpful in evaluating thyroid nodules and masses; however, their results are rarely conclusive. Needle biopsy of the thyroid gland is used as an outpatient procedure to make a diagnosis of thyroid cancer, to differentiate cancerous thyroid nodules from noncancerous nodules, and to stage the cancer if detected. The procedure is safe and usually requires only a local anesthetic. Patients who undergo the procedure are followed closely, however, because cancerous tissues may be missed during the procedure. A second type of aspiration or biopsy uses a large-bore needle rather than the fine needle used in standard biopsy; it may be used when the results of the standard biopsy are inconclusive, or with rapidly growing tumours. Additional diagnostic studies include ultrasound, MRI, CT scans, thyroid scans, radioactive iodine uptake studies, and thyroid suppression tests.

Medical Management

The treatment of choice for thyroid carcinoma is surgical removal. Total or near-total thyroidectomy is performed when possible. Modified neck dissection or more extensive radical neck dissection is performed if there is lymph node involvement.

SURGICAL MANAGEMENT

Efforts are made to spare parathyroid tissue to reduce the risk for postoperative hypocalcemia and tetany. After surgery, ablation procedures are carried out with radioactive iodine to eradicate residual thyroid tissue if the tumour is radiosensitive. Radioactive

TYPE OF THYROID CANCER	INCIDENCE (%)	CHARACTERISTICS
Papillary adenocarcinoma	70	Most common and least aggressive Asymptomatic nodule in a normal gland Starts in childhood or early adult life, remains localized Metastasizes along the lymphatics if untreated More aggressive in the elderly
Follicular adenocarcinoma	15	Appears after 40 years of age Encapsulated; feels elastic or rubbery on palpation Spreads through the bloodstream to bone, liver, and lung Prognosis is not as favourable as for papillary adenocarcinoma
Medullary	5	Appears after 50 years of age Occurs as part of multiple endocrine neoplasia (MEN) Hormone-producing tumour causing endocrine dysfunction symptoms Metastasizes by lymphatics and bloodstream Moderate survival rate
Anaplastic	5	50% of anaplastic thyroid carcinomas occur in patients older than 60 years Hard, irregular mass that grows quickly and spreads by direct invasion to adjacent tissues May be painful and tender Survival for patients with anaplastic cancer is usually less than 6 months
Thyroid lymphoma	5	Appears after age 40 years May have history of goitre, hoarseness, dyspnea, pain, and pressure Good prognosis

Table 42-3 • **Types of Thyroid Cancers**

Chart 42-6 Radiation-Induced Thyroid Damage and Cancer

The thyroid gland has a very efficient mechanism to remove iodine from the bloodstream and concentrate or "trap" it for subsequent synthesis of thyroid hormone. The effectiveness of this mechanism to concentrate iodide is reflected in a concentration of iodide 20 to 40 times the concentration of iodide in the plasma.

If milk and other food sources become contaminated with radio-activity as a result of a nuclear detonation or a nuclear power plant incident or mishap, the radioactive iodide would become concentrated in the thyroid gland at a very high concentration and would irradiate the thyroid gland, increasing the risk for thyroid gland cancer. Therefore, in communities exposed to increased radioactivity, attempts have been made to block the uptake of radioactive iodide by flooding or saturating the thyroid gland with nonradioactive iodide.

Administration of potassium iodide (KI) or other iodide preparations as soon as possible after exposure almost completely inhibits thyroid absorption of the radioactive iodide and promotes rapid excretion of any that is absorbed. In 2001, the Food and Drug Administration (FDA) issued a statement recommending KI administration in advance of exposure to radioactive iodine—that is, when exposure is imminent (FDA, 2001).

---

the skin, anorexia, and fatigue (see Chap. 16 for a discussion of these side effects of radiation). Chemotherapy is infrequently used to treat thyroid cancer.

Patients whose thyroid cancer is detected early and who are appropriately treated usually do very well. Patients who have had papillary cancer, the most common and least aggressive tumour, have a 10-year survival rate greater than 90%. Long-term survival is also common in follicular cancer, a more aggressive form of thyroid cancer (Tierney et al., 2001). Continued thyroid hormone therapy and periodic follow-up and diagnostic testing, however, are important to ensure the patient's well-being (Thyroid Carcinoma Guidelines, 2001).

Postoperatively, the patient is instructed to take exogenous thyroid hormone to prevent hypothyroidism. Later follow-up includes clinical assessment for recurrence of nodules or masses in the neck and signs of hoarseness, dysphagia, or dyspnea. Total-body scans are performed 2 to 4 months after surgery to detect residual thyroid tissue or metastatic disease. Thyroid hormones are stopped for about 6 weeks before the tests. Care must be taken to avoid iodine-containing foods and contrast agents. A repeat scan is done 1 year after the initial surgery. If measurements are stable, a final scan is obtained in 3 to 5 years.

FT_4, TSH, serum calcium, and phosphorus levels are monitored to determine whether the thyroid hormone supplementation is adequate and to note whether calcium balance is maintained.

Although local and systemic reactions to radiation may occur and may include neutropenia or thrombocytopenia, these complications are rare when radioactive iodine is used. Patients who undergo surgery that is combined with radioiodine have a higher survival rate than those undergoing surgery alone. Patient teaching emphasizes the importance of taking prescribed medications and following recommendations for follow-up monitoring. The patient who is undergoing radiation therapy is also instructed in how to assess and manage side effects of treatment.

Partial or complete **thyroidectomy** may be carried out as primary treatment of thyroid carcinoma, hyperthyroidism, or

---

iodine also maximizes the chance of discovering thyroid metastasis at a later date if total-body scans are carried out.

After surgery, thyroid hormone is administered in suppressive doses to lower the levels of TSH to a euthyroid state (Thyroid Carcinoma Guidelines, 2001). If remaining thyroid tissue is inadequate to produce sufficient thyroid hormone, thyroxine is required permanently.

Several routes are available for administering radiation to the thyroid or tissues of the neck, including oral administration of radioactive iodine and external administration of radiation therapy. The patient who receives external sources of radiation therapy is at risk for mucositis, dryness of the mouth, dysphagia, redness of

---

NURSING RESEARCH PROFILE 42-1
Thyroid Cancer: Patients' Experiences

Stajduhar, K. I., Neithercut, J., Chu, E., Pham, P., Rohde, J., Sicotte, A., & Young, K. (2000). Thyroid cancer: Patients' experiences of receiving iodine-131 therapy. *Oncology Nursing Forum, 27*(8), 1213–1218.

Purpose
Examination of quality of life and patient experiences for prevalent cancers is well documented in the literature. However, for cancers with low incidence rates, such as thyroid cancer, little information exists. This study examines the experiences of patients who received ^{131}I treatment for thyroid cancer. It explores the patients' perspective of educational needs related to treatment.

Study Sample and Design
Patients who had received ^{131}I therapy treatment within the previous 2 years were recruited from an oncology/acute care medical unit in a large tertiary medical centre. Unstructured focus groups, telephone interviews, and field notes were used in data collection. Five men and 22 women ages 18 to 80 years (mean 38) were asked to respond to an open-ended prompt, such as, "Tell me about your experiences when you were a patient on our unit." Tape recordings were made during each contact and transcribed verbatim. Thematic analysis was used to identify emerging themes.

Findings
Four major themes were elicited from the analysis: recognizing the totality of the cancer experience, recognizing the totality of the treat-

ment experiences, being isolated, and understanding barriers to treatment. Participants reported that health care providers did not understand the totality of their experience and that the experiences were often unrecognized or minimized. Isolation left many participants feeling uncared for and ignored. Effective communication by health care providers was identified as an important part of the support needed by patients. Information provided by caregivers was inconsistent, leaving the patients feeling confused and concerned that nurses and other care providers were unaware of the implications of receiving ^{131}I therapy.

Nursing Implications
Patients receiving ^{131}I therapy share many of the fears and concerns expressed by those receiving treatment for more prevalent forms of cancer. Effective communication is an essential component in addressing the psychosocial and physical needs of these patients. Comprehensive education programs for staff and patients prior to therapy are critical in providing consistent quality care. These programs must address the fears resulting from a lack of understanding and the implications associated with ^{131}I therapy treatment to address the totality of the experience.

hyperparathyroidism. The type and extent of the surgery depend on the diagnosis, goal of surgery, and prognosis. Thyroidectomy may be the treatment of choice for patients with symptomatic hyper-parathyroidism (see later discussion), kidney stones, or bone disease.

The patient undergoing surgery for treatment of hyperthyroidism is given appropriate medications to return the thyroid hormone levels and metabolic rate to normal and to reduce the risk for thyroid storm and hemorrhage during the postoperative period. Medications that may prolong clotting (eg, aspirin) are stopped several weeks before surgery to minimize the risk for postoperative bleeding.

Nursing Management

Important preoperative goals are to gain the patient's confidence and reduce anxiety. Often, the patient's home life has become tense because of his or her restlessness, irritability, and nervousness secondary to hyperthyroidism. Efforts are necessary to protect the patient from such tension and stress to avoid precipitating thyroid storm. If the patient reports increased stress when with family or friends, suggestions are made to limit contact with them. Quiet and relaxing forms of recreation or occupational therapy may be helpful.

PROVIDING PREOPERATIVE CARE

The nurse instructs the patient about the importance of eating a diet high in carbohydrates and proteins. A high daily caloric intake is necessary because of the increased metabolic activity and rapid depletion of glycogen reserves. Supplementary vitamins, particularly thiamine and ascorbic acid, may be prescribed. The patient is reminded to avoid tea, coffee, cola, and other stimulants.

The nurse also informs the patient about the purpose of preoperative tests, if they are to be performed, and explains what preoperative preparations to expect. The information should help to reduce the patient's anxiety about the surgery. In addition, special efforts are made to ensure a good night's rest before surgery, although many patients are admitted to the hospital on the day of surgery.

Preoperative teaching includes demonstrating to the patient how to support the neck with the hands after surgery to prevent stress on the incision. This involves raising the elbows and placing the hands behind the neck to provide support and reduce strain and tension on the neck muscles and the surgical incision.

PROVIDING POSTOPERATIVE CARE

The nurse periodically assesses the surgical dressings and reinforces them when necessary. When the patient is in a recumbent position, the nurse observes the sides and the back of the neck as well as the anterior dressing for bleeding. In addition to monitoring the pulse and blood pressure for any indication of internal bleeding, it is also important to be alert for complaints of a sensation of pressure or fullness at the incision site. Such symptoms may indicate hemorrhage and hematoma formation subcutaneously and should be reported.

Difficulty in respiration occurs as a result of edema of the glottis, hematoma formation, or injury to the recurrent laryngeal nerve. This complication requires that an airway be inserted. Therefore, a tracheostomy set is kept at the bedside at all times, and the surgeon is summoned at the first indication of respiratory distress. If the respiratory distress is due to hematoma, surgical evacuation is required.

The intensity of pain is assessed and analgesic agents are administered as prescribed for pain. The nurse should anticipate apprehension in the patient and should inform him or her that oxygen will assist breathing. When moving and turning the pa-

tient, the nurse carefully supports the head and avoids tension on the sutures. The most comfortable position is the semi-Fowler's position, with the head elevated and supported by pillows.

Intravenous fluids are administered during the immediate postoperative period. Water may be given by mouth as soon as nausea subsides. Usually, there is a little difficulty in swallowing; initially, cold fluids and ice may be taken better than other fluids. Often, patients prefer a soft diet to a liquid diet in the immediate postoperative period.

The patient is advised to talk as little as possible to reduce edema to the vocal cords, but when the patient does speak, any voice changes are noted because they might indicate injury to the recurrent laryngeal nerve, which lies just behind the thyroid next to the trachea.

An overbed table may be used to provide easy access to items that are needed frequently, such as paper tissues, water pitcher and glass, and a small emesis basin. These are kept within easy reach so that the patient will not need to turn the head to reach for them. It is also convenient to use this table when vapor-mist inhalations are prescribed for the relief of excessive mucous secretions.

The patient is usually permitted out of bed as soon as possible and is encouraged to eat foods that are easily eaten. A well-balanced, high-calorie diet may be prescribed to promote weight gain. Sutures or skin clips are usually removed on the second day. The patient is usually discharged from the hospital the day of surgery or soon afterward if the postoperative course is uncomplicated.

MONITORING AND MANAGING POTENTIAL COMPLICATIONS

Hemorrhage, hematoma formation, edema of the glottis, and injury to the recurrent laryngeal nerve are complications that have been reviewed previously in this chapter. Occasionally in thyroid surgery the parathyroid glands are injured or removed, producing a disturbance in calcium metabolism. As the blood calcium level falls, hyperirritability of the nerves occurs, with spasms of the hands and feet and muscle twitching. This group of symptoms is termed tetany, and the nurse must immediately report its appearance because laryngospasm, although rare, may occur and obstruct the airway. Tetany of this type is usually treated with intravenous calcium gluconate. This calcium abnormality is usually temporary after thyroidectomy.

PROMOTING HOME AND COMMUNITY-BASED CARE

Teaching Patients Self-Care. The patient may be discharged the evening of surgery or within 1 or 2 days. Therefore, the patient and family need to be knowledgeable about the signs and symptoms of the complications that may occur and those that should be reported. Strategies are suggested for managing postoperative pain at home and for increasing humidification. The nurse explains to the patient and family the need for rest, relaxation, and nutrition. The patient is permitted to resume his or her former activities and responsibilities completely once recovered from surgery.

Continuing Care. If indicated, a referral to home care is made. The home care nurse assesses the patient's recovery from surgery. The nurse also assesses the surgical incision and reinforces instruction about limiting activities that put strain on the incision and sutures. Family responsibilities and factors relating to the home environment that produce emotional tension have often been implicated as precipitating causes of thyrotoxicosis. A home visit provides an opportunity to evaluate these factors and to suggest ways to improve the home and family environment. The nurse gives specific instructions regarding follow-up visits to the physician or the clinic, which are important for monitoring the thyroid status.

Management of Patients With Parathyroid Disorders

The parathyroid glands (normally four) are situated in the neck and embedded in the posterior aspect of the thyroid gland (Fig. 42-5). These small glands are easily overlooked and can be removed inadvertently during thyroid surgery. Inadvertent surgical removal is the most common cause of hypoparathyroidism.

PARATHYROID FUNCTION

Parathormone, the protein hormone from the parathyroid glands, regulates calcium and phosphorus metabolism. Increased secretion of parathormone results in increased calcium absorption from the kidney, intestine, and bones, thereby raising the blood calcium level. Some actions of this hormone are increased by the presence of vitamin D. Parathormone also tends to lower the blood phosphorus level.

Excess parathormone can result in markedly elevated levels of serum calcium, a potentially life-threatening situation. When the product of serum calcium and serum phosphorus (calcium × phosphorus) rises, calcium phosphate may precipitate in various organs of the body and cause tissue calcification.

The serum level of ionized calcium regulates the output of parathormone. Increased serum calcium results in decreased parathormone secretion, creating a negative feedback system.

HYPERPARATHYROIDISM

Hyperparathyroidism, which is caused by overproduction of parathyroid hormone by the parathyroid glands, is characterized by bone decalcification and the development of renal calculi (kidney stones) containing calcium.

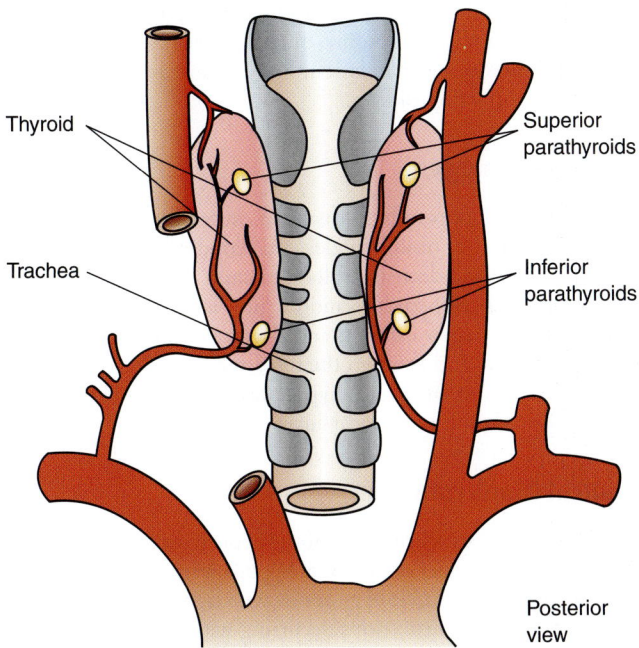

Thyroid

Trachea

Superior parathyroids

Inferior parathyroids

Posterior view

FIGURE 42-5 The parathyroid glands are located behind the thyroid gland. The parathyroids may be embedded in the thyroid tissue.

Primary hyperparathyroidism occurs two to four times more often in women than in men and is most common in patients between 60 and 70 years of age. The disease is rare in children younger than 15 years, but the incidence increases tenfold between the ages of 15 and 65 years. Half of the patients diagnosed with hyperparathyroidism do not have symptoms.

Secondary hyperparathyroidism, with manifestations similar to those of primary hyperparathyroidism, occurs in patients with chronic renal failure and so-called renal rickets as a result of phosphorus retention, increased stimulation of the parathyroid glands, and increased parathyroid hormone secretion.

Clinical Manifestations

The patient may have no symptoms or may experience signs and symptoms resulting from involvement of several body systems. Apathy, fatigue, muscle weakness, nausea, vomiting, constipation, hypertension, and cardiac dysrhythmias may occur; all are attributable to the increased concentration of calcium in the blood. Psychological manifestations may vary from irritability and neurosis to psychoses caused by the direct effect of calcium on the brain and nervous system. An increase in calcium produces a decrease in the excitation potential of nerve and muscle tissue.

The formation of stones in one or both kidneys, related to the increased urinary excretion of calcium and phosphorus, is one of the important complications of hyperparathyroidism and occurs in 55% of patients with primary hyperparathyroidism. Renal damage results from the precipitation of calcium phosphate in the renal pelvis and parenchyma, resulting in renal calculi (kidney stones), obstruction, pyelonephritis, and renal failure.

Musculoskeletal symptoms accompanying hyperparathyroidism may result from demineralization of the bones or bone tumours composed of benign giant cells resulting from overgrowth of osteoclasts. The patient may develop skeletal pain and tenderness, especially of the back and joints; pain on weight bearing; pathologic fractures; deformities; and shortening of body stature. Bone loss attributable to hyperparathyroidism increases the risk for fracture.

The incidence of peptic ulcer and pancreatitis is increased with hyperparathyroidism and may be responsible for many of the gastrointestinal symptoms that occur.

Assessment and Diagnostic Findings

Primary hyperparathyroidism is diagnosed by persistent elevation of serum calcium levels and an elevated level of parathormone. Radioimmunoassays for parathormone are sensitive and differentiate primary hyperparathyroidism from other causes of hypercalcemia in more than 90% of patients with elevated serum calcium levels. An elevated serum calcium level alone is a nonspecific finding because serum levels may be altered by diet, medications, and renal and bone changes. Bone changes may be detected on x-ray or bone scans in advanced disease. The double antibody parathyroid hormone test is used to distinguish between primary hyperparathyroidism and malignancy as a cause of hypercalcemia. Ultrasound, MRI, thallium scan, and fine-needle biopsy have been used to evaluate the function of the parathyroids and to localize parathyroid cysts, adenomas, or hyperplasia.

Complications: Hypercalcemic Crisis

Acute hypercalcemic crisis can occur with extreme elevation of serum calcium levels. Serum calcium levels higher than 3.7 mmol/L result in neurologic, cardiovascular, and renal symptoms that can be life-threatening. Treatment includes rehydration with large volumes of intravenous fluids, diuretic agents to promote renal excretion of excess calcium, and phosphate therapy to correct hypophosphatemia and decrease serum calcium levels by promoting calcium deposit in bone and reducing the gastrointestinal absorption of calcium. Cytotoxic agents (mithramycin), calcitonin, and dialysis may be used in emergency situations to decrease serum calcium levels quickly.

 NURSING ALERT The patient in acute hypercalcemic crisis requires close monitoring for life-threatening complications and prompt treatment to reduce serum calcium levels.

A combination of calcitonin and corticosteroids has been administered in emergencies to reduce the serum calcium level by increasing calcium deposition in bone. Other agents that may be administered to decrease serum calcium levels include bisphosphonates (eg, etidronate [Didronel], pamidronate).

The patient requires expert assessment and care to minimize complications and reverse the life-threatening hypercalcemia. Medications are administered with care, and attention is given to fluid balance to promote return of normal fluid and electrolyte balance. Supportive measures are necessary for the patient and family.

Medical Management

The insidious onset and chronic nature of hyperparathyroidism and its diverse and commonly vague symptoms may result in depression and frustration. The family may have considered the patient's illness to be psychosomatic. An awareness of the course of the disorder and an understanding approach by the nurse may help the patient and family to deal with their reactions and feelings. The recommended treatment of primary hyperparathyroidism is the surgical removal of abnormal parathyroid tissue. In some patients without symptoms and with only mildly elevated serum calcium levels and normal renal function, surgery may be delayed and the patient followed closely for worsening of hypercalcemia, bone deterioration, renal impairment, or the development of kidney stones.

HYDRATION THERAPY

Because kidney involvement is possible, patients with hyperparathyroidism are at risk for renal calculi. Therefore, a fluid intake of 2000 mL or more is encouraged to help prevent calculus formation. Cranberry juice is suggested because it may lower the urinary pH. It can be added to juices and ginger ale for variety. The patient is instructed to report other manifestations of renal calculi, such as abdominal pain and hematuria. Thiazide diuretics are avoided because they decrease the renal excretion of calcium and further elevate serum calcium levels. Because of the risk of hypercalcemic crisis, the patient is instructed to avoid dehydration and to seek immediate health care if conditions that commonly produce dehydration (eg, vomiting, diarrhea) occur.

MOBILITY

Mobility of the patient, with walking or use of a rocking chair for those with limited mobility, is encouraged as much as possible because bones subjected to normal stress give up less calcium. Bed rest increases calcium excretion and the risk for renal calculi. Oral phosphates lower the serum calcium level in some patients. Long-term use is not recommended because of the risk for ectopic calcium phosphate deposits in soft tissues.

DIET AND MEDICATIONS

Nutritional needs are met, but the patient is advised to avoid a diet with restricted or excess calcium. If the patient has a coexisting peptic ulcer, prescribed antacids and protein feedings are necessary. Because anorexia is common, efforts are made to improve the appetite. Prune juice, stool softeners, and physical activity, along with increased fluid intake, help to offset constipation, which is common postoperatively.

Nursing Management

The nursing management of the patient undergoing parathyroidectomy is essentially the same as that of a patient undergoing thyroidectomy. However, the previously described precautions about dehydration, immobility, and diet are particularly important in the patient awaiting and recovering from parathyroidectomy. Although not all parathyroid tissue is removed during surgery in an effort to control the calcium–phosphorus balance, the nurse closely monitors the patient to detect symptoms of tetany (which may be an early postoperative complication). Most patients quickly regain function of the remaining parathyroid tissue and experience only mild, transient postoperative hypocalcemia. In patients with significant bone disease or bone changes, a more prolonged period of hypocalcemia should be anticipated. The nurse reminds the patient and family about the importance of follow-up to ensure return of serum calcium levels to normal (Chart 42-7).

HYPOPARATHYROIDISM

The most common cause of hypoparathyroidism is inadequate secretion of parathyroid hormone after interruption of the blood supply or surgical removal of parathyroid gland tissue during thyroidectomy, parathyroidectomy, or radical neck dissection. Atrophy of the parathyroid glands of unknown cause is a less common cause of hypoparathyroidism.

Pathophysiology

Symptoms of hypoparathyroidism are caused by a deficiency of parathormone that results in elevated blood phosphate (hyperphosphatemia) and decreased blood calcium (hypocalcemia) levels. In the absence of parathormone, there is decreased intestinal absorption of dietary calcium and decreased resorption of calcium from bone and through the renal tubules. Decreased renal excretion of phosphate causes hypophosphaturia, and low serum calcium levels result in hypocalciuria.

Clinical Manifestations

Hypocalcemia causes irritability of the neuromuscular system and contributes to the chief symptom of hypoparathyroidism—tetany. Tetany is a general muscle hypertonia, with tremor and spasmodic or uncoordinated contractions occurring with or without efforts to make voluntary movements. Symptoms of latent tetany are numbness, tingling, and cramps in the extremities, and the patient complains of stiffness in the hands and feet. In overt tetany, the

Chart 42-7
Home Care Checklist • The Patient With Hyperparathyroidism

At the completion of the home care instruction, the patient or caregiver will be able to:	Patient	Caregiver
• State present and potential effects of hyperparathyroidism on the body	✓	✓
• State precipitating factors and interventions for complications	✓	✓
• State importance of regular follow-up visits with health care provider	✓	✓
• Describe potential benefits and risks of parathyroidectomy	✓	✓
• State the purpose, dose, route, schedule, side effects, and precautions of prescribed medications (loop diuretics, phosphate, calcitonin, mithramycin)	✓	✓
• State the need to contact health care provider before taking over-the-counter medication containing calcium	✓	✓
• State need to take pain medications on a scheduled basis	✓	✓
• Describe nonpharmacologic methods of pain management	✓	✓
• Identify safety hazards and methods of injury prevention	✓	✓
• Identify areas of activity limitations and impact on lifestyle	✓	✓
• State need for increased fluid intake and diet low in calcium and vitamin D	✓	✓

signs include bronchospasm, laryngeal spasm, carpopedal spasm (flexion of the elbows and wrists and extension of the carpophalangeal joints), dysphagia, photophobia, cardiac dysrhythmias, and seizures. Other symptoms include anxiety, irritability, depression, and even delirium. ECG changes and hypotension also may occur.

Assessment and Diagnostic Findings

A positive Trousseau's sign or a positive Chvostek's sign suggests latent tetany. **Trousseau's sign** is positive when carpopedal spasm is induced by occluding the blood flow to the arm for 3 minutes with a blood pressure cuff. **Chvostek's sign** is positive when a sharp tapping over the facial nerve just in front of the parotid gland and anterior to the ear causes spasm or twitching of the mouth, nose, and eye (see Chap. 14).

The diagnosis of hypoparathyroidism often is difficult because of the vague symptoms, such as aches and pains. Therefore, laboratory studies are especially helpful. Tetany develops at serum calcium levels of 1.2 to 1.5 mmol/L or lower. Serum phosphate levels are increased, and x-rays of bone show increased density. Calcification is detected on x-rays of the subcutaneous or paraspinal basal ganglia of the brain.

Medical Management

The goal of therapy is to raise the serum calcium level to 2.2 to 2.5 mmol/L and to eliminate the symptoms of hypoparathyroidism and hypocalcemia. When hypocalcemia and tetany occur after a thyroidectomy, the immediate treatment is to administer calcium gluconate intravenously. If this does not decrease neuromuscular irritability and seizure activity immediately, sedative agents such as pentobarbital may be administered.

Parenteral parathormone can be administered to treat acute hypoparathyroidism with tetany. The high incidence of allergic reactions to injections of parathormone, however, limits its use to acute episodes of hypocalcemia. The patient receiving parathormone is monitored closely for allergic reactions and changes in serum calcium levels.

Because of neuromuscular irritability, the patient with hypocalcemia and tetany requires an environment that is free of noise, drafts, bright lights, or sudden movement. Tracheostomy or mechanical ventilation may become necessary, along with bronchodilating medications, if the patient develops respiratory distress.

Therapy for the patient with chronic hypoparathyroidism is determined after serum calcium levels are obtained. A diet high in calcium and low in phosphorus is prescribed. Although milk, milk products, and egg yolk are high in calcium, they are restricted because they also contain high levels of phosphorus. Spinach also is avoided because it contains oxalate, which would form insoluble calcium substances. Oral tablets of calcium salts, such as calcium gluconate, may be used to supplement the diet. Aluminum hydroxide gel or aluminum carbonate (Gelusil, Amphojel) also is administered after meals to bind phosphate and promote its excretion through the gastrointestinal tract.

Variable dosages of a vitamin D preparation—dihydrotachysterol (AT 10 or Hytakerol), ergocalciferol (vitamin D), cholecalciferol (vitamin D)—are usually required and enhance calcium absorption from the gastrointestinal tract.

Nursing Management

Nursing management of the patient with possible acute hypoparathyroidism includes the following:

- Care of postoperative patients having thyroidectomy, parathyroidectomy, and radical neck dissection is directed toward detecting early signs of hypocalcemia and anticipating signs of tetany, seizures, and respiratory difficulties.
- Calcium gluconate is kept at the bedside, with equipment necessary for intravenous administration. If the patient has a cardiac disorder, is subject to dysrhythmias, or is receiving digitalis, calcium gluconate is administered slowly and cautiously.
- Calcium and digitalis increase systolic contraction and also potentiate each other; this may produce potentially fatal dysrhythmias. Consequently, the cardiac patient requires continuous cardiac monitoring and careful assessment.

An important aspect of nursing care is teaching about medications and diet therapy. The patient needs to know the reason for high calcium and low phosphate intake and the symptoms of hypocalcemia and hypercalcemia; he or she should know to contact the physician immediately if these symptoms occur (Chart 42-8).

Management of Patients With Adrenal Disorders

There are two adrenal glands in the human, each attached to the upper portion of a kidney. Each adrenal gland is, in reality, two endocrine glands with separate, independent functions. The adrenal medulla at the centre of the gland secretes catecholamines, and the outer portion of the gland, the adrenal cortex, secretes steroid hormones (Fig. 42-6). The secretion of hormones from the adrenal cortex is regulated by the hypothalamic-pituitary-adrenal axis. The hypothalamus secretes corticotropin-releasing hormone (CRH), which in turn stimulates the pituitary gland to secrete ACTH. ACTH then stimulates the adrenal cortex to secrete glucocorticoid hormone (cortisol). Increased levels of the adrenal hormone then inhibit the production or secretion of CRH and ACTH. This system is an example of a negative feedback mechanism.

ADRENAL FUNCTION

Adrenal Medulla

The adrenal medulla functions as part of the autonomic nervous system. Stimulation of preganglionic sympathetic nerve fibres, which travel directly to the cells of the adrenal medulla, causes release of the catecholamine hormones epinephrine and norepinephrine. About 90% of the secretion of the human adrenal medulla is epinephrine (also called adrenaline). Catecholamines regulate metabolic pathways to promote catabolism of stored fuels to meet caloric needs from endogenous sources. The major effects of epinephrine release are to prepare to meet a challenge (fight-or-flight response). Secretion of epinephrine causes decreased blood flow to tissues that are not needed in emergency situations, such as the gastrointestinal tract, and causes increased

A **B**

FIGURE 42-6 (**A**) The adrenal glands sit on top of each kidney. (**B**) Each gland is composed of the outer cortex and the inner medulla. Each area secretes specific hormones. The adrenal medulla secretes catecholamines, epinephrine, and norepinephrine; the adrenal cortex secretes glucocorticoids, mineralocorticoids, and sex hormones. From Porth, C. (2002). *Pathophysiology: Concepts of altered health states* (6th ed.). Philadelphia: Lippincott Williams & Wilkins.

blood flow to tissues that are important for effective fight or flight, such as cardiac and skeletal muscle. Catecholamines also induce the release of free fatty acids, increase the basal metabolic rate, and elevate the blood glucose level.

Adrenal Cortex

A functioning adrenal cortex is necessary for life; adrenocortical secretions make it possible for the body to adapt to stress of all kinds. The three types of steroid hormones produced by the adrenal cortex are **glucocorticoids**, the prototype of which is hydrocortisone; **mineralocorticoids**, mainly aldosterone; and sex hormones, mainly **androgens** (male sex hormones). Without the adrenal cortex, severe stress would cause peripheral circulatory failure, circulatory shock, and prostration. Survival in the absence of a functioning adrenal cortex is possible only with nutritional, electrolyte, and fluid replacement and appropriate replacement with exogenous adrenocortical hormones.

GLUCOCORTICOIDS

The glucocorticoids are so named because they have an important influence on glucose metabolism: increased hydrocortisone secretion results in elevated blood glucose levels. However, the glucocorticoids have major effects on the metabolism of almost all organs of the body. Glucocorticoids are secreted from the adrenal cortex in response to the release of ACTH from the anterior lobe of the pituitary gland. This system represents an example of negative feedback. The presence of glucocorticoids in the blood inhibits the release of corticotropin-releasing factor from the hypothalamus and also inhibits ACTH secretion from the pituitary. The resultant decrease in ACTH secretion causes diminished release of glucocorticoids from the adrenal cortex.

Glucocorticoids (in the form of **corticosteroids**) are administered frequently to inhibit the inflammatory response to tissue injury and suppress allergic manifestations. Their side effects include the development of diabetes mellitus, osteoporosis, peptic ulcer, increased protein breakdown resulting in muscle wasting and poor wound healing, and redistribution of body fat.

Large amounts of exogenously administered glucocorticoids in the blood inhibit the release of ACTH and endogenous glucocorticoids. Because of this, the adrenal cortex can atrophy. If exogenous glucocorticoid administration is discontinued suddenly, adrenal insufficiency results because of the inability of the atrophied cortex to respond adequately.

MINERALOCORTICOIDS

Mineralocorticoids exert their major effects on electrolyte metabolism. They act principally on the renal tubular and gastrointestinal epithelium to cause increased sodium ion absorption in exchange for excretion of potassium or hydrogen ions. ACTH only minimally influences aldosterone secretion. It is primarily secreted in response to the presence of angiotensin II in the bloodstream. Angiotensin II is a substance that elevates the blood pressure by constricting arterioles. Its concentration is increased when renin is released from the kidney in response to decreased perfusion pressure. The resultant increased aldosterone levels promote sodium reabsorption by the kidney and the gastrointestinal tract, which tends to restore blood pressure to normal. The release of aldosterone is also increased by hyperkalemia. Aldosterone is the primary hormone for the long-term regulation of sodium balance.

ADRENAL SEX HORMONES (ANDROGENS)

Androgens, the third major type of steroid hormones produced by the adrenal cortex, exert effects similar to those of male sex hormones. The adrenal gland may also secrete small amounts of some estrogens, or female sex hormones. ACTH controls the secretion of adrenal androgens. When secreted in normal amounts, the adrenal androgens probably have little effect, but when secreted in excess, in certain inborn enzyme deficiencies, masculinization may result. This is termed the **adrenogenital syndrome**.

PHEOCHROMOCYTOMA

Pheochromocytoma is a tumour that is usually benign and originates from the chromaffin cells of the adrenal medulla. In 80% to 90% of patients (O'Connell, 1999), the tumour arises in the medulla; in the remaining patients, it occurs in the extra-adrenal chromaffin tissue located in or near the aorta, ovaries, spleen, or other organs. Pheochromocytoma may occur at any age, but its peak incidence is between ages 40 and 50 years (Rakel & Bope, 2001). It affects men and women equally. Because of the high incidence of pheochromocytoma in family members, the patient's family members should be alerted and screened for this tumour. Ten percent of the tumours are bilateral, and 10% are malignant.

Pheochromocytoma is the cause of high blood pressure in 0.2% of patients with new onset of hypertension (O'Connell, 1999). Although it is uncommon, it is one form of hypertension that is usually cured by surgery; without detection and treatment, it is usually fatal. Pheochromocytoma may occur in the familial form as part of multiple endocrine neoplasia type 2; therefore, it should be considered a possibility in patients with medullary thyroid carcinoma and parathyroid hyperplasia or tumour.

Clinical Manifestations

The nature and severity of symptoms of functioning tumours of the adrenal medulla depend on the relative proportions of epinephrine and norepinephrine secretion. The typical triad of symptoms comprises headache, diaphoresis, and palpitations (Matthews et al., 1999). Hypertension and other cardiovascular disturbances are common. The hypertension may be intermittent or persistent. Only half of patients with pheochromocytoma, however, have sustained or persistent hypertension. If the hypertension is sustained, it may be difficult to distinguish from other causes of hypertension. Other symptoms may include tremor, headache, flushing, and anxiety. Hyperglycemia may result from conversion of liver and muscle glycogen to glucose by epinephrine secretion; insulin may be required to maintain normal blood glucose levels.

The clinical picture in the paroxysmal form of pheochromocytoma is usually characterized by acute, unpredictable attacks lasting seconds or several hours. During these attacks, the patient is extremely anxious, tremulous, and weak. The patient may experience headache, vertigo, blurring of vision, tinnitus, air hunger, and dyspnea. Other symptoms include polyuria, nausea, vomiting, diarrhea, abdominal pain, and a feeling of impending doom. Palpitations and tachycardia are common. Blood pressures exceeding 250/150 mm Hg have been recorded. Such blood pressure elevations are life-threatening and may cause severe complications, such as cardiac dysrhythmias, dissecting aneurysm, stroke, and acute renal failure. Postural hypotension occurs in 70% of patients with untreated pheochromocytoma.

Assessment and Diagnostic Findings

Pheochromocytoma is suspected if signs of sympathetic nervous system overactivity occur in association with marked elevation of blood pressure. These signs can be associated with the "five Hs": hypertension, headache, hyperhidrosis (excessive sweating), hypermetabolism, and hyperglycemia. The presence of these signs has a 93.8% specificity and a 90.9% sensitivity for pheochromocytoma. Absence of hypertension excludes pheochromocytoma with a 99% certainty. Paroxysmal symptoms of pheochromocytoma commonly develop in the fifth decade of life.

Measurements of urine and plasma levels of catecholamines are the most direct and conclusive tests for overactivity of the adrenal medulla. Measurements of urinary catecholamine metabolites (metanephrines [MN] and vanillylmandelic acid [VMA]) or free catecholamines are the standard diagnostic tests used in the diagnosis of pheochromocytoma. Levels can be as high as three times normal limits (O'Connell, 1999). A 24-hour specimen of urine is collected for determining free catecholamines, MN, and VMA; the use of combined tests increases the diagnostic accuracy of testing. A number of medications and foods (eg, coffee, tea, bananas, chocolate, vanilla, aspirin) may alter the results of these tests; therefore, careful instructions to avoid restricted items must be given to the patient. Urine collected over a 2- or 3-hour period after an attack of hypertension can be assayed for catecholamine content.

Total plasma catecholamine (epinephrine and norepinephrine) concentration is measured with the patient supine and at rest for 30 minutes. To prevent elevation of catecholamine levels by the stress of venipuncture, a butterfly needle, scalp vein needle, or venous catheter may be inserted 30 minutes before the blood specimen is obtained.

Factors that may elevate catecholamine levels must be controlled to obtain valid results; these factors include consumption of coffee or tea, use of tobacco, emotional and physical stress, and use of many prescription and over-the-counter medications (eg, amphetamines, nose drops or sprays, decongestant agents, and bronchodilators).

Normal plasma values of epinephrine are 590 pmol/L; normal values of norepinephrine are generally less than 590 to 3,240 pmol/L. Values of epinephrine greater than 2,180 pmol/L or norepinephrine values greater than 11,800 pmol/L are considered diagnostic of pheochromocytoma. Values that fall between normal values and those diagnostic of pheochromocytoma indicate the need for further testing.

A clonidine suppression test may be performed if the results of plasma and urine tests of catecholamines are inconclusive. Clonidine (Catapres) is a centrally acting, antiadrenergic medication that suppresses the release of neurogenically mediated catecholamines. The suppression test is based on the principle that catecholamine levels are normally increased through the activity of the sympathetic nervous system. In pheochromocytoma, increased catecholamine levels result from the diffusion of excess catecholamines into the circulation, bypassing normal storage and release mechanisms. Therefore, in patients with pheochromocytoma, clonidine does not suppress the release of catecholamines.

The results of the test are considered normal if 2 to 3 hours after a single oral dose of clonidine, the total plasma catecholamine value decreases at least 40% from baseline. Patients with pheochromocytoma exhibit no change in catecholamine levels. False-positive results, however, may occur in patients with primary hypertension.

Imaging studies, such as CT scans, MRI, and ultrasound, may also be carried out to localize the pheochromocytoma and to determine whether more than one tumour is present. Use of ^{131}I-metaiodobenzylguanidine (MIBG) scintigraphy may be required to determine the location of the pheochromocytoma and to detect metastatic sites outside the adrenal gland. MIBG is a specific isotope for catecholamine-producing tissue. It has been helpful in identifying tumours not detected by other tests or procedures. MIBG scintigraphy is a noninvasive, safe procedure that has increased the accuracy of diagnosis of adrenal tumours.

Other diagnostic studies may focus on evaluating the function of other endocrine glands because of the association of pheochromocytoma in some patients with other endocrine tumours.

Medical Management

During an episode or attack of hypertension, tachycardia, anxiety, and the other symptoms of pheochromocytoma, the patient is placed on bed rest with the head of the bed elevated to promote an orthostatic decrease in blood pressure.

PHARMACOLOGIC THERAPY

The patient may be moved to the intensive care unit for close monitoring of ECG changes and careful administration of alpha-adrenergic blocking agents (eg, phentolamine [Regitine]) or smooth muscle relaxants (eg, sodium nitroprusside [Nipride]) to lower the blood pressure quickly.

Phenoxybenzamine (Dibenzyline), a long-acting alpha-blocker, may be used when the blood pressure is stable to prepare the patient for surgery. Beta-adrenergic blocking agents, such as propranolol (Inderal), may be used in patients with cardiac dysrhythmias or those not responsive to alpha-blockers. Alpha-adrenergic and beta-adrenergic blocking agents must be used with caution because patients with pheochromocytoma may have increased sensitivity to them. Still other medications that may be used preoperatively are catecholamine synthesis inhibitors, such as alpha-methyl-p-tyrosine (metyrosine). These are occasionally used when adrenergic blocking agents do not reduce the effects of catecholamines.

SURGICAL MANAGEMENT

The definitive treatment of pheochromocytoma is surgical removal of the tumour, usually with **adrenalectomy**. Bilateral adrenalectomy may be necessary if tumours are present in both adrenal glands. Patient preparation includes control of blood pressure and blood volumes; usually this is carried out over 7 to 10 days. Phentolamine or phenoxybenzamine (Dibenzyline) may be used safely without causing undue hypotension. Other medications (metyrosine [Demser] and prazosin [Minipress]) have been used to treat pheochromocytoma. The patient needs to be well hydrated before, during, and after surgery to prevent hypotension.

Manipulation of the tumour during surgical excision may cause release of stored epinephrine and norepinephrine, with marked increases in blood pressure and changes in heart rate. Therefore, use of sodium nitroprusside (Nipride) and alpha-adrenergic blocking agents may be required during and after surgery. Exploration of other possible tumour sites is frequently undertaken to ensure removal of all tumour tissue. As a result, the patient is subject to the stress and effects of a long surgical procedure, which may increase the risk of hypertension postoperatively.

Corticosteroid replacement is required if bilateral adrenalectomy has been necessary. Corticosteroids may also be necessary for the first few days or weeks after removal of a single adrenal gland. Intravenous administration of corticosteroids (methylprednisolone sodium succinate [Solu-Medrol]) may begin the evening before surgery and continue during the early postoperative period to prevent adrenal insufficiency. Oral preparations of corticosteroids (prednisone) will be prescribed after the acute stress of surgery diminishes.

Hypotension and hypoglycemia may occur in the postoperative period because of the sudden withdrawal of excessive amounts of catecholamines. Therefore, careful attention is directed toward monitoring and treating these changes. Blood pressure is expected to return to normal with treatment; however, one third of patients continue to be hypertensive after surgery. This may result if not all pheochromocytoma tissue was removed, if pheochromocytoma recurs, or if the blood vessels were damaged by severe and prolonged hypertension. Several days after surgery, urine and plasma levels of catecholamines and their metabolites are measured to determine whether surgery was successful.

Nursing Management

The patient who has undergone surgery to treat pheochromocytoma has experienced a stressful preoperative and postoperative course and may remain fearful of repeated attacks. Although it is usually expected that all pheochromocytoma tissue has been removed, there is a possibility that other sites were undetected and that attacks may recur. The patient is monitored for several days in the intensive care unit with special attention given to ECG changes, arterial pressures, fluid and electrolyte balance, and blood glucose levels. Several intravenous lines are inserted for administration of fluids and medications.

PROMOTING HOME AND COMMUNITY-BASED CARE

Teaching Patients Self-Care.   During the preoperative and postoperative phases of care, the nurse informs the patient about the importance of follow-up monitoring to ensure that pheochromocytoma does not recur undetected. After adrenalectomy, use of corticosteroids may be needed. Therefore, the nurse instructs the patient about their purpose, the medication schedule, and the risks of skipping doses or stopping their administration abruptly.

It is important to teach the patient and family how to measure the patient's blood pressure and when to notify the physician about changes in blood pressure. Additionally, the nurse provides verbal and written instructions about the procedure for collecting 24-hour urine specimens to monitor urine catecholamine levels.

Continuing Care.   A follow-up visit from a home care nurse may be indicated to assess the patient's postoperative recovery, surgical incision, and compliance with the medication schedule. This may help to reinforce previous teaching about management and monitoring. The home care nurse also obtains blood pressure measurements and assists the patient in preventing or dealing with problems that may result from long-term use of corticosteroids.

Because of the risk of recurrence of hypertension, periodic checkups are required, especially in young patients and in patients whose families have a history of pheochromocytoma. The patient is scheduled for periodic follow-up appointments to observe for return of normal blood pressure and plasma and urine levels of catecholamines.

ADRENOCORTICAL INSUFFICIENCY (ADDISON'S DISEASE)

Pathophysiology

Addison's disease, or adrenocortical insufficiency, results when adrenal cortex function is inadequate to meet the patient's need for cortical hormones. Autoimmune or idiopathic atrophy of the adrenal glands is responsible for 80% of cases (Rakel & Bope, 2001). Other causes include surgical removal of both adrenal glands or infection of the adrenal glands. Tuberculosis and histoplasmosis are the most common infections that destroy adrenal gland tissue. Although autoimmune destruction has replaced tuberculosis as the principal cause of Addison's disease, tuberculosis should be considered in the diagnostic workup because of its increasing incidence. Inadequate secretion of ACTH from the pituitary gland also results in adrenal insufficiency because of decreased stimulation of the adrenal cortex.

Therapeutic use of corticosteroids is the most common cause of adrenocortical insufficiency (Coursin & Wood, 2002). The symptoms of adrenocortical insufficiency may also result from the sudden cessation of exogenous adrenocortical hormonal therapy, which suppresses the body's normal response to stress and interferes with normal feedback mechanisms. Treatment with daily administration of corticosteroids for 2 to 4 weeks may suppress function of the adrenal cortex; therefore, adrenal insufficiency should be considered in any patient who has been treated with corticosteroids.

Clinical Manifestations

Addison's disease is characterized by muscle weakness, anorexia, gastrointestinal symptoms, fatigue, emaciation, dark pigmentation of the skin, knuckles, knees, elbows, and mucous membranes, hypotension, and low blood glucose levels, low serum sodium levels, and high serum potassium levels. Mental status changes such as depression, emotional lability, apathy, and confusion are present in 60% to 80% of patients. In severe cases, the disturbance of sodium and potassium metabolism may be marked by depletion of sodium and water and severe, chronic dehydration.

With disease progression and acute hypotension, the patient develops **addisonian crisis**, which is characterized by cyanosis and the classic signs of circulatory shock: pallor, apprehension, rapid and weak pulse, rapid respirations, and low blood pressure. In addition, the patient may complain of headache, nausea, abdominal pain, and diarrhea and show signs of confusion and restlessness. Even slight overexertion, exposure to cold, acute infections, or a decrease in salt intake may lead to circulatory collapse, shock, and death if untreated. The stress of surgery or dehydration resulting from preparation for diagnostic tests or surgery may precipitate an addisonian or hypotensive crisis.

Assessment and Diagnostic Findings

Although the clinical manifestations presented appear specific, the onset of Addison's disease usually occurs with nonspecific symptoms. The diagnosis is confirmed by laboratory test results. Laboratory findings include decreased blood glucose (hypoglycemia) and sodium (hyponatremia) levels, an increased serum potassium (hyperkalemia) level, and an increased white blood cell count (leukocytosis).

The diagnosis is confirmed by low levels of adrenocortical hormones in the blood or urine and decreased serum cortisol levels. If the adrenal cortex is destroyed, baseline values are low, and ACTH administration fails to cause the normal rise in plasma cortisol and urinary 17-hydroxycorticosteroids. If the adrenal gland is normal but not stimulated properly by the pituitary, a normal response to repeated doses of exogenous ACTH is seen, but no response follows the administration of metyrapone, which stimulates endogenous ACTH.

Medical Management

Immediate treatment is directed toward combating circulatory shock: restoring blood circulation, administering fluids and corticosteroids, monitoring vital signs, and placing the patient in a recumbent position with the legs elevated. Hydrocortisone (Solu-Cortef) is administered intravenously, followed with 5% dextrose in normal saline. Vasopressor amines may be required if hypotension persists.

Antibiotics may be administered if infection has precipitated adrenal crisis in a patient with chronic adrenal insufficiency. Additionally, the patient is assessed closely to identify other factors, stressors, or illnesses that led to the acute episode.

Oral intake may be initiated as soon as tolerated. Gradually, intravenous fluids are decreased when oral fluid intake is adequate to prevent hypovolemia. If the adrenal gland does not regain function, the patient needs lifelong replacement of corticosteroids and mineralocorticoids to prevent recurrence of adrenal insufficiency. The patient will require additional supplementary therapy with glucocorticoids during stressful procedures or significant illnesses to prevent addisonian crisis (Coursin & Wood, 2002). Additionally, the patient may need to supplement dietary intake with added salt during times of gastrointestinal losses of fluids through vomiting and diarrhea.

Nursing Management

ASSESSING THE PATIENT

The health history and examination focus on the presence of symptoms of fluid imbalance and on the patient's level of stress. To detect inadequate fluid volume, the nurse monitors the blood pressure and pulse rate as the patient moves from a lying to a standing position. The nurse assesses the skin colour and turgor for changes related to chronic adrenal insufficiency and hypovolemia. Other key assessments include checking for weight changes, muscle weakness, and fatigue and investigating any illness or stress that may have precipitated the acute crisis.

MONITORING AND MANAGING ADDISONIAN CRISIS

The patient at risk is monitored for signs and symptoms indicative of addisonian crisis. These symptoms are often the manifestations of shock: hypotension; rapid, weak pulse; rapid respiratory rate; pallor; and extreme weakness. The patient with addisonian crisis is at risk for circulatory collapse and shock (see Chap. 15 for management of the patient in shock); therefore, physical and psychological stressors must be avoided. These include exposure to cold, overexertion, infection, and emotional distress.

The patient with addisonian crisis requires immediate treatment with intravenous administration of fluid, glucose, and electrolytes, especially sodium; replacement of missing steroid hormones; and vasopressors. During acute addisonian crisis, the patient must avoid exertion; therefore, the nurse anticipates the patient's needs and takes measures to meet them.

Careful monitoring of symptoms, vital signs, weight, and fluid and electrolyte status is essential to monitor the patient's progress and return to a precrisis state. To reduce the risk of future episodes of addisonian crisis, efforts are made to identify and reduce the factors that may have led to the crisis.

RESTORING FLUID BALANCE

To provide information about fluid balance and the adequacy of hormone replacement, the nurse assesses the patient's skin turgor, mucous membranes, and weight while instructing the patient to report increased thirst, which may indicate impending fluid imbalance. Lying, sitting, and standing blood pressures also provide information about fluid status. A decrease in systolic pressure (20 mm Hg or more) may indicate depletion of fluid volume, especially if accompanied by symptoms. The nurse encourages the patient to consume foods and fluids that will assist in restoring and maintaining fluid and electrolyte balance; along with the dietitian, the nurse assists the patient to select foods high in sodium during gastrointestinal disturbances and very hot weather.

The nurse instructs the patient and family to administer hormone replacement as prescribed and to modify the dosage during illness and other stressful occasions. Written and verbal instructions are provided about the administration of mineralocorticoid (Florinef) or corticosteroid (prednisone) as prescribed.

IMPROVING ACTIVITY TOLERANCE

Until the patient's condition is stabilized, the nurse takes precautions to avoid unnecessary activity and stress that could precipitate another hypotensive episode. Efforts are made to detect signs of infection or the presence of other stressors. Even minor events or stressors may be excessive in patients with adrenal insufficiency. During the acute crisis, the nurse maintains a quiet, nonstressful environment and performs all activities (eg, bathing, turning) for the patient. Explaining all procedures to the patient and family will reduce their anxiety. Explaining the rationale for minimizing stress during the acute crisis assists the patient to increase activity gradually.

PROMOTING HOME AND COMMUNITY-BASED CARE

Teaching Patients Self-Care. Because of the need for lifelong replacement of adrenal cortex hormones to prevent addisonian crises, the patient and family members receive explicit verbal and written instructions about the rationale for replacement therapy and proper dosage. Additionally, they are instructed about how to modify the medication dosage and increase salt intake in times of illness, very hot weather, and other stressful situations. The patient also learns how to modify diet and fluid intake to help maintain fluid and electrolyte balance.

The patient and family are frequently prescribed preloaded, single-injection syringes of corticosteroid for use in emergencies. Careful instructions about how and when to use the injection are also provided. It is important to instruct the patient to inform other health care providers, such as dentists, about the use of corticosteroids, to wear a medical alert bracelet, and to carry information at all times about the need for corticosteroids. If the patient with Addison's disease requires surgery, careful administration of fluids and corticosteroids is necessary before, during, and after surgery to prevent addisonian crisis.

The patient and family need to know the signs of excessive or insufficient hormone replacement. The development of edema or weight gain may signify too high a dose of hormone; postural hypotension (decrease in systolic blood pressure, lightheadedness, dizziness on standing) and weight loss frequently signify too low a dose (Chart 42-9).

Continuing Care. Although most patients can return to their job and family responsibilities soon after hospital discharge, others cannot do so because of concurrent illnesses or incomplete recovery from the episode of adrenal insufficiency. In these circumstances, a referral for home care enables the home care nurse to assess the patient's recovery, monitor hormone replacement, and evaluate stress in the home. The nurse assesses the patient's and family's knowledge about medication therapy and dietary modifications. A home visit also allows the nurse to assess the patient's plans for follow-up visits to the clinic or physician's office. The nurse reminds the patient and family about the importance of participating in health promotion activities and health screening.

CUSHING'S SYNDROME

Cushing's syndrome results from excessive, rather than deficient, adrenocortical activity. The syndrome may result from excessive administration of corticosteroids or ACTH or from hyperplasia of the adrenal cortex.

Pathophysiology

Cushing's syndrome is commonly caused by use of corticosteroid medications and is infrequently due to excessive corticosteroid production by the adrenal cortex (Tierney et al., 2001). However, overproduction of endogenous corticosteroids may be caused by several mechanisms, including a tumour of the pituitary gland that produces ACTH and stimulates the adrenal cortex to increase its hormone secretion despite adequate amounts being produced. Primary hyperplasia of the adrenal glands in the absence of a pituitary tumour is less common. Another less common cause of Cushing's syndrome is the ectopic production of ACTH by malignancies; bronchogenic carcinoma is the most common type of these malignancies. Regardless of the cause, the normal feedback mechanisms that control the function of the adrenal cortex become ineffective, and the usual diurnal pattern of cortisol is lost.

The signs and symptoms of Cushing's syndrome are primarily a result of oversecretion of glucocorticoids and androgens (sex hormones), although mineralocorticoid secretion also may be affected.

Clinical Manifestations

When overproduction of the adrenal cortical hormone occurs, arrest of growth, obesity, and musculoskeletal changes occur along with glucose intolerance. The classic picture of Cushing's syndrome in the adult is that of central-type obesity, with a fatty "buffalo hump" in the neck and supraclavicular areas, a heavy trunk, and relatively thin extremities. The skin is thin, fragile, and easily traumatized; ecchymoses (bruises) and striae develop. The patient complains of weakness and lassitude. Sleep is disturbed because of altered diurnal secretion of cortisol.

Excessive protein catabolism occurs, producing muscle wasting and osteoporosis. Kyphosis, backache, and compression fractures of the vertebrae may result. Retention of sodium and water occurs as a result of increased mineralocorticoid activity, producing hypertension and heart failure.

The patient develops a "moon-faced" appearance and may experience increased oiliness of the skin and acne. There is increased susceptibility to infection. Hyperglycemia or overt diabetes may develop. The patient may also report weight gain, slow healing of minor cuts, and bruises.

Women ages 20 to 40 years are five times more likely than men to develop Cushing's syndrome. In females of all ages, virilization may occur as a result of excess androgens. Virilization is characterized by the appearance of masculine traits and the recession of feminine traits. There is an excessive growth of hair on the face (hirsutism), the breasts atrophy, menses cease, the clitoris enlarges, and the voice deepens. Libido is lost in men and women.

Changes occur in mood and mental activity; psychosis may develop. Distress and depression are common and are increased by the severity of the physical changes that occur with this syndrome. If Cushing's syndrome is a consequence of pituitary tumour, visual disturbances may occur because of pressure of the growing tumour on the optic chiasm. Chart 42-10 summarizes the changes associated with Cushing's syndrome.

Chart 42-9

Home Care Checklist • The Patient With Adrenal Insufficiency (Addison's Disease)

At the completion of the home care instruction, the patient or caregiver will be able to:	Patient	Caregiver
• State present and potential effects of adrenal insufficiency on the body	✓	✓
• State warning signs of adrenal crisis and need for emergency care	✓	✓
• Explain components of an emergency kit and indications for their use; demonstrate how to use them	✓	✓
• State strategies for dealing with stress and avoiding adrenal crisis	✓	✓
• State the purpose, dose, route, schedule, side effects, and precautions of prescribed medications (corticosteroid replacement)	✓	✓
• State that compliance with medical regimen is lifelong	✓	✓
• State importance of regular follow-up visits with health care provider	✓	✓
• Recognize the need for dosage adjustment during times of stress	✓	✓
• State need to wear medical alert identification and carry medical information card	✓	✓
• State need to notify health care providers about disease before treatment or procedure	✓	✓
• State need to avoid strenuous activity in hot, humid weather	✓	✓
• State need for increased fluid intake and salt with excessive perspiration	✓	✓
• State need for high-carbohydrate, high-protein diet with adequate sodium intake	✓	✓
• Identify needed activity limitations and impact on lifestyle	✓	✓

Chart 42-10   Clinical Manifestations of Cushing's Syndrome

Ophthalmic
Cataracts
Glaucoma

Cardiovascular
Hypertension
Heart failure

Endocrine/Metabolic
Truncal obesity
Moon face
Buffalo hump
Sodium retention
Hypokalemia
Metabolic alkalosis
Hyperglycemia
Menstrual irregularities
Impotence
Negative nitrogen balance
Altered calcium metabolism
Adrenal suppression

Immune Function
Decreased inflammatory
  responses
Impaired wound healing
Increased susceptibility to
  infections

Skeletal
Osteoporosis
Spontaneous fractures
Aseptic necrosis of femur
Vertebral compression
  fractures

Gastrointestinal
Peptic ulcer
Pancreatitis

Muscular
Myopathy
Muscle weakness

Dermatologic
Thinning of skin
Petechiae
Ecchymoses
Striae
Acne

Psychiatric
Mood alterations
Psychoses

This woman with Cushing's syndrome has several classic signs, including facial hair, buffalo hump, and moon face. From Rubin, E. & Farber, J. L. (1999). *Pathology* (3rd ed.). Philadelphia: Lippincott Williams & Wilkins.

Assessment and Diagnostic Findings

Indicators of Cushing's syndrome include an increase in serum sodium and blood glucose levels and a decreased serum concentration of potassium, a reduction in the number of blood eosinophils, and disappearance of lymphoid tissue. Measurements of plasma and urinary cortisol levels are obtained. Several blood samples may be collected to determine whether the normal diurnal variation in plasma levels is present; this variation is frequently absent in adrenal dysfunction. If several blood samples are required, they must be collected at the times specified and the time of collection must be noted on the requisition slip.

An overnight dexamethasone suppression test is the most widely used screening test for diagnosis of pituitary and adrenal causes of Cushing's syndrome. It can be performed on an outpatient basis. Dexamethasone (1 mg) is administered orally at 11 pm, and a plasma cortisol level is obtained at 8 the next morning. Suppression of cortisol to less than 138 nmol/L indicates that the hypothalamic-pituitary-adrenal axis is functioning properly. Stress, obesity, depression, and medications such as antiseizure agents, estrogen, and rifampin can falsely elevate cortisol levels. Other diagnostic studies include a 24-hour urinary free cortisol level and a high-dose or low-dose dexamethasone suppression test. High-dose and low-dose suppression tests are similar to the overnight test but vary in dosage and timing.

Measurement of plasma ACTH by radioimmunoassay is used in conjunction with the high-dose suppression test to distinguish pituitary tumours from ectopic sites of ACTH production as the cause of Cushing's syndrome. Elevation of both ACTH and cortisol level indicates pituitary or hypothalamic disease. Low ACTH with a high cortisol level indicates adrenal disease. A CT scan, ultrasound, or MRI may be performed to localize adrenal tissue and detect tumours of the adrenal gland.

Medical Management

If Cushing's syndrome is caused by pituitary tumours rather than tumours of the adrenal cortex, treatment is directed at the pituitary gland. Surgical removal of the tumour by transsphenoidal hypophysectomy (see Chap. 61) is the treatment of choice and has a 90% success rate (Rakel & Bope, 2001). Radiation of the pituitary gland also has been successful, although it may take several months for control of symptoms. Adrenalectomy is the treatment of choice in patients with primary adrenal hypertrophy.

Postoperatively, symptoms of adrenal insufficiency may begin to appear 12 to 48 hours after surgery because of reduction of the high levels of circulating adrenal hormones. Temporary replacement therapy with hydrocortisone may be necessary for several months until the adrenal glands begin to respond normally to the body's needs. If both adrenal glands have been removed (bilateral adrenalectomy), lifetime replacement of adrenal cortex hormones is necessary.

Adrenal enzyme inhibitors (eg, metyrapone, aminoglutethimide, mitotane, ketoconazole) may be used to reduce hyperadrenalism if the syndrome is caused by ectopic ACTH secretion by a tumour that cannot be eradicated. Close monitoring is necessary because symptoms of inadequate adrenal function may result and because of possible side effects of these medications.

If Cushing's syndrome is a result of the administration of corticosteroids, an attempt is made to reduce or taper the medication to the minimum dosage needed to treat the underlying disease process (eg, autoimmune and allergic diseases and rejection of transplanted organs). Frequently, alternate-day therapy decreases the symptoms of Cushing's syndrome and allows recovery of the adrenal glands' responsiveness to ACTH.

NURSING PROCESS: THE PATIENT WITH CUSHING'S SYNDROME

Assessment

The health history and examination focus on the effects on the body of high concentrations of adrenal cortex hormones and on the inability of the adrenal cortex to respond to changes in cortisol and aldosterone levels. The history includes information about the patient's level of activity and ability to carry out routine and self-care activities. The skin is observed and assessed for trauma, infection, breakdown, bruising, and edema. Changes in physical appearance are noted, and the patient's responses to these changes are elicited. The nurse assesses the patient's mental function, including mood, responses to questions, awareness of environment, and level of depression. The family is often a good source of information about gradual changes in the patient's physical appearance as well as emotional status.

Diagnosis

NURSING DIAGNOSES

Based on all the assessment data, the major nursing diagnoses of the patient with Cushing's syndrome include the following:

- Risk for injury related to weakness
- Risk for infection related to altered protein metabolism and inflammatory response
- Self-care deficit related to weakness, fatigue, muscle wasting, and altered sleep patterns
- Impaired skin integrity related to edema, impaired healing, and thin and fragile skin
- Disturbed body image related to altered physical appearance, impaired sexual functioning, and decreased activity level
- Disturbed thought processes related to mood swings, irritability, and depression

COLLABORATIVE PROBLEMS/ POTENTIAL COMPLICATIONS

Based on assessment data, potential complications may include the following:

- Addisonian crisis
- Adverse effects of adrenocortical activity

Planning and Goals

The major goals for the patient include decreased risk for injury, decreased risk for infection, increased ability to carry out self-care activities, improved skin integrity, improved body image, improved mental function, and absence of complications.

Nursing Interventions

DECREASING RISK FOR INJURY

Establishing a protective environment will help to prevent falls, fractures, and other injuries to bones and soft tissues. The patient who is very weak may require assistance from the nurse in ambulating to prevent falls or bumping into sharp corners of furniture. Foods high in protein, calcium, and vitamin D are recommended to minimize muscle wasting and osteoporosis. Referral to a dietitian may assist the patient in selecting appropriate foods that are also low in sodium and calories.

DECREASING RISK FOR INFECTION

The patient should avoid unnecessary exposure to others with infections. The nurse frequently assesses the patient for subtle signs of infection because the anti-inflammatory effects of corticosteroids may mask the common signs of inflammation and infection.

PREPARING THE PATIENT FOR SURGERY

The patient is prepared for adrenalectomy, if indicated, and the postoperative course (see later discussion in this chapter). If Cushing's syndrome is a result of a pituitary tumour, a transsphenoidal hypophysectomy may be performed (see Chap. 61). Diabetes mellitus and peptic ulcer are common in the patient with Cushing's syndrome. Therefore, insulin therapy and medication to treat peptic ulcer may be initiated if needed. Before, during, and after surgery, blood glucose monitoring and assessment of stools for blood are carried out to monitor for appropriate intervention. If the patient has other symptoms of Cushing's syndrome, these are considered in the preoperative preparation. For example, if the patient has experienced weight gain, special instruction is given about postoperative breathing exercises.

ENCOURAGING REST AND ACTIVITY

Weakness, fatigue, and muscle wasting make it difficult for the patient with Cushing's syndrome to carry out normal activities. Yet the nurse should encourage moderate activity to prevent complications of immobility and promote increased self-esteem. Insomnia often contributes to the patient's fatigue. It is important to help the patient plan and space rest periods throughout the day. Efforts are made to promote a relaxing, quiet environment for rest and sleep.

PROMOTING SKIN INTEGRITY

Meticulous skin care is necessary to avoid traumatizing the patient's fragile skin. Use of adhesive tape is avoided because it can irritate the skin and tear the fragile tissue when the tape is removed. The nurse frequently assesses the skin and bony prominences and encourages and assists the patient to change positions frequently to prevent skin breakdown.

IMPROVING BODY IMAGE

If the cause of Cushing's syndrome can be treated successfully, the major physical changes disappear in time. The patient may benefit from discussion of the effect the changes have had on his or her self-concept and relationships with others. Weight gain and edema may be modified by a low-carbohydrate, low-sodium diet, and a high-protein intake may reduce some of the other bothersome symptoms.

IMPROVING THOUGHT PROCESSES

Explanations to the patient and family members about the cause of emotional instability are important in helping them cope with the mood swings, irritability, and depression that may occur. Psychotic behaviour may occur in a few patients and should be reported. The nurse encourages the patient and family members to verbalize their feelings and concerns.

MONITORING AND MANAGING POTENTIAL COMPLICATIONS

Addisonian Crisis

The patient with Cushing's syndrome whose symptoms are treated by withdrawing corticosteroids, by adrenalectomy, or by removing a pituitary tumour is at risk for adrenal hypofunction and addisonian crisis. If high levels of circulating adrenal hormones have suppressed the function of the adrenal cortex, atrophy of the adrenal cortex is likely. If the circulating hormone level is decreased rapidly because of surgery or by abruptly stopping corticosteroid agents, manifestations of adrenal hypofunction and addisonian crisis may develop. Therefore, the patient with Cushing's syndrome is monitored closely for hypotension; rapid, weak pulse; rapid respiratory rate; pallor; and extreme weakness. Efforts are made to identify factors that may have led to the crisis.

The patient with Cushing's syndrome who experiences highly stressful events, such as trauma or emergency surgery, is at increased risk for addisonian crisis because of long-term suppression of the adrenal cortex. The patient may require intravenous administration of fluid and electrolytes and corticosteroids before, during, and after treatment or surgery. If addisonian crisis occurs, the patient is treated for circulatory collapse and shock (see Chap. 15 for management of the patient in shock).

Adverse Effects of Adrenocortical Activity

The nurse assesses fluid and electrolyte status by monitoring laboratory values and daily weights. Because of the increased risk for glucose intolerance and hyperglycemia, blood glucose monitoring is initiated. The nurse reports elevated blood glucose levels to the physician so that treatment can be prescribed if indicated.

PROMOTING HOME AND COMMUNITY-BASED CARE

Teaching Patients Self-Care

The patient with Cushing's syndrome and the patient's family require teaching and support to enable them to prevent problems associated with the syndrome and to manage those that cannot be prevented. The nurse presents information verbally and in writing. If the disorder is a result of corticosteroid use for treatment of a chronic disease, the patient and family need to understand that stopping the corticosteroid use abruptly and without medical supervision is likely to result in acute adrenal insufficiency and reappearance of the underlying symptoms of the chronic disease. The nurse emphasizes the need to ensure an adequate supply of the corticosteroid, because running out of the medication and skipping doses can precipitate addisonian crisis. Refer to the later discussion, Therapeutic Uses of Corticosteroids, for more information.

The nurse stresses the need for dietary modifications to ensure adequate calcium intake without increasing the risk for hypertension, hyperglycemia, and weight gain. The patient and family may be taught to monitor blood pressure, blood glucose levels, and weight. Wearing a medical alert bracelet and notifying other health providers (eg, dentist) are important to alert others that the patient has Cushing's syndrome (Chart 42-11).

Continuing Care

The need for follow-up depends on the origin and duration of the disease and its management. The patient who has been treated by adrenalectomy or removal of a pituitary tumour requires close monitoring to ensure that adrenal function has returned to normal and to ensure adequacy of circulating adrenal hormones. The patient who requires continued corticosteroid therapy is monitored to ensure understanding of the medications and the need for a dosage that treats the underlying disorder while minimizing the side effects. Home care referral may be indicated to ensure a safe environment that minimizes stress and risk for falls and other side effects. The home care nurse assesses the patient's physical and psychological status and reports changes to the physician. The nurse also assesses the patient's understanding of the medication regimen and the patient's compliance with the regimen, and reinforces previous teaching about the medications and the importance of taking them as prescribed. The nurse emphasizes the importance of regular medical follow-up, the side effects and toxic effects of medications, and the need to wear medical identification with Addison's and Cushing's disease. Additionally, the nurse reminds the patient and family about the importance of health promotion activities and recommended health screening, including bone mineral density testing.

Evaluation

EXPECTED PATIENT OUTCOMES

Expected patient outcomes may include:

1. Decreases risk for injury
   a. Is free of fractures or soft tissue injuries
   b. Is free of ecchymotic areas
2. Decreases risk for infection
   a. Experiences no temperature elevation, redness, pain, or other signs of infection and inflammation
   b. Avoids contact with others who have infections

Chart 42-11
Home Care Checklist • The Patient With Cushing's Syndrome

At the completion of the home care instruction, the patient or caregiver will be able to:	Patient	Caregiver
• State present and potential effects of Cushing's syndrome on the body	✓	✓
• Identify signs and symptoms of excessive and insufficient adrenal hormone	✓	✓
• State the relationship between adrenal hormones, emotional state, and stress	✓	✓
• Identify methods for managing labile emotions	✓	✓
• Describe protective skin care measures and use of protective devices and practices	✓	✓
• State the importance of regular follow-up visits with primary health care provider	✓	✓
• State the purpose, dose, route, schedule, side effects, and precautions for prescribed medications (adrenocortical inhibitors)	✓	✓
• Identify need to wear medical alert identification and carry medical information card	✓	✓
• State importance of compliance with medical regimen	✓	✓
• State the need to contact health care provider before taking over-the-counter medications	✓	✓
• Identify foods high in potassium and low in sodium, calories, and carbohydrates	✓	✓
• Identify areas of activity limitations and impact on lifestyle	✓	✓

3. Increases participation in self-care activities
   a. Plans activities and exercises to allow alternating periods of rest and activity
   b. Reports improved well-being
   c. Is free of complications of immobility
4. Attains/maintains skin integrity
   a. Has intact skin, without evidence of breakdown or infection
   b. Exhibits decreased edema in extremities and trunk
   c. Changes position frequently and inspects bony prominences daily
5. Achieves improved body image
   a. Verbalizes feelings about changes in appearance, sexual function, and activity level
   b. States that physical changes are a result of excessive corticosteroids
6. Exhibits improved mental functioning
7. Absence of complications
   a. Exhibits normal vital signs and weight and is free of symptoms of addisonian crisis
   b. Identifies signs and symptoms of adrenocortical hypofunction that should be reported and measures to take in case of severe illness and stress
   c. Identifies strategies to minimize complications of Cushing's syndrome
   d. Complies with recommendations for follow-up appointments and health screening.

PRIMARY ALDOSTERONISM

The principal action of aldosterone is to conserve body sodium. Under the influence of this hormone, the kidneys excrete less sodium and more potassium and hydrogen. Excessive production of aldosterone, which occurs in some patients with functioning tumours of the adrenal gland, causes a distinctive pattern of biochemical changes and a corresponding set of clinical manifestations that are diagnostic of this condition.

Clinical Manifestations

Patients with aldosteronism exhibit a profound decline in the serum levels of potassium (hypokalemia) and hydrogen ions (alkalosis), as demonstrated by an increase in pH and serum bicarbonate level. The serum sodium level is normal or elevated depending on the amount of water reabsorbed with the sodium. Hypertension is the most prominent and almost universal sign of aldosteronism, although it is the primary cause in less than 1% of cases of hypertension (Tierney et al., 2001).

Hypokalemia is responsible for the variable muscle weakness, cramping, and fatigue in patients with aldosteronism, as well as an inability on the part of the kidneys to acidify or concentrate the urine. Accordingly, the urine volume is excessive, leading to polyuria. Serum, by contrast, becomes abnormally concentrated, contributing to excessive thirst (polydipsia) and arterial hypertension. A secondary increase in blood volume and possible direct effects of aldosterone on nerve receptors, such as the carotid sinus, are other factors producing the hypertension.

Hypokalemic alkalosis may decrease the ionized serum calcium level and predispose the patient to tetany and paresthesias. Trousseau's and Chvostek's signs can be used to assess neuromuscular irritability before overt paresthesia and tetany occur.

Glucose intolerance may occur because hypokalemia interferes with insulin secretion from the pancreas.

Assessment and Diagnostic Findings

In addition to a high or normal serum sodium level and low serum potassium level, diagnostic studies indicate high serum aldosterone levels and low serum renin levels. The measurement of the aldosterone excretion rate after salt loading is a useful diagnostic test for primary aldosteronism. The renin–aldosterone stimulation test and bilateral adrenal venous sampling are useful in differentiating the cause of primary aldosteronism. Antihypertensive medication may be discontinued up to 2 weeks prior to testing.

Medical Management

Treatment of primary aldosteronism usually involves surgical removal of the adrenal tumour through adrenalectomy. Hypokalemia resolves for all patients after surgery, but hypertension may persist. Spironolactone may be prescribed to control hypertension.

SURGICAL MANAGEMENT: ADRENALECTOMY

Adrenalectomy may be used in treating adrenal tumours, primary Cushing's syndrome, and aldosteronism. For adrenal tumours, all of the endocrine disturbances associated with a hypersecreting tumour of the adrenal cortex or medulla can be relieved completely by surgical removal of the involved gland.

Adrenalectomy is performed through an incision in the flank or the abdomen. In general, the postoperative care resembles that for other abdominal surgery. However, the patient is susceptible to fluctuations in adrenocortical hormones and requires administration of corticosteroids, fluids, and other agents to maintain blood pressure and prevent acute complications. If the adrenalectomy is bilateral, replacement of corticosteroids will be lifelong; if one adrenal gland is removed, replacement therapy may be temporarily necessary because of suppression of the remaining adrenal gland by high levels of adrenal hormones. A normal serum glucose level is maintained with insulin, appropriate intravenous fluids, and dietary modifications.

Nursing management in the postoperative period includes frequent assessment of vital signs to detect early signs and symptoms of adrenal insufficiency and crisis or hemorrhage. Explaining all treatments and procedures, providing comfort measures, and providing rest periods can reduce the patient's stress and anxiety level.

Corticosteroid Therapy

Corticosteroids are used extensively for adrenal insufficiency and are also widely used in suppressing inflammation and autoimmune reactions, controlling allergic reactions, and reducing the rejection process in transplantation. Commonly used corticosteroid preparations are listed in Table 42-4. Their antiinflammatory and antiallergy actions make corticosteroids effective in treating rheumatic or connective tissue diseases, such as rheumatoid arthritis and systemic lupus erythematosus. They are also frequently used in the treatment of asthma, multiple sclerosis, and other autoimmune disorders.

High doses appear to allow patients to tolerate high degrees of stress. Such antistress action may be caused by the ability of corticosteroids to aid circulating vasopressor substances in keeping

Table 42-4 • Commonly Used Corticosteroid Preparations

GENERIC NAMES	TRADE NAMES
Hydrocortisone	Cortisol, Cortef, Hydrocortone, Solu-Cortef
Cortisone	Cortone, Cortate, Cortogen
Dexamethasone	Decadron, Dexameth, Deronil, Delalone, Dexasone, Dexone, Hexadrol
Prednisone	Meticorten, Deltasone, Orasone, Panasol, Novo-prednisone
Prednisolone	Meticortelone, Delta-Cortef, Prelone, Predalone
Methylprednisolone	Medrol, Solu-Medrol, Meprolone
Triamcinolone	Aristocort, Kenacort, Kenalog, Cenocort, Azmacort, Aristospan
Beclomethasone	Beconase, Beclovent, Vanceril, Vancenase, Propaderm
Betamethasone	Celestone, Betameth, Betnesol, Betnelan

the blood pressure elevated; other effects, such as maintenance of the serum glucose level, also may keep blood pressure elevated.

SIDE EFFECTS

Although the synthetic corticosteroids are safer for some patients because of relative freedom from mineralocorticoid activity, most natural and synthetic corticosteroids produce similar kinds of side effects. The dose required for anti-inflammatory and anti-allergy effects also produces metabolic effects, pituitary and adrenal gland suppression, and changes in the function of the central nervous system. Thus, although corticosteroids are highly effective therapeutically, they may also be very dangerous. Dosages of these medications are frequently altered to allow high concentrations when necessary and then tapered in an attempt to avoid undesirable effects. This requires that patients be observed closely for side effects and that the dose be reduced when high doses are no longer required. Suppression of the adrenal cortex may persist up to a year after a course of corticosteroids of only 2 weeks' duration.

THERAPEUTIC USES OF CORTICOSTEROIDS

The dosage of corticosteroids is determined by the nature and chronicity of the illness as well as the patient's other medical problems. Rheumatoid arthritis, bronchial asthma, and multiple sclerosis are chronic disorders that corticosteroids do not cure; however, these medications may be useful when other measures do not provide adequate control of symptoms. In addition, corticosteroids may be used to treat acute exacerbations of these disorders.

In such situations, the adverse effects of corticosteroids are weighed against the patient's current problems. These medications may be used for a period but then are gradually reduced or tapered as the symptoms subside. The nurse plays an important role in providing encouragement and understanding during the times the patient may experience (or is apprehen-

sive about experiencing) recurrence of symptoms while taking smaller doses.

Treatment of Acute Conditions

Acute flare-ups and crises are treated with large doses of corticosteroids. Examples include emergency treatment for bronchial obstruction in status asthmaticus and septic shock from septicemia caused by gram-negative bacteria. Other measures, such as anti-infective agents or medications, are also used with corticosteroids to treat shock and other major symptoms. At times, corticosteroids are continued past the acute flare-up stage to prevent serious complications.

Eye Treatment

A different problem exists when corticosteroids are used in treating eye infections. Outer eye infection can be treated by topical application of eye drops because these do not cause systemic toxicity. However, long-term application may cause an increase in intraocular pressure, which leads to glaucoma in some patients. In some patients, prolonged use of corticosteroids leads to cataract formation.

Dermatologic Disorders

Topical administration of corticosteroids in the form of creams, ointments, lotions, and aerosols is especially effective in many dermatologic disorders. It may be more effective in some conditions to use occlusive dressings around the affected part to achieve maximum absorption of the medication. Penetration and absorption are also increased if the medication is applied when the skin is hydrated or moist (eg, immediately after bathing).

Absorption of topical agents varies with body location. For example, absorption is greater through the layers of skin on the scalp, face, and genital area than on the forearm; as a result, use of topical agents on these sites increases the risk for side effects of the medication. The availability of over-the-counter topical corticosteroids increases the risk for side effects in patients who are unaware of their potential risks. Excessive use of these agents, especially on large surface areas of inflamed skin, can lead to decreased therapeutic effects and increased side effects.

DOSAGE

Attempts have been made to determine the best time to administer pharmacologic doses of steroids. When symptoms have been controlled on a 6-hour or 8-hour program, a once-daily or every-other-day schedule may be implemented. In keeping with the natural secretion of cortisol, the best time of the day for the total corticosteroid dose is in the early morning from 0700 to 0800 hours. Large-dose therapy at 0800 hours, when the gland is most active, produces maximal suppression of the gland. A large 0800 hours dose is more physiologic because it allows the body to escape effects of the steroids from 1600 to 1800 hours, when serum levels are normally low, hence minimizing cushingoid effects. If symptoms of the disorder being treated are suppressed, alternate-day therapy is helpful in reducing pituitary-adrenal suppression in patients requiring prolonged therapy. Some patients report discomfort associated with symptoms of their primary illness on the second day; therefore, it is important to explain to patients that this regimen is necessary to minimize side effects and suppression of adrenal function.

TAPERING

Corticosteroid dosages are reduced gradually (tapered) to allow normal adrenal function to return and to prevent steroid-induced adrenal insufficiency. Up to 1 year or more after use of corticosteroids, the patient is still at risk for adrenal insufficiency in times of stress. For example, if surgery for any reason is necessary, the patient is likely to require intravenous corticosteroids during and after surgery to reduce the risk for acute adrenal crisis. Patients receiving corticosteroids must have an adequate supply of medication on hand, so that they do not miss a scheduled dose and increase their risk for adrenal insufficiency. Table 42-5 provides an overview of the effects of corticosteroid therapy and their nursing implications.

Table 42-5 • Side Effects of Corticosteroid Therapy and Implications for Practice

SIDE EFFECTS	COLLABORATIVE INTERVENTIONS
Cardiovascular Effects	
Hypertension	Monitor for elevated blood pressure.
Thrombophlebitis	Assess for positive Homans' signs.
Thromboembolism	Remind patient to avoid positions and situations that restrict blood
Accelerated atherosclerosis	flow (eg, crossing legs, prolonged sitting in same position).
	Encourage foot and leg exercises when recumbent.
	Encourage low sodium intake.
	Encourage limited intake of fat.
Immunologic Effects	
Increased risk of infection and masking of signs of infection	Assess for subtle signs of infection and inflammation.
	Encourage patient to avoid exposure to others with upper respiratory infection.
	Monitor patient for fungal infections.
	Encourage hand washing.
Eye Changes	
Glaucoma	Encourage frequent eye examinations.
Corneal lesions	Refer patient to ophthalmologist if changes in visual acuity are detected.
Musculoskeletal Effects	
Muscle wasting	Encourage high protein intake.
Poor wound healing	Encourage diet high in calcium and vitamin D or calcium and
Osteoporosis with vertebral compression fractures, pathologic fractures of long bones, aseptic necrosis of head of the femur	vitamin D supplementation if indicated.
	Take measures to avoid falls and other trauma.
	Use caution in moving and turning patient.
	Encourage postmenopausal women on corticosteroids to consider bone mineral density testing and treatment, if indicated.
	Instruct patient to rise slowly from bed or chair to avoid falling due to postural hypotension.
Metabolic Effects	
Alterations in glucose metabolism	Monitor blood glucose levels at periodic intervals.
Steroid withdrawal syndrome	Instruct patient about medications, diet, and exercise prescribed to control blood glucose level.
	Report signs of adrenal insufficiency.
	Administer corticosteroids and mineralocorticoids as prescribed.
	Monitor fluid and electrolyte balance.
	Administer fluids and electrolytes as prescribed.
	Instruct patient about importance of taking corticosteroids as prescribed without abruptly stopping therapy.
	Encourage patient to obtain and wear a medical identification bracelet.
	Advise patient to notify all health care providers (eg, dentist) about need for corticosteroid therapy.
Changes in Appearance	
Moon face	Encourage low-calorie, low-sodium diet.
Weight gain	Assure patient that most changes in appearance are temporary and
Acne	will disappear if and when corticosteroid therapy is no longer necessary.

Critical Thinking Exercises

1. Your patient has just been diagnosed with hyperthyroidism. Because she is wary of radioactive substances and unwilling to take radioactive iodine, she has been scheduled for a thyroidectomy in 6 weeks. Prior to surgery, she will receive antithyroid medication to control her symptoms. What preoperative teaching is needed for the patient and her family? What nursing interventions are warranted preoperatively and during the postoperative period?

2. Your 70-year-old patient has a diagnosis of bronchogenic carcinoma. He reports that his voiding has decreased in frequency and volume recently and he is being evaluated for possible syndrome of inappropriate antidiuretic hormone secretion (SIADH). The patient and his family are asking for explanations about the syndrome and about methods of managing it. What nursing interventions and patient and family teaching are warranted when caring for this patient?

3. Your 24-year-old patient has been receiving corticosteroids for treatment of ulcerative colitis. She is distraught about the changes in her appearance related to corticosteroids and is talking about stopping the corticosteroids because of the weight gain and other symptoms she has experienced. What interventions are appropriate at this time? What teaching should be provided to the patient and her family about the use of corticosteroids?

4. A 46-year-old patient received radiation therapy 5 years ago for treatment of thyroid cancer. She is being seen for her annual gynecologic examination. What questions are important in assessing her to evaluate her thyroid status? Identify the rationale for each area of assessment and how it relates to thyroid function.

5. Your patient, a 30-year-old woman with two small children, lives within 2 miles of a nuclear power plant. She expresses anxiety and concern about the risks to herself and her children if there is a terrorist attack on the plant. What intervention is warranted? Provide your rationale and describe the explanation you would give to the woman.

6. Your patient has pheochromocytoma and is scheduled to undergo adrenalectomy. What preoperative and postoperative nursing priorities are important in his care? What assessment parameters are important during the pre- and postoperative periods?

REFERENCES AND SELECTED READINGS

Books

Braunwald, E., Fauci, A. S., Kasper, D. L., Hauser, S. L., Longo, D. L., & Jameson, J. L. (Eds.). (2001). *Harrison's principles of internal medicine* (15th ed.). New York: McGraw-Hill.

Canadian Cancer Society/National Cancer Institute of Canada. (2005). *Canadian cancer statistics 2005.* Toronto: Canada.

Grenvik, A., Ayres, S. M., Holbrook, P. R., & Shoemaker, W. C. (Eds.). (2000). *Textbook of critical care* (4th ed.). Philadelphia: W. B. Saunders.

Kacsho, B. (2000). *Endocrine physiology.* New York: McGraw-Hill.

Porth, C. (2002). *Pathophysiology: Concepts of altered health states* (6th ed.). Philadelphia: Lippincott Williams & Wilkins.

Rakel, R. E., & Bope, E. T. (Eds.). (2001). *Conn's current therapy.* Philadelphia: W. B. Saunders.

Tierney, L. M., McPhee, S. J., & Papadakis, M. A. (Eds.). (2001). *Current medical diagnosis and treatment.* New York: Lange Medical Books/McGraw-Hill.

Journals

Adrenal Disorders

Baker, S., Kenward, D., & White, K. G. (2001). Addison's disease: After 40 years much remains the same. *British Medical Journal, 322*(7284), 494.

Boscaro, M., Dbarzon, L., & Sonino, N. (2000). The diagnosis of Cushing's syndrome: Atypical presentation and laboratory shortcomings. *Archives of Internal Medicine, 160*(20), 3045–3053.

Carson, P., & Kearney, K. (2000). Emergency: Adrenal crisis. *American Journal of Nursing, 100*(7), 49–50.

Coursin, D. B., & Wood, K. E. (2002). Corticosteroid supplementation for adrenal insufficiency. *Journal of the American Medical Association, 287*(2), 236–240.

Gafni, R. I., Papanicolaou, D. A., & Nieman, L. K. (2000). Nighttime salivary cortisol measurement as a simple, noninvasive, outpatient screening test for Cushing's syndrome in children and adolescents. *Journal of Pediatrics, 137*(1), 30–35.

Goldberg, M. (2000). The diagnostic challenge: Hyperaldosteronism caused by bilateral adrenal hyperplasia. *Emergency Medicine, 32*(3), 55–56.

Hilditch, K. (2000). My Addison's disease. *British Medical Journal, 321*(7261), 645.

Kearney, K. (2000). Adrenal crisis: It looks like the flu, but it's actually life-threatening. *American Journal of Nursing, 100*(7), 49–50.

Krasner, A. S. (1999). Glucocorticoid-induced adrenal insufficiency. *Journal of the American Medical Association, 282*(7), 671–676.

Lee, L. W., & Glenn, M. B. (2000). Adrenal insufficiency masquerading as sepsis in a patient with tetraparesis: A case report. *Archives of Physical Medicine and Rehabilitation, 81*(6), 830–833.

Lenders, J. W. M., Pacak, K., Walther, M. M., et al. (2000). Biochemical diagnosis of pheochromocytoma—which test is best? *Journal of American Medical Association, 287*(11), 1427–1434.

Matthews, M. R., Al-kasspooles, M. F., Caruso, D. M., Phillips, B. J., Malone, J. M., & Canulla, M. V. (1999). Management of a trauma patient with incidental pheochromocytoma. *Journal of Trauma: Injury, Infection, and Critical Care, 46*(4), 738–740.

O'Connell, C. (1999). Case study: A young woman with palpitations and diaphoresis. *Physician Assistant, 23*(4), 84–96.

Sheahan, W. T. (1999). Case and comment. Anxiety and a severe headache. *Patient Care, 33*(15), 112.

Takao, T., Mimoto, T., Yamamoto, M., & Hashimoto, K. (2001). Preclinical Cushing disease. *Archives of Internal Medicine, 161*(6), 892–893.

Parathyroid Disorders

Bilezikian, J. P., & Silverberg, S. J. (2000). Parathyroid hormone: Does it have a role in the pathogenesis of osteoporosis? *Clinics in Laboratory Medicine, 20*(3), 559–567.

Capriotti, T. (2000). Nursing pharmacology. Pharmacologic prevention and treatment of osteoporosis in women. *MedSurg Nursing, 9*(2), 86–90.

Irvin, G. L. III, & Carneio, D. M. (2000). Contemporary updates: Linking evidence and experience. Management changes in primary hyperparathyroidism. *Journal of the American Medical Association, 284*(8), 934–936.

Koea, J. B., & Shaw, J. H (1999). Parathyroid cancer: Biology and management. *Surgical Oncology, 8*(3), 155–165.

Steffensrud, S. (2000). Parathyroids: The forgotten glands. *Neonatal Network: Journal of Neonatal Nursing, 19*(1), 9–16.

Vestergaard, P., Mollerup, C. L., Frokjaer, V. G., Christeansen, P., Blichert-Toft, M., & Mosekilde, L. (2000). Cohort study of risk of fracture before and after surgery for primary hyperparathyroidism. *British Medical Journal, 321*(7261), 598–602.

Pituitary Disorders

Sachse, D. (2001). Acromegaly. *American Journal of Nursing, 101*(1), 69–77.

Terpstra, T. L., & Terpstra, T. L. (2000). Syndrome of inappropriate antidiuretic hormone secretion: Recognition and management. *Med-Surg Nursing, 9*(2), 61–68.

Thyroid Disorders

Argueta, R., & Whitaker, M. D. (2000). When a thyroid abnormality is palpable: What it means and what you should do. *Postgraduate Medicine, 107*(1), 100–110.

Ayala, A. R., Danese, M. D., & Landenson, P. W. (2000). When to treat mild hypothyroidism. *Endocrinology and Metabolism Clinics of North America, 29*(2), 399–415.

Castro, M. R., & Gharib, H. (2000). Thyroid nodules and cancer: When to wait and watch, when to refer. *Postgraduate Medicine, 107*(1), 113–124.

Cooper, D. S. (2001). Subclinical hypothyroidism. *New England Journal of Medicine, 345*(4), 260–264.

Elliott, B. (2000). Case report. Diagnosing and treating hypothyroidism. *Nurse Practitioner: American Journal of Primary Health Care, 25*(3), 92–94.

Food and Drug Administration. (2001). Potassium iodide as a thyroid blocking agent in radiation emergencies. U.S. Department of Health and Human Services, Washington, DC. http://www.fda.gov/cder/guidance/index.htm.

Fatourechi, V. (2000). Demystifying autoimmune thyroid disease: Which disorders require treatment? *Postgraduate Medicine, 107*(1), 127–134.

Goldsmith, C. (1999). Clinical snapshot: Hypothyroidism. *American Journal of Nursing, 99*(6), 42–43.

Ladenson, P. W., Singer, P. A., Ain, K. B., Bagchi, N., Bigos, S. T., Levy, E. G., Smith, S. A., & Daniels, G. H. (2000). American Thyroid Association guidelines for detection of thyroid dysfunction. *Archives of Internal Medicine, 160*(11), 1573–1575.

Larson, J., Anderson, E. H., & Koslawy, M. (2000). Thyroid disease: A review for primary care. *Journal of the American Academy of Nurse Practitioners, 12*(6), 226–232.

Malchiodi, L. (2002). Thyroid storm. *American Journal of Nursing, 102*(5), 33–35.

Mettler, F. A. Jr., & Voelz, G. L. (2002). Major radiation exposure: What to expect and how to respond. *New England Journal of Medicine, 346*(20), 1554–1561.

Orzeck, E. A., & Yin, J. M. (2000). Primary care updates: Brief summaries for clinical practice. Thyroid hormone resistance. *Consultant, 40*(6), 1149–1151.

Ringel, M. D. (2001). Management of hypothyroidism and hyperthyroidism in the intensive care unit. *Critical Care Clinics, 17*(1), 59–74.

Smallridge, R. C. (2000). Disclosing subclinical thyroid disease: An approach to mild laboratory abnormalities and vague or absent symptoms. *Postgraduate Medicine, 107*(1), 143–152.

Stajduhar, K. I., Neithercut, J., Chu, E., Pham, P., Rohde, J., Sicotte, A., & Young, K. (2000). Thyroid cancer: Patients' experiences of receiving iodine-131 therapy. *Oncology Nursing Forum, 27*(8), 1213–1218.

Tate, J., & Tasota, F. J. (2001). Eye on diagnostics. Assessing thyroid function with serum tests. *Nursing, 31*(1), 22.

Thyroid Carcinoma Task Force. (2001). AACE/AAES Medical/Surgical guidelines for clinical practice: Management of thyroid carcinoma. *Endocrine Practice, 7*(3), 202–220.

Toft, A. D. I (2001). Subclinical hyperthyroidism. *New England Journal of Medicine, 345*(7), 512–516.

Tunbridge, W., M., & Vanderpump, M. P. J. (2000). Population screening for autoimmune thyroid disease. *Endocrinology and Metabolism Clinics of North America, 29*(2), 239–253.

RESOURCES AND WEBSITES

Canadian Association of Genetic Counsellors (CAGC); www.cagc-accg.ca.

Canadian Cancer Society/Société canadienne du cancer, National Office, Suite 200, 10 Alcorn Avenue, Toronto, ON M4V 3B1; (416) 961-7223; fax: (416) 961-4189; www.cancer.ca.

Canadian Directory of Genetic Support Groups, Support Group Directory, Regional Medical Genetics Centre, Children's Hospital of Western Ontario, 800 Commissioner's Road East, London ON N6C 2V5; (519) 685-8453; in Ontario only 1-800-243-8416; fax: (519) 685-8214; www.lhsc.on.ca/programs/medgenet.

Canadian Genetic Disease Network, Suite 201, 2150 Western Parkway, Vancouver BC V6T 1V6; (604) 221-7300; fax: (604) 221-0778; e-mail: info@cgdn.ca; www.cgdn.ca.

Canadian Organization for Rare Disorders (CORD), P.O. Box 814, Coaldale, AB T1M 1M7; (403) 345-4544; toll-free: 1-877-302-7273; fax: (403) 345-3948; www.cord.ca.

Cushing's Support and Research Foundation, 65 East India Row, Suite 22B, Boston, MA 02110; (617) 723-3674; e-mail: CSRF@world.std.com; http://world.std.com/~CSRF.

GeneTests, 9725 Third Avenue NE, Suite 602, Seattle, WA 98115 USA; (206) 616-4033; fax: (206) 221-4679; e-mail: genetests@genetests.org; www.genetests.org.

Genetic Alliance, 4301 Connecticut Avenue NW, Suite 404, Washington, DC 20008-2369 USA; (202) 966-5557; fax: (202) 966-8553; e-mail: info@geneticalliance.org; www.geneticalliance.org.

National Adrenal Disease Foundation, 505 Northern Boulevard, Suite 200, Great Neck, NY 11021; (516) 487-4992.

National Adrenal Diseases Foundation, 505 Northern Boulevard, Great Neck, NY 11021; (516) 487-4992; http://www.medhelp.org/nadf.

National Cancer Institute of Canada/Institut National du Cancer du Canada, Suite 200, 10 Alcorn Avenue, Toronto, ON M4V 3B1; (416) 961-7223; fax: (416) 961-4189; www.ncic.cancer.ca.

National Organization for Rare Disorders (NORD), P.O. Box 1968 (55 Kenosia Ave.), Danbury, CT 06813; (203) 744-0100; http://www.rarediseases.org.

National Heart, Lung, and Blood Institute (NHBLI), National Institutes of Health, Bldg., 32, Rm. 4A21, Bethesda, MD 20892; (301) 592-8573; (800) 575-WELL (9355); http://www.nhlbi.nih.gov.

OMIM Online Mendelian Inheritance in Man; www.ncbi.nlm.nih.gov/entrez/query.fcgi?db=OMIM.

The Genetics Society of Canada; http://life.biology.mcmaster.ca/GSC.

Thyroid Foundation of Canada, 797 Princess Street, Suite 304; Kingston, ON K7L 1G1; (613) 544-8364; toll-free (in Canada) 1-800-267-8822; fax: (613) 544-9731; www.thyroid.ca.

Renal and Urinary Tract Function

Applying Concepts from NANDA, NIC, and NOC

Mrs. Martinez is a 44-year-old woman with no significant medical history. She has three children. During her annual physical examination, she tells the women's health nurse practitioner that when she jogs, coughs, or sneezes, she experiences an involuntary loss of small amounts of urine. The patient's urinalysis is normal. On physical examination, the nurse finds that Mrs. Martinez has a moderate cystocele and that her bladder feels mildly distended, although she had just voided to provide a urine sample. The nurse catheterizes Mrs. Martinez to check for postvoid residual urine and obtains 120 mL of clear urine. The concept map demonstrates the relationships that exist among the nursing diagnoses, interventions, and outcomes for Mrs. Martinez's clinical problem.

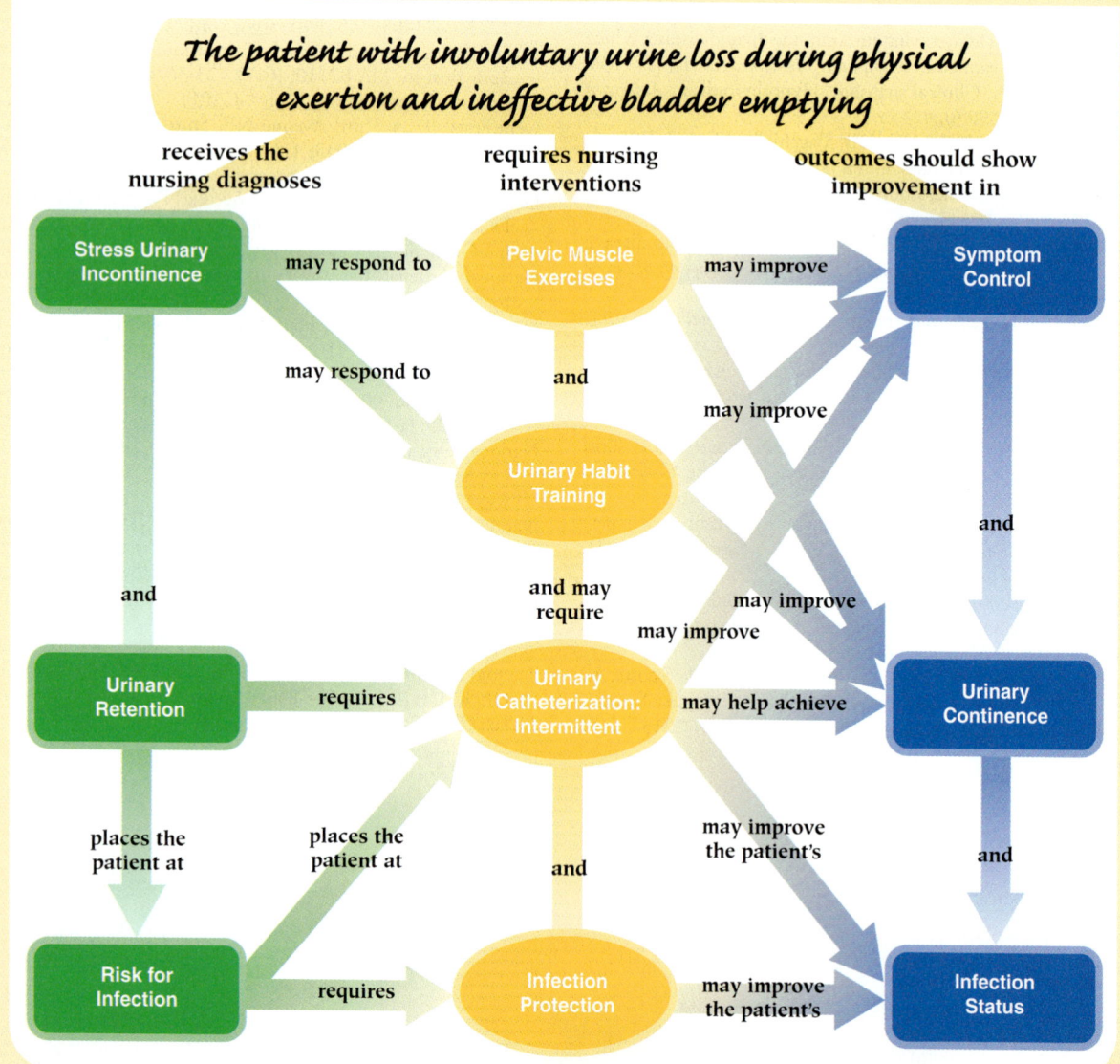

The patient with involuntary urine loss during physical exertion and ineffective bladder emptying

Nursing Classifications and Languages

NANDA
Nursing Diagnoses

Stress Urinary Incontinence—Loss of less than 50 mL of urine occurring with increased abdominal pressure

Urinary Retention—Incomplete emptying of the bladder

Risk for Infection—At increased risk for being invaded by pathogenic organisms

NIC
Nursing Interventions*

Pelvic Muscle Exercises—Strengthening and training the levator ani and urogenital muscles through voluntary, repetitive contraction to decrease stress, urge, or mixed types of urinary incontinence

Urinary Habit Training—Establishing a predictable pattern of bladder emptying to prevent incontinence for persons who have urge stress or functional incontinence

Urinary Catheterization: Intermittent—Regular periodic use of a catheter to empty the bladder

Infection Protection—Prevention and early detection of infection in a patient at risk

NOC
Nursing Outcomes†

Return to functional baseline status, stabilization of, or improvement in

Symptom Control—Personal actions to minimize perceived changes in physical and emotional functioning

Urinary Continence—Control of the elimination of urine

Infection Status—Presence and extent of infection

NANDA, North American Nursing Diagnosis Association; NIC, Nursing Interventions Classification; NOC, Nursing Outcomes Classification.

*Iowa Intervention Project © 2000. In McCloskey, J. C., & Bulechek, G. M. (2000). *Nursing interventions classification (NIC)* (3rd ed.). St. Louis: Mosby.

†Iowa Outcomes Project © 2000. In Johnson, M., Maas, M., & Moorhead, S. (2000). *Nursing outcomes classification (NOC)* (3rd ed.). St. Louis: Mosby.

Assessment of Renal and Urinary Tract Function

Adapted by Jill Milne

LEARNING OBJECTIVES ⬤

On completion of this chapter, the learner will be able to:

1. Describe the anatomy and physiology of the upper and lower urinary tracts.

2. Identify the assessment parameters used for determining the status of upper and lower urinary tract function.

3. Describe the diagnostic studies used to determine upper and lower urinary tract function.

4. Initiate education and preparation for patients undergoing assessment of the urinary system.

5. Discuss the role of the kidney in regulating fluid and electrolyte balance, acid–base balance, and blood pressure.

*P*roper function of the urinary system is essential to life. Dysfunction of the kidneys and lower urinary tract is common and may occur at any age and with varying levels of severity. Assessment of upper and lower urinary tract function is part of every health examination and necessitates an understanding of the anatomy and physiology of the urinary system as well as of the effect of changes in the system on other physiologic functions.

Anatomic and Physiologic Overview

The urinary system comprises the kidneys, ureters, bladder, and urethra. A thorough understanding of the urinary system is necessary for assessing individuals with acute or chronic urinary dysfunction and implementing appropriate nursing care.

ANATOMY OF THE UPPER AND LOWER URINARY TRACTS

The urinary system—the structures of which precisely maintain the internal chemical environment of the body—perform various excretory, regulatory, and secretory functions.

Kidneys

The kidneys are a pair of brownish-red structures located retroperitoneally (behind and outside the peritoneal cavity) on the posterior wall of the abdomen from the 12th thoracic vertebra to the 3rd lumbar vertebra in the adult (Fig. 43-1). An adult kidney weighs 120 to 170 g and is 12 cm long, 6 cm wide, and 2.5 cm thick. The kidneys are well protected by the ribs, muscles, Gerota's fascia, perirenal fat, and the renal capsule, which surround each kidney.

The kidney consists of two distinct regions, the renal parenchyma and the renal pelvis. The renal parenchyma is divided into the cortex and the medulla. The cortex contains the glomeruli, proximal and distal tubules, and cortical collecting ducts and their adjacent peritubular capillaries. The medulla resembles conical pyramids. The pyramids are situated with the base facing the concave surface of the kidney and the apex facing the hilum, or

pelvis. Each kidney contains approximately 8 to 18 pyramids. The pyramids drain into 4 to 13 minor calices that, in turn, drain into 2 to 3 major calices that open directly into the renal pelvis.

The hilum, or pelvis, is the concave portion of the kidney through which the renal artery enters and the renal vein exits. The renal artery (arising from the abdominal aorta) divides into smaller and smaller vessels, eventually forming the afferent arteriole. The afferent arteriole branches to form the **glomerulus**, which is the capillary bed responsible for glomerular filtration. Blood leaves the glomerulus through the efferent arteriole and flows back to the inferior vena cava through a network of capillaries and veins.

Each kidney contains about 1 million **nephrons**, the functional units of the kidney. Each kidney is capable of providing adequate renal function if the opposite kidney is damaged or becomes nonfunctional. The nephron consists of a glomerulus containing afferent and efferent arterioles, Bowman's capsule, proximal tubule, loop of Henle, distal tubule, and collecting ducts (Fig. 43-2). Collecting ducts converge into papillae, which empty into the minor calices, which drain into three major calices that open directly into the renal pelvis.

Nephrons are structurally divided into two types: cortical and juxtamedullary. Cortical nephrons are found in the cortex of the kidney, and juxtamedullary nephrons sit adjacent to the medulla. The juxtamedullary nephrons are distinguished by their long loops of Henle and the vasa recta, long capillary loops that dip into the medulla of the kidney.

The glomerulus is composed of three filtering layers: the capillary endothelium, the basement membrane, and the epithelium. The glomerular membrane normally allows filtration of fluid and small molecules yet limits passage of larger molecules, such as blood cells and albumin. Kidney function begins to decrease at a rate of approximately 1% each year beginning at approximately age 30.

Ureters, Bladder, and Urethra

Urine, which is formed within the nephrons, flows into the ureter, a long fibromuscular tube that connects each kidney to the bladder. The ureters are narrow, muscular tubes, each 24 to 30 cm long, that originate at the lower portion of the renal pelvis and terminate

Glossary

aldosterone: hormone synthesized and released by the adrenal cortex; causes the kidneys to reabsorb sodium

antidiuretic hormone (ADH): hormone secreted by the posterior pituitary gland; causes the kidneys to reabsorb more water

anuria: total urine output less than 50 mL in 24 hours

bacteriuria: bacteria in the urine; bacterial count higher than 100,000 colonies/mL

clearance: volume of plasma that the kidneys can clear of a specific solute (eg, creatinine); expressed in millilitres per minute

creatinine: endogenous waste product of muscle energy metabolism

dysuria: painful or difficult urination

frequency: voiding more frequently than every 3 hours

glomerulus: tuft of capillaries forming part of the nephron through which filtration occurs

glomerular filtration rate (GFR): volume of plasma filtered at the glomerulus into the kidney tubules each minute; normal rate is approximately 120 mL/min

hematuria: red blood cells in the urine

micturition: urination or voiding

nephron: structural and functional unit of the kidney responsible for urine formation

nocturia: awakening at night to urinate

oliguria: total urine output less than 400 mL in 24 hours

osmolality: number of particles dissolved per kilogram of urine; expression of the degree of concentration of the urine

proteinuria: protein in the urine

pyuria: pus in the urine

specific gravity: reflects the weight of particles dissolved in the urine; expression of the degree of concentration of the urine

tubular reabsorption: movement of a substance from the kidney tubule into the blood in the peritubular capillaries or vasa recta

tubular secretion: movement of a substance from the blood in the peritubular capillaries or vasa recta into the kidney tubule

urea nitrogen: nitrogenous end product of protein metabolism

urinary incontinence: involuntary loss of urine

Valsalva leak-point pressure (VLPP): amount of abdominal pressure against the bladder that causes the urethra to open and leak urine

vesicoureteral reflux: backflow of urine from the bladder into the ureters

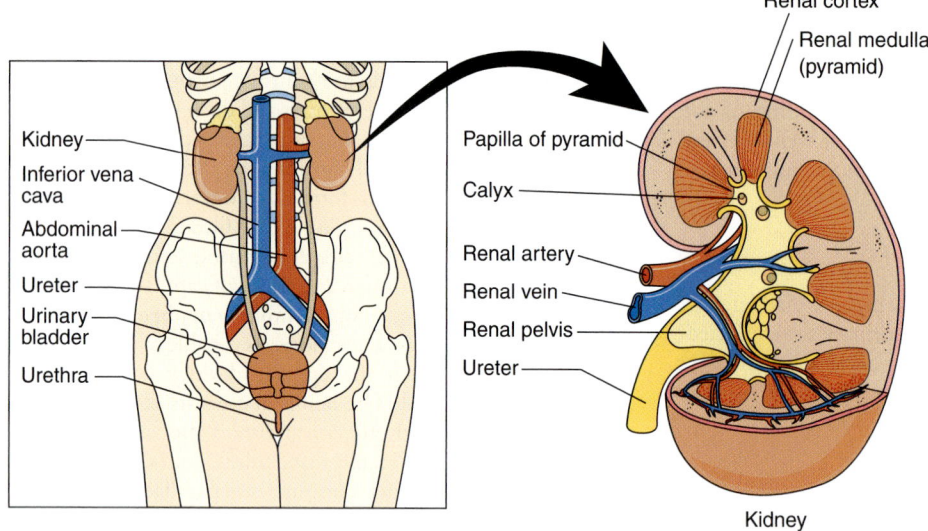

FIGURE 43-1 The urinary tract includes the kidneys (enlargement at right), ureters, and bladder.

in the trigone of the bladder wall. There are three narrowed areas of each ureter: the ureteropelvic junction, the ureteral segment near the sacroiliac junction, and the ureterovesical junction.

The angling of the ureterovesical junction is the primary means of providing antegrade, or downward, movement of urine, also referred to as efflux of urine. This angling prevents **vesicoureteral**

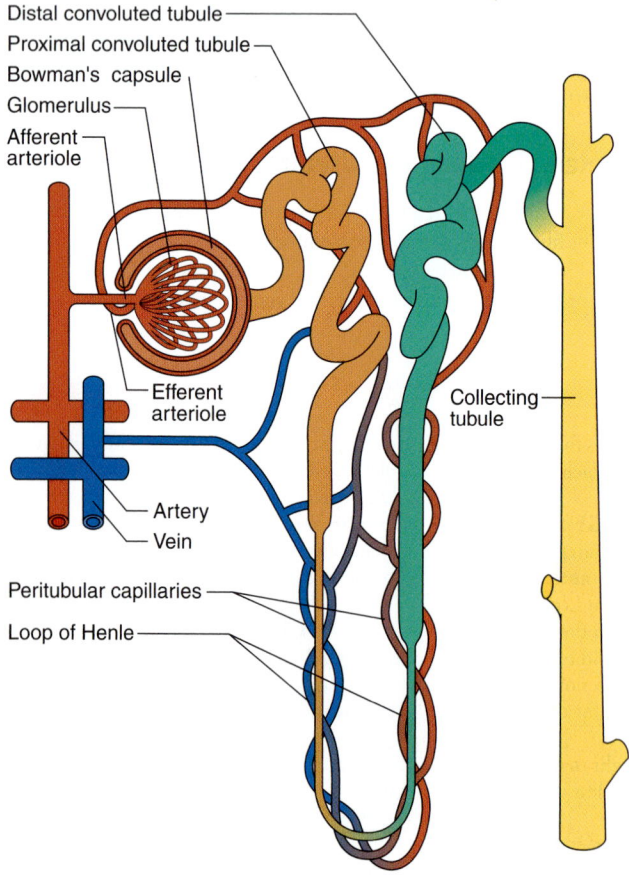

FIGURE 43-2 Representation of a nephron. Each kidney has about 1 million nephrons, which take two forms: cortical and juxtamedullary. Cortical nephrons are located in the cortex of the kidney; juxtamedullary nephrons are adjacent to the medulla.

reflux, which is the retrograde, or backward, movement of urine from the bladder, up the ureter, toward the kidney. During voiding (**micturition**), increased intravesical pressure keeps the ureterovesical junction closed and keeps urine within the ureters. As soon as micturition is completed, intravesical pressure returns to its normal low baseline value, allowing efflux of urine to resume. Therefore, the only time that the bladder is completely empty is in the last seconds of micturition before efflux of urine resumes.

The three areas of narrowing within the ureters have a propensity toward obstruction because of renal calculi (kidney stones) or stricture. Obstruction of the ureteropelvic junction is the most serious because of its close proximity to the kidney and the risk of associated kidney dysfunction. The left ureter is slightly shorter than the right. The lining of the ureters is made up of transitional cell epithelium called urothelium. As in the bladder, the urothelium prevents reabsorption of urine. The movement of urine from the renal pelves through the ureters into the bladder is facilitated by peristaltic waves (occurring about one to five times per minute) from contraction of the smooth muscle in the ureter wall (Walsh, Retik, Vaughan & Wein, 1998).

The urinary bladder is a muscular, hollow sac located just behind the pubic bone. Adult bladder capacity is about 300 to 600 mL of urine. In infancy, the bladder is found within the abdomen. In adolescence and through adulthood, the bladder assumes its position in the true pelvis. The bladder is characterized by its central, hollow area called the vesicle, which has two inlets (the ureters) and one outlet (the urethrovesical junction), which is surrounded by the bladder neck. The wall of the bladder comprises four layers. The outermost layer is the adventitia, which is made up of connective tissue. Immediately beneath the adventitia is a smooth muscle layer known as the detrusor. Beneath the detrusor is a smooth muscle tunic known as the lamina propria, which serves as an interface between the detrusor and the innermost layer, the urothelium. The urothelium layer is specialized, transitional cell epithelium, containing a membrane that is impermeable to water. The urothelium prevents the reabsorption of urine stored in the bladder. The bladder neck contains bundles of involuntary smooth muscle that form a portion of the urethral sphincter known as the internal sphincter. The portion of the sphincteric mechanism that is under voluntary control is the external urinary sphincter at the anterior urethra, the segment most distal from the bladder (Walsh et al., 1998).

The urethra arises from the base of the bladder: In the male, it passes through the penis; in the female, it opens just anterior to the vagina. In the male, the prostate gland, which lies just below the bladder neck, surrounds the urethra posteriorly and laterally.

PHYSIOLOGY OF THE UPPER AND LOWER URINARY TRACTS

The urinary system performs various roles that are essential for normal bodily homeostasis (Chart 43-1). These functions include urine formation; excretion of waste products; regulation of electrolyte, acid, and water excretion; and autoregulation of blood pressure.

Urine Formation

Urine is formed in the nephrons through a complex three-step process: glomerular filtration, **tubular reabsorption,** and **tubular secretion**. Figure 43-3 illustrates the three processes of urine formation and typical values of water and electrolytes associated with each process. The various substances normally filtered by the glomerulus, reabsorbed by the tubules, and excreted in the urine include sodium, chloride, bicarbonate, potassium, glucose, urea, creatinine, and uric acid. Within the tubule, some of these substances are selectively reabsorbed into the blood. Others are secreted from the blood into the filtrate as it travels down the tubule. Some substances, such as glucose, are completely reabsorbed in the tubule and normally do not appear in the urine. Amino acids and glucose are usually filtered at the level of the

glomerulus and reabsorbed so that neither is excreted in the urine. Glucose, however, appears in the urine (glycosuria) if the amount of glucose in the blood and glomerular filtrate exceeds the amount that the tubules are able to reabsorb. Normally, glucose is completely reabsorbed when the blood glucose level is less than 11 mmol/L. In diabetes, when the blood glucose level exceeds the kidneys' reabsorption capacity, glucose appears in the urine. Glycosuria is also common in pregnancy.

Protein molecules are also generally not found in the urine; however, low-molecular-weight proteins (globulins and albumin) may periodically be excreted in small amounts. Transient **proteinuria** in amounts less than 8 mmol/L is considered normal and does not require further evaluation. Persistent proteinuria usually signifies damage to the glomeruli.

Chart 43-1	**Functions of the Kidney**

- Urine formation
- Excretion of waste products
- Regulation of electrolytes
- Regulation of acid–base balance
- Control of water balance
- Control of blood pressure
- Renal clearance
- Regulation of red blood cell production
- Synthesis of vitamin D to active form
- Secretion of prostaglandins

 ## Physiology/Pathophysiology

FIGURE 43-3 Urine is formed in the nephrons in a three-step process: filtration, reabsorption, and excretion. Water, electrolytes, and other substances, such as glucose and creatinine, are filtered by the glomerulus; varying amounts of these are reabsorbed in the renal tubule, or excreted in the urine. Typical normal volumes of these substances during the steps of urine formation appear above. Wide variations may occur in the values depending on diet.

The steps of urine formation are:

- Glomerular filtration: The normal blood flow through the kidneys is about 1,200 mL/min. As blood flows into the glomerulus from an afferent arteriole, filtration occurs. The filtered fluid, also known as filtrate or ultrafiltrate, then enters the renal tubules. Under normal conditions, about 20% of the blood passing through the glomeruli is filtered into the nephron, amounting to about 180 L/day of filtrate. The filtrate normally consists of water, electrolytes, and other small molecules, because water and small molecules are allowed to pass, whereas larger molecules stay in the bloodstream. Efficient filtration depends on adequate blood flow maintaining a consistent pressure through the glomerulus. Many factors can alter this blood flow and pressure, including hypotension, decreased oncotic pressure in the blood, and increased pressure in the renal tubules from an obstruction.

- Tubular reabsorption and tubular secretion: The second and third steps of urine formation occur in the renal tubules and are called tubular reabsorption and tubular secretion. In tubular reabsorption, a substance moves from the filtrate back into the peritubular capillaries or vasa recta. In tubular secretion, a substance moves from the peritubular capillaries or vasa recta into tubular filtrate. Of the 180 L of filtrate that the kidneys produce each day, 99% is reabsorbed into the bloodstream, resulting in 1,000 to 1,500 mL of urine each day. Although most reabsorption occurs in the proximal tubule, reabsorption occurs along the entire tubule. Reabsorption and secretion in the tubule frequently involve passive and active transport and may require the use of energy. Filtrate becomes concentrated in the distal tubule and collecting ducts under the influence of **antidiuretic hormone (ADH)** and becomes urine, which then enters the renal pelvis.

Excretion of Waste Products

The kidney functions as the body's main excretory organ, eliminating the body's metabolic waste products. The major waste product of protein metabolism is urea, of which about 25 to 30 g is produced and excreted daily. All of this urea must be excreted in the urine; otherwise it will accumulate in body tissues. Other waste products of metabolism that must be excreted are creatinine, phosphates, and sulfates. Uric acid, formed as a waste product of purine metabolism, is also eliminated in the urine. The kidneys serve as the primary mechanism for excreting drug metabolites.

Regulation of Electrolyte Excretion

When the kidneys are functioning normally, the volume of electrolytes excreted per day is exactly equal to the amount ingested. For example, the average Canadian daily diet contains 6 to 8 g each of sodium chloride (salt) and potassium chloride. Nearly all of this is excreted in the urine. Electrolyte excretion includes sodium and potassium.

SODIUM

More than 99% of the water and sodium filtered at the glomeruli is reabsorbed into the blood by the time the urine leaves the body. Water from the filtrate follows the reabsorbed sodium to maintain osmotic balance. By regulating the amount of sodium (and therefore water) reabsorbed, the kidney can regulate the volume of body fluids. If more sodium is excreted than ingested, dehydration results; if less sodium is excreted than ingested, fluid retention results.

The regulation of sodium volume excreted depends on **aldosterone,** a hormone synthesized and released from the adrenal cortex. With increased aldosterone in the blood, less sodium is excreted in the urine because aldosterone fosters renal reabsorption of sodium. Release of aldosterone from the adrenal cortex is largely under the control of angiotensin II. Angiotensin II levels are in turn controlled by renin, an enzyme that is released from specialized cells in the kidneys (Fig. 43-4). This complex system is activated when pressure in the renal arterioles falls below normal levels, as occurs with shock, dehydration, or decreased sodium chloride delivery to the tubules. Activation of this system increases the retention of water and expansion of intravascular fluid volume.

POTASSIUM

Potassium is the most abundant intracellular ion, with about 98% of the total-body potassium located intracellularly. To maintain a normal potassium balance in the body, the kidneys are responsible for excreting more than 90% of the total daily potassium intake. Several factors influence potassium loss through the kidneys. Aldosterone causes the kidney to excrete potassium, in contrast to aldosterone's effects on sodium described previously. Acid–base balance, the amount of dietary potassium intake, and the flow rate of the filtrate in the distal tubule also influence the amount of potassium secreted into the urine. Retention of potassium is the most life-threatening effect of renal failure.

Regulation of Acid Excretion

The catabolism, or breakdown, of proteins results in the production of acid compounds, in particular phosphoric and sulfuric acids. The normal daily diet also includes a certain amount of acid materials. Unlike carbon dioxide (CO_2), phosphoric and sulfuric acids are nonvolatile and cannot be eliminated by the lungs. Because accumulation of these acids in the blood would lower its pH (making the blood more acidic) and inhibit cell function, they must be excreted in the urine. A person with normal kidney function excretes about 70 mmol/L of acid each day. The kidney is able to excrete some of this acid directly into the urine until the urine pH reaches 4.5, which is 1,000 times more acidic than blood.

More acid, however, usually needs to be eliminated from the body than can be excreted directly as free acid in the urine. These excess acids are bound to chemical buffers so they can be excreted in the urine. Two important chemical buffers are phosphate ions and ammonia (NH_3). When buffered with acid, ammonia becomes ammonium (NH_4). Phosphate is present in the glomerular filtrate, and ammonia is produced by the cells of the renal tubules and secreted into the tubular fluid. Through the buffering process, the kidney is able to excrete large quantities of acid in a bound form, without further lowering the pH of the urine.

Regulation of Water Excretion

Regulation of the amount of water excreted is also an important function of the kidney. With high fluid intake, a large volume of dilute urine is excreted. Conversely, with a low fluid intake, a small volume of concentrated urine is excreted. A person normally ingests about 1 to 2 L of water per day, and normally all but 400 to 500 mL of this fluid is excreted in the urine. The remainder is lost from the skin, from the lungs during breathing, and in the feces.

OSMOLALITY

The degree of dilution or concentration of the urine can be measured in terms of **osmolality**, the number of particles (electrolytes

Physiology/Pathophysiology

FIGURE 43-4 Renin–angiotensin system. GFR, glomerular filtration rate; ADH, antidiuretic hormone.

and other molecules) dissolved per kilogram of urine. The filtrate in the glomerular capillary normally has the same osmolality as the blood, with a value of about 300 mmol/L. As the filtrate passes through the tubules and collecting ducts, the osmolality may vary from 50 to 1,200 mmol/L, reflecting the maximal diluting and concentrating abilities of the kidney. When a person is dehydrated or retaining fluid, less water is excreted, and proportionately more particles are present in the urine, giving the urine a concentrated appearance and a high osmolality. When a person excretes a large volume of water, the particles are diluted. The urine appears dilute and the osmolality is low. Certain substances can alter the volume of water excreted and are described as osmotically active. When these substances are filtered, they pull water across the glomeruli and tubules and increase the volume of urine. Glucose and proteins are two examples of osmotically active molecules. Urine osmolality normally ranges from 300 to 1,100 mmol/kg; however, after a 12-hour fluid restriction, that range narrows to 500 to 850 mmol/kg. This wide range of normal makes the test valuable only when the kidneys' concentrating and diluting abilities are questioned.

SPECIFIC GRAVITY

Specific gravity is a measurement of the kidney's ability to concentrate urine. It compares the weight of urine (weight of particles) to the weight of distilled water, which has a specific gravity of 1.000. Normal urine specific gravity is 1.010 to 1.025 when fluid intake is normal. Factors that may interfere with an accurate urine

specific gravity reading include radiopaque contrast agents, glucose, and proteins. Cold urine specimens may also produce a falsely high reading. Several methods can be used to measure specific gravity:

- Multiple-test dipstick (most common method), with a specific reagent area for specific gravity
- Urinometer (least accurate method), in which urine is placed in a small cylinder, and the urinometer is floated in the urine; a specific gravity reading is obtained at the meniscus level of the urine
- Refractometer, an instrument used in a laboratory setting, which measures differences in the speed of light passing through air and the urine sample

Urine specific gravity depends largely on hydration status. When fluid intake decreases, specific gravity normally increases. With high fluid intake, specific gravity decreases. In patients with kidney disease, urine specific gravity does not vary with fluid intake, and the patient's urine is said to have a fixed specific gravity. Disorders or conditions that cause a low urine specific gravity include diabetes insipidus, glomerulonephritis, and severe renal damage. Those that can cause an increased specific gravity include diabetes mellitus, nephrosis, and excessive fluid loss.

ANTIDIURETIC HORMONE

ADH (also known as vasopressin) regulates water excretion and urine concentration in the tubule by varying the amount of water that is reabsorbed. ADH is a hormone that is secreted by the posterior part of the pituitary gland in response to changes in osmolality of the blood. With decreased water intake, blood osmolality tends to rise and stimulate ADH release. ADH then acts on the kidney, increasing reabsorption of water and thereby returning the osmolality of the blood to normal. With excess water intake, the secretion of ADH by the pituitary is suppressed; therefore, less water is reabsorbed by the kidney tubule. This latter situation leads to increased urine volume (diuresis).

A dilute urine with a fixed specific gravity (about 1.010) or fixed osmolality (about 300 mmol/L) indicates an inability to concentrate and dilute the urine, a common early sign of kidney disease.

Autoregulation of Blood Pressure

Regulation of blood pressure is also a function of the kidney. Specialized vessels of the kidney called the vasa recta constantly monitor blood pressure as blood begins its passage into the kidney. When the vasa recta detect a decrease in blood pressure, specialized juxtaglomerular cells near the afferent arteriole, distal tubule, and efferent arteriole secrete the hormone renin. Renin converts angiotensinogen to angiotensin I, which is then converted to angiotensin II, the most powerful vasoconstrictor known. The vasoconstriction causes the blood pressure to increase. The adrenal cortex secretes aldosterone in response to stimulation by the pituitary gland, which in turn is in response to poor perfusion or increasing serum osmolality. The result is an increase in blood pressure. When the vasa recta recognize the increase in blood pressure, renin secretion stops. Failure of this feedback mechanism is one of the primary causes of hypertension.

Renal Clearance

Renal **clearance** refers to the ability of the kidneys to clear solutes from the plasma. A 24-hour collection of urine is the primary test of renal clearance used to evaluate how well the kidney performs this important excretory function. Clearance depends on several factors: how quickly the substance is filtered across the glomerulus, how much of the substance is reabsorbed along the tubules, and how much of the substance is secreted into the tubules. It is possible to measure the renal clearance of any substance, but the one measure that is particularly useful is the creatinine clearance.

Creatinine is an endogenous waste product of skeletal muscle that is filtered at the glomerulus, passed through the tubules with minimal change, and excreted in the urine. Hence, creatinine clearance is a good measure of the **glomerular filtration rate (GFR).** To calculate creatinine clearance, a 24-hour urine specimen is collected. Midway through the collection, the serum creatinine level is measured. The following formula is then used to calculate the creatinine clearance:

$$\frac{(\text{Volume of urine }[\text{mL/min}]\times\text{urine creatinine }[\text{mmol/L}])}{\text{serum creatinine }(\text{mmol/L})}$$

The normal adult GFR is about 100 to 120 mL/min (1.67 to 2.0 mL/sec). Creatinine clearance is an excellent measure of renal function; as renal function declines, creatinine clearance decreases.

Regulation of Red Blood Cell Production

When the kidneys sense a decrease in the oxygen tension in renal blood flow, they release erythropoietin. Erythropoietin stimulates the bone marrow to produce red blood cells (RBCs), thereby increasing the amount of hemoglobin available to carry oxygen.

Vitamin D Synthesis

The kidneys are also responsible for the final conversion of inactive vitamin D to its active form, 1,25-dihydroxycholecalciferol. Vitamin D is necessary for maintaining normal calcium balance in the body.

Secretion of Prostaglandins

The kidneys also produce prostaglandin E (PGE) and prostacyclin (PGI), which have a vasodilatory effect and are important in maintaining renal blood flow.

Urine Storage

The bladder is the reservoir for urine. Both bladder filling and emptying are mediated by coordinated sympathetic and parasympathetic nervous system control mechanisms involving the detrusor muscle and the bladder outlet. In an infant, bladder filling and emptying are mediated within the micturition centre in the pons area of the brain stem. By the time a child is 3 to 4 years old, the cerebral cortex is mature enough to cause a conscious awareness of bladder filling. This conscious awareness of bladder filling occurs as a result of sympathetic neuronal pathways that travel via the spinal cord to the level of T10-12, where peripheral, hypogastric nerve innervation allows for continued bladder filling. As bladder filling continues, stretch receptors in the bladder wall are activated, coupled with the desire to void. This information from the detrusor muscle is relayed back to the cerebral cortex via the parasympathetic pelvic nerves at the level of S2 through S4. Normally, the pressure in the bladder remains low even as the urine accumulates, due to the bladder's compliance, or ability to expand with increasing urine volumes (Appell, 1999).

Bladder compliance is due in part to the smooth muscle lining of the bladder and collagen deposits within the wall of the bladder, as well as to neuronal mechanisms that inhibit the detrusor muscle from contracting (specifically, adrenergic receptors that mediate relaxation). To maintain adequate kidney filtration rates, bladder pressure during filling must remain lower than 40 cm H_2O. Ordinarily, the first sensation of bladder filling occurs when there is approximately 100 to 150 mL of urine in the bladder. The first sensation of bladder fullness is transmitted to the central nervous system when the bladder has reached approximately half of its capacity, about 200 to 300 mL in adults, and an initial desire to void occurs. A marked sense of fullness with a strong desire to void usually occurs when the bladder contains 350 mL or more of urine ("functional capacity"). During anesthesia, the average adult bladder under pressure of 60 cm H_2O can hold 1,500 to 2,000 mL ("anatomic capacity"). During normal circumstances, with appropriate bladder wall innervation, capacity would never reach this level because of the tremendous pain and pressure that such fullness would cause. Neurologic changes to the bladder at the level of the supraspinal, spinal, or bladder wall itself can cause abnormally high volumes of urine to be stored due to a decreased or absent urge to void. Under normal circumstances with average fluid intake of approximately 1,500 to 2,000 mL per day, the bladder should be able to store urine for periods of 2 to 4 hours at a time during the day. At night, the release of vasopressin in response to decreased fluid intake causes less production of urine that is more concentrated. This phenomenon usually allows the bladder to continue filling for periods of 6 to 8 hours in adolescents and adults. In older individuals, decreasing bladder compliance and vasopressin levels cause nighttime bladder filling to decrease to periods ranging from 3 to 6 hours (Appell, 1999).

Bladder Emptying

Micturition (voiding) normally occurs approximately eight times in a 24-hour period. It is activated via the micturition reflex arc within the sympathetic and parasympathetic nervous system, which causes a coordinated sequence of events. Initiation of voiding occurs when the efferent pelvic nerve, which originates in S2 to S4, stimulates the bladder to contract, resulting in complete relaxation of the striated urethral sphincter and followed by a fall in urethral pressure, contraction of the detrusor muscle, opening of the vesicle neck and proximal urethra, and flow of urine. This coordinated effort by the parasympathetic system is mediated by muscarinic and, to a lesser extent, cholinergic receptors within the detrusor muscle. The pressure generated in the bladder during micturition is about 20 to 40 cm H_2O in females. It is somewhat higher and more variable in males ages 45 and older due to the normal hyperplasia of the cells of the middle lobes of the prostate gland that surround the proximal urethra. An obstruction of the bladder outlet, such as in advanced benign prostatic hyperplasia (BPH), results in abnormally high voiding pressure with a slow, prolonged flow of urine. In females, gravity drains any urine remaining in the urethra; in males, voluntary muscle contractions expel the urine (Wein, 2001).

If the spinal pathways from the brain to the urinary system are destroyed (eg, after a spinal cord injury), reflex contraction of the bladder is maintained, but voluntary control over the process is lost. In both situations, the detrusor muscle can contract and expel urine, but the contractions are generally insufficient to empty the bladder completely, so residual urine (urine left in the bladder after voiding) remains. Normally, residual urine amounts to no more than 50 mL in the middle-aged adult and less than 50 to 100 mL in the older adult. Chronic urine retention is more prevalent in older men and women (Gray, 2000b).

Assessment

Obtaining a comprehensive health history, which includes an assessment of risk factors, is the first step in assessing a patient with upper or lower urinary tract dysfunction. Various diseases or clinical situations can place a patient at increased risk for urinary tract dysfunction. Data collection about previous health problems or diseases provides the health care team with useful information for evaluating the patient's current urinary status. Risk factors for specific disorders and kidney and lower urinary tract dysfunction are discussed in Chart 43-2 and in Chapters 44 and 45.

HEALTH HISTORY

Obtaining a urologic health history requires excellent communication skills because many patients are embarrassed or uncomfortable discussing genitourinary function or symptoms. It is important to use language the patient can understand and to avoid medical jargon. It is also important to review risk factors, particularly with those at risk. For example, the nurse needs to be aware that multiparous women delivering their children vaginally are at high risk for stress **urinary incontinence**. Elderly women and persons with neurologic disorders such as diabetic neuropathy, multiple sclerosis, or Parkinson's disease often have incomplete emptying of the bladder with urinary stasis, which may result in urinary tract infection or increasing bladder pressure leading to overflow incontinence, hydronephrosis, pyelonephritis, or renal insufficiency.

Persons with a family history of urinary tract problems are at increased risk for renal disorders. Persons with diabetes who have consistent hypertension are at risk for renal dysfunction (Bakris, Williams, Dworkin et al., 2000). Older men are at risk for pros-

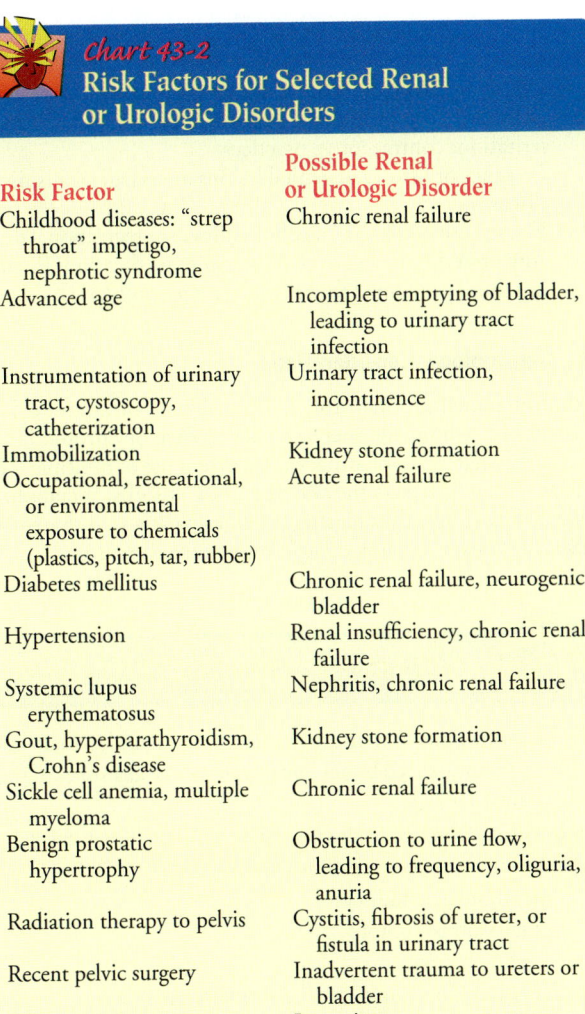

Chart 43-2
Risk Factors for Selected Renal or Urologic Disorders

Risk Factor	Possible Renal or Urologic Disorder
Childhood diseases: "strep throat" impetigo, nephrotic syndrome	Chronic renal failure
Advanced age	Incomplete emptying of bladder, leading to urinary tract infection
Instrumentation of urinary tract, cystoscopy, catheterization	Urinary tract infection, incontinence
Immobilization	Kidney stone formation
Occupational, recreational, or environmental exposure to chemicals (plastics, pitch, tar, rubber)	Acute renal failure
Diabetes mellitus	Chronic renal failure, neurogenic bladder
Hypertension	Renal insufficiency, chronic renal failure
Systemic lupus erythematosus	Nephritis, chronic renal failure
Gout, hyperparathyroidism, Crohn's disease	Kidney stone formation
Sickle cell anemia, multiple myeloma	Chronic renal failure
Benign prostatic hypertrophy	Obstruction to urine flow, leading to frequency, oliguria, anuria
Radiation therapy to pelvis	Cystitis, fibrosis of ureter, or fistula in urinary tract
Recent pelvic surgery	Inadvertent trauma to ureters or bladder
Obstetric injury, tumours	Incontinence
Spinal cord injury	Neurogenic bladder, urinary tract infection, incontinence

tatic enlargement, which causes urethral obstruction and which can result in urinary tract infections and renal failure (Degler, 2000). Moreover, many persons with a history of systemic lupus erythematosus (SLE) develop lupus nephritis (Smith, Fortune-Faulkner & Spurbeck, 2000). When obtaining the health history, the nurse should inquire about the following:

- The patient's chief concern or reason for seeking health care, the onset of the problem, and its effect on the patient's quality of life
- The location, character, and duration of pain, if present, and its relationship to voiding; factors that precipitate pain, and those that relieve it
- History of urinary tract infections, including past treatment or hospitalization for urinary tract infection
- Fever or chills
- Previous renal or urinary diagnostic tests or use of indwelling urinary catheters
- **Dysuria** and when it occurs during voiding (at initiation or termination of voiding)
- Hesitancy, straining, or pain during or after urination
- Urinary incontinence (stress incontinence, urge incontinence, overflow incontinence, or functional incontinence)
- Hematuria or change in colour or volume of urine
- **Nocturia** and its date of onset

- Renal calculi (kidney stones), passage of stones or gravel in urine
- Female patients: number and type (vaginal or cesarean) of deliveries; use of forceps; vaginal infection, discharge, or irritation; contraceptive practices
- Presence or history of genital lesions or sexually transmitted diseases
- Habits: use of tobacco, alcohol, caffeine or recreational drugs
- Any prescription and over-the-counter medications (including those prescribed for renal or urinary problems)

Gerontologic Considerations

A thorough medication history is especially important for elderly patients, for whom the increased occurrence of chronic illness often necessitates polypharmacy (concurrent use of multiple medications). Aging affects the way the body absorbs, metabolizes, and excretes drugs, thus placing the elderly patient at risk for adverse reactions, including compromised renal function.

Other key information to obtain while gathering the health history includes an assessment of the patient's psychosocial status, level of anxiety, perceived threats to body image, available support systems, and sociocultural patterns. Obtaining this information during the initial and subsequent nursing assessments enables the nurse to uncover special needs, misunderstandings, lack of knowledge, and need for patient teaching. Pain, changes in voiding, and gastrointestinal symptoms are particularly suggestive of urinary tract disease. Dysfunction of the kidney can produce a complex array of symptoms throughout the body.

Unexplained Anemia

Gradual kidney dysfunction can be insidious in its presentation, although fatigue is a common symptom. Fatigue, shortness of breath, and exercise intolerance all result from the condition known as "anemia of chronic disease." Although hematocrit has been the blood test of choice when assessing a patient for anemia, the 2001 Kidney Disease Outcomes Quality Initiative: Management of Anemia

GENETICS IN NURSING PRACTICE—Urinary Tract Disorders

Various conditions that affect the renal system and urinary tract function are influenced by genetic factors. Some examples of these genetic disorders are:

- Congenital absence of the vas deferens (caused by CFTR gene mutation for cystic fibrosis)
- Cystic, dysplastic kidneys
- Familial Wilms' tumour
- Horseshoe kidney
- Polycystic kidney (autosomal dominant gene)
- Nephrosis of later onset
- Renal cystic disease in tuberous sclerosis complex

NURSING ASSESSMENTS

FAMILY HISTORY

- Inquire about other family members with renal and/or urinary tract malformations.
- Ask about family history of kidney disease with onset in third to fifth decade (polycystic kidney, autosomal dominant gene).
- Identify family history of male infertility and cystic fibrosis (congenital absence of vas deferens).
- Be alert for family members with history of early-onset renal (Wilms' tumour) or other cancers.

PHYSICAL ASSESSMENT

- Be alert for signs and symptoms of renal disease at an early age (hematuria, hypertension, abdominal mass).
- Assess for clinical findings suggesting that renal disease is a component of a genetic syndrome (eg, seizures, mental retardation, skin involvement).

MANAGEMENT ISSUES SPECIFIC TO GENETICS

- Inquire whether DNA mutation or other genetic testing has been performed on an affected family member.
- If indicated, refer for genetic counselling and evaluation so that the family can discuss concerns regarding inheritance, risks to other family members, availability of genetic testing, and gene-based interventions.

- Offer appropriate genetic information and resources (eg, Genetic Alliance web site).
- Provide support to families newly diagnosed with genetic-related renal and/or kidney disease.

GENETICS RESOURCES FOR NURSES AND THEIR PATIENTS ON THE WEB

Canadian Association of Genetic Counsellors (CAGC) http://www.cagc-accg.ca—a listing of genetic centres across Canada

Canadian Cancer Society http://www.cancer.ca—a source of information on genetic factors/risk and genetic testing

Canadian Directory of Genetic Support Groups http://www.lhsc.on.ca/programs/medgenet—a resource guide for families and professionals

Canadian Genetic Disease Network http://www.cgdn.ca—a group with the stated mission to be the primary catalyst in advancing Canada's scientific and commercial competitiveness in genetic research and the application of genetic discoveries to the prevention, diagnosis, and treatment of human disease

Canadian Organization for Rare Disorders (CORD) http://www.cord.ca—a source of information on over 6,000 rare disorders; links individuals/families with the same rare disorder

Genetic Alliance http://www.geneticalliance.org—an organization that increases the capacity of genetic advocacy groups to achieve their missions and leverages the voices of millions of individuals and families living with genetic conditions

The Genetics Society of Canada (GSC); http://life.biology.mcmaster.ca/GSC—a group that promotes research and communicates the results and implications of genetics to the public

GeneTests http://www.genetests.org—a publicly funded medical genetics information resource developed for physicians, other healthcare providers, and researchers

OMIM Online Mendelian Inheritance in Man http://www.ncbi.nlm.nih.gov/entrez/query.fcgi?db=OMIM—a catalogue of human genes and genetic disorders

Guidelines recommend that anemia be quantified using hemoglobin level rather than hematocrit, because that measurement is a better assessment of circulating oxygen (Eschbach, 2001).

Pain

Genitourinary pain is usually caused by distention of some portion of the urinary tract because of obstructed urine flow or inflammation and swelling of tissues. Severity of pain is related to the sudden onset rather than the extent of distention.

Table 43-1 lists the various types of genitourinary pain, characteristics of the pain, associated signs and symptoms, and possible causes. However, kidney disease does not always involve pain. It tends to be diagnosed because of other symptoms that cause a patient to seek health care, such as pedal edema, shortness of breath, and changes in urine elimination (Kuebler, 2001).

Changes in Voiding

Voiding (micturition) is normally a painless function occurring approximately eight times in a 24-hour period. The average person voids 1,200 to 1,500 mL of urine in 24 hours, although this amount varies depending on fluid intake, sweating, environmental temperature, vomiting, or diarrhea. Common problems associated with voiding include frequency, urgency, dysuria, hesitancy, incontinence, enuresis, polyuria, oliguria, and hematuria. These problems and others are described in Table 43-2. Increased urinary urgency and frequency coupled with decreasing urine volumes strongly suggest urine retention. Depending on the acuity of the onset of these symptoms, immediate bladder emptying via catheterization and evaluation are necessary to prevent kidney dysfunction (Gray, 2000a).

Gastrointestinal Symptoms

Gastrointestinal symptoms may occur with urologic conditions because of shared autonomic and sensory innervation and renointestinal reflexes. The anatomic relation of the right kidney to the colon, duodenum, head of the pancreas, common bile duct, liver, and gallbladder may cause gastrointestinal disturbances. The proximity of the left kidney to the colon (splenic flexure), stomach, pancreas, and spleen may also result in intestinal symptoms. The most common signs and symptoms include nausea, vomiting, diarrhea, abdominal discomfort, and abdominal distention. Urologic symptoms can mimic such disorders as appendicitis, peptic ulcer disease, or cholecystitis, thus making diagnosis difficult, especially in the elderly, because of decreased neurologic innervation to this area (Kuebler, 2001; Wade-Elliot, 1999).

PHYSICAL EXAMINATION

Several body systems can affect upper and lower urinary tract dysfunction, and that dysfunction can affect several end organs; therefore, a head-to-toe assessment is indicated. Areas of emphasis include the abdomen, suprapubic region, genitalia and lower back, and lower extremities.

Direct palpation of the kidneys may help determine their size and mobility. The correct position for palpation is presented in Figure 43-5. It may be possible to feel the smooth, rounded lower pole of the kidney between the hands, although the right kidney is easier to feel because it is somewhat lower than the left one. In obese patients, palpation of the kidneys is generally more difficult.

Renal dysfunction may produce tenderness over the costovertebral angle, which is the angle formed by the lower border of the 12th, or bottom, rib and the spine. The abdomen (just slightly to the right and left of midline in both upper quadrants) is auscultated to assess for bruits (low-pitched murmurs that indicate renal artery stenosis or an aortic aneurysm). The abdomen is also assessed for the presence of peritoneal fluid, which may occur with kidney dysfunction.

The bladder should be percussed after the patient voids to check for residual urine. Percussion of the bladder begins at the midline just above the umbilicus and proceeds downward. The sound changes from tympanic to dull when percussing over the bladder. The bladder, which can be palpated only if it is moderately distended, feels like a smooth, firm, round mass rising out of the abdomen, usually at midline (Fig. 43-6). Dullness to percussion of the bladder following voiding indicates incomplete bladder emptying.

Table 43-1 • Identifying Characteristics of Genitourinary Pain

TYPE	LOCATION	CHARACTER	ASSOCIATED SIGNS AND SYMPTOMS	POSSIBLE ETIOLOGY
Kidney	Costovertebral angle, may extend to umbilicus	Dull constant ache; if sudden distention of capsule, pain is severe, sharp, stabbing, and colicky in nature	Nausea and vomiting, diaphoresis, pallor, signs of shock	Acute obstruction, kidney stone, blood clot, acute pyelonephritis, trauma
Bladder	Suprapubic area	Dull, continuous pain, may be intense with voiding, may be severe if bladder full	Urgency, pain at end of voiding, painful straining	Overdistended bladder, infection, interstitial cystitis; tumour
Ureteral	Costovertebral angle, flank, lower abdominal area, testis, or labium	Severe, sharp, stabbing pain, colicky in nature	Nausea and vomiting, paralytic ileus	Ureteral stone, edema or stricture, blood clot
Prostatic	Perineum and rectum	Vague discomfort, feeling of fullness in perineum, vague back pain	Suprapubic tenderness, obstruction to urine flow; frequency, urgency, dysuria, nocturia	Prostatic cancer, acute or chronic prostatitis
Urethral	Male: along penis to meatus; female: urethra to meatus	Pain variable, most severe during and immediately after voiding	Frequency, urgency, dysuria, nocturia, urethral discharge	Irritation of bladder neck, infection of urethra, trauma, foreign body in lower urinary tract

Table 43-2 • **Problems Associated With Changes in Voiding**

PROBLEM	DEFINITION	POSSIBLE ETIOLOGY
Frequency	Frequent voiding—more than every 2 hours	Infection, obstruction of lower urinary tract leading to residual urine and overflow, anxiety, diuretics, benign prostatic hyperplasia, urethral stricture, diabetic neuropathy
Urgency	Strong desire to void	Infection, chronic prostatitis, urethritis, obstruction of lower urinary tract leading to residual urine and overflow, anxiety, diuretics, benign prostatic hyperplasia, urethral stricture, diabetic neuropathy
Dysuria	Painful or difficult voiding	Lower urinary tract infection, inflammation of bladder or urethra, acute prostatitis, stones, foreign bodies, tumours in bladder
Hesitancy	Delay, difficulty in initiating voiding	Benign prostatic hyperplasia, compression of urethra, outlet obstruction, neurogenic bladder
Nocturia	Excessive urination at night	Decreased renal concentrating ability, heart failure, diabetes mellitus, incomplete bladder emptying, excessive fluid intake at bedtime, nephrotic syndrome, cirrhosis with ascites
Incontinence	Involuntary loss of urine	External urinary sphincter injury, obstetric injury, lesions of bladder neck, detrusor dysfunction, infection, neurogenic bladder, medications, neurologic abnormalities
Enuresis	Involuntary voiding during sleep	Delay in functional maturation of central nervous system (bladder control usually achieved by 5 years of age), obstructive disease of lower urinary tract, genetic factors, failure to concentrate urine, urinary tract infection, psychological stress
Polyuria	Increased volume of urine voided	Diabetes mellitus, diabetes insipidus, use of diuretics, excess fluid intake, lithium toxicity, some forms of kidney disease (hypercalcemic and hypokalemic nephropathy)
Oliguria	Urine output less than 400 mL/day	Acute or chronic renal failure (see Chap. 45), inadequate fluid intake
Anuria	Urine output less than 50 mL/day	Acute or chronic renal failure (see Chap. 45), complete obstruction
Hematuria	Red blood cells in the urine	Cancer of genitourinary tract, acute glomerulonephritis, renal stones, renal tuberculosis, blood dyscrasia, trauma, extreme exercise, rheumatic fever, hemophilia, leukemia, sickle cell trait or disease
Proteinuria	Abnormal amounts of protein in the urine	Acute and chronic renal disease, nephrotic syndrome, vigourous exercise, heat stroke, severe heart failure, diabetic nephropathy, multiple myeloma

In older men, benign prostatic hyperplasia (BPH) is a common cause of urinary dysfunction. Because the signs and symptoms of prostate cancer can mimic those of BPH, the prostate gland is palpated by digital rectal examination (DRE) as part of the yearly physical examination in men ages 50 and older (45 if there is a family history of prostate cancer). In addition, a blood specimen is obtained to test the prostate specific antigen (PSA) level annually; the results of the DRE and PSA are then correlated. Blood is drawn for PSA before the DRE because manipulation of the prostate can cause the PSA level to rise temporarily. The inguinal area is examined for enlarged nodes, an inguinal or femoral hernia, or varicocele (varicose veins of the spermatic cord) (American Foundation for Urological Disease, 2000; Degler, 2001).

In women, the vulva, urethral meatus, and vagina are examined. The urethra is palpated for diverticula and the vagina is assessed for adequate estrogen effect and any of five types of herniation (Goolsby, 2001). Urethrocele is the bulging of the anterior vaginal wall into the urethra. Cystocele is the herniation of the bladder wall into the vaginal vault. The cervix bulging into the vaginal vault is referred to as pelvic prolapse. Enterocele is herniation of the bowel into the posterior vaginal wall, and rectocele is the herniation of the rectum into the vaginal wall. These prolapses are graded depending on the degree of herniation (see Chap. 47 for more information).

The woman is asked to cough and perform a Valsalva manoeuvre to assess the urethra's system of muscular and ligament support. If urine leakage occurs, the index and middle fingers of the examiner's gloved hand are used to support either side of the urethra as the woman is asked to repeat these manoeuvres. This is called the Marshall-Boney manoeuvre.

If no urine leakage is detected when external support is provided to the urethra, poor pelvic floor support—referred to as urethral hypermobility—is identified as the suspected cause of the urinary incontinence. Stress urinary incontinence (SUI) is graded based on its severity. Grade 1 and Grade 2 SUI relate to the degree of urethral hypermobility. Grade 3, the most severe form of SUI, refers to the inability of the urethral walls to remain compressed with abdominal pressure such as a cough or Valsalva manoeuvre. Grade 3 is referred to as intrinsic sphincter deficiency (ISD) (Albaugh, 1999).

If some residual leakage of urine is noted despite support, ISD is suspected. Urethral hypermobility may be suspected when Q-tip test results are positive. The Q-tip test involves gently placing a well-lubricated Q-tip into the urethra until resistance is no longer noted, then gently pulling back on the Q-tip until resistance is felt. The female patient is asked to cough and perform the Valsalva manoeuvre. If there is an upward (positive deflection) of the visible part of the Q-tip, urethral hypermobility is at least one of the causes for the type of incontinence referred to as stress incontinence (see Chap. 44) (Albaugh, 1999).

The patient is assessed for edema and changes in body weight. Edema may be observed, particularly in the face and dependent parts of the body, such as the ankles and sacral areas, and suggests fluid retention. An increase in body weight commonly accompanies edema. A 1-kg weight gain equals approximately 1,000 mL of fluid.

FIGURE 43-5 Technique for palpating the right kidney (**top**). Place one hand under the patient's back with the fingers under the lower rib. Place the palm of the other hand anterior to the kidney with fingers above the umbilicus. Push the hand on top forward as the patient inhales deeply. The left kidney (**bottom**) is palpated similarly by reaching over to the patient's left side and placing the right hand beneath the patient's lower left rib. From Weber, J. W., & Kelley, J. (2003). *Health assessment in nursing.* Philadelphia: Lippincott Williams & Wilkins.

The deep tendon reflexes of the knee are assessed for quality and symmetry. This is an important part of testing for neurological causes of bladder dysfunction because the sacral area, which innervates the lower extremities, is the same peripheral nerve area responsible for urinary continence. The gait pattern of the individual with bladder dysfunction is also noted, as well as the patient's ability to walk toe-to-heel. These tests evaluate possible supraspinal causes for urinary incontinence (Appell, 1999).

 Gerontologic Considerations

Upper and lower urinary tract function changes with age. The GFR decreases with age starting between ages 35 and 40. A yearly decline of about 1 mL/min continues thereafter. Tubular function, including reabsorption and concentrating ability, is also reduced with increasing age. Although renal function usually remains adequate despite these changes, renal reserve is decreased and may reduce the kidneys' ability to respond effectively to drastic or sudden physiologic changes. This steady decrease in glomerular filtration, combined with the use of multiple medications whose metabolites clear the body via the kidneys, puts the older individual at higher risk for adverse drug effects and drug-to-drug interactions (Schafer, 2001).

Structural or functional abnormalities that occur with aging may prevent complete emptying of the bladder. This may be due

to decreased bladder wall contractility, due to myogenic or neurogenic causes, or structurally, related to bladder outlet obstruction, as in BPH. Vaginal and urethral tissues atrophy (become thinner) in aging women due to decreased estrogen levels. This causes decreased blood supply to the urogenital tissues, causing urethral and vaginal irritation and urinary incontinence.

Urinary incontinence is the most common reason for admission to skilled nursing facilities. Many older individuals and their families are unaware that urinary incontinence stems from many causes. The nurse needs to inform the patient and family that with appropriate evaluation, urinary incontinence can often be managed at home and in many cases can be eliminated (Degler, 2000). Many treatments are available for urinary incontinence in the elderly, including noninvasive, behavioural interventions that the individual or the caregiver can carry out (Kincade, Peckous & Busby-Whitehead, 2001). Treatment modalities for urinary incontinence are described in further detail in Chapter 44.

Preparation of the elderly patient for diagnostic tests must be managed carefully to prevent dehydration, which might precipitate renal failure in a patient with marginal renal reserve. Limitations in mobility may affect an elderly patient's ability to void adequately or to consume an adequate volume of fluids. The patient may limit fluid intake to minimize the frequency of voiding or the risk of incontinence. Teaching the patient and family about the dangers of an inadequate fluid intake is an important role of the nurse caring for the elderly patient.

Diagnostic Evaluation

URINALYSIS AND URINE CULTURE

The urinalysis provides important clinical information on kidney function and helps diagnose other diseases, such as diabetes. The urine culture determines if bacteria are present in the urine, as well as their strains and concentration. Urine culture and sensitivity also identify the antimicrobial therapy that is best suited for the particular strains identified, taking into consideration the antibiotics that have the best rate of resolution in that particular geographic region. Appropriate evaluation of any abnormality can assist in detecting serious underlying diseases.

Urine examination includes the following:

- Urine colour (Table 43-3)
- Urine clarity and odour
- Urine pH and specific gravity
- Tests to detect protein, glucose, and ketone bodies in the urine (proteinuria, glycosuria, and ketonuria, respectively)
- Microscopic examination of the urine sediment after centrifuging to detect RBCs (**hematuria**), white blood cells, casts (cylindruria), crystals (crystalluria), pus (**pyuria**), and bacteria (**bacteriuria**)

Significance of Findings

Several abnormalities, such as hematuria and proteinuria, produce no symptoms but may be detected during a routine urinalysis using a dipstick. Normally, about 1 million RBCs pass into the urine daily, which is equivalent to one to three RBCs per high-power field. Hematuria (more than three RBCs per high-power field) can develop from an abnormality anywhere along the genitourinary tract. Common causes include acute infection (cystitis, urethritis, or prostatitis), renal calculi, and neoplasm. Other causes include systemic disorders, such as bleeding disorders; malignant lesions; and medications, such as warfarin (Coumadin)

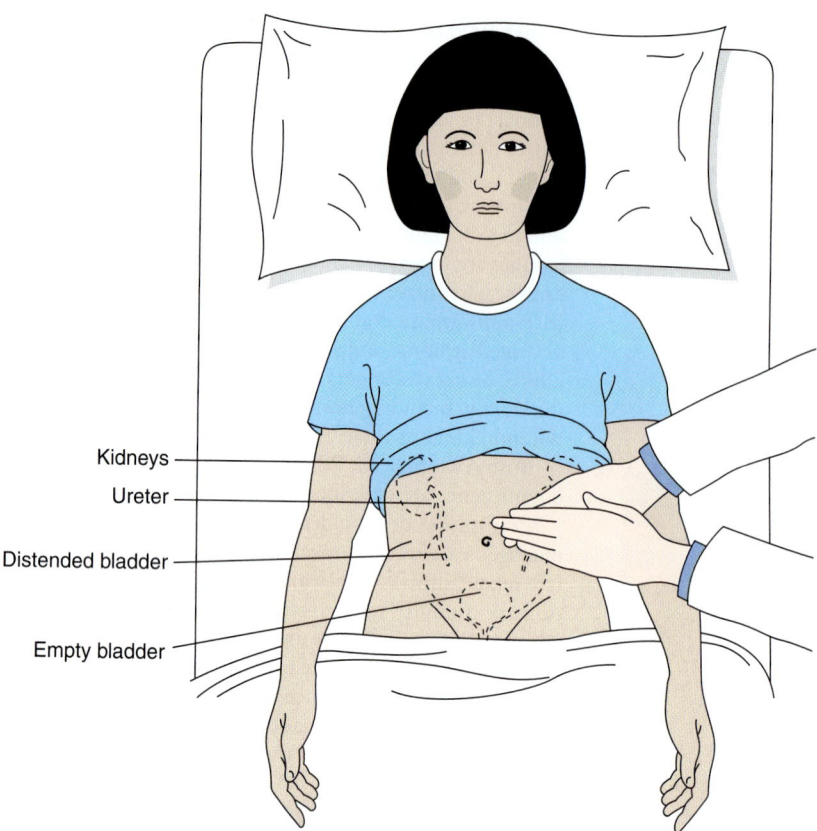

Kidneys

Ureter

Distended bladder

Empty bladder

FIGURE 43-6 Palpation of the bladder.

and heparin. Although hematuria may initially be detected using a dipstick test, further microscopic evaluation is necessary (National Institute of Diabetes & Digestive & Kidney Diseases [NIDDK], 1999).

Protein in the urine (proteinuria) may be a benign finding, or it may signify serious disease. Occasional loss of up to 150 mg/day of protein in the urine, primarily albumin and Tamm-Horsfall protein, is considered normal and usually does not require further evaluation. A dipstick examination, which can detect from 1.6 to 55 mmol/L of protein, should be used as a screening test only, because urine concentration, pH, hematuria, and radiocontrast materials all affect the results. Because dipstick analysis does not detect protein concentrations of less than 1.6 mmol/L, the test cannot be used for early detection of diabetic nephropathy. Micro-albuminuria (excretion of 1.1 to 11 mmol/L of protein in the urine) is an early sign of diabetic nephropathy. Common benign causes of transient proteinuria are fever, strenuous exercise, and prolonged standing.

Causes of persistent proteinuria include glomerular diseases, malignancies, collagen diseases, diabetes mellitus, preeclampsia, hypothyroidism, heart failure, exposure to heavy metals, and use of medications, such as nonsteroidal anti-inflammatory drugs (NSAIDs) and angiotensin-converting enzyme inhibitors (NIDDK, 2000).

RENAL FUNCTION TESTS

Renal function tests are used to evaluate the severity of kidney disease and to assess the patient's clinical progress. These tests also provide information on the effectiveness of the kidney in carrying out its excretory function. Renal function test results may be within normal limits until the GFR is reduced to less than 50%

of normal. Renal function can be assessed most accurately if several tests are performed and their results analyzed together. Common tests of renal function include renal concentration tests, creatinine clearance, and serum creatinine and blood urea nitrogen levels. Table 43-4 describes the purpose and normal ranges for each. Other helpful tests for evaluating renal function are serum electrolyte levels.

X-RAY FILMS AND OTHER IMAGING MODALITIES

Kidney, Ureter, and Bladder Studies

An x-ray study of the abdomen or kidney, ureters, and bladder (KUB) may be performed to delineate the size, shape, and position of the kidneys and to reveal any abnormalities, such as calculi (stones) in the kidneys or urinary tract, hydronephrosis (distention of the pelvis of the kidney), cysts, tumours, or kidney displacement by abnormalities in surrounding tissues.

General Ultrasonography

Ultrasonography is a noninvasive procedure that uses sound waves passed into the body through a transducer to detect abnormalities of internal tissues and organs. Structures of the urinary system create characteristic ultrasonographic images. Abnormalities such as fluid accumulation, masses, congenital malformations, changes in organ size, or obstructions can be identified. During the test, the lower abdomen and genitalia may need to be exposed. Ultrasonography requires a full bladder; therefore, fluid intake should be encouraged before the procedure. Because of its sensitivity, ultra-

NURSING RESEARCH PROFILE 43-1

Diary-Keeping as a Predictor of Urinary Incontinence Treatment Success

Kincade, J. E., Peckous, B. K., & Busby-Whitehead, J. (2001). A pilot study to determine predictors of behavioural treatment completion for urinary incontinence. *Urologic Nursing, 21*(1), 39–44.

Purpose

Urinary incontinence (UI) affects approximately 13 million Americans. The usual behavioural interventions include a program of pelvic muscle strengthening. Despite the well-documented safety and efficacy of this intervention, high rates of patient withdrawal have been reported. The purpose of this study was to determine the characteristics that best predict completion of behavioural treatment for UI in an outpatient setting.

Study Sample and Design

The sample for this descriptive study was obtained from a university-affiliated clinic that provided community-based care for adults with UI. To be eligible for inclusion in the study, subjects had to be 50 years old or older. They also had to complete an initial clinic visit and perform pelvic floor exercises augmented with biofeedback prescribed by the clinician. Data collected by review of clinic records for the study included demographic data (age, gender, race, and education level), incontinence-related variables (initial treatment goal; frequency, amount, and duration of urine loss; type of incontinence and presence of nocturia), service-related variables (distance to clinic, source of referral to the UI clinic, previous efforts to get provider help for UI, and completion of a 7-day bladder diary), and health-related variables (number of comorbidities and of prescription medications). Program completion was the study's dependent variable.

Findings

Of the 156 patients in the UI clinic, 98 met the study criteria. The majority of participants were older, Caucasian, well-educated women with mainly urge and mixed urinary incontinence of many years' duration. Over half (55.1%) of the patients completed the treatment program. The only characteristic that differed significantly ($p \leq 0.0001$) in those who completed the program and those who did not was completion of a 7-day bladder diary. Those who completed the 7-day bladder diary before the program study was initiated were much more likely to complete the program than those who did not complete the diary.

Nursing Implications

Completion of a 7-day voiding diary before beginning a behavioural continence program is usually considered pivotal for an accurate record of day-to-day bladder status, and the data obtained from the review are important in assessing the effectiveness of the treatment. Clinicians need to assess the patient's reasons for unwillingness or inability to complete the diary. Protocols or treatment strategies should be developed for this subset of patients so that they can benefit from this noninvasive, effective treatment modality for UI.

Table 43-3 • Changes in Urine Colour and Possible Causes

URINE COLOUR	POSSIBLE CAUSE
Colourless to pale yellow	Dilute urine due to diuretics, alcohol consumption, diabetes insipidus, glycosuria, excess fluid intake, renal disease
Yellow to milky white	Pyuria, infection, vaginal cream
Bright yellow	Multiple vitamin preparations
Pink to red	Hemoglobin breakdown, red blood cells, gross blood, menses, bladder or prostate surgery, beets, blackberries, medications (phenytoin, rifampin, phenothiazine, cascara, senna products)
Blue, blue green	Dyes, methylene blue, *Pseudomonas* species organisms, medications (amitriptyline, triamterene, phenylsalicylate)
Orange to amber	Concentrated urine due to dehydration, fever, bile, excess bilirubin or carotene, medications (phenazopyridium HCl, nitrofurantoin, sulfasalazine, ducusate calcium, thiamine)
Brown to black	Old red blood cells, urobilinogen, bilirubin, melanin, porphyrin, extremely concentrated urine due to dehydration, medications (cascara, metronidazole, iron preparations, quinine, senna products, methyldopa, nitrofurantoin)

catheterization during the initial stages of an intermittent catheterization training program. Portable, battery-operated devices are available for bedside use. The scan head is placed on the patient's abdomen and directed toward the bladder. The device automatically calculates and displays urine volume.

Computed Tomography and Magnetic Resonance Imaging

Computed tomography (CT) and magnetic resonance imaging (MRI) are noninvasive techniques that provide excellent cross-sectional views of the kidney and urinary tract. They are used in evaluating genitourinary masses, nephrolithiasis, chronic renal infections, renal or urinary tract trauma, metastatic disease, and soft tissue abnormalities. The nurse should explain to the patient that a sedative may be prescribed. Claustrophobia is often a problem, especially with MRI. Patient preparation for the MRI includes removal of any metallic objects, such as jewelry or clothing with metallic clasps. Credit cards should be kept away from the MRI area because of their magnetic strips. MRI is contraindicated in patients with pacemakers, surgical clips, or any metallic objects anywhere in the body. Occasionally, an oral or intravenous radiopaque contrast material is used in CT scanning to enhance visualization. Nursing care guidelines for patient preparation and test precautions for any imaging procedure requiring a contrast agent (also called contrast medium) are explained in Chart 43-3.

sonography has replaced many other tests as the initial diagnostic procedure.

Bladder Ultrasonography

Bladder ultrasonography is a noninvasive method of measuring urine volume in the bladder. It may be indicated for urinary frequency, inability to void after removal of an indwelling urinary catheter, measurement of postvoiding residual urine volume, inability to void postoperatively, or assessment of the need for

Table 43-4 • Renal Function Tests

TEST	PURPOSE	NORMAL VALUES		
Renal Concentration Tests				
Specific gravity	Evaluates ability of kidneys to concentrate solutes in urine.	1.010–1.025		
Urine osmolality	Concentrating ability is lost early in kidney disease; hence, these test findings may disclose early defects in renal function.	300–900 mmol/kg/24 h, 50–1,200 mmol/kg random sample		
24-Hour Urine Test				
Creatinine clearance	Detects and evaluates progression of renal disease. Test measures volume of blood cleared of endogenous creatinine in 1 minute, which provides an approximation of the glomerular filtration rate. Sensitive indicator of renal disease used to follow progression of renal disease.	Measured in mL/minute/1.73 m²		
		Age	Male	Female
		Under 30	88–146	81–134
		30–40	82–140	75–128
		40–50	75–133	69–122
		50–60	68–126	64–116
		60–70	61–120	58–110
		70–80	55–113	52–105
Serum Tests				
Creatinine level	Measures effectiveness of renal function. Creatinine is end product of muscle energy metabolism. In normal function, level of creatinine, which is regulated and excreted by the kidneys, remains fairly constant in body.	50–110 μmol/L		
Urea nitrogen (blood urea nitrogen [BUN])	Serves as index of renal function. Urea is nitrogenous end product of protein metabolism. Test values are affected by protein intake, tissue breakdown, and fluid volume changes.	.4–1.0 mmol/L Patients over age 60 years: .4–1.1 mmol/L		
BUN to creatinine ratio	Evaluates hydration status. An elevated ratio is seen in hypovolemia; a normal ratio with an elevated BUN and creatinine is seen with intrinsic renal disease.	About 10 : 1		

Chart 43-3

Patient Care During Urologic Testing With Contrast Agents

For some patients, contrast agents are nephrotoxic and allergenic. The following guidelines can help the nurse and other caregivers respond quickly in the event of a problem.

Nursing Actions for Room Preparation

- Have emergency equipment and medications available in case the patient has an anaphylactic reaction to the contrast agent. Emergency supplies include epinephrine, corticosteroids, and vasopressors; oxygen; and airway and suction equipment.

Nursing Actions for Patient Preparation

- Obtain the patient's allergy history with emphasis on allergy to iodine, shellfish, and other seafood, because many contrast agents contain iodine.
- Notify physician and radiologist if the patient is allergic or suspected to be allergic to iodine.
- Obtain health history. Contrast agents should be used with caution in older patients and patients who have diabetes mellitus, multiple myeloma, renal insufficiency, or volume depletion.
- Inform the patient that he or she may experience a temporary feeling of warmth, flushing of the face, and an unusual flavor (seafood) in the mouth when the contrast agent is infused.
- Monitor patient closely for allergic reaction and monitor urine output.

Nuclear Scans

Nuclear scans require injection of a radioisotope (technetium-99m–labelled compound or iodine-131 hippurate) into the circulatory system; the isotope is then monitored as it moves through the blood vessels of the kidneys. A scintillation camera is placed behind the kidney with the patient in a supine, prone, or seated position. Hypersensitivity to the radioisotope is rare. The technetium scan provides information about kidney perfusion; the hippurate scan provides information about kidney function.

Nuclear scans are used to evaluate acute and chronic renal failure, renal masses, and blood flow before and after kidney transplantation. The radioisotope is injected at a specified time before the study to achieve the proper concentration in the kidneys. After the procedure is completed, the patient is encouraged to drink fluids to promote excretion of the radioisotope by the kidneys.

Intravenous Urography

Intravenous urography includes various tests such as excretory urography, intravenous pyelography (IVP), and infusion drip pyelography. A radiopaque contrast agent is administered intravenously. An IVP, or intravenous urogram, shows the kidneys, ureter, and bladder via x-ray imaging as dye moves through the upper and then lower urinary system. A nephrotomogram may be carried out as part of the study to visualize different layers of the kidney and the diffuse structures within each layer and to differentiate solid masses or lesions from cysts in the kidneys or urinary tract.

Intravenous urography may be used as the initial assessment of any suspected urologic problem, especially lesions in the kidneys and ureters. It also provides a rough estimate of renal function. After the contrast agent (sodium diatrizoate or meglumine diatrizoate) is administered intravenously, multiple x-rays are obtained to visualize drainage structures.

Infusion drip pyelography requires an intravenous infusion of a large volume of a dilute contrast agent to opacify the renal parenchyma and fill the urinary tract. This examination method is useful when prolonged opacification of the drainage structures is desired so that tomograms (body-section radiography) can be made. Images are obtained at specified intervals after the start of the infusion. These images show the filled and distended collecting system. The patient preparation is the same as for excretory urography, except that fluids are not restricted.

Retrograde Pyelography

In retrograde pyelography, catheters are advanced through the ureters into the renal pelvis by means of cystoscopy. A contrast agent is then injected. Retrograde pyelography is usually performed if intravenous urography provides inadequate visualization of the collecting systems. It may also be used before extracorporeal shock-wave lithotripsy or in patients with urologic cancer who need follow-up and are allergic to intravenous contrast agents. Possible complications include infection, hematuria, and perforation of the ureter. Retrograde pyelography is used infrequently because of improved techniques in excretory urography.

Cystography

Cystography aids in evaluating vesicoureteral reflux (backflow of urine from the bladder into one or both ureters) and assessing the patient for bladder injury. A catheter is inserted into the bladder, and a contrast agent is instilled to outline the bladder wall. The contrast agent may leak through a small bladder perforation stemming from bladder injury, but such leakage is usually harmless. Cystography can also be performed with simultaneous pressure recordings inside the bladder.

Voiding Cystourethrography

Voiding cystourethrography uses fluoroscopy to visualize the lower urinary tract and assess urine storage in the bladder. It is commonly used as a diagnostic tool to identify vesicoureteral reflux (between bladder and ureter). A urethral catheter is inserted, and a contrast agent is instilled into the bladder. When the bladder is full and the patient feels the urge to void, the catheter is removed, and the patient voids. Retrograde urethrography, in which a contrast agent is injected retrograde into the urethra, is always performed before urethral catheterization if urethral trauma is suspected.

Renal Angiography

A renal angiogram, or renal arteriogram, provides an image of the renal arteries. The femoral (or axillary) artery is pierced with a needle, and a catheter is threaded up through the femoral and iliac arteries into the aorta or renal artery. A contrast agent is injected to opacify the renal arterial supply. Angiography is used to evaluate renal blood flow in suspected renal trauma, to differentiate renal cysts from tumours, and to evaluate hypertension. It is used preoperatively for renal transplantation. Before the procedure, a laxative may be prescribed to evacuate the colon so that unobstructed x-rays can be obtained. Injection sites (groin for femoral approach or axilla for axillary approach) may be shaved. The peripheral pulse sites (radial, femoral, and dorsalis pedis) are marked for easy access during postprocedural assessment. The patient is informed that there may be a brief sensation of heat along the course of the vessel when the contrast agent is injected.

After the procedure, vital signs are monitored until stable. If the axillary artery was the injection site, blood pressure measurements are taken on the opposite arm. The injection site is examined for swelling and hematoma. Peripheral pulses are palpated, and the colour and temperature of the involved extremity are noted and compared with those of the uninvolved extremity. Cold compresses may be applied to the injection site to decrease edema and pain. Possible complications include hematoma formation, arterial thrombosis or dissection, false aneurysm formation, and altered renal function.

UROLOGIC ENDOSCOPIC PROCEDURES

Endourology, or urologic endoscopic procedures, can be performed in one of two ways: using a cystoscope inserted into the urethra, or percutaneously, through a small incision.

The cystoscopic examination is used to directly visualize the urethra and bladder. The cystoscope, which is inserted through the urethra into the bladder, has a self-contained optical lens system that provides a magnified, illuminated view of the bladder (Fig. 43-7). The use of a high-intensity light and interchangeable lenses allows excellent visualization and permits still and motion pictures to be taken. The cystoscope is manipulated to allow complete visualization of the urethra and bladder as well as the ureteral orifices and prostatic urethra. Small ureteral catheters can be passed through the cystoscope, allowing assessment of the ureters and the pelvis of each kidney.

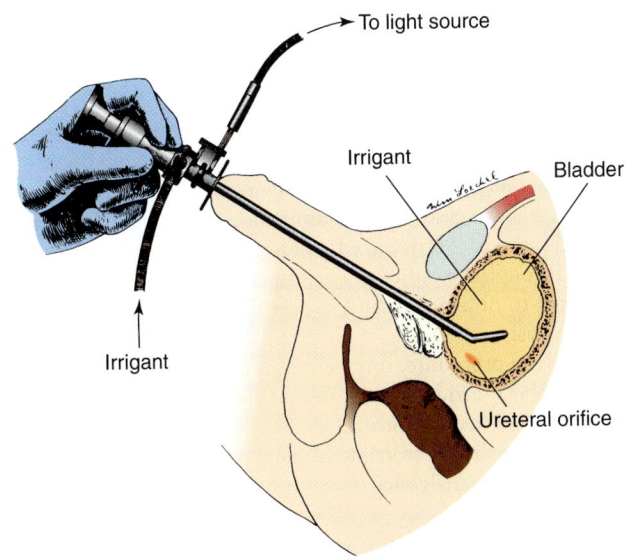

FIGURE 43-7 Cystoscopic examination. A cystoscope is introduced into the bladder. The upper cord is an electric line for the light at the distal end of the cystoscope. The lower tubing leads from a reservoir of sterile irrigant that is used to inflate the bladder.

The cystoscope also permits the urologist to obtain a urine specimen from each kidney to evaluate its function. Cup forceps can be inserted through the cystoscope for biopsy. Calculi may be removed from the urethra, bladder, and ureter using cystoscopy. If a lower tract cystoscopy is performed, the patient is usually awake and the procedure is usually no more uncomfortable than a catheterization. To minimize post-test urethral discomfort, viscous lidocaine is usually injected several minutes prior to the study. If the cystoscopy includes examination of the upper tracts, a sedative may be administered before the procedure. General anesthesia is usually administered to ensure that there are no involuntary muscle spasms when the scope is being passed through the ureters or kidney.

The nurse describes the examination to the patient and family to prepare them and to allay their fears. If an upper cystoscopy is to be performed, the patient is usually kept NPO (nothing by mouth) for several hours beforehand, unless the examination is being done to assess structural integrity following trauma.

Postprocedural management is directed at relieving any discomfort resulting from the examination. Some burning on voiding, blood-tinged urine, and urinary frequency from trauma to the mucous membrane can be expected. Moist heat to the lower abdomen and warm sitz baths are helpful in relieving pain and relaxing the muscles.

After a cystoscopic examination, the patient with obstructive pathology may experience urine retention if the instruments used during the examination caused edema. The nurse carefully monitors the patient with prostatic hyperplasia for urine retention. Warm sitz baths and antispasmodic medication, such as flavoxate (Urispas), may be prescribed to relieve temporary urine retention due to poor relaxation of the urinary sphincter; however, intermittent catheterization may be necessary for a few hours after the examination. The nurse monitors the patient for signs and symptoms of urinary tract infection. Because edema of the urethra secondary to local trauma may obstruct urine flow, the patient is also monitored for signs and symptoms of obstruction (NIDDK, 2001a).

BIOPSY

Renal and Ureteral Brush Biopsy

Brush biopsy techniques provide specific information when abnormal x-ray findings of the ureter or renal pelvis raise questions about whether the defect is a tumour, a stone, a blood clot, or an artefact. First, a cystoscopic examination is conducted. Then, a ureteral catheter is introduced, followed by a biopsy brush that is passed through the catheter. The suspected lesion is brushed back and forth to obtain cells and surface tissue fragments for histologic analysis.

After the procedure, intravenous fluids may be administered to help clear the kidneys and prevent clot formation. Urine may contain blood (usually clearing in 24 to 48 hours) from oozing at the brushing site. Postoperative renal colic occasionally occurs and responds to analgesics.

Kidney Biopsy

Biopsy of the kidney is used in diagnosing and evaluating the extent of kidney disease. Indications for biopsy include unexplained acute renal failure, persistent proteinuria or hematuria, transplant rejection, and glomerulopathies. A small section of renal cortex is obtained either percutaneously (needle biopsy) or by open biopsy through a small flank incision. Before the biopsy is carried out, coagulation studies are conducted to identify any risk for postbiopsy bleeding. Contraindications to a kidney biopsy include bleeding tendencies, uncontrolled hypertension, and a solitary kidney.

PROCEDURE

The patient may be placed on a fasting regimen 6 to 8 hours before the test. An intravenous line is established. A urine specimen is obtained and saved for comparison with the postbiopsy specimen.

If a needle biopsy is to be performed, the patient is instructed to breathe in and hold that breath (to prevent the kidney from moving) while the needle is being inserted. The sedated patient is placed in a prone position with a sandbag under the abdomen. The skin at the biopsy site is infiltrated with a local anesthetic. The biopsy needle is introduced just inside the renal capsule of the outer quadrant of the kidney. The location of the needle may be confirmed by fluoroscopy or by ultrasound, in which case a special probe is used.

With open biopsy, a small incision is made over the kidney, allowing direct visualization. Preparation for an open biopsy is similar to that for any major abdominal surgery (NIDDK, 2001b).

NURSING INTERVENTIONS

After the tissue specimen is obtained, pressure is applied to the biopsy site. The patient may be kept in a prone position immediately after biopsy and on bed rest for 6 to 8 hours to minimize the risk of bleeding.

Monitoring and Managing Potential Complications. Potential postbiopsy complications include persistent hematuria, fistula or aneurysm formation, or laceration of organs or blood vessels adjacent to the kidney. The nurse monitors the patient closely for hematuria, which may appear soon after biopsy. The kidney is a highly vascular organ, and about one fourth of the entire cardiac output circulates through it in about 1 minute. The passage of the biopsy needle punctures the kidney capsule, and bleeding can occur in the perirenal space. Usually the bleeding subsides on its own, but a large amount of blood can accumulate in this space in a short time without noticeable signs until cardiovascular collapse is evident.

Nursing interventions after a kidney biopsy include:

- Monitor vital signs every 5 to 15 minutes for the first hour to detect early signs of bleeding, and then with decreasing frequency as indicated.
- Be alert for signs and symptoms that suggest bleeding, including a rise or fall in blood pressure, tachycardia, anorexia, vomiting, and the development of a dull, aching discomfort in the abdomen.
- Immediately report any symptoms of backache, shoulder pain, or dysuria.

Flank pain may occur but usually represents bleeding into the muscle rather than around the kidney. Colicky pain similar to that of ureteral colic may develop when a clot is present in the ureter; there may be excruciating, sharp flank pain that radiates to the groin.

All urine that the patient voids is inspected for evidence of bleeding and compared with the prebiopsy specimen and subsequent voiding samples. If bleeding persists, as indicated by an enlarging hematoma, the abdomen should not be palpated or manipulated.

Hematocrit and hemoglobin levels are obtained within 8 hours to assess for changes; decreasing levels may indicate bleeding. Usually, the fluid intake is maintained at 3,000 mL/day unless the patient has renal insufficiency. If bleeding occurs, the patient is prepared for blood component therapy and surgical intervention to control the hemorrhage; surgical drainage or, rarely, nephrectomy (removal of the kidney) may be needed.

Patient Teaching. Because hemorrhage can occur up to several days after the biopsy, the patient is instructed to avoid strenuous activities, sports, and heavy lifting for at least 2 weeks. The patient and family are instructed to notify the physician or clinic if any of the following occur: flank pain, hematuria, light-headedness and fainting, rapid pulse, or any other signs and symptoms of bleeding.

URODYNAMIC TESTS

Urodynamic tests provide an accurate evaluation of voiding problems, thus assisting in diagnosis. Urodynamic studies are useful in evaluating changes in bladder filling and bladder emptying. Chart 43-4 outlines patient education for all basic urodynamic tests. The following urodynamic test procedures and measurements are the most common and are often performed simultaneously (Albaugh, 1999; Appell, 1999).

Uroflowmetry

Uroflowmetry (flow rate) is the record of the volume of urine passing through the urethra per time unit (millilitres per second). The flow rate reflects the combined activity of the detrusor muscle and the bladder neck and the degree of relaxation of the urethral sphincter. Because this test depends on the amount voided, the patient is instructed to arrive for the test with a strong urge to void, but not have an overly full bladder. When urethral sphincter competency is being evaluated, uroflowmetry is combined with electromyographic (EMG) measurement of the external urethral sphincter via surface wire or needle electrodes placed at the level of the sphincter, on either side of the urethra. Uroflowmetry is often combined with cystometrography, in which case the bladder is filled as the intravesical pressure is being monitored before the voiding phase of the study.

Cystometrography

A cystometrogram (CMG) is a graphic recording of the pressures in the bladder during bladder filling and emptying. It is the major diagnostic portion of urodynamic testing. During the test, the amount of fluid instilled into the bladder and the patient's sensations of bladder fullness and urge to void are recorded. These are then compared with the pressures measured in the bladder during bladder emptying. A urethral catheter is connected to a water manometer, and sterile solution of either normal saline or water is allowed to flow into the bladder, usually at the rate of 1 mL/sec. The patient informs the examiner when the first sensation of bladder filling is felt, when mild urgency is noted, and again when the bladder feels full. The degree of bladder filling at these points is recorded. The pressures above the zero level at the symphysis pubis are measured, and the pressures and volumes within the bladder are plotted and recorded. This test measures bladder sensation, compliance of the bladder wall during filling, and functional capacity. It also evaluates any phasic or sharp increases in bladder pressure, which may or may not be associated with incontinence of the infused fluid.

Throughout and at the end of bladder filling, the degree of abdominal pressure against the bladder, which could potentially cause leaking (stress incontinence), is measured. This measurement is referred to as the **Valsalva leak-point pressure (VLPP)**. The terms VLPP and abdominal leak-point pressure can be used interchangeably.

While in a sitting or standing position, the patient is asked to cough or perform a Valsalva manoeuvre to assess whether urine leaks. Before this test is performed, it is important to determine if the patient is prone to vasovagal reactions and to alert the urodynamicist. A competent sphincter will not allow for any loss of

---

Chart 43-4 • PATIENT EDUCATION
Before and After Urodynamic Testing

In preparing the patient for urodynamic testing, the nurse instructs the patient about how urodynamic procedures are performed, what is expected of the patient, and what sensations the patient can expect afterward. The nurse reassures the patient that staff will be present during the procedure, but privacy and comfort will be maintained. Additional information for the patient follows:

- An in-depth interview will be conducted. Questions related to your urologic symptoms and voiding habits will be asked by the staff.
- You will be asked to describe sensations felt during the procedure.
- During the procedure, you might be asked to change positions (for example, from supine to sitting or standing).
- You may be asked to cough or perform the Valsalva manoeuvre (bear down) during the procedure.
- You will probably need to have one or two urethral catheters inserted so that bladder pressure and bladder filling can be measured. Another catheter may be placed in the rectum or vagina to measure abdominal pressure.
- You may also have electrodes (surface, wire, or needle) placed in the perianal area for electromyography (EMG). This may be

uncomfortable initially during insertion and later during position changes.
- Your bladder will be filled through the urethral catheter one or more times during the procedure.
- After the procedure, you may experience urinary frequency, urgency, or dysuria from the urethral catheters. Avoid caffeinated, carbonated, and alcoholic beverages after the procedure because these can further irritate the bladder. These symptoms usually decrease or subside by the day after the procedure.
- You might notice a slight hematuria (blood-tinged urine) right after the procedure (especially in men with benign prostatic hyperplasia). Drinking fluids will help to clear the hematuria.
- If the urinary meatus is irritated, a warm sitz bath may be helpful.
- Be alert for signs of a urinary tract infection after the procedure. Contact your physician if you experience fever, chills, lower back pain, or continued dysuria and hematuria.
- If you receive an antibiotic medication before the procedure, you should continue taking the complete course of medication after the procedure. This is a measure to prevent infection.

urine even with a full bladder and manoeuvres such as a cough, laugh, or position change. When minimal weakness of the urethral sphincter causes a small amount of incontinence (currently considered leakage at or above a bladder pressure of 100 cm H_2O), urethral hypermobility is the cause. When leakage occurs with a cough or the Valsalva manoeuvre at bladder pressures less than 100 cm H_2O, intrinsic sphincter deficiency is believed to contribute to the incontinence. During the cystometrogram portion of the urodynamic study, if any urine leakage is noted when the patient coughs or performs a Valsalva manoeuvre, regardless of the amount of abdominal force that caused the leaking, a diagnosis of "genuine stress urinary incontinence" is made. The VLPP determines the severity of SUI.

Urinary Pressure Flow

Urinary pressure flow is a study that is performed immediately after the filling phase of the CMG and simultaneously with the voiding CMG. Bladder pressure, urine flow, and sphincter electromyography are measured simultaneously. This allows for a detailed picture of voiding function.

Electromyography

Electromyography (EMG) involves the placement of electrodes in the pelvic floor musculature or over the area of the anal sphincter to evaluate the neuromuscular function of the lower tract. It is usually performed simultaneously with the CMG.

Videofluorourodynamic Study

The videofluorourodynamic study is considered the optimal urodynamic evaluation. This test combines a study of the filling and voiding phases of the CMG and the EMG with a simultaneous visualization of the lower urinary tract via a radiopaque filling agent in place of sterile water or saline. It allows for a complete and detailed assessment of the voiding dysfunction, which may be due in part to anatomic dysfunction.

Urethral Pressure Profile

The urethral pressure profile measures the amount of urethral pressure along the length of the urethra needed to maintain continence. Gas or fluid is instilled through a catheter that is withdrawn while the pressures along the urethral wall are obtained.

Nursing Implications

Most patients undergoing urologic testing or imaging studies are apprehensive, even those who have had these tests in the past. Patients frequently feel discomfort and embarrassment about such a private and personal function as voiding. Voiding in the presence of others can frequently cause guarding, a natural reflex that inhibits voiding due to situational anxiety. Because the outcomes of these studies determine the plan of care, the nurse must help the patient relax by providing as much privacy and explanation about the procedure as possible.

NURSING DIAGNOSIS

Potential nursing diagnoses for the patient undergoing assessment of urinary or renal function include the following:

- Deficient knowledge about the procedures and diagnostic tests
- Acute pain related to renal infection, edema, obstruction, or bleeding along the urinary tract, or to invasive diagnostic procedures
- Fear related to possible diagnosis of serious illness, altered renal function, and embarrassment secondary to discussion of urinary function, and exposure and invasion of genitalia

PLANNING, IMPLEMENTATION, AND EVALUATION

The goals, nursing interventions and rationale, and expected outcomes are discussed in greater detail in the Plan of Nursing Care. Patient and family education is essential to help the patient understand the purpose of the procedure and what to expect before, during, and after it. Pertinent home care considerations can be discussed at this time.

Promoting Home and Community-Based Care

TEACHING PATIENTS SELF-CARE

Many procedures and tests used to evaluate upper and lower urinary tract function are carried out in outpatient or short-procedure settings. Therefore, family members or other caregivers in the home may be called upon to provide postprocedural care. They need clear explanations about the procedures and tests, how to prepare for them, and what precautions, if any, need to be taken afterward. The patient and family members are provided with verbal and written explanations about monitoring that may be necessary at home and are instructed about steps to take if complications occur.

CONTINUING CARE

Follow-up telephone calls made to the patient and family at home provide an opportunity for them to ask questions and to report on the patient's status. Teaching is reinforced, and the patient is reminded of the importance of keeping follow-up appointments with primary health care providers.

 Critical Thinking Exercises

1. Following the removal of an indwelling catheter 2 days after a complete abdominal hysterectomy, your patient complains of abdominal pain. An abdominal examination confirms a distended bladder on visual observation, dullness to percussion over the suprapubic area, and pain with light palpation to this area. You confirm your suspicions of acute urine retention when a review of the urine output over the past 12 hours shows no output and the patient confirms that she has not voided since the catheter was removed. What should be your next course of action? Review the possible causes, and describe the actions you could take and the rationale for each action.

2. A 65-year-old man with newly diagnosed type 2 diabetes comes to the primary care clinic for his quarterly lab work and urinalysis. He states that he has been following the dietitian's recommendations for his diabetic diet. Results of a urinalysis demonstrate a protein level greater than 13.5 mmol/L and a glucose level greater than 22.0 mmol/L. Explain the appropriate patient education in regard to these findings in relation to the management of his diabetes.

Plan of Nursing Care
Care of the Patient Undergoing Diagnostic Testing of the Renal-Urologic System

Nursing Interventions	Rationale	Expected Patient Outcomes

Nursing Diagnosis: Deficient knowledge about procedures and diagnostic tests
Goal: Patient demonstrates understanding of the procedure and tests and expected behaviours.

Nursing Interventions	Rationale	Expected Patient Outcomes
1. Assess patient's level of understanding of planned diagnostic tests.	1. Provides basis for teaching and gives indication of patient's perception of tests	• States rationale for planned diagnostic tests and what tasks and behaviours are expected during the procedure
2. Provide a factual description of tests in language the patient can understand.	2. Understanding what is expected enhances patient compliance and cooperation.	• Complies with urine collection, fluid modifications, or other procedures required for diagnostic evaluation
3. Assess patient's understanding of test results after their completion.	3. Apprehension may interfere with patient's ability to understand information and results provided by health care team.	• Restates in own words results of diagnostic tests
4. Reinforce information provided to patient about test results and implications for follow-up care.	4. Provides opportunity for patient to clarify information and anticipate follow-up care	• Asks for clarification of terms and procedures
		• Explains rationale for follow-up care
		• Participates in follow-up care

Nursing Diagnosis: Acute pain related to infection, edema, obstruction, or bleeding along urinary tract or to invasive diagnostic tests
Goal: Patient reports decrease in pain and absence of discomfort.

Nursing Interventions	Rationale	Expected Patient Outcomes
1. Assess level of pain: dysuria, burning on urination, abdominal or flank pain, bladder spasm.	1. Provides baseline for evaluation of pain relief strategies and progression of dysfunction	• Reports decreasing levels of pain
2. Encourage fluid intake (unless contraindicated).	2. Promotes dilute urine and flushing of the lower urinary tract	• Reports absence of local symptoms
3. Encourage warm sitz baths.	3. Relieves local discomfort and promotes relaxation	• States ability to start and stop urinary stream without discomfort
4. Report increased pain to physician.	4. May indicate progression or recurrence of dysfunction, or untoward signs (eg, bleeding, calculi)	• Consumes increased fluid intake if indicated
5. Administer analgesics and antispasmodics for pain and spasm as prescribed.	5. Prescribed to relieve pain or spasm	• Uses sitz bath as indicated
6. Assess voiding patterns and hygiene practices and provide instructions about recommended voiding patterns and hygienic practices.	6. Delayed emptying of the bladder and poor hygiene may contribute to pain secondary to renal or urinary tract dysfunction.	• Identifies signs and symptoms to be reported to the health care provider
		• Takes medications as prescribed
		• Does not delay in emptying bladder
		• Uses appropriate hygienic measures, avoids use of bubble bath, uses appropriate hygiene after bowel movements

Nursing Diagnosis: Fear related to potential alteration in renal function and embarrassment secondary to discussion of urinary function and invasion of genitalia
Goal: Patient appears relaxed and reports decreased fear and anxiety.

Nursing Interventions	Rationale	Expected Patient Outcomes
1. Assess patient's level of fear and apprehension.	1. A high level of fear or apprehension can interfere with learning and cooperation.	• Appears relaxed with a low level of fear or apprehension
2. Explain all procedures and tests to patient.	2. Knowledge about what is expected helps reduce fear and apprehension.	• States rationale for tests and procedures in a calm, relaxed manner
3. Provide privacy and respect patient's modesty by closing doors and keeping patient covered. Keep urinal and bedpan covered and out of sight.	3. Communicates that you are aware of and accept patient's need for privacy and modesty	• Maintains usual privacy and modesty
4. Use correct terminology in a factual manner when questioning patient about urinary tract dysfunction.	4. Conveys that you are comfortable discussing patient's urinary dysfunction and symptoms with patient	• Discusses own urinary tract dysfunction using correct terminology without overt indications of embarrassment or discomfort
5. Assess patient's fears about perceived changes associated with tests and other procedures.	5. May uncover fears and misconceptions of the patient that can be alleviated by correct understanding	• Relates fears and concerns
6. Instruct patient in relaxation techniques.	6. Promotes relaxation and assists the patient in coping with uncertainty about outcomes	• Demonstrates correct understanding of procedures and possible outcomes
		• Appears relaxed with low level of fear and apprehension

3. A 50-year-old patient with suspected renal artery stenosis stops by his family physician's office for a scheduled blood pressure check. He states that despite a recent discussion with his physician about the possible need for referral to a urologist for a renal artery stent, he does not understand what his kidneys have to do with his blood pressure. Describe the patient teaching you would provide regarding the role of the kidneys in blood pressure management, based on your knowledge of renal physiology.

4. You make a home visit to a patient recently discharged from the hospital after treatment for heart failure. Your patient explains that she has not voided for about 18 hours. Upon abdominal assessment, you find that her bladder is not distended. Identify other assessment information that is important for you to obtain to determine which actions to take. Provide the rationale for obtaining the information, and explain how it will be used in determining subsequent actions.

REFERENCES AND SELECTED READINGS

Books

Agency for Health Care Policy and Research, Public Health Service, U.S. Department of Health and Human Services (1996). *Urinary incontinence in adults: acute and chronic management.* Clinical Practice Guideline (AHCPR Pub. No. 96-0682). Washington, DC: U.S. Government Printing Office.

American Academy of Clinical Endocrinologists. (1999). Medical guidelines for clinical practice for management of menopause. http://www.aace.com/clin/guidelines/menopause.pdf.

American Foundation for Urological Disease. (1999–2000). Resource guide: Prostate cancer, Part 2: Overview of the prostate and prostate cancer. http://www.afud.org/pca/pcaindex.html.

Bickley, L. S. & Szilagyi, P. G. (2003). *Bates' guide to physical examination and history taking* (8th ed.). Philadelphia: Lippincott Williams & Wilkins.

Eschbach, J. W. (2001). National Kidney Foundation–Dialysis outcomes quality initiative clinical practice guidelines: Treatment of anemia of chronic kidney disease. http://www.kidney.org/professionals/doqi/guidelines/doqi_upex.html.

Karlowicz, K., & Meredith, C. (Eds.). (2001). *Urologic nursing: A study guide* (2nd ed.). Pitman, NJ: Society of Urologic Nurses and Associates, Inc.

Lancaster, L. (1995). *American Nephrology Nurses Association core curriculum for nephrology nursing* (3rd ed.). Pitman, NJ: American Nephrology Nurses Association.

Metheny, N. (2000). *Fluid and electrolyte balance: Nursing considerations* (4th ed.). Philadelphia: Lippincott Williams & Wilkins.

National Institute of Diabetes & Digestive & Kidney Diseases (NIDDKD). (1999). Hematuria (blood in the urine). NIH Publication #99-4559, 1999, http://www.niddk.nih.gov/health/urolog/summary/hematuri/index.htm.

National Institute of Diabetes & Digestive & Kidney Diseases (NIDDKD). (2000). Proteinuria. NIH Publication #01-4732, June 2000, http://www.niddk.nih.gov/health/kidney/pubs/proteinuria/proteinuria.htm.

National Institute of Diabetes & Digestive & Kidney Diseases (NIDDKD). (2001*a*). Cystoscopy and ureteroscopy. NIH Publication #01-4800, April 2001, http://www.niddk.nih.gov/health/kidney/pubs/cystoscopy/cystoscopy.htm#info.

National Institute of Diabetes & Digestive & Kidney Diseases (NIDDKD). (2001*b*). Kidney biopsy. NIH Publication #01-4763. May, 2001, http://www.niddk.nih.gov/health/kidney/pubs/kidney-biopsy/biopsy.htm.

National Kidney Foundation. (2001). Executive summary–K/DOQI clinical practice guidelines. http://www.kidney.org/professionals/doqi/guidelines/doqiupex.html.

Parker, J. (1998). *Contemporary nephrology nursing.* Pitman, NJ: Anthony J. Janetti, Inc.

Rose, B., & Post, T. (2000). *Clinical physiology of acid-base and electrolyte disorders.* New York: McGraw-Hill Text.

Tanagho, E. A., & McAnich, J. W. (Eds.). (2000). *Smith's general urology* (15th ed.). New York: McGraw-Hill Professional Publishing.

U.S. Department of Health and Human Services (2000). *Healthy people 2010. Understanding and improving health.* Washington, DC: U.S. Government Printing Office.

Walsh, P., Retik, A., Vaughan, E., & Wein, A. (Eds.). (1998). *Campbell's urology* (7th ed.). Philadelphia: W. B. Saunders.

Journals

Asterisks denote nursing research articles.

Albaugh, J. (1999). Unlocking the mystery of urodynamics. *Urologic Nursing, 19*(3), 202–208.

Appell, R. A. (1999). Pathophysiology of urge incontinence. *Contemporary Urology,* Supplement: 1–6.

Bakris, G. L., Williams, M., Dworkin, L., et al. (2000). Preserving renal function in adults with hypertention and diabetes: A consensus approach. *American Journal of Kidney Disease, 36*(3), 646–661.

Degler, M. (2001). Prostate cancer: What are your risks? Available at: http://www.MyBladder.com. Protocol Driven Healthcare Incorporated.

Degler, M. (1999). Types of urinary incontinence. Available at: http://www.MyBladder.com. Protocol Driven Healthcare Incorporated.

Degler, M. (2000). Urinary incontinence: Caring for the caregiver. Available at: http://www.MyBladder.com. Protocol Driven Healthcare Incorporated.

Goolsby, M. J. (2001). Clinical practice guidelines: Management of menopause. *Journal of the American Academy of Nurse Practitioners, 13*(4), 147–151.

Gray, M. (2000a). Urinary retention: Management in the acute care setting, Part 1. *American Journal of Nursing, 100*(7), 40–48.

Gray, M. (2000b). Urinary retention: Management in the acute care setting, Part 2. *American Journal of Nursing, 100*(8), 36–44.

Hoffman, E. (2001). Overactive bladder: Diagnosis of a hidden disorder. *Patient Care for the Nurse Practitioner,* Spring Supplement, 15–21.

*Kincade, J. E., Peckous, B. K., & Busby-Whitehead, J. (2001). A pilot study to determine predictors of behavioral treatment completion for urinary incontinence. *Urologic Nursing, 21*(1), 39–44.

Klingman, L. (1999). Assessing the male genitalia. *American Journal of Nursing, 99*(7), 47–50.

Kuebler, K. K. (2001). Palliative nursing care for the patient experiencing end-stage renal failure. *Urologic Nursing, 21*(3), 167–178.

*Lillibridge, J., & Watt, E. (2000) Timing of urinary catheter removal: A descriptive study. *Urologic Nursing, 20*(6), 375–380.

Litwiller, S. E., Frohman, E. M., & Zimmern, P. E. (1999). Multiple sclerosis and the urologist. *Journal of Urology, 161*(3), 743–757.

Schafer, S. L. (2001). Prescribing for seniors: It's a balancing act. *Journal of the American Academy of Nurse Practitioners, 13*(3), 108–112.

Smith, D. M., Fortune-Faulkner, E. M., & Spurbeck, B. L. (2000, April). Lupus nephritis: Pathophysiology, diagnosis, and collaborative management. *Nephrology Nursing Journal, 27*(2), 199–211.

Steinberg, E. P., Eknoyan, G., Levin, N. W., Eschbach, J. W., et al. (2000). Methods used to evaluate the quality of evidence underlying the National Kidney Foundation-Dialysis Outcomes Quality Initiative Clinical Practice Guidelines: Description, findings, and implications. *American Journal of Kidney Disease, 36*(1), 1–11.

Wade-Elliott, R. (1999). Caring for the elderly with renal failure: Gastrointestinal changes. *ANNA Journal, 26*(6), 563–571.

Wein, A. J. (2001). Putting overactive bladder into clinical perspective. *Patient Care for the Nurse Practitioner,* Spring Supplement, 1–5.

RESOURCES AND WEBSITES

Canadian Association of Genetic Counsellors (CAGC); www.cagc-accg.ca.

Canadian Cancer Society/Société canadienne du cancer, National Office, Suite 200, 10 Alcorn Avenue, Toronto, ON M4V 3B1; (416) 961-7223; fax: (416) 961-4189; www.cancer.ca.

Canadian Directory of Genetic Support Groups, Support Group Directory, Regional Medical Genetics Centre, Children's Hospital of Western Ontario, 800 Commissioner's Road East, London, ON N6C 2V5; (519) 685-8453; in Ontario only: 1-800-243-8416; fax: (519) 685-8214; www.lhsc.on.ca/programs/medgenet.

Canadian Genetic Disease Network, Suite 201, 2150 Western Parkway, Vancouver, BC V6T 1V6; (604) 221-7300; fax: (604) 221-0778; e-mail: info@cgdn.ca; www.cgdn.ca.

Canadian Organization for Rare Disorders (CORD), PO Box 814, Coaldale, AB T1M 1M7; (403) 345-4544; toll-free: 1-877-302-7273; fax: (403) 345-3948; www.cord.ca.

GeneTests, 9725 Third Avenue NE, Suite 602, Seattle, WA 98115; (206) 616-4033; fax: (206) 221-4679; e-mail: genetests@genetests.org; www.genetests.org.

Genetic Alliance, 4301 Connecticut Avenue NW, Suite 404, Washington, DC 20008-2369; (202) 966-5557; fax: (202) 966-8553; e-mail: info@geneticalliance.org; www.geneticalliance.org.

The Genetics Society of Canada; http://life.biology.mcmaster.ca/GSC.

OMIM Online Mendelian Inheritance in Man; www.ncbi.nlm.nih.gov/entrez/query.fcgi?db=OMIM.

Management of Patients With Upper or Lower Urinary Tract Dysfunction

Adapted by Jill Milne

LEARNING OBJECTIVES

On completion of this chapter, the learner will be able to:

1. Explain the different types of urinary incontinence and their causes.

2. Compare and contrast urinary retention and urinary incontinence in terms of their clinical manifestations, complications, and medical and nursing management.

3. Describe the sequence of events leading to urinary tract infection in a patient with an indwelling urinary catheter.

4. Outline the principles of management of a patient with an indwelling urinary catheter.

5. Compare and contrast hemodialysis and peritoneal dialysis in terms of underlying principles, procedures, complications, and nursing considerations.

6. Describe nursing management of the hospitalized dialysis patient.

7. Use the nursing process as a framework for care of patients undergoing kidney surgery.

*P*atients with disorders of the upper or lower urinary tract often exhibit similar problems, regardless of the underlying disorder. This chapter provides an overview of common problems that these patients experience, such as fluid and electrolyte imbalances and dysfunctional voiding patterns. Interdisciplinary medical and surgical management strategies (eg, catheterization, dialysis, and surgery) for various urologic diseases and disorders are also discussed.

Fluid and Electrolyte Imbalances in Renal Disorders

Patients with renal disorders commonly experience fluid and electrolyte imbalances and require astute assessment and close monitoring for signs of potential problems. The fluid intake and output record, a key monitoring tool, is used to document important fluid parameters, including the amount of fluid taken in (orally or parenterally), the volume of urine excreted, and other fluid losses (diarrhea, vomiting, diaphoresis).

These records and changes in the patient's weight are essential for determining the daily fluid allowance and indicating signs of fluid overload or deficit. The patient whose fluid intake exceeds the ability of the kidneys to excrete fluid is said to have a fluid overload. If fluid intake is inadequate, the patient is said to be volume-depleted and may show signs and symptoms of fluid volume deficit.

 NURSING ALERT The most accurate indicator of fluid loss or gain in an acutely ill patient is weight. An accurate daily weight must be obtained and recorded. A 1-kg weight gain is equal to 1,000 mL of retained fluid.

Glossary

arteriovenous graft: type of surgically created vascular access for dialysis by which a piece of biologic, semibiologic, or synthetic graft material is connected to the patient's artery and vein

catheterization: insertion of a tube into the urinary bladder to permit drainage of urine

continuous ambulatory peritoneal dialysis (CAPD): method of peritoneal dialysis whereby a patient performs four or five complete dialysis exchanges or cycles throughout the day

continuous arteriovenous hemodialysis (CAVHD): form of continuous renal replacement therapy that results in removal of fluid and waste products; arterial blood is circulated through a hemofilter (surrounded by dialysate fluid) and returned to the patient through a venous catheter

continuous arteriovenous hemofiltration (CAVH): form of continuous renal replacement therapy that primarily results in removal of fluid; arterial blood circulates through a hemofilter and returns to the patient through a venous catheter

continuous cyclic peritoneal dialysis (CCPD): method of peritoneal dialysis in which a peritoneal dialysis machine (cycler) automatically performs dialysis exchanges, usually while the patient sleeps

continuous renal replacement therapy (CRRT): variety of methods used to replace normal kidney function by circulating the patient's blood through a hemofilter

continuous venovenous hemodialysis (CVVHD): form of continuous renal replacement therapy that results in removal of fluid and waste products; venous blood circulates through a hemofilter and returns to the patient

continuous venovenous hemofiltration (CVVH): form of continuous renal re-

placement therapy that primarily results in removal of fluid; venous blood circulates through a hemofilter and returns to the patient

dialysate: dialysis solution that circulates through the dialyzer in hemodialysis and through the peritoneal membrane in peritoneal dialysis

dialyzer: "artificial kidney" or dialysis machine; contains semipermeable membrane through which particles of a certain size can pass

diffusion: movement of solutes (waste products) from an area of higher concentration to an area of lower concentration

fistula: type of vascular access for dialysis; created by surgically connecting an artery to a vein

functional incontinence: lower urinary tract function is intact, but other factors such as severe cognitive impairment make it difficult for the person to identify the need to void or physical impairment make it impossible for the person to reach the toilet in time for voiding.

hemodialysis: circulation of the patient's blood through a dialyzer to remove waste products and excess fluid

nephrostomy: procedure in which a tube is inserted through the skin and subcutaneous tissue into the renal pelvis for drainage

micturition: voiding

mixed incontinence: presence of several types of urinary incontinence, usually a combination of stress and urge incontinence.

neurogenic bladder: bladder dysfunction that results from a disorder or dysfunction of the nervous system; may result in either urinary retention or bladder overactivity, resulting in urinary urgency and urge incontinence

osmosis: movement of water through a semipermeable membrane from an area of

lower solute concentration to an area of higher solute concentration

overactive bladder syndrome (OAB): a range of symptoms, including urgency, frequency, nocturia, and/or urge incontinence, that are associated with a sudden and strong desire to void.

overflow incontinence: involuntary urine loss associated with overdistention of the bladder due to mechanical or anatomic bladder outlet obstruction

peritoneal dialysis: form of dialysis in which the patient's peritoneal membrane is used as the semipermeable membrane for exchange of fluid and solutes

peritonitis: inflammation of the peritoneal membrane (lining of the peritoneal cavity)

reflex bladder: bladder empties on reflex with a loss-of-conscious sensation or voluntary inhibition.

reflex incontinence: involuntary loss of urine due to hyperreflexia or involuntary urethral relaxation in the absence of normal sensations; usually associated with micturition (voiding)

residual urine: urine that remains in the bladder after voiding

stress incontinence: the complaint of involuntary leakage of urine on effort or exertion, sneezing, or coughing.

suprapubic catheter: a urinary catheter that is inserted through a suprapubic incision into the bladder

ultrafiltration: process whereby water is removed from the blood by means of a pressure gradient between the patient's blood and the dialysate

urge incontinence: the complaint of involuntary leakage of urine accompanied or immediately preceded by urgency.

urinary incontinence: the complaint of any involuntary leakage of urine.

Clinical Manifestations

The signs and symptoms of common fluid and electrolyte disturbances that can occur in patients with renal disease are listed in Table 44-1, as are general management strategies. The nurse should continually assess, monitor, and inform appropriate members of the health care team if the patient exhibits any of these signs. Management strategies for fluid and electrolyte disturbances in renal disease are discussed in greater depth later in this chapter (see also Chap. 14).

Dysfunctional Voiding Patterns

Dysfunctional voiding presents in the form of complaints of urinary incontinence or urine retention. **Urinary incontinence** is defined as any involuntary loss of urine (Abrams, Cardoza, Fall et al., 2002). Urinary continence relies on intact urinary, neurologic, and musculoskeletal systems. Continence is maintained via a complex communication system of suprasacral, sacral, and local nerve-mediated loops of information, all of which must be functioning efficiently and synergistically. Any break in these loops of communication (for

Table 44-1 • Common Fluid and Electrolyte Disturbances in Renal Disease

DISTURBANCE	MANIFESTATIONS	GENERAL MANAGEMENT STRATEGIES
Fluid volume deficit	Acute weight loss ≥5%, decreased skin turgor, dry mucous membranes, oliguria or anuria, increased hematocrit, blood urea nitrogen (BUN) level increased out of proportion to creatinine level, hypothermia	Fluid challenge, fluid replacement orally or parenterally
Fluid volume excess	Acute weight gain ≥5%, edema, crackles, shortness of breath, decreased BUN, decreased hematocrit, distended neck veins	Fluid and sodium restriction, diuretics, dialysis
Sodium deficit	Nausea, malaise, lethargy, headache, abdominal cramps, apprehension, seizures	Diet, normal saline or hypertonic saline solutions
Sodium excess	Dry, sticky mucous membranes, thirst, rough dry tongue, fever, restlessness, weakness, disorientation	Fluids, diuretics, dietary restriction
Potassium deficit	Anorexia, abdominal distention, paralytic ileus, muscle weakness, ECG changes, dysrhythmias	Diet, oral or parenteral potassium replacement therapy
Potassium excess	Diarrhea, colic, nausea, irritability, muscle weakness, ECG changes	Dietary restriction, diuretics, IV glucose, insulin and sodium bicarbonate, cation exchange resin, calcium gluconate, dialysis
Calcium deficit	Abdominal and muscle cramps, stridor, carpopedal spasm, hyperactive reflexes, tetany, positive Chvostek's or Trousseau's sign, tingling of fingers and around mouth, ECG changes	Diet, oral or parenteral calcium salt replacement
Calcium excess	Deep bone pain, flank pain, muscle weakness, depressed deep tendon reflexes, constipation, nausea and vomiting, confusion, impaired memory, polyuria, polydipsia, ECG changes	Fluid replacement, etidronate, pamidronate, mithramycin, calcitonin, glucocorticoids, phosphate salts
Bicarbonate deficit	Headache, confusion, drowsiness, increased respiratory rate and depth, nausea and vomiting, warm flushed skin	Bicarbonate replacement, dialysis
Bicarbonate excess	Depressed respirations, muscle hypertonicity, dizziness, tingling of fingers and toes	Fluid replacement if volume depleted; ensure adequate chloride
Protein deficit	Chronic weight loss, emotional depression, pallor, fatigue, soft flabby muscles	Diet, dietary supplements, hyperalimentation, albumin
Magnesium deficit	Dysphagia, muscle cramps, hyperactive reflexes, tetany, positive Chvostek's or Trousseau's sign, tingling of fingers, dysrhythmias, vertigo	Diet, oral or parenteral magnesium replacement therapy
Magnesium excess	Facial flushing, nausea and vomiting, sensation of warmth, drowsiness, depressed deep tendon reflexes, muscle weakness, respiratory depression, cardiac arrest	Calcium gluconate, mechanical ventilation, dialysis
Phosphorus deficit	Deep bone pain, flank pain, muscle weakness and pain, paresthesia, apprehension, confusion, seizures	Diet, oral or parenteral phosphorus supplementation therapy
Phosphorus excess	Tetany, tingling of fingers and around mouth, muscle spasms, soft tissue calcification	Diet restriction, phosphate binders, normal saline solution, IV dextrose solution, and insulin

example, an upper or lower neuron lesion, spinal stenosis, or bladder outlet obstruction) can cause some degree of urinary dysfunction. Depending on the location of the insult, both incontinence and incomplete bladder emptying can occur. Anatomic integrity of the upper and lower urinary system must be intact; otherwise, urine extravasation into the peritoneal or perivesical cavity (as seen in acute trauma) or extraurethral incontinence (as seen in some forms of congenital malformations) will occur. Genitourinary fistula formation between the bladder wall and other areas, such as the vagina, will result in extraurethral incontinence. The etiology of dysfunctional voiding can be congenital or acquired in adulthood. Each is reviewed separately.

CONGENITAL VOIDING DYSFUNCTION

Congenital anomalies usually result in voiding dysfunction early in life and are usually partially or completely surgically corrected. When voiding dysfunction occurs in adults, it may affect only the lower urinary system (eg, the bladder and urethra); when voiding dysfunction occurs in children, it commonly involves damage to the upper urinary system (ie, the ureters and kidneys) as well. Many congenital anomalies are discovered early in utero because of prenatal care measures such as ultrasound. The urinary system begins developing days after conception, and anomalies can be seen on a sonogram as early as 20 weeks. Depending on the anomaly, intrauterine surgery may be performed on the fetus. Because the urinary system may be only one of several organ systems that are abnormal due to genetic disorders, any defects not noted during gestation should be immediately apparent at birth. Such anomalies include renal agenesis (complete absence of one or both kidneys), ectopic ureter, and Eagle-Barrett syndrome (also known as prune-belly syndrome), with exstrophy of the bladder. On the other hand, voiding dysfunction can be discovered insidiously (for example, during toilet training). At times congenital anomalies, such as posterior urethral valves, typically seen only in males, may escape detection until early adolescence or adulthood,

when the voiding dysfunction or its sequelae cause the individual to seek a urologic evaluation. Although pediatric in nature, these disorders may affect urinary tract function when the patient becomes an adult.

ADULT VOIDING DYSFUNCTION

Both neuropathic (Table 44-2) and non-neuropathic disorders can cause adult voiding dysfunction. The **micturition** (voiding) process involves several highly coordinated neurologic responses that mediate bladder function. A functional urinary system allows for appropriate bladder filling and complete bladder emptying (see Chap. 43). If voiding dysfunction goes undetected and untreated, the upper urinary system may be compromised. Chronic incomplete bladder emptying from poor detrusor pressure results in recurrent bladder infection. Incomplete bladder emptying due to bladder outlet obstruction (such as benign prostatic hyperplasia), causing high-pressure detrusor contractions, can result in hydronephrosis from the high detrusor pressure that radiates up the ureters to the renal pelves.

URINARY INCONTINENCE

More than 1.5 million Canadians are estimated to have urinary incontinence, including one in every four women and approximately 15% of all men (Canadian Continence Foundation, 2001). Despite widespread media coverage, urinary incontinence remains underdiagnosed and underreported. Patients may be too embarrassed to seek help, causing them to ignore or conceal symptoms. Many patients resort to using absorbent pads or other devices without having their condition properly diagnosed and treated. Health care providers must be alert to subtle cues of urinary incontinence and stay informed about current management strategies.

A variety of nursing literature relates to incontinence: historical review of nursing and medical literature from 1850–1976 (Moore & Paul, 1997), products and devices used in continence manage-

Table 44-2 • **Conditions Contributing to Neuropathic Voiding Dysfunction**

CONDITION	COMMON VOIDING DYSFUNCTION	TREATMENT
Cerebellar ataxia	Incontinence *and/or* detrusor-sphincter dyssynergia	Timed voiding, anticholinergics
Cerebrovascular accident	Retention for several weeks, then detrusor overactivity and urge incontinence	Intermittent catheterization as necessary. Anticholinergics, pelvic floor muscle exercises, bladder training, urge inhibition
Dementia	Reflex incontinence	Prompted voiding, anticholinergics
Diabetes mellitus	Hesitancy, slow stream, decreased detrusor contractility, increased bladder capacity or detrusor overactivity and urge incontinence	Timed voiding, EMG/biofeedback, electrical stimulation, intermittent catheterization / Anticholinergics for overactivity
Multiple sclerosis	Detrusor overactivity and urge incontinence with or without detrusor-sphincter dyssynergia *or* areflexia and retention	Timed voiding, pelvic floor muscle exercises, urge inhibition, electrical stimulation, anticholinergics
Parkinson's disease	Detrusor overactivity and urge incontinence	Anticholinergics, pelvic floor muscle exercise, bladder training
Acute spinal cord injury	Urinary retention	Intermittent/indwelling catheterization
Degenerative disease	Incontinence and/or incomplete bladder emptying	Electrical stimulation, pelvic floor muscle exercise, biofeedback, anticholinergics

ment (Lekan-Routledge, Doughty, Moore, et al., 2003), continence care services worldwide (Milne & Moore, 2003), catheters and catheterization (Moore, 1995; Moore, Kelm, Sinclair, et al., 1993; Moore & Rayome, 1995), treatment in men (McCallum, Moore, & Griffiths, 2001; Moore & Dorey, 1999; Moore & Gray, 2004), and penile clamps (Moore, Schlieman, Ackerman, et al., 2004).

The costs of care for patients with urinary incontinence are not limited to the dollars spent for absorbent products, medications, and surgical or nonsurgical treatment modalities. The psychosocial costs of urinary incontinence are also significant: embarrassment, loss of self-esteem, and social isolation are common outcomes. Urinary incontinence in elderly patients often decreases their ability to maintain an independent lifestyle. This increases dependence on caregivers and often leads to institutionalization.

Urinary incontinence affects people of all ages but is particularly common among the elderly. It has been reported that more than half of all nursing home residents have urinary incontinence. Although urinary incontinence is not a normal consequence of aging, age-related changes in the urinary tract predispose the older person to incontinence.

Although urinary incontinence is commonly regarded as a condition that occurs in older multiparous women, it is also common in young nulliparous women, especially during vigourous high-impact activity. Age, gender, and number of vaginal deliveries are established risk factors (Chart 44-1); they explain, in part, the increased incidence in women. Urinary incontinence is a symptom with many possible causes.

Clinical Manifestations: Types of Incontinence

There are two major categories of urinary incontinence: transient and persistent. Transient incontinence is so-named because its causes (as identified by the mnemonic DIAPPERS, Chart 44-2) are outside the urinary system; addressing the causes will resolve the incontinence. For example, alpha-adrenergic agents taken to lower blood pressure adversely affect the alpha receptors responsible for bladder neck closing pressure. As a result, the bladder neck may relax to allow leakage with only minimal increase in intra-abdominal pressure, thus mimicking stress incontinence. As soon as the medication is discontinued, the transient incontinence generally resolves (Reilly, 2001). Transient incontinence may be responsible for as much as 50% of urinary incontinence among

Chart 44-2 — Causes of Transient Incontinence: DIAPPERS

Delirium
Infection of urinary tract
Atrophic vaginitis, urethritis
Pharmacologic agents (anticholinergics, sedatives, alcohol, analgesics, diuretics, muscle relaxants, adrenergic agents)
Psychological factors (depression, regression)
Excessive urine production (increased intake, diabetes insipidus, diabetic ketoacidosis)
Restricted activity
Stool impaction

older adults in acute care settings and should be ruled out before proceeding to other assessment and treatment modalities. Types of persistent incontinence include stress, urge, mixed, reflex, and overflow.

Stress incontinence is the involuntary loss of urine associated with an increase in intra-abdominal pressure (sneezing, coughing, or changing position) (Abrams, Cardozo, Fall, et al., 2002). It predominantly affects women who have had vaginal deliveries and is thought to be the result of decreasing ligament and pelvic floor support of the urethra and decreasing or absent estrogen levels within the urethral walls and bladder base. In men, stress incontinence is often experienced after a radical prostatectomy for prostate cancer primarily as a result of intrinsic sphincter deficiency that can co-exist with new or recurring detrusor overactivity (Hunter, Moore, & Cody, et al., 2004), as well as loss of urethral compression that the prostate had supplied before the surgery (Reilly, 2001; Sueppel, Kreder, & See, 2001). (See Nursing Research Profile 44-1.)

Urge incontinence is the involuntary loss of urine associated with a strong urge to void that cannot be suppressed. The patient is aware of the need to void but is unable to reach a toilet in time. An uninhibited detrusor contraction is the precipitating factor. This can occur in a patient with neurologic dysfunction that impairs inhibition of bladder contraction or in a patient without overt neurologic dysfunction (Chancellor, 1999).

Overactive bladder syndrome (OAB) is the term that has recently been applied to the range of symptoms, including urgency, frequency, nocturia, and/or urge incontinence, that are associated with a sudden and strong desire to void (Gray, 2005). Approximately 60% of people with OAB experience distressing symptoms but are not incontinent (Canadian Continence Foundation, 2001). Although its causes are not fully understood, OAB appears to be neuropathic or idiopathic. Neurogenic lesions associated with conditions such as cerebrovascular accident, Parkinson's disease, spinal trauma, multiple sclerosis, and diabetes mellitus interrupt the neural pathways, although symptoms vary depending on the site and severity of the pathology. Spinal cord lesions cause neurogenic detrusor overactivity and may lead to **reflex bladder**, whereby the bladder empties on reflex with loss of conscious sensation or voluntary inhibition. Approximately 50% of patients with multiple sclerosis also experience incomplete bladder emptying due to detrusor-external sphincter dyssynergia, or uncoordinated contraction/relaxation of the detrusor and sphincter muscles. Idiopathic OAB is associated with increased bladder sensations or sensory urgency in the presence or absence of detrusor overactivity (Gray, 2005).

Reflex incontinence is the involuntary loss of urine due to hyperreflexia in the absence of normal sensations usually associated

Chart 44-1 — Risk Factors for Urinary Incontinence

Pregnancy: vaginal delivery, episiotomy
Menopause
Genitourinary surgery
Pelvic floor muscle weakness
Incompetent urethra due to trauma or sphincter relaxation
Immobility
High-impact exercise
Diabetes mellitus
Stroke
Age-related changes in the urinary tract
Morbid obesity
Cognitive disturbances: dementia, Parkinson's disease
Medications: diuretics, sedatives, hypnotics, opioids
Caregiver or toilet unavailable

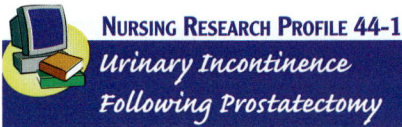

NURSING RESEARCH PROFILE 44-1
Urinary Incontinence Following Prostatectomy

McCallum, T. J., Moore, K. N. & Griffiths, D. (2001). Urinary incontinence after radical prostatectomy: Implications and urodynamics. *Urologic Nursing, 21*(2), 113–119.

Purpose

Urinary incontinence is debilitating for some men after radical prostatectomy. Previous research shows that men with preoperative symptoms of urinary urgency, frequency, and nocturia are more likely to have persistent incontinence than men without preoperative symptoms. The objective of this study was to evaluate urine loss, quality of life, and urodynamic findings in men with persistent urinary incontinence 12 months after radical prostatectomy.

Study Sample and Design

One hundred eighty men from a previous study on quality of life (QOL) and treatment for post-prostatectomy incontinence were asked to participate. Sixty-three men who were still incontinent participated in the study and were asked to complete a 24-hour pad test, a frequency/volume chart, and a QOL questionnaire at 2, 3, 6, and 8 months after radical prostatectomy. Persistent incontinence was defined as more than 10 g of urine loss on a 24-hour pad test at 8 months after surgery. Of the original 63 men, 21 were identified as still being incontinent. A second researcher then contacted these men for enrolment for video urodynamic testing. Sixteen of the 21 agreed to participate and underwent video urodynamic testing.

Findings

Four of the 16 men in the final sample reported preoperative urinary urgency, frequency, and nocturia. These 4 as well as 3 others (7), demonstrated objective evidence of overactive bladder (detrusor instability) on urodynamics. Four of these 7 had demonstrable stress incontinence as well (mixed incontinence). One other study participant demonstrated stress incontinence without associated detrusor instability. Although the retrospective nature of the questionnaire is a limitation of the study, the findings suggest that preoperative symptoms may be a risk factor for postoperative incontinence.

Nursing Implications

Men who have postoperative symptoms of stress incontinence may well have unrecognized detrusor dysfunction that, if recognized, could be treated, although symptoms of stress incontinence may persist. Preoperative identification of men with detrusor dysfunction could result in an altered postoperative plan of care to increase the overall level of continence and improved quality of life.

with voiding. This commonly occurs in patients with spinal cord injury because they have neither neurologically mediated motor control of the detrusor nor sensory awareness of the need to void.

Overflow incontinence is the involuntary loss of urine associated with overdistention of the bladder. Such overdistention results from the bladder's inability to empty normally, despite frequent urine loss. Both neurologic abnormalities (eg, spinal cord lesions) and factors that obstruct the outflow of urine (eg, tumours, strictures, and prostatic hyperplasia) can cause overflow incontinence (Reilly, 2001).

Functional incontinence refers to those instances in which lower urinary tract function is intact but other factors, such as severe cognitive impairment (eg, Alzheimer's dementia), make it difficult for the patient to identify the need to void or physical impairments make it difficult or impossible for the patient to reach the toilet in time for voiding. There is some controversy over the use of the term functional incontinence, since those affected likely share causes of transient incontinence and dealing with these causes, including mobility issues, may resolve the condition (Fonda, Benvenuti, Cottendam, et al., 2002).

Some patients have several types of urinary incontinence. This **mixed incontinence** is usually a combination of stress and urge incontinence.

Only with appropriate recognition of the problem, assessment, and referral for diagnostic evaluation and treatment can the outcome of incontinence be determined. All people with incontinence should be considered for evaluation and treatment.

Assessment and Diagnostic Findings

Once incontinence is recognized, a thorough history is necessary. This includes a detailed description of the problem and a history of medication use. The patient's medical and surgical history, a bladder diary with a record of fluid intake (type and volume), the amount and timing of voids, and any episodes of incontinence for a 3- or 7-day period, and bedside tests (ie, **residual urine,** stress manoeuvres) may be used to help determine the type of urinary incontinence involved. Extensive urodynamic tests may be performed; see Chapter 43. Urinalysis and urine culture are performed to identify hematuria (from infection, cancer, or a kidney stone), glycosuria (causes polyuria), pyuria, and bacteriuria (bacteria in the urine), all of which may identify transient causes of urinary incontinence.

Management depends on the type of urinary incontinence and its causes. The use of clinical practice guidelines is encouraged (Roe & Moore, 2001). Management of urinary incontinence not considered transient or reversible falls into three categories: pharmacologic, surgical, and behavioural.

 ### Gerontologic Considerations

Many older individuals experience transient episodes of incontinence that tend to be abrupt in onset. When this occurs, the nurse should question the patient, as well as the family if possible, about the onset of symptoms and any signs or symptoms of a change in other organ systems.

Acute urinary tract infection, infection elsewhere in the body, constipation, decreased fluid intake, a change in a chronic disease pattern, such as elevated blood glucose levels in patients with diabetes or decreased estrogen levels in menopausal women, can provoke the onset of urinary incontinence. If the cause is identified and modified or eliminated early at the onset of incontinence, the incontinence itself may be eliminated. Although the older bladder is more vulnerable to unstable detrusor activity, age alone is not a risk factor for urinary incontinence (Suchinski et al., 1999).

Medical Management

Treatment of urinary incontinence depends on the underlying cause. Before appropriate treatment can be initiated, however, the problem and the cause must be identified.

BEHAVIOURAL THERAPY

Behavioural therapies are always the first choice to decrease or eliminate urinary incontinence. In using these techniques, clinicians help patients avoid potential adverse effects of pharmacologic or surgical interventions (The Canadian Continence Foundation, 2001; Roberts, 2001) (Chart 44-3).

Chart 44-3 Behavioural Interventions for Urinary Incontinence

Behavioural strategies are largely carried out, coordinated, and monitored by the nurse. These interventions may or may not be augmented by the use of medications.

Fluid Management

One of the most common approaches is fluid management because adequate daily fluid intake of approximately 1,500 to 2,000 mL, taken as small increments between breakfast and the evening meal, helps to reduce urinary urgency related to concentrated urine production, decreases the risk of urinary tract infection, and maintains bowel functioning.

Constipation, resulting from inadequate daily fluid intake, can increase urinary urgency and/or urine retention. The best fluid is water. Fluids containing caffeine, carbonation, alcohol, or artificial sweetener should be avoided because they irritate the bladder wall, and may cause urinary urgency. Some individuals who have coexisting medical diagnoses, such as heart failure or end-stage renal disease, need to discuss their daily fluid limit with their primary health care provider.

Standardized Voiding Frequency

After establishing a patient's natural voiding and urinary incontinence tendencies, using a bladder or diary, urinary voiding on a schedule can be very effective in both cognitively intact and cognitively impaired patients, although cognitively impaired patients require assistance with this technique from nursing personnel or family members. The object is to purposely empty the bladder before the bladder reaches the critical volume that would cause an urge or stress incontinence episode. This approach involves the following strategies that vary in their requirement of patient/caregiver involvement and motivation. Timed voiding and habit training are initiated to pre-empt episodes of incontinence rather than to modify client behaviour (Ostaszkiewicz, Johnston, & Roe, 2004). In contrast, prompted voiding and bladder training share a requirement for active client participation. Prompted voiding programs are, however, initiated and maintained by the caregiver, whereas bladder training relies on the motivation of the individual with incontinence.

- **Timed voiding,** also known as scheduled toileting, may be the most common form of toileting assistance provided in institutional settings. It is less labour intensive because schedules are not individualized. Instead, caregivers toilet patients according to a fixed schedule, often every 2 hours. Timed voiding most commonly involves the patient or resident as a passive-care recipient, although the patient may choose to "void by the clock."
- **Habit retraining** is generally more labour intensive than timed voiding. Caregivers identify a patient's individual voiding pattern (both continent and incontinent voids) by completing a 3-day bladder diary. They then initiate a schedule of toileting to reflect but adapt that pattern, thereby pre-empting involuntary urine loss. Intervals between toileting may increase or decrease as necessary.
- **Prompted voiding** aims to change patient behaviour by increasing self-initiated requests for toileting (Eustice, Roe, & Paterson, 2004). Patients are approached according to individualized schedules (most commonly every 2 hours while awake), asked to report whether they are wet or dry, and prompted to use the toilet. Verbal praise is offered for correct reporting of dryness/wetness and successful toileting. The patient, therefore, maintains a prominent role in prompted voiding. However, since the therapy is generally targeted towards ambulatory patients with cognitive impairment, caregiver participation and motivation are critical to outcome.
- **Bladder training** aims to restore a normal voiding pattern by progressively lengthening the interval between voids. Individu-

als, particularly those who experience frequency, urgency, and urge incontinence, are taught to void at regular intervals throughout the day and to otherwise suppress the urge to void using strategies such as distraction and relaxation. Regimens may be individualized following assessment of a client's usual voiding pattern, but often begin with hourly schedules that are extended by 15 to 30 minutes at a time until an acceptable voiding interval is reached. Since positive outcome relies on active patient participation, motivation and the cognitive/physical ability to adhere to a progressive schedule are essential.

Pelvic Floor Muscle Exercise (PFME)

Also known as Kegel exercises, PFME aims to strengthen the voluntary muscles that assist in bladder and bowel continence in both men and women particularly following radical prostatectomy; however, recent evidence suggests they also play a role in the inhibition of involuntary contractions associated with OAB (Berghmans, van Waalwijk van Doorne, Hieman, et al, 2000). Research shows that written and/or verbal instruction alone is usually inadequate to teach an individual how to identify and strengthen the pelvic floor for sufficient bladder and bowel control (Sueppel, et al, 2001; Joseph & Chang, 2000). Biofeedback-assisted PFME uses either electromyography or manometry to help the individual identify the pelvic muscles as he or she attempts to learn which muscle group is involved when performing PFME. The biofeedback method also allows assessment of the strength of this muscle area while the exercise is taking place. When visual biofeedback is not available, the nurse may gently insert one or two fingers intravaginally, and then ask the female patient to squeeze around the finger(s). This helps the patient to identify the correct muscle and allows the nurse to assess pelvic floor muscle strength. Men who are contracting the correct musculature will notice the penis drawing slightly upward and inward.

Pelvic floor muscle exercises can be taught by all nurses at the primary care level (Canadian Continence Foundation, 2001). The recommended number and frequency of contractions vary. The patient generally starts with a few contractions (3 to 5) several times a day, gradually increasing their number and duration. Contractions should be held for a minimum of 6 to 8 seconds to recruit both fast- and slow-twitch muscle fibres (Wilson, Bo, Hay-Smith, et al., 2002), with each contraction followed by a minimum 10-second rest period. To be effective, these exercises need to be performed for at least 6 weeks, and possibly for longer periods in elderly patients.

Vaginal Cone Retention Exercises

Vaginal cone retention exercises are an adjunct to the Kegel exercises. Vaginal cones of varying weight are inserted intravaginally twice a day. The patient tries to retain the cone for 15 minutes by contracting the pelvic muscles. Cone weight is gradually increased over time.

Transvaginal or Transrectal Electrical Stimulation

Commonly used to treat urinary incontinence, electrical stimulation is known to elicit a passive contraction of the pelvic floor musculature, thus re-educating these muscles to provide enhanced levels of continence. This modality is often used with biofeedback-assisted pelvic muscle exercise training and voiding schedules. At high frequencies, it is effective for stress incontinence. At low frequencies, electrical stimulation can also relieve symptoms of urinary urgency, frequency, and urge incontinence. Intermediate ranges are used for mixed incontinence (AHCPR, 1996; Bernier & Davila, 2000).

Neuromodulation

Neuromodulation via transvaginal or transrectal nerve stimulation of the pelvic floor inhibits detrusor overactivity and hypersensory bladder signals and strengthens weak sphincter muscles.

PHARMACOLOGIC THERAPY

Pharmacologic therapy works best when used as an adjunct to behavioural interventions (Taylor, 2005). Anticholinergic agents (oxybutynin [Ditropan], and tolterodine [Detrol]) inhibit bladder contraction and are considered first-line medications for urge incontinence and OAB. Trospium chloride (Santura), solifenacin (Vesicare), and darifenacin (Enablux) will soon be available in Canada. Several tricyclic antidepressant medications (imipramine, doxepin, desipramine, and nortriptyline) also decrease bladder contractions as well as increase bladder neck resistance. These antidepressants can have serious adverse effects and with the advent of the newer anticholinergics, they are rarely prescribed for urinary incontinence. Stress incontinence may be treated using pseudoephedrine (eg, Sudafed). Estrogen (taken orally, transdermally, or topically as an intravaginal cream) has been shown to be beneficial for all types of urinary incontinence. Estrogen decreases obstruction to urine flow by restoring the mucosal, vascular, and muscular integrity of the urethra.

Gerontologic Considerations

Elderly individuals may experience cognitive decline when taking short-acting anticholinergic medications. The long-acting forms of anticholinergic medications such as oxybutynin (Ditropan XL) and tolterodine (Detrol LA) have a significantly lower incidence of adverse effects in all populations, including the elderly (Roberts, 2001).

SURGICAL MANAGEMENT

Surgical correction may be indicated in patients who have not achieved continence using behavioural and pharmacologic therapy. Surgical options vary according to the underlying anatomy and the physiologic problem. Most procedures involve lifting and stabilizing the bladder or urethra to restore the normal urethrovesical angle or to lengthen the urethra.

Women with stress incontinence may have an anterior vaginal repair, retropubic suspension, or needle suspension to reposition the urethra. Procedures to compress the urethra and increase resistance to urine flow include sling procedures and placement of periurethral bulking agents such as artificial collagen.

Periurethral bulking is a semipermanent procedure in which small amounts of artificial collagen are placed within the walls of the urethra to enhance the closing pressure of the urethra. This procedure takes only 10 to 20 minutes and may be performed under local anesthesia or moderate sedation. A cystoscope is inserted into the urethra. An instrument is inserted through the cystoscope to deliver a small amount of collagen into the urethral wall at locations selected by the urologist. The patient is usually discharged home after voiding. There are no restrictions following the procedure, although occasionally more than one collagen bulking session may be necessary if the initial procedure did not halt the stress urinary incontinence. Collagen placement anywhere in the body is considered semipermanent because its durability averages between 12 and 24 months, until the body absorbs the material. Periurethral bulking with collagen offers an alternative to surgery, as in a frail, elderly individual. It is also an option for individuals who are seeking help with stress urinary incontinence who prefer to avoid surgery and who do not have access to biofeedback and electrical stimulation.

A modified artificial sphincter that uses a silicone-rubber balloon as a self-regulating pressure mechanism can be used to close the urethra. Electronic stimulation of the pelvic floor by means of a miniature pulse generator with electrodes mounted on an intra-anal plug is another method of controlling stress incontinence.

Men with overflow or OAB symptoms may undergo a transurethral resection to relieve symptoms of prostatic enlargement. An artificial sphincter can be used after prostatic surgery for sphincter incompetence (Fig. 44-1). After surgery, periurethral bulking agents can be injected into the periurethral area to increase compression of the urethra.

Nursing Management

Nursing management is based on the premise that incontinence is not inevitable with illness or aging and that it is often reversible and treatable. The nursing interventions are determined in part by the type of treatment that is undertaken. For behavioural therapy to be effective, the nurse must provide support and encouragement, because it is easy for the patient to become discouraged if therapy does not quickly improve the level of continence. Patient teaching regarding the bladder program is important and should be provided verbally and in writing (Chart 44-4). The patient is assisted to develop and use a bladder diary and a log to record timing of Kegel exercises, changes in bladder function with treatment, and episodes of incontinence.

If pharmacologic treatment is used, its purpose is explained to the patient and family. If surgical correction is undertaken, the procedure and its desired outcomes are described to the patient and family. Follow-up contact with the patient enables the nurse to answer the patient's questions and to provide reinforcement and encouragement. Patients who have mixed incontinence (both stress and urge incontinence) need to understand that anticholinergic and antispasmodic agents can help decrease urinary urgency and frequency and urge incontinence, but they do not decrease the urinary incontinence related to stress incontinence.

PROMOTING HOME AND COMMUNITY-BASED CARE

Modifying the home environment is a simple and effective way to treat urinary incontinence. In adapting the home environment to provide easy, safe access to the bathroom, the patient may need to remove barriers, such as throw rugs or other objects, from the route. Other modifications that the nurse may recommend include installing support bars in the bathroom and placing a bedpan or urinal within easy reach. Leaving a light on in the bedroom and bathroom and wearing clothing that is easy to remove when using the toilet are other recommendations (see Chart 44-4).

FIGURE 44-1 Male artificial urinary sphincter. An inflatable cuff is inserted surgically around the urethra or neck of the bladder. To empty the bladder, the cuff is deflated by squeezing the control pump located in the scrotum.

Chart 44-4 • PATIENT EDUCATION
Strategies for Managing Urinary Incontinence

Review the following recommendations with patients who are coping with urinary incontinence:

- Increase your awareness of the amount and timing of all fluid intake.
- Avoid taking diuretics after 4 PM.
- Avoid bladder irritants, such as caffeine, alcohol, and aspartame (NutraSweet).
- Take steps to avoid constipation: drink adequate fluids, eat a well-balanced diet high in fibre, exercise regularly, and take stool softeners if recommended.
- Void regularly, 5 to 8 times a day (about every 2 to 3 hours):
    First thing in the morning
    Before each meal
    Before retiring to bed
    Once during night if necessary
- Perform all pelvic floor muscle exercises as prescribed, every day.
- Stop smoking (smokers usually cough frequently, which increases incontinence).

 ### Gerontologic Considerations

If nurses and other health care providers accept incontinence as an inevitable part of illness or aging or consider it irreversible and untreatable at any age, it cannot be treated successfully. Collaborative, interdisciplinary efforts are essential in assessing and effectively treating urinary incontinence.

URINARY RETENTION

Urinary retention is the marked accumulation of urine due to the inability to empty the bladder completely during attempts to void. Chronic urine retention often leads to overflow incontinence (from the pressure of the retained urine in the bladder). Residual urine is urine that remains in the bladder after voiding. In a healthy adult younger than age 60, complete bladder emptying should occur with each voiding. In adults older than age 60, 50 to 100 mL of residual urine may remain after each void because of the decreased contractility of the detrusor muscle.

Urinary retention can occur postoperatively in any patient, particularly if the surgery affected the perineal or anal regions and resulted in reflex spasm of the sphincters. General anesthesia reduces bladder muscle innervation and suppresses the urge to void, impeding bladder emptying (Gray, 2000a, 2000b).

Pathophysiology

Urinary retention may result from diabetes, prostatic enlargement, urethral pathology (infection, tumour, calculus), trauma (pelvic injuries), pregnancy, or neurologic disorders such as cerebrovascular accident, spinal cord injury, multiple sclerosis, or Parkinson's disease.

Some medications cause urinary retention, either by inhibiting bladder contractility or by increasing bladder outlet resistance. Medications that cause retention by inhibiting bladder contractility include anticholinergic agents (atropine sulfate, dicyclomine hydrochloride [Antispas, Bentyl]), antispasmodic agents (oxybutynin chloride [Ditropan], tolterodine (Detrol), belladonna, and opioid suppositories), and tricyclic antidepressant medications (imipramine [Tofranil], doxepin [Sinequan]). Medications that cause urine retention by increasing bladder outlet resistance include alpha-adrenergic agents (ephedrine sulfate, pseudoephedrine), beta-adrenergic blockers (propranolol), and estrogens.

Assessment and Diagnostic Findings

The assessment of a patient for urinary retention is multifaceted because the signs and symptoms may be easily overlooked. The following questions serve as a guide in assessment:

- What was the time of the last voiding, and how much urine was excreted?
- Is the patient voiding small amounts of urine frequently?
- Is the patient dribbling urine?
- Does the patient complain of pain or discomfort in the lower abdomen? (Discomfort may be relatively mild if the bladder distends slowly.)
- Is the pelvic area rounded and swollen (could indicate urine retention and a distended bladder)?
- Does percussion of the suprapubic region elicit dullness (possibly indicating urine retention and a distended bladder)?
- Are other indicators of urinary retention present, such as restlessness and agitation?
- Does a postvoid bladder ultrasound test reveal residual urine?

The patient may verbalize an awareness of bladder fullness and a sensation of incomplete bladder emptying. The nurse also assesses the patient for signs and symptoms of urinary tract infection, such as hematuria and dysuria. A series of urodynamic studies, described in Chapter 43, may be performed to identify the type of bladder dysfunction and to aid in determining appropriate treatment. The patient may complete a bladder diary to provide a written record of the amount of urine voided and the frequency of voiding.

Postvoid residual urine can be measured accurately without the need for postvoid straight **catheterization** using a portable ultrasound bladder scanner (see Nursing Research Profile 44-2). The scanner is operated by gently pressing a wand-like scan head that detects fluid over the bladder. If the scanner detects more than 100 mL of urine after a patient voids, the need for a postvoid catheterization should be considered to reduce the risks of urinary tract infection and bladder overdistention (Phillips, 2000; Schott-Baer & Reaume, 2001). Comprehensive urodynamics may also be performed.

Complications

Urine retention can lead to chronic infection. Infections that are unresolved predispose the patient to calculi, pyelonephritis, and sepsis. The kidney may also eventually deteriorate if large volumes of urine are retained, causing backward pressure on the upper urinary tract. In addition, urine leakage can lead to perineal skin breakdown, especially if regular hygiene measures are neglected.

Nursing Management

Management strategies are instituted to prevent overdistention of the bladder and to treat infection or correct obstruction. Many problems, however, can be prevented with careful nursing assessment and appropriate nursing interventions. The nurse should explain why normal voiding is not occurring and should monitor

NURSING RESEARCH PROFILE 44-2

Ultrasound as a Predictor of Postvoid Residual Volume

Schott-Baer, F. D., & Reaume, L. (2001). Accuracy of ultrasound esti-mates of urine volume. *Urologic Nursing, 21*(3), 193–195.

Purpose
UTIs following catheterization are the leading cause of infection in hospitalized patients and can lead to sepsis in this population. Therefore, it is important to avoid catheterization when possible while ensuring adequate emptying of the bladder. The purpose of this study was to compare urine volumes obtained with ultrasound bladder scanning to actual bladder volumes obtained from inter-mittent catheterization.

Study Sample and Design
Forty-eight patients on general surgery and rehabilitation units were included in the sample. The bladder scanner used for this study was the Diagnostic Ultrasound Corporation BVI 2500, a portable, battery-operated ultrasonic device intended for the non-invasive measurement of bladder volume. Subjects included all patients on whom a postvoid catheterization measurement was or-dered by their physician, following the removal of an indwelling catheter. Each patient's actual catheterized volume provided the comparison data. The catheterization was performed immediately after the bladder scan was completed.

Findings
Mean bladder ultrasound volumes and urinary catheterization vol-umes were essentially equal. Only 10% of the sample had scan vol-umes that differed by more than 100 mL from the actual volume.

Implications
The results of this study demonstrate that bladder ultrasound vol-ume is a relatively accurate prediction of actual postvoid residual volume. This technology is an acceptable alternative to postvoid catheterization for determining residual volume and avoids the risks of infection associated with catheterization procedures. Use of ultrasound bladder scanning may increase patient comfort, de-crease length of stay, decrease nursing time, and decrease the inci-dence of nosocomial infections associated with catheterization.

---

urine output closely. The nurse should also provide reassurance about the temporary nature of retention and successful manage-ment strategies.

PROMOTING NORMAL URINARY ELIMINATION
Nursing measures to encourage voiding include providing pri-vacy, ensuring an environment and a position conducive to void-ing, and assisting the patient with the use of the bathroom or commode, rather than a bedpan, to provide a more natural setting for voiding. The male patient may stand beside the bed while using the urinal; most men find this position more comfortable and natural.

Additional measures include applying warmth to relax the sphincters (ie, sitz baths, warm compresses to the perineum, showers), giving the patient hot tea, and offering encouragement and reassurance. Simple trigger techniques, such as turning on the water faucet while the patient is trying to void, may also be used. Other examples of trigger techniques are stroking the ab-domen or inner thighs, tapping above the pubic area, and dipping the patient's hands in warm water. A combination of techniques may be necessary to initiate voiding.

After surgery, the prescribed analgesic should be administered because pain in the incisional area can make voiding difficult.

To enhance bladder emptying, the individual may try "double voiding." After each voiding, the individual remains on the toilet, relaxes for 1 to 2 minutes, and then attempts to void again in an effort to further empty the bladder. This can be effective in patients with disorders characterized by neurogenic bladder (eg, multiple sclerosis) (Halper, 1998).

Use of timed, or habit, voiding is also considered. For example, a 2-hour voiding schedule may be established to prevent over-distention. A bladder training program may also be effective in treating urine retention (Davies et al., 2000; Joseph, 1999).

PHARMACOLOGIC THERAPY
Parasympathomimetic medications, such as bethanechol (Ure-choline), may help to increase the contraction of the detrusor muscle.

SURGICAL MANAGEMENT
In some cases, surgery may be carried out to correct bladder neck contractures or vesicoureteral reflux or to perform some type of urinary diversion procedure.

CATHETERIZATION
In patients with a urologic disorder or with marginal kidney func-tion, care must be taken to ensure that urinary drainage is ade-quate and that kidney function is preserved. When urine cannot be eliminated naturally and must be drained artificially, catheters may be inserted directly into the bladder, the ureter, or the renal pelvis. Catheters vary in size, shape, length, material, and config-uration. The type of catheter used depends on its purpose.

 NURSING ALERT Latex catheters and drainage systems must not be used with patients who have known or possible latex allergy.

Catheterization is performed to achieve the following:

- Relieve urinary tract obstruction
- Assist with postoperative drainage in urologic and other surgeries
- Provide a means to monitor accurate urine output in criti-cally ill patients
- Promote urinary drainage in patients with neurogenic blad-der dysfunction or urine retention
- Prevent urinary leakage in patients with stage III to IV pres-sure ulcers

A patient should be catheterized only if necessary because catheterization commonly leads to urinary tract infection. In ad-dition, urinary catheters have been associated with other compli-cations, such as bladder spasms, urethral strictures, and pressure necrosis.

Indwelling Devices and Infections. When an indwelling cath-eter cannot be avoided, a closed drainage system is essential. This drainage system is designed to prevent any disconnections, thereby reducing the risk of contamination. One common system consists of an indwelling catheter, a connecting tube, and a collecting bag with an antireflux chamber emptied by a drainage spout. Another common system has a triple-lumen indwelling urethral catheter attached to a closed sterile drainage system. With the triple-lumen catheter, urinary drainage occurs through one channel. The re-tention balloon of the catheter is inflated with water or air through the second channel, and the bladder is continuously irrigated with sterile irrigating solution through the third channel. Triple-lumen catheters are commonly used after transurethral prostate surgery.

An indwelling catheter can lead to infection. Bacterial colonization (bacteriuria) occurs within 2 weeks in half of catheterized patients and within 4 to 6 weeks in almost all patients after insertion of a catheter—even if recommendations for infection control and catheter care are followed carefully.

Urinary tract infections are the most commonly occurring nosocomial infections, accounting for 40% of them. Every year, about 1 million patients in acute-care hospitals in the United States develop nosocomial urinary tract infections, and about 80% of these are associated with the use of indwelling urinary catheters (Phillips, 2000). Most urinary tract infections follow instrumentation of the urinary tract, usually catheterization (Moore, Day, & Albers, 2002). The pathogens responsible for catheter-associated urinary tract infections include *Escherichia coli* and *Klebsiella, Proteus, Pseudomonas, Enterobacter, Serratia,* and *Candida* species. Many of these organisms are part of the patient's endogenous or normal bowel flora or are acquired through cross-contamination by patients or health care personnel or through exposure to nonsterile equipment.

Catheters impede most of the natural defenses of the lower urinary tract by obstructing the periurethral ducts, irritating the bladder mucosa, and providing an artificial route for organisms to enter the bladder. Organisms may be introduced from the urethra into the bladder during catheterization, or they may migrate along the epithelial surface of the urethra or external surface of the catheter.

The spout of the urinary drainage bag can become contaminated when opened to drain the bag. Bacteria enter the urinary drainage bag, multiply rapidly, and then migrate to the drainage tubing, catheter, and bladder. Scanning electron microscopy has demonstrated that thick layers (biofilms) of organisms often colonize the internal surfaces of catheters and drainage systems (Doyle et al., 2001; Godfrey & Evans, 2000; Phillips, 2000).

Suprapubic Catheterization. Suprapubic catheterization allows bladder drainage by inserting a catheter or tube into the bladder through a suprapubic (above the pubis) incision or puncture (Fig. 44-2). It may be a temporary measure to divert the flow of urine from the urethra when the urethral route is impassable (because of injuries, strictures, prostatic obstruction), after gynecologic or other abdominal surgery when bladder dysfunction is likely to occur, and occasionally after pelvic fractures. Suprapubic catheters may also be used on a long-term basis for women with urethral destruction secondary to long-term indwelling urethral catheters (Addison, 1999a, 1999b).

For insertion of the suprapubic catheter, the patient is placed in a supine position and the bladder distended by administering oral or intravenous fluids or by instilling sterile saline solution into the bladder through a urethral catheter. These measures make it easier to locate the bladder. The suprapubic area is prepared as for surgery and the puncture site located about 5 cm (2 in) above the symphysis pubis. The bladder is entered through an incision or through a puncture made by a small trocar (pointed instrument). The catheter or suprapubic drainage tube is threaded into the bladder and secured with sutures or tape; the area around the catheter is covered with a sterile dressing. The catheter is connected to a sterile closed drainage system, and the tubing is secured to prevent tension on the catheter.

Suprapubic bladder drainage may be maintained continuously for several weeks. When the patient's ability to void is to be tested, the catheter is clamped for 4 hours, during which time the patient attempts to void. After the patient voids, the catheter is unclamped, and the residual urine (the amount of urine remaining) is mea-

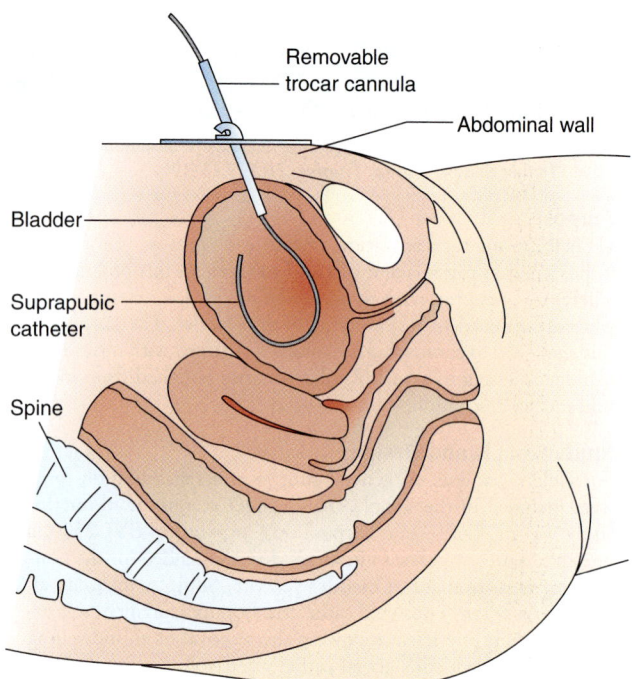

FIGURE 44-2 Suprapubic bladder drainage. A trocar cannula is used to puncture the abdominal and bladder walls. The catheter is threaded through the trocar cannula, which is then removed, leaving the catheter in place. The catheter is secured by tape or sutures to prevent unintentional removal.

sured. If the amount of residual urine is less than 100 mL on two separate occasions (morning and evening), the catheter is usually removed. If the patient complains of pain or discomfort, however, the suprapubic catheter is usually left in place until the patient can void successfully. When a suprapubic catheter remains in place indefinitely, it is changed regularly at 6- to 12-week intervals (Gujral et al., 1999).

Suprapubic drainage offers certain advantages. Patients can usually void sooner after surgery than those with urethral catheters, and they may be more comfortable. The catheter allows greater mobility, permits measurement of residual urine without urethral instrumentation, and presents less risk of bladder infection. The suprapubic catheter is removed when it is no longer necessary, and a sterile dressing is placed over the site.

The patient requires liberal amounts of fluid to prevent encrustation around the catheter. Other potential problems include the formation of bladder stones, acute and chronic infections, and problems collecting urine. An enterostomal therapist may be consulted to assist the patient and family in selecting the most suitable urine collection system and to teach them about its use and care.

Nursing Management During Catheterization

ASSESSING THE PATIENT AND THE SYSTEM

For patients with indwelling catheters, the nurse assesses the drainage system to ensure that it provides adequate urinary drainage. The colour, odour, and volume of urine are also monitored. An accurate record of fluid intake and urine output provides essential information about the adequacy of renal function and urinary drainage (Moore & Rayome, 1995).

The nurse observes the catheter to make sure that it is properly anchored, to prevent pressure on the urethra at the penoscrotal junction in male patients, and to prevent tension and traction on the bladder in both male and female patients.

Patients at high risk for urinary tract infection from catheterization need to be identified and monitored carefully. These include women, older adults, and patients who are debilitated, malnourished, chronically ill, immunosuppressed, or diabetic. They are observed for signs and symptoms of urinary tract infection: cloudy malodourous urine, hematuria, fever, chills, anorexia, and malaise. The area around the urethral orifice is observed for drainage and excoriation. Urine cultures provide the most accurate means of assessing a patient for infection.

Bladder ultrasonography can be used for noninvasive measurement of bladder volume. A portable bladder scan can be performed to assess the volume of urine in the bladder, the degree of bladder emptying, and therefore the need for catheterization (Phillips, 2000; Schott-Baer & Reaume, 2001).

ASSESSING FOR AGE-RELATED COMPLICATIONS
Elderly patients with an indwelling catheter may not exhibit the typical signs and symptoms of infection. Therefore, any subtle change in physical condition or mental status must be considered a possible indication of infection and promptly investigated because sepsis may occur before the infection is diagnosed. Figure 44-3 summarizes the sequence of events leading to infection and leakage of urine that often follow long-term use of an indwelling catheter in elderly patients.

PREVENTING INFECTION
Certain principles of care are essential to prevent infection in patients with a closed urinary drainage system (Chart 44-5). The catheter is a foreign body in the urethra and produces a reaction in the urethral mucosa with some urethral discharge. Vigorous cleaning of the meatus while the catheter is in place is discouraged, however, because the cleaning action can move the catheter to and fro, increasing the risk of infection. To remove obvious encrustations from the external catheter surface, the area can be washed gently with soap during the daily bath. The catheter is anchored as securely as possible to prevent it from moving in the urethra. Encrustations arising from urinary salts may serve as a nucleus for stone formation; however, using silicone catheters results in significantly less crust formation.

A liberal fluid intake, within the limits of the patient's cardiac and renal reserve, and an increased urine output must be ensured to flush the catheter and to dilute urinary substances that might form encrustations.

> **NURSING ALERT** Hand hygiene is essential when moving from one patient to another to provide care and before and after handling any part of the catheter or drainage system.

Urine cultures are obtained as prescribed or indicated in monitoring the patient for infection; many catheters have an aspiration (puncture) port from which a specimen can be obtained.

Controversy exists about the usefulness of taking cultures and treating bacteriuria in patients who have symptoms of infection and who have indwelling catheters. Bacteriuria is considered to be inevitable, and overtreatment may lead to resistant strains of bacteria (Suchinski et al., 1999).

MINIMIZING TRAUMA
Trauma to the urethra can be minimized by:

- Using an appropriate-sized catheter
- Lubricating the catheter adequately with a water-soluble lubricant during insertion
- Inserting the catheter far enough into the bladder to prevent trauma to the urethral tissues when the retention balloon of the catheter is inflated

Manipulation of the catheter is the most common cause of trauma to the bladder mucosa in the catheterized patient. Infection then inevitably occurs when urine invades the damaged mucosa.

The catheter is secured properly to prevent it from moving, causing traction on the urethra, or being unintentionally removed, and care is taken to ensure that the catheter position permits leg movement. In male patients, the drainage tube (not the catheter) is taped laterally to the thigh to prevent pressure on the urethra at the penoscrotal junction, which can eventually lead to formation of a urethrocutaneous fistula. In female patients, the drainage tubing attached to the catheter is taped to the thigh to prevent tension and traction on the bladder.

Care is taken to ensure that any patient who is confused does not remove the catheter with the retention balloon still inflated. This could cause bleeding and considerable injury to the urethra (Phillips, 2000).

TRAINING THE BLADDER
When an indwelling urinary catheter is in place, the detrusor muscle does not actively contract the bladder wall to stimulate emptying, because urine is continuously draining from the bladder. As a result, the detrusor may not immediately respond to bladder filling when the catheter is removed, resulting in either urine retention or urinary incontinence. This condition, known as postcatheterization detrusor instability, can be managed with bladder training (Chart 44-6).

Immediately after the indwelling catheter is removed, the patient is placed on a timed voiding schedule, usually every 2 to 3 hours. At the given time interval, the patient is instructed to void. The bladder is then scanned using a portable ultrasonic bladder scanner. If 100 mL or more of urine remains in the bladder, straight catheterization may be performed for complete bladder emptying. After a few days, as the nerve endings in the bladder wall become aware of bladder filling and emptying, bladder function usually returns to normal. If the individual has had an indwelling catheter in place for an extended period, bladder training will take much longer; in some cases, function may never return to normal. If this occurs, long-term intermittent catheterization may become necessary (Phillips, 2000).

ASSISTING WITH INTERMITTENT SELF-CATHETERIZATION
Intermittent self-catheterization provides periodic drainage of urine from the bladder. By promoting drainage and eliminating excessive residual urine, intermittent catheterization protects the kidneys, reduces the incidence of urinary tract infections, and improves continence (Moore, 1995). It is the treatment of choice in patients with spinal cord injury and other neurologic disorders, such as multiple sclerosis, when the ability to empty the bladder is impaired. Self-catheterization promotes independence, results in few complications, and enhances self-esteem and quality of life.

When teaching the patient how to perform self-catheterization, the nurse must use aseptic technique to minimize the risk of cross-contamination. The patient, however, may use a "clean" (nonsterile) technique at home, where the risk of cross-contamination is reduced. Either antibacterial liquid soap or povidone-iodine (Betadine) solution is recommended for cleaning urinary catheters at home. The catheter is thoroughly rinsed with tap water after soaking in the cleaning solution. It must dry before reuse.

Physiology/Pathophysiology

CAUSES

Catheterization

Bacterial ascension

Bacterial colonization

Permanent bacteriuria

Manipulations of catheter
Change of catheter
Irrigation
Unintentional removal

Bacterial invasion

Damaged mucosa

PATHOPHYSIOLOGY

Bladder infection

Damaged and inflamed mucosa

Detrusor irritation

Detrusor spasms

Inflammatory cells   Fibrin
Red blood cells   Other glutinous products

MANIFESTATIONS

Adherence to the catheter

Leakage

CLINICAL SIGNS

Encrustation   Distention
Obstruction   Leakage

URINALYSIS

Leukocytes   Urothelial cells
Erythrocytes

FIGURE 44-3 Pathophysiology and manifestations of bladder infection in long-term catheterized patients.

Chart 44-5 · Guidelines for Preventing Infection in the Catheterized Patient

- Use scrupulous aseptic technique during insertion of the catheter. Use a preassembled, sterile, closed urinary drainage system.
- To prevent contamination of the closed system, *never* disconnect the tubing. The drainage bag must *never* touch the floor. The bag and collecting tubing are changed if contamination occurs, if urine flow becomes obstructed, or if tubing junctions start to leak at the connections.
- If the collection bag must be raised above the level of the patient's bladder, clamp the drainage tube. This prevents backflow of contaminated urine into the patient's bladder from the bag.
- Ensure a free flow of urine to prevent infection. Improper drainage occurs when the tubing is kinked or twisted, allowing pools of urine to collect in the tubing loops.
- To reduce the risk of bacterial proliferation, empty the collection bag at least every 8 hours through the drainage spout—more frequently if there is a large volume of urine.
- Avoid contamination of the drainage spout. A receptacle in which to empty the bag is provided for each patient.

- Never irrigate the catheter routinely. If the patient is prone to obstruction from clots or large amounts of sediment, use a three-way system with continuous irrigation.
- Never disconnect the tubing to obtain urine samples, to irrigate the catheter, or to ambulate or transport the patient.
- Never leave the catheter in place longer than is necessary.
- Avoid routine catheter changes. The catheter is changed only to correct problems such as leakage, blockage, or encrustations.
- Avoid unnecessary handling or manipulation of the catheter by the patient or staff.
- Carry out hand hygiene before and after handling the catheter, tubing, or drainage bag.
- Wash the perineal area with soap and water at least twice a day; avoid a to-and-fro motion of the catheter. Dry the area well, but avoid applying powder because it may irritate the perineum.
- Monitor the patient's voiding when the catheter is removed. The patient must void within 8 hours; if unable to void, the patient may require catheterization with a straight catheter.
- Obtain a urine specimen for culture at the first sign of infection.

It should be kept in its own container, such as a plastic food-storage bag.

In teaching the patient, the nurse emphasizes the importance of frequent catheterization and emptying the bladder at the prescribed time. The average daytime clean intermittent catheterization schedule is every 4 to 6 hours and just before bedtime. If the patient is awakened at night with an urge to void, catheterization may be performed after an attempt to void (Reilly, 2001).

The female patient assumes a Fowler's position and uses a mirror to help locate the urinary meatus. She inserts the catheter 7.5 cm into the urethra, in a downward and backward direction. The male patient assumes a Fowler's or sitting position, lubricates the catheter and retracts the foreskin of the penis with one hand while grasping the penis and holding it at a right angle to the body. (This manoeuvre straightens the urethra and makes it easier to insert the catheter.) He inserts the catheter 15 to 25 cm until urine begins to flow. After removal, the catheter is cleaned, rinsed, and wrapped in a paper towel or placed in a plastic bag or case. Patients following this routine should consult a primary health care provider at regular intervals to assess urinary function and to detect complications.

If the patient cannot perform intermittent self-catheterization, a family member may be taught to carry out the procedure at regular intervals during the day.

Another self-catheterization option is creation of the Mitrofanoff umbilical appendicovesicostomy, which provides easy access to the bladder. In this procedure, the bladder neck is closed and the appendix is used to gain access to the bladder from the skin surface. A submucosal tunnel is created with the appendix; one end of the appendix is brought to the skin surface and used as a stoma and the other end is tunnelled into the bladder. The appendix may be used as an artificial urinary sphincter when an alternative is necessary to empty the bladder. In children, the most common reason for the procedure is spina bifida. In adults, a surgically prepared continent urine reservoir with a sphincter mechanism is required in cases of bladder cancer, severe interstitial cystitis, or in males, bladder exstrophy-epispadias complex when a radical cystectomy (surgical removal of the bladder) is necessary. This procedure for surgically creating a sphincter, which is attached to an internal pouch reservoir that can be catheterized, is possible only in individuals who have a healthy appendix (Kajbafzadeh & Chubak, 2001; Uygur et al., 2001).

Dialysis

Dialysis is used to remove fluid and uremic waste products from the body when the kidneys cannot do so. It may also be used to treat patients with edema that does not respond to treatment, hepatic coma, hyperkalemia, hypercalcemia, hypertension, and uremia. Methods of therapy include **hemodialysis**, continuous renal replacement therapy (CRRT; discussed later), and various forms of **peritoneal dialysis**. The need for dialysis may be acute or chronic.

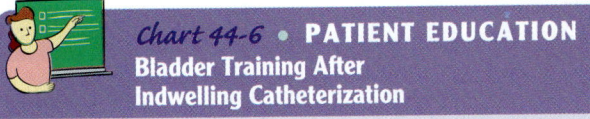

Chart 44-6 · PATIENT EDUCATION
Bladder Training After Indwelling Catheterization

- Instruct the patient to drink a measured amount of fluid from 8 AM to 10 PM to avoid bladder overdistention. Offer no fluids (except sips) after 10 PM.
- At specified times, ask the patient to void by applying pressure over the bladder, tapping the abdomen, or stretching the anal sphincter with a finger to trigger the bladder.
- Immediately after the voiding attempt, catheterize the patient to determine the amount of residual urine.
- Measure the volumes of urine voided and obtained by catheterization.
- Palpate the bladder at repeated intervals to assess for distention.
- Instruct the patient without usual sensation to be alert for any signs that indicate a full bladder, such as perspiration, cold hands or feet, and feelings of anxiety.
- Lengthen the intervals between catheterizations as the volume of residual urine decreases. Catheterization is usually discontinued when the volume of residual urine is at an acceptable level.

Acute dialysis is indicated when there is a high and rising level of serum potassium, fluid overload, or impending pulmonary edema, increasing acidosis, pericarditis, and severe confusion. It may also be used to remove certain medications or other toxins (poisoning or medication overdose) from the blood.

Chronic or maintenance dialysis is indicated in chronic renal failure, known as end-stage renal disease (ESRD), in the following instances: the presence of uremic signs and symptoms affecting all body systems (nausea and vomiting, severe anorexia, increasing lethargy, mental confusion), hyperkalemia, fluid overload not responsive to diuretics and fluid restriction, and a general lack of well-being. An urgent indication for dialysis in patients with chronic renal failure is pericardial friction rub.

Patients with no renal function can be maintained by dialysis for years. Although the costs of dialysis are usually reimbursable, limitations on the patient's ability to work resulting from illness and dialysis usually impose a great financial burden on patients and families.

The decision to initiate dialysis should be reached only after thoughtful discussion among the patient, family, physician, and others as appropriate. Many potentially life-threatening issues are associated with the need for dialysis. The nurse can assist the patient and family by answering their questions, clarifying the information provided, and supporting their decision. The lifestyle changes that patients needing hemodialysis eventually need to make are often overwhelming. Sometimes the news that a donor kidney is available for transplantation can be so disruptive to the changes in lifestyle that were made to accommodate hemodialysis that the patient may stall the process required for transplantation or refuse the kidney when it becomes available, choosing instead to continue with hemodialysis.

No "gold standard" is available to assess the compliance of hemodialysis patients (Kaveh & Kimmel, 2001), and methods to do so vary from one dialysis facility to the next. Therefore, it is difficult to assess how many deaths are due to natural causes and how many are due to patients' noncompliance with treatment.

Successful kidney transplantation eliminates the need for dialysis. Not only is the quality of life much improved in patients with ESRD who undergo transplantation, but physiologic function, such as heart rate variability, is improved as well (Hathaway, Wicks, Cashion, et al., 2000). Patients who undergo renal transplantation from living donors before dialysis is initiated generally have longer survival of the transplanted kidney than patients who receive transplantation after dialysis treatment is initiated (Mange, Joffe & Feldman, 2001).

HEMODIALYSIS

Hemodialysis is the most commonly used method of dialysis. In 2001, approximately 13,000 Canadians were on hemodialysis (Canadian Organ Replacement Register, 2003). It is used for patients who are acutely ill and require short-term dialysis (days to weeks) and for patients with ESRD who require long-term or permanent therapy. A **dialyzer** (once referred to as an artificial kidney) serves as a synthetic semipermeable membrane, replacing the renal glomeruli and tubules as the filter for the impaired kidneys.

For patients with chronic renal failure, hemodialysis prevents death, although it does not cure renal disease and does not compensate for the loss of endocrine or metabolic activities of the kidneys. Patients receiving hemodialysis must undergo treatment for the rest of their lives or until they undergo a successful kidney transplant. Treatments usually occur three times a week for at least 3 to 4 hours per treatment (some patients undergo short-daily he-

modialysis; Chart 44-7). Patients receive chronic or maintenance dialysis when they require dialysis therapy for survival and control of uremic symptoms. The trend in managing ESRD is to initiate treatment before the signs and symptoms associated with uremia become severe.

Principles of Hemodialysis

The objectives of hemodialysis are to extract toxic nitrogenous substances from the blood and to remove excess water. In hemodialysis, the blood, laden with toxins and nitrogenous wastes, is diverted from the patient to a machine, a dialyzer, in which the blood is cleansed and then returned to the patient.

Diffusion, **osmosis**, and **ultrafiltration** are the principles on which hemodialysis is based. The toxins and wastes in the blood are removed by diffusion—that is, they move from an area of higher concentration in the blood to an area of lower concentration in the **dialysate**. The dialysate is a solution made up of all the important electrolytes in their ideal extracellular concentrations. The electrolyte level in the patient's blood can be brought under control by properly adjusting the dialysate bath. The semipermeable membrane impedes the diffusion of large molecules, such as red blood cells and proteins.

Excess water is removed from the blood by osmosis, in which water moves from an area of higher solute concentration (the blood) to an area of lower solute concentration (the dialysate bath). Ultrafiltration is defined as water moving under high pressure to an area of lower pressure. This process is much more efficient at water removal than osmosis. Ultrafiltration is accomplished by applying negative pressure or a suctioning force to the dialysis membrane. Because patients with renal disease usually cannot excrete water, this force is necessary to remove fluid to achieve fluid balance.

The body's buffer system is maintained using a dialysate bath made up of bicarbonate (most common) or acetate, which is metabolized to form bicarbonate. The anticoagulant heparin is administered to keep blood from clotting in the dialysis circuit. Cleansed blood is returned to the body. By the end of the dialysis

Chart 44-7   Short, Daily Hemodialysis

With an increasing number of individuals receiving hemodialysis, cost issues continue to be of concern. Some think that daily hemodialysis may improve clinical outcomes and reduce hospital days, thereby justifying the cost of daily dialysis. Daily dialysis can be safely delivered in the clinical setting by health professionals or in the home setting by patients and family members trained in the procedure. Although short, daily hemodialysis was originally described in 1969, it lost favour when large clinical dialysis centres emerged in the 1970s.

Daily hemodialysis can be completed by the short, high-efficiency method or the slow, nocturnal method. To date, there are no studies demonstrating that one method is superior to the other. Patients in both groups have a higher success rate than those receiving three traditional hemodialysis treatments per week, and quality of life is significantly increased as well. Anemia is reduced, thus decreasing the need for Epogen. Blood pressure and volume management is better with daily dialysis. Although the economic impact of daily dialysis is yet unknown, the general premise appears to be that the higher dialysis costs will be offset by lower morbidity rates, including fewer acute hospitalizations and lower overall medication costs (Fagugli et al., 2001; Lindsay & Kortas, 2001; Mohr et al., 2001).

treatment, many waste products have been removed, the electrolyte balance has been restored to normal, and the buffer system has been replenished.

Equipment: Dialyzers

Most dialyzers, or artificial kidneys, are either flat-plate dialyzers or hollow-fibre artificial kidneys that contain thousands of tiny cellophane tubules that act as semipermeable membranes. The blood flows through the tubules, while a solution (the dialysate) circulates around the tubules. The exchange of wastes from the blood to the dialysate occurs through the semipermeable membrane of the tubules (Fig. 44-4).

Dialyzers have undergone many technological changes. The difference between flat-plate dialyzers and hollow-fibre dialyzers lies in performance and biocompatibility. Biocompatibility refers to the ability of the dialyzer to accomplish its objectives without causing hypersensitive, allergic, or adverse reactions. Some dialyzers remove middle-weight molecules at a faster rate and ultrafiltrate at higher rates, which is thought to reduce neuropathy of the lower extremities, a complication of long-term hemodialysis. In general, the more efficient the dialyzer, the higher the cost.

Another technological advance is high-flux dialysis, which uses highly permeable membranes that increase the clearance of low- and mid-molecular-weight molecules. These special membranes are used with higher-than-traditional rates of flow for the blood entering and exiting the dialyzer (500 to 800 mL/min). High-flux dialysis requires the use of precise volumetric ultrafiltration control systems, and not every dialysis unit can perform this type of dialysis. High-flux dialysis increases the efficiency of treatments while shortening their duration and reducing the need for heparin.

Because of the costs associated with hemodialysis, hemodialyzers are commonly reused in dialysis centres in Canada and the United States. Recent studies have raised concerns about the mortality risks associated with some hemodialyzer reuse practices. Results from the United States Renal Data System (USRDS) Dialysis Morbidity and Mortality Study demonstrated differences in mortality rate with the reuse of certain hemodialyzers. Among all membranes, mortality is lowest for patients treated with high-flux synthetic membranes. The bleaching process to reuse high-flux synthetic membrane dialyzers may account for the lower mortality rate: with this process, clearance of larger molecules is still possible, even though the hemodialyzer is not new. These findings are important because high-flux hemodialyzers are very efficient and are used in most dialysis centres (Port, Wolfe, Hulbert-Shearson et al., 2001).

Vascular Access

Access to the patient's vascular system must be established to allow blood to be removed, cleansed, and returned to the patient's vascular system at rates between 200 and 800 mL/minute. Several types of access are available.

SUBCLAVIAN, INTERNAL, JUGULAR, AND FEMORAL CATHETERS

Immediate access to the patient's circulation for acute hemodialysis is achieved by inserting a double-lumen or multilumen catheter into the subclavian, internal jugular, or femoral vein. Although this method of vascular access involves some risk (eg, hematoma, pneumothorax, infection, thrombosis of the subclavian vein, and inadequate flow), it can be used for several weeks. The catheters

FIGURE 44-4 Hemodialysis system. (**A**) Blood from an artery is pumped into (**B**) a dialyzer where it flows through the cellophane tubes, which act as the semipermeable membrane (*inset*). The dialysate, which has the same chemical composition as the blood except for urea and waste products, flows in around the tubules. The waste products in the blood diffuse through the semipermeable membrane into the dialysate.

are removed when no longer needed, because the patient's condition has improved or another type of access has been established. Double-lumen, cuffed catheters may also be surgically inserted into the subclavian vein of patients requiring a central venous catheter for dialysis (Fig. 44-5).

FISTULA

A more permanent access, known as a **fistula**, is created surgically (usually in the forearm) by joining (anastomosing) an artery to a vein, either side to side or end to side (Fig. 44-6). Needles are inserted into the vessel to obtain blood flow adequate to pass through the dialyzer. The arterial segment of the fistula is used for arterial flow and the venous segment for reinfusion of the dialyzed blood. The fistula takes 4 to 6 weeks to mature before it is ready for use. This gives time for healing and for the venous segment of the fistula to dilate to accommodate two large-bore (14- or 16-gauge) needles. The patient is encouraged to perform exercises to increase the size of these vessels (ie, squeezing a rubber ball for forearm fistulas) and thereby to accommodate the large-bore needles used in hemodialysis.

GRAFT

An **arteriovenous graft** can be created by subcutaneously interposing a biologic, semibiologic, or synthetic graft material between an artery and vein (see Fig. 44-6). The most commonly used synthetic graft material is expanded polytetrafluoroethylene (PTFE). Usually, a graft is created when the patient's vessels are not suitable for a fistula. Patients with compromised vascular systems (eg, from diabetes) often need to have a graft to undergo hemodialysis. Grafts are usually placed in the forearm, upper arm,

or upper thigh. Infection and thrombosis are the most common complications of arteriovenous grafts.

> **NURSING ALERT** Failure of the permanent dialysis access (fistula or graft) accounts for most hospital admissions of patients undergoing chronic hemodialysis. Thus, protection of the access is of high priority.

Complications of Hemodialysis

Although hemodialysis can prolong life indefinitely, it does not alter the natural course of the underlying kidney disease, nor does it completely replace kidney function. The patient is subject to a number of problems and complications. One leading cause of death among patients undergoing maintenance hemodialysis is atherosclerotic cardiovascular disease. Disturbances of lipid metabolism (hypertriglyceridemia) appear to be accentuated by hemodialysis. Heart failure, coronary heart disease and anginal pain, stroke, and peripheral vascular insufficiency may occur and may incapacitate the patient. Anemia and fatigue contribute to diminished physical and emotional well-being, lack of energy and drive, and loss of interest, although the use of erythropoietin (Epogen) before the start of dialysis has been shown to have a significant effect on hematocrit values for the first 19 months after starting dialysis (Fink et al., 2001). Increased dialyzer clotting may occur, which is prevented by adjusting heparin doses, and dialyzer solute clearances may decrease slightly (Eschbach & Adamson, 1989).

Gastric ulcers and other gastrointestinal problems occur from the physiologic stress of chronic illness, medication, and related problems. Disturbed calcium metabolism leads to renal osteodystrophy that produces bone pain and fractures. Other problems include fluid overload associated with heart failure, malnutrition, infection, neuropathy, and pruritus.

Up to 85% of people undergoing hemodialysis experience major sleep problems that further complicate their overall health status. Recent studies suggest that early-morning or late-afternoon dialysis may be a risk factor for developing sleep abnormalities. Researchers suggest such interventions as changing the temperature

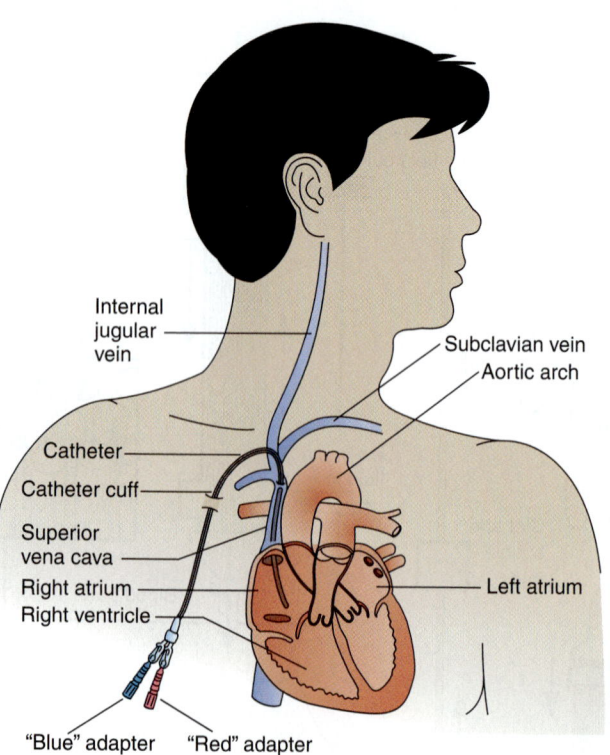

FIGURE 44-5 Double-lumen, cuffed hemodialysis catheter used in acute hemodialysis. The red adapter is attached to a blood line through which blood is pumped from the patient to the dialyzer. After the blood passes through the dialyzer (artificial kidney), it returns to the patient through the blue adapter.

FIGURE 44-6 An internal arteriovenous fistula (*top*) is created by a side-to-side anastomosis of the artery and vein. A graft (*bottom*) can also be established between the artery and vein.

of the dialysate bath to prevent temperature elevation and limiting napping during dialysis as strategies to reduce sleep problems in individuals receiving hemodialysis (Parker et al., 2000). Other complications of dialysis treatment may include the following:

- Hypotension may occur during the treatment as fluid is removed. Nausea and vomiting, diaphoresis, tachycardia, and dizziness are common signs of hypotension.
- Painful muscle cramping may occur, usually late in dialysis as fluid and electrolytes rapidly leave the extracellular space.
- Exsanguination may occur if blood lines separate or dialysis needles accidentally become dislodged.
- Dysrhythmias may result from electrolyte and pH changes or from removal of antiarrhythmic medications during dialysis.
- Air embolism is rare but can occur if air enters the vascular system.
- Chest pain may occur in patients with anemia or arteriosclerotic heart disease.
- Dialysis disequilibrium results from cerebral fluid shifts. Signs and symptoms include headache, nausea and vomiting, restlessness, decreased level of consciousness, and seizures. It is more likely to occur in acute renal failure or when blood urea nitrogen levels are very high (exceeding 150 mg/dL).

Long-Term Management

During dialysis, the patient, the dialyzer, and the dialysate bath require constant monitoring because numerous complications are possible, including air embolism, inadequate or excessive ultrafiltration (hypotension, cramping, vomiting), blood leaks, contamination, and access complications. The nurse in the dialysis unit has an important role in monitoring, supporting, assessing, and educating the patient. Nursing care of the patient and maintenance of the access device are discussed under "Care of the Hospitalized Dialysis Patient."

Pharmacologic Therapy

Just as many medications are excreted wholly or in part by the kidneys, many medications are removed from the blood during hemodialysis; therefore, the physician may need to adjust the dosage. Metabolites of drugs that are bound to protein are not removed during dialysis. Removal of other drug metabolites depends on the weight and size of the molecule.

Patients undergoing hemodialysis who require medications (eg, cardiac glycosides, antibiotic agents, antiarrhythmic medications, antihypertensive agents) are monitored closely to ensure that blood and tissue levels of these medications are maintained without toxic accumulation.

In patients receiving dialysis, all medications and their dosages must be carefully evaluated. Antihypertensive therapy, often part of the dialysis patient's regimen, is one example in which communication, teaching, and evaluation can make a difference in patient outcomes. The patient must know when and when not to take the medication. For example, if an antihypertensive agent is taken on a dialysis day, a hypotensive effect may occur during dialysis, causing dangerously low blood pressure. Many medications that are taken once daily can be held until after the dialysis treatment.

Nutritional and Fluid Therapy

When damaged kidneys cannot excrete end products of metabolism, these substances accumulate in the serum as toxins. The resulting symptoms, collectively known as uremic symptoms or uremic syndrome, affect every body system. The more toxins that accumulate, the more severe the symptoms.

Diet is an important factor for patients on hemodialysis because of the effects of uremia. Goals of nutritional therapy are to minimize uremic symptoms and fluid and electrolyte imbalances; to maintain good nutritional status through adequate protein, calorie, vitamin, and mineral intake; and to enable the patient to eat a palatable and enjoyable diet. Restricting dietary protein decreases the accumulation of nitrogenous wastes, reduces uremic symptoms, and may even postpone the initiation of dialysis for a few months. Restriction of fluid is also part of the dietary prescription because fluid accumulation may occur, leading to weight gain, heart failure, and pulmonary edema.

With the initiation of hemodialysis, the patient's dietary intake usually still requires some restriction of dietary protein, sodium, potassium, and fluid intake. Protein intake is restricted to about 1 g/kg ideal body weight per day; therefore, protein must be of high biologic quality and consist of the essential amino acids to prevent poor protein use and to maintain a positive nitrogen balance. Examples of foods high in biologic protein content include eggs, meat, milk, poultry, and fish. Sodium is usually restricted to 2 to 3 g/day; fluids are restricted to an amount equal to the daily urine output plus 500 mL/day. The goal for hemodialysis patients is to keep their interdialytic (between dialysis treatments) weight gain under 1.5 kg. Potassium restriction (average 1.5 to 2.5 g/day) depends on the amount of residual renal function and the frequency of dialysis (National Kidney Foundation, 2000).

Dietary restriction is an unwelcome change in lifestyle for many patients with chronic renal failure. Patients often feel stigmatized in social situations because there may be few food selections available for their diet. If the restrictions are ignored, life-threatening complications, such as hyperkalemia and pulmonary edema, may result. Thus, the patient may feel punished for responding to basic human drives to eat and drink. The nurse who encounters a patient with symptoms or complications resulting from dietary indiscretion must avoid harsh, judgmental, or punitive tones when communicating with him or her.

Nursing Management

Patients requiring long-term hemodialysis are often concerned about the unpredictability of the illness and the disruption of their lives. They often have financial problems, difficulty holding a job, waning sexual desire and impotence, depression from being chronically ill, and fear of dying. Younger patients worry about marriage, having children, and the burden that they bring to their families. The regimented lifestyle that frequent dialysis treatments and restrictions in food and fluid intake impose is often demoralizing to the patient and family.

MEETING PSYCHOSOCIAL NEEDS

Dialysis alters the lifestyle of the patient and family. The amount of time required for dialysis and physician visits and being chronically ill can create conflict, frustration, guilt, and depression. It may be difficult for the patient, spouse, and family to express anger and negative feelings.

The nurse needs to give the patient and family the opportunity to express feelings of anger and concern over the limitations that the disease and treatment impose and over possible financial problems and job insecurity. If anger is not expressed, it may be directed inward and lead to depression, despair, and attempts at suicide (suicide is more prevalent in dialysis patients); however, if anger is projected outward to other people, it may destroy already threatened family relationships.

Although normal in this situation, these feelings are often profound and overwhelming. Counselling and psychotherapy may be necessary. Depression may require treatment with antidepressant agents. Referring the patient and family to a mental health provider with expertise in the care of patients receiving dialysis may also be helpful. Clinical nurse specialists, psychologists, and social workers may be helpful in assisting the patient and family to cope with the changes brought about by renal failure and its treatment.

The sense of loss that the patient experiences cannot be underestimated because every aspect of a "normal life" is disrupted. Some patients use denial to deal with the overwhelming array of medical problems (eg, infections, hypertension, anemia, neuropathy). Staff who are tempted to label the patient as noncompliant must consider the impact of renal failure and its treatment on the patient and family and the coping strategies that they may use. The nurse helps the patient to identify safe, effective coping strategies to cope with these ever-present problems and fears (Tonelli et al., 2001).

PROMOTING HOME AND COMMUNITY-BASED CARE

Preparing a patient for hemodialysis is challenging. Often the patient does not fully comprehend the impact of dialysis, and learning needs may go unrecognized. Good communication between the dialysis staff (in the hospital and outpatient clinic), unit staff, and home care nurses is essential for providing sound, continuous care.

Teaching Patients Self-Care. Assessment helps identify the learning needs of the patient and family members. In many cases, the patient is home before learning needs and readiness to learn can be thoroughly evaluated; therefore, hospital-based nurses, dialysis staff, and home care nurses must work together to provide appropriate teaching that meets the patient's and family's changing needs and readiness to learn.

The diagnosis of chronic renal failure and the need for dialysis often overwhelm the patient and family. In addition, many patients with ESRD have depressed mentation, a shortened attention span, a decreased level of concentration, and altered perceptual states. Therefore, teaching must occur in brief, 10- to 15-minute sessions, with time added for clarification, repetition, reinforcement, and questions from the patient and family. The nurse needs to convey a nonjudgmental attitude to enable the patient and family to discuss options and their feelings about those options. Team conferences are helpful for sharing information and providing every team member the opportunity to discuss the needs of the patient and family.

Teaching Patients About Hemodialysis. Although most patients who require hemodialysis undergo the procedure in an outpatient setting, home hemodialysis is an option for some. Home hemodialysis requires a highly motivated patient who is willing to take responsibility for the procedure and is able to adjust each treatment to meet the body's changing needs. It also requires the commitment and cooperation of a family member to assist the patient. Many patients, however, are not comfortable imposing on others in that way and do not wish to subject family members to the feeling that their home is being turned into a clinic.

The health care team should never force a patient into using home hemodialysis. Because this treatment requires many significant changes in the home and family, home hemodialysis must be the patient's and family's decision.

The patient undergoing home hemodialysis and the caregiver assisting that patient must be trained to prepare, operate, and disassemble the dialysis machine; maintain and clean the equipment; administer medications (eg, heparin) into the machine lines; and handle emergency problems (hemodialysis dialyzer rupture, electrical or mechanical problems, hypotension, shock, and seizures). Because home hemodialysis places primary responsibility for the treatment on the patient and the family member, they must understand and be capable of performing all aspects of the hemodialysis procedure (Chart 44-8).

Before home hemodialysis is initiated, the home environment, household and community resources, and ability and willingness of the patient and family to carry out this treatment are assessed.

Chart 44-8
Home Care Checklist • Hemodialysis

At the completion of the home care instruction, the patient or caregiver will be able to:	Patient	Caregiver
• Discuss renal failure and its effects on the body.	✓	✓
• Describe the cause of renal failure and why hemodialysis is necessary.	✓	✓
• Describe the basic principles of hemodialysis.	✓	✓
• Discuss common problems that may occur during hemodialysis and their prevention and management.	✓	✓
• Demonstrate knowledge about prescribed medications and the reason for their use, potential side effects, guidelines on when to notify physician, and the schedule of medications on dialysis and nondialysis days.	✓	✓
• Acknowledge dietary and fluid restrictions, rationale, and consequences of noncompliance.	✓	✓
• Describe commonly measured laboratory values, results, and implications.	✓	✓
• List guidelines for prevention and detection of fluid overload, meaning of "dry" weight, and how to weigh self.	✓	✓
• Demonstrate vascular access care, how to check patency, signs and symptoms of infection, prevention of complications.	✓	✓
• Discuss strategies for detection, management, and relief of pruritus, neuropathy, and other complications of renal failure.	✓	✓
• Develop strategies to manage or reduce anxiety and maintain independence.	✓	✓
• Coordinate financial arrangements for dialysis and strategies to identify and obtain resources.	✓	✓

The home is surveyed to see if electrical outlets, plumbing facilities, and storage space are adequate. Modifications may be needed to enable the patient and assistant to perform dialysis safely and to deal with emergencies.

Once home dialysis is initiated, the home care nurse must visit periodically to evaluate compliance with the recommended techniques, to assess the patient for complications, to reinforce previous teaching, and to provide reassurance.

Continuing Care. The health care team's goal in treating patients with chronic renal failure is to maximize their vocational potential, functional status, and quality of life. To facilitate renal rehabilitation, appropriate follow-up and monitoring by members of the health care team (physicians, dialysis nurses, social workers, psychologist, home care nurses, and others as appropriate) are essential to identify and resolve problems early on. Many patients with chronic renal failure can resume relatively normal lives, doing the things that are important to them: traveling, exercising, working, or actively participating in family activities. If appropriate interventions are available early in the course of dialysis, the potential for better health improves, and the patient can remain active in family and community life. Chart 44-9 outlines the essential elements identified by the Life Options Rehabilitation Advisory Council for the rehabilitation of dialysis patients. Outcome goals for renal rehabilitation include employment for those able to work, improved physical functioning of all patients, improved understanding about adaptation and options for living well, increased control over the effects of kidney disease and dialysis, and resumption of activities enjoyed before dialysis.

CONTINUOUS RENAL REPLACEMENT THERAPIES

Several types of **continuous renal replacement therapy (CRRT)** are available and are widely used in critical care units. CRRT may be indicated for patients who have acute or chronic renal failure and who are too clinically unstable for traditional hemodialysis,

for patients with fluid overload secondary to oliguric (low urine output) renal failure, and for patients whose kidneys cannot handle their acutely high metabolic or nutritional needs. CRRT does not produce rapid fluid shifts, does not require dialysis machines or dialysis personnel to carry out the procedures, and can be initiated quickly in hospitals without dialysis facilities.

CRRT methods are similar to hemodialysis methods in that they require access to the circulation and blood to pass through an artificial filter. A hemofilter (an extremely porous blood filter containing a semipermeable membrane) is used in all CRRT methods, which are described below (Astle, 2001).

Continuous Arteriovenous Hemofiltration

Continuous arteriovenous hemofiltration (CAVH) was first used in 1977 to treat fluid overload. Blood is circulated through a small-volume, low-resistance filter, using the patient's arterial pressure rather than that of the blood pump as is used in hemodialysis. Blood flows from an artery (usually by an arterial catheter in the femoral artery) to a hemofilter. A pressure gradient is necessary for optimal filtration; cannulation of the femoral artery and vein provides the necessary gradient (difference) in arterial and venous pressures. The filtered blood then returns to the patient's circulation through a venous catheter. Intravenous fluids may be administered to replace fluid removed by the procedure. With CAVH, there is no concentration gradient, so only fluid is filtered. Electrolytes are eliminated only as they are pulled along and removed with the fluid. Ultrafiltrate is collected in a drainage bag, measured, and discarded. CAVH is usually set up and initiated by trained dialysis staff and then maintained and monitored by critical care personnel.

Continuous Arteriovenous Hemodialysis

Continuous arteriovenous hemodialysis (CAVHD) has many of the characteristics of CAVH but offers the advantage of a concentration gradient for faster clearance of urea. This is accomplished by the circulation of dialysate on one side of a semipermeable membrane. The blood flow through the system depends on the patient's arterial pressure, as in CAVH; a blood pump is not used as it is in standard hemodialysis. CAVHD is usually set up and initiated by trained dialysis staff and then maintained and monitored by critical care personnel.

Continuous Venovenous Hemofiltration

Continuous venovenous hemofiltration (CVVH) is increasingly being used in managing acute renal failure. Blood from a double-lumen venous catheter is pumped (using a small blood pump) through a hemofilter and then returned to the patient through the same catheter (Fig. 44-7). CVVH provides continuous slow fluid removal (ultrafiltration); therefore, hemodynamic effects are mild and better tolerated by patients with unstable conditions. CVVH has several other benefits over CAVH in that no arterial access is required and critical care nurses can set up, initiate, maintain, and terminate the system.

Continuous Venovenous Hemodialysis

Continuous venovenous hemodialysis (CVVHD) is similar to CVVH. Blood is pumped from a double-lumen venous catheter through a hemofilter and returned to the patient through the same catheter. In addition to the benefits of ultrafiltration, CVVHD

> ### Chart 44-9   The Five Es: Bridges to Renal Rehabilitation
>
> **Encouragement:** Patients, families, and staff need encouragement to adopt a positive attitude toward rehabilitation.
>
> **Education:** Patients need to understand their disease. They need to learn strategies for successful adaptation to dialysis and how to maximize functional status, among many other subjects. Parents, staff, and employers require education about the many positive life options of dialysis patients.
>
> **Exercise:** Exercise is critical to rehabilitation, just as with heart disease. Many levels of activity to fit the different abilities of renal patients are helpful, from vigorous workouts to stretching exercises.
>
> **Employment:** The primary goal is to allow dialysis patients to keep their current jobs whenever possible. If not possible, vocational rehabilitation counselling should be used.
>
> **Evaluation:** Systematic evaluation of rehabilitation outcomes is necessary to identify and measure which interventions have made an impact.
>
> ---
>
> Adapted from Life Options Rehabilitation Advisory Council (1994). *Renal rehabilitation: Bridging the barriers.* Madison, WI: Medical Education Institute.

FIGURE 44-7 Continuous venovenous hemofiltration (CVVH) removes fluid (ultrafiltrate) slowly from the blood.

uses a concentration gradient to facilitate the removal of uremic toxins. Therefore, no arterial access is required, hemodynamic effects are usually mild, and critical care nurses can set up, initiate, maintain, and terminate the system.

PERITONEAL DIALYSIS

The goals of peritoneal dialysis are to remove toxic substances and metabolic wastes and to re-establish normal fluid and electrolyte balance. Peritoneal dialysis may be the treatment of choice for patients with renal failure who are unable or unwilling to undergo hemodialysis or renal transplantation. Patients who are susceptible to the rapid fluid, electrolyte, and metabolic changes that occur during hemodialysis experience fewer of these problems with the slower rate of peritoneal dialysis. Therefore, patients with diabetes or cardiovascular disease, many older patients, and those who may be at risk for adverse effects of systemic heparin are likely candidates for peritoneal dialysis. Additionally, severe hypertension, heart failure, and pulmonary edema not responsive to usual treatment regimens have been successfully treated with peritoneal dialysis.

Peritoneal dialysis can be performed using several different approaches: acute, intermittent peritoneal dialysis; **continuous am-**

bulatory peritoneal dialysis (CAPD); and **continuous cyclic peritoneal dialysis (CCPD)**. These three methods are discussed later in this chapter. As with other forms of treatment, the decision to begin peritoneal dialysis is made by the patient and family in consultation with the physician.

Although specific patient populations do benefit from peritoneal dialysis, it is not as efficient as hemodialysis (Lindsay & Kortas, 2001). Because cardiovascular disease is the cause of death in half of all patients with ESRD, the adequacy of dialysis must be defined, in part, by its potential to reduce cardiovascular disease. Blood pressure, volume, left ventricular hypertrophy, and dyslipidemias are the major causes of morbidity and mortality in patients undergoing peritoneal dialysis (Chatoth, Golper & Gokal, 1999).

Underlying Principles

In peritoneal dialysis, the peritoneum, a serous membrane that covers the abdominal organs and lines the abdominal wall, serves as the semipermeable membrane. The surface of the peritoneum constitutes a body surface area of about 22,000 cm². Sterile dialysate fluid is introduced into the peritoneal cavity through an abdominal catheter at intervals (Fig. 44-8). Urea and creatinine,

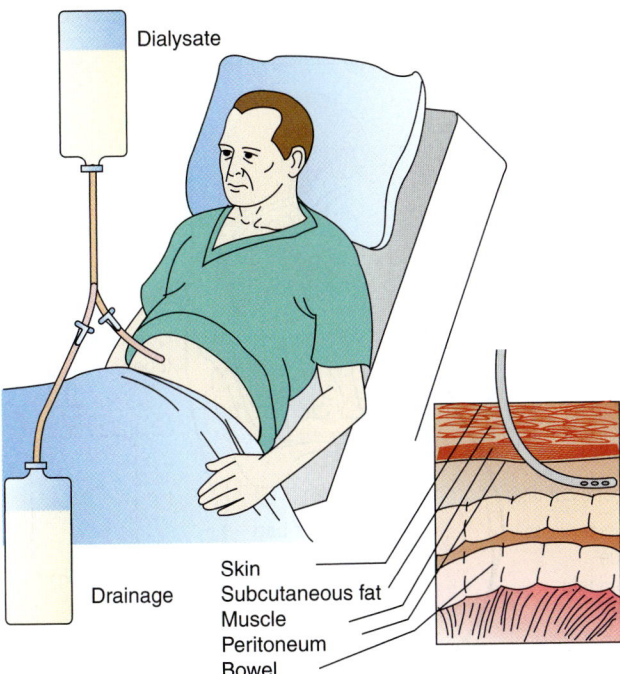

Dialysate

Drainage

Skin
Subcutaneous fat
Muscle
Peritoneum
Bowel

FIGURE 44-8 In peritoneal dialysis and in acute intermittent peritoneal dialysis, dialysate is infused into the peritoneal cavity by gravity, after which the clamp on the infusion line is closed. After a dwell time (when the dialysate is in the peritoneal cavity), the drainage tube is unclamped and the fluid drains from the peritoneal cavity, again by gravity. A new container of dialysate is infused as soon as drainage is complete. The duration of the dwell time depends on the type of peritoneal dialysis.

metabolic end products normally excreted by the kidneys, are cleared from the blood by diffusion and osmosis as waste products move from an area of higher concentration (the peritoneal blood supply) to an area of lower concentration (the peritoneal cavity) across a semipermeable membrane (the peritoneal membrane). Urea is cleared at a rate of 15 to 20 mL/min, whereas creatinine is removed at a slower rate. It usually takes 36 to 48 hours to achieve with peritoneal dialysis what hemodialysis accomplishes in 6 to 8 hours. Ultrafiltration (water removal) occurs in peritoneal dialysis through an osmotic gradient created by using a dialysate fluid with a higher glucose concentration.

Procedure

The patient undergoing peritoneal dialysis may be acutely ill, thus requiring short-term treatment to correct severe disturbances in fluid and electrolyte status, or may have chronic renal failure and need to receive ongoing treatments.

PREPARING THE PATIENT

The nurse's preparation of the patient and family for peritoneal dialysis depends on the patient's physical and psychological status, level of alertness, previous experience with dialysis, and understanding of and familiarity with the procedure.

The nurse explains the procedure to the patient and obtains signed consent for it. Baseline vital signs, weight, and serum electrolyte levels are recorded. The patient is encouraged to empty the bladder and bowel to reduce the risk of puncturing internal organs. The nurse also assesses the patient's anxiety about the procedure and provides support and instruction. Broad-spectrum

antibiotic agents may be administered to prevent infection. If the peritoneal catheter is to be inserted in the operating room, this is explained to the patient and family.

PREPARING THE EQUIPMENT

In addition to assembling the equipment for peritoneal dialysis, the nurse consults with the physician to determine the concentration of dialysate to be used and the medications to be added to it. Heparin may be added to prevent blood clotting and resultant occlusion of the peritoneal catheter. Potassium chloride may be prescribed to prevent hypokalemia. Antibiotics may be added to treat peritonitis. Insulin may be added for diabetic patients; a larger-than-normal dose may be needed, however, because about 10% of the insulin binds to the dialysate container. All medications are added immediately before the solution is instilled. Aseptic technique is crucial.

Before medications are added, the dialysate is warmed to body temperature to prevent patient discomfort and abdominal pain and to dilate the vessels of the peritoneum to increase urea clearance. Solutions that are too cold cause pain and vasoconstriction and reduce clearance. Solutions that are too hot burn the peritoneum. Dry heating is recommended (heating cabinet, incubator, or heating pad). Microwave heating of the fluid is not recommended because of the danger of burning the peritoneum.

Immediately before initiating dialysis, the nurse assembles the administration set and tubing. The tubing is filled with the prepared dialysate to reduce the amount of air entering the catheter and peritoneal cavity, which could increase abdominal discomfort and interfere with instillation and drainage of the fluid.

INSERTING THE CATHETER

Ideally, the peritoneal catheter is inserted in the operating room to maintain surgical asepsis and minimize the risk of contamination. In some circumstances, however, the physician inserts the catheter at the bedside under strict asepsis.

A rigid stylet catheter is inserted for acute peritoneal dialysis use only. Before the procedure, the skin is prepared with a local antiseptic to reduce skin bacteria and the risk of contamination and infection. The physician anesthetizes the site with a local anesthetic agent before making a small incision or stab wound in the lower abdomen, 3 to 5 cm below the umbilicus. Because this area is relatively free from large blood vessels, little bleeding occurs. A trocar is used to puncture the peritoneum as the patient tightens the abdominal muscles by raising the head. The catheter is threaded through the trocar and positioned. Previously prepared dialysate is infused into the peritoneal cavity, pushing the omentum (peritoneal lining extending from the abdominal organs) away from the catheter. The physician may then secure the catheter with a purse-string suture and apply antibacterial ointment and a sterile dressing over the site.

Catheters for long-term use (Tenckhoff, Swan, Cruz) are usually made of silicone and are radiopaque to permit visualization on x-ray. These catheters have three sections: (1) an intraperitoneal section, with numerous openings and an open tip to let dialysate flow freely; (2) a subcutaneous section that passes from the peritoneal membrane and tunnels through muscle and subcutaneous fat to the skin; and (3) an external section for connection to the dialysate system. Most of these catheters have two cuffs, which are made of Dacron polyester. The cuffs stabilize the catheter, limit movement, prevent leaks, and provide a barrier against microorganisms. One cuff is placed just distal to the peritoneum, and the other cuff is placed subcutaneously. The subcutaneous tunnel (5 to 10 cm long) further protects against bacterial infection (Fig. 44-9).

FIGURE 44-9 Continuous ambulatory peritoneal dialysis. (**A**) The peritoneal catheter is implanted through the abdominal wall. (**B**) Dacron cuffs and a subcutaneous tunnel provide protection against bacterial infection. (**C**) Dialysate flows by gravity through the peritoneal catheter into the peritoneal cavity. After a prescribed period of time, the fluid is drained by gravity and discarded. Additional solution is then infused into the peritoneal cavity until the next drainage period. Dialysis thus continues on a 24-hour-a-day basis during which the patient is free to move around and engage in his or her usual activities.

PERFORMING THE EXCHANGE

Peritoneal dialysis involves a series of exchanges or cycles. An exchange is defined as the infusion, dwell, and drainage of the dialysate. This cycle is repeated throughout the course of the dialysis. The dialysate is infused by gravity into the peritoneal cavity. A period of about 5 to 10 minutes is usually required to infuse 2 L of fluid. The prescribed dwell, or equilibration, time allows diffusion and osmosis to occur. Diffusion of small molecules, such as urea and creatinine, peaks in the first 5 to 10 minutes of the dwell time. At the end of the dwell time, the drainage portion of the exchange begins. The tube is unclamped and the solution drains from the peritoneal cavity by gravity through a closed system. Drainage is usually completed in 10 to 30 minutes. The drainage fluid is normally colourless or straw-coloured and should not be cloudy. Bloody drainage may be seen in the first few exchanges after insertion of a new catheter but should not occur after that time. The entire exchange (infusion, dwell time, and drainage) takes 1 to 4 hours, depending on the prescribed dwell time. The number of cycles or exchanges and their frequency are prescribed based on the patient's physical status and acuity of illness.

The removal of excess water during peritoneal dialysis is achieved by using a hypertonic dialysate with a high dextrose concentration that creates an osmotic gradient. Dextrose solutions of 1.5%, 2.5%, and 4.25% are available in several volumes, from 500 mL to 3,000 mL, allowing the dialysate selection to fit the patient's tolerance, size, and physiologic needs. The higher the dextrose concentration, the greater the osmotic gradient and the more water removed. Selection of the appropriate solution is based on the patient's fluid status.

Complications of Peritoneal Dialysis

Peritoneal dialysis is not without complications. Most are minor, but several, if unattended, can have serious consequences.

PERITONITIS

Peritonitis (inflammation of the peritoneum) is the most common and most serious complication of peritoneal dialysis. The organism responsible for peritoneal dialysis-related peritonitis is an important factor in clinical outcome and the basis of treatment guidelines. *Staphylococcus aureus* and *Staphylococcus epidermidis* remain the most common Gram-positive organisms responsible for peritonitis, although the rates of each have decreased. *Pseudomonas aeruginosa, E. coli,* and *Klebsiella* species are the most common causes of Gram-negative peritonitis. Resistance to antibacterial agents (ie, ciprofloxacin, methicillin) used in their treatment increased dramatically from 1991 to 1998 (Zelenitsky et al., 2000).

Peritonitis is characterized by cloudy dialysate drainage, diffuse abdominal pain, and rebound tenderness. Hypotension and other signs of shock may occur if *S. aureus* is the responsible organism. The patient with peritonitis may be treated as an inpatient or outpatient (most common), depending on the severity of the infection and the patient's clinical status. Initially, one to three rapid exchanges with a 1.5% dextrose solution without added medications are completed to wash out mediators of inflammation and to reduce abdominal pain. Drainage fluid is examined for cell count, and Gram's stain and culture are used to identify the organism and guide treatment. Antibiotic agents (aminoglycosides or cephalosporins) are usually added to subsequent exchanges until the Gram's stain or culture results are available for appropriate antibiotic determination. Intraperitoneal administration of antibiotics is as effective as intravenous administration. Antibiotic therapy continues for 10 to 14 days. Careful calculation of the antibiotic dosage helps prevent nephrotoxicity and further compromise of renal function.

Heparin (500 to 1,000 U/L) may be added to the dialysate to prevent fibrin clot formation; oral administration of low-dose warfarin (Coumadin) is also effective in decreasing coagulation factors and preventing thrombosis without increasing the risk of bleeding (Kim, Lee, Park et al., 2001).

Peritonitis that is unresolved after 4 days of appropriate therapy necessitates catheter removal. The patient is maintained on hemodialysis for about 1 month before a new catheter is inserted. In patients with fungal peritonitis, the peritoneal catheter must be removed if there is no response to therapy in 4 to 7 days. Tunnel infections and fecal peritonitis also necessitate catheter removal. Systemic antibiotics should continue for 5 to 7 days after catheter removal.

Regardless of which organism causes peritonitis, the patient with peritonitis loses large amounts of protein through the peritoneum. Acute malnutrition and delayed healing may result. Therefore, attention must be given to detecting and promptly treating the infections.

LEAKAGE
Leakage of dialysate through the catheter site may occur immediately after the catheter is inserted. Usually, the leak stops spontaneously if dialysis is withheld for several days to give the incision and exit site time to heal. During this time, it is important to reduce factors that might delay healing, such as undue abdominal muscle activity and straining during bowel movement. Leakage through the exit site or into the abdominal wall can occur for months or years after catheter placement. In many cases, leakage can be avoided by using small volumes (100 to 200 mL) of dialysate, gradually increasing the volume up to 2,000 mL.

BLEEDING
A bloody effluent (drainage) may be observed occasionally, especially in young, menstruating women. (The hypertonic fluid pulls blood from the uterus, through the opening in the fallopian tubes, and into the peritoneal cavity.) Bleeding is common during the first few exchanges after a new catheter insertion because some blood exists in the abdominal cavity from the procedure. In many cases, no cause can be found for the bleeding, although catheter displacement from the pelvis has occasionally been associated with bleeding. Some patients have had bloody effluent after an enema or from minor trauma. Invariably, bleeding stops in 1 to 2 days and requires no specific intervention. More frequent exchanges during this time may be necessary to prevent blood clots from obstructing the catheter.

LONG-TERM COMPLICATIONS
Hypertriglyceridemia is common in patients undergoing long-term peritoneal dialysis, suggesting that this therapy may accelerate atherogenesis. Despite this, the use of cardioprotective medications is relatively low, and many patients have suboptimal blood pressure control. Given the high burden of disease in these patients, beta-blockers and angiotensin-converting enzyme inhibitors should be used to control hypertension or protect the heart; the use of aspirin and statins should be considered. In general, health care providers need to be better educated in this area of dialysis management (Tonelli et al., 2001).

Other complications that may occur with long-term peritoneal dialysis include abdominal hernias (incisional, inguinal, diaphragmatic, and umbilical), probably resulting from continuously increased intra-abdominal pressure. The persistently elevated intra-abdominal pressure also aggravates symptoms of hiatal hernia and hemorrhoids. Low back pain and anorexia from fluid in the abdomen and a constant sweet taste related to glucose absorption may also occur.

Mechanical problems occasionally occur and may interfere with instillation or drainage of the dialysate. Formation of clots in the peritoneal catheter and constipation are factors that may contribute to these problems.

Acute Intermittent Peritoneal Dialysis

Indications for acute intermittent peritoneal dialysis, a variation of peritoneal dialysis, include uremic signs and symptoms (nausea, vomiting, fatigue, altered mental status), fluid overload, acidosis, and hyperkalemia. Although peritoneal dialysis is not as efficient as hemodialysis in removing solute and fluid, it permits a more gradual change in the patient's fluid volume status and in waste product removal. Therefore, it may be the treatment of choice for the hemodynamically unstable patient. It can be carried out manually (the nurse warms, spikes, and hangs each container of dialysate) or by a cycler machine. Exchange times range from 30 minutes to 2 hours. A common routine is hourly exchanges consisting of a 10-minute infusion, a 30-minute dwell time, and a 20-minute drain time.

Maintaining the peritoneal dialysis cycle is a nursing responsibility. Strict aseptic technique is maintained when changing solution containers and emptying drainage containers. Vital signs, weight, intake and output, laboratory values, and patient status are frequently monitored. The nurse uses a flow sheet to document each exchange and records vital signs, dialysate concentration, medications added, exchange volume, dwell time, dialysate fluid balance for the exchange (fluid lost or gained), and cumulative fluid balance. The nurse also carefully assesses skin turgor and mucous membranes to evaluate fluid status and monitor the patient for edema.

If the peritoneal fluid does not drain properly, the nurse can facilitate drainage by turning the patient from side to side or raising the head of the bed. The catheter should never be pushed in. Other measures to promote drainage include checking the patency of the catheter by inspecting for kinks, closed clamps, or an air lock. The nurse always monitors for complications, including peritonitis, bleeding, respiratory difficulty, and leakage of peritoneal fluid. Abdominal girth may be measured periodically to determine if the patient is retaining large amounts of dialysis solution. Additionally, the nurse must ensure that the peritoneal dialysis catheter remains secure and that the dressing remains dry. Physical comfort measures, frequent turning, and skin care are provided. The patient and family are educated about the procedure and are kept informed about progress (fluid loss, weight loss, laboratory values). Emotional support and encouragement are given to the patient and family during this stressful and uncertain time.

Continuous Ambulatory Peritoneal Dialysis

CAPD is a form of dialysis used for many patients with ESRD. CAPD is performed at home by the patient or a trained caregiver, who is usually a family member; the procedure allows the patient reasonable freedom and control of daily activities (Chart 44-10).

Chart 44-10 • ASSESSMENT

Assessing Suitability for CAPD

Although CAPD is not suitable for all patients with end-stage renal disease (ESRD), it is a viable therapy for those who can perform self-care and exchanges and who can fit therapy into their own routines. Often, patients report having more energy and feeling healthier once they begin CAPD. Nurses can be instrumental in helping patients with ESRD find the dialysis therapy that best suits their lifestyle. Those considering CAPD need to investigate the advantages and disadvantages along with the indications and contraindications for this form of therapy.

Advantages
- Freedom from a dialysis machine
- Control over daily activities
- Opportunities to avoid dietary restrictions, increase fluid intake, raise serum hematocrit values, improve blood pressure control, avoid venipuncture, and gain a sense of well-being.

Disadvantages
- Continuous dialysis 24 hours a day, 7 days a week

Indications
- Patient's willingness, motivation, and ability to perform dialysis at home
- Strong family or community support system (essential for success), particularly if the patient is an older adult
- Special problems with long-term hemodialysis, such as dysfunctional or failing vascular access devices, excessive thirst, severe

hypertension, postdialysis headaches, and severe anemia requiring frequent transfusion
- Interim therapy while awaiting kidney transplantation
- ESRD secondary to diabetes because hypertension, uremia, and hyperglycemia are easier to manage with CAPD than with hemodialysis

Contraindications
- Adhesions from previous surgery (adhesions reduce clearance of solutes) or systemic inflammatory disease
- Chronic backache and preexisting disk disease, which could be aggravated by the continuous pressure of dialysis fluid in the abdomen
- Risk of complications, for example, in patients receiving immunosuppressive medications, which impede healing of the catheter site, and in patients with a colostomy, ileostomy, nephrostomy, or ileal conduit because of the risk of peritonitis. The risk for complications is not an absolute contraindication for CAPD therapy.
- Diverticulitis because CAPD has been associated with rupture of the diverticulum
- Severe arthritis or poor hand strength necessitating assistance in performing the exchange. However, blind or partially blind patients and those with other physical limitations can learn to perform CAPD.

UNDERLYING PRINCIPLES

CAPD works on the same principles as other forms of peritoneal dialysis: diffusion and osmosis. Less extreme fluctuations in the patient's laboratory results occur with CAPD than with intermittent peritoneal dialysis or hemodialysis because the dialysis is constantly in progress. The serum electrolyte levels usually remain in the normal range.

PROCEDURE

The patient performs exchanges four or five times a day, 24 hours a day, 7 days a week, at intervals scheduled throughout the day (before meals and bedtime). After infusing the dialysate into the peritoneal cavity through the catheter (over about 10 minutes), the patient can fold the bag and tuck it underneath the clothing during the dwell time. This provides the patient with some freedom and reduces the number of connections and disconnections necessary at the catheter end of the tubing, thereby reducing the risk of contamination and peritonitis.

The longer the dwell time, the better the clearance of middle-sized molecules. It is thought that these molecules may be significant uremic toxins. At the end of the dwell time, the dialysate is drained from the peritoneal cavity by unfolding the empty bag, opening the clamp, and placing the bag lower than the abdomen near the floor. This allows the peritoneal fluid to drain out by gravity. When drainage ends, the patient repeats the procedure by spiking a new bag containing dialysate and infusing the solution into the peritoneal cavity. Other systems are available that allow the catheter to be clamped, disconnected, and capped, thus allowing the patient freedom from wearing an empty dialysate bag. Before the next exchange, however, an empty drainage bag must be attached to permit drainage of the dwell solution.

COMPLICATIONS

To reduce the risk of peritonitis, the patient takes meticulous care to avoid contaminating the catheter, fluid, or tubing and accidentally disconnecting the catheter from the tubing. The catheter is protected from manipulation, and the catheter entry site is meticulously cared for according to a standardized protocol.

Nursing Management

In addition to the complications of peritoneal dialysis previously described, patients who elect to use CAPD may experience altered body image because of the abdominal catheter and the bag and tubing. Waist size increases from 1 to 2 inches (or more) with fluid in the abdomen. This affects clothing selection and may make the patient feel "fat." Body image may be so altered that patients do not want to look at or care for the catheter for days or weeks. The nurse may arrange for the patient to talk with other patients who have adapted well to CAPD. Although some patients have no psychological problems with the catheter—they think of it as their lifeline and as a life-sustaining device—other patients feel they are doing exchanges all day long and have no free time, particularly in the beginning. They may experience depression because they feel overwhelmed with the responsibility of self-care.

Patients undergoing CAPD may also experience altered sexuality patterns and sexual dysfunction. The patient and partner may be reluctant to engage in sexual activities, partly because of the catheter being psychologically "in the way" of sexual performance. The peritoneal catheter, drainage bag, and about 2 L of dialysate may interfere with the patient's sexual function and body image as well. Although these problems may resolve with time, some problems may warrant special counselling. Questions by the nurse about concerns related to sexuality and sexual function often provide the patient with a welcome opportunity to discuss these issues and a first step toward their resolution.

PROMOTING HOME AND COMMUNITY-BASED CARE

Teaching Patients Self-Care. Patients are taught as inpatients or outpatients to perform CAPD once their condition is medically stable. Training usually takes 5 days to 2 weeks. Patients are taught according to their own learning ability and knowledge level, and only as much at one time as they can handle without feeling uncomfortable or becoming overwhelmed. Education topics for the patient and family who will be performing peritoneal dialysis at home are described in Chart 44-11.

Because of protein loss with continuous peritoneal dialysis, patients are instructed to eat a high-protein, well-balanced diet. They are also encouraged to increase their daily fibre intake to help prevent constipation, which can impede the flow of dialysate into or out of the peritoneal cavity. Many patients gain 1.5 to 2.5 kg within a month of initiating CAPD, so they may be asked to limit their carbohydrate intake to avoid excessive weight gain. Potassium, sodium, and fluid restrictions are not usually needed. Patients commonly lose about 2 L of fluid over and above the 8 L of dialysate infused into the abdomen during a 24-hour period, permitting a normal fluid intake even in an anephric patient (a patient without kidneys). Greater small-solute clearances are associated with better dietary intake and better nutrition (Wang, Sea, Ip et al., 2001).

Continuing Care. Follow-up care through phone calls, visits to the outpatient department, and continuing home care assists patients in the transition to home and promotes their active participation in their own health care. Patients often depend on checking with the nurse to see if they are making the right choices about dialysate or control of blood pressure, or simply to discuss a problem.

Patients may be seen by the CAPD team as outpatients once a month or more often if needed. The exchange procedure is evaluated at that time to see that strict aseptic technique is being used. The CAPD nurse may change the tubing used to instill the dialysate every 4 to 8 weeks. Long-life tubing now lasts up to 6 months before tubing changes are necessary. Infrequent tubing changes decrease the risk of contamination. Blood chemistry values are followed closely to make certain the therapy is adequate for the patient.

If a referral is made for home care, the home care nurse assesses the home environment and suggests modifications to accommodate the equipment and facilities needed to carry out CAPD. In addition, the nurse assesses the patient's and family's understanding of CAPD and their use of safe technique in performing CAPD. Additional assessments include checking for changes related to renal disease, complications such as peritonitis, and treatment-related problems such as heart failure, inadequate drainage, and weight gain or loss. The nurse continues to reinforce and clarify teaching about CAPD and renal disease and assesses the patient's and family's progress in coping with the procedure. In addition, the patient is reminded about the need to participate in health promotion activities and health screening.

Due to the projected high numbers of elderly patients who will develop ESRD in the future, the nursing home or extended-care facility will become an increasingly important site for both rehabilitation and long-term management of patients with renal failure. Although few such sites currently provide dialysis, highly structured educational programs for personnel in these environments by nephrology staff will likely make these effective sites of care for patients requiring continuous peritoneal dialysis (Carey, Chorney, Pherson et al., 2001).

Chart 44-11
Home Care Checklist • Peritoneal Dialysis (CAPD or CCPD)

At the completion of the home care instruction, patient or caregiver will be able to:	Patient	Caregiver
• Discuss basic information about normal kidney function.	✓	✓
• Discuss basic information about the disease process.	✓	✓
• Discuss the basic principles of peritoneal dialysis.	✓	✓
• Demonstrate catheter and exit site care.	✓	✓
• Demonstrate measurement of vital signs and weight measurement.	✓	✓
• Discuss monitoring and management of fluid balance.	✓	✓
• Discuss basic principles of aseptic technique.	✓	✓
• Demonstrate the CAPD exchange procedure using aseptic technique (CCPD patients should also demonstrate exchange procedure in case of failure or unavailability of cycling machine).	✓	✓
• Demonstrate cycler set-up procedure and maintenance if on CCPD.	✓	✓
• Discuss complications of peritoneal dialysis; prevention, recognition, and management of complications.	✓	✓
• Demonstrate procedure for adding medications to the dialysis solution.	✓	✓
• Demonstrate procedure for obtaining sterile dialysis fluid samples.	✓	✓
• Discuss routine laboratory tests needed and implications of results.	✓	✓
• Discuss dietary restrictions.	✓	✓
• Discuss medications: name of medications, their actions, potential side effects, and when to contact physician.	✓	✓
• Discuss ordering, storage, and inventory of dialysis supplies.	✓	✓
• Describe plan for follow-up continuing care.	✓	✓
• Demonstrate maintenance of home dialysis records.	✓	✓
• Describe actions in case of emergency.	✓	✓

Continuous Cyclic Peritoneal Dialysis

CCPD combines overnight intermittent peritoneal dialysis with a prolonged dwell time during the day. The peritoneal catheter is connected to a cycler machine every evening, and the patient receives three to five 2-L exchanges during the night. In the morning, the patient caps off the catheter after infusing 1 to 2 L of fresh dialysate. This dialysate remains in the abdominal cavity until the tubing is reattached to the cycler machine at bedtime. Because the machine is very quiet, the patient can sleep. Moreover, the extra-long tubing allows the patient to move and turn normally during sleep.

CCPD has a lower infection rate than other forms of peritoneal dialysis because there are fewer opportunities for contamination with bag changes and tubing disconnections. It also allows the patient to be free from exchanges throughout the day, making it possible to work more freely and carry out activities of daily living.

SPECIAL CONSIDERATIONS: CARE OF THE HOSPITALIZED DIALYSIS PATIENT

Whether undergoing hemodialysis or peritoneal dialysis, the patient may be hospitalized for treatment of complications related to the dialysis treatment, the underlying renal disorder, or health problems not related to renal dysfunction or its treatment.

Nursing Management

PROTECTING THE VASCULAR ACCESS
When the hemodialysis patient is hospitalized for any reason, care must be taken to protect the vascular access from damage. The nurse assesses the vascular access for patency and takes precautions to ensure that the extremity with the vascular access is not used for measuring blood pressure or for obtaining blood specimens; tight dressings, restraints, or jewelry over the vascular access are to be avoided as well.

The bruit, or "thrill," over the venous access site must be evaluated at least every 8 hours. Absence of a palpable thrill or audible bruit may indicate blockage or clotting in the access device. Clotting can occur if the patient has an infection anywhere in the body (serum viscosity is increased) or if the blood pressure has dropped. When blood flow is reduced through the access for any reason (hypotension, application of blood pressure cuff or tourniquet), the access can clot or become infected. The nurse observes the patient for signs and symptoms of infection, such as redness, swelling, drainage from the site, and fever. Patients with renal disease are more prone to infection; therefore, infection control measures must be used for all procedures.

TAKING PRECAUTIONS DURING INTRAVENOUS THERAPY
When the patient needs intravenous therapy, the rate of administration must be as slow as possible and should be strictly controlled by a volumetric infusion pump. Because dialysis patients cannot excrete water, rapid or excessive administration of intravenous fluid can result in pulmonary edema. Accurate intake and output records are essential.

MONITORING SYMPTOMS OF UREMIA
As metabolic end products accumulate, uremic symptoms worsen. Patients whose metabolic rate accelerates (those on corticosteroid medications or parenteral nutrition, those with infections or bleeding disorders, those undergoing surgery) accumulate waste products more quickly and may require daily dialysis. These same patients are more likely to experience complications than other dialysis patients.

DETECTING CARDIAC AND RESPIRATORY COMPLICATIONS
Cardiac and respiratory assessment must be conducted frequently. As fluid builds up, fluid overload, heart failure, and pulmonary edema develop. Crackles in the bases of the lungs may indicate pulmonary edema.

Pericarditis may result from the accumulation of uremic toxins. If not detected and treated promptly, this serious complication may progress to pericardial effusion and cardiac tamponade. Pericarditis is detected by the patient's report of substernal chest pain (if the patient can communicate), low-grade fever (often overlooked), and pericardial friction rub. A pulsus paradoxus (a decrease in blood pressure of more than 10 mm Hg during inspiration) is often present. When pericarditis progresses to effusion, the friction rub disappears, heart sounds become distant and muffled, electrocardiographic waves show very low voltage, and the pulsus paradoxus worsens.

The effusion may progress to life-threatening cardiac tamponade, noted by narrowing of the pulse pressure in addition to muffled or inaudible heart sounds, crushing chest pain, dyspnea, and hypotension. Although pericarditis, pericardial effusion, and cardiac tamponade can be detected by chest x-ray, they should also be detected through astute nursing assessment. Because of their clinical significance, assessment of the patient for cardiac complications is a priority.

CONTROLLING ELECTROLYTE LEVELS AND DIET
Electrolyte alterations are common, and potassium changes can be life threatening. All intravenous solutions and medications to be administered are evaluated for their electrolyte content. Serum laboratory values are assessed daily. If blood transfusions are required, they may be administered during hemodialysis, if possible, so that excess potassium can be removed. Dietary intake must also be monitored. The patient's frustrations related to dietary restrictions typically increase if the hospital food is unappetizing. The nurse needs to recognize that this may lead to dietary indiscretion and hyperkalemia.

Hypoalbuminemia is an indicator of malnutrition in patients undergoing long-term or maintenance dialysis. Although some patients can be treated with adequate nutrition alone, some patients remain hypoalbuminemic for reasons that are poorly understood.

MANAGING DISCOMFORT AND PAIN
Complications such as pruritus and pain secondary to neuropathy must be managed. Antihistamine agents, such as diphenhydramine hydrochloride (Benadryl), are commonly used, and analgesic medications may be prescribed. Because elimination of the metabolites of medications occurs through dialysis rather than through renal excretion, however, medication dosages may need to be adjusted. Keeping the skin clean and well moisturized using bath oils, superfatted soap, and creams or lotions helps to promote comfort and reduce itching. Teaching the patient to keep the nails trimmed to avoid scratching and excoriation and to rub lotion into the skin instead of scratching also promotes comfort.

MONITORING BLOOD PRESSURE
Hypertension in renal failure is common. It is usually the result of fluid overload and, in part, oversecretion of renin. Many dialysis

patients receive some form of antihypertensive therapy and require intense teaching about its purpose and adverse effects. The trial-and-error approach that may be necessary to identify the most effective antihypertensive agent and dosage may confuse or alarm the patient if no explanation is provided. Antihypertensive agents must be withheld on dialysis days to avoid hypotension due to the combined effect of the dialysis and the medication.

Typically these patients require single or multiple antihypertensive agents to achieve normal blood pressure, thus adding to the total number of medications needed on an ongoing basis. Research has demonstrated that by maintaining strict volume control via absolute dietary salt restrictions, thorough explanation of the rationale behind the sodium restriction to the patient and family, and increased ultrafiltration by using more hypertonic peritoneal dialysis solution, most persons can maintain a normal blood pressure without the use of antihypertensive agents (Gunal, Duman, Ozkahya et al., 2001).

PREVENTING INFECTION

Patients with ESRD commonly have low white blood cell counts (and decreased phagocytic ability), low red blood cell counts (anemia), and impaired platelet function. Together, these pose a high risk for infection and potential for bleeding after even minor trauma. Preventing and controlling infection are essential because the incidence of infection is high. Infection of the vascular access site and pneumonia are common.

CARING FOR THE CATHETER SITE

Patients receiving CAPD usually know how to care for the catheter site; however, the hospital stay should be an opportunity to assess compliance with recommended catheter care and to correct any misperceptions or deviations from correct technique. Recommended daily or three-or-four-times-weekly routine catheter site care is typically performed during showering or bathing. The exit site should not be submerged in bath water. The most common cleaning method is soap and water; liquid soap is recommended. During care, the nurse and patient need to make sure that the catheter remains secure to avoid tension and trauma. The patient may wear a gauze or semitransparent dressing over the exit site.

ADMINISTERING MEDICATIONS

The medications prescribed for any dialysis patient must be closely monitored to avoid those that are toxic to the kidneys and may threaten remaining renal function. All medications must be monitored, and alterations in dosages may be necessary to prevent either toxic effects on the kidney or overdosage because of impaired renal excretion. Care must be taken to evaluate all problems and symptoms that the patient reports without automatically attributing them to renal failure or to dialysis therapy.

PROVIDING PSYCHOLOGICAL SUPPORT

Patients undergoing dialysis for a while may begin to re-evaluate their status, the treatment modality, their satisfaction with life, and the impact of these factors on their families and support systems. Nurses must provide opportunities for these patients to express their feelings and reactions and to explore options.

The decision to begin dialysis does not require that dialysis be continued indefinitely, and it is not uncommon for patients to consider discontinuing treatment. These feelings and reactions must be taken seriously, and the patient should have the opportunity to discuss them with the dialysis team as well as with a psychologist, psychiatrist, psychiatric nurse, trusted friend, or spiritual advisor. The patient's informed decision about discontinuing treatment, after thoughtful deliberation, should be respected.

Kidney Surgery

A patient may undergo surgery to remove obstructions that affect the kidney (tumours or calculi), to insert a tube for draining the kidney (**nephrostomy**, ureterostomy), or to remove the kidney involved in unilateral kidney disease, renal carcinoma, or kidney transplantation.

PREOPERATIVE CONSIDERATIONS

Surgery is performed only after a thorough evaluation of renal function. Patient preparation to ensure that optimal renal function is maintained is mandatory. Fluids are encouraged to promote increased excretion of waste products before surgery, unless contraindicated because of preexisting renal or cardiac dysfunction. If kidney infection is present preoperatively, wide-spectrum antimicrobial agents may be prescribed to prevent bacteremia. Antibiotic agents must be given with extreme care because many are toxic to the kidneys. Coagulation studies (prothrombin time, partial thromboplastin time, platelet count) may be indicated if the patient has a history of bruising and bleeding. The general preoperative preparation is similar to that described in Chapter 18.

Because many patients facing kidney surgery are apprehensive, the nurse encourages the patient to recognize and express any feelings of anxiety. Confidence is reinforced by establishing a relationship of trust and by providing expert care. Patients faced with the prospect of losing a kidney may think that they will be dependent on dialysis for the rest of their life. It is important to teach the patient and family that normal function may be maintained by a single healthy kidney.

PERIOPERATIVE CONCERNS

Renal surgery requires various patient positions to expose the surgical site adequately. Three surgical approaches are common: flank, lumbar, and thoracoabdominal (Fig. 44-10). During surgery, plans are carried out for managing altered urinary drainage and drainage systems. Plans may include inserting a nephrostomy or other drainage tube or using ureteral stents.

POSTOPERATIVE MANAGEMENT

Because the kidney is a highly vascular organ, hemorrhage and shock are the chief complications of renal surgery. Fluid and blood component replacement is frequently necessary in the immediate postoperative period to treat intraoperative blood loss.

Abdominal distention and paralytic ileus are fairly common after renal and ureter surgery and are thought to be due to a reflex paralysis of intestinal peristalsis and manipulation of the colon or duodenum during surgery. Abdominal distention is relieved by decompression through a nasogastric tube (see Chap. 38 for treatment of paralytic ileus). Oral fluids are permitted when the passage of flatus is noted.

If infection occurs, antibiotic agents are prescribed after a culture reveals the causative organism. The toxic effects that antibiotic agents have on the kidneys (nephrotoxicity) must be kept in mind when assessing the patient. Low-dose heparin therapy may be initiated postoperatively to prevent thromboembolism in patients who had any type of urologic surgery.

Drainage Tubes

Almost all patients undergoing kidney and urologic surgery, as well as patients with other kidney and urologic disturbances, have drains, tubes, or catheters in place. All catheters and tubes must

A Flank approach	**B** Lumbar approach	**C** Thoracoabdominal approach

FIGURE 44-10 Patient positioning and incisional approaches (**A**, flank; **B**, lumbar; **C**, thoracoabdominal) for kidney surgery are associated with significant postoperative discomfort.

be kept patent (eg, draining) to prevent obstruction by blood clots, which can cause infection, kidney damage, or severe pain (similar to renal colic) when they pass along the ureter.

Nephrostomy Drainage

A nephrostomy tube is inserted directly into the kidney for temporary or permanent urinary diversion. It can be inserted either percutaneously or through a surgical incision. A single tube or a self-retaining U loop or circular nephrostomy tube may be used and is attached to a closed drainage system or to a urostomy appliance. Nephrostomy drainage may be required to provide drainage from the kidney after surgery or to bypass an obstruction in the ureter or lower urinary tract. Permanent nephrostomy tubes are usually changed every 3 months.

Percutaneous nephrostomy is the insertion of a tube through the skin into the renal pelvis. This procedure is performed to provide external drainage of urine from an obstructed ureter, to create a route for inserting a ureteral stent (see following discussion), to dilate strictures, to close fistulas, to administer medications, to allow insertion of a brush biopsy instrument and nephroscope, or to perform selected surgical procedures.

The skin site is prepared and anesthetized, and the patient is asked to inhale and hold his or her breath while a spinal needle is advanced into the renal pelvis. Urine is aspirated for culture, and a contrast agent may be injected into the pyelocalyceal system. An angiographic catheter guide wire is introduced through the needle to the kidney. The needle is withdrawn and the tract dilated by the passage of tubes or guide wires. The nephrostomy tube is introduced and positioned within the kidney or ureter, fixed by skin sutures, and connected to a closed drainage system.

Before a percutaneous nephrostomy tube is inserted, several precautions should be taken. The patient should receive a broad-spectrum antibiotic to prevent infection. Bleeding disorders and uncontrolled hypertension should be corrected. Also, anticoagulant agents and aspirin should be discontinued and bleeding study results (prothrombin time, partial thromboplastin time,

platelet count) should be normal to decrease the chance of developing a perirenal hematoma or renal hemorrhage. Chart 44-12 describes postsurgical nursing care of the patient with a nephrostomy tube (also see Chart 44-13).

Ureteral Stents

A ureteral stent is a self-retaining tubular device that helps maintain the position and patency of the ureter. Stents are used to maintain urine flow in patients with ureteral obstruction (from edema, stricture, fibrosis, calculi, or tumours), to divert urine, to promote healing, and to maintain the calibre and patency of the

---

Chart 44-12 | **Patient Care After a Nephrostomy**

- Assess patient for complications: bleeding at nephrostomy site (main complication) or hematuria, fistula formation, infection.
- Assess skin at nephrostomy exit site for bleeding, signs of inflammation or infection, leakage of urine, and skin irritation.
- Ensure unobstructed drainage of nephrostomy tube or catheter. Obstruction causes pain, trauma, pressure, infection, and stress on suture lines.
- If the tube dislodges, report immediately. The surgeon must replace the tube immediately to prevent the opening from contracting.
- *Never* clamp a nephrostomy tube, which could cause obstruction and resultant pyelonephritis.
- *Never* irrigate a nephrostomy tube without specific orders.
- Encourage fluid intake to promote natural flushing of the kidney and nephrostomy tube.
- Using aseptic technique, apply dry dressing at nephrostomy exit site; replace dressing as needed.
- Measure urine output from the nephrostomy tube. If both kidneys have a tube in place, measure output from each tube separately.

Chart 44-13 • PATIENT EDUCATION
Caring for Nephrostomy Equipment at Home

Review the following recommendations with patients going home with a percutaneous nephrostomy tube:
- Drink at least 8 glasses of water a day (unless otherwise directed by the physician).
- Avoid kinking, clamping, or twisting the nephrostomy tube.
- Always keep the drainage bag below the waist.
- During the day, connect the nephrostomy tube to a leg bag (*left*) and wear it under clothing. At night, connect it to a large bedside drainage bag.
- When connecting to the leg bag or large drainage bag (*right*), wear gloves and clean the ends of the nephrostomy tube and connecting tube with alcohol.

- Change the dressing around the nephrostomy tube at least once a week. It may be changed daily if preferred.
- Avoid getting the dressing wet during showering or bathing.
- Clean the drainage tube and bag daily after each use with warm soapy water. Rinse well to remove the soap. The bag may be disinfected and deodourized using a solution of 1 tablespoon bleach and 2 cups water.
- Notify the physician immediately if the nephrostomy tube comes out, if large amounts of urine leak around the tube, if urine volume decreases, or if fever, back pain, or cloudy, foul-smelling urine develops.

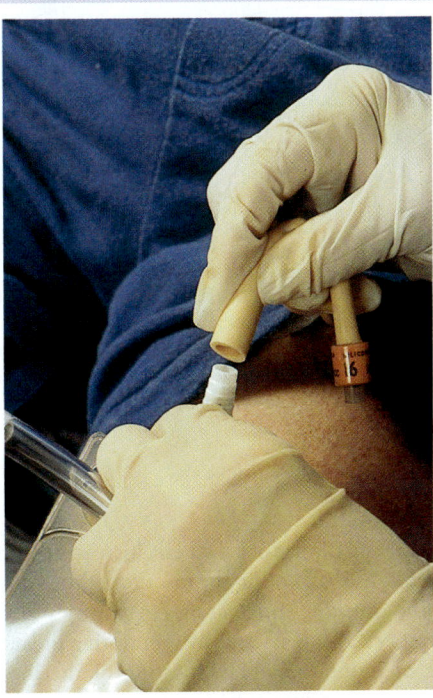

ureter after surgery (Fig. 44-11). Stents are usually removed 4 to 6 weeks after surgery in an outpatient setting without the need for general anesthesia or risk of ureteral injury.

The stent, usually made of soft, flexible silicone, may be inserted through a cystoscope or nephrostomy tube or by open surgery. Complications include infection, inflammation secondary to a foreign body in the genitourinary tract, tube encrustation, bleeding or clot obstruction within the stent, and migration or displacement of the stent (Lehmann & Dietz, 2002).

Several stents are designed to avoid some of these problems. The double-J ureteral stent has a J-shaped curve molded into each end that prevents upward or downward migration. This stent can be used in place of a nephrostomy for short- or long-term urinary drainage. The double-pigtail ureteral stent has a pigtail coil at each end; this permits placement of the upper coil (pigtail) in the renal pelvis, with the lower coil at the ureteral orifice. The coils prevent the stent from moving and allow free body movement.

Nursing interventions related to the care of a patient with a ureteral stent include monitoring the patient for bleeding, assess-

ing and measuring urine output, assessing the patient for signs of urinary tract infection or retroperitoneal infection from leakage of urine, and monitoring the patient for stent displacement, which is evidenced by colicky pain and a decrease in urine output. An indwelling stent may produce a local ureteral reaction, including mucosal edema, which can cause temporary obstruction of the ureter and intense pain.

NURSING PROCESS:
THE PATIENT UNDERGOING KIDNEY SURGERY

Assessment

Immediate care of the patient who has undergone surgery of the kidney includes assessment of all body systems. Respiratory and circulatory status, pain level, fluid and electrolyte status, and patency and adequacy of urinary drainage systems are assessed.

FIGURE 44-11 Ureteral stents. (**A**) Retrograde passage of ureteral stent. The double-J ureteral stent is shaped to resist migration. The proximal J hooks into the lower calix or renal pelvis, and the distal J curves into the bladder. (**B**) Open surgical placement of double-J stent before ureteral anastomosis. Courtesy of Medical Engineering Corporation, Racine, Wisconsin.

RESPIRATORY STATUS

As with any surgery, the use of anesthesia increases the risk of respiratory complications. Noting the location of the surgical incision assists the nurse in anticipating respiratory problems and pain. Respiratory status is assessed by monitoring the rate, depth, and pattern of respirations. The location of the incision frequently causes pain on inspiration and coughing; therefore, the patient tends to splint the chest wall and take shallow respirations. Auscultation is performed to assess normal and adventitious breath sounds.

CIRCULATORY STATUS AND BLOOD LOSS

The vital signs and arterial or central venous pressure are monitored. Skin colour and temperature and urine output provide information about circulatory status. The surgical incision and drainage tubes are observed frequently to help detect unexpected blood loss and hemorrhage.

PAIN

Postoperative pain is a major problem for the patient because of the location of the surgical incision and the position the patient assumed on the operating table to permit access to the kidney. The location and severity of pain are assessed before and after analgesic medications are administered. Abdominal distention, which increases discomfort, is also noted.

URINARY DRAINAGE

Urine output and drainage from tubes inserted during surgery are monitored for amount, colour, and type or characteristics. Decreased or absent drainage is promptly reported to the physician

because it may indicate obstruction that could cause pain, infection, and disruption of the suture lines.

Diagnosis

NURSING DIAGNOSES

Based on the history and assessment data and the type of surgical procedure performed, some major nursing diagnoses for the patient include the following (additional diagnoses and interventions appear in the Plan of Nursing Care):

- Ineffective airway clearance related to the location of the surgical incision
- Ineffective breathing pattern related to surgical incision and general anesthesia
- Acute pain related to the location of the surgical incision, the position the patient assumed on the operating table during surgery, and abdominal distention
- Urine retention related to pain, immobility, and anesthesia

COLLABORATIVE PROBLEMS/POTENTIAL COMPLICATIONS

Based on assessment data, potential complications that may develop include the following:

- Bleeding
- Pneumonia
- Infection
- Fluid disturbances (deficit or excess)
- Deep vein thrombosis

Planning and Goals

The major goals for the patient include maintenance of effective airway clearance and breathing pattern, relief of pain and discomfort, maintenance of urinary elimination, and absence of complications.

Nursing Interventions

MAINTAINING AIRWAY CLEARANCE AND BREATHING PATTERNS

The surgical approaches to the kidney predispose the patient to respiratory complications and paralytic ileus. If the pleural cavity has been entered during surgery, a pneumothorax may occur, necessitating insertion of a chest tube. The incision is generally close to the diaphragm, and with a substernal incision, the nerves may be stretched and bruised. These factors can lead to pain and limited chest movement during inspiration; breathing patterns are altered or ineffective when the chest cannot fully expand. If the patient cannot generate an effective cough, either because of pain at the incision site and restricted movement or because of anesthesia, ineffective airway clearance may result.

Adequate use of analgesic medications is necessary to relieve pain so that the patient can take deep breaths and cough. When the analgesia is administered at regular, frequent intervals, the patient can perform deep-breathing and coughing exercises more effectively. The incentive spirometer (see Chap. 25) may be used to help maximize lung inflation. The patient is encouraged to cough after each deep breath to loosen secretions.

RELIEVING PAIN

In addition to pain at the incision site, the patient may experience pain and discomfort from distention of the renal capsule (by tumour or blood clot), ischemia (from occlusion of blood vessels),

Plan of Nursing Care
Care of the Patient Undergoing Kidney Surgery

Nursing Interventions	Rationale	Expected Outcomes
Nursing Diagnosis: Ineffective airway clearance related to pain of high abdominal or flank incision, abdominal discomfort, and immobility; risk for ineffective breathing pattern related to high abdominal incision **Goal:** Relief of pain and discomfort		
1. Administer analgesics as prescribed. 2. Splint incision with hands or pillow to assist patient in coughing. 3. Assist patient to change positions frequently. 4. Encourage use of incentive spirometer if indicated or prescribed. 5. Assist with and encourage early ambulation.	1. Enables patient to take deep breaths and cough 2. Splints incision and promotes adequate cough and prevention of atelectasis 3. Promotes drainage and inflation of all lobes of the lungs 4. Encourages adequate deep breaths 5. Mobilizes pulmonary secretions	• Takes deep breaths and coughs adequately when encouraged and assisted • Exhibits respiratory rate of 12–18 breaths/min • Exhibits normal breath sounds without adventitious sounds • Exhibits full thoracic excursion without shallow respirations • Uses incentive spirometer with encouragement • Splints incision while taking deep breaths and coughing • Reports progressively less pain and discomfort with coughing and deep breaths • Exhibits normal blood gas levels and chest x-ray • Exhibits normal body temperature with no signs of atelectasis or pneumonia on assessment
Nursing Diagnosis: Acute pain and discomfort related to surgical incision, positioning, and stretching of muscles during kidney surgery **Goal:** Relief of pain and discomfort		
1. Assess level of pain. 2. Administer analgesics as prescribed. 3. Apply moist heat and massage to areas with muscular aches and discomfort. 4. Splint incision with hands or pillow during movement or deep breathing and coughing exercises. 5. Assist and encourage early ambulation.	1. Provides baseline for later evaluation of pain relief strategies 2. Promotes pain relief 3. Promotes relaxation and relief of muscle pain and discomfort 4. Minimizes sensation of pulling or tension on incision and provides sense of support to the patient 5. Promotes resumption of muscle activity exercise	• Reports relief of severe pain and discomfort • Takes analgesia as prescribed • States rationale for use of moist heat and massage • Exercises aching muscles within recommendations • Gradually increases physical activity and exercise • Uses distraction, relaxation exercises, and imagery to relieve pain • Exhibits no behavioural manifestations of pain and discomfort (eg, restlessness, perspiration, verbal expressions of pain) • Participates in deep-breathing and coughing exercises
Nursing Diagnosis: Fear and anxiety related to diagnosis, outcome of surgery, and alteration in urinary function **Goal:** Reduction of fear and anxiety		
1. Assess patient's anxiety and fear before surgery if possible. 2. Assess patient's knowledge about procedure and expected surgical outcome preoperatively. 3. Evaluate the meaning alterations resulting from surgical procedure have for patient and family or partner.	1. Provides a baseline for postoperative assessment 2. Provides a basis for further teaching 3. Enables understanding of patient's reactions and responses to expected and unexpected results of surgery	• Verbalizes reactions and feelings to staff • Shares reactions and feelings with family or partner • Grieves appropriately for self and for changes in role and function • Identifies information needed to promote own adaptation and coping • Participates in activities and events in immediate environment

(continued)

Plan of Nursing Care

Care of the Patient Undergoing Kidney Surgery (Continued)

Nursing Interventions	Rationale	Expected Outcomes
4. Encourage patient to verbalize reactions, feelings, and fears. 5. Encourage patient to share feelings with spouse or partner. 6. Offer and arrange for visit from member of support group (eg, ostomy group, if indicated).	4. Affirms patient's understanding of and ultimate resolution of feelings and fears 5. Enables patient and partner to receive mutual support and reduces sense of isolation from each other 6. Provides support from another person who has encountered the same or a similar surgical procedure and an example of how others have coped with the alteration	• Accepts visit from support person or participates in support group • Identifies support person from own experience and peer group

Nursing Diagnosis: Impaired urinary elimination related to urinary drainage; risk for infection related to altered urinary drainage

Goal: Maintenance of urinary elimination; infection-free urinary tract

1. Assess urinary drainage system immediately. 2. Assess adequacy of urinary output and patency of drainage system. 3. Use asepsis and hand hygiene when providing care and manipulating drainage system. 4. Maintain closed urinary drainage system. 5. If irrigation of the drainage system is necessary, use gloves and sterile irrigating solution and a closed drainage and irrigation system. 6. If irrigation is necessary and prescribed, carry it out gently with sterile saline and the prescribed amount of irrigating fluid. 7. Assist patient in turning and moving in bed and when ambulating to prevent displacement or inadvertent removal of urinary stent or ureteral catheters if in place. 8. Observe urine colour, volume, odour, and components. 9. Minimize trauma and manipulation of catheter, drainage system, and urethra. 10. Clean catheter gently with soap during bath, avoiding any to-and-fro movement of catheter. 11. Anchor drainage tube. 12. Maintain adequate fluid intake. 13. Assist with and encourage early ambulation while ensuring placement of urinary drainage system.	1. Provides basis for further assessment and action 2. Provides baseline 3. Prevents or reduces risk of contamination of urinary drainage system 4. Reduces risk of bacterial contamination and infection 5. Permits irrigation when necessary while maintaining closed drainage system, minimizing risk of infection 6. Maintains patency of the catheter or drainage system and prevents sudden increases in pressure in the urinary tract that may cause trauma, pressure on sutures or urinary tract structures, and pain 7. Prevents trauma from accidental displacement of urinary stent or ureteral catheter necessitating repeated instrumentation of the urinary tract (eg, cystoscopy) to replace them 8. Provides information about adequacy of urine output, condition and patency of drainage system, and debris in urine 9. Reduces risk of contamination of drainage system and eliminates site of bacterial invasion 10. Removes debris and encrustations without causing trauma to or contamination of urethra 11. Prevents movement or slipping of drainage tube, minimizing trauma to and contamination of urethra or catheter 12. Promotes adequate urine output and prevents urinary stasis 13. Minimizes cardiovascular and pulmonary complications while preventing loss, dislodging, or disruption of drainage system	• Exhibits adequate urinary output and patent drainage system • Exhibits urinary output consistent with fluid intake • Demonstrates normal laboratory values: blood urea nitrogen and creatinine levels, urine specific gravity, and osmolality • Exhibits sterile urine on urine culture • Exhibits clear, dilute urine without debris or encrustation in the drainage system • States rationale for avoiding manipulation of catheter, drainage, or irrigation system • Exhibits normal placement of urinary stent or ureteral catheters until removed by physician • Maintains closed urinary drainage system • Exhibits normal body temperature without signs or symptoms of urinary tract infection • Cleans catheter with soap and water • Consumes adequate fluid intake (6 to 8 glasses of water or more per day, unless contraindicated) • Urinary drainage system remains in place until physician removes or discontinues it • Maintains urinary drainage system without infection or obstruction • Maintains urinary diversion as instructed • Maintains self-care so that environment is odour-free • States rationale for close follow-up and maintains recommended schedule of appointments with health care providers

(continued)

Plan of Nursing Care
Care of the Patient Undergoing Kidney Surgery *(Continued)*

Nursing Interventions	Rationale	Expected Outcomes
14. If patient is to be discharged with urinary drainage system (catheter) in place or a urinary diversion, instruct patient and family member in care.	14. Knowledge and understanding of the drainage system or urinary diversion are essential to prevent infection and other complications	

Nursing Diagnosis: Risk for imbalanced fluid volume related to surgical fluid loss, altered urinary output, parenteral fluid administration

Goal: Normal fluid balance will be maintained.

1. Weigh patient daily.	1. Daily weight is the most sensitive indicator of fluid loss or gain	• Patient's weight will be within 1–1.5 kg of normal.
2. Take accurate intake and output measurements.	2. Detects fluid retention due to poor cardiac or renal output	• Intake that exceeds output will be detected early.
3. Place all parenteral therapy on an infusion pump.	3. Ensures that the patient does not receive excess or insufficient intravenous fluids	• The exact amount of solution is infused with no adverse effects resulting from overinfusion or underinfusion.
4. Monitor amount and characteristics of urine.	4. Assists in early detection of possible complications of surgery or tube insertion	• Urine is clear and absent of blood, pus, or any foreign substances.
5. Monitor vital signs: temperature, pulse, respirations, and blood pressure.	5. When fluid volume or cardiac output is altered, vital signs are affected	• Temperature, pulse, respiration, and blood pressure are normal.
6. Auscultate heart and lungs every shift.	6. When fluid volume is increased because of poor cardiac or renal output, fluid accumulates in the lungs. Also, heart sounds change as heart failure develops; frequent auscultation ensures early detection.	• Normal heart and lung sounds are present.

and stretching of the intrarenal blood vessels. Muscle aches and pain stemming from the position the patient assumed on the operating table, which places anatomic and physiologic stresses on the body, are also common. Massage, moist heat, and analgesic medications provide relief. Patient-controlled analgesia may be effective in controlling pain and enabling the patient to ambulate, cough, and breathe deeply (see Chap. 13 for discussion of patient-controlled analgesia).

PROMOTING URINARY ELIMINATION

The nurse closely monitors urine output and drainage to identify complications and to preserve and protect remaining kidney function (by preventing obstruction and infection). The output from each urinary drainage tube is recorded separately; accurate output measurements are essential in monitoring renal function and ensuring the patency of the urinary drainage system.

Strict asepsis is used when manipulating the drainage catheter and tube. Hand hygiene is mandatory before and after touching any parts of the system. Use of closed drainage systems is essential to avoid contamination of the system and infection. Urinary drainage is monitored closely for changes in volume, colour, odour, and components. Urinalysis and urine cultures are indicated to follow the patient's progress. Care is taken to ensure that the collection bag is suspended below the bladder to prevent reflux of urine into the urinary tract. The bag must be kept off the floor to prevent contamination.

Most urinary drainage systems do not require routine irrigation. If irrigation is necessary and prescribed, however, it should be performed carefully, with the use of sterile solution; with minimal pressure, consistent with the physician's instructions; and with strict asepsis without interruption of the closed drainage system.

MONITORING AND MANAGING POTENTIAL COMPLICATIONS

Bleeding is a major complication of kidney surgery. If undetected and untreated, bleeding can result in hypovolemia and hemorrhagic shock. The nurse's role is to observe for these complications, to report their signs and symptoms, and to administer prescribed parenteral fluids and blood and blood components if complications occur. Monitoring of vital signs, skin condition, urinary drainage system, surgical incision, and level of consciousness is necessary to detect evidence of bleeding, decreased circulating blood, and fluid volume and cardiac output. Frequent monitoring of vital signs (initially monitored at least at hourly intervals) and urinary output is necessary for early detection of these complications.

If bleeding goes undetected or is late in being detected, the patient may lose significant amounts of blood and may experience hypoxemia. In addition to hypovolemic shock due to hemorrhage, this type of blood loss may precipitate a myocardial infarction or transient ischemic attack. Bleeding may be suspected when the patient experiences fatigue and when urine output is less than 30 mL per hour. As bleeding persists, late signs of hypovolemia occur, such as cool skin, flat neck veins, and change in level of consciousness or responsiveness. Transfusions of blood components are indicated, along with surgical repair of the bleeding vessel.

Pneumonia may be prevented through use of an incentive spirometer, adequate pain control, and early ambulation. Early signs of pneumonia include fever, increased heart and respiratory rates, and adventitious breath sounds.

Preventing infection is the rationale for using asepsis when changing dressings and preparing catheters, other drainage tubes, central venous catheters, and intravenous catheters for administration of fluids. Insertion sites are monitored closely for signs and symptoms of inflammation: redness, drainage, heat, and pain. Special care must be taken to prevent urinary tract infection, which is associated with the use of indwelling urinary catheters. Catheters and other invasive tubes are removed as soon they are no longer needed.

Antibiotic agents are commonly administered postoperatively to prevent infection. If antibiotic agents are prescribed, serum creatinine and blood urea nitrogen levels must be monitored closely because many antibiotic agents are toxic to the kidney or can accumulate to toxic levels if renal function is decreased.

Preventing fluid imbalance is critical when caring for a patient undergoing kidney surgery, because both fluid loss and fluid excess are possible adverse effects of the surgery. Fluid loss may occur during surgery as a result of excessive urinary drainage when the obstruction is removed, or it may occur if diuretic agents are used. Such loss may also occur with gastrointestinal losses, with diarrhea resulting from antibiotic use or with nasogastric drainage. When postoperative intravenous therapy is inadequate to match the output or fluids lost, a fluid deficit results. Fluid excess, or overload, may result from cardiac effects of anesthesia, administration of excessive amounts of fluids, or the patient's inability to excrete fluid because of changes in renal function. Decreased urine output may be an indication of fluid excess.

Astute assessment skills are needed to detect early signs of fluid excess (such as weight gain, pedal edema, urine output below 30 mL/h, and slightly elevated pulmonary wedge pressure, if available) before they become severe (appearance of adventitious breath sounds, shortness of breath).

Fluid excess may be treated with fluid restriction and administration of furosemide (Lasix) or other diuretic agents. If renal insufficiency is present, these medications may prove ineffective; therefore, dialysis may be necessary to prevent heart failure and pulmonary edema.

Deep vein thrombosis may occur postoperatively because of surgical manipulation of the iliac vessels during surgery. Elastic compression stockings are applied, and the patient is monitored closely for signs and symptoms of thrombosis and encouraged to exercise the legs. Heparin may be administered postoperatively to reduce the risk of thrombosis. Specific nursing interventions for the patient undergoing kidney surgery are presented in the Plan of Nursing Care.

PROMOTING HOME AND COMMUNITY-BASED CARE

Teaching Patients Self-Care

If the patient has a drainage system in place, measures are taken to ensure that both patient and family understand the importance of maintaining the system correctly at home and preventing infection. Verbal and written instructions and guidelines are provided to the patient and family at the time of hospital discharge. The patient may be asked to demonstrate management of the drainage system to ensure understanding. The importance of strategies to prevent postoperative complications (urinary tract infection and obstruction, deep vein thrombosis, atelectasis, and pneumonia) is stressed to the patient and family. Those signs, symptoms, problems, and questions that should be referred to the physician or other primary health care provider are reviewed by the nurse with the patient and family.

Continuing Care

The need for postoperative assessment and care after renal surgery continues regardless of setting: the home, subacute care unit, outpatient clinic or office, or rehabilitation setting. Referral for home care is indicated for the patient going home with a urinary drainage system in place. During the home visit, the home care nurse reviews the instructions and guidelines given to the patient at hospital discharge. The nurse assesses the patient's ability to carry out the instructions in the home and answers questions that the patient or family has about management of the drainage system and the surgical incision.

Additionally, the home care nurse obtains vital signs and assesses the patient for signs and symptoms of urinary tract infection and obstruction. The nurse also ensures that pain is adequately controlled and that the patient is complying with recommendations. The home care nurse encourages adequate fluid intake and increased levels of activity. Together the nurse, patient, and family review the signs, symptoms, problems, and questions that should be referred to the physician or other primary health care provider. If the patient has a drainage tube in place, the nurse assesses the site and the patency of the system and monitors the patient for complications, such as deep vein thrombosis, bleeding, or pneumonia.

Because it is easy for the patient, family, and health care team to focus on the patient's immediate disorder to the exclusion of other health issues, reminding the patient and family about the importance of participating in health promotion activities, including health screening, is key.

Evaluation

EXPECTED PATIENT OUTCOMES

Expected patient outcomes may include:

1. Achieves effective airway clearance
   a. Exhibits clear and normal breath sounds, normal respiratory rate, and unrestricted thoracic excursion
   b. Performs deep-breathing exercises, coughs every 2 hours, and uses the incentive spirometer as directed
   c. Demonstrates normal temperature and vital signs
2. Reports progressive decrease in pain
   a. Requires analgesic medications at less frequent intervals
   b. Turns, coughs, and takes deep breaths as suggested
   c. Ambulates progressively
3. Maintains urinary elimination
   a. Demonstrates unobstructed urine flow from drainage tubes
   b. Exhibits normal fluid and electrolyte balance (normal skin turgor, serum electrolyte levels within normal range, absence of symptoms of imbalances)
   c. Reports no increase in pain, tenderness, or pressure at drainage site
   d. Exhibits cautious handling of drainage system
   e. Uses hand hygiene before and after handling drainage system, and handles it only when necessary
   f. States rationale for use and maintenance of a closed drainage system
4. Participates in self-care activities
5. Experiences no complications
   a. Demonstrates normal vital signs and arterial and central venous pressures, normal skin turgor, temperature, and colour

b. Exhibits no signs or symptoms of bleeding, shock, or hypovolemia (eg, decreased urine output, restlessness, rapid pulse)

c. Exhibits no signs or symptoms of infection (eg, fever or pain) or evidence of deep vein thrombosis (tenderness or redness of calves)

d. Maintains normal fluid balance, without rapid weight gain or loss

e. Has clear breath sounds and no shortness of breath

f. Excretes urine at a rate of at least 30 mL per hour

Critical Thinking Exercises

1. A 50-year-old woman comes in for her annual pelvic checkup with complaints of occasional urinary urgency, sometimes with "near incontinence" just as she is reaching the toilet. She denies intake of any potentially bladder-irritating substances, such as beverages containing caffeine or synthetic sweeteners. She also mentions that she is having difficulty with decreased lubrication during intercourse and that her menses are very irregular. On physical examination, you notice some thinning of the vaginal mucosa. Based on your understanding of the major role that estrogen plays in maintaining continence, discuss your plan for patient education.

2. You are a staff nurse in an outpatient dialysis facility. A middle-aged man with renal failure secondary to poorly controlled diabetes is scheduled to be seen in the clinic; it is anticipated that he will need dialysis in the near future. The physician has asked you to teach the patient and his wife about his dialysis options. Describe how you would develop a teaching plan to explain the different types of dialysis, their goals, and the level of involvement on the part of the patient and family. How would you modify your approach if the patient is distraught and does not seem to hear what you are saying?

3. A 45-year-old married woman with three teenage children visits the nephrology department to discuss options for dealing with her ESRD. Her healthy twin sister has begun the workup to donate one of her kidneys to her sister, and the preliminary reports show that a match is possible. The patient states that she does not want her sister to go through the process of kidney donation if dialysis is a possibility. As the nurse educator, you know that research demonstrates much higher rates of allograft success in individuals who have never undergone dialysis. Discuss the emotional aspects that are important to address in communication with this woman.

4. You are taking phone triage as one of the nurses in a busy urology practice. A 62-year-old man who has just been seen in consultation for increasing urinary frequency, including several awakenings at night, phones to report increasing abdominal pain. He notes that he has not voided for over 12 hours, although he has made several unsuccessful attempts. Based on your understanding of benign prostatic hyperplasia, explain the instructions you would provide to him. What medical and nursing interventions would you anticipate?

REFERENCES AND SELECTED READINGS

Books

Agency for Health Care Policy and Research (AHCPR). *Overview: Urinary Incontinence in adults, clinical practice guideline update—1996.* Rockville, MD: US Public Health Services. AHCPR #396-0682). Available online: http:www.ahrq.gov/clinic/uiovervw.htm.

Appell, R. A. (Ed.) (2000). *Voiding dysfunction: Diagnosis and treatment (Current Clinical Urology).* Totawa, NJ: Humana Press.

Bickley, L. S. (2003). *Bates' guide to physical examination and history taking* (8th ed.). Philadelphia: Lippincott Williams & Wilkins.

Brown, E. A., & Parfrey, P. S. (Eds.) (1999). *Complications of long-term dialysis.* New York: Oxford University Press, Inc.

Daugirdas, J. T., & Blake, P. G. (Eds.) (2000). *Handbook of dialysis.* New York: Little Brown & Co.

Gutch, C. F., Stoner, M. H., & Corea, A. L. (1999). *Review of hemodialysis for nurses and dialysis personnel* (6th ed.). St. Louis: Mosby, Inc.

Karlowicz, K. (1995). *Urologic nursing: Principles and practice.* Philadelphia: J. B. Lippincott.

Karlowicz, K., & Meredith, C. (Eds.) (2001). *Urologic nursing: A study guide* (2d ed.). Pitman, NJ: Society of Urologic Nurses and Associates, Inc.

Life Options Rehabilitation Advisory Council and the American Association of Kidney Patients (1997). *New life, new hope: A book for families and friends of renal patients.* Amgen Inc.

Lancaster, L. (1995). *Core curriculum for nephrology nursing* (3rd ed.). Pitman, NJ: Anthony J. Janetti.

Metheny, N. (2000). *Fluid and electrolyte balance: Nursing considerations* (4th ed.). Philadelphia: Lippincott Williams & Wilkins.

National Kidney Foundation (2000). *K/DOQI guidelines, 2000: Adult guidelines, maintenance dialysis: Management of protein and energy intake.* Guideline Number 15.

Reilly, N. J. (Ed.) (2001). *Urologic nursing: A study guide* (2d ed.). Pitman, NJ: Society of Urologic Nurses and Associates, Inc.

Walsh, P., Retik, A., Vaughan, E., & Wein, A. (Eds.) (1998). *Campbell's urology* (7th ed.). Philadelphia: W. B. Saunders.

Journals

Asterisks indicate nursing research articles.

General

Abrams, P., Cardoza, L., Fall, M., et al. (2002). The standardization of terminology of lower urinary tract function: A report from the standardization sub-committee of the International Continence Society. *Neurourology and Urodynamics, 21*, 167–178.

Berghmans, L. C. M., van Waalwijk van Doorne, E. S. C., Hieman, F., et al. (2000). Efficacy of extramural physical therapy modalities in women with proven bladder overactivity: A randomized clinical trial. *Neurourology and Urodynamics, 19*, 496–497.

*Bernier, F., & Davila, G. W. (2000). The treatment of nonobstructive urinary retention with high frequency transvaginal stimulation. *Urologic Nursing, 20*(4), 261–264.

Doyle, B., Mawii, Z., Horgan, M., et al. (2001). Decreasing nosocomial urinary tract infection in a large academic community hospital. *Lippincott's Case Management, 6*(3), 127–136.

Halper, J. (1998). New strategies, new hope: Meeting the challenge of multiple sclerosis, Part II. *American Journal of Nursing, 98*(11), 39–48.

Godfrey, H., & Evans, A. (2000). Catheterization and urinary tract infections: Microbiology. *British Journal of Nursing, 9*(11), 682–690.

Gray, M. (2000a). Urinary retention: Management in the acute care setting, Part 1. *American Journal of Nursing, 100*(7), 40–48.

Gray, M. (2000b). Urinary retention: Management in the acute care setting, Part 2. *American Journal of Nursing, 100*(8), 36–44.

Gray, M. (2005). Overactive bladder: An overview. *Journal of Wound Ostomy and Continence Nursing, 32*(Supplement 1), S1–S4.

Kajbafzadeh, A. M., & Chubak, N. (2001). Simultaneous Malone antegrade continent enema and Mitrofanoff principle using the divided appendix: Report of a new technique for prevention of stoma complications. *Journal of Urology, 165*(6 Pt 2), 2404–2409.

Moore, K. N. (1995). Intermittent self-catheterisation: Research-based practice. *British Journal of Nursing 4*(18), 1057–1058, 1060, 1062–1063.

*Moore, K. N., Day, R. A., & Albers, M. (2002). Pathogenesis of urinary tract infections: A review. *Journal of Clinical Nursing 11*(5), 568–574.

*Moore, K. N., Kelm, M., Sinclair, O., et al. (1993). Bacteriuria in intermittent catheterization users: The effect of sterile versus clean reused catheters. *Rehabilitation Nursing 18*(5), 306–309, 355–356.

Moore, K. N., & Rayome R. G. (1995). Problem solving and troubleshooting: The indwelling catheter. *Journal of Wound, Ostomy, and Continence Nursing, 22*(5), 242–247.

*Moore, K. N., Schlieman, S., Ackerman, T., et al. (2004). Assessing comfort, safety, and patient satisfaction with three commonly used penile compression devices. *Urology 63*(1), 150–154.

Newman, D. K., & Giovannini, D. (2002). The overactive bladder: A nursing perspective. *American Journal of Nursing, 102*(6), 36–45.

Newton, M., Hanney Kosier, J., & Smith, D. (2000). Treatments for overactive bladder. *Urologic Nursing, 20*(4), 267–268.

*Phillips, J. K. (2000). Integrating bladder ultrasound into a urinary infection reduction project. *American Journal of Nursing, 100*(3), 3–11.

*Schott-Baer, F. D., & Reaume, L. (2001). Accuracy of ultrasound estimates of urine volume. *Urologic Nursing, 21*(3), 193–195.

Taylor, P. (2005). Pharmacologic management of overactive bladder. *Journal of Wound, Ostomy, and Continence Nursing, 32*(Supplement 1), S16–S24.

Uygur, M. C., Altug, U., Ozgur, M., & Erol, D. (2001). The application of appendiceal Mitrofanoff principle to Stanford pouch. *Journal of Urology, 8*(1), 1193–1198.

Wade-Elliott, R. (1999). Caring for the elderly with renal failure: Gastrointestinal changes. *ANNA Journal, 26*(6), 563–571.

Dialysis

Alexander, G. C., & Sehgal, A. R. (2001). Why hemodialysis patients fail to complete the transplantation process. *American Journal of Kidney Diseases, 37*(2), 321–328.

Astle, S. M. (July 2001). A new direction for dialysis. *RN, 64*(7), 56–62.

Bliwise, D. L., Kutner, N. G., Zhang, R., & Parker, P. K. (2001). Survival by time of day of hemodialysis in an elderly cohort. *Journal of the American Medical Association, 286*(21), 2690–2694.

Carey, H. B., Chorney, W., Pherson, K., et al. (2001). Continuous peritoneal dialysis and the extended care facility. *American Journal of Kidney Diseases, 37*(3), 580–587.

Chatoth, D. K., Golper, T. A. & Gokal, R. (1999). Morbidity and mortality in redefining adequacy of peritoneal dialysis: A step beyond the National Kidney Foundation Dialysis Outcomes Quality Initiative. *American Journal of Kidney Diseases, 33*(4), 617–632.

Dirkes, S. M. (2000). Continuous renal replacement therapy: Dialytic therapy for acute renal failure in intensive care. *Nephrology Nursing Journal, 27*(6), 581–590.

Eschbach, J. W., & Adamson, J. W. (1989). Guidelines for recombinant human erythropoietin therapy. *American Journal of Kidney Diseases, 14*(2 Supp; 1), 2–8.

Fagugli, G. R., Reboldi, G., Quintaliani, G., et al. (2001). Short daily hemodialysis: Blood pressure control and left ventricular mass reduction in hypertensive hemodialysis patients. *American Journal of Kidney Diseases, 38*(2), 371–376.

Fink, J. C., Blahut, S. A., Reddy, M., & Light, P. D. (2001). Use of erythropoietin before the initiation of dialysis and its impact on mortality. *American Journal of Kidney Diseases, 37*(2), 348–355.

Graves, G. D. (2001). Arterial and venous pressure monitoring during hemodialysis. *Nephrology Nursing Journal, 28*(1), 23–28.

Gunal, A. I., Duman, S., Ozkahya, M., et al. (2001). Strict volume control normalizes hypertension in peritoneal dialysis. *American Journal of Kidney Diseases, 37*(3), 588–593.

*Hathaway, D. K., Wicks, M. N., Cashion, A. K., et al. (2000). Post-transplant improvement in heart rate variability correlates with improved quality of life. *Western Journal of Nursing Research. 22*(6), 749–768.

Headley, C. M., & Wall, B. (2000). Advanced practice nurses: Roles in the hemodialysis unit. *Nephrology Nursing Journal, 27*(2), 177–184.

Kaplow, R. & Barry, R. (2002). Continuous renal replacement therapies. *American Journal of Nursing, 102*(11), 26–33.

Kaveh, K., & Kimmel, P. L. (2001). Compliance in hemodialysis patients: Multidimensional measures in search of a gold standard. *American Journal of Kidney Diseases, 37*(2), 244–266.

Kim, S. B., Lee, S. K., Park, J. S., et al. (2001). Effects of fixed low-dose warfarin on hemostatic factors in continuous ambulatory peritoneal dialysis. *American Journal of Kidney Diseases, 37*(2), 343–347.

Lacson, E., Teng, M., Lazarus, M., et al. (2001). Limitations of the facility-specific standardized mortality ratio for profiling health care quality in dialysis. *American Journal of Kidney Diseases, 37*(2), 267–275.

Lindsay, R. M., & Kortas, C. (2001). Hemeral (daily) hemodialysis. *Advanced Renal Replacement Therapy, 8*(4), 236–249.

Mange, K. C., Joffe, M. M., & Feldman, H. I. (2001). Effect of the use or nonuse of long-term dialysis on the subsequent survivor of renal transplants from living donors. *New England Journal of Medicine, 344*(10), 726–731.

Mohr, P. E., Neuman, P. J., Franco, S. J., et al. (2001). The case for daily dialysis: Its impact on costs and quality of life. *American Journal of Kidney Diseases, 37*(4), 777–789.

Moss, A. H., Hozayen, O., King, K., et al. (2001). Attitudes of patients toward cardiopulmonary resuscitation in the dialysis unit. *American Journal of Kidney Diseases, 38*(4), 847–852.

*Parker, K. P., Bliwise, D. L., & Rye, D. B. (2000). Hemodialysis disrupts basic sleep regulatory mechanisms: Building hypotheses. *Nursing Research, 49*(6), 327–332.

Port, F. K., Wolfe, R. A., Hulbert-Shearon, T. E., et al. (2001). Mortality risk by hemodialyzer reuse practice and dialyzer membrane characteristics: Results from the USRDS Dialysis Morbidity and Mortality Study. *American Journal of Kidney Diseases, 37*(2), 276–286.

Tonelli, M., Bohm, C., Pandeya, S., et al. (2001). Cardiac risk factors and the use of cardioprotective medications in patients with chronic renal insufficiency. *American Journal of Kidney Diseases, 37*(3), 484–489.

van der Sande, F. M., Kooman, J. P., Burema, J. H. G. A., et al. (1999). Effect of dialysate temperature on energy balance during hemodialysis: Quantification of extracorporeal energy transfer. *American Journal of Kidney Diseases, 33*(6), 1115–1121.

Wade-Elliott, R. (1999). Caring for the elderly with renal failure: Gastrointestinal changes. *ANNA Journal, 26*(6), 563–571.

Wang, A. Y., Sea, M. M., Ip, R., et al. (2001). Independent effects of residual renal function and dialysis adequacy on actual dietary protein, calorie, and other nutrient intake in patients on continuous ambulatory peritoneal dialysis. *Journal of the American Society of Nephrology, 12*, 2450–2457.

Zelenitsky, S., Barns, L., Findlay, I., et al. (2000). Analysis of microbiological trends in peritoneal dialysis-related peritonitis from 1991 to 1998. *American Journal of Kidney Diseases, 36*(5), 1009–1013.

Incontinence

*Bush, A. B., Castellucci, D. T., & Phillips, C. (2001). Exploring women's beliefs regarding urinary incontinence. *Urologic Nursing, 21*(3), 211–218.

Canadian Continence Foundation. (2001). Promoting a collaborative consumer-focused approach to continence care in Canada. Available at: http://www.continence-fdn.ca. Retrieved June 13, 2005.

Chancellor, M. (1999). Managing the urge incontinent bladder: Competent therapies help restore quality of life. *Contemporary Urology Supplement, 7*–13.

Davies, J. A., Hosker, G., Lord, J., & Smith, A. R. (2000). An evaluation of the efficacy of in-patient bladder retraining. *International Urogynecology Journal & Pelvic Floor Dysfunction, 11*(5), 271–276.

Degler, M. (1999). Types of urinary incontinence. Available at: http://www.MyBladder.com. Protocol Driven Healthcare Incorporated.

Degler, M. (2000). Reversible causes of urinary incontinence. Available at: http://www.MyBladder.com. Protocol Driven Healthcare Incorporated.

*Eustice, S., Roe, B., & Paterson, J. (2004). Prompted voiding for the management of urinary incontinence in adults. [Systemic review]. Cochrane Incontinence Group. *Cochrane Database of Systematic Reviews, 4.*

Fonda, D., Benvenuti, A., DuBeau, C., et al. (2002). Urinary incontinence and bladder dysfunction in older persons. In P. Abrams, L. Cardozo, S. Khoury, et al. (Eds.), *Incontinence* (pp. 627–695). Plymouth, UK: Health Publication Ltd.

*Gray, M., McClain, R., Peruggia, M., Patrie, J., & Steers, W. D. (2001). A model for predicting motor urge urinary incontinence. *Nursing Research, 50*(2), 116–126.

*Hunter, K. F., Moore, K. N., Cody, D. J., et al. (2004). Conservative management of postprostatectomy urinary incontinence. [System review]. Cochrane Incontinence Group. *Cochrane Database of Systematic Reviews, 4.*

*Joseph, A., & Chang, M. (2000). Comparison of behavior therapy methods for urinary incontinence following prostate surgery: A pilot study. *Urologic Nursing, 20*(3), 203–210.

Joseph, A. C. (1999). The challenge of developing the nursing clinical practice guideline: Neurogenic bladder management. *Urologic Nursing, 19*(3), 195–201.

*Kincade, J. E., Peckous, B. K., & Busby-Whitehead, J. (2001). A pilot study to determine predictors of behavioral treatment completion for urinary incontinence. *Urologic Nursing, 21*(1), 39–44.

Lekan-Routledge, D., Doughty, D., Moore, K. N., et al. (2003). Promoting social continence: Products and devices in the management of urinary continence. *Urologic Nursing 23*(6), 416–429.

Madersbacher, H., Wyndaele, J., Igawa, Y., et al. (2002). Conservative management in neuropathic urinary incontinence. In P. Abrams, L. Cardozo, S. Khoury, et al. (Eds.), *Incontinence* (pp. 699–754). Plymouth, UK: Health Publication Ltd.

McCallig Bates, P. (2000). Helping women manage urinary incontinence. *Advances in Skin & Wound Care: The Journal for Prevention and Healing, 13*(6), 285–289.

*McCallum, T. J., Moore, K. N., & Griffiths, D. (2001). Urinary incontinence after radical prostatectomy: Implications and urodynamics. *Urologic Nursing 21*(2), 113–119.

*Milne, J. L., & Moore, K. N. (2003). An exploratory study of continence care services worldwide. *International Journal of Nursing Studies 40*(3), 235–247.

Moore, K. N. (1994). Electrical stimulation for the treatment of urinary incontinence: Do we know enough to accept it as part of our practice? *Journal of Advanced Nursing 20*(6) 1018–1022.

Moore, K. N. (1999). A review of the anatomy of the male continence mechanism and the cause of urinary incontinence after prostatectomy. *Journal of Wound Ostomy Continence Nursing, 26*(2), 86–93.

Moore, K. N. (2000). Treatment of urinary incontinence in men with electrical stimulation: Is practice evidenced-based? *Journal of Wound Ostomy Continence Nursing, 27*(1), 20–31.

Moore, K. N., & Dorey, G. F. (1999). Conservative treatment of urinary incontinence in men: A review of the literature. *Physiotherapy 85*(2), 77–87.

Moore, K. N., & Gray, M. (2004). Urinary incontinence in men: Current status and future directions. *Nursing Research 53*(6S), S36–S41.

*Moore, K. N., & Jensen, L. (2000). Testing of the Incontinence Impact Questionnaire (IIQ-7) with men after radical prostatectomy. *Journal of Wound Ostomy Continence Nursing, 27*(6), 304–312.

Moore, K. N., & Paul, P. (1997). A historical review of selected nursing and medical literature on urinary incontinence between 1850 and 1976. *Journal of Wound Ostomy Continence Nursing, 24*(2), 106–122.

*Ostaszkiewicz, J., Johnston, L., & Roe, B. (2004). Habit retraining for the management of urinary incontinence in adults. *Cochrane Database of Systematic Reviews, 2.*

Resnick, N. (1984). Urinary incontinence in the elderly. *Medical Grand Rounds*, 3, 281–290.

Roberts, R. (2001). Current management strategies for overactive bladder. *Patient Care for the Nurse Practitioner Supplement*, 22–30.

Roe, B., & Moore, K. N. (2001). Utilization of incontinence clinical practice guidelines. *Journal of Wound Ostomy Continence Nursing, 28*(6), 297–304.

Suchinski, G. A., Piano, M. R., Rosenberg, N., & Zerwic, J. J. (1999). Treating urinary tract infections in the elderly. *DCCN—Dimensions of Critical Care Nursing, 18*(1), 21–27.

*Sueppel, C., Kreder, K., & See, W. (2001). Improved continence outcomes with preoperative pelvic floor muscle strengthening exercises. *Urologic Nursing, 21*(3), 201–210.

Wilson, P., Bo, K., Hay-Smith, J., et al. (2002). Conservative treatment in women. In P. Abrams, L. Cardozo, S. Khoury, et al. (Eds.), *Incontinence* (pp. 573–624). Plymouth, UK: Health Publication Ltd.

Renal Surgery

Batler, R. A., Campbell, S. C., Funk, G. T., et al. (2001). Hand-assisted vs. retroperitoneal laparoscopic nephrectomy. *Journal of Endourology, 15*(9), 899–902.

Fishman, M., Seigne, J. & Antonia, S. (2001). Novel therapies for renal cell carcinoma. *Expert Opinion on Investigational Drugs, 10*(6), 1033–1044.

Lehmann, S., & Dietz, C. (2002). Double-J stents. They're not trouble free. *RN, 65*(1), 54–59.

Sullivan, M., & Frydenberg, M. (2001). Nephron-sparing surgery for small incidental renal cell carcinoma. *ANZ Journal of Surgery, 71*(16), 349–353.

Transplantation

Canadian Institute of Health Information. (2003). *Canadian organ replacement register*. Available at: http://www.cihi.ca. Retrieved June 15, 2005.

Cohen, D., & Galbraith, C. (2001). General health management and long-term care of the renal transplant recipient. *American Journal of Kidney Disease, 38*(6 Suppl 6), 510–524.

Hariharan, S. (2001). Long-term kidney transplant survival. *American Journal of Kidney Disease, 38*(6 Suppl 6), 544–550.

Howard, A. D. (2001). Long-term management of the renal transplant recipient: Optimizing the relationship between the transplant center and the community nephrologist. *American Journal of Kidney Disease, 38*(6 Suppl 6), 551–557.

Urinary Catheters

Addison, R. (1999*a*). Changing a suprapubic catheter: Part 1. *Nursing Times, 95*(42), Suppl 1-2, Oct. 20–26.

Addison, R. (1999*b*). Changing a suprapubic catheter: Part 2. *Nursing Times, 95*(43), Suppl 1-2, Oct. 27–Nov. 2.

Addison, R. (1999*c*). Changing a suprapubic catheter: Part 3. *Nursing Times, 95*(44), Suppl 1-2, Nov. 3–9.

Gujral, S., Kirkwood, L. & Hinchliffe, A. (1999). Suprapubic catheterization: A suitable procedure for clinician nurse specialists in selected patients. *British Journal of Urology International, 83*(9), 954–956.

*Lillibridge, J., & Watt, E. (2000). Timing of urinary catheter removal: A descriptive study. *Urologic Nursing, 20*(6), 375–380.

Montagnino, B. (2000). The LoFric catheter: New technology improves an old technique. *Urologic Nursing, 20*(4), 247–253.

RESOURCES AND WEBSITES

Association de la C.I. du Quebec, 14 Grand-Côteau, Sainte-Julie QC J3E 2X4; (450) 922-6498; fax: (450) 922-6498; www.cystiteinterstitielle.org.

Canadian Association of Nephrology Nurses, 336 Yonge Street, Suite 322, Barrie, ON L4N 4C8; (705) 720-2819; fax: (705) 720-1451; email: cannt@cannt.ca; www.cannt.ca.

Canadian Continence Foundation, P.O. Box 30, Victoria Branch, Westmount, QC H3Z 2V4; (514) 488-9999, Montreal area: 1-800-265-9575; email: help@continence-fdn.ca; www.continence-fdn.ca.

Kidney Foundation of Canada, 300-5165 Sherbrooke Street West, Montreal, QC H4A 1T6; (514) 369-4806/1-800-361-7494; fax: (514) 369-2472; www.kidney.ca.

National Institute of Diabetes and Digestive and Kidney Diseases, National Institutes of Health, Bethesda, MD 20892; http://www.niddk.nih.gov.

National Kidney and Urologic Diseases Information Clearinghouse, Box NKUDIC, 9000 Rockville Pike, Bethesda, MD 20892; (301) 654-4415; http://www.niddk.nih.gov.

North American Society for Dialysis and Transplantation, c/o Wadi N. Suki, MD, 6550 Fannin, Suite 1273, Houston, TX 77030; (713) 790-3275.

Urology Nurses of Canada; www.unc.org.

Wound, Ostomy and Continence Nurses Society, 1500 S. Coast Highway, Suite 201, Laguna Beach, CA 94651; (888) 224WOCN; http://www.wocn.org.

Management of Patients With Urinary Disorders

Adapted by Jill Milne

On completion of this chapter, the learner will be able to:

1. Identify factors contributing to urinary tract infections.
2. Develop a teaching plan for the patient with urinary tract infection.
3. Compare and contrast pyelonephritis, glomerulonephritis, and the nephrotic syndrome: causes, pathophysiologic changes, clinical manifestations, management, and nursing care.
4. Describe causes of acute and chronic renal failure.
5. Use the nursing process as a framework for the care of patients with acute renal failure.
6. Use the nursing process as a framework for the care of patients with chronic renal failure.
7. Develop a postoperative plan of nursing care and teaching plan for the patient undergoing kidney transplantation.
8. Describe management strategies for renal calculi (kidney stones).
9. Develop a teaching plan for the patient undergoing treatment for renal calculi (kidney stones).
10. Formulate preoperative and postoperative nursing diagnoses for the patient undergoing surgery for urinary diversion.
11. Describe interstitial cystitis and its physical and psychological effects on the patient.

$\mathcal{D}$isorders of the lower and upper urinary tracts range from easily treated infections to life-threatening disorders that necessitate organ replacement or long-term treatment with dialysis. Recent advances in pharmacotherapeutics and technology have improved the diagnostic and treatment possibilities for these disorders. Additionally, many disorders that once required surgical intervention and prolonged recuperation can now be treated with noninvasive, nonsurgical techniques.

Infections of the Urinary Tract

Urinary tract infections (UTIs) are caused by pathogenic microorganisms in the urinary tract (the normal urinary tract is sterile above the urethra). UTIs are generally classified as infections involving the upper or lower urinary tract (Chart 45-1).

Lower UTIs include bacterial **cystitis** (inflammation of the urinary bladder), bacterial **prostatitis** (inflammation of the prostate gland), and bacterial **urethritis** (inflammation of the urethra). There can be acute or chronic nonbacterial causes of inflammation in any of these areas that can be misdiagnosed as bacterial infections. Upper UTIs are much less common and include acute or chronic **pyelonephritis** (inflammation of the renal pelvis), **interstitial nephritis** (inflammation of the kidney), and renal abscesses. Upper and lower UTIs are further classified as uncomplicated or complicated, depending on other patient-related conditions (for example, whether the UTI is recurrent and the duration of the infection). Most uncomplicated UTIs are community-acquired. Complicated UTIs usually occur in people with urologic abnormalities or recent catheterization and are often hospital-acquired. Bacteriuria and UTIs are more common in persons older than 65 years of age than in younger adults. Conservative estimates suggest that 20% to 25% of ambulatory women and 10% of men in this age group have asymptomatic bacteriuria; the incidence rises to 50% in women over the age of 80 (Gomolin & McCue, 2000).

Urinary tract infections are among the most frequently encountered of all infections and account for considerable morbidity, disruption to work time, and health-related costs each year (Stamm & Raz, 1999). Women are more likely to develop a UTI than men; over 500,000 Canadian women visit the doctor each year because of a UTI (Kidney Foundation of Canada, 2004). The urinary tract is also the most common site of nosocomial infection, accounting for greater than 40% of the total number reported by hospitals (Foxman, 2002). In most of these hospital-acquired UTIs, instrumentation of the urinary tract or catheterization is the precipitating cause. The prevalence of UTIs in long-term care may be as high as 50% (Nicolle, 1994).

LOWER URINARY TRACT INFECTIONS

Several mechanisms maintain the sterility of the bladder: the physical barrier of the urethra, urine flow, ureterovesical junction competence, various antibacterial enzymes and antibodies, and antiadherent effects mediated by the mucosal cells of the bladder. Abnormalities or dysfunctions of these mechanisms are contributing factors to lower UTIs (Chart 45-2).

Chart 45-1 | Classifying Urinary Tract Infections

Urinary tract infections (UTIs) are classified by location: the lower urinary tract (which includes the bladder and structures below the bladder) or the upper urinary tract (which includes the kidneys and ureters). They can also be classified as uncomplicated or complicated UTI.

Lower UTI
Cystitis, prostatitis, urethritis

Upper UTI
Acute pyelonephritis, chronic pyelonephritis, renal abscess, interstitial nephritis, perirenal abscess

Uncomplicated Lower or Upper UTI
Community-acquired infection; common in young women

Complicated Lower or Upper UTI
Often nosocomial (acquired in the hospital) and related to catheterization; occurs in patients with urologic abnormalities, pregnancy, immunosuppression, diabetes mellitus, obstructions

---

Glossary

acute tubular necrosis: type of acute renal failure in which there is actual damage to the kidney tubules

bacteriuria: more than 10^5 colonies of bacteria per millilitre of urine

continent urinary diversion (Koch, Indiana, Charleston pouch): transplantation of the ureters to a segment of bowel with construction of an effective continence mechanism or valve

cutaneous ureterostomy: procedure in which the distal ureter is detached from the bladder, brought through the abdominal wall, and attached to an opening in the skin

cystectomy: removal of the urinary bladder

cystitis: inflammation of the urinary bladder

end-stage renal disease (ESRD): progressive, irreversible deterioration in renal function that results in retention of uremic waste products

glomerulonephritis: inflammation of the glomerular capillaries

ileal conduit: transplantation of the ureters to an isolated section of the terminal ileum, with one end of the ureters brought to the abdominal wall

interstitial cystitis: inflammation of the bladder wall that eventually causes disintegration of the lining and loss of bladder elasticity

interstitial nephritis: inflammation of the renal interstitial tissue, often due to use of medications or exposure to chemicals

nephrosclerosis: hardening, or sclerosis, of the arteries of the kidney due to prolonged hypertension

nephrotic syndrome: disorder characterized by proteinuria, edema, hypoalbuminuria, and hyperlipidemia

prostatitis: inflammation of the prostate gland

pyelonephritis: inflammation of the renal pelvis

pyuria: white blood cells in the urine

urethritis: inflammation of the urethra

ureterosigmoidostomy: transplantation of the ureters into the sigmoid colon, allowing urine to flow through the colon and out the rectum

ureterovesical or **vesicoureteral reflux:** backward flow of urine from the bladder into one or both ureters

urethrovesical reflux: backward flow of urine from the urethra into the bladder

urinary casts: protein plugs secreted by damaged kidney tubules

Chart 45-2
Risk Factors for Urinary Tract Infection

General risk factors for urinary tract infection (UTI) include the following:

Inability or failure to empty the bladder completely

Obstructed urinary flow, from congenital anomalies, urethral strictures, contracture of the bladder neck, bladder tumours, calculi (stones) in the ureters or kidneys, compression of the ureters, and neurologic abnormalities

Decreased natural host defenses or immunosuppression

Instrumentation of the urinary tract (eg, catheterization, cystoscopic procedures)

Inflammation or abrasion of the urethral mucosa

Contributing conditions (certain populations of patients are more prone to UTIs than others), including those with:

Diabetes mellitus (increased urinary glucose levels create an infection-prone environment in the urinary tract), pregnancy, neurologic disorders, gout, and other altered states characterized by incomplete emptying of the bladder and urinary stasis

Pathophysiology

For infection to occur, bacteria must gain access to the bladder, attach to and colonize the epithelium of the urinary tract to avoid being washed out with voiding, evade host defense mechanisms, and initiate inflammation (Moore, Day, & Albers, 2002). Most UTIs result from fecal organisms that ascend from the perineum to the urethra and the bladder and then adhere to the mucosal surfaces.

BACTERIAL INVASION OF THE URINARY TRACT

By increasing the normal slow shedding of bladder epithelial cells (resulting in bacteria removal), the bladder can clear itself of even large numbers of bacteria. Glycosaminoglycan (GAG), a hydrophilic protein, normally exerts a nonadherent protective effect against various bacteria. The GAG molecule attracts water molecules, forming a water barrier that serves as a defensive layer between the bladder and the urine. GAG may be impaired by certain agents (cyclamate, saccharin, aspartame, and tryptophan metabolites). The normal bacterial flora of the vagina and urethral area also interfere with adherence of *Escherichia coli* (the most common microorganism causing UTI). Urinary immunoglobulin A (IgA) in the urethra may also provide a barrier to bacteria.

REFLUX

An obstruction to free-flowing urine is a problem known as **urethrovesical reflux**, which is the reflux (backward flow) of urine from the urethra into the bladder (Fig. 45-1). With coughing, sneezing, or straining, the bladder pressure rises, which may force urine from the bladder into the urethra. When the pressure returns to normal, the urine flows back into the bladder, bringing into the bladder bacteria from the anterior portions of the urethra. Urethrovesical reflux is also caused by dysfunction of the bladder neck or urethra. The urethrovesical angle and urethral closure pressure may be altered with menopause, increasing the incidence of infection in postmenopausal women. Reflux is most often noted, however, in young children. Treatment is based on its severity.

Ureterovesical or **vesicoureteral reflux** refers to the backward flow of urine from the bladder into one or both ureters (see Fig. 45-1). Normally, the ureterovesical junction prevents urine from traveling back into the ureter. The ureters tunnel into the

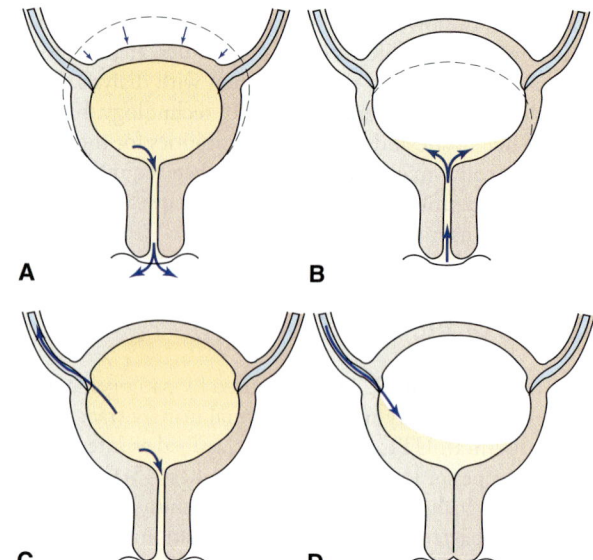

FIGURE 45-1 Mechanisms of urethrovesical and ureterovesical reflux may cause urinary tract infection. **Urethrovesical reflux:** With coughing and straining, bladder pressure rises, which may force urine from the bladder into the urethra (**A**). When bladder pressure returns to normal, the urine flows back to the bladder (**B**), which introduces bacteria from the urethra to the bladder. **Ureterovesical reflux:** With failure of the ureterovesical valve, urine moves up the ureters during voiding (**C**) and flows into the bladder when voiding stops (**D**). This prevents complete emptying of the bladder. It also leads to urinary stasis and contamination of the ureters with bacteria-laden urine.

bladder wall so that the bladder musculature compresses a small portion of the ureter during normal voiding. When the ureterovesical valve is impaired by congenital causes or ureteral abnormalities, the bacteria may reach and eventually destroy the kidneys.

UROPATHOGENIC BACTERIA

Bacteriuria is generally defined as more than 10^5 colonies of bacteria per millilitre of urine. Because urine samples (especially in women) are commonly contaminated by the bacteria normally present in the urethral area, a bacterial count exceeding 10^5 colonies/mL of clean-catch midstream urine is the measure that distinguishes true bacteriuria from contamination. In men, contamination of the collected urine sample occurs less frequently; hence, bacteriuria can be defined as 10^4 colonies/mL urine. Community-acquired UTIs are among the most common bacterial infections in women (Gupta, Hooton & Stamm, 2001).

The organisms most frequently responsible for UTIs are those normally found in the lower gastrointestinal (GI) tract. In a large-scale study of the types and prevalence of organisms of patients with UTIs in both the community and hospital setting, *E. coli* was responsible for 54.7% of urinary tract infections. Isolation of *E. coli* is decreasing in comparison to previous observations, especially in males and in patients with indwelling bladder catheters, who instead had higher rates of *Pseudomonas* and *Enterococcus* organisms than females and noncatheterized patients (Bonadio, Meini, Spitaleri & Gigli, 2001).

ROUTES OF INFECTION

There are three well-recognized routes by which bacteria enter the urinary tract: up the urethra (ascending infection), through the bloodstream, (hematogenous spread), or by means of a fistula from the intestine (direct extension).

The most common route of infection is transurethral, in which bacteria (often from fecal contamination) colonize the periurethral area and subsequently enter the bladder by means of the urethra. In women, the short urethra offers little resistance to the movement of uropathogenic bacteria. Sexual intercourse or massage of the urethra forces the bacteria up into the bladder. This accounts for the increased incidence of UTIs in sexually active women. Bacteria may also enter the urinary tract by means of the blood (hematogenous spread) from a distant site of infection or through direct extension by way of a fistula from the intestinal tract.

Clinical Manifestations

A variety of signs and symptoms are associated with UTI. About half of all patients with bacteriuria have no symptoms. Signs and symptoms of uncomplicated lower UTI (cystitis) include frequent pain and burning on urination, frequency, urgency, nocturia, incontinence, and suprapubic or pelvic pain. Hematuria and back pain may also be present. In older individuals, these typical symptoms are seldom noted (see Gerontologic Considerations, below).

Signs and symptoms of upper UTI (pyelonephritis) include fever, chills, flank or low back pain, nausea and vomiting, headache, malaise, and painful urination. Physical examination for tenderness begins by palpating with the fingertips over the area of the costovertebral angles (CVA), which are the angles formed on each side of the body by the bottom rib of the rib cage and the vertebral column (Fig. 45-2). This will be enough pressure to detect tenderness or pain in some patients. If no pain is elicited, the examiner places the ball of one hand over each CVA in turn, and strikes that hand with the ulnar side of the other fist, hard enough to jar the patient.

In patients with complicated UTIs, such as those with indwelling catheters, manifestations can range from asymptomatic bacteriuria to a gram-negative sepsis with shock. Complicated UTIs often are due to a broader spectrum of organisms, have a lower response rate to treatment, and tend to recur. Many patients with catheter-associated UTIs are asymptomatic; however, any patient who suddenly develops signs and symptoms of septic shock should be evaluated for urosepsis.

Assessment and Diagnostic Findings

Results of various tests, such as colony counts, cellular studies, and urine cultures, help confirm the UTI diagnosis. Pregnant women are generally screened for asymptomatic bacteriuria because the bladder may not empty as well as it usually does. In an uncomplicated UTI, the strain of bacteria will determine the antibiotic of choice.

COLONY COUNTS

UTI is diagnosed by bacteria in the urine. A colony count of at least 10^5 colony-forming units (CFU) per millilitre of urine on a clean-catch midstream or catheterized specimen is a major criterion for infection. However, UTI and subsequent sepsis have occurred with lower bacterial colony counts. About one third of women with symptoms of acute infections have negative midstream urine culture results and may go untreated if 10^5 CFU/mL is used as the criterion for infection. The presence of any bacteria in specimens obtained by suprapubic needle aspiration of the urinary bladder or catheterization is considered indicative of infection.

CELLULAR STUDIES

Microscopic hematuria (greater than 4 red blood cells [RBCs] per high-power field) is present in about half of patients with acute infection. **Pyuria** (greater than 4 white blood cells [WBCs] per high-power field) occurs in all patients with UTI; however, it is not specific for bacterial infection. Pyuria can also be seen with kidney stones, interstitial nephritis, and renal tuberculosis.

URINE CULTURES

Urine cultures remain the gold standard in documenting a UTI and can identify the specific organism present. Because of the high probability that the organism in young women with their first UTI is *E. coli,* cultures are often omitted. The following groups of patients should have urine cultures obtained when bacteriuria is present:

- All men (because of the likelihood of structural or functional abnormalities)
- All children
- Women with a history of compromised immune function or renal problems
- Patients with diabetes mellitus
- Patients who have undergone recent instrumentation (including catheterization) of the urinary tract
- Patients who were hospitalized recently
- Patients with prolonged or persistent symptoms
- Patients with three or more UTIs in the past year
- Pregnant women
- Postmenopausal women
- Women who are sexually active or have new partners

TESTING METHODS

Multistrip dipstick testing for WBCs, known as the leukocyte esterase test, and nitrite testing (nitrate reduction test) are common. If the leukocyte esterase test is positive, it is assumed that the patient has pyuria (WBCs in the urine) and should be treated. The

Left kidney

Costovertebral angle

12th rib

Right kidney

FIGURE 45-2 Location of the costovertebral angle.

nitrate reduction test is considered positive if bacteria that reduce normal urinary nitrates to nitrites are present.

Tests for sexually transmitted diseases (STDs) may be performed because acute urethritis caused by sexually transmitted organisms (ie, *Chlamydia trachomatis, Neisseria gonorrhoeae,* herpes simplex) or acute vaginitis infections (caused by *Trichomonas* or *Candida* species) may be responsible for symptoms similar to those of UTI. Therefore, evaluation for STDs may be performed (see Chap. 70).

Historically, intravenous pyelography (IVP) was used to detect abnormalities in patients at high risk for complicated or recurring UTI. Today, diagnostic studies such as computed tomography (CT) and ultrasonography are preferred detection methods for several reasons: CT scans may detect areas of pyelonephritis or abscesses, and ultrasonography is extremely sensitive for detecting obstruction, abscesses, tumours, and cysts. Transrectal ultrasonography (to assess the prostate and bladder) is the procedure of choice for men with recurrent or complicated UTIs. An IVP may be indicated to visualize the ureters or to detect strictures or stones and is necessary for an accurate diagnosis of reflux nephropathy. It is generally accepted that the first episode of UTI in women does not require urologic evaluation (Hooton, Scholes, Stapleton et al., 2000).

 Gerontologic Considerations

The incidence of bacteriuria in the elderly differs from that in younger adults. Bacteriuria increases with age and disability, and women are affected more frequently than men. UTI is the most common cause of acute bacterial sepsis in patients older than 65 years of age, in whom gram-negative sepsis carries a mortality rate exceeding 50%. Urologists see many asymptomatic older patients with bacteriuria, and these individuals represent 20% of women over the age of 65. In the nursing home environment, up to 50% of females have asymptomatic bacteriuria (Foxman, 2002).

In the elderly population at large, structural abnormalities and neurogenic bladder secondary to strokes or autonomic neuropathy of diabetes may prevent complete emptying of the bladder and increase the risk for UTI. When indwelling catheters are used, the risk for UTI rises dramatically as two or more different strains of bacteria can be found in the urine of catheterized patients: in the urine itself, and on the surface of the catheter. Elderly women often have incomplete emptying of the bladder and urinary stasis. In the absence of estrogen, postmenopausal women are susceptible to colonization and increased adherence of bacteria to the vagina and urethra. Oral or topical estrogen has been used to restore the glycogen content of vaginal epithelial cells and an acidic pH for some postmenopausal women with recurrent cystitis. Local estrogen replacement may reduce the rate of UTIs in postmenopausal women with recurrent UTIs (Raz, 2001).

The antibacterial activity of prostatic secretions that protects men from bacterial colonization of the urethra and bladder decreases with aging. Although UTIs are rare in men, the prevalence of infection in men older than 50 years of age approaches that of women in the same age group. The dramatic rise in UTI in men as they age is due largely to prostatic hyperplasia or carcinoma, strictures of the urethra, and neuropathic bladder. The use of catheterization or cystoscopy in evaluation or treatment may contribute further to the higher incidence of UTI. The incidence of bacteriuria rises in men with confusion, dementia, or bowel or bladder incontinence. The most common cause of recurrent UTI in the elderly male patient is chronic bacterial prostatitis.

Transurethral resection of the prostate gland may help to reduce its incidence (see Chap. 49).

In elderly patients in institutions, such as nursing homes, infecting pathogens are often resistant to many antibiotics. Factors that may contribute to UTI include: high incidence of chronic illness; frequent use of antimicrobial agents; infected pressure ulcers; immobility and incomplete emptying of the bladder; and use of a bedpan rather than a commode or toilet (Chart 45-3).

Diligent hand hygiene, careful perineal care, and frequent toileting may decrease the incidence of UTIs in patients in nursing homes. The organisms responsible for UTIs in the elderly in institutions may differ from those found in patients residing in the community; this is thought to be due in part to the frequent use of antibiotic agents by patients in nursing homes. *E. coli* is the most common organism seen in elderly patients in the community or hospital. Patients with indwelling catheters, however, are more likely to be infected with *Proteus, Klebsiella, Pseudomonas,* or *Staphylococcus* species. Patients who have been previously treated with antibiotics may be infected with *Enterococcus* species. Frequent reinfections are common in older adults.

The most common subjective presenting symptom of UTI in older adults is generalized fatigue. The most common objective finding is a change in cognitive functioning, especially in those with dementia, because these patients usually exhibit even more profound cognitive changes with the onset of a UTI.

 NURSING ALERT Elderly patients often lack the typical symptoms of UTI and sepsis. Although frequency, urgency, and dysuria may occur, nonspecific symptoms, such as altered sensorium, lethargy, anorexia, new incontinence, hyperventilation, and low-grade fever, may be the only clues.

Medical Management

Management of UTIs typically involves pharmacologic therapy and patient education. The nurse is a key figure in teaching the patient about medication regimens and infection prevention measures.

Controversy continues about the need for treatment of asymptomatic bacteriuria in elderly patients in institutions because resulting antibiotic-resistant organisms and sepsis may be greater threats to the patient. Most experts now recommend withholding antibiotics unless symptoms develop. Treatment regimens, however, are generally the same as those for younger adults, although age-related changes in the intestinal absorption of medications and decreased renal function and hepatic flow may necessitate alterations in the antimicrobial regimen. Renal function must be monitored and the dosage of medications altered accordingly.

 Gerontologic Considerations

Factors Contributing to Urinary Tract Infection in Older Adults

- Higher incidence of chronic illness
- Frequent use of antimicrobial agents
- Presence of infected pressure ulcers
- Immobility and incomplete emptying of bladder
- Use of a bedpan rather than a commode or toilet

ACUTE PHARMACOLOGIC THERAPY

The ideal treatment of UTI is an antibacterial agent that eradicates bacteria from the urinary tract with minimal effects on fecal and vaginal flora, thereby minimizing the incidence of vaginal yeast infections. (Yeast vaginitis occurs in as many as 25% of patients treated with antimicrobial agents that affect vaginal flora. Yeast vaginitis often causes more symptoms and is more difficult and costly to treat than the original UTI.) Additionally, the antibacterial agent should be affordable and should produce few adverse effects and low resistance. Because the organism in initial, uncomplicated UTIs in women is most likely *E. coli* or other fecal flora, the agent should be effective against these organisms. Various treatment regimens have been successful in treating uncomplicated lower UTIs in women: single-dose administration, short-course (3 to 4 days) medication regimens, or 7- to 10-day therapeutic courses. The trend is toward a shortened course of antibiotic therapy for uncomplicated UTIs because about 80% of cases are cured after 3 days of treatment.

In a complicated UTI (ie, pyelonephritis), the general treatment of choice is usually a cephalosporin or an ampicillin/aminoglycoside combination. Patients in institutional settings may require 7 to 10 days of medication for the treatment to be effective. Other commonly used medications include trimethoprim-sulfamethoxazole (TMP-SMZ, Bactrim, Septra) and nitrofurantoin (Macrodantin, Furadantin). Occasionally, medications such as ampicillin or amoxicillin are used, but *E. coli* organisms have developed resistance to these agents. Recent clinical trials comparing the use of TMP-SMZ and the fluoroquinolone ciprofloxacin (Cipro) found ciprofloxacin to be significantly more effective in community-based patients and in residents in nursing homes (Gomolin & McCue, 2000; Talan et al., 2000).

Levofloxacin (Levaquin), another fluoroquinolone, is a good choice for short-course therapy of uncomplicated, mild to moderate UTI. Clinical trial data show high patient compliance with the 3-day regimen (95.6%) and a high eradication rate for all pathogens (96.4%). Before using levofloxacin in patients with complicated UTIs, the causative pathogen should be identified. Levofloxacin is used only when generic and less costly antibiotics are likely to be ineffective (Bonapace et al., 2000).

Nitrofurantoin should not be used in patients with renal insufficiency because it is ineffective at glomerular filtration rates (GFRs) of less than 50 mL/min and may cause peripheral neuropathy. Phenazopyridine (Pyridium), a urinary analgesic, may be prescribed to relieve the discomfort associated with the infection.

Regardless of the regimen prescribed, the patient is instructed to take all the doses prescribed, even if relief of symptoms occurs promptly. Longer medication courses are indicated for men, pregnant women, and women with pyelonephritis and other types of complicated UTIs. In pregnant women, amoxicillin, ampicillin, or an oral cephalosporin is used for 7 to 10 days.

LONG-TERM PHARMACOLOGIC THERAPY

Although brief pharmacologic treatment of UTI for 3 days is usually adequate in women, infection recurs in about 20% of women treated for uncomplicated UTI. Infections that recur within 2 weeks after therapy (referred to as a relapse) do so because organisms of the original offending strain remain in the vagina. Relapses suggest that the source of bacteriuria may be the upper urinary tract or that initial treatment was inadequate or administered for too short a time. Recurrent infections in men are usually due to persistence of the same organism; further evaluation and treatment are indicated (Gupta et al., 2001; Hooton et al., 2000; Stamm, 2001).

Reinfection of the female patient with new bacteria is the reason for more than 90% of recurrent UTIs in women. If the diagnostic evaluation reveals no structural abnormalities in the urinary tract, the woman with recurrent UTIs may be instructed to begin treatment on her own whenever symptoms occur and to contact the health care provider only when symptoms persist, fever occurs, or the number of treatment episodes exceeds four in a 6-month period. This patient may be taught to use dip-slide culture devices to detect bacteria.

If infection recurs after completing antimicrobial therapy, another short course (3 to 4 days) of full-dose antimicrobial therapy followed by a regular bedtime dose of an antimicrobial agent may be prescribed. If there is no recurrence, medication is taken every other night for 6 to 7 months. Other options include a dose of an antimicrobial agent after sexual intercourse, a dose at bedtime, or a dose every other night or three times per week. Long-term use of antimicrobial agents decreases the risk of reinfection and may be indicated in patients with recurrent infections.

If recurrence is caused by persistent bacteria from preceding infections, the cause (ie, kidney stone, abscess), if known, must be treated. After treatment and sterilization of the urine, low-dose preventive therapy (trimethoprim with or without sulfamethoxazole) each night at bedtime is often prescribed.

There is evidence that cranberry products can significantly reduce the incidence of UTIs (Jepson, Mihaljevic, & Craig, 2005). Although the exact mechanism of action is unknown, cranberries contain two antiadherence compounds that help to prevent *E. coli* from adhering to uroepithelial cells (Raz, Chazan, & Dan, 2004). No evidence exists, however, to support the use of cranberries in the treatment of UTIs (Jepson, Mihaljevic, & Craig, 2005).

NURSING PROCESS: THE PATIENT WITH LOWER URINARY TRACT INFECTION

Nursing care of the patient with lower UTI focuses on treating the underlying infection and preventing its recurrence.

Assessment

A history of signs and symptoms related to UTI is obtained from the patient with a suspected UTI. The presence of pain, frequency, urgency, and hesitancy and changes in urine are assessed, documented, and reported. The patient's usual pattern of voiding is assessed to detect factors that may predispose him or her to UTI. Infrequent emptying of the bladder, the association of symptoms of UTI with sexual intercourse, contraceptive practices, and personal hygiene are assessed. The patient's knowledge about prescribed antimicrobial medications and preventive health care measures is also assessed. Additionally, the urine is assessed for volume, colour, concentration, cloudiness, and odour, all of which are altered by bacteria in the urinary tract.

Diagnosis

NURSING DIAGNOSES

Based on the assessment data, the nursing diagnoses may include the following:

- Acute pain related to inflammation and infection of the urethra, bladder, and other urinary tract structures
- Deficient knowledge related to factors predisposing the patient to infection and recurrence, detection and prevention of recurrence, and pharmacologic therapy

COLLABORATIVE PROBLEMS/ POTENTIAL COMPLICATIONS

Based on assessment data, the following complications may develop:

- Renal failure due to extensive damage of kidney
- Sepsis

Planning and Goals

Major goals for the patient may include relief of pain and discomfort; increased knowledge of preventive measures and treatment modalities; and absence of complications.

Nursing Interventions

RELIEVING PAIN

The pain associated with UTI is quickly relieved once effective antimicrobial therapy is initiated. Antispasmodic agents may also be useful in relieving bladder irritability and pain. Aspirin and applying heat to the perineum help relieve pain and spasm. The patient is encouraged to drink liberal amounts of fluids (water is the best choice) to promote renal blood flow and to flush the bacteria from the urinary tract. Urinary tract irritants (eg, coffee, tea, citrus, spices, colas, alcohol) are avoided. Frequent voiding (every 2 to 3 hours) is encouraged to empty the bladder completely because this can significantly lower urine bacterial counts, reduce urinary stasis, and prevent reinfection.

MONITORING AND MANAGING POTENTIAL COMPLICATIONS

Early recognition of UTI and prompt treatment are essential to prevent recurrent infection and the possibility of complications, such as renal failure and sepsis. The goal of treatment is to prevent infection from progressing and causing permanent renal damage and renal failure. Thus, the patient must be taught to recognize early signs and symptoms, to test for bacteriuria, and to initiate treatment as prescribed. Appropriate antimicrobial therapy, liberal fluid intake, frequent voiding, and hygienic measures are commonly prescribed for managing UTI. The patient is instructed to notify the physician if fatigue, nausea, vomiting, or pruritus occurs. Periodic monitoring of renal function (creatinine clearance, blood urea nitrogen [BUN], and serum creatinine levels) may be indicated for patients with repeated UTIs. If extensive renal damage does occur, dialysis may be necessary.

Patients with UTI, especially catheter-associated infection, are at increased risk for Gram-negative sepsis. Indwelling catheters should be avoided if possible and removed at the earliest opportunity (Thees & Dreblow, 1999). If an indwelling catheter is necessary, however, specific nursing interventions are initiated to prevent infection (see Chap. 44). These include the following:

- Using strict aseptic technique during insertion of the smallest catheter possible
- Securing the catheter with tape to prevent movement
- Frequently inspecting urine colour, odour, and consistency
- Performing meticulous daily perineal care with soap and water
- Maintaining a closed system
- Using the catheter's port to obtain urine specimens

Careful assessment of vital signs and level of consciousness may warn of impending sepsis. Blood cultures that are positive for infection and elevated WBC counts are reported to the physician. At the same time, appropriate antibiotic therapy and increased fluid intake are prescribed (intravenous antibiotic therapy and fluids may be required). Preventing sepsis is key because the mortality rate for Gram-negative sepsis is significant, especially in elderly patients.

PROMOTING HOME AND COMMUNITY-BASED CARE

Teaching Patients Self-Care

In helping patients learn about and prevent or manage a recurrent UTI, the nurse needs to implement teaching that meets individual patient needs. For a detailed discussion of patient teaching interventions, see Chart 45-4.

Evaluation

EXPECTED PATIENT OUTCOMES

Expected patient outcomes may include:

1. Experiences relief of pain
   a. Reports absence of pain, urgency, dysuria, or hesitancy on voiding
   b. Takes analgesic and antibiotic agents as prescribed
2. Explains UTIs and their treatment
   a. Demonstrates knowledge of preventive measures and prescribed treatments
   b. Drinks 8 to 10 glasses of fluids daily
   c. Voids every 2 to 3 hours
   d. Voids urine that is clear and odourless
3. Experiences no complications
   a. Reports no symptoms of infection (fever, dysuria, frequency) or renal failure (nausea, vomiting, fatigue, pruritus)
   b. Has normal BUN and serum creatinine levels, negative urine and blood cultures
   c. Exhibits normal vital signs and temperature; no signs or symptoms of sepsis
   d. Maintains adequate urine output of more than 30 mL per hour

UPPER URINARY TRACT INFECTION: ACUTE PYELONEPHRITIS

Pyelonephritis is a bacterial infection of the renal pelvis, tubules, and interstitial tissue of one or both kidneys. Upper UTIs are associated with the antibody coating of the bacteria in the urine. (This occurs in the renal medulla; when the bacteria are excreted in the urine, the immunofluorescent test can detect the antibody coating.) Bacteria reach the bladder by means of the urethra and ascend to the kidney. Although the kidneys receive 20% to 25% of the cardiac output, bacteria rarely reach the kidneys from the blood: fewer than 3% of cases are due to hematogenous spread (Warren et al., 1999).

Pyelonephritis is frequently secondary to ureterovesical reflux, in which an incompetent ureterovesical valve allows the urine to back up (reflux) into the ureters (see Fig. 45-1). Urinary tract obstruction (which increases the susceptibility of the kidneys to infection), bladder tumours, strictures, benign prostatic hyperplasia, and urinary stones are some of the other causes. Pyelonephritis may be acute or chronic.

Patients with acute pyelonephritis usually have enlarged kidneys with interstitial infiltrations of inflammatory cells. Abscesses may be noted on the renal capsule and at the corticomedullary junction. Eventually, atrophy and destruction of tubules and the glomeruli may result. When pyelonephritis becomes chronic, the kidneys become scarred, contracted, and nonfunctioning.

Chart 45-4 • PATIENT EDUCATION
Preventing Recurrent Urinary Tract Infections

An objective of teaching about recurrent urinary tract infections (UTIs) is their prevention. Health-related behaviours that help prevent recurrent UTIs include implementing careful personal hygiene, increasing fluid intake to promote voiding and dilution of urine, urinating regularly and more frequently, and adhering to the therapeutic regimen.

Hygiene
- Shower rather than bathe in tub because bacteria in the bath water may enter the urethra.
- After each bowel movement, clean the perineum and urethral meatus from front to back. This will help reduce concentrations of pathogens at the urethral opening and, in women, the vaginal opening.

Fluid Intake
- Drink liberal amounts of fluids daily to flush out bacteria.
- Avoid coffee, tea, colas, alcohol, aspartame sweetener, and other fluids that are urinary tract irritants.

Voiding Habits
- Void every 2 to 3 hours during the day and completely empty the bladder. This prevents overdistention of the bladder and compromised blood supply to the bladder wall. Both predispose the patient to UTI. Precautions expressly for women include the following: Void immediately after sexual intercourse.
  Take the prescribed single dose of an oral antimicrobial agent after sexual intercourse.

Therapy
- Take medication *exactly* as prescribed.
- If bacteria continue to appear in the urine, long-term antimicrobial therapy may be required to prevent colonization of the periurethral area and recurrence of infection. The medication should be taken after emptying the bladder just before going to bed to ensure adequate concentration of the medication during the overnight period.
- For recurrent infection, consider acidification of the urine through ascorbic acid (vitamin C), 1,000 mg daily, or cranberry juice.
- If prescribed, collect a midstream urine specimen as follows:
  1. Wash around the urethral meatus, moving from front to back several times, using a different washcloth or wipes each time.
  2. Keep the cleansed labia separated with one hand.
  3. Pass a small amount of urine into the toilet. Stop the stream.
  4. Pass urine into the specimen cup. Stop the stream.
  5. Pass remaining urine into the toilet.
  6. Carefully cover the specimen.
  7. Take the specimen to your doctor's office or medical laboratory as directed.
- If prescribed, test urine for bacteria with recommended test devices, such as dip sticks, as follows:
  1. Wash the urethral meatus moving from front to back several times, using a different washcloth or wipes each time.
  2. Collect a midstream urine specimen, as above.
  3. Remove a dip stick from its container, dip it into the urine sample, and return it to the container.
  4. Incubate the dip stick at room temperature according to product directions.
  5. Read the results by comparing the dip stick with the colony density chart provided with the product.
  6. Begin therapy as directed, and complete the full prescribed course of medication.
  7. Notify the health care provider if fever occurs or if signs and symptoms persist.
- Consult the health care provider regularly for follow-up, recurrence of symptoms, or infections nonresponsive to treatment.

Clinical Manifestations

The patient with acute pyelonephritis appears acutely ill with chills and fever, leukocytosis, bacteriuria and pyuria, flank pain, and CVA tenderness. In addition, symptoms of lower urinary tract involvement, such as dysuria and frequency, are common.

Assessment and Diagnostic Findings

An ultrasound study or a CT scan may be performed to locate any obstruction in the urinary tract. Relief of obstruction is essential to save the kidney from destruction. An IVP is rarely indicated during acute pyelonephritis because findings are normal in up to 75% of patients. Radionuclide imaging with gallium citrate and indium-111 (In[111])–labelled WBCs may be useful to identify sites of infection that may not be visualized on CT scan or ultrasound. Urine culture and sensitivity tests are performed to determine the causative organism so that appropriate antimicrobial agents can be prescribed.

Medical Management

Patients with acute uncomplicated pyelonephritis are usually treated as outpatients if they are not dehydrated, not experiencing nausea or vomiting, and not showing signs or symptoms of sepsis. In addition, they must be responsible and reliable to ensure that all medications are taken as prescribed. Other patients, including all pregnant women, may be hospitalized for at least 2 or 3 days of parenteral therapy. Oral agents may be substituted once the patient is afebrile and showing clinical improvement.

PHARMACOLOGIC THERAPY

For outpatients, a 2-week course of antibiotics is recommended because renal parenchymal disease is more difficult to eradicate than mucosal bladder infections. Commonly prescribed agents include TMP-SMZ, ciprofloxacin, gentamicin with or without ampicillin, or a third-generation cephalosporin (Warren et al., 1999). These medications must be used with great caution if the patient has renal or liver dysfunction.

A possible problem in acute pyelonephritis treatment is a chronic or recurring symptomless infection persisting for months or years. After the initial antibiotic regimen, the patient may need antibiotic therapy for up to 6 weeks if evidence of a relapse is seen. A follow-up urine culture is done 2 weeks after completion of antibiotic therapy to document clearing of the infection.

UPPER URINARY TRACT INFECTION: CHRONIC PYELONEPHRITIS

Repeated bouts of acute pyelonephritis may lead to chronic pyelonephritis. Recent evidence suggests that chronic pyelonephritis is decreasing as a common cause of **end-stage renal disease (ESRD),** while renovascular disease is increasing as one of the most common causes for ESRD (Fatica, Port & Young, 2001).

Clinical Manifestations

The patient with chronic pyelonephritis usually has no symptoms of infection unless an acute exacerbation occurs. Noticeable signs and symptoms may include fatigue, headache, poor appetite, polyuria, excessive thirst, and weight loss. Persistent and recurring infection may produce progressive scarring of the kidney, with renal failure the end result.

Assessment and Diagnostic Findings

The extent of the disease is assessed by an intravenous urogram and measurements of creatinine clearance and BUN and creatinine levels. Bacteria, if detected in the urine, are eradicated if possible.

Complications

Complications of chronic pyelonephritis include ESRD (from progressive loss of nephrons secondary to chronic inflammation and scarring), hypertension, and formation of kidney stones (from chronic infection with urea-splitting organisms).

Medical Management

The choice of antimicrobial agent is based on which pathogen is identified through urine culture. If the urine cannot be made bacteria-free, nitrofurantoin or TMP-SMZ may be used to suppress bacterial growth. Impaired renal function alters the excretion of antimicrobial agents and necessitates careful monitoring of renal function, especially if the medications are potentially toxic to the kidneys.

Nursing Management

The patient may require hospitalization or may be treated as an outpatient. When the patient is hospitalized, fluid intake and output are carefully measured and recorded. Unless contraindicated, fluids are encouraged (3 to 4 L/day) to dilute the urine, decrease burning on urination, and prevent dehydration. The nurse assesses the patient's temperature every 4 hours and administers antipyretic and antibiotic agents as prescribed. Often the patient is more comfortable on bed rest during the acute phase of the illness.

Patient teaching focuses on prevention of UTIs by consuming adequate fluids, emptying the bladder regularly, and performing recommended perineal hygiene. The importance of taking antimicrobial medications exactly as prescribed is stressed to the patient, as is the need for keeping follow-up appointments.

Primary Glomerular Diseases

A variety of diseases can affect the glomerular capillaries, including acute and chronic glomerulonephritis, rapidly progressive glomerulonephritis, and nephrotic syndrome. In all of these disorders, the glomerular capillaries are primarily involved. Antigen–antibody complexes form in the blood and become trapped in the glomerular capillaries (the filtering portion of the kidney), inducing an inflammatory response. IgG, the major immunoglobulin (antibody) found in the blood, can be detected in the glomerular capillary walls. The major clinical manifestations of glomerular injury include proteinuria, hematuria, decreased glomerular filtration rate, and alterations in excretion of sodium (leading to edema and hypertension).

ACUTE GLOMERULONEPHRITIS

Glomerulonephritis is an inflammation of the glomerular capillaries. Acute glomerulonephritis is primarily a disease of children older than 2 years of age, but it can occur at nearly any age.

Pathophysiology

In most cases of acute glomerulonephritis, a group A beta-hemolytic streptococcal infection of the throat precedes the onset of glomerulonephritis by 2 to 3 weeks (Fig. 45-3). It may also follow impetigo (infection of the skin) and acute viral infections (upper respiratory tract infections, mumps, varicella zoster virus, Epstein-Barr virus, hepatitis B, and human immunodeficiency virus infection). In some patients, antigens outside the body (eg, medications, foreign serum) initiate the process, resulting in antigen-antibody complexes being deposited in the glomeruli. In other patients, the kidney tissue itself serves as the inciting antigen.

Clinical Manifestations

The primary presenting feature of acute glomerulonephritis is hematuria (blood in the urine), which may be microscopic (identifiable through microscopic examination) or macroscopic or gross (visible to the eye). The urine may appear cola-coloured because of RBCs and protein plugs or casts. (RBC casts indicate glomerular injury.) Glomerulonephritis may be so mild, however, that hema-

Physiology/Pathophysiology

Antigen (group A beta-hemolytic streptococcus)

↓

Antigen-antibody product

↓

Deposition of antigen–antibody complex in glomerulus

↓

Increased production of epithelial cells lining the glomerulus

↓

Leukocytes infiltrate the glomerulus

↓

Thickening of the glomerular filtration membrane

↓

Scarring and loss of glomerular filtration membrane

↓

Decreased glomerular filtration rate (GFR)

FIGURE 45-3 Sequence of events in acute glomerulonephritis.

turia is discovered incidentally through a routine microscopic urinalysis, or the disease may be so severe that the patient has acute renal failure with oliguria. Acute glomerulonephritis typically has an abrupt onset preceded by a latent period between the streptococcal infection and the first indications of renal involvement averaging 10 days.

Proteinuria (primarily albumin), which is present, is due to the increased permeability of the glomerular membrane. BUN and serum creatinine levels may rise as urine output drops. The patient may be anemic.

Some degree of edema and hypertension is noted in 75% of patients. In the more severe form of the disease, the patient also complains of headache, malaise, and flank pain. Tenderness over the costovertebral angles (CVA) is common. Elderly patients may experience circulatory overload with dyspnea, engorged neck veins, cardiomegaly, and pulmonary edema. Atypical symptoms include confusion, somnolence, and seizures, which are often confused with the symptoms of a primary neurologic disorder.

Assessment and Diagnostic Findings

In acute glomerulonephritis, the kidneys become large, swollen, and congested. All renal tissues—glomeruli, tubules, and blood vessels—are affected to varying degrees. Electron microscopy and immunofluorescent analysis help identify the nature of the lesion; however, a kidney biopsy may be needed for definitive diagnosis.

Serial determinations of antistreptolysin O or anti-DNase B titers are usually elevated in poststreptococcal glomerulonephritis. Serum complement levels may be decreased but generally return to normal within 2 to 8 weeks. More than half of patients with IgA nephropathy (the most common type of primary glomerulonephritis) have an elevated serum IgA and a normal complement level.

If the patient improves, the amount of urine increases and the urinary protein and sediment diminish. Usually, more than 90% of children recover. The percentage of adults who recover is not well established but is probably about 70%. Some patients become severely uremic within weeks and require dialysis for survival. Others, after a period of apparent recovery, insidiously develop chronic glomerulonephritis.

Complications

Complications of acute glomerulonephritis include hypertensive encephalopathy, heart failure, and pulmonary edema. Hypertensive encephalopathy is considered a medical emergency, and therapy is directed toward reducing the blood pressure without impairing renal function (Tonelli et al., 2001). Although rare, optic neuropathy in uremia is a medical emergency requiring the immediate institution of dialysis, corticosteroid therapy, and correction of anemia (Winkelmayer et al., 2001).

Rapidly progressive glomerulonephritis is a rapid and progressive decline in renal function. Without treatment, it results in ESRD in a matter of weeks or months. Signs and symptoms are similar to those of acute glomerulonephritis (hematuria and proteinuria), but the course of the disease is more severe and rapid. Crescent-shaped cells accumulate in Bowman's space, disrupting the filtering surface. Plasma exchange (plasmapheresis) and treatment with high-dose corticosteroids and cytotoxic agents have been used to reduce the inflammatory response. Dialysis is initiated in acute glomerulonephritis if signs and symptoms of uremia are severe. With aggressive treatment, the prognosis for patients with rapidly progressive glomerulonephritis is greatly improved.

Medical Management

Management consists primarily of treating symptoms, attempting to preserve kidney function, and treating complications promptly. Pharmacologic therapy depends on the cause of acute glomerulonephritis. If residual streptococcal infection is suspected, penicillin is the agent of choice; however, other antibiotic agents may be prescribed. Corticosteroids and immunosuppressant medications may be prescribed for patients with rapidly progressive acute glomerulonephritis, but in most cases of poststreptococcal acute glomerulonephritis, these medications are of no value and may actually worsen the fluid retention and hypertension.

Dietary protein is restricted when renal insufficiency and nitrogen retention (elevated BUN) develop. Sodium is restricted when the patient has hypertension, edema, and heart failure. Loop diuretic medications and antihypertensive agents may be prescribed to control hypertension. Prolonged bed rest has little value and does not alter long-term outcomes.

Nursing Management

Although most patients with acute uncomplicated glomerulonephritis are treated as outpatients, nursing care is important no matter what the setting. In a hospital setting, carbohydrates are given liberally to provide energy and reduce the catabolism of protein. Intake and output are carefully measured and recorded. Fluids are given according to the patient's fluid losses and daily body weight. Insensible fluid loss through the respiratory and GI tracts (500 to 1,000 mL) is considered when estimating fluid loss. Diuresis begins about 1 week after the onset of symptoms with a decrease in edema and blood pressure. Proteinuria and microscopic hematuria may persist for many months, and some patients may go on to develop chronic glomerulonephritis. Other nursing interventions focus primarily on patient education for safe and effective self-care at home.

PROMOTING HOME AND COMMUNITY-BASED CARE

Teaching Patients Self-Care. Patient education is directed toward maintaining kidney function and preventing complications. Fluid and diet restrictions must be reviewed with the patient to avoid worsening of edema and hypertension. The patient is instructed to notify the physician if symptoms of renal failure occur (eg, fatigue, nausea, vomiting, diminishing urine output) or at the first sign of any infection. Information is given verbally and in writing.

Continuing Care. The importance of follow-up evaluations of blood pressure, urinalysis for protein, and serum BUN and creatinine levels to determine if the disease has progressed is stressed to the patient. A referral for home care may be indicated; a visit from a home care nurse provides an opportunity for careful assessment of the patient's progress and detection of early signs and symptoms of renal insufficiency. If corticosteroids, immunosuppressant agents, or antibiotic medications are prescribed, the home care nurse or nurse in the outpatient setting uses the opportunity to review the dosage, desired actions, and adverse effects of medications and the precautions to be followed.

CHRONIC GLOMERULONEPHRITIS

Pathophysiology

Chronic glomerulonephritis may be due to repeated episodes of acute glomerulonephritis, hypertensive nephrosclerosis, hyperlipidemia, chronic tubulointerstitial injury, or hemodynamically mediated glomerular sclerosis. The kidneys are reduced to as little as one-fifth their normal size (consisting largely of fibrous tissue). The cortex shrinks to a layer 1 to 2 mm thick or less. Bands of scar tissue distort the remaining cortex, making the surface of the kidney rough and irregular. Numerous glomeruli and their tubules become scarred, and the branches of the renal artery are thickened. The result is severe glomerular damage that results in ESRD.

Clinical Manifestations

The symptoms of chronic glomerulonephritis vary. Some patients with severe disease have no symptoms at all for many years. Their condition may be discovered when hypertension or elevated BUN and serum creatinine levels are detected. The diagnosis may be suggested during a routine eye examination when vascular changes or retinal hemorrhages are found. The first indication of disease may be a sudden, severe nosebleed, a stroke, or a seizure. Many patients report that their feet are slightly swollen at night. Most patients also have general symptoms, such as loss of weight and strength, increasing irritability, and an increased need to urinate at night (nocturia). Headaches, dizziness, and digestive disturbances are common.

As chronic glomerulonephritis progresses, signs and symptoms of renal insufficiency and chronic renal failure may develop. The patient appears poorly nourished, with a yellow-grey pigmentation of the skin and periorbital and peripheral (dependent) edema. Blood pressure may be normal or severely elevated. Retinal findings include hemorrhage, exudate, narrowed tortuous arterioles, and papilledema. Mucous membranes are pale because of anemia. Cardiomegaly, a gallop rhythm, distended neck veins, and other signs and symptoms of heart failure may be present. Crackles can be heard in the lungs.

Peripheral neuropathy with diminished deep tendon reflexes and neurosensory changes occurs late in the disease. The patient becomes confused and demonstrates a limited attention span. An additional late finding includes evidence of pericarditis with a pericardial friction rub and pulsus paradoxus (difference in blood pressure during inspiration and expiration of greater than 10 mm Hg).

Assessment and Diagnostic Findings

A number of laboratory abnormalities occur. Urinalysis reveals a fixed specific gravity of about 1.010, variable proteinuria, and **urinary casts** (protein plugs secreted by damaged kidney tubules). As renal failure progresses and the GFR falls below 50 mL/min, the following changes occur:

- Hyperkalemia due to decreased potassium excretion, acidosis, catabolism, and excessive potassium intake from food and medications
- Metabolic acidosis from decreased acid secretion by the kidney and inability to regenerate bicarbonate
- Anemia secondary to decreased erythropoiesis (production of RBCs)

- Hypoalbuminemia with edema secondary to protein loss through the damaged glomerular membrane
- Increased serum phosphorus level due to decreased renal excretion of phosphorus
- Decreased serum calcium level (calcium binds to phosphorus to compensate for elevated serum phosphorus levels)
- Hypermagnesemia from decreased excretion and inadvertent ingestion of antacids containing magnesium
- Impaired nerve conduction due to electrolyte abnormalities and uremia

Chest x-rays may show cardiac enlargement and pulmonary edema. The electrocardiogram may be normal or may indicate left ventricular hypertrophy associated with hypertension and signs of electrolyte disturbances, such as tall, tented (or peaked) T waves associated with hyperkalemia. Serum markers, including vascular endothelial growth factor and thrombospondin-1, are being evaluated for their reliability in assessing renal disease (Kang et al., 2001).

Medical Management

Symptoms guide the course of treatment for the patient with chronic glomerulonephritis. If the patient has hypertension, the blood pressure is reduced with sodium and water restriction, antihypertensive agents, or both. Weight is monitored daily, and diuretic medications are prescribed to treat fluid overload. Proteins of high biologic value (dairy products, eggs, meats) are provided to promote good nutritional status. Adequate calories are also important to spare protein for tissue growth and repair. UTIs must be treated promptly to prevent further renal damage.

Initiation of dialysis is considered early in the course of the disease to keep the patient in optimal physical condition, prevent fluid and electrolyte imbalances, and minimize the risk of complications of renal failure. The course of dialysis is smoother if treatment begins before the patient develops significant complications.

Nursing Management

If the patient is hospitalized or seen by the nurse in the home, the nurse observes the patient for changes in fluid and electrolyte status and for signs and symptoms of deterioration of renal function. Changes in fluid and electrolyte status and in cardiac and neurologic status are reported promptly to the physician. Anxiety levels are often extremely high for both the patient and family. Throughout the course of the disease and treatment, the nurse gives emotional support by providing opportunities for the patient and family to verbalize their concerns, have their questions answered, and explore their options.

PROMOTING HOME AND COMMUNITY-BASED CARE

Teaching Patients Self-Care. The nurse has a major role in teaching the patient and family about the prescribed treatment plan and the risks associated with noncompliance. Instructions to the patient include explanations and scheduling for follow-up evaluations: blood pressure, urinalysis for protein and casts, and blood studies of BUN and creatinine levels. If long-term dialysis is needed, the patient and family are taught about the procedure, how to care for the access site, dietary restrictions, and other necessary lifestyle modifications. See Chapter 44 for a detailed checklist of teaching topics for the dialysis patient.

Periodic hospitalization, visits to the outpatient clinic or office, and home care referrals provide the nurse in each setting with the opportunity for careful assessment of the patient's progress and continued education about changes to report to the primary health care provider (worsening signs and symptoms of renal failure, such as nausea, vomiting, and diminished urine output). Specific teaching may include explanations about recommended diet and fluid modifications and medications (purpose, desired effects, adverse effects, dosage, and administration schedule).

Continuing Care. Periodic evaluation of creatinine clearance and serum BUN and creatinine levels is carried out to assess residual renal function and the need for dialysis or transplantation. If dialysis is initiated, the patient and family will require considerable assistance and support in dealing with therapy and its long-term implications. See Chapter 44 for a discussion of dialysis. (Kidney transplantation is discussed later in this chapter.) The patient and family are reminded of the importance of participation in health promotion activities, including health screening. The patient is instructed to inform all health care providers about the diagnosis of glomerulonephritis so that all medical management, including pharmacologic therapy, is based on altered renal function.

NEPHROTIC SYNDROME

Nephrotic syndrome is a primary glomerular disease characterized by the following:

- Marked increase in protein in the urine (proteinuria)
- Decrease in albumin in the blood (hypoalbuminemia)
- Edema

- High serum cholesterol and low-density lipoproteins (hyperlipidemia)

The syndrome is apparent in any condition that seriously damages the glomerular capillary membrane and results in increased glomerular permeability.

Pathophysiology

Nephrotic syndrome can occur with almost any intrinsic renal disease or systemic disease that affects the glomerulus. Although generally considered a disorder of childhood, nephrotic syndrome does occur in adults, including the elderly. Causes include chronic glomerulonephritis, diabetes mellitus with intercapillary glomerulosclerosis, amyloidosis of the kidney, systemic lupus erythematosus, multiple myeloma, and renal vein thrombosis.

Nephrotic syndrome is characterized by the loss of plasma protein, particularly albumin, in the urine. Although the liver is capable of increasing the production of albumin, it cannot keep up with the daily loss of albumin through the kidneys. Thus, hypoalbuminemia results (Fig. 45-4).

Clinical Manifestations

The major manifestation of nephrotic syndrome is edema. It is usually soft and pitting and most commonly occurs around the eyes (periorbital), in dependent areas (sacrum, ankles, and hands), and in the abdomen (ascites). Other symptoms, including malaise, headache, irritability, and fatigue, are common (Fogo, 2000).

  ## Physiology/Pathophysiology

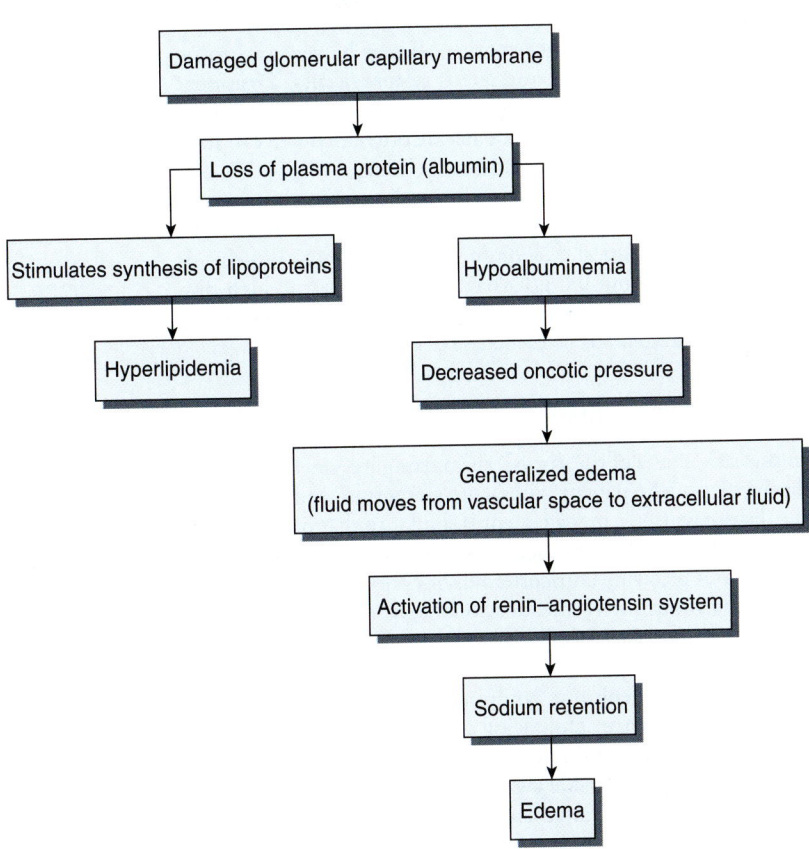

FIGURE 45-4 Sequence of events in nephrotic syndrome.

Assessment and Diagnostic Findings

Proteinuria (predominately albumin) exceeding 3 to 3.5 g/day is sufficient for the diagnosis of nephrotic syndrome. Protein electrophoresis and immunoelectrophoresis may be performed on the urine to categorize the type of proteinuria. The urine may also contain increased WBCs as well as granular and epithelial casts. A needle biopsy of the kidney may be performed for histologic examination of renal tissue to confirm the diagnosis. Recent studies have confirmed the usefulness of serum markers as a means of assessing the disease process. Anti-C1q antibodies are the most reliable markers for assessing disease activity in lupus nephritis (Moroni et al., 2001).

Complications

Complications of nephrotic syndrome include infection (due to a deficient immune response), thromboembolism (especially of the renal vein), pulmonary emboli, acute renal failure (due to hypovolemia), and accelerated atherosclerosis (due to hyperlipidemia).

Medical Management

The objective of management is to preserve renal function. Diuretic agents may be prescribed for the patient with severe edema; however, caution must be used because of the risk of reducing the plasma volume to the point of impaired circulation with subsequent prerenal acute renal failure. The use of angiotensin-converting enzyme (ACE) inhibitors in combination with diuretics often reduces the degree of proteinuria but may take 4 to 6 weeks to be effective.

Other medications used in treating nephrotic syndrome include antineoplastic agents (cyclophosphamide [Cytoxan]) or immunosuppressant medications (azathioprine [Imuran], chlorambucil [Leukeran], or cyclosporine). It may be necessary to repeat treatment with corticosteroids if relapse occurs. Treatment of the associated hyperlipidemia is controversial. The usual medications used to treat hyperlipidemia are often ineffective or have serious consequences, including muscle injury.

The patient may be placed on a low-sodium, liberal-potassium diet to enhance the sodium/potassium pump mechanism, thereby assisting in elimination of sodium to reduce edema. Protein intake should be about 0.8 g/kg/day, with emphasis on high biologic proteins (dairy products, eggs, meats), and the diet should be low in saturated fats (Deschenes & Doucet, 2000).

Nursing Management

In the early stages of the disease, the nursing management is similar to that of the patient with acute glomerulonephritis, but as the disease worsens, management is similar to that of the patient with chronic renal failure (see the section that follows). The patient who is receiving corticosteroids or cyclosporine requires instructions about the medications and signs and symptoms that should be reported to the physician. Dietary instructions may also be necessary.

Patients with nephrotic syndrome need adequate instruction about the importance of following all medication and dietary regimens so that their condition can remain stable as long as possible. The patient must be made aware of the importance of communicating any health-related change to the health care provider as soon as possible so that appropriate medication and dietary changes can be made before further changes occur within the

glomeruli. When indications of an acute infection, such as an acute respiratory tract infection, are first apparent, increased doses of maintenance corticosteroids have been found to decrease the risk of relapse (Mattoo & Mahmoud, 2000).

Renal Failure

Renal failure results when the kidneys cannot remove the body's metabolic wastes or perform their regulatory functions. The substances normally eliminated in the urine accumulate in the body fluids as a result of impaired renal excretion, leading to a disruption in endocrine and metabolic functions as well as fluid, electrolyte, and acid–base disturbances. Renal failure is a systemic disease and is a final common pathway of many different kidney and urinary tract diseases. The number of patients being treated for renal failure increased by 2006 between 1997 and 2001 (Canadian Institute of Health Information, 2001).

ACUTE RENAL FAILURE
Pathophysiology

Acute renal failure (ARF) is a sudden and almost complete loss of kidney function (decreased GFR) over a period of hours to days. Although ARF is often thought of as a problem seen only in hospitalized patients, it may occur in the outpatient setting as well. ARF manifests with oliguria, anuria, or normal urine volume. Oliguria (less than 400 mL/day of urine) is the most common clinical situation seen in ARF; anuria (less than 50 mL/day of urine) and normal urine output are not as common. Regardless of the volume of urine excreted, the patient with ARF experiences rising serum creatinine and BUN levels and retention of other metabolic waste products (azotemia) normally excreted by the kidneys.

CATEGORIES OF ACUTE RENAL FAILURE

Three major categories of conditions cause ARF: prerenal (hypoperfusion of kidney), intrarenal (actual damage to kidney tissue), and postrenal (obstruction to urine flow).

- Prerenal conditions occur as a result of impaired blood flow that leads to hypoperfusion of the kidney and a drop in the GFR. Common clinical situations are volume-depletion states (hemorrhage or GI losses), impaired cardiac performance (myocardial infarction, heart failure, or cardiogenic shock), and vasodilation (sepsis or anaphylaxis).
- Intrarenal causes of ARF are the result of actual parenchymal damage to the glomeruli or kidney tubules. Conditions such as burns, crush injuries, and infections, as well as nephrotoxic agents, may lead to **acute tubular necrosis** and cessation of renal function. With burns and crush injuries, myoglobin (a protein released from muscle when injury occurs) and hemoglobin are liberated, causing renal toxicity, ischemia, or both. Severe transfusion reactions may also cause intrarenal failure; hemoglobin is released through hemolysis, filters through the glomeruli, and becomes concentrated in the kidney tubules to such a degree that precipitation of hemoglobin occurs. Medications may also predispose a patient to intrarenal damage, especially nonsteroidal anti-inflammatory drugs (NSAIDs) and ACE inhibitors. These medications interfere with the normal autoregulatory mechanisms of the kidney and may cause hypoperfusion and eventual ischemia. Other potential causes of intrarenal or intrinsic

ARF include rhabdomyolysis, which results in accumulation of myoglobin in the glomeruli secondary to damage to skeletal muscle, and nephrotoxicity secondary to herbal remedies (Myhre, 2000).

- Postrenal causes of ARF are usually the result of an obstruction somewhere distal to the kidney. Pressure rises in the kidney tubules; eventually, the GFR decreases.

Common causes of ARF are summarized in Chart 45-5.

Although the exact pathogenesis of ARF and oliguria is not always known, many times there is a specific underlying problem. Some of the factors may be reversible if identified and treated promptly, before kidney function is impaired. This is true of the following conditions that reduce blood flow to the kidney and impair kidney function: (1) hypovolemia; (2) hypotension; (3) reduced cardiac output and heart failure; (4) obstruction of the kidney or lower urinary tract by tumour, blood clot, or kidney stone; and (5) bilateral obstruction of the renal arteries or veins. If these conditions are treated and corrected before the kidneys are permanently damaged, the increased BUN and creatinine levels, oliguria, and other signs associated with ARF may be reversed.

Although not a common cause of ARF, some types of renal stones may increase the risk for ARF more than others. Hereditary stone diseases (cystinuria, primary hyperoxaluria, Dent's disease), primary struvite stones, and infection-related urolithiasis associated with anatomic and functional urinary tract anomalies and spinal cord injury may cause recurrent bouts of obstruction as well as crystal-specific effects on tubular epithelial cells and interstitial renal cells. This in turn may activate the fibrogenic cascade responsible for the loss of renal parenchyma (Gambaro, Favaro & D'Angelo, 2001).

PHASES OF ACUTE RENAL FAILURE

There are four clinical phases of ARF: initiation, oliguria, diuresis, and recovery. The initiation period begins with the initial insult and ends when oliguria develops. The oliguria period is accompanied by a rise in the serum concentration of substances usually excreted by the kidneys (urea, creatinine, uric acid, organic acids, and the intracellular cations [potassium and magnesium]). The minimum amount of urine needed to rid the body of normal metabolic waste products is 400 mL. In this phase uremic symptoms first appear and life-threatening conditions such as hyperkalemia develop.

Some patients have decreased renal function with increasing nitrogen retention, yet actually excrete normal amounts of urine (2 L/day or more). This is the nonoliguric form of renal failure and occurs predominantly after nephrotoxic antibiotic agents are administered to the patient; it may occur with burns, traumatic injury, and the use of halogenated anesthetic agents.

In the diuresis period, the third phase, the patient experiences gradually increasing urine output, which signals that glomerular filtration has started to recover. Laboratory values stop rising and eventually decrease. Although the volume of urinary output may reach normal or elevated levels, renal function may still be markedly abnormal. Because uremic symptoms may still be present, the need for expert medical and nursing management continues. The patient must be observed closely for dehydration during this phase; if dehydration occurs, the uremic symptoms are likely to increase.

The recovery period signals the improvement of renal function and may take 3 to 12 months. Laboratory values return to the patient's normal level. Although a permanent 1% to 3% reduction in the GFR is common, it is not clinically significant.

Clinical Manifestations

Almost every system of the body is affected when there is failure of the normal renal regulatory mechanisms. The patient may appear critically ill and lethargic, with persistent nausea, vomiting, and diarrhea. The skin and mucous membranes are dry from dehydration, and the breath may have the odour of urine (uremic fetor). Central nervous system signs and symptoms include drowsiness, headache, muscle twitching, and seizures. Table 45-1 summarizes common clinical findings for all three categories of ARF.

Assessment and Diagnostic Findings

CHANGES IN URINE

Urine output varies (scanty to normal volume), hematuria may be present, and the urine has a low specific gravity (1.010 or less, compared with a normal value of 1.015 to 1.025). Patients with

---

Chart 45-5 **Causes of Acute Renal Failure**

Prerenal Failure
- Volume depletion resulting from:
  Hemorrhage
  Renal losses (diuretics, osmotic diuresis)
  Gastrointestinal losses (vomiting, diarrhea, nasogastric suction)
- Impaired cardiac efficiency resulting from:
  Myocardial infarction
  Heart failure
  Dysrhythmias
  Cardiogenic shock
- Vasodilation resulting from:
  Sepsis
  Anaphylaxis
  Antihypertensive medications or other medications that cause vasodilation

Intrarenal Failure
- Prolonged renal ischemia resulting from:
  Pigment nephropathy (associated with the breakdown of blood cells containing pigments that in turn occlude kidney structures)
  Myoglobinuria (trauma, crush injuries, burns)
  Hemoglobinuria (transfusion reaction, hemolytic anemia)
- Nephrotoxic agents such as:
  Aminoglycoside antibiotics (gentamicin, tobramycin)
  Radiopaque contrast agents
  Heavy metals (lead, mercury)
  Solvents and chemicals (ethylene glycol, carbon tetrachloride, arsenic)
  Nonsteroidal anti-inflammatory drugs (NSAIDs)
  Angiotensin-converting enzyme inhibitors (ACE inhibitors)
- Infectious processes such as:
  Acute pyelonephritis
  Acute glomerulonephritis

Postrenal Failure
- Urinary tract obstruction, including:
  Calculi (stones)
  Tumours
  Benign prostatic hyperplasia
  Strictures
  Blood clots

Table 45-1 • Comparing Types of Acute Renal Failure

CHARACTERISTICS	TYPES		
	Prerenal	Intrarenal	Postrenal
Etiology	Hypoperfusion	Parenchymal damage	Obstruction
Blood urea nitrogen value	Increased (out of normal 20:1 proportion to creatinine)	Increased	Increased
Creatinine	Increased	Increased	Increased
Urine output	Decreased	Varies, often decreased	Varies, may be decreased, or sudden anuria
Urine sodium	Decreased to <20 mmol/L	Increased to >40 mmol/L	Varies, often decreased to 20 mmol/L or less
Urinary sediment	Normal, few hyaline casts	Abnormal casts and debris	Usually normal
Urine osmolality	Increased to 500 mmol	About 350 mmol similar to serum	Varies, increased or equal to serum
Urine specific gravity	Increased	Low normal, 1.010	Varies

prerenal azotemia have a decreased amount of sodium in the urine (below 20 mmol/L) and normal urinary sediment. Patients with intrarenal azotemia usually have urinary sodium levels greater than 40 mmol/L with casts and other cellular debris. Urinary casts are mucoproteins secreted by the renal tubules whenever inflammation is present.

CHANGE IN KIDNEY CONTOUR

Ultrasonography is a critical component of the evaluation of both acute and chronic renal failure. Although many sonographic findings are nonspecific, their diagnostic utility is greatly enhanced by a familiarity with the clinical presentation and a thorough understanding of renal pathophysiology (O'Neill, 2000).

INCREASED BUN AND CREATININE LEVELS (AZOTEMIA)

The BUN level rises steadily at a rate dependent on the degree of catabolism (breakdown of protein), renal perfusion, and protein intake. Serum creatinine rises in conjunction with glomerular damage. Serum creatinine levels are useful in monitoring kidney function and disease progression.

HYPERKALEMIA

With a decline in the GFR, the patient cannot excrete potassium normally. Patients with oliguria and anuria are at greater risk for hyperkalemia than those without oliguria. Protein catabolism results in the release of cellular potassium into the body fluids, causing severe hyperkalemia (high serum K^+ levels). Hyperkalemia may lead to dysrhythmias and cardiac arrest. Sources of potassium include normal tissue catabolism, dietary intake, blood in the GI tract, or blood transfusion and other sources (intravenous infusions, potassium penicillin, and extracellular shift in response to metabolic acidosis).

METABOLIC ACIDOSIS

Patients with acute oliguria cannot eliminate the daily metabolic load of acid-type substances produced by the normal metabolic processes. In addition, normal renal buffering mechanisms fail. This is reflected by a fall in the serum CO_2-combining power and blood pH. Thus, progressive metabolic acidosis accompanies renal failure.

CALCIUM AND PHOSPHORUS ABNORMALITIES

There may be an increase in serum phosphate concentrations; serum calcium levels may be low in response to decreased absorption of calcium from the intestine and as a compensatory mechanism for the elevated serum phosphate levels.

ANEMIA

Anemia inevitably accompanies ARF due to reduced erythropoietin production, uremic GI lesions, reduced RBC life span, and blood loss, usually from the GI tract. With use of the parenteral form of erythropoietin (Epogen), anemia is not the major problem it once was.

Prevention

A careful history is obtained to determine whether the patient has been taking potentially nephrotoxic antibiotic agents or has been exposed to environmental toxins. The kidneys are especially susceptible to the adverse effects of medications because the kidneys are repeatedly exposed to substances in the blood. They receive a large blood flow (25% of the cardiac output at rest; the entire blood volume circulates through the kidneys about 14 times a minute). In addition, the kidney is the major excretory organ for many toxic substances, and during the normal urine concentration process, these substances increase in concentration and can be toxic to the kidneys. Therefore, in patients taking potentially nephrotoxic medications (aminoglycosides, gentamicin, tobramycin, colistimethate, polymyxin B, amphotericin B, vancomycin, amikacin, cyclosporine), renal function should be monitored closely. Serum BUN and creatinine levels should be obtained at baseline by 24 hours after initiation of these medications and at least twice a week while the patient is receiving them.

Any agent that reduces renal blood flow (eg, chronic analgesic use) may cause renal insufficiency. Chronic analgesic use, particularly with NSAIDs, may cause interstitial nephritis and papillary necrosis. Patients with heart failure or cirrhosis with ascites are at particular risk for NSAID-induced renal failure. Increased age, preexisting renal disease, and the administration of several nephrotoxic agents simultaneously increase the risk for kidney damage.

Management of ARF is expensive and complex, and even when optimal, the mortality rate remains high. Therefore, prevention of ARF is key (Chart 45-6).

Medical Management

The kidney has a remarkable ability to recover from insult. Therefore, the objectives of treatment of ARF are to restore normal chemical balance and prevent complications until repair of renal tissue and restoration of renal function can take place. Any possible cause of damage is identified, treated, and eliminated. Prerenal azotemia is treated by optimizing renal perfusion, whereas postrenal failure is treated by relieving the obstruction. Treatment of intrarenal azotemia is supportive, with removal of causative agents, aggressive management of prerenal and postrenal failure, and avoidance of associated risk factors. Shock and infection, if present, are treated promptly. Overall, medical management includes maintaining fluid balance, avoiding fluid excesses, or possibly performing dialysis.

Maintenance of fluid balance is based on daily body weight, serial measurements of central venous pressure, serum and urine concentrations, fluid losses, blood pressure, and the clinical status of the patient. The parenteral and oral intake and the output of urine, gastric drainage, stools, wound drainage, and perspiration are calculated and are used as the basis for fluid replacement. The insensible fluid lost through the skin and lungs and produced through the normal metabolic processes is also considered in fluid management.

Fluid excesses can be detected by the clinical findings of dyspnea, tachycardia, and distended neck veins. The lungs are auscultated for moist crackles. Because pulmonary edema may be caused by excessive administration of parenteral fluids, extreme caution must be used to prevent fluid overload. The development of generalized edema is assessed by examining the presacral and pretibial areas several times daily. Mannitol, furosemide, or ethacrynic acid may be prescribed to initiate a diuresis and prevent or minimize subsequent renal failure.

Adequate blood flow to the kidneys in patients with prerenal causes of ARF may be restored by intravenous fluids or blood product transfusions. If ARF is caused by hypovolemia secondary to hypoproteinemia, an infusion of albumin may be prescribed. Dialysis may be initiated to prevent serious complications of ARF, such as hyperkalemia, severe metabolic acidosis, pericarditis, and pulmonary edema. Dialysis corrects many biochemical abnormalities; allows for liberalization of fluid, protein, and sodium intake; diminishes bleeding tendencies; and may help wound healing. Hemodialysis, peritoneal dialysis, or any of the new continuous renal replacement therapies may be performed. These forms of dialysis are discussed in Chapter 44, which presents treatment modalities for patients with renal dysfunction.

PHARMACOLOGIC THERAPY

Because hyperkalemia is the most life-threatening of the fluid and electrolyte disturbances, the patient is monitored for hyperkalemia through serial serum electrolyte levels (potassium value more than 5.5 mmol/L), electrocardiogram changes (tall, tented, or peaked T waves), and changes in clinical status.

The elevated potassium levels may be reduced by administering cation-exchange resins (sodium polystyrene sulfonate [Kayexalate]) orally or by retention enema. Kayexalate works by exchanging a sodium ion for a potassium ion in the intestinal tract. Sorbitol is often administered in combination with Kayexalate to induce a diarrhea-type effect (it induces water loss in the GI tract).

If a retention enema is administered (the colon is the major site for potassium exchange), a rectal catheter with a balloon may be used to facilitate retention if necessary. The patient should retain the resin 30 to 45 minutes to promote potassium removal. Afterward, a cleansing enema may be prescribed to remove the Kayexalate resin as a precaution against fecal impaction.

> **Chart 45-6**
> ## Preventing Acute Renal Failure
>
> 1. Provide adequate hydration to patients at risk for dehydration:
>   Surgical patients before, during, and after surgery
>   Patients undergoing intensive diagnostic studies requiring fluid restriction and contrast agents (eg, barium enema, intravenous pyelograms), especially elderly patients who may not have adequate renal reserve
>   Patients with neoplastic disorders or disorders of metabolism (ie, gout) and those receiving chemotherapy
> 2. Prevent and treat shock promptly with blood and fluid replacement.
> 3. Monitor central venous and arterial pressures and hourly urine output of critically ill patients to detect the onset of renal failure as early as possible.
> 4. Treat hypotension promptly.
> 5. Continually assess renal function (urine output, laboratory values) when appropriate.
> 6. Take precautions to ensure that the appropriate blood is administered to the correct patient in order to avoid severe transfusion reactions, which can precipitate renal failure.
> 7. Prevent and treat infections promptly. Infections can produce progressive renal damage.
> 8. Pay special attention to wounds, burns, and other precursors of sepsis.
> 9. Give meticulous care to patients with indwelling catheters to prevent infections from ascending in the urinary tract. Remove catheters as soon as possible.
> 10. To prevent toxic drug effects, closely monitor dosage, duration of use, and blood levels of all medications metabolized or excreted by the kidneys.

> **NURSING ALERT** A patient with a high and rising level of serum potassium often requires immediate dialysis.

> **NURSING ALERT** Intravenous glucose and insulin or calcium gluconate may be used as emergency and temporary measures to treat hyperkalemia. Glucose and insulin drive potassium into the cells, thereby lowering serum potassium levels temporarily. Potassium will move out of the cells and rise again to a dangerous level unless removed by dialysis. The administration of calcium gluconate helps protect the heart from the effects of the high potassium levels.

> **NURSING ALERT** Sodium bicarbonate may be administered to elevate the plasma pH. Sodium bicarbonate increases the pH, which causes potassium to move into the cell, and the result is lowering of the serum potassium level. This is short-term therapy and is used with other long-term measures, such as dietary restriction and dialysis.

NURSING ALERT All external sources of potassium (foods, salt substitutes, medications) are eliminated or reduced.

Because many medications are eliminated through the kidneys, medication dosages must be reduced when a patient has ARF. Examples of commonly used medications that require adjustment are antibiotic agents (especially aminoglycosides), digoxin, ACE inhibitors, and medications containing magnesium.

Many medications have been used in patients with ARF in an attempt to improve patient outcomes. Diuretic agents are often used to control fluid volume, but they have not been shown to hasten the recovery from ARF.

Low-dose dopamine (1 to 3 g/kg) is often used to dilate the renal arteries through stimulation of dopaminergic receptors; however, research has not definitely demonstrated that dopamine prevents ARF or improves outcome in patients with established renal failure.

Atrial natriuretic peptide (ANP), an endogenous hormone synthesized by the cardiac atria, has been shown to improve renal function in multiple animal models of ARF. It has also decreased the need for dialysis in patients with oliguric acute tubular necrosis in a multisite clinical trial of patients. Patients with nonoliguric acute tubular necrosis did not benefit (Lewis, Salem, Chertow et al., 2000). Further research on ANP use is underway.

In patients with severe acidosis, the arterial blood gases or serum bicarbonate levels (CO_2-combining power) must be monitored because the patient may require sodium bicarbonate therapy or dialysis. If respiratory problems develop, appropriate ventilatory measures must be instituted. The elevated serum phosphate level may be controlled with phosphate-binding agents (aluminum hydroxide). These agents help prevent a continuing rise in serum phosphate levels by decreasing the absorption of phosphate from the intestinal tract.

NUTRITIONAL THERAPY

ARF causes severe nutritional imbalances (because nausea and vomiting contribute to inadequate dietary intake), impaired glucose use and protein synthesis, and increased tissue catabolism. The patient is weighed daily and can be expected to lose 0.2 to 0.5 kg daily if the nitrogen balance is negative (ie, the patient's caloric intake falls below caloric requirements). If the patient gains or does not lose weight or develops hypertension, fluid retention should be suspected.

Dietary proteins are limited to about 1 g/kg during the oliguric phase to minimize protein breakdown and to prevent accumulation of toxic end products. Caloric requirements are met with high-carbohydrate meals because carbohydrates have a protein-sparing effect (ie, in a high-carbohydrate diet, protein is not used for meeting energy requirements but is "spared" for growth and tissue healing). Foods and fluids containing potassium or phosphorus (bananas, citrus fruits and juices, coffee) are restricted. Potassium intake is usually restricted to 40 to 60 mmol/day, and sodium is usually restricted to 2 g/day. The patient may require parenteral nutrition.

The oliguric phase of ARF may last 10 to 20 days and is followed by the diuretic phase, at which time urine output begins to increase, signaling that kidney function is returning. Blood chemistry evaluations are made to determine the amounts of sodium, potassium, and water needed for replacement, along with assessment for overhydration or underhydration. After the diuretic phase, the patient is placed on a high-protein, high-calorie diet and is encouraged to resume activities gradually.

Nursing Management

The nurse has an important role in caring for the patient with ARF. In addition to directing attention to the patient's primary disorder (which may be a factor in the development of ARF), the nurse monitors for complications, participates in emergency treatment of fluid and electrolyte imbalances, assesses progress and response to treatment, and provides physical and emotional support. Additionally, the nurse keeps family members informed about the patient's condition, helps them understand the treatments, and provides psychological support. Although the development of ARF may be the most serious problem, the nurse must continue to include in the plan of care those nursing measures indicated for the primary disorder (eg, burns, shock, trauma, obstruction of the urinary tract).

MONITORING FLUID AND ELECTROLYTE BALANCE

Because of the serious fluid and electrolyte imbalances that can occur with ARF, the nurse monitors the patient's serum electrolyte levels and physical indicators of these complications during all phases of the disorder. Hyperkalemia is the most immediate life-threatening imbalance seen in ARF. Parenteral fluids, all oral intake, and all medications are screened carefully to ensure that hidden sources of potassium are not inadvertently administered or consumed. Intravenous solutions must be carefully selected according to the patient's fluid and electrolyte status. The patient's cardiac function and musculoskeletal status are monitored closely for signs of hyperkalemia.

The nurse monitors fluid status by paying careful attention to fluid intake (intravenous medications should be administered in the smallest volume possible), urine output, apparent edema, distention of the jugular veins, alterations in heart sounds and breath sounds, and increasing difficulty in breathing. Accurate daily weights, as well as intake and output records, are essential.

Indicators of deteriorating fluid and electrolyte status are reported immediately to the physician, and preparation is made for emergency treatment. Hyperkalemia is treated with glucose and insulin, calcium gluconate, cation-exchange resins (Kayexalate), or dialysis. Fluid and other electrolyte disturbances are often treated with hemodialysis, peritoneal dialysis, or other continuous renal replacement therapies.

REDUCING METABOLIC RATE

The nurse also directs attention to reducing the patient's metabolic rate during the acute stage of renal failure to reduce catabolism and the subsequent release of potassium and accumulation of endogenous waste products (urea and creatinine). Bed rest may be indicated to reduce exertion and the metabolic rate during the most acute stage of the disorder. Fever and infection, both of which increase the metabolic rate and catabolism, are prevented or treated promptly.

PROMOTING PULMONARY FUNCTION

Attention is given to pulmonary function, and the patient is assisted to turn, cough, and take deep breaths frequently to prevent atelectasis and respiratory tract infection. Drowsiness and lethargy may prevent the patient from moving and turning without encouragement and assistance.

PREVENTING INFECTION

Asepsis is essential with invasive lines and catheters to minimize the risk of infection and increased metabolism. An indwelling urinary catheter is avoided whenever possible because of the high risk for UTI associated with its use.

PROVIDING SKIN CARE

The skin may be dry or susceptible to breakdown as a result of edema; therefore, meticulous skin care is important. Additionally, excoriation and itching of the skin may result from the deposit of irritating toxins in the patient's tissues. Massaging bony prominences, turning the patient frequently, and bathing the patient with cool water are often comforting and prevent skin breakdown.

PROVIDING SUPPORT

The patient with ARF requires treatment with hemodialysis, peritoneal dialysis, or continuous renal replacement therapies to prevent serious complications (see Chap. 44); the length of time that these treatments are necessary varies with the cause and extent of damage to the kidneys. The patient and family need assistance, explanation, and support during this time. The purpose and rationale of the treatments are explained to the patient and family by the physician. High levels of anxiety and fear, however, may necessitate repeated explanation and clarification by the nurse. The family members may initially be afraid to touch and talk to the patient during the procedure but should be encouraged and assisted to do so.

Although many of the nurse's functions are devoted to the technical aspects of the procedure, the psychological needs and concerns of the patient and family cannot be ignored. Continued assessment of the patient for complications of ARF and of its precipitating cause is essential.

CHRONIC RENAL FAILURE (END-STAGE RENAL DISEASE)

Chronic renal failure, or ESRD, is a progressive, irreversible deterioration in renal function in which the body's ability to maintain metabolic and fluid and electrolyte balance fails, resulting in uremia or azotemia (retention of urea and other nitrogenous wastes in the blood).

Recent data from the Canadian Institute for Health Information (2005) suggest that the number of Canadians being treated for ESRD increased by 20% between 1997 and 2001.

ESRD may be caused by systemic diseases, such as diabetes mellitus (leading cause); hypertension; chronic glomerulonephritis; pyelonephritis; obstruction of the urinary tract; hereditary lesions, as in polycystic kidney disease; vascular disorders; infections; medications; or toxic agents.

Autosomal dominant polycystic disease accounts for 8% to 10% of cases of ESRD in the United States and Europe (Perrone, Ruthazer, & Terrin, 2001). Approximately 27,000 Canadians are affected by polycystic kidney disease (Kidney Foundation of Canada, 2005). Comorbid conditions that develop during chronic renal insufficiency contribute to the high morbidity and mortality among patients with ESRD (Kausz, et al., 2001).

Environmental and occupational agents that have been implicated in chronic renal failure include lead, cadmium, mercury, and chromium. Dialysis or kidney transplantation eventually becomes necessary for patient survival. Dialysis is an effective means of correcting metabolic toxicities at any age, although the mortality rate in infants and young children is greater than adults in the presence of other, nonrenal diseases and in the presence of anuria or oliguria (Wood et al., 2001).

Pathophysiology

As renal function declines, the end products of protein metabolism (which are normally excreted in urine) accumulate in the blood. Uremia develops and adversely affects every system in the body. The greater the buildup of waste products, the more severe the symptoms. There are three well-recognized stages of chronic renal disease: reduced renal reserve, renal insufficiency, and ESRD (Chart 45-7).

The rate of decline in renal function and progression of chronic renal failure is related to the underlying disorder, the urinary excretion of protein, and the presence of hypertension. The disease tends to progress more rapidly in patients who excrete significant amounts of protein or have elevated blood pressure than in those without these conditions.

Clinical Manifestations

Because virtually every body system is affected by the uremia of chronic renal failure, patients exhibit a number of signs and symptoms. The severity of these signs and symptoms depends in part on the degree of renal impairment, other underlying conditions, and the patient's age.

CARDIOVASCULAR MANIFESTATIONS

Hypertension (due to sodium and water retention or from activation of the renin–angiotensin–aldosterone system), heart failure and pulmonary edema (due to fluid overload), and pericarditis (due to irritation of the pericardial lining by uremic toxins) are among the cardiovascular problems manifested in ESRD. Strict fluid volume control has been found to normalize hypertension in patients receiving peritoneal dialysis (Gunal, Duman, Ozkahya et al., 2001).

Cardiovascular disease is the predominant cause of death in patients with ESRD. In chronic hemodialysis patients, approximately 45% of overall mortality is attributable to cardiac disease, and about 20% of these cardiac deaths are due to acute myocardial infarction (USRDS, 2001).

DERMATOLOGIC SYMPTOMS

Severe itching (pruritus) is common. Uremic frost, the deposit of urea crystals on the skin, is uncommon today because of early and aggressive treatment of ESRD with dialysis.

Chart 45-7 Stages of Chronic Renal Disease

Stage 1
Reduced renal reserve, characterized by a 40% to 75% loss of nephron function. The patient usually does not have symptoms because the remaining nephrons are able to carry out the normal functions of the kidney.

Stage 2
Renal insufficiency occurs when 75% to 90% of nephron function is lost. At this point, the serum creatinine and blood urea nitrogen rise, the kidney loses its ability to concentrate urine and anemia develops. The patient may report polyuria and nocturia.

Stage 3
End-stage renal disease (ESRD), the final stage of chronic renal failure, occurs when there is less than 10% nephron function remaining. All of the normal regulatory, excretory, and hormonal functions of the kidney are severely impaired. ESRD is evidenced by elevated creatinine and blood urea nitrogen levels as well as electrolyte imbalances. Once the patient reaches this point, dialysis is usually indicated. Many of the symptoms of uremia are reversible with dialysis.

OTHER SYSTEMIC MANIFESTATIONS

GI signs and symptoms are common and include anorexia, nausea, vomiting, and hiccups. Neurologic changes, including altered levels of consciousness, inability to concentrate, muscle twitching, and seizures, have been observed. The precise mechanisms for many of these diverse signs and symptoms have not been identified. It is generally thought, however, that the accumulation of uremic waste products is the probable cause. Chart 45-8 summarizes the signs and symptoms often seen in chronic renal failure.

Assessment and Diagnostic Findings

GLOMERULAR FILTRATION RATE

Decreased GFR can be detected by obtaining a 24-hour urinalysis for creatinine clearance. As glomerular filtration decreases (due to nonfunctioning glomeruli), the creatinine clearance value decreases, whereas the serum creatinine and BUN levels increase. Serum creatinine is the more sensitive indicator of renal function because of its constant production in the body. The BUN is affected not only by renal disease but also by protein intake in the diet, catabolism (tissue and RBC breakdown), parenteral nutrition, and medications such as corticosteroids.

SODIUM AND WATER RETENTION

The kidney cannot concentrate or dilute the urine normally in ESRD. Appropriate responses by the kidney to changes in the daily intake of water and electrolytes, therefore, do not occur. Some patients retain sodium and water, increasing the risk for edema, heart failure, and hypertension. Hypertension may also result from activation of the renin–angiotensin–aldosterone axis and the concomitant increased aldosterone secretion. Other patients have a tendency to lose salt and run the risk of developing hypotension and hypovolemia. Episodes of vomiting and diarrhea may produce sodium and water depletion, which worsens the uremic state.

ACIDOSIS

With advanced renal disease, metabolic acidosis occurs because the kidney cannot excrete increased loads of acid. Decreased acid secretion primarily results from inability of the kidney tubules to excrete ammonia (NH_3^-) and to reabsorb sodium bicarbonate (HCO_3^-). There is also decreased excretion of phosphates and other organic acids.

ANEMIA

Anemia develops as a result of inadequate erythropoietin production, the shortened life span of RBCs, nutritional deficiencies,

---

Chart 45-8 • ASSESSMENT

Signs and Symptoms of Chronic Renal Failure

Neurologic
Weakness and fatigue; confusion; inability to concentrate; disorientation; tremors; seizures; asterixis; restlessness of legs; burning of soles of feet; behaviour changes

Integumentary
Grey-bronze skin colour; dry, flaky skin; pruritus; ecchymosis; purpura; thin, brittle nails; coarse, thinning hair

Cardiovascular
Hypertension; pitting edema (feet, hands, sacrum); periorbital edema; pericardial friction rub; engorged neck veins; pericarditis; pericardial effusion; pericardial tamponade; hyperkalemia; hyperlipidemia

Pulmonary
Crackles; thick, tenacious sputum; depressed cough reflex; pleuritic pain; shortness of breath; tachypnea; Kussmaul-type respirations; uremic pneumonitis; "uremic lung"

Gastrointestinal
Ammonia odour to breath ("uremic fetor"); metallic taste; mouth ulcerations and bleeding; anorexia, nausea, and vomiting; hiccups; constipation or diarrhea; bleeding from gastrointestinal tract

Hematologic
Anemia; thrombocytopenia

Reproductive
Amenorrhea; testicular atrophy; infertility; decreased libido

Musculoskeletal
Muscle cramps; loss of muscle strength; renal osteodystrophy; bone pain; bone fractures; foot drop

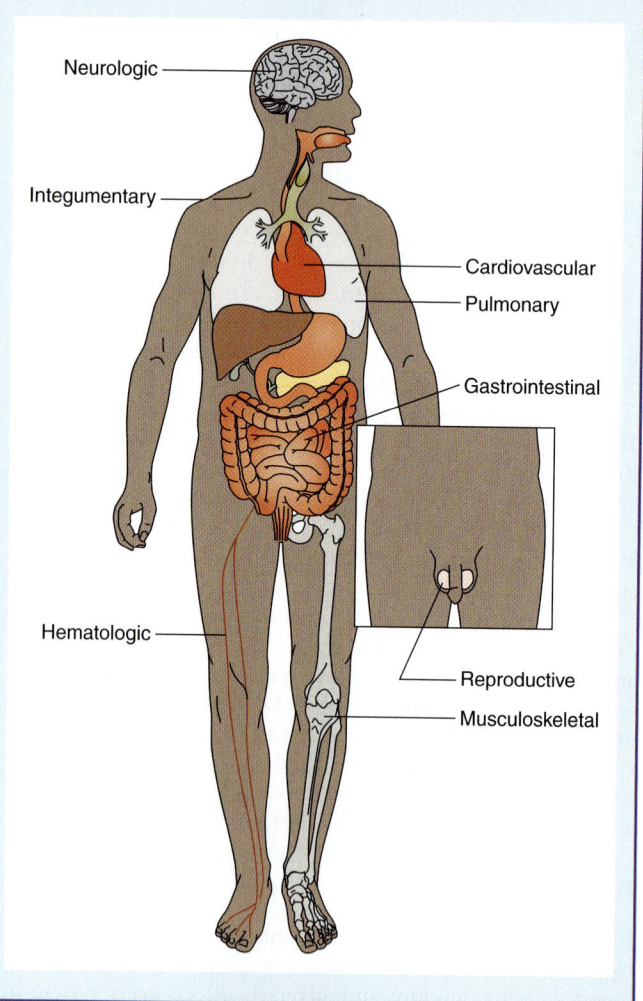

and the patient's tendency to bleed, particularly from the GI tract. Erythropoietin, a substance normally produced by the kidney, stimulates bone marrow to produce RBCs. In renal failure, erythropoietin production decreases and profound anemia results, producing fatigue, angina, and shortness of breath.

CALCIUM AND PHOSPHORUS IMBALANCE

Another major abnormality seen in chronic renal failure is a disorder in calcium and phosphorus metabolism. Serum calcium and phosphate levels have a reciprocal relationship in the body: as one rises, the other decreases. With decreased filtration through the glomerulus of the kidney, there is an increase in the serum phosphate level and a reciprocal or corresponding decrease in the serum calcium level. The decreased serum calcium level causes increased secretion of parathormone from the parathyroid glands. In renal failure, however, the body does not respond normally to the increased secretion of parathormone; as a result, calcium leaves the bone, often producing bone changes and bone disease. In addition, the active metabolite of vitamin D (1,25-dihydroxycholecalciferol) normally manufactured by the kidney decreases as renal failure progresses. Uremic bone disease, often called renal osteodystrophy, develops from the complex changes in calcium, phosphate, and parathormone balance (Barnas, Schmidt, Seidl et al., 2001).

Complications

Potential complications of chronic renal failure that concern the nurse and that necessitate a collaborative approach to care include the following:

- Hyperkalemia due to decreased excretion, metabolic acidosis, catabolism, and excessive intake (diet, medications, fluids)
- Pericarditis, pericardial effusion, and pericardial tamponade due to retention of uremic waste products and inadequate dialysis
- Hypertension due to sodium and water retention and malfunction of the renin–angiotensin–aldosterone system
- Anemia due to decreased erythropoietin production, decreased RBC life span, bleeding in the GI tract from irritating toxins, and blood loss during hemodialysis
- Bone disease and metastatic calcifications due to retention of phosphorus, low serum calcium levels, abnormal vitamin D metabolism, and elevated aluminum levels

Medical Management

The goal of management is to maintain kidney function and homeostasis for as long as possible. All factors that contribute to ESRD and all factors that are reversible (eg, obstruction) are identified and treated. Management is accomplished primarily with medications and diet therapy, although dialysis may also be needed to decrease the level of uremic waste products in the blood (Fink et al., 2001).

PHARMACOLOGIC THERAPY

Complications can be prevented or delayed by administering prescribed antihypertensives, erythropoietin (Epogen), iron supplements, phosphate-binding agents, and calcium supplements.

Antacids. Hyperphosphatemia and hypocalcemia are treated with aluminum-based antacids that bind dietary phosphorus in the GI tract. However, concerns about the potential long-term toxicity of aluminum and the association of high aluminum levels with neurologic symptoms and osteomalacia have led some physicians to prescribe calcium carbonate in place of high doses of aluminum-based antacids. This medication also binds dietary phosphorus in the intestinal tract and permits the use of smaller doses of antacids. Both calcium carbonate and phosphorus-binding antacids must be administered with food to be effective. Magnesium-based antacids must be avoided to prevent magnesium toxicity.

Antihypertensive and Cardiovascular Agents. Hypertension is managed by intravascular volume control and a variety of antihypertensive agents. Heart failure and pulmonary edema may also require treatment with fluid restriction, low-sodium diets, diuretic agents, inotropic agents such as digitalis or dobutamine, and dialysis. The metabolic acidosis of chronic renal failure usually produces no symptoms and requires no treatment; however, sodium bicarbonate supplements or dialysis may be needed to correct the acidosis if it causes symptoms (Tonelli et al., 2001).

Antiseizure Agents. Neurologic abnormalities may occur, so the patient must be observed for early evidence of slight twitching, headache, delirium, or seizure activity. If seizures occur, the onset of the seizure is recorded along with the type, duration, and general effect on the patient. The physician is notified immediately. Intravenous diazepam (Valium) or phenytoin (Dilantin) is usually administered to control seizures. The side rails of the bed should be padded to protect the patient. The nursing management of the patient with seizures is discussed in Chapter 61.

Erythropoietin. Anemia associated with chronic renal failure is treated with recombinant human erythropoietin (Epogen). Anemic patients (hematocrit less than 30%) present with nonspecific symptoms, such as malaise, general fatigability, and decreased activity tolerance. Epogen therapy is initiated to achieve a hematocrit of 33% to 38%, which generally alleviates the symptoms of anemia. Epogen is administered either intravenously or subcutaneously three times a week. It may take 2 to 6 weeks for the hematocrit to rise; therefore, Epogen is not indicated for patients who need immediate correction of severe anemia. Adverse effects seen with Epogen therapy include hypertension (especially during early stages of treatment), increased clotting of vascular access sites, seizures, and depletion of body iron stores (Fink et al., 2001).

The patient receiving Epogen may experience influenza-like symptoms with initiation of therapy; these tend to subside with repeated doses. Management involves adjustment of heparin to prevent clotting of the dialysis lines during hemodialysis treatments, frequent monitoring of hematocrit, and periodic assessment of serum iron and transferrin levels. Because adequate stores of iron are necessary for an adequate response to erythropoietin, supplementary iron may be prescribed. In addition, the patient's blood pressure and serum potassium level are monitored to detect hypertension and rising serum potassium levels, which may occur with therapy and the increasing RBC mass. The occurrence of hypertension requires initiation or adjustment of the patient's antihypertensive therapy. Hypertension that cannot be controlled is a contraindication to recombinant erythropoietin therapy.

Patients who have received Epogen have reported decreased levels of fatigue, an increased feeling of well-being, better tolerance of dialysis, higher energy levels, and improved exercise tolerance. Additionally, this therapy has decreased the need for transfusion and its associated risks, including bloodborne infectious disease, antibody formation, and iron overload (Fink et al., 2001).

NUTRITIONAL THERAPY

Dietary intervention is necessary with deterioration of renal function and includes careful regulation of protein intake, fluid intake to balance fluid losses, sodium intake to balance sodium losses, and some restriction of potassium. At the same time, adequate caloric intake and vitamin supplementation must be ensured. Protein is restricted because urea, uric acid, and organic acids—the breakdown products of dietary and tissue proteins—accumulate rapidly in the blood when there is impaired renal clearance. The allowed protein must be of high biologic value (dairy products, eggs, meats). High-biologic-value proteins are those that are complete proteins and supply the essential amino acids necessary for growth and cell repair.

Usually, the fluid allowance is 500 to 600 mL more than the previous day's 24-hour urine output. Calories are supplied by carbohydrates and fat to prevent wasting. Vitamin supplementation is necessary because a protein-restricted diet does not provide the necessary complement of vitamins. Additionally, the patient on dialysis may lose water-soluble vitamins from the blood during the dialysis treatment.

OTHER THERAPY: DIALYSIS

Hyperkalemia is usually prevented by ensuring adequate dialysis treatments with potassium removal and careful monitoring of all medications, both oral and intravenous, for their potassium content. The patient is placed on a potassium-restricted diet. Occasionally, Kayexalate, a cation-exchange resin, administered orally, may be needed. The patient with increasing symptoms of chronic renal failure is referred to a dialysis and transplantation centre early in the course of progressive renal disease. Dialysis is usually initiated when the patient cannot maintain a reasonable lifestyle with conservative treatment. The details of dialysis treatment can be found in Chapter 44.

Nursing Management

The patient with chronic renal failure requires astute nursing care to avoid the complications of reduced renal function and the stresses and anxieties of dealing with a life-threatening illness. Examples of potential nursing diagnoses for these patients include the following:

- Excess fluid volume related to decreased urine output, dietary excesses, and retention of sodium and water
- Imbalanced nutrition: less than body requirements related to anorexia, nausea and vomiting, dietary restrictions, and altered oral mucous membranes
- Deficient knowledge regarding condition and treatment regimen
- Activity intolerance related to fatigue, anemia, retention of waste products, and dialysis procedure
- Low self-esteem related to dependency, role changes, changes in body image, and sexual dysfunction

Nursing care is directed toward assessing fluid status and identifying potential sources of imbalance, implementing a dietary program to ensure proper nutritional intake within the limits of the treatment regimen, and promoting positive feelings by encouraging increased self-care and greater independence. It is extremely important to provide explanations and information to the patient and family concerning ESRD, treatment options, and potential complications. A great deal of emotional support is needed by the patient and family because of the numerous changes experienced. Specific interventions, along with rationale

and evaluation criteria, are presented in more detail in the Plan of Nursing Care.

PROMOTING HOME AND COMMUNITY-BASED CARE

Teaching Patients Self-Care. The nurse plays an extremely important role in teaching the patient with ESRD. Because of the extensive teaching needed, the home care nurse, dialysis nurse, and nurse in the outpatient setting all provide ongoing education and reinforcement while monitoring the patient's progress and compliance with the treatment regimen.

A nutritional referral and explanations of nutritional needs are helpful because of the numerous dietary changes required. The patient is taught how to check the vascular access device for patency and how to take precautions, such as avoiding venipunctures and blood pressure measurements on the arm with the access device.

Additionally, the patient and family require considerable assistance and support in dealing with the need for dialysis and its long-term implications. For instance, they need to know what problems to report to the health care provider, including the following:

- Worsening signs and symptoms of renal failure (nausea, vomiting, change in usual urine output [if any], ammonia odour on breath)
- Signs and symptoms of hyperkalemia (muscle weakness, diarrhea, abdominal cramps)
- Signs and symptoms of access problems (clotted fistula or graft, infection)

These signs and symptoms of decreasing renal function, in addition to increasing BUN and serum creatinine levels, may indicate a need to alter the dialysis prescription. The dialysis nurses also provide ongoing education and support at each treatment visit.

Continuing Care. The importance of follow-up examinations and treatment is stressed to the patient and family because of changing physical status, renal function, and dialysis requirements. Referral for home care provides the home care nurse with the opportunity to assess the patient's environment, emotional status, and the coping strategies used by the patient and family to deal with the changes in family roles often associated with chronic illness.

The home care nurse also assesses the patient for further deterioration of renal function and signs and symptoms of complications resulting from the primary renal disorder, the resulting renal failure, and effects of treatment strategies (eg, dialysis, medications, dietary restrictions). Many patients need ongoing education and reinforcement on the multiple dietary restrictions required, including fluid, sodium, potassium, and protein restriction. Reminders about the need for health promotion activities and health screening are an important part of nursing care for the patient with renal failure.

🍂 Gerontologic Considerations

Changes in kidney function with normal aging increase the susceptibility of elderly patients to kidney dysfunction and renal failure. Because alterations in renal blood flow, glomerular filtration, and renal clearance increase the risk for medication-associated changes in renal function, precautions are indicated with all

(text continues on page 1339)

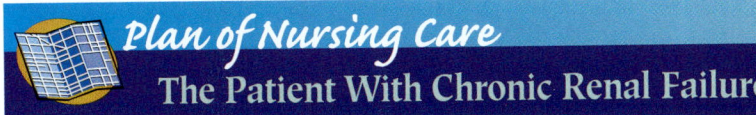

Plan of Nursing Care
The Patient With Chronic Renal Failure

Nursing Interventions	Rationale	Expected Outcomes

Nursing Diagnosis: Excess fluid volume related to decreased urine output, dietary excesses, and retention of sodium and water

Goal: Maintenance of ideal body weight without excess fluid

Nursing Interventions	Rationale	Expected Outcomes
1. Assess fluid status: a. Daily weight b. Intake and output balance c. Skin turgor and presence of edema d. Distention of neck veins e. Blood pressure, pulse rate, and rhythm f. Respiratory rate and effort 2. Limit fluid intake to prescribed volume. 3. Identify potential sources of fluid: a. Medications and fluids used to take medications: oral and intravenous b. Foods 4. Explain to patient and family rationale for restriction. 5. Assist patient to cope with the discomforts resulting from fluid restriction. 6. Provide or encourage frequent oral hygiene.	1. Assessment provides baseline and ongoing database for monitoring changes and evaluating interventions. 2. Fluid restriction will be determined on basis of weight, urine output, and response to therapy. 3. Unrecognized sources of excess fluids may be identified. 4. Understanding promotes patient and family cooperation with fluid restriction. 5. Increasing patient comfort promotes compliance with dietary restrictions. 6. Oral hygiene minimizes dryness of oral mucous membranes.	• Demonstrates no rapid weight changes • Maintains dietary and fluid restrictions • Exhibits normal skin turgor without edema • Exhibits normal vital signs • Exhibits no neck vein distention • Reports no difficulty breathing or shortness of breath • Performs oral hygiene frequently • Reports decreased thirst • Reports decreased dryness of oral mucous membranes

Nursing Diagnosis: Imbalanced nutrition; less than body requirements related to anorexia, nausea, vomiting, dietary restrictions, and altered oral mucous membranes

Goal: Maintenance of adequate nutritional intake

Nursing Interventions	Rationale	Expected Outcomes
1. Assess nutritional status: a. Weight changes b. Laboratory values (serum electrolyte, BUN, creatinine, protein, transferrin, and iron levels) 2. Assess patient's nutritional dietary patterns: a. Diet history b. Food preferences c. Calorie counts 3. Assess for factors contributing to altered nutritional intake: a. Anorexia, nausea, or vomiting b. Diet unpalatable to patient c. Depression d. Lack of understanding of dietary restrictions e. Stomatitis 4. Provide patient's food preferences within dietary restrictions. 5. Promote intake of high biologic value protein foods: eggs, dairy products, meats. 6. Encourage high-calorie, low-protein, low-sodium, and low-potassium snacks between meals.	1. Baseline data allow for monitoring of changes and evaluating effectiveness of interventions. 2. Past and present dietary patterns are considered in planning meals. 3. Information about other factors that may be altered or eliminated to promote adequate dietary intake is provided. 4. Increased dietary intake is encouraged. 5. Complete proteins are provided for positive nitrogen balance needed for growth and healing. 6. Reduces source of restricted foods and proteins and provides calories for energy, sparing protein for tissue growth and healing.	• Consumes protein of high biologic value • Chooses foods within dietary restrictions that are appealing • Consumes high-calorie foods within dietary restrictions • Explains in own words rationale for dietary restrictions and relationship to urea and creatinine levels • Takes medications on schedule that does not produce anorexia or feeling of fullness • Consults written lists of acceptable foods • Reports increased appetite at meals • Exhibits no rapid increases or decreases in weight • Demonstrates normal skin turgor without edema; healing and acceptable plasma albumin levels

(continued)

Plan of Nursing Care
The Patient With Chronic Renal Failure *(Continued)*

Nursing Interventions	Rationale	Expected Outcomes
7. Alter schedule of medications so that they are not given immediately before meals.	7. Ingestion of medications just before meals may produce anorexia and feeling of fullness.	
8. Explain rationale for dietary restrictions and relationship to kidney disease and increased urea and creatinine levels.	8. Promotes patient understanding of relationships between diet and urea and creatinine levels to renal disease.	
9. Provide written lists of foods allowed and suggestions for improving their taste without use of sodium or potassium.	9. Lists provide a positive approach to dietary restrictions and a reference for patient and family to use when at home.	
10. Provide pleasant surroundings at mealtimes.	10. Unpleasant factors that contribute to patient's anorexia are eliminated.	
11. Weigh patient daily.	11. Allows monitoring of fluid and nutritional status.	
12. Assess for evidence of inadequate protein intake: a. Edema formation b. Delayed healing c. Decreased serum albumin levels	12. Inadequate protein intake can lead to decreased albumin and other proteins, edema formation, and delay in healing.	

Nursing Diagnosis: Deficient knowledge regarding condition and treatment
Goal: Increased knowledge about condition and related treatment

Nursing Interventions	Rationale	Expected Outcomes
1. Assess understanding of cause of renal failure, consequences of renal failure, and its treatment: a. Cause of patient's renal failure b. Meaning of renal failure c. Understanding of renal function d. Relationship of fluid and dietary restrictions to renal failure e. Rationale for treatment (hemodialysis, peritoneal dialysis, transplantation)	1. Provides baseline for further explanations and teaching.	• Verbalizes relationship of cause of renal failure to consequences • Explains fluid and dietary restrictions as they relate to failure of kidney's regulatory functions • States in own words relationship of renal failure and need for treatment • Asks questions about treatment options, indicating readiness to learn • Verbalizes plans to continue as normal a life as possible • Uses written information and instructions to clarify questions and seek additional information
2. Provide explanation of renal function and consequences of renal failure at patient's level of understanding and guided by patient's readiness to learn.	2. Patient can learn about renal failure and treatment as he or she becomes ready to understand and accept the diagnosis and consequences.	
3. Assist patient to identify ways to incorporate changes related to illness and its treatment into lifestyle.	3. Patient can see that his or her life does not have to revolve around the disease.	
4. Provide oral and written information as appropriate about: a. Renal function and failure b. Fluid and dietary restrictions c. Medications d. Reportable problems, signs, and symptoms e. Follow-up schedule f. Community resources g. Treatment options	4. Provides patient with information that can be used for further clarification at home.	

(continued)

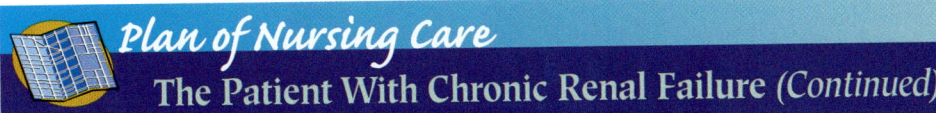

Plan of Nursing Care
The Patient With Chronic Renal Failure (Continued)

Nursing Interventions	Rationale	Expected Outcomes

Nursing Diagnosis: Activity intolerance related to fatigue, anemia, retention of waste products, and dialysis procedure
Goal: Participation in activity within tolerance

1. Assess factors contributing to fatigue:
  a. Anemia
  b. Fluid and electrolyte imbalances
  c. Retention of waste products
  d. Depression
2. Promote independence in self-care activities as tolerated; assist if fatigued.
3. Encourage alternating activity with rest.
4. Encourage patient to rest after dialysis treatments.
	1. Indicates factors contributing to severity of fatigue.
	
	2. Promotes improved self-esteem
	
	3. Promotes activity and exercise within limits and adequate rest.
	4. Adequate rest is encouraged after dialysis treatments, which are exhausting to many patients.
		• Participates in increasing levels of activity and exercise
		• Reports increased sense of well-being
		• Alternates rest and activity
		• Participates in selected self-care activities

Nursing Diagnosis: Disturbed self-esteem related to dependency, role changes, change in body image, and change in sexual function
Goal: Improved self-concept

1. Assess patient's and family's responses and reactions to illness and treatment.
2. Assess relationship of patient and significant family members.
3. Assess usual coping patterns of patient and family members.
 	
4. Encourage open discussion of concerns about changes produced by disease and treatment:
  a. Role changes
  b. Changes in lifestyle
  c. Changes in occupation
  d. Sexual changes
  e. Dependence on health care team
5. Explore alternate ways of sexual expression other than sexual intercourse.
6. Discuss role of giving and receiving love, warmth, and affection.
	1. Provides data about problems encountered by patient and family in coping with changes in life.
	2. Identifies strengths and supports of patient and family.
	3. Coping patterns that may have been effective in past may be harmful in view of restrictions imposed by disease and treatment.
	4. Encourages patient to identify concerns and steps necessary to deal with them.
	
	5. Alternative forms of sexual expression may be acceptable.
	6. Sexuality means different things to different people, depending on stage of maturity.
		• Identifies previously used coping styles that have been effective and those no longer possible due to disease and treatment (alcohol or drug use; extreme physical exertion)
		• Patient and family identify and verbalize feelings and reactions to disease and necessary changes in their lives
		• Seeks professional counselling, if necessary, to cope with changes resulting from renal failure
		• Reports satisfaction with method of sexual expression

Collaborative Problems: Hyperkalemia; pericarditis, pericardial effusion, and pericardial tamponade; hypertension; anemia; bone disease and metastatic calcifications
Goal: Patient experiences an absence of complications

Hyperkalemia

1. Monitor serum potassium levels and notify physician if level greater than 5.5 mmol/L. 2. Assess patient for muscle weakness, diarrhea, ECG changes (tall-tented T waves and widened QRS).	1. Hyperkalemia causes potentially life-threatening changes in the body. 2. Cardiovascular signs and symptoms are characteristic of hyperkalemia.	• Patient has normal potassium level • Experiences no muscle weakness or diarrhea. • Exhibits normal ECG pattern • Vital signs are within normal limits

(continued)

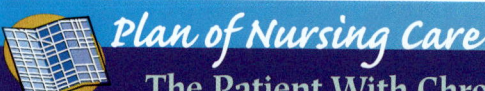
Plan of Nursing Care
The Patient With Chronic Renal Failure (Continued)

Nursing Interventions	Rationale	Expected Outcomes

Pericarditis, Pericardial Effusion, and Pericardial Tamponade

1. Assess patient for fever, chest pain, and a pericardial friction rub (signs of pericarditis) and, if present, notify physician.
2. If patient has pericarditis, assess for the following every 4 hours:
   a. Paradoxical pulse > 10 mm Hg
   b. Extreme hypotension
   c. Weak or absent peripheral pulses
   d. Altered level of consciousness
   e. Bulging neck veins

3. Prepare patient for cardiac ultrasound to aid in diagnosis of pericardial effusion and cardiac tamponade.
4. If cardiac tamponade develops, prepare patient for emergency pericardiocentesis.

1. About 30%–50% of chronic renal failure patients develop pericarditis due to uremia; fever, chest pain, and a pericardial friction rub are classic signs.
2. Pericardial effusion is a common fatal sequela of pericarditis. Signs of an effusion include a paradoxical pulse (> 10 mm Hg drop in blood pressure during inspiration) and signs of shock due to compression of the heart by a large effusion. Cardiac tamponade exists when the patient is severely compromised hemodynamically.
3. Cardiac ultrasound is useful in visualizing pericardial effusions and cardiac tamponade.
4. Cardiac tamponade is a life-threatening condition, with a high mortality rate. Immediate aspiration of fluid from the pericardial space is essential.

- Has strong and equal peripheral pulses
- Absence of a paradoxical pulse
- Absence of pericardial effusion or tamponade on cardiac ultrasound
- Patient has normal heart sounds

Hypertension

1. Monitor and record blood pressure as indicated.

2. Administer antihypertensive medications as prescribed.

3. Encourage compliance with dietary and fluid restriction therapy.

4. Teach patient to report signs of fluid overload, vision changes, headaches, edema, or seizures.

1. Provides objective data for monitoring. Elevated levels may indicate nonadherence to the treatment regimen.
2. Antihypertensive medications play a key role in treatment of hypertension associated with chronic renal failure.
3. Adherence to diet and fluid restrictions and dialysis schedule prevents excess fluid and sodium accumulation.
4. These are indications of inadequate control of hypertension and need to alter therapy.

- Blood pressure within normal limits
- Reports no headaches, visual problems, or seizures
- Edema is absent
- Demonstrates compliance with dietary and fluid restrictions

Anemia

1. Monitor RBC count, hemoglobin, and hematocrit levels as indicated.
2. Administer medications as prescribed, including iron and folic acid supplements, Epogen, and multivitamins.
3. Avoid drawing unnecessary blood specimens.
4. Teach patient to prevent bleeding: avoid vigourous nose blowing and contact sports, and use a soft toothbrush.
5. Administer blood component therapy as indicated.

1. Provides assessment of degree of anemia.
2. RBCs need iron, folic acid, and vitamins to be produced. Epogen stimulates the bone marrow to produce RBC.
3. Anemia is worsened by drawing numerous specimens.
4. Bleeding from anywhere in the body worsens anemia.

5. Blood component therapy may be needed if the patient has symptoms.

- Patient has a normal colour without pallor
- Exhibits hematology values within acceptable limits
- Experiences no bleeding from any site

Bone Disease and Metastatic Calcifications

1. Administer the following medications as prescribed: phosphate binders, calcium supplements, vitamin D supplements.
2. Monitor serum lab values as indicated (calcium, phosphorus, aluminum levels) and report abnormal findings to physician.
3. Assist patient with an exercise program.

1. Chronic renal failure causes numerous physiologic changes affecting calcium, phosphorus, and vitamin D metabolism.
2. Hyperphosphatemia, hypocalcemia, and excess aluminum accumulation are common in chronic renal failure.

3. Bone demineralization increases with immobility.

- Exhibits serum calcium, phosphorus, and aluminum levels within acceptable ranges
- Exhibits no symptoms of hypocalcemia
- Has no bone demineralization on bone scan
- Discusses importance of maintaining activity level and exercise program

medications. This is because of the frequent use of multiple-prescription and over-the-counter medications by elderly patients. The incidence of systemic diseases, such as atherosclerosis, hypertension, heart failure, diabetes, and cancer, increases with advancing age, predisposing older adults to renal disease associated with these disorders. Therefore, nurses in all settings need to be alert for signs and symptoms of renal dysfunction in elderly patients.

With age, the kidney is less able to respond to acute fluid and electrolyte changes. Therefore, acute problems need to be prevented if possible or recognized and treated quickly to avoid kidney damage. When the elderly patient must undergo extensive diagnostic tests, or when new medications (eg, diuretic agents) are added, precautions must be taken to prevent dehydration, which can compromise marginal renal function and lead to ARF.

The elderly patient may develop atypical and nonspecific signs and symptoms of disturbed renal function and fluid and electrolyte imbalances. Recognition of these problems is further hampered by their association with preexisting disorders and the misconception that they are normal changes of aging.

ACUTE RENAL FAILURE IN OLDER ADULTS

The incidence of ARF is increasing in older, hospitalized patients. About half of patients who develop ARF during hospitalization for a medical or surgical problem are older than 60 years of age. Evidence also demonstrates that ARF is often seen in the community setting. Nurses in the ambulatory setting need to be cognizant of the risk for ARF in their elderly patients, especially those undergoing diagnostic testing or procedures that can result in dehydration. The mortality rate is slightly higher for ARF in elderly patients than for their younger counterparts.

The etiology of ARF in older adults includes prerenal causes, such as dehydration, and intrarenal causes, such as nephrotoxic agents (medications, contrast agents). Diabetes mellitus increases the risk for contrast agent-induced renal failure because of preexisting renal insufficiency and the imposed fluid restriction needed for many tests. Suppression of thirst, enforced bed rest, lack of drinking water, and confusion all contribute to the older patient's failure to consume adequate fluids and may lead to dehydration and compromise of already decreased renal function.

CHRONIC RENAL FAILURE IN OLDER ADULTS

Historically, the age of patients developing ESRD steadily rose each year, but it appears to have stabilized since 1993 at a mean age of 60 years. In the past, rapidly progressive glomerulonephritis, membranous glomerulonephritis, and nephrosclerosis were the most common causes of chronic renal failure in the elderly. Today, however, diabetes mellitus and hypertension are the leading causes of chronic renal failure in the elderly (Bakris et al., 2000). Other common causes of chronic renal failure in the elderly population are interstitial nephritis and urinary tract obstruction. The signs and symptoms of renal disease in the elderly are commonly nonspecific. The occurrence of symptoms of other disorders (heart failure, dementia) can mask the symptoms of renal disease and delay or prevent diagnosis and treatment. The patient often develops signs and symptoms of nephrotic syndrome, such as edema and proteinuria.

Hemodialysis and peritoneal dialysis have been used effectively in treating elderly patients (Carey et al., 2001). Although there is no specific age limitation for renal transplantation, concomitant disorders (ie, coronary artery disease, peripheral vascular disease) have made it a less common treatment for the elderly.

The outcome, however, is comparable to that of younger patients. Some elderly patients elect not to participate in these treatment strategies. Conservative management, including nutritional therapy, fluid control, and medications, such as phosphate binders, may be considered in patients who are not suitable for or elect not to participate in dialysis or transplantation.

Kidney Transplantation

Kidney transplantation has become the treatment of choice for most patients with ESRD. During the past 40 years, more than 380,000 kidney transplantations have been performed worldwide. In 1999, 1010 Canadians underwent kidney transplants: 631 from deceased donors, 287 from living related donors, and 92 from living unrelated donors. Approximately 3,000 others were awaiting a kidney transplant in 2001 (Canadian Organ Replacement Register, 2001). Patients choose kidney transplantation for various reasons, such as the desire to avoid dialysis or to improve their sense of well-being and the wish to lead a more normal life. Additionally, the cost of maintaining a successful transplantation is one-third the cost of treating a dialysis patient.

Kidney transplantation involves transplanting a kidney from a living donor or human cadaver to a recipient who has ESRD (Chart 45-9). Kidney transplants from well-matched living donors who are related to the patient (those with compatible ABO and HLA antigens) are slightly more successful than those from cadaver donors. The success rate increases if kidney transplantation from a living donor is performed before dialysis is initiated (Mange, Joffe & Feldman, 2001). Due to the overwhelming numbers of persons on kidney transplant waiting lists, new techniques for matching nonrelated living donors are being developed (Gridelli & Remuzzi, 2000).

A nephrectomy of the patient's own native kidneys may be performed before transplantation. The transplanted kidney is placed in the patient's iliac fossa anterior to the iliac crest. The ureter of the newly transplanted kidney is transplanted into the bladder or anastomosed to the ureter of the recipient (Fig. 45-5).

Chart 45-9	**Organ Donation**

An inadequate number of available kidneys remains the greatest limitation to treating patients with end-stage renal disease successfully. For those interested in donating a kidney, the National Kidney Foundation provides written information describing the organ donation program and a card specifying the organs to be donated in the event of death.

The organ donation card is signed by the donor and two witnesses and should be carried by the donor at all times. Procurement of an adequate number of kidneys for potential recipients is still a major problem, despite national legislation that requires relatives of deceased patients or patients declared brain-dead to be asked if they would consider organ donation.

In Canada, drivers can indicate their desire to be organ donors on their driver's license application or renewal.

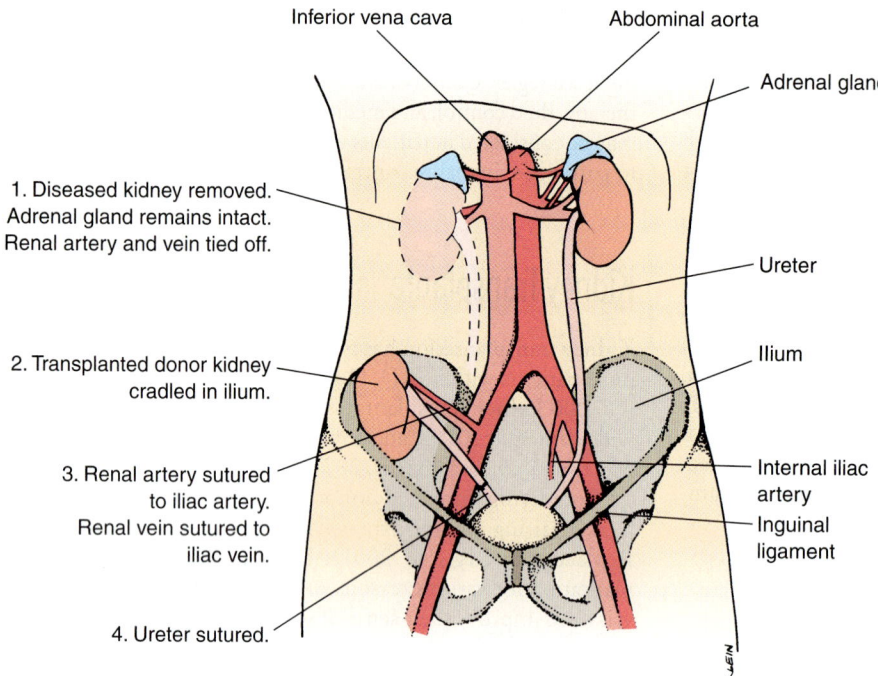

Inferior vena cava

Abdominal aorta

Adrenal gland

1. Diseased kidney removed. Adrenal gland remains intact. Renal artery and vein tied off.

Ureter

Ilium

2. Transplanted donor kidney cradled in ilium.

3. Renal artery sutured to iliac artery. Renal vein sutured to iliac vein.

Internal iliac artery

Inguinal ligament

4. Ureter sutured.

FIGURE 45-5 Renal transplantation: (1) The diseased kidney may be removed and the renal artery and vein tied off. (2) The transplanted kidney is placed in the iliac fossa. (3) The renal artery of the donated kidney is sutured to the iliac artery, and the renal vein is sutured to the iliac vein. (4) The ureter of the donated kidney is sutured to the bladder or to the patient's ureter.

PREOPERATIVE MANAGEMENT

Preoperative management goals include bringing the patient's metabolic state to a level as close to normal as possible, making sure that the patient is free of infection, and preparing the patient for surgery and the postoperative course.

Medical Management

A complete physical examination is performed to detect and treat any conditions that could cause complications after transplantation. Tissue typing, blood typing, and antibody screening are performed to determine compatibility of the tissues and cells of the donor and recipient. Other diagnostic tests must be completed to identify conditions requiring treatment before transplantation. The lower urinary tract is studied to assess bladder neck function and to detect ureteral reflux.

The patient must be free of infection at the time of renal transplantation because after surgery the patient will receive medications to prevent transplant rejection. These medications suppress the immune response, leaving the patient immunosuppressed and at risk for infection. Therefore, the patient is evaluated and treated for any infections, including gingival (gum) disease and dental caries.

A psychosocial evaluation is conducted to assess the patient's ability to adjust to the transplant, coping styles, social history, social support available, and financial resources. A history of psychiatric illness is important to ascertain because psychiatric conditions are often aggravated by the corticosteroids needed for immunosuppression after transplantation.

Hemodialysis is often performed the day before the scheduled transplantation procedure to optimize the patient's physical status if a dialysis routine had already been established. However, it is preferable to avoid initiation of dialysis before transplantation when a donor kidney is available (Mange et al., 2001).

Nursing Management

The nursing aspects of preoperative care are similar to those for patients undergoing other elective abdominal surgery. Preoperative teaching can be conducted in a variety of settings, including the outpatient preadmission area, the hospital, or the transplantation clinic during the preliminary workup phase. Patient teaching addresses postoperative pulmonary hygiene, pain management options, dietary restrictions, intravenous and arterial lines, tubes (indwelling catheter and possibly a nasogastric tube), and early ambulation. The patient who receives a kidney from a living related donor may be concerned about the donor and how the donor will tolerate the surgical procedure.

Most patients have been on dialysis for months or years before transplantation. Many have waited months to years for a kidney transplant and are anxious about the surgery, possible rejection, and the need to return to dialysis. Helping the patient to deal with these concerns is part of the nurse's role in preoperative management, as is teaching the patient about what to expect after surgery.

POSTOPERATIVE MANAGEMENT

The goal of care is to maintain homeostasis until the transplanted kidney is functioning well. The patient whose kidney functions immediately has a more favourable prognosis than the patient whose kidney does not.

Immunosuppressive Therapy

The survival of a transplanted kidney depends on the ability to block the body's immune response to the transplanted kidney. To overcome or minimize the body's defense mechanism, immunosuppressant agents such as azathioprine (Imuran), corticosteroids (prednisone), cyclosporine, and orthoclone OKT-3 (a monoclonal antibody) are administered (Shapiro, 2000b).

Cyclosporine is available in a microemulsion form (Neoral), which delivers the medication reliably, thus producing a steady-state serum concentration. Tacrolimus (Prograf, formerly called FK-506) is similar to cyclosporine and about 100 times more potent. Mycophenolate (CellCept, RS-61433) has been approved by Health Canada solely for the prevention of renal transplant rejection. It may be used in patients who have failed to respond to the standard corticosteroid pulse therapy or orthoclone OKT-3. Antilymphocyte globulin is occasionally used to modify the immune response. Leukapheresis, lymph drainage, and cyclophosphamide (Cytoxan) are other methods of immunosuppression, but they are rarely used.

Treatment with combinations of these new agents has dramatically improved survival rates. The newest class of agents, the first of which is sirolimus, is called target of rapamycin (TOR) inhibitors; these agents are used with cyclosporine for maintenance therapy. Immunosuppressive drug therapy after kidney transplantation continues to evolve (Chan, Gaston & Hariharan, 2001).

Doses of immunosuppressant agents are gradually reduced (tapered) over a period of several weeks, depending on the patient's immunologic response to the transplant. The patient will, however, take some form of antirejection medication for the entire time that he or she has the transplanted kidney (Chart 45-10).

The clinical profile of neurotoxicity caused by immunosuppression has changed. When toxic levels are reached, both cyclosporine and tacrolimus may produce a clinical spectrum that varies from tremor and acute confusional state to status epilepticus and major speech or language abnormalities. Coma has become an unusual manifestation (Baan et al., 2001; Shapiro, 2000; Wijdicks, 2001).

Chart 45-10 — Renal Transplant Rejection and Infection

Renal graft rejection and failure may occur within 24 hours (hyperacute), within 3 to 14 days (acute), or after many years (chronic). It is not uncommon for rejection to occur during the first year after transplantation.

Detecting Rejection
Ultrasonography may be used to detect enlargement of the kidney; percutaneous renal biopsy (most reliable) and x-ray techniques are used to evaluate transplant rejection. If the body rejects the transplanted kidney, the patient needs to return to dialysis. The rejected kidney may or may not be removed, depending on when the rejection occurs (acute versus chronic) and the risk for infection if the kidney is left in place.

Potential Infection
About 75% of kidney transplant recipients have at least one episode of infection in the first year after transplantation because of immunosuppressant therapy. Immunosuppressants of the past made the transplant recipient more vulnerable to opportunistic infections (candidiasis, cytomegalovirus, *Pneumocystis carinii* pneumonia) and infection with other relatively nonpathogenic viruses, fungi, and protozoa, which can be a major hazard. Cyclosporine therapy has reduced the incidence of opportunistic infections because it selectively exerts its effect, sparing T cells that protect the patient from life-threatening infections. In addition, combination immunosuppressant therapy and improved clinical care have produced 1-year patient survival rates approaching 100% and graft survival exceeding 90%. Infections, however, remain a major cause of death at all points in time for kidney transplant recipients (Chan, Gaston & Hariharan, 2001).

Postoperative Nursing Management

ASSESSING THE PATIENT FOR TRANSPLANT REJECTION

After kidney transplantation, the nurse assesses the patient for signs and symptoms of transplant rejection: oliguria, edema, fever, increasing blood pressure, weight gain, and swelling or tenderness over the transplanted kidney or graft. Patients receiving cyclosporine may not exhibit the usual signs and symptoms of acute rejection. In these patients, the only sign may be an asymptomatic rise in the serum creatinine level (more than a 20% rise is considered acute rejection).

The results of blood chemistry tests (BUN and creatinine) and leukocyte and platelet counts are monitored closely because immunosuppression depresses the formation of leukocytes and platelets. The patient is closely monitored for infection because of susceptibility to impaired healing and infection related to immunosuppressive therapy and complications of renal failure.

 NURSING ALERT A distinction must be made between infection and rejection because impaired renal function and fever are evidence of both infection and rejection, and their treatments differ.

Clinical manifestations of infection include shaking chills, fever, rapid heartbeat and respirations (tachycardia and tachypnea), and either an increase or a decrease in WBCs (leukocytosis or leukopenia).

PREVENTING INFECTION

Infection may be introduced through the urinary tract, the respiratory tract, the surgical site, or other sources. Urine cultures are performed frequently because of the high incidence of bacteriuria during early and late stages of transplantation. Any type of wound drainage should be viewed as a potential source of infection because drainage is an excellent culture medium for bacteria. Catheter and drain tips may be cultured when removed by cutting off the tip of the catheter or drain (using aseptic technique) and placing the cut portion in a sterile container to be taken to the laboratory for culture.

The nurse ensures that the patient is protected from exposure to infection by hospital staff, visitors, and other patients with active infections. Careful hand hygiene is imperative; face masks may be worn by hospital staff and visitors to reduce the risk for transmitting infectious agents while the patient is receiving high doses of immunosuppressants.

MONITORING URINARY FUNCTION

The vascular access for hemodialysis is monitored to ensure patency and to evaluate for evidence of infection. After successful renal transplantation, the vascular access device may clot, possibly from improved coagulation with the return of renal function. Hemodialysis may be necessary postoperatively to maintain homeostasis until the transplanted kidney is functioning well.

A kidney from a living donor related to the patient usually begins to function immediately after surgery and may produce large quantities of dilute urine. A kidney from a cadaver donor may undergo acute tubular necrosis and therefore may not function for 2 or 3 weeks, during which time anuria, oliguria, or polyuria may be present. During this stage, the patient may experience significant changes in fluid and electrolyte status. Therefore, careful monitoring is indicated. The output from the urinary catheter (connected to a closed drainage system) is measured every hour. Intravenous fluids are administered on the basis of urine volume and serum electrolyte levels and as prescribed by the physician.

Hemodialysis may be required if fluid overload and hyperkalemia occur (Gridelli & Remuzzi, 2000).

ADDRESSING PSYCHOLOGICAL CONCERNS

The rejection of a transplanted kidney remains a matter of great concern to the patient, the family, and the health care team for many months. The fears of kidney rejection and the complications of immunosuppressive therapy (Cushing's syndrome, diabetes, capillary fragility, osteoporosis, glaucoma, cataracts, acne) place tremendous psychological stresses on the patient. Anxiety and uncertainty about the future and difficult posttransplantation adjustment are often sources of stress for the patient and family.

An important nursing function is the assessment of the patient's stress and coping. The nurse uses each visit with the patient to determine if the patient and family are coping effectively and the patient is complying with the prescribed medication regimen. If indicated or requested, the nurse refers the patient for counselling.

MONITORING AND MANAGING POTENTIAL COMPLICATIONS

The patient undergoing kidney transplantation is at risk for the postoperative complications that are associated with any surgical procedure. In addition, the patient's physical condition may be compromised because of the complications associated with long-standing renal failure and its treatment. Therefore, careful assessment for the complications related to renal failure and those associated with a major surgical procedure are important aspects of nursing care. Strategies to promote surgical recovery (breathing exercises, early ambulation, care of the surgical incision) are important aspects of postoperative care.

GI ulceration and corticosteroid-induced bleeding may occur. Fungal colonization of the GI tract (especially the mouth) and urinary bladder may occur secondary to corticosteroid and antibiotic therapy. Closely monitoring the patient and notifying the physician about the occurrence of these complications are important nursing interventions. In addition, the patient is monitored closely for signs and symptoms of adrenal insufficiency if the treatment has included use of corticosteroids.

PROMOTING HOME AND COMMUNITY-BASED CARE

Teaching Patients Self-Care. The nurse works closely with the patient and family to be sure that they understand the need for continuing the immunosuppressive therapy as prescribed. Additionally, the patient and family are instructed to assess for and report signs and symptoms of transplant rejection, infection, or significant adverse effects of the immunosuppressant regimen. These include decreased urine output; weight gain; malaise; fever; respiratory distress; tenderness over the transplanted kidney; anxiety; depression; changes in eating, drinking, or other habits; and changes in blood pressure readings. The patient is instructed to inform other health care providers (eg, dentist) about the kidney transplant and the use of immunosuppressive agents.

Continuing Care. The patient needs to know that follow-up care after transplantation is a lifelong necessity. Individual verbal and written instructions are provided concerning diet, medication, fluids, daily weight, daily measurement of urine, management of intake and output, prevention of infection, resumption of activity, and avoidance of contact sports in which the transplanted kidney may be injured. Because of the risk of other potential complications, the patient is followed closely. Cardiovascular dis-

ease is now the major cause of morbidity and mortality after transplantation, due in part to the increasing age of transplantation patients. An additional problem is possible malignancy; patients receiving long-term immunosuppressive therapy have been found to develop cancers more frequently than the general population. Because of the usual need for health promotion along with the increased risks for malignancy because of immunosuppressive therapy, the patient is reminded of the importance of health promotion and health screening.

The Kidney Foundation of Canada and its provincial branches provide information and support to patients with kidney disease and their families.

Urolithiasis

Urolithiasis refers to stones (calculi) in the urinary tract. Stones are formed in the urinary tract when urinary concentrations of substances such as calcium oxalate, calcium phosphate, and uric acid increase. This is referred to as supersaturation and is dependent on the amount of the substance, ionic strength, and pH of the urine.

Pathophysiology

Stones can also form when there is a deficiency of substances that normally prevent crystallization in the urine, such as citrate, magnesium, nephrocalcin, and uropontin. The fluid volume status of the patient (stones tend to occur more often in dehydrated patients) is another factor playing a key role in stone development.

Calculi may be found anywhere from the kidney to the bladder. They vary in size from minute granular deposits, called sand or gravel, to bladder stones as large as an orange. The different sites of calculi formation in the urinary tract are shown in Figure 45-6.

FIGURE 45-6 Various sites of calculi formation in the urinary tract (urolithiasis).

Certain factors favour the formation of stones, including infection, urinary stasis, and periods of immobility (slows renal drainage and alters calcium metabolism). In addition, increased calcium concentrations in blood and urine promote precipitation of calcium and formation of stones (about 75% of all renal stones are calcium-based). Causes of hypercalcemia (high serum calcium) and hypercalciuria (high urine calcium) include the following:

- Hyperparathyroidism
- Renal tubular acidosis
- Cancers
- Granulomatous diseases (sarcoidosis, tuberculosis), which may cause increased vitamin D production by the granulomatous tissue
- Excessive intake of vitamin D
- Excessive intake of milk and alkali
- Myeloproliferative diseases (leukemia, polycythemia vera, multiple myeloma), which produce an unusual proliferation of blood cells from the bone marrow

For patients with stones containing uric acid, struvite, or cystine, a thorough physical examination and metabolic workup are indicated because of associated disturbances contributing to the stone formation. Uric acid stones (5% to 10% of all stones) may be seen in patients with gout or myeloproliferative disorders. Struvite stones account for 15% of urinary calculi and form in persistently alkaline, ammonia-rich urine caused by the presence of urease-splitting bacteria such as *Proteus, Pseudomonas, Klebsiella, Staphylococcus,* or *Mycoplasma* species. Predisposing factors for struvite stones (commonly called infection stones) include neurogenic bladder, foreign bodies, and recurrent UTIs. Cystine stones (1% to 2% of all stones) occur exclusively in patients with a rare inherited defect in renal absorption of cystine (an amino acid).

Urinary stone formation may also occur with inflammatory bowel disease and in patients with an ileostomy or bowel resection because these patients absorb more oxalate. Some medications that are known to cause stones in some patients include antacids, acetazolamide (Diamox), vitamin D, laxatives, and high doses of aspirin. In many patients, however, no cause may be found.

Urinary stones account for about 328,000 hospital admissions each year in the United States. The occurrence of urinary stones occurs predominantly in the third to fifth decades of life and affects men more than women. About half of patients with a single renal stone have another episode within 5 years. Most stones contain calcium or magnesium in combination with phosphorus or oxalate. Most stones are radiopaque and can be detected by x-ray studies (Bihl & Meyers, 2001).

Clinical Manifestations

Signs and symptoms of stones in the urinary tract depend on obstruction, infection, and edema. When the stones block the flow of urine, obstruction develops, producing an increase in hydrostatic pressure and distending the renal pelvis and proximal ureter. Infection (pyelonephritis and cystitis with chills, fever, and dysuria) can occur from constant irritation by the stone. Some stones cause few, if any, symptoms while slowly destroying the functional units (nephrons) of the kidney; others cause excruciating pain and discomfort.

Stones in the renal pelvis may be associated with an intense, deep ache in the costovertebral region. Hematuria is often present; pyuria may also be noted. Pain originating in the renal area radiates anteriorly and downward toward the bladder in the female and toward the testis in the male. If the pain suddenly becomes acute, with tenderness over the costovertebral area, and nausea and vomiting appear, the patient is having an episode of renal colic. Diarrhea and abdominal discomfort may occur. These GI symptoms are due to renointestinal reflexes and the anatomic proximity of the kidneys to the stomach, pancreas, and large intestine.

Stones lodged in the ureter (ureteral obstruction) cause acute, excruciating, colicky, wavelike pain, radiating down the thigh and to the genitalia. Often, the patient has a desire to void, but little urine is passed, and it usually contains blood because of the abrasive action of the stone. This group of symptoms is called ureteral colic. Colic is mediated by prostaglandin E, a substance that increases ureteral contractility and renal blood flow and that leads to increased intraureteral pressure and pain. In general, the patient spontaneously passes stones 0.5 to 1 cm in diameter. Stones larger than 1 cm in diameter usually must be removed or fragmented (broken up by lithotripsy) so that they can be removed or passed spontaneously.

Stones lodged in the bladder usually produce symptoms of irritation and may be associated with UTI and hematuria. If the stone obstructs the bladder neck, urinary retention occurs. If infection is associated with a stone, the condition is far more serious, with sepsis threatening the patient's life.

Assessment and Diagnostic Findings

The diagnosis is confirmed by x-ray films of the kidneys, ureter, and bladder (KUB) or by ultrasonography, intravenous urography, or retrograde pyelography. Blood chemistries and a 24-hour urine test for measurement of calcium, uric acid, creatinine, sodium, pH, and total volume are part of the diagnostic workup. Dietary and medication histories and family history of renal stones are obtained to identify factors predisposing the patient to the formation of stones.

When stones are recovered (stones may be freely passed by the patient or removed through special procedures), chemical analysis is carried out to determine their composition. Stone analysis can provide a clear indication of the underlying disorder. For example, calcium oxalate or calcium phosphate stones usually indicate disorders of oxalate or calcium metabolism, whereas urate stones suggest a disturbance in uric acid metabolism.

Medical Management

The basic goals of management are to eradicate the stone, to determine the stone type, to prevent nephron destruction, to control infection, and to relieve any obstruction that may be present. The immediate objective of treatment of renal or ureteral colic is to relieve the pain until its cause can be eliminated. Opioid analgesics are administered to prevent shock and syncope that may result from the excruciating pain. NSAIDs may be as effective as other analgesics in treating renal stone pain. They provide specific pain relief because they inhibit the synthesis of prostaglandin E.

Hot baths or moist heat to the flank areas may also be useful. Unless the patient is vomiting or has heart failure or any other condition requiring fluid restriction, fluids are encouraged. This increases the hydrostatic pressure behind the stone, assisting it in its downward passage. A high, around-the-clock fluid intake reduces the concentration of urinary crystalloids, dilutes the urine, and ensures a high urine output.

Nutritional therapy plays an important role in preventing renal stones. Fluid intake is the mainstay of most medical therapy for renal stones. Unless contraindicated, any patient with renal stones should drink at least eight 227-g glasses of water daily to keep the urine dilute. A urine output exceeding 2 L a day is advisable (Chart 45-11).

Calcium Stones. Historically, patients with calcium-based renal stones were advised to restrict calcium in their diet. Recent evidence, however, has questioned the advisability of this practice, except for patients with type II absorptive hypercalciuria (half of all patients with calcium stones), in whom stones are clearly due to excess dietary calcium. Current research supports a liberal fluid intake along with dietary restriction of protein and sodium. It is thought that a high-protein diet is associated with increased urinary excretion of calcium and uric acid, thereby causing a supersaturation of these substances in the urine. Similarly, a high sodium intake has been shown in some studies to increase the amount of calcium in the urine. The urine may be acidified by use of medications such as ammonium chloride or acetohydroxamic acid (Lithostat) (Trinchieri, Zanetti, Curro & Lizzano, 2001; Williams, Child, Hudson et al., 2001).

Cellulose sodium phosphate (Calcibind) may be effective in preventing calcium stones. It binds calcium from food in the intestinal tract, reducing the amount of calcium absorbed into the circulation. If increased parathormone production (resulting in increased serum calcium levels in blood and urine) is a factor in the formation of stones, therapy with thiazide diuretics may be beneficial in reducing the calcium loss in the urine and lowering the elevated parathormone levels.

Uric Acid Stones. For uric acid stones, the patient is placed on a low-purine diet to reduce the excretion of uric acid in the urine. Foods high in purine (shellfish, anchovies, asparagus, mushrooms, and organ meats) are avoided, and other proteins may be limited. Allopurinol (Zyloprim) may be prescribed to reduce serum uric acid levels and urinary uric acid excretion. The urine is alkalinized. For cystine stones, a low-protein diet is prescribed, the urine is alkalinized, and penicillamine is administered to reduce the amount of cystine in the urine.

Oxalate Stones. For oxalate stones, a dilute urine is maintained and the intake of oxalate is limited. Many foods contain oxalate; however, only certain foods have been proved to increase the urinary excretion of oxalate significantly. These include spinach, strawberries, rhubarb, chocolate, tea, peanuts, and wheat bran.

SURGICAL MANAGEMENT

If the stone is not passed spontaneously or if complications occur, treatment modalities may include surgical, endoscopic, or other procedures—for example, ureteroscopy, extracorporeal shock wave lithotripsy (ESWL), or endourologic (percutaneous) stone removal.

Ureteroscopy (Fig. 45-7) involves first visualizing the stone and then destroying it. Access to the stone is accomplished by inserting a ureteroscope into the ureter and then inserting a laser, electrohydraulic lithotriptor, or ultrasound device through the ureteroscope to fragment and remove the stones. A stent may be inserted and left in place for 48 hours or more after the procedure to keep the ureter patent. Hospital stays are generally brief, and some patients can be treated as outpatients.

ESWL is a noninvasive procedure used to break up stones in the calyx of the kidney (see Fig. 45-7B). After the stones are fragmented to the size of grains of sand, the remnants of the stones are spontaneously voided. In ESWL, a high-energy amplitude of pressure, or shock wave, is generated by the abrupt release of energy and transmitted through water and soft tissues. When the shock wave encounters a substance of different intensity (a renal stone), a compression wave causes the surface of the stone to fragment. Repeated shock waves focused on the stone eventually reduce it to many small pieces. These small pieces are excreted in the urine, usually without difficulty.

The need for anesthesia for the procedure depends on the type of lithotriptor used, which determines the number and intensity of shock waves delivered. An average treatment comprises between 1,000 and 3,000 shocks. The first-generation lithotriptors required use of either regional or general anesthesia. Second- and third-generation lithotriptors, many of which also employ ultrasound guidance, require little to no anesthesia (Tombolini, Ruoppolo, Bellorofonte et al., 2000).

Although the shock waves usually do not damage other tissue, discomfort from the multiple shocks may occur. The patient is observed for obstruction and infection resulting from blockage of the urinary tract by stone fragments. All urine is strained after the procedure; voided gravel or sand is sent to the laboratory for chemical analysis. Several treatments may be necessary to ensure disintegration of stones. Although lithotripsy is a costly treatment, the length of hospital stay is decreased, as is expense, because an invasive surgical procedure to remove the renal stone is avoided.

Endourologic methods of stone removal (see Fig. 45-7C) may be used to extract renal calculi that cannot be removed by other procedures. A percutaneous nephrostomy or a percutaneous nephrolithotomy (which are similar procedures) may be performed, and a nephroscope is introduced through the dilated percutaneous tract into the renal parenchyma. Depending on its size, the stone may be extracted with forceps or by a stone retrieval basket. Alternatively, an ultrasound probe may be introduced through the nephrostomy tube. Then, ultrasonic waves are used to pulverize the stone. Small stone fragments and stone dust are irrigated and suctioned out of the collecting system. Larger stones may be further reduced by ultrasonic disintegration and then removed with forceps or a stone retrieval basket (Streem, 2000).

Electrohydraulic lithotripsy is a similar method in which an electrical discharge is used to create a hydraulic shock wave to break up the stone. A probe is passed through the cystoscope, and

---

Chart 45-11

Dietary Recommendations for Prevention of Kidney Stones

- Restricting protein to 60 g/day is recommended to decrease urinary excretion of calcium and uric acid.
- A sodium restriction of 3–4 g/day is recommended. Table salt and high-sodium foods should be reduced because sodium competes with calcium for reabsorption in the kidneys.
- Low-calcium diets are not generally recommended, except for true absorptive hypercalciuria. Evidence shows that limiting calcium, especially in women, can lead to osteoporosis and does not prevent renal stones.
- Oxalate-containing foods (spinach, strawberries, rhubarb, tea, peanuts, wheat bran) may be restricted.

FIGURE 45-7 Methods of treating renal stones. (**A**) During a cystoscopy, which is used for removing small renal stones located close to the bladder, a ureteroscope is inserted into the ureter to visualize the stone. The stone is then fragmented or captured and removed. (**B**) Extracorporeal shock wave lithotripsy (ESWL) is used for most symptomatic nonpassable upper urinary tract stones. Electromagnetically generated shock waves are focused over the area of the renal stone. The high-energy dry shock waves pass through the skin and fragment the stone. (**C**) Percutaneous nephroli-thotomy is used to treat larger stones. A percutaneous tract is formed and a nephroscope is inserted through it. Then the stone is extracted or pulverized.

the tip of the lithotriptor is placed near the stone. The strength of the discharge and pulse frequency can be varied. This procedure is performed under topical anesthesia. After the stone is extracted, the percutaneous nephrostomy tube is left in place for a time to ensure that the ureter is not obstructed by edema or blood clots. The most common complications are hemorrhage, infection, and urinary extravasation. After the tube is removed, the nephrostomy tract closes spontaneously.

Chemolysis, stone dissolution using infusions of chemical solutions (eg, alkylating agents, acidifying agents) for the purpose of dissolving the stone, is an alternative treatment sometimes used in patients who are at risk for complications of other types of therapy, who refuse to undergo other methods, or who have stones (struvite) that dissolve easily. A percutaneous nephrostomy is performed, and the warm irrigating solution is allowed to flow continuously onto the stone. The irrigating solution exits the renal collecting system by means of the ureter or the nephrostomy tube. The pressure inside the renal pelvis is monitored during the procedure.

Several of these treatment modalities may be used in combination to ensure removal of the stones (Bihl & Meyers, 2001; Joshi, Kumar & Timoney, 2001; Liou & Streem, 2001).

Surgical removal was the major mode of therapy before the advent of lithotripsy. Today, however, surgery is performed in only 1% to 2% of patients. Surgical intervention is indicated if the stone does not respond to other forms of treatment. It may also be performed to correct anatomic abnormalities within the kidney to improve urinary drainage. If the stone is in the kidney, the surgery performed may be a nephrolithotomy (incision into the kidney with removal of the stone) or a nephrectomy, if the kidney is nonfunctional secondary to infection or hydronephrosis. Stones in the kidney pelvis are removed by a pyelolithotomy, those in the ureter by ureterolithotomy, and those in the bladder by cystotomy. If the stone is in the bladder, an instrument may be inserted through the urethra into the bladder, and the stone is crushed in the jaws of this instrument. Such a procedure is called a cystolitholapaxy (Maheshwari, Oswal & Bansal, 1999; Monga & Oglevie, 2000; Streem, 2000). Nursing management following kidney surgery is discussed in Chapter 44.

NURSING PROCESS:
THE PATIENT WITH KIDNEY STONES

Assessment

The patient with suspected renal stones is assessed for pain and discomfort as well as associated symptoms, such as nausea, vomiting, diarrhea, and abdominal distention. The severity and location of pain are determined, along with any radiation of the pain. Nursing assessment also includes observing for signs and symptoms of UTI (chills, fever, dysuria, frequency, and hesitancy) and obstruction (frequent urination of small amounts, oliguria, or anuria). The urine is inspected for blood and is strained for stones or gravel.

The history focuses on factors that predispose the patient to urinary tract stones or that may have precipitated the current episode of renal or ureteral colic. Predisposing factors include family history of stones, the presence of cancer or bone marrow disorders or the use of chemotherapeutic agents, inflammatory bowel disease, or a diet high in calcium or purines. Factors that may precipitate stone formation in the patient predisposed to renal calculi include episodes of dehydration, prolonged immobilization, and infection. The patient's knowledge about renal stones and measures to prevent their occurrence or recurrence is also assessed.

Diagnosis

NURSING DIAGNOSES

Based on the assessment data, the nursing diagnoses in the patient with renal stones may include the following:

- Acute pain related to inflammation, obstruction, and abrasion of the urinary tract
- Deficient knowledge regarding prevention of recurrence of renal stones

COLLABORATIVE PROBLEMS/
POTENTIAL COMPLICATIONS

Based on assessment data, potential complications that may develop include the following:

- Infection and sepsis (from UTI and pyelonephritis)
- Obstruction of the urinary tract by a stone or edema with subsequent acute renal failure

Planning and Goals

The major goals for the patient may include relief of pain and discomfort, prevention of recurrence of renal stones, and absence of complications.

Nursing Interventions

RELIEVING PAIN

Immediate relief of the severe pain from renal or ureteral colic is accomplished with the administration of opioid analgesic agents (intravenous or intramuscular administration may be prescribed to provide rapid relief) or NSAIDs (ie, ketorolac). The patient is encouraged and assisted to assume a position of comfort. If activity brings some pain relief, the patient is assisted to ambulate. The pain level is monitored closely, and increases in severity are reported promptly to the physician so that relief can be provided and additional treatment initiated. The patient is prepared for other treatment (eg, lithotripsy, percutaneous stone removal, ureteroscopy, or surgery) if severe pain is unrelieved and the stone is not passed spontaneously.

MONITORING AND MANAGING
POTENTIAL COMPLICATIONS

Because renal stones increase the risk for infection, sepsis, and obstruction of the urinary tract, the patient is instructed to report decreased urine volume and bloody or cloudy urine. The total urine output and patterns of voiding are monitored. Increased fluid intake is encouraged to prevent dehydration and increase hydrostatic pressure within the urinary tract to promote passage of the stone. If the patient cannot take adequate fluids orally, intravenous fluids are prescribed. Ambulation is encouraged as a means of moving the stone through the urinary tract.

Patients with calculi require frequent nursing observation to detect the spontaneous passage of a stone. All urine is strained through gauze because uric acid stones may crumble. Any blood clots passed in the urine should be crushed and the sides of the urinal and bedpan inspected for clinging stones. The patient is instructed to report any sudden increases in pain immediately because of the possibility of a stone fragment obstructing a ureter. Analgesic medications are administered as prescribed for the relief of pain and discomfort.

Vital signs, including temperature, are monitored closely to detect early signs of infection. UTIs may be associated with renal stones due to an obstruction from the stone or from the stone itself. All infections should be treated with the appropriate antibiotic agent before efforts are made to dissolve the stone (DeLeskey & Massi-Ventura, 2000).

PROMOTING HOME AND COMMUNITY-BASED CARE

Teaching Patients Self-Care

Because the risk of recurring renal stones is high, the nurse provides education about the causes of kidney stones and ways to prevent their recurrence (Chart 45-12). The patient is encouraged to follow a regimen to avoid further stone formation. One facet of prevention is to maintain a high fluid intake because stones form more readily in concentrated urine. A patient who has shown a tendency to form stones should drink enough fluid to excrete greater than 2,000 mL of urine every 24 hours (preferably 3,000 to 4,000 mL), should adhere to the prescribed diet, and should avoid sudden increases in environmental temperatures, which may cause a fall in urinary volume. Occupations and activities that produce excessive sweating can lead to severe temporary dehydration; therefore, fluid intake should be increased. Sufficient fluids should be taken in the evening to prevent urine from becoming too concentrated at night.

Urine cultures may be performed every 1 to 2 months the first year and periodically thereafter. Recurrent UTI is treated vigorously. Because prolonged immobilization slows renal drainage and alters calcium metabolism, increased mobility is encouraged whenever possible. In addition, excessive ingestion of vitamins (especially vitamin D) and minerals is discouraged.

If lithotripsy, percutaneous stone removal, ureteroscopy, or other surgical procedures for stone removal have been performed, the patient is instructed about the signs and symptoms of complications that need to be reported to the physician. The importance of follow-up to assess kidney function and to ensure the eradication or removal of all kidney stones is emphasized to the patient and family.

If the patient underwent ESWL, the nurse must provide instructions for home care and necessary follow-up. The patient is encouraged to increase fluid intake to assist in the passage of stone fragments, which may occur for 6 weeks to several months after the procedure. The patient and family are instructed about signs and symptoms that indicate complications, such as fever, decreasing urine output, and pain. It is also important to tell the patient to expect hematuria (it is anticipated in all patients), but it should disappear within 4 to 5 days. If the patient has a stent in the ureter,

hematuria may be expected until it is removed. The patient is instructed to notify the physician if nausea or vomiting, a temperature greater than 38°C, or pain unrelieved by the prescribed medication occurs. The patient is also informed that a bruise may be observed on the treated side of the back.

Continuing Care

The patient is monitored closely in follow-up care to ensure that treatment has been effective and that no complications, such as obstruction, infection, renal hematoma, or hypertension, have developed. During the patient's visits to the clinic or physician's office, the nurse has the opportunity to assess the patient's understanding of ESWL and possible complications. Additionally, the nurse has the opportunity to assess the patient's understanding of factors that increase the risk for recurrence of renal calculi and strategies to reduce those risks.

The patient's ability to monitor urinary pH and interpret the results is assessed during follow-up visits to the clinic or physician's office. Because of the high risk for recurrence, the patient with renal stones needs to understand the signs and symptoms of stone formation, obstruction, and infection and the importance of reporting these signs promptly. If medications are prescribed for the prevention of stone formation, the actions and importance of the medications are explained to the patient.

Evaluation

EXPECTED PATIENT OUTCOMES

Expected patient outcomes may include:

1. Reports relief of pain
2. States increased knowledge of health-seeking behaviours to prevent recurrence
   a. Consumes increased fluid intake (at least eight 227-g glasses of fluid per day)
   b. Participates in appropriate activity
   c. Consumes diet prescribed to reduce dietary factors predisposing to stone formation
   d. Recognizes symptoms to be reported to health care provider (fever, chills, flank pain, hematuria)
   e. Monitors urinary pH as directed
   f. Takes prescribed medication as directed to reduce stone formation
3. Experiences no complications
   a. Reports no signs or symptoms of sepsis or infection
   b. Voids 200 to 400 mL per voiding of clear urine without evidence of bleeding
   c. Experiences absence of dysuria, frequency, and hesitancy
   d. Maintains normal body temperature

Genitourinary Trauma

Various types of injuries of the flank, back, or upper abdomen may result in trauma to the kidney, ureter, bladder, or urethra. Trauma to the kidney accounts for about half of all cases of genitourinary trauma (Dreitlein, Suner & Basler, 2001).

RENAL TRAUMA

Normally, the kidneys are protected by the rib cage and musculature of the back posteriorly and by a cushion of abdominal

---

Chart 45-12 • PATIENT EDUCATION
Avoiding Recurrent Kidney Stones

- Follow prescribed diet closely.
- During the day, drink fluids (ideally water) every 1 to 2 hours.
- Drink two glasses of water at bedtime and an additional glass at each nighttime awakening to prevent urine from becoming too concentrated during the night.
- Avoid activities that cause excessive sweating and dehydration.
- Avoid sudden increases in environmental temperatures that may cause excessive sweating and dehydration.
- Contact primary health care provider at the first sign of a urinary tract infection.

wall and viscera anteriorly. They are highly mobile and are fixed only at the renal pedicle (stem of renal blood vessels and the ureter). With traumatic injury, the kidney can be thrust against the lower ribs, resulting in contusion and rupture. Rib fractures or fractures of the transverse process of the upper lumbar vertebrae may be associated with renal contusion or laceration. Injuries may be blunt (automobile and motorcycle crashes, falls, athletic injuries, assaults) or penetrating (gunshot wounds, stabbings). Failure to wear seat belts contributes to the incidence of renal trauma in motor vehicle crashes. Up to 80% of patients with renal trauma have associated injuries of other internal organs.

Renal trauma may be classified by the mechanism of injury: blunt or penetrating. Blunt renal trauma accounts for 80% to 90% of all renal injuries; penetrating renal trauma accounts for the remaining 10% to 20% (Bayerstock, Simons & McLoughlin, 2001). Blunt renal trauma is classified into one of four groups, as follows:

- Contusion: bruises or hemorrhages under the renal capsule; capsule and collecting system intact
- Minor laceration: superficial disruption of the cortex; renal medulla and collecting system are not involved
- Major laceration: parenchymal disruption extending into cortex and medulla, possibly involving the collecting system
- Vascular injury: tears of renal artery or vein

The most common renal injuries are contusions, lacerations, ruptures, and renal pedicle injuries or small internal lacerations of the kidney (Fig. 45-8). The kidneys receive half of the blood flow from the abdominal aorta; therefore, even a fairly small renal laceration can produce massive bleeding. About 70% of patients

are in shock when admitted to the hospital (Dreitlein et al., 2001).

Clinical manifestations include pain, renal colic (due to blood clots or fragments obstructing the collecting system), hematuria, mass or swelling in the flank, ecchymoses, and lacerations or wounds of the lateral abdomen and flank. Hematuria is the most common manifestation of renal trauma; its presence after trauma suggests renal injury. There is no relationship between the degree of hematuria and the degree of injury. Hematuria may not occur, or it may be detectable only on microscopic examination. Signs and symptoms of hypovolemia and shock are likely with significant hemorrhage.

URETERAL TRAUMA

Penetrating trauma and unintentional injury during surgery are the major causes of trauma to the ureters. Gunshot wounds account for 95% of ureteral injuries, which may range from contusions to complete transection. Unintentional injury to the ureter may occur during gynecologic or urologic surgery (Mathevet, Valencia, Cousin et al., 2001; Perez-Brayfield, Keane, Krishnan et al., 2001). There are no specific signs or symptoms of ureteral injury; many traumatic injuries are discovered during exploratory surgery. If the ureteral trauma is not detected and urine leakage continues, fistulas are likely to develop.

Intravenous urography detects 90% of ureteral injuries and can be performed on the operating table in patients undergoing emergent surgery. Surgical repair with placement of stents (to divert urine away from the anastomoses) is usually necessary.

BLADDER TRAUMA

Injury to the bladder may occur with pelvic fractures and multiple trauma or from a blow to the lower abdomen when the bladder is full. Blunt trauma may result in contusion evident as an ecchymosis—a large, discoloured bruise resulting from escape of blood into the tissues and involving a segment of the bladder wall—or in rupture of the bladder extraperitoneally, intraperitoneally, or both. Complications from these injuries include hemorrhage, shock, sepsis, and extravasation of blood into the tissues, which must be treated promptly (Morey, Iverson, Swan et al., 2001).

URETHRAL TRAUMA

Urethral injuries usually occur with blunt trauma to the lower abdomen or pelvic region. Many patients also have associated pelvic fractures. The classic triad of symptoms comprises blood at the urinary meatus, inability to void, and a distended bladder (Jordan, Jezior & Rosenstein, 2001).

Medical Management

The goals of management in patients with genitourinary trauma are to control hemorrhage, pain, and infection; to preserve and restore renal function; and to maintain urinary drainage. In renal trauma, all urine is saved and sent to the laboratory for analysis to detect RBCs and to evaluate the course of bleeding. Hematocrit and hemoglobin levels are monitored closely; decreasing values indicate hemorrhage.

The patient is monitored for oliguria and signs of hemorrhagic shock because a pedicle injury or shattered kidney can lead to

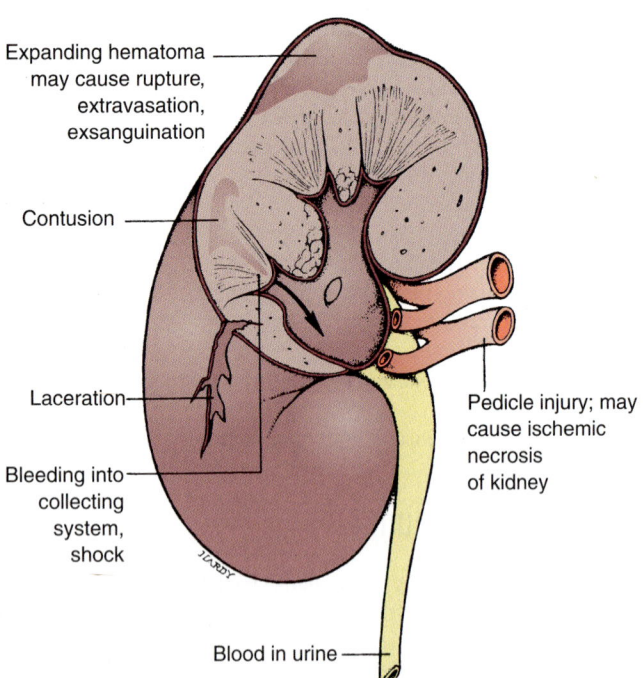

FIGURE 45-8 Types and pathophysiologic effects of renal injuries: contusions, lacerations, rupture, and pedicle injury.

Expanding hematoma may cause rupture, extravasation, exsanguination

Contusion

Laceration

Bleeding into collecting system, shock

Pedicle injury; may cause ischemic necrosis of kidney

Blood in urine

rapid exsanguination (lethal blood loss). An expanding hematoma may cause rupture of the kidney capsule. To detect hematoma, the area around the lower ribs, upper lumbar vertebrae, flank, and abdomen is palpated for tenderness. A palpable flank or abdominal mass with local tenderness, swelling, and ecchymosis suggests renal hemorrhage. The area of the original mass can be outlined with a marking pencil so that the examiner can evaluate the area for change.

Renal trauma is often associated with other injuries to the abdominal organs (liver, colon, small intestines); therefore, the patient is assessed for skin abrasions, lacerations, and entry and exit wounds of the upper abdomen and lower thorax because these may be associated with renal injury.

With renal trauma, such as a contusion of the kidney, healing may take place with conservative measures. If the patient has microscopic hematuria and a normal intravenous urogram, outpatient management is possible. If gross hematuria or a minor laceration is present, the patient is hospitalized and kept on bed rest until hematuria clears. Antimicrobial medications may be prescribed to prevent infection from perirenal hematoma or urinoma (a cyst containing urine). Patients with retroperitoneal hematomas may develop low-grade fever as absorption of the clot takes place.

SURGICAL MANAGEMENT

In renal trauma, any sudden change in the patient's condition may indicate hemorrhage and requires surgical intervention.

 NURSING ALERT Vital signs, urine output, and level of consciousness are monitored to detect bleeding and shock. Opioid analgesia is avoided because this may mask accompanying abdominal symptoms.

 NURSING ALERT The patient is prepared for immediate surgery in cases of increasing pulse rate, hypotension, and impending shock.

Depending on the patient's condition and the nature of the injury, major lacerations may be treated through surgical intervention or conservatively (bed rest, no surgery). Vascular injuries require immediate exploratory surgery because of the high incidence of involvement of other organ systems and the serious complications that may result if these injuries are untreated. The patient is often in shock and requires aggressive fluid resuscitation. The damaged kidney may have to be removed (nephrectomy).

Early postoperative complications (within 6 months) include rebleeding, perinephritic abscess formation, sepsis, urine extravasation, and fistula formation. Other complications include stone formation, infection, cysts, vascular aneurysms, and loss of renal function. Hypertension can be a complication of any renal surgery but usually is a late complication of renal injury.

In bladder trauma, treatment for rupture of the bladder involves immediate exploratory surgery and repair of the laceration, suprapubic drainage of the bladder and the perivesical space (around the bladder), and insertion of an indwelling urinary catheter. In addition to the usual care following urologic surgery, the drainage systems (suprapubic, indwelling urethral catheter, and perivesical drains) are closely monitored to ensure adequate drainage until healing takes place. The patient with a ruptured bladder may have gross bleeding for several days after repair.

In urethral trauma, unstable patients who need monitoring of urine output may need a suprapubic catheter inserted.

 NURSING ALERT If blood is seen at the urinary meatus, urethral catheterization should not be attempted until an emergency retrograde urethrogram can be performed.

The patient is catheterized after urethrography is performed to minimize the risk of urethral disruption and extensive, long-term complications, such as stricture, incontinence, and impotence. Surgical repair may be performed immediately or at a later time. Delayed surgical repair tends to be the favoured procedure because it is associated with fewer long-term complications, such as impotence, strictures, and incontinence. After surgery, an indwelling urinary catheter may remain in place for up to 1 month.

Nursing Management

The patient with genitourinary trauma (particularly renal trauma) should be assessed frequently during the first few days after injury to detect flank and abdominal pain, muscle spasm, and swelling over the flank.

During this time, patients can be instructed about care of the incision and the importance of an adequate fluid intake. In addition, instructions about changes that should be reported to the physician, such as fever, hematuria, flank pain, or any signs and symptoms of decreasing kidney function, are provided. Guidelines for increasing activity gradually, lifting, and driving are also provided in accordance with the physician's prescription.

Follow-up nursing care includes monitoring the blood pressure to detect hypertension and advising the patient to restrict activities for about 1 month after trauma to minimize the incidence of delayed or secondary bleeding. The patient should be advised to schedule periodic follow-up assessments of renal function (creatinine clearance, serum BUN and creatinine analyses). If a nephrectomy was necessary, the patient is advised to wear medical identification.

Urinary Tract Cancers

The Canadian Cancer Society and National Cancer Institute of Canada (2005) estimate that death rates from urinary tract cancers have levelled off over the last 5 years while incidence of these cancers shows a very slight downward trend. The incidence of bladder cancer for males shows a slower decrease of 22.7 per 100,000 in 2001 to 22.0 per 100,000 in 2005. The highest rate for this cancer in males was also reached in 1984 at 31.7 per 100,000. The male rate for bladder cancer deaths has stabilized at 7.2 per 100,000 for the last five years, down from 8.6 per 100,000 in the early 1980s. Urinary tract cancers include those of the urinary bladder, kidney and renal pelvis, ureter, and other urinary structures, such as the prostate. Prostate cancer is discussed in Chapter 49. Tobacco use continues to be a leading cause of all urinary tract cancers.

CANCER OF THE KIDNEY

Cancer of the kidney accounts for about 3% of all cancers in adults in Canada. It affects almost twice as many men as women. The most common type of renal tumour is renal cell or renal adenocarcinoma, accounting for more than 85% of all kidney tumours (Hock et al., 2002). These tumours may metastasize early to the lungs, bone, liver, brain, and contralateral kidney. One third of patients have metastatic disease at the time of diagnosis. The incidence of all stages of kidney cancer has increased in the last two decades in Canada. Although enhanced imaging techniques account for improved detection of early-stage kidney cancer, it is unknown why the rate of late-stage kidney cancers is higher (Hock, Lynch & Balaji, 2002) (Chart 45-13).

Clinical Manifestations

Many renal tumours produce no symptoms and are discovered on a routine physical examination as a palpable abdominal mass. The classic triad of signs and symptoms, which occurs in only 10% of patients, comprises hematuria, pain, and a mass in the flank. The usual sign that first calls attention to the tumour is painless hematuria, which may be either intermittent and microscopic or continuous and gross. There may be a dull pain in the back from the pressure produced by compression of the ureter, extension of the tumour into the perirenal area, or hemorrhage into the kidney tissue. Colicky pains occur if a clot or mass of tumour cells passes down the ureter. Symptoms from metastasis may be the first manifestations of renal tumour and may include unexplained weight loss, increasing weakness, and anemia.

Assessment and Diagnostic Findings

The diagnosis of a renal tumour may require intravenous urography, cystoscopic examination, nephrotomograms, renal angiograms, ultrasonography, or a CT scan. These tests may be exhausting for patients already debilitated by the systemic effects of a tumour as well as for elderly patients and those who are anxious about the diagnosis and outcome. The nurse assists the patient to prepare physically and psychologically for these procedures and monitors carefully for signs and symptoms of dehydration and exhaustion.

Medical Management

The goal of management is to eradicate the tumour before metastasis occurs (Kirkali, Tuzel & Munga, 2002).

SURGICAL MANAGEMENT

A radical nephrectomy is the preferred treatment if the tumour can be removed. This includes removal of the kidney (and tumour), adrenal gland, surrounding perinephric fat and Gerota's fascia, and lymph nodes. Radiation therapy, hormonal therapy, or chemotherapy may be used along with surgery. Immunotherapy may also be helpful. For patients with bilateral tumours or cancer of a functional single kidney, nephron-sparing surgery (partial nephrectomy) may be considered. Favourable results have been achieved in patients with small local tumours and a normal contralateral kidney.

Nephron-sparing surgery is increasingly being used to treat patients with solid renal lesions. The technical success rate of

Chart 45-13

Risk Factors for Renal Cancer

- Gender: Affects men more than women
- Tobacco use
- Occupational exposure to industrial chemicals, such as petroleum products, heavy metals, and asbestos
- Obesity
- Unopposed estrogen therapy
- Polycystic kidney disease

nephron-sparing surgery is excellent, and operative morbidity and mortality are low. For renal cell carcinoma, long-term cancer-free survival is comparable to that after radical nephrectomy, particularly for low-stage disease (Uzzo & Novick, 2001). Although laparoscopic nephroureterectomy is a lengthier surgical procedure, it has the same efficacy and is better tolerated by patients than open nephroureterectomy for upper tract transitional cell carcinoma. As more experience is gained with this type of surgery, surgical time will be reduced (Chen & Bagley, 2000; Jabbour, Desgrandchamps, Cazin et al., 2000; Shalhav, Dunn, Portis et al., 2000).

Renal Artery Embolization. In patients with metastatic renal carcinoma, the renal artery may be occluded to impede the blood supply to the tumour and thus kill the tumour cells. After angiographic studies are completed, a catheter is advanced into the renal artery, and embolizing materials (Gelfoam, autologous blood clot, steel coils) are injected into the artery and carried with the arterial blood flow to occlude the tumour vessels mechanically. This decreases the local blood supply, making removal of the kidney (nephrectomy) easier. It also stimulates an immune response because infarction of the renal cell carcinoma releases tumour-associated antigens that enhance the patient's response to metastatic lesions. The procedure may also reduce the number of tumour cells entering the venous circulation during surgical manipulation.

After renal artery embolization and tumour infarction, a characteristic symptom complex called postinfarction syndrome occurs, lasting 2 to 3 days. The patient has pain localized to the flank and abdomen, elevated temperature, and GI symptoms. Pain is treated with parenteral analgesic agents, and acetaminophen is administered to control fever. Antiemetic medications, restriction of oral intake, and intravenous fluids are used to treat the GI symptoms.

PHARMACOLOGIC THERAPY

Currently, no pharmacologic agents are in widespread use for treating renal cell carcinoma. Depending on the stage of the tumour, percutaneous partial or radical nephrectomy may be followed by treatment with chemotherapeutic agents. The use of biologic response modifiers such as interleukin-2 (IL-2) and topical instillation of bacillus Calmette-Guerin (BCG) in the renal pelvis continue to be studied, with both treatments currently used in clinical practice (Hvarness, Krarup & Eldrup, 2001; Nonomura, Ono, Nozawa et al., 2000; Okubo, Ichioka, Matsuta et al., 2001).

Patients may be treated with IL-2, a protein that regulates cell growth. This may be used alone or in combination with lymphokine-activated killer cells, which are WBCs that have been stimulated by IL-2 to increase their ability to kill cancer cells. Interferon, another biologic response modifier, appears to have a direct antiproliferative effect on renal tumours. The study of these biologic agents and new biologic response modifiers is a priority because nearly half of all patients with renal cell carcinoma die within 5 years of diagnosis (Pizza, De Vinci, LoConte et al., 2001).

Nursing Management

The patient with a renal tumour usually undergoes extensive diagnostic and therapeutic procedures, including surgery, radiation therapy, and medication (or systemic) therapy. After surgery, the patient usually has catheters and drains in place to maintain a patent urinary tract, to remove drainage, and to permit accurate measurement of urine output. Because of the location of the surgical incision, the position of the patient during surgery, and the nature of the surgical procedure, pain and muscle soreness are common.

The patient requires frequent analgesia during the postoperative period and assistance with turning. Turning, coughing, use of incentive spirometry, and deep breathing are encouraged to prevent atelectasis and other pulmonary complications. The patient and family require assistance and support to cope with the diagnosis and uncertainties about the prognosis. (See Chap. 44 for a discussion of postoperative care of the patient undergoing kidney surgery and Chap. 16 for discussion of care of the patient with cancer.)

PROMOTING HOME AND COMMUNITY-BASED CARE

Teaching Patients Self-Care. The patient is taught to inspect and care for the incision and perform other general postoperative care. Additionally, the patient learns about activity and lifting restrictions, driving, and use of pain medications. Instructions are provided about follow-up care and when to notify the physician about problems (fever, breathing difficulty, wound drainage, blood in the urine, pain or swelling of the legs).

The patient is encouraged to eat a well-balanced diet and to drink adequate liquids to avoid constipation and to maintain an adequate urine volume. Education and emotional support are provided related to the disease process, treatment plan, and continuing care because many patients are concerned about the loss of the other kidney, the possible need for dialysis, or the recurrence of cancer.

Continuing Care. Follow-up care is essential to detect signs of metastases and to reassure the patient and family about the patient's status and well-being. The patient who has had surgery for renal carcinoma should have a yearly physical examination and chest x-ray because late metastases are not uncommon. All subsequent symptoms should be evaluated with possible metastases in mind.

If follow-up chemotherapy is necessary, the patient and family are informed about the entire treatment plan or chemotherapy protocol, what to expect with each visit, and how to notify the physician. Periodic evaluation of remaining renal function (creatinine clearance, serum BUN and creatinine levels) may also be carried out periodically. A home care nurse may monitor the patient's physical status and psychological well-being and coordinate other services and resources needed by the patient.

CANCER OF THE BLADDER

Cancer of the urinary bladder is more common in people aged 50 to 70 years. It affects men more than women (3:1) and is more common in whites than in people of African descent. Bladder cancer is the fourth most prevalent type of cancer in Canadian men, accounting for 1150 deaths in Canada in 2005 (Canadian Cancer Society/National Cancer Institute of Canada, 2005). Bladder cancer has a high worldwide incidence (Amling, 2001). Bladder tumours account for nearly 3.4% of cancers diagnosed in Canada. There are two forms of bladder cancer: superficial (which tends to recur) and invasive. About 80% to 90% of all bladder cancers are transitional cell (which means they arise from the transitional cells of the bladder); the remaining types of tumours are squamous cell and adenocarcinoma. Research has demonstrated that many individuals with bladder cancer for which a total cystectomy is required go on to develop upper urinary tract tumours (Amling, 2001; Huguet-Perez, Palui, Millan-Rodriguez et al., 2001).

The predominant cause of bladder cancer today is cigarette smoking. Cancers arising from the prostate, colon, and rectum in males and from the lower gynecologic tract in females may metastasize to the bladder (Chart 45-14).

Clinical Manifestations

Bladder tumours usually arise at the base of the bladder and involve the ureteral orifices and bladder neck. Visible, painless hematuria is the most common symptom of bladder cancer. Infection of the urinary tract is a common complication, producing frequency, urgency, and dysuria. Any alteration in voiding or change in the urine, however, may indicate cancer of the bladder. Pelvic or back pain may occur with metastasis.

Assessment and Diagnostic Findings

The diagnostic evaluation includes cystoscopy (the mainstay of diagnosis), excretory urography, a CT scan, ultrasonography, and bimanual examination with the patient anesthetized. Biopsies of the tumour and adjacent mucosa are the definitive diagnostic procedures. Transitional cell carcinomas and carcinomas in situ shed recognizable cancer cells. Cytologic examination of fresh urine and saline bladder washings provide information about the prognosis, especially for patients at high risk for recurrence of primary bladder tumours (Amling, 2001).

Although mainstay diagnostic tools such as cytology and CT scanning have a high detection rate, they are costly. Newer diagnostic indicators are being studied. Bladder tumour antigens, nuclear matrix proteins, adhesion molecules, cytoskeletal proteins, and growth factors are being studied to support the early detection and diagnosis of bladder cancer. There are an increasing number of molecular assays available for the detection of bladder cancer (Saad, Hanbury, McNicholas et al., 2001).

Medical Management

Treatment of bladder cancer depends on the grade of the tumour (the degree of cellular differentiation), the stage of tumour growth (the degree of local invasion and the presence or absence of metastasis), and the multicentricity (having many centres) of the tumour. The patient's age and physical, mental, and emotional status are considered when determining treatment modalities.

SURGICAL MANAGEMENT

Transurethral resection or fulguration (cauterization) may be performed for simple papillomas (benign epithelial tumours). These procedures, described in more detail in Chapter 49, eradicate the

Chart 45-14
Risk Factors for Bladder Cancer

- Cigarette smoking: risk proportional to number of packs smoked daily and number of years of smoking
- Environmental carcinogens: dyes, rubber, leather, ink, or paint
- Recurrent or chronic bacterial infection of the urinary tract
- Bladder stones
- High urinary pH
- High cholesterol intake
- Pelvic radiation therapy
- Cancers arising from the prostate, colon, and rectum in males

tumours through surgical incision or electrical current with the use of instruments inserted through the urethra. After this bladder-sparing surgery, intravesical administration of BCG is the treatment of choice.

Management of superficial bladder cancers presents a challenge because there are usually widespread abnormalities in the bladder mucosa. The entire lining of the urinary tract, or urothelium, is at risk because carcinomatous changes can occur in the mucosa of the bladder, renal pelvis, ureter, and urethra. About 25% to 40% of superficial tumours recur after transurethral resection or fulguration. Patients with benign papillomas should undergo cytology and cystoscopy periodically for the rest of their lives because aggressive malignancies may develop from these tumours.

A simple **cystectomy** (removal of the bladder) or a radical cystectomy is performed for invasive or multifocal bladder cancer. Radical cystectomy in men involves removal of the bladder, prostate, and seminal vesicles and immediate adjacent perivesical tissues. In women, radical cystectomy involves removal of the bladder, lower ureter, uterus, fallopian tubes, ovaries, anterior vagina, and urethra. It may include removal of pelvic lymph nodes. Removal of the bladder requires a urinary diversion procedure.

Although radical cystectomy remains the standard of care for invasive bladder cancer in Canada, researchers are exploring trimodality therapy: transurethral resection of the bladder tumour, radiation, and chemotherapy. This is in an effort to spare patients the need for cystectomy. A trimodality approach to transitional cell bladder cancer mandates lifelong surveillance with cystoscopy. Although most completely responding patients retain their bladders free from invasive relapse, one quarter develop superficial disease. This may be managed with transurethral resection of the bladder tumour and intravesical therapies but carries an additional risk that late cystectomy will be required (Zietman, Grocela & Zehr, 2001; Zietman, Shipley & Kaufman, 2000).

PHARMACOLOGIC THERAPY

Chemotherapy with a combination of methotrexate, 5-fluorouracil, vinblastine, doxorubicin (Adriamycin), and cisplatin has been effective in producing partial remission of transitional cell carcinoma of the bladder in some patients. Intravenous chemotherapy may be accompanied by radiation therapy. The development of new chemotherapeutic agents such as gemcitabine and the taxanes has opened up promising new perspectives in the treatment of bladder cancer. However, the preliminary phase II data must be confirmed in adequately conducted phase III trials (Bellmunt & Albiol, 2001).

Topical chemotherapy (intravesical chemotherapy or instillation of antineoplastic agents into the bladder, resulting in contact of the agent with the bladder wall) is considered when there is a high risk for recurrence, when cancer in situ is present, or when tumour resection has been incomplete. Topical chemotherapy delivers a high concentration of medication (thiotepa, doxorubicin, mitomycin, ethoglucid, and BCG) to the tumour to promote tumour destruction. BCG is now considered the most effective intravesical agent for recurrent bladder cancer because it enhances the body's immune response to cancer.

Intravesical BCG is an immunotherapeutic agent that is given intravesically and is effective in the treatment of superficial transitional cell carcinoma. BCG has a 43% advantage in preventing tumour recurrence, a significantly better rate than the 16% to 21% advantage of intravesical chemotherapy. In addition, BCG is particularly effective in the treatment of carcinoma in situ, eradicating it in more than 80% of cases. In contrast to intravesical

chemotherapy, BCG has also been shown to decrease the risk of tumour progression.

The optimal course of BCG appears to be a 6-week course of weekly instillations, followed by a 3-week course at 3 months in tumours that do not respond. In high-risk cancers, maintenance BCG administered for 3 weeks every 6 months may limit recurrence and prevent progression (Amling, 2001). The adverse effects associated with this prolonged therapy, however, may limit its widespread applicability.

The patient is allowed to eat and drink before the instillation procedure, but once the bladder is full, the patient must retain the intravesical solution for 2 hours before voiding. At the end of the procedure, the patient is encouraged to void and to drink liberal amounts of fluid to flush the medication from the bladder.

RADIATION THERAPY

Radiation of the tumour may be performed preoperatively to reduce microextension of the neoplasm and viability of tumour cells, thus reducing the chances that the cancer may recur in the immediate area or spread through the circulatory or lymphatic systems. Radiation therapy is also used in combination with surgery or to control the disease in patients with an inoperable tumour. The transitional cell variety of bladder cancer responds poorly to chemotherapy. Cisplatin, doxorubicin, and cyclophosphamide have been administered in various doses and schedules and appear most effective.

Bladder cancer may also be treated by direct infusion of the cytotoxic agent through the bladder's arterial blood supply to achieve a higher concentration of the chemotherapeutic agent with fewer systemic toxic effects. For more advanced bladder cancer or for patients with intractable hematuria (especially after radiation therapy), a large, water-filled balloon placed in the bladder produces tumour necrosis by reducing the blood supply of the bladder wall (hydrostatic therapy). The instillation of formalin, phenol, or silver nitrate relieves hematuria and strangury (slow and painful discharge of urine) in some patients.

INVESTIGATIONAL THERAPY

The use of photodynamic techniques in treating superficial bladder cancer is under investigation. This procedure involves systemic injection of a photosensitizing material (hematoporphyrin), which the cancer cell picks up. A laser-generated light then changes the hematoporphyrin in the cancer cell into a toxic medication. This process is being investigated for patients in whom intravesical chemotherapy or immunotherapy has failed (Amling, 2001).

Urinary Diversions

Urinary diversion procedures are performed to divert urine from the bladder to a new exit site, usually through a surgically created opening (stoma) in the skin. These procedures are primarily performed when a bladder tumour necessitates removal of the entire bladder (cystectomy). Urinary diversion has also been used in managing pelvic malignancy, birth defects, strictures, trauma to ureters and urethra, neurogenic bladder, chronic infection causing severe ureteral and renal damage, and intractable interstitial cystitis and as a last resort in managing incontinence.

Controversy exists about the best method of establishing permanent diversion of the urinary tract. New techniques are frequently introduced in an effort to improve patient outcomes and quality of life. The age of the patient, condition of the bladder, body build, degree of obesity, degree of ureteral dilation, status of renal function, and the patient's learning ability and willingness to participate in postoperative care are all taken into consideration when determining the appropriate surgical procedure. Creating a reliable continence mechanism for a continent reservoir is a great challenge. The ability of urinary diversions to be continent devices for both ease of emptying and better quality of life has been the focus of research during recent years (Abol-Enein & Ghoneim, 2001; Deliveliotis, Alargoff, Skolarikos et al., 2001; Kane, 2000; Yachia & Erlich, 2001; Zinman, 1999).

The extent to which the patient accepts urinary diversion depends to a large degree on the location or position of the stoma, whether the drainage device (pouch or bag) establishes a watertight seal to the skin, and the patient's ability to manage the pouch and drainage apparatus. Paying attention to these considerations helps to promote a positive outcome (Kane, 2000).

There are two categories of urinary diversion: cutaneous urinary diversion, in which urine drains through an opening created in the abdominal wall and skin (Fig. 45-9), and **continent urinary diversion**, in which a portion of the intestine is used to create a new reservoir for urine (Fig. 45-10).

CUTANEOUS URINARY DIVERSIONS

Ileal Conduit (Ileal Loop)

The **ileal conduit,** the oldest of the urinary diversion procedures, is considered the gold standard because of the low number of complications and surgeons' familiarity with the procedure. In an ileal conduit, the urine is diverted by implanting the ureter into

A

Conventional ileal conduit. The surgeon transplants the ureters to an isolated section of the terminal ileum (ileal conduit), bringing one end to the abdominal wall. The ureter may also be transplanted into the transverse sigmoid colon (colon conduit) or proximal jejunum (jejunal conduit).

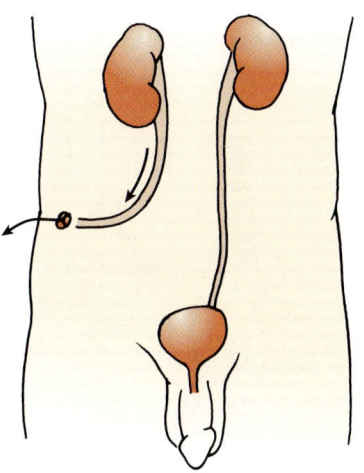

B

Cutaneous ureterostomy. The surgeon brings the detached ureter through the abdominal wall and attaches it to an opening in the skin.

C

Vesicostomy. The surgeon sutures the bladder to the abdominal wall and creates an opening (stoma) through the abdominal and bladder walls for urinary drainage.

D

Nephrostomy. The surgeon inserts a catheter into the renal pelvis via an incision into the flank or, by percutaneous catheter placement, into the kidney.

FIGURE 45-9 Types of cutaneous diversions include (**A**) the conventional ileal conduit, (**B**) cutaneous ureterostomy, (**C**) vesicostomy, and (**D**) nephrostomy.

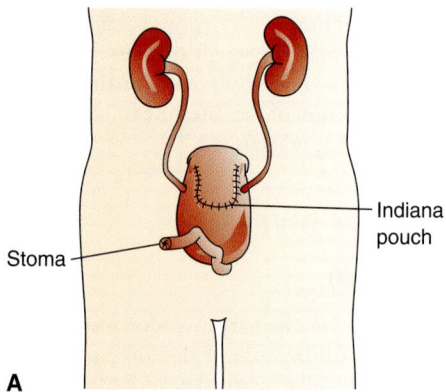

A

Indiana pouch. The surgeon introduces the ureters into a segment of ileum and cecum. Urine is drained periodically by inserting a catheter into the stoma.

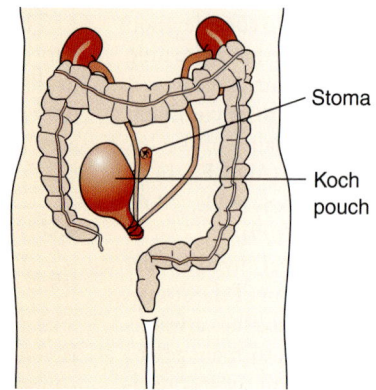

B

Continent ileal urinary diversions (Koch pouch). The surgeon transplants the ureters to an isolated segment of small bowel, ascending colon, or ileocolonic segment and develops an effective continence mechanism or valve. Urine is drained by inserting a catheter into the stoma.

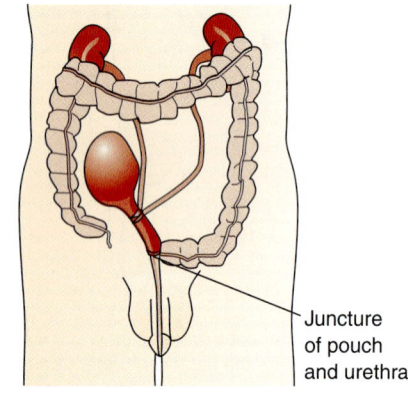

C

In male patients, the *Koch pouch* can be modified by attaching one end of the pouch to the urethra, allowing more normal voiding. The female urethra is too short for this modification.

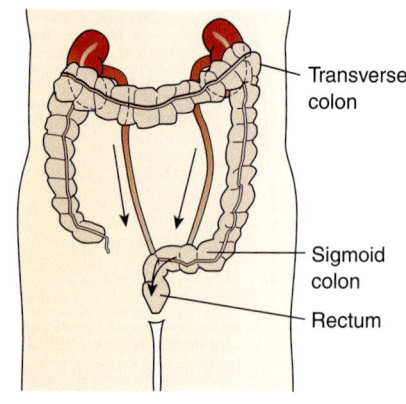

D

Ureterosigmoidostomy. The surgeon introduces the ureters into the sigmoid, thereby allowing urine to flow through the colon and out of the rectum.

FIGURE 45-10 Types of continent urinary diversions include (**A**) the Indiana pouch, (**B** and **C**) the Koch pouch, also called a continent ileal diversion, and (**D**) a ureterosigmoidostomy.

a 12-cm loop of ileum that is led out through the abdominal wall. This loop of ileum is a simple conduit (passageway) for urine from the ureters to the surface. A loop of the sigmoid colon may also be used. An ileostomy bag is used to collect the urine. The resected (cut) ends of the remaining intestine are anastomosed (connected) to provide an intact bowel.

Stents, usually made of thin, pliable tubing, are placed in the ureters to prevent occlusion secondary to postsurgical edema. The bilateral ureteral stents allow urine to drain from the kidney to the stoma and provide a method for accurate measurement of urine output. They may be left in place 10 to 21 days postoperatively. Jackson-Pratt tubes or other types of drains are inserted to prevent the accumulation of fluid in the space created by removal of the bladder.

After surgery, a skin barrier and a transparent, disposable urinary drainage bag are applied around the conduit and connected to drainage. A custom-cut appliance is used until the edema subsides and the stoma shrinks to normal size. The clear bag allows the stoma to be seen and the patency of the stent and the urine output to be monitored. The ileal bag drains urine constantly (not feces). The appliance (bag) usually remains in place as long as it is watertight; it is changed when necessary to prevent leakage of urine.

Complications that may follow placement of an ileal conduit include wound infection or wound dehiscence, urinary leakage, ureteral obstruction, hyperchloremic acidosis, small bowel obstruction, ileus, and stomal gangrene. Delayed complications include ureteral obstruction, contraction or narrowing of the stoma (stomal stenosis), renal deterioration due to chronic reflux, pyelonephritis, and renal calculi.

Nursing Management

In the immediate postoperative period, urine volumes are monitored hourly. An output below 30 mL/h may indicate dehydration or an obstruction in the ileal conduit, with possible backflow or leakage from the ureteroileal anastomosis. Throughout the patient's hospitalization, the nurse monitors closely for complications, reports signs and symptoms of them promptly, and intervenes quickly to prevent their progression.

PROMOTING URINE OUTPUT

A catheter may be inserted through the urinary conduit if prescribed to monitor the patient for possible stasis or residual urine from a constricted stoma. Urine may drain through the bilateral ureteral stents as well as around the stents. If the ureteral stents are not draining, the nurse may be instructed to irrigate them with 5 to 10 mL of sterile normal saline solution. It is important to avoid any tension on the stents because this may dislodge them. Hematuria may be noted in the first 48 hours after surgery but usually resolves spontaneously.

PROVIDING STOMA AND SKIN CARE

Because the patient requires specialized care, a consultation is initiated with an enterostomal therapist or clinical nurse specialist in skin care. The stoma is inspected frequently for colour and viability. A healthy stoma is beefy red. A change from this normal colour to a dark purplish colour suggests that the vascular supply may be compromised. If cyanosis and a compromised blood supply persist, surgical intervention may be necessary. The stoma is not sensitive to touch, but the skin around the stoma becomes sensitive if urine or the appliance irritates it. The skin is inspected for (1) signs of irritation and bleeding of the stomal mucosa, (2) encrustation and skin irritation around the stoma (from alkaline urine coming in contact with exposed skin), and (3) wound infections.

TESTING URINE AND CARING FOR THE OSTOMY

Moisture in bed linens or clothing or the odour of urine around the patient should alert the nurse to the possibility of leakage from the appliance, potential infection, or a problem in hygienic management. Because severe alkaline encrustation can accumulate rapidly around the stoma, the urine pH is kept below 6.5 by administration of ascorbic acid by mouth. Urine pH can be determined by testing the urine draining from the stoma, not from the collecting appliance. A properly fitted appliance is essential to prevent exposure of the peristomal skin (skin around the stoma) to urine. If the urine is foul-smelling, the stoma is catheterized, if prescribed, to obtain a urine specimen for culture and sensitivity testing.

ENCOURAGING FLUIDS AND RELIEVING ANXIETY

Because mucous membrane is used in forming the conduit, the patient may excrete a large amount of mucus mixed with urine. This causes many patients to feel anxious. To help relieve this anxiety, the nurse reassures the patient that this is a normal occurrence after an ileal conduit procedure. The nurse encourages adequate fluid intake to flush the ileal conduit and decrease the accumulation of mucus.

SELECTING THE OSTOMY APPLIANCE

Various urine collection appliances are available, and the nurse is instrumental in selecting an appropriate one. The urinary appliance may consist of one or two pieces and may be disposable (usually used once and discarded) or reusable. The choice of appliance is determined by the location of the stoma and by the patient's normal activity, manual dexterity, visual function, body build, economic resources, and preference.

> **! NURSING ALERT** All patients should be assessed for possible latex allergy. Latex appliances and drainage systems must not be used with patients with known or suspected latex allergy.

A reusable appliance has a faceplate that is attached to the skin surface with cement or adhesive. Either reusable pouches or disposable pouches may be used with the reusable faceplate. Disposable appliances have the advantages of having a surface that is already prepared for application to the skin and of being lightweight and easy to conceal. A skin barrier must be used to protect the skin from excoriation due to exposure to the urine.

PROMOTING HOME AND COMMUNITY-BASED CARE

Teaching Patients Self-Care. Patient education begins in the hospital but continues into the home setting because patients are usually discharged within days of surgery. The nurse teaches the patient how to assess and manage the urinary diversion as well as how to deal with body image changes. An enterostomal therapist is invaluable in consulting with the nurse on various aspects of care and patient education.

Changing the Appliance. The patient and family are taught to apply and change the appliance so that they are comfortable carrying out the procedure and can do so proficiently. Ideally, the appliance system is changed before the system leaks and at a time that is convenient for the patient. Many patients find early morning most convenient because the urine output is reduced. A variety of appliances are available; an average collecting appliance lasts 3 to 7 days before leakage occurs.

Regardless of the type of appliance used, a skin barrier is essential to protect the skin from irritation and excoriation. To maintain peristomal skin integrity, a skin barrier or leaking pouch is never patched with tape to prevent accumulation of urine under the skin barrier or faceplate. The patient is instructed to avoid moisturizing soaps when cleaning the area because they interfere with the adhesion of the pouch. Because the degree to which the stoma protrudes is not the same in all patients, there are various accessories and custom-made appliances to solve individual problems. Guidelines for applying reusable and disposable systems are presented in Chart 45-15.

Controlling Odour. The patient is instructed to avoid foods that give the urine a strong odour (eg, asparagus, cheese, eggs). Today, most appliances contain odour barriers, but a few drops of liquid deodourizer or diluted white vinegar may be introduced through the drain spout into the bottom of the pouch with a syringe or eyedropper to reduce odours. Ascorbic acid by mouth helps acidify the urine and suppress urine odour. Patients should be cautioned about putting aspirin tablets in the pouch to control odour because they may ulcerate the stoma. Also, the patient is reminded that odour will develop if the pouch is worn too long and not cared for properly.

Managing the Ostomy Appliance. The patient is instructed to empty the pouch by means of a drain valve when it is one-third full because the weight of the urine will cause the pouch to separate from the skin if filled more. Some patients prefer wearing a leg bag attached with an adapter to the drainage apparatus. To promote uninterrupted sleep, a collecting bottle and tubing (one unit) are snapped onto an adapter that connects to the ileal appliance. A small amount of urine is left in the bag when the adapter is attached to prevent the bag from collapsing against itself. The tubing may be threaded down the pajama or pants leg to prevent kinking. The collecting bottle and tubing are rinsed daily with cool water and once a week with a 3:1 solution of water and white vinegar.

Cleaning and Deodourizing the Appliance. Usually, the reusable appliance is rinsed in warm water and soaked in a 3:1 solution of water and white vinegar or a commercial deodourizing solution for

Chart 45-15 • PATIENT EDUCATION
Using Urinary Diversion Collection Appliances

Applying a Reusable Pouch System

1. Gather all necessary supplies.
2. Prepare new appliance according to the manufacturer's directions.
   - Apply double-faced adhesive disk that has been properly sized to fit the reusable pouch faceplate. Remove paper backing and lay pouch aside. *or:*
   - Apply thin layer of contact cement to one side of the reusable pouch faceplate. Lay pouch aside.
3. Remove soiled pouch gently. Lay aside to clean later.
4. Clean peristomal skin with small amount of soap and water. Rinse thoroughly and dry. If a film of soap remains on the skin and the site does not dry, the appliance will not adhere adequately.
5. Use a wick (rolled gauze pad or tampon) on top of the stoma to absorb urine and keep the skin dry throughout the appliance change.
6. Inspect peristomal skin (skin around stoma) for irritation.
7. A skin protector wipe or barrier ring may be applied before centreing the faceplate opening directly over the stoma.
8. Position appliance over stoma and press gently into place.
9. If desired, use a pouch cover or apply cornstarch under the pouch to prevent perspiration and skin irritation.
10. Clean soiled pouch and prepare for reuse.

Applying a Disposable Pouch System

1. Gather all necessary supplies.
2. Measure stoma and prepare an opening in the skin barrier about 1.6 mm larger than the stoma and the same shape as the stoma.
3. Remove paper backing from skin barrier and set aside.
4. Gently remove old appliance and set aside.
5. Clean peristomal skin with warm water and dry thoroughly.
6. Inspect peristomal skin (skin around stoma) for irritation.
7. Use a wick (rolled gauze pad or tampon) on top of the stoma to absorb urine and keep the skin dry during the appliance change.

8. Centre opening of skin barrier over stoma and apply with firm, gentle pressure to attain a watertight seal.
9. If using a two-piece system, snap pouch onto the flanged wafer that adheres to skin.
10. Close drainage tap or spout at bottom of pouch.
11. A pouch cover can be used or cornstarch applied under pouch to prevent perspiration and skin irritation.
12. Apply hypoallergenic tape around the skin barrier in a picture-frame manner.
13. Dispose of soiled appliance.

---

30 minutes. It is rinsed with tepid water and air-dried away from direct sunlight. (Hot water and exposure to direct sunlight dry the pouch and increase the incidence of cracking.) After drying, the appliance may be powdered with cornstarch and stored. Two appliances are necessary—one to be worn while the other is air-drying.

Continuing Care. Follow-up care is essential to determine how the patient has adapted to the body image changes and lifestyle changes. Referral for home care is indicated to determine how well the patient and family are coping with the changes necessitated by altered urinary drainage. The home care nurse assesses the patient's physical status and emotional response to urinary diversion. Additionally, the nurse assesses the ability of the patient and family to manage the urinary diversion and appliance, reinforces previous teaching, and provides additional information (eg, community resources, sources of ostomy supplies, insurance coverage for supplies).

As the postoperative edema subsides, the home care nurse assists in determining the appropriate changes needed in the ostomy appliance. The stoma opening is recalibrated every 3 to 6 weeks for the first few months postoperatively. The correct appliance size is determined by measuring the widest part of the stoma with a ruler. The permanent appliance should be no more than 1.6 mm larger than the diameter of the stoma and the same shape as the stoma to prevent contact of the skin with drainage.

The nurse encourages the patient and family to contact the United Ostomy Association of Canada and local ostomy association for visits, reassurance, and practical information. In addition, the local division of the Canadian Cancer Society can provide medical equipment and supplies and other resources for the patient who has undergone ostomy surgery for cancer.

The home care nurse also assesses the patient for potential long-term complications, such as ureteral obstruction, stomal stenosis, hernias, or deterioration of renal function, and reinforces previous teaching about these complications.

The nurse also needs to remind the patient who has had surgery for carcinoma to have a yearly physical examination and chest x-ray to assess for metastases. Periodic evaluation of remaining renal function (creatinine clearance, serum BUN and creatinine levels) is also essential. Long-term monitoring for anemia is performed to identify a vitamin B deficiency that may occur when a significant portion of the terminal ileum is removed. This may take several years to develop and can be treated with vitamin B injections. Additionally, the patient is reminded of the importance of participating in health promotion activities and recommended health screening.

Cutaneous Ureterostomy

A **cutaneous ureterostomy** (see Fig. 45-9), in which the ureters are directed through the abdominal wall and attached to an opening in the skin, is used for selected patients with ureteral obstruction (advanced pelvic cancer); for poor-risk patients, because it requires less extensive surgery than other urinary diversion procedures; and for patients who have had previous abdominal irradiation.

A urinary appliance is fitted immediately after surgery. The management of the patient with a cutaneous ureterostomy is similar to the care of the patient with an ileal conduit, although the stomas are usually flush with the skin or retracted.

Other Cutaneous Urinary Diversions

Other cutaneous urinary diversions are used less frequently and are most often used to bypass obstructions. Suprapubic bladder drainage (cystostomy) and nephrostomy are discussed further in Chapter 44.

CONTINENT URINARY DIVERSIONS

Continent Ileal Urinary Reservoir (Indiana Pouch)

The most common continent urinary diversion is the Indiana pouch, created for patients whose bladder is removed or can no longer function (neurogenic bladder). The Indiana pouch uses a segment of the ileum and cecum to form the reservoir for urine (see Fig. 45-10A). The ureters are tunnelled through the muscular bands of the intestinal pouch and anastomosed. The reservoir is made continent by narrowing the efferent portion of the ileum and sewing the terminal ileum to the subcutaneous tissue, forming a continent stoma flush with the skin. The pouch is sewn to the anterior abdominal wall around a cecostomy tube. Urine can collect in the pouch until a catheter is inserted and the urine is drained.

The pouch must be drained at regular intervals by a catheter to prevent absorption of metabolic waste products from the urine, reflux of urine to the ureters, and UTI. Postoperative nursing care of the patient with a continent ileal urinary pouch is similar to nursing care of the patient with an ileal conduit. However, these patients usually have additional drainage tubes (cecostomy catheter from the pouch, stoma catheter exiting from the stoma, ureteral stents, Penrose drain, as well as a urethral catheter), as depicted in Figure 45-11. All drainage tubes must be carefully monitored for patency and amount and type of drainage. The cecostomy tube is irrigated two or three times daily to remove mucus from the pouch and prevent blockage.

Other variations of continent urinary reservoirs include the Kock pouch (U-shaped pouch constructed of ileum, with a nipple-like one-way valve; see Fig. 45-10B and C) and the Charleston pouch (uses the ileum and ascending colon as the pouch, with the appendix and colon junction serving as the one-way valve mechanism). With both of these methods, the pouch must be drained at regular intervals by a catheter.

Line of incision

Penrose drain

Urethral catheter

Cecostomy catheter

Collection bags for drainage from ureteral stents and for bile

Stomal catheter drainage

FIGURE 45-11 After surgery to create a continent ileal urinary reservoir (Indiana pouch), the patient will have many drains and catheter devices in place.

Ureterosigmoidostomy

Ureterosigmoidostomy, another form of continent urinary diversion, is an implantation of the ureters into the sigmoid colon (see Fig. 45-10D). It is usually performed in patients who have had extensive pelvic irradiation, previous small bowel resection, or coexisting small bowel disease.

After surgery, voiding occurs from the rectum (for life), and an adjustment in lifestyle will be necessary because of urinary frequency (as often as every 2 hours). Drainage has a consistency equivalent to watery diarrhea, and the patient has some degree of nocturia. Patients usually need to plan activities around the frequent need to urinate, which in turn may affect the patient's social life. Patients have the advantage, however, of urinary control without having to wear an external appliance.

Nursing Management

In addition to the usual preoperative regimen, the patient may be placed on a liquid diet for several days preoperatively to reduce residue in the colon. Antibiotic agents (neomycin, kanamycin) are administered to disinfect the bowel. Ureterosigmoidostomy requires a competent anal sphincter, adequate renal function, and active renal peristalsis. The degree of anal sphincter control may be determined by assessing the patient's ability to retain enemas.

The postoperative regimen initially includes placing a catheter in the rectum to drain the urine and prevent reflux of urine into the ureters and kidneys. The tube is taped to the buttocks, and special skin care is given around the anus to prevent excoriation. Irrigations of the rectal tube may be prescribed, but force is never used because of the danger of introducing bacteria into the newly implanted ureters.

MONITORING FLUID AND ELECTROLYTES

In ureterosigmoidostomy, larger areas of the bowel mucosa are exposed to urine and electrolyte reabsorption. As a result, electrolyte imbalance and acidosis may occur. Potassium and magnesium in the urine may cause diarrhea. Fluid and electrolyte balance is maintained in the immediate postoperative period by closely monitoring the serum electrolyte levels and administering appropriate intravenous infusions. Acidosis may be prevented by placing the patient on a low-chloride diet supplemented with sodium potassium citrate.

The patient should be instructed never to wait longer than 2 to 3 hours before emptying urine from the intestine. This keeps rectal pressure low and minimizes the absorption of urinary constituents from the colon. It is essential to teach the patient about the symptoms of UTI: fever, flank pain, and frequency.

RETRAINING THE ANAL SPHINCTER

After the rectal catheter is removed, the patient learns to control the anal sphincter through special sphincter exercises. At first, urination is frequent. With reassurance and encouragement and the passage of time, the patient gains greater control and learns to differentiate between the need to void and the need to defecate.

PROMOTING DIETARY MEASURES

Specific dietary instructions include avoidance of gas-forming foods (flatus can cause stress incontinence and offensive odours). Other ways to avoid gas are to avoid chewing gum, smoking, and any other activity that involves swallowing air. Salt intake may be restricted to prevent hyperchloremic acidosis. Potassium intake is increased through foods and medication because potassium may be lost in acidosis.

MONITORING AND MANAGING POTENTIAL COMPLICATIONS

Pyelonephritis (upper UTI) due to reflux of bacteria from the colon is fairly common. Long-term antibiotic therapy may be prescribed to prevent infection. A late complication is adenocarcinoma of the sigmoid colon, possibly from cellular changes due to exposure of the colonic mucosa to urine.

Urinary carcinogens promote late malignant transformation of the colon after a ureterosigmoidostomy. Therefore, diligent patient teaching regarding the need for life-long medical follow-up is essential (Guy et al, 2001; Huang & McPherson, 2000).

OTHER URINARY DIVERSION PROCEDURES

Variations on urinary diversion surgical procedures are devised frequently in an effort to identify and perfect procedures that will improve patient outcomes and reduce the incidence of postoperative problems. These include cecal, patched cecal, and Mainz reservoirs. These techniques involve isolating a part of the large intestine to form a reservoir for urine and creating an abdominal stoma. Another surgical procedure, the Camey procedure, uses a portion of the ileum as a bladder substitute. In this procedure, the isolated ileum serves as the reservoir for urine; it is anastomosed directly to the portion of the remaining urethra after cystectomy. This procedure permits emptying of the bladder through the urethra. The Camey procedure, however, applies only to men because the entire urethra is removed when a cystectomy is performed in women.

NURSING PROCESS: THE PATIENT UNDERGOING URINARY DIVERSION SURGERY

Preoperative Assessment

The following are key preoperative nursing assessment concerns:

- Cardiopulmonary function assessments are performed because patients undergoing cystectomy (excision of the urinary bladder) are often older people who may not be able to tolerate a lengthy, complex surgical procedure.
- A nutritional status assessment is important because of possible poor nutritional intake related to underlying health problems.
- Learning needs are assessed to evaluate the patient's and the family's understanding of the procedure and the changes in physical structure and function that result from the surgery. The patient's self-concept and self-esteem are assessed, in addition to methods for coping with stress and loss. The patient's mental status, manual dexterity and coordination, and preferred method of learning are noted because they will affect postoperative self-care.

Preoperative Nursing Diagnoses

Based on the assessment data, the preoperative nursing diagnoses for the patient undergoing urinary diversion surgery may include the following:

- Anxiety related to anticipated losses associated with the surgical procedure
- Imbalanced nutrition, less than body requirements related to inadequate nutritional intake
- Deficient knowledge about the surgical procedure and postoperative care

Preoperative Planning and Goals

The major goals for the patient may include relief of anxiety, improved preoperative nutritional status, and increased knowledge about the surgical procedure, expected outcomes, and postoperative care.

Preoperative Nursing Interventions

RELIEVING ANXIETY

The threat of cancer and removal of the bladder create fears related to body image and security. The patient faces problems in adapting to an external appliance, a stoma, a surgical incision, and altered toileting habits. The male patient must also adapt to sexual impotency. (A penile implant is considered if the patient is a candidate for the procedure.) Women also fear altered appearance, body image, and self-esteem. A supportive approach, both physical and psychosocial, is needed and includes assessing the patient's self-concept and manner of coping with stress and loss; helping the patient to identify ways to maintain his or her lifestyle and independence with as few changes as possible; and encouraging the patient to express fears and anxieties about the ramifications of the upcoming surgery. A visitor from the United Ostomy Association of Canada can provide emotional support and make adaptation easier both before and after surgery.

ENSURING ADEQUATE NUTRITION

In addition to cleansing the bowel to minimize fecal stasis, decompress the bowel, and minimize postoperative ileus, a low-residue diet is prescribed and antibiotic medications are administered to reduce pathogenic flora in the bowel and to reduce the risk of infection. Because the patient undergoing a urinary diversion procedure for cancer may be severely malnourished due to the tumour, radiation enteritis, and anorexia, enteral or parenteral nutrition may be prescribed to promote healing. Adequate preoperative hydration is imperative to ensure urine flow during surgery and to prevent hypovolemia during the prolonged surgical procedure.

EXPLAINING SURGERY AND ITS EFFECTS

An enterostomal therapist is invaluable in preoperative teaching and in planning postoperative care. Explanations of the surgical procedure, the appearance of the stoma, the rationale for preoperative bowel preparation, the reasons for wearing a collection device, and the anticipated effects of the surgery on sexual functioning are part of patient teaching. The placement of the stoma site is planned preoperatively with the patient standing, sitting, or lying down to locate the stoma away from bony prominences, skin creases, and fat folds. The stoma should also be placed away from old scars, the umbilicus, and the belt line.

For ease of self-care, the patient must be able to see and reach the site comfortably. The site is marked with indelible ink so that it can be located easily during surgery. The patient is assessed for allergies or sensitivity to tape or adhesives. (Patch testing of certain appliances may be necessary before the ostomy equipment is selected. This is particularly important if the patient may be or is allergic to latex.) It may be helpful to have the patient practice wearing an appliance partially filled with water before surgery (Krupski & Theodorescu, 2001).

Preoperative Evaluation

To measure the effectiveness of care, the nurse evaluates the preoperative patient's anxiety level and nutritional status as well as his or her knowledge and expectations of surgery.

EXPECTED PATIENT OUTCOMES

Expected patient outcomes may include:

1. Exhibits reduced anxiety about surgery and expected losses
   a. Verbalizes fears with health care team and family
   b. Expresses positive attitude about outcome of surgery
2. Exhibits adequate nutritional status
   a. Maintains adequate intake before surgery
   b. Maintains body weight
   c. States rationale for enteral or parenteral nutrition if needed
   d. Exhibits normal skin turgor, moist mucous membranes, adequate urine output, and absence of excessive thirst
3. Demonstrates knowledge about the surgical procedure and postoperative course
   a. Identifies limitations expected after surgery
   b. Discusses expected immediate postoperative environment (tubes, machines, nursing surveillance)
   c. Practices deep breathing, coughing, and foot exercises

Postoperative Assessment

The role of the nurse in the immediate postoperative period is to prevent complications and to assess the patient carefully for any signs and symptoms of complications. The catheters and any drainage devices are monitored closely. Urine volume, patency of the drainage system, and colour of the drainage are assessed. A sudden decrease in urine volume or increase in drainage is reported promptly to the physician because these may indicate obstruction of the urinary tract, inadequate blood volume, or bleeding. In addition, the patient's needs for pain control are assessed (Colwell, Goldberg & Cramel, 2001).

Postoperative Diagnosis

NURSING DIAGNOSES

Based on the assessment data, the major postoperative nursing diagnoses for the patient following urinary diversion surgery may include the following:

- Risk for impaired skin integrity related to problems in managing the urine collection appliance
- Acute pain related to surgical incision
- Disturbed body image related to urinary diversion
- Potential for sexual dysfunction related to structural and physiologic alterations
- Deficient knowledge about management of urinary function

Collaborative Problems/ Potential Complications

Potential complications may include the following:

- Peritonitis due to disruption of anastomosis
- Stomal ischemia and necrosis due to compromised blood supply to stoma
- Stoma retraction and separation of mucocutaneous border due to tension or trauma

Postoperative Planning and Goals

The major goals for the patient may include maintaining peristomal skin integrity, relieving pain, increasing self-esteem, developing appropriate coping mechanisms to accept and deal with altered urinary function and sexuality, increasing knowledge about management of urinary function, and preventing potential complications (Krupski & Theodorescu, 2001; O'Shea, 2001).

Postoperative Nursing Interventions

Postoperative management focuses on monitoring urinary function, preventing postoperative complications (infection and sepsis, respiratory complications, fluid and electrolyte imbalances, fistula formation, and urine leakage), and promoting patient comfort. Catheters or drainage systems are observed, and urine output is monitored carefully. A nasogastric tube is inserted during surgery to decompress the GI tract and to relieve pressure on the intestinal anastomosis. It is usually kept in place for several days after surgery. As soon as bowel function resumes, as indicated by bowel sounds, the passage of flatus, and a soft abdomen, oral fluids are permitted. Until that time, intravenous fluids and electrolytes are administered. The patient is assisted to ambulate as soon as possible to prevent complications of immobility.

MAINTAINING PERISTOMAL SKIN INTEGRITY

Strategies to promote skin integrity begin with reducing and controlling those factors that increase the patient's risk for poor nutrition and poor healing. As indicated previously, meticulous skin care and management of the drainage system are provided by the nurse until the patient can manage them and is comfortable doing so. Care is taken to keep the drainage system intact to protect the skin from exposure to drainage. Supplies must be readily available to manage the drainage in the immediate postoperative period. Consistency in implementing the skin care program throughout the postoperative period will result in maintenance of skin integrity and patient comfort. Additionally, maintenance of skin integrity around the stoma will enable the patient and family to adjust more easily to the alterations in urinary function and will help them to learn skin care techniques.

RELIEVING PAIN

Analgesic medications are administered liberally postoperatively to relieve pain and promote comfort, thereby allowing the patient to turn, cough, and do deep-breathing exercises. Patient-controlled analgesia and administration of analgesic agents regularly around the clock are two options that may be used to ensure adequate pain relief. A pain-intensity scale is used to evaluate the adequacy of the medication and the approach to pain management.

IMPROVING BODY IMAGE

The patient's ability to cope with the changes associated with the surgery depends to some degree on his or her body image and self-esteem before the surgery and the support and reaction of others. Allowing the patient to express concerns and anxious feelings can help, especially in adjusting to the changes in toileting habits. The nurse can also help improve the patient's self-concept by teaching the skills needed to be independent in managing the urinary drainage devices. Education about ostomy care is conducted in a private setting to encourage the patient to ask questions without fear of embarrassment. Explaining why the nurse must wear gloves when performing ostomy care can prevent the patient from misinterpreting the use of gloves as a sign of aversion to the stoma.

EXPLORING SEXUALITY ISSUES

Patients who experience altered sexual function as a result of the surgical procedure may mourn for this loss. Encouraging the patient and partner to share their feelings about this loss with each other and acknowledging the importance of sexual function and expression may encourage the patient and partner to seek sexual counselling and to explore alternative ways of expressing sexuality. A visit from another "ostomate" who is functioning fully in society and family life may also assist the patient and family in recognizing that full recovery is possible.

MONITORING AND MANAGING POTENTIAL COMPLICATIONS

Complications are not unusual because of the complexity of the surgery, the underlying reason (cancer, trauma) for the urinary diversion procedure, and the patient's frequently less-than-optimal nutritional status. Complications may include the usual postoperative complications (eg, respiratory problems, such as atelectasis, fluid and electrolyte imbalances) as well as breakdown of the anastomoses, sepsis, fistula formation, fecal or urine leakage, and skin irritation. If these occur, the patient will remain hospitalized for an extended length of time and will probably require parenteral nutrition, GI decompression by means of nasogastric suction, and further surgery. The goals of management are to establish drainage, provide adequate nutrition for healing to occur, and prevent sepsis.

Peritonitis

Peritonitis can occur postoperatively if urine leaks at the anastomosis. Signs and symptoms include abdominal pain and distention, muscle rigidity with guarding, nausea and vomiting, paralytic ileus (absence of bowel sounds), fever, and leukocytosis.

Urine output must be monitored closely because a sudden decrease in amount with a corresponding increase in drainage from the incision or drains may indicate urine leakage. In addition, the urine drainage device is observed for leakage. The pouch is changed if a leak is observed. Small leaks in the anastomosis may seal themselves, but surgery may be needed for larger leaks.

Vital signs (blood pressure, pulse and respiratory rates, temperature) are monitored. Changes in vital signs, as well as increasing pain, nausea and vomiting, and abdominal distention, are reported to the physician and may indicate peritonitis.

Stomal Ischemia and Necrosis

The stoma is monitored because stomal ischemia and necrosis can result from tension on the mesentery blood vessels, twisting of the bowel segment (conduit) during surgery, or arterial insufficiency. The new stoma must be inspected at least every 4 hours to assess the adequacy of its blood supply. The stoma should be red or pink. If the blood supply to the stoma is compromised, the colour changes to purple, brown, or black. These changes are reported immediately to the physician. The physician or enterostomal therapist may insert a small, lubricated tube into the stoma and shine a flashlight into the lumen of the tube to assess for superficial ischemia or necrosis. A necrotic stoma requires surgical intervention. If the ischemia is superficial, the dusky stoma is observed and may slough its outer layer in several days.

Stomal Retraction and Separation

Stoma retraction and separation of the mucocutaneous border can occur as a result of trauma or tension on the internal bowel segment used for creation of the stoma. In addition, mucocutaneous separation can occur if the stoma does not heal as a result of accumulation of urine on the stoma and mucocutaneous border. Using a collection drainage pouch with an antireflux valve is helpful because the valve prevents urine from pooling on the stoma and mucocutaneous border. Meticulous skin care to keep the area around the stoma clean and dry promotes healing. If a separation of the mucocutaneous border occurs, surgery is not usually needed. The separated area is protected by applying karaya powder, stoma adhesive paste, and a properly fitted skin barrier and pouch. By protecting the separation, healing is promoted. If the stoma retracts into the peritoneum, surgical intervention is mandatory.

If surgery is needed to manage these complications, the nurse provides explanations to the patient and family. The need for additional surgery is usually perceived as a setback by the patient and family. Emotional support of the patient and family is provided along with physical preparation of the patient for surgery.

PROMOTING HOME AND COMMUNITY-BASED CARE

Teaching Patients Self-Care
A major postoperative objective is to assist the patient to achieve the highest level of independence and self-care possible. The primary nurse and enterostomal therapist work closely with the patient and family to instruct and assist them in all phases of managing the ostomy. Adequate supplies and complete instruction are necessary to enable the patient and a family member to develop competence and confidence in their skills. Written and verbal instructions are provided, and the patient is encouraged to contact the nurse or physician with follow-up questions. Follow-up telephone calls from the nurse to the patient and family after discharge may provide added support and provide another opportunity to answer their questions. Follow-up visits and reinforcement of correct skin care and appliance management techniques also promote skin integrity. Specific techniques for managing the appliance are described in Chart 45-15.

The patient is encouraged to participate in decisions regarding the type of collecting appliance and the time of day to change the appliance. The patient is assisted and encouraged to look at and touch the stoma early to overcome any fears. The patient and family need to know the characteristics of a normal stoma, as follows:

- Pink and moist, like the inside of the mouth
- Insensitive to pain because it has no nerve endings
- Vascular and may bleed when cleaned

Additionally, if a segment of the GI tract was used to create the urinary diversion, mucus may be visible in the urine. By learning what is normal, the patient and family become familiar with what signs and symptoms they should report to the physician or nurse and what problems they can handle themselves.

Information provided to the patient and the extent of involvement in self-care are determined by the patient's physical recovery and ability to accept and acquire the knowledge and skill needed for independence. Verbal and written instructions are provided, and the patient is given the opportunity to practice and demonstrate the knowledge and skills needed to manage urinary drainage.

Continuing Care
Follow-up care is essential to determine how the patient has adapted to the body image changes and lifestyle adjustments. Visits from a home care nurse are important to assess the patient's adaptation to the home setting and management of the ostomy. Teaching and reinforcement may assist the patient and family to cope with altered urinary function. It is also necessary to assess for long-term complications that may occur, such as pouch leakage

or rupture, stone formation, stomal stenosis, deterioration in renal function, or incontinence (Baker, 2001).

The following procedures are recommended for patients with a continent urinary diversion: pouch-o-gram (x-rays taken after a radioactive agent is instilled into the pouch) between 3 and 6 months, 9 and 12 months, 24 months, then every other year; renal function tests (BUN, serum creatinine) 1 month, 3 months, 6 months, then twice yearly; and pouchoscopy (endoscopic examination of the pouch) every year starting 5 to 7 years after surgery (Colwell, Goldberg & Cramel, 2001). The patient who has had surgery for carcinoma should have a yearly physical examination and chest x-ray to assess for metastases. In addition, the patient and family are reminded of the importance of participating in health promotion activities and recommended health screening.

Long-term monitoring for anemia is performed to identify vitamin B deficiency, which may occur when a significant portion of the terminal ileum is removed. This may take several years to develop and can be treated with vitamin B injections. The patient and family are informed of the United Ostomy Association of Canada and any local ostomy support groups to provide ongoing support, assistance, and education.

Postoperative Evaluation

EXPECTED PATIENT OUTCOMES
Expected patient outcomes may include:

1. Maintains skin integrity
   a. Maintains intact peristomal skin and demonstrates skill in managing drainage system and appliance
   b. Reports absence of pain or discomfort in peristomal area
   c. States actions to take if skin excoriation occurs
2. Exhibits increased knowledge about managing urinary function
   a. Participates in managing urinary system and skin care
   b. Verbally describes anatomic alteration due to surgery
   c. Revises daily routine to accommodate urinary drainage management
   d. Identifies potential problems, reportable signs and symptoms, and subsequent measures to take
3. Exhibits improved self-concept as evidenced by the following:
   a. Voices acceptance of urinary diversion, stoma, and appliance
   b. Demonstrates increasingly independent self-care, including hygiene and grooming
   c. States acceptance of support and assistance from family members, health care providers, and other ostomates
4. Copes with sexuality issues
   a. Verbalizes concern about possible alterations in sexuality and sexual function
   b. Reports discussion of sexual concerns with partner and appropriate counsellor
5. Demonstrates knowledge needed for self-care
   a. Performs self-care and proficient management of urinary diversion and appliance
   b. Asks questions relevant to self-management and prevention of complications
   c. Identifies signs and symptoms needing care from physician or other health care providers
6. Absence of complications as evidenced by the following:
   a. Reports absence of pain or tenderness in abdomen
   b. Has temperature within normal range

    c. Reports no urine leakage from incision or drains
    d. Has urine output within desired volume limits
    e. Maintains stoma that is red or pink, moist, and appropriately "budded"
    f. Has intact and healed stomal border

Other Urinary Tract Disorders

NEPHROSCLEROSIS

Nephrosclerosis is hardening, or sclerosis, of the arteries of the kidney due to prolonged hypertension. This causes decreased blood flow to the kidney and patchy necrosis of the renal parenchyma. Eventually, fibrosis occurs and glomeruli are destroyed. Nephrosclerosis is a major cause of ESRD (Segura, Campo, Rodicio & Ruilope, 2001).

Pathophysiology

There are two forms of nephrosclerosis: malignant (accelerated) and benign. Malignant nephrosclerosis is often associated with malignant hypertension (diastolic blood pressure higher than 130 mm Hg). It usually occurs in young adults, and men are affected twice as often as women. The disease process progresses rapidly. Without dialysis, more than half of patients die from uremia in a few years. Benign nephrosclerosis is usually found in older adults and is often associated with atherosclerosis and hypertension.

Assessment and Diagnostic Findings

Symptoms are rare early in the disease, even though the urine usually contains protein and occasional casts. Renal insufficiency and associated signs and symptoms occur late in the disease.

Medical Management

Treatment of nephrosclerosis is aggressive antihypertensive therapy. In hypertensive nephrosclerosis, therapy containing an ACE inhibitor, alone or in combination with other antihypertensive medications, significantly reduces the incidence of renal events. This effect is independent of blood pressure control (Segura et al., 2001).

HYDRONEPHROSIS

Hydronephrosis is dilation of the renal pelvis and calyces of one or both kidneys due to an obstruction.

Pathophysiology

Obstruction to the normal flow of urine causes the urine to back up, resulting in increased pressure in the kidney. If the obstruction is in the urethra or the bladder, the back pressure affects both kidneys, but if the obstruction is in one of the ureters because of a stone or kink, only one kidney is damaged.

Partial or intermittent obstruction may be caused by a renal stone that has formed in the renal pelvis but has moved into the ureter and blocked it. The obstruction may be due to a tumour pressing on the ureter or to bands of scar tissue resulting from an abscess or inflammation near the ureter that pinches it. The disorder may be due to an odd angle of the ureter as it leaves the renal pelvis or to an unusual position of the kidney, favouring a

ureteral twist or kink. In elderly men, the most common cause is urethral obstruction at the bladder outlet by an enlarged prostate gland. Hydronephrosis can also occur in pregnancy because of the enlarged uterus. High pressure in the bladder during the filling phase, generally 15 cm H_2O or higher, has been found to result in hydronephrosis, due to the high pressure radiating to one or both kidneys via the ureter (Ghobish, 2001).

Whatever the cause, as the urine accumulates in the renal pelvis, it distends the pelvis and its calyces. In time, atrophy of the kidney results. As one kidney undergoes gradual destruction, the other kidney gradually enlarges (compensatory hypertrophy). Ultimately, renal function is impaired.

Clinical Manifestations

The patient may not have symptoms if the onset is gradual. Acute obstruction may produce aching in the flank and back. If infection is present, dysuria, chills, fever, tenderness, and pyuria may occur. Hematuria and pyuria may be present. If both kidneys are affected, signs and symptoms of chronic renal failure may develop.

Medical Management

The goals of management are to identify and correct the cause of the obstruction, to treat infection, and to restore and conserve renal function. To relieve the obstruction, the urine may have to be diverted by nephrostomy (see Chap. 44) or another type of diversion. The infection is treated with antibiotic agents because residual urine in the calyces leads to infection and pyelonephritis. The patient is prepared for surgical removal of obstructive lesions (calculus, tumour, obstruction of the ureter). If one kidney is severely damaged and its function is destroyed, nephrectomy (removal of the kidney) may be performed.

URETHRITIS

Urethritis (inflammation of the urethra) is usually an ascending infection and may be classified as gonococcal or nongonococcal. Both conditions may be present in the same patient. Gonococcal urethritis and nongonococcal urethritis are the most common STDs in men in developed countries (Centers for Disease Control and Prevention, 2001).

Gonococcal urethritis is caused by *N. gonorrhoeae* and is transmitted by sexual contact. In men, inflammation of the urethral meatus or orifice occurs, with burning on urination. A purulent urethral discharge appears 3 to 14 days (or longer) after sexual exposure, although the disease is asymptomatic in up to 10% of men. The infection involves the tissues around the urethra, causing periurethritis, prostatitis, epididymitis, and urethral stricture. Sterility may occur as a result of vasoepididymal obstruction. Gonorrhea in women is frequently not diagnosed and reported because a urethral discharge is not always present and the disease may be asymptomatic. Treatment of gonorrhea is discussed and patient education information is provided in Chapter 70.

Nongonococcal urethritis is usually caused by *C. trachomatis* or *Ureaplasma urealyticum*. Male patients with symptoms usually complain of mild to severe dysuria and scant to moderate urethral discharge. Nongonococcal urethritis requires prompt treatment with tetracycline or doxycycline. In patients who do not respond to or who are allergic to the tetracyclines, erythromycin may be substituted. Follow-up care is necessary to make certain that a cure is achieved. All sexual partners of patients with nongonococcal urethritis should be examined for STDs and treated.

RENAL ABSCESS

Renal abscesses may be localized to the renal cortex (renal carbuncle) or extend into the fatty tissue around the kidney (perinephric abscess). The incidence of renal abscesses ranges from 1 to 10 cases per 10,000 hospital admissions in the United States.

Pathophysiology

A renal abscess may be caused by an infection of the kidney (pyelonephritis) or may occur as a hematogenous (spread through the bloodstream) infection originating elsewhere in the body. Offending organisms include *Staphylococcus* and *Proteus* species and *E. coli.* Occasionally, infection spreads from adjacent areas, such as with diverticulitis or appendicitis.

Clinical Manifestations

The manifestations of a perinephritic abscess often are acute in onset, with chills, fever, leukocytosis, a dull ache or palpable mass in the flank, abdominal pain with guarding, and CVA tenderness on palpation. The patient usually appears seriously ill.

Assessment and Diagnostic Findings

The patient with a renal abscess may report a recent history of a cutaneous boil or carbuncle and may complain of malaise, fever, chills, anorexia, weight loss, and a dull pain over the kidney. Leukocytosis and sterile urine (no microorganisms seen because the infection does not extend into the urinary collection system) are present with renal abscesses localized to the renal cortex. The CT examination results are important both in the diagnostic phase to establish the extent of the lesions and in the follow-up phase to assess the effectiveness of treatment (Dalla Palma, Pozzi-Mucelli & Ene, 1999).

Management

Small localized abscesses are usually cured by intravenous antibiotic medications alone but may require incision and drainage. Perinephritic abscesses require percutaneous drainage of the abscess. Culture and sensitivity tests are performed, and appropriate antibiotic therapy is prescribed. Drains are usually inserted and left in the perinephric space until all significant drainage has ceased. Because the drainage is often profuse, frequent changes of the outer dressings may be necessary. As in treating an abscess in any site, the patient is monitored for sepsis, fluid intake and output, and general response to treatment. Surgery may be indicated for extensive perinephritic abscesses.

TUBERCULOSIS OF THE URINARY TRACT

Pathophysiology

Tuberculosis of the urinary tract is caused by the organism *Mycobacterium tuberculosis* and is relatively rare in developed countries. The organism usually travels from the lungs by means of the bloodstream to the kidneys. On arrival in the kidney, the microorganism

may lie dormant for years. After the organism reaches the kidney, a low-grade inflammation and the characteristic tubercles are seen. If the organism continues to multiply, the tubercles enlarge to form cavities, with eventual destruction of parenchymal tissue. The organism spreads down the urinary tract into the bladder and may also infect the prostate, epididymis, and testicles in men.

Clinical Manifestations

At first, the signs and symptoms of renal tuberculosis are mild; there is usually a slight afternoon fever, weight loss, night sweats, loss of appetite, and general malaise. Hematuria (microscopic or gross) and pyuria may be present. Pain, dysuria, and urinary frequency, when they occur, are due to bladder involvement. Cavity formations and calcifications may be noted on an intravenous urogram.

Assessment and Diagnostic Findings

A search for tuberculosis elsewhere in the body is conducted when tuberculosis of the kidney or urinary tract is found. The patient is asked about possible exposure to tuberculosis. Three or more clean-catch, first-morning urine specimens are obtained for culture for *M. tuberculosis.* The erythrocyte sedimentation rate is usually elevated and is helpful in monitoring response to treatment.

Other diagnostic studies include intravenous urography, biopsy, and urine culture for acid-fast bacilli. Recent studies have shown that the polymerase chain reaction (PCR) provides a much faster diagnosis of urinary *M. tuberculosis.* It is a rapid, sensitive, and specific diagnostic method and avoids a delay in starting treatment (Hemal, Gupta, Rajeev et al., 2000).

Medical Management

The goal of treatment is to eradicate the offending organism. Combinations of ethambutol, isoniazid, and rifampin are used to delay the emergence of resistant organisms. Shorter-course chemotherapy (4 months) has been effective in eradicating the organism and in penetrating renal tissue. Surgical intervention may be necessary to treat obstruction and to remove an extensively diseased kidney. Because renal tuberculosis is a manifestation of a systemic disease, all measures to promote the general health of the patient are taken, including proper nutrition, adequate rest, and good hygiene practices. A scrotal support may be used by male patients with genital swelling.

Nursing Management

For the most part, nursing interventions focus on patient education to promote effective self-care at home and to prevent active recurrence or transmission of disease.

Instructions are provided about taking prescribed medications properly, recognizing adverse effects, and understanding the importance of completing the course of therapy. Instructions are also given regarding the nature of tuberculosis; its cause, spread, and treatment; and necessary follow-up care. Men are instructed to use condoms during sexual intercourse to prevent spread of the organisms; those with penile or urethral tuberculosis are instructed to abstain from intercourse during treatment. The patient is encouraged to maintain a healthy lifestyle with a well-balanced diet, adequate intake of fluids, and exercise.

Follow-up care is essential to reinforce the importance of taking medications exactly as prescribed (many patients do not take them correctly). The patient is counselled about the need for follow-up examinations (urine cultures, intravenous urograms), usually for 1 year. Treatment is reinstituted if a relapse occurs and the tubercle bacilli again invade the genitourinary tract. Because ureteral stenosis or bladder contractures may develop during healing, the patient is monitored for these complications.

URETHRAL STRICTURES

A urethral stricture is a narrowing of the lumen of the urethra as a result of scar tissue and contraction.

Pathophysiology

Common causes of strictures are urethral injury (caused by insertion of surgical instruments during transurethral surgery, indwelling catheters, or cystoscopic procedures), straddle injuries, and injuries associated with automobile crashes, untreated gonorrheal urethritis, and congenital abnormalities.

Assessment and Diagnostic Findings

The patient reports that the force and volume of the urinary stream are diminished, and symptoms of urinary infection and retention occur. Stricture causes urine to back up, resulting in cystitis, prostatitis, and pyelonephritis.

Prevention

An important element of prevention is to treat all urethral infections promptly. Prolonged urethral catheter drainage should be avoided and the utmost care taken in any type of instrumentation involving the urethra, including catheterization.

Medical Management

Treatment may include gradual dilation of the narrowed area (with metal sounds or bougies) or surgery (internal urethrotomy). If the stricture prevents the passage of a catheter, the urologist uses several small filiform bougies in search of the opening. When one bougie passes beyond the stricture into the bladder, it is fixed in place, and urine drains from the bladder. The opening then can be dilated, bypassing a larger sound (a dilating instrument), with the filiform then acting as a guide. After dilation, hot sitz baths and nonopioid analgesic agents are administered to control pain. Antibiotic medications are prescribed for several days after dilation to prevent infection.

Surgical excision or urethroplasty may be necessary for severe cases. A suprapubic cystostomy may be necessary in some patients. The postoperative management for cystostomy is described earlier in this chapter. Research studies using the diode laser to treat urethral strictures suggest that it is safe and reliable, especially as the first line of treatment (Kamal, 2001).

RENAL CYSTS

Renal cysts are abnormal, fluid-filled sacs that arise from the kidney tissue. They may be genetic in origin, acquired, or associated with a host of unrelated conditions. Cysts of the kidney may be single or multiple (polycystic), involving one or both kidneys. Polycystic disease of the adult is inherited as an autosomal dominant trait and affects men and women equally.

Autosomal Dominant Polycystic Kidney Disease

Autosomal dominant polycystic kidney disease is a common inherited condition, occurring in between 1 in 200 and 1 in 1,000 of the population. After diagnosis, patients are usually treated by nephrologists because of the risk of progression to ESRD. Almost two thirds (64%) of people with adult polycystic kidney disease also develop hematuria. Most episodes are due to UTIs and rupture of renal cysts that relate to the underlying anatomic abnormalities. The symptoms are usually short-lived and resolve with conservative measures such as rest and antibiotic treatment. Renal stone disease is also common, occurring in 20% of patients. Frank hematuria is also a presenting symptom of common, but unrelated, disorders that may occur coincidentally. These patients must be evaluated to rule out a genitourinary cancer because hematuria is also a presenting symptom of urinary tract cancer. Simple noninvasive diagnostic studies such as transabdominal ultrasound and urine cytology may demonstrate additional pathology that needs treatment to reduce further morbidity (Dedi, Bhandari, Turney et al., 2001).

Polycystic renal disease is also associated with cystic diseases of other organs (liver, pancreas, spleen) and aneurysms of the cerebral arteries. It has long been recognized that patients on long-term dialysis (both hemodialysis and peritoneal dialysis) develop multiple cysts on their nonfunctioning kidneys. Many of these cysts contain cancer cells.

Acquired Cystic Kidney Disease

An acquired form of polycystic disease occurring as a result of ESRD associated with dialysis is called acquired cystic kidney disease. While most of the cysts remain benign, serious complications can develop. Acquired cystic kidney disease has been associated with cyst infection, cyst hemorrhage, retroperitoneal hemorrhage, and spontaneous rupture of the kidney; therefore, it is important for the nurse to be aware of this variation of cystic kidney disease (Dedi, Bhandari, Turney et al., 2001; Headley & Wall, 1999).

Clinical Manifestations

The kidney gradually enlarges, with signs and symptoms becoming apparent in the fourth or fifth decade of life. The patient reports abdominal or lumbar pain. Hematuria, hypertension, palpable renal masses, and recurrent UTIs are additional manifestations. Renal insufficiency and failure usually develop in the end stages. Diagnosis of renal cysts is confirmed either by intravenous urography or CT scan.

Management

Because there is no specific treatment for polycystic renal disease, patient care focuses on relief of pain, symptoms, and complications. Hypertension and UTIs are treated aggressively. Dialysis (see Chap. 44) is initiated when signs and symptoms of renal insufficiency and failure occur. Genetic counselling is part of management with polycystic kidney disease that is genetic in origin. The patient is advised to avoid sports and occupations that present a risk for trauma to the kidney. Simple cysts of the kidney usually occur unilaterally and differ clinically and pathophysiologically from polycystic kidney disease. In such cases, the cyst may be drained percutaneously.

CONGENITAL ANOMALIES

Congenital anomalies of the kidney are not uncommon. Occasionally, there is fusion of the two kidneys, forming what is called a horseshoe kidney. One kidney may be small and deformed and is often nonfunctioning. The patient may have a double ureter or congenital stricture of the ureter. Treating these anomalies is necessary only if they cause symptoms, but it is essential to determine that the other kidney is present and functioning before surgery is undertaken.

INTERSTITIAL CYSTITIS

Interstitial cystitis, a chronic inflammatory condition of the bladder wall, frequently remains undiagnosed. The cause is unknown and no treatment is effective for all patients, although several treatments are available and most patients obtain some relief. More than 150,000 Canadians have interstitial cystitis (Association de la C.I. du Quebec, 2005). It can occur at any age and in all ethnic groups and both genders, although 90% of those affected are women. The average age at onset is 40, although one in four people affected is under age 30 at onset of symptoms. Preliminary results of studies of men with nonbacterial prostatitis indicate that many of them may also have interstitial cystitis (Interstitial Cystitis Association, 2001).

Pathophysiology

Although no single theory can explain the disorder, several pathophysiologic mechanisms may cause it, including changes in epithelial permeability, pelvic floor dysfunction, mastocytosis, activation of C-fibres, increase of nerve growth factors, and bradykinin. A decrease in the glycosaminoglycan (GAG) layer on the urothelium is thought to be a possible cause (Doggweiler-Wiygul, Blankenship & MacDiarmid, 2001).

Clinical Manifestations

Interstitial cystitis is characterized by severe, irritable voiding symptoms (day and night frequency, nocturia, urgency), pain and discomfort (suprapubic pressure, pain with bladder filling, suprapubic or perineal pain and pressure), and a markedly diminished bladder capacity. Some patients void more than 60 times a day. Sexual intercourse is often painful (Doggweiler-Wiygul et al., 2001).

Patients commonly present with multiple health problems that may be difficult to diagnose and may be associated with changes in the immune system. Patients with chronic fatigue syndrome, fibromyalgia, and temporomandibular disorder share many clinical illness features such as myalgia, fatigue, sleep disturbances, and impaired ability to perform activities of daily living as a consequence of these symptoms. Research findings suggest that various other chronic illnesses and pain syndromes may be associated with interstitial cystitis, including irritable bowel syndrome and chronic tension-type headache (Aaron, Burke & Buchwald, 2000).

Assessment and Diagnostic Findings

The diagnosis is made by excluding other causes of the symptoms. Diagnosis is complicated because there are no definitive diagnostic criteria. As a result, several years may pass and patients see an average of four or five physicians before the definitive diagnosis is made. The lack of more specific diagnostic criteria does not mean that interstitial cystitis is psychologically based; rather, it is a physical disorder with psychological consequences. Many patients have difficulty coping with the lack of a diagnosis, the inability of health care professionals to provide an explanation for their symptoms, and the persistence of symptoms.

Medical Management

Treatment strategies include use of medications that target pain and discomfort. Other therapies are used with the goal of repairing the bladder wall or their anti-inflammatory effects.

PHARMACOLOGIC THERAPY

Health Canada has approved the use of a bladder protectant, pentosan polysulfate sodium (Elmiron), which is given orally. Since its introduction, Elmiron has been the most effective agent; it is the only oral agent in its class. Intrabladder instillation of various compounds (eg, silver nitrate, dimethyl sulfoxide, oxychlorosene [Clorpactin]) may provide relief. About 50% of patients respond favourably to intravesicular instillation of dimethyl sulfoxide. Antispasmodic agents, such as oxybutynin (Ditropan), and urinary mucosal anesthetic agents, such as phenazopyridine (Pyridium), may be useful. Intravesicular heparin has some effect in decreasing symptoms in half of patients. Patients must be able to self-catheterize to instill the heparin on a daily basis initially, then three or four times weekly. Tricyclic antidepressant medications (doxepin and amitriptyline), which have central and peripheral anticholinergic actions, may decrease the excitability of smooth muscle in the bladder and reduce pain and discomfort.

OTHER THERAPY

Other treatments include transcutaneous electrical nerve stimulation (TENS) and destruction of ulcers with laser photoirradiation. Percutaneous sacral nerve stimulation is a means of neuromodulation to decrease the pelvic area pain and irritable bladder symptoms. Some women with intractable interstitial cystitis respond favourably to percutaneous sacral stimulation, with a significant improvement in pelvic pain, daytime frequency, nocturia, urgency, and average voided volume. Permanent sacral implantation can be an effective treatment modality in refractory interstitial cystitis; further long-term evaluation is required, although initial results are promising (Interstitial Cystitis Association, 2001).

Nursing Management

Often, the patient has experienced symptoms for a prolonged time. These symptoms prevent the patient from carrying out normal activities of daily living. The patient has usually been treated by a number of health care providers, often with little relief of symptoms. As a consequence, the patient may feel depressed, anxious, distrustful, and skeptical about proposed treatments.

 Critical Thinking Exercises

1. As the head nurse in a nursing home, you are approached by the daughter of one of the patients. She requests that her mother, who can ambulate with assistance, have an indwelling urinary catheter inserted "for convenience sake." Based on your knowledge regarding the effects of long-term indwelling catheter use, what would be your response?

2. Your patient is a 50-year-old woman who has been on hemodialysis for 7 years. On her baseline renal ultrasound, three small cysts were noted. She was recently started on anticoagulation therapy to maintain the patency of her venous access. This morning she presents for dialysis with severe flank pain. Identify possible causes of her pain and laboratory tests that would be indicated. What nursing assessment and interventions should you take at this time? What explanations would you give the patient while awaiting the results of laboratory tests?

3. Your 60-year-old patient has undergone a cystectomy and continent urinary diversion surgery. Your responsibility is to assist the patient in learning to manage the urinary diversion. Describe the postoperative patient teaching that you will provide to the patient and family. How will you modify the postoperative teaching if the patient and family have limited understanding of English? If the patient is blind?

4. A 35-year-old woman presents to the urinary clinic with complaints of frequent daytime urination with nearly constant voiding urgency without any incontinence, postcoital suprapubic discomfort, and nocturia (averaging three times a night). A urinalysis is negative for bacteria but reveals microscopic hematuria. A urodynamic study and office cystoscopy are scheduled to assess for interstitial cystitis. Outline the patient teaching you will provide to her about the diagnostic workup and about management of interstitial cystitis.

In such situations, the nurse assesses the patient's ability to cope with the disorder and provides psychological support. The nurse must convey a sense of acceptance to the patient and acknowledge the severity of the symptoms and their effect on the patient's lifestyle. The nurse also teaches the patient about diagnostic tests and treatment regimens (Degler, 2000).

REFERENCES AND SELECTED READINGS

Books

Brown, E. A., & Parfrey, P. S. (Eds.) (1999). *Complications of long-term dialysis.* New York: Oxford University Press.
Danovitch, G. M. (Ed.) (2000). *Handbook of kidney transplantation.* Philadelphia: Lippincott Williams & Wilkins.
Daugirdas, J. T., & Blake, P. G. (Eds.) (2000). *Handbook of dialysis.* New York: Little Brown & Co.
Gutch, C. F., Stoner, M. H., & Corea, A. L. (1999). *Review of hemodialysis for nurses and dialysis personnel* (6th ed.). St. Louis: Mosby.
Johnson, R. J., & Feehally, J. (2000). *Comprehensive clinical nephrology.* St. Louis: Mosby-Year Book.
Karlowicz, K. (1995). *Urologic nursing: Principles and practice.* Philadelphia: W. B. Saunders.
Metheny, N. (2000). *Fluid and electrolyte balance: Nursing considerations* (4th ed.). Philadelphia: Lippincott Williams & Wilkins.
Nicolle, L. (1994). Urinary tract infection. In P. O'Donnell (Ed.). *General urology* (pp. 399–412). Boston: Little, Brown, & Co.
Parker, J. (1998). *Contemporary nephrology nursing.* Pitman, NJ: Anthony J. Janetti.
Reilly, N. J. (Ed.) (2001). *Urologic nursing: A study guide* (2nd ed.). Pitman, NJ: Society of Urologic Nurses and Associates, Inc.
Schrier, R. W. (Ed.) (2000). *Manual of nephrology.* Philadelphia: Lippincott Williams & Wilkins.
Schwab, S. J. (Ed.) (2000). *2000 yearbook of nephrology, hypertension and mineral metabolism.* St. Louis: Mosby-Year Book.
Shapiro, R. (2000a). *Decision making in nephrology.* St. Louis: Mosby-Year Book.
Walsh, P., Retik, A., Vaughan, E., & Wein, A. (Eds.) (1997). *Campbell's urology* (7th ed.). Philadelphia: W. B. Saunders.

Journals

Asterisks indicate nursing research articles.
General
Bakris, G. L., Williams, M., Dworkin, L., et al. (2000). Special report: Preserving renal function in adults with hypertention and diabetes: A consensus approach. *American Journal of Kidney Diseases, 36*(3), 646–661.
Cely, C. M., & Contreras, G. (2001). Approach to the patient with hypertention, unexplained hypokalemia and metabolic alkalosis. *American Journal of Kidney Diseases, 37*(3), pE24.
Centers for Disease Control and Prevention. (2001). Evaluation of sexually transmitted disease control practices for male patients with urethritis at a large group practice affiliated with a managed care organization, Massachusetts, 1995–1997. *MMWR Morbidity & Mortality Weekly Report, 500*(22), 460–462
Criner, J. A., Appelt, M., Coker, C., et al. (2002). Rhabdomyolysis: The hidden killer. *MedSurg Nursing, 11*(3), 138–143, 155.
Dalla Palma, L., Pozzi-Mucelli, F., & Ene, V. (1999). Medical treatment of renal and perirenal abscesses: CT evaluation. *Clinical Radiology, 54*(12), 792–797.
Fink, J. C., Blahut, S. A., Reddy, M., & Light, P. D. (2001). Use of erythropoietin before the initiation of dialysis and its impact on mortality. *American Journal of Kidney Diseases, 37*(2), 348–355.
Ghobish, A. G. (2001). Storage detrusor pressure in bilateral hydroureteronephrosis. *European Urology, 39*(5), 571–574.
Hemal, A. K., Gupta, N. P., Rajeev, T. P., et al. (2000). Polymerase chain reaction in clinically suspected genitourinary tuberculosis: Comparison with intravenous urography, bladder biopsy, and urine acid-fast bacilli culture. *Urology, 56*(4), 570–574.
Kamal, B. A. (2001). The use of the diode laser for treating urethral strictures. *British Journal of Urology International, 877*(9), 831–833.
Kang, D. H., Anderson, S., Kim, Y. G., et al. (2001). Impaired angiogenesis in the aging kidney: Vascular endothelial growth factor and thrombospondin-1 in renal disease. *American Journal of Kidney Diseases, 37*(3), 601–611.
Myhre, M. J. (2000). Herbal remedies, nephropathies and renal disease. *Nephrology Nursing Journal, 27*(5), 473–478.
Nzerue, C. M., Hewan-Lowe, K., & Riley, Jr., L. J. (2000). Cocaine and the kidney: A synthesis of pathophysiologic and clinical perspectives. *American Journal of Kidney Diseases, 35*(5), 783–795.
O'Neill, W. C. (2000). Sonographic evaluation of renal failure. *American Journal of Kidney Diseases, 35*(6), 1021–1038.
Scolari, F., Tardanico, R., Zani, R., et al. (2000). Cholesterol crystal embolism: A recognizable cause of renal disease. *American Journal of Kidney Diseases, 36*(3), 1089–1109.
Segura, J., Campo, C., Rodicio, J. L., & Ruilope, L. M. (2001). ACE inhibitors and appearance of renal events in hypertensive nephrosclerosis. *Hypertension, 38*(3 Pt 2), 645–649.
Acute Renal Failure
Dillon, J. (1999). Continuous renal replacement therapy or hemodialysis for acute renal failure? *International Journal of Artificial Organs, 22*(3), 125–127.
Dirkes, S. M. (2000). Continuous renal replacement therapy: Dialytic therapy for acute renal failure in intensive care. *Nephrology Nursing Journal, 27*(6), 581–590.
Gambaro, G., Favaro, S., & D'Angelo, A. (2001). Risk for renal failure in nephrolithiasis. *American Journal of Kidney Diseases, 37*(2), 233–243.
Haas, M., Spargo, B. H., Wit, E. C., & Meehan, S. M. (2000). Etiologies and outcome of acute renal insufficiency in older adults: A renal biopsy study of 259 cases. *American Journal of Kidney Diseases, 35*(3), 433–447.

Lewis, J., Salem, M. M., Chertow, G. M., et al. (2000). Atrial natriuretic factor in oliguric acute renal failure. *American Journal of Kidney Diseases, 36*(4), 767–774.

Chronic Renal Failure

Barnas, U., Schmidt, A., Seidl, G., et al. (2001). A comparison of quantitative computed tomography and dual X-ray absorptiometry for evaluation of bone mineral density in patients on chronic hemodialysis. *American Journal of Kidney Diseases, 37,* 1247–1252.

Carey, H. B., Chorney, W., Pherson, K., et al. (2001). Continuous peritoneal dialysis and the extended care facility. *American Journal of Kidney Diseases, 37*(3), 580–587.

Fatica, R. A., Port, F. K., & Young, E. W. (2001). Incidence trends and mortality in end-stage renal disease attributed to renovascular disease in the United States. *American Journal of Kidney Diseases, 37*(6), 1184–1190.

Fink, J. C., Burdick, R. A., Kurth, S. J., et al. (1999). Significance of serum creatinine values in new end-stage renal disease. *American Journal of Kidney Diseases, 34*(4), 694–701.

Fored, C. M., Ejerblad, E., Lindblad, P., et al. (2001). Acetaminophen, aspirin, and chronic renal failure. *New England Journal of Medicine, 345*(25), 1801–1808.

Gunal, A. I., Duman, S., Ozkahya, M., et al. (2001). Strict volume control normalizes hypertension in peritoneal dialysis. *American Journal of Kidney Diseases, 37*(3), 588–593.

Headley, C. M., & Wall, B. (1999). Acquired cystic kidney disease in ESRD. *Nephrology Nursing Journal, 26*(4), 381–388.

Hou, S. (1999). Pregnancy in chronic renal insufficiency and end-stage renal disease. *American Journal of Kidney Diseases, 33*(2), 235–252.

Kalo, Z., Jarey, J., & Nagy, J. (2001). Economic evaluation of kidney transplantation versus hemodialysis in patients with end-stage renal disease. *Progress in Transplantation, 11*(3), 188–193.

Kausz, A. T., Khan, S. S., Abichandani, R., et al. (2001). Management of patients with chronic renal insufficiency in the Northeastern United States. *Journal of the American Society of Nephrology, 12*(7), 1501–1507.

McCoy, K. L., Goldstein, D. R., Gahtan, V., et al. (2001). Peripheral vascular disease intervention in patients with end-stage renal disease: Few complications in those treated with peritoneal dialysis. *Southern Medical Journal, 94*(10), 997–1001.

O'Neill, W. C. (2000). Sonographic evaluation of renal failure. *American Journal of Kidney Diseases, 35*(6), 1021–1038.

Perrone, R. D., Ruthazer, R., & Terrin, N. C. (2001). Survival after end-stage renal disease in autosomal dominant polycystic kidney disease: Contribution of extrarenal complications to mortality. *American Journal of Kidney Diseases, 38*(4), 777–784.

U.S. Renal Data System (2001). *USRDS 2001 Annual Data Report: Atlas of End-Stage Renal Disease in the United States.* National Institutes of Health, National Institute of Diabetes and Digestive and Kidney Diseases, Bethesda, MD.

Winkelmayer, W. C., Glynn, R. G., Levin, R., et al. (2001). Determinants of delayed nephrologist referral in patients with chronic kidney disease. *American Journal of Kidney Diseases, 38*(6), 1178–1184.

Wood, E. G., Hand, M., Briscoe, D. M., et al. (2001). Risk factors for mortality in infants and young children on dialysis. *American Journal of Kidney Diseases, 37*(3), 573–579.

Disorders of the Kidney

Canadian Institute of Health Information. (2004). *End-stage renal disease continues to climb among Canada's seniors, reports CIHI.* Available at: http://secure.cihi.ca/cihiweb/dispPage.jsp?cw_page=media_21jan2004_e. Retrieved May 29, 2005.

Dedi, R., Bhandari, S., Turney, J. H., et al. (2001). Causes of haematuria in adult polycystic kidney disease. *British Medical Journal, 323*(8), 386–387.

Deschenes, G., & Doucet, A. (2000). Collecting duct Na+/K+-ATPase activity is correlated with urinary sodium excretion in rat nephritic syndromes. *Journal of the American Society of Nephrology, 11*(4), 604–615.

Dunn, M. D., Portis, A. J., Elbahnasy, A. M., et al. (2000). Laparoscopic nephrectomy in patients with end-stage renal disease and

autosomal dominant polycystic kidney disease. *American Journal of Kidney Diseases, 35*(4), 720–725.

Fogo, A. (2000). Nephrotic syndrome: Molecular and genetic basis. *Nephron, 85*(1), 8–13.

Grampsas, S. A., Chandhoke, P. S., Fan, J., et al. (2000). Anatomic and metabolic risk factors for nephrolithiasis in patients with autosomal dominant polycystic kidney disease. *American Journal of Kidney Diseases, 36*(1), 53–57.

Kidney Foundation of Canada. (2002). *Polycystic kidney disease.* Available at: http://www.kidney.ca/english/publications/brochures/polycystic/polycystic.htm. Retrieved May 27, 2005.

Mattoo, T. K., & Mahmoud, M. A. (2000). Increased maintenance corticosteroids during upper respiratory infection decrease the risk of relapse in nephrotic syndrome.*Nephron, 85*(4), 343–345.

Moroni, G., Trendelenburg, M., Del Papa, N., et al. (2001). Anti-C1q antibodies may help in diagnosing a renal flare in lupus nephritis. *American Journal of Kidney Diseases, 37*(3), 490–498.

Winkelmayer, W. C., Eigner, M., Berger, O., et al. (2001). Optic neuropathy in uremia: An interdisciplinary emergency. *American Journal of Kidney Diseases, 37*(3), E23.

Genitourinary Trauma

Bayerstock, R., Simons, R., & McLoughlin, M. (2001). Severe blunt trauma: A 7-year retrospective review from a provinicial trauma centre. *Canadian Journal of Urology, 8*(5), 1372–1376.

Dreitlein, D. A., Suner, S., & Basler, J. (2001). Genitourinary trauma. *Emergency Medicine Clinics of North America, 19*(3), 569–590.

Jordan, G. H., Jezior, J. R., & Rosenstein, D. I. (2001). Injury to the genitourinary tract and functional reconstruction of the urethra. *Current Opinion in Urology, 11*(3), 257–261.

Mathevet, P., Valencia, P., Cousin, C., et al. (2001). Operative injuries during vaginal hysterectomy. *European Journal of Obstetrics Gynecology and Reproductive Biology, 97*(1), 71–75.

Morey, A. F., Iverson, A. J., Swan, A., et al. (2001). Bladder rupture after blunt trauma: Guidelines for diagnostic imaging. *Journal of Trauma, 51*(4), 683–686.

Perez-Brayfield, M. R., Keane, T. E., Krishnan, A., et al. (2001). Gunshot wounds to the ureter: A 40-year experience at Grady Memorial Hospital. *Journal of Urology, 166*(1), 119–121.

Interstitial Cystitis

Aaron, L. A., Burke, M. M., & Buchwald, D. (2000). Overlapping conditions among patients with chronic fatigue syndrome, fibromyalgia, and temporomandibular disorder. *Archives of Internal Medicine, 160*(2), 121–127.

Association de la C.I. du Quebec (2005). *Cystite interstitielle.* Available at: www.cystiteinterstitielle.org. Retrieved May 29, 2005.

Degler, M. (2000). Understanding interstitial cystitis. Protocol Driven Healthcare, Inc. Available at: http://www.MyBladder.com

Doggweiler-Wiygul, R., Blankenship, J., & MacDiarmid, S. A. (2001). Review on chronic pelvic pain from a urological point of view. *World Journal of Urology, 19*(3), 160–165.

Driscoll, A., & Teichman, J. M. H. (2001). How do patients with interstitial cystitis present? *Journal of Urology, 166*(6), 2118–2120.

Erickson, D. R., Morgan, K. C., Ordille, S., et al. (2001). Non-bladder related symptoms in patients with interstitial cystitis. *Journal of Urology, 166*(2), 557–562.

Interstitial Cystitis Association. (2001). Interstitial Cystitis Fact Sheet. Available at: http://www.ichelp.org/whatisic/welcome.html

Lutgendorf, S. K., Kreder, K. J., Rothrock, N. E., et al. (2000). Stress and symptomatology in patients with interstitial cystitis: A laboratory stress model. *Journal of Urology, 164*(4), 1265–1269.

Metts, J. F. (2001). Interstitial cystitis: Urgency and frequency syndrome. *American Family Physician, 64*(7), 1199–1206.

Michael, Y. L., Kawachi, I., Stampfer, M. J., et al. (2000). Quality of life among women with interstitial cystitis. *Journal of Urology, 164*(2), 423–427.

Kidney Transplantation

Baan, C. C., van Riemsdijk-Van Overbeeke, I. C., Balk, A. H., et al. (2001). Conversion from cyclosporin A to tacrolimus is safe and decreases blood pressure, cholesterol levels and TGF-beta1 type I receptor expression. *Clinical Transplantation, 5*(4), 276–283.

Canadian Organ Replacement Register/Canadian Institute for Health Information (2001). *CORR report—dialysis and renal transplantation, 2001.* Available at: http://secure.cihi.ca/cihiweb/dispPage.jsp?cw_page=PG_31_E&cw_topic=31&cw_rel=AR_5_E. Retrieved May 29, 2005.

Chan, L., Gaston, R., & Hariharan, S. (2001). Evolution of immunosuppression and continued importance of acute rejection in renal transplantation. *American Journal of Kidney Diseases, 38*(6 Suppl. 6), 2S–9S.

Cohen, D., & Galbraith, C. (2001). General health management and long-term care of the renal transplant recipient. *American Journal of Kidney Diseases, 38*(6 Suppl. 6), 10S–24S.

Gridelli, B., & Remuzzi, G. (2000). Strategies for making more organs available for transplantation. *New England Journal of Medicine, 343*(6), 404–410.

Hariharan, S., Johnson, C. P., Bresnahan, B. A., et al. (2000). Improved graft survival after renal transplantation in the United States, 1988 to 1996. *New England Journal of Medicine, 342*(9), 605–612.

*Hathaway, D. K., Wicks, M. N., Cashion, A. K., et al. (2000). Post-transplant improvement in heart rate variability correlates with improved quality of life. *Western Journal of Nursing Research, 22,* 749–768.

Heeger, P. S., & Hricik, D. (2002). Immune monitoring in kidney transplant recipients revisited. *Journal of the American Society of Nephrology, 13*(1), 288–290.

Hjelmesæth, J., Hartmann, A., Kofstad, J., et al. (2001). Tapering off prednisolone and cyclosporin the first year after renal transplantation: the effect on glucose tolerance. *Nephrology Dialysis Transplantation, 16*(4), 829–835.

Hricik, D. E., Halbert, R. J., Barr, M. L., et al. (2001). Life satisfaction in renal transplant recipients: Preliminary results from the Transplant Learning Center. *American Journal of Kidney Disease, 38*(3), 580–587.

Kalo, Z., Jarey, J., & Nagy, J. (2001). Economic evaluation of kidney transplantation verses hemodialysis in patients with end-stage renal disease. *Progress in Transplantation, 11*(3), 188–193.

Kouli, F., Morrell, C. H., Ratner, L. E., & Kraus, E. S. (2001). Impact of donor/recipient traits independent of rejection on long-term renal function. *American Journal of Kidney Diseases, 37*(2), 356–365.

Mange, K. C., Joffe, M. M., & Feldman, H. I. (2001). Effect of the use or nonuse of long-term dialysis on the subsequent survivor of renal transplants from living donors. *New England Journal of Medicine, 344*(10), 726–731.

McLaughlin, K., Manns, B., Culleton, B., et al. (2001). An economic evaluation of early versus late referral of patients with progressive renal insufficiency. *American Journal of Kidney Diseases, 38*(5), 1122–1128.

Najafian, N., Salama, A. D., Fedoseyeva, E. V., et al. (2002). Enzyme-linked immunosorbent spot assay analysis of peripheral blood lymphocyte reactivity to donor HLA-DR peptides: Potential novel assay for prediction of outcomes for renal transplant recipients. *Journal of the American Society of Nephrology, 13*(1), 252–259.

Shapiro, R. (2000b). Tacrolimus in renal transplatation. *Graft, 3*(2), 64–80.

Transplant Patient DataSource. United Network for Organ Sharing. http://www.unos.org.

Wijdicks, E. F. (2001). Neurotoxicity of immunosuppressive drugs. *Liver Transplantation, 7*(11), 937–942.

Tumours of the Urinary System and Urinary Diversions

Abol-Enein, H., & Ghoneim, M. A. (2001). Functional results of orthotopic ileal neobladder with serous-lined extramural ureteral reimplantation: Experience with 450 patients. *Journal of Urology, 165*(5), 1427–1432.

Amling, C. L. (2001). Diagnosis and management of superficial bladder cancer. *Current Problems in Cancer, 25*(4), 219–278.

Baker, C. P. (2001). The WOC nurse in home care. *Journal of Wound Ostomy Continence Nursing, 28*(6), 270–273.

Benson, M., & Olsson, C. (1999). Continent urinary diversion. *Urologic Clinics of North America, 26*(1), 125–147.

Bellmunt, J., & Albiol, S. (2001). New chemotherapy combinations for advanced bladder cancer. *Current Opinion in Urology, 11*(5), 517–522.

Canadian Cancer Society/National Cancer Institute of Canada (2005). *Canadian cancer statistics.* Available at: www.cancer.ca. Retrieved June 6, 2005.

Chang, S. S., Baumgartner, R. G., Wells, N., et al. (2002). Causes of increased hospital stay after radical cystectomy in a clinical pathway setting. *Journal of Urology, 167*(1), 208–211.

Chen, G. L., & Bagley, D. H. (2000). Ureteroscopic management of upper tract transitional cell carcinoma in patients with normal contralateral kidneys. *Journal of Urology, 164*(4), 1173–1176.

Colwell, J. C., Goldberg, M., & Cramel, J. (2001). The state of the standard diversion. *Journal of Wound Ostomy Continence Nursing, 28*(1), 6–17.

Deliveliotis, C., Alargoff, E., Skolarikos, A., et al. (2001). Modified ileal neobladder for continent urinary diversion: Experience and results. *Urology, 58*(5), 712–716.

*Floruta, C. V. (2001). Dietary choices of people with ostomies. *Journal of Wound Ostomy Continence Nursing, 28*(1), 28–31.

Guy, R. J., Handa, A., Traill, Z., & Mortensen, N. J. (2001). Rectosigmoid carcinoma at previous ureterosigmoidostomy site in a renal transplant recipient: Report of a case. *Diseases of the Colon & Rectum, 44*(10), 1534–1536.

Hara, I., Miyake, H., Hara, S., et al. (2002). Health-related quality of life after radical cystectomy for bladder cancer: A comparison of ileal conduit and orthotopic bladder replacement. *British Journal of Urology International, 89,* (1), 10–13.

Hart, S., Skinner, E. C., Meyerowitz, B. E., et al. (1999). Quality of life after radical cystectomy for bladder cancer in patients with an ileal conduit, cutaneous or urethral Koch pouch. *Journal of Urology, 162*(1), 77–81.

Hisataki, T., Miyao, N., Masumori, N., et al. (2001). Risk factors for multiple intravesical recurrences of superficial bladder cancer. *Urology, 58*(6), 935–939.

Hock, L. M., Lynch, J., & Balaji, K. C. (2002). Increasing incidence of all stages of kidney cancer in the last 2 decades in the United States: An analysis of surveillance, epidemiology and end results program data. *Journal of Urology, 167*(1), 57–60.

Huang, A., & McPherson, G. A. (2000). Colonic carcinoma after ureterosigmoidostomy. *Postgraduate Medical Journal, 76*(899), 579–581.

Huguet-Perez, J., Palou, J., Millan-Rodriguez, F., et al. (2001). Upper tract transitional cell carcinoma following cystectomy for bladder cancer. *European Urology, 40*(3), 318–323.

Hvarness, H., Krarup, T. & Eldrup, L. (2001). Long-term remission of transitional cell carcinoma after Bacillus Calmette-Guerin instillation in the renal pelvis. *Journal of Urology, 166*(5), 1829.

Jabbour, M. E., Desgrandchamps, F., Cazin, S., et al. (2000). Percutaneous management of grade II upper urinary tract transitional cell carcinoma: The long-term outcome. *Journal of Urology, 163*(4), 1105–1107.

Kane, A. M. (2000). Criteria for successful neobladder surgery: Patient selection and surgical construction. *Urologic Nursing, 20*(3), 182–188.

Kirkali, Z., Tuzel, E., & Munga, U. (2002). Recent advances in kidney cancer and metastatic disease. *British Journal of Urology International, 88*(8), 818–824.

Krupski, T., & Theodorescu, D. (2001). Orthotopic neobladder following cystectomy: Indications, management, and outcomes. *Journal of Wound Ostomy Continence Nursing, 28*(1), 37–46.

Matthews, S. D. & Courts, N. F. (2001). Orthotopic neobladder surgery. *American Journal of Nursing*, 101(7), 24AA–24GG.

Nonomura, N., Ono, Y., Nozawa, M., et al. (2000). Bacillus Calmette-Guerin perfusion therapy for the treatment of transitional cell carcinoma in situ of the upper urinary tract. *European Urology, 38*(6), 701–705.

Okubo, K., Ichioka, K., Matsuta, T. N., et al. (2001). Intrarenal Bacillus Calmette-Guerin therapy for carcinoma in situ of the upper urinary tract: Long-term follow-up and natural course in cases of failure. *British Journal of Urology International, 88*(4), 343–347.

O'Shea, H. S. (2001). Teaching the adult ostomy patient. *Journal of Wound Ostomy Continence Nursing, 28*(1), 47–54.

Pizza, G., De Vinci, C., LoConte, G., et al. (2001). Immunotherapy of metastatic kidney cancer. *International Journal of Cancer, 94*(1), 109–120.

Saad, A., Hanbury, D. C., McNicholas, T. A., et al. (2001). The early detection and diagnosis of bladder cancer: A critical review of the options. *European Urology, 39*(6), 619–633.

Shalhav, A. L., Dunn, M. D., Portis, A. J., et al. (2000). Laparoscopic nephroureterectomy for upper tract transitional cell cancer: The Washington University experience. *Journal of Urology, 163*(4), 1100–1104.

Uzzo, R. L., & Novick, A. C. (2001). Nephron-sparing surgery for renal tumors: Indications, techniques and outcomes. *Journal of Urology, 166*(1), 6–18.

Yachia, D., & Erlich, N. (2001). The Hadera continent reservoir: A new appendico-umbilical continent stoma mechanism for urinary diversion. *Journal of Urology, 165*(5), 1423–1426.

Zietman, A. L., Grocela, J., Zehr, E., et al. (2001). Selective bladder conservation using transurethral resection, chemotherapy, and radiation: Management and consequences of TA, T1, and TIS recurrence within the retained bladder. *Urology, 58*(3), 380–385.

Zietman, A. L., Shipley, W. U., & Kaufman, D. S. (2000). Organ-conserving approaches to muscle-invasive bladder cancer: Future alternatives to radical cystectomy. *Annals of Medicine, 32*(1), 34–42.

Zinman, L. (1999). Changing concepts in orthotopic urinary diversion. *Journal of Urology, 161*(6), 1807–1808.

Urinary Calculi

Assimos, D. G. (2001). Anatrophic nephrolithotomy. *Urology, 57*(1), 161–165.

Bihl, G., & Meyers, A. (2001). Recurrent renal stone disease: Advances in pathogenesis and clinical management. *Lancet, 358*(9282), 651–656.

DeLeskey, K. L., & Massi-Ventura, G. (2000). Management of the extracorporeal shock wave lithotripsy patient. *Journal of Perianesthesia Nursing, 15*(2), 94–101.

Gambaro, G., Favaro, S., & D'Angelo, A. (2001). Risk for renal failure in nephrolithiasis. *American Journal of Kidney Diseases, 37*(2), 233–243.

Joshi, H. B., Kumar, P. V., & Timoney, A. G. (2001). Citric acid (solution R) irrigation in the treatment of refractory infection (struvite) stone disease: Is it useful? *European Urology, 39*(5), 586–590.

Liou, L. S., & Streem, S. B. (2001). Long-term renal functional effects of shock wave lithotripsy, percutaneous nephrolithotomy and combination therapy: A comparative study of patients with solitary kidney. *Journal of Urology, 166*(1), 36–37.

Maheshwari, P. N., Oswal, A. T., & Bansal, M. (1999). Percutaneous cystolithotomy for vesical calculi: A better approach. *Technical Urology, 5*(1), 40–42.

Monga, M., & Oglevie, S. (2000). Minipercutaneous nephrolithotomy. *Journal of Endourology, 14*(5), 419–421.

Ryan, C., Hedgepeth, R. C., Yang, L., et al. (2001). Expression of proteins that inhibit calcium oxalate crystallization in vitro in the urine of normal and stone-forming individuals. *American Journal of Kidney Diseases, 37*(1), 104–112.

Streem, S. B. (2000). Percutaneous endopyelotomy. *Urology Clinics of North America, 27*(4), 685–693.

Tawfiek, E., & Bagley, D. (1999). Management of upper urinary tract calculi with ureteroscopic techniques. *Urology, 53*(1), 25–31.

Tombolini, P., Ruoppolo, M., Bellorofonte, C., et al. (2000). Lithotripsy in the treatment of urinary lithiasis. *Journal of Nephrology, 13*(suppl 3), S71–82.

Trinchieri, A., Zanetti, G., Curro, A., & Lizzano, R. (2001). Effect of potential renal acid load of foods on calcium metabolism of renal calcium stone formers. *European Urology, 39*(suppl 2), 33–37.

Williams, C. P., Child, D. F., Hudson, P. R., et al. (2001). Why oral calcium supplements may reduce renal stone disease: Report of a clinical pilot study. *Journal of Clinical Pathology, 54*(1), 54–62.

Urinary Tract Infections

Bonadio, M., Meini, M., Spitaleri, P., & Gigli, C. (2001). Current microbiological and clinical aspects of urinary tract infections. *European Urology, 40*(4), 439–445.

Bradley, S. F. (2002). *Staphylococcus aureus* infections and antibiotic resistance in older adults. *Clinical Infectious Disease, 34*(2), 211–216.

Foxman, B. (2002). Epidemiology of urinary tract infections: Incidence, morbidity, and economic costs. *American Journal of Medicine, 113* (Suppl. 1A), 5S–13S.

Gomolin, I. H., & McCue, J. D. (2000). Urinary tract infection in the elderly patient. *Infections in Urology, 13*(5A), s7–s13.

Gupta, K., Hooton, T. M., & Stamm, W. E. (2001). Increasing antimicrobial resistance and the management of uncomplicated community-acquired urinary tract infections. *Annals of Internal Medicine, 135*(1), 41–50.

Hooton, T. M., Scholes, D., Stapleton, A. E., et al. (2000). A prospective study of asymptomatic bacteriuria in sexually active young women. *New England Journal of Medicine, 343*(14), 992–997.

Jepson, R. G., Mihaljevic, L., & Craig, J. C. (2005). Cranberries for preventing urinary tract infections. Cochrane Renal Group. *Cochrane Database of Systematic Reviews, 4.*

Kidney Foundation of Canada, Northern Alberta and the Territories Branch. (2004). *Urinary tract infections (UTIs).* Available at: http://www.kidney.ab.ca/kidneys/utis.html. Retrieved May 26, 2005.

Lawrenson, R. A., & Logie, J. W. (2001). Antibiotic failure in the treatment of urinary tract infections in young women. *Journal of Antimicrobial Chemotherapy, 48*(6), 895–901.

Moore, K., Day, R.A., & Albers, M. (2002). Pathogenesis of urinary tract infections: A review. *Journal of Clinical Nursing, 11*, 568–574.

Raz, R. (2001). Postmenopausal women with recurrent UTI. *International Journal of Antimicrobial Agents, 17*(4), 269–271.

Raz, R., Chazan, B., & Dan, M. (2004). Cranberry juice and urinary tract infection. *Clinical Infectious Diseases, 38*, 1413–1419.

Raz, R., Gennesin, Y., Wasser, J., et al. (2000). Recurrent urinary tract infections in postmenopausal women. *Clinical Infectious Disease, 30*(1), 152–156.

Ronald, A. R., Nicolle, L. E., Stamm, E., et al. (2001). Urinary tract infection in adults: Research priorities and strategies. *International Journal of Antimicrobial Agents, 17*(4), 343–348.

Sabbuba, N., Hughes, G., & Stickler, D. J. (2002). The migration of *Proteus mirabilis* and other urinary tract pathogens over Foley catheters. *British Journal of Urology International, 89*(1), 55–60.

Stamm, W. E. (2001). An epidemic of urinary tract infections? *New England Journal of Medicine, 345*(14), 1055–1057.

Stamm, W., & Raz, R. (1999). Factors contributing to susceptibility of postmenopausal women to recurrent urinary tract infections. *Clinical Infectious Diseases, 28*, 723–725.

Talan, D. A., Stamm, W. E., & Hooton, T. M. (2000). Comparison of ciprofloxan (7 days) and trimethoprim-sulfamethoxazole (14 days) for acute uncomplicated pyelonephritis in women: A randomized trial. *Journal of the American Medical Association, 283*(12), 1583–1590.

Thees, K., & Dreblow, L. (1999). Trial of voiding: What's the verdict? *Urologic Nursing, 19*(1), 20–22.

Warren, J. W., Abrutyn, E., Hebel, R. J., et al. (1999). Guidelines for antimicrobial treatment of uncomplicated acute bacterial cystitis and acute pyelonephritis in women. *Clinical Infectious Diseases, 29*(4), 745–758.

Zandi-Nejad, K., & Brown, P. D. (2001). Diagnostic investigation of pyelonephritis. *Current Infectious Disease Reports, 3*(6), 529–533.

RESOURCES AND WEBSITES

American Association of Kidney Patients, 3505 E. Frontage Rd., Suite 315, Tampa, FL 33607; (800) 749-2257; http://www.aakp.org.

American Association of Nephrology Nurses, North Woodbury Road, Box 56, Pitman NJ 08071; (609) 589-2187; http://www.annanurse.com.

American Cancer Society, 1599 Clifton Rd. NE, Atlanta, GA 30329; (800) ACS-2345; http://www.cancer.org.

American Kidney Fund, 6110 Executive Blvd., Suite 1010, Rockville, MD 20852; (800) 638-8299; http://www.arbon.com/kidney.

Association de la C.I. du Quebec, 14 Grand-Coteau, Sainte-Julie, QC J3E 2X4; 450-922-6498; www.cystiteinterstitielle.org.

Canadian Association of Enterostomal Therapy, PO Box 48069, 60 Dundas Street E., Mississauga, ON L5A 1W4; www.caet.ca.

Canadian Association of Nephrology Nurses, 336 Yonge Street, Suite 322, Barrie, ON L4N 4C8; 705-720-2819; www.cannt.ca.

Canadian Association of Transplantation, University Campus, London Health Centre, 339 Windermere Road, London, ON N6A 5A5; www.transplant.ca.

Canadian Cancer Society and National Cancer Institute of Canada, 10 Alcorn Avenue, Suite 200, Toronto, ON M4V 3B1; 416-961-7223; www.cancer.ca.

Canadian Continence Foundation, PO Box 30, Victoria Branch, Westmount, QC H3Z 2V4; toll free: 800-265-9575; 514-488-9999; www.continence-fdn.ca.

Interstitial Cystitis Association, P.O. Box 1553, Madison Square Garden Station, New York, NY 10159; (212) 979-6057; http://www.ichelp.com.

Kidney Foundation of Canada, 300-5165 Sherbrooke Street West, Montreal, QC H4A 1T6; toll free: 800-361-7494; 514-369-4806; wwww.kidney.ca.

National Association for Patients on Hemodialysis and Transplantation, 211 East 43rd Street, Suite 301, New York, NY 10017; (212) 867-4486.

National Institute of Diabetes & Digestive and Kidney Diseases (NIDDK), National Institutes of Health, Building 31, Bethesda, MD 20892; http://www.niddk.nih.gov/index.htm.

National Kidney Foundation, 30 East 33rd St., New York, NY 10016; (212) 889-2210; http://www.kidney.org.

National Kidney and Urologic Diseases Information Clearinghouse, Box NKUDIC, 3 Information Way, Bethesda, MD, 20892; (800) 891-5390; (301) 654-4415; http://www.niddk.nih.gov/health/kidney/nkudic.htm.

United Ostomy Association of Canada, P.O. Box 825-50, Charles Street East, Toronto, ON M4Y 2N7; 416-595-5452; toll free: 1-888-969-9698; www.ostomycanada.ca.

Urology Nurses of Canada; www.unc.ca.

Wound, Ostomy and Continence Nurses Society (WOCN), 2755 Bristol Street, Suite 110, Costa Mesa, CA 92626; (714) 476-0268; http://www.wocn.org.

Reproductive Function

Applying Concepts from NANDA, NIC, and NOC

Mrs. Gates is a 43-year-old woman who has been undergoing cancer staging after positive breast biopsy results. The surgeon has informed her that she has stage IIB infiltrating ductal carcinoma. Her surgeon has informed her of the two different surgical approaches—breast conserving or modified radical mastectomy (MRM). If she chooses MRM, Mrs. Gates must decide whether she will undergo breast reconstruction or use a breast prosthesis. The nurse notes that Mrs. Gates is trembling and near tears. Mrs. Gates tells the nurse that she is uncertain about how her husband will respond if she chooses MRM. She is also concerned that she will not feel feminine after MRM but states she is very frightened about anything less since a friend died of metastatic breast cancer. The concept map illustrates the relationships that exist among selected nursing diagnoses, interventions, and outcomes for Mrs. Gates.

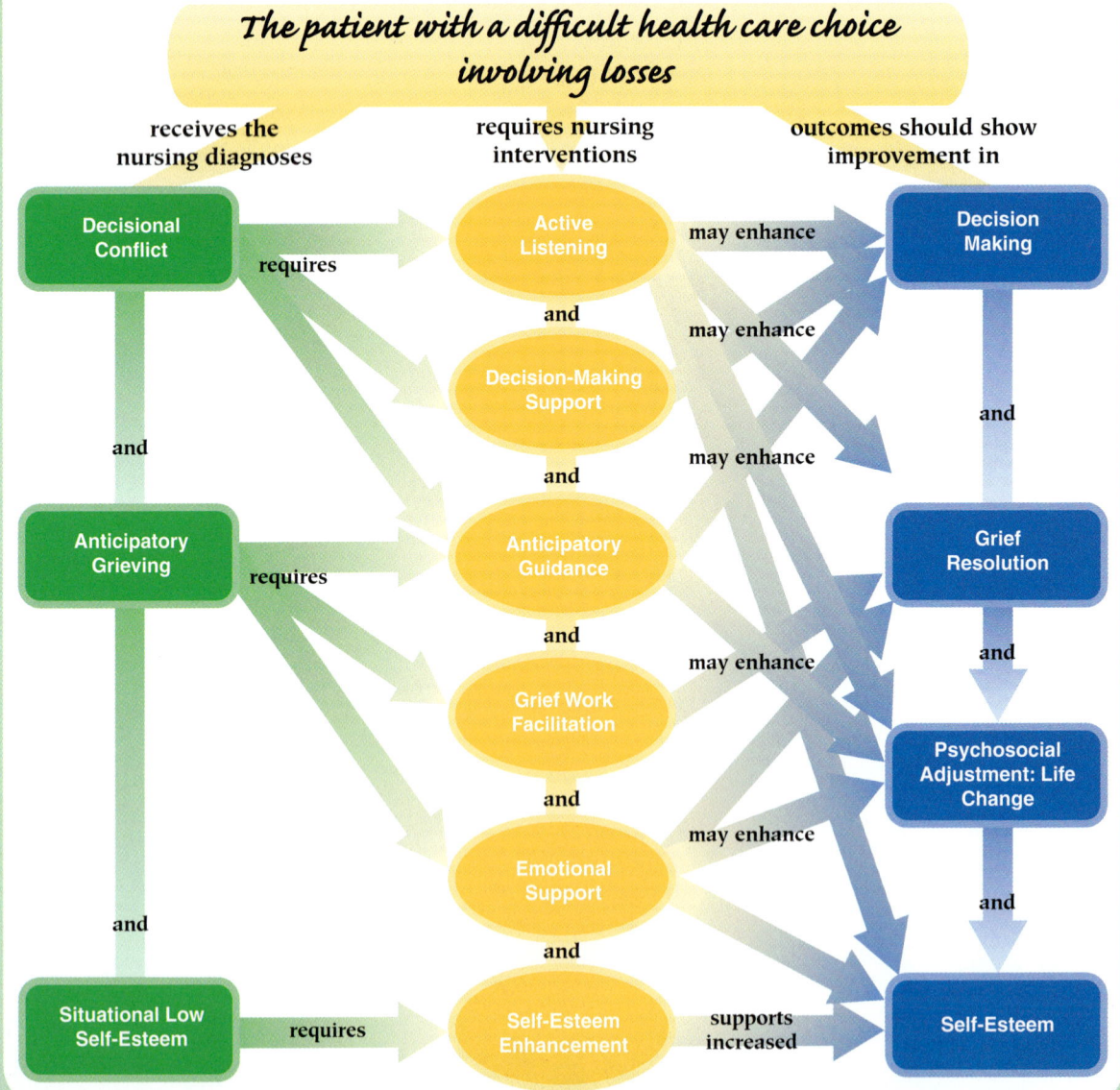

The patient with a difficult health care choice involving losses

Nursing Classifications and Languages

NANDA
Nursing Diagnoses

Decisional Conflict—Uncertainty about course of action to be taken when choice among competing actions involves risk, loss, or challenge to personal life values

Anticipatory Grieving—Intellectual and emotional responses and behaviours by which individuals, families, and communities work through the process of modifying self-concept based on the perception of potential loss

Situational Low Self-Esteem—Development of a negative perception of self-worth in response to a current situation (possible disfiguring surgery)

NIC
Nursing Interventions*

Active Listening—Attending closely to and attaching significance to a patient's verbal and nonverbal messages

Decision-Making Support—Providing information and support for a patient who is making a decision regarding health care

Anticipatory Guidance—Preparation of a patient for an anticipated developmental and/or situational crisis

Grief Work Facilitation—Assistance with the resolution of a significant loss

Emotional Support—Provision of reassurance, acceptance and encouragement during times of stress

Self-Esteem Enhancement—Assisting a person to increase his/her personal judgment of self-worth

NOC
Nursing Outcomes†

Return to functional baseline status, stabilization of, or improvement in

Decision Making—Ability to choose between two or more alternatives

Grief Resolution—Adjustment to actual or impending loss

Psychosocial Adjustment: Life Change—Psychosocial adaptation of an individual to a life change

Self-Esteem—Personal judgment of self-worth

NANDA, North American Nursing Diagnosis Association; NIC, Nursing Interventions Classification; NOC, Nursing Outcomes Classification.

*Iowa Intervention Project © 2000. In McCloskey, J. C., & Bulechek, G. M. (2000). *Nursing interventions classification (NIC)* (3rd ed.). St. Louis: Mosby.

†Iowa Outcomes Project © 2000. In Johnson, M., Maas, M., & Moorhead, S. (2000). *Nursing outcomes classification (NOC)* (3rd ed.). St. Louis: Mosby.

Assessment and Management of Female Physiologic Processes

Adapted by Jean Chow and Rene A. Day

LEARNING OBJECTIVES

On completion of this chapter, the learner will be able to:

1. Describe female reproductive function.
2. Describe approaches to effective sexual assessment.
3. Describe indicators of domestic violence and abuse of women and methods of identifying and treating women who are survivors of abuse.
4. Identify the diagnostic examinations and tests used to determine alteration in female reproductive function and describe the nurse's role before, during, and after these examinations and procedures.
5. Identify factors that cause disturbances of menstruation and related nursing implications.
6. Describe nursing care for patients with premenstrual syndrome.
7. Develop a teaching plan for women experiencing menopause.
8. Describe methods of contraception and implications for health care and education.
9. Describe the nursing management of the patient having an abortion.
10. Describe the causes and management of infertility.
11. Use the nursing process to plan for the care of patients with ectopic pregnancies.

Women's health is a unique specialty of health care. In addition to understanding normal female anatomy and physiology, the nurse needs to understand the physical, developmental, psychological, and social-cultural influences on women's health and use of health care. Health assessment, maintenance, and promotion across the life span must address growth and development, sexuality, contraception, preconception care, conception, prenatal care, effects of pregnancy on health, aging, perimenopause, menopause, and disorders that affect women. Further, the effects of disability on women's access to health care and the effect of disabilities and chronic illness on their health status must also be considered. Because women use the health care system more often than men and make up the majority of health care workers, addressing women's health needs and concerns will improve quality and access for all people.

Role of Nurses in Women's Health

As their presence in the labour market has increased, women have faced major changes in their roles, lifestyles, and family patterns. Moreover, they have encountered environmental hazards and stress, prompting them to focus greater attention on health and health-promoting practices. As a result, some women are taking a greater interest in and responsibility for their own health care. Many others do not have the time, finances, or other resources to do so.

Other changes over the years have included delaying pregnancy and childbearing until well after a career is established. Various methods of contraception have made this option possible. Advances in the treatment of infertility have enabled many women previously unable to have children to become pregnant and have extended the period of possible childbearing for couples well beyond their 40s. As women exercise greater control over their health care options, nurses are becoming more knowledgeable about preventive care for women, particularly with regard to their unique needs. The nurse encourages women to determine their own health goals and behaviours, teaches about health and illness, offers interventional strategies, and provides support, counselling, and ongoing monitoring. Areas of special interest in health promotion include the following:

- Personal hygiene
- Strategies for detecting and preventing disease, especially sexually transmitted diseases (STDs), including human immunodeficiency virus (HIV) infection
- Issues related to sexuality and sexual function, such as contraception; preconceptional, prenatal, and postnatal care; sexual satisfaction; and menopause
- Diet, exercise, and other health-promoting practices that maintain and enhance health
- Avoidance of stressful and abusive situations that are detrimental to health and well-being
- Maintaining a normal weight for height and avoiding substance abuse and smoking
- Avoidance of unhealthy lifestyle and risk behaviours

Nurses who promote healthy ways of living also need to model that lifestyle for their patients.

An important role of the nurse is promoting positive practices and behaviours related to the reproductive and sexual health of each patient, including the following:

- Providing information about scheduling regular examinations to promote health, detect health problems at an early

Glossary

adnexa: the fallopian tubes and ovaries

amenorrhea: absence of menstrual flow

androgens: hormones produced by the ovaries and adrenals that affect many aspects of female health, including follicle development, libido, oiliness of hair and skin, and hair growth

cervix: bottom (inferior) part of the uterus that is located in the vagina

chandelier sign: pain on gentle movement of the cervix; associated with pelvic infection

corpus luteum: site of a follicle that changes after ovulation to produce progesterone

cystocele: weakness of the anterior vaginal wall that allows the bladder to protrude into the vagina

dysmenorrhea: painful menstruation

dyspareunia: difficult or painful sexual intercourse

endometriosis: condition in which endometrial tissue implants in other areas of the pelvis; may produce dysmenorrhea or infertility

endometrium: mucous membrane lining the uterus

estrogen: hormone that develops and maintains the female reproductive system

follicle-stimulating hormone (FSH): hormone released by the pituitary gland

to stimulate estrogen production and ovulation

fornix: upper part of the vagina

fundus: body of the uterus

graafian follicle: cystic structure that develops on the ovary as ovulation begins

hymen: tissue that covers the vaginal opening partially or completely before vaginal penetration

hysteroscopy: a procedure performed using a long telescope-like instrument inserted through the cervix to diagnose uterine problems

introitus: opening to the vagina on the perineum

luteal phase: stage in the menstrual cycle in which the endometrium becomes thicker and more vascular

luteinizing hormone (LH): hormone released by the pituitary gland that stimulates progesterone production

menarche: beginning of menstrual function

menopause: permanent cessation of menstruation resulting from the loss of ovarian follicular activity

menstruation: sloughing and discharge of the lining of the uterus if conception does not take place

osteoporosis: a disorder in which bones lose density and become porous and fragile

ovaries: almond-shaped reproductive organs that produce eggs at ovulation and play a major role in hormone production

ovulation: discharge of a mature ovum from the ovary

perimenopause: the period immediately prior to menopause and the first year after menopause

polyp (cervical or endometrial): growth of tissue on the cervix or endometrial lining; usually benign

progesterone: hormone produced by the corpus luteum

proliferative phase: stage in the menstrual cycle before ovulation when the endometrium proliferates

rectocele: weakness of the posterior vaginal wall that allows the rectal cavity to protrude into the submucosa of the vagina

secretory phase: stage of the menstrual cycle in which the endometrium becomes thickened, more vascular, and edematous

uterine prolapse: relaxation of pelvic tone that allows the cervix and uterus to descend into the lower vagina stage, assess problems related to gynecologic and reproductive function, and discuss questions or concerns related to sexual function and sexuality

- Providing an open, nonjudgmental environment; this is crucial if the patient is to feel comfortable discussing personal issues. The nurse must convey understanding and sensitivity when discussing these issues and must assess their effects on the patient and the patient's partner.
- Recognizing signs and symptoms of abuse and screening all patients in a private and safe environment
- Recognizing cultural differences and beliefs and respecting sexual orientation and concerns related to both

Anatomic and Physiologic Overview

ANATOMY OF THE FEMALE REPRODUCTIVE SYSTEM

The female reproductive system consists of external and internal structures. Other anatomic structures that affect the female reproductive system include the hypothalamus and pituitary gland of the endocrine system.

External Genitalia

The external genitalia (the vulva) include two thick folds of tissue called the labia majora and two smaller lips of delicate tissue called the labia minora, which lie within the labia majora. The upper portions of the labia minora unite, forming a partial covering for the clitoris, a highly sensitive organ composed of erectile tissue. Between the labia minora, below and posterior to the clitoris, is the urinary meatus. This is the external opening of the female urethra and is about 3 cm long. The openings of Skene's (paraurethral) glands are on either side of the urethral meatus in a posterior position. Below the urinary meatus is a larger opening, the vaginal orifice or **introitus** (Fig. 46-1). On each side of the vaginal orifice is a vestibular (Bartholin's) gland, a bean-sized structure that empties its mucous secretion through a small duct. The opening of the duct lies within the labia minora, external to the hymen. The area between the vagina and rectum is called the perineum.

Internal Reproductive Structures

The internal structures consist of the vagina, uterus, ovaries, and fallopian or uterine tubes (Fig. 46-2).

VAGINA

The vagina, a canal lined with mucous membrane, is 7.5 to 10 cm long and extends upward and backward from the vulva to the cervix. Anterior to it are the bladder and the urethra, and posterior to it lies the rectum. The anterior and posterior walls of the vagina normally touch each other. The upper part of the vagina, the **fornix**, surrounds the **cervix** (the inferior part of the uterus).

UTERUS

The uterus, a pear-shaped muscular organ, is about 7.5 cm long and 5 cm wide at its upper part. Its walls are about 1.25 cm thick. The size of the uterus varies, depending on parity (number of viable births) and uterine abnormalities (eg, fibroids, which are a type of tumour that may distort the uterus). A nulliparous woman (one who has not completed a pregnancy to the stage of fetal viability) usually has a smaller uterus than a multiparous woman (one who has completed two or more pregnancies to the stage of fetal viability). The uterus lies posterior to the bladder and is held in position by several ligaments. The round ligaments extend anteriorly and laterally to the internal inguinal ring and down the inguinal canal, where they blend with the tissues of the labia majora. The broad ligaments are folds of peritoneum extending from the lateral pelvic walls and enveloping the fallopian tubes. The uterosacral ligaments extend posteriorly to the sacrum. The uterus has two parts: the cervix, which projects into the vagina, and a larger upper part, the **fundus** or body, which is covered posteriorly and partly anteriorly by peritoneum. The triangular inner portion of the fundus narrows to a small canal in the cervix that has constrictions at each end, referred to as the external os and internal os. The upper lateral parts of the uterus are called the cornua. From here, the oviducts or fallopian (or uterine) tubes extend outward, and their lumina are internally continuous with the uterine cavity.

OVARIES

The **ovaries** lie behind the broad ligaments, behind and below the fallopian tubes. They are oval bodies about 3 cm long. At birth, they contain thousands of tiny egg cells, or ova. The ovaries and the fallopian tubes together are referred to as the **adnexa**.

FUNCTION OF THE FEMALE REPRODUCTIVE SYSTEM

Ovulation

At puberty (usually between ages 12 and 14, but earlier for some; 10 or 11 years of age is not uncommon), the ova begin to mature. During a period known as the follicular phase, an ovum enlarges as a type of cyst called a **graafian follicle** until it reaches the sur-

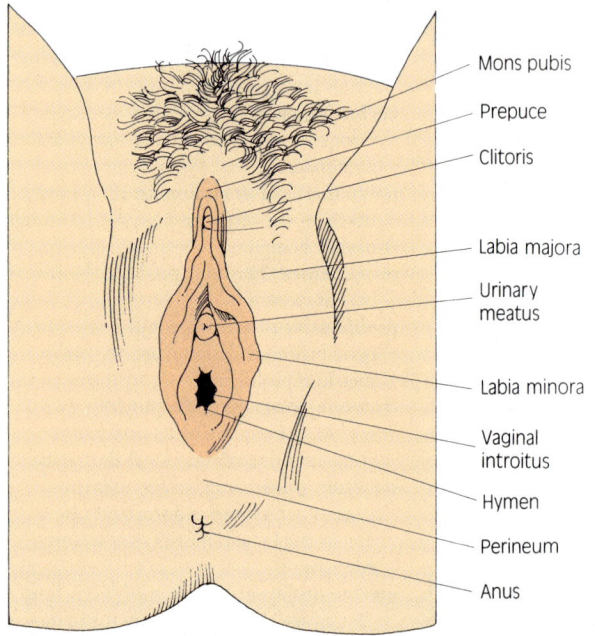

FIGURE 46-1 External female genitalia.

Mons pubis
Prepuce
Clitoris
Labia majora
Urinary meatus
Labia minora
Vaginal introitus
Hymen
Perineum
Anus

FIGURE 46-2 Internal female reproductive structures.

face of the ovary, where transport occurs. The ovum (or oocyte) is discharged into the peritoneal cavity. This periodic discharge of matured ovum is referred to as **ovulation**. The ovum usually finds its way into the fallopian tube, where it is carried to the uterus. If it meets a spermatozoon, the male reproductive cell, a union occurs and conception takes place. After the discharge of the ovum, the cells of the graafian follicle undergo a rapid change. Gradually, they become yellow (**corpus luteum**) and produce **progesterone**, a hormone that prepares the uterus for receiving the fertilized ovum. Ovulation usually occurs 2 weeks prior to the next menstrual period.

The Menstrual Cycle

The menstrual cycle is a complex process involving the reproductive and endocrine systems. The ovaries produce steroid hormones, predominantly estrogens and progesterone. Several different **estrogens** are produced by the ovarian follicle, which consists of the developing ovum and its surrounding cells. The most potent of the ovarian estrogens is estradiol. Estrogens are responsible for developing and maintaining the female reproductive organs and the secondary sex characteristics associated with the adult female. Estrogens play an important role in breast development and in monthly cyclic changes in the uterus.

Progesterone is also important in regulating the changes that occur in the uterus during the menstrual cycle. It is secreted by the corpus luteum, which is the ovarian follicle after the ovum has been released. Progesterone is the most important hormone for conditioning the **endometrium** (the mucous membrane lining the uterus) in preparation for implantation of a fertilized ovum. If pregnancy occurs, the progesterone secretion becomes largely a function of the placenta and is essential for maintaining a normal pregnancy. In addition, progesterone, working with estrogen, prepares the breast for producing and secreting milk. **Androgens** are also produced by the ovaries, but only in small amounts. These

hormones are involved in the early development of the follicle and also affect the female libido.

Two gonadotropic hormones are released by the pituitary gland: FSH and LH. **Follicle-stimulating hormone** (FSH) is primarily responsible for stimulating the ovaries to secrete estrogen. **Luteinizing hormone** (LH) is primarily responsible for stimulating progesterone production. Feedback mechanisms, in part, regulate FSH and LH secretion. For example, elevated estrogen levels in the blood inhibit FSH secretion but promote LH secretion, whereas elevated progesterone levels inhibit LH secretion. In addition, gonadotropin-releasing hormone (GnRH) from the hypothalamus affects the rate of FSH and LH release.

The secretion of ovarian hormones follows a cyclic pattern that results in changes in the uterine endometrium and in **menstruation** (Fig. 46-3; Table 46-1). This cycle is typically 28 days in length, but there are many normal variations (21 to 42 days). In the **proliferative phase** at the beginning of the cycle (just after menstruation), FSH output increases, stimulating estrogen secretion. This causes the endometrium to thicken and become more vascular. In the **secretory phase** near the middle portion of the cycle (day 14 in a 28-day cycle), LH output increases, stimulating ovulation. Under the combined stimulus of estrogen and progesterone, the endometrium reaches the peak of its thickening and vascularization. The **luteal phase** begins after ovulation and is characterized by the secretion of progesterone from the corpus luteum.

If the ovum is fertilized, estrogen and progesterone levels remain high and the complex hormonal changes of pregnancy follow. If the ovum has not been fertilized, FSH and LH output diminishes, estrogen and progesterone secretion falls, the ovum disintegrates, and the endometrium, which has become thick and congested, becomes hemorrhagic. The product consisting of old blood, mucus, and endometrial tissue is discharged through the cervix and into the vagina. After the menstrual flow stops, the cycle begins again; the endometrium proliferates and thickens from estrogenic stimulation, and ovulation recurs.

Physiology/Pathophysiology

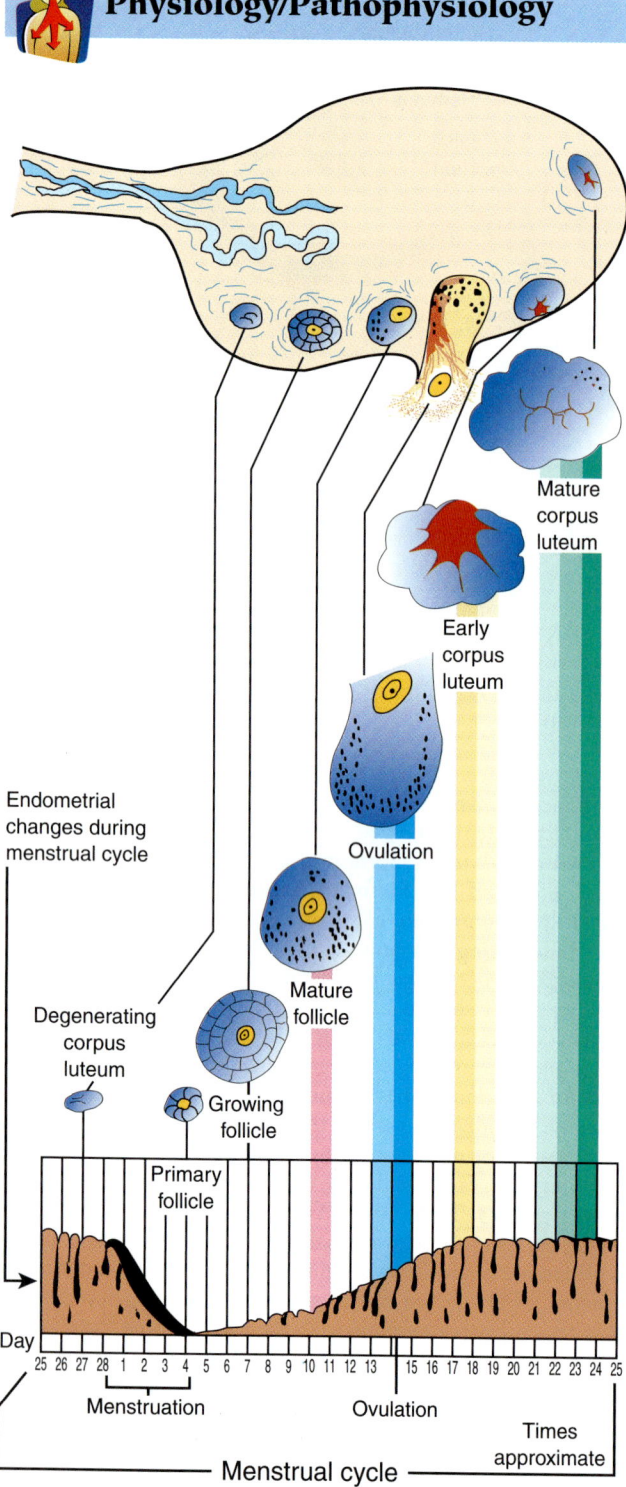

FIGURE 46-3 One menstrual cycle and the corresponding changes in the endometrium.

Menopausal Period

The menopausal period marks the end of a woman's reproductive capacity. It usually occurs between the ages of 45 and 52 years but may occur as early as age 42 or as late as age 55; the median age is 51. **Menopause** is not a pathologic phenomenon but a normal part of aging and maturation. Menstruation ceases, and because the ovaries are no longer active, the reproductive organs become smaller. No more ova mature; therefore, no ovarian hormones are produced. (An artificial menopause may occur earlier if the ovaries are surgically removed or are destroyed by radiation or chemotherapy.) Besides changes in the reproductive system that reduce estrogen levels, multifaceted changes occur throughout the woman's body. These changes include neuroendocrinologic, biochemical, and metabolic alterations related to normal maturation or aging (Table 46-2).

Assessment

The nurse who is obtaining information from the patient for the health history and performing physical assessment is in an ideal position to discuss the woman's general health issues, health promotion, and health-related concerns. Topics that are relevant would include fitness, nutrition, cardiovascular risks, health screening, sexuality, abuse, health risk behaviours, and immunizations. Recommendations for health screening are summarized in Chart 46-1.

HEALTH HISTORY AND CLINICAL MANIFESTATIONS

In addition to obtaining a general health history, the nurse asks about past illnesses and experiences that are specific to women's health. Data should be collected about the following:

- Menstrual history (including **menarche**, length of cycles, length and amount of flow, presence of cramps or pain, bleeding between periods or after intercourse, bleeding after menopause)
- History of pregnancies (number of pregnancies, outcomes of pregnancies)
- History of exposure to medications (diethylstilbestrol [DES], immunosuppressive agents, others)
- Pain with menses (**dysmenorrhea**), pain with intercourse (**dyspareunia**), pelvic pain
- History of vaginal discharge and odour or itching
- History of problems with urinary function (ie, frequency or urgency); may be related to STDs or pregnancy
- History of problems with bowel or bladder control
- Sexual history
- History of sexual abuse or physical abuse
- History of surgery or other procedures on reproductive tract structures (including female genital mutilation or female circumcision)
- History of chronic illness or disability that may affect health status, reproductive health, need for health screening, or access to health care
- History of genetic disorder

In collecting data related to reproductive health, the nurse is in a unique position to teach patients about normal physiologic processes, such as menstruation and menopause, and to assess possible abnormalities. Many problems experienced by young or middle-aged women can be corrected easily. If allowed to go untreated, however, they may result in anxiety and health problems. Issues related to sexuality and sexual function are typically brought more often to the attention of the gynecologic or women's health care provider than other health care providers; any nurse, however, should consider these issues to be part of routine health assessment.

Table 46-1 • Hormonal Changes During the Menstrual Cycle

(TIMES APPROXIMATE) PHASE	MENSTRUAL	FOLLICULAR	OVULATION	LUTEAL	PREMENSTRUAL
Days	1 2 3 4 5 6 7 8	9 10 11 12 13 14	15 16 17 18	19 20 21 22 23 24	25 26 27 28 1 2
Ovary	Degenerating corpus luteum; beginning follicular development	Growth and maturation of follicle	Ovulation	Active corpus luteum	Degenerating corpus luteum
Estrogen Production	Low	Increasing	High	Declining, then a secondary rise	Decreasing
Progesterone Production	None	Low	Low	Increasing	Decreasing
FSH Production	Increasing	High, then declining	Low	Low	Increasing
LH Production	Low	Low, then increasing	High	High	Decreasing
Endometrium	Degeneration and shedding of superficial layer. Coiled arteries dilate, then constrict again.	Reorganization and proliferation of superficial layer	Continued growth	Active secretion and glandular dilation; highly vascular; edematous	Vasoconstriction of coiled arteries; beginning degeneration

Table 46-2 • Age-Related Changes in Female Reproductive System

	PHYSIOLOGIC CHANGES	SIGNS AND SYMPTOMS
Cessation of ovarian function and decreased estrogen production	Decreased ovulation	Decreased/loss of ability to conceive; increased infertility
	Onset of menopause	Irregular menses with eventual cessation of menses
	Vasomotor instability and hormonal fluctuations	Hot flashes or flushing; night sweats, sleep disturbances; mood swings; fatigue
	Decreased bone formation	Bone loss and increased risk for osteoporosis and osteoporotic fractures; loss of height
	Decreased vaginal lubrication	Dyspareunia, resulting in lack of interest in sex
	Thinning of urinary and genital tracts	Increased risk for urinary tract infection
	Increased pH of vagina	Increased incidence of bacterial infections (atrophic vaginitis) with discharge, itching, and vulvar burning
	Thinning of pubic hair and shrinking of labia	
Relaxing of pelvic musculature	Prolapse of uterus, cystocele, rectocele	Dyspareunia, incontinence, feelings of perineal pressure

Chart 46-1 Summary of Health Screening and Counselling Issues for Women

Ages 19–39

Sexuality and Reproductive Issues

Annual pelvic examination
Annual clinical breast exam
Breast self-examination monthly
Contraceptive options
High-risk sexual behaviours

Health and Risk Behaviours

Hygiene
Injury prevention
Nutrition, including requirements for calcium and vitamin D. Folic acid to be taken prior to pregnancy and for 3 months
Exercise patterns
Risk for domestic abuse
Use of tobacco, drugs, and alcohol
Life stresses
Immunizations

Diagnostic Testing*

Pap smear
STD screening as indicated

Ages 40–64

Sexuality and Reproductive Issues

Annual pelvic examination
Annual clinical breast exam
Breast self-examination monthly
Contraceptive options
High-risk sexual behaviours
Menopausal concerns

Health and Risk Behaviours

Hygiene
Bone loss and injury prevention
Nutrition, including requirements for calcium and vitamin D
Exercise patterns
Risk for domestic abuse

Use of tobacco, drugs, and alcohol
Life stresses
Immunizations

Diagnostic Testing*

Pap smear
Mammography
Cholesterol and lipid profile
Colorectal cancer screening
Bone mineral density testing
Thyroid-stimulating hormone testing
Hearing and eye examinations

Ages 65 and Over

Sexuality and Reproductive Issues

Annual pelvic examination
Annual clinical breast exam
Breast self-examination
High-risk sexual behaviours

Health and Risk Behaviours

Hygiene
Injury prevention
Nutrition, including requirement for calcium and vitamin D
Exercise patterns
Risk for domestic abuse
Use of tobacco, drugs, and alcohol
Life stresses
Immunizations

Diagnostic Testing*

Pap smear
Mammography
Cholesterol and lipid profile
Colorectal cancer screening
Bone mineral density testing
Thyroid-stimulating hormone testing
Hearing and eye examinations

*Each individual's risks (family history, personal history) influence the need for specific assessments and their frequency.

Sexual History

A sexual assessment includes both subjective and objective data. Health and sexual histories, physical examination findings, and laboratory results are all part of the database. The purpose of a sexual history is to obtain information that provides a picture of the woman's sexuality and sexual practices and promotes sexual health. The sexual history may enable the patient to discuss sexual matters openly and to discuss sexual concerns with an informed health professional. This information can be obtained with the health history after the gynecologic-obstetric or genitourinary history is completed. By incorporating the sexual history into the general health history, the nurse can move from areas of lesser sensitivity to areas of greater sensitivity after establishing initial rapport.

Taking the sexual history becomes a dynamic process reflecting an exchange of information between the patient and the nurse and provides the opportunity to clarify myths and explore areas of concern that the patient may not have felt comfortable discussing in the past. In obtaining a sexual history, the nurse must not assume the patient's sexual preference until clarified. When asking about sexual health, the nurse also cannot assume that the patient is married or unmarried. Asking a woman to label herself as single, married, widowed, or divorced may be seen as an inappropriate inquiry by the patient. Asking about a partner or about current meaningful relationships may be a less offensive way to initiate a sexual history.

The PLISSIT (Permission, Limited Information, Specific Suggestions, Intensive Therapy) model of sexual assessment and intervention may be used to provide a framework for nursing interventions (Annon, 1976). The assessment begins by introducing the topic and asking the woman for permission to discuss issues of sexual functioning with her.

The nurse can begin by explaining the purpose of obtaining a sexual history (eg, "I ask all my patients about their sexual health. May I ask you some questions about this?"). History taking continues by inquiring about present sexual activity and sexual orientation (eg, "Are you currently having sex with a man, a woman, or both?"). Inquiries about possible sexual dysfunction may include, "Are you having any problems related to your current sexual activity?" Such problems may be related to medication, life changes, disability, or the onset of physical or emotional illness. Patients can be asked about their thoughts on what is causing the current problem.

Limited information about sexual function may be provided to the patient. As the discussion progresses, the nurse may offer specific suggestions for interventions. For some women, a professional who specializes in sex therapy may provide more intensive therapy as needed. By initiating an assessment about sexual concerns, the nurse communicates to the patient that issues about changes in sexual functioning are valid health topics for discus-

GENETICS IN NURSING PRACTICE—Reproductive Disorders

Various reproductive disorders are influenced by genetic factors. Some examples are:

- Hereditary breast or ovarian cancer syndromes
- Hereditary nonpolyposis colon cancer syndrome (risk for uterine cancer)
- Müllerian aplasia
- 21-Hydroxylase deficiency (female masculinization)
- Turner syndrome (45,XO)
- Klinefelter syndrome (47,XXY)

NURSING ASSESSMENTS

FAMILY HISTORY ASSESSMENT

- Assess family history for other family members with similar reproductive problems/abnormalities.
  - Inquire about ethnic background (eg, Ashkenazi Jewish populations and hereditary breast/ovarian cancer mutations).
  - Inquire about relatives with other cancers, including early-onset ovarian, uterine, renal, prostate cancers.

PHYSICAL ASSESSMENT

- In females with delayed puberty or primary amenorrhea, assess for clinical features of Turner syndrome (short stature, webbing of the neck, widely spaced nipples).
- In males with delayed puberty or infertility, assess for clinical features of Klinefelter syndrome (tall stature, gynecomastia, learning disabilities).
- Assess for other congenital anomalies in females with Müllerian defect, including renal and vertebral anomalies.

MANAGEMENT ISSUES SPECIFIC TO GENETICS

- Inquire whether genetic testing (DNA chromosomal, metabolic) has been carried out on affected family member(s).
  - If indicated, refer for further genetic counselling and evaluation so that family members can discuss inheritance, risk to other family members, availability of genetic testing, and gene-based interventions.
  - Offer appropriate genetics information and resources.
  - Assess patient's understanding of genetics information.

- Provide support to families with newly diagnosed gene-related reproductive disorders.
- Participate in management and coordination of care of patients with genetic conditions, individuals predisposed to develop or pass on a genetic condition.

GENETICS RESOURCES FOR NURSES AND THEIR PATIENTS ON THE WEB

Canadian Association of Genetic Counsellors (CAGC): http://www.cagc-accg.ca—a listing of genetic centres across Canada

Canadian Cancer Society: http://www.cancer.ca—a source of information on genetic factors/risk and genetic testing

Canadian Directory of Genetic Support Groups: http://www.lhsc.on.ca/programs/medgenet—a resource guide for families and professionals

Canadian Genetic Disease Network: http://www.cgdn.ca—a group with the stated mission to be the primary catalyst in advancing Canada's scientific and commercial competitiveness in genetic research and the application of genetic discoveries to the prevention, diagnosis, and treatment of human disease

Canadian Organization for Rare Disorders (CORD): http://www.cord.ca—a source of information on over 6,000 rare disorders; links individuals/families with the same rare disorder

Genetic Alliance: http://www.geneticalliance.org—an organization that increases the capacity of genetic advocacy groups to achieve their missions and leverages the voices of millions of individuals and families living with genetic conditions

The Genetics Society of Canada (GSC): http://life.biology.mcmaster.ca/GSC—a group that promotes research and communicates the results and implications of genetics to the public

GeneTests: http://www.genetests.org—a publicly funded medical genetics information resource developed for physicians, other health care providers, and researchers

OMIM Online Mendelian Inheritance in Man: http://www.ncbi.nlm.nih.gov/entrez/query.fcgi?db=OMIM—a catalogue of human genes and genetic disorders

---

sion and provides a safe environment for discussing these sensitive topics.

Risk for STDs can be assessed by asking about number of partners in the past year or in the patient's lifetime. An open-ended question related to the patient's need for further information should be included (eg, "Do you have any questions or concerns about your sexual health?"). Nurses should be aware that some women and men are using the Internet to seek partners; obtaining sexual partners this way has been associated with an increased risk for STDs (McFarlane, Bull & Rietmeijer, 2000; U.S. Department of Health and Human Services, 2001).

Young women may be apprehensive about irregular periods, may be concerned about STDs, or may need contraception. They may want information on using tampons, emergency contraception, or issues related to pregnancy. Perimenopausal women may have concerns about irregular menses; menopausal women may be concerned about vaginal dryness and burning with inter-

course. Women of any age may have concerns about sexual satisfaction, orgasm, or anorgasmia (lack of orgasm).

Female Genital Mutilation

Female genital mutilation (FGM) refers to the partial or total removal of the external female genitalia or other injury to female organs. Individuals from some cultures believe that FGM promotes hygiene, protects virginity and family honour, prevents promiscuity, improves female attractiveness and male sexual pleasure, and enhances fertility. It is viewed in some cultures as a rite of passage to womanhood. Many organizations (eg, World Health Organization, Amnesty International) are working to end this practice.

Four types of FGM are known: excision of the clitoral prepuce; total excision of the clitoral prepuce and glans with partial or total excision of the labia minora; excision of part or all of the external genitalia and stitching or narrowing of the vaginal opening (referred to as infibulation); and unclassified, which includes pricking, piercing, or incision of the clitoris, the labia, or both, stretching of the clitoris or surrounding tissues, and introduction of corrosive substances into the vagina (American College of Obstetricians and Gynecologists [ACOG] Committee Opinion #151, 1995). FGM is usually performed between 4 and 10 years of age; hemorrhage and infection may be consequences.

A growing number of women entering the Canadian health care system underwent FGM before coming to this country. Others have undergone FGM since they arrived in Canada. Because FGM can affect sexual function, menstrual hygiene, and bladder function, the possibility of FGM is included in the sexual history, particularly for women from cultures and countries where the practice is common.

Long-term complications of FGM include urinary problems, chronic vaginitis and pelvic infections, inability to undergo pelvic examination, painful intercourse, impaired sexual response, anemia, increased risk for HIV infection due to tearing of scar tissue, and psychological and psychosexual sequelae (Chalmers & Hashi, 2000). Nurses who care for patients who have undergone FGM need to be sensitive, empathetic, knowledgeable, and nonjudgmental.

Domestic Violence

Domestic violence is a broad term that includes child abuse, elder abuse, and abuse of women and men. Abuse can be emotional, physical, sexual, or economic. Battering involves repeated physical or sexual assault in a context of coercive control and, more broadly, emotional degradation, threats, and intimidation. Nurses need to

be aware of the prevalence of abuse and violence directed against women in our society. Abuse is related to the need to maintain control of a partner and involves fear of one partner by another and control by threats, intimidation, and physical abuse. Violence is rarely a one-time occurrence in a relationship; it usually continues and escalates in severity. This is an important point to emphasize when a woman states that her partner has hurt her but has promised to change. Batterers can change their behaviour, but not without extensive counselling and motivation. If a woman states that she is being hurt, sensitive care is required (Chart 46-2). Because three in every ten women in Canada will be battered by a male partner each year (MacLeod, 1995), battered women are encountered daily in nursing practice. By knowing about this major public health problem, being alert to abuse-related problems, and learning how to elicit information from women about abuse in their lives, nurses can offer intervention for a problem that might otherwise go undetected. Asking each woman about violence in her life in a safe environment (ie, a private room with the door closed) is part of a comprehensive assessment and universal screening. The Abuse Assessment Screen has been found effective in identifying the presence of abuse and should be included in the health history of all women (Chart 46-3).

No specific signs or symptoms are diagnostic of battering; however, nurses may see an injury that does not fit the account of how it happened (eg, a bruise on the side of the upper arm after "I walked into a door"). Manifestations of abuse may involve suicide attempts, drug and alcohol abuse, frequent emergency department visits, vague pelvic pain, and depression. However, there may be no obvious signs or symptoms. Women in abusive

---

 Chart 46-2

GUIDELINES FOR Managing Reported Domestic Abuse

NURSING ACTION	RATIONALE
1. Reassure the woman that she is not alone.	Many women are hurt by their partners, and nurses see them daily. Let the woman know that no one deserves to be abused.
2. Express your belief that no one should be hurt, that abuse is the fault of the batterer and is against the law.	
3. Assure the woman that her information is confidential, although it does become part of her medical record. **If children are suspected of being abused or are being abused, the law requires that this be reported to the authorities.** (If nurses are in doubt, they need to check with their local or provincial domestic violence agency.)	Women are often afraid that their information will be reported to the police or protective services and their children may be taken away.
4. Document the woman's statement of abuse and take photographs of any visible injuries *if* written formal consent has been obtained. (Emergency departments usually have a camera available if one is not on the nursing unit.)	Provide documentation of injuries that may be needed for later legal or criminal proceedings.
5. Provide teaching: • Inform the woman that shelters are available to ensure safety for her and her children. (Lengths of stay in shelters vary by province but are often up to 21 days. Staff often assist with housing, jobs, and the emotional distress that accompanies the break-up of the family.) Provide list of shelters. • Inform woman that violence gets worse, not better. • If the woman chooses to go to a shelter, let her make the call. • If she chooses to return to the abuser, remain nonjudgmental and provide information that will make her safer than she was before disclosing her situation. • Make sure that she has a 24-hour hotline telephone number that provides information and support, police number, and 911. • Assist her to set up a safety plan in case she decides to return home. (A safety plan is an organized plan for departure with packed bags and important papers hidden in a safe spot.)	These options may be life-saving for the woman and her children.

The Abuse Assessment Screen consists of the following three questions:
1. In the past year, have you been hit, slapped, kicked, or otherwise physically hurt by someone?
2. If pregnant, since you have been pregnant, have you been hit, slapped, kicked, or otherwise physically hurt by someone?
3. Have you ever been forced into sexual activity?

situations often report that they do not feel well, due to the stress of fear and anticipation of abuse. Nurses need to be knowledgeable about abuse, ask every woman patient about abuse in her life, provide resources, and follow written protocols within their institution to ensure comprehensive care.

Incest and Childhood Sexual Abuse

Among adult Canadians, 53% of women were sexually abused as children (Public Health Agency of Canada, 2005), so nurses frequently encounter women who have been sexually traumatized. It has been reported that female survivors of sexual abuse have more health problems and undergo more surgery than women who were not victimized. Victims of childhood sexual abuse are reported to experience more chronic depression, posttraumatic stress disorder, morbid obesity, marital instability, gastrointestinal problems, and headaches, as well as greater use of health care services, than persons who were not victims. Chronic pelvic pain in women is often associated with physical violence, emotional neglect, and sexual abuse in childhood (ACOG Educational Bulletin #259, 2001). Women who have experienced rape or sexual abuse may have difficulty with pelvic examinations, labour, pelvic or breast irradiation, or any treatment or examination that involves hands-on treatment or requires removal of clothing. Nurses should be prepared to offer support and referral to psychologists, community resources, and self-help groups.

Rape and Sexual Assault

One half of all Canadian women have experienced at least one incidence of sexual or physical violence (Public Health Agency of Canada, 2005). Men, women, and children may be victims of sexual assault. Sexual assault nurse examiners, emergency department staff, and gynecologists perform the painstaking collection of forensic evidence that is needed for criminal prosecution. Oral, anal, and genital tissue is examined for evidence of trauma, semen, or infection. Saliva, hair, and fingernail evidence is also collected. Cultures are obtained for STDs, and prophylactic antibiotics are prescribed. HIV testing is offered and is repeated in 3 to 6 months. HIV prophylaxis is not universally recommended but is considered when mucosal exposure to contamination has occurred. Prophylaxis against chlamydia and gonorrhea are provided (Kaplan, Feinstein, Fisher et al., 2001). Emergency contraception is provided if requested. Emotional counselling is provided, and follow-up treatment visits are arranged. Rape trauma syndrome is the emotional reaction to a sexual assault and may consist of shock, sleep disturbances, nightmares, flashbacks, anxiety, anger, mood swings, and depression. It is important for survivors to discuss the experience and to obtain professional counselling.

Screening for abuse, rape, and violence should be part of routine assessment because women often do not report or seek treatment for assault. Often, the assailant is a partner, husband, or date. Nurses may encounter women with infections or pregnancies related to sexual assault that were never treated.

Health Issues of Women With Disabilities

Studies have shown that women with disabilities receive less primary health care and preventive health screening than other women, often because of access problems and health care providers' focus on the causes of disability rather than on general health issues of concern to all women. To address these issues, the history should include questions about barriers to health care experienced by disabled women and the effect of their disability on their health status and health care. Other issues to be addressed are identified in Chart 46-4. If the patient has hearing loss, vision loss, or another disability, the nurse may need to obtain the assistance of a signer or interpreter. The nurse assessing a person with a disability may require additional time and the assistance of others to be certain that accurate information is obtained from the patient. Extra time may be needed to conduct the assessment in a sensitive and unhurried manner (Kirschner, Gill, Reis & Welner, 1998; Smeltzer, 2000).

PHYSICAL ASSESSMENT

Periodic examinations and routine cancer screening are important for all women. An annual breast and pelvic examination is important for all women age 18 or older and for those who are sexually active, regardless of age. The patient deserves understanding and support because of the emotional and physical considerations associated with gynecologic examinations. Women may be sensitive or embarrassed by the usual questions asked by a gynecologist or women's health care provider. Because gynecologic conditions are of a personal and private nature to most women, such information is shared only with those directly involved in patient care (as is true with all patient information).

Throughout the examination, the nurse explains the procedures to be performed. This not only encourages the woman to relax but also provides an opportunity for her to ask questions and minimizes the negative feelings that many women associate with gynecologic examinations.

The first pelvic examination is often anxiety-producing for women; the nurse can alleviate many of these feelings with explanations and teaching (Chart 46-5). Before the examination begins, the patient is asked to empty her bladder and to provide a urine specimen if urine tests are part of the total assessment. Voiding ensures patient comfort and eases the examination because a full bladder can make palpation of pelvic organs uncomfortable for the patient and difficult for the examiner.

Positioning

Although several positions may be used for the pelvic examination, the supine lithotomy position is used most commonly, although the upright lithotomy position (in which the woman assumes a semisitting posture) may also be used. This position offers several advantages:

- It is more comfortable for some women.
- It allows better eye contact between patient and examiner.
- It may provide an easier means for the examiner to carry out the bimanual examination.
- It enables the woman to use a mirror to see her anatomy (if she chooses) to visualize any conditions that require treatment or to learn about using certain types of contraceptive methods.

Chart 46-4 • ASSESSMENT

Assessing a Woman With a Disability

Health History

Address questions directly to the woman herself rather than to persons accompanying her.

Self-care limitations resulting from her disability (ability to feed and dress self, use of assistive devices, transportation requirements, other assistance needed)

Sensory limitations (lack of sensation, low vision, deaf or hard of hearing)

Accessibility issues (ability to get to health care provider, transfer to examination table, accessibility of office/clinic of health care provider, previous experiences with health care providers, health screening practices; her understanding of physical examination)

Cognitive or developmental changes that affect understanding

Limitations secondary to disability that affect general health issues and reproductive health and health care

Sexual function and concerns (those of all women and those that may be affected by the presence of a disabling condition)

Menstrual history and menstrual hygiene practices

Physical, sexual, or psychological abuse (including abuse by care providers)

Presence of secondary disabilities (ie, those resulting from the patient's primary disability: pressure ulcers, spasticity, osteoporosis, etc.)

Health concerns related to aging with a disability

Physical Assessment

Provide instructions directly to the woman herself rather than to persons accompanying her; provide written or audiotaped instructions.

Ask the woman what assistance she needs for the physical examination and provide assistance if needed:

—Undressing and dressing

—Providing a urine specimen

—Standing on scale to be weighed (provide alternative means of obtaining weight if she is unable to stand on scale)

—Moving on and off the examination table

—Assuming, changing, and maintaining positions

Consider the fatigue experienced by the woman during a lengthy exam and allow rest.

Provide assistive devices and other aids/methods needed to allow adequate communication with the patient (interpreters, signers, large-print written materials).

Complete examination that would be indicated for any other woman; having a disability is *never* justification for omitting parts of the physical examination, including the pelvic examination.

In the supine lithotomy position, the patient lies on the table with her feet on foot rests or stirrups. She is encouraged to relax so that her buttocks are positioned at the edge of the examination table, and she is asked to relax and spread her thighs as widely apart as possible.

If the patient is too ill, disabled, or neurologically impaired to lie safely on the examination table or cannot maintain the supine lithotomy position, the Sims' position may be used. In Sims' position, the patient lies on her left side with her right leg bent at a 90-degree angle. The right labia may be retracted to gain adequate access to the vagina. Other positions for pelvic examination for disabled women make the examination easier for the woman and the clinician. The presence of a disability does not justify skipping any parts of the physical assessment, including the pelvic examination.

The following equipment is obtained and readily available: a good light source; a vaginal speculum; clean examination gloves; lubricant, spatula, cytobrush, glass slides, fixative solution or spray; and diagnostic testing supplies for screening for occult rectal blood if the woman is older than 40. Latex-free gloves should be available if the patient or clinician is allergic to latex. This allergy is becoming more prevalent in nurses and other health care providers and patients and is potentially life-threatening. Patients should be questioned about previous reactions to latex. (See Chap. 18 for a latex screening form and Chap. 53 for more information on latex allergy.)

Chart 46-5 ## Patient Education: The Pelvic Examination

The nurse should explain the following to the patient:

- A pelvic examination includes assessment of the appearance, size, and shape of the vulva, vagina, uterus, and ovaries to ensure reproductive health and absence of illness.
- A pelvic examination should never hurt except in the presence of a pelvic infection. Women often describe a feeling of fullness or pressure but should not feel pain. Some women who are very tense feel discomfort, so relaxation is important.
- It is normal to feel uncomfortable and apprehensive.
- A narrow, warmed speculum will be inserted to visualize the cervix.
- A Papanicolaou (Pap) smear will be obtained and should not be uncomfortable.
- The patient may watch the examination with a mirror if she chooses.
- The examination usually takes no longer than 5 minutes.
- Draping will be used to minimize exposure (despite appropriate draping, some women feel uncomfortable or embarrassed during the examination).

Inspection

After the patient is prepared, the examiner inspects the labia majora and minora, noting the epidermal tissue of the labia majora; the skin fades to the pink mucous membrane of the vaginal introitus. Lesions of any type (eg, venereal warts, pigmented lesions [melanoma]) are evaluated. In the nulliparous woman, the labia minora come together at the opening of the vagina. In women who have delivered children vaginally, the labia minora may gape and vaginal tissue may protrude.

Trauma to the anterior vaginal wall during childbirth may have resulted in incompetency of the musculature, and a bulge caused by the bladder protruding into the submucosa of the anterior vaginal wall (**cystocele**) may be seen. Childbirth trauma may also have affected the posterior vaginal wall, producing a bulge caused by rectal cavity protrusion (**rectocele**). The cervix may descend under pressure through the vaginal canal and be seen at the introitus (**uterine prolapse**). See Chapter 47 for a discussion of these structural changes. To identify such protrusions, the examiner asks the patient to "bear down."

The introitus should be free of superficial mucosal lesions. The labia minora may be separated by the fingers of the gloved hand and the lower part of the vagina palpated. In virgins, a **hymen** of variable thickness may be felt circumferentially within 1 or 2 cm of the vaginal opening. The hymenal ring usually permits the insertion of one finger. Rarely, the hymen totally occludes the vaginal entrance (imperforate hymen).

In women who are not virgins, a rim of scar tissue representing the remnants of the hymenal ring may be felt circumferentially around the vagina near its opening. The greater vestibular glands (Bartholin's glands) lie between the labia minora and the remnants of the hymenal ring. An abscess of the Bartholin's gland can cause discomfort and requires incision and drainage.

Speculum Examination

The bivalved speculum, either metal or plastic, is available in many sizes. Metal specula are soaked, scrubbed, and sterilized between patients. Some clinicians and some patients prefer plastic specula, which permit one-time use. The speculum should be warmed with a heating pad or warm water to make insertion more comfortable for the patient. The speculum is not lubricated because commercial lubricants interfere with cervical cytology (Papanicolaou [Pap] smear) findings.

The metal speculum has two set-screws. The one along the handle, holding the two valves of the speculum together, is kept tightened. The screw that holds the thumb rest in place is loosened. The speculum is grasped in the dominant hand, with the thumb against the back of the thumb rest to keep the tips of the valves closed. The speculum is rotated slightly counterclockwise, and the vaginal orifice is held open by the thumb and the forefinger of the gloved nondominant hand by some examiners. Other examiners find that straight insertion of a speculum with downward pressure on the vagina is more comfortable for the patient. The speculum is gently inserted into the posterior portion of the introitus and slowly advanced to the top of the vagina; this should not be painful or uncomfortable for the woman. The tip of the speculum may then be elevated and the speculum rotated to a transverse position. The speculum is then slowly opened and the set-screw of the thumb rest is tightened to hold the speculum open (Fig. 46-4).

CERVIX

The cervix is inspected. In nulliparous women, the cervix usually is 2 to 3 cm wide and smooth. Women who have borne children may have a laceration, usually transverse, giving the cervical os a "fishmouth" appearance. Epithelium from the endocervical canal may have grown onto the surface of the cervix, appearing as beefy-red surface epithelium circumferentially around the os. Occasionally, the cervix of a woman whose mother took DES has a hooded appearance (a peaked aspect superiorly or a ridge of tissue surrounding it); this is evaluated by colposcopy when identified.

ABNORMAL GROWTH

Malignant changes may not be obviously differentiated from the rest of the cervical mucosa. Small, benign cysts may appear on the cervical surface. These are usually bluish or white and are called nabothian cysts. A **polyp** of endocervical mucosa may protrude through the os and usually is dark red. Polyps can cause irregular bleeding; they are rarely malignant and usually are removed easily in an office or clinic setting. A carcinoma may appear as a cauliflower-like growth that bleeds easily when touched. Bluish colouration of the cervix is a sign of early pregnancy (Chadwick's sign).

PAP SMEAR

During the pelvic examination, a Pap smear is obtained by rotating a small spatula at the os, followed by a cervical brush rotated in the os. The tissue obtained is spread on a glass slide and sprayed or fixed immediately, or inserted into a liquid. A small broom-like device can also be used to obtain specimens for the Pap smear.

A specimen of any purulent material appearing at the cervical os is obtained for culture. A sterile applicator is used to obtain the specimen, which is immediately placed in an appropriate medium for transfer to a laboratory. In patients at high risk for infection, routine cultures for gonococcal and chlamydial organisms are recommended because of the high incidence of both diseases and the high risk for pelvic infection, fallopian tube damage, and subsequent infertility.

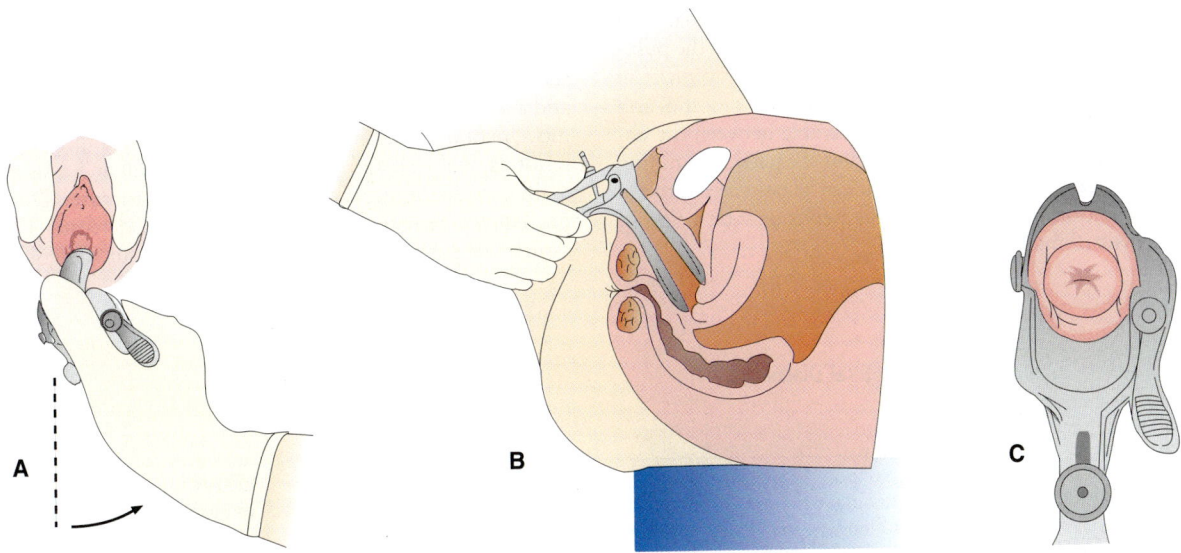

FIGURE 46-4 Technique for speculum examination of the vagina and cervix. (**A**) The labia are spread apart with a gloved left hand, while the speculum is grasped in the right hand and turned counterclockwise before being inserted into the vagina. Once the speculum is inserted, the blades are then spread apart (**B**) to reveal the cervical os (**C**).

Vaginal discharge, which may be normal or may result from vaginitis, may be present. Discharge caused by bacteria (bacterial vaginosis) usually appears grey and purulent. Discharge caused by *Trichomonas* species infection is usually frothy, copious, and malodourous. Discharge caused by *Candida* species infection is usually thick and white-yellow and has a cottage-cheese appearance. Table 46-3 summarizes the characteristics of vaginal discharge found in different conditions.

The vagina is inspected as the examiner withdraws the speculum. It is smooth in young girls and thickens after puberty, with many rugae (folds) and redundancy in the epithelium. In menopausal women, the vagina thins and has fewer rugae because of decreased estrogen.

Bimanual Palpation

To complete the pelvic examination, the examiner performs a bimanual examination from a standing position. The examination is performed with the forefinger and middle finger of the gloved and lubricated hand. These fingers are placed in the vaginal orifice, while the other fingers are held tightly out of the way, with the thumb completely adducted. The fingers are advanced vertically along the vaginal canal, and the vaginal wall is palpated. It is important to assess the strength of pelvic muscles by asking the patient to squeeze the examiner's fingers as tightly and for as long as possible. If the squeeze is tight around the examiner's fingers and lasts for at least 3 seconds, then full strength of the pelvic muscles is present. Weakness of the muscles may be related to urinary stress incontinence (Bickley & Szilagyi, 2003). Any firm part of the vaginal wall may represent old scar tissue from childbirth trauma but may also require further evaluation.

CERVICAL PALPATION

The cervix is palpated and assessed for its consistency, mobility, size, and position. The normal cervix is uniformly firm but not hard. Softening of the cervix is a finding in early pregnancy. Hardness and immobility of the cervix may reflect invasion by a neoplasm. Pain on gentle movement of the cervix is called a positive **chandelier sign** or positive cervical motion tenderness (recorded as +CMT) and usually indicates a pelvic infection.

UTERINE PALPATION

To palpate the uterus, the examiner places the opposite hand on the abdominal wall halfway between the umbilicus and the pubis and presses firmly toward the vagina (Fig. 46-5). Movement of the abdominal wall causes the body of the uterus to descend, and the pear-shaped organ becomes freely movable between the abdominal examining hand and the fingers of the pelvic examining hand. Uterine size, mobility, and contour can be estimated through palpation. Fixation of the uterus in the pelvis may be a sign of **endometriosis** or malignancy.

FIGURE 46-5   Technique for the bimanual examination of the pelvis.

The body of the uterus is normally twice the diameter and twice the length of the cervix, curving anteriorly toward the abdominal wall. Some women have a retroverted or retroflexed uterus, which tips posteriorly toward the sacrum, whereas others have a uterus that is neither anterior nor posterior but is midline.

ADNEXAL PALPATION

Next, the right and left adnexal areas are palpated to evaluate the fallopian tubes and ovaries. The fingers of the hand examining the pelvis are moved first to one side, then to the other, while the hand palpating the abdominal area is moved correspondingly to either side of the abdomen and downward. The adnexa (ovaries and fallopian tubes) are trapped between the two hands and palpated for an obvious mass, tenderness, and mobility. Commonly, the ovaries are slightly tender, and the patient is informed that slight discomfort on palpation is normal.

VAGINAL AND RECTAL PALPATION

Bimanual palpation of the vagina and cul-de-sac is accomplished by placing the index finger in the vagina and the middle finger in the rectum. To prevent cross-contamination between the vaginal and rectal orifices, the examiner puts on new gloves. A gentle movement of these fingers toward each other compresses the posterior vaginal wall and the anterior rectal wall and assists the examiner in identifying the integrity of these structures. During this procedure, the patient may sense an urge to defecate. The nurse assures the patient that this is unlikely to occur. Ongoing expla-

---

Table 46-3 • Characteristics of Vaginal Discharge

CAUSE OF DISCHARGE	SYMPTOMS	ODOUR	CONSISTENCY/COLOUR
Physiologic	None	None	Mucus/white
Candida species infection	Itching, irritation	Yeast odour or none	Thin to thick, curdlike/white
Bacterial vaginosis	Odour	Fishy, often noticed after intercourse	Thin/greyish or yellow
Trichomonas species infection	Irritation, odour	Malodourous	Copious, often frothy/yellow-green
Atrophic	Vulvar or vaginal dryness	Occasional mild malodour	Usually scant and mucoid/may be blood-tinged

nations are provided to reassure and educate the patient about the procedure.

 ### Gerontologic Considerations

Yearly examinations can help prevent problems of the reproductive tract in aging women. Some older women do not have regular gynecologic examinations. If a woman delivered her children at home, she may never have had a pelvic examination. Some regard it as an embarrassing and unpleasant procedure. An important role of the nurse is to encourage an annual gynecologic examination for all women. The nurse can make the examination a time for education and reassurance rather than a time of embarrassment.

Perineal pruritus is common in elderly women and should be evaluated because it may indicate a disease process (diabetes or malignancy). It may also indicate vulvar dystrophy, a thickened or whitish discolouration of tissue that needs biopsy to rule out abnormal cells. Topical cortisone and hormone creams may be prescribed for symptomatic relief.

With relaxing pelvic musculature, uterine prolapse and relaxation of the vaginal walls can occur. Appropriate evaluation and surgical repair can provide relief if the patient is a candidate for surgery. After surgery, the patient needs to know that tissue repair and healing may require additional time. Pessaries (latex devices that provide support) are often used if surgery is contraindicated or before surgery to see if surgery can be avoided. They are fitted by a health care provider and may reduce discomfort and pressure. Use of a pessary requires the patient to have routine gynecologic examinations to monitor for irritation or infection.

Diagnostic Evaluation

CYTOLOGIC TEST FOR CANCER (PAP SMEAR)

The Pap smear is performed to detect cervical cancer. Before 1940, cervical cancer was the most common cause of cancer death in women. Dr. George Papanicolaou discovered the value of examining exfoliated cells for malignancy in the 1930s. Due to the effectiveness of the Pap smear as a screening method, cervical cancer is now less common than breast or ovarian cancer.

Cervical secretions are gently removed from the cervical os (Fig. 46-6), gently transferred to a glass slide, and fixed immediately by spraying with a fixative. A Thin-prep Pap specimen is immersed in a solution rather than being placed on a slide. This method allows for human papillomavirus (HPV) testing if the Pap smear result is abnormal (see Chap. 47 for further discussion of HPV, a commonly transmitted STD that can cause venereal warts or cervical changes).

The patient should be instructed not to douche before this examination to avoid washing away cellular material. The Pap smear should be performed when the patient is not menstruating because blood usually interferes with interpretation. The proper technique for obtaining a cervical specimen for cytologic study is described in Chart 46-6. False-negative Pap smear results may occur, as may false positives.

The Bethesda Classification system (Chart 46-7) has been developed to promote consistency in reporting Pap smear results and to assist in standardizing management guidelines (Solomon, Davey, Kurman et al., 2001). Terminology includes the following categories:

- Low-grade squamous intraepithelial lesion (LSIL), which is equivalent to cervical intraepithelial neoplasia (CIN 1) and to mild changes related to exposure to HPV

- High-grade squamous intraepithelial lesion (HSIL), which equates to moderate and severe dysplasia, carcinoma in situ (CIS), and CIN 2 and CIN 3

These terms seen on Pap smear findings encompass the precursors to invasive carcinoma of the cervix.

Pap smears that reveal mild inflammation or atypical squamous cells are usually repeated in 3 to 6 months, with findings often returning to normal. Patients are apprehensive because many women incorrectly assume that an abnormal Pap smear means cancer. If a specific infection is causing inflammation, it is treated appropriately, and the Pap smear is repeated. If the repeat Pap smear reveals atypical squamous cells, then a colposcopy is appropriate.

Thin-prep Pap specimens that show atypical cells can also be used to determine the presence of HPV DNA. If HPV DNA is present, it is more likely that HSIL is present.

If the Pap smear results are abnormal, prompt notification, evaluation, and treatment are crucial. Notification of patients is often done by nurses in women's health care. Pap smear follow-up is crucial as it can prevent cervical cancer. Many women do not adhere to recommendations—particularly young women, those of low socioeconomic status, minorities, women who have difficulty coping with the diagnosis, and those without social support. Fear, lack of understanding, and childcare responsibilities have all been identified by women as reasons for poor follow-up. Women with a history of abuse, obese women, and women who had a negative gynecologic experience may also find returning for follow-up difficult (Wee, McCarthy, Davis & Phillips, 2000). Interventions are tailored to meet the needs of the particular group. Intensive telephone counselling, tracking systems, brochures, videos, and financial incentives have all been used to encourage follow-up. Nurses can provide clear explanations and emotional support along with a carefully designed follow-up protocol designed to meet the needs of their specific patient population (DeRemer Abercrombie, 2001).

COLPOSCOPY AND CERVICAL BIOPSY

All suspicious Pap smears should be evaluated by colposcopy. The colposcope is a portable microscope (magnification from 10× to 25×) that allows the examiner to visualize the cervix and obtain a sample of abnormal tissue for analysis. Nurse practitioners and gynecologists require special training in this diagnostic technique.

After inserting a speculum and visualizing the cervix and vaginal walls, the examiner applies acetic acid to the cervix. Subsequent abnormal findings that indicate the need for biopsy include leukoplakia (white plaque visible before applying acetic acid), acetowhite tissue (white epithelium after applying acetic acid), punctation (dilated capillaries occurring in a dotted or stippled pattern), mosaicism (a tile-like pattern), and atypical vascular patterns.

An endocervical curettage may be performed during colposcopy if a problem is suspected based on Pap smear findings. This analysis of tissue from the cervical canal is used to determine whether abnormal changes have occurred in the cervical canal. If these biopsy specimens show premalignant cells or CIN, the patient usually needs cryotherapy, laser therapy, or a cone biopsy (excision of an inverted tissue cone from the cervix) (Public Health Agency of Canada, 1998).

CRYOTHERAPY AND LASER THERAPY

Cryotherapy (freezing cervical tissue with nitrous oxide) and laser treatment are used in the outpatient setting. Cryotherapy may result in cramping and occasional feelings of faintness (vasovagal

FIGURE 46-6 Method of using a wooden Ayre spatula to obtain cervical secretions for cytology. (**A**) Speculum in place and the Ayre spatula in position at the cervical os. (**B**) The tip of the spatula is placed in the cervical os and the spatula rotated 360 degrees, firmly but nontraumatically. (**C**) Cellular material clinging to the spatula is then smeared gently and smoothly on a glass slide. (**D**) Cytobrush is rotated in the cervical os and rolled onto a glass slide. Smear is then sprayed with fixative. *Note:* Thin-prep (liquid-based) Pap smears are collected in the same way with a spatula and a brush, but then both are swirled separately in a bottle of Thin-prep solution and sent to the laboratory.

response). A watery discharge is normal for a few weeks after the procedure as the cervix heals.

CONE BIOPSY AND LEEP

If the endocervical curettage findings indicate abnormal changes or if the lesion extends into the canal, the patient may undergo a cone biopsy. This can be performed surgically or with a procedure called LEEP (loop electrosurgical excision procedure), which uses a laser beam.

Usually performed in the outpatient setting, LEEP is associated with a high success rate in removal of abnormal cervical tissue and has a low incidence of complications (Health Canada, 1998). The gynecologist excises a small amount of cervical tissue, and the pathologist examines the borders of the specimen to determine if they are free of disease. A patient anesthetized for a surgical cone

biopsy is advised to rest for 24 hours after the procedure and to leave any vaginal packing in place until the physician removes it (usually the next day). The patient is instructed to report any excessive bleeding.

Guidelines regarding postoperative sexual activity, bathing, and other activities are provided by the nurse or the physician. Because open tissue may be potentially exposed to HIV and other pathogens, the patient is usually cautioned to avoid intercourse until healing is complete and verified at follow-up. Cervical stenosis can be a complication of this procedure.

ENDOMETRIAL (ASPIRATION) BIOPSY

A tissue sample obtained through biopsy permits diagnosis of cellular changes in the endometrium. Endometrial biopsy, a method of obtaining endometrial tissue, is performed during the pelvic ex-

Chart 46-6

GUIDELINES FOR Obtaining an Optimal Pap Smear

NURSING ACTION	RATIONALE
1. Do not obtain a Pap smear if the woman is menstruating or has other frank bleeding (exception: high suspicion of neoplasia).	Blood obscures a proper reading of cells.
2. If performing more than one test (eg, Pap and GC), obtain the Pap smear first.	By performing the Pap smear first, the chance of a bloody smear is avoided.
3. Label the frosted end of the slide with the patient's name in pencil or label Thin-prep Pap bottle.	Ink may rub off or blur. Labelling with a pencil prevents improper identification.
4. Put on gloves before gently inserting the unlubricated speculum. (Speculum may be moistened with warm water.)	Gloves provide protection and warm water prevents discomfort. Lubricants may obscure cells on Pap smear.
5. Place the longer end of the Ayre spatula in the cervical canal and rotate it in a full circle to obtain a sample from the exocervix. Gently spread the material obtained onto the Pap smear slide.	This technique obtains a sampling of the exocervix and squamo-columnar junction. This prevents damaging the cells.
6. Insert a cytobrush 2 cm into the cervical canal and rotate 180 degrees. Roll the brush gently onto the Pap smear slide. (With Thin-prep Pap smears, the brushings are not spread onto a slide. The spatula and brush are placed in a bottle of fixative and swirled.)	This obtains endocervical cells and may sample cells from the squamocolumnar junction if it is high in the canal.
7. In women who have had a hysterectomy, use a cotton applicator moistened with saline solution to obtain a sampling of cells from the vaginal cuff or posterior vagina.	Saline solution prevents drying, which makes interpretation difficult for the cytologist and prevents absorption of cells into the cotton, increasing the yield on the slide.
8. Immediately spray the slide or, if a Thin-prep, swirl the brush and spatula in the solution.	Exposure to air or light causes distortion of cells.

amination when indicated as an outpatient procedure. Women undergoing this procedure may experience slight discomfort. Usually, the procedure can be performed without anesthesia; however, a paracervical block or a small injection of lidocaine into the uterus is effective if required. The examiner may apply a tenaculum (a clamp-like instrument that stabilizes the uterus) after the pelvic examination and then inserts a thin, hollow, flexible suction tube (pipelle or sampler) through the cervix into the uterus.

Endometrial biopsy is usually indicated in cases of midlife irregular bleeding, postmenopausal bleeding, and infertility (to identify changes in the uterine lining after ovulation). Women who are bleeding irregularly while receiving hormone replacement

Chart 46-7

The 2001 Bethesda System for Cytologic Classification of Pap Smears

Negative for Intraepithelial Lesion or Malignancy
Organisms
Trichomonas vaginalis
Fungal organisms morphologically consistent with *Candida* species
Shift in flora suggestive of bacterial vaginosis
Bacteria morphologically consistent with *Actinomyces* species
Cellular changes consistent with herpes simplex virus

Other Non-Neoplastic Findings (list not comprehensive)
Reactive cellular changes associated with
—Inflammation (includes typical repair)
—Radiation
—Intrauterine contraceptive device (IUD)
Glandular cells status posthysterectomy
Atrophy

Epithelial Cell Abnormalities
Squamous Cell
Atypical squamous cells (ASC)
—Of undetermined significance (ASC-US)
—Cannot exclude HSIL (ASC-H)
Low-grade squamous intraepithelial lesion (LSIL) encompassing:
HPV/mild dysplasia/cervical intraepithelial neoplasia (CIN) 1

High-grade squamous intraepithelial lesion (HSIL) encompassing:
moderate and severe dysplasia, carcinoma in situ, CIN 2 and CIN 3
—With features suspicious for invasion
Squamous cell carcinoma

Glandular Cell
Atypical (AGC)
 Endocervical cells
 Endometrial cells
 Glandular cells
Atypical
 Endocervical cells, favour neoplastic
 Glandular cells, favour neoplastic
Endocervical adenocarcinoma in situ (AIS)
Adenocarcinoma
 Endocervical
 Endometrial
 Extrauterine
 Not otherwise specified (NOS)

Other Malignant Neoplasms

Source: Solomon, D., Davey, D., Kurman, R., Moriarty, A., O'Connor, D., Prey, M., et al. (2001). The 2001 Bethesda System: Terminology for reporting results of cervical cytology. Consensus Statement. *Journal of the American Medical Association, 287*(16), 2114–2119.

therapy or who experience any bleeding while taking tamoxifen are usually advised to undergo endometrial biopsy.

Findings on aspiration may include normal endometrial tissue, hyperplasia, or endometrial cancer. Simple hyperplasia is an overgrowth of the uterine lining and is usually treated with progesterone. Complex hyperplasia is a risk factor for uterine cancer and is treated with progesterone and careful follow-up. Women who are overweight, who are over 45, who have a history of nulliparity and infertility, and who have a family history of colon cancer seem to be at higher risk for hyperplasia (Farquhar, Lethaby, Sowter et al., 1999). Endometrial cancer is discussed in Chapter 47.

DILATION AND CURETTAGE

A dilation and curettage (D & C) may be diagnostic (identifies the cause of irregular bleeding) or therapeutic (often temporarily stops irregular bleeding). The cervical canal is widened with a dilator and the uterine endometrium is scraped with a curette. The purpose of the procedure is to secure endometrial or endocervical tissue for cytologic examination, to control abnormal uterine bleeding, and as a therapeutic measure for incomplete abortion.

Because this procedure is usually carried out under anesthesia and requires surgical asepsis, it is usually performed in the operating room. However, it may take place in the outpatient setting with the patient receiving a local anesthetic supplemented with diazepam (Valium), midazolam (Versed), or meperidine (Demerol). The patient who receives these medications is carefully monitored until she has fully recovered.

The nurse provides an explanation of the procedure as well as physical and psychological preparation, informing the patient about what the procedure involves and what to expect in terms of postoperative discomfort and bleeding. The perineum is not shaved, but the patient is instructed to void before the procedure. The patient is placed in the lithotomy position, the cervix is dilated with a dilating instrument, and endometrial scrapings are

obtained by a curette. A perineal pad is placed over the perineum after the procedure, and excessive bleeding is reported. No restrictions are placed on dietary intake. If pelvic discomfort or low back pain occurs, mild analgesics usually provide relief. The physician indicates when sexual intercourse may be safely resumed. To reduce the risk of infection and bleeding, most physicians advise no vaginal penetration or use of tampons for 2 weeks.

ENDOSCOPIC EXAMINATIONS

Laparoscopy (Pelvic Peritoneoscopy)

A laparoscopy involves inserting a laparoscope (a tube about 10 mm wide and similar to a small periscope) into the peritoneal cavity through a 2-cm incision below the umbilicus to allow visualization of the pelvic structures (Fig. 46-7). Laparoscopy may be used for diagnostic purposes (eg, in cases of pelvic pain when no cause can be found) or treatment. Laparoscopy also facilitates many surgical procedures, such as tubal sterilization, ovarian biopsy, myomectomy, and lysis of adhesions (scar tissue that can cause pelvic discomfort). A surgical instrument (intrauterine sound or cannula) may be positioned inside the uterus to permit manipulation or movement during laparoscopy, affording better visualization. The pelvic organs can be visualized after the injection of a prescribed amount of carbon dioxide intraperitoneally into the cavity. Called insufflation, this technique separates the intestines from the pelvic organs. If the patient is undergoing sterilization, the fallopian or uterine tubes may be electrocoagulated, sutured, or ligated and a segment removed for histologic verification (clips are an alternative device for occluding the tubes).

After the laparoscopy is completed, the laparoscope is withdrawn, carbon dioxide is allowed to escape through the outer cannula, the small skin incision is closed with sutures or a clip, and the incision is covered with an adhesive bandage. The patient is carefully monitored for several hours to detect any untoward signs indicating bleeding (most commonly from vascular injury

FIGURE 46-7 Laparoscopy. The laparoscope (*right*) is inserted through a small incision in the abdomen. A forceps is inserted through the scope to grasp the fallopian tube. To improve the view, a uterine cannula (*left*) is inserted into the vagina to push the uterus upward. Insufflation of gas creates an air pocket (pneumoperitoneum), and the pelvis is elevated (note the angle), which forces the intestines higher in the abdomen.

to the hypogastric vessels), bowel or bladder injury, or burns from the coagulator. These complications are rare, making laparoscopy a cost-effective and safe short-stay procedure. The patient may experience abdominal or shoulder pain related to the use of carbon dioxide gas.

Hysteroscopy

Hysteroscopy (transcervical intrauterine endoscopy) allows direct visualization of all parts of the uterine cavity by means of a lighted optical instrument. The procedure is best performed about 5 days after menstruation stops, in the estrogenic phase of the menstrual cycle. The vagina and vulva are cleansed, and a paracervical anesthetic block is performed or lidocaine spray is used. The instrument used for the procedure, a hysteroscope, is passed into the cervical canal and advanced 1 or 2 cm under direct vision. Uterine-distending fluid (normal saline solution or 5% dextrose in water) is infused through the instrument to dilate the uterine cavity and enhance visibility.

Hysteroscopy is most commonly indicated as an adjunct to a D & C and laparoscopy in cases of infertility, unexplained bleeding, retained intrauterine device (IUD), and recurrent early pregnancy loss. Treatment for some conditions (eg, fibroid tumours) can be accomplished during this procedure. Hysteroscopy is contraindicated in patients with cervical or endometrial carcinoma or acute pelvic inflammation. Endometrial ablation (destruction of the uterine lining) is performed with a hysteroscope and laser beam in cases of severe bleeding not responsive to other therapies. Performed in an outpatient setting, this rapid procedure is an alternative to hysterectomy for some patients. Hysteroscopy, a safe procedure with few complications, has been found to be useful for evaluating endometrial pathology. Uterine perforation can occur.

OTHER DIAGNOSTIC PROCEDURES

Many diagnostic procedures are helpful in evaluating pelvic conditions. These may include x-rays, barium enemas, gastrointestinal x-ray series, intravenous urography, and cystography studies. Additionally, because the uterus, ovaries, and fallopian tubes are near the kidneys, ureters, and bladder, urologic diagnostic studies, such as the KUB (kidney, ureter, and bladder) and pyelography are used, as are angiography and radioisotope scanning, if needed. Other diagnostic procedures include hysterosalpingography and computed tomography (CT) scanning.

Hysterosalpingography or Uterotubography

Hysterosalpingography is an x-ray study of the uterus and the fallopian tubes after injection of a contrast agent. The diagnostic procedure is performed to evaluate infertility or tubal patency and to detect any abnormal condition in the uterine cavity. Sometimes the procedure is therapeutic because the flowing contrast agent flushes debris or loosens adhesions.

In preparation for hysterosalpingography, the intestinal tract is cleansed with cathartics and an enema so that gas shadows do not distort the x-ray findings. An analgesic agent may be prescribed. The patient is placed in the lithotomy position and the cervix is exposed with a bivalved speculum. A cannula is inserted into the cervix and the contrast agent is injected into the uterine cavity and the fallopian tubes. X-rays are taken to show the path and the distribution of the contrast agent.

Some patients experience nausea, vomiting, cramps, and faintness. After the test, the patient is advised to wear a perineal pad for several hours because the radiopaque agent may stain clothing.

CT Scan

CT scanning has several advantages over ultrasonography (described below), even though it involves radiation exposure and is more costly. It is more effective than ultrasonography for obese patients or patients with a distended bowel. A CT scan can also demonstrate a tumour and any extension into the retroperitoneal lymph nodes and skeletal tissue, although it has limited value in diagnosing other gynecologic abnormalities.

Ultrasonography

Ultrasonography (or ultrasound) is a useful adjunct to the physical examination, particularly in the obstetric patient or the patient with abnormal pelvic examination findings. It is a simple procedure based on sound wave transmission that uses pulsed ultrasonic waves at frequencies exceeding 20,000 Hz (formerly cycles per second). A transducer placed in contact with the abdomen (abdominal scan) or a vaginal probe (vaginal ultrasound) converts mechanical energy into electrical impulses, which in turn are amplified and recorded on an oscilloscope screen while a photograph or video recording of the patterns is taken. The entire procedure takes about 10 minutes and involves no ionizing radiation and no discomfort other than a full bladder, which is necessary for good visualization during an abdominal scan. (A vaginal ultrasound or sonogram does not require a full bladder.) Saline may be instilled into the uterus (saline infusion sonogram) to help delineate endometrial polyps or fibroids. Polyps are a frequent benign cause of bleeding in older women and can be removed by polypectomy.

Magnetic Resonance Imaging

Magnetic resonance imaging (MRI) produces patterns that are finer and more definitive than other imaging procedures without exposing the patient to radiation. MRI, however, is more costly.

Management of Normal and Altered Female Physiologic Processes

Many health concerns of women are related to normal changes or abnormalities of the menstrual cycle. Many result from women's lack of understanding of the menstrual cycle, developmental changes, and factors that may affect the pattern of the menstrual cycle. Educating women about the menstrual cycle and changes over time is an important aspect of the nurse's role in providing quality care to women. Teaching should begin early, so that menstruation and the lifelong changes in the menstrual cycle can be anticipated and accepted as a normal part of life.

MENSTRUATION

Menstruation, a cyclic vaginal flow of tissue that lines the uterus, occurs about every 28 days during the reproductive years, although normal cycles can vary from 21 to 42 days. The flow usually lasts 4 to 5 days, during which time 50 to 60 mL of blood are lost.

A perineal pad is generally used to absorb menstrual discharge; deodourant-treated pads are available, but some women are allergic or sensitive to the deodourants. Tampons are also used extensively; there is no significant evidence of untoward effects from their use, provided that there is no difficulty in inserting them. However, tampons should not be used for more than 4 to 6 hours, nor should superabsorbent tampons be used because of the association with toxic shock syndrome (see Chap. 47 for more about this syndrome). If a tampon is hard to remove, the vagina feels dry, or the tampon shreds when removed, less absorbent tampons should be used. If the string breaks or retracts, a woman should squat in a comfortable position, insert one finger into the vagina, try to locate the tampon, and remove it. If the woman feels uncomfortable attempting this manoeuvre or if she cannot remove the tampon, she should consult a health care provider.

Psychosocial Considerations

Girls who are approaching menarche (the onset of menstruation) should be instructed about the normal process of the menstrual cycle before it occurs. Psychologically, it is much healthier to refer to this event as a "period" rather than as "being sick." With adequate nutrition, rest, and exercise, most women feel little discomfort, although some report breast tenderness and a feeling of fullness 1 or 2 days before menstruation begins. Others report fatigue and some discomfort in the lower back, legs, and pelvis on the first day and temperament or mood changes. Slight deviations from a usual pattern of daily living are considered normal, but excessive deviation may require evaluation. Regular exercise and a low-fat vegetarian diet have been found to decrease discomfort. Heating pads may be very effective for cramps, as may nonsteroidal anti-inflammatory drugs (NSAIDs). The patient with excessive cramping or dysmenorrhea is referred to a gynecologist; oral contraceptives may be prescribed following evaluation.

Cultural Considerations

Canada is becoming more culturally diverse. Culture can be defined as the thoughts, communications, actions, customs, beliefs, and values of a racial, ethnic, religious, or social group. These aspects of culture affect many health care encounters, and these encounters can be positive if nurses understand the various cultures of their patients.

Differing cultural views and beliefs on menstruation exist. Some women believe that it is detrimental to change a pad or tampon too frequently; they think that allowing the discharge to accumulate increases the flow, which is considered desirable. Some women believe they are vulnerable to illness during menstruation. Others feel it is harmful to swim, shower, have their hair permed, have their teeth filled, or eat certain foods during menstruation. They may also avoid using contraception.

In such situations, the nurse is in a position to provide women with facts in an accepting and culturally sensitive manner. The objective is to be mindful of these unexpressed, deep-rooted beliefs and to provide the facts with care. Aspects of gynecologic problems cannot always be expressed easily. The nurse needs to convey confidence and openness and to offer facts to facilitate communication. Suggestions to improve care include overcoming language barriers, providing language-appropriate materials, asking about traditional beliefs and dietary practices, and asking patients about their fears regarding care (Mattson, 2000). Patience, sensitivity, and a desire to learn about other cultures and groups will enhance the nursing care of all women (Chart 46-8).

PERIMENOPAUSE

Perimenopause is the period extending from the first signs of menopause—usually hot flashes, vaginal dryness, and irregular menses—to beyond the complete cessation of menses. It has also been defined as the period around menopause, lasting up to 1 year after the last menstrual period. Women often have varied beliefs about aging, and these must be considered by the nurse caring for or educating perimenopausal patients.

Nursing Management

Perimenopausal women often benefit from information about the subtle physiologic changes they are experiencing. Perimenopause has been described as an opportune time for teaching women about health promotion and disease prevention strategies. When discussing health-related concerns with midlife women, nurses should consider the following issues:

• Sexuality, fertility, contraception, STDs

Chart 46-8 **Lesbian Health Care**

Lesbians can generally be defined as women who have sex with or primary emotional partnerships with women, but there is no universally accepted definition; variability exists in relationships and sexual preferences. Lesbians are found in every ethnic group and socioeconomic class. They can be single, celibate, divorced, teens, and seniors. Most experts believe that sexual orientation is not a conscious choice.

Lesbians have often encountered insensitivity in health care encounters. When they are asked if they are sexually active and respond affirmatively, contraception is immediately urged as health care providers may assume incorrectly that they practice heterosexual intercourse. Similar to many other marginalized groups of women, they often underuse health care. Some health care providers are homophobic, and discrimination against lesbians has been found in health care (Blackwell & Blackwell, 1999). Nurses need to consider lesbian-

ism within the continuum of human sexual behaviour and need to use gender-neutral questions and terms that are non-judgmental and accepting. Lesbian teens are at risk for suicide and STDs. Many lesbians do participate in heterosexual activity and often consider themselves at low risk for STDs. Because HPV, herpes infections, and other organisms implicated in STDs are transmitted by secretions and contact, they may need information on STDs and contraception. If sex toys are used and not cleaned, pelvic infections can occur.

Lesbians may smoke and drink more alcohol, may have a higher body mass index, may bear fewer or no children, and often have fewer health preventive screenings than heterosexual women (Carroll, 1999). These factors may predispose them to colon, lung, endometrial, ovarian, and breast cancer, as well as cardiovascular disease and diabetes. Nurses need to understand the unique needs of this population and provide appropriate and sensitive care.

- Unintended pregnancy (this is possible if contraception is not used)
- Oral contraceptive use. Oral contraceptives provide perimenopausal women with protection against uterine cancer, ovarian cancer, anemia, pregnancy, and fibrocystic breast changes as well as relief from perimenopausal symptoms. This option should be discussed with perimenopausal women. (Women who smoke and who are 35 or older should not take oral contraceptives because of an increased risk for cardiovascular disease.)
- Breast health. About 16% of cases of breast cancer occur in this group of women, so breast self-examination, routine physical examinations, and mammograms are essential.

Women need to be aware that diet and exercise are crucial to their health. The Women's Health Initiative study has found that the risks of long-term use of hormone replacement therapy (HRT) outweigh the benefits. Although HRT decreases hot flashes and reduces the risk for osteoporotic fractures and colorectal cancer, it increases the risk for breast cancer, heart attack, stroke, and blood clots (Writing Group for Women's Health Initiative Investigators, 2002). (It has been suggested that the term "menopausal hormone therapy" be used in place of HRT.)

MENOPAUSE

Menopause is the permanent physiologic cessation of menses associated with declining ovarian function; during this time, reproductive function diminishes and ends. Postmenopause is the period beginning from about 1 year after menses cease. Menopause is associated with some atrophy of breast tissue and genital organs, loss in bone density, and vascular changes.

Menopause starts gradually and is usually signaled by changes in menstruation. The monthly flow may increase, decrease, become irregular, and finally cease. Often, the interval between periods is longer; a lapse of several months between periods is not uncommon.

Changes signaling menopause begin to occur as early as the late 30s, when ovulation occurs less frequently, estrogen levels fluctuate, and FSH levels rise in an attempt to stimulate estrogen production.

Clinical Manifestations

Because of these hormonal changes, some women notice irregular menses, breast tenderness, and mood changes long before menopause occurs. The hot or warm flashes and night sweats reported by some women are directly attributable to hormonal changes. Hot flashes, which denote vasomotor instability, may vary in intensity from a barely perceptible warm feeling to a sensation of extreme warmth accompanied by profuse sweating, causing discomfort, sleep disturbances and subsequent fatigue, and embarrassment.

Other physical changes may include atrophic changes and **osteoporosis** (decreased bone density), resulting in decreased stature and bone fractures. Osteoporotic fractures will occur in one in six Canadian women over 50 years of age (Cheung, Feig, Kapral, et al., 2004). The entire genitourinary system is affected by the reduced estrogen level. Changes in the vulvovaginal area may include a gradual thinning of pubic hair and a slow shrink-

age of the labia. Vaginal secretions decrease, and the woman may report dyspareunia (discomfort during intercourse). The vaginal pH rises during menopause, predisposing the woman to bacterial infections (atrophic vaginitis). Discharge, itching, and vulvar burning may result.

Some women report fatigue, dizziness, forgetfulness, weight gain, irritability, trouble sleeping, feeling "blue," and feelings of panic. Menopausal complaints need to be evaluated carefully as they may indicate other disorders.

Psychological Considerations

Women's reactions and feelings related to loss of reproductive capacity may vary (Jacob's Institute of Women's Health, 2000). For women with grown families, menopause may result in role confusion or feelings of sexual and personal freedom. Women may be relieved that the childbearing phase of their lives is over. Each woman's circumstances will affect her response and must be considered on an individual basis. Nurses need to be aware of and sensitive to all possibilities and take their cues from the patient.

Medical Management

As stated earlier, menopause may be characterized by decreased vaginal secretions, hot flashes, changes in the urinary tract, and mood swings. Decreased vaginal lubrication may cause dyspareunia in the menopausal woman; this may be prevented by the use of a water-soluble lubricant (eg, K-Y jelly, Replens, Astro-Glide, or contraceptive foam or jelly). A vaginal cream containing estrogen or an estrogen-containing vaginal ring may be prescribed.

Women approaching menopause often have many concerns about their health. Some have concerns based on a family history of heart disease, osteoporosis, or breast cancer. Each woman should discuss her concerns and feelings with her primary health care provider so that she can make an informed decision about managing menopausal symptoms and maintaining her health.

PHARMACOLOGIC THERAPY

Hormone Replacement Therapy. HRT reduces or eliminates persistent and severe hot flashes, reduces bone loss, decreases the risk for colon cancer, and improves lipoproteins and lowers fibrinogen levels (Hulley, Grady, Bush, et al., 1998). Despite these findings, the more recent Women's Health Initiative controlled trial of HRT in over 16,600 women demonstrated that the risks of HRT outweigh the benefits (Writing Group of the Women's Health Initiative Investigators, 2002). This study was halted after 5.2 years rather than continuing it for the planned duration of 8.5 years because women receiving HRT had a higher risk for invasive breast cancer than the group receiving placebo. Although the absolute risk of breast cancer is low for an individual woman taking HRT, the risks were considered contrary to its intended effect, which is to preserve health and prevent disease. Because of these findings, many women have elected to discontinue HRT, and many of those who previously would have taken HRT have refused or are reluctant to consider it. Some women and their health care providers have elected to begin or continue use of HRT to treat menopausal symptoms because of its benefits. Nurses need to be knowledgeable about the issues associated with

HRT use if they are to provide appropriate health care to perimenopausal and menopausal women.

Risks and Benefits of HRT.
The changes that occur during menopause have adverse effects on women, placing them at increased risk for atherosclerosis, angina, and coronary artery disease. The effectiveness of HRT in reducing the risk for some of these conditions has not been supported, and the Heart and Stroke Foundation of Canada has recommended against initiating HRT for primary and secondary prevention of cardiovascular disease or stroke (Abramson, Dzerko, Lalonde, et. al, 2002). HRT is contraindicated in women with a history of breast cancer, vascular thrombosis, active liver disease or chronically impaired liver function, some cases of uterine cancer, and undiagnosed abnormal vaginal bleeding. The risk of thromboembolic phenomena is slightly elevated. Women who elect to take HRT despite these risks should be taught the signs and symptoms of deep vein thrombosis and pulmonary embolism and should be instructed to report these signs and symptoms immediately. Nurses should assess for leg redness, tenderness, chest pain, and shortness of breath in patients who take HRT. Further, women taking HRT need to be informed about the need for follow-up and monitoring. For women who decide to take HRT, regular follow-up care, including a yearly physical examination and mammogram, is important. An endometrial biopsy is indicated for women with any irregular bleeding during treatment. Because the risk of complications increases the longer HRT is used, HRT should be used for the shortest time necessary (Abramson et al., 2002).

Making a Decision About HRT.
The decision of whether to use HRT has been a difficult one for many women. Although the results of the Women's Health Initiative trial may make the decision easier for some women, it is likely to remain a difficult decision for those who may benefit from its use because of very disruptive symptoms of menopause and evidence of bone loss. Women often want to learn about alternatives to HRT use; therefore, nurses should address other strategies that women can use to promote their health in the perimenopausal period.

Method of HRT Administration.
There are several different approaches for use of hormone replacement. Some women take both estrogen and progestin daily; others take estrogen for 25 consecutive days each month, with progestin taken in cycles (eg, 10 to 14 days of the month). Progestin is taken to prevent proliferation of the uterine lining and hyperplasia in women who have not had their uterus removed. Women who take hormones for 25 days often experience bleeding after completing the progestin. Other women take estrogen and progesterone every day and usually experience no bleeding. They occasionally have irregular spotting, which should be evaluated by their health care provider.

Estrogen patches, which are replaced once or twice weekly, are another option but require a progestin along with them if the woman still has a uterus. Vaginal treatment with an estrogen cream, suppository, or an estradiol vaginal ring (Estring) may be used for vaginal dryness or atrophic vaginitis. Estring is a small, flexible vaginal ring that slowly releases estrogen in small doses over 3 months.

Alternatives to HRT.
Women may benefit from learning about alternatives to HRT, including diet, vitamins, and exercise. They need to know that these approaches to menopause have not been examined thoroughly through research. Osteoporosis, a disease characterized by low bone mass and microarchitectural deterio-

ration of bone tissue, occurs with menopause and leads to enhanced bone fragility and increased risk for fracture. Other factors that increase a woman's risk for osteoporosis include a thin body frame, race (Caucasian or Asian), family history of osteoporosis, nulliparity, early menopause, moderate to heavy alcohol ingestion, smoking, caffeine use, sedentary lifestyle, and a diet low in calcium. Women should be advised to remain active or to begin an exercise program of weight-bearing activity, such as walking; to take a calcium supplement and vitamin D_3; to decrease or stop smoking; and to discuss the use of pharmacologic agents (bisphosphonates, calcitonin, parathyroid hormone, HRT) to reduce bone loss with their health care provider (Brown & Josse, 2002). Selective estrogen receptor modulators (SERMs) such as raloxifene (Evista) provide another alternative to HRT for the prevention and treatment of osteoporosis. These medications do not appear to increase the risk for breast cancer; indeed, the risk of breast and uterine cancer may be reduced. Their use may increase hot flashes. No long-term studies exist on these medications because of their recent development. Osteoporosis and its treatment are described in detail in Chapter 68.

Problematic hot flashes have been treated with venlafaxine (Effexor), paroxetine (Paxil), gabapentin (Neurontin), and clonidine (Catapres). These medications have been found to reduce hot flashes and are alternatives for women who do not wish to use HRT. The web site of the North American Menopause Society (http://www.menopause.org) provides additional suggestions.

Vitamin B in doses of less than 200 mg has been found to relieve some distressing menopausal symptoms. Vitamin E has been effective in decreasing hot flashes for many women. Some women are interested in alternative treatments (eg, natural estrogens and progestins, black cohosh, ginseng, dong quai, soy products, and several other herbal preparations); however, few scientific data exist about the safety or effectiveness of these remedies. Assessment of menopausal patients should include their use of complementary and alternative therapies and supplements. Medications, including alendronate (Fosamax), raloxifene (Evista), and calcitonin, for the treatment of osteoporosis have given women another option in preventing or treating this major health problem.

The Heart and Stroke Foundation of Canada (Abramson et al., 2002) suggests the use of established methods of treatment to lower heart disease risk in women. These include lifestyle changes and behavioural strategies. Pharmacologic therapy (eg, aspirin, beta blockers, statins, angiostatin-converting enzyme inhibitors) may be indicated in women who have cardiovascular disease or are at high risk for it. See Chapter 26 for a more detailed discussion of treatment and prevention of cardiovascular disease.

BEHAVIOURAL STRATEGIES
Regular physical exercise, including weight-bearing exercise, raises the heart rate, increases high-density lipoprotein (HDL) levels, and helps to maintain bone mass. It may also reduce stress, enhance well-being, and improve self-image. Loss of muscle tissue is mediated by exercise; weight-bearing exercise (eg, walking, jogging) at least four times a week is recommended.

NUTRITIONAL THERAPY
Women should also be encouraged to decrease caloric intake, decrease fat intake, and increase intake of whole grains, fibre, fruit, and vegetables. Women of all ages are urged to include high-calcium food in their diets daily. For example, 250 mL of milk contains about 300 mg of calcium, and 250 mL of nonfat yogurt provides

415 mg of calcium. Other sources of dietary calcium include most green leafy vegetables, seafood, and calcium-fortified foods.

Calcium supplementation may be helpful in reducing bone loss and preventing the morbidity associated with fractures secondary to osteoporosis. Bones serve as a storehouse of the body's calcium, and bone density decreases with age. When calcium levels in the blood are low, the bones give up calcium to maintain homeostasis. Women of all age groups often ingest less than the recommended amount of calcium. The average calcium intake is 300 to 500 mg/day, whereas the recommended amount is 1,300 mg/day for adolescents and young adults, 1,000 mg/day for adults 19 to 50 years of age, and 1,500 mg/day for adults 51 years of age and older. Due to low sun exposure, Canadians require vitamin D_3 (cholecalciferol) supplements. Daily intake for children to age 18 years is 200–400 IU (International Units) (Holick, 1998); for those 19–50 years, 400–600 IU; and those 51 and older require 800 IU per day (Brown & Josse, 2002).

Nursing Management

Nurses can encourage women to view menopause as a natural change resulting in freedom from menses and symptoms related to hormonal changes. No relationship exists between menopause and mental health problems; however, social circumstances (eg, adolescent children, ill partners, and dependent or ill parents) that usually coincide with menopause may produce stress.

Measures should be taken to promote general health. The nurse can explain to the patient that cessation of menses is a physiologic function that is rarely accompanied by nervous symptoms or illness. The current expected life span after menopause for the average woman is 30 to 35 years, which may encompass as many years as the childbearing phase of her life. Menopause is not a complete change of life, however. Normal sexual urges continue, and women retain their usual response to sex long after menopause. Many women enjoy better health after menopause than before, especially those who have experienced dysmenorrhea. The individual woman's evaluation of herself and her worth, now and in the future, is likely to affect her emotional reaction to menopause. Patient teaching and counselling regarding healthy lifestyles, health promotion, and health screening are of paramount importance (Chart 46-9).

PREMENSTRUAL SYNDROME

Premenstrual syndrome (PMS) is a combination of symptoms that occur before the menses and subside with the onset of menstrual flow (Chart 46-10). The cause is unknown, but serotonin

---

Chart 46-9
Home Care Checklist • The Woman Approaching Menopause

At the completion of the home care instruction, the patient or caregiver will be able to:	Patient	Caregiver
• Describe menopause as a normal period in a woman's life.	✓	✓
• State that fatigue and stress may worsen hot flashes.	✓	✓
• State that a nutritious diet and weight control will enhance physical and emotional well-being.	✓	✓
• State the importance of exercising for 30 minutes three or four times a week to maintain good health.	✓	✓
• Describe involvement in outside activities as beneficial in reducing anxiety and tension.	✓	✓
• Identify the following as changes that often occur in midlife: departure of children, aging, dependence of parents, possible loss of loved ones.	✓	✓
• Describe this phase of life as having the potential for intellectual growth, personal accomplishment, and initiation of new activities.	✓	✓
• State the following points about sexual activity: Frequent sexual activity helps to maintain the elasticity of the vagina. Contraception is advised until 1 year passes without menses. Safer sex is important at any age. Sexual functioning may be enhanced at midlife.	✓	
• Identify the importance of an annual physical examination to screen for problems and to promote general health.	✓	
• Identify strategies and methods to prevent or manage the following problems: Itching or burning of vulvar areas: see primary health care provider to rule out dermatologic abnormalities and, if appropriate, to obtain a prescription for a lubricating or hormonal cream.	✓	
Dyspareunia (painful intercourse) due to vaginal dryness; use a water-soluble lubricant, such as K-Y Jelly, Astro-Glide, Replens, hormone cream, or contraceptive foam.	✓	
Decreased perineal muscle tone and bladder control: practice Kegel exercises daily (contract the perineal muscles as though stopping urination; hold for 5–10 seconds and release; repeat frequently during the day).	✓	
Dry skin: use mild emollient skin cream and lotions to prevent dry skin.	✓	
Weight control: join a weight-reduction support group such as Weight Watchers or a similar group if appropriate, or consult a registered dietitian for guidance about the tendency to gain weight, particularly around the hips, thighs, and abdomen.	✓	
Osteoporosis: observe recommended calcium and vitamin D intake, including supplements, if indicated, to slow the process of osteoporosis; avoid smoking, alcohol, and excessive caffeine, all of which increase bone loss. Perform weight-bearing exercises. Have bone density testing when appropriate.	✓	
Risk for urinary tract infection (UTI): drink 6 to 8 glasses of water daily and take vitamin C (500 mg) as a possible way to reduce the incidence of UTI related to atrophic changes of the urethra.	✓	
Vaginal bleeding: report any bleeding after 1 year of no menses to a primary health care provider *immediately, no matter how minimal.*	✓	

Chart 46-10   **Causes, Manifestations, and Treatment of Premenstrual Syndrome**

Cause

Unknown; may be related to hormonal changes combined with other factors (diet, stress, and lack of exercise)

Many women have some symptoms related to menses, but PMS affects 2% to 5% of women and is a complex of symptoms that result in dysfunction.

Physical Symptoms

Fluid retention (eg, bloating, breast tenderness)

Headache

Swelling

Affective Symptoms

Depression

Anger

Irritability

Anxiety

Confusion

Withdrawal

Symptoms begin in the 5 days preceding menses and relief is within 4 days of onset of menses. Dysfunction usually occurs in relationships, parenting, work, or school.

Treatment

Use of social support and family resources

Nutritious diet consisting of whole grains, fruits, and vegetables; increased water intake may help.

Serotonin reuptake inhibitors

Alprazolam (Xanax) has been effective but is addictive.

Spironolactone, a diuretic, may be effective in treating fluid retention.

Initiation/maintenance of exercise program.

Stress reduction techniques.

---

regulation is currently the most plausible theory. Other hormones may also be involved. Dietary factors may play a role because carbohydrates may affect serotonin. Severe symptoms have been labelled as premenstrual dysphoric disorder (DiCarlo, Palomba, Tommaselli et al., 2001; Morse, 1999). This severe form of PMS, which interferes with the woman's schoolwork, job, or social or family life, is uncommon.

Clinical Manifestations

Major symptoms of PMS include headache, fatigue, low back pain, painful breasts, and a feeling of abdominal fullness. General irritability, mood swings, fear of losing control, binge eating, and crying spells may also occur. Symptoms vary widely from one woman to another and from one cycle to the next in the same person. Great variability is found in the degree of symptoms. Many women are affected to some degree, but few are severely affected. Many women are not bothered at all, whereas some experience severe and disabling symptoms (Morse, 1999).

A generally stressful life and problematic relationships may be related to the intensity of physical symptoms. Some women report moderate to severe life disruption secondary to PMS that negatively affects their interpersonal relationships. PMS may also be a factor in reduced productivity, work-related accidents, and absenteeism.

Identifying the time when these symptoms occur helps in determining the diagnosis. Symptoms recur regularly at the same phase of each menstrual cycle, usually 1 week to a few days before menses, and subside once the menstrual flow starts.

Medical Management

Because there is no single treatment or known cure for PMS, the woman should chart her symptoms so she can possibly anticipate and therefore cope with them. Exercise is encouraged for all patients as noncontrolled studies have shown a benefit. Many practitioners advise women to avoid caffeine, high-fat foods, and refined sugars, but there is little research to demonstrate the efficacy of dietary changes. Alternative therapies that women have used include vitamins B and E, magnesium, and oil of evening primrose capsules. No studies have evaluated the effectiveness of these therapies.

PHARMACOLOGIC THERAPY

Pharmacologic remedies include selective serotonin reuptake inhibitors (eg, fluoxetine [Prozac, Sarafem]), gonadotropin-releasing hormone agonists, prostaglandin inhibitors (eg, ibuprofen and naproxen [Anaprox]), and antianxiety agents. Some clinicians prescribe analgesic agents, diuretic medications, and natural and synthetic progesterones, although the long-term risks of progesterone use are unknown. Many women find over-the-counter carbohydrate products useful; they provide complex carbohydrates along with vitamins and minerals. Ratios of serum levels of tryptophan to other amino acids are elevated in patients who use tryptophan. It may relieve psychological symptoms and food cravings. Calcium (1,200 mg/day) has been found to be effective, as has magnesium (200 to 400 mg/day).

Nursing Management

The nurse should establish rapport with the patient and obtain a health history, noting the time when symptoms began and their nature and intensity. The nurse then determines whether the onset of symptoms occurs before or shortly after the menstrual flow begins. Additionally, the nurse can show the patient how to develop a chart to record the timing and intensity of symptoms. A nutritional history is also elicited to determine if the diet is high in salt, caffeine, or alcohol or low in essential nutrients.

The patient's goals may include reduction of anxiety (mood swings, crying, binge eating, fear of losing control), ability to cope with day-to-day stressors and relationships with family and co-workers, and increased knowledge about PMS with improved use of control measures.

Positive coping measures are facilitated. Partners can be advised to assist by offering support and increased involvement with childcare. The patient can try to plan her working time to accommodate the days she will be less productive because of PMS. The nurse encourages the patient to use exercise, meditation, imagery, and creative activities to reduce stress. The nurse also encourages the patient to take medications as prescribed and provides instructions about the desired effects of the medications. Enrolling in a PMS group that meets to discuss problems may help the patient learn that others recognize and understand what she is experiencing.

If the patient has severe symptoms of PMS or premenstrual dysphoric disorder, the nurse assesses her for suicidal, uncontrollable, and violent behaviour. Any suggestions of suicidal tendencies must be evaluated by psychiatric consultation immediately. Uncontrollable behaviour may lead to violence toward family members. If abuse of children or other members of the patient's family is suspected, reporting protocols are implemented and followed. Referral is made for immediate psychiatric or psychological care and counselling.

DYSMENORRHEA

Primary dysmenorrhea is painful menstruation, with no identifiable pelvic pathology. It occurs at the time of menarche or shortly thereafter. It is characterized by crampy pain that begins before or shortly after the onset of menstrual flow and continues for 48 to 72 hours. Pelvic examination findings are normal. Dysmenorrhea is thought to result from excessive production of prostaglandins, which causes painful contraction of the uterus and arteriolar vasospasm. Psychological factors, such as anxiety and tension, may also contribute to dysmenorrhea. As women grow older, dysmenorrhea often decreases and frequently completely resolves after childbirth.

In secondary dysmenorrhea, pelvic pathology such as endometriosis, tumour, or pelvic inflammatory disease (PID) exists. Patients with secondary dysmenorrhea frequently have pain that occurs several days before menses, with ovulation, and occasionally with intercourse.

Assessment and Diagnostic Findings

A complete pelvic examination is performed to rule out possible abnormalities, such as strictures of the cervix or vagina, an imperforate hymen, or other conditions, such as endometriosis, PID, adenomyosis, and fibroid uterus. A laparoscopy is usually required to identify organic causes.

Management

In primary dysmenorrhea, the reason for the discomfort is explained, and the patient is assured that menstruation is a normal function of the reproductive system. If the patient is young and accompanied by her mother, the mother may also need reassurance. Many young women expect to have painful periods if their mothers did. The discomfort of cramps can be treated once anxiety and concern over its cause are dispelled by adequate explanation. Symptoms usually subside with appropriate medication. Aspirin, a mild prostaglandin inhibitor, may be taken at recommended doses every 4 hours. Other useful prostaglandin antagonists include NSAIDs such as ibuprofen (Motrin), naproxen (Aleve, Anaprox, Naprosyn), and mefenamic acid (Ponstel). If one medication does not provide relief, another may be recommended. Usually these medications are well tolerated, but some women experience gastrointestinal side effects. Contraindications include allergy, peptic ulcer history, sensitivity to aspirin-like medications, asthma, and pregnancy. Low-dose oral contraceptives provide relief in more than 90% of patients and are indi-

cated in women with dysmenorrhea who are sexually active but do not desire a pregnancy.

Continuous low-level local heat has recently been found to be effective in treating primary dysmenorrhea and may be as effective as medication (Akin, Weingand, Hengehold et al., 2001). The mechanism is not clear, but heat may counteract the activity of hormones that cause the uterus to contract. Heat is a vasodilator that increases blood flow and may counteract constriction and muscle contraction. Heat therapy and medication have been found to work well in combination.

The patient is encouraged to continue her usual activities and to increase physical exercise if possible, as this seems to relieve discomfort for some women. Taking analgesic agents before cramps start, in anticipation of discomfort, is advised.

Management of secondary dysmenorrhea is directed at diagnosis and treatment of the underlying cause (eg, endometriosis or PID). The same analgesic agents used for primary dysmenorrhea may be part of the management of secondary dysmenorrhea due to endometriosis.

AMENORRHEA

Amenorrhea (absence of menstrual flow) is a symptom of a variety of disorders and dysfunctions. Primary amenorrhea (delayed menarche) refers to the situation in which a young woman older than 16 has not begun to menstruate but otherwise shows evidence of sexual maturation, or when a young woman has not begun to menstruate and has not begun to show development of secondary sex characteristics by 14 years of age. Amenorrhea may be of considerable concern but is usually due to minor variations in body build, heredity, environment, and physical, mental, and emotional development.

The nurse allows the patient to express her concerns and anxiety about this problem, because the patient may feel that she is different from her peers. A complete physical examination, careful health history, and simple laboratory tests help to rule out possible causes, such as physiologic disorders, metabolic or endocrine difficulties, and systemic diseases. Treatment is directed toward correcting any abnormalities.

Secondary amenorrhea (an absence of menses for three cycles or 6 months after a normal menarche) may be caused by pregnancy, tension, emotional upset, or stress. In an adolescent, secondary amenorrhea is usually caused by minor emotional upset related to being away from home, attending college, tension due to schoolwork, or interpersonal problems. The second most common cause, however, is pregnancy, so a pregnancy test is almost always indicated.

Secondary nutritional disturbances may also be factors. Obesity can result in anovulation and subsequent amenorrhea. Eating disorders, such as anorexia and bulimia, are characterized by lack of menses because the decrease in body fat and caloric intake affects hormonal function. Competitive female athletes typically experience amenorrhea and are frequently placed on HRT to prevent bone loss related to low estrogen levels. On occasion, a pituitary or thyroid dysfunction may cause amenorrhea. These dysfunctions can be treated successfully by treatment of the underlying endocrine disorder. Infrequent periods (oligomenorrhea) may be related to thyroid disorders, polycystic ovarian syndrome, or premature ovarian failure. Again, evaluation by a primary health care provider is necessary.

ABNORMAL UTERINE BLEEDING

Dysfunctional uterine bleeding is abnormal bleeding that does not have a known organic cause. This can occur at any age but is most common at opposite ends of the reproductive life span. Dysfunctional uterine bleeding is defined as irregular, painless bleeding of endometrial origin that may be excessive, prolonged, or without pattern. It is usually secondary to anovulation (lack of ovulation) and is common in adolescents and women approaching menopause. Adolescents account for many cases of abnormal uterine bleeding since they often do not ovulate as their pituitary-ovarian axis matures. Perimenopausal women also experience this condition due to irregular ovulation because of their decreasing ovarian hormone production. The remaining causes are often related to cysts, obesity, or hypothalamic dysfunction.

Abnormal or unusual vaginal bleeding that is atypical in time or amount must be evaluated because it may be a manifestation of a major, life-threatening disorder. Physical examination is performed and the patient is evaluated for conditions such as pregnancy, neoplasm, infection, anatomic abnormalities, endocrine disorders, trauma, blood dyscrasias, platelet dysfunction, and hypothalamic disorders. Women of any age require evaluation for a specific cause of uterine bleeding. Pregnancy testing and hormonal evaluation are usually part of the initial assessment. Treatment usually consists of hormones or oral contraceptives.

Menorrhagia

Menorrhagia is defined as prolonged or excessive bleeding at the time of the regular menstrual flow. In early life the cause is usually related to endocrine disturbance, whereas in later life it usually results from inflammatory disturbances, tumours of the uterus, or hormonal imbalance. Emotional disturbances may also affect bleeding.

The nurse encourages a woman with menorrhagia to see her primary health care provider and to describe the amount of bleeding by pad count and saturation (ie, absorbency of perineal pad or tampon and number saturated hourly). Persistent heavy bleeding can result in anemia.

Metrorrhagia

Metrorrhagia (vaginal bleeding between regular menstrual periods) is probably the most significant form of menstrual dysfunction because it may signal cancer, benign tumours of the uterus, or other gynecologic problems. This condition warrants early diagnosis and treatment. Although bleeding between menstrual periods by a woman taking oral contraceptives is usually not serious, irregular bleeding by a woman taking HRT should be evaluated. Menometrorrhagia is heavy vaginal bleeding between and during periods and requires evaluation.

Postmenopausal Bleeding

Bleeding 1 year after menses cease at menopause must be investigated, and a malignant condition must be considered until proved otherwise. An endometrial biopsy or a D & C is indicated. A vaginal ultrasound can also be used in postmenopausal bleeding to measure the thickness of the endometrial lining. The uterine lining in postmenopausal women should be thin because of low estrogen levels. A lining thicker than 5 mm usually warrants evaluation by endometrial biopsy.

Management of Normal and Altered Female Reproductive Function

DYSPAREUNIA

Dyspareunia (difficult or painful intercourse) is increasing in incidence and can be superficial, deep, primary, or secondary. This problem can be embarrassing for women to discuss because they may believe that it is their problem if their partner is not experiencing discomfort. Dyspareunia may occur at the beginning of, during, or after intercourse and may be related to injury during childbirth, lack of lubrication, a history of incest, sexual abuse, or assault, endometriosis, pelvic infection, vaginal atrophy with menopause, gastrointestinal disorders, fibroids, urinary tract infection, STDs, or vulvodynia (vulvar pain that affects women of all ages without any discernible physical cause). Because dyspareunia is often due to lack of vaginal lubrication, use of vaginal lubricants can be suggested. Depending on the cause of dyspareunia, antidepressants may be prescribed in selected patients, and surgery to expand or repair the vaginal opening is occasionally needed.

CONTRACEPTION

Adolescents are more likely to experience pregnancy complications and are more prone to have low-birthweight babies. Teen mothers are less likely to obtain a high school diploma and are more likely to live in poverty. Of women undergoing abortions, many did not use contraception in the month they became pregnant, while others never use any method. It seems that women often fail to use effective methods consistently or at all. Nurses can assist with information and support. Women sometimes fear that they will get cancer and fear other risks from contraception. Women often report using their contraceptive method inconsistently, which makes all methods less effective.

Many women who are sexually active or who are considering becoming sexually active can benefit from learning about contraception. Fewer unwanted pregnancies may reduce the number of abortions, abused children, stressed families, and infant mortality and morbidity. It is important that women receive unbiased and nonjudgmental information, understand the benefits and risks of each method, learn about alternatives and how to use them, and receive positive reinforcement and acceptance of their choice.

Nurses involved in helping patients make contraceptive choices need to listen, educate, spend time answering questions, and assist patients in choosing the method they prefer. Methods and practices to prevent unwanted or unplanned pregnancies and births are described in subsequent sections of this chapter.

Abstinence

Abstinence, or celibacy, is the only completely effective means of preventing pregnancy. Abstinence may not be a desired or available option for many women because of cultural expectations and their own and their partner's values and sexual needs.

Sterilization

After abstinence, sterilization by bilateral tubal occlusion or vasectomy is the most effective means of contraception. Both procedures must be considered permanent because neither is easily reversible. Women and men who choose these methods should be certain that they have completed their childbearing, no matter how the circumstances in their life may change. Often, decisions are made that may be regretted later. Some gynecologists suggest a waiting period to ensure that the patient is certain about a potentially irreversible decision. See Chapter 49 for a discussion of vasectomy (male sterilization).

TUBAL LIGATION

Female sterilization by tubal ligation is one of the most common operations performed on women. Surveys of Canadian women aged 18 to 49 were conducted in 1984 (5315 women) and 1995 (3220 women). Tubal ligations decreased from 24% in 1984 to 17% in 1995. However, there was an increase in the proportion of women sterilized for reasons other than contraception from 1984 to 1995 (Martin & Wu, 2000). Tubal ligation is usually performed as a same-day surgical procedure. The procedure is carried out by laparoscopy, with the patient receiving a general or local anesthetic. The laparoscope, a small periscope-like optical instrument, is inserted through a small umbilical incision. Carbon dioxide is introduced to lift other abdominal organs away from the tubal area. The fallopian tubes are visualized and may be coagulated, sutured (Pomeroy procedure), or ligated with a rubber band or a spring clip, thereby disrupting their patency. Many sterilizations are performed with bipolar coagulation. Silicone bands and spring clips are also being used. Spring clips have the highest rate of pregnancy following sterilization. A new procedure, selective tubal occlusion procedure, uses a 1.5-cm metal coil or spring that is inserted into the fallopian tubes through the cervix, thus avoiding the need for laparoscopy or a surgical incision (Association of Reproductive Health Professionals, 2002). This method works by inducing obstruction of the tubes by scar tissue.

Despite a very high rate of effectiveness, any woman who has undergone tubal ligation but misses a period should be tested for pregnancy because ectopic and intrauterine pregnancies, although rare, may occur. Ovulation and menstruation are not affected by sterilization, although some women report heavier menstrual bleeding and more cramping after tubal ligation. Vasectomy and laparoscopic tubal ligation are compared in Chart 46-11.

Before undergoing tubal ligation, the patient should be informed that an IUD, if present, will be removed. If the patient is taking oral contraceptives, she usually continues them up to the time of the procedure. Postoperatively, women may experience abdominal or shoulder discomfort for a few days, related to the carbon dioxide gas and the manipulation of organs. The woman is instructed to report heavy bleeding, fever, or pain that persists or increases. The patient should avoid intercourse, strenuous exercise, and lifting for 2 weeks. Risks of the procedure are minimal and are more often related to the anesthesia than to the surgery itself. Risk is increased in women with diabetes, previous abdominal or pelvic surgery, or obesity.

Oral Contraceptives

Oral contraceptive preparations of synthetic estrogen (estradiol) and progesterone (desogestrel, ethynodiol diacetate, levonorgestrel, norethindrone, norethindrone acetate or norgestrel) are currently used by many women. They block ovarian stimulation by preventing the release of FSH from the anterior pituitary gland. In the absence of FSH, a follicle does not ripen, and ovulation does not occur. This is the mechanism of action of oral contraceptives. Progestins (synthetic forms of progesterone) suppress the LH surge, prevent ovulation, and also render the cervical mucus impenetrable to sperm. Synthetic estrogens and progestin, found in the many oral contraceptive variations available, differ in androgenic activity (Chart 46-12).

BENEFITS AND RISKS

In general, no definite long-term undesirable effects have been observed with prolonged oral contraceptive use. Resumption of normal menses is delayed 2 to 3 months in about 20% of oral contraceptive users. Venous thromboembolism has occurred with use of oral contraceptives, but it occurs less now than years ago, when estrogen concentrations in oral contraceptives were higher. Venous thromboembolism is less than half as likely to occur with oral contraceptives than with pregnancy. Desogestrel, a new pro-

---

Chart 46-11 **Comparison of Sterilization Methods**

Vasectomy

Advantages
- Highly effective
- Relieves the female of the contraceptive burden
- Inexpensive in the long run
- Permanent
- Highly acceptable procedure to most clients
- Very safe
- Quickly performed

Disadvantages
- Serious long-term effects suggested (although currently unproved)
- Permanent (although reversal is possible, it is expensive and requires a highly technical and major surgery, and its results cannot be guaranteed)
- Regret in 5%–10% of patients
- No protection against STDs, including HIV
- Not effective until sperm remaining in the reproductive system are ejaculated

Laparoscopic Tubal Sterilization

Advantages
- Low incidence of complications
- Short recovery
- Leaves small scar
- Quickly performed

Disadvantages
- Permanent
- Reversal difficult and expensive
- Sterilization procedures technically difficult
- Requires surgeon, operating room (aseptic conditions), trained assistants, medications, surgical equipment
- If failure, high probability of ectopic pregnancy
- No protection against STDs, including HIV

Chart 46-12 • PHARMACOLOGY
Comparison of Oral Contraceptives

There are two kinds of oral contraceptives: *combined* and *progestin only*. Combined pills consist of an estrogen and a progestin. The result of both types of medications is a lighter-than-normal menstrual flow after the contraceptives are taken for 21 days and then stopped for 7 days. The flow is actually withdrawal bleeding from discontinuing hormones because a normal period occurs only with ovulation. Most women using oral contraceptives take the combination medication.

Combined Preparations
- Each dose contains estrogen and progestin.
- Monophasic preparations supply a constant dose of estrogen and progestin.
- Biphasic preparations are available; they contain a constant amount of estrogen, with an increase in the progestin on day 10.
- Triphasic preparations are available; they provide varying low doses of estrogen along with progesterone during the 21-day cycle. This variation provides an effective contraceptive that mimics the normal cycle and has enough progesterone to prevent ovulation and spotting.

Progestin-Only "Mini" Preparations
- Each dose contains progestin only (estrogen is not contained in a progestin-only preparation).
- Preparation provides less protection against conception than combined preparations.
- About 40% of women taking progestin only have ovulatory cycles.
- Progestin only is useful for women who have had estrogen-related side effects on combination pills (eg, headaches, hypertension, leg pain, chloasma or skin discolouration, weight gain, or nausea).
- Progestin-only preparations are useful for lactating women who need a hormonal contraceptive method.

gestin, may be slightly more likely to be associated with venous thromboembolism, but the risk is still very low. Gallbladder problems (eg, cholestasis) may occur. Fetal anomalies do not appear to be a concern, and normal reproductive tract function and fertility are restored after oral contraceptive use is discontinued. However, most health care providers recommend that women use a barrier contraceptive method for 1 to 2 months after stopping the pill before becoming pregnant so that the accurate date of the last menstrual period is available to date the pregnancy.

Some of the benefits of using oral contraceptives include a reduction in the incidence of benign breast disease, improvement in acne, reduced risk of uterine and ovarian cancers, anemia, and pelvic infection.

> **NURSING ALERT** Patients need to be aware that oral contraceptives protect them from pregnancy but not from STDs or HIV infection. In addition, sex with multiple partners or sex without a condom may also result in chlamydial and other infections, including HIV infection.

A few patients experience adverse reactions when using oral contraceptives. These include nausea, depression, headache, weight gain, leg cramps, and breast soreness. Usually, these symptoms subside after 3 or 4 months. Because such symptoms are sometimes related to sodium and water retention caused by estrogen, a smaller dose of the hormone or a different hormonal combination may alleviate the problem. Many patients experi-

ence spotting in the first month taking the pill or if they take it irregularly, so they need to be reassured and advised to take a pill every 24 hours, as prescribed. Chart 46-13 describes the benefits and risks of oral contraceptive use.

CONTRAINDICATIONS

Absolute contraindications include current or past thromboembolic disorder, cerebrovascular disease, or artery disease; known or suspected breast cancer; known or suspected current or past estrogen-dependent neoplasia; pregnancy; current or past benign or malignant liver tumour; impaired liver function; congenital hyperlipidemia; and undiagnosed abnormal vaginal bleeding.

Relative contraindications include hypertension, bile-induced jaundice, acute phase of mononucleosis, and sickle cell disease. Women older than 35 who smoke are at risk for cardiac problems and should not use oral contraceptives. Occasionally, neuro-ocular complications arise, but a cause-and-effect relationship has not been established. If visual disturbances occur, oral contraceptives should be discontinued (Chart 46-14).

Some gynecologists allow patients with migraine headaches to take oral contraceptives if the headaches do not worsen with use or so long as the patient has no neurologic symptoms. (A young woman who has blurred vision with a migraine will probably be discouraged from taking oral contraceptives.) Diabetes is also problematic, although some diabetes specialists allow their patients to use oral contraceptives with careful glucose monitoring. Leiomyomas (fibroid tumours) of the uterus can enlarge with oral contraceptive use. Patients with this condition are advised and monitored carefully; if fibroids enlarge, they are advised to discontinue oral contraceptives and choose another contraceptive method.

Injectable Contraceptives

DEPO-PROVERA

An intramuscular injection of Depo-Provera, a long-acting progestin, every 3 months inhibits ovulation and provides a reliable

Chart 46-13 • PHARMACOLOGY
Benefits and Risks of Oral Contraceptives

Benefits
- Decreased cramps and bleeding
- Regular bleeding cycle
- Decreased incidence of anemia
- Decrease in acne with some formulations
- Protection from uterine and ovarian cancer
- Decreased incidence of ectopic pregnancy
- Protection from benign breast disease
- Decreased incidence of pelvic infection

Risks
- Rare in healthy women
- Bothersome side effects (eg, breakthrough bleeding, breast tenderness)
- Nausea, weight gain, mood changes
- Small increased risk of developing blood clots, stroke, or heart attack, related more to smoking than to oral contraceptive use alone
- Possible increased incidence of benign liver tumours and gallbladder problems
- No protection from STDs (possible increased risk with unsafe sex)

and convenient contraceptive method. It can be used by lactating women and those with hypertension, liver disease, migraine headaches, heart disease, and hemoglobinopathies. Women who use this method must be prepared for irregular or no bleeding. With continued use, irregular bleeding episodes and spotting decrease, and amenorrhea usually occurs.

Advantages include reduction of menorrhagia, dysmenorrhea, and anemia. It may reduce the risk of pelvic infection and has been associated with improvement in hematologic status in women with anemia due to heavy menstrual bleeding and women with sickle cell disease; it has also been associated with a reduced frequency of seizures in women with seizure disorders. It also reduces the risk of endometrial cancer (ACOG Technical Bulletin #198, 1995).

Potential disadvantages include irregular menstrual bleeding, bloating, headaches, hair loss, decreased sex drive, and weight loss or weight gain. Fertility may be delayed when women discontinue this method; therefore, other methods of contraception may be more appropriate for the woman who wishes to conceive within a year of discontinuing contraception.

Depo-Provera is contraindicated in women who are pregnant and those who have abnormal vaginal bleeding of unknown cause, breast or pelvic cancer, or sensitivity to synthetic progestin. The long-term effects on the infant of a nursing mother who uses Depo-Provera are unknown but are thought to be negligible. Depo-Provera does not protect against STDs. Bone density is decreased while using this method and the bone mineral density loss may be significant (Health Canada, 2004). It is not known if the use of Depo-Provera during adolescence or early adulthood will increase the risk of osteoporotic fractures in later life.

Implant Contraceptive

The Norplant system was a reversible, low-dose, progestin-only contraceptive device consisting of several soft Silastic capsules or implants that were inserted under the skin of the woman's upper arm. The implant released the progestin levonorgestrel over 5 years, thereby inhibiting ovulation. Health Canada discontinued the use of Norplant in 2002. However, additional implant contraceptives are expected to become available in the near future. Contraindications to using these systems are acute liver disease or liver tumours, pregnancy, unexplained vaginal bleeding, breast cancer, and a history of thrombophlebitis or pulmonary embolism.

New Hormonal Methods of Contraception

Two new hormonal methods of contraception are Ortho Evra and NuvaRing. Ortho Evra is a thin, beige, matchbook-sized square that releases an estrogen and a progestin continuously. It is

changed every week for 3 weeks. The fourth week is patch-free, producing withdrawal bleeding. The effectiveness of Ortho Evra is comparable to that of oral contraceptives. Its risks are similar to those of oral contraceptives and include an increased risk of blood clots. The patch may be applied to the torso, chest, arms, or thighs; it should not be applied to the breasts.

NuvaRing is a vaginal ring that is inserted in the vagina for 3 weeks and then removed, resulting in withdrawal bleeding. It is as effective as oral contraceptives and has the same risks. It is flexible, does not require sizing or fitting, and is effective when placed anywhere in the vagina.

Although both of these contraceptive methods increase the options for women, neither protects against STDs. Women using these methods should be instructed not to smoke. Chart 46-15 lists hormonal methods of birth control approved by Health Canada.

Intrauterine Device

An IUD is a small plastic device, usually T-shaped, that is inserted into the uterine cavity to prevent pregnancy. A string attached to the IUD is visible and palpable at the cervical os. An IUD prevents conception by causing a local inflammatory reaction that is toxic to spermatozoa and blastocysts, thus preventing fertilization. The IUD does not work by causing abortion.

Mirena is a plastic IUD that releases levonorgestrel, a synthetic progestin used in oral contraceptives, and has been found to reduce heavy bleeding. Limited studies show that IUDs may prevent the need for hysterectomy in some women by reducing bleeding, may be an adjunct in HRT, may protect women from endometrial cancer, and may prevent cervical cancer.

The IUD method is effective over a long time, appears to have no systemic effects, and reduces the possibility of patient error. This reversible method of birth control is as effective as oral contraceptives and more effective than barrier methods.

Disadvantages include possible excessive bleeding, cramps, and backaches and a slight risk of tubal pregnancy, pelvic infection, displacement of the device, and, rarely, perforation of the cervix and uterus. If a pregnancy occurs with an IUD in place, the device is removed immediately to avoid infection. Spontaneous abortion (miscarriage) may occur on removal. An IUD is not usually used in women who have not had children because the nulliparous uterus may be too small to tolerate it. Women with multiple partners, women with heavy or crampy periods, or those with a history of ectopic pregnancy or pelvic infection are encouraged to use other methods. Some clinicians test for chlamydia and gonorrhea prior to insertion to prevent PID.

Mechanical Barriers

DIAPHRAGM

The diaphragm is an effective contraceptive device that consists of a round, flexible spring (50 to 90 mm wide) covered with a dome-like latex rubber cup. A spermicidal (contraceptive) jelly or cream is used to coat the concave side of the diaphragm before it is inserted deep into the vagina, covering the cervix. The diaphragm is a spermicide holder; the spermicide inhibits spermatozoa from entering the cervical canal. The diaphragm is not felt by the user or her partner when properly fitted and inserted. Because women vary in size, the diaphragm must be sized and fitted by an experienced clinician. The woman is instructed in using and caring for the device. A return demonstration ensures that the woman can insert the diaphragm correctly and that it covers the cervix.

Each time that the woman uses the diaphragm, she should examine it carefully. By holding it up to a bright light, she can ensure that there are no pinpoint holes, cracks, or tears in the diaphragm. Spermicidal jelly or cream is applied, and the diaphragm is then positioned to cover the cervix completely. The diaphragm should remain in place at least 6 hours (but no more than 12 hours) after coitus. Additional spermicide is applied if more than 6 hours have passed before intercourse occurs and before each act of intercourse. On removal, the diaphragm is cleansed thoroughly with mild soap and water, rinsed, and dried before it is stored in its original container.

Disadvantages include allergic reactions in those who are sensitive to latex and an increased incidence of urinary tract infections. Toxic shock syndrome has been reported in some diaphragm users.

> **!** **NURSING ALERT** The nurse must assess the woman for possible latex allergy because use of latex barrier methods may cause severe allergic reactions, including anaphylaxis, in patients with latex allergy.

CERVICAL CAP

The cervical cap is much smaller (22 to 35 mm) than the diaphragm and covers only the cervix; it is used with a spermicide. If a woman can feel her cervix, she can usually learn to use a cervical cap. The chief advantage is that the cap may be left in place for 2 days.

Although convenient to use, the cervical cap may cause cervical irritation; therefore, before fitting a cap, most clinicians obtain a Pap smear and repeat the smear after 3 months. The cap can stay in place for 48 hours and does not require additional spermicide for repeated acts of intercourse.

FEMALE CONDOM

The female condom was developed to provide women with protection from STDs and HIV as well as pregnancy. The female condom (Reality) consists of a cylinder of polyurethane enclosed at one end by a closed ring that covers the cervix and at the other end by an open ring that covers the perineum (Fig. 46-8). Advantages include some degree of protection from STDs (HPV, herpes simplex virus, and HIV). Disadvantages include the inability to use the female condom with some coital positions (ie, standing).

SPERMICIDES

Spermicides are available over the counter as foams, gels, and inserts and on condoms. Spermicides are effective, relatively inexpensive chemical contraceptives when used with condoms. When used alone, spermicide is better than no contraception at all; it can be used without a partner's cooperation and may provide pro-

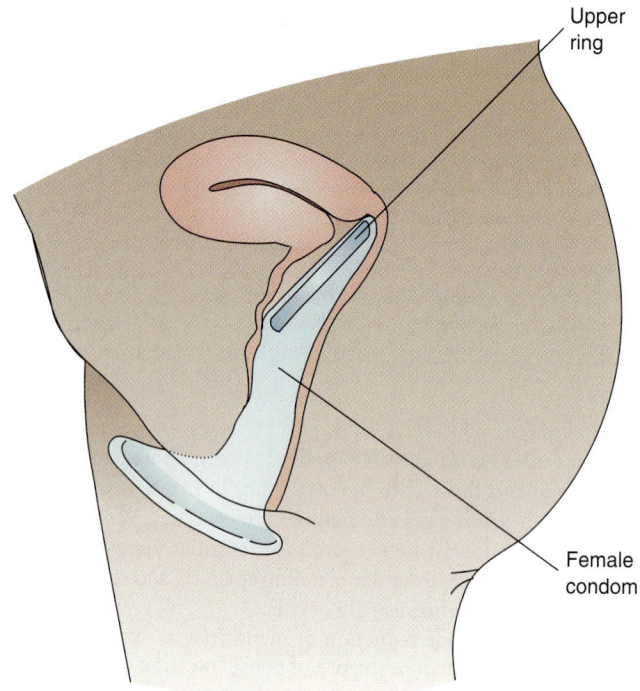

FIGURE 46-8 Female condom. The upper ring keeps the condom in place.

tection from gonorrhea and chlamydia. Burning, a rash, or irritation can develop in either partner and is usually temporary. Changing to another brand of spermicide often alleviates the problem. Spermicides are made from nonoxynol-9 or octoxynol. Nonoxynol-9 has been found to be associated with minute tears in vaginal tissue with frequent use, possibly increasing the possibility of contracting HIV from an infected partner (Stephenson, 2000). It also may increase the risk of latex allergy when used with a condom by leaching out a natural rubber protein from the latex (Greydanus, Patel & Rimsza, 2001).

MALE CONDOM

The male condom is an impermeable, snug-fitting cover applied to the erect penis before it enters the vaginal canal. The tip of the condom is pinched while being applied to leave space for ejaculate. If no space is left, ejaculation may cause a tear or hole in the condom and reduce its effectiveness. The penis, with the condom held in place, is removed from the vagina while still erect to prevent the ejaculate from leaking.

The condom is an effective method when used with contraceptive foam. The latex condom also creates a barrier against transmission of STDs, especially gonorrhea, chlamydial infection, and HIV. Natural condoms (those made from animal tissue), however, do not protect against HIV infection. The nurse needs to reassure women that they have a right to insist on their male partner using a condom and a right to refuse sex without condoms, although women in abusive relationships may increase their risk for abuse by doing so. Some women are buying and carrying condoms with them to be certain that one is available. Nurses should be familiar and comfortable with instructions about using a condom because many women need to know about this way of protecting themselves from HIV and other STDs.

During patient teaching about barrier methods of contraception, nurses need to consider the possibility of latex allergy for themselves and their patients. Contact dermatitis is often the first symptom of latex allergy. Swelling and itching can also occur. Possible warning signs of latex allergy include oral itching after blowing up a balloon or eating kiwis, bananas, pineapples, passion fruits, avocados, or chestnuts. Because many contraceptives are made of latex, patients who experience burning or itching while using a latex contraceptive are instructed to see their primary health care provider. Alternatives to latex condoms may include the female (Reality) and male (Avanti) condoms made of polyurethane.

Condoms do not provide complete protection from STDs, as the HPV virus may be transmitted by skin-to-skin contact. Other STDs may be transmitted if any abraded skin is exposed to body fluids. This information should be included in patient teaching.

Coitus Interruptus

Coitus interruptus (removing the penis from the vagina before ejaculation) requires careful control by the male. Although it is a frequently used method of preventing pregnancy, it is considered an unreliable method of contraception.

Rhythm and Natural Methods

Natural family planning is any method of conception regulation that is based on awareness of signs and symptoms of fertility during a menstrual cycle. The advantages of natural contraceptive methods include the following: (1) they are not hazardous to health, (2) they are inexpensive, and (3) they are approved by some religions. The disadvantage is that they require discipline by the couple, who must monitor the menstrual cycle and abstain from sex during the fertile phase. In addition, the rhythm method of contraception can be difficult to use because it relies on the woman determining her time of ovulation and on avoiding intercourse during the fertile period. The fertile phase (which requires sexual abstinence) is estimated to occur about 14 days before menstruation, although it may occur between the 10th and 17th days. Spermatozoa can fertilize an ovum up to 72 hours after intercourse, and the ovum can be fertilized for 24 hours after leaving the ovary. The pregnancy rate with the rhythm method is about 40% yearly.

Women who carefully determine their "safe period," based on a precise recording of menstrual dates for at least 1 year, and who follow a carefully worked-out formula may achieve very effective protection. A long abstinence period during each cycle is required. These prerequisites require more time and control than many couples have. Changes in cervical mucus and basal body temperature due to hormonal changes related to ovulation form the scientific basis for the symptothermal method of ovulatory timing. Courses in natural family planning are offered at many Catholic hospitals and some family planning clinics.

Ovulation detection methods (eg, Ovulindex) are available in most pharmacies. The presence of the enzyme guaiacol peroxidase in cervical mucus signals ovulation 6 days beforehand and also affects mucosal viscosity. Test kits are available over the counter and are easy to use and reliable, but they can be expensive. Ovulation prediction kits are more effective for planning conception than for avoiding it.

Emergency Contraception

DOSE OF ESTROGEN/PROGESTIN

A properly timed, adequate dose of progestin or estrogen and a progestin after intercourse without birth control, or when a method has failed, can prevent pregnancy by inhibiting or delaying ovulation. This method does not interrupt an established pregnancy. Nurses should be aware of this option and the indications for its use and educate women about it to reduce unwanted pregnancies and abortions. This method obviously is not suitable for long-term contraception because it is not as effective as daily oral contraceptives or other reliable methods used regularly. However, it is valuable in emergency situations such as rape, a defective or torn condom or diaphragm, unprotected intercourse, ejaculation onto genitals, coitus interruptus, more than TWO missed oral contraceptive pills or pills started more than 2 days late, condom alone, or spermicide alone plus recent teratogen exposure (eg, Accutane) (Canadian Paediatric Society, 2003, p. 4-5).

In Canada, Plan B (levonorgestrel, 0.75 mg), which contains only progestin, can be dispensed by a pharmacist without a prescription. Plan B is appropriate for adolescent girls who have menstrual periods, who meet the criteria for oral contraceptives, and who have had unprotected intercourse or contraceptive failure. Ideally Plan B should be started within 24 hours of unprotected intercourse or contraceptive failure but can be started up to 72 hours after intercourse or even up to 5 days later (Rodrigues, Grou, & Joly, 2001). Usually, one tablet is taken as soon as possible. The second tablet is taken 12 hours later. However, taking both tablets at once is equally effective and improves compliance (Canadian Paediatric Society, 2003). There is evidence that Plan B is more effective than the combined form (Preven) and causes less nausea and vomiting (Task Force on Postovulatory Methods of Fertility Regulation, 1998). The term "morning after pill" should not be used because it conveys the inaccurate message that this emergency contraception can only be used the next day rather than up to 3 days. Some adolescent girls or women may avoid seeking emergency contraception immediately after intercourse (thinking it is too soon) or will think that after 24 hours it is too late (Canadian Paediatric Society, Adolescent Health Committee, 2003).

The combined form of estrogen and progestin (Preven), in which two pills are taken and then two more are taken 12 hours later, does require a prescription. Similar guidelines apply to taking the first dose within 72 hours after intercourse. Nausea is a common side effect and can be minimized by taking an antiemetic such as dimenhydrinate (Gravol, 50 mg) 1 hour before taking the combined form.

Other side effects, such as breast soreness and irregular bleeding, may occur but are transient. Any woman using emergency contraception needs to be advised of the 1.6% failure rate and counselled about other contraceptive methods. There are no known contraindications to the use of this method (Morris & Young, 2000).

If the woman is breastfeeding, a progestin-only formulation is prescribed. To avoid exposing the infant to synthetic hormones through breast milk, she can manually express milk and bottle-feed for 24 hours after treatment.

The woman's next menstrual period may begin a few days earlier or a few days later than expected, and she needs to be informed of this. The patient must have a pregnancy test if she has not had a menstrual period in 3 weeks and should be offered information about a regular method of contraception if she does not have one currently. The Canadian Paediatric Society recommends that a supply of Plan B be readily available at doctors' offices and organizations such as Planned Parenthood and the like. Adolescent girls and women who use condoms as their only method of birth control should have Plan B on hand in case of an emergency.

POSTCOITAL IUD INSERTION

Postcoital IUD insertion, another form of emergency contraception, involves insertion of a copper-bearing IUD within 5 days of exposure in women who want this method of contraception; however, it may be inappropriate for some women or if other contraindications exist. The mechanism of action is unknown, but it is thought that the IUD interferes with fertilization (Morris & Young, 2000). The patient may experience discomfort on insertion and heavier menstrual periods and increased cramping. Contraindications include a confirmed or suspected pregnancy or any contraindication to regular copper IUD use. The patient must be informed that there is a risk that insertion of an IUD may disrupt a pregnancy that is already present.

NURSING MANAGEMENT

Patients who use emergency contraception may be anxious, embarrassed, and lacking information about birth control. Nurses must be supportive and nonjudgmental and provide facts and appropriate patient teaching. If a patient repeatedly uses this method of birth control, she should be informed that the failure rate with this method is higher than with a regularly used method.

ABORTION

Interruption of pregnancy or expulsion of the product of conception before the fetus is viable is called abortion. The fetus is generally considered to be viable any time after the fifth to sixth month of gestation. The term "premature labour" is used when a woman experiences labour after this point in the pregnancy.

Spontaneous Abortion

It is estimated that 1 of every 5 to 10 conceptions results in spontaneous abortion. Most of these occur because an abnormality in the fetus makes survival impossible. Other causes may include systemic diseases, hormonal imbalance, or anatomic abnormalities. If a pregnant woman experiences bleeding and cramping, a threatened abortion is diagnosed because an actual abortion is usually imminent. Spontaneous abortion occurs most commonly in the second or third month of gestation.

There are various kinds of spontaneous abortion, depending on the nature of the process (threatened, inevitable, incomplete, or complete). In a threatened abortion, the cervix does not dilate. With bed rest and conservative treatment, the abortion may be prevented. If it cannot, an abortion is imminent. If only some of the tissue is passed, the abortion is referred to as incomplete. If the fetus and all related tissue are spontaneously evacuated, the abortion is complete.

HABITUAL ABORTION

Habitual or recurrent abortion is defined as successive, repeated, spontaneous abortions of unknown cause. As many as 60% of abortions may result from chromosomal anomalies. After two consecutive abortions, patients are referred for genetic counselling and testing, and other possible causes are explored. If bleeding occurs in these patients, conservative measures, such as bed rest and administering progesterone to support the endometrium, are tried in an attempt to save the pregnancy. Supportive counselling is crucial in this stressful condition. Bed rest, sexual abstinence, a light diet, and no straining on defecation are recommended in an effort to prevent spontaneous abortion. If infection is suspected, antibiotics may be prescribed.

In the condition known as incompetent or dysfunctional cervix, the cervix dilates painlessly in the second trimester of pregnancy, often resulting in a spontaneous abortion. In such cases, a surgical procedure called cervical cerclage may be used to prevent the cervix from dilating prematurely. The procedure involves placing a purse-string suture around the cervix at the level of the internal os. Bed rest is usually advised to keep the weight of the uterus off the cervix.

The patient and her health care providers must be informed that such a suture is in place in this high-risk pregnancy. About 2 to 3 weeks before term or the onset of labour, the suture is cut. Delivery is usually by cesarean section.

MEDICAL MANAGEMENT

After a spontaneous abortion, all tissue passed vaginally is saved for examination. The patient and all personnel caring for her are alerted to save any discharged material. In the rare case of heavy bleeding, the patient may require blood component transfusions and fluid replacement. An estimate of the bleeding volume can be determined by recording the number of perineal pads and the degree of saturation over 24 hours. When an incomplete abortion occurs, oxytocin may be prescribed to cause uterine contractions before dilation and evacuation (D & E) or uterine suctioning.

NURSING MANAGEMENT

Because patients experience loss and anxiety, emotional support and understanding are important aspects of nursing care. The response of the woman who desperately wants a baby is very different from that of the woman who does not want to be pregnant but may be frightened by the possible consequences of an abortion.

The nurse must be aware that the woman having a spontaneous abortion often experiences a grieving period. The grieving may be delayed and may cause other problems until resolved. The many reasons for a delayed grief reaction include the following: friends may not have known the woman was pregnant; the woman may not have seen the lost fetus and can only imagine the gender, size, and characteristics of the child who never developed; there is usually no burial service; and those who know about the loss (family, friends, caregivers) may encourage denial by rarely talking about the loss or by discouraging the woman from crying.

Providing opportunities for the patient to talk and express her emotions helps and also provides clues for the nurse in planning more specific care. Those closest to the woman are encouraged to give emotional support and to allow her to talk and freely express her grief. Unresolved grief may manifest itself in persistent vivid memories of the events surrounding the loss, persistent sadness or anger, and episodes of overwhelming emotion when recalling the loss. Dysfunctional grief may require the assistance of a skilled therapist.

Elective Abortion

A voluntary induced termination of pregnancy is called an elective abortion and is performed by skilled health care providers. Abortion is legal in Canada and was removed from the Criminal Code in 1988. Since health is a provincial matter in Canada, differences are present across the country in terms of women's access to elective abortion and whether the cost of the abortion is covered. Abortions performed in hospitals generally are free for women covered by government health insurance. Abortions are also free of charge at clinics in British Columbia, Alberta, Ontario, and Newfoundland. In the other provinces, women have to pay for part of the cost of an abortion at a clinic. Freestanding clinics will perform abortions for teenagers without a parent's permission, providing the teenager is clear about what she is doing. Some hospitals may require parental consent for teenagers.

Women do not have to give a reason for needing an abortion and their identity is kept confidential. The Supreme Court of Canada ruled in 1989 that a woman's decision to have an abortion cannot be altered by the "biological father."

The rate of abortion rose from 14.6 to 15.5 between 1990 and 1995 (Public Health Agency of Canada, 2002). There is aproximately one abortion for every three to four live births. In 1995, 20% of the abortions were obtained by women under 20 years of age. Most abortions occur in pregnancies under 12 weeks. There is a need for nurses to provide contraceptive education and counselling. Elective abortions may be carried out in different ways (Chart 46-16).

MEDICAL MANAGEMENT

Before the procedure is performed, a nurse or counselor trained in pregnancy counselling explores with the patient her fears, feelings, and options. After the patient's choice is identified (ie, continuing pregnancy and parenthood; continuing pregnancy followed by adoption; or terminating pregnancy by abortion), a pelvic examination is performed to determine uterine size. Laboratory studies before an abortion must include a pregnancy test to confirm the pregnancy, hematocrit to rule out anemia, Rh determination, and an STD screen. A patient with anemia may need an iron supplement, and an Rh-negative patient may require RhoGAM to prevent isoimmunization. Before the procedure, all patients should be screened for STDs to prevent introducing pathogens upward through the cervix during the procedure.

NURSING MANAGEMENT

Patient teaching is an important aspect of care for women who elect to terminate a pregnancy. A woman undergoing elective abortion is informed about what the procedure entails and the expected course after the procedure. The patient is scheduled for a follow-up appointment 2 weeks after the procedure and is instructed in recognizing and reporting signs and symptoms of complications (ie, fever, heavy bleeding, or pain).

Available contraceptive methods are reviewed with the patient at this time. Effectiveness depends on the method used and the extent to which the woman and her partner follow the instructions for use. The woman who has used any method of birth control should be assessed for her understanding of the method and its potential side effects and her satisfaction with the method. If the patient was not using contraception, the nurse explains all methods and their benefits and risks and assists the patient in making a contraceptive choice for use after abortion. An increasingly important related teaching issue is the need to use barrier contraceptive devices (ie, condoms) for protection against transmission of STDs and HIV infection.

Psychological support is another important aspect of nursing care. Nurses need to be aware that women terminate pregnancies for many reasons. Some women terminate pregnancies because of severe genetic defects. Many women who have been raped or impregnated in incestuous relationships or by an abusive partner elect to terminate their pregnancies. Infertility patients may elect to undergo selective termination if they become pregnant with multiple fetuses. In pregnancies with multiple gestation, adverse outcomes are directly proportional to the number of fetuses in the uterus. Such multifetal reductions are specialized procedures that are stressful and difficult for the parents; therefore, psychological support and understanding are required. The care of women undergoing termination of pregnancy is stressful, and assistance needs to be provided in a safe and nonjudgmental way. Nurses have the right to refuse to participate in a procedure that is against their religious beliefs but are professionally obligated not to impose their beliefs or judgments on their patients.

> **NURSING ALERT** Some women resort to using unskilled attempts to end a pregnancy. The methods usually include administering large amounts of various toxic agents (effects are toxic, and the uterus is never fully evacuated) or performing a curettage, with the associated risks of uterine rupture, hemorrhage, or infection. If a woman who has had a septic abortion receives proper medical attention early enough and is treated with broad-spectrum antibiotics, the prognosis is excellent. Fluid and blood component replacement may be required before careful attempts are made to evacuate the uterus.

Patients may opt for a type of aborption that ends a pregnancy by using medication rather than surgery. Methotrexate and miso-

---

> ### Chart 46-16 — Types of Elective Abortions
>
> #### Vacuum Aspiration
> - The cervix is dilated manually with instrumentation or by laminaria (small suppositories made of seaweed that swells as it absorbs water).
> - A uterine aspirator is introduced.
> - Suction is applied, and tissue is removed from the uterus.
>
> This is the most common type of termination procedure and is used in pregnancy, up to 20–22 weeks. Laminaria may be used to soften and dilate the cervix prior to the procedure.
>
> #### Dilation and Evacuation
> Cervical dilation with laminaria followed by vacuum aspiration
>
> #### Labour Induction
> These procedures account for less than 1% of all terminations and generally take place in an inpatient setting.
> 1. Installation of saline or urea results in uterine contractions.
>   - Although rare, serious complications can occur, including cardiovascular collapse, cerebral edema, pulmonary edema, renal failure, and disseminated intravascular coagulopathy (DIC).
> 2. Prostaglandins
>   - Prostaglandins are introduced into the amniotic fluid or by vaginal suppository or intramuscular injection in later pregnancy.
>   - Strong uterine contractions begin within 4 hours and usually result in abortion.
>   - Gastrointestinal side effects (eg, nausea, vomiting, diarrhea, and abdominal cramping) and fever can occur.
> 3. Intravenous oxytocin
>   Used for later abortions for genetic indications. Requires patient to go through labour.
>
> #### Medical Abortion
> *Mifepristone*
> - Mifepristone (known as RU-486 or the "abortion pill") is a progesterone antagonist that prevents implantation of the ovum.
> - As of June 1, 2005, Mifepristone is not available in Canada.
>
> *Methotrexate and Misoprostol combined*
> - Methotrexate is a teratogen that is lethal to the fetus. Misoprostol is a synthetic prostaglandin analog that produces cervical effacement and uterine contractions.
> - Methotrexate/Misoprostol is available in some clinics in Canada and has a high effectiveness rating. It is only used in pregnancies up to 49 days from the last menstrual period.

prostol are combined and are used in early pregnancy (up to 49 days from the last menstrual period). This treatment is the only medication available in Canada for a nonsurgical abortion and can be obtained at some clinics.

Infertility

Infertility is defined as a couple's inability to achieve pregnancy after 1 year of unprotected intercourse. Primary infertility refers to a couple who has never had a child. Secondary infertility means that at least one conception has occurred, but currently the couple cannot achieve a pregnancy. In Canada, infertility is a major medical and social problem. Women's infertility may be related to anovulation, uterine or cervical factors, blocked fallopian tubes, or endometriosis, while men's infertility is related to sperm quality or sperm production. For infertile women who wish to bear children, infertility may have a profound emotional toll (Gonzalez, 2000; Hart, 2002).

Pathophysiology

Possible causes of infertility include uterine displacement by tumours, congenital anomalies, and inflammation. For an ovum to become fertilized, the vagina, fallopian tubes, cervix, and uterus must be patent and the mucosal secretions of the cervix must be receptive to sperm. Semen and cervical secretions are alkaline, whereas normal vaginal secretions are acidic. Often more than one factor is responsible for the problem. Identifying the causes may require the services of a gynecologist, urologist, and endocrinologist.

Assessment and Diagnostic Findings

Careful evaluation includes physical examination, endocrinologic investigation, and consideration of psychosocial factors. Three complete histories (one of each partner and one of the couple), physical examination, and laboratory studies are performed on both partners to rule out such causative factors as previous STDs, anomalies, injuries, tuberculosis, mumps orchitis, impaired sperm production, endometriosis, DES exposure, or antisperm antibodies. Five factors are considered basic to infertility: ovarian, tubal, cervical, uterine, and semen conditions.

OVARIAN FACTORS

Studies performed to determine if there is regular ovulation and if progestational endometrium is adequate for implantation may include a basal body temperature chart for at least four cycles, an endometrial biopsy, serum progesterone level, and ovulation index. The ovulation index involves a urine-stick test that determines if the surge in LH that precedes follicular rupture has occurred.

TUBAL FACTORS

Hysterosalpingography is used to rule out uterine or tubal abnormalities. Laparoscopy permits direct visualization of the tubes and other pelvic structures and can assist in identifying conditions that may interfere with fertility (eg, endometriosis).

CERVICAL FACTORS

The cervical mucus can be examined at ovulation and after intercourse to determine whether proper changes occur that promote sperm penetration and survival. A postcoital cervical mucus test (Sims-Huhner test) is performed 2 to 8 hours after intercourse. Cervical mucus is aspirated with a medicine dropper–like instrument. Aspirated material is placed on a slide and examined under the microscope for the presence and viability of sperm cells. The woman is instructed not to bathe or douche between coitus and the examination.

UTERINE FACTORS

Fibroids, polyps, and congenital malformations are possible conditions in this category. Their presence may be determined by pelvic examination, hysteroscopy, saline sonogram (a variation of a sonogram), and hysterosalpingography.

SEMEN FACTORS

After 2 to 3 days of sexual abstinence, a specimen of ejaculate is collected in a clean container, kept warm, and examined within 1 hour for the number of sperm (density), percentage of moving forms, quality of forward movement (forward progression), and morphology (shape and form). From 2 to 6 mL of watery alkaline semen is normal; a normal count is 60 million to 100 million sperm/mL, although the incidence of impregnation is lessened only when the count drops below 20 million sperm/mL. A normal semen analysis should show the following (Angard, 1999):

- Volume: more than 1 mL
- Concentration: more than 20 million/mL
- Motility: more than 50% of the forms should be moving
- Morphology: more than 60% of sperm should have normal forms
- No sperm clumping, significant red or white blood cells, or thickening of seminal fluid (hyperviscosity)

MISCELLANEOUS FACTORS

Men may also be affected by varicoceles, varicose veins around the testicle, which decrease semen quality by increasing testicular temperature. Retrograde ejaculation or ejaculation into the bladder is assessed by urinalysis after ejaculation.

Blood tests for male partners may include measuring testosterone; FSH and LH (both of which are involved in maintaining testicular function); and prolactin levels and antisperm antibodies (treated with corticosteroids).

Immunologic factors also are being investigated. Some cases of recurrent early pregnancy loss or recurrent natural abortion are the result of an abnormal response by the woman to antigens on fetal or placental tissues. Some women have been treated with infusions of their partner's lymphocytes with some success, but this treatment remains experimental and the long-term effects are unknown.

Medical Management

Infertility is often difficult to treat because it frequently results from a combination of factors. Couples undergoing an infertility evaluation may conceive without the cause of infertility ever identified. Likewise, although some couples undergo all tests, the cause of the problem may remain undiscovered and infertility persists. Between these extremes, many problems, both simple and complex, can be discovered and corrected. Patients may need assisted reproductive technology to conceive; the methods are described below. Therapy may require surgery to correct a malfunction or anomaly, hormonal supplements, attention to proper timing, and recognition and correction of psychological or emotional factors.

PHARMACOLOGIC THERAPY

Pharmacologically induced ovulation is undertaken when women do not ovulate on their own or ovulate irregularly. Various medications are used, depending on the primary cause of infertility (Chart 46-17). Clomiphene citrate (Clomid) is the most common medication used. Although Clomid's precise action is un-

Chart 46-17 • PHARMACOLOGY
Medications That Induce Ovulation

Clomifene (Clomid)
Clomifene is used when the hypothalamus is not stimulating the pituitary gland to release FSH and LH. This oral medication stimulates follicles in the ovary. It is usually taken for 5 days beginning on the fifth day of the menstrual cycle. Ovulation should occur 4 to 8 days after the last dose. Patients receive instructions about timing intercourse to facilitate fertilization.

Menotropin (Pergonal)
Menotropin, a combination of FSH and LH, given intramuscularly, is used for women with deficiencies in these hormones. Pergonal stimulates the ovaries, so monitoring by ultrasound and hormone levels is essential because overstimulation may occur.

Urofollitropin (Metrodin)
Urofollitropin, containing FSH with a small amount of LH, is given intramuscularly in some disorders (eg, polycystic ovarian syndrome) to stimulate follicle growth. Clomid is then used to stimulate ovulation.

Chorionic Gonadotropin
Chorionic gonadotropin is given subcutaneously to stimulate release of the egg from the ovary and may be used in combination with the above medications.

known, it enhances the release of pituitary gonadotropins, resulting in follicular rupture or ovulation.

Another mode of pharmacotherapy for anovulatory women includes the use of pulsatile gonadotropin-releasing hormone (GnRH). The woman wears an infusion pump attached to an intravenous or subcutaneous catheter for up to 21 days. Administration of GnRH can result in ovulation in some women with low hormone levels. This option can reduce cycle monitoring and the incidence of multiple gestation (ACOG Technical Bulletin #197, ACOG Compendium, 2001).

Human menopausal gonadotropin may also be used as it stimulates the ovaries to produce eggs. Blood tests and ultrasounds are used to monitor ovulation. Multiple pregnancies may occur with these medications. Ovarian hyperstimulation syndrome (OHSS) may also occur. This condition is characterized by enlarged multicystic ovaries and is complicated by a shift of fluid from the intravascular space into the abdominal cavity. It is iatrogenic and preventable and develops after ovarian stimulation. The fluid shift can result in ascites, pleural effusion, and edema; hypovolemia may also result. Risk factors include younger age, history of polycystic ovarian syndrome, high serum estradiol levels, a larger number of follicles, and pregnancy. If the woman is pregnant, she is producing human chorionic gonadotropin, which can worsen OHSS. Symptoms include abdominal discomfort, distention, weight gain, and ovarian enlargement. This condition may be moderate, severe, or critical. Severe OHSS may result in acute respiratory distress syndrome (ARDS). It is prevented by careful monitoring and adjustment of medication dosage.

Management in mild and moderate cases of OHSS consists of decreased activity, monitoring of urine output, and frequent office visits as designated by the reproductive endocrinologist. The patient with severe OHSS is hospitalized for monitoring and treatment. Severe OHSS is characterized by clinical ascites, hypovolemia, oliguria, hemoconcentration, electrolyte imbalance, and ovarian size greater than 10 cm. Treatment of severe OHSS includes use of an indwelling catheter for strict monitoring of fluid intake and output and daily measurements of weight and abdominal circumference. Intravenous fluids and heparin are administered as prescribed. The patient is permitted to ambulate as tolerated. Critical OHSS is life-threatening and is characterized by tense ascites that may be accompanied by hydrothorax, renal failure, and ARDS. Volume expanders, diuretic agents, hemodialysis, and intubation may be required (Copeland, 2000).

ARTIFICIAL INSEMINATION

Depositing semen into the female genital tract by artificial means is called artificial insemination. If the sperm cannot penetrate the cervical canal normally, artificial insemination using the partner's semen (AIH, or artificial insemination with sperm from the husband or partner) may be considered. In azoospermia (lack of sperm in the semen), semen from carefully selected donors may be used (AID, or artificial insemination with sperm from donor).

Indications for using artificial insemination include: (1) the man's inability to deposit semen in the vagina, which may be due to premature ejaculation, pronounced hypospadias (a displaced male urethra), or dyspareunia (painful intercourse experienced by the woman), (2) inability of semen to be transported from the vagina to the uterine cavity (this is usually due to faulty chemical conditions and may occur with an abnormal cervical discharge), and (3) a single woman's desire to have a child.

The woman may have received clomifene (Clomid) and menotropins (Pergonal) to stimulate ovulation before insemination. Ultrasounds and blood studies of varying hormone levels are used to pinpoint the best time for insemination and to monitor for OHSS. The recipient is placed in the lithotomy position on the examination table, a speculum is inserted, and the vagina and cervix are swabbed with a cotton-tipped applicator to remove any excess secretions. Semen is drawn into a sterile syringe, and a cannula is attached. The semen is then directed to the external os. Semen may also be placed into the uterine cavity (intrauterine insemination). In this procedure, the sperm are washed before insertion to remove biochemicals and to select the most active sperm. This is indicated when mucus is inadequate, when antibodies are present, or when the sperm count is low. After careful withdrawal of the cannula, the patient remains in a supine position for 30 minutes.

The success rate for artificial insemination varies. Three to six inseminations may be required over 2 to 4 months. Because artificial insemination is likely to be a stressful and difficult situation for couples, nursing support and strategies to promote coping are crucial.

Cannula With Partner's Semen. Certain conditions need to be established before semen is transferred to the vagina. The woman must have no abnormalities of the genital system, the fallopian tubes must be patent, and ova must be available. In the male, sperm need to be normal in shape, amount, motility, and endurance. The time of ovulation should be determined as accurately as possible so that the 2 or 3 days during which fertilization is possible each month can be targeted for treatment. Fertilization seldom occurs from a single insemination. Usually, insemination is attempted between days 10 and 17 of the cycle; three different attempts may be made during one cycle. Semen is collected by masturbation; alternatively, a perforated sheath is worn over the penis during intercourse by couples who object to masturbation. Withdrawal and using condoms for sperm collection are considered unsatisfactory by many infertility specialists because some sperm may be lost or adversely affected.

Insemination With Donor Semen. When the sperm of the woman's partner is defective or absent or when there is a risk of transmitting a genetic disease, donor sperm may be used. Safeguards are put in place to address legal, ethical, emotional, and religious issues. Written consent is obtained to protect all parties involved, including the woman, the donor, and the resulting child. The donor's semen is frozen and the donor is evaluated to ensure that he is free of genetic disorders and STDs, including HIV infection.

IN VITRO FERTILIZATION

In vitro fertilization (IVF) involves ovarian stimulation, egg retrieval, fertilization, and embryo transfer. This procedure is accomplished by first stimulating the ovary to produce multiple eggs or ova, usually with medications, because success rates are greater with more than one early embryo. Many different protocols exist for inducing ovulation with one or more agents. Patients are carefully selected and evaluated, and cycles are carefully monitored using ultrasound and estradiol levels. At the appropriate time, the ova are recovered by transvaginal ultrasound retrieval. Sperm and eggs are coincubated for up to 36 hours, and the embryos are transferred about 48 hours after retrieval. Implantation should occur in 3 to 5 days.

Gamete intrafallopian transfer (GIFT), a variation of IVF, is the treatment of choice for patients with ovarian failure. Success rates vary from 20% to 30%. The ovaries are stimulated with gonadotropin derivatives, and follicles are observed with vaginal ultrasound. Once the oocyte is mature, it is retrieved by laparoscopy or transvaginally with ultrasound guidance. The oocyte (unfertilized egg) is removed and drawn into a catheter, where it is mixed with sperm that was obtained shortly before the oocyte retrieval. The most motile fraction of sperm is selected by a washing process. The oocyte and sperm are then inserted into the fallopian tube, where fertilization occurs. The latter method avoids anesthesia. GIFT is the technique of choice for nontubal causes of infertility and for older infertile women.

Zygote intrafallopian transfer (ZIFT) consists of oocyte retrieval and fertilization in vitro; the zygotes are placed into the fallopian tubes via laparoscopy.

The most common indications for IVF and GIFT are irreparable tubal damage, endometriosis, immunologic problems, unexplained infertility, inadequate sperm, and exposure to DES.

OTHER ASSISTED REPRODUCTIVE TECHNOLOGIES

In intracytoplasmic sperm injection (ICSI), an ovum is retrieved as described previously, and a single sperm is injected through the zona pellucida, through the egg membrane, and into the cytoplasm of the oocyte. The fertilized egg is then transferred back to the donor. ICSI is the treatment of choice in severe male factor infertility.

Women who cannot produce their own eggs (ie, premature ovarian failure) have the option of using the eggs of a donor after stimulation of the donor's ovaries. The recipient also receives hormones in preparation for these procedures. Couples may also choose this modality if the female partner has a genetic disorder that may be passed on to children.

Nursing Management

Nursing interventions appropriate when working with couples during infertility evaluations include the following: assist in reducing stress in the relationship, encourage cooperation, protect privacy, foster understanding, and refer the couple to appropriate resources when necessary. Because infertility workups are expensive, time-consuming, invasive, stressful, and not always successful, couples need support in working together to deal with this endeavour.

Infertility Awareness Association of Canada is a nonprofit self-help group that provides information and support for infertile patients. The literature on infertility that is produced by this group is an important resource for patients and professionals. Most areas across the country have local support groups. More information can be obtained by writing to the Infertility Awareness Association of Canada (see the address at the end of this chapter).

Smoking is strongly discouraged because it has an adverse effect on the success of assisted reproduction. Diet, exercise, stress reduction techniques, health maintenance, and disease prevention are being emphasized in many infertility programs.

ECTOPIC PREGNANCY

The incidence of ectopic pregnancy is on the rise: it occurs in 2% of pregnancies (Lemus, 2000). It occurs when a fertilized ovum (a blastocyst) becomes implanted on any tissue other than the uterine lining (eg, the fallopian tube, ovary, abdomen, or cervix; Fig. 46-9). The most common site of ectopic implantation is the fallopian tube.

Possible causes include salpingitis, peritubal adhesions (after pelvic infection, endometriosis, appendicitis), structural abnormalities of the fallopian tube (rare and usually related to DES exposure), previous ectopic pregnancy (after one ectopic pregnancy, the risk of recurrence is 7% to 15%; Lemus, 2000), previous tubal surgery, multiple previous induced abortions (particularly if followed by infection), tumours that distort the tube, and IUD and progestin-only contraceptives. PID appears to be the major risk factor for ectopic pregnancy. Improved antibiotic therapy for PID usually prevents total tubal closure but may leave a stricture or narrowing, predisposing the woman to ectopic implantation. The odds of recurrent ectopic pregnancy are three times higher if an infectious pathology was the cause of the first one. If a woman has a second ectopic pregnancy, assisted reproduction is considered.

The rate of tubal pregnancies has increased in disproportion to population growth. Ectopic pregnancies are being diagnosed sooner and more often because of advanced diagnostic techniques. Moreover, they are being treated conservatively before emergency rupture and hemorrhage occur. It may be that the increased numbers result from better diagnostic techniques. Conservative treatment makes ectopic pregnancy less life-threatening than previously, but this condition persists as the leading cause of pregnancy-related death in the first trimester and the second leading cause of maternal mortality. Ectopic pregnancy is also a complication of IVF.

Clinical Manifestations

Early intervention decreases rupture, minimizes tubal damage, and usually avoids the need for surgery. Signs and symptoms vary depending on whether tubal rupture has occurred. Delay in menstruation from 1 to 2 weeks followed by slight bleeding (spotting) or a report of a slightly abnormal period suggests the possibility of an ectopic pregnancy. Symptoms may begin late, with vague soreness on the affected side, probably due to uterine contractions and distention of the tube. Typically, the patient experiences sharp, colicky pain. Most patients experience pelvic or abdominal

NURSING RESEARCH PROFILE 46-1
The Experience of Premature Ovarian Failure

Orshan, S. A., Furniss, K. K., Forst, C., & Santoro, N. (2001). The lived experience of premature ovarian failure. *JOGNN, 30*(2), 202–207.

Purpose
Premature ovarian failure (POF), the premature cessation of function of the ovaries, affects 1% to 5% of women below the age of 40. Little is known about the impact of POF on women who experience it and their reactions to the diagnosis. The purpose of this study was to describe the experiences of women diagnosed with idiopathic POF.

Study Sample and Design
A qualitative research study using phenomenology was used. Six women who experienced idiopathic POF before the age of 35 were asked to describe the meaning of POF to them. The subjects ranged in age from 25 to 41 at the time of the interview; mean age was 36.7 years. Five of the women were Caucasian; one was African American. Four of the six women had ceased menstruating between 5 and 10 years before the interview. Interviews were conducted in private settings; the women were asked to share what it had been like to live with POF and to describe the reactions of their family and friends to the diagnosis of POF. Audiotapes of the interviews were transcribed and analyzed.

Findings
Four major themes emerged from analysis of the interview data: 1) being treated as a diagnosis rather than as a person, 2) grieving for death of a dream for the future, 3) existing in a world with others, most of whom are fertile, and 4) being too young to be so old. The women in the study reported feeling robbed of their ability to have children and robbed of their youth with the premature onset of menopause. Women reported reacting to the diagnosis of POF with feelings of anger, depression, grief, and mourning.

Nursing Implications
Nurses need to be sensitive to the impact that POF has on women and need to create a supportive environment for women who experience premature menopause. While POF is not a common diagnosis, women who experience it might benefit from health care providers who listen to their concerns, provide support, teach, and make appropriate referrals. Recognizing the impact the diagnosis has on women is important for nurses caring for women with POF.

pain and some spotting or bleeding. Gastrointestinal symptoms, dizziness, or lightheadedness is common. The patient frequently thinks the abnormal bleeding is a menstrual period, especially if a recent period occurred and was normal.

If implantation occurs in the fallopian tube, the tube becomes more and more distended and can rupture if the ectopic pregnancy remains undetected for 4 to 6 weeks or longer after conception. When the tube ruptures, the ovum is discharged into the abdominal cavity.

When tubal rupture occurs, the woman experiences agonizing pain, dizziness, faintness, and nausea and vomiting. These symptoms are related to the peritoneal reaction to blood escaping from the tube. Air hunger and symptoms of shock may occur, and the signs of hemorrhage—rapid and thready pulse, decreased blood pressure, subnormal temperature, restlessness, pallor, and sweating—are evident. Later, the pain becomes generalized in the abdomen and radiates to the shoulder and neck because of accumulating intraperitoneal blood that irritates the diaphragm.

Assessment and Diagnostic Findings

During vaginal examination, a large mass of clotted blood that has collected in the pelvis behind the uterus or a tender adnexal mass may be palpable. If an ectopic pregnancy is suspected, the patient is evaluated by sonography and the beta subunit of human chorionic gonadotropin (hCG) levels. If the ultrasound results are inconclusive, the beta-hCG test is repeated to evaluate the rate of rise in the level. The levels of hCG (the diagnostic hormone of pregnancy) double in early normal pregnancies every 3 days but are reduced in abnormal or ectopic pregnancies. A less-than-normal increase is cause for suspicion. Serum progesterone levels are also measured. Levels under 16 nmol/L are considered abnormal; levels over 80 nmol/L are associated with a normally developing pregnancy. Urine tests for pregnancy are not helpful in ectopic pregnancies.

Ultrasound can detect a pregnancy between 5 and 6 weeks from the last menstrual period. Detectable fetal heart movement outside the uterus on ultrasound is firm evidence of an ectopic pregnancy. On occasion, an ultrasound study is not definitive and the diagnosis must be made with combined diagnostic aids (hCG level, ultrasound, pelvic examination, and clinical judgment). Studies using ultrasound with Doppler flow, in which colour indicates perfusion, are helpful.

Occasionally, the clinical picture makes the diagnosis relatively easy. However, when the clinical signs and symptoms are questionable, which is often the case, other procedures have value. Laparoscopy is used because the physician can visually detect an unruptured tubal pregnancy and thereby circumvent the risk of its rupture.

Medical Management

SURGICAL MANAGEMENT
When surgery is performed early, almost all patients recover rapidly; if tubal rupture occurs, mortality increases. The type of surgery is determined by the size and extent of local tubal damage. Conservative surgery would include "milking" an ectopic pregnancy from the tube. Resection of the involved fallopian tube with end-to-end anastomosis may be effective. Some surgeons attempt to salvage the tube with a salpingostomy, which involves opening and evacuating the tube and controlling bleeding. More extensive surgery includes removing the tube alone (salpingectomy) or with the ovary (salpingo-oophorectomy). Depending on the amount of blood lost, blood component therapy and treatment of hemorrhagic shock may be necessary before and during surgery. Surgery may also be indicated in women unlikely to comply with close monitoring or those who live too far away from a health care facility to obtain the monitoring needed with nonsurgical management.

Methotrexate, a chemotherapeutic agent and folic acid antagonist, is used after surgery to treat any remaining embryonic or early pregnancy tissue, as indicated by a persistent or rising beta-hCG level. The beta-hCG test is repeated 2 weeks after surgery to ensure a falling level.

PHARMACOLOGIC THERAPY
Another option is the use of methotrexate without surgery. Because this medication stops the pregnancy from progressing by interfering with DNA synthesis and the multiplication of cells, it interrupts early, small, unruptured tubal pregnancies. Patients must be hemodynamically stable, have no active renal or hepatic disease, have no evidence of thrombocytopenia or leukopenia, and have a very small, unruptured tubal pregnancy on ultrasound. The medication

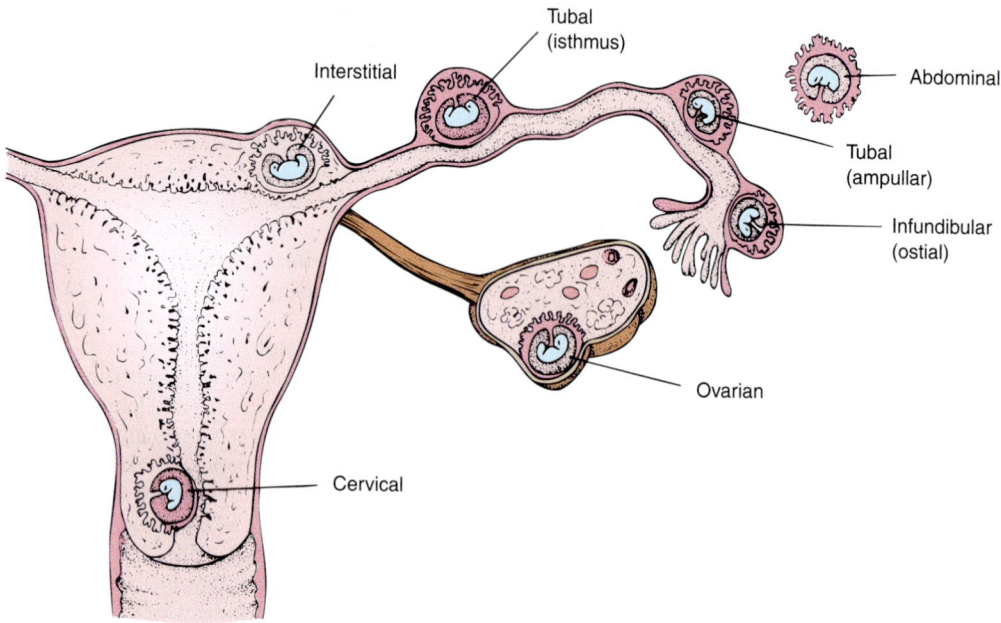

FIGURE 46-9 Sites of ectopic pregnancy.

is administered intramuscularly or intravenously. Some patients may be treated with intratubal injection of methotrexate. Complete blood count, blood typing, and tests of liver and renal function are conducted to monitor the patient. The patient is advised to refrain from alcohol, intercourse, and vitamins with folic acid until the pregnancy is resolved because these may exacerbate the adverse effects of methotrexate. Abdominal pain may occur within 5 to 10 days and may indicate termination of the pregnancy. This requires careful assessment by the health care provider. Serum levels of hCG are monitored carefully, and these levels should gradually decrease. Ultrasounds may also be used for monitoring. Side effects of methotrexate include stomatitis and diarrhea, bone marrow suppression, impaired liver function, dermatitis, and pleuritis.

NURSING PROCESS:
THE PATIENT WITH AN
ECTOPIC PREGNANCY

Assessment

The health history includes the menstrual pattern and any (even slight) bleeding since the last menstrual period. The nurse elicits the patient's description of pains and their location. The nurse asks the patient whether any sharp, colicky pains have occurred. Then the nurse notes whether pain radiates to the shoulder and neck (possibly caused by rupture and pressure on the diaphragm).

The nurse monitors vital signs, level of consciousness, and nature and amount of vaginal bleeding. If possible, the nurse assesses how the woman is coping with the loss of a pregnancy.

Diagnosis

NURSING DIAGNOSES

Based on the assessment data, the patient's major nursing diagnoses may include the following:

- Acute pain related to the progression of the tubal pregnancy
- Anticipatory grieving related to the loss of pregnancy and effect on future pregnancies

- Deficient knowledge related to the treatment and effect on future pregnancies

COLLABORATIVE PROBLEMS/
POTENTIAL COMPLICATIONS

Based on the assessment data, major complications may include the following:

- Hemorrhage
- Hemorrhagic shock

Planning and Goals

The major goals for the patient may include relief of pain; acceptance and resolution of grief and pregnancy loss; increased knowledge about ectopic pregnancy, its treatment, and its outcome; and absence of complications.

Nursing Interventions

RELIEVING PAIN

The abdominal pain associated with ectopic pregnancy may be described as cramping or severe continuous pain. If the patient is to have surgery, preanesthetic medications may provide pain relief. Postoperatively, analgesic agents are administered liberally; this promotes early ambulation and enables the patient to cough and take deep breaths.

SUPPORTING THE GRIEVING PROCESS

Patients' distress levels vary. If the pregnancy is wanted, loss may or may not be expressed verbally by the patient and her partner. The impact may not be fully realized until much later. The nurse should be available to listen and provide support. The patient's partner, if appropriate, should participate in this process. Even if the pregnancy was unplanned, a loss has been experienced, and a grief reaction may follow. Severe and persistent psychological distress may require referral for psychological counselling.

MONITORING AND MANAGING POTENTIAL COMPLICATIONS

Potential complications of ectopic pregnancy are hemorrhage and shock. Careful assessment is essential to detect the development of these complications. Continuous monitoring of vital signs, level of consciousness, amount of bleeding, and intake and output provides information about the possibility of hemorrhage and the need to prepare for intravenous therapy. Bed rest is indicated. Hematocrit, hemoglobin, and blood gas levels are monitored to assess hematologic status and adequacy of tissue perfusion. Significant deviations in these laboratory values are reported immediately, and the patient is prepared for possible surgery. Blood component therapy may be required if blood loss has been rapid and extensive. If hypovolemic shock occurs, the treatment is directed toward re-establishing tissue perfusion and adequate blood volume. See Chapter 15 for a discussion of the intravenous fluids and medications used in treating shock.

PROMOTING HOME AND COMMUNITY-BASED CARE

Teaching Patients Self-Care

If the patient has experienced life-threatening hemorrhage and shock, these complications are addressed and treated before any in-depth teaching can begin. At this time, the patient's and the nurse's attention is focused on the crisis, not on learning. Therefore, it may be later that the patient begins to ask questions about what has happened and why certain procedures were performed. Procedures are explained in terms that a distressed and apprehensive patient can understand. The patient's partner is included in teaching and explanations when possible. After the patient recovers from postoperative discomforts, it may be more appropriate to address any questions and concerns that the patient and her partner have, including the effect of this pregnancy or its treatment on future pregnancies. Patients should be advised that ectopic pregnancies may recur. It is important to review signs and symptoms with the patient and instruct her to report an abnormal menstrual period promptly. Patient teaching is based on the needs of the patient and her partner and must take into consideration their distress and grief. The patient is informed about possible complications and instructed to report early signs and symptoms.

Continuing Care

Because of the risk of subsequent ectopic pregnancies, the patient is advised to seek preconception counselling before considering future pregnancies and to seek early prenatal care. Psychological support and counselling may be advisable for women and their partners to help them deal with the loss of the pregnancy. Follow-up contact enables the nurse to answer questions and clarify information for the woman and her partner. In addition, it provides an opportunity to assess their ability to cope with the loss of the pregnancy.

Evaluation

EXPECTED PATIENT OUTCOMES

Expected patient outcomes may include:

1. Experiences relief of pain
   a. Reports a decrease in pain and discomfort
   b. Ambulates as prescribed; performs coughing and deep breathing
2. Begins to accept loss of pregnancy and expresses grief by verbalizing feelings and reactions to loss
3. Verbalizes an understanding of the causes of ectopic pregnancy

4. Experiences no complications
   a. Exhibits no signs of bleeding, hemorrhage, or shock
   b. Has decreased amounts of discharge (on perineal pad)
   c. Has normal skin colour and turgor
   d. Exhibits stable vital signs and adequate urine output
   e. Levels of beta-hCG return to normal

Critical Thinking Exercises

1. A 25-year-old woman is having a complete physical examination for the first time and is extremely apprehensive. How would you approach the history and physical examination with her? How would you modify your approach if the woman had significant physical and developmental/cognitive disabilities?

2. A 57-year-old woman with osteoporosis has been taking hormone replacement therapy (HRT) for 9 years to treat hot flashes and to prevent further bone loss. She has recently read about the results of the Women's Health Initiative study suggesting that the risks of HRT outweigh the benefits. She is concerned not only about her risk for breast cancer based on those results, but also about the return of hot flashes and further bone loss if she stops the HRT. How would you advise her? What resources would you recommend to her?

3. An 18-year-old woman comes to the clinic for a gynecologic examination because she anticipates having sex with her new boyfriend. She asks you for advice about oral contraceptives versus barrier methods of contraception. What advice would you give her? How would you teach her about using a barrier method of contraception if that is what she chooses? How would you modify your teaching if she informed you that her new boyfriend has AIDS? What general health promotion teaching would you provide to her?

4. You are working in an infertility practice and are responsible for orienting couples beginning an evaluation for infertility to the procedures and services of the practice. A 40-year-old woman and her 48-year-old husband are eager to learn about the process. During your initial conversation with them, you learn that they both have high levels of stress and high-pressure jobs. While the woman is eager to begin the process, her husband is uncertain about wanting to proceed with the workup because of concerns about privacy, confidentiality, costs, and possible disappointment. How would you proceed in your explanations of the process and procedures? What information about your assessment of the couple's readiness to undergo the evaluation would you report to the physician or nurse practitioner?

5. During a checkup at the clinic where you work, a 43-year-old patient tells you that she has met a new partner and is not concerned about sexual risks of STDs because she is a lesbian and has never had a sexual relationship with a man. How would you address the educational needs of this patient?

6. At a health clinic, you meet a 48-year-old woman with spina bifida who uses a cane at home and a wheelchair outside the home. She is approaching menopause and is concerned about how her limitations secondary to spina bifida might affect her health related to menopause. Describe what health promotion issues would be relevant and the actions, including patient teaching, that are warranted.

REFERENCES AND SELECTED READINGS

Books

American College of Obstetricians and Gynecologists (ACOG). *2001 Compendium of selected publications.* Washington, DC: Author.

Andrews, M., & Boyle, J. (Eds.) (2001). *Transcultural concepts in nursing care* (3rd ed.). Philadelphia: Lippincott William & Wilkins.

Annon, J. S. (1976). *Behavioral treatment of sexual problems: Brief therapy.* Hagerstown, MD: Harper & Row.

AWHONN (1999). *Women's health at midlife and beyond: Nursing practice for wellness promotion and disease prevention. Monograph 1: Postmenopausal health risks and the importance of prevention. A CE Self-Study Series for Nurses.* Washington, DC: Author.

Canadian Pharmacists Association. (2003). *CPhA guidelines for the provision of Plan B (levonorgestrel 0.75 mg) as a Schedule II product.* Ottawa: Author.

Cooper, J., Osmond, B., & Rantucci, M. (2000). *Emergency contraceptive pills: Questions and answers.* Ottawa: Canadian Pharmacists Association.

Copeland, L. (2000). *Textbook of gynecology* (2nd ed.). Philadelphia: W. B. Saunders.

Goldman, M., & Hatch, M. (2000). *Women and health.* San Diego: Academic Press.

Hawkins, J., Roberto-Nichols, D., & Stanley-Haney, J. (1999). *Protocols for nurse practitioners in gynecologic setttings* (7th ed.). New York: Tiresias Press.

Kirschner, K. L., Gill, C. J., Reis, J. P., & Welner, S. (1998). Health issues for women with disabilities. In J. A. DeLisa & B. M. Gans, *Rehabilitation medicine: Principles and practice* (3d ed.). Philadelphia: Lippincott-Raven.

National Osteoporosis Foundation. (1999). *Physician's guide to prevention and treatment of osteoporosis.* Washington, DC: Author.

North American Menopause Society (2000). *Menopause core curriculum study guide.* Cleveland: Author (http://www.menopause.org).

Northrup, C. (1998). *Women's bodies, women's wisdom: Creating physical and emotional health and healing.* New York: Bantam.

U.S. Department of Health and Human Services. (2001). *Surgeon general's call to action to promote sexual health and responsible sexual behavior.* Washington, DC: U.S. Government Printing Office.

Toubia, N. (1999). *Caring for women with circumcision.* New York: Rainbow.

Varicchio, C. (1997). *A cancer source book for nurses* (7th ed.). Atlanta: American Cancer Society.

Journals

Asterisks indicate nursing research articles.
General

ACOG (2001). Antibiotic prophylaxis for gynecologic procedures. ACOG Practice Bulletin #23. *Obstetrics & Gynecology, 97*(4), 1–13.

Asch-Goodkin, J. (2001). Caring for the postmenopausal woman: Complete care of the older woman. *Patient Care for the Nurse Practitioner, 4*(5), 15–22.

Asch-Goodkin, J. (2001). Complete care of the older woman. *Patient Care, 35*(9), 23–34.

Centers for Disease Control and Prevention (CDC). (2002). Sexually transmitted diseases treatment guidelines, 2002. *MMWR-Morbidity and Mortality Weekly Report, 51*(RR-6), 1–85.

Charney, P. (2000). Women's health: An evolving mosaic. *Journal of General Internal Medicine, 15*(8), 600–602.

Holick, M. F. (1998). *How much vitamin D is enough?* Available at: http://www.mcmaster.ca/inabis98/arkinson/holick0835/two.html.

Kopac, C., Fritz, J., & Holt, R. (1998). Gynecologic and reproductive services for women with developmental disabilities. *Clinical Excellence for Nursing Practice, 2*(2), 88–95.

*Lamp, J. Alteneder, R., & Lee, C. (2000). Nurses' knowledge, attitude and skills related to sexuality. *Journal of Nursing Scholarship, 32*(4), 391.

McFarlane, M., Bull, S., & Rietmeijer, C. (2000) The Internet as a newly emerging risk environment for sexually transmitted diseases. *Journal of the American Medical Association, 284*(4), 443–446.

Muscari, M. E. (1999). Adolescent health: The first gynecologic exam. *American Journal of Nursing, 99*(1), 66–67.

Peck, S. A. (2001). The importance of the sexual health history in the primary care setting. *Journal of Obstetric, Gynecologic and Neonatal Nursing, 30*(3), 269–274.

Sandelowski, M. (2000). "This most dangerous instrument": Propriety, power and the vaginal speculum. *JOGNN, 29*(1), 73–82.

Smeltzer, S. C. (2000). Double jeopardy: Women with disabilities. *American Journal of Nursing, 100*(8), 11.

Abortion

Abortion surveillance: preliminary analysis—United States, 1997. (2000). *MMWR, Morbidity & Mortality Weekly Reports, 48*(51/52), 1171–1174, 1191.

ACOG Committee on Practice Bulletins—Gynecology. (2001). Medical management of abortion. Clinical management guidelines for obstetrician-gynecologists. ACOG Practice Bulletin #26. *Obstetrics & Gynecology, 97*(4), suppl 1–13.

ACOG (2000). Mifepristone for medical pregnancy termination. ACOG Committee on Gynecologic Practice Committee Opinion #245. *Obstetrics & Gynecology, 96*(6), 1–2.

Borgatta, L., Burnhill, M., Tyson, J., et al. (2001). Early medical abortion with methotrexate and misoprostol. *Obstetrics & Gynecology, 97*(1), 11–16.

Christin-Maitre, S., Bouchard, P., & Spitz, I., (2000). Medical termination of pregnancy. *New England Journal of Medicine, 342*(13), 946–955.

Goldberg, A., Greenberg, M., & Darney, P. (2001). Drug therapy: Misoprostol and pregnancy. *New England Journal of Medicine, 344*(1), 38–47.

Hale, R., & Zinberg, S. (2001). Use of misoprostol in pregnancy. *New England Journal of Medicine, 344*(1), 59–60.

Robinson, D., Dollins, A., & O'Shaughnessy, L. (2000). Care of the woman before and after an elective abortion. *American Journal for Nursing Practice, 4*(3), 17–29.

Williams, G. (2000). Grief after elective abortion. *AWHONN Lifelines, 4*(2), 37–40.

Zapka, J., Lemon, S., Peerson, et al. (2001). The silent consumer: Women's reports and ratings of abortion services. *Medical Care, 39*(1), 50–60.

Conception Control

ACOG (2001). Managing the anovulatory state: medical induction of ovulation. ACOG Technical Bulletin #197. *ACOG 2001 Compendium of Selected Publications,* 596–601.

ACOG (1995). Hormonal contraception. ACOG Technical Bulletin #198. *International Journal of Gynecology & Obstetrics, 48*(1), 115–126.

ACOG Committee on Ethics. (1999). Sterilization of women, including those with mental disabilities. ACOG Committee Opinion # 216. *International Journal of Gynecology & Obstetrics, 65*(3), 317–320.

Barron, M., & Daly, K. (2001). Expert in fertility appreciation: The Creighton model practitioner. *Journal of Obstetric, Gynecologic and Neonatal Nursing, 30*(4), 386–391.

Canadian Paediatric Society, Adolescent Health Committee. (2003). Emergency contraception. *Paediatric and Child Health, 8*(3), 181–183. Reference No. AH03-01. Available at: www.cps.ca/english/statement/AM/ah03-01.htm.

CDC (1999). Achievements in public health, 1990–1999: Family planning. *MMWR, Morbidity & Mortality Weekly Reports, 48,* 1073–1080.

Christman, G., & Uechi, H. (May 2000). Female sterilization. *Female Patient, 25*(5), 29–35.

———(2000). Evolution and revolution; the past, present and future of contraception. *Contraception Report, 10*(6), 15–25.

Farrington, A. (2001). Today's contraceptive options: Finding the right fit. *Health and Sexuality, 6*(3), 4–6.

Grabrick, D., Hartman, L., Cerhan, J., et al. (2000). Risk of breast cancer with oral contraceptive use in women with a family history of breast cancer. *Journal of the American Medical Association, 284*(14), 1791–1798.

Grimes, D., & Raymond, E. (1999). Bundling a pregnancy test with the Yupze regimen of emergency contraception. *Obstetrics & Gynecology, 94*(3), 471–473.

Grydanus, D., Patel, D., & Rimsza, M. (2001). Contraception in the adolescent: An update. *Pediatrics, 107*(3), 562–573.

Health Canada. (2004). *Health Canada–endorsed important safety information on DEPO-PROVERA* (medroxyprogesterone acetate)*. Available at: www.hc-sc.gc.ca/hpfb-dgpsa/tpd-dpt/depo-provera_hpc_e.html.

Jamieson, D., Hillis, S., Duerr, A., et al. (2000). Complications of interval laparoscopic tubal sterilization: Findings from the United States Collaborative Review of Sterilization. *Obstetrics & Gynecology, 96*(6), 997–1002.

Martin, K., & Wu, Z. (2000). Contraceptive use in Canada: 1984–1995. *Family Planning Perspective, 32*(2), 65–73.

Morris, B. J., & Young, C. (2000). Emergency contraception. *American Journal of Nursing, 100*(9), 46–48.

Peterson, H. B., Xia, Z., Wilcox, L. S., et al. (2001). Collaborative Review of Sterilization Working Group. Pregnancy after tubal sterilization with silicone rubber band and spring clip application. *Obstetrics & Gynecology, 97*(2), 205–210.

Rawlins, S., Burkman, R., & Schwarz, B. (2000). The power of the pill: Making evidence-based decisions. *American Journal of Nursing Practice, 4*(1), 25–40.

Rodrigues, I., Grou, F., & Joly, J. (2001). Effectiveness of emergency contraceptive pills between 72 and 120 hours after unprotected sexual intercourse.[see comment]. *American Journal of Obstetrics & Gynecology, 184*(4), 531–537.

Schnare, S. (2000). Emergency postcoital contraception. *American Journal of Nursing Practice, 4*(2), 15–22.

Stephenson, J. (2000). Widely used spermicide may increase, not decrease risk of HIV transmission. *Journal of the American Medical Association, 284*(8), 949.

Task Force on Postovulatory Methods of Fertility Regulation. (1998). Randomised controlled trial of levonorgestrel versus the Yuzpe regimen of combined oral contraceptives for emergency contraception. *Lancet, 352*(9126), 428–433.

Cultural Differences in Health Care of Women

ACOG Committee on Health Care for Underserved Women (1998). Cultural competency in health care. ACOG Committee Opinion #201. *International Journal of Gynecology & Obstetrics, 62*(1), 96–99.

Blackwell, D., & Blackwell, J. (1999). Building alternative families: Helping lesbian couples find the path to parenthood. *AWHONN Lifelines, 3*(5), 45–48.

Carroll, N. (1999). Optimal gynecologic and obstetric care for lesbians. *Obstetrics & Gynecology, 93*(4), 611–613.

Cesario, S. (2001) Care of the native American woman: Strategies for practice education and research. *Journal of Obstetric, Gynecologic and Neonatal Nursing, 30*(1), 13–18.

Cochran, S. D., Mays, V. M., Bowen, D., et al. (2001). Cancer-risk risk indicators and preventive screening behaviors among lesbians and bisexual women. *American Journal of Public Health, 91*(4), 591–597.

Mattson, S. (2000) Providing culturally competent care: Strategies and approaches for perinatal clients. *AWHONN Lifelines, 4*(5), 37–39.

Sinclair, B. (2000). Putting cultural competence into practice. *AWHONN Lifelines, 4*(2), 7–8.

Diagnostic Techniques and Treatments

ACOG (1997). Operative laparoscopy. ACOG Educational Bulletin #239. *International Journal of Gynecology & Obstetrics, 59*(3), 265–268.

Farquhar, C., Lethaby, A., Sowter, M., et al. (1999). An evaluation of risk factors for endometrial hyperplasia in premenopausal women with abnormal menstrual bleeding. *American Journal of Obstetrics & Gynecology, 181*(3), 525–529.

Klein, A., & Schwartz, M. (2001). Uterine artery embolization of uterine fibroids: An outpatient procedure. *American Journal of Obstetrics & Gynecology, 184*(7), 1556–1563.

Public Health Agency of Canada. (1998). Programmatic guidelines for cancer of the cervix screening in Canada. Available at: www.phac-aspc.gc.ca/dpg_e.html#cancer.

Soriano, D., Ajaj, S. Chuong, T., et al. (2000). Lidocaine spray and out-patient hysteroscopy: Randomized placebo controlled trial. *Obstetrics & Gynecology, 96*(5, Part 1), 661–664.

Suh-Burghman, E., Whall-Strojwas, D., Chang, Y., et al. (2000). Risk factors for cervical stenosis after loop electrocautery excision procedure. *Obstetrics & Gynecology, 96*(5, Part 1), 657–660.

Tjarks, M., & Van Voorhis, B. (2000). Treatment of endometrial polyps. *Obstetrics & Gynecology, 96*(6), 886–889.

Ectopic Pregnancy

Buster, J., & Heard, M. (2000). Current issues in medical management of ectopic pregnancy. *Current Opinion in Obstetrics & Gynecology, 12*(6), 525–527.

Garcia, C., & Barnhart, K. (2001). Diagnosing ectopic pregnancy: Decision analysis comparing six strategies. *Obstetrics & Gynecology, 97*(3), 464–470.

Lemus, J. (2000). Ectopic pregnancy: An update. *Current Opinion in Obstetrics & Gynecology, 12*(5), 369–375.

Lipscomb, G., Stovall, T., & Ling, F. (2000). Primary care: Non-surgical treatment of ectopic pregnancy. *New England Journal of Medicine, 343*(18), 1325–1329.

Morlock, R., Lafata, J., & Eisenstein, D. (2000). Cost-effectiveness of single-dose methotrexate compared with laparoscopic treatment of ectopic pregnancy. *Obstetrics & Gynecology, 95*(3), 407–412.

Infertility

ACOG (2000). Infertility. ACOG Technical Bulletin #125. *2001 Compendium of Selected Publications Compendium*, 556–561.

Angard, N. (1999). Diagnosis: Infertility. *AWHONN Lifelines, 3*(3), 22–29.

Cramer, D., Liberman, J., Powers, D., et al. (2000). Recent trends in assisted reproductive techniques and associated outcomes. *Obstetrics & Gynecology, 95*(1), 61–66.

DeMaio, C. (Spring 2000). Clomiphene for infertility? When to refer. *Conversations in Counseling, 2*(1), 4–6.

Gonzalez, L. O. (2000). Infertility as a transformational process: A framework for psychotherapeutic support of infertile women. *Issues in Mental Health Nursing, 21*(6), 619–633.

Guermandi, E., Vegetti, W., Massimiliano, M. et al. (2001). Reliability of ovulation tests in infertile women. *Obstetrics & Gynecology, 97*(1), 92–96.

Hart, V. A. (2002). Infertility and the role of psychotheraphy. *Issues in Mental Health Nursing, 23*(1), 31–41.

Van Voorhis, B., & Syrop, C. (2000). Cost-effective treatment of the couple with infertility. *Clinical Obstetrics and Gynecology, 43*(4), 958–973.

Menstruation, Irregular Bleeding, Perimenopause, PMS, and Menopause

Abramson, B., Dzerko, C., Lalonde, A., et al. (2002). Hormone replacement therapy and cardiovascular disease. Available at: www.ccs.ca/download/HRT_Statement_2.pdf.

Akin, M., Weingand, K., Hengehold, D., et al. (2001). Continuous low-level topical heat in the treatment of dysmenorrhea. *Obstetrics & Gynecology, 97*(3), 343–349.

American Association of Clinical Endocrinologists (1999). Medical guidelines for clinical practice for management of menopause. *Endourinology Practice, 5*(6), 355–366.

Bachmann, G. (2001). Physiologic aspects of natural and surgical menopause. *Journal of Reproductive Medicine, 46*(3 Suppl), 307–315.

Barnard, N., Scialli, A., Hurlock, D., & Bertron, P. (2000) Diet and sex-hormone binding globulin, dysmenorrhea and premenstrual symptoms. *Obstetrics & Gynecology, 95*(2), 245–250.

Brown, J. P., Josse, R. G., & The Scientific Advisory Council of the Osteoporosis Society of Canada. (2002). 2002 clinical practice guidelines for the diagnosis and management of osteoporosis in Canada. *CMAJ: Canadian Medical Association Journal, 167*(10 Suppl), S1–S34.

Cheung, A. M., Feig, D. S., Kapral, M., et al. (2004). Prevention of osteoporosis and osteoporotic fractures in postmenopausal women: recommendation statement from the Canadian Task Force on Preventive Health Care. *CMAJ: Canadian Medical Association Journal, 170*(11), 1665–1667.

Dell, D., Moskowitz, D., & Sondheimer, S. (2001). PMS and PMDD: Identification and treatment. *Contemporary Obstetrics & Gynecology, 46*(4), 15–24.

DeMasters, J. (2000). HRT and menopause: A clinician's guide to understanding the dilemma. *AWHONN Lifelines, 4*(2), 26–35.

DiCarlo, C., Palomba, S., Tommaselli, G., et al. (2001). Use of leuprolide acetate plus tibolone in the treatment of severe premenstrual syndrome. *Fertility & Sterility, 75*(2), 380–384.

Finkel, M. L., Cohen, M., & Mahoney, H. (2001). Treatment options for the menopausal woman. *Nurse Practitioner, 26*(2), 5–7, 11–17.

Goolsby, M. J. (2001). Clinical practice guidelines. Management of menopause. *Journal of the American Academy of Nursing Practice, 13*(4), 147–151.

Grady, D., Brown, J., Vittinghoff, E., et al. (2001). Postmenopausal hormones and incontinence: The heart and estrogen/progestin replacement study. *Obstetrics & Gynecology, 97*(1), 116–120.

Hulley, S., Grady, D., Bush, T., et al. (1998). Randomized trial of estrogen plus progestin for secondary prevention of coronary heart disease in postmenopausal women. Heart and Estrogen/progestin Replacement Study (HERS) Research Group. *Journal of the American Medical Association, 280*(7), 605–613.

Kessenich, C. (2000). Osteoporosis in primary care: Role of biochemical markers and diagnostic imaging. *American Journal of Nursing Practice, 4*(2), 24–29.

Manson, J., & Martin, K. (2001). Post-menopausal hormone-replacement therapy. *New England Journal of Medicine, 345*(1), 34–40.

Mishell, D. (2000). Oral contraceptives: Making evidence-based decisions. *International Journal of Fertility, 45*(Suppl 2), 99–150.

Morse, G. (1999). Positively reframing perceptions of the menstrual cycle among women with premenstrual syndrome. *Journal of Obstetric, Gynecologic and Neonatal Nursing, 28*(2), 165–174.

Mosca, L., Collins, P., Herrington, D., et al. (2001). Hormone replacement therapy and cardiovascular disease: A statement for health care professionals from the American Heart Association. *Circulation, 104*(4), 499–503.

North American Menopause Society (2000). Consensus opinion: Clinical challenges of perimenopause. *Menopause, 7*(1), 5–13.

Penckofer, S., & Schertz, D. (2001). Hormone replacement therapy: Primary and secondary prevention. *Journal of Cardiovascular Nursing, 15*(3), 1–25.

Pilon, D., Castilloux, A., & Lelorier, J. (2001). Estrogen replacement therapy: Determinants of persistence with treatment. *Obstetrics & Gynecology, 97*(1), 97–100.

Sawaya, G., Grady, D., Kerlikowske, K., et al. (2000). The positive predictive value of cervical smears in previously screened postmenopausal women: The heart and estrogen/progestin replacement study (HERS). *Annals of Internal Medicine, 133*(12), 942–950.

*Schott-Baer, D., & Kotal, B. (2000). Frequency and effectiveness of self-care actions and menopause symptoms of middle-aged working women. *MedSurg Nursing, 9*(6), 302–308.

Sharts-Hopko, N. C. (2001). Hysterectomy for nonmalignant conditions. *American Journal of Nursing, 101*(9), 32–40.

Taylor, M. (2001). Psychological consequences of surgical menopause. *Journal of Reproductive Medicine, 46*(3 Suppl), 317–324, 333–336.

Utian, W., & Boggs, P. (1999). The North American Menopause Society 1998 Menopause Survey. Part 1. Postmenopausal women's perceptions about menopause and midlife. *Menopause, 6,* 122–128.

Vandenakker, C. B., & Glass, D. D. (February 2001). Menopause and aging with disability. *Physical and Medical Rehabilitation Clinics of North America, 12*(1), 133–151.

Writing Group for Women's Health Initiative Investigators. (2002). Risks and benefits of estrogen plus progestin in healthy postmenopausal women: Principal results from the Women's Health Initiative randomized controlled trial. *Journal of the American Medical Association, 288*(3), 321–333.

Mutilation, Domestic Violence, Physical and Sexual Assault

ACOG Committee on Gynecologic Practice and Committee on International Affairs. (1995). Female genital mutilation. ACOG Committee Opinion #151.

ACOG (2000). Educational Bulletin #259. Adult manifestations of childhood sexual abuse. Clinical management guidelines for obstetricians-gynecologists. *International Journal of Gynecology & Obstetrics, 74*(3), 311–320.

Affara, F. (August 2000). When tradition maims. *American Journal of Nursing, 100*(8), 52–60.

Chalmers, B., & Hashi, K. O. (2000). 432 Somali women's birth experiences in Canada after earlier female genital mutilation. *Birth, 27*(4), 227–234.

Fourcroy, J. L. (1999). Female circumcision. *American Family Physician, 60*(2), 657–658.

Garcia-Moreno, C. (2000). Violence against women: International perspectives. *American Journal of Preventive Medicine, 19*(4), 330–333.

Kaplan, D., Feinstein, R., Fisher, M., et al. (2001). Care of the adolescent sexual assault victim. *Pediatrics, 107*(6), 1476–1479.

Lampe, A., Solder, E., Ennemoser, A., et al. (2000). Chronic pelvic pain and previous sexual abuse. *Obstetrics & Gynecology, 96*(6), 929–932.

*McFarlane, J., Soeken, K., & Wiist, W. (2000). An evaluation of interventions to decrease intimate partner violence to pregnant women. *Public Health Nursing, 17*(6), 443–451.

Public Health Agency of Canada. (2005). *Child sexual abuse.* Available at: www.phac-aspc.gc.ca/ncfv-cnivf/familyviolence/html/nfntsxagrsexe.html.

Salber, P., & McCaw, B. (2000). Barriers to screening for intimate partner violence: Time to reframe the question. *American Journal of Preventive Medicine, 19*(4), 276–278.

Pap Smears

ACOG Committee on Primary Care. (2000). Primary and preventive care: Periodic assessments. *International Journal of Gynaecology & Obstetrics, 70*(3), 393–399.

ACOG Committee on Gynecology Practice Committee (2000). Routine cancer screening. Committee Opinion #247. *Obstetrics & Gynecology, 96*(6), insert 1–5.

Association of Reproductive Health Professionals. (2002). Clinical update on transcervical sterilization. *ARHP Clinical Proceedings,* pp. 1–25.

DeRemer Abercrombie, P. (2001). Improving adherence to abnormal Pap smear follow-up. *Journal of Obstetric, Gynecologic and Neonatal Nursing, 30*(1), 80–88.

Franco, E., Duarte-Franco, E., & Ferenczy, A. (2001). Cervical cancer: Epidemiology, prevention and the role of human papillomavirus infection. *Canadian Medical Association Journal, 164*(7), 1017–1025.

Hopman, E. H., Rozendaal, L., Voorhorst, F. J., et al. (2000). High-risk human papillomavirus in women with normal cervical cytology prior to the development of abnormal cytology and colposcopy. *British Journal of Obstetrics & Gynaecology, 107*(5), 600–604.

Sawaya, G. F., Brown, A. D., Washington, A. E., & Garber, A. M. (2001). Clinical practice. Current approaches to cervical-cancer screening. *New England Journal of Medicine, 344*(21), 1603–1607.

Sawaya, G. F., Kerlikowske, K., Lee, N. C., et al. (2000). Frequency of cervical smear abnormalities within 3 years of normal cytology. *Obstetrics & Gynecology, 96*(2), 219–223.

Solomon, D., Davey, D., Kurman, R., Moriarty, A., O'Connor, D., Prey, M., et al. (2001). The 2001 Bethesda System: Terminology for reporting results of cervical cytology. Consensus Statement. *Journal of the American Medical Association, 287*(16), 2114–2119.

Sung, H., Kearny, K., Miller, M., et al. (2000). Papanicolaou smear history and diagnosis of invasive cervical carcinoma among members of a large prepaid health plan. *Cancer, 88*(10), 2283–2289.

Wee, C., McCarthy, E., Davis, R., & Phillips, R. (2000). Screening for cervical and breast cancer: Is obesity an unrecognized barrier to preventive care? *Annals of Internal Medicine, 132*(9), 697–704.

Wright, T. C., Jr., Cox, J. T., Massad, L. S., Twiggs, L. B., & Wilkinson, E. J. (2002). ASCCP-Sponsored Consensus Conference. 2001 Consensus Guidelines for the management of women with cervical cytological abnormalities. *Journal of the American Medical Association, 287*(16), 2120–2129.

RESOURCES AND WEBSITES

American College of Obstetricians and Gynecologists (ACOG), 409 12th St. SW, P.O. Box 96920, Washington, DC 20090-6920; http://www.acog.org.

Amnesty International, 322 Eighth Ave., New York, NY 10001 (212) 807-8400; http://www.amnesty.org/ailib/intcam/femgen/fgm10.htm (resource for activists to end female genital mutilation).

Association of Women's Health, Obstetrical and Neonatal Nurses (AWHONN, formerly NAACOG), 2000 L Street NW, Suite 740, Washington, DC 20036; (800) 673-8499; http://www.awhonn.org.

Canadian Association of Genetic Counsellors (CAGC); www.cagc-accg.ca.

Canadian Cancer Society/Société canadienne du cancer, National Office, Suite 200, 10 Alcorn Avenue, Toronto, ON M4V 3B1; (416) 961-7223; fax: (416) 961-4189; www.cancer.ca.

Canadian Directory of Genetic Support Groups, Support Group Directory, Regional Medical Genetics Centre, Children's Hospital of Western Ontario, 800 Commissioner's Road East, London, ON N6C 2V5; (519) 685-8453; in Ontario only: 1-800-243-8416; fax: (519) 685-8214; www.lhsc.on.ca/programs/medgenet.

Canadian Genetic Disease Network, Suite 201, 2150 Western Parkway, Vancouver, BC V6T 1V6; (604) 221-7300; fax: (604) 221-0778; e-mail: info@cgdn.ca; www.cgdn.ca.

Canadian Fertility and Andrology Society, 2065 Alexandre de Sève, Suite 409, Montreal, QC H2L 2W5; (514) 524-9009; fax: (514) 524-2163; e-mail: info@cfas.ca; www.cfas.ca.

Canadian Organization for Rare Disorders (CORD), PO Box 814, Coaldale, AB T1M 1M7; (403) 345-4544; toll-free: 1-877-302-7273; fax: (403) 345-3948; www.cord.ca.

Canadian Paediatric Society, 2305 St. Laurent Boulevard, Ottawa, ON K1G 4J8; (613) 526-9397; fax: (613) 526-3332; www.cps.ca.

Canadian Pharmacists Association, 1785 Alta Vista Drive, Ottawa, ON KIG 3Y6; 1-800-919-9489; e-mail: cpha@pharmacists.ca; www.pharmacists.ca.

Canadian Public Health Association, 400-1565 Carling Avenue, Ottawa, ON K1Z 8R1; (613) 725-3769; fax: (613) 725-9826; e-mail: info@cpha.ca; www.cpha.ca.

DAWN Canada (Disabled Women's Network Canada), Box 1138, North Bay, ON P1B 8K4; (705) 474-4242; fax: (705) 474-9622; TTY: (705) 474-7435; www.dawncanada.net.

Department of Adolescent Health, American Medical Association, 515 North State St., Chicago, IL 60610; Adolescent Health on Line at http://www.ama-assn.org/ama/pub/category/1947.html.

DES Action Canada, 5890 Monkland Avenue, Suite 107, Montreal, QC H4A 1G2; (514) 482-3204, 1-800-482-1-DES (Canada and USA); www.web.net/~desact.

Emergency Contraception; Office of Population Research, Princeton University, Princeton, NJ 08540; (888) Not-2-Late; http://opr.princeton.edu/ec.

Family Violence Prevention Fund, 383 Rhode Island St., Suite 304, San Francisco, CA 94103; (415) 252-8900; http://www.fvpf.org.

Female Genital Mutilation Education and Networking Project, http://www.fgmnetwork.org; e-mail: fgm@fgmnetwork.org.

GeneTests, 9725 Third Avenue NE, Suite 602, Seattle, WA 98115; (206) 616-4033; fax: (206) 221-4679; e-mail: genetests@genetests.org; www.genetests.org.

Genetic Alliance, 4301 Connecticut Avenue NW, Suite 404, Washington, DC 20008-2369; (202) 966-5557; fax: (202) 966-8553; e-mail: info@geneticalliance.org; www.geneticalliance.org.

The Genetics Society of Canada; http://life.biology.mcmaster.ca/GSC.

Infertility Awareness Association of Canada (IAAC), 2100 Marlowe Avenue, Suite 39, Montreal, QC H4A 3L5; (514) 484-2891, toll-free info line: 1-800-263-2929; fax: (514) 484-0454; e-mail: info@iaac.ca; http://iaac.ca.

Jacob's Institute of Women's Health, 409 12th St SW, Washington, DC; (202) 863-4990; http://www.jiwh.org.

MenopauseCanada; www.menopausecanada.com.

The National Action Committee on the Status of Women (NAC), 234 Eglinton Avenue East, Suite 203, Toronto, ON M4P 1K5; (416) 932-1718; fax: (416) 932-0646; e-mail: nac@web.net; www.nac-cca.ca.

National Association of Nurse Practitioners in Women's Health (NPWH); (202) 543-9693; e-mail: info@npwh.org; http://www.npwh.org/index.html.

National Cancer Institute of Canada/Institut national du cancer du Canada, 10 Alcorn Avenue, Suite 200; Toronto, ON M4V 3B1; (416) 961-7223; fax: (416) 961-4189; www.ncic.cancer.ca.

National Coalition Against Domestic Violence, 503 Capitol Court, NE, Suite 300, Washington, DC 20002.

Nursing Network on Violence Against Women International, 1801 H Street, Suite B5-165, Modesto, CA 95354; (888) 909-9993.

OMIM Online Mendelian Inheritance in Man; www.ncbi.nlm.nih.gov/entrez/query.fcgi?db=OMIM.

Osteoporosis Society of Canada, 33 Laird Drive, Toronto, ON M4G 3S8; (416) 696-2663; toll-free (English): 1-800-463-6842 (in Canada only); toll-free (French): 1-800-977-1778 (in Canada only); fax: (416) 696-2673; e-mail: osc@osteoporosis.ca; www.osteoporosis.ca.

Planned Parenthood Federation of Canada, 1 Nicholas Street, Suite 430, Ottawa, ON K1N 7B7; (613) 241-4474; www.ppfc.ca.

Research, Action and Information Network for the Bodily Integrity of Women (RAINBO), 915 Broadway, Suite 1109, New York, NY 10010-7108; (212) 477-3318; e-mail: Info@rainbow.org; http://www.rainbo.org.

Sex Information and Education Council of Canada (SIECCAN), 850 Coxwell Avenue, Toronto, ON M4C 5R1; (416) 466-5304; fax: (416) 778-0785; e-mail: sieccan@web.net; www.sieccan.org.

World Health Organization Department of Women's Health; 525 23 St. NW, Washington, DC 20037; (202) 974-3000; e-mail: whd@who.co; http://www.who.int/frh-whd/fgm/index.htm.

Management of Patients With Female Reproductive Disorders

Adapted by Jean Chow

LEARNING OBJECTIVES

On completion of this chapter, the learner will be able to:

1. Compare the various types of vaginal infections and the signs, symptoms, and treatments of each.
2. Develop a teaching plan for the patient with a vaginal infection.
3. Use the nursing process as a framework for care of the patient with a vulvovaginal infection.
4. Use the nursing process as a framework for care of the patient with genital herpes.
5. Describe medical and nursing management for the patient with toxic shock syndrome.
6. Discuss the signs and symptoms, management, and nursing care implications of malignant disorders of the female reproductive tract.
7. Use the nursing process as a framework for care of the patient undergoing a hysterectomy.
8. Describe indications for a wide excision of the vulva, or vulvectomy, and the preoperative and postoperative nursing interventions.
9. Compare nursing interventions indicated for the patient undergoing radiation therapy and chemotherapy for cancer of the female reproductive tract.

*D*isorders of the female reproductive system are relatively common. Some disorders are self-limited and cause only minor inconvenience to the woman; others are life-threatening and require immediate attention and long-term therapy. Many disorders are managed by the patient at home, whereas others require hospitalization and surgical intervention. All disorders require understanding and skill in patient teaching on the part of the nurse. The nurse must also be sensitive to women's concerns and their possible, even probable, discomfort in discussing and dealing with these disorders.

Vulvovaginal Infections

The vagina is protected against infection by its normally low pH (3.5 to 4.5), which is maintained in part by the actions of *Lactobacillus acidophilus,* the dominant bacteria in a healthy vaginal ecosystem. These bacteria suppress the growth of anaerobes and produce lactic acid, which maintains normal pH. They also produce hydrogen peroxide, which is toxic to anaerobes. The risk of infection rises if a woman's resistance is reduced by stress or illness, if the pH is altered, or if a pathogen is introduced.

Vulvovaginal infections are common problems, and nurses have an important role in providing information that may prevent their occurrence. To prevent these infections, women need to understand their own anatomy and vulvovaginal hygiene measures. In addition, continued research into causes and treatments is needed, along with better ways to encourage growth of **lactobacilli**.

The epithelium of the vagina is highly responsive to estrogen, which induces glycogen formation. The subsequent breakdown of glycogen into lactic acid assists in producing a low vaginal pH. When estrogen decreases during lactation and menopause, glycogen also decreases. With reduced glycogen formation, infections may occur. In addition, as estrogen production ceases during the perimenopausal and postmenopausal periods, the vagina and labia may atrophy (thin), making the vaginal area more susceptible to infection. When patients are treated with antibiotics, the normal vaginal flora are reduced. This results in altered pH and growth of fungal organisms. Other factors that may initiate infections include sexual intercourse with an infected partner and wearing tight, nonabsorbent, and heat-retaining clothing (Chart 47-1).

Vaginitis (inflammation of the vagina) occurs when *Candida* or *Trichomonas* species or other bacteria invade the vagina. The normal vaginal discharge, which may occur in slight amounts during ovulation or just before the onset of menstruation, becomes more profuse when vaginitis occurs. Urethritis may accompany

Glossary

abscess: a collection of purulent material

acquired immunodeficiency syndrome (AIDS): a disease transmitted by body fluids that results in impaired immune response

Bartholin's cyst: a cyst in a paired vestibular gland in the vulva

brachytherapy: radiation delivered by an internal device placed close to the tumour

candidiasis: infection caused by *Candida* species or yeast; also referred to as monilial vaginitis or yeast infection

chancre: painless lesion caused by syphilis

choriocarcinoma: a type of gestational neoplasm

colporrhaphy: repair of the vagina

condylomata: warty growths indicative of the human papillomavirus (HPV)

conization: procedure in which a cone-shaped piece of cervical tissue is removed as a result of detection of abnormal cells; also called cone biopsy

cryotherapy: destruction of tissue by freezing (eg, with liquid nitrogen)

cystocele: bulging of the bladder downward into the vagina

dermoid cyst: ovarian tumour of undefined origin that consists of undifferentiated embryonal cells

douche: rinsing the vaginal canal with fluid

dysplasia: term related to abnormal cell changes found on Pap smear and cervical biopsy reports

endocervicitis: inflammation of the mucosa and the glands of the cervix

endometrial ablation: procedure performed through a hysteroscope in which the lining of the uterus is burned away or ablated to treat abnormal uterine bleeding

endometriosis: endometrial tissue in abnormal locations; causes pain with menstruation, scarring, and possible infertility

fibroid tumour: usually benign tumour of the uterus that may cause irregular bleeding; also called myoma or leiomyoma

fistula: abnormal opening between two organs or sites (ie, vesicovaginal, between bladder and vagina; rectovaginal, between rectum and vagina)

hydatidiform mole: a type of gestational trophoblastic neoplasm

hyphae: microscopic findings that indicate monilia

hysterectomy: surgical removal of the uterus

lactobacilli: vaginal bacteria that limit the growth of other bacteria by producing hydrogen peroxide

laparoscope: surgical device inserted through a periumbilical incision to facilitate surgical visualization and procedures

lichen sclerosus: benign disorder of the vulva that usually occurs when estrogen levels are low; characterized by itching

liposomal therapy: chemotherapy delivered in a liposome, a nontoxic drug carrier

loop electrocautery excision procedure (LEEP): procedure in which laser energy is used to remove a portion of cervical tissue after abnormal biopsy findings

mucopurulent cervicitis (MCP): inflammation of the cervix with exudate; almost always related to a chlamydial infection

myomectomy: removal of uterine fibroids though an abdominal incision

oophorectomy: surgical removal of an ovary

pelvic exenteration: major surgical procedure in which the pelvic organs are removed

pelvic inflammatory disease (PID): infection of uterus and fallopian tubes, usually from a sexually transmitted disease

perineorrhaphy: surgical repair of perineal lacerations

rectocele: bulging of the rectum into the vagina

salpingo-oophorectomy: removal of the ovary and its fallopian tube (removal of the fallopian tube alone is a salpingectomy)

salpingitis: inflammation of the fallopian tube

Skene's duct cyst: a cyst in a paired paraurethral gland located posterior to and on either side of the urinary meatus.

toxic shock syndrome (TSS): a rare but potentially life-threatening infection caused by a toxin produced by *Staphylococcus aureus;* commonly associated with, but not exclusive to, use of superabsorbent tampons

vaginal vault: term used to describe the vagina following a hysterectomy, which involves removal of the uterus including the cervix

vaginitis: inflammation of the vagina, usually secondary to infection

vestibulitis: inflammation of the vulvar vestibule, or tissue around the opening of the vagina, that causes pain often with intercourse (dyspareunia)

vulvar dystrophy: thickening or lesions of the vulva; usually causes itching and may require biopsy to exclude malignancy

vulvectomy: removal of the tissue of the vulva

vulvitis: inflammation of the vulva, usually secondary to infection or irritation

vulvodynia: painful condition that affects the vulva

Chart 47-1
Risk Factors for Vulvovaginal Infections

Premenarche
Pregnancy
Perimenopause/Menopause
Poor personal hygiene
Tight undergarments
Synthetic clothing
Frequent douching
Allergies
Use of oral contraceptives
Use of broad-spectrum antibiotics
Diabetes mellitus
Low estrogen levels
Intercourse with infected partner
Oral–genital contact (yeast can inhabit the mouth and intestinal tract)
HIV infection

vaginitis because of the proximity of the urethra to the vagina. Discharge that occurs with vaginitis may produce itching, odour, redness, burning, or edema, which may be aggravated by voiding and defecation. After the causative organism has been identified, appropriate treatment (discussed later) is prescribed. This may include oral medication or local medication that may be inserted into the vagina using an applicator.

CANDIDIASIS

Vulvovaginal **candidiasis** is a fungal or yeast infection caused by strains of Candida (Table 47-1). *Candida albicans* accounts for most cases, but other strains, such as *Candida glabrata,* may also be implicated. Many women with a healthy vaginal ecosystem harbour *Candida* but are asymptomatic. Certain conditions favour the change from an asymptomatic state to colonization with symptoms. For example, use of antibiotics decreases bacteria, thereby altering the natural protective organisms usually present in the vagina. Clinical infection may occur during pregnancy, with a systemic condition such as diabetes mellitus or human

Table 47-1 • Vaginal Infections and Vaginitis

INFECTION	CAUSE	CLINICAL MANIFESTATIONS	MANAGEMENT STRATEGIES
Candidiasis	*Candida albicans, glabrata,* or *tropicalis*	Inflammation of vaginal epithelium, producing itching, reddish irritation White, cheeselike discharge clinging to epithelium	Eradicate the fungus by administering an antifungal agent. Frequently used brand names of vaginal creams and suppositories are Monistat, Femstat, Terazol, and Gyne-Lotrimin. Review other causative factors (eg, antibiotic therapy, nylon underwear, tight clothing, pregnancy, oral contraceptives). Assess for diabetes and HIV infection in patients with recurrent monilia.
Gardnerella-associated bacterial vaginosis	*Gardnerella vaginalis* and vaginal anaerobes	Usually no edema or erythema of vulva or vagina Grey-white to yellow-white discharge clinging to external vulva and vaginal walls	Administer metronidazole (Flagyl), with instructions about avoiding alcohol while taking this medication. If infection is recurrent may treat partner.
Trichomonas vaginalis vaginitis (STD)	*Trichomonas vaginalis*	Inflammation of vaginal epithelium, producing burning and itching Frothy yellow-white or yellow-green vaginal discharge	Relieve inflammation, restore acidity, and reestablish normal bacterial flora; provide oral metronidazole for patient and partner.
Bartholinitis (infection of greater vestibular gland)	*Escherichia coli* *Trichomonas vaginalis* Staphylococcus Streptococcus Gonococcus	Erythema around vestibular gland Swelling and edema Abscessed vestibular gland	Drain the abscess; provide antibiotic therapy; excise gland of patients with chronic bartholinitis.
Cervicitis: acute and chronic	Chlamydia Gonorrhea Streptococcus Many pathogenic bacteria	Profuse purulent vaginal discharge Backache Urinary frequency and urgency	Determine the cause: perform cytologic examination of cervical smear and appropriate cultures. Eradicate the gonococcal organism, if present: penicillin (as directed) or spectinomycin or tetracycline, if patient is allergic to penicillin. Tetracycline, doxycycline (Vibramycin) to eradicate chlamydia. Eradicate other causes.
Atrophic vaginitis	Lack of estrogen; glycogen deficiency	Discharge and irritation with alkaline pH of vaginal secretions	Provide topical vaginal estrogen therapy; improve nutrition if necessary; relieve dryness through use of moisturizing medications.

immunodeficiency virus (HIV) infection, or in a patient taking corticosteroids or oral contraceptives.

Clinical Manifestations

Clinical manifestations include a vaginal discharge that causes pruritus (itching) and subsequent irritation. The discharge may be watery or thick but has a white, cottage cheese-like appearance. Symptoms are usually more severe just before menstruation and are usually less responsive to treatment during pregnancy. Diagnosis is made by microscopic identification of spores and **hyphae** on a glass slide prepared from a discharge specimen mixed with potassium hydroxide. With candidiasis, the pH is 4.5 or less.

Medical Management

The goal of management is to eliminate symptoms. Treatments include antifungal agents such as miconazole (Monistat), nystatin (Mycostatin), clotrimazole (Gyne-Lotrimin), and terconazole (Terazol) cream. These agents are inserted into the vagina with an applicator at bedtime and may be applied to the vulvar area for pruritus. There are 1-night, 3-night, or 7-night treatment courses available. Oral medication is also available (fluconazole [Diflucan]). Fluconazole is given in a one-pill dose; relief should be noted within 3 days.

Vaginal creams are available without a prescription; however, patients are cautioned to use these creams only if they are certain that they have a yeast or monilial infection. Many patients use these remedies for problems other than yeast infections. If the patient is uncertain about the cause of her symptoms or has not obtained relief after using these creams, she is instructed to seek health care promptly. Yeast infections can sometimes become recurrent and may be related to cell-mediated immunity or to an allergic response. Boric acid capsules (made by a compounding pharmacist) inserted into the vagina at bedtime for a number of weeks and then slowly tapered off to once a week may be helpful in resistant cases. Women with recurrent yeast infections benefit from a comprehensive gynecologic workup.

SEMINAL PLASMA PROTEIN ALLERGY

Women with this condition develop an immunologic response to human semen, resulting in vaginal inflammation. Symptoms vary from local inflammation and pruritus to rare systemic anaphylaxis after exposure. Diagnosis is usually based on the absence of symptoms with condom use. Treatment may include cromolyn vaginal cream and immunotherapy. The success rate of treatment varies, and referral to an immunologist may be warranted.

BACTERIAL VAGINOSIS

Bacterial vaginosis is caused by an overgrowth of anaerobic bacteria and *Gardnerella vaginalis* normally found in the vagina and an absence of lactobacilli (see Table 47-1). It is characterized by a fish-like odour that is particularly noticeable after sexual intercourse or during menstruation as a result of a rise in the vaginal pH. It is usually accompanied by a heavier-than-normal discharge. Risk factors include douching, smoking, and increased sexual activity.

Bacterial vaginosis can occur throughout the menstrual cycle and does not produce local discomfort or pain. More than half of women with bacterial vaginosis do not notice any symptoms. Discharge, if noticed, is grey to yellowish white. The fish-like odour can be detected readily by adding a drop of potassium hydroxide to a glass slide with a sample of vaginal discharge, which releases amines. Under the microscope, vaginal cells are coated with bacteria and are described as "clue cells." The pH of the discharge is usually above 4.7 because of the amines that result from enzymes from anaerobes. Lactobacilli, a natural host defense, are usually absent. Bacterial vaginosis is usually not a serious condition, but it has been associated with premature labour, endometritis, and recurrent urinary tract infection.

Medical Management

Metronidazole (Flagyl), administered orally twice a day for 1 week, is effective; a vaginal gel is also available. Clindamycin (Cleocin) vaginal cream or ovules (oval suppositories) are also effective. If the infection recurs, the patient's partner may require treatment. Patients with recurrent bacterial vaginosis should be tested for gonorrhea and chlamydia.

TRICHOMONIASIS

Trichomonas vaginalis is a flagellated protozoan that causes a common, usually sexually transmitted vaginitis that is often called "trich." It may be transmitted by an asymptomatic carrier who harbours the organism in the urogenital tract (see Table 47-1). It may increase the risk of contracting HIV from an infected partner.

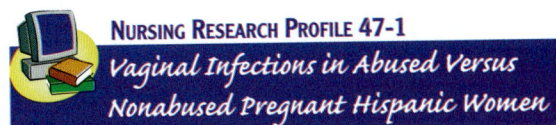

NURSING RESEARCH PROFILE 47-1
Vaginal Infections in Abused Versus Nonabused Pregnant Hispanic Women

King., E. A., Britt, R., McFarlane, J. M., & Hawkins, C. (2000). Bacterial vaginosis and *Chlamydia trachomatis* among pregnant abused and nonabused Hispanic women. *JOGNN, 29*(6), 606–612.

Purpose

The purpose of this study was to examine the prevalence of bacterial vaginosis (BV) and *Chlamydia trachomatis* (CT) in a cohort of abused and nonabused pregnant Hispanic women.

Study Sample and Design

The sample consisted of 233 pregnant, abused Hispanic women and 468 pregnant, nonabused Hispanic women from three urban prenatal clinics of a public health department in the southwestern United States. The women's status regarding abuse (abused vs. nonabused) was determined for a previous study by self-report using the Abuse Assessment Screen. Chart review was undertaken to determine the prevalence of BV and CT in both groups. Evidence of BV and CT in the women's medical records was based on standard ACOG criteria.

Findings

The combined prevalence of BV and CT in the group of abused women was significantly higher ($p < .05$) than that for nonabused women. There was no difference in prevalence of CT alone, but the prevalence of BV was significantly higher ($p < .05$) for abused women. There were no significant differences in the two groups in terms of marital status, age, gestational age, or number of prenatal visits.

Nursing Implications

Although the findings are limited to one ethnic group in an urban public clinic setting, they do suggest the need for targeted screening of all abused pregnant women for BV. Detection and treatment of women with BV may prevent premature rupture of membranes and premature delivery in this high-risk group of pregnant women.

Clinical Manifestations

Clinical manifestations include a vaginal discharge that is thin (sometimes frothy), yellow to yellow-green, malodourous, and very irritating. An accompanying vulvitis may result, with vulvovaginal burning and itching. Diagnosis is made by microscopic detection of the pear-shaped, mobile, flagellate organisms. Inspection with a speculum often reveals vaginal and cervical erythema (redness) with multiple small petechiae ("strawberry spots"). pH testing of a trichomonal discharge will demonstrate a pH greater than 4.5.

Medical Management

The most effective treatment for trichomoniasis is metronidazole (Flagyl). Both partners receive a one-time loading dose or a smaller dose three times a day for 1 week. The one-time dose is more convenient; consequently, compliance tends to be greater. The weeklong treatment has occasionally been noted to be more effective. Some patients complain of an unpleasant but transient metallic taste when taking metronidazole. Nausea and vomiting, as well as a hot, flushed feeling, occur when this medication is taken with an alcoholic beverage (disulfiram-like reaction). In view of these side effects, the patient is strongly advised to abstain from alcohol while taking the medication.

Metronidazole therapy is contraindicated in patients with some blood dyscrasias or central nervous system diseases, in the first trimester of pregnancy, and in women who are breastfeeding. It is not prescribed without examination.

Gerontologic Considerations

After menopause, the vaginal mucosa becomes thinner and may atrophy. This condition can be complicated by infection from pyogenic bacteria, resulting in atrophic vaginitis (see Table 47-1). Leukorrhea (vaginal discharge) may cause itching and burning. Management is similar to that for bacterial vaginosis if bacteria are present. Estrogenic hormones, either taken orally or inserted into the vagina in a cream form, can also be effective in restoring the epithelium.

NURSING PROCESS: THE PATIENT WITH A VULVOVAGINAL INFECTION

Assessment

The woman with vulvovaginal symptoms should be examined as soon as possible after the onset of symptoms. She is instructed not to **douche** because doing so removes the vaginal discharge needed to make the diagnosis. The area is observed for erythema, edema, excoriation, and discharge. Each of the infection-producing organisms produces its own characteristic discharge and effect (see Table 47-1). The patient is asked to describe any discharge and other symptoms, such as odour, itching, or burning. Dysuria often occurs as a result of local irritation of the urinary meatus. A urinary tract infection may need to be ruled out by obtaining a urine specimen for culture and sensitivity testing.

The patient is asked about the occurrence of factors that may contribute to vulvovaginal infection:

- Physical and chemical factors, such as constant moisture from tight or synthetic clothing, perfumes and powders, soaps, bubble bath, poor hygiene, and use of feminine hygiene products

- Psychogenic factors (eg, stress, fear of STDs, abuse)
- Medical conditions or endocrine factors, such as a predisposition to vulvar involvement in a patient who has diabetes or is elderly
- Use of medications such as antibiotics, which may alter the vaginal flora and allow an overgrowth of monilial organisms
- New sex partner, multiple sex partners, previous vaginal infection

The patient is also asked about other factors that could contribute to infection, including hygiene practices (tampons, douching), use or nonuse of condoms, and use of chemicals such as nonoxynol-9 with barrier methods of birth control.

The nurse may prepare a vaginal smear (wet mount) to assist in diagnosing the infection. A common method for preparing the smear is to collect vaginal secretions with an applicator and place the secretions on two separate glass slides. A drop of saline solution is added to one slide and a drop of 10% potassium hydroxide is added to another slide for examination under a microscope. If bacterial vaginosis is present, the slide with normal saline solution added shows epithelial cells dotted with bacteria (clue cells). If *Trichomonas* species is present, small motile cells are seen. In the presence of yeast, the potassium hydroxide slide reveals typical characteristics. Discharge associated with bacterial vaginosis produces a strong odour when mixed with potassium hydroxide. This is called a positive "whiff test." Testing the pH of the discharge with Nitrazine paper assists in proper diagnosis.

Diagnosis

NURSING DIAGNOSES

Based on the nursing assessment and other data, the patient's major nursing diagnoses may include the following:

- Discomfort related to burning, odour, or itching from the infectious process
- Anxiety related to stressful symptoms
- Risk for infection or spread of infection
- Deficient knowledge about proper hygiene and preventive measures

Planning and Goals

The major goals for the patient may include relief of discomfort, reduction of anxiety related to stress symptoms, prevention of reinfection or infection of sexual partner, and acquisition of knowledge about methods for preventing vulvovaginal infections and managing self-care.

Nursing Interventions

RELIEVING DISCOMFORT

Treatment with the appropriate medication usually relieves discomfort. Sitz baths are occasionally recommended.

REDUCING ANXIETY

Although vulvovaginal infections are upsetting and require treatment, they are not life-threatening. The patient who experiences such an infection, however, may be anxious and fearful about the significance of the symptoms and possible causes. Explaining the cause of symptoms may reduce anxiety related to fear of a more serious illness. Discussing ways to help prevent vulvovaginal infections may help the patient adopt specific strategies to decrease infection and the related symptoms.

PREVENTING REINFECTION OR SPREAD OF INFECTION

There is a risk of another episode of the same infection or spread of the infection to sexual partners. The patient needs to be informed about these risks and the importance of adequate treatment of herself and her partner, if indicated. Other strategies to prevent persistence or spread of infection include abstaining from sexual intercourse when infected, treatment of sexual partners, and minimizing irritation of the affected area. When medications such as antibiotic agents are prescribed for any infection, the nurse instructs the patient about the usual precautions related to using these agents. If vaginal itching occurs, the patient can be reassured that this is usually not an allergic reaction but may be a yeast or monilial infection resulting from altered vaginal bacteria. Treatment for monilial infection is prescribed. For women susceptible to yeast infections and who require antibiotic therapy, using antifungal cream in the vagina and applied to the vulva while on the antibiotic may prevent another yeast infection.

Another goal of treatment is to reduce tissue irritation caused by scratching or wearing tight clothing. The area needs to be kept clean by daily bathing and adequate hygiene after voiding and defecation. The use of a cool-air hairdryer after bathing, and wearing cotton underwear and loose-fitting clothes (no jeans) may be useful to keep the area dry and minimize irritation.

When teaching the patient about medications such as suppositories and devices such as applicators to dispense cream or ointment, the nurse may demonstrate the procedure by using a plastic model of the pelvis and vagina. The nurse should also stress the importance of hand washing before and after each administration of medication. To prevent the medication from escaping from the vagina, the patient should recline for 30 minutes after it is inserted, if possible. The patient is informed that seepage of medication may occur, and the use of a perineal pad may be helpful.

PROMOTING HOME AND COMMUNITY-BASED CARE

Teaching Patients Self-Care

Vulvovaginal conditions are treated on an outpatient basis, unless the patient has other medical problems. Patient teaching, tact, and reassurance are important aspects of nursing care. Women may express embarrassment, guilt, or anger and may be concerned that the infection may be serious (causing infertility) or that it may have been acquired from a sex partner. In some instances, treatment plans include the partner.

In addition to reviewing ways of relieving discomfort and preventing reinfection, the nurse assesses each patient's learning needs relative to the immediate problem. The patient needs to know the characteristics of normal as opposed to abnormal discharge. Questions often arise about douching. Normally, douching and use of feminine hygiene sprays are unnecessary because daily baths or showers and proper hygiene after voiding and defecating keep the perineal area clean. Douching tends to eliminate normal flora, reducing the body's ability to ward off infection. In addition, repeated douching may result in vaginal epithelial breakdown and chemical irritation and has been associated with other pelvic disorders.

Therapeutic douching, however, may be recommended and prescribed to reduce unpleasant, abnormal odours; to remove excessive discharge; to change the pH (eg, vinegar douches); and to serve as an antiseptic irrigating solution. The procedure is reviewed with the patient, as is the care and cleaning of equipment so that it is properly disinfected.

In the case of recurrent yeast infections, the perineum should be kept as dry as possible. Loose-fitting cotton instead of tight-fitting synthetic, nonabsorbent, heat-retaining underwear is recommended. The patient is instructed to perform a monthly inspection of the vulvar region for changes.

Evaluation

EXPECTED PATIENT OUTCOMES

Expected patient outcomes may include:

1. Experiences reduced discomfort
   a. Cleans the perineum as instructed
   b. Reports that itching is relieved
   c. Maintains urine output within normal limits and without dysuria
2. Experiences relief of anxiety
3. Remains free from infection
   a. Has no signs of inflammation, pruritus, odour, or dysuria
   b. Notes that vaginal discharge appears normal (thin, clear, not frothy)
4. Participates in self-care
   a. Takes medication as prescribed
   b. Wears absorbent underwear
   c. Avoids unprotected sexual intercourse
   d. Douches only as prescribed

HUMAN PAPILLOMAVIRUS

Human papillomavirus (HPV) infection is sexually transmitted and is the most common sexually transmitted disease (STD) among young, sexually active persons. In an Ontario study, cervical samples were collected from 995 women 15 to 49 years of age (Sellors, et al., 2000). The incidence of HPV was highest at 24% in women 20 to 24 years of age and decreased progressively in older age groups. The prevalence of HPV in Canadian women ranges from 20% to 33% (cancer and noncancer causing). There is an 11% to 25% prevalence when only the cancer-causing HPV types were examined (Public Health Agency of Canada, 2000). More than 80 strains exist, some of which are associated with cervical abnormalities, including dysplasia and cancer. Infections can be latent (asymptomatic and detected only by DNA hybridization tests for HPV), subclinical (visualized only after application of acetic acid followed by inspection under magnification), or clinical (visible condylomata acuminata). The most common strains, 6 and 11, usually cause **condylomata** (warty growths) on the vulva. These are often visible or may be palpable by the patient. Condylomata are rarely premalignant but are an outward manifestation of the virus. Strains 6 and 11 are associated with a low risk for cervical cancer. Some strains may not cause condylomata but affect the cervix, resulting in abnormal Pap smear results. For example, strains 16, 18, 31, 33, 35, and 45 affect the cervix. Their effects are usually invisible on examination but may be seen on colposcopy. They may cause cervical changes that may appear as koilocytosis on Pap smear or abnormal smear results. These strains are associated with a higher risk for cervical cancer (Public Health Agency of Canada, 2000).

The incidence of HPV in young, sexually active women is high. Risk factors include being sexually active, having multiple sex partners, and having sex with a partner who has or has had multiple partners. Alcohol consumption and drug use are risk factors, as both impair careful decision making, judgment, and self-care (Association of Reproductive Health Practitioners, 2001).

Medical Management

Treatment of external genital warts includes topical application of trichloroacetic acid, podophyllin (Podofin, Podocon), and chemotherapeutic agents. Interferon injections are also used in treatment. These agents are applied by the health care provider. Topical agents that can be applied by the patient to external lesions include podofilox (Condylox) and imiquimod (Aldara). Because the safety of podophyllin, imiquimod, and podofilox during pregnancy has not been determined, these agents should not be used to treat pregnant women. Electrocautery and laser therapy are alternative therapies that may be indicated for patients with a large number or area of genital warts (Health Canada 2004).

Treatment usually eradicates perineal warts or condylomata. However, they may resolve spontaneously without treatment and may also recur even with treatment.

If the treatment includes application of the topical agent by the patient, she needs to be carefully instructed in the use of the agent prescribed and must be able to identify the warts and be able to apply the medication to them. The patient is instructed to anticipate mild pain or local irritation with the use of these agents.

Patients with HPV should have regular Pap smears, possibly every 6 months for several years, because of the propensity of HPV to cause **dysplasia** (changes in cervical cells).

Much remains unknown about the subclinical disease and latent phase of the disease. Women are often exposed to this virus by a partner who is unknowingly a carrier. Condoms can prevent transmission, but transmission can also occur during skin-to-skin contact in areas not covered by condoms. In many cases, patients are angry about having warts or HPV and do not know who infected them because the incubation period can be long and partners may have no symptoms. Acknowledging the emotional distress that occurs when an STD is diagnosed and providing support and facts are important nursing actions.

HERPESVIRUS TYPE 2 INFECTION (HERPES GENITALIS, HERPES SIMPLEX VIRUS)

Herpes genitalis is a recurrent, life-long viral infection that causes herpetic lesions (blisters) on the cervix, vagina, and external genitalia. It is an STD but may also be transmitted asexually from wet surfaces or by self-transmission (ie, touching a cold sore and then touching the genital area). The initial infection is usually very painful and lasts about 1 week, but it can also be asymptomatic. Recurrences are less painful and usually produce minor itching and burning. Some patients have few or no recurrences, whereas others have frequent bouts. Recurrences are often associated with stress, sunburn, dental work, or inadequate rest or nutrition. The incidence of herpes infection is increasing. The prevalence of other STDs has decreased slightly, possibly due to increased condom use, but herpes can be transmitted by contact with skin not covered by a condom. Transmission is possible even when the carrier does not have symptoms (subclinical shedding). Lesions increase vulnerability to HIV infection and other STDs. Vaccines for this virus are in clinical trials.

Pathophysiology

Of the known herpesviruses, six affect humans: (1) herpes simplex type 1 (HSV-1), which usually causes cold sores of the lips; (2) herpes simplex type 2 (HSV-2), or genital herpes; (3) varicella zoster, or shingles; (4) Epstein-Barr virus; (5) cytomegalovirus; and (6) human B-lymphotrophic virus. HSV-2 appears to be the

cause of about 80% of genital and perineal lesions; HSV-1 may cause about 20%.

There is considerable overlap between HSV-1 and HSV-2, which are clinically indistinguishable. Close human contact by the mouth, oropharynx, mucosal surface, vagina, or cervix appears necessary to acquire the infection. Other susceptible sites are skin lacerations and conjunctivae. Usually, the virus is killed at room temperature by drying. When viral replication diminishes, the virus ascends the peripheral sensory nerves and remains inactive in the nerve ganglia. Another outbreak may occur when the host is subjected to stress. In pregnant women with active herpes, babies delivered vaginally may become infected with the virus. There is a risk for fetal morbidity and mortality if this occurs; therefore, a cesarean delivery may be performed if the virus recurs near the time of delivery.

Clinical Manifestations

Itching and pain accompany the process as the infected area becomes red and swollen (edematous). The vesicular state often appears as a blister, which later coalesces, ulcerates, and encrusts. In women, the labia are the usual primary site, although the cervix, vagina, and perianal skin may be affected. In men, the glans penis, foreskin, or penile shaft is typically affected. Influenza-like symptoms may occur 3 or 4 days after the lesions appear. Inguinal lymphadenopathy (swollen lymph nodes in the groin), minor temperature elevation, malaise, headache, myalgia (aching muscles), and dysuria (pain on urination) are often noted. Pain is evident during the first week and then decreases. The lesions subside in about 2 weeks unless secondary infection occurs.

Rarely, complications may arise from extragenital spread, such as to the buttocks, upper thighs, or even the eyes as a result of touching lesions and then touching other areas. Patients should be advised to wash their hands after contact with lesions. Other potential problems are aseptic meningitis and severe emotional stress related to the diagnosis.

Medical Management

There is currently no cure for HSV-2 infection, but treatment is aimed at relieving the symptoms. Management goals are preventing the spread of infection, making the patient comfortable, decreasing potential health risks, and initiating a counselling and education program. Acyclovir (Zovirax), valacyclovir (Valtrex), and famciclovir (Famvir) are antiviral agents that can suppress symptoms and shorten the course of the infection. Other antiviral agents are also available. All of them are effective at reducing the duration of lesions and preventing recurrences. Resistance and long-term side effects do not appear to be major problems. Recurrent episodes are much milder than the initial episode.

NURSING PROCESS: THE PATIENT WITH A GENITAL HERPESVIRUS INFECTION

Assessment

The health history and a physical and pelvic examination are important in establishing the nature of the infectious condition. Additionally, the patient is assessed for risk for STDs. The perineum is inspected for painful lesions. Inguinal nodes are assessed because they often are enlarged and tender during an occurrence of HSV.

Diagnosis

NURSING DIAGNOSES
Based on the assessment data, the patient's major nursing diagnoses may include the following:

- Acute pain related to the genital lesions
- Risk for infection or spread of infection
- Anxiety related to the diagnosis
- Deficient knowledge about the disease and its management

Planning and Goals
The major goals for the patient may include relief of pain and discomfort, control of infection and its spread, relief of anxiety, knowledge of and adherence to the treatment regimen and self-care, and knowledge about implications for the future.

Nursing Interventions

RELIEVING PAIN
The lesions should be kept clean, and proper hygiene practices are advocated. Sitz baths ease discomfort. Clothing should be clean, loose, soft, and absorbent. Aspirin and other analgesics are usually effective in controlling pain. Occlusive ointments and powders are avoided because they prevent the lesions from drying.

If there is considerable pain and malaise, bed rest may be required. The patient is encouraged to increase fluid intake, to be alert for possible bladder distention, and to contact her primary health care provider immediately if she cannot void because of discomfort. Painful voiding may occur if urine comes in contact with the herpes lesions. Discomfort with urination can be reduced by pouring warm water over the vulva during voiding or by sitz baths. When oral acyclovir or other antiviral agents are prescribed, the patient is instructed about when to take the medication and what side effects to note, such as rash and headache. Rest, fluids, and a nutritious diet are recommended to promote recovery.

PREVENTING INFECTION AND ITS SPREAD
The risk of reinfection and spread of infection to others or to other structures of the body can be reduced by hand washing, use of barrier methods with sexual contact, and adherence to prescribed medication regimens. Avoidance of contact when obvious lesions are present does not eliminate the risk because the virus can be shed in the absence of symptoms, and lesions may not be visible to the woman. Avoiding stress, sunburn, and other stress-producing situations may decrease the episodes of recurrence.

RELIEVING ANXIETY
Concern about the presence of herpes infection, future occurrences of lesions, and the impact of the infection on future relationships and childbearing may cause considerable anxiety in the patient. The nurse can be an important support, listening to the patient's concerns and providing information and instruction. The patient may be angry with her partner if her partner is the probable source of the infection. She may need assistance and support in discussing the infection and its implications with her current sexual partner and in future sexual relationships. The

nurse can refer the patient to a support group to assist in coping with the diagnosis (see Resources at the end of the chapter).

INCREASING KNOWLEDGE ABOUT THE DISEASE AND ITS TREATMENT
Patient teaching is an essential part of nursing care of the patient with a genital herpes infection. This includes an adequate explanation about the infection and how it is transmitted, management and treatment strategies, strategies to minimize spread of infection, the importance of adherence to the treatment regimen, and self-care strategies. Because of the increased risk of HIV and other STDs in the presence of skin lesions, an important part of patient education involves instructing the patient to protect herself from exposure to HIV and other STDs. Further details are included in Chart 47-2.

PROMOTING HOME AND COMMUNITY-BASED CARE

Teaching Patients Self-Care
Genital herpes causes physical pain and emotional distress. Usually, the patient is upset on learning the diagnosis. Therefore, when counselling the patient, the nurse should explain the causes of the condition and the manner in which it can be managed. Questions are encouraged because they may indicate that the patient is receptive to learning.

The nurse can provide reassurance that the lesions will heal and that recurrences can be minimized by adopting a healthful lifestyle and by taking prescribed medications. Self-care measures for the person with genital herpes appear in Chart 47-2.

Evaluation

EXPECTED PATIENT OUTCOMES
Expected patient outcomes may include:

1. Experiences a reduction in pain and discomfort
2. Keeps infection under control
   a. Demonstrates proper hygiene techniques
   b. Takes medication as prescribed
   c. Consumes adequate fluids
   d. Adopts healthy lifestyle (diet, adequate fluid intake, safer sex practices, stress management)
3. Uses strategies to reduce anxiety
   a. Verbalizes issues and concerns related to genital herpes infection
   b. Discusses strategies to deal with issues and concerns with current and future sexual partner
   c. Initiates contact with support group if indicated
4. Demonstrates knowledge about genital herpes and strategies to control and minimize recurrences
   a. Identifies methods of transmission of herpes infection and strategies to prevent transmission to others
   b. Discusses strategies to reduce recurrence of lesions
   c. Takes medications as prescribed
   d. Reports no recurrence of lesions

TOXIC SHOCK SYNDROME

Toxic shock syndrome (TSS) is a life-threatening, multisystem disease caused by response to the toxins produced by strains of the bacterium *S. aureus* in susceptible patients. This rare condition is associated with menstruation (although the incidence of menstrual TSS has dramatically decreased due to public awareness, the number of nonmenstrual cases of TSS has not declined).

Approximately 1% of women carry strains of staphylococcus capable of producing the responsible toxin. Nonmenstrual TSS occurs after childbirth, after abortion, and in persons with bone and skin infections, postoperative infections, burns, mastitis, and varicella-related cellulitis. Sinusitis, tracheitis, pneumonia, and the presence of foreign bodies (eg, nasal packing, IUDs, contraceptive sponges) have been associated with nonmenstrual TSS.

Clinical Manifestations

In an otherwise healthy person, the onset of TSS occurs with a sudden fever (temperature is always at least 38.9° C), chills, malaise, and muscle pain. Vomiting, diarrhea, hypotension, headache, and signs suggesting early septic shock may develop. A red, macular rash similar to sunburn (diffuse, macular erythroderma) is a classic sign of TSS. In some patients, this rash appears first on the torso; in others, it is first seen on the hands (palms and fingers) and feet (soles and toes). Inflammation of mucous membranes also may occur. In 7 to 10 days, it desquamates (becomes scaly or peels). Myalgia and dizziness are common. Severe cases can result in acute respiratory distress syndrome (ARDS), and cardiac dysfunction may occur.

Assessment and Diagnostic Findings

Urine output decreases, and the blood urea nitrogen level increases, often resulting in disorientation. Laboratory tests also reveal leukocytosis and elevated bilirubin. Uncontrollable hypotension and disseminated intravascular coagulopathy (DIC) may also occur. The clinical picture of septic shock (described in Chap. 15) results. Respiratory distress may develop as a result of pulmonary edema. If ARDS occurs, the outlook is grave. About 2% to 3% of patients with TSS die of complications.

Medical Management

Treatment includes elimination of the source of the infection; administration of fluids, vasopressors, and antibiotic agents; and irrigation of the presumed site of infection. The patient is placed on bed rest, and the treatment plan is directed primarily at controlling the infection and restoring circulating blood volume.

Antibiotic therapy is based on the results of blood, urine, and other cultures. Antistaphylococcal agents are prescribed. Antibiotic therapy has not been found to affect the course of TSS but to prevent recurrence.

In cases of respiratory distress, oxygen therapy is instituted; if signs of acidosis appear, sodium bicarbonate is administered. Calcium is prescribed for hypocalcemia. A Swan-Ganz catheter (for hemodynamic monitoring) and intravenous dopamine may be used to manage shock. The entire treatment plan, including strategies directed toward emotional and psychological concerns, is adjusted according to each patient's condition, which may vary from mild to acute.

Nursing Management

The patient with suspected TSS is assessed for factors known to be associated with it: use of tampons (high absorbency, length of time a tampon was retained before changing it, trauma that may have occurred with its insertion) or diaphragms and the presence of other risk factors. Additionally, the patient is assessed and treated for complications associated with TSS (DIC and septic shock). The patient is observed for hematomas, petechiae, oozing from needle and infusion sites, cyanosis, and coolness of the nose, fingertips, and toes. The patient is further observed for skin changes and fluid intake and loss; these data assist in evaluating hydration and kidney function. The patient with TSS is usually critically ill and is cared for in the intensive care unit to facilitate constant monitoring and assessment for the onset of complications and response to treatment. Because of the likelihood of severe septic shock, the patient is monitored closely for changes in vital signs, level of consciousness and responsiveness to stimuli, and laboratory values, including arterial blood gases. The patient's response to prescribed medications and fluids is also evaluated. See Chapter 15 for more information about management of shock.

Teaching Patients Self-Care. Because of the lengthy period that is required for recovery from TSS, the patient must be prepared to increase participation in self-care activities gradually. The patient and caregiver need instructions about detection and prevention of the complications associated with immobility. The nurse also explains the possible causes of TSS and steps to take to prevent its recurrence. Because use of tampons during menstruation has been linked with TSS, women who have had TSS should not use tampons. If a diaphragm is used, it should not be left in place longer than 8 to 10 hours. Using the diaphragm or cervical cap during menses or in the first 3 months postpartum is also discouraged. The risk of developing TSS increases any time a woman bleeds vaginally (ie, during menses and postpartum). Because of the risk of TSS, all women who use tampons should be informed that they must be changed frequently (every 4 hours) and inserted carefully to avoid abrasions (applicators with rough edges should be avoided). Use of superabsorbent tampons is not recommended.

ENDOCERVICITIS AND CERVICITIS

Endocervicitis is an inflammation of the mucosa and the glands of the cervix that may occur when organisms gain access to the cervical glands after intercourse and, less often, after procedures such as abortion, intrauterine manipulation, or vaginal delivery. If untreated, the infection may extend into the uterus, fallopian tubes, and pelvic cavity. Inflammation can irritate the cervical tissue, resulting in spotting or bleeding and **mucopurulent cervicitis**.

CHLAMYDIA AND GONORRHEA

Chlamydia and gonorrhea are the most common causes of endocervicitis, although Mycoplasma may also be involved. In 2000, women accounted for more than two thirds of the 46,000 reported chlamydia cases in Canada (Public Health Agency of Canada, 2003); it is most commonly found in young, sexually active people with more than one partner and is transmitted through sexual intercourse. It can result in serious complications, including pelvic infection, an increased risk for ectopic pregnancy, and infertility. Fifteen percent of infertility is caused by pelvic inflammatory disease (PID; Wong, Singh, Mann, et al., 2004). Chlamydial infections of the cervix often produce no symptoms, but cervical discharge, dyspareunia, dysuria, and bleeding may occur. Other complications include conjunctivitis and perihepatitis. If a pregnant woman is infected, stillbirth, neonatal death, and premature labour may occur. Infants born to infected mothers may experience prematurity, conjunctivitis, and pneumonia.

Chlamydial infection and gonorrhea often coexist. As many as 25% of females who have chlamydial infections also have gonorrhea. The inflamed cervix that results from this infection may leave a woman more vulnerable to HIV transmission from an infected partner. Gonorrhea is also a major cause of PID, tubal infertility, ectopic pregnancy, and chronic pelvic pain. Fifty percent of women with gonorrhea have no symptoms, but without treatment 40% may develop PID. In males, urethritis and epididymitis may occur. Diagnosis can be confirmed by culture, smear, or other methods, using a swab to obtain a sample of cervical discharge or penile discharge from the patient's partner.

Medical Management

The Centers for Disease Control and Prevention (CDC) recommends treating chlamydia with doxycycline for 1 week or with a single dose of azithromycin. Because of the high incidence of coinfection with chlamydia and gonorrhea, treatment for gonorrhea should include treatment for chlamydia as well (CDC, 2002). Partners must also be treated. Pregnant women are cautioned not to take tetracycline because of potential adverse effects on the fetus. In these cases, erythromycin may be prescribed. Results are usually good if treatment begins early. Possible complications from delayed treatment are tubal disease, ectopic pregnancy, PID, and infertility.

Cultures for chlamydia and other STDs should be obtained from all patients who have been sexually assaulted when they first seek medical attention; patients are treated prophylactically. Cultures should then be repeated in 2 weeks. Annual screening for chlamydia is recommended for all sexually active women 20 to 25 years of age and older women with new sex partners or multiple partners (CDC, 2002).

Nursing Management

All sexually active women may be at risk for chlamydia, gonorrhea, and other STDs, including HIV. Nurses can assist patients in assessing their own risk. Recognition of risk is a first step before changes in behaviour occur. Patients should be discouraged from assuming that a partner is "safe" without open, honest discussion. Nonjudgmental attitudes, educational counselling, and role playing may all be helpful.

Because chlamydia, gonorrhea, and other STDs may have a serious effect on future health and fertility and because many STDs can be prevented by the use of condoms and spermicides and careful choice of partners, the nurse can play a major role in talking with patients about how to make sex as safe as possible. Exploring options with patients, determining their use of safer sex practices and their knowledge deficits, and correcting misinformation may prevent morbidity and mortality.

PROMOTING HOME AND COMMUNITY-BASED CARE

Teaching Patients Self-Care. Nurses can educate women and help them to develop communication skills and to initiate discussions about sex with their partners. Communicating with partners about sex, risk, postponing intercourse, and using safer sex behaviours, including use of condoms, may be lifesaving. Some young women report having sex with someone but not being comfortable enough to discuss sexual risk issues. The nurse can pose the question, "If you are uncomfortable talking about sex with this person, how do you feel about having a sexual relationship with this person?"

Reinforcing the need for annual screening for chlamydia and other STDs is an important part of patient teaching. Instructions also include the need for the patient to abstain from sexual intercourse until all of her sex partners are treated (CDC, 2002). The CDC has revised its guidelines and recommends rescreening of all women with chlamydial infections 3 to 4 months after treatment is completed; this is in an effort to protect young women from infertility.

PELVIC INFECTION (PELVIC INFLAMMATORY DISEASE)

Pelvic inflammatory disease (PID) is an inflammatory condition of the pelvic cavity that may begin with cervicitis and may involve the uterus (endometritis), fallopian tubes (**salpingitis**), ovaries (oophoritis), pelvic peritoneum, or pelvic vascular system. Infection, which may be acute, subacute, recurrent, or chronic and localized or widespread, is usually caused by bacteria but may be attributed to a virus, fungus, or parasite. Gonorrheal and chlamydial organisms are the most likely causes (Ronald & Peeling, 1993). Cytomegalovirus (CMV) has also been implicated. This condition can result in the fallopian tubes becoming narrowed and scarred, which increases the risk for ectopic pregnancy (fertilized eggs become trapped in the tube), infertility, recurrent pelvic pain, tuboovarian **abscess**, and recurrent disease. Rupture of a tubo-ovarian abscess has a 5% to 10% mortality rate and usually necessitates a complete hysterectomy. About 10% of Canadian women have at least one episode of PID in their lifetime (Ronald & Peeling, 1993). Of concern is the fact that 15% of women are infertile after only one episode of PID and 30% are infertile after two episodes. Since reporting of PID is not required in Canada, all data come from hospital discharge data (Public Health Agency of Canada, 1998), thus missing those cases that were less severe or were asymptomatic (Ross, 2001). Across Canada, hospital discharges for PID decreased by 55.5% over a 10-year period. Using 1994-95 hospital discharge results (Canadian Institute for Health Information & Statistics Canada, 1999), women 25 to 34 years of age had the highest rate of PID (125.5 cases per 100,000 females). The second highest age group was 20 to 24 years at 120.7 per 100.000. Young women aged 15 to 19 showed a 60.7% drop in 10 years and had a rate of 98.2 per 100,000. The age group 35 to 44 had the lowest rate of 96.6 per 100,000 women. The sequelae of PID includes infertility, ectopic pregnancy, or chronic pelvic pain (Rein, Kasler, Irwin, & Rabiee, 2000).

Pathophysiology

The exact pathogenesis of PID has not been determined, but it is presumed that organisms usually enter the body through the vagina, pass through the cervical canal, colonize the endocervix, and move upward into the uterus. Under various conditions, the organisms may proceed to one or both fallopian tubes and ovaries and into the pelvis. In bacterial infections that occur after childbirth or abortion, pathogens are disseminated directly through the tissues that support the uterus by way of the lymphatics and blood vessels (Fig. 47-1). In pregnancy, the increased blood supply required by the placenta provides more pathways for infection. These postpartum and postabortion infections tend to be unilateral. Infections can cause perihepatic inflammation when the organism invades the peritoneum.

In gonorrheal infections, the gonococci pass through the cervical canal and into the uterus, where the environment, especially during menstruation, allows them to multiply rapidly and spread to the fallopian tubes and into the pelvis (see Fig. 47-1). The infection is usually bilateral. In rare instances, organisms (eg, tuberculosis) gain access to the reproductive organs by way of the bloodstream from the lungs (see Fig. 47-1). One of the most common causes of salpingitis (inflammation of the fallopian tube) is chlamydia, possibly accompanied by gonorrhea.

Pelvic infection is most commonly caused by sexual transmission but can also occur with invasive procedures such as endometrial biopsy, surgical abortion, hysteroscopy, or IUD insertion. Bacterial vaginosis, a vaginal infection, may predispose women to pelvic infection. Risk factors include early age at first intercourse, multiple sexual partners, frequent intercourse, intercourse without condoms, sex with a partner with an STD, and a history of STDs or previous pelvic infection.

Clinical Manifestations

Symptoms of pelvic infection usually begin with vaginal discharge, dyspareunia, lower abdominal pelvic pain, and tenderness that occurs after menses. Pain may increase while voiding or with defecation. Other symptoms include fever, general malaise, anorexia, nausea, headache, and possibly vomiting. On pelvic examination, intense tenderness may be noted on palpation of the uterus or movement of the cervix (cervical motion tenderness). Symptoms may be acute and severe or low-grade and subtle.

Complications

Pelvic or generalized peritonitis, abscesses, strictures, and fallopian tube obstruction may develop. Obstruction may cause an ectopic pregnancy in the future if a fertilized egg cannot pass a tubal stricture, or scar tissue may occlude the tubes, resulting in sterility. Adhesions are common and often result in chronic pelvic pain; they eventually may require removal of the uterus, fallopian tubes, and ovaries. Other complications include bacteremia with septic shock and thrombophlebitis with possible embolization.

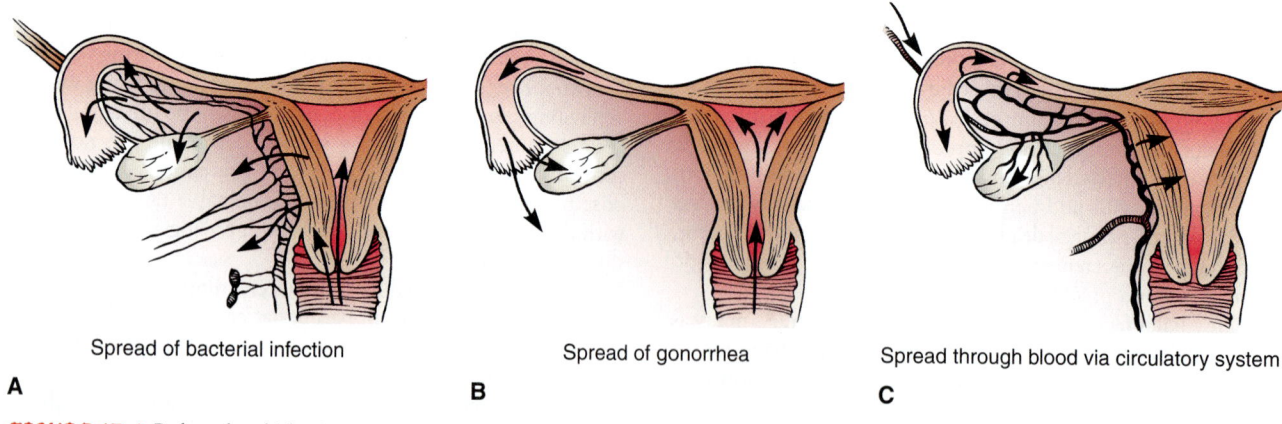

Spread of bacterial infection

Spread of gonorrhea

Spread through blood via circulatory system

A **B** **C**

FIGURE 47-1 Pathway by which microorganisms spread in pelvic infections. (**A**) Bacterial infection spreads up the vagina into the uterus and through the lymphatics. (**B**) Gonorrhea spreads up the vagina into the uterus and then to the tubes and ovaries. (**C**) Bacterial infection can reach the reproductive organs through the bloodstream (hematogenous spread).

Medical Management

Broad-spectrum antibiotic therapy is prescribed. Women with mild infections may be treated as outpatients (Ness, Soper, Holley et al., 2002*c*), but hospitalization may be necessary. Intensive therapy includes bed rest, intravenous fluids, and intravenous antibiotic therapy. If the patient has abdominal distention or ileus, nasogastric intubation and suction are initiated. Carefully monitoring vital signs and symptoms assists in evaluating the status of the infection. Treating sexual partners is necessary to prevent reinfection.

Nursing Management

Infection takes a toll, both physically and emotionally. The patient may feel well one day and experience vague symptoms and discomfort the next. She may also suffer from constipation and menstrual difficulties.

The hospitalized patient is maintained on bed rest and is usually placed in the semi-Fowler's position to facilitate dependent drainage. Accurate recording of vital signs and the characteristics and amount of vaginal discharge is necessary as a guide to therapy.

The nurse administers analgesic agents as prescribed for pain relief. Heat applied safely to the abdomen may also provide some pain relief and comfort.

The nurse minimizes the transmission of infection to others by carefully handling perineal pads with gloves, discarding the soiled pad according to hospital guidelines for disposal of biohazardous material, and performing meticulous hand hygiene.

PROMOTING HOME AND COMMUNITY-BASED CARE

Teaching Patients Self-Care. The patient must be informed of the need for precautions and must be encouraged to take part in procedures to prevent infecting others and protecting herself from reinfection. If a partner is not well known or has had other sexual partners recently, use of condoms may prevent life-threatening infection and its sequelae. If reinfection occurs or if the infection spreads, symptoms may include abdominal pain, nausea and vomiting, fever, malaise, malodourous purulent vaginal discharge, and leukocytosis. Patient teaching consists of explaining how pelvic infections occur, how they can be controlled and avoided, and their signs and symptoms. Guidelines and instructions provided to the patient are summarized in the accompanying Home Care Checklist (Chart 47-3).

All patients who have had PID need to be informed of the signs and symptoms of ectopic pregnancy (pain, abnormal bleed-ing, delayed menses, faintness, dizziness, and shoulder pain) because they are prone to this complication. (See Chap. 46 for a discussion of ectopic pregnancy.)

HUMAN IMMUNODEFICIENCY VIRUS INFECTION AND ACQUIRED IMMUNODEFICIENCY SYNDROME

Any discussion of vulvovaginal infections must include the topic of HIV and **acquired immunodeficiency syndrome (AIDS)**, described in Chapter 52.

The incidence of HIV infection and AIDS is increasing in women. Females represent the fastest-growing segment of the AIDS epidemic. More than half are intravenous (or injecting) drug users, whereas the other half have been exposed through sexual contact with HIV-infected partners. Women who exchange sex for drugs are at high risk, as are women who engage in anal intercourse. Heterosexual transmission is the leading cause of new HIV infection in women. Women are nine times more likely to get HIV from men than men are from women. Factors that may account for this difference include a higher quantity of HIV in semen as compared with vaginal secretions, a larger inoculum on ejaculation, retention of HIV-infected semen in the vagina, and traumatic microscopic mucosal injury during intercourse. The presence of genital ulcers or a friable cervix increases risk. Intercourse during menses may also increase risk. Additionally, any break in skin integrity increases the possibility of infection (eg, a herpetic lesion or syphilitic **chancre** could provide a portal of entry). Nurses need to inform women about the dangers of unprotected sex (Hader, Smith, Moore & Holmberg, 2001; *Healthy People 2010, 2000*).

Syphilis appears to accelerate in HIV-positive patients and proceeds directly from primary to tertiary disease in some patients. Chlamydia is associated with a high risk for HIV (which may be related to inflammatory changes of the cervix, providing entry sites). HIV-positive women have a higher rate of HPV, and this risk increases as their CD4 cell count decreases. Infections with HPV and HIV together increase the risk of malignant transformation and cervical cancer. This risk also increases as the CD4 cell count decreases. Thus, women with HIV infection should have frequent Pap smears. HIV-positive women also have larger and more painful herpes lesions with more recurrences, probably related to immunosuppression from their disease. Treatment with acyclovir or other antiviral agents is appropriate for such patients. Pneumonitis, esophagitis, and disseminated skin involvement are common in this population. Candidiasis also occurs frequently in this population; oral candidiasis

---

Chart 47-3
Home Care Checklist • The Patient With Pelvic Inflammatory Disease

At the completion of the home care instruction, the patient or caregiver will be able to:	Patient	Caregiver
• State that any pelvic pain and/or abnormal discharge, particularly after sexual exposure, childbirth, or pelvic surgery, should be evaluated as soon as possible.	✓	✓
• State that antibiotics may be prescribed after insertion of intrauterine devices (IUDs).	✓	✓
• Describe proper perineal care procedures (wiping from front to back after defecation or urination).	✓	✓
• State that douching reduces the natural flora that combat infecting organisms and may introduce bacteria upward.	✓	✓
• Identify the importance of consulting a health care provider if unusual vaginal discharge or odour is noted.	✓	✓
• Discuss the importance of following health practices (ie, proper nutrition, exercise, and weight control), and safer sex practices (ie, using condoms, avoiding multiple sexual partners).	✓	✓
• Explain the importance of consistent use of condoms before intercourse or any penile–vaginal contact if there is any chance of transmitting infection.	✓	✓
• State that a gynecologic examination should be performed at least once a year.	✓	✓

may signal rapidly advancing disease. Many HIV-infected women have gynecologic disorders, including candidiasis, PID, anogenital warts, and cervical dysplasia (*Healthy People 2010*, 2000).

Women with HIV and women with partners who have HIV must be counselled about safer sex. Consistent use of condoms with an HIV-infected partner can keep seroconversion rates to about 1%, but inconsistent use results in an annual 7.2% seroconversion rate. Because there is a 25% to 30% chance of perinatal transmission, decisions to conceive or to use contraception must be based on teaching and care. (The use of antiretroviral agents by pregnant women has been shown to decrease perinatal transmission of HIV infection significantly. Therefore, the use of these agents during pregnancy must also be discussed.) For those who choose to avoid conception, condoms or condoms with oral contraceptives are possible choices.

Women who are at risk for HIV should be offered testing after informed consent by a trained nurse or counsellor. Because patients may be reluctant to discuss risk-taking behaviour, routine screening should be offered to all women. Early detection permits early treatment to delay progression of the disease. The nurse plays a crucial role in educating patients about HIV and prevention of HIV infection and AIDS.

Structural Disorders

FISTULAS OF THE VAGINA

A **fistula** is an abnormal, tortuous opening between two internal hollow organs or between an internal hollow organ and the exterior of the body. The name of the fistula indicates the two areas that are connected abnormally: a vesicovaginal fistula is an opening between the bladder and the vagina, and a rectovaginal fistula is an opening between the rectum and the vagina (Fig. 47-2). Fistulas may be congenital in origin. In adults, however, breakdown usually occurs because of tissue damage resulting from injury sustained during surgery, vaginal delivery, radiation therapy, or disease processes such as carcinoma.

Clinical Manifestations

Symptoms depend on the specific defect. For example, in the patient with a vesicovaginal fistula, urine escapes continuously into the vagina. With a rectovaginal fistula, there is fecal incontinence,

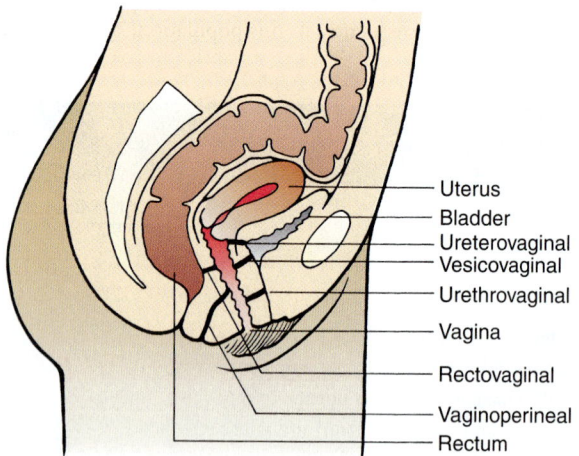

FIGURE 47-2 Common sites for vaginal fistulas: *Vesicovaginal*—bladder and vagina. *Urethrovaginal*—urethra and vagina. *Vaginoperineal*—vagina and perineal area. *Ureterovaginal*—ureter and vagina. *Rectovaginal*—rectum and vagina.

and flatus is discharged through the vagina. The combination of fecal discharge with leukorrhea results in malodour that is difficult to control.

Assessment and Diagnostic Findings

A history of the symptoms experienced by the patient is important to identify the structural alterations and to assess the impact of the symptoms on the patient's quality of life. In addition, the use of methylene blue dye helps delineate the course of the fistula. In vesicovaginal fistula, the dye is instilled into the bladder and appears in the vagina. After a negative methylene blue test result, indigo carmine is injected intravenously; the appearance of the dye in the vagina indicates a ureterovaginal fistula. Cystoscopy or intravenous pyelography may then be used to determine the exact location.

Medical Management

The goal is to eliminate the fistula and to treat infection and excoriation. A fistula may heal without surgical intervention, but surgery is often required. If the primary care provider determines that a fistula will heal without surgical intervention, care is planned to relieve discomfort, prevent infection, and improve the patient's self-concept and self-care abilities. Measures to effect healing include proper nutrition, cleansing douches and enemas, rest, and administration of prescribed intestinal antibiotic agents. A rectovaginal fistula heals faster when the patient eats a low-residue diet and when the affected tissue drains properly. Warm perineal irrigations and controlled heat-lamp treatments promote healing.

Sometimes a fistula does not heal on its own and cannot be surgically repaired. In this situation care must be planned and implemented on an individual basis. Cleanliness, frequent sitz baths, and deodourizing douches are required, as are perineal pads and protective undergarments. Meticulous skin care is necessary to prevent excoriation. Applying specifically designed skin care products may be soothing. Additionally, attending to the patient's social and psychological needs is an essential aspect of care.

If the patient will have a fistula repaired surgically, preoperative treatment of any existing vaginitis is important to ensure success. Usually, the vaginal approach is used to repair vesicovaginal and urethrovaginal fistulas; the abdominal approach is used to repair fistulas that are large or complex. Fistulas that are difficult to repair or that are very large may require surgical repair with a urinary or fecal diversion.

Because fistulas usually are related to obstetric, surgical, or radiation trauma, occurrence in a patient without previous vaginal delivery or a history of surgery must be evaluated carefully. Crohn's disease or lymphogranuloma venereum may be the cause.

Despite the best surgical intervention, fistulas may recur. After surgery, medical follow-up continues for at least 2 years to monitor for a possible recurrence.

PELVIC ORGAN PROLAPSE: CYSTOCELE, RECTOCELE, ENTEROCELE

Time and gravity can put strain on the ligaments and structures that make up the female pelvis. Childbirth can result in tears of the levator sling musculature, resulting in structural weakness. Hormone deficiency also may play a role.

Cystocele is a downward displacement of the bladder toward the vaginal orifice (Fig. 47-3) resulting from damage to the anterior vaginal support structures. It usually results from injury and strain during childbirth. The condition usually appears some years later

FIGURE 47-3 Diagrammatic representation of the three most common types of pelvic floor relaxation: **(A)** cystocele, **(B)** rectocele, and **(C)** enterocele. *Arrows* depict sites of maximum protrusion.

when genital atrophy associated with aging occurs, but younger, multiparous, premenopausal women may also be affected.

Rectocele and perineal lacerations may affect the muscles and tissues of the pelvic floor and may occur during childbirth. Because of muscle tears below the vagina, the rectum may pouch upward, thereby pushing the posterior wall of the vagina forward. This structural abnormality is called a **rectocele**. Sometimes the lacerations may completely sever the fibres of the anal sphincter (complete tear). An enterocele is a protrusion of the intestinal wall into the vagina. Prolapse (if complete prolapse occurs, it may also be referred to as procidentia) results from a weakening of the support structures of the uterus itself; the cervix drops and may protrude from the vagina.

Clinical Manifestations

Because a cystocele causes the anterior vaginal wall to bulge downward, the patient may report a sense of pelvic pressure, fatigue, and urinary problems such as incontinence, frequency, and urgency. Back pain and pelvic pain may occur as well. The symptoms of rectocele resemble those of cystocele, with one exception: instead of urinary symptoms, the patient may experience rectal pressure. Constipation, uncontrollable gas, and fecal incontinence may occur in patients with complete tears. Prolapse can result in feelings of pressure and ulcerations and bleeding. Dyspareunia may occur with these disorders.

Medical Management

Kegel exercises, which involve contracting or tightening the vaginal muscles, are prescribed to help strengthen these weakened muscles. The exercises are more effective in the early stages of a cystocele. Kegel exercises are easy to do and are recommended for all women, including those with strong pelvic floor muscles (Chart 47-4).

Pessaries can be used to avoid surgery. This device is inserted into the vagina and positioned to keep an organ, such as the bladder, uterus, or intestine, properly aligned when a cystocele, rectocele, or prolapse has occurred. Pessaries are usually ring-shaped or doughnut-shaped and are made of various materials, such as rubber or plastic (Fig. 47-4). Rubber pessaries must be avoided in women with latex allergy. The size and type of pessary are selected and fitted by a gynecologic health care provider. The patient should have the pessary removed, examined, and cleaned by her health care provider at prescribed intervals. At this checkup, vaginal walls are examined for pressure points or signs of irritation. Normally, the patient experi-

ences no pain, discomfort, or discharge with a pessary, but if chronic irritation occurs, alternative measures may be needed.

SURGICAL MANAGEMENT

In many cases, surgery helps to correct structural abnormalities. The procedure to repair the anterior vaginal wall is called anterior **colporrhaphy**, repair of a rectocele is called a posterior colporrhaphy, and repair of perineal lacerations is called a **perineorrhaphy**. These repairs are frequently performed laparoscopically, resulting in short hospital stays and good outcomes. A **laparoscope** is inserted through a small abdominal incision, the pelvis is visualized, and surgical repairs are performed.

UTERINE PROLAPSE

Usually, the uterus and the cervix lie at right angles to the long axis of the vagina and with the body of the uterus inclined slightly forward. The uterus is normally freely movable upon examination. Individual variations may result in an anterior, middle, or posterior uterine position. A backward positioning of the uterus, known as retroversion and retroflexion, is not uncommon (Fig. 47-5).

Chart 47-4 • PATIENT EDUCATION
Performing Kegel (Pelvic Muscle) Exercises

Purposes: To strengthen and maintain the tone of the pubococcygeal muscle, which supports the pelvic organs; reduce or prevent stress incontinence and uterine prolapse; enhance sensation during sexual intercourse; and hasten postpartum healing

1. Become aware of pelvic muscle function by "drawing in" the perivaginal muscles and anal sphincter as if to control urine or defecation, but not contracting the abdominal, buttock, or inner thigh muscles.
2. Sustain contraction of the muscles for up to 10 seconds, followed by at least 10 seconds of relaxation. Another variation is to include several sets of rapid contraction and relaxation each day.
3. Perform these exercises 30–80 times a day in supine, sitting, and standing positions.
4. Since these exercises can be done inconspicuously, perform them with other daily activities (eg, brushing teeth, in a car or bus, talking on the telephone, standing in line) as well as before rising from bed and after retiring at night.

Training and exercise should be individualized for each patient.

FIGURE 47-4 Examples of pessaries. (**A**) Various shapes and sizes of pessaries available. (**B**) Insertion of one type of pessary.

FIGURE 47-5 Positions of the uterus. (**A**) The most common position of the uterus detected on palpation. (**B**) In *retroversion* the uterus turns posteriorly as a whole unit. (**C**) In *retroflexion* the fundus bends posteriorly. (**D**) In *anteversion* the uterus tilts forward as a whole unit. (**E**) In *anteflexion* the uterus bends anteriorly.

If the structures that support the uterus weaken (typically from childbirth), the uterus may work its way down the vaginal canal (prolapse) and even appear outside the vaginal orifice (procidentia) (Fig. 47-6). As the uterus descends, it may pull the vaginal walls and even the bladder and rectum with it. Symptoms include pressure and urinary problems (incontinence or retention) from displacement of the bladder. The problems are aggravated when the woman coughs, lifts a heavy object, or stands for a long time. Normal activities, even walking up stairs, may aggravate the problem.

Medical Management

Pessaries and surgery are two options for treatment. If surgery is the method of treatment used, the uterus is sutured back into place and repaired to strengthen and tighten the muscle bands. In postmenopausal women, the uterus may be removed (**hysterectomy**). For elderly women or those who are too ill to withstand the strain of surgery, pessaries may be the treatment of choice.

Nursing Management

IMPLEMENTING PREVENTIVE MEASURES

Some problems related to "relaxed" pelvic muscles (cystocele, rectocele, and uterine prolapse) may be prevented. During pregnancy, early visits to the health care provider permit early detection of problems. During the postpartum period, the woman can be taught to perform Kegel exercises to strengthen the muscles that support the uterus.

Delays in obtaining evaluation and treatment may result in complications such as infection, cervical ulceration, cystitis, and hemorrhoids. The nurse encourages the patient to obtain prompt treatment for these structural disorders.

IMPLEMENTING PREOPERATIVE NURSING CARE

Before surgery, the patient needs to know the extent of the proposed surgery, the expectations for the postoperative period, and the effect of surgery on future sexual function. In addition, the patient having a rectocele repair needs to know that before surgery, a laxative and a cleansing enema may be prescribed. She may be asked to administer these at home the day before surgery. A perineal shave may be prescribed as well. The patient is usually placed in a lithotomy position for surgery, with special attention given to moving both legs in and out of the stirrups simultaneously to prevent muscle strain and excess pressure on the legs and thighs. Other preoperative interventions are similar to those described in Chapter 18.

INITIATING POSTOPERATIVE NURSING CARE

Immediate postoperative goals include preventing infection and pressure on any existing suture line. This may require perineal care and may preclude using dressings. The patient is encouraged to void within a few hours after surgery for cystocele and complete tear. If the patient does not void within this period and reports discomfort or pain in the bladder region after 6 hours, she will need to be catheterized. Some physicians prefer to leave an indwelling catheter in place for 2 to 4 days, so some women may return home with a catheter in place. Various other bladder care methods are described in Chapter 44. After each voiding or bowel movement, the perineum is cleansed with warm, sterile saline solution and dried with sterile absorbent material if a perineal incision has been made.

After an external perineal repair, several methods are used in caring for the sutures. In one method, the sutures are left alone until healing occurs (in 5 to 10 days). Thereafter, daily vaginal douches with sterile saline solution may be administered during recovery. In another method—the wet method—small, sterile saline douches are administered twice daily, beginning on the day after surgery and continuing throughout recovery. A heat lamp or hair dryer may be used to help dry the area and promote healing. Commercially available sprays containing combined antiseptic and anesthetic solutions are soothing and effective, and an ice pack applied locally may relieve discomfort. However, the weight of the ice bag must rest on the bed and not on the patient.

Routine postoperative care is similar to that given after abdominal surgery. The patient is positioned in bed with the head and knees elevated slightly. The patient may go home the day of or the day after surgery; the duration of the hospital stay depends on the surgical approach used.

After surgery for a complete perineal laceration (through the rectal sphincter), special care and attention are required. The bladder is drained through the catheter to prevent strain on the sutures. Throughout recovery, stool-softening agents are administered nightly after the patient begins a soft diet.

PROMOTING HOME AND COMMUNITY-BASED CARE

Teaching Patients Self-Care. Predischarge instructions include information pertaining to the gynecologist's postoperative instructions related to douching, using mild laxatives, performing exercise as recommended, and avoiding lifting heavy objects or standing for prolonged periods. The patient is reminded to return to the gynecologist for a follow-up visit and to consult with the physician about when it is safe to resume sexual intercourse.

The patient is instructed to report any pelvic pain, unusual discharge, inability to carry out personal hygiene, and vaginal bleeding. She is advised to continue with perineal exercises, which are recommended to improve muscle strength and tone.

Benign Disorders

Vulvitis, an inflammation of the vulva, may occur with other disorders, such as diabetes, dermatologic problems, or poor hygiene, or it may be secondary to irritation from a vaginal discharge related to a specific vaginitis.

FIGURE 47-6 Complete prolapse of the uterus through the introitus.

Vulvodynia is a chronic syndrome of vulvar discomfort. Symptoms may include burning, stinging, irritation or excoriation. It has been described as primary, with onset at first tampon insertion or sexual experience, or secondary, beginning months or years after first tampon insertion or sexual experience. It may be classified as organic if it has a known cause (infection, trauma, or irritants) or idiopathic if no cause is known. It seems to be similar to a peripheral neuralgia and may respond to treatment with tricyclic antidepressants.

Cyclic vulvitis is a subset of vulvodynia and is characterized by episodes of vulvar discomfort. Typical complaints are recurrent itching and burning, often worsening with menses and after sexual intercourse. Erythema and swelling may occur. It is often related to candidal infection, and fungal cultures are often positive.

Vulvar **vestibulitis** is a chronic persistent syndrome of severe pain on touch to the vestibular area or attempted vaginal entry, and physical findings of vestibular erythema. Treatment methods vary. Research is ongoing to identify treatment for vulvar vestibulitis, but topical treatments (ie, estrogens, corticosteroids, trichloroacetic acid), surgery, and interferon have been used. Biofeedback has also been used.

VULVAR CYSTS

Bartholin's cyst results from the obstruction of a duct in one of the paired vestibular glands located in the posterior third of the vulva, near the vestibule. This cyst is the most common of vulvar tumours. A simple cyst may be asymptomatic, but an infected cyst or abscess causes pain, labial swelling, erythema, and heat. The duct opening may be reddened and pus may be observed (Bickley & Szilagyi, 2003). Infection may be due to a gonococcal organism, *Escherichia coli, Chlamydia trachomatis,* or *S. aureus* and can cause an abscess with or without involving the inguinal lymph nodes. The openings of the paraurethral (Skene's) glands are located posterior to and on each side of the urethral meatus. A **Skene's duct cyst** may result in pressure, dyspareunia, altered urinary stream, and pain, especially if infection is present. If inflammation of the paraurethral glands is suspected, the nurse places an index finger in the vagina, pushes upward, and "milks the urethra gently from inside outward" (Bickley & Szilagyi, 2003, p. 400). This action may result in discharge appearing at or around the urinary meatus, which should be cultured. Vestibular cysts, located inferior to the hymen, may also occur.

Medical Management

The usual treatment for a Bartholin's cyst is incision and drainage followed by antibiotic therapy. If a cyst is asymptomatic, treatment is unnecessary. Moist heat or sitz baths may promote drainage and resolution. If surgery is necessary, a Word Bartholin gland catheter is usually used. This catheter, a short latex stem with an inflatable bulb at the distal end, creates a tract that preserves the gland and allows for drainage. A nonopioid analgesic agent may be administered before this outpatient procedure. A local anesthetic agent is injected, and the cyst is incised or lanced and irrigated with normal saline; the catheter is inserted and inflated with 2 to 3 mL of water. The catheter stem is then tucked into the vagina to allow freedom of movement. The catheter is left in place for 4 to 6 weeks until the tract re-epithelializes. The patient is informed that discharge should be expected, as the catheter allows drainage of the cyst. She is instructed to contact her primary health care provider if pain occurs because the bulb may be too large for the cavity and fluid may need to be removed. Routine hygiene is encouraged.

Skene's duct cysts can be excised or drained with a Word catheter. Vestibular cysts are excised if symptomatic.

VULVAR DYSTROPHY

Vulvar dystrophy is a condition found in older women that causes dry, thickened skin on the vulva or slightly raised, whitish papules, fissures, or macules. Symptoms usually consist of varying degrees of itching, but some patients have no symptoms. A few patients with vulvar cancer have associated dystrophy (vulvar cancer is discussed later in this chapter). Biopsy with careful follow-up is the standard intervention. Benign dystrophies include lichen planus, simplex chronicus, **lichen sclerosus**, squamous cell hyperplasia, vulvar vestibulitis, and other dermatoses (Chart 47-5).

Medical Management

Topical corticosteroids (ie, hydrocortisone suppositories) are the usual treatment for lichen planus. Petrolatum jelly may relieve pruritus. Use is decreased as symptoms abate. Topical corticosteroids are effective in treating squamous cell hyperplasia. Treatment is often complete in 2 to 3 weeks; this condition is not likely to recur after treatment is complete.

If malignant cells are detected on biopsy, local excision, laser therapy, local chemotherapy, and immunologic treatment are used. Vulvectomy is avoided, if possible, to spare the patient from the stress of disfigurement and possible sexual dysfunction.

Nursing Management

Key nursing responsibilities for patients with vulvar dystrophies focus on teaching. Important topics include hygiene and self-monitoring for signs and symptoms of complications.

Chart 47-5 **Types of Benign Vulvar Disorders**

Lichen Planus and Simplex Chronicus
- Chronic vulvar and vaginal disorders that are diagnosed by biopsy
- May appear as mild inflammation or as severe erosion
- Result in redness, lesions, pain, and dyspareunia

Lichen Sclerosus
- A benign epithelial disorder that is most common in prepubertal and postmenopausal females
- A familial tendency toward this condition may exist.
- Epithelial thinning, edema, and fibrosis occur, and the vulva appears white and paper thin.
- Bleeding and pruritus may occur, and intercourse may be difficult.
- Diagnosis is confirmed by biopsy.

Squamous Cell Hyperplasia
- A benign epithelial disorder that may look like lichen sclerosus but is not inflamed
- Causes itching and plaquelike excoriated skin
- Must be differentiated from vulvar intraepithelial neoplasia or carcinoma in situ by biopsy

Vulvar Vestibulitis
- An inflammatory process associated with vulvodynia and possibly interstitial cystitis
- Causes pain during and after intercourse; discomfort may also preclude intercourse
- Onset of symptoms may be related to vaginal infection, laser treatment, history of sexual abuse, or excessive washing with irritant soaps.
- Examination reveals redness, inflammation, and tenderness.

Teaching Patients Self-Care. Instructions for patients with benign vulvar dystrophies include the importance of maintaining good personal hygiene and keeping the vulva dry. Lanolin or hydrogenated vegetable oil is recommended for relief of dryness. Sitz baths may help but should not be overused because dryness may result or increase. The patient is instructed to notify her primary health care provider about any change or ulceration because biopsy may be necessary to rule out squamous cell carcinoma.

By encouraging all patients to perform genital self-examinations regularly and have any itching, lesions, or unusual symptoms assessed by a health care provider, nurses can help prevent complications and progression of vulvar lesions.

OVARIAN CYSTS

The ovary is a common site for cysts, which may be simple enlargements of normal ovarian constituents, the graafian follicle, or the corpus luteum, or they may arise from abnormal growth of the ovarian epithelium.

Dermoid cysts are tumours that are thought to arise from parts of the ovum that normally disappear with ripening (maturation). Their origin is undefined, and they consist of undifferentiated embryonal cells. They grow slowly and are found during surgery to contain a thick, yellow, sebaceous material arising from the skin lining. Hair, teeth, bone, and many other tissues are found in a rudimentary state within these cysts. Dermoid cysts are only one type of lesion that may develop. Many other types can occur, and treatment usually depends on the type.

The patient may or may not report acute or chronic abdominal pain. Symptoms of a ruptured cyst mimic various acute abdominal emergencies, such as appendicitis or ectopic pregnancy. Larger cysts may produce abdominal swelling and exert pressure on adjacent abdominal organs.

Polycystic ovary syndrome, a complex endocrine condition involving a disorder in the hypothalamic-pituitary and ovarian network or axis resulting in anovulation, occurs in women of childbearing age. Symptoms are related to androgen excess. Irregular periods resulting from lack of regular ovulation, obesity, and hirsutism may be presenting complaints. Cysts form in the ovaries because the hormonal milieu cannot cause ovulation on a regular basis. Onset may occur at menarche or later. When pregnancy is desired, medications to stimulate ovulation are often effective. Women with polycystic ovary syndrome may develop insulin resistance and may be at higher risk for cardiac disorders in later life.

Medical Management

The treatment of large ovarian cysts is usually surgical removal. For cysts that are small and appear to be fluid-filled or physiologic in a young, healthy patient, however, oral contraceptives may be used to suppress ovarian activity and resolve the cyst. Oral contraceptives are also usually prescribed to treat polycystic ovary syndrome. About 98% of cysts that occur in women aged 29 years and younger are benign. In women older than 50 years of age, only half of these cysts are benign. The postoperative nursing care after surgery to remove an ovarian cyst is similar to that after abdominal surgery, with one exception. The marked decrease in intra-abdominal pressure resulting from removal of a large cyst usually leads to considerable abdominal distention. This complication may be prevented to some extent by applying a snug-fitting abdominal binder.

Some surgeons discuss the option of a hysterectomy when a woman is undergoing a bilateral ovary removal because of a sus-

picious mass because it may increase life expectancy, avoid a later second surgery, and save on health care costs. It is preventive in that future cancer is avoided, as is benign disease that might require hysterectomy. Patient preference is a priority in determining its appropriateness.

BENIGN TUMOURS OF THE UTERUS: FIBROIDS (LEIOMYOMAS, MYOMAS)

Myomatous or **fibroid tumours** of the uterus are estimated to occur in 25% of women over age 30. Some women are genetically predisposed. They are a common reason for hysterectomy as they often result in menorrhagia that can be difficult to control. They arise from the muscle tissue of the uterus and can be found in the lining (intracavitary), muscle wall (intramural), and outside surface (serosal) of the uterus. They develop slowly in women between the ages of 25 and 40 and may become large. Fibroids may cause no symptoms, or they may produce abnormal vaginal bleeding. Other symptoms are due to pressure on the surrounding organs and include pain, backache, constipation, and urinary problems. Menorrhagia (excessive bleeding) and metrorrhagia (irregular bleeding) may occur because fibroids may distort the uterine lining (Fig. 47-7).

Medical Management

The treatment of uterine fibroids depends to a large extent on their size, symptoms, and location. The patient with minor symptoms is closely monitored. If she plans to have children, treatment is as conservative as possible. As a rule, large tumours that produce pressure symptoms should be removed (**myomectomy**). The uterus may be removed (hysterectomy) if symptoms are bothersome and childbearing is completed (see later discussion of nursing care for a patient having a hysterectomy).

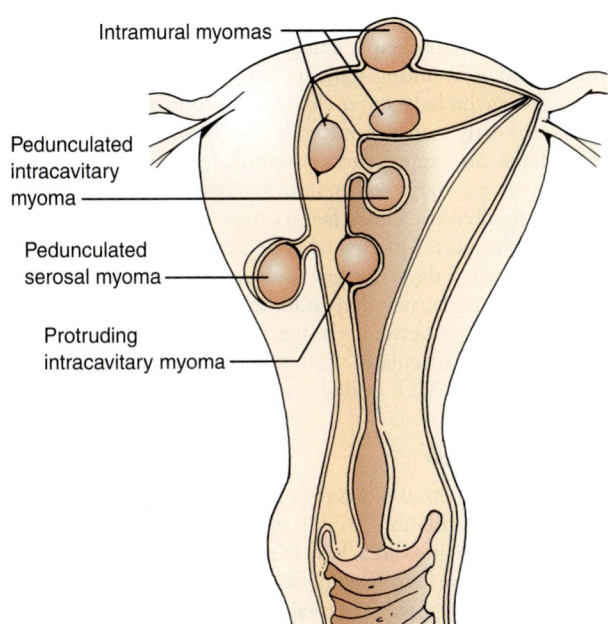

FIGURE 47-7 Myomas (fibroids) that impinge on the uterine cavity are called intracavitary myomas.

Several other alternatives to hysterectomy have been developed for the treatment of excessive bleeding due to fibroids. These include:

- Hysteroscopic resection of myomas: a laser is used through a hysteroscope passed through the cervix; no incision or overnight stay is needed
- Laparoscopic myomectomy: removal of a fibroid through a laparoscope inserted through a small abdominal incision
- Laparoscopic myolysis: a laser or electrical needles are used to cauterize and shrink the fibroid
- Laparoscopic cryomyolysis: electric current is used to coagulate the fibroid
- Uterine artery embolization: polyvinyl alcohol particles are injected into the blood vessels that supply the fibroid, shrinking it; this procedure may result in serious complications such as pain, infection, and bleeding

Fibroids usually shrink and disappear during menopause, when estrogen is no longer produced. Medications (eg, leuprolide [Lupron]) or other GnRH analogs that induce medical menopause may be prescribed to shrink the tumours. This treatment consists of monthly injections, which may cause hot flashes and vaginal dryness. This treatment is usually short term (ie, before surgery) to shrink the fibroids, allowing easier surgery, and to alleviate anemia, which may coexist due to heavy menstrual flow. Antifibrotic agents are under investigation for long-term treatment of fibroids.

ENDOMETRIOSIS

In **endometriosis**, a benign lesion or lesions with cells similar to those lining the uterus grow aberrantly in the pelvic cavity outside the uterus. Often, extensive endometriosis causes few symptoms, whereas an isolated lesion may produce severe symptoms. It is a major cause of chronic pelvic pain and infertility (Olive & Pritts, 2001). In order of frequency, pelvic endometriosis involves the ovary, uterosacral ligaments, cul-de-sac, rectovaginal septum, uterovesical peritoneum, cervix, outer surface of the uterus, umbilicus, laparotomy scar tissue, hernial sacs, and appendix.

Endometriosis has been diagnosed more frequently as a result of the increased use of laparoscopy. Before laparoscopy, major surgery was necessary before a diagnosis could be made. There is a high incidence among patients who bear children late and among those who have fewer children. In countries where tradition favours early marriage and early childbearing, endometriosis is rare. There also appears to be a familial predisposition to endometriosis; it is more common in women whose close female relatives are affected. Other factors that may suggest increased risk include a shorter menstrual cycle (less than every 27 days), flow longer than 7 days, outflow obstruction, and younger age at menarche. Characteristically, endometriosis is found in young, nulliparous women between the ages of 25 and 35 years. It is also found in teens, particularly those with dysmenorrhea that does not respond to NSAIDs or oral contraceptives.

Pathophysiology

Misplaced endometrial tissue responds to and depends on ovarian hormonal stimulation. During menstruation, this ectopic tissue bleeds, mostly into areas having no outlet, which causes pain and adhesions. The lesions are typically small and puckered, with a blue/brown/grey powder-burn appearance and brown or blue-black appearance, indicating concealed bleeding. They may also have an atypical appearance as red, white, petechial, and reddish-brown implants.

Endometrial tissue contained within an ovarian cyst has no outlet for the bleeding; this formation is referred to as a pseudo-cyst or chocolate cyst. Adhesions, cysts, and scar tissue may result, causing pain and infertility.

Currently the best-accepted theory regarding the origin of endometrial lesions is the transplantation theory, which suggests that a backflow of menses (retrograde menstruation) transports endometrial tissue to ectopic sites through the fallopian tubes. Transplantation of tissue can also occur during surgery if endometrial tissue is transferred inadvertently by way of surgical instruments. Retrograde menstruation has been found to occur in many women, not just those with endometriosis. Why some women develop this condition and others do not is unknown. Endometrial tissue can also be spread by lymphatic or venous channels.

Clinical Manifestations

Symptoms vary but include dysmenorrhea, dyspareunia, and pelvic discomfort or pain. Dyschezia (pain with bowel movements) and radiation of pain to the back or leg may occur. Depression, loss of work due to pain, and relationship difficulties may result. Infertility may occur because of fibrosis and adhesions or because of a variety of substances (prostaglandins, cytokines, other factors) produced by the implants (Olive & Pritts, 2001).

Assessment and Diagnostic Findings

A health history, including an account of the menstrual pattern, is necessary to elicit specific symptoms. On bimanual pelvic examination, fixed tender nodules are sometimes palpated and uterine mobility may be limited, indicating adhesions. Laparoscopic examination confirms the diagnosis and helps to stage the disease. In stage 1, the patient has superficial or minimal lesions; stage 2, mild involvement; stage 3, moderate involvement; and stage 4, deep involvement and dense adhesions, with obliteration of the cul-de-sac.

Medical Management

Treatment depends on the symptoms, the patient's desire for pregnancy, and the extent of the disease. If the woman does not have symptoms, routine examination may be all that is required. Other therapy for varying degrees of symptoms may be NSAIDs, oral contraceptives, GnRH agonists, or surgery. Pregnancy often alleviates symptoms because neither ovulation nor menstruation occurs.

PHARMACOLOGIC THERAPY

Palliative measures include use of medications, such as analgesic agents and prostaglandin inhibitors, for pain. Hormonal therapy is effective in suppressing endometriosis and relieving dysmenorrhea (menstrual pain). Oral contraceptives are used frequently. Side effects that may occur with oral contraceptives include fluid retention, weight gain, or nausea. These can usually be managed by changing brands or formulations. Depo-Provera, an injectable contraceptive agent, may also be used.

Several types of hormonal therapy are also available in addition to the oral contraceptives. A synthetic androgen, danazol (Cyclomen), causes atrophy of the endometrium and subsequent amenorrhea. The medication inhibits the release of gonadotropin with minimal overt sex hormone stimulation. The drawbacks of this medication are that it is expensive and may cause troublesome side effects such as fatigue, depression, weight gain, oily skin, decreased breast size, mild acne, hot flashes, and vaginal atrophy. GnRH agonists decrease estrogen production and cause subsequent amenorrhea. Side effects are related to low estrogen levels (eg, hot flashes and vaginal dryness). Loss of bone density is often offset by concurrent use of estrogen. Leuprolide (Lupron), another medication, is injected monthly to suppress hormones, induce an artificial menopause, and thereby avoid menstrual effects and relieve endometriosis. Some clinicians prescribe a combination of therapies. Most women continue treatment despite side effects, and symptoms diminish for 80% to 90% of women with mild to moderate endometriosis.

Assisted reproductive techniques may be warranted and effective in women with infertility secondary to endometriosis (Olive & Pritts, 2002). Hormonal medications are not used, however, in patients with a history of abnormal vaginal bleeding or liver, heart, or kidney disease. Bone density is followed carefully because of the risk of bone loss; hormone therapy is usually short-term.

SURGICAL MANAGEMENT

If conservative measures are not helpful, surgery may be necessary to relieve pain and enhance the possibility of pregnancy. Surgery may be combined with use of medical therapy. The procedure selected depends on the patient. Laparoscopy may be used to fulgurate (cut with high-frequency current) endometrial implants and to release adhesions. Laser surgery is another option made possible by laparoscopy. Laser therapy vaporizes or coagulates the endometrial implants, thereby destroying this tissue. Other surgical options include endocoagulation and electrocoagulation, laparotomy, abdominal hysterectomy, **oophorectomy**, bilateral **salpingo-oophorectomy**, and appendectomy. For women older than 35 or those willing to sacrifice reproductive capability, total hysterectomy is an option. Endometriosis recurs in many women.

Nursing Management

The health history and physical examination focus on specific symptoms (eg, pain) and when and how long they have been bothersome, the effect of prescribed medications, and the woman's reproductive plans. This information helps in determining the treatment plan. Explaining the various diagnostic procedures may help to alleviate the patient's anxiety. Patient goals include relief of pain, dysmenorrhea, dyspareunia, and avoidance of infertility.

As the treatment progresses, the woman with endometriosis and her partner may find that pregnancy is not easily possible, and the psychosocial impact of this realization must be recognized and addressed. Alternatives, such as in vitro fertilization or adoption, may be discussed at an appropriate time and referrals offered.

The nurse's role in patient education is to dispel myths and encourage the patient to seek care if dysmenorrhea or dyspareunia occurs. The Endometriosis Association (listed at the end of this chapter) is a helpful resource for patients seeking further information and support for this condition, which can cause disabling pain and severe emotional distress.

ADENOMYOSIS

In adenomyosis, the tissue that lines the endometrium invades the uterine wall. The incidence is highest in women ages 40 to 50. Symptoms include hypermenorrhea (excessive and prolonged bleeding), acquired dysmenorrhea, polymenorrhea (abnormally frequent bleeding), and premenstrual staining. Physical examination findings on palpation include an enlarged, firm, and tender uterus. Treatment depends on the severity of bleeding and pain. Hysterectomy may offer greater relief than more conservative therapies.

Malignant Conditions

In Canada, gynecologic tumours (cancers of the endometrium, ovaries, vulva, vagina, placenta, and adnexa) account for 11% of malignant tumours in women and 81% of genital cancers (Public Health Agency of Canada, 2003). Endometrial cancer accounts for 43% of genital cancer, but the prognosis is good since diagnosis occurs in early stages of the disease. The incidence of ovarian cancer in Canada is similar to endometrial cancer, but the survival is poor because greater than 70% of ovarian cases are diagnosed in late stages of the disease. Cancer involving the vulva and vagina are rare.

Although some cancers are difficult to detect or prevent, yearly pelvic examination with a Pap smear is a painless and relatively inexpensive method of early detection. Health care providers can encourage women to follow this health practice by providing nonstressful examinations that are educational and supportive and offering an opportunity for the patient to ask questions and clarify misinformation. If more women understood that the pelvic examination and Pap smear do not have to be uncomfortable or embarrassing, early detection rates would undoubtedly improve, and lives would be saved.

CANCER OF THE CERVIX

Carcinoma of the cervix is predominantly squamous cell cancer (10% are adenocarcinomas). Cervical cancer ranks as the 12th most common malignancy for Canadian women (Public Health Agency of Canada, 2002). It is the 3rd most common malignancy for women aged 20 to 49. The incidence and mortality rates have decreased substantially in Canada due to early detection of cell changes by Papanicolaou (Pap) smear. Cervical cancer occurs most commonly in women ages 30 to 45, but it can occur as early as age 18. Risk factors include multiple sex partners, early age at first coitus, short interval between menarche and first coitus, sexual contact with men whose partners have had cervical cancer, exposure to the HPV virus, and smoking (Chart 47-6).

Clinical Manifestations

There are several different types of cervical cancer. Most cancers originate in squamous cells, while the remainder are adenocarcinomas or mixed adenosquamous carcinomas. Adenocarcinomas begin in mucus-producing glands and are often due to HPV infection. Most cervical cancers, if not detected and treated, spread to regional pelvic lymph nodes, and local recurrence is not uncommon. Early cervical cancer rarely produces symptoms. If symptoms are present, they may go unnoticed as a thin watery vaginal discharge often noticed after intercourse or douching. When symptoms such as discharge, irregular bleeding, or bleeding after sexual intercourse occur, the disease may be advanced. Advanced disease should not occur if all women have access to gynecologic care and avail themselves of it. The nurse's role in access and utilization is crucial and may prevent the delay of detection of cervical cancer until the advanced stage.

In advanced cervical cancer, the vaginal discharge gradually increases and becomes watery and, finally, dark and foul-smelling from necrosis and infection of the tumour. The bleeding, which occurs at irregular intervals between periods (metrorrhagia) or after menopause, may be slight (just enough to spot the undergarments) and occurs usually after mild trauma or pressure (eg, intercourse,

Chart 47-6
Risk Factors for Cervical Cancer

Risk Factors
Sexual activity:
    Multiple sex partners
    Early age (younger than 20) at first coitus (exposes the vulnerable young cervix to potential carcinogens from a partner)
Early childbearing
Exposure to human papillomavirus
HIV infection
Smoking
Exposure to diethylstilbestrol (DES) in utero
Low socioeconomic status (may be related to early marriage and early childbearing)
Nutritional deficiencies (folate, beta-carotene, and vitamin C levels are lower in women with cervical cancer than in women without it)
Chronic cervical infection

Preventive Measures
Regular pelvic examinations and Pap tests for all women, especially older women past childbearing age (decreases the chance of dying from cervical cancer from 1 in 250 to 1 in 2,000 women)
Education related to reproductive health and safer sex
Smoking cessation

douching, or bearing down during defecation). As the disease continues, the bleeding may persist and increase. Leg pain, dysuria, rectal bleeding, and edema of extremities signal advanced disease.

As the cancer advances, it may invade the tissues outside the cervix, including the lymph glands anterior to the sacrum. In one third of patients with invasive cervical cancer, the disease involves the fundus. The nerves in this region may be affected, producing excruciating pain in the back and the legs that is relieved only by large doses of opioid analgesic agents. If the disease progresses, it often produces extreme emaciation and anemia, usually accompanied by fever due to secondary infection and abscesses in the ulcerating mass, and by fistula formation. Because the survival rate for in situ cancer is 100% and the rate for women with more advanced stages of cervical cancer decreases dramatically, early detection is essential.

Assessment and Diagnostic Findings

Diagnosis may be made on the basis of abnormal Pap smear results, followed by biopsy results identifying severe dysplasia (cervical intraepithelial neoplasia type III [CIN III], high-grade squamous intraepithelial lesions [HGSIL] [also referred to as HSIL], or carcinoma in situ; see below). HPV infections are usually implicated in these conditions. Biopsy results may indicate carcinoma in situ. Carcinoma in situ is technically classified as severe dysplasia and is defined as cancer that has extended through the full thickness of the epithelium of the cervix, but not beyond. This is often referred to as preinvasive cancer.

In its very early stages, invasive cervical cancer is found microscopically by Pap smear. In later stages, pelvic examination may reveal a large, reddish growth or a deep, ulcerating lesion. The patient may report spotting or bloody discharge.

When the patient has been diagnosed with invasive cervical cancer, clinical staging estimates the extent of the disease so that treatment can be planned more specifically and prognosis rea-

sonably predicted. The International Classification adopted by the International Federation of Gynecology and Obstetrics and included in the NIH Consensus Conference on Cervical Cancer (1996) (Table 47-2) is the most widely used staging system; the TNM (tumour, nodes, and metastases) classification is also used in describing cancer stages. In this system, T refers to the extent of the primary tumour, N to lymph node involvement, and M to metastasis, or spread of the disease.

Signs and symptoms are evaluated, and x-rays, laboratory tests, and special examinations, such as punch biopsy and colposcopy, are performed. Depending on the stage of the cancer, other tests and procedures may be performed to determine the extent of disease and appropriate treatment. These tests include dilation and curettage (D & C), computed tomography (CT) scan, magnetic resonance imaging (MRI), intravenous urography, cystography, and barium x-ray studies.

Medical Management

PRECURSOR OR PREINVASIVE LESIONS

When precursor lesions, such as low-grade squamous intraepithelial lesion (LGSIL), which is also referred to as LSIL (CIN I and II or mild to moderate dysplasia), are found by colposcopy

Table 47-2 • International Classification of Carcinoma of the Uterine Cervix	
STAGE OF LESION	SIZE AND DESCRIPTION
Preinvasive	
Stage 0	**Carcinoma in situ; cancer limited to epithelial layer; no evidence of invasion**
Invasive	
Stage I	**Carcinoma strictly confined to cervix**
Stage Ia	Microinvasive; identified only microscopically
Stage Ia1	Invasion no greater than 3 mm in depth and no wider than 7 mm
Stage Ia2	Invasion > 3 mm and no greater than 5 mm and no wider than 7 mm
Stage Ib	Clinical lesions confined to cervix or preclinical lesions > stage Ia
Stage Ib1	Clinical lesions no greater than 4 cm in size
Stage Ib2	Clinical lesions > 4 cm in size
Stage II	**Carcinoma extends beyond the cervix but not onto the pelvic wall**
Stage IIa	Vaginal extension only
Stage IIb	Paracervical extension with or without vaginal involvement
Stage III	**Carcinoma extends to one or both pelvic walls** Involves lower third of vagina. One or both ureters obstructed by the tumour on IV urogram
Stage IIIa	No extension onto the pelvic wall
Stage IIIb	Extension onto the pelvic wall or hydronephrosis or nonfunctioning kidney, or both
Stage IV	**Extension of carcinoma beyond the true pelvis** Clinical involvement of the mucosa of the bladder or rectum
Stage IVa	Spread of carcinoma to adjacent organs
Stage IVb	Spread to distant organs

National Institutes of Health (NIH) (1996). *NIH Consensus Statement: Cervical Cancer.* 14(1),1–38.

and biopsy, careful monitoring by frequent Pap smears or conservative treatment is possible. Conservative treatment may consist of monitoring, **cryotherapy** (freezing with nitrous oxide), or laser therapy. A **loop electrocautery excision procedure (LEEP)** may also be used to remove abnormal cells. In this procedure, a thin wire loop with laser is used to cut away a thin layer of cervical tissue. LEEP is an outpatient procedure usually performed in a gynecologist's office; it takes only a few minutes. Analgesia is given before the procedure, and a local anesthetic agent is injected into the area. This procedure allows the pathologist to examine the removed tissue sample to determine if the borders of the tissue are disease-free. Another procedure called a cone biopsy or **conization** (removing a cone-shaped portion of the cervix) is performed when biopsy findings demonstrate CIN III or HGSIL, equivalent to severe dysplasia and carcinoma in situ.

If preinvasive cervical cancer (carcinoma in situ) occurs when a woman has completed childbearing, a hysterectomy is usually recommended. If a woman has not completed childbearing and invasion is less than 1 mm, a cone biopsy may be sufficient. Frequent re-examinations are necessary to monitor for recurrence.

A newly developed procedure called a radical trachelectomy is an alternative to hysterectomy in women with cervical cancer who are young and want to have children (Dargent, Martin, Sacchetoni & Mathevet, 2000). In this procedure the cervix is gripped with retractors and pulled into the vagina until it is visible. The affected tissue is excised while the rest of the cervix and uterus remain intact. A drawstring suture is placed to close the cervix.

Patients who have precursor or premalignant lesions need reassurance that they do not have invasive cancer. However, the importance of close follow-up is emphasized because the condition, if untreated for a long time, may progress to cancer. Patients with cervical cancer in situ also need to know that this is usually a slow-growing and nonaggressive type of cancer that is not expected to recur after appropriate treatment.

INVASIVE CANCER

Treatment of invasive cervical cancer depends on the stage of the lesion, the patient's age and general health, and the judgment and experience of the physician. Surgery and radiation treatment (intracavitary and external) are most often used. When tumour invasion is less than 3 mm, a hysterectomy is often sufficient. Invasion exceeding 3 mm usually requires a radical hysterectomy with pelvic node dissection and aortic node assessment. Stage 1B1 tumours are treated with radical hysterectomy and radiation. Stage 1B2 tumours are treated individually because no single correct course has been determined, and many variable options may be seen clinically (Chart 47-7). Frequent follow-up after surgery by a gynecologic oncologist is imperative because the risk of recurrence is 35% after treatment for invasive cervical cancer. Recurrence usually occurs within the first 2 years. Recurrences are often in the upper quarter of the vagina, and ureteral obstruction may be a sign. Weight loss, leg edema, and pelvic pain may be signs of lymphatic obstruction and metastasis.

Radiation, which is often part of treatment to reduce recurrent disease, may be delivered by an external beam or by **brachytherapy** (method by which the radiation source is placed near the tumour) or both. The field to be irradiated and dose of radiation are determined by stage, volume of tumour, and lymph node involvement. Treatment can be administered daily for 4 to 6 weeks followed by one or two treatments of intracavitary radiation. Interstitial therapy may be used when vaginal placement has become impossible due to tumour or stricture.

> ### Chart 47-7 **Surgical Procedures for Cervical Cancer**
>
> Surgical procedures that may be carried out to treat cervical cancer include the following:
> - Total hysterectomy—removal of the uterus, cervix, and ovaries
> - Radical hysterectomy—removal of the uterus, ovaries, fallopian tubes, proximal vagina, and bilateral lymph nodes through an abdominal incision (*Note:* "radical" indicates that an extensive area of the paravaginal, paracervical, parametrial, and uterosacral tissues is removed with the uterus.)
> - Radical vaginal hysterectomy—vaginal removal of the uterus, ovaries, fallopian tubes, and proximal vagina
> - Bilateral pelvic lymphadenectomy—removal of the common iliac, external iliac, hypogastric, and obturator lymphatic vessels and nodes
> - Pelvic exenteration—removal of the pelvic organs, including the bladder or rectum and pelvic lymph nodes, and construction of diversional conduit, colostomy, and vagina
> - Radical trachelectomy—removal of the cervix and selected nodes to preserve childbearing capacity in a woman of reproductive age with cervical cancer

Platinum-based agents are being used to treat advanced cervical cancer. They are often used in combination with radiation therapy, surgery, or both. Studies are ongoing to find the best approach to treat advanced cervical cancer. Vaginal stenosis is a frequent side effect of radiation. Sexual activity with lubrication is preventive, as is use of a vaginal dilator to avoid severe permanent vaginal stenosis.

Some patients with recurrences of cervical cancer are considered for **pelvic exenteration**, in which a large portion of the pelvic contents is removed. Unilateral leg edema, sciatica, and ureteral obstruction indicate likely disease progression. Patients with these symptoms have advanced disease and are not considered candidates for this major surgical procedure. Surgery is often complex because it is performed close to the bowel, bladder, ureters, and great vessels. Complications can be considerable and include pulmonary emboli, pulmonary edema, myocardial infarction, cerebrovascular accident, hemorrhage, sepsis, small bowel obstruction, fistula formation, urinary obstruction of ileal conduit, bladder dysfunction, and pyelonephritis, most often in the first 18 months. Vein constriction must be avoided postoperatively. Patients with varicose veins or a history of thromboembolic disease may be treated prophylactically with heparin. Pneumatic compression stockings are prescribed to reduce the risk for deep vein thrombosis. Nursing care of these patients is complex and requires coordination and care by experienced health care professionals. This is a complex, extensive surgical procedure that is reserved for those with a high likelihood of cure.

PREGNANCY-RELATED NEOPLASM

Hydatidiform mole is a type of gestational trophoblastic neoplasm that occurs in 1 in 1,000 pregnancies. Delayed menses with spotting is the most common sign. Hyperemesis and uterine enlargement beyond that expected for gestational dates are also indicative. Moles can be partial or complete. Complete moles are more likely to be associated with medical complications. Pregnancy-induced hypertension (formerly called preeclampsia), a pregnancy-related complex of symptoms that may include edema, hypertension, and proteinuria, may occur. Treatment consists of suction curettage followed by monitoring serial beta-human chorionic gonadotropin (HCG) levels, which usually take about 2.5 months to return to normal. This condition may recur. Moles can be invasive also.

Choriocarcinoma, another gestational neoplasm that usually occurs in the postpartum period, is a placental site trophoblastic tumour. These malignancies are being diagnosed more readily and treated more effectively today due to the availability of testing for HCG, a sensitive marker that can be used for monitoring. Ultrasound is also used for making the diagnosis. These malignancies are usually found in obstetric patients and are described in detail in obstetric and oncologic textbooks. Nurses need to be aware that these conditions are traumatic, anxiety-producing, and often very stressful for the patient since they are often associated with pregnancy loss.

CANCER OF THE UTERUS (ENDOMETRIUM)

Cancer of the uterine endometrium (fundus or corpus) has increased in incidence, partly because people are living longer and because reporting is more accurate. Most uterine cancers are endometrioid (that is, originating in the lining of the uterus). After breast, colorectal, and lung cancer, endometrial cancer is the fourth most common cancer in women and the most common pelvic neoplasm. Cumulative exposure to estrogen is considered the major risk factor (Chart 47-8). This exposure occurs with the use of estrogen replacement therapy without the use of progestin, early menarche, late menopause, never having children, and anovulation. Other risk factors include infertility, diabetes, hypertension, gallbladder disease, and obesity (Canadian Cancer Society, 2005). Tamoxifen may also cause proliferation of the uterine lining, and women receiving this medication for treatment or prevention of breast cancer are monitored by their oncologists. Another less common type of cancer of the uterus is not estrogen-dependent and is found in multiparous, thin women.

Assessment and Diagnostic Findings

All women should be encouraged to have annual checkups, including a gynecologic examination. Any woman who is experiencing irregular bleeding should be evaluated promptly. If a menopausal or perimenopausal woman experiences bleeding, an endometrial aspiration or biopsy is performed to rule out hyperplasia, a possible precursor of endometrial cancer. The procedure is quick and painless. Ultrasonography can also be used to measure the thickness of the endometrium. (Postmenopausal women should have a very thin endometrium due to low levels of estro-

gen; a thicker lining warrants further investigation.) A biopsy or aspiration is diagnostic.

Medical Management

Treatment of endometrial cancer consists of total hysterectomy (discussed later in this chapter) and bilateral salpingo-oophorectomy and node sampling. Depending on the stage, the therapeutic approach is individualized and is based on stage, type, differentiation, degree of invasion, and node involvement. Whole pelvis radiotherapy is used if there is any spread beyond the uterus. Preoperative and postoperative treatments for stage II and beyond may include pelvic, abdominal, and vaginal intracavitary radiation. Recurrent cancer usually occurs inside the **vaginal vault** or in the upper vagina, and metastasis usually occurs in lymph nodes or the ovary. Recurrent lesions in the vagina are treated with surgery and radiation. Recurrent lesions beyond the vagina are treated with hormonal therapy or chemotherapy. Progestin therapy is used frequently. Patients should be prepared for such side effects as nausea, depression, rash, or mild fluid retention with this therapy.

CANCER OF THE VULVA

Primary cancer of the vulva represents 3% to 5% of all gynecologic malignancies and is seen mostly in postmenopausal women, although its incidence in younger women is increasing. The median age for cancer limited to the vulva is 44 years, whereas the median age for invasive vulvar cancer is 61 years. Possible risk factors include hypertension, obesity, diabetes, and immunosuppression. Squamous cell carcinoma accounts for most primary vulvar tumours. Less common are Bartholin's gland cancer and malignant melanoma. Little is known about what causes this disease; however, increased risk may be related to chronic vulvar irritation, vulvar disorders, HPV, and smoking.

Clinical Manifestations

Long-standing pruritus and soreness are the most common symptoms of vulvar cancer. Itching occurs in half of all patients with vulvar malignancy. Bleeding, foul-smelling discharge, and pain may also be present and are usually signs of advanced disease. Cancerous lesions of the vulva are visible and accessible and grow relatively slowly. Early lesions appear as a chronic dermatitis; later, the patient may note a lump that continues to grow and becomes a hard, ulcerated, cauliflower-like growth. Biopsy should be performed on any vulvar lesion that persists, ulcerates, or fails to heal quickly with proper therapy. Vulvar malignancies may appear as a lump or mass, redness, or a lesion that fails to heal.

The nurse is in an ideal position to encourage a woman to perform vulvar self-examination regularly. Using a mirror, the patient can see what constitutes normal female anatomy and learn about changes that should be reported (eg, lesions, ulcers, masses, and persistent itching). The nurse must urge women to seek health care if they notice anything abnormal because this is one of the most curable of all malignant conditions.

Medical Management

Vulvar intraepithelial lesions are preinvasive and are also called vulvar carcinoma in situ. They may be treated by local excision, laser ablation, chemotherapeutic creams (ie, 5-fluorouracil), or cryosurgery.

Chart 47-8
Risk Factors for Uterine Cancer

- Age: at least 55 years; median age, 61 years
- Postmenopausal bleeding
- Obesity that results in increased estrone levels (related to excess weight) resulting from conversion of androstenedione to estrone in body fat, which exposes the uterus to unopposed estrogen
- Unopposed estrogen therapy (estrogen used without progesterone, which offsets the risk of unopposed estrogen)
- Other: nulliparity, truncal obesity, late menopause (after 52 years of age) and, possibly, use of tamoxifen

When invasive vulvar carcinoma exists, primary treatment may include wide excision or removal of the vulva (**vulvectomy**). An effort is made to individualize treatment, depending on the extent of the disease. A wide excision is performed only if lymph nodes are normal. More pervasive lesions require vulvectomy with deep pelvic node dissection. Vulvectomy is very effective at prolonging life but is frequently followed by complications (ie, scarring, wound breakdown, leg swelling, vaginal stenosis, or rectocele). To reduce complications, only necessary tissue is removed.

Radiation is used to treat unresectable tumours or cancer that has spread to the lymph nodes. If a widespread area is involved or the disease is advanced, a radical vulvectomy with bilateral groin dissection may be performed. Excision and evaluation of the sentinel node, which drains the primary tumour, may be performed. If negative, full groin dissection may be omitted (Duffy, 2001). Antibiotic and heparin prophylaxis may be prescribed preoperatively and continued postoperatively to prevent infection, deep vein thrombosis, and pulmonary emboli. Elastic compression stockings are applied to reduce the risk for deep vein thrombosis.

Clinical trials to determine the most effective treatment are difficult to conduct, as there are few patients with this condition. Morbidity with recurrence of the disease is high. Patterns can vary in patients.

NURSING PROCESS: THE PATIENT UNDERGOING VULVAR SURGERY

Assessment

The health history is a valuable tool for establishing rapport with the patient. The reason the patient is seeking health care is apparent. What the nurse can tactfully elicit is the reason why a delay, if any, occurred, in seeking health care—for example, because of modesty, economics, denial, neglect, or fear (abusive partners sometimes prevent women from seeking health care). Factors involved in any delay in seeking health care and treatment may also affect the patient's recovery. The patient's health habits and lifestyle are assessed, and her receptivity to teaching is evaluated. Psychosocial factors are also assessed. Preoperative preparation and psychological support begin at this time.

Diagnosis

NURSING DIAGNOSES

Based on all the assessment data, the patient's major nursing diagnoses may include the following:

- Anxiety related to the diagnosis and surgery
- Acute pain related to the surgical incision and subsequent wound care
- Impaired skin integrity related to the wound and drainage
- Sexual dysfunction related to change in body image
- Self-care deficit related to lack of understanding of perineal care and general health status

COLLABORATIVE PROBLEMS/ POTENTIAL COMPLICATIONS

Based on assessment data, potential complications may include the following:

- Wound infection and sepsis
- Deep vein thrombosis
- Hemorrhage

Planning and Goals

The major goals for the patient may include acceptance of and preparation for surgical intervention, relief of pain, maintenance of skin integrity, recovery of optimal sexual function, ability to perform adequate and appropriate self-care, and absence of complications.

Preoperative Nursing Interventions

RELIEVING ANXIETY

The patient must be allowed time to talk and ask questions. Fear often decreases when a woman of childbearing age who is to undergo wide excision of the vulva or vulvectomy learns that the possibility for subsequent sexual relations is good and that pregnancy is possible after a wide excision. The nurse must know what information the physician has given the patient about the surgery to reinforce that information and address the patient's questions and concerns.

PREPARING SKIN FOR SURGERY

Skin preparation may include cleansing the lower abdomen, inguinal areas, upper thighs, and vulva with a detergent germicide for several days before the surgical procedure. The patient may be instructed to do this at home.

Postoperative Nursing Interventions

RELIEVING PAIN

Because of the wide excision, the patient may experience severe pain and discomfort even with minimal movement. Inadequate pain relief will inhibit the patient's mobility and increase the likelihood of complications. Therefore, analgesic agents are administered preventively (ie, around the clock at designated times) to relieve pain and increase the patient's comfort level. Patient-controlled analgesia may be used to provide pain relief and promote patient comfort. Careful positioning using pillows usually increases comfort, as do soothing back rubs. A low Fowler's position or, occasionally, a pillow placed under the knees will reduce pain by relieving tension on the incision; however, efforts must be made to avoid pressure behind the knees, which increases the risk for deep vein thrombosis. Positioning the patient on her side, with pillows between her legs and against the lumbar region, provides comfort and reduces tension on the surgical wound.

IMPROVING SKIN INTEGRITY

The patient may be confined to bed for several days to promote healing of the surgical and donor sites (if skin grafts were used). A pressure-reducing mattress may be used to prevent pressure ulcers. Moving from one position to another requires time and effort; use of an overbed trapeze bar may help the patient to move herself more easily. Ambulation may be attempted on the second day.

The extent of the surgical incision and the type of dressing are considered when choosing strategies to promote skin integrity. Intact skin needs to be protected from drainage and moisture, and dressings must be changed as needed to ensure patient comfort, to perform wound care and irrigation (if prescribed), and to permit observation of the surgical site. When the patient returns from the operating room, perineal dressings are more likely to remain in place and be comfortable if a T-binder is used.

A skin graft from the buttocks may have been performed if the edges of the excision could not be approximated, and drains may have been put in place as well. A pressure stent may be applied to the grafted site to promote adhesion. Nursing care includes monitoring for suppuration (accumulation of purulent material) under the graft and assisting the patient to keep the perineal area clean and dry.

The wound is cleansed daily with warm, normal saline irrigations or other antiseptic solutions as prescribed. A transparent dressing or Xeroform gauze may be in place over the wound to minimize exposure to the air and subsequent pain. The appearance of the surgical site and the characteristics of drainage are assessed and documented. After the dressings are removed, a bed cradle may be used to keep the bed linens away from the surgical site. The nurse must protect the patient from exposure when visitors arrive or someone else enters the room.

SUPPORTING POSITIVE SEXUALITY AND SEXUAL FUNCTION

The patient who undergoes vulvar surgery usually experiences concerns about the effects of the surgery on her body image, sexual attractiveness, and functioning. Establishing a trusting nurse–patient relationship is important for the patient to feel comfortable expressing her concerns and fears. The patient is encouraged to share and discuss her concerns with her sexual partner.

Because alterations in sexual sensation and functioning depend on the extent of surgery, the nurse needs to know about any structural and functional changes resulting from the surgery. Consulting with the surgeon will clarify which changes to expect, and referring the patient and her partner to a sex counselor may help them address these changes and resume satisfying sexual activity.

MONITORING AND MANAGING POTENTIAL COMPLICATIONS

Infection

The location and extent of the surgical site and incision put the patient at risk for contamination of the site and infection and sepsis. The patient is monitored closely for local and systemic signs and symptoms of infection: purulent drainage, redness, increased pain, fever, and an increased white blood cell count. The nurse assists in obtaining tissue specimens for culture if infection is suspected and administers antibiotic agents as prescribed. Hand hygiene, always a crucial infection-preventing measure, is of particular importance whenever there is an extensive area of exposed tissue. Catheters, drains, and dressings are handled carefully and with gloves to avoid cross-contamination. A low-residue diet prevents straining on defecation and wound contamination. Sitz baths are discouraged after a wide excision because of the risk for infection.

Deep Vein Thrombosis

The patient is at risk for deep vein thrombosis because of the positioning required during surgery, postoperative edema, and the usually prolonged immobility needed to promote healing. Elastic compression stockings are applied, and the patient is encouraged and reminded to perform ankle exercises to minimize venous pooling, which leads to deep vein thrombosis. The patient is encouraged and assisted in changing position by using the overhead trapeze. Pressure behind the knees is avoided when positioning the patient because this may increase venous pooling. The patient is assessed for signs and symptoms of deep vein thrombosis (leg pain, redness, warmth, positive Homans' sign) and pulmonary embolism (chest pain, tachycardia, dyspnea). Fluid intake is encouraged to prevent dehydration, which also increases the risk for deep vein thrombosis.

Hemorrhage

The extent of the surgical incision and possibly wide excision of tissue increase the risk of postoperative bleeding and hemorrhage. Although the pressure dressings that are applied after surgery minimize the risk, the patient must be monitored closely for signs of hemorrhage and resulting hypovolemic shock. These signs may include decreased blood pressure, increased pulse rate, decreased urine output, decreased mental status, and cold, clammy skin.

If hemorrhage and shock occur, interventions include fluid replacement, blood component therapy, and vasopressor medications. Laboratory results (eg, hematocrit and hemoglobin levels) and hemodynamic monitoring are used to assess the patient's response to treatment. Depending on the specific cause of hemorrhage, the patient may be returned to the operating room. The patient who experiences hemorrhage is anxious and apprehensive. Providing brief explanations of the procedures being performed and offering reassurance that the problem has been identified and is being taken care of may reduce the anxiety and fears of the patient and her family.

PROMOTING HOME AND COMMUNITY-BASED CARE

Teaching Patients Self-Care

Preparing the patient for hospital discharge begins before hospital admission. The patient and family are informed about what to expect during the immediate postoperative and recovery periods. Posthospital care requires giving complete instructions to a family member or significant other who will help care for the patient at home and to the home care nurse who will provide follow-up care. Depending on the changes resulting from the surgery, the patient and her family may need instruction about wound care, urinary catheterization, and possible complications. The patient is encouraged to share her concerns and to assume increasing responsibility for her own care. She is encouraged and assisted in learning to care for the surgical wound.

Continuing Care

Shortened hospital stays may result in the patient's discharge during the early postoperative recovery stage. Thus, home care referral or discharge to a subacute facility may be indicated. During this phase, the patient's physical status and psychological responses to the surgery are assessed. Additionally, the patient is assessed for complications and healing of the surgical site. During home visits, the patient's environment is assessed to determine if modifications are needed to facilitate patient care. The home care nurse uses the home visit to reinforce previous teaching and to assess the patient's and the family's understanding of and adherence to the prescribed treatment strategies. Follow-up phone calls by the nurse to the patient between home visits are usually reassuring to the patient and family, who may be responsible for performing complex care procedures. Attention to the patient's psychological responses is important because the patient may become discouraged and depressed because of alterations in body image and a slow recovery. Communication between the nurse involved in the patient's immediate postoperative care and the home care nurse is essential to ensure continuity of care.

Evaluation

EXPECTED PATIENT OUTCOMES

Expected patient outcomes may include:

1. Adjusts to the trauma of the surgical experience
   a. Uses available resources in coping with and alleviating emotional stress

b. Asks questions related to postoperative expectations
c. Demonstrates willingness to discuss alternative approaches to sexual expression
2. Obtains pain relief
   a. Reports progressive decline in pain and discomfort
   b. Assumes position of comfort
3. Maintains skin integrity
   a. States rationale for use of a special mattress or other device
   b. Uses overhead trapeze to change position frequently
   c. Exhibits healing of surgical site without excoriated skin
   d. Cares for incision and surgical site as instructed
4. Exhibits positive outlook about sexuality and sexual functioning
   a. Verbalizes concerns and anxieties about sexual functioning
   b. Discusses options and alternative approaches to sexual intercourse
5. Increases participation in self-care activities
   a. Demonstrates self-care activities as instructed
   b. Identifies signs and symptoms of complications that should be reported to the nurse or physician
   c. Properly cleans the surgical site after voiding and defecation
6. Absence of complications
   a. Is free of any signs and symptoms of infection: has normal vital signs (temperature, blood pressure, pulse rate); has no purulent discharge
   b. Identifies activities to prevent deep vein thrombosis: avoids crossing legs or sitting with pressure against knees; exercises ankles and legs
   c. Exhibits no signs or symptoms of deep vein thrombosis (leg pain, redness, edematous or swollen extremities)
   d. Demonstrates no signs or symptoms of hemorrhage

CANCER OF THE VAGINA

Cancer of the vagina usually results from metastasized choriocarcinoma or from cancer of the cervix or adjacent organs (eg, uterus, vulva, bladder, or rectum). Primary cancer of the vagina is squamous in origin.

Risk factors include previous cervical cancer, in utero exposure to diethylstilbestrol (DES), previous vaginal or vulvar cancer, previous radiation therapy, history of HPV, or pessary use. Any patient with previous cervical cancer should be examined regularly for vaginal lesions.

Before 1970, vaginal cancer occurred primarily in postmenopausal women. In the 1970s, it was shown that maternal ingestion of DES affected female offspring who were exposed in utero. Benign genital tract abnormalities have occurred in some of these young women. Vaginal adenosis (abnormal tissue growth) may also occur. The risk for clear cell tumour related to DES exposure is 0.14 to 1.4 in 1,000 women. Colposcopy is indicated for all women exposed to this medication in utero. If colposcopic examination discloses adenosis or a significant cervical lesion, follow-up is essential.

Vaginal pessaries, used to support prolapsed tissues, have been associated with vaginal cancer only if the devices were not cared for properly (ie, regularly cleaned and the vagina examined by a health care professional) because pessaries can be a source of chronic irritation.

Patients often do not have symptoms but may report slight bleeding after intercourse, spontaneous bleeding, vaginal discharge, pain, and urinary or rectal symptoms (or both). Diagnosis is often by Pap smear of the vagina.

Medical Management

Treatment of early lesions may be local excision or administration of a chemotherapeutic cream (ie, 5-fluorouracil applied with a tampon or a diaphragm). Cotton balls placed at the introitus lessen spillage, which otherwise can result in perineal irritation. Laser therapy is a common treatment option in early vaginal and vulvar cancer. Radiation, another treatment option, is delivered by external beam to the pelvis, by vaginal intracavitary radiation using a tandem and colpostats, or by interstitial vaginal implants using an obturator and vaginal template. For a tumour located in the lower third of the vagina, radical node dissection is followed by radiation.

Encouraging close follow-up by health care providers is the prime focus of nursing interventions with women who were exposed to DES in utero. Because DES was used only from the 1940s to the 1970s, the incidence will decrease with each subsequent year. Emotional support for mothers and daughters is essential. For young women who have had vaginal reconstructive surgery, specific vagina-dilating procedures may be initiated and taught. Water-soluble lubricants are helpful in reducing painful intercourse (dyspareunia). If a lesion requiring treatment develops, all aspects and effects of radiation therapy, chemotherapy, or surgery need to be explored on an individual basis.

CANCER OF THE FALLOPIAN TUBES

Malignancies of the fallopian tube are rare and are the least common type of genital cancer. Symptoms include a profuse, watery discharge and a colicky lower abdominal pain or abnormal vaginal bleeding. An enlarged fallopian tube may be found on examination. Surgery followed by radiation therapy is the usual treatment.

CANCER OF THE OVARY

Ovarian cancer causes more deaths than any other cancer of the female reproductive system. About 75% of cases are detected at a late stage (Duffy, 2001). The ovary is a common site of primary as well as metastatic lesions from other cancers. Most cases affect women ages 50 to 59. The incidence of ovarian cancer is highest in industrialized countries, except for Japan, where its incidence is low.

A woman with ovarian cancer has a threefold to fourfold increased risk for breast cancer, and women with breast cancer have an increased risk for ovarian cancer. No definitive causative factors have been determined, but oral contraceptives appear to provide a protective effect. Heredity plays a part, and many physicians advocate pelvic examinations every 6 months for women who have one or two relatives with ovarian cancer. Despite careful examination, ovarian tumours are often difficult to detect because they are usually deep in the pelvis. No early screening mechanism exists at present, although tumour markers are being explored. Transvaginal ultrasound and Ca-125 antigen testing are helpful in those at high risk for this condition. Tumour-associated antigens are helpful in follow-up care after diagnosis and treatment but not in early general screening.

Advances in our knowledge of genetics are changing the approaches to detecting and treating breast and ovarian cancer. Some families have specific genes that predispose them to various cancers. BRCA-1 is a genetic mutation that results in an increased risk for breast and ovarian cancer. BRCA-2 is another genetic mutation that may result in increased risk for both female and male breast cancers and for ovarian cancer (Duffy, 2001). Other mutations are also under study. Testing for susceptibility is in the early stages at centres that have expertise in genetics, testing, and counselling. Testing is indicated when a family history of three or more cases of closely related members includes premenopausal breast cancer or ovarian cancer. One member with cancer is tested, and if the results are positive, other members without cancer may undergo testing.

Much more needs to be learned about the risks associated with some mutations, the reliability of testing, and the efficacy of follow-up. Confidentiality and insurance risks are ethical issues that need clarification. Because there are no primary methods of preventing breast or ovarian cancer, emotional distress is also a problem. Patients with concerns about their family history should be referred to a cancer genetics centre to obtain information and testing, if indicated. Women with inherited types of ovarian cancer tend to be younger when the diagnosis is made than the average age of 59 years at the time of diagnosis.

Risk factors also include nulliparity and infertility. Older age is a major risk factor because the incidence of this disease peaks in the eighth decade of life. High dietary fat intake, mumps before menarche, use of talc in the perineal area, and family history are suspected to increase risk, while multiparity, oral contraceptive use, breastfeeding, and anovulatory disorders may be protective. Survival rates depend on the stage of the cancer at diagnosis.

Fifteen percent of all new cases of ovarian tumours have low malignancy potential (LMP tumours). These borderline tumours resemble ovarian cancer but have much more favourable outcomes. Women diagnosed with this type of cancer tend to be younger, in their early 40s. A conservative surgical approach is now used. The affected ovary is removed, but the uterus and the contralateral ovary may remain. Adjuvant therapy may not be warranted for these tumours.

Clinical Manifestations

Symptoms are nonspecific and include increased abdominal girth, pelvic pressure, bloating, indigestion, flatulence, increased waist size, leg pain, and pelvic pain. Symptoms are often vague, and many women ignore the symptoms. Ovarian cancer is often silent, but enlargement of the abdomen from an accumulation of fluid is the most common sign. Any woman with gastrointestinal symptoms and without a known diagnosis must be evaluated with ovarian cancer in mind. Flatulence, fullness after a light meal, and increasing abdominal girth are significant symptoms.

Vague, undiagnosed, persistent gastrointestinal symptoms should alert the nurse to the possibility of an early ovarian malignancy. A palpable ovary in a woman who has gone through menopause is investigated because ovaries normally become smaller and less palpable after menopause.

Assessment and Diagnostic Findings

Any enlarged ovary must be investigated. Pelvic examination often does not detect early ovarian cancer, and pelvic imaging techniques are not always definitive. About 75% of ovarian cancers have metastasized by the time of diagnosis; about 60% have spread beyond the pelvis. Of the many different ovarian cancer cell types, epithelial tumours constitute 90%. Germ cell tumours and stromal tumours make up the other 10%.

Medical Management

SURGICAL MANAGEMENT

Surgical staging, exploration, and reduction of tumour mass are the basics of treatment. Surgical removal is the treatment of choice; the preoperative workup includes a barium enema or colonoscopy, upper gastrointestinal series, chest x-rays, and intravenous urography. CT scans and immunoscintigraphy, the use of radioactive antibodies, may be used preoperatively to rule out intra-abdominal metastasis. Staging the tumour is important to guide treatment (Chart 47-9). A total abdominal hysterectomy with removal of the fallopian tubes and ovaries and the omentum (bilateral salpingo-oophorectomy and omentectomy) is the standard procedure for early disease.

PHARMACOLOGIC THERAPY

Chemotherapy often follows surgery, usually with cyclophosphamide (Cytoxan), doxorubicin (Adriamycin), cisplatin (Platinol-AQ), carboplatin (Paraplatin), or paclitaxel (Taxol). Hexamethylmelamine (Hexalen), ifosfamide (Ifex), bone marrow transplantation, and peripheral blood stem cell support may also be used. Paclitaxel, cisplatin, and carboplatin are most often used because of their excellent clinical benefits and manageable toxicity. Leukopenia, neurotoxicity, and fever may occur.

Paclitaxel, an agent derived from the Pacific yew tree, works by causing microtubules within the cells to gather and prevents the breakdown of these threadlike structures. In general, cells cannot function when they are clogged with microtubules and cannot divide. Because this medication often causes leukopenia, the patient may need to take granulocyte colony-stimulating factor as well.

Paclitaxel is contraindicated in patients with hypersensitivity to medications formulated in polyoxyethylated castor oil and in patients with baseline neutropenia. Because of possible adverse cardiac effects, paclitaxel is not used in patients with cardiac disorders. Hypotension, dyspnea, angioedema, and urticaria indicate severe reactions that usually occur soon after the first and second doses are administered. The nurse must be prepared to assist in treating anaphylaxis. The patient should be prepared for inevitable hair loss.

Cisplatin is used frequently in chemotherapeutic treatment of ovarian cancer, both alone and in combination with other agents, and in intraperitoneal applications. Patients may require bone marrow transplantation or stem cell transplantation to treat ovarian cancer. Care for these patients is described in Chapter 16. Intraperitoneal chemotherapy with cisplatin may provide a promising mode of treatment.

Carboplatin may be used in the initial treatment of advanced ovarian cancer in combination with other chemotherapeutic agents. It may also be used in patients with recurrence of ovarian cancer after other chemotherapy, including cisplatin. It must be used with caution in patients with renal impairment.

Chart 47-9 Stages of Ovarian Cancer

I—Growth limited to the ovaries
II—Growth involves one or both ovaries with pelvic extension
III—Growth involves one or both ovaries with metastases outside the pelvis or positive retroperitoneal or inguinal nodes
IV—Growth involves one or both ovaries with distant metastases

Other medications include topotecan (Hycamtin), irinotecan (Camptosar), gemcitabine (Gemzar), vinorelbine (Navelbine), liposomal doxorubicin (Doxil), and docetaxel (Taxotere). Different combinations, different regimens, different routes, and use of growth factors are being investigated.

Liposomal therapy, delivery of chemotherapy in a liposome, allows the highest possible dose of chemotherapy to the tumour target with a reduction in adverse effects. Liposomes are used as drug carriers because they are nontoxic, biodegradable, easily available, and relatively inexpensive. This encapsulated chemotherapy allows increased duration of action and better targeting. The encapsulation of doxorubicin lessens the incidence of nausea, vomiting, and alopecia. The patient must be monitored for bone marrow suppression. Gastrointestinal and cardiac effects may also occur. These medications are administered by oncology nurses as a slow intravenous infusion over 60 to 90 minutes.

Genetic engineering and identification of cancer genes may make gene therapy a future possibility. Gene therapy is under investigation. Radiation may be helpful and is more useful in some types of ovarian cancer than others.

After adjunct therapies are completed, a second-look laparoscopy or a laparotomy may be performed in some clinical centres to evaluate the treatment results and to obtain multiple tissue samples for biopsy. Occasionally, catheters are left in place if radioactive agents are to be used postoperatively. Chemotherapy is the most common form of treatment in advanced disease.

Nursing Management

Nursing measures include those related to the patient's treatment plan, be it surgery, chemotherapy, radiation, or palliation. Emotional support, comfort measures, and information, plus attentiveness and caring, are meaningful aids to the patient and her family.

Nursing interventions after pelvic surgery to remove the tumour are similar to those after other abdominal surgeries. If ovarian cancer occurs in a young woman and the tumour is unilateral, it is removed. Childbearing, if desired, is encouraged in the near future. After childbirth, surgical re-exploration may be performed and the remaining ovary may be removed. If both ovaries are involved, surgery is performed and chemotherapy follows.

Patients with advanced ovarian cancer may develop ascites and pleural effusion. Nursing care may include administering intravenous therapy to alleviate fluid and electrolyte imbalances, initiating parenteral nutrition to provide adequate nutrition, providing postoperative care after intestinal bypass to alleviate an obstruction, and providing pain relief and managing drainage tubes. These conditions are complex and often require assistance and support from an oncology nurse specialist. Comfort measures for women with ascites may include providing small frequent meals, decreasing fluid intake, administering diuretic agents, and providing rest. Patients with pleural effusion may experience shortness of breath, hypoxia, pleuritic chest pain, and cough. Thoracentesis is usually performed.

Hysterectomy

A total hysterectomy involves removing the uterus and the cervix. This procedure is performed for many conditions other than cancer, including dysfunctional uterine bleeding, endometriosis, nonmalignant growths, pelvic relaxation and prolapse, and previous injury to the uterus. Malignant conditions often require a total abdominal hysterectomy and bilateral salpingo-oophorectomy (removal of fallopian tubes and ovaries).

Laparoscopically assisted hysterectomy is performed by some physicians with excellent results and rapid recovery. This method is most often used for vaginal hysterectomy and is performed as a short-stay procedure or ambulatory surgery in carefully selected patients. Patients have a short hospital stay and a low incidence of postoperative infection.

In Canada, 22% of Canadian women aged 35 years and older (1.8 million) have had a hysterectomy. This rate is double those of Norway, England, Sweden, and the Netherlands (Canadian Women's Health Network, 2004). Newer techniques such as ablation therapy, embolization, and myomectomy exist, which may decrease the rate of hysterectomies.

PREOPERATIVE MANAGEMENT

The physical preparation of a patient undergoing a hysterectomy differs little from that of a patient undergoing a laparotomy. The lower half of the abdomen and the pubic and perineal regions may be shaved, and these areas are cleaned with soap and water (some surgeons do not require that the patient be shaved). The intestinal tract and the bladder need to be empty before the patient is taken to the operating room to prevent contamination and injury to the bladder or intestinal tract. An enema and antiseptic douche may be prescribed the evening before surgery, and the patient may be instructed to administer these treatments at home. Preoperative medications administered before surgery may help the patient relax.

POSTOPERATIVE MANAGEMENT

The principles of general postoperative care for abdominal surgery apply, with particular attention given to peripheral circulation to prevent thrombophlebitis and deep vein thrombosis (noting varicosities, promoting circulation with leg exercises, and using elastic compression stockings). Major risks are infection and hemorrhage. In addition, because the surgical site is close to the bladder, voiding problems may occur, particularly after a vaginal hysterectomy.

Edema or nerve trauma may cause temporary loss of bladder tone (bladder atony), and an indwelling catheter may be inserted. During surgery, the handling of the bowel may cause paralytic ileus and interfere with bowel functioning.

NURSING PROCESS: THE PATIENT UNDERGOING A HYSTERECTOMY

Assessment

The health history and the physical and pelvic examination are completed, and laboratory studies are performed. Additional assessment data include the patient's psychosocial responses, because the need for a hysterectomy may elicit strong emotional reactions. If the hysterectomy is performed to remove a malignant tumour, anxiety related to fear of cancer and its consequences adds to the stress of the patient and her family. These women may be at greater risk for psychological symptoms, physical symptoms, postmenopausal syndrome, and increased use of health care postoperatively. Other women note improved physical and mental health after hysterectomy.

Diagnosis

NURSING DIAGNOSES

Based on all the assessment data, the patient's major nursing diagnoses may include the following:

- Anxiety related to the diagnosis of cancer, fear of pain, possible perception of loss of femininity, and disfigurement
- Disturbed body image related to altered fertility and fears about sexuality and relationships with partner and family
- Acute pain related to surgery and other adjuvant therapy
- Deficient knowledge of the perioperative aspects of hysterectomy and postoperative self-care

COLLABORATIVE PROBLEMS/POTENTIAL COMPLICATIONS

Based on assessment data, potential complications may include the following:

- Hemorrhage
- Deep vein thrombosis
- Bladder dysfunction

Planning and Goals

The major goals for the patient may include relief of anxiety, acceptance of loss of the uterus, absence of pain or discomfort, increased knowledge of self-care requirements, and absence of complications.

Nursing Interventions

RELIEVING ANXIETY

Anxiety stems from several factors: unfamiliar environment, the effects of surgery on body image and reproductive ability, fear of pain and other discomfort, and, possibly, feelings of embarrassment about exposure of the genital area in the perioperative period. Conflicts between medical treatment and religious beliefs may arise as well. In such cases, the nurse needs to determine what the experience means to the patient and how to assist her in expressing her feelings. Throughout the pre- and postoperative and recovery periods, explanations are given about physical preparations and procedures that are performed.

Patient education addresses the outcomes of surgery, possible feelings of loss, and options for management of symptoms of menopause. Women vary in their preferences; many want a choice of treatment options, a part in decision making, accurate and useful information at the appropriate time, support from their health care providers, and access to professional and lay support systems.

Recent findings from the Women's Health Initiative study of hormone replacement therapy (HRT) have indicated that HRT does not have long-term cardiac benefits and may increase the risk for breast cancer (Humphries & Gill, 2003). Although HRT has some positive effects on bone density in women, many clinicians and women have concluded that the risks of HRT outweigh the benefits. If prescribed, HRT should be used for the shortest possible time interval (Women's Health Initiative, 2002). If the patient is considering beginning HRT, risks and benefits are discussed preoperatively and medication is started following surgery. Teaching is provided and the need for monitoring is emphasized.

IMPROVING BODY IMAGE

The patient may have strong emotional reactions to having a hysterectomy and strong personal feelings related to the diagnosis, views of significant others who may be involved (family, partner), religious beliefs, and fears about prognosis. Concerns such as the inability to have children and the effect on femininity may surface, as may questions about the effects of surgery on sexual relationships, function, and satisfaction. The patient needs reassurance that she will still have a vagina and that she can experience sexual intercourse after a temporary postoperative abstinence while tissues heal. Information that sexual satisfaction and orgasm arise from clitoral stimulation rather than from the uterus reassures many women. Most women note some change in sexual feelings after hysterectomy, but they vary in intensity. In some cases, the vagina is shortened by surgery, and this may affect sensitivity or comfort.

When a woman's hormonal balance is upset, as usually occurs in reproductive system disturbances, the patient may experience depression and heightened emotional sensitivity to people and situations. The nurse needs to approach and evaluate each patient individually in light of these factors. The nurse who exhibits interest, concern, and willingness to listen to the patient's fears will assist in the patient's progress throughout the surgical experience.

RELIEVING PAIN

A hysterectomy may be performed abdominally or vaginally. The surgeon bases this decision on the diagnosis and the size of the uterus. An abdominal approach is used when the patient has cancer or when the uterus is enlarged. Resultant pain and abdominal discomfort are common. Analgesic agents are administered as prescribed to relieve pain and promote movement and ambulation.

In some circumstances, a nasogastric tube may be inserted before the patient leaves the operating room to relieve discomfort from abdominal distention, especially if excessive handling of the viscera was required or if a large tumour was removed. Excision of a large tumour could cause edema because of the sudden release of pressure. In the postoperative period, fluids and food may be restricted for 1 or 2 days. If the patient has abdominal distention or flatus, a rectal tube and application of heat to the abdomen may be prescribed. When abdominal auscultation reveals return of bowel sounds and peristalsis, additional fluids and a soft diet are permitted. Early ambulation facilitates the return of normal peristalsis.

MONITORING AND MANAGING POTENTIAL COMPLICATIONS

Hemorrhage

Vaginal bleeding and hemorrhage may occur after hysterectomy. To detect these complications early, the nurse counts the perineal pads used, assesses the extent of saturation with blood, and monitors vital signs. Abdominal dressings are monitored for drainage if an abdominal surgical approach was used. In preparation for hospital discharge, the nurse gives prescribed guidelines for activity restrictions to promote healing and to prevent postoperative bleeding.

Deep Vein Thrombosis

Because of positioning during surgery, postoperative edema, and immobility, the patient is at risk for deep vein thrombosis and pulmonary embolus. To minimize the risk, elastic compression stockings are applied. Additionally, the patient is encouraged and assisted to change positions frequently, although pressure under patient will receive directions about safe times and distances related to care provision to ensure that their occupational exposure is as low as reasonably achievable (*Radiation Safety Institute of Canada*). Other instructions vary but may include the following:

- Wear film badges or pocket ion chambers to monitor exposure.
- Wear rubber gloves to dispose of any soiled matter that may be contaminated. (These gloves, however, do not provide protection from sealed radiation sources.)
- Provide specific laundry and housekeeping directions.
- Keep the patient restricted to her room and allow no visitors who are or may be pregnant or who are younger than 18 years of age.
- Explain that a discharge survey is usually performed by *Radiation Safety Institute of Canada* personnel before the patient leaves the room. The survey ensures that all sources of radiation have been removed.

NURSING PRIORITIES FOR PATIENT CARE
Of the many nursing concerns, primary concerns involve providing the patient with emotional support and physical comfort and not dislodging the applicator. Although the radiation oncologist takes steps to secure the internal applicator in place and nursing personnel need not be preoccupied with the fear that the applicator will be prematurely extruded, they should monitor to see that the applicator or the radioactive sources have not been dislodged. Should this happen, the nurse should avoid touching the radioactive object and notify the *Radiation Safety Institute of Canada* at once.

The nurse needs to explain that during the treatment, the patient must stay on absolute bed rest. She may move from side to side with her back supported by a pillow, and the head of the bed may be raised to 15 degrees. She should be encouraged to practice deep-breathing and coughing exercises and to flex and extend the feet to stretch the calf muscles, promoting circulation and venous return. Elastic compression stockings are important. Back care, though appreciated by the patient, needs to be performed within the minimal time allowed at the bedside.

Usually the patient receives a low-residue diet to prevent frequent bowel movements. In addition, a urinary catheter will be in place and must be inspected frequently to ensure that it drains properly. The chief hazard of improper drainage is that the bladder may become distended and its walls exposed to radiation. Although perineal care is not performed at this time, any profuse discharge should be reported immediately to the radiation oncologist or gynecologic surgeon.

Additional nursing interventions include observing the patient for temperature elevation, nausea, and vomiting. These symptoms should be reported because they may indicate such complications as infection or perforation.

Patient teaching includes informing the patient that abdominal fullness, cramping, backache, and the urge to void are normal feelings during therapy. Severe pain should not occur. Administering mild opioid agents, muscle relaxants, or sedative medications may be helpful.

APPLICATOR REMOVAL
The radiation oncologist calculates precisely the radiation dose. At the end of the prescribed period, the nurse may be requested to assist the physician in removing the applicator. Because the sources are afterloaded, they can be removed by the physician in the same manner as they were inserted. This does not require

local or general anesthesia and is performed in the patient's room. Medicating the patient with a mild sedative agent may be required, however, before the applicator is removed.

POST-TREATMENT CARE
Progressive ambulation is recommended after any period of enforced bed rest. Diet may be offered as tolerated. The patient may shower as soon as she wishes but should be instructed not to douche after removal of the applicator. Because the cervix may have been dilated, any chance of bacterial contamination should be minimized.

Both before and after treatment, nurses caring for patients undergoing radiation therapy need to assess any misconceptions about this mode of treatment that the patient and family may have. The oncology clinical nurse specialist may be a valuable resource for information and problem solving, if necessary. Resources for further clinical and patient information are listed at the end of Chapter 16.

Critical Thinking Exercises

1. Your 42-year-old patient has not received gynecologic care for the last 15 years but is currently seeking care for intermittent vaginal bleeding. When obtaining a history from her, you learn that her mother received diethylstilbestrol (DES) during her pregnancies. What implications does this have for care and follow-up of this patient?

2. A 22-year-old graduate student seeks care because of severe pelvic pain, fever, and vaginal discharge. She reports having multiple sex partners and says she never uses a condom during sex because she uses oral contraceptives. Her physician has informed her that her symptoms are those of pelvic inflammatory disease (PID), and she is admitted to the hospital for intravenous antibiotic agents. What nursing care is important for her to minimize the risk for complications and to prevent transmission to others? Design a teaching plan to address the short- and long-term implications of the diagnosis of PID.

3. Your 48-year-old patient is scheduled for a total hysterectomy. She tells you that she has a family history of breast cancer and both her mother and sister have osteoporosis. She asks you for advice about beginning hormone replacement therapy (HRT) because of her osteoporosis risk and to prevent hot flashes. How would you proceed, and what information would you give her?

4. A 68-year-old woman is undergoing surgery to treat cervical cancer. While she is in the operating room, her husband reveals his concerns that he and his wife will never be able to have sexual relations again because of her diagnosis and treatment. What approach would you take in discussing this with the patient and with her husband?

5. A 45-year-old woman is scheduled for surgery to repair a rectovaginal fistula. Twenty years ago she experienced a spinal cord injury that resulted in paralysis below the waist. Explain how you will modify pre- and postoperative nursing care in view of her disability. What discharge planning will be important for her?

REFERENCES AND SELECTED READINGS

Books

ACOG (2001). Compendium of Selected Publications. Washington, DC: Author.

American Cancer Society. (2002). *Cancer facts and figures.* Atlanta: Author.

Barakat, R., Bevers, M., Gershenson, D., & Hoskins, W. (2000). *M. D. Anderson Cancer Center and Memorial Sloan-Kettering Cancer Center handbook of gynecologic oncology.* London: Dunitz.

Bickley, L. S., & Szilagyi, P. (2003). *Bates' guide to physical examination and history taking* (8th ed.). Philadelphia: Lippincott Williams & Wilkins.

Canadian Cancer Society. (2005). *Uterine cancer: What do you need to know.* Toronto: Author.

Emans, J., Laufer, M., & Goldstein, D. (1998). *Pediatric and adolescent gynecology* (4th ed.). Philadelphia: Lippincott-Raven.

Goldman, J., & Hatch, M. (Eds.) (2000). *Women and health.* San Diego: Academic Press.

Holmes, K. K., Maidli, P. A., et al. (2000). *Sexually transmitted diseases.* New York: McGraw-Hill.

Kiviat, N., Kousky, L. A., et al. (2000). In K. K. Holmes, P. A. Maidli, et al. *Sexually transmitted diseases.* New York: McGraw-Hill.

Lenhard, R., Osteen, R., & Gansler, T. (2001). *American Cancer Society's clinical oncology.* Atlanta: American Cancer Society.

Moore-Higgs, G. (2000). *Women and cancer* (2nd ed.). Sudbury: Jones and Bartlett.

Public Health Agency of Canada. (2003). *Women's health surveillance report.* Ottawa: Canadian Institute for Health Information.

Public Health Agency of Canada. (2000). *Cervical cancer screening in Canada: 1998 surveillance report.* Ottawa: Author. Available at: www.phac-aspc.gc.ca/publicat/ccsic-dccuac/index.html. Retrieved December 1, 2005.

Public Health Agency of Canada. (1998). Sexually transmitted disease surveillance in Canada. 1995 Annual Report. *Canadian Communicable Disease Report, 24S1.* Available at: www.phac-aspc.gc.ca/publicat/ccdr-rmtc/98vol24/24sl/index.html. Retrieved December 1, 2005.

Ronald, A. R., & Peeling, R. W. (1993). Sexually transmitted infection: Their manifestations and links to infertility and reproductive illness. In *Understanding infertility: Risk factors affecting infertility* (pp. 1-131). Ottawa: Minister of Supply and Services.

Journals

Asterisks indicate nursing research articles.

General

Centers for Disease Control and Prevention (CDC) (2002). Sexually transmitted diseases treatment guidelines, 2002. *MMWR, Morbidity and Mortality Weekly Report, 51*(RR-6), 1–85.

*Czerwinski, B. (2000). Variation in feminine hygiene practices as a function of age. *JOGNN, 29*(6), 625–633.

Nelson, H. D., Hymprey, L. L., Nygren, P. et al. (2002). Postmenopausal hormone replacement therapy: Scientific review. *Journal of the American Medical Association, 288*(7), 872–881.

Public Health Agency of Canada. (2000). What everyone should know about human papillomavirus (HPV): Questions and answers. *STD Epi Updates.* Available at: www.phac-aspc.gc.ca/publicat/epiu-aepi/std-mts/hpv_e.html. Retrieved December 1, 2005.

Rein, D., Kasler, W., Irwin, K., & Rabiee, L. (2000). Direct medical cost of pelvic inflammatory disease and its sequelae: Decreasing but still substantial. *Obstetrics & Gynecology, 95*(3), 397–402.

Templeman, C., Fallat, M., Blinchevsky, A., & Hertweck, P. (2000). Noninflammatory ovarian masses in girls and young women. *Obstetrics & Gynecology, 96*(2), 229–233.

VanZandt, S. (2000). Pelvic pain in women. *Clinician Reviews, 10*(9), 51–64.

Women's Health Initiative (2002). Risks and benefits of estrogen plus progestin in healthy postmenopausal women: Principal results from the Women's Health Initiative randomized controlled trial. *Journal of the American Medical Association, 288*(3), 321–333.

Benign Vulvar Disorders

Haefner, H., & Pearlman, J. (1999). Diagnosing and managing vulvodynia. *Contemporary Obstetrics & Gynecology, 44*(2), 110–121.

Scrimmin, F., Rustja, S., Radillo, O., et al. (2000). Vulvar lichen sclerosus: An immunologic study. *Obstetrics & Gynecology, 95*(1), 147–150.

Endometriosis

American College of Obstetricians and Gynecologists. ACOG Committee on Practice Bulletins (2000). Medical management of endometriosis. *International Journal of Gynaecology & Obstetrics, 71*(2), 183–96.

Olive, D. L., & Pritts, E. A. (2001). Treatment of endometriosis. *New England Journal of Medicine, 345*(4), 266–275.

Propst, A., & Laufer, M. (1999). Diagnosing and treating adolescent endometriosis. *Contemporary Obstetrics & Gynecology, 44*(12), 52–59.

Winkel, C. (1999). Laparoscopy plus GnRH analogs: A practical approach to endometriosis. *Contemporary Obstetrics & Gynecology, 44*(4), 99–109.

Fibroids/Myomas

Chiaffarino, F., Parazzini, F., laVecchia, C., Chatenoud, L., & DeCintio, E. (1999). Diet and uterine myomas. *Obstetrics & Gynecology, 94*(3), 395–402.

Lethaby, A., Vollenhoven, B., & Sowter, M. (2000). Pre-operative gonadotropin-releasing hormone analogue before hysterectomy or myomectomy for uterine fibroids. *The Cochrane Library,* Issue 2: Oxford.

Lethaby, A., Shepperd, S., Cooke, I., & Farquhar, C. (2000). Endometrial resection and ablation versus hysterectomy for heavy menstrual bleeding. *The Cochrane Library,* Issue 2: Oxford.

Stringer, N. (2000). Pirfenidone and tibolone: Innovations in drug therapy for uterine fibroids. *Female Patient, 25*(5), 12–18.

Gynecologic Cancers (General)

Chan, Y. M., Ngan, H. Y., Yip, P. S., et al. (2001). Psychosocial adjustment in gynecologic cancer survivors: A longitudinal study on risk factors for maladjustment. *Gynecologic Oncology, 80*(3), 387–394.

Chan, Y. M., Ngan, H. Y., Li, B. Y., et al. (2001). A longitudinal study on quality of life after gynecologic cancer treatment. *Gynecologic Oncology, 83*(1), 10–19.

*Chan, C. W., Molassiotis, A., Yam, B. M., et al. (2001). Traveling through the cancer trajectory: Social support perceived by women with gynecologic cancer in Hong Kong. *Cancer Nursing, 24*(5), 387–394.

Dargent, D. F. (2001). Laparoscopic surgery in gynecologic oncology. *Surgical Clinics of North America, 81*(4), 949–964.

Dargent, D., Martin, X., Sacchetoni, A., & Mathevet, P. (2000). Laparoscopic vaginal radical trachelectomy: A treatment to preserve the fertility of cervical carcinoma patients. *Cancer, 88*(8), 1877–1882.

Duffy, M. S. (2001). Recent surgical approaches to gynecologic oncology. *Nursing Clinics of North America, 36*(3), 603–615.

*Foxall, M. J., Barron, C. R., & Houfek, J. F. (2001). Ethnic influences on body awareness, trait anxiety, perceived risk, and breast and gynecologic cancer screening practices. *Oncology Nursing Forum, 28*(4), 727–738.

Grigsby, P. W. (2002). Vaginal cancer. *Current Treatment Options in Oncology, 3*(2), 125–130.

*Kwekkeboom, K. L. (2001). Pain management strategies used by patients with breast and gynecologic cancer with postoperative pain. *Cancer Nursing, 24*(5), 378–386.

Mendez, L. E. (2001). Iatrogenic injuries in gynecologic cancer surgery. *Surgical Clinics of North America, 81*(4), 897–923.

Nordin, A. J., Chinn, D. J., & Moloney, I., et al. (2001). Do elderly cancer patients care about cure? Attitudes to radical gynecologic oncology surgery in the elderly. *Gynecologic Oncology, 81*(3), 447–455.

Pasacreta, J. V., Jabobs, L. & Cataldo, J. K. (2002). Genetic testing for breast and ovarian cancer risk: The psychosocial issues. *American Journal of Nursing, 102*(12), 40–47.

Pignata, S., Ballatori, E., Favalli, G., & Scambia, G. (2001). Quality of life: Gynaecological cancers. *Annals of Oncology, 12*(Suppl 3), S37-S42.

Plante, M., & Roy, M. (2001). New approaches in the surgical management of early-stage cervical cancer. *Current Opinion in Obstetrics and Gynecology, 13*(1), 41–46.

Sevin, B. U., & Koechli, O. R. (2001). Pelvic exenteration. *Surgical Clinics of North America, 81*(4), 771–779.

Shepherd, J. H., Mould, T., & Oram, D. H. (2001). Radical trachelectomy in early-stage carcinoma of the cervix: Outcome as judged by recurrence and fertility rates. *BJOG: International Journal of Obstetrics & Gynaecology, 108*(8), 882–885.

Swisher, E. M., Cohn, D. E., Goff, B. A., et al. (2002). Use of complementary and alternative medicine among women with gynecologic cancers. *Gynecologic Oncology, 84*(3), 363–367.

*Velji, K., & Fitch, M. (2001). The experience of women receiving brachytherapy for gynecologic cancer. *Oncology Nursing Forum, 28*(4), 743–751.

Herpes

Burkhart, C., & Burkhart, K. (2000). Primary care update: Brief summaries for clinical practice. How to cope with genital herpes. *Consultant, 40*(7), 1298–1301.

McClain, N., Cheung, K., Giardet, R., et al. (2000). Practice guidelines: Screening and treatment of sexually transmitted diseases: Part 2: trichomonas, human papillomavirus infection and genital herpes simplex virus. *Journal of Pediatric Health Care, 14*(3), 130–132.

Steben, M., & Sacks, S. L. (1997). Genital herpes: The epidemiology and control of a common sexually transmitted disease. *The Canadian Journal of Human Sexuality, 6*(2). Available at: www.hc-sc.gc.ca/hpb/lcdc/publicat/cjhs/cjhs5.html.

Swanson, J. (1999). The biopsychosocial burden of genital herpes: evidence-based and other approaches to care. *Dermatology Nursing, 11*(4), 257–270.

Swanson, J., Dibble, S., & Chapman, L. (1999). Effects of psychoeducational interventions on sexual health risks and psychosocial adaptation in young adults with genital herpes. *Journal of Advanced Nursing, 29*(4), 840–851.

Human Papillomavirus and HIV Infection

Davies, J. E. (2000). Hide and seek. Make sure HPV infection doesn't escape diagnosis. *Advance for Nurse Practitioners, 8*(9), 39–43.

Dell, D., Chen, H., Ahmad, F., & Stewart, D. (2000). Knowledge about human papillomavirus among adolescents. *Obstetrics & Gynecology, 96*(5, Part 1), 653–656.

French, L., Nashelsky, J., & White D. (2002). What is the most effective treatment for external genital warts? *Journal of Family Practice, 51*(4), 313.

Hader, S. L., Smith, D. K., Moore, J. S., & Holmberg, S. D. (2001). HIV infection in the United States: Status at the millennium. *Journal of the American Medical Association, 285*(9), 1186–1192.

Health Canada. (2004). *Human papillomavirus (HPV). It's your health.* Available at: www.hc-sc.gc.ca/english/iyh/diseases/hpv-vph_e.html. Retrieved December 1, 2005.

Mosicki, A. B., Hills, N., Shiboski, S., et al. (2001). Risks for incident human papillomavirus infection and low-grade squamous intraepithelial lesion development in young females. *Journal of the American Medical Association, 285*(23), 2995–3002.

Naomi, J., & Moscicki, A. (2000). Human papillomavirus infections in women with HIV disease: Prevalence, risk and management. *The AIDS Reader, 10*(11), 659–668.

Sellors, J. W., Mahony, J. B., Kaczorowski, J., et al. (2000). Prevalence and predictors of human papillomavirus infection in women in Ontario, Canada. *CMAJ: Canadian Medical Association Journal, 163*(5), 503–508.

Hysterectomy

Broder, M., Kanouse, D., Mittman, B., & Bernstein, S. (2000). The appropriateness of recommendations for hysterectomy. *Obstetrics & Gynecology, 95*(2), 199–204.

Brooks-Brunn, J. (2000). Risk factors associated with postoperative pulmonary complications following total abdominal hysterectomy. *Clinical Nursing Research, 9*(1), 27–46.

Kjerulff, K., Langenberg, P., Rhodes, J., et al. (2000). Effectiveness of hysterectomy. *Obstetrics & Gynecology, 95*(3), 319–326.

Lewis, C., Groff, J., Herman, C., et al. (2000). Overview of women's decision making regarding elective hysterectomy, oophorectomy and hormone replacement therapy. *Journal of Women's Health and Gender-Based Medicine, 9*(Suppl 2), 5–14.

Moreira, V. (2000). Learning curve: Hysterectomy, nursing the physical and emotional wounds. *Nursing Times, 96*(20), 41–42.

*Wade, J., Pletsch, P., Morgan, S., & Menting, S. (2000). Hysterectomy: What do women need and want to know? *JOGNN, 29*(1), 33–42.

Winston, K. (2000). Reflections on women's health. In my shoes: a story about hysterectomy. *AWHONN Lifelines, 4*(2), 64–66.

Pelvic Inflammatory Disease (PID)

*Champion, J. D., Piper, J. N., Shain, R. N., et al. (2001). Minority women with sexually transmitted diseases: Sexual abuse and risk for pelvic inflammatory disease. *Research in Nursing & Health, 24*(1), 38–43.

Molitor, L. (2001). A 26-year-old woman with right shoulder pain. *Journal of Emergency Nursing, 27*(4), 404–405.

Ness, R. B., Soper, D. E., Holley, R. L., et al. (2001*a*). Douching and endometritis: Results from the PID evaluation and clinical health (PEACH) study. *Sexually Transmitted Diseases, 28*(4), 240–245.

Ness, R. B., Soper, D. E., Holley, R. L., et al. (2001*b*). Hormonal and barrier contraception and risk of upper genital tract disease in the PID Evaluation and Clinical Health (PEACH) study. *American Journal of Obstetrics & Gynecology, 185*(1), 121–127.

Ness, R. B., Soper, D. E., Holley, R. L., et al. (2001*c*). Effectiveness of inpatient and outpatient treatment strategies for women with pelvic inflammatory disease: Results from the Pelvic Inflammatory Disease Evaluation and Clinical Health (PEACH) Randomized Trial. *American Journal of Obstetrics & Gynecology. 186*(5), 929–937.

Peipert, J. F., Ness, R. B., Blume, J., et al. (2001). Clinical predictors of endometritis in women with symptoms and signs of pelvic inflammatory disease. *American Journal of Obstetrics & Gynecology, 184*(5), 856–863.

Ross, J. (2001). Pelvic inflammatory disease. *British Medical Journal, 322*(7287), 658–659.

Wong, T., Singh, A., Mann J., et al. (2004). Gender differences in bacterial STIs in Canada. *BMC Women's Health 2004, 4* (Suppl 1): S26.

Reproductive Malignancy

American College of Obstetricians and Gynecologists. (2001). ACOG committee opinion: Tamoxifen and endometrial cancer. *International Journal of Gynaecology & Obstetrics. 73*(1), 77–79.

American College of Obstetricians and Gynecologists. (2000). ACOG committee opinion: Breast-ovarian cancer screening. *International Journal of Gynaecology & Obstetrics. 75*(3), 339–340.

Cottreau, C., Ness, R., & Kriska, A. (2000). Physical activity and reduced risk of ovarian cancer. *Obstetrics & Gynecology, 96*(4), 609–614.

Furniss, K. (2000). Tomatoes, Pap smears and tea? Adopting behaviors that may prevent reproductive cancers and improve health. *JOGNN, 29*(6), 641–652.

Humphries K. H., Gill, S. (2003). Risk and benefits of hormone replacement therapy: The evidence speaks. *Canadian Medical Association Journal, 168*(8), 1001–1010.

Lammers, S., Schaefer, K., Ladd, E., & Echenberg, R. (2000). Caring for women living with ovarian cancer: Recommendations for advanced practice nurses. *JOGNN, 29*(6), 567–573.

Lowdermilk, D., & Germino, B. (2000). Helping women and their families cope with the impact of gynecologic cancer. *JOGNN, 29*(6), 653–660.

Marchbanks, P., Hoyt, W., Bastos, E., et al. (2000). Cigarette smoking and epithelial ovarian cancer by histologic type. *Obstetrics & Gynecology, 95*(2), 255–260.

Massad, L., Abu-Rustum, N., Lee, S., & Renta, V. (2000). Poor compliance with postmolar surveillance and treatment protocols by indigent women. *Obstetrics and Gynecology, 96*(6), 940–944.

Montz, F. (2000). Management of high-grade cervical intraepithelial neoplasia and low-grade squamous intraepithelial lesion and potential complications. *Clinical Obstetrics & Gynecology, 43*(2), 394–409.

National Institutes of Health (NIH) (1996). *NIH consensus statement: Cervical cancer. 14*(1), 1–38.

Olopade, O., & Cummings, S. (2000). Breast and ovarian cancer: Counseling patients about risk. *Consultant, 40*(11), 1930–1940.

Santoso, J., Canada, T., Latson, B., et al. (2000). Prognostic nutritional index in relation to hospital stay in women with gynecologic cancer. *Obstetrics and Gynecology, 95*(6 Pt 1), 844–846.

Toxic Shock Syndrome

Hajjeh, R., Reingold, A., Weil, A., et al., (1999). Toxic shock syndrome in the United States: Surveillance update, 1979–1996. *Emerging Infectious Diseases, 5*(6), 807–810.

Nakase, J. (2000). Update on emerging infections from the Centers for Disease Control and Prevention. *Annals of Emergency Medicine, 36*(3), 269–270.

Vaginitis and Vulvovaginal Infections

Cullins, V., Dominguez, L., Guberski, T., et al. (1999). Treating vaginitis. *Nursing Practice, 24*(10), 46–50.

Harmanli, O., Cheng, G., Nyirjesy, P., et al. (2000). Urinary tract infections in women with bacterial vaginosis. *Obstetrics & Gynecology, 95*(5), 710–712.

Hutti, M., & Hoffman, C. (2000). Pearls for practice: Cytolytic vaginosis: An overlooked cause of cyclic vaginal itching and burning. *Journal of the American Academy of Nursing Practice, 12*(2), 55–57.

*Lowe, N., & Ryan-Wenger, N. (2000). A clinical test of women's self-diagnosis of genitourinary infections. *Clinical Nursing Research, 9*(2), 144–160.

Paavonen, J., Mangioni, C., Martin, M., & Wajszcuk, C. (2000). Vaginal clindamycin and oral metronidazole for bacterial vaginosis: A randomized trial. *Obstetrics & Gynecology, 96*(2), 256–260.

Sobel, J. (2000). Managing vulvovaginal candidiasis. *Female Patient, 5*(5), 20–23.

Witkin, S., & Giraldo, P. (2000). The quandary of recurrent vaginal candidiasis. *Patient Care, 34*(2), 123–126.

RESOURCES AND WEBSITES

American Social Health Association, P.O. Box 13827, Research Triangle Park, NC 27709; (800) 227-8922; http://www.ashastd.org/std/std.html; teen website: http://www.iwannaknow.org.

American Social Health Association Herpes Hotline; (919) 361-8488; www.ashastd.org/hotlines/herphotline.html.

Association of Reproductive Health Professionals, 2401 Pennsylvania Avenue, Suite 350, Washington, DC 20037-1718; (202) 466-3825; http://www.arhp.org.

AWHONN: Association of Women's Health, Obstetrical and Neonatal Nurses, 2000 L St., NW, Suite 7400, Washington, DC 20036; http://www.awhonn.org.

Canadian Cancer Society/Société Canadienne du Cancer, National Office, Suite 200, 10 Alcorn Avenue, Toronto, ON M4V 3B1; (416) 961-7223; fax: (416) 961-4189; www.cancer.ca.

Canadian HIV/AIDS Information Centre; www.aidssida.cpha.ca.

Cancer Journey: Issues for Survivors. A leader's guide and videotape available from the National Cancer Institute (1-800-4-CANCER)

Centers for Disease Control and Prevention, Office of Women's Health, 1600 Clifton Road, MS: D-51, Atlanta, GA 30033; (404) 639-7230; http://www.cdc.gov/od/owh/whstd.htm.

Endometriosis Association, International Headquarters, 8585 N. 76th Place, Milwaukee, WI 53223 USA; (414) 355-2200; fax: (414) 355-6065; www.endometriosisassn.org.

Endometriosis Support Network, London, Inc.; http://endosisters.ca.

Gay and Lesbian Medical Association, 459 Fulton St., Suite 107, San Francisco, CA 94102; (415) 225-4547; http://www.glma.org/home.html.

Gay and Lesbian Medical Association (GLMA); www.glma.org.

Health Canada, Bureau of Women's Health and Gender Analysis; www.hc-sc.gc.ca/english/women.

Healthy People 2010; www.healthypeople.gov.

Herpes Hotline: (919) 361-8488.

Herpetics Engaged in Living Productively (HELP), 260 Sheridan Avenue, Palo Alto, CA 94306.

Infertility Awareness Association of Canada (IAAC), 2100 Marlowe Avenue, Suite 39 Montreal, QC H4A 3L5; (514) 484-2891; fax: (514) 484-0454; toll-free info line: 1-800-263-2929; email: info@iaac.ca; http://iaac.ca.

National Cancer Institute of Canada/Institut National du Cancer du Canada, 10 Alcorn Avenue, Suite 200, Toronto, ON M4V 3B1; (416) 961-7223; fax: (416) 961-4189; www.ncic.cancer.ca.

Planned Parenthood Federation of Canada, 1 Nicholas Street, Suite 430, Ottawa, ON K1N 7B7; (613) 241-4474; www.ppfc.ca.

Provincial and territorial STI/HIV/AIDS helpline telephone numbers; www.phac-aspc.gc.ca/std-mts/phone_e.html.

Radiation Safety Institute of Canada, National Education Centre–Toronto, 1120 Finch Avenue West, Suite 607, Toronto, ON M3J 3H7; (416) 650-9090; toll-free: 1-800-263-5803; fax: (416) 650-9920; www.radiationsafety.ca.

Sunnybrook and Women's College Health Sciences Centre, Women's Health Matters; www.womenshealthmatters.ca.

The College of Family Physicians of Canada Patient Information: *STIs (Sexually Transmitted Infections–Common STIs and tips on prevention*; www.cfpc.ca/English/cfpc/programs/patient%20education/sti/default.asp?s=1.

The Society of Obstetricians and Gynaecologists of Canada; http://sogc.medical.org/sogcnet/index_e.shtml.

Assessment and Management of Patients With Breast Disorders

Adapted by Jean Chow

LEARNING OBJECTIVES

On completion of this chapter, the learner will be able to:

1. Develop a teaching plan for breast self-examination for patients and consumer groups.
2. Describe the diagnostic tests used to detect breast disorders.
3. Use the nursing process as a framework for care of the patient with breast cancer.
4. Compare the therapeutic effectiveness of chemotherapy, surgery, and radiation therapy in treating breast cancer.
5. Describe the physical, psychosocial, and rehabilitative needs of the patient who has had breast surgery for the treatment of breast cancer.

In many cultures, the breast plays a significant role in a woman's sexuality and identification of herself as female. Although advances in the diagnosis and treatment of breast disorders are changing the prognosis for breast disease and cancer, women's responses to possible breast disease include fear of disfigurement and loss of sexual attractiveness and fear of death. The woman with breast disease may undergo diagnostic testing, surgery, radiation therapy, chemotherapy, and hormonal therapy. Thus, nurses caring for patients with breast disease must have an in-depth understanding of these treatment modalities and expert assessment and clinical skills to address the physical and psychological needs of patients facing breast disorders, and their families.

Anatomic and Physiologic Overview

In males and females, the breasts are the same until puberty, when estrogen and other hormones initiate breast development in females. This development usually occurs at about age 10 years and continues until about age 16 years, although the range can vary from 9 to 18 years. Stages of breast development are described as Tanner stages 1 through 5. Stage 1 describes a prepubertal breast. Stage 2 is breast budding, the first sign of puberty in a female. Stage 3 involves further enlargement of breast tissue and the areola (a darker tissue ring around the nipple), and stage 4 occurs when the nipple and areola form a secondary mound on top of the breast tissue. Stage 5 is the continued development of a larger breast with a single contour.

The breast contains glandular (parenchyma) and ductal tissue, along with fibrous tissue that binds the lobes together and fatty tissue in and between the lobes. These paired mammary glands are located between the second and sixth ribs over the pectoralis major muscle from the sternum to the midaxillary line. An area of breast tissue, called the tail of Spence, extends into the axilla. Cooper's ligaments, which are fascial bands, support the breast on the chest wall. Figure 48-1 shows the anatomy of the fully developed breast.

Each breast consists of 12 to 20 cone-shaped lobes that are made up of lobules containing clusters of acini, small structures ending in a duct. All of the ducts in each lobule empty into an ampulla, which then opens onto the nipple after narrowing. About 85% of the breast is fat.

Glossary

atypical hyperplasia: abnormal increase in the number of cells in a specific area within the ductal or lobular areas of the breast; this abnormal proliferation increases the risk for cancer

benign proliferative breast disease: various types of atypical, yet noncancerous, breast tissue that increase the risk for breast cancer

BRCA-1: gene on chromosome 17 that, when damaged or mutated, places a woman at greater risk for breast or ovarian cancer, or both, compared with women who do not have the mutation

BRCA-2: gene on chromosome 17 that, when damaged or mutated, places a woman at greater risk for breast cancer (though less so than BRCA-1) compared with women who do not have the mutation

breast-conservation therapy: surgery to remove a breast tumour and a margin of tissue around the tumour without removing any other part of the breast; may include an axillary lymph node dissection, radiation therapy, or both

breast self-examination (BSE): technique for checking one's own breasts for lumps or suspicious changes

ductal carcinoma in situ (DCIS): cancer cells that start in the ductal system of the breast but have not penetrated the surrounding tissue

estrogen and progesterone receptor assay: test to determine whether the breast tumour is nourished by hormones; this information is useful in making a prognosis and determining treatment

fibrocystic breast changes: term used to describe certain benign changes in the breast, typically associated with palpable nodularity, lumpiness, swelling, or pain

fine-needle aspiration (FNA): the removal of fluid for diagnostic analysis from a cyst or cells from a mass using a needle and syringe

galactography: use of mammography after an injection of radiopaque dye to diagnose problems in the ductal system of the breast

gynecomastia: overdeveloped breast tissue typically seen in adolescent boys

lobular carcinoma in situ (LCIS): an atypical change and proliferation of the lobular cells of the breast; previously considered a premalignant condition but now considered a marker of increased risk for invasive breast cancer

lymphatic mapping and sentinel node biopsy: procedure using radiopaque dye and nuclear medicine techniques to identify and analyze the first draining lymph node from the breast within the axillary region

lymphedema: chronic swelling of an extremity due to interrupted lymphatic circulation, typically from an axillary dissection

mammography: an x-ray of the breast; the principal method of screening for and detection of breast cancer in women

mammoplasty: surgical procedure to reconstruct or change the size or shape of the breast; can be done for reduction or augmentation

mastalgia: breast pain, usually related to hormonal fluctuations or irritation of a nerve

mastitis: inflammation or infection of the breast

medullary carcinoma: special type of infiltrating breast cancer in which the tumour is well defined, with obvious boundaries

modified radical mastectomy: removal of the breast tissue, nipple–areola complex, and a portion of the axillary lymph nodes

Paget's disease: form of breast cancer that begins in the ductal system and involves the nipple, areola, and surrounding skin

prophylactic mastectomy: removal of the breast to reduce the risk for or to prevent the development of breast cancer in women considered at high risk

stereotactic biopsy: computer-guided method of core needle biopsy that is useful when masses in the breast cannot be felt but can be visualized using mammography

surgical biopsy: procedure in which tissue samples or the entire specimen is removed for examination under a microscope by a pathologist

tissue expander with permanent implant: series of surgical procedures used to reconstruct the breast after a mastectomy; involves stretching the skin and muscle before inserting the permanent implant

total mastectomy: removal of the breast tissue and nipple–areola complex, typically used as one type of treatment for DCIS

transverse rectus abdominis myocutaneous flap (TRAM flap): method of breast reconstruction in which adipose tissue and muscle from the lower abdomen, along with their circulatory structures, are transferred to the mastectomy site

ultrasonography: imaging method using high-frequency sound waves to diagnose whether masses are solid or fluid-filled

wire needle localization: procedure used to perform a breast biopsy when the lump is difficult to palpate but can be visualized using mammography; a wire is inserted into the breast tissue under mammographic visualization, and the surgeon then removes the tissue surrounding the wire

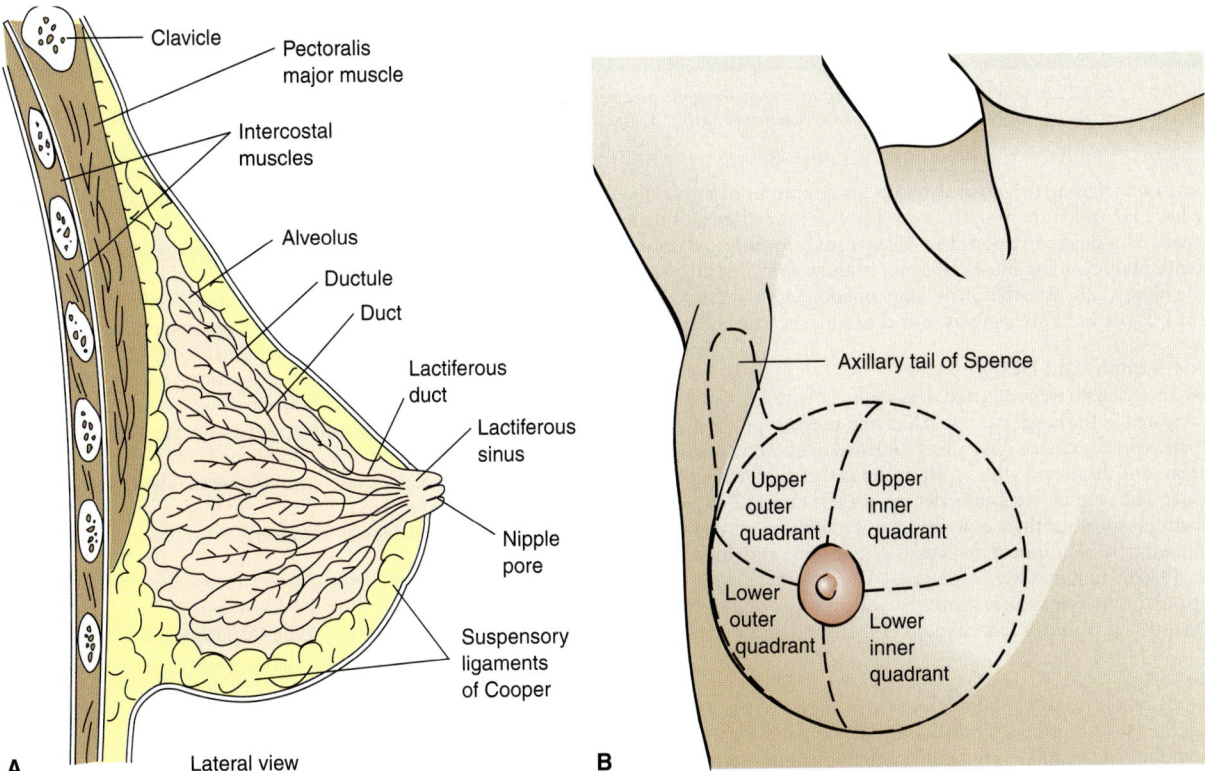

FIGURE 48-1 (**A**) Anatomy of the breast. (**B**) Areas of breast, including the tail of Spence. Adapted from Weber, J., & Kelley, J. (2003). *Health assessment in nursing* (2nd ed). Philadelphia: Lippincott Williams & Wilkins.

Assessment

HEALTH HISTORY AND CLINICAL MANIFESTATIONS

When assessing a patient who describes a breast problem, the nurse should ask the woman when she noted the problem and how long it has been present. Other questions include: Is pain associated with the symptom, and can you feel any areas in your breast that are of concern? What are your **breast self-examination** (BSE) practices? Have you had a mammogram or any other screening or diagnostic tests? If so, when? What follow-up recommendations were made?

The woman is asked about her reproductive history because of its relationship to risk for breast disorders. Questions should include the woman's age at menarche, last menstrual period, cycle regularity, and use of oral contraceptives or other hormone products. Other necessary information includes her history of pregnancies, live births, abortions, or miscarriages, and breastfeeding. If the patient is postmenopausal, her age at menopause and any symptoms she experienced and current or previous use of hormone replacement therapy are also addressed.

General health assessment includes the patient's use of tobacco and alcohol. Her medical and surgical history is important to obtain, along with any family history of diseases, particularly cancer. Social information, such as marital status, occupation, and the availability of resources and support persons, should also be elicited.

Psychosocial Implications of Breast Disease

Because of the significant role of the breast in a woman's sexuality, responses to any actual or suspected disease may include fear, anxiety, and depression. Specific responses may include fears of

disfigurement, loss of sexual attractiveness, abandonment by her partner, and death. These fears may cause some women to delay seeking health care for evaluation of a possible breast problem. Alternatively, in some women anxiety or fear regarding breast cancer may cause them to seek the services of a health care provider for the slightest change or problem.

In response to these reactions, the nurse's role is to identify the patient's concerns, anxieties, and fears. Patient education and psychosocial support become key nursing interventions. Assessment of the woman's concerns related to breast care and her responses to a potential problem is important whether the problem is benign or potentially malignant. Nurses can help women through the potentially frightening visit to the primary health care provider or surgeon. Because of underlying fears about a breast problem, anxiety management is a valuable intervention, and the nurse's calm, caring demeanor, along with astute listening skills and concrete direction and guidance, can decrease a woman's anxiety during the process.

PHYSICAL ASSESSMENT: FEMALE BREAST

Examination of the female breast can be conducted during any general physical or gynecologic examination or whenever the patient suspects, reports, or fears breast disease. A clinical breast examination is recommended at least every 3 years for women ages 20 to 40 years, and then annually. A thorough breast examination, including instruction in BSE, takes at least 10 minutes.

Inspection

Examination begins with inspection. The patient disrobes to the waist and sits in a comfortable position facing the examiner. The breasts are inspected for size and symmetry. A slight variation in

NURSING RESEARCH PROFILE 48-1

Undergoing Diagnosis for Breast Disease

Poole, K., & Lyne, P. A. (2000). The 'cues' to diagnosis: Describing the monitoring activities of women undergoing diagnostic investigations for breast disease. *Journal of Advanced Nursing, 31*(4), 752–758.

Purpose

Women undergoing diagnostic workup for symptoms of breast disease have identified the process as very stressful for them and their partners. This qualitative portion of a larger study investigated the experience of undergoing fine-needle biopsy and waiting for the results of the biopsy. The transactional theory of stress, appraisal, and coping of Lazarus and Folkman served as the framework for the study.

Study Sample and Design

Focus interviews were conducted with a subset of the 235 women who participated in the larger study and had fine-needle aspirations at two outpatient breast clinics. The subset consisted of 40 women; 20 of the women were diagnosed with breast cancer and 20 with benign breast disease. The women were interviewed in their homes 2 to 3 weeks post-diagnosis about their experiences from discovery of their breast abnormality to the time of diagnosis. The interviews, which ranged from 30 to 90 minutes, were audiotaped. Categories of themes emerging from the interviews were generated: the discovery of the breast abnormality and women's reflections after receiving biopsy results.

Findings

Analysis of the transcripts revealed four different types of threat-related cues during the diagnostic period: temporal, interpersonal, procedural, and spatial. Temporal cues identified by women in the study were those related to time. For example, the amount of time from referral by the primary care practitioner to the specialist breast unit was perceived by women as an indicator of the urgency of their problem; the quicker the referral, the greater urgency they perceived their problem to have. Interpersonal cues identified by the women were words, actions, gestures, or pauses in conversation by health care personnel. Active identification and interpretation of interpersonal cues by women were linked to uncertainty and lack of control during the diagnostic process. Procedural cues were those associated with the aspects of how the biopsy and other diagnostic procedures were performed. For example, the need to repeat an x-ray or the refusal of the radiologist to let the patient see the mammogram were taken as cues of a likely diagnosis of cancer. Spatial cues were those in which women interpreted usually uneventful aspects in the environment as indicative of their diagnosis. For example, one women interpreted the actions of health care personnel in arranging the chairs in the room in a certain way as she entered as indicative of the fact that they were about to inform her of a diagnosis of cancer.

Nursing Implications

These findings, described by the researchers as monitoring activities on the part of women undergoing diagnostic assessment for breast cancer, suggest the need women have to know their diagnosis and to reduce their uncertainty about the diagnosis. The stress associated with misinterpretation of these cues suggests the need for nurses and other health care providers to provide women with accurate and timely information to minimize their possible misinterpretation of behaviours. Nurses can help patients understand what time frames exist within the institution and explain the routines involved with the process of undergoing evaluation for a breast lump.

---

the size of each breast is common and generally normal. The skin is inspected for colour, venous pattern, and thickening or edema. Erythema (redness) may indicate benign local inflammation or superficial lymphatic invasion by a neoplasm. A prominent venous pattern can signal increased blood supply required by a tumour. Edema and pitting of the skin may result from a neoplasm blocking lymphatic drainage and giving the skin an orange-peel appearance (peau d'orange), a classic sign of advanced breast cancer. Examples of abnormal breast findings can be found in Chart 48-1.

Although the appearance of the nipple–areola complex varies greatly between patients, for individual women the two are generally similar in size and shape. Inversion of one or both is not uncommon and is a significant finding only when of recent origin. Ulceration, rashes, or spontaneous nipple discharge requires evaluation. To elicit a dimpling or retraction that may otherwise go undetected, the examiner instructs the patient to raise both arms overhead. This manoeuvre normally elevates both breasts equally. Next, the patient is instructed to place her hands at her waist and push in. These movements, causing contraction of the pectoral muscles, do not normally alter the breast contour or nipple direction. Any dimpling or retraction during these position changes may suggest a potential malignancy. Then with the patient bending forward, the examiner looks for asymmetry or retraction. The skin beneath the breast is inspected for rashes or excoriation. The clavicular and axillary regions are inspected for swelling, discolouration, lesions, or enlarged lymph nodes.

Palpation

Palpation of the clavicular and axillary areas is easily performed with the patient seated. Using finger pads (top one third of fingers), the examiner palpates the infraclavicular nodes below the clavicle in the 1st interspace on each side, and then the supraclavicular nodes above the clavicle bilaterally. To examine the axillary lymph nodes, the examiner slightly abducts the patient's arm from the thorax. The patient's left forearm is grasped gently and supported with the examiner's left hand. The right hand is then free to palpate the axillae and note any lymph nodes that may be lying against the thoracic wall. The positions are reversed for the right axilla. The finger pads are used to gently palpate the areas of the central, lateral, subscapular, and pectoral nodes (Fig. 48-2). Usually, these lymph nodes are not palpable, but if they are enlarged, their size, location, mobility, consistency, and tenderness are noted. Patients with large breasts are again asked to bend forward. The examiner performs a bimanual examination by palpating each breast between her or his hands.

The patient is then assisted to a supine position with no pillow under the head. A small pillow or folded towel is placed under the patient's shoulder on the side to be examined to balance the breast on the chest wall. Some examiners use a pillow under the shoulder only if the breast is large and needs to be spread more evenly over the chest. Systematic palpation includes the entire surface of the breast and the axillary tail from below the clavicles to 3 cm below the breasts, and from the midaxillary line to midsternal line. The examiner uses the flat part of the four fingers to make small circles while staying in contact with the skin. One approach is to move in imaginary rows horizontally or vertically over the area (Bickley & Szilagyi, 2003). This provides the most systematic examination for detecting breast masses. The examiner may choose to proceed in a clockwise direction, following imaginary concentric circles from the outer limits of the breast toward the nipple or palpate from each number on the face of the clock toward the nipple in a clockwise fashion (Fig. 48-3).

Chart 48-1 • ASSESSMENT

Abnormal Breast Findings

Retraction Signs
- Signs include skin dimpling, creasing, or changes in the contour of the breast or nipple
- Secondary to fibrosis or scar tissue formation in the breast
- Retraction signs may appear only with position changes or with breast palpation.

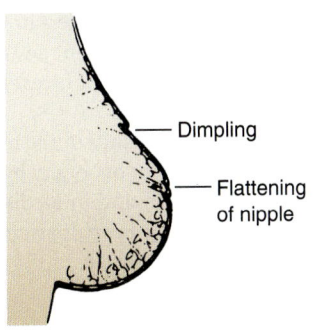

Dimpling

Flattening of nipple

Retraction signs   Retraction with compression

Breast Cancer Mass (Malignant Tumour)
- Usually occurs as a single mass (lump) in one breast
- Usually nontender
- Irregular shape
- Firm, hard, embedded in surrounding tissue
- Referral and biopsy indicated for definitive diagnosis

Breast cancer mass

Breast Cyst (Benign Mass of Fibrocystic Disease)
- Occur as single or multiple lumps in one or both breasts
- Usually tender (omitting caffeine reduces tenderness); tenderness increases during premenstrual period
- Round shape
- Soft or firm, mobile
- Referral and biopsy indicated for definitive diagnosis, especially for first mass; later masses may be evaluated over time by a specialist

Breast cysts

Fibroadenoma (Benign Breast Lump)
- Usually occurs as a single mass in women aged 15–35 years
- Usually nontender
- May be round or lobular
- Firm, mobile, and not fixed to breast tissue or chest wall
- No premenstrual changes
- Referral and biopsy indicated for definitive diagnosis

Fibroadenoma

Increased Venous Prominence
- Associated with breast cancer if unilateral
- Unilateral localized increase in venous pattern associated with malignant tumours
- Normal with breast enlargement associated with pregnancy and lactation if bilateral and bilateral symmetry

Increased venous prominence

Peau d'Orange (Edema)
- Associated with breast cancer
- Caused by interference with lymphatic drainage
- Breast skin has orange peel appearance
- Skin pores enlarge
- May be noted on the areola
- Skin becomes thick, hard, immobile
- Skin discolouration may occur

Peau d'orange

Nipple Inversion
- Considered normal if long-standing
- Associated with fibrosis and malignancy if recent development

Nipple inversion

Acute Mastitis (Inflammation of the Breasts)
- Associated with lactation but may occur at any age
- Nipple cracks or abrasions noted
- Breast skin reddened and warm to touch
- Tenderness
- Systemic signs include fever and increased pulse

Paget's Disease (Malignancy of Mammary Ducts)
- Early signs: erythema of nipple and areola
- Late signs: thickening, scaling, and erosion of the nipple and areola

Paget's disease

FIGURE 48-2 Palpating for central axillary nodes.

During palpation, the examiner notes tissue consistency, patient-reported tenderness, or masses. If a mass is detected, it is described by its location (eg, left breast, 2 cm from the nipple at 2 o'clock position). Size, shape, consistency, border delineation, and mobility are included in the description. Then the nipple and aureola are gently palpated. Squeezing the areola to detect discharge or secretion is not generally recommended.

The breast tissue of the adolescent is usually firm and lobular, whereas that of the postmenopausal woman is more likely to feel thinner and more granular. During pregnancy and lactation, the breasts are firmer and larger, with lobules that are more distinct. Hormonal changes cause the areola to darken. Cysts are commonly found in menstruating women and are usually well defined and freely movable. Premenstrually, cysts may be larger and more tender. Malignant tumours, on the other hand, tend to be hard, the consistency of a pencil eraser, poorly defined, fixed to the skin or underlying tissue, and usually nontender. A physician should evaluate any abnormalities detected during inspection and palpation.

PHYSICAL ASSESSMENT: MALE BREAST

Because breast cancer can occur in men, examination of the male breast and axillae is an important part of physical assessment. The nipple and areola are inspected for masses. Most cancers in men are found at a later stage, possibly because men are not aware of their risk for developing breast cancer. Treatment of breast cancer in males is similar as well.

Gynecomastia (overdeveloped mammary glands in the male) is differentiated from the soft, fatty enlargement of obesity by the firm enlargement of glandular tissue beneath and immediately surrounding the areola. The same procedure for palpating the female axillae is used when assessing the male axillae.

Diagnostic Evaluation

BREAST SELF-EXAMINATION

BSE instruction can be performed during assessment as part of the physical examination; it can be taught in any setting, either to individuals or groups. Instructions about BSE are provided to men if they have a family history of breast cancer because these men may be at higher risk for male breast cancer.

Variations in breast tissue occur during the menstrual cycle, pregnancy, and menopause. Therefore, expected changes must be distinguished from those that may signal disease. Most women notice increased tenderness and lumpiness before their menstrual period; therefore, BSE is best performed 7 days from the start of the last menstrual period, when less fluid is retained. Also, many women have grainy-textured breast tissue, but these areas are usually less nodular after menses.

Because women themselves detect many breast cancers, priority is given to teaching all women how and when to examine their breasts (Chart 48-2). It is estimated that only 25% to 30% of women perform BSE proficiently and regularly each month.

FIGURE 48-3 Breast palpation parameters: Below clavicle to 3 cm below breast; midaxillary line to midsternal line on each side. Breast palpation patterns: Palpate in small circles along horizontal strips, vertical strips, circular lines, and wedge strips. Adapted from Weber, J. & Kelley, J. (2003). *Health assessment in nursing* (2nd ed.). Philadelphia: Lippincott Williams & Wilkins, and Skillen, D. L., & Day, R. A. (Eds.). (2004). *A syllabus for adult health assessment*. Edmonton, AB: Faculty of Nursing, University of Alberta.

Chart 48-2 • PATIENT EDUCATION
Breast Self-Examination (BSE)

Step 1
1. Stand before a mirror.
2. Check both breasts for anything un-usual.
3. Look for discharge from the nipple, puckering, dimpling, or scaling of the skin.

The next two steps are done to check for any changes in the contour of your breasts. As you do them, you should be able to feel your muscles tighten.

Step 2
1. Watch closely in the mirror as you clasp your hands behind your head and press your hands together.
2. Note any change in the contour of your breasts.

Step 4
1. Raise your left arm.
2. Use the flat part (top one third of finger) of four fingers of your right hand to feel the left side of your chest and your left breast firmly, carefully, and thoroughly.
3. Beginning below your collarbone at the middle of your chest, press the flat part of your fingers in small circles, moving back and forth across the chest or up and down the chest along imaginary lines.
4. Be sure to cover from below collarbone to 3 cm below breast, from the centre of your chest to the opposite side. This includes all the breast tissue and the nipple.
5. Pay special attention to the area between the breast and the underarm, including the underarm itself.
6. Feel for any unusual lumps or masses under the skin.
7. If you have any spontaneous discharge during the month—whether or not it is during your BSE—see your doctor.
8. Repeat the examination on your right breast.

Step 3
1. Next, press your hands firmly on your hips and bow slightly toward the mirror as you pull your shoulders and elbows forward.
2. Note any change in the contour of your breasts.
3. Bend forward and check contour of your breast
4. Lift each breast and check condition of skin.

Some women do the next part of the examination in the shower. Your fingers will glide easily over soapy skin, so you can concentrate on feeling for changes inside the breast.

Step 5
1. Step 4 should be repeated lying down.
2. Lie flat on your back with your left arm over your head and a pillow or folded towel under your left shoulder. (This position flattens your breast and makes it easier to check.)
3. Use the same circular motion described above and cover the same areas.
4. Repeat on your right breast.

Adapted from U.S. Department of Health and Human Services, Public Health Service, *What you need to know about breast cancer.* Bethesda, MD: National Institutes of Health, and Skillen, D.L., & Day, R. A. (Eds.). (2004). *A syllabus for adult health assessment.* Edmonton, AB: Faculty of Nursing, University of Alberta.

Younger women, who have normal lumps in their breasts, find it particularly difficult to perform BSE because they have a harder time distinguishing normal from abnormal lumps and are not sure of what they are feeling due to the density of their breast tissue. Even women who perform BSE may delay seeking medical attention because of fear, economic factors, lack of education, reluctance to act if no pain is involved, psychological factors, and modesty.

Women should begin practicing BSE at the time of their first gynecologic examination, which usually occurs in their late teens or early 20s. All health care providers, aware of these implications, should encourage women to examine their own breasts and teach them to recognize early changes that may indicate problems. The nurse plays a pivotal role in preventive education. Almost all settings lend themselves to teaching, providing information, and encouraging appropriate care for prevention, detection, and treatment of breast problems. An individual teaching session with the patient can increase the frequency with which she practices BSE.

A lesson in BSE should include the following: optimal timing for BSE (7 days from the start of the last menstrual period for premenopausal women and once monthly for postmenopausal women), a demonstration of examination techniques, a review of what normal breast tissue feels like, a discussion on identification of breast changes, and a return demonstration on the patient and a breast model. Patients who have had breast surgery for the treatment of breast cancer are carefully instructed to examine themselves for any nodules or changes in their breasts or along the chest wall that may indicate a recurrence of the disease.

Pamphlets about BSE in different languages can be obtained from local chapters of the Canadian Cancer Society.

MAMMOGRAPHY

Mammography is a breast-imaging technique that can detect nonpalpable lesions and assist in diagnosing palpable masses. The procedure takes about 20 minutes and can be performed in an x-ray department or independent imaging centre. Two views are taken of each breast: a craniocaudal view and a mediolateral oblique view. For these views, the breast is mechanically compressed from top to bottom and side to side (Fig. 48-4). Women may experience some fleeting discomfort because maximum compression is necessary for proper visualization. The current mammograms are compared with previous mammograms, and any changes indicate a need for further investigation. Mammography may detect a breast tumour before it is clinically palpable (ie, smaller than 1 cm); however, it has limitations and is not foolproof. The false-negative rate ranges between 5% and 10%; it is generally greater in younger women with greater density of breast tissue. Some patients have very dense breast tissue, making it difficult to detect lesions with mammography.

Patients scheduled for a mammogram may voice concern about exposure to radiation. The radiation exposure is equivalent to about 1 hour of exposure to sunlight, so patients would have to have many mammograms in a year to increase their cancer risk. The benefits of this test outweigh the risks. Because the quality of mammography varies widely from one setting to the next, it is important for women to find accredited breast care centres that produce reliable mammograms.

Current mammographic screening guidelines from the Canadian Cancer Society recommend a mammogram every two years between 50 and 69 years of age. Younger women who are identified as at a higher risk for breast cancer by family history should seek the opinion of a breast specialist about when to begin screen-

A   **B**

FIGURE 48-4 The mammography procedure (**A**) relies on x-ray imaging to produce the mammogram (**B**), which in this case reveals a breast lump.

ing mammograms. Several studies suggest that screening for high-risk women should begin about 10 years before the age of diagnosis of the family member with breast cancer (Hartmann, Sellers, Schaid et al., 1999). In families with a history of breast cancer, a downward shift in age of diagnosis of about 10 years is seen (eg, grandmother diagnosed with breast cancer at age 48, mother diagnosed with breast cancer at age 38, then daughter should begin screening at age 28). Nurses need to provide teaching about screening guidelines for women in the general population and those at high risk so that these women can make informed choices about screening.

The combination of screening mammography, physical examination, and BSE has reduced overall mortality from breast cancer by 63% among women ages 40 to 69 years (Tabar, Vitak, Tony et al., 2001). Women with fewer resources (eg, elderly, poor, minority women) often do not have the means to undergo mammography or the resources for follow-up treatment when lesions are detected. Recent studies have shown that social support contributes to adherence to mammographic screening guidelines (Anderson, Urban & Etzioni, 1999; Faccione, 1999; Lauver, Kane, Bodden et al., 1999). Many nurses direct their efforts at educating women about the benefits of mammography. Working to overcome barriers to screening mammography, especially among the elderly and women with disabilities, is an important nursing intervention in the community, and nurses have an important role in the development of educational materials targeted to specific literacy levels and ethnic groups.

Galactography

Galactography is a mammographic diagnostic procedure that involves injection of less than 1 mL of radiopaque material through a cannula inserted into a ductal opening on the areola, followed by a mammogram. It is performed when the patient has a bloody nipple discharge on expression, spontaneous nipple discharge, or a solitary dilated duct noted on mammography. These symptoms may indicate a benign lesion or a cancerous one.

ULTRASONOGRAPHY

Ultrasonography (ultrasound) is used in conjunction with mammography to distinguish fluid-filled cysts from other lesions. A transducer is used to transmit high-frequency sound waves through the skin and into the breast, and an echo signal is measured. The echo waves are interpreted electronically and then displayed on a screen. This technique is 95% to 99% accurate in diagnosing cysts but does not definitively rule out a malignant lesion.

For women with dense breasts, the introduction of screening ultrasound examinations has been researched during this past decade. The addition of ultrasonography to breast cancer screening can increase the sensitivity of screening for this population of women, who tend to be either young or on hormone replacement therapy. The largest study showed an increase in cancer detection by 17% with the addition of screening ultrasonography (Kolb, Lichy & Newhouse, 1998). Further research will help provide information on the usefulness of ultrasound as a screening modality.

MAGNETIC RESONANCE IMAGING

Magnetic resonance imaging (MRI) of the breast is a promising tool for use in diagnosing breast conditions. It is a highly sensitive, although not specific, test and serves as an adjunct to mammography. A coil is placed around the breast, and the patient is placed inside the MRI machine for about 2 minutes. An injection of gadolinium, a contrast dye, is given intravenously. MRI of the breast can be helpful in determining the exact size of a lesion or the presence of multiple foci more precisely than mammography. It also can determine more precisely than a CT scan if a lesion is fixed to the chest wall. Other uses include identifying occult (undetectable) breast cancer, determining the tumour's response to chemotherapy, and determining the integrity of saline or silicone breast implants. The cost of breast MRI, however, is high; therefore, it is not currently used for routine screening. However, the sensitivity of the MRI may be beneficial for cancer detection in higher-risk women, and the results from preliminary studies are encouraging (Schnall, 2001).

PROCEDURES FOR TISSUE ANALYSIS

Fine-Needle Aspiration

Fine-needle aspiration (FNA) is an outpatient procedure usually initiated when mammography, ultrasonography, or palpation detects a lesion. A surgeon performs the procedure when there is a palpable lesion, or a radiologist performs it under x-ray guidance for nonpalpable lesions. Injection of a local anesthetic may or may not be used, but most times the surgeon or radiologist inserts a 21- or 22-gauge needle attached to a syringe into the site to be sampled. The syringe is then used to withdraw tissue or fluid into the needle. This cytologic material is spread on a slide and sent to the laboratory for analysis. FNA is less expensive than other diagnostic methods, and results are usually available quickly; however, this diagnostic test is often not 100% accurate, and the false-negative rate is substantial. False-negative or false-positive results are possible, and clinical follow-up depends on the level of suspicion about the breast lesion.

Stereotactic Biopsy

Stereotactic biopsy, also an outpatient procedure, is performed for nonpalpable lesions found on mammography. The patient lies prone on a special table, and the breast is positioned through an opening in the table and compressed for a mammogram. The lesion to be sampled is then located with the aid of a computer. Next, a local anesthetic is injected into the entry site on the breast,

a core needle is inserted, and samples of the tissue are taken for pathologic examination. If the lesion is small, a clip is placed at the site of the biopsy, so that a specific area can be visualized again as another mammogram is performed. This technique allows accurate diagnosis and often allows the patient to avoid a surgical biopsy, although some patients may end up needing a surgical biopsy, depending on the pathologic diagnosis.

Surgical Biopsy

Surgical biopsy is the most common outpatient surgical procedure. Eight of 10 lesions are benign on biopsy. The procedure is usually done using local anesthesia, moderate sedation, or both. The biopsy involves excising the lesion and sending it to the laboratory for pathologic examination.

EXCISIONAL BIOPSY

Excisional biopsy is the usual procedure for any palpable breast mass. The entire lesion, plus a margin of surrounding tissue, is removed. This type of biopsy may also be referred to as a lumpectomy. Depending on the clinical situation, a frozen section may be done at the time of the biopsy (a small piece of the mass or lesion is given a provisional diagnosis by the pathologist), so that the surgeon can provide the patient with a diagnosis in the recovery room.

INCISIONAL BIOPSY

Incisional biopsy is performed when tissue sampling alone is required; this is done both to confirm a diagnosis and to determine the hormonal receptor status. Complete excision of the area may not be possible or immediately beneficial to the patient, depending on the clinical situation. This procedure is often performed in women with locally advanced breast cancer or in cancer patients with a suspicion of recurrent disease, whose treatment may depend on the tumour's estrogen and progesterone receptor status. These receptors are identified during pathologic examination of the tissue.

TRU-CUT CORE BIOPSY

In a Tru-Cut core biopsy, the surgeon uses a special large-lumen needle to remove a core of tissue. This procedure is used when a tumour is relatively large and close to the skin surface and the surgeon strongly suspects that the lesion is a carcinoma. If cancer is diagnosed, the tissue is also tested for hormone receptor status.

WIRE NEEDLE LOCALIZATION

Wire needle localization is a technique used when mammography detects minute, pinpoint calcifications (indicating a potential malignancy) or nonpalpable lesions and a biopsy is necessary. A long, thin wire is inserted, usually painlessly, through a needle before the excisional biopsy under mammographic guidance to ensure that the wire tip designates the area to undergo biopsy. The wire remains in place after the needle is withdrawn to ensure a precise biopsy. The patient is then taken to the operating room, where the surgeon follows the wire down and excises the area around the wire tip. The tissue removed is x-rayed at the time of the procedure; these specimen x-rays, along with follow-up mammograms taken several weeks later (after the site has healed), verify that the area of concern was located and removed.

Nursing Care of the Patient Undergoing a Breast Biopsy

Breast biopsies are one of the most common ambulatory surgical procedures performed, with 80% of the results negative for malignancy (Norris, 2001). Prior to the procedure, the nurse's role is to provide instruction; however, it is important for the nurse to first assess how the woman is coping with her need for the procedure and her ability to process information about the procedure and the possible implications of the biopsy results. Anxiety and fear are normal responses to the need for a breast biopsy, but these responses may interfere with the woman's ability to recall and understand the information that is provided prior to the procedure. Therefore, written information and booklets are used to reinforce teaching. The nurse also must give the patient an opportunity to address issues and concerns related to the biopsy.

The nurse instructs the patient to avoid use of agents that can interfere with blood clotting and increase the risk for bleeding. Among these agents are nonsteroidal anti-inflammatory drugs, vitamin E supplements, herbal substances (such as gingko biloba and garlic supplements), warfarin, and products containing aspirin. The patient may be instructed not to eat or drink after midnight, depending on the type of biopsy planned. Most breast biopsy procedures today are performed with the use of moderate sedation and local anesthesia; thus, the recovery period is relatively brief.

Postoperative assessment includes monitoring the effects of the anesthesia and inspection of the dressing covering the incision. Prior to discharge from the ambulatory surgery centre or office, the patient must be able to tolerate fluids or food, ambulate, and void. The patient should be accompanied home by a family member or friend. At discharge, the nurse reviews with the patient the care of the biopsy site, pain management, and activity restrictions. The dressing covering the incision is usually removed on the second day, but use of a supportive bra is encouraged immediately after the procedure for 3 to 7 days to limit movement of the breast and reduce discomfort. Steri-strips applied over the incision are left in place until they start to come off, usually a couple of weeks after the procedure. A follow-up telephone call to the patient by the nurse 24 to 48 hours after the procedure is standard care and provides an opportunity for the nurse to answer any questions the patient might have.

Most women return to their usual activities the day after the procedure but are encouraged to avoid jarring or high-impact activities for 1 week to promote healing of the biopsy site. Discomfort is usually minimal from the procedure and most women find acetaminophen sufficient for pain relief; however, a mild opioid may be prescribed, if needed.

Follow-up after the biopsy includes a return visit to the surgeon for discussion of the final pathology report and assessment of the healing of the biopsy site. Depending on the results of the biopsy, the nurse's role varies. If the pathology report is negative for cancer, the nurse reviews incision care and explains what to expect as the biopsy site heals (ie, changes in sensation may occur weeks or months after the biopsy due to injury to the nerves within the breast tissue). If a diagnosis of cancer is made, the nurse's role changes dramatically; this is discussed in depth later in this chapter.

Overview of Breast Conditions and Diseases

Not all disorders of the breast are cancerous. Some disorders are structural, such as fissure, or infection-related, such as mastitis. Some conditions may progress from a benign to a malignant condition, such as benign proliferative breast disease, and some conditions are clearly cancer of various kinds in various stages.

Conditions Affecting the Nipple

FISSURE

A fissure is a longitudinal ulcer that tends to develop in breast-feeding women. If the nipple becomes irritated, a painful, raw area may form and become a site of infection. Daily washing with water, massage with breast milk or lanolin, and exposure to air are helpful. Breastfeeding can continue with a nipple shield, if necessary. If the fissure is severe or extremely painful, the woman is advised to stop breastfeeding; a breast pump can be used until the breastfeeding can be resumed. Persistent ulceration requires further diagnosis and therapy. Guidance with breastfeeding from a nurse or lactation consultant may be helpful because nipple irritation can result from improper positioning (ie, the infant has not grasped the areola fully).

BREAST DISCHARGE

Breast discharge in a woman who is not lactating may be related to many causes. Carcinoma, papilloma, pituitary adenoma, cystic breasts, and various medications can result in a discharge of fluid from the nipple. Oral contraceptives, pregnancy, hormone replacement therapy, chlorpromazine-type medications, and frequent breast stimulation may be contributing factors. In some athletic women, breast discharge may occur during running or aerobic exercises. Breast discharge should be evaluated by the health care provider, but it is not often a cause for alarm. One in three women have clear discharge on expression, which is usually normal. Causes for concern are green discharge, which usually indicates infection, and brown or red discharge, which is indicative of a disorder. Spontaneous discharge should always be evaluated because it is not normal unless a woman is lactating. The discharge is examined for fat globules to determine if it is breast milk. It is also tested for occult blood because malignancy must be considered.

BLEEDING OR BLOODY NIPPLE DISCHARGE

At times, a bloody discharge may be produced when pressure is placed on one area at the edge of the areola. Although a bloody discharge can signal a malignancy, it usually results from a wart-like, benign epithelial tumour or papilloma growing in one of the large collecting ducts just at the edge of the areola or in an area of cystic disease. Bleeding occurs with any trauma, and the blood collects in the duct until it is pressed out at the nipple. Treatment includes excision of the duct with the papilloma. Such a lesion is usually benign, but it should be evaluated histologically after it is removed to rule out malignancy.

Breast Infections

MASTITIS

Mastitis, an inflammation or infection of breast tissue, occurs most commonly in breastfeeding women, although it may also occur in nonlactating women. The infection may result from a transfer of microorganisms to the breast by the patient's hands or those of others or from a breastfed infant with an oral, eye, or skin infection. Mastitis may also be caused by bloodborne organisms. As inflammation progresses, an infection of the ducts results, causing milk to stagnate in one or more of the lobules. The breast texture becomes tough or doughy, and the patient complains of dull pain in the infected region. A nipple that is discharging purulent material, serum, or blood needs to be investigated.

Treatment consists of antibiotics and local heat. A broad-spectrum antibiotic agent may be prescribed for 7 to 10 days. The patient should wear a snug bra and perform personal hygiene carefully. Adequate rest and hydration are important aspects of management.

LACTATIONAL ABSCESS

A breast abscess may develop as a consequence of acute mastitis. In such a case, the area affected becomes tender and red. Purulent matter can usually be expressed from the nipple, and incision and drainage are usually required. At the time of drainage, specimens are obtained for culture.

Benign Conditions of the Breast

Benign breast lesions include fibrocystic changes, fibroadenomas, and cysts.

FIBROCYSTIC BREAST CHANGES

Fibrocystic breast changes occur as ducts dilate and cysts form. This condition occurs most commonly in women ages 30 to 50 years. Although the cause is unknown, estrogen appears to be a factor because cysts usually disappear after menopause. Cystic

areas often fluctuate in size, depending on the menstrual cycle. They are usually larger premenstrually and smaller postmenstrually because of the retention of fluid in the days preceding the menstrual period. The cysts may be painless or may become very tender premenstrually. Occasionally, a patient may report breast pain, which is usually intermittent and can be shooting or a dull ache (Table 48-1 describes various breast masses). Breast pain (**mastalgia**) is usually related to hormonal fluctuations and their effect on the breasts or is stimulated by irritation of a nerve in the chest wall from an activity such as weight training.

Medical Management

If pain and tenderness are severe, danazol (Cyclomen) may be prescribed; this agent has an antiestrogenic effect, therefore decreasing breast pain and nodularity. Danazol is used only in severe cases because of its potential side effects, which include flushing, vaginitis, and androgenic changes (virilization).

Nursing Management

The nurse may recommend that the patient wear a supportive bra both day and night for a week except during bathing, decrease her salt and caffeine intake, and take ibuprofen (Motrin, Advil) as needed for its anti-inflammatory actions. Vitamin E supplements or oil of evening primrose (an over-the-counter herbal preparation) may also be helpful, but this recommendation is based on anecdotal information from patients, not on research.

Table 48-1 • Variations in Breast Masses

The most common breast masses are due to fibrocystic changes, fibroadenomas, or malignancy. Biopsy is usually needed for confirmation, but the following characteristics are diagnostic clues:

CHARACTERISTICS	FIBROCYSTIC CHANGES	FIBROADENOMAS	MALIGNANCY
(Illustrations show how the lump may feel because it is usually not visible.)			
Age	30–60 years, regress after menopause except with use of estrogen therapy	Puberty to menopause	30–90 years; most common, 40–80 years
Number	Single or multiple	Usually single	Usually single
Shape	Round	Round, disk, or lobular	Irregular or stellate
Consistency	Soft to firm, usually elastic	Usually firm	Firm or hard
Mobility	Mobile	Mobile	May be fixed to skin or underlying tissues
Tenderness	Usually tender	Usually nontender	Usually nontender
Retraction signs	Absent	Absent	May be present

If diuretic agents or oral contraceptives are prescribed, the patient should know that symptoms usually recur after these medications are discontinued. Patients should also be reassured that breast pain is rarely indicative of cancer in its early stages. If the pain is not relieved after menses begins, however, the woman should see her primary health care provider.

FIBROADENOMAS

Fibroadenomas are firm, round, movable, benign tumours of the breast that usually affect women in their late teens to late 30s. These masses are nontender and are sometimes removed for diagnostic certainty.

OTHER BENIGN CONDITIONS

Cystosarcoma phyllodes is a fibroepithelial lesion that tends to grow rapidly. It is rarely malignant and is surgically excised. If it is malignant, mastectomy may follow. *Fat necrosis* is a rare condition of the breast that is often related to trauma from a blow; however, it may be indistinguishable from carcinoma, and the entire mass is usually excised.

Gigantomastia or macromastia (overly large breasts) is a problem for some women. Weight loss and various medications have been tried to little avail. Reduction mammoplasty (discussed later in this chapter) is an elective procedure for the patient who is physically or emotionally distressed by this condition. *Superficial thrombophlebitis* of the breast (Mondor's disease) is an uncommon condition that is usually associated with pregnancy, trauma, or breast surgery. Pain and redness occur as a result of a superficial thrombophlebitis in the vein that drains the outer part of the breast. The mass is usually linear, tender, and erythematous. Treatment consists of analgesics and heat.

BENIGN PROLIFERATIVE BREAST DISEASE

The two most common diagnoses of **benign proliferative breast disease** found on biopsy are atypical hyperplasia and lobular carcinoma in situ. Both of these diagnoses increase a woman's risk for the development of breast cancer. **Atypical hyperplasia** is an abnormal increase in the ductal or lobular cells in the breast and is usually found incidentally in mammographic abnormalities. Atypical hyperplasia increases a woman's risk for breast cancer about 10% to 20% over a period of 10 years; the risk is greater for premenopausal women and decreases significantly after menopause (Hulka & Moorman, 2001). **Lobular carcinoma in situ** (LCIS) is usually an incidental finding in breast tissue because it cannot be seen on mammography and does not form a palpable lump. Historically, LCIS was considered a premalignant condition, and treatment consisted of a bilateral prophylactic mastectomy; however, current research indicates that LCIS is a marker for the risk for invasive breast cancer, which can either be ductal or lobular in origin and can develop in either breast. LCIS increases a woman's risk for breast cancer by about 25% to 40% over a period of 25 years, and the risk does not diminish with time (Frykberg, 1999).

For women at higher risk, a newer technique called ductal lavage may be used. It involves inserting a microcatheter through the nipple while instilling saline and retrieving the fluid for analysis. It has been shown to identify atypical cells in this population (Dooley, Ljung, Veronisi et al., 2001), providing women with more information regarding their risk. This procedure, which is done in the office and is well tolerated, was found to be more useful at detecting cellular changes within the breast tissue. Continued research is needed to determine its benefit in screening and early detection for women at high risk.

Medical Management

After a woman has been diagnosed with a benign proliferative condition such as atypical hyperplasia or LCIS, she has three treatment options: long-term surveillance (observation), bilateral prophylactic mastectomy (a risk-reducing surgical procedure), or chemoprevention (using a medication to decrease the risk of developing breast cancer). Each of these options may be offered by a breast specialist, usually associated with a comprehensive breast centre. Most women choose surveillance and attempt to modify certain risk factors, such as diet, exercise, and alcohol consumption. For some women, however, prophylactic mastectomy may be an option (see discussion later in this chapter); taking tamoxifen (Nolvadex) may be an option for others. Tamoxifen has recently been shown to decrease the incidence of invasive breast cancer for high-risk women by 49% (Fisher, Constantino, Wickerham et al., 1998). The risks and benefits of each of these options must be explained so that the woman can make a careful decision.

Malignant Conditions of the Breast

Breast cancer is a major health problem in Canada. At present, there is no cure for breast cancer. Breast cancer is the most frequently diagnosed cancer for Canadian women (Canadian Breast Cancer Foundation, 2005). In 2005, 21,600 women and 150 men in Canada were diagnosed with breast cancer and 5,300 women and 45 men died.

Current statistics indicate that a woman's lifetime risk for developing breast cancer is 1 in 8.8, but this risk is not the same for all age groups. For example, the risk for developing breast cancer by age 35 years is 1 in 622; the risk for developing breast cancer by age 60 years is 1 in 23. Approximately 80% of breast cancers are diagnosed after the age of 50. Since 1986, there has been a decrease of 20% in the mortality rate due to lifestyle choices such as not smoking, healthy eating, and physical fitness.

CARCINOMA IN SITU (NONINVASIVE)

In situ carcinoma of the breast is being detected more frequently with the widespread use of screening mammography. Since the introduction of widespread mammographic screening over the past two decades, **ductal carcinoma in situ** (DCIS) has accounted for approximately 20% of diagnosed breast cancers (Winchester, Jeske & Goldschmidt, 2000). This disease is characterized by the proliferation of malignant cells within the ducts and lobules, without invasion into the surrounding tissue; therefore, it is a noninvasive form of cancer and is considered stage 0 breast cancer. There are two types of in situ carcinoma: ductal and lobular.

Ductal Carcinoma in Situ

DCIS, the more common of the two types, is divided histologically into two major subtypes (comedo and noncomedo), but there are many different forms of noncomedo DCIS. Because DCIS has the capacity to progress to invasive cancer, the most traditional treatment is total or simple mastectomy (removal of the breast only), with a cure rate of 98% to 99% (Winchester et al., 2000). The use of breast-conserving surgery for invasive cancer led to the use of **breast-conservation therapy** (limited surgery followed by radiation) for patients with DCIS, and this option is appropriate for localized lesions. More than half of cases of DCIS are now being treated with breast-conservation therapy; however, the rate of local recurrence is 15% to 20% (Solin, Fourquet, Vicini et al., 2001). In some cases, lumpectomy alone is an option, but this is decided on a case-by-case basis. In 1999, a large study demonstrated that tamoxifen (Nolvadex) significantly reduced local recurrence rates (Fisher, Dignam, Wolmark et al., 1999). It is usually prescribed for 5 years.

Lobular Carcinoma in Situ

LCIS is characterized by proliferation of cells within the breast lobules. LCIS is usually an incidental finding discovered on pathologic evaluation of a breast biopsy for a breast change noted during physical examination or on screening mammography. It is commonly associated with multicentric disease and is rarely associated with invasive cancer. Historically, treatment was bilateral **total mastectomy**, but current thinking that LCIS is a marker of increased risk for the development of an invasive cancer (rather than an actual malignancy) has changed this approach. Long-term surveillance is one appropriate option. Another option is a bilateral prophylactic mastectomy to decrease risk; current research (Hartmann et al., 1999) suggests that a 90% reduction in risk is possible with this option. (Prophylactic mastectomy is discussed in more detail at the end of this chapter.) The other treatment option for LCIS is chemoprevention. Tamoxifen has been used as a chemopreventive agent but, as with any drug, tamoxifen has both benefits and risks, along with possible side effects.

INVASIVE CARCINOMA
Infiltrating Ductal Carcinoma

Infiltrating ductal carcinomas are the most common histologic type of breast cancer and account for 75% of all breast cancers. These tumours are notable because of their hardness on palpation. They usually metastasize to the axillary nodes. Prognosis is poorer than for other cancer types.

Infiltrating Lobular Carcinoma

Infiltrating lobular carcinoma accounts for 5% to 10% of breast cancers. These tumours typically occur as an area of ill-defined thickening in the breast, as compared with the infiltrating ductal types. They are most often multicentric; that is, several areas of thickening may occur in one or both breasts. Infiltrating ductal and infiltrating lobular carcinomas usually spread to bone, lung, liver, or brain, whereas lobular carcinomas may metastasize to meningeal surfaces or other unusual sites.

Medullary Carcinoma

Medullary carcinoma constitutes about 6% of breast cancers and grows in a capsule inside a duct. This type of tumour can become large, but the prognosis is often favourable.

Mucinous Cancer

Mucinous cancer accounts for about 3% of breast cancers. A mucin producer, it is also slow-growing and thus has a more favourable prognosis than many other types.

Tubular Ductal Cancer

Tubular ductal cancer accounts for only 2% of cancers. Because axillary metastases are uncommon with this histology, prognosis is usually excellent.

Inflammatory Carcinoma

Inflammatory carcinoma is a rare type of breast cancer (1% to 2%) with symptoms different from those of other breast cancers. The localized tumour is tender and painful, and the skin over it is red and dusky. The breast is abnormally firm and enlarged. Often, edema and nipple retraction occur. These symptoms rapidly grow more severe and usually prompt the woman to seek health care sooner than the woman with a small breast mass. The disease can spread to other parts of the body rapidly; chemotherapeutic agents play a major role in attempting to control the progression of this disease. Radiation and surgery are also used to control spread.

Paget's Disease

Paget's disease of the breast accounts for 1% of diagnosed breast cancer cases. A scaly lesion and burning and itching around the nipple–areola complex are frequent symptoms. The neoplasm is ductal and may be in situ alone or may also have invasive cancer cells. Often, a tumour mass cannot be palpated underneath the nipple where this disease arises. Mammography may be the only diagnostic test that detects the tumour, but results of the mammogram are often negative, making biopsy of the lesion the only definitive test.

Current Research in Breast Cancer

Because of the incidence, significant mortality, and lack of a cure, breast cancer survivors, advocates, and activists have brought social and political attention to this disease and put it in the national spotlight. Activists have demanded and obtained increased federal funding for a national program aimed at finding a cure for breast cancer.

Preventing the development of cancer through the use of medications is a relatively new and exciting area of research. In April 1998, the results of the Breast Cancer Prevention Trial were released to the general public. This nationwide, U.S. randomized, double-blind, placebo-controlled clinical trial evaluated tamoxifen (Nolvadex) versus a placebo in more than 13,000 women considered to be at high risk for the development of breast cancer. The women who received tamoxifen had a 45% reduction in the incidence of breast cancer (Fisher et al., 1998). These results suggested that tamoxifen was an effective chemopreventive agent. Much attention has been focused on this medication. Clinicians are still unclear, however, about who should receive the medication, and no consensus exists. Nurses can provide information to patients on the benefits, risks, and possible side effects of tamoxifen to help women in considering this option.

Another agent that shows promise for chemoprevention is raloxifene (Evista). This medication is used for the prevention of osteoporosis; however, in the studies that have been performed, incidental findings indicated that fewer of the women who received raloxifene developed breast cancer (Cummings, Eckert, Kreuger et al., 1999). This has led to the hypothesis that this drug may also be an effective chemopreventive agent. Researchers are conducting another nationwide, U.S. randomized clinical trial, the Study of Tamoxifen and Raloxifene, which is comparing these two agents in postmenopausal women for the prevention of breast cancer. Twenty-two thousand women are needed for this trial, so results will not be available until later in the decade.

Prophylactic Mastectomy

Some women who are at high risk for breast cancer may elect to undergo **prophylactic mastectomy**. This procedure can reduce the risk for cancer by 90% (Hartmann et al., 1999; Meijers-Heijboer, van Geel, van Putten et al., 2001), so a more appropriate term for this surgery is "risk-reducing" mastectomy. The procedure, performed by a breast surgeon, consists of a total mastectomy (removal of breast tissue only). Possible candidates are women with a strong family history of breast cancer, a diagnosis of LCIS or atypical hyperplasia, a diagnosis of BRCA-1 or BRCA-2 gene mutation (see following discussion), an extreme fear of cancer ("cancer phobia"), or previous cancer in one breast. Many women opt for immediate reconstruction with the mastectomy.

The woman needs to understand that this surgery is elective and not emergent. To be sure that she understands the implications of surgery, the woman should be offered a consultation with a plastic surgeon, a genetic counselling session, and a psychological evaluation. Women who make an informed decision tend to demonstrate more satisfaction with the cosmetic results (Rowland, Desmond, Meyerowitz et al., 2000).

Nursing interventions for the woman considering a risk-reducing mastectomy include ensuring that the patient has information about reconstructive options and providing referrals to the plastic surgeon, genetic counsellor, and psychological counsellor. Many women need time to think over the procedure, and the nurse can be helpful in answering questions about the procedure and its implications and in assisting the patient to decide whether the surgery is an appropriate option. The woman considering this option may wish to talk with a woman who has had the procedure.

Breast Cancer

There is no single, specific cause of breast cancer; rather, a combination of hormonal, genetic, and possibly environmental events may contribute to its development.

Etiology

Hormones produced by the ovaries have an important role in breast cancer. Two key ovarian hormones, estradiol and progesterone, are altered in the cellular environment by a variety of factors, and these may affect growth factors for breast cancer.

HORMONES

The role of hormones and their relationship to breast cancer remain controversial. Research suggests that a relationship exists between estrogen exposure and the development of breast cancer. In laboratory studies, tumours grow much faster when exposed to estrogen, and epidemiologic research suggests that women who have longer exposure to estrogen have a higher risk for breast cancer. Early menarche, nulliparity, childbirth after 30 years of age, and late menopause are known but minor risk factors. The assumption is that these factors are all associated with prolonged exposure to estrogen because of menstruation. The theory is that each cycle (which has high levels of endogenous estrogen) provides the cells of the breast another chance to mutate, increasing the chance for cancer to develop. Estrogen itself does not cause breast cancer, but it is associated with its development.

GENETICS

Growing evidence indicates that genetic alterations are associated with the development of breast cancer. These genetic alterations include changes or mutations in normal genes and the influence of proteins that either promote or suppress the development of breast cancer. Genetic alterations may be somatic (acquired) or germline (inherited). To date, two gene mutations have been identified that may play a role in the development of breast cancer. A mutation in the **BRCA-1** gene has been linked to the development of breast and ovarian cancer, whereas a mutation in the **BRCA-2** gene identifies risk for breast cancer, but less so for ovarian cancer (Houshmand, Campbell, Briggs et al., 2000). These gene mutations may also play a role in the development of colon, prostate, and pancreatic cancer, but this is far from clear at present. It has been estimated that 1 of 600 women in the general population has either a BRCA-1 or BRCA-2 gene mutation. For women who carry either mutation, the risk for developing breast cancer can range from 50% to 90% (Kauff, Satagopan, Robson et al., 2002).

At present, only 5% to 10% of all breast cancers are estimated to be associated with the BRCA-1 or BRCA-2 gene mutations. It is thought, however, that breast cancer is genetic and that up to 80% of women diagnosed with breast cancer before age 50 years have a genetic component to their disease (Boyd, 1996). This is believed to be linked to either unidentified BRCA-1 or BRCA-2 carriers or less penetrating genes that have yet to be identified through genetics research. A woman's risk for either BRCA-1 or BRCA-2 should be interpreted with caution and with an exhaustive look at all her other risk factors; this is usually carried out by a genetics counsellor.

Abnormalities in either of the two genes can be identified by a blood test; however, women should be counselled about the risks and benefits before actually undergoing genetic testing. The risks and benefits of a positive or negative result should be explored. Treatment options for a positive result are long-term surveillance, bilateral prophylactic mastectomy, or chemoprevention with tamoxifen, as discussed previously. A positive result can cause tremendous anxiety and fear, can unleash potential discrimination in employment and insurability, and can cause a woman to search for answers that may not be available. A negative result can produce survivor guilt in a person with a strong family history of cancer. For these women, the risk for breast cancer is similar to that of the general population, and routine screening guidelines should be followed. The decision to pursue genetic testing must be made carefully, and women should be asked what they will do differently after they know the results. Furthermore, because testing is relatively new and health care providers have yet to determine a true benefit from a positive or negative result, genetic testing should be done under the auspices of clinical research protocols to protect the patient (because these data are kept separate from the patient's medical record). Nurses play a role in educating patients and their family members about the implications of genetic testing. Ethical issues related to genetic testing include possible employment discrimination, bias in insurability and possibly with insurance rates, and family members' concerns (eg, effect on siblings, children).

Risk Factors

Although there are no specific known causes of breast cancer, researchers have identified a cluster of risk factors (Chart 48-3). These factors are important in helping to develop prevention programs. However, nearly 60% of women diagnosed with breast cancer have no identifiable risk factors other than their hormonal environment (Vogel, 2000). Thus, all women are considered at risk for developing breast cancer during their lifetime. Nonetheless, identifying risk factors provides a means for identifying women who may benefit from increased surveillance and early treatment. In addition, further research into risk factors will help in developing strategies to prevent or modify breast cancer in the future.

A high-fat diet was once thought to increase the risk of breast cancer. Epidemiologic studies of American and Japanese women showed that American women had a fivefold higher rate of breast cancer. Japanese women who moved to the United States were shown to have breast cancer rates similar to their Caucasian counterparts. Recent cohort studies show only weak or inconclusive relationships between a high-fat diet and breast cancer (Brown et al., 2001). Because fat intake is implicated in colon cancer and heart disease, however, women may benefit from lowering their intake of fat.

Oral contraceptives were once thought to increase the risk for breast cancer. Currently, no association is thought to exist in women in the general population, but there are no data about the effect on women considered to be at high risk.

The role of smoking in breast cancer remains unclear. Most studies suggest that smoking does not increase a woman's risk for breast cancer. Some studies, however, suggest that smoking does increase the risk for breast cancer and that the earlier a woman begins smoking, the higher her risk. Smoking does increase the risk for lung cancer, which is the leading cause of death in women with cancer (breast cancer is second). Smoking cessation is part of a healthy lifestyle, and nurses have a key role in providing women with information about smoking cessation programs.

Silicone breast implants can be associated with fibrous capsular contraction, and some women and medical professionals have claimed an association with certain immune disorders. There is no evidence, however, that breast implants are associated with an increased risk of breast cancer.

Protective Factors

Certain factors may be protective in relation to the development of breast cancer. Regular, vigorous exercise has been shown to decrease risk, perhaps because it can delay menarche, suppress menstruation, and, like pregnancy, reduce the number of ovulatory menstrual cycles. Also, exercise decreases body fat, where estrogens are stored and produced from other steroid hormones. Thus, decreased body fat can decrease extended exposure to estrogen.

Chart 48-3
Risk Factors for Breast Cancer

BRCA-1 or BRCA-2 genetic mutation
Women with gene mutation have a 50% to 90% chance of developing breast cancer and a 50/50 possibility of developing breast cancer before 50 years of age

Increasing age
Greatest risk for breast cancer occurs after age 50.

Personal or family history of breast cancer
Risk of developing breast cancer in the other breast increases about 1% per year.
Risk increases twofold if first-degree female relatives (sister, mother, or daughter) had breast cancer
Risk increases if the mother was affected with cancer before 60 years of age.
Risk increases four to six times if breast cancer occurred in two first-degree relatives.

Early menarche
Menses beginning before 12 years of age

Nulliparity and late maternal age at first birth
Women having their first child after 30 years of age have twice the risk for breast cancer as women having first child before 20 years of age.

Late menopause
Menopause after 55 years of age but women with bilateral oophorectomy before 35 years of age have one third the risk.

History of benign proliferative breast disease
Risk doubles in women with benign tumours with proliferative epithelial changes; risk quadruples with atypical hyperplasia or LCIS.

Exposure to ionizing radiation between puberty and 30 years of age
Risk doubles; exposure to radiation causes potential aberrations while the breast cells are developing.

Obesity
Weak risk among obese postmenopausal women: estrogen is stored in body adipose tissue, and dietary fat increases pituitary prolactin, thus increasing estrogen production. Obese women diagnosed with breast cancer have a higher mortality rate, which may be related to these hormonal influences or perhaps a delayed diagnosis.

Hormone replacement therapy
Reported risk for breast cancer related to hormone replacement therapy varies.
Older women taking estrogen supplements for more than 5 years *may* have an increased risk; addition of progesterone to estrogen replacement decreases the incidence of endometrial cancer, but it does not decrease the risk of breast cancer.

Alcohol intake
As a risk factor, alcohol use remains controversial; however, a slightly increased risk is found in women who consume even one drink daily. The risk doubles among women drinking three drinks daily. In countries where wine is consumed daily (eg, France and Italy), the rate is slightly higher. Some research findings suggest that young women who drink alcohol are more vulnerable in later years.

Breastfeeding is also thought to decrease risk because it prevents the return of menstruation, again decreasing exposure to endogenous estrogen. Having had a full-term pregnancy before the age of 30 years is also thought to be protective. Protective hormones are released after delivery of the fetus, with the purpose of reverting to normal the proliferation of cells in the breast that occur with pregnancy.

Clinical Manifestations

Breast cancers occur anywhere in the breast, but most are found in the upper outer quadrant, where most breast tissue is located. Generally, the lesions are nontender rather than painful, fixed rather than mobile, and hard with irregular borders rather than encapsulated and smooth. Complaints of diffuse breast pain and tenderness with menstruation are usually associated with benign breast disease. Marked pain at presentation, however, may be associated with breast cancer in the later stages.

With the increased use of mammography, more women are seeking treatment at an earlier stage of disease. These women may have no symptoms and no palpable lump, but abnormal lesions are detected on mammography. Unfortunately, many women with advanced disease seek initial treatment only after ignoring symptoms. For example, they may seek attention for dimpling or for a peau d'orange (orange-peel) appearance of the skin (a condition caused by swelling that results from obstructed lymphatic circulation in the dermal layer). Nipple retraction and lesions fixed to the chest wall may also be evident. Involvement of the skin is manifested by ulcerating and fungating lesions. These classic signs and symptoms characterize breast cancer in the late stages. A high index of suspicion should be maintained with any breast abnormality, and abnormalities should be promptly evaluated.

Assessment and Diagnostic Findings

Techniques to determine the histology and tissue diagnosis of breast cancer include FNA, excisional (or open) biopsy, incisional biopsy, needle localization, core biopsy, and stereotactic biopsy (all described previously). In addition to the staging criteria described below, other pathologic features and prognostic tests are used to identify different patient groups that may benefit from adjuvant treatment. Histologic examination of the cancer cells helps determine the prognosis and leads to a better understanding of how the disease progresses.

Breast Cancer Staging

Staging involves classifying the cancer by the extent of disease (see Fig. 48-5). Staging of any cancer is important because it helps the health care team identify and recommend the best treatment available, offer a prognosis, and compare the results of various treatment regimens. Several diagnostic tests and procedures are performed in the staging of the disease. These may include chest x-rays, bone scans, and liver function tests. Clinical staging involves the physician's estimate of the size of the breast tumour and the extent of axillary node involvement by physical examination (palpable nodes may indicate progression of the disease) and mammography. After the diagnostic workup and the definitive surgical treatment, the breast cancer is staged according to the TNM system (Greene, Page, Fleming, et al., 2002), which evaluates the size of the tumour, number of nodes involved, and evidence of distant metastasis. Pathologic staging based on histology provides information for a more accurate prognosis. Table 48-2 lists typical treatment guidelines by stage at diagnosis (see the following management section for details regarding these treatments).

Prognosis

Several features of breast tumours contribute to the prognosis. Generally, the smaller the tumour, the better the prognosis. Carcinoma of the breast is not a pathologic entity that develops overnight. It starts with a genetic alteration in a single cell. It can take about 16 doubling times for a carcinoma to become 1 cm or larger, at which point it becomes clinically apparent. Assuming that it takes at least 30 days for each doubling time, it would take a minimum of 2 years for a carcinoma to become palpable. This

Stage I: Tumours are less than 2 cm in diameter and confined to breast.

Stage II: Tumours are less than 5 cm, or tumours are smaller with mobile axillary lymph node involvement.

Stage IIIa: Tumours are greater than 5 cm, or tumours are accompanied by enlarged axillary lymph nodes fixed to one another or to adjacent tissue.

Stage IIIb: More advanced lesions with satellite nodules, fixation to the skin or chest wall, ulceration, edema, or with supraclavicular or intraclavicular nodal involvement.

Stage IV: All tumours with distant metastases.

FIGURE 48-5 Stages of breast cancer.

Table 48-2 • Breast Cancer Treatment Guidelines by Stage at Diagnosis

STAGE	TUMOUR	SURGERY	CHEMOTHERAPY	RADIATION
0	DCIS	TM or lumpectomy	Tamoxifen	For lumpectomy
I	0–2 cm	BCT or MRM	Considered for all invasive tumours	For BCT
II	2–5 cm	BCT or MRM	Regimen depends on tumour size and nodal status	For BCT
III	>5 cm	MRM	Postoperative and possibly preoperative	To chest wall and possibly axillae after MRM
IV	Metastatic disease	Possible lumpectomy or MRM	To control progression and/or palliation	To control progression and/or palliation

DCIS, ductal carcinoma in situ; TM, total mastectomy; BCT, breast-conservation treatment (lumpectomy and axillary dissection); MRM, modified radical mastectomy.

concept is important for nurses in teaching and counselling patients because once breast cancer is diagnosed, women have a safe period of several weeks to make a decision regarding treatment.

The prognosis also depends on whether the cancer has spread. For example, the overall 5-year survival rate is greater than 98% when the tumour is confined to the breast (ACS, 2002). When the cancer cells have spread to the regional lymph nodes, however, the overall 5-year survival rate falls to 76%. The 5-year survival rate for women diagnosed with metastatic disease is 16%. At diagnosis, about 37% of patients have evidence of regional or distant spread or metastasis. The most common route of regional spread is to the axillary lymph nodes. Table 48-3 describes the relationship between positive axillary lymph nodes and the risk for breast cancer recurrence. Other sites of lymphatic spread include the internal mammary and supraclavicular nodes (Fig. 48-6). Distant metastasis can affect any organ, but the most common sites are bone (71%), lung (69%), liver (65%), pleura (51%), adrenals (49%), skin (30%), and brain (20%) (Winchester & Cox, 1998).

In addition to tumour size, nodal involvement, evidence of metastasis, and histologic type, other measures help in determining prognosis. The presence of estrogen and progesterone receptor proteins indicates retention of regulatory controls of the mammary epithelium. The presence of both receptor proteins is associated with an improved prognosis; their absence is associated with a poorer prognosis. Similarly, a tumour with a high degree of differentiation is associated with a better prognosis than a poorly differentiated anaplastic tumour. The assessment of a tumour's proliferative rate (S-phase fraction) and DNA content (ploidy) by laboratory assay may help to determine prognosis because these two factors are strongly correlated with other prognostic factors, and research is ongoing to examine how helpful these two factors may actually be. Tumours classified as diploid (normal DNA content) are associated with a better prognosis than are tumours classified as aneuploid (abnormal DNA content).

Table 48-3 • Relationship Between Positive Axillary Lymph Nodes and Risk for Breast Cancer Recurrence*

NO. OF POSITIVE AXILLARY LYMPH NODES	RISK FOR BREAST CANCER RECURRENCE (%)
0	<10
1–3	12–20
4–9	30–35
>10	>50

*At 5 years' follow-up.

Medical Management

CHANGING APPROACHES

In 1990, the National Institutes of Health Consensus Development Conference on Breast Cancer issued its third statement on the management of breast cancer. Based on worldwide data, breast-conserving surgery (such as lumpectomy), along with radiation therapy, was found to result in a survival rate equal to that of modified radical mastectomy. In addition, recommendations were made for systemic treatment with chemotherapy based on the patient's menopausal status and the presence of hormone receptors. For a premenopausal woman without involvement of the lymph nodes, adjuvant chemotherapy was recommended if the woman was at high risk for recurrence. For a postmenopausal woman without involvement of the lymph nodes, adjuvant chemotherapy was not recommended regardless of hormonal receptor status. For a premenopausal woman with involvement of the nodes, adjuvant chemotherapy was recommended. In a postmenopausal woman, hormone therapy was recommended if the woman had an estrogen receptor-positive tumour. The section on hormonal therapy later in this chapter describes this in more depth.

In 1991, the National Cancer Institute issued a clinical alert that altered the recommendations of the 1990 Consensus Development Conference Statement. This alert recommended that all premenopausal, node-negative women at high risk for recurrent disease receive adjuvant chemotherapy. This clinical alert was issued before the results of clinical trials were published, creating confusion among clinicians and patients alike. The 2000 Consensus Development Conference Statement stated that all women with invasive breast cancer should consider systemic chemotherapy, not just women with tumours larger than 1 cm (NIH, 2000).

Decisions regarding local treatment with either mastectomy or breast-conserving surgery with radiation still vary widely. Mastectomy is still performed in many cases, and rates for breast-conserving surgery are higher in metropolitan areas with teaching and research hospitals and medical centres. In the past, women have not routinely been presented with the option of breast-conserving surgery by their physicians. Thus, women have not uniformly had the opportunity to exercise informed choice in their options for local treatment, but this is changing as women become more knowledgeable about breast cancer and its treatment. A second opinion regarding treatment options is usually helpful to women diagnosed with breast cancer.

SURGICAL MANAGEMENT

The main goal of surgical treatment is to eradicate the local presence of the cancer. The procedures most often used for the local

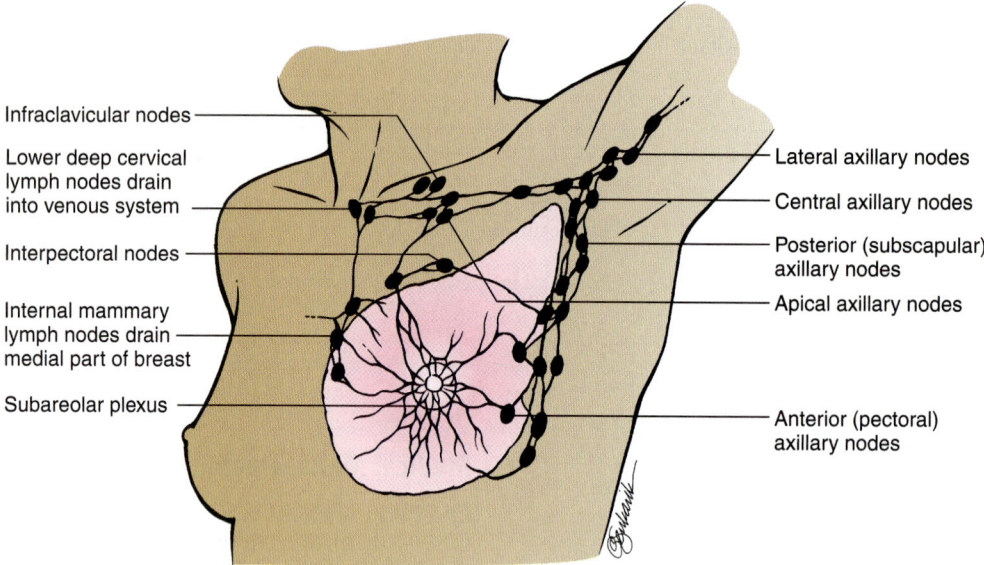

FIGURE 48-6 Lymphatic drainage of the breast.

management of invasive breast cancer are mastectomy with or without reconstruction and breast-conserving surgery combined with radiation therapy. These procedures are described below. Surgical treatment options are summarized in Table 48-4. For patients who undergo total mastectomy for the treatment of DCIS or as prophylactic surgery for the treatment for LCIS, the nursing care is similar to that of a modified radical mastectomy (described later in the text). However, total mastectomy does not involve the removal of axillary lymph nodes; therefore, mobility of the arm on the affected side is regained much quicker, and there is no risk for lymphedema. Women still face the same psychosocial issues involving the diagnosis of cancer and the loss of the breast, and the nurse needs to address these in a similar manner.

Modified Radical Mastectomy.

Modified radical mastectomy is removal of the entire breast tissue, along with axillary lymph nodes. The pectoralis major and pectoralis minor muscles remain intact. Before surgery, the surgeon plans an incision that will provide maximum opportunity to remove the tumour and the affected nodes. At the same time, efforts are made to avoid a scar that will be visible and restrictive. An objective of surgical treatment is to maintain or restore normal function to the hand, arm, and shoulder girdle on the affected side. Skin flaps and tissue are handled with great care to ensure proper viability, hemostasis, and drainage. If reconstructive surgery is planned, a consultation is made with a plastic surgeon before the mastectomy is performed.

After the tumour is removed, bleeding points are ligated and the skin is closed over the chest wall. Skin grafting is performed if the skin flaps are too small to close the wound. A nonadherent dressing (Adaptic) may be applied and covered by a pressure dressing. Two drainage tubes may be placed in the axilla and beneath the superior skin flap, and portable suction devices may be used; these remove the blood and lymph fluid that collect after surgery. The dressing may be held in place by wide elastic bandages or a surgical bra.

Breast-Conserving Surgery.

Breast-conserving surgery consists of lumpectomy, wide excision, partial or segmental mastectomy, or quadrantectomy (resection of the involved breast quadrant) and removal of the axillary nodes (axillary lymph node dissection) for tumours with an invasive component, followed by a course of radiation therapy to treat residual, microscopic disease.

The goal of breast conservation is to remove the tumour completely with clear margins while achieving an acceptable cosmetic result. The axillary lymph nodes are also removed through a separate semicircular incision under the hair-bearing portion of the axilla. A drain is inserted into the axilla through a separate stab

Table 48-4 • Surgical Treatment of Breast Cancer	
SURGICAL PROCEDURE	DESCRIPTION

Breast-conserving procedures:
  Lumpectomy
  Wide excision
  Partial mastectomy
  Segmental mastectomy
  Quadrantectomy
	Relatively synonymous terms to describe removal of varying amounts of breast tissue, including the malignant tissue and some surrounding tissue to ensure clear margins; axillary lymph nodes are also removed with these procedures, if the cancer was of the invasive type

Axillary lymph node dissection	Removal of some or all fat-enmeshed axillary lymph nodes for determination of extent of disease spread; the single most important determinant for prognosis and for need for adjuvant treatment
Total mastectomy	Removal of the breast tissue only; this procedure is generally done for the treatment of carcinoma in situ, typically ductal
Modified radical mastectomy	Removal of the breast tissue and an axillary lymph node dissection; the pectoralis major and minor muscles remain intact
Radical mastectomy	Removal of the breast tissue along with pectoralis major and minor muscles in conjunction with an axillary lymph node dissection

wound to remove blood and lymph fluid. A dressing is applied over the breast and under the arm and is secured with wide elastic bandages or a surgical bra.

Survival rates after breast-conserving surgery are equivalent to those after modified radical mastectomy. The risk for local recurrence, however, is greater, at 1% per year after surgery (Winchester & Cox, 1998). If the patient experiences a local recurrence, standard treatment is a completion or salvage mastectomy, in which the rest of the breast tissue is removed. Survival rates after this procedure are equivalent to those after mastectomy, but because the skin has been irradiated, the choices for reconstruction remain limited, and the woman should be informed of this possibility at the time of diagnosis and when considering her treatment options.

Postoperative Issues. The postoperative care of the patient undergoing a modified radical mastectomy or breast-conserving surgery is similar because both procedures involve an alteration to the breast and removal of lymph nodes from the axillary region. As with any surgical patient, the immediate focus is recovery from general anesthesia and pain management. In addition, the patient who has had breast surgery may experience both physical and psychological effects. Possible complications include the accumulation of blood (hematoma) at the incision site, infection, and late accumulation of serosanguineous fluid (seroma) after drain removal. Most patients who undergo breast surgery are discharged home with a drainage collection device in place. The nurse teaches the patient and family members to manage the drainage system.

Nerve trauma with resultant phantom breast sensations, numbness, tingling, or burning sensations may also occur and may persist for months or possibly years after surgery. Impaired arm and shoulder mobility can result from the axillary dissection. The disruption of lymphatic and venous drainage can leave the patient at risk for **lymphedema** (chronic swelling of the affected extremity) at any point after surgery (discussed later in this chapter). Psychological sequelae may include an altered body image or self-concept as a result of the alteration or loss of the breast. Other major psychosocial concerns include uncertainty about the future, fear of recurrence, and the effects of breast cancer and its treatment on family and work roles.

Lymphatic Mapping and Sentinel Node Biopsy. In the mid 1990s, a new procedure was introduced for use in patients undergoing breast surgery for the treatment of invasive breast cancer. Approximately 60% of patients who undergo an axillary lymph node dissection to determine the extent of the disease have negative nodes (Veronesi, Galimberti, Zurrida et al., 2001). The use of **lymphatic mapping and sentinel node biopsy** is changing the way these patients are treated because it provides the same prognostic information as the axillary dissection. A radiocolloid and/or blue dye is injected into the tumour site; the patient then undergoes the surgical procedure. The surgeon uses a hand-held probe to locate the sentinel node (the primary drainage site from the breast) and excises it, and it is examined by the pathologist. If the sentinel node is negative for metastatic breast cancer, a standard axillary dissection is not needed, thus sparing the patient the sequelae of the procedure (surgical drain, altered mobility of the extremity, paresthesias, risk for lymphedema). If the sentinel node is positive, the patient undergoes the standard axillary dissection. Reported results of this technique suggest a success rate of more than 90% in correctly identifying the sentinel node and correctly predicting axillary metastases (Hsueh, Hansen & Guiliano, 2000), and many centres have incorporated this procedure into stan-

dards of care. Short-term follow-up demonstrates that the rate of lymphedema is approximately 1% for women who undergo sentinel lymph node biopsy.

Nursing issues for this procedure focus on informing the patient about the expectations and possible implications. Because patients with a negative node are spared the axillary dissection, they may be discharged home the same day. Research is needed on the technique's sequelae, however. Questions to be addressed include: Do patients experience similar sensations in the affected arm as those who had an axillary dissection? Do patients demonstrate impaired mobility? Do these patients develop axillary seromas after the procedure? What is the risk for lymphedema? Initial nursing research on patient care issues related to sentinel node biopsy demonstrates that women who have sentinel node biopsy alone do have neuropathic sensations similar to those who undergo an axillary dissection, although the prevalence, severity, and distress are less so (Baron, Fey, Raboy et al., 2002).

RADIATION THERAPY

With breast-conserving surgery, a course of external-beam radiation therapy usually follows excision of the tumour mass to decrease the chance of local recurrence and to eradicate any residual microscopic cancer cells. Radiation treatment is necessary to obtain results equal to those of removal of the breast. If radiation therapy is contraindicated, mastectomy is the patient's only option (Chart 48-4).

Radiation treatment typically begins about 6 weeks after the surgery to allow the incision to heal. If systemic chemotherapy is indicated, radiation therapy usually begins after completion of the chemotherapy. External-beam irradiation provided by a linear accelerator using photons is delivered on a daily basis over 5 to 7 weeks to the entire breast region. In addition, a concentrated radiation dose or "boost" is administered to the primary site by means of electrons. Before radiation therapy begins, the patient undergoes a planning session for radiation treatment that will serve as the model for daily treatments. Small permanent ink markings are used to identify the breast tissue to be irradiated. Patients need reassurance about the procedure and self-care instructions related to side effects and their management.

Postoperative radiation after mastectomy is not common today but is still used in certain cases: when tumours have spread regionally (chest wall involvement, four or more positive nodes, or tumours larger than 5 cm). Occasionally, patients who have had a mastectomy require radiation treatment to the chest wall, generally after completion of systemic chemotherapy. Treatment usually consists of a course of external-beam irradiation to the area

Chart 48-4

Contraindications to Breast-Conservation Treatment

Note: Breast-conservation treatment includes both surgery and radiation.

Absolute Contraindications
- First or second trimester of pregnancy
- Presence of multicentric disease in the breast
- Prior radiation to the breast or chest region

Relative Contraindications
- History of collagen vascular disease
- Large tumour-to-breast ratio
- Tumour beneath nipple

for a period of several weeks, but the time frame is determined by the radiation oncologist. Some studies suggest that survival may be enhanced for high-risk premenopausal women who receive chest wall irradiation after mastectomy.

Another approach to radiation therapy is the use of intraoperative radiation therapy (IORT), in which a single dose of radiation is delivered to the lumpectomy site immediately after the surgeon has performed the lumpectomy. The dosage is limited to the tumour area, as any errant cells are most likely to be within the approximate area. The typical side effects of skin changes and fatigue are minimized with this approach. It may be as effective as the standard 5- to 7-week radiation course, but long-term data are still needed to determine the effect on local recurrence and survival rates.

Postirradiation Reaction. Generally, radiation therapy is well tolerated. Side effects are temporary and usually consist of mild to moderate skin reaction and fatigue. Fatigue usually occurs about 2 weeks after treatment and may last for several weeks after the treatments are completed. Fatigue can be depressing, as can the frequent trips to the radiation oncology unit or department for treatment. The patient needs to be reassured that the fatigue is normal and not a sign of recurrence. Rare complications of radiation therapy to the breast include pneumonitis, rib fracture, and breast fibrosis.

Postirradiation Nursing Management. Self-care instructions for patients receiving radiation are based on maintaining skin integrity during and after radiation therapy:

- Use mild soap with minimal rubbing.
- Avoid perfumed soaps or deodorants.
- Use hydrophilic lotions (Lubriderm, Eucerin, Aquaphor) for dryness.
- Use a nondrying, antipruritic soap (Aveeno) if itching occurs.
- Avoid tight clothes, underwire bras, excessive temperatures, and ultraviolet light.

Patients may note increased redness and, rarely, skin breakdown at the booster site (tissue site that received concentrated radiation). Important aspects of follow-up care include teaching patients to minimize exposure of the treated area to the sun for 1 year and reassurance that minor twinges and shooting pain in the breast are normal reactions after radiation treatment.

CHEMOTHERAPY

Chemotherapy is administered to eradicate the micrometastatic spread of the disease. An overview of chemotherapy is presented in Chapter 16. Although chemotherapy is generally initiated after breast surgery, no single standard exists for the sequencing of systemic chemotherapy and radiation therapy. Ongoing clinical trials may help to determine which treatment sequence produces the best outcomes.

Chemotherapy regimens for breast cancer combine several agents to increase tumour cell destruction and to minimize medication resistance. The chemotherapeutic agents most often used in combination are cyclophosphamide (Cytoxan) (C), methotrexate (M), fluorouracil (F), and doxorubicin (Adriamycin) (A). Paclitaxel (Taxol) (T) has been recently introduced into the adjuvant chemotherapy setting, and the data from clinical trials suggest a slight survival benefit with its use (Norton, 2001). Additionally, a newer taxane, docetaxel (Taxotere) (T), is being used more frequently, but research remains limited on its difference. The combination regimen of CMF or CAF is a common treatment protocol. AC, ACT (AC given first followed by T), and ATC, with all three agents given together, are other regimens that may be used (Levine, 2001). A new anthracycline agent, epirubicin (Ellence), which has been used more in Europe, is being used in certain regimens and protocols. Decisions regarding the chemotherapeutic protocol are based on the patient's age, physical status, and disease status and whether she is participating in a clinical trial. Chemotherapy treatment modalities are summarized in Table 48-5.

Reactions to Chemotherapy. Anticipatory anxiety is a common response among patients facing chemotherapy. Today, however, side effects can be managed well, with many women continuing their daily work and routine schedules. This has occurred in large measure because of the meticulous educational and psychological preparation provided to patients and their families by oncology nurses, oncologists, social workers, and other members of the health care team. The other factor is the availability of medication regimens that can alleviate the side effects of nausea and vomiting.

Common physical side effects of chemotherapy for breast cancer include nausea, vomiting, taste changes, alopecia (hair loss), mucositis, dermatitis, fatigue, weight gain, and bone marrow suppression. In addition, premenopausal women may experience temporary or permanent amenorrhea leading to sterility.

Less common side effects include hemorrhagic cystitis and conjunctivitis. Although its cause is unknown, weight gain of more than 10 pounds occurs in about half of all patients. Aerobic exercise and its anxiety-alleviating effects may be helpful to decrease weight gain and elevate mood. Side effects may vary with the chemotherapeutic agent used. CMF is generally well tolerated with only minimal side effects. Doxorubicin can be toxic to tissue if it infiltrates the vein, so it is usually diluted and infused through a large vein. Nausea and vomiting can occur. Antiemetics and tranquilizers may provide relief, as may visual imagery and relaxation exercises. Doxorubicin and paclitaxel usually cause alopecia, so obtaining a wig before hair loss occurs may prevent some of the associated emotional trauma. The patient needs reassurance that new hair will grow when treatment is completed, although the colour and texture of the hair may differ. It is helpful to provide a list of wig suppliers in the patient's geographic region and to become familiar with creative ways to use scarves and turbans to reduce the patient's reactions to hair loss. Look Good, Feel Better (a registered charity) can provide workshops, literature, and information on makeup, hair alternatives, and skin and nail care.

Nursing Management in Chemotherapy. Nurses working with patients receiving chemotherapy play an important role in assisting those who have difficulty with the side effects of treatment. Encouraging the use of medications to limit nausea, vomiting, and mouth sores reduces discomfort during chemotherapy. Some patients may receive granulocyte colony-stimulating factor (G-CSF), a synthetic growth-stimulating factor injected subcutaneously daily for 10 days, which boosts the white blood cell count to prevent nadir fever (a fever that occurs with infection when the blood cell counts are at their lowest level) and infections. The nurse instructs the patient and family on injection technique and about symptoms that require follow-up with a physician (Chart 48-5).

Taking time to explain side effects and possible solutions may alleviate some of the anxiety of women who feel uncomfortable asking questions. The more informed a patient is about the side effects of chemotherapy and how to manage them, the better she can anticipate and deal with them.

Table 48-5 • Chemotherapy and Hormonal Therapy for Breast Cancer

TYPE OF TREATMENT	GOALS OF THERAPY	POSSIBLE SIDE EFFECTS	NURSING INTERVENTIONS
Chemotherapy	Destroy neoplastic cells Decrease or prevent metastasis		
doxorubicin (Adriamycin) (A)		ECG changes, tachycardia, nausea, vomiting, stomatitis, hair loss, severe cellulitis if infiltration occurs	*Nausea and vomiting:* Administer antiemetics as prescribed; monitor fluid intake and output
cyclophosphamide (Cytoxan) (C)		Nausea, vomiting, anorexia, menstrual abnormalities, hemorrhagic cystitis	*Anorexia:* Assist patient and family to identify appetizing foods; provide frequent small meals if better tolerated than three regular meals; refer to dietitian for assistance in planning palatable, nutritious meals
methotrexate (M)		Stomatitis, CNS changes, hair loss	
5-fluorouracil (F)		CNS changes, neurotoxicity, nausea, vomiting, constipation, stomatitis	*Stomatitis:* Avoid commercial mouthwashes; use baking soda, salt and water rinses, or oral anesthetic agents
paclitaxel (Taxol) (T)		Hypersensitivity, peripheral neuropathy, nausea, vomiting, diarrhea, stomatitis, hair loss	*Hair loss:* Avoid brushing, blow drying, frequent shampooing; encourage use of turbans and scarves; encourage patient to obtain wig before hair loss occurs
epirubicin (Ellence) (E)		Myelosuppression; cardiac toxicity; nausea, vomiting, and mucositis	*CNS changes:* Monitor for weakness, malaise, fatigue, seizures, change in cognitive status; assist with activities of daily living if fatigue and malaise occur
docetaxel (Taxotere) (T)		Hypersensitivity; neurosensory disturbances; nausea, vomiting, stomatitis	*Neurotoxicity:* Monitor deep tendon reflexes, assess gait and muscle strength, monitor for changes in sensory function
Combination therapy: CMF CAF AC ACT CEF		Side effects of all agents used	*Fluid retention:* Monitor weight, fluid intake and output, skin turgor *Cardiac changes:* Monitor ECG, cardiac rate and rhythm; notify physician of dysrhythmias *Hypercalcemia:* Monitor serum calcium levels, monitor cardiac rate and rhythm *Constipation:* Monitor bowel function; consider that constipation may be indicative of neurotoxicity; administer stool softeners, laxatives as prescribed; encourage adequate intake of fluids and fibre *Anxiety:* Administer tranquilizers as prescribed; encourage use of strategies to minimize anxiety (imagery, relaxation)
Hormonal Therapy			
Androgens fluorymesterone (Halotestin)	Suppress estrogens	Masculinization, fluid retention, cholestatic jaundice, hypercalcemia	*Hormonal instability:* Observe for changes (hot flashes, vaginal bleeding, flare); facial hirsutism, deepening of voice; fluid retention, Cushing's syndrome (fullness of face, lower extremity edema, weight gain); increased blood pressure; assess for thrombophlebitis; monitor serum calcium levels; educate patient on symptom management of hot flashes and assure patient that most changes are temporary
Estrogens diethylstilbestrol (DES)	Suppress FSH and LH	Nausea, vomiting, anorexia, dizziness, headache	
Corticosteroids prednisone	Suppress estrogen production by the adrenals and decrease urinary estrogen metabolites	Cushing's syndrome: fullness of face, weight gain, edema of lower extremities	
Antihormonal agents tamoxifen (Nolvadex)	Estrogen antagonist; effective in decreasing risk for cancer recurrence in postmenopausal women and as a palliative treatment for recurrent cancer	Weight gain, hot flashes, nausea, anorexia, lethargy	
megestrol acetate (Megace)	Progestational agent; may decrease number of estrogen receptors in breast tissue	Weight gain, hot flashes, vaginal bleeding, increased blood pressure, peripheral edema, depression, tumour flare	
aminoglutethimide (Cytadren)	Enzyme antagonist that inhibits estrogen synthesis	CNS changes: dizziness, clumsiness, drowsiness, depression, headache	
anastrazole (Arimidix)	Aromatase inhibitor; blocks production of estrogen in peripheral tissues	Asthenia, nausea, headache, hot flashes, back pain	

*This listing of medications, side effects, and nursing interventions is not meant to be exhaustive but is rather a sample of frequently used chemotherapeutic agents for breast cancer.
FSH, follicle-stimulating hormone; LH, luteinizing hormone.

Chemotherapy may negatively affect the patient's self-esteem, sexuality, and sense of well-being. Combined with the stress of a potentially life-threatening diagnosis, these changes can be overwhelming. Because many women are distressed by financial concerns and time spent away from the family, nursing support and teaching can reduce emotional distress during treatment. Important aspects of nursing care include communicating, facilitating support groups, encouraging patients to ask questions, and promoting trust in health care providers. Adequate time must be scheduled for clinical appointments to allow discussion and questions. Most women with breast cancer today are treated in a multidisciplinary environment, and referrals to the dietitian, social worker, psychiatrist, or spiritual advisor can assist in dealing with many of the issues of cancer treatment. In addition, numerous community supports and advocacy groups are available to these patients and their families.

HORMONAL THERAPY

Decisions about hormonal therapy for breast cancer are based on the outcome of an **estrogen and progesterone receptor assay** of tumour tissue taken during the initial biopsy. The tissue requires special handling by laboratory technicians with expertise in assessment techniques. Normal breast tissue contains receptor sites for estrogen. About two thirds of breast cancers are estrogen dependent, or ER-positive (ER+). An ER+ assay indicates that tumour growth depends on estrogen supply; therefore, measures that reduce hormone production may limit the progression of the disease, and these receptors can be considered prognostic indicators. ER+ tumours may grow more slowly in general than those that do not depend on estrogen (ER−); thus, having an ER+ tumour indicates a better prognosis. A value less than 3 fmol/mg is considered negative. Values of 3 to 10 are questionable, and values greater

NURSING RESEARCH PROFILE 48-2
Menopausal Symptoms During Breast Cancer Treatment

McPhail, G., & Smith, L. N. (2000). Acute menopausal symptoms during adjuvant systemic treatment for breast cancer. *Cancer Nursing, 6*(23), 430–443.

Purpose
Early detection and improved treatment of breast cancer have increased the life expectancy of women who reach menopause after the diagnosis of breast cancer to near-normal. It has been suggested that menopause experienced by women receiving treatment for breast cancer may differ from natural menopause, although no empirical study has addressed this issue. The purpose of this study was to determine if menopausal symptoms in women who were undergoing systemic chemotherapy differed from those in women who experience a natural menopause.

Study Sample and Design
The sample in this case-control study comprised two groups of women ranging from 50 to 64 years of age: 200 women undergoing treatment for breast cancer with tamoxifen or chemotherapy and a control group of 200 women who had undergone breast screening and had no diagnosis of breast cancer. A self-report questionnaire addressed general health and menstrual history, breast cancer treatment and associated symptoms, and menopause and menopausal symptoms. The women with breast cancer completed all portions of the questionnaire, while women without breast cancer completed only the third section, which included the Greene Climacteric Scale, an established scale for menopausal symptoms. Questionnaires were mailed to the 400 women, and 238 completed and returned the questionnaires. The final sample included 139 women with breast cancer and 99 women without a diagnosis of breast cancer. Most of the women in both groups were perimenopausal or postmenopausal at the time of the study. Statistical

procedures were used to describe study results and to examine differences between the two groups.

Findings
Women with breast cancer were more likely than those without cancer to report that they were currently experiencing menopause symptoms ($p = 0.04$) and were more likely to have a greater severity of symptoms as assessed by the Greene Climacteric Scale. Women who were receiving adjuvant systematic treatment for breast cancer perceived their menopause symptoms as a significant source of distress, with hot flushes second to tiredness as a side effect attributed to cancer treatment. Women receiving chemotherapy were more likely to report tiredness, and women receiving tamoxifen were more likely to report hot flushes. The group undergoing treatment and the control group differed on four specific symptoms: tiredness, hot flushes, night sweats, and headaches. The women undergoing breast cancer treatment reported more severe tiredness, hot flushes, and night sweats than the control group. The control group experienced more severe headaches.

Nursing Implications
Nurses who care for patients undergoing systemic chemotherapy for treatment of breast cancer need to be aware of the greater potential for distressing side effects related to menopause. Management of these side effects is important to assist the woman through the treatment. Providing suggestions about strategies to manage fatigue and minimize hot flushes is an important nursing intervention.

than 10 are considered positive. The greater the value, the more beneficial the anticipated effect from hormone suppression can be. Patients with tumours that are positive for both estrogen and progesterone (PR+) generally have a more favourable prognosis than patients with tumours that are ER– and PR–. Most progesterone-receptive tumours also have a positive estrogen receptor status. The loss of progesterone receptors can be a sign of advancing disease. Premenopausal women and perimenopausal women are more likely to have non–hormone-dependent lesions; postmenopausal women are likely to have hormone-dependent lesions.

Hormonal therapy may include surgery to remove endocrine glands (eg, the ovaries, pituitary, or adrenal glands) with the goal of suppressing hormone secretion. Oophorectomy (removal of the ovaries) is one treatment option for premenopausal women with estrogen-dependent tumours. Tamoxifen is the primary hormonal agent used in breast cancer treatment today. Anastrazole (Arimidex), letrozole (Femara), leuprolide (Lupron), megestrol (Megace), diethylstilbestrol (DES), fluoxymesterone (Halotestin), and aminoglutethimide (Cytadren) are other hormonal agents used to suppress hormone-dependent tumours. Most of these agents may be associated with menopausal symptoms such as vasomotor changes. Hypercalcemia may also occur and may necessitate discontinuing the agent. These hormonal agents are described in Table 48-5.

BONE MARROW TRANSPLANTATION

Bone marrow transplantation (BMT) involves removing bone marrow from the patient and then administering high-dose chemotherapy. The patient's bone marrow, spared from the effects of chemotherapy, is then reinfused intravenously. This procedure is usually performed in specialized transplantation centres, and specific patient preparation, education, and support must be given throughout the treatment course. In 1999, scientific misconduct was discovered in the only study that showed a benefit (Hagmann, 2000), casting doubt on the role that BMT may play in breast cancer treatment. The use remains controversial outside of clinical trials, since studies are not clear as to the true benefits in comparison to standard high-dose chemotherapy (Antman, 2001). BMT is described more fully in Chapter 16.

INVESTIGATIONAL THERAPY: THE FUTURE

Research is underway to develop chemotherapeutic agents that modify multidrug resistance and agents that enhance or modify standard chemotherapy. Research in breast cancer treatment includes the following areas: peripheral stem cell transplants, oncogenes (tumour genes that control cell growth), growth factors (substances released by cancer cells to make the environment more conducive to growth), monoclonal antibodies (synthetic antibodies that fight cancer cells), biologic response modifiers (substances that help increase the body's immune system response), and vaccine studies.

Another treatment modality that has shown promise is trastuzumab (Herceptin). This monoclonal antibody was engineered from mouse antibodies and closely resembles a human antibody. Herceptin binds with the HER2 protein, and this protein regulates cell growth, thus inhibiting tumour cell growth. For women with metastatic breast cancer, about 25% to 30% of tumours overproduce HER2, and this monoclonal antibody can slow growth and possibly stimulate the immune response. Herceptin is approved by Health Canada. Research is ongoing, but the addition of this agent to traditional chemotherapy has shown improved survival rates in clinical trials (Capriotti, 2001). Further

research and clinical experience will demonstrate the potential of this drug in the treatment of breast cancer, particularly on the role of Herceptin for women undergoing adjuvant therapy.

Special Issues in Breast Cancer Management

RECONSTRUCTIVE SURGERY

After mastectomy, some women elect to have reconstructive surgery, which provides considerable psychological benefit. Support groups and classes provide education and peer support for patients who are candidates for and interested in breast reconstruction. Some concerns that women may have about reconstructive surgery are cost, safety, and timing—whether to undergo reconstruction immediately (at the time of mastectomy) or delay it (6 months to 1 year after surgery). Cost to the patient may vary depending on her health insurance, but because reconstruction is considered rehabilitative surgery, it is often covered.

In regard to safety, there are the usual surgical risks for infection and reaction to anesthesia, as well as the risk for a cosmetically unsatisfactory result. Reconstructive surgery is contraindicated if a woman has locally advanced, metastatic, or inflammatory breast cancer. Otherwise, most women with either in situ or early-stage breast cancer are candidates for immediate reconstruction. Breast reconstruction does not interfere with systemic treatment, nor does it affect the risk of cancer recurrence.

If a woman decides to have reconstructive surgery at the time of mastectomy, she avoids future surgery, although the total operative time increases. Some women find that immediate reconstruction lessens the feelings of loss and disfigurement. Occasionally, reconstruction cannot be performed because skin and muscles are too tight. Loose, supple skin and subcutaneous tissue with a sufficient blood supply contribute to reconstructive success. Some women benefit by waiting until later because initially they are not sure about their choice. Reconstructive surgery is discussed in more detail later in this chapter.

PROSTHETICS

Not all women desire reconstruction, nor are all women candidates for reconstructive surgery. In these instances, patients may need information about prostheses (molds made of silicone shaped in the form of a breast) and the names of shops where they can be fitted for a prosthesis. The Canadian Cancer Society's Reach to Recovery program can provide women with the names and addresses of local establishments where they can be fitted. Women should be encouraged to find a shop that has a comfortable, supportive atmosphere and employs a certified prosthetics consultant. Generally, medical supply shops are not recommended because they often do not have the appropriate resources to ensure the proper fit of a prosthesis.

Before the patient is discharged from the hospital (following a day-surgery procedure or an overnight hospital stay), the nurse usually provides the patient with a temporary cotton fluff that can be worn until the surgical incision is well healed (4 to 6 weeks). At that time, the woman can be fitted for a prosthesis. Insurance generally covers the cost of a prosthesis and the special bras that hold it in place. Women should be encouraged to wear the prosthesis because it provides a sense of psychological restoration and wholeness. The prosthesis also assists the woman in resuming proper posture, because it helps to balance the weight of the remaining breast.

QUALITY OF LIFE AND BREAST CANCER

Despite current treatment, there has been only a slight overall improvement in survival for breast cancer patients. Consequently, quality-of-life considerations have become important issues in treatment and recovery. Quality of life is a multidimensional construct that includes functional (self-care) status, social and family functioning, and psychological and spiritual well-being. These parameters are important indicators of how well a patient is functioning after diagnosis and treatment.

Breast cancer is the most frequently investigated cancer in quality-of-life studies. Early psychosocial studies emphasized that the loss of the breast was the single most important factor in women's adjustment, especially in Western cultures. Thus, it is not surprising that studies of women's adjustment to breast cancer found similar results. A growing body of research, however, indicates that concerns related to uncertainty about the future, day-to-day issues in work and family relationships, and demands of illness are more important factors in adjusting to having breast cancer than the loss of the breast alone. For example, younger women are more vulnerable to issues of psychosocial adjustment than many older women (Hoskins & Haber, 2000). They worry about their jobs and whether they will be able to keep their employer-paid health care benefits. They are concerned about their work productivity and career advancement (Wonghongkul, Moore, Musil et al., 2000). They face many family concerns related to whether they can have children, whether they will live to see their children grow up, and whether their disease will recur and incapacitate them (Horden, 2000). Middle-aged women worry about their disease in relation to their family and work (Walker, Nail & Croyle, 1999). They also worry about their aging parents and whether they will be able to care for them in the future. They are increasingly concerned about their daughters' risk for breast cancer. Older women are more vulnerable to chronic health problems. Living an average of 6 years longer than men, older women face loss of their social circles, must deal with the potential for other diseases, and worry about whether they will have the resources to pay for medications.

These concerns are intertwined with the effects of breast cancer on the family. Studies indicate that up to 35% of families of breast cancer patients experience significant changes in family functioning. More than 25% of children also experience problems related to their mothers' breast cancer (Hilton, Crawford & Tarko, 2000). In addition, families shoulder substantial costs in caring for family members with advanced breast cancer. These out-of-pocket, unreimbursed expenses include lost wages and salaries and lost opportunities.

When faced with any life-threatening illness, spiritual and existential concerns usually surface. Patients with breast cancer often express the need to talk about the uncertainties of their future and their hope and faith that they will be able to manage whatever crisis or challenge comes their way.

PREGNANCY AND BREAST CANCER

From 2% to 5% of breast cancers occur in relation to pregnancy (Dow, 2000; Moore & Foster, 2000). The potent hormones released during pregnancy (1,000 times greater than those during a menstrual cycle) stimulate changes in breast tissue (Gemignani & Petrek, 1999). Thus, detecting masses is more difficult during pregnancy. An important aspect of health promotion is to encourage BSE throughout pregnancy.

NURSING RESEARCH PROFILE 48-3
Breast Cancer Survivorship

Utley, R. (1999). The evolving meaning of cancer for long-term survivors of breast cancer. *Oncology Nursing Forum, 26*(9), 1519–1523.

Purpose
While the incidence of cancer is highest in women over 65 years of age, the highest survival rates also occur in this group, with a survival rate of 97% for localized breast cancer. Little is known about the experience of survivorship of women with breast cancer. Thus, the purpose of this study was to describe the different meanings of cancer for older women who were long-term survivors of breast cancer.

Study Sample and Design
A descriptive qualitative study was conducted to explore the experience of long-term survivors of breast cancer. The sample comprised eight women whose survival following treatment for breast cancer ranged from 5.5 to 29 years. Their ages at the time of the study ranged from 65 to 77 years. Four of the women had lumpectomy with radiation and chemotherapy, and one had lumpectomy with radiation only as her treatment. Three women had undergone mastectomy and one of them had received oral chemotherapy. Two of the women had positive axillary lymph nodes, and they had lumpectomy combined with radiation and chemotherapy.

Interviews lasting 60 to 90 minutes were conducted with the women in their homes; three life history interviews were conducted with each woman and audiotaped. The interviews were then transcribed and coded for themes and patterns. In addition, the researcher used a methodology log and reflexive journal.

Findings
Three meanings of cancer emerged from the data: cancer as sickness and death, cancer as an obstacle, and cancer as transforming. Cancer as sickness and death was the initial perspective of the women at the time of diagnosis and during the early phases of their treatment. Cancer as obstacle reflected the women's perspective that breast cancer was an obstacle that was intrusive or in the way of their life path that they had to deal with before moving on. Cancer as transforming described the change in women's outlooks about life and their own strength as they put their diagnosis in perspective. They viewed their cancer treatment as past and moved on to renewing their interactions with their surroundings.

Nursing Implications
Nurses need a better understanding of and sensitivity to the experience of women with breast cancer as they move beyond their disease and its treatment. By asking open-ended questions, the nurse can help women explore their experience so they can begin to shift their view of breast cancer from an experience of sickness and death to a surmountable challenge.

If a mass is found during pregnancy, ultrasound is the preferred diagnostic method because it involves no exposure to radiation, although mammography with appropriate shielding, fine-needle aspiration, and biopsy may also be indicated. Treatment is basically the same as in other women, although radiation is contraindicated in pregnancy. Some oncologists begin chemotherapy as early as the 16th week of pregnancy because fetal organs are already formed at this point. If systemic treatment is necessary, a cesarean section may be performed as soon as maturation of the fetus allows. If aggressive disease is detected early in pregnancy and chemotherapy is advised, termination of the pregnancy is an issue that some patients must face. If a mass is found while a woman is breastfeeding, she is urged to stop breastfeeding to allow the breast to involute (return to its baseline state) before any type of surgery is performed.

After a woman has completed treatment for breast cancer, she may consider having children. In this case, individual issues must be addressed, including the patient and her partner's desire for children and family, disease and prognostic concerns, age, fertility and infertility issues, and social, financial, ethical, and quality-of-life issues. Although recommendations vary, most women are advised to wait 2 years before becoming pregnant after completing treatment for breast cancer. Most retrospective studies indicate that pregnancy after treatment for breast cancer does not appear to increase the risk of the disease recurring (Gemignani & Petrek, 1999); however, prospective studies are needed to confirm this. Counselling, providing accurate information, and active listening and caring are important nursing interventions when patients are involved in making difficult personal decisions about treatment options, childbearing, or termination of pregnancy.

NURSING PROCESS:
THE PATIENT WITH BREAST CANCER

Assessment

The health history includes an assessment of the patient's reaction to the diagnosis and her ability to cope with it. Pertinent questions include the following:

- How is the patient responding to the diagnosis?
- What coping mechanisms does she find most helpful?
- What psychological or emotional supports does she have and use?
- Is there a partner, family member, or friend available to assist her in making treatment choices?
- What are the most important areas of information she needs?
- Is the patient experiencing any discomfort?

Diagnosis

PREOPERATIVE NURSING DIAGNOSES

Based on the health history and other assessment data, the patient's major preoperative nursing diagnoses may include the following:

- Deficient knowledge about breast cancer and treatment options
- Anxiety related to cancer diagnosis
- Fear related to specific treatments, body image changes, or possible death
- Risk for ineffective coping (individual or family) related to the diagnosis of breast cancer and related treatment options
- Decisional conflict related to treatment options

POSTOPERATIVE NURSING DIAGNOSES

Based on the health history and other assessment data, the patient's major postoperative nursing diagnoses may include the following:

- Acute pain related to surgical procedure
- Impaired skin integrity due to surgical incision
- Risk for infection related to surgical incision and presence of surgical drain
- Disturbed body image related to loss or alteration of the breast related to the surgical procedure
- Risk for impaired adjustment related to the diagnosis of cancer, surgical treatment, and fear of death
- Self-care deficit related to partial immobility of upper extremity on operative side
- Disturbed sensory perception (kinesthesia) related to sensations in affected arm, breast, or chest wall

- Risk for sexual dysfunction related to loss of body part, change in self-image, and fear of partner's responses
- Deficient knowledge: drain management after breast surgery
- Deficient knowledge: arm exercises to regain mobility of affected extremity
- Deficient knowledge: hand and arm care after an axillary lymph node dissection

COLLABORATIVE PROBLEMS/
POTENTIAL COMPLICATIONS

Based on the assessment data, potential complications may include the following:

- Lymphedema
- Hematoma formation
- Infection

Planning and Goals

The major goals for the patient may include increased knowledge about the disease and its treatment; reduction of preoperative and postoperative fears, anxiety, and emotional stress; improvement of decision-making ability; pain management; maintenance of skin integrity; improved self-concept; improved sexual function; and the absence of complications.

Preoperative Nursing Interventions

EXPLAINING BREAST CANCER AND TREATMENT OPTIONS
The patient confronting the diagnosis of breast cancer reacts with fear, dread, and anxiety. In view of the usually overwhelming emotional reactions to the diagnosis, the patient must be given time to absorb the significance of the diagnosis and any information that will help her to evaluate treatment options.

The nurse caring for the woman who has just received a diagnosis of breast cancer needs to be knowledgeable about current treatment options and able to discuss them with the patient. The nurse should be aware of the information that has been given to the patient by the physician.

Information about the surgery, the location and extent of the tumour, and postoperative treatments involving radiation therapy and chemotherapy are details that the patient needs to enable her to make informed decisions. As appropriate, the nurse discusses with the patient medications, the extent of treatment, management of side effects, possible reactions after treatment, frequency and duration of treatment, and treatment goals. Methods to compensate for physical changes related to mastectomy (eg, prostheses and plastic surgery) are also discussed and planned. The amount and timing of the information provided are based on the patient's responses, coping ability, and readiness to learn.

REDUCING FEAR AND ANXIETY
AND IMPROVING COPING ABILITY
The patient's emotional preparation begins when the tentative diagnosis of cancer is made. Patients who have lost close relatives to breast cancer (or any cancer) may have difficulty coping with the possible diagnosis of breast cancer because memories of loss and death can emerge during their own crisis.

The patient may have the diagnostic procedure performed in the surgeon's office or in the hospital when she is admitted for ambulatory or same-day surgery for a biopsy. Fears and concerns are common and are discussed with the patient. If she will undergo a mastectomy, information about various resources and options is provided. Such services include prostheses, reconstructive surgery, and groups such as Reach to Recovery. Discussion with a plastic surgeon about the various options for reconstructive surgery can be a valuable source of information and support.

The nurse provides anticipatory teaching and counselling at each stage of the process and identifies the sensations that can be expected during additional diagnostic procedures. The nurse also discusses the implications of each treatment option and how it may affect various aspects of the patient's treatment course and lifestyle. The patient is introduced to other members of the oncology team (eg, radiation oncologist, medical oncologist, oncology nurse, and social worker) and is acquainted with the role of each in her care. After the treatment plan has been established, the nurse needs to promote preoperative physical, psychological, social, and nutritional well-being. The patient usually prefers to be active in her care and decision making. Some women find it helpful and reassuring to talk to a breast cancer survivor, someone who has completed treatment and has been trained as a volunteer to talk with newly diagnosed patients.

PROMOTING DECISION-MAKING ABILITY

At times, a patient may demonstrate behaviour that indicates she cannot make a decision about treatment. Careful guidance and supportive counselling are the interventions the nurse can use to help such a patient. Also, encouraging the patient to take one step of the treatment process at a time can be helpful. The advanced practice nurse or oncology social worker can be helpful for patients and family members in discussing some of the personal issues that may arise in relation to treatment. Some patients may need a mental health consultation before surgery to assist them in coping with the diagnosis and impending treatment. Such patients may have had a history of psychiatric problems or demonstrate behaviour that leads the surgeon or nurse to initiate a referral to the psychiatrist, psychologist, or psychiatric clinical nurse specialist.

Postoperative Nursing Interventions

RELIEVING PAIN AND DISCOMFORT

Ongoing nursing assessment of pain and discomfort is important because patients experience differing degrees of pain intensity. Some women may have more generalized pain and discomfort of the chest wall, affected breast, or affected arm. Moderate elevation of the involved extremity is one means of relieving pain because it decreases tension on the surgical incision, promotes circulation, and prevents venous congestion in the affected extremity. Intravenous or intramuscular opioid analgesic agents are another method to manage pain in the initial postoperative phase. After the patient is taking fluids and food and the anesthesia has cleared sufficiently (usually by the next morning), oral analgesic agents can be effective in relieving pain. Patient teaching before discharge then becomes important in managing discomfort after

surgery because pain intensity varies widely. Patients should be encouraged to take analgesic agents (opioid or nonopioid analgesic medications such as acetaminophen) before exercises or at bedtime and also to take a warm shower twice daily (usually allowed on the second postoperative day) to alleviate the discomfort that comes from referred muscle pain.

MAINTAINING SKIN INTEGRITY AND PREVENTING INFECTION

In the immediate postoperative period, the patient will have a snug but not tight dressing or a surgical bra packed with gauze over the surgical site and one or more drainage tubes in place. A particular concern is preventing fluid from accumulating under the chest wall incision or in the axilla by maintaining the patency of the surgical drains. The dressings and drains should be inspected for bleeding and the extent of drainage monitored regularly.

If a hematoma develops, it usually occurs within the first 12 hours after surgery; thus, monitoring the incision is important. A hematoma could cause necrosis of the surgical flaps, although this complication is rare in breast surgery patients. If either of these complications occurs, the surgeon should be notified, and the patient should have an Ace wrap placed around the incision and an ice pack applied. Initially, the fluid in the surgical drain appears bloody, but it gradually changes to a serosanguineous and then a serous fluid during the next several days. The drain is usually left in place for 7 to 10 days and is then removed after the output is less than 30 mL in a 24-hour period. The patient is discharged home with the drains in place; therefore, teaching of the patient and family is important to ensure correct management of the drainage system (Chart 48-6).

Dressing changes present an opportunity for the nurse and patient to discuss the incision, particularly how it looks and feels and the progressive changes in its appearance. The nurse explains the care of the incision, sensations to expect, and the possible signs and symptoms of an infection. Generally, the patient may shower on the second postoperative day and wash the incision and drain site with soap and water to prevent infection. A dry dressing should be applied to the incision each day for 7 days. The patient needs to know that sensation is decreased in the operative area because the nerves were disrupted during surgery and that gentle care is needed to avoid injury. After the incision is completely healed (usually 4 to 6 weeks), lotions or creams may be applied to the area to increase skin elasticity. After the incision is fully healed, the patient may again use deodorant on the affected side, although many women note that they no longer perspire as much as before the surgery.

PROMOTING POSITIVE BODY IMAGE

During teaching sessions, the nurse can address the patient's perception of the body image changes and physical alteration of the

---

Chart 48-6
Home Care Checklist • Surgical Breast Cancer Patient with a Drainage Device

At the completion of the home care instruction, the patient or caregiver will be able to:	Patient	Caregiver
• Demonstrate how to empty and measure fluid from the drainage device	✓	✓
• Demonstrate how to strip or milk clots through the tubing of the drainage device	✓	✓
• State observations that require contacting the physician or nurse (eg, sudden drainage colour change, sudden cessation of drainage, signs or symptoms of an infection)	✓	✓
• Care for the drain site as per surgeon's recommendation	✓	✓
• Identify when the drain is ready for removal (usually when draining less than 30 mL for a 24-hour period)	✓	✓

breast. Patients may initially be uncomfortable looking at the surgical incision. No matter how prepared a patient may be, the view of her incision and absence of her breast is often difficult for her. Exploring this sensitive area must be a careful nursing action, and cues provided by the patient must be respected and sensitively handled. Privacy is a consideration when assisting the woman to view her incision fully for the first time and allows the patient to express her feelings safely to the nurse. Asking the patient what she perceives, acknowledging her feelings, and allowing her to express her emotions are important nursing actions. Explaining that her feelings are a normal response to breast cancer surgery may be reassuring to the patient. Ideally, she will see the incision for the first time when she is with the nurse or another health care provider who is available for support. With short hospital stays, many women will view the incision for the first time with the home care nurse or ambulatory care nurse at the time of postoperative follow-up visits.

PROMOTING POSITIVE ADJUSTMENT AND COPING

Ongoing assessment of the patient's concerns related to the diagnosis of cancer, the consequences of surgical treatment, and fear of death is important in determining her progress in adjusting and the effectiveness of her coping strategies. Assisting the patient in identifying and mobilizing her support systems is important. The patient's spouse or partner may need guidance, support, and education as well. The patient and spouse may benefit from a wide network of available community resources, including the Canadian Cancer Society, Canadian Breast Cancer Foundation, Canadian Cancer Society's Reach to Recovery Program, advocacy groups, or a spiritual advisor. Encouraging the patient to discuss issues and concerns with other patients who have had breast cancer may help her to understand that her feelings are normal and that other women who have had breast cancer can provide invaluable support and understanding.

Another important aspect of promoting the patient's adjustment and coping includes answering questions and addressing her concerns about the treatment options that may follow surgery. After the surgery has been completed, thoughts about what lies in the future in terms of additional treatment are normal, and this topic can cause understandable anxiety. Refocusing the patient on the recovery from surgery, while addressing her concerns and answering her questions, can be helpful. Being knowledgeable about the plan of care and encouraging the patient to ask questions of the appropriate members of the health care team will also promote coping during recovery.

A few women require additional support to adjust to the diagnosis and the changes that it brings. If a woman displays ineffective coping, counselling or consultation with a mental health practitioner may be indicated.

Table 48-6 summarizes the needs of and nursing interventions for patients and their partners at various stages of the breast can-

Table 48-6 • Needs and Nursing Interventions for Patients and Partners

DIAGNOSTIC PHASE	POSTSURGICAL PHASE	ADJUVANT THERAPY PHASE	ONGOING RECOVERY PHASE
Needs and Interventions Related to the Health Care System			
Minimize uncertainty: • correct misinformation • discuss surgical options • explore resources • explain health care system logistics	Establish confidence in health care: • encourage questions • provide information on postoperative care • promote a sense of control	Develop a supportive network: • clarify information • discuss side effects and management • assist in decision making	Maintain association with professionals: • encourage regular follow-up exams, changes in diet and exercise • teach early detection skills • provide realistic reassurance
Needs and Interventions Related to Physical Well-Being			
Prevent disease advancement: • expedite early treatment • reduce anxiety through timely care	Promote physical well-being: • provide information on the healing process • discuss self-care	Minimize adverse physical outcomes: • promote recovery from surgery • teach side effects management	Maintain a positive outlook: • assess perception of physical change • encourage healthful behaviours
Needs and Interventions Related to Psychological Well-Being			
Protect emotional well-being: • alter perceptions of the illness • foster active participation in health care • identify ways to reduce anxiety	Develop a framework of expectations: • describe the treatment process • discuss potential emotional sequelae • support a positive self-image • help to accept altered roles	Manage stress: • identify feelings of vulnerability • provide information on adjuvant therapies and potential side effects • encourage communication of needs	Redefine self and partner: • normalize activities of daily living • reprioritize values, needs, and expectations • incorporate health-promoting behaviours
Needs and Interventions Related to Social Support			
Establish trusting communication: • explore the meaning of the diagnosis • examine treatment options • foster the ability to ask for help	Establish a supportive network: • consider sources of emotional support	Understand family members' responses: • interpret others' reactions	Cultivate ongoing support: • promote an understanding of how to live as a cancer survivor

Reproduced with permission from Hoskins, C. N., & Haber, J. (2000). Adjusting to breast cancer. *American Journal of Nursing, 100*(4), 26–32.

cer experience. Chart 48-7 provides insights into ways to initiate conversations with patients and their partners in different phases of therapy.

PROMOTING PARTICIPATION IN CARE

Ambulation is encouraged when the patient is free of postanesthesia nausea and is tolerating fluids. The nurse supports the patient on the nonoperative side. Exercises (hand, shoulder, arm, and respiratory) are initiated on the second postoperative day, although instruction occurs on the first postoperative day. The goals of the exercise regimen are to increase circulation and muscle strength, prevent joint stiffness and contractures, and restore full range of motion. Hand exercises are also important for the same reasons.

<table>
<tr><td>**Chart 48-7**</td><td>**Talking with Patients & Partners**</td></tr>
</table>

For patients in the diagnostic phase: We've talked about your recent breast cancer diagnosis. It's natural for you to be full of feelings, concerns, and fears about yourself and your family. Sometimes it's hard to find someone to speak freely with. Would you share what you've been thinking, feeling, and worrying about recently?

For partners in the diagnostic phase: We've talked about your partner's recent breast cancer diagnosis. It's natural for you to have a lot of feelings, concerns, and fears about your partner, yourself, and your family. Partners often feel that they have to be strong for the patient or for others and that they aren't entitled to express their own concerns. Would you share what you've been thinking about, feeling, or worrying about recently?

For patients in the postsurgical phase: Many women who have had breast surgery, especially mastectomy or extensive lumpectomy are concerned not only with their own loss, but with how their partner will accept it. How have you felt about losing [part of] your breast? How has it changed your body image? Your sense of your sexuality? Your desire for intimacy?

For partners in the postsurgical phase: Many partners of women who have had breast surgery are concerned, as are the women themselves, about how they'll respond to the loss. How have you felt about your partner's losing [part of] her breast? How has it changed her attractiveness for you? Your sexual feelings toward her? Your desire for intimacy?

For patients in the adjuvant therapy phase: Given the type of therapy (radiation, chemotherapy, hormone therapy) you're going to have, what side effects do you anticipate? What do you know about them? Let's talk about ways to reduce and handle potential side effects.

For partners in the adjuvant therapy phase: Given the type of therapy (radiation, chemotherapy, hormone therapy) your partner is going to have, what side effects do you anticipate? What do you know about them? Let's talk about ways to reduce and handle potential side effects, and how it might help you to be familiar with them.

For patients in the ongoing recovery phase: As you plan your return to a full work schedule, what measures—setting priorities, delegating responsibility, managing stress—might help you make the necessary physical and emotional adjustments? What have you learned about balancing work, family, and play in your life?

For partners in the ongoing recovery phase: As your partner plans her return to a full work-schedule, what strategies have you thought about using to make your own physical and emotional adjustments, so that you don't continue to be overburdened at work and at home?

Reproduced with permission from Hoskins, C. N., & Haber, J. (2000). Adjusting to breast cancer. *American Journal of Nursing, 100*(4), 26–32.

Postmastectomy exercises (Chart 48-8) are usually performed three times daily for 20 minutes at a time until full range of motion is restored (generally 4 to 6 weeks). Showering before exercising loosens stiff muscles, and taking an analgesic agent 30 minutes before beginning exercise increases the patient's ability to comply with the regimen. Also, self-care activities, such as brushing the teeth, washing the face, and combing and brushing the hair, are physically and emotionally therapeutic because they aid in restoring arm function and a sense of normalcy for the patient.

The nurse encourages the patient to use the muscles in both arms and to maintain proper posture. If a patient is favouring or splinting the affected side, or not standing up straight, any exercise will be ineffective. If a patient has skin grafts, a tense, tight surgical incision, or immediate reconstruction, exercises may need to be prescribed specifically and introduced gradually. Most patients find that after the drain is removed, range of motion returns quickly if they have been compliant with their exercise programs. This reinforcement may be provided in the outpatient setting by the ambulatory care nurse or the home care nurse.

Patients are instructed regarding activity limitations while healing postoperatively. Generally, heavy lifting is avoided, although normal household and work-related activities are promoted to maintain muscle tone. Driving may begin after the drain is removed and when the patient has full range of motion and is no longer taking opioid analgesic agents. General guidelines for activity focus on gradually introducing previous activities (eg, bowling, weight-training) when fully healed, although checking with the physician beforehand is usually indicated.

Transient edema in the affected extremity is common during the healing period, and women are encouraged to elevate the arm above the level of the heart on a pillow for 45 minutes at a time three times daily to promote circulation. Performing the prescribed exercises also assists in reducing the transient edema. Prevention of lymphedema is taught to patients before discharge. Hand and arm care after an axillary lymph node dissection focuses on the prevention of injury or trauma to the affected extremity, which increases the likelihood of developing lymphedema (Chart 48-9).

MANAGING POSTOPERATIVE SENSATIONS

Because nerves in the skin are cut during breast surgery, patients experience a variety of sensations. Common sensations are tightness, pulling, burning, and tingling along the chest wall, in the axilla, and along the inside aspect of the upper arm. They tend to become more noticeable and increase as the patient begins to heal. They usually persist for several months up to a year and then begin to diminish. Explaining to the patient that this is a normal part of healing helps to reassure her that these sensations are not indicative of a problem. Performing the exercises may decrease the sensations. Acetaminophen (Tylenol), taken as needed, also assists in managing the discomfort. Many breast surgery patients report these sensations as one of the most bothersome aspects of having the surgery.

IMPROVING SEXUAL FUNCTION

Most breast surgery patients are physically allowed to engage in sexual activity once discharged from the hospital. However, any change in the patient's body image and self-esteem or the partner's response may increase the couple's anxiety level and may affect sexual function. Some partners may have difficulty looking at the incision, whereas others appear to be unaffected and comfortable. Either response affects the patient's self-image, sexuality, and acceptance. Open discussion and clear communication about how the patient sees herself and about possible decreased libido related to fatigue, anxiety, or nausea may help to clarify issues for her and her partner. Encouraging discussion about fears,

Chart 48-8 • PATIENT EDUCATION
Exercises After Breast Surgery

1. *Wall handclimbing.* Stand facing the wall with feet apart and toes as close to the wall as possible. With elbows slightly bent, place the palms of the hand on the wall at shoulder level. By flexing the fingers, work the hands up the wall until arms are fully extended. Then reverse the process, working the hands down to the starting point.

3. *Rod or broomstick lifting.* Grasp a rod with both hands, held about 61 cm apart. Keeping the arms straight, raise the rod over the head. Bend elbows to lower the rod behind the head. Reverse manoeuvre, raising the rod above the head, then return to the starting position.

2. *Rope turning.* Tie a light rope to a doorknob. Stand facing the door. Take the free end of the rope in the hand on the side of surgery. Place the other hand on the hip. With the rope-holding arm extended and held away from the body (nearly parallel with the floor), turn the rope, making as wide swings as possible. Begin slowly at first; speed up later.

4. *Pulley tugging.* Toss a light rope over a shower curtain rod or doorway curtain rod. Stand as nearly under the rope as possible. Grasp an end in each hand. Extend the arms straight and away from the body. Pull the left arm up by tugging down with the right arm, then the right arm up and the left down in a see-sawing motion.

Chart 48-9 • PATIENT EDUCATION
Hand and Arm Care After Axillary Dissection

- Avoid blood pressures, injections, and blood draws in affected extremity.
- Use sunscreen (higher than 15 SPF) for extended exposure to sun.
- Apply insect repellent to avoid bug bites.
- Wear gloves for gardening.
- Use cooking mitt for removing objects from oven.
- Avoid cutting cuticles; push them back during manicures.
- Use electric razor for shaving armpit.
- Avoid lifting objects greater than 2.5–4.5 kg.
- If a trauma or break in the skin occurs, wash the area with soap and water, and apply an over-the-counter antibacterial ointment (Bacitracin or Neosporin).
- Observe the area and extremity for 24 hours; if redness, swelling, or a fever occurs, call the surgeon or nurse.

needs, and desires may reduce the couple's stress. Suggestions regarding varying the time of day for sexual activity (when the patient is less tired) or assuming positions that are more comfortable can be helpful, as are other options for expressing affection (eg, hugging, kissing, manual stimulation).

Most patients and their partners adjust with minimal difficulty if they openly discuss their concerns; however, if problems develop or persist, referral to a psychosocial resource (psychologist, psychiatrist, or psychiatric clinical nurse specialist, social worker, or sex therapist) can be helpful for the woman and her partner. To identify difficulty in sexual relationships, the ambulatory care nurse and home care nurse must be sensitive to this issue following treatment for breast cancer and must initiate discussion with the patient.

MONITORING AND MANAGING POTENTIAL COMPLICATIONS

Lymphedema

Lymphedema can occur any time after an axillary lymph node dissection. Lymphedema results if functioning lymphatic channels are inadequate to ensure a return flow of lymph fluid to the general circulation. After removal of axillary nodes, collateral or auxiliary circulation must take over their function. Transient edema in the postoperative period occurs until this collateral circulation has fully assumed functioning for the removed nodes, which generally occurs within a month by moving and exercising the affected arm. Patients need reassurance that this transient swelling is not lymphedema. Education about how to prevent lymphedema is an important part of hand and arm care after an axillary dissection. Lymphedema occurs in about 10% to 20% of patients who undergo an axillary dissection. Risk factors for lymphedema are increasing age, obesity, presence of extensive axillary disease, radiation treatment, and injury or infection to the extremity. Patients should follow these guidelines to prevent injury to the affected extremity because lymphedema is subsequently associated with a trauma of some type.

If lymphedema occurs, the patient should contact the surgeon or nurse to discuss management because she may need a course of antibiotics or specific exercises to decrease the swelling. Emphasis should be placed on early intervention because lymphedema can be manageable if treated early; however, if allowed to progress without treatment, the swelling can become painful and difficult to reverse. Management consists of arm elevation with the elbow above the shoulder and the hand higher than the elbow, along with specific exercises, such as hand pumps. A referral to a

physical therapist or rehabilitation specialist may be necessary for a custom-made elastic sleeve, exercises, manual lymph drainage, or a special pump to decrease swelling.

Prior to 1996, there was the belief that strenuous upper-body exercises after breast cancer treatment would result in lymphedema. In 1996, a group of 24 women between the ages of 31 and 62 years who were all survivors of breast cancer began training as a dragon boating team. The group worked on stretching, strengthening, and resistance exercises along with cardiopulmonary activities. The team "Abreast in a Boat" competed in Vancouver at a large dragon boat racing festival. They demonstrated that dragon boating was an excellent physical, mental, and support activity for women after breast cancer and that lymphedema did not occur. The team members became role models in promoting health and raising awareness of breast cancer; they were fit, had improved well-being, better body image, and were confident. A manual was developed to guide other women's dragon boating teams, and the movement has spread across Canada and around the world (McKenzie, 1998). June 2005 marks the 10th anniversary of a "breast cancer survivor category" being included in dragon boat competitions.

Hematoma Formation

Hematoma formation may occur after either mastectomy or breast conservation. The nurse monitors the surgical site for excessive swelling and monitors the drainage device, if present. Gross swelling or output from the drain may indicate hematoma formation, and the surgeon should be notified promptly. Depending on the surgeon's assessment, an Ace wrap may be applied for compression of the surgical site along with ice packs for 24 hours, or the patient may be returned to surgery to identify the source of bleeding. The nurse monitors the site and reassures the patient that this complication is rare but does occur and that she will be assisted through its management. A calm demeanor on the part of the nurse helps prevent anxiety and panic on the part of the patient.

Infection

Infection follows breast surgery in about 1 in 100 patients. Infection can occur for a variety of reasons, including concurrent conditions (diabetes, immune disorders, advanced age) and exposure to pathogens. In addition, cellulitis may occur after breast surgery. Both preoperatively and before discharge, patients are taught to monitor for signs and symptoms of infection (redness, foul-smelling drainage, temperature greater than 38°C) and to contact the surgeon or nurse for evaluation. Treatment consists of oral or intravenous antibiotics for 1 or 2 weeks, depending on the severity of the infection. Cultures are taken of any foul-smelling discharge. Infections are a serious threat to women who have had breast reconstruction because they may lose the breast mound if the infection persists; there is a risk of lymphedema in women who develop an infection and have had an axillary lymph node dissection.

PROMOTING HOME AND COMMUNITY-BASED CARE

Teaching Patients Self-Care

Patients who undergo breast surgery receive a tremendous amount of information before and after surgery. Additional teaching is necessary to prepare the patient and family to manage aspects of care after home discharge. Even though the ambulatory care nurse prepares the patient for what to expect postoperatively, the details often appear less important to the patient in light of the diagnosis of breast cancer. Thus, teaching may need to be repeated and reinforced postoperatively. Most patients are discharged either the same day or 1 to 2 days after the surgery with the drains in place. The inpatient nurse assesses the patient's readiness to assume self-care and focuses on teaching the patient incision care; signs to report, such as an infection; pain management; arm exercises; hand and arm care; and management of the drainage system at home. Family members may be included in the discharge teaching, and many women find it reassuring and helpful to have another person assist them with management of the drainage system. The ambulatory care nurse reinforces teaching by telephone follow-up and during postoperative visits in the office.

Continuing Care

Referral for home care may be indicated to assist the patient and family caregiver with postoperative care at home. The home care nurse assesses the patient's incision and drainage system, physical and psychological status, adequacy of pain management, and adherence to the exercise plan. In addition, the home care nurse reinforces previous teaching and communicates important physiologic findings or psychosocial issues to the patient's primary care provider, nurse, or surgeon.

Follow-up visits to the physician after diagnosis and treatment of breast cancer depend on the individual and on postoperative treatments, stage of disease at diagnosis, late effects from cancer, and the patient's adaptation. Visits every 3 months for 2 years, followed by every 6 months up to 5 years, may be then extended to annual examinations, depending on the patient's progress and the physician's preference. A disease-free state for as long as possible is the goal. Patients are also encouraged to do BSE on the remaining breast (and operative side if breast-conserving surgery was done) and the chest wall (after mastectomy) between appointments because the risk for cancer in the remaining breast (or recurrence in the operative breast) is about 1% per year after the original diagnosis. Additional screening is done with annual mammography. Ultrasound and MRI are being used more commonly with women who have survived breast cancer. Because it is common to ignore routine health care when a major health issue arises, the woman is reminded of the importance of participating in health promotion activities and other health screening. Because some problems with coping may not occur until the woman has returned to more usual routines, the ambulatory care nurse needs to be sensitive to this issue and encourage discussion throughout the recovery period.

Evaluation

EXPECTED PREOPERATIVE PATIENT OUTCOMES

Expected preoperative patient outcomes may include:

1. Exhibits knowledge about diagnosis and treatment options
   a. Asks relevant questions about diagnosis and available treatments
   b. States rationale for surgery and other treatment options
   c. Describes advantages and disadvantages of treatment options
2. Verbalizes willingness to deal with anxiety and fears related to the diagnosis and the effects of surgery on self-image and sexual functioning
3. Demonstrates ability to cope with diagnosis and treatment
   a. Verbalizes feelings appropriately and recognizes normalcy of mood lability
   b. Proceeds with treatment in timely fashion
   c. Discusses impact of diagnosis and treatment on family and work
4. Demonstrates ability to make decisions regarding treatment options in timely fashion

EXPECTED POSTOPERATIVE PATIENT OUTCOMES

Expected postoperative patient outcomes may include:

1. Reports that pain has decreased and states pain and discomfort management strategies are effective

2. Exhibits clean, dry, and intact surgical incisions without signs of inflammation or infection
3. Lists the signs and symptoms of infection to be reported to the nurse or surgeon
4. Verbalizes feelings regarding change in body image
5. Discusses meaning of the diagnosis, surgical treatment, and fears (especially of death) appropriately
6. Participates actively in self-care activities
   a. Performs exercises as prescribed
   b. Participates in self-care activities as prescribed
7. Recognizes that postoperative sensations are normal and identifies management strategies
8. Discusses issues of sexuality and resumption of sexual relations
9. Demonstrates knowledge of postdischarge recommendations and restrictions
   a. Describes follow-up care and activities
   b. Demonstrates appropriate care of incisions and drainage system
   c. Demonstrates arm exercises and describes exercise regimen and activity limitations during postoperative period
   d. Describes care of affected arm and hand and lists indications to contact the surgeon or nurse
10. Experiences no complications
    a. Identifies signs and symptoms of reportable complications (ie, redness, heat, pain, edema)
    b. Describes side effects of chemotherapy and strategies to cope with possible side effects
    c. Explains how to contact appropriate health care providers in case of complications

Care of the patient with breast cancer is summarized in the Plan of Nursing Care.

RECURRENT BREAST CANCER

The recurrence of breast cancer can be very difficult for patients and family members. Depending on the clinical presentation, progression of the disease can have different meanings. Generally, the longer the disease-free interval, the better the prognosis. Local recurrence either in the affected breast or along the chest wall can be treated, generally with surgery, radiation, or hormonal manipulation, although a metastatic disease workup may be in order to look for further evidence of disease. Although metastatic spread of the breast cancer (to the bone, lungs, brain, or liver) cannot be cured, a variety of treatments are available (chemotherapy, radiation treatment, hormonal manipulation, or possibly some form of surgery). In some patients, metastases progress very slowly and life functioning is generally not affected, whereas in others the disease progresses rapidly despite treatment, and death from the complications of metastatic disease is inevitable.

The patient with advanced breast cancer is monitored closely for signs that the tumour has recurred or that metastasis has occurred. The following studies are conducted to monitor for spread of disease: metastatic x-ray series (chest, skull, long bones, and pelvis); liver function tests (alkaline phosphatase, aspartate aminotransferase [AST] or serum glutamic-pyruvic transaminase [ALT] lactate dehydrogenase); mammogram of contralateral breast and ipsilateral breast (if breast-conserving surgery was originally performed); and bone, liver, and brain imaging. In half of all patients with recurrent disease, the cancer reappears locally (on the chest wall or in the conserved breast) or regionally in the remaining

(text continues on page 1484)

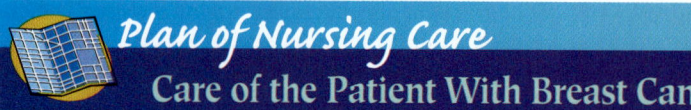

Plan of Nursing Care
Care of the Patient With Breast Cancer

Nursing Interventions	Rationale	Expected Outcomes

Nursing Diagnosis: Fear and ineffective coping related to the diagnosis of breast cancer, its treatment, and prognosis
Goal: Reduction of emotional stress, fear, and anxiety

1. Begin emotional preparation of the patient (and partner) as soon as she is informed of tentative diagnosis.	1. This enables the patient to initiate coping responses.	• Displays reduced emotional stress and anxiety and exhibits an ability to cope with the problem
2. Assess: a. Personal experience with and knowledge about breast cancer b. Coping mechanisms in crisis c. Support systems d. Emotional reaction to diagnosis	2. These factors strongly affect the patient's behaviour and ability to deal with the diagnosis, surgery, and follow-up treatment. If a patient has lost close relatives or friends to breast cancer, she will probably react differently from a patient who has friends surviving with an excellent quality of life.	• Participates in the treatment plan and asks questions relating to the best choice for her particular needs • States that anger, anxiety, depression, denial, and withdrawal are normal reactions • Responds positively to the information she has received
3. Inform the patient of recent research and new treatment modalities for breast cancer.	3. Increasing options and improved results both statistically and cosmetically greatly reduce the fear and promote acceptance of the treatment plan.	• Describes the value of social support of family, friends, and women who have had breast surgery in coping with a stressful experience
4. Describe the experiences the patient will face and encourage her questions.	4. Decreases fear of the unknown.	• Is aware that partner has been advised and prepared with regard to supportive role
5. Acquaint her with available resources to facilitate her recovery.	5. The information about new prosthetics, reconstruction specialists, and other resources confirms that a great deal of attention is being given to newer treatment methods for breast cancer.	• Reads literature provided

Nursing Diagnosis: Disturbed body image related to nature of surgery and side effects of radiation and/or chemotherapy
Goal: Realistic adaptation to changes that will occur relative to treatment modalities

1. Confirm with the physician the nature of the treatment anticipated.	1. This sets the basis for a cooperative therapeutic plan that will prevent conflicting information from reaching the patient.	• Decides on the treatment plan after discussion with physician and family • Verbalizes that grief must run its course
2. Explain that it is normal to experience grief at the loss of a body part.	2. With this understanding, the patient can then be free to move to the next level of coping.	• Uses her support system effectively; plans future activities with them
3. Encourage visits by loved ones and understanding friends.	3. Support systems that are meaningful to the patient are more endurable than those from relative strangers.	• Eventually looks at her incision site and participates in dressing changes
4. Explain that it is normal not to want herself or partner to view the incision (do not refer to this as a "scar"); further reinforce the fact that each day the site will look better.	4. This reduces the feeling that she will never be able to adjust to her altered body.	• Expresses an understanding of the long-term benefits of chemotherapy/radiation (if prescribed) even though there may be uncomfortable side effects
5. Discuss the use of prosthesis, reconstruction possibilities, and clothing adjustment as realistic and attainable expectations.	5. The emphasis on the positive and the availability of adaptations will enhance her self-concept and promote positive acceptance of the treatment plan.	

Nursing Diagnosis: Acute pain related to tissue trauma from incision(s)
Goal: Absence of pain and discomfort

1. Assess intensity, nature, and location of pain.	1. Provides baseline to assess effectiveness of pain relief measures	• Reports when pain is worsening and accepts prescribed pain medication
2. Administer analgesia by IM, oral, or IV route as prescribed.	2. Promotes pain relief	• Adjusts her position to relieve discomfort; uses small pillows effectively

(continued)

Plan of Nursing Care

Care of the Patient With Breast Cancer *(Continued)*

Nursing Interventions	Rationale	Expected Outcomes
3. Collaborate with physician about use of patient-controlled analgesia (PCA).	3. Patient-controlled analgesia results in pain relief and increased comfort and maintains patient's sense of control.	• Exercises frequently; moves affected arm gently and shows progress in moving from passive to active exercises
4. Explain that analgesics are available for pain relief.	4. Analgesics and opioids can interrupt nerve pathways to the brain and spinal cord.	• Describes home-related activities that will provide the required range of motion of the affected arm
5. Proper body positioning will promote comfort, such as semi-Fowler's position and elevation of the arm of the affected side.	5. Stress on the incision site is reduced; gravity reduces fluid accumulation in the arm. (Squeezing ball and wrist flexion begin in first 24 hours.)	• Relates procedures to follow if injury is sustained
6. Promote passive and then active exercises of the hand, arm, and shoulder of the affected side.	6. This will stimulate circulation, promote neurovascular competence, and prevent stasis and subsequent stiffening of the shoulder girdle.	• Orders medical identification tags when arm lymphedema is diagnosed
7. Encourage protection and the avoidance of anything that can break through the skin barrier to impose stress on the arm and shoulder (cuts, burns, strong detergents, infections, carrying a heavy bag or purse).	7. Impaired circulation and weakened muscles are vulnerable to sudden or prolonged stress.	
8. Suggest application of an effective cream several times a day.	8. This practice will keep the skin healthy, intact, pliable, and resistant to break-down.	
9. Instruct patient to contact the physician if the arm or incision site becomes painful, swollen, or red.	9. Early treatment of possible infection or injury will avoid further discomfort and complications.	
10. Suggest wearing a medical identification tag if there is a potential for injury or edema.	10. A recognized medical identification tag will serve as a precaution against injury to the affected arm.	

Nursing Diagnosis: Dressing/grooming, bathing/hygiene self-care deficit related to partial immobility of upper extremity on side of breast surgery

Goal: Avoidance of impaired mobility and achievement of self-care to the fullest possible level

1. Encourage patient's active participation in postoperative care.	1. Patient involvement enhances and facilitates the recovery process.	• Participates in dressing change; expresses interest in working with rehabilitative team, including physical therapist
2. Encourage patient's socialization, particularly with others who have successfully recovered in similar circumstances.	2. Humans thrive more effectively when they are able to relate to others socially.	• Expresses concern about her appearance and accepts suggestions from rehabilitation support groups
3. Make progressive modifications in the patient's exercise program as dictated by comfort and tolerance levels.	3. There is lessened strain on tissues; improvement is consistent.	• Participates in self-care (ie, dressing, bathing, grooming)
4. Provide positive reinforcement when ingenuity and creativity are in evidence, such as an attractive hairstyle or make-up application.	4. Psychological well-being complements the effects of optimal physical good health.	• Verbalizes anticipation and enjoyment of partner's visits and relates her progress

Nursing Diagnosis: Possible sexual dysfunction related to loss of body part and fear of partner's reaction to this loss

Goal: Identification of alternative satisfying/acceptable sexual experiences

1. Become comfortable in discussing sexuality; display a caring, nonjudgmental, supportive attitude.	1. The patient will easily sense insincerity, insecurity, lack of knowledge, and inexperience. Nurses new to this area can obtain assistance from the oncology clinical nurse specialist.	• Responds by conveying trust and a desire to obtain assistance; asks appropriate questions.
		• Includes partner in discussion of issues that concern both.

(continued)

Plan of Nursing Care
Care of the Patient With Breast Cancer (Continued)

Nursing Interventions	Rationale	Expected Outcomes
2. Encourage, at the appropriate time, both partners to discuss their concerns; this can be done before and after major treatment.	2. The patient will not feel that she is alone in facing issues that may concern both partners.	• Verbalizes concerns about sexuality issues
3. Arrange for privacy when discussing personal issues with the patient.	3. Sensitive personal issues are not revealed when people not close to the patient are present.	• Accepts the incision site as evidenced by assisting with dressings and using an appropriate prescribed emollient such as cocoa butter
4. Describe the incision site and its appearance to the partner before partner actually sees it.	4. Partner will know what to expect and not likely register shock in front of the patient.	• Expresses awareness that any adjustments take time but that with patience and understanding, the desired goals can be approached and possibly reached
5. Emphasize that behavioural changes take time and should not be interpreted as rejection.	5. Undergoing any surgery takes time for acceptance, recuperation, and perhaps altered lifestyle.	

Collaborative Problem: Infection, injury, lymphedema, neurovascular deficits
Goal: Avoidance of complications

1. Encourage elevation of the arm, if not contraindicated, with each joint positioned higher than the more proximal joint.	1. Edema is reduced and there is less pressure on the nerves and blood vessels; pain and discomfort are reduced.	• Demonstrates positioning pillows so that proper elevation of arm is maintained
2. Instruct patient to avoid injury, strenuous activity, or infection.	2. These can produce fluid accumulation and compromise the neurovasculature of the arm.	• Describes strategies for avoiding injury and infection
3. Describe and demonstrate exercises in a step-up fashion from simple to more complex.	3. A graduated exercise program will improve muscle tone and hasten full range of activities with avoidance of impairment, such as a frozen shoulder.	• Gradually moves the arm freely so that hair combing and "climbing the wall" can be achieved with no discomfort. Avoids the discomfort of a frozen shoulder.
4. Recommend physical therapy and a weight-reduction program if indicated.	4. Properly prescribed activities and exercise plus diet modification are general health measures that enhance well-being and reduce risk for complications.	• Acquires good health habits and avoids complications

lymph nodes, and in one fourth other organs become involved. Bone metastasis is the most common site for spread of the disease, usually involving the hips, spine, ribs, or pelvis. Other sites for metastatic spread are the brain, lungs, and liver.

Medical Management

Regression or relief of the symptoms is the goal of nursing and medical management, and quality of survival time is an important focus of nursing intervention. Assessing the patient's physical and psychosocial status is a challenge for the nurse. Information from family members and significant others is valuable and should be included in planning care for the patient with advanced disease.

Palliative treatment, if indicated, is also an important aspect of care. Comfort and a pain-free existence, even if the disease cannot be eradicated, enhance the quality of remaining life. Palliative surgery may be offered if the patient has a fungating or necrotic tumour in the breast; the most common procedure is a modified radical mastectomy. In patients with bone metastases that cause pain or produce pathologic fractures, reparative or restorative surgery may also be an option; however, this may not

be indicated depending on the patient's medical status and personal choices. Hospice and home health care may be indicated as alternatives. Regardless, specific arrangements for these services should be discussed and planned early, before the actual need arises, to decrease patient distress. Severe anxiety and depression may occur. Treatment modes vary and depend on the patient's condition, the modalities available, and the patient's preferences for end-of-life care. Chapter 16 provides more information on the general care of the patient with advanced cancer. Chapter 17 discusses end-of-life care.

Reconstructive Breast Surgery

Because the breast plays such an important part in self-image of many women, a perceived abnormality may lead to a request for **mammoplasty** (plastic surgery of the breast in which size, shape, or position is altered). Variations in the size of the breasts are a common reason for women to seek information about reconstructive breast surgery. Reduction mammoplasty is performed to reduce the size of the breast, whereas augmentation mammoplasty is performed to increase the size of the breast. Other women desire surgery to reconstruct their breasts after mastectomy. There are several different procedures used for this type of reconstructive surgery. In addition, some women choose to undergo prophylactic (risk-reducing) mastectomy if they are at high risk for breast cancer. This type of mastectomy is included in this discussion because it is considered elective.

REDUCTION MAMMOPLASTY

Reduction mammoplasty is usually performed on women who have breast hypertrophy (excessively large breasts). If the enlargement occurs early in life, it is called virginal breast hypertrophy. The condition is usually bilateral but may affect just one breast. Hypertrophy in later life almost always affects both breasts.

Tenderness, diffuse pain, and fatigue are common complaints of women with hypertrophy. Premenstrual tenderness and pain are marked. The weight of the enlarged breasts causes a dragging sensation in the shoulder, and support is commonly futile, despite use of the most supportive bra. Many women have deep grooves in their shoulders from the weight borne by bra straps. Poor posture, discomfort, and embarrassment when wearing bathing suits and participating in athletic events may limit the woman's social life. As a result, insecurity may develop from poor self-image.

After a surgical or plastic surgery consultation, a reduction mammoplasty may be performed under general anesthesia. One approach is an incision in the skin of the anterior breast in the shape of a keyhole or an anchor if a large amount of tissue needs to be removed. Another approach is through an incision around the areola complex. The surgeon then removes the excess tissue and transplants the nipple to a new location. Skin edges are approximated with sutures, and the nipple is secured with sutures. Drains are placed in the incision, where they remain for 1 to 2 days. Simple gauze dressings are applied, without pressure.

Postoperative Nursing Management

After mammoplasty, the usual postoperative care is indicated. Patients are ambulatory fairly quickly and typically describe their surgery as nontraumatic, possibly because of the relief they experience. Hypertrophy does not recur, but if the patient gains weight, the breasts may enlarge. The newly transplanted nipple most likely becomes covered with a scab. As the nipple regains a new blood supply, the scab falls off, and the appearance approximates normal. Lactation may be impossible after this type of surgery, although half of women who have this surgery can breastfeed successfully. Sensory changes, such as numbness, are normal after this surgery but resolve after several months, although diminished sensation in the nipples can persist. Postoperatively, the woman may feel a mixture of euphoria, relief, sorrow over loss of a body part, and anxiety over these feelings. Providing reassurance is an important nursing measure.

AUGMENTATION MAMMOPLASTY

Augmentation mammoplasty is requested frequently by women desiring larger or fuller breasts. It is performed through an incision along the undermargin of the breast, in the axilla, or at the border of the areola. The breast is then elevated, and a pocket is formed between the breast and the chest wall into which various types of synthetic materials are inserted to enlarge and uplift the breast. The subpectoral approach is preferred because it interferes less with clinical breast examinations or mammography than do subglandular implants. These procedures may be performed on an outpatient basis with local anesthesia. Infection, an immediate complication that can occur, may require removal of the implant. A delayed complication, which usually occurs years after the surgery, is a capsular contracture (scar formation around the implant); further surgery may be needed to correct this problem.

Saline implants are typically used for augmentation mammography. Silicone implants were used in the past; however, because of the reported systemic complications associated with their use, they have been removed from the market. They are now available only to women enrolled in controlled clinical trials designed to study specific safety questions. Long-term risks associated with their use are also being studied. Women with breast implants need to be aware that accurate mammograms are more difficult, and they should seek radiologists at specialized breast centres who are familiar with reading mammograms of women who have breast implants.

RECONSTRUCTIVE PROCEDURES AFTER MASTECTOMY

When a woman undergoes a mastectomy (either total or modified radical) for the treatment of breast cancer, she may desire to have immediate reconstruction at the time of surgery, or delayed reconstruction may be an option at a later point after all treatments have been completed. About 75% of women with breast cancer undergoing mastectomy elect immediate reconstruction. A consultation with the surgeon may assist women in deciding whether reconstruction is something that they desire at the time of surgery. It is important for women to understand that reconstruction does not interfere with the treatment of their breast cancer, and they should also understand that although a good cosmetic result can be obtained, the reconstructed breast will never be what they once had. Another key point for women to understand is that reconstruction is a three-stage process that occurs over a period of months: the first is creation of the breast mound, the second is achieving symmetry with the contralateral breast, and the third is creation of the nipple–areola complex (described later). Women who undergo reconstruction with realistic expectations tend to be more pleased with the cosmetic result. Also, women who have mastectomy with immediate reconstruction may demonstrate a more positive adjustment afterward.

The choice of the surgical procedure is based on the patient's wishes, the condition of the overlying skin and underlying muscle, and any previous scars that may be present, because they may limit possible reconstructive options. Another important factor is any secondary medical conditions that may affect the healing process (eg, hypertension, diabetes mellitus, tobacco use, or obesity).

Tissue Expanders With Permanent Implants

One method of reconstruction is the **tissue expander with permanent implant** (Fig. 48-7). After the surgeon has completed the mastectomy, the plastic surgeon creates a pocket inside the pectoralis muscle and inserts a partially filled Silastic expander and a drainage device. Then, over a period of weeks, the patient comes to the office for injections of additional saline into the expander through a port that is under the skin; this temporary expander stretches the skin and muscle. When the implant is fully expanded (usually one third larger than the other breast to create a natural crease and droop to match the contralateral breast), the patient has the temporary implant exchanged for a permanent implant. This is usually performed as outpatient surgery. It may be done 4 to 6 months later to allow the tissue to soften and become more pliable before the permanent implant is inserted.

FIGURE 48-7 Breast reconstruction with tissue expander. (**A**) After mastectomy, a tissue expander is inserted to prepare for reconstruction. (**B**) The expander is gradually filled with saline solution through a tube to stretch the skin enough to accept an implant beneath the chest muscle. (**C**) The breast mound is restored. Although permanent, scars will fade with time. The nipple and areola are reconstructed later. Adapted from "Breast Reconstruction," American Society of Plastic and Reconstructive Surgeons, Arlington Heights, IL.

Postoperative care is similar to that of the patient undergoing breast surgery, although more discomfort can be expected due to the additional surgery. Nausea may take longer to clear because there was a greater period under general anesthesia. Patients receive instruction just as any other surgical breast cancer patient would, but usually they are not allowed to shower until the drain is removed.

Tissue Transfer Procedures

Another method of reconstruction is using the patient's own tissue and transferring it to the mastectomy site. These flap surgeries can use the **transverse rectus abdominis myocutaneous flap** (TRAM flap) (Fig. 48-8), gluteal muscle, or latissimus dorsi muscle (Fig. 48-9). The plastic surgeon transfers the muscle flap with attached circulatory structures, skin, and fatty tissue, rotates it to the operative site, and molds it to create a mound that simulates the breast. These procedures are far more extensive and involve greater operative time (about 8 to 10 hours total time for the mastectomy and reconstruction) and duration of general anesthesia than does the tissue expander procedure. The risk for potential complications is greater (infection, bleeding, flap necrosis), but the benefits are a more natural-looking breast and avoidance of synthetic material. The recovery period is greater, and activity restrictions are different due to the cut muscles.

The TRAM flap is the most commonly used tissue transfer procedure, and postoperative care involves drain management and monitoring the operative site for changes in circulation. During the immediate postoperative period, patients are more limited in their activity and are at greater risk for respiratory complications, so pulmonary hygiene is essential. Measures to reduce tension on the incisions include elevating the head of the bed by 30 degrees and flexing the patient's knees to reduce tension on the abdominal incision. Antiemetic agents are administered to control nausea and vomiting, and analgesic medications are administered to reduce pain and discomfort. Assessing circulation by observing the colour and temperature of the newly constructed breast area is an important nursing function. Mottling or an obvious decrease in skin temperature is reported to the surgeon immediately. Excessive drainage should also be reported.

During ambulation, the patient usually protects the surgical incision by splinting. Gradually, she will achieve a more upright position. The patient is instructed to avoid tight and underwire bras until the surgeon indicates that no injury will result. Elevating the arms above the shoulder and lifting more than 2 kg of weight are avoided for 1 month after surgery to avoid stress on the incision.

Nipple–Areola Reconstruction

After the breast mound has been created and the site has healed, some women choose to have a nipple–areola reconstruction. This consists of minor surgical procedures carried out either in the physician's office or as outpatient surgery. A nipple is created using a skin graft from the inner thigh or labia because this skin has darker pigmentation than the skin on the reconstructed breast. After the nipple graft has healed, the areolar complex is usually completed with micropigmentation (tattooing). The surgeon can usually match the reconstructed nipple–areola complex with that of the contralateral breast for an acceptable cosmetic result.

FIGURE 48-8 Breast reconstruction: TRAM flap. (**A**) The flap of the transrectus abdominal muscle is tunnelled through the abdomen to the breast area. In some cases a breast implant may not be needed if enough skin and muscle can be transferred. (**B**) Scarring will fade substantially over time. Adapted from "Breast Reconstruction," American Society of Plastic and Reconstructive Surgeons, Arlington Heights, IL.

FIGURE 48-9 Breast reconstruction: latissimus dorsi flap. (**A**) Tissue taken from the back is tunnelled to the front of the chest wall to support the reconstructed breast. (**B**) The transported tissue forms a flap that can hold a breast implant if there is not enough tissue to form a breast mound, or (**C**) tissue may be taken from the abdomen and tunnelled to the breast or surgically transplanted to form a new breast mound. Adapted from "Breast Reconstruction," American Society of Plastic and Reconstructive Surgeons, Arlington Heights, IL.

Diseases of the Male Breast

GYNECOMASTIA

Gynecomastia, or overdeveloped breast tissue, is the most common breast condition in the male. Adolescent boys can be affected by this condition because of hormones secreted by the testes. Gynecomastia usually subsides in 1 or 2 years, but it can occur before or after puberty and in elderly men. It is usually unilateral and presents as a firm, tender mass underneath the areola. In adult men, gynecomastia may be diffuse and related to medications (ie, digitalis, reserpine, ergotamine, ranitidine, and phenytoin). Pain and tenderness are initial symptoms. Treatment depends on the man's feelings and preference. Observation is acceptable because it may resolve on its own; surgical removal of the tissue through an incision around the areola is another option. Liposuction of the tissue done by a plastic surgeon, another option, yields a positive cosmetic result.

MALE BREAST CANCER

Cancer of the male breast in 2005 accounted for 45 deaths and 150 new cases (Canadian Breast Cancer Foundation, 2005). Symptoms can include a painless lump beneath the areola, nipple retraction, nipple discharge, or skin ulceration. Diagnostic tests and treatment modalities are similar to those used for women. The average age of the patient at the time of diagnosis is 60 years, but it can occur in younger men, especially if there is a genetic link to the disease, because there may be a relationship to BRCA-2 in men with breast cancer. Risk factors may include a history of mumps orchitis, radiation exposure, and Klinefelter's syndrome (a chromosomal condition reflecting decreased testosterone levels).

Detection usually occurs well into the disease because cancer of the breast is not a common concern among men. Therefore, treatment generally consists of a modified radical mastectomy. If the pectoralis muscles are involved, a radical mastectomy is indicated. Radiation therapy may be used postoperatively. Prognosis varies depending on the stage of disease at diagnosis. Bone and soft tissue are the most common sites of advanced disease and metastasis. Orchiectomy (removal of the testes), adrenalectomy (removal of the adrenal gland), and hypophysectomy (removal of the pituitary gland) may be used in advanced disease, but antihormonal agents are preferable because they are less invasive and disfiguring.

 Critical Thinking Exercises

1. You are caring for a patient who had breast augmentation surgery 10 years ago. When you ask her how often she examines her breasts, she states that she does not do so because she would be unable to detect masses because of her previous surgery. She also states that she does not think it is appropriate to touch her own breasts and that her physician performs a clinical breast examination each year when she has a Pap smear. How would you address the issues she has raised? Describe the teaching approach you would use.

2. Your 40-year-old patient has been diagnosed with breast cancer. Her mother, aunt, and one of her sisters have all had breast cancer. She is very worried about her two daughters' risks for breast cancer and asks if they should undergo genetic testing. She also asks about the need for her daughters to have mammograms performed. What guidelines would you give to this patient about mammography and genetic testing that might be considered for her daughters? What issues must be taken into account when someone is considering genetic testing for breast cancer?

3. A 46-year-old woman reports to you that she wants to undergo mastectomy and oophorectomy because she has a positive family history of breast cancer and is terrified of developing breast or ovarian cancer. Describe the benefits and risks of these surgeries for prophylactic management in women at risk for breast cancer. What postoperative care and teaching are indicated if she has both mastectomy and oophorectomy performed to reduce her risks for breast and ovarian cancer?

4. Two weeks after having a mastectomy to treat breast cancer, a 37-year-old patient calls you. She is distraught because her husband, who moved out of their bedroom immediately after her discharge so that he did not disturb her, has refused to sleep in the same bed or same room with her. How would you address this issue? What resources would you use to address the problem, and what resources would you provide to the patient and her spouse?

5. A 59-year-old woman with a history of cardiac disease is scheduled for a modified radical mastectomy and breast reconstruction surgery. Describe the preoperative and postoperative care of this patient, including discharge planning.

REFERENCES AND SELECTED READINGS

Books

Bickley, L. S., & Szilagyi, P. G. (2003). *Bates' guide to physical examination and history taking* (8th ed.). Philadelphia: Lippincott Williams & Wilkins.

Bland, K. I., & Copeland, E. M. III (Eds.). (1998). *The breast: Comprehensive management of benign and malignant diseases.* Philadelphia: W. B. Saunders.

Canadian Breast Cancer Foundation. (2005). *Breast cancer facts.* Available at: http://www.cbcf.org/what/breast_cancer_facts.html. Retrieved December 1, 2005.

Canadian Cancer Society. (2005). *Canadian cancer statistics 2005.* Toronto: Canadian Cancer Society.

Dow, K. H. (1999). *Pocket guide to breast cancer.* Boston: Jones & Bartlett.

Dow, K. H. (Ed.) (1996). *Contemporary issues in breast cancer.* Boston: Jones & Bartlett.

Greene, F. L., Page, D. L., Fleming, I. D., et al. (2002). *AJCC cancer staging manual* (6th ed.). New York: Springer-Verlag.

Harris, J. R., Lippman, M. E., Morrow, M., & Hellman, S. (Eds.) (1996). *Diseases of the breast.* Philadelphia: Lippincott-Raven.

Holland, J. C. (Ed.) (1998). *Psycho-oncology.* New York: Oxford University Press.

Love, S. M. (2000). *Dr. Susan Love's breast book.* Reading, MA: Addison-Wesley.

Moore, G. (Ed.). (2000). *Women and cancer: A gynecologic oncology nursing perspective* (2d ed.). Boston: Jones & Bartlett.

National Institutes of Health. (2000). *NIH consensus statement: Adjuvant therapy for early-stage breast cancer, 17*(4), 1–35.

National Institutes of Health. (1997). *NIH consensus statement: Breast cancer screening for women ages 40-49. 15*(1), 1–35

National Institutes of Health. (1990). *NIH consensus statement: Treatment of early-stage breast cancer, 8*(6), 1–19.

Runowicz, C. D., Petrek, J. A., & Gansler, T. S. (1999). *Women and cancer.* Atlanta: American Cancer Society.

Weber, J., & Kelley, J. (2003). *Health assessment in nursing* (2d ed.). Philadelphia: Lippincott Williams & Wilkins.

Yarbro, C. H., Frogge, M. H., Goodman, M., & Groenwald, S. (Eds.) (2000). *Cancer nursing: Principles and practices* (5th ed.). Sudbury, MA: Jones & Bartlett.

Journals

Asterisks indicate nursing research articles.

Breast Cancer Risk and Prevention

Chlebowksi, R. T. (2000). Reducing the risk of breast cancer. *Primary Care, 343*(3), 191–198.

Cummings, S. R., Eckert, S., Krueger, K. A., et al. (1999). The effect of raloxifene on risk of breast cancer in postmenopausal women: Results from the MORE randomized trial. *Journal of American Medical Association, 281*(23), 2189–2197.

Dooley, W. C., Ljung, B. M., Veronisi, U., et al. (2001). Ductal lavage for detection of cellular atypia in women at high risk for breast cancer. *Journal of the National Cancer Institute, 93*(21), 1624–1632.

Fisher, B., Constantino, J. P., Wickerham, D. L., et al. (1998). Tamoxifen for prevention of breast cancer. Report of the National Surgical Adjuvant Breast and Bowel Project P-1 Study. *Journal of National Cancer Institute, 90*(18), 1371–1388.

Frykberg, E. R. (1999). Lobular carcinoma in situ of the breast. *Breast Journal, 5*(5), 296–303.

Gail, M. H., Costantino, J. P., Bryant, J., et al. (1999). Weighing the risks and benefits of tamoxifen treatment for preventing breast cancer. *Journal of National Cancer Institute, 91*(21), 1829–1846.

Gross, R. E., (2000). Breast cancer: Risk factors, screening, and prevention. *Seminars in Oncology Nursing, 16*(3), 176–184.

Hartmann, L. C., Sellers, T. A., Schaid, D. J., et al. (1999). Clinical options for women at high risk for breast cancer. *Surgical Clinics of North America, 79*(5), 1189–1206.

Hartmann, L. C., Schaid, D. J., Woods, J. E., et al. (1999). Efficacy of bilateral prophylactic mastectomy in women with a family history of breast cancer. *New England Journal of Medicine, 340*(2), 77–84.

Hulka, B. S., & Moorman, P. G. (2001). Breast cancer: hormones and other risk factors. *Maturitas, 38*(1), 103–113.

MacDonald, D. J. (2002). Women's decisions regarding management of breast cancer risk. *MedSurg Nursing, 11*(4), 183–186.

*Machia, J. (2001). Breast cancer: Risk, prevention, and tamoxifen. *American Journal of Nursing, 101*(4), 26–35.

Meijers-Heijboer, H., van Geel, B., van Putten, W. L. J., et al. (2001). Breast cancer after prophylactic bilateral mastectomy in women with a BRCA1 or BRCA2 mutation. *New England Journal of Medicine, 345*(3), 159–164.

Newman, L. A., Keurer, H. M., Hung, K. K., et al. (2000). Prophylactic mastectomy. *Journal of the American College of Surgeons, 191*(3), 322–330.

Vogel, V. (2000). Breast cancer prevention: A review of the current evidence. *CA: A Cancer Journal for Clinicians, 50*(2), 156–170.

Cancer

Brown, J., Byers, T., & Thompson, K. (2001). Nutrition during and after cancer treatment: A guide for informed choices by cancer survivors. *CA: A Cancer Journal for Clinicians, 51*(3), 153–187.

English, J. C., Middleton, C., Patterson, J. W., et al. (2000). Cancer of the male breast. *International Journal of Dermatology, 39*(12), 881–886.

Fisher, B., Dignam, J., Wolmark, N., et al. (1999). Tamoxifen in the treatment of intraductal breast cancer: National Surgical Adjuvant Breast and Bowel Project B-24 randomised controlled trial. *Lancet, 353*(9169), 1993–2000.

Mautner, B. D., Schmidt, K. V., & Brennan, M. B. (2000). New diagnostic techniques and treatments for early breast cancer. *Seminars in Oncology Nursing, 16*(3), 185–196.

*Samarel, N., Fawcett J., Tulman, L., et al. (1999). A resource kit for women with breast cancer: Development and evaluation. *Oncology Nursing Forum, 26*(3), 611–618.

Solin, L. J., Kurtz, J., Fourquet, A., et al. (1996). Fifteen-year results of breast conserving and definitive breast irradiation for the treatment of ductal carcinoma in situ of the breast. *Journal of Clinical Oncology, 14,* 754–763.

Smith, T. J., Davidson, N. E., Schapira, D. V. et al. (1999). American Society of Clinical Oncology 1998 update of recommended breast cancer surveillance guidelines. *Journal of Clinical Oncology, 17*(3), 1080–1082.

Weber, E. S. (1997). Questions and answers about breast cancer diagnosis. *American Journal of Nursing, 97*(10), 34–38.

Winchester, D. P., & Cox, J. D. (1998). Standards for diagnosis and management of invasive breast carcinoma. *CA: A Cancer Journal for Clinicians, 48*(2), 83–107.

Winchester, D. P., Jeske, J. M., & Goldschmidt, R. A. (2000). The diagnosis and management of ductal carcinoma in situ of the breast. *CA: The Cancer Journal for Clinicians, 50*(2), 184–200.

Chemotherapy

Antman, K. H. (2001). Randomized trials of high dose chemotherapy for breast cancer. *Biochimica et Biophyic Acta (BBA/Reviews in Cancer), 1471*(3), 89–98.

Barse, P. M. (2000). Issues in the treatment of metastatic breast cancer. *Seminars in Oncology Nursing, 16*(3), 197–205.

*Berger, A. M., & Higginbotham, P. (2000). Correlates of fatigue during and following adjuvant breast cancer chemotherapy: A pilot study. *Oncology Nursing Forum, 27*(9), 1443–1448.

Capriotti, T. (2001). Monoclonal antibodies: Drugs that combine pharmacology and biotechnology. *MedSurg Nursing, 10*(2), 89–95.

Cloutier, A. O. (2000). Advanced breast cancer: Recent developments in hormonal therapy. *Seminars in Oncology Nursing, 16*(3), 206–213.

Frankel, C. (2000). Nursing management considerations with trastuzumab (Herceptin). *Seminars in Oncology Nursing, 16*(4), 23–28.

Hagmann, M. (2000). Scientific misconduct: Cancer researcher sacked for alleged fraud. *Science, 287*(5460), 1901–1902.

Levine, M. (2001). Clinical practice guidelines for the care and treatment of breast cancer: Adjuvant systemic therapy for node-negative breast cancer (summary of the 2001 update). *Canadian Medical Association Journal, 164*(2), 213.

Levine, M. (2001). Clinical practice guidelines for the care and treatment of breast cancer: Adjuvant systemic therapy for node-positive breast cancer (summary of the 2001 update). *Canadian Medical Association Journal, 164*(5), 644–646.

McGinn, K., & Moore, J. (2001). Metastatic breast cancer: Understanding current management options. *Oncology Nursing Forum, 28*(3), 507–512.

*McPhail, G., & Smith, L. N. (2000). Acute menopause symptoms during adjuvant systemic treatment for breast cancer: A case-control study. *Cancer Nursing, 23*(6), 430–443.

Norton, L. (2001). Theoretical concepts and the emerging role of taxanes in adjuvant therapy. *Oncologist, 6*, Suppl 3, 30–35.

Pasacretta, J. V., & McCorkle, R. (1998). Providing accurate information to women about tamoxifen therapy for breast cancer: Current indications, effects, and controversies. *Oncology Nursing Forum, 25*(9), 1577–1583.

Tyler, T. (1998). The medical management of breast cancer. *Lippincott's Primary Care Practice, 2*(2), 176–183.

Genetics

Boyd, J. (1996). BRCA2 as a low penetrance cancer gene. *Journal of the National Cancer Institute, 88*(19), 1408–1409.

Houshmand, S. L., Campbell, C. T., Briggs, S. E., et al. (2000). Prophylactic mastectomy and genetic testing: an update. *Oncology Nursing Forum, 27*(10), 1537–1547.

Nogueira, S. M., & Appling, S. E. (2000). Breast cancer: Genetics, risks, and strategies. *Nursing Clinics of North America, 35*(3), 663–669.

Press, N., Fishman, J. R., Koenig, B. A. (2000). Collective fear, individualized risk: The social and cultural context of genetic testing for breast cancer. *Nursing Ethics, 7*(3), 237–249.

Schrag, D., Kuntz, K. M., Garber, E., & Weeks, J. C. (1997). Decision analysis: Effects of prophylactic mastectomy and oophorectomy on life expectancy among women with BRCA1 and BRCA2 mutations. *New England Journal of Medicine, 335*(20), 1401–1408.

Zimmerman, V. L. (2002). BRCA gene mutations and cancer. Preventive strategies benefit patients at risk. *American Journal of Nursing, 102*(8), 28–36.

Geriatrics

Kimmick, G. G., & Muss, H. B. (2001). Systemic therapy for older women with breast cancer. *Oncology, 15*(3), 280–291.

Nattinger, A. B. (2000). Older women, mammography, and mortality from breast cancer. *American Journal of Medicine, 108*(2), 174–175.

*Utley, R. (1999). The evolving meaning of cancer for long-term survivors of breast cancer. *Oncology Nursing Forum, 26*(9), 1519–1523.

Zoorob, R., Anderson, R., Cefalu, C., et al. (2001). Cancer screening guidelines. *American Family Physician, 63*(6), 1101–1112.

Lymphedema

*Coward, D. D. (1999). Lymphedema prevention and management knowledge in women treated for breast cancer. *Oncology Nursing Forum, 26*(6), 1047–1053.

Erickson, V. S., Pearson, M. L., Ganz, P. A., et al. (2001). Arm edema in breast cancer patients. *Journal of the National Cancer Institute, 93*(2), 96–111.

Hull, M. M. (2000). Lymphedema in women treated for breast cancer. *Seminars in Oncology Nursing, 16*(3), 226–237.

McKenzie, D. C. (1998). Abreast in a boat–A race against breast cancer. *Canadian Medical Association Journal, 159*(4), 376–378.

Petrek, J. A., Pressman, P. I., & Smith, R. A. (2000). Lymphedema: Current issues in research and management. *CA: Cancer Journal for Clinicians, 50*(5), 292–307.

Plastic and Reconstructive Surgery

Alderman, A. K., Wilkins, E. G., Lowery, J. C., et al. (2000). Determinants of patient satisfaction in postmastectomy breast reconstruction. *Plastic and Reconstructive Surgery, 106*(4), 769–776.

Malata, C. M., McIntosh, S. A., & Purushotham, A. D. (2000). Immediate breast reconstruction after mastectomy for cancer. *British Journal of Surgery, 87*(11), 1455–1472.

*Neill, K. M., Armstrong, N., & Burnett, C. B. (1998). Choosing reconstruction after mastectomy: A qualitative analysis. *Oncology Nursing Forum, 25*(4), 743–750.

Reaby, L. L. (1999). Breast restoration decision making. *Plastic Surgical Nursing, 19*(1), 22–29.

Resnick, B., & Belcher, A. E. (2002). Breast reconstruction: Options, answers, and support for patients making a difficult personal decision. *American Journal of Nursing, 102*(4), 26–33.

Rowland, J. H., Desmond, K. A., Meyerowitz, B. E., et al. (2000). Role of breast reconstructive surgery in physical and emotional outcomes among breast cancer survivors. *Journal of the National Cancer Institute, 92*(17), 1422–1429.

Sandau, K. E. (2002). Free TRAM flap breast reconstruction. *American Journal of Nursing, 102*(4), 36–43.

Pregnancy and Breast Cancer

Dow, K. H. (2000). Pregnancy and breast cancer. *Journal of Obstetrical & Gynecologic Neonatal Nursing, 29*(6), 634–640.

Gelber, S., Coates, A. S., Goldhirsch, A., et al. (2001). Effects of pregnancy on overall survival after diagnosis of early-stage breast cancer. *Journal of Clinical Oncology, 19*(6), 1671–1675.

Gemignani, M. L., & Petrek, J. A. (1999). Pregnancy after breast cancer. *Cancer Control, 6*(3), 272–276.

Moore, H. C., & Foster, R. S. (2000). Breast cancer and pregnancy. *Seminars in Oncology, 27*(6), 646–653.

Psychological Aspects of Breast Cancer

Gray, R. E., Goel, V., Fitch, M. I., et al. (2000). Utilization of professional care services by women with breast cancer. *Breast Cancer Research & Treatment, 64*(3), 253–258.

*Hilton, B. A., Crawford, J. A., & Tarko, M. A. (2000). Men's perspectives on individual and family coping with their wives' breast cancer and chemotherapy. *Western Journal of Nursing Research, 22*(4), 438–459.

*Holmberg, S. K., Scott, L. L., Alexy, W., et al. (2001). Relationship issues of women with breast cancer. *Cancer Nursing, 24*(1), 53–60.

*Horden, A. (2000). Intimacy and sexuality for the woman with breast cancer. *Cancer Nursing, 23*(3), 230–236.

Hoskins, C. N., & Haber, J. (2000). Adjusting to breast cancer. *American Journal of Nursing, 100*(4), 26–32.

Utley, R. (1999). The evolving meaning of cancer for long-term survivors of breast cancer. *Oncology Nursing Forum, 26*(9), 1519–1523.

*Walker, B. L., Nail, L. M., & Croyle, R. T. (1999). Does emotional expression make a difference in reactions to breast cancer? *Oncology Nursing Forum, 26*(6), 1025–1032.

Woodward, V., & Webb, C. (2001). Women's anxieties surrounding breast disorders: A systematic review of the literature. *Journal of Advanced Nursing, 33*(1), 29–41.

*Wonghongkul, T., Moore, S. M., Musil, C., et al. (2000). The influence of uncertainty in illness, stress appraisal, and hope on coping in survivors of breast cancer. *Cancer Nursing, 23*(6), 422–429.

Radiation

*Dow, K. H., & Lafferty, P. (2000). Quality of life, survivorship, and psychosocial adjustment of young women with breast cancer after breast-conserving surgery and radiation therapy. *Oncology Nursing Forum, 27*(10), 1555–1564.

*Kolcaba, K., & Fox, C. (1999). The effects of guided imagery on comfort of women with early-stage breast cancer undergoing radiation therapy. *Oncology Nursing Forum, 26*(1), 67–72.

Morrow, M., White, J., Moughan, J., et al. (2001). Factors predicting the use of breast-conserving therapy in stage I and stage II breast carcinoma. *Journal of Clinical Oncology, 19*(8), 2254–2262.

Screening, BSE, and Mammography

Anderson, M. R., Urban, N., & Etzioni, R. (1999). Community attitudes and mammography use: Does it really matter what other people think? *Women Health, 29*(3), 83–95.

Center for Disease Control Database. (2000). *National Center for Health Statistics (via the Internet:* http://www.cdc.gov/hchs).

Clarke, V. A., & Savage, S. A. (1999). Breast self-examination training: A brief review. *Cancer Nursing, 22*(4), 320–326.

Cole, C. F. (1998). Issues in breast imaging. *Lippincott's Primary Care Practice, 2*(2), 141–148.

*Faccione, N. C. (1999). Breast cancer screening in relation to access to health services. *Oncology Nursing Forum, 26*(4), 689–696.

Gail, M. H., & Rimer, B. K. (1998). Risk-based recommendations for mammographic screening for women in their forties. *Journal of Clinical Oncology, 16*(9), 3105–3114.

Kolb, T. M., Lichy, J., & Newhouse, J. H. (1998). Occult cancer in women with dense breasts: Detection with screening US: diagnostic yield and tumor characteristics. *Radiology, 207*(1), 191–199.

*Lauver, D. R., Kane J., Bodden, J., et al. (1999). Engagement in breast cancer screening behaviors. *Oncology Nursing Forum, 26*(3), 545–554.

National Institutes of Health. (1997). *Consensus statement: Breast cancer screening for women ages 40–49.*

Norris, T. G. (2001). Benign breast disease. *Radiology Technology, 72*(3), 245–267.

Schnall, M. D. (2001). Application of magnetic resonance imaging to early detection of breast cancer. *Breast Cancer Research & Treatment, 3*(1), 17–21.

Tabar, L., Vitak, B., Tony, H. H., et al. (2001). Beyond randomized controlled trials: Organized mammographic screening substantially reduces breast carcinoma mortality. *Cancer, 91*(9), 1724–1731.

*Yarbrough, S. S., & Braden, C. J. (2001). Utility of health belief model as guide for explaining or predicting breast cancer screening behaviors. *Journal of Advanced Nursing, 33*(5), 677–688.

Surgical Treatment of Breast Cancer

Baron, R. H. (1999). Sentinel lymph node biopsy in breast cancer and the role of the oncology nurse. *Clinical Journal of Oncology Nursing, 3*(1), 17–22.

Baron, R. H., Fey, J. V., Raboy, S., et al. (2002). Eighteen sensations after breast cancer surgery: A comparison of sentinel lymph node biopsy and axillary lymph node dissection. *Oncology Nursing Forum, 29*(4), 651–659.

*Burke, C. C., Zabka, C. L., McCarver, K. J., & Singletary, S. E. (1997). Patient satisfaction with 23-hour "short-stay" observation following breast cancer surgery. *Oncology Nursing Forum, 24*, 645–651.

Dell, D. D. (1997). Common questions about ductal carcinoma in situ. *American Journal of Nursing, 97*(5), 61–65.

Gross, R. E. (1998). Current issues in the surgical treatment of early stage breast cancer. *Clinical Journal of Oncology Nursing, 2*(2), 55–63.

Hsueh, E. C., Hansen, N., & Giuliano, A. E. (2000). Intraoperative lymphatic mapping and sentinel lymph node dissection in breast cancer. *CA: Cancer Journal for Clinicians, 50*(5), 279–291.

Kauff, N., Satagopan, J. M., Robson, M. E., et al. (2002). Risk-reducing salpingo-oophorectomy in women with a BRCA1 or BRCA2 mutation. *New England Journal of Medicine, 346*(21), 1609–1615.

*Poole, K., & Lyne, P. A. (2000). The 'cues' to diagnosis: Describing the monitoring of activities of women undergoing diagnostic investigations for breast disease. *Journal of Advanced Nursing, 31*(4), 752–758.

Rebbeck, T. R., Lynch, H. T., Neuhausen, S. L., et al. (2002). Prophylactic oophorectomy in carriers of BRCA1 and BRCA2 mutations. *New England Journal of Medicine, 346*(21), 1616–1622.

Solin, L. J., Fourquet, A., Vicini, F. A., et al. (2001). Mammographically detected ductal carcinoma in situ of the breast treated with breast-conserving surgery and definitive breast irradiation: Long-term outcome and prognostic significance of patient age and margin status. *International Journal of Radiation Oncology and Biologic Physics, 50*(4), 991–1002.

Strozzo, M. D. (1998). An overview of surgical management of stage I and stage II breast cancer for the primary care provider. *Lippincott's Primary Care Practice, 2*(2), 160–169.

Veronesi, U., Galimberti, V., Zurrida, S., et al. (2001). Sentinel lymph node biopsy as an indicator for axillary dissection in early breast cancer. *European Journal of Cancer, 37*(4), 454–458.

RESOURCES AND WEBSITES

Agencies

Breast Cancer Prevention Coalition, 23 Lynden Hill, Crescent, Brantford, ON N3P 1R1 (519) 751-2560, www.stopcancer.org.

Canadian Association of Nurses in Oncology, CANO Head Office, 570 West 7th Ave, Suite 402, Vancouver, B.C. V5Z 1B3; (604) 874-4322; email: cano@malachite-mgmt.com; http://www.cos.ca/cano.

Canadian Association of Psychosocial Oncology, 365 Blloor Street East, Suite 1807, Toronto, ON M4W 3L4; (416) 968-9424; email: capo@funnel.ca; http://www.capo.ca.

Canadian Breast Cancer Foundation, 790 Bay Street, Suite 1000, Toronto, ON M5G IW8; 1-800-389-9816; http://www.cbcf.org.

Canadian Breast Cancer Research Alliance; 790 Bay St., Suite 1000, Toronto, ON M5G IN8; (416) 596-6598; email-info@cbcra.ca; http://www.breast.cancer.ca.

Canadian Cancer Society, Suite 200, 10 Alcorn Ave., Toronto, ON M4V 3B1; (416) 961-7223; http://www.cancer.ca.

Canadian Society of Plastic Surgeons, 1469 St., Joseph Blvd. E#4, Montreal, QC H2J IM6; (514) 843-5415; http://www.plasticsurgery.ca.

Look Good Feel Better, 420 Britannia Road East, Suite 102, Mississauga, ON L4Z 3L5; 1-800-914-5665; www.lookgoodfeelbetter.ca.

Lymphovenous Canada; email: info@lymphovenous-canada.ca; http://www.lymphovenous-canada.ca.

Websites

cancernet.nci.gov (produced jointly by the International Cancer Information Center, NCI, and the Office of Cancer Communications).

mskcc.org (information on Memorial Sloan-Kettering Cancer Center's programs and services for the prevention, cure, and control of cancer).

nysernet.org/bcic (serves as a clearinghouse for information on breast cancer).

oncolink.upenn.edu (University of Pennsylvania's educational resource for patients with cancer).

access.digex.net/~mkragen/index.html (a guide to cancer resources).

cancercareinc.org (produced by Cancer Care, Inc., an organization supported through educational grants and private contributions that provides telephone services and sponsors free teleconference seminars in addition to its Web-based services).

Assessment and Management of Problems Related to Male Reproductive Processes

Adapted by Jill Milne

On completion of this chapter, the learner will be able to:

1. Describe structures and function of the male reproductive system.
2. Discuss nursing assessment of the male reproductive system and identify diagnostic tests that complement assessment.
3. Discuss the causes and management of male sexual dysfunction.
4. Compare the types of prostatectomy with regard to advantages and disadvantages.
5. Use the nursing process as a framework for care of the patient undergoing prostatectomy.
6. Describe the nursing management of patients with testicular cancer.
7. Describe the various conditions affecting the penis, including pathophysiology, clinical manifestations, and management.

Disorders of the male reproductive system include a wide variety of conditions that usually affect both the urinary and reproductive systems. Because these disorders focus on the genitalia and in some instances sexuality, the patient may experience anxiety and embarrassment. Nurses must recognize the patient's need for privacy as well as his need for education. This requires an openness to discuss critical and sensitive issues with the patient as well as effective assessment, management, and communication on the part of the nurse.

Anatomic and Physiologic Overview

In the male, several organs serve as parts of both the urinary tract and the reproductive system. Disorders in the male reproductive organs may interfere with the functions of one or both of these systems. As a result, diseases of the male reproductive system are usually treated by a urologist. The structures in the male reproductive system are the testes, the vas deferens (ductus deferens) and the seminal vesicles, the penis, and certain accessory glands, such as the prostate gland and Cowper's gland (bulbourethral gland) (Fig. 49-1).

TESTICULAR DEVELOPMENT

The **testes** are formed in the embryo within the abdominal cavity near the kidney. During the last month of fetal life, they descend posterior to the peritoneum and pierce the abdominal wall in the groin. Later, they progress along the inguinal canal into the scrotum. In this descent, they are accompanied by blood vessels, lymphatics, nerves, and ducts, which support the tissue and make up the spermatic cord. This cord extends from the internal inguinal ring through the abdominal wall and the inguinal canal to the scrotum. As the testes descend into the scrotum, a tubular extension of peritoneum accompanies them. Normally, this tissue is obliterated during fetal development, the only remaining portion being that which covers the testes, the tunica vaginalis. (When this peritoneal process is not obliterated but remains open into the abdominal cavity, a potential sac remains into which abdominal contents may enter to form an indirect inguinal hernia.)

The testes are encased in the scrotum, which keeps them at a slightly lower temperature than the rest of the body to facilitate **spermatogenesis** (production of sperm). The testes consist of numerous seminiferous tubules in which the spermatozoa form. Collecting tubules transmit the spermatozoa into the epididymis,

Glossary

benign prostatic hyperplasia (BPH): noncancerous enlargement or hypertrophy of the prostate. BPH is the most common pathologic condition in older men and the second most common cause of surgical intervention in men older than age 60 years.

Bowen's disease: form of squamous cell carcinoma in situ of the penile shaft

circumcision: excision of the foreskin, or prepuce, of the glans penis

cryosurgery of the prostate: localized treatment of the prostate by application of freezing temperatures

cryptorchidism: most common congenital defect, characterized by failure of one or both of the testes to descend into the scrotum

epididymitis: infection of the epididymis that usually descends from an infected prostate or urinary tract; also may develop as a complication of gonorrhea

erectile dysfunction: also called impotence; the inability to either achieve or maintain an erection sufficient to accomplish sexual intercourse

hydrocele: a collection of fluid, generally in the tunica vaginalis of the testis, although it also may collect within the spermatic cord

nocturia: urination during the night

orchiectomy: surgical removal of one or both of the testes

orchitis: inflammation of the testes (testicular congestion) caused by pyogenic, viral, spirochetal, parasitic, traumatic, chemical, or unknown factors

penile cancer: represents about 0.5% of malignancies in men in the United States; can involve the glans, the body of the penis, the urethra, and regional or distant lymph nodes

penis: male organ for copulation and urination; consists of glans penis, body, and root

Peyronie's disease: buildup of fibrous plaques in the sheath of the corpus cavernosum, causing curvature of the penis when it is erect

phimosis: condition in which the foreskin is constricted so that it cannot be retracted over the glans; can occur congenitally or from inflammation and edema

priapism: an uncontrolled, persistent erection of the penis occurring from either neural or vascular causes, including medications, sickle cell thrombosis, leukemic cell infiltration, spinal cord tumours, and tumour invasion of the penis or its vessels

prostate cancer: the most common cancer in men; risk factors include increasing age, African American race, and possibly a higher-fat diet; the genetic association of prostate cancer and the increased incidence within certain families is being investigated

prostate gland: gland that lies just below the neck of the bladder, surrounds the urethra, and is traversed by the ejaculatory duct, a continuation of the vas deferens; produces a secretion that is chemically and physiologically suitable to the needs of the spermatozoa in their passage from the testes

prostate-specific antigen (PSA): substance that is produced by the prostate gland and measured in a blood specimen; PSA levels are increased with prostate cancer; the PSA test is used in combination with digital rectal examination to detect prostate cancer

prostatism: obstructive and irritative symptom complex that includes increased frequency and hesitancy in starting urination, a decrease in the volume and force of the urinary stream, acute urinary retention, and recurrent urinary tract infections

prostatitis: inflammation of the prostate gland caused by infectious agents (bacteria, fungi, mycoplasma) or various other problems (eg, urethral stricture, prostatic hyperplasia)

spermatogenesis: production of sperm in the testes

testes: the ovoid sex glands encased in the scrotum; the testes produce sperm

testicular cancer: the most common cancer in men 15 to 35 years of age and the second most common malignancy in those 35 to 39 years of age; its cause is unknown

testosterone: male sex hormone secreted by the testes; induces and preserves the male sex characteristics

transurethral resection of the prostate (TUR or TURP): resection of the prostate through endoscopy; the surgical and optical instrument is introduced directly through the urethra to the prostate, and the gland is then removed in small chips with an electrical cutting loop

varicocele: an abnormal dilation of the veins of the pampiniform venous plexus in the scrotum (the network of veins from the testis and the epididymis, which constitute part of the spermatic cord)

vasectomy: also called male sterilization; ligation and transection of part of the vas deferens, with or without removal of a segment of the vas to prevent the passage of the sperm from the testes

FIGURE 49-1 Structures of the male reproductive system. Adapted from Willis, M. C. (1996). *Medical terminology: The language of health care.* Baltimore: Williams & Wilkins.

a hoodlike structure lying on the testes and containing winding ducts that lead into the vas deferens. This firm, tubular structure passes upward through the inguinal canal to enter the abdominal cavity behind the peritoneum. It then extends downward toward the base of the bladder. An outpouching from this structure is the seminal vesicle, which acts as a reservoir for testicular secretions. The tract is continued as the ejaculatory duct, which passes through the prostate gland to enter the urethra. Testicular secretions take this pathway when they exit the penis during ejaculation.

GLANDULAR FUNCTION

The testes have a dual function: the formation of spermatozoa from the germinal cells of the seminiferous tubules and the secretion of the male sex hormone **testosterone**, which induces and preserves the male sex characteristics.

The **prostate gland** lies just below the neck of the bladder. It surrounds the urethra and is traversed by the ejaculatory duct, a continuation of the vas deferens. This gland produces a secretion that is chemically and physiologically suitable to the needs of the spermatozoa in their passage from the testes.

Cowper's gland lies below the prostate within the posterior aspect of the urethra. This gland empties its secretions into the urethra during ejaculation, providing lubrication. The **penis** has a dual function: it is the organ for copulation and for urination. Anatomically, it consists of the glans penis, body, and root. The glans penis is the soft, rounded portion at the distal end of the penis. The urethra, the tube that carries urine, opens at the tip of the glans. The glans is naturally covered or protected by elongated

penile skin—the foreskin—which may be retracted to expose the glans. However, many men have had the foreskin removed (circumcision) as newborns. The body of the penis is composed of erectile tissues containing numerous blood vessels that become distended, leading to an erection during sexual excitement. The urethra, which passes through the penis, extends from the bladder through the prostate to the distal end of the penis.

Assessment

HEALTH HISTORY AND CLINICAL MANIFESTATIONS

Assessment of male reproductive function begins with an evaluation of urinary function and symptoms. This assessment also includes a focus on sexual function as well as manifestations of sexual dysfunction. The patient is asked about his usual state of health and any recent change in general physical and sexual activity. Any symptoms or changes in function are explored fully and described in detail. These symptoms may include those associated with an obstruction caused by an enlarged prostate gland: increased urinary frequency, decreased force of urine stream, "double" or "triple" voiding (the patient needs to urinate two or three times over a period of several minutes to completely empty his bladder). The patient is also assessed for dysuria, hematuria, and hematospermia (blood in the ejaculate).

Assessment of sexual function and dysfunction is an essential part of every health history. The extent of the history will depend on the patient's presenting symptoms and the presence of factors that may affect sexual function: chronic illnesses (eg, diabetes, multiple sclerosis, stroke, cardiac disease), use of medications that affect sexual function (eg, many antihypertensive and anticholesterolemic medications, psychotropic agents), stress, and alcohol use.

Discussing sexuality with patients with an illness or who have a disability can be uncomfortable for nurses and other health care providers. Health care professionals may unconsciously have stereotypes related to sexuality (eg, ill or persons with a disability are asexual or should remain sexually inactive). In addition, patients are often embarrassed to initiate a discussion about these issues with their health care providers (Hughes, 2000). Because changes in sexual functioning are a common concern of patients, it is important to address these issues when obtaining the health history. By initiating an assessment about sexual concerns, the nurse demonstrates that changes in sexual functioning are valid topics for discussion and provides a safe environment for discussing these sensitive topics. The PLISSIT (permission, limited information, specific suggestions, intensive therapy) model of sexual assessment and intervention may be used to provide a framework for nursing interventions (Annon, 1976). This model begins by asking the patient's permission to discuss sexual functioning. Limited information about sexual function may then be provided to the patient. As the discussion progresses, the nurse may offer specific suggestions for interventions. For some individuals, a professional who specializes in sex therapy may provide more intensive therapy as needed.

PHYSICAL ASSESSMENT

In addition to the customary aspects of the physical examination, two essential components address disorders of the male genital or reproductive system: the digital rectal examination and the testicular examination.

Digital Rectal Examination

The digital rectal examination (DRE) is recommended as part of the regular health checkup for every man older than 40 years of age; it is invaluable in screening for cancer of the prostate gland. The DRE enables the examiner to assess the size, shape, and consistency of the prostate gland (Fig. 49-2). Tenderness of the prostate gland on palpation and the presence and consis-

tency of any nodules are noted. Although having this examination may be embarrassing for the patient, it is an important screening tool.

Testicular Examination

The male genitalia are inspected for abnormalities and palpated for masses. The scrotum is palpated carefully for nodules, masses, or inflammation. Examining the scrotum can reveal such disorders as hydrocele, hernia, or tumour of the testis. The penis is inspected and palpated for ulcerations, nodules, inflammation, and discharge. The testicular examination provides an excellent opportunity to instruct the patient about techniques for testicular self-examination and its importance in early detection of testicular cancer (discussed later in this chapter). This self-examination should begin during adolescence.

Gerontologic Considerations

As men age, the prostate gland enlarges, prostate secretion decreases, the scrotum hangs lower, the testes become smaller and more firm, and pubic hair becomes sparser and stiffer. Changes in gonadal function include a decline in plasma testosterone levels and reduced production of progesterone (Table 49-1). Other changes include decreasing sexual function, slower sexual responses, an increased incidence of genitourinary tract cancer, and urinary incontinence for various reasons.

Male reproductive capability is maintained with advancing age. Although degenerative changes occur in the seminiferous tubules, spermatogenesis (production of sperm) continues. Sexual function, however, involving libido (desire) and potency, decreases. Vascular problems cause about half of the cases of impotence in men older than 50 years of age.

Hypogonadism occurs in up to one fourth of older men. The relationship of hypogonadism to impotence is uncertain. This decline is more evident in men older than 70 years but is also noted in men in their 60s. In older men, the sexual response slows. Erection takes longer in men older than 50 years of age, and full erections may not be attained until orgasm. Sexual function is affected by several factors, such as psychological problems, illnesses, and medications. In general, the sexual act takes longer. In older men, ejaculatory control increases; however, if the erection is partially

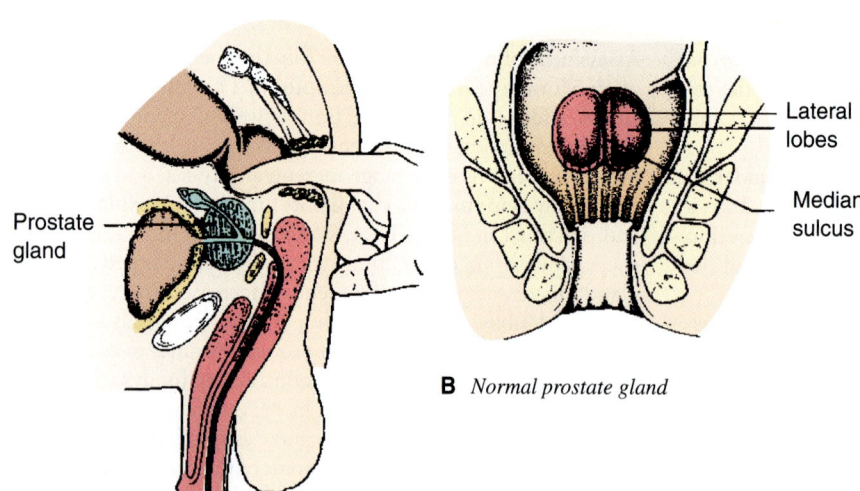

B *Normal prostate gland*

Lateral lobes

Median sulcus

Prostate gland

A

FIGURE 49-2 (**A**) Palpation of the prostate gland during digital rectal examination (DRE) enables the examiner to assess the size, shape, and texture of the gland. (**B**) The prostate is round, with a palpable median sulcus or groove separating the two lobes. It should feel rubbery and free of nodules and masses.

Table 49-1 • Age-Related Changes in Male Reproductive System

AGE-RELATED CHANGES	PHYSIOLOGIC CHANGES	MANIFESTATIONS
Decrease in sex hormone secretion, especially testosterone	Decreased muscle strength and sexual energy	Changes in sexual response: prolonged time to reach full erection, rapid penile detumescence and prolonged refractory period Decrease in number of viable sperm
	Shrinkage and loss of firmness of testes; thickening of seminiferous tubules	Smaller testes
	Fibrotic changes of corpora cavernosa	Erectile dysfunction
	Enlargement of prostate gland	Weakening of prostatic contractions Hyperplasia of prostate gland Signs and symptoms of obstruction of lower urinary tract (urgency, frequency, nocturia)

lost, there may be difficulty in attaining a full erection again, and resolution may occur without orgasm. Sexual activity is closely correlated with the man's sexual activity of his earlier years; if he was more active than average as a young man, he will most likely continue to be more active than average in his later years.

Cancers of the kidney, bladder, prostate, and penis all have increased incidence in men older than 50 years of age. DRE and screening tests for hematuria may uncover a higher percentage of malignancies at earlier stages.

Urinary incontinence in the elderly man may have many causes, including medications and age-related conditions, such as neurologic diseases or **benign prostatic hyperplasia** (BPH; also referred to as hypertrophy and called an enlarged prostate by the lay public). Diagnostic tests are performed to exclude reversible causes of urinary incontinence. For some patients with severe incontinence, augmentation cystoplasty (repair of the bladder) with placement of an artificial urinary sphincter may help alleviate this problem.

Diagnostic Evaluation

Diagnostic studies that relate to the male reproductive organs and the ability to participate in sexual activity include the following.

PROSTATE-SPECIFIC ANTIGEN TEST

The prostate gland produces a substance known as **prostate-specific antigen (PSA)**. It can be measured in a blood specimen, and levels increase with prostate cancer. Many factors can increase PSA levels, including BPH, prostate cancer, and infections of the prostate and urinary tract. PSA levels are measured in nanograms per millilitre (ng/mL). The PSA test and DRE are used to detect prostate cancer (Smith, Cokkinides, von Eschenbach, et al., 2002).

The range of values considered normal is 0.2 to 4.0 ng/mL. Values over 4.0 are considered elevated. An elevated PSA level is not a specific indicator of prostate cancer. A number of conditions (eg, BPH, transurethral resection of the prostate, acute urinary retention, and acute prostatitis) can also cause an elevated PSA level in the absence of prostate cancer. Despite these limitations, in combination with other procedures, PSA is useful in identifying men at risk and in monitoring patients following treatment for cancer of the prostate (Barry, 2001). The Canadian Cancer Society recommends that men 50 years of age and older discuss the early detection of prostate cancer with PSA testing and DRE. Those at risk, including African Canadian men and those with a family history of prostate cancer, should discuss the tests with their doctor at a younger age.

ULTRASONOGRAPHY

Transrectal ultrasound (TRUS) studies may be performed in patients with abnormalities detected by DRE or those with elevated PSA levels. After DRE, a lubricated, condom-covered, rectal probe transducer is inserted into the rectum along the anterior wall. Water may be introduced to the condom to help transmit sound waves to the prostate. TRUS may be used in detecting nonpalpable prostate cancers and in staging localized prostate cancer. Needle biopsies of the prostate are commonly guided by TRUS.

PROSTATE FLUID OR TISSUE ANALYSIS

Specimens of prostate fluid or tissue may be obtained for culture when disease or inflammation of the prostate gland is suspected. A biopsy of the prostate gland may be necessary to obtain tissue for histologic examination. This may be performed at the time of prostatectomy or by means of a perineal or transrectal needle biopsy.

TESTS OF MALE SEXUAL FUNCTION

If the patient cannot engage in sexual intercourse to his satisfaction, a detailed history is obtained. Nocturnal penile tumescence tests may be conducted in a sleep laboratory to monitor changes in penile circumference during sleep (using a mercury strain gauge placed around the penis); the results help to identify the cause of erectile dysfunction. Arterial blood flow to the penis is measured with the Doppler probe. Nerve conduction tests and psychological evaluations are also part of the diagnostic workup and are usually conducted by a specialized team of health care providers.

Disorders of Male Sexual Function

ERECTILE DYSFUNCTION

Erectile dysfunction, also called impotence, is the inability to achieve or maintain an erection sufficient to accomplish intercourse. The man may report decreased frequency of erections, inability to achieve a firm erection, or rapid detumescence (subsiding of erection). Incidence ranges from 25% to 50% in men older than 65 years of age. The physiology of erection and ejaculation is complex and involves sympathetic and parasympathetic components. At the time of erection, pelvic nerves carry parasympathetic impulses that dilate the smaller blood vessels of the region and increase blood flow to the penis, expanding the corpora cavernosa.

Erectile dysfunction has both psychogenic and organic causes. Psychogenic causes include anxiety, fatigue, depression, and pressure to perform sexually. Organic impotence, however, may account for more impotence than previously realized. Organic causes include occlusive vascular disease, endocrine disease (diabetes, pituitary tumours, hypogonadism with testosterone deficiency, hyperthyroidism, and hypothyroidism), cirrhosis, chronic renal failure, genitourinary conditions (radical pelvic surgery), hematologic conditions (Hodgkin's disease, leukemia), neurologic disorders (neuropathies, parkinsonism, spinal cord injury, multiple sclerosis), trauma to the pelvic or genital area, alcohol, medications (Chart 49-1), and drug abuse.

Assessment and Diagnostic Findings

The diagnosis of erectile dysfunction requires a sexual and medical history; an analysis of presenting symptoms; a physical examination, including a neurologic examination; a detailed assessment of all medications, alcohol, and drugs used; and various laboratory studies. Nocturnal penile tumescence tests are conducted in sleep laboratories to monitor changes in penile circumference. In healthy men, nocturnal penile erections closely parallel rapid eye movement (REM) sleep in occurrence and duration. Organically impotent men show inadequate sleep-related erections that correspond to their waking performance. The nocturnal penile tumescence test can help to determine whether erectile impotence has an organic or psychological cause. Arterial blood flow to the penis is measured using a Doppler probe. In addition, nerve conduction tests and extensive psychological evaluations are carried out. Figure 49-3 describes the evaluation and treatment of men with erectile dysfunction.

Chart 49-1 • PHARMACOLOGY
Classes of Medications Associated With Erectile Dysfunction

Antiadrenergics and antihypertensives: guanethidine (Ismelin), clonidine (Catapres), hydralazine (Apresoline), metoprolol (Lopressor)

Anticholinergics and phenothiazines: prochlorperazine (Compazine), trihexyphenidyl (Artane)

Anti-seizure agents: carbamazepine (Tegretol)

Antifungals: ketoconazole (Nizoral)

Antihormone (prostate cancer treatment): flutamide (Eulexin), leuprolide (Lupron)

Antipsychotics: haloperidol (Haldol), chlorpromazine (Thorazine)

Antispasmodics: oxybutynin (Ditropan)

Anxiolytics, sedative–hypnotics, tranquilizers: lorazepam (Ativan), triazolam (Halcion)

Beta-blockers: nadolol (Corgard)

Calcium channel blockers: nifedipine (Adalat, Procardia)

Carbonic anhydrase inhibitors: acetazolamide (Diamox)

H_2 antagonists: nizatidine (Axid)

Nonsteroidal anti-inflammatory drugs: naproxen (Naprosyn)

Thiazide diuretics: hydrochlorothiazide (HydroDIURIL)

Tricyclic antidepressants: amitriptyline (Elavil), desipramine (Norpramin)

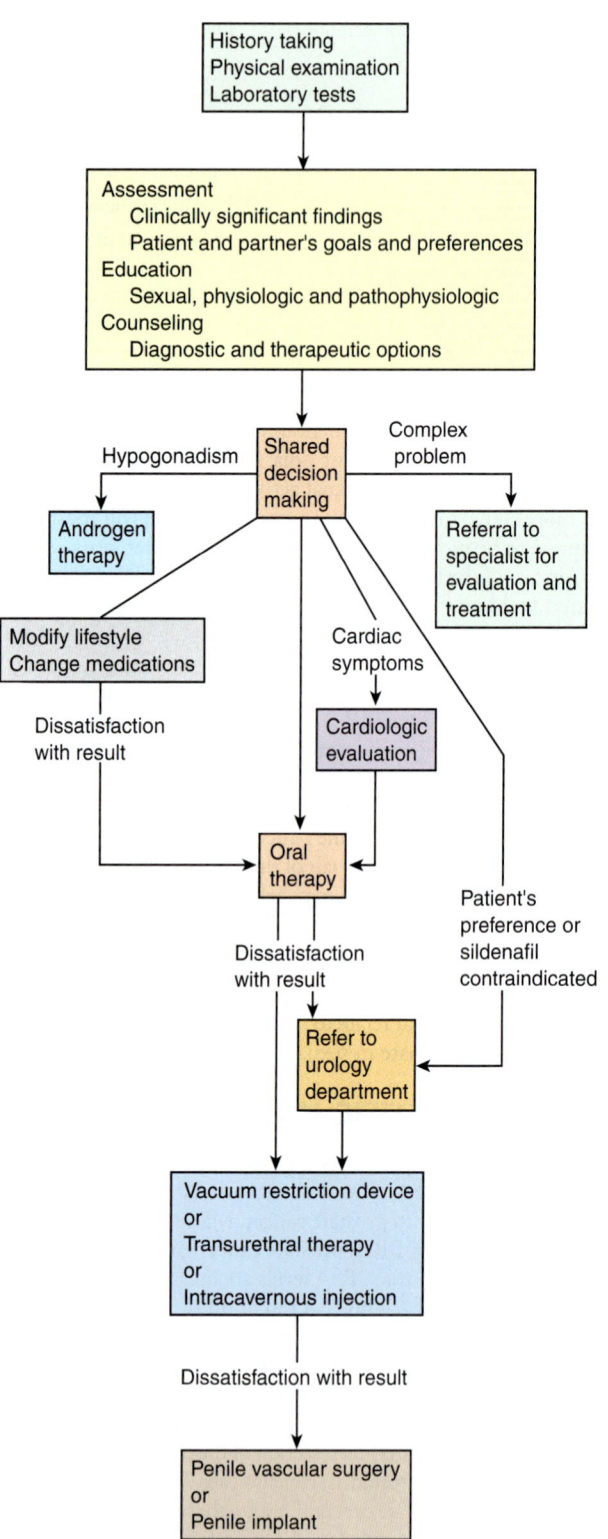

FIGURE 49-3 Evaluation and treatment of men with erectile dysfunction. From Lue, T. F. (2000). Erectile dysfunction. *New England Journal of Medicine, 342*(24), 1807. © 2000 Massachusetts Medical Society. All rights reserved. Used with permission.

Medical Management

Treatment, which depends on the cause, can be medical, surgical, or both (Table 49-2). Nonsurgical therapy includes treating associated conditions, such as alcoholism, and readjusting hypertensive agents or other medications. Endocrine therapy may be instituted for erectile dysfunction secondary to hypothalamic-pituitary-gonadal dysfunction and may reverse the condition. Insufficient penile blood flow may be treated with vascular surgery. Patients with erectile dysfunction from psychogenic causes are referred to a health care provider or therapist specializing in sexual dysfunction. Patients with erectile dysfunction secondary to organic causes may be candidates for penile implants.

PHARMACOLOGIC THERAPY

Sildenafil (Viagra) is an oral medication for erectile dysfunction (Eid, 2000). When it is taken about 1 hour before sex, an erection can occur with stimulation; the erection can last about 60 to 120 minutes. Despite the effectiveness of this medication, it does have side effects: headache, flushing, and dyspepsia. Sildenafil is contraindicated in patients who take organic nitrates and should be used with caution in patients with retinopathy, especially those with diabetic retinopathy (Chart 49-2).

Other pharmacologic measures to induce erections include injecting vasoactive agents, such as alprostadil, papaverine, and phentolamine, directly into the penis. Complications include **priapism** (a persistent abnormal erection) and development of fibrotic plaques at the injection sites. Alprostadil is also formulated in a gel pellet that can be inserted into the urethra to create an erection.

PENILE IMPLANTS

Penile implants are available in two types: the semirigid rod and the inflatable prosthesis. The semirigid rod (eg, the Small-Carrion prosthesis) leaves the man with a permanent semierection. The inflatable prosthesis simulates natural erections and natural flaccidity. Complications after implantation include infection, erosion of the prosthesis through the skin (more common with the semirigid rod than with the inflatable prosthesis), and persistent pain, which may require removal of the implant. Cystoscopic surgery, such as **transurethral resection of the prostate** (TUR or TURP), is more difficult with a semirigid rod than with the inflatable prosthesis. Factors to consider in choosing a prosthesis are the patient's activities of daily living and social activities and the expectations of the patient and his partner. Ongoing counselling for the patient and his partner is usually necessary to help them in adapting to the prosthesis.

NEGATIVE-PRESSURE DEVICES

Negative-pressure (vacuum) devices may also be used to induce an erection. A plastic cylinder is placed over the flaccid penis, and negative pressure is applied. When an erection is attained, a constriction band is placed around the base of the penis to maintain the erection. Although many men find this method satisfactory, others experience premature loss of penile rigidity or pain when applying suction or during intercourse.

Nursing Management

Personal satisfaction and the ability to sexually satisfy a partner are common concerns of patients. Men with illnesses and disabilities may need the assistance of a sex therapist to find, implement, and integrate their sexual beliefs and behaviours into a healthy and satisfying lifestyle. The nurse can inform patients that support groups for men with erectile dysfunction and their partners have been established. Information about Impotence Anonymous for patients and I-Anon for their partners can be found at the end of this chapter.

EJACULATION PROBLEMS

Premature ejaculation occurs when a man cannot control the ejaculatory reflex and, once aroused, reaches orgasm before or shortly after intromission. It is the most common dysfunction in men. Inhibited or retarded ejaculation is the involuntary inhibition of the ejaculatory reflex. The spectrum of responses includes occasional ejaculation through intercourse or self-stimulation or the complete inability to ejaculate under any circumstances.

Treatment modalities depend on the nature and severity of the ejaculation problem. Behavioural therapies may be indicated for people with premature ejaculation; these therapies often involve the man and his sexual partner. "Homework" assignments are often given to the couple to encourage them to identify their sexual needs and to communicate those needs to each other. In some cases, pharmacologic and behavioural therapy together may be effective.

Neurologic disorders (eg, spinal cord injury, multiple sclerosis, neuropathy secondary to diabetes), surgery (prostatectomy), and medications are the most common causes of inhibited ejaculation. Chemical, vibratory, and electrical stimulation have been used with some success. Treatment is usually multidisciplinary and addresses the physical and psychological factors that are often involved in inhibited ejaculation (Lue, 2000).

For men with retrograde ejaculation, the urine may be collected after ejaculation; sperm is then collected from the urine for use in artificial insemination. In men with spinal cord injury, electroejaculation may be used to obtain sperm for artificial insemination.

The effects of trauma, chronic illness, and physical disability on sexual function can be profound. In addition to psychogenic factors, the physical changes associated with illness and injury can impair sexual function.

Infections of the Male Genitourinary Tract

Acute uncomplicated cystitis in adult men is uncommon but occasionally occurs in men whose sexual partners have vaginal infections with *Escherichia coli*. Asymptomatic bacteriuria may also occur from genitourinary manipulation, catheterization, or instrumentation. Urinary tract infections in the male are discussed in Chapter 45.

The incidence of sexually transmitted diseases (STDs) is increasing in men and women. STDs are most common in young, sexually active people, with the incidence higher in men than women (U.S. Surgeon General, 2001). STDs affect people from all walks of life—from all social, educational, economic, and racial backgrounds. Several diseases are classified as STDs: urethritis (gonococcal and nongonococcal), genital ulcers (genital herpes infections, primary syphilis, chancroid, granuloma inguinale, and lymphogranuloma venereum), genital warts (human papillomavirus [HPV]), scabies, pediculosis pubis, molluscum contagiosum, hepatitis and enteric infections, proctitis, and acquired immunodeficiency syndrome (AIDS). Trichomoniasis and STDs characterized by genital ulcers are thought to increase susceptibility to human immunodeficiency virus (HIV) infection. Trichomoniasis is associated with nonchlamydial, nongonococcal urethritis.

Table 49-2 • Treatments for Erectile Dysfunction

METHOD	DESCRIPTION	ADVANTAGES AND DISADVANTAGES	DURATION
Penile implants • Semirigid rod • Inflatable Penile implant	Surgically implanted into corpus cavernosum	Reliable Requires surgery Healing takes up to 3 weeks Subsequent cystoscopic surgery is difficult Semirigid rod results in permanent semierection	Indefinite Inflatable prosthesis: saline returns from penile receptacle to reservoir
Negative-pressure (vacuum) devices Penile vacuum pump	Induction of erection with vacuum; maintained with constriction band around base of penis	Few side effects Cumbersome to use before intercourse Vasocongestion of penis can cause pain or numbness	To prevent penile injury, constriction band must not be left in place for longer than 1 hour
Pharmacologic therapy • Oral medication (sildenafil [Viagra]) Oral medication	Smooth muscle relaxant causing blood to flow into penis	Can cause headache and diarrhea Contraindicated for men taking organic nitrates Used with caution in patients with retinopathy, especially diabetic retinopathy	Taken orally 1 hour before intercourse Stimulation is required to achieve erection Erection can last 1 hour
• Injection (alprostadil, papaverine, phentolamine) Penile injection	Smooth muscle relaxant causing blood to flow into penis	Firm erections are achievable in more than 50% of cases Pain at injection site; plaque formation, risk of priapism	Injection 20 minutes before intercourse Erection can last up to 1 hour

(continued)

Table 49-2 • Treatments for Erectile Dysfunction (Continued)

METHOD	DESCRIPTION	ADVANTAGES AND DISADVANTAGES	DURATION
• Urethral suppository (alprostadil)	Smooth muscle relaxant causing blood to flow into penis	May be used twice a day Not recommended with pregnant partners	Inserted 10 minutes before intercourse Erection can last up to 1 hour

Penile suppository

Treatment of STDs must be targeted at the patient as well as his or her sexual partners and sometimes the unborn child. A thorough history that includes a sexual history is crucial to identify patients at risk and to direct care and teaching. Partners of men with STDs must also be examined, treated, and counselled to prevent reinfection and complications in both partners and to limit the spread of the disease. Sexual abstinence during treatment and recovery is advised to prevent the transmission of STDs (CDC, 2002). Using latex condoms for at least 6 months after completion of treatment is recommended to decrease transmission of HPV infections as well as other STDs. Because patients with one STD may also have another STD, it is important to

---

Chart 49-2 • PATIENT EDUCATION
Questions and Answers About Viagra

What Is Viagra?
It is a pill that is taken by mouth to restore erectile function in men with impotence. Viagra will not restore desire or sex drive.

How Does Viagra Work?
Viagra works by relaxing the penis, thus increasing the efficiency of the erection. The enzyme that the medication specifically works on is a type 5 phosphodiesterase (PDE-5), which is found almost exclusively in the penis.

How Do I Take Viagra?
Take 1 hour before intercourse. The peak action occurs between 30 and 120 minutes. *You must have sexual stimulation to create the erection.* If you fall asleep or need to go out in public, you will have no erection if you have no stimulation.

What Happens If I Don't Have Stimulation in the First Hour?
The beneficial effect can be seen as late as 8 hours, but most of the effectiveness is within the first 4 hours.

How Often May I Use Viagra?
The recommended frequency is once a day. If you take it more than once a day, you may experience back and leg aches as well as nausea and vomiting. Taking Viagra more than once a day will not improve its effects. You may take it 7 days a week if you desire, but it does not build up in your blood. Remember, only take it when you want to have intercourse.

What Are the Side Effects of Viagra?
  Mild headache—but not bad enough to prevent taking the drug or enjoying its effects

  Facial flushing—your face may get red
  Indigestion—very mild upset stomach, which can be severe if you take more than one pill a day
  Runny nose
  Visual disturbance ("blue haze")—a transient, or temporary change in your vision that makes everything appear blue for about an hour; this will happen if you take more than the highest dose available (100 mg).

Are There Any Interactions With Other Medications?
You should not take Viagra if you are taking any nitrate medications:
  Nitroglycerin   Isordil
  Nitro-bid   Ismo
  Any nitro medication   Indur
If you are unsure about your medications, it is important that you ask your doctor or pharmacist. You do not need to worry about blood pressure medications or anti-diabetic medications.

Can I Use Viagra with MUSE or Penile Injections?
The use of Viagra with other forms of therapy has not been tested and should be avoided.

Is There More Than One Dose of Viagra?
The doses available are 25 mg, 50 mg, and 100 mg. Your first prescription will be for two tablets of each dose. Use the 25-mg dose first. If the 25-mg dose does not work, then try the 50-mg tablet. If this is not strong enough, then try the 100-mg tablet. *Do not take more than one tablet per day of any one dose.* When you find a dose that works for you, call your physician or provider, and a long-term prescription will be sent to you.

Used with permission of John Rieke, MD, Virginia Mason Division of Radiation Oncology.

examine and test for other STDs. Use of spermicides with nonoxynol 9 ("N-9") is discouraged as they do not protect against HIV infection and may increase the risk for transmission of the virus (van Damme, 2000; CDC, 2002). See Chapters 52 and 70 for more detailed discussions of HIV infection and AIDS and other STDs.

Conditions of the Prostate

PROSTATITIS

Prostatitis is an inflammation of the prostate gland caused by infectious agents (bacteria, fungi, mycoplasma) or other conditions (eg, urethral stricture, prostatic hyperplasia). *E. coli* is the most commonly isolated organism. Microorganisms are usually carried to the prostate from the urethra. Prostatitis may be classified as bacterial or abacterial, depending on the presence or absence of microorganisms in the prostatic fluid.

Clinical Manifestations

Symptoms of prostatitis may include perineal discomfort, burning, urgency, frequency, and pain with or after ejaculation. Prostatodynia (pain in the prostate) is manifested by pain on voiding or perineal pain without evidence of inflammation or bacterial growth in the prostate fluid.

Acute bacterial prostatitis may produce sudden fever and chills and perineal, rectal, or low back pain. Urinary symptoms, such as dysuria, frequency, urgency, and **nocturia** (urination during the night), may occur. Some patients do not have symptoms. Chronic bacterial prostatitis is a major cause of relapsing urinary tract infection in men. Symptoms are usually mild, consisting of frequency, dysuria, and occasionally urethral discharge. High temperature and chills are uncommon.

Complications of prostatitis may include swelling of the prostate gland and urinary retention. Other complications include epididymitis, bacteremia, and pyelonephritis.

Assessment and Diagnostic Findings

The diagnosis of prostatitis requires a careful history, culture of prostate fluid or tissue, and occasionally a histologic examination of the tissue. To locate the source of a lower genitourinary infection (bladder neck, urethra, prostate), it is necessary to collect a divided urinary specimen for segmental urine culture. After cleaning the glans penis and retracting the foreskin (if present), the patient voids 10 to 15 mL of urine into a container. This represents urethral urine. Without interrupting the urinary stream, he collects 50 to 75 mL of urine in a second container; this represents bladder urine.

If the patient does not have acute prostatitis, the physician immediately performs a prostatic massage and collects any prostatic fluid that is expressed into a third container. If it is not possible to collect prostatic fluid, the patient voids a small quantity of urine. The specimen may contain the bacteria present in the prostatic fluid. Urinalysis after prostate examination commonly reveals many white blood cells.

Medical Management

The goal of therapy for acute bacterial prostatitis is to avoid the complications of abscess formation and septicemia. A broad-spectrum antibiotic agent (to which the causative organism is sen-

sitive) is administered for 10 to 14 days. Intravenous administration of the agent may be necessary to achieve high serum and tissue levels; the agent may be administered at home. The patient is encouraged to remain on bed rest to alleviate symptoms quickly. Comfort is promoted with analgesic agents (to relieve pain), antispasmodic medications and bladder sedatives (to relieve bladder irritability), sitz baths (to relieve pain and spasm), and stool softeners (to prevent pain from straining).

Chronic bacterial prostatitis is difficult to treat because most antibiotics diffuse poorly from the plasma into the prostatic fluid. Nevertheless, antibiotics may be prescribed, including trimethoprim-sulfamethoxazole (TMP-SMZ) or a fluoroquinolone. Continuous therapy with low-dose antibiotics to suppress the infection may also be indicated. The patient is advised that the urinary tract infection may recur and is taught to recognize its symptoms. In addition, treatment for chronic prostatitis may include reducing the retention of prostatic fluid by ejaculation through sexual intercourse or masturbation. Other treatments include antispasmodics, sitz baths, stool softeners, and evaluation of sexual partners to reduce the possibility of cross-infection. The treatment of nonbacterial prostatitis is directed toward relieving symptoms.

Nursing Management

If the patient experiences symptoms of acute prostatitis (fever, severe pain and discomfort, inability to urinate, malaise), he may be hospitalized for intravenous antibiotic therapy. Nursing management includes administration of prescribed antibiotics and provision of comfort measures, including prescribed analgesic agents and sitz baths.

The patient with chronic prostatitis is usually treated on an outpatient basis and needs to be instructed about the importance of continuing antibiotic therapy.

PROMOTING HOME AND COMMUNITY-BASED CARE

Teaching Patients Self-Care. The nurse instructs the patient to complete the prescribed course of antibiotics. If intravenous antibiotics are to be administered at home, the nurse instructs the patient and family about correct and safe administration. Arrangements for home care to oversee administration may be needed. Hot sitz baths (10 to 20 minutes) may be taken several times daily. Fluids are encouraged to satisfy thirst but are not "forced" because an effective medication level must be maintained in the urine. Foods and liquids that have diuretic action or that increase prostatic secretions, such as alcohol, coffee, tea, chocolate, cola, and spices, should be avoided. During periods of acute inflammation, sexual arousal and intercourse should be avoided.

To minimize discomfort, the patient should avoid sitting for long periods. Medical follow-up is necessary for at least 6 months to 1 year because prostatitis caused by the same or different organisms can recur.

BENIGN PROSTATIC HYPERPLASIA (ENLARGED PROSTATE)

In many patients older than 50 years, the prostate gland enlarges, extending upward into the bladder and obstructing the outflow of urine by encroaching on the vesical orifice. This condition is known as benign prostatic hyperplasia (BPH), the enlargement, or hypertrophy, of the prostate. BPH is one of the most common pathologic conditions in older men (McConnell, 1998).

Clinical Manifestations

Examination reveals a prostate gland that is large, rubbery, and nontender. The cause is uncertain, but evidence suggests that hormones initiate hyperplasia of the supporting stromal tissue and the glandular elements in the prostate (McConnell, 1998). The hypertrophied lobes may obstruct the vesical neck or prostatic urethra, causing incomplete emptying of the bladder and urinary retention. As a result, a gradual dilation of the ureters (hydroureter) and kidneys (hydronephrosis) can occur. Urinary tract infections may result from urinary stasis, because some urine remains in the urinary tract and serves as a medium for infective organisms.

Assessment and Diagnostic Findings

The obstructive and irritative symptom complex (referred to as **prostatism**) includes increased frequency of urination, nocturia, urgency, hesitancy in starting urination, abdominal straining with urination, a decrease in the volume and force of the urinary stream, interruption of the urinary stream, dribbling (urine dribbles out after urination), a sensation that the bladder has not been completely emptied, acute urinary retention (when more than 60 mL of urine remains in the bladder after urination), and recurrent urinary tract infections. Ultimately, azotemia (accumulation of nitrogenous waste products) and renal failure can occur with chronic urinary retention and large residual volumes. Generalized symptoms may also be noted, including fatigue, anorexia, nausea, vomiting, and epigastric discomfort. Other disorders producing similar symptoms include urethral stricture, prostate cancer, neurogenic bladder, and urinary bladder stones.

A physical examination with DRE and diagnostic studies may be performed to determine the degree to which the prostate is enlarged, the presence of any changes in the bladder wall, and the efficiency of renal function. These tests may include urinalysis and urodynamic studies to assess urine flow. Renal function tests, including serum creatinine levels, may be performed to determine if there is renal impairment from prostatic back-pressure and to evaluate renal reserve. Complete blood studies are performed. Because hemorrhage is a major complication of prostate surgery, all clotting defects must be corrected. A high percentage of patients with BPH have cardiac or respiratory complications, or both, because of their age; therefore, cardiac and respiratory function is also assessed.

Medical Management

The treatment plan depends on the cause of BPH, the severity of the obstruction, and the patient's condition. If the patient is admitted on an emergency basis because he cannot void, he is immediately catheterized. The ordinary catheter may be too soft and pliable to advance through the urethra into the bladder. In such cases, a thin wire called a stylet is introduced (by a urologist) into the catheter to prevent the catheter from collapsing when it encounters resistance. In severe cases, metal catheters with a pronounced prostatic curve may be used. Sometimes an incision is made into the bladder (a suprapubic cystostomy) to provide drainage.

Although prostatectomy (described later in the chapter) to remove the hyperplastic prostatic tissue is frequently performed, other treatment options are available. These include "watchful waiting," transurethral incision of the prostate (TUIP), balloon dilation, alpha-blockers, 5-alpha-reductase inhibitors, transurethral laser resection, transurethral needle ablation, and microwave thermotherapy (Lepor, 1998; Mebust, 1998; McCullough, 1998). Watchful waiting is the appropriate treatment for many patients because the likelihood of progression of the disease or the development of complications is unknown. Patients are monitored periodically for severity of symptoms, physical findings, laboratory tests, and diagnostic urologic tests.

Alpha-adrenergic receptor blockers (eg, terazosin [Hytrin]) relax the smooth muscle of the bladder neck and prostate. These agents help to reduce obstructive symptoms in many patients.

Because the hormonal component of BPH has been identified, one method of treatment involves hormonal manipulation with antiandrogen agents, such as finasteride (Proscar). In clinical studies, 5-alpha-reductase inhibitors such as finasteride have been effective in preventing the conversion of testosterone to dihydrotestosterone (DHT). With decreased levels of DHT, suppression of glandular cell activity and decreases in prostate size have been demonstrated. Side effects of these medications include gynecomastia (breast enlargement), erectile dysfunction, and flushing.

With ultrasound guidance, resection of the prostate can be accomplished with lasers. The treated tissue either vaporizes or becomes necrotic and sloughs. This treatment is delivered in the outpatient setting and generally results in less postoperative bleeding than a traditional surgical prostatectomy.

Transurethral needle ablation uses low-level radiofrequencies to produce localized heat to destroy prostate tissue while sparing the urethra, nerves, muscles, and membranes. The radiofrequencies are delivered by thin needles placed into the prostate gland from a catheter. The body then resorbs the dead tissue.

In microwave thermotherapy, heat is applied to the hypertrophied prostatic tissue. A transurethral probe is inserted into the urethra, and microwaves are carefully directed to the prostate tissue. A water-cooling system helps to minimize damage to the urethra and decreases the discomfort from the procedure. The tissue becomes necrotic and sloughs.

Saw palmetto is a botanical remedy used for symptoms of mild to moderate BPH such as urinary frequency and decreased force of urine stream (Gerber, 2000; Marks, Partin, Epstein et al., 2000; Wilt, Ishani, Stark et al., 1998). It is theorized that saw palmetto works by interfering with the conversion of testosterone to DHT. In addition, saw palmetto may directly block the ability of DHT to stimulate prostate cell growth. It should not be used with finasteride or medications containing estrogen.

CANCER OF THE PROSTATE

Prostate cancer is the most common form of cancer in Canadian men, affecting one in every seven some time during their lives. The Canadian Cancer Society (2005) estimates that 20,500 men will be diagnosed with prostate cancer in 2005 and that 4,300 will die of the disease. Prostate cancer rates are twice as high in African Canadian men than in Caucasian men, and African Canadian men are more likely to die of prostate cancer than men in any other racial or ethnic group. To address this issue, Agho and Lewis (2001) assessed knowledge of prostate cancer and the use of prostate cancer screening services among 108 African American men. The men were unable to answer most of the 21 questions on the test with more than 70% accuracy, although individuals younger than 40 years of age were more knowledgeable than older men. Despite their increased risk for prostate cancer, only 47% of the men in the sample who were 40 years or older had prostate cancer screening as part of their annual physical examination. Knowledge about prostate cancer was found to be negatively correlated with education, age, and income. A culturally sensitive promotional campaign has been identified as an important strategy to increase awareness of the racial disparities in the incidence of prostate cancer and mortality rates. Nurses are in an ideal position to use these research findings to improve the health of African Canadian men by teaching and counselling them about prostate cancer, screening, and treatment.

Risk factors for prostate cancer include increasing age: the incidence of prostate cancer increases rapidly after the age of 50 years, and more than 70% of cases occur in men over 65 years of age. African American men have the highest incidence of prostate cancer in the world. Prostate cancer is common in Canada, the United States and northwestern Europe but is rare in Asia, Africa, Central America, and South America. A familial predisposition may occur in 5% to 10% of cases of prostate cancer. Having a father or brother with prostate cancer doubles the risk; the risk increases further if several relatives have had prostate cancer and if the relatives were young at diagnosis. A diet high in red meat and fat increases the risk for prostate cancer (American Cancer Society, 2002, Canadian Cancer Society, 2005). Large-scale studies are in progress to determine if prostate cancer can be prevented by use of selected supplements or finasteride (Proscar).

Clinical Manifestations

Cancer of the prostate in its early stages rarely produces symptoms. The symptoms that develop from urinary obstruction occur late in the disease. This cancer tends to vary in its course. If the neoplasm is large enough to encroach on the bladder neck, signs and symptoms of urinary obstruction occur: difficulty and frequency of urination, urinary retention, and decreased size and force of the urinary stream. Other symptoms may include blood in the urine or semen and painful ejaculation. Hematuria may result if the cancer invades the urethra or bladder, or both. Prostate cancer can metastasize to bone and lymph nodes. Symptoms related to metastases include backache, hip pain, perineal and rectal discomfort, anemia, weight loss, weakness, nausea, and oliguria (decreased urine output). Unfortunately, these symptoms may be the first indications of prostate cancer.

Assessment and Diagnostic Findings

When prostate cancer is detected early, the likelihood of cure is high. Every man older than 40 years of age should have a DRE as part of his regular health checkup. Routine repeated rectal palpation of the gland (preferably by the same examiner) is important because early cancer may be detected as a nodule within the substance of the gland or as an extensive hardening in the posterior lobe. The more advanced lesion is "stony hard" and fixed. DRE also provides useful clinical information about the rectum, anal sphincter, and quality of stool.

NURSING RESEARCH PROFILE 49-1
Impact of Prostate Cancer

Fitch, M. I., Gray, R., Franssen, E., & Johnson, B. (2000). Men's perspectives on the impact of prostate cancer: Implications for oncology nurses. *Oncology Nursing Forum, 27*(8), 1255–1263.

Purpose
This study was conducted to describe the experience of and support used by men with prostate cancer and to compare those with recurrent prostate cancer and those without recurrent disease.

Study Sample and Design
This was a descriptive study of men with prostate cancer: 120 men with recurrent prostate cancer and 845 men without recurrent cancer living in Canada. Consecutive subjects were recruited through urology offices and self-help groups. A 52-item survey developed by the researchers was used to obtain information from the subjects.

Descriptive data analysis addressed demographic characteristics, problems experienced, assistance received for problems, factors surrounding emotional support (eg, satisfaction with communication, satisfaction with information received, benefits of self-help groups), and impact of illness and treatment on lifestyle (including relationships with partners, children, and friends; employment opportunities and work life; financial status; leisure time activities; mental health; and household responsibilities). The two groups were compared on relevant variables.

Findings
Men in both groups reported physical and psychological problems, although the incidence of these problems was higher in men with recurrent disease. Sexual dysfunction was the most frequently identified problem in both groups, but among those with recurrent disease, a significantly higher percentage reported problems with side effects, pain, and anger. Although few men reported having difficulty talking with their health care providers, 10% of men with recurrent disease

had trouble doing so compared to 2% of those without recurrent disease ($p < 0.025$). The percentage of men with recurrent disease who reported dissatisfaction with the information that was provided was higher in the areas of possible side effects or symptoms (31% vs. 14%, $p < 0.005$) and medical condition (25% vs. 10%, $p < 0.005$) than that of men without recurrent disease. Men in both groups indicated that they received inadequate help with problems such as side effects, incontinence, sexual dysfunction, and pain.

Overall, family and friends were the most frequent sources of support when men needed to talk, followed by medical professionals and self-help groups. The subjects also identified the need for more information about possible emotional reactions to the disease, how to arrange to speak to another man with prostate cancer, alternative therapies, diet and nutrition.

Nursing Implications
Nurses should conduct early and ongoing comprehensive patient assessments, including physical as well as psychosocial components, to determine patient needs so that they can provide timely and effective interventions. Patients at high risk of experiencing psychosocial difficulties include those who do not have the social networks available to discuss their experiences. To enhance coping with the consequences of prostate cancer and its treatment, particularly in those with recurrent disease, nurses need to teach patients about the disease and provide an opportunity for them to discuss their concerns. In addition, assessment findings will help guide the creation and provision of effective interventions. Referral to self-help groups may be indicated, particularly in the absence of social support from family and friends.

The diagnosis of prostate cancer is confirmed by a histologic examination of tissue removed surgically by transurethral resection, open prostatectomy, or transrectal needle biopsy. Fine-needle aspiration is a quick, painless method of obtaining prostate cells for cytologic examination. The procedure is helpful for determining the stage of disease as well.

Most prostate cancers are diagnosed when a man seeks medical attention for symptoms of urinary obstruction or after abnormalities are found by DRE. Incidentally detected cancer with transurethral resection of the prostate for clinically benign disease and prostatism occurs in 10% to 20% of patients. Rarely do patients have other signs and symptoms, such as azotemia (nitrogen compounds in the blood), weakness, anemia, or bone pain.

PSA, a neutral serine protease, is produced by the normal and neoplastic ductal epithelium of the prostate and secreted into the glandular lumen (Brawer, Cheli, Neaman et al., 2000; Kalish & McKinlay, 1999). A simple blood test can be used to measure PSA levels. The concentration of PSA in the blood is proportional to the total prostatic mass. Although the PSA level indicates the presence of prostate tissue, it does not necessarily indicate malignancy. PSA testing is routinely used to monitor the patient's response to cancer therapy and to detect local progression and early recurrence of prostate cancer. The combination of DRE and PSA testing appears to be a cost-effective method for detecting prostate cancer. The Canadian Cancer Society recommends that, beginning at age 50, an annual DRE and PSA measurement be offered to men who have a life expectancy of at least 10 years and to younger men (age 45 years or older) who are at high risk. Risk factors include strong familial predisposition (two or more affected primary relatives) and African American race (Smith et al., 2000).

Transrectal ultrasound (TRUS) studies are indicated for men who have elevated PSA levels and abnormal DRE findings. TRUS studies help in detecting nonpalpable prostate cancers and assist with staging localized prostate cancer. Needle biopsies of the prostate are commonly guided by TRUS.

Other tests include bone scans to detect metastatic bone disease, skeletal x-rays to identify bone metastases, excretory urography to detect changes caused by ureteral obstruction, renal function tests, and computed tomography (CT) scans or lymphangiography to identify metastases in the pelvic lymph nodes.

The radiolabelled monoclonal antibody Capromab Pendetide with Indium-111 (ProstaScint) is an antibody that is attracted to the prostate-specific membrane antigen found on prostate cancer cells (Narayan et al., 2000). The radioactive element attached to the antibody is then visible with scanning, allowing detection of disease spread. This study is used to detect spread of prostate cancer in the lymph nodes or other parts of the body in newly diagnosed men who have apparently localized prostate cancer and who are thought to be at high risk for metastasis. In addition, men who have undergone a prostatectomy and who develop a rising PSA level may also be evaluated with this study.

Sexual Complications

Men with prostate cancer commonly experience sexual dysfunction before the diagnosis is made. Each treatment (see discussion that follows) for prostate cancer further increases the incidence of sexual problems. With nerve-sparing radical prostatectomy, the chance of recovering erections is better for men who are younger and in whom both neurovascular bundles are spared. Hormonal therapy also affects the central nervous system mechanisms that mediate sexual desire and arousability.

Sildenafil (Viagra) has been found to be effective for treating erectile dysfunction in younger men after radical retropubic pros-

tatectomy, especially if the neurovascular bundles were preserved (Zagaja, Mhoon, Aikens et al., 2000). In addition, sildenafil can improve erectile function in men with partial or moderate erectile dysfunction following radiation therapy for localized prostate cancer (Zelefsky, 1999).

Medical Management

Treatment is based on the stage of the disease and the patient's age and symptoms. Partin and associates (1997) combined PSA level with the clinical stage and pathologic grade of the tumour to create a nomogram to predict the pathologic stage of localized prostate cancer. This nomogram can be useful in making treatment decisions and predicting treatment outcomes. Nursing care of the patient with cancer of the prostate is summarized in the Plan of Nursing Care.

SURGICAL MANAGEMENT

A radical prostatectomy (removal of the prostate and seminal vesicles) remains the standard surgical procedure for patients who have early-stage, potentially curable disease and a life expectancy of 10 years or more (Carroll et al., 2001). Sexual impotence follows radical prostatectomy, and 5% to 10% of patients have various degrees of urinary incontinence (Bishoff, Motley, Optenberg et al., 1998).

RADIATION THERAPY

If prostate cancer is detected in its early stage, the treatment may be curative radiation therapy: either teletherapy with a linear accelerator or interstitial irradiation (implantation of radioactive seeds of iodine or palladium), also referred to as brachytherapy (Carroll et al., 2001). Teletherapy involves about 6 to 7 weeks of daily (5 days/week) radiation treatments. Interstitial seed implantation is performed under anesthesia. About 80 to 100 seeds are placed with ultrasound guidance, and the patient returns home after the procedure. Exposure of others to radiation is minimal, but close contact with pregnant women and infants should be avoided for up to 2 months. Radiation safety guidelines include straining urine for seeds and using a condom during sexual intercourse for 2 weeks after implantation to catch seeds that may pass through the urethra.

Side effects, which usually are transitory, include inflammation of the rectum, bowel, and bladder (proctitis, enteritis, and cystitis) due to their proximity to the prostate and the radiation doses (Horwitz & Hanks, 2000; Krumholtz et al., 2000; Ragde, Grado, Nadir et al., 2000). Irritation of the bladder and urethra from radiation therapy can cause pain with urination and during ejaculation until the irritation subsides. There is a greater preservation of sexual potency, however, with radiation therapy than with surgery. For locally advanced prostate cancer, hormonal treatments before and during radiation therapy are frequently used to improve local control and disease-free survival (Lue, 2000).

HORMONAL THERAPY

Hormonal therapy is one method used to control rather than cure prostate cancer (Carroll et al., 2001). In the early 1940s, it was determined that most prostate cancers were androgen-dependent and could be controlled by androgen withdrawal. Hormonal therapy for advanced prostate cancer suppresses androgenic stimuli to the prostate by decreasing the circulating plasma testosterone levels or interrupting the conversion to or

(text continues on page 1507)

Plan of Nursing Care
The Patient With Prostate Cancer

Nursing Interventions	Rationale	Expected Outcomes

Nursing Diagnosis: Anxiety related to concern and lack of knowledge about the diagnosis, treatment plan, and prognosis

Goal: Reduced stress and improved ability to cope

Nursing Interventions	Rationale	Expected Outcomes
1. Obtain health history to determine the following: a. Patient's concerns b. His level of understanding of his health problem c. His past experience with cancer d. Whether he knows his diagnosis of malignancy and its prognosis e. His support systems and coping methods	1. Nurse clarifies information and facilitates patient's understanding and coping.	• Appears relaxed • States that anxiety has been reduced or relieved • Demonstrates understanding of illness and treatment when questioned • Engages in open communication with others
2. Provide education about diagnosis and treatment plan: a. Explain in simple terms what diagnostic tests to expect, how long they will take, and what will be experienced during each test. b. Review treatment plan and allow patient to ask questions.	2. Helping the patient to understand the diagnostic tests and treatment plan will help decrease his anxiety and promote cooperation.	
3. Assess his psychological reaction to his diagnosis/prognosis and how he has coped with past stresses.	3. This information provides clues in determining appropriate measures to facilitate coping.	
4. Provide information about institutional and community resources for coping with prostate cancer: social services, support groups, community agencies	4. Institutional and community resources can help the patient and family cope with the illness and treatment on an ongoing basis.	

Nursing Diagnosis: Urinary retention related to urethral obstruction secondary to prostatic enlargement or tumour and loss of bladder tone due to prolonged distention/retention

Goal: Improved pattern of urinary elimination

Nursing Interventions	Rationale	Expected Outcomes
1. Determine patient's usual pattern of urinary function.	1. Provides a baseline for comparison and goal to work toward	• Voids at normal intervals • Reports absence of frequency, urgency, or bladder fullness • Displays no palpable suprapubic distention after voiding • Maintains balanced intake and output
2. Assess for signs and symptoms of urinary retention: amount and frequency of urination, suprapubic distention, complaints of urgency and discomfort.	2. Voiding 20 to 30 mL frequently and output less than intake suggests retention.	
3. Catheterize patient to determine amount of residual urine.	3. Determines amount of urine remaining in bladder after voiding	
4. Initiate measures to treat retention: a. Encourage assuming normal position for voiding. b. Recommend using Valsalva manoeuvre. c. Administer prescribed cholinergic agent. d. Monitor effects of medication.	4. Promotes voiding a. Usual position provides relaxed conditions conducive to voiding. b. Valsalva manoeuvre exerts pressure to force urine out of bladder. c. Stimulates bladder contraction d. If unsuccessful, another measure may be required.	
5. Consult with physician regarding intermittent or indwelling catheterization; assist with procedure as required.	5. Catheterization will relieve urinary retention until the specific cause is determined; it may be an obstruction that can be corrected only surgically.	
6. Monitor catheter function; maintain sterility of closed system; irrigate as required.	6. Adequate functioning of catheter is to be ensured to empty bladder and to prevent infection.	
7. Prepare patient for surgery if indicated.	7. Surgical removal of obstruction may be necessary.	

(continued)

Plan of Nursing Care
The Patient With Prostate Cancer (Continued)

Nursing Interventions	Rationale	Expected Outcomes

Nursing Diagnosis: Deficient knowledge related to the diagnosis of: cancer, urinary difficulties, and treatment modalities
Goal: Understanding of the diagnosis and ability to care for self

Nursing Interventions	Rationale	Expected Outcomes
1. Encourage communication with the patient.	1. This is designed to establish rapport and trust.	• Discusses his concerns and problems freely
2. Review the anatomy of the involved area.	2. Orientation to one's anatomy is basic to understanding its function.	• Asks questions and shows interest in his condition
3. Be specific in selecting information that is relevant to the patient's particular treatment plan.	3. This is based on the treatment plan; as it varies with each patient, individualization is desirable.	• Describes activities that help or hinder recovery • Identifies ways of attaining/maintaining bladder control

4. Identify ways to reduce pressure on the operative area after prostatectomy:
  a. Avoid prolonged sitting (in a chair, long automobile rides), standing, walking.
  b. Avoid straining, such as during exercises, bowel movement, lifting, and sexual intercourse.
	4. This is to prevent bleeding; such precautions are in order for 6 to 8 weeks postoperatively.	• Demonstrates satisfactory technique and understanding of catheter care
		• Lists signs and symptoms that must be reported should they occur

5. Familiarize patient with ways of attaining/maintaining bladder control.
 	
  a. Encourage urination every 2 to 3 hours; discourage voiding when supine.
  b. Avoid drinking cola and caffeine beverages; urge a cutoff time in the evening for drinking fluids to minimize frequent voiding during the night.
  c. Describe pelvic floor muscle exercises to be performed two to three times a day (see page 1513).
  d. Develop a schedule with patient that will fit into his routine.
	5. These measures will help control frequency and dribbling and aid in preventing retention.
	  a. By sitting or standing, patient is more likely to empty his bladder.
	  b. Spacing the kind and amount of liquid intake will help to prevent frequency.
	
	  c. Exercises will assist him in starting and stopping the urinary stream.
	
	  d. A schedule will assist in developing a workable pattern of normal activities.	

6. Demonstrate catheter care; encourage his questions; stress the importance of position of urinary receptacle.	6. By requiring a return demonstration of care, collection, and emptying of the device, he will become more independent and also can prevent backflow of urine, which can lead to infection.	

Nursing Diagnosis: Imbalanced nutrition: less than body requirements related to decreased oral intake because of anorexia, nausea, and vomiting caused by cancer or its treatment
Goal: Maintain optimal nutritional status

Nursing Interventions	Rationale	Expected Outcomes
1. Assess the amount of food eaten.	1. This assessment will help determine nutrient intake.	• Responds positively to his favourite foods
2. Routinely weigh patient.	2. Weighing the patient on the same scale under similar conditions can help monitor changes in weight.	• Assumes responsibility for his oral hygiene • Notes increase in weight after improved appetite
3. Elicit patient's explanation of why he is unable to eat more.	3. His explanation may present easily corrected practices.	
4. Cater to his individual food preferences (eg, avoiding foods that are too spicy or too cold).	4. He will be more likely to consume larger servings if food is palatable and appealing.	
5. Recognize effect of medication or radiation therapy on appetite.	5. Many chemotherapeutic agents and radiation therapy promote anorexia.	

(continued)

Plan of Nursing Care
The Patient With Prostate Cancer (Continued)

Nursing Interventions	Rationale	Expected Outcomes
6. Inform patient that alterations in taste can occur.	6. Aging and the disease process can reduce taste sensitivity. In addition, smell and taste can be altered as a result of the body's absorption of byproducts of cellular destruction (brought on by malignancy and its treatment).	
7. Use measures to control nausea and vomiting: a. Administer prescribed antiemetics, around the clock if necessary. b. Provide oral hygiene after vomiting episodes. c. Provide rest periods after meals.	7. Prevention of nausea and vomiting can stimulate appetite.	
8. Provide frequent small meals and a comfortable and pleasant environment.	8. Smaller portions of food are less overwhelming to the patient.	
9. Assess patient's ability to obtain and prepare foods.	9. Disability or lack of social support can hinder the patient's ability to obtain and prepare foods.	

Nursing Diagnosis: Sexual dysfunction related to effects of therapy: chemotherapy, hormonal therapy, radiation therapy, surgery
Goal: Ability to resume/enjoy modified sexual functioning

Nursing Interventions	Rationale	Expected Outcomes
1. Determine from nursing history what effect patient's medical condition is having on his sexual functioning.	1. Usually decreased libido and, later, impotence may be experienced.	• Describes the reasons for changes in sexual functioning
2. Inform patient of the effects of prostate surgery, orchiectomy (when applicable), chemotherapy, irradiation, and hormonal therapy on sexual function.	2. Treatment modalities may alter sexual function, but each is evaluated separately with regard to its effect on a particular patient.	• Discusses with appropriate health care personnel alternative approaches and methods of sexual expression
3. Include his partner in developing understanding and in discovering alternative, satisfying close relations with each other.	3. Often the bonds between a couple are strengthened with new appreciation and support that had not been evident before the current illness.	• Includes partner in discussions related to changes in sexual function

Nursing Diagnosis: Pain related to progression of disease and treatment modalities
Goal: Relief of pain

Nursing Interventions	Rationale	Expected Outcomes
1. Evaluate nature of patient's pain, its location and intensity using pain rating scale.	1. Determining nature and causes of pain and its intensity helps to select proper relief modality and provide baseline for later comparison.	• Reports relief of pain
2. Avoid activities that aggravate or worsen pain.	2. Bumping the bed is an example of an action that can intensify the patient's pain.	• Expects exacerbations, reports their quality and intensity, and obtains relief
3. Because pain is usually related to bone metastasis, ensure that patient's bed has a bed board on a firm mattress. Also, protect the patient from falls/injuries.	3. This will provide added support and is more comfortable. Protecting the patient from injury protects him from additional pain.	• Uses pain relief strategies appropriately and effectively
4. Provide support for affected extremities.	4. More support, coupled with reduced movement of the part, helps in pain control.	• Identifies strategies to avoid complications of analgesic use
5. Prepare patient for radiation therapy if prescribed.	5. Radiation therapy may be effective in controlling pain.	
6. Administer analgesics or opioids at regularly scheduled intervals as prescribed.	6. Analgesics alter perception of pain and provide comfort. Regularly scheduled analgesics around the clock rather than PRN provide more consistent pain relief.	
7. Initiate bowel program to prevent constipation.	7. Opioid analgesics and inactivity contribute to constipation.	

(continued)

Plan of Nursing Care
The Patient With Prostate Cancer (*Continued*)

Nursing Interventions	Rationale	Expected Outcomes
Nursing Diagnosis: Impaired physical mobility and activity intolerance related to tissue hypoxia, malnutrition, and exhaustion and to spinal cord or nerve compression from metastases **Goal:** Improved physical mobility		
1. Assess for factors causing limited mobility (eg, pain, hypercalcemia, limited exercise tolerance). 2. Provide pain relief by administering prescribed medications. 3. Encourage use of assistive devices: cane, walker. 4. Involve significant others in helping patient with range-of-motion exercises, positioning, and walking. 5. Provide positive reinforcement for achievement of small gains. 6. Assess nutritional status.	1. This information offers clues to the cause; if possible, cause is treated. 2. Analgesics/opioids allow the patient to increase his activity more comfortably. 3. Support may offer the security needed to become mobile. 4. Assistance from partner or others encourages patient to repeat activities and achieve goals. 5. Encouragement stimulates improvement of performance. 6. See Nursing Diagnosis: Imbalanced nutrition: less than body requirements.	• Achieves improved physical mobility • Relates that short-term goals are encouraging him because they are attainable
Collaborative Problems: Hemorrhage, infection, bladder neck obstruction **Goal:** Absence of complications		

1. Alert the patient to changes that may occur (after discharge) and that need to be reported:
   a. Continued bloody urine; passing blood clots
   b. Pain; burning around the catheter
 	
   c. Frequency of urination
 	
   d. Diminished urinary output
 	
   e. Increasing loss of bladder control
	1. Certain changes signal beginning complications, which call for nursing and medical interventions.
	   a. Hematuria with or without blood clot formation may occur postoperatively.
	   b. Indwelling urinary catheters may be a source of infections.
	   c. Urinary frequency may be caused by urinary tract infections or by bladder neck obstruction, resulting in incomplete voiding.
	   d. Bladder neck obstruction decreases the amount of urine that is voided.
	   e. Urinary incontinence may be a result of urinary retention.
		• Experiences no bleeding or passage of blood clots
		 • Reports no pain around the catheter
		 • Experiences normal frequency of urination
		 • Reports normal urinary output
		 • Maintains bladder control

binding of dihydrotestosterone. As a result, the prostatic epithelium atrophies (decreases). This effect is accomplished either by **orchiectomy** (removal of the testes) or by the administration of medications.

Orchiectomy lowers plasma testosterone levels because about 93% of circulating testosterone is of testicular origin (7% is from the adrenal glands). As a result, the testicular stimulus required for continued prostatic growth is removed, resulting in prostatic atrophy. Although orchiectomy does not cause the side effects associated with other hormonal therapies, it carries a significant emotional impact.

Estrogen therapy, usually in the form of diethylstilbestrol (DES), has long been used to inhibit the gonadotropins responsible for testicular androgenic activity, thereby removing the androgenic hormone that promotes the growth of the malignancy. DES relieves symptoms of advanced prostate cancer, reduces tumour size, decreases pain from metastatic nodules, and pro-

motes well-being. However, DES significantly increases the risk for thromboembolism, pulmonary embolism, myocardial infarction, and stroke. Other side effects of estrogen therapy include impotence, decreased libido, difficulty in achieving orgasm, decreased sperm production, and gynecomastia (enlargement of breasts in men).

Newer hormonal therapies include the luteinizing hormone–releasing hormone (LH-RH) agonists (leuprolide [Lupron] and goserelin [Zoladex]) and antiandrogen agents, such as flutamide (Eulexin). LH-RH suppresses testicular androgen, whereas flutamide causes adrenal androgen suppression (Carroll et al., 2001). Cyproterone acetate is a synthetic progesterone derivative that provides effective, competitive inhibition of androgens at the target cells. In contrast to estrogen, the newer hormonal agents are associated with a lower incidence of cardiovascular side effects, gynecomastia, and decreased sexual function. Hot flushing can occur with orchiectomy or LH-RH agonist therapy because these agents increase hypothalamic activity, which stimulates the thermoregulatory centres of the body.

OTHER THERAPIES

Cryosurgery of the prostate is used to ablate prostate cancer in patients who could not physically tolerate surgery or in those with recurrent prostate cancer. Transperineal probes are inserted into the prostate under ultrasound guidance to freeze the tissue directly. Chemotherapy, such as doxorubicin, cisplatin, and cyclophosphamide, may also be used.

Keeping the urethral passage patent may require repeated transurethral resections. When this is impractical, catheter drainage is instituted by way of the suprapubic or transurethral route.

For men with advanced prostate cancer, palliative measures are indicated. Although cure is unlikely with advanced prostate cancer, many men survive for long intervals apparently free of metastatic disease. If prostate cancer metastasizes to the bones, these bone lesions can be very painful. Opioid and nonopioid medications are used to control the pain. In addition, external-beam radiation therapy can be delivered to skeletal lesions to relieve pain. Radiopharmaceuticals, such as strontium-89 and samarium-153, can also be intravenously injected to treat multiple sites of bone metastases (Cherney, 2000). Antiandrogen therapies are used in an effort to reduce the circulating androgens. If antiandrogen therapies are not effective, medications such as prednisone and mitoxantrone have been effective in reducing pain and improving quality of life. With advanced prostate cancer, blood transfusions are administered to maintain adequate hemoglobin levels when bone marrow is replaced by tumour.

THE PATIENT UNDERGOING PROSTATE SURGERY

Prostate surgery may be indicated for the patient with BPH or prostate cancer. The objectives before prostate surgery are to assess the patient's general health status and to establish optimal renal function. Prostate surgery should be performed before acute urinary retention develops and damages the upper urinary tract and collecting system or, in the case of prostate cancer, before cancer progresses.

Surgical Procedures

Several approaches can be used to remove the hypertrophied portion of the prostate gland: transurethral resection of the prostate (TURP), suprapubic prostatectomy, perineal prostatectomy, retropubic prostatectomy, and transurethral incision of the prostate (TUIP) (Table 49-3). In these approaches, the surgeon removes all hyperplastic tissue, leaving behind only the capsule of the prostate. The transurethral approaches (TURP, TUIP) are closed procedures; the other three are open procedures (ie, a surgical incision is required). The procedure chosen depends on the underlying disorder, the patient's age and physical status, and patient preference.

TRANSURETHRAL RESECTION OF THE PROSTATE

TURP, the most common procedure used, can be carried out through endoscopy. The surgical and optical instrument is introduced directly through the urethra to the prostate, which can then be viewed directly. The gland is removed in small chips with an electrical cutting loop (Fig. 49-4A). This procedure, which requires no incision, may be used for glands of varying size and is

ideal for patients who have small glands and those who are considered poor surgical risks.

This approach usually requires an overnight hospital stay. Strictures are more frequent, and repeated procedures may be necessary because the residual prostatic tissue can grow back. TURP rarely causes erectile dysfunction, but it may cause retrograde ejaculation because removing the prostatic tissue at the bladder neck can cause the seminal fluid to flow backward into the bladder rather than forward through the urethra during ejaculation.

SUPRAPUBIC PROSTATECTOMY

Suprapubic prostatectomy is one method of removing the gland through an abdominal incision. An incision is made into the bladder, and the prostate gland is removed from above (see Fig. 49-4B). Such an approach can be used for a gland of any size, and few complications occur, although blood loss may be greater than with the other methods. Another disadvantage is the need for an abdominal incision, with the concomitant hazards of any major abdominal surgical procedure.

PERINEAL PROSTATECTOMY

Perineal prostatectomy involves removing the gland through an incision in the perineum (see Fig. 49-4C). This approach is practical when other approaches are not possible and is useful for an open biopsy. Postoperatively, the wound may easily become contaminated because the incision is near the rectum. Incontinence, impotence, and rectal injury are more likely with this approach.

RETROPUBIC PROSTATECTOMY

Retropubic prostatectomy, another technique, is more common than the suprapubic approach. The surgeon makes a low abdominal incision and approaches the prostate gland between the pubic arch and the bladder without entering the bladder (see Fig. 49-4D). This procedure is suitable for large glands located high in the pelvis. Although blood loss can be better controlled and the surgical site is easier to visualize, infections can readily start in the retropubic space.

TRANSURETHRAL INCISION OF THE PROSTATE

Transurethral incision of the prostate (TUIP) is another procedure used in treating BPH. An instrument is passed through the urethra (see Fig. 49-4E). One or two incisions are made in the prostate and prostate capsule to reduce the prostate's pressure on the urethra and to reduce urethral constriction. TUIP is indicated when the prostate gland is small (30 g or less) and is an effective treatment for many cases of BPH. TUIP can be performed on an outpatient basis and has a lower complication rate than other invasive prostate procedures (Mebust, 1998).

LAPAROSCOPIC RADICAL PROSTATECTOMY

Laparoscopic radical prostatectomy is a method recently developed in France. Although not yet widespread in Canada, it is anticipated that this procedure will be widely used in place of more extensive surgery for patients with localized prostate cancer. The laparoscopic approach provides better visualization of the surgical site and surrounding areas. Preliminary data suggest that patients who undergo this procedure have less bleeding and reduced need for blood transfusion, a shorter hospital stay, less postoperative pain, a shorter duration of in-dwelling catheterization, and more rapid return to normal activity compared to open radical prostatectomy (Rassweiler, Sentker, Seemann et al., 2001). Further research is needed to assess long-term outcomes.

Table 49-3 • Comparing Surgical Approaches for Treatment of Prostate Disorders

The surgical approach of choice depends on (1) the size of the gland, (2) the severity of the obstruction, (3) the age of the patient, (4) the condition of patient, and (5) the presence of associated diseases.

SURGICAL APPROACH	ADVANTAGES	DISADVANTAGES	NURSING IMPLICATIONS
Transurethral Resection (TUR or TURP) (removal of prostatic tissue by instrument introduced through urethra)	Avoids abdominal incision Safer for surgical-risk patient Shorter hospitalization and recovery periods Lower morbidity rate Causes less pain	Requires highly skilled surgeon Recurrent obstruction, urethral trauma, and stricture may develop. Delayed bleeding may occur.	Monitor for hemorrhage. Observe for symptoms of urethral stricture (dysuria, straining, weak urinary stream).
Open Surgical Removal Suprapubic approach	Technically simple Offers wide area of exploration Permits exploration for cancerous lymph nodes Allows more complete removal of obstructing gland Permits treatment of associated bladder lesions	Requires surgical approach through the bladder Control of hemorrhage difficult Urine may leak around the suprapubic tube. Recovery may be prolonged and uncomfortable.	Monitor for indications of hemorrhage and shock. Give meticulous aseptic care to the area around suprapubic tube.
Perineal approach	Offers direct anatomic approach Permits gravity drainage Particularly effective for radical cancer therapy Allows hemostasis under direct vision Low mortality rate Lower incidence of shock Ideal for very old, frail, and poor-surgical-risk patient with large prostate	Higher postoperative incidence of impotence and urinary incontinence Possible damage to rectum and external sphincter Restricted operative field Greater potential for infection	Avoid using rectal tubes or thermometers and enemas after perineal surgery. Use drainage pads to absorb excess urinary drainage. Provide foam rubber ring for patient comfort in sitting. Anticipate urinary leakage around the wound for several days after the catheter is removed.
Retropubic approach	Avoids incision into the bladder Permits surgeon to see and control bleeders Shorter recovery period Less bladder sphincter damage	Cannot treat associated bladder disease Increased incidence of hemorrhage from prostatic venous plexus; pubic osteitis	Monitor for hemorrhage. Anticipate posturinary leakage for several days after removing the catheter.
Transurethral Incision (TUIP)	Results comparable to TURP Lower incidence of erectile dysfunction No bladder neck contracture Lower incidence of retrograde ejaculation	Requires highly skilled surgeon Recurrent obstruction and urethral trauma Delayed bleeding	Monitor for hemorrhage.

Complications

Complications depend on the type of prostatectomy performed and may include hemorrhage, clot formation, catheter obstruction, and sexual dysfunction. All prostatectomies carry a risk of impotence because of potential damage to the pudendal nerves. In most instances, sexual activity may be resumed in 6 to 8 weeks, the time required for the prostatic fossa to heal. During ejaculation, the seminal fluid goes into the bladder and is excreted with the urine. (The anatomic changes in the posterior urethra lead to retrograde ejaculation.) A vasectomy may be performed during surgery to prevent infection from spreading from the prostatic urethra through the vas and into the epididymis.

After total prostatectomy (usually for cancer), impotence almost always results. For the patient who does not want to give up sexual activity, options are available to produce erections sufficient for sexual intercourse: prosthetic penile implants, negative-pressure (vacuum) devices, and pharmacologic interventions (see earlier discussion in this chapter).

NURSING PROCESS: THE PATIENT UNDERGOING PROSTATECTOMY

Assessment

The nurse assesses how the underlying disorder (BPH or prostate cancer) has affected the patient's lifestyle. Has he been reasonably active for his age? What is his presenting urinary problem (described in his own words)? Has he experienced decreased force of urinary flow, decreased ability to initiate voiding, urgency, frequency, nocturia, dysuria, urinary retention, hematuria? Does the patient report associated problems, such as back pain, flank pain, and lower abdominal or suprapubic discomfort? If he reports such discomfort, possible causes include infection, retention, and renal colic. Has he experienced erectile dysfunction or changes in frequency or enjoyment of sexual activity?

The nurse obtains further information about the patient's family history of cancer and heart or kidney disease, including

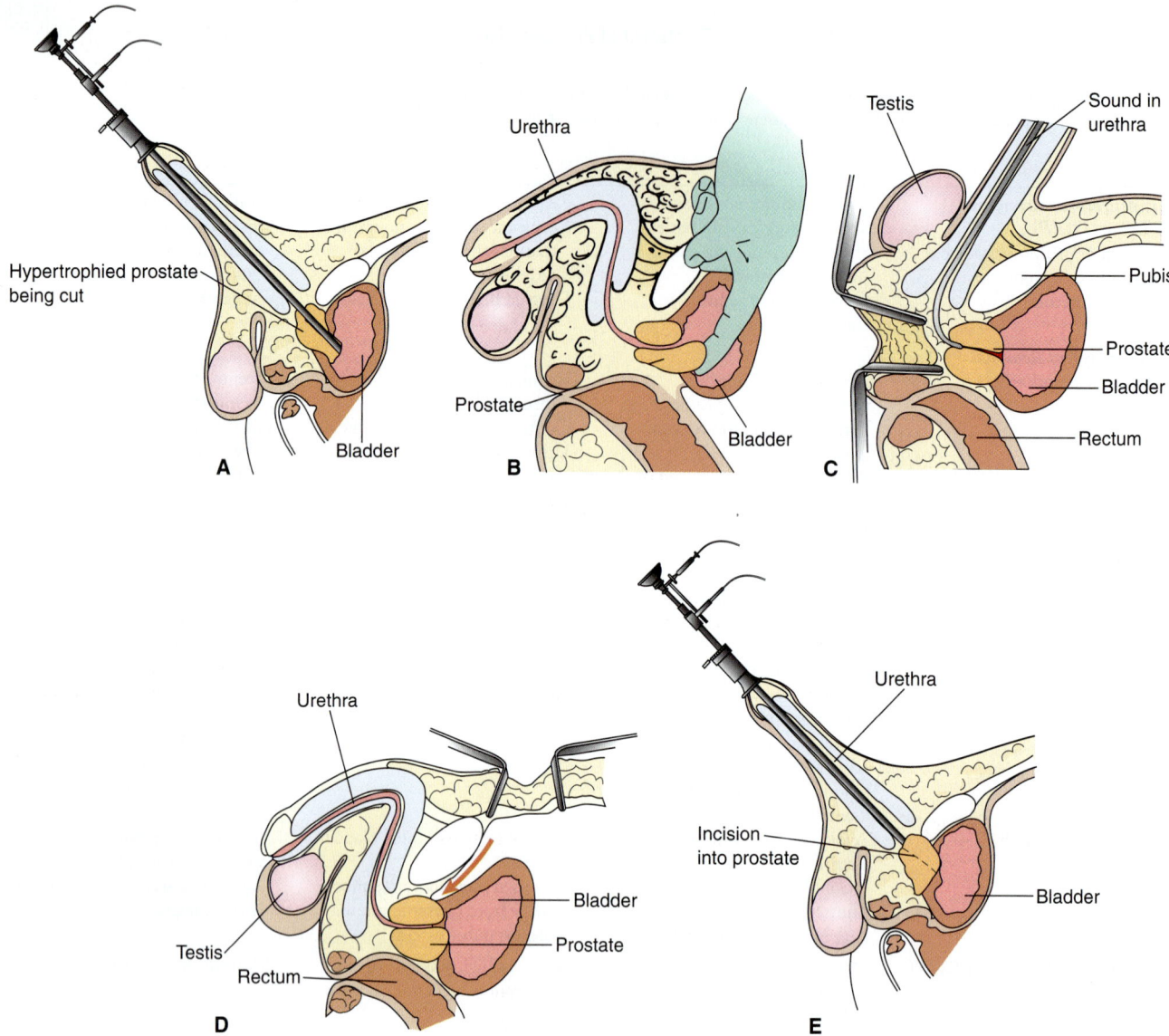

FIGURE 49-4 Prostate surgery procedures. (**A**) Transurethral resection (TUR). A loop of wire connected with a cutting current is rotated in the cystoscope to remove shavings of prostate at the bladder orifice. (**B**) Suprapubic prostatectomy. With an abdominal approach, the prostate is shelled out of its bed. (**C**) Perineal prostatectomy. Two retractors on the left spread the perineal incision to provide a view of the prostate. (**D**) Retropubic prostatectomy is performed through a low abdominal incision. Note two abdominal retractors and *arrow* pointing to the prostate gland. (**E**) Transurethral incision of prostate (TUIP) involves one or two incisions into the prostate to reduce pressure on the urethra.

hypertension. Has he lost weight? Does he appear pale? Can he raise himself out of bed and return to bed without assistance? Can he perform usual activities of daily living? This information will help in determining how soon he will return to normal activities after prostatectomy.

Diagnosis

Based on the assessment data, the patient's major nursing diagnoses may include the following.

PREOPERATIVE NURSING DIAGNOSES

- Anxiety about surgery and its outcome
- Acute pain related to bladder distention
- Deficient knowledge about factors related to the disorder and the treatment protocol

POSTOPERATIVE NURSING DIAGNOSES

- Acute pain related to the surgical incision, catheter placement, and bladder spasms
- Deficient knowledge about postoperative care and management

COLLABORATIVE PROBLEMS/POTENTIAL COMPLICATIONS

Based on the assessment data, the potential complications may include the following:

- Hemorrhage and shock
- Infection
- Deep vein thrombosis
- Catheter obstruction
- Sexual dysfunction

Planning and Goals

The major preoperative goals for the patient may include reduced anxiety and learning about his prostate disorder and the perioperative experience. The major postoperative goals may include maintenance of fluid volume balance, relief of pain and discomfort, ability to perform self-care activities, and absence of complications.

Preoperative Nursing Interventions

REDUCING ANXIETY

The patient is frequently admitted to the hospital on the morning of surgery. Because contact with the patient may be limited before surgery, the nurse must establish communication with the patient to assess his understanding of the diagnosis and of the planned surgical procedure. The nurse clarifies the nature of the surgery and expected postoperative outcomes. In addition, the nurse familiarizes the patient with the pre- and postoperative routines and initiates measures to reduce anxiety. Because the patient may be sensitive and embarrassed discussing problems related to the genitalia and sexuality, the nurse provides privacy and establishes a trusting and professional relationship. Guilt feelings often surface if the patient falsely assumes a cause-and-effect relationship between sexual practices and his current problems. He is encouraged to verbalize his feelings and concerns.

RELIEVING DISCOMFORT

If discomfort is present before the day of surgery, the patient is placed on bed rest, analgesic agents are administered, and measures to relieve anxiety are initiated. If the patient is hospitalized, the nurse monitors the patient's voiding patterns, watches for bladder distention, and assists with catheterization if indicated. An indwelling catheter is inserted if the patient has continuing urinary retention or if laboratory test results indicate azotemia (accumulation of nitrogenous waste products in the blood). The catheter can help to decompress the bladder gradually over several days, especially if the patient is elderly and hypertensive and has diminished renal function or an excessive amount of urinary retention that has existed for many weeks. For a few days after the bladder begins draining, the blood pressure may fluctuate and renal function may decline. If the patient cannot tolerate a urinary catheter, he is prepared for a cystostomy (see Chaps. 44 and 45).

PROVIDING INSTRUCTION

Before surgery, the nurse reviews with the patient the anatomy of the affected parts and their function in relation to the urinary and reproductive system, using diagrams and other teaching aids if indicated. This is often done either during the preadmission testing visit or in the urologist's office. The nurse explains what will take place as the patient is prepared for diagnostic tests and then for surgery (depending on the kind of prostatectomy planned). The nurse describes the type of incision, which varies with the type of surgical approach (directly over the bladder, low on the abdomen, or in the perineal area; in the case of a transurethral procedure, no incision will be made). The patient is informed about the type of urinary drainage system that is expected, the type of anesthesia, and the recovery room procedure. The amount of information given is based on the patient's needs and questions. Procedures expected during the immediate perioperative period are explained, questions are answered, and support is provided. In addition, the patient is instructed about postoperative use of medications for pain management.

PREPARING THE PATIENT

When the patient is scheduled for a prostatectomy, the preoperative preparation described in Chapter 18 is provided. Elastic compression stockings are applied before surgery and are particularly important for prevention of deep vein thrombosis if the patient is placed in a lithotomy position during surgery. An enema is usually administered at home the evening before surgery or the morning of surgery to prevent postoperative straining, which can induce bleeding.

Postoperative Nursing Interventions

MAINTAINING FLUID BALANCE

During the postoperative period, the patient is at risk for imbalanced fluid volume because of the irrigation of the surgical site during and after surgery. With irrigation of the urinary catheter to prevent its obstruction by blood clots, fluid may be absorbed through the open surgical site and retained, increasing the risk for excessive fluid retention, fluid imbalance, and water intoxication. The urine output and the amount of fluid used for irrigation must be closely monitored to determine if irrigation fluid is being retained and to ensure an adequate urine output. The patient also is monitored for electrolyte imbalances (ie, hyponatremia), rising blood pressure, confusion, and respiratory distress. The risk for fluid and electrolyte imbalance is increased in elderly patients with preexisting cardiovascular or respiratory disease. These signs and symptoms are documented and reported to the surgeon.

RELIEVING PAIN

After a prostatectomy, the patient is assisted to sit and dangle his legs over the side of the bed on the day of surgery. The next morning, he is assisted to ambulate. If pain occurs, the cause and location are determined. It may be related to the incision or may be the result of excoriation of the skin at the catheter site. It may be in the flank area, indicating a kidney problem, or it may be due to bladder spasms. Bladder irritability can initiate bleeding and result in clot formation, leading to urinary retention.

Patients experiencing bladder spasms may note an urgency to void, a feeling of pressure or fullness in the bladder, and bleeding from the urethra around the catheter. Medications that relax the smooth muscles can help to ease the spasms, which can be intermittent and severe; these medications include flavoxate (Urispas) and oxybutynin (Ditropan). Warm compresses to the pubis or sitz baths may also relieve the spasms.

The nurse monitors the drainage tubing and irrigates the system as prescribed to relieve any obstruction that may cause discomfort. Usually, the catheter is irrigated with 50 mL of irrigating fluid at a time. It is important to make sure that the same amount is recovered in the drainage receptacle. Securing the catheter drainage tubing to the leg or abdomen can help to decrease tension on the catheter and prevent bladder irritation. Discomfort may be caused by dressings that are too snug, saturated with drainage, or improperly placed. Analgesic agents are administered as prescribed.

When ambulatory, the patient is encouraged to walk but not to sit for prolonged periods because this increases intra-abdominal pressure and the possibility of discomfort and bleeding. Prune juice and stool softeners are provided to ease bowel movements and to prevent excessive straining. An enema, if prescribed, is administered with caution to avoid rectal perforation.

MONITORING AND MANAGING POTENTIAL COMPLICATIONS

After prostatectomy, the patient is monitored for major complications such as hemorrhage, infection, deep vein thrombosis, catheter obstruction, and sexual dysfunction.

Hemorrhage

The immediate dangers after a prostatectomy are bleeding and hemorrhagic shock. This risk is increased with BPH because a hyperplastic prostate gland is very vascular. Bleeding may occur from the prostatic bed. Bleeding may also result in the formation of clots, which then obstruct urine flow. The drainage normally begins as reddish-pink and then clears to a light pink within 24 hours after surgery. Bright-red bleeding with increased viscosity and numerous clots usually indicates arterial bleeding. Venous blood appears darker and less viscous. Arterial hemorrhage usually requires surgical intervention (eg, suturing of bleeders or transurethral coagulation of bleeding vessels), whereas venous bleeding may be controlled by applying prescribed traction to the catheter so that the balloon holding the catheter in place applies pressure to the prostatic fossa. The surgeon applies traction by securely taping the catheter to the patient's thigh.

Nursing management includes strategies to stop the bleeding and to prevent or reverse hemorrhagic shock. If blood loss is extensive, fluids and blood component therapy may be administered. If hemorrhagic shock occurs, treatments described in Chapter 15 are initiated.

Nursing interventions include close monitoring of vital signs; administering medications, intravenous fluids, and blood component therapy as prescribed; maintaining an accurate record of intake and output; and careful monitoring of drainage to ensure adequate urine flow and patency of the drainage system. The patient who experiences hemorrhage and his family are often anxious and benefit from explanations and reassurance about the event and the procedures that are performed.

Infection

After perineal prostatectomy, the surgeon usually changes the dressing on the first postoperative day. Further dressing changes may become the nurse's responsibility. Careful aseptic technique is used because the possibility for infection is great. Dressings can be held in place by a double-tailed, T-binder bandage or a padded athletic supporter. The tails cross over the incision to give double thickness, and then each tail is drawn up on either side of the scrotum to the waistline and fastened.

Rectal thermometers, rectal tubes, and enemas are avoided because of the risk for injury to and bleeding in the prostatic fossa. After the perineal sutures are removed, the perineum is cleansed as indicated. A heat lamp may be directed to the perineal area to promote healing. The scrotum is protected with a towel while the heat lamp is in use. Sitz baths are also used to promote healing.

Urinary tract infections and epididymitis are possible complications after prostatectomy. The patient is assessed for their occurrence; if they occur, the nurse administers antibiotics as prescribed.

Because the risk for infection continues after discharge from the hospital, the patient and family need to be instructed to monitor for signs and symptoms of infection (fever, chills, sweats, myalgias, dysuria, urinary frequency, and urgency). The patient and family are instructed to contact the urologist if these symptoms occur.

Deep Vein Thrombosis

Because patients undergoing prostatectomy have a high incidence of deep vein thrombosis (DVT) and pulmonary embolism, the physician may prescribe prophylactic (preventive) low-dose heparin

therapy. The nurse assesses the patient frequently after surgery for manifestations of DVT and applies elastic compression stockings to reduce the risk for DVT and pulmonary embolism. Nursing and medical management of DVT and pulmonary embolism are detailed in Chapters 31 and 23, respectively. The patient who is receiving heparin must be closely monitored for excessive bleeding.

Obstructed Catheter

After a TUR, the catheter must drain well; an obstructed catheter produces distention of the prostatic capsule and resultant hemorrhage. Furosemide (Lasix) may be prescribed to promote urination and initiate postoperative diuresis, thereby helping to keep the catheter patent.

The nurse observes the lower abdomen to ensure that the catheter has not become blocked. An overdistended bladder presents a distinct, rounded swelling above the pubis.

The drainage bag, dressings, and incisional site are examined for bleeding. The colour of the urine is noted and documented; a change in colour from pink to amber indicates reduced bleeding. Blood pressure, pulse, and respirations are monitored and compared with baseline preoperative vital signs to detect hypotension. The nurse also observes the patient for restlessness, cold sweats, pallor, any drop in blood pressure, and an increasing pulse rate.

Drainage of the bladder may be accomplished by gravity through a closed sterile drainage system. A three-way drainage system is useful in irrigating the bladder and preventing clot formation (Fig. 49-5). Continuous irrigation may be used with TUR. Some urologists leave an indwelling catheter attached to a dependent drainage system. Gentle irrigation of the catheter may be prescribed to remove any obstructing clots.

If the patient complains of pain, the tubing is examined. The drainage system is irrigated, if indicated and prescribed, to clear any obstruction. Usually, the catheter is irrigated with 50 mL of irrigating fluid at a time. The amount of fluid recovered in the

FIGURE 49-5 A three-way system for bladder irrigation.

drainage bag must equal the amount of fluid injected. Over-distention of the bladder is avoided because it can induce secondary hemorrhage by stretching the coagulated blood vessels in the prostatic capsule.

The nurse maintains an intake and output record, including the amount of fluid used for irrigation.

The drainage tube (not the catheter) is taped to the shaved inner thigh to prevent traction on the bladder. If a cystostomy catheter is in place, it is taped to the abdomen. The nurse explains the purpose of the catheter to the patient and assures him that the urge to void results from the presence of the catheter and from bladder spasms. He is cautioned not to pull on the catheter because this causes bleeding and subsequent catheter blockage, which leads to urinary retention.

Complications With Catheter Removal

After the catheter is removed (usually when the urine appears clear), urine may leak around the wound for several days in patients who have undergone perineal, suprapubic, and retropubic surgery. The cystostomy tube may be removed before or after the urethral catheter is removed. Some urinary incontinence may occur after catheter removal, and the patient is informed that this is likely to subside in time.

Sexual Dysfunction

Depending on the type of surgery, the patient may experience sexual dysfunction related to erectile dysfunction, decreased libido, and fatigue. These issues may become a concern of the patient soon after surgery or in the weeks to months during rehabilitation. Erectile dysfunction may occur following prostate surgery. Several options to restore erectile function are discussed with the patient by the surgeon or urologist. These options may include medications, surgically placed implants, or negative-pressure devices. A decrease in libido may also occur following surgery and is usually related to the impact of the surgery on the man's body. Reassurance that the usual level of libido will return following recuperation from surgery is often helpful to the patient and his partner. The patient may also experience fatigue during rehabilitation from surgery. This fatigue may also decrease his libido and alter his enjoyment of usual activities.

Nursing interventions include assessing for the presence of sexual dysfunction following surgery. Providing a private and confidential environment to discuss issues of sexuality is important. The emotional challenges of prostate surgery and its consequences need to be carefully explored with the patient and his partner. Providing the opportunity to discuss these issues can be very beneficial to the patient. For patients who demonstrate significant problems adjusting to their sexual dysfunction, a referral to a sex therapist may be indicated.

PROMOTING HOME AND COMMUNITY-BASED CARE

Teaching Patients Self-Care

The patient undergoing prostatectomy may be discharged within several days. The length of the hospital stay depends on the type of prostatectomy performed. Patients undergoing a perineal prostatectomy are hospitalized for 3 to 5 days. If a retropubic or suprapubic prostatectomy is performed, the hospital stay is 5 to 7 days. The patient and family require instructions about how to manage the drainage system, how to assess for complications, and how to promote recovery. Verbal and written instructions are provided about the need to maintain the drainage system and to monitor urinary output, about wound care, and about strategies to prevent complications, such as infection, bleeding, and thrombosis. They are informed about signs and symptoms that should be reported to the physician (eg, blood in urine, decreased urine output, fever, change in wound drainage, calf tenderness).

As the patient recovers and drainage tubes are removed, he may become discouraged and depressed because he cannot regain bladder control immediately. Moreover, urinary frequency and burning may occur after the catheter is removed. Teaching the following exercises, known as pelvic floor muscle exercises, may help the patient regain urinary control:

- Tighten the pelvic floor by tensing the muscles around the rectum as if trying to stop from passing gas. The buttocks, thighs, and stomach should stay relaxed. If the penis twitches and contracts inwards slightly, the patient is tightening the correct muscles.
- Squeeze firmly for 5 to 10 seconds per contraction.
- Try to perform 10 to 12 contractions two to three times a day, relaxing the muscle for 10 to 20 seconds between each contraction (Moore & Vandall-Walker, 2000).

Pelvic floor muscle exercises should continue until the patient gains full urinary control. The patient is instructed to urinate as soon as he feels the first urge to do so. It is important for the patient to know that regaining urinary control is a gradual process; he may continue to "dribble" after being discharged from the hospital, but the dribbling should gradually diminish (within up to 1 year). Lining underwear with absorbent pads can help to minimize embarrassing stains on clothing. The urine may be cloudy for several weeks after surgery but should clear as the prostate area heals.

While the prostatic fossa heals (6 to 8 weeks), the patient should avoid activities that produce Valsalva effects (straining at stool, heavy lifting) because this increases venous pressure and may produce hematuria. He should avoid long motor trips and strenuous exercise, which increase the tendency to bleed. He should also know that spicy foods, alcohol, and coffee may cause bladder discomfort. The patient is cautioned to drink enough fluids to avoid dehydration, which increases the tendency for a blood clot to form and obstruct the flow of urine. Signs of complications, such as bleeding, passage of blood clots, a decrease in the urinary stream, urinary retention, or urinary tract infection symptoms, should be reported to the physician (Chart 49-3).

Through research, nurses are gaining more knowledge about the aftermath of prostatectomy, including early postoperative concerns (Moore & Estey, 1999), after effects (Moore, 2000), patient evaluation of a discharge program (Davison, Moore, MacMillan, et al., 2004), incontinence and management (Hunter, Moore, Cody, et al., 2005; McCallum, Moore & Griffiths, 2001; Moore, 1999), and testing of the Incontinence Impact Questionnaire (Moore & Jensen, 2000).

Continuing Care

Referral for home care may be indicated if the patient is elderly or has other health problems, if the patient and family cannot provide care in the home, or if the patient lives alone without available supports. The home care nurse assesses the patient's physical status (cardiovascular and respiratory status, fluid and nutritional status, patency of the urinary drainage system, wound and nutritional status) and provides catheter and wound care, if indicated. The nurse reinforces previous teaching and assesses the ability of the patient and family to manage required care. The home care nurse encourages the patient to ambulate and to carry out pelvic floor muscle exercises as prescribed. The patient may need to be reminded that return of bladder control may take time.

The patient is reminded about the importance of participating in routine health screening and other health promotion activities. If the prostatectomy was performed to treat prostate cancer, the patient and family are also instructed about the importance of follow-up and monitoring with the physician.

> **Chart 49-3**
> **Home Care Checklist • Postprostatectomy Care**
>
> *At the completion of the home care instruction, the patient or caregiver will be able to:*
>
> | | Patient | Caregiver |
> | --- | :---: | :---: |
> | • Demonstrate appropriate measures to control postoperative pain and discomfort | ✓ | ✓ |
> | • Demonstrate appropriate care of urinary catheter and collection receptacle | ✓ | ✓ |
> | • Demonstrate appropriate wound care | ✓ | ✓ |
> | • Demonstrate performance of pelvic floor muscle exercises to facilitate bladder control | ✓ | |
> | • Demonstrate increased activity and ambulation | ✓ | |
> | • Identify activities to avoid, such as lifting heavy objects | ✓ | ✓ |
> | • Identify signs and symptoms of complications that should be reported to surgeon | ✓ | ✓ |

Evaluation

EXPECTED PREOPERATIVE PATIENT OUTCOMES

Expected preoperative patient outcomes may include:

1. Demonstrates reduced anxiety
2. States that pain and discomfort are decreased
3. Relates understanding of the surgical procedure and postoperative course and practices pelvic floor muscle exercises and other techniques useful in facilitating bladder control

EXPECTED POSTOPERATIVE PATIENT OUTCOMES

Expected postoperative patient outcomes may include:

1. Relates relief of discomfort
2. Exhibits fluid and electrolyte balance
   a. Irrigation fluid and urinary output are within parameters determined by surgeon.
   b. Experiences no signs or symptoms of fluid retention
3. Participates in self-care measures
   a. Increases activity and ambulation daily
   b. Produces urine output within normal ranges and consistent with intake
   c. Performs pelvic floor muscle exercises and interrupts urinary stream to promote bladder control
   d. Avoids straining and lifting heavy objects
4. Is free of complications
   a. Maintains vital signs within normal limits
   b. Exhibits wound healing, without signs of inflammation or hemorrhage
   c. Maintains acceptable level of urinary elimination
   d. Maintains optimal drainage of catheter and other drainage tubes
   e. Reports understanding of changes in sexual function

Conditions Affecting the Testes and Adjacent Structures

UNDESCENDED TESTIS (CRYPTORCHIDISM)

Cryptorchidism is a congenital condition characterized by failure of one or both of the testes to descend into the scrotum. One or both testes may be absent. The testis may be located in the abdominal cavity or inguinal canal. If the testis does not descend as the boy matures, a surgical procedure known as orchiopexy is performed to position it properly. An incision is made over the inguinal canal, and the testis is brought down and anchored in the scrotum.

ORCHITIS

Orchitis is an inflammation of the testes (testicular congestion) caused by pyogenic, viral, spirochetal, parasitic, traumatic, chemical, or unknown factors. Mumps is one such factor. Mumps vaccination is recommended for postpubertal men who have not been infected. When postpubertal men contract mumps, about one in five develops some form of orchitis 4 to 7 days after the jaw and neck swell. The testis may show some atrophy. In the past, sterility and impotence often resulted. Today, a man who has never had mumps and who is exposed to the disease receives gamma-globulin immediately; the disease is likely to be less severe, with minimal or no complications.

Medical Management

If the cause of orchitis is bacterial, viral, or fungal, therapy is directed at the specific infecting organism. Rest, elevation of the scrotum, ice packs to reduce scrotal edema, antibiotics, analgesic agents, and anti-inflammatory medications are recommended.

EPIDIDYMITIS

Epididymitis is an infection of the epididymis that usually descends from an infected prostate or urinary tract. It may also develop as a complication of gonorrhea. In men younger than age 35, the major cause of epididymitis is *Chlamydia trachomatis*. The infection passes upward through the urethra and the ejaculatory duct and then along the vas deferens to the epididymis.

The patient complains of unilateral pain and soreness in the inguinal canal along the course of the vas deferens and then develops pain and swelling in the scrotum and the groin. The epididymis becomes swollen and extremely painful; the patient's temperature is elevated. The urine may contain pus (pyuria) and bacteria (bacteriuria), and the patient may experience chills and fever.

Medical Management

If the patient is seen within the first 24 hours after onset of pain, the spermatic cord may be infiltrated with a local anesthetic agent to relieve pain. If the epididymitis is from a chlamydial infection, the patient and his sexual partner must be treated with antibiotics. The patient is observed for abscess formation as well. If no improvement occurs within 2 weeks, an underlying testicular tumour should be considered. An epididymectomy (excision of the epididymis from the testis) may be performed for patients with recurrent, incapacitating episodes of epididymitis or for those with chronic, painful conditions. With long-term epididymitis, the passage of sperm may be obstructed. If the obstruction is bilateral, infertility may result.

Nursing Management

The patient is placed on bed rest, and the scrotum is elevated with a scrotal bridge or folded towel to prevent traction on the spermatic cord and to promote venous drainage and relieve pain. Antimicrobial agents are administered as prescribed until the acute inflammation subsides. Intermittent cold compresses to the scrotum may help ease the pain. Later, local heat or sitz baths may help resolve the inflammation. Analgesic medications are administered for pain relief as prescribed.

The nurse instructs the patient to avoid straining, lifting, and sexual stimulation until the infection is under control. He should continue taking analgesic agents and antibiotics as prescribed and using ice packs if necessary to relieve discomfort. He needs to know that it may take 4 weeks or longer for the epididymis to return to normal.

TESTICULAR CANCER

Testicular cancer is the most common cancer in men 15 to 35 years of age. Although testicular cancer occurs most often between the ages of 15 and 40, it can occur in males of any age. It is a highly treatable and usually curable form of cancer. Approximately 850 Canadian men will be diagnosed with testicular cancer in 2005 and 30 will die from it (Canadian Cancer Society/National Cancer Institute of Canada, 2005).

The testicles contain several types of cells, each of which may develop into one or more types of cancer. The type of cancer determines the appropriate treatment and affects the prognosis. Testicular cancers are classified as germinal or nongerminal (stromal); secondary testicular cancers may also occur.

Germinal Tumours

Over 90% of all cancers of the testicle are germinal; geminal tumours may be further classified as seminomas or nonseminomas. About half of all geminal tumours are seminomas, or tumours that develop from the sperm-producing cells of the testes. Nonseminoma germinal cell tumours tend to develop earlier in life than seminomas, usually occurring in men in their 20s. Examples of nonseminomas include teratocarcinomas, choriocarcinomas, yolk sac carcinomas, and embryonal carcinomas. Seminomas tend to remain localized, whereas nonseminomatous tumours grow quickly.

Nongerminal Tumours

Testicular cancer may also develop in the supportive and hormone-producing tissues, or stroma, of the testicles. These tumours account for about 4% of testicular tumours in adults and 20% of testicular tumours in children. The two main types of stromal tumours are Leydig cell tumours and Sertoli cell tumours. Although these tumours infrequently spread beyond the testicle, a small number of these tumours metastasize and tend to be resistant to chemotherapy and radiation therapy.

Secondary Testicular Tumours

Secondary testicular tumours are those that have metastasized to the testicle from other organs. Lymphoma is the most common cause of secondary testicular cancer. Cancers may also spread to the testicles from the prostate gland, lung, skin (melanoma), kidney, and other organs. The prognosis for these cancers is usually poor because these cancers generally also spread to other organs. Treatment depends on the specific type of cancer (American Cancer Society, 2002).

Risk Factors

The risk for testicular cancer is several times greater in men with any type of undescended testis than in the general population (Bosl, Bajorin, Scheinfeld et al., 2001). Risk factors include a family history of testicular cancer and cancer of one testicle, which increases the risk for the other testicle. Race and ethnicity have been identified as risk factors. For example, in the U.S., Caucasian American men have a five times greater risk than that of African American men and more than double the risk of Asian American men. Occupational hazards, including exposure to chemicals encountered in mining, oil and gas production, and leather processing, have been suggested as possible risk factors. Prenatal exposure to DES may also be a risk factor, but evidence is not strong (American Cancer Society, 2002). Vasectomy, once considered a possible risk factor, has been shown in recent studies not to be a risk factor (Cox, Sneyd, Paul et al., 2002).

Clinical Manifestations

The symptoms appear gradually, with a mass or lump on the testicle and generally painless enlargement of the testis. The patient may complain of heaviness in the scrotum, inguinal area, or lower abdomen. Backache (from retroperitoneal node extension), abdominal pain, weight loss, and general weakness may result from metastasis. Enlargement of the testis without pain is a significant diagnostic finding. Testicular tumours tend to metastasize early, spreading from the testis to the lymph nodes in the retroperitoneum and to the lungs.

Assessment and Diagnostic Findings

Monthly testicular self-examinations (TSEs) are effective in detecting testicular cancer (Chart 49-4). Teaching men of all ages to perform TSE is an important health promotion intervention for early detection of testicular cancer. Since testicular cancer occurs most often in young adults, testicular self-examination should begin during adolescence.

Human chorionic gonadotropin and alpha-fetoprotein are tumour markers that may be elevated in patients with testicular cancer. (Tumour markers are substances synthesized by the tumour cells and released into the circulation in abnormal amounts.) Tumour marker levels in the blood are used for diagnosis, staging, and monitoring the response to treatment. Other diagnostic tests include intravenous urography to detect any ureteral deviation caused by a tumour mass; lymphangiography to assess the extent of tumour spread to the lymphatic system; ultrasound to determine the presence and size of the testicular mass; and CT scan of the chest, abdomen, and pelvis to determine the extent of the disease in the lungs, retroperitoneum, and pelvis. Microscopic analysis of tissue is the only definitive way to determine if

Chart 49-4 • PATIENT EDUCATION
Testicular Self-Examination

Testicular self-examination (TSE) is to be performed once a month. The test is neither difficult nor time-consuming. A convenient time is usually after a warm bath or shower when the scrotum is more relaxed.

1. Use both hands to palpate the testis. The normal testicle is smooth and uniform in consistency.
2. With the index and middle fingers under the testis and the thumb on top, roll the testis gently in a horizontal plane between the thumb and fingers (**A**).
3. Feel for any evidence of a small lump or abnormality.
4. Follow the same procedure and palpate upward along the testis (**B**).

5. Locate and palpate the epididymis (**C**), a cord-like structure on the top and back of the testicle that stores and transports sperm. Also locate and palpate the spermatic cord.
6. Repeat the examination for the other testis, epididymis, and spermatic cord. It is normal to find that one testis is larger than the other.
7. If you find any evidence of a small, pea-like lump or if the testis is swollen (possibly from an infection or tumour), consult your physician.

cancer is present but is usually performed at the time of surgery rather than as a part of the diagnostic workup to reduce the risk of promoting spread of the cancer (American Cancer Society, 2000).

Medical Management

Testicular cancer is one of the most curable solid tumours. The goals of management are to eradicate the disease and achieve a cure. Treatment selection is based on the cell type and the anatomic extent of the disease. The testis is removed by orchiectomy through an inguinal incision with a high ligation of the spermatic cord. A gel-filled prosthesis can be implanted. After unilateral orchiectomy for testicular cancer, most patients experience no impairment of endocrine function. Other patients, however, have decreased hormonal levels, suggesting that the unaffected testis is not functioning at normal levels. Retroperitoneal lymph node dissection to prevent lymphatic spread of the cancer may be performed after orchiectomy. Although libido and orgasm are usually unimpaired after retroperitoneal lymph node

dissection, the patient may develop ejaculatory dysfunction with resultant infertility. Thus, sperm banking before surgery may be considered (Agarwa, 2000; Zapzalka et al., 1999).

Postoperative irradiation of the lymph nodes from the diaphragm to the iliac region is used in treating seminomas. Radiation is delivered only to the affected side; the other testis is shielded from radiation to preserve fertility. Radiation is also used for patients whose disease does not respond to chemotherapy or for whom lymph node surgery is not recommended. Lymphangiograms and CT scans are used to determine spread of the disease to the lymph nodes.

Testicular carcinomas are highly responsive to chemotherapy. (Bosl et al., 2001) Chemotherapy with cisplatin-based regimens results in a high percentage of complete remissions. Good results may be obtained by combining different types of treatment, including surgery, radiation therapy, and chemotherapy. Even with disseminated testicular cancer, the prognosis is favourable, and the disease is probably curable because of advances in diagnosis and treatment.

A patient with a history of one testicular tumour has a greater chance of developing subsequent tumours. Follow-up studies include chest x-rays, excretory urography, radioimmunoassay of human chorionic gonadotropins and alpha-fetoprotein levels, and examination of lymph nodes to detect recurrent malignancy.

Long-term side effects associated with treatments for testicular cancer include kidney damage, hearing problems, gonadal damage, neurological changes, and rarely secondary cancers (Kollmannsberger, Kuzcyk, Mayer et al., 1999). Research on treatment regimens with less toxicity and the use of cytoprotectants is ongoing.

Nursing Management

Nursing management includes assessment of the patient's physical and psychological status and monitoring the patient for response to and possible effects of surgery, chemotherapy, and radiation therapy (see Chap. 16). Pre- and postoperative care is described in Chapters 18 and 19, respectively. In addition, because the patient may have difficulty coping with his condition, issues related to body image and sexuality are addressed. He needs encouragement to maintain a positive attitude during what may be a long course of therapy. He also needs to know that radiation therapy will not necessarily prevent him from fathering children, nor does unilateral excision of a testis necessarily decrease virility. The nurse reminds the patient about the importance of performing TSE and keeping follow-up appointments with the physician. The patient is also encouraged to participate in health promotion and health screening activities.

HYDROCELE

A **hydrocele** is a collection of fluid, generally in the tunica vaginalis of the testis, although it may also collect within the spermatic cord. The tunica vaginalis becomes widely distended with fluid. Hydrocele can be differentiated from a hernia by transillumination; a hydrocele transmits light, whereas a hernia does not. Hydrocele may be acute or chronic. Acute hydrocele may occur in association with acute infectious diseases of the epididymis or as a result of local injury or systemic infectious diseases, such as mumps. The cause of chronic hydrocele is unknown.

Usually, therapy is not required. Treatment is necessary only if the hydrocele becomes tense and compromises testicular circulation or if the scrotal mass becomes large, uncomfortable, or embarrassing. In the surgical treatment of hydrocele, an incision is made through the wall of the scrotum down to the distended tunica vaginalis. The sac is resected or, after being opened, is sutured together to collapse the wall. Postoperatively, the patient wears an athletic supporter for comfort and support. The major complication is hematoma in the loose scrotal tissues.

VARICOCELE

A **varicocele** is an abnormal dilation of the veins of the pampiniform venous plexus in the scrotum (the network of veins from the testis and the epididymis that constitute part of the spermatic cord). Varicoceles usually occur in the veins on the upper portion of the left testicle in adults. In some men, a varicocele has been associated with infertility. Few, if any, subjective symptoms may be produced by the enlarged spermatic vein, and no treatment is required unless fertility is a concern. Symptomatic varicocele (pain, tenderness, and discomfort in the inguinal region) is corrected surgically by ligating the external spermatic vein at the inguinal area. An ice pack may be applied to the scrotum for the first few hours after surgery to relieve edema. The patient then wears a scrotal supporter.

VASECTOMY

Vasectomy, or male sterilization, is the ligation and transection of part of the vas deferens, with or without removal of a segment of the vas deferens. To prevent the passage of the sperm from the testes, the vas deferens is exposed through a surgical opening in the scrotum or a puncture using a sharp, curved hemostat (Fig. 49-6). The severed ends are occluded with ligatures or clips, or the lumen of each vas deferens is sealed by cautery. The spermatozoa, which are manufactured in the testes, cannot travel up the vas deferens after this surgery.

Because seminal fluid is manufactured predominantly in the seminal vesicles and prostate gland, which are unaffected by vasectomy, no noticeable decrease occurs in the amount of ejaculate even though it contains no spermatozoa. Because the sperm cells have no exit, they are resorbed into the body. This procedure has no effect on sexual potency, erection, ejaculation, or production of male hormones and provides no protection against sexually transmitted diseases.

Couples who were worried about pregnancy resulting from contraceptive failure often report a decrease in concern and an increase in spontaneous sexual arousal after vasectomy. Concise and factual preoperative explanations may minimize or relieve the patient's concerns related to masculinity. Although a relationship between vasectomy and autoimmune disorders and prostatic cancer has been suggested, there is no clinical evidence of either.

The patient is advised that he will be sterile but that potency will not be altered after a bilateral vasectomy. As with any surgical procedure, a surgical consent form must be signed. On rare occasions, a spontaneous reanastomosis of the vas deferens occurs, making it possible to impregnate a partner.

Complications of vasectomy include scrotal ecchymoses and swelling, superficial wound infection, vasitis (inflammation of the vas deferens), epididymitis or epididymo-orchitis, hematomas, and spermatic granuloma. A spermatic granuloma is an inflammatory response to the collection of sperm leaking into the scrotum from the severed end of the proximal vas deferens. This can initiate recanalization of the vas deferens, making pregnancy possible.

FIGURE 49-6 A vasectomy is a resection of the vas deferens to prevent passage of sperm from the testes to the urethra during ejaculation. (**A**) An incision or small puncture is made to expose the vas deferens. (**B**) The vas deferens is isolated and severed. (**C**) The severed ends are occluded with ligatures or clips, or the lumen of each vas is sealed by electrocautery and the incision is sutured closed. (Suturing may not be required if a puncture approach has been used.)

Nursing Management

Ice bags are applied intermittently to the scrotum for several hours after surgery to reduce swelling and to relieve discomfort. The nurse advises the patient to wear cotton, Jockey-type briefs for added comfort and support. He may become greatly concerned about the discolouration of the scrotal skin and superficial swelling. These are temporary conditions that occur frequently after vasectomy and may be relieved by sitz baths.

Sexual intercourse may be resumed as desired, although fertility remains for a varying time after vasectomy until the spermatozoa stored distal to the severed vas deferens have been evacuated. Other methods of contraception should be used until infertility is confirmed by an examination of ejaculate. Some physicians examine a specimen 4 weeks after the vasectomy to determine sterility; others examine two consecutive specimens 1 month apart; and still others consider a patient sterile after 36 ejaculations.

Vasovasostomy (Sterilization Reversal)

Microsurgical techniques are used to reverse a vasectomy (vasovasostomy), thus restoring patency to the vas deferens. Many men have sperm in their ejaculate after a reversal, and 40% to 75% can impregnate a partner.

Banking Sperm

Storing fertile semen in a sperm bank before a vasectomy is an option for men who face an unforeseen life event that may cause them to want to father a child at a later time. In addition, if a man is about to undergo a procedure or treatment (eg, radiation therapy to the pelvis or chemotherapy) that may affect his fertility, sperm banking may be considered. This procedure usually requires several visits to the facility where the sperm is stored under hypothermic conditions. The semen is produced by masturbation and collected in a sterile container for storage.

Conditions Affecting the Penis

HYPOSPADIAS AND EPISPADIAS

Hypospadias and epispadias are congenital anomalies of the urethral opening. In hypospadias, the urethral opening is a groove on the underside of the penis. In epispadias, the urethral opening is on the dorsum. These anatomic abnormalities may be repaired by various types of plastic surgery, usually when the boy is very young.

PHIMOSIS

Phimosis, a condition in which the foreskin is constricted so that it cannot be retracted over the glans, can occur congenitally or from inflammation and edema. With the trend away from routine circumcision of newborns, early instruction should be given about cleansing the prepuce. If the preputial area is not cleaned, normal secretions accumulate, causing inflammation (balanitis), which can lead to adhesions and fibrosis. The thickened secretions become encrusted with urinary salts and calcify, forming calculi in the prepuce. In elderly men, penile carcinoma may develop. Phimosis is corrected by circumcision (see later discussion).

Paraphimosis is a condition in which the foreskin is retracted behind the glans and, because of narrowness and subsequent edema, cannot be returned to its usual position (covering the glans). Paraphimosis is treated by firmly compressing the glans to reduce its size and then pushing the glans back while simultaneously moving the prepuce forward (manual reduction). Circumcision is usually indicated after the inflammation and edema subside.

CANCER OF THE PENIS

Penile cancer occurs in men older than age 60 and represents about 0.5% of malignancies in men in the United States (Stadler, Vogelzang, Elwell & Jones, 2000). In some countries, however, the incidence is 10% to 12%. Since most penile cancers occur in uncircumcised men, it has been suggested that the etiology of this cancer may be the irritative effect of smegma and poor hygiene. However, the "protective" effect of circumcision is seen only in males who are circumcised in the neonatal period; circumcision that occurs at puberty or after does not confer the same benefit (Herr et al., 2001). Cancer of the penis appears on the skin of the penis as a painless, wartlike growth or ulcer. Cancer of the penis can involve the glans, the coronal sulcus under the prepuce, the corporal bodies, the urethra, and regional or distant lymph nodes. **Bowen's disease** is a form of squamous cell carcinoma in situ of the penile shaft. Typically, a man delays seeking treatment for more than a year, probably because of guilt, embarrassment, or ignorance.

Prevention

Circumcision in infancy almost eliminates the possibility of penile cancer because chronic irritation and inflammation of the glans penis predispose to penile tumours (Herr et al., 2001; Pettaway & Dinney, 2001; Schoen et al., 2000). In uncircumcised men, personal hygiene is an important preventive measure.

Medical Management

Smaller lesions involving only the skin may be controlled by excision (Herr et al., 2001). Topical chemotherapy with 5-fluorouracil cream is an option in selected patients. Radiation therapy is used to treat small squamous cell carcinomas of the penis or for palliation in advanced tumours or lymph node metastasis. Partial penectomy (removal of the penis) is preferred to total penectomy if possible; about 40% of patients can then participate in sexual intercourse and stand for urination. The shaft of the penis can still respond to sexual arousal with an erection and has the sensory capacity for orgasm and ejaculation. Total penectomy is indicated when the tumour is not amenable to conservative treatment. After a total penectomy, the patient may still experience orgasm with stimulation of the perineum and scrotal area.

PRIAPISM

Priapism is an uncontrolled, persistent erection of the penis that causes the penis to become large, hard, and painful. It occurs from either neural or vascular causes, including sickle cell thrombosis, leukemic cell infiltration, spinal cord tumours or injury, and tumour invasion of the penis or its vessels. It may also occur with use of medications that affect the central nervous system, antihypertensive agents, antidepressant medications, and substances injected into the penis to treat erectile dysfunction. This condition may result in gangrene and often results in impotence, whether treated or not.

Priapism is a urologic emergency. The goal of therapy is to improve venous drainage of the corpora cavernosa to prevent ischemia, fibrosis, and impotence. The initial treatment is directed at relieving the erection and includes bed rest and sedation. The corpora may be irrigated with an anticoagulant, which allows stagnant blood to be aspirated. Shunting procedures to divert the blood from the turgid corpora cavernosa to the venous system (corpora cavernosa–saphenous vein shunt) or into the corpus spongiosum–glans penis compartment may be attempted.

PEYRONIE'S DISEASE

Peyronie's disease involves the buildup of fibrous plaques in the sheath of the corpus cavernosum. These plaques are not visible when the penis is relaxed. When erect, however, curvature of the penis occurs that can be painful and can make sexual intercourse difficult or impossible. Peyronie's disease primarily occurs in middle-aged and older men. Although the plaques may shrink over time, surgical removal of the plaques may be necessary.

URETHRAL STRICTURE

Urethral stricture is a condition in which a section of the urethra is narrowed. It can occur congenitally or from a scar along the urethra. Traumatic injury to the urethra (for example, from instrumentation or infections) can result in strictures. Treatment involves dilation of the urethra or, in severe cases, urethrotomy (surgical removal of the stricture).

CIRCUMCISION

Circumcision is the excision of the foreskin, or prepuce, of the glans penis. It is usually performed in infancy. In adults, it is part of the treatment for phimosis, paraphimosis, and recurrent infections of the glans and foreskin and may be performed at the personal desire of the patient.

Postoperatively, a petrolatum (Vaseline) gauze dressing is applied and changed as indicated. The patient is observed for bleeding. Because considerable pain may occur after circumcision, analgesic agents are administered as needed.

 Critical Thinking Exercises

1. During a community health fair, you are approached by a 49-year-old African Canadian man who asks you about his risks for prostate cancer. Develop a plan to address this issue with him at the health fair and provide the rationale for your plan. How would your responses differ if you saw the patient during an office visit to follow up an elevated PSA test result?

2. One of your patients, a 44-year-old man with multiple sclerosis, asks you about Viagra. What information would you give him about Viagra, and what teaching approach would you use? How would your approach differ if your patient were a 56-year-old man with long-standing diabetes? If your patient were a 68-year-old man with coronary artery disease?

3. You are caring for two patients who have undergone prostatectomy. One has had surgery to treat BPH and the other to treat prostate cancer. How would your care differ for these two patients? How would the patient's underlying disorder alter your hospital care and your discharge planning?

4. A 34-year-old man is seeking treatment for an STD. When you are obtaining the health history, he reports that this is his fifth or sixth episode of STD. In addition to assisting with medical management and follow-up, what other interventions would you consider for this patient? What strategies would you suggest to him to reduce his risk for subsequent STDs and the risk of transmitting an STD to his sexual partner? How would your teaching differ if the patient revealed that he had sex with men only?

5. During a routine pre-employment physical examination, a 23-year-old man is found to have a mass in the left testicle. He dismisses its significance, saying that it is nothing to be concerned about and that he cannot interrupt his plans to have it evaluated, as he will be getting married in a month and beginning a new job. What information would you provide to the patient at this time? What explanation would you give to him about the evaluation of the testicular mass and possible outcomes?

REFERENCES AND SELECTED READINGS

Books

American Cancer Society (2002). *Cancer facts and figures 2002.* Atlanta: American Cancer Society.

Annon, J. S. (1976). *Behavioral treatment of sexual problems: Brief therapy.* Hagerstown, MD: Harper & Row.

Bosl, G. J., Bajorin, D. F., Scheinfeld, J., et al. (2001). Cancer of the testis. In V. T. DeVita, S. Hellman, & S. A. Rosenberg (Eds.). *Cancer: Principles and practice of oncology* (6th ed.). Philadelphia: Lippincott Williams & Wilkins.

Bruner, D. W., & Iwamoto, R. R. (1999). Altered sexual health. In C. H. Yarbro, M. H. Frogge, & M. Goodman (Eds.). *Cancer symptom management* (2nd ed.). Boston: Jones & Bartlett.

Campbell, M. F., Retik, A. B., Vaughn, E. D., & Walsh, P. C. (Eds.). (1998). *Campbell's urology* (7th ed.). Philadelphia: W. B. Saunders.

Canadian Cancer Society (2005). *What causes prostate cancer?* Available at: www.cancer.ca/ccs/internet/standard/0,3182,3172_10175_272747_langId-en,00.html. Retrieved June 6, 2005.

Canadian Cancer Society/National Cancer Institute of Canada (2005). *Canadian cancer statistics 2005.* [Monograph.] Available at: www.cancer.ca. Retrieved June 6, 2005.

Carroll, P. R., Lee, K. L., Fuks, Z. Y., & Kantoff, P. W. (2001). Cancer of the prostate. In V. T. DeVita, S. Hellman, & S. A. Rosenberg (Eds.). *Cancer: Principles and practice of oncology* (6th ed.). Philadelphia: Lippincott Williams & Wilkins.

Dodd, P. M., & Kelly, W. K. (2001). Testicular cancer. In R. E. Lenhard, R. T. Osteen, & T. Gansler (Eds.). *Clinical oncology.* Atlanta: American Cancer Society.

Ducharme, S. H., & Gill, K. M. (1997). Management of other male sexual dysfunctions. In M. L. Sipski & C. J. Alexander. *Sexual function in people with disability and chronic illness.* Gaithersburg, MD: Aspen.

Fosså, S. D., Aass, N., Roghavan, D., & Vogelzang, N. J. (2000). Late toxicity after chemotherapy of germ cell testis cancer. In N. J. Vogelzang, P. T. Scardino, W. U. Shipley & D. S. Coffey (Eds.). *Comprehensive textbook of genitourinary oncology* (2d ed.). Philadelphia: Lippincott Williams & Wilkins.

Greene, F. L., Page, D. L., Fleming, I. D., et al. (2002). *AJCC cancer staging manual* (6th ed.). New York: Springer-Verlag.

Herr, H. W., Dalbagni, G., Bajorin, D. F., & Shipley, W. U. (2001). Cancer of the urethra and penis. In V. T. DeVita, S. Hellman & S. A. Rosenberg (Eds.). *Cancer: Principles and practice of oncology* (6th ed.). Philadelphia: Lippincott Williams & Wilkins.

Hinman, F. (Ed.). (1998). *Atlas of urologic surgery* (2nd ed.). Philadelphia: W. B. Saunders.

Kantoff, P. W., Carroll, A. V., & D'Amico, A. V. (Eds.) (2002). *Prostate cancer: Principles and practice.* Philadelphia: Lippincott Williams & Wilkins.

Kelly, W. K., & Dodd, P. M. (2001). Prostate cancer. In R. E. Lenhard, R. T. Osteen & T. Gansler (Eds.). *Clinical oncology.* Atlanta: American Cancer Society.

Lepor, H. (1998). Natural history, evaluation, and nonsurgical management of benign prostatic hyperplasia. In M. F. Campbell, A. B. Retik, E. D. Vaughn & P. C. Walsh (Eds.). *Campbell's urology* (7th ed.). Philadelphia: W. B. Saunders.

Leung, A. C., Kadmon, D., & Fair, W. (2000). Prevention of prostate cancer. In N. J. Vogelzang, P. T. Scardino, W. U. Shipley & D. S. Coffey (Eds.). *Comprehensive textbook of genitourinary oncology* (2d ed.) Philadelphia: Lippincott Williams & Wilkins.

McCullough, D. L. (1998). Minimally invasive treatment of benign prostatic hyperplasia. In M. F. Campbell, A. B. Retik, E. D. Vaughn, & P. C. Walsh (Eds.). *Campbell's urology* (7th ed.). Philadelphia: W. B. Saunders.

McConnell, J. D. (1998). Epidemiology, etiology, pathophysiology, and diagnosis of benign prostatic hyperplasia. In M. F. Campbell, A. B. Retik, E. D. Vaughn, & P. C. Walsh (Eds.). *Campbell's urology* (7th ed.). Philadelphia: W. B. Saunders.

Mebust, W. K. (1998). Transurethral surgery. In M. F. Campbell, A. B. Retik, E. D. Vaughn & P. C. Walsh (Eds.). *Campbell's urology* (7th ed.). Philadelphia: W. B. Saunders.

Moore, K., & Vandall-Walker, V. (2000). *Before and after your radical prostatectomy.* Montreal: The Canadian Continence Foundation.

Narayan, P., Yu, K. K., Patel, M., & Hricak, H. (2000) Imaging in prostate cancer. In N. J. Vogelzang, P. T. Scardino, W. U. Shipley & D. S. Coffey (Eds.). *Comprehensive textbook of genitourinary oncology* (2d ed.) Philadelphia: Lippincott Williams & Wilkins.

Oliver, R. T. D. (2000). Epidemiology of testis cancer: A clinical perspective. In N. J. Vogelzang, P. T. Scardino, W. U. Shipley & D. S. Coffey (Eds.). *Comprehensive textbook of genitourinary oncology* (2d ed.) Philadelphia: Lippincott Williams & Wilkins.

Pettaway, C. A., & Dinney, C. P. N. (2001). Penile and urethral cancer. In R. E. Lenhard, R. T. Osteen & T. Gansler (Eds.). *Clinical oncology.* Atlanta: American Cancer Society.

Sipski, M. L., & Alexander, C. J. (Eds.). (1997). *Sexual function in people with disability and chronic illness: A health professional's guide.* Gaithersburg, MD: Aspen.

Stadler, W. M., Vogelzang, N. J., Elwell, C. M., & Jones, W. G. (2000) Penile cancer: Overview. In N. J. Vogelzang, P. T. Scardino, W. U. Shipley & D. S. Coffey (Eds.). *Comprehensive textbook of genitourinary oncology* (2d ed.) Philadelphia: Lippincott Williams & Wilkins.

Thomas, G. M., & Williams, S. D. (1998). Testis. In C. A. Perez & L. W. Brady (Eds.). *Principles and practices of radiation oncology* (3rd ed.). Philadelphia: Lippincott-Raven.

U.S. Surgeon General (2001). *U.S. Surgeon General's call to action to promote sexual health and responsible sexual behavior.* Washington DC: United States Public Health Service.

Journals

Asterisks indicate nursing research articles.
General

Centers of Disease Control and Prevention (2000). CDC statement on study results of products containing nonoxynol-9. *Journal of the American Medical Association, 284*(11), 1376.

Centers for Disease Control and Prevention (CDC). (2002). Sexually transmitted diseases treatment guidelines, 2002. *MMWR-Morbidity and Mortality Weekly Report, 51*(RR-6), 1–85.

*Davison, B. J., Moore, K. N., MacMillan, H., et al. (2004). Patient evaluation of a discharge program following a radical prostatectomy. *Urologic Nursing, 24*(6), 483–489.

Eckert, J. K., & Rubinstein, R. L. (1999). Older men's health: Sociocultural and ecological perspectives. *Medical Clinics of North America, 83*(5), 1151.

*Hunter, K. F., Moore, K. N., Cody, D. J., et al. (2005). *The Cochrane Library, 2.* ID #CD001843.

Johnson, T. M. II, & Ouslander, J. G. (1999). Urinary incontinence in the older man. *Medical Clinics of North America, 83*(5), 1247.

McCallum, T. J., Moore, K. N., & Griffiths, D. (2001). Urinary incontinence after radical prostatectomy: Implications and urodynamics. *Urologic Nursing, 21*(2), 113–119.

Millon-Underwood, S., & Sanders, E. (1990). Factors contributing to health promotion behaviors among African-American men. *Oncology Nursing Forum, 17*(5), 707–712.

Moore, K. N. (1999). A review of the anatomy of the male continence mechanism and the cause of urinary incontinence after prostatectomy. *Journal of Wound, Ostomy and Continence Nursing, 26*(2), 86–93.

*Moore, K. N. (2000). After effects: Tackling the morbidity of prostate cancer treatment. *Journal of Wound, Ostomy and Continence Nursing, 27*(3), 188–190.

*Moore, K. N., & Estey, A. (1999). The early post-operative concerns of men after radical prostatectomy. *Journal of Advanced Nursing, 29*(5), 1121–1129.

*Moore, K. N., & Jensen, L. (2000). Testing the Incontinence Impact Questionnaire (IIQ-7) with men after radical prostatectomy. *Journal of Wound, Ostomy and Continence Nursing, 27*(6), 304–312.

Schoen, E. J., Oehrli, M., Colby, C., & Machin, G. (2000) The highly protective effect of newborn circumcision against invasive penile cancer. *Pediatrics, 105*(3), E36.

Van Damme, L. (2000). *Advances in topical microbicides.* Presented at the XIII International AIDS Conference, July 9–14, 2000, Durban, South Africa.

Watson, J., & Fried, L. P. (1999). Frailty and the older man. *Medical Clinics of North America, 83*(5), 1173.

Assessment of Function and Dysfunction of Male Reproductive System

Bakshi, S., & Miller, D. K. (1999). Assessment of the aging man. *Medical Clinics of North America, 83*(5), 1131–1147.

Hughes, M. K. (2000). Sexuality and the cancer survivor: A silent coexistence. *Cancer Nursing, 23*(6), 477–482.

Penson, R. T., Gallagher, J., Gioiella, M. E., et al. (2000). Sexuality and cancer: Conversation comfort zone. *Oncologist, 5*(4), 336–344.

Eid, J. F. (2000). Sildenafil citrate: Current clinical experience. *International Journal of Impotence Research, 12*Suppl 4, S62-S66.

Goldstein, I., Lue, T. F., Padma-Nathan, H., et al. (1998). Oral sildenafil in the treatment of erectile dysfunction. Sildenafil Study Group. *New England Journal of Medicine, 338*(20), 1397–1404.

Kaiser, F. E. (1999). Erectile dysfunction in the aging man. *Medical Clinics of North America, 83*(5), 1267.

Klingman, L. (1999). Assessing the male genitalia. *American Journal of Nursing, 99*(7), 47–50.

Korenman, S. G. (1998). New insights into erectile dysfunction: A practical approach. *American Journal of Medicine, 105*(2), 135–144.

Lue, T. F. (2000). Erectile dysfunction. *New England Journal of Medicine, 342*(24), 1802–1813.

National Institutes of Health Consensus Development Panel on Impotence. (1993). Impotence. *Journal of the American Medical Association, 270*(1), 83–90.

Padma-Nathan, H., Hellstrom W. J., Kaiser, F. E., et al. (1997). Treatment of men with erectile dysfunction with transurethral alprostadil. Medicated Urethral System for Erection (MUSE) Study Group. *New England Journal of Medicine, 336*(1), 1–7.

Sundaram, C. P., Thomas, W., Pryor, L. E., et al. (1997). Long-term follow-up of patients receiving injection therapy for erectile dysfunction. *Urology, 49*(6), 932–935.

Benign Prostatic Hyperplasia

Barry, M. J., Fowler, F. J. Jr., Bin, L., et al. (1997). The natural history of patients with benign prostatic hyperplasia as diagnosed by North American urologists. *Journal of Urology, 157*(1), 10–15.

Gerber, G. S. (2000). Saw palmetto for the treatment of men with lower urinary tract symptoms. *Journal of Urology, 163*(5), 1408–1412.

(1999) Saw palmetto for benign prostatic hyperplasia. *Medical Letter on Drugs and Therapeutics, 41*(1046), 18.

Marks, L. S., Partin, A. W., Epstein, J. L., et al. (2000). Effects of a saw palmetto herbal blend in men with symptomatic benign prostatic hyperplasia. *Journal of Urology, 163*(5), 1451–1456.

Medina, J. J., Parra, R. O., & Moore, R. G. (1999). Benign prostatic hyperplasia (the aging prostate). *Medical Clinics of North America, 83*(5), 1213.

Ramsey, E. W., Miller, P. D., Parsons, K., et al. (1997). A novel transurethral microwave thermal ablation system to treat benign prostatic hyperplasia: Results of a prospective multicenter clinical trial. *Journal of Urology, 158*(1), 112–119.

Reilly, N. J. (1997). Benign prostatic hyperplasia in older men. *Lippincott's Primary Care Practice, 1*(4), 421–430.

Roper, W. G. (1998). The etiology of benign prostatic hypertrophy. *Medical Hypotheses, 50*(1), 61–65.

Wilt, T. J., Ishani, A., Stark, G., et al. (1998), Saw palmetto extracts for treatment of benign prostatic hyperplasia: A systematic review. *Journal of the American Medical Association, 280*(18), 1604–1609.

Prostate Cancer

*Agho, A. O., & Lewis, M. A. (2001). Correlates of actual and perceived knowledge of prostate cancer among African Americans. *Cancer Nursing, 24*(3), 165–171.

Barry, M. J. (2001). Clinical practice. Prostate-specific-antigen testing for early diagnosis of prostate cancer. *New England Journal of Medicine, 344*(18), 1373–1377.

Bickert, D., & Frickel, D. (2002). Laparoscopic radical prostatectomy. *AORN Journal, 75*(4), 762–780.

Bishoff, J. T., Motley, G., Optenberg, S. A., et al. (1998). Incidence of fecal and urinary incontinence following radical perineal and retropubic prostatectomy in a national population. *Journal of Urology, 160*, 454–458.

Brawer, M. K., Cheli, C. D., Neaman, I. E., et al. (2000). Complexed prostate specific antigen provides significant enhancement of specificity compared with total prostate specific antigen for detecting prostate cancer. *Journal of Urology, 163*(5), 1476–1480.

Bruner, D. W., Pickett, M., Joseph, A., & Burgraff, V. (2000). Prostate cancer elder alert (Part I): Epidemiology, screening, and early detection. *Journal of Gerontological Nursing, 26*(1), 6–15

Cash, J. C., & Dattoli, M. J. (1997). Management of patients receiving transperineal palladium-103 prostate implants. *Oncology Nursing Forum, 24*(8), 1361–1367.

Cherney, N. I. (2000). The management of cancer pain. *CA Cancer Journal for Clinicians, 50*, 70–116.

*Collins, M. (1997). Increasing prostate cancer awareness in African American men. *Oncology Nursing Forum, 24*(1), 91–95.

D'Amico, A. V., Schultz, D., Loffredo, M., et al. (2000). Biochemical outcome following external beam radiation therapy with or without androgen suppression therapy for clinically localized prostate cancer. *Journal of the American Medical Association, 284*(10), 1280–1283.

Denis, L. J., & Griffiths, K. (2000). Endocrine treatment in prostate cancer. *Seminars in Surgical Oncology, 18*, 52–74.

*Esper, P., Hampton, J. N., Smith, D. C., et al. (1999). Quality-of-life evaluation in patients receiving treatment for advanced prostate cancer. *Oncology Nursing Forum, 26*(1), 107–112.

*Fitch, M. I., Gray, R. E., Franssen, E., et al. (2000). Men's perspectives on the impact on prostate cancer: Implications for oncology nurses. *Oncology Nursing Forum, 27*(8), 1255–1263.

*Gelfand, D. E., Panzuchowski, S., Cort, M., et al. (1995). Digital rectal examinations and prostate cancer screening: Attitudes of African American men. *Oncology Nursing Forum, 22*(8), 1253–1263.

Gerard, M. J., & Frank-Stromborg, M. (1998). Screening for prostate cancer in asymptomatic men: Clinical, legal, and ethical implications. *Oncology Nursing Forum, 25*(9), 1561–1569.

Greenlee, R. T., Murray, T., Bolden, S., et al. (2001). Cancer statistics 2001. *CA: A Cancer Journal for Clinicians, 51*(1), 15–36.

Hahnfeld, L. E., & Moon, T. D. (1999). Prostate cancer. *Medical Clinics of North America, 83*(5), 1231.

Herr, H. W., & O'Sullivan M. (2000). Quality of life for men with prostate cancer on androgen deprivation therapy. *Journal of Urology, 163*, 1743–1746.

Horwitz, E. M., & Hanks, G. E. (2000). External beam radiation therapy for prostate cancer. *CA: Cancer Journal for Clinicians, 50*(6), 349–375.

*Jakobsson, L., Loven, L., & Hallberg, I. R. (2001). Sexual problems in men with prostate cancer in comparison with men with benign prostatic hyperplasia and men from the general population. *Journal of Clinical Nursing, 10*(4), 573–582.

Kalish, L. A., & McKinlay, J. B. (1999). Serum prostate-specific antigen levels (PSA) in men without clinical evidence of prostate cancer: Age-specific reference ranges for total PSA, free PSA, and percent free PSA. *Urology, 54*(6), 1022–1027.

Kestin, L. L., et al. (2000). Matched-pair analysis of conformal high-dose-rate brachytherapy boost versus external-beam radiation therapy alone for locally advanced prostate cancer. *Journal of Clinical Oncology, 18*(15), 2869–2880.

Krumholtz, J. S., Michalski, M. J., & Sundaram, C. P. (2000). Health-related quality of life and morbidity in patients receiving brachytherapy for clinically localized prostate cancer. *Journal of Endourology, 14*(4), 371–374.

*Maliski, S. L. Heilemann, M. V., & McCorkle, R. (2002). From "death sentence" to "good cancer": Couples' transformation of a prostate cancer diagnosis. *Nursing Research, 51*(6), 391–397.

Mettlin, C. (1997). National patterns of prostate cancer detection and treatment. The American Cancer Society National Prostate Cancer Detection Project. *CA: A Cancer Journal for Clinicians, 47*(5), 365–372.

Middleton, R. G. (1996). The management of clinically localized prostate cancer: guidelines from the American Urological Association. *CA: A Cancer Journal for Clinicians, 46*(4), 249–253.

*O'Rourke, M. E., & Germino, B. B. (1998). Prostate cancer treatment decisions: A focus group exploration. *Oncology Nursing Forum, 25*(1), 97–104.

Partin, A. W., Kattan, M. W., Subong, E. N., et al. (1997). Combination of prostate-specific antigen, clinical stage, and Gleason score to predict pathological stage of localized prostate cancer. A multi-institutional update. *Journal of the American Medical Association, 277*(18), 1445–1451.

Pickett, M., Bruner, D. W., Joseph, A., & Burgraff, V. (2000). Prostate cancer elder alert (Part II): Living with treatment choices and outcomes. *Journal of Gerontological Nursing, 26*(2), 22–34.

Pollack, A., Zogars, G. K., Smith, L. G., et al. (2000). Preliminary results of a randomized radiotherapy dose-escalation study comparing 70 Gy with 78 Gy for prostate cancer. *Journal of Clinical Oncology, 18*, 3904–3911.

Ragde, H., Grado, G. L., Nadir, B., et al. (2000). Modern prostate brachytherapy. *CA: A Cancer Journal for Clinicians, 50*(6), 380–393.

Rassweiler, J., Sentker, L., Seemann, O., et al. (2001). Laparoscopic radical prostatectomy with the Heilbronn technique: An analysis of the first 180 cases. *Journal of Urology, 166*(6), 2101–2108.

Smith, R. A., Cokkinides, V., von Eschenbach, A. C., et al. (2002). American Cancer Society Guidelines for the early detection of cancer. *CA: Cancer Journal for Clinicians, 52*(1), 8–22.

Society of Surgical Oncology. (1997). Prostate cancer surgical practice guidelines. *Oncology, 11*(6), 907–912.

Tarman, G. J., Kane, C. J., Moul, J. W., et al. (2000). Impact of socioeconomic status and race on clinical parameters of patients undergoing radical prostatectomy in an equal access healthcare system. *Urology, 56*, 1016–1020.

von Eschenbach, A., Ho, R., Murphy, G. P., et al. (1997). American Cancer Society guidelines for the early detection of prostate cancer: Update 1997. *CA: A Cancer Journal for Clinicians, 47*(5), 261–264.

*Weinrich, S. P., Weinrich, M. C., Boyd, M. D., et al. (1998). The impact of prostate cancer knowledge on cancer screening. *Oncology Nursing Forum, 25*(3), 527–534.

*Weinrich, S. P., Reynolds, W. A., Jr., Tingen, M. S., & Starr, C. R. (2000). Barriers to prostate cancer screening. *Cancer Nursing, 23*(2), 117–121.

*Yarbro, C. H., & Ferrans, C. E. (1998). Quality of life of patients with prostate cancer treated with surgery or radiation therapy. *Oncology Nursing Forum, 25*(4), 685–693.

Zagaja, G. P., Mhoon, D. A., Aikens, J. E., et al. (2000). Sildenafil in the treatment of erectile dysfunction after radical prostatectomy. *Urology, 56*(4), 631–634.

Zelefsky, M. J. (1999). Efficacy of oral sildenafil in patients with erectile dysfunction after radiotherapy for carcinoma of the prostate. *Urology, 53*(4), 775–778.

*Zimmerman, S. M. (1997). Factors influencing Hispanic participation in prostate cancer screening. *Oncology Nursing Forum, 24*(3), 499–504.

Testicular Cancer

Agarwa, A. (2000). Semen banking in patients with cancer: 20-year experience. *International Journal of Andrology, 23,* Suppl 2, 16–19.

American Cancer Society (2000). American Cancer Society web site. Available at: http://www.americancancer.org. Retrieved Aug. 12, 2002.

Cox, B., Sneyd, M. J., Paul, C., et al. (2002). Vasectomy and risk of prostate cancer. *Journal of the American Medical Association, 287*(23), 3110–3115.

Kollmannsberber, C., Kuzcyk, M., Mayer, F., et al. (1999). Late toxicity following curative treatment of testicular cancer. *Seminars in Surgical Oncology, 17*(4), 275–281.

National Cancer Institute web site (2002). Available at: http://cis.nci.nih.gov/asp/FactSheetPub/FactSheetList.asp. Retrieved Aug. 12, 2002.

*Sandén, I., Larsson, U. S., & Ericksson, C. (2000). An interview study of men discovering testicular cancer. *Cancer Nursing, 23*(4), 304–309.

Zapzalka, D. M., Redmon, J. B., & Pryor, J. L. (1999). A survey of oncologists regarding sperm cryopreservation and assisted reproductive techniques for male cancer. *Cancer, 86*(9), 1812–1817.

RESOURCES AND WEBSITES

Agencies

American Cancer Society, 1599 Clifton Road, NE, Atlanta, GA 30326; (800) ACS-2345; Man to Man Support Group; http://www.cancer.org.

American Foundation for Urologic Disease, Prostate Cancer Support Network, 300 West Pratt, Suite 401, Baltimore, MD 21201-2463; (800) 828-7866; http://www.afud.org.

Canadian Cancer Society/Société canadienne du cancer, National Office, Suite 200, 10 Alcorn Avenue, Toronto, ON M4V 3B1; (416) 961-7223; fax: (416) 961-4189; www.cancer.ca.

Canadian Continence Foundation, P.O. Box 30, Victoria Branch, Westmount, QC H3Z 2V4; (514) 488-9999; Montreal area, 1-800-265-9575; email: help@continence-fdn.ca; www.continence-fdn.ca.

Canadian Prostate Cancer Network, P.O. Box 1253, Lakefield, ON K0L 2H0; (705) 652-9200; 1-866-810-CPCN (2726); 1-800-363-0063 (francais); fax: (705) 652-0663; email: cpcn@nexicom.net; www.cpcn.org.

Canadian Prostate Health Council, P.O. Box 7600, Dorval, QC H94 4P8; www.canadian-prostate.com.

CancerCare: 275 7th Ave., New York, NY 10001; (800) 813 HOPE (4673); http://www.cancercareinc.org/campaigns/prostate1.htm.

Impotence Anonymous and I-Anon, Impotence World Association, P.O. Box 410, Bowie, MD 20718-0410; (800) 669-1603; http://www.impotenceworld.org.

National Cancer Institute, Office of Cancer Communications, Building 31, Room 10A24, Bethesda, MD 20892; (800) 4-CANCER; http://www.nci.nih.gov.

National Prostate Cancer Coalition, 1158 Fifteenth St. NW, Washington, D.C. 20005; (888) 245-9455; http://www.4npcc.org.

Prostate Cancer At-A-Glance-Centers for Disease Control: http://www.cdc.gov/cancer/prostate/.

Prostate Cancer Information (Health Canada and the Department of Urology, Dalhousie University); www.caprostate.com.

Prostate Cancer Support Group: Canadian Cancer Society; 1-888-939-3333.

The Prostate Cancer InfoLink: http://www.comed.com/prostate.

Urology Nurses of Canada. Prostate Cancer–A Medical Education Program; www.unc.org/prostate/introduction.ht.

US Too International, Inc., Prostate Cancer Survivor Support Group, 930 North York Road, Suite 50, Hinsdale, IL 60521-2993; (800) 80-US-TOO; http://www.ustoo.com.

Patient Resources

Alterowitz, R., & Alterowitz, B. (1999). *The lovin' ain't over: The couple's guide to better sex after prostate disease.* Westbury, NY: Health Education Literary Publisher.

Bostwick, D. G., MacLennan, G. T., & Larson, T. R. (Eds.) (1999). *The American Cancer Society: Prostate Cancer* (revised ed.). New York: Villard Books.

Bostwick, D. G., MacLennan, G. T., & Larson, T. R. (1999). *Prostate cancer: What every man and his family needs to know.* Atlanta: American Cancer Society.

Marks, S. (1999). *Prostate and cancer: A family guide to diagnosis, treatment and survival.* Tucson, AZ: Fisher Books.

National Cancer Institute (1998). *Understanding prostate changes: A health guide for all men.* Bethesda, MD: National Cancer Institute (NIH Pub no. 98-4303).

Oesterling, J. E., & Moyad, M. A. (1997). *The ABC's of prostate cancer.* Lanham: Madison Books.

Rous, S. (2002). *The prostate book* (2nd ed.). New York: W. W. Norton.

Schultz, R. E., & Oliver, A. W. (2000). *Humanizing prostate cancer: A physician-patient perspective.* White Stone, VA: Brandylane Publishers.

Wainrib, B. R., Haber, S., & Maguire, J. (2000). *Men, women and prostate cancer* (2d ed.). Oakland, CA: New Harbinger Publications.

Walsh, P. C., & Worthington, J. F. (1997). *The prostate: A guide for men and the women who love them.* New York: Warner Books.

Walsh, P. C., & Worthington, J. F. (2002). *Dr. Patrick Walsh's guide to surviving prostate cancer.* New York: Warner Books.

Immunologic Function

Applying Concepts from NANDA, NIC, and NOC

Mrs. Miller is a 41-year-old mother of three with severe rheumatoid arthritis. She has been taking prednisone 10 mg daily for 6 months as part of a treatment plan that will also include nonsteroidal anti-inflammatory drugs (NSAIDs) and disease-modifying antirheumatic drugs (DMARDs). Although her physician has tried to taper the prednisone, each time the dose is reduced Mrs. Miller experiences a painful flare-up of her rheumatoid arthritis and symptoms of steroid withdrawal. Mrs. Miller states that when her symptoms flare, she takes an extra dose of prednisone. She has had oral candidal disease twice in the preceding 3 months and has had frequent upper respiratory tract infections. The concept map illustrates the relationships that exist among selected nursing diagnoses, interventions, and outcomes for Mrs. Miller's immunosuppression and history of oral infections.

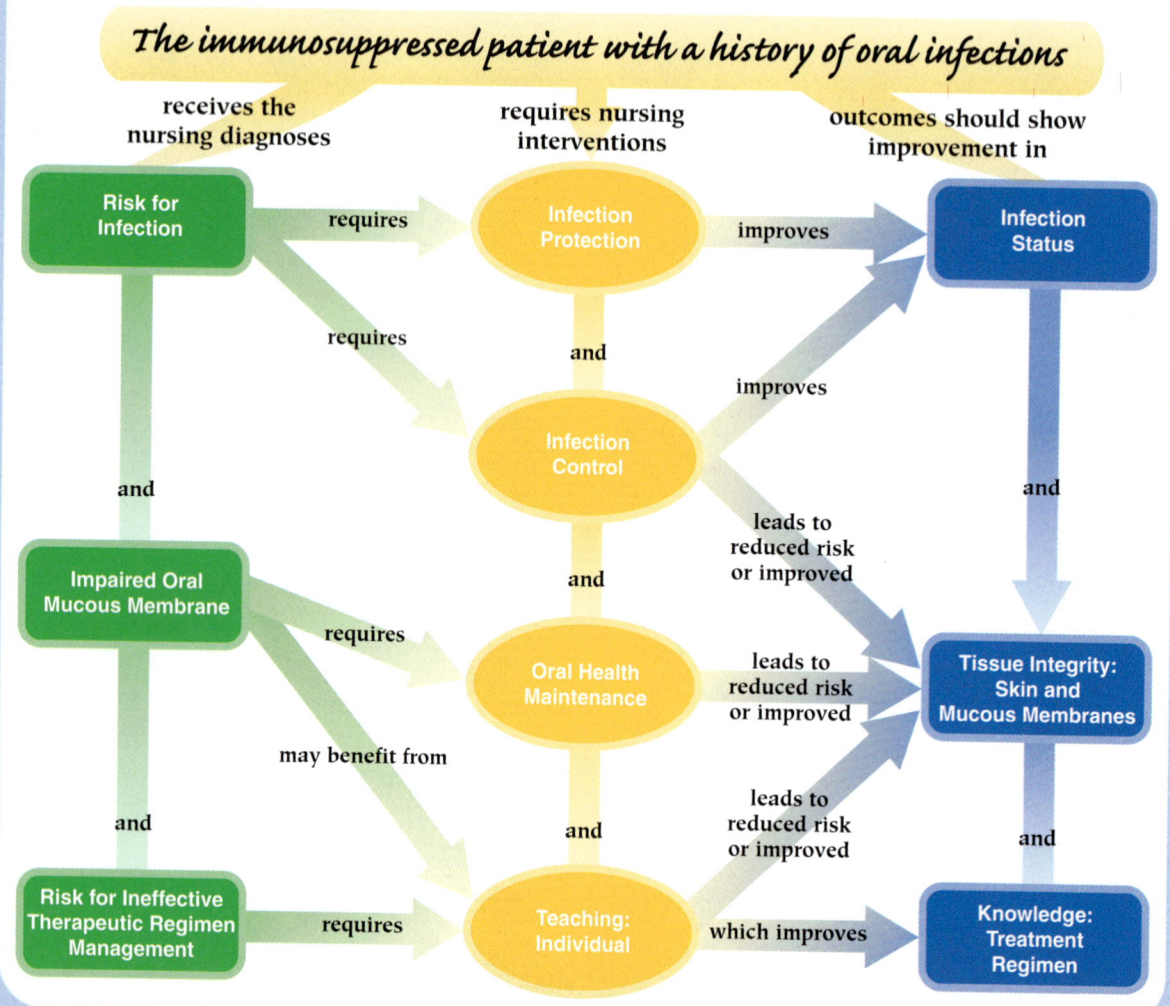

The immunosuppressed patient with a history of oral infections

receives the nursing diagnoses	requires nursing interventions	outcomes should show improvement in

Risk for Infection — requires → Infection Protection — improves → Infection Status

Risk for Infection — requires → Infection Control

and

Impaired Oral Mucous Membrane — requires → Oral Health Maintenance

Infection Control — improves → Infection Status

and

Oral Health Maintenance — leads to reduced risk or improved → Tissue Integrity: Skin and Mucous Membranes

Impaired Oral Mucous Membrane — may benefit from → Teaching: Individual

and

Risk for Ineffective Therapeutic Regimen Management — requires → Teaching: Individual

Teaching: Individual — leads to reduced risk or improved → Tissue Integrity: Skin and Mucous Membranes

Teaching: Individual — which improves → Knowledge: Treatment Regimen

Nursing Classifications and Languages

NANDA
Nursing Diagnoses

Risk for Infection—At risk for being invaded by pathogenic organisms

Impaired Oral Mucous Membrane—Description of the lips and soft tissues of the oral cavity

Risk for Ineffective Therapeutic Regimen Management—Having the potential for developing a pattern of regulating and integrating into daily living a program for treatment of illness and the sequelae of illness that is unsatisfactory for meeting specific health goals

NIC
Nursing Interventions*

Infection Protection—Prevention and early detection of infection in a patient at risk

Infection Control—Minimizing the acquisition and transmission of infectious agents

Oral Health Maintenance—Maintenance and promotion of oral hygiene and dental health for the patient at risk for developing oral or dental lesions

Teaching: Individual—Planning, implementation, and evaluation of a teaching program designed to address a patient's particular needs

NOC
Nursing Outcomes†

Return to functional baseline status, stabilization of, or improvement in

Infection Status—Presence and extent of infection

Tissue Integrity: Skin and Mucous Membranes—Structural intactness and normal physiological function of skin and mucous membranes

Knowledge: Treatment Regimen—Extent of understanding conveyed about a specific treatment regimen

NANDA, North American Nursing Diagnosis Association; NIC, Nursing Interventions Classification; NOC, Nursing Outcomes Classification.

*Iowa Intervention Project © 2000. In McCloskey, J. C., & Bulechek, G. M. (2000). *Nursing interventions classification (NIC)* (3rd ed.). St. Louis: Mosby.

†Iowa Outcomes Project © 2000. In Johnson, M., Maas, M., & Moorhead, S. (2000). *Nursing outcomes classification (NOC)* (3rd ed.). St. Louis: Mosby.

Assessment of Immune Function

Adapted by Wanda Pierson

LEARNING OBJECTIVES

On completion of this chapter, the learner will be able to:

1. Describe the body's general immune responses.
2. Discuss the stages of the immune response.
3. Differentiate between cellular and humoural immune responses.
4. Describe the effects of the following variables on function of the immune system: age, gender, nutrition, psychoneuroimmunology, concurrent illness, cancer, medications, and radiation.
5. Use assessment parameters for determining the status of immune function.

The immune system functions as the body's defense mechanism against invasion. The term **immunity** refers to the body's specific protective response to an invading foreign agent or organism. Immune function is affected by age and by a variety of other factors, such as central nervous system function, emotional status, medications, the stress of illness, trauma, and surgery. Dysfunctions involving the immune system occur across the life span. Many are genetically based; others are acquired. The term **immunopathology** refers to the study of diseases resulting from dysfunctions within the immune system. Disorders of the immune system may stem from excesses or deficiencies of immunocompetent cells, alterations in the function of these cells, immunologic attack on self-antigens, or inappropriate or exaggerated responses to specific antigens (Table 50-1).

To gain insight into immunopathology and the growing number of immunologic-based disorders and to assess and care for people with immunologic disorders, the nurse needs a sound knowledge base of the immune system and how it functions.

Anatomic and Physiologic Overview

ANATOMY OF THE IMMUNE SYSTEM

The immune system comprises cells and molecules with specialized roles in defending against infection and invasion by other organisms. Its major components include the bone marrow, the white blood cells (WBCs) produced by the bone marrow, and the lymphoid tissues. Lymphoid tissues include the thymus gland, the spleen, the lymph nodes, the tonsils and adenoids, and similar tissues in the gastrointestinal, respiratory, and reproductive systems (Fig. 50-1).

Bone Marrow

The bone marrow is the production site of the WBCs involved in immunity (Fig. 50-2). Like other blood cells, lymphocytes are generated from stem cells, which are undifferentiated cells. Descendants of **stem cells** become lymphocytes, the B lymphocytes (**B cells**), and the T lymphocytes (T cells) (Fig. 50-3). B lymphocytes mature in the bone marrow and then enter the circulation. T lymphocytes move from the bone marrow to the thymus, where they mature into several kinds of cells capable of different functions.

Lymphoid Tissues

The spleen, composed of red and white pulp, acts somewhat like a filter. The red pulp is the site where old and injured red blood cells are destroyed. The white pulp contains concentrations of lymphocytes. The lymph nodes are distributed throughout the body. They are connected by lymph channels and capillaries, which remove foreign material from the lymph before it enters the bloodstream. The lymph nodes also serve as centres for immune cell proliferation. The remaining lymphoid tissues, such as the tonsils and adenoids and other mucoid lymphatic tissues,

Table 50-1 • Immune System Disorders

DISORDER	DESCRIPTION
Autoimmunity	Normal protective immune response paradoxically turns against or attacks the body, leading to tissue damage
Hypersensitivity	Body produces inappropriate or exaggerated responses to specific antigens
Gammopathies	Immunoglobulins are overproduced
Immune deficiencies	
Primary	Deficiency results from improper development of immune cells or tissues, usually with a genetic basis
Secondary	Deficiency results from some interference with an already developed immune system

Glossary

agglutination: clumping effect occurring when an antibody acts as a cross-link between two antigens

antibody: a protein substance developed by the body in response to and interacting with a specific antigen

antigen: substance that induces the production of antibodies

apoptosis: programmed cell death that results from the digestion of DNA by endonucleases

B cells: cells that are important in producing circulating antibodies

cellular immune response: the immune system's third line of defense, involving the attack of pathogens by T cells

complement: series of enzymatic proteins in the serum that, when activated, destroy bacteria and other cells

cytokines: generic term for non-antibody proteins that act as intercellular mediators, as in the generation of immune response

cytotoxic T cells: lymphocytes that lyse cells infected with virus; also play a role in graft rejection

genetic engineering: emerging technology designed to enable replacement of missing or defective genes

helper T cells: lymphocytes that attack foreign invaders (antigens) directly

humoural immune response: the immune system's second line of defense; often termed the antibody response

immunity: the body's specific protective response to an invading foreign agent or organism

immunopathology: study of diseases resulting in dysfunctions within the immune system

immunoregulation: complex system of checks and balances that regulates or controls immune responses

interferons: proteins formed when cells are exposed to viral or foreign agents; capable of activating other components of the immune system

lymphokines: substances released by sensitized lymphocytes when they contact specific antigens

memory cells: cells that are responsible for recognizing antigens from previous exposure and mounting an immune response

natural killer cells (NK cells): lymphocytes that defend against microorganisms and malignant cells

null lymphocytes: lymphocytes that destroy antigens already coated with the antibody

opsonization: the coating of antigen—antibody molecules with a sticky substance to facilitate phagocytosis

phagocytic cells: cells that engulf, ingest, and destroy foreign bodies or toxins

phagocytic immune response: the immune system's first line of defense, involving white blood cells that have the ability to ingest foreign particles

stem cells: precursors of all blood cells; reside primarily in bone marrow

suppressor T cells: lymphocytes that decrease B-cell activity to a level at which the immune system is compatible with life

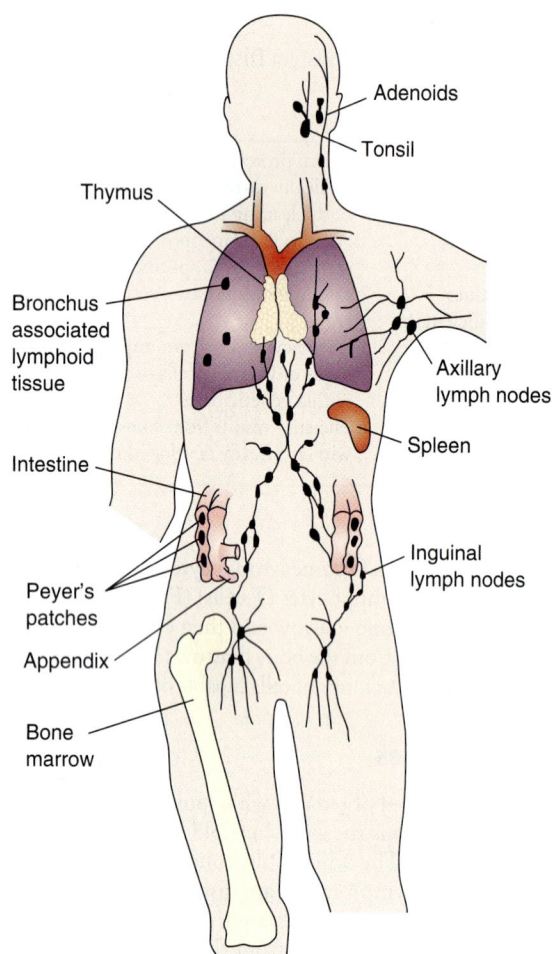

FIGURE 50-1 Central and peripheral lymphoid organs and tissues. From Porth, C. M. (2002). *Pathophysiology: Concepts of altered health states* (6th ed.). Philadelphia: Lippincott Williams & Wilkins.

contain immune cells that defend the body's mucosal surfaces against microorganisms.

IMMUNE FUNCTION: DEFENSES AND RESPONSES

There are two general types of immunity: natural (innate) and acquired (adaptive). Natural immunity is a nonspecific immunity present at birth. Acquired or specific immunity develops after birth. Natural immune responses to a foreign invader are very similar from one encounter to the next regardless of the number of times the invader is encountered; in contrast, acquired responses increase in intensity with repeated exposure to the invading agent (Delves & Roitt, 2000a). Although each type of immunity plays a distinct role in defending the body against harmful invaders, the various components usually act in an interdependent manner.

Natural Immunity

Natural (innate) immunity provides a nonspecific response to any foreign invader, regardless of the invader's composition. The basis of natural defense mechanisms is the ability to distinguish between friend and foe or "self" and "nonself." Such natural mechanisms

include physical and chemical barriers, the action of WBCs, and inflammatory responses.

PHYSICAL AND CHEMICAL BARRIERS

Physical surface barriers include intact skin and mucous membranes, which prevent pathogens from gaining access to the body, and the cilia of the respiratory tract along with coughing and sneezing responses, which act to filter and clear pathogens from the upper respiratory tract before they can invade the body further. Chemical barriers, such as acidic gastric secretions, mucus, enzymes in tears and saliva, and substances in sebaceous and sweat secretions, act in a nonspecific way to destroy invading bacteria and fungi. Viruses are countered by other means, such as interferon. **Interferon**, one type of biologic response modifier, is a nonspecific viricidal protein naturally produced by the body that is capable of activating other components of the immune system.

WHITE BLOOD CELL ACTION

WBCs, or leukocytes, participate in both the natural and the acquired immune responses. Granular leukocytes, or granulocytes (so called because of granules in their cytoplasm), fight invasion by foreign bodies or toxins by releasing cell mediators, such as histamine, bradykinin, and prostaglandins, and engulfing the foreign bodies or toxins. Granulocytes include neutrophils, eosinophils, and basophils.

Neutrophils (also called polymorphonuclear leukocytes, or PMNs, because their nuclei have multiple lobes) are the first cells to arrive at the site where inflammation occurs. Eosinophils and basophils, other types of granulocytes, increase in number during allergic reactions and stress responses. Nongranular leukocytes include monocytes or macrophages (referred to as histiocytes when they enter tissue spaces) and lymphocytes. Monocytes also function as **phagocytic cells**, engulfing, ingesting, and destroying greater numbers and quantities of foreign bodies or toxins than granulocytes. Lymphocytes, consisting of B cells and T cells, play major roles in humoural and cell-mediated immune responses. About 60% to 70% of lymphocytes in the blood are T cells, and about 10% to 20% are B cells (Porth, 2002).

INFLAMMATORY RESPONSE

The inflammatory response is a major function of the natural (nonspecific or innate) immune system elicited in response to tissue injury or invading organisms. Chemical mediators assist this response by minimizing blood loss, walling off the invading organism, activating phagocytes, and promoting formation of fibrous scar tissue and regeneration of injured tissue. (The inflammatory response is discussed further in Chap. 6.)

Dysfunction of the natural immune system can occur when the immune components are inactivated or when they remain active long after their effects are beneficial. Immunodeficiencies are characterized by inactivation or impairment of immune components, and disorders with an inflammatory component (eg, asthma, allergy, arthritis) are characterized by persistent inflammatory responses (Medahitov & Janeway, 2000). The immune system's recognition of one's own tissues as "foreign" rather than as self is the basis for many autoimmune disorders.

Acquired Immunity

Acquired (adaptive) immunity—immunologic responses acquired during life but not present at birth—usually develops as a result of prior exposure to an antigen through immunization (vaccination) or by contracting a disease, both of which generate a protective

Physiology/Pathophysiology

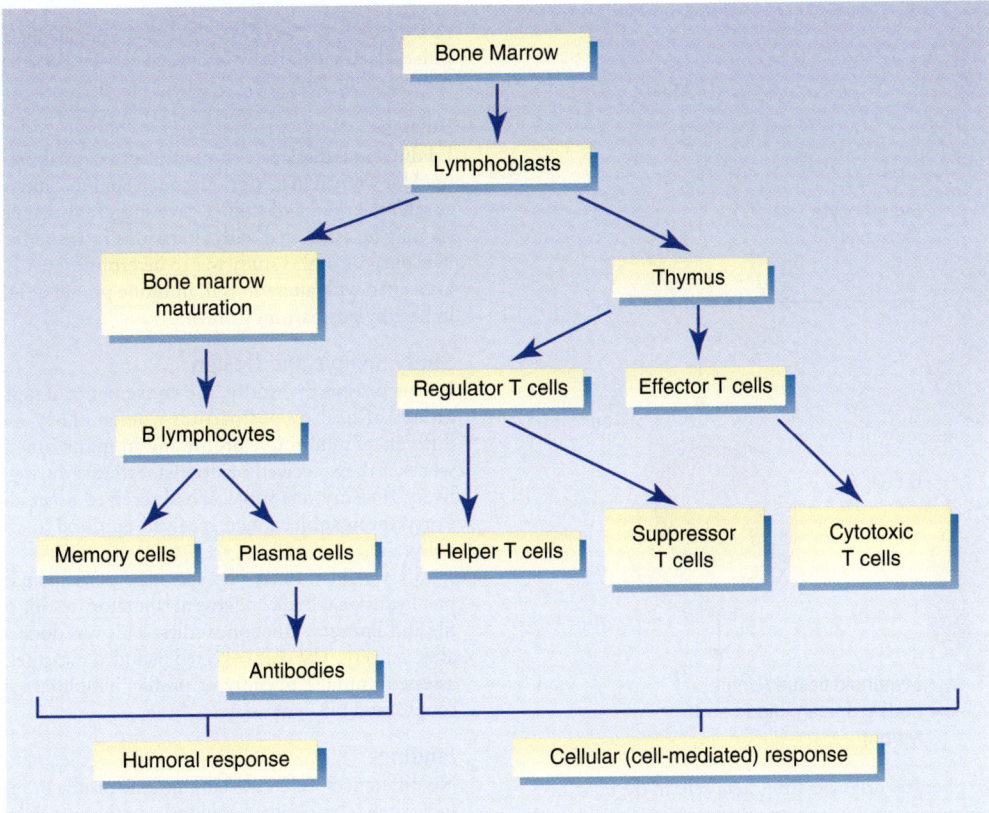

FIGURE 50-2 Development of cells of the immune system.

immune response. Weeks or months after exposure to the disease or vaccine, the body produces an immune response that is sufficient to defend against the disease upon re-exposure to it.

The two types of acquired immunity are known as active and passive. In active acquired immunity, the immunologic defenses are developed by the person's own body. This immunity generally lasts many years or even a lifetime.

Passive acquired immunity is temporary immunity transmitted from another source that has developed immunity through previous disease or immunization. For example, immune globulin and antiserum, obtained from the blood plasma of people with acquired immunity, are used in emergencies to provide immunity to diseases when the risk for contracting a specific disease is great and there is not enough time for a person to develop adequate active immunity. For example, immune globulin may be administered to those exposed to hepatitis. Immunity resulting from the transfer of antibodies from the mother to an infant in utero or through breastfeeding is another example of passive immunity. Active and passive acquired immunity involve humoral and cellular (cell-mediated) immunologic responses (described later in this chapter) (Ada, 2001).

Response to Invasion

When the body is invaded or attacked by bacteria, viruses, or other pathogens, it has three means of defending itself:

- The phagocytic immune response
- The humoral or antibody immune response
- The cellular immune response

The first line of defense, the **phagocytic immune response**, involves the WBCs (granulocytes and macrophages), which have the ability to ingest foreign particles. These cells move to the point of attack, where they engulf and destroy the invading agents. Phagocytes also remove the body's own dying or dead cells. Cells in necrotic tissue that are dying release substances that trigger an inflammatory response. **Apoptosis**, or programmed cell death, is the body's way of destroying unwanted cells such as cancer cells or cells that die a natural death. Apoptosis involves the digestion of DNA by endonucleases, resulting in the cells being targeted for phagocytosis (Delves & Roitt, 2000a).

Unlike macrophages, eosinophils are only weakly phagocytic. On activation, eosinophils probably kill parasites by releasing specific chemical mediators into the extracellular fluid. Additionally, they secrete leukotrienes, prostaglandins, and various cytokines (Delves & Roitt, 2000a).

A second protective response, the **humoral immune response** (sometimes called the **antibody** response), begins with the B lymphocytes, which can transform themselves into plasma cells that manufacture antibodies. These antibodies, highly specific proteins, are transported in the bloodstream and attempt to disable

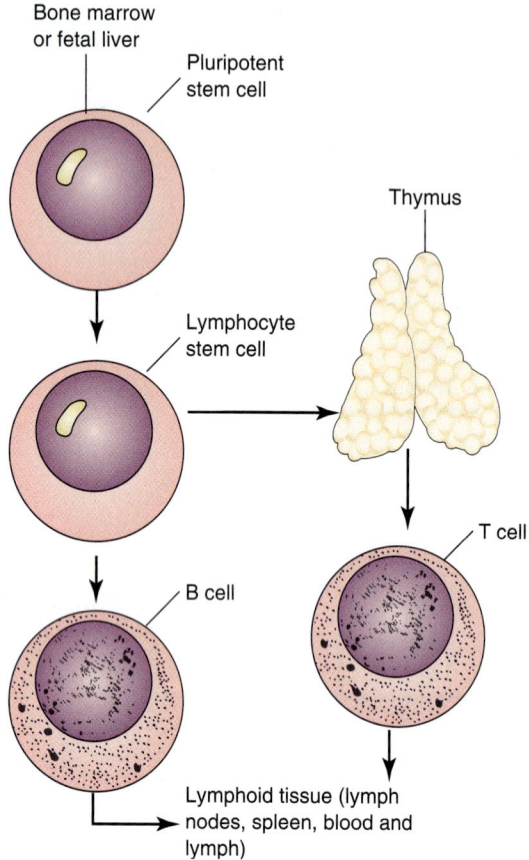

FIGURE 50-3 Lymphocytes originate from stem cells in the bone marrow. B-lymphocytes mature in the bone marrow before entering the bloodstream, whereas T lymphocytes mature in the thymus, where they also differentiate into cells with various functions. From Porth, C. M. (2002). *Pathophysiology: Concepts of altered health states* (6th ed.). Philadelphia: Lippincott Williams & Wilkins.

NURSING RESEARCH PROFILE 50-1
Epidural Anesthesia and Immune Response in Postpartum Women

Fehder, W. P., & Gennaro, S. G. (1998). Immune alterations associated with epidural anesthesia for labour and delivery. *Maternal Child Health Nursing, 23*(6), 292–299

Purpose
Epidural anesthesia is a common form of analgesia and anesthesia used for women in labour. Although epidural anesthesia is regarded as safe, the results of studies have suggested that epidural anesthesia may be associated with alterations in white blood cell counts. The purpose of this study was to determine if epidural anesthesia is associated with alterations in immune profile or immune function in healthy postpartum women.

Study Sample and Design
In this prospective study, the convenience sample included two groups of healthy postpartum women. They were assessed for differences in immune profile and immune function based upon whether they received epidural anesthesia during labour and delivery. Twenty-one subjects had received no epidural anesthesia. Forty-seven subjects had received epidural anesthesia for their deliveries.

Sixty-eight women who agreed to participate in the study and met inclusion criteria underwent laboratory testing for immune profile and immune function studies. This was done within 24 hours after delivery. The data collected included measures that specifically assessed immune phenotypic profile, lymphocyte proliferative response, and NK lysis assays.

Findings
No differences were noted in immune profile or immune function in women who received epidural anesthesia in labour versus those who did not.

Nursing Implications
This study demonstrated that white blood cell count and other phenotypic measures of leukocytes are not affected by epidural anesthesia. It is suggested that the epidural anesthesia technique does not alter immune response in postpartum women, although studies with larger samples are warranted. Efforts to support the immune response in women who receive epidural anesthesia should be comparable to women who do not receive epidural anesthesia.

---

the invaders. The third mechanism of defense, the **cellular immune response**, also involves the T lymphocytes, which can turn into special cytotoxic (or killer) T cells that can attack the pathogens themselves.

The part of the invading or attacking organism that is responsible for stimulating antibody production is called an **antigen** (or an immunogen). For example, an antigen can be a small patch of proteins on the outer surface of the microorganism. Not all antigens are naturally immunogenic and must be coupled to other molecules to stimulate the immune response. A single bacterium, even a single large molecule, such as a toxin (diphtheria or tetanus toxin), may have several such antigens, or markers, on its surface, thus inducing the body to produce a number of different antibodies. Once produced, an antibody is released into the bloodstream and carried to the attacking organism. There it combines with the antigen, binding with it like an interlocking piece of a jigsaw puzzle (Fig. 50-4). There are four well-defined stages in an immune response: recognition, proliferation, response, and effector.

RECOGNITION STAGE
Recognition of antigens as foreign, or nonself, by the immune system is the initiating event in any immune response. The body must first recognize invaders as foreign before it can react to them. The body accomplishes recognition using lymph nodes and lymphocytes for surveillance. Lymph nodes are widely distributed internally throughout the body and in the circulating blood, and externally near the body's surfaces. They continuously discharge small lymphocytes into the bloodstream. These lymphocytes patrol the tissues and vessels that drain the areas served by that node.

Lymphocytes recirculate from the blood to lymph nodes and from the lymph nodes back into the bloodstream, in a never-ending series of patrols. Some circulating lymphocytes can survive for decades. Some of these small, hardy cells maintain their solitary circuits for the person's lifetime.

The exact way in which circulating lymphocytes recognize antigens on foreign surfaces is not known; however, recognition is thought to depend on specific receptor sites on the surface of the lymphocytes. Macrophages play an important role

Physiology/Pathophysiology

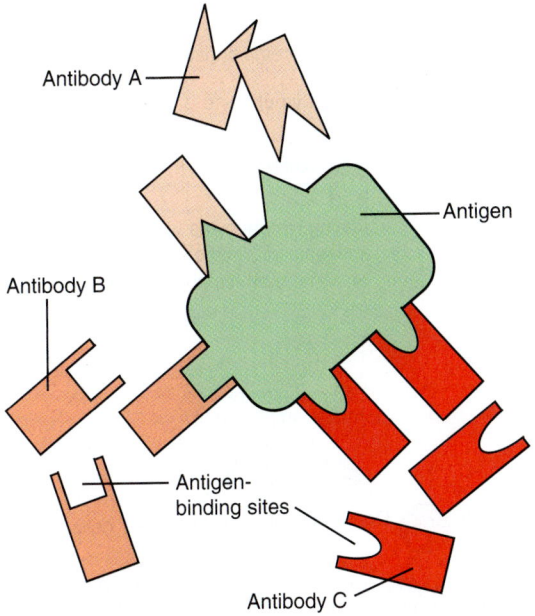

FIGURE 50-4 Antibody specificity. Antibodies are produced by B-cell lymphocytes to bind with specific antigens.

in helping the circulating lymphocytes process the antigens. Both macrophages and neutrophils have receptors for antibodies and complement; as a result, the coating of microorganisms with antibodies, complement, or both enhances phagocytosis. The engulfed microorganisms are then subjected to a wide range of toxic intracellular molecules. When foreign materials enter the body, a circulating lymphocyte comes into physical contact with the surfaces of these materials. Upon contact, the lymphocyte, with the help of macrophages, either removes the antigen from the surface or in some way picks up an imprint of its structure, which comes into play with subsequent re-exposure to the antigen.

In a streptococcal throat infection, for example, the streptococcal organism gains access to the mucous membranes of the throat. A circulating lymphocyte moving through the tissues of the neck comes in contact with the organism. The lymphocyte, familiar with the surface markers on the cells of its own body, recognizes the antigens on the microbe as different (nonself) and the streptococcal organism as antigenic (foreign). This triggers the second stage of the immune response—proliferation.

PROLIFERATION STAGE
The circulating lymphocyte containing the antigenic message returns to the nearest lymph node. Once in the node, the sensitized lymphocyte stimulates some of the resident dormant T and B lymphocytes to enlarge, divide, and proliferate. T lymphocytes differentiate into cytotoxic (or killer) T cells, whereas B lymphocytes produce and release antibodies. Enlargement of the lymph nodes in the neck in conjunction with a sore throat is one example of the immune response.

RESPONSE STAGE
In the response stage, the changed lymphocytes function either in a humoural or a cellular fashion. The production of antibodies by the B lymphocytes in response to a specific antigen begins the humoural response. Humoural refers to the fact that the antibodies are released into the bloodstream and so reside in the plasma (fluid fraction of the blood).

With the initial cellular response, the returning sensitized lymphocytes migrate to areas of the lymph node (other than those areas containing lymphocytes programmed to become plasma cells). Here, they stimulate the residing lymphocytes to become cells that will attack microbes directly rather than through the action of antibodies. These transformed lymphocytes are known as cytotoxic (killer) T cells. The T stands for thymus, signifying that during embryologic development of the immune system, these T lymphocytes spent time in the thymus of the developing fetus, where they were genetically programmed to become T lymphocytes rather than the antibody-producing B lymphocytes. Viral rather than bacterial antigens induce a cellular response. This response is manifested by the increasing number of T lymphocytes (lymphocytosis) seen in the blood smears of people with viral illnesses, such as infectious mononucleosis. (Cellular immunity is discussed in further detail later in this chapter.)

Most immune responses to antigens involve both humoural and cellular responses, although one usually predominates. For example, during transplantation rejection, the cellular response predominates, whereas in the bacterial pneumonias and sepsis, the humoural response plays the dominant protective role (Chart 50-1).

EFFECTOR STAGE
In the effector stage, either the antibody of the humoural response or the cytotoxic (killer) T cell of the cellular response reaches and couples with the antigen on the surface of the foreign invader. The coupling initiates a series of events that in most instances results in the total destruction of the invading microbes or the complete neutralization of the toxin. The events involve an interplay of antibodies (humoural immunity), complement, and action by the cytotoxic T cells (cellular immunity). Figure 50-5 summarizes the stages of the immune response.

 Role of Cellular and Humoural Immune Responses

Whereas B-cell antibodies are distinctive components of the humoural immune response, cytotoxic T cells are distinguishing components of the cellular immune response. Some specific roles of B cells and T cells are as follows:

Humoural Responses (B Cells)
- Bacterial phagocytosis and lysis
- Anaphylaxis
- Allergic hay fever and asthma
- Immune complex disease
- Bacterial and some viral infections

Cellular Responses (T Cells)
- Transplant rejection
- Delayed hypersensitivity (tuberculin reaction)
- Graft-versus-host disease
- Tumour surveillance or destruction
- Intracellular infections
- Viral, fungal, and parasitic infections

Physiology/Pathophysiology

FIGURE 50-5 Stages of the immune response. (**I**) In the *recognition stage,* antigens are recognized by circulating lymphocytes and macrophages. (**II**) In the *proliferation stage,* the dormant lymphocytes proliferate and differentiate into cytotoxic (killer) T cells or B cells responsible for formation and release of antibodies. (**III**) In the *response stage,* the cytotoxic T cells and the B cells perform cellular and humoral functions, respectively. (**IV**) In the *effector stage,* antigens are destroyed or neutralized through the action of antibodies, complement, macrophages, and cytotoxic T cells.

Humoural Immune Response

The humoural response is characterized by production of antibodies by the B lymphocytes in response to a specific antigen. Although the B lymphocyte is ultimately responsible for the production of antibodies, both the macrophages of natural immunity and the special T-cell lymphocytes of cellular immunity are involved in recognizing the foreign substance and in producing antibodies.

ANTIGEN RECOGNITION

Several theories exist about the mechanisms by which the B lymphocytes recognize the invading antigen and respond by producing antibodies. This is probably because the B lymphocytes recognize invading antigens in more than one way and respond in several ways as well. Additionally, the B lymphocytes appear to respond to some antigens by triggering antibody formation directly. In response to other antigens, however, they need the assistance of T cells to trigger antibody formation.

T cells (or T lymphocytes), part of a surveillance system dispersed throughout the body, recycle through the general circulation, tissues, and lymphatic system. With the assistance of macrophages, the T lymphocytes are believed to recognize the antigen of a foreign invader. The T lymphocyte picks up the antigenic message, or "blueprint," of the antigen and returns to the nearest lymph node with that message.

Production of B Lymphocytes. B lymphocytes stored in the lymph nodes are subdivided into thousands of clones, each responsive to a single group of antigens having almost identical characteristics. When the antigenic message is carried back to the lymph node, specific clones of the B lymphocyte are stimulated to enlarge, divide, proliferate, and differentiate into plasma cells capable of producing specific antibodies to the antigen. Other B lymphocytes differentiate into B-lymphocyte clones with a memory for the antigen. These memory cells are responsible for the more exaggerated and rapid immune response in a person who is repeatedly exposed to the same antigen.

ROLE OF ANTIBODIES

Antibodies are large proteins called immunoglobulins because they are found in the globulin fraction of the plasma proteins. All immunoglobulins are glycoproteins and contain a certain amount of carbohydrate. The carbohydrate concentration, which ranges from approximately 3% to 13%, is dependent upon the class of the antibody. Each antibody molecule consists of two subunits, each of which contains a light and a heavy peptide chain (Fig. 50-6). The subunits are held together by a chemical link composed of disulfide bonds. Each subunit has a portion that serves as a binding site for a specific antigen referred to as the Fab fragment. This site provides the "lock" portion that is highly specific for an antigen. An additional portion, known as the Fc fragment, allows the antibody molecule to take part in the complement system.

Antibodies defend against foreign invaders in several ways, and the type of defense employed depends on the structure and composition of both the antigen and the immunoglobulin. The antibody molecule has at least two combining sites, or Fab fragments. One antibody can act as a cross-link between two antigens, causing them to bind or clump together. This clumping effect, referred to as **agglutination**, helps clear the body of the invading organism by facilitating phagocytosis. Some antibodies assist in removing offending organisms through **opsonization**. In this process, the antigen–antibody molecule is coated with a sticky substance that also facilitates phagocytosis.

Antibodies also promote the release of vasoactive substances, such as histamine and slow-reacting substance, two of the chemical mediators of the inflammatory response.

Antibodies do not function in isolation but rather mobilize other components of the immune system to defend against the invader. Their usual role is to focus components of the natural immune system on the invader. This includes activation of the complement system and activation of phagocytosis (Delves & Roitt, 2000a).

Types of Immunoglobulins. The body can produce five different types of immunoglobulins. (Immunoglobulins are commonly designated by the abbreviation Ig.) Each of the five types, or classes, is identified by a specific letter of the alphabet (IgA, IgD, IgE, IgG, and IgM). Classification is based on the chemical structure and biologic role of the individual immunoglobulin. The following list summarizes major characteristics of the immunoglobulins:

IgG (75% of Total Immunoglobulin)
- Appears in serum and tissues (interstitial fluid)
- Assumes a major role in bloodborne and tissue infections
- Activates the complement system
- Enhances phagocytosis
- Crosses the placenta

IgA (15% of Total Immunoglobulin)
- Appears in body fluids (blood, saliva, tears, breast milk, and pulmonary, gastrointestinal, prostatic, and vaginal secretions)
- Protects against respiratory, gastrointestinal, and genitourinary infections
- Prevents absorption of antigens from food
- Passes to neonate in breast milk for protection

IgM (10% of Total Immunoglobulin)
- Appears mostly in intravascular serum
- Appears as the first immunoglobulin produced in response to bacterial and viral infections
- Activates the complement system

IgD (0.2% of Total Immunoglobulin)
- Appears in small amounts in serum
- Possibly influences B-lymphocyte differentiation, but role is unclear

IgE (0.004% of Total Immunoglobulin)
- Appears in serum
- Takes part in allergic and some hypersensitivity reactions
- Combats parasitic infections

ANTIGEN–ANTIBODY BINDING

The portion of the antigen involved in binding with the antibody is referred to as the antigenic determinant. The binding of the Fab fragment (antibody-binding site) to the antigenic determinant can be likened to a lock-and-key situation (Fig. 50-7). The most efficient immunologic responses occur when the antibody and antigen fit exactly. Poor fit can occur with an antibody that was produced in response to a different antigen. This phenomenon is known as cross-reactivity. For example, in acute rheumatic fever, the antibody produced against *Streptococcus pyogenes* in the upper respiratory tract may cross-react with the patient's heart tissue, leading to heart valve damage.

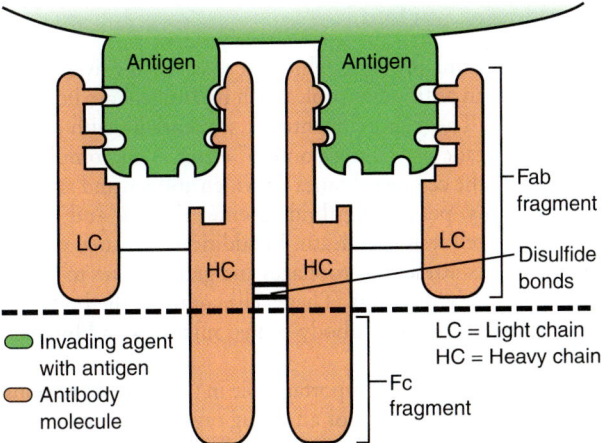

FIGURE 50-6 An antibody molecule. The Fab fragment serves as the binding site for a specific antigen. The Fc fragment initiates classic complement activation.

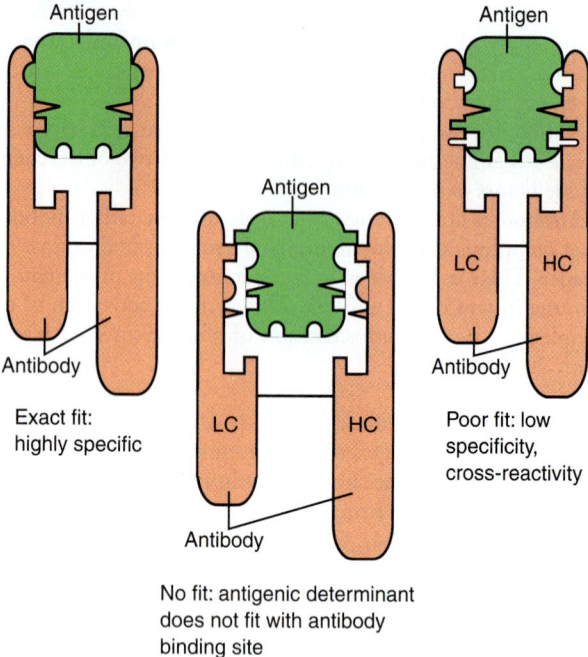

FIGURE 50-7 Antigen–antibody binding. (*Left*) A highly specific antigen–antibody complex. (*Middle*) No match and therefore, no immune response. (*Right*) Poor fit or match with low specificity; antibody reacts to antigen with similar characteristics, producing cross-reactivity.

Cellular Immune Response

Whereas the B lymphocytes are responsible for humoural immunity, the T lymphocytes (or T cells) are primarily responsible for cellular immunity. Stem cells continuously migrate from the bone marrow to the thymus gland, where they develop into T cells. T cells continue to develop in the thymus gland, despite partial degeneration of the thymus gland that occurs at puberty (Delves & Roitt, 2000a). By spending time in the thymus, these cells are programmed to become T cells rather than antibody-producing B lymphocytes. Several types of T cells exist, each with designated roles in the defense against bacteria, viruses, fungi, parasites, and malignant cells. T cells attack foreign invaders directly rather than by producing antibodies.

Cellular reactions are initiated by the binding of an antigen with an antigen receptor located on the surface of a T cell. This may occur with or without the assistance of macrophages. The T cells then carry the antigenic message, or blueprint, to the lymph nodes, where the production of other T cells is stimulated. Some T cells remain in the lymph nodes and retain a memory for the antigen. Other T cells migrate from the lymph nodes into the general circulatory system and ultimately to the tissues, where they remain until they either come in contact with their respective antigens or die.

ROLE OF T LYMPHOCYTES

Two major categories of effector T cells are helper T cells and cytotoxic T cells. These cells participate in destroying foreign organisms. Other T cells include suppressor T cells and memory T cells. T cells interact closely with B cells, indicating that humoural and cellular immune responses are not separate, unrelated processes but rather branches of the immune response that can and do affect each other.

Helper T cells are activated upon recognition of antigens and stimulate the rest of the immune system. When activated, helper T cells secrete **cytokines** that attract and activate B cells, cytotoxic T cells, natural killer cells, macrophages, and other cells of the immune system. Separate subpopulations of helper T cells produce different types of cytokines and determine whether the immune response will be the production of antibodies or a cell-mediated immune response. Helper T cells produce **lymphokines**, one category of cytokines. These lymphokines activate other T cells (interleukin-2 [IL-2]), natural and cytotoxic T cells (interferon-gamma), and other inflammatory cells (tumour necrosis factor). Helper T cells produce IL-4 and IL-5, lymphokines that activate B cells to grow and differentiate (Table 50-2).

Cytotoxic T cells (killer T cells) attack the antigen directly by altering the cell membrane and causing cell lysis (disintegration) and releasing cytolytic enzymes and cytokines. Lymphokines can recruit, activate, and regulate other lymphocytes and WBCs. These cells then assist in destroying the invading organism. Delayed-type hypersensitivity is an example of an immune reaction that protects the body from antigens through the production and release of lymphokines and is discussed in more detail later.

Another type of cell, the **suppressor T cell**, has the ability to decrease B-cell production, thereby keeping the immune response at a level that is compatible with health (eg, sufficient to fight infection adequately without attacking the body's healthy tissues). **Memory cells** are responsible for recognizing antigens from previous exposure and mounting an immune response (Table 50-3).

ROLES OF NULL LYMPHOCYTES AND NATURAL KILLER CELLS

Null lymphocytes and natural killer (NK) cells are other lymphocytes that assist in combating organisms. These are distinct from B cells and T cells and lack the usual characteristics of B cells and T cells. **Null lymphocytes**, a subpopulation of lymphocytes, destroy antigens already coated with antibody. These cells have special Fc receptor sites on their surfaces that allow them to couple with the Fc end of antibodies (antibody-dependent, cell-mediated cytotoxicity).

Natural killer cells, another subpopulation of lymphocytes, defend against microorganisms and some types of malignant cells. NK cells are capable of directly killing invading organisms and producing cytokines. The helper T cells contribute to the differentiation of null and NK cells.

Complement System

Circulating plasma proteins, which are made in the liver and activated when an antibody couples with its antigen, are known as **complement**. These proteins interact sequentially with one another in a cascade or "falling domino" effect. This complement cascade alters the cell membranes on which antigen and antibody complex forms, permitting fluid to enter the cell and leading eventually to cell lysis and death. In addition, activated complement molecules attract macrophages and granulocytes to areas of antigen–antibody reactions. These cells continue the body's defense by devouring the antibody-coated microbes and by releasing bacterial agents.

Complement plays an important role in the immune response. Destruction of an invading or attacking organism or toxin is not achieved merely by the binding of the antibody and antigens; it also requires activation of complement, the arrival of killer T cells, or the attraction of macrophages. Complement has three major physiologic functions: defending the body against bacterial infection,

Table 50-2 • Cytokines and Their Biologic Effects

CYTOKINE*	ACTION
Interleukin-1	Promotes differentiation of T and B cells, natural killer (NK) cells, and null cells
Interleukin-2	Stimulates growth of T cells and special activated killer lymphocytes (known as lymphocyte-activated killer cells [LAK cells])
Interleukin-3	Stimulates growth of mast cells and other blood cells
Interleukin-4	Stimulates growth of T and B cells, mast cells, and macrophages
Interleukin-5	Stimulates antibody responses
Interleukin-6	Stimulates growth and function of B cells and antibodies
Interleukin-7	Stimulates growth of pre-B, CD4, and CD8, T cells and activates mature T cells
Interleukin-8	Promotes chemotaxis and activation of neutrophils
Interleukin-9	Stimulates growth and proliferation of T cells
Interleukin-10	Inhibits interferon-gamma and mononuclear cell inflammation
Interleukin-11	Promotes induction of acute-phase proteins
Interleukin-12	Introduces helper T cells
Interleukin-13	Inhibits mononuclear phagocyte inflammation and promotes differentiation of B cells
Interleukin-16	Promotes chemotaxis CD4 T cells and eosinophils
Permeability factor	Increases vascular permeability, allowing white cells into area
Interferon	Interferes with viral growth, stopping the spread of viral infection
Migration inhibitory factor	Suppresses movement of macrophages, keeping macrophages in area of foreign cells
Skin reactive factor	Induces inflammatory response
Cytotoxic factor (lymphotoxin)	Kills certain antigenic cells
Macrophage chemotactic factor	Attracts macrophages into the area
Lymphocyte blastogenic factor	Stimulates more lymphocytes, recruiting additional lymphocytes into the area
Macrophage aggregation factor	Causes clumping of macrophages and lymphocytes
Macrophage activation factor	Allows macrophages to adhere to surfaces more readily
Proliferation inhibitor factor	Inhibits growth of certain antigenic cells
Cytophilic antibody	Binds to an Fc receptor on macrophages, thereby permitting macrophages to bind to antigens
Tumour necrosis factor (alpha)	Stimulates inflammation, wound healing, and tissue remodeling
Tumour necrosis factor (beta)	Mediates inflammation and graft rejection

*Cytokines are biologically active substances released by cells to regulate growth and function of other cells within the immune system. Lymphocytes produce lymphokines, and monocytes and macrophages produce monokines. This table lists some of the cytokines that play a role in immune system functioning.

bridging natural and acquired immunity, and disposing of immune complexes and the byproducts associated with inflammation (Walport, 2001a). Complement-mediated immune responses are summarized in Table 50-4.

There are several ways to activate the complement system: the classic pathway, the alternate pathway, and the lectin pathway (Delves & Roitt, 2000a).

CLASSIC PATHWAY OF COMPLEMENT ACTIVATION

The classic pathway (the first method discovered) is activated by antigen–antibody complexes; it begins when antibody binds to a cell surface and ends with lysis of the cell. It involves the reaction of the first of the circulating complement proteins (C_1) with the receptor site of the Fc portion of an antibody molecule after formation of an antigen–antibody complex. The activation of the first complement component then activates all the other components in the following sequence: C_4, C_2, C_3, C_5, C_6, C_7, C_8, and C_9. (The components are named in the sequence in which they were discovered.)

ALTERNATE AND LECTIN PATHWAYS

The alternate and lectin pathways of complement activation are activated without the formation of antigen–antibody complexes. These pathways can be initiated by the release of bacterial products, such as endotoxins. When complement is activated without the formation of antigen–antibody complexes, the process bypasses the first three components (C_1, C_4, and C_2) and begins with C_3. Whatever the method of activation, once activated, the complement destroys cells by altering or damaging the cell membrane of the antigen, by chemically attracting phagocytes to the antigen (chemotaxis), and by rendering the antigen more vulnerable to phagocytosis (opsonization). The complement system enhances the inflammatory response by releasing vasoactive substances.

Complement components, prostaglandins, leukotrienes, and other inflammatory mediators all contribute to the recruitment of inflammatory cells, as do chemokines, a group of cytokines. The activated neutrophils pass through the vessel walls to accumulate at the site of infection, where they phagocytose complement-coated microbes (Delves & Roitt, 2000a).

This response is usually therapeutic and can be lifesaving if the cell attacked by the complement system is a true foreign invader, such as a streptococcal or staphylococcal organism. If that cell, however, is in reality part of the person—a cell of the brain or liver, the tissue lining the blood vessels, or the cells of a transplanted organ or skin graft, for example—the result can be devastating disease and even death. The result of the immune response—the vigorous attack on any material identified as foreign, the deadliness of the struggle—is obvious in the purulent material, or pus (the remains of microbes, granulocytes, macrophages, T-cell lymphocytes, plasma proteins, complement, and antibodies), that accumulates in wound infections and abscesses. In addition, many autoimmune diseases (ie, systemic lupus erythematosus) and disorders characterized by chronic infection

Porth, C. M. (2002). *Pathophysiology: Concepts of altered health states* (6th ed.). Philadelphia: Lippincott Williams & Wilkins

Table 50-3 • Lymphocytes Involved in Immune Responses

CELL TYPE	FUNCTION	TYPE OF IMMUNE RESPONSE
B cell	Produces antibodies or immunoglobulins (IgA, IgD, IgE, IgG, IgM)	Humoural
T cell		Cellular
Helper T4	Attacks foreign invaders (antigens) directly	
	Initiates and augments inflammatory response	
Helper T_1	Increases activated cytotoxic T cells	
Helper T_2	Increases B-cell antibody production	
Suppressor T	Suppresses the immune response	
Memory T	Remembers contact with an antigen and on subsequent exposures mounts an immune response	
Cytotoxic T (killer T)	Lyses cells infected with virus; plays a role in graft rejection	
Non-T or non-B lymphocytes		Nonspecific
Null cells	Destroys antigens already coated with antibody	
Natural killer (NK) (granular lymphocyte)	Defends against microorganisms and some types of malignant cells; produces cytokines	

(ie, hepatitis C, bacterial endocarditis) and necrosis (myocardial infarction, stroke) are thought to be due in part to continued or chronic activation of complement, which in turn causes chronic inflammation (Walport, 2001b).

The red blood cells (erythrocytes) and platelets (thrombocytes) also have a role in the immune response. Red blood cells

Table 50-4 • Complement-Mediated Immune Responses

RESPONSE	EFFECTS
Cytolysis	Lysis and destruction of cell membranes of body cells or pathogens
Opsonization	Targeting of the antigen so that it can be easily engulfed and digested by the macrophages and other phagocytic cells
Chemotaxis	Chemical attraction of neutrophils and phagocytic cells to the antigen
Anaphylaxis	Activation of mast cells and basophils with release of inflammatory mediators that produce smooth muscle contraction and increased vascular permeability

and platelets have complement receptors and as a result play an important role in the clearance of immune complexes that consist of antigen, antibody, and components of the complement system (Delves & Roitt, 2000a).

Role of Interferons

Biologic response modifiers, such as the interferons, are under investigation to determine their roles in the immune system and their potential therapeutic effects in disorders characterized by disturbed immune responses. Interferons have antiviral and antitumour properties. In addition to responding to viral infection, they are produced by T lymphocytes, B lymphocytes, and macrophages in response to antigens. They are thought to modify the immune response by suppressing antibody production and cellular immunity. They also facilitate the cytolytic role of macrophages and NK cells. Interferons are undergoing extensive testing to evaluate their effectiveness in treating tumours and acquired immunodeficiency syndrome (AIDS). Some interferons are already used to treat immune-related disorders (eg, multiple sclerosis) and chronic inflammatory conditions (eg, chronic hepatitis).

Advances in Immunology

GENETIC ENGINEERING

One of the more remarkable technologies that is evolving is **genetic engineering**, which involves the use of recombinant DNA technology. Two facets exist with this technology. The first permits scientists to combine genes from one type of organism with genes of a second organism. This type of technology allows cells and microorganisms to manufacture proteins, monokines and lymphokines, which can alter and enhance immune system function. The second facet of recombinant DNA technology involves gene therapy. For example, if a particular gene is abnormal or missing, a recombinant gene can be inserted onto a virus particle. When the virus splices its genes, it will automatically insert the missing gene, which theoretically will correct the situation and revitalize the immune system in an immune deficiency disorder. These genes can be carried via harmless viruses, inactivated retroviruses, grafted onto a protein carrier, or hidden in fat globules that are known as liposomes (Delves & Roitt, 2000b). Extensive research into recombinant DNA technology and gene therapy is ongoing.

STEM CELLS

Stem cell research also is under way. The stem cell is known as a precursor cell that continually replenishes the body's entire supply of both red and white cells. Stem cells represent only a small portion of all types of bone marrow cells. Research conducted with mouse models has demonstrated that once the immune system has been destroyed experimentally, it can be completely restored with the implantation of just a few purified stem cells. Stem cell transplantation has been carried out in humans with certain types of immune dysfunction, such as severe combined immunodeficiency (SCID) (Parslow, Stites, Terr & Imboden, 2001). Clinical trials using stem cells are underway in patients with a variety of disorders with an autoimmune component, including systemic lupus erythematosus, rheumatoid arthritis, scleroderma, and multiple sclerosis (Davidson & Diamond, 2001).

IMMUNOREGULATION

A successful immune response eliminates the inciting antigen. Once the antigen that has stimulated the immune response is eliminated, the response returns to a nearly normal level. This process, known as **immunoregulation**, balances and counterbalances the immune response. For example, autoimmune diseases can be better controlled by suppressing areas of the immune system that are overactive and boosting those areas that are underactive. Immunoregulation research holds the promise of preventing graft rejection and aiding the body in dispersing cells that are cancerous or infected (Delves & Roitt, 2000b).

Assessment

An assessment of immune function begins with a health history and physical examination. The history should note the patient's age along with information about past and present conditions and events that may provide clues to the status of the patient's immune system. Areas to be addressed include nutritional status; infections and immunizations; allergies; disorder and disease states, such as autoimmune disorders, cancer, and chronic illnesses; surgery; medications; and blood transfusions. Physical assessment includes palpation of the lymph nodes and examination of the skin, mucous membranes, and respiratory, gastrointestinal, genitourinary, cardiovascular, and neurosensory systems (Chart 50-2).

HEALTH HISTORY

Age

Age is an important factor to elicit from the patient as people at the extremes of the life span are more likely to develop problems related to immune system functioning than are those in their middle years (Table 50-5).

 Gerontological Considerations

The frequency and severity of infections are increased in elderly people, possibly due to a decreased ability to respond adequately to invading organisms. Both the production and the function of T and B lymphocytes may be impaired. Responses to antigen stimulation may be altered, with increasing proportions of lymphocytes becoming unresponsive with age (Porth, 2002). The incidence of autoimmune diseases also increases with aging, possibly from a decreased ability of antibodies to differentiate between self and nonself. Failure of the surveillance system to recognize mutant, or abnormal, cells may be responsible for the high incidence of cancer associated with increasing age.

Declining function of various organ systems associated with increasing age also contributes to impaired immunity. Decreased gastric secretions and motility allow normal intestinal flora to proliferate and produce infection, causing gastroenteritis and diarrhea. Decreased renal circulation, filtration, absorption, and excretion contribute to risk for urinary tract infections. Moreover, prostatic enlargement and neurogenic bladder can impede urine passage and subsequently bacterial clearance through the urinary system. Urinary stasis, common in elderly people, permits the growth of microorganisms. Exposure to tobacco and environmental toxins impairs pulmonary function. Prolonged exposure to these agents decreases the elasticity of lung tissue, the effec-

Chart 50-2 • ASSESSMENT

Indications of Immune Dysfunction

Respiratory System
- Changes in respiratory rate
- Cough (dry or productive)
- Abnormal lung sounds (wheezing, crackles, rhonchi)
- Rhinitis
- Hyperventilation
- Bronchospasm

Cardiovascular System
- Hypotension
- Tachycardia
- Dysrhythmia
- Vasculitis
- Anemia

Gastrointestinal System
- Hepatosplenomegaly
- Colitis
- Vomiting
- Diarrhea

Genitourinary System
- Frequency and burning on urination
- Hematuria
- Discharge

Skin
- Rashes
- Lesions
- Dermatitis
- Hematomas or purpura
- Edema or urticaria
- Inflammation
- Discharge

Neurosensory System
- Cognitive dysfunction
- Hearing loss
- Visual changes
- Headaches and migraines
- Ataxia
- Tetany

tiveness of cilia, and the ability to cough effectively. These impairments hinder the removal of infectious organisms and toxins, increasing the elderly person's susceptibility to pulmonary infections and cancers.

Finally, with aging, the skin becomes thinner and less elastic. Peripheral neuropathy and the accompanying decreased sensation and circulation may lead to stasis ulcers, pressure ulcers, abrasions, and burns. Impaired skin integrity predisposes the aging person to infection from organisms that are part of normal skin flora.

Nutrition

The nurse assesses the patient's nutritional status, including caloric intake as well as the type of calories that the patient is consuming. Adequate nutrition is essential for optimal functioning of the immune system. Inadequate intake of vitamins that are essential for DNA and protein synthesis may lead to protein-calorie deficiency and subsequently to impaired immune function. Vitamins also

Table 50-5 • Age-Related Changes in Immunologic Function

BODY SYSTEM	CHANGES	CONSEQUENCES
Immune system	Impaired function of B and T lymphocytes Failure of lymphocytes to recognize mutant or abnormal cells Decreased antibody production Failure of immune system to differentiate "self" from "non-self" Suppressed phagocytic immune response	Suppressed responses to pathogenic organisms with increased risk for infection Increased incidence of cancers Anergy (lack of response to antigens applied to the skin [PPD, allergens]) Increased incidence of autoimmune diseases Absence of typical signs and symptoms of infection and inflammation Dissemination of organisms usually destroyed or suppressed by phagocytes (reactivation or spread of TB)
Gastrointestinal system	Decreased gastric secretions and motility Decreased phagocytosis by the liver's Kupffer cells Altered nutritional intake with inadequate protein intake	Proliferation of intestinal organisms resulting in gastroenteritis and diarrhea Increased incidence and severity of hepatitis B; increased incidence of liver abscesses Suppressed immune response
Urinary system	Decreased kidney function and changes in lower urinary tract function (enlargement of prostate gland, neurogenic bladder). Altered genitourinary tract flora.	Urinary stasis and increased incidence of urinary tract infections
Pulmonary system	Impaired ciliary action due to exposure to smoke and environmental toxins	Impaired clearance of pulmonary secretions; increased incidence of respiratory infections
Integumentary system	Thinning of skin with less elasticity; loss of adipose tissue	Increased risk of skin injury, breakdown and infection
Circulatory system	Impaired microcirculation	Stasis and pressure ulcers
Neurologic function	Decreased sensation and slowing of reflexes	Increased risk of injury (ulcers, abrasions, burns)

help in the regulation of cell proliferation and maturation of immune cells. Excess or deficiency of trace elements (ie, copper, iron, manganese, selenium, or zinc) in the diet generally suppresses immune function.

Fatty acids are the building blocks that make up the structural components of cell membranes. Lipids are precursors of vitamins A, D, E, and K as well as cholesterol. Both excess and deficiency of fatty acids have been found to suppress immune function.

Depletion of protein reserves results in atrophy of lymphoid tissues, depression of antibody response, reduction in the number of circulating T cells, and impaired phagocytic function. As a result, susceptibility to infection is greatly increased. During periods of infection and serious illness, nutritional requirements may be exaggerated further, potentially contributing to depletion of protein, fatty acid, vitamin, and trace elements and an even greater risk of impaired immune response and sepsis.

Infection and Immunization

The patient is asked about immunizations (including those received recently and those received in childhood) and the usual childhood diseases. Known past or present exposure to tuberculosis is assessed, and the dates and results of any tuberculin tests (purified protein derivative [PPD] or tine test) and chest x-rays are obtained. Recent patient exposure to any infections and the exposure dates are elicited. It is important for the nurse to assess whether the patient has been exposed to any sexually transmitted diseases and bloodborne pathogens such as hepatitis A, B, C, D, and E infections, and HIV infection. A history of sexually transmitted diseases, such as gonorrhea, syphilis, HPV infection, and chlamydia, can alert the nurse that the patient may have been exposed to HIV infection or hepatitis. A history of past and present infections and the dates and types of treatments that were used,

along with a history of any multiple persistent infections, fevers of unknown origin, lesions or sores, or any type of drainage, are obtained.

Allergy

The patient is asked about history of any allergies, including types of allergens (pollens, dust, plants, cosmetics, food, medications, vaccines), the symptoms experienced, and seasonal variations in occurrence or severity in the symptoms. A history of testing and treatments that the patient has received or is currently receiving for these allergies and the effectiveness of the treatments is obtained. All medication and food allergies are listed on an allergy alert sticker and placed on the front of the patient's health record or chart to alert others to the possibility of these allergies. Continued assessment for potential allergic reactions in this patient is vital.

Disorders and Diseases

AUTOIMMUNE DISORDERS

The patient is asked about any autoimmune disorders, such as lupus erythematosus, rheumatoid arthritis, or psoriasis. The onset, severity, remissions and exacerbations, functional limitations, treatments that the patient has received or is currently receiving, and the effectiveness of the treatments are described. Although most autoimmune disorders are individually rare, together they affect approximately 5% of the U.S. population. The occurrence of different autoimmune diseases within a family strongly suggests a genetic predisposition to more than one autoimmune disease (Davidson & Diamond, 2001).

In general, autoimmune disorders are more common in females than in males. This is believed to be the result of the activity of the sex hormones. The ability of sex hormones to modulate immunity has been well established. There is evidence that estrogen modulates the activity of T lymphocytes (especially suppressor cells), whereas androgens act to preserve IL-2 production and suppressor cell activity. The effects of sex hormones on B cells are less pronounced. Estrogen activates the autoimmune-associated B-cell population that expresses the CD5 marker (an antigenic marker on the B cell). Estrogen tends to enhance immunity, whereas androgen tends to be immunosuppressive.

NEOPLASTIC DISEASE

A history of cancer in the patient is obtained, along with the type of cancer and date of diagnosis. Dates and results of any cancer screening tests are also obtained.

Immunosuppression contributes to the development of cancers; however, cancer itself is immunosuppressive. Large tumours can release antigens into the blood, and these antigens combine with circulating antibodies and prevent them from attacking the tumour cells. Furthermore, tumour cells may possess special block-

ing factors that coat tumour cells and prevent destruction by killer T lymphocytes. During the early development of tumours, the body may fail to recognize the tumour antigens as foreign and subsequently fail to initiate destruction of the malignant cells. Hematologic cancers, such as leukemia and lymphoma, are associated with altered production and function of WBCs and lymphocytes.

All treatments that the patient has received or is currently receiving, such as radiation or chemotherapy, are identified and documented in the health history. Radiation destroys lymphocytes and decreases the population of cells required to replace them. The size or extent of the irradiated area determines the extent of immunosuppression. Whole-body irradiation may leave the patient totally immunosuppressed. Chemotherapy also destroys immune cells and causes immunosuppression.

A family history of cancer is obtained. If there is a family history of cancer, the type of cancer, age of onset, and relationship (maternal or paternal) of the patient to the affected family member is noted. (See Genetics in Nursing Practice.)

GENETICS IN NURSING PRACTICE—Immunologic Disorders

IMMUNOLOGIC DISORDERS INFLUENCED BY GENETIC FACTORS

- Ankylosing spondylitis
- Ataxia-telangiectasia
- Bloom syndrome
- Common variable immunodeficiency
- Fanconi anemia
- Rheumatoid arthritis
- Systemic lupus erythematosus (SLE)
- Severe combined immune deficiency (SCID)

NURSING ASSESSMENTS

FAMILY HISTORY ASSESSMENT

- Inquire about rheumatic diseases such as rheumatoid arthritis, ankylosing spondylitis, and systemic lupus erythematosus in other family members in several generations.
- Inquire about ethnic background (eg, Bloom syndrome is common among individuals of Ashkenazi heritage).
- Assess family history for closely related members with immune deficiency.
- Determine the age of onset of symptoms in affected family members (eg, for SCID, symptoms of pneumonia and unresponsive candidiasis are evident within the first 3 months of life).

PHYSICAL ASSESSMENT

- In children, assess for other clinical signs of immune dysfunction, including failure to thrive, growth retardation, developmental delays, pallor, irritability.
- Assess skin for cutaneous telangiectases (spider-like blood vessels in ataxia telangiectasia, or as in Bloom syndrome in a butterfly pattern on the nose and cheeks).
- Assess for hyperpigmentation, short stature, and other organ involvement seen in Fanconi anemia.

MANAGEMENT ISSUES SPECIFIC TO GENETICS

- Inquire whether DNA mutation or other genetic testing has been performed on affected family members.

- If indicated, refer for further genetic counselling and evaluation so that family members can discuss inheritance, risk to other family members, availability of genetic testing and gene-based interventions.
- Offer appropriate genetics information and resources.
- Assess patient's understanding of genetics information.
- Provide support to families with newly diagnosed genetic-related immune disorders.
- Participate in management and coordination of care of patients with genetic conditions and individuals predisposed to develop or pass on a genetic condition.

GENETIC RESOURCES FOR NURSES AND THEIR PATIENTS ON THE WEB

Genetic Alliance http://www.geneticalliance.org—a directory of support groups for patients and families with genetic conditions

Gene Clinics http://www.geneclinics.org—a listing of common genetic disorders with clinical summaries, genetic counselling and testing information

Genes and Diseases http://www.ncbi.nlm.nih.gov/books/bv.fcgi?rid=gnd—information about each chromosome and about diseases associated with each chromosome

Immune Deficiency Foundation http://www.primaryimmune.org—offers general information, peer support, and other resources for families with immune disorders

Medicine and the New Genetics http:www.ornl.gov/sci/techresources/Human_Genome/medicine/medicine.shtml—information on the Human Genome project and gene testing and genetic counselling

National Organization of Rare Disorders http://www.rarediseases.org—a directory of support groups and information for patients and families with rare genetic disorders

OMIM: Online Mendelian Inheritance in Man http://www.ncbi.nlm.nih.gov/omim/stats/html—a complete listing of inherited genetic conditions

CHRONIC ILLNESS AND SURGERY

The health assessment includes a history of chronic illnesses, such as diabetes mellitus, renal disease, or chronic obstructive pulmonary disease. The onset and severity of illnesses, as well as treatment that the patient is receiving for the illness, are obtained. Chronic illness may contribute to immune system impairments in various ways. Renal failure is associated with a deficiency in circulating lymphocytes. In addition, immune defenses may be altered by acidosis and uremic toxins. In diabetes, an increased incidence of infection has been associated with vascular insufficiency, neuropathy, and poor control of serum glucose levels. Recurrent respiratory tract infections are associated with chronic obstructive pulmonary disease as a result of altered inspiratory and expiratory function and ineffective airway clearance. Additionally, a history of surgical removal of the spleen, lymph nodes, or thymus or a history of organ transplantation is noted because these conditions may place the patient at risk for impaired immune function.

SPECIAL PROBLEMS

Conditions such as burns and other forms of injury and infection may contribute to altered immune system function. Major burns or other factors cause impaired skin integrity and compromise the body's first line of defense. Loss of large amounts of serum with burn injuries depletes the body of essential proteins, including immunoglobulins. The physiologic and psychological stressors associated with surgery or injury stimulate cortisol release from the adrenal cortex; increased serum cortisol also contributes to suppression of normal immune responses.

Medications and Blood Transfusions

A list of past and present medications is obtained. In large doses, antibiotics, corticosteroids, cytotoxic agents, salicylates, nonsteroidal anti-inflammatory drugs (NSAIDs), and anesthetics can cause immune suppression (Table 50-6).

A history of blood transfusions is obtained because previous exposure to foreign antigens through transfusion may be associated with abnormal immune function. Additionally, although the risk of human immunodeficiency virus (HIV) transmission through blood transfusion is extremely low in patients who received a transfusion after 1985 (the year that testing of blood for HIV was initiated in the United States), a risk still exists.

The patient is also asked about use of herbal agents and over-the-counter medications. Because many of these products have not been subjected to rigorous testing, not all of their effects have been identified. It is important, therefore, to ask patients about their use of these substances and to document their use.

Lifestyle and Other Factors

Like any other body system, the immune system functions depend on other body systems. A detailed history of smoking, alcohol consumption, dietary intake and nutritional status, amount of perceived stress, injection drug use, sexual practices, sexually transmitted diseases, and occupational or residential exposure to radiation or pollutants is obtained. Poor nutritional status, smoking, excessive consumption of alcohol, injection drug use, sexually transmitted diseases, and exposure to environmental radiation and pollutants have been associated with impaired immune function and are assessed in the patient history.

Table 50-6 • Selected Medications and Effects on the Immune System

DRUG CLASSIFICATION (AND EXAMPLES)	EFFECTS ON THE IMMUNE SYSTEM
Antibiotics (in large doses)	***Bone Marrow Suppression***
ceftriaxone (Rocefin)	Eosinophilia, hemolytic anemia, hypoprothrombinemia, neutropenia, thrombocytopenia
cefuroxime sodium (Ceftin)	Eosinophilia, hemolytic anemia, hypoprothrombinemia, neutropenia, thrombocytopenia
chloramphenicol (Chloromycetin)	Leukopenia, aplastic anemia
dactinomycin (Cosmogen)	Agranulocytosis, neutropenia
fluoroquinolones (Cipro, Levaquin, Tequin)	Hemolytic anemia, methemoglobinemia, eosinophilia, leukopenia, pancytopenia
gentamicin sulfate (Garamycin)	Agranulocytosis, granulocytosis
macriolides (erythromycin, Zithromax, Biaxin)	Neutropenia, leukopenia
penicillins	Agranulocytosis
streptomycin	Leukopenia, neutropenia, pancytopenia
vancomycin (Vancocin, Vancoled)	Transient leukopenia
Antithyroid Drugs	
propylthiouracil (PTU)	Agranulocytosis, leukopenia
Nonsteroidal Anti-inflammatory Drugs (NSAIDs) (in large doses)	***Inhibit Prostaglandin Synthesis or Release***
aspirin	Agranulocytosis
cox-2 inhibitors (Vioxx, Celebrex, Bextra)	Anemia, allergy, no major other adverse affects to the immune system
ibuprofen (Advil, Motrin)	Leukopenia, neutropenia
indomethacin (Indocid, Indocin)	Agranulocytosis, leukopenia
phenylbutazone	Pancytopenia, agranulocytosis, aplastic anemia
Adrenal Corticosteroids	***Immunosuppression***
prednisone	
Antineoplastic Agents (Cytotoxic Agents)	***Immunosuppression***
alkylating agents	Leukopenia
cyclophosphamide (Cytoxan)	Leukopenia, neutropenia
mechlorethamine HCl (Mustargen)	Agranulocytosis, neutropenia
cyclosporine	Leukopenia, inhibits T-cell function
Antimetabolites	***Immunosuppression***
fluorouracil (pyrimidine antagonist)	Leukopenia, eosinophilia
methotrexate (folic acid antagonist)	Leukopenia, aplastic bone marrow
mercaptopurine (6-MP) (purine antagonist)	Leukopenia, pancytopenia

PSYCHONEUROIMMUNOLOGIC FACTORS

The assessment also addresses psychoneuroimmunologic factors. It is thought that the immune response is regulated and modulated in part by neuroendocrine influences. Lymphocytes and macrophages have receptors capable of responding to neurotransmitters and endocrine hormones. Lymphocytes can produce and secrete adrenocorticotropic hormone and endorphin-like compounds. Neurons in the brain, especially in the hypothalamus, can recognize prostaglandins, interferons, and interleukins as well as histamine and serotonin, which are released during the inflammatory process. Like all other biologic systems functioning in the interest of homeostasis, the immune system is integrated with other psychophysiologic processes and is subject to regulation and modulation by the brain.

Conversely, the immune processes can affect neural and endocrine function, including behaviour. Thus, the interaction of the nervous system and immune system appears to be bidirectional. Growing evidence indicates that measurable immune system parameters can be influenced by biobehavioural strategies involving self-regulation. Examples of these strategies are relaxation and imagery techniques, biofeedback, humour, hypnosis, and conditioning. The assessment should address the patient's general psychological status and the patient's use of these strategies.

PHYSICAL EXAMINATION

On physical examination (see Chart 50-2), the skin and mucous membranes are assessed for lesions, dermatitis, purpura (subcutaneous bleeding), urticaria, inflammation, or any discharge. Any signs of infection are noted. The patient's temperature is recorded, and the patient is observed for chills and sweating. The anterior and posterior cervical, axillary, and inguinal lymph nodes are palpated for enlargement; if palpable nodes are detected, the location, size, consistency, and reports of tenderness upon palpation are noted. Joints are assessed for tenderness and swelling and for limited range of motion. The patient's respiratory, cardiovascular, gastrointestinal, genitourinary, and neurosensory status is evaluated for signs and symptoms indicative of immune dysfunction. The patient's nutritional status, level of stress, and coping ability are also assessed, along with his or her age and any functional limitations or disabilities.

Diagnostic Evaluation

A series of blood tests and skin tests and a bone marrow biopsy may be performed to evaluate the patient's immune competence. Specific laboratory and diagnostic tests are discussed in greater detail along with specific disease processes in subsequent chapters in this unit. Laboratory and diagnostic tests used to evaluate immune competence are summarized in Chart 50-3.

Nursing Management

The nurse needs to be aware that patients undergoing evaluation for possible immune system disorders experience not only physical pain and discomfort with certain types of diagnostic procedures, but many psychological reactions as well. For example, patients may fear test results that demonstrate decreased immune function that makes them more prone to certain infections, cancers, and other disorders. It is the nurse's role to counsel, educate, and support patients throughout the diagnostic process. Further, many patients may be extremely anxious about the results of diagnostic tests and the possible implications of those results for their employment, insurance, and personal relationships. This is an opportune time for the nurse to provide counselling and education should these interventions be warranted.

Chart 50-3   Selected Tests for Evaluating Immunologic Status

Various laboratory tests may be performed to assess immune system activity or dysfunction. The studies assess leukocytes and lymphocytes, humoural immunity, cellular immunity, phagocytic cell function, complement activity, hypersensitivity reactions, specific antigen–antibodies, or HIV infection.

Leukocytes and Lymphocyte Tests
- White blood cell count and differential
- Bone marrow biopsy

Humoural (Antibody-Mediated) Immunity Tests
- B-cell quantification with monoclonal antibody
- In vivo immunoglobulin synthesis with T-cell subsets
- Specific antibody response
- Total serum globulins and individual immunoglobulins (by electrophoresis, immunoelectrophoresis, single radial immunodiffusion, nephelometry, isohemagglutinin techniques)

Cellular (Cell-Mediated) Immunity Tests
- Total lymphocyte count
- T-cell and T-cell subset quantification with monoclonal antibody
- Delayed hypersensitivity skin test
- Cytokine production
- Lymphocyte response to mitogens, antigens, and allogenic cells
- Helper and suppressor T-cell functions

Phagocytic Cell Function Tests
- Nitroblue tetrazolium reductase assay

Complement Component Tests
- Total serum hemolytic complement
- Individual complement component titrations
- Radial immunodiffusion
- Electroimmunoassay
- Radioimmunoassay
- Immunonephelometric assay
- Immunoelectrophoresis

Hypersensitivity Tests
- Scratch test
- Patch test
- Intradermal test
- Radioallergosorbent test (RAST)

Specific Antigen-antibody Tests
- Radioimmunoassay
- Immunofluorescence
- Agglutination
- Complement fixation test

HIV Infection Tests
- Enzyme-linked immunosorbent assay (ELISA)
- Western blot
- CD4 and CD8 cell counts
- P24 antigen test
- Polymerase chain reaction (PCR)

Critical Thinking Exercises

1. An 18-year-old man presents for a physical examination to enter college. His mother asks if her son should receive a vaccination to prevent meningococcal meningitis. How would you respond? What recommendations would you give her, and why?

2. A 68-year-old woman is hospitalized for a heart transplant, and immune suppressant medications are given. Describe the parameters you would use to assess her immune function. How would altered immune function affect the care that you provide?

3. An 84-year-old woman who lives alone and has a long history of use of corticosteroids to treat rheumatoid arthritis is hospitalized with pneumonia. Discuss the changes in her immune status due to aging that need to be considered in her care. Identify the assessment strategies that are indicated.

REFERENCES AND SELECTED READINGS

Books

Abbas, A. K., & Lichtman, A. H. (2001). *Basic immunology: Functions and disorders of the immune system*. Philadelphia: W. B. Saunders Co.

Buttaro, T. M., Trybulski, J., Bailey, P. P., & Sandberg-Cook, J. (1999). *Primary care: A collaborative practice*. St. Louis, MO: Mosby, Inc.

Eisenhauer, L., Nichols, L. W., Spencer, R. T., & Bergan, F. W. (1998). *Clinical pharmacology and nursing management* (5th ed.). Philadelphia: Lippincott-Raven.

Goroll, A. H., & Mulley, A. G. Jr. (2000). *Primary care medicine* (4th ed.). Philadelphia: Lippincott Williams & Wilkins.

Huether, S. E., & McCance, K. L. (2000). *Understanding pathophysiology* (2d ed.). St. Louis, MO: Mosby, Inc.

Molony, S. L., Waszynski, C. M., & Lyder, C. H. (1999). *Gerontological nursing: An advanced practice approach*. Stamford, CT: Appleton & Lange.

Parkinson, C. F. (2000). *Study guide and workbook for understanding pathophysiology* (2d ed.). St. Louis, MO: Mosby, Inc.

Parslow, T. G., Stites, D. P., Terr, A. K., & Imboden, J. B. (2001). *Medical immunology* (10th ed.). New York: McGraw-Hill.

Porth, C. M., (2002). *Pathophysiology: Concepts of altered health states*. Philadelphia: Lippincott Williams & Wilkins.

Rich, R. (Ed.) (2001). *Clinical immunology: Principles and practice* (Vol. II). Philadelphia: Mosby.

Roitt, I., & Delves, P. J. (2001). *Roitt's essential immunology*. Malden, MA: Blackwell Science.

Journals

Asterisks indicate nursing research articles.

Ada, G. (2001). Vaccines and vaccination. *New England Journal of Medicine, 345*(14), 1042–1053.

Davidson, A., & Diamond, B. (2001). Advances in immunology: Autoimmune diseases. *New England Journal of Medicine, 345*(5), 340–350.

Delves, P. J., & Roitt, I. M. (2000*a*). Advances in immunology: The immune system (first of two parts). *New England Journal of Medicine, 343*(1), 37–49.

Delves, P. J., & Roitt, I. M. (2000*b*). Advances in immunology: The immune system (second of two parts). *New England Journal of Medicine, 343*(2), 108–117.

Fehder, W. P., & Douglas, S. D. (2001). Interactions between the nervous and immune systems. *Seminars in Clinical Neuropsychiatry, 6*(4), 229–240.

*Fehder, W. P., & Gennaro, S. (1998). Immune alterations associated with epidural analgesia for labor and delivery. *Maternal Child Health Nursing, 23*(6), 292–299.

Luster, A. D. (1998). Chemokines—chemotactic cytokines that mediate inflammation. *New England Journal of Medicine, 338*(7), 436–445.

Medahitov, R., & Janeway C. Jr. (2000). Innate immunity. *New England Journal of Medicine, 343*(5), 338–344.

Walport, M. J. (2001*a*). Advances in immunology: Complement (first of two parts). *New England Journal of Medicine, 344*(14), 1058–1066.

Walport, M. J. (2001*b*). Advances in immunology: Complement (second of two parts). *New England Journal of Medicine, 344*(14), 1140–1144.

RESOURCES AND WEBSITES

Canadian Institute for Health Information, 377 Dalhousie Street, Suite 200, Ottawa ON, K1N 9N8; (613) 241-7860; http://www.cihi.ca.

Centers for Disease Control and Prevention, 1600 Clifton Road, Atlanta, GA 30333; (404) 639-3311, (800) 311-3435; http://www.cdc.gov.

National Institute of Allergy and Infectious Disease, Office of Communication and Public Liaison, Building 31, Room 7A-50, 31 Center Drive MSC 2520, Bethesda, MD, 20892-2520; http://www.niaid.nih.gov/.

National Institutes of Health, Bethesda, Maryland; http://nih.gov. For toll-free information line for NIH departments: http://www.nih.gov/health/infoline.htm.

The Canadian Allergy, Asthma and Immunology Foundation, 774 Echo Drive, Ottawa, ON K1S 5N8; (613) 730-6272; http://www.allergyfoundation.ca.

The Canadian Society of Allergy and Clinical Immunology, 774 Echo Drive, Ottawa, ON K1S 5N8; (613) 730-6272; http://csaci.medical.org.

Management of Patients With Immunodeficiency

Adapted by Wanda Pierson

On completion of this chapter, the learner will be able to:

1. Compare the different types of primary immunodeficiency disorders, addressing causes, clinical manifestations, management, possible complications, and available treatments.
2. Discuss the possible management of patients with immunodeficiency disorders.
3. Describe the nursing management of the patient with an immunodeficiency.
4. Identify the teaching points necessary for a patient with an immunodeficiency.

*I*mmunodeficiency disorders may be caused by a defect or deficiency in phagocytic cells, B lymphocytes, T lymphocytes, or the complement system. The specific symptoms and their severity, age of onset, and prognosis depend on the immune system components affected and their degree of functional impairment. Regardless of the underlying cause, the cardinal symptoms of immunodeficiency include chronic or recurrent severe infections, infections caused by unusual organisms or organisms that are normal body flora, poor response to treatment of infections, and chronic diarrhea. In addition, the patient is susceptible to a variety of secondary disorders, including cancer (Buckley, 2000).

Immunodeficiencies may be classified as either primary or secondary and by the components of the immune system that are affected. Primary immunodeficiency diseases are genetic in origin and are caused by intrinsic defects in the cells of the immune system. This is in contrast to secondary immunodeficiencies such as AIDS, caused by infection with human immunodeficiency virus (HIV). Knowledge of the immune system and of the possibility of secondary disorders, skillful assessment and management, and sensitivity and responsiveness to the learning needs of the patient and caregiver are the essential elements for effective nursing care.

Primary Immunodeficiencies

Primary immunodeficiencies, rare disorders with genetic origins, are seen primarily in infants and young children. To date, more than 95 immunodeficiencies of genetic origin have been identified (Buckley, 2000). Symptoms usually develop early in life after protection from maternal antibodies decreases. Without treatment, infants and children with these disorders seldom survive to adulthood. These disorders may involve one or more components of the immune system. Symptoms of immune deficiency diseases are related to the role that the deficient component normally plays (Table 51-1).

PHAGOCYTIC DYSFUNCTION
Pathophysiology

A variety of primary defects of phagocytes may occur; nearly all of them are genetic in origin and affect the innate immune system. In some types of phagocytic disorders, the neutrophils are impaired so that they cannot exit the circulation and travel to sites of infection. As a result the patient cannot mount a normal inflammatory response against pathogenic organisms (Lekstrom-Himes & Gallin, 2002). In some disorders, the neutrophil count may be very low; in others, it may be very high because the neutrophils remain in the vascular system.

Clinical Manifestations

Phagocytic cell disorders are manifested by an increased incidence of bacterial and fungal infections due to normally nonpathogenic organisms (Lekstrom-Himes & Gallin, 2002). People with these disorders may also develop fungal infections from Candida organisms and viral infections from herpes simplex or herpes zoster virus. These patients experience recurrent furunculosis, cutaneous abscesses, chronic eczema, bronchitis, pneumonia, chronic otitis media, and sinusitis. In one type of phagocytic disorder, hyper-immunoglobulinemia E (HIE) syndrome, formerly known as Job syndrome, white blood cells cannot produce an inflammatory response to the skin infections; this results in deep-seated cold abscesses that lack the classic signs and symptoms of inflammation (redness, heat, and pain).

While patients with phagocytic cell disorders may be asymptomatic, severe neutropenia may be accompanied by deep and painful mouth ulcers, gingivitis, stomatitis, and cellulitis. Death from overwhelming infection occurs in about 10% of patients with severe neutropenia. Chronic granulomatous disease, another type of primary phagocytic disorder, produces recurrent or persistent infections of the soft tissues, lungs, and other organs; these are resistant to aggressive treatment with antibiotics (Lekstrom-Himes & Gallin, 2002).

Assessment and Diagnostic Findings

Diagnosis is based on the history, signs and symptoms, and laboratory analysis of the cytocidal (causing the death of cells) activity of the phagocytic cells by the nitroblue tetrazolium reductase test (see Chart 50-3 in Chap. 50). A history of recurrent infection and fever in a child and occasionally in an adult is an important key to the diagnosis. Failure of an infection to resolve with usual treatment is also an important indicator (Lekstrom-Himes & Gallin, 2002). See Chart 51-1 for a summary of warning signs of primary immunodeficiency disorders.

Medical Management

Because the signs and symptoms of infection are often blunted because of an impaired inflammatory response, early diagnosis and treatment of infectious complications can be lifesaving (Lekstrom-Himes & Gallin, 2002). Management of phagocytic cell disorders includes treating bacterial infections with prophylactic antibiotic therapy. Additional treatment for fungal and viral infections is often needed. Granulocyte transfusions, although used, are seldom successful because of the short half-life of the cells. Treatment with granulocyte-macrophage colony-stimulating factor (GM-CSF) or granulocyte colony-stimulating factor (G-CSF) may

Glossary

agammaglobulinemia: disorder marked by an almost complete lack of immunoglobulins or antibodies

angioneurotic edema: condition marked by development of urticaria and an edematous area of skin, mucous membranes, or viscera

ataxia: uncoordinated muscle movement

ataxia-telangiectasia: autosomal recessive disorder affecting T- and B-cell immunity primarily seen in children and resulting in a degenerative brain disease

hypogammaglobulinemia: lack of one or more of the five immunoglobulins; caused by B-cell deficiency

immunocompromised host: person with a secondary immunodeficiency and associated immunosuppression

panhypoglobulinemia: general lack of immunoglobulins in the blood

severe combined immunodeficiency disease (SCID): disorder involving a complete absence of humoural and cellular

immunity resulting from an X-linked or autosomal genetic abnormality

telangiectasia: vascular lesions caused by dilated blood vessels

thymic hypoplasia: T-cell deficiency that occurs when the thymus gland fails to develop normally during embryogenesis; also known as DiGeorge syndrome

Wiskott-Aldrich syndrome: immunodeficiency characterized by thrombocytopenia and the absence of T and B cells

Table 51-1 • Selected Primary Immunodeficiency Disorders

IMMUNE COMPONENT	DISORDER	MAJOR SYMPTOMS	TREATMENT
Phagocytic cells	Hyperimmunoglobulinemia E (HIE) syndrome	Bacterial, fungal, and viral infections; deep-seated cold abscesses	Antibiotic therapy and treatment for viral and fungal infections Granulocyte-macrophage colony-stimulating factor (GM-CSF); granulocyte colony-stimulating factor (G-CSF)
B lymphocytes	Sex-linked agammaglobulinemia (Bruton's disease)	Severe infections soon after birth	Passive pooled plasma or gamma-globulin
	Common variable immuno-deficiency (CVID)	Bacterial infections, infection with *Giardia lamblia*	IV immunoglobulin Metronidazole (Flagyl) Quinacrine HCl (Atabrine)
		Pernicious anemia Chronic respiratory infections	Vitamin B$_{12}$ Antimicrobial therapy
	Immunoglobulin A (IgA) deficiency	Predisposition to recurrent infections, adverse reactions to blood transfusions or immunoglobulin, autoimmune diseases, hypothyroidism	None
	IgC$_2$ deficiency	Heightened incidence of infectious diseases	Pooled immunoglobulin
T lymphocytes	Thymic hypoplasia (DiGeorge syndrome)	Recurrent infections; hypoparathyroidism; hypocalcemia, tetany, convulsions; congenital heart disease; possible renal abnormalities; abnormal facies	Thymus graft

	Chronic mucocutaneous candidiasis	*Candida albicans* infections of mucous membrane, skin, and nails; endocrine abnormalities (hypoparathyroidism, Addison's disease)	Antifungal agents:
			  Topical: miconazole
			  Oral: clotrimazole, ketoconazole
			  IV: amphotericin B

B and T lymphocytes	Ataxia-telangiectasia	Ataxia with progressive neurologic deterioration; telangiectasia (vascular lesions); recurrent infections; malignancies	Antimicrobial therapy; management of presenting symptoms; fetal thymus transplant, IV immunoglobulin
	Nezelof's syndrome	Severe infections; malignancies	Antimicrobial therapy; IV immunoglobulin, bone marrow transplantation; thymus transplantation; thymus factors
	Wiskott-Aldrich syndrome	Thrombocytopenia, resulting in bleeding; infections; malignancies	Antimicrobial therapy; splenectomy with continuous antibiotic prophylaxis; IV immunoglobulin and bone marrow transplantation
	Severe combined immuno-deficiency disease (SCID)	Overwhelming severe fatal infections soon after birth (also includes opportunistic infections)	Antimicrobial therapy; IV immunoglobulin and bone marrow transplantation
Complement system	Angioneurotic edema	Episodes of edema in various parts of the body, including respiratory tract and bowels	Pooled plasma, androgen therapy
	Paroxysmal nocturnal hemoglobinuria (PNH)	Lysis of erythrocytes due to lack of decay-accelerating factor (DAF) on erythrocytes	None

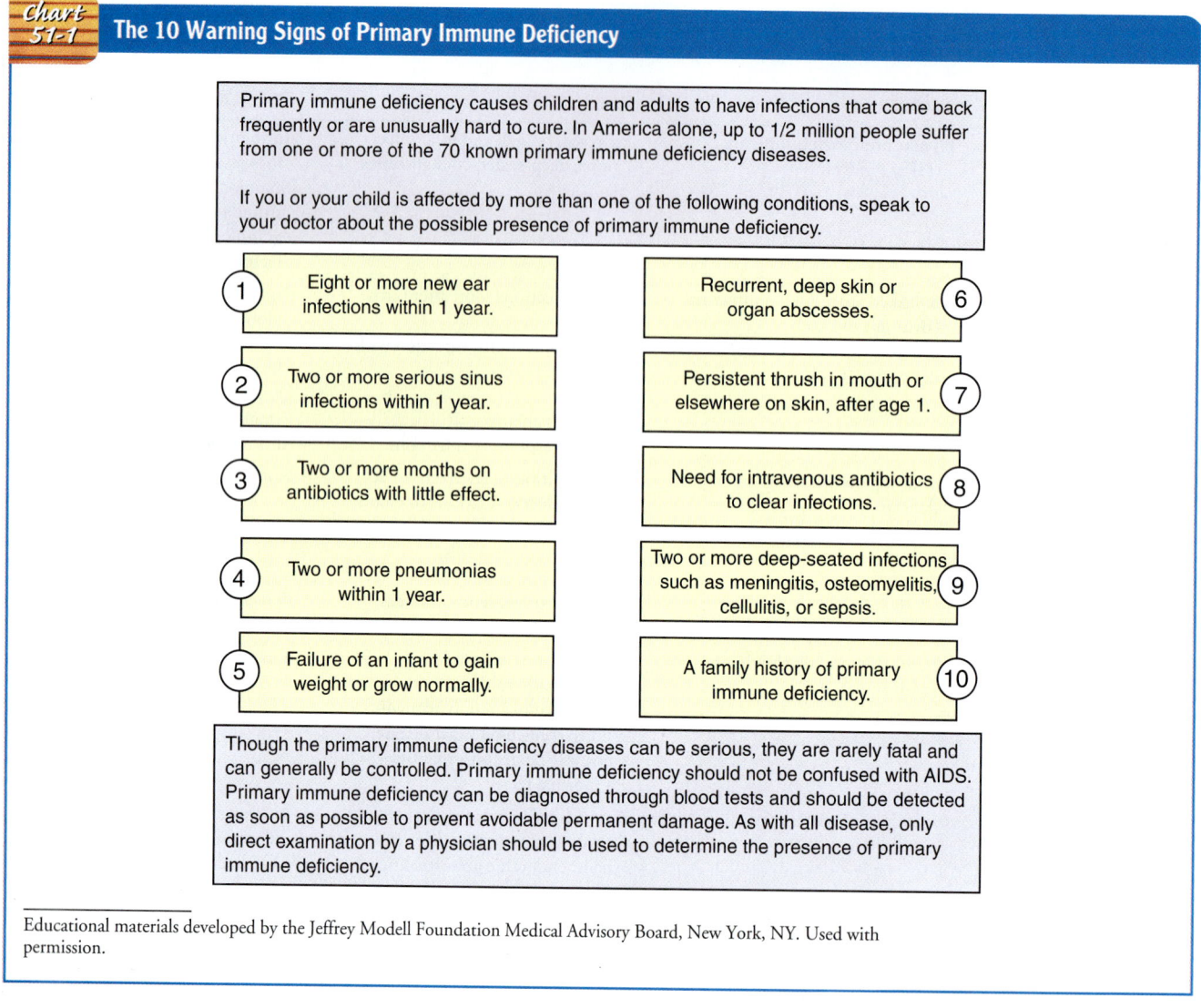

Chart 51-1 **The 10 Warning Signs of Primary Immune Deficiency**

Primary immune deficiency causes children and adults to have infections that come back frequently or are unusually hard to cure. In America alone, up to 1/2 million people suffer from one or more of the 70 known primary immune deficiency diseases.

If you or your child is affected by more than one of the following conditions, speak to your doctor about the possible presence of primary immune deficiency.

1. Eight or more new ear infections within 1 year.
2. Two or more serious sinus infections within 1 year.
3. Two or more months on antibiotics with little effect.
4. Two or more pneumonias within 1 year.
5. Failure of an infant to gain weight or grow normally.
6. Recurrent, deep skin or organ abscesses.
7. Persistent thrush in mouth or elsewhere on skin, after age 1.
8. Need for intravenous antibiotics to clear infections.
9. Two or more deep-seated infections such as meningitis, osteomyelitis, cellulitis, or sepsis.
10. A family history of primary immune deficiency.

Though the primary immune deficiency diseases can be serious, they are rarely fatal and can generally be controlled. Primary immune deficiency should not be confused with AIDS. Primary immune deficiency can be diagnosed through blood tests and should be detected as soon as possible to prevent avoidable permanent damage. As with all disease, only direct examination by a physician should be used to determine the presence of primary immune deficiency.

Educational materials developed by the Jeffrey Modell Foundation Medical Advisory Board, New York, NY. Used with permission.

prove successful because these proteins draw nonlymphoid stem cells from the bone marrow and hasten their maturation.

B-CELL DEFICIENCIES
Pathophysiology

Two types of inherited B-cell deficiencies exist. The first type results from lack of differentiation of B-cell precursors into mature B cells. As a result, plasma cells are lacking, and the germinal centres from all lymphatic tissues disappear, leading to a complete lack of antibody production against invading bacteria, viruses, and other pathogens. Infants born with this disorder suffer from severe infections starting soon after birth. This syndrome is called sex-linked **agammaglobulinemia** (Bruton's disease) because all antibodies disappear from the patient's plasma. B cells in the peripheral blood and the immunoglobulins IgG, IgM, IgA, IgD, and IgE are low or absent. The prevalence of this disorder is approximately 1 case per 100,000 population (Parslow, Stites, Terr & Imboden, 2001).

The second type of B-cell deficiency results from a lack of differentiation of B cells into plasma cells. Only diminished an-

tibody production occurs with this disorder. Although plasma cells are the most vigourous producers of antibodies, affected patients have normal lymph follicles and many B lymphocytes that produce some antibodies. This syndrome, called **hypogammaglobulinemia**, is a frequently occurring immunodeficiency. It is also called common variable immunodeficiency (CVID), a term that encompasses a variety of defects ranging from immunoglobulin A (IgA) deficiency, in which only the plasma cells that produce IgA are lacking, to the other extreme, in which there is severe **panhypoglobulinemia** (general lack of immunoglobulins in the blood).

CVID is the most common primary immunodeficiency seen in adults; it can occur in either gender. Although it can occur at any age, its onset is most often in the second decade of life. The vast majority of patients do not become symptomatic until 15 to 35 years of age. The major immunologic features of CVID include recurrent pyogenic infections, an increased incidence of autoimmune diseases, and a decreased level of total immunoglobulins, with IgG below 250 mg/dL. The B-cell numbers usually remain normal. The etiology of this disorder is unknown and believed to be multifactorial. The prevalence of CVID is about 1 case per 50,000 population in Canada (Greenberg, 2005).

Clinical Manifestations

Infants with sex-linked agammaglobulinemia usually become symptomatic after the natural loss of maternally transmitted immunoglobulins, which occurs at about 5 to 6 months of age. Symptoms of recurrent pyogenic infections usually occur by 5 to 6 months of age.

More than half of patients with CVID develop pernicious anemia. Lymphoid hyperplasia of the small intestine and spleen and gastric atrophy detected by biopsy of the stomach are common findings. Other autoimmune diseases, such as arthritis and hypothyroidism, frequently develop in patients with CVID. Those who develop late-onset disease also have an increased incidence of chronic lung disease, hepatitis, gastric cancer, and malabsorption that results in chronic diarrhea (Porth, 2002). CVID must be distinguished from secondary immunodeficiency diseases caused by protein-losing enteropathy, nephrotic syndrome, or burns.

Patients with CVID are susceptible to infections with encapsulated bacteria, such as *Haemophilus influenzae, Streptococcus pneumoniae,* and *Staphylococcus aureus.* Frequent respiratory tract infections typically lead to chronic progressive bronchiectasis and pulmonary failure. Commonly, infection with *Giardia lamblia* occurs. Opportunistic infections with *Pneumocystis carinii,* however, are seen only in patients who have a concomitant deficiency in T-cell immunity.

Assessment and Diagnostic Findings

Sex-linked agammaglobulinemia may be diagnosed by the marked deficiency or complete absence of all serum immunoglobulins. The diagnosis of CVID is based on the history of bacterial infections, quantification of B-cell activity, and reported signs and symptoms. The number of B lymphocytes and the total and specific immunoglobulin levels are measured. Total serum globulin level alone is an inadequate measure because a compensatory overproduction of one globulin may mask the loss of a missing globulin or one present in very low amounts. Antibody titers to confirm successful childhood vaccination are determined by specific serologic tests. Previous successful childhood immunization indicates that B cells were functioning adequately earlier in life. If the patient exhibits signs and symptoms suggestive of pernicious anemia, hemoglobin and hematocrit levels are also obtained.

Medical Management

Patients with primary phagocytic disorders may be treated with intravenous immunoglobulin (IVIG). Those who are receiving adequate treatment with IVIG usually do not require prophylactic antibiotics unless they also have chronic respiratory disease. Antimicrobial therapy is prescribed for respiratory infections to prevent complications such as pneumonia, sinusitis, and otitis media. Intestinal infestation with *G. lamblia* is treated with a 10-day course of metronidazole (Flagyl) or a 7-day course of quinacrine hydrochloride (Atabrine) (Parslow et al., 2001). Patients with pernicious anemia receive parenteral injections of vitamin B_{12} at monthly intervals. Management may also include physical therapy with postural drainage for patients with chronic lung disease or bronchiectasis (Parslow et al., 2001).

T-CELL DEFICIENCIES
Pathophysiology

Defects in T cells lead to opportunistic infections. Most primary T-cell immunodeficiencies are genetic in origin. An increased susceptibility to infection is common. Symptoms can vary considerably depending on the type of T-cell defect. Because the T cells play a regulatory role in immune system function, the loss of T-cell function is usually accompanied by some loss of B-cell activity.

DiGeorge syndrome, or **thymic hypoplasia**, is one example of a primary T-cell immunodeficiency. This rare congenital disease results from the absence of several genes on chromosome 22 (Porth, 2002). The variation in symptoms is a result of differences in the amount of genetic material affected. T-cell deficiency occurs when the thymus gland fails to develop normally during embryogenesis. DiGeorge syndrome is one of the few immunodeficiency disorders with symptoms that present almost immediately following birth (Parslow et al., 2001).

Chronic mucocutaneous candidiasis with or without endocrinopathy is another T-cell disorder associated with a selective defect in T-cell immunity; it is thought to be caused by an autosomal recessive inheritance, affecting both males and females. It is considered an autoimmune disorder in which the thymus and other endocrine glands are involved in the autoimmune process. The disease causes extensive morbidity resulting from endocrine dysfunction.

Clinical Manifestations

Infants born with DiGeorge syndrome have hypoparathyroidism with resultant hypocalcemia resistant to standard therapy, congenital heart disease, characteristic facial features, and possibly renal abnormalities. These infants, susceptible to yeast, fungal, protozoan, and viral infections, are particularly susceptible to childhood diseases (chickenpox, measles, and rubella), which are usually severe and may be fatal. Many of these infants are also born with congenital heart defects, which can result in congestive heart failure. The most frequent presenting sign in patients with DiGeorge syndrome is hypocalcemia that is resistant to standard therapy. It usually occurs within the first 24 hours of life (Parslow et al., 2001).

The initial presentation of chronic mucocutaneous candidiasis may be either chronic candidal infection or idiopathic endocrinopathy. Patients may survive to the second or third decade of life. Problems may include hypocalcemia and tetany secondary to hypofunction of the parathyroid glands. Hypofunction of the adrenal cortex (Addison's disease) is the major cause of death in these patients; it may develop suddenly and without any history of previous symptoms.

Assessment and Diagnostic Findings

The status of T cells can be evaluated by peripheral blood lymphocyte counts. Because T cells constitute 65% to 85% of peripheral blood lymphocytes, lymphopenia may signify a T-cell deficit. Dermal sensitization of the patient or stimulation of the patient's T cells in vitro may be conducted to determine if the T cells are capable of producing the expected responses. Immunoglobulin evaluation is not useful in infants because of the presence of maternally transmitted immunoglobulin (Parslow et al., 2001).

Medical Management

Patients with T-cell deficiency should receive *P. carinii* prophylaxis. General care includes management of hypocalcemia and correction of cardiac abnormalities. Hypocalcemia is controlled by oral calcium supplementation in conjunction with vitamin D or parathyroid hormone administration. Congenital heart disease frequently results in heart failure, and these patients may require immediate surgical intervention in a tertiary pediatric centre. Transplantation of the fetal thymus, postnatal thymus, and human leukocyte antigen (HLA)-matched bone marrow has been used for permanent reconstitution of T-cell immunity. IVIG therapy may be used if an antibody deficiency exists. This therapy may also be used to control recurrent infections. Prolonged survival has been reported following the successful transplantation of the thymus gland or spontaneous remission of immunodeficiency, which occurs in some patients (Parslow et al., 2001).

COMBINED B-CELL AND T-CELL DEFICIENCIES
Pathophysiology

Combined B-cell and T-cell deficiencies are those disorders of the immune system that have elements of dysfunction of both the B cells and T cells. A variety of inherited (autosomal recessive and X-linked) conditions fit this description. These conditions have in common disruption of the normal communication system of B cells and T cells and impairment of the immune response (Porth, 2002). These conditions generally appear early in life. Examples of these deficiencies are discussed below.

Ataxia-telangiectasia is an autosomal recessive disorder affecting both T- and B-cell immunity. In 40% of patients with this disease, a selective IgA deficiency exists. IgA and IgG subclass deficiencies, along with IgE deficiencies, have been identified. Variable degrees of T-cell deficiencies are observed and become more severe with advancing age. The disease is associated with neurologic, vascular, endocrine, hepatic, and cutaneous abnormalities. It is accompanied by progressive cerebellar ataxia, telangiectasias, recurrent bacterial infection of the sinuses and lungs, and an increased incidence of cancer (Buckley, 2000).

Both B and T cells are missing in **severe combined immunodeficiency disease (SCID)**. SCID is a phenotypic term that is used for a wide variety of congenital and hereditary immunologic defects that are characterized by early onset of infections, defects in both B- and T-cell systems, lymphoid aplasia, and thymic dysplasia. Inheritance of this disorder can be X-linked, autosomal-recessive, or sporadic. The exact incidence of SCID is unknown; it is recognized as a rare disease in most population groups, with an incidence of about 1 case in 1,000,000. This illness occurs in all racial groups and both genders (Parslow et al., 2001). **Wiskott-Aldrich syndrome** is a variation of SCID compounded by thrombocytopenia (loss of platelets). The prognosis is generally poor because most affected infants develop overwhelming fatal infections.

Clinical Manifestations

The onset of **ataxia** (uncoordinated muscle movement) **telangiectasia** (vascular lesions caused by dilated blood vessels) usually occurs in the first 4 years of life of those with ataxia-telangiectasia. Many patients, however, remain symptom-free for 10 years or longer. As patients approach the second decade of life, chronic lung disease, mental retardation, neurologic symptoms, and physical disability become severe. Long-term survivors develop progressive deterioration of immunologic and neurologic functions. Some affected patients have reached the fifth decade of life. The primary causes of death in these patients are overwhelming infection and lymphoreticular or epithelial cancer.

The onset of symptoms occurs within the first 3 months of life in the majority of patients with SCID with respiratory infections, pneumonia (often secondary to *P. carinii*), thrush, diarrhea, and failure to thrive. Many of these infections are resistant to treatment. Shedding of viruses such as respiratory syncytial virus or cytomegalovirus from the respiratory and gastrointestinal tracts is persistent. Maculopapular and erythematous skin rashes may occur. Vomiting, fever, and a persistent diaper rash are also common manifestations (Parslow et al., 2001).

Medical Management

Treatment of ataxia-telangiectasia includes early management of infections with antimicrobial therapy, management of chronic lung disease with postural drainage and physical therapy, and management of other presenting symptoms. Other treatments include transplantation of fetal thymus tissue and IVIG administration (Chart 51-2).

Treatment options for SCID include stem cell and bone marrow transplantation. The ideal donor is an HLA-identical sibling (Parslow et al., 2001). Other treatment regimens include IVIG replacement, administration of thymus-derived factors, and thymus gland transplantation. Gene therapy has been used, but the results have thus far been disappointing. As treatment improves, an increased number of those who previously would have died in infancy may live to adulthood.

Nursing Management

As many patients require immunosuppression to ensure engraftment of depleted bone marrow during certain transplantation procedures, nursing care must be exquisite, with attention to preventing the transmission of infection to patients. Use of standard precautions and meticulous hand hygiene is essential in caring for these patients. Reverse isolation procedures, where nurses protect the patient by donning gowns, gloves, caps, and so on, is essential. The patient's condition must be monitored at all times as a certain number of patients experience reactions to transplantation that can be fatal.

DEFICIENCIES OF THE COMPLEMENT SYSTEM

The complement system is an integral part of the immune system, and alterations in normal components of complement can result in increased susceptibility to infectious diseases and to immune-mediated disorders (Porth, 2002). Improved techniques to identify the individual components of the complement system have led to a steady increase in the number of deficiencies identified. Disorders of the complement system can be primary or secondary.

Chart 51-2 • PHARMACOLOGY
Managing an IV Immunoglobulin Infusion

Previously available only for intramuscular injection, immunoglobulin can now be administered for replacement therapy as an IV infusion in greater, more effective doses without painful side effects.

How Supplied
Immunoglobulin is supplied in a 5% solution or a lyophilized powder with a reconstituting diluent prepared from Cohn fraction II obtained from pools of 1,000 to 10,000 donors. Currently, a number of different IV preparations are approved for use and have been shown to be effective and safe by the U.S. Food and Drug Administration.

Dosage
The optimal dose is that determined by the patient's response. In most instances, an IV dose of 100 to 400 mg/kg of body weight is administered monthly or more frequently to ensure adequate serum IgG levels.

Adverse Effects
- Complaints of flank pain, shaking chills, and tightness in the chest, terminating with a slight rise in body temperature
- Hypotension (possible with severe reactions)
- Anaphylactic reactions

Guidelines for Nursing Management
- Weigh the patient before treatment.
- Obtain vital signs before, during, and after treatment.
- Administer the prescribed pretreatment prophylactic aspirin or IV antihistamine, such as diphenhydramine (Benadryl).
- Be aware that corticosteroids may be used to prevent possible severe reactions.
- Administer the IV infusion at a slow rate, not to exceed 3 mL/minute.
- Assess the patient for adverse reactions, including the early signs of anaphylactic shock; prepare to slow the infusion rate if necessary.
- Be aware that patients with low gammaglobulin levels have more severe reactions than those with normal levels (eg, patients who receive gammaglobulin for thrombocytopenia or Kawasaki disease).
- Keep in mind that patients who have an immunoglobulin A (IgA) deficiency have IgE antibodies to IgA, which requires administration of plasma or immunoglobulin replacement from IgA-deficient patients. Because all IV immunoglobulin preparations contain some IgA, they may cause an anaphylactic reaction in patients with IgE anti-IgA antibodies.
- Remember that the risk for transmission of hepatitis, HIV, or other known viruses is extremely low.

C2 and C3 component deficiencies result in diminished resistance to bacterial infections. **Angioneurotic edema** is caused by an inherited deficiency of the inhibitor of C1 esterase, which opposes the release of inflammatory mediators. A deficiency of this inhibitor results in frequent episodes of urticaria and edema in various parts of the body.

Patients with paroxysmal nocturnal hemoglobinuria (PNH) lack decay-accelerating factor (DAF), which is found on erythrocytes (red blood cells). DAF normally protects the erythrocytes from lysis (disintegration). In PNH, the complement component C3b accumulates on the CR1 molecule on the erythrocyte, acts as a binding site for the late-acting component, and allows lysis to occur.

Secondary Immunodeficiencies

Secondary immunodeficiencies are more common than primary immunodeficiencies and frequently occur as a result of underlying disease processes or from the treatment of these diseases. Common causes of secondary immunodeficiencies include malnutrition, chronic stress, burns, uremia, diabetes mellitus, certain autoimmune disorders, certain viruses, exposure to immunotoxic medications and chemicals, and self-administration of recreational drugs and alcohol. AIDS, the most common secondary immunodeficiency disorder, is discussed in detail in Chapter 52. Patients with secondary immunodeficiencies have immunosuppression and are often referred to as **immunocompromised hosts**.

Medical Management

Management of secondary immunodeficiencies includes diagnosis and treatment of the underlying disease process. Interventions include eliminating the contributing factors, treating the underlying condition, and using sound principles of infection control.

Nursing Management for Patients With Immunodeficiencies

Nursing management includes assessment, patient teaching, and supportive care. Assessment of the patient for infection and for response to treatment is important if it is to be effective. Nursing care of patients with primary and secondary immunodeficiencies depends on the underlying cause of the immunodeficiency, the type of immunodeficiency, and its severity. Because immunodeficiencies result in a compromised immune system and high risk for infection, careful assessment of the patient's immune status is essential. The assessment focuses on history of past infections, particularly the type and frequency of infection; signs and symptoms of any current skin, respiratory, gastrointestinal, or genitourinary infection; and measures that prevent infection. The nurse monitors the patient for signs and symptoms of infection: fever; chills; cough with or without sputum; shortness of breath; difficulty breathing; difficulty swallowing; white patches in the oral cavity; swollen lymph nodes; nausea; vomiting; persistent diarrhea; frequency, urgency, or pain on urination; redness, swelling, or drainage from skin wounds; lesions on the face, lips, or perianal area; persistent vaginal discharge with or without perianal itching; and persistent abdominal pain.

Because the inflammatory response may be blunted, the patient is monitored for subtle and unusual signs and changes in physical status. Vital signs and the development of pain, neurologic signs, cough, and skin lesions are monitored and reported. Pulse rate and respiratory rate should be counted for a full minute, as even subtle changes can signal deterioration in the patient's clinical status. Thorough auscultation and assessment of the breath sounds are also key in detecting changes in respiratory status. Any unusual response to treatment and any significant change in the patient's clinical condition are promptly reported to the physician.

Fehder, W. P., Sachs, J., Uvaydova, M., & Douglas, S. D. (1997). Substance P as an immune modulator of anxiety. *Neuroimmunomodulation, 4*(1), 42–48.

Purpose

Proinflammatory peptide substance P (SP), a protein that is widely distributed in the central and peripheral nervous systems, has been implicated in modulation of the immune and hematopoietic systems. Studies have demonstrated that peripheral blood concentrations of SP have increased in response to psychological anxiety in humans. The purposes of this study were to 1) examine changes in SP levels in peripheral blood in response to anxiety over time, and 2) correlate changes in percentages of CD8-expressing T lymphocytes with alterations in measures of anxiety and SP.

Study Sample and Design

Two groups of patients were included in the sample in an effort to have two groups of patients receiving similar diagnostic procedures but with different levels of anxiety. Subjects (n = 11) in one group underwent colonoscopy with sedation and subjects (n = 12) in the second group underwent sigmoidoscopy without sedation. It was expected that the patients who received sedation would have lower levels of anxiety than the nonsedated group. Anxiety was assessed by the Multiple Affect Adjective Checklist-Revised state forms (MAACL-R), which were administered to patients prior to the diagnostic procedure, after the diagnostic procedure, and at a home visit 3 days after the procedure. At the same times that the MAACL-R was administered, blood samples were collected. A competitive solid-phase, enzyme-linked immunoabsorbent assay was used to measure blood levels of SP. Flow cytometry was used to express the percentage of mononuclear cells bearing the specific marker.

Data from the two groups were compared using repeated-measure analysis of variance (ANOVA) with post-hoc t test and Pearson's correlation coefficients. A p value of < 0.05 was used to determine statistical significance.

Findings

Data analysis revealed no significant differences between the anxiety levels of the two groups of patients before, immediately after, and 3 days after the procedures. As patients in both groups experienced high levels of preprocedure anxiety, the researchers divided the subjects into anxiety groups on the basis of the initial anxiety scores using a median split technique. SP levels were then examined by high and low levels of anxiety by repeated-measures ANOVA. The high-anxiety group had significantly higher SP levels than the low-anxiety group. Post-hoc t tests revealed SP levels were significantly elevated in the high-anxiety group compared with the low-anxiety group both before and after the procedures. Blood levels of SP, once elevated, remained elevated after the cause of the initial anxiety was removed. Levels of SP in the peripheral blood were found to be significantly correlated with the percent and absolute numbers of CD8 and T lymphocytes.

Nursing Implications

This study demonstrated that peripheral blood levels of SP may be influenced by levels of anxiety. These findings suggest that patients' anxiety level may have an effect on their immune system; therefore, nurses need to monitor anxiety levels in patients preparing for diagnostic and other procedures and design and implement measures to alleviate such anxiety-provoking situations. Such interventions may prevent changes in the immune system secondary to anxiety.

The nurse also monitors laboratory values (ie, white blood cell count and differential cell count) for changes indicating infection. Culture and sensitivity reports from wound drainage, lesions, sputum, stool, urine, and blood are monitored to identify pathogenic organisms and appropriate antimicrobial therapy. Changes in laboratory results and subtle changes in clinical status must be reported to the physician because the immunocompromised patient may not develop typical signs and symptoms of infection.

Assessment also focuses on nutritional status; stress level and coping skills; use of alcohol, drugs, or tobacco; and general hygiene, all of which may affect immune function. Strategies the patient has used to reduce risk for infection are identified.

Other aspects of nursing care are directed toward reducing the patient's risk for infection, assisting with medical measures aimed at improving immune status and treating infection, improving the nutritional status, and maintaining bowel and bladder function. These include careful hand hygiene, encouraging the patient to cough and perform deep-breathing exercises at regular intervals, and protecting the integrity of the skin and mucous membranes. All health care personnel must use strict aseptic technique when performing invasive procedures, such as dressing changes, venipunctures, and bladder catheterizations.

Other aspects of nursing care include assisting the patient in managing stress and in adopting a lifestyle that enhances immune system function.

If the patient is a candidate for any of the newer or experimental therapies (gene therapy, bone marrow transplantation, immunomodulators such as interferon gamma), the patient or parents (if the patient is a child) must be informed about the potential risks and benefits of the treatment regimen. A major role of the nurse is to assist the patient and family to understand the treatment options and to cope with the uncertainties of treatment outcomes.

PROMOTING HOME AND COMMUNITY-BASED CARE

Teaching Patients Self-Care. The patient and the caregivers are instructed about the signs and symptoms that indicate infection. The nurse explains that the immunosuppressed patient may also have atypical symptoms secondary to underlying immunosuppression. Patients should be advised that they know themselves best; therefore, whenever they experience a symptom that is not typical for them, they should contact their health care provider. The health care provider will then determine and initiate indicated therapy. The patient and caregiver need instruction about any prophylactic medication regimen, including dosage, indications, times, actions, and side effects. The patient is instructed about the importance of avoiding others with infections and avoiding crowds. The patient and family also need to learn about other ways to prevent infection (Chart 51-3).

The patient who is to receive IVIG at home will need information about the expected benefits and outcomes of the treatment as well as expected adverse reactions and their management (Chart 51-4). Patients who can perform self-infusion at home are instructed in sterile technique, medication dosages, administration rate, and detection and management of adverse reactions.

Chart 51-3

Home Care Checklist • Infection Prevention for the Patient With Immunodeficiency

At the completion of the home care instruction, the patient or caregiver will be able to:	Patient	Caregiver
• Identify signs and symptoms of infection to report to the health care provider, such as fever, chills; wet or dry cough; breathing problems; white patches in the mouth; swollen glands; nausea; vomiting; persistent abdominal pain; persistent diarrhea; problems with urination; red, swollen, or draining wounds; sores or lesions on the body; and persistent vaginal discharge with or without itching.	✓	✓
• Demonstrate correct handwashing procedure.	✓	✓
• State rationale for thorough handwashing before eating, after using the bathroom, and before and after performing health care procedures.	✓	✓
• State rationale for use of cream and emollients to prevent or manage dry, chafed, or cracked skin.	✓	✓
• Demonstrate recommended personal hygiene in bathing and foot care to prevent bacterial and fungal diseases.	✓	✓
• State rationale for avoiding contact with people who have known illness or who have recently been vaccinated.	✓	✓
• Verbalize understanding of ways to maintain a well-balanced diet and adequate calories.	✓	✓
• State the reason for avoiding the eating of raw fruits and vegetables, cooking all foods thoroughly, and immediately refrigerating all leftover food.	✓	✓
• Identify the rationale for frequent cleaning of kitchen and bathroom surfaces with disinfectant.	✓	✓
• Identify rationale and benefits of avoiding alcohol, tobacco, and unprescribed medications.	✓	✓
• State rationale for taking prescribed medications as directed.	✓	✓
• Verbalize ways to cope with stress successfully, plans for regular exercise, and rationale for obtaining adequate rest.	✓	✓

The patient and family must be instructed to monitor for subtle changes in physical status and must be informed of the importance of seeking immediate health care if changes occur. Patients and their families are also instructed about the importance of continuing the treatment regimen and assisted in incorporating it into their lives.

Continuing Care. The importance of follow-up appointments is emphasized to the patient and family. They are urged to notify the primary health care provider about early signs and symptoms of infection, including any subtle changes. The importance of continuing disease-prevention strategies is stressed because these strategies need to be followed lifelong. The patient should be encouraged to have recommended health screening because of the increased susceptibility for cancer secondary to the immune suppression.

If the patient's treatment includes IVIG and the patient or family cannot administer it, a referral for home care or an infusion service may be warranted.

Critical Thinking Exercises

1. Intravenous immunoglobulin (IVIG) infusions have been prescribed for your patient, who has an immunodeficiency. He tells you that he is very fearful that he may contract hepatitis, HIV infection, AIDS, and other blood-borne diseases from the infusion. How would you respond to these fears and concerns?

2. You are scheduled to make a home care visit to a patient who was recently discharged from the hospital for an opportunistic infection secondary to AIDS. Upon arrival at the patient's home, you note a very unkempt environment, with many cats roaming around and several other unsanitary conditions. Explain the course of action that you would take to address these issues, given the patient's diagnosis and condition.

Chart 51-4

Home Care Checklist • Home Infusion of Intravenous Immunoglobulin (IVIG)

At the completion of the home care instruction, the patient or caregiver will be able to:	Patient	Caregiver
• Identify the benefits and expected outcome of IVIG.	✓	✓
• Demonstrate how to check for patency of IV access device.	✓	✓
• Demonstrate how to prepare IVIG.	✓	✓
• Demonstrate how to infuse IVIG.	✓	✓
• Demonstrate how to clean and maintain IV equipment.	✓	✓
• Identify side effects and adverse effects of IVIG.	✓	✓
• State rationale for prophylactic use of aspirin and an antihistamine before treatment begins.	✓	✓
• Verbalize understanding of emergency measures for anaphylactic shock.	✓	✓

3. Describe the teaching plan you would use to instruct a patient with an immunodeficiency disorder about prevention and management of infection. How would you modify your approach if the patient did not believe in medications or vaccinations? Are vaccinations recommended in a patient with an underlying immunodeficiency disease? If not, why not?

REFERENCES AND SELECTED READINGS

Books

Abbas, A. K., & Lichtman, A. H. (2001). *Basic immunology.* Philadelphia: W. B. Saunders.

Antel, P., Birnbaum, G., & Hartung, H. P. (1998). *Clinical neuroimmunology.* Malden, MA: Blackwell Scientific.

Delves, P. J. (1998). *Encyclopedia of immunology* (2nd ed.). San Diego: Academic Press.

Descotes, J., & Bernard, C. (1999). *An introduction to immunotoxicology.* Philadelphia: Taylor & Francis.

Nakamura, R. M., et al. (Eds.) (1998). *Clinical diagnostic immunology: Protocols in quality assurance and standardization.* Malden, MA: Blackwell Scientific.

Parslow, G. G., Stites, D. P., Terr, A. I., & Imboden, J. B. (2001). *Medical immunology.* New York: McGraw-Hill.

Porth, C. M. (2002). *Pathophysiology: Concepts of altered health states.* Philadelphia: Lippincott Williams & Wilkins.

Rich, R. R., Fleisher, T. A., Schwartz, B. D., et al. (2001). *Clinical immunology: Principles and practice* (2d ed.). St. Louis: Mosby, Inc.

Roitt, I. M., & Delves, P. J. (2001). *Roitt's essential immunology.* Malden, MA: Blackwell Science.

Seidel, H. M., Ball, J. W., Dains, J. E., & Benedict, G. W. (1999). *Mosby's guide to physical examination* (4th ed). St. Louis: Mosby, Inc.

Tierney, L. M. Jr., McPhee, S. J., & Papadakis, M. A. (2001). *Current medical diagnosis and treatment.* Stamford, CT: Appleton & Lange.

Virella, G. (Ed.). (2001). *Medical immunology.* New York: Marcel Dekker.

Journals

Asterisks indicate nursing research articles.

Alcoser, P. W., & Burchett, B. A. (1999). Bone marrow transplantation. Immune system suppression and reconstitution. *American Journal of Nursing, 99*(6), 26–31.

Buckley, R. H., Schiff, S. E., Schiff, R. I., et al. (1999). Hematopoietic stem-cell transplantation for the treatment of severe combined immunodeficiency. *New England Journal of Medicine, 340*(7), 508–516.

Buckley, R. H. (2000). Primary immunodeficiency diseases due to defects in lymphocytes. *New England Journal of Medicine, 343*(18), 1313–1324.

Davis, J., Krasnewich, D., & Puck, J. M. (2000). Genetic testing and screening in pediatric populations. *Nursing Clinics of North America, 35*(3), 643–650.

*Fehder, W. P. (1999). Alterations in immune response associated with anxiety in surgical patients. *CRNA: Clinical Forum for Nurse Anesthetists, 10*(3), 124–129.

*Fehder, W. P., Sachs, J., Uvaydova, M., & Douglas, S. D. (1997). Substance P as an immune modulator of anxiety. *Neuroimmunomodulation, 4*(1), 42–48.

Fleisher, T. A. (1997). Introduction to diagnostic laboratory immunology. *Journal of American Medical Association, 278*(22), 1823–1834.

Greenberg, S. (2005). Hypogammaglobulinemia. Available at: http://www.utoronto.ca/kids. Retrieved May 15, 2005.

Huston, D. P. (1997). The biology of the immune system. *Journal of American Medical Association, 278*(22), 1804–1822.

Lekstrom-Himes, J. A., & Gallin, J. I. (2002). Immunodeficiency diseases caused by defects in phagocytes. *New England Journal of Medicine, 343*(23), 1703–1714.

Smith, J. K., Krishnaswamy, G. H., Dykes, R., et al. (1997). Clinical manifestations of IgE hypogammaglobulinemia. *Annals of Allergy, Asthma, and Immunology, 78*(3), 313–318.

RESOURCES AND WEBSITES

Canadian Institute for Health Information, 377 Dalhousie Street, Suite 200, Ottawa ON K1N 9N8; (613) 241-7860; http://www.cihi.ca.

Canadian Immunodeficiency Patient Organization; http://cipo.ca/english/home.htm.

Centers for Disease Control and Prevention, 1600 Clifton Road, Atlanta, GA 30333; (404) 639-3311 or (800) 311-3435; http://www.cdc.gov.

Genetic Information and Patient Services; http://icomm.ca/geneinfo/agamprin.htm.

National Institute of Allergy and Infectious Disease, NIAID Office of Communications and Public Liaison, NIH, Building #31, Room 7A50, 31 Center Drive, MSC 2520, Bethesda, MD 20892-2520; (301) 496-5717, http://www.niaid.nih.gov.

National Institutes of Health, 9000 Rockville Pike, Bethesda, MD 20892; (301) 496-4000, http://www.nih.gov.

National Library of Medicine, 8600 Rockville Pike, Bethesda, MD 20894; (888) FIND-NLM, (888) 346-3656, (301) 594-5983; http://www.nlm.nih.gov.

The Canadian Allergy, Asthma and Immunology Foundation, 774 Echo Drive, Ottawa, ON K1S 5N8; (613) 730-6272; http://www.allergyfoundation.ca.

The Canadian Society of Allergy and Clinical Immunology, 774 Echo Drive, Ottawa, ON K1S 5N8; (613) 730-6272; http://csaci.medical.org.

Management of Patients With HIV Infection and AIDS

Adapted by Jean Groft and Judy Mill

LEARNING OBJECTIVES

On completion of this chapter, the learner will be able to:

1. Describe the modes of transmission of HIV infection.
2. Describe the pathophysiology of HIV infection.
3. Explain the physiology underlying the clinical manifestations of HIV infection.
4. Describe the management of patients with HIV infection.
5. Discuss the nursing interventions appropriate for patients with HIV infection and AIDS.
6. Use the nursing process as a framework for care of the patient with AIDS.

Although progress has been made in treating HIV infection and AIDS, the epidemic remains a critical public health issue in all communities across the country and around the world. Prevention, early detection, and ongoing treatment remain important aspects of care for people with HIV infection and AIDS. Nurses in all settings encounter people with this disease; thus, nurses need an understanding of the disorder, knowledge of the physical and psychological consequences associated with the diagnosis, and expert assessment and clinical management skills to provide optimal care for people with HIV infection and AIDS.

In 1987, just 6 years after the first cases of AIDS were reported, the U.S. Food and Drug Administration (FDA) approved the first antiretroviral agent; in 1988 the first randomized controlled trial of primary prophylaxis of *Pneumocystis carinii* pneumonia appeared in the literature; and in 1995 protease inhibitors joined the growing number of antiretroviral agents. Improved treatment of HIV and AIDS has resulted in declining death rates in Canada, from a peak of 1500 reported deaths in 1995 to 93 reported deaths in 2003 (Health Canada, 2004a). However, the annual number of positive HIV tests has been gradually increasing since 2001, with an estimated 30% of infected individuals unaware of their sero-

positive status (Public Health Agency of Canada [PHAC], 2005). HIV disease remains a serious issue in this country.

HIV Infection and AIDS

Since acquired immunodeficiency syndrome (AIDS) was first recognized more than 25 years ago, remarkable progress has been made in improving the quality and duration of life of persons with HIV infection. During the first decade, this progress was associated with recognition of opportunistic disease processes, more effective therapy for complications, and introduction of prophylaxis against common **opportunistic infections** (OIs). The second decade has witnessed progress in developing highly active antiretroviral therapies (HAART) as well as continuing progress in treating OIs (Masur, Kaplan & Holmes, 1999). Canadian scientists continue to participate in research on new types of antiretroviral drugs and vaccine development during the third decade of the epidemic (Canadian Legal HIV/AIDS Network, 2002). Since the HIV serologic test (enzyme immunoassay [EIA], formerly enzyme-linked immunosorbent assay [ELISA]), became available in 1984, allowing early diagnosis of the infection before onset of symptoms, HIV in-

Glossary

alpha-interferon: protein substance that the body produces in response to infection

anergy: loss or weakening of the body's immunity to an irritating agent or antigen

B-cell lymphoma: common malignancy in patients with HIV/AIDS

candidiasis: yeast infection of skin or mucous membrane

CCR5: cell surface molecule that is needed along with the CD4 molecule to fuse with the membranes of the host's immune system cells

cytomegalovirus: a species-specific herpes virus that may cause retinitis in people with AIDS

EIA (enzyme immunoassay): a blood test that determines the presence of antibodies to HIV in the blood or saliva; also referred to as **enzyme-linked immunosorbent assay (ELISA).** Positive results must be validated, usually with Western blot test.

HIV-1: retrovirus isolated and recognized as the etiologic agent of AIDS

HIV-2: virus closely related to HIV-1 that has also been found to cause AIDS

HIV encephalopathy: degenerative neurologic condition characterized by a group of clinical presentations including loss of coordination, mood swings, loss of inhibitions, and widespread cognitive dysfunctions; formerly referred to as AIDS dementia complex (ADC)

human papillomavirus (HPV): virus that causes venereal warts

Kaposi's sarcoma: malignancy that involves the epithelial layer of blood and lymphatic vessels

macrophage: large immune cell that devours invading pathogens and other intruders. Can harbour large quantities of HIV without being killed, acting as a reservoir of the virus.

monocyte: large white blood cell that ingests microbes or other cells and foreign particles. When a monocyte enters tissues, it develops into a macrophage.

Mycobacterium avium complex (MAC): opportunistic infection caused by mycobacterial organisms that commonly causes a respiratory illness but can also infect other body systems

opportunistic infection (OI): illness caused by various organisms, some of which usually do not cause disease in persons with normal immune systems

p24 antigen: blood test that measures viral core protein; accuracy of test is limited because the p24 antibody binds with the antigen and makes it undetectable

peripheral neuropathy: disorder characterized by sensory loss, pain, muscle weakness, and wasting of muscles in the hands or legs and feet

Pneumocystis carinii pneumonia (PCP): common opportunistic lung infection caused by an organism, initially thought to be a protozoan but now believed to be a fungus based on its structure

polymerase chain reaction (PCR): a sensitive laboratory technique that can detect and quantify HIV in a person's blood or lymph nodes

primary infection: 4- to 7-week period of rapid viral replication immediately follow-

ing infection; also known as acute HIV infection

progressive multifocal leukoencephalopathy (PML): opportunistic infection that infects brain tissue and causes damage to the brain and spinal cord

protease inhibitor: medication that inhibits the function of protease, an enzyme needed for HIV replication

provirus: viral genetic material in the form of DNA that has been integrated into the host genome. When it is dormant in human cells, HIV is in a proviral form.

retrovirus: a virus that carries genetic material in RNA instead of DNA and contains reverse transcriptase

reverse transcriptase: enzyme that transforms single-stranded RNA into a double-stranded DNA

viral load test: measures the quantity of HIV RNA in the blood

viral set point: amount of virus present in the blood after the initial burst of viremia and the immune response that follows

wasting syndrome: involuntary weight loss of 10% of baseline body weight with chronic diarrhea or chronic weakness and documented fever.

Western blot assay: a blood test that identifies antibodies to HIV and is used to confirm the results of an EIA (ELISA) test

window period: time from infection with HIV until seroconversion detected on HIV antibody test fection has been best managed as a chronic disease and most appropriately managed in an outpatient care setting (Gallant, 2001).

Epidemiology

In fall 1982, the Centers for Disease Control and Prevention (CDC) in the United States issued a case definition of AIDS after the first 100 cases were reported. Since then, the CDC has revised the case definition a number of times (1985, 1987, and 1993). In Canada, the most recent revision confirms a case of AIDS in the presence of a positive HIV test and a definitive diagnosis of one or more of the specified indicator diseases (Health Canada, 2000). As of May 2003, HIV infection became legally notifiable in all Canadian provinces and territories (PHAC, 2005). All jurisdictions voluntarily report positive HIV tests to the Centre for Infectious Disease Prevention and Control (CIDPC). Three types of HIV tests may be available in Canada, depending on the province or territory where testing occurs: Nominal, Non-Nominal, and Anonymous (PHAC, 2005). Nominal, or name-based testing, means that the test is ordered using the name of the person being tested. A non-nominal, or non-identifying test is requested using a code or the initials of the person being tested. An anonymous test uses a code known only to the person being tested. This process offers the highest degree of confidentiality and may encourage more people to come forward for testing (Jürgens, 2001). However, anonymous testing is available in only eight provinces currently (PHAC, 2005).

Between 1979 and June 30, 2004, there were 19,468 cases of AIDS reported to the CIDPC; 56,523 positive HIV tests have been reported between 1985 and June 30, 2004 (PHAC, 2005). The annual number of positive tests continues to increase, from 2,112 in 2000 to 2,499 in 2003 (Health Canada, 2004b).

Unprotected sex and sharing of injection drug use equipment are the major means of transmission of HIV. A total of 469 AIDS cases were diagnosed in 2003 (Health Canada, 2004a). Among reported cases of AIDS in adult males in 2003, 47% were in the exposure category of men who have sex with men; 17%, injection drug use; and 32%, heterosexual contact. Among women during the same time period, 20% reported injection drug use and 80% heterosexual contact. Aboriginal and Black Canadians, overrepresented among reported AIDS cases, account for 20.7% and 14.4% respectively, with injection drug use and heterosexual exposure the leading risk categories (PHAC, 2005).

The number of people living with HIV is not evenly distributed throughout Canada. Provinces with the highest number of reported HIV infections in 2003 were Ontario (1,104), Quebec (621), and British Columbia (436) (Health Canada, 2004a).

AIDS has reached epidemic proportions in some other parts of the world. According to the Joint United Nations Programme on HIV/AIDS (UNAIDS), more than 20 million people worldwide have died of AIDS and 38 million people are infected with HIV, with 4.9 million people newly infected with HIV in 2004 alone (UNAIDS, 2004a, 2004b). As of December 2003, 50% of all people living with HIV were women, and young people (15 to 24 years of age) account for almost half of all new infections worldwide (UNAIDS, 2004a). UNAIDS (2001) reports that since the epidemic began, more than 60 million people have been infected with the virus, making it the most devastating disease ever.

The earliest confirmed case of HIV infection was found in blood drawn from an African man in 1959 (Stephenson, 1998).

Although factors associated with the spread of HIV in Africa remain unknown, possibilities include the reuse of unsterilized needles in large-scale vaccination campaigns that began in Africa in the 1960s; however, social changes such as easier access to transportation, increasing population density, and more frequent sexual contacts may have been more important (Stephenson, 1998).

HIV Transmission

HIV-1 is transmitted in body fluids containing HIV and/or infected CD4+ (or CD4) T lymphocytes. These fluids include blood, seminal fluid, vaginal secretions, amniotic fluid, and breast milk. Mother-to-child transmission of HIV-1 may occur in utero, at the time of delivery, or through breastfeeding, but transmission frequency during each period has been difficult to determine (Nduati et al., 2000). Any behaviour that results in breaks in the skin or mucosa results in the increased probability of exposure to HIV (Chart 52-1). Since HIV is harboured within lymphocytes, a type of white blood cell, any exposure to infected blood results in a significant risk of infection. The amount of virus and infected cells in the body fluid is associated with the risk of new infections.

Blood and blood products can transmit HIV to recipients. However, the risk associated with transfusions has been virtually eliminated as a result of voluntary self-deferral, serologic testing, heat treatment of clotting factor concentrates, and more effective virus inactivation methods. Blood donor screening tests detect antibodies to HIV-1 and **HIV-2**, and **p24 antigen** testing has been added as an interim measure. In 2001, the Canadian Blood Services began using nucleic acid amplification testing to test directly for viral nucleic acids rather than evidence of antibody production by the individual's immune system (Canadian Blood Services, 2001). This test reduces the size of the window period, indicating the presence of HIV 11 to 13 days after infection as compared with the 16-day window period associated with antibody tests. However, blood donated during the **window period** will be infectious but will test negative for HIV antibodies. The window period is the period of time between exposure to the virus and seroconversion, during which screening tests will be falsely negative. Although antibodies will usually be detected within days or weeks of infection, the window period can last up to a year (Busch, Kleinman, & Nemo, 2003; Cilsielski & Metler, 1997; McGill University, 2005).

Chart 52-1
Risk Factors for HIV Infection and AIDS

In Canada, most people with HIV/AIDS have engaged in high-risk behaviours, such as the following:

- Intravenous or injection drug use (the term "*intravenous drug user*" has been replaced by the term "*injecting (or injection) drug user,*"). This term includes people who inject drugs intravenously as well as those who inject drugs intradermally. This method is sometimes referred to as "skin popping."
- Sexual relations with infected individuals (both male and female)

Also at risk are people who received blood or blood products contaminated with HIV (especially before blood screening was instituted in 1985) and children born to mothers with HIV infection.

Prevention of HIV Infection

Until an effective vaccine is developed, preventing HIV by eliminating or reducing risk behaviours is essential. Primary prevention efforts through effective educational programs are vital for control and prevention. HIV is not transmitted by casual contact.

PREVENTIVE EDUCATION

Effective educational programs have been initiated to educate the public regarding safer sexual practices to decrease the risk of transmitting HIV-1 infection to sexual partners (Chart 52-2). Latex condoms should be used during vaginal or anal intercourse. Nonlatex condoms are available for people with latex allergy. A condom should be used for oral contact with the penis, and dental dams (a piece of latex used by dentists to isolate a tooth for treatment) should be used for oral contact with the vagina or rectum. Because nonoxynol-9 (N-9), a spermicide, has been shown to cause irritation and trauma to the vaginal mucosa, its use as a method to prevent HIV transmission is not recommended (Health Canada, 2003). The World Health Organization (WHO, 2003) suggests that N-9 may increase the risk of contracting HIV in people who use the chemical frequently.

Other topics important in preventive education include the importance of avoiding sexual practices that might cut or tear the lining of the rectum, penis, or vagina and avoiding sexual contact with multiple partners or people who are known to be HIV positive or injection drug users. In addition, people who are HIV positive or use injection drugs should be instructed not to donate blood or share drug equipment with others. Increasingly, needle exchange programs are available to enable injection drug users to obtain sterile drug equipment at no cost.

Extensive research has demonstrated that needle exchange programs do not promote increased drug use; on the contrary, they have been found to decrease the incidence of blood-borne infections in persons who use injection drugs (Trzcianowska & Mortensen, 2001). In the absence of needle exchange programs, injection drug users should be instructed on methods to clean their syringes and to avoid sharing cotton and other drug use equipment.

RELATED REPRODUCTIVE EDUCATION

Because HIV infection in women usually occurs during the child-bearing years, family planning issues need to be addressed. Attempts to achieve pregnancy by couples in which one partner has HIV and the other does not expose the unaffected partner to the virus. Efforts at artificial insemination using processed semen from an HIV-infected partner are underway. Studies are needed because HIV has been found in the spermatozoa of patients with AIDS, with possible HIV replication in the male germ cell. Women considering pregnancy need to have adequate information about the risks of transmitting HIV infection to themselves, their partner, and their future children and about the benefits of antiretroviral agents in reducing perinatal HIV transmission. Other than abstinence, the condom has been the only method that has proved to decrease the risk of sexual transmission of HIV infection.

Certain contraceptive methods may pose additional health risks for women. Estrogen in oral contraceptives may increase a women's risk for HIV infection. In addition, women infected with HIV who use estrogen oral contraceptives have shown increased shedding of HIV in vaginal and cervical secretions. The intrauterine contraceptive device (IUD) may also increase the risk for HIV transmission because the device's string may serve as a means to transmit HIV infection. It also can cause penile abrasions. The female condom is as effective in preventing pregnancy as other barrier methods, such as the diaphragm and the male condom. Unlike the diaphragm, the female condom is also effective in preventing the transmission of HIV infection and sexually transmitted diseases (STDs). The female condom has the distinction of being the first barrier method that can be controlled by women (see Chap. 46).

Transmission to Health Care Providers

STANDARD PRECAUTIONS

In 1987, following the recommendations of the Centers for Disease Control in the United States, the Laboratory Centre for Disease Control endorsed and published these recommendations to guide practice in Canada (Health Canada, 1997b). By 1996, efforts to standardize procedures and reduce the risk for exposure resulted in the development of Standard Precautions. Standard Precautions incorporate the major features of Universal Precautions (designed to reduce the risk of transmission of blood-borne pathogens) and Body Substance Isolation (designed to reduce the risk of transmission of pathogens from moist body substances); they are applied to all patients receiving care in hospitals regardless of their diagnosis or presumed infectious status (Chart 52-3). Standard Precautions apply to blood; all body fluids, secretions, and excretions, except sweat, regardless of whether they contain visible blood; nonintact skin; and mucous membranes (Health Canada, 1997a).

The primary goal of Standard Precautions is to prevent the transmission of nosocomial infection. The first tier, referred to as Standard Precautions, was developed to reduce the risk for all rec-

Chart 52-2

Health Promotion and Illness Prevention
Safer Sex and Safer Behaviours

- Practice abstinence.
- Reduce the number of sexual partners to one.
- Always use latex condoms; if allergic to latex, use female condoms (nonlatex).
- Do not reuse condoms.
- Do not use cervical caps or diaphragms without using a condom as well.
- Always use dental dams for oral female genital or anal stimulation.
- Avoid anal intercourse because this practice may injure tissues.
- Avoid manual–anal intercourse ("fisting").
- Do not ingest urine or semen.
- Engage in nonpenetrative sex such as body massage, social kissing (dry), mutual masturbation, fantasy, and sex films.
- Inform prospective sexual and drug-using partners of your HIV-positive status.
- Notify previous and present sexual partners if you learn that you are HIV seropositive.
- If you are HIV seropositive, do not have unprotected sex with another HIV-seropositive person, because cross-infection with another HIV strain can increase the severity of the disease.
- Do not share needles, razors, toothbrushes, sex toys, or other blood-contaminated articles.
- If you are HIV seropositive, do not donate blood, plasma, body organs, or sperm.

Standard Precautions

The following guidelines were developed to prevent the transmission of infection during patient care for all patients, regardless of known or unknown infectious status.

Hand Washing/Hand Hygiene
- Wash hands/perform hand hygiene after touching blood, body fluids, secretions, excretions, and contaminated items, whether or not gloves are worn.
- Wash hands/perform hand hygiene immediately after gloves are removed, between patient contacts, and when otherwise indicated to avoid transfer of microorganisms to other patients or environments.
- Wash hands/perform hand hygiene between tasks and procedures on the same patient to prevent cross-contamination of different body sites.
- Use a plain (nonantimicrobial) soap or alcohol-based hand rub for routine hand washing.
- Use an antimicrobial agent or waterless antiseptic agent for specific circumstances (control of outbreaks or hyperendemic infections). (See Contact Precautions.)

Gloves
- Wear clean, nonsterile gloves when touching blood, body fluids, secretions, excretions, and contaminated items.
- Put on clean gloves just before touching mucous membranes and nonintact skin.
- Change gloves between tasks and procedures on the same patient after contact with materials that may contain a high concentration of microorganisms.
- Remove gloves promptly after use, before touching noncontaminated items and environmental surfaces, and before going to another patient.
- Wash hands/perform hand hygiene immediately after removing gloves.

Mask, Eye Protection, Face Shield
- Wear a mask and eye protection or a face shield to protect mucous membranes of the eyes, nose, and mouth during procedures and patient care activities that are likely to generate splashes or sprays of blood, body fluids, secretions, or excretions.

Gown
- Wear a clean, nonsterile gown to protect skin and prevent soiling of clothing during procedures and patient care activities that are likely to generate splashes or sprays of blood, body fluids, secretions, or excretions.
- Select a gown that is appropriate for the activity and amount of fluid likely to be encountered.
- Remove a soiled gown as promptly as possible and wash hands/perform hand hygiene to prevent the transfer of microorganisms to other patients or environments.

Patient Care Equipment
- Handle used patient care equipment soiled with blood, body fluids, secretions, and excretions in a manner that prevents skin and mucous membrane exposures, contamination of clothing, and transfer of microorganisms to other patients and environments.
- Ensure that reusable equipment is not used for the care of another patient until it has been cleaned and reprocessed appropriately.
- Ensure that single-use items are discarded properly.

Environmental Control
- Ensure that the hospital has adequate procedures for the routine care, cleaning, and disinfection of environmental surfaces, beds, bed rails, bedside equipment, and other frequently touched surfaces.
- Ensure that procedures are being followed.

Linen
- Handle, transport, and process used linen soiled with blood, body fluids, secretions, and excretions in a manner that prevents skin and mucous membrane exposures and contamination of clothing and that avoids transfer of microorganisms to other patients and environments.

Occupational Health and Bloodborne Pathogens
- Take care to prevent injuries when using needles, scalpels, and other sharp instruments or devices:
    - When handling sharp instruments after procedures
    - When cleaning used instruments
    - When disposing of used needles
- Never recap used needles or otherwise manipulate them by using both hands or use any technique that involves directing the point of the needle toward any part of the body.
- Use either a one-handed scoop technique or a mechanical device designed for holding the needle sheath.
- Do not remove used needles from disposable syringes by hand and do not bend, break, otherwise manipulate used needles by hand.
- Place used disposable syringes and needles, scalpel blades, and other sharp items in appropriate puncture-resistant containers as close as practical to the area in which the items were used.
- Place reusable syringes and needles in a puncture-resistant container for transport to the reprocessing area.
- Use mouthpieces, resuscitation bags, or other ventilation devices as an alternative to mouth-to-mouth resuscitation methods in areas where the need for resuscitation is predictable.

Patient Placement
- Place a patient who contaminates the environment or who does not or cannot be expected to assist in maintaining appropriate hygiene or environmental control in a private room.
- If a private room is not available, consult with infection control professionals regarding patient placement or other alternatives.

Adapted from Health Canada. (1997b). *Infection control guidelines: Preventing the transmission of bloodborne pathogens in health care and public service settings.* Ottawa, ON: Health Canada.

---

ognized or unrecognized sources of infections in hospitals. A second tier for infection control precautions for specified conditions, called Transmission-Based Precautions, was designed for use in addition to Standard Precautions for patients with documented or suspected infections involving highly transmissible pathogens. The three types of Transmission-Based Precautions are referred to as Airborne Precautions, Droplet Precautions, and Contact Precautions. They can be used singularly or in combination, but they are always to be used in addition to Standard Precautions (Health Canada, 1999).

Large-scale studies of exposed health care workers continue to be conducted by the Public Health Agency of Canada and other groups. In 2000, the Canadian Needle Stick Surveillance Network was implemented by Health Canada to monitor health care workers exposed to blood and body fluids (Public Health Agency of Canada, 2003).

POSTEXPOSURE PROPHYLAXIS FOR HEALTH CARE PROVIDERS

Postexposure prophylaxis in response to exposure of health care personnel to blood or other body fluids has been proven to reduce the risk for HIV infection (Worthington, 2001) (see Chart 52-4). Health care providers who have sustained a significant exposure to HIV should be counselled and offered anti-HIV postexposure prophylaxis, if appropriate (Health Canada, 1997a). Some clinicians are considering using postexposure prophylaxis for patients exposed to HIV from high-risk sexual behaviour or possible contact through injection drug use. This use of postexposure prophylaxis is controversial because of concern that it may be substituted for safer sex practices and safer injection drug use. Postexposure prophylaxis should not be considered an acceptable method of preventing HIV infection.

The medications recommended for postexposure prophylaxis are those used to treat established HIV infection. Ideally, prophylaxis needs to start immediately after exposure; therapy started more than 72 hours after exposure is thought to offer no benefit.

The recommended course of therapy involves taking the prescribed mediations for 4 weeks. Those who choose postexposure prophylaxis must be prepared for the side effects of the medications and must be willing to face the unknown long-term risks, because HIV often becomes resistant to the medications used to treat it. If the person becomes infected despite prophylaxis, viral drug resistance may reduce future treatment options.

Pathophysiology

Since HIV infection is an infectious disease, it is important to understand how HIV integrates itself into a person's immune system and how immunity plays a role in the course of infection. This knowledge is also essential for understanding drug therapy and vaccine development.

Viruses are intracellular parasites. HIV belongs to a group of viruses known as **retroviruses**. These viruses carry their genetic material in the form of ribonucleic acid (RNA) rather than deoxyribonucleic acid (DNA). As can be seen in Figure 52-1, HIV consists of a viral core containing the viral RNA that is surrounded by an envelope consisting of glycoproteins (gp) that protrude. For HIV to enter the targeted cell, the membrane of the viral envelope must be fused with the plasma membrane of the cell, a process mediated by the envelope glycoproteins of HIV (Wyatt & Sodroski, 1998).

The HIV life cycle is complex and consists of a number of steps (Fig. 52-2). First, the HIV GP120 and GP41 attach to the uninfected CD4 cell surface (receptor) and fuse with the cell membrane. Second, the viral core contents are emptied into the host cell, a process known as uncoating. Third, HIV enzyme **reverse transcriptase** copies the viral genetic material from RNA into double-stranded DNA. Fourth, double-stranded DNA is spliced into the cellular DNA by the action of another HIV enzyme integrase. Fifth, using the integrated DNA or **provirus** as a blueprint, the cell makes new viral proteins and viral RNA. Sixth, HIV protease cleaves the new proteins (polyproteins). Seventh, the new proteins join the viral RNA into new viral particles. Finally, new viral particles bud from the cell and start the process all over (Porth, 2002).

Perhaps the least understood aspects of the HIV life cycle are the events that occur immediately after entry of the viral core into the host CD4 cell. The process of viral assembly is intimately linked to its subsequent reversal (disassembly). Interactions occur between viral proteins and cellular factors in the cells that produce virus and frequently influence events at the next round of infection (Emerman & Malim, 1998). In resting (nondividing) cells, HIV can apparently survive in a latent state as an integrated provirus that produces few or no viral particles. These resting CD4 T cells can be prodded to churn out new particles if something reactivates them (Mellors, 1998). When a T cell that harbours this integrated DNA (also known as provirus) becomes activated against HIV or other microbes, the cell replicates and also unwittingly begins to

Chart 52-4 Postexposure Prophylaxis for Health Care Providers

If you sustain a needlestick injury, take the following actions immediately:

- Wash the area with soap and water.
- Alert your supervisor and initiate the injury-reporting system used in the setting.
- Identify the source patient, who may need to be tested for HIV, hepatitis B, and hepatitis C. (State laws will determine if written informed consent must be obtained from the source patient prior to his or her testing.)
- Report to the employee health services, the emergency department, or other designated treatment facility.
- Give consent for baseline testing for HIV, hepatitis B, and hepatitis C.
- Get postexposure prophylaxis for HIV in accordance with CDC guidelines. Start the prophylaxis medications within 2 hours after exposure. Make sure that you are being monitored for symptoms of toxicity. Practice safer sex until follow-up testing is complete.
- Follow up with postexposure testing at 6 weeks, 3 months, and 6 months and perhaps 1 year.
- Document the exposure in detail for your own records as well as for the employer.

Worthington, K. (2001). You've been stuck: What do you do? *American Journal of Nursing, 101*(3); 104.

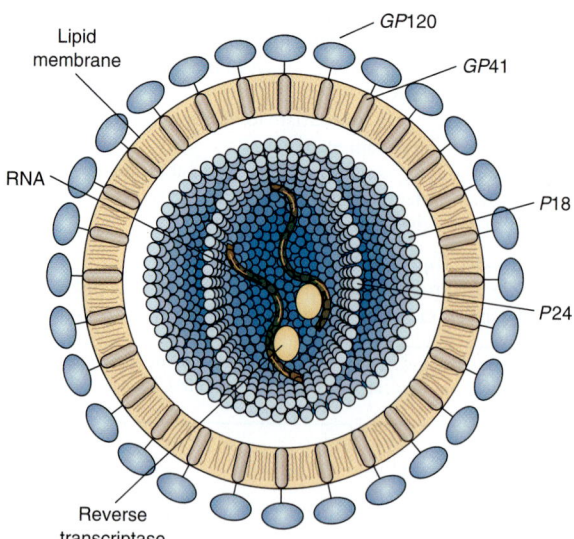

FIGURE 52-1 Structure of the HIV-1 virus. A glycoprotein envelope surrounds the virus, which carries its genetic material in RNA. Knobs, consisting of protein GP120 and GP41, protrude from the envelope. These proteins are essential for binding the virus to the CD4+ T lymphocyte. From Porth, C. (2002). *Pathophysiology: Concepts of altered health states* (6th ed.). Philadelphia: Lippincott Williams & Wilkins.

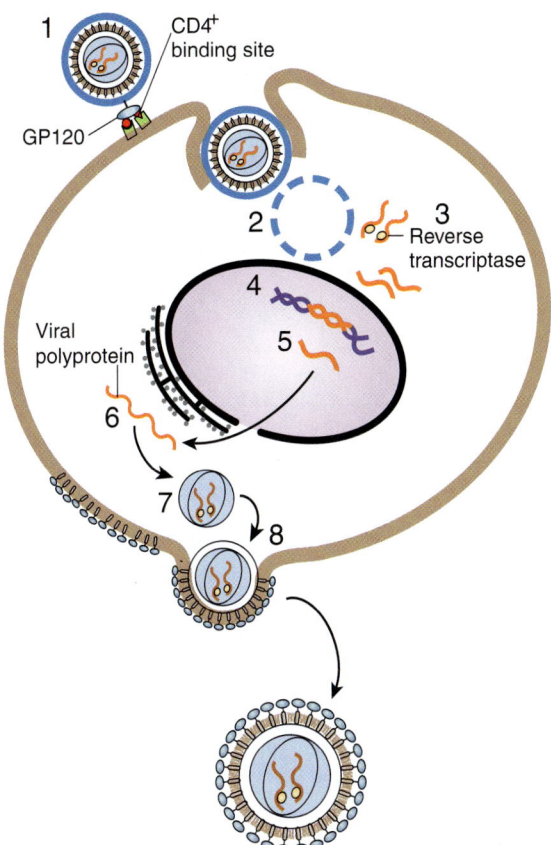

FIGURE 52-2 Life cycle of the HIV-1: (1) Attachment of the HIV virus to CD4+ receptor; (2) internalization and uncoating of the virus with viral RNA and reverse transcriptase; (3) reverse transcription, which produces a mirror image of the viral RNA and double-stranded DNA molecule; (4) integration of viral DNA into host DNA using the integrase enzyme; (5) transcription of the inserted viral DNA to produce viral messenger RNA; (6) translation of viral messenger RNA to create viral polyprotein; (7) cleavage of viral polyprotein into individual viral proteins that make up the new virus; and (8) assembly and release of the new virus from the host cell. From Porth, C. (2002). *Pathophysiology: Concepts of altered health states* (6th ed.). Philadelphia: Lippincott Williams & Wilkins.

produce new copies of both RNA and viral proteins (Bartlett & Moore, 1998). Activation of the infected cell may be achieved by antigens, mitogens, select cytokines (tumour necrosis factor-alpha or interleukin-1), or virus gene products of such viruses as **cytomegalovirus** (CMV), Epstein-Barr virus, herpes simplex virus, and hepatitis. Consequently, whenever the infected T4 cell is activated, HIV replication and budding occur, which often destroys the host cell. Newly formed HIV is then released into the blood plasma and infects other CD4+ cells (see Fig. 52-1).

HIV-1 mutates quickly, at a relatively constant rate, with about 1% of the virus's genetic material changing annually. Over the years, 10 distinct subtypes of HIV-1 have emerged, designated A through J. Subtype B is the dominant subtype in North America and Europe, while subtype D predominates in Africa (Stephenson, 1998).

All viruses target specific cells. Lymphocytes consist of three major populations: T cells, B cells, and natural killer cells (Huston, 1997). Mature T cells are phenotypically composed of two major subpopulations defined by cell surface reciprocal expression of CD4 or CD8 (Huston, 1997). Approximately two thirds of peripheral blood T cells are CD4 and approximately one third are CD8. Most people have about 700 to 1,000 CD4 cells/mm³,

but as low as 500/mm³ can be considered "normal." HIV targets cells with the CD4 glycoprotein, which is expressed on the surface of T lymphocytes, **monocytes**, dendritic cells, and brain microglia (Wyatt & Sodroski, 1998). A major function of CD4 binding is to induce conformational changes in the GP120 glycoprotein of the HIV envelope that contribute to the formation or exposure of the binding site for the chemokine receptors (Wyatt & Sodroski, 1998). Most primary clinical isolates of HIV use the chemokine receptor **CCR5** for entry. HIV-1 isolates arising later in the course of infection often use other chemokine receptors such as CXCR4 in addition to CCR5 (Wyatt & Sodroski, 1998). HIV must attach to both the CD4 and CCR5 binding sites in order to infect CD4+ cells. CD4 fits into a recessed pocket in the viral envelope GP120 that may simply be too deep to be easily accessed by antibodies (Balter, 1998). A mutation of CCR5 was identified that is common among Caucasians but not other ethnic groups. About 1% of Caucasians lack functional CCR5 and are highly protected against HIV infection even if exposed (although protection is not absolute); about 18% are not markedly protected against infection but if infected demonstrate significantly slower rates of disease progression (Collman, 1997).

Stages of HIV Disease

The stage of HIV disease is based on clinical history, physical examination, laboratory evidence of immune dysfunction, signs and symptoms, and infections and malignancies. The Health Canada standard case definition of AIDS categorizes HIV infection and AIDS in adults and adolescents on the basis of clinical conditions associated with HIV infection and CD4+ T-cell counts (Health Canada, 2000). The classification system (Table 52-1) groups clinical conditions into one of three categories denoted as A, B, or C.

PRIMARY INFECTION (ALSO KNOWN AS ACUTE HIV INFECTION OR ACUTE HIV SYNDROME)

The period from infection with HIV to the development of antibodies to HIV is known as **primary infection**. During this period, there is intense viral replication and widespread dissemination of HIV throughout the body. Symptoms associated with the viremia range from none to severe flu-like symptoms. During the primary infection period, the window period occurs because a person is infected with HIV but tests negative on the HIV antibody blood test. Although antibodies to the HIV envelope glycoproteins typically can be detected in the sera of HIV-infected individuals by 2 to 3 weeks after infection, most of these antibodies lack the ability to inhibit virus infection. By the time neutralizing antibodies are detected, HIV-1 is firmly established in the host (Wyatt & Sodroski, 1998). During this period, there are high levels of viral replication and the killing of CD4 T cells, resulting in high levels of HIV in the blood and a dramatic drop in CD4 T cell counts from the normal level of at least 800 cells/mm³ of blood. About 3 weeks into this acute phase, individuals may display symptoms reminiscent of mononucleosis, such as fever, enlarged lymph nodes, rash, muscle aches, and headaches. These symptoms resolve within another 1 to 3 weeks as the immune system begins to gain some control over the virus. That is, the CD4 T-cell population responds in ways that spur other immune cells, such as CD8 lymphocytes, to increase their killing of infected, virus-producing cells. The body produces antibody molecules in an effort to contain the virus; they bind to free HIV particles (outside cells) and assist in their removal (Bartlett & Moore, 1998). This balance between the amount of HIV in the body and the immune response is referred to as the **viral set point** and

Table 52-1 • Classification System for HIV Infection and Expanded AIDS Surveillance Case Definition for Adolescents and Adults

DIAGNOSTIC CATEGORIES	CLINICAL CATEGORIES		
CD4+ T-Cell Categories	A Asymptomatic, Acute (Primary) HIV or PGL	B Symptomatic, Not (A) or (C) Conditions	C AIDS-Indicator Conditions
(1) ≥500/μL	A1	B1	C1
(2) 200–499/μL	A2	B2	C2
(3) <200/μL AIDS-indicator T-cell count	A3	B3	C3

People with AIDS-indicator conditions (clinical category C) and those in categories A3 or B3 are considered to have AIDS.

Clinical Category A

Includes one or more of the following in an adult or adolescent with confirmed HIV infection and without conditions in clinical categories B and C:

- Asymptomatic HIV infection
- Persistent generalized lymphadenopathy (PGL)
- Acute (primary) HIV infection with accompanying illness or history of acute HIV infection

Clinical Category B

Examples of conditions in clinical category B include, but are not limited to, the following:

- Bacillary angiomatosis
- Candidiasis, oropharyngeal (thrush) or vulvovaginal (persistent, frequent, or poorly responsive to therapy)
- Cervical dysplasia (moderate or severe)/cervical carcinoma in situ
- Constitutional symptoms, such as fever (38.5°C) or diarrhea exceeding 1 month in duration
- Hairy leukoplakia, oral
- Herpes zoster (shingles), involving at least two distinct episodes or more than one dermatome
- Idiopathic thrombocytopenic purpura
- Listeriosis
- Pelvic inflammatory disease, particularly if complicated by tuboovarian abscess
- Peripheral neuropathy

Clinical Category C

Examples of conditions in adults and adolescents include the following:

- Candidiasis of bronchi, trachea, or lungs; esophagus
- Cervical cancer, invasive
- Coccidioidomycosis, disseminated or extrapulmonary
- Cryptococcosis, extrapulmonary
- Cryptosporidiosis, chronic intestinal (exceeding 1 month's duration)
- Cytomegalovirus disease (other than liver, spleen, or lymph nodes)
- Cytomegalovirus retinitis (with loss of vision)
- Encephalopathy, HIV-related
- Herpes simplex: chronic ulcer(s) (exceeding 1 month's duration); or bronchitis, pneumonitis, or esophagitis
- Histoplasmosis, disseminated or extrapulmonary
- Isosporiasis, chronic intestinal (exceeding 1 month's duration)
- Kaposi's sarcoma
- Lymphoma, Burkitt's (or equivalent term); immunoblastic (or equivalent term); primary, of brain
- *Mycobacterium avium* complex or *M. kansasii,* disseminated or extrapulmonary
- *Mycobacterium tuberculosis,* any site (pulmonary or extrapulmonary)
- *Mycobacterium,* other species or unidentified species, disseminated or extrapulmonary
- *Pneumocystis carinii* pneumonia
- Pneumonia, recurrent
- Progressive multifocal leukoencephalopathy
- *Salmonella* septicemia, recurrent
- Toxoplasmosis of brain
- Wasting syndrome due to HIV

Adapted from Centers for Disease Control, U.S. Department of Health and Human Services. (1992). 1993 revised classification system for HIV infection and expanded surveillance case definition for AIDS among adolescents and adults. *MMWR CDC Recommendations and Reports, 41* (RR 17), 1–19.

results in a steady state of infection. During this steady state, which can last for years, the amount of virus in circulation and the number of infected cells equal the rate of viral clearance (Ropka & Williams, 1998).

Primary HIV infection, the time during which the viral burden set point is achieved, includes the acute symptomatic and early infection phases. During this initial stage, viral replication is associated with dissemination in lymphoid tissue and a distinct immunologic response. The final level of the viral set point is inversely correlated with disease prognosis; that is, the higher the viral set point, the poorer the prognosis (Cates, Chesney & Cohen, 1997). The primary infection stage is part of CDC category A.

HIV ASYMPTOMATIC (CDC CATEGORY A: MORE THAN 500 CD4+ T LYMPHOCYTES/MM³)

On reaching a viral set point, a chronic, clinically asymptomatic state begins. Despite its best efforts, the immune system rarely if ever fully eliminates the virus. By about 6 months, the rate of viral

replication reaches a lower but relatively steady state that is reflected in the maintenance of viral levels at a kind of "set point." This set point varies greatly from patient to patient and dictates the subsequent rate of disease progression; on average, 8 to 10 years pass before a major HIV-related complication develops. In this prolonged, chronic stage, patients feel well and show few if any symptoms (Bartlett & Moore, 1998). Apparent good health continues because CD4 T-cell levels remain high enough to preserve defensive responses to other pathogens.

HIV SYMPTOMATIC (CDC CATEGORY B: 200 TO 499 CD4+ T LYMPHOCYTES/MM³)

Over time, the number of CD4 T cells gradually falls. Category B consists of symptomatic conditions in HIV-infected patients that are not included in the conditions listed in category C. These conditions must also meet one of the following criteria: (1) the condition is due to HIV infection or a defect in cellular immunity, or (2) the condition must be considered to have a clinical course or require management that is complicated by HIV infection. If an individual was once treated for a category B condition and has not developed a category C disease but is now symptom-free, that person's illness would be considered category B.

AIDS (CDC CATEGORY C: LESS THAN 200 CD4+ T LYMPHOCYTES/MM³)

When CD4 T-cell levels drop below 200 cells/mm³ of blood, patients are said to have AIDS. As levels fall below 100, the immune system is significantly impaired (Bartlett & Moore, 1998). Once a patient has had a category C condition, he or she remains in category C. This classification has implications for entitlements (ie, disability benefits, housing, and food stamps) since these programs are often linked to an AIDS diagnosis. Although the revised classification emphasizes CD4+ T-cell counts, it allows for CD4+ percentages (percentage of CD4+ T cells of total lymphocytes). The CD4+ percentage is less subject to variation on repeated measurements than is the absolute CD4+ T-cell count. Less than 14% of the CD4+ T cells of the total lymphocytes is consistent with an AIDS diagnosis. The percentage, as compared to the absolute number of CD4+ T cells, becomes particularly important when the patient has a heightened immune response to infections in addition to HIV. One complication of advanced HIV infection is anemia, which may be caused by HIV, opportunistic diseases, and medications (Collier et al., 2001).

Assessment and Diagnostic Findings

During the first stage of HIV infection, the patient may be asymptomatic or may exhibit various signs and symptoms. The patient history should alert the health care provider about the need for HIV screening based on the patient's sexual practices, injection drug use, and receipt of blood transfusions. Additionally, exposure to body fluids containing infected blood while providing care to others with HIV infection, such as through needlesticks, should alert health care providers to possible HIV infection. Patients who are in later stages of HIV infection may have a variety of symptoms related to their immunosuppressed state.

Several screening tests are used to diagnose HIV infection. Others are used to assess the stage and severity of the infection. Table 52-2 identifies common blood tests.

HIV ANTIBODY TESTS

In 1985, the FDA licensed an HIV-1 antibody assay, which is used to screen all blood and plasma donations. When an individual is infected with HIV, the immune system responds by producing antibodies against the virus, usually within 3 to 12 weeks after infection. This delay in the production of antibody helps to explain why a person may be infected but not test antibody-positive during primary infection. The ability to document HIV antibodies in the blood has permitted screening of blood products and facilitated identification of individuals with HIV infection. Before an HIV antibody test is performed, the meaning of the test and possible test results are explained, and informed consent for the test is obtained from the patient. When results of the HIV antibody testing are received, they are carefully explained to the patient in private (Chart 52-5). All test results are kept confidential. Education and counselling about the test results and disease transmission are essential.

Blood samples are tested with two different blood tests to determine the presence of antibodies to HIV. The **EIA (enzyme immunoassay),** formerly referred to as the **ELISA (enzyme-linked immunosorbent assay)** test, identifies antibodies directed specifically against HIV. The **Western blot assay** is used to confirm seropositivity when the EIA is positive. People whose blood contains antibodies for HIV are seropositive. Saliva can also be tested using the EIA antibody test.

The FDA approved a rapid HIV antibody screening test in November 2002. Using less than a drop of blood, this new test can quickly (approximately 20 minutes) and reliably (99.6% accuracy) detect antibodies to HIV-1. It is anticipated that the newly approved HIV test, the OraQuick Rapid HIV-1 Antibody Test, will allow more rapid notification of individuals about their HIV status so that they can obtain care early in the course of HIV infection and take measures to help prevent the spread.

Patients' psychological responses to seropositive test results may include feelings of panic, depression, and hopelessness. The social and interpersonal consequences of a positive test result can be devastating. Patients may lose their sexual partners and their health insurance because of disclosure; they may experience discrimination in employment and housing as well as social ostracism. For these reasons and others, patients who test positive may need ongoing counselling as well as referrals for social, financial, medical, and psychological support services. Patients whose test results are seronegative may develop a false sense of security, possibly resulting in continued high-risk behaviours or feelings that they are immune to the virus. They may need ongoing counselling to help them modify high-risk behaviours and to return for repeated testing. Other patients may experience anxiety regarding the uncertainty of their status.

Home-based testing for HIV antibodies using a small amount of blood was first proposed in 1985 but not approved by the FDA until 1995. Although home testing kits are commercially available, they do raise concerns because of the lack of counselling and

TEST	FINDINGS IN HIV INFECTION
EIA (enzyme immunoassay), formerly referred to as ELISA (enzyme-linked immunosorbent assay)	Antibodies are detected, resulting in positive results and marking the end of the window period.
Western blot	Also detects antibodies to HIV; used to confirm EIA
Viral load	Measures HIV RNA in the plasma
CD4/CD8 ratio	These are lymphocytes. HIV kills CD4 cells, which results in a significantly impaired immune system.

Table 52-2 • **Selected Laboratory Tests for Diagnosing and Tracking HIV and Assessing Immune Status**

Chart 52-5 • PATIENT EDUCATION
HIV Test Results: Implications for Patients

Interpretation of Positive Test Results
- Antibodies to HIV are present in the blood (the patient has been infected with the virus, and the body has produced antibodies).
- HIV is active in the body, and the patient can transmit the virus to others.
- Despite HIV infection, the patient does not necessarily have AIDS.
- The patient is not immune to AIDS (the antibodies do not indicate immunity).

Interpretation of Negative Test Results
- Antibodies to HIV are not present in the blood at this time, which can mean that the patient has not been infected with HIV or, if infected, the body has not yet produced antibodies (which takes from 3 weeks to 6 months or longer).
- The patient should continue taking precautions. The test result does not mean that the patient is immune to the virus, nor does it mean the patient is not infected; it just means that the body may not have produced antibodies yet.

the possibility of inaccurate results, including both false-positive and false-negative results (Lewis, 2001).

VIRAL LOAD TESTS

Target amplification methods quantify HIV RNA or DNA levels in the plasma and have replaced p24 antigen capture assays. Target amplification methods include reverse transcriptase **polymerase chain reaction** (RT-PCR) or nucleic acid sequence-based amplification (NASBA). A widely used **viral load test** measures plasma HIV RNA levels. Currently, these tests are used to track viral load and response to treatment for HIV infection. RT-PCR is also used to detect HIV in high-risk seronegative people before the development of antibodies, to confirm a positive EIA, and to screen neonates. HIV culture or quantitative plasma culture and plasma viremia are additional tests that measure viral burden, but they are used infrequently. Viral load is a better predictor of the risk of HIV disease progression than the CD4 count. The lower the viral load, the longer the time to AIDS diagnosis and the longer the survival time.

Treatment of HIV Infection

Protocols of how to treat HIV disease change relatively often. Yearly a team of physicians from throughout the United States evaluates the latest evidence and makes recommendations that are widely disseminated, and monthly a subgroup evaluates available evidence (Panel on Clinical Practices for Treatment of HIV Infection [Panel], 2004, cited by McGill University, 2005). These recommendations are generally used by Canadian health care providers to guide treatment protocols. Treatment decisions for an individual patient are based on three factors: HIV RNA (viral load); CD4 T-cell count; and the clinical condition of the patient (Panel, 2000). Treatment should be offered to all patients with the primary infection (acute HIV syndrome, as previously described). In general, treatment should be offered to individuals with a T-cell count of less than 350 or plasma HIV RNA levels exceeding 55,000 copies/mL (RT-PCR assay)(McGill University, 2005).

The increasing number of antiretroviral agents (Table 52-3) and the rapid evolution of new information have introduced ex-

traordinary complexity into the treatment of HIV-infected persons (Panel, 2000). Adherence rates among persons living with HIV and AIDS are no different from those of patients with other chronic diseases (Williams, 2001). Antiretroviral regimens are complex, have major side effects, pose difficulties with regard to adherence, and carry serious potential consequences from the development of viral resistance due to lack of adherence to the drug regimen or suboptimal levels of antiretroviral agents (Panel, 2000). The goals of treatment are maximal and durable suppression of viral load, restoration and/or preservation of immunologic function, improved quality of life, and reduction of HIV-related morbidity and mortality. The Panel's guidelines recommend viral load testing at diagnosis and every 3 to 4 months thereafter in the untreated person; T-cell counts should be measured at diagnosis and generally every 3 to 6 months thereafter.

It is difficult to predict which patients will adhere to medication regimens (Holzemer, Corless, Nokes, et al., 1999). Perceived engagement with the health care provider has been associated with greater adherence to HIV medication regimens (Bakken et al., 2000). Individualized plans of care that take into consideration housing and social support issues in addition to health indicators are essential.

Results of therapy are evaluated with viral load tests (Panel, 2000). Viral load levels should be measured immediately prior to and again at 2 to 8 weeks after initiation of antiretroviral therapy, since in most patients adherence to a regimen of potent antiretroviral agents should result in a large decrease in the viral load by 2 to 8 weeks. The viral load should continue to decline over the following weeks and in most individuals will drop below detectable levels (currently defined as less than 50 RNA copies/mL) by 16 to 20 weeks. The rate of viral load decline toward undetectable levels is affected by the baseline T-cell count, the initial viral load, the potency of the medication, adherence of the patient to the medication regimen, prior exposure to antiretroviral agents, and the presence of any OIs (Panel, 2000). The confirmed absence of a viral load response should prompt the health care team to re-evaluate the regimen.

All approved anti-HIV drugs attempt to block viral replication within cells by inhibiting either reverse transcriptase or the HIV protease (Bartlett & Moore, 1998). A treatment duration of 5 to 7 years of continuous therapy is difficult because of the complexity, toxicity, and cost of the current drug regimens, especially when the concept of maintenance therapy with a simplified regimen does not seem viable (Ho, 1998). Medication side effects can make life difficult and are one of the main reasons people miss doses of the medications or stop taking them completely (Horn & Pieribone, 1999).

All medications have toxic side effects. The nurse can obtain Web-based information to remain current about medications used to treat HIV/AIDS. The NIH (National Institutes of Health) maintains an AIDS drug line Website (see resources at the end of this chapter). Increasing numbers of patients with HIV infection receiving medications are presenting with metabolic complications such as increases in cholesterol and triglyceride levels, hyperglycemia, and altered body habitus (NIAID, 2001). Toxicity to cell mitochondria may be involved in many of the side effects of HIV medications, including peripheral neuropathy, myopathy and cardiomyopathy, lactic acidosis and hepatic steatosis (fatty degeneration of liver), pancreatitis, osteopenia and osteoporosis, and bone marrow suppression. Fat redistribution (lipodystrophy syndrome, also known as pseudo-Cushing's syndrome [Panel, 2001]) is one of the most frequent systemic side effects. Many people who have lipodystrophy experience an increase in fat loss

MEDICATION	SIDE/ADVERSE EFFECTS	COMMENTS	COMBINATION PREPARATIONS
Nucleoside analog reverse transcriptase inhibitors (NRTIs)			

Act by becoming part of HIV's DNA and derail its building process. As a result, the damaged viral DNA cannot take control of the host cell's DNA (Gracia Jones, 2001). Possible adverse reactions associated with medications that act through this mechanism include peripheral neuropathy, pancreatitis, lactic acidosis, bone marrow suppression, neutropenia, anemia, arthralgia, myopathy, kidney dysfunction, hepatomegaly, liver failure, vision changes, neuropathy, hypersensitivity reaction, abdominal pain, fever, chills, sore throat, oral ulcers, dry mouth, muscle and joint pain, irritability, anxiety, nervousness (Gracia Jones, 2001). Lactic acidosis with hepatic steatosis (fatty degeneration of the liver) is a rare but potentially life-threatening toxicity with this classification of medications (Panel on Clinical Practices, 2000, 2001).

MEDICATION	SIDE/ADVERSE EFFECTS	COMMENTS	COMBINATION PREPARATIONS
zidovudine (AZT, Retrovir)	Bone marrow suppression: anemia, neutropenia. Subjective complaints: GI intolerance, appetite loss, fatigue, headaches, insomnia, asthenia, pain	Take without regard to meals.	Combination agents containing AZT: zidovudine/lamivudine (Combivir); Retrovir, Epivir, and Ziagen (Trizivir)
lamivudine (3TC, Epivir)	Minimal toxicity; anemia, fatigue, hair loss, headache, nausea, peripheral neuropathy	Take without regard to meals.	Combination agents containing lamivudine: zidovudine/lamivudine (Combivir); Retrovir, Epivir, and Ziagen (Trizivir)
d4t (Zerit, stavudine)	Peripheral neuropathy, pancreatitis, facial wasting, fungal infections, nausea	Take without regard to meals.	
ddi (Videx, didanosine, Videx EC (enteric-coated/delayed-release)	Diarrhea, nausea, oral ulcers, pancreatitis (fatal and non-fatal); peripheral neuropathy	Take ½ hour before or 1 hour after meals; avoid alcohol.	
ddc (Hivid, zalcitabine)	Peripheral neuropathy; stomatitis (mouth ulcers), nausea, more rarely pancreatitis	Take without regard to meals.	
abacavir (Ziagen)	Hypersensitivity reaction (can be fatal); fever, rash, nausea, vomiting, malaise or fatigue, insomnia, loss of appetite	Discontinue drug as soon as hypersensitivity reaction is suspected, and do not restart.	Combination agent containing abacavir: Retrovir, Epivir, and Ziagen (Trizivir)

Non-nucleoside reverse transcriptase inhibitors (NNRTIs)

Act by attaching to the reverse transcriptase enzyme, which prevents it from converting HIV RNA into HIV DNA (Gracia Jones, 2001). Possible adverse reactions for this group of agents include abnormal liver function test results, hepatitis, stomatitis, numbness, muscle pain, drowsiness, changes in dreams, trouble concentrating, severe psychiatric symptoms in rare cases (severe depression, suicidal thoughts, angry behaviour) (Gracia Jones, 2001). Rare cases of Stevens-Johnson syndrome have been reported with the use of this class of medications (Panel on Clinical Practices, 2000, 2001). Drug resistance develops very easily, which makes adherence essential.

MEDICATION	SIDE/ADVERSE EFFECTS	COMMENTS	COMBINATION PREPARATIONS
nevirapine (Viramune)	Skin rash, increased transaminase levels, hepatitis, fever, headache, nausea, stomach upset	Take without regard to meals.	
delavirdine (Rescriptor)	Skin rash, increased transaminase levels, headache, diarrhea, fatigue, stomach upset	Take without regard to meals.	
efavirenz (Sustiva)	Unusual dreams, poor concentration, anxiety, CNS symptoms including dizziness, drowsiness, increased transaminase levels, nausea, false-positive cannabinoid test	Avoid taking after high-fat meals.	
tenofovir (Viread)	Generally well tolerated. Adverse effect data not available at this point. Mild to moderate GI side effects (nausea, diarrhea, vomiting, flatulence)	Take with food. Monitor for lactic acidosis and hepatomegaly.	

Protease inhibitors

Work at a later stage in the HIV replication process by preventing the protease enzyme from cutting HIV viral proteins into the viral particles that infect new CD4 T4 cells. As a result, new copies of HIV are defective and unable to infect new host cells (Gracia Jones, 2001). Possible adverse reactions include hemolytic anemia, paresthesia, kidney stones, asymptomatic hyperbilirubinemia, dyspepsia, numbness (of lips, hands, or feet), altered taste, drowsiness, mood alterations (Gracia Jones, 2001); in patients with hemophilia, there are possible increased bleeding episodes (Panel on Clinical Practices, 2000, 2001).

(continued)

Table 52-3 • Antiretroviral Agents (Continued)

DRUG	SIDE/ADVERSE EFFECTS	COMMENTS	COMBINATION PREPARATIONS
nelfinavir (Viracept)	Diarrhea, hyperglycemia, fat redistribution and lipid abnormalities	Take with meal or snack.	
ritonavir (Norvir)	Peripheral neuropathy, liver toxicity (hepatitis), GI intolerance, nausea, vomiting, diarrhea, paraesthesias (circumoral and extremities), asthenia, taste perversion. Triglycerides can increase more than 200%, transaminase elevation, elevated CPK and uric acid, hyperglycemia. Fat redistribution and lipid abnormalities.	Take with food if possible to increase tolerability. Refrigerate capsules; do not refrigerate oral solution.	
saquinavir (Invirase, Fortovase)	Fatigue, GI intolerance, nausea, diarrhea, headache, elevated transaminase enzymes, hyperglycemia, fat redistribution and lipid abnormalities	No food effect for Invirase when taken with ritonavir; take Fortovase with a large meal. Refrigerate Fortovase or store at room temperature up to 3 months.	Combination agent containing ritonavir: lopinavir and ritonavir (Kaletra). Additional side effects: insomnia, abdominal pain, rash. Take with food.
indinavir (Crixivan)	Kidney stones (nephrolithiasis), GI intolerance, nausea, increased indirect bilirubinemia, headache, asthenia, blurred vision, dizziness, rash, metallic taste, thrombocytopenia, hyperglycemia, fat redistribution and lipid abnormalities	Take 1 hour before or 2 hours after meals; may take with skim milk or low-fat meal. Store in original container, which contains desiccant— without this, it is stable for only 3 days. Drink a large volume of water.	
amprenavir (Agenerase)	Diarrhea, nausea, oral tingling and numbness, rash, vomiting	Avoid taking with high-fat meal.	

in the legs, arms, and face and/or a buildup of fat around the abdomen and at the base of the neck. Patients may also experience an increase in breast size. These changes in body image can be very disturbing to persons living with HIV/AIDS and have been reported to occur in 6% to 80% of patients receiving HAART (see following discussion). Hepatotoxicity associated with certain protease inhibitors may limit the use of these agents, especially in patients with underlying liver dysfunction (Panel, 2000).

Combination therapy is defined as a regimen containing any combination of two antiretroviral agents; HAART is defined as a regimen consisting of two nucleoside reverse transcriptase inhibitors plus a **protease inhibitor** or a non-nucleoside reverse transcriptase inhibitor, or two protease inhibitors and one other antiretroviral agent (Agins, 2000). As new medications are developed, the number of combinations continues to increase. Safety and efficacy data on many of the combination therapies are limited. Use of three- and four-drug combination regimens has become more widespread, starting earlier in the course of infection, with careful monitoring by viral load measures. In some patients receiving three-drug regimens, viral levels are so low that they are no longer detectable. Future therapy may be individualized based on the viral strain and resistance to antiretroviral drugs. Initially, HAART consisting of a triple-drug regimen (a protease inhibitor

and two non-nucleoside reverse transcriptase inhibitors) is recommended. Drawbacks of HAART are the inability of some patients to adhere to the regimen, the need to take multiple medications on different dosing schedules, and the risk for drug interactions. The duration of therapy needed to control acute HIV infection is unknown, but therapy may continue for several years or for life. Combination therapy with different types of fusion and entry inhibitors (such as T-20) may be synergistic against HIV. These agents fall into a new category of HIV medications called fusion inhibitors and target the GP120 during the initial stage of the HIV life cycle, which is cell fusion (Saag, 2001).

Drug Resistance

Drug resistance can be broadly defined as the ability of pathogens to withstand the effects of medications intended to be toxic to them. Resistance develops as a result of spontaneous genetic mutation of the pathogens or in response to exposure to the medication (Esch & Frank, 2001). Factors associated with the development of drug resistance include serial monotherapy (taking one medication at a time), inadequate suppression of virus replication with suboptimal treatment regimens, difficulty with adherence to complex and toxic regimens, and initiation of therapy late in the course of HIV infection (Boden et al., 1999). HIV-1 may find refuge in organ sanctuaries such as behind the blood–brain barrier, where diminished drug concentrations in the central nervous system (CNS) might induce the development of drug-resistant mutants (Cavert & Haase, 1998). HIV-1 persists in lymphoid tissue even in individuals who appear to have responded well to antiviral therapy (Letvin, 1998). Deciding whether the medication regimen is effective or ineffective is a complex phenomenon. Some individuals experience an optimal response to treatment, as shown by effective viral suppression and ensuing immune recovery; others experience increasing CD4+ cell counts in the presence of ongoing viral replication or blunted immune recovery despite viral control, and finally complete treatment failure (Perrin & Telenti, 1998).

Central to the complexity of HIV drug resistance are the phenomenon of HIV quasi-species (the simultaneous presence in a patient of multiple viral variants), the extent of cross-resistance among antiviral agents, the existence in each individual of archival HIV DNA copies representing all viruses that emerged under the patient's previous treatment, and the preexistence of resistant variants even without prior exposure to the medication (Perrin & Telenti, 1998). Measurement of HIV drug susceptibility for management of HIV infection is now practical using recombinant DNA technology (Hirsch et al., 2000). Although available data support a role for HIV drug resistance testing in selecting medications in many clinical situations, these test results should not be used as the principal criterion for decisions on initiating or changing antiretroviral therapy. Such decisions should be based primarily on the patient's plasma HIV viral load. Several factors in addition to resistance testing must be considered in choosing medications for a new regimen once the prior regimen has failed. These factors include the patient's past treatment history, viral load, medication tolerance, the likelihood of the patient adhering to the medication regimen, and concomitant medical conditions or medications (Hirsch et al., 2000). Blood specimens should be obtained for resistance testing before the failing drug regimen is stopped (Hirsch et al., 2000).

Structured Intermittent Therapy

Because of drug toxicities, drug resistance, difficulties with adherence, and the high cost of medications, the complex medication regimen is often difficult for patients to follow. In an effort to determine if alternative treatment approaches are possible, a study is underway to examine patients' responses to stopping HAART therapy by monitoring their immune status and viral load (Dybul et al., 2001). This would allow patients to move from a continuous regimen of anti-HIV therapy to a strategy in which they discontinue therapy for a specific period of time (ie, 7 days) and then resume therapy for 7 days. This approach is known as structured intermittent therapy. While preliminary results of the study are promising, larger studies are needed to determine the effectiveness of these alternative medication regimens.

IMMUNOMODULATOR THERAPY

Combating HIV infection requires not only agents that will inhibit viral growth but also those that will restore or augment the damaged immune system. New therapies are needed to restore immune function, and immunologic markers need to be identified to predict the success of therapy (NIAID, 2001). Current research is testing the effectiveness of interleukin-2, interleukin-12, and other cytokines and lymphokines (NIAID, 2001).

VACCINES

HIV-1 is a uniquely difficult target for the development of vaccines (Burton, 2005). Since HIV-1 was discovered, researchers have been working to develop a vaccine. A vaccine is a substance that triggers the production of antibodies to destroy the offending organism. Most vaccines activate the humoral arm of the immune system, which stimulates the production of protective antibodies. In addition to antibodies, B lymphocytes take the form of memory B cells. These cells do not produce antibodies immediately but respond vigorously to subsequent exposure. Vaccines that stimulate the cellular arm of the immune system are being developed. Since 1995, there have been a variety of vaccines under study using different strategies to prevent HIV infection in animals and humans. Some researchers are exploring whether different immunization schedules, different schedules of boosters, or a combination of several vaccines will result in stronger or more durable responses. Creation of an HIV vaccine is feasible, but a worldwide commitment is needed. Cooperation between all nations is necessary to develop and commit the resources to develop the vaccine and to create and support the infrastructure needed to facilitate testing of vaccine immunogens (Letvin, Bloom & Hoffman, 2001).

The Canadian HIV Trials Network (CTN) is a partnership of physicians, nurses, people living with HIV, pharmaceutical companies, and others who are committed to developing treatments, vaccines, and a cure for HIV disease and AIDS through the conduct of scientifically sound and ethical clinical trials. Development of antiretroviral drugs as well as a vaccine are two foci of the Network's activities, and clinical trials are under way in various parts of the country. For more information, see the CTN website: http://www.hivnet.ubc.ca/e/home/index.html.

Clinical Manifestations

Treatment of specific manifestations of HIV infection and AIDS in the person with advanced disease targets specific symptoms. These are discussed later in this chapter.

Patients with HIV/AIDS experience a number of symptoms related to the disease as well as the effects of treatment. Nurses need to understand the causes, signs and symptoms, and interventions to enhance the quality of life of patients with HIV across the illness trajectory (Ropka & Williams, 1998; Sherman, 1999). The clinical manifestations of HIV/AIDS are widespread and may affect virtually any organ system. Diseases associated with HIV infection and AIDS result from infections, malignancies, or the direct effect of HIV on body tissues. Symptom assessment tools developed for research purposes could be useful in clinical practice to assess symptom intensity and severity (Holzemer, Henry, Nokes, et al., 1999; Nokes, Wheeler & Kendrew, 1994; Nokes & Bakken, 2002).

RESPIRATORY MANIFESTATIONS

Shortness of breath, dyspnea (laboured breathing), cough, chest pain, and fever are associated with various OIs, such as those caused by *Pneumocystis carinii*, *Mycobacterium avium-intracellulare*, CMV, and *Legionella* species. The most common infection in people with AIDS is **Pneumocystis carinii pneumonia** (PCP), one of the first OIs described in association with AIDS.

PCP. PCP is the most common OI resulting in an AIDS diagnosis. Without prophylactic therapy (discussed below), PCP will develop in 80% of all HIV-infected individuals. *P. carinii* was originally classified as a protozoan; however, studies and analysis of its ribosomal RNA structure suggest that it is a fungus. Its structure and antimicrobial sensitivity are very different from other disease-causing fungi. *P. carinii* causes disease only in immunocompromised hosts, invading and proliferating within the pulmonary alveoli with resultant consolidation of the pulmonary parenchyma.

The clinical presentation of PCP in HIV infection is generally less acute than in people who are immunosuppressed as a result of other conditions. The time between the onset of symptoms and the actual documentation of disease may be weeks to months. Patients with AIDS initially develop nonspecific signs and symptoms, such as nonproductive cough, fever, chills, shortness of breath, dyspnea, and occasionally chest pain. PCP may be present despite the absence of crackles. Arterial oxygen concentrations in patients breathing room air may be mildly decreased, indicating minimal hypoxemia.

Untreated, PCP eventually progresses and causes significant pulmonary impairment and, ultimately, respiratory failure. A few patients have a dramatic onset and fulminant course involving severe hypoxemia, cyanosis, tachypnea, and altered mental status. Respiratory failure can develop within 2 to 3 days of initial symptoms.

PCP can be diagnosed definitively by identifying the organism in lung tissue or bronchial secretions. This is accomplished by such procedures as sputum induction, bronchial-alveolar lavage, and transbronchial biopsy (by fibreoptic bronchoscopy).

Mycobacterium avium Complex.

Mycobacterium avium complex (MAC) disease is a leading OI in people with AIDS. Organisms belonging to MAC include *M. avium, M. intracellulare,* and *M. scrofulaceum.* MAC, comprising a group of acid-fast bacilli, usually causes respiratory infection but is also commonly found in the GI tract, lymph nodes, and bone marrow. Most patients with AIDS who have T-cell counts less than 100 have widespread disease at diagnosis and are usually debilitated. MAC infections are associated with rising mortality rates.

Tuberculosis.

Mycobacterium tuberculosis tends to occur in injection drug users and other groups with a preexisting high prevalence of tuberculosis (TB) infection. Unlike other OIs, TB tends to occur early in the course of HIV infection, usually preceding the diagnosis of AIDS. This early occurrence is associated with the development of caseating granulomas (dry, cheeselike masses of granulation tissue), which should raise the suspicion of TB. At this stage, TB responds well to antituberculosis therapy.

TB that occurs late in HIV infection is characterized by absence of an immune response to a tuberculin skin test response. This is known as **anergy** and results because the compromised immune system can no longer respond to the TB antigen. In the later stages of HIV infection, TB is associated with dissemination to extrapulmonary sites such as the CNS, bone, pericardium, stomach, peritoneum, and scrotum. Multiple drug-resistant strains of the bacillus have emerged and are often associated with noncompliance with antituberculosis therapy.

GI MANIFESTATIONS

The GI manifestations of AIDS include loss of appetite, nausea, vomiting, oral and esophageal candidiasis, and chronic diarrhea. Diarrhea is a problem in 50% to 90% of all AIDS patients. GI symptoms may be related to the direct effect of HIV on the cells lining the intestines. Some of the enteric pathogens that occur most frequently, identified by stool cultures or intestinal biopsy, include *Cryptosporidium muris, Salmonella* species, *Isopora belli, Giardia lamblia,* CMV, *Clostridium difficile,* and *M. avium-*

intracellulare. In patients with AIDS, the effects of diarrhea can be devastating in terms of profound weight loss (more than 10% of body weight), fluid and electrolyte imbalances, perianal skin excoriation, weakness, and inability to perform the usual activities of daily living.

Oral Candidiasis.

Candidiasis, a fungal infection, occurs in nearly all patients with AIDS and AIDS-related conditions. Commonly preceding other life-threatening infections, it is characterized by creamy-white patches in the oral cavity. Untreated, oral candidiasis progresses to involve the esophagus and stomach. Associated signs and symptoms include difficult and painful swallowing and retrosternal pain. Some patients also develop ulcerating oral lesions and are particularly susceptible to dissemination of candidiasis to other body systems.

Wasting Syndrome.

Wasting syndrome is part of the category C case definition for AIDS. Diagnostic criteria include profound involuntary weight loss exceeding 10% of baseline body weight and either chronic diarrhea for more than 30 days or chronic weakness and documented intermittent or constant fever in the absence of any concurrent illness that could explain these findings. This protein-energy malnutrition is multifactorial. In some AIDS-associated illnesses, patients experience a hypermetabolic state in which excessive calories are burned and lean body mass is lost. This state is similar to that seen in sepsis and trauma and can lead to organ failure. A distinction between cachexia (wasting) and malnutrition or between cachexia and simple weight loss is important because the metabolic derangement seen in wasting syndrome may not be modified by nutritional support alone.

Anorexia, diarrhea, GI malabsorption, and lack of nutrition in chronic disease all contribute to wasting syndrome. Progressive tissue wasting, however, may occur with only modest GI involvement and without diarrhea. Tumour necrosis factor (TNF) and interleukin-1 (IL-1) are cytokines that play important roles in AIDS-related wasting syndrome. Both act directly on the hypothalamus to cause anorexia. Cytokine-induced fever accelerates the body's metabolism by 14% for every 1°F increase in temperature. TNF causes inefficient use of lipids by reducing enzymes that are needed for fat metabolism, whereas IL-1 triggers the release of amino acids from muscle tissue. People with AIDS generally experience increased protein metabolism in relation to fat metabolism, which results in significant decreases in lean body mass due to muscle and protein breakdown.

Hypertriglyceridemia, seen in people with AIDS and attributed to chronically elevated cytokine levels, can persist in people with AIDS for months without tissue wasting and loss of lean body mass. It is believed that infections and sepsis lead to transient rises in TNF, IL-1, and other cell mediators above the chronically elevated levels generally seen. These transient rises in TNF and IL-1 trigger muscle wasting.

ONCOLOGIC MANIFESTATIONS

Patients with AIDS have a higher than usual incidence of cancer, possibly related to HIV stimulation of developing cancer cells or to the immune deficiency allowing cancer-causing substances, such as viruses, to transform susceptible cells into malignant cells. Kaposi's sarcoma, certain types of B-cell lymphomas, and invasive cervical carcinoma are included in the CDC classification of AIDS-related malignancies. Carcinomas of the skin, stomach, pancreas, rectum, and bladder also occur more frequently than expected in people with AIDS.

Kaposi's Sarcoma. **Kaposi's sarcoma** (KS), the most common HIV-related malignancy, is a disease involving the endothelial layer of blood and lymphatic vessels. It is associated with human herpes virus 8 (HHV-8) transmission (USPHS/IDSA, 2002). When first noted in 1872 by Dr. Moritz Kaposi, KS characteristically presented as lower-extremity skin lesions in elderly men of Eastern European ancestry. This form, referred to as classic Kaposi's sarcoma, was slow to progress and easily treated. An endemic form of KS, found in children and young men in equatorial Africa, is more virulent than the classic form. Acquired KS occurs in patients who are treated with immunosuppressive agents and commonly occurs in patients who have undergone organ transplantation. In such patients, acquired KS usually resolves once the dose of the immunosuppressive medication is decreased or discontinued. In people with AIDS, epidemic KS is most often seen in male homosexuals and bisexuals.

Although the histopathology of all forms of KS is virtually identical, the clinical manifestations differ: AIDS-related KS exhibits a more variable and aggressive course, ranging from localized cutaneous lesions to disseminated disease involving multiple organ systems. Cutaneous signs may be the first manifestations of HIV, appearing in more than 90% of HIV-infected patients as immune function deteriorates. These skin signs correlate to low CD4 counts. Some disorders, such as Kaposi's sarcoma, oral hairy leukoplakia, facial molluscum contagiosum, dry skin, and oral candidiasis, indicate CD4 counts at or below 200 to 300.

Cutaneous lesions appearing anywhere on the body are usually brownish pink to deep purple. They may be flat or raised and surrounded by ecchymoses (hemorrhagic patches) and edema (Fig. 52-3). Rapid development of lesions involving large areas of skin is associated with extensive disfigurement. The location and size of some lesions can lead to venous stasis, lymphedema, and pain. Ulcerative lesions disrupt skin integrity and increase discomfort and susceptibility to infection. The most common sites of visceral involvement include the lymph nodes, GI tract, and lungs. Involvement of internal organs may eventually lead to organ failure, hemorrhage, infection, and death.

Diagnosis of KS is confirmed by biopsy of suspected lesions. Prognosis depends on the extent of the tumour, presence of constitutional symptoms, and CD4 count. Death may result from

FIGURE 52-3 Lesions of the AIDS-related Kaposi's sarcoma. Whereas some patients may have lesions that remain flat, others experience extensively disseminated, raised lesions with edema. From DeVita, V. T. Jr., Hellman, S., & Rosenberg, S. (Eds.). *AIDS: Etiology, diagnosis, treatment, and prevention* (4th ed.). Philadelphia: Lippincott Williams & Wilkins.

tumour progression. More often, however, it results from other complications of HIV infection.

B-Cell Lymphomas. **B-cell lymphomas** are the second most common malignancy occurring in people with AIDS. Lymphomas associated with AIDS usually differ from those occurring in the general population. Patients with AIDS are generally much younger than the usual population affected by non-Hodgkin's lymphoma. In addition, AIDS-related lymphomas tend to develop outside the lymph nodes, most commonly in the brain, bone marrow, and GI tract. These types of lymphomas are characteristically of a higher grade, indicating aggressive growth and resistance to treatment. The course of AIDS-related lymphomas includes multiple sites of organ involvement and complications related to OIs. Although aggressive combination chemotherapy is frequently successful in non-Hodgkin's lymphoma not associated with HIV infection, it is less successful in people with AIDS because of the severe hematologic toxicity and complications of OIs that occur from treatment.

NEUROLOGIC MANIFESTATIONS

An estimated 80% of all patients with AIDS experience some form of neurologic involvement during the course of HIV infection. Many neuropathologic disorders are underreported because patients may have neurologic involvement without overt signs or symptoms. Neurologic complications involve central, peripheral, and autonomic functions.

Neurologic dysfunction results from the direct effects of HIV on nervous system tissue, OIs, primary or metastatic neoplasms, cerebrovascular changes, metabolic encephalopathies, or complications secondary to therapy. Immune system response to HIV infection in the CNS includes inflammation, atrophy, demyelination, degeneration, and necrosis.

HIV Encephalopathy. **HIV encephalopathy** was formerly referred to as AIDS dementia complex. It is a clinical syndrome characterized by a progressive decline in cognitive, behavioural, and motor functions. Substantial evidence exists that HIV encephalopathy is a direct result of HIV infection. HIV has been found in the brain and cerebrospinal fluid (CSF) of patients with HIV encephalopathy. The brain cells infected by HIV are predominantly the CD4 cells of monocyte-**macrophage** lineage. HIV infection is thought to trigger the release of toxins or lymphokines that result in cellular dysfunction or interference with neurotransmitter function rather than cellular damage.

Signs and symptoms may be subtle and difficult to distinguish from fatigue, depression, or the adverse effects of treatment for infections and malignancies. Early manifestations include memory deficits, headache, difficulty concentrating, progressive confusion, psychomotor slowing, apathy, and ataxia. Later stages include global cognitive impairments, delay in verbal responses, a vacant stare, spastic paraparesis, hyperreflexia, psychosis, hallucinations, tremor, incontinence, seizures, mutism, and death.

Confirming the diagnosis of HIV encephalopathy may be difficult. Extensive neurologic evaluation includes a computed tomography (CT) scan, which may indicate diffuse cerebral atrophy and ventricular enlargement. Other tests that may detect abnormalities include magnetic resonance imaging (MRI), analysis of CSF through lumbar puncture, and brain biopsy.

Cryptococcus neoformans. A fungal infection, *Cryptococcus neoformans,* is another common OI among patients with AIDS and causes neurologic disease. Cryptococcal meningitis is characterized by symptoms such as fever, headache, malaise, stiff neck, nausea, vomiting, mental status changes, and seizures. Diagnosis is confirmed by CSF analysis.

Progressive Multifocal Leukoencephalopathy. Progressive multifocal leukoencephalopathy is a demyelinating CNS disorder that affects the oligodendroglia. It occurs in about 3% of AIDS patients. Clinical manifestations often begin with mental confusion and rapidly progress to include blindness, aphasia, paresis (slight paralysis), and death. Treatments have greatly reduced the threat of mortality associated with this disorder.

Other Neurologic Disorders. Other common infections involving the nervous system include *Toxoplasma gondii,* CMV, and *M. tuberculosis.* Additional neurologic manifestations include both central and peripheral neuropathies. Vascular myelopathy is a degenerative disorder affecting the lateral and posterior columns of the spinal cord, resulting in progressive spastic paraparesis, ataxia, and incontinence. HIV-related **peripheral neuropathy** is thought to be a demyelinating disorder; it is associated with pain and numbness in the extremities, weakness, diminished deep tendon reflexes, orthostatic hypotension, and impotence.

DEPRESSIVE MANIFESTATIONS

The prevalence of depression among people with HIV infection is unknown. The causes of depression are multifactorial and may include a history of preexisting mental illness, neuropsychiatric disturbances, and psychosocial factors. Depression also occurs in people with HIV infection in response to the physical symptoms, including pain and weight loss, and the lack of someone to talk with about their concerns. People with HIV/AIDS who are depressed may experience irrational guilt and shame, loss of self-esteem, feelings of helplessness and worthlessness, and suicidal ideation.

INTEGUMENTARY MANIFESTATIONS

Cutaneous manifestations are associated with HIV infection and the accompanying OIs and malignancies. KS (described above) and OIs such as herpes zoster and herpes simplex are associated with painful vesicles that disrupt skin integrity. *Molluscum contagiosum* is a viral infection characterized by deforming plaque formation. Seborrheic dermatitis is associated with an indurated, diffuse, scaly rash involving the scalp and face. Patients with AIDS may also exhibit a generalized folliculitis associated with dry, flaking skin or atopic dermatitis, such as eczema or psoriasis. Up to 60% of patients treated with trimethoprim-sulfamethoxazole (TMP-SMZ) develop a drug-related rash that is pruritic with pinkish-red macules and papules. Regardless of the origin of these rashes, patients experience discomfort and are at increased risk for additional infection from disrupted skin integrity.

ENDOCRINE MANIFESTATIONS

The endocrine manifestations of HIV infection are not completely understood. At autopsy, endocrine glands show infiltration and destruction from OIs or neoplasms. Endocrine function may also be affected by therapeutic agents.

GYNECOLOGIC MANIFESTATIONS

Persistent, recurrent vaginal candidiasis may be the first sign of HIV infection in women. Past or present genital ulcer disease is a risk factor for the transmission of HIV infection. Women with HIV infection are more susceptible to and have increased rates and recurrence of genital ulcer disease and venereal warts. Ulcerative STDs such as chancroid, syphilis, and herpes are more severe in women with HIV infection. **Human papillomavirus** causes

venereal warts and is a risk factor for cervical intraepithelial neoplasia, a cellular change that is frequently a precursor to cervical cancer. Women with HIV are 10 times more likely to develop cervical intraepithelial neoplasia than are those not infected with HIV. There is a strong association between abnormal Pap smears and HIV seropositivity. HIV-seropositive women with cervical carcinoma present with a more advanced stage of disease and have more persistent and recurrent disease and a shorter interval to recurrence and death than women who do not have HIV infection.

A significant percentage of women who require hospitalization for pelvic inflammatory disease (PID) have HIV infection. Women with HIV are at increased risk for PID, and the inflammation associated with PID may potentiate the transmission of HIV infection. Moreover, women with HIV appear to have a higher incidence of menstrual abnormalities, including amenorrhea or bleeding between periods, than women without HIV infection. The failure of health care providers to consider HIV infection in women may lead to a later diagnosis, thereby denying women appropriate treatment.

 ## Gerontologic Considerations

As of June 2004, 11.8% of AIDS cases in Canada were among persons 50 years of age or older, with more than 90% of these cases occurring in men (Public Health Agency of Canada, 2005). HIV infection in middle-aged and older populations may be under-reported and underdiagnosed because health care professionals erroneously believe they are not at risk for HIV infection. Many older adults are sexually active but do not use condoms, viewing them only as a means of unneeded birth control and not considering themselves at risk for HIV infection. Many older gay men who grew up and lived in an era when disclosure of their sexual orientation was not acceptable have lost long-time partners and may turn to younger males for sexual gratification. Older adults may also be injection drug users or may have received HIV-infected blood through transfusions before 1985. As a result, they may be at risk for HIV infection.

Normal age-related changes include a reduction in immune system function similar to that of HIV infection. Older adults are normally at greater risk for infections, cancer, and autoimmune disorders. Many older adults also experience the loss of loved ones, resulting in depression and bereavement, factors that are also associated with depressed immune function. HIV-related dementia in the older adult may mimic Alzheimer's disease and may be misdiagnosed. There are at least three major differences between older (age 50 and up) and younger persons with HIV/AIDS: presence of comorbidities such as diabetes or high blood pressure; number of persons to whom HIV status was disclosed; and physical functioning ability (Nokes et al., 2000) (Nursing Research Profile 52-1). Limited research has demonstrated that the virologic efficacy of HAART in older patients is comparable to that in younger patients; however, the recovery of the immune system is slower and more blunted in older patients (Manfredi, 2004). There is an urgent need for research to document the efficacy of HAART, examine frequency and severity of side effects, and explore issues of adherence in the older population (Manfredi, 2004).

Medical Management

TREATMENT OF INFECTIONS

General Infections. Trimethoprim-sulfamethoxazole (TMP-SMZ; Bactrim, Septra) is an antibacterial agent for treating various organisms causing infection. Persons with HIV infection who have

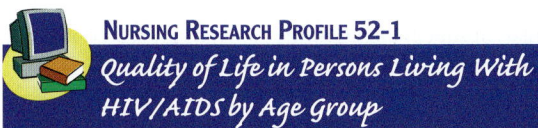

Nokes, K., Holzemer, W., Corless, I., et al. (2000). Health-related quality of life in persons younger and older than 50 who are living with HIV/AIDS. *Research on Aging, 22*(3), 290–310.

NURSING RESEARCH PROFILE 52-1
Quality of Life in Persons Living With HIV/AIDS by Age Group

Purpose
Although HIV/AIDS affects individuals across the age spectrum, it is often perceived as a disease that affects younger persons. As a result, there is little information about people living with HIV/AIDS who are older than 50 years of age. The purpose of this study was to explore health-related quality of life (QOL) for people with HIV and to explore differences in QOL in those 50 or older and in those younger than 50.

Study Sample and Design
A descriptive survey design was used to identify differences in variables predicting health-related QOL. The conceptual model of QOL of Wilson and Cleary was used as the framework for the study. This model describes measures of health on a continuum of increasing biologic, social, and psychological complexity. The convenience sample consisted of 640 people with HIV disease younger than 50 years of age and 73 who were 50 or older. Data analyzed in this study were collected in a national study of persons living with HIV/AIDS who were recruited from a variety of clinical and community-based sites throughout the United States. Various instruments were used to assess HIV disease severity and comorbidities, symptom status, general health perceptions, and overall QOL. In addition, data on individual and environmental characteristics were collected. Individual characteristics included personality/motivation and values/preferences; environmental characteristics examined included psychological support, social and economic support, professional support, and nonmedical factors.

Findings
Older subjects reported significantly more medical conditions and more physical limitations than the younger subjects. They disclosed their HIV status to fewer people than subjects in the younger age group. No significant differences were found between the two groups on any other variables.

Nursing Implications
Although few differences were found in the two groups, the ones that were detected may be clinically relevant. Nurses need to be aware of and address the effect of other medical conditions and physical limitations on self-care in older patients with HIV/AIDS. The fact that older persons had disclosed their HIV status to fewer people than the younger age group may affect the availability of others to assist in their care. Nursing assessment of self-care and the availability of support from others is an important aspect of care of the older person with HIV/AIDS.

---

a T-cell count of less than 200 should receive chemoprophylaxis against PCP with TMP-SMZ. PCP prophylaxis can be safely discontinued in patients responding to HAART with a sustained increase in T lymphocytes. Its use also confers cross-protection against toxoplasmosis and some common respiratory bacterial infections (USPHS/IDSA, 2002). Patients with AIDS who are treated with TMP-SMZ experience a high incidence of adverse effects, such as fever, rashes, leukopenia, thrombocytopenia, and renal dysfunction. Reintroduction of TMP-SMZ using a gradual increase in dose (desensitization) may be successful in up to 70% of patients.

PCP. In the past several years, there have been many advances in the treatment of PCP. TMP-SMZ, the drug of choice for PCP in patients with AIDS and in immunocompromised patients without HIV infection, is available in both intravenous (IV) and oral preparations. Pentamidine (Pentacarinat, Pentam 300, NebuPent), an antiprotozoal medication, is used as an alternative agent for combating PCP. If adverse effects develop or if patients do not improve clinically when treated with TMP-SMZ, the health care provider may recommend pentamidine. Intramuscular administration is avoided because of the potential for painful sterile abscess formation. Also, IV pentamidine may cause severe hypotension if administered too rapidly. Other adverse effects include impaired glucose metabolism (with diabetes mellitus), renal damage, hepatic dysfunction, and neutropenia. Initially, the success of aerosolized pentamidine led to its use as a treatment for mild to moderate PCP. However, it has proved to be less effective and more costly than TMP-SMZ, and early relapses are common. Because of these limitations, the inhalant form of pentamidine is usually reserved for patients with mild to moderate PCP who are intolerant of other treatments. The combination of TMP-SMZ and pentamidine has shown no additional benefit and is avoided because of the cumulative toxic effects that may result.

MAC. Chemoprophylaxis against disseminated MAC disease is indicated for HIV-infected persons with T-cell counts less than 50 (USOHS/IDSA, 2002). Treatment for MAC infections involves use of either clarithromycin (Biaxin) or azithromycin (Zithromax). The combination of azithromycin with rifabutin (Mycobutin) is more effective but the additional cost, increased occurrence of adverse effects, potential for drug interactions, and absence of differences in survival do not warrant the recommendation of both medications (USPHS/IDSA, 2002). Secondary prophylaxis for disseminated MAC may be discontinued in patients with sustained increases (eg, longer than 6 months) in CD4 counts greater than 100 in response to HAART, if they have completed 12 months of MAC therapy and have no signs or symptoms attributable to MAC. Primary prophylaxis for disseminated MAC may be discontinued in patients who have responded to HAART with CD4 counts of 100 or more for at least 3 months and reintroduced if counts decrease to 50 to 100 (USPHS/IDSA, 2002).

Meningitis. Current primary therapy for cryptococcal meningitis is IV amphotericin B with or without oral flucytosine (5-FC, Ancobon) or fluconazole (Diflucan). Serious potential adverse effects of amphotericin B include anaphylaxis, renal and hepatic impairment, electrolyte imbalances, anemia, fever, and severe chills. Intrathecal administration of amphotericin B has been used in place of or in combination with IV administration in patients who have failed to respond to the latter. Until fluconazole, an antifungal agent, was approved and used for lifelong suppressive therapy, frequent relapses and high mortality rates often necessitated prolonged therapy with amphotericin B. In some instances, the patient continues to receive IV amphotericin in the home setting. Oral fluconazole is used as suppressive therapy when the CSF tests negative for the organism. This medication is less toxic and better tolerated than amphotericin B.

Cytomegalovirus Retinitis. Retinitis caused by CMV is a leading cause of blindness in patients with AIDS. Prophylaxis with oral ganciclovir may be considered for HIV-infected persons with T-cell counts of less than 50. Two antiviral agents, ganciclovir

(DHPG, Cytovene, Vitrasert) and foscarnet (Foscavir), offer effective treatment but not a cure for CMV retinitis. Because ganciclovir and foscarnet do not kill the virus but rather control its growth, they must be taken lifelong. Relapse rates of the two agents are similar. Discontinuation of the medication is associated with the relapse of retinitis within 1 month.

A common adverse reaction to ganciclovir is severe neutropenia, which limits the concomitant use of zidovudine (AZT, Compound S, Retrovir). For patients who cannot tolerate systemic ganciclovir because of severe neutropenia, infection at the venous access site, or the need to take zidovudine, intravitreal injections of ganciclovir have been effective. Zidovudine can be given with foscarnet (Foscavir). Common adverse reactions to foscarnet are nephrotoxicity, including acute renal failure, and electrolyte imbalances, including hypocalcemia, hyperphosphatemia, and hypomagnesemia, which can be life-threatening. Other common adverse effects include seizures, GI disturbances, anemia, phlebitis at the infusion site, and low back pain. Possible bone marrow suppression (producing a decrease in white blood cell and platelet counts), oral candidiasis, and liver and renal impairments require close patient monitoring.

Other Infections. Oral acyclovir, famciclovir, or valacyclovir can be used to treat infections caused by herpes simplex or herpes zoster. Esophageal or oral candidiasis is treated topically with clotrimazole (Mycelex) oral troches or nystatin suspension. Chronic refractory infection with candidiasis (thrush) or esophageal involvement is treated with ketoconazole (Nizoral) or fluconazole (Diflucan).

ANTIDIARRHEAL THERAPY

Although many forms of diarrhea respond to treatment, it is not unusual for this condition to recur and become a chronic problem for the patient. Therapy with octreotide acetate (Sandostatin), a synthetic analog of somatostatin, has been shown to be effective in managing chronic severe diarrhea. High concentrations of somatostatin receptors have been found in the GI tract and other tissues. Somatostatin inhibits many physiologic functions, including GI motility and intestinal secretion of water and electrolytes.

CHEMOTHERAPY

Kaposi's Sarcoma. Management of KS is usually difficult because of the variability of symptoms and the organ systems involved. KS is rarely life-threatening except when there is pulmonary or GI involvement. The treatment goal is reduction of symptoms by decreasing the size of the skin lesions, reducing discomfort associated with edema and ulcerations, and controlling symptoms associated with mucosal or visceral involvement. No one treatment has been shown to increase survival. Localized treatment includes surgical excision of the lesions or application of liquid nitrogen to local skin lesions and injections of intraoral lesions with dilute vinblastine. Injection of intraoral lesions has been associated with local pain and skin irritation. Radiation therapy is effective as a palliative measure to relieve localized pain due to tumour mass (especially in the legs) or for KS lesions that are in sites such as the oral mucosa, conjunctiva, face, and soles of the feet.

Interferon is known for its antiviral and antitumour effects. Patients with cutaneous KS treated with **alpha-interferon** have experienced tumour regression and improved immune system function. Positive responses have been observed in 30% to 50% of patients, with the best responses seen in those with limited disease and no OIs. Alpha-interferon is administered by the IV,

intramuscular, or subcutaneous route. Patients may self-administer interferon at home or receive it in an outpatient setting.

Lymphoma. Successful treatment of AIDS-related lymphomas has been limited because of the rapid progression of these malignancies. Combination chemotherapy and radiation therapy regimens may produce an initial response, but it is usually short-lived. Because standard regimens for non-AIDS lymphomas have been ineffective, many clinicians suggest that AIDS-related lymphomas be studied as a separate group in clinical trials.

ANTIDEPRESSANT THERAPY

Treatment for depression in people with HIV infection involves psychotherapy integrated with pharmacology. If depressive symptoms are severe and of sufficient duration, treatment with antidepressants may be initiated. Antidepressants such as imipramine (Tofranil), desipramine (Norpramin), and fluoxetine (Prozac) may be used because these medications also alleviate the fatigue and lethargy that are associated with depression. A psychostimulant such as methylphenidate (Ritalin) may be used in low doses in patients with neuropsychiatric impairment. Electroconvulsive therapy may be an option for patients with severe depression that has not responded to pharmacologic interventions.

NUTRITION THERAPY

Malnutrition increases the risk for infection and may also increase the incidence of OIs. Nutrition therapy should be integrated into the overall management plan and should be tailored to meet the nutritional needs of the patient, from oral diet to enteral tube feedings through parenteral nutritional support if needed. As with all patients, a healthy diet is essential for the patient with HIV infection. Calorie counts should be obtained for all patients with AIDS with unexplained weight loss to evaluate nutritional status and to initiate appropriate therapy. The goal is to maintain the ideal weight and, when necessary, to increase weight.

Appetite stimulants have been successfully used in patients with AIDS-related anorexia. Megestrol acetate (Megace), a synthetic oral progesterone preparation used to treat breast cancer, promotes significant weight gain and inhibits cytokine IL-1 synthesis. In patients with HIV infection, it increases body weight primarily by increasing body fat stores. Dronabinol (Marinol), synthetic tetrahydrocannabinol (THC), the active ingredient in marijuana, has been used to relieve nausea and vomiting associated with cancer chemotherapy. Preliminary results show that after beginning Marinol therapy, almost all patients with HIV infection experience a modest weight gain. The effects on body composition are unknown.

Oral supplements may be used to supplement diets deficient in calories and protein. Ideally, oral supplements should be lactose-free (many people with HIV infection are intolerant to lactose), high in calories and easily digestible protein, low in fat with the fat easily digestible, palatable, inexpensive, and tolerated without causing diarrhea. Advera is a nutritional supplement that has been developed specifically for people with HIV infection and AIDS. Parenteral nutrition is the final option because of the costs and associated risks, including infections.

Complementary and Alternative Modalities

Traditional Western medicine focuses on the treatment of disease. These treatments or interventions are taught in medical schools and are used by physicians in the care of patients. Complementary and alternative therapies are often viewed as unconventional and unorthodox treatments or interventions not traditionally taught in medical schools. Alternative therapy stresses the need to treat the whole person, recognizing the interaction of the body, mind, and spirit. What is considered to be an alternative therapy in one culture may actually be a traditional therapy in another. For example, one Canadian study (Mill, 2000) found that Aboriginal women's views about the etiology of, and treatment for, their HIV illness was different from the conventional biomedical view of HIV disease. The women used a combination of biomedical, traditional, and alternative treatments for their illness (see Nursing Research Profile 52-2). Persons with HIV infection report substantial use of complementary and alternative medical therapies for symptom management (Canadian AIDS Treatment Information Exchange [CATIE], 2004). The use of alternative therapy in HIV infection and AIDS has resulted from disillusionment with standard medical treatment, which to date has provided no cure. Used with traditional therapies, alternative therapies may improve the patient's overall well-being.

Alternative therapies can be divided into four categories:

- Spiritual or psychological therapies may include humour, hypnosis, faith healing, guided imagery, and positive affirmations.
- Nutritional therapies may include vegetarian or macrobiotic diets, vitamin C or beta-carotene supplements, and turmeric, which contains curcumin, a food spice supplement. Chinese herbs, such as traditional herbal mixtures, as well as compound Q (a Chinese cucumber extract) and *Monmordica charantia* (bitter melon), which is given as an enema, are also used.
- Drug and biologic therapies include medicines not approved by the FDA. Examples of these include N-acetylcysteine, pentoxifylline (Trental), and 1-chloro-2, 4-dinitrobenzene. Also included in this category are oxygen therapy, ozone therapy, and urine therapy.
- Treatment with physical forces and devices may include acupuncture, acupressure, massage therapy, reflexology, therapeutic touch, yoga, and crystals.

Although there is insufficient research on the effects of alternate therapies, there is a growing body of literature reporting benefits in the areas of nutrition, exercise, psychosocial treatment, and Chinese medicine. Clinical trials are in progress to examine the effect of Chinese herbal treatments of HIV-associated symptoms related to inadequate nutrition, such as fatigue, nausea, vomiting, painful or difficult swallowing, altered taste sensation, and diarrhea. At present there are no definitive study results that indicate that these treatments are effective, but some appear promising.

Many patients who use these alternative therapies do not report their use to their health care providers. To obtain a complete health history, the nurse should ask about the patient's use of alternative therapies. Patients may need to be encouraged to report their use to their primary health care provider. Problems may arise when patients are using alternative therapies while they are participating in clinical drug trials. They may have significant adverse side effects, making it difficult to assess the effects of the medications in the clinical trial. The nurse needs to become familiar with the potential adverse side effects of alternative therapies. The nurse who suspects that the alternative therapy is causing a side effect needs to discuss this with the patient, the alternative therapy provider, and the primary health care provider. It is important for the nurse to view alternative therapies with an open mind and to try to understand the importance of this treatment to the patient. Doing so will improve communication with the patient and reduce conflict, so that all involved in care can meet the patient's needs.

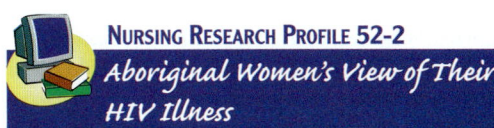

NURSING RESEARCH PROFILE 52-2
Aboriginal Women's View of Their HIV Illness

Mill, J. E. (2000). Describing an explanatory model of HIV illness in Aboriginal women. *Holistic Nursing Practice, 15*(1), 42–56.

Purpose
Despite progress in limiting the spread of HIV infection in some subgroups of the population, the epidemic is of growing concern for women. The purpose of this study was to describe Aboriginal women's view of their HIV illness using Kleinman's explanatory model framework.

Study Sample and Design
A qualitative research design was selected for the study and in-depth interviews were the primary data collection methods. The interviews were open ended to enable all aspects of the women's views of their illness to be elicited and to promote an in-depth understanding of their experiences. Fifteen interviews were completed with eight First Nations women, the majority of whom lived in an urban setting. There was a 2- to 3-week interval between the first and second interview, with the seven women interviewed twice. The data were analyzed simultaneously with data collection. The transcriptions were read and reread to identify emergent themes, and the NUD*IST software program was used to assist with the storage and retrieval of data.

Findings
There was a strong feeling among most of the participants that they had become HIV positive for a reason. Some felt that the disease had come to them as a teaching from the Creator, whereas others believed that they had become HIV positive as a payment for their previous behaviour. The valuing of Aboriginal traditions was common to all participants, regardless of whether they were from urban or rural areas. In relation to treatment, most of the participants emphasized the importance of staying healthy. For some of the participants, the decision about when to seek treatment was based on their assessment of whether they felt "sick." In general, there was a reticence among the participants to engage in some of the recommended biomedical treatments and to take pills, based on their concerns regarding side effects of the medications and their history of drug use. Most of the participants had used traditional treatments, including sweat lodges, healing circles, dancing, smudging, and visiting an elder, to treat their illness. About half of the women had taken antiretrovirals and/or alternative treatments (herbs, vitamins, Reiki).

Nursing Implications
Despite the small sample interviewed in this study, several themes provide insights that are germane to the planning of culturally sensitive HIV prevention and treatment programs. The narratives described by the women suggest that they continue to be influenced by their traditional cultural beliefs and that these beliefs are reflected in their explanatory model of HIV illness. Evidence of the belief that "a disease must be felt" before the assistance of a healer is sought may mean that some Aboriginal clients seek treatment at a much later stage of the disease. Aboriginal clients are interested in biomedical, traditional Aboriginal, and alternative treatments for their HIV illness; therefore, treatment programs for HIV illness in Aboriginal individuals and communities must provide a range of options and treatment modalities.

Supportive Care

Patients who are weak and debilitated as a result of chronic illness associated with HIV infection typically require many kinds of supportive care. Nutritional support may be as simple as providing assistance in obtaining or preparing meals. For patients with more advanced nutritional impairment that results from decreased intake, wasting syndrome, or GI malabsorption associated with diarrhea, parenteral feedings may be required. Imbalances that result from nausea, vomiting, and profuse diarrhea often necessitate IV fluid and electrolyte replacement.

Skin breakdown associated with KS, perianal skin excoriation, and immobility is managed with thorough and meticulous skin care involving regular turning, cleansing, and applying medicated ointments and dressings.

Pain associated with skin breakdown, abdominal cramping, peripheral neuropathy, or KS is managed by analgesics given at regular intervals around the clock. Relaxation and guided imagery may be helpful in reducing pain and anxiety.

Pulmonary symptoms, such as dyspnea and shortness of breath, may be related to infection, KS, or fatigue. For these patients, oxygen therapy, relaxation training, and energy conservation techniques may be helpful. Patients with severe respiratory dysfunction may require mechanical ventilation. Before placing a patient on mechanical ventilation, the procedure is explained to the patient and the caregiver. The patient may elect not to be placed on mechanical ventilation, and the patient's wishes should be followed. Ideally, the patient has prepared an advanced directive identifying preferences for treatments and end-of-life care, including hospice care. If the patient has not identified preferences in advance, treatment options are described so that the patient can make informed decisions and have those wishes respected.

NURSING PROCESS:
THE PATIENT WITH AIDS

The nursing care of patients with AIDS is challenging because of the potential for any organ system to be the target of infections or cancer. In addition, this disease is complicated by many emotional, social, and ethical issues. The plan of care for the patient with AIDS is individualized to meet the needs of the patient (see Plan of Nursing Care). Care includes many of the interventions and concerns cited in the supportive care section.

Assessment

Nursing assessment includes identification of potential risk factors, including a history of risky sexual practices and injection drug use. The patient's physical status and psychological status are assessed. All factors affecting immune system functioning are thoroughly explored.

NUTRITIONAL STATUS

Nutritional status is assessed by obtaining a dietary history and identifying factors that may interfere with oral intake, such as anorexia, nausea, vomiting, oral pain, or difficulty swallowing. In addition, the patient's ability to purchase and prepare food is assessed. Weight, anthropometric measurements, and blood urea nitrogen (BUN), serum protein, albumin, and transferrin levels provide objective measurements of nutritional status.

SKIN INTEGRITY

The skin and mucous membranes are inspected daily for evidence of breakdown, ulceration, or infection. The oral cavity is monitored for redness, ulcerations, and the presence of creamy-white patches indicative of candidiasis. Assessment of the perianal area for excoriation and infection in patients with profuse diarrhea is important. Wounds are cultured to identify infectious organisms.

RESPIRATORY STATUS

Respiratory status is assessed by monitoring the patient for cough, sputum production, shortness of breath, orthopnea, tachypnea, and chest pain. The presence and quality of breath sounds are investigated. Other measures of pulmonary function include chest x-ray results, arterial blood gas values, pulse oximetry, and pulmonary function test results.

NEUROLOGIC STATUS

Neurologic status is determined by assessing level of consciousness; orientation to person, place, and time; and memory lapses. Mental status is assessed as early as possible to provide a baseline (Chart 52-6). The patient is also assessed for sensory deficits (visual changes, headache, or numbness and tingling in the extremities) and motor involvement (altered gait, paresis, or paralysis) and seizure activity.

FLUID AND ELECTROLYTE BALANCE

Fluid and electrolyte status is assessed by examining the skin and mucous membranes for turgor and dryness. Increased thirst, decreased urine output, low blood pressure or a decrease in systolic blood pressure between 10 and 15 mm Hg with a concurrent rise in pulse rate when the patient sits up or stands, weak and rapid pulse, and urine specific gravity of 1.025 or more may indicate dehydration. Electrolyte imbalances, such as decreased serum sodium, potassium, calcium, magnesium, and chloride, typically result from profuse diarrhea. The patient is assessed for signs and symptoms of electrolyte deficits, including decreased mental status (see Chart 52-6), muscle twitching, muscle cramps, irregular pulse, nausea and vomiting, and shallow respirations.

KNOWLEDGE LEVEL

The patient's level of knowledge about the disease and the modes of disease transmission is evaluated. In addition, the level of knowledge of family and friends is assessed. The patient's psychological reaction to the diagnosis of HIV infection or AIDS is important to explore. Reactions vary among patients and may include denial, anger, fear, shame, withdrawal from social interactions, and depression. It is often helpful to gain an understanding of how the patient has dealt with illness and major life stress in the past. The patient's resources for support are also identified.

Diagnosis

NURSING DIAGNOSES

The list of potential nursing diagnoses is extensive because of the complex nature of this disease. Based on assessment data, however, major nursing diagnoses for the patient may include the following:

- Impaired skin integrity related to cutaneous manifestations of HIV infection, excoriation, and diarrhea
- Diarrhea related to enteric pathogens or HIV infection
- Risk for infection related to immunodeficiency
- Activity intolerance related to weakness, fatigue, malnutrition, impaired fluid and electrolyte balance, and hypoxia associated with pulmonary infections
- Disturbed thought processes related to shortened attention span, impaired memory, confusion, and disorientation associated with HIV encephalopathy
- Ineffective airway clearance related to PCP, increased bronchial secretions, and decreased ability to cough related to weakness and fatigue

(text continues on page 1578)

Plan of Nursing Care
Care of the Patient With AIDS

Nursing Interventions	Rationale	Expected Patient Outcomes

Nursing Diagnosis: Diarrhea related to enteric pathogens or HIV infection
Goal: Resumption of usual bowel habits

Nursing Interventions	Rationale	Expected Patient Outcomes

1. Assess patient's normal bowel habits.
2. Assess for diarrhea: frequent, loose stools; abdominal pain or cramping, volume of liquid stools, and exacerbating and alleviating factors.
3. Obtain stool cultures and administer antimicrobial therapy as prescribed.
4. Initiate measures to reduce hyperactivity of bowel:
  a. Maintain food and fluid restrictions as prescribed. Suggest BRAT diet (*b*ananas, *r*ice, *a*pplesauce, *t*ea and *t*oast).
  b. Discourage smoking.
 	
  c. Avoid bowel irritants such as fatty or fried foods, raw vegetables, and nuts. Offer small, frequent meals.
5. Administer anticholinergic antispasmodics and opioids or other medications as prescribed.
6. Maintain fluid intake of at least 3 L unless contraindicated.
	1. Provides baseline for evaluation
	2. Detects changes in status, quantifies loss of fluid, and provides basis for nursing measures
	
	3. Identifies pathogenic organism; therapy targets specific organism
	4. Promotes bowel rest, which may decrease acute episodes
	  a. Reduces stimulation of bowel
	
	  b. Eliminates nicotine, which acts as bowel stimulant
	  c. Prevents stimulation of bowel and abdominal distention and promotes adequate nutrition
	5. Decreases intestinal spasms and motility
	
	6. Prevents hypovolemia
		• Exhibits return to normal bowel patterns
		• Reports decreasing episodes of diarrhea and abdominal cramping
		• Identifies and avoids foods that irritate the gastrointestinal tract
		• Appropriate therapy is initiated as prescribed.
		• Exhibits normal stool cultures
		• Maintains adequate fluid intake
		• Maintains body weight and reports no additional weight loss
		• States rationale for avoiding smoking
		• Enrolls in program to stop smoking
		• Uses medication as prescribed
		• Maintains adequate fluid status
		• Exhibits normal skin turgor, moist mucous membranes, adequate urine output, and absence of excessive thirst

Nursing Diagnosis: Risk for infection related to immunodeficiency
Goal: Absence of infection

Nursing Interventions	Rationale	Expected Patient Outcomes

1. Monitor for infection: fever, chills, and diaphoresis; cough; shortness of breath; oral pain or painful swallowing; creamy-white patches in oral cavity; urinary frequency, urgency, or dysuria; redness, swelling, or drainage from wounds; vesicular lesions on face, lips, or perianal area.
2. Teach patient or caregiver about need to report possible infection.
3. Monitor white blood cell count and differential.
4. Obtain cultures of wound drainage, skin lesions, urine, stool, sputum, mouth, and blood as prescribed. Administer antimicrobial therapy as prescribed.
5. Instruct patient in ways to prevent infection:
  a. Clean kitchen and bathroom surfaces with disinfectants.
  b. Clean hands thoroughly after exposure to body fluids.
  c. Avoid exposure to others' body fluids or sharing eating utensils.
  d. Turn, cough, and deep breathe, especially when activity is decreased.
  e. Maintain cleanliness of perianal area.
  f. Avoid handling pet excreta or cleaning litter boxes, bird cages, or aquariums.
  g. Cook meat and eggs thoroughly.
	1. Allows for early detection of infection, essential for prompt initiation of treatment. Repeated and prolonged infections contribute to patient's debilitation.
	
	2. Allows early detection of infection
	
	3. Identifies elevated WBC possibly associated with infection
	4. Assists in determining offending organism to initiate appropriate treatment
	
	5. Minimizes exposure to infection and transmission of HIV infection to others
		• Identifies reportable signs and symptoms of infection
		• Reports signs and symptoms of infection if present
		• Exhibits and reports absence of fever, chills, and diaphoresis
		• Exhibits normal (clear) breath sounds without adventitious breath sounds
		• Maintains weight
		• Reports adequate energy level without excessive fatigue
		• Reports absence of shortness of breath and cough
		• Exhibits pink, moist oral mucous membranes without fissures or lesions
		• Takes appropriate therapy as prescribed
		• Experiences no infection
		• States rationale for strategies to avoid infection
		• Modifies activities to reduce exposure to infection or infectious persons
		• Practices "safer sex"
		• Avoids sharing eating utensils and toothbrush
		• Exhibits normal body temperature
		• Uses recommended techniques to maintain cleanliness of skin, skin lesions, and perianal area

(continued)

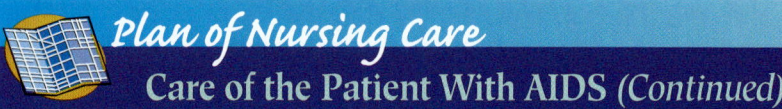

Plan of Nursing Care
Care of the Patient With AIDS (Continued)

Nursing Interventions	Rationale	Expected Patient Outcomes
6. Maintain aseptic technique when performing invasive procedures such as venipunctures, bladder catheterizations, and injections.	6. Prevents hospital-acquired infections	• Has others handle pet excreta and cleanup • Uses recommended cooking techniques

Nursing Diagnosis: Ineffective airway clearance related to Pneumocystis carinii pneumonia, increased bronchial secretions, and decreased ability to cough related to weakness and fatigue

Goal: Improved airway clearance

Nursing Interventions	Rationale	Expected Patient Outcomes

1. Assess and report signs and symptoms of altered respiratory status, tachypnea, use of accessory muscles, cough, colour and amount of sputum, abnormal breath sounds, dusky or cyanotic skin colour, restlessness, confusion, or somnolence.
2. Obtain sputum sample for culture prescribed. Administer antimicrobial therapy as prescribed.
3. Provide pulmonary care (cough, deep breathing, postural drainage, and vibration) every 2 to 4 hours.
4. Assist patient in attaining semi- or high Fowler's position.
5. Encourage adequate rest periods.
6. Initiate measures to decrease viscosity of secretions:
  a. Maintain fluid intake of at least 3 L per day unless contraindicated.
  b. Humidify inspired air as prescribed.
  c. Consult with physician concerning use of mucolytic agents delivered through nebulizer or IPPB treatment.
7. Perform tracheal suctioning as needed.
8. Administer oxygen therapy as prescribed.
9. Assist with endotracheal intubation; maintain ventilator settings as prescribed.
	1. Indicates abnormal respiratory function
	
	2. Aids in identification of pathogenic organisms
	
	3. Prevents stasis of secretions and promotes airway clearance
	4. Facilities breathing and airway clearance
	5. Maximizes energy expenditure and prevents excessive fatigue
	6. Facilitates expectoration of secretions; prevents stasis of secretions
	
	7. Removes secretions if patient is unable to do so
	8. Increases availability of oxygen
	9. Maintains ventilation
		• Maintains normal airway clearance: Respiratory rate <20 breaths/min Unlaboured breathing without use of accessory muscles and flaring nares (nostrils) Skin colour pink (without cyanosis) Alert and aware of surroundings Arterial blood gas values normal Normal breath sounds without adventitious breath sounds
		• Begins appropriate therapy
		• Takes medication as prescribed
		• Reports improved breathing
		• Maintains clear airway
		• Coughs and takes deep breaths every 2–4 hours as recommended
		• Demonstrates appropriate positions and practices postural drainage every 2–4 hours
		• Reports reduced breathing difficulty when in semi- or high Fowler's position
		• Practices energy-conserving strategies and alternates rest with activity
		• Demonstrates reduction in thickness (viscosity) of pulmonary secretions
		• Reports increased ease in coughing up sputum
		• Uses humidified air or oxygen as prescribed and indicated
		• Indicates need for assistance with removal of pulmonary secretions
		• Understands need for and cooperates with endotracheal intubation and use of a mechanical ventilator
		• Verbalizes concerns about respiratory difficulty, intubation, and mechanical ventilation

Nursing Diagnosis: Imbalanced nutrition, less than body requirements, related to decreased oral intake

Goal: Improvement of nutritional status

Nursing Interventions	Rationale	Expected Patient Outcomes
1. Assess for malnutrition with height, weight, age, BUN, serum protein, and albumin, transferrin levels, hemoglobin, hematocrit, and cutaneous anergy. 2. Obtain dietary history, including likes and dislikes and food intolerances. 3. Assess factors that interfere with oral intake.	1. Provides objective measurement of nutritional status 2. Defines need for nutritional education; helps individualize interventions 3. Provides basis and directions for interventions	• Identifies factors limiting oral intake and uses resources to promote adequate dietary intake • Reports increased appetite • States understanding of nutritional needs • Identifies ways to reduce factors that limit oral intake • Rests before meals • Eats in pleasant, odour-free environment

(continued)

Plan of Nursing Care
Care of the Patient With AIDS *(Continued)*

Nursing Interventions	Rationale	Expected Patient Outcomes
4. Consult with dietitian to determine patient's nutritional needs.	4. Facilitates meal planning	• Arranges meals to coincide with visitors' visits

5. Reduce factors limiting oral intake:
  a. Encourage patient to rest before meals.
 	
  b. Plan meals so that they do not occur immediately after painful or unpleasant procedures.
  c. Encourage patient to eat meals with visitors or others when possible.
  d. Encourage patient to prepare simple meals or to obtain assistance with meal preparation if possible.
  e. Serve small, frequent meals: 6 per day.
  f. Limit fluids 1 hour before meals and with meals.
	5. Addresses factors limiting intake:
	  a. Minimizes fatigue, which can decrease appetite
	  b. Decreases noxious stimuli
	
	  c. Limits social isolation
	
	  d. Limits energy expenditure
	
	  e. Prevents overwhelming patient
	  f. Reduces satiety
		• Reports increased dietary intake
		• Uses oral hygiene before meals
		• Takes analgesics before meals as prescribed
		• Identifies ways to increase protein and caloric intake
		• Identifies foods high in protein and calories
		• Consumes foods high in protein and calories
		• Reports decreased rate of weight loss.
		• Maintains adequate intake
		• States rationale for enteral or parenteral nutrition if needed
		• Demonstrates skill in preparing alternate sources of nutrition

6. Instruct patient in ways to supplement nutrition: consume protein-rich foods (meat, poultry, fish) and carbohydrates (pasta, fruit, breads).	6. Provides additional proteins and calories	
7. Consult with physician and dietitian about alternative feeding (enteral or parenteral nutrition).	7. Provides nutritional support if patient is unable to take sufficient amounts by mouth	
8. Consult with social worker or community liaison about financial assistance if patient cannot afford food.	8. Increases availability of resources and nutrition	

Nursing Diagnosis: Deficient knowledge related to means of preventing HIV transmission
Goal: Increased knowledge concerning means of preventing disease transmission

1. Instruct patient, family, and friends about routes of transmission of HIV.	1. Knowledge about disease transmission can help prevent spread of disease; may also alleviate fears.	• Patient, family, and friends state means of transmission. • Reports and demonstrates practices to reduce exposure of others to HIV • Avoids intravenous drug use • Demonstrates knowledge of safer sexual practices • Identifies means of preventing disease transmission • States that sexual partners are informed about positive HIV antibodies in blood • Avoids IV/injection drug use and sharing of drug equipment with others

2. Instruct patient, family, and friends about means of preventing transmission of HIV:
  a. Avoid sexual contact with multiple partners, and use precautions if sexual partner's HIV status is not certain.
 	
  b. Use condoms during sexual intercourse (vaginal, anal, oral–genital); avoid mouth contact with the penis, vagina, or rectum; avoid sexual practices that can cause cuts or tears in the lining of the rectum, vagina, or penis.
  c. Avoid sex with sex trade workers and others at high risk.
 	
  d. Do not use injection drugs; if addicted and unable or unwilling to change behaviour, use clean needles and syringes.
 	
  e. Women who may have been exposed to AIDS through sexual or drug practices should consult with a physician before becoming pregnant; consider use of antiretroviral agents if pregnant.
	2. Reduces transmission risk
	
	  a. The risk of infection increases with the number of sexual partners, male or female, and sexual contact with those who engage in high-risk behaviours.
	  b. Risk of HIV transmission is reduced.
	
	  c. Many sex trade workers are infected with HIV through sexual contact with multiple partners or IV/injection drug use.
	  d. Clean needles and syringes are the only way to prevent HIV transmission for those who continue to use drugs. Taking precautions is important for those who are antibody positive to prevent transmitting HIV.
	  e. AIDS can be transmitted from mother to child in utero; use of antiretroviral agents during pregnancy significantly reduces perinatal transmission of HIV.	

(continued)

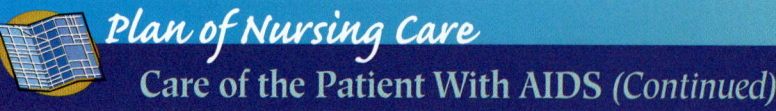

Plan of Nursing Care
Care of the Patient With AIDS *(Continued)*

Nursing Interventions	Rationale	Expected Patient Outcomes

Nursing Diagnosis: Social isolation related to stigma of the disease, withdrawal of support systems, isolation procedures, and fear of infecting others
Goal: Decreased sense of social isolation

1. Assess patient's usual patterns of social interaction.	1. Establishes basis for individualized interventions	• Shares with others the need for valued social interaction
2. Observe for behaviours indicative of social isolation, such as decreased interaction with others, hostility, noncompliance, sad affect, and stated feelings of rejection or loneliness.	2. Promotes early detection of social isolation, which may be manifested in several ways	• Demonstrates interest in events, activities, and communication • Verbalizes feelings and reactions to diagnosis, prognosis, and life changes • Identifies modes of transmission of AIDS
3. Provide instruction concerning modes of transmission of HIV.	3. Provides accurate information, corrects misconceptions, and alleviates anxiety	• States ways of preventing transmission of AIDS virus to others while maintaining contact with valued friends and relatives
4. Assist patient to identify and explore resources for support and positive mechanisms for coping (eg, contact with family, friends, AIDS task force).	4. Enables mobilization of resources and supports	• Reveals AIDS diagnosis to others when appropriate • Identifies resources (ie, family, friends, and support groups)
5. Allow time to be with patient other than for medications and procedures.	5. Promotes feelings of self-worth and provides social interaction	• Uses resources when appropriate • Accepts offers of assistance and support
6. Encourage participation in diversional activities such as reading, television, or hand crafts.	6. Provides distraction	• Reports decreased sense of isolation • Maintains contacts with those of importance to him or her • Develops or continues hobbies that effectively serve as diversion or distraction

Collaborative Problems: Opportunistic infections; impaired breathing; wasting syndrome and fluid and electrolyte imbalances; adverse reaction to medications
Goal: Absence of complications

Opportunistic Infections

1. Monitor vital signs.	1. Changes in vital signs such as increases in pulse rate, respirations, blood pressure, and temperature may indicate infection.	• Exhibits stable vital signs • Experiences control of infection • Identifies signs and symptoms correctly and experiences no complications
2. Obtain laboratory specimens and monitor test results.	2. Smears and cultures can identify causative agents such as bacteria, fungi, and protozoa, and sensitivity studies can identify antibiotics or other medications effective against the causative agent.	• Identifies signs and symptoms that are reportable to the physician • Takes medications as prescribed
3. Instruct the patient and caregiver about signs and symptoms of infection and the need to report them early.	3. Early recognition of symptoms facilitates prompt treatment and avoids extra complications.	

Impaired Breathing

1. Monitor respiratory rate and pattern.	1. Rapid shallow breathing, diminished breath sounds, and shortness of breath may indicate respiratory failure resulting in hypoxia.	• Maintains stable respiratory rate and pattern within the normal limits • Exhibits no adventitious lung sounds; normal breath sounds
2. Auscultate the chest for breath sounds and abnormal lung sounds.	2. Crackles and wheezes may indicate fluid in the lungs, which disrupts respiratory function and alters the blood's oxygen-carrying capacity.	• Has stable pulse rate and blood pressure within normal limits, and exhibits no evidence of hypoxia
3. Monitor pulse rate, blood pressure, and oxygen saturation levels.	3. Changes in pulse rate, blood pressure, and oxygen levels may indicate the development of respiratory or cardiac failure.	• Oxygen saturation levels within acceptable range

(continued)

Plan of Nursing Care
Care of the Patient With AIDS (Continued)

Nursing Interventions	Rationale	Expected Patient Outcomes
Wasting Syndrome and Fluid and Electrolyte Disturbances 1. Monitor weight and laboratory values for nutritional status. 2. Monitor intake and output and laboratory values for fluid and electrolyte imbalance (potassium, sodium, calcium, phosphorus, magnesium, and zinc). 3. Monitor for and report signs and symptoms of dehydration.	1. Weight loss, malnutrition, and anemia are common in HIV infection and increase risk for superinfection. 2. Chronic diarrhea, inadequate oral intake, vomiting, and profuse sweating deplete electrolytes. Small intestine inflammation may impair the absorption of fluids and electrolytes. 3. Fluid loss results in decreased circulating volume leading to tachycardia, dry skin and mucous membranes, poor skin turgor, elevated urine specific gravity, and thirst. Early detection allows early treatment.	• Maintains stable weight • Eats a nutritious diet • Attains and maintains hemoglobin, hematocrit, and ferritin levels within normal limits • Sustains fluid–electrolytes balance within normal limits • Exhibits no signs and symptoms of dehydration
Reactions to Medications 1. Monitor for medication interactions. 2. Monitor for and promptly report side effects from antiretroviral agents. 3. Instruct the patient and caregiver in the medication regimen.	1. People with HIV infection receive many medications for HIV and for disease complications. Early detection of medication interactions is necessary to prevent complications. 2. Side effects from antiretroviral agents can be life-threatening. Serious side effects include anemia, pancreatitis, peripheral neuropathy, mental confusion, and persistent nausea and vomiting. Corrective measures need to be instituted. 3. Knowledge of the medication purpose, correct administration, side effects, and strategies to manage or prevent side effects promote safety and greater compliance with treatment.	• Experiences no serious side effects or complications from medications • Correctly describes medication regimen and complies with therapy, including adaptations in eating routines and type of food used with prescribed medications

Chart 52-6 • ASSESSMENT
Mental Status in HIV Infection

Assessment	Function	Selected Descriptors
Appearance	Physical characteristics, grooming, dress	Obese, cachectic, emaciated, poor eye contact, clean, disheveled, inappropriate dress for weather, slumped posture
Behaviour	Motor activity	Restless, agitated, lethargic, hyperactive, rigid, repetitive
Speech	Verbal communication	Intelligible, clear, slurred, rapid, slowed, pressured, repetitive, perseveration, mute
Mood	General feeling tone	Friendly, fearful, hostile, euphoric, despondent, labile
Affect	Emotional expression	Appropriate, bizarre, flat, blunted, apathetic, overly dramatic
Cognition	Memory and orientation	Oriented (to time, place, and person), confused, disoriented, distractible, short attention span, intact remote and immediate memory, forgetful
Comprehension	Intellectual functioning	Able to abstract, concrete, poor judgment, lacks insight, unable to compute, lacks general knowledge, able to learn
Thought process	Expression of thoughts	Goal oriented, tangential, delusional, looseness of associations, confabulation, obsessive, ritualistic
Perception	Perspective of world	Presence of auditory, visual, olfactory, or kinesthetic hallucinations

- Pain related to impaired perianal skin integrity secondary to diarrhea, KS, and peripheral neuropathy
- Imbalanced nutrition, less than body requirements, related to decreased oral intake
- Social isolation related to stigma of the disease, withdrawal of support systems, isolation procedures, and fear of infecting others
- Anticipatory grieving related to changes in lifestyle and roles and unfavourable prognosis
- Deficient knowledge related to HIV infection, means of preventing HIV transmission, and self-care

COLLABORATIVE PROBLEMS/ POTENTIAL COMPLICATIONS

Based on the assessment data, possible complications may include the following:

- Opportunistic infections
- Impaired breathing or respiratory failure
- Wasting syndrome and fluid and electrolyte imbalance
- Adverse reaction to medications

Planning and Goals

Goals for the patient may include achievement and maintenance of skin integrity, resumption of usual bowel habits, absence of infection, improved activity tolerance, improved thought processes, improved airway clearance, increased comfort, improved nutritional status, increased socialization, expression of grief, increased knowledge regarding disease prevention and self-care, and absence of complications.

Nursing Interventions

PROMOTING SKIN INTEGRITY

The skin and oral mucosa are assessed routinely for changes in appearance, location and size of lesions, and evidence of infection and breakdown. The patient is encouraged to maintain a balance between rest and mobility whenever possible. Patients who are immobile are assisted to change position every 2 hours. Devices such as alternating-pressure mattresses and low-air-loss beds are used to prevent skin breakdown. Patients are encouraged to avoid scratching, to use nonabrasive, nondrying soaps, and to apply nonperfumed skin moisturizers to dry skin surfaces. Regular oral care is also encouraged.

Medicated lotions, ointments, and dressings are applied to affected skin surfaces as prescribed. Adhesive tape is avoided. Skin surfaces are protected from friction and rubbing by keeping bed linens free of wrinkles and avoiding tight or restrictive clothing. Patients with foot lesions are advised to wear cotton socks and shoes that do not cause the feet to perspire. Antipruritic, antibiotic, and analgesic agents are administered as prescribed.

The perianal region is assessed frequently for impairment of skin integrity and infection. The patient is instructed to keep the area as clean as possible. The perianal area is cleaned after each bowel movement with nonabrasive soap and water to prevent further excoriation and breakdown of the skin and infection. If the area is very painful, soft cloths or cotton sponges may prove to be less irritating than washcloths. In addition, sitz baths or gentle irrigation may facilitate cleaning and promote comfort. The area is dried thoroughly after cleaning. Topical lotions or ointments may be prescribed to promote healing. Wounds are cultured if infection is suspected so that the appropriate antimicrobial treatment can be initiated. Debilitated patients may require assistance in maintaining hygienic practices.

PROMOTING USUAL BOWEL HABITS

Bowel patterns are assessed for diarrhea. The nurse monitors the frequency and consistency of stools and reports of abdominal pain or cramping associated with bowel movements. Factors that exacerbate frequent diarrhea are also assessed. The quantity and volume of liquid stools are measured to document fluid volume losses. Stool cultures are obtained to identify pathogenic organisms.

The patient is counselled about ways to decrease diarrhea. The physician may recommend restriction of oral intake to rest the bowel during periods of acute inflammation associated with severe enteric infections. As the patient's dietary intake is increased, foods that act as bowel irritants, such as raw fruits and vegetables, popcorn, carbonated beverages, spicy foods, and foods of extreme temperatures, should be avoided. Small, frequent meals help to prevent abdominal distention. The physician may prescribe medications such as anticholinergic antispasmodics or opioids, which decrease diarrhea by decreasing intestinal spasms and motility. Administering antidiarrheal agents on a regular schedule may be more beneficial than administering them on an as-needed basis. Antibiotics and antifungal agents may also be prescribed to combat pathogens identified by stool cultures. The nurse should also assess the self-care strategies being used by the patient to control diarrhea (Henry et al., 1999).

PREVENTING INFECTION

The patient and caregivers are instructed to monitor for signs and symptoms of infection: fever; chills; night sweats; cough with or without sputum production; shortness of breath; difficulty breathing; oral pain or difficulty swallowing; creamy-white patches in the oral cavity; unexplained weight loss; swollen lymph nodes; nausea; vomiting; persistent diarrhea; frequency, urgency, or pain on urination; headache; visual changes or memory lapses; redness, swelling, or drainage from skin wounds; and vesicular lesions on the face, lips, or perianal area. The nurse also monitors laboratory values that indicate infection, such as the white blood cell count and differential. The physician may decide to culture specimens of wound drainage, skin lesions, urine, stool, sputum, mouth, and blood to identify pathogenic organisms and the most appropriate antimicrobial therapy. The patient is instructed to avoid others with active infections such as upper respiratory infections.

IMPROVING ACTIVITY TOLERANCE

Activity tolerance is assessed by monitoring the patient's ability to ambulate and perform activities of daily living. Patients may be unable to maintain their usual levels of activity because of weakness, fatigue (see Nursing Research Profile 52-3), shortness of breath, dizziness, and neurologic involvement. Assistance in planning daily routines that maintain a balance between activity and rest may be necessary. In addition, patients benefit from instructions about energy conservation techniques, such as sitting while washing or while preparing meals. Personal items that are frequently used should be kept within the patient's reach. Measures such as relaxation and guided imagery may be beneficial because they decrease anxiety, which contributes to weakness and fatigue.

Collaboration with other members of the health care team may uncover other factors associated with increasing fatigue and strategies to address them. For example, if fatigue is related to anemia, administering epoetin alfa (Epogen) as prescribed may relieve fatigue and increase activity tolerance.

MAINTAINING THOUGHT PROCESSES

The patient is assessed for alterations in mental status that may be related to neurologic involvement, metabolic abnormalities, infection, side effects of treatment, and coping mechanisms. Manifestations of neurologic impairment may be difficult to distinguish from psychological reactions to HIV infection, such as anger and depression.

Family members are instructed to speak to the patient in simple, clear language and give the patient sufficient time to respond to questions. Family members are instructed to orient the patient to the daily routine by talking about what is taking place during daily activities. They are encouraged to provide the patient with a regular daily schedule for medication administration, grooming, meal times, bedtimes, and awakening times. Posting the schedule in a prominent area (eg, on the refrigerator), providing nightlights for the bedroom and bathroom, and planning safe leisure activities allow the patient to maintain a regular routine in a safe manner. Activities that the patient previously enjoyed are encouraged. These should be easy to accomplish and fairly short in duration. The nurse encourages the family to remain calm and not to argue with the patient while protecting the patient from injury. Around-the-clock supervision may be necessary, and strategies can be implemented to prevent the patient from engaging in potentially dangerous activities, such as driving, using the stove, or mowing the lawn. Strategies for improving or maintaining functional abilities and for providing a safe environment are used for patients with HIV encephalopathy (Chart 52-7).

IMPROVING AIRWAY CLEARANCE

Respiratory status, including rate, rhythm, use of accessory muscles, and breath sounds; mental status; and skin colour must be assessed at least daily. Any cough and the quantity and characteristics of sputum are documented. Sputum specimens are analyzed for infectious organisms. Pulmonary therapy (coughing, deep breathing, postural drainage, percussion, and vibration) is provided as often as every 2 hours to prevent stasis of secretions and to promote airway clearance. Because of weakness and fatigue, many patients require assistance in attaining a position (such as a high Fowler's or semi-Fowler's position) that facilitates breathing and airway clearance. Adequate rest is essential to maximize energy expenditure and prevent excessive fatigue. The fluid volume status is evaluated so that adequate hydration can be maintained. Unless contraindicated by renal or cardiac disease, an intake of 3 L of fluid daily is encouraged. Humidified oxygen may be prescribed, and nasopharyngeal or tracheal suctioning, intubation, and mechanical ventilation may be necessary to maintain adequate ventilation.

RELIEVING PAIN AND DISCOMFORT

The patient is assessed for the quality and severity of pain associated with impaired perianal skin integrity, the lesions of KS, and peripheral neuropathy. In addition, the effects of pain on elimination, nutrition, sleep, affect, and communication are explored, along with exacerbating and relieving factors. Cleaning the perianal area as previously described can promote comfort. Topical anesthetics or ointments may be prescribed. Use of soft cushions or foam pads may increase comfort while sitting. The patient is instructed to avoid foods that act as bowel irritants. Antispasmodics and antidiarrheal medications may be prescribed to reduce the discomfort and frequency of bowel movements. If necessary, systemic analgesic agents may also be prescribed.

Pain from KS is frequently described as a sharp, throbbing pressure and heaviness if lymphedema is present. Pain management

NURSING RESEARCH PROFILE 52-3

Assessing Fatigue in Persons Living With HIV/AIDS

Bormann, J., Shively, M., Smith, T. L., & Gifford, A. (2001). Measurement of fatigue in HIV-positive adults: Reliability and validity of the Global Fatigue Index. *Journal of Association of Nurses in AIDS Care, 12*(3), 75–83.

Purpose

Fatigue is often cited by people living with HIV/AIDS as one of the most bothersome and frequently reported symptoms. Fatigue is a complex construct that consists of cognitive, emotional, and physical components, so its assessment can be challenging. The purpose of this study was to refine an assessment tool that could be used by nurses in clinical practice and research.

Study Sample and Design

The Global Fatigue Index (GFI) was taken from the Multidimensional Assessment of Fatigue instrument, which was developed in patients with rheumatoid arthritis. The GFI consists of 15 items and assesses 5 dimensions of fatigue: degree; severity; distress; impact on activities of daily living; and timing, which addresses the frequency of fatigue and changes in degree of fatigue over the past week. A Likert scale is used for each item, and a single score of fatigue is calculated. Data were collected from 209 symptomatic HIV-positive persons living in San Diego, California, who were participating in an 8-week longitudinal descriptive study.

Findings

The nonrandom sample included 183 men and 26 women. Their mean age was 40.8 ± 8.3; their ages ranged from 26 to 70 years. Fifty percent of the sample reported a diagnosis of AIDS; 71.8% of them reported taking highly active antiretroviral therapy (HAART). Almost 88% of the sample reported fatigue. Internal consistency reliability of the GFI was assessed at 0.96. Test–retest reliability of the assessment tool was demonstrated by lack of significant changes in scores over 8 weeks. Construct validity was analyzed through principal components factor analysis and demonstrated two factors. Construct validity was determined by examining the correlation of GFI scores and more established, widely used scales that assess health distress, depression, stress levels, and measures of physical and mental health. Significant correlations with these measures indicated construct validity of the GFI.

There were no significant bivariate correlations between GFI scores and patient characteristics (age, gender, ethnicity, education, employment, and types of antiretroviral therapy). There was no significant relationship between fatigue as measured by the GFI and viral load as measured by HIV-RNA levels or CD4T4 cell.

Nursing Implications

The GFI is a practical, patient-centred instrument with evidence of reliability and validity. It takes only about 5 minutes to complete and can be used by nurses to assess baseline fatigue, to monitor the course of fatigue over time and in relation to changes in patients' HIV disease status and treatment plans, and to identify the need for more in-depth assessments of psychosocial, physical, and sleep status. The GFI can also be used by patients to monitor their fatigue scores to assess the effectiveness of different strategies.

may include using nonsteroidal anti-inflammatory drugs (NSAIDs) and opioids plus nonpharmacologic approaches such as relaxation techniques. When NSAIDs are used in patients receiving zidovudine, hepatic and hematologic status must be monitored.

The patient with pain related to peripheral neuropathy frequently describes it as burning, numbness, and "pins and needles." Pain management measures may include opioids, tricyclic

Chart 52-7 **Care of the Patient With HIV Encephalopathy**

Disturbed Thought Processes
- Assess mental status and neurologic functioning.
- Monitor for medication interactions, infections, electrolyte imbalance, and depression.
- Frequently orient the patient to time, place, person, reality, and the environment.
- Use simple explanations.
- Teach the patient to perform tasks in incremental steps.
- Provide memory aids (clocks and calendars).
- Provide memory aids for medication administration.
- Post activity schedule.
- Give positive feedback for appropriate behaviour.
- Teach caretakers how to orient patient to time, place, person, reality, and the environment.
- Encourage the patient to designate a responsible person to assume power of attorney.

Disturbed Sensory Perception
- Assess sensory impairment.
- Decrease amount of stimuli in the patient's environment.
- Correct inaccurate perceptions.
- Provide reassurance and safety if the patient displays fear.
- Provide a secure and stable environment.
- Teach caregivers how to recognize inaccurate sensory perceptions.
- Teach caregivers techniques to correct inaccurate perceptions.
- Teach the patient and caregivers to report any changes in the patient's vision to the patient's health care provider.

Risk for Injury
- Assess the patient's level of anxiety, confusion, or disorientation.
- Assess the patient for delusions or hallucinations.
- Remove potentially dangerous objects from the patient's environment.
- Structure the environment for safety (ensure adequate lighting, avoid clutter, provide bed rails if needed).
- Supervise smoking.
- Do not let the patient drive a car if confusion is present.
- Instruct the patient and caregiver in home safety.
- Provide assistance as needed for ambulation and in getting in and out of bed.
- Pad headboard and side rails if the patient has seizures.

Self-Care Deficits
- Encourage activities of daily living within the patient's level of ability.
- Encourage independence but assist if the patient cannot perform an activity.
- Demonstrate any activity that the patient is having difficulty accomplishing.
- Monitor food and fluid intake.
- Weigh patient weekly.
- Encourage the patient to eat, and offer nutritious meals, snacks, and adequate fluids.
- If patient is incontinent, establish a routine toileting schedule.
- Teach caregivers how to meet the patient's self-care needs.

---

antidepressants, and elastic compression stockings to equalize pressure. Tricyclic antidepressants have been found helpful in controlling the symptoms of neuropathic pain. They also potentiate the actions of opioids and can be used to relieve pain without increasing the dose of the opioid.

IMPROVING NUTRITIONAL STATUS
Nutritional status is assessed by monitoring weight; dietary intake; anthropometric measurements; and serum albumin, BUN, protein, and transferrin levels. The patient is also assessed for factors that interfere with oral intake, such as anorexia, oral and esophageal candidal infection, nausea, pain, weakness, fatigue, and lactose intolerance. Based on the results of assessment, the nurse can implement specific measures to facilitate oral intake. The dietitian is consulted to determine the patient's nutritional requirements.

Control of nausea and vomiting with antiemetic medications administered on a regular basis may increase the patient's dietary intake. Inadequate food intake resulting from pain caused by mouth sores or a sore throat may be managed by administering prescribed opioids and viscous lidocaine (the patient is instructed to rinse the mouth and swallow). Additionally, the patient is encouraged to eat foods that are easy to swallow and to avoid rough, spicy, or sticky food items and foods that are excessively hot or cold. Oral hygiene before and after meals is encouraged.

When fatigue and weakness interfere with intake, the nurse encourages the patient to rest before meals. If the patient is hospitalized, meals should be scheduled so that they do not occur immediately after painful or unpleasant procedures. The patient with diarrhea and abdominal cramping is encouraged to avoid foods that stimulate intestinal motility and abdominal distention (eg, fibre-rich food or lactose if the patient is intolerant to lactose).

The patient is instructed about ways to enhance the nutritional value of meals. Adding eggs, butter, margarine, and fortified milk (powdered skim milk is added to milk to increase the caloric content) to gravies, soups, or milkshakes can provide additional calories and protein. Commercial supplements such as puddings, powders, milkshakes, and Advera (a nutritional product specifically designed for people with HIV infection or AIDS) may also be useful. Patients who cannot maintain their nutritional status through oral intake may require enteral feedings or parenteral nutrition.

DECREASING THE SENSE OF ISOLATION
Individuals with AIDS are at risk for double stigmatization. They have what society refers to as a "dread disease," and they may have a lifestyle that differs from what is considered acceptable by many people. Many people with AIDS are young adults at a developmental stage usually associated with establishing intimate relationships and personal and career goals and having and raising children. Their focus changes as they are faced with a disease that threatens their life expectancy with no cure. In addition, they may be forced to reveal hidden lifestyles or behaviours to family, friends, coworkers, and health care providers. As a result, people with HIV infection may be overwhelmed with emotions such as anxiety, guilt, shame, and fear. They also may be faced with multiple losses, such as rejection by family and friends and loss of sexual partners, family, and friends; financial security; normal roles and functions; self-esteem; privacy; ability to control bodily functions; ability to interact meaningfully with the environment; and sexual functioning. Some patients may harbour feelings of guilt because of their lifestyle or because they may have infected others in current or previous relationships. Other patients may feel anger toward sexual partners who transmitted the virus. Infection

control measures used in the hospital or at home may further contribute to the patient's emotional isolation. Any or all of these stressors may cause the patient with AIDS to withdraw both physically and emotionally from social contact.

Nurses are in a key position to provide an atmosphere of acceptance and understanding of people with AIDS and their families and partners. The patient's usual level of social interaction is assessed as early as possible to provide a baseline for monitoring changes in behaviour indicative of social isolation (eg, decreased interaction with staff or family, hostility, noncompliance). Patients are encouraged to express feelings of isolation and loneliness, with the assurance that these feelings are not unique or abnormal.

Providing information about how to protect themselves and others may help patients avoid social isolation. Patients, family, and friends must be assured that AIDS is not spread through casual contact. Educating ancillary personnel, nurses, and physicians will help to reduce factors that might contribute to patients' feelings of isolation. Patient care conferences that address the psychosocial issues associated with AIDS may help sensitize the health care team to patients' needs.

COPING WITH GRIEF

The nurse can help patients verbalize feelings and explore and identify resources for support and mechanisms for coping, especially when the patient is grieving about anticipated losses. Patients are encouraged to maintain contact with family, friends, and coworkers and to use local or national AIDS support groups and hotlines. If possible, losses are identified and addressed. The patient is encouraged to continue usual activities whenever possible. Consultations with mental health counsellors are useful for many patients.

MONITORING AND MANAGING POTENTIAL COMPLICATIONS

Opportunistic Infections

Patients who are immunosuppressed are at risk for OIs. Therefore, anti-infective agents may be prescribed and laboratory tests obtained to monitor their effect. Signs and symptoms of OIs, including fever, malaise, difficulty breathing, nausea or vomiting, diarrhea, difficulty swallowing, and any occurrences of swelling or discharge, should be reported.

Respiratory Failure

Impaired breathing is a major complication that increases the patient's discomfort and anxiety and may lead to respiratory and cardiac failure. The respiratory rate and pattern are monitored and the lungs are auscultated for abnormal breath sounds. The patient is instructed to report shortness of breath and increasing difficulty in carrying out usual activities. Pulse rate and rhythm, blood pressure, and oxygen saturation are monitored. Suctioning and oxygen therapy may be prescribed to ensure an adequate airway and to prevent hypoxia. Mechanical ventilation may be necessary for a patient who cannot maintain adequate ventilation as a result of pulmonary infection, fluid and electrolyte imbalance, or respiratory muscle weakness. Arterial blood gas values are used to guide ventilator settings. If the patient is intubated, a method must be established to allow communication with the nurse and others. Attention must be given to assisting the patient on mechanical ventilation to cope with the stress associated with intubation and ventilator assistance. The possible need for mechanical ventilation in the future should be discussed early in the course of the disease, when the patient is able to make his or her desires about treatment known. The use of mechanical ventilation should be consistent with the patient's decisions about end-of-life treatment. (Further discussion of end-of-life care can be found in Chap. 17.)

Cachexia and Wasting

Wasting syndrome and fluid and electrolyte disturbances, including dehydration, are common complications of HIV infection and AIDS. The patient's nutritional and electrolyte status is evaluated by monitoring weight gains or losses, skin turgor, ferritin levels, hemoglobin and hematocrit values, and electrolyte levels. Fluid and electrolyte status is monitored on an ongoing basis; fluid intake and output and urine specific gravity may be monitored daily if the patient is hospitalized with complications. The skin is assessed for dryness and adequate turgor. Vital signs are monitored for decreased systolic blood pressure or increased pulse rate upon sitting or standing. Signs and symptoms of electrolyte disturbances, such as muscle cramping, weakness, irregular pulse, decreased mental status, nausea, and vomiting, are documented and reported to the physician. Serum electrolyte values are monitored and abnormalities reported.

The nurse helps the patient select foods that will replenish electrolytes, such as oranges and bananas (potassium) and cheese and soups (sodium). A fluid intake of 3 L or more, unless contraindicated, is encouraged to replace fluid lost with diarrhea, and measures to control diarrhea are initiated. If fluid and electrolyte imbalances persist, the nurse may administer IV fluids and electrolytes as prescribed. Effects of parenteral therapy are monitored.

Side Effects of Medications

Adverse reactions are of concern in patients who receive many medications to treat HIV infection or its complications. Many medications can cause severe toxic effects. Information about the purpose of the medications, correct administration, side effects, and strategies to manage or prevent side effects is provided. Patients and their caregivers need to know which signs and symptoms of side effects should be reported immediately to their primary health care provider (see Table 52-3).

In addition to medications used to treat HIV infection, other medications that may be required include opioids, tricyclics, and NSAIDs for pain relief; medications for treatment of OIs; antihistamines (diphenhydramine) for relief of pruritus (itching); acetaminophen or aspirin for management of fever; and antiemetic agents for control of nausea and vomiting. Concurrent use of many of these medications may cause many drug interactions, including hepatic and hematologic abnormalities. Therefore, careful laboratory monitoring for these abnormalities is warranted.

During each contact with the patient, it is important for the nurse to ask not only about side effects but also how well the patient is managing the medication regimen. The nurse may be able to assist the patient in organizing and planning the medication schedule to promote adherence to the medication regimen.

PROMOTING HOME AND COMMUNITY-BASED CARE

Teaching Patients Self-Care

Patients, families, and friends are instructed about the routes of transmission of HIV. The nurse discusses precautions to prevent transmitting HIV, including using condoms during vaginal or anal intercourse (Chart 52-8); using dental dams or avoiding oral contact with the penis, vagina, or rectum; avoiding sexual practices that might cut or tear the lining of the rectum, vagina, or penis; and avoiding sexual contact with multiple partners, individuals

Chart 52-8 • PATIENT EDUCATION
The Right Way to Use a Male Condom

1. Put on a new condom before any kind of sex.
2. Hold the condom by the tip to squeeze out the air.

3. Unroll the condom all the way over the erect penis.

4. Have sex.
5. Hold the condom so it cannot come off the penis.
6. Pull out.
7. Use a new condom if you want to have sex again or if you want to have sex in a different place (eg, in the anus and then in the vagina).
Keep condoms cool and dry. Never use skin lotions, baby oil, petroleum jelly, or cold cream with condoms. The oil in these products will cause the condom to break. You may use products made with water (like K-Y jelly or glycerin).

known to be HIV infected, people who use injection drugs, and sexual partners of people who inject drugs.

Patients and their families or caregivers must receive instructions about how to prevent disease transmission, including handwashing techniques, and in methods for safely handling items soiled with body fluids. Caregivers in the home are taught how to administer medications, including IV preparations.

The medication regimens used for patients with HIV infection and AIDS are often complex and expensive. Patients receiving combination therapies for treatment of HIV infection and its complications require careful teaching about the importance of taking medications as prescribed and explanations and assistance in fitting the medication regimen into their lives (Chart 52-9).

Guidelines about infection and infection control, follow-up care, diet, rest, and activity are also necessary. Patient teaching also includes strategies to avoid infection. The importance of personal hygiene is emphasized. Kitchen and bathroom surfaces should be cleaned regularly with disinfectants to prevent fungal and bacterial growth. Patients with pets are instructed to have another person clean areas soiled by animals, such as bird cages and litter boxes. If this is not possible, the patient should use gloves to clean up after pets. Patients are advised to avoid exposure to others who are sick or who have been recently vaccinated. Patients with AIDS and their sexual partners are strongly urged to avoid exposure to body fluids during sexual activities and to use condoms for any form of sexual intercourse. Injection drug use is strongly discouraged because of the risk to the patient of other infections and transmission of HIV infection to others. Patients infected with HIV are urged to avoid exposure to bodily fluids (through sexual contact or injection drug use) to prevent exposure to other HIV strains. The importance of avoiding smoking and maintaining a balance between diet, rest, and exercise is also emphasized.

If the patient requires enteral or parenteral nutrition, instruction is provided to patients and families about how to administer nutritional therapies at home. Home care nurses provide ongoing teaching and support for the patient and family.

Chart 52-9
Home Care Checklist • Adhering to Medication Therapy for HIV

At the completion of the home care instruction, the patient or caregiver will be able to:	Patient	Caregiver
• Verbalize knowledge of each medication name.	✓	✓
• State the action of each medication.	✓	✓
• State the correct times that medications are to be taken.	✓	✓
• Identify special guidelines to follow when taking medications (eg, with meals, on an empty stomach, medications that are not to be taken together).	✓	✓
• Demonstrate methods of keeping track of the medication regimen and storage of the prescribed medications.	✓	✓
• Identify specific laboratory tests that are necessary for the prescribed medication regimen.	✓	✓
• List expected side effects of each medication.	✓	✓
• Identify side effects that should be reported to health care providers.	✓	✓
• Explain the importance of and necessity for adherence with prescribed medication regimen.	✓	✓
• Demonstrate correct disposal of sharps and of parenteral medication according to Standard Precautions guidelines.	✓	✓
• Demonstrate correct administration of IM, SC, or IV medications.	✓	✓
• Demonstrate correct use and safe disposal of needles, syringes, and other IV equipment.	✓	✓
• Discuss with health care providers any problems that he or she is having with side effects and adherence.	✓	✓
• Report any episodes of nonadherence to the medication regimen.	✓	✓

Patients who are HIV positive or who inject drugs are instructed not to donate blood. Injection drug users who are unwilling to stop using drugs are advised to avoid sharing drug equipment with others.

Continuing Care

Many people with AIDS remain in their community and continue their usual daily activities, whereas others can no longer work or maintain their independence. Families or caregivers may need assistance in providing supportive care. There are many community-based organizations that provide a variety of services for people living with HIV infection and AIDS; nurses can help identify these services.

Community health nurses, home care nurses, and hospice nurses are in an excellent position to provide the support and guidance so often needed in the home setting. As hospital costs continue to rise and insurance coverage continues to decline, the complexity of home care increases. Home care nurses are key in the administration of parenteral antibiotics, chemotherapy, and nutrition in the home.

During home visits, the nurse assesses the patient's physical and emotional status and home environment. The patient's adherence to the therapeutic regimen is assessed, and strategies are suggested to assist with adherence. The patient is assessed for progression of disease and for adverse side effects of medications. Previous teaching is reinforced, and the importance of keeping follow-up appointments is stressed.

Complex wound care or respiratory care may be required in the home. Patients and families are often unable to meet these skilled care needs without assistance. Nurses may refer patients to community programs that offer a range of services for patients, friends, and families, including help with housekeeping, hygiene, and meals; transportation and shopping; individual and group therapy; support for caregivers; telephone networks for the homebound; and legal and financial assistance. These services are typically provided by both professional and nonprofessional volunteers. A social worker may be consulted to identify sources of financial support, if needed.

Home care and hospice nurses are increasingly called on to provide physical and emotional support to patients and families as patients with AIDS enter the terminal stages of disease. This support takes on special meaning when people with AIDS lose friends and when family members fear the disease or feel anger concerning the patient's lifestyle. The nurse encourages the patient and family to discuss end-of-life decisions and to ensure that care is consistent with those decisions, all comfort measures are employed, and the patient is treated with dignity at all times.

Evaluation

EXPECTED PATIENT OUTCOMES

Expected patient outcomes may include:

1. Maintains skin integrity
2. Resumes usual bowel habits
3. Experiences no infections
4. Maintains adequate level of activity tolerance
5. Maintains usual level of thought processes
6. Maintains effective airway clearance
7. Experiences increased sense of comfort, less pain
8. Maintains adequate nutritional status
9. Experiences decreased sense of social isolation
10. Progresses through grieving process
11. Reports increased understanding of AIDS and participates in self-care activities as possible
12. Remains free of complications

Emotional and Ethical Concerns

Nurses in all settings will be called on to provide care for patients with HIV infection. In doing so, they encounter not only the physical challenges of this epidemic but also emotional and ethical concerns. The concerns raised by health care professionals involve issues such as fear of infection, responsibility for giving care, values clarification, confidentiality, developmental stages of patients and caregivers, and poor prognostic outcomes.

Many patients with HIV infection have engaged in "stigmatized" behaviours. Because these behaviours challenge some traditional religious and moral values, nurses may feel reluctant to care for these patients. In addition, health care providers may still have fear and anxiety about disease transmission despite education concerning infection control and the low incidence of transmission to health care providers (Chart 52-10). Nurses are encouraged to examine their personal beliefs and use the process of values clarification to approach controversial issues. The Canadian Nurses Association Code of Ethics for Registered Nurses (see Chapter 3) (http://cna-aiic.ca/CNA/practice/ethics/code/default_e.aspx) can also be used to help resolve ethical dilemmas that might affect the quality of care given to HIV-infected patients.

Nurses are responsible for protecting the patient's right to privacy by safeguarding confidential information. Inadvertent disclosure of confidential patient information may result in personal, financial, and emotional hardships for HIV-infected individuals. The controversy surrounding confidentiality concerns the circumstances in which information can be disclosed to others. Health care team members need accurate patient information to conduct assessment, planning, implementation, and evaluation of patient care. Failure to disclose HIV status could compromise the quality of patient care. Sexual partners of HIV-infected patients should know about the potential for infection and the need to engage in safer sex practices, as well as the possible need for testing and medical care. Nurses are advised to discuss concerns about confidentiality with nurse administrators and professional nursing organizations such as the Canadian Association of Nurses in AIDS Care (http://www.canac.org/), and to consult legal experts in their provincial/territorial jurisdiction to identify the most appropriate course of action.

AIDS has had a high mortality rate, but advances in antiretroviral and multidrug therapy have demonstrated promise in slowing or controlling disease progression. It is not known whether current treatment regimens will remain effective, because viral drug resistance has developed with most previous medications. Most nurses in Canada have never faced an epidemic in which young and middle-aged adults experience serious illness and may die during the usual course of the disease process. Nurses may struggle with the value and meaning of their professional roles as they witness repeated instances of deterioration. Exposure to so many deaths in a population that is at the same developmental stage as many nurses can create feelings of stress. Contributing to this stress are personal fears of contagion or disapproval of the patient's lifestyle and behaviours. Unlike cancer or other diseases, AIDS is associated with controversies challenging our legal and political systems as

Chart 52-10 • Ethics and Related Issues
Revealing One's HIV Status

Should all people who are infected with HIV be required to reveal this status to all their sexual and/or needle-sharing contacts?

Situation

The human immunodeficiency virus (HIV) causes HIV infection, which progresses to AIDS, a disease that is currently incurable and ultimately fatal. Many HIV-positive people are aware that they carry the virus but refuse to share this information with others, especially their sexual partners or injecting drug contacts. Because sexual contacts and needle-sharing partners are at risk for developing the disease, would a policy that requires notification of contacts infringe on the liberty and privacy of the known HIV-infected person?

Dilemma

The person's right to privacy conflicts with notifying all people who are contacts either through sexual or needle-sharing behaviour (autonomy versus justice). The person's right to privacy conflicts with society's need to contain the deadly virus and stem a deadly epidemic (autonomy versus justice).

Discussion

What arguments would you offer in favour of notifying all the person's contacts?

What arguments would you offer against notifying all or some of the person's contacts?

Each provincial/territorial jurisdiction has various laws that pertain to whether contacts can be notified and who is responsible for notifying contacts. Is there a law for contact notification in the provincial/territorial jurisdiction in which you live? If there is such a law in your provincial/territorial jurisdiction, who is responsible for contact notification?

What would you do if the person responsible for contact notification refuses to do so based on his own beliefs for confidentiality of HIV infection status?

---

well as religious and personal beliefs. Nurses who feel stressed and overburdened may experience physical and mental distress in the form of fatigue, headache, changes in appetite and sleep patterns, helplessness, irritability, apathy, negativity, and anger.

Many strategies have been used by nurses to cope with the stress associated with caring for AIDS patients. Education and provision of up-to-date information help to alleviate apprehension and prepare nurses to deliver safe, high-quality patient care. Interdisciplinary meetings allow participants to support one another and provide comprehensive patient care. Staff support groups give nurses an opportunity to solve problems and explore values and feelings about caring for AIDS patients and their families; they also provide a forum for grieving. Other sources of support include nursing administrators, peers, and spiritual advisors.

Critical Thinking Exercises

1. A 27-year-old man who was tested for HIV infection when he volunteered as a blood donor has been identified as HIV positive. He does not believe the results, says he cannot be HIV positive, and becomes angry when you attempt to explain the test results to him. How should you respond to

---

the patient, and what further testing or treatment would you anticipate? How would you modify your approach if the patient seemed suicidal?

2. You are making a home visit to a patient with HIV encephalopathy. Describe the aspects of the home environment you would assess to ensure safety and adequate care. How would you modify your assessment if the patient lived alone in a third-floor apartment without an elevator? If the patient lived in a rural setting?

3. You are the nurse manager of a surgical department. A new graduate working in the operating room was inadvertently stuck with a needle used to administer medication to a patient who is HIV positive. She is frightened about contracting HIV infection. What actions should you take as nurse manager? What do you tell the new graduate about possible risks and consequences related to her needlestick? What testing, treatment, and counselling are warranted?

4. The partner of a patient hospitalized with AIDS asks you directly, "Does my partner have AIDS?" He demands a response, saying he has a legal right to know. How would you respond to him? What ethical and legal issues are involved here?

5. You are caring for a 26-year-old woman who is HIV positive and has two young children who are HIV negative. She tells you that she has recently remarried and that she and her new husband are considering having a child. She asks you what the likelihood is that her third child will also be HIV negative. What information and knowledge do you need to discuss pregnancy and childbearing with her? What counselling and teaching are warranted for the patient and her spouse?

6. One of your patients is hospitalized in the advanced stages of HIV disease with major complications and hepatitis C. The patient has brief episodes of disorientation. He has refused to prepare or even discuss an advance directive, although his family would like him to do so. What is the impact of lack of an advance directive on his care if he lapses into a coma? If he cannot participate in making decisions about his health care?

REFERENCES AND SELECTED READINGS

Books

Agins, B. (2000). *Clinical management of HIV infection: Quality of care performance in New York State: 1996–1998.* New York State Department of Health.

Bartlett, J., & Finkbeiner, A. (2001). *The guide to living with HIV infection.* Baltimore: MD: Johns Hopkins University Press.

Bradley-Springer, L. (1999). *HIV/AIDS and nursing care plans.* Albany, NY: Delmar Press.

Burton, D. R. (2005, May 13). *Neutralizing antibodies and HIV vaccine design.* Paper presented at the 14th Annual Canadian Conference on HIV/AIDS Research, Vancouver, BC.

Canadian AIDS Treatment Information Exchange. (2004). *A practical guide to complementary therapies for people living with HIV* (rev. ed.). Toronto, ON: Author.

Canadian Blood Services. (2001). *Nucleic acid amplification testing (NAT) for hepatitis C.* Available at: http://www.bloodservices.ca/CentreApps/Internet/UW_V502_MainEngine.nsf/page/NATFAQs?OpenDocument. Retrieved December 19, 2005.

Canadian Legal HIV/AIDS Network. (2002). *Current state of HIV vaccine research.* Available at: http://www.aidslaw.ca/Maincontent/issues/vaccines.htm.

DeVita, V. T. Jr., Hellman, S., & Rosenberg, S. (Eds.). (1997). *AIDS: Etiology, diagnosis, treatment, and prevention* (4th ed.). Philadelphia: Lippincott-Raven.

Gallant, J. (2001). The seropositive patient: The initial encounter. *HIV/AIDS Clinical Management Modules,* Medscape, Inc.

Health Canada. (1999). *Routine practices and additional precautions for preventing the transmission of infection in health care: Revision of isolation precautions and techniques.* Ottawa, ON: Author.

Health Canada. (2000). *Case definitions for diseases under national surveillance.* Ottawa, ON: Author.

Health Canada. (2003). *HIV/AIDS epi updates, April.* Ottawa, ON: Author.

Health Canada. (2004a). *HIV and AIDS in Canada: Surveillance report to December 31, 2003.* Ottawa, ON: Author.

Health Canada. (2004b). *HIV and AIDS in Canada: Surveillance report to June 30, 2004.* Ottawa, ON: Author.

Horn, T., & Pieribone, D. (1999). *Managing drug side effects.* New York: Community Research Initiative on AIDS.

Joint United Nations Programme on HIV/AIDS. (2004a). *2004 report on the global AIDS epidemic.* Geneva, Switzerland: Author.

Joint United Nations Programme on HIV/AIDS. (2004b). *AIDS epidemic update: December 2004.* Geneva, Switzerland: Author.

Jürgens, R. (2001). *HIV testing and confidentiality: The final report* (2nd ed.). Montreal, QC: Canadian HIV/AIDS Legal Network and the Canadian AIDS Society.

Mantell, J. E., DiVittis, A. T., & Auerbach, M. I. (1997). *Evaluating HIV prevention interventions.* New York: Plenum Press.

McGill University. (2005). *Understanding concepts in HIV/AIDS: From the science to the clinical setting.* [CD-ROM]. Montreal, QC: Author.

Porth, C. (2002). *Pathophysiology: Concepts of altered health states* (6th ed.). Philadelphia: Lippincott Williams & Wilkins.

Public Health Agency of Canada. (2005). *HIV/AIDS epi updates, May 2005.* Ottawa, ON: Author.

Ropka, M., & Williams, A. (1998). *HIV nursing and symptom management.* Sudbury, MA: Jones & Bartlett.

Sande, M., & Volberding, P. (1999). *The medical management of AIDS.* (6th ed.). Philadelphia: W. B. Saunders.

Smith, R. (2001). *Encyclopedia of AIDS: A social, political, cultural, and scientific record of the HIV epidemic.* New York: Penguin Books.

UNAIDS (2001). *AIDS epidemic update, December 2001.* UNAIDS & World Health Organization.

Ungvarski, P. J., & Flaskerud, J. H. (Eds.). (1999). *HIV/AIDS: A guide to primary care management* (4th ed.). Philadelphia: W. B. Saunders.

World Health Organization. (2003). *WHO/CONRAD technical consultation on nonoxynol-9.* Geneva, Switzerland: Author.

Journals

Asterisks indicate nursing research articles.

AIDS Institute (9/21/00). Information update: AIDS Institute discontinues recommendation of intra-vaginal application of N-9 as method of HIV risk reduction. Corning Tower, Albany, NY.

American Red Cross (2001). This month's HIV/AIDS facts. http://www.redcross.org/services/hss/tips/july/answer98.html

*Bakken, S., Holzemer, W., Brown, M. A., et al. (2000). Relationships between perception of engagement with health care provider and demographic characteristics, health status, and adherence to therapeutic regimen in persons with HIV/AIDS. *AIDS Patient Care and STDs, 14*(4), 189–197.

Balter, M. (1998). Revealing HIV's T cell passkey. *Science, 280*(5371), 1833–1834.

Bartlett, J., & Moore, R. (1998). Improving HIV therapy. *Scientific American, 279*(1), 84–87.

Boden, D., Hurley, A., Zhang, L., et al. (1999). HIV-1 drug resistance in newly infected individuals. *Journal of American Medical Association, 282*(12), 1135–1141.

Bradley-Springer, L. (2001). HIV prevention: What works? *American Journal of Nursing, 101*(6), 45–50.

Busch, M. P., Kleinman, S. H., & Nemo, G. J. (2003). Current and emerging infectious risks of blood transfusions. *Journal of the American Medical Association, 289*(8), 959–962.

Cates, W., Chesney, M. & Cohen, M. (1997). Primary HIV infection: A public health opportunity. *American Journal of Public Health, 87*(12), 1928–1930.

Cavert, W., & Haase, A. (1998). A national tissue bank to track HIV eradication and immune reconstitution. *Science, 280*(5371), 1865–1866.

Centers for Disease Control and Prevention (2002). Guideline for hand hygiene in healthcare settings. *MMWR CDC Recommendations and Reports, 51* (RR-16), 1–45.

Centers for Disease Control and Prevention (2000). *HIV/AIDS Surveillance Report, 12*(1), 1–41.

Centers for Disease Control and Prevention (2002). *HIV/AIDS Surveillance Report, 13*(2), 1–44.

Centers for Disease Control and Prevention. Hospital Infection Control Practices Advisory Committee (1997). Part I. Evolution of Isolation Practices. http://www.cdc.gov/hcidod/hip/isolat/isopart1.htm

Centers for Disease Control and Prevention. Hospital Infection Control Practices Advisory Committee (1997). Part II. Recommendations for Isolation Precautions in Hospitals. http://www.cdc.gov/hcidod/hip/isolat/isopart2.htm

Centers for Disease Control and Prevention. (1998). Appendix: First-line drugs for HIV postexposure prophylaxis. *MMWR CDC Recommendation and Reports, 47*(RR-7), 29–30.

Centers for Disease Control and Prevention. (1998). Public health service guidelines for the management of health-care worker exposure to HIV and recommendations for postexposure prophylaxis. *MMWR CDC Recommendations and Reports, 47*(RR-7), 1–28.

Centers for Disease Control and Prevention, U.S. Department of Health and Human Services. (1998). Report of the NIH panel to define principles of therapy of HIV infection and guidelines for the use of antiretroviral agents in HIV infected adults and adolescents. *MMWR CDC Recommendations and Reports, 24*(RR-5), 1–82.

Centers for Disease Control and Prevention, U.S. Department of Health and Human Services. (1992). 1993 revised classification system for HIV infection and expanded surveillance case definition for AIDS among adolescents and adults. *MMWR CDC Recommendations and Reports, 41*(RR-17), 1–19.

Cilsielski, C. A., & Metler, R. P. (1997). Duration of time between exposure and seroconversion in healthcare workers with occupationally acquired infection with human immunodeficiency virus. *American Journal of Medicine, 102*(Suppl. 5B), 115–116.

Collier, A. & the Viral Activation Transfusion Study Group (2001). Leukocyte-reduced red blood cell transfusions in patients with anemia and HIV infection: The Viral Activation Transfusion study: A randomized control trial. *Journal of American Medical Association, 285*(12), 1592–1601.

Collman, R. (1997). Effect of CCR2 and CCR5 variants on HIV disease. *Journal of American Medical Association, 278*(23), 2113–2114.

Coyne, P. J., Lyne, M. E., & Watson, A. C. (2002). Symptom management in people with AIDS. *American Journal of Nursing, 102*(9), 48–56.

Daughtry, L., Bankston, J., & Deshotels, J. (2002). HIV meds: Keeping trouble at bay. *RN, 65*(2), 31–35.

Dybul, M., et al. (2001). Short cycle structured intermittent treatment of chronic HIV infection with highly active antiretroviral therapy: Effects of virologic, immunologic, and toxicity parameters. *Proceedings of the National Academy of Sciences, Early Edition.* Online, Dec. 4, 2001.

Emerman, M., & Malim, M. (1998). HIV-1 regulatory/accessory genes: Keys to unraveling viral and host cell biology. *Science, 280*(5371), 1880–1884.

Esch, J., & Frank, S. (2001). Drug resistance and nursing practice. *American Journal of Nursing, 101*(6), 30–36.

Gracia Jones, S. (2001). Taking HAART: How to support patients with HIV/AIDS. *Nursing 2001, 31*(12), 36–41.

Havlir, D. V., & Barnes, P. F. (1999). Tuberculosis in patients with human immunodeficiency virus infection. *New England Journal of Medicine, 340*(5), 367–372.

Health Canada. (1997a). An integrated protocol to manage health care workers exposed to bloodborne pathogens. *Canada Communicable Disease Report, 23*(Suppl 2).

Health Canada. (1997b). Infection control guidelines: Preventing the transmission of bloodborne pathogens in health care and public service settings. *Canada Communicable Disease Report, 23*(Suppl 3).

*Henry, S., Holzemer, W., Weaver, K., & Stotts, N. (1999). Quality of life and self-care management strategies of PLWAs with chronic diarrhea. *Journal of Association of Nurses in AIDS Care, 10*(2), 46–54.

Hirsch, M., Brun-Vezinet, F., D'Aquila, R., et al. (2000). Antiretrovrial drug resistance testing in adult HIV-1 infection: Recommendations of an International AIDS Society-USA Panel. *Journal of American Medical Association, 283*(18), 2417–2426.

Hirschfeld, S. (1998). Pain as a complication of HIV disease. *AIDS Patient Care and STDs, 12*(2), 91–108.

Ho, D. (1998). Toward HIV eradication or remission: The tasks ahead. *Science, 280*(5371), 1866–1867.

*Holzemer, W. L., Henry, S. B., & Reilly, C. A. (1998). Assessing and managing pain in AIDS care: The patient perspective. *Journal of the Association of Nurses in AIDS Care, 9*(1), 22–30.

*Holzemer, W., Corless, I., Nokes, K., et al. (1999). Predictors of self-reported adherence in persons living with HIV disease. *AIDS Patient Care and STDs, 13*(3), 185–197.

*Holzemer, W., Henry, S., Nokes, K., et al. (1999). Validation of the Sign and Symptom Checklist for Persons with HIV Disease. *Journal of Advanced Nursing 30*(5), 1041–1049.

Huston, D. (1997). The biology of the immune system. *Journal of the American Medical Association, 278*(22), 1804–1814.

International Perinatal HIV Group. (1999). The mode of delivery and the risk of vertical transmission of human immunodeficiency virus type I. *New England Journal of Medicine, 340*(13), 977–987.

Jemmott, J. B. III, Jemmott, L. S., & Fong, G. T. (1998). Abstinence and safer sex HIV risk-reduction interventions for African American adolescents: A randomized controlled trial. *Journal of American Medical Association, 279*(19), 1529–1536.

Keithley, J. K., & Swanson, B. (1998). Minimizing HIV/AIDS malnutrition. *MedSurg Nursing, 7*(5), 256–267.

Kirton, C. A., Ferri, R. S., & Eleftherakis, V. (1999). Primary care and case management of persons with HIV/AIDS. *Nursing Clinics of North America, 34*(1), 71–94.

Lee, L., Karon, J., Selik, R., et al. (2001). Survival after AIDS diagnosis in adolescents and adults during the treatment era, United States, 1984–1997. *Journal of American Medical Association, 285*(10), 1308–1315.

Lewis, C. (2001). Home diagnostic tests: The ultimate house call? US Food and Drug Administration. *FDA Consumer Magazine* Nov.–Dec., 1–6.

Letvin, N. (1998). Progress in the development of an HIV-1 vaccine. *Science, 280*(5371), 1875–1880.

Letvin, N., Bloom, B., & Hoffman, S. (2001). Prospects for vaccines to protect against AIDS, tuberculosis, and malaria. *Journal of the American Medical Association, 285*(5), 606–611.

MacIntyre, R. C., & Holzemer, W. L. (1997). Complementary and alternative medicine and HIV/AIDS. II. Selected literature review. *Journal of the Association of Nurses in AIDS Care, 8*(2), 25–38.

Manfredi, R. (2004). HIV infection and advanced age: Emerging epidemiological, clinical, and management issues. *Ageing Research Reviews, 3*, 31–4.

Masur, H., Kaplan, J., & Holmes, K. (1999). 1999 USPHS/IDSA guidelines for the prevention of opportunistic infections in persons infected with human immunodeficiency virus. *MMWR,* August 20, 1999/48(R10), 1–59.

Mellors, J. (1998). Viral-load tests provide valuable answers. *Scientific American, 279*(1), 90–93.

*Mill, J. (2000). Describing an explanatory model of HIV illness among Aboriginal women. *Holistic Nursing Practice, 15*(1), 42–6.

National Institutes of Health. (2002). New HIV vaccine holds promise of global effectiveness. [News release]. http://www.nih.gov/pr/nov2002/niaid-13.htm

Nduati, R., John, G., Mbori-Ngacha, D., et al. (2000). Effect of breast-feeding and formula feeding on transmission of HIV-1: A randomized clinical trial. *Journal of American Medical Association, 283*(9), 1167–1174.

NIAID (2001). HIV research. http://www.niaid.nih.gov/daids/therapeutics/research/hivpriorities.htm

*Nokes, K., & Bakken, S. (2002). Issues associated with measuring symptoms status: HIV/AIDS case illustration. *Journal of the New York State Nurses Association, 33*(2), 17–21.

*Nokes, K., Holzemer, W., Corless, I., et al. (2000). Health-related quality of life in persons younger and older than 50 who are living with HIV/AIDS. *Research on Aging, 22*(3), 290–310.

*Nokes, K., Wheeler, K. & Kendrew, J. (1994). Development of an HIV assessment tool. *Image: Journal of Nursing Scholarship, 26*(2), 133–138.

Perrin, L., & Telenti, A. (1998). HIV treatment failure: Testing for HIV resistance in clinical practice. *Science, 280*(5371), 1871–1873.

Public Health Agency of Canada. (2005). *HIV/AIDS epi update: Centre for Infectious Disease Prevention and Control.* Available at: http://www.phac-aspc.gc.ca. Retrieved June 21, 2005.

Public Health Agency of Canada. (2003). Update—Surveillance of health care workers exposed to blood, body fluids and bloodborne pathogens in Canadian hospital settings, 1 April, 2000 to 31 March, 2002. *Canadian Communicable Disease Report, 29*(24), 209–213.

Saag, M. (2001). Eighth conference on retroviruses and opportunistic infections, Chicago: Feb. 4-8, 2001. HIV Information Network, FAX Newsletter. Feb. 8, 2001.

Schutz, M., & Wendrow, A. (1/3/02). Quick reference guide to antiretrovirals. HIV/AIDS Treatment Updates. http://hiv.medscape.com/Medscape/HIV/Treatment_Update/1998/tu01/eng/pnt-eng.tu01.html

Sherman, D. (1999). Essential information for providing quality care to patients with HIV/AIDS. *Journal of New York State Nurses Association, 30*(2), 8–19.

*Sowell, R. L., Phillips, K. D., & Grier, J. (1998). Restructuring life to face the future: The perspective of men after a positive response to protease inhibitor therapy. *AIDS Patient Care and STDs, 12*(1), 33–41.

Stephenson, J. (1998). Studies reveal early impact of HIV infection, effects of treatment. *Journal of American Medical Association, 279*(9), 641–642.

Swanson, J., Keithley, J., Zeller, J., & Cronin-Stubbs, D. (2000). Complementary and alternative therapies to manage HIV-related symptoms. *Journal of Association of Nurses in AIDS Care, 11*(5), 40–60.

Trzcianowska, H., & Mortensen, E. (2001). HIV and AIDS: Separating fact from fiction. *American Journal of Nursing, 101*(6), 53–59.

*Ungvarski, P. J. (1997). Adherence to prescribed HIV-1 protease inhibitors in the home setting. *Journal of Association of Nurses in AIDS Care, 8*(Suppl). 37–45.

*Ungvarski, P. J., & Rottner, J. E. (1997). Errors in prescribing HIV-1 protease inhibitors. *Journal of the Association of Nurses in AIDS Care, 8*(4), 55–61.

U.S. Food and Drug Administration. (2002). FDA approves new rapid HIV test kit. [News release]. http://www.fda.gov/bbs/topics/NEWS/2002/NEW00852.html

Williams, A. B. (1999). Adherence to a highly active antiretroviral therapy. *Nursing Clinics of North America, 34*(1), 113–129.

Williams, A. (2001). Adherence to HIV regimens: 10 vital lessons. *American Journal of Nursing, 101*(6), 37–44.

Worthington, K. (2001). You've been stuck: What do you do? *American Journal of Nursing, 101*(3), 104.

Wyatt, R., & Sodroski, J. (1998). The HIV-1 envelope glycoproteins: Fusogens, antigens, and immunogens. *Science, 280*(5371), 1884–1888.

RESOURCES AND WEBSITES

AIDS Education and Training Centers (ETCs) Program, 5600 Fishers Lane, Room 9A-39, Rockville, MD 20857; (301) 443-6364; Fax (301) 433-9887.

AIDS Action Council, 875 Connecticut NW, Suite 700, Washington, DC 20003; (202) 986-1300; Fax (202) 986-1345; http://www.aidsaction.org.

AIDS Treatment Information Service: (800) 448-0440 (Spanish available); Fax (800) 519-3739; e-mail: atis@hivtis.org.

AIDS Clinical Trials Information Service, P.O. 621, Rockville, MD 20849-6421; (800) HIV-0440; http://www.hivatis.org.

American Red Cross: http://www.redcross.org.

American Social Health Association, P.O. Box 13827, Research Triangle Park, NC 27709; (919) 361-8400; fax (919) 361-8425; http://www.afhastd.org.

British Columbia Centre for Excellence in HIV/AIDS, 608-1081 Burrard Street, Vancouver, B.C V6Z 1Y6; (604) 806-8515; fax (604) 806-9044; http://www.cfenet.ubc.ca/index.php#.

Canadian AIDS Society, 309 Cooper Street, 4th Floor, Ottawa, ON K2P 0G5; (613) 230-3580; fax: (613) 563-4998; http://www.cdnaids.ca/.

Canadian AIDS Treatment Information Exchange, 555 Richmond Street West, Suite 505, Box 1104, Toronto, ON M5V 3B1; (416) 203-7122 or 1-800-263-1638; fax: (416) 203-8284; http://www.catie.ca/.

Canadian Association for HIV Research, University of British Columbia, 201-1200 Burrard Street, Vancouver, BC V6Z 2C7; (604) 642-6429 x307; fax: (604) 642-6419; http://www.cahr-acrv.ca.

Canadian Association of Nurses in AIDS Care, 9 Huntley Street, Toronto, ON M4Y 2K8; fax: (416) 962-5147; http://www.canac.org.

Canadian Blood Services, 1800 Alta Vista Drive, Ottawa, ON K1G 4J5; (613) 739-2300; fax: (613) 731-1411; http://www.bloodservices.ca/.

Canadian Harm Reduction Network, 666 Spadina Avenue, Suite 1904, Toronto, ON M5S 2H8; (416) 928-0279 or 1-800-728-1293; fax: (416) 966-9512; http://www.canadianharmreduction.com/.

Canadian HIV/AIDS Information Centre, 400-1565 Carling Avenue, Ottawa, ON K1Z 8R1; (613) 725-3434 or 1-877-999-7740; fax: (613) 725-1205; http://www.aidssida.cpha.ca/.

Canadian HIV/AIDS Legal Network, 417 Saint-Pierre Street, Suite 408, Montreal, QC H2Y 2M4; (514) 397-6828; fax: (514) 397-8570; http://www.aidslaw.ca/.

Canadian HIV Trials Network, 620-1081 Burrard Street, Vancouver, BC V6Z 1Y6; (604) 806-8327 or 1-800-661-4664; fax: (604) 806-8210; http://www.hivnet.ubc.ca/e/home/.

Canadian Hospice Palliative Care Association, Annex B, Saint-Vincent Hospital, 60 Cambridge Street North, Ottawa, ON K1R 7A5; (613) 241-3663 or 1-800-668-2785; fax: (613) 241-3986; http://www.chpca.net/home.htm.

Canadian Institutes of Health Research, 160 Elgin Street, 9th Floor, Address Locator 4809A, Ottawa, ON K1A 0W9; (613) 941-2672 or 1-888-603-4178; fax: (613) 954-1800; http://www.cihr-irsc.gc.ca/.

Canadian International Development Agency, 200 Promenade du Portage, Gatineau, QC K1A 0G4; (819) 997-5006 or 1-800-230-6349; fax: (819) 953-6088; http://www.acdi-cida.gc.ca/index-e.htm.

Canadian Nurses Association, 50 Driveway, Ottawa, ON K2P 1E2; (613) 237-2133 or 1-800-361-8404; fax: (613) 237-3520; http://www.cna-nurses.ca/cna/.

Canadian Public Health Association, 400-1565 Carling Avenue, Ottawa ON, K1Z 8R1; (613) 725-3769; fax: (613) 725-9826; http://www.cpha.ca/.

Centers for Disease Control and Prevention, 1600 Clifton Rd., Atlanta, GA 30333; (404) 639-3311; http://www.cdc.gov.

Centers for Disease Control and Prevention. AIDS Hotline: (800) 342-2437; Spanish: (800) 344-7432; http://www.cdc.gov.

Community Research Initiative on AIDS, 230 W. 38th St., 17th floor, New York, NY 10018; (212) 924-3934; fax (212) 924-3936; http://www.criany.org.

Gay Men's Health Crisis Network, 119 W. 24th St., New York, NY 10011; (800) AIDS-NYC (800-243-7692); http://www.gmhc.org.

Health Canada, AL 0900C2, Ottawa, ON K1A 0K9; (613) 957-2991 or 1-866-225-0709; fax: (613) 941-5366; http://www.hc-sc.gc.ca.

Hemophilia and AIDS/HIV Network for the Dissemination of Information, The National Hemophilia Foundation, 116 W. 32nd St., 11th Floor, New York, NY 10001; (212) 328-3700; (800) 42-HANDI; fax (212) 328-3777; http://www.hemophilia.org.

HIV Community-Based Research Network, Suite 122, 1628 West 1st Ave, Vancouver, BC V6J1G1; http://cbr.cbrc.net/.

HRSA National Clinician's Post-exposure prophylaxis hotline (health care providers only): (888) HIV-4911.

HRSA National HIV Telephone Consultation Service: (800) 933-3413.

International Council of Nurses, 3, Place Jean Marteau, 1201 - Geneva, Switzerland; 41-22-908-0100; fax: 41-22-908-0101; http://www.icn.ch/.

International Development Research Centre, PO Box 8500, Ottawa, ON, K1G 3H9; (613) 236-6163; fax: (613) 238-7230; http://www.idrc.ca/.

Joint United Nations Programme on HIV/AIDS, 20, avenue Appia, CH-1211 Geneva 27, Switzerland; 41-22-791-3666; fax: 41-22-791-4187; http://www.unaids.org/en/default.asp.

Living with HIV/AIDS. http://www.cdc.gov/hiv/pubs/brochure/livingwith hiv.htm.

National Association of People With AIDS, 1413 K Street, N.W., 7th Floor, Washington, DC 20005; (202) 898-0414; fax (202) 898-0435; http://www.natwa.org.

National Pediatric and Family HIV Resource Center, University of Medicine and Dentistry, 30 Bergen St., ADMC #4, Newark, NJ 07103; (973) 972-0410; http://www.pedhivaids.org.

Office of Minority Health Resource Center, P.O. Box 37337, Washington, DC 20013; (800) 444-6472; TDD (301) 230-7199; public inquiries (404) 639-3534; (800) 311-3435; http://www.omhrc.org.

National Pediatric HIV Resource Center: (800) 362-0071

Pharmaceutical Research and Manufacturers of America, 1100 Fifteenth St, NW, Washington, DC 20005; (202) 835-3400; http://www.phrma.org.

Public Health Agency of Canada, Centre for Infectious Disease Prevention and Control, Postal Locator: 0602B, Ottawa, ON K1A 0K9; (613) 954-5159; fax: (613) 946-8695; http://www.phac-aspc.gc.ca.

Treatment Information Service. AIDS*info*. PO Box 6303, Rockville, MD 20849-6303, USA; (800) HIV-0440; outside US: (301) 519-0459; www.aidsinfo.nih.gov. Glossary of HIV/AIDS-related terms.

United Nations Association in Canada, Suite 300, 309 Cooper Street, Ottawa, ON K2P 0G5; (613) 232-5751; fax: (613) 563-2455; http://www.unac.org/en/index.asp.

World Health Organization, Avenue Appia 20, 1211 Geneva 27, Switzerland; 41-22-791-2111; fax: 41-22-791-3111; http://www.who.int/en/.

Assessment and Management of Patients With Allergic Disorders

Adapted by Wanda Pierson

LEARNING OBJECTIVES

On completion of this chapter, the learner will be able to:

1. Explain the physiologic events involved with allergic reactions.
2. Describe the types of hypersensitivity.
3. Describe the management of patients with allergic disorders.
4. Describe measures to prevent and manage anaphylaxis.
5. Use the nursing process as a framework for care of the patient with allergic rhinitis.
6. Discuss the different allergic disorders according to type.

*T*he human body is menaced by a host of potential invaders—allergens as well as microbial organisms—that constantly threaten its surface defenses. After penetrating those defenses, these allergens and organisms compete with the body for its nutrients and, if allowed to flourish unimpeded, disrupt its enzyme systems and destroy its vital tissues. To protect against these agents, the body is equipped with an elaborate defense system.

The epithelial cells coating the skin and making up the lining of the respiratory, gastrointestinal, and genitourinary tracts provide the first line of defense. The structure and continuity of these surfaces and the resistance to penetration are initial deterrents to invaders.

One of the most effective defense mechanisms is the body's capacity to equip itself rapidly with weapons (antibodies) individually designed to meet each new invader, namely specific protein antigens. Antibodies react with antigens in a variety of ways: (1) by coating the antigens' surfaces if they are particular substances, (2) by neutralizing the antigens if they are toxic, and (3) by precipitating the antigens out of solution if they are dissolved.

The antibodies prepare the antigens so that the phagocytic cells of the blood and the tissues can dispose of them. In some cases, however, the body produces inappropriate or exaggerated responses to specific antigens, and the result is an allergic or hypersensitivity disorder.

Allergic Reaction: Physiologic Overview

An allergic reaction is a manifestation of tissue injury resulting from interaction between an antigen and an antibody. **Allergy** is an inappropriate and often harmful response of the immune system to normally harmless substances. In this case, the substance is termed an **allergen**. **Atopy** refers to allergic reactions characterized by the action of IgE antibodies and a genetic predisposition to allergic reactions.

When the body is invaded by an **antigen**, usually a protein that the body's defenses recognize as foreign, a series of events occurs in an attempt to render the invader harmless, destroy it, and remove it from the body. When lymphocytes respond to the antigen, **antibodies** (protein substances that protect against antigens) are produced. Common allergic reactions occur when the immune system of a susceptible person responds aggressively to a substance that is normally harmless (eg, dust, weeds, pollen, dander). Chemical mediators released in allergic reactions may produce symptoms ranging from mild to life-threatening.

The many cells and organs of the immune system secrete various substances important in the immune response. These parts of the immune system must work together to ensure adequate defense against invaders (ie, virus, bacteria, other foreign substances) without destroying the body's own tissues by an overly aggressive reaction.

FUNCTION AND PRODUCTION OF IMMUNOGLOBULINS

Antibodies formed by lymphocytes and plasma cells in response to an immunogenic stimulus constitute a group of serum proteins called **immunoglobulins**. Grouped into five classes (IgE, IgD, IgG, IgM, and IgA), antibodies can be found in the lymph nodes, tonsils, appendix, and Peyer's patches of the intestinal tract or circulating in the blood and lymph. Each antibody molecule is composed of two identical heavy (H) chains and two identical light (L) chains. Each chain contains one variable region and one or more constant regions. The constant regions determine the class (IgE, IgD, etc.) of each antibody and allow each class of antibody to interact with specific effector cells and molecules. The variable regions contain antigen-binding sites (Porth, 2002). Antibodies are capable of binding with a wide variety of antigens, which include macromolecules and small chemicals (Abbas & Lichtman, 2001). Antibodies of the IgM, IgG, and IgA classes have definite and well-established protective functions. These include neutralization of toxins and viruses and precipitation, agglutination, and lysis of bacteria and other foreign cellular material. (See Chap. 50 for further discussion of these functions.)

Immunoglobulins of the IgE class are involved in allergic disorders and some parasitic infections, evidenced by elevation of IgE levels. IgE-producing cells are located in the respiratory and intestinal mucosa. Two or more IgE molecules bind together to an allergen and trigger **mast cells** or basophils to release chemical mediators, such as histamine, serotonin, kinins, slow-reacting substance of anaphylaxis (SRS-A), and the neutrophil factor, which produces allergic skin reactions, asthma, and hay fever.

Glossary

allergen: substance that causes manifestations of allergy

allergy: inappropriate and often harmful immune system response to substances that are normally harmless

anaphylaxis: clinical response to an immediate immunologic reaction between a specific antigen and antibody

angioneurotic edema: condition characterized by urticaria and diffuse swelling of the deeper layers of the skin

antibody: protein substance developed by the body in response to and interacting with a specific antigen

antigen: substance that induces the production of antibodies

antihistamine: medication that opposes the action of histamine

atopic dermatitis: type I hypersensitivity involving inflammation of the skin evidenced by itching, redness, and a variety of skin lesions

atopy: term often used to describe IgE-mediated diseases; genetically determined allergic disorders

B lymphocyte: cells that are important in producing circulating antibodies

bradykinin: polypeptide that stimulates nerve fibres and causes pain

eosinophil: granular leukocyte

epitope: an immunologically active site on an antigen; a single antigen can have several different epitopes that elicit responses from different antibodies

erythema: diffuse redness of the skin

hapten: incomplete antigen

histamine: substance in the body that causes increased gastric secretion, dilation of capillaries, and constriction of the bronchial smooth muscle

hypersensitivity: abnormal heightened reaction to a stimulus of any kind

immunoglobulins: a family of closely related proteins capable of acting as antibodies

leukotrienes: a group of chemical mediators that initiate the inflammatory response

lymphokines: substances released by sensitized lymphocytes when they contact specific antigens

mast cell: connective tissue cells that contain heparin and histamine in their granules

prostaglandins: unsaturated fatty acids that have a wide assortment of biologic activity

rhinitis: inflammation of the nasal mucosa

serotonin: chemical mediator that acts as a potent vasoconstrictor and bronchoconstrictor

T lymphocyte: cells that can cause graft rejection, kill foreign cells, or suppress production of antibodies

urticaria: hives

Antibodies combine with antigens in a special way, likened to keys fitting into a lock. Antigens (the keys) only fit certain antibodies (the locks). Hence, the term "specificity" refers to the specific reaction of an antibody to an antigen. There are many variations and complexities in these patterns. The strength with which one antigen-binding surface of an antibody binds to one **epitope**, an immunologically active site on an antigen, is known as the affinity of the interaction (Abbas & Lichtman, 2001).

Antibody molecules are bivalent; that is, they have two combining sites. Therefore, the antibody easily becomes a cross-link between two antigen groups, causing them to clump together (agglutination). By this action, foreign invaders are cleared from the bloodstream. Agglutination is the means for determining blood group in laboratory tests.

Role of B Cells

The B cell, or **B lymphocyte**, is programmed to produce one specific antibody. On encountering a specific antigen, a B cell stimulates production of plasma cells, the site of antibody production. The result is the outpouring of antibodies for the purpose of destroying and removing the antigen.

Role of T Cells

The T cell, or **T lymphocyte**, assists the B cells in producing antibodies. T cells secrete substances known as **lymphokines** that encourage cell growth, promote cell activation, direct the flow of cell activity, destroy target cells, and stimulate the macrophages. Macrophages present the antigen to the T cells and initiate the immune response. They also digest antigens and assist in removing cells and other debris. The antigen-binding site of a T cell has a structure much like that of an immunoglobulin. It recognizes epitopes through complementary interactions. Unlike a specific antibody, a T cell does not bind free antigens (Parslow, Stites, Terr & Imboden, 2001).

FUNCTION OF ANTIGENS

Antigens are divided into two groups: complete protein antigens and low-molecular-weight substances. Complete protein antigens, such as animal dander, pollen, and horse serum, stimulate a complete humoural response. (See Chap. 50 for a discussion of humoural

immunity.) Low-molecular-weight substances, such as medications, function as **haptens** (incomplete antigens), binding to tissue or serum proteins to produce a carrier complex that initiates an antibody response. The term "hapten" is derived from the Greek word *haptien* (to fasten). The proteins or other immunogens that haptens are fastened to are known as carriers (Parslow et al., 2001).

In an allergic reaction, the production of antigen-specific IgE antibodies requires active communication between macrophages, T cells, and B cells. When the allergen is absorbed through the respiratory tract, gastrointestinal tract, or skin, allergen sensitization occurs. The macrophage processes the antigen and presents it to the appropriate T cell. B cells that are influenced by the T cell mature into an allergen-specific IgE immunoglobulin-secreting plasma cell that synthesizes and secretes antigen-specific IgE antibody.

FUNCTION OF CHEMICAL MEDIATORS

Mast cells, which have a major role in IgE-mediated immediate hypersensitivity, are located in the skin and mucous membranes. When mast cells are stimulated by antigens, powerful chemical mediators are released that cause a sequence of physiologic events resulting in symptoms of immediate hypersensitivity (Fig. 53-1). There are two types of chemical mediators: primary, which are preformed and found in mast cells or basophils, and secondary, which are inactive precursors formed or released in response to primary mediators. The most prevalent known primary and secondary mediators are described next. Table 53-1 summarizes the actions of primary and secondary chemical mediators.

Primary Mediators

IgE-mediated inflammation occurs when an antigen binds to the IgE antibodies that occupy certain receptors on mast cells. Within minutes, this binding causes the mast cell to degranulate, releasing certain preformed mediators. A two-phase response results. There is an initial immediate effect on blood vessels, smooth muscle, and glandular secretion. This is followed a few hours later by cellular infiltration of the involved site. This type of inflammatory response is commonly known as an immediate hypersensitivity response (Parslow et al., 2001).

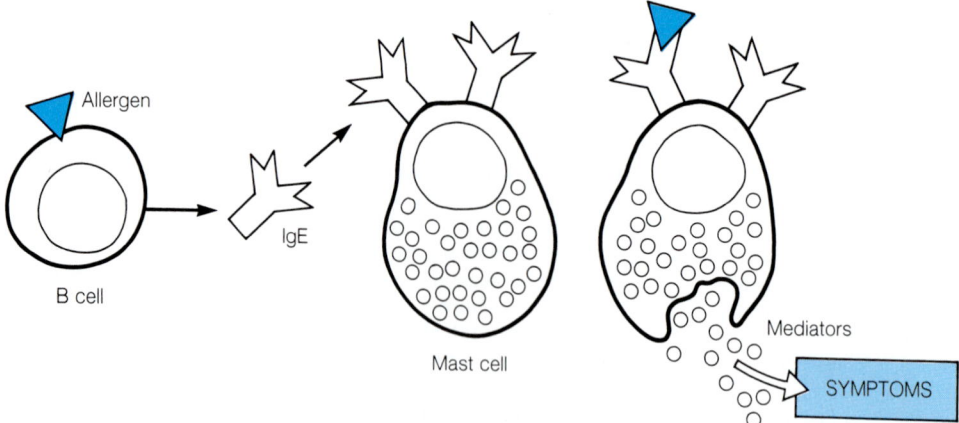

FIGURE 53-1 Allergen triggers B cell to make IgE antibody, which attaches to mast cell. When that allergen reappears, it binds to the IgE and triggers the mast cell to release its chemicals. Courtesy of U.S. Dept. of Health and Human Services, National Institutes of Health.

Table 53-1 • **Chemical Mediators of Hypersensitivity**

MEDIATORS	ACTION
Primary Mediators (Preformed and found in mast cells or basophils)	
Histamine (preformed in mast cells)	Vasodilation Smooth muscle contraction, increased vascular permeability, increased mucus secretions
Eosinophil chemotactic factor of anaphylaxis (ECF-A) (preformed in mast cells)	Attracts eosinophils
Platelet-activating factor (PAF) (requires synthesis by mast cells, neutrophils, and macrophages)	Smooth muscle contraction Incites platelets to aggregate and release serotonin and histamine
Prostaglandins (chemically derived from arachidonic acid; require synthesis by cells)	D and F series → bronchoconstriction E series → bronchodilation D, E, and F series → vasodilation
Basophil kallikrein (preformed in mast cells)	Frees bradykinin, which causes bronchoconstriction, vasodilation, and nerve stimulation
Secondary Mediators (Inactive precursors formed or released in response to primary mediators)	
Bradykinin (derived from precursor kininogen)	Smooth muscle contraction, increased vascular permeability, stimulates pain receptors, increased mucus production
Serotonin (preformed in platelets)	Smooth muscle contraction, increased vascular permeability
Heparin (preformed in mast cells)	Anticoagulant
Leukotrienes (derived from arachidonic acid and activated by mast cell degranulation) C, D, and E or slow-reacting substance of anaphylaxis (SRS-A)	Smooth muscle contraction, increased vascular permeability

HISTAMINE

Histamine plays an important role in the immune response. Histamine is released from mast cell granules where it is stored. Maximal intensity is reached within about 15 minutes after antigen contact (Parslow et al., 2001). The effects of histamine release include erythema; localized edema in the form of wheals; pruritus; contraction of bronchial smooth muscle, resulting in wheezing and bronchospasm; dilation of small venules and constriction of larger vessels; and increased secretion of gastric and mucosal cells, resulting in diarrhea. Histamine action results from stimulation of histamine-1 (H_1) and histamine-2 (H_2) receptors found on different types of lymphocytes, particularly T-lymphocyte suppressor cells and basophils. H_1 receptors are found predominantly on bronchiolar and vascular smooth muscle cells. H_2 receptors are found on gastric parietal cells.

Certain medications are categorized by their action at these receptors. Diphenhydramine (Benadryl) is an example of an **antihistamine**, which is a medication displaying an affinity for H_1 receptors; cimetidine (Tagamet) and ranitidine (Zantac) are examples of other pharmacologic agents that target H_2 receptors to inhibit gastric secretions in peptic ulcer disease.

EOSINOPHIL CHEMOTACTIC FACTOR OF ANAPHYLAXIS

Preformed in the mast cells, this chemotactic factor, which affects movement of **eosinophils** (granular leukocytes) to the site of allergens, is released upon degranulation to inhibit the action of leukotrienes and histamine.

PLATELET-ACTIVATING FACTOR

Platelet-activating factor (PAF) is responsible for initiating platelet aggregation at sites of immediate hypersensitivity reactions. It also causes bronchoconstriction and increased vascular permeability. PAF also activates factor XII, or Hageman factor, which induces the formation of bradykinin.

PROSTAGLANDINS

Prostaglandins, composed of unsaturated fatty acids, produce smooth muscle contraction as well as vasodilation and increased capillary permeability. The fever and pain that occur with inflammation are due in part to the prostaglandins.

Secondary Mediators

LEUKOTRIENES

Leukotrienes are chemical mediators that initiate the inflammatory response. They are metabolites released by mucosal mast cells. They collectively make up what was once termed "slow-reacting substance of anaphylaxis" (SRS-A). Leukotrienes cause smooth muscle contraction, bronchial constriction, mucus secretion in the airways, and the typical wheal and flare reaction of the skin (Parslow et al., 2001). Compared with histamine, leukotrienes are 100 to 1,000 times more potent in causing bronchospasm. Many manifestations of inflammation can be attributed in part to leukotrienes. Medications categorized as leukotriene antagonists or modifiers (zileuton [Zyflo], zafirlukast [Accolate], montelukast [Singulair]) block the synthesis or action of leukotrienes and prevent the signs and symptoms associated with asthma.

BRADYKININ

Bradykinin is a polypeptide with the ability to cause increased vascular permeability, vasodilation, hypotension, and contraction of many types of smooth muscle, such as the bronchi (Parslow et al., 2001). Increased permeability of the capillaries results in edema. Bradykinin stimulates nerve cell fibres and produces pain.

SEROTONIN

Serotonin is released during platelet aggregation, acting as a potent vasoconstrictor and causing contraction of bronchial smooth muscle.

HYPERSENSITIVITY

Although the immune system defends the host against infections and foreign antigens, immune responses can themselves cause tissue injury and disease. An immune response to an antigen may result in sensitivity to challenge with that antigen; **hypersensitivity** is a reflection of excessive or aberrant immune responses (Abbas & Lichtman, 2001).

A hypersensitivity reaction is an abnormal, heightened reaction to any type of stimuli. It usually does not occur with the first exposure to an allergen. Rather, the reaction follows a re-exposure after sensitization in a predisposed individual. Sensitization initiates the humoural response or buildup of antibodies. To promote understanding of the immunopathogenesis of disease, hypersensitivity reactions have been classified into four specific types of re-

actions (Fig. 53-2). Most allergies are identified as either type I or type IV hypersensitivity reactions.

Anaphylactic (Type I) Hypersensitivity

The most severe form of a hypersensitivity reaction is **anaphylaxis**. This systemic reaction is characterized by edema in many tissues, including the larynx, and is often accompanied by hypotension (Abbas & Lichtman, 2001). Type I or anaphylactic hypersensitivity is an immediate reaction beginning within minutes of exposure to an antigen. This reaction is mediated by IgE antibodies rather than IgG or IgM antibodies. Type I hypersensitivity requires previous exposure to the specific antigen. In turn, the plasma cells produce IgE antibodies in the lymph nodes, where helper T cells aid in promoting this reaction. The IgE antibodies

Type I

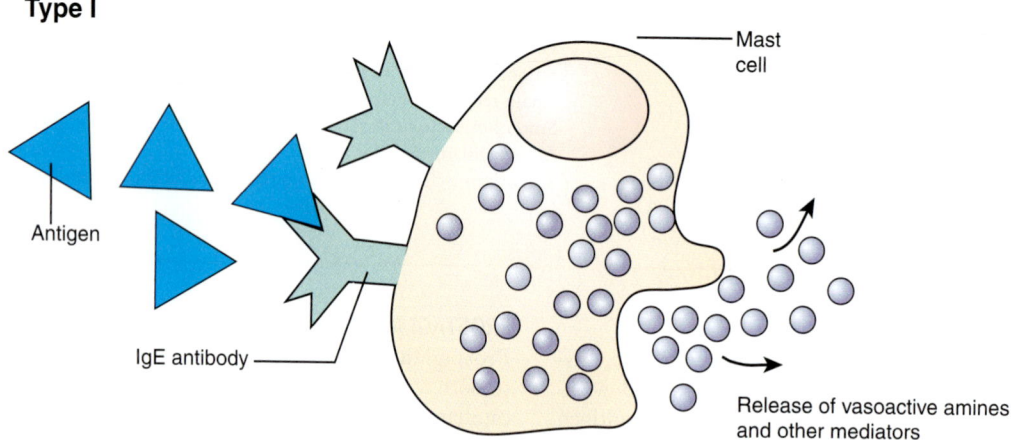

Type I. An anaphylactic reaction is characterized by vasodilation, increased capillary permeability, smooth muscle contraction, and eosinophilia. Systemic reactions may involve laryngeal stridor, angioedema, hypotension, and bronchial, GI, or uterine spasm; local reactions are characterized by hives. Examples of type I reactions include extrinsic asthma, allergic rhinitis, systemic anaphylaxis, and reactions to insect stings.

Type II

Type II. A cytotoxic reaction, which involves the binding of either the IgG or IgM antibody to a cell-bound antigen, may lead to eventual cell and tissue damage. The reaction is the result of mistaken identity when the system identifies a normal constituent of the body as foreign and activates the complement cascade. Examples of type II reactions are myasthenia gravis, Goodpasture's syndrome, pernicious anemia, hemolytic disease of the newborn, transfusion reaction, and thrombocytopenia.

FIGURE 53-2 Four types of hypersensitivity reactions.

bind to membrane receptors on mast cells found in connective tissue and basophils. During re-exposure, the antigen binds to adjacent IgE antibodies, activating a cellular reaction that triggers degranulation and the release of chemical mediators (histamine, leukotrienes, and eosinophil chemotactic factor of anaphylaxis [ECF-A]).

Primary chemical mediators are responsible for the symptoms of type I hypersensitivity because of their effects on the skin, lungs, and gastrointestinal tract. When chemical mediators continue to be released, a delayed reaction may occur lasting for up to 24 hours. Clinical symptoms are determined by the amount of the allergen, the amount of mediator released, the sensitivity of the target organ, and the route of allergen entry. Type I hypersensitivity reactions may include both local and systemic anaphylaxis.

Cytotoxic (Type II) Hypersensitivity

Type II, or cytotoxic, hypersensitivity occurs when the system mistakenly identifies a normal constituent of the body as foreign. This reaction may be a result of a cross-reacting antibody, possibly leading to cell and tissue damage. Type II hypersensitivity involves the binding of either IgG or IgM antibody to the cell-bound antigen. The result of antigen–antibody binding is activation of the complement cascade (see Chap. 50) and destruction of the cell to which the antigen is bound.

A type II hypersensitivity reaction is associated with several disorders. For example, in myasthenia gravis, the body mistakenly generates antibodies against normal nerve ending receptors. In Goodpasture syndrome, antibodies against lung and renal tissue are generated, producing lung damage and renal failure.

Type III. An immune complex reaction is marked by acute inflammation resulting from formation and deposition of immune complexes. The joints and kidneys are particularly susceptible to this kind of reaction, which is associated with systemic lupus erythematosus, serum sickness, nephritis and rheumatoid arthritis. Some signs and symptoms include urticaria, joint pain, fever, rash, and adenopathy (swollen glands).

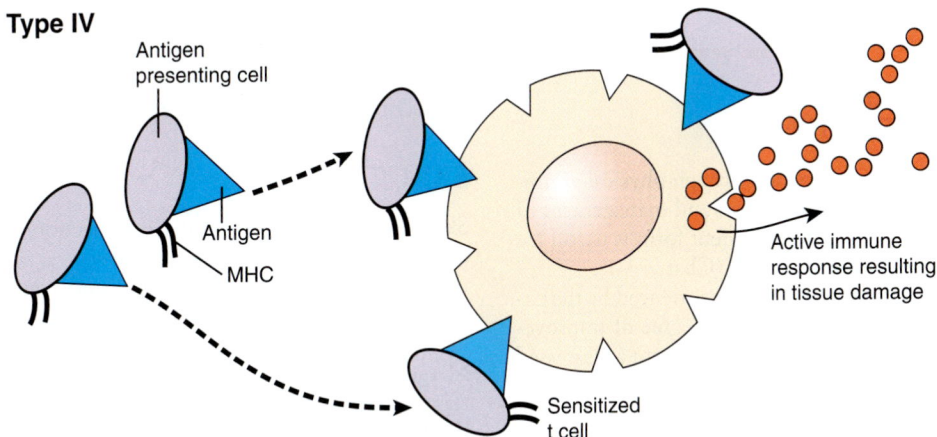

Type IV. A delayed, or cellular, reaction occurs 1 to 3 days after exposure to an antigen. The reaction, which results in tissue damage, involves activity by lymphokines, macrophages, and lysozymes. Erythema and itching are common; a few examples include contact dermatitis, graft-versus-host disease, Hashimoto's thyroiditis, and sarcoidosis.

FIGURE 53-2 (Continued)

A type II hypersensitivity reaction resulting in red blood cell destruction is associated with drug-induced immune hemolytic anemia, Rh-hemolytic disease of the newborn, and incompatibility reactions in blood transfusions (see Chap. 33).

Immune Complex (Type III) Hypersensitivity

Type III, or immune complex, hypersensitivity involves immune complexes formed when antigens bind to antibodies. These complexes are then cleared from the circulation by phagocytic action. When these type III complexes are deposited in tissues or vascular endothelium, two factors contribute to injury: the increased amount of circulating complexes and the presence of vasoactive amines. As a result, there is an increase in vascular permeability and tissue injury. The joints and kidneys are particularly susceptible to this type of injury. Type III hypersensitivity is associated with systemic lupus erythematosus, rheumatoid arthritis, certain types of nephritis, and some types of bacterial endocarditis. These are discussed elsewhere in this text.

Delayed-Type (Type IV) Hypersensitivity

Type IV, or delayed-type hypersensitivity, also known as cellular hypersensitivity, occurs 24 to 72 hours after exposure to an allergen. It is mediated by sensitized T cells and macrophages. An example of this reaction is the effect of an intradermal injection of tuberculin antigen or purified protein derivative (PPD). Sensitized T cells react with the antigen at or near the injection site. Lymphokines are released and attract, activate, and retain macrophages at the site. These macrophages then release lysozymes, causing tissue damage. Edema and fibrin are responsible for the positive tuberculin reaction.

An example of a type IV hypersensitivity reaction is contact dermatitis resulting from exposure to allergens such as cosmetics, adhesive tape, topical medications, medication additives, and plant toxins. The primary exposure results in sensitization. Reexposure causes a hypersensitivity reaction composed of low-molecular-weight molecules (haptens) that bind with proteins or carriers and are then processed by Langerhans cells in the skin. The symptoms that occur include itching, erythema, and raised lesions.

Assessment

HEALTH HISTORY AND CLINICAL MANIFESTATIONS

A comprehensive allergy history and a thorough physical examination provide useful data for the diagnosis and management of patients with allergic disorders. An assessment form is useful for obtaining and organizing this information (Chart 53-1).

The degree of difficulty and discomfort experienced by the patient because of allergic symptoms and the degree of improvement in those symptoms with and without treatment are assessed and documented. The relationship of symptoms to exposure to possible allergens is noted.

Diagnostic Evaluation

Diagnostic evaluation of the patient with allergic disorders commonly includes blood tests, smears of body secretions, skin tests, and the radioallergosorbent test (RAST). Results of laboratory blood studies provide supportive data for various diagnostic possibilities; however, they are not the major criteria for the diagnosis of allergic disease.

COMPLETE BLOOD COUNT WITH DIFFERENTIAL

The white blood cell (WBC) count is usually normal except with infection. Eosinophils, granular leukocytes, normally make up 1% to 3% of the total number of WBCs. A level between 5% and 15% is nonspecific but does suggest allergic reaction. Higher levels are considered moderate and severe. In moderate eosinophilia, 15% to 40% of blood leukocytes as eosinophils are found in patients with allergic disorders as well as in patients with malignancy, immunodeficiencies, parasitic infections, and congenital heart disease, and those receiving peritoneal dialysis. In severe eosinophilia, 50% to 90% of blood leukocytes as eosinophils are found in the idiopathic hypereosinophilic syndrome.

EOSINOPHIL COUNT

An actual count of eosinophils may be obtained from blood samples or smears of secretions. A total eosinophil count can be obtained from a blood sample by using special diluting fluids that hemolyze erythrocytes and stain the eosinophils. During symptomatic episodes, smears obtained from nasal secretions, conjunctival secretions, and sputum of atopic patients usually reveal eosinophils, indicative of an active allergic response.

TOTAL SERUM IMMUNOGLOBULIN E LEVELS

High total serum IgE levels support the diagnosis of atopic disease. A normal IgE level, however, does not exclude the diagnosis of an allergic disorder. IgE levels are not as sensitive as the paper radioimmunosorbent test (PRIST) and the enzyme-linked immunosorbent assay (ELISA). Indications for determining IgE levels include the following:

- Evaluation of immunodeficiency
- Evaluation of drug reactions
- Initial laboratory screening for allergic bronchopulmonary aspergillosis
- Evaluation of allergy among children with bronchiolitis
- Differentiation of atopic and nonatopic eczema
- Differentiation of atopic and nonatopic asthma and rhinitis

SKIN TESTS

Skin testing entails the intradermal injection or superficial application (epicutaneous) of solutions at several sites. Depending on the suspected cause of allergic signs and symptoms, several different solutions may be applied at several separate sites. These solutions contain individual antigens representing an assortment of allergens, including pollen, most likely to be implicated in the patient's disease. Positive reactions (wheal and flare) are clinically significant when correlated with the history, physical findings, and results of other laboratory tests.

The results of skin tests complement the data obtained from the history. They indicate which of several antigens are most likely to provoke symptoms and provide some clue to the intensity of the patient's sensitization. The dosage of the antigen (allergen) injected is also important. Most patients are hypersensitive

Chart 53-1 • ASSESSMENT

Allergy Assessment Form

Name _____ Age _____ Sex _____ Date _____

- I. Chief complaint: _____
- II. Present illness: _____
- III. Collateral allergic symptoms: _____

  Eyes: Pruritus _____ Burning _____ Lacrimation _____
             Swelling _____ Injection _____ Discharge _____

  Ears: Pruritus _____ Fullness _____ Popping _____
             Frequent infections _____

  Nose: Sneezing _____ Rhinorrhea _____ Obstruction _____
             Pruritus _____ Mouth-breathing _____
             Purulent discharge _____

  Throat: Soreness _____ Postnasal discharge _____
             Palatal pruritus _____ Mucus in the morning _____

  Chest: Cough _____ Pain _____ Wheezing _____
             Sputum _____ Dyspnea _____
             Colour _____ Rest _____
             Amount _____ Exertion _____

  Skin: Dermatitis _____ Eczema _____ Urticaria _____

- IV. Family allergies
- V. Previous allergic treatment or testing: _____
  Prior skin testing: _____

  Medications: Antihistamines   Improved _____ Unimproved _____
               Bronchodilators   Improved _____ Unimproved _____
               Nose drops   Improved _____ Unimproved _____
               Hyposensitization Improved _____ Unimproved _____
                  Duration _____
                  Antigens _____
                  Reactions _____
               Antibiotics   Improved _____ Unimproved _____
               Corticosteroids   Improved _____ Unimproved _____

- VI. Physical agents and habits: _____

  Bothered by:

  Tobacco for _____ years   Alcohol _____   Air cond. _____
  Cigarettes _____ packs/day Heat _____   Muggy weather _____
  Cigars _____ per day   Cold _____   Weather changes _____
  Pipes _____ per day   Perfumes _____   Chemicals _____
  Never smoked _____ Paints _____   Hair spray _____
  Bothered by smoke _____ Insecticides _____ Newspapers _____
                           Cosmetics _____   Latex _____

- VII. When symptoms occur: _____
  Time and circumstances of 1st episode: _____
  Prior health: _____
  Course of illness over decades: progressing _____ regressing _____
  Time of year: _____ Exact dates: _____
      Perennial _____
      Seasonal _____
      Seasonally exacerbated _____
  Monthly variations (menses, occupation): _____
  Time of week (weekends vs. weekdays): _____
  Time of day or night: _____
  After insect stings: _____
- VIII. Where symptoms occur: _____
  Living where at onset: _____
  Living where since onset: _____
  Effect of vacation or major geographic change: _____
  Symptoms better indoors or outdoors: _____
  Effect of school or work: _____
  Effect of staying elsewhere nearby: _____
  Effect of hospitalization: _____
  Effect of specific environments: _____
  Do symptoms occur around:
      old leaves _____ hay _____ lakeside _____ barns _____
      summer homes _____ damp basement _____ dry attic _____
      lawnmowing _____ animals _____ other _____

(continued)

Chart 53-1 • ASSESSMENT (Continued)

Allergy Assessment Form

Do symptoms occur after eating:

cheese _____ mushrooms _____ beer _____ melons _____

bananas _____ fish _____ nuts _____ citrus fruits _____

other foods (list) _____

Home: city _____ rural _____

house _____ age _____

apartment _____ basement _____ damp _____ dry _____

heating system _____

pets (how long) _____ dog _____ cat _____ other _____

Bedroom:	Type	Age	*Living room:*	Type	Age
Pillow	____	____	Rug	____	____
Mattress	____	____	Matting	____	____
Blankets	____	____	Furniture	____	____
Quilts	____	____			
Furniture	____	____			

Anywhere in home symptoms are worse: _____

IX. What does patient think makes symptoms worse? _____

X. Under what circumstances is patient free of symptoms? _____

XI. Summary and additional comments: _____

---

to more than one pollen. Under testing conditions, they may not react (although they usually do) to the specific pollens that induce their attacks.

In cases of doubt about the validity of the skin tests, a RAST or a provocative challenge test may be performed. If a skin test is indicated, there is a reasonable suspicion that a specific allergen is producing symptoms in an allergic patient. Several precautionary steps, however, must be observed before skin testing with allergens:

- Testing is not performed during periods of bronchospasm.
- Epicutaneous tests (scratch or prick tests) are performed before other testing methods in an effort to minimize the risk of systemic reaction.
- Emergency equipment must be readily available to treat anaphylaxis.

Types of Skin Tests

The methods of skin testing include prick skin tests, scratch tests, and intradermal skin testing (Fig. 53-3). After prick or scratch tests, intradermal skin testing is performed with allergens that did not elicit positive reactions. Because a larger antigen challenge is being used, local or systemic reactions could occur if the same antigens that produced positive skin or scratch reactions are used. The back is the most suitable area of the body for skin testing because it permits the performance of many tests. The multitest applicator is a commercially available device with multiple test heads that allows simultaneous administration of antigens by multiple punctures at different sites.

Interpretation of Skin Test Results

Familiarity with and consistent use of a grading system are essential. The grading system used should be identified on a skin test sheet for later interpretation. A positive reaction, evidenced by the appearance of an urticarial wheal (round, reddened skin elevation) (Fig. 53-4), localized **erythema** (diffuse redness) in the area of inoculation or contact, or pseudopodia (irregular projec-

tion at the end of a wheal) with associated erythema is considered indicative of sensitivity to the corresponding antigen.

There may be false-negative results due to improper technique, outdated allergen solutions, and prior use of medications that suppress skin reactivity. Corticosteroids and antihistamines, including allergy medications, suppress skin test reactivity and are usually withheld 48 to 96 hours before testing, depending on the duration of their activity. False-positive skin tests may result from improper preparation or administration of allergen solutions.

Interpretation of positive or negative skin tests must be based on the history, physical examination, and other laboratory test

FIGURE 53-3 Intradermal testing. A 0.5-mL or 1-mL sterile syringe with a 26/27 gauge intradermal needle is used to inject 0.02 to 0.03 mL of intradermal allergen. The needle is inserted with the bevel facing upward and the syringe parallel to the skin. The skin is penetrated superficially, and a small amount of the allergen solution is injected to create a bleb (raised area) approximately 5 mm in diameter. A separate sterile syringe and needle are used for each injection. From Taylor, C., Lillis C., & LeMone, P. (2001). *Fundamentals of nursing: The art and science of nursing care* (4th ed.). Philadelphia; Lippincott Williams & Wilkins.

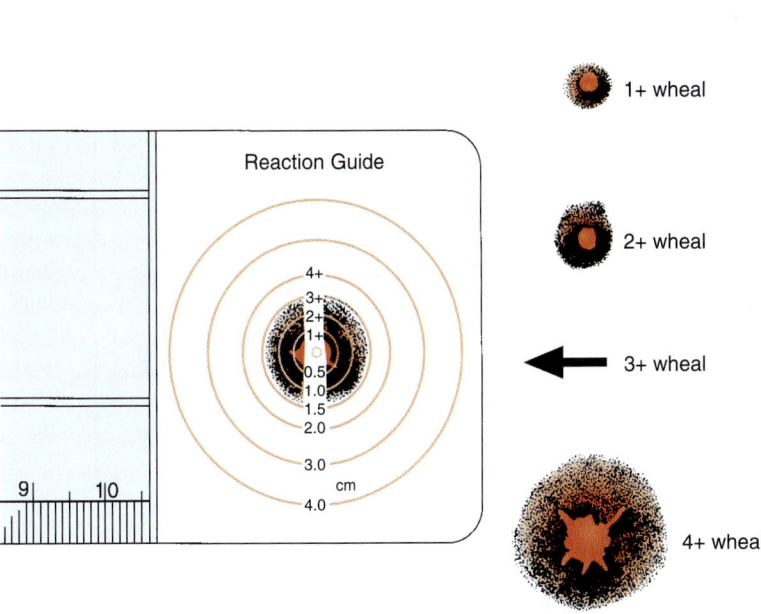

Negative wheal

1+ wheal

2+ wheal

3+ wheal

4+ wheal

Reaction Guide

4+
3+
2+
1+
0.5
1.0
1.5
2.0
3.0   cm
4.0

9   10

FIGURE 53-4 Interpretation of reactions: Negative = wheal soft with minimal erythema. 1+ = wheal present (5–8 mm) with associated erythema. 2+ = wheal (7–10 mm) with associated erythema. 3+ = wheal (9–15 mm), slight pseudopodia possible with associated erythema. 4+ = wheal (12 mm+) with pseudopodia and diffuse erythema.

results. The following guidelines are used for the interpretation of skin test results:

- Skin tests are more reliable for diagnosing atopic sensitivity in patients with allergic rhinoconjunctivitis than in patients with asthma.
- Positive skin tests correlate highly with food allergy.
- The use of skin tests to diagnose immediate hypersensitivity to medications is limited because metabolites of medications, not the medications themselves, are usually responsible for causing hypersensitivity.

PROVOCATIVE TESTING

Provocative testing involves the direct administration of the suspected allergen to the sensitive tissue, such as the conjunctiva, nasal or bronchial mucosa, or gastrointestinal tract (by ingestion of the allergen) with observation of target organ response. This type of testing is helpful in identifying clinically significant allergens in patients with a large number of positive tests. Major disadvantages of this type of testing are the limitation of one antigen per session and the risk of producing severe symptoms, particularly bronchospasm, in patients with asthma.

RADIOALLERGOSORBENT TEST

RAST is a radioimmunoassay that measures allergen-specific IgE. A sample of the patient's serum is exposed to a variety of suspected allergen particle complexes. If antibodies are present, they will combine with radiolabelled allergens. After the serum is centrifuged, radioimmunoassay detects the allergen-specific IgE antibody. Test results are then compared with control values. In addition to detecting an allergen, RAST indicates the quantity of allergen necessary to evoke an allergic reaction. Values are reported on a scale from 0 to 5. Values of 2+ or greater are considered significant. The major advantages of RAST over other tests include decreased risk of systemic reaction, stability of antigens, and lack of dependence on skin reactivity modified by medica-

tions. The major disadvantages include the limited allergen selection, reduced sensitivity compared with intradermal skin tests, lack of immediate results, and cost.

Allergic Disorders

There are two types of IgE-mediated allergic reactions: atopic and nonatopic disorders. While the underlying immunologic reactions of the two types of disorders are the same, predisposing factors and manifestations are different. The atopic disorders are characterized by a hereditary predisposition and production of a local reaction to IgE antibodies produced in response to common environmental allergens (Kay, 2001a). The nonatopic disorders lack the genetic component and organ specificity of the atopic disorders (Porth, 2002). Examples of atopic disorders are allergic rhinitis, allergic asthma, and atopic dermatitis (Kay, 2001a).

A type I hypersensitivity response results in atopic (allergic) diseases, which affect 10% to 20% of the U.S. population. Genetic factors play a role in susceptibility to these diseases. Disorders characterized as atopic include anaphylaxis, allergic rhinoconjunctivitis, atopic dermatitis, urticaria and angioedema, gastrointestinal allergy, and asthma. Latex allergy may be a type I or type IV hypersensitivity reaction, although true latex allergy is considered to be a type I hypersensitivity reaction (Brehler & Kütting, 2001). Latex allergy is discussed later in this chapter. Contact dermatitis is considered a type IV hypersensitivity reaction.

ANAPHYLAXIS

Anaphylaxis is a clinical response to an immediate (type I hypersensitivity) immunologic reaction between a specific antigen and an antibody. The reaction results from IgE antibody. An anaphylactic reaction can be triggered by exposure to an antigen through inhalation, injection, ingestion, or skin contact. It is a severe, life-threatening allergic reaction. It is estimated that 3.3 to 43 million persons in the United States (1.24% to 16.8% of the population) are at risk for anaphylaxis (Neugut, Ghatak & Miller, 2001). In Canada it is estimated that 1% to 2% of Canadians are at risk of an anaphylactic reaction (Anaphylaxis Canada, 2005).

Pathophysiology

Anaphylaxis is caused by the interaction of a foreign antigen with specific IgE antibodies found on the surface membrane of mast cells and peripheral blood basophils. The subsequent release of histamine and other bioactive mediators causes activation of platelets, eosinophils, and neutrophils and the coagulation cascade. Smooth muscle spasm, bronchospasm, mucosal edema and inflammation, and increased capillary permeability result. These systemic changes characteristically produce clinical manifestations within seconds or minutes of antigen exposure (Neugut et al., 2001). Closely related to anaphylaxis is an anaphylactoid (anaphylaxis-like) reaction, which is described in Chart 53-2.

Substances that most commonly cause anaphylaxis include foods, medications, insect stings, and latex (Chart 53-3). Foods that are common causes of anaphylaxis include peanuts, tree nuts, shellfish, fish, milk, eggs, soy, and wheat. Many medications have been implicated in anaphylaxis. Those that are most frequently reported include antibiotics (including penicillin), radiocontrast agents, intravenous anesthetics, aspirin and other nonsteroidal anti-inflammatory drugs (NSAIDs), and opioids. Antibiotics and radiocontrast agents cause the most serious anaphylactic reactions, producing reactions in about 1 of every 5,000 exposures. Penicillin is the most common cause of anaphylaxis and accounts for about 75% of fatal anaphylactic reactions in the U.S. each year (Neugut et al., 2001).

Clinical Manifestations

Anaphylactic reactions may be categorized as mild, moderate, and severe systemic reactions. The time from exposure to the antigen to onset of symptoms is a good indicator of the severity of the reaction: the faster the onset, the more severe the reaction (Neugut et al., 2001).

Mild systemic reactions consist of peripheral tingling and a sensation of warmth, possibly accompanied by fullness in the mouth and throat. Nasal congestion, periorbital swelling, pruritus, sneezing, and tearing of the eyes can also be expected. Onset of symptoms begins within the first 2 hours of exposure.

Moderate systemic reactions may include flushing, warmth, anxiety, and itching in addition to any of the above symptoms.

Chart 53-2 Anaphylactoid (Anaphylaxis-Like) Reaction

Closely related to anaphylaxis is an anaphylactoid (anaphylaxis-like) reaction, caused by the release of mast cell and basophil mediators triggered by non–IgE-mediated events. An anaphylactoid reaction may occur with medications, food, exercise, and cytotoxic antibody transfusions. The reaction may be local or systemic. Local reactions usually involve urticaria and angioedema at the site of the antigen exposure. Although possibly severe, anaphylactoid reactions are rarely fatal. Systemic reactions occur within about 30 minutes of exposure involving cardiovascular, respiratory, gastrointestinal, and integumentary organ systems. For the most part, an anaphylactoid reaction and its treatment are identical to that of anaphylaxis (Neugut et al., 2001).

Chart 53-3 Common Causes of Anaphylaxis

Foods
Peanuts, tree nuts (walnuts, pecans, cashews, almonds, etc.), shellfish (shrimp, lobster, crab, etc.), fish, milk, eggs, soy, wheat

Medications
Antibiotics, especially penicillin and sulfa antibiotics, allopurinol, radiocontrast agents, anesthetic agents (lidocaine, procaine), vaccines, hormones (insulin, vasopressin, ACTH), aspirin, nonsteroidal anti-inflammatory drugs (NSAIDs)

Other Pharmaceutical/Biologic Agents
Animal serums (tetanus antitoxin, snake venom antitoxin, rabies antitoxin), antigens used in skin testing

Insect Stings
Bees, wasps, hornets, yellow jackets, ants, including fire ants

Latex
Medical and nonmedical products containing latex

More serious reactions include bronchospasm and edema of the airways or larynx with dyspnea, cough, and wheezing. The onset of symptoms is the same as for a mild reaction.

Severe systemic reactions have an abrupt onset with the same signs and symptoms described above. These progress rapidly to bronchospasm, laryngeal edema, severe dyspnea, cyanosis, and hypotension. Dysphagia (difficulty swallowing), abdominal cramping, vomiting, diarrhea, and seizures can also occur. Cardiac arrest and coma may follow.

Prevention

Strict avoidance of potential allergens is an important preventive measure for the patient at risk for anaphylaxis (Neugut et al., 2001). Patients at risk for anaphylaxis from insect stings should avoid areas populated by insects and should use appropriate clothing, insect repellent, and caution to avoid further stings.

If avoidance of exposure to allergens is impossible, administration of epinephrine is a critical measure to prevent an anaphylactic reaction. People sensitive to insect bites and stings, those who have experienced food or medication reactions, and those who have experienced idiopathic or exercise-induced anaphylactic reactions should always carry an emergency kit that contains epinephrine. The EpiPen from Dey Pharmaceuticals is a commercially available first-aid device that delivers premeasured doses of 0.3 mg (Epipen) and 0.15 mg (Epipen Jr.) of epinephrine (Fig. 53-5). The autoinjection system requires no preparation, and the self-administration technique is uncomplicated. The patient must be given an opportunity to demonstrate the correct technique for use; an Epipen training device is available. Verbal and written information about the emergency kit, as well as strategies to avoid exposure to threatening allergens, must also be provided.

Screening for allergies before a medication is prescribed or first administered is an important preventive measure. A careful history of any sensitivity to suspected antigens must be obtained before administering any medication, particularly in parenteral form, because this route is associated with the most severe anaphylaxis. Nurses caring for patients in any setting (hospital, home, outpatient diagnostic testing sites, long-term care facilities) must assess patients' risk for anaphylactic reactions. The patient is asked about previous exposure to contrast agents used for diag-

FIGURE 53-5 The EpiPen and EpiPen Jr. (for children up to 15 kg). Autoinjectors are commercially available first-aid devices that administer premeasured doses of epinephrine. An EpiPen training device is available for patients to practice correct self-injection technique. Courtesy of Dey Pharmaceuticals, Napa, CA.

nostic tests and any allergic reactions, as well as reactions to any medications, foods, insect stings, and latex. Persons predisposed to anaphylaxis should wear some form of identification, such as a medical alert bracelet, naming allergies to medications, food, and other substances.

People who are allergic to insect venom may require venom immunotherapy, which is used as a control measure and not a cure. Immunotherapy following an insect sting is very effective in reducing the risk of anaphylaxis from future stings (Neugut et al., 2001). Insulin-allergic diabetic patients and penicillin-sensitive patients may require desensitization. Desensitization is based on controlled anaphylaxis, with a gradual release of mediators. Patients who undergo desensitization are cautioned that there should be no lapses in therapy, because this may lead to the reappearance of an allergic reaction when the medication is reinstituted.

Medical Management

Management depends on the severity of the reaction. Initially, respiratory and cardiovascular functions are evaluated. If the patient is in cardiac arrest, cardiopulmonary resuscitation is instituted. Oxygen is provided in high concentrations during cardiopulmonary resuscitation or when the patient is cyanotic, dyspneic, or wheezing. Epinephrine, in a 1:1,000 dilution, is administered subcutaneously in the upper extremity or thigh and may be followed by a continuous intravenous infusion. Antihistamines and corticosteroids may also be given to prevent recurrences of the reaction and to treat urticaria and angioedema. To maintain blood pressure and normal hemodynamic status, IV fluids (ie, normal saline solution), volume expanders, and vasopressor agents are given. In patients with episodes of bronchospasm or a history of bronchial asthma or chronic obstructive pulmonary disease, aminophylline and corticosteroids may also be administered to improve airway patency and function. If hypotension is unresponsive to vasopressors, intravenous glucagon may be given for its acute inotropic and chronotropic effects. Patients with severe reactions are observed closely for 12 to 14 hours. Because of the potential for recurrence, patients with even mild reactions must be educated concerning this risk.

Nursing Management

If a patient is experiencing an allergic response, the nurse's initial action is to assess the patient for signs and symptoms of anaphylaxis. The nurse assesses the airway, breathing pattern, and other vital signs. The patient is observed for signs of increasing edema and respiratory distress. Prompt notification of the physician and preparation for initiation of emergency measures (intubation, administration of emergency medications, insertion of intravenous lines, fluid administration, oxygen administration) are important to reduce the severity of the reaction and to restore cardiovascular function. The nurse documents the interventions used and the patient's response to treatment, vital signs, and laboratory values.

The patient who has recovered from anaphylaxis needs an explanation of what occurred and instruction about avoiding future exposure to antigens and administering emergency medications to treat anaphylaxis. The patient must be instructed about antigens that should be avoided and about other strategies to prevent recurrence of anaphylaxis. All patients who have experienced an anaphylactic reaction should receive a prescription for preloaded syringes of epinephrine. The nurse instructs the patient and family in their use and has the patient and family demonstrate correct administration (Chart 53-4).

ALLERGIC RHINITIS

Allergic **rhinitis** (inflammation of nasal mucosa; hay fever, chronic allergic rhinitis, pollinosis) is the most common form of respiratory allergy presumed to be mediated by an immediate (type I hypersensitivity) immunologic reaction. It affects about 8% to 10% of the U.S. population (20% to 30% of adolescents). The symptoms are similar to viral rhinitis but are usually more persistent and demonstrate seasonal variation (Tierney, McPhee & Papadakis, 2001). It often occurs with other conditions, such as allergic conjunctivitis, sinusitis, and asthma. Allergic rhinitis is associated with impaired work and school performance and decreased quality of life (Ratner, Ehrlich, Fineman et al., 2002). When untreated, many complications may result, such as allergic asthma, chronic nasal obstruction, chronic otitis media with hearing loss, anosmia (absence of the sense of smell), and, in children, orofacial dental deformities. Early diagnosis and adequate treatment are essential to reduce complications and relieve symptoms.

Because allergic rhinitis is induced by airborne pollens or molds, it is characterized by the following seasonal occurrences:

- Early spring—tree pollen (oak, elm, poplar)
- Early summer—rose pollen (rose fever), grass pollen (Timothy, red-top)
- Early fall—weed pollen (ragweed)

Each year, attacks begin and end at about the same time. Airborne mold spores require warm, damp weather. Although there is no rigid seasonal pattern, these spores appear in early spring, are rampant during the summer, and taper off and disappear by the first frost.

Pathophysiology

Sensitization begins by ingestion or inhalation of an antigen. On re-exposure, the nasal mucosa reacts by the slowing of ciliary action, edema formation, and leukocyte (primarily eosinophil) infiltration. Histamine is the major mediator of allergic reactions in the nasal mucosa. Tissue edema results from vasodilation and increased capillary permeability.

Chart 53-4 • PATIENT EDUCATION
Self-Administration of Epinephrine

The patient is taught how to inject epinephrine in the event of an anaphylactic reaction. The patient should be encouraged to practice this technique using a training device.

1. Carefully uncap the Epipen device, holding it so that the injecting end is upright.

2. Position the device at the middle portion of the thigh.

3. Push the device into the thigh as far as possible. The Epipen device will autoinject a premeasured dose of epinephrine into the subcutaneous tissue.

Clinical Manifestations

Typical signs and symptoms of allergic rhinitis include nasal congestion; clear, watery nasal discharge; intermittent sneezing; and nasal itching. Itching of the throat and soft palate is common. Drainage of nasal mucus into the pharynx initiates multiple attempts to clear the throat and results in a dry cough or hoarseness. Headache, pain over the paranasal sinuses, and epistaxis can accompany allergic rhinitis. The symptoms of this chronic condition depend on environmental exposure and intrinsic host responsiveness. Allergic rhinitis may affect quality of life by also producing fatigue, loss of sleep, and poor concentration (Ratner et al., 2002).

Assessment and Diagnostic Findings

Diagnosis of seasonal allergic rhinitis is based on history, physical examination, and diagnostic test results. Diagnostic tests include nasal smears, peripheral blood counts, total serum IgE, epicutaneous and intradermal testing, RAST, food elimination and challenge, and nasal provocation tests. Results indicative of allergy as the cause of rhinitis include increased IgE and eosinophil levels and positive reactions on allergen testing. False-positive and false-negative responses to these tests, particularly skin testing and provocation tests, may occur.

Medical Management

The goal of therapy is to provide relief from symptoms. Therapy may include one or all of the following interventions: avoidance therapy, pharmacotherapy, and immunotherapy (Kay, 2001b). Verbal instructions must be reinforced by written information. Knowledge of general concepts regarding assessment and therapy in allergic diseases is important so that patients can learn to manage certain conditions as well as prevent severe reactions and illnesses.

AVOIDANCE THERAPY

In avoidance therapy, every attempt is made to remove the allergens that act as precipitating factors. Simple measures and environmental controls are often effective in decreasing symptoms. Examples include use of air conditioners, air cleaners, humidifiers and dehumidifiers, and smoke-free environments. In many cases, it is impossible to avoid exposure to all environmental allergens, so pharmacologic therapy or immunotherapy is needed.

PHARMACOLOGIC THERAPY

Antihistamines. Antihistamines, now classified as H_1-receptor antagonists (or H_1-blockers), are used in managing mild allergic disorders. (H_2-receptor antagonists are used to treat gastric and duodenal ulcers.) H_1-blockers bind selectively to H_1 receptors, preventing the actions of histamines at these sites. They do not prevent the release of histamine from mast cells or basophils. The H_1-antagonists have no effect on H_2-receptors, but they do have the ability to bind to nonhistaminic receptors. The ability of certain antihistamines to bind to and block muscarinic receptors underlies several of the prominent anticholinergic side effects of these medications.

Oral antihistamines, which are readily absorbed, are most effective when given at the first occurrence of symptoms because they prevent the development of new symptoms by blocking the actions of histamine at the H_1-receptors. The effectiveness of these medications is limited to certain patients with hay fever, vasomotor rhinitis, **urticaria** (hives), and mild asthma. They are rarely effective in other conditions or in any severe conditions.

Antihistamines are the major class of medications prescribed for the symptomatic relief of allergic rhinitis. The major side effect is sedation, although histamine H_1 antagonists are less sedating than earlier antihistamines (Kay, 2001b). Additional side effects include nervousness, tremors, dizziness, dry mouth, palpitations, anorexia, nausea, and vomiting. Antihistamines are contraindicated during the third trimester of pregnancy; for nursing mothers and newborns; in children and elderly people; and in patients whose conditions can be aggravated by muscarinic blockade (ie, asthma, urinary retention, open-angle glaucoma, hypertension, and prostatic hyperplasia).

Newer antihistamines are called second-generation or nonsedating H_1-receptor antagonists. Unlike first-generation H_1-receptor antagonists, they do not cross the blood–brain barrier and do not bind to cholinergic, serotonin, or alpha-adrenergic receptors. They bind to peripheral rather than central nervous system H_1-receptors, causing less sedation. Examples of these medications are loratadine (Claritin), cetirizine (Zyrtec), and fexofenadine (Allegra). These are summarized in Table 53-2.

Adrenergic Agents. Adrenergic agents, vasoconstrictors of mucosal vessels, are used topically (nasal and ophthalmic) in addition to the oral route. The topical route (drops and sprays) causes fewer side effects than oral administration; however, the use of drops and sprays should be limited to a few days to avoid rebound congestion. Adrenergic nasal decongestants are used for the relief of nasal congestion when applied topically to the nasal mucosa. They activate the alpha-adrenergic receptor sites on the smooth muscle of the nasal mucosal blood vessels, reducing local blood flow, fluid exudation, and mucosal edema. Topical ophthalmic drops are used for symptomatic relief of eye irritations due to allergies. Potential side effects include hypertension, dysrhythmias, palpitations, central nervous system stimulation, irritability, tremor, and tachyphylaxis (acceleration of hemodynamic status). Examples of adrenergic decongestants and their routes of administration are found in Table 53-3.

Mast Cell Stabilizers. Intranasal cromolyn sodium (Nasalcrom) is a spray that acts by stabilizing the mast cell membrane, thus reducing the release of histamine and other mediators of the allergic response. In addition, it inhibits macrophages, eosinophils, monocytes, and platelets involved in the immune response (Ratner et al., 2002). Cromolyn interrupts the physiologic response to nasal antigens and is used prophylactically before exposure to

---

Table 53-2 • **Chemical Classes of H_1 Antihistamines**

CLASSIFICATION AND EXAMPLE	MAJOR SIDE EFFECTS	NURSING IMPLICATIONS
Sedating		
Ethanolamines Ex: diphenhydramine (Benadryl)	Drowsiness, confusion	Teach patient to avoid alcohol, driving, or engaging in any hazardous activities until CNS response to drug treatment is stabilized.
	Dry mouth, nausea, vomiting	Suggest sucking on hard candy or ice chips for relief of dry mouth.
	Photosensitivity	Encourage use of sunscreen and hat while outdoors.
	Urinary retention	Assess for urinary retention; monitor urinary output.
Piperazines Ex: hydroxyzine (Atarax)	Dulls mental alertness; drowsiness	Teach patient to avoid alcohol, driving, or engaging in any hazardous activities until CNS response to drug treatment is stabilized.
	Dry mouth	Suggest sucking on hard candy or ice chips for relief of dry mouth.
Alkylamines Ex: chlorpheniramine (Chlor-Trimeton)	Less CNS depression than other groups; best class for daytime use	Teach patient to avoid alcohol, driving, or engaging in any hazardous activities until CNS response to drug treatment is stabilized.
Ethylenediamines Ex: tripelennamine (PBZ)	Gastrointestinal upset	Administer medication with food or milk to decrease GI distress. Increase fluid intake.
	Drowsiness	Teach patient to avoid alcohol, driving, or engaging in any hazardous activities until CNS response to drug treatment is stabilized.
	Palpitations	Instruct patient to sit and relax a few minutes before activity.
Phenothiazines Ex: promethazine (Phenergan)	Heavy sedation and drowsiness	Teach patient to avoid alcohol, driving, or engaging in any hazardous activities until CNS response to drug treatment is stabilized.
	Nasal congestion	Encourage use of humidification at home.
	Hypotension	Instruct patient to rise from a sitting position slowly.
Nonsedating		
loratadine (Claritin)	Gastrointestinal upset	Counsel patient to take the medication on an empty stomach.
fexofenadine (Allegra)	Occasional drowsiness and fatigue	Teach patient to avoid alcohol, driving, or engaging in any hazardous activities until CNS response to drug treatment is stabilized.
cetirizine (Zyrtec)	Drowsiness, dry mouth	Teach patient to avoid alcohol, driving, or engaging in any hazardous activities until CNS response to drug treatment is stabilized.

Table 53-3 • Adrenergic Decongestants and Their Routes of Administration

ADRENERGIC DECONGESTANT	TRADE NAME	ROUTE OF ADMINISTRATION
naphazoline hydrochloride	Privine	Topical
oxymetazoline hydrochloride	Afrin, Dristan long-lasting, Neo-Synephrine 12 hour, Sinex long-lasting	Topical
phenylephrine hydrochloride	Neo-Synephrine	Topical
pseudoephedrine hydrochloride	Sudafed	Oral
tetrahydrozoline hydrochloride	Collyrium, Murine Plus, Visine	Topical ophthalmic and nasal preparations
xylometazoline hydrochloride	Neo-Synephrine II, Otrivin	Topical

allergens to prevent the onset of symptoms and to treat symptoms once they occur. It is also used therapeutically in chronic allergic rhinitis. This spray is as effective as antihistamines but less effective than intranasal corticosteroids in the treatment of seasonal allergic rhinitis. Patients must be informed that the beneficial effects of the medication may take a week or so to occur. The medication is of no benefit in the treatment of nonallergic rhinitis. Adverse effects (ie, sneezing, local stinging, and burning sensations) are usually mild.

Corticosteroids. Intranasal corticosteroids are indicated in more severe cases of allergic and perennial rhinitis that cannot be controlled by more conventional medications such as decongestants, antihistamines, and intranasal cromolyn. These medications include beclomethasone (Beconase, Vancenase), budesonide (Rhinocort), dexamethasone (Decadron Phosphate Turbinaire), flunisolide (Nasalide), fluticasone (Cutivate, Flonase), and triamcinolone (Nasacort).

Because of their anti-inflammatory actions, these medications are equally effective in preventing or suppressing the major symptoms of allergic rhinitis. Corticosteroids are administered by metered-spray devices. If the nasal passages are blocked, a topical decongestant can be used to clear the passages before the administration of the intranasal corticosteroid. Patients must be aware that full benefit may not be achieved for several days to 2 weeks. Adverse effects of intranasal corticosteroids are mild and include drying of the nasal mucosa and burning and itching sensations caused by the vehicle used to administer the medication. Systemic effects are more likely with dexamethasone. Recommended use of this medication is limited to 30 days. Beclomethasone, budesonide, flunisolide, fluticasone, and triamcinolone are deactivated rapidly after absorption, so they do not achieve significant blood levels. Corticosteroids suppress host defenses, so they must be used with caution in patients with tuberculosis or untreated bacterial infections of the lungs. Patients on corticosteroids are at risk for infection and for suppression of typical manifestations of inflammation because host defenses are compromised. Inhaled corticosteroids do not affect the immune system to the same degree as systemic corticosteroids (ie, oral corticosteroids). As corticosteroids are inhaled into the upper respiratory tract, tuberculosis or untreated bacterial infections of the lungs may become apparent and progress. Whenever possible, patients with tuberculosis and other bacterial infections of the lungs should avoid inhaled corticosteroids.

Oral and parenteral corticosteroids are used when conventional therapy has failed and symptoms are severe and of short duration. They can control symptoms of allergic reactions such as hay fever, medication-induced allergies, and allergic reactions to insect stings. Because the response to corticosteroids is delayed, they have little or no value in acute therapy for severe reactions such as anaphylaxis. Patients who receive corticosteroids must be cautioned not to stop taking the medication suddenly or without specific instructions from the physician. The patient is also instructed about side effects, which include fluid retention, weight gain, hypertension, gastric irritation, glucose intolerance, and adrenal suppression. Further discussion of corticosteroids is provided in Chapter 42.

IMMUNOTHERAPY

Allergen desensitization (allergen immunotherapy, hyposensitization) is primarily used to treat IgE-mediated diseases by injections of allergen extracts. This type of therapy provides an adjunct to symptomatic pharmacologic therapy and can be used when allergen avoidance is not possible (Parslow et al., 2001). Specific immunotherapy has been used in the treatment of allergic disorders for about 100 years. It consists of administering increasing concentrations of extracts of specific allergens over a long period (Kay, 2001b). Goals of immunotherapy include reducing the level of circulating IgE, increasing the level of blocking antibody IgG, and reducing mediator cell sensitivity. Immunotherapy has been most effective for ragweed pollen; however, treatment for grass, tree pollen, cat, and house dust mite allergens has also been effective.

Correlation of a positive skin test with a positive allergy history is an indication for immunotherapy if the allergen cannot be avoided. The value has been fairly well established in instances of allergic rhinitis and bronchial asthma that are clearly due to sensitivity to one of the common pollens, molds, and household dust. Although helpful in most patients, immunotherapy does not cure the condition. Before immunotherapy is initiated, the patient must understand what to expect and the importance of continuing therapy for several years. When skin tests are performed, the results are correlated with clinical manifestations; treatment is based on the patient's needs rather than on skin tests.

The most common method of treatment is the serial injection of one or more antigens that are selected in each particular case on the basis of skin tests. This method provides a simple and efficient technique for identifying IgE antibodies to specific antigens. Specific treatment consists of injecting extracts of the pollens or mold spores that cause symptoms in a particular patient. Injections begin with very small amounts and are gradually increased, usually at weekly intervals, until a maximum tolerated dose is attained. Maintenance booster injections are given at 2- to 4-week intervals, frequently for a period of several years, before maximum benefit is achieved.

There are three methods of injection therapy: coseasonal, preseasonal, and perennial. When treatment is given on a coseasonal basis, therapy is initiated during the season in which the patient experiences symptoms. This method has been proved ineffective and is used infrequently. Also, there is an increased risk of systemic reactions. Preseasonal therapy injections are given 2 to 3 months before symptoms are expected, allowing time for hyposensitization to occur. This treatment is discontinued after the season begins. Perennial therapy is administered all year round, usually on a monthly basis, and is the preferred method because it has more effective, longer-lasting results.

Any patient who receives specific immunotherapy is at risk for general, and potentially fatal, anaphylaxis. This occurs most frequently at the induction or "up-dosing" phase. Attempts have been made to minimize the risk of systemic reactions by pretreating allergen extracts with agents such as formaldehyde. This approach decreases the binding of the allergen by IgE, but it also results in decreased immunogenicity (Kay, 2001b).

> **! NURSING ALERT** Because the injection of an allergen may induce systemic reactions, such injections are given only in a setting (ie, physician's office, clinic) where epinephrine is immediately available.

Because of the risk for anaphylaxis, injections should not be given by a lay person or by the patient. The patient remains in the office or clinic for at least 30 minutes after the injection and is observed for possible systemic symptoms. If a large, local swelling develops at the injection site, the next dose should not be increased, because this may be a warning sign of a possible systemic reaction.

Therapeutic failure is evident when a patient does not experience a decrease of symptoms within 12 to 24 months, fails to develop increased tolerance to known allergens, and cannot decrease the use of medications to reduce symptoms. Potential causes of treatment failure include misdiagnosis of allergies, inadequate doses of allergen, newly developed allergies, and inadequate environmental controls.

NURSING PROCESS:
THE PATIENT WITH ALLERGIC RHINITIS

Assessment

The examination and history of the patient reveal sneezing, often in paroxysms, thin and watery nasal discharge, itching eyes and nose, lacrimation, and occasionally headache. The health history includes a personal or family history of allergy. The allergy assessment identifies the nature of antigens, seasonal changes in symptoms, and medication history. The nurse also obtains subjective data about how the patient feels just before symptoms become obvious, such as the occurrence of pruritus, breathing problems, and tingling sensations. In addition to these symptoms, hoarseness, wheezing, hives, rash, erythema, and edema are noted. Any relationship between emotional problems or stress and the triggering of allergy symptoms is assessed.

Diagnosis

NURSING DIAGNOSES

Based on the assessment data, the patient's major nursing diagnoses may include the following:

- Ineffective breathing pattern related to allergic reaction

- Deficient knowledge about allergy and the recommended modifications in lifestyle and self-care practices
- Ineffective individual coping with chronicity of condition and need for environmental modifications

COLLABORATIVE PROBLEMS/ POTENTIAL COMPLICATIONS

Based on assessment data, potential complications may include the following:

- Anaphylaxis
- Impaired breathing
- Nonadherence to the therapeutic regimen

Planning and Goals

The goals for the patient may include restoration of normal breathing pattern, increased knowledge about the causes and control of allergic symptoms, improved coping with alterations and modifications, and absence of complications.

Nursing Interventions

IMPROVING BREATHING PATTERN

The patient is instructed and assisted to modify the environment to reduce the severity of allergic symptoms or to prevent their occurrence. The patient is instructed to reduce exposure to people with upper respiratory infections (URIs). If a URI occurs, the patient is encouraged to take deep breaths and cough frequently to ensure adequate gas exchange and prevent atelectasis. The patient is instructed to seek medical attention because allergy symptoms along with a URI may compromise adequate lung function. Compliance with medications and other treatment regimens is encouraged and reinforced.

PROMOTING UNDERSTANDING OF ALLERGY AND ALLERGY CONTROL

Instruction includes strategies to minimize exposure to allergens, desensitization procedures, and correct use of medications. The nurse informs and reminds the patient of the importance of keeping appointments for desensitization procedures because usually dosages are adjusted on a weekly basis, and missed appointments may interfere with the dosage adjustment.

Patients also need to understand that medications for allergy control should be used only when the allergy is apparent. This is usually on a seasonal basis. Continued use of medications when not required may cause an increased tolerance to the medication, with the result that the medication is not effective when needed.

COPING WITH A CHRONIC DISORDER

Although allergic reactions are infrequently life-threatening, they require constant vigilance to avoid allergens and modification of the lifestyle or environment to prevent recurrence of symptoms. Allergic symptoms are often present year-round and create discomfort and inconvenience for the patient. Although patients may not feel ill during allergy seasons, they often do not feel well either. The need to be alert for possible allergens in the environment may be tiresome, placing a burden on the patient's ability to lead a normal life. Stress related to these difficulties may in turn increase the frequency or severity of symptoms.

To assist the patient in adjusting to these modifications, the nurse must have an appreciation of the difficulties encountered by the patient. The patient is encouraged to verbalize feelings and concerns in a supportive environment and to identify strategies to deal with them effectively.

MONITORING AND MANAGING POTENTIAL COMPLICATIONS

Anaphylaxis and Impaired Breathing

Respiratory and cardiovascular functioning can be significantly altered during allergic reactions by the reaction itself or by the medications used to treat reactions. The respiratory status is evaluated by monitoring the respiratory rate and pattern and by assessing for breathing difficulties or abnormal lung sounds. The pulse rate and rhythm and blood pressure are monitored to assess cardiovascular status regularly or any time the patient reports symptoms such as itching or difficulty breathing. In the event of signs and symptoms suggestive of anaphylaxis, emergency medications and equipment must be available for immediate use.

Nonadherence to Therapeutic Regimen

Knowing about the treatment regimen does not ensure adherence. Having the patient identify potential barriers and explore acceptable solutions for effective management of the condition (eg, installing tile floors rather than carpet, not gardening in the spring) can increase adherence to the treatment regimen.

PROMOTING HOME AND COMMUNITY-BASED CARE

Teaching Patients Self-Care

The patient is instructed about strategies to minimize exposure to allergens, the actions and adverse effects of medications, and the correct use of medications. The patient should know the names, dose, frequency, actions, and side effects of all medications taken.

Instruction about strategies to control allergic symptoms is based on the needs of the patient as determined by the results of tests, the severity of symptoms, and the motivation of the patient and family to deal with the condition. Suggestions for patients sensitive to dust and mold in the home are given in Chart 53-5.

If the patient is to undergo immunotherapy, the nurse reinforces the physician's explanation regarding the purpose and procedure. Instructions are given regarding the series of injections, usually given initially every week and then at 2- to 4-week intervals. These instructions include remaining in the physician's office or the clinic at least 30 minutes after the injection so that emergency treatment may be given if the patient has a reaction; avoiding rubbing or scratching the injection site; and continuing with the series for the period of time required. In addition, the patient and family are instructed about emergency treatment of severe allergic symptoms.

Because antihistamines often produce drowsiness, the patient is cautioned about this and other side effects of the particular medication. Operating machinery, driving a car, and performing activities requiring intense concentration should be postponed. The patient is also informed about the dangers of drinking alcohol when taking these medications because they tend to exaggerate the effects of alcohol.

The patient must be aware of the effects caused by overuse of the sympathomimetic agents in nose drops or sprays. A condition referred to as rhinitis medicamentosa may result (Fig. 53-6). After topical application of the medication, a rebound period may occur in which the nasal mucous membranes become more edematous and congested than they were before the medication was used. Such a reaction encourages the use of more medication, and a cyclical pattern results. The topical agent must be discontinued immediately and completely to correct this problem.

Chart 53-5
Home Care Checklist • Allergy Management

At the completion of the home care instruction, the patient or caregiver will be able to:	Patient	Caregiver
• Verbalize how to maintain a dust-free environment by removing drapes, curtains, and venetian blinds and replacing them with pull shades; covering the mattress with a hypoallergenic cover that can be zipped; and removing rugs and replacing them with wood flooring or linoleum.	✓	✓
• Identify rationale for washing the floor and dusting and vacuuming daily.	✓	✓
• Identify rationale for replacing stuffed furniture with wood pieces that can easily be dusted.	✓	✓
• State rationale for wearing a mask whenever cleaning is being done.	✓	✓
• Identify rationale for avoiding use of tufted bedspreads, stuffed toys, and feather pillows and replacing them with washable cotton material.	✓	✓
• State rationale for avoiding the use of any clothing that causes itching.	✓	✓
• Verbalize ways to reduce dust in the house as a whole by using steam or hot water for heating rather than air and using air filters or air conditioning.	✓	✓
• Verbalize ways to reduce exposure to pollens or molds by identifying seasons of the year when pollen counts are high; wearing a mask at times of increased exposure (windy days and when grass is being cut); and avoiding contact with weeds, dry leaves, and freshly cut grass.	✓	✓
• State rationale for seeking air-conditioned areas at the height of the allergy season.	✓	✓
• State rationale for avoiding sprays and perfumes.	✓	✓
• State rationale for use of hypoallergenic cosmetics.	✓	✓
• State rationale for taking prescribed medications as ordered.	✓	✓
• Identify specific foods that may cause allergic symptoms. (Examples of foods that can cause allergic reactions are fish, nuts, eggs, and chocolate.)	✓	✓
• Develop a list of foods to avoid.	✓	✓

FIGURE 53-6 Rhinitis medicamentosa. This cyclic pattern results from overuse of sympathomimetic nose drops or sprays.

Continuing Care

Follow-up telephone calls to the patient are often reassuring to the patient and family and provide an opportunity for the nurse to answer any questions. The patient is reminded to keep follow-up appointments and is informed about the importance of continuing with treatment. The importance of participating in health promotion activities and health screening is emphasized to the patient.

Evaluation

EXPECTED PATIENT OUTCOMES

Expected patient outcomes may include:

1. Exhibits normal breathing patterns
   a. Demonstrates lungs clear on auscultation
   b. Exhibits absence of adventitious breath sounds (crackles, rhonchi, wheezing)
   c. Has a normal respiratory rate and pattern
   d. Reports no complaints of respiratory distress (shortness of breath, difficulty on inspiration or expiration)
2. Demonstrates knowledge about allergy and strategies to control symptoms
   a. Identifies causative allergens, if known
   b. States methods of avoiding allergens and controlling indoor and outdoor precipitating factors
   c. Removes from the environment items that retain dust
   d. Wears a dampened mask if dust or mold may be a problem
   e. Avoids smoke-filled rooms and dust-filled or freshly sprayed areas
   f. Uses air conditioning for a major part of the day
   g. Takes antihistamines as prescribed; participates in hyposensitization program, if applicable
   h. Describes name, purpose, side effects, and method of administration of prescribed medications
   i. Identifies when to seek immediate medical attention for severe allergic responses
   j. Describes activities that are possible, including ways to participate in activities without activating the allergies
3. Experiences relief of discomfort while adapting to the inconveniences of an allergy
   a. Relates the emotional aspects of the allergic response
   b. Demonstrates use of measures to cope positively with allergy
4. Absence of complications
   a. Exhibits vital signs within normal limits

b. Reports no symptoms or episodes of anaphylaxis (urticaria, itching, peripheral tingling, fullness in the mouth and throat, flushing, or difficulty swallowing) or coughing, wheezing, or difficulty breathing
   c. Demonstrates correct procedure to self-administer emergency medications to treat severe allergic reaction
   d. Correctly states medication names, dose and frequency of administration, and medication actions
   e. Correctly identifies side effects and untoward signs and symptoms to report to physician
   f. Discusses acceptable lifestyle changes and solutions for identified potential barriers for compliance with treatment and medication regimen

CONTACT DERMATITIS

Contact dermatitis (dermatitis venenata), a type IV delayed hypersensitivity reaction, is an acute or chronic skin inflammation that results from direct skin contact with chemicals or allergens. There are four basic types: allergic, irritant, phototoxic, and photoallergic (Table 53-4). Eighty percent of cases are due to excessive exposure to or additive effects of irritants (eg, soaps, detergents, organic solvents) (Tierney et al., 2001). Skin sensitivity may develop after brief or prolonged periods of exposure, and the clinical picture may appear hours or weeks after the sensitized skin has been exposed.

Clinical Manifestations

Symptoms include itching, burning, erythema, skin lesions (vesicles), and edema, followed by weeping, crusting, and finally drying and peeling of the skin. In severe responses, hemorrhagic bullae may develop. Repeated reactions may be accompanied by thickening of the skin and pigmentary changes. Secondary invasion by bacteria may develop in skin abraded by rubbing or scratching. Usually, there are no systemic symptoms unless the eruption is widespread.

Assessment and Diagnostic Findings

The location of the skin eruption and the history of exposure aid in determining the condition. In cases of obscure irritants or an unobservant patient, however, diagnosis may be extremely difficult, often involving many trial-and-error procedures before the cause is determined. Patch tests on the skin with suspected offending agents may clarify the diagnosis.

ATOPIC DERMATITIS

Atopic dermatitis is a type I immediate hypersensitivity disorder. A family history is common. The incidence of atopic dermatitis is highest in infants and children. Atopic dermatitis (eczema) affects 10% to 20% of children in Western populations (Kay, 2001b). Most patients have significant elevations of serum IgE and peripheral eosinophilia. Pruritus and hyperirritability of the skin are the most consistent features of atopic dermatitis and are related to large amounts of histamine in the skin. Excessive dryness of the skin with resultant itching is related to changes in lipid content, sebaceous gland activity, and sweating. In response to stroking of the skin, immediate redness appears on the skin and is followed in 15 to 30 seconds by pallor, which persists for

Table 53-4 • Types, Testing, and Treatment of Contact Dermatitis

TYPE	ETIOLOGY	CLINICAL PRESENTATION	DIAGNOSTIC TESTING	TREATMENT
Allergic	Results from contact of skin and allergenic substance. Has a sensitization period of 10–14 days.	Vasodilation and perivascular infiltrates on the dermis Intracellular edema Usually seen on dorsal aspects of hand	Patch testing (contraindicated in acute, widespread dermatitis)	Avoidance of offending material Burow's solution or cool water compress Systemic corticosteroids (prednisone) for 7–10 days Topical corticosteroids for mild cases Oral antihistamines to relieve pruritus
Irritant	Results from contact with a substance that chemically or physically damages the skin on a nonimmunologic basis. Occurs after first exposure to irritant or repeated exposures to milder irritants over an extended time.	Dryness lasting days to months Vesiculation, fissures, cracks Hands and lower arms most common areas	Clinical picture Appropriate negative patch tests	Identification and removal of source of irritation Application of hydrophilic cream or petrolatum to soothe and protect Topical corticosteroids and compresses for weeping lesions Antibiotics for infection and oral antihistamines for pruritus
Phototoxic	Resembles the irritant type but requires sun and a chemical in combination to damage the epidermis.	Similar to irritant dermatitis	Photopatch test	Same as for allergic and irritant dermatitis
Photoallergic	Resembles allergic dermatitis but requires light exposure in addition to allergen contact to produce immunologic reactivity.	Similar to allergic dermatitis	Photopatch test	Same as for allergic and irritant dermatitis

1 to 3 minutes. Lesions develop secondary to the trauma of scratching and appear in areas of increased sweating and hypervascularity. Atopic dermatitis is chronic, with remissions and exacerbations. This condition has a tendency to recur, with remission from adolescence to age 20 (Tierney et al., 2001). Treatment must be individualized.

Medical Management

Guidelines for treatment include decreasing itching and scratching by wearing cotton fabrics, washing with a mild detergent, humidifying dry heat in winter, maintaining room temperature at 20°C to 22.2°C, using antihistamines such as diphenhydramine (Benadryl), and avoiding animals, dust, sprays, and perfumes. Keeping the skin moisturized with daily baths to hydrate the skin and topical skin moisturizers is encouraged. Topical corticosteroids are used to prevent inflammation, and any infection is treated with antibiotics to eliminate *Staphylococcus aureus* when indicated. Use of low doses of cyclosporine (Neoral, Sandimmune), an immunosuppressive agent, may be effective (Kay, 2001b).

Nursing Management

Patients who experience atopic dermatitis and their families require assistance and support from the nurse to cope with the disorder. The symptoms are often disturbing to the patient and disruptive to the family. The appearance of the skin may affect the patient's self-esteem and may affect the patient's willingness to interact with others. Instructions and counselling about strategies to incorporate preventive measures and treatments into the lifestyle of the family may be helpful.

Patients and family members need to be aware of signs of secondary infection and of the need to seek treatment if infection occurs. The nurse also teaches the patient and family about the side effects of medications used in treatment.

DERMATITIS MEDICAMENTOSA (DRUG REACTIONS)

Dermatitis medicamentosa, a type I hypersensitivity disorder, is the term applied to skin rashes induced by the internal administration of certain medications. Although individuals react differently to each medication, certain medications tend to induce eruptions of similar types. Rashes are among the most common adverse reactions to medications and occur in approximately 2% to 3% of hospitalized patients (Tierney et al., 2001).

In general, drug reactions appear suddenly, have a particularly vivid colour, present with characteristics that are more intense than the somewhat similar eruptions of infectious origin, and, with the exception of bromide and the iodide rashes, disappear rapidly after the medication is withdrawn. Rashes may be accompanied by systemic or generalized symptoms. Upon discovery of a medication allergy, patients are warned that they have a hypersensitivity to a particular medication and are advised not to take it again. Information identifying the hypersensitivity should be carried with them at all times.

Skin eruptions related to medication therapy suggest more serious hypersensitivities. Frequent assessment and prompt reporting of the appearance of any eruptions are important so that early treatment can be initiated. Some cutaneous drug reactions may be associated with a clinical complex that involves other organs. These are known as complex drug reactions (Tierney et al., 2001).

URTICARIA AND ANGIONEUROTIC EDEMA

Urticaria (hives) is a type I hypersensitive allergic reaction of the skin characterized by the sudden appearance of pinkish, edematous elevations that vary in size and shape and itch and cause local discomfort. They may involve any part of the body, including the mucous membranes (especially those of the mouth), the larynx (occasionally with serious respiratory complications), and the gastrointestinal tract.

Each hive remains for a few minutes to several hours before disappearing. For hours or days, clusters of these lesions may come, go, and return episodically. If this sequence continues for longer than 6 weeks, the condition is called chronic urticaria (Tierney et al., 2001).

Angioneurotic edema involves the deeper layers of the skin, resulting in more diffuse swelling rather than the discrete lesions characteristic of hives. On occasion, this reaction covers the entire back. The skin over the reaction may appear normal but often has a reddish hue. The skin does not pit on pressure, as ordinary edema does. The regions most often involved are the lips, eyelids, cheeks, hands, feet, genitalia, and tongue; the mucous membranes of the larynx, the bronchi, and the gastrointestinal canal may also be affected, particularly in the hereditary type (see section that follows). Swellings may appear suddenly, in a few seconds or minutes, or slowly, in 1 or 2 hours. In the latter case, their appearance is often preceded by itching or burning sensations. Seldom does more than a single swelling appear at one time, although one may develop while another is disappearing. Infrequently, swelling recurs in the same region. Individual lesions usually last 24 to 36 hours. On rare occasions, swelling may recur with remarkable regularity at intervals of 3 to 4 weeks.

HEREDITARY ANGIOEDEMA

Hereditary angioedema, although not an immunologic disorder in the usual sense, is included because of its resemblance to allergic angioedema and because of the seriousness of the condition. Symptoms are due to edema of the skin, the respiratory tract, or the digestive tract. Attacks may be precipitated by trauma or may seem to occur spontaneously.

Clinical Manifestations

When skin is involved, the swelling is usually diffuse, does not itch, and is usually not accompanied by urticaria. Gastrointestinal edema may cause abdominal pain severe enough to suggest the need for surgery. Typically, attacks last 1 to 4 days and are gener-

ally harmless. Occasionally, attacks affect the subcutaneous and submucosal tissues in the region of the upper airway and can be associated with respiratory obstruction and asphyxiation. This disorder is inherited as an autosomal dominant trait. Approximately 85% of patients with this disorder have one nonproductive gene; the other 15% have a gene mutation (Parslow et al., 2001).

Medical Management

Attacks usually subside within 3 to 4 days, but during this time the patient should be observed carefully for signs of laryngeal obstruction, which may necessitate tracheostomy as a life-saving measure. Epinephrine, antihistamines, and corticosteroids are usually used in treatment, but their success is limited.

FOOD ALLERGY

IgE-mediated food allergy, a type I hypersensitivity reaction, occurs in 0.1% to 7.0% of the population. Almost any food can cause allergic symptoms. Any food can contain an allergen that results in anaphylaxis. The most common offenders are seafood (lobster, shrimp, crab, clams, fish), legumes (peanuts, tree nuts, peas, beans, licorice), seeds (sesame, cottonseed, caraway, mustard, flaxseed, and sunflower seeds), nuts, berries, egg white, buckwheat, milk, and chocolate (Parslow et al., 2001). Peanut and tree nut (ie, cashew, walnut) allergies are responsible for most severe food allergy reactions (Sicherer, Munoz-Furlong, Burks et al., 1999).

One of the dangers of food allergens is that they may be hidden in other foods and not apparent to those susceptible to the allergen. For example, peanuts and peanut butter are often used in salad dressings and Asian, African, and Mexican cooking and may result in severe allergic reactions, including anaphylaxis. Previous contamination of equipment with allergens (ie, peanuts) during preparation of another food product (ie, chocolate cake) is enough to produce anaphylaxis in those with severe allergy.

Clinical Manifestations

Clinical symptoms are classic allergic symptoms (itching, urticaria, atopic dermatitis, wheezing, cough, laryngeal edema, angioedema) and gastrointestinal symptoms (swelling of lips, tongue, and palate; abdominal pain; nausea; cramps; vomiting; and diarrhea).

Assessment and Diagnostic Findings

A careful diagnostic workup is required in any patient with a suspected food hypersensitivity. Included are a detailed allergy history, a physical examination, and pertinent diagnostic tests. When testing for allergy, skin testing is used to identify the source of symptoms and is useful in identifying specific foods as causative agents.

Medical Management

Therapy for food hypersensitivity includes elimination of the food responsible for the hypersensitivity (Chart 53-6). Pharmacologic therapy is necessary in patients who cannot avoid exposure to offending foods or patients with multiple food sensitivities not responsive to elimination measures. Medication therapy involves the use of H_1- and H_2-blockers, antihistamines, adrenergic agents, corticosteroids, and cromolyn sodium.

Chart 53-6

Home Care Checklist • Managing Food Allergies

At the completion of the home care instruction, the patient or caregiver will be able to:	Patient	Caregiver
• Verbalize understanding of the need to maintain an allergen-free diet.	✓	✓
• Demonstrate reading of food labels to identify hidden allergens in food.	✓	✓
• Identify ways to manage an allergen-free diet when eating away from home.	✓	✓
• State the need to wear a medical alert medallion or bracelet.	✓	✓
• List symptoms of food allergy.	✓	✓
• Demonstrate emergency administration of epinephrine.	✓	✓
• State the importance of prompt treatment and health care follow-up.	✓	✓

Many food allergies disappear with time, particularly in children. About one third of proven allergies disappear in 1 to 2 years if the patient carefully avoids the offending food.

Nursing Management

In addition to participating in management of the allergic reaction, the nurse focuses on preventing future exposure of the patient to the food allergen. If a severe allergic or anaphylactic reaction to food allergens has occurred, the nurse must instruct the patient and family about strategies to prevent its recurrence. The patient is instructed about the importance of carefully assessing food prepared by others for obvious as well as hidden sources of food allergens and of avoiding locations and facilities where those allergens are likely to be present. The patient and family must be knowledgeable about early signs and symptoms of allergic reactions and must be proficient in emergency administration of epinephrine if a reaction occurs. The nurse also advises the patient to wear a medical alert bracelet or to carry identification and emergency equipment at all times.

SERUM SICKNESS

The illness known as serum sickness is an example of an immune complex type III hypersensitivity. It has traditionally resulted from the administration of therapeutic antisera of animal sources for the treatment or prevention of infectious diseases, such as tetanus, pneumonia, rabies, diphtheria, botulism, and venomous snake and black widow spider bites. With the advent of human antitetanus serum and antibiotics, classic serum sickness is much less common now. However, various medications (primarily penicillin) may cause a serum sickness–like reaction similar to that caused by foreign sera.

Clinical Manifestations

Symptoms are due to a reaction and immunologic attack on the serum or medication. Antibodies appear to be of the IgE and IgM classes. Early manifestations, beginning 6 to 10 days after the administration of the medication, include an inflammatory reaction at the site of injection of the medication, followed by regional and generalized lymphadenopathy. There is usually a skin rash, which may be urticarial or purpuric. Joints are frequently tender and swollen. Vasculitis may occur in any organ but is most commonly observed in the kidney, resulting in proteinuria and, occasionally, casts in the urine. There may be mild to severe cardiac involvement. Peripheral neuritis may cause temporary paralysis of the upper extremities or may be widespread, causing Guillain-Barré syndrome.

Medical Management

The usual course lasts for several days to a few weeks if untreated, but the patient responds promptly and completely if treated with antihistamines and corticosteroids. Aggressive therapy, including ventilator support, may be necessary if peripheral neuritis and Guillain-Barré syndrome occur.

Nursing Management

See Chapter 64 for nursing management of Guillain-Barré syndrome.

LATEX ALLERGY

Latex allergy, the allergic reaction to natural rubber proteins, has been implicated in rhinitis, conjunctivitis, contact dermatitis, urticaria, asthma, and anaphylaxis. Latex allergy and hypersensitivity were first reported in 1927 (Parslow et al., 2001). Although the prevalence of latex allergy is unknown, since 1989 the number of cases of latex allergy has steadily increased (Parslow et al., 2001). This increase may be due to the widespread use of latex gloves with implementation of universal and now standard precautions in response to the AIDS epidemic, changes in the manufacturing of gloves to speed the process to meet the increased demand for gloves, and greater awareness about latex allergy and its signs and symptoms.

Natural rubber latex is derived from the sap of the rubber tree (*Hevea brasiliensis*). The conversion of the liquid rubber latex into a finished product entails the addition of more than 200 chemicals. The proteins in the natural rubber latex (Hevea proteins) or the various chemicals that are used in the manufacturing process are thought to be the source of the allergic reactions. Not all objects composed of latex have the same ability to stimulate an allergic response. For example, the antigenicity of latex gloves can differ widely depending on their manufacturing method.

Populations at risk include health care workers, patients with atopic allergies or multiple surgeries, people working in factories manufacturing latex products, females, and patients with spina bifida. Because more food handlers, hairdressers, auto mechanics, and police are now wearing latex gloves, they may also be at risk for latex allergy. It is estimated that 1% to 3% of the general population has an allergy to latex and that 10% to 17% of health care workers are sensitized. Patients are at risk for anaphylactic reactions due to contact with latex during medical treatments, especially surgical procedures. About 19% of anaphylactic reactions associated with anesthesia are caused by allergy to latex (Brehler & Kütting, 2001).

Food that has been handled by individuals wearing latex gloves may stimulate an allergic response. Cross-reactions have been reported in people who are allergic to certain food products, such as kiwis, bananas, pineapples, passion fruits, avocados, and chestnuts.

Routes of exposure to latex products can be cutaneous, percutaneous, mucosal, parenteral, and aerosol. The most frequent source of exposure is cutaneous, which usually involves the wearing of natural latex gloves. The powder used to facilitate putting on latex gloves can become a carrier of latex proteins from the gloves; when the gloves are put on or removed, the particles become airborne and can be inhaled or can settle on skin, mucous membranes, or clothing. Mucosal exposure can occur from the use of latex condoms, catheters, airways, and nipples. Parenteral exposure can occur from intravenous lines or hemodialysis equipment. In addition to latex-derived medical devices, many household items also contain latex. Examples of medical and household items containing latex and a list of alternative products are found in Table 53-5. It is estimated that over 40,000 medical devices and nonmedical products contain latex (Brehler & Kütting, 2001).

Clinical Manifestations

Several different types of reactions to latex are possible. Irritant contact dermatitis, a nonimmunologic response, may be due to mechanical skin irritation or an alkaline pH associated with latex gloves. Common symptoms of irritant dermatitis include erythema and pruritus. These symptoms can be eliminated by changing glove brands or using powder-free gloves. Use of hand lotion before donning latex gloves may worsen the symptoms because lotions may leach latex proteins from the gloves, increasing skin exposure and the risk of developing true allergic reactions (Burt, 1998).

Delayed hypersensitivity to latex, a type IV allergic reaction mediated by T cells in the immune system, is localized to the area of exposure and is characterized by symptoms of contact dermatitis, including vesicular skin lesions, papules, pruritus, edema, erythema, and crusting and thickening of the skin. These symptoms usually appear on the back of the hands. This reaction is thought to be due to chemicals that are used for manufacturing latex products. It is the most common allergic reaction to latex. Although not usually life-threatening, delayed hypersensitivity

Table 53-5 • Selected Products Containing Natural Rubber Latex and Latex-Free Alternatives

PRODUCTS CONTAINING LATEX	EXAMPLES OF LATEX-SAFE ALTERNATIVES*
Hospital Environment	
Ace bandage (brown)	Ace bandage, white, all cotton
Adhesive bandages, Band-Aid dressing, Telfa	Cotton pads and plastic or silk tape, Active Strip (3M), Duoderm
Anesthesia equipment	Neoprene anesthesia kit (King)
Blood pressure cuff, tubing, and bladder	Clean Cuff, single-use nylon or vinyl blood pressure cuffs or wrap with stockinette or apply over clothing
Catheters	All-silicone or vinyl catheters
Catheter leg bag straps	Velcro straps
Crutch axillary pads and hand grips, tips	Cover with cloth, tape
ECG pads	Baxter, Red Dot 3M ECG pads
Elastic compression stockings	Kendall SCD stockings with stockinette
Gloves	Dermaprene, Neoprene, polymer, or vinyl gloves
IV catheters	Jelko, Deseret IV catheters
IV rubber injection ports	Cover Y-sites and ports; do not puncture. Use three-way stopcocks on plastic tubing.
Levin tube	Salem sump tube
Medication vials	Remove rubber stopper.
Penrose drains	Jackson-Pratt, Zimmer hemovac drains
Prepackaged enema kits	Theravac, Fleet Ready-to-use
Pulse oximeters	Nonin oximeters
Resuscitation bags	Laerdal, Puritan Bennett, *certain* Ambu
Stethoscope tubing	PVC tubing; cover with latex-free stockinette
Syringes—single use (Monoject, B & D)	Terumo syringes, Abbott PCA Abboject
Suction tubing	PVC (Davol, Laerdal)
Tapes	Dermicel, Micropore
Thermometer probes	Diatec probe covers
Tourniquets	X-Tourn straps (Avcor)
Theraband	New Thera-band Exercisers, plastic tubing
Home Environment	
Balloons	Mylar balloons
Diapers, incontinence pads	Huggies, Always, *some* Attends
Condoms, diaphragms	Polyurethane products, Durex/Avanti and Reality products (female condom)
Feminine hygiene pad	Kimberly-Clark products
Wheelchair cushions	ROHO cushions, Sof Care bed/chair cushions

*Confirmation is essential to verify that all items are latex-free before using, especially if risk of latex allergy.

NURSING RESEARCH PROFILE 53-1
Barrier Effectiveness of Latex and Non-latex Gloves

Korniewicz, D., el-Masri, M., Broyles, J. M., Martin, C. D., & O'Connell, K. P. (2002). Performance of latex and nonlatex medical examination gloves during simulated use. *American Journal of Infection Control, 30*(2), 133–138.

Purpose

In recent years, a variety of non-latex gloves have been used in health care in response to the increasing incidence of allergic reactions to latex, which has occurred with the increased use of gloves to protect health care personnel from exposure to body fluids. However, little research data about the barrier quality of these new synthetic gloves are available. The purpose of this study was to examine the effects of glove stress, type of material, and manufacturer on the barrier effectiveness of medical examination gloves.

Study Design and Sample

The sample consisted of 5,510 medical examination gloves: 1,464 nitrile, 1,052 latex, 1,006 copolymer, and 1,988 vinyl gloves. Eleven brands of gloves from five manufacturers were tested for barrier effectiveness. The gloves were divided into two groups: stressed and unstressed. Unstressed gloves were tested by the FDA 1989 water-leak test in which the gloves were filled with 1,000 mL of water, hung for 2 minutes, and observed for leaks. The gloves were rated as ineffective barriers if a water leak was detected. The remaining gloves were subjected to a laboratory and clinical stress protocol that mimics the stresses on gloves that occur during clinical use. Visible water leaks or leakage on the FDA water-leak test indicated barrier ineffectiveness. Chi-square analyses were used to test the differences between the frequencies of failure across glove material, manufacturer, and the stressed vs. nonstressed conditions.

Findings

Nitrile gloves had the lowest rate of failure, followed by latex gloves. Copolymer and vinyl gloves had the highest rates of failure. The failure rates were significantly different ($p < 0.001$). Subjecting gloves to the stress protocol increased the failure rate significantly ($p < 0.002$). Failure rates were also significantly different by glove manufacturer ($p < 0.001$). The data demonstrated that glove material, manufacturer, and stress are important factors that influence the barrier effectiveness of medical examination gloves.

Nursing Implications

The research findings suggest that nitrile medical examination gloves are an acceptable alternative to latex gloves and that vinyl and copolymer gloves provide less protection to the wearer. These findings suggest the need for health care providers and facilities to use care in selecting the type and manufacturer of gloves to protect the wearer during patient care. The researchers indicated that studies using larger samples are warranted and should address other variables that may affect the barrier effectiveness of gloves during use, including duration of use, presence of powder, glove size, hand dominance, complexity of tasks performed while wearing gloves, and the use of instruments.

---

reactions often require major changes in the patient's home and work environment to avoid further exposure.

Immediate hypersensitivity, a type I allergic reaction, is mediated by the IgE mast cell system. Symptoms can include rhinitis, conjunctivitis, asthma, and anaphylaxis. The term "latex allergy" is usually used to describe the type I reaction. Clinical manifestations have a rapid onset and can include urticaria, wheezing, dyspnea, laryngeal edema, bronchospasm, tachycardia, angioedema, hypotension, and cardiac arrest.

Localized itching, erythema, or local urticaria within minutes after exposure to latex are often the initial symptoms. Symptoms of subsequent reactions can include generalized urticaria, angioedema, rhinitis, conjunctivitis, asthma, and anaphylactic shock minutes after dermal or mucosal exposure to latex. An increasing number of individuals allergic to latex experience severe reactions characterized by generalized urticaria, bronchospasm, and hypotension (Brehler & Kütting, 2001).

Diagnostic Testing

The diagnosis of latex allergy is based on the history and diagnostic test results (Parslow et al., 2001). Sensitization is detected by skin testing, RAST, or ELISA. Skin tests have been unreliable because of variability in the techniques used; however, a new standardized skin testing reagent is expected to be available in the near future. Skin tests should be done only by clinicians who have expertise in their administration and interpretation and who have the necessary equipment available to treat local or systemic allergic reactions to the reagent (Hamilton & Adkinson, 1998). Nasal challenge and dipstick tests may be useful in the future as screening tests for latex allergy.

Medical Management

The best treatment available for latex allergy is the avoidance of latex products, but this is often difficult because of the widespread use of latex-based products. Patients who have experienced an anaphylactic reaction to latex should be instructed to wear medical identification. Antihistamines and an emergency kit containing epinephrine should be provided to these patients, along with instructions about emergency management of latex allergy symptoms. Patients should be counselled to notify all health care workers as well as local paramedic and ambulance companies about their allergy. Warning labels can be attached to car windows to alert police and paramedics about the driver's or passenger's latex allergy in case of a motor vehicle crash. Individuals with latex allergy should be provided with a list of alternative products and referred to local support groups; they are also urged to carry their own supply of nonlatex gloves.

People with type I latex sensitivity may be unable to continue to work if a latex-free environment is not possible. This may occur with surgeons, dentists, operating room personnel, or intensive care nurses. Occupational implications for employees with type IV latex sensitivity are usually easier to manage by changing to nonlatex gloves and avoiding direct contact with latex-based medical equipment. Although latex-specific immunotherapy has been reported, this method of treatment remains experimental (Brehler & Kütting, 2001).

Nursing Management

The nurse can assume a pivotal role in the management of both patients and staff with latex allergies. All patients should be asked about latex allergy, although special attention should be given to those at particularly high risk (eg, patients with spina bifida, patients who have undergone multiple surgical procedures). Every time an invasive procedure must be performed, the nurse should consider the possibility of latex allergies. Nurses working in operating rooms, intensive care units, short procedure units, and emergency departments need to pay particular attention to latex allergy. See Chapter 19 for a latex allergy screening form.

Although the type I reaction is the most significant of the reactions to latex, care must be taken in the presence of irritant contact dermatitis and delayed hypersensitivity reaction to avoid further exposure of the individual to latex. Patients with latex allergy are advised to notify their health care providers and to wear a medical information bracelet. Patients must become knowledgeable about what products contain latex and what products are safe, nonlatex alternatives. They must also become knowledgeable about signs and symptoms of latex allergy and emergency treatment and self-injection of epinephrine in case of allergic reaction.

Nurses can be instrumental in establishing and participating in multidisciplinary committees to address latex allergy and to promote a latex-free environment. Latex allergy protocols and education of staff about latex allergy and precautions are important strategies to reduce this growing problem and to ensure assessment and prompt treatment of affected individuals.

New Approaches to Treatment of Allergic Diseases

Although allergen-specific immunotherapy reduces symptoms for several years after it is discontinued, this approach to management is limited in terms of usefulness because of its potential adverse effects, particularly anaphylaxis, and the relatively crude allergen extracts involved. Newer approaches to the treatment of allergic diseases to overcome these limitations are being evaluated and include the use of substances such as naturally occurring isoforms of allergens from plants and trees. These isoforms are less likely to stimulate anaphylactic reactions. Use of recombinant allergens is expected to eliminate variation between batches of allergen. Other experimental approaches include the use of DNA vaccines and monoclonal antibodies and other strategies to block IgE or its synthesis (Kay, 2001b).

Critical Thinking Exercises

1. A 45-year-old man arrives at the emergency department where you are employed. He states that he is severely allergic to bees and was stung by a wasp approximately 10 minutes ago. He tells you that he has been in anaphylactic shock in the past as a result of bee stings. He tells you that he received allergy injections for bee allergy approximately 10 years ago. Upon assessing the patient, you note that he has generalized hives and urticaria on his body, and he is complaining of his throat swelling. What would be your immediate course of action?

2. A patient with severe allergies is to receive instructions about self-administration of epinephrine if she experiences anaphylaxis. Develop a teaching plan for this patient and identify outcomes to measure the effectiveness of your

teaching. How would you modify your teaching if the patient reports a severe fear of injection? If the patient has a profound hearing loss? If the patient is visually impaired?

3. A 28-year-old man has a surgical procedure for a varicocele. A Penrose drain is inserted into his scrotum during the surgical procedure in the operating room. The patient develops erythema and significant edema of the scrotum inconsistent with the procedure that was performed. The circulating nurse had noted on the operative checklist that the patient was allergic to latex. What would be your immediate course of action? How could you ensure that a similar situation would not occur in the future? What course of action could you take to ensure a latex-free environment for patients who require such an environment?

REFERENCES AND SELECTED READINGS

Books

Abbas, A. K., & Lichtman, A. H. (2001). *Basic immunology: Functions and disorders of the immune system.* Philadelphia: W. B. Saunders.

Antel, P., Birnbaum, G., & Hartung, H. P. (1998). *Clinical neuroimmunology.* Malden, MA: Blackwell Scientific.

Buttaro, T. M., Trybulski, J., Bailey, P. P., & Sandberg-Cook, J. (1999). *Primary care: A collaborative practice.* St. Louis, MO: Mosby, Inc.

Delves, P. J. (1998). *Encyclopedia of immunology* (2nd ed.). San Diego: Academic Press.

Goroll, A. H., & Mulley Jr., A. G. (2000). *Primary care medicine* (4th ed.). Philadelphia: Lippincott Williams & Wilkins.

Huether, S. E., & McCance, K. L. (2000). *Understanding pathophysiology* (2d ed.). St. Louis, MO: Mosby, Inc.

Middleton, E. Jr (Ed.). (1998). *Allergy: Principles and practice.* St. Louis: C. V. Mosby.

Parkinson, C. F. (2000). *Study guide and workbook for understanding pathophysiology* (2d ed.). St. Louis, MO: Mosby, Inc.

Parslow, T. G., Stites, D. P., Terr, A. I., & Imboden, J. B. (2001). *Medical immunology.* New York: McGraw-Hill.

Porth, C. M. (2002). *Pathophysiology: Concepts of altered health states* (6th ed.). Philadelphia: Lippincott Williams & Wilkins.

Roitt, I. M. & Delves, P. J. (2001). *Roitt's essential immunology.* Malden, MA: Blackwell Science.

Tierney Jr., L. M., McPhee, S. J., & Papadakis, M. A. (Eds.). (2001). *Current medical diagnosis and treatment.* Stamford, CT: Appleton & Lange.

Virella, G. (Ed.). (2001). *Medical immunology.* New York: Marcel Dekker.

Journals

Asterisks indicate nursing research articles.

Anaphylaxis Canada. (2005). Welcome to anaphylaxis Canada. Available at: http://www.anaphylaxis.ca/. Retrieved February 16, 2006.

Barbarito, C. (1999). Anaphylaxis. *American Journal of Nursing, 99*(1), 33.

Becker, H. S. (2000). An analysis of the epidemiology of latex allergy: Implications for primary prevention. *MedSurg Nursing, 9*(3), 135–143.

Brehler, R., & Kütting, B. (2001). Natural rubber latex allergy: A problem of interdisciplinary concern in medicine. *Archives of Internal Medicine, 161*(8), 1057–1064.

Burt, S. (1998). What you need to know about latex allergy. *Nursing, 28*(10), 33–39.

Gehring, L. L., & Ring, P. (1999). Latex allergy: Creating a safe environment. *MedSurg Nursing, 8*(6), 358–362.

Gritter, M. (1998). The latex threat. *American Journal of Nursing, 98*(9), 26–32.

Hamilton, R. G., & Adkinson, N. F., Jr. (1998). Diagnosis of natural rubber latex allergy: Multicenter latex skin testing efficacy study. *Journal of Allergy and Clinical Immunology, 102*(3), 482–490.

Kay, A. B. (2001*a*). Advances in immunology: Allergy and allergic diseases (first of two parts). *New England Journal of Medicine, 344*(1), 30–37.

Kay, A. B. (2001*b*). Advances in immunology: Allergy and allergic diseases (second of two parts). *New England Journal of Medicine, 344*(2), 109–113.

*Korniewicz, D., el-Masri, M., Broyles, J. M., Martin, C. D., & O'Connell, K. P. (2002). Performance of latex and nonlatex medical examination gloves during simulated use. *American Journal of Infection Control, 30*(2), 133–138.

*Korniewicz, D. M., Garzon, L., Seltzer, J., et al. (2001). Implementing a nonlatex surgical glove study in the OR. *AORN Journal, 73*(2), 435–445.

Lilley, L. L., & Gaunci, R. (1999). Cross sensitivities: Medication errors waiting to happen. *American Journal of Nursing, 99*(2), 12.

Neugut, A. I., Ghatak, A. T., & Miller, R. L. (2001). Anaphylaxis in the United States: An investigation into its epidemiology. *Archives of Internal Medicine, 161*(1), 15–21.

Ratner, P. H., Ehrlich, P. M., Fineman, S. M., et al. (2002). Use of intranasal cromolyn sodium for allergic rhinitis. *Mayo Clinic Proceedings, 77*(4), 350–354.

Sicherer, S. H., Munoz-Furlong, A., Burks, A. W., et al. (1999). Prevalence of peanut and tree nut allergy in the U.S. determined by a random digit dial telephone survey. *Journal of Allergy and Clinical Immunology, 103*(4), 559–562.

Silkoff, P. E., Robbins, R. A., Gaston, B., et al. (2000). Endogenous nitric oxide in allergic airway disease. *Journal of Allergy and Clinical Immunology, 105*(3), 438–448.

Walker, S., & Sheikh, A. (2002). Rhinitis. *British Medical Journal, 324*(7334), 403.

Williams, L. W., & Bock, S. A. (1999). Skin testing and food challenges in allergy and immunology practice. *Clinical Reviews in Allergy and Immunology, 17*(3), 323–338.

RESOURCES AND WEBSITES

American Academy of Allergy, Asthma and Immunology, 611 East Wells Street, Milwaukee, WI 53202; (800) 822-ASMA; http://www.aaai.org.

The Canadian Allergy, Asthma and Immunology Foundation, 774 Echo Drive, Ottawa, ON K1S 5N8; (613) 730-6272; http://www.allergyfoundation.ca and http://www.allergyfoundation.ca/anapschools.htm.

The Canadian Society of Allergy and Clinical Immunology, 774 Echo Drive, Ottawa, ON K1S 5N8; (613) 730-6272; http://csaci.medical.org.

Canadian Institute for Health Information, 377 Dalhousie Street, Suite 200, Ottawa ON, K1N 9N8; (613) 241-7860; http://www.cihi.ca.

Centers for Disease Control and Prevention, 1600 Clifton Road, Atlanta, GA 30333; (404) 639-3311 or (800) 311-3435; http://www.cdc.gov.

Food Allergy & Anaphylaxis Network, 10400 Eaton Place, Suite 107, Fairfax, VA 22030; (800) 929-4040; http://www.foodallergy.org; e-mail: faan@foodallergy.org.

National Institute of Allergy and Infectious Disease, NIAID Office of Communications and Public Liaison, NIH, Bldg. 31, Room 7A50, 31 Center Drive, MSC 2520, Bethesda, MD 20893; (301) 496-5717; http://www.niaid.nih.gov/.

National Institutes of Health, 9000 Rockville Pike, Bethesda, MD 20892; (301) 496-4000; http://www.nih.gov.

Spina Bifida Association of America, 4590 MacArthur Blvd NW, Suite 250, Washington, DC 20007; (800) 621-3141; http://www.sbaa.org.

Assessment and Management of Patients With Rheumatic Disorders

Adapted by Wanda Pierson

LEARNING OBJECTIVES

On completion of this chapter, the learner will be able to:

1. Explain the processes of inflammation and degradation in the development of rheumatic diseases.
2. Describe the assessment and diagnostic findings that may be evidenced by patients with a suspected diagnosis of rheumatic disease.
3. Discuss appropriate nursing interventions based on nursing diagnoses and collaborative problems that commonly occur with rheumatic disorders.
4. Apply the nursing process as a framework for the care of the patient with a rheumatic disease, such as connective tissue disease or osteoarthritis.
5. Describe the systemic effects of a connective tissue disease.
6. Devise a teaching plan for the patient with newly diagnosed rheumatic disease.
7. Identify modifications in interventions to accommodate changes in patients' functional ability that may occur with disease progression.

Rheumatic diseases include common disorders such as osteoarthritis or rarer conditions such as systemic lupus erythematosus or scleroderma. These conditions can be life-threatening or minor illnesses. The problems caused by the rheumatic diseases include not only the obvious limitations in mobility and activities of daily living but also the subtler systemic effects that can lead to organ failure and death or result in problems such as pain, fatigue, altered self-image, and sleep disturbances. The rheumatic disease may be the patient's primary health problem or a secondary diagnosis. Thus, thorough understanding of rheumatic diseases and their effects on the patient's function and well-being is the key to developing an appropriate plan of care.

Rheumatic Diseases

Commonly called arthritis (inflammation of a joint) and thought of as one condition, the rheumatic diseases are actually more than 100 different types of disorders that primarily affect skeletal muscles, bones, cartilage, ligaments, tendons, and joints of males and females of all ages. Some disorders are more likely to occur at a particular time of life or to affect one gender more than the other. The onset of these conditions may be acute or insidious, with a course possibly marked by periods of remission (a period when disease symptoms are reduced or absent) and exacerbation (a period when symptoms occur or increase). Treatment can be simple, aimed at localized relief, or it can be complex, directed toward relieving systemic effects. Permanent changes may result from the disease.

There are several approaches to the classification of rheumatic diseases. One basic system is to classify disease as either monoarticular (affects a single joint) or polyarticular (affects multiple joints) and then to further classify it as either inflammatory or noninflammatory (Klippel, 2001). Conditions that may secondarily affect the musculoskeletal structure are also included, emphasizing the diversity of the rheumatic diseases.

Pathophysiology

Understanding the normal anatomy and physiology of the **diarthrodial** or **synovial** joints is key to understanding the pathophysiology of the rheumatic diseases. The function of the synovial joints is movement. Each synovial joint has a given range of motion, although range of motion of movable joints varies between individuals.

In a normal synovial joint, a smooth, nearly friction-free, resilient surface for movement is provided by articular cartilage, which covers the bone end of the joint. Lining the inner surface of the fibrous capsule is the synovial membrane, which secretes fluid into the space between the bone ends. The synovial fluid functions as a shock absorber and a lubricant, allowing the joint to move freely.

The joint is the area most commonly affected by the inflammation and degeneration seen in rheumatic diseases. Despite the diversity of rheumatic diseases, from localized involvement of one joint to systemic, multisystem disorders, they all involve some degree of inflammation and degeneration, which may occur simultaneously. Inflammation is manifested in the joints as synovitis. In inflammatory rheumatic diseases, the primary process is inflammation as a result of the immune response. Degeneration occurs as a secondary process, resulting from the effect of **pannus** (proliferation of newly formed synovial tissue infiltrated with inflammatory cells). The inflammation is a result of altered immune function.

Conversely, in degenerative rheumatic diseases, inflammation occurs as a secondary process. This synovitis is usually milder, is more likely to be seen in advanced disease, and represents a reactive process. The synovitis is thought to result from mechanical irritation from cartilage **matrix** products.

INFLAMMATION

Inflammation involves a series of related steps. With the triggering event, the **antigen** stimulus activates monocytes and T lymphocytes (also called T cells). Next, the immunoglobulin antibodies form immune complexes with antigens. Phagocytosis of the immune complexes is initiated, generating an inflammatory reaction (joint effusion, pain, and edema) (Fig. 54-1).

During the next step, the normal immune response deviates. Phagocytosis produces chemicals such as leukotrienes and prostaglandins. **Leukotrienes** contribute to the inflammatory process by attracting other white blood cells to the area. **Prostaglandins** act as modifiers to inflammation. In some cases, they increase inflammation; in other cases, they slow it down. Leukotrienes and prostaglandins produce enzymes such as collagenase that break down collagen, a vital part of a normal joint. The release of these enzymes in the joint causes edema, proliferation of synovial membrane and pannus formation, destruction of cartilage, and erosion of bone.

The immunologic inflammatory process begins when antigens are presented to T lymphocytes, leading to a proliferation of T and B cells. B cells are a source for **antibody**-forming cells, or plasma cells. In response to specific antigens, plasma cells produce and release antibodies. Antibodies combine with corresponding

Glossary

ankylosis: fixation or immobility of a joint

antibody: a protein substance developed by the body in response to and interacting with a specific antigen

antigen: a substance that induces production of antibodies

arthroplasty: replacement of a joint

complement: a plasma protein associated with immunologic reactions

cytokines: generic term for nonantibody proteins that act as intercellular mediators, as in the generation of immune response

diarthrodial: a joint with two freely moveable parts

hemarthrosis: bleeding into the joint

joint effusion: the escape of fluid from the blood vessels or lymphatics into the joint space

leukotrienes: chemical mediators formed from constituents (ie, arachidonic acid) of cell membranes; they initiate and mediate the inflammatory response

matrix: noncellular component of tissue

osteophyte: a bony outgrowth or protuberance; spur

pannus: newly formed synovial tissue infiltrated with inflammatory cells

prostaglandins: lipid-soluble molecules synthesized from constituents (ie, arachidonic acid) from cell membranes; they mediate the inflammatory process

subchondral bone: bony plate that supports the articular cartilage

synovial: pertaining to the joint-lubricating fluid

tophi: accumulation of crystalline deposits in articular surfaces, bones, soft tissue, and cartilage

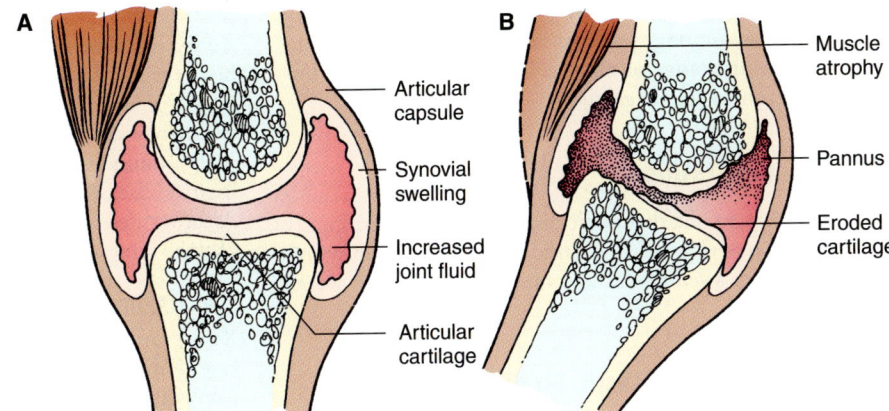

FIGURE 54-1 (**A**) Synovial swelling and fluid accumulation. (**B**) Pannus (a proliferation of synovial tissue), eroded articular cartilage, and joint space narrowing—all of which contribute to muscle atrophy and ankylosis (joint rigidity and immobility).

antigens to form pairs, or immune complexes. The immune complexes build up and are deposited in synovial tissue or other organs in the body, triggering the inflammatory reaction that can ultimately damage the involved tissue.

The systemic nature of the rheumatic disease category known as the diffuse connective tissue diseases is reflected in the resultant widespread inflammatory process. Although focused in the joints, inflammation also involves other areas. The blood vessels (vasculitis and arteritis), lungs, heart, and kidneys may also be affected by the inflammation. In the joints, this inflammatory response is manifested as pannus extending throughout the joint space and, if persistent, eroding the articular cartilage, causing secondary degenerative changes to the joint.

DEGENERATION

Although the cause for degeneration of the articular cartilage is poorly understood, the process is known to be metabolically active and therefore more accurately called "degradation." One theory of degradation is that genetic or hormonal influences, mechanical factors, or prior joint damage causes cartilage failure. Degradation of cartilage ensues and increased mechanical stress on bone ends causes stiffening of bone tissue. Another theory is that bone stiffening occurs and results in increased mechanical stress on cartilage, which in turn initiates the processes of degradation.

Articular cartilage plays two essential mechanical roles in joint physiology. First, the articular cartilage provides a remarkably smooth weight-bearing surface and, with synovial fluid, provides extremely low friction during movement. Second, the cartilage transmits load or pressure to the bone, dissipating the mechanical stress. Specific factors have been implicated in association with degenerative joint changes.

Mechanical Stress. Articular cartilage is highly resistant to wear under conditions of repeated movement. However, repetitive impact loading (velocity at which the force is applied) rapidly leads to joint failure at the cartilage level. When a person walks, three to four times the body weight is transmitted through the knee. A deep knee bend transmits up to nine times the body weight through the patellofemoral joint. As a joint undergoes repeated mechanical stress, the elasticity of the joint capsule, articular cartilage, and ligaments is reduced. The articular plate (**subchondral bone**) thins, and its ability to absorb shock decreases. The joint space narrows, accompanied by a loss of stability. When the articular plate disappears, bony spurs (**osteophytes**) form at the edges of the joint surfaces, and the capsule and synovial mem-

branes thicken. The joint cartilage degenerates and atrophies (shrinks), the bones harden and hypertrophy (thicken) at their articular surfaces, and the ligaments calcify. As a result, sterile **joint effusions** (fluid escaping from the blood vessels or lymphatics into the joint cavity) and secondary synovitis may be present (Fig. 54-2).

Altered Lubrication. In addition to the changes in the articular cartilage and subchondral bone, lubrication of the joint is also a factor in joint degeneration. With joint loading (forces carried through the joint), lubrication depends on a film of interstitial fluid squeezed out of the cartilage upon compression of the opposing surfaces of the joint. The mechanisms that normally operate under high weight loads to produce this lubricating film may be affected.

Immobility. Immobilization of a joint is another factor that can produce degenerative changes in articular cartilage. Although these changes are more marked and appear earlier in areas of contact, they also occur in areas not subject to mechanical compression. Cartilage degeneration due to joint immobility may result from loss of the pumping action of lubrication that occurs with joint movement. By 3 weeks after remobilization of the joint, the

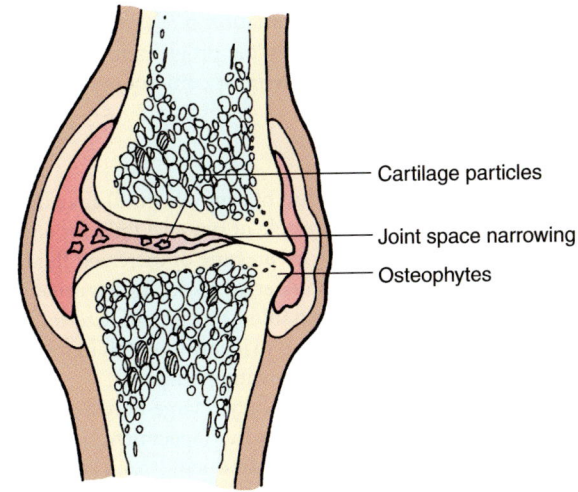

FIGURE 54-2 Joint space narrowing and osteophytes (bone spurs) are characteristic of degenerative changes in joints.

cartilage abnormalities are reversed. However, impact exercising (activities such as running) prevents reversal of the atrophy. Instead, slow, gradual range of motion is thought to be very important in preventing cartilage injury.

Clinical Manifestations

Pain is the symptom of a rheumatic disease that most commonly causes a person to seek medical attention. Other common symptoms include joint swelling, limited movement, stiffness, weakness, and fatigue.

Assessment and Diagnostic Findings

Assessment begins with a general health history, which includes the onset of symptoms and how they evolved, family history, past health history, and any other contributing factors. Because many of the rheumatic diseases are chronic conditions, the health history should also include information about the patient's perception of the problem, previous treatments and their effectiveness, the patient's support systems, and the patient's current knowledge base and the source of that information. A complete health history is followed by a complete physical assessment.

Assessment for rheumatic diseases combines the physical examination with a functional assessment. Inspection of the patient's general appearance occurs during initial contact. Gait, posture, and general musculoskeletal size and structure are observed. Gross deformities and abnormalities in movement are noted. The symmetry, size, and contour of other connective tissues, such as the skin and adipose tissue, are also noted and recorded. Chart 54-1 outlines the important areas for consideration during the physical assessment. The functional assessment is a combination of history (what the patient reports that he or she can and cannot do) and examination (observation of activities: the patient demonstrates what he or she can and cannot do, such as dressing and getting in and out of a chair). Observation also includes the adaptations and adjustments the patient may have made (sometimes without awareness); for example, with shoulder or elbow involvement, the individual may bend over to reach the fork to the mouth rather than raising the fork to the mouth.

The history and physical assessment data are supplemented by supportive or confirming diagnostic test findings. In some instances, tests are used to follow the course of the disease. For example, the erythrocyte sedimentation rate (ESR) reflects inflammatory activity and indirectly the progression or remission of disease. The following tests are most commonly used for patients with rheumatic diseases.

ARTHROCENTESIS

Arthrocentesis (needle aspiration of synovial fluid) may be performed not only to obtain a sample of synovial fluid for analysis but also to relieve pain caused by pressure of increased fluid volume, usually in the knee or shoulder. Synovial fluid is usually analyzed in cases such as suspected joint infection to determine the presence of inflammatory cells and to identify crystals in suspected gout or the presence of blood following trauma.

After the joint is anesthetized locally, a large-bore needle is inserted into the joint space to obtain a fluid specimen. Because this procedure has the potential for introducing bacteria into the joint, aseptic technique is essential. After the procedure, the patient is observed for signs of infection and **hemarthrosis** (bleeding into the joint).

Normally, synovial fluid is clear, viscous, straw-coloured, and scanty in volume, with few cells. In inflammatory joint disease, however, the fluid may become cloudy, milky, or dark yellow and may contain numerous inflammatory cells, such as leukocytes (white blood cells) and **complement** (a plasma protein associated with immunologic reactions). The viscosity is reduced in inflammatory disease, and copious amounts of fluid may be present. Arthrocentesis is diagnostically a valuable test, but arthrocentesis of small joints (ie, fingers or wrist) to obtain fluid may be difficult.

X-RAY STUDIES

X-rays are often used in evaluating patients with rheumatic disease. The timing of the studies influences their usefulness: it is unlikely that a patient with a 2-month history of joint inflammation will have demonstrable changes on an x-ray study, but someone with long-standing disease may show severe joint degeneration. X-rays can also be used to monitor disease activity and progression, demonstrating the loss of cartilage and narrowing of the joint space over time. In addition, x-rays can demonstrate cartilage abnormalities, joint erosions, abnormal bony growth, and osteopenia (decreased bone mineralization).

Arthrography. Arthrography is a diagnostic procedure used to detect connective tissue disorders. A radiopaque substance or air is injected into the joint cavity, especially the knee or shoulder, to outline the contour of the joint. The joint is then put through passive range of motion while several x-rays are obtained. The radiopaque substance is absorbed systemically, and joint swelling consequently subsides. After the procedure, the patient is observed for signs of infection and hemarthrosis.

BONE AND JOINT SCANS

A bone scan reflects the degree to which the crystal lattice of bone takes up or absorbs a bone-seeking radioactive isotope. An area demonstrating increased uptake, such as a joint, is considered abnormal. A joint scan, the most sensitive study, allows determination of joint damage throughout the body. Because bone and joint scans are not the most cost-effective methods for detecting early disease, they are not done routinely at the time of diagnosis.

TISSUE BIOPSIES

A muscle biopsy, carried out to examine skeletal muscle, is useful in diagnosing myositis. Following administration of local anesthesia under sterile conditions in an outpatient setting or in an operating room, a surgical incision is made to obtain the desired specimen, which is sent to the laboratory for microscopic analysis. A pressure dressing is applied, and the affected extremity is immobilized for 12 to 24 hours.

An arterial biopsy may be performed to examine a specimen of an arterial wall using a procedure similar to that for a muscle biopsy. Most frequently the temporal artery is selected, but other arteries may be used as indicated. Arterial biopsy most often confirms inflammation of the vessel wall, or arteritis, a type of vasculitis.

A skin biopsy may be performed to confirm inflammatory connective tissue diseases such as lupus erythematosus or scleroderma. A specimen may be lightly scraped from the skin without causing discomfort. Deeper skin biopsies may be needed when scraping is insufficient.

BLOOD TESTS

In general, laboratory studies in rheumatology are based on the assumption that most rheumatic diseases are autoimmune disorders. Although many of the tests are highly complex and

Chart 54-1 • ASSESSMENT

Rheumatic Diseases

In addition to the head-to-toe assessment or systems review, the following are important areas of consideration to be noted when performing the complete physical assessment of a patient with a known or suspected rheumatic disease.

Manifestation	Significance
Skin (inquire and inspect)	
Rash, lesions	• Associated with lupus erythematosus, vasculitis, adverse effect of medication
Increased bruising	• Associated with several rheumatic diseases and adverse effect of medication
Erythema	• Sign of inflammation
Thinning	• Adverse effect of medication
Warmth	• Sign of inflammation
Photosensitivity	• Associated with systemic lupus erythematosus (SLE), dermatomyositis, adverse effect of medication
Hair (inquire and inspect)	
Alopecia or thinning	• Associated with rheumatic diseases or adverse effect of medication
Eye (inquire and inspect)	
Dryness, grittiness	• Associated with Sjögren's syndrome (commonly occurring with rheumatoid arthritis [RA] and LE)
Decreased acuity or blindness	• Associated with temporal arteritis, medication complications
Cataracts	• Adverse effect of medication
Decreased peripheral vision	• Adverse effect of medication
Conjunctivitis, uveitis	• Associated with ankylosing spondylitis and Reiter's syndrome
Ear (inquire)	
Tinnitus	• Adverse effect of medication
Decreased acuity	• Adverse effect of medication
Mouth (inquire and inspect)	
Buccal, sublingual lesions	• Associated with vasculitis, dermatomyositis, adverse effect of medication
Altered sense of taste	• Adverse effect of medication
Dryness	• Associated with Sjögren's syndrome
Dysphagia	• Associated with myositis
Difficulty chewing	• Associated with decreased range of motion of jaw
Chest (inspect and inquire)	
Pleuritic pain	• Associated with RA and SLE
Decreased chest expansion	• Associated with ankylosing spondylitis
Activity intolerance (dyspnea)	• Associated with pulmonary hypertension in scleroderma
Cardiovascular system (inquire, inspect, palpate)	
Blanching of fingers on exposure to cold	• Associated with Raynaud's phenomenon
Peripheral pulses	• Deficit may indicate vascular involvement or edema associated with medication effect or rheumatic diseases, especially SLE or scleroderma
Abdomen (inquire and palpate)	
Altered bowel habits	• Associated with scleroderma, spondylosis, ulcerative colitis, decreased physical mobility, medication effect
Nausea, vomiting, bloating, and pain	• Adverse effect of medication
Weight change (measure)	• Associated with RA (decreased), adverse effect of medication (increased or decreased)
Genitalia (inquire and inspect)	
Dryness, itching	• Associated with Sjögren's syndrome
Abnormal menses	• Adverse effect of medication
Altered sexual performance	• Fear of pain (or of pain caused by partner) and limitation of motion may affect sexual mobility.
Hygiene	• Poor hygiene may be related to limitations in activities of daily living.
Urethritis, dysuria	• Associated with ankylosing spondylitis and Reiter's syndrome
Lesions	• Associated with vasculitis
Neurologic (inquire and inspect)	
Paresthesias of extremities; abnormal reflex pattern	• Nerve compressions associated with carpal tunnel syndrome, spinal stenosis, etc.
Headaches	• Associated with temporal arteritis, adverse effect of medication
Musculoskeletal (inspect and palpate)	
Joint redness, warmth, swelling, tenderness, deformity—location of first joint involved, pattern of progression, symmetry, acute vs chronic nature	• Signs of inflammation
Joint range of motion	• Decreased range of motion may indicate severity or progression of disease.
Surrounding tissue findings	
Muscle atrophy, subcutaneous nodules, popliteal cyst	• Extra-articular manifestations
Muscle strength (grip)	• Muscle strength decreases with increased disease activity.

1617

technical, no single test used in isolation sufficiently supports a diagnosis of a rheumatic disease. Some of the most common blood studies are listed with their corresponding normal ranges and primary indications in Table 54-1. Because many of the tests require special laboratory techniques, they may not be used in every health care facility. The physician determines which tests are necessary based on the symptoms, stage of disease, and cost and likely benefit of the test.

IMPLICATIONS

Diagnosis of a specific rheumatic disease may or may not be relatively simple and clear-cut. Commonly, observation of clinical signs and symptoms over time is needed to make the diagnosis. The combination of history, assessment, testing, and evolving manifestations of the disease may require explanation and interpretation to the patient with early disease. This is especially true for patients with multisystem rheumatic disease, such as one of the connective tissue diseases.

The presence of crystals or bacteria in the synovial fluid is specifically diagnostic for gout or infectious arthritis, respectively. Diagnosis, however, may be more presumptive in the case of the older person who is thought to have osteoarthrosis (OA) based on single joint involvement, supportive x-ray findings, and no evidence of other disease processes (Altman et al., 2000).

Many forms of rheumatic disease can be accurately diagnosed by the primary health care provider, but patients with more complicated signs and symptoms may need referral to a rheumatologist (a physician who specializes in diagnosing and treating rheumatic disease). Patients should know which type of rheumatic disease they have, not just that they have "arthritis" or "arthritis of the knee."

Gerontologic Considerations

Although people of all ages, from infancy through childhood, adolescence, and maturity, may be affected, rheumatic disease is commonly thought of by the patient, family, and society as a whole as an inevitable consequence of aging. Many older people expect and accept the immobility and self-care problems related to the rheumatic diseases and do not seek help, thinking that nothing can be done. Careful diagnosis and appropriate treatment can improve the quality of life for older people. However, the rheumatic diseases do have some special implications for the older adult.

In elderly patients, other medical conditions may take precedence over the rheumatic disease, which commonly becomes a secondary diagnosis and concern. Identifying the effects of the rheumatic disease on the patient's lifestyle, independence, and other chronic or acute conditions is important.

The frequency, pattern of onset, clinical features, severity, and effects on function of the rheumatic disease in elderly patients may be different in very elderly patients. Some of the rheumatic diseases, such as OA, are more prevalent with aging (Altman et al., 2000). One disease, polymyalgia rheumatica, is exclusive to the elderly (Gonzalez-Gay et al., 1999), whereas some disorders may be less severe for elderly people than for younger patients. However, OA, the most prevalent activity-limiting condition among elderly people, may account for more total disability among elderly patients than many diseases, such as stroke or cancer, that are considered more serious.

In some instances, the age of the patient and coexisting health problems may make diagnosis difficult. A missed diagnosis is not unusual because of the assumption that most older people with joint problems have OA. In addition, it may be difficult to differentiate problems associated with aging from those caused by a rheumatic disease. For example, rheumatoid arthritis (RA) that begins in the later years has been shown to differ prognostically and therapeutically from RA that begins in childhood or early adulthood. In the elderly patient with initial RA, the onset is more likely to be abrupt, but the clinical course does not appear to differ from that of RA with an insidious onset. Moreover, patients with elderly-onset RA are less likely to have subcutaneous nodules or rheumatoid factor at disease onset (Ruddy et al., 2001).

For the elderly person who has had a diffuse connective tissue disease, the risk for osteoporosis is increased. Pain, loss of mobility, diminished self-image, and increasing morbidity can result from progressive osteoporosis. Thus, diagnosis and treatment for osteoporosis should not be overlooked in this population. Exercise, postural assistance, analgesic agents, modification of activities of daily living, and psychological support can be useful.

Other conditions (eg, soft tissue problems such as bursitis) usually are not problematic by themselves. When combined with other health problems and the normal physiologic processes of aging, however, these conditions may significantly reduce the patient's quality of life. In fact, the effects of most forms of rheumatic disease may lead to considerable changes in the individual's lifestyle, possibly threatening his or her independence. Decreased vision and altered balance, often present in elderly people, may be problematic if rheumatic disease in the lower extremities affects locomotion. Also, the combination of poor hearing, diminished vision, memory loss, and depression contributes to nonadherence to the treatment regimen in elderly patients. Special techniques for promoting patient safety, self-management, and strategies such as memory aids for medications may be necessary.

Partly because of the more frequent contact of the elderly with the health care system for a variety of health issues, overtreatment or inappropriate treatment is possible. Complaints of pain may be met with a prescription for an opioid analgesic rather than instructions for rest, use of an assistive device, and local comfort measures such as heat or cold. Acetaminophen may be appropriate and worth trying before using other medications that pose a greater chance of side effects. Intra-articular corticosteroid injections, with their usually rapid relief of symptoms, may be requested by the patient who is unaware of the consequences of too-frequent use. In addition to these factors, exercise programs may not be instituted or may be ineffective because the patient expects results to occur quickly or fails to appreciate the effectiveness of a program of exercise.

Pharmacologic treatment of rheumatic disease in older patients is more difficult than it is in younger patients. If the medications used have an effect on the senses (hearing, cognition), this effect is intensified in the elderly. The cumulative effect of medications is accentuated because of the physiologic changes of aging. For example, decreased renal function in the elderly alters the metabolism of certain medications, such as nonsteroidal anti-inflammatory drugs (NSAIDs). Elderly patients are more prone to such side effects as gastroduodenal ulceration or bleeding, and they are more likely to use nonprescription remedies, to try many different medications (polypharmacy), and to be susceptible to unproven treatment methods (Michocki, 2001).

Elderly patients with rheumatic disease may accept or endure pain, loss of ambulation, and difficulty with activities of daily living unnecessarily. The need to view oneself as capable of managing life independently despite increasing age may take considerable energy. The body image and self-esteem of the elderly person with rheumatic disease, combined with underlying depression, may interfere with the use of assistive devices such as canes. Use of adaptive equipment such as long-handled reachers or tongs may be viewed as evidence of aging rather than as a means of increasing independence.

Table 54-1 • **Common Blood Studies for Rheumatic Diseases**

TEST	NORMAL VALUE	SIGNIFICANCE
Serum		
Creatinine Metabolic waste excreted through the kidneys	0.7–1.2 mg/dL (62–106 µmol/L)	Increase may indicate renal damage in SLE, scleroderma, and polyarteritis.
Erythrocyte Sedimentation Rate (ESR) Measures the rate at which red blood cells settle out of unclotted blood in 1 hour	Female 0–20mm Male 0–10mm	Increase is usually seen in inflammatory connective tissue diseases. An increase indicates rising inflammation, resulting in clustering of RBCs, which makes them heavier than normal. The higher the ESR, the greater the inflammatory activity.
Hematocrit Measures the size, capacity, and number of cells present in blood	*Men:* 42–52% *Women:* 35–47%	Decrease can be seen in chronic inflammation (anemia of chronic disease); also, blood loss through bowel due to medication.
Red Blood Cell Count Measures circulating erythrocytes	*Men:* Average 4.8 million/µL *Women:* Average 4.3 million/µL	Decrease can be seen in RA, SLE.
White Blood Cell Count Measures circulating leukocytes	5,000–10,000 cells/mm³	Decrease may be seen in SLE.
VDRL (Venereal Disease Research Laboratory) Measures antibody to syphilis	Nonreactive	False-positive results are sometimes found with SLE.
Uric Acid Measures level of uric acid in serum	2.5–8 mg/dL (0.15–0.5 mmol/L)	Increase is seen with gout.
Serum Immunology		
Antinuclear Antibody (ANA) Measures antibodies that react with a variety of nuclear antigens If antibodies are present, further testing determines the type of ANA circulating in the blood (anti-DNA, anti-RNP).	Negative A few healthy adults have a positive ANA.	Positive test is associated with SLE, RA, scleroderma, Raynaud's disease, Sjögren's syndrome, necrotizing arteritis. The higher the titer, the greater the inflammation. The pattern of immunofluorescence (speckled, homogeneous, or nucleolar) helps determine the diagnosis.
Anti-DNA, DNA binding Titer measurement of antibody to double-stranded DNA	Negative	High titer is seen in SLE; increases in titer may indicate increase in disease activity.
Complement levels—C_3, C_4 Complement is a protein substance that binds with antigen–antibody complexes for the purpose of lysis. When the number of complexes increases markedly, complement is used for lysis, thus depleting the amount available in the blood.	C_3: 55–120 mg/dL (550–1,200 mg/L) C_4: 11–40 mg/dL (110–400 mg/L)	Decrease may be seen in RA and SLE. Decrease indicates autoimmune and inflammatory activity.
C-Reactive Protein Test (CRP) Shows presence of abnormal glycoprotein due to inflammatory process	Trace–6 µg/mL	A positive reading indicates active inflammation. Often is positive for RA, disseminated lupus erythematosus
Immunoglobulin Electrophoresis Measures the values of immunoglobulins	IgA 50–300 mg/dL (0.5–3 g/L) IgG 635–1,400 mg/dL (6.35–14 g/L) IgM 40–280 mg/dL (0.4–238 g/L)	Increased levels are found in people who have autoimmune disorders.
Rheumatoid Factor (RF) Determines the presence of abnormal antibodies seen in connective tissue disease	Negative	Positive titer > 1 : 80 Present in 80% of those with RA Positive RF may also suggest SLE, Sjögren's syndrome, or mixed connective tissue disease. The higher the titer (number at right of colon), the greater the inflammation.
Tissue Typing		
HLA-B27 Antigen Measures presence of HLA antigens, which are used for tissue recognition	Negative	Found in 80%–90% of those with ankylosing spondylitis and Reiter's syndrome.

The elderly person usually has a lifelong pattern of dealing with the stresses of daily life. Depending on the success of that pattern, the elderly person can often maintain a positive attitude and self-esteem when faced with a rheumatic disease, especially when support is available. Previous stress management strategies are assessed. If these strategies have been effective, the patient is encouraged and supported in their use. If the strategies were ineffective, the nurse assists the patient in identifying alternative strategies, encourages use of new strategies, and assesses their effectiveness.

Medical Management

A treatment program involving the interdisciplinary team, including the patient, is the basis for managing the rheumatic diseases. The chronic nature of most of these diseases mandates that the patient understand the disease, have the information necessary to make good self-management decisions, and be presented with a therapeutic program that is compatible with his or her lifestyle. Table 54-2 outlines the goals and strategies of basic rheumatic disease management.

PHARMACOLOGIC THERAPY

Medications are used with the rheumatic diseases to manage symptoms, control inflammation, and in some instances to modify the disease. Useful medications include the salicylates, NSAIDs, and disease-modifying antirheumatic drugs. Table 54-3 reviews the medications often used.

Controlling the inflammation related to the disease process will help in managing pain, but this is often a delayed response. Nonopioid medications are often used for pain management, especially early in the treatment program, until other measures can be instituted (Burckhardt, 2001a). Short-term use of low-dose antidepressant medications, such as amitriptyline, may be prescribed to reestablish adequate sleep patterns and improve pain management (Wegner, 2001).

NONPHARMACOLOGIC PAIN MANAGEMENT

Nonpharmacologic methods of pain management are important. Methods used include therapeutic heat or cold and devices such as a cane or a wrist splint to protect and support the joint. A combination of methods may be required because different methods often work better at different times.

Exercise and Activity

The ongoing nature of most rheumatic diseases makes it important to maintain and, when possible, improve joint mobility and overall functional status. The individualized exercise program is crucial to movement. Table 54-4 summarizes the exercises appropriate for patients with rheumatic diseases. Appropriate programs of exercise have been shown to decrease pain and improve function. A mild analgesic may be suggested prior to exercise for a patient starting a program of exercise. Acute or prolonged pain associated with exercise should be reported to a health care provider for evaluation (Minor & Westby, 2001).

The major challenge for the patient and the health care provider is the need to adjust all aspects of treatment according to the activity of the disease. Especially for the patient with an active diffuse connective tissue disease, such as RA or systemic lupus erythematosus (SLE), activity levels may vary from day to day and even within the day itself.

NURSING PROCESS: THE PATIENT WITH A RHEUMATIC DISEASE

Assessment

The depth and focus of the nursing assessment depend on several factors: the health care setting (clinic or office, home, extended care facility, or hospital), the role of the nurse (home care nurse; nurse practitioner; hospital, clinic, or office nurse), and the needs of the patient. The nurse is often the first of the health care team members to come in contact with the patient. This enables the nurse to assess the patient's perceptions of the disorder and situation, actions taken to relieve symptoms, plans for treatment, and expectations. The nurse's assessment may lead to identifying issues and concerns that can be addressed by nursing interventions and, through collaboration with other team members, to achieving the expected patient outcomes.

The health history and physical assessment focus on current and past symptoms, such as fatigue, weakness, pain, stiffness, fever, or anorexia, and the effects of these symptoms on the patient's lifestyle and self-image. Because the rheumatic diseases affect many body systems, the history and physical assessment include a review and examination of all systems, with particular attention given to those areas most commonly affected, including the musculoskeletal system (see Chart 54-1).

The patient's psychological and mental status and social support systems are also assessed, as is his or her ability to participate in daily activities, comply with the treatment regimen, and manage self-care. The information obtained can give insight into the patient's understanding of the medication regimen and may reveal misuse of medications, noncompliance, or use of potentially harmful unproven remedies. Additional areas assessed include the patient's understanding, motivation, knowledge, coping abilities, past experiences, preconceptions, and fears. The effects of the disease on the patient's self-concept and coping abilities are also assessed. The patient's perception of the condition and its impact influences the decisions, choices, and actions associated with treatment recommendations.

Table 54-2 • **Goals and Strategies for Rheumatic Diseases**	
MAJOR GOALS	MANAGEMENT STRATEGY
Suppress inflammation and the autoimmune response	Optimize pharmacologic therapy (anti-inflammatory and disease-modifying agents)
Control pain	Protect joints; ease pain with splints, thermal modalities, relaxation techniques
Maintain or improve joint mobility	Implement exercise programs for joint motion and muscle strengthening and overall health
Maintain or improve functional status	Make use of adaptive devices and techniques
Increase patient's knowledge of disease process	Provide and reinforce patient teaching
Promote self-management by patient compatible with the therapeutic regimen	Emphasize compatibility of therapeutic regimen and lifestyle

Table 54-3 • Medications Used in Rheumatic Diseases

MEDICATION	ACTION, USE, AND INDICATION	NURSING CONSIDERATIONS
Salicylates *Acetylated* aspirin *Nonacetylated* choline magnesium trisalicylate (Trilisate) choline salicylate (Arthropan) diflunisal (Dolobid) salsalate (Disalcid) sodium salicylate	*Action:* anti-inflammatory, analgesic, antipyretic Acetylated salicylates are platelet aggregation inhibitors. Anti-inflammatory doses will produce blood salicylate levels of 20–30 mg/dL.	Administer with meals to prevent gastric irritation. Assess for tinnitus, gastric intolerance, GI bleeding, and purpura. Monitor for possible confusion in the elderly.
Nonsteroidal Anti-inflammatory Drugs (NSAIDs) diclofenac (Voltaren) etodolac (Lodine) flurbiprofen (Ansaid) ibuprofen (Motrin) indomethacin (Indocin) ketoprofen (Orudis, Oruvail) meclofenamate (Meclomen) meloxicam (Mobic) nabumatone (Relafen) naproxen (Naprosyn) oxaprozin (DayPro) piroxicam (Feldene) sulindac (Clinoril) tolmetin sodium (Tolectin)	*Action:* anti-inflammatory, analgesic, antipyretic, platelet aggregation inhibitor Anti-inflammatory effect occurs 2–4 weeks after initiation. All NSAIDs are useful for short-term treatment of acute gout attack. NSAIDs are alternative to salicylates for first-line therapy in several rheumatic diseases.	Administer NSAIDs with food. Monitor for GI, CNS, cardiovascular, renal, hematologic, and dermatologic adverse effects. Avoid salicylates; use acetaminophen for additional analgesia. Watch for possible confusion in the elderly.
COX-2 inhibitors celocoxib (Celebrex) rofecoxib (Vioxx) valdecoxib (Bextra)	*Action:* Inhibit only cyclooxygenase-2 (COX-2) enzymes, which are produced during inflammation and spare COX-1 enzymes, which can be protective to the stomach and kidneys	Monitoring the same as for other NSAIDs Appropriate for the elderly and patients who are at high risk for gastric ulcers
Disease-Modifying Antirheumatic Drugs (DMARDs) Antimalarials hydroxychloroquine (Plaquenil) chloroquine (Aralen)	*Action:* Anti-inflammatory, inhibits lysosomal enzymes Slow-acting, onset may take 2–4 months Useful in RA and SLE	Administer concurrently with NSAIDs. Assess for visual changes, GI upset, skin rash, headaches, photosensitivity, bleaching of hair. Emphasize need for ophthalmologic exams (every 6–12 months).
Gold-containing compounds aurothioglucose (Solganol) gold sodium thiomalate (Myochrysine) auranofin (Ridaura)	*Action:* Inhibits T- and B-cell activity, suppresses synovitis during active stage of rheumatoid disease Slow-acting, onset may take 3–6 months IM preparations are given weekly for about 6 months, then every 2–4 weeks	Administer concurrently with NSAIDs. Assess for stomatitis, diarrhea, dermatitis, proteinuria, hematuria, bone marrow suppression (decreased WBCs and/or platelets), CBC and urinalysis with every other injection
sulfasalazine (Azulfidine)	*Action:* Anti-inflammatory, reduces lymphocyte response, inhibits angiogenesis Useful in RA, seronegative spondyloarthropathies	Administer concurrently with NSAIDs. Do not use in patients with allergy to sulfa medications or salicylates. Emphasize adequate fluid intake. Assess for GI upset, skin rash, headache, liver abnormalities, anemia.
penicillamine (Cuprimine)	*Action:* Anti-inflammatory, inhibits T-cell function, impairs antigen presentation Slow-acting, onset may take 2–3 months Useful in RA and systemic sclerosis	Administer concurrently with NSAIDs. Assess for GI irritation, decreased taste, skin rash or itching, bone marrow suppression, proteinuria with CBC, and urinalysis every 2–4 weeks.
Immunosuppressives methotrexate (Rheumatrex) azathioprine (Imuran) cyclophosphamide (Cytoxan)	*Action:* Immune suppression, effects DNA synthesis and other cellular effects Have teratogenic potential; azathioprine and cyclophosphamide reserved for more aggressive or unresponsive disease Methotrexate is "gold standard" for RA treatment; also useful in SLE.	Assess for bone marrow suppression, GI ulcerations, skin rashes, alopecia, bladder toxicity, increased infections. Monitor CBC, liver enzymes, creatinine every 2–4 weeks. Advise patient of contraceptive measures because of teratogenicity.

(continued)

Table 54-3 • Medications Used in Rheumatic Diseases (Continued)

MEDICATION	ACTION, USE, AND INDICATION	NURSING CONSIDERATIONS
cyclosporine (Neoval)	*Action:* Immunomodulator Used for severe, progressive RA, unresponsive to other DMARDs Used in combination with methotrexate	Assess slow dose titration upward until response noted or toxicity occurs. Assess for toxic effects: bleeding gums, fluid retention, hair growth, tremors. Monitor blood pressure and creatinine every 2 weeks until stable.
Immunomodulators leflunomide (Arava)	*Action:* Inhibit pyrimidine synthesis; anti-inflammatory May be used alone or in combination with other DMARDs. Used in moderate to severe RA.	Long half-life; requires loading dose followed by daily administration. Assess for diarrhea, nausea, rash, alopecia. Contraindicated in pregnancy. Monitor liver function tests.
etanercept (Enbrel)	*Action:* Binds to tumour necrosis factor, a cytokine involved in inflammatory and immune responses. Used in moderate to severe RA unresponsive to methotrexate.	Teach patient subcutaneous self-injection to be administered 2×/week. Monitor for injection site reactions. Educate patient about increased potential for infection and to withhold medication if fever occurs.
infliximab (Remicade)	May be used in combination with methotrexate	
Corticosteroids prednisone prednisolone hydrocortisone intra-articular injections	*Action:* Anti-inflammatory, analgesic Used for shortest duration and at lowest dose possible to minimize adverse effects Useful for unremitting RA, SLE, polymyalgia rheumatica, myositis, arteritis Fast-acting; onset in days Injections useful for joints unresponsive to NSAIDs	Assess for toxicity: cataracts, GI irritation, hyperglycemia, hypertension, fractures, avascular necrosis, hirsutism, psychosis. Joints most amenable to injections include ankles, knees, hips, shoulders, and hands. Repeated injections can cause joint damage.
Topical Analgesics capsaicin (Zostrix)	*Action:* analgesic	Teach patient to apply sparingly, avoid areas of open skin, avoid contact with eyes and mucous membranes. Wash hands carefully after application. Assess for local skin irritation.

DMARDs, disease-modifying antirheumatic drugs.

Diagnosis

NURSING DIAGNOSES

Although many nursing diagnoses are appropriate for the patient with a rheumatic disease, a few of the most common include the following:

- Acute and chronic pain related to inflammation and increased disease activity, tissue damage, fatigue, or lowered tolerance level
- Fatigue related to increased disease activity, pain, inadequate sleep/rest, deconditioning, inadequate nutrition, emotional stress/depression
- Disturbed sleep pattern related to pain, depression, and medications
- Impaired physical mobility related to decreased range of motion, muscle weakness, pain on movement, limited endurance, lack of or improper use of ambulatory devices
- Self-care deficits related to contractures, fatigue, or loss of motion
- Disturbed body image related to physical and psychological changes and dependency imposed by chronic illness
- Ineffective coping related to actual or perceived lifestyle or role changes

COLLABORATIVE PROBLEMS/ POTENTIAL COMPLICATIONS

Based on assessment data, potential complications may include the following:

- Adverse effects of medications

Planning and Goals

The major goals for the patient may include relief of pain and discomfort, relief of fatigue, increased mobility, maintenance of self-care, improved body image, effective coping, and absence of complications.

Table 54-4 • Suggested Exercises to Promote Mobility

INFLAMMATORY PROCESS (PAIN)	RECOMMENDED EXERCISE	PATIENT PERFORMANCE LEVEL
Acute exacerbation; severe pain	Passive range of motion (ROM)	Unable to perform exercises alone
Subacute; moderate or minimal pain	Active assistive or active ROM within pain tolerance	Can perform with help from another person or an assistive mechanical device
Inactive; remission; minimal pain or absence of pain	Active ROM: isometrics	Can perform alone

Nursing Interventions

An understanding of the underlying disease process (ie, degeneration or inflammation, including degeneration resulting from inflammation or vice versa) guides the nurse's critical thinking processes. In addition, knowledge about whether the condition is localized or more widely systemic influences the scope of the nursing activity.

Some rheumatic diseases (eg, OA) are more localized alterations in which control of symptoms such as pain or stiffness is possible. Others (eg, gout) have a known cause and specific treatment to control the symptoms. The diseases that usually present the greatest challenge are those with systemic manifestations, such as the diffuse connective tissue diseases. The Plan of Nursing Care details the nursing interventions to be considered for each nursing diagnosis.

RELIEVING PAIN AND DISCOMFORT

Medications are used on a short-term basis to relieve acute pain. Because the pain may be persistent, nonopioid analgesics such as acetaminophen are often used. After administering medications, the nurse needs to reassess pain levels at intervals. With persistent pain, assessment findings should be compared with baseline measurements and evaluations. Additional measures include exploring coping skills and strategies that have worked in the past.

The patient needs to understand the importance of taking medications, such as NSAIDs and disease-modifying agents, exactly as prescribed to achieve maximum benefits. These benefits include relief of pain and anti-inflammatory action as the disease is brought under control. Because disease control and pain relief are delayed, the patient may mistakenly believe the medication is ineffective or may think of the medication as merely "pain pills," taking them only sporadically and failing to achieve control over the disease activity. Alternately, the patient may not understand the need to continue the medication for its anti-inflammatory actions once pain control has been achieved.

A weight reduction program may be recommended to relieve stress on painful joints. Heat applications are also helpful in relieving pain, stiffness, and muscle spasm. Superficial heat may be applied in the form of warm tub baths or showers and warm moist compresses. Paraffin baths (dips), which offer concentrated heat, are helpful to patients with wrist and small-joint involvement. Maximum benefit is achieved within 20 minutes of application. More frequent use for shorter lengths of time is most beneficial. Therapeutic exercises can be carried out more comfortably and effectively after heat has been applied.

In some patients, however, heat may actually increase pain, muscle spasm, and synovial fluid volume. If the inflammatory process is acute, cold applications in the form of moist packs or an ice bag may be tried. Both heat and cold are analgesic to nerve pain receptors and can relax muscle spasms. Safe use of heat and cold must be evaluated and taught, particularly to patients with impaired sensation.

The use of braces, splints, and assistive devices for ambulation, such as canes, crutches, and walkers, eases pain by limiting movement or stress from weight bearing on painful joints. Acutely inflamed joints can be rested by applying splints to limit motion. Splints also support the joint to relieve spasm. Canes and crutches can relieve stress from inflamed and painful weight-bearing joints while promoting safe ambulation. Cervical collars may be used to support the weight of the head and limit cervical motion. A metatarsal bar or special pads may be put into shoes if foot pain or deformity is present.

Other strategies for decreasing pain include muscle relaxation techniques, imagery, self-hypnosis, and distraction.

DECREASING FATIGUE

Fatigue related to rheumatic disease can be both acute (brief and relieved by rest or sleep) and chronic. Chronic fatigue, related to the disease process, is persistent, cumulative, and not eliminated by rest but is influenced by biologic, psychological, social, and personal factors.

Disease-related factors that may influence the amount and severity of fatigue include persistent pain, sleep disturbance, impaired physical activity, and disease duration. Pain increases fatigue by requiring additional physical and emotional energy to deal with it. It may also cause the patient to expend more energy to do tasks in a way that causes less pain. Pain may also interfere with sleep, thereby increasing the fatigue level (Aaronson et al., 1999; Wolfe & Skevington, 2000).

Efforts are aimed at modifying and reducing the fatigue. Energy may be regained by using rest periods. The patient's needs determine the type and amount of rest needed. Naps or nighttime sleep can provide systemic rest. Splints can provide articular rest by limiting motion and stress on the joints. Relaxation techniques can provide emotional rest. Inactivity may lead to deconditioning and fatigue, so measures to build endurance should be instituted. Conditioning exercise, such as walking, swimming, or biking, requires gradual progression of activity and monitoring of disease activity.

Psychosocial factors with an effect on fatigue include depression, learned helplessness, and perceived social support (Belza, 2001; Parker et al., 2001). These factors affect the patient's perception and evaluation of the fatigue. Improvement of functional status can improve mood. The patient is taught strategies to conserve energy, such as planning and grouping activities to minimize the number of times the patient needs to climb the stairs each day and sitting down to prepare meals.

PROMOTING RESTORATIVE SLEEP

Restful sleep is important in helping the patient to cope with pain, minimize physical fatigue, and deal with the changes necessitated by a chronic disease. In patients with acute disease, sleep time is frequently reduced and fragmented by prolonged awakenings. Stiffness, depression, and medications may also compromise the quality of sleep and increase daytime fatigue. A sleep-inducing routine, medication, and comfort measures may help improve the quality of sleep.

INCREASING MOBILITY

Proper body positioning is essential to minimize stress on inflamed joints and prevent deformities that limit mobility. All joints should be supported in a position of optimal function. When in bed, the patient should lie flat on a firm mattress, with feet positioned against a footboard and with only one pillow under the head because of the risk of dorsal kyphosis. A pillow should not be placed under the knees because this promotes flexion contracture. The patient should lie prone several times daily to prevent hip flexion contracture.

Active range-of-motion exercises are encouraged because they prevent joint stiffness. If the patient cannot actively exercise the joints, passive range of motion should be performed.

Measures to reinforce proper body posture and increase mobility include walking erect and using chairs with straight backs. When seated, the patient should rest the feet flat on the floor and the shoulders and hips against the back of the chair.

(text continues on page 1626)

Nursing Interventions	Rationale	Expected Patient Outcomes

Nursing Diagnosis: Acute and chronic pain related to inflammation and increased disease activity, tissue damage, or lowered tolerance level

Goal: Improvement in comfort level; incorporation of pain management techniques into daily life

1. Provide variety of comfort measures
  a. Application of heat or cold
  b. Massage, position changes, rest
  c. Foam mattress, supportive pillow, splints
  d. Relaxation techniques, diversional activities
2. Administer anti-inflammatory, analgesic, and slow-acting antirheumatic medications as prescribed.
3. Individualize medication schedule to meet patient's need for pain management.
4. Encourage verbalization of feelings about pain and chronicity of disease.
5. Teach pathophysiology of pain and rheumatic disease, and assist patient to recognize that pain often leads to unproved treatment methods.
6. Assist in identification of pain that leads to use of unproven methods of treatment.
7. Assess for subjective changes in pain.
	1. Pain may respond to non-pharmacologic interventions such as joint protection, exercise, relaxation, and thermal modalities.
	
	2. Pain of rheumatic disease responds to individual or combination medication regimens.
	3. Previous pain experiences and management strategies may be different from those needed for persistent pain.
	4. Verbalization promotes coping.
	5. Knowledge of rheumatic pain and appropriate treatment may help patient avoid unsafe, ineffective therapies.
	6. The impact of pain on an individual's life often leads to misconceptions about pain and pain management techniques.
	7. The individual's description of the pain sensation is a more reliable indicator than objective measurements such as change in vital signs, body movement, and facial expression.
		• Identifies factors that exacerbate or influence pain response
		• Identifies and uses pain management strategies
		• Verbalizes decrease in pain
		• Reports signs and symptoms of side effects in timely manner to prevent additional problems
		• Verbalizes that pain is characteristic of rheumatic disease
		• Establishes realistic pain-relief goals
		• Verbalizes that pain often leads to the use of nontraditional and unproved self-treatment methods
		• Identifies changes in quality or intensity of pain

Nursing Diagnosis: Fatigue related to increased disease activity, pain, inadequate sleep/rest, deconditioning, inadequate nutrition, and emotional stress/depression

Goal: Incorporates as part of daily activities strategies necessary to modify fatigue

1. Provide instruction about fatigue
 	
  a. Describe relationship of disease activity to fatigue.
  b. Describe comfort measures while providing them.
  c. Develop and encourage a sleep routine (warm bath and relaxation techniques that promote sleep).
  d. Explain importance of rest for relieving systematic, articular, and emotional stress.
  e. Explain how to use energy conservation techniques (pacing, delegating, setting priorities).
  f. Identify physical and emotional factors that can cause fatigue.
 	
2. Facilitate development of appropriate activity/rest schedule.
3. Encourage adherence to the treatment program.
4. Refer to and encourage a conditioning program.
5. Encourage adequate nutrition, including source of iron from food and supplements.
	1. The patient's understanding of fatigue will affect his or her actions.
	  a. The amount of fatigue is directly related to the activity of the disease.
	  b. Relief of discomfort can relieve fatigue.
	
	  c. Effective bedtime routine promotes restorative sleep.
	
	  d. Different kinds of rest are needed to relieve fatigue and are based on patient need and response.
	  e. A variety of measures can be used to conserve energy.
	
	  f. Awareness of the various causes of fatigue provides the basis for measures to modify the fatigue.
	2. Alternating rest and activity conserves energy while allowing most productivity.
	3. Overall control of disease activity can decrease the amount of fatigue.
	4. Deconditioning resulting from lack of mobility, understanding, and disease activity contributes to fatigue.
	5. A nutritious diet can help counteract fatigue.
		• Self-evaluates and monitors fatigue pattern
		• Verbalizes the relationship of fatigue to disease activity
		• Uses comfort measures as appropriate
		• Practices effective sleep hygiene and routine
		• Makes use of various assistive devices (splints, canes) and strategies (bed rest, relaxation techniques) to ease different kinds of fatigue
		• Incorporates time management strategies in daily activities
		• Uses appropriate measures to prevent physical and emotional fatigue
		• Has an established plan to ensure well-paced, therapeutic activity schedule
		• Adheres to therapeutic program
		• Follows a planned conditioning program
		• Consumes a nutritious diet consisting of appropriate food groups and recommended daily allowance of vitamins and minerals

(continued)

Plan of Nursing Care
Care of the Patient With a Rheumatic Disease *(Continued)*

Nursing Interventions	Rationale	Expected Patient Outcomes

Nursing Diagnosis: Impaired physical mobility related to decreased range of motion, muscle weakness, pain on movement, limited endurance, lack of or improper use of ambulatory devices

Goal: Attains and maintains optimal functional mobility

Nursing Interventions	Rationale	Expected Patient Outcomes
1. Encourage verbalization regarding limitations in mobility.	1. Mobility is not necessarily related to deformity. Pain, stiffness, and fatigue may temporarily limit mobility. The degree of mobility is not synonymous with the degree of independence. Decreased mobility may influence a person's self-concept and lead to social isolation.	• Identifies factors that interfere with mobility • Describes and uses measures to prevent loss of motion • Identifies environmental (home, school, work, community) barriers to optimal mobility • Uses appropriate techniques and/or assistive equipment to aid mobility • Identifies community resources available to assist in managing decreased mobility

2. Assess need for occupational or physical therapy consultation:
  a. Emphasize range of motion of affected joints.
  b. Promote use of assistive ambulatory devices.
  c. Explain use of safe footwear.
  d. Use individual appropriate positioning/posture.
	2. Therapeutic exercises, proper footwear, and/or assistive equipment may improve mobility. Correct posture and positioning are necessary for maintaining optimal mobility.	

3. Assist to identify environmental barriers.	3. Furniture and architectural adaptations may enhance mobility.	

4. Encourage independence in mobility and assist as needed.
  a. Allow ample time for activity
  b. Provide rest period after activity.
  c. Reinforce principles of joint protection and work simplification.
	4. Changes in mobility may lead to a decrease in personal safety.	

5. Initiate referral to community health agency.	5. The degree of mobility may be slow to improve or may not improve with intervention.	

Nursing Diagnosis: Self-care deficits related to contractures, fatigue, or loss of motion

Goal: Achieves self-care independently or with the use of resources

Nursing Interventions	Rationale	Expected Patient Outcomes
1. Assist patient to identify self-care deficits and factors that interfere with ability to perform self-care activities.	1. The ability to perform self-care activities is influenced by the disease activity and the accompanying pain, stiffness, fatigue, muscle weakness, loss of motion, and depression.	• Identifies factors that interfere with the ability to perform self-care activities • Identifies alternative methods for meeting self-care needs • Uses alternative methods for meeting self-care needs • Identifies and uses other health care resources for meeting self-care needs

2. Develop a plan based on the patient's perceptions and priorities on how to establish and achieve goals to meet self-care needs, incorporating joint protection, energy conservation, and work simplification concepts.
  a. Provide appropriate assistive devices.
  b. Reinforce correct and safe use of assistive devices.
  c. Allow patient to control timing of self-care activities.
  d. Explore with the patient different ways to perform difficult tasks or ways to enlist the help of someone else.
	2. Assistive devices may enhance self-care abilities. Effective planning for changes must include the patient who must accept and adopt the plan.	

3. Consult with community health care agencies when individuals have attained a maximum level of self-care yet still have some deficits, especially regarding safety.	3. Individuals differ in ability and willingness to perform self-care activities. Changes in ability to care for self may lead to a decrease in personal safety.	

(continued)

Plan of Nursing Care
Care of the Patient With a Rheumatic Disease (Continued)

Nursing Interventions	Rationale	Expected Patient Outcomes

Nursing Diagnosis: Disturbed body image related to physical and psychological changes and dependency imposed by chronic illness

Goal: Adapts to physical and psychological changes imposed by the rheumatic disease

Nursing Interventions	Rationale	Expected Patient Outcomes

1. Help patient identify elements of control over disease symptoms and treatment.
2. Encourage patient's verbalization of feelings, perceptions, and fears.
  a. Help to assess present situation and identify problems.
  b. Assist to identify past coping mechanisms.
  c. Assist to identify effective coping mechanisms.
	1. The individual's self-concept may be altered by the disease or its treatment.
	2. The individual's coping strategies reflect the strength of his or her self-concept.
		• Verbalizes an awareness that changes taking place in self-concept are normal responses to rheumatic disease and other chronic illnesses
		• Identifies strategies to cope with altered self-concept

Nursing Diagnosis: Ineffective coping related to actual or perceived lifestyle or role changes

Goal: Use of effective coping behaviours for dealing with actual or perceived limitations and role changes

Nursing Interventions	Rationale	Expected Patient Outcomes
1. Identify areas of life affected by disease. Answer questions and dispel possible myths. 2. Develop plan for managing symptoms and enlisting support of family and friends to promote daily function.	1. The effects of disease may be more or less manageable once identified and explored reasonably. 2. By taking action and involving others appropriately, patient develops or draws on coping skills and community support.	• Names functions and roles affected and not affected by disease process • Describes therapeutic regimen and states actions to take to improve, change, or accept a particular situation, function, or role

Collaborative Problems: Complications secondary to effects of medications

Goal: Experiences absence or resolution of complications

Nursing Interventions	Rationale	Expected Patient Outcomes
1. Perform periodic clinical assessment and laboratory evaluation. 2. Instruct in correct self-administration, side effects, and importance of monitoring. 3. Counsel regarding methods to reduce side effects and manage symptoms. 4. Administer medications in modified doses as prescribed if complications occur.	1. Skillful assessment helps detect early symptoms of side effects of medications. 2. The patient needs accurate information about medications and side effects to avoid or manage them. 3. Appropriate identification and early intervention may minimize complications. 4. Modifications may help minimize side effects or other complications.	• Complies with monitoring procedures and experiences minimal side effects • Takes medication as prescribed and lists potential side effects • Identifies strategies to reduce or manage side effects • Reports that side effects or complications have subsided

Care must be taken so that splinting for comfort does not restrict mobility later. The knee is splinted at full extension and the wrist at slight dorsiflexion. Because of the predominant strength of flexor muscles, the joints should not be permitted to "freeze" in positions of flexion. This can be prevented by regularly removing the splint and exercising the joint through a range of motion. Splint modification may be needed when changes occur in joint structure.

Additionally, assistive devices may be necessary for mobility. They should be properly fitted and the patient should be instructed in their correct and safe use. A cane, long enough to allow for only a slight bend of the elbow, should be held in the hand opposite the affected side. Forearm-trough style crutches (platform crutches) may be needed to protect the upper extremities if the disease also involves the hands and wrists. This is especially important for the patient undergoing rehabilitation after lower extremity joint reconstructive surgery. Assistive devices can mean the difference between dependence and independence in mobility; however, they may also alter the patient's body image, which can become a barrier to compliance with treatment.

FACILITATING SELF-CARE

Adaptive equipment may increase the patient's independence. When introducing adaptive equipment, however, the nurse should be sensitive to the patient's feelings by demonstrating acceptance and positive attitudes about using these devices. The nurse needs to keep in mind that a patient's deformity does not necessarily equate with the severity of limitations or disability. For example, swollen hands may be more limiting than deformed hands. The nurse in the hospital or in the extended care facility can help preserve the patient's independence in these settings by making available adaptive equipment for eating, toileting, bathing, and dressing. In the home, the nurse can encourage use of these devices. Again, by relieving pain, stiffness, and fatigue, the nurse may increase the patient's ability to perform self-care (Luck, 2001).

IMPROVING BODY IMAGE AND COPING

All aspects of the patient's life, including perception of self, work role, social life, sexual function, and financial status, may be altered because of the unpredictability and uncertainty of the course of a rheumatic disease. Body image changes may cause social isolation and depression. The nurse and the family need to empathize with the patient's emotional reactions to the disease. Communication should be encouraged so that the patient and family verbalize feelings, perceptions, and fears related to the disease. The nurse helps the patient and family identify areas in which they have some control over disease symptoms and treatment. The nurse also encourages commitment to the treatment program, which is a key to positive outcomes, as well as use of effective coping strategies.

MONITORING AND MANAGING POTENTIAL COMPLICATIONS

Medications used for treating rheumatic diseases have the potential for serious and adverse effects. Thus, an important aspect of care is avoiding medication-induced complications. The physician bases the prescribed medication regimen on clinical findings and past medical history, then monitors for side effects with periodic clinical assessments and laboratory testing. The nurse has a major role in working with the physician and pharmacist to help the patient recognize and deal with side effects from medications. These side effects may include gastrointestinal bleeding or irritation, bone marrow suppression, kidney or liver toxicity, infection, mouth sores, rashes, and changes in vision. Other signs and symptoms include bruising, breathing problems, dizziness, jaundice, dark urine, black or bloody stools, diarrhea, nausea and vomiting, and headaches. Systemic and local infections, which can often be masked by high doses of corticosteroids, need close monitoring (see Table 54-3 for more information about administration considerations).

Patient instruction also includes teaching correct techniques of self-administration of medications, methods of reducing side effects, and measures to ensure regular monitoring. The nurse can be available for consultation between physician visits. If side effects occur, the medication may need to be stopped or the dose reduced. The patient may experience an increase in symptoms while the complication is being resolved or a new medication is being initiated. In such cases, the nurse's counselling regarding symptom management may relieve potential anxiety and distress.

PROMOTING HOME AND COMMUNITY-BASED CARE

Teaching Patients Self-Care

Patient teaching is an essential aspect of nursing care of the patient with rheumatic disease to enable the patient to maintain as much independence as possible, to take medications accurately and safely, and to use adaptive devices correctly. Patient teaching focuses on the disorder itself, the possible changes related to the disorder, the therapeutic regimen prescribed to treat it, the side effects of medications, strategies to maintain independence and function, and patient safety in the home (Chart 54-2).

The patient and family are encouraged to verbalize their concerns and ask questions. Pain, fatigue, and depression can interfere with the patient's ability to learn and should be addressed before initiating teaching. Various educational strategies may then be used, depending on the patient's previous knowledge base, interest level, degree of comfort, social or cultural influences, and readiness to learn. The nurse instructs the patient about basic disease management and necessary adaptations in lifestyle. Because suppression of inflammation and autoimmune responses requires the use of anti-inflammatory, disease-modifying antirheumatic and immunosuppressive agents, the patient is taught about prescribed medications, including type, dosage, rationale, side effects, self-administration, and required monitoring procedures. If hospitalized, the patient is encouraged to practice new self-management skills with support from caregivers and significant others. The nurse then reinforces disease management skills during each patient contact. Barriers to compliance are assessed and measures are taken to promote adherence to medications and the treatment program.

Continuing Care

Depending on the severity of the disorder and the patient's resources and supports, referral for home care may or may not be warranted. However, the patient who is elderly or frail, has a rheumatic disorder that limits function significantly, and lives alone may need a referral for home care.

Chart 54-2
Home Care Checklist • The Patient with Rheumatic Disease

At the completion of the home care instruction, the patient or caregiver will be able to:	Patient	Caregiver
• Explain the nature of the disease and principles of disease management.	✓	✓
• Describe the medication regimen (name of medications, dosage, schedule of administration, precautions, side effects, and desired effects).	✓	✓
• Identify monitoring procedures and strategies that should be implemented.	✓	✓
• Identify sources of additional information, if necessary.	✓	✓
• Demonstrate accurate and safe self-administration of medications.	✓	✓
• Describe and demonstrate use of pain management techniques.	✓	✓
• Demonstrate use of joint protection techniques in activities of daily living (ADLs).	✓	✓
• Demonstrate ability to perform self-care activities independently or with assistive devices.	✓	
• Demonstrate a safe exercise program.	✓	
• Demonstrate a relaxation technique.	✓	

The impact of rheumatic disease on everyday life is not always evident when the patient is seen in the hospital or an ambulatory care setting. The increased frequency with which nurses see patients in the home provides opportunities for recognizing problems and implementing interventions aimed at improving the quality of life of patients with rheumatic disorders. The patient encountered in the home setting often has a rheumatic disease that is secondary to the primary reason for the visit. In such cases, the problems caused by the rheumatic disease may interfere with the treatment of the primary condition. For example, the patient who is recovering from coronary artery surgery may have been instructed to exercise but is unable or only partially able to do so because of the rheumatic disease. Conversely, treatment of the primary condition may cause or increase problems related to the rheumatic disease. For example, the cardiac patient who has been instructed to walk long distances every day may find that doing so increases the symptoms of OA in the knees.

During home visits, the nurse has the opportunity to assess the home environment and its adequacy for patient safety and management of the disorder. Compliance with the treatment program can be more easily monitored in the home setting, where physical and social barriers to adherence are more readily identified. For example, the patient with diabetes who requires insulin may be unable to fill the syringe accurately or administer the insulin because of impaired joint mobility. Appropriate adaptive equipment needed for increased independence is often identified more readily when the nurse sees how the patient functions in the home. Any barriers to compliance can be identified and appropriate referrals made.

For patients at risk for impaired skin integrity, the home care nurse can closely monitor skin status and also instruct, provide, or supervise the patient and family in preventive skin care measures. The nurse also assesses the patient's need for assistance in the home and supervises home health aides, who may meet many of the needs of the patient with a rheumatic disease. Referrals to physical and occupational therapists may be made as problems are identified and limitations increase. A home care nurse can visit the home to make sure the patient can function as independently as possible despite mobility problems and can safely manage treatments and pharmacotherapy. The patient and family should be alerted to support services such as Meals on Wheels and local Arthritis Society programs such as the Arthritis Self-Management Program.

Because many of the medications to suppress inflammation are injectable, the nurse may administer the medication to the patient or teach self-injection procedure. These frequent contacts allow the nurse to reinforce other disease management techniques.

The nurse also assesses the patient's physical and psychological status, adequacy of symptom management, and adherence to the management plan. Previous teaching is reinforced with emphasis on side effects of medications and changes in physical status indicating disease progression and the need to contact the health care provider for reevaluation; otherwise, patients may wait until their next appointment. The importance of follow-up appointments is emphasized to the patient and family.

Patients with chronic disorders often neglect general health issues if they are focused on their chronic disorder; therefore, the patient and family should be reminded about the importance of participating in other health promotion activities and health screening (eg, immunizations, cholesterol screening, bone density testing, gynecologic examinations, mammography, colonoscopy).

Evaluation

EXPECTED PATIENT OUTCOMES

Expected patient outcomes may include:

1. Experiences relief of pain or improved comfort level
   a. Identifies factors that cause or increase pain
   b. Identifies realistic goals for pain relief
   c. Uses pain management strategies safely and effectively
   d. Reports decreased pain and increased comfort level
2. Experiences reduction in level of fatigue
   a. Identifies factors that contribute to fatigue
   b. Verbalizes the relationship of fatigue to disease activity
   c. Schedules periodic rest periods and identifies and uses other measures to prevent or modify fatigue
   d. Reports decreased level of fatigue
   e. Practices energy conservation strategies
3. Improves sleep patterns
   a. Reports fewer night-time awakenings
   b. Adheres to sleep-inducing routine
   c. Reports feeling rested upon awakening
4. Increases or maintains level of mobility
   a. Identifies factors that impede mobility
   b. Participates in activities and exercises that promote or maintain mobility
   c. Uses assistive devices appropriately and safely
   d. Demonstrates normal or acceptable body alignment and posture
5. Maintains self-care activities
   a. Participates in self-care activities within capabilities
   b. Uses adaptive equipment and alternative methods to increase participation in self-care activities
   c. Maintains self-care at highest possible level
6. Experiences improved body image and coping
   a. Verbalizes concerns about the impact of rheumatic disease on appearance and function
   b. Sets and achieves meaningful goals
   c. States acceptance of self-worth
   d. Adapts to body image changes caused by disease
   e. Identifies and uses effective coping strategies
7. Experiences absence of complications
   a. Takes medications as prescribed
   b. States potential side effects of medications and names reportable side effects
   c. Verbalizes understanding of rationale for monitoring
   d. Complies with recommendations for monitoring
   e. Identifies strategies to reduce risks of side effects

Diffuse Connective Tissue Diseases

Diffuse connective tissue disease refers to a group of disorders that are chronic in nature and characterized by diffuse inflammation and degeneration in the connective tissues. These disorders share similar clinical features and may affect some of the same organs. The characteristic clinical course is one of exacerbations and remissions. Although the diffuse connective tissue diseases have unknown causes, they are thought to be the result of immunologic abnormalities. They include RA, SLE, scleroderma, polymyositis, and polymyalgia rheumatica.

RHEUMATOID ARTHRITIS

Pathophysiology

RA is commonly used as the prototype for inflammatory arthritis. The incidence rate is approximately 3%, with a two to three times greater incidence in women (Ruddy et al., 2001). In RA, the autoimmune reaction (Fig. 54-3) primarily occurs in the synovial tissue. Phagocytosis produces enzymes within the joint. The enzymes break down collagen, causing edema, proliferation of the synovial membrane, and ultimately pannus formation. Pannus destroys cartilage and erodes the bone. The consequence is loss of articular surfaces and joint motion. Muscle fibres undergo degenerative changes. Tendon and ligament elasticity and contractile power are lost.

Clinical Manifestations

Clinical manifestations of RA vary, usually reflecting the stage and severity of the disease. Joint pain, swelling, warmth, erythema, and lack of function are classic. Palpation of the joints reveals spongy or boggy tissue. Often fluid can be aspirated from the inflamed joint. Characteristically, the pattern of joint involvement begins with the small joints in the hands, wrists, and feet. As the disease progresses, the knees, shoulders, hips, elbows, ankles, cervical spine, and temporomandibular joints are involved. The onset of symptoms is usually acute. Symptoms are usually bilateral and symmetric. In addition to joint pain and swelling, another classic sign of RA is joint stiffness, especially in the morning, lasting for more than 30 minutes (Klippel, 2001).

In the early stages of disease, even before bony changes occur, limitation in function can occur when there is active inflammation in the joints. Joints that are hot, swollen, and painful are not easily moved. The patient tends to guard or protect these joints through immobilization. Immobilization for extended periods can lead to contractures, creating soft tissue deformity.

Deformities of the hands and feet are common in RA (Fig. 54-4). The deformity may be caused by misalignment resulting from swelling, progressive joint destruction, or the subluxation (partial dislocation) that occurs when a bone slips over another and eliminates the joint space.

RA is a systemic disease with multiple extra-articular features. Most common are fever, weight loss, fatigue, anemia, lymph node enlargement, and Raynaud's phenomenon (cold- and

 ## Physiology/Pathophysiology

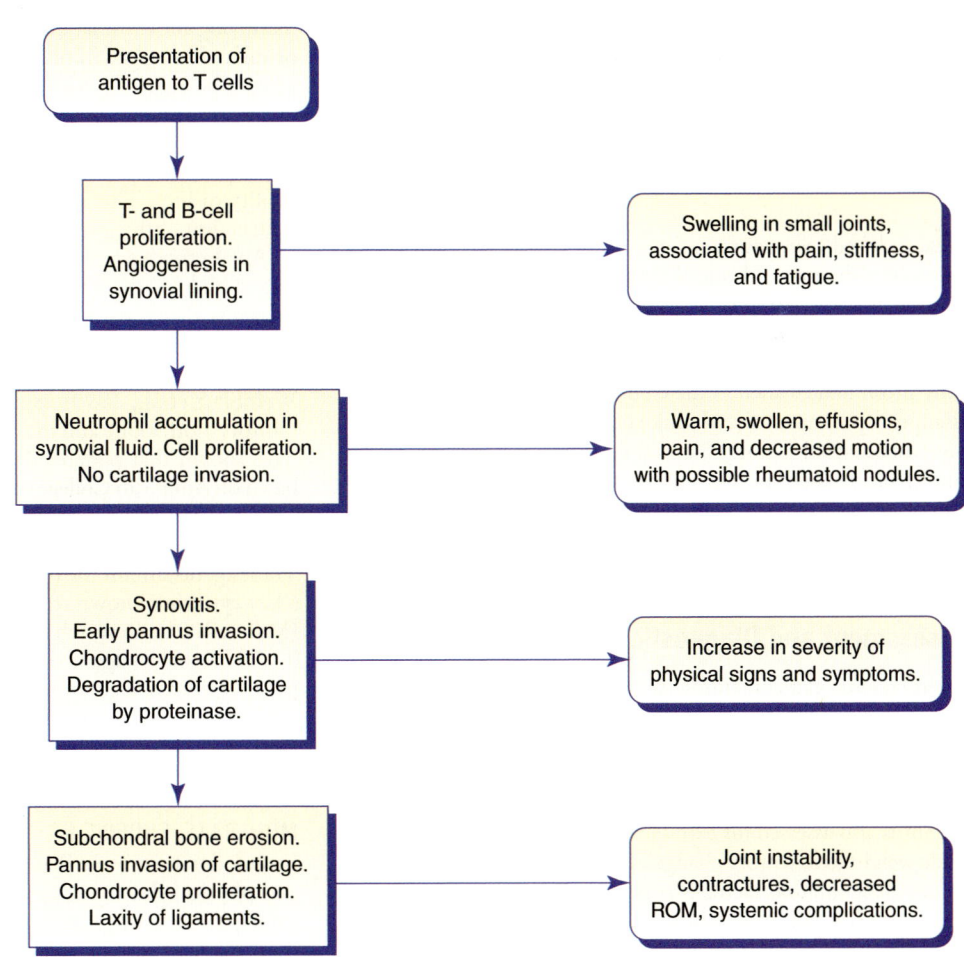

FIGURE 54-3 Pathophysiology and associated physical signs of rheumatoid arthritis.

FIGURE 54-4 Rheumatoid arthritis. (**A**) Early. (**B**) Advanced.

stress-induced vasospasm causing episodes of digital blanching or cyanosis). Rheumatoid nodules may be noted in patients with more advanced RA and develop at some time in up to half of patients (Klippel, 2001). These nodules are usually nontender and movable in the subcutaneous tissue. They usually appear over bony prominences such as the elbow, are varied in size, and can disappear spontaneously. Nodules occur only in individuals who have rheumatoid factor. The nodules often are associated with rapidly progressive and destructive disease. Other extra-articular features include arteritis, neuropathy, scleritis, pericarditis, spleno-megaly, and Sjögren's syndrome (dry eyes and dry mucous membranes).

Assessment and Diagnostic Findings

Several factors can contribute to a diagnosis of RA: rheumatoid nodules, joint inflammation detected on palpation, and certain laboratory findings. The history and physical examination address manifestations such as bilateral and symmetric stiffness, tenderness, swelling, and temperature changes in the joints. The patient is also assessed for extra-articular changes; these often include weight loss, sensory changes, lymph node enlargement, and fatigue. Rheumatoid factor is present in more than 80% of patients with RA, but its presence alone is not diagnostic of RA. The erythrocyte sedimentation rate (ESR) is significantly elevated with RA. The red blood cell count and C4 complement component are decreased. C-reactive protein and antinuclear antibody test results may also be positive. Arthrocentesis shows synovial

fluid that is cloudy, milky, or dark yellow and contains numerous inflammatory components, such as leukocytes and complement.

X-ray studies, performed to help diagnose and monitor the progression of disease, show characteristic bony erosions and narrowed joint spaces occurring later in the disease.

Medical Management

EARLY-STAGE RA

In patients with early RA, treatment begins with education, a balance of rest and exercise, and referral to community agencies for support. Medical management begins with therapeutic doses of salicylates or NSAIDs. When used in full therapeutic dosages, these medications provide both anti-inflammatory and analgesic effects. Taking medications as prescribed to maintain a consistent blood level is necessary to optimize the effectiveness of the anti-inflammatory medication.

Several COX-2 inhibitors, another class of NSAIDs, have been approved for treatment of RA. COX (cyclooxygenase) is an enzyme involved in the inflammatory process. COX-2 inhibitors block the enzyme involved in inflammation while leaving intact the enzyme involved in protecting the stomach lining. As a result, COX-2 inhibitors are less likely to cause gastric irritation and ulceration than other NSAIDs (Bombardier et al., 2000).

The trend in management is toward a more aggressive pharmacologic approach earlier in the disease. A window of opportunity for symptom control and improved disease management occurs within the first 2 years of disease onset. Therefore, the disease-modifying antirheumatic agents (antimalarials, gold, penicillamine, or sulfasalazine) are initiated early in treatment. If symptoms appear to be aggressive (ie, early bony erosions as seen on x-rays), methotrexate may be considered. Methotrexate is currently the gold standard in the treatment of RA because of its success in improving disease parameters (ie, pain, tender and swollen joints, quality of life). The goals are to control symptoms and prevent destruction of the joints (Koopman, 2001).

An alternative treatment approach for RA has emerged in the area of biologic therapies. Biologic response modifiers are a group of agents that consist of molecules produced by cells of the immune system or by cells that participate in the inflammatory reactions (Koopman, 2001). Recent studies (Moreland et al., 1999; Weinblatt et al., 1999) using tumour necrosis factor-alpha inhibitors, both alone and in combination with other medications, have shown that patients demonstrate significant improvement based on American College of Rheumatology criteria (Felson et al., 1995). Two examples of biologic response modifiers that are currently available are enatercept (Enbrel) and infliximab (Remicade). These agents inhibit the function of tumour necrosis factor-alpha, a key **cytokine** known to play a role in the disease process in RA (Miller, 2001). Research in this area is ongoing.

Additional analgesia may be prescribed for periods of extreme pain. Opioid analgesics are avoided because of the potential for continuing need for pain relief. Nonpharmacologic pain management techniques (eg, relaxation techniques, heat and cold applications) are taught.

MODERATE, EROSIVE RA

For moderate, erosive RA, a formal program with occupational and physical therapy is prescribed to educate the patient about principles of joint protection, pacing activities, work simplification, range of motion, and muscle-strengthening exercises. The patient is encouraged to participate actively in the management program. The medication program is reevaluated periodically, and appropriate changes are made if indicated. Cyclosporine, an immunomodulator, may be added to enhance the disease-modifying effect of methotrexate.

PERSISTENT, EROSIVE RA

For persistent, erosive RA, reconstructive surgery and corticosteroids are often used. Reconstructive surgery is indicated when pain cannot be relieved by conservative measures. Surgical procedures include synovectomy (excision of the synovial membrane), tenorrhaphy (suturing a tendon), arthrodesis (surgical fusion of the joint), and **arthroplasty** (surgical repair and replacement of the joint). Surgery is not performed during disease flares.

Systemic corticosteroids are used when the patient has unremitting inflammation and pain or needs a "bridging" medication while waiting for the slower disease-modifying antirheumatic agent (eg, methotrexate) to begin working. Low-dose corticosteroid therapy is prescribed for the shortest time necessary to minimize side effects. Joints that are severely inflamed and fail to respond promptly to the measures outlined previously may be treated by local injection of a corticosteroid (Ruddy et al., 2001).

ADVANCED, UNREMITTING RA

For advanced, unremitting RA, immunosuppressive agents are prescribed because of their ability to affect the production of antibodies at the cellular level. These include high-dose methotrexate (Rheumatrex), cyclophosphamide (Cytoxan), and azathioprine (Imuran). These medications, however, are highly toxic and can produce bone marrow suppression, anemia, gastrointestinal disturbances, and rashes.

Through all stages of RA, depression and sleep deprivation may require the short-term use of low-dose antidepressant medications, such as amitriptyline (Elavil), paroxetine (Paxil), or sertraline (Zoloft), to reestablish an adequate sleep pattern and to manage chronic pain better.

The FDA has approved a medical device for use in treating patients with more severe and longstanding cases of RA who have failed to respond to or are intolerant of disease-modifying antirheumatic drugs. The device, a protein A Immunoadsorption column (Prosorba), is used in 12 weekly 2-hour apheresis treatments to bind IgG (ie, circulating immune complex). In this unique population of patients, a significant improvement using the American College of Rheumatology Criteria for Improvement has been demonstrated in several studies using the Prosorba column (Felson et al., 1999; Gendreau, 2001).

Nutrition Therapy

Patients with RA frequently experience anorexia, weight loss, and anemia. A dietary history identifies usual eating habits and food preferences. Food selection should include the daily requirements from the basic food groups, with emphasis on foods high in vitamins, protein, and iron for tissue building and repair. For the extremely anorexic patient, small, frequent feedings with increased protein supplements may be prescribed. Some medications (ie, oral corticosteroids) used in RA treatment stimulate the appetite and, when combined with decreased activity, may lead to weight gain. Therefore, patients may need to be counselled about eating a healthy, calorie-restricted diet.

Nursing Management

Nursing care of the patient with RA follows the basic plan of care presented earlier in the chapter. The most common issues for the patient with RA include pain, sleep disturbance, fatigue,

altered mood, and limited mobility. The patient with newly diagnosed RA needs information about the disease to make daily self-management decisions and to cope with having a chronic disease.

Because of repeated contact with the patient, the nurse has the opportunity to assess and intervene in patient concerns and issues that occur with the diagnosis of a chronic illness such as RA. Because the disease commonly affects young women, major concerns may be related to the effects of the disease on childbearing potential, caring for family, or work responsibilities. The patient with a chronic illness may seek a "cure" or have questions about alternative therapies. Frequently, however, patients are hesitant to share their concerns with health care professionals (American College of Rheumatology, 1998).

SYSTEMIC LUPUS ERYTHEMATOSUS

The overall prevalence of SLE is estimated to be 100 per 100,000 persons. It occurs 10 times more frequently in women than in men and approximately three times more frequently in the African-American population than in Caucasians (Ruddy et al., 2001).

Pathophysiology

SLE is a result of disturbed immune regulation that causes an exaggerated production of autoantibodies. This immunoregulatory disturbance is brought about by some combination of genetic, hormonal (as evidenced by the usual onset during the childbearing years), and environmental factors (sunlight, thermal burns). Certain medications, such as hydralazine (Apresoline), procainamide (Pronestyl), isoniazid (INH), chlorpromazine (Thorazine), and some antiseizure medications, have been implicated in chemical or drug-induced SLE.

In SLE, the increase in autoantibody production is thought to result from abnormal suppressor T-cell function, leading to immune complex deposition and tissue damage. Inflammation stimulates antigens, which in turn stimulate additional antibodies, and the cycle repeats.

Clinical Manifestations

The onset of SLE may be insidious or acute. For this reason, SLE may remain undiagnosed for many years. Clinical features of SLE involve multiple body systems.

SYSTEMIC MANIFESTATIONS

SLE is an autoimmune systemic disease that can affect any body system. Involvement of the musculoskeletal system, with arthralgias and arthritis (synovitis), is a common presenting feature of SLE. Joint swelling, tenderness, and pain on movement are also common. Frequently, these are accompanied by morning stiffness.

Several different types of skin manifestations may occur in patients with SLE, including subacute cutaneous lupus erythematosus, which involves papulosquamous or annular polycyclic lesions, and discoid lupus erythematosus, which is a chronic rash that has erythematous papules or plaques and scaling and can cause scarring and pigmentation changes. The most familiar skin manifestation (but occurring in fewer than half of patients with SLE) is an acute cutaneous lesion consisting of a butterfly-shaped rash across the bridge of the nose and cheeks (Fig. 54-5). In some cases of discoid lupus erythematosus, only skin involvement may occur. In some SLE patients, the initial skin involvement may be

FIGURE 54-5 The characteristic butterfly rash of systemic lupus erythematosus.

the precursor to more systemic involvement. The lesions often worsen during exacerbations (flares) of the systemic disease and possibly are provoked by sunlight or artificial ultraviolet light. Oral ulcers, which may accompany skin lesions, may involve the buccal mucosa or the hard palate. The ulcers occur in crops and are often associated with exacerbations.

Pericarditis is the most common cardiac manifestation. Women who have SLE are also at risk for early atherosclerosis.

Serum creatinine levels and urinalysis are used in screening for renal involvement. Early detection allows for prompt treatment so that renal damage can be prevented. Renal involvement may lead to hypertension, which also requires careful monitoring and management.

Central nervous system involvement is widespread, encompassing the entire range of neurologic disease. The varied and frequent neuropsychiatric presentations of SLE are now widely recognized. These are generally demonstrated by subtle changes in behaviour patterns or cognitive ability. Depression and psychosis are common (Klippel, 2001; Petri, 2000; Ruddy et al., 2001).

Assessment and Diagnostic Findings

Diagnosis of SLE is based on a complete history, physical examination, and blood tests. In addition to the general assessment performed for any patient with a rheumatic disease, assessment for known or suspected SLE has special features. The skin is inspected for erythematous rashes. Cutaneous erythematous plaques with an adherent scale may be observed on the scalp, face, or neck. Areas of hyperpigmentation or depigmentation may be noted, depending on the phase and type of the disease. The patient should be questioned about skin changes (because these may be transitory) and specifically about sensitivity to sunlight or artificial ultraviolet light. The scalp should be inspected for alopecia and the mouth and throat for ulcerations reflecting gastrointestinal involvement.

Cardiovascular assessment includes auscultation for pericardial friction rub, possibly associated with myocarditis and accompanying pleural effusions. The pleural effusions and infiltrations, which reflect respiratory insufficiency, are demonstrated by abnormal lung sounds. Papular, erythematous, and purpuric lesions developing on the fingertips, elbows, toes, and extensor surfaces of the forearms or lateral sides of the hand that may become necrotic suggest vascular involvement.

Joint swelling, tenderness, warmth, pain on movement, stiffness, and edema may be detected on physical examination. The joint involvement is often symmetric and similar to that found in RA.

Typically, assessment reveals classic symptoms, including fever, fatigue, and weight loss and possibly arthritis, pleurisy, and pericarditis. Interactions with the patient and family may provide further evidence of systemic involvement. The neurologic assessment is directed at identifying and describing any central nervous system changes. The patient and family members are asked about any behavioural changes, including manifestations of neuroses or psychosis. Signs of depression are noted, as are reports of seizures, chorea, or other central nervous system manifestations.

No single laboratory test confirms SLE; rather, blood testing reveals moderate to severe anemia, thrombocytopenia, leukocytosis, or leukopenia and positive antinuclear antibodies. Other diagnostic immunologic tests support but do not confirm the diagnosis. Hematuria may be found on urinalysis.

Medical Management

Treatment of SLE includes management of acute and chronic disease. Although SLE can be life-threatening, advances in its treatment have led to improved survival and reduced morbidity. Acute disease requires interventions directed at controlling increased disease activity or exacerbations that may involve any organ system. Disease activity is a composite of clinical and laboratory features that reflect active inflammation secondary to SLE. Management of the more chronic condition involves periodic monitoring and recognition of meaningful clinical changes requiring adjustments in therapy (Ruddy et al., 2001).

The goals of treatment include preventing progressive loss of organ function, reducing the likelihood of acute disease, minimizing disease-related disabilities, and preventing complications from therapy. Management of SLE involves regular monitoring to assess disease activity and therapeutic effectiveness.

PHARMACOLOGIC THERAPY

Medication therapy for SLE is based on the concept that local tissue inflammation is mediated by exaggerated or heightened immune responses, which can vary widely in intensity and require different therapies at different times. The NSAIDs used for minor clinical manifestations are often used along with corticosteroids in an effort to minimize corticosteroid requirements.

Corticosteroids are the single most important medication available for treatment. They are used topically for cutaneous manifestations, in low oral doses for minor disease activity, and in high doses for major disease activity. Intravenous administration of corticosteroids is an alternative to traditional high-dose oral use. Antimalarial medications are effective for managing cutaneous, musculoskeletal, and mild systemic features of SLE. Immunosuppressive agents (alkylating agents and purine analogs) are used because of their effect on immune function. These medications are generally reserved for patients who have serious forms of SLE and who have not responded to conservative therapies (Kimberly, 2001; National Institutes of Health, 1998; Ruddy et al., 2001).

Nursing Management

The nursing care of the patient with SLE is based on the basic plan presented earlier in the chapter. The most common problems include fatigue, impaired skin integrity, body image disturbance, and lack of knowledge for self-management decisions. The disease or its treatment may produce dramatic changes in appearance and considerable distress for the patient. The changes and the unpredictable course of SLE necessitate expert assessment skills and nursing care and sensitivity to the psychological reactions of the patient. Patients may benefit from participation in support groups by receiving disease information, daily management tips, and social support. Because sun and ultraviolet light exposure can increase disease activity or cause an exacerbation, patients should be taught to avoid exposure or to protect themselves with sunscreen and clothing.

Because of the increased risk for involvement of multiple organ systems, patients should understand the need for routine periodic screenings as well as health promotion activities. A dietary consultation may be indicated to ensure that the patient is knowledgeable about dietary recommendations, given the increased risk for cardiovascular disease, including hypertension and atherosclerosis. The nurse instructs the patient about the importance of continuing prescribed medications and addresses the changes and side effects that are likely with their use. The patient is reminded of the importance of monitoring because of the increased risk for systemic involvement, including renal and cardiovascular effects.

SCLERODERMA

Scleroderma ("hard skin") is a relatively rare disease that is poorly understood; the cause is unknown. Its incidence is 18 to 20 persons per million per year (Ruddy et al., 2001).

Pathophysiology

Like other diffuse connective tissue diseases, scleroderma (also known as systemic sclerosis) has a variable course with remissions and exacerbations. Its prognosis is not as optimistic as that of SLE. The disease commonly begins with skin involvement. Mononuclear cells cluster on the skin and stimulate lymphokines to stimulate procollagen. Insoluble collagen is formed and accumulates excessively in the tissues. Initially, the inflammatory response causes edema formation, with a resulting taut, smooth, and shiny skin appearance. The skin then undergoes fibrotic changes, leading to loss of elasticity and movement. Eventually, the tissue degenerates and becomes nonfunctional. This chain of events, from inflammation to degeneration, also occurs in blood vessels, major organs, and body systems (Klippel, 2001).

Clinical Manifestations

Scleroderma starts insidiously with Raynaud's phenomenon and swelling in the hands. The skin and the subcutaneous tissues become increasingly hard and rigid and cannot be pinched up from the underlying structures. Wrinkles and lines are obliterated. The skin is dry because sweat secretion over the involved region is suppressed. The extremities stiffen and lose mobility. The condition

spreads slowly; for years, these changes may remain localized in the hands and the feet. The face appears masklike, immobile, and expressionless, and the mouth becomes rigid.

The changes within the body, although not visible directly, are vastly more important than the visible changes. The left ventricle of the heart is involved, resulting in heart failure. The esophagus hardens, interfering with swallowing. The lungs become scarred, impeding respiration. Digestive disturbances occur because of hardening (sclerosing) of the intestinal mucosa. Progressive renal failure may occur.

The patient may manifest a variety of symptoms referred to as the CREST syndrome. CREST stands for calcinosis (calcium deposits in the tissues), Raynaud's phenomenon, esophageal hardening and dysfunctioning, sclerodactyly (scleroderma of the digits), and telangiectasis (capillary dilation that forms a vascular lesion).

Assessment and Diagnostic Findings

Assessment focuses on the sclerotic changes in the skin, contractures in the fingers, and colour changes or lesions in the fingertips. Assessment of systemic involvement requires a systems review with special attention to gastrointestinal, pulmonary, renal, and cardiac symptoms. Limitations in mobility and self-care activities should be assessed, along with the impact the disease has had (or will have) on body image.

There is no one conclusive test to diagnose scleroderma. A skin biopsy is performed to identify cellular changes specific to scleroderma. Pulmonary studies show ventilation-perfusion abnormalities. Echocardiography identifies pericardial effusion (often present with cardiac involvement). Esophageal studies demonstrate decreased motility in 75% of patients with scleroderma. Blood tests may detect antinuclear antibodies, indicating a connective tissue disorder and possibly distinguishing the subgroup of scleroderma. A positive antinuclear antibody test result is common in patients with scleroderma.

Medical Management

Treatment of scleroderma depends on the clinical manifestations. All patients require counselling, during which realistic individual goals may be determined. Support measures include strategies to decrease pain and limit disability. A moderate exercise program is encouraged to prevent joint contractures. Patients are advised to avoid extreme temperatures and to use lotion to minimize skin dryness.

PHARMACOLOGIC THERAPY

No medication regimen has proved effective in modifying the disease process in scleroderma, but various medications are used to treat organ system involvement. Calcium channel blockers and other antihypertensive agents may provide improvement in symptoms of Raynaud's phenomenon. Anti-inflammatory medications can be used to control arthralgia, stiffness, and general musculoskeletal discomfort (Klippel, 2001; Ramsey-Goldman, 2001).

Nursing Management

The nursing care of the patient with scleroderma is based on the basic plan of nursing care presented earlier in the chapter. The most common nursing diagnoses of the patient with scleroderma include impaired skin integrity; self-care deficits; imbalanced nutrition, less than body requirements; and disturbed body image. The patient with advanced disease may also have problems with impaired gas exchange, decreased cardiac output, impaired swallowing, and constipation.

Providing meticulous skin care and preventing the effects of Raynaud's phenomenon are major nursing challenges. Patient teaching must include the importance of avoiding cold and protecting the fingers with mittens in cold weather and when shopping in the frozen-food section of the grocery store. Warm socks and properly fitting shoes are helpful in preventing ulcers. Careful, frequent inspection for early ulcers is important. Smoking cessation is critical.

POLYMYOSITIS

Polymyositis is one of a group of diseases termed idiopathic inflammatory myopathies. It is a rare condition with an incidence that is estimated to be from fewer than one to eight cases per million (Ruddy et al., 2001).

Pathophysiology

Polymyositis is classified as autoimmune because autoantibodies are present. However, these antibodies do not cause damage to muscle cells, indicating only an indirect role in tissue damage. The pathogenesis is multifactorial, and a genetic predisposition is likely. Drug-induced disease is rare. Some evidence suggests a viral link.

Clinical Manifestations

The onset varies from sudden onset with rapid progression to a very slow, insidious onset. Proximal muscle weakness is typically a first symptom. Muscle weakness is usually symmetric and diffuse. Dermatomyositis, a related condition, is most commonly identified by an erythematous smooth or scaly lesion found over the joint surface.

Assessment and Diagnostic Findings

A complete history and physical examination help to exclude other muscle-related disorders. As with other diffuse connective tissue disorders, no one test confirms polymyositis. An electromyogram is performed to rule out degenerative muscle disease. A muscle biopsy may reveal inflammatory infiltrate in the tissue. Serum studies indicate increased muscle enzyme activity.

Medical Management

Management involves high-dose corticosteroid therapy initially, followed by a gradual dosage reduction over several months as muscle enzyme activity decreases. Patients who do not respond to corticosteroids require the addition of an immunosuppressive agent. For patients who are unresponsive to corticosteroids and immunosuppressive medications, plasmapheresis, lymphapheresis, and total-body irradiation have been used. Skin rashes may respond to the antimalarial drug hydroxychloroquine. Physical therapy is initiated slowly with range-of-motion exercises to maintain joint mobility, followed by gradual strengthening exercises (Klippel, 2001).

Nursing Management

Nursing care is based on the basic plan of nursing care presented earlier in the chapter. The most frequent nursing diagnoses for the patient with polymyositis include impaired physical mobility, fatigue, self-care deficit, and insufficient knowledge of self-management techniques.

Patients with polymyositis may have symptoms similar to those of other inflammatory diseases. However, proximal muscle weakness is characteristic, making activities such as combing hair, reaching overhead, and using stairs difficult. Therefore, use of assistive devices may be recommended and referral to occupational or physical therapy may be warranted.

POLYMYALGIA RHEUMATICA

Pathophysiology

The underlying mechanism involved with polymyalgia rheumatica is unknown. This disease occurs predominately in Caucasians and often in first-degree relatives. An association with the genetic marker HLA-DR4 suggests a familial predisposition. Immunoglobulin deposits in the walls of inflamed temporal arteries also suggest an autoimmune process.

Clinical Manifestations

Polymyalgia rheumatica is characterized by severe proximal muscle discomfort with mild joint swelling. Severe aching in the neck, shoulder, and pelvic muscles is common. Stiffness is noticeable most often in the morning and after periods of inactivity. Systemic features include low-grade fever, weight loss, malaise, anorexia, and depression. Because polymyalgia rheumatica generally occurs in people 50 years of age and older, it may be confused with, or disregarded as, an inevitable consequence of aging.

Giant cell arteritis, sometimes associated with polymyalgia rheumatica, may cause headaches, changes in vision, and jaw claudication. These symptoms should be evaluated immediately because of the potential for a sudden and permanent loss of vision if untreated. Polymyalgia rheumatica and giant cell arteritis generally have a self-limited course, lasting several months to several years (Paget, 2001).

Assessment and Diagnostic Findings

Polymyalgia rheumatica and giant cell arteritis are found almost exclusively in people over 50 years of age. Giant cell arteritis has a reported incidence of 18 cases per 100,000, and polymyalgia rheumatica has an annual incidence rate of 52 cases per 100,000 over age 50 (Loeslie, 2000; Ruddy et al., 2001).

Assessment focuses on musculoskeletal tenderness, weakness, and decreased function. Careful attention should be directed toward assessing the head (for changes in vision, headaches, and jaw claudication).

Often diagnosis is difficult because of the lack of specificity of tests. A markedly high ESR is a screening test but is not definitive. Diagnosis is more likely to be made by eliminating other potential diagnoses, but this is highly dependent on the skills and experience of the diagnostician. The dramatic and immediate response to treatment with corticosteroids is considered by some to be diagnostic.

Medical Management

Polymyalgia rheumatica (without giant cell arteritis) is treated with moderate doses of corticosteroids. NSAIDs are sometimes used for mild disease. For patients with giant cell arteritis, rapid initiation of and strict adherence to a regimen of corticosteroids are essential to avoid the complication of blindness.

Nursing Management

The nursing care of the patient with polymyalgia rheumatica is based on the basic plan of nursing care presented earlier in the chapter. The most common nursing diagnoses include pain and insufficient knowledge of the medication regimen.

A management concern is that the patient will take the prescribed medication, frequently corticosteroids, until symptoms improve and then discontinue the medication. The decision to discontinue the medication should be based on clinical and laboratory findings. Nursing implications are related to helping the patient prevent and monitor side effects from medications (eg, infections, diabetes mellitus, gastrointestinal problems, and depression) and adjust to side effects that cannot be prevented (eg, increased appetite and altered body image).

 NURSING ALERT The nurse must emphasize to the patient the need for continued adherence to the prescribed medication regimen to avoid complications of giant cell arteritis such as blindness.

The loss of bone mass with corticosteroid use increases the risk for osteoporosis in this already at-risk population. Interventions to promote bone health such as adequate dietary calcium and vitamin D, weight-bearing exercise, and smoking cessation, if indicated, should be emphasized (Buckley et al., 2001; Loeslie, 2000).

Degenerative Joint Disease (Osteoarthritis)

OA, also known as degenerative joint disease or osteoarthrosis (even though inflammation may be present), is the most common and frequently disabling of the joint disorders. OA is both over-diagnosed and trivialized; it is frequently overtreated or under-treated. The functional impact of OA on quality of life, especially for elderly patients, is often ignored.

OA has been classified as primary (idiopathic), with no prior event or disease related to the OA, and secondary, resulting from previous joint injury or inflammatory disease. The distinction between primary and secondary OA is not always clear.

Increasing age directly relates to the degenerative process in the joint, as the ability of the articular cartilage to resist micro-fracture with repetitive low loads diminishes. OA often begins in the third decade of life and peaks between the fifth and sixth decades. By age 75 years, 85% of the population has either x-ray or clinical evidence of OA, but only 15% to 25% of these people experience significant symptoms (Ruddy et al., 2001).

Pathophysiology

OA may be thought of as the end result of many factors combining in a generalized predisposition to the disease. OA affects the articular cartilage, subchondral bone (the bony plate that supports the articular cartilage), and synovium. A combination of cartilage degradation, bone stiffening, and reactive inflammation of the synovium occurs. The basic degenerative process in the joint exemplified in OA is presented in Figure 54-6. Understanding of OA has been greatly expanded beyond what previously was thought of as simply "wear and tear" related to aging. Risk factors for OA are summarized in Chart 54-3.

Congenital and developmental disorders of the hip are well known for predisposing a person to OA of the hip. These include congenital subluxation–dislocation of the hip, acetabular dysplasia, Legg-Calvé-Perthes disease, and slipped capital femoral epiphysis.

 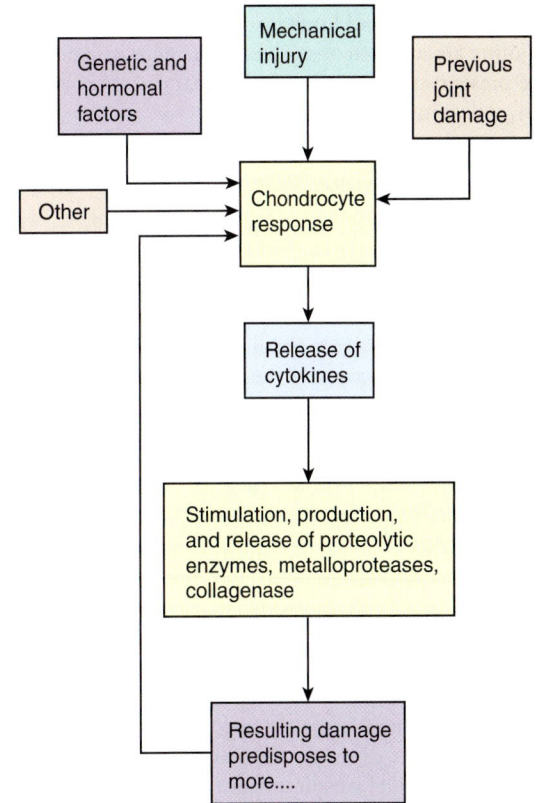

FIGURE 54-6 Pathophysiology of osteoarthritis.

Obesity is now a well-recognized risk factor for the development of OA (USDHHS, 2001). Being overweight or obese also increases the pain and discomfort associated with the disease (Altman et al., 2000; Coggon et al., 2001).

Clinical Manifestations

The primary clinical manifestations of OA are pain, stiffness, and functional impairment. The pain is due to an inflamed synovium, stretching of the joint capsule or ligaments, irritation of nerve endings in the periosteum over osteophytes, trabecular micro-fracture, intraosseous hypertension, bursitis, tendinitis, and muscle spasm. Stiffness, which is most commonly experienced in the morning or after awakening, usually lasts less than 30 minutes

Chart 54-3
Risk Factors for Osteoarthritis

- Increased age
- Obesity
- Previous joint damage
- Repetitive use (occupational or recreational)
- Anatomic deformity
- Genetic susceptibility

and decreases with movement. Functional impairment is due to pain on movement and limited motion caused by structural changes in the joints.

Although OA occurs most often in weight-bearing joints (hips, knees, cervical and lumbar spine), the proximal and distal finger joints are also often involved. Characteristic bony nodes may be present; on inspection and palpation, these are usually painless, unless inflammation is present.

Assessment and Diagnostic Findings

Diagnosis of OA is complicated because only 30% to 50% of patients with changes seen on x-rays report symptoms. Physical assessment of the musculoskeletal system reveals tender and enlarged joints. Inflammation, when present, is not the destructive type seen in the connective tissue diseases such as RA. OA is characterized by a progressive loss of the joint cartilage, which appears on x-ray as a narrowing of joint space. In addition, reactive changes occur at the joint margins and on the subchondral bone in the form of osteophytes (or spurs) as the cartilage attempts to regenerate. Neither the presence of osteophytes nor joint space narrowing alone is specific for OA; however, when combined, these are sensitive and specific findings. In early or mild OA, there is only a weak correlation between joint pain and synovitis. Blood tests are not useful in the diagnosis of OA.

Medical Management

Although no treatment halts the degenerative process, certain preventive measures can slow the progress if undertaken early enough. These include weight reduction, prevention of injuries, perinatal screening for congenital hip disease, and ergonomic modifications.

Conservative treatment measures include the use of heat, weight reduction, joint rest and avoidance of joint overuse, orthotic devices to support inflamed joints (splints, braces), isometric and postural exercises, and aerobic exercise. Occupational and physical therapy can help the patient adopt self-management strategies.

PHARMACOLOGIC THERAPY

Pharmacologic management of OA is directed toward symptom management and pain control. Medications are used in conjunction with nonpharmacologic strategies, which are the mainstay of OA management (Altman et al., 2000). In most patients with OA, the initial analgesic therapy is acetaminophen. Some patients respond to the nonselective NSAIDs, and patients who are at increased risk for gastrointestinal complications, especially gastrointestinal bleeding, have been managed effectively with COX-2 inhibitors (Altman et al., 2000; Beehrle & Evans, 1999; Bombardier et al., 2000; Pasero & McCaffery, 2001; Ruddy et al., 2001). Selection of medication is based on the patient's needs, the stage of disease, and the risk for side effects. Other medications that may be considered are the opioids and intra-articular corticosteroids. Topical analgesics such as capsaicin and methylsalicylate are also recommended (Altman et al., 2000; Ruddy et al., 2001).

Newer therapeutic approaches include glucosamine and chondroitin, which are thought to improve tissue function and retard breakdown of cartilage (Altman et al., 2000; McAlindon et al., 2000). Viscosupplementation, the intra-articular injection of hyaluronic acid, is thought to improve cartilage function and retard degradation; it may also have some anti-inflammatory effects (Huskisson & Donnelly, 1999; Watterson & Esdaile, 2000; Wright et al., 2000). Glucosamine and chondroitin and visco-

supplementation, although approved by the U.S. FDA, are still undergoing intensive investigation for safety and efficacy (Brandt et al., 2000).

SURGICAL MANAGEMENT

In moderate to severe OA, when pain is severe or because of loss of function, surgical intervention may be used. Procedures most commonly used are osteotomy (to alter the force distribution in the joint) and arthroplasty. In arthroplasty, diseased joint components are replaced with artificial products (see Chap. 67).

Other procedures include viscosupplementation (the reconstitution of synovial fluid viscosity). Hyaluronic acid (Hyalgan, Synvisc), a glycosaminoglycan that acts as a lubricant and shock-absorbing fluid in the joint, may be used in this procedure. Hyaluronic acid stimulates the production of synoviocytes, possibly providing better and more prolonged pain control. A series of three to five weekly intra-articular injections are given. Pain relief may last for 6 months (Kellick et al., 1998).

Tidal irrigation (lavage) of the knee involves the introduction and then removal of a large volume of saline into the joint through cannulas. In some cases it provides pain relief for up to 6 months (Klippel, 2001; Lozada & Altman, 2001).

Nursing Management

The nursing management of the patient with OA includes both pharmacologic and nonpharmacologic approaches. The nonpharmacologic interventions are used first and continued with the addition of pharmacologic agents. Pain management and optimizing functional ability are major goals of nursing intervention. Patients' understanding of their disease process and symptom pattern is critical to a plan of care. Because patients with OA are older, they may have other health problems. Commonly they are overweight, and they may have a sedentary lifestyle. Weight loss and an increase in aerobic activity such as walking, with special attention to quadriceps strengthening, are important approaches to pain management (Altman et al., 2000; Bautch et al., 1997; Ettinger et al., 1997). A referral for physical therapy or to an exercise program for individuals with similar problems may be very helpful. Canes or other assistive devices for ambulation should be considered. Exercises such as walking should be begun in moderation and increased gradually. Patients should plan their daily exercise for a time when the pain is least severe or should plan to use an analgesic, if appropriate, before exercising. Adequate pain management is important for the success of an exercise program.

Spondyloarthropathies

The spondyloarthropathies are another category of systemic inflammatory disorders of the skeleton. The spondyloarthropathies include ankylosing spondylitis, reactive arthritis (Reiter's syndrome), and psoriatic arthritis. Spondyloarthritis is also associated with inflammatory bowel diseases such as regional enteritis (Crohn's disease) and ulcerative colitis.

These rheumatic diseases share several clinical features. The inflammation tends to occur peripherally at the sites of attachment—at tendons, joint capsules, and ligaments. Periosteal inflammation may be present. Many patients have arthritis of the sacroiliac joints. Onset tends to occur during young adulthood, with the disease affecting men more often than women. There is a strong tendency for these conditions to occur in families. Frequently, the HLA-B27 genetic marker is found.

NURSING RESEARCH PROFILE 54-1
Older Women With Osteoarthritis

Baird, C. L. (2000). Living with hurting and difficulty doing: Older women with osteoarthritis. *Clinical Excellence for Nurse Practitioners,* 4(4), 231–237.

Purpose
Osteoarthritis (OA), the most common rheumatic disorder in older adults, presents a major challenge to individuals' independence. A greater understanding of patient experiences is necessary to develop appropriate needs-based interventions to help patients maintain independence. The purpose of this study was to develop an understanding of how OA affects individuals' lives and to provide data on which to base nursing interventions.

Study Sample and Design
A qualitative research design was used. After informed written consent was obtained from eligible participants, semistructured interviews were conducted. The interviews were recorded for transcription and analysis. Data analyzed included the transcriptions of the interviews and the investigator's field notes of observations and impressions.

The sample comprised 18 women, 65 to 92 years of age, who reported having OA and who participated in an Area Council on Aging Centre or were referred by other study participants. Data were continuously compared throughout data gathering and analysis. A process of deconstructing and reconstructing the data into several levels of categories was carried out.

Findings
Subjects reported a continuous condition of "living with OA" and "living with hurting." Hurting characterized the participants' experience because of its chronicity and the participants' persistent discomfort and pain. The hurting was reported as being prominent during activities such as walking, attending to personal care, and managing tasks for independent living. This finding resulted in a second category: "living with difficulty doing." The state of "living with difficulty doing" was characterized by being unable to carry out activities because of pain, stiffness, and instability. Personal care and completing household tasks became difficult and often impossible to accomplish.

Nursing Implications
The findings of this study demonstrate the need for health care providers to understand the problems associated with living with OA and to assess the impact of OA on activities of daily living. Further, the findings emphasize the need to help patients with OA to obtain pain relief and to develop alternative strategies to deal with pain and to accomplish tasks important to them. These strategies include helping patients to learn how to pace themselves and to use nonpharmacologic modalities along with pharmacologic therapies for pain relief.

ANKYLOSING SPONDYLITIS

Ankylosing spondylitis affects the cartilaginous joints of the spine and surrounding tissues. Occasionally, the large synovial joints, such as hips, knees, or shoulders, may be involved. Ankylosing spondylitis is usually diagnosed in the second or third decade of life. The disease is not usually as severe in females as in males, in whom the disease is more prevalent and likely to include significant systemic involvement. Back pain is the characteristic feature. As the disease progresses, ankylosis of the entire spine may occur, leading to respiratory compromise and complications.

REACTIVE ARTHRITIS (REITER'S SYNDROME)

This disease process is called reactive because the arthritis occurs following an infection. It affects young adult males and is characterized primarily by urethritis, arthritis, and conjunctivitis. Dermatitis and ulcerations of the mouth and penis may also be present. Low back pain is common.

PSORIATIC ARTHRITIS

Psoriatic arthritis is characterized by synovitis, polyarthritis, and spondylitis. Both psoriasis and arthritis are common conditions, and one theory suggests that the overlap of the two conditions is a chance occurrence. However, epidemiologic data suggest that the prevalence of arthritis in patients with psoriasis is 7% to 42%, exceeding the rate in the general population. Similarly, the prevalence of psoriasis in persons with arthritis is 2.6% to 7.0%, compared with 0.1% to 2.8% in the general population, supporting the theory that these two processes occur together in a unique disease process (Ruddy et al., 2001).

Medical Management of Spondyloarthropathies

Medical management of spondyloarthropathies focuses on treating pain and maintaining mobility by suppressing inflammation. For the patient with ankylosing spondylitis, good body positioning and posture are essential, so that if **ankylosis** (fixation) does occur, the patient is in the most functional position. Maintaining range of motion with a regular exercise and muscle-strengthening program is especially important.

PHARMACOLOGIC THERAPY
Salicylates, NSAIDs, and corticosteroids often produce marked improvement in back, skin, and joint symptoms. Methotrexate is also used to control psoriasis as well as joint inflammation.

SURGICAL MANAGEMENT
Surgical management may include total hip replacement (see Chap. 67).

Nursing Management of Spondyloarthropathies

Major nursing interventions in the spondyloarthropathies are related to symptom management and maintaining optimal functioning. This population is unique in rheumatology, because patients are primarily young men. Their major concerns are often related to prognosis and job modification, especially among those who perform physical work.

Metabolic and Endocrine Diseases Associated With Rheumatic Disorders

Metabolic and endocrine diseases may be associated with rheumatic disorders. These include biochemical abnormalities (amyloidosis and scurvy), endocrine diseases (diabetes mellitus and acromegaly), immunodeficiency diseases (HIV infection, AIDS), and other hereditary disorders (hypermobility syndromes). The most common conditions, however, are the crystal-induced arthropathies in which crystals, such as monosodium urate (gout) or calcium pyrophosphate (calcium pyrophosphate dihydrate disease [CPPD] or pseudogout), are deposited within joints and other tissues.

GOUT

Gout is a heterogeneous group of conditions related to a genetic defect of purine metabolism resulting in hyperuricemia. Oversecretion of uric acid or a renal defect resulting in decreased excretion of uric acid, or a combination of both, occurs. The prevalence of gout is reported to be 1.6 to 13.6 per thousand. The incidence increases with age and body mass index. It occurs more commonly in males than females (Ruddy et al., 2001).

In primary hyperuricemia, elevated serum urate levels or manifestations of urate deposition appear to be consequences of faulty uric acid metabolism. Primary hyperuricemia may be due to severe dieting or starvation, excessive intake of foods that are high in purines (shellfish, organ meats), or heredity. In secondary hyperuricemia, gout is a clinical feature secondary to any of a number of genetic or acquired processes, including conditions in which there is an increase in cell turnover (leukemia, multiple myeloma, some types of anemias, psoriasis) and an increase in cell breakdown. Altered renal tubular function, either as a major action or as an unintended side effect of certain pharmacologic agents (diuretics such as thiazides and furosemide), low-dose salicylates, and ethanol can contribute to uric acid underexcretion.

Pathophysiology

Hyperuricemia (serum concentration greater than 7 mg/dL [0.4 fmol/L]) can but does not always cause monosodium urate crystal deposition. However, as uric acid levels rise, risk increases (Ruddy et al., 2001). Attacks of gout appear to be related to sudden increases or decreases of serum uric acid levels. When the urate crystals precipitate within a joint, an inflammatory response occurs and an attack of gout begins. With repeated attacks, accumulations of sodium urate crystals, called **tophi**, are deposited in peripheral areas of the body, such as the great toe, the hands, and the ear. Renal urate lithiasis (kidney stones) with chronic renal disease secondary to urate deposition may develop.

The finding of urate crystals in the synovial fluid of asymptomatic joints suggests that factors other than crystals may be related to the inflammatory reaction. Recovered monosodium urate crystals are coated with immunoglobulins that are mainly immunoglobulin G (IgG). IgG enhances crystal phagocytosis, thereby demonstrating immunologic activity.

Clinical Manifestations

Manifestations of the gout syndrome include acute gouty arthritis (recurrent attacks of severe articular and periarticular inflammation), tophi (crystalline deposits accumulating in articular tissue, osseous tissue, soft tissue, and cartilage), gouty nephropathy (renal impairment), and uric acid urinary calculi. Four stages of gout can be identified: asymptomatic hyperuricemia, acute gouty arthritis, intercritical gout, and chronic tophaceous gout. The subsequent development of gout is directly related to the duration and magnitude of the hyperuricemia. Therefore, the commitment to lifelong pharmacologic treatment of hyperuricemia is deferred until there is an initial attack of gout.

For hyperuricemic people who are going to develop gout, acute arthritis is the most common early clinical manifestation. The metatarsophalangeal joint of the big toe is the most commonly affected (75% of patients). The tarsal area, ankle, or knee may also be affected. Less commonly, the wrists, fingers, and elbows may be affected. The acute attack may be triggered by trauma, alcohol ingestion, dieting, medications, surgical stress, or illness. The abrupt onset often occurs at night, awakening the patient with severe pain, redness, swelling, and warmth of the affected joint. Early attacks tend to subside spontaneously over 3 to 10 days even without treatment. The attack is followed by a symptom-free period (the intercritical stage) until the next attack, which may not come for months or years. With time, however, attacks tend to occur more frequently, involve more joints, and last longer.

Tophi are generally associated with more frequent and severe inflammatory episodes. Higher serum concentrations of uric acid are also associated with more extensive tophus formation. Tophi most commonly occur in the synovium, olecranon bursa, subchondral bone, infrapatellar and Achilles tendons, subcutaneous tissue on the extensor surface of the forearms, and overlying joints. They have also been found in the aortic walls, heart valves, nasal and ear cartilage, eyelids, cornea, and sclerae. Joint enlargement may cause a loss of joint motion. Uric acid deposits may cause renal stones and kidney damage.

Medical Management

A definitive diagnosis of gouty arthritis is established by polarized light microscopy of the synovial fluid of the involved joint. Uric acid crystals are seen within the polymorphonuclear leukocytes within the fluid. Colchicine (oral or parenteral) or an NSAID such as indomethacin is used to relieve an acute attack of gout. Management of hyperuricemia, tophi, joint destruction, and renal disorders is usually initiated after the acute inflammatory process has subsided. Uricosuric agents, such as probenecid, correct hyperuricemia and dissolve deposited urate. Allopurinol is also effective, but its use is limited because of the risk for toxicity. When reduction of the serum urate level is indicated, the uricosuric agents are the medications of choice. When the patient has, or is at risk for, renal insufficiency or renal calculi (kidney stones), allopurinol is the medication of choice. Corticosteroids may be used in resistant cases. If the individual experiences several acute episodes or there is evidence of tophi formation, prophylactic treatment is considered. Specific treatment is based on serum uric acid level, 24-hour urinary uric acid excretion, and renal function (Table 54-5).

Nursing Management

Historically, gouty arthritis was thought to be a condition of the royalty and the very rich, with the disease attributed to "high living." This has not been shown to be entirely true. While severe dietary restriction is not necessary, patients should be encouraged to restrict consumption of foods high in purines, especially organ meats, and to limit alcohol intake. Maintenance of normal body weight should be encouraged. In an acute episode of gouty arthritis, pain management is essential. During the intercritical period, the patient feels well and may abandon preventive behaviours, which may result in an acute attack. Acute attacks are most effectively treated if therapy is begun early in the course.

Table 54-5 • Medications Used to Treat Gout

MEDICATION	ACTIONS AND USE	NURSING IMPLICATIONS
colchicine	Lowers the deposition of uric acid and interferes with leukocytes and kinin formation, thus reducing inflammation; does not alter serum or urine levels of uric acid; used in acute and chronic management	*Acute management:* Administer when attack begins; dosage increased until pain relieved or diarrhea develops *Chronic management:* Prolonged use may decrease vitamin B_{12} absorption; causes GI upset in most patients
probenecid (Benemid)	Uricosuric agent; inhibits renal reabsorption of urates and increases the urinary excretion of uric acid; prevents tophi formation	Be alert for nausea, rash, and constipation.
allopurinol (Zyloprim)	Xanthine oxidase inhibitor; interrupts the breakdown of purines before uric acid is formed; inhibits xanthinoxidase because it blocks uric acid formation	Monitor for side effects, including bone marrow depression, vomiting, and abdominal pain.

Fibromyalgia

Fibromyalgia is a common syndrome that involves chronic fatigue, generalized muscle aching, and stiffness. It is estimated that approximately 900,000 Canadians may have fibromyalgia (Arthritis Society, 2003). Although criteria for the classification of fibromyalgia have been established (Wolfe & Skevington, 1990), controversy exists as to whether this diagnosis represents a unique syndrome. The cause is unknown and no pathologic characteristics have been identified that are specific for the condition. Treatment consists of attention to the specific symptoms reported by the patient. NSAIDs may be used to treat the diffuse muscle aching and stiffness. Tricyclic antidepressants are used to improve or restore normal sleep patterns, and individualized programs of exercise are used to decrease muscle weakness and discomfort and to improve the general deconditioning that occurs in these individuals (American College of Rheumatology Fact Sheet, 2000; Burckhardt, 2001b; Clark et al., 2001).

Nursing Management

Typically, patients with fibromyalgia have endured their symptoms for a long period of time. They may feel as if their symptoms have not been taken seriously. Nurses need to pay special attention to supporting these individuals and providing encouragement as they begin their program of therapy. Patient support groups may be helpful. Careful listening to patients' descriptions of their concerns and symptoms is essential to helping them make changes necessary to improve their quality of life (Anderson & Burckhardt, 1999).

Arthritis Associated With Infectious Organisms

Arthritis, tenosynovitis, and bursitis can be associated with infectious organisms. Some inflammation of joints, tendons, and bursae is directly related to infection caused by bacterial, viral, fungal, or parasitic agents. Bacterial arthritis is the most rapidly destructive form of infectious arthritis. There are two major classes of bacterial arthritis: arthritis caused by *Neisseria gonorrhoeae* and nongonococcal bacterium. The most prevalent of the nongonococcal organisms include *Staphylococcus aureus* and the various streptococcal variants. Less common pathogens are related to syphilis, tuberculosis, leprosy, fungi (particularly coccidioidomycosis), mycoplasmas, and viral agents, such as rubella, parvovirus, and hepatitis B.

Clinical Manifestations

The characteristic symptom is acute onset of a warm, swollen joint. Culture of the bacterium from the synovial fluid confirms the diagnosis. The patient often immobilizes the joint and elevates the affected extremity because of pain and swelling. Fever may be high or it may be absent. Signs of systemic infection may be lacking in elderly patients, those with diabetes, and those with suppressed immune systems. Diagnosis and treatment may be delayed by patients with pre-existing arthritic conditions if they attribute the symptoms to a flare-up of arthritis.

Management

This condition is a medical emergency necessitating early diagnosis and appropriate treatment to eliminate the causative organism; otherwise, the joint may be destroyed relatively quickly. Treatment consists of parenteral antibiotics and drainage of the joint. The results of cultures are used to determine the appropriate antibiotic therapy. Immobilization of the joint and repeated joint aspirations may be necessary along with intravenous antibiotics. Nursing management focuses on providing pain relief, administering antibiotics, and assisting the patient with self-care activities. If the patient is sent home on intravenous antibiotics, the nurse arranges home care and instructs the patient and care providers in safe administration and changes to report to a health care provider.

Neoplasms and Neurovascular, Bone, and Extra-Articular Disorders

Primary neoplasms of joints, tendon sheaths, and bursae are rare. Most neoplasms are benign, arising from the synovium. These benign tumours include lipoma, hemangioma, and fibroma and tumour-like lesions such as ganglion, bursitis, and synovial cyst. Malignant tumours include primary tumours, such as synovial and bone sarcomas, and secondary involvement as manifestations of joint invasion by leukemia, lymphoma, and myeloma or metastasis. Neoplasms may present as back or neck pain.

Neurovascular disorders include the compression syndromes, such as those with peripheral entrapment (carpal tunnel syndrome), radiculopathy, and spinal stenosis. Raynaud's phenomenon or disease and erythromelalgia (throbbing and burning pain often affecting the hands and feet) are also included in this category.

Bone and cartilage disorders include osteoporosis, osteomalacia, hypertrophic osteoarthropathy, diffuse idiopathic skeletal hyperostosis, Paget's disease, osteonecrosis, avascular necrosis, costochondritis, osteolysis or chondrolysis, and biomechanical or anatomic abnormalities. Notably, these conditions involve resorption, destruction, infection, or remodeling of bone.

Extra-articular rheumatism is a descriptive term for a group of conditions affecting structures other than the joints. Included are general and regional pain syndromes, low back pain and intervertebral disk disorders, tendonitis and bursitis, and ganglion cysts.

Miscellaneous Disorders

The last category in the classification of the rheumatic diseases is aptly labelled miscellaneous disorders because it contains a mix of disorders frequently associated with arthritis and other conditions. These disorders include the direct result of trauma (including internal derangement and loose bodies of joints), pancreatic disease (related to avascular necrosis or osteonecrosis), sarcoidosis (a multisystem disorder particularly of the lymph nodes and lungs), and palindromic rheumatism (an uncommon variety of recurring and acute arthritis and periarthritis that in some may progress to RA but is characterized by symptom-free periods of days to months). Other conditions include villonodular synovitis, chronic active hepatitis, and drug-related rheumatic syndromes. The nursing interventions related to these varied conditions are specific to the multisystemic problems experienced by the patient. However, the musculoskeletal components should not be neglected or overlooked. Further information about these rare disorders can be found in specialty references.

Critical Thinking Exercises

1. Your 28-year-old, newly married patient has recently been informed that she has SLE. Although she is undergoing extensive testing to determine the systemic effects of SLE, she states that she feels fine and cannot understand the reasons for the testing. What explanations would you provide? Explain the relationship of SLE to possible systemic effects of the disorder.

2. A 68-year-old woman is admitted for surgery to treat a bowel obstruction; it is anticipated that she will have a colostomy. She has advanced rheumatoid arthritis that has affected all four extremities and her cervical spine. How will the rheumatoid arthritis affect her immediate postoperative care? What modifications are necessary to enable her to manage her colostomy, given the effects of arthritis on her hands?

3. A 57-year-old patient with a long history of osteoarthritis comes to the emergency department with severe pain and swelling of his right knee of 10 days' duration. His knee is

hot to the touch and he has a fever. He explains that he thought his symptoms were due to a flare-up of his osteoarthritis. It is suspected that he has infectious arthritis. Explain the possible consequences of this form of arthritis and the medical and nursing interventions you would anticipate. What are the possible consequences of the delay in seeking treatment?

4. NSAIDs and corticosteroids have been prescribed for your patient's rheumatic disorder. How do the actions of these medications differ, and what instructions and recommendations would you give to the patient to ensure their safe administration?

REFERENCES AND SELECTED READINGS
Books

Belza, B. (2001). Fatigue. In L. Robbins, C. S. Burckhardt, M. T. Hannan, & R. J. DeHoratius (Eds.), *Clinical care in the rheumatic diseases* (pp. 251–254). Atlanta: Association of Rheumatology Health Professionals.

Burckhardt, C. (2001a). Pain management. In L. Robbins, C. S. Burckhardt, M. T. Hannan, & R. J. DeHoratius (Eds.), *Clinical care in the rheumatic diseases* (pp. 245–249). Atlanta: Association of Rheumatology Health Professionals.

Burckhardt, C. S. (2001b). Fibromyalgia. In L. Robbins, C. S. Burckhardt, M. T. Hannan, & R. J. DeHoratius (Eds.), *Clinical care in the rheumatic diseases* (pp. 135–139). Atlanta: Association of Rheumatology Health Professionals.

Klippel, J. H. (Ed.) (2001). *Primer on the rheumatic diseases* (12th ed.). Atlanta: Arthritis Foundation.

Lozada, C. J., & Altman, R. D. (2001). Osteoarthritis. In L. Robbins, C. S. Burckhardt, M. T. Hannan, & R. J. DeHoratius (Eds.), *Clinical care in the rheumatic diseases* (pp. 97–103). Atlanta: Association of Rheumatology Health Professionals.

Luck, J. N. (2001). Enhancing functional ability. In L. Robbins, C. S. Burckhardt, M. T. Hannan, & R. J. DeHoratius (Eds.), *Clinical care in the rheumatic diseases* (pp. 197–202). Atlanta: Association of Rheumatology Health Professionals

Michocki, R. J. (2001). Polypharmacy and principles of drug therapy. In A. M. Adelman & M. P. Daly (Eds.), *20 common problems in geriatrics.* New York: McGraw-Hill.

Miller, D. R. (2001). Pharmacologic interventions in the 21st century. In L. Robbins, C. S. Burckhardt, M. T. Hannan, & R. J. DeHoratius (Eds.), *Clinical care in the rheumatic diseases* (pp. 169–177). Atlanta: Association of Rheumatology Health Professionals.

Minor, M. A., & Westby, M. D. (2001). Rest and exercise. In L. Robbins, C. S. Burckhardt, M. T. Hannan, & R. J. DeHoratius (Eds.), *Clinical care in the rheumatic diseases* (pp. 179–184). Atlanta: Association of Rheumatology Health Professionals.

Nadler, S. (1997). Arthritis and other connective tissue diseases. In M. L. Sipski & C. J. Alexander (Eds.), *Sexual function in people with disability and chronic illness.* Gaithersburg, MD: Aspen.

Paget, S. A. (2001). Polymyalgia rheumatica. In L. Robbins, C. S. Burckhardt, M. T. Hannan, & R. J. DeHoratius (Eds.), *Clinical care in the rheumatic diseases* (pp. 151–153). Atlanta: Association of Rheumatology Health Professionals.

Parker, J. C., Wright, G. E., & Smarr, K. L. (2001). Psychological assessment. In L. Robbins, C. S. Burckhardt, M. T. Hannan, & R. J. DeHoratius (Eds.), *Clinical care in the rheumatic diseases* (pp. 69–73). Atlanta: Association of Rheumatology Health Professionals.

Ramsey-Goldman, R. (2001). Connective tissue diseases. In L. Robbins, C. S. Burckhardt, M. T. Hannan, & R. J. DeHoratius (Eds.), *Clinical care in the rheumatic diseases* (pp. 97–103). Atlanta: Association of Rheumatology Health Professionals.

Ruddy, S., Harris, E. D., & Sledge, C. B. (Eds.) (2001). *Kelley's textbook of rheumatology.* Philadelphia: W. B. Saunders.

U.S. Department of Health and Human Services. (2001). *The Surgeon General's call to action to prevent and decrease overweight and obesity.* Rockville, MD: U.S. Department of Health and Human Services, Public Health Service.

Wegner, S. T. (2001). Sleep problems. In L. Robbins, C. S. Burckhardt, M. T. Hannan, & R. J. DeHoratius (Eds.), *Clinical care in the rheumatic diseases* (pp. 255–259). Atlanta: Association of Rheumatology Health Professionals.

Journals

Asterisks indicate nursing research articles.

General

American College of Rheumatology. (1998). Position statement: "Complementary" and "alternative" therapies for rheumatic diseases: http://www.rheumatology.org/position/alternative.html.

*Aaronson, L. S., Teel, C. S., Cassmeyer, V., et al. (1999). Defining and measuring fatigue. *Image: Journal of Nursing Scholarship, 31*(1), 45–50.

*Anderson, K. L., & Burckhardt, C. S. (1999). Conceptualization and measurement of quality of life as an outcome variable for health care intervention and research. *Journal of Advanced Nursing, 29*(2), 298–306.

Beehrle, D. M., & Evans, D. (1999). A review of NSAID complications: Gastrointestinal and more. *Lippincott's Primary Care Practice, 3*(3), 305–315.

Bello, C. E., & Garrett, S. D. (1999). Therapeutic issues in oral glucocorticoid use. *Lippincott's Primary Care Practice, 3*(3), 333–341.

*Belza, B., Topolski, T., Kinne S., et al. (2002). Does adherence make a difference? Results from a community-based aquatic exercise program. *Nursing Research, 51*(5), 285–291.

Buckley, L., Greenwald, M., Hochberg, M., et al. (2001). Recommendations for the prevention and treatment of glucocorticoid-induced osteoporosis. *Arthritis & Rheumatism, 44*(7), 1496–1503.

Capriotti, T. (2000). The new NSAIDs: COX-2 inhibitors. *MedSurg Nursing, 9*(6), 313–317.

Davidson, A., & Diamond, B. (2002). Advances in immunology. Autoimmune diseases. *New England Journal of Medicine, 345*(5), 340–350.

*Jakobsson, U., & Hallberg, I. R. (2002). Pain and quality of life among older people with rheumatoid arthritis and/or osteoarthritis: A literature review. *Journal of Clinical Nursing, 11*(4), 430–443.

Rheumatoid Arthritis

*Ailinger, R. L., & Dear, M. R. (1997). An examination of the self-care needs of clients with rheumatoid arthritis. *Rehabilitation Nursing, 22*(3), 135–140.

*Allaire, S. H., Anderson, J. J., & Meenan, R. F. (1996). Reducing work disability associated with rheumatoid arthritis: Identification of additional risk factors and persons likely to benefit from intervention. *Arthritis Care Research, 9*(5), 349–357.

Bombardier, C., Laine, L., Reicin, A., et al. (2000). Comparison of upper gastrointestinal toxicity of Rofecoxib and Naproxen in patients with rheumatoid arthritis. *New England Journal of Medicine, 343*(21), 1520–1528.

Felson, D. T., LaValley, M. P., Baldassare, A. R., et al. (1999). The Prosorba column for treatment of refractory rheumatoid arthritis: a randomized, double-blind, sham-controlled trial. *Arthritis & Rheumatism, 42*(10), 2153–2159.

Felson, D. T., Anderson, J. J., Boers, M., et al. (1995). American College of Rheumatology preliminary definition of improvement in rheumatoid arthritis. *Arthritis & Rheumatism, 38*(6), 727–735.

Gendreau, R. M. (2001). A randomized double-blind sham-controlled trial of the Prosorba column for treatment of refractory rheumatoid arthritis. *Therapeutic Apheresis, 5*(2), 79–83.

Kellick, K. A., Martins-Richards, J., & Chow, C. (1998). Management of arthritis. *Lippincott's Primary Care Practice, 2*(1), 66–80.

Koopman, W. J. (2001). Prospects for autoimmune disease: Research advances in rheumatoid arthritis. *Journal of the American Medical Association, 285*(5), 648–650.

MacLean, C. H., Rachel, L., et al. (2000). Quality of care for patients with rheumatoid arthritis. *Journal of the American Medical Association, 284*(8), 984–992.

Moreland, L. W., Schiff, M. H., Baumgartner, S. W., et al. (1999). Etanercept therapy in rheumatoid arthritis. *Annals of Internal Medicine, 130*(6), 476–486.

Multon, K. D., Parker, J. C., Smarr, K. L., et al. (2001). Effects of stress management on pain behavior in rheumatoid arthritis. *Arthritis Care & Research, 45*(2), 122–128.

Ramsburg, K. K. (2000). Rheumatoid arthritis. *American Journal of Nursing, 100*(11), 40–43.

Weinblatt, M. E., Kremer, J. M, Bankhurst, A. D., et al. (1999). A trial of etanercept, a recombinant tumor necrosis factor receptor: Fc fusion protein, in patients with rheumatoid arthritis receiving methotrexate. *New England Journal of Medicine, 340*(4), 253–259.

Osteoarthritis

Altman, R., Asch, E., Bloch, et al. (1986). Development of criteria for the classification and reporting of osteoarthritis: Classification of osteoarthritis of the knee. *Arthritis & Rheumatism, 29*(8), 1039–1049.

Altman, R. D., Hochberg, M. C., Moskowitz, R. W., & Schnitzer, T. J. (2000). Recommendations for the medical management of osteoarthritis of the hip and knee. *Arthritis & Rheumatism, 43*(9), 1905–1915.

American College of Rheumatology. (2000). Recommendations for the medical management of osteoarthritis of the hip and knee. *Arthritis & Rheumatism, 43*(9), 1905–1915.

*Baird, C. L. (2000). Living with hurting and difficulty doing: Older women with osteoarthritis. *Clinical Excellence for Nurse Practitioners, 4*(4), 231–237.

*Bautch, J. C., Malone, D. G., & Vailas, A. C. (1997). Effects of exercise on knee joints with osteoarthritis: A pilot study of biologic markers. *Arthritis Care Research, 10*(1), 48–55.

Brandt, K. D., Smith, G. N., Jr, & Simon, L. S. (2000). Intraarticular injection of hyaluronan as treatment for knee osteoarthritis: What is the evidence? *Arthritis & Rheumatism, 43*(6), 1192–1203.

Coggon, D., Reading, I., Croft, P., et al. (2001). Knee osteoarthritis and obesity. *International Journal of Obesity and Related Metabolic Disorders, (5)*, 622–627.

*Davis, G. C., Hiemenz, M. L., & White, T. L. (2002). Barriers to managing chronic pain of older adults with arthritis. *Journal of Nursing Scholarship, 34*(2), 121–126.

Ettinger, W. H., Burns, R., et al. (1997). A randomized trial comparing aerobic exercise and resistance exercise with a health education program in older adults with knee osteoarthritis: The Fitness Arthritis and Seniors Trial (FAST). *Journal of the American Medical Association, 277*(1), 25–31.

*Gaines, J. M., Talbot, L. A., & Metter, E. J. (2002). The relationship of arthritis self-efficacy to functional performance in older men and women with osteoarthritis of the knee. *Geriatric Nursing, 23*(3), 167–170.

Gonzalez-Gay, M. A., Garcia-Porrua, C., Salvarani, C., & Hunder, G. G. (1999). Diagnostic approach in a patient presenting with polymyalgia. *Clinical and Experimental Rheumatology, 17*(3), 276–278.

Huskisson, E. C., & Donnelly, S. (1999). Hyaluronic acid in the treatment of osteoarthritis of the knee. *Rheumatology, 38*(7), 602–607.

McAlindon, T. E., LaValley, M. P., Gulin, J. P., & Felson, D. T. (2000). Glucosamine and chondroitin for treatment of osteoarthritis. *Journal of the American Medical Association, 283*(11), 1469–1475.

Pasero, C., & McCaffery, M. (2001). Selective COX-2 inhibitors. *American Journal of Nursing, 101*(4), 55–56.

Watterson, J. R., & Esdaile, J. M. (2000). Viscosupplementation: Therapeutic mechanisms and clinical potential in osteoarthritis of the knee. *Journal of the American Academy of Orthopedic Surgery, 8*(5), 277–284.

Wright, K. E., Maurer, S. G., & DiCesare, P. E. (2000). Viscosupplementation for osteoarthritis. *American Journal of Orthopedics, 29*(2), 80–89.

Systemic Lupus Erythematosus

Johnson, B. (1999). Systemic lupus erythematosus. *American Journal of Nursing, 99*(1), 40–41.

National Institutes of Health, National Institute of Arthritis and Musculoskeletal and Skin Diseases. *Handout on Health–Systemic Lupus Erythematosus,* 1998.

Kimberly, R. P. (2001). Research advances in systemic lupus erythematosus. *Journal of the American Medical Association, 285*(5), 650–652.

Petri, M. (2000). Systemic lupus erythematosus: Women's health issues. *Bulletin on the Rheumatic Diseases, 49*(8), 1–3.

Wolfe, F., & Skevington, S. M. (2000). Measuring the epidemiology of distress: The rheumatology distress index. *Journal of Rheumatology, 27*(8), 2000–2009.

Other Specific Rheumatic Diseases

ACR Fact Sheet. (2002). Fibromyalgia. Available at: http://www.rheumatology.org/patients/factsheet/fibromya.html.

Arthritis Society. (2003). Fibromyalgia. Available at: http://www.arthritis.ca. Retrieved May 15, 2005.

Clark, S. R., Jones, K. D., Burckhardt, C. S., & Bennett, R. (2001). Exercise for patients with fibromyalgia: Risks versus benefits. *Current Rheumatology Reports, 3*(2), 135–140.

Khan, M. A. (2002). Update on spondyloarthropathies. *Annals of Internal Medicine, 136*(12), 896–907.

Loeslie, V. (2000). Pain in the elderly: Polymyalgia rheumatica. *Clinical Excellence for Nurse Practitioners, 4*(6), 345–348.

Wolfe, F., Smythe, H. A., Yunus, M. B., et al. (1990). The American College of Rheumatology 1990 criteria for the classification of fibromyalgia: report of the multicenter criteria committee. *Arthritis & Rheumatism, 33,* 160–172.

RESOURCES AND WEBSITES

American Fibromyalgia Syndrome Association, Inc., 6380 E. Tanque Verde, Suite D, Tucson, AZ 85615; (520) 733-1570; http://www.afsafund.org.

American College of Rheumatology and Association of Rheumatology Health Professionals, 1800 Century Place, Suite 250, Atlanta, GA 30345; (404) 633-3777; http://www.rheumatology.org.

Arthritis Foundation, P.O Box 7669, Atlanta, GA 30309; (404) 872-7100 or (800) 283-7800 (information line); http://www.arthritis.org.

Arthritis Society; http://www.arthritis.ca.

Fibromyalgia Network; http://www.fmnetnews.com.

Joints in Motion; http://www.canada.com/national/features/arthritis2003/index.htm.

Lupus Foundation of America, Inc., 1300 Picard Drive, Suite 200, Rockville, MD 20850-4303; (800) 558-0121; http://www.lupus.org/lupus.

National CFS and Fibromyalgia Association, PO Box 18426, Kansas City, MO 64133; (816) 313-2000; http://www.ncfsfa.org.

National Institute of Arthritis and Musculoskeletal and Skin Diseases, National Institutes of Health, Building 31, MSC 2350, 31 Center Drive, Bethesda, MD 20892-2350; (301) 496-8188, http://www.nih.gov/niams.

Sjögren's Syndrome Foundation, Inc., 333 N. Broadway, Jericho, NY 11753; (516) 933-6365; http://www.sjogrens.com.

Spondylitis Association of America, 14827 Ventura Blvd. #222, Sherman Oaks, CA 91403; (800) 777-8189; e-mail: info@spondylitis.org

United Scleroderma Foundation, Inc., P.O. Box 399, Watsonville, CA 95077; (408) 728-2202; http://www.scleroderma.com.

Integumentary Function

Applying Concepts from NANDA, NIC, and NOC

Mr. Reynolds is an 82-year-old man who lives with his wife at an assisted living residence. He filled a basin of water to soak his feet and immersed his left foot in the basin before checking the water temperature. He sustained a deep partial thickness burn on his foot and ankle and has been admitted to the residence's skilled nursing unit. The nurse notes that the skin of his left foot is bright red and there are three 2- to 4-cm blisters on the dorsum. The burn is quite painful and Mr. Reynolds cannot bear weight on his foot. His wife states that she is concerned because he is not eating his meals. The concept map illustrates the relationships that exist among selected nursing diagnoses, interventions, and outcomes for Mr. Reynolds' thermal injury.

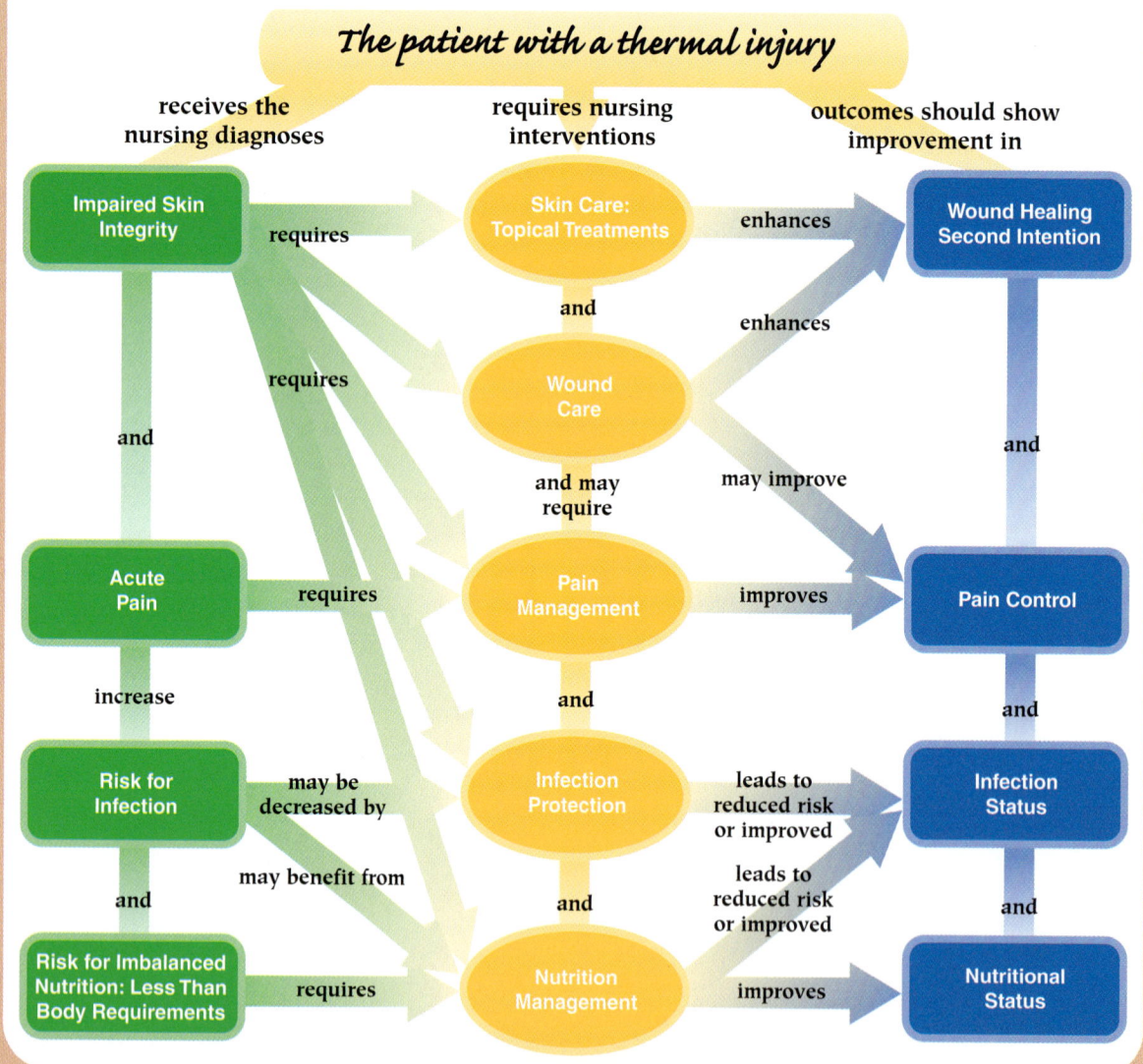

The patient with a thermal injury

receives the nursing diagnoses | requires nursing interventions | outcomes should show improvement in

Impaired Skin Integrity — requires → Skin Care: Topical Treatments — enhances → Wound Healing Second Intention

and

requires → Wound Care — enhances → (Wound Healing Second Intention)

and may require → may improve → Pain Control

Acute Pain — requires → Pain Management — improves → Pain Control

increase

Risk for Infection — may be decreased by → Infection Protection — leads to reduced risk or improved → Infection Status

and — may benefit from → leads to reduced risk or improved

and

Risk for Imbalanced Nutrition: Less Than Body Requirements — requires → Nutrition Management — improves → Nutritional Status

and

Nursing Classifications and Languages

NANDA
Nursing Diagnoses

Impaired Skin Integrity—Altered epidermis and/or dermis

Acute Pain—Unpleasant sensory and emotional experience arising from actual or potential tissue damage or described in terms of such damage; sudden or slow onset of any intensity from mild to severe with an anticipated or predictable end and a duration of less than 6 months

Risk for Infection—At risk for being invaded by pathogenic organisms

Risk for Imbalanced Nutrition: Less Than Body Requirements—At risk for intake of nutrients insufficient to meet metabolic needs

NIC
Nursing Interventions*

Skin Care: Topical Treatments—Application of topical substances or manipulation of devices to promote skin integrity and minimize skin breakdown

Wound Care—Prevention of wound complications and promotion of wound healing

Pain Management—Alleviation of pain or reduction in pain to a level of comfort that is acceptable to the patient

Infection Protection—Prevention and early detection of infection in a patient at risk

Nutrition Management—Assisting with or providing a balanced dietary intake of foods and fluids

NOC
Nursing Outcomes†

Return to functional baseline status, stabilization of, or improvement in

Wound Healing Secondary Intention—The extent to which cells and tissues in an open wound have regenerated

Pain Control—Personal actions to control pain

Infection Status—Presence and extent of infection

Nutritional Status—Extent to which nutrients are available to meet metabolic needs

---

NANDA, North American Nursing Diagnosis Association; NIC, Nursing Interventions Classification; NOC, Nursing Outcomes Classification

*Iowa Intervention Project © 2000. In McCloskey, J. C., & Bulechek, G. M. (2000). *Nursing interventions classification (NIC)* (3rd ed.). St. Louis: Mosby.

†Iowa Outcomes Project © 2000. In Johnson, M., Maas, M., & Moorhead, S. (2000). *Nursing outcomes classification (NOC)* (3rd ed.). St. Louis: Mosby.

Assessment of Integumentary Function

Adapted by Tracey Stephen

LEARNING OBJECTIVES

On completion of this chapter, the learner will be able to:

1. Identify the structures and functions of the skin.
2. Differentiate the composition and function of each skin layer: epidermis, dermis, and subcutaneous tissue.
3. Identify and describe primary and secondary skin lesions and their pattern and distribution.
4. Recognize common skin eruptions and manifestations associated with systemic disease.
5. Describe the normal aging process of the skin and skin changes common to elderly patients.
6. List appropriate questions that will help elicit information during an assessment of the skin.
7. Describe the components of physical assessment most useful when examining the skin, hair, and nails.
8. Discuss common skin tests and procedures used in diagnosing skin and related disorders.

Skin disorders are encountered frequently in nursing practice. Because the skin mirrors the general condition of the patient, many systemic conditions may be accompanied by dermatologic manifestations (Fleischer et al., 2000).

The psychological stress of illness or various personal and family problems is commonly exhibited outwardly as dermatologic problems. Any hospitalized patient may suddenly develop itching and a rash from the treatment regimen. In certain systemic conditions, such as hepatitis and some cancers, dermatologic manifestations may be the first sign of the disorder.

Anatomic and Physiologic Overview

The largest organ system of the body, the skin is indispensable for human life. Skin forms a barrier between the internal organs and the external environment and participates in many vital body functions. The skin is contiguous with the mucous membrane at the external openings of the digestive, respiratory, and urogenital systems. Because skin disorders are readily visible, dermatologic complaints are commonly the primary reason for a patient to seek health care.

ANATOMY OF THE SKIN, HAIR, NAILS, AND GLANDS OF THE SKIN

The skin is composed of three layers: epidermis, dermis, and subcutaneous tissue (Fig. 55-1). The epidermis is an outermost layer of stratified epithelial cells and composed predominantly of keratinocytes. It ranges in thickness from about 0.1 mm on the eyelids to about 1 mm on the palms of the hands and soles of the feet. Four distinct layers compose the epidermis, from innermost to outermost: stratum germinativum, stratum granulosum, stratum lucidum, and stratum corneum. Each layer becomes more differentiated (ie, mature and with more specific functions) as it rises from the basal stratum germinativum layer to the outermost stratum corneum layer.

Epidermis

The epidermis, which is contiguous with the mucous membranes and the lining of the ear canals, consists of live, continuously dividing cells covered on the surface by dead cells that were originally deeper in the dermis but were pushed upward by the newly developing, more differentiated cells underneath. This external layer is almost completely replaced every 3 to 4 weeks. The dead cells contain large amounts of **keratin**, an insoluble, fibrous protein that forms the outer barrier of the skin and has the capacity to repel pathogens and prevent excessive fluid loss from the body. Keratin is the principal hardening ingredient of the hair and nails.

Melanocytes are the special cells of the epidermis that are primarily involved in producing the pigment **melanin**, which colours the skin and hair. The more melanin in the tissue, the darker is the colour. Most of the skin of dark-skinned people and the darker areas of the skin on light-skinned people (eg, the nipple) contain larger amounts of this pigment. Normal skin colour depends on race and varies from pale; almost ivory, to deep brown, almost pure black. Systemic disease affects skin colour as well. For example, the skin appears bluish when there is insufficient oxygenation of the blood, yellow-green in people with jaundice, or red or flushed when there is inflammation or fever (Table 55-1).

Production of melanin is controlled by a hormone secreted from the hypothalamus of the brain called *melanocyte-stimulating hormone.* It is believed that melanin can absorb ultraviolet light in sunlight.

Two other cells are common to the epidermis: Merkel and Langerhans cells. **Merkel cells** are receptors that transmit stimuli to the axon through a chemical synapse. Langerhans cells are believed to play a significant role in cutaneous immune system reactions. These accessory cells of the afferent immune system process invading antigens and transport the antigens to the lymph system to activate the T lymphocytes.

The epidermis is modified in different areas of the body. It is thickest over the palms of the hands and soles of the feet and contains increased amounts of keratin. The thickness of the epidermis can increase with use and can result in calluses forming on the hands or corns forming on the feet.

The junction of the epidermis and dermis is an area of many undulations and furrows called **rete ridges**. This junction anchors the epidermis to the dermis and permits the free exchange of essential nutrients between the two layers. This interlocking between the dermis and epidermis produces ripples on the surface of the skin. On the fingertips, these ripples are called *fingerprints.* They are a person's most individual characteristic, and they rarely change.

Glossary

alopecia: loss of hair from any cause

anagen phase: active phase of hair growth

dermatosis: any abnormal skin condition

erythema: redness of the skin caused by congestion of the capillaries

hirsutism: the condition of having excessive hair growth

hyperpigmentation: increase in the melanin of the skin, resulting in an increase in pigmentation

hypopigmentation: decrease in the melanin of the skin, resulting in a loss of pigmentation

keratin: an insoluble, fibrous protein that forms the outer layer of skin

lichenification: leathery thickening of the skin

Merkel cells: cells of the epidermis that play a role in transmission of sensory messages

melanin: the substance responsible for colouration of the skin

melanocytes: cells of the skin that produce melanin

petechiae: pinpoint red spots that appear on the skin as a result of blood leakage into the skin

rete ridges: undulations and furrows that appear at the dermis–epidermis junction and are responsible for cementing together the two layers

sebaceous glands: glands that exist within the epidermis and secrete sebum to keep the skin soft and pliable

sebum: fatty secretion of the sebaceous glands

striae: bandlike streaks on the skin, distinguished by colour, texture, depression, or elevation from the tissue in which they are found; usually purplish or white

telangiectases: red marks on the skin caused by distention of the superficial blood vessels

vitiligo: a localized or widespread condition characterized by destruction of the melanocytes in circumscribed areas of the skin, resulting in white patches

Wood's light: a blue light used for diagnosing skin conditions

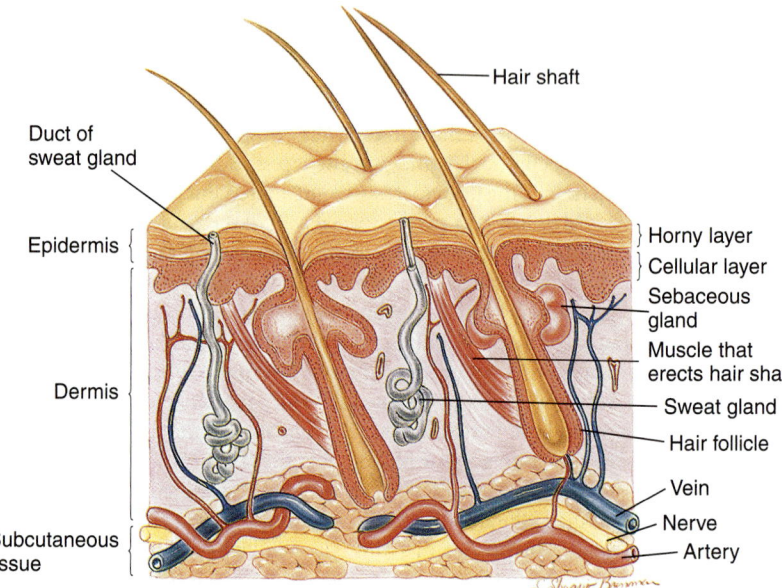

FIGURE 55-1 Anatomic structures of the skin. From Bickley, L. S., & Szilagyi, P. G. (2003). *Bates' guide to physical examination and history taking,* 8th ed. Philadelphia: Lippincott Williams & Wilkins.

Dermis

The dermis makes up the largest portion of the skin, providing strength and structure. It is composed of two layers: papillary and reticular. The papillary dermis lies directly beneath the epidermis and is composed primarily of fibroblast cells capable of producing one form of collagen, a component of connective tissue. The reticular layer lies beneath the papillary layer and also produces collagen and elastic bundles. The dermis is also made up of blood and lymph vessels, nerves, sweat and sebaceous glands, and hair roots. The dermis is often referred to as the "true skin."

Subcutaneous Tissue

The subcutaneous tissue, or hypodermis, is the innermost layer of the skin. It is primarily adipose tissue, which provides a cushion between the skin layers, muscles, and bones. It promotes skin mobility, molds body contours, and insulates the body. Fat is deposited and distributed according to the person's gender and in part accounts for the difference in body shape between men and women. Overeating results in increased deposition of fat beneath the skin. The subcutaneous tissues and amount of fat deposited are important factors in body temperature regulation.

Hair

An outgrowth of the skin, hair is present over the entire body except for the palms and soles. The hair consists of a root formed in the dermis and a hair shaft that projects beyond the skin. It grows in a cavity called a *hair follicle.* Proliferation of cells in the bulb of the hair causes the hair to form (see Fig. 55-1).

Hair follicles undergo cycles of growth and rest. The rate of growth varies; beard growth is the most rapid, followed by hair on the scalp, axillae, thighs, and eyebrows. The growth or **anagen phase** may last up to 6 years for scalp hair, whereas the telogen or resting phase lasts for approximately 4 months. During telogen, hair sheds from the body. The hair follicle recycles into the growing phase spontaneously, or it can be induced by plucking out hairs. Growing and resting hair can be found side by side on all parts of the body. About 90% of the 100,000 hair follicles on a normal scalp are in the growing phase at any one time, and 50 to 100 scalp hairs are shed each day.

There is a small bulge on the side of the hair follicle that houses the stem cells that migrate down to the follicle root and begin the cycle of reproducing the hair shaft. It was discovered that these bulges also contain the stem cells that migrate upward to reproduce skin (Jaworski & Gilliam, 1999). The location of these cells on the side of the hair shaft rather than at the base is a factor in hair loss. In conditions in which inflammation causes damage to the root of the hair, regrowth is possible. However, if inflammation causes damage to the bulge on the side, stem cells are destroyed and hair does not grow.

In certain locations on the body, hair growth is controlled by sex hormones. The most vivid example is the growth of hair on the face (ie, beard and mustache), chest, and back, which is controlled by the male hormones known as androgens. Some women with higher levels of testosterone have hair in the areas generally thought of as masculine, such as the face, chest, and lower abdomen. This is often a normal genetic variation; if it appears along with irregular menses and weight changes it may indicate a hormonal imbalance.

Hair in different parts of the body serves different functions. The hairs of the eyes (ie, eyebrows and lashes), nose, and ears filter out dust, bugs, and airborne debris. The hair of the skin provides thermal insulation in lower animals. This function is enhanced during cold or fright by piloerection (ie, hairs standing on end), caused by contraction of the tiny erector muscles attached to the hair follicle. The piloerector response that occurs in humans is probably vestigial (ie, rudimentary).

Hair colour is supplied by various amounts of melanin within the hair shaft. Grey or white hair reflects the loss of pigment. Hair quantity and distribution can be affected by endocrine conditions. For example, Cushing's syndrome causes **hirsutism** (ie, excessive hair growth, especially in women), and hypothyroidism (ie, underactive thyroid) causes changes in hair texture. In many cases, chemotherapy and radiation therapy cause hair thinning or weakening of the hair shaft, resulting in partial or complete **alopecia** (ie, hair loss) from the scalp and other parts of the body.

Table 55-1 • Select Cutaneous Manifestations of Systemic Diseases

Common cutaneous manifestations of systemic diseases include *pruritus* (itching), which may result from chronic renal disease, scabies, pediculosis (lice), obstructive biliary disease with jaundice, Hodgkin's or non-Hodgkin's lymphoma, or medication reactions; *pallor,* which suggests anemia or a cardiopulmonary disorder; and *skin thickening and hardening,* such as that which occurs with scleroderma and dermatomyositis.

	MANIFESTATION	SYSTEMIC DISEASE
Scale 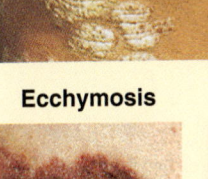	Plaques with scales (on the front of a knee)	Psoriasis
Ecchymosis **Purpura** 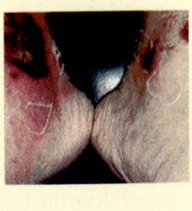	Ecchymosis (bruise) and purpura (bleeding into the skin)	Platelet disorder, vessel fragility
Urticaria 	Urticaria (wheals or hives)	Infections, allergic reactions
Plaque **Nodule** 	Cutaneous lesions: blue-red or dark brown plaques and nodules	Kaposi's sarcoma
Café-au-lait spot 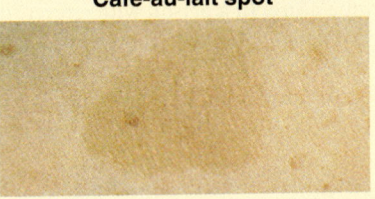	Macular, tan *café-au-lait* spots	Neurocutaneous disorders, such as neuro-fibromatosis (von Recklinghausen's disease)
Ulcerated lesion 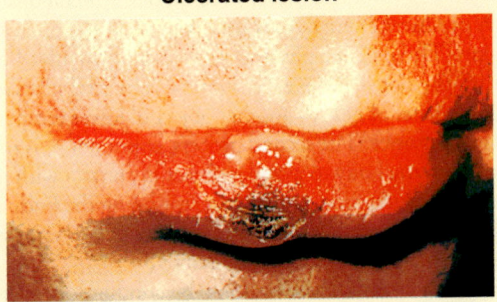	Painless chancre or ulcerated lesion	Syphilis

Nails

On the dorsal surface of the fingers and toes, a hard, transparent plate of keratin, called the *nail,* overlies the skin. The nail grows from its root, which lies under a thin fold of skin called the cuticle. The nail protects the fingers and toes by preserving their highly developed sensory functions, such as for picking up small objects.

Nail growth is continuous throughout life, with an average growth of 0.1 mm daily. Growth is faster in fingernails than toenails and tends to slow with aging. Complete renewal of a fingernail takes about 170 days, whereas toenail renewal takes 12 to 18 months.

Glands of the Skin

There are two types of skin glands: sebaceous glands and sweat glands (see Fig. 55-1). The **sebaceous glands** are associated with hair follicles. The ducts of the sebaceous glands empty **sebum** (ie, oily secretion) onto the space between the hair follicle and the hair shaft. For each hair there is a sebaceous gland, the secretions of which lubricate the hair and render the skin soft and pliable.

Sweat glands are found in the skin over most of the body surface. They are heavily concentrated in the palms of the hands and soles of the feet. Only the glans penis, the margins of the lips, the external ear, and the nail bed are devoid of sweat glands. Sweat glands are subclassified into two categories: eccrine and apocrine.

The eccrine sweat glands are found in all areas of the skin. Their ducts open directly onto the skin surface. The thin, watery secretion called *sweat* is produced in the basal coiled portion of the eccrine gland and is released into its narrow duct. Sweat is composed of predominantly water and contains about one half of the salt content of the blood plasma. Sweat is released from eccrine glands in response to elevated ambient temperature and elevated body temperature. The rate of sweat secretion is under the control of the sympathetic nervous system. Excessive sweating of the palms and soles, axillae, forehead, and other areas may occur in response to pain and stress.

The apocrine sweat glands are larger, and unlike eccrine glands, their secretion contains parts of the secretory cells. They are located in the axillae, anal region, scrotum, and labia majora. Their ducts generally open onto hair follicles. The apocrine glands become active at puberty. In women, they enlarge and recede with each menstrual cycle. Apocrine glands produce a milky sweat that is sometimes broken down by bacteria to produce the characteristic underarm odour. Specialized apocrine glands called *ceruminous glands* are found in the external ear, where they produce cerumen (ie, wax).

FUNCTIONS OF THE SKIN

Protection

The skin covering most of the body is no more than 1 mm thick, but it provides very effective protection against invasion by bacteria and other foreign matter. The thickened skin of the palms and soles protects against the effects of the constant trauma that occurs in these areas.

The epidermis is the outermost layer of the skin and is composed of several layers of keratinocytes that change character as they migrate to the surface. The stratum corneum, the outer layer of the epidermis, provides the most effective barrier to epidermal water loss and penetration of environmental factors such as chemicals, microbes, and insect bites.

Various lipids are synthesized in the stratum corneum and are the basis for the barrier function of this layer. These are long-chain lipids that are better suited than phospholipids for water resistance. The presence of these lipids in the stratum corneum creates a relatively impermeable barrier for water egress and for the entry of toxins, microbes, and other substances that come in contact with the surface of the skin.

Some substances do penetrate the skin but meet resistance in trying to move through the channels between the cell layers of the stratum corneum. Microbes and fungi, which are part of the body's normal flora, cannot penetrate unless there is a break in the skin barrier.

The dermis–epidermis junction is the basal layer, which is composed of collagen. The basal layer serves four functions. It acts as a scaffold for tissue organization and a template for regeneration; it provides selective permeability for filtration of serum; it is a physical barrier between different types of cells; and it adheres the epithelium to underlying cell layers.

Sensation

The receptor endings of nerves in the skin allow the body to constantly monitor the conditions of the immediate environment. The primary functions of the receptors in the skin are to sense temperature, pain, light touch, and pressure (or heavy touch). Different nerve endings respond to each of the different stimuli. Although the nerve endings are distributed over the entire body, they are more concentrated in some areas than in others. For example, the fingertips are more densely innervated than the skin on the back.

Fluid Balance

The stratum corneum (ie, outermost layer of the epidermis) has the capacity to absorb water, thereby preventing an excessive loss of water and electrolytes from the internal body and retaining moisture in the subcutaneous tissues. When skin is damaged, as occurs with a severe burn, large quantities of fluids and electrolytes may be lost rapidly, possibly leading to circulatory collapse, shock, and death.

The skin is not completely impermeable to water. Small amounts of water continuously evaporate from the skin surface. This evaporation, called *insensible perspiration,* amounts to approximately 600 mL daily in a normal adult. Insensible water loss varies with the body and ambient temperature. In a person with a fever, the loss can increase. During immersion in water, the skin can accumulate water up to three or four times its normal weight, such as swelling of the skin that occurs after prolonged bathing.

Temperature Regulation

The body continuously produces heat as a result of the metabolism of food, which produces energy. This heat is dissipated primarily through the skin. Three major physical processes are involved in loss of heat from the body to the environment. The first process, radiation, is the transfer of heat to another object of lower temperature situated at a distance. The second process, conduction, is the transfer of heat from the body to a cooler object in contact with it. Heat transferred by conduction to the air surrounding the body is removed by the third process, convection, which consists of movement of warm air molecules away from the body.

Evaporation from the skin aids heat loss by conduction. Heat is conducted through the skin into water molecules on its surface, causing the water to evaporate. The water on the skin surface may be from insensible perspiration, sweat, or the environment.

Normally, all of these mechanisms for heat loss are used. When the ambient temperature is very high, however, radiation and convection are ineffective, and evaporation becomes the only means for heat loss.

Under normal conditions, metabolic heat production is balanced by heat loss, and the internal temperature of the body is maintained constant at approximately 37°C. The rate of heat loss depends primarily on the surface temperature of the skin, which is a function of the skin blood flow. Under normal conditions, the total blood circulated through the skin is approximately 450 mL per minute, or 10 to 20 times the amount of blood required to provide necessary metabolites and oxygen. Blood flow through these skin vessels is controlled primarily by the sympathetic nervous system. Increased blood flow to the skin results in more heat delivered to the skin and a greater rate of heat loss from the body. In contrast, decreased skin blood flow decreases the skin temperature and helps conserve heat for the body. When the temperature of the body begins to fall, as occurs on a cold day, the blood vessels of the skin constrict, thereby reducing heat loss from the body.

Sweating is another process by which the body can regulate the rate of heat loss. Sweating does not occur until the core body temperature exceeds 37°C, regardless of skin temperature. In extremely hot environments, the rate of sweat production may be as high as 1 L per hour. Under some circumstances (eg, emotional stress), sweating may occur as a reflex and may be unrelated to the need to lose heat from the body.

Vitamin Production

Skin exposed to ultraviolet light can convert substances necessary for synthesizing vitamin D_3 (cholecalciferol). Vitamin D is essential for preventing rickets, a condition that causes bone deformities and results from a deficiency of vitamin D, calcium, and phosphorus. Canada's northern geographical location affects the amount of exposure to ultraviolet light, resulting in inadequate ultraviolet exposure for portions of the year. In Edmonton, for example, there is inadequate ultraviolet exposure between the months of October and March to stimulate vitamin D synthesis in the skin; therefore, dietary vitamin D is recommended. Vitamin D_3 (cholecalciferol) is recommended over D_2. Infants living in northern Canada require 400 IU of vitamin D if bottle-fed and 800 IU if breast-fed. The recommended daily intake for children up to 18 years of age is 200 to 400 IU (Holick, 1998). For 19 to 50 year olds, the recommended vitamin D intake is 400 IU and could be increased to 600 IU per day. Over 50 years of age, men and women require 800 IU per day (Brown, et al., 2002).

Immune Response Function

Research findings (Demis, 1998) indicate that several dermal cells (ie, Langerhans cells, interleukin-1–producing keratinocytes, and subsets of T lymphocytes) and three varieties of human leukocyte antigen (ie, protein marker on white blood cells indicating the type of cell) are important components of the immune system. Ongoing research is expected to more clearly define the role of these dermal cells in immune function.

Gerontologic Considerations

The skin undergoes many physiologic changes associated with normal aging. A lifetime of excessive sun exposure, systemic dis-

eases, poor nutrition, and certain medications (eg, antihistamines, diuretics) can enhance the range of skin problems and the rapidity with which they appear. The outcome is an increasing vulnerability to injury and to certain diseases. Skin problems are common among older people.

Before conducting a skin assessment, the nurse needs to be aware of significant changes that occur with aging. The major changes in the skin of older people include dryness, wrinkling, uneven pigmentation, and various proliferative lesions. Cellular changes associated with aging include a thinning at the junction of the dermis and epidermis. This results in fewer anchoring sites between the two skin layers, so that even minor injury or stress to the epidermis can cause it to shear away from the dermis. This phenomenon of aging may account for the increased vulnerability of aged skin to trauma. With increasing age, the epidermis and dermis thin and flatten, causing wrinkles, sags, and overlapping skin folds (Fig. 55-2).

Loss of the subcutaneous tissue substances of elastin, collagen, and subcutaneous fat diminishes the protection and cushioning of underlying tissues and organs, decreases muscle tone, and results in the loss of the insulating properties of fat.

Cellular replacement slows as a result of aging. As the dermal layers thin, the skin becomes fragile and transparent. The blood supply to the skin also changes with age. Vessels, especially the capillary loops, decrease in number and size. These vascular changes contribute to the delayed wound healing commonly seen in the elderly patient. Sweat and sebaceous glands decrease in number and functional capacity, leading to dry and scaly skin. Reduced hormonal levels of androgens are thought to contribute to declining sebaceous gland function.

Hair growth gradually diminishes, especially over the lower legs and dorsum of the feet. Thinning is common in the scalp, axilla, and pubic areas. Other functions affected with normal aging include the barrier function of skin, sensory perception, and thermoregulation.

Photoaging, or damage from excessive sun exposure, has detrimental effects on the normal aging of skin. A lifetime of outdoor work or outdoor activities (eg, construction work, lifeguarding, sunbathing) without prudent use of sunscreens can lead to profound wrinkling; increased loss of elasticity; mottled, pigmented areas; cutaneous atrophy; and benign or malignant lesions.

Many skin lesions are part of normal aging. Recognizing these lesions enables the examiner to assist the patient to feel less anx-

FIGURE 55-2 Hands with wrinkling and overlapping folds common to aging skin.

ious about changes in skin. Chart 55-1 summarizes some skin lesions that are expected to appear as the skin ages. These are normal and require no special attention unless the skin becomes infected or irritated.

Assessment

HEALTH HISTORY AND CLINICAL MANIFESTATIONS

When caring for patients with dermatologic disorders, the nurse obtains important information through the health history and direct observations. The nurse's skill in physical assessment and an understanding of the anatomy and function of the skin can ensure that deviations from normal are recognized, reported, and documented.

During the health history interview, the nurse asks about any family and personal history of skin allergies, allergic reactions to food, medications, chemicals, previous skin problems, and skin cancer. The names of cosmetics, soaps, shampoos, and other personal hygiene products are obtained if there have been any recent skin problems noticed with the use of these products. The health history contains specific information about the onset, signs and symptoms, location, and duration of any pain, itching, rash, or other discomfort experienced by the patient. The accompanying assessment chart lists selected questions useful in obtaining appropriate information (Chart 55-2).

PHYSICAL ASSESSMENT

Assessment of the skin involves the entire skin area, including the mucous membranes, scalp, hair, and nails. The skin is a reflection of a person's overall health, and alterations commonly correspond to disease in other organ systems. Inspection and palpation are techniques commonly used in examining the skin. The room must be well lighted and warm. A penlight may be used to highlight lesions. The patient completely disrobes and is adequately draped. Gloves are worn during skin examination if rash or lesions are to be palpated. However, it is important to avoid making the patient feel as if he or she cannot be touched. Touching skin lesions indicates a level of acceptance of the patient.

Chart 55-1

Benign Changes in Elderly Skin

- Cherry angiomas (bright red "moles")
- Diminished hair, especially on scalp and pubic area
- Dyschromias (colour variations)
    Solar lentigo (liver spots)
    Melasma (dark discolouration of the skin)
    Lentigines (freckles)
- Neurodermatitis (itchy spots)
- Seborrheic keratoses (crusty brown "stuck-on" patches)
- Spider angiomas
- Telangiectasias (red marks on skin caused by stretching of the superficial blood vessels)
- Wrinkles
- Xerosis (dryness)
- Xanthelasma (yellowish waxy deposits on upper and lower eyelids)

Assessing General Appearance

The general appearance of the skin is assessed by observing colour, temperature, moisture or dryness, skin texture (rough or smooth), lesions, vascularity, mobility, and the condition of the hair and nails. Skin turgor, possible edema, and elasticity are assessed by palpation.

Skin colour varies from person to person and ranges from ivory to deep brown to almost pure black. The skin of exposed portions of the body, especially in sunny, warm climates, tends to be more pigmented than the rest of the body. The vasodilation that occurs with fever, sunburn, and inflammation produces a pink or reddish hue to the skin. Pallor is an absence of or a decrease in normal skin colour and vascularity and is best observed in the conjunctivae or around the mouth.

The bluish hue of cyanosis indicates cellular hypoxia and is easily observed in the extremities, nail beds, lips, and mucous membranes. Jaundice, a yellowing of the skin, is directly related to elevations in serum bilirubin and is often first observed in the sclerae and mucous membranes (Fig. 55-3).

Erythema

Erythema is redness of the skin caused by the congestion of capillaries. In light-skinned people, it is easily observed at any location where it appears. To determine possible inflammation, the skin is palpated for increased warmth and for smoothness (ie, edema) or hardness (ie, intracellular infiltration). Because dark skin tends to assume a purple-grey cast when an inflammatory process is present, it may be difficult to detect erythema.

Rash

In instances of pruritus (ie, itching), the patient should be asked to indicate which areas of the body are involved. The skin is then stretched gently to decrease the reddish tone and make the rash stand out. Pointing a penlight laterally across the skin may effectively highlight the rash. The differences in skin texture are then assessed by running the tips of the fingers lightly over the skin. The borders of the rash may be palpable. The patient's mouth and ears are included in the examination. (Sometimes rubeola, or measles, causes a red cast to appear on the tip of the ears.) The patient's temperature is assessed, and the lymph nodes are palpated.

Cyanosis

Cyanosis is the bluish discolouration that results from a lack of oxygen in the blood. It appears with shock or with respiratory or circulatory compromise. In people with light skin, cyanosis manifests as a bluish hue to the lips, fingertips, and nail beds. Other indications of decreased tissue perfusion include cold, clammy skin; a rapid, thready pulse; and rapid, shallow respirations. The conjunctivae of the eyelids are examined for pallor and **petechiae** (ie, pinpoint red spots that appear on the skin as a result of blood leakage into the skin).

In a person with dark skin, the skin usually assumes a greyish cast. To detect cyanosis, the areas around the mouth and lips and over the cheekbones and earlobes should be observed.

Colour Changes

Almost every process that occurs on the skin causes some colour change. For example, **hypopigmentation** (ie, decrease in the melanin of the skin, resulting in a loss of pigmentation) may be

GENETICS IN NURSING PRACTICE—Integumentary Conditions

Examples of integumentary conditions influenced by genetic factors include the following:

- Albinism
- Eczema
- Hypohidrotic ectodermal dysplasia
- Incontinentia pigmenti
- Neurofibromatosis type 1
- Pseudoxanthoma elasticum
- Psoriasis

NURSING ASSESSMENTS

FAMILY HISTORY ASSESSMENT

- Assess for other closely related family members with integumentary impairment or abnormalities.
- Inquire about the nature and type of skin lesions and age at onset (eg, skin involvement with incontinentia pigmenti occurs in the first few weeks of life with blistering of the skin, whereas lesions of neurofibromatosis type 1 may appear in early childhood through adulthood).
- Note gender of affected individuals (eg, mostly females with incontinentia pigmenti, mostly males with hypohidrotic ectodermal dysplasia).
- Inquire about the presence of other clinical features, such as unusual hair, teeth, or nails; thrombocytopenia; recurrent infections.

PHYSICAL ASSESSMENT

- Assess for related clinical features, such as sparse eyebrows and eyelashes, abnormally shaped teeth, alopecia, nail abnormalities (eg, hypohidrotic ectodermal dysplasia).
- Assess for related alterations in vision, such as nystagmus, strabismus; albinism; retinal abnormalities (eg, pseudoxanthoma elasticum); Lisch nodules and/or optic glioma (neurofibromatosis type 1).

MANAGEMENT ISSUES SPECIFIC TO GENETICS

- Inquire whether DNA mutation or other genetic testing has been performed on affected family members.
- If indicated, refer for further genetic counselling and evaluation so that family members can discuss inheritance, risk to other family members, availability of genetic testing, and gene-based interventions.
- Offer appropriate genetics information and resources.
- Assess patient's understanding of genetics information.
- Provide support to families with newly diagnosed genetic-related integumentary conditions.
- Participate in management and coordination of care for patients with genetic conditions and for individuals predisposed to develop or pass on a genetic condition.

GENETICS RESOURCES FOR NURSES AND THEIR PATIENTS ON THE WEB

Canadian Association of Genetic Counsellors (CAGC)—a listing of genetic centres across Canada; www.cagc-accg.ca

Canadian Cancer Society—information on the genetic factors/risks and genetic testing; www.cancer.ca

Canadian Directory of Genetic Support Groups—a resource guide for families and professionals; www.lhsc.on.ca/programs/medgenet

Canadian Genetic Disease Network—its stated mission to be the primary catalyst in advancing Canada's scientific and commercial competitiveness in genetic research and the application of genetic discoveries to the prevention, diagnosis and treatment of human disease; www.cgdn.ca

Canadian Organization for Rare Disorders (CORD)—information on over 6,000 rare disorders and links individuals/families together with the same rare disorder; www.cord.ca

GeneTests—a publicly funded medical genetics information resource developed for physicians, other health care providers, and researchers; www.genetests.org

Genetic Alliance—increases the capacity of genetic advocacy groups to achieve their missions and leverages the voices of millions of individuals and families living with genetic conditions; www.geneticalliance.org

OMIM Online Mendelian Inheritance in Man—a catalogue of human genes and genetic disorders; www.ncbi.nlm.nih.gov/entrez/query.fcgi?db=OMIM

The Genetics Society of Canada (GSC)—promotes research and communicates the results and implications of genetics to the public; http://life.biology.mcmaster.ca/GSC

---

caused by a fungal infection, eczema, or **vitiligo** (ie, condition characterized by destruction of the melanocytes in circumscribed areas of the skin, resulting in white patches). **Hyperpigmentation** (ie, increase in the melanin of the skin, resulting in increased pigmentation) may occur after disease or injury to the skin (ie, postinflammatory), after sun injury, or as a result of aging.

Changes in skin colour in people with dark skin are more noticeable and may cause more concern because the discolouration is more readily visible. Some variation in skin pigment levels is considered normal. Examples include the pigmented crease across the bridge of the nose, pigmented streaks in the nails, and pigmented spots on the sclera of the eye. Many variations of colour are genetically determined.

ASSESSING PATIENTS WITH DARK SKIN

The colour gradations that occur in people with dark skin are largely determined by genetic transmission; they may be described as light, medium, or dark. In people with dark skin, melanin is produced at a faster rate and in larger quantities than in people with light skin. Healthy dark skin has a reddish base or undertone. The buccal mucosa, tongue, lips, and nails normally are pink. The degree of pigmentation of the patient's skin may affect the appearance of a lesion. Lesions may be black, purple, or grey instead of the tan or red seen in patients with light skin. Dark pigment responds with discolouration after injury or inflammation, and patients with dark skin more often experience postinflammatory hyperpigmentation than those with lighter skin. The hyperpigmentation eventually fades but may require months to a year to do so.

Chart 55-2 • ASSESSMENT

Patient History of Skin Disorders

Patient history relevant to skin disorders may be obtained by asking the following questions:

When did you first notice this skin problem? (Also investigate duration and intensity.)

Has it occurred previously?

Are there any other symptoms?

What site was first affected?

What did the rash or lesion look like when it first appeared?

Where and how fast did it spread?

Do you have any itching, burning, tingling, or crawling sensations?

Is there any loss of sensation?

Is the problem worse at a particular time or season?

How do you think it started?

Do you have a history of hay fever, asthma, hives, eczema, or allergies?

Who in your family has skin problems or rashes?

Did the eruptions appear after certain foods were eaten? Which foods?

When the problem occurred, had you recently consumed alcohol?

What relation do you think there may be between a specific event and the outbreak of the rash or lesion?

What medications are you taking?

What topical medication (ointment, cream, salve) have you put on the lesion (including over-the-counter medications)?

What skin products or cosmetics do you use?

What is your occupation?

What in your immediate environment (plants, animals, chemicals, infections) might be precipitating this disorder? Is there anything new, or are there any changes in the environment?

Does anything touching your skin cause a rash?

How has this affected you (or your life)?

Is there anything else you wish to talk about in regard to this disorder?

In general, people with dark skin suffer the same skin conditions as those with light skin. They are less likely to have skin cancer but more likely to have keloid or scar formation and disorders resulting from occlusion or blockage of hair follicles.

Table 55-2 provides an overview of colour changes in light-skinned and dark-skinned people, and the following section provides specific guidelines for assessing dark and light skin.

ASSESSING SKIN LESIONS

Skin lesions are the most prominent characteristics of dermatologic conditions. They vary in size, shape, and cause and are clas-

sified according to their appearance and origin. Skin lesions can be described as primary or secondary. Primary lesions are the initial lesions and are characteristic of the disease itself. Secondary lesions result from external causes, such as scratching, trauma, infections, or changes caused by wound healing. Depending on the stage of development, skin lesions are further categorized according to type and appearance (Chart 55-3).

A preliminary assessment of the eruption or lesion should help to identify the type of **dermatosis** (ie, abnormal skin condition) and indicate whether the lesion is primary or secondary. At the same time, the anatomic distribution of the eruption should be observed, because certain diseases affect certain sites of the body and are distributed in characteristic patterns and shapes (Figs. 55-4 and 55-5). To determine the extent of the regional distribution, the left and right sides of the body should be compared while the colour and shape of the lesions are assessed. After observation, the lesions are palpated to determine their texture, shape, and border and to see if they are soft and filled with fluid or hard and fixed to the surrounding tissue.

A metric ruler is used to measure the size of the lesions so that any further extension can be compared with this baseline measurement. The dermatosis is documented on the patient's health record; it should be described clearly and in detail, using precise terminology.

After the characteristic distribution of the lesions has been determined, the following information should be obtained and described clearly and in detail:

- Colour of the lesion
- Any redness, heat, pain, or swelling
- Size and location of the involved area
- Pattern of eruption (eg, macular, papular, scaling, oozing, discrete, confluent)
- Distribution of the lesion (eg, bilateral, symmetric, linear, circular)

If acute open wounds or lesions are found on inspection of the skin, a comprehensive assessment should be made and documented in the patient's record. This assessment should address several issues:

- Wound bed: Inspect for necrotic and granulation tissue, epithelium, exudate, colour, and odour.
- Wound edges and margins: Observe for undermining (ie, extension of the wound under the surface skin), and evaluate for condition.
- Wound size: Measure in millimeters or centimeters, as appropriate, to determine diameter and depth of the wound and surrounding erythema.
- Surrounding skin: Assess for colour, suppleness and moisture, irritation, and scaling.

Assessing Vascularity and Hydration

After the colour of the skin has been evaluated and lesions have been inspected, an assessment of vascular changes in the skin is performed. A description of vascular changes includes location, distribution, colour, size, and the presence of pulsations. Common vascular changes include petechiae, ecchymoses, **telangiectases** (ie, red marks on the skin caused by stretching of the superficial blood vessels), angiomas, and venous stars.

Skin moisture, temperature, and texture are assessed primarily by palpation. The elasticity (ie, turgor) of the skin, which decreases in normal aging, may be a factor in assessing the hydration status of a patient.

FIGURE 55-3 Examples of skin colour changes: the bluish tint of cyanosis (*left*) and the yellow hue of jaundice (*right*).

Table 55-2 • Colour Changes in Light and Dark Skin

ETIOLOGY	LIGHT SKIN	DARK SKIN
Pallor		
Anemia—decreased hematocrit Shock—decreased perfusion, vasoconstriction	Generalized pallor	Brown skin appears yellow-brown, dull; black skin appears ashen grey, dull. (Observe areas with least pigmentation: conjunctivae, mucous membranes.)
Local arterial insufficiency	Marked localized pallor (lower extremities, especially when elevated)	Ashen grey, dull; cool to palpation
Albinism—total absence of pigment melanin	Whitish pink	Tan, cream, white
Vitiligo—a condition characterized by destruction of the melanocytes in circumscribed areas of the skin (may be localized or widespread)	Patchy, milky white spots, often symmetric bilaterally	Same
Cyanosis		
Increased amount of unoxygenated hemoglobin:	Dusky blue	Dark but dull, lifeless; only severe cyanosis is apparent in skin. (Observe conjunctivae, oral mucosa, nail beds.)
Central—chronic heart and lung disease cause arterial desaturation	Nail beds dusky	
Peripheral—exposure to cold, anxiety		
Erythema		
Hyperemia—increased blood flow through engorged arterial vessels, as in inflammation, fever, alcohol intake, blushing	Red, bright pink	Purplish tinge, but difficult to see. (Palpate for increased warmth with inflammation, taut skin, and hardening of deep tissues.)
Polycythemia—increased red blood cells, capillary stasis	Ruddy blue in face, oral mucosa, conjunctivae, hands and feet	Well concealed by pigment. (Observe for redness in lips.)
Carbon monoxide poisoning	Bright, cherry red in face and upper torso	Cherry red nail beds, lips, and oral mucosa
Venous stasis—decreased blood flow from area, engorged venules	Dusky rubor of dependent extremities (a prelude to necrosis with pressure ulcer)	Easily masked. (Use palpation to identify warmth or edema.)
Jaundice		
Increased serum bilirubin concentration (>2–3 mg/100 mL) due to liver dysfunction or hemolysis, as after severe burns or some infections	Yellow first in sclerae, hard palate, and mucous membranes; then over skin	Check sclerae for yellow near limbus; do not mistake normal yellowish fatty deposits in the periphery under eyelids for jaundice. (Jaundice is best noted at junction of hard and soft palate, on palms.)
Carotenemia—increased level of serum carotene from ingestion of large amounts of carotene-rich foods	Yellow-orange tinge in forehead, palms and soles, and nasolabial folds, but no yellowing in sclerae or mucous membranes	Yellow-orange tinge in palms and soles
Uremia—renal failure causes retained urochrome pigments in the blood	Orange-green or grey overlying pallor of anemia; may also have ecchymoses and purpura	Easily masked. (Rely on laboratory and clinical findings.)
Brown-Tan		
Addison's disease—cortisol deficiency stimulates increased melanin production	Bronzed appearance, an "external tan"; most apparent around nipples, perineum, genitalia, and pressure points (inner thighs, buttocks, elbows, axillae)	Easily masked. (Rely on laboratory and clinical findings.)
Café-au-lait spots—caused by increased melanin pigment in basal cell layer	Tan to light brown, irregularly shaped, oval patch with well-defined borders often not visible in the very dark skinned person	

Assessing the Nails and Hair

A brief inspection of the nails includes observation of configuration, colour, and consistency. Many alterations in the nail or nail bed reflect local or systemic abnormalities in progress or resulting from past events (Fig. 55-6). Transverse depressions known as Beau's lines in the nails may reflect retarded growth of the nail matrix because of severe illness or, more commonly, local trauma. Ridging, hypertrophy, and other changes may also be visible with local trauma. Paronychia, an inflammation of the skin around the nail, is usually accompanied by tenderness and erythema. The angle between the normal nail and its base is 160 degrees. When palpated, the nail base is usually firm. Clubbing is manifested by a straightening of the normal angle (180 degrees or greater) and softening of the nail base. The softened area feels spongelike when palpated.

(text continues on page 1658)

Chart 55-3 **Primary and Secondary Skin Lesions**

PRIMARY SKIN LESIONS

Primary skin lesions are original lesions arising from previously normal skin. Secondary lesions can originate from primary lesions and are the progression of the primary disease to a different appearance.

Macule

Patch

Macule, Patch
Flat, nonpalpable skin colour change (colour may be brown, white, tan, purple, red)
- *Macule:* <1 cm, circumscribed border
- *Patch:* >1 cm, may have irregular border

Examples:
Freckles, flat moles, petechia, rubella, vitiligo, port wine stains, ecchymosis

Papule

Plaque

Papule, Plaque
Elevated, palpable, solid mass
Circumscribed border
Plaque may be coalesced papules with flat top
- *Papule:* <0.5 cm
- *Plaque:* >0.5 cm

Examples:
Papules: Elevated nevi, warts, lichen planus
Plaques: Psoriasis, actinic keratosis

Tumour

Nodule, Tumour
Elevated, palpable, solid mass
Extends deeper into the dermis than a papule
- *Nodule:* 0.5–2 cm; circumscribed
- *Tumour:* >1–2 cm; tumours do not always have sharp borders

Examples:
Nodules: Lipoma, squamous cell carcinoma, poorly absorbed injection, dermatofibroma
Tumours: Larger lipoma, carcinoma

Bulla

Vesicle

Vesicle, Bulla
Circumscribed, elevated, palpable mass containing serous fluid
- *Vesicle:* <0.5 cm
- *Bulla:* >0.5 cm

Examples:
Vesicles: Herpes simplex/zoster, chickenpox, poison ivy, second-degree burn (blister)
Bulla: Pemphigus, contact dermatitis, large burn blisters, poison ivy, bullous impetigo

Wheal

Wheal
- Elevated mass with transient borders
- Often irregular
- Size and colour vary
- Caused by movement of serous fluid into the dermis
- Does not contain free fluid in a cavity (as, for example, a vesicle does)

Examples:
Urticaria (hives), insect bites

Pustule

Pustule
- Pus-filled vesicle or bulla

Examples:
Acne, impetigo, furuncles, carbuncles

Cyst

Cyst
- Encapsulated fluid-filled or semisolid mass
- In the subcutaneous tissue or dermis

Examples:
Sebaceous cyst, epidermoid cysts

(continued)

Chart 55-3   **Primary and Secondary Skin Lesions (Continued)**

SECONDARY SKIN LESIONS

Secondary skin lesions result from changes in primary lesions.

Erosion

Erosion
- Loss of superficial epidermis
- Does not extend to dermis
- Depressed, moist area

Examples:
Ruptured vesicles, scratch marks

Ulcer
- Skin loss extending past epidermis
- Necrotic tissue loss
- Bleeding and scarring possible

Examples:
Stasis ulcer of venous insufficiency, pressure ulcer

Ulcer

Fissure
- Linear crack in the skin
- May extend to dermis

Examples:
Chapped lips or hands, athlete's foot

Fissure

Scales
- Flakes secondary to desquamated, dead epithelium
- Flakes may adhere to skin surface
- Colour varies (silvery, white)
- Texture varies (thick, fine)

Examples:
Dandruff, psoriasis, dry skin, pityriasis rosea

Scales

Crust
- Dried residue of serum, blood, or pus on skin surface
- Large, adherent crust is a scab

Examples:
Residue left after vesicle rupture: impetigo, herpes, eczema

Crust

Scar (Cicatrix)
- Skin mark left after healing of a wound or lesion
- Represents replacement by connective tissue of the injured tissue
- Young scars: red or purple
- Mature scars: white or glistening

Examples:
Healed wound or surgical incision

Scar

Keloid
- Hypertrophied scar tissue
- Secondary to excessive collagen formation during healing
- Elevated, irregular, red
- Greater incidence among African Americans

Example:
Keloid of ear piercing or surgical incision

Keloid

Atrophy
- Thin, dry, transparent appearance of epidermis
- Loss of surface markings
- Secondary to loss of collagen and elastin
- Underlying vessels may be visible

Examples:
Aged skin, arterial insufficiency

Atrophy

Lichenification
- Thickening and roughening of the skin
- Accentuated skin markings
- May be secondary to repeated rubbing, irritation, scratching

Example:
Contact dermatitis

Lichenification

(continued)

Chart 55-3 | **Primary and Secondary Skin Lesions (Continued)**

VASCULAR SKIN LESIONS

Petechiae

Petechia (*pl.* petechiae)
- Round red or purple macule
- Small: 1–2 mm
- Secondary to blood extravasation
- Associated with bleeding tendencies or emboli to skin

Spider angioma

Spider Angioma
- Red, arteriole lesion
- Central body with radiating branches
- Noted on face, neck, arms, trunk
- Rare below the waist
- May blanch with pressure
- Associated with liver disease, pregnancy, vitamin B deficiency

Ecchymoses

Ecchymosis (*pl.* ecchymoses)
- Round or irregular macular lesion
- Larger than petechia
- Colour varies and changes: black, yellow, and green hues
- Secondary to blood extravasation
- Associated with trauma, bleeding tendencies

Telangiectasia

Telangiectasia (Venous Star)
- Shape varies: spider-like or linear
- Colour bluish or red
- Does not blanch when pressure is applied
- Noted on legs, anterior chest
- Secondary to superficial dilation of venous vessels and capillaries
- Associated with increased venous pressure states (varicosities)

Cherry angioma

Cherry Angioma
- Papular and round
- Red or purple
- Noted on trunk, extremities
- May blanch with pressure
- Normal age-related skin alteration
- Usually not clinically significant

The hair assessment is carried out by inspecting and palpating. Gloves are worn, and the examination room should be well lighted. Separating the hair so that the condition of the skin underneath can be easily seen, the nurse assesses colour, texture, and distribution. Any abnormal lesions, evidence of itching, inflammation, scaling, or signs of infestation (ie, lice or mites) are documented.

COLOUR AND TEXTURE
Natural hair colour ranges from white to black. Hair colour begins to grey with age, initially appearing during the third decade of life, when the loss of melanin begins to become apparent. However, it is not unusual for the hair of younger people to turn grey as a result of hereditary traits. The person with albinism (ie, partial or complete absence of pigmentation) has a genetic predisposition to white hair from birth. The natural state of the hair can be altered by using hair dyes, bleaches, and curling or relaxing products. The types of products used are identified during the assessment.

The texture of scalp hair ranges from fine to coarse, silky to brittle, oily to dry, and shiny to dull, and hair can be straight, curly, or kinky. Dry, brittle hair may result from overuse of hair dyes, hair dryers, and curling irons or from endocrine disorders, such as thyroid dysfunction. Oily hair is usually caused by increased secretion from the sebaceous glands close to the scalp. If the patient reports a recent change in hair texture, the underlying reason is pursued; the alteration may arise simply from the overuse of commercial hair products or from changing to a new shampoo.

DISTRIBUTION
Body hair distribution varies with location. Hair over most of the body is fine, except in the axillae and pubic areas, where it is coarse. Pubic hair, which develops at puberty, forms a diamond shape extending up to the umbilicus in boys and men. Female pubic hair resembles an inverted triangle. If the pattern found is more characteristic of the opposite gender, it may indicate an endocrine problem and further investigation is in order. Racial differences in hair are expected, such as straight hair in Asians and curly, coarser hair in people of African descent.

Men tend to have more body and facial hair than women. Loss of hair, or alopecia, can occur over the entire body or be confined to a specific area. Scalp hair loss may be localized to patchy areas or may range from generalized thinning to total

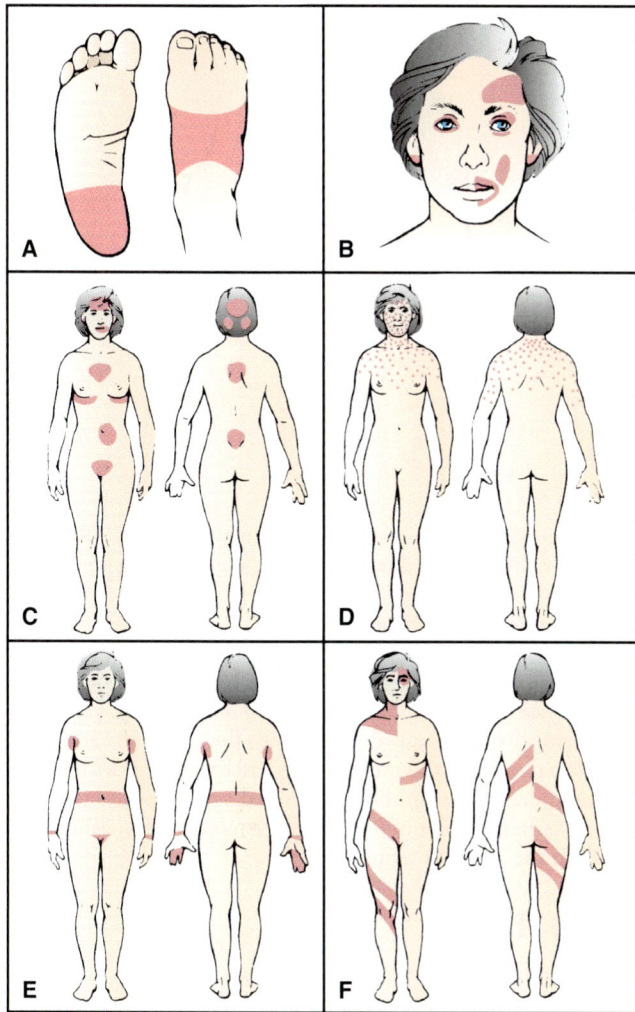

FIGURE 55-4 Anatomic distribution of common skin disorders. (**A**) Contact dermatitis (shoes). (**B**) Contact dermatitis (cosmetics, perfumes, earrings). (**C**) Seborrheic dermatitis. (**D**) Acne. (**E**) Scabies. (**F**) Herpes zoster (shingles).

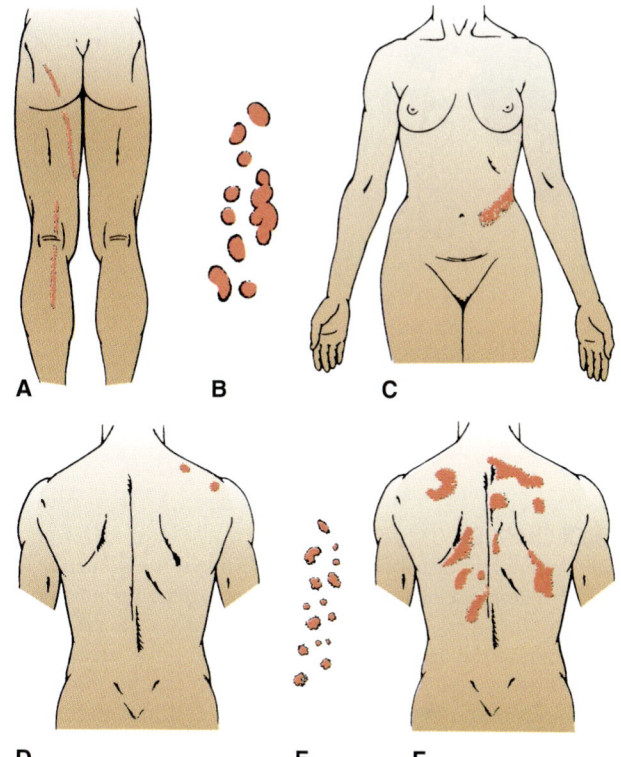

FIGURE 55-5 Skin lesion configurations. (**A**) Linear (in a line). (**B**) Annular and arciform (circular or arcing). (**C**) Zosteriform (linear along a nerve route). (**D**) Grouped (clustered). (**E**) Discrete (separate and distinct). (**F**) Confluent (merged). From Weber, J. W., & Kelley, J. (2003). *Health assessment in nursing* (2nd ed.). Philadelphia: Lippincott Williams and Wilkins.

baldness. When assessing scalp hair loss, it is important to investigate the underlying cause with the patient. Patchy hair loss may be from habitual hair pulling or twisting; from excessive traction on the hair (eg, braiding too tightly); excessive use of dyes, straighteners, and oils; chemotherapeutic agents (eg, doxorubicin, cyclophosphamide); fungal infection; or moles or lesions on the scalp. Regrowth may be erratic, and distribution may never attain the previous thickness.

HAIR LOSS

The most common cause of hair loss is male pattern baldness, which affects more than one half of the male population and is believed to be related to heredity, aging, and androgen (male hormone) levels. Androgen is necessary for male pattern baldness to develop. The pattern of hair loss begins with receding of the hairline in the frontal-temporal area and progresses to gradual thinning and complete loss of hair over the top of the scalp and crown. Figure 55-7 illustrates the typical male pattern hair loss.

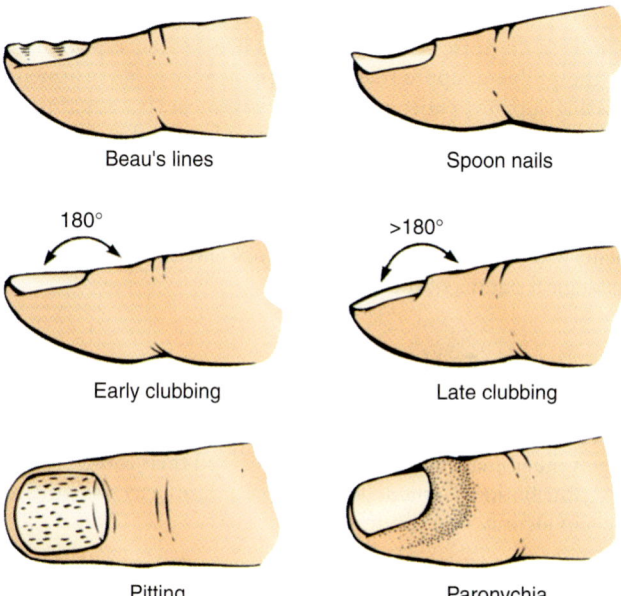

FIGURE 55-6 Common nail disorders. From Weber, J. W., & Kelley, J. (2003). *Health assessment in nursing* (2nd ed.). Philadelphia: Lippincott Williams and Wilkins.

FIGURE 55-7 The progression of male pattern baldness.

OTHER CHANGES

Male pattern hair distribution may be seen in some women at the time of menopause, when the hormone estrogen is no longer produced by the ovaries. In women with hirsutism, excessive hair may grow on the face, chest, shoulders, and pubic area. When menopause is ruled out as the underlying cause, hormonal abnormalities related to pituitary or adrenal dysfunction must be investigated.

Because patients with skin conditions may be viewed negatively by others, these patients may become distraught and avoid interaction with people. Skin conditions can lead to disfigurement, isolation, job loss, and economic hardship.

Some conditions may subject the patient to a protracted illness, leading to feelings of depression, frustration, self-consciousness, poor self-image, and rejection. Itching and skin irritation, features of many skin diseases, may be a constant annoyance. The results of these discomforts may be loss of sleep, anxiety, and depression, all of which reinforce the general distress and fatigue that frequently accompany skin disorders.

For patients suffering such physical and psychological discomforts, the nurse needs to provide understanding, explanations of the problem, appropriate instructions related to treatment, nursing support, patience, and encouragement. It takes time to help patients gain insight into their problems and resolve their difficulties. It is imperative to overcome any aversion that may be felt when caring for patients with unattractive skin disorders. The nurse should show no sign of hesitancy when approaching patients with skin disorders. Such hesitancy only reinforces the psychological trauma of the disorder.

Diagnostic Evaluation

In addition to obtaining the patient's history, the examiner inspects the primary and secondary lesions and their configuration and distribution. Certain diagnostic procedures may also be used to help identify skin conditions.

SKIN BIOPSY

Performed to obtain tissue for microscopic examination, a skin biopsy may be obtained by scalpel excision or by a skin punch instrument that removes a small core of tissue. Biopsies are performed on skin nodules, plaques, blisters, and other lesions to rule out malignancy and to establish an exact diagnosis.

IMMUNOFLUORESCENCE

Designed to identify the site of an immune reaction, immunofluorescence testing combines an antigen or antibody with a fluorochrome dye. Antibodies can be made fluorescent by attaching them to a dye. Direct immunofluorescence tests on skin are techniques to detect autoantibodies directed against portions of the skin. The indirect immunofluorescence test detects specific antibodies in the patient's serum.

PATCH TESTING

Performed to identify substances to which the patient has developed an allergy, patch testing involves applying the suspected allergens to normal skin under occlusive patches. The development of redness, fine bumps, or itching is considered a weak positive reaction; fine blisters, papules, and severe itching indicate a moderately positive reaction; and blisters, pain, and ulceration indicate a strong positive reaction (see Chap. 53).

SKIN SCRAPINGS

Tissue samples are scraped from suspected fungal lesions with a scalpel blade moistened with oil so that the scraped skin adheres to the blade. The scraped material is transferred to a glass slide, covered with a coverslip, and examined microscopically.

TZANCK SMEAR

The Tzanck smear is a test used to examine cells from blistering skin conditions, such as herpes zoster, varicella, herpes simplex, and all forms of pemphigus. The secretions from a suspected lesion are applied to a glass slide, stained, and examined.

WOOD'S LIGHT EXAMINATION

Wood's light is a special lamp that produces long-wave ultraviolet rays, which result in a characteristic dark purple fluorescence. The colour of the fluorescent light is best seen in a darkened room, where it is possible to differentiate epidermal from dermal lesions and hypopigmented and hyperpigmented lesions from normal skin. The patient is reassured that the light is not harmful to skin or eyes. Lesions that still contain melanin almost disappear under ultraviolet light, whereas lesions that are devoid of melanin increase in whiteness with ultraviolet light.

CLINICAL PHOTOGRAPHS

Photographs are taken to document the nature and extent of the skin condition and are used to determine progress or improvement resulting from treatment.

Critical Thinking Exercises

1. In thinking about the skin as the first line of defense for homeostasis, identify some of the threats to skin integrity that should be assessed when admitting a patient to the hospital. What impact does the type of skin care delivered have on skin integrity? How would skin assessment of an elderly patient differ from that of a young adult?

2. An elderly African Canadian woman is admitted to the hospital for treatment of diabetes. What concerns should be addressed relative to the skin and circulation in a patient with diabetes? How will your assessment of the skin of this patient differ from the assessment of the skin of a Caucasian patient?

REFERENCES AND SELECTED READINGS

Books

Bickley, L. S., & Szilagyi, P. G. (2003). *Bates' guide to physical examination and history taking* (8th ed.). Philadelphia: Lippincott Williams & Williams.

Champion, R. H., Burton, J. L., Burns, D. A., & Breathnach, S. M. (1998). *Rook/Wilkinson/Ebling textbook of dermatology* (6th ed.). Boston: Blackwell Science.

Demis, D. J. (Ed.). (1998). *Clinical dermatology.* Philadelphia: Lippincott-Raven.

Fitzpatrick, T. B., et al. (1997). *Color atlas & synopsis of clinical dermatology* (3rd ed.). New York: McGraw-Hill.

Freedberg, I. M., Eisen, A. Z., Austen, K. F., Goldsmith, S. I., Katz, S., & Fitzpatrick, T. B. (1999). *Fitzpatrick's dermatology in general medicine* (5th ed.). New York: McGraw-Hill.

Holick, M. F. (1998). *How much vitamin D is enough?* Available at: http://www.mcmaster.ca/inabis98/arkinson/holick0835/two.html. Retrieved December 15, 2005.

Odom, R. B., James, W. D., & Berger, T. G. (2000). *Andrews' diseases of the skin* (9th ed.). Philadelphia: W. B. Saunders.

Weber, J. W., & Kelley, J. (2003). *Health assessment in nursing* (2nd ed.). Philadelphia: Lippincott Williams & Wilkins.

Journals

Brown, J., et al. (2002). Clinical practice guidelines for the diagnosis and management of osteoporosis in Canada. *Canadian Medical Association Journal, 167*(10 suppl), S1–S34.

Draelos, Z. D. (1997). Understanding African-American hair. *Dermatology Nursing, 9*(4), 227–231.

Fleischer, A. B., Feldman, S. R., & Rapp, S. R. (2000). The magnitude of skin disease in the United States. *Dermatologic Clinics, 17*(2), 322–327.

Jaworski, C., & Gilliam, A. C. (1999). Immunopathology of the hair follicle. *Dermatologic Clinics, 17*(3), 561–568.

Kang, S. (2001). Photoaging: Pathogenesis, prevention and treatment. *Clinical Geriatric Medicine, 17*(4), 643–659.

Sun-protection behaviors used by adults for their children: U.S. (1998). *Morbidity and Mortality Weekly Report, 47*(23), 48–52.

Weinstock, M. A., & Rossi, J. S. (1998). The Rhode Island Sun Smart Project: A scientific approach to skin cancer prevention. *Clinical Dermatology, 16*(4), 411–413.

RESOURCES AND WEBSITES

Canadian Alopecia Areata Association, Box 42084, RPO Millbourne, Edmonton, AB T6K 4C4; (780) 454-2326; www.kumc.edu/gec/support/alopecia.html.

Canadian Association of Genetic Counsellors (CAGC); www.cagc-accg.ca.

Canadian Cancer Society/Société canadienne du cancer, National Office, Suite 200, 10 Alcorn Avenue, Toronto, ON M4V 3B1;(416) 961-7223; fax: (416) 961-4189; www.cancer.ca.

Canadian Directory of Genetic Support Groups: Support Group Directory, Regional Medical Genetics Centre, Children's Hospital of Western Ontario, 800 Commissioner's Road East, London, ON N6C 2V5; (519) 685-8453; Ontario only: 1-800-243-8416; fax: (519) 685-8214; www.lhsc.on.ca/programs/medgenet.

Canadian Genetic Disease Network, Suite 201, 2150 Western Parkway, Vancouver, BC V6T 1V6; (604) 221-7300; fax: (604) 221-0778; email: info@cgdn.ca; www.cgdn.ca.

Canadian Organization for Rare Disorders (CORD), PO Box 814, Coaldale, AB T1M 1M7; (403) 345-4544; toll free: 1-877-302-7273; fax: (403) 345-3948; www.cord.ca.

Dermatology online atlas, a cooperation between the Department of Clinical Social Medicine (University of Heidelberg) and the Department of Dermatology (University of Erlangen); http://www.dermis.net.

Eczema Society of Canada, 24 Park Road, Whitby, ON L1M 1G7; (905) 655-9232; 1-866-432-0362; www.eczemacanada.ca.

Foundation for Ichthyosis and Related Skin Types, 650 N. Cannon Avenue, Suite 17, Lansdale, PA 19446; 215-631-1411; http://www.scalyskin.org.

GeneTests, 9725 Third Avenue NE, Suite 602, Seattle, WA 98115, USA; (206) 616-4033; fax: (206) 221-4679; genetests@genetests.org; www.genetests.org.

Genetic Alliance, 4301 Connecticut Ave NW, Suite 404, Washington, DC 20008-2369, USA; (202) 966-5557; fax: (202) 966-8553; info@geneticalliance.org; www.geneticalliance.org.

Health Canada, AL 0900C2, Ottawa ON K1A 0K9; (866) 225-0709; www.healthcanada.ca/nutrition.

Lupus Canada, 590 Alden Road, Suite 211 Markham ON L3R 8N2; 1-800-661-1468; www.lupuscanada.org.

Medscape online sources for medical information; http://www.medscape.com.

National Organization for Albinism and Hypopigmentation, P.O. Box 959, East Hampstead, NH 03826-0959; 800-473-2310; http://www.albinism.org.

National Vitiligo Foundation, 611 South Fleishel Ave., Tyler, TX 75701; 903-531-0074; http://www.nvfi.org.

Neutrogena and Orthopharmaceuticals Products: 1-800-582-4048; http://www.neutrogena.com.

New Zealand Dermatology Society; http://www.dermnetnz.org.

OMIM Online Mendelian Inheritance in Man; www.ncbi.nlm.nih.gov/entrez/query.fcgi?db=OMIM.

Psoriasis Society of Canada, National Office, PO Box 25015, Halifax, NS B3M 4H4; 1-800-656-4494; www.psoriasissociety.org.

Rosacea Awareness Program, 368 Notre Dame Street West, Montreal QC H2Y 1T9; 1-888-767-2232; www.about-rosacea.com; www.rosacea.org.

Skin Cancer Foundation, 575 Park Ave. S., New York, NY 10016; 1-800-SKIN-490; http://www.skincancer.org.

The Canadian Association of Wound Care, PO Box 85557, 1048 Eglinton Avenue, West Toronto, ON M6C 4A8; (877) 288-7018; www.cawc.net.

The Genetics Society of Canada; http://life.biology.mcmaster.ca/GSC.

Management of Patients With Dermatologic Problems

Adapted by Tracey Stephen

LEARNING OBJECTIVES ●

On completion of this chapter, the learner will be able to:

1. Describe the general management of the patient with an abnormal skin condition.
2. Use the nursing process as a framework for care of the patient with psoriasis.
3. Describe the health education needs of the patient with infections of the skin and parasitic skin diseases.
4. Use the nursing process as a framework for care of patients with noninfectious, inflammatory dermatoses.
5. Describe the management and nursing care of the patient with skin cancer.
6. Use the nursing process as a framework for care of the patient with malignant melanoma.
7. Describe characteristics of the various types of Kaposi's sarcoma.
8. Compare the various types of dermatologic and plastic reconstructive surgeries.
9. Use the nursing process as a framework for care of the patient undergoing facial reconstructive surgery.

Nursing care for patients with dermatologic problems includes administering topical and systemic medications, managing wet dressings and other special dressings, and providing therapeutic baths. The four major objectives of therapy are to prevent additional damage, prevent secondary infection, reverse the inflammatory process, and relieve the symptoms.

Skin Care for Patients With Skin Conditions

Some skin problems are markedly aggravated by soap and water, and bathing routines are modified according to the condition. Denuded skin, whether the area of desquamation is large or small, is excessively prone to damage by chemicals and trauma. The friction of a towel, if applied with vigour, is sufficient to produce a brisk inflammatory response that causes any existing lesion to flare up and extend.

Protecting the Skin

The essence of skin care and protection in bathing a patient with skin problems is as follows: a mild, lipid-free soap or soap substitute is used; the area is rinsed completely and blotted dry with a soft cloth; and deodorant soaps are avoided.

Special care is necessary when changing dressings. Pledgets saturated with oil, sterile saline, or another prescribed solution help to loosen crusts, remove exudates, or free an adherent dry dressing.

Preventing Secondary Infection

Potentially infectious skin lesions should be regarded strictly as such, and proper precautions should be observed until the diagnosis is established. Most lesions with pus contain infectious material. The nurse and physician must adhere to standard precautions and wear gloves when inspecting the skin or changing the dressing. Proper disposal of any contaminated dressing is carried out according to Canadian Centre for Occupational Health and Safety (CCOHS) regulations.

Reversing the Inflammatory Process

The type of skin lesion (eg, oozing, infected, or dry) usually determines the type of local medication or treatment that is prescribed. As a rule, if the skin is acutely inflamed (ie, hot, red, and swollen) and oozing, it is best to apply wet dressings and soothing lotions. For chronic conditions in which the skin surface is dry and scaly, water-soluble emulsions, creams, ointments, and pastes are used. The therapy is modified as the responses of the skin indicate. The patient and the nurse should note whether the medication or dressings seem to irritate the skin. The success or failure of therapy usually depends on adequate instruction and motivation of the patient and the interest of and support by the health care personnel.

Wound Care for Skin Conditions

There are three major classifications of dressings for skin conditions: wet, moisture-retentive, and occlusive. During the 1980s and 1990s, new product development quadrupled the available choices for wound care, especially within the moisture-retentive dressing classification. Products classified as moisture-retentive dressings include hydrogels, foams, and alginates. Biologicals and biosynthetics containing collagen and growth factor are being researched and will soon be available. Chart 56-1 lists generic wound care products. Consultation with a wound care specialist can be very helpful in choosing the product most appropriate for the patient.

Dressings and Rules of Wound Care

Even with the increased availability of dressings, an appropriate selection can be made if certain principles are maintained, referred to as the five rules of wound care (Krastner, et al, 2002).

Rule 1: Categorization. The nurse should learn about dressings by generic category and compare new products with those that already make up the category. As hundreds of choices become available, the nurse should become familiar with the generic categories and develop a systematic approach to product selection. The nurse should become familiar with indications, contraindications, and side effects. The best dressing may be created by combining products in different categories to achieve several goals at the same time. These categories are discussed in subsequent sections.

Rule 2: Selection. The nurse should select the safest and most effective, user-friendly, and cost-effective dressing possible. In

Glossary

acantholysis: separation of epidermal cells from each other due to damage or abnormality of the intracellular substance
balneotherapy: a bath with therapeutic additives
carbuncle: localized skin infection involving several hair follicles
cheilitis: dry, cracking, inflamed skin at the corners of the mouth
comedones: the primary lesions of acne, caused by sebum blockage in the hair follicle
débridement: removal of necrotic or dead tissue by mechanical, surgical, or autolytic means

dermatitis: any inflammation of the skin
dermatosis: any abnormal skin lesion
epidermopoiesis: development of epidermal cells
furuncle: localized skin infection of a single hair follicle
hydrophilic: a material that absorbs moisture
hydrophobic: a material that repels moisture
hygroscopic: a material that absorbs moisture from the air
lichenification: thickening of the horny layer of the skin
liniments: lotions with added oil for increased softening of the skin

plasmapheresis: removal of whole blood from the body, separation of its cellular elements by centrifugation, and reinfusion of them suspended in saline or some other plasma substitute, thereby depleting the body's own plasma without depleting its cells
Propionibacterium acnes: bacteria that live on the skin; the primary causative agent of acne
pyodermas: bacterial skin infections
suspensions: liquid preparations in which powder is suspended, requiring shaking before use
tinea: a superficial fungal infection on the skin or scalp

Chart 56-1 Wound Care Products

adhesives	creams or skin	lubricating, stimu-
adhesive removers	protectant	lating sprays
adhesive skin	pastes	moisturizers
closures	dressing covers	moisture barrier
adhesive tapes	enzyme débriding	ointments
alginate dressings	agents	ointments
antibiotics	foam dressings	perineal cleansers
antimicrobials	gauze dressings	skin sealants
antiseptics	growth factors	transparent film
bandages	hydrocolloid	dressings
biosynthetic	dressings	wound fillers:
dressings	hydrogel dressings	pastes, powders,
cleansers	leg ulcer wraps,	beads, etc.
collagen dressings	compression	wound pouches
composite dressings	bandages or	
contact layers	wraps	

many cases, nurses carry out the physician's prescriptions for dressings, but they should be prepared to give the physician feedback about the dressing's effect on the wound, ease of use for the patient, and other considerations when applicable.

Rule 3: Change. The nurse changes dressings based on patient, wound, and dressing assessments, not on standardized routines. Traditional nursing care plans recommended changing dressings on a routine schedule, often three or four times each day.

NURSING ALERT It is believed that the natural wound-healing process should not be disrupted. Unless the wound is infected or has a heavy discharge, it is common to leave chronic wounds covered for 48 to 72 hours and acute wounds for 24 hours.

Rule 4: Evolution. As the wound progresses through the phases of wound healing, the dressing protocol is altered to optimize wound healing. It is rare, especially in cases of chronic wounds, that the same dressing material is appropriate throughout the healing process. The rule assumes that the nurse and the patient or family have access to a wide variety of products and knowledge about their use. The nurse teaches the patient or family caregiver about wound care and ensures that the family has access to appropriate dressing choices.

Rule 5: Practice. Practice with dressing material is required for the nurse to learn the performance parameters of the particular dressing. Refining the skills of applying appropriate dressings correctly and learning about new dressing products are essential nursing responsibilities. Dressing changes should not be delegated to assistive personnel; these techniques require the knowledge base and assessment skills of professional nurses.

Wet Dressings

Wet dressings (ie, wet compresses applied to the skin) were traditionally used for acute, weeping, inflammatory lesions. They have become almost obsolete in light of the many newer products available for wound care. Wet dressings are sterile or nonsterile (clean), depending on the skin disorder. They are used to reduce inflammation by producing constriction of the blood vessels

(thereby decreasing vasodilation and local blood flow in inflammation); to clean the skin of exudates, crusts, and scales; to maintain drainage of infected areas; and to promote healing by facilitating the free movement of epidermal cells across the involved skin so that new granulation tissue forms. Wet dressings can be used for vesicular, bullous, pustular, and ulcerative disorders, as well as for inflammatory conditions.

Before applying these dressings, the nurse performs hand hygiene and puts on sterile or clean gloves. The open dressing requires frequent changes because evaporation is rapid. The closed dressing is changed less frequently, but there is always a danger that the closed dressing may cause not only softening and but actual maceration of the underlying skin. Wet-to-dry dressings are used to remove exudate from erosions or ulcers. The dressing remains in place until it dries. It is then removed without soaking so that crusts, exudate, or pus from the skin lesion adhere to the dressing and are removed with it.

Moisture-Retentive Dressings

Newer, commercially produced moisture-retentive dressings can perform the same functions as wet compresses but are more efficient at removing exudate because of their higher moisture-vapor transmission rate; some have reservoirs that can hold excessive exudate. There is also evidence that moist wound healing results in wound resurfacing 40% faster than with air exposure. A number of moisture-retentive dressings are already impregnated with saline solution, petrolatum, zinc-saline solution, hydrogel, or antimicrobial agents, thereby eliminating the need to coat the skin to avoid maceration. The main advantages of moisture-retentive dressings over wet compresses are reduced pain, fewer infections, less scar tissue, gentle autolytic débridement, and decreased frequency of dressing changes. Depending on the product used and the type of dermatologic problem encountered, most moisture-retentive dressings may remain in place from 12 to 24 hours; some can remain in place as long as a week. Table 56-1 is a guide to wound dressing functions and categories.

Hydrogels are polymers with a 90% to 95% water content. They are available in impregnated sheets or as gel in a tube. Their high moisture content makes them ideal for autolytic débridement of wounds. They are semitransparent, allowing for wound inspection without dressing removal. They are comfortable and soothing for the painful wound. They have no inherent adhesive and require a secondary dressing to keep them in place. Hydrogels are appropriate for superficial wounds with high serous output, such as abrasions, skin graft sites, and draining venous ulcers.

Hydrocolloids are composed of a water-impermeable, polyurethane outer covering separated from the wound by a hydrocolloid material. They are adherent and nonpermeable to water vapour and oxygen. As it evaporates over the wound, water is absorbed into the dressing, which softens and discolours with the increased water content. The dressing can be removed without damage to the wound. As the dressing absorbs water, it produces a foul-smelling, yellowish covering over the wound. This is a normal chemical interaction between the dressing and wound exudate and should not be confused with purulent drainage from the wound. Unfortunately, most of the hydrocolloid dressings are opaque, limiting inspection of the wound without removal of the dressing.

Available in sheets and in gels, hydrocolloids are a good choice for exudative wounds and for acute wounds. Easy to use and comfortable, hydrocolloid dressings promote débridement and formation of granulation tissue. They do not have to be removed for bathing. Most can be left in place for up to 7 days.

Table 56-1 • Quick Guide to Wound Dressing Function and Categories

FUNCTION	ACTION	EXAMPLE
Absorption	Absorbs exudate	Alginates, composite dressings, foams, gauze, hydrocolloids, hydrogels
Cleansing	Removes purulent drainage, foreign debris, and devitalized tissue	Wound cleansers
Débridement	*Autolytic;* covers a wound and allows enzymes to self-digest sloughed skin	Absorption beads, pastes, powders; alginates; composite dressings; foams; hydrate gauze; hydrogels; hydrocolloids; transparent films; wound care systems
	Chemical or enzymatic; applied topically to break down devitalized tissue	Enzymatic débridement agents
	Mechanical; removes devitalized tissue with mechanical force	Wound cleansers, gauze (wet to dry), whirlpool
Diathermy	Produces electrical current to promote warmth and new tissue growth	
Hydration	Adds moisture to a wound	Gauze (saturated with saline) solution, hydrogels, wound care systems, fibrous fleece dressings
Maintain moist environment	Manages moisture levels in a wound and maintains a moist environment	Composites, contact layers, foams, gauze (impregnated or saturated), hydogels, hydrocolloids, transparent films, wound care systems
Manage high-output wounds	Manages excessive quantities of exudate	Pouching systems
Pack or fill dead space	Prevents premature wound closure or fills shallow areas and provides absorption	Absorbent beads, powders, pastes; alginates, composites, foams, gauze (impregnated and non-impregnated)
Protect and cover wound	Provides protection from the external environment	Composites, compression bandages/wraps, foams, gauze dressings, hydrogels, hydrocolloids, transparent film dressings
Protect periwound skin	Prevents moisture and mechanical trauma from damaging delicate tissue around wound	Composites, foams, hydrocolloids, pouching systems, skin sealants, transparent film dressings
Provide therapeutic compression	Provides appropriate levels of support to the lower extremities in venous stasis disease	Compression bandages, wraps

Foam dressings consist of microporous polyurethane with an absorptive **hydrophilic** (ie, water-absorbing) surface that covers the wound and a **hydrophobic** (ie, water-resistant) backing to block leakage of exudate. They are nonadherent and require a secondary dressing to keep them in place. Moisture is absorbed into the foam layer, decreasing maceration of surrounding tissue. A moist environment is maintained, and removal of the dressing does not damage the wound. The foams are opaque and must be removed for wound inspection. Foams are a good choice for exudative wounds. They are especially helpful over bony prominences because they provide contoured cushioning.

Calcium alginates are derived from seaweed and consist of tremendously absorbent calcium alginate fibres. They are hemostatic and bioabsorbable and can be used as sheets, mats, or ropes of absorbent material. As the exudate is absorbed, the fibres turn into a viscous hydrogel. They are quite useful in areas where the tissue is more irritated or macerated. The alginate dressing forms a moist pocket over the wound while the surrounding skin stays dry. They also react with wound fluid to form a foul-smelling coating. Alginates work well when packed into a deep cavity, wound, or sinus tract with heavy drainage (Krastner et al, 2002). They are nonadherent and require a secondary dressing.

Occlusive Dressings

Occlusive dressings may be commercially produced or made inexpensively from sterile or nonsterile gauze squares or wrap. Occlusive dressings cover topical medication that is applied to a **dermatosis** (ie, abnormal skin lesion). The area is kept airtight by using plastic film (eg, plastic wrap). Plastic film is thin and readily adapts to all sizes, body shapes, and skin surfaces. Plastic surgical tape containing a corticosteroid in the adhesive layer can be cut to size and applied to individual lesions. Generally, plastic wrap should be used no more than 12 hours each day.

AUTOLYTIC DÉBRIDEMENT

Autolytic **débridement** is a process that uses the body's own digestive enzymes to break down necrotic tissue. The wound is kept moist with occlusive dressings. Eschar and necrotic debris are softened, liquefied, and separated from the bed of the wound.

Several commercially available products contain the same enzymes that the body produces naturally. These are called enzymatic débriding agents; examples include Accu Zyme, Granulex, and Zymase. Currently, none of these products is available in Canada. Application of these products speeds the rate at which necrotic tissue is removed. This method is still slower and no more effective than surgical débridement. When enzymatic débridement is being used under an occlusive dressing, a foul odour is produced by the breakdown of cellular debris. This odour does not indicate that the wound is infected. The nurse should expect this reaction, and help the patient understand the reason for the odour.

Advances in Wound Treatment

Increasing understanding of how skin heals has led to several advances in therapy. Growth factors are cytokines or proteins that have potent mitogenic activity (Valencia et al., 2001). Low levels of cytokines circulate in the blood continuously, but activated platelets release increased amounts of preformed growth factors into a wound. This increase in cytokines in the wound stimulates cellular growth and granulation of skin. Regranex gel contains becaplermin, a platelet-derived growth factor, which is applied to the wound to stimulate healing. Apligraf is a skin construct (ie, bioengineered skin substitute) imbedded in a dressing that also contains cytokines and fibroblasts. When applied to wounds, these agents stimulate platelet activity and potentially decrease wound healing time (Paquette & Falanga, 2002).

Some oral medications are being investigated for their benefits in healing chronic venous ulcers of the lower legs. Pentoxifylline (Trental) increases peripheral blood flow by decreasing the viscosity of blood. It has some fibrinolytic action and decreases leukocyte adhesion to the wall of the blood vessels. Enteric-coated aspirin has also been shown to be of value, although its exact mechanism is still not clear (Valencia et al., 2001).

Medical Management

THERAPEUTIC BATHS (BALNEOTHERAPY) AND MEDICATIONS

Baths or soaks, known as **balneotherapy**, are useful when large areas of skin are affected. The baths remove crusts, scales, and old medications and relieve the inflammation and itching that accompany acute dermatoses. The water temperature should be comfortable, and the bath should not exceed 20 to 30 minutes because of the tendency of baths and soaks to produce skin maceration. Table 56-2 lists the different types of therapeutic baths and their uses.

PHARMACOLOGIC THERAPY

Because skin is easily accessible and therefore easy to treat, topical medications are often used. High concentrations of some medications can be applied directly to the affected site with little systemic absorption and therefore with few systemic side effects. However, some medications are readily absorbed through the skin and can produce systemic effects. Because topical preparations may induce allergic contact **dermatitis** (ie, inflammation of the skin) in sensitive patients, any untoward response should be reported immediately and the medication discontinued.

Medicated lotions, creams, ointments, and powders are frequently used to treat skin lesions. In general, moisture-retentive dressings, with or without medication, are used in the acute stage; lotions and creams are reserved for the subacute stage; and ointments are used when inflammation has become chronic and the skin is dry with scaling or **lichenification** (ie, leathery thickening).

With all types of topical medication, the patient is taught to apply the medication gently but thoroughly and, when necessary, to cover the medication with a dressing to protect clothing. Table 56-3 lists some commonly used topical preparations.

Lotions. Lotions are of two types: suspensions and liniments. **Suspensions** consist of a powder in water, requiring shaking before application, and clear solutions, containing completely dissolved active ingredients. Lotions are usually applied directly to the skin, but a dressing soaked in the lotion can be placed on the affected area. A suspension such as calamine lotion provides a rapid cooling and drying effect as it evaporates, leaving a thin, medicinal layer of powder on the affected skin. Lotions are frequently used to replenish lost skin oils or to relieve pruritus. Lotions must be applied every 3 or 4 hours for sustained therapeutic effect. If left in place for a longer period, they may crust and cake on the skin. **Liniments** are lotions with oil added to prevent crusting. Because lotions are easy to use, therapeutic compliance is generally high.

Powders. Powders usually have a talc, zinc oxide, bentonite, or cornstarch base and are dusted on the skin with a shaker or with cotton sponges. Although their therapeutic action is brief, powders act as **hygroscopic** agents that absorb and retain moisture from the air and reduce friction between skin surfaces and clothing or bedding.

Table 56-2 • Types of Therapeutic Baths

BATH SOLUTION	EFFECTS AND USES	NURSING INTERVENTIONS
Water	Same effect as wet dressings	• Fill the tub half full.
Saline	Used for widely disseminated lesions	• Keep the water at a comfortable temperature.
Colloidal (Aveeno, oatmeal)	Antipruritic, soothing	• Do not allow the water to cool excessively.
Sodium bicarbonate (baking soda)	Cooling	• Use a bath mat—*medications added to bath can cause the tub to be slippery.*
Starch	Soothing	• Apply an emollient cream to damp skin after the bath if lubrication is desired.
Medicated tars	Psoriasis and chronic eczema	• Because tars are volatile, the bath area should be well ventilated.
Bath oils	Antipruritic and emollient action; acute and subacute generalized eczematous eruptions	• Dry by gently blotting with a towel.
		• Keep room warm to minimize temperature fluctuations.
		• Encourage the patient to wear light, loose clothing after the bath.

Table 56-3 • Common Topical Preparations and Medications

PREPARATION	PRODUCT NAME
Bath preparations	
With tar	Balnetar, Doak Oil, Lavatar
With colloidal oatmeal	Aveeno Oilated Bath Powder
With oatmeal and mineral oil	Aveeno Bath Oil, Nutra Soothe
With mineral oil	Nutraderm Bath Oil, Lubath, Alpha-Keri Bath Oil
Moisturizer creams	Acid Mantle Cream, Curel Cream, Dermasil, Eucerin, Lubriderm, Noxzema Skin Cream
Moisturizer ointments	Aquaphor Ointment, Eutra Swiss Skin Cream, Vaseline Ointment
Topical anesthetics	lidocaine (Xylocaine) of various strengths in the form of spray, ointment, gel; EMLA cream (lidocaine 2.5% and prilocaine 2.5%)
Topical antibiotics	bacitracin, Polysporin (bacitracin and polymixin B), Bactroban ointment or cream (mupirocin 2%), erythromycin 2% (Emgel, Eryderm Solution), clindamycin phosphate 1% (Cleocin cream, gel, solution), gentamicin sulfate 1% (Garamycin cream or ointment), 1% silver sulfadiazine cream (Silvadene)

Creams. Creams may be suspensions of oil in water or emulsions of water in oil, with additional ingredients to prevent bacterial and fungal growth. Both may cause an allergic reaction such as contact dermatitis. Oil-in-water creams are easily applied and usually are the most cosmetically acceptable to the patient. Although they can be used on the face, they tend to have a drying effect. Water-in-oil emulsions are greasier and are preferred for drying and flaking dermatoses. Creams usually are rubbed into the skin by hand. They are used for their moisturizing and emollient effects.

Gels. Gels are semisolid emulsions that become liquid when applied to the skin or scalp. They are cosmetically acceptable to the patient because they are not visible after application, and they are greaseless and nonstaining. The newer water-based gels appear to penetrate the skin more effectively and cause less stinging on application. They are especially useful for acute dermatitis in which there is weeping exudate (eg, poison ivy).

Pastes. Pastes are mixtures of powders and ointments and are used in inflammatory blistering conditions. They adhere to the skin and may be difficult to remove without using an oil (eg, olive oil, mineral oil). Pastes are applied with a wooden tongue depressor or gloved hand.

Ointments. Ointments retard water loss and lubricate and protect the skin. They are the preferred vehicle for delivering medication to chronic or localized dry skin conditions, such as eczema or psoriasis. Ointments are applied with a wooden tongue depressor or by hand (gloved).

Sprays and Aerosols. Spray and aerosol preparations may be used on any widespread dermatologic condition. They evaporate on contact and are used infrequently.

Corticosteroids. Corticosteroids are widely used in treating dermatologic conditions to provide anti-inflammatory, antipruritic, and vasoconstrictive effects. The patient is taught to apply this medication according to strict guidelines, using it sparingly but rubbing it into the prescribed area thoroughly. Absorption of topical corticosteroid is enhanced when the skin is hydrated or the affected area is covered by an occlusive or moisture-retentive dressing. Inappropriate use of topical corticosteroids can result in local and systemic side effects, especially when the medication is absorbed through inflamed and excoriated skin, under occlusive dressings, or when used for long periods on sensitive areas. Local side effects may include skin atrophy and thinning, striae (ie, band-like streaks), and telangiectasia. Thinning of the skin results from the ability of corticosteroids to inhibit skin collagen synthesis (Odom et al., 2000). The thinning process can be reversed by discontinuing the medication, but striae and telangiectasia are permanent. Systemic side effects may include hyperglycemia and symptoms of Cushing's syndrome. Caution is required when applying corticosteroids around the eyes because long-term use may cause glaucoma or cataracts, and the anti-inflammatory effect of corticosteroids may mask existing viral or fungal infections.

Concentrated (fluorinated) corticosteroids are never applied on the face or intertriginous areas (ie, axilla and groin), because these areas have a thinner stratum corneum and absorb the medication much more quickly than areas such as the forearm or legs. Persistent use of concentrated topical corticosteroids in any location may produce acnelike dermatitis, known as steroid-induced acne, and hypertrichosis (ie, excessive hair growth). Because some topical corticosteroid preparations are available without prescription, patients should be cautioned about prolonged and inappropriate use. Table 56-4 lists topical corticosteroid preparations according to potency.

Intralesional Therapy. Intralesional therapy consists of injecting a sterile suspension of medication (usually a corticosteroid) into or just below a lesion. Although this treatment may have an anti-inflammatory effect, local atrophy may result if the medication is injected into subcutaneous fat. Skin lesions treated with intralesional therapy include psoriasis, keloids, and cystic acne. Occasionally, immunotherapeutic and antifungal agents are administered as intralesional therapy.

Systemic Medications. Systemic medications are also prescribed for skin conditions. These include corticosteroids for short-term therapy for contact dermatitis or for long-term treatment of a chronic dermatosis, such as pemphigus vulgaris. Other frequently used systemic medications include antibiotics, antifungals, antihistamines, sedatives, tranquilizers, analgesics, and cytotoxic agents.

Nursing Management

Management begins with a health history, direct observation, and a complete physical examination. Chapter 55 provides a description of integumentary assessment. Because of its visibility, a skin condition is usually difficult to ignore or conceal from others and may therefore cause the patient some emotional distress. The major goals for the patient may include maintenance of skin integrity, relief of discomfort, promotion of restful sleep, self-acceptance, knowledge about skin care, and avoidance of complications.

Table 56-4 • Potency: Topical Corticosteroids

POTENCY	TOPICAL CORTICOSTEROID	PREPARATIONS
OTC	0.5–1.0% hydrocortisone	cr, lot, oint*
Lowest	dexamethasone 0.1% (Decaderm)	cr, oint, aerosol, gel
	alclometasone 0.05% (Aclovate)	cr, oint
	hydrocortisone 2.5% (Hytone)	cr, lot, oint
Low–medium	desonide 0.05% (DesOwen, Tridesilon)	cr, lot, oint
	fluocinolone acetonide 0.025% (Synalar)	cr, solution
	hydrocortisone valerate 0.2% (Westcort)	cr, solution
	betamethasone valerate 0.1% (Valisone)	cr, oint
	fluticasonepropionate 0.05% (Cutivate)	cr, oint
Medium–high	triamcinolone acetonide 0.1–0.5% (Aristocort)	cr, oint, lot
	fluocinonide 0.05% (Lidex)	cr, oint, gel
	desoximetasone 0.05–0.25% (Topicort)	cr, oint, gel
	fluocinolone 0.2% (Synalar)	cr, oint
	diflorasone diacetate 0.05% (Psorcon)	cr, oint
Very high	clobetasol propionate 0.05% (Temovate)	cr, oint, gel
	betamethasone dipropionate 0.05% (Diprolene)	cr, oint, gel
	halobetasole propionate 0.05% (Ultravate)	cr, oint

*cr, cream; lot, lotion; oint, ointment; OTC, over the counter

Nursing management for patients who must perform self-care for skin problems, such as applying medications and dressings, focuses mainly on teaching the patient how to wash the affected area and pat it dry, apply medication to the lesion while the skin is moist, cover the area with plastic (eg, Telfa pads, plastic wrap, vinyl gloves, plastic bag) if recommended, and cover it with an elastic bandage, dressing, or paper tape to seal the edges. Dressings that contain or cover a topical corticosteroid should be removed for 12 of every 24 hours to prevent skin thinning (ie, atrophy), striae, and telangiectasia (ie, small, red lesions caused by dilation of blood vessels).

Other forms of dressings, such as those used to cover topical medications, include soft cotton cloth and stretchable cotton dressings (eg, Surgitube, TubeGauz) that can be used for fingers, toes, hands, and feet. The hands can be covered with disposable polyethylene or vinyl gloves sealed at the wrists; the feet can be wrapped in plastic bags covered by cotton socks. Gloves and socks that are already impregnated with emollients, making application to the hands and feet more convenient, are also available. When large areas of the body must be covered, cotton cloth topped by an expandable stockinette can be used. Disposable diapers or cloths folded in diaper fashion are useful for dressing the groin and the

perineal areas. Axillary dressings can be made of cotton cloth, or a commercially prepared dressing may be used and taped in place or held by dress shields. A turban or plastic shower cap is useful for holding dressings on the scalp. A face mask, made from gauze with holes cut out for the eyes, nose, and mouth, may be held in place with gauze ties looped through holes cut in the four corners of the mask. See the Plan of Nursing Care 56-1 for more information.

Pruritus

GENERAL ITCHING

Pruritus (ie, itching) is one of the most common symptoms of patients with dermatologic disorders. Itch receptors are unmyelinated, penicillate (ie, brushlike) nerve endings that are found exclusively in the skin, mucous membranes, and cornea. Although pruritus is usually caused by primary skin disease with resultant rash or lesions, it may occur without a rash or lesion. This is referred to as essential pruritus, which generally has a rapid onset, may be severe, and interferes with normal daily activities.

Pruritus may be the first indication of a systemic internal disease such as diabetes mellitus, blood disorders, or cancer. It may also accompany renal, hepatic, and thyroid diseases (Chart 56-2). Some common oral medications such as aspirin, antibiotics, hormones (ie, estrogens, testosterone, or oral contraceptives), and opioids (ie, morphine or cocaine) may cause pruritus directly or by increasing sensitivity to ultraviolet light. Certain soaps and chemicals, radiation therapy, prickly heat (ie, miliaria), and contact with woolen garments are also associated with pruritus. Pruritus may also be caused by psychological factors, such as excessive stress in family or work situations.

Pathophysiology

Scratching the itchy area causes the inflamed cells and nerve endings to release histamine, which produces more pruritus, generating a vicious itch–scratch cycle. If the patient responds to an itch by scratching, the integrity of the skin may be altered, and excoriation, redness, raised areas (ie, wheals), infection, or changes in pigmentation may result. Pruritus usually is more severe at night and is less frequently reported during waking hours, probably because the person is distracted by daily activities. At night, when there are few distractions, the slightest pruritus cannot be easily ignored. Severe itching is debilitating.

Gerontologic Considerations

Pruritus occurs frequently in elderly people as a result of dry skin. Elderly people are also more likely to have a systemic illness that triggers pruritus, are at higher risk for occult malignancy, and are more likely to be on multiple medications than is the younger population. All of these factors increase the incidence of pruritus.

Medical Management

A thorough history and physical examination usually provide clues to the underlying cause of the pruritus, such as hay fever, allergy, recent administration of a new medication, or a change of cosmetics or soaps. After the cause has been identified, treatment of the condition should relieve the pruritus. Signs of infection and environmental clues, such as warm, dry air or irritating bed linens, should be identified. In general, washing with soap and hot water

(text continues on page 1672)

Plan of Nursing Care
Patients With Dermatoses (Abnormal Skin Conditions)

Nursing Interventions	Rationale	Expected Outcomes

Nursing Diagnosis: Impaired skin integrity related to changes in the barrier function of the skin
Goal: Maintenance of skin integrity

1. Protect healthy skin from maceration (excessive hydration of stratum corneum) when applying wet dressings.	1. Maceration of healthy skin can cause skin breakdown and extension of the primary condition.	• Maintains skin integrity • Absence of maceration • No signs of thermal injury • Absence of infection • Applies prescribed topical medication • Takes prescribed medication on schedule
2. Remove moisture from skin by blotting gently and avoiding friction.	2. Friction and maceration play a major role in some skin diseases.	
3. Guard carefully against risks of thermal injuries from excessively hot wet dressings and from subtle heat injuries (heating pads, radiators).	3. Patients with dermatoses may have decreased sensitivity to heat.	
4. Advise patient to use sunscreening agents.	4. Many cosmetic problems and virtually all cutaneous malignancies can be attributed to chronic skin damage.	

Nursing Diagnosis: Acute pain and itching related to skin lesions
Goal: Relief of discomfort

1. Examine area of involvement.	1. Understanding the extent and characteristics of the skin involved helps in planning interventions.	• Achieves relief of discomfort • Verbalizes that itching has been relieved • Demonstrates absence of skin excoriation from scratching • Complies with prescribed treatment • Keeps skin hydrated and lubricated • Demonstrates intact skin; skin regaining healthy appearance
a. Attempt to discover cause of discomfort.	a. Helps to identify appropriate comfort measures.	
b. Record observations in detail, using descriptive terminology.	b. An accurate description of a cutaneous lesion is necessary for diagnosis and treatment. Many skin conditions appear similar but have different etiologies. Cutaneous inflammatory response may be muted in elderly patients.	
c. Anticipate possible allergic reaction; obtain a medication history.	c. A generalized rash, particularly of sudden onset, may indicate a medication allergy.	
2. Control environmental and physical factors.	2. Itching is aggravated by heat, chemicals, and physical irritants.	
a. Keep humidity about 60%; use a humidifier.	a. At low humidity, the skin loses water.	
b. Maintain a cool environment.	b. Coolness deters itching.	
c. Use mild soap for sensitive skin (Dove, Cetaphil, Aveeno).	c. These contain no detergents, dyes, fragrances, or hardening agents.	
d. Remove excess clothing or bedding.	d. Promotes cool environment.	
e. Wash bed linens and clothing with mild fragrance-free soap.	e. Strong soaps and laundry additives can cause skin irritation.	
f. Stop repeated exposures to detergents, cleansers, and solvents.	f. Any substance that removes water, lipids, or protein from the epidermis alters the skin's barrier function.	
3. Use skin care measures to maintain skin integrity and promote comfort.	3. The skin is an important barrier that must be maintained intact to function properly.	
a. Provide tepid cooling baths or cool dressings for itching.	a. Gradual evaporation of water from dressings cools the skin and relieves pruritus.	
b. Treat dryness (xerosis) as prescribed.	b. Dry skin can produce areas of dermatitis with redness, itching, scaling, and, in more severe forms, swelling, blistering, cracking, and weeping.	
c. Apply skin lotion or cream immediately after bathing.	c. Effective hydration of the stratum corneum prevents compromise of the barrier layer of the skin.	

(continued)

Plan of Nursing Care
Patients With Dermatoses (Abnormal Skin Conditions) *(Continued)*

Nursing Interventions	Rationale	Expected Outcomes
d. Keep nails trimmed.	d. Trimming decreases skin damage from scratching.	
e. Apply prescribed topical therapy.	e. This helps to relieve symptoms.	
f. Help the patient accept possibly prolonged treatment.	f. Effective coping measures usually promote comfort.	
g. Advise the patient to refrain from using salves or lotions that are commercially available.	g. The patient's problem may be aggravated by self-medication.	

Nursing Diagnosis: Disturbed sleep pattern related to pruritus
Goal: Achievement of restful sleep

1. Prevent and treat dry skin.	1. Nocturnal pruritus interferes with normal sleep.	• Achieves restful sleep
		• Reports relief of itching
a. Advise patient to keep bedroom well ventilated and humidified.	a. Dry air will make skin feel itchy. A comfortable environment promotes relaxation.	• Maintains appropriate environmental conditions
		• Avoids caffeine in late afternoon and evening
b. Keep skin moisturized.	b. This prevents water loss. Dry, itchy skin can usually be controlled but not cured.	• Identifies measures to promote sleep
		• Experiences satisfactory rest/sleep pattern
c. Bathe/shower only as necessary if skin is excessively dry. Use no soap or only mild soap. Apply skin lotion/cream immediately after bathing while skin is damp.	c. These measures preserve skin moisture.	
2. Advise patient of the following measures that may be helpful in promoting sleep:		
a. Keep a regular schedule for sleeping. Go to bed at the same time; get up at the same time.	a. Regularity of sleep schedule is important in maintaining sleep.	
b. Avoid caffeinated drinks in the evening.	b. Caffeine has peak effect 2–4 hours after being consumed.	
c. Exercise regularly, particularly in late afternoon.	c. Exercise at this time appears to have beneficial sleep effect.	
d. Use a bedtime routine or ritual.	d. This eases transition from wakefulness to sleep.	
e. Use an antihistamine at bedtime if prescribed.	e. Antihistamines decrease itching and promote sleep.	

Nursing Diagnosis: Disturbed body image related to unsightly skin appearance
Goal: Development of increasing self-acceptance

1. Assess patient for disturbance of self-image (avoidance of eye contact, self-negating verbalizations, expression of disgust about skin condition).	1. Disturbance of body image may accompany any disease or condition that is apparent to the patient. An impression of one's own body has an effect on self-concept.	• Develops increasing acceptance of own body
		• Follows through and participates in self-care measures
2. Identify psychosocial stage of development.	2. There is a relationship between development stage, self-image, and the patient's reaction to and understanding of skin condition.	• Reports feeling in control of situation
		• Gives self positive reinforcement
		• Verbalizes a more healthful self-regard
		• Appears less self-conscious; is not afraid to socialize and be seen by others
3. Provide opportunity for expression. Listen (in an open, nonjudgmental way) to expressions of grief/anxiety about changes in body image.	3. The patient needs the experience of being heard and understood.	• Uses concealing and highlighting techniques to enhance appearance

(continued)

Plan of Nursing Care
Patients With Dermatoses (Abnormal Skin Conditions) *(Continued)*

Nursing Interventions	Rationale	Expected Outcomes
4. Assess the patient's concerns and fears. Assist anxious patient to develop insight and identify and cope with problems.	4. This gives health care personnel opportunity to neutralize undue anxiety and restore reality to the situation. Fear is destructive to adaptation.	
5. Support patient's efforts to improve body image (participation in skin treatments; grooming), develop self-acceptance, socialize with others, and use cosmetics to conceal disfigurement.	5. A positive approach and suggestions about cosmetic techniques are often helpful in promoting self-acceptance and socialization.	

Nursing Diagnosis: Deficient knowledge about skin care and methods of treating skin ailment
Goal: Understanding of skin care

Nursing Interventions	Rationale	Expected Outcomes
1. Determine what the patient knows (understands and misunderstands) about the condition.	1. Provides baseline data for developing the teaching plan.	• Acquires understanding of skin care
2. Keep the patient informed; correct misconceptions/misinformation.	2. Patients need to have a sense that there is something they can do. Most patients benefit from explanations and reassurance.	• Follows treatment as prescribed and can verbalize rationale for measures taken
3. Demonstrate application of prescribed therapy (wet compresses; topical medication).	3. Allows patient the opportunity to observe the correct way to perform therapies.	• Carries out prescribed baths, soaks, wet dressings
4. Advise the patient to keep skin moist and flexible with hydration and application of skin cream and lotion.	4. The stratum corneum needs water to stay flexible. Application of skin cream or lotion to damp skin prevents dry, rough, cracked, and scaly skin.	• Uses topical medication appropriately
5. Encourage the patient to attain a healthy nutritional status.	5. The appearance of the skin reflects a person's general health. Changes may signal abnormal nutrition.	• Understands importance of nutrition to skin health

Collaborative Problems: Infection
Goal: Absence of complications

Nursing Interventions	Rationale	Expected Outcomes
1. Have a high index of suspicion for an infection in patients with compromised immune systems.	1. Any condition that compromises the immune status increases the risk of cutaneous infection.	• Remains free of infection
2. Instruct the patient clearly and in detail about the therapeutic regimen.	2. Effective patient education is dependent on the interpersonal skills of the health professionals and on giving clear instructions reinforced through written instructions.	• Describes skin care measures that promote cleanliness and prevent skin breakdown
3. Apply intermittent wet dressings as prescribed to reduce intensity of inflammation.	3. A wet dressing produces evaporative cooling, causing constriction of superficial cutaneous vessels and thereby decreasing erythema and serum production. Wet dressings help in débridement of vesicles and crusts and control inflammatory processes.	• Identifies signs and symptoms of infection to report
4. Provide tub baths and soaks as prescribed.	4. Loosens exudates and scales.	• Identifies adverse effects of medications that should be reported to health care personnel
5. Administer prescribed antimicrobial agents.	5. Kills or prevents the growth of the infectious organism.	• Participates in skin care measures (eg, dressing changes, soaks)

(continued)

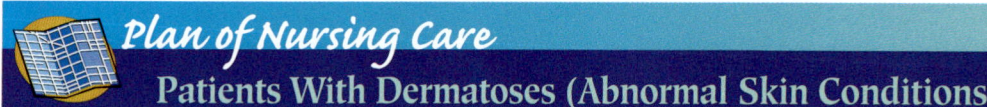

Plan of Nursing Care
Patients With Dermatoses (Abnormal Skin Conditions) *(Continued)*

Nursing Interventions	Rationale	Expected Outcomes

6. Use topical medications containing corticosteroids as prescribed and as indicated.
  a. Observe lesion periodically for changes in response to therapy.
  b. Instruct the patient about possible adverse effects of long-term use of fluorinated topical corticosteroids.
7. Advise patient to stop using any skin agent that makes the problem worse.
	6. Corticosteroids have an anti-inflammatory action, resulting in part from their ability to induce vasoconstriction of the small vessels in the upper dermis. Extensive prolonged use of topical corticosteroids can lead to antiproliferative effects on epidermal cells (loss of hair in area used; thinning of the skin).
	7. A contact dermatitis or allergic reaction may develop from any ingredient in the medication.	

is avoided. Bath oils (eg, Lubath, Alpha-Keri) containing a surfactant that makes the oil mix with bath water may be sufficient for cleaning. However, an elderly patient or a patient with unsteady balance should avoid adding oil because it increases the danger of slipping in the bathtub. A warm bath with a mild soap followed by application of a bland emollient to moist skin can control xerosis (ie, dry skin). Applying a cold compress, ice cube, or cool agents that contain menthol and camphor (which constrict blood vessels) may also help relieve pruritus.

PHARMACOLOGIC THERAPY

Topical corticosteroids may be beneficial as anti-inflammatory agents to decrease itching. Oral antihistamines are even more effective because they can overcome the effects of histamine release from damaged mast cells. An antihistamine, such as diphenhydramine (Benadryl) or hydroxyzine (Atarax), prescribed in a sedative dose at bedtime is effective in producing a restful and comfortable sleep. Nonsedating antihistamine medications such

as fexofenadine (Allegra) should be used to relieve daytime pruritus. Tricyclic antidepressants, such as doxepin (Sinequan), may be prescribed for pruritus of neuropsychogenic origin. If pruritus continues, further investigation of a systemic problem is advised.

Nursing Management

The nurse reinforces the reasons for the prescribed therapeutic regimen and counsels the patient on specific points of care. If baths have been prescribed, the patient is reminded to use tepid (not hot) water and to shake off the excess water and blot between intertriginous areas (ie, body folds) with a towel. Rubbing vigorously with the towel is avoided because this overstimulates the skin and causes more itching. It also removes water from the stratum corneum. Immediately after bathing, the skin should be lubricated with an emollient to trap moisture.

The patient is instructed to avoid situations that cause vasodilation (ie, expansion of the blood vessels). Examples include exposure to an overly warm environment and ingestion of alcohol or hot foods and liquids. All can induce or intensify itching. Using a humidifier is helpful if environmental air is dry. Activities that result in perspiration should be limited because perspiration may irritate and promote pruritus. If the patient is troubled at night with itching that interferes with sleep, the nurse can advise wearing cotton clothing next to the skin rather than synthetic materials. The room should be kept cool and humidified. Vigorous scratching should be avoided, and nails kept trimmed to prevent skin damage and infection. When the underlying cause of pruritus is unknown and further testing is required, the nurse explains each test and the expected outcome.

PERINEAL AND PERIANAL ITCHING

Pruritus of the genital and anal regions may be caused by small particles of fecal material lodged in the perianal crevices or attached to anal hairs or by perianal skin damage caused by scratching, moisture, and decreased skin resistance as a result of corticosteroid or antibiotic therapy. Other possible causes of perianal itching include local irritants such as scabies and lice, local lesions such as hemorrhoids, fungal or yeast infections, and pinworm infestation. Conditions such as diabetes mellitus, anemia, hyperthyroidism, and pregnancy may also result in pruritus. Occasionally, no cause can be identified.

Chart 56-2
Systemic Disorders Associated With Generalized Pruritus

Chronic renal disease
Obstructive biliary disease (primary biliary cirrhosis, extrahepatic biliary obstruction, drug-induced cholestasis)
Endocrine disease (thyrotoxicosis, hypothyroidism, diabetes mellitus)
Psychiatric disorders (emotional stress, anxiety, neurosis, phobias)
Malignancies (polycythemia vera, Hodgkin's disease, lymphoma, leukemia, multiple myeloma, mycosis fungoides, and cancers of the lung, breast, central nervous system, and gastrointestinal tract)
Neurologic disorders (multiple sclerosis, brain abscess, brain tumour)
Infestations (scabies, lice, other insects)
Pruritus of pregnancy (pruritic urticarial papules of pregnancy [PUPP], cholestasis of pregnancy, pemphigoid of pregnancy)
Folliculitis (bacterial, candidiasis, dermatophyte)
Skin conditions (seborrheic dermatitis, folliculitis, iron deficiency anemia, atopic dermatitis)

Management

The patient is instructed to follow proper hygiene measures and to discontinue home and over-the-counter remedies. The perineal or anal area should be rinsed with lukewarm water and blotted dry with cotton balls. Premoistened tissues may be used after defecation. Cornstarch can be applied in the skinfold areas to absorb perspiration.

As part of health teaching, the nurse instructs the patient to avoid bathing in water that is too hot and to avoid using bubble baths, sodium bicarbonate, and detergent soaps, all of which aggravate dryness. To keep the perineal or perianal skin area as dry as possible, patients should avoid wearing underwear made of synthetic fabrics. Local anesthetic agents should not be used because of possible allergic effects. The patient should also avoid vasodilating agents or stimulants (eg, alcohol, caffeine) and mechanical irritants such as rough or woolen clothing. A diet that includes adequate fibre may help maintain soft stools and prevent minor trauma to the anal mucosa.

Secretory Disorders

The main secretory function of the skin is performed by the sweat glands, which help to regulate body temperature. These glands excrete perspiration that evaporates, thereby cooling the body. The sweat glands are located in various parts of the body and respond to different stimuli. Those on the trunk generally respond to thermal stimulation; those on the palms and soles respond to nervous stimulation; and those in the axillae and on the forehead respond to both kinds of stimulation. Normal perspiration has no odour. Body odour is produced by the increase in bacteria on the skin and the interaction of bacterial waste products with the chemicals of perspiration.

As a rule, moist skin is warm, and dry skin is cool, but this is not always true. It is not unusual to observe warm, dry skin in a dehydrated patient and very hot, dry skin in some febrile states.

Normally, sweat can be controlled with the use of antiperspirants and deodorants. Most antiperspirants are aluminum salts that block the opening to the sweat duct. Pure deodorants inhibit bacterial growth and block the metabolism of sweat; they have no antiperspirant effect. Fragrance-free deodorants are available for those with sensitive skin (Odom et al., 2000).

HYDRADENITIS SUPPURATIVA

A condition called hydradenitis suppurativa can occur in certain individuals. The cause is unknown.

Pathophysiology

Abnormal blockage of the sweat glands causes recurring inflammation, nodules, and draining sinus tracts. Eventually, hypertrophic bands of scar tissue form in the area of the sweat glands.

Clinical Manifestations

The condition occurs more frequently in the axilla but also appears in inguinal folds, on the mons pubis, and around the buttocks. The patients can be extremely uncomfortable with multiple suppurative lesions within a small area. This condition does not appear before puberty and does appear to have a genetic basis.

Management

Management is difficult. Hot compresses and oral antibiotics are used frequently. Isotretinoin (Accutane) or etretinate can be tried; careful monitoring for side effects is important. Incision and drainage of large suppurating areas with gauze packs inserted to facilitate drainage is often necessary. Rarely, the entire area is excised, removing the scar tissue and any infection. This surgery is drastic and attempted only as a last resort (Hall, 2000).

SEBORRHEIC DERMATOSES

Seborrhea is excessive production of sebum (ie, secretion of sebaceous glands) in areas where sebaceous glands are normally found in large numbers, such as the face, scalp, eyebrows, eyelids, sides of the nose and upper lip, malar regions (ie, cheeks), ears, axillae, under the breasts, groin, and gluteal crease of the buttocks. Seborrheic dermatitis is a chronic inflammatory disease of the skin with a predilection for areas that are well supplied with sebaceous glands or lie between skin folds, where the bacteria count is high.

Clinical Manifestations

Two forms of seborrheic dermatoses can occur, an oily form and a dry form. Either form may start in childhood and continue throughout life. The oily form appears moist or greasy. There may be patches of sallow, greasy skin, with or without scaling, and slight erythema (ie, redness), predominantly on the forehead, nasolabial fold, beard area, scalp, and between adjacent skin surfaces in the regions of the axillae, groin, and breasts. Small pustules or papulopustules resembling acne may appear on the trunk. The dry form, consisting of flaky desquamation of the scalp with a profuse amount of fine, powdery scales, is commonly called dandruff. The mild forms of the disease are asymptomatic. When scaling occurs, it is often accompanied by pruritus, which may lead to scratching and secondary infections and excoriation.

Seborrheic dermatitis has a genetic predisposition. Hormones, nutritional status, infection, and emotional stress influence its course. The remissions and exacerbations of this condition should be explained to the patient. If a person has not previously been diagnosed with this condition and suddenly appears with a severe outbreak, a complete history and physical examination should be considered.

Medical Management

Because there is no known cure for seborrhea, the objective of therapy is to control the disorder and allow the skin to repair itself. Seborrheic dermatitis of the body and face may respond to a topically applied corticosteroid cream, which allays the secondary inflammatory response. However, this medication should be used with caution near the eyelids, because it can induce glaucoma and cataracts in predisposed patients. Patients with seborrheic dermatitis may develop a secondary candidal (yeast) infection in body creases or folds. To avoid this, patients should be advised to ensure maximum aeration of the skin and to clean carefully areas where there are creases or folds in the skin. Patients with persistent candidiasis should be evaluated for diabetes.

The mainstay of dandruff treatment is proper, frequent shampooing (daily or at least three times weekly) with medicated shampoos. Two or three different types of shampoo should be used in rotation to prevent the seborrhea from becoming resistant to a particular shampoo. The shampoo is left on at least 5 to 10 minutes. As the condition of the scalp improves, the treatment can be less frequent. Antiseborrheic shampoos include those containing selenium sulfide suspension, zinc pyrithione, salicylic acid or sulfur compounds, and tar shampoo that contains sulfur or salicylic acid.

Nursing Management

A person with seborrheic dermatitis is advised to avoid external irritants, excessive heat, and perspiration; rubbing and scratching prolong the disorder. To avoid secondary infection, the patient should air the skin and keep skin folds clean and dry.

Instructions for using medicated shampoos are reinforced for those with dandruff that requires treatment. Frequent shampooing is contrary to some cultural practices; the nurse should be sensitive to these differences when teaching the patient about home care.

The patient is cautioned that seborrheic dermatitis is a chronic problem that tends to reappear. The goal is to keep it under control. Patients need to be encouraged to adhere to the treatment program. Those who become discouraged and disheartened by the effect on body image should be treated with sensitivity and an awareness of their need to express their feelings.

ACNE VULGARIS

Acne vulgaris is a common follicular disorder affecting susceptible hair follicles, most commonly found on the face, neck, and upper trunk. It is characterized by **comedones** (ie, primary acne lesions), both closed and open, and by papules, pustules, nodules, and cysts.

Acne is the most commonly encountered skin condition in adolescents and young adults between ages 12 and 35. Both genders are affected equally, although onset is slightly earlier for girls. This may be because girls reach puberty at a younger age than boys. Acne becomes more marked at puberty and during adolescence because the endocrine glands that influence the secretions of the sebaceous glands are functioning at peak activity. Acne appears to stem from an interplay of genetic, hormonal, and bacterial factors. In most cases, there is a family history of acne.

Pathophysiology

During childhood, the sebaceous glands are small and virtually nonfunctioning. These glands are under endocrine control, especially by the androgens. During puberty, androgens stimulate the sebaceous glands, causing them to enlarge and secrete a natural oil, sebum, which rises to the top of the hair follicle and flows out onto the skin surface. In adolescents who develop acne, androgenic stimulation produces a heightened response in the sebaceous glands so that acne occurs when accumulated sebum plugs the pilosebaceous ducts. This accumulated material forms comedones.

Clinical Manifestations

The primary lesions of acne are comedones. Closed comedones (ie, whiteheads) are obstructive lesions formed from impacted lipids or oils and keratin that plug the dilated follicle. They are small, whitish papules with minute follicular openings that generally cannot be seen. These closed comedones may evolve into open comedones, in which the contents of the ducts are in open communication with the external environment. The colour of open comedones (ie, blackheads) results not from dirt, but from an accumulation of lipid, bacterial, and epithelial debris.

Although the exact cause is unknown, some closed comedones may rupture, resulting in an inflammatory reaction caused by leakage of follicular contents (eg, sebum, keratin, bacteria) into the dermis. This inflammatory response may result from the action of certain skin bacteria, such as ***Propionibacterium acnes***, that live in the hair follicles and break down the triglycerides of the sebum into free fatty acids and glycerin. The resultant inflammation is seen clinically as erythematous papules, inflammatory pustules, and inflammatory cysts. Mild papules and cysts drain and heal on their own without treatment. Deeper papules and cysts may result in scarring of the skin. Acne is usually graded as mild, moderate, or severe based on the number and type of lesions (eg, comedones, papules, pustules, cysts).

Assessment and Diagnostic Findings

The diagnosis of acne is based on the history and physical examination, evidence of lesions characteristic of acne, and age. Acne does not occur until puberty. The presence of the typical comedones (ie, whiteheads and blackheads) along with excessively oily skin is characteristic. Oiliness is more prominent in the midfacial area; other parts of the face may appear dry. When there are numerous lesions, some of which are open, the person may exude a distinct sebaceous odour. Women may report a history of flare-ups a few days before menses. Biopsy of lesions is seldom necessary for a definitive diagnosis.

Medical Management

The goals of management are to reduce bacterial colonies, decrease sebaceous gland activity, prevent the follicles from becoming plugged, reduce inflammation, combat secondary infection, minimize scarring, and eliminate factors that predispose the person to acne. The therapeutic regimen depends on the type of lesion (eg, comedonal, papular, pustular, cystic).

There is no predictable cure for the disease, but combinations of therapies are available that can effectively control its activity. Topical treatment may be all that is needed to treat mild to moderate lesions and superficial inflammatory lesions (ie, papular or pustular).

NUTRITION AND HYGIENE THERAPY

Although food restrictions have been recommended from time to time in treating acne, diet is not believed to play a major role in therapy. However, the elimination of a specific food or food product associated with a flare-up of acne, such as chocolate, cola, fried foods, or milk products, should be promoted. Maintenance of good nutrition equips the immune system for effective action against bacteria and infection.

For mild cases of acne, washing twice each day with a cleansing soap may be all that is required. These soaps can remove the excessive skin oil and the comedo in most cases. Providing positive reassurance, listening attentively, and being sensitive to the feelings of the patient with acne are essential contributors to the patient's psychological well-being and understanding of the disease and treatment plan. Over-the-counter acne medications contain salicylic acid and benzoyl peroxide, both of which are very effective at removing the sebaceous follicular plugs. However, the skin of some people is sensitive to these products, which can cause irritation or excessive dryness, especially when used with some prescribed topical medications. The patient should be instructed to discontinue their use if severe irritation occurs. Oil-free cosmetics and creams should be chosen. These products are usually designated as useful for acne-prone skin. The duration of treatment depends on the extent and severity of the acne. In severe cases, treatment may extend over years.

TOPICAL PHARMACOLOGIC THERAPY

Benzoyl Peroxide. Benzoyl peroxide preparations are widely used because they produce a rapid and sustained reduction of inflammatory lesions. They depress sebum production and promote breakdown of comedo plugs. They also produce an antibacterial effect by suppressing *P. acnes*. Initially, benzoyl peroxide causes redness and scaling, but the skin usually adjusts quickly to its use. Typically, the patient applies a gel of benzoyl peroxide once daily. In many instances, this is the only treatment needed. Benzoyl peroxide, benzoyl erythromycin, and benzoyl sulfur combinations are available over the counter and by prescription. Vitamin A acid (tretinoin) applied topically is used to clear the keratin plugs from the pilosebaceous ducts. Vitamin A acid speeds the cellular turnover, forces out the comedones, and prevents new comedones.

The patient should be informed that symptoms may worsen during early weeks of therapy because inflammation may occur during the process. Erythema and peeling also frequently result. Improvement may take 8 to 12 weeks. Some patients cannot tolerate this therapy. The patient is cautioned against sun exposure while using this topical medication because it may cause an exaggerated sunburn. Package insert directions should be followed carefully.

Topical Antibiotics. Topical antibiotic treatment for acne is common. Topical antibiotics suppress the growth of *P. acnes;* reduce superficial free fatty acid levels; decrease comedones, papules, and pustules; and produce no systemic side effects. Common topical preparations include tetracycline, clindamycin, and erythromycin.

SYSTEMIC PHARMACOLOGIC THERAPY

Antibiotics. Oral antibiotics, such as tetracycline, doxycycline, and minocycline, administered in small doses over a long period are very effective in treating moderate and severe acne, especially when the acne is inflammatory and results in pustules, abscesses, and scarring. Therapy may continue for months to years. The tetracycline family of antibiotics is contraindicated in children younger than age 12 and in pregnant women. Although these medications are considered safe for long-term use in most cases, administration during pregnancy can affect the development of teeth, causing enamel hypoplasia and permanent discolouration of teeth in infants. Side effects of tetracyclines include photosensitivity, nausea, diarrhea, cutaneous infection in either gender, and vaginitis in women. In some women, broad-spectrum antibiotics may suppress normal vaginal bacteria and predispose the patient to candidiasis, a fungal infection.

Oral Retinoids. Synthetic vitamin A compounds (ie, retinoids) are used with dramatic results in patients with nodular cystic acne unresponsive to conventional therapy. One compound is isotretinoin (Accutane). Isotretinoin is also used for active inflammatory papular pustular acne that has a tendency to scar. Isotretinoin reduces sebaceous gland size and inhibits sebum production. It also causes the epidermis to shed (ie, epidermal desquamation), thereby unseating and expelling existing comedones.

The most common side effect, experienced by almost all patients, is **cheilitis** (ie, inflammation of the lips). Dry and chafed skin and mucous membranes are frequent side effects. These changes are reversible with the withdrawal of the medication. Most important, isotretinoin, like other vitamin A metabolites, is teratogenic in humans, meaning that it can have an adverse effect on a fetus, causing central nervous system and cardiovascular defects and structural abnormalities of the face. Contraceptive measures for women of childbearing age are mandatory during treatment and for about 4 to 8 weeks thereafter. To avoid additive toxic effects, patients are cautioned not to take vitamin A supplements while taking isotretinoin (Odom et al., 2000).

Hormone Therapy. Estrogen therapy (including progesterone–estrogen preparations) suppresses sebum production and reduces skin oiliness. It is usually reserved for young women when the acne begins somewhat later than usual and tends to flare up at certain times in the menstrual cycle. Estrogen in the form of estrogen-dominant oral contraceptive compounds may be administered on a prescribed cyclic regimen. Estrogen is not administered to male patients because of undesirable side effects such as enlargement of the breasts and decrease in body hair.

SURGICAL MANAGEMENT

Surgical treatment of acne consists of comedo extraction, injections of corticosteroids into the inflamed lesions, and incision and drainage of large, fluctuant (ie, moving in palpable waves), nodular cystic lesions. Cryosurgery (ie, freezing with liquid nitrogen) may be used for nodular and cystic forms of acne. Patients with deep scars may be treated with deep abrasive therapy (ie, dermabrasion), in which the epidermis and some superficial dermis are removed down to the level of the scars.

Comedones may be removed with a comedo extractor. The site is first cleaned with alcohol. The opening of the extractor is then placed over the lesion, and direct pressure is applied to cause extrusion of the plug through the extractor. Removal of comedones leaves erythema, which may take several weeks to subside. Recurrence of comedones after extraction is common because of the continuing activity of the pilosebaceous glands.

Table 56-5 summarizes the treatment modalities for acne vulgaris.

Nursing Management

Nursing care of patients with acne consists largely of monitoring and managing potential complications of skin treatments. Major nursing activities include patient education, particularly in proper skin care techniques, and managing potential problems related to the skin disorder or therapy.

PREVENTING SCARRING

Prevention of scarring is the ultimate goal of therapy. The chance of scarring increases as the grade of acne increases. Grades III and IV (25 to more than 50 comedones, papules, or pustules) usually require longer-term therapy with systemic antibiotics or isotretinoin. Patients should be warned that discontinuing these medications can exacerbate acne, lead to more flare-ups, and increase the chance of deep scarring. Moreover, manipulation of the comedones, papules, and pustules increases the potential for scarring.

When acne surgery is prescribed to extract deep-seated comedones or inflamed lesions or to incise and drain cystic lesions, the intervention itself may result in further scarring. Dermabrasion, which levels existing scar tissue, can also increase scar formation. Hyperpigmentation or hypopigmentation also may affect the tis-

Table 56-5 • Commonly Prescribed Treatments of Acne Vulgaris	
TYPE OF THERAPY	**PRESCRIBED TREATMENT AGENT**
Topical	benzoyl peroxide wash, gel
	benzoyl peroxide and erythromycin (Benzamycin gel)
	benzoyl peroxide and sulfur (Benzulfoid cream)
	resorcinol (as ingredient in other preparations)
	salicylic acid (as ingredient in other preparations)
	sulfur (as ingredient in other preparations)
	tretinoin (Retin A, Avita)
	other comedogenics (adapalene [Differen], azelaic acid [Azelex], tazorotene [Tazorac])
	topical antibiotics
Systemic	oral antibiotics (erythromycin, tetracycline, doxycycline, minocin, penicillins)
	isotretinoin (Accutane)
	hormones:
	corticosteroids
	high dose for anti-inflammatory action
	low dose to suppress androgenic action
	intralesional for anti-inflammatory action
	antiandrogens
	oral contraceptives (women only)
Surgical	extraction of comedo contents
	drainage of pustules and cysts
	excision of sinus tracts and cysts
	intralesional corticosteroids for anti-inflammatory action
	cryotherapy
	dermabrasion for scars
	laser resurfacing of scars

Treatments listed are common but do not include all available forms of therapy.

sue involved. The patient should be informed of these potential outcomes before choosing surgical intervention for acne.

PREVENTING INFECTION

Female patients receiving long-term antibiotic therapy with tetracycline should be advised to watch for and report signs and symptoms of oral or vaginal candidiasis, a yeastlike fungal infection.

PROMOTING HOME AND COMMUNITY-BASED CARE

Teaching Patients Self-Care. In addition to receiving instructions for taking prescribed medications, patients are instructed to wash the face and other affected areas with mild soap and water twice each day to remove surface oils and prevent obstruction of the oil glands. They are cautioned to avoid scrubbing the face; acne is not caused by dirt and cannot be washed away.

Mild abrasive soaps and drying agents are prescribed to eliminate the oily feeling that troubles many patients. At the same time, patients are cautioned to avoid excessive abrasion because it makes acne worse. Excessive abrasion causes minute scratches on the skin surface and increases possible bacterial contamination. Soap itself can irritate the skin.

All forms of friction and trauma are avoided, including propping the hands against the face, rubbing the face, and wearing tight collars and helmets. Patients are instructed to avoid manipulation of pimples or blackheads. Squeezing merely worsens the problem, because a portion of the blackhead is pushed down into the skin, which may cause the follicle to rupture. Because cosmetics, shaving creams, and lotions can aggravate acne, these substances are best avoided unless the patient is advised otherwise. There is no evidence that a particular food can cause or aggravate acne. In general, eating a nutritious diet helps the body maintain a strong immune system.

Bacterial Infections: Pyodermas

Also called **pyodermas**, pus-forming bacterial infections of the skin may be primary or secondary. Primary skin infections originate in previously normal-appearing skin and are usually caused by a single organism. Secondary skin infections arise from a preexisting skin disorder or from disruption of the skin integrity from injury or surgery. In either case, several microorganisms may be implicated (eg, *Staphylococcus aureus,* group A streptococci). The most common primary bacterial skin infections are impetigo and folliculitis. Folliculitis may lead to furuncles or carbuncles.

IMPETIGO

Impetigo is a superficial infection of the skin caused by staphylococci, streptococci, or multiple bacteria. Bullous impetigo, a more deep-seated infection of the skin caused by *S. aureus,* is characterized by the formation of bullae (ie, large, fluid-filled blisters) from original vesicles. The bullae rupture, leaving raw, red areas.

The exposed areas of the body, face, hands, neck, and extremities are most frequently involved. Impetigo is contagious and may spread to other parts of the patient's skin or to other members of the family who touch the patient or use towels or combs that are soiled with the exudate of the lesions.

Although impetigo is seen at all ages, it is particularly common among children living in poor hygienic conditions. It often follows pediculosis capitis (head lice), scabies (itch mites), herpes simplex, insect bites, poison ivy, or eczema. Chronic health problems, poor hygiene, and malnutrition may predispose an adult to impetigo. Some people have been identified as asymptomatic carriers of *S. aureus,* usually in the nasal passages.

Clinical Manifestations

The lesions begin as small, red macules, which quickly become discrete, thin-walled vesicles that soon rupture and become covered with a loosely adherent honey-yellow crust (Fig. 56-1). These crusts are easily removed to reveal smooth, red, moist surfaces on which new crusts soon develop. If the scalp is involved, the hair is matted, which distinguishes the condition from ringworm.

Medical Management

Systemic antibiotic therapy is the usual treatment. It reduces contagious spread, treats deep infection, and prevents acute glomerulonephritis (ie, kidney infection), which may occur as an aftermath of streptococcal skin diseases. In nonbullous impetigo, benzathine penicillin or oral penicillin may be prescribed. Bullous impetigo is treated with a penicillinase-resistant penicillin (eg, cloxacillin,

FIGURE 56-1 Impetigo of the nostril.

dicloxacillin). In penicillin-allergic patients, erythromycin is an effective alternative.

Topical antibacterial therapy (eg, mupirocin) may be prescribed when the disease is limited to a small area. However, topical therapy requires that the medication be applied to the lesions several times daily for a week. The treatment regimen may be impossible for some patients or their caregivers to follow. Topical antibiotics generally are not as effective as systemic therapy in eradicating or preventing the spread of streptococci from the respiratory tract, thereby increasing the risk for developing glomerulonephritis.

When topical therapy is prescribed, lesions are soaked or washed with soap solution to remove the central site of bacterial growth, giving the topical antibiotic an opportunity to reach the infected site. After the crusts are removed, a topical medication (eg, Polysporin, bacitracin) may be applied. Gloves are worn when providing patient care. An antiseptic solution, such as povidone-iodine (Betadine) may be used to clean the skin, reduce bacterial content in the infected area, and prevent spread.

Nursing Management

The nurse instructs the patient and family members to bathe at least once daily with bactericidal soap. Cleanliness and good hygiene practices help prevent the spread of the lesions from one skin area to another and from one person to another. Each person should have a separate towel and washcloth. Because impetigo is a contagious disorder, infected people should avoid contact with other people until the lesions heal.

FOLLICULITIS, FURUNCLES, AND CARBUNCLES

Folliculitis is an infection of bacterial or fungal origin that arises within the hair follicles. Lesions may be superficial or deep. Single or multiple papules or pustules appear close to the hair follicles. Folliculitis commonly affects the beard area of men who shave and women's legs. Other areas include the axillae, trunk, and buttocks.

Pseudofolliculitis barbae (ie, shaving bumps) are an inflammatory reaction that occurs predominately on the faces of African Canadian and other curly-haired men as a result of shaving. The sharp ingrowing hairs have a curved root that grows at a more acute angle and pierces the skin, provoking an irritative reaction. The only entirely effective treatment is to avoid shaving. Other treatments include using special lotions or antibiotics or using a hand brush to dislodge the hairs mechanically. If the patient must

remove facial hair, a depilatory cream or electric razor may be more appropriate than a straight razor.

A **furuncle** (ie, boil) is an acute inflammation arising deep in one or more hair follicles and spreading into the surrounding dermis. It is a deeper form of folliculitis. Furunculosis refers to multiple or recurrent lesions. Furuncles may occur anywhere on the body but are more prevalent in areas subjected to irritation, pressure, friction, and excessive perspiration, such as the back of the neck, the axillae, and the buttocks.

A furuncle may start as a small, red, raised, painful pimple. Frequently, the infection progresses and involves the skin and subcutaneous fatty tissue, causing tenderness, pain, and surrounding cellulitis. The area of redness and induration represents an effort of the body to keep the infection localized. The bacteria (usually staphylococci) produce necrosis of the invaded tissue. The characteristic pointing of a boil follows in a few days. When this occurs, the centre becomes yellow or black, and the boil is said to have "come to a head."

A **carbuncle** is an abscess of the skin and subcutaneous tissue that represents an extension of a furuncle that has invaded several follicles and is large and deep seated. It is usually caused by a staphylococcal infection. Carbuncles appear most commonly in areas where the skin is thick and inelastic. The back of the neck and the buttocks are common sites. In carbuncles, the extensive inflammation frequently prevents a complete walling off of the infection; absorption may occur, resulting in high fever, pain, leukocytosis, and even extension of the infection to the bloodstream.

Furuncles and carbuncles are more likely to occur in patients with underlying systemic diseases, such as diabetes or hematologic malignancies, and in those receiving immunosuppressive therapy for other diseases. Both are more prevalent in hot climates, especially on skin beneath occlusive clothing.

Medical Management

In treating staphylococcal infections, it is important not to rupture or destroy the protective wall of induration that localizes the infection. The boil or pimple should never be squeezed.

Follicular disorders, including folliculitis, furuncles, and carbuncles, are usually caused by staphylococci; although if the immune system is impaired, the causative organisms may be gram-negative bacilli. Systemic antibiotic therapy, selected by sensitivity study, is generally indicated. Oral cloxacillin, dicloxacillin, and flucloxacillin are first-line medications. Cephalosporins and erythromycin are also effective. Bed rest is advised for patients who have boils on the perineum or in the anal region, and a course of systemic antibiotic therapy is indicated to prevent the spread of the infection.

When the pus has localized and is fluctuant, a small incision with a scalpel can speed resolution by relieving the tension and ensuring direct evacuation of the pus and slough. The patient is instructed to keep the draining lesion covered with a dressing.

Nursing Management

Intravenous fluids, fever reduction, and other supportive treatments are indicated for patients who are very ill or suffering with toxicity. Warm, moist compresses increase vascularization and hasten resolution of the furuncle or carbuncle. The surrounding skin may be cleaned gently with antibacterial soap, and an antibacterial ointment may be applied. Soiled dressings are handled according to standard precautions. Nursing personnel should carefully follow isolation precautions to avoid becoming carriers of staphylococci. Disposable gloves are worn when caring for these patients.

> **! NURSING ALERT** Nurses must take special precautions in caring for boils on the face, because the skin area drains directly into the cranial venous sinuses. Sinus thrombosis with fatal pyemia can develop after manipulating a boil in this location. The infection can travel through the sinus tract and penetrate the brain cavity, causing brain abscess.

PROMOTING HOME AND COMMUNITY-BASED CARE

Teaching Patients Self-Care. To prevent and control staphylococcal skin infections such as boils and carbuncles, the staphylococcal pathogen must be eliminated from the skin and environment. Efforts must be made to increase the patient's resistance and provide a hygienic environment. If lesions are actively draining, the mattress and pillow should be covered with plastic material and wiped off with disinfectant daily; the bed linens, towels, and clothing should be laundered after each use; and the patient should use an antibacterial soap and shampoo for an indefinite period, often for several months.

Recurrent infection is prevented with the use of prescribed antibiotic therapy (eg, a daily dose of oral clindamycin to be taken continuously for about 3 months). The patient must take the full dose for the time prescribed. The purulent exudate (ie, pus) is a source of reinfection or transmission of infection to caregivers. When the patient has a history of recurrent infections, a carrier state may exist, which should be investigated and treated with an antibacterial cream such as mupirocin.

Viral Skin Infections

HERPES ZOSTER

Herpes zoster, also called shingles, is an infection caused by the varicella-zoster virus, a member of a group of DNA viruses. The viruses causing chickenpox and herpes zoster are indistinguishable, hence the name varicella-zoster virus. The disease is characterized by a painful vesicular eruption along the area of distribution of the sensory nerves from one or more posterior ganglia. It is assumed that herpes zoster represents a reactivation of latent varicella virus infection and reflects lowered immunity. After a case of chickenpox runs its course, it is thought that the varicella-zoster viruses responsible for the outbreak lie dormant inside nerve cells near the brain and spinal cord. Later, when these latent viruses are reactivated, they travel by way of the peripheral nerves to the skin, where the viruses multiply and create a red rash of small, fluid-filled blisters. About 10% of adults get shingles during their lifetimes, usually after age 50 years. There is an increased frequency of herpes zoster infections among patients with weakened immune systems and cancers, especially leukemias and lymphomas (Odom et al., 2000).

Clinical Manifestations

The eruption is usually accompanied or preceded by pain, which may radiate over the entire region supplied by the affected nerves. The pain may be burning, lancinating (ie, tearing or sharply cutting), stabbing, or aching. Some patients have no pain, but itching and tenderness may occur over the area. Sometimes, malaise and gastrointestinal disturbances precede the eruption. The

patches of grouped vesicles appear on the red and swollen skin. The early vesicles, which contain serum, later may become purulent, rupture, and form crusts. The inflammation is usually unilateral, involving the thoracic, cervical, or cranial nerves in a bandlike configuration. The blisters are usually confined to a narrow region of the face or trunk (Fig. 56-2). The clinical course varies from 1 to 3 weeks. If an ophthalmic nerve is involved, the patient may have eye pain. Inflammation and a rash on the trunk may cause pain with the slightest touch. The healing time varies from 7 to 26 days.

Herpes zoster in healthy adults is usually localized and benign. However, in immunosuppressed patients, the disease may be severe and the clinical course acutely disabling.

Medical Management

The goals of herpes zoster management are to relieve the pain and to reduce or avoid complications, which include infection, scarring, and postherpetic neuralgia and eye complications. Pain is controlled with analgesics, because adequate pain control during the acute phase helps prevent persistent pain patterns. Systemic corticosteroids may be prescribed for patients older than age 50 years to reduce the incidence and duration of postherpetic neuralgia (ie, persistent pain of the affected nerve after healing). Healing usually occurs sooner in those who have been treated with corticosteroids. Triamcinolone (Aristocort, Kenacort, Kenalog) injected subcutaneously under painful areas is effective as an anti-inflammatory agent.

There is evidence that infection is arrested if oral antiviral agents such as acyclovir (Zovirax), valacyclovir (Valtrex), or famciclovir (Famvir) are administered within 24 hours of the initial eruption. Intravenous acyclovir, if started early, is effective in significantly reducing the pain and halting the progression of the disease. In older patients, the pain from herpes zoster may persist as postherpetic neuralgia for months after the skin lesions disappear (Hall, 2000).

Ophthalmic herpes zoster occurs when an eye is involved. This is considered an ophthalmic emergency, and the patient should be referred to an ophthalmologist immediately to prevent the possible sequelae of keratitis, uveitis, ulceration, and blindness.

FIGURE 56-2 Herpes zoster (shingles).

People who have been exposed to varicella (ie, chickenpox) by primary infection or by vaccination are not at risk for infection after exposure to patients with herpes zoster.

Nursing Management

The nurse assesses the patient's discomfort and response to medication and collaborates with the physician to make necessary adjustments to the treatment regimen. The patient is taught how to apply wet dressings or medication to the lesions and to follow proper hand hygiene techniques to avoid spreading the virus.

Diversionary activities and relaxation techniques are encouraged to ensure restful sleep and to alleviate discomfort. A caregiver may be required to assist with dressings, particularly if the patient is elderly and unable to apply them. Relatives, neighbours, or a home care nurse may need to help with dressing changes and food preparation for patients who cannot care for themselves or prepare nourishing meals.

HERPES SIMPLEX

Herpes simplex is a common skin infection. There are two types of the causative virus, which are identified by viral typing. Generally, herpes simplex type 1 occurs on the mouth and type 2 in the genital area, but both viral types can be found in both locations. About 85% of adults worldwide are seropositive for herpes type 1. The prevalence of type 2 is lower; type 2 usually appears at the onset of sexual activity. Serologic testing shows that many more people are infected than have a history of clinical disease.

Herpes simplex is classified as a true primary infection, a nonprimary initial episode, or a recurrent episode. True primary infection is the initial exposure to the virus. A nonprimary initial episode is the initial episode of type 1 or type 2 in a person previously infected with the other type. Recurrent episodes are subsequent episodes of the same viral type.

OROLABIAL HERPES

Orolabial herpes, also called fever blisters or cold sores, consists of erythematous-based clusters of grouped vesicles on the lips. A prodrome of tingling or burning with pain may precede the appearance of the vesicles by up to 24 hours. Certain triggers, such as sunlight exposure or increased stress, may cause recurrent episodes. Fewer than 1% of people with primary orolabial herpes infections develop herpetic gingivostomatitis. This complication occurs more in children and young adults. The onset is often accompanied by high fever, regional lymphadenopathy, and generalized malaise. Another complication of orolabial herpes is the development of erythema multiforme, an acute inflammation of the skin and mucous membranes with characteristic lesions that have the appearance of targets.

GENITAL HERPES

Genital herpes, or type 2 herpes simplex, manifests with a broad spectrum of clinical signs. Minor infections may produce no symptoms at all; severe primary infections with type 1 can cause systemic flulike illness. Lesions appear as grouped vesicles on an erythematous base initially involving the vagina, rectum, or penis. New lesions can continue to appear for 7 to 14 days. Lesions are symmetric and usually cause regional lymphadenopathy. Fever and flulike symptoms are common. Typical recurrences begin with a prodrome of burning, tingling, or itching about 24 hours before the vesicles appear. As the vesicles rupture, erosions and ulcerations begin to appear. Severe infections can cause extensive erosions of the vaginal or anal canal. For further information see Chapter 47.

Assessment and Diagnostic Findings

Herpes simplex infections are confirmed in several ways. Generally, the appearance of the skin eruption is strongly suggestive. Viral cultures and rapid assays are available, and the type of test used depends on lesion morphology. Acute vesicular lesions are more likely to react positively to the rapid assay, whereas older, crusted patches are better diagnosed with viral culture. In all cases, it is imperative to obtain enough viral cells for testing, and careful collection methods are therefore important. All crusts should be gently removed or vesicles gently unroofed. A sterile cotton swab premoistened in viral culture preservative is used to swab the base of the vesicle to obtain a specimen for analysis.

Complications

Eczema herpeticum is a condition in which patients with eczema contract herpes that spreads throughout the eczematous areas. The same type of spread of herpes can occur in severe seborrhea, scabies, and other chronic skin conditions.

Herpes Whitlow is an infection of the pulp of a fingertip with herpes type 1 or 2. There is tenderness and erythema of the lateral fold of the cuticle. Deep-seated vesicles appear within 24 hours.

Most cases of neonatal infection with herpes occur during delivery by contact of the infant with the mother's active ulcerations. Rarely, in mothers who have primary infections during pregnancy, intrauterine neonatal infections occur. Fetal anomalies include skin lesions, microcephaly, encephalitis, and intracerebral calcifications.

Medical Management

In many patients, recurrent orolabial herpes represents more of a nuisance than a disease. Because sun exposure is a common trigger, those with recurrent orolabial herpes should use a sunscreen liberally on the lips and face. Topical treatment with drying agents may accelerate healing. In more severe outbreaks or in patients who have identified a trigger, intermittent treatment with 200 mg of acyclovir administered five times each day for 5 days is often started as soon as the earliest symptoms occur.

Treatment of genital herpes depends on the severity, the frequency, and the psychological impact of recurrences and on the infectious status of the sexual partner. For people who have mild or rare outbreaks, no treatment may be required. For those who have more severe outbreaks, but for whom outbreaks are still infrequent, intermittent treatment as described for oral lesions can be used. Because intermittent treatment reduces the duration of the infection by only 24 to 36 hours, it should be initiated as early as possible.

Patients who have more than six recurrences per year may benefit from suppressive therapy. Use of acyclovir, valacyclovir, or famciclovir suppresses 85% of recurrences, and 20% of patients are free of recurrences during suppressive therapy. Suppressive therapy also reduces viral shedding by almost 95%, making the person less contagious. Treatment with suppressive doses of oral antiviral medications prevents recurrent erythema multiforme.

Eczema herpeticum is managed with oral or intravenous acyclovir.

Management of genital herpes in pregnancy is controversial. Routine prenatal cultures do not predict shedding at the time of delivery. The use of scalp electrodes during delivery should be avoided because they increase the risk for infection in the newborn. Because the risk for neonatal herpes is greater in women with their initial episode during pregnancy, suppression therapy should be started in these women to reduce outbreaks during the third trimester. All women with active lesions at the time of delivery undergo cesarean section.

In immunocompromised patients, suppression therapy should be considered. In severe infections of the hospitalized patient, intravenous acyclovir is prescribed.

Fungal (Mycotic) Infections

Fungi, tiny members of a subdivision of the plant kingdom that feed on organic matter, are responsible for various common skin infections. In some cases, they affect only the skin and its appendages (ie, hair and nails). In other cases, the internal organs are involved, and this disease may be life-threatening. Superficial infections, however, rarely cause even temporary disability and respond readily to treatment. Secondary infection with bacteria, *Candida,* or both organisms may occur.

The most common fungal skin infection is **tinea,** which is also called ringworm because of its characteristic appearance of ring or rounded tunnel under the skin. Tinea infections affect the head, body, groin, feet, and nails. Table 56-6 summarizes the tinea infections.

To obtain a specimen for diagnosis, the lesion is cleaned, and a scalpel or glass slide is used to remove scales from the margin of the lesion. The scales are dropped onto a slide to which potassium hydroxide has been added. The diagnosis is made by examination of the infected scales microscopically for spores and hyphae or by isolating the organism in culture. Under Wood's light, a specimen of infected hair appears fluorescent; this may be helpful in diagnosing some cases of tinea capitis.

TINEA PEDIS: ATHLETE'S FOOT

Tinea pedis (ie, athlete's foot) is the most common fungal infection. It is especially prevalent in those who use communal showers or swimming pools (Odom et al., 2000).

Clinical Manifestations

Tinea pedis may appear as an acute or chronic infection on the soles of the feet or between the toes. The toenail may also be involved. Lymphangitis and cellulitis occur occasionally when bacterial superinfection occurs. Sometimes, a mixed infection involving fungi, bacteria, and yeast occurs.

Medical Management

During the acute, vesicular phase, soaks of Burow's solution or potassium permanganate solutions are used to remove the crusts, scales, and debris and to reduce the inflammation. Topical antifungal agents (eg, miconazole, clotrimazole) are applied to the infected areas. Topical therapy is continued for several weeks because of the high rate of recurrence.

Nursing Management

Footwear provides a favourable environment for fungi, and the causative fungus may be in the shoes or socks. Because moisture encourages the growth of fungi, the patient is instructed to keep the feet as dry as possible, including the areas between the toes.

Table 56-6 • **Tinea (Ringworm) Infections**

TYPE AND LOCATION	CLINICAL MANIFESTATIONS	TREATMENT
Tinea capitis (head) Contagious fungal infection of the hair shaft	• Common in children • Oval, scaling, erythematous patches • Small papules or pustules on the scalp • Brittle hair that breaks easily	• Griseofulvin for 6 weeks • Shampoo hair 2 or 3 times with Nizoral or selenium sulfide shampoo.
Tinea corporis (body)	• Begins with red macule, which spreads to a ring of papules or vesicles with central clearing • Lesions found in clusters • Many spread to the hair, scalp, or nails • Very pruritic • An infected pet may be the source.	• Mild conditions: topical antifungal creams • Severe conditions: griseofulvin or terbinafine
Tinea cruris (groin area; "jock itch")	• Begins with small, red scaling patches, which spread to form circular elevated plaques • Very pruritic • Clusters of pustules may be seen around borders.	• Mild conditions: topical antifungal creams • Severe conditions: griseofulvin or terbinafine
Tinea pedis (foot; "athlete's foot")	• Soles of one or both feet have scaling and mild redness with maceration in the toe webs. • More acute infections may have clusters of clear vesicles on dusky base.	• Soak feet in vinegar and water solution. • Resistant infections: griseofulvin or terbinafine • Terbinafine (Lamisil) daily for 3 months
Tinea ungum (toenails; affects about 50% of adults)	• Nails thicken, crumble easily, and lack luster • Whole nail may be destroyed.	• Itraconazole (Sporanox) in pulses of 1 week a month for 3 months

Small pieces of cotton can be placed between the toes at night to absorb moisture. Socks should be made of cotton, and hosiery should have cotton feet, because cotton is an effective absorber of perspiration.

For people whose feet perspire excessively, perforated shoes permit better aeration of the feet. Plastic- or rubber-soled footwear should be avoided. Talcum powder or antifungal powder applied twice daily helps to keep the feet dry. Several pairs of shoes should be alternated so that they can dry completely before being worn again.

TINEA CORPORIS: RINGWORM OF THE BODY

In tinea corporis (ie, ringworm of the body), the typical ringed lesion appears on the face, neck, trunk, and extremities (Fig. 56-3). Animal (nonhuman) varieties are known to cause an intense inflammatory reaction in humans because they are not adapted to living on human hosts. Humans make contact with animal varieties through contact with pets or objects that have been in contact with an animal.

Medical Management

Topical antifungal medication may be applied to small areas. Oral antifungal agents are used only in extensive cases. Side effects of oral antifungal agents include photosensitivity, skin rashes, headache, and nausea. Newer antifungal agents, including itraconazole, fluconazole, and terbinafine, have been more effective with fewer systemic side effects than griseofulvin in patients with chronic fungal (dermatophyte) infections.

Nursing Management

The patient is instructed to use a clean towel and washcloth daily. Because fungal infections thrive in heat and moisture, all skin areas and skin folds that retain moisture must be dried thoroughly. Clean cotton clothing should be worn next to the skin.

TINEA CAPITIS: RINGWORM OF THE SCALP

Ringworm of the scalp is a contagious fungal infection of the hair shafts and a common cause of hair loss in children. Any child with scaling of the scalp should be considered to have tinea capitis until proven otherwise. Clinical examination reveals one or several round, red scaling patches. Small pustules or papules may

FIGURE 56-3 Tinea corporis (ringworm) of the face.

be seen at the edges of such patches. As the hairs in the affected areas are invaded by the fungi, they become brittle and break off at or near the surface of the scalp, leaving bald patches or the classic sign of black dots, which are the broken ends of hairs. Because most cases of tinea capitis heal without scarring, the hair loss is only temporary.

Medical Management

Griseofulvin, an antifungal agent, is prescribed for patients with tinea capitis. Topical agents do not provide an effective cure because the infection occurs within the hair shaft and below the surface of the scalp. However, topical agents can be used to inactivate organisms already on the hair. This minimizes contagion and eliminates the need to clip the hair. Infected hairs break off anyway, and noninfected ones may remain in place. The hair should be shampooed two or three times weekly, and a topical antifungal preparation should be applied to reduce dissemination of the organisms.

Nursing Management

Because tinea capitis is contagious, the patient and family should be instructed to set up a hygiene regimen for home use. Each person should have a separate comb and brush and should avoid exchanging hats and other headgear. All infected members of the family must be examined because familial infections are relatively common. Household pets should also be examined.

TINEA CRURIS: RINGWORM OF THE GROIN

Tinea cruris (ie, jock itch) is ringworm infection of the groin, which may extend to the inner thighs and buttock area. It occurs most frequently in young joggers, obese people, and those who wear tight underclothing. The incidence of tinea cruris is increased among people with diabetes.

Management

Mild infections may be treated with topical medication such as clotrimazole, miconazole, or terbinafine for at least 3 to 4 weeks to ensure eradication of the infection. Oral antifungal agents may be required for more severe infections. Heat, friction, and maceration (from sweating) predispose the patient to the infection. The nurse instructs the patient to avoid excessive heat and humidity as much as possible and to avoid wearing nylon underwear, tight-fitting clothing, and a wet bathing suit. The groin area should be cleaned, dried thoroughly, and dusted with a topical antifungal agent such as tolnaftate (Tinactin) as a preventive measure, because the infection is likely to recur.

TINEA UNGUIUM: ONYCHOMYCOSIS

Tinea unguium (ie, ringworm of the nails) is a chronic fungal infection of the toenails or, less commonly, the fingernails. It is usually caused by *Trichophyton* species (*T. rubrum*, *T. mentagrophytes*) or *Candida albicans*. It is usually associated with long-standing fungal infection of the feet. The nails become thickened, friable (ie, easily crumbled), and lusterless. In time, debris accumulates under the free edge of the nail. Ultimately, the nail plate separates. Because of the chronicity of this infection, the entire nail may be destroyed.

Management

An oral antifungal agent is prescribed for 6 weeks when the fingernails are involved and 12 weeks when the toenails are involved. Selection of the antifungal agent depends on the causative fungus. Candidal infections are treated with fluconazole (Diflucan) or itraconazole (Sporanox). Griseofulvin is no longer considered effective therapy because of its long treatment course and poor cure rate. Response to oral antifungal agents in treating infections of the toenails is poor at best. Frequently, when the treatment stops, the infection returns.

Parasitic Skin Infestation

PEDICULOSIS: LICE INFESTATION

Lice infestation affects people of all ages. Three varieties of lice infest humans: *Pediculus humanus capitis* (ie, head louse), *Pediculus humanus corporis* (ie, body louse), and *Phthirus pubis* (ie, pubic louse or crab louse). Lice are called ectoparasites because they live on the outside of the host's body. They depend on the host for their nourishment, feeding on human blood approximately five times each day. They inject their digestive juices and excrement into the skin, which causes severe itching.

PEDICULOSIS CAPITIS

Pediculosis capitis is an infestation of the scalp by the head louse. The female louse lays her eggs (ie, nits) close to the scalp. The nits become firmly attached to the hair shafts with a tenacious substance. The young lice hatch in about 10 days and reach maturity in 2 weeks.

Clinical Manifestations

Head lice are found most commonly along the back of the head and behind the ears. The eggs are visible to the naked eye as silvery, glistening oval bodies that are difficult to remove from the hair. The bite of the insect causes intense itching, and the resultant scratching often leads to secondary bacterial infection, such as impetigo or furunculosis. The infestation is more common in children and people with long hair. Head lice may be transmitted directly by physical contact or indirectly by infested combs, brushes, wigs, hats, and bedding.

Medical Management

Treatment involves washing the hair with a shampoo containing lindane (Kwell) or pyrethrin compounds with piperonyl butoxide (RID or R&C Shampoo). The patient is instructed to shampoo the scalp and hair according to the product directions. After the hair is rinsed thoroughly, it is combed with a fine-toothed comb dipped in vinegar to remove any remaining nits or nit shells freed from the hair shafts. They are extremely difficult to remove and may have to be picked off one by one with the fingernails.

All articles, clothing, towels, and bedding that may have lice or nits should be washed in hot water—at least 54°C—or dry-cleaned to prevent re-infestation. Upholstered furniture, rugs, and floors should be vacuumed frequently. Combs and brushes are also disinfected with the shampoo. All family members and close contacts are treated. Complications such as severe pruritus, pyoderma, and dermatitis are treated with antipruritics, systemic antibiotics, and topical corticosteroids.

Nursing Management

The nurse informs the patient that head lice may infest anyone and are not a sign of uncleanliness. Because the condition spreads rapidly, treatment must be started immediately. School epidemics may be managed by having all of the students shampoo their hair on the same night. Students should be warned not to share combs, brushes, and hats. Each family member should be inspected for head lice daily for at least 2 weeks. The patient should be instructed that lindane may be toxic to the central nervous system when used improperly.

PEDICULOSIS CORPORIS AND PUBIS

Pediculosis corporis is an infestation of the body by the body louse. This is a disease of unwashed people or those who live in close quarters and do not change their clothing. Pediculosis pubis is extremely common. The infestation is generally localized in the genital region and is transmitted chiefly by sexual contact.

Clinical Manifestations

Chiefly involved are those areas of the skin that come in closest contact with the underclothing (ie, neck, trunk, and thighs). The body louse lives primarily in the seams of underwear and clothing, to which it clings as it pierces the skin with its proboscis. Its bites cause characteristic minute hemorrhagic points. Widespread excoriation may appear as a result of intense itching and scratching, especially on the trunk and neck. Among the secondary lesions produced are parallel linear scratches and a slight degree of eczema. In long-standing cases, the skin may become thick, dry, and scaly, with dark pigmented areas.

Itching is the most common symptom of pediculosis pubis, particularly at night. Reddish brown dust (ie, excretions of the insects) may be found in the patient's underclothing. The pubic area should be examined with a magnifying glass for lice crawling down a hair shaft or nits cemented to the hair or at the junction with the skin. Infestation by pubic lice may coexist with sexually transmitted diseases such as gonorrhea, herpes, or syphilis. There may also be infestation of the hairs of the chest, armpit, beard, and eyelashes. Grey-blue macules may sometimes be seen on the trunk, thighs, and axillae as a result of either the reaction of the insects' saliva with bilirubin (converting it to biliverdin) or an excretion produced by the salivary glands of the louse.

Medical Management

The patient is instructed to bathe with soap and water, after which lindane (Kwell) or 5% permethrin (Elimite) is applied to affected areas of the skin and to hairy areas, according to the product directions. An alternative topical therapy is an over-the-counter strength of permethrin (1% Nix). If the eyelashes are involved, petrolatum may be thickly applied twice daily for 8 days, followed by mechanical removal of any remaining nits.

Complications, such as severe pruritus, pyoderma, and dermatitis, are treated with antipruritics, systemic antibiotics, and topical corticosteroids. Body lice can transmit epidemic rickettsial disease to humans such as epidemic typhus, relapsing fever, and trench fever. The causative organism may be in the gastrointestinal tract of the insect and may be excreted on the skin surface of the infested person.

Nursing Management

All family members and sexual contacts must be treated and educated in personal hygiene and methods to prevent or control infestation. The patient and partner must also be scheduled for a diagnostic workup for coexisting sexually transmitted disease. All clothing and bedding should be machine washed in hot water or dry-cleaned.

SCABIES

Scabies is an infestation of the skin by the itch mite *Sarcoptes scabiei*. The disease may be found in people living in substandard hygienic conditions, but it is also common in very clean individuals and among the sexually active, although infestations do not depend on sexual activity. The mites frequently involve the fingers, and hand contact may produce infection. In children, overnight stays with friends or the exchange of clothes may be a source of infection. Health care personnel who have prolonged hands-on physical contact with an infected patient may likewise become infected.

The adult female burrows into the superficial layer of the skin and remains there for the rest of her life. With her jaws and the sharp edges of the joints of her forelegs, the mite extends the burrow, laying two or three eggs daily for up to 2 months. She then dies. The larvae hatch from the eggs in 3 to 4 days and progress through larval and nymphal states to form adult mites in about 10 days.

Clinical Manifestations

It takes approximately 4 weeks from the time of contact for the patient's symptoms to appear. The patient complains of severe itching caused by a delayed type of immunologic reaction to the mite or its fecal pellets. During examination, the patient is asked where the itch is most severe. A magnifying glass and a penlight are held at an oblique angle to the skin while a search is made for the small, raised burrows. The burrows may be multiple, straight or wavy, brown or black, threadlike lesions, most commonly observed between the fingers and on the wrists. Other sites are the extensor surfaces of the elbows, the knees, the edges of the feet, the points of the elbows, around the nipples, in the axillary folds, under pendulous breasts, and in or near the groin or gluteal fold, penis, or scrotum. Red, pruritic eruptions usually appear between adjacent skin areas. The burrow, however, is not always visible. Any patient with a rash may have scabies.

One classic sign of scabies is the increased itching that occurs at night, perhaps because the increased warmth of the skin has a stimulating effect on the parasite. Hypersensitivity to the organism and its products of excretion also may contribute to the itching. If the infection has spread, other members of the family and close friends also complain of itching about a month later.

Secondary lesions are quite common and include vesicles, papules, excoriations, and crusts. Bacterial superinfection may result from constant excoriation of the burrows and papules.

Assessment and Diagnostic Findings

The diagnosis is confirmed by recovering *S. scabiei* or the mites' byproducts from the skin. A sample of superficial epidermis is scraped off the top of the burrows or papules with a small scalpel blade. The scrapings are placed on a microscope slide and examined through a low-powered microscope to demonstrate the mite at any stage (eg, egg, egg casing, larva, nymph, adult) and fecal pellets.

Gerontologic Considerations

Elderly patients living in long-term care facilities are more susceptible to outbreaks of scabies because of close living quarters, poor hygiene due to limited physical ability, and the potential for incidental spread of the organisms by nursing staff.

Although the older patient itches severely, the vivid inflammatory reaction seen in younger people seldom occurs. Scabies may not be recognized in the elderly person; the itching may erroneously be attributed to the dry skin of old age or to anxiety.

Health care personnel in extended-care facilities should wear gloves when providing hands-on care for a patient suspected of having scabies until the diagnosis is confirmed and treatment accomplished. It is advisable to treat all residents, staff, and families of patients at the same time to prevent reinfection. Because geriatric patients may be more sensitive to side effects of the scabicides, they should be closely observed for reactions.

Medical Management

The patient is instructed to take a warm, soapy bath or shower to remove the scaling debris from the crusts and then to dry thoroughly and allow the skin to cool. A prescription scabicide, such as lindane (Kwell), crotamiton (Eurax), or 5% permethrin (Elimite), is applied thinly to the entire skin from the neck down, sparing only the face and scalp (which are not affected in scabies). The medication is left on for 12 to 24 hours, after which the patient is instructed to wash thoroughly. One application may be curative, but it is advisable to repeat the treatment in 1 week.

 NURSING ALERT The patient must understand medication instructions, because application of a scabicide immediately after bathing and before the skin dries and cools increases percutaneous absorption of the scabicide and the potential for central nervous system abnormalities such as seizures.

Nursing Management

The patient should wear clean clothing and sleep between freshly laundered bed linens. All bedding and clothing should be washed in hot water and dried on the hot dryer cycle, because the mites can survive up to 36 hours in linens. If bed linens or clothing cannot be washed in hot water, dry-cleaning is advised.

After treatment is completed, the patient should apply an ointment, such as a topical corticosteroid, to skin lesions because the scabicide may irritate the skin. The patient's hypersensitivity does not cease on destruction of the mites. Itching may continue for several weeks as a manifestation of hypersensitivity, particularly in atopic (allergic) people. This is not a sign that the treatment has failed. The patient is instructed not to apply more scabicide because it will cause more irritation and increased itching and advised not to take frequent hot showers because they can dry the skin and produce itching. Oral antihistamines such as diphenhydramine (Benadryl) or hydroxyzine (Atarax) can help control the itching.

All family members and close contacts should be treated simultaneously to eliminate the mites. Some scabicides are approved for use in infants and pregnant women. If scabies is sexually transmitted, the patient may require treatment for coexisting sexually transmitted disease. Scabies may also coexist with pediculosis.

Contact Dermatitis

Contact dermatitis is an inflammatory reaction of the skin to physical, chemical, or biologic agents. The epidermis is damaged by repeated physical and chemical irritations. Contact dermatitis may be of the primary irritant type, in which a nonallergic reaction results from exposure to an irritating substance, or it may be allergic (ie, allergic contact dermatitis), resulting from exposure of sensitized people to contact allergens. Allergic dermatoses are discussed in Chapter 53. Common causes of irritant dermatitis are soaps, detergents, scouring compounds, and industrial chemicals. Predisposing factors include extremes of heat and cold, frequent contact with soap and water, and a preexisting skin disease (Chart 56-3).

Clinical Manifestations

The eruptions begin when the causative agent contacts the skin. The first reactions include itching, burning, and erythema, followed closely by edema, papules, vesicles, and oozing or weeping. In the subacute phase, these vesicular changes are less marked, and they alternate with crusting, drying, fissuring, and peeling. If repeated reactions occur or if the patient continually scratches the skin, lichenification and pigmentation occur. Secondary bacterial invasion may follow.

Medical Management

The objectives of management are to rest the involved skin and protect it from further damage. The distribution pattern of the reaction is determined to differentiate between allergic and irritant contact dermatitis. A detailed history is obtained. If indicated, the offending irritant is removed. Local irritation should be avoided, and soap is not generally used until healing occurs.

Chart 56-3 • PATIENT EDUCATION
Strategies for Avoiding Contact Dermatitis

The following precautions may help prevent repeated cases of contact dermatitis. Follow these instructions for at least 4 months after your skin appears to be completely healed.

- Study the pattern and location of your dermatitis and think about which things have touched your skin and which things may have caused the problem.
- Try to avoid contact with these materials.
- Avoid heat, soap, and rubbing, all of which are external irritants.
- Choose bath soaps, laundry detergents, and cosmetics that do not contain fragrance.
- Avoid using a fabric softener dryer sheet (Bounce, Cling). Fabric softeners that are added to the washer may be used.
- Avoid topical medications, lotions, or ointments, except those specifically prescribed for your condition.
- Wash your skin thoroughly immediately after exposure to possible irritants.
- When wearing gloves (for example, for washing dishes or general cleaning), be sure they are cotton-lined. Do not wear them more than 15 or 20 minutes at a time.

Many preparations are advocated for relieving dermatitis. In general, a bland, unmedicated lotion is used for small patches of erythema (ie, red, inflamed skin). Cool, wet dressings also are applied over small areas of vesicular dermatitis. Finely cracked ice added to the water often enhances its antipruritic effect.

Wet dressings usually help clear the oozing eczematous lesions. A thin layer of cream or ointment containing a corticosteroid then may be used. Medicated baths at room temperature are prescribed for larger areas of dermatitis. For severe, widespread conditions, a short course of systemic corticosteroids may be prescribed.

Noninfectious Inflammatory Dermatoses

PSORIASIS

Psoriasis is a chronic noninfectious inflammatory disease of the skin in which epidermal cells are produced at a rate that is about six to nine times faster than normal. The cells in the basal layer of the skin divide too quickly, and the newly formed cells move so rapidly to the skin surface that they become evident as profuse scales or plaques of epidermal tissue. The psoriatic epidermal cell may travel from the basal cell layer of the epidermis to the stratum corneum (ie, skin surface) and be cast off in 3 to 4 days, which is in sharp contrast to the normal 26 to 28 days. As a result of the increased number of basal cells and rapid cell passage, the normal events of cell maturation and growth cannot take place. This abnormal process does not allow the normal protective layers of the skin to form.

One of the most common skin diseases, psoriasis affects over 1 million Canadians, appearing more often in people who have a European ancestry. It is thought that the condition stems from a hereditary defect that causes overproduction of keratin. Although the primary cause is unknown, a combination of specific genetic makeup and environmental stimuli may trigger the onset of disease. There is some evidence that the cell proliferation is mediated by the immune system. Periods of emotional stress and anxiety aggravate the condition. Trauma, infections, and seasonal and hormonal changes also are trigger factors. The onset may occur at any age but is most common between the ages of 15 and 50 years. Psoriasis has a tendency to improve and then recur periodically throughout life (Champion et al., 1998).

Clinical Manifestations

Lesions appear as red, raised patches of skin covered with silvery scales. The scaly patches are formed by the buildup of living and dead skin resulting from the vast increase in the rate of skin-cell growth and turnover (Fig. 56-4). If the scales are scraped away, the dark red base of the lesion is exposed, producing multiple bleeding points. These patches are not moist and may be pruritic. One variation of this condition is called guttate psoriasis because the lesions remain about 1 cm wide and are scattered like raindrops over the body. This variation is believed to be associated with a recent streptococcal throat infection. Psoriasis may range in severity from a cosmetic source of annoyance to a physically disabling and disfiguring disorder.

Particular sites of the body tend to be affected most by this condition; they include the scalp, the extensor surface of the elbows and knees, the lower part of the back, and the genitalia. Bilateral symmetry is a feature of psoriasis. In approximately one fourth to one half of patients, the nails are involved, with pitting, discolouration, crumbling beneath the free edges, and separation of the nail plate. When psoriasis occurs on the palms and soles, it can cause pustular lesions called palmar pustular psoriasis.

FIGURE 56-4 Psoriasis. Courtesy of Roche Laboratories.

Complications

The disease may be associated with asymmetric rheumatoid factor–negative arthritis of multiple joints. The arthritic development can occur before or after the skin lesions appear. The relation between arthritis and psoriasis is not understood. Another complication is an exfoliative psoriatic state in which the disease progresses to involve the total body surface, called erythrodermic psoriasis. In this case, the patient is more acutely ill, with fever, chills, and an electrolyte imbalance. Erythrodermic psoriasis often appears in people with chronic psoriasis after infections or after exposure to certain medications, including withdrawal of systemic corticosteroids (Champion et al., 1998).

Assessment and Diagnostic Findings

The presence of the classic plaque-type lesions generally confirms the diagnosis of psoriasis. Because the lesions tend to change histologically as they progress from early to chronic plaques, biopsy of the skin is of little diagnostic value. There are no specific blood tests helpful in diagnosing the condition. When in doubt, the health professional should assess for signs of nail and scalp involvement and for a positive family history.

Medical Management

The goals of management are to slow the rapid turnover of epidermis, to promote resolution of the psoriatic lesions, and to control the natural cycles of the disease. There is no known cure.

The therapeutic approach should be one that the patient understands; it should be cosmetically acceptable and not too disruptive of lifestyle. Treatment involves the commitment of time and effort by the patient and possibly the family. First, any precipitating or aggravating factors are addressed. An assessment is made of lifestyle, because psoriasis is significantly affected by stress. The patient is informed that treatment of severe psoriasis can be time consuming, expensive, and aesthetically unappealing at times.

The most important principle of psoriasis treatment is gentle removal of scales. This can be accomplished with baths. Oils (eg, olive oil, mineral oil, Aveeno Oilated Oatmeal Bath) or coal tar preparations (eg, Balnetar) can be added to the bath water and a soft brush used to scrub the psoriatic plaques gently. After bathing, the application of emollient creams containing alpha-hydroxy acids (eg, Lac-Hydrin, Penederm) or salicylic acid will continue to soften thick scales. The patient and family should be encouraged to establish a regular skin care routine that can be maintained even when the psoriasis is not in an acute stage.

PHARMACOLOGIC THERAPY

Three types of therapy are standard: topical, intralesional, and systemic (Table 56-7).

Topical Agents. Topically applied agents are used to slow the overactive epidermis without affecting other tissues. Medications include tar preparations, anthralin, salicylic acid, and corticosteroids. Two topical treatments introduced within the last few years are a vitamin D preparation, calcipotriene (Dovonex), and

Table 56-7 • Current Treatments for Psoriasis

TOPICAL AGENTS	USE	SELECTED AGENTS
Topical corticosteroids	Mild to moderate lesions Moderate to severe lesions Severe lesions Lesions on face and groin	Aristocort, Kenalog, Valisone Lidex, Psorcon, Cutivate Temovate, Diprolene, Ultravate Aclovate, DesOwen, Hytone 2.5%
Topical nonsteroidals	Mild to severe	Retinoids such as tazarotene (Tazorac) Vitamin D₂ derivative calcipotriene (Dovonex)
Coal tar products	Mild to moderate lesions	Coal tar and salicylic acid ointment (Aquatar, Estar gel, Fototar, Zetar); anthralin (AnthraDerm, Dritho-Cream); Neutrogena T-Derm, Psori Gel
Medicated shampoos	Scalp lesions	Neutrogena T-Gel, T-Sal, Zetar, Head & Shoulders, Desenex, Selsun Blue, Bakers P&S (emulsifying agent with phenol, saline solution, and mineral oil)
Intralesional therapy	Thick plaques and nails	Kenalog, Cordran-impregnated tape, Fluoroplex
Systemic therapy	Extensive lesions and nails	Methotrexate (Folex, Mexate); hydrourea (Hydrea); retinoic acid (Tegison) (not to be used in women of childbearing age)
	Psoriatic arthritis	Oral gold (auranofin), etrentinate, methotrexate
Photochemotherapy	Moderate to severe lesions	UVA or UVB light with or without topical medications PUVA (combines UVA light with oral psoralens, or topical tripsoralen)

a retinoid compound, tazarotene (Tazorac). Treatment with these agents tends to suppress **epidermopoiesis** (ie, development of epidermal cells) and cause sloughing of the rapidly growing epidermal cells.

Topical formulations include lotions, ointments, pastes, creams, and shampoos. Older treatments, including tar baths and application of tar preparations on involved skin, are rarely used. Tar and anthralin cause irritation of the skin at the sites of application, are malodourous and difficult to apply, and do not give reliable results. Newer preparations that cause less irritation and have more consistent results are becoming more widely used.

Topical corticosteroids may be applied for their antiinflammatory effect. Choosing the correct strength of corticosteroid for the involved site and choosing the most effective vehicle base are important aspects of topical treatment. In general, highpotency topical corticosteroids should not be used on the face and intertriginous areas, and their use on other areas should be limited to a 4-week course of twice-daily applications. A 2-week break should be taken before repeating treatment with the high-potency corticosteroids. For long-term therapy, moderate-potency corticosteroids are used. On the face and intertriginous areas, only low-potency corticosteroids are appropriate for long-term use (see Table 56-4).

Occlusive dressings may be applied to increase the effectiveness of the corticosteroid. For the hospitalized patient, large plastic bags may be used—one for the upper body with openings cut for the head and arms and one for the lower body with openings for the legs. This leaves only the extremities to wrap. In some dermatologic units, large rolls of tubular plastic are used, such as those used by dry-cleaners. For patients being treated at home, a vinyl jogging suit may be used. The medication is applied, and the suit is put on over it. The hands can be wrapped in gloves, the feet in plastic bags, and the head in a shower cap. Occlusive dressings should not remain in place longer than 8 hours. The nurse should very carefully inspect the skin for the appearance of atrophy and telangiectasias which are side effects of corticosteroids.

> **! NURSING ALERT** When plastic substances are used, the nurse needs to check for flammability. Some thin plastic films burn slowly (if touched by a lighted cigarette), whereas others burst rapidly into flame. The patient should be cautioned not to smoke while wrapped in plastic dressing.

When psoriasis involves large areas of the body, topical corticosteroid treatment can become expensive and involve some systemic risk. Some potent corticosteroids, when applied to large areas of the body, have the potential to cause adrenal suppression through percutaneous absorption of the medication. In this event, other treatment modalities (eg, nonsteroidal topical medications, ultraviolet light) may be used instead or in combination to decrease the need for corticosteroids.

Newer nonsteroidal topical preparations are available and effective for many patients. Calcipotriene 0.05% (Dovonex) is a derivative of vitamin D_2. It works to decrease the mitotic turnover of the psoriatic plaques. Its most common side effect is local irritation, and the intertriginous areas and face should be avoided when using this medication. Patients should be monitored for symptoms of hypercalcemia. It is available as a cream for use on the body and a solution for the scalp. Calcipotriene is not recommended for use by elderly patients because of their more fragile skin or for pregnant or lactating women.

The second advance in topical treatment of psoriasis is tazarotene (Tazorac). Tazarotene, a retinoid, causes sloughing of the scales

covering psoriatic plaques. As with other retinoids, it causes increased sensitivity to sunlight, so patients should be cautioned to use an effective sunscreen and avoid other photosensitizers (eg, tetracycline, antihistamines). Tazarotene is listed as a Category X drug in pregnancy; reports indicate evidence of fetal risk, and the risk of use in pregnant women clearly outweighs any possible benefits. A negative result on a pregnancy test should be obtained before initiating this medication, and an effective contraceptive should be continued during treatment. Side effects of tazarotene include burning, erythema, or irritation at the site of application and worsening of psoriasis.

Intralesional Agents. Intralesional injections of triamcinolone acetonide (Aristocort, Kenalog-10, Trymex) can be administered directly into highly visible or isolated patches of psoriasis that are resistant to other forms of therapy. Care must be taken to ensure that normal skin is not injected with the medication.

Systemic Agents. Although systemic corticosteroids may cause rapid improvement of psoriasis, their usual risks and the possibility of triggering a severe flare-up on withdrawal limit their use. Systemic cytotoxic preparations, such as methotrexate, have been used in treating extensive psoriasis that fails to respond to other forms of therapy. Other systemic medications in current use include hydroxyurea (Hydrea) and cyclosporine A (CyA).

Methotrexate appears to inhibit DNA synthesis in epidermal cells, thereby reducing the turnover time of the psoriatic epidermis. However, the medication can be toxic, especially to the liver, which can suffer irreversible damage. Laboratory studies must be monitored to ensure that the hepatic, hematopoietic, and renal systems are functioning adequately. Bone marrow suppression is another potential side effect. The patient should avoid drinking alcohol while taking methotrexate, because alcohol ingestion increases the possibility of liver damage. The medication is teratogenic (ie, producing physical defects in the fetus) and should not be administered to pregnant women.

Hydroxyurea also inhibits cell replication by affecting DNA synthesis. The patient is monitored for signs and symptoms of bone marrow depression.

Cyclosporine A, a cyclic peptide used to prevent rejection of transplanted organs, has shown some success in treating severe, therapy-resistant cases of psoriasis. Its use, however, is limited by side effects such as hypertension and nephrotoxicity.

Oral retinoids (ie, synthetic derivatives of vitamin A and its metabolite, vitamin A acid) modulate the growth and differentiation of epithelial tissue. Etretinate is especially useful for severe pustular or erythrodermic psoriasis. Etretinate is a teratogen with a very long half-life; it cannot be used in women with childbearing potential.

PHOTOCHEMOTHERAPY

One treatment for severely debilitating psoriasis is a psoralen medication combined with ultraviolet-A (PUVA) light therapy. Ultraviolet light is the portion of the electromagnetic spectrum containing wavelengths ranging from 180 to 400 nm. In this treatment, the patient takes a photosensitizing medication (usually 8-methoxypsoralen) in a standard dose and is subsequently exposed to long-wave ultraviolet light as the medication plasma levels peak. Although the mechanism of action is not completely understood, it is thought that when psoralen-treated skin is exposed to ultraviolet-A light, the psoralen binds with DNA and decreases cellular proliferation. PUVA is not without its hazards;

it has been associated with long-term risks of skin cancer, cataracts, and premature aging of the skin.

The PUVA unit consists of a chamber that contains high-output black-light lamps and an external reflectance system. The exposure time is calibrated according to the specific unit in use and the anticipated tolerance of the patient's skin. The patient is usually treated two or three times each week until the psoriasis clears. An interim period of 48 hours between treatments is necessary because it takes this long for any burns resulting from PUVA therapy to become evident.

After the psoriasis clears, the patient begins a maintenance program. Once little or no disease is active, less potent therapies are used to keep minor flare-ups under control.

Ultraviolet-B (UVB) light therapy is also used to treat generalized plaques. UVB light ranges from 270 to 350 nm, although research has shown that a narrow range, 310 to 312 nm, is the action spectrum. It is used alone or combined with topical coal tar. Side effects are similar to those of PUVA therapy. A new development in light therapy is the narrow-band UVB, which ranges from 311 to 312 nm, decreasing exposure to harmful ultraviolet energy while providing more intense, specific therapy (Shelk & Morgan, 2000).

If access to a light treatment unit is not feasible, the patient can expose himself or herself to sunlight. The risks of all light treatments are similar and include acute sunburn reaction; exacerbation of photosensitive disorders such as lupus, rosacea, and polymorphic light eruption; and other skin changes such as increased wrinkles, thickening, and an increased risk for skin cancer.

Excimer lasers have come into use in treating psoriasis. These lasers function at 308 nm. Studies show that medium-sized psoriatic plaques clear in four to six treatments and remain clear for up to 9 months. A laser can be more effective on the scalp or on other hard-to-treat areas, because the laser can be aimed very specifically on the plaque (Lebwohl, 2000). Table 56-7 summarizes the treatment plans.

NURSING PROCESS:
CARE OF THE PATIENT WITH PSORIASIS

Assessment

The nursing assessment focuses on how the patient is coping with the psoriatic skin condition, appearance of the normal skin, and appearance of the skin lesions, as described previously. The notable manifestations are red, scaling papules that coalesce to form oval, well-defined plaques. Silver-white scales may also be present. Adjacent skin areas show red, smooth plaques with a macerated surface. It is important to examine the areas especially prone to psoriasis: elbows, knees, scalp, gluteal cleft, fingers, and toenails (for small pits).

Psoriasis may cause despair and frustration for the patient; observers may stare, comment, ask embarrassing questions, or even avoid the person. The disease can eventually exhaust the patient's resources, interfere with his or her job, and make life miserable in general. Teenagers are especially vulnerable to the psychological effects of this disorder. The family, too, is affected, because time-consuming treatments, messy salves, and constant shedding of scales may disrupt home life and cause resentment. The patient's frustrations may be expressed through hostility directed at health care personnel and others.

The nurse assesses the impact of the disease on the patient and the coping strategies used for conducting normal activities and interactions with family and friends. Many patients need reassurance that the condition is not infectious, not a reflection of poor personal hygiene, and not skin cancer.

Diagnosis

NURSING DIAGNOSES

Based on the nursing assessment data, the patient's major nursing diagnoses may include the following:

- Deficient knowledge about the disease process and treatment
- Impaired skin integrity related to lesions and inflammatory response
- Disturbed body image related to embarrassment over appearance and self-perception of uncleanliness

COLLABORATIVE PROBLEMS/
POTENTIAL COMPLICATIONS

Based on the assessment data, potential complications include the following:

- Infection
- Psoriatic arthritis

Planning and Goals

Major goals for the patient may include increased understanding of psoriasis and the treatment regimen, achievement of smoother skin with control of lesions, development of self-acceptance, and absence of complications.

Nursing Interventions

PROMOTING UNDERSTANDING

The nurse explains with sensitivity that, although there is no cure for psoriasis and lifetime management is necessary, the condition can usually be controlled. The pathophysiology of psoriasis is reviewed, as are the factors that provoke it—irritation or injury to the skin (eg, cut, abrasion, sunburn), current illness (eg, pharyngeal streptococcal infection), and emotional stress. It is emphasized that repeated trauma to the skin and an unfavourable environment (eg, cold) or a specific medication (eg, lithium, beta-blockers, indomethacin) may exacerbate psoriasis. The patient is cautioned about taking any nonprescription medications because some may aggravate mild psoriasis.

Reviewing and explaining the treatment regimen are essential to ensure compliance. For example, if the patient has a mild condition confined to localized areas, such as the elbows or knees, application of an emollient to maintain softness and minimize scaling may be all that is required. However, if the patient uses anthralin, the dosage schedule, possible side effects, and problems to report to the nurse or physician should be explained.

Most patients need a comprehensive plan of care that ranges from using topical medications and shampoos to more complex and lengthy treatment with systemic medications and photochemotherapy, such as PUVA therapy. Patient education materials that include a description of the therapy and specific guidelines are helpful but cannot replace face-to-face discussions of the treatment plan.

INCREASING SKIN INTEGRITY

To avoid injuring the skin, the patient is advised not to pick at or scratch the affected areas. Measures to prevent dry skin are encouraged because dry skin worsens psoriasis. Too-frequent washing produces more soreness and scaling. Water should be warm, not hot, and the skin should be dried by patting with a towel rather than by rubbing. Emollients have a moisturizing effect, providing an occlusive film on the skin surface so that normal water loss through the skin is halted and allowing the trapped water to hydrate the stratum corneum. A bath oil or emollient cleansing agent can comfort sore and scaling skin. Softening the skin can prevent fissures (see Plan of Nursing Care 56-1).

IMPROVING SELF-CONCEPT AND BODY IMAGE

A therapeutic relationship between health care professionals and the patient with psoriasis is one that includes education and support. After the treatment regimen is established, the patient should begin to feel more confident and empowered in carrying it out and in using coping strategies that help deal with the altered self-concept and body image brought about by the disease. Introducing the patient to successful coping strategies used by others with psoriasis and making suggestions for reducing or coping with stressful situations at home, school, and work can facilitate a more positive outlook and acceptance of the chronicity of the disease.

MONITORING AND MANAGING POTENTIAL COMPLICATIONS

Psoriatic Arthritis

The diagnosis of psoriasis, especially when it is accompanied by the complication of arthritis, is usually difficult to make. Psoriatic arthritis involving the sacroiliac and distal joints of the fingers may be overlooked, especially if the patient has the typical psoriatic lesions. However, patients who complain of mild joint discomfort and some pitting of the fingernails may not be diagnosed with psoriasis until the more obvious cutaneous lesions appear.

The complaint of joint discomfort in the patient with psoriasis should be noted and evaluated. The symptoms of psoriatic arthritis can mimic the symptoms of Reiter's disease and ankylosing spondylitis, and a definitive diagnosis must be made. Treatment of the condition usually involves joint rest, application of heat, and salicylates.

The patient requires education about the care and treatment of the involved joints and the need for compliance with therapy. The incidence of psoriatic arthropathy is unknown because the symptoms are so variable. It is believed, however, that when the psoriasis is extensive and a family history of inflammatory arthritis is elicited, the chance that the patient will develop psoriatic arthritis increases substantially. It is recommended that a rheumatologist be consulted to assist in the diagnosis and treatment of the arthropathy.

PROMOTING HOME AND COMMUNITY-BASED CARE

Teaching Patients Self-Care

Printed patient education materials may be provided to reinforce face-to-face discussions about treatment guidelines and other con-

siderations. For example, the patient and the family caregiver may need to know that the topical agent anthralin leaves a brownish purple stain on the skin but that the discolouration subsides after anthralin treatment stops. The patient should also be instructed to cover lesions treated with anthralin with gauze, stockinette, or other soft coverings to avoid staining clothing, furniture, and bed linens.

Patients using topical corticosteroid preparations repeatedly on the face and around the eyes should be aware that cataract development is possible. Strict guidelines for applying these medications should be emphasized because overuse can result in skin atrophy, striae, and medication resistance.

Photochemotherapy (PUVA), which is reserved for moderate to severe psoriasis, produces photosensitization, which means that the skin is sensitive to the sun until methoxsalen has been excreted from the body in about 6 to 8 hours. Patients undergoing PUVA treatments should avoid exposure to the sun. If exposure is unavoidable, the skin must be protected with sunscreen and clothing. Grey- or green-tinted, wraparound sunglasses should be worn to protect the eyes during and after treatment, and ophthalmologic examinations should be performed on a regular basis. Nausea, which may be a problem in some patients, is lessened when methoxsalen is taken with food. Lubricants and bath oils may be used to help remove scales and prevent excessive dryness. No other creams or oils are to be used except on areas that have been shielded from ultraviolet light. Contraceptives should be used by sexually active women of reproductive age, because the teratogenic effect of PUVA has not been determined. The patient is kept under constant and careful supervision and is encouraged to recognize unusual changes in the skin.

If indicated, referral may be made to a mental health professional who can help to ease emotional strain and give support. Belonging to a support group may also help patients acknowledge that they are not alone in experiencing life adjustments in response to a visible, chronic disease. The National Psoriasis Foundation publishes periodic bulletins and reports about new and relevant developments in this condition.

Chart 56-4 is a Home Care Checklist for the patient with psoriasis.

Evaluation

EXPECTED PATIENT OUTCOMES

Expected patient outcomes may include the following:

1. Demonstrates knowledge and understanding of disease process and its treatment
   a. Describes psoriasis and the prescribed therapy
   b. Verbalizes that trauma, infection, and emotional stress may be trigger factors

---

Chart 56-4
Home Care Checklist • The Patient With Psoriasis

At the completion of the home care instruction, the patient or caregiver will be able to:	Patient	Caregiver
• Describe the etiology of psoriasis.	✓	✓
• Describe optimal skin maintenance practices to maintain moisture of skin and prevent infection.	✓	✓
• Demonstrate proper application of prescribed topical medications.	✓	✓
• Describe common side effects of oral medication, if prescribed.	✓	✓
• Demonstrate appropriate therapeutic bath technique, if prescribed.	✓	✓
• Verbalize optimism about condition.	✓	
• Identify a support person with whom to discuss feelings and concerns.	✓	

c. Maintains control with appropriate therapy
d. Demonstrates proper application of topical therapy
2. Achieves smoother skin and control of lesions
   a. Exhibits no new lesions
   b. Keeps skin lubricated and soft
3. Develops self-acceptance
   a. Identifies someone with whom to discuss feelings and concerns
   b. Expresses optimism about outcomes of treatment
4. Absense of complications
   a. Has no joint discomfort
   b. Reports control of cutaneous lesions with no extension of disease

EXFOLIATIVE DERMATITIS

Exfoliative dermatitis is a serious condition characterized by progressive inflammation in which erythema and scaling occur in a more or less generalized distribution. It may be associated with chills, fever, prostration, severe toxicity, and an itchy scaling of the skin. There is a profound loss of stratum corneum (ie, outermost layer of the skin), which causes capillary leakage, hypoproteinemia, and negative nitrogen balance. Because of widespread dilation of cutaneous vessels, large amounts of body heat are lost, and exfoliative dermatitis has a marked effect on the entire body.

Exfoliative dermatitis has a variety of causes. It is considered to be a secondary or reactive process to an underlying skin or systemic disease. It may appear as a part of the lymphoma group of diseases and may precede the appearance of lymphoma. Preexisting skin disorders that have been implicated as a cause include psoriasis, atopic dermatitis, and contact dermatitis. It also appears as a severe reaction to many medications, including penicillin and phenylbutazone. The cause is unknown in approximately 25% of cases (Odom et al., 2000).

Clinical Manifestations

This condition starts acutely as a patchy or a generalized erythematous eruption accompanied by fever, malaise, and occasionally gastrointestinal symptoms. The skin colour changes from pink to dark red. After a week, the characteristic exfoliation (ie, scaling) begins, usually in the form of thin flakes that leave the underlying skin smooth and red, with new scales forming as the older ones come off. Hair loss may accompany this disorder. Relapses are common. The systemic effects include high-output heart failure, intestinal disturbances, breast enlargement, elevated levels of uric acid in the blood (ie, hyperuricemia), and temperature disturbances.

Medical Management

The objectives of management are to maintain fluid and electrolyte balance and to prevent infection. The treatment is individualized and supportive and should be initiated as soon as the condition is diagnosed.

The patient may be hospitalized and placed on bed rest. All medications that may be implicated are discontinued. A comfortable room temperature should be maintained because the patient does not have normal thermoregulatory control as a result of temperature fluctuations caused by vasodilation and evaporative water loss. Fluid and electrolyte balance must be maintained because there is considerable water and protein loss from the skin surface. Plasma volume expanders may be indicated.

Nursing Management

Continual nursing assessment is carried out to detect infection. The disrupted, erythematous, moist skin is susceptible to infection and becomes colonized with pathogenic organisms, which produce more inflammation. Antibiotics, prescribed if infection is present, are selected on the basis of culture and sensitivity.

 NURSING ALERT The nurse observes the patient for signs and symptoms of heart failure because hyperemia and increased cutaneous blood flow can produce high-output cardiac failure.

Hypothermia may occur because increased blood flow in the skin, coupled with increased water loss through the skin, leads to heat loss by radiation, conduction, and evaporation. Changes in vital signs are closely monitored and reported.

As in any acute dermatitis, topical therapy is used to provide symptomatic relief. Soothing baths, compresses, and lubrication with emollients are used to treat the extensive dermatitis. The patient is likely to be extremely irritable because of the severe itching. Oral or parenteral corticosteroids may be prescribed when the disease is not controlled by more conservative therapy. When a specific cause is known, more specific therapy may be used. The patient is advised to avoid all irritants in the future, particularly medications.

Blistering Diseases

Blisters of the skin have many origins, including bacterial, fungal, or viral infections; allergic contact reactions; burns; metabolic disorders; and immunologically mediated reactions. Some of these have been discussed previously (eg, herpes simplex and zoster infections, contact dermatitis). Immunologically mediated diseases are autoimmune reactions and represent a defect of IgM, IgE, IgG, and C3. Some of these conditions are life-threatening; others become chronic problems.

The diagnosis is always made by histologic examination of a biopsy specimen by a dermatopathologist. A specimen from the blister and surrounding skin demonstrates **acantholysis** (ie, separation of epidermal cells from each other because of damage to or an abnormality of the intracellular substance). Circulating antibodies may be detected by immunofluorescent studies of the patient's serum.

PEMPHIGUS

Pemphigus is a group of serious diseases of the skin characterized by the appearance of bullae (ie, blisters) of various sizes on apparently normal skin (Fig. 56-5) and mucous membranes. Available evidence indicates that pemphigus is an autoimmune disease involving immunoglobulin G. It is thought that the pemphigus antibody is directed against a specific cell-surface antigen in epidermal cells. A blister forms from the antigen–antibody reaction. The level of serum antibody is predictive of disease severity. Genetic factors may also play a role in its development, with the highest incidence among those of Jewish or Mediterranean descent. This disorder usually occurs in men and women in middle and late adulthood. The condition may be associated with penicillins and captopril and with myasthenia gravis.

FIGURE 56-5 Vesicles on the chin (in pemphigus). Sauer, G. C. (1985). *Manual of Skin Diseases.* Philadelphia: J. B. Lippincott.

Clinical Manifestations

Most patients present with oral lesions appearing as irregularly shaped erosions that are painful, bleed easily, and heal slowly. The skin bullae enlarge, rupture, and leave large, painful eroded areas that are accompanied by crusting and oozing. A characteristic offensive odour emanates from the bullae and the exuding serum. There is blistering or sloughing of uninvolved skin when minimal pressure is applied (ie, Nikolsky's sign). The eroded skin heals slowly, and huge areas of the body eventually are involved. Bacterial superinfection is common.

Complications

The most common complications of pemphigus vulgaris arise when the disease process is widespread. Before the advent of corticosteroid and immunosuppressive therapy, patients were very susceptible to secondary bacterial infection. Skin bacteria have relatively easy access to the bullae as they ooze, rupture, and leave denuded areas that are open to the environment. Fluid and electrolyte imbalance results from the loss of both fluid and protein as the bullae rupture. Hypoalbuminemia is common when the disease process includes extensive areas of the body skin surface and mucous membranes.

Management

The goals of therapy are to bring the disease under control as rapidly as possible, to prevent loss of serum and the development of secondary infection, and to promote re-epithelization (ie, renewal of epithelial tissue).

Corticosteroids are administered in high doses to control the disease and keep the skin free of blisters. The high dosage level is maintained until remission is apparent. In some cases, corticosteroid therapy must be maintained for life.

Corticosteroids are administered with or immediately after a meal and may be accompanied by an antacid as prophylaxis against gastric complications. Essential to therapeutic management are daily evaluations of body weight, blood pressure, blood glucose levels, and fluid balance. High-dose corticosteroid therapy has its own serious toxic effects (see Chap. 42).

Immunosuppressive agents (eg, azathioprine, cyclophosphamide, gold) may be prescribed to help control the disease and reduce the corticosteroid dose. **Plasmapheresis** (ie, plasma exchange) temporarily decreases the serum antibody level and has been used with variable success, although it is generally reserved for life-threatening cases.

BULLOUS PEMPHIGOID

Bullous pemphigoid is an acquired disease of flaccid blisters appearing on normal or erythematous skin. It appears more often on the flexor surfaces of the arms, legs, axilla, and groin. Oral lesions, if present, are usually transient and minimal. When the blisters break, the skin has shallow erosions that heal fairly quickly. Pruritus can be intense, even before the appearance of the blisters. Bullous pemphigoid is common in the elderly, with a peak incidence at about 60 years of age. There is no gender or racial predilection, and the disease can be found throughout the world.

Management

Medical treatment includes topical corticosteroids for localized eruptions and systemic corticosteroids for widespread involvement. Systemic prednisone may be continued for months, in alternate-day doses. The patient needs to understand the implications of long-term corticosteroid therapy, including loss of bone mass, osteoporosis, cataracts, peptic ulcers, psychotic reactions, increased risk for infection, weight gain from fluid retention, and the potential for adrenal suppression.

DERMATITIS HERPETIFORMIS

Dermatitis herpetiformis is an intensely pruritic, chronic disease that manifests with small, tense blisters that are distributed symmetrically over the elbows, knees, buttocks, and nape of the neck. It is most common between the ages of 20 and 40 years but can appear at any age. Most patients with dermatitis herpetiformis have a subclinical defect in gluten metabolism.

Management

Most patients respond to dapsone (combination of tetracycline and nicotinamide) and to a gluten-free diet. All patients should be screened for glucose-6-phosphate dehydrogenase deficiency, because dapsone can induce severe hemolysis in those with this deficiency. Patients benefit from dietary counselling because the dietary restrictions are lifelong, and a gluten-free diet is often difficult to follow. They need emotional support as they deal with the process of learning new habits and accepting major changes in their life.

HERPES GESTATIONIS

Herpes gestationis is a disease that occurs during or shortly after pregnancy. It shares several clinical features with bullous pemphigoid, and despite its name, it has no relation to the herpes virus. This disease is uncommon, with an incidence of approximately 1 case in every 50,000 pregnancies. It appears in the second or third trimester. It begins with urticarial papules on the abdomen and spreads to the trunk and extremities. It usually resolves within a few weeks of delivery but can recur in subsequent pregnancies, with menses, or with the use of oral contraceptives (Odom et al., 2000).

Management

Herpes gestationis is best managed with systemic corticosteroids. There is debate about whether there is any risk for fetal morbidity or mortality in babies born to mothers with herpes gestationis. As in other blistering diseases, special attention is required to prevent secondary infection.

NURSING PROCESS: CARE OF THE PATIENT WITH BLISTERING DISEASES

Assessment

Patients with blistering disorders may experience significant disability. There is constant itching and possible pain in the denuded areas of skin. There may be drainage from the denuded areas, which may be malodourous. Effective assessment and nursing management become a challenge.

Disease activity is monitored clinically by examining the skin for the appearance of new blisters. Areas where healing has occurred may show signs of hyperpigmentation. Particular attention is given to assessing for signs and symptoms of infection.

Diagnosis

NURSING DIAGNOSES

Based on nursing assessment data, the patient's major nursing diagnoses may include the following:

- Acute pain of skin and oral cavity related to blistering and erosions
- Impaired skin integrity related to ruptured bullae and denuded areas of the skin
- Anxiety and ineffective coping related to the appearance of the skin and no hope of a cure
- Deficient knowledge about medications and side effects

COLLABORATIVE PROBLEMS/ POTENTIAL COMPLICATIONS

Based on the assessment data, potential complications include the following:

- Infection and sepsis related to loss of protective barrier of skin and mucous membranes
- Fluid volume deficit and electrolyte imbalance related to loss of tissue fluids

Planning and Goals

The major goals for the patient may include relief of discomfort from lesions, skin healing, reduced anxiety and improved coping capacity, and absence of complications.

Nursing Interventions

RELIEVING ORAL DISCOMFORT

The patient's entire oral cavity may be affected with erosions and denuded surfaces. A necrotic slough may develop over these areas, adding to the patient's discomfort and interfering with food intake. Weight loss and hypoproteinemia may result. Meticulous oral hygiene is important to keep the oral mucosa clean and allow the epithelium to regenerate. Frequent rinsing of the mouth is prescribed to rid the mouth of debris and to soothe ulcerated areas. Commercial mouthwashes are avoided. The lips are kept moist with lanolin, petrolatum, or lip balm. Cool mist therapy helps to humidify environmental air.

ENHANCING SKIN INTEGRITY AND RELIEVING DISCOMFORT

Cool, wet dressings or baths are protective and soothing. The patient with painful and extensive lesions should be premedicated with analgesics before skin care is initiated. Patients with large

areas of blistering have a characteristic odour that decreases when secondary infection is controlled. After the patient's skin is bathed, it is dried carefully and dusted liberally with nonirritating powder, which enables the patient to move freely in bed. Fairly large amounts are necessary to keep the patient's skin from sticking to the sheets. Tape should never be used on the skin because it may produce more blisters. Hypothermia is common, and measures to keep the patient warm and comfortable are priority nursing activities. The nursing management of patients with bullous skin conditions is similar to that for patients with extensive burns (see Chap. 57).

REDUCING ANXIETY

Attention to the psychological needs of the patient requires listening to the patient, being available, giving expert nursing care, and educating the patient and the family. The patient is encouraged to express freely anxieties, discomfort, and feelings of hopelessness. Arranging for a family member or a close friend to spend more time with the patient can be supportive. When patients receive information about the disease and its treatment, uncertainty and anxiety are reduced, and the patient's capacity to act on his or her own behalf is enhanced. Referral for psychological counselling may assist the patient in dealing with fears, anxiety, and depression.

MONITORING AND MANAGING POTENTIAL COMPLICATIONS

Infection and Sepsis

The patient is susceptible to infection because the barrier function of the skin is compromised. Bullae are also susceptible to infection, and sepsis may follow. The skin is cleaned to remove debris and dead skin and to prevent infection.

Secondary infection may be accompanied by an offensive odour from skin or oral lesions. *C. albicans* of the mouth (ie, thrush) commonly affects patients receiving high-dose corticosteroid therapy. The oral cavity is inspected daily, and any changes are reported. Oral lesions are slow to heal.

Infection is the leading cause of death in patients with blistering diseases. Particular attention is given to assessment for signs and symptoms of local and systemic infection. Seemingly trivial complaints or minimal changes are investigated, because corticosteroids can mask or alter typical signs and symptoms of infection. The patient's vital signs are taken, and temperature fluctuations are monitored. The patient is observed for chills, and all secretions and excretions are monitored for changes suggesting infection. Results of culture and sensitivity tests are monitored. Antimicrobial agents are administered as prescribed, and response to treatment is assessed. Health care personnel must perform effective hand hygiene and wear gloves.

In the hospitalized patient, environmental contamination is reduced as much as possible. Protective isolation measures and standard precautions are warranted.

Fluid and Electrolyte Imbalance

Extensive denudation of the skin leads to fluid and electrolyte imbalance because of significant loss of fluids and sodium chloride from the skin. This sodium chloride loss is responsible for many of the systemic symptoms associated with the disease and is treated by intravenous administration of saline solution.

A large amount of protein and blood is lost from the denuded skin areas. Blood component therapy may be prescribed to maintain the blood volume, hemoglobin level, and plasma protein concentration. Serum albumin, protein, hemoglobin, and hematocrit values are monitored.

The patient is encouraged to maintain adequate oral fluid intake. Cool, nonirritating fluids are encouraged to maintain hydration. Small, frequent meals or snacks of high-protein, high-calorie foods (eg, Ensure, Sustacal, eggnog, milkshakes) help maintain nutritional status. Parenteral nutrition is considered if the patient cannot eat an adequate diet.

Evaluation

EXPECTED PATIENT OUTCOMES

Expected patient outcomes may include the following:

1. Achieves relief from pain of oral lesions
   a. Identifies therapies that reduce pain
   b. Uses mouthwashes and anesthetic or antiseptic aerosol mouth spray
   c. Drinks chilled fluids at 2-hour intervals
2. Achieves skin healing
   a. States purpose of therapeutic regimen
   b. Cooperates with soaks and bath regimen
   c. Reminds caregivers to use liberal amounts of nonirritating powder on bed linens
3. Is less anxious and better able to cope
   a. Verbalizes concerns about condition, self, and relationships with others
   b. Participates in self-care
4. Experiences no complications
   a. Has cultures from bullae, skin, and orifices that are negative for pathogenic organisms
   b. Has no purulent drainage
   c. Shows signs that skin is clearing
   d. Has normal temperature
   e. Keeps intake record to ensure adequate fluid intake and normal fluid and electrolyte balance
   f. Verbalizes the rationale for intravenous infusion therapy
   g. Has urine output within normal limits
   h. Has serum chemistry and hemoglobin and hematocrit values within normal limits

TOXIC EPIDERMAL NECROLYSIS AND STEVENS-JOHNSON SYNDROME

Toxic epidermal necrolysis (TEN) and Stevens-Johnson syndrome (SJS) are potentially fatal skin disorders and the most severe form of erythema multiforme. The mortality rate from TEN approaches 30%. Both conditions are triggered by a reaction to medications or result from a viral infection. Antibiotics, antiseizure agents, butazones, and sulfonamides are the most frequent medications implicated in TEN and SJS (Odom et al., 2000).

Clinical Manifestations

TEN and SJS are characterized initially by conjunctival burning or itching, cutaneous tenderness, fever, cough, sore throat, headache, extreme malaise, and myalgias (ie, aches and pains). These signs are followed by a rapid onset of erythema involving much of the skin surface and mucous membranes, including the oral mucosa, conjunctiva, and genitalia. In severe cases of mucosal involvement, there may be danger of damage to the larynx, bronchi, and esophagus from ulcerations. Large, flaccid bullae develop in

some areas; in other areas, large sheets of epidermis are shed, exposing the underlying dermis. Fingernails, toenails, eyebrows, and eyelashes may be shed along with the surrounding epidermis. The skin is excruciatingly tender, and the loss of skin leaves a weeping surface similar to that of a total-body, partial-thickness burn; hence the condition is also referred to as scalded skin syndrome.

These conditions occur in all ages and both genders. The incidence is increased in older people because of their use of many medications. People with HIV, particularly those with acquired immunodeficiency syndrome (AIDS), and others who are immunocompromised are at higher risk for SJS and TEN. Although the incidence of TEN and SJS in the general population is about 3 cases per 1 million person-years, the risk associated with sulfonamides in HIV-positive individuals may approach 1 case per 1000 (Odom et al., 2000). Most patients with TEN have an abnormal metabolism of the culprit medication, and the mechanism leading to TEN seems to be a cell-mediated cytotoxic reaction (Wolkenstein, 2000).

Complications

Sepsis and keratoconjunctivitis are complications of TEN and SJS. Unrecognized and untreated sepsis can be life-threatening. Keratoconjunctivitis can impair vision and result in conjunctival retraction, scarring, and corneal lesions.

Assessment and Diagnostic Findings

Histologic studies of frozen skin cells from a fresh lesion and cytodiagnosis of collections of cellular material from a freshly denuded area are performed. A history of ingestion of medications known to precipitate TEN or SJS may confirm medication reaction as the underlying cause.

Immunofluorescent studies may be performed to detect atypical epidermal autoantibodies. A genetic predisposition to erythema multiforme has been suggested but is not confirmed for all cases.

Medical Management

The goals of treatment include control of fluid and electrolyte balance, prevention of sepsis, and prevention of ophthalmic complications. Supportive care is the mainstay of treatment.

All nonessential medications are discontinued immediately. If possible, the patient is treated in a regional burn centre, because aggressive treatment similar to that for severe burns is required. Skin loss may approach 100% of the total body surface area. Surgical débridement or hydrotherapy in a Hubbard tank (ie, large, steel tub) may be performed to remove involved skin.

Tissue samples from the nasopharynx, eyes, ears, blood, urine, skin, and unruptured blisters are obtained for culture to identify pathogenic organisms. Intravenous fluids are prescribed to maintain fluid and electrolyte balance, especially in the patient who has severe mucosal involvement and who cannot easily take oral nourishment. Because an indwelling intravenous catheter may be a site of infection, fluid replacement is carried out by nasogastric tube and then orally as soon as possible.

Initial treatment with systemic corticosteroids is controversial. Some experts argue for early high-dose corticosteroid treatment. However, in most cases, the risk for infection, the complication of fluid and electrolyte imbalance, the delay in the healing process, and the difficulty in initiating oral corticosteroids early in the course of the disease outweigh the perceived benefits. In patients with TEN thought to result from a medication reaction, corticosteroids may be administered; however, the patients should be closely monitored for the previously stated adverse effects.

One report stated that intravenous administration of immunoglobulin (IVIG) to 10 patients led to improvement within 48 hours and skin healing within 1 week. This response is dramatically better than that obtained with immunosuppressives, and IVIG may soon become the treatment of choice (Rutter & Luger, 2001).

Protecting the skin with topical agents is crucial. Various topical antibacterial and anesthetic agents are used to prevent wound sepsis and to assist with pain management. Systemic antibiotic therapy is used with extreme caution. Temporary biologic dressings (eg, pigskin, amniotic membrane) or plastic semipermeable dressings (eg, Vigilon) may be used to reduce pain, decrease evaporation, and prevent secondary infection until the epithelium regenerates. Meticulous oropharyngeal and eye care is essential when there is severe involvement of the mucous membranes and the eyes.

NURSING PROCESS:
CARE OF THE PATIENT WITH TOXIC EPIDERMAL NECROLYSIS

Assessment

A careful inspection of the skin is made, including its appearance and the extent of involvement. The normal skin is closely observed to determine if new areas of blisters are developing. Seepage from blisters is monitored for amount, colour, and odour. Inspection of the oral cavity for blistering and erosive lesions is performed daily; the patient is assessed daily for itching, burning, and dryness of the eyes. The patient's ability to swallow and drink fluids, as well as speak normally, is determined.

The patient's vital signs are monitored, and special attention is given to the presence and character of fever and the respiratory rate, depth, rhythm, and cough. The characteristics and amount of respiratory secretions are reviewed. Assessment for high fever, tachycardia, and extreme weakness and fatigue is essential, because these factors indicate the process of epidermal necrosis, increased metabolic needs, and possible gastrointestinal and respiratory mucosal sloughing. Urine volume, specific gravity, and colour are monitored. The insertion sites of intravenous lines are inspected for signs of local infection. Daily body weights are recorded.

The patient is asked to describe fatigue and pain levels. An attempt is made to evaluate the patient's level of anxiety. The patient's basic coping mechanisms are assessed, and effective coping strategies are identified.

Diagnosis

NURSING DIAGNOSES

Based on the assessment data, the patient's major nursing diagnoses may include the following:

- Impaired tissue integrity (ie, oral, eye, and skin) related to epidermal shedding
- Deficient fluid volume and electrolyte losses related to loss of fluids from denuded skin
- Risk for imbalanced body temperature (ie, hypothermia) related to heat loss secondary to skin loss
- Acute pain related to denuded skin, oral lesions, and possible infection

- Anxiety related to the physical appearance of the skin and prognosis

COLLABORATIVE PROBLEMS/ POTENTIAL COMPLICATIONS

Based on the assessment data, potential complications include the following:

- Sepsis
- Conjunctival retraction, scars, and corneal lesions

Planning and Goals

The major goals for the patient may include skin and oral tissue healing, fluid balance, prevention of heat loss, relief of pain, reduced anxiety, and absence of complications.

Nursing Interventions

MAINTAINING SKIN AND MUCOUS MEMBRANE INTEGRITY

The local care of the skin is an important area of nursing management. The skin denudes easily, even when the patient is lifted and turned; it may be necessary to place the patient on a circular turning frame. The nurse applies the prescribed topical agents that reduce the bacterial population of the wound surface. Warm compresses, if prescribed, should be applied gently to denuded areas. The topical antibacterial agent may be used in conjunction with hydrotherapy in a tank, bathtub, or shower. The nurse monitors the patient's condition during the treatment and encourages the patient to exercise the extremities during hydrotherapy.

The painful oral lesions make oral hygiene difficult. Careful oral hygiene is performed to keep the oral mucosa clean. Prescribed mouthwashes, anesthetics, or coating agents are used frequently to rid the mouth of debris, soothe ulcerative areas, and control foul mouth odour. The oral cavity is inspected several times each day, and any changes are documented and reported. Petrolatum or a prescribed ointment is applied to the lips.

ATTAINING FLUID BALANCE

The vital signs, urine output, and sensorium are observed for indications of hypovolemia. Mental changes from fluid and electrolyte imbalance, sensory overload, or sensory deprivation may occur. Laboratory test results are evaluated, and abnormal results are reported. The patient is weighed daily (with a bed scale if necessary).

The nurse regulates intravenous fluids at prescribed infusion rates and assesses for systemic (ie, overinfusion or underinfusion) and local (eg, infection) complications. Oral lesions may result in dysphagia, making tube feeding or parenteral nutrition necessary. Prescribed enteral nourishment or enteral supplements can be administered by tube feeding until oral ingestion can be tolerated. A daily calorie count and accurate recording of all intake and output are essential.

PREVENTING HYPOTHERMIA

The patient with TEN is prone to chilling. Dehydration may be made worse by exposing the denuded skin to a continuous current of warm air. The patient is usually sensitive to room temperature changes. Measures implemented for a burn patient, such as cotton blankets, ceiling-mounted heat lamps, and heat shields, are useful in maintaining body temperature. To minimize shivering and heat loss, the nurse should work rapidly and efficiently when large wounds are exposed for wound care. The patient's temperature is monitored frequently.

RELIEVING PAIN

The nurse assesses the patient's pain, its characteristics, any factors that influence the pain, and the patient's behavioural responses. Prescribed analgesics are administered, and the nurse documents pain relief and any side effects. Analgesics are administered before painful treatments are performed. Providing thorough explanations and speaking calmly to the patient during treatments can allay the anxiety that may intensify pain. Offering emotional support and reassurance and implementing measures that promote rest and sleep are basic in achieving pain control. As the pain diminishes and the patient has more physical and emotional energy, self-management techniques for pain relief, such as progressive muscle relaxation and imagery, may be taught.

REDUCING ANXIETY

Because the lifestyle of patients with TEN has been abruptly changed to one of complete dependence, an assessment of their emotional state may reveal anxiety, depression, and fear of dying. Patients can be reassured that these reactions are normal. They also need nursing support, honest communication, and hope that their situation can improve. They are encouraged to express their feelings to someone they trust. Listening to their concerns and being readily available with skillful and compassionate care are important anxiety-relieving interventions. Emotional support by a psychiatric nurse, chaplain, psychologist, or psychiatrist may be helpful to promote coping during the long recovery period.

MONITORING AND MANAGING POTENTIAL COMPLICATIONS

Sepsis

The major cause of death from TEN is infection, and the most common sites of infection are the skin and mucosal surfaces, lungs, and blood. The organisms most often involved are *S. aureus, Pseudomonas, Klebsiella, Escherichia coli, Serratia,* and *Candida.* Monitoring vital signs closely and noticing changes in respiratory, renal, and gastrointestinal function may quickly detect the beginning of an infection. Strict asepsis is always maintained during routine skin care measures. Hand hygiene and wearing sterile gloves when carrying out procedures are necessary. When the condition involves a large portion of the body, the patient should be in a private room to prevent possible cross-infection from other patients. Visitors should wear protective garments and wash their hands before and after coming into contact with the patient. People with any infectious disease should not visit the patient until they are no longer a danger to the patient.

Conjunctival Retraction, Scars, and Corneal Lesions

The eyes are inspected daily for signs of itching, burning, and dryness, which may indicate progression often to keratoconjunctivitis, the principal eye complication. Applying a cool, damp cloth over the eyes may relieve burning sensations. The eyes are kept clean and observed for signs of discharge or discomfort, and the progression of symptoms is documented and reported. Administering an eye lubricant, when prescribed, may alleviate dryness and prevent corneal abrasion. Using eye patches or reminding the patient to blink periodically may also counteract dryness. The patient is instructed to avoid rubbing the eyes or putting any medication into the eyes that has not been prescribed or approved by the physician.

Evaluation

EXPECTED PATIENT OUTCOMES

Expected patient outcomes may include the following:

1. Achieves increasing skin and oral tissue healing
   a. Demonstrates areas of healing skin
   b. Swallows fluids and speaks clearly
2. Attains fluid balance
   a. Demonstrates laboratory values within normal ranges
   b. Maintains urine volume and specific gravity within acceptable range
   c. Shows stable vital signs
   d. Increases intake of oral fluids without discomfort
   e. Gains weight, if appropriate
3. Attains thermoregulation
   a. Registers body temperature within normal range
   b. Reports no chills
4. Achieves pain relief
   a. Uses analgesics as prescribed
   b. Uses self-management techniques for relief of pain
5. Appears less anxious
   a. Discusses concerns freely
   b. Sleeps for progressively longer periods
6. Absence of complications, such as sepsis and impaired vision
   a. Body temperature within normal range
   b. Laboratory values within normal ranges
   c. Has no abnormal discharges or signs of infection
   d. Continues to see objects at baseline acuity level
   e. Shows no signs of keratoconjunctivitis

Ulcerations

Superficial loss of surface tissue as a result of death of the cells is called an ulceration. A simple ulcer, such as the kind found in a small, superficial, partial-thickness burn, tends to heal by granulation (ie, new tissue granules) if kept clean and protected from injury. If it is exposed to the air, the serum that escapes will dry and form a scab, under which the epithelial cells will grow and cover the surface completely. Certain diseases cause characteristic ulcers; tuberculous ulcers and syphilitic ulcers are examples.

Ulcers related to problems with arterial circulation are seen in patients with peripheral vascular disease, arteriosclerosis, Raynaud's disease, and frostbite. In these patients, treatment of the ulcers is concurrent with treatment of the arterial disease (see Chap. 31). Nursing management includes the use of the dressings discussed at the beginning of this chapter. If nursing interventions are instituted early in the progression of an ulcer, the condition can often be effectively improved. Surgical amputation of an affected limb is a last resort.

Pressure ulcers involve breakdown of the skin due to prolonged pressure and insufficient blood supply, usually at bony prominences. Information about these ulcers is presented in chapter 11.

Benign Tumours of the Skin

CYSTS

Cysts of the skin are epithelium-lined cavities that contain fluid or solid material. Epidermal cysts (ie, epidermoid cysts) occur frequently and may be described as slow-growing, firm, elevated tumours found most frequently on the face, neck, upper chest, and back. Removal of the cysts provides a cure.

Pilar cysts (ie, trichilemmal cysts), formerly called sebaceous cysts, are most frequently found on the scalp. They originate from the middle portion of the hair follicle and from the cells of the outer hair root sheath. The treatment is surgical removal.

ACTINIC AND SEBORRHEIC KERATOSES

Seborrheic keratoses are benign, wartlike lesions of various sizes and colours, ranging from light tan to black. They are usually located on the face, shoulders, chest, and back and are the most common skin tumours seen in middle-aged and elderly people. They may be cosmetically unacceptable to the patient. A black keratosis may be erroneously diagnosed as malignant melanoma. The treatment is removal of the tumour tissue by excision, electrodesiccation and curettage, or application of carbon dioxide or liquid nitrogen. However, there is no harm in allowing these growths to remain, because there is no medical significance to their presence.

Actinic keratoses are premalignant skin lesions that develop in chronically sun-exposed areas of the body. They appear as rough, scaly patches with underlying erythema. A small percentage of these lesions gradually transform into cutaneous squamous cell carcinoma; they are usually removed by cryotherapy or shave excision.

VERRUCAE: WARTS

Warts are common, benign skin tumours caused by infection with the human papillomavirus, which belongs to the DNA virus group. All age groups may be affected, but the condition occurs most frequently between ages 12 and 16 years. There are many types of warts.

As a rule, warts are asymptomatic, except when they occur on weight-bearing areas, such as the soles of the feet. They may be treated with locally applied laser therapy, liquid nitrogen, salicylic acid plasters, or electrodesiccation (ie, destruction of skin lesions by monopolar high-frequency electric current).

Warts occurring on the genitalia and perianal areas are known as condylomata acuminata. They may be transmitted sexually and are treated with liquid nitrogen, cryosurgery, electrosurgery, topically applied trichloracetic acid, and curettage. Condylomata (see Chapter 47) that affect the uterine cervix predispose the patient to cervical cancer.

ANGIOMAS

Angiomas are benign vascular tumours that involve the skin and the subcutaneous tissues. They are present at birth and may occur as flat, violet-red patches (ie, port-wine angiomas) or as raised, bright-red, nodular lesions (ie, strawberry angiomas). The latter tend to involute spontaneously within the first few years of life, but port-wine angiomas usually persist indefinitely. Most patients use masking cosmetics (ie, Covermark or Dermablend) to camouflage the lesion. The argon laser is being used on various angiomas with some success. Treatment of strawberry angiomas is more successful if undertaken as soon after birth as possible (Odom et al., 2000).

PIGMENTED NEVI: MOLES

Moles are common skin tumours of various sizes and shades, ranging from yellowish brown to black. They may be flat, macular lesions or elevated papules or nodules that occasionally contain hair. Most pigmented nevi are harmless lesions. However, in rare cases, malignant changes occur, and a melanoma develops at the site of the nevus. Some authorities believe that all congenital moles should be removed, because they may have a higher incidence of malignant change. However, depending on the quantity and location, this may be impractical. Nevi that show a change in colour or size or become symptomatic (eg, itch) or develop irregular borders should be removed to determine if malignant changes have occurred. Moles that occur in unusual places should be examined carefully for any irregularity and for notching of the border and variation in colour. Early melanomas may display some redness and irritation and areas of bluish pigmentation where the pigment-containing cells have spread deeper into the skin. Late melanomas have areas of paler colour, where pigment cells have stopped producing melanin. Nevi larger than 1 cm should be examined carefully. Excised nevi should be examined histologically.

KELOIDS

Keloids are benign overgrowths of fibrous tissue at the site of a scar or trauma. They appear to be more common among dark-skinned people. Keloids are asymptomatic but may cause disfigurement and cosmetic concern. The treatment, which is not always satisfactory, consists of surgical excision, intralesional corticosteroid therapy, and radiation.

DERMATOFIBROMA

A dermatofibroma is a common, benign tumour of connective tissue that occurs predominantly on the extremities. It is a firm, dome-shaped papule or nodule that may be skin coloured or pinkish brown. Excisional biopsy is the recommended method of treatment.

NEUROFIBROMATOSIS: VON RECKLINGHAUSEN'S DISEASE

Neurofibromatosis is a hereditary condition manifested by pigmented patches (ie, café-au-lait macules), axillary freckling, and cutaneous neurofibromas that vary in size. Developmental changes may occur in the nervous system, muscles, and bone. Malignant degeneration of the neurofibromas occurs in some patients.

Malignant Tumours of the Skin: Skin Cancer

Skin cancer is the most common cancer in Canada, accounting for approximately one-third of all newly diagnosed cancers (Canadian Cancer Society, 2005) (Chart 56-5). Because the skin is easily inspected, skin cancer is readily seen and detected and is the most successfully treated type of cancer (Odom et al., 2000).

Exposure to the sun is the leading cause of skin cancer; incidence is related to the total amount of exposure to the sun. Sun damage is cumulative, and harmful effects may be severe by age 20 years. The increase in skin cancer probably reflects changing lifestyles and the emphasis on sunbathing and related activities in light of changes in the environment, such as holes in the Earth's ozone layer. Protective measures should be used throughout life, and nurses need to inform patients about risk factors associated with skin cancer.

Chart 56-5
Risk Factors for Skin Cancer

Changes in the ozone layer from the effects of worldwide industrial air pollutants, such as chlorofluorocarbons, have prompted concern that the incidence of skin cancers, especially malignant melanoma, will increase. The ozone layer, a stratospheric blanket of bluish, explosive gas formed by the sun's ultraviolet radiation, varies in depth with the seasons and is thickest at the North and South Poles and thinnest at the equator. Scientists believe that it helps protect the earth from the effects of solar ultraviolet radiation. Proponents of this theory predict an increase in skin cancers as a consequence of changes in the ozone layer. Other skin cancer risk factors follow:

- Fair-skinned, fair-haired, blue-eyed people, particularly those of Celtic origin, with insufficient skin pigmentation to protect underlying tissues
- People who sustain sunburn and who do not tan
- Long-time sun exposure (farmers, fishermen, construction workers)
- Exposure to chemical pollutants (industrial workers in arsenic, nitrates, coal, tar and pitch, oils and paraffins)
- Sun-damaged skin (elderly people)
- History of x-ray therapy for acne or benign lesions
- Scars from severe burns
- Chronic skin irritations
- Immunosuppression
- Genetic factors

FIGURE 56-6 Basal cell carcinoma (*left*) and squamous cell carcinoma (*right*). Reprinted by permission from *New England Journal of Medicine, 326,* 169–170, 1992.

BASAL CELL AND SQUAMOUS CELL CARCINOMA

The most common types of skin cancer are basal cell carcinoma (BCC) and squamous cell (epidermoid) carcinoma (SCC). The third most common type, malignant melanoma, is discussed separately. Skin cancer is diagnosed by biopsy and histologic evaluation.

Clinical Manifestations

BCC is the most common type of skin cancer. It generally appears on sun-exposed areas of the body and is more prevalent in regions where the population is subjected to intense and extensive exposure to the sun. The incidence is proportional to the age of the patient (average age of 60 years) and the total amount of sun exposure, and it is inversely proportional to the amount of melanin in the skin.

BCC usually begins as a small, waxy nodule with rolled, translucent, pearly borders; telangiectatic vessels may be present. As it grows, it undergoes central ulceration and sometimes crusting (Fig. 56-6). The tumours appear most frequently on the face. BCC is characterized by invasion and erosion of contiguous (adjoining) tissues. It rarely metastasizes, but recurrence is common. However, a neglected lesion can result in the loss of a nose, an ear, or a lip. Other variants of BCC may appear as shiny, flat, grey or yellowish plaques.

SCC is a malignant proliferation arising from the epidermis. Although it usually appears on sun-damaged skin, it may arise from normal skin or from preexisting skin lesions. It is of greater concern than BCC because it is a truly invasive carcinoma, metastasizing by the blood or lymphatic system.

Metastases account for 75% of deaths from SCC. The lesions may be primary, arising on the skin and mucous membranes, or

they may develop from a precancerous condition, such as actinic keratosis (ie, lesions occurring in sun-exposed areas), leukoplakia (ie, premalignant lesion of the mucous membrane), or scarred or ulcerated lesions. SCC appears as a rough, thickened, scaly tumour that may be asymptomatic or may involve bleeding (see Fig. 56-6). The border of an SCC lesion may be wider, more infiltrated, and more inflammatory than that of a BCC lesion. Secondary infection can occur. Exposed areas, especially of the upper extremities and of the face, lower lip, ears, nose, and forehead, are common sites (Odom et al., 2000).

Prognosis

The prognosis for BCC is usually good. Tumours remain localized, and although some require wide excision with resultant disfigurement, the risk for death from BCC is low. The prognosis for SCC depends on the incidence of metastases, which is related to the histologic type and the level or depth of invasion. Usually, tumours arising in sun-damaged areas are less invasive and rarely cause death, whereas SCC that arises without a history of sun or arsenic exposure or scar formation appears to have a greater chance for spread. Regional lymph nodes should be evaluated for metastases (Odom et al., 2000).

Medical Management

The goal of treatment is to eradicate the tumour. The treatment method depends on the tumour location; the cell type, location, and depth; the cosmetic desires of the patient; the history of previous treatment; whether the tumour is invasive, and whether metastatic nodes are present. The management of BCC and SCC includes surgical excision, Mohs' micrographic surgery, electrosurgery, cryosurgery, and radiation therapy.

SURGICAL MANAGEMENT

The primary goal is to remove the tumour entirely. The best way to maintain cosmetic appearance is to place the incision properly along natural skin tension lines and natural anatomic body lines. In this way, scars are less noticeable. The size of the incision depends on the tumour size and location but usually involves a length-to-width ratio of 3 : 1.

The adequacy of the surgical excision is verified by microscopic evaluation of sections of the specimen. When the tumour is large, reconstructive surgery with use of a skin flap or skin grafting may be required. The incision is closed in layers to enhance cosmetic effect. A pressure dressing applied over the wound provides support. Infection after a simple excision is uncommon if proper surgical asepsis is maintained.

Mohs' Micrographic Surgery. Mohs' micrographic surgery is the technique that is most accurate and that best conserves normal tissue. When the surgical technique was introduced, the excision followed an application of zinc chloride paste to the tumour, but Mohs' surgery is now performed without the initial chemosurgery component. The procedure removes the tumour layer by layer. The first layer excised includes all evident tumour and a small margin of normal-appearing tissue. The specimen is frozen and analyzed by section to determine if all the tumour has been removed. If not, additional layers of tissue are shaved and examined until all tissue margins are tumour free. In this manner, only the tumour and a safe, normal-tissue margin are removed. Mohs' surgery is the recommended tissue-sparing procedure, with cure rates for BCC and SCC approaching 99%. It is the treatment of choice and the most effective for tumours around the eyes, nose, upper lip, and auricular and periauricular areas (Odom et al., 2000).

Electrosurgery. Electrosurgery is the destruction or removal of tissue by electrical energy. The current is converted to heat, which then passes to the tissue from a cold electrode. Electrosurgery may be preceded by curettage (ie, excising the skin tumour by scraping its surface with a curette). Electrodesiccation is then implemented to achieve hemostasis and to destroy any viable malignant cells at the base of the wound or along its edges. Electrodesiccation is useful for lesions smaller than 1 to 2 cm in diameter.

This method takes advantage of the fact that the tumour in each instance is softer than surrounding skin and therefore can be outlined by a curette, which "feels" the extent of the tumour. The tumour is removed and the base cauterized. The process is repeated twice. Usually, healing occurs within a month.

Cryosurgery. Cryosurgery destroys the tumour by deep freezing the tissue. A thermocouple needle apparatus is inserted into the skin, and liquid nitrogen is directed to the centre of the tumour until the tumour base is −40°C to −60°C. Liquid nitrogen has the lowest boiling point of all cryogens tried, is inexpensive, and is easy to obtain. The tumour tissue is frozen, allowed to thaw, and then refrozen. The site thaws naturally and then becomes gelatinous and heals spontaneously. Swelling and edema follow the freezing. The appearance of the lesion varies. Normal healing, which may take 4 to 6 weeks, occurs faster in areas with a good blood supply.

RADIATION THERAPY

Radiation therapy is frequently performed for cancer of the eyelid, the tip of the nose, and areas in or near vital structures (eg, facial nerve). It is reserved for older patients, because x-ray changes may be seen after 5 to 10 years, and malignant changes in scars may be induced by irradiation 15 to 30 years later.

The patient should be informed that the skin may become red and blistered. A bland skin ointment prescribed by the physician may be applied to relieve discomfort. The patient should also be cautioned to avoid exposure to the sun.

Nursing Management

Because many skin cancers are removed by excision, patients are usually treated in outpatient surgical units. The role of the nurse is to teach the patient about prevention of skin cancer and about self-care after treatment (Chart 56-6).

PROMOTING HOME AND COMMUNITY-BASED CARE

Teaching Patients Self-Care. The wound is usually covered with a dressing to protect the site from physical trauma, external irritants, and contaminants. The patient is advised when to report for a dressing change or is given written and verbal information on how to change dressings, including the type of dressing to purchase, how to remove dressings and apply fresh ones, and the importance of hand washing before and after the procedure.

The patient is advised to watch for excessive bleeding and tight dressings that compromise circulation. If the lesion is in the perioral area, the patient is instructed to drink liquids through a straw and limit talking and facial movement. Dental work should be avoided until the area is completely healed.

After the sutures are removed, an emollient cream may be used to help reduce dryness. Applying a sunscreen over the wound is advised to prevent postoperative hyperpigmentation if the patient spends time outdoors.

Chart 56-6
Health Promotion: Preventing Skin Cancer

Because skin cancer rates are rising, taking preventive measures such as the ones outlined below may help individuals avoid increasing their skin cancer risk.

- Do not try to tan if your skin burns easily, never tans, or tans poorly.
- Avoid unnecessary exposure to the sun, especially during the time of day when ultraviolet radiation (sunlight) is most intense (10 AM to 3 PM).
- Avoid sunburn.
- Apply sunscreen before being in the sun; sunscreens block harmful sun rays.
- Use a sunscreen with an SPF of 15 or higher. Sunscreens are rated in strength from 4 (weakest) to 50 (strongest). The SPF indicates the solar protection factor, or how much longer you can stay in the sun before getting burned. Look for sunscreens that protect against both ultraviolet-A (UVA) and ultraviolet-B (UVB) light.
- Reapply water-resistant sunscreens after swimming, if heavily sweating, and every 2 to 3 hours during prolonged periods of sun exposure.
- Avoid oils. Applied before or during sun exposure, oils do not protect against sunlight or sun damage.
- Use a lip balm that contains a sunscreen with the highest SPF number.
- Wear protective clothing, such as a broad-brimmed hat and long sleeves.
- Remember that up to 50% of ultraviolet rays can penetrate loosely woven clothing.
- Remember that ultraviolet light can penetrate a cloud cover, and a sunburn can still occur.
- Do not use sun lamps for indoor tanning, and avoid commercial tanning booths. These rays are just as harmful.
- Teach children to avoid all but modest sun exposure and to use a sunscreen regularly for lifelong protection.

Follow-up examinations should be at regular intervals, usually every 3 months for a year, and should include palpation of the adjacent lymph nodes. The patient should also be instructed to seek treatment for any moles that are subject to repeated friction and irritation, and to watch for indications of potential malignancy in moles as described previously. The importance of lifelong follow-up evaluations should be emphasized.

Teaching About Prevention. Studies show that regular daily use of a sunscreen with a solar protection factor (SPF) of at least 15 can reduce the recurrence of skin cancer by as much as 40%. The sunscreen should be applied to head, neck, arms, and hands every morning at least 30 minutes before leaving the house and reapplied every 4 hours if the skin perspires. Discretionary application (ie, applied only when sun exposure is anticipated) has not shown the same preventive response (Barton, 2001).

MALIGNANT MELANOMA

A malignant melanoma is a cancerous neoplasm in which atypical melanocytes (ie, pigment cells) are present in the epidermis and the dermis (and sometimes the subcutaneous cells). It is the most lethal of all the skin cancers and is responsible for about 2% of all cancer deaths (Odom et al., 2000).

It can occur in one of several forms: superficial spreading melanoma, lentigo-maligna melanoma, nodular melanoma, and acral-lentiginous melanoma. These types have specific clinical and histologic features as well as different biologic behaviours. Most melanomas arise from cutaneous epidermal melanocytes, but some appear in preexisting nevi (ie, moles) in the skin or develop in the uveal tract of the eye. Melanomas occasionally appear simultaneously with cancer of other organs.

The worldwide incidence of melanoma doubles every 10 years, a rise that is probably related to increased recreational sun exposure and better methods of early detection. Peak incidence occurs between ages 20 and 45. The incidence of melanoma is increasing faster than that of almost any other cancer, and the mortality rate is increasing faster than that of any other cancer except lung cancer. The estimated number of new cases in 2005 is 4,400 and the number of deaths is 880 (Canadian Cancer Society, 2005).

Risk Factors

The cause of malignant melanoma is unknown, but ultraviolet rays are strongly suspected, based on indirect evidence such as the increased incidence of melanoma in countries near the equator and in people younger than age 30 who have used a tanning bed more than 10 times per year. In general, 1 in 100 Caucasians will get melanoma every year. Up to 10% of melanoma patients are members of melanoma-prone families who have multiple changing moles (ie, dysplastic nevi) that are susceptible to malignant transformation. Patients with dysplastic nevus syndrome have been found to have unusual moles, larger and more numerous moles, lesions with irregular outlines, and pigmentation located all over the skin. Microscopic examination of dysplastic moles shows disordered, faulty growth. Chart 56-7 lists risk factors for malignant melanoma.

Research has identified a gene that resides on chromosome 9p, the absence of which increases the likelihood that potentially mutagenic DNA damage will escape repair before cell division. The absence of this gene can be identified in melanoma-prone families (Piepkorn, 2000).

Chart 56-7
Risk Factors for Malignant Melanoma

- Fair-skinned or freckled, blue-eyed, light-haired people of Celtic or Scandinavian origin
- People who burn and do not tan or who have a significant history of severe sunburn
- Environmental exposure to intense sunlight
- History of melanoma (personal or family)
- Skin with giant congenital nevi

Clinical Manifestations

Superficial spreading melanoma occurs anywhere on the body and is the most common form of melanoma. It usually affects middle-aged people and occurs most frequently on the trunk and lower extremities. The lesion tends to be circular, with irregular outer portions. The margins of the lesion may be flat or elevated and palpable (Fig. 56-7). This type of melanoma may appear in a combination of colours, with hues of tan, brown, and black mixed with grey, blue-black, or white. Sometimes a dull pink rose colour can be seen in a small area within the lesion.

LENTIGO-MALIGNA MELANOMAS

Lentigo-maligna melanomas are slowly evolving, pigmented lesions that occur on exposed skin areas, especially the dorsum of the hand, the head, and the neck in elderly people. Often, the lesions are present for many years before they are examined by a physician. They first appear as tan, flat lesions, but in time, they undergo changes in size and colour.

NODULAR MELANOMA

Nodular melanoma is a spherical, blueberry-like nodule with a relatively smooth surface and a relatively uniform, blue-black colour (see Fig. 56-7). It may be dome shaped with a smooth surface. It may have other shadings of red, grey, or purple. Sometimes, nodular melanomas appear as irregularly shaped plaques. The patient may describe this as a blood blister that fails to resolve. A nodular melanoma invades directly into adjacent dermis (ie, vertical growth) and therefore has a poorer prognosis.

ACRAL-LENTIGINOUS MELANOMA

Acral-lentiginous melanoma occurs in areas not excessively exposed to sunlight and where hair follicles are absent. It is found on

FIGURE 56-7 Two forms of malignant melanoma: superficial spreading (*left*) and nodular (*right*). From Bickley, L. S., & Szilagyi, P. (2003). *Bates' guide to physical examination and history taking* (8th ed.). Philadelphia: Lippincott Williams & Wilkins.

the palms of the hands, on the soles, in the nail beds, and in the mucous membranes in dark-skinned people. These melanomas appear as irregular, pigmented macules that develop nodules. They may become invasive early.

Assessment and Diagnostic Findings

Biopsy results confirm the diagnosis of melanoma. An excisional biopsy specimen provides histologic information on the type, level of invasion, and thickness of the lesion. An excisional biopsy specimen that includes a 1-cm margin of normal tissue and a portion of underlying subcutaneous fatty tissue is sufficient for staging a melanoma in situ or an early, noninvasive melanoma. Incisional biopsy should be performed when the suspicious lesion is too large to be removed safely without extensive scarring. Biopsy specimens obtained by shaving, curettage, or needle aspiration are not considered reliable histologic proof of disease.

A thorough history and physical examination should include a meticulous skin examination and palpation of regional lymph nodes that drain the lesional area. Because melanoma occurs in families, a positive family history of melanoma is investigated so that first-degree relatives, who may be at high risk for melanoma, can be evaluated for atypical lesions. After the diagnosis of melanoma has been confirmed, a chest x-ray, complete blood cell count, liver function tests, and radionuclide or computed tomography scans are usually ordered to stage the extent of disease.

Prognosis

The prognosis for long-term (5-year) survival is considered poor when the lesion is more than 1.5 mm thick or there is regional lymph node involvement. A person with a thin lesion and no lymph node involvement has a 3% chance of developing metastases and a 95% chance of surviving 5 years. If regional lymph nodes are involved, there is a 20% to 50% chance of surviving 5 years. Patients with melanoma on the hand, foot, or scalp have a better prognosis; those with lesions on the torso have an increased chance of metastases to the bone, liver, lungs, spleen, and central nervous system. Men and elderly patients also have poor prognoses (Demis, 1998).

Medical Management

Treatment depends on the level of invasion and the depth of the lesion. Surgical excision is the treatment of choice for small, superficial lesions. Deeper lesions require wide local excision, after which skin grafting may be needed. Regional lymph node dissection is commonly performed to rule out metastasis, although new surgical approaches call for only sentinel node biopsy. This technique is used to sample the nodes nearest the tumour and spares the patient the long-term sequelae of extensive removal of lymph nodes if the sample node is negative (Wagner, 2000).

Immunotherapy has had varied success. Immunotherapy modifies immune function and other biologic responses to cancer. Several forms of immunotherapy (eg, bacillus Calmette-Guérin [BCG] vaccine, *Corynebacterium parvum,* levamisole) offer encouraging results. Some investigational therapies include biologic response modifiers (eg, interferon-alpha, interleukin-2), adaptive immunotherapy (ie, lymphokine-activated killer cells), and monoclonal antibodies directed at melanoma antigens. One of these, proleukin, shows promise in preventing recurrence of melanoma (Demis, 1998). Under investigation is the laboratory assay of tyrosinase, an enzyme believed to be produced only by melanoma cells (Demis, 1998). Several other studies are attempting to develop

autologous immunization against specific tumour cells. These studies are still in the early experimental stage but show promise of producing a vaccine against melanoma (Piepkorn, 2000).

Current treatments for metastatic melanoma are largely unsuccessful, with cure generally impossible. Further surgical intervention may be performed to debulk the tumour or to remove part of the organ involved (eg, lung, liver, or colon). The rationale for more extensive surgery, however, is for relief of symptoms, not for cure. Chemotherapy for metastatic melanoma may be used; however, only a few agents (eg, dacarbazine, nitrosoureas, cisplatin) have been effective in controlling the disease.

When the melanoma is located in an extremity, regional perfusion may be used; the chemotherapeutic agent is perfused directly into the area that contains the melanoma. This approach delivers a high concentration of cytotoxic agents while avoiding systemic, toxic side effects. The limb is perfused for 1 hour with high concentrations of the medication at temperatures of 39°C to 40°C with a perfusion pump. Inducing hyperthermia enhances the effect of the chemotherapy so that a smaller total dose can be used. It is hoped that regional perfusion can control the metastasis, especially if it is used in combination with surgical excision of the primary lesion and with regional lymph node dissection.

NURSING PROCESS: CARE OF THE PATIENT WITH MALIGNANT MELANOMA
Assessment

Assessment of the patient with malignant melanoma is based on the patient's history and symptoms. The patient is asked specifically about pruritus, tenderness, and pain, which are not features of a benign nevus. The patient is also questioned about changes in preexisting moles or the development of new, pigmented lesions. People at risk are assessed carefully.

A magnifying lens and good lighting are needed for inspecting the skin for irregularity and changes in the mole. Signs that suggest malignant changes are referred to as the ABCDEs of moles (Chart 56-8).

Common sites of melanomas are the skin of the back, the legs (especially in women), between the toes, and on the feet, face, scalp, fingernails, and backs of hands. In dark-skinned people, melanomas are most likely to occur in less pigmented sites: palms, soles, subungual areas, and mucous membranes. Satellite lesions (ie, those situated near the mole) are inspected.

Diagnosis
NURSING DIAGNOSES
Based on the nursing assessment data, the patient's major nursing diagnoses may include the following:

- Acute pain related to surgical excision and grafting
- Anxiety and depression related to possible life-threatening consequences of melanoma and disfigurement
- Deficient knowledge about early signs of melanoma

COLLABORATIVE PROBLEMS/ POTENTIAL COMPLICATIONS
Based on the assessment data, potential complications include the following:

- Metastasis
- Infection of the surgical site

Chart 56-8 • ASSESSMENT

The ABCDEs of Moles

A for Asymmetry
- The lesion does not appear balanced on both sides. If an imaginary line were drawn down the middle, the two halves would not look alike.
- The lesion has an irregular surface with uneven elevations (irregular topography) either palpable or visible. A change in the surface may be noted from smooth to scaly.
- Some nodular melanomas have a smooth surface.

B for Irregular Border
- Angular indentations or multiple notches appear in the border
- The border is fuzzy or indistinct, as if rubbed with an eraser.

C for Variegated Colour
- Normal moles are usually a uniform light to medium brown. Darker colouration indicates that the melanocytes have penetrated to a deeper layer of the dermis.
- Colours that may indicate malignancy if found together within a single lesion are shades of red, white, and blue; shades of blue are ominous.
- White areas within a pigmented lesion are suspicious.
- Some malignant melanomas, however, are not variegated but are uniformly coloured (bluish-black, bluish-grey, bluish-red).

D for Diameter
- A diameter exceeding 6 mm (about the size of a pencil eraser) is considered more suspicious, although this finding without other signs is not significant. Many benign skin growths are larger than 6 mm, whereas some early melanomas may be smaller.

E for Elevation (Bickley & Szilagyi, 2003) **or Evolving** (Skin Cancer Foundation, n.d.)
- The lesion is elevated (some melanomas are flat or slightly elevated).
- Mole is suddenly increasing in size.
- Additional colours may appear.
- Mole that was flat or slightly elevated shows rapid increase in height.
- Skin surrounding a mole is reddened.
- Surface of mole changes from smooth to scaly, crusting, oozing.
- Itching is the most common early symptom.

Planning and Goals

The major goals for the patient may include relief of pain and discomfort, reduced anxiety and depression, knowledge of early signs of melanoma, and absence of complications.

Nursing Interventions

RELIEVING PAIN AND DISCOMFORT

Surgical removal of melanoma in different locations (eg, head, neck, eye, trunk, abdomen, extremities, central nervous system) presents different challenges, taking into consideration the removal of the primary melanoma, the intervening lymphatic vessels, and the lymph nodes to which metastases may spread. Nursing management of the patient having surgery in these regions is discussed in the appropriate chapters.

Nursing intervention after surgery for a malignant melanoma centres on promoting comfort, because wide excision surgery may be necessary. A split-thickness or full-thickness skin graft may be necessary when large defects are created by surgical removal of a melanoma. Anticipating the need for and administering appropriate analgesic medications are important.

REDUCING ANXIETY AND DEPRESSION

Psychological support is essential when disfiguring surgery is performed. Support includes allowing patients to express feelings about the seriousness of this cutaneous neoplasm, understanding their anger and depression, and conveying understanding of these feelings. During the diagnostic workup and staging of the depth, type, and extent of the tumour, the nurse answers questions, clarifies information, and helps clarify misconceptions. Learning that they have a melanoma can cause patients considerable fear and anguish. Pointing out patients' resources, past effective coping mechanisms, and social support systems helps them to cope with the problems associated with diagnosis, treatment, and continuing follow-up. The patient's family should be included in all discussions to clarify the information presented, ask questions that the patient might be reluctant to ask, and provide emotional support.

MONITORING AND MANAGING POTENTIAL COMPLICATIONS

Metastasis

The prognosis for malignant melanoma is related to metastasis: the deeper and thicker (more than 4 mm) the melanoma, the greater is the likelihood of metastasis. If the melanoma is growing radially (ie, horizontally) and is characterized by peripheral growth with minimal or no dermal invasion, the prognosis is favourable. When the melanoma progresses to the vertical growth phase (ie, dermal invasion), the prognosis is poor. Lesions with ulceration have a poor prognosis. Melanomas of the trunk appear to have a poorer prognosis than those of other sites, perhaps because the network of lymphatics in the trunk permits metastasis to regional lymph nodes.

The role of the nurse in caring for the patient with metastatic disease is holistic. The nurse must be knowledgeable about the most effective current therapies and must deliver supportive care, provide and clarify information about the therapy and the rationale for its use, identify potential side effects of therapy and ways to manage them, and instruct the patient and family about the expected outcomes of treatment. The nurse monitors and documents symptoms that may indicate metastasis: lung (eg, difficulty breathing, shortness of breath, increasing cough), bone (eg, pain, decreased mobility and function, pathologic fractures), and liver (eg, change in liver enzyme levels, pain, jaundice). Nursing care is based on the patient's symptoms.

Although the chance of a cure for malignant melanoma that has metastasized is poor, the nurse encourages the patient to have hope in the therapy employed while maintaining a realistic perspective about the disease and ultimate outcome. Moreover, the nurse provides time for the patient to express fears and concerns regarding future activities and relationships, offers information about support groups and contact people, and arranges palliative and hospice care if appropriate (see Chap. 17).

PROMOTING HOME AND COMMUNITY-BASED CARE

Teaching Patients Self-Care

The best hope of controlling the disease lies in educating patients about the early signs of melanoma. According to the Canadian Dermatology Association's website (2005), "at least 50% of all malignant melanomas are discovered by skin self-examination." Patients at risk are taught to examine their skin and scalp monthly in a systematic manner (Chart 56-9). The nurse also points out that a key factor in the development of malignant melanoma is exposure to sunlight. Because melanoma is thought to be genetically linked, the family and the patient should be taught sun-avoiding measures.

Chart 56-9 • **PATIENT EDUCATION**
How to Examine Your Skin

Step 1
Make sure the room is well lighted, and that you have nearby a full-length mirror, a hand-held mirror, a hand-held blow dryer, and two chairs or stools. Undress completely.

Step 2
Hold your hands with the palms face up, as shown in the drawing. Look at your palms, fingers, spaces between the fingers, and forearms. Then turn your hands over and examine the backs of your hands, fingers, spaces between the fingers, fingernails and forearms.

Step 3
Now position yourself in front of the full-length mirror. Hold up your arms, bent at the elbows, with your palms facing you in the mirror, look at the backs of your forearms and elbows.

Step 4
Again using the full-length mirror, observe the entire front of your body. In turn, look at your face, neck, and arms. Turn your palms to face the mirror and look at your upper arms. Then look at your chest and abdomen; pubic area; thighs and lower legs.

Step 5
Still standing in front of the mirror, lift your arms over your head with the palms facing each other. Turn so that your right side is facing the mirror and look at the entire side of your body, your hands and arms, underarms, sides of your trunk, thighs and lower legs. Then turn, and repeat the process with your left side.

Step 6
With your back toward the full-length mirror, look at your buttocks and the backs of your thighs and lower legs.

Step 7
Now pick up the hand-held mirror. With your back still to the full-length mirror, examine the back of your neck, and your back and buttocks. Also examine the backs of your arms in this way. Some areas are hard to see, and you may find it helpful to ask your spouse or a friend to assist you.

Step 8
Use the hand-held mirror and the full-length mirror to look at your scalp. Because the scalp is difficult to examine, we suggest you also use a hand-held blow dryer turned to a cool setting, to lift the hair from the scalp. While some people find it easy to hold the mirror in one hand and the dryer in the other, while looking in the full-length mirror, many do not. For the scalp examination in particular, then, you might ask your spouse or a friend to assist you.

(continued)

Chart 56-9 • PATIENT EDUCATION
How to Examine Your Skin (Continued)

Step 9
Sit down and prop up one leg on a chair or stool in front of you as shown. Using the hand-held mirror, examine the inside of the propped-up leg, beginning at the groin area and moving the mirror down the leg to your foot. Repeat the procedure for your other leg.

Step 10
Still sitting, cross one leg over the other. Use the hand-held mirror to examine the top of your foot, the toes, toenails, and spaces between the toes. Then look at the sole or bottom of your foot. Repeat the procedure for the other foot.

Source: American Cancer Society, Inc., Atlanta, GA; 1-800-ACS-2345.

Evaluation

EXPECTED PATIENT OUTCOMES

Expected patient outcomes may include the following:

1. Experiences relief of pain and discomfort
   a. States pain is diminishing
   b. Exhibits healing of surgical scar without heat, redness, or swelling
2. Is less anxious
   a. Expresses fears and fantasies
   b. Asks questions about medical condition
   c. Requests repetition of facts about melanoma
   d. Identifies support and comfort provided by family member or significant other
3. Demonstrates understanding of the means for detecting and preventing melanoma
   a. Demonstrates how to conduct self-examination of skin on a monthly basis
   b. Verbalizes the following danger signals of melanoma: change in size, colour, shape, or outline of mole, mole surface, or skin around mole
   c. Identifies measures to protect self from exposure to sunlight
4. Experiences absence of complications
   a. Recognizes abnormal signs and symptoms that should be reported to physician
   b. Complies with recommended follow-up procedures and prevention strategies

METASTATIC SKIN TUMOURS

The skin is an important, although not a common, site of metastatic cancer. All types of cancer may metastasize to the skin, but carcinoma of the breast is the primary source of cutaneous metastases in women. Other sources include cancer of the large intestine, ovaries, and lungs. In men, the most common primary sites are the lungs, large intestine, oral cavity, kidneys, or stomach. Skin metastases from melanomas are found in both genders. The clinical appearance of metastatic skin lesions is not distinctive, except perhaps in some cases of breast cancer in which diffuse, brawny hardening of the skin of the involved breast is seen. In most instances, metastatic lesions occur as multiple cutaneous or subcutaneous nodules of various sizes that may be skin coloured or different shades of red.

Other Malignancies of the Skin

KAPOSI'S SARCOMA

First described by Moritz Kaposi in 1872, Kaposi's sarcoma (KS) has received renewed attention since its association with HIV infection and AIDS. Its occurrence with AIDS involves a more varied and aggressive form of KS than was seen previously. Before the AIDS epidemic, KS was considered a rare malignancy. It was subdivided into three categories: classic KS, African (endemic) KS, and KS associated with immunosuppressant therapy. Classic KS occurs predominantly in men of Mediterranean or Jewish ancestry between the ages of 40 and 70 years. Most patients have nodules or plaques on the lower extremities that rarely metastasize beyond the lower extremities. This KS is chronic, relatively benign, and rarely fatal.

African KS affects people predominantly in the eastern half of Africa near the equator. Men are affected more often than women, and children can be affected as well. The disease may resemble classic KS, or it may infiltrate and progress to lymphadenopathic forms.

KS associated with immunosuppressive therapy, as in transplant recipients, is characterized by local skin lesions and disseminated visceral and mucocutaneous diseases. The greater the degree of immunosuppression, the higher is the incidence of KS.

AIDS-related KS was identified in the early 1980s as distinctly different from previously described types of KS. Typically, it is an aggressive tumour that involves multiple body organs. Its presentation resembles that of KS associated with immunosuppressive therapy. Most patients are between the ages of 20 and 40 years (Odom et al., 2000). More information on this topic can be found in Chapter 52.

BASAL AND SQUAMOUS CELL CARCINOMAS IN THE IMMUNOCOMPROMISED POPULATION

The incidence of basal cell carcinoma and squamous cell carcinoma is increased in all immunocompromised individuals, including those infected with HIV. Clinically, the tumours have the same appearance as in non–HIV-infected people; however, in HIV patients, the tumours may grow more rapidly and recur more frequently. These tumours are managed the same as for the general population. Frequent follow-up (every 4 to 6 months) is recommended to monitor for recurrence.

Dermatologic and Plastic Reconstructive Surgery

The word *plastic* comes from a Greek word meaning *to form*. Plastic or reconstructive surgery is performed to reconstruct or alter congenital or acquired defects to restore or improve the body's form and function. Often, the terms plastic and reconstructive are used interchangeably. This type of surgery includes closure of wounds, removal of skin tumours, repair of soft tissue injuries or burns, correction of deformities, and repair of cosmetic defects. Plastic surgery can be used to repair many parts of the body and numerous structures, such as bone, cartilage, fat, fascia, mucous membrane, muscle, nerve, and cutaneous structures. Bone inlays and transplants for deformities and nonunion can be performed, muscle can be transferred, nerves can be reconstructed and spliced, and cartilage can be replaced. As important as any of these measures is the reconstruction of the cutaneous tissues around the neck and the face; this is usually referred to as aesthetic or cosmetic surgery.

WOUND COVERAGE: GRAFTS AND FLAPS

Various surgical techniques, including skin grafts and flaps, are used to cover skin wounds.

Skin Grafts

Skin grafting is a technique in which a section of skin is detached from its own blood supply and transferred as free tissue to a distant (recipient) site. Skin grafting can be used to repair almost any type of wound and is the most common form of reconstructive surgery.

Skin grafts are commonly used to repair defects that result from excision of skin tumours, to cover areas denuded of skin (e.g., burns), and to cover wounds in which insufficient skin is available to permit wound closure. They are also used when primary closure of the wound increases the risk for complications or when primary wound closure would interfere with function.

Skin grafts may be classified as autografts, allografts, or xenografts. An autograft is tissue obtained from the patient's own skin. An allograft is tissue obtained from a donor of the same species. These grafts are also called allogeneic or homograft. A xenograft or heterograft is tissue from another species.

Grafts are also referred to by their thickness. A skin graft may be a split-thickness (ie, thin, intermediate, or thick) or full-thickness graft, depending on the amount of dermis included in the specimen. A split-thickness graft can be cut at various thicknesses and is commonly used to cover large wounds or defects for which a full-thickness graft or flap is impractical (Fig. 56-8). A full-thickness graft consists of epidermis and the entire dermis without the underlying fat. It is used to cover wounds that are too large to be closed directly.

DONOR SITE

The donor site is selected with several criteria in mind:

- Achieving the closest possible colour match
- Matching the texture and hair-bearing qualities
- Obtaining the thickest possible skin graft without jeopardizing the healing of the donor site (Fig. 56-9)
- Considering the cosmetic effects of the donor site after healing, so that it is in an inconspicuous location

FIGURE 56-8 Layers of skin appropriate for split-thickness and full-thickness graft.

■ Split-thickness grafts

■ Full-thickness grafts

■ Fat-dermal grafts

FIGURE 56-9 Common donor skin graft sites. Blue skin areas are appropriate for full-thickness grafts; green areas are used for split-thickness grafts; rose sites are used for fat-dermal grafts.

DONOR SITE CARE

Detailed attention to the donor site is just as important as the care of the recipient area. The donor site heals by re-epithelization of the raw, exposed dermis. Usually, a single layer of nonadherent, fine-mesh gauze is placed directly over the donor site. Absorbent gauze dressings are then placed on top to absorb blood or serum from the wound. A membrane dressing (eg, Op-Site) may be used and provides certain advantages. It is transparent and allows the wound to be observed without disturbing the dressing, and it permits the patient to shower without fear of saturating the dressing with water.

After healing, the patient is instructed to keep the donor site soft and pliable with cream (eg, lanolin, olive oil). Extremes in temperature, external trauma, and sunlight are to be avoided for donor sites and grafted areas because these areas are sensitive, especially to thermal injuries.

GRAFT APPLICATION

A graft is obtained by a variety of instruments: razor blades, skin-grafting knives, electric- or air-powered dermatomes, or drum dermatomes. The skin graft is taken from the donor or host site and applied to the desired site, called the recipient site or graft bed.

For a graft to survive and be effective, certain conditions must be met:

- The recipient site must have an adequate blood supply so that normal physiologic function can resume.
- The graft must be in close contact with its bed to avoid accumulation of blood or fluid.
- The graft must be fixed firmly (immobilized) so that it remains in place on the recipient site.
- The area must be free of infection.

The graft, when applied to the recipient site, may be sutured in place. It may be slit and spread apart to cover a greater area. The process of revascularization (ie, establishing the blood supply) and reattachment of a skin graft to a recipient bed is referred to as a "take." After a skin graft is put in place, it may be left exposed (in areas that are impossible to immobilize) or covered with a light dressing or a pressure dressing, depending on the area.

Nursing Interventions

The nurse instructs the patient to keep the affected part immobilized as much as possible. For a facial graft, strenuous activity must be avoided. A graft on the hand or arm may be immobilized with a splint. When a graft is placed on a lower extremity, the part is kept elevated because the new capillary connections are fragile and excess venous pressure may cause rupture. When ambulation is permitted, the patient wears an elastic stocking to counterbalance venous pressure.

The nurse instructs the patient, family member, or other caregiver to inspect the dressing daily. Unusual drainage or an inflammatory reaction around the wound margin suggests infection and should be reported to the physician. Any fluid, purulent drainage, blood, or serum that has collected is gently evacuated by the surgeon, because accumulation of this material would cause the graft to separate from its bed.

When the graft appears pink, it is vascularized. After 2 to 3 weeks, mineral oil or a lanolin cream is massaged into the wound to moisten the graft. Because there may be loss of feeling or sensation in the grafted area for a prolonged period, the application of heating pads and exposure to sun are avoided to prevent burns and further skin trauma.

Flaps

Another form of wound coverage is provided by flaps. A flap is a segment of tissue that remains attached at one end (ie, a base or pedicle) while the other end is moved to a recipient area. Its survival depends on functioning arterial and venous blood supplies and lymphatic drainage in its pedicle or base. A flap differs from a graft in that a portion of the tissue is attached to its original site and retains its blood supply. An exception is the free flap, which is described later.

Flaps may consist of skin, mucosa, muscle, adipose tissue, omentum, and bone. They are used for wound coverage and provide bulk, especially when bone, tendon, blood vessels, or nerve tissue is exposed. Flaps are used to repair defects caused by congenital deformity, trauma, or tumour ablation (ie, removal, usually by excision) in an adjacent part of the body.

Flaps offer an aesthetic solution because a flap retains the colour and texture of the donor area, is more likely to survive than a graft, and can be used to cover nerves, tendons, and blood vessels. However, several surgical procedures are usually required to advance a flap. The major complication is necrosis of the pedicle or base as a result of failure of the blood supply.

Free Flaps

A striking advance in reconstructive surgery is the use of free flaps or free-tissue transfer achieved by microvascular techniques. A free flap is completely severed from the body and transferred to another site. A free flap receives early vascular supply from microvascular anastomosis (ie, attachment) with vessels at the recipient site. The procedure usually is completed in one step, eliminating the need for a series of surgical procedures to move the flap. Microvascular surgery allows surgeons to use a variety of donor sites for tissue reconstruction.

CHEMICAL FACE PEELING

Chemical face peeling, a technique that involves applying a chemical mixture to the face for superficial destruction of the epidermis and the upper layers of the dermis, treats fine wrinkles, keratoses, and pigment problems. It is especially useful for wrinkles at the upper and lower lip, forehead, and periorbital areas.

Pretreatment may consist of cleansing the face and hair for several days before the procedure with a hexachlorophene detergent. Pretreatment medication (ie, analgesic and tranquilizer for moderate sedation) may be prescribed to alleviate apprehension and control pain. This permits the patient to be sedated but conscious during the procedure, although some patients request general anesthesia.

The type of chemical used depends on the planned depth of the peel. A phenol-based chemical in an oil–water emulsion is commonly used because it produces a controlled, predictable chemical burn. The chemical is applied systematically to the face with cotton-tipped applicators. The conscious patient feels a burning sensation at this time. A mask of waterproof adhesive may then be applied directly to the skin and molded closely to the contours of the face, thereby acting as an occlusive dressing that increases the chemical penetration and action. Some surgeons believe that equally good results can be obtained with occlusive tape. After the tape mask is applied, the burning sensation continues, and the tape mask remains in place for 12 to 24 hours. Frequent small doses of analgesics and tranquilizers are prescribed to keep the patient comfortable.

Complications

Complications may arise when control of the chemically induced burn cannot be sustained. Complications include pigment changes, infection, milia (ie, small inclusion cysts that disappear after several months), scarring, atrophy, sensitivity changes, and long-term (4 to 5 months) erythema or pruritus.

Management

Because chemical face peeling is performed in the physician's office or in an outpatient surgical department, most care takes place in the home. After 6 to 8 hours, the face becomes edematous and the eyelids usually swell shut. The patient should be reassured that this reaction is expected and normal. The patient is cautioned to move the mouth as little as possible so that the tape continues to adhere to the skin. The head of the bed is elevated, and liquids are administered through a straw. Most of the burning sensation and discomfort subside after the first 12 to 24 hours.

By the second day, the patient may feel moisture under the dressings as serous exudate seeps from the chemically exfoliated skin. Dressings are usually removed 24 to 48 hours after treatment, exposing skin resembling a second-degree burn. The patient may be alarmed by the appearance of the skin and should be reassured. After the tape mask is removed, some surgeons dust the treated skin surface with thymol-iodine powder for its drying and bacteriostatic effects. Application of triple-antibiotic ointment may be substituted in some cases. The skin surface is left uncovered to dry. The patient may be permitted to wash the face with lukewarm water or advised to shower several times daily to help remove any remaining facial crusting. An ointment is prescribed to cover the face and soften and loosen the crust between washings.

The nurse reinforces the physician's explanation that the redness of the skin will gradually subside over the next 4 to 12 weeks. Although a line between treated and untreated skin may be seen, makeup is usually permitted after the first few weeks. The patient is cautioned to avoid exposure to direct or reflected sunlight, because the treatment reduces the natural protection of the skin from sun. The skin will probably never tan evenly again. Blotchy pigmentation can occur with exposure to the sun.

DERMABRASION

Dermabrasion is a form of skin abrasion used to correct acne scarring, aging, and sun-damaged skin. A special instrument (ie, motor-driven wire brush, diamond-impregnated disk, or serrated wheel) is used in the procedure. The epidermis and some superficial dermis are removed, while enough of the dermis is preserved to allow re-epithelization of the treated areas. Results are best in the face because it is rich in intradermal epithelial elements.

Preparation and Procedure

The primary reason for undergoing dermabrasion is to improve appearance. The surgeon explains to the patient what can be expected from dermabrasion. The patient should also be informed about the nature of the postoperative dressing, what discomfort may be experienced, and how long it will be before the tissues look normal.

Dermabrasion may be performed in the physician's office, the operating room, or an outpatient setting. It is performed under local or general anesthesia. During the procedure, some surgeons use refrigerant anesthetics to turn the skin into a numb, solid mass of rigid tissue and to provide a momentarily bloodless surgical field. During and after planing, the area is irrigated with copious amounts of saline solution to remove debris and allow the surgeon to see the area. A dressing impregnated with ointment is usually applied to the abraded surface.

Management

The nurse instructs the patient about postoperative effects. Edema occurs during the first 48 hours and may cause the eyelids to close. The head of the bed is elevated to hasten fluid drainage. Erythema occurs and can last for weeks or months. After 24 hours, the dressing may be removed if the physician approves. When the serum oozing from the skin begins to gel, the patient applies the prescribed ointment to the face several times each day to prevent hard crusting and to keep the abraded areas soft and flexible. With the physician's approval, clear-water cleansing or soaking of the face is started to remove crusts from the healing skin.

The patient is advised to avoid extreme cold and heat and excessive straining or lifting, which may bruise delicate new capillaries. Direct or reflected sunlight should be avoided for 3 to 6 months and a sunscreen used.

FACIAL RECONSTRUCTIVE SURGERY

Reconstructive procedures on the face are individualized to the patient's needs and desired outcomes. They are performed to repair deformities or restore normal function as much as possible. They may vary from closure of small defects to complicated procedures involving implantation of prosthetic devices to conceal a large defect or reconstruct a lost part of the face (eg, nose, ear, jaw). Each surgical procedure is customized and involves a variety of incisions, flaps, and grafts.

In correcting a primary defect, the surgeon may have to create a secondary defect. Although the procedure may restore some function, such as eating or talking, the cosmetic or aesthetic results may be limited. The original appearance of a patient who has severe damage to soft tissue and bone structure can seldom be restored. Multiple surgical procedures may be required. The process of facial reconstruction is usually slow and tedious.

NURSING PROCESS: CARE OF THE PATIENT WITH FACIAL RECONSTRUCTION

Assessment

The face is a part of the body that every person desires to keep at its best or improve, because most human interactions involve the face. When the face loses its appearance and function by injury or disease, significant emotional reactions often occur. Changes in appearance frequently cause anxiety and depression. Patients with facial changes frequently mourn for the lost part, suffer a loss of self-esteem because of reactions or rejection by others, and withdraw and isolate themselves. Health care personnel can acknowledge that anxiety and depression are appropriate for what the patient is experiencing.

The nurse assesses the patient's emotional responses and identifies strengths as well as usual coping mechanisms to determine how the patient will handle the surgical procedure. Any area in which the patient and family need extra support is identified.

The preoperative assessment determines the extent of disfigurement and improvement that can be anticipated, as well as the patient's understanding and acceptance of these limitations. The nurse is in a better position to reinforce facts and clarify misconceptions after the surgeon has fully informed the patient about the procedure, the functional defects that may result, the possible need for a tracheostomy or other prosthesis, and the probability of additional surgery. The nurse instructs the patient about various postoperative measures: intravenous therapy, the use of a nasogastric tube to allow gastric decompression and prevent vomiting, and the frequent and lengthy periods that may be required to care for wounds, flaps, and skin grafts and to change dressings. Extra time is needed when presenting this information to anxious patients because they may not hear, concentrate, or comprehend what is being said.

Diagnosis

NURSING DIAGNOSES

Based on the nursing assessment data, the patient's major postoperative nursing diagnoses may include the following:

- Ineffective airway clearance related to tracheobronchial secretions
- Acute pain related to facial edema and effects of the procedure
- Imbalanced nutrition: less than body requirements related to altered physiology of oral cavity, drooling, impaired chewing and swallowing, or excision affecting the tongue
- Impaired verbal communication related to trauma or surgery producing anatomic and physiologic abnormalities of speech
- Disturbed body image related to disfigurement

- Interrupted family processes related to grief reaction and disruption of family life

COLLABORATIVE PROBLEMS/ POTENTIAL COMPLICATIONS

Based on the assessment data, potential complications that may develop include.

- Infection

Planning and Goals

The major goals for the patient may include a patent airway and adequate pulmonary function, increased comfort, adequate nutritional status, an effective communication method, positive self-concept, effective family coping, and absence of infection.

Nursing Interventions

MAINTAINING AIRWAY AND PULMONARY FUNCTION

The immediate concern after facial reconstruction is maintenance of an adequate airway. If the patient has regained consciousness, mental confusion with combative, anxious behaviour is a sign of hypoxia (ie, reduced oxygen supply to tissues). Sedatives or opioids are not prescribed in this situation because they may impair oxygenation. If the patient shows signs of restlessness, the airway is carefully inspected to detect laryngeal edema or accumulation of tracheobronchial mucus. Secretions are suctioned as necessary until the patient can manage the secretions without help. If the patient has a tracheostomy, suctioning is performed with sterile technique to prevent infection and cross-contamination. Chapter 25 provides information on care of the patient with a tracheostomy.

RELIEVING PAIN AND ACHIEVING COMFORT

Facial edema is an uncomfortable but natural consequence of facial reconstructive surgery. The patient's head and upper torso are kept slightly elevated (if the blood pressure is stable) to help reduce facial edema. Catheters attached to closed drainage may be in place to keep the tissue in close apposition and to remove serous discharge. If extensive reconstruction has been performed, the patient's head should be properly aligned and supported so that minimal stress is placed on the suture line.

Analgesics are prescribed to relieve pain. If bone grafts have been used for reconstruction, there is usually considerable pain in the donor area. If the patient has head and neck cancer and increasing levels of pain, comprehensive nursing management is required (see Chap. 13).

MAINTAINING ADEQUATE NUTRITION

Fluids may be offered to the patient after oral and pharyngeal edema diminish, the incisional areas and flaps heal, and the patient can swallow saliva. Gradually, soft foods are added as tolerated. If the patient cannot meet nutritional needs by the oral route, parenteral nutrition (ie, infusion of nutrients, water, and vitamins into the stomach or proximal small intestine through a tube) is initiated. The formula strength and feeding rate are gradually increased until the desired daily caloric level is attained. Chapter 36 provides information about nursing management of the patient requiring enteral feedings. Patients who have had radical surgery for large, encroaching neoplasms may have difficulty resuming eating. Positive nutrition is reflected in weight gain, and nutritional status is monitored by measuring body weight daily and assessing serum protein and electrolyte levels periodically.

ENHANCING COMMUNICATION

Communication problems may range from minimal difficulty to the loss of oral speech. Some tumours and injuries require extensive surgery involving the larynx, tongue, and mandible. Paper, pen or pencil, and a firm writing surface should be provided. If the patient cannot write, a pictograph board may be used. Referral to a speech therapist may be necessary for the patient who has undergone structural changes. The family may become frustrated by the patient's inability to communicate. The patient soon senses this, and both parties may withdraw. Allowing the family to vent their feelings and fears (away from the patient) is important.

IMPROVING SELF-CONCEPT

Success in rehabilitating the patient undergoing reconstructive surgery depends on the relationships among the patient and the nurse, the physician, and other health care personnel. Mutual trust, respect, and clear lines of communication are essential. Unhurried care provides emotional reassurance and support.

The kinds of dressings worn, the unusual positions to be maintained, and the temporary incapacity experienced can upset the most stable person. Reinforcement of the patient's successful coping strategies improves self-esteem. If prosthetic devices are used, the patient is taught how to use and care for them to gain a sense of greater independence. Once involved in self-care activities, the patient may feel some control over what was previously an overwhelming situation.

Patients with severe disfigurement are encouraged to socialize to experience the reactions of others in a more protected environment. Gradually, they can widen their sphere of contact. Every effort is made to cover or mask defects. Patients may require support by members of the mental health team to accept their changed appearance.

PROMOTING FAMILY COPING

The family is informed about the patient's appearance after surgery, the supportive equipment, and the ways that the equipment aids recovery. It is helpful to join the family for a few minutes during their first postoperative visit to help them cope with the changes they will see.

A major role of the nurse is to support the family in their decision to participate (or not to participate) in the patient's treatment. Nursing interventions also include helping the family members communicate by suggesting ways to reduce anxiety and stress and to promote problem solving and decision making. These activities encourage family members and promote growth.

MONITORING AND MANAGING POTENTIAL COMPLICATIONS

Infection

Secondary infection is a primary concern after reconstructive surgery. The source of infection depends on the location and extent of the procedure, the suture line, and the pedicle flap.

The mouth is inspected to determine the location of sutures (when present) so that they are not accidentally disturbed during the cleaning process. The mouth is cleaned according to protocol several times daily. Loose blood clots may be removed with gentle swabbing. The patient is advised not to loosen clots with the tongue because this may cause fresh bleeding. The patient is instructed not to use fingers to clean or remove blood clots because this may introduce organisms that cause infection.

The suture line remains under stress for several days after surgery because of edema, increased drainage, and hematoma formation. The nurse assesses the suture line carefully for signs of increased tension and infection (ie, elevated temperature, increasing edema, redness, bleeding, and increased pain) with each dressing change. Dressings may need to be changed many times each day until the drainage begins to decrease. Drainage and edema are expected after reconstructive surgery; however, both should decrease, and the process is hastened by using properly placed, functioning suction devices and elevating the head of the bed about 45 degrees. The nurse inspects the suction devices, empties them promptly, and documents the amount and consistency of drainage, as well as any unusual odour. When drainage is not removed or if saturated dressings are left unchanged for long periods, infection is likely to occur. Strict asepsis must be maintained in wound care.

A pedicle flap used in reconstruction may become a source of infection if its circulation becomes compromised. Poor circulation may result from a hematoma forming beneath the flap and causing increased pressure on the underlying vasculature. The nurse inspects the flap for changes in colour and temperature indicative of poor circulation. Signs of necrosis, increased drainage, or an odour may be a warning of an infection and should be reported promptly. Reinforcing preoperative teaching about wound healing, the need for strict sterile technique, good personal hygiene, and the need to restrict movement and stress on the operative site is an important part of the nurse's role in postoperative care and in the prevention of secondary infection.

Evaluation

EXPECTED PATIENT OUTCOMES

Expected patient outcomes may include the following:

1. Maintains patent airway
   a. Demonstrates respiratory rate within normal limits
   b. Exhibits normal breath sounds
   c. Demonstrates no signs of choking or aspiration
2. Achieves increasing comfort
   a. Reports decreasing pain
   b. Follows instructions on proper positioning
   c. Avoids movements that stress the operative site
3. Attains adequate nutrition
   a. Consumes adequate amounts of food and fluids
   b. Maintains weight within normal range or progressively regains weight lost in the early postoperative period
   c. Maintains serum protein and electrolyte levels within normal range
4. Communicates effectively
   a. Uses appropriate aids to enhance communication
   b. Interacts with health care team members, family, and other support people using new communication strategies
5. Develops positive self-image
   a. Expresses positive feelings about surgical changes
   b. Demonstrates increasing independence in self-care activities
   c. Uses prosthetic devices independently (when appropriate)
   d. Verbalizes plans for resuming usual activities (eg, work, recreation)
6. Family members cope with situation
   a. Demonstrate decreasing anxiety and conflict
   b. Verbalize what to expect
7. Absence of complications
   a. Demonstrates vital signs within normal limits
   b. Undergoes normal wound healing without signs of infection or sepsis

c. Lists signs of infection that should be reported
d. Understands the need for asepsis (ie, sterile procedures) and good personal hygiene

FACE LIFT

Rhytidectomy (ie, face lift) is a surgical procedure that removes soft tissue folds and minimizes cutaneous wrinkles on the face. It is performed to create a more youthful appearance.

Psychological preparation requires that the patient recognize the limitations of surgery and the fact that miraculous rejuvenation will not occur. The patient is informed that the face may appear bruised and swollen after the dressings are removed and that several weeks may pass before the edema subsides.

The procedure is performed under local or general anesthesia, often in the outpatient setting. The incisions are concealed in natural skin folds and creases and areas hidden by hair. The loose skin, separated from underlying muscle, is pulled upward and backward. Excess skin that overlaps the incision line is removed. Liposuction-assisted rhytidectomy is being performed more frequently. In this procedure, fat is suctioned from the body through a cannula inserted through a small incision.

Management

The nurse encourages the patient to rest quietly for the first 2 postoperative days until the dressings are removed. The head of the bed is elevated, and neck flexion is discouraged to avoid compromising the circulation and the suture line. The patient may feel some tightness of the face and neck from pressure created by the newly tightened muscles, fascia, and skin. Analgesics may be prescribed to relieve discomfort. A liquid diet may be given by means of straws, and a soft diet is permitted if chewing is not too uncomfortable.

When the dressings are removed, the skin is gently cleaned of crusting and oozing and coated with the prescribed topical ointment. Any hair matted with drainage may be combed with warm water and a wide-toothed comb.

The patient is advised not to lift or bend for 7 to 10 days because this activity may increase edema and provoke bleeding. Activities are gradually resumed. When all sutures are removed, the hair may be shampooed and blown dry with warm, not hot, air to avoid burning the ears, which may be numb for a while.

The patient needs to know that a face lift will not stop the aging process and that, with time, the tissues will resume the downward drift. Some patients have two or more face lifts.

Sudden pain indicates that blood is accumulating underneath the skin flaps; it should be reported to the surgeon immediately. Complications include sloughing of the skin, deformities of the face and neck, and partial facial paralysis. Cigarette smoking has been implicated as a cause of skin slough in some patients.

Laser Treatment of Cutaneous Lesions

Lasers are devices that amplify or generate highly specialized light energy. They can mobilize immense heat and power when focused at close range and are valuable tools in surgical procedures. The argon laser, carbon dioxide (CO_2) laser, and tunable pulse-dye laser are used in dermatologic surgery. Each type of laser emits its own wavelength within the colour spectrum.

ARGON LASER

The argon laser produces a visible blue-green light that is absorbed by vascular tissue and is therefore useful in treating vascular lesions: port-wine stains, telangiectases, vascular tumours, and pigmented lesions. The argon beam can penetrate approximately 1 mm of skin and reach the pigmented layer, causing protein coagulation in this area. An immediate effect is that tiny blood vessels under the skin coagulate, causing the area to turn a much lighter colour. A crust forms within a few days.

During the procedure, the patient may require local anesthesia (lidocaine) but only if the lesion, such as a port-wine stain, is wider than 0.5 cm. Laser beams, regardless of type, are reflected and scattered in all directions during the treatment. Laser radiation is hazardous to the eye, and the eyes of the patient and all personnel involved in the surgical procedure and those who are within the immediate surgical environment must be protected with orange, argon light–absorbing safety goggles.

Management

Cold compresses are usually applied over the treatment area for approximately 6 hours to minimize edema, exudate, and loss of capillary permeability. The nurse advises the patient that swelling will subside in 1 to 2 days and will be followed by a crust that will last 7 to 10 days. The nurse instructs the patient to avoid picking at the crust, to apply an antibacterial ointment sparingly until the crust separates, to avoid applying makeup until the wound heals, and to avoid exposure to the sun. Sunscreen is to be used when exposure is unavoidable.

CARBON DIOXIDE LASER

The CO_2 laser emits invisible light in the infrared spectrum that is absorbed at the skin surface because of the high water content of the skin and the long wavelength of the CO_2 light. As the laser beam strikes tissue, it is absorbed by the intracellular and extracellular water, which vaporizes, destroying the tissue. The CO_2 laser is a precise surgical instrument that vaporizes and excises tissue with minimal damage. Because the beam can seal blood and lymphatic vessels, it creates a dry surgical field that makes many procedures easier and quicker. It is therefore safe to use on patients with bleeding disorders or those receiving anticoagulant therapy. It is useful for removing epidermal nevi, tattoos, certain warts, skin cancer, ingrown toenails, and keloids. Incisions made with the laser beam heal and scar much like those made by a scalpel.

In addition to wearing safety goggles, the patient and personnel wear laser-grade surgical masks to avoid inhaling the byproduct smoke, referred to as a plume.

Management

Immediately after undergoing CO_2 laser surgery, the treated area turns a charcoal colour. The wound is covered with antibacterial ointment and a nonadhesive dressing. The patient is instructed to keep the wound dry except for gentle cleansing with mild soap several times each day. After the skin is cleaned, a prescribed ointment and light dressing are applied.

Because nerve endings and lymphatic vessels are sealed by the laser, less edema and pain follow the laser procedure than follow conventional surgery. A mild analgesic is sufficient to maintain patient comfort. Wound healing occurs by secondary intention, with granulation tissue appearing within a week; complete healing occurs in several weeks. Sun exposure to the area should be avoided for approximately 6 months. Application of a sunscreen with an SPF value of at least 15 is recommended. People at high risk for skin cancer from sun exposure are advised to use a sunscreen with an SPF greater than 15 to block ultraviolet-B and ultraviolet-A light.

PULSE-DYE LASER

The tunable pulse-dye laser with various wavelengths is the latest laser available for dermatologic surgery. It is especially useful in treating cutaneous vascular lesions such as port-wine stains and telangiectasia. Eye protection used for the argon and CO_2 lasers is insufficient when the pulse-dye laser is in use. Special eyeglasses, such as those made of didymium glass, are required for the patient and all personnel. The procedure is generally painless. For procedures requiring anesthesia, lidocaine without epinephrine is sufficient because local vasoconstriction (which epinephrine induces) is unnecessary.

Management

The patient should be informed that there may be stinging in the treated area for several hours. Applying ice to the area and a light antibacterial ointment followed by a nonstick dressing (eg, Telfa) usually eases discomfort.

NURSING ALERT Telfa pads contain latex and should not be used on patients who are latex sensitive. Other dressings such as petrolatum-impregnated gauze should be used to prevent the dressing from adhering to the wound.

If crusting occurs, the patient is advised to wash the area gently with soap and water and reapply the antibacterial cream twice daily until the crust disappears. The nurse also advises the patient to avoid wearing makeup until all crust is removed. Sun exposure should be avoided as well; sunscreens with an SPF value of 15 or greater should be used for 3 to 4 months after the treatment. Complete removal of the lesion at one session, especially a port-wine stain, is rare. The patient should be informed that several treatments may be necessary.

Critical Thinking Exercises

1. A patient is admitted with generalized psoriasis in an acute flare. About 70% of his skin is involved. What type of treatment will you be expected to administer? What nursing interventions would you anticipate in caring for this man? Explain the physiologic basis for these interventions.

2. You are caring for an elderly man who has had surgery. He is a regular resident of a long-term care facility. When giving him a bath, you find two ulcerations on his buttocks. What are some of the considerations in taking care of this man? What will help prevent further breakdown of the skin?

Which dressings may be appropriate for his wounds? What other hospital resources can you consult in making a care plan for this patient?

3. A middle-aged woman is admitted to same-day surgery for a wide excision of a melanoma on her back. She is very anxious about the cause of this cancer and about her prognosis. What issues would you address in helping her diminish her anxiety? What should she be told about sun exposure? What should she tell her children about their risk for melanoma?

REFERENCES AND SELECTED READINGS

American Cancer Society. (2002). *Cancer facts and figures.* Atlanta, GA: (Author)

Barton, S. (Ed.). (2001) *Clinical evidence* (5th ed.). London: BJM Publishing.

Bickley, L. S., & Szilagyi, P. (2003). *Bates' guide to physical examination and history taking* (8th ed.). Philadelphia: Lippincott Williams & Wilkins.

Canadian Cancer Society. (2005). *Canadian cancer statistics 2005.* Ottawa, ON: Author.

Champion, R. H., Burton, J. L., Burns, D. A., & Breathnach, S. M. (1998). *Rook/Wilkinson/Ebling textbook of dermatology* (6th ed.). Boston: Blackwell Science.

Demis, D. J. (Ed.). (1998). *Clinical dermatology.* Philadelphia: Lippincott-Raven.

Fitzpatrick, T. B., et al. (1997). *Color atlas & synopsis of clinical dermatology* (3rd ed.). New York: McGraw-Hill.

Freedberg, I. M., Eisen, A. Z., Austen, K. F., Goldsmith, S. I., Katz, S., & Fitzpatrick, T. B. (1999). *Fitzpatrick's dermatology in general medicine* (5th ed.). New York: McGraw-Hill.

Hall, J. (Ed.). (2000). *Sauer's manual of skin diseases* (8th ed.). Philadelphia: Lippincott Williams & Wilkins.

Krastner, D. L., Rodeheaver, G. O., & Sibbald, R. G. (2002). *Chronic wound care: A clinical source book for healthcare professionals* (3rd ed.). Wayne, PA: HMP Communications.

Murphy, J. L. (Ed.) (2002). *Nurse practitioners' prescribing reference.* New York: Prescribing Reference.

Odom, R. B., James, W. D., & Berger, T. G. (Eds.). (2000). *Andrews' diseases of the skin* (9th ed.). Philadelphia: W. B. Saunders.

Skin Cancer Foundation. (n.d.). *What to look for: The ABCD's of moles and melanoma.* Available at: http://www.skincancer.org/self_exam/look_for.php. Retrieved June 15, 2005.

Journals

Aly, R., Forney, R., & Bayles, C. (2001). Treatments for common superficial fungal infections. *Dermatology Nursing, 2,* 91–101.

Bryant, R. A., & Rolstad, B. S. (2001). Examining threats to skin integrity. *Ostomy Wound Management, 47*(6), 18–27.

Choucair, M. M., & Fivenson, D. P. (2001). Leg ulcer diagnosis and management. *Dermatologic Clinics, 19*(4), 52–56.

Crissey, J. T. (1998). Common dermatophyte infections: A simple diagnostic test and current management. *Postgraduate Medicine, 103*(2), 191–205.

Crutchfield, C. E. (1998). The causes and treatment of pseudofolliculitis barbae. *Cutis, 61*(6), 351–356.

Fleischer, A. B., Feldman, S. R., & Rapp, S. R. (2000). The magnitude of skin disease in the United States. *Dermatologic Clinics, 18*(2), 76–81.

Goolsby, M. J. (1998). The elusive itch: Assessment, diagnosis, and management of pruritus. *Advance for Nurse Practitioners, 6,* 61–64.

Gritter, M. (1998). The latex threat. *American Journal of Nursing, 98*(9), 26–33.

Halder, R. M. (2000). New and emerging therapies for vitiligo. *Dermatologic Clinics, 18*(1), 79–89, ix.

Harrigan, E. (1999). Atopic dermatitis. *Immunology and Allergy Clinics of North America, 19*(2), 383–396.

Hilton, D. C., Williams, L. C., & Nesbitt, L. T. (2000). Systemic glucocorticosteroid therapy in dermatology. *Dermatology Nursing, 12*(4), 258–263.

Joe, E. K., Li, V. W., Magro, C. M., Arndt, K. A., & Bowers, K. E. (1999). Diagnostic clues to dermatitis artefacta. *Cutis, 63*(4), 209–214.

Koo, J. Y., Lowe, N. J., Lew-Kaya, D. A., Vasilopoulos, A. L., Lue, J. C., Sefton, J., & Gibson, J. R. (2000). Tazarotene plus UV-B phototherapy in the treatment of psoriasis. *Journal of the American Academy of Dermatology, 43*(5 Pt. 1), 821–828.

Kunimoto, B. (2001). Management and prevention of venous leg ulcers: A literature-guided approach. *Ostomy Wound Management, 47*(2), 36–46, 48–50.

Landi, G., & Landi, C. (2001). The sentinel node biopsy in melanoma patients. *Dermatology Nursing, 13*(6), 429–434.

Lebwohl, M. (2000). Advances in psoriasis therapy. *Dermatologic Clinics, 18*(1), 62–66.

Lee, S. W., Li, H., Strong, T. V., et al. (2000). Development of a polynucleotide vaccine from melanoma antigen recognized by T cells-1 and recombinant protein from melanoma antigen recognized by T cells-1 for melanoma vaccine clinical trials. *Journal of Immunotherapy, 23*, 379–386.

Levin, N., & Greer, K. E. (2000). Cutaneous manifestations of endocrine disorders. *Dermatology Nursing, 13*(3), 185–195.

Leung, D. Y. (2000). Atopic dermatitis: New insights and opportunities for therapeutic intervention. *Journal of Allergy and Clinical Immunology, 105*, 860–876.

Lim, H. W., et al. (2001). American Academy of Dermatology Consensus Conference on UVA Protection of Sunscreens: Summary and recommendations. *Journal of American Academy of Dermatology, 44*(3), 505–508.

McCowan, C. B. (1998). Systemic lupus erythematosus. *Journal of the American Academy of Nurse Practitioners, 10*(5), 225–231.

Mercurio, M. G. (1998). Managing the patient with hirsutism. *Hospital Medicine, 34*(9), 45–51.

Mutasim, D. F. (2002). Bullous diseases in the elderly. *Clinics in Geriatric Medicine, 18*(1), 43–58.

Nall, L., Gulliver, W., Charmley, P., & Farber, E. M. (1999). Search for the psoriasis susceptibility gene: The Newfoundland Study. *Cutis, 64*(5), 323–330.

Nilsson, T. N., Klang, B., & Berg, M. (1999). Patient education for adults with chronic eczema. *Dermatology Nursing, 11*(2), 117–122.

Noble, S. L., Forbes, R. C., & Stamm, P. L. (1998). Diagnosis and management of common tinea infections. *American Family Physician, 58*(1), 163–178.

Paquette, D., & Falanga, V. (2002). Geriatric dermatology. Part II. Leg ulcers. *Clinics in Geriatric Medicine, 18*(1), 154–162.

Piepkorn, M. (2000). Melanoma genetics: An update with focus on the CDKN2A(p16)/ARF tumor suppressors. *Journal of the American Academy of Dermatology, 43*(2), 705–722.

Pullen, R. L. (2001). Managing subacute cutaneous lupus erythematosus. *Dermatology Nursing, 13*(6), 419–426.

Raza, A., Rutledge, F., & Bayles, C. (2001). Treatments for common superficial fungal infections. *Dermatology Nursing, 2*, 91–100.

Robinson, J. K. (2000). Early detection and treatment of melanoma: Update 2000. *Dermatology Nursing, 12*(6), 397–402.

Rodgers, P. (2001). Treating onychomycosis. *American Family Physician, 63*(4), 663–672.

Romero, P., & Alster T. (2001). Skin rejuvenation with cool touch 1320 nm Nd:YAG laser: The nurse's role. *Dermatology Nursing, 13*(2), 122–127.

Rousseau, R. F., Hirschmann-Jax, C., Takahashi, S., & Brenner, M. K. (2001). Cancer vaccines. *Hematology/Oncology Clinics of North America, 15*(4), 741–773.

Rutter, A., & Luger, T. A. (2001). Clinical review: High dose intravenous immunoglobulins. *Journal of the American Academy of Dermatology, 44*(6), 213–219.

Shaw, J. C. (2001). Hormonal therapy in dermatology. *Dermatologic Clinics, 19*(1), 169–178.

Shelk, J., & Morgan, P. (2000). Narrow band UVB: A practical approach. *Dermatology Nursing, 12*(6), 407–411.

Shindl, A., & Neumann, R. (1999). Low-intensity laser therapy is an effective treatment for recurrent herpes simplex infections. *Journal of Investigative Dermatology, 113*(2), 221–223.

Talarico, L. D. (1998). Aging skin: Best approaches to common problems. *Patient Care Nurse Practitioner, 1*(5), 28–40.

Valencia, I. C., Falabella, A., Dirsner, R. S., & Eaglestein, W. H. (2001). Chronic venous insufficiency and venous leg ulcers. *Journal of the American Academy of Dermatology, 44*(3), 401–421.

Wachsmuth, R. C. (1998). The atypical mole syndrome and predisposition to melanoma. *New England Journal of Medicine, 339*(5), 348–349.

Wagner, J. D. (2000). Sentinel lymph node biopsy for melanoma: Experience with 234 consecutive procedures. *Plastic Reconstruction Surgery, 105*(6), 1956–1966.

Williams, L. C. (2001). Update on systemic glucocorticosteroids in dermatology. *Dermatologic Clinics, 19*(1), 63–77.

Wolkenstein, P. (2000). Toxic epidermal necrolysis. *Dermatologic Clinics, 18*(3), 485–495.

Wolkenstein, P. E., Roujeau, J. C., & Revuz, J. (1998). Drug-induced toxic epidermal necrolysis. *Clinical Dermatology, 16*(3), 399–408.

RESOURCES AND WEBSITES

Canadian Alopecia Areata Association, Box 42084, RPO Millbourne, Edmonton, AB T6K 4C4; (780) 454-2326; http://www.kumc.edu/gec/support/alopecia.html.

Canadian Cancer Society/Société canadienne du cancer, National Office, Suite 200, 10 Alcorn Avenue, Toronto, ON M4V 3B1; (416) 961-7223; fax: (416) 961-4189; http://www.cancer.ca.

Canadian Dermatology Association, 1385 Bank Street, Suite 425, Ottawa, ON K1H 8N4; (613) 738-1748 or 1-800-267-3376; fax: (613) 738-4695; e-mail: cda@dermatology.ca; http://www.dermatology.ca.

Canadian Directory of Genetic Support Groups, Support Group Directory, Regional Medical Genetics Centre, Children's Hospital of Western Ontario, 800 Commissioner's Road East, London, ON N6C 2V5; (519) 685-8453; (in Ontario only) 1-800-243-8416; fax: (519) 685-8214; e-mail: Database Administrator; www.lhsc.on.ca/programs/medgenet.

Canadian Genetic Disease Network, Suite 201, 2150 Western Parkway, Vancouver, BC V6T 1V6; (604) 221-7300; fax: (604) 221-0778; e-mail: info@cgdn.ca; http://www.cgdn.ca.

Canadian Organization for Rare Disorders (CORD), PO Box 814, Coaldale, AB T1M 1M7; (403) 345-4544; toll-free: 1-877-302-7273; fax: (403) 345-3948; http://www.cord.ca.

Dermatology online atlas, a cooperation between the Department of Clinical Social Medicine (University of Heidelberg) and the Department of Dermatology (University of Erlangen); http://www.dermis.net.

Eczema Society of Canada, 24 Park Road, Whitby, ON L1M 1G7; (905) 655-9232, 1-866-432-0362; http://www.eczemacanada.ca.

Foundation for Ichthyosis & Related Skin Types, 650 N. Cannon Avenue, Suite 17, Lansdale, PA 19446; 215-631-1411; http://www.scalyskin.org.

GeneTests, 9725 Third Avenue NE, Suite 602, Seattle, WA 98115; (206) 616-4033; fax: (206) 221-4679; e-mail: genetests@genetests.org; http://www.genetests.org.

Genetic Alliance, 4301 Connecticut Avenue NW, Suite 404, Washington, DC 20008-2369; (202) 966-5557; fax: (202) 966-8553; e-mail: info@geneticalliance.org; http://www.geneticalliance.org.

Health Canada, AL 0900C2, Ottawa, ON K1A 0K9; (866) 225-0709; http://www.healthcanada.ca.

Lupus Canada, 590 Alden Road, Suite 211, Markham, ON L3R 8N2; 1-800-661-1468; http://www.lupuscanada.org.

National Organization for Albinism and Hypopigmentation, PO Box 959, East Hampstead, NH 03826-0959; 1-800-473-2310; http://www.albinism.org.

National Vitiligo Foundation, 611 South Fleishel Ave., Tyler, TX 75701; 903-531-0074; http://www.nvfi.org.

New Zealand Dermatology Society; http://www.dermnetnz.org.

OMIM Online Mendelian Inheritance in Man; http://www.ncbi.nlm.nih.gov/entrez/query.fcgi?db=OMIM.

Psoriasis Society of Canada, National Office, PO Box 25015, Halifax, NS B3M 4H4; 1-800-656-4494; http://www.psoriasissociety.org.

Rosacea Awareness Program, 368 Notre Dame Street West, Montreal, QC H2Y 1T9; 1-888-767-2232; http://www.about-rosacea.com; http://www.rosacea.org.

The Canadian Association of Wound Care; PO Box 85557, 1048 Eglinton Avenue West, Toronto, ON M6C 4A8; (877) 288-7018; http://www.cawc.net.

The Genetics Society of Canada; http://life.biology.mcmaster.ca/GSC.

The Skin Cancer Foundation, 245 5th Avenue, Suite 1403, New York, NY 10016; 1-800-SKIN-490; fax: 212-725-5751; e-mail: info@skincancer.org; http://www.skincancer.org.

Management of Patients With Burn Injury

Adapted by F. Margaret Milner

On completion of this chapter, the learner will be able to:

1. Discuss the classification system used for burn injuries.
2. Describe the local and systemic effects of a major burn injury.
3. Describe the three phases of burn care and the priorities of care for each phase.
4. Compare and contrast the potential fluid and electrolyte alterations of the emergent/resuscitative and acute phases of burn management.
5. Describe the goals of the following aspects of burn wound care and the nurse's role in each: wound cleaning, topical antibacterial therapy, wound dressing, dressing changes, wound débridement, and wound grafting
6. Describe the nurse's role in the following areas of management: pain management, restrictions of activity and joint motion, psychological support of the patient and family, nutritional support, pulmonary care, and patient and family education.
7. Use the nursing process as a framework for care of the patient during the three phases of burn care.

*T*he nurse who cares for a patient with a burn injury requires a high level of knowledge about the physiologic changes that occur after a burn, as well as astute assessment skills to detect subtle changes in the patient's condition. In addition, the nurse must be able to provide sensitive, compassionate care to patients who are critically ill and must initiate rehabilitation early in the course of care. The nurse must also be able to communicate effectively with burn patients, distraught family members, and members of the entire interdisciplinary burn management team. This will ensure quality care, which increases the likelihood of the patient's survival and promotes optimal quality of life.

Incidence of Burn Injury

The incidence of burn injuries has been declining during the past several decades. Approximately 2 million people require medical attention for burn injury in the United States each year (Kao & Garner, 2000). Of this group, 51,000 require acute hospital admission. About 4,500 people die from burns and related inhalation injuries annually (American Burn Association, 2000). The risk of death increases significantly if the patient has sustained both a cutaneous burn injury and a smoke inhalation injury.

Young children and elderly people are at particularly high risk for burn injury. The skin in people in these two age groups is thin and fragile; therefore, even a limited period of contact with a source of heat can create a full-thickness burn. The National Center for Injury Prevention and Control lists "fire/burn" among the categories of the 1998 Unintentional Injuries and Adverse Effects. Chart 57-1 presents the ranking of "fire/burn" as cause of death by age group.

Most burn injuries occur in the home, usually in the kitchen while cooking and in the bathroom by means of scalds or improper use of electrical appliances around water sources (Gordon & Goodwin, 1997). Careless cooking is one of the leading causes of household fires in the United States. The U.S. Fire Administration reports that nearly one third of all residential fires begin in the kitchen. The major factors contributing to cooking fires include unattended cooking, grease, and combustible materials on the stovetop.

Burns can also occur from work-related injuries. Education to prevent burn injuries in the workplace should include safe handling of chemicals and chemical products and increasing awareness of the potential for injuries caused by hot objects and substances. The National Institute for Burn Medicine, which collects statistical data from burn centres throughout the United States, notes that most patients (75%) are victims of their own actions. Contributing to the statistics are scalds in toddlers, school-age children playing with matches, electrical injury in teenage boys, and smoking in adults combined with the use of drugs and alcohol. One of the major culprits of burn injuries is the inappropriate use of gasoline. The U.S. Home Product Report, 1993–1997 (2000), indicated that there were over 140,000 gasoline-related fires and approximately 500 people died from gasoline-related injuries during this period.

Many burns can be prevented. Nurses can play an active role in preventing fires and burns by teaching prevention concepts and promoting legislation related to fire safety (Chart 57-2). Promoting the use of smoke alarms has had the greatest impact on decreasing fire deaths in the United States.

There are four major goals relating to burns:

1. Prevention
2. Institution of lifesaving measures for the severely burned person

Chart 57-1	**Ranking of "Fire/Burn" as Cause of Death by Age Group**
Age	Rank
1–4	3
5–9	3
10–14	3
15–24	7
25–34	6
35–44	5
45–54	5
55–64	6
65–85+	6
All ages, all races, both sexes	7

Unintentional Injuries and Adverse Effects, from the National Center for Injury Prevention and Control, 1998.

Glossary

Alloderm: processed dermis from human cadaver skin; can be used as dermal layer for skin grafts

autograft: a graft derived from one part of a patient's body and used on another part of that same patient's body

Biobrane: synthetic dressing composed of a nylon, Silastic membrane combined with a collagen derivative

carboxyhemoglobin: a compound of carbon monoxide and hemoglobin, formed in the blood with exposure to carbon monoxide

collagen: a protein present in skin, tendon, bone, cartilage, and connective tissue

contracture: shrinkage of burn scar through collagen maturation

cultured epithelial autografts (CEA): autologous epidermal cells that proliferate in culture and then are grafted onto the patient

dermis: the second layer of skin containing sweat glands, hair follicles, and nerves

débridement: removal of foreign material and devitalized tissue until surrounding healthy tissue is exposed

donor site: the area from which skin is taken to provide a skin graft for another part of the body

epidermis: the outermost layer of skin

eschar: devitalized tissue resulting from a burn

escharotomy: a linear excision made through eschar to release constriction of underlying tissue

excision: surgical removal of tissue

fasciotomy: an incision made through the fascia to release constriction of underlying muscle

heterograft: graft obtained from an animal of a species (ie, pigskin) other than that of the recipient; also called a xenograft

homograft: a graft transferred from one human (living or cadaveric) to another human; also called allograft

hydrotherapy: cleansing of wounds through use of bath, shower, shower cart table, or immersion

hypertrophic scar: excessive scar formation that rises above the level of the skin

Integra: synthetic dermal substitute

rule of nines: method for calculating body surface area burned by dividing the body into multiples of nine

Chart 57-2

Burn Prevention Tips

- Keep matches and lighters out of the reach of children.
- Never leave children unattended around fire or in bathroom/bathtub.
- Install and maintain smoke detectors in the home.
- Develop and practice a home exit fire drill with all members of the household.
- Set the water heater temperature no higher than 48.9°C.
- Do not smoke in bed. Do not fall asleep while smoking.
- Do not throw flammable liquids onto an already burning fire.
- Do not use flammable liquids to start fires.
- Do not remove radiator cap from a hot engine.
- Watch for overhead electrical wires and underground wires when working outside.
- Never store flammable liquids near a fire source, such as a pilot light.
- Use caution when cooking.
- Keep a working fire extinguisher in your home.

3. Prevention of disability and disfigurement through early, specialized, individualized treatment
4. Rehabilitation through reconstructive surgery and rehabilitative programs

Outlook for Survival and Recovery

Great strides in research have helped to increase the survival rate of burn victims. Mortality has fallen to levels never thought possible. Hunt et al. (2000) reported that survival following large burns based on total body surface area (TBSA) appears to have leveled off. Persons older than 70 years are surviving burns of 30% TBSA; those 60 to 70 years of age, 50% TBSA; those 20 to 30 years of age, 80% TBSA; and those 2 to 5 years of age, 75% TBSA. Research in areas such as fluid resuscitation, emergent burn treatment, inhalation injury treatment, and changes in wound care practice with early **débridement** and **excision** have contributed greatly to the decrease in burn deaths. Additionally, a better understanding of the importance of adequate nutritional support has contributed to increased survival rates. Very young and very old people have a high risk of death after burn injuries due to immature and stressed immunologic systems and pre-existing medical conditions, respectively. Chances of survival are greater in children older than age 5 and in adults younger than age 40. Inhalation injuries in combination with cutaneous burns worsen the prognosis. Outcome depends on the depth and extent of the burn as well as on the pre-injury health status and age of the patient. Acute care of patients with burn injuries has improved to the point at which survival is expected for most patients, and the burn team has shifted its focus to long-term outcomes for these patients.

 ### Gerontologic Considerations

Reduced mobility, changes in vision and cognitive function, and decreased sensation in the feet and hands place elderly people at higher risk for burn injury; scalds and flames are the leading causes. These changes also place older people at risk for suffering a severe burn because they have difficulty in extinguishing the fire and removing themselves from the burn source.

Morbidity and mortality rates associated with burns are usually greater in elderly patients than in younger patients. Thinning

and loss of elasticity of the skin in the elderly predispose them to a deep injury from a thermal insult that might cause a less severe burn in a younger person. Moreover, chronic illnesses decrease the older person's ability to withstand the multisystem stresses imposed by burn injury.

An important goal of nurses in community and home settings is preventing burn injury, especially among the elderly. Nurses need to assess an elderly patient's ability to perform activities of daily living safely, assist elderly patients and families to modify the environment to ensure safety, and make referrals as needed.

Pathophysiology of Burns

Burns are caused by a transfer of energy from a heat source to the body. Heat may be transferred through conduction or electromagnetic radiation. Burns are categorized as thermal (which includes electrical burns), radiation, or chemical. Tissue destruction results from coagulation, protein denaturation, or ionization of cellular contents. The skin and the mucosa of the upper airways are the sites of tissue destruction. Deep tissues, including the viscera, can be damaged by electrical burns or through prolonged contact with a heat source. Disruption of the skin can lead to increased fluid loss, infection, hypothermia, scarring, compromised immunity, and changes in function, appearance, and body image.

The depth of the injury depends on the temperature of the burning agent and the duration of contact with the agent. For example, in the case of scald burns in adults, 1 second of contact with hot tap water at 68.9°C may result in a burn that destroys both the **epidermis** and the **dermis**, causing a full-thickness (third-degree) injury. Fifteen seconds of exposure to hot water at 56.1°C results in a similar full-thickness injury. Temperatures less than 43.9°C are tolerated for long periods without injury.

CLASSIFICATION OF BURNS

Burn injuries are described according to the depth of the injury and the extent of body surface area injured.

Burn Depth

Burns are classified according to the depth of tissue destruction as superficial partial-thickness injuries, deep partial-thickness injuries, or full-thickness injuries. Burn depth determines whether epithelialization will occur. Determining burn depth can be difficult even for the experienced burn care provider. See Chapter 56 for discussion and a diagram of the skin layers; see also Table 57-1. (The categories of superficial partial-thickness, deep partial-thickness, and full-thickness burns are similar to, but not the same as, first-, second-, and third-degree burns.)

In a superficial partial-thickness burn, the epidermis is destroyed or injured and a portion of the dermis may be injured. The damaged skin may be painful and appear red and dry, as in sunburn, or it may blister.

A deep partial-thickness burn involves destruction of the epidermis and upper layers of the dermis and injury to deeper portions of the dermis. The wound is painful, appears red, and exudes fluid. Capillary refill follows tissue blanching. Hair follicles and other dermal appendages remain intact. Deep partial-thickness burns take longer to heal and are more likely to result in hypertrophic scars.

A full-thickness burn involves total destruction of epidermis and dermis and, in some cases, underlying tissue as well. Wound colour ranges widely from white to red, brown, or black. The burned area

Table 57-1 • Characteristics of Burns According to Depth

DEPTH OF BURN AND CAUSES	SKIN INVOLVEMENT	SYMPTOMS	WOUND APPEARANCE	RECUPERATIVE COURSE
Superficial Partial-Thickness (Similar to First Degree)				
Sunburn Low-intensity flash	Epidermis; possibly a portion of dermis	Tingling Hyperesthesia (supersensitivity) Pain that is soothed by cooling	Reddened; blanches with pressure; dry Minimal or no edema Possible blisters	Complete recovery within a week; no scarring Peeling
Deep Partial-Thickness (Similar to Second Degree)				
Scalds Flash flame	Epidermis, upper dermis, portion of deeper dermis	Pain Hyperesthesia Sensitive to cold air	Blistered, mottled red base; broken epidermis; weeping surface Edema	Recovery in 2 to 4 weeks Some scarring and depigmentation contractures Infection may convert it to full thickness
Full-Thickness (Similar to Third Degree)				
Flame Prolonged exposure to hot liquids Electric current Chemical	Epidermis, entire dermis, and sometimes subcutaneous tissue; may involve connective tissue, muscle, and bone	Pain free Shock Hematuria (blood in the urine) and possibly hemolysis (blood cell destruction) Possible entrance and exit wounds (electrical burn)	Dry; pale white, leathery, or charred Broken skin with fat exposed Edema	Eschar sloughs Grafting necessary Scarring and loss of contour and function; contractures Loss of digits or extremity possible

is painless because nerve fibres are destroyed. The wound appears leathery; hair follicles and sweat glands are destroyed (Fig. 57-1).

The following factors are considered in determining the depth of the burn:

- How the injury occurred
- Causative agent, such as flame or scalding liquid
- Temperature of the burning agent
- Duration of contact with the agent
- Thickness of the skin

Extent of Body Surface Area Injured

Various methods are used to estimate the TBSA affected by burns; among them are the rule of nines, the Lund and Browder method, and the palm method.

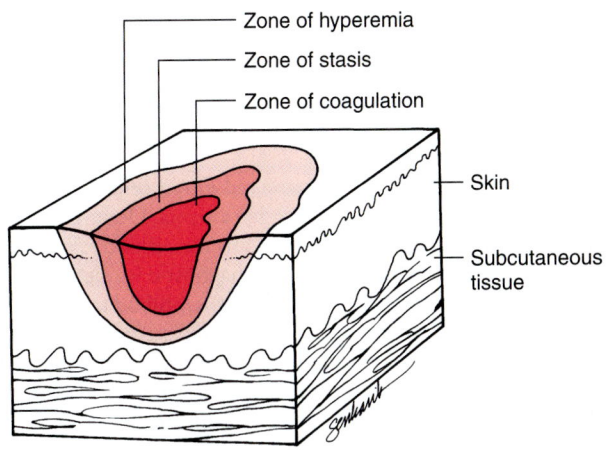

FIGURE 57-1 Zones of burn injury. Each burned area has three zones of injury. The inner zone (known as the area of coagulation, where cellular death occurs) sustains the most damage. The middle area, or zone of stasis, has a compromised blood supply, inflammation, and tissue injury. The outer zone—the zone of hyperemia—sustains the least damage.

Labels in figure: Zone of hyperemia; Zone of stasis; Zone of coagulation; Skin; Subcutaneous tissue

RULE OF NINES

An estimation of the TBSA involved in a burn is simplified by using the **rule of nines** (Fig. 57-2). The rule of nines is a quick way to calculate the extent of burns. The system assigns percentages in multiples of nine to major body surfaces.

LUND AND BROWDER METHOD

A more precise method of estimating the extent of a burn is the Lund and Browder method, which recognizes that the percentage of TBSA of various anatomic parts, especially the head and legs, and changes with growth. By dividing the body into very small areas and providing an estimate of the proportion of TBSA accounted for by such body parts, one can obtain a reliable estimate of the TBSA burned. The initial evaluation is made on the patient's arrival at the hospital and is revised on the second and third post-burn days because the demarcation usually is not clear until then.

PALM METHOD

In patients with scattered burns, a method to estimate the percentage of burn is the palm method. The size of the patient's palm is approximately 1% of TBSA.

LOCAL AND SYSTEMIC RESPONSES TO BURNS

Burns that do not exceed 25% TBSA produce a primarily local response. Burns that exceed 25% TBSA may produce both a local and a systemic response and are considered major burn injuries. This systemic response is due to the release of cytokines and other mediators into the systemic circulation. The release of local mediators and changes in blood flow, tissue edema, and infection can cause progression of the burn injury.

Pathophysiologic changes resulting from major burns during the initial burn-shock period include tissue hypoperfusion and organ hypofunction secondary to decreased cardiac output, followed by a hyperdynamic and hypermetabolic phase. The incidence, magnitude, and duration of pathophysiologic changes in

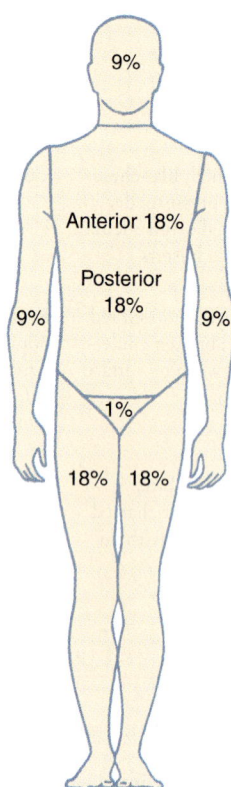

FIGURE 57-2 The rule of nines: Estimated percentage of total body surface area (TBSA) in the adult is arrived at by sectioning the body surface into areas with a numerical value related to nine. (Note: The anterior and posterior head total 9% of TBSA.) In burn victims, the total estimated percentage of TBSA injured is used to calculate the patient's fluid replacement needs.

burns are proportional to the extent of burn injury, with a maximal response seen in burns covering 60% or more TBSA.

The initial systemic event after a major burn injury is hemodynamic instability, resulting from loss of capillary integrity and a subsequent shift of fluid, sodium, and protein from the intravascular space into the interstitial spaces. Figure 57-3 illustrates the pathophysiologic processes in acute major burns. Hemodynamic instability involves cardiovascular, fluid and electrolyte, blood volume, pulmonary, and other mechanisms.

Cardiovascular Response

Hypovolemia is the immediate consequence of fluid loss resulting in decreased perfusion and oxygen delivery. Cardiac output decreases before any significant change in blood volume is evident. As fluid loss continues and vascular volume decreases, cardiac output continues to fall and blood pressure drops. This is the onset of burn shock. In response, the sympathetic nervous system releases catecholamines, resulting in an increase in peripheral resistance (vasoconstriction) and an increase in pulse rate. Peripheral vasoconstriction further decreases cardiac output. Myocardial contractility may be suppressed by the release of inflammatory cytokine necrosis factor (Wolf, Prough & Herndon, 2002).

Prompt fluid resuscitation maintains the blood pressure in the low-normal range and improves cardiac output. Despite adequate fluid resuscitation, cardiac filling pressures (central venous pressure, pulmonary artery pressure, and pulmonary artery wedge pres-

sure) remain low during the burn-shock period. If inadequate fluid resuscitation occurs, distributive shock will occur (see Chap. 15).

Generally, the greatest volume of fluid leak occurs in the first 24 to 36 hours after the burn, peaking by 6 to 8 hours. As the capillaries begin to regain their integrity, burn shock resolves and fluid returns to the vascular compartment. As fluid is reabsorbed from the interstitial tissue into the vascular compartment, blood volume increases. If renal and cardiac function is adequate, urinary output increases. Diuresis continues for several days to 2 weeks.

Burn Edema

Local swelling due to thermal injury is often extensive. Edema is defined as the presence of excessive fluid in the tissue spaces (Lund, 1999). As previously noted, in burns involving less than 25% TBSA, the loss of capillary integrity and shift of fluid are localized to the burn itself, resulting in blister formation and edema only in the area of injury. Patients with more severe burns develop massive systemic edema. Edema is usually maximal after 24 hours. It begins to resolve 1 to 2 days post-burn and usually is completely resolved in 7 to 10 days post-injury. Edema in burn wounds can be reduced by avoiding excessive fluid during the early post-burn period. Unnecessary over-resuscitation will increase edema formation in both burn tissue and non-burn tissue.

As edema increases in circumferential burns, pressure on small blood vessels and nerves in the distal extremities causes an obstruction of blood flow and consequent ischemia. This complication is known as compartment syndrome. The physician may need to perform an **escharotomy**, a surgical incision into the **eschar** (devitalized tissue resulting from a burn), to relieve the constricting effect of the burned tissue.

Effects on Fluids, Electrolytes, and Blood Volume

Circulating blood volume decreases dramatically during burn shock. In addition, evaporative fluid loss through the burn wound may reach 3 to 5 L or more over a 24-hour period until the burn surfaces are covered.

During burn shock, serum sodium levels vary in response to fluid resuscitation. Usually hyponatremia (sodium depletion) is present. Hyponatremia is also common during the first week of the acute phase, as water shifts from the interstitial to the vascular space.

Immediately after burn injury, hyperkalemia (excessive potassium) results from massive cell destruction. Hypokalemia (potassium depletion) may occur later with fluid shifts and inadequate potassium replacement.

At the time of burn injury, some red blood cells may be destroyed and others damaged, resulting in anemia. Despite this, the hematocrit may be elevated due to plasma loss. Blood loss during surgical procedures, wound care, and diagnostic studies and ongoing hemolysis further contribute to anemia. Blood transfusions are required periodically to maintain adequate hemoglobin levels for oxygen delivery. Abnormalities in coagulation, including a decrease in platelets (thrombocytopenia) and prolonged clotting and prothrombin times, also occur with burn injury.

Pulmonary Response

Inhalation injury is the leading cause of death in fire victims. It is estimated that half of these deaths could have been prevented with use of a smoke detector. Often, burn victims make it out of

Physiology/Pathophysiology

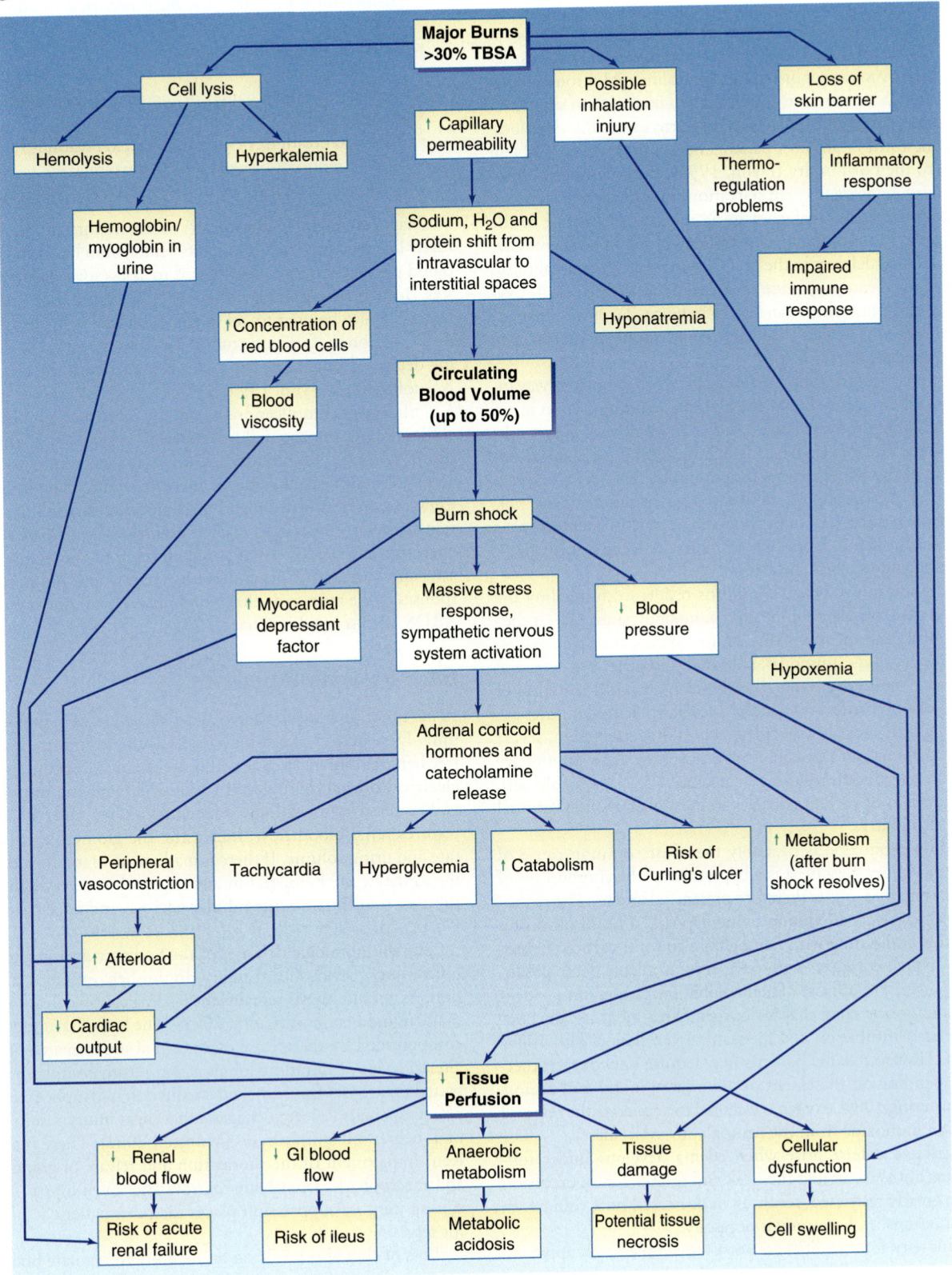

FIGURE 57-3 Overview of physiologic changes that occur after major burn.

a burning home safely. However, once they are outside, they may realize that their loved ones, pets, or valuable items are still inside the burning home. They then re-enter the burning home and are overcome with toxic smoke and fumes and become disoriented or unconscious.

Inhalation injury has a significant impact on survivability of a burn patient. Deterioration in severely burned patients can occur without evidence of a smoke inhalation injury. Bronchoconstriction caused by release of histamine, serotonin, and thromboxane, a powerful vasoconstrictor, as well as chest constriction secondary to circumferential full-thickness chest burns causes this deterioration. One third of all burn patients have a pulmonary problem related to the burn injury (Flynn, 1999). Even without pulmonary injury, hypoxia (oxygen starvation) may be present. Early in the postburn period, catecholamine release in response to the stress of the burn injury alters peripheral blood flow, thereby reducing oxygen delivery to the periphery. Later, hypermetabolism and continued catecholamine release lead to increased tissue oxygen consumption, which can lead to hypoxia. To ensure that adequate oxygen is available to the tissues, supplemental oxygen may be needed.

Pulmonary injuries fall into several categories: upper airway injury; inhalation injury below the glottis, including carbon monoxide poisoning; and restrictive defects. Upper airway injury results from direct heat or edema. It is manifested by mechanical obstruction of the upper airway, including the pharynx and larynx. Because of the cooling effect of rapid vaporization in the pulmonary tract, direct heat injury does not normally occur below the level of the bronchus. Upper airway injury is treated by early nasotracheal or endotracheal intubation.

Inhalation injury below the glottis results from inhaling the products of incomplete combustion or noxious gases. These products include carbon monoxide, sulfur oxides, nitrogen oxides, aldehydes, cyanide, ammonia, chlorine, phosgene, benzene, and halogens. The injury results directly from chemical irritation of the pulmonary tissues at the alveolar level. Inhalation injuries below the glottis cause loss of ciliary action, hypersecretion, severe mucosal edema, and possibly bronchospasm. The pulmonary surfactant is reduced, resulting in atelectasis (collapse of alveoli). Expectoration of carbon particles in the sputum is the cardinal sign of this injury.

Carbon monoxide is probably the most common cause of inhalation injury because it is a byproduct of the combustion of organic materials and is therefore present in smoke. The pathophysiologic effects are due to tissue hypoxia, a result of carbon monoxide combining with hemoglobin to form **carboxyhemoglobin**, which competes with oxygen for available hemoglobin-binding sites. The affinity of hemoglobin for carbon monoxide is 200 times greater than that for oxygen. Treatment usually consists of early intubation and mechanical ventilation with 100% oxygen. However, some patients may require only oxygen therapy, depending on the extent of pulmonary injury and edema. Administering 100% oxygen is essential to accelerate the removal of carbon monoxide from the hemoglobin molecule.

Restrictive defects arise when edema develops under full-thickness burns encircling the neck and thorax. Chest excursion may be greatly restricted, resulting in decreased tidal volume. In such situations, escharotomy is necessary.

Pulmonary abnormalities are not always immediately apparent. More than half of all burn victims with pulmonary involvement do not initially demonstrate pulmonary signs and symptoms. Any patient with possible inhalation injury must be observed for at least 48 hours for respiratory complications. Airway obstruction may

occur very rapidly or develop in hours. Decreased lung compliance, decreased arterial oxygen levels, and respiratory acidosis may occur gradually over the first 5 days after a burn.

Indicators of possible pulmonary damage include the following:

- History indicating that the burn occurred in an enclosed area
- Burns of the face or neck
- Singed nasal hair
- Hoarseness, voice change, dry cough, stridor, sooty sputum
- Bloody sputum
- Laboured breathing or tachypnea (rapid breathing) and other signs of reduced oxygen levels (hypoxemia)
- Erythema and blistering of the oral or pharyngeal mucosa

Diagnosis of inhalation injury is an important priority for many burn victims. Serum carboxyhemoglobin levels and arterial blood gas levels are frequently used to assess for inhalation injuries. Bronchoscopy and xenon-133 (^{133}Xe) ventilation-perfusion scans can also be used to aid diagnosis in the early postburn period. Pulmonary function studies may also be useful in diagnosing decreased lung compliance or obstructed airflow (Fitzpatrick & Cioffi, 2002; Flynn, 1999).

Pulmonary complications secondary to inhalation injuries include acute respiratory failure and acute respiratory distress syndrome (ARDS). Respiratory failure occurs when impairment of ventilation and gas exchange is life-threatening. The immediate intervention is intubation and mechanical ventilation. If ventilation is impaired by restricted chest excursion, immediate chest escharotomy is needed. ARDS may develop in the first few days after the burn injury secondary to systemic and pulmonary responses to the burn and inhalation injury. Respiratory failure and ARDS are discussed in Chapter 23.

Other Systemic Responses

Renal function may be altered as a result of decreased blood volume. Destruction of red blood cells at the injury site results in free hemoglobin in the urine. If muscle damage occurs (eg, from electrical burns), myoglobin is released from the muscle cells and excreted by the kidney. Adequate fluid volume replacement restores renal blood flow, increasing the glomerular filtration rate and urine volume. If there is inadequate blood flow through the kidneys, the hemoglobin and myoglobin occlude the renal tubules, resulting in acute tubular necrosis and renal failure (see Chap. 45).

The immunologic defenses of the body are greatly altered by burn injury. Serious burn injury diminishes resistance to infection. As a result, sepsis remains the leading cause of death in thermally injured patients (Cioffi, 2001). The loss of skin integrity is compounded by the release of abnormal inflammatory factors, altered levels of immunoglobulins and serum complement, impaired neutrophil function, and a reduction in lymphocytes (lymphocytopenia). Research suggests that burn injury results in loss of T-helper cell lymphocytes (Munster, 2002). There is a significant impairment of the production and release of granulocytes and macrophages from bone marrow after burn injury. The resulting immunosuppression places the burn patient at high risk for sepsis.

Loss of skin also results in an inability to regulate body temperature. Burn patients may therefore exhibit low body temperatures in the early hours after injury. Then, as hypermetabolism resets core temperatures, burn patients become hyperthermic for much of the postburn period, even in the absence of infection.

Two potential gastrointestinal complications may occur: paralytic ileus (absence of intestinal peristalsis) and Curling's ulcer. Decreased peristalsis and bowel sounds are manifestations of paralytic ileus resulting from burn trauma. Gastric distention and nausea may lead to vomiting unless gastric decompression is initiated. Gastric bleeding secondary to massive physiologic stress may be signaled by occult blood in the stool, regurgitation of "coffee ground" material from the stomach, or bloody vomitus. These signs suggest gastric or duodenal erosion (Curling's ulcer).

Management of the Patient With a Burn Injury

Burn care must be planned according to the burn depth and local response, the extent of the injury, and the presence of a systemic response. Burn care then proceeds through three phases: emergent/resuscitative phase, acute/intermediate phase, and rehabilitation phase. Although priorities exist for each of the phases, the phases overlap, and assessment and management of specific problems and complications are not limited to these phases but take place throughout burn care. The three phases and the priorities for care are summarized in Table 57-2.

EMERGENT/RESUSCITATIVE PHASE OF BURN CARE

On-the-Scene Care

Anyone who encounters a burn victim for the first time may feel overwhelmed. The burned person's appearance can be frightening at first. It can be difficult not to get caught up with the appearance of the person and instead to concentrate on the burn wounds. However, the burn wound is not the first priority at the scene: the first priority of on-the-scene care for a burn victim is to prevent injury to the rescuer. If needed, fire and emergency medical services should be requested at the first opportunity. Additional emergency procedures are highlighted in Chart 57-3.

AIRWAY, BREATHING, CIRCULATION

Although the local effects of a burn are the most evident, the systemic effects pose a greater threat to life. Therefore, it is important to remember the ABCs of all trauma care during the early postburn period:

- Airway
- Breathing
- Circulation; cervical spine immobilization for patients with high-voltage electrical injuries and if indicated for other injuries; cardiac monitoring for patients with all electrical injuries for at least 24 hours after cessation of dysrhythmia

Some practitioners include "DEF" in the trauma assessment: disability, exposure, and fluid resuscitation (Weibelhaus & Hansen, 2001).

 NURSING ALERT Breathing must be assessed and a patent airway established immediately during the initial minutes of emergency care. Immediate therapy is directed toward establishing an airway and administering humidified 100% oxygen. If such a high concentration of oxygen is not available under emergency conditions, oxygen by mask or nasal cannula is given initially. If qualified personnel and equipment are available and if the victim has severe respiratory distress or airway edema, the rescuers can insert an endotracheal tube and initiate manual ventilation.

The circulatory system must also be assessed quickly. Apical pulse and blood pressure are monitored frequently. Tachycardia (abnormally rapid heart rate) and slight hypotension are expected soon after the burn. The neurologic status is assessed quickly in the patient with extensive burns. Often the burn patient is awake and alert initially, and vital information can be obtained at that time. A secondary head-to-toe survey of the patient is carried out to identify other potentially life-threatening injuries. (The E and F parameters of trauma assessment are discussed in detail later.) Preventing shock in a burn patient is imperative.

 NURSING ALERT No food or fluid is given by mouth, and the patient is placed in a position that will prevent aspiration of vomitus because nausea and vomiting typically occur due to paralytic ileus resulting from the stress of injury.

Usually, rescue workers will cool the wound, establish an airway, supply oxygen, and insert at least one large-bore intravenous line.

Table 57-2 • **Phases of Burn Care**		
PHASE	**DURATION**	**PRIORITIES**
Emergent or immediate resuscitative	From onset of injury to completion of fluid resuscitation	• First aid • Prevention of shock • Prevention of respiratory distress • Detection and treatment of concomitant injuries • Wound assessment and initial care
Acute	From beginning of diuresis to near completion of wound closure	• Wound care and closure • Prevention or treatment of complications, including infection • Nutritional support
Rehabilitation	From major wound closure to return to individual's optimal level of physical and psychosocial adjustment	• Prevention of scars and contractures • Physical, occupational, and vocational rehabilitation • Functional and cosmetic reconstruction • Psychosocial counselling

Chart 57-3 — Emergency Procedures at the Burn Scene

- **Extinguish the flames.** When clothes catch fire, the flames can be extinguished if the victim falls to the floor or ground and rolls ("drop and roll"); anything available to smother the flames, such as a blanket, rug, or coat, may be used. Standing still forces the victim to breathe flames and smoke, and running fans the flames. If the burn source is electrical, the electrical source must be disconnected.
- **Cool the burn.** After the flames are extinguished, the burned area and adherent clothing are soaked with *cool* water, briefly, to cool the wound and halt the burning process. Once a burn has been sustained, the application of cool water is the best first-aid measure. Soaking the burn area intermittently in cool water or applying cool towels gives immediate and striking relief from pain and limits local tissue edema and damage. However, *never* apply ice directly to the burn, *never* wrap burn victims in ice, and *never* use cold soaks or dressings for longer than several minutes; such procedures may worsen the tissue damage and lead to hypothermia in patients with large burns.
- **Remove restrictive objects.** If possible, remove clothing immediately. Adherent clothing may be left in place once cooled. Other clothing and all jewelry should be removed to allow for assessment and to prevent constriction secondary to rapidly developing edema.
- **Cover the wound.** The burn should be covered as quickly as possible to minimize bacterial contamination and decrease pain by preventing air from coming into contact with the injured surface. Sterile dressings are best, but any clean, dry cloth can be used as an emergency dressing. Ointments and salves should *not* be used. Other than the dressing, no medication or material should be applied to the burn wound.
- **Irrigate chemical burns.** Chemical burns resulting from contact with a corrosive material are irrigated immediately. Most chemical laboratories have a high-pressure shower for such emergencies. If such an injury occurs at home, brush off the chemical agent, remove clothes immediately, and rinse all areas of the body that have come in contact with the chemical. Rinsing can occur in the shower or any other source of continuous running water. Flushing/rinsing should be done for *at least* 20 minutes. If a chemical gets in or near the eyes, the eyes should be flushed with cool, clean water immediately. Outcomes for the patient with chemical burns are significantly improved by rapid, sustained flushing of the injury at the scene.

Emergency Medical Management

The patient is transported to the nearest emergency department. The hospital and physician are alerted that the patient is en route to the emergency department so that life-saving measures can be initiated immediately by a trained team.

Initial priorities in the emergency department remain airway, breathing, and circulation. For mild pulmonary injury, inspired air is humidified and the patient is encouraged to cough so that secretions can be removed by suctioning. For more severe situations, it is necessary to remove secretions by bronchial suctioning and to administer bronchodilators and mucolytic agents. If edema of the airway develops, endotracheal intubation may be necessary. Continuous positive airway pressure and mechanical ventilation may also be required to achieve adequate oxygenation.

After adequate respiratory status and circulatory status have been established, the patient is assessed for cervical spinal injuries or head injury if the patient was involved in an explosion, a fall, a jump, or an electrical injury. Once the patient's condition is stable, attention is directed to the burn wound itself. All clothing and jewelry are removed. For chemical burns, flushing of the exposed areas is continued. The patient is checked for contact lenses. These are removed immediately if chemicals have contacted the eyes or if facial burns have occurred.

It is important to validate an account of the burn scenario provided by the patient, witnesses at the scene, and paramedics. Information needs to include time of the burn injury, source of the burn, place where the burn occurred, how the burn was treated at the scene, and any history of falling with the injury. A history of preexisting diseases, allergies, and medications and the use of drugs, alcohol, and tobacco is obtained at this point to plan care. A large-bore (16- or 18-gauge) intravenous catheter should be inserted in a non-burned area (if not inserted earlier). Most patients have a central venous catheter inserted so that large amounts of intravenous fluids can be given quickly and central venous pressures can be monitored. If the burn exceeds 25% TBSA or if the patient is nauseated, a nasogastric tube should be inserted and connected to suction to prevent vomiting due to paralytic ileus (absence of peristalsis).

The physician evaluates the patient's general condition, assesses the burn, determines the priorities of care, and directs the individualized plan of treatment, which is divided into systemic management and local care of the burned area. Nonsterile gloves, caps, and gowns are worn by personnel while assessing the exposed burned areas. Clean technique is maintained while assessing burn wounds.

Assessment of both the TBSA burned and the depth of the burn is completed after soot and debris have been gently cleansed from the burn wound. Careful attention is paid to keeping the burn patient warm during wound assessment and cleansing. Assessment is repeated frequently throughout burn wound care. Photographs may be taken of the burn areas initially and periodically throughout treatment; in this way, the initial injury and burn wound can be documented. Such documentation is invaluable for insurance and legal claims. Clean sheets are placed under and over the patient to protect the area from contamination, maintain body temperature, and reduce pain caused by air currents passing over exposed nerve endings.

An indwelling urinary catheter is inserted to permit more accurate monitoring of urine output and renal function for patients with moderate to severe burns. Baseline height, weight, arterial blood gases, hematocrit, electrolyte values, blood alcohol level, drug panel, urinalysis, and chest x-rays are obtained. If the patient is elderly or has an electrical burn, a baseline electrocardiogram is obtained. Because burns are contaminated wounds, tetanus prophylaxis is administered if the patient's immunization status is not current or is unknown.

Although the major focus of care during the emergent phase is physical stabilization, the nurse must also attend to the patient's and family's psychological needs. Burn injury is a crisis, causing variable emotional responses. The patient's and family's coping abilities and available supports are assessed. Circumstances surrounding the burn injury should be considered when providing care. Individualized psychosocial support must be given to the patient and family. Because the emergent burn patient is usually anxious and in pain, those in attendance should provide reassurance and support, explanations of procedures, and adequate pain relief. Because poor tissue perfusion accompanies burn injuries, only intravenous pain medication (usually morphine) is given, titrated for the patient. If the patient wishes to see a spiritual advisor, one is notified.

TRANSFER TO A BURN CENTRE

The depth and extent of the burn are considered in determining whether the patient should be transferred to a burn centre. Patients with major burns, those who are at the extremes of the age continuum, those with coexisting health problems that may affect recovery, and those with circumstances that increase their risk for acute and long-term complications are transferred to a burn centre. Chart 57-4 lists the American Burn Association's criteria for burn centre referral after initial assessment and management.

If the patient is to be transported to a burn centre, the following measures are instituted before transfer:

- A secure intravenous catheter is inserted with lactated Ringer's solution infusing at the rate required to maintain a urine output of at least 30 mL per hour.
- A patent airway is ensured.
- Adequate pain relief is attained.
- Adequate peripheral circulation is established in any burned extremity.
- Wounds are covered with a clean, dry sheet, and the patient is kept comfortably warm.

All assessments and treatments are documented, and this information is provided to the burn centre personnel. The transferring facility must relay accurate intake and output totals to

burn centre personnel so that adequate fluid resuscitation measures continue.

MANAGEMENT OF FLUID LOSS AND SHOCK

Next to handling respiratory difficulties, the most urgent need is preventing irreversible shock by replacing lost fluids and electrolytes. As mentioned previously, survival of burn victims depends on adequate fluid resuscitation. Table 57-3 summarizes the fluid and electrolyte changes in the emergent phase of burn care. Intravenous lines and an indwelling urinary catheter must be in place before implementing fluid resuscitation. Baseline weight and laboratory test results are obtained as well. These parameters must be monitored closely in the immediate post-burn (resuscitation) period. Controversy continues regarding the definition of adequate resuscitation and the optimal fluid type for resuscitation. Refinement of resuscitation techniques remains an active area of burn research.

Fluid Replacement Therapy. The total volume and rate of intravenous fluid replacement are gauged by the patient's response. The adequacy of fluid resuscitation is determined by following urine output totals, an index of renal perfusion. Output totals of 30 to 50 mL/hour have been used as goals. Other indicators of adequate fluid replacement are a systolic blood pressure exceeding 100 mm Hg and/or a pulse rate less than 110/minute.

 NURSING ALERT Clinical parameters are far more important in resuscitation than any formula. Indeed, the patient's individual response is the key to assessing the adequacy of fluid resuscitation.

Additional gauges of fluid requirements and response to fluid resuscitation include hematocrit and hemoglobin and serum sodium levels. If the hematocrit and the hemoglobin levels decrease or if the urinary output exceeds 50 mL/hour, the rate of intravenous fluid administration may be decreased. The goal is to maintain serum sodium levels in the normal range during fluid replacement.

Appropriate resuscitation endpoints for burn patients remain controversial. Research in this area has led to the study of hemodynamic and oxygen transport resuscitation endpoints. When these endpoints were used, massive fluid resuscitation volumes were administered that could have deleterious effects. Successful resuscitation is associated with increased delivery of oxygen and consumption of oxygen with declining serum lactate levels (Holm et al., 2000). Attention has been directed recently toward other indicators of adequate resuscitation: base deficit and serum lactate levels. Measurement of serum lactate levels does not appear useful in the treatment of burn patients because of the large amounts of lactate released from burned tissue; however, metabolism of lactate is unaltered. Elevated levels occur despite adequate fluid resuscitation (Yowler & Fratianne, 2000). Factors that are associated with the increased fluid requirements include delayed resuscitation, scald burn injuries, inhalation injuries, high-voltage electrical injuries, hyperglycemia, alcohol intoxication, and chronic diuretic therapy. Second 24-hour post-burn fluid infusion rates incorporate both the maintenance amount of fluid and any additional fluid needs secondary to evaporative water loss through the burn wound.

Fluid Requirements. The projected fluid requirements for the first 24 hours are calculated by the clinician based on the extent of the burn injury. Some combination of fluid categories may be used: colloids (whole blood, plasma, and plasma expanders) and crystalloids/electrolytes (physiologic sodium chloride or lactated

---

Chart 57-4 **Burn Unit Referral Criteria**

A burn unit may treat adults or children or both. Burn injuries that should be referred to a burn unit include the following:

1. Partial-thickness burns greater than 10% total body surface area (TBSA)
2. Burns that involve the face, hands, feet, genitalia, perineum, or major joints
3. Third-degree burns in any age group
4. Electrical burns, including lightning injury
5. Chemical burns
6. Inhalation injury
7. Burn injury in patients with preexisting medical disorders that could complicate management, prolong recovery, or affect mortality
8. Any patients with burns and concomitant trauma (such as fractures) in which the burn injury poses the greatest risk of morbidity or mortality. In such cases, if the trauma poses the greater immediate risk, the patient may be initially stabilized in a trauma centre before being transferred to a burn unit. Physician judgment will be necessary in such situations and should be in concert with the regional medical control plan and triage protocols.
9. Burned children in hospitals without qualified personnel or equipment for the care of children
10. Burn injury in patients who will require special social, emotional, or long-term rehabilitative intervention

Reprinted from *Resources for optimal care of the injured patient, Chapter 14: Committee on Trauma.* American College of Surgeons. (1999). Retrieved from the American Burn Association. Available at http://www.ameriburn.org/pub/guidelinesops.pdf. Retrieved May 29, 2005.

Table 57-3 • Fluid and Electrolyte Changes in the Emergent/Resuscitative Phase

Fluid accumulation phase (shock phase)
Plasma → interstitial fluid (edema at burn site)

OBSERVATION	EXPLANATION
Generalized dehydration	Plasma leaks through damaged capillaries.
Reduction of blood volume	Secondary to plasma loss, fall of blood pressure, and diminished cardiac output
Decreased urinary output	Secondary to: Fluid loss Decreased renal blood flow Sodium and water retention caused by increased adrenocortical activity (Hemolysis of red blood cells, causing hemoglobinuria and myonecrosis or myoglobinuria)
Potassium (K^+) excess	Massive cellular trauma causes release of K^+ into extracellular fluid (ordinarily, most K^+ is intracellular).
Sodium (Na^+) deficit	Large amount of Na^+ is lost in trapped edema fluid and exudate and by shift into cells as K^+ is released from cells (ordinarily most Na^+ is extracellular).
Metabolic acidosis (base-bicarbonate deficit)	Loss of bicarbonate ions accompanies sodium loss.
Hemoconcentration (elevated hematocrit)	Liquid blood component is lost into extravascular space.

Ringer's solution). Adequate fluid resuscitation results in slightly decreased blood volume levels during the first 24 post-burn hours and restores plasma levels to normal by the end of 48 hours. Oral resuscitation can be successful in adults with less than 20% TBSA and children with less than 10% to 15% TBSA.

Formulas have been developed for estimating fluid loss based on the estimated percentage of burned TBSA and the weight of the patient. Length of time since burn injury occurred is also very important in calculating estimated fluid needs. Formulas must be adjusted so that initiation of fluid replacement reflects the time of injury. Resuscitation formulas are approximations only and are individualized to meet the requirements of each patient. The various formulas are discussed below and summarized in Chart 57-5.

As early as 1978, the NIH Consensus Development Conference on Supportive Therapy in Burn Care established that salt and water are required in burn patients, but that colloid may or may not be useful during the first 24 to 48 post-burn hours. The consensus formula provides for the volume of balanced salt solution to be administered in the first 24 hours in a range of 2 to 4 mL/kg per percent burn. In general, 2 mL/kg per percent burn of lactated Ringer's solution may be used initially for adults. This is the most common fluid replacement formula in use today. As with the other formulas, half of the calculated total should be given over the first 8 post-burn hours, and the other half should be given over the next 16 hours. The rate and volume of the infusion must be regulated according to the patient's response by changing the

---

Chart 57-5 • Guidelines and Formulas for Fluid Replacement in Burn Patients

Consensus Formula
Lactated Ringer's solution (or other balanced saline solution): 2–4 mL × kg body weight × % total body surface area (TBSA) burned. Half to be given in first 8 hours; remaining half to be given over next 16 hours.

Evans Formula
1. Colloids: 1 mL × kg body weight × % TBSA burned
2. Electrolytes (saline): 1 mL × body weight × % TBSA burned
3. Glucose (5% in water): 2,000 mL for insensible loss
Day 1: Half to be given in first 8 hours; remaining half over next 16 hours
Day 2: Half of previous day's colloids and electrolytes; all of insensible fluid replacement
Maximum of 10,000 mL over 24 hours. Second- and third-degree (partial- and full-thickness) burns exceeding 50% TBSA are calculated on the basis of 50% TBSA.

Brooke Army Formula
1. Colloids: 0.5 mL × kg body weight × % TBSA burned
2. Electrolytes (lactated Ringer's solution): 1.5 mL × kg body weight × % TBSA burned
3. Glucose (5% in water): 2,000 mL for insensible loss

Day 1: Half to be given in first 8 hours; remaining half over next 16 hours
Day 2: Half of colloids; half of electrolytes; all of insensible fluid replacement.
Second- and third-degree (partial- and full-thickness) burns exceeding 50% TBSA are calculated on the basis of 50% TBSA.

Parkland/Baxter Formula
Lactated Ringer's solution: 4 mL × kg body weight × % TBSA burned
Day 1: Half to be given in first 8 hours; half to be given over next 16 hours
Day 2: Varies. Colloid is added.

Hypertonic Saline Solution
Concentrated solutions of sodium chloride (NaCl) and lactate with concentration of 250–300 mEq of sodium per litre, administered at a rate sufficient to maintain a desired volume of urinary output. Do not increase the infusion rate during the first 8 postburn hours. Serum sodium levels must be monitored closely. Goal: Increase serum sodium level and osmolality to reduce edema and prevent pulmonary complications.

hourly infusion rates. Fluid boluses are recommended only in the presence of marked hypotension, not low urine output. Typical fluid rate changes should involve an increase or decrease in flow rate by no more than 25% to 33% (Yowler & Fratianne, 2000).

Studies demonstrate that with large burns, there is a failure of the sodium-potassium pump (a physiologic mechanism involved in fluid–electrolyte balance) at the cellular level. Thus, patients with very large burns may need proportionately more millilitres of fluid per percent of burn than those with smaller burns. Also, patients with electrical injury, pulmonary injury, and delayed fluid resuscitation and those who were burned while intoxicated may need additional fluids.

The following example illustrates use of the formula in a 70-kg patient with a 50% TBSA burn:

1. Consensus formula: 2 to 4 mL/kg/% TBSA
2. $2 \times 70 \times 50 = 7,000$ mL/24 hours
3. Plan to administer: First 8 hours = 3,500 mL, or 437 mL/hour; next 16 hours = 3,500 mL, or 219 mL/hour

Most fluid replacement formulas use isotonic electrolyte solutions. Regardless of which standard replacement formula is used, the patient receives approximately the same fluid volume and sodium replacement during the first 48 hours.

Another fluid replacement method requires hypertonic electrolyte solutions. This method uses concentrated solutions of sodium chloride and lactate (a balanced salt solution) so that the resulting fluid has a concentration of 250 to 300 mEq of sodium. The rationale for this replacement method is that by increasing serum osmolality, fluid will be pulled back into the vascular space from the interstitial space. Reduced systemic and pulmonary edema has been reported after administering hypertonic solutions.

> **! NURSING ALERT** Formulas are only a guide. The patient's response, evidenced by heart rate, blood pressure, and urine output, is the primary determinant of actual fluid therapy and must be assessed at least hourly. Patient outcomes are improved by optimal fluid resuscitation.

Gerontologic Considerations

Decreased function of the cardiovascular, renal, and pulmonary systems increases the need for close observation of elderly patients with even relatively minor burns during the emergent and acute phases. Acute renal failure is much more common in elderly patients than in those younger than age 40. The margin of difference between hypovolemia and fluid overload is very small. Suppressed immunologic response, a high incidence of malnutrition, and an inability to withstand metabolic stressors (eg, a cold environment) further compromise the elderly person's ability to heal. As a result of these issues in elderly patients who sustain burn injury, close monitoring and prompt treatment of complications are mandatory.

Nursing Management: Emergent/Resuscitative Phase

Assessment data obtained by prehospital providers (rescuers such as emergency medical technicians) are shared with the physician and nurse in the emergency department. Nursing assessment in the emergent phase of burn injury focuses on the major priorities for any trauma patient; the burn wound is a secondary consider-

ation. Aseptic management of the burn wounds and invasive lines continues.

The nurse monitors vital signs frequently. Respiratory status is monitored closely, and apical, carotid, and femoral pulses are evaluated. Cardiac monitoring is indicated if the patient has a history of cardiac disease, electrical injury, or respiratory problems, or if the pulse is dysrhythmic or the rate is abnormally slow or rapid.

If all extremities are burned, determining blood pressure may be difficult. A sterile dressing applied under the blood pressure cuff will protect the wound from contamination. Because increasing edema makes blood pressure difficult to auscultate, a Doppler (ultrasound) device or a noninvasive electronic blood pressure device may be helpful. In severe burns, an arterial catheter is used for blood pressure measurement and for collecting blood specimens. Peripheral pulses of burned extremities are checked hourly; the Doppler device is useful for this. Elevation of burned extremities is crucial to decrease edema. Elevation of the lower extremities on pillows and of the upper extremities on pillows or by suspension using intravenous poles may be helpful.

Large-bore intravenous catheters and an indwelling urinary catheter are inserted, and the nurse's assessment includes monitoring fluid intake and output. Urine output, an indicator of renal perfusion, is monitored carefully and measured hourly. The amount of urine first obtained when the urinary catheter was inserted is recorded. This may assist in determining the extent of preburn renal function and fluid status. Urine specific gravity, pH, and glucose, acetone, protein, and hemoglobin levels are assessed frequently.

Burgundy-coloured urine suggests the presence of hemochromogen and myoglobin resulting from muscle damage. This is associated with deep burns caused by electrical injury or prolonged contact with flames. Glucosuria, a common finding in the early postburn hours, results from the release of stored glucose from the liver in response to stress.

Although not responsible for calculating the patient's fluid requirements, the nurse needs to know the maximum volume of fluid the patient should receive. Infusion pumps and rate controllers are used to deliver a complex regimen of prescribed intravenous fluids. Administering and monitoring intravenous therapy are major nursing responsibilities.

Body temperature, body weight, preburn weight, and history of allergies, tetanus immunization, past medical and surgical problems, current illnesses, and use of medications are assessed. A head-to-toe assessment is performed, focusing on signs and symptoms of concomitant illness, injury, or developing complications. Patients with facial burns should have their eyes examined for potential injury to the corneas. An ophthalmologist is consulted for complete assessment via fluorescent staining.

Assessing the extent of the burn wound continues and is facilitated with anatomic diagrams (described previously). In addition, the nurse works with the physician to assess the depth of the wound and areas of full- and partial-thickness injury. Assessment of the circumstances surrounding the injury is important. Obtaining a history of the burn injury can help to plan the care for the patient. Assessment should include the time of injury, mechanism of burn, whether the burn occurred in a closed space, the possibility of inhalation of noxious chemicals, and any related trauma.

The neurologic assessment focuses on the patient's level of consciousness, psychological status, pain and anxiety levels, and behaviour. The patient's and family's understanding of the injury and treatment is assessed as well.

Nursing care of the patient during the emergent/resuscitative phase of burn injury is detailed in the Plan of Nursing Care.

(text continues on page 1727)

Plan of Nursing Care

Care of the Patient During the Emergent/Resuscitative Phase of Burn Injury

Nursing Interventions	Rationale	Expected Outcomes

Nursing Diagnosis: Impaired gas exchange related to carbon monoxide poisoning, smoke inhalation, and upper airway obstruction

Goal: Maintenance of adequate tissue oxygenation

Nursing Interventions	Rationale	Expected Outcomes
1. Provide humidified oxygen.	1. Humidified oxygen provides moisture to injured tissues; supplemental oxygen increases alveolar oxygenation.	• Absence of dyspnea • Respiratory rate between 12 and 20 breaths/min • Lungs clear on auscultation • Arterial oxygen saturation >96% by pulse oximetry • Arterial blood gas levels within normal limits
2. Assess breath sounds, and respiratory rate, rhythm, depth, and symmetry. Monitor patient for signs of hypoxia.	2. These factors provide baseline data for further assessment and evidence of increasing respiratory compromise.	

3. Observe for the following:
  a. Erythema or blistering of lips or buccal mucosa
  b. Singed nostrils
  c. Burns of face, neck, or chest
  d. Increasing hoarseness
  e. Soot in sputum or tracheal tissue in respiratory secretions
	3. These signs indicate possible inhalation injury and risk of respiratory dysfunction.	

4. Monitor arterial blood gas values, pulse oximetry readings, and carboxyhemoglobin levels.	4. Increasing PCO_2 and decreasing PO_2 and O_2 saturation may indicate need for mechanical ventilation.	
5. Report laboured respirations, decreased depth of respirations, or signs of hypoxia to physician immediately.	5. Immediate intervention is indicated for respiratory difficulty.	
6. Prepare to assist with intubation and escharotomies.	6. Intubation allows airway patency and mechanical ventilation. Escharotomy enables chest excursion in circumferential chest burns.	
7. Monitor mechanically ventilated patient closely.	7. Monitoring allows early detection of decreasing respiratory status or complications of mechanical ventilation.	

Nursing Diagnosis: Ineffective airway clearance related to edema and effects of smoke inhalation

Goal: Maintain patent airway and adequate airway clearance

Nursing Interventions	Rationale	Expected Outcomes
1. Maintain patent airway through proper patient positioning, removal of secretions, and artificial airway if needed.	1. A patent airway is crucial to respiration.	• Patent airway • Respiratory secretions are minimal, colourless, and thin • Respiratory rate, pattern, and breath sounds normal
2. Provide humidified oxygen.	2. Humidity liquefies secretions and facilitates expectoration.	
3. Encourage patient to mobilize, turn, cough, and deep breathe. Encourage patient to use incentive spirometry. Suction as needed.	3. These activities promote mobilization and removal of secretions.	

Nursing Diagnosis: Fluid volume deficit related to increased capillary permeability and evaporative losses from the burn wound

Goal: Restoration of optimal fluid and electrolyte balance and perfusion of vital organs

Nursing Interventions	Rationale	Expected Outcomes
1. Observe vital signs (including central venous pressure or pulmonary artery pressure, if indicated) and urine output, and be alert for signs of hypovolemia or fluid overload.	1. Hypovolemia is a major risk immediately after the burn injury. Overresuscitation might cause fluid overload.	• Serum electrolytes within normal limits • Urine output between 0.5 and 1.0 mL/kg/hr • Blood pressure higher than 90/60 mm Hg • Heart rate less than 120 beats/min • Exhibits clear sensorium • Voids clear yellow urine with specific gravity within normal limits
2. Monitor urine output at least hourly and weigh patient daily.	2. Output and weight provide information about renal perfusion, adequacy of fluid replacement, and fluid requirement and fluid status.	

(continued)

Plan of Nursing Care

Care of the Patient During the Emergent/Resuscitative Phase of Burn Injury *(Continued)*

Nursing Interventions	Rationale	Expected Outcomes
3. Maintain IV lines and regulate fluids at appropriate rates, as prescribed.	3. Adequate fluids are necessary to maintain fluid and electrolyte balance and perfusion of vital organs.	
4. Observe for symptoms of deficiency or excess of serum sodium, potassium, calcium, phosphorus, and bicarbonate.	4. Rapid shifts in fluid and electrolyte status are possible in the postburn period.	
5. Elevate head of patient's bed and elevate burned extremities.	5. Elevation promotes venous return.	
6. Notify physician immediately of decreased urine output, blood pressure, central venous, pulmonary artery, or pulmonary artery wedge pressures, or increased pulse rate.	6. Because of the rapid fluid shifts in burn shock, fluid deficit must be detected early so that distributive shock does not occur.	

Nursing Diagnosis: Hypothermia related to loss of skin microcirculation and open wounds
Goal: Maintenance of adequate body temperature

1. Provide a warm environment through use of heat shield, space blanket, heat lights, or blankets.	1. A stable environment minimizes evaporative heat loss.	• Body temperature remains 36.1° to 38.3°C
2. Work quickly when wounds must be exposed.	2. Minimal exposure minimizes heat loss from wound.	• Absence of chills or shivering
3. Assess core body temperature frequently.	3. Frequent temperature assessments help detect developing hypothermia.	

Nursing Diagnosis: Pain related to tissue and nerve injury and emotional impact of injury
Goal: Control of pain

1. Use pain intensity scale to assess pain level (ie, 1 to 10). Differentiate from hypoxia.	1. Pain level provides baseline for evaluating effectiveness of pain relief measures. Hypoxia can cause similar signs and must be ruled out before analgesic medication is administered.	• States pain level is decreased
		• Absence of nonverbal cues of pain
2. Administer intravenous opioid analgesics as prescribed. Observe for respiratory depression in the patient who is not mechanically ventilated. Assess response to analgesic.	2. Intravenous administration is necessary because of altered tissue perfusion from burn injury.	
3. Provide emotional support and reassurance.	3. Emotional support is essential to reduce fear and anxiety resulting from burn injury. Fear and anxiety increase the perception of pain.	

Nursing Diagnosis: Anxiety related to fear and the emotional impact of burn injury
Goal: Minimization of patient's and family's anxiety

1. Assess patient's and family's understanding of burn injury, coping skills, and family dynamics.	1. Previous successful coping strategies can be fostered for use in the present crisis. Assessment allows planning of individualized interventions.	• Patient and family verbalize understanding of emergent burn care
		• Able to answer simple questions
2. Individualize responses to the patient's and family's coping level.	2. Reactions to burn injury are extremely variable. Interventions must be appropriate to the patient's and family's present level of coping.	
3. Explain all procedures to the patient and the family in clear, simple terms.	3. Increased understanding alleviates fear of the unknown. High levels of anxiety may interfere with understanding of complex explanations.	

(continued)

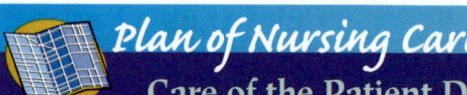

Plan of Nursing Care

Care of the Patient During the Emergent/Resuscitative Phase of Burn Injury *(Continued)*

Nursing Interventions	Rationale	Expected Outcomes
4. Maintain adequate pain relief.	4. Pain increases anxiety.	
5. Consider administering prescribed anti-anxiety medications if the patient remains extremely anxious despite nonpharmacologic interventions.	5. Anxiety levels during the emergent phase may exceed the patient's coping abilities. Medication decreases physiologic and psychological anxiety responses.	

Collaborative Problems: Acute respiratory failure, distributive shock, acute renal failure, compartment syndrome, paralytic ileus, Curling's ulcer
Goal: Absence of complications

Acute Respiratory Failure

1. Assess for increasing dyspnea, stridor, changes in respiratory patterns.	1. Such signs reflect deteriorating respiratory status.	• Arterial blood gas values within acceptable limits: $PO_2 >80$ mm Hg, $PCO_2 <50$ mm Hg
2. Monitor pulse oximetry, arterial blood gas values for decreasing PO_2 and oxygen saturation, and increasing PCO_2.	2. Such signs reflect decreased oxygenation status.	• Breathes spontaneously with adequate tidal volume
3. Monitor chest x-ray results.	3. X-ray may disclose pulmonary injury.	• Chest x-ray findings normal
4. Assess for restlessness, confusion, difficulty attending to questions, or decreasing level of consciousness.	4. Such manifestations may indicate cerebral hypoxia.	• Absence of cerebral signs of hypoxia
5. Report deteriorating respiratory status immediately to physician.	5. Acute respiratory failure is life-threatening, and immediate intervention is required.	
6. Prepare to assist with intubation or escharotomies as indicated.	6. Intubation allows mechanical ventilation. Escharotomies allow improved chest excursion with respirations.	

Distributive Shock

1. Assess for decreasing urine output, pulmonary artery and pulmonary artery wedge pressures, blood pressure, and cardiac output, or increasing pulse.	1. Such signs and symptoms may indicate distributive shock and inadequate intravascular volume.	• Urine output between 0.5 and 1.0 mL/kg/hr
2. Assess for progressive edema as fluid shifts occur.	2. As fluid shifts into the interstitial spaces in burn shock, edema occurs and may compromise tissue perfusion.	• Blood pressure within patient's normal range (usually >90/60 mm Hg)
		• Heart rate within patient's normal range (usually <110/min)
3. Adjust fluid resuscitation in collaboration with the physician in response to physiologic findings.	3. Optimal fluid resuscitation prevents distributive shock and improves patient outcomes.	• Pressures and cardiac output remain within normal limits

Acute Renal Failure

1. Monitor urine output and blood urea nitrogen (BUN) and creatinine levels.	1. These values reflect renal function.	• Adequate urine output
2. Report decreased urine output or increased BUN and creatinine values to physician.	2. These laboratory values indicate possible renal failure.	• BUN and creatinine values remain normal
3. Assess urine for hemoglobin or myoglobin.	3. Hemoglobin or myoglobin in the urine points to an increased risk of renal failure.	
4. Administer increased fluids as prescribed.	4. Fluids help to flush out hemoglobin and myoglobin from renal tubules, decreasing the potential for renal failure.	

Compartment Syndrome

1. Assess peripheral pulses hourly with Doppler ultrasound device.	1. Assessment with Doppler device substitutes for auscultation and indicates characteristics of arterial blood flow.	• Absence of paresthesias or symptoms of ischemia of nerves and muscles
2. Assess warmth, capillary refill, sensation, and movement of extremity hourly. Compare affected with unaffected extremity.	2. These assessments indicate characteristics of peripheral perfusion.	• Peripheral pulses detectable by Doppler

(continued)

Plan of Nursing Care

Care of the Patient During the Emergent/Resuscitative Phase of Burn Injury (Continued)

Nursing Interventions	Rationale	Expected Outcomes
3. Remove blood pressure cuff after each reading.	3. Cuff may act as a tourniquet as extremities swell.	
4. Elevate burned extremities.	4. Elevation reduces edema formation.	
5. Report loss of pulse or sensation or presence of pain to physician immediately.	5. These signs and symptoms may indicate inadequate tissue perfusion.	
6. Prepare to assist with escharotomies.	6. Escharotomies relieve the constriction caused by swelling under circumferential burns and improve tissue perfusion.	
Paralytic Ileus		• Absence of abdominal distention
1. Maintain nasogastric tube on low intermittent suction until bowel sounds resume.	1. This measure relieves gastric and abdominal distention, also prevents vomiting.	• Normal bowel sounds within 48 hours
2. Auscultate for bowel sounds, abdominal distention.	2. As bowel sounds resume, feeding may be slowly initiated. Abdominal distention reflects inadequate decompression.	
Curling's Ulcer		• Absence of abdominal distention
1. Assess gastric aspirate for pH and blood.	1. Acidic pH indicates need for antacids or histamine blockers. Blood indicates possible gastric bleeding.	• Normal bowel sounds within 48 hours • Gastric aspirate and stools do not contain blood
2. Assess stools for occult blood.	2. Blood in stools may indicate gastric or duodenal ulcer.	
3. Administer histamine blockers and antacids as prescribed.	3. Such medications reduce gastric acidity and risk of ulceration.	

ACUTE OR INTERMEDIATE PHASE OF BURN CARE

The acute or intermediate phase of burn care follows the emergent/resuscitative phase and begins 48 to 72 hours after the burn injury. During this phase, attention is directed toward continued assessment and maintenance of respiratory and circulatory status, fluid and electrolyte balance, and gastrointestinal function. Infection prevention, burn wound care (ie, wound cleaning, topical antibacterial therapy, wound dressing, dressing changes, wound débridement, and wound grafting), pain management, and nutritional support are priorities at this stage and will be discussed in detail.

Airway obstruction caused by upper airway edema can take as long as 48 hours to develop. Changes detected by x-ray and arterial blood gases may occur as the effects of resuscitative fluid and the chemical reaction of smoke ingredients with lung tissues become apparent. The arterial blood gas values and other parameters determine the need for intubation or mechanical ventilation.

As capillaries regain integrity, at 48 or more postburn hours, fluid moves from the interstitial to the intravascular compartment and diuresis begins (Table 57-4). If cardiac or renal function is inadequate, for instance in the elderly patient or in the patient with preexisting cardiac disease, fluid overload occurs and symptoms of congestive heart failure may result (see Chap. 30). Early detection allows for early intervention and carefully calculated fluid intake. Vasoactive medications, diuretics, and fluid restriction may be used to support circulatory function and prevent congestive heart failure and pulmonary edema.

Cautious administration of fluids and electrolytes continues during this phase of burn care because of the shifts in fluid from the interstitial to intravascular compartments, losses of fluid from large burn wounds, and the patient's physiologic responses to the burn injury. Blood components are administered as needed to treat blood loss and anemia.

Fever is common in burn patients after burn shock resolves. A resetting of the core body temperature in severely burned patients

Table 57-4 • Fluid and Electrolyte Changes in the Acute Phase

Fluid remobilization phase (state of diuresis)
Interstitial fluid → plasma

OBSERVATION	EXPLANATION
Hemodilution (decreased hematocrit)	Blood cell concentration is diluted as fluid enters the intravascular compartment; loss of red blood cells destroyed at burn site
Increased urinary output	Fluid shift into intravascular compartment increases renal blood flow and causes increased urine formation.
Sodium (Na^+) deficit	With diuresis, sodium is lost with water; existing serum sodium is diluted by water influx.
Potassium (K^+) deficit (occurs occasionally in this phase)	Beginning on the fourth or fifth postburn day, K^+ shifts from extracellular fluid into cells.
Metabolic acidosis	Loss of sodium depletes fixed base; relative carbon dioxide content increases.

results in a body temperature a few degrees higher than normal for several weeks after the burn. Bacteremia and septicemia also cause fever in many patients. Acetaminophen (Tylenol) and hypothermia blankets may be required to maintain body temperature in a range of 37.2° to 38.3°C to reduce metabolic stress and tissue oxygen demand.

Central venous, peripheral arterial, or pulmonary artery thermodilution catheters may be required for monitoring venous and arterial pressures, pulmonary artery pressures, pulmonary capillary wedge pressures, or cardiac output. Generally, however, invasive vascular lines are avoided unless essential because they provide an additional port for infection in an already greatly compromised patient.

Infection progressing to septic shock is the major cause of death in patients who have survived the first few days after a major burn. The immunosuppression that accompanies extensive burn injury places the patient at high risk for sepsis. The infection that begins within the burn site may spread to the bloodstream.

Infection Prevention

Despite aseptic precautions and the use of topical antimicrobial agents, the burn wound is an excellent medium for bacterial growth and proliferation. Bacteria such as *Staphylococcus, Proteus, Pseudomonas, Escherichia coli,* and *Klebsiella* find optimal conditions for growth within the burn wound. The burn eschar is a nonviable crust with no blood supply; therefore, neither polymorphonuclear leukocytes or antibodies nor systemic antibiotics can reach the area. Phenomenal numbers of bacteria—more than 1 billion per gram of tissue—may appear and subsequently spread to the bloodstream or release their toxins, which reach distant sites. Staphylococci and enterococci are the organisms responsible for more than 50% of nosocomial bloodstream infections in patients with burn injuries. Fungi such as *Candida albicans* also grow easily in burn wounds.

When the burn wound is healing through spontaneous re-epithelialization or is being prepared for skin grafting, it must be protected from sepsis. Burn wound sepsis has these characteristics:

- $\geq 10^5$ bacteria per gram of tissue
- Inflammation
- Sludging and thrombosis of dermal blood vessels

The primary source of bacterial infection appears to be the patient's intestinal tract, the source of most microbes. The intestinal mucosa normally serves as a barrier to keep the internal environment free from a variety of pathogens. After a severe burn injury, the intestinal mucosal barrier becomes markedly permeable. Because of this impaired intestinal mucosal barrier, the disturbed microbial flora and endotoxins found in the intestinal lumen pass freely into the systemic circulation, finally causing infection. If the intestinal mucosa receives some type of protection against permeability change, infection could be avoided. Early enteral feeding is one step to help avoid this increased intestinal permeability and prevent early endotoxin translocation (Cioffi, 2000; Peng, Yuan & Ziao, 2001).

Infection impedes burn wound healing by promoting excessive inflammation and damaging tissue. A major secondary source of pathogenic microbes is the environment. Infection control is a major role of the burn team in providing appropriate burn wound care. Cap, gown, mask, and gloves are worn while caring for the patient with open burn wounds. Clean technique is used when caring directly for burn wounds.

Tissue specimens are obtained for culture regularly to monitor colonization of the wound by microbial organisms. These may be swab, surface, or tissue biopsy cultures. Swab or surface cultures are noninvasive, simple, and painless. However, data obtained from such cultures apply only to the area sampled; therefore, invasive wound biopsy cultures may be required. Antibiotics are seldom prescribed prophylactically because of the risk of promoting resistant strains of bacteria. Systemic antibiotics are administered when there is documentation of burn wound sepsis or other positive cultures such as urine, sputum, or blood. Sensitivity of the organisms to the prescribed antibiotics should be determined before administration. Several parenteral antimicrobial agents may be given together to treat the infection. Careful attention is paid to antibiotic use in the burn unit because inappropriate use of antibiotics significantly affects the microbial flora present in the unit.

Wound Cleaning

Various measures are used to clean the burn wound. **Hydrotherapy** in the form of shower carts, individual showers, and bed baths can be used to clean the wounds. Total immersion hydrotherapy is performed in some settings. Because of the high risk of infection and sepsis, the use of plastic liners and thorough decontamination of hydrotherapy equipment and wound care areas are necessary to prevent cross-contamination. Tap water alone can be used for burn wound cleansing. The temperature of the water is maintained at 37.8°C, and the temperature of the room should be maintained between 26.6° and 29.4°C. Hydrotherapy, in whatever form, should be limited to a 20- to 30-minute period to prevent chilling of the patient and additional metabolic stress.

During the bath, the patient is encouraged to be as active as possible. Hydrotherapy provides an excellent opportunity for exercising the extremities and cleaning the entire body. When the patient is removed from the tub after the bath, any residue adhering to the body is washed away with a clear water spray or shower. Unburned areas, including the hair, must be washed regularly as well. At the time of wound cleaning, all skin is inspected for any hints of redness, breakdown, or local infection. Hair in and around the burn area, except the eyebrows, should be clipped short. Intact blisters may be left, but the fluid should be aspirated with a needle and syringe and discarded.

Conscientious management of the burn wound is essential. When nonviable loose skin is removed, aseptic conditions must be established. Wound cleaning is usually performed at least daily in wound areas that are not undergoing surgical intervention. When the eschar begins to separate from the viable tissue beneath (approximately 1.5 to 2 weeks after the burn), more frequent cleaning and débridement may be in order.

After the burn wounds are cleaned, they are gently patted with towels and the prescribed method of wound care is performed. Physician preferences, the availability of skilled nursing staff, and resources in terms of number of personnel, supplies, and time must be considered in choosing the best method for a given patient. Whatever the method, the goal is to protect the wound from overwhelming proliferation of pathogenic organisms and invasion of deeper tissues until either spontaneous healing or skin grafting can be achieved.

Patient comfort and ability to participate in the prescribed treatment are also important considerations. Wound care procedures, particularly tub baths, are metabolically stressful. Therefore, the patient is assessed for signs of chilling, fatigue, changes in hemodynamic status, and pain unrelieved by analgesic medications or relaxation techniques.

Topical Antibacterial Therapy

There is general agreement that some form of antimicrobial therapy applied to the burn wound is the best method of local care in extensive burn injury. Topical antibacterial therapy does not sterilize the burn wound; it simply reduces the number of bacteria so that the overall microbial population can be controlled by the body's host defense mechanisms. Topical therapy promotes conversion of the open, dirty wound to a closed, clean one.

Criteria for choosing a topical agent include the following:

- It is effective against gram-negative organisms, *Pseudomonas aeruginosa, Staphylococcus aureus,* and even fungi.
- It is clinically effective.
- It penetrates the eschar but is not systemically toxic.
- It does not lose its effectiveness, allowing another infection to develop.
- It is cost-effective, available, and acceptable to the patient.
- It is easy to apply, minimizing nursing care time.

The three most commonly used topical agents are silver sulfadiazine (Silvadene), silver nitrate, and mafenide acetate (Sulfamylon). These agents are described in Table 57-5. Many other topical agents are available, including povidone–iodine ointment 10% (Betadine), gentamicin sulfate, nitrofurazone (Furacin), Dakin's solution, acetic acid, miconazole, and chlortrimazole. Bacitracin or polysporin may be used for facial burns or on skin grafts initially.

A newer product used in burn wound care is Acticoat Antimicrobial Barrier dressing. Acticoat is a silver-coated dressing approved for treatment of burn wounds and **donor sites**. This dressing is kept moist with water for a controlled, sustained release of silver over the wound to provide an antimicrobial barrier. Acticoat has been shown to have a better antimicrobial performance than the traditional silver-based products commonly used in burn wound treatment. Acticoat is also cost-effective. The dressing can be left in place for up to 5 days, decreasing patient discomfort, the cost of dressing supplies, and nursing time for dressing changes. The dressing has been shown clinically to be very effective for prevention of burn wound infection (Yin, Langford & Burrell, 1999).

No single topical medication is universally effective. Using different agents at different times in the postburn period may be necessary. Bacteriologic cultures are required to monitor the effect of topical medications. Prudent use and alternation of antimicrobial agents result in less resistant strains of bacteria, greater effectiveness of the agents, and a decreased risk of sepsis.

Before a topical agent is reapplied, the previously applied topical agent must be thoroughly removed. The number of times the dressings are changed and soaked is planned to promote optimal therapeutic use of the topical agent.

Table 57-5 • **Overview of Topical Antibacterial Agents Used for Burn Wounds**

AGENT	INDICATION	APPLICATION	NURSING IMPLICATIONS
Silver sulfadiazine 1% (Silvadene) water-soluble cream	• Most bactericidal agent • Minimal penetration of eschar	Apply 1.6 mm layer of cream with a sterile glove 1–3 times daily.	• Watch for leukopenia 2–3 days after initiation of therapy. (Leukopenia usually resolves within 2–3 days.) • Anticipate formation of pseudoeschar (proteinaceous gel), which is removed easily after 72 hours.
Mafenide acetate 5% to 10% (Sulfamylon) hydrophilic-based cream	• Effective against gram-negative and gram-positive organisms • Diffuses rapidly through eschar • In 10% strength, it is the agent of choice for electrical burns because of its ability to penetrate thick eschar.	Apply thin layer with sterile glove twice a day and leave open as prescribed. Or if the wound is dressed, change the dressing every 6–12 hours as prescribed.	• Monitor arterial blood gas levels and discontinue as prescribed, if acidosis occurs. Mafenide acetate is a strong carbonic anhydrase inhibitor that may reduce renal buffering and cause metabolic acidosis. • Premedicate the patient with an analgesic before applying mafenide acetate because this agent causes severe burning pain for up to 20 minutes after application.
Silver nitrate 0.5% aqueous solution	• Bacteriostatic and fungicidal • Does *not* penetrate eschar	Apply solution to gauze dressing and place over wound. Keep the dressing wet but covered with dry gauze and dry blankets to decrease vaporization. Remoisten every 2 hours, and redress wound twice a day.	• Monitor serum sodium (Na^+) and potassium (K^+) levels and replace as prescribed. Silver nitrate solution is hypotonic and acts as wick for sodium and potassium. • Protect bed linen and clothing from contact with silver nitrate, which stains everything it touches black.
Acticoat	• Effective against gram-negative and gram-positive organisms and some yeasts and molds • Delivers a uniform, antimicrobial concentration of silver to the burn wound	Moisten with sterile water only (*never* use normal saline). Apply directly to wound. Cover with absorbent secondary dressing. Remoisten every 3–4 hours with sterile water.	• Do not use oil-based products or topical antimicrobials with Acticoat burn dressing. Keep Acticoat moist, not saturated. May produce a "pseudoeschar" from silver after application. • Can be left in place for 3–5 days. Now available in Acticoat 7, which can be left in place for up to 7 days without the need to change the dressing.

Wound Dressing

When the wound is clean, the burned areas are patted dry and the prescribed topical agent is applied; the wound is then covered with several layers of dressings. A light dressing is used over joint areas to allow for motion (unless the particular area has a graft and motion is contraindicated). A light dressing is also applied over areas for which a splint has been designed to conform to the body contour for proper positioning. Circumferential dressings should be applied distally to proximally. If the hand or foot is burned, the fingers and toes should be wrapped individually to promote adequate healing.

Burns to the face may be left open to air once they have been cleaned and the topical agent has been applied. Careful attention must be given to burns left exposed to ensure that they do not dry out and convert to a deeper burn.

Close communication and cooperation among the patient, surgeon, nurse, and other health care team members are essential for optimal burn wound care. Different wound areas on a given patient may require a variety of wound care techniques. Diagrams posted at the bedside are useful to inform staff of the current prescription for wound care, splints to be applied over dressings, and the exercise regimen to be followed before dressings are reapplied.

OCCLUSIVE METHOD

There is a role for occlusive dressings in treating specific wounds. An occlusive dressing is a thin gauze that is impregnated with a topical antimicrobial agent or that is applied after topical antimicrobial application. Occlusive dressings are most often used over areas with new skin grafts. Their purpose is to protect the graft, promoting an optimal condition for its adherence to the recipient site. Ideally, these dressings remain in place for 3 to 5 days, at which time they are removed for examination of the graft.

When these dressings are applied, precautions are taken to prevent two body surfaces from touching, such as fingers or toes, ear and scalp, the areas under the breasts, any point of flexion, or between the genital folds. Functional body alignment positions are maintained by using splints or by careful positioning of the patient.

Dressing Changes

Dressings are changed in the patient's unit, hydrotherapy room, or treatment area approximately 20 minutes after an analgesic agent is administered. They may also be changed in the operating room after the patient is anesthetized. A mask, goggles, hair cover, disposable plastic apron or cover gown, and gloves are worn by health care personnel when removing the dressings. The outer dressings are slit with blunt scissors, and the soiled dressings are removed and disposed of in accordance with established procedures for contaminated materials.

Dressings that adhere to the wound can be removed more comfortably if they are moistened with tap water or if the patient is allowed to soak for a few moments in the tub. The remaining dressings are carefully and gently removed. The patient may participate in removing the dressings, providing some degree of control over this painful procedure. The wounds are then cleaned and débrided to remove debris, any remaining topical agent, exudate, and dead skin. Sterile scissors and forceps may be used to trim loose eschar and encourage separation of devitalized skin. During this procedure, the wound and surrounding skin are carefully inspected. The colour, odour, size, exudate, signs of re-epithelialization, and other characteristics of the wound and the eschar and any changes from the previous dressing change are noted.

Wound Débridement

As debris accumulates on the wound surface, it can retard keratinocyte migration, thus delaying the epithelialization process. Débridement, another facet of burn wound care, has two goals:

- To remove tissue contaminated by bacteria and foreign bodies, thereby protecting the patient from invasion of bacteria
- To remove devitalized tissue or burn eschar in preparation for grafting and wound healing

There are three types of débridement—natural, mechanical, and surgical.

NATURAL DÉBRIDEMENT

With natural débridement, the dead tissue separates from the underlying viable tissue spontaneously. After partial- and full-thickness burns, bacteria that are present at the interface of the burned tissue and the viable tissue underneath gradually liquefy the fibrils of **collagen** that hold the eschar in place for the first or second postburn week. Proteolytic and other natural enzymes cause this phenomenon. Using antibacterial topical agents, however, tends to slow this natural process of eschar separation. It is advantageous to the patient to speed this process through other means, such as mechanical or surgical débridement, thereby reducing the time during which bacterial invasion and other iatrogenic problems may arise.

MECHANICAL DÉBRIDEMENT

Mechanical débridement involves using surgical scissors and forceps to separate and remove the eschar. This technique can be performed by skilled physicians, nurses, or physical therapists and is usually done with daily dressing changes and wound cleaning procedures. Débridement by these means is carried out to the point of pain and bleeding. Hemostatic agents or pressure can be used to stop bleeding from small vessels.

Dressings are also useful débriding agents. Coarse-mesh dressings applied dry or wet-to-dry (applied wet and allowed to dry) will slowly débride the wound of exudate and eschar when they are removed. Topical enzymatic débridement agents are available to promote débridement of the burn wounds. Because such agents do not have antimicrobial properties, they should be used with topical antibacterial therapy to protect the patient from bacterial invasion.

SURGICAL DÉBRIDEMENT

Early surgical excision to remove devitalized tissue along with early burn wound closure is now being recognized as one of the most important factors contributing to survival in a patient with a major burn injury. Aggressive surgical wound closure has reduced the incidence of burn wound sepsis, thus improving survival rates (Gibran & Heimbach, 2000). Early excision is carried out before the natural separation of eschar is allowed to occur.

Surgical débridement is an operative procedure involving either primary excision (surgical removal of tissue) of the full thickness of the skin down to the fascia (tangential excision) or shaving the burned skin layers gradually down to freely bleeding, viable tissue. Surgical excision is initiated early in burn wound management. This may be performed a few days after the burn or as soon as the patient is hemodynamically stable and edema has decreased.

Ideally, the wound is then covered immediately with a skin graft, if needed, and an occlusive dressing. If the wound bed is not ready for a skin graft at the time of excision, a temporary biologic dressing may be used until a skin graft can be applied during subsequent surgery.

The use of surgical excision carries with it risks and complications, especially with large burns. The procedure creates a high risk of extensive blood loss (as much as 100 to 125 mL of blood per percent body surface excised) and lengthy operating and anesthesia time. However, when conducted in a timely and efficient manner, surgical excision results in shorter hospital stays and possibly a decreased risk of complications from invasive burn wound sepsis.

Gerontologic Considerations

Eschar separation in full-thickness burns is typically delayed in elderly patients, and older patients are frequently poor risks for surgical excision. Therefore, prolonged hospitalization, immobilization, and associated problems may be common. If the elderly patient can tolerate surgery, early excision with skin grafting is the treatment of choice because it decreases the mortality rate in this population. Prevention of complications of prolonged hospitalization, immobility, and surgery is essential in the care of the elderly burn patient.

Grafting the Burn Wound

If wounds are deep (full-thickness) or extensive, spontaneous re-epithelialization is not possible. Therefore, coverage of the burn wound is necessary until coverage with a graft of the patient's own skin (**autograft**) is possible. The purposes of wound coverage are to decrease the risk for infection; prevent further loss of protein, fluid, and electrolytes through the wound; and minimize heat loss through evaporation. Several methods of wound coverage are available; some are temporary until grafting with permanent coverage is possible. Wound coverage may consist of biologic, biosynthetic, synthetic, and autologous methods or a combination of these approaches.

The main areas for skin grafting include the face (for cosmetic and psychological reasons); functional areas, such as the hands and feet; and areas that involve joints. Grafting permits earlier functional ability and reduces **contractures** (shrinkage of burn scar through collagen maturation). When burns are very extensive, the chest and abdomen may be grafted first to reduce the burn surface.

Granulation tissue fills the space created by the wound, creates a barrier to bacteria, and serves as a bed for epithelial cell growth. Richly vascular granulation tissue is pink, firm, shiny, and free of exudate and debris. It should have a bacterial count of less than 100,000 per gram of tissue to optimize graft take. If the wound is not ready for skin grafting, the burn wound is excised and allowed to granulate. Once the wound is excised, a wound covering is applied to keep the wound bed moist and promote the granulation process.

BIOLOGIC DRESSINGS (HOMOGRAFTS AND HETEROGRAFTS)

Biologic dressings have several uses. In extensive burns, they save lives by providing temporary wound closure and protecting the granulation tissue until autografting is possible. Biologic dressings are commonly used in patients with large areas of burn and little remaining normal skin donor sites. Biologic dressings may also be used to débride wounds after eschar separation. With each biologic dressing change, débridement occurs. Once the biologic dressing appears to be "taking," or adhering to the granulating surface with minimal underlying exudation, the patient is ready for an autograft.

Biologic dressings also provide temporary immediate coverage for clean, superficial burns and decrease the wound's evaporative water and protein loss. They decrease pain by protecting nerve endings and are an effective barrier against water loss and entry of bacteria. When applied to superficial partial-thickness wounds, they seem to speed healing. Biologic materials can be left open or covered. They stay in place for varying lengths of time but are removed in instances of infection or rejection.

Biologic dressings consist of **homografts** (or allografts) and **heterografts** (or xenografts). Homografts are skin obtained from living or recently deceased humans. The amniotic membrane (amnion) from the human placenta may also be used as a biologic dressing. Heterografts consist of skin taken from animals (usually pigs). Most biologic dressings are used as temporary coverings of burn wounds and are eventually rejected because of the body's immune reaction to them as foreign.

Homografts tend to be the most expensive biologic dressings. They are available from skin banks in fresh and cryopreserved (frozen) forms. Homografts are thought to provide the best infection control of all the biologic or biosynthetic dressings available. Revascularization occurs within 48 hours, and the graft may be left in place for several weeks. Cost, availability, and the possibility of transmission of disease limit the use of homografts.

Amnion is less expensive and is available in hospitals with burn centres and specialized tissue banks, which obtain and process it in cooperation with obstetric services. However, amnion grafts do not become vascularized by the patient's vessels and can be left in place only for short periods.

Pigskin is available from commercial suppliers. It is available fresh, frozen, or lyophilized (freeze-dried) for longer shelf life. Pigskin impregnated with a topical antibacterial agent such as silver nitrate is also available. Pigskin is widely used for temporary covering of clean wounds such as superficial partial-thickness wounds and donor sites. Although pigskin does not vascularize, it will adhere to clean superficial wounds and provides excellent pain control while the underlying wound epithelializes.

BIOSYNTHETIC AND SYNTHETIC DRESSINGS

Problems with availability, sterility, and cost have prompted the search for biosynthetic and synthetic skin substitutes, which may eventually replace biologic dressings as temporary wound coverings. Currently the most widely used synthetic dressing is **Biobrane**, which is composed of a nylon, Silastic membrane combined with a collagen derivative. The material is semitransparent and sterile. It has an indefinite shelf life and is less costly than homograft or pigskin. Like biologic dressings, Biobrane protects the wound from fluid loss and bacterial invasion.

Biobrane adheres to the wound fibrin, which binds to the nylon–collagen material. Within 5 days, cells migrate into the nylon mesh. Generally, adherence to the wound surface correlates directly with low bacterial counts. When the Biobrane dressing adheres to the wound, the wound remains stable and the Biobrane can remain in place for 3 to 4 weeks. Biobrane dressings (Fig. 57-4) readily adhere to donor sites and meticulously clean débrided partial-thickness wounds; they will remain until spontaneous epithelialization and wound healing occur. Biobrane can be laid on top of a wide-meshed autograft to protect the wound until the autograft epithelium grows out to close the interstices.

FIGURE 57-4 (**A**) Use of Biobrane dressing for full-thickness burn wound. Biobrane dressing applied to lower extremity partial-thickness burn. (**B**) Healed full-thickness burn wound after use of Biobrane. Used with permission. Bertek Pharmaceuticals, Research Triangle Park, North Carolina.

As the Biobrane gradually separates, it is trimmed, leaving a healed wound.

Biobrane is also useful for intermediate or long-term closure of a surgically excised wound until an autograft becomes available. Like biologic dressings, Biobrane should not be used over grossly contaminated or necrotic wounds. Removal of Biobrane after several weeks is similar to but easier than removal of a vascularized allograft and leaves a bleeding granulation bed that readily accepts an autograft.

Another fairly new temporary wound covering is BCG Matrix. This dressing combines beta-glucan, a complex carbohydrate, with collagen in a meshed reinforced wound dressing. Beta-glucan is known to stimulate macrophages, which are vital in the inflammatory process of healing. BCG Matrix is a temporary wound covering intended for use with partial-thickness burns and donor sites. It is applied immediately after cleaning and débridement. If the burn wound surface remains free of infection, BCG Matrix can be left in place until healing is complete.

Several other synthetic dressings are available for burn wound care. Op-Site, a thin, transparent, polyurethane elastic film, can be used to cover clean partial-thickness wounds and donor sites. This dressing is occlusive and waterproof but permeable to water vapor and air; this permeability not only provides protection from microbial contamination but also allows for the exchange of gases, which occurs much more quickly in a moist environment. Other synthetic dressings used for burn wounds include Tegaderm, N-Terface, and DuoDerm.

Burns that are between superficial and deep partial thickness in depth can be treated with a promising new temporary biologic covering, TransCyte, a material composed of human newborn fibroblasts, which are cultured on the nylon mesh of Biobrane. The thin silicone membrane bonded to the mesh provides a moisture vapor barrier for the wound. TransCyte is used to treat burns in which the depth is indeterminate. TransCyte delivers a variety of biologically active proteins, which may benefit the wound healing process. Research has shown that wounds treated with TransCyte healed more quickly and with less hypertrophic scarring than burns treated with the traditional silver sulfadiazine protocols (Noordenbos, Dore & Hansbrough, 1999).

DERMAL SUBSTITUTES

In an attempt to develop the ideal burn wound covering product, dermal substitutes have been created. Two such products are Integra Artificial Skin and Alloderm.

Artificial skin (**Integra**) is the newest type of dermal substitute. A dermal analog, Integra is composed of two main layers. The epidermal layer, consisting of Silastic, acts as a bacterial barrier and prevents water loss from the dermis. The dermal layer is composed of animal collagen. It interfaces with the open wound surface and allows migration of fibroblasts and capillaries into the material. This "neodermis" becomes a permanent structure. The artificial dermis is biodegraded and reabsorbed. The outer silicone membrane is removed 2 to 3 weeks after application and is replaced with the patient's own skin in the form of a thin epidermal skin graft. Long-term effects of Integra include minimal contracture formation. The graft site is very pliable, almost eliminating the need for repeated cosmetic surgery. Most importantly, Integra has resulted in less hypertrophic scarring (Fig. 57-5), thus eliminating the need for compression devices once the burn wound has healed. The use of Integra is increasing the survivability of burns and improving the functional and cosmetic qualities of the healed burn (Winfrey, Cochran & Hegarty, 1999).

Another promising dermal substitute is **Alloderm**. It is processed dermis from human cadaver skin, which can be used as the dermal layer for skin grafts. When a donor site (the area from which skin is taken to provide a skin graft for another part of the body) is harvested for an autologous skin graft, both the epidermal and dermal layers of skin are removed from the donor site. Alloderm provides a permanent dermal layer replacement. Its use allows the burn surgeon to harvest a thinner skin graft consisting of the epidermal layer only. The patient's epidermal layer is placed directly over the dermal base (Alloderm). The new graft is then treated according to the burn unit's protocol. Use of Alloderm has also resulted in less scarring and contractures with healed grafts; donor sites heal much more quickly than conventional donor sites because only the epidermal layer has been harvested. This is important when donor sites are limited because of extensive burns (Luterman, 2000).

AUTOGRAFTS

Autografts remain the preferred material for definitive burn wound closure following excision. Autografts are the ideal means of covering burn wounds because the grafts are the patient's own skin and thus are not rejected by the patient's immune system. They can be split-thickness, full-thickness, pedicle flaps, or epithelial grafts. Full-thickness and pedicle flaps are commonly used for reconstructive surgery, months or years after the initial injury.

Split-thickness autografts can be applied in sheets or in postage stamp–like pieces, or they can be expanded by meshing so that they can cover 1.5 to 9 times more than a given donor site

FIGURE 57-5 Comparison of Integra template site (right leg) to split thickness autograft site (left leg). Used with permission from Glenn Warden, MD.

area. Skin meshers enable the surgeon to cut tiny slits into a sheet of donor skin, making it possible to cover large areas with smaller amounts of donor skin. These expanded grafts adhere to the recipient site more easily than sheet grafts and prevent the accumulation of blood, serum, air, or purulent material under the graft. However, any kind of graft other than a sheet graft will contribute to scar formation as it heals. Using expanded grafts may be necessary in large wounds but should be viewed as a compromise in terms of cosmesis.

If blood, serum, air, fat, or necrotic tissue lies between the recipient site and the graft, there may be partial or total loss of the graft. Infection and mishandling of the graft, as well as trauma during dressing changes, account for most other instances of graft loss. Using split-thickness grafts allows the remaining donor site to retain sweat glands and hair follicles and minimizes donor site healing time.

Use of **cultured epithelial autograft** (CEA) is common at several burn centres. This involves a biopsy of the patient's skin in an unburned area. Keratinocytes are then isolated and epithelial cells are cultured in a laboratory. The original epithelial cell sample can multiply to 10,000 times its original size over 30 days. These cells are then attached to the burn wound. Varying degrees of success have been reported, and results are encouraging. However, the disadvantages of the CEA are that the grafts are thin and fragile and can shear easily. Research has shown that the outcomes of use of CEA are not as positive as once thought. The quality of burn scars is better, but patients have longer hospital stays and higher hospital costs and require more surgical procedures than those treated by traditional methods. In addition, patients require more reconstructive procedures in the first 1 to 2 years postinjury. Therefore, CEA use is very limited and reserved for burn patients whose donor sites are limited (Noordenbos et al., 1999).

Care of the Patient with an Autograft. Occlusive dressings are commonly used initially after grafting to immobilize the graft. Occupational therapists may be helpful in constructing splints to immobilize newly grafted areas to prevent dislodging the graft. Homografts, heterografts, or synthetic dressings may also be used to protect grafts. The graft may be left open with skin staples to immobilize it, which allows close observation of progress.

The first dressing change is usually performed 3 to 5 days after surgery, or earlier in the case of purulent drainage or a foul odour. If the graft is dislodged, sterile saline compresses will help prevent drying of the graft until the physician reapplies it.

The patient is positioned and turned carefully to avoid disturbing the graft or putting pressure on the graft site. If an extremity has been grafted, it is elevated to minimize edema. The patient begins exercising the grafted area 5 to 7 days after grafting.

Care of Donor Site. A moist gauze dressing is applied at the time of surgery to maintain pressure and to stop any oozing. A thrombostatic agent such as thrombin or epinephrine may be applied directly to the site as well. The donor site may be treated in several ways, from single-layer gauze impregnated with petrolatum, scarlet red, or bismuth to new biosynthetic dressings such as Biobrane or BCG Matrix. Some burn centres are using the Acticoat dressing on donor sites. Despite the type of donor site covering, donor sites must remain clean, dry, and free from pressure. Because a donor site is usually a partial-thickness wound, it will heal spontaneously within 7 to 14 days with proper care. Donor sites are painful, and additional pain management must be a part of the patient's care.

Pain Management

Pain is inevitable during recovery from any burn injury. Pain in the burn patient has been described as a tormenting consequence of burn injury and wound healing (Jonsson, Holmsten, Dahlstrom & Jonsson, 1998). Burn pain is thought to have both nociceptive and neuropathic pain components. Management of the often-severe pain is one of the most difficult challenges facing the burn team. Many factors contribute to the burn patient's pain experience. These factors include but are not limited to the severity of the pain, the adequacy of the health care provider's assessment of the pain, the appropriateness and adequacy of pharmacologic treatment of pain, the multiple procedures involved in burn care (ie, wound care, rehabilitative exercises), and appropriate evaluation of the effectiveness of pain relief measures. The outstanding features of burn pain are its intensity and long duration. Further, necessary wound care carries with it the anticipation of pain and anxiety.

In partial-thickness burns, the nerve endings are exposed, resulting in excruciating pain with exposure to air currents. Although nerve endings are destroyed in full-thickness burns, the margins of the burn wound are hypersensitive to pain, and there is pain in adjacent structures. Healing of full-thickness burns creates significant discomfort as regenerating nerve endings become entrapped in scar formation. Most severe burns are a combination of partial-thickness and full-thickness burns.

Burn patients have been described as having three types of pain: background or resting pain, procedural pain, and breakthrough pain. Background pain is pain that exists on a 24-hour basis. Procedural pain is pain caused by procedures such as burn wound care or range of motion exercises. Breakthrough pain occurs when blood levels of analgesic agents fall below the level required to control background pain. The patient's pain level must be assessed throughout the day because each type of pain is different and various pain management strategies may be needed to address different types of pain (McCaffrey & Pasaro, 1999).

The primary pain from the burn itself is intense in the initial acute postburn phase. In the next few weeks thereafter, until the skin heals or skin grafts are applied and heal, the pain intensity remains high because of treatment-induced pain. Wound cleaning, dressing changes, débridement, and physical therapy can all cause intense pain. Donor sites may be intensely painful for several days. Discomfort related to tissue healing, such as itching, tingling, and tightness of contracting skin and joints, adds to the duration, if not the intensity, of pain over weeks or months. Because pain cannot be eliminated short of complete anesthesia, the goal is to minimize the pain with analgesic agents to an acceptable goal set by the patient.

Opioid administration via the intravenous (IV) route, particularly in the emergent and acute phases of burn management, remains the mainstay for pharmacologic management of burn pain. Use of opioids is complicated by the fluctuation in the bioavailability of drugs, protein binding of the drug, and the drug clearance related to the hemodynamic and fluid volume shifts that occur with a burn injury. Absorption of the opioid also may be affected. Titrating analgesic agents to obtain pain relief while minimizing side effects is crucial. The burn patient's requirements for analgesia are often high, but fear of addiction on the part of the patient and health care provider hamper adequate opioid administration.

Morphine sulfate remains the analgesic of choice for treatment of acute burn pain. It is titrated to obtain pain relief based on the patient's self-report of pain using a standardized pain rating scale.

Fentanyl is another useful opioid for burn pain, particularly procedural burn pain. It has been shown to be effective for management of intense pain of short duration. Fentanyl has a rapid onset, high potency, and short duration, all of which make it effective for use with burn wound procedures. Appropriate cardiac and respiratory monitoring must be carried out during its administration.

Patient-controlled analgesia (PCA), in which a pump is used to self-administer a continuous infusion of an opioid, maintains a steady level of opioid for pain relief. Use of continuous infusion requires close monitoring of the patient's responses.

Sustained-release opioids, such as MS Contin or oxycodone (OxyContin), have also been used successfully in the treatment of burn pain. These medications can effectively treat the resting pain that is often associated with burn injury. Additional medications must be prescribed with these medications to cover breakthrough pain.

Some burn units use self-administered nitrous oxide during burn wound procedures. Proper ventilation and monitoring equipment and availability of qualified personnel to administer nitrous oxide limit its use.

Short-acting anesthetic agents (eg, propofol), that cause conscious sedation or general anesthesia, are being used for the management of procedural pain associated with major dressing changes and initial surgical dressing removal. Anesthetic agents are given in combination with narcotic analgesics by a qualified anesthetist. Continuous patient cardiac monitoring is required, with emergency resuscitation equipment readily at hand.

Anxiety and pain go hand in hand for burn patients. The entire burn experience can produce severe anxiety, which can, in turn, exacerbate pain. Therefore, the ideal pain management regimen must incorporate the treatment of pain and anxiety and must be individualized for each patient. Sedation with anxiolytic medications such as lorazepam (Ativan) and midazolam (Versed) may be indicated in addition to the administration of opioids.

The use of nonpharmacologic measures has also proven effective in the management of burn pain. These measures include relaxation techniques, deep breathing exercises, distraction, guided imagery, hypnosis, therapeutic touch, humour, information giving, and music therapy (McCaffrey & Pasaro, 1999).

Music therapy has gained interest recently in the treatment of pain. Researchers have found that music affects both the physiologic and psychological aspects of the pain experience. Music diverts the patient's attention from the painful stimulus; provides reality orientation, distraction, and sensory stimulation; and allows for patient self-expression (Fratianne et al., 2001; Prensner et al., 2001).

Nutritional Support

Burn injuries produce profound metabolic abnormalities fueled by the exaggerated stress response to the injury. The body's response has been classified as hyperdynamic, hypermetabolic, and hypercatabolic. Hypermetabolism can affect morbidity and mortality by increasing the risk of infection and slowing the healing rate. Patients' metabolic demands vary with the extent of the burn injury. Hypermetabolism is evident immediately after a burn injury. The degree of the response depends on the size of the burn and the patient's age, body composition, size, and genetic response to insult. Persistent hypermetabolism may last up to 1 year after burn injury (Hart et al., 2000).

Major metabolic abnormalities seen after a burn injury include increased catabolic hormones (cortisol and catechols); decreased anabolic hormones (human growth factor and testosterone); a marked increase in the metabolic rate; a sustained increase in body temperature; a marked increase in glucose demands; rapid skeletal muscle breakdown with amino acids serving as the energy source; lack of ketosis, indicating that fat is not a major source of calories; and catabolism that does not respond to nutrient intake (Demling & Seigne, 2000). Metabolic measures using indirect calorimetry provide more accurate assessments of energy expenditure and caloric demand. Therefore, it is essential to control the stress response by increasing the anabolic process through adequate nutrition and increased muscle activity, decreasing heat loss from wounds, and maintaining a warm environment. Controlling secondary stress, such as pain and anxiety, also helps to control the stress response.

The most important of these interventions is to provide adequate nutrition and calories to decrease catabolism. Nutritional support with optimized protein intake can decrease protein losses by approximately 50% (Cioffi, 2000). Healing of the burn wound consumes large quantities of energy. Effective nutrition management depends on how well the energy expenditure due to the burn injury can be estimated and matched with appropriate amounts of micronutrients, carbohydrates, lipids, and protein. The goal of nutritional support is to promote a state of positive nitrogen balance by optimizing nutrition to match nutrient utilization. The nutritional support required is based on the patient's preburn status and the TBSA burned.

Several formulas exist for estimating the daily metabolic expenditure and caloric requirements of patients with burn injuries. The most commonly used formulas include the Curreiri formula, which uses body weight and percent burn, and a variation of the Harris-Bennedict equation, which determines basal energy requirements based on stress and burn size (Demling & Seigne, 2000). Protein requirements may range from 1.5 to 4.0 g of protein per kilogram of body weight every 24 hours. Lipids are included in the nutritional support of every burn patient because of their importance for wound healing, cellular integrity, and absorption of fat-soluble vitamins. Carbohydrates are included to meet caloric requirements as high as 5,000 calories per day and to spare protein, which is essential for wound healing. The patient also needs adequate vitamins and minerals. Existing formulas may underestimate the daily metabolic expenditures associated with burns. The formulas fail to account for added stressors such as pain, anxiety, daily dressing changes, and decreased activity levels. These must be considered when estimating appropriate nutritional support. Research findings have brought about changes in specific guidelines for estimating energy expenditure during the various phases of postburn recovery. The proportions of fat, protein, and carbohydrate must be carefully planned for maximal use (Demling & Seigne, 2000).

The enteral route of feeding is far superior to the parenteral route. Enteral feedings preserve the intestinal barrier function and absorption of peptides and amino acids, which leads to higher nitrogen retention. Feedings are started as soon as possible. If a feeding tube is used, placement into the duodenum is ideal to prevent aspiration and to allow for continuous, uninterrupted feedings during surgical procedures. If the oral route is used, high-protein, high-calorie meals and supplements are given. Dietary consultations are useful in helping patients meet their nutritional needs. Daily calorie counts aid in assessing the adequacy of nutritional intake. Overfeeding must be avoided because it increases metabolism, O_2 consumption, and CO_2 production.

Patients lose a great deal of weight during recovery from severe burns. Reserve fat deposits are catabolized, fluids are lost, and caloric intake may be limited. Because a burn injury lowers the patient's resistance to infection and disease, the nutritional status must be improved and maintained although the patient has a poor appetite and is weak.

Indications for parenteral nutrition include weight loss greater than 10% of normal body weight, inadequate intake of enteral nutrition due to clinical status, prolonged wound exposure, and malnutrition or debilitated condition before injury. The risk of infection at the site of the central venous catheter required for parenteral nutrition must be considered. Moreover, the risk of Curling's ulcer continues in the acute phase.

DISORDERS OF WOUND HEALING

Disorders of wound healing in the burn patient result from excessive abnormal healing or inadequate new tissue formation. Hypertrophic scarring and keloid formation result from excessive abnormal healing.

Scars

One of the most devastating sequelae of a burn injury is the formation of **hypertrophic scars**. Clinicians cannot reliably predict or prevent the formation of hypertrophic scars. Hypertrophic scars are more common in children, in people with dark skin, and in areas of stretch or motion. The pathophysiology behind these scars is not completely understood, but they are characterized by an overabundant matrix formation, especially collagen.

Hypertrophic scars and wound contractures are more likely to occur if the initial burn injury extends below the level of the deep dermis. Healing of such deep wounds results in the replacement of normal integument with highly metabolically active tissues that lack the normal architecture of the skin. In the collagen layer beneath the epithelium, many fibroblasts proliferate gradually. Myofibroblasts, cells that have the ability to contract, are also present in immature wounds. As the myofibroblasts contract, the collagen fibres, which normally lie in flat bundles, tend to form a wavy pattern. Eventually the collagen bundles take on a super-coiled appearance and collagen nodules develop. The scar becomes red (because of its hypervascular nature), raised, and hard.

Burn personnel must be proactive in the prevention and management of scar formation. Compression measures are instituted early in burn wound treatment. Ace wraps are used initially to help promote adequate circulation, but they can also be used as the first form of compression. Scar management occurs mainly in the rehabilitative phase, after the wounds are closed. Hypertrophic scarring may cause severe contracture across involved joints. Therefore, prevention and management of this type of scarring is essential (see "Prevention of Hypertrophic Scarring" in the rehabilitation phase discussion). However, these scars are limited to the area of injury and gradually regress over time.

Keloids

A large, heaped-up mass of scar tissue, a keloid, may develop and extend beyond the wound surface. Keloids tend to be found in people with darkly pigmented skin, tend to grow outside of wound margins, and are likely to recur after surgical excision.

Failure to Heal

Failure of the wound to heal may result from many factors, including infection and inadequate nutrition. A serum albumin level of less than 2 g/dL is usually a factor in impaired healing in the burn patient.

Contractures

Contractures are another concern as wounds heal. The burn wound tissue shortens because of the force exerted by the fibroblasts and the flexion of muscles in natural wound healing. An opposing force provided by splints, traction, and purposeful movement and positioning must be used to counteract deformity in burns affecting joints.

NURSING PROCESS: CARE OF THE PATIENT DURING THE ACUTE PHASE

Assessment

Continued assessment of the burn patient during the early weeks after the burn injury focuses on hemodynamic alterations, wound healing, pain and psychosocial responses, and early detection of complications. Assessment of respiratory and fluid status remains the highest priority for detection of potential complications.

The nurse assesses vital signs frequently. Continued assessment of peripheral pulses is essential for the first few postburn days while edema continues to increase, potentially damaging peripheral nerves and restricting blood flow. Observation of the electrocardiogram may give clues to cardiac dysrhythmias resulting from potassium imbalance, preexisting cardiac disease, or the effects of electrical injury or burn shock.

Assessment of residual gastric volumes and pH in the patient with a nasogastric tube is also important. Blood in the gastric fluid or the stools must also be noted and reported.

Assessment of the burn wound requires an experienced eye, hand, and sense of smell. Important wound assessment features include size, colour, odour, eschar, exudate, abscess formation under the eschar, epithelial buds (small pearl-like clusters of cells on the wound surface), bleeding, granulation tissue appearance, status of grafts and donor sites, and quality of surrounding skin. Any significant changes in the wound are reported to the physician, because they usually indicate burn wound or systemic sepsis and require immediate intervention.

Other significant and ongoing assessments focus on pain and psychosocial responses, daily body weights, caloric intake, general hydration, and serum electrolyte, hemoglobin, and hematocrit levels. Assessment for excessive bleeding from blood vessels adjacent to areas of surgical exploration and débridement is necessary as well. The Plan of Nursing Care provides an outline of nursing activities in the acute phase of burn care.

Diagnosis

NURSING DIAGNOSES

Based on the assessment data, priority nursing diagnoses in the acute phase of burn care may include the following:

- Excessive fluid volume related to resumption of capillary integrity and fluid shift from the interstitial to intravascular compartment
- Risk for infection related to loss of skin barrier and impaired immune response
- Imbalanced nutrition, less than body requirements, related to hypermetabolism and wound healing needs
- Impaired skin integrity related to open burn wounds
- Acute pain related to exposed nerves, wound healing, and treatments

- Impaired physical mobility related to burn wound edema, pain, and joint contractures
- Ineffective coping related to fear and anxiety, grieving, and forced dependence on health care providers
- Interrupted family processes related to burn injury
- Deficient knowledge about the course of burn treatment

COLLABORATIVE PROBLEMS/ POTENTIAL COMPLICATIONS

Based on the assessment data, potential complications that may develop in the acute phase of burn care may include:

- Heart failure and pulmonary edema
- Sepsis
- Acute respiratory failure
- Acute respiratory distress syndrome
- Visceral damage (electrical burns)

Planning and Goals

The major goals for the patient may include restoration of normal fluid balance, absence of infection, attainment of anabolic state and normal weight, improved skin integrity, reduction of pain and discomfort, optimal physical mobility, adequate patient and family coping, adequate patient and family knowledge of burn treatment, and absence of complications. Achieving these goals requires a collaborative, interdisciplinary approach to patient management.

Nursing Interventions

RESTORING NORMAL FLUID BALANCE

To reduce the risk of fluid overload and consequent congestive heart failure, the nurse closely monitors IV and oral fluid intake, using IV infusion pumps to minimize the risk of rapid fluid infusion. To monitor changes in fluid status, careful intake and output and daily weights are obtained. Changes in pulmonary artery, wedge, and central venous pressures, as well as in blood pressure and pulse rate, are reported to the physician. Low-dose dopamine to increase renal perfusion and diuretics may be prescribed to promote increased urine output. The nurse's role is to administer these medications as prescribed and to monitor the patient's response.

PREVENTING INFECTION

A major part of the nurse's role during the acute phase of burn care is detecting and preventing infection. The nurse is responsible for providing a clean and safe environment and for closely scrutinizing the burn wound to detect early signs of infection. Culture results and white blood cell counts are monitored.

Clean technique is used for wound care procedures. Aseptic technique is used for any invasive procedures, such as insertion of IV lines and urinary catheters or tracheal suctioning. Meticulous hand hygiene before and after each patient contact is also an essential component of preventing infection, even though gloves are worn to provide care.

The nurse protects the patient from sources of contamination, including other patients, staff members, visitors, and equipment. Invasive lines and tubing must be routinely changed according to recommendations of the Centers for Disease Control and Prevention. Tube feeding reservoirs, ventilator circuits, and drainage containers are replaced regularly. Fresh flowers, plants, or fresh

(text continues on page 1741)

Plan of Nursing Care
Care of the Patient During the Acute Phase of Burn Injury

Nursing Interventions	Rationale	Expected Outcomes

Nursing Diagnosis: Fluid volume excess related to resumption of capillary integrity and fluid shift from interstitial to intravascular compartment

Goal: Maintenance of optimal fluid balance

Nursing Interventions	Rationale	Expected Outcomes
1. Monitor vital signs, intake and output, weight. Assess for edema, jugular vein distention (JVD), crackles, increased arterial pressures.	1. These signs reflect fluid status.	• Intake, output, and body weight correlate with expected pattern
2. Notify physician of urine output <30 mL/hr, weight gain, JVD, crackles, increased arterial pressures.	2. These indicate increased fluid volume.	• Vital signs and arterial pressures remain within designated limits
3. Maintain intravenous fluids on pumps or rate controllers.	3. Regulation prevents unintentional fluid bolus.	• Urine output increases in response to diuretic and vasoactive medications
4. Administer dopamine or diuretics as prescribed. Assess response.	4. Dopamine increases renal perfusion, which increases urine output. Diuretics promote increased urine formation and urine output and decrease intravascular volume.	

Nursing Diagnosis: Risk for infection related to loss of skin barrier and impaired immune response

Goal: Absence of localized or systemic infection

Nursing Interventions	Rationale	Expected Outcomes
1. Use asepsis in all aspects of patient care: a. Meticulous hand hygiene before and after patient care. b. Use clean or sterile gloves for wound care. c. Wear isolation gown or protective plastic apron for patient care. d. Wear mask and hair cover when wounds are exposed and during sterile procedures. e. Change invasive lines and tubings as recommended by CDC.	1. Aseptic techniques minimize risk of cross-contamination and spread of bacterial contamination.	• Wound cultures show minimal bacteria • Negative blood, urine, and sputum cultures • Urine output and vital signs within acceptable range • Absence of signs and symptoms of infection and sepsis
2. Screen visitors for respiratory, gastrointestinal, or integumentary infections. Provide isolation gowns for visitors without active infection and instruct in hand hygiene.	2. Avoiding known infecting agents prevents introduction of additional microorganisms.	
3. Exclude plants and flowers in water from patient's room.	3. Stagnant water is a potential source of bacterial growth.	
4. Inspect wound for signs of infection, purulent drainage, or discolouration.	4. Such signs indicate localized infection.	
5. Monitor white blood cell (WBC) count, culture and sensitivity results.	5. Increased WBC count indicates infection. Culture and sensitivity indicate microorganisms present and appropriate antibiotics to be used.	
6. Administer antibiotics as prescribed.	6. Antibiotics reduce bacteria.	
7. Provide regular linen changes and assist patient with personal hygiene.	7. These measures reduce potential bacterial colonization of burn wound.	
8. Report to physician decreased bowel sounds, tachycardia, decreased blood pressure, decreased urine output, fever, and flushing, confusion or sudden disorientation.	8. These signs may indicate sepsis.	
9. Administer fluids and vasoactive medications as prescribed. Assess response.	9. These agents are used to maintain tissue perfusion in sepsis.	

(continued)

Plan of Nursing Care

Care of the Patient During the Acute Phase of Burn Injury (Continued)

Nursing Interventions	Rationale	Expected Outcomes

Nursing Diagnosis: Altered nutrition, less than body requirements, related to hypermetabolism and wound healing
Goal: Attainment of anabolic nutritional status

1. Provide high-calorie, high-protein diet; include patient preferences and home-made food. Provide nutritional supplements as prescribed.	1. The patient needs sufficient nutrients for wound healing and increased metabolic requirements.	• Gains weight daily after initial loss • Exhibits no signs of protein, vitamin, or mineral deficiencies • Meets required nutritional needs entirely by oral intake • Participates in selection of diet with prescribed nutrients • Serum protein levels within acceptable range
2. Monitor patient's daily weight and calorie count.	2. These measures assist in determining whether dietary needs are being met.	
3. Administer supplemental vitamins and minerals as prescribed.	3. These help meet additional nutritional needs; adequate vitamins and minerals are necessary for wound healing and cellular function.	
4. Administer enteral or parenteral nutrition per protocol if dietary needs are not met through oral intake.	4. Nutritional techniques ensure that nutritional needs are met.	
5. Report abdominal distention, large gastric residual volumes, or diarrhea to physician.	5. These signs may indicate intolerance of route or type of feeding.	

Nursing Diagnosis: Impaired skin integrity related to open burn wounds
Goal: Demonstration of improved skin integrity

1. Clean wounds, body, and hair daily.	1. Daily cleaning reduces potential bacterial colonization.	• Skin is generally intact, and free of signs of infection, pressure, and trauma • Open wounds are pink, reepithelializing, and free of infection • Donor sites are clean and reepithelializing • Healed wounds are soft and smooth • Skin is lubricated and elastic
2. Provide wound care as prescribed.	2. Care promotes wound healing.	
3. Apply topical antibacterial agents and dressing as prescribed.	3. Wound care regimen reduces bacterial colonization and promotes healing.	
4. Prevent pressure, infection, and mobilization of skin grafts.	4. These measures promote graft take and healing.	
5. Provide donor site care.	5. Care promotes healing of donor site.	
6. Provide adequate nutritional support.	6. Adequate nutrition is essential for normal granulation and healing.	
7. Assess wound and graft sites. Report signs of poor healing, poor graft take, or trauma to physician.	7. Early intervention for poor wound healing or graft take is essential. Grafted or healed burn wounds are susceptible to trauma.	

Nursing Diagnosis: Pain related to exposed nerves, wound healing, and treatments
Goal: Reduction or control of pain

1. Assess pain level using pain intensity scale. Observe for nonverbal indicators of pain: grimacing, tachycardia, clenched fists.	1. Pain assessment data provide baseline for assessing response to interventions.	• Requests analgesics for specific wound care procedures or physical therapy activities • States pain is minimal • Gives no physiologic or nonverbal cues of moderate or severe pain • Uses pain control measures such as nitrous oxide, relaxation, imagery, and distraction techniques to assist with coping with pain • Can sleep without being disturbed by pain • Reports skin is comfortable with no itching or tightness
2. Educate the patient about the usual pain trajectory in burn recovery and options for pain control. Allow patient as much control as possible regarding pain management.	2. Knowledge reduces fear of the unknown and provides some measure of control to the patient.	
3. Offer analgesics approximately 20 minutes before painful procedures.	3. Premedication allows time for therapeutic response.	
4. Provide analgesia before pain becomes severe.	4. Pain is more easily controlled before it becomes severe.	
5. Instruct and assist patient in relaxation, imagery, distraction techniques.	5. Nonpharmacologic pain measures provide multiple interventions to decrease pain sensation.	

(continued)

Plan of Nursing Care
Care of the Patient During the Acute Phase of Burn Injury *(Continued)*

Nursing Interventions	Rationale	Expected Outcomes
6. Assess and document the patient's response to interventions.	6. Patient's responses assist in ascertaining best pain control techniques for the patient.	
7. Administer antianxiety and antipruritic agents as indicated.	7. These medications help to increase patient's comfort.	
8. Lubricate healing burn wounds with water- or silica-based lotion.	8. These preparations decrease sensation of skin tightness.	

Nursing Diagnosis: Impaired physical mobility related to burn wound edema, pain, and joint contractures
Goal: Achievement of optimal physical mobility

1. Position patient carefully to prevent flexed position in burned areas.	1. Proper positioning reduces risk of flexion contractures.	• Improves range of motion of joints daily • Demonstrates preinjury range of motion of all joints
2. Implement range-of-motion (ROM) exercises several times daily.	2. ROM exercises minimize muscle atrophy.	• Absence of signs of periarticular calcification
3. Assist with early sitting and ambulation.	3. Early mobility encourages increased use of muscles.	• Participates in activities of daily living
4. Use splints and exercise devices recommended by occupational and physical therapists.	4. Such devices encourage activity while maintaining proper position of joints.	
5. Encourage self-care to the extent of the patient's ability.	5. Self-care promotes both independence and increased activity.	

Nursing Diagnosis: Ineffective individual coping related to fear and anxiety, grieving, and forced dependence on health care providers
Goal: Use of appropriate coping strategies to deal with postburn problems

1. Assess patient for coping abilities and previous successful coping strategies.	1. Psychosocial data provide baseline for planning care.	• Verbalizes reactions to burns, therapeutic procedures, losses
2. Demonstrate acceptance of patient. Provide positive feedback and support.	2. Acceptance encourages self-esteem and continued progress toward independence.	• Identifies effective coping strategies used previously in stressful situations
3. Assist patient to set achievable short-term goals for increased independence in activities of daily living.	3. Short-term goal setting leads to pattern of success for patient. Long-term goals may seem unrealistic or unattainable to patient.	• Accepts dependency on health care providers during acute illness • Resolves grief over losses resulting from burn injury
4. Use multidisciplinary approach to promote mobility and independence.	4. Communication among disciplines provides consistent approach.	• Participates in decision making regarding care
5. Consult with health care team members for assistance with regressive or maladaptive behaviours.	5. Collaboration uses the expertise of others.	• Has hopeful attitude toward future

Nursing Diagnosis: Altered family processes related to burn injury
Goal: Achievement of appropriate patient/family processes

1. Assess patient and family's perception of impact of burn injury on family functioning.	1. Assessment data provide baseline from which to plan care.	• Patient verbalizes feelings regarding alteration in family interactions
2. Demonstrate willingness to listen. Provide realistic support.	2. Empathetic attitude promotes verbalizing of concerns.	• Family can emotionally support the patient during hospitalization
3. Refer family to social services and other resources as needed.	3. Collaboration assists to address concerns comprehensively.	• Family states that needs are met
4. Explain the burn patient's coping patterns to family. Discuss ways that they can support the patient.	4. Explanations help decrease anxiety about the unknown and promote appropriate support of patient by family.	

(continued)

Plan of Nursing Care

Care of the Patient During the Acute Phase of Burn Injury (Continued)

Nursing Interventions	Rationale	Expected Outcomes

Nursing Diagnosis: Knowledge deficit about the course of burn treatment
Goal: Verbalization of understanding of the course of burn treatment by patient and family

Nursing Interventions	Rationale	Expected Outcomes
1. Assess readiness of patient and family to learn.	1. Limit education to patient's and family's ability to process information.	• States rationale for different aspects of treatment
2. Explore patient's and family's previous experience with hospitalization and illness.	2. This information provides a baseline for explanations and indication of patient's and family's expectations.	• States realistic time period for recovery • Patient and family participate in management plans as appropriate
3. Review general course of burn treatment with patient and family.	3. Knowing what to expect prepares patient and family for upcoming events.	
4. Explain importance of patient participation in care for optimal results.	4. This information provides specific direction to patient.	
5. Realistically explain length of time involved in burn recovery.	5. Honesty promotes realistic expectations.	

Collaborative Problems: Congestive heart failure, pulmonary edema, sepsis, acute respiratory failure, ARDS, visceral damage (electrical burns)
Goal: Absence of complications

Congestive Heart Failure (CHF) and Pulmonary Edema

Nursing Interventions	Rationale	Expected Outcomes
1. Assess for decreased urine output, JVD, or an S_3 or S_4 heart sound.	1. These signs may indicate decreased cardiac output and the onset of CHF.	• Lungs clear to auscultation
2. Monitor for increases in arterial pressures or decrease in cardiac output.	2. Increased pressures indicate increased preload and intravascular volumes. Decreasing cardiac output reflects less oxygen and nutrients available to the tissues and may indicate the onset of CHF.	• Absence of dyspnea, orthopnea, JVD, and S_3 or S_4 heart sounds • Urine output, arterial pressures, and cardiac output within normal limits
3. Assess for crackles on lung auscultation, dyspnea, orthopnea, or decreased oxygenation detected by pulse oximetry or arterial blood gas values.	3. Such signs may indicate progression of CHF to pulmonary edema.	
4. Report the above mentioned signs and symptoms to the physician.	4. Prompt medical intervention is needed.	
5. Position patient with the head of bed up 45° to 90° as tolerated.	5. Elevation facilitates gas exchange.	
6. Administer diuretics as prescribed. Assess patient's response.	6. Diuretics increase urine output and decrease cardiac preload and intravascular volumes.	

Sepsis

Nursing Interventions	Rationale	Expected Outcomes
1. Assess for fever, increased pulse, widened pulse pressure, and flushed, dry skin in unburned areas. Watch trends and notify physician if noted.	1. Such signs may indicate impending sepsis.	• Negative blood, sputum, and urine cultures
2. Monitor wound and blood cultures and notify physician of positive cultures.	2. Positive cultures indicate infection and possible sepsis.	• Absence of tachycardia, widening pulse pressure, and flushed, dry skin in unburned areas
3. Administer fluids, vasoactive medications and antibiotics as prescribed. Monitor for therapeutic response. Check that infecting organisms are sensitive to prescribed antibiotics.	3. Antibiotics kill susceptible bacteria. Intravenous fluids and vasoactive medications maintain intravascular volume and blood pressure.	
4. Monitor for therapeutic serum antibiotic levels.	4. Antibiotics are most effective at therapeutic levels. Excessive levels can cause organ damage.	

(continued)

Plan of Nursing Care
Care of the Patient During the Acute Phase of Burn Injury *(Continued)*

Nursing Interventions	Rationale	Expected Outcomes
Acute Respiratory Failure/ARDS 1. Assess for respiratory distress, changes in respiratory patterns, or onset of adventitious breath sounds. Report to physician. 2. Monitor pulse oximetry and arterial blood gas levels for decreasing oxygen saturation and PO_2. Report to physician. 3. Monitor the mechanically ventilated patient for decreased spontaneous tidal volumes and lung compliance. 4. In collaboration with the physician and respiratory therapist, administer positive end-expiratory pressure and pressure support. Assess patient's response.	1. Such problems indicate possible acute respiratory failure. Pulmonary complications may not appear for 24 to 48 hours after the burn injury. 2. Decreasing oxygenation indicates deteriorating respiratory status. Medical intervention is needed. 3. Respiratory problems reflect increased difficulty with ventilation and may indicate the onset of ARDS. 4. These measures optimize diffusion of oxygen across the alveolar capillary membrane.	• Arterial blood gases within normal limits • Normal lung compliance • Absence of respiratory distress • Improved PO_2 level
Visceral Damage (Electrical Burns) 1. Assess patient for signs of deep pain. Focus on areas between entrance and exit wounds of burn. 2. Monitor ECG rhythm. 3. Report to the physician any complaints of deep pain or dysrhythmias.	1. Pain may reflect visceral damage. 2. The patient with electrical burns is at risk for dysrhythmias. 3. Visceral damage requires immediate intervention.	• Absence of visceral organ damage • Stable cardiac rhythm

fruit baskets are not permitted in the patient's room because of the risk of microorganism growth. Visitors are screened to avoid exposing the immunocompromised burn patient to pathogens.

Patients can inadvertently promote migration of microorganisms from one burned area to another by touching their wounds or dressings. Bed linens also can spread infection through either colonization with wound microorganisms or fecal contamination. Regularly bathing unburned areas and changing linens can help prevent infection.

MAINTAINING ADEQUATE NUTRITION

Oral fluids should be initiated slowly when bowel sounds resume. The patient's tolerance is noted. If vomiting and distention do not occur, fluids may be increased gradually and the patient may advance to a normal diet or to tube feedings.

The nurse collaborates with the dietitian or nutrition support team to plan a protein- and calorie-rich diet that is acceptable to the patient. Family members may be encouraged to bring nutritious and favourite foods to the hospital. Milkshakes and sandwiches made with meat, peanut butter, and cheese may be offered as snacks between meals and late in the evening. Nutritional supplements such as Ensure and Resource may be provided. Caloric intake must be documented. Vitamin and mineral supplements may be prescribed.

If caloric goals cannot be met by oral feeding, a feeding tube is inserted and used for continuous or bolus feedings of specific formulas. The volume of residual gastric secretions should be checked to ensure absorption. Parenteral nutrition may also be required but should be used only if gastrointestinal function is compromised (see Chap. 36).

Patients should be weighed each day and their weights graphed. Patients can use this information to set goals for their own nutritional intake and to monitor weight loss and gain. Ideally, the patient will lose no more than 5% of preburn weight if aggressive nutritional management is implemented.

The patient with anorexia requires encouragement and support from the nurse to increase food intake. The patient's surroundings should be as pleasant as possible at mealtime. Catering to food preferences and offering high-protein, high-vitamin snacks are ways of encouraging the patient to increase intake.

PROMOTING SKIN INTEGRITY

Wound care is usually the single most time-consuming element of burn care after the emergent phase. The physician will prescribe the desired topical antibacterial agents and specific biologic, biosynthetic, or synthetic wound coverings and will plan for surgical excision and grafting. The nurse needs to make astute assessments of wound status, to use creative approaches to wound dressing, and to support the patient during the emotionally distressing and very painful experience of wound care.

The nurse serves as the coordinator of the complex aspects of wound care and dressing changes for the patient. The nurse must be aware of the rationale and nursing implications for the various wound management approaches. Nursing functions include assessing and recording any changes or progress in wound healing and keeping all members of the health care team informed of changes in the wound or treatment. A diagram, updated daily by the nurse responsible for the patient's care, helps to inform all those concerned about the latest wound care procedures in use for the patient.

The nurse also assists the patient and family by providing instruction, support, and encouragement to take an active part in dressing changes and wound care when appropriate. Discharge planning needs for wound care are anticipated early in the course of burn management, and the strengths of the patient and family are assessed and used in preparing for eventual discharge and home care.

RELIEVING PAIN AND DISCOMFORT

Pain measures discussed earlier are continued during the acute phase of burn recovery. Analgesic agents and anxiolytic medications are administered as prescribed. Frequent assessment of pain and discomfort is essential. To increase its effectiveness, analgesic medication is provided before the pain becomes severe. Nursing interventions such as teaching the patient relaxation techniques, giving the patient some control over wound care and analgesia, and providing frequent reassurance are helpful. Guided imagery may be effective in altering the patient's perceptions of and responses to pain. Other pain-relieving approaches include distraction through video programs or video games, hypnosis, biofeedback, and behavioural modification.

The nurse works quickly to complete treatments and dressing changes to reduce pain and discomfort. The patient is encouraged to take analgesic medications before painful procedures. The patient's response to the medication and other interventions is assessed and documented.

Healing burn wounds are typically described by patients as itchy and tight. Oral antipruritic agents, a cool environment, frequent lubrication of the skin with water or a silica-based lotion, exercise and splinting to prevent skin contracture, and diversional activities all help to promote comfort in this phase.

PROMOTING PHYSICAL MOBILITY

An early priority is to prevent complications resulting from immobility. Deep breathing, turning, and proper repositioning are essential nursing practices that prevent atelectasis and pneumonia, control edema, and prevent pressure ulcers and contractures. These interventions are modified to meet the patient's needs. Low-air-loss and rotation beds may be useful, and early sitting and ambulation are encouraged. Whenever the lower extremities are burned, elastic pressure bandages should be applied before the patient is placed in an upright position. These bandages promote venous return and minimize swelling.

The burn wound is in a dynamic state for a year or more after wound closure. During this time, aggressive efforts must be made to prevent contracture and hypertrophic scarring. Both passive and active range-of-motion exercises are initiated from the day of admission and are continued after grafting, within prescribed limitations. Splints or functional devices may be applied to extremities for contracture control. The nurse monitors the splinted areas for signs of vascular insufficiency and nerve compression.

STRENGTHENING COPING STRATEGIES

In the acute phase of burn care, the patient is facing the reality of the burn trauma and is grieving over obvious losses. Depression, regression, and manipulative behaviour are common responses of

---

NURSING RESEARCH PROFILE 57-1

Burn Pain and Anxiety

Beyers, J. F., Bridges, S., Kijek, J., & LaBorde, P. J. (2001). Burn patients' pain and anxiety experiences. *Journal of Burn Care and Rehabilitation, 22*(2), 144–149.

Purpose

Pain associated with burns and treatment of burn wounds is common and often excruciating. Its management is important in patient care and is often a nursing challenge. The purpose of this study was to examine burn patients' experiences with pain and anxiety during rest and during painful wound care procedures.

Study Sample and Design

A descriptive study was conducted; the sample included 23 acutely burned adults in a southeastern level I trauma centre who were undergoing wound care and who had not had previous surgery to treat their burn wounds. Ages ranged from 18 to 75 with a mean age of 33 ± 13.2. Data on pain and anxiety levels were collected in three phases: at the time of recruitment of subjects, at baseline (defined as at least 8 hours after the last procedure), and during burn wound care procedures (within 5 minutes of scrubbing/débridement/before dressings were reapplied).

Subjects completed the Visual Analogue Scale (VAS-pain) to assess the level of pain they considered acceptable, with possible scores ranging from no pain to worst pain possible. The Short-Form McGill (SF-M) questionnaire was used to measure the sensory and affective dimensions of pain, as well as the patient's present pain on a Likert-type scale (0 = no pain; 5 = excruciating). A Visual Analogue Scale (VAS-anxiety) was used to measure anxiety, with scores ranging along a continuum from no anxiety to worse anxiety possible. Subjects were asked to mark both VAS instruments with an X, indicating the severity of their pain and anxiety. Other data collected included demographic data, analgesic and sedative use, and use of nonpharmacologic

methods as distraction techniques during procedures. Descriptive and nonparametric statistical tests were used to analyze data.

Findings

Results showed that burn patients report higher levels of pain during procedures than when at rest. A strong positive relationship between pain and anxiety was found. The most frequently reported pain descriptor on the SF-M was "tender" during baseline measurements. Frequent descriptors during procedures included "throbbing," "hot-burning," and "aching." There were no significant differences in anxiety between resting conditions and procedural dressing changes ($p > 0.16$). There were significant differences between burn patients' acceptable level, resting level, and procedural pain levels ($p = 0.01$). Patients reported their baseline pain as less than their acceptable level of pain. Other findings noted that family presence during procedure was related to decreased procedural pain and decreased use of medications prescribed for relief of anxiety.

Nursing Implications

Because burn patients describe burn wound care procedures to be the most painful experience, efforts should be made to identify strategies that are effective in reducing pain intensity. Also, since pain and anxiety were linked, strategies need to be developed to decrease both. The researchers suggested that use of both pharmacologic and nonpharmacologic interventions during wound care procedures may be warranted to help patients cope with anxiety, resting pain, and pain associated with wound care procedures. Future studies of the effect of different pharmacologic interventions with larger and more diverse samples are needed.

patients who have burn injuries. Withdrawal from participation in required treatments and regression must be viewed with an understanding that such behaviour helps the patient cope with an enormously stressful event. Much of the patient's energy goes into maintaining vital physical functions and wound healing in the early postburn weeks, leaving little emotional energy for coping in a more effective manner. Nurses can assist patients to develop effective coping strategies by setting specific expectations for behaviour, promoting truthful communication to build trust, helping patients practice appropriate strategies, and giving positive reinforcement when appropriate. Most importantly, the nurse and all members of the health care team must demonstrate acceptance of the patient.

The patient frequently vents feelings of anger. At times the anger may be directed inward because of a sense of guilt, perhaps for causing the fire or even for surviving when loved ones perished. The anger may reach outward toward those who escaped unharmed or to those who are now providing care. One way to help the patient handle these emotions is to enlist someone to whom the patient can vent feelings without fear of retaliation. A nurse, social worker, psychiatric liaison nurse, or clergy member who is not involved in direct care activities may fill this role successfully.

Burn patients are very dependent on health care team members during the long period of acute illness. However, even when physically unable to contribute much to self-care, they can be included in decisions regarding care and encouraged to assert their individuality in terms of preferences and recognition of their unique identities. As patients improve in mobility and strength, the nurse works with them to set realistic expectations for self-care, including self-feeding, assistance with wound care procedures, exercise, and planning for the future. Many patients respond positively to the use of contractual agreements and other strategies that recognize their independence and their specific role as part of the health care team moving toward the goal of self-care.

SUPPORTING PATIENT AND FAMILY PROCESSES

Family functioning is disrupted with burn injury. One of the nurse's responsibilities is to support the patient and family and to address their spoken and unspoken concerns. Family members need to be instructed about ways that they can support the patient as adaptation to burn trauma occurs. The family also needs support by the health care team. The burn injury has tremendous psychological, economic, and practical impact on the patient and family. Referrals for social services or psychological counselling should be made as appropriate. This support continues into the rehabilitation phase.

Burn patients are commonly sent to burn centres far from home. Because burn injuries are not anticipated, family roles are disrupted. Therefore, both the patient and the family need thorough information about the patient's burn care and expected course of treatment. Patient and family education begins at the initiation of burn management. Barriers to learning are assessed and considered in teaching. The preferred learning styles of both the patient and family are assessed. This information is used to tailor teaching activities. The nurse assesses the ability of the patient and family to grasp and cope with the information. Verbal information is supplemented by videos, models, or printed materials if available. Patient and family education is a priority in the rehabilitation phase.

MONITORING AND MANAGING POTENTIAL COMPLICATIONS

Heart Failure and Pulmonary Edema

The patient is assessed for fluid overload, which may occur as fluid is mobilized from the interstitial compartment back into the intravascular compartment. If the cardiac and renal systems can-

not compensate for the excess vascular volume, congestive heart failure and pulmonary edema may result. The patient is assessed for signs of heart failure, including decreased cardiac output, oliguria, jugular vein distention, edema, and the onset of an S_3 or S_4 heart sound. Increasing central venous, pulmonary artery, and wedge pressures indicate increased fluid volume.

Crackles in the lungs and increased difficulty with respiration may indicate a fluid buildup in the lungs, which is reported promptly to the physician. In the meantime, the patient is positioned comfortably, with the head of the bed raised (if not contraindicated because of other treatments or injuries) to promote lung expansion and gas exchange. Management of this complication includes providing supplemental oxygen, administering IV diuretic agents, carefully assessing the patient's response, and providing vasoactive medications, if indicated.

Sepsis

The signs of early systemic sepsis are subtle and require a high index of suspicion and very close monitoring of changes in the patient's status. Early signs of sepsis may include confusion, increased temperature, increased pulse rate, widened pulse pressure, and flushed dry skin in unburned areas. As with many observations of the burn patient, one needs to look for patterns or trends in the data. (See Chap. 15 for a more detailed discussion of septic shock.)

Wound and blood cultures are performed as prescribed, and results are reported to the physician immediately. The nurse also observes for and reports early signs of sepsis and promptly intervenes, administering prescribed IV fluids and antibiotics to prevent septic shock, a complication with a high mortality rate. Antibiotics must be given as scheduled to maintain proper blood concentrations. Serum antibiotic levels are monitored for evidence of maximal effectiveness, and the patient is monitored for toxic side effects.

Acute Respiratory Failure and Acute Respiratory Distress Syndrome

The patient's respiratory status is monitored closely for increased difficulty breathing, change in respiratory pattern, and onset of adventitious (abnormal) sounds. Typically at this stage, signs and symptoms of injury to the respiratory tract become apparent. Respiratory failure may follow. As described previously, signs of hypoxia (decreased O_2 to the tissues), decreased breath sounds, wheezing, tachypnea, stridor, and sputum tinged with soot (or in some cases containing sloughed tracheal tissue) are among the many possible findings. Patients receiving mechanical ventilation must be assessed for a decrease in tidal volume and lung compliance. The key sign of the onset of ARDS is hypoxemia while receiving 100% oxygen, decreased lung compliance, and significant shunting. The physician should be notified immediately of deteriorating respiratory status.

Medical management of the patient with acute respiratory failure requires intubation and mechanical ventilation (if not already in use). If ARDS has developed, higher oxygen levels, positive end-expiratory pressure, and pressure support are used with mechanical ventilation to promote gas exchange across the alveolar–capillary membrane.

Visceral Damage

The nurse must be alert to signs of necrosis of visceral organs due to electrical injury. Tissues affected are usually between the entrance and exit wounds of the electrical burn. All patients with electrical burns should undergo electrocardiographic monitoring, with dysrhythmias being reported to the physician. Careful attention must also be paid to signs or reports of pain related to deep muscle ischemia. To minimize the severity of complications, visceral ischemia must be detected as early as possible. The physician can perform **fasciotomies** to relieve the swelling and ischemia in the muscles and fascia and to promote oxygenation of the injured tissues. Because of the deep incisions involved with fasciotomies, the patient must be monitored carefully for signs of excessive blood loss and hypovolemia.

Evaluation

EXPECTED PATIENT OUTCOMES

Expected patient outcomes may include:

1. Achieves optimal fluid balance
   a. Maintains intake and output and body weight that correlate with expected pattern
   b. Exhibits vital signs and central venous, pulmonary artery, and pulmonary artery wedge pressures within designated limits
   c. Demonstrates increased urine output in response to diuretic and vasoactive medications
   d. Has heart rate less than 110 beats/min in normal sinus rhythm
2. Has no localized or systemic infection
   a. Has wound culture results showing minimal bacteria
   b. Has normal urine and sputum culture results
3. Demonstrates anabolic nutritional status
   a. Gains weight daily after initial loss secondary to fluid diuresis and no oral intake of food or fluid
   b. Shows no signs of protein, vitamin, or mineral deficiencies
   c. Meets required nutritional needs entirely by oral intake
   d. Participates in selecting diet containing prescribed nutrients
   e. Exhibits normal serum protein levels
4. Demonstrates improved skin integrity
   a. Sustains generally intact skin that remains free of infection, pressure, and injury
   b. Demonstrates remaining open wound areas that are pink, re-epithelializing, and free of infection
   c. Demonstrates donor graft sites that are clean and healing
   d. Has healed wounds that are soft and smooth
   e. Demonstrates skin that is lubricated and elastic
5. Has minimal pain
   a. Requests analgesic agents for specific wound care procedures or physical therapy activities
   b. Reports minimal or tolerable pain
   c. Gives no physiologic, verbal, or nonverbal cues that pain is moderate or severe
   d. Uses pain control measures such as nitrous oxide, relaxation, imagery, and distraction techniques to cope with and alleviate pain and discomfort
   e. Can sleep without being disturbed by pain
   f. Reports skin is comfortable, with no itching or tightness
6. Demonstrates optimal physical mobility
   a. Improves range of motion of joints daily
   b. Demonstrates preinjury range of motion of all joints
   c. Has no signs of calcification around the joints
   d. Participates in activities of daily living
7. Uses appropriate coping strategies to deal with postburn problems
   a. Verbalizes reactions to burns, therapeutic procedures, losses
   b. Identifies coping strategies used effectively in previous stressful situations
   c. Accepts dependency on health care providers during acute phase
   d. Verbalizes realistic view of problems resulting from burn injury and plans for future
   e. Cooperates with health care providers in required therapy
   f. Participates in decision making regarding care
   g. Resolves grief over losses resulting from burn injury and circumstances surrounding injury (eg, death of others, damage to home or other property)
   h. States realistic objectives for plastic surgery, further medical intervention, and results
   i. Verbalizes realistic abilities and goals
   j. Displays hopeful attitude toward future
8. Relates appropriately in patient/family processes
   a. Patient and family verbalize feelings regarding change in family interactions
   b. Family emotionally supports the patient during the hospitalization
   c. Family states that own needs are met
9. Patient and family verbalize understanding of the treatment course
   a. States rationale for different aspects of treatment
   b. States realistic time period for recovery
10. Absence of complications
    a. Lungs clear on auscultation
    b. Exhibits no dyspnea or orthopnea and can breathe easily when standing, sitting, and lying down
    c. Exhibits no S_3 or S_4 heart sounds or jugular venous distention
    d. Exhibits urine output; central venous, pulmonary artery, and pulmonary artery wedge pressures; and cardiac output within normal or acceptable limits
    e. Exhibits normal blood, sputum, and urine culture results
    f. Maintains arterial blood gas values within normal or acceptable limits
    g. Has normal lung compliance
    h. Has no visceral organ damage
    i. Has stable cardiac rhythm

REHABILITATION PHASE OF BURN CARE

Although long-term aspects of burn care are discussed last in this chapter, rehabilitation begins immediately after the burn has occurred—as early as the emergent period—and often extends for years after injury. In the aftermath of the acute stages of injury, the burn patient increasingly focuses on the alterations in self-image and lifestyle that may occur. Wound healing, psychosocial support, and restoring maximal functional activity remain priorities. The focus on maintaining fluid and electrolyte balance and improving nutritional status continues. Reconstructive surgery to improve body appearance and function may be needed.

Burn injuries can have a major impact on quality of life. Changes in physical activity and social, psychological, and employment status may occur. Therefore, psychological and vocational counselling and referral to support groups may be helpful to promote recovery and quality of life. Family members also need support and guidance in assisting the patient to return to optimal health.

Prevention of Hypertrophic Scarring

The wound is in a dynamic state for 1.5 to 2 years after the burn occurs. If appropriate measures are instituted during this active period, the scar tissue loses its redness and softens. Healed areas that are prone to hypertrophic scarring require the patient to wear a pressure garment (Fig. 57-6). These devices are especially useful for partial-thickness wounds that required more than 2 weeks to heal and for the edges of grafted skin. Applying elastic pressure garments loosens collagen bundles and encourages parallel orientation of the collagen to the skin surface, with the disappearance of the dermal nodules. As pressure continues over time, there is a restructuring of the collagen and a decrease in vascularity and cellularity (Serghiou, Young, Ott et al., 2002).

The physical therapist, occupational therapist, or a representative of the manufacturer of elastic pressure garments measures the patient for correct fit. While awaiting the arrival of the garment, soft, tubular, knitted elastic pressure bandages can be used to help desensitize the patient's skin, protect healing areas, apply pressure, and promote venous return. Patients must be instructed about the need for lubrication and protection of the healing skin and the need for pressure garments for at least a year after the injury. A program including elastic pressure garments, splints, and exercise under the supervision of an experienced physical and occupational therapy team is recommended for optimal functional and cosmetic results.

NURSING PROCESS: CARE OF THE PATIENT DURING THE REHABILITATION PHASE

Assessment

Information about the patient's educational level, occupation, leisure activities, cultural background, religion, and family interactions is obtained early. The patient's self-concept, mental status, emotional response to the injury and hospitalization, level of intellectual functioning, previous hospitalizations, response to pain and pain relief measures, and sleep pattern are also essential components of a comprehensive assessment. Information about the patient's general self-concept, self-esteem, and coping strategies in the past will be valuable in addressing emotional needs.

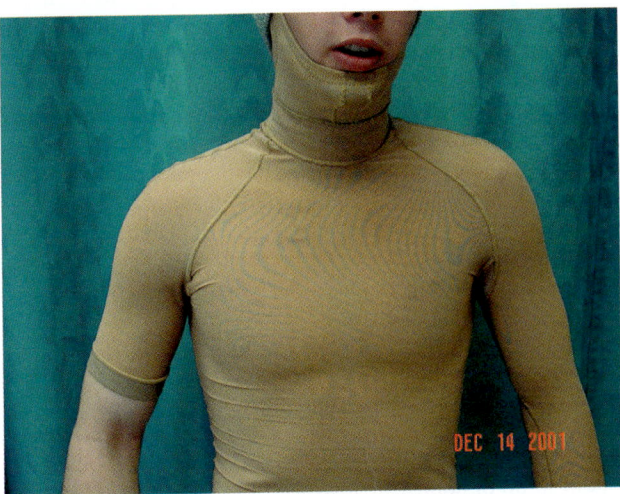

FIGURE 57-6 Elastic pressure garments. Application of pressure garments helps prevent hypertrophic burn scarring. Used with permission of Jobst Institute, Inc., Toledo, Ohio.

Ongoing physical assessments related to rehabilitation goals include range of motion of affected joints, functional abilities in activities of daily living, early signs of skin breakdown from splints or positioning devices, evidence of neuropathies (neurologic damage), activity tolerance, and quality or condition of healing skin. The patient's participation in care and ability to demonstrate self-care in such areas as ambulation, eating, wound cleaning, and applying pressure wraps are documented on a regular basis. In addition to these assessment parameters, specific complications and treatments require additional specific assessments; for example, the patient undergoing primary excision requires postoperative assessment.

Recovery from burn injury involves every system of the body. Therefore, assessment of the burn patient must be comprehensive and continuous. Priorities will vary at different points during the rehabilitation phase. Understanding the pathophysiologic responses to burn injury forms the framework for detecting early progress or signs and symptoms of complications. Early detection leads to early intervention and enhances the potential for successful rehabilitation.

Diagnosis

NURSING DIAGNOSES

Based on the assessment data, priority nursing diagnoses in the long-term rehabilitation phase of burn care may include the following:

- Activity intolerance related to pain on exercise, limited joint mobility, muscle wasting, and limited endurance
- Disturbed body image related to altered physical appearance and self-concept
- Deficient knowledge about postdischarge home care and follow-up needs

COLLABORATIVE PROBLEMS/ POTENTIAL COMPLICATIONS

Based on the assessment data, potential complications that may develop in the rehabilitation phase include:

- Contractures
- Inadequate psychological adaptation to burn injury

Planning and Goals

The major goals for the patient include increased participation in activities of daily living; increased understanding of the injury, treatment, and planned follow-up care; adaptation and adjustment to alterations in body image, self-concept, and lifestyle; and absence of complications.

Nursing Interventions

PROMOTING ACTIVITY TOLERANCE

Nursing interventions that must be carried out according to a strict regimen and the pain that accompanies movement take their toll on a burn patient. The patient may become confused and disoriented and lack the energy to participate optimally in care. The nurse must schedule care in such a way that the patient has periods of uninterrupted sleep. A good time for planned patient rest is after the stress of dressing changes and exercise, while pain interventions and sedatives may still be effective. This plan must be communicated to family members and other care providers.

Burn patients may have insomnia related to frequent nightmares about the burn injury or to other fears and anxieties about the outcome of the injury. The nurse listens to and reassures the patient and administers hypnotic agents, as prescribed, to promote sleep.

Reducing metabolic stress by relieving pain, preventing chilling or fever, and promoting the physical integrity of all body systems will help the patient conserve energy for therapeutic activities and wound healing.

The nurse incorporates physical therapy exercises in the patient's care to prevent muscle atrophy and to maintain the mobility required for daily activities. The patient's activity tolerance, strength, and endurance will gradually increase if activity occurs over increasingly longer periods. Fatigue, fever, and pain tolerance are monitored and used to determine the amount of activity to be encouraged on a daily basis. Activities such as family visits and recreational or play therapy (eg, video games, radio, TV) can provide diversion, improve the patient's outlook, and increase tolerance for physical activity.

IMPROVING BODY IMAGE AND SELF-CONCEPT

Burn patients frequently suffer profound losses. These include not only a loss of body image due to disfigurement but also losses of personal property, homes, loved ones, and ability to work. They lack the benefit of anticipatory grief often seen in a patient approaching surgery or a person dealing with the terminal illness of a loved one.

As care progresses, the patient who is recovering from burns becomes aware of daily improvement and begins to exhibit basic concerns: Will I be disfigured? How long will I be in the hospital? What about my job and family? Will I ever be independent again? How can I pay for my care? Was my burn the result of my carelessness? As the patient expresses such concerns, the nurse must take time to listen and to provide realistic support. The nurse can refer patients to a support group, such as those usually available at regional burn centres or through organizations such as the Phoenix Society. Through participation in such groups, patients will meet others with similar experiences and learn coping strategies to help them deal with their losses. Interaction with other burn survivors allows the patient to see that adaptation to the burn injury is possible. If a support group is not available, visits from burn survivors can be helpful to the patient coping with such a traumatic injury.

A major responsibility of the nurse is to assess constantly the patient's psychosocial reactions. What are the patient's fears and concerns? Does the patient fear loss of control of care, independence, or sanity itself? Is the patient afraid of rejection by family and loved ones? Does he or she fear being unable to cope with pain or physical appearance? Does the patient have concerns about sexuality, including sexual function? Being aware of these anxieties and understanding the basis of the patient's fears enable the nurse to provide support and to cooperate with other members of the health care team in developing a plan to help the patient deal with these feelings.

When caring for burn patients, the nurse needs to be aware that there are prejudices and misunderstandings in society about those who are viewed as different. Opportunities and accommodations available to others are often denied those who are disfigured. Such amenities include social participation, employment, prestige, various roles, and status. The health care team must actively promote a healthy body image and self-concept in burn survivors so that they can accept or challenge others' perceptions of those who are disfigured. Survivors themselves must show others who they are, how they function, and how they want to be treated.

The nurse can help patients practice their responses to people who may stare or inquire about their injury once they are discharged from the hospital. The nurse can help patients build self-

esteem by recognizing their uniqueness—for example, with small gestures such as providing a birthday cake, combing the patient's hair before visiting hours, giving information about the availability of a cosmetician to enhance appearance, and teaching the patient ways to direct attention away from a disfigured body to the self within. Consultants such as psychologists, social workers, vocational counsellors, and teachers are valuable participants in assisting burn patients to regain their self-esteem.

MONITORING AND MANAGING POTENTIAL COMPLICATIONS

Contractures

With early and aggressive physical and occupational therapy, contractures are rarely a long-term complication. However, surgical intervention is indicated if a full range of motion in the burn patient is not achieved. (See Chap. 11 for a discussion of prevention of contractures.)

Impaired Psychological Adaptation to the Burn Injury

Some patients, particularly those with limited coping skills or psychological function or a history of psychiatric problems before the burn injury, may not achieve adequate psychological adaptation to the burn injury. Psychological counselling or psychiatric referral may be made to assess the patient's emotional status, to help the patient develop coping skills, and to intervene if major psychological issues or ineffective coping is identified.

PROMOTING HOME AND COMMUNITY-BASED CARE

Teaching Patients Self-Care

As the inpatient phase of recovery becomes shorter, the focus of rehabilitative interventions is directed toward outpatient care or care in a rehabilitation centre. In the long term, much of the care of healing burns will be performed by the patient and others at home. Throughout the phases of burn care, efforts are made to prepare the patient and family for the care that will continue at home. Thus, they are instructed about the measures and procedures that they will need to perform. For example, patients commonly have small areas of clean, open wounds that are healing slowly. They are instructed to wash these areas daily with mild soap and water and to apply the prescribed topical agent or dressing.

In addition to instructions about wound care, patients and families require careful written and verbal instructions about prevention of complications, pain management, and nutrition. Information about specific exercises and use of pressure garments and splints is reviewed with both the patient and family; written instructions are provided for reference. They are taught to recognize abnormal signs and instructed to report them to the physician. All of this information will enable patients to progress successfully through the rehabilitative phase of burn management. The patient and family are assisted in planning for the patient's continued care by identifying and acquiring supplies and equipment that are needed at home (Chart 57-6).

Continuing Care

Follow-up care by an interdisciplinary burn care team will be necessary. Preparations should begin during the early stages of care. Patients who receive care in a burn centre usually return to the burn clinic or centre periodically for evaluation by the burn team, modification of home care instructions, and planning for reconstructive surgery. Other patients receive ongoing care from the general or plastic surgeon who cared for them during the acute phase of their management. Still other patients require the services

Chart 57-6
Home Care Checklist • The Patient with a Burn Injury

At the completion of the home care instruction, the patient or caregiver will be able to:	Patient	Caregiver
Mental Health		
Identify strategies to promote own mental health; for example:		
• Remember that changes in lifestyle take time.	✓	✓
• Resume previous interests and activities gradually.	✓	
• Take one day at a time to regain physical and mental strength.	✓	
• Be aware of own feelings and fears and discuss them with selected others.	✓	✓
• Expect concerns, frustrations, and depression about changes in appearance.	✓	✓
• Be honest with self, family, and friends about needs, hopes, and fears.	✓	✓
• Realize that emotional adjustment to the burn injury will occur with time.	✓	✓
Burn Skin Precautions and Wound Care		
Identify the following skin precautions and wound care:		
• Cover burned skin with light clothing or wear sun block with the highest SPF possible to protect burned skin from the sun.	✓	
• Avoid further trauma to burned skin; leave unbroken blisters that may form.	✓	✓
• Lubricate healed burned skin with mild lotion (as prescribed); avoid scratching.	✓	
• Wear wide-brimmed hats if face has been burned to protect the area from the sun.	✓	
• Use only mild soap and lotion (ie, products without perfume) on burned areas.	✓	✓
Exercise		
Describe the following guidelines for exercise:		
• Do as much for self as possible.	✓	
• Adhere to the exercise regimen given by the therapist.	✓	
• Participate in exercise every day, several times a day, even when "not feeling like it."	✓	
Nutrition		
Identify the following guidelines for nutrition:		
• Eat a diet high in calories and protein.	✓	
• Drink adequate volume of fluids to prevent constipation associated with use of analgesic medications.	✓	
Pain Management		
Describe the following steps for managing pain:		
• Take analgesic medication as prescribed.	✓	
• Avoid situations that require alertness (analgesic agents may produce drowsiness).	✓	
• Use analgesic medication as prescribed (30 minutes before painful procedures such as dressing changes).	✓	✓
• Use relaxation and distraction to relieve pain and discomfort.	✓	
Thermoregulation		
Identify strategies to compensate for inability to regulate body temperature:		
• Dress to accommodate cold and hot weather or environment.	✓	
• Avoid extremes of temperature.	✓	
Clothing Considerations		
State the following strategies in selection of clothing to wear:		
• Avoid tight clothing over burned areas.	✓	
• Select white cotton, loose-fitting clothing so that dyes in coloured clothes do not irritate healing skin.	✓	
• Wear clothing and gloves to protect healing skin from unnecessary bruises, bumps, and scratches.	✓	
Management of Burn Scar		
Describe the following strategies to manage burn scar:		
• Massage and stretch skin to maintain/increase its elasticity.	✓	✓
• Use lotion for massage as recommended by therapist.	✓	✓
• Wear compression garments 23 hours a day.	✓	
Resumption of Sexual Relations		
Identify the following guidelines regarding resumption of sexual relationships:		
• Realize that resumption of sexual relationships is the rule rather than the exception.	✓	✓
• Expect sensitivity of and around the genital area for several months if these areas were burned.	✓	
• Resume sexual activity slowly; endurance will increase with time.	✓	

Adapted with permission from Orlando Regional Medical Center Burn Unit's *Personal Guide to Burn Care.*

of a rehabilitation centre and may be transferred to such a centre for aggressive rehabilitation before going home. Many patients require outpatient physical or occupational therapy, often several times weekly. It is often the nurse who is responsible for coordinating all aspects of care and ensuring that the patient's needs are met. Such coordination is an important aspect in assisting a burn victim to achieve independence.

Patients who return home after a severe burn injury, those who cannot manage their own burn care, and those with inadequate support systems will need referral for home care. During visits to the patient at home, the home care nurse assesses the patient's physical and psychological status as well as the adequacy of the home setting for safe and adequate care. The nurse monitors the patient's progress and adherence to the plan of care and notes any problems that interfere with the patient's ability to carry out the care. During the visit, the nurse assists the patient and family with wound care and exercises. Patients with severe or persistent depression or difficulty adjusting to changes in their social and/or occupational roles are identified and referred to the burn team for possible referral to a psychologist, psychiatrist, or vocational counsellor.

The burn team or home care nurse identifies community resources that may be helpful for the patient and family. Several burn patient support groups and other organizations offer services for burn victims. They provide caring people (often recovered burn victims) who can visit a burn patient in the hospital or home or telephone the patient and family periodically to provide support and counselling about skin care, cosmetics, and problems related to psychosocial adjustment. Such organizations sponsor group meetings and social functions at which outpatients are welcome. Some also provide school-reentry programs and are active in burn prevention activities. If more information is needed regarding burn prevention, the American Burn Association can help locate the nearest burn centre (including locations in Canada) and offer current burn prevention tips (see Chart 57-2).

Because so much attention is given to the burn wound and the treatments that are necessary to treat the burn wound and to prevent complications, the patient, family, and health care providers may inadvertently ignore the patient's ongoing needs for health promotion and screening. Thus, the patient and family are reminded of the importance of periodic health screening and preventive care (eg, gynecologic examinations, dental care).

Evaluation

EXPECTED PATIENT OUTCOMES
Expected patient outcomes may include:

1. Demonstrates activity tolerance required for desired daily activities
   a. Obtains sufficient sleep daily
   b. Reports absence of nightmares or sleep disturbances
   c. Shows gradually increasing tolerance and endurance in physical activities
   d. Can concentrate during conversations
   e. Has energy available to sustain desired daily activities
2. Adapts to altered body image
   a. Verbalizes accurate description of alterations in body image and accepts physical appearance
   b. Demonstrates interest in resources that may improve body appearance and function
   c. Uses cosmetics, wigs, and prostheses as desired to achieve acceptable appearance
   d. Socializes with significant others, peers, and usual social group
   e. Seeks and achieves return to role in family, school, and community as a contributing member
3. Demonstrates knowledge of required self-care and follow-up care
   a. Describes surgical procedures and treatments accurately
   b. Verbalizes detailed plan for follow-up care
   c. Demonstrates ability to perform wound care and prescribed exercises
   d. Returns for follow-up appointments as scheduled
   e. Identifies resource people and agencies to contact for specific problems
4. Exhibits no complications
   a. Demonstrates full range of motion
   b. Shows no signs of withdrawal or depression
   c. Displays no psychotic behaviours

Burn Care in the Home

More and more burns are being treated exclusively in outpatient settings, including wound clinics, physicians' offices, and emergency department clinics. The outpatient setting is appropriate for the care of minor burns and most moderate burns. However, a number of factors must be considered in determining the appropriate site of care. These factors include the age of the patient, the extent and depth of the burn, the availability of family support systems and community resources to assist the patient, the patient's adherence to the prescribed plan of care, and the distance from home to the outpatient setting.

Initially, looking at and touching the burn wound may be difficult and even frightening to some family members and patients. However, with encouragement and support, most can handle burn wound care with little need for daily professional care. Instructions, both verbal and written, are given to the patient about burn wound care, pain management strategies, the need for adequate nutrition, and the importance of exercise and rest. Instruction is also given about signs and symptoms of infection that should be reported to the physician. The importance of notifying the physician about complications early and of keeping follow-up appointments is emphasized to the patient and family.

 Gerontologic Considerations

Nursing assessment of the elderly burn patient should include particular attention to pulmonary function, response to fluid resuscitation, and signs of mental confusion or disorientation. A careful history of preburn medications and preexisting illnesses is essential.

Nursing care promotes early mobilization, aggressive pulmonary care, and attention to preventing complications. Because of lowered resistance, burn wound sepsis and lethal systemic septicemia are more likely in elderly patients. Moreover, fever may not be present in the elderly to signal such events. Therefore, surveillance for other signs of infection becomes even more important.

Rehabilitation must take into account preexisting functional abilities and limitations, such as arthritis and low activity tolerance. Elderly patients commonly lack family members who can provide home care, so social services and community nursing services must be contacted to provide optimal care and supervision after hospital discharge.

Critical Thinking Exercises

1. A 60-year-old man weighing 50 kg is transferred to the emergency department after his tractor caught on fire, burning both of his legs circumferentially, his anterior chest, and his entire right upper extremity. Using the rule of nines chart, estimate the percent of TBSA burned. What are the emergent priorities for this patient? What are the fluid resuscitation requirements for this patient based on his percent burn and his weight? What assessment parameters would you be monitoring closely?

2. Your 25-year-old patient received burns over 60% of her body, including her upper extremities and face, as a result of a kitchen fire 2 weeks ago. She is depressed and distraught about the pain associated with wound care and the changes in her appearance. What assessments are important in her care, and what nursing interventions would be appropriate for her at this time?

3. Your 26-year-old burn patient is scheduled for surgery. The burn physician plans on using Integra on his upper extremity burns after débridement and to apply Acticoat to the superficial burns. What patient education would you give this patient about Integra and Acticoat? Explain what these two products are, their purpose, and the benefits of their use. Explain how the implications for nursing care differ for the two products.

4. Your 41-year-old patient, an attorney, is expected to be discharged from the hospital in a week following 6 weeks of treatment for severe burns to the lower part of her body. She has used a wheelchair for the last 20 years as a result of a spinal cord injury. The burns occurred when she was lighting a candle at home and it fell onto her clothing. What preparation would be important in making arrangements for referral and home care if she lives alone? What specific safety precautions should be included in discharge teaching for her?

REFERENCES AND SELECTED READINGS

Books

Caine, R. M., & Lefcourt, N. D. (1996). Patients with burns. In J. M. Clochesy, et al. (Eds.), *Critical care nursing* (2nd ed.). Philadelphia: W. B. Saunders.

Carrougher, G. J. (1998). *Burn care and therapy.* St. Louis: Mosby.

Fitzpatrick, J. C., & Cioffi, W. G. (2002). Diagnosis and treatment of inhalation injury. In D. N. Herndon (Ed.), *Total burn care* (2d ed.). Philadelphia: W. B. Saunders.

Herndon, D. N. (2002). *Total burn care.* Philadelphia: W. B. Saunders.

Hudak, C. M., Gallo, B. M., & Morton, P. G. (1997). *Critical care nursing: A holistic approach.* Philadelphia: Lippincott Williams & Wilkins.

LaBorde, P. J., & Willis, J. M. (2001). Burns. In M. L. Sole et al. (Eds.), *Introduction to critical care nursing* (3d ed.). Philadelphia: W. B. Saunders.

McCaffrey, M., & Pasaro, C. (1999). *Pain: Clinical manual* (2d ed.). St. Louis: Mosby.

Molter, N. C., et al. (1997). Burns. In J. Hartshorn, M. Lamborn, & M. L. Noll (Eds.), *Introduction to critical care nursing.* Philadelphia: W. B. Saunders.

Munster, A. M. (2002). The immunological response and strategies for intervention. In D. N. Herndon (Ed.), *Total burn care* (2d ed.). London: W. B. Saunders.

Serghiou, M. A., Young, E. B., Ott, S., et al. (2002). Comprehensive rehabilitation of the burned patient. In D. N. Herndon (Ed.), *Total burn care* (2d ed.). London: W. B. Saunders.

Wolf, S., Prough, D. S., & Herndon, D. N. (2002). Critical care in the severely burned: Organ support and management of complications. In D. H. Herndon (Ed.), *Total burn care* (2d ed.). London: W. B. Saunders.

Journals

Asterisks indicate nursing research articles.

Ahrns, K. S., & Harkins, D. R. (1997). Initial resuscitation after burn injury: Therapies, strategies, and controversies. *AACN Clinical Issues, 10*(1), 46–60.

American Burn Association (2000). Burn incidence and treatment in the US: 2000 fact sheet. Available online: http:www.ameriburn.org/pub/factsheet.htm.

Arturson, G. (2000). Forty years in burn research: The postburn inflammatory response. *Burns, 26*(7), 599–604.

Ashworth, H. L., Cubison, T. C., Gilbert, P. M., & Sim, K. M. (2001). Treatment before transfer: The patient with burns. *Emergency Medical Journal, 18*(5), 349–351.

Atkinson, A. (1998). Nursing burn wounds on general wards. *Nursing Standard, 12*(41), 58, 61–64, 67.

Brigham, P. A., & McLoughlin, E. (1996). Burn incidence and medical care use in the United States: Estimates, trends, and data sources. *Journal of Burn Care & Rehabilitation, 17*(2), 95–107.

*Byers, J. F., Bridges, S., Kijek, J., & LaBorde, P. J. (2001). Burn patients' pain and anxiety experiences. *Journal of Burn Care & Rehabilitation, 22*(2), 144–149.

Cioffi, W. G. (2001). What's new in burns and metabolism. *Journal of American College of Surgeons, 192*(2), 241–254.

Cortiella, J., & Marvin, J. A. (1997). Management of the pediatric burn patient. *Nursing Clinics of North America, 32*(2), 311–329.

Cumming, J., Purdue, G. F., Hunt, J. L., & O'Keefe, G. E. (2001). Objective estimates of the incidence and consequences of multiple organ dysfunction and sepsis after burn trauma. *Journal of Trauma Injury, Infection and Critical Care, 50*(3), 510–515.

Delatte, S. J., Evans, J., Hebra, A., et al. (2001). Effectiveness of beta-glucan collagen for treatment of partial-thickness burns in children. *Journal of Pediatric Surgery, 36*(1), 113–118.

Demling, R. H., & Seigne, P. (2000). Metabolic management of patients with severe burns. *World Journal of Surgery, 24*(6), 673–680.

DeSanti, L., Lincoln, L., Egan, F., & Demling, R. (1998). Development of a burn rehabilitation unit: Impact on burn center length of stay and functional outcome. *Journal of Burn Care & Rehabilitation, 19*(5), 414–419.

De-Souza, D. A., & Greene, L. J. (1998). Pharmacological nutrition after burn injury. *Journal of Nutrition, 128*(5), 797–803.

Essex, T. L. (1999). Burn tragedy. *Rehabilitation Nursing, 24*(1), 5–6.

*Flynn, M. B. (1999). Identifying and treating inhalation injuries in fire victims. *Dimensions of Critical Care Nursing, 18*(4), 18–23.

Forjuoh, S. N. (1998). The mechanisms, intensity of treatment, and outcomes of hospitalized burns: Issues for prevention. *Journal of Burn Care and Rehabilitation, 19*(5), 456–460.

Fowler, A. (1998). Nursing management of minor burn injuries. *Nursing Standard, 12*(49), 47–52.

Fratianne, R. B., & Brandt, C. P. (1997). Determining when care for burns is futile. *Journal of Burn Care & Rehabilitation, 18*(3), 262–267.

*Fratianne, R. B., Prensner, J. D., Hutson, M. J., et al. (2001). The effect of music-based imagery and musical alternate engagement on the burn débridement process. *Journal of Burn Care and Rehabilitation, 22*(1), 47–53.

Garvin, C. G., & Brown, R. O. (2001). Nutritional support in the intensive care unit: Are patients receiving what is prescribed? *Critical Care Medicine, 29*(1), 204–205.

Gibran, N. S., & Heimbach, D. M. (2000). Current status of burn wound pathophysiology. *Clinics in Plastic Surgery, 27*(1), 11–22.

Gilboa, D. (2001). Long-term psychosocial adjustment after burn injury. *Burns, 27*(4), 335–341.

*Gordon, M., Greenfield, E., Marvin, J., et al. (1998). Use of pain assessment tools: Is there a preference? *Journal of Burn Care and Rehabilitation, 19*(5), 451–454.

Gordon, M., & Goodwin, C. W. (1997). Burn management: Initial assessment, management and stabilization. *Nursing Clinics of North America, 32*(2), 237–249.

Greenfield, E., & McManus, A. T. (1997). Infectious complications: Prevention and strategies for their control. *Nursing Clinics of North America, 32*(2), 297–309.

Gueugniaud, P. Y., Carsin, H., Bertin-Maghit, M., & Petit, P. (2000). Current advances in the initial management of major thermal injuries. *Intensive Care Medicine, 26*(7), 848–856.

Hart, D. W., Wolf, S. E., Chinkes, D. L., et al. (2000). Determinants of skeletal muscle catabolism after severe burn. *Annals of Surgery, 232*(4), 455–456.

Hedderich, R., & Ness, T. J. (1999). Analgesia for trauma and burns. *Critical Care Clinics, 15*(1), 167–184.

Hermans, M. H. (1998). Results of a survey on the use of different treatment options for partial- and full-thickness burns. *Burns, 24*(6), 539–551.

Holm, C., Melcer, B., Horbrand, F., et al. (2000). The relationship between oxygen delivery and oxygen consumption during fluid resuscitation of burn related shock. *Journal of Burn Care & Rehabilitation, 21*(2), 147–154.

Hunt, J. L., Calvert, C. T., Peck, M. D., & Meyer, A. A. (2000). Occupation-related burn injuries. *Journal of Burn Care & Rehabilitation, 21*(4), 327–332.

Istre, G. R., McCoy, M. A., Osborn, L., et al. (2001). Deaths and injuries from house fires. *New England Journal of Medicine, 344*(25), 1911–1916.

Jain, S., & Bandi, V. (1999). Electrical and lightning injuries. *Critical Care Clinics, 15*(2), 319–331.

Jonsson, C. E., Holmsten, A., Dahlstrom, L., & Jonsson, K. (1998). Background pain in burn patients: Routine measurement and recording of pain intensity in burn unit. *Burns, 24*(5), 448–454.

Jordan, R. B., Daher, J., & Wasil, K. (2000). Splints and scar management for acute and reconstructive burn care. *Clinics in Plastic Surgery, 27*(1), 71–85.

Jordon, B. S., & Harrington, D. T. (1997). Management of the burn wound. *Nursing Clinics of North America, 32*(2), 251–273.

Kao, C. C., & Garner, W. L. (2000). Acute burns. *Plastic Reconstructive Surgery, 105*(7), 2482–2493.

Katz, W. A. (1998). The needs of a patient in pain. *American Journal of Medicine, 105*(1B), 2S–7S.

*Keane, A., Jepson, C., Pickett, M., Robinson, L., & McCorkle, R. (1996). Demographic characteristics, fire experiences, and distress of residential fire survivors. *Issues in Mental Health Nursing, 17*(5), 487–501.

*Keane, A., Brennan, A. M., & Pickett, M. (2000). A typology of residential fire survivors' multidimensional needs. *Western Journal of Nursing Research, 22*(3), 263–278.

Koschel, M. J. (2002). Where there's smoke, there may be cyanide. *American Journal of Nursing, 102*(8), 39–42.

Koupil, J., Brychta, P., Rihova, H., & Kincova S. (2001). Special features of burn injuries in elderly patients. *Acta Chirurgiae Plasticae, 43*(2), 57–60.

Leistikow, B. N., Martin, D. C., & Milano, C. E. (2000). Fire injuries, disasters, and costs from cigarettes and cigarette lights: A global overview. *Preventive Medicine, 31*, 91–99.

Lim, J. J., Rehmar, S. G., & Elmore, P. (1998). Rapid response: Care of burn victims. *AAOHN Journal, 46*(4), 169–178.

Linneman, P. K., Terry, B. E., & Burd, R. S. (2000). The efficacy and safety of fentanyl for the management of severe procedural pain in patients with burn injuries. *Journal of Burn Care & Rehabilitation, 21*(6), 519–522.

Long, T. D., Cathers, T. A., Twillman, R., et al. (2001). Morphine-infused silver sulfadiazine (MISS) cream for burn analgesia: A pilot study. *Journal of Burn Care & Rehabilitation, 22*(2), 118–123.

Loss, M., Wedler, V., Kunzi, W., et al. (2000). Artificial skin, split-thickness autograft and cultured autologous keratinocytes combined to treat a serious burn injury of 93% TBSA. *Burns, 26*(7), 644–652.

Lund, T. L. (1999). The 1999 Everett Idris Evans memorial lecture. Edema generation following thermal injury: An update. *Journal of Burn Care & Rehabilitation, 20*(6), 445–451.

Luterman, A. (2000). Burns and metabolism. *Journal of American College of Surgeons, 190*(2), 104–114.

Martinez-Herz, S. P., Thurber, C. A., & Patterson, D. R. (2000). Psychological principles of burn wound pain in children. II: Treatment application. *Journal of Burn Care & Rehabilitation, 21*(5), 458–472.

Matheson, J. D., Clayton, J., & Muller, J. (2001). The reduction of itch during burn wound healing. *Journal of Burn Care & Rehabilitation, 22*(1), 76–81.

McCain, D., & Sutherland, S. (1998). Nursing essentials: Skin grafts for patients with burns. *American Journal of Nursing, 98*(7), 34–38.

Mertens, D. M., Jenkins, M. E., & Warden, G. D. (1997). Outpatient burn management. *Nursing Clinics of North America, 32*(2), 343–364.

Muller, M. J., Pegg, S. P., & Rule, M. R. (2001). Determinants of death following burn injury. *British Journal of Surgery, 88*(4), 583–587.

National Association of State Fire Marshalls Cooking Fires Taskforce Association of Home Appliance Manufacturers Safety Cooking Campaign. (July 1996). *Executive Summary.*

Noordenbos, J., Dore, C. & Hansbrough, J. F. (1999). Safety and efficacy of TransCyte for the treatment of partial-thickness burns. *Journal of Burn Care & Rehabilitation, 20*(4), 275–281.

Pal, S. K., Cortiella, J., & Herndon, D. (1997). Adjunctive methods of pain control in burns. *Burns, 23*(5), 404–412.

Parsons, L. (1997). Office management of minor burns. *Lippincott's Primary Care Practice, 1*(1), 40–49.

Patterson, D. R. (1996). Non-opioid-based approaches to burn pain. *Journal of Burn Care & Rehabilitation, 17*(4), 372–375.

Patterson, D. R., Ptacek, J. T., Cromes, F., et al. (2000). The 2000 Clinical Research Award. Describing and predicting distress and satisfaction with life for burn survivors. *Journal of Burn Care & Rehabilitation, 21*(6), 490–498.

Peng, Y. Z., Yuan, Z. Q., & Xiao, G. X. (2001). Effects of early enteral feeding on the prevention of enterogenic infection in severely burned patients. *Burns, 27*(2), 145–149.

Pessina, M., & Ellis, S. M. (1997). Rehabilitation. *Nursing Clinics of North America, 32*(2), 365–374.

Polko, L. E., & McMahon, M. J. (1998). Burns in pregnancy. *Obstetrical and Gynecological Survey, 53*(1), 50–56.

Prensner, J. D., Yowler, C. J., Smith, L. F., et al. (2001). Music therapy for assistance with pain and anxiety management in burn treatment. *Journal of Burn Care & Rehabilitation, 22*(1), 83–88.

Ptacek, J. P., Patterson, D. R., & Doctor, J. (2000). Describing and predicting the nature of procedural pain after thermal injuries: Implication for research. *Journal of Burn Care & Rehabilitation, 21*(4), 318–326.

Purna, S. K., & Babu, M. (2000). Collagen-based dressings: A review. *Burns, 26*(1), 54–62.

Ramzy, P. I., Barret, J. P., & Herndon, D. N. (1999). Thermal injury. *Critical Care Clinics, 15*(2), 333–352.

Raymond, I., Nielsen, T. A., Lavigne, G., et al. (2001). Quality of sleep and its relationship to pain intensity in hospitalized adult burn patients. *Pain, 92*, 381–388.

Richard, R. (1999). Assessment and diagnosis of burn wounds. *Advances in Wound Care, 12*(9). 468–471.

Richard, R., Staley, M., Miller, S., & Warden, G. (1997). To splint or not to splint: Past philosophy and present practice: Part III. *Journal of Burn Care & Rehabilitation, 18*(3), 251–254.

Rose, J. K., & Herndon, D. N. (1997). Advances in treatment of burn patients. *Burns, 23*(Suppl 1), S19–S26.

Shakespeare, P. G. (1999). Cost effectiveness of skin substitutes. *Burns, 25*(2), 179–181.

Schiller, W. R., Bay, R. C., Garren, R. L., et al. (1997). Hyperdynamic resuscitation improves survival in patients with life-threatening burns. *Journal of Burn Care and Rehabilitation, 18*(1), 10–16.

Sheridan, R. L., Ryan, C. M, Yin, L. M., et al. (1998). Death in burn unit: Sterile multiple organ failure. *Burns, 24*(4), 307–311.

Sheridan, R. L., & Tompkins, R. G. (1999). Skin substitutes in burns. *Burns, 25*(2), 179–181.

Sheridan, R. L., & Moreno, C. (2001). Skin substitutes in burns. *Burns, 27*(1), 92.

Stewart, R., Bhagwanjee, A. M., Mbakaza, Y., & Binase, T. (2000). Pressure garment adherence in adult patients with burn injuries: An analysis of patient and clinician perceptions. *American Journal of Occupational Therapy, 54*(6), 598–606.

Still, J. M., & Law, E. J. (2000). Primary excision of the burn wound. *Clinics in Plastic Surgery, 27*(1), 23–47.

Tassiopoulos, A. K. (1999). Nutritional support of the patient with severe burn injury. *Nutrition, 15*(11–12), 956–957.

The U.S. Home Product Report, 1993–1997, Flammable or Combustible Liquids. (August 2000). National Fire Protection Association, Fire Analysis and Research Division. Quincy, MA.

Thurber, C. A., Martin-Herz, S. P., & Patterson, D. R. (2000). Psychological principles of burn wound pain in children. I: Theoretical framework. *Journal of Burn Care & Rehabilitation, 21*(4), 376–387.

*Turner, J. G., Clark, A. J., Gauthier, D. K, & Williams, M. (1998). The effect of therapeutic touch on pain and anxiety in burn patients. *Journal of Advanced Nursing, 28*(1), 10–20.

Wainright, D., Madden, M., Luterman, A., et al. (1996). Clinical evaluation of an acellular allograft dermal matrix in full-thickness burns. *Journal of Burn Care and Rehabilitation, 17*(2), 124–136.

Wall-Alonso, E., Schoeller, D. A., Schecter, L., & Guttileb, L. J. (1999). Measured total energy requirements of adult patients with burns. *Journal of Burn Care and Rehabilitation, 20*(4), 329–337.

Weibelhaus, P., & Hansen, S. L. (2001). Another choice for burn victims. *RN, 64*(9), 34–37.

Weinbren, M. J. (1999). Pharmacokinetics of antibiotics in burn patients. *Journal of Antimicrobial Chemotherapy, 44*(3), 319–327.

Wibbenmeyer, L. A., Amelon, M. J., Morgan, L. J., et al. (2001). Predicting survival in an elderly burn population. *Burns, 27*(6), 583–590.

Wiebelhaus, P., & Hansen, S. L. (2001). What should you know about managing burn emergencies? *Nursing, 31*(1), 36–41.

Winfree, J., & Barillo, D. J. (1997). Nonthermal injuries. *Nursing Clinics of North America, 32*(2), 275–296.

Winfrey, M. E., Cochran, M., & Hegarty, M. (1999). A new technology in burn therapy: Integra artificial skin. *Dimensions in Critical Care Nursing, 18*(1), 14–20.

Wysocki, A. B. (1999). Skin anatomy, physiology, and pathophysiology. *Nursing Clinics of North America, 34*(4), 777–797.

Yin, H. Q., Langford, R., & Burrell, D. E. (1999). Comparative evaluation of the antimicrobial activity of Acticoat Antimicrobial Barrier dressing. *Journal of Burn Care and Rehabilitation, 20*(3), 195–200.

Yowler, C. J., & Fratianne, R. B. (2000). Current status of burn resuscitation. *Clinics in Plastic Surgery, 27*(1), 1–10.

Yu, Y. M., Tompkins, R. G., Ryan, C. M., & Young, V. R. (1999). The metabolic basis of the increase in energy expenditure in severely burned patients. *JPEN: Journal of Parenteral and Enteral Nutrition, 23*(3), 160–168.

Also see issues of *The Journal of Burn Care and Rehabilitation* and *Burns—The Journal of the International Society for Burn Injuries.*

RESOURCES AND WEBSITES

Alisa Ann Ruch Burn Foundation, 20944 Sherman Way, Suite 115, Canoga Park, CA 91303; (818) 883-7700; http://www.aarbf.org.

American Burn Association, 625 N. Michigan Ave., Suite 1530, Chicago, IL 60611; (800) 548-BURN; http://www.ameriburn.org.

American Red Cross. P.O. Box 37243, Washington, DC 20013; (800) HELPNOW; http://www.redcross.org.

Association of Home Appliance Manufacturers. Suite 402, 111 19th Street, NW, Washington, DC 20036; (202) 872-5955; http://www.aham.org.

Burn Children Recovery Foundation, P.O. Box 246, Arlington, VA 98223; (800) 799-BURN; http://www.burnchildrenrecovery.org.

Burn Foundation, 1128 Walnut St., Philadelphia, PA 19107; (215) 629-9200; e-mail: burnctrs@aol.com.

Burn Institute, 3702 Ruffin Rd. #101, San Diego, CA 92123-1812; (619) 541-2277; http://www.burninstitute.com.

Burn Prevention, (610) 481-9810; http://www.burnprevention.org.

Burn Survivor Newsletter: http://www.interlog.com.

Burn Survivors On-Line: http://www.alpha-tek.com/burn/.

Center for Injury Prevention: http://www.bucklebear.com.

Chemical Educational Foundation, 1560 Wilson Boulevard, Suite 1250, Arlington, VA 22209. (703) 527-6223; http://www.chemed.org. Cool the Burn: http://www.cooltheburn.com.

Firefighters Pacific Burn Institute, 3101 Stockton Blvd., Sacramento, CA 95820; (916) 739-8525; http://www.ffpbi.org.

Integra Life Sciences Corporation, P.O. Box 688, 105 Morgan Lane, Plainsboro, NJ 08536; (800) 654-2873; fax: (609) 799-3297; http://www.integra-ls.com.

International Association of Fire Fighters Burn Foundation, 1750 New York Ave., NW, Washington, DC 20006; (202) 737-8484; http://www.iaff.org.

International Society for Burn Injuries; Dr. Keith Judkins, ISBI Secretary/Treasurer, Medical Director for Burn Care, Pinderfields Hospital, Aberford Road, Wakefield, WFI 4DG, England. Phone: +44 1924 212331; http://www.worldburn.org.

Lifecell Corporation, 3606 Research Forest Dr., The Woodlands, TX 77381; (800) 367-5737; http://www.lifecell.com.

Phoenix Society for Burn Survivors, 11 Rust Hill Rd., Levittown, PA 19056; (215) 946-BURN; (800) 888-BURN; http://www.phoenix-society.org.

Sensorineural Function

Applying Concepts from NANDA, NIC, and NOC

Mr. Littlefield is a 64-year-old man who has had several strokes. Ophthalmologic testing reveals that he has homonymous hemianopsia of the left visual field and visual spatial neglect; this means that he has limited vision in the left visual fields of both eyes. He has difficulty in many areas, such as bumping into objects and ignoring the left side of his body. The concept map shows the relationships among selected nursing diagnoses, interventions, and outcomes for Mr. Littlefield's visual problems.

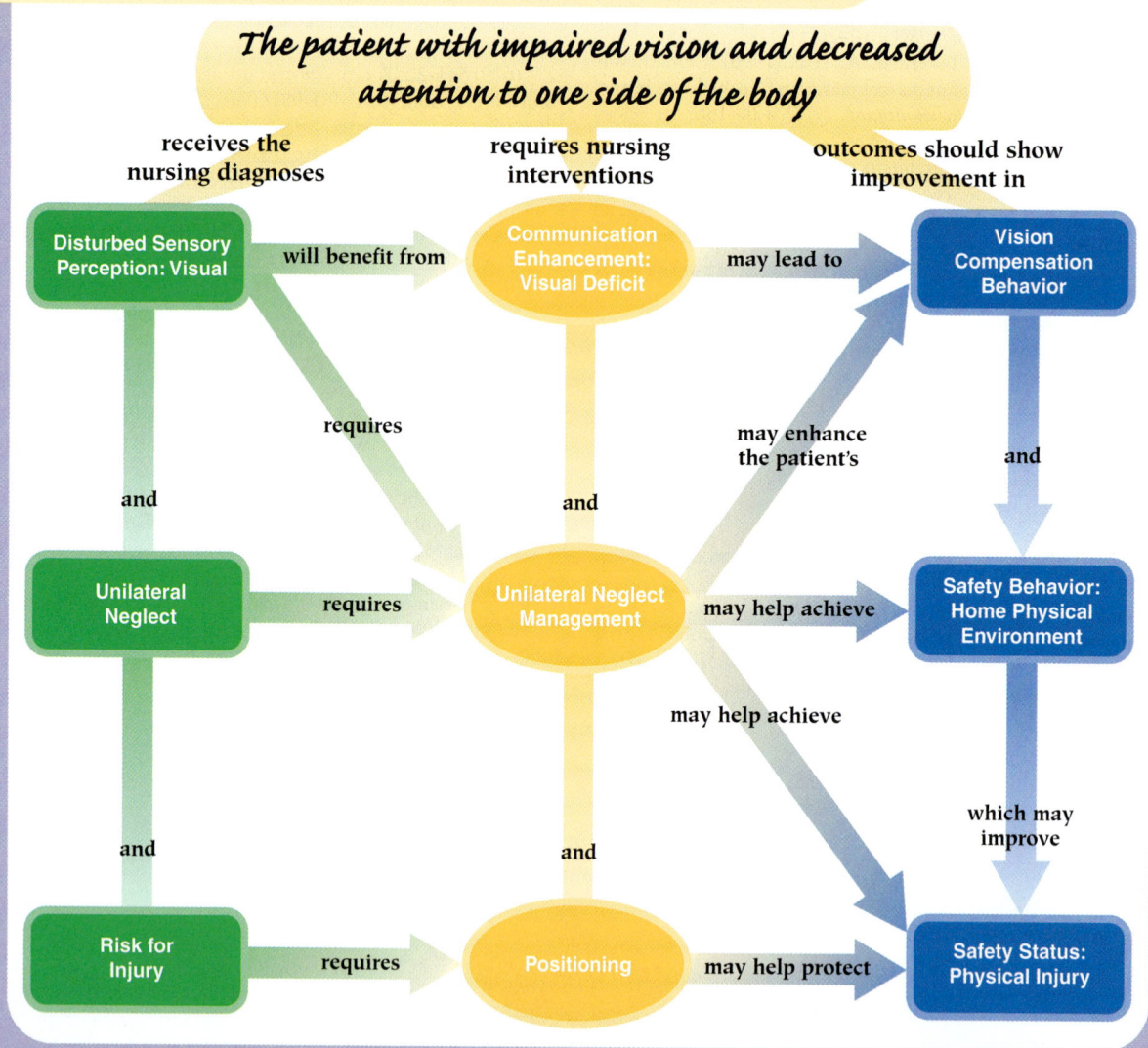

The patient with impaired vision and decreased attention to one side of the body

Nursing Classifications and Languages

NANDA
Nursing Diagnoses

Disturbed Sensory Perception: Visual—Change in the amount or patterning of incoming stimuli accompanied by a diminished, exaggerated, distorted, or impaired response to such stimuli

Unilateral Neglect—Lack of awareness and attention to one side of the body

Risk for Injury—At risk for injury as a result of environmental conditions interacting with the individual's adaptive and defensive resources

NIC
Nursing Interventions*

Communication Enhancement: Visual Deficit—Assistance in accepting and learning alternative methods for living with diminished vision

Unilateral Neglect Management—Protecting and safely reintegrating the affected part of the body while helping the patient adapt to disturbed perceptual abilities

Positioning—Deliberative placement of the patient or a body part to promote physiological and/or psychological well-being

NOC
Nursing Outcomes†

Return to functional baseline status, stabilization of, or improvement in

Vision Compensation Behaviour—Actions to compensate for visual impairment

Safety Behaviour: Home Physical Environment—Individual or caregiver actions to minimize environmental factors that might cause physical harm or injury in the home

Safety Status: Physical Injury—Severity of injuries from trauma

NANDA, North American Nursing Diagnosis Association; NIC, Nursing Interventions Classification; NOC, Nursing Outcomes Classification

*Iowa Intervention Project © 2000. In McCloskey, J. C., & Bulechek, G. M. (2000). *Nursing interventions classification (NIC)* (3rd ed.). St. Louis: Mosby.

†Iowa Outcomes Project © 2000. In Johnson, M., Maas, M., & Moorhead, S. (2000). *Nursing outcomes classification (NOC)* (3rd ed.). St. Louis: Mosby.

Assessment and Management of Patients With Eye and Vision Disorders

Adapted by Tracey Stephen

LEARNING OBJECTIVES

On completion of this chapter, the learner will be able to:

1. Identify significant eye structures and describe their functions.
2. Identify diagnostic tests for assessment of vision and evaluation of visual disabilities.
3. Discuss clinical features of ocular disorders, diagnostic assessment and examinations, medical or surgical management, and patient care.
4. Describe therapeutic effects of ophthalmic medications.
5. Define low vision and blindness and differentiate between functional and visual impairment.
6. List and describe assessment and management strategies for low vision.
7. Demonstrate orientation and mobility techniques for low-vision patients in a hospital setting.
8. Demonstrate instillation of eye drops and ointment.
9. Discuss general discharge instructions for patients after ocular surgery.

*T*he ability to see the world clearly can easily be taken for granted. The eye is a sensitive, highly specialized sense organ subject to various disorders, many of which lead to impaired vision. Impaired vision affects an individual's independence in self-care, work and lifestyle choices, sense of self-esteem, safety, ability to interact with society and the environment, and overall quality of life. Many of the leading causes of visual impairment are associated with aging (eg, cataracts, glaucoma, macular degeneration), and two thirds of the visually impaired population is older than 65 years of age. Younger people are also at risk for eye disorders, particularly traumatic injuries.

Although most people with eye disorders are treated in an ambulatory care setting, many patients receiving health care have an eye disease as a comorbid condition. In addition to understanding the prevention, treatment, and consequences of eye disorders, nurses in all settings should assess visual acuity in those at risk (eg, patients who are elderly, those with diabetes or acquired immunodeficiency syndrome [AIDS]), refer patients to eye care specialists as appropriate, implement measures to prevent further visual loss, and help patients adapt to impaired vision.

Anatomic and Physiologic Overview

Unlike most organs of the body, the eye is available for external examination, and its anatomy is more easily assessed than many other body parts (Fig. 58-1). The eyeball, or globe, sits in a protective bony structure known as the orbit. Lined with muscle and

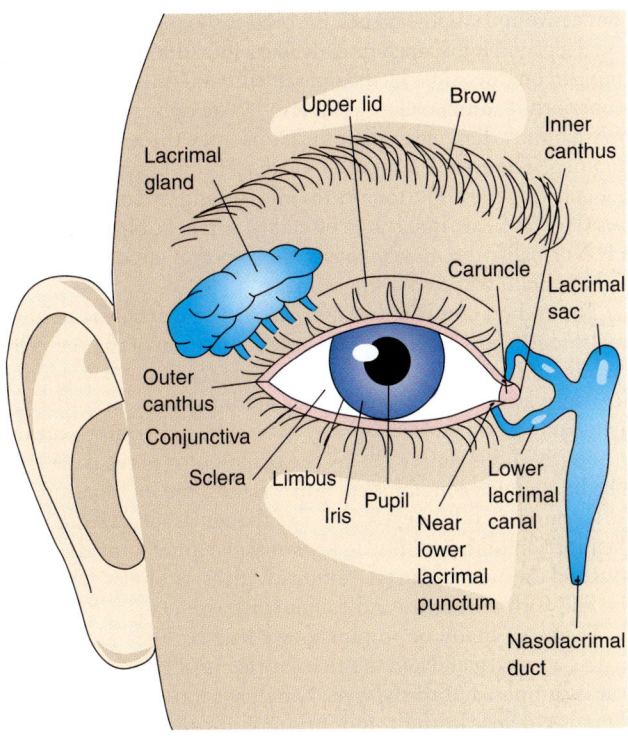

FIGURE 58-1 External structures of the eye and position of the lacrimal structures.

Glossary

accommodation: process by which the eye adjusts for near distance (eg, reading) by changing the curvature of the lens to focus a clear image on the retina

anterior chamber: space in the eye bordered anteriorly by the cornea and posteriorly by the iris and pupil

aphakia: absence of the natural lens

astigmatism: refractive error in which light rays are spread over a diffuse area rather than sharply focused on the retina, a condition caused by differences in the curvature of the cornea and lens

binocular vision: normal ability of both eyes to focus on one object and fuse the two images into one

blindness: inability to see, usually defined as corrected visual acuity of 20/400 or less, or a visual field of no more than 20 degrees in the better eye

chemosis: edema of the conjunctiva

cones: retinal photoreceptor cells essential for visual acuity and colour discrimination

diplopia: seeing one object as two; double vision

emmetropia: absence of refractive error

enucleation: complete removal of the eyeball and part of the optic nerve

exenteration: surgical removal of the entire contents of the orbit, including the eyeball and lids

evisceration: removal of the intraocular contents through a corneal or scleral incision; the optic nerve, sclera, extraocular muscles, and sometimes, the cornea are left intact

hyperemia: "red eye" resulting from dilation of the vasculature of the conjunctiva

hyperopia: farsightedness; a refractive error in which the focus of light rays from a distant object is behind the retina

hyphema: blood in the anterior chamber

hypopyon: collection of inflammatory cells that has the appearance of a pale layer in the inferior anterior chamber of the eye

injection: congestion of blood vessels

keratoconus: cone-shaped deformity of the cornea

keratopathy, bullous: corneal edema with painful blisters in the epithelium due to excessive corneal hydration

limbus: junction of the cornea and sclera

miotics: medications that cause pupillary constriction

mydriatics: medications that cause pupillary dilation

myopia: nearsightedness; a refractive error in which the focus of light rays from a distant object is anterior to the retina

neovascularization: growth of abnormal new blood vessels

nystagmus: involuntary oscillation of the eyeball

papilledema: swelling of the optic disc due to increased intracranial pressure

photophobia: ocular pain on exposure to light

posterior chamber: space between the iris and vitreous

proptosis: downward displacement of the eyeball resulting from an inflammatory condition of the orbit or a mass within the orbital cavity

ptosis: drooping eyelid

refraction: determination of the refractive errors of the eye and correction by lenses

rods: retinal photoreceptor cells essential for bright and dim light

scotomas: blind or partially blind areas in the visual field

strabismus: a condition in which there is deviation from perfect ocular alignment

sympathetic ophthalmia: an inflammatory condition created in the fellow eye by the affected eye (without useful vision): the condition may become chronic and result in blindness (of the fellow eye)

trachoma: a bilateral chronic follicular conjunctivitis of childhood that leads to blindness during adulthood, if left untreated

vitreous humour: gelatinous material (transparent and colourless) that fills the eyeball behind the lens

Note: Common abbreviations related to vision and eye health are OD (ocular dexter, right eye), OS (ocular sinister, left eye), and OU (ocular uterque, both eyes).

connective and adipose tissues, the orbit is about 4 cm high, wide, and deep, and it is shaped roughly like a four-sided pyramid, surrounded on three sides by the sinuses: ethmoid (medially), frontal (superiorly), and maxillary (inferiorly). The optic nerve and the ophthalmic artery enter the orbit at its apex through the optic foramen. The eyeball is moved though all fields of gaze by the extraocular muscles. The four rectus muscles and two oblique muscles (Fig. 58-2) are innervated by cranial nerves (CN) III, IV, and VI. Normally, the movements of the two eyes are coordinated, and the brain perceives a single image.

The eyelids, composed of thin elastic skin that covers striated and smooth muscles, protect the anterior portion of the eye. The eyelids contain multiple glands, including sebaceous, sweat, and accessory lacrimal glands, and they are lined with conjunctival material. The upper lid normally covers the uppermost portion of the iris and is innervated by the oculomotor nerve (CN III). The lid margins contain meibomian glands, the inferior and superior puncta, and the eyelashes. The triangular spaces formed by the junction of the eyelids are known as the inner or medial canthus and the outer or lateral canthus. With every blink of the eyes, the lids wash the cornea and conjunctiva with tears.

Tears are vitally important to eye health. They are formed by the lacrimal gland and the accessory lacrimal glands. A healthy tear is composed of three layers: lipoid, aqueous, and mucoid. If there is a defect in the composition of any of these layers, the integrity of the cornea may be compromised. Tears are secreted in response to reflex or emotional stimuli.

The conjunctiva, a mucous membrane, provides a barrier to the external environment and nourishes the eye. The goblet cells of the conjunctiva secrete lubricating mucus. The bulbar conjunctiva covers the sclera, whereas the palpebral conjunctiva lines the inner surface of the upper and lower eyelids. The junction of the two portions is known as the fornix.

The sclera, commonly known as the white of the eye, is a dense, fibrous structure that comprises the posterior five sixths of the eye (Fig. 58-3). The sclera helps to maintain the shape of the eyeball and protects the intraocular contents from trauma. The sclera may have a slightly bluish tinge in young children, a dull white colour in adults, and a slightly yellowish colour in the elderly. Externally, it is overlaid with conjunctiva, which is a thin, transparent, mucous membrane that contains fine blood vessels. The conjunctiva meets the cornea at the **limbus** on the outermost edge of the iris.

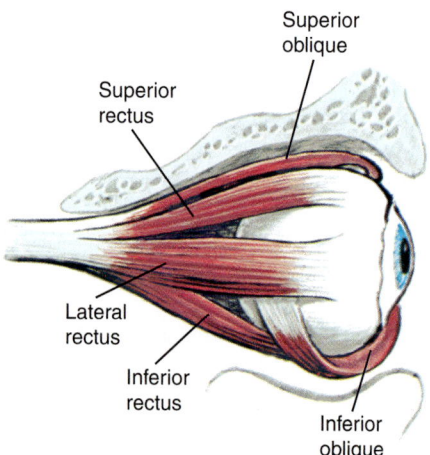

FIGURE 58-2 The extraocular muscles responsible for eye movement. The medial rectus muscle (not shown) is responsible for opposing the movement of the lateral rectus muscle.

The cornea (Fig. 58-4), a transparent, avascular, domelike structure, forms the most anterior portion of the eyeball and is the main refracting surface of the eye. It is composed of five layers: epithelium, Bowman's membrane, stroma, Descemet's membrane, and endothelium. The epithelial cells are capable of rapid replication and are completely replaced every 7 days.

Behind the cornea lies the **anterior chamber**, filled with a continually replenished supply of clear aqueous humour, which nourishes the cornea. The aqueous humour is produced by the ciliary body, and its production is related to the intraocular pressure (IOP). Normal pressure is 10 to 21 mm Hg.

The uvea consists of the iris, the ciliary body, and the choroid. The iris, or coloured part of the eye, is a highly vascularized, pigmented collection of fibres surrounding the pupil. The pupil is a space that dilates and constricts in response to light. Normal pupils are round and constrict symmetrically when a bright light shines on them. About 20% of the population has pupils that are slightly unequal in size but that respond equally to light. Dilation and constriction are controlled by the sphincter and dilator pupillae muscles. The dilator muscles are controlled by the sympathetic nervous system, whereas the sphincter muscles are controlled by the parasympathetic nervous system.

Directly behind the pupil and iris lies the lens, a colourless and almost completely transparent, biconvex structure held in position by zonular fibres. It is avascular and has no nerve or pain fibres. The lens enables focusing for near vision and refocusing for distance vision. The ability to focus and refocus is called **accommodation**. The lens is suspended behind the iris by the zonules and is connected to the ciliary body. The ciliary body controls accommodation through the zonular fibres and the ciliary muscles. The aqueous humour is anterior to the lens; posterior to the lens is the **vitreous humour**. All cells formed throughout life are retained by the lens, which makes the cell structure of the lens susceptible to the degenerative effects of aging. The lens continues to grow throughout life, laying down fibres in concentric rings. This gradual thickening becomes evident in the fifth decade of life and eventually results in an increasingly dense core or nucleus, which can limit accommodative powers.

The **posterior chamber** is a small space between the vitreous and the iris. Aqueous fluid is manufactured in the posterior chamber by the ciliary body. This aqueous fluid flows from the posterior chamber into the anterior chamber, from which it drains through the trabecular meshwork into the canal of Schlemm.

The choroid lies between the retina and the sclera. It is a vascular tissue, supplying blood to the portion of the sensory retina closest to it.

The ocular fundus is the largest chamber of the eye and contains the vitreous humour, a clear, gelatinous substance, composed mostly of water and encapsulated by a hyaloid membrane. The vitreous humour occupies about two thirds of the eye's volume and helps maintain the shape of the eye. As the body ages, the gel-like characteristics are gradually lost, and various cells and fibres cast shadows that the patient perceives as "floaters." The vitreous is in continuous contact with the retina and is attached to the retina by scattered collagenous filaments. The vitreous shrinks and shifts with age.

The innermost surface of the fundus is the retina. The retina is composed of 10 microscopic layers and has the consistency of wet tissue paper. It is neural tissue, an extension of the optic nerve. Viewed through the pupil, the landmarks of the retina are the optic disc, the retinal vessels, and the macula. The point of entrance of the optic nerve into the retina is the optic disc. The optic disc is oval or circular, is pink, and has sharp margins. In

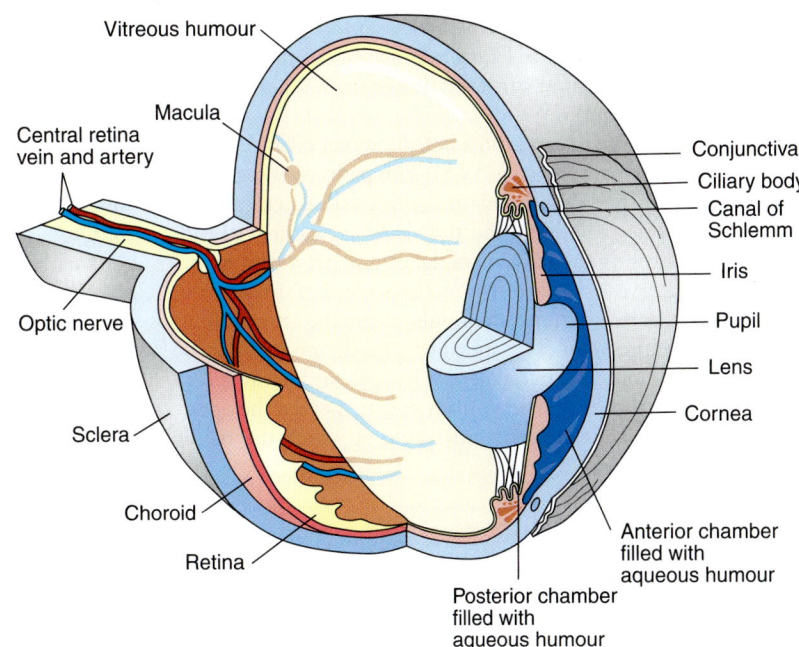

FIGURE 58-3 Three-dimensional cross-section of the eye.

the disc, a physiologic depression or cup is present centrally, with the retinal blood vessels emanating from it. The retinal tissues arise from the optic disc and line the inner surface of the vitreous chamber. The retinal vessels also enter the eye through the optic nerve, branching out through the retina and forming superior and inferior arcades. The area of the retina responsible for central vision is the macula. The rest of the retina is responsible for peripheral vision. In the centre of the macula is the most sensitive area, the fovea, which is avascular and surrounded by the superior and inferior vascular arcades. Two important layers of the retina are the retinal pigment epithelium (RPE) and the sensory retina. A single layer of cells constitutes the RPE, and these cells have numerous functions, including the absorption of light. The sensory retina contains the photoreceptor cells: **rods** and **cones**. Rods and cones are long, narrow cells shaped like rods or cones. The rods are mainly responsible for night vision or vision in low

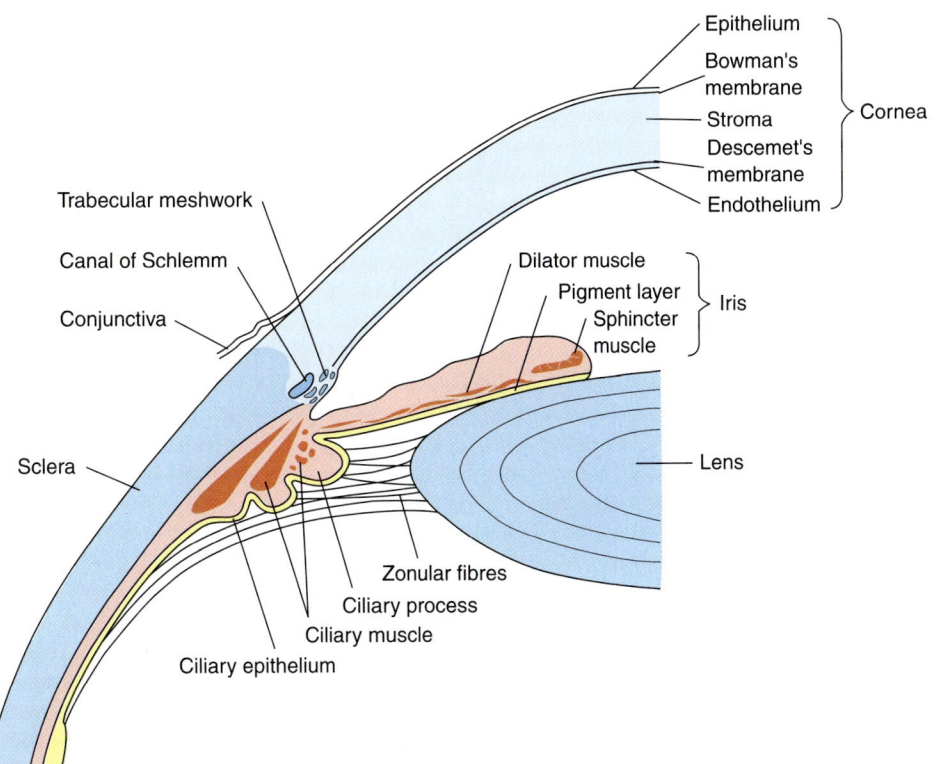

FIGURE 58-4 Internal structures of the eye. From Goldblum, K. (Ed.) (1997). *Core curriculum for ophthalmic nursing, American Society of Ophthalmic Registered Nurses.* Dubuque, IA: Kendall/ Hall Publishing.

light, whereas the cones provide the best vision for bright light, colour vision, and fine detail. Cones are distributed throughout the retina with their greatest concentration in the fovea. Rods are absent in the fovea.

Good visual acuity depends on a healthy, functioning eyeball and an intact visual pathway (Fig. 58-5). This pathway is made up of the retina, optic nerve, optic chiasm, optic tracks, lateral geniculate bodies, optic radiations, and the visual cortex area of the brain. The pathway is an extension of the central nervous system.

The optic nerve is also known as the second cranial nerve (CN II). Its purpose is to transmit impulses from the retina to the occipital lobe of the brain. The optic nerve head, or optic disc, is the physiologic blind spot in each eye. The optic nerve leaves the eye and then meets the optic nerve from the other eye at the optic chiasm. The chiasm is the anatomic point at which the nasal

fibres from the nasal retina of each eye cross to the opposite side of the brain. The nerve fibres from the temporal retina of each eye remain uncrossed. Fibres from the right half of each eye, which would be the left visual field, therefore carry impulses to the right occipital lobe. Fibres from the left half of each eye, or the right visual field, carry impulses to the left occipital lobe. Beyond the chiasm, these fibres are known as the optic tract. The optic tract continues on to the lateral geniculate body. The lateral geniculate body leads to the optic radiations and then to the cortex of the occipital lobe of the brain.

Assessment

The health care provider, through careful questioning, elicits the necessary information that can lead to the diagnosis of an ophthalmic condition. Pertinent questions to ask during the interview can be found in Chart 58-1.

OCULAR EXAMINATION

After the patient's chief complaint or concern has been identified and the history has been obtained, visual acuity should be assessed. This is an essential part of the eye examination and a measure against which all therapeutic outcomes are based.

Visual Acuity

Most health care providers are familiar with the standard Snellen chart. This chart is composed of a series of progressively smaller rows of letters and is used to test distance vision. The fraction 20/20 is considered the standard of normal vision. Most people can see the letters on the line designated as 20/20 from a distance of 20 feet. A person whose vision is 20/200 can see an object from 20 feet away that a person whose vision is 20/20 can see from 200 feet away.

The patient is positioned at the prescribed distance, usually 20 feet, from the chart and is asked to read the smallest line that he or she can see. The patient should wear distance correction (eye-

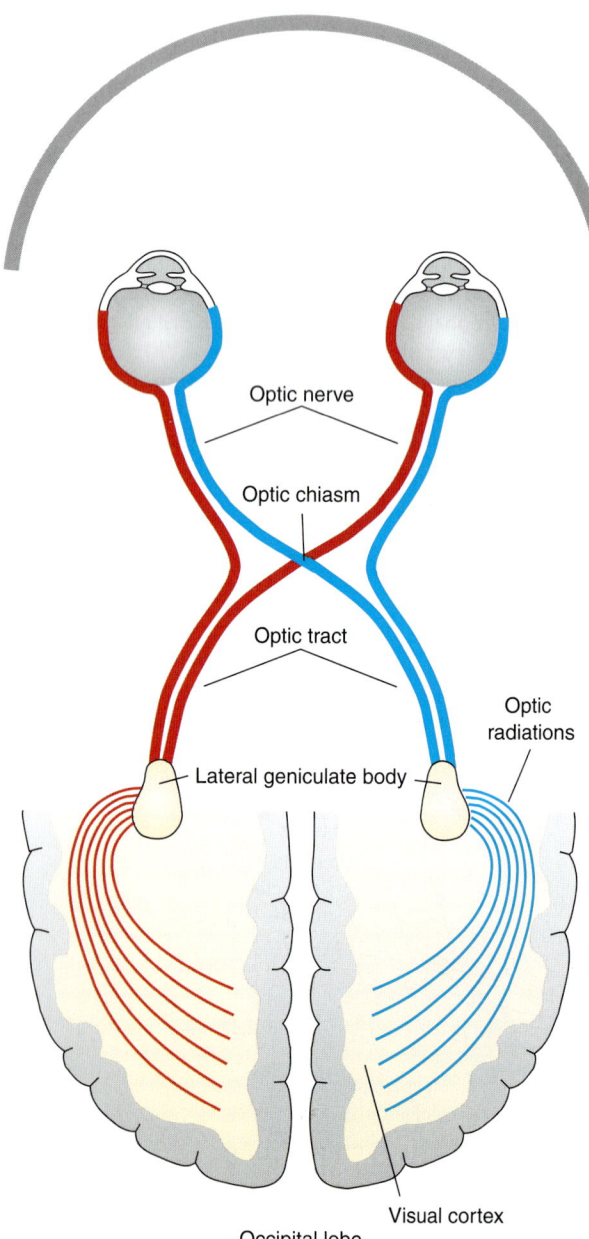

Optic nerve

Optic chiasm

Optic tract

Optic radiations

Lateral geniculate body

Visual cortex

Occipital lobe

FIGURE 58-5 The visual pathway. From Goldblum, K. (Ed.) (1997). *Core curriculum for ophthalmic nursing, American Society of Ophthalmic Registered Nurses.* Dubuque, IA: Kendall/Hall Publishing.

Chart 58-1 • ASSESSMENT

Taking an Ocular History

- What does the patient perceive to be the problem?
- Is visual acuity diminished?
- Does the patient experience blurred, double, or distorted vision?
- Is there pain; is it sharp or dull; is it worse when blinking?
- Is the discomfort an itching sensation or more of a foreign body sensation?
- Are both eyes affected?
- Is there a history of discharge? If so, question colour, consistency, odour.
- What is the duration of the problem?
- Is this a recurrence of a previous condition?
- How has the patient self-treated?
- What makes the symptoms improve or worsen?
- Are there any systemic diseases? What medications are used in their treatment?
- What concurrent ophthalmic conditions does the patient have?
- Is there an ophthalmic surgery history?
- Have other family members had the same symptoms or condition?

glasses or contact lenses) if required, and each eye should be tested separately. The right eye is commonly tested first. The patient is asked to cover the left eye while the right eye is being tested. Patients should be encouraged to read every letter possible and to guess, if necessary. If the patient successfully reads the line, the examiner encourages the patient to attempt the next line of smaller letters. The smallest line in which the patient can successfully identify more than half the letters is recorded as the visual acuity for the eye being tested. This procedure is then repeated for the left eye, with the right eye covered, and then both eyes are tested together. If a patient is unable to read the English alphabet, a Snellen E Chart is available.

The visual acuity (VA) is recorded in the following way. If the patient reads all five letters from the 20/20 line with the right eye (OD) and three of the five letters on the 20/15 line with the left eye (OS), the examiner writes OD 20/20, OS 20/15-2, or VA 20/20, 20/15-2.

If the patient is unable to read the largest letter on the chart (the 20/200 line), the patient should be moved toward the chart or the chart moved toward the patient, until the patient is able to identify the largest letter on the chart. If the patient can recognize only the letter E on the top line at a distance of 10 feet, the visual acuity would be recorded as 10′/200. If the patient is unable to see the letter E at any distance, the examiner should determine if the patient can count fingers (CF). The examiner holds up a random number of fingers and asks the patient to count the number he or she sees. If the patient correctly identifies the number of fingers at 3 feet, the examiner would record CF/3′.

If the patient is unable to count fingers, the examiner raises one hand up and down or moves it side to side and asks in which direction the hand is moving. This level of vision is known as hand motions (HM). A patient who can perceive only light is described as having light perception (LP). The vision of a patient who is unable to perceive light is described as no light perception (NLP).

The External Eye Examination

After the visual acuity has been recorded, an external eye examination is performed. The position of the eyelids is noted. Commonly, the upper 2 mm of the iris is covered by the upper lid. The patient is examined for **ptosis** (ie, drooping eyelid) and for lid retraction (ie, too much of the eye exposed). Sometimes, the upper or lower lid turns out, affecting closure. The lid margins and lashes should have no edema, erythema, or lesions. The examiner looks for scaling or crusting, and the sclera is inspected. A normal sclera is opaque and white. Lesions on the conjunctiva, discharge, and tearing or blinking are noted.

The room should be darkened so that the pupils can be examined. The pupillary response should be checked with a penlight to be certain that the pupils are equally reactive and regular. A normal pupil is black. An irregular pupil may result from trauma, previous surgery, or a disease process.

The patient's eyes are observed in primary or direct gaze, and any head tilt is noted. A tilt may indicate cranial nerve palsy. The patient is asked to stare at a target; each eye is covered and uncovered quickly while the examiner looks for any shift in gaze. The examiner observes for **nystagmus** (ie, oscillating movement of the eyeball). The extraocular movements of the eyes are simply tested by having the patient follow the examiner's finger or penlight through the six cardinal directions of gaze (right, right upward, right downward, left, left upward, and left downward). (Fig. 58-6). This is especially important when screening patients for ocular trauma or for neurologic disorders.

FIGURE 58-6 Testing extraocular movements. From Skillen, D. L. & Day, R. A. (Eds.) (2004). *A syllabus for adult health assessment.* Edmonton, AB: Faculty of Nursing, University of Alberta.

Diagnostic Evaluation

DIRECT OPHTHALMOSCOPY

A direct ophthalmoscope is a hand-held instrument with various plus and minus lenses. The lenses can be rotated into place, enabling the examiner to bring the cornea, lens, and retina into focus sequentially. The examiner holds the ophthalmoscope in the right hand and uses the right eye to examine the patient's right eye. The examiner switches to the left hand and left eye when examining the patient's left eye. During this examination, the room should be darkened, and the patient's eye should be on the same level as the examiner's eye. The patient and the examiner should be comfortable, and both should breathe normally. The patient is given a target to gaze on and is encouraged to keep both eyes open and steady.

When the fundus is examined, the vasculature comes into focus first. The veins are larger in diameter than the arteries. The examiner should focus on a large vessel and then follow it toward the midline of the body, which leads to the optic nerve. The central depression in the disc is known as the cup. The normal cup is about one third of the disc. The size of the physiologic optic cup should be estimated. Are the disc margins sharp, or are they blurred? Do the veins have a silvery or coppery appearance? The periphery of the retina can be examined by having the patient shift his or her gaze. The last area of the fundus to be examined should be the macula, because this area is the most light sensitive. The retina of a young person often has a glistening effect, which is sometimes referred to as a cellophane reflex.

The healthy fundus should be free of any lesions. The examiner should look for intraretinal hemorrhages, which may appear as red smudges or, if the patient has hypertension, may look somewhat flame shaped. Lipid may be present in the retina of patients with hypercholesterolemia or diabetes. This lipid has a yellowish appearance. Soft exudates that have a fuzzy, white appearance (ie, cotton-wool spots) should be noted. The examiner looks for microaneurysms, which look like little red dots, and nevi. Drusen (ie, small, hyaline, globular growths), commonly found in macular degeneration, appear to be yellowish areas with indistinct edges. Small drusen have a more distinct edge. The examiner should sketch the fundus and document any abnormalities.

INDIRECT OPHTHALMOSCOPY

The indirect ophthalmoscope is an instrument commonly used by the ophthalmologist. It produces a bright and intense light. The light source is affixed with a pair of binocular lenses, which are mounted on the examiner's head. The ophthalmoscope is used with a hand-held, 20-diopter lens. This instrument enables the examiner to see larger areas of the retina, although in an unmagnified state.

SLIT-LAMP EXAMINATION

The slit lamp is a binocular microscope mounted on a table. This instrument enables the user to examine the eye with magnification of 10 to 40 times the real image. The illumination can be varied from a broad to a narrow beam of light for different parts of the eye. For example, by varying the width and intensity of the light, the anterior chamber can be examined for signs of inflammation. Cataracts may be evaluated by changing the angle of the light. When a hand-held contact lens, such as a three-mirror lens, is used with the slit lamp, the angle of the anterior chamber may be examined, as may the ocular fundus.

COLOUR VISION TESTING

The ability to differentiate colours has a dramatic effect on the activities of daily living. For example, the inability to differentiate between red and green can compromise traffic safety. Some careers (eg, commercial art, colour photography, airline pilot, electrician) may be closed to people with significant colour deficiencies. The photoreceptor cells responsible for colour vision are the cones, and the greatest area of colour sensitivity is in the macula, the area of densest cone concentration.

A screening test, such as the polychromatic plates discussed in the next paragraph, can be used to establish whether a person's colour vision is within normal range. Colour vision deficits can be inherited. For example, red/green colour deficiencies are inherited in an X-linked manner, affecting approximately 8% of men and 0.4% of women. Acquired colour vision losses may be caused by medications (eg, digitalis toxicity) or pathology such as cataracts. A simple test, such as asking a patient if the red top on a bottle of eye drops appears redder to one eye than the other, can be an effective tool. Changes in the appreciation of the gradations of the colour red can indicate macular or optic nerve disease.

Because alteration in colour vision is sometimes indicative of conditions of the optic nerve, colour vision testing is often performed in a neuro-ophthalmologic workup. The most common colour vision test is performed using Ishihara polychromatic plates. These plates are bound together in a booklet. On each plate of this booklet are dots of primary colours that are integrated into a background of secondary colours. The dots are arranged in simple patterns, such as numbers or geometric shapes. Patients with diminished colour vision may be unable to identify the hidden shapes. Patients with central vision conditions (eg, macular degeneration) have more difficulty identifying colours than those with peripheral vision conditions (eg, glaucoma) because central vision identifies colour.

AMSLER GRID

The Amsler grid is a test often used for patients with macular problems, such as macular degeneration. It consists of a geometric grid of identical squares with a central fixation point. The grid should be viewed by the patient wearing normal reading glasses. Each eye is tested separately. The patient is instructed to stare at the central fixation spot on the grid and report any distortion in the squares of the grid itself. For patients with macular problems, some of the squares may look faded, or the lines may be wavy. Patients with age-related macular degeneration are commonly given

these Amsler grids to take home. The patient is encouraged to check them frequently, as often as daily, to detect any early signs of distortion that may indicate the development of a neovascular choroidal membrane, an advanced stage of macular degeneration characterized by the growth of abnormal choroidal vessels.

ULTRASONOGRAPHY

Lesions in the globe or the orbit may not be directly visible and are evaluated by ultrasonography. A probe placed against the eye aims the beam of sound. High-frequency sound waves emitted from a special transmitter are bounced back from the lesion and collected by a receiver that amplifies and displays the sound waves on a special screen. Ultrasonography can be used to identify orbital tumours, retinal detachment, and changes in tissue composition.

COLOUR FUNDUS PHOTOGRAPHY

Fundus photography is a technique used to detect and document retinal lesions. The patient's pupils are widely dilated during the procedure, and visual acuity is diminished for about 30 minutes due to retinal "bleaching" by the intense flashing lights.

FLUORESCEIN ANGIOGRAPHY

Fluorescein angiography evaluates clinically significant macular edema, documents macular capillary nonperfusion, and identifies retinal and choroidal **neovascularization** (ie, growth of abnormal new blood vessels) in age-related macular degeneration. It is an invasive procedure in which fluorescein dye is injected, usually into an antecubital area vein. Within 10 to 15 seconds, this dye can be seen coursing through the retinal vessels. Over a 10-minute period, serial black-and-white photographs are taken of the retinal vasculature. The dye may impart a gold tone to the skin of some patients, and urine may turn deep yellow or orange. This discolouration usually disappears in 24 hours.

TONOMETRY

Tonometry measures IOP by determining the amount of force necessary to indent or flatten (applanate) a small anterior area of the globe of the eye. The principle involved is that a soft eye is dented more easily than a hard eye. Pressure is measured in millimeters of mercury (mm Hg). High readings indicate high pressure; low readings, low pressure. The three most common types of tonometers are indentation, applanation, and noncontact. The procedure is noninvasive and is usually painless. A topical anesthetic eye drop is instilled in the lower conjunctival sac, and the tonometer is then used to measure the IOP.

GONIOSCOPY

Gonioscopy visualizes the angle of the anterior chamber to identify abnormalities in appearance and measurements. The gonioscope uses a refracting lens that can be a direct or indirect lens. The indirect lens views the mirror image of the opposite anterior chamber angle and can be used only with a slit lamp. The direct gonioscopic lens gives a direct view of the angle and its structures.

PERIMETRY TESTING

Perimetry testing evaluates the field of vision. A visual field is the area or extent of physical space visible to an eye in a given position. Its average extent is 65 degrees upward, 75 degrees downward, 60 degrees inward, and 95 degrees outward when the eye is in the primary gaze (ie, looking directly forward). It is a three-dimensional contour representing areas of relative retinal sensitivity. Visual acuity is sharpest at the very top of the field and declines progressively toward the periphery. Visual field testing (ie, perimetry) helps to identify which parts of the patient's central and peripheral visual fields have useful vision. It is most helpful in detecting central **scotomas** (ie, blind areas in the visual field) in macular degeneration and the peripheral field defects in glaucoma and retinitis pigmentosa.

The two methods of perimetric testing are manual and automated perimetry. Manual perimetry involves the use of moving (kinetic) or stationary (static) stimuli or targets. An example of kinetic manual perimetry is the tangent screen. A tangent screen is a black felt material mounted on a wall that has a series of concentric circles dissected by straight lines emanating from the centre. It tests the central 30 degrees of the visual field. Automated perimetry uses stationary targets, which are harder to detect than moving targets. In this test, a computer projects light randomly in different areas of a hollow dome while the patient looks through a telescopic opening and depresses a button whenever he or she detects the light stimulus. Automated perimetry is more accurate than manual perimetry.

Impaired Vision

REFRACTIVE ERRORS

In refractive errors, vision is impaired because a shortened or elongated eyeball prevents light rays from focusing sharply on the retina. Blurred vision from refractive error can be corrected with eyeglasses or contact lenses. The appropriate eyeglass or contact lens is determined by **refraction**. Refraction ophthalmology consists of placing various types of lenses in front of the patient's eyes to determine which lens best improves the patient's vision.

The depth of the eyeball is important in determining refractive error (Fig. 58-7). Patients for whom the visual image focuses precisely on the macula and who do not need eyeglasses or contact lenses are said to have **emmetropia** (normal vision). People who have **myopia** are said to be nearsighted. They have deeper eyeballs; the distant visual image focuses in front of, or short of, the retina. Myopic people experience blurred distance vision. When people have a shorter depth to their eyes, the visual image focuses beyond the retina; the eyes are shallower and are called hyperopic. People with **hyperopia** are farsighted. These patients experience near vision blurriness, whereas their distance vision is excellent.

Another important cause of refractive error is **astigmatism**, an irregularity in the curve of the cornea. Because astigmatism causes a distortion of the visual image, acuity of distance and near vision can be decreased. Eyeglasses with a cylinder correction or rigid or soft toric contact lenses are appropriate for these patients.

LOW VISION AND BLINDNESS

Low vision is a general term describing visual impairment that requires patients to use devices and strategies in addition to corrective lenses to perform visual tasks. Low vision is defined as a best corrected visual acuity (BCVA) of 20/70 to 20/200 (Table 58-1).

Blindness is defined as a BCVA of 20/400 to no light perception. The clinical definition of absolute blindness is the absence of light perception. Legal blindness is a condition of impaired vision in which an individual has a BCVA that does not exceed 20/200 in the better eye or whose widest visual field diameter is 20 degrees or less. This definition does not equate with functional

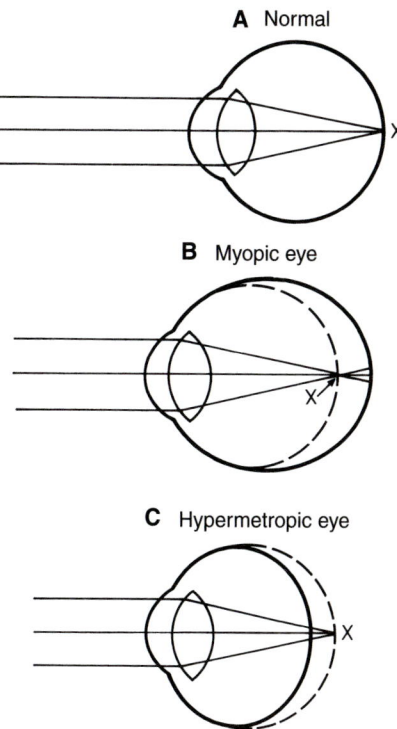

FIGURE 58-7 Eyeball shape determines visual acuity in refractive errors. (**A**) Normal eye. (**B**) Myopic eye. (**C**) Hypermetropic eye.

ability, nor does it classify the degrees of visual impairment. Legal blindness ranges from an inability to perceive light to having some vision remaining. An individual who meets the criteria for legal blindness may obtain government financial assistance. There are approximately 105,000 legally blind Canadians, with the largest

Table 58-1 • Categories of Visual Impairment

CATEGORY OF VISUAL IMPAIRMENT	VISUAL ACUITY (BEST CORRECTED)
Low vision	
1	6/18
	3/10 (0.3)
	20/70
2	6/60
	1/10 (0.1)
	20/200
Blindness	
3	3/60 (finger counting at 3 m)
	1/20 (0.05)
	20/400
4	1/60 (finger counting at 1 m)
	1/50 (0.02)
	5/300
5	No light perception

Visual Field
Patients with a visual field radius no greater than 10 degrees but greater than 5 degrees around central fixation should be placed in category 3, and patients with a field no greater than 5 degrees around central fixation in category 4—even if the central acuity is not impaired.

Adapted from the *International Classification of Diseases*, World Health Organization, 1977; and from Vaughn, D. G., Asbury, T., & Riorda-Eva, P. (Eds.). (1999). *General ophthalmology*. Stamford, CT: Appleton & Lange.

portion of this group being over 65 years of age. Five percent are children and 64% are seniors. The number of Canadians who are blind or visually impaired is estimated to increase to 187,000 by 2015 (Canadian National Institute for the Blind, 2005b).

Impaired vision is accompanied by difficulty in performing functional activities. Individuals with visual acuity of 20/80 to 20/100 with a visual field restriction of 60 degrees to greater than 20 degrees can read at a nearly normal level with optical aids. Their visual orientation is near normal but requires increased scanning of the environment (ie, systematic use of head and eye movements). In a visual acuity range of 20/200 to 20/400 with a 20-degree to greater than 10-degree visual field restriction, the individual can read slowly with optical aids. His or her visual orientation is slow, with constant scanning of the environment; individuals in this category have travel vision. Individuals with hand motion vision or no vision may benefit from the use of mobility devices (eg, cane, guide dog) and should be encouraged to learn Braille and to use computer aids.

The most common causes of blindness and visual impairment among adults 40 years of age or older are diabetic retinopathy, macular degeneration, glaucoma, and cataracts, (Preshel & Prevent Blindness America, 2002). Macular degeneration is more prevalent among Caucasians, whereas glaucoma is more prevalent among African Canadians. Age-related changes in the eye are described in Table 58-2.

Low-Vision Assessment

The assessment of low vision includes a thorough history and the examination of distance and near visual acuity, visual field, contrast sensitivity, glare, colour perception, and refraction. Specially designed, low-vision visual acuity charts are used to evaluate patients.

PATIENT INTERVIEW

During history taking, the cause and duration of the patient's visual impairment are identified. Patients with retinitis pigmentosa,

for example, have a genetic abnormality. Patients with diabetic macular edema typically have fluctuating visual acuity. Patients with macular degeneration have central acuity problems. Central acuity problems cause difficulty in performing activities that require finer vision, such as reading. People with peripheral field defects have more difficulties with mobility. The patient's customary activities of daily living, medication regimen, habits (eg, smoking), acceptance of the physical limitations brought about by the visual impairment, and realistic expectations of low-vision aids must also be identified. These aspects of the patient's activities are important indicators for planning care that will include guidelines for safety and referrals to social services.

ASSESSMENT

Contrast-sensitivity testing measures visual acuity in different degrees of contrast. The initial test may take the form of simply turning on the lights while testing the distance acuity. If the patient can read better with the lights on, the patient can benefit from magnification. Glare testing enables the examiner to obtain a more realistic evaluation of the patient's ability to function in his or her environment. Glare can reduce a person's ability to see, especially in patients with cataracts. Devices that test glare, such as the Brightness Acuity Tester, produce three degrees of bright light to create a dazzle effect while the patient is viewing a target, such as Snellen letters on the wall. The lights have been calibrated to imitate certain objects that create glare, such as the brightness of a car's headlights at night.

Medical Management

Managing low vision involves magnification and image enhancement through the use of low-vision aids and strategies and through referrals to social services and community agencies serving the visually impaired. The goals are to enhance visual function and assist patients with low vision to perform customary activities. Low-vision aids include optical and nonoptical devices

Table 58-2 • Age-Related Changes in the Eye

THE EXTERNAL EYE	STRUCTURAL CHANGE	FUNCTIONAL CHANGE	HISTORY & PHYSICAL FINDINGS
Eyelids and lacrimal structures	Loss of skin elasticity and orbital fat, decreased muscle tone; wrinkles develop	Lid margins turn in causing lashes to irritate cornea and conjunctiva (entropian); or lid margins may turn out, resulting in increased corneal exposure (ectropian)	Reports of burning, foreign body sensation, increased tearing (epiphoria); injection, inflammation, and ulceration may occur
Refractive changes; presbyopia	Loss of accommodative power in the lens with age	Reading materials must be held at increasing distance in order to focus	Patient reports, "Arms are too short!"; need for increased light; reading glasses or bifocals needed
Cataract	Opacities in the normally crystalline lens	Interference with the focus of a sharp image on the retina	Patients report increased glare, decreased vision, changes in colour values (blue and yellow especially affected)
Posterior vitreous detachment	Liquefaction and shrinkage of vitreous body	May lead to retinal tears and detachment	Reports light flashes, cobwebs, floaters
Age-related macular degeneration (AMD)	Drusen (yellowish aging spots in the retina) appear and coalesce in the macula. Abnormal choroidal blood vessels may lead to formation of fibrotic disciform scars in the macula	Central vision is affected; onset is more gradual in dry AMD, more rapid in wet AMD; distortion and loss of central vision may occur	Reading vision is affected; words may be missing letters, faded areas appear on the page, straight lines may appear wavy; drusen, pigmentary changes in retina; abnormal submacular choroidal vessels

GENETICS IN NURSING PRACTICE—Eye and Vision Disorders

SELECTED EYE AND VISION DISORDERS INFLUENCED BY GENETIC FACTORS
- Albinism
- Aniridia
- Colour blindness
- Glaucoma
- Homocystinuria
- Isolated familial congenital cataracts
- Leber hereditary optic neuropathy
- Marfan syndrome
- Retinitis pigmentosa

NURSING ASSESSMENTS
FAMILY HISTORY ASSESSMENT
- Assess history of family members with glaucoma, cataracts, night blindness (retinitis pigmentosa), colour blindness, or other vision impairment.
- Inquire about family members with other disorders that may include visual impairment, such as cutaneous, metabolic, connective tissue disorders, and hearing loss.

PHYSICAL ASSESSMENT
- Assess for other systemic and/or clinical features such as cutaneous or skeletal conditions, or hearing loss.

MANAGEMENT ISSUES SPECIFIC TO GENETICS
- Inquire whether DNA gene mutation or other genetic testing has been performed on any affected family members.
- If indicated, refer for further genetic counselling and evaluation so that family members can discuss inheritance, risk to other family members, availability of genetic testing, and gene-based interventions.
- Offer appropriate genetics information and resources.
- Assess patient's understanding of genetics information.
- Provide support to families with newly diagnosed genetic-related sensorineural disorders.

- Participate in management and coordination of care of patients with genetic conditions and individuals predisposed to develop or pass on a genetic condition

GENETICS RESOURCES
Canadian Association of Genetic Counsellors (CAGC)—a listing of genetic centres across Canada; www.cagc-accg.ca

Canadian Cancer Society—information on the genetic factors/risk and genetic testing; www.cancer.ca

Canadian Directory of Genetic Support Groups—a resource guide for families and professionals; www.lhsc.on.ca/programs/medgenet

Canadian Genetic Disease Network—its stated mission is to be the primary catalyst in advancing Canada's scientific and commercial competitiveness in genetic research and the application of genetic discoveries to the prevention, diagnosis, and treatment of human disease; www.cgdn.ca

Canadian Organization for Rare Disorders (CORD)—information on over 6,000 rare disorders and links individuals/families together with the same rare disorder; www.cord.ca

Genetic Alliance—increases the capacity of genetic advocacy groups to achieve their missions and leverages the voices of millions of individuals and families living with genetic conditions; www.geneticalliance.org

The Genetics Society of Canada (GSC)—promotes research and communicates the results and implications of genetics to the public; http://life.biology.mcmaster.ca/GSC

GeneTests—a publicly funded medical genetics information resource developed for physicians, other health care providers, and researchers; www.genetests.org

OMIM Online Mendelian Inheritance in Man—a catalogue of human genes and genetic disorders; www.ncbi.nlm.nih.gov/entrez/query.fcgi?db=OMIM

(Table 58-3). The optical devices include convex lens aids, such as magnifiers and spectacles; telescopic devices; anti-reflective lenses that diminish glare; and electronic reading systems, such as closed-circuit television and computers with large print. Continuing advances in computer software provide very useful products for patients with low vision. Scanners teamed with the appropriate software enable the user to scan printed data into the computer and have it read by computer voice or to increase the magnification for reading. Magnifiers can be hand-held or attached to a stand with or without illumination. Telescopic devices can be spectacle telescopes or clip-on or hand-held loupes.

Nonoptical aids include large-print publications and a variety of writing aids. The Internet continues to expand, and a telephone system has been developed that allows access to the Internet and e-mail using voice commands (see Chart 58-2).

Strategies that enhance the performance of visual tasks include modification of body movements and illumination and training for independent living skills. Head movements and positions can be modified to place images in functional areas of the visual field. Illumination is an added feature in magnifiers.

Adjusting the lighting helps with reading and other activities. Simple optical and nonoptical aids are available in low-vision clinics.

Referrals to community agencies may be necessary for low-vision patients living alone who are unable to self-administer their medications. Community agencies, such as The Lighthouse National Centre for Vision and Aging, offer services to low-vision patients that include training in independent living skills and the provision of occupational and recreational activities and a wide variety of assistive devices for vision enhancement and orientation and mobility.

VISION RESTORATION FOR THE BLIND
Ophthalmologists have worked toward visual restoration for blind individuals for years, and computer technology now provides opportunities for restoring sight. For example, a multiple-unit artificial retina chipset (MARC) has been devised for implanting within the eye. The MARC can be enabled to receive signals from an external camera mounted in a glasses frame. The acquired image is wirelessly transmitted to the chip, which provides

Table 58-3 • Activities Affected by Visual Impairment and Visual Aids

ACTIVITY	OPTICAL AIDS	NONOPTICAL AIDS
Shopping	Hand magnifier	Lighting, colour cues
Fixing a snack	Bifocals	Colour cues, consistent storage plan
Eating out	Hand magnifier	Flashlight, portable lamp
Identifying money	Bifocals, hand magnifier	Arrange paper money in wallet compartments
Reading print	High-power spectacle, bifocals, hand magnifier, stand magnifier, closed-circuit television	Lighting, high-contrast print, large print, reading slit
Writing	Hand magnifier, focusable telescope, closed-circuit television	Lighting, bold-tip pen, black ink
Using a telephone	Hand magnifier	Large print dial or touch tone buttons, hand-printed directory
Crossing streets	Telescope	Cane, ask directions
Finding taxis and bus signs	Telescope	
Reading medication labels	Hand magnifier	Colour codes, large print
Reading stove dials	Hand magnifier	Colour codes, raised dots
Adjusting the thermostat	Hand magnifier	Enlarged print model
Using a computer	Spectacles	High-contrast colour, large-print program
Reading signs	Spectacles	Move closer
Watching sporting event	Telescope	Sit in front rows

Adapted from Vaughn, D. G., Asbury, T., & Riorda-Eva, P. (Eds.). (1999). *General ophthalmology.* Stamford, CT: Appleton & Lange.

a type of artificial vision and which, with training, allows the patient to achieve some useful vision. Although the device is still experimental, some work has been done with patients who have lost vision from retinitis pigmentosa and age-related macular degeneration (Humayan et al., 1999).

Nursing Management

Coping with blindness involves three types of adaptation: emotional, physical, and social. The emotional adjustment to blindness or severe visual impairment determines the success of the physical and social adjustments of the patient. Successful emotional adjustment means acceptance of blindness or severe visual impairment.

PROMOTING COPING EFFORTS

Effective coping may not occur until the patient recognizes the permanence of the blindness. Clinging to false hopes of regaining vision hampers effective adaptation to blindness. A newly blind patient and his or her family members (especially those who

Chart 58-2 **Web Access for the Visually Impaired**

People with impaired vision need not be left behind in the computer age. Various technologies are available. A list of general equipment needs follows:
- Computer: typically with IBM- or MAC-compatible software and a Windows operating system
- Internet service provider (eg, AOL, Netscape, Earthlink, Hotmail)
- Screen-reader program: converts text on the computer screen to synthesized speech (eg, JAWS for Windows, Window-Eyes, Slimware Window Bridge, outspoken); cost varies between $500 and $800
- Browser program to navigate the World Wide Web (eg, Microsoft Internet Explorer, IBM Home Page Reader)

live with the patient) undergo the various steps of grieving: denial and shock, anger and protest, restitution, loss resolution, and acceptance. The ability to accept the changes that must come with visual loss and willingness to adapt to those changes influence the successful rehabilitation of the patient who is blind. Additional aspects to consider are value changes, independence–dependence conflicts, coping with stigma, and learning to function in social settings without visual cues and landmarks.

PROMOTING SPATIAL ORIENTATION AND MOBILITY

People who are blind detect and incorporate less information about their environment than do sighted people. The blind person relies on egocentric, sequential, and positional information, which centres on the person and his or her relationship to the objects in the environment. For example, the topographic concepts of front, back, left, right, above, and below and measures of distances are most useful in determining the exact position, sequence, and location of objects in relation to the person who is blind. Although their basis of information may be different from that of sighted people, people who are blind can comprehend spatial concepts.

The goal of orientation and mobility training is to foster independence in the environment. Training may be accomplished by using auditory and tactile cues and by providing anticipatory information. Having a concept of the spatial composition of the environment (ie, cognitive map) enhances independence of those who are blind. Orientation and mobility training programs are offered by community agencies serving the blind or visually impaired. Training includes using mobility devices for travel, the long cane, electronic travel aids, dog guides, and orientation aids. The basic orientation and mobility techniques used by a sighted person to assist a person who is blind or visually impaired to ambulate safely and efficiently are called sighted-guide techniques.

Spatial Orientation and Mobility in Institutional Settings.
A blind or severely visually impaired patient requires strategies for adapting to the environment. The monocular postoperative patient whose functioning eye is restricted by a surgical patch or by post-

operative inflammation requires early ambulation just like any postoperative patient. The activities of daily living, such as walking to a chair from a bed, require spatial concepts. The patient needs to know where he or she is in relation to the rest of the room, to understand the changes that may occur, and how to approach the desired location safely. This requires a collaborative effort between the patient and the nurse, who serves as the sighted guide.

Patients whose visual impairment results from a chronic progressive eye disorder, such as glaucoma, have better cognitive mapping skills than the suddenly blinded patient. They have developed the use of spatial and topographic concepts early and gradually; hence, remembering a room layout is easier for them. Suddenly blinded patients have more difficulty in adjusting; and emotional and behavioural issues of coping with blindness may hinder their learning. These patients require intensive emotional support. The nurse must assess the degree of physical assistance the patient with a visual deficit requires and communicate this to other health care personnel.

The food tray's composition is likened to the face of a clock. For example, the main plate may be described as being at 12 o'clock or the coffee cup at 3 o'clock. In the hospital, the bedside table and the call button must always be within reach. The parts of the call button are explained, and the patient is encouraged to touch and press the buttons or dials until the activity is mastered. The patient must be familiarized with the location of the telephone, water pitcher, and other objects on the bedside table. All articles and furniture must be replaced in the same positions. Introducing oneself on entering a patient's room is always a polite gesture and helps in the orientation of a blind patient.

The nurse should be aware of the importance of technique in providing physical assistance, developing independence, and ensuring safety. The readiness of the patient and his or her family to learn must be assessed before initiating orientation and mobility training.

PROMOTING HOME AND COMMUNITY-BASED CARE

Teaching Patients Self-Care. The nurse, social workers, family, and others collaborate to assess the patient's home condition and support system. If available, a low-vision specialist should be consulted before discharge, particularly for patients for whom identifying and administering medications pose problems. The level of visual acuity and patient preference help to determine appropriate interventions. For example, a plastic pill container with dividers that has been prefilled with a week's supply of medication can make medication administration easier for some patients, whereas others may prefer to have medication bottles marked with textured paints. Many patients require referral to social services. Patients with habits that may jeopardize safety, such as smoking, need to be cautioned and assisted to make their environment safe.

In Canada, laws such as the Canadian Charter of Human Rights and Freedoms, Access to Information Act, and the Canadian Human Rights Act support assistance of the blind. Governmental services include income assistance and health insurance through Family and Community Services, support services through programs such as the Canadian National Institute for the Blind and the Alliance for Equality of Blind Canadians, tax exemptions and tax deductions, educational services through programs such as the Canadian Association Disability Service Providers in Post Secondary Education and National Educational Association of Disabled Students, reduced or free postage for Braille materials through the Canada Post Corporation Act, and assistance for veterans

through Veteran Affairs Canada. Other resources and services are identified in "Resources and Websites" at the end of this chapter.

Glaucoma

Glaucoma is a group of ocular conditions characterized by optic nerve damage. The optic nerve damage is related to the IOP caused by congestion of aqueous humour in the eye. There is a range of pressures that have been considered "normal" but that may be associated with vision loss in some patients. Glaucoma is one of the leading causes of irreversible blindness in the world and affects 1 in 100 Canadians over the age of 40 (Canadian National Institute for the Blind, 2005c). It usually occurs in older people but can occur in people of any age. Approximately 13 percent of the population over the age of 60 years will be affected by glaucoma (Canadian National Institute for the Blind, 2005c). It is estimated that glaucoma affects at least 300,000 Canadians, with approximately half of them unaware of their disease. Glaucoma is more prevalent among people older than 40 years of age, and the incidence increases with age. It is also more prevalent among men than women and in the African Canadian and Asian populations (Chart 58-3). There is no cure for glaucoma, but research continues.

Aqueous Humour and Intraocular Pressure

Aqueous humour flows between the iris and the lens, nourishing the cornea and lens. Most (90%) of the fluid then flows out of the anterior chamber, draining through the spongy trabecular meshwork into the canal of Schlemm and the episcleral veins (Fig. 58-8). About 10% of the aqueous fluid exits through the ciliary body into the suprachoroidal space and then drains into the venous circulation of the ciliary body, choroid, and sclera. Unimpeded outflow of aqueous fluid depends on an intact drainage system and an open angle (about 45 degrees) between the iris and the cornea. A narrower angle places the iris closer to the trabecular meshwork, diminishing the angle. The amount of aqueous humour produced tends to decrease with age, in systemic diseases such as diabetes, and in ocular inflammatory conditions.

IOP is determined by the rate of aqueous production, the resistance encountered by the aqueous humour as it flows out of the passages, and the venous pressure of the episcleral veins that drain into the anterior ciliary vein. When aqueous fluid production and drainage are in balance, the IOP is between 10 and 21 mm Hg. When aqueous fluid is inhibited from flowing out, pressure builds up within the eye. Fluctuations in IOP occur with time of day, exertion, diet, and medications. It tends to increase with

Chart 58-3
Risk Factors for Glaucoma

- Family history of glaucoma
- African American race
- Older age
- Diabetes
- Cardiovascular disease
- Migraine syndromes
- Nearsightedness (myopia)
- Eye trauma
- Prolonged use of topical or systemic corticosteroids

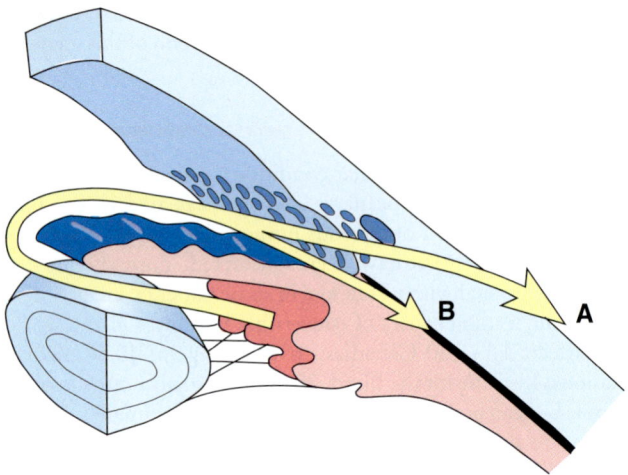

FIGURE 58-8 Normal outflow of aqueous humour. (**A**) Trabecular meshwork. (**B**) Uveoscleral route. From Kanski, J. J. (1999). *Clinical ophthalmology.* Oxford: Butterworth-Heinemann Ltd.

blinking, tight lid squeezing, and upward gazing. Systemic conditions such as hypertension and intraocular conditions such as uveitis and retinal detachment have been associated with elevated IOP. Exposure to cold weather, alcohol, a fat-free diet, heroin, and marijuana have been found to lower IOP.

Pathophysiology

There are two accepted theories regarding how increased IOP damages the optic nerve in glaucoma. The direct mechanical theory suggests that high IOP damages the retinal layer as it passes through the optic nerve head. The indirect ischemic theory suggests that high IOP compresses the microcirculation in the optic nerve head, resulting in cell injury and death. Some glaucomas appear as exclusively mechanical, and some are exclusively ischemic types. Typically, most cases are a combination of both.

Regardless of the cause of damage, glaucomatous changes typically evolve through clearly discernible stages:

1. *Initiating events:* precipitating factors include illness, emotional stress, congenital narrow angles, long-term use of corticosteroids, and **mydriatics** (ie, medications causing pupillary dilation). These events lead to the second stage.
2. *Structural alterations in the aqueous outflow system:* tissue and cellular changes caused by factors that affect aqueous humour dynamics lead to structural alterations and to the third stage.
3. *Functional alterations:* conditions such as increased IOP or impaired blood flow create functional changes that lead to the fourth stage.
4. *Optic nerve damage:* atrophy of the optic nerve is characterized by loss of nerve fibres and blood supply, and this fourth stage inevitably progresses to the fifth stage.
5. *Visual loss:* progressive loss of vision is characterized by visual field defects.

Classification of Glaucoma

There are several types of glaucoma. Whether glaucoma is known as *open-angle* or *angle-closure* glaucoma depends on which mechanisms cause impaired aqueous outflow. Glaucoma can be pri-

mary or secondary, depending on whether associated factors contribute to the rise in IOP.

Although glaucoma classification is changing as knowledge increases, current clinical forms of glaucoma are open-angle glaucomas, angle-closure glaucomas (also called pupillary block), congenital glaucomas, and glaucomas associated with other conditions, such as developmental anomalies, corticosteroid use, and other ocular conditions. The two common clinical forms of glaucoma encountered in adults are open-angle and angle-closure glaucoma. Table 58-4 explains the general characteristics of the different types of open-angle and angle-closure glaucomas.

Clinical Manifestations

Glaucoma is often called the silent thief of sight because most patients are unaware that they have the disease until they have experienced visual changes and vision loss. The patient may not seek health care until he or she experiences blurred vision or "halos" around lights, difficulty focusing, difficulty adjusting eyes in low lighting, loss of peripheral vision, aching or discomfort around the eyes, and headache.

Assessment and Diagnostic Findings

The purpose of a glaucoma workup is to establish the diagnostic category, assess the optic nerve damage, and formulate a treatment plan. The patient's ocular and medical history must be detailed to investigate the history of predisposing factors. There are four major types of examinations used in glaucoma evaluation, diagnosis, and management: tonometry to measure the IOP, ophthalmoscopy to inspect the optic nerve, gonioscopy to examine the filtration angle of the anterior chamber, and perimetry to assess the visual fields.

The changes in the optic nerve significant for the diagnosis of glaucoma are pallor and cupping of the optic nerve disc. The pallor of the optic nerve is caused by a lack of blood supply that results from cellular destruction. Cupping is characterized by exaggerated bending of the blood vessels as they cross the optic disc, resulting in an enlarged optic cup that appears more basin-like compared with a normal cup. The progression of cupping in glaucoma is caused by the gradual loss of retinal nerve fibres accompanied by the loss of blood supply, resulting in increased pallor of the optic disc.

As the optic nerve damage increases, visual perception in the area is lost. The localized areas of visual loss (ie, scotomas) represent loss of retinal sensitivity and are measured and mapped by perimetry. The results are mapped on a graph. In patients with glaucoma, the graph has a distinct pattern that is different from other ocular diseases and is useful in establishing the diagnosis. Figure 58-9 shows the progression of visual field defects caused by glaucoma.

Medical Management

The aim of all glaucoma treatment is prevention of optic nerve damage through medical therapy, laser or nonlaser surgery, or a combination of these approaches. Lifelong therapy is almost always necessary because glaucoma cannot be cured. Although treatment cannot reverse optic nerve damage, further damage can be controlled. The treatment goal is to maintain an IOP within a range unlikely to cause further damage.

Table 58-4 • Glaucoma Types, Clinical Manifestation, and Treatment

TYPES OF GLAUCOMA	CLINICAL MANIFESTATIONS	TREATMENT
Open-Angle Glaucomas Usually bilateral, but one eye may be more severely affected than the other. In all three types of open-angle glaucoma, the anterior chamber angle is open and appears normal.		
Chronic open-angle glaucoma (COAG)	Optic nerve damage, visual field defects, IOP >21 mm Hg. May have fluctuating IOPs. Usually no symptoms but possible ocular pain, headache, and halos.	Decrease IOP 20% to 50%. Additional topical and oral agents added as necessary. If medical treatment is unsuccessful, laser trabeculoplasty (LT) can provide a 20% drop in intraocular pressure. Glaucoma filtering surgery if continued optic nerve damage despite medication therapy and LT.
Normal tension glaucoma	IOP ≤ 21 mm Hg. Optic nerve damage, visual field defects.	Treatment similar to COAG, however, the best management for normal tension glaucoma management is yet to be established. Goal is to lower the IOP by at least 30%.
Ocular hypertension	Elevated IOP. Possible ocular pain or headache.	Lower IOP by at least 20%.
Angle-Closure (Pupillary Block) Glaucomas Obstruction in aqueous humour outflow due to the complete or partial closure of the angle from the forward shift of the peripheral iris to the trabecula. The obstruction results in an increased IOP.		
Acute angle-closure glaucoma (AACG)	Rapidly progressive visual impairment, periocular pain, conjunctival hyperemia, and congestion. Pain may be associated with nausea, vomiting, bradycardia, and profuse sweating. Reduced central visual acuity, severely elevated IOP, corneal edema. Pupil is vertically oval, fixed in a semi-dilated position, and unreactive to light and accommodation.	Ocular emergency; administration of hyperosmotics, azetazolamide, and topical ocular hypotensive agents, such as pilocarpine and beta-blockers (betaxolol). Possible laser incision in the iris (iridotomy) to release blocked aqueous and reduce IOP. Other eye is also treated with pilocarpine eye drops and/or surgical management to avoid a similar spontaneous attack.
Subacute angle-closure glaucoma	Transient blurring of vision, halos around lights; temporal headaches and/or ocular pain; pupil may be semi-dilated.	Prophylactic peripheral laser iridotomy. Can lead to acute or chronic angle-closure glaucoma if untreated.
Chronic angle-closure glaucoma	Progression of glaucomatous cupping and significant visual field loss; IOP may be normal or elevated; ocular pain and headache.	Management similar to that for COAG: includes laser iridotomy and medications.

IOP, intraocular pressure.

The initial target for IOP among patients with elevated IOP and those with low-tension glaucoma with progressive visual field loss is typically set at 30% lower than the current pressure. The patient is monitored for the stability of the optic nerve. If there is evidence of progressive damage, the target IOP is again lowered until the optic nerve shows stability.

Treatment focuses on achieving the greatest benefit at the least risk, cost, and inconvenience to the patient. All treatment options have potential complications, especially surgery, which yields the best success rates. In Canada, medical management is utilized in conjunction with surgical treatment, depending on the severity and type of glaucoma. In the United States, medical management is the common approach, and surgical management is the last resort. In Great Britain, the initial treatment of choice is surgery (Fechtner & Singh, 2001).

PHARMACOLOGIC THERAPY

Medical management of glaucoma relies on systemic and topical ocular medications that lower IOP. Periodic follow-up examinations are essential to monitor IOP, appearance of the optic nerve,

visual fields, and side effects of medications. In considering a therapeutic regimen, the ophthalmologist aims for the greatest effectiveness with the least side effects, inconvenience, and cost. Therapy takes into account the patient's health and stage of glaucoma. Comfort, affordability, convenience, lifestyle, and personality are factors to consider in the patient's compliance with the medical regimen.

The patient is usually started on the lowest dose of topical medication and then advanced to increased concentrations until the desired IOP level is reached and maintained. Because of their efficacy, minimal dosing (can be used once each day), and low cost, beta-blockers are the preferred initial topical medications. One eye is treated first, with the other eye used as a control in determining the efficacy of the medication; once efficacy has been established, treatment of the fellow eye is started. If the IOP is elevated in both eyes, both are treated. When results are not satisfactory, a new medication is substituted. The main markers of the efficacy of the medication in glaucoma control are lowering of the IOP to the target pressure, appearance of the optic nerve head, and the visual field.

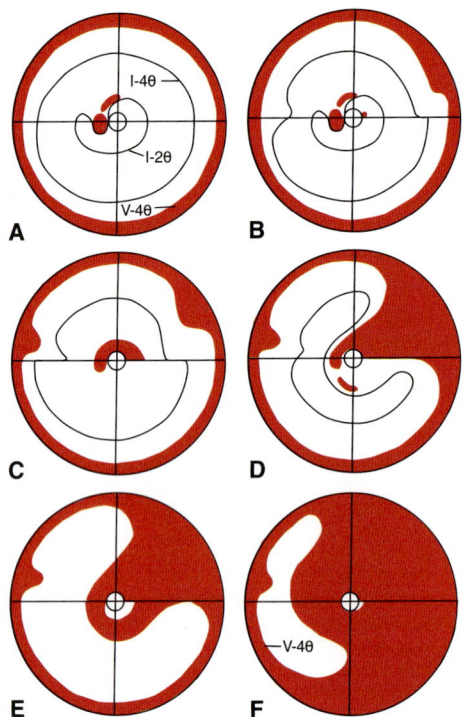

FIGURE 58-9 Progression of glaucomatous visual field defects. A central scotoma at 10 to 20 degrees of fixation near the blind spot is the initial significant finding (**A, B**). As the glaucoma progresses, the scotomas enlarge and deepen, resulting in peripheral vision loss. (**C**) Defect within 5 degrees of fixation point nasally. (**D**) Peripheral involvement enlarges. (**E**) Ringlike scotoma. (**F**) Eventually, vision is lost. The resulting "island of vision" becomes the characteristic visual field appearance of glaucoma and correlates with the "tunnel vision," in which peripheral vision is lost. From Kanski, J. J. (1999). *Clinical ophthalmology.* Oxford: Butterworth-Heinemann Ltd.

Several types of ocular medications are used to treat glaucoma (Table 58-5), including **miotics** (ie, cause pupillary constriction), adrenergic agonists (ie, sympathomimetic agents), beta-blockers, alpha$_2$-agonists (ie, adrenergic agents), carbonic anhydrase inhibitors, and prostaglandins. Cholinergics (ie, miotics) increase the outflow of the aqueous humour by affecting ciliary muscle contraction and pupil constriction, allowing flow through a larger opening between the iris and the trabecular meshwork. Adrenergic agonists increase aqueous outflow but primarily decrease aqueous production with an action similar to beta-blockers and carbonic anhydrase inhibitors.

SURGICAL MANAGEMENT

In *laser trabeculoplasty* for glaucoma, laser burns are applied to the inner surface of the trabecular meshwork to open the intra-trabecular spaces and widen the canal of Schlemm, thereby promoting outflow of aqueous humour and decreasing IOP. The procedure is indicated when IOP is inadequately controlled by medications; it is contraindicated when the trabecular meshwork cannot be fully visualized because of narrow angles. A serious complication of this procedure is a transient rise in IOP (usually 2 hours after surgery) that may become persistent. IOP assessment in the immediate postoperative period is essential.

In *laser iridotomy* for pupillary block glaucoma, an opening is made in the iris to eliminate the pupillary block. Laser iridotomy is contraindicated in patients with corneal edema, which interferes with laser targeting and strength. Potential complications

are burns to the cornea, lens, or retina; transient elevated IOP; closure of the iridotomy; uveitis; and blurring. Pilocarpine is usually prescribed to prevent closure of the iridotomy.

Filtering procedures for chronic glaucoma are used to create an opening or fistula in the trabecular meshwork to drain aqueous humour from the anterior chamber to the subconjunctival space into a bleb, thereby bypassing the usual drainage structures. This allows the aqueous humour to flow and exit by different routes (ie, absorption by the conjunctival vessels or mixing with tears). *Trabeculectomy* is the standard filtering technique used to remove part of the trabecular meshwork. Complications include hemorrhage, an extremely low (hypotony) or elevated IOP, uveitis, cataracts, bleb failure, bleb leak, and endophthalmitis. Unlike other surgical procedures, the filtering procedure's goal in glaucoma treatment is to achieve incomplete healing of the surgical wound. The outflow of aqueous humour in a newly created drainage fistula is circumvented by the granulation of fibrovascular tissue or scar tissue formation on the surgical site. Scarring is inhibited by using antifibrosis agents such as the antimetabolites fluorouracil (Efudex) and mitomycin (Mutamycin). Like all antineoplastic agents, they require special handling procedures before, during, and after the procedure. Fluorouracil can be administered intraoperatively and by subconjunctival injection during follow-up; mitomycin is much more potent and is administered only intraoperatively.

Drainage implants or shunts are open tubes implanted in the anterior chamber to shunt aqueous humour to an attached plate in the conjunctival space. A fibrous capsule develops around the episcleral plate and filters the aqueous humour, thereby regulating the outflow and controlling IOP.

Nursing Management

TEACHING PATIENTS ABOUT GLAUCOMA CARE

The medical and surgical management of glaucoma slows the progression of glaucoma but does not cure it. The lifelong therapeutic regimen mandates patient education. The nature of the disease and the importance of strict adherence to the medication regimen must be explained to help ensure compliance. A thorough patient interview is essential to determine systemic conditions, current systemic and ocular medications, family history, and problems with compliance to glaucoma medications. Then the medication program can be discussed, particularly the interactions of glaucoma-control medications with other medications. For example, the diuretic effect of acetazolamide has an additive effect on the diuretic effects of other antihypertensive medications and can result in hypokalemia. The effects of glaucoma-control medications on vision must also be explained. Miotics and sympathomimetics result in altered focus; therefore, patients need to be cautious in navigating their surroundings. Information about instilling ocular medication and preventing systemic absorption with punctal occlusion is described in the section on ophthalmic medications.

Nurses in all settings encounter patients with glaucoma. Even patients with long-standing disease and those with glaucoma as a secondary diagnosis should be assessed for knowledge level and compliance with the therapeutic regimen. Chart 58-4 contains points to review with glaucoma patients.

CONTINUING GLAUCOMA CARE AT HOME

For patients with severe glaucoma and impaired function, referral to services that assist the patient in performing customary ac-

Table 58-5 • Medications Used in the Management of Glaucoma

MEDICATION	ACTION	SIDE EFFECTS	NURSING IMPLICATIONS
Cholinergics (miotics) (pilocarpine, carbachol)	Increases aqueous fluid outflow by contracting the ciliary muscle and causing miosis (constriction of the pupil) and opening of trabecular meshwork	Periorbital pain, blurry vision, difficulty seeing in the dark	Caution patients about diminished vision in dimly lit areas
Adrenergic agonists (dipivefrin, epinephrine)	Reduces production of aqueous humour and increases outflow	Eye redness and burning; can have systemic effects, including palpitations, elevated blood pressure, tremor, headaches, and anxiety	Teach patients punctal occlusion to limit systemic effects (described in Chart 58–10.)
Beta-blockers (betaxolol, timolol)	Decreases aqueous humour production	Can have systemic effects, including bradycardia, exacerbation of pulmonary disease, and hypotension	Contraindicated in patients with asthma, chronic obstructive pulmonary disease, second- or third-degree heart block, bradycardia, or cardiac failure; teach patients punctal occlusion to limit systemic effects
Alpha-adrenergic agonists (apraclonidine, brimonidine)	Decreases aqueous humour production	Eye redness, dry mouth and nasal passages	Teach patients punctal occlusion to limit systemic effects
Carbonic anhydrase inhibitors (acetazolamide, methazolamide, dorzolamide)	Decreases aqueous humour production	Oral medications (acetazolamide and methazolamide) associated with serious side effects, including anaphylactic reactions, electrolyte loss, depression, lethargy, gastrointestinal upset, impotence, and weight loss; topical form (dorzolamide) side effects include topical allergy	Do not administer to patients with sulfa allergies; monitor electrolyte levels
Prostaglandin analogs (latanoprost)	Increases uveoscleral outflow	Darkening of the iris, conjunctival redness, possible rash	Instruct patients to report any side effects

tivities may be needed. The loss of peripheral vision impairs mobility the most. These patients need to be referred to low-vision and rehabilitation services. Patients who meet the criteria for legal blindness should be offered referrals to agencies that assist in obtaining federal assistance.

Reassurance and emotional support are important aspects of care. A lifelong disease involving a possible loss of sight has psychological, physical, social, and vocational ramifications. The family must be integrated into the plan of care, and because the disease has a familial tendency, family members should be encouraged to undergo examinations at least once every 2 years to detect glaucoma early.

Cataracts

A cataract is a lens opacity or cloudiness (Fig. 58-10). Cataracts rank only behind arthritis and heart disease as a leading cause of disability in older adults. Each year, over 1.5 million cataract surgeries are performed in North America, with that number expected to increase yearly (Canadian Ophthalmological Society, 2003). According to the World Health Organization, cataract is the leading cause of blindness in the world (Preshel & Prevent Blindness America, 2002).

Pathophysiology

Cataracts can develop in one or both eyes at any age for a variety of causes (Chart 58-5). Visual impairment normally progresses at the same rate in both eyes over many years or in a matter of months. The three most common types of senile (age-related) cataracts are defined by their location in the lens: nuclear, cortical, and posterior subcapsular. The extent of visual impairment depends on the size, density, and location in the lens. More than one type can be present in one eye.

A nuclear cataract is associated with myopia (ie, nearsightedness), which worsens when the cataract progresses. If dense, the cataract severely blurs vision. Periodic changes in prescription eyeglasses help manage this problem.

A cortical cataract involves the anterior, posterior, or equatorial cortex of the lens. A cataract in the equator or periphery of the cortex does not interfere with the passage of light through the centre of the lens and has little effect on vision. Cortical cataracts progress at a highly variable rate. Vision is worse in very bright light. Studies show that people with the highest levels of sunlight exposure have twice the risk of developing cortical cataracts than those with low-level sunlight exposure (West et al., 1998).

Posterior subcapsular cataracts occur in front of the posterior capsule. This type typically develops in younger people and, in some cases, is associated with prolonged corticosteroid use,

Chart 58-4 • PATIENT EDUCATION
Managing Glaucoma

- Know your intraocular pressure (IOP) measurement and the desired range.
- Be informed about the extent of your vision loss and optic nerve damage.
- Keep a record of your eye pressure measurements and visual field test results to monitor your own progress.
- Review all your medications (including over-the-counter and herbal medications) with your ophthalmologist, and mention any side effects each time you visit.
- Ask about potential side effects and drug interactions of your eye medications.
- Ask whether generic or less costly forms of your eye medications are available.
- Review the dosing schedule with your ophthalmologist and inform him or her if you have trouble complying with the schedule.
- Participate in the decision-making process. Let your doctor know what dosing schedule works for you and other preferences regarding your eye care.
- Have the nurse observe you instilling eye medication to determine whether you are administering it properly.
- Be aware that glaucoma medications can cause adverse effects if used inappropriately. Eyedrops are to be administered as prescribed, not when eyes feel irritated.
- Ask your ophthalmologist to send a report to your primary care physician after each appointment.
- Keep all follow-up appointments.

Chart 58-5
Risk Factors for Cataract Formation

Aging
- Loss of lens transparency
- Clumping or aggregation of lens protein (which leads to light scattering)
- Accumulation of a yellow-brown pigment due to the breakdown of lens protein
- Decreased oxygen uptake
- Increase in sodium and calcium
- Decrease in levels of vitamin C, protein, and glutathione (an antioxidant)

Associated Ocular Conditions
- Retinitis pigmentosa
- Myopia
- Retinal detachment and retinal surgery
- Infection (eg, herpes zoster, uveitis)

Toxic Factors
- Corticosteroids, especially at high doses and in long-term use
- Alkaline chemical eye burns, poisoning
- Cigarette smoking
- Calcium, copper, iron, gold, silver, and mercury, which tend to deposit in the pupillary area of the lens

Nutritional Factors
- Reduced levels of antioxidants
- Poor nutrition
- Obesity

Physical Factors
- Dehydration associated with chronic diarrhea, use of purgatives in anorexia nervosa, and use of hyperbaric oxygenation
- Blunt trauma, perforation of the lens with a sharp object or foreign body, electric shock
- Ultraviolet radiation in sunlight and x-ray

Systemic Diseases and Syndromes
- Diabetes mellitus
- Down syndrome
- Disorders related to lipid metabolism
- Renal disorders
- Musculoskeletal disorders

inflammation, or trauma. Near vision is diminished, and the eye is increasingly sensitive to glare from bright light (eg, sunlight, headlights).

Clinical Manifestations

Painless, blurry vision is characteristic of cataracts. The patient perceives that surroundings are dimmer, as if glasses need cleaning. Light scattering is common, and the individual experiences reduced contrast sensitivity, sensitivity to glare, and reduced visual acuity. Other effects include myopic shift, astigmatism, monocular **diplopia** (ie, double vision), colour shift (ie, the aging lens becomes progressively more absorbent at the blue end of the spectrum), brunescens (ie, colour values shift to yellow-brown), and reduced light transmission.

Assessment and Diagnostic Findings

Decreased visual acuity is directly proportionate to cataract density. The Snellen visual acuity test, ophthalmoscopy, and slit-lamp biomicroscopic examination are used to establish the degree of cataract formation. The degree of lens opacity does not always correlate with the patient's functional status. Some patients can perform normal activities despite clinically significant cataracts. Others with less lens opacification have a disproportionate decrease in visual acuity; hence, visual acuity is an imperfect measure of visual impairment.

Medical Management

No nonsurgical treatment cures cataracts. Ongoing studies are investigating ways to slow cataract progression, such as intake of antioxidants (eg, vitamin C, beta-carotene, vitamin E) (Age-Related

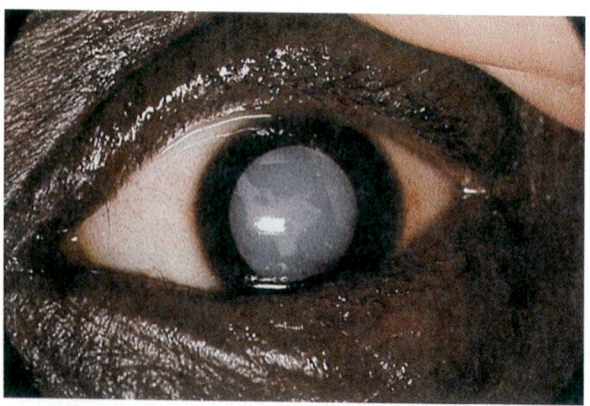

FIGURE 58-10 A cataract is a cloudy or opaque lens. On visual inspection, the lens appears grey or milky. From Rubin, E., & Farber, J. L. (1999). *Pathology* (3rd ed.). Philadelphia: Lippincott Williams & Wilkins.

Eye Disease Research Study Group, 2001). In the early stages of cataract development, glasses, contact lenses, strong bifocals, or magnifying lenses may improve vision. Reducing glare with proper light and appropriate lighting can facilitate reading. Mydriatics can be used as short-term treatment to dilate the pupil and allow more light to reach the retina, although this increases glare.

SURGICAL MANAGEMENT

Fewer than 15% of people with cataracts suffer vision problems severe enough to require surgery. In general, if reduced vision from cataract does not interfere with normal activities, surgery may not be needed. However, in deciding when cataract surgery is to be performed, the patient's functional and visual status should be a primary consideration. Surgery is performed on an outpatient basis and usually takes less than 1 hour, with the patient being discharged in 30 minutes or less afterward. Although complications from cataract surgery are uncommon, they can have significant

effects on vision (Table 58-6). Restoration of visual function through a safe and minimally invasive procedure is the surgical goal, which is achieved with advances in topical anesthesia, smaller wound incision (ie, clear cornea incision), and lens design (ie, foldable and more accurate intraocular lens measurements).

Topical anesthesia, such as lidocaine gel applied to the surface of the eye, eliminates the hazards of regional anesthesia, such as ocular perforation, retrobulbar hemorrhage, optic injuries, diplopia, and ptosis, and is ideal for patients receiving anticoagulants. Moreover, patients can communicate and cooperate during surgery.

When both eyes have cataracts, one eye is treated first, with at least several weeks, preferably months, separating the two operations. Because cataract surgery is performed to improve visual functioning, the delay for the other eye gives time for the patient and the surgeon to evaluate whether the results from the first surgery are adequate enough to preclude the need for a second operation. The delay also provides time for the first eye to recover;

Table 58-6 • **Potential Complications of Cataract Surgery**

COMPLICATION	EFFECTS	MANAGEMENT AND OUTCOME
Immediate Preoperative Retrobulbar hemorrhage: can result from retrobulbar infiltration of anesthetic agents if the short ciliary artery is located by the injectia	Increased IOP, proptosis, lid tightness, and subconjunctival hemorrhage with or without edema	Emergent lateral canthotomy (slitting of the canthus) is performed to stop central retinal perfusion when the IOP is dangerously elevated. If this procedure fails to reduce IOP, a puncture of the anterior chamber with removal of fluid is considered. The patient must be closely monitored for at least a few hours. Postponement of cataract surgery for 2 to 4 weeks is advised. Complications such as iris prolapse, vitreous loss, and choroidal hemorrhage could result in a catastrophic visual outcome.
Intraoperative Complications Rupture of the posterior capsule Suprachoroidal (expulsive) hemorrhage: profuse bleeding into the suprachoroidal space	May result in loss of vitreous Extrusion of intraocular contents from the eye or opposition of retinal surfaces	Anterior vitrectomy is required if vitreous loss occurs. Closure of the incision and administration of a hyperosmotic agent to reduce IOP or corticosteroids to reduce intraocular inflammation. Vitrectomy is performed 1 to 2 weeks later. Visual prognosis is poor; some useful vision may be salvaged on rare occasions.
Early Postoperative Complications Acute bacterial endophthalmitis: devastating complication that occurs in about 1 in 1000 cases; the most common causative organisms are *Staphylococcus epidermitus, S. aureus, Pseudomonas* and *Proteus* species	Characterized by marked visual loss, pain, lid edema, hypopyon, corneal haze, and chemosis	Managed by aggressive antibiotic therapy. Broad-spectrum antibiotics are administered while awaiting culture and sensitivity results. Once results are obtained, the appropriate antibiotics are administered via intravitreal injection. Corticosteroid therapy is also administered.
Late Postoperative Complications Suture-related problems	Toxic reactions or mechanical injury from broken or loose sutures	Suture removal relieves the symptoms. Topical corticosteroids are used when the incision is not healed and sutures cannot be removed.
Malposition of the IOL	Results in astigmatism, sensitivity to glare, or appearance of halos	Miotics are used for mild cases, whereas IOL removal and replacement are necessary for severe cases.
Chronic endophthalmitis	Persistent, low-grade inflammation and granuloma	Corticosteroids and antibiotics are administered systemically. If the condition persists, removal of the IOL and capsular bag, vitrectomy, and intravitreal injection of antibiotics are required.
Opacification of the posterior capsule (most common late complication of extracapsular cataract extraction)	Visual acuity is diminished.	YAG laser is used to create a hole in the posterior capsule. Blurred vision is cleared immediately.

IOP, intraocular pressure.

if there are any complications, the surgeon may decide to perform the second procedure differently.

Intracapsular Cataract Extraction.

From the late 1800s until the 1970s, the technique of choice for cataract extraction was intracapsular cataract extraction (ICCE). The entire lens (ie, nucleus, cortex, and capsule) is removed, and fine sutures close the incision. ICCE is infrequently performed today; however, it is indicated when there is a need to remove the entire lens, such as with a subluxated cataract (ie, partially or completely dislocated lens).

Extracapsular Surgery.

Extracapsular cataract extraction (ECCE) achieves the intactness of smaller incisional wounds (less trauma to the eye) and maintenance of the posterior capsule of the lens, reducing postoperative complications, particularly aphakic retinal detachment and cystoid macular edema. In ECCE, a portion of the anterior capsule is removed, allowing extraction of the lens nucleus and cortex. The posterior capsule and zonular support are left intact. An intact zonular-capsular diaphragm provides the needed safe anchor for the posterior chamber intraocular lens (IOL). After the pupil has been dilated and the surgeon has made a small incision on the upper edge of the cornea, a viscoelastic substance (clear gel) is injected into the space between the cornea and the lens. This prevents the space from collapsing and facilitates insertion of the IOL.

Phacoemulsification.

This method of extracapsular surgery uses an ultrasonic device that liquefies the nucleus and cortex, which are then suctioned out through a tube. The posterior capsule is left intact. Because the incision is even smaller than the standard ECCE, the wound heals more rapidly, and there is early stabilization of refractive error and less astigmatism. Hardware and software advances in ultrasonic technology—including new phaco needles that are used to cut and aspirate the cataract—permit safe and efficient removal of nearly all cataracts through a clear cornea incision that is as small or smaller than required for available foldable lenses. Ultimately, advances in technology will achieve an injectable IOL.

Lens Replacement.

After removal of the crystalline lens, the patient is referred to as *aphakic* (ie, without lens). The lens, which focuses light on the retina, must be replaced for the patient to see clearly. There are three lens replacement options: aphakic eyeglasses, contact lenses, and IOL implants.

Aphakic glasses are effective but heavy. Objects are magnified by 25%, making them appear closer than they actually are. Objects are magnified unequally, creating distortion. Peripheral vision is also limited, and **binocular vision** (ie, ability of both eyes to focus on one object and fuse the two images into one) is impossible if the other eye is phakic (normal).

Contact lenses provide patients with almost normal vision, but because contact lenses need to be removed occasionally, the patient also needs a pair of aphakic glasses. Contact lenses are not advised for patients who have difficulty inserting, removing, and cleaning them. Frequent handling and improper disinfection increase the risk for infection.

Insertion of IOLs during cataract surgery is the usual approach to lens replacement. After ICCE, the surgeon implants an anterior chamber IOL in front of the iris. Posterior chamber lenses, generally used in ECCE, are implanted behind the iris. ECCE and posterior chamber IOLs are associated with a relatively low incidence of complications (eg, hyphema, macular edema, secondary glaucoma, damage to the corneal endothelium). IOL implantation is contraindicated in patients with recurrent uveitis, proliferative diabetic retinopathy, neovascular glaucoma, or rubeosis iridis. Like any device, IOLs can malfunction and cause complications.

Nursing Management

The patient with cataracts should receive the usual preoperative care for ambulatory surgical patients undergoing eye surgery. According to the study on Medical Testing for Cataract Surgery, routine preoperative testing before cataract surgery does not improve health or clinical outcomes. Hence, the standard battery of preoperative tests should be prescribed only when they would have been indicated by the patient's medical history (Schein et al., 2000).

PROVIDING PREOPERATIVE CARE

To reduce the risk for retrobulbar hemorrhage (after retrobulbar injection), any anticoagulation therapy that the patient is receiving is withheld, if medically appropriate. Aspirin should be withheld for 5 to 7 days, nonsteroidal anti-inflammatory medications (NSAIDs) for 3 to 5 days, and warfarin (Coumadin) until the prothrombin time of 1.5 is almost reached.

Dilating drops are administered every 10 minutes for four doses at least 1 hour before surgery. Additional dilating drops may be administered in the operating room (immediately before surgery) if the affected eye is not fully dilated. Antibiotic, corticosteroid, and NSAID drops may be administered prophylactically to prevent postoperative infection and inflammation.

PROVIDING POSTOPERATIVE CARE

After recovery from anesthesia, the patient receives verbal and written instruction regarding how to protect the eye, administer medications, recognize signs of complications, and obtain emergency care. Activities to be avoided are identified in Chart 58-6. The nurse also explains that there is minimal discomfort after surgery and instructs the patient to take a mild analgesic agent, such as acetaminophen, as needed. Antibiotic, anti-inflammatory, and corticosteroid eye drops or ointments are prescribed postoperatively. A clinical pathway for the care of patients undergoing ambulatory cataract surgery is presented in Appendix A at the end of the book.

PROMOTING HOME AND COMMUNITY-BASED CARE

Teaching Patients Self-Care. To prevent accidental rubbing or poking of the eye, the patient wears a protective eye patch for 24 hours after surgery, followed by eyeglasses worn during the day and a metal shield worn at night for 1 to 4 weeks. The nurse instructs the patient and family in applying and caring for the eye shield. Sunglasses should be worn while outdoors during the day because the eye is sensitive to light.

Slight morning discharge, some redness, and a scratchy feeling may be expected for a few days. A clean, damp washcloth may be used to remove slight morning eye discharge. Because cataract surgery increases the risk for retinal detachment, the patient must know to notify the surgeon if new floaters (ie, dots) in vision, flashing lights, decrease in vision, pain, or increase in redness occurs.

Continuing Care. The eye patch is removed after the first follow-up appointment. Patients may experience blurring of vision for several days to weeks. Sutures left in the eye alter the curvature of the cornea, resulting in temporary blurring and some astigmatism. Vision gradually improves as the eye heals. Patients with IOL implants have visual improvement faster than those waiting for aphakic glasses or contact lenses. Vision is stabilized when the eye is completely healed, usually within 6 to 12 weeks, when final corrective prescription is completed. Visual correction is needed for any remaining nearsightedness or farsightedness (even in patients with IOL implants).

Chart 58-6
Home Care Checklist • Intraocular Lens Implant

At the completion of the home care instruction, the patient or caregiver will be able to:	Patient	Caregiver
• Wear glasses or metal eye shield at all times following surgery as instructed by the physician.	✓	
• Always wash hands before touching or cleaning the postoperative eye.	✓	✓
• Clean postoperative eye with a clean tissue; wipe the closed eye with a single gesture from the inner canthus outward.	✓	✓
• Bathe or shower; shampoo hair cautiously or seek assistance.	✓	
• Avoid lying on the side of the affected eye the night after surgery.	✓	
• Keep activity light (eg, walking, reading, watching television). Resume the following activities only as directed by the physician: driving, sexual activity, unusually strenuous activity.	✓	
• Remember not to lift, push, or pull objects heavier than 7 kg.	✓	
• Avoid bending or stooping for an extended period.	✓	
• Be careful when climbing or descending stairs.	✓	
• Know when to call the physician.*	✓	✓

*Call the physician immediately if any of the following problems occur before the next physician's appointment: (1) vision changes; (2) continuous flashing lights appear to the affected eye; (3) redness, swelling, or pain increase in the eye; (4) the amount or type of eye drainage changes; (5) the eye is injured in any way; (6) significant pain is not relieved by acetaminophen.

Corneal Disorders

CORNEAL DYSTROPHIES

Corneal dystrophies are inherited as autosomal dominant traits and manifest when the person is about 20 years of age. They are characterized by deposits in the corneal layers. Decreased vision is caused by the irregular corneal surface and corneal deposits. Corneal endothelial decompensation leads to corneal edema and blurring of vision. Persistent edema leads to **bullous keratopathy**, which is formation of blisters that cause pain and discomfort on rupturing. This condition is usually associated with primary open-angle glaucoma.

A bandage contact lens is used to flatten the bullae, protect the exposed corneal nerve endings, and relieve discomfort. Symptomatic treatments, such as hypertonic drops or ointment (5% sodium chloride), may reduce epithelial edema; lowering the IOP also reduces stromal edema. Penetrating keratoplasty has a high success rate in advanced cases (see "Corneal Surgeries"). For diffuse bullous keratopathy, amniotic membrane transplantation may become the procedure of choice for patients with limited visual potential (Rapuano, 2000).

KERATOCONUS

Keratoconus is a condition characterized by a conical protuberance of the cornea with progressive thinning on protrusion and irregular astigmatism. The hereditary condition has a higher incidence among women. Onset occurs at puberty; the condition may progress for more than 20 years and is bilateral. Corneal scarring occurs in severe cases. Blurred vision is a prominent symptom. Rigid, gas-permeable contact lenses correct irregular astigmatism and improve vision. Advances in contact lens design have reduced the need for surgery. Penetrating keratoplasty is indicated when contact lens correction is no longer effective.

CORNEAL SURGERIES

Among the surgical procedures used to treat diseased corneal tissue are phototherapeutic keratectomy (PTK) and keratoplasty.

Phototherapeutic Keratectomy

PTK is a laser procedure that is used to treat diseased corneal tissue by removing or reducing corneal opacities and smoothing the anterior corneal surface to improve functional vision. PTK is a safer, more effective (when indicated) alternative than penetrating or lamellar keratoplasty. PTK is contraindicated in patients with active herpetic keratitis because the ultraviolet rays may reactivate latent virus. Common side effects are induced hyperopia and stromal haze. Complications are delayed re-epithelialization (particularly in patients with diabetes) and bacterial keratitis. Postoperative management consists of oral analgesics for eye pain. Re-epithelialization is promoted with a pressure patch or therapeutic soft contact lens. Antibiotic and corticosteroid ointment and NSAIDs are prescribed postoperatively. Follow-up examinations are required for up to 2 years.

Keratoplasty

Keratoplasty (ie, corneal transplantation or corneal grafting) involves replacing abnormal host tissue with a healthy donor corneal tissue. Common indications are keratoconus, corneal dystrophy, corneal scarring from herpes simplex keratitis, and chemical burns.

Several factors affect the success of the graft: ocular structures (eg, lids, conjunctiva), tear film function, adequacy of blinking, and viability of the donor endothelium. Tissue that is the possible source of disease transmission from donor to recipient or cornea with functionally compromised endothelium is typically not used for grafting (Chart 58-7), nor is corneal tissue used from donors who have undergone laser-assisted in situ keratomileusis (LASIK) because the cornea is no longer intact. Conditions such as glaucoma, retinal disease, and **strabismus** (ie, deviation in ocular alignment) can negatively influence the outcome. Promising experimental therapies include stem cell transplants (Rongé, 2001) and autologous limbal epithelial cell transplants (Tsai et al., 2000).

The surgeon determines the graft size before the procedure, and the appropriate size is marked on the surface of the cornea. The surgeon prepares the donor cornea and the recipient bed,

Contraindications to the Use of Donor Tissue for Corneal Transplantation: Donor Characteristics

Systemic Disorders
- Death from unknown cause
- Creutzfeldt-Jakob disease
- AIDS or high risk for HIV infection
- Hepatitis
- Eye infection, systemic infection

Intrinsic Eye Disease
- Retinoblastoma
- Ocular inflammation
- Malignant tumours of anterior segment
- Disorders of the conjunctiva or corneal surface involving the optical zone of the cornea

Other
- History of eye trauma
- Corneal scars
- Previous surgical procedure
- Corneal graft
- LASIK eye surgery

removes the diseased cornea, places the donor cornea on the recipient bed, and sutures it in place. Sutures remain in place for 12 to 18 months. Potential complications include early graft failure due to poor quality of donor tissue, surgical trauma, acute infection, and persistently increased IOP and late graft failure due to rejection.

Postoperatively, the patient receives mydriatic medications (2 weeks) and topical corticosteroids (12 months; daily doses for 6 months and tapered doses thereafter). Patients typically describe a sensation of postoperative eye discomfort rather than acute pain.

Nursing Management

The nurse reinforces the surgeon's recommendations and instructions regarding visual rehabilitation and visual improvement by explaining why a technically successful graft may initially produce disappointing results because the procedure has produced a new optical surface and only after several months do patients start seeing the natural and true colours of their environment. Correction of a resultant refractive error with eyeglasses or contact lenses determines the final visual outcome. The nurse assesses the patient's support system and his or her ability to comply with long-term follow-up, which includes frequent clinic visits for several months for tapering of topical corticosteroid therapy, selective suture removal, and ongoing evaluation of the graft site and visual acuity. The nurse also initiates appropriate referral to community services when indicated.

Because graft failure is an ophthalmic emergency that can occur at any time, the primary goal of nursing care is to teach the patient to identify signs and symptoms of graft failure. The early symptoms are blurred vision, discomfort, tearing, or redness of the eye. Decreased vision results after graft destruction. Patients must contact the ophthalmologist as soon as symptoms occur. Treatment of graft rejection is prompt administration of hourly topical corticosteroids and periocular corticosteroid injections. Systemic immunosuppressive agents may be necessary for severe, resistant cases.

REFRACTIVE SURGERIES

Refractive surgeries are cosmetic, elective procedures performed to reshape corneal tissue and correct refractive errors so that eyeglasses or contact lenses are no longer needed. Current procedures include radial keratotomy, photorefractive keratectomy (PFK), and LASIK.

Refractive surgery alters the major optical function of the eye and thereby carries certain surgical risks. The patient must fully understand benefits, potential risks and complications, common side effects, and limitations of the procedure. Refractive surgery does not alter the normal aging process of the eye. If the reason for the procedure is occupational vision requirements, the results must satisfy both the patient and the employer. Precise visual outcome cannot be guaranteed with certainty. Typically, patients must be at least 18 years of age.

The corneal structure must be normal and refractive error stable. Patients are required to discontinue using contact lenses for a period before the procedure (ie, 2 to 3 weeks for soft lenses and 4 weeks for hard lenses). Patients with conditions that are likely to adversely affect corneal wound healing (eg, corticosteroid use, immunosuppression, elevated IOP) are not good candidates for the procedure. Any superficial eye disease must be diagnosed and fully treated before a refractive procedure.

Radial Keratotomy

Radial keratotomy (RK) is indicated for low myopia (less than 8D). The procedure involves making four to eight, deep, radial incisions in the paracentral and peripheral cornea with a metal or diamond blade. The corneal contour then becomes flatter. Glare, photosensitivity, fluctuations of vision during the day, and occasional diplopia are common side effects. As the popularity of laser refractive surgery grows, RK procedures decrease.

Laser Vision Correction Photorefractive Keratectomy

Laser vision correction photorefractive keratectomy (PRK) is a procedure used to treat myopia and hyperopia with or without astigmatism. The 193-mm argon fluoride excimer laser is applied directly to the cornea according to carefully calculated measurements. For myopia, the relative curvature is decreased; for hyperopia, the relative curvature is increased. A bandage contact lens is placed over the cornea to promote epithelial healing and reduce pain similar to that of severe corneal abrasion. PRK requires a longer visual recovery period than RK, but PRK provides more predictable and stable results. Except for the side effect of corneal haze and night vision problems, PRK has not been associated with the two major disadvantages of RK: hyperopic drift and weakening of the structural integrity of the cornea.

Laser-Assisted In Situ Keratomileusis (LASIK)

An improvement over PRK, particularly for correcting high (severe) myopia, LASIK involves flattening the anterior curvature of the cornea by removing a stromal lamella or layer. The surgeon creates a corneal flap with a microkeratome, which is an automatic corneal shaper similar to a carpenter's plane. The surgeon retracts a flap of corneal tissue less than one third of the thickness of a human hair to access the corneal stroma and then uses the excimer laser on the stromal bed to reshape the cornea according to calculated measurements (Fig. 58-11). The corneal flap, a naturally adhering bandage, is rolled back and repositioned. LASIK

FIGURE 58-11 LASIK combines delicate surgical procedures and laser treatment. A flap is surgically created and lifted to one side. A laser is then applied to the cornea to reshape it. With permission from The Wilmer Laser Vision Center, Lutherville, MD.

also appears to be an effective, predictable, stable, and safe procedure for correcting residual myopia after cataract surgery (Ayala et al., 2001).

LASIK causes less postoperative discomfort, has fewer side effects, and is safer than PRK. The patient has no corneal haze and requires less postoperative care. With LASIK, however, the cornea has been invaded at a deeper level, and any complications are more significant than those that can occur with PRK.

PERIOPERATIVE COMPLICATIONS

Ablation-Related Complications. Ablation complications of LASIK include an elevated area within the corneal treatment ablation zone (ie, central island). Signs and symptoms of this complication include ghosting, blurred vision, halo formation around lights, decreased visual activity, and contrast sensitivity in low light. Most of the island formations resolve over time; reablation is considered only after the island appears stable after repeated examinations for at least 3 months.

Diffuse Lamellar Keratitis. As LASIK increases in popularity and is performed more often, the vision-threatening complication known as diffuse lamellar keratitis (DLK) is reported more often. DLK is a peculiar, noninfectious, inflammatory reaction in the lamellar interface after LASIK. DLK is characterized by a white, granular, diffuse, culture-negative lamellar keratitis occurring in the first week after surgery. Studies suggest that, because no single agent appears to be solely the cause of DLK, the cause is multifactorial (Holland et. al., 2000).

DLK is diagnosed by identifying cells in the lamellar interface by slit-lamp examination from postoperative day 1. Depending on the severity of the condition, treatment methods range from administering corticosteroid drops to intervening surgically.

Central Islands and Decentred Ablations. Decentred or eccentric ablation involves a shift of the centre of the ablation pattern from the pupil or visual axis to a more eccentric location. Symptoms include decreased visual acuity, halos, glare, and ghosting, especially in low-light settings.

LASIK Enhancements

LASIK enhancements are surgical options from improved technology and software used to treat a wider range of myopia, hyperopia, and astigmatism in eyes with a history of LASIK surgery.

Astigmatic keratotomy continues to work well for patients with significant regular astigmatism. A newer procedure, Intacs implantation, is performed for patients left with significant myopia but who have thin corneas. Hyperopic excimer laser enhancements are indicated for patients who have undergone myopic LASIK and have consecutive hyperopia.

IMPLANTABLE DEVICES

Because the results of refractive surgery on high (severe) myopia, hyperopia, and astigmatism are less predictable, there has been increasing interest in the use of phakic IOLs. Anterior and posterior chamber IOLs are now in use, and design improvements continue to be made. Phakic IOL implantation does not compromise the central optical zone and retains the normal aspheric contour of the cornea. Most importantly, it is reversible. Early research results on vision quality favour phakic IOL over LASIK. Potential complications include cataract, iritis or uveitis, endothelial cell loss, and increased IOP.

Intacs is an implantable intrastromal corneal ring used to correct mild to moderate myopia. The intrastromal corneal ring segments are placed in the corneal stroma outside of the central optical zone and reshape the anterior surface of the cornea.

Management

Patient satisfaction is the ultimate goal; therefore, patient education and counselling about potential risks, complications, and postoperative follow-up are critical. Minimal postoperative care includes topical corticosteroid drops. The length of postoperative follow-up depends on the refractive procedure, with PRK requiring a longer course, followed by RK and then LASIK.

Retinal Disorders

Although the retina is composed of multiple microscopic layers, the two innermost layers, the sensory retina and the retinal pigment epithelium (RPE), are the most relevant to common retinal disorders. Just as the film in a camera captures an image, so does the retina, the neural tissue of the eye. The rods and cones, the photoreceptor cells, are found in the sensory layer of the retina. Beneath the sensory layer lies the RPE, the pigmented layer. When the rods and cones are stimulated by light, an electrical impulse is generated, and the image is transmitted to the brain.

RETINAL DETACHMENT

Retinal detachment refers to the separation of the RPE from the sensory layer. The four types of retinal detachment are rhegmatogenous, traction, a combination of rhegmatogenous and traction, and exudative. *Rhegmatogenous detachment* is the most common form. In this condition, a hole or tear develops in the sensory retina, allowing some of the liquid vitreous to seep through the sensory retina and detach it from the RPE (Fig. 58-12). People at risk for this type of detachment include those with high myopia or **aphakia** after cataract surgery. Trauma may also play a role in rhegmatogenous retinal detachment. Between 5% and 10% of all rhegmatogenous retinal detachments are associated with proliferative retinopathy, a retinopathy associated with diabetic neovascularization (see Chap. 41).

Tension, or a pulling force, is responsible for *traction retinal detachment*. An ophthalmologist must ascertain all of the areas of retinal break and identify and release the scars or bands of fibrous material providing traction on the retina. Generally, patients with

Detached retina

Retinal tear

Lens

Fluid

Vitreous humour

FIGURE 58-12 Retinal detachment.

Scleral buckle
encircles globe

Buckle holds sclera
against the retina

Repaired
tear

FIGURE 58-13 Scleral buckle.

this condition have developed fibrous scar tissue from conditions such as diabetic retinopathy, vitreous hemorrhage, or the retinopathy of prematurity. The hemorrhages and fibrous proliferation associated with these conditions exert a pulling force on the delicate retina.

Patients can have both rhegmatogenous and traction retinal detachment. *Exudative retinal detachments* are the result of the production of a serous fluid under the retina from the choroid. Conditions such as uveitis and macular degeneration may cause the production of this serous fluid.

Clinical Manifestations

Patients may report the sensation of a shade or curtain coming across the vision of one eye, cobwebs, bright flashing lights, or the sudden onset of a great number of floaters. Patients do not complain of pain.

Assessment and Diagnostic Findings

After visual acuity is determined, the patient must have a dilated fundus examination using an indirect ophthalmoscope and a Goldmann three-mirror examination. This examination is detailed and prolonged, and it can be very uncomfortable for the patient. Many patients describe this as looking directly into the sun. All retinal breaks, all fibrous bands that may be causing traction on the retina, and all degenerative changes must be identified. A detailed retinal drawing is made by the ophthalmologist.

Surgical Management

In rhegmatogenous detachment, an attempt is made to reattach the sensory retina to the RPE surgically. The retinal surgeon compresses the sclera (often with a scleral buckle or a silicone band; Fig. 58-13) to indent the scleral wall from the outside of the eye and bring the two retinal layers in contact with each other. Gas bubbles, silicone oil, or perfluorocarbon and liquids may also be injected into the vitreous cavity to help push the sensory retina up against the RPE. Argon laser photocoagulation or cryotherapy is also used to "spot-weld" small holes.

In traction retinal detachment, a vitrectomy is performed. A vitrectomy is an intraocular procedure in which 1- to 4-mm incisions are made at the pans plana. One incision allows the introduction of a light source (ie, endoilluminator), and another incision serves as the portal for the vitrectomy instrument. The surgeon dissects preretinal membranes under direct visualization while the retina is stabilized by an intraoperative vitreous substitute. Technologic advances, including the use of operating microscopes, microinstrumentation, irrigating contact lenses, and instruments that combine vitreous cutting, aspiration, and illumination capabilities into one device, have allowed tremendous progress in vitreoretinal surgery. The techniques of vitreoretinal surgery can be used in various procedures, including the removal of foreign bodies, vitreous opacities such as blood, and dislocated lenses. Traction on the retina may be relieved through vitrectomy and may be combined with scleral buckling to repair retinal breaks. Treatment of macular holes includes vitrectomy, laser photocoagulation, air-fluid-gas exchanges, and the use of growth factor.

Nursing Management

For the most part, nursing interventions consist of educating the patient and providing supportive care.

PROMOTING COMFORT

If gas tamponade is used to flatten the retina, the patient may have to be specially positioned to make the gas bubble float into the best position. Some patients must lie face down or on their side for days. Patients and family members should be made aware of these special needs beforehand, so that the patient can be made as comfortable as possible.

TEACHING ABOUT COMPLICATIONS

In many cases, vitreoretinal procedures are performed on an outpatient basis, and the patient is seen the next day for a follow-up examination and closely monitored thereafter as required. Postoperative complications in these patients may include increased IOP, endophthalmitis, development of other retinal detachments, development of cataracts, and loss of turgor of the eye. Patients must be taught the signs and symptoms of complications, particularly of increasing IOP and postoperative infection.

RETINAL VASCULAR DISORDERS

Loss of vision can occur from occlusion of a retinal artery or vein. Such occlusions may result from atherosclerosis, cardiac valvular disease, venous stasis, hypertension, or increased blood viscosity.

Central Retinal Vein Occlusion

Blood supply to and from the ocular fundus is provided by the central retinal artery and vein. Patients who have suffered a central retinal vein occlusion report decreased visual acuity, which may range from mild blurring to vision that is limited to only hand-motion vision.

Direct ophthalmoscopy of the retina shows optic disc swelling, venous dilation and tortuousness, retinal hemorrhages, cotton-wool spots, and a "blood and thunder" (extremely bloody) appearance of the retina. The better the initial visual acuity, the better the general prognosis.

Fluorescein angiography may show extensive areas of capillary closure. The patient should be monitored carefully over the ensuing several months for signs of neovascularization and neovascular glaucoma. Laser panretinal photocoagulation may be necessary to treat the abnormal neovascularization. Neovascularization of the iris may cause neovascular glaucoma, which may be difficult to control.

Branch Retinal Vein Occlusion

Some patients with branch retinal vein occlusions are symptom free, whereas others complain of a sudden loss of vision if the macular area is involved. A more gradual loss of vision may occur if macular edema associated with the branch retinal vein occlusion develops.

On examination, the ocular fundus appears similar to that found with central retinal vein occlusion; however, only those portions of the retina affected by the obstructive veins have what is known as a "blood and thunder" appearance. The diagnostic evaluation and follow-up assessments are the same as for central retinal vein occlusion. Potential complications are similar. Potential associated conditions include glaucoma, systemic hypertension, diabetes mellitus, hyperlipidemia, and hyperviscosity syndrome.

Central Retinal Artery Occlusion

The patient with central retinal artery occlusion presents with a sudden loss of vision. Visual acuity is reduced to counting the examiner's fingers, or the field of vision is tremendously restricted. A relative afferent pupillary defect is present. Examination of the ocular fundus reveals a pale retina with a cherry-red spot at the fovea. The retinal arteries are thin, and emboli are occasionally seen in the central retinal artery or its branches. Central retinal artery occlusion is a true ocular emergency. Various treatments are used, including ocular massage, anterior chamber paracentesis, intravenous administration of hyperosmotic agents such as acetazolamide, and high concentrations of oxygen.

FIGURE 58-14 Retina showing drusen and AMD.

MACULAR DEGENERATION

Macular degeneration is the most common cause of severe vision loss in Canadians, especially among the elderly, responsible for 1 in 3 cases of reported vision loss (Canadian National Institute for the Blind, 2005d). Commonly called age-related macular degeneration (AMD), it is characterized by tiny, yellowish spots called drusen (Fig. 58-14) beneath the retina. Most people older than 60 years of age have at least a few small drusen. There is a wide range of visual loss in patients with macular degeneration, but most patients do not experience total blindness. Central vision is generally the most affected, with most patients retaining peripheral vision (Fig. 58-15). There are two types of AMD, commonly known as the dry type and wet type.

Between 85% and 90% of people with AMD have the dry or nonexudative type in which the outer layers of the retina slowly break down (Fig. 58-16). With this breakdown comes the appearance of drusen. When the drusen occur outside of the macular area, patients generally have no symptoms. When the drusen occur within the macula, there is a gradual blurring of vision that patients may notice when they try to read. There is no known treatment that can slow or cure this type of AMD.

The second type of AMD, the wet or exudative type, may have an abrupt onset. Patients complain that straight lines appear crooked and distorted or that letters in words appear broken up.

FIGURE 58-15 Visual loss associated with macular degeneration.

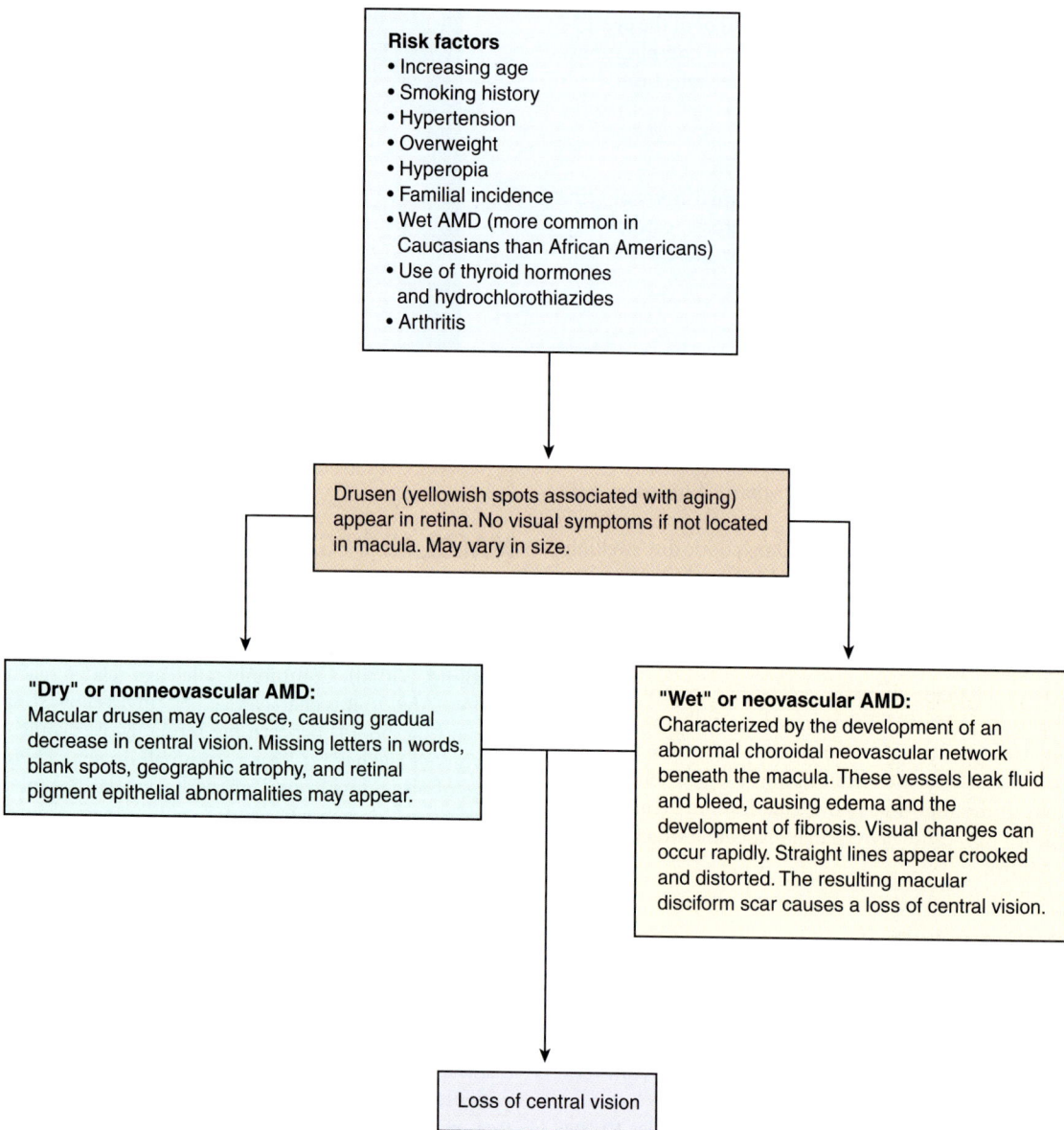

FIGURE 58-16 Progression of age-related macular degeneration (AMD): pathways to vision loss.

This effect results from proliferation of abnormal blood vessels growing under the retina, within the choroid layer of the eye, a condition known as choroidal neovascularization (CNV). The affected vessels can leak fluid and blood, elevating the retina. Some patients can be treated with the laser to stop the leakage from these vessels. This treatment is not ideal because vision may be affected by the laser treatment and abnormal vessels often grow back after treatment.

Medical Management

PHOTODYNAMIC THERAPY
Visual loss from CNV lesions in AMD is a growing problem. With the growth of these new vessels from the choriocapillar layer, fibrous tissue develops that can, over months, destroy central vision. Laser treatment has been used to close these abnormal vessels, but the very process of photocoagulation carries with it some level of retinal destruction, albeit less than the natural scarring that would occur in the untreated eye. Photodynamic therapy (PDT)

has been developed in an attempt to ameliorate the CNV while causing minimal damage to the retina. The Treatment of Age-Related Macular Degeneration With Photodynamic Therapy (TAP) study group (1999) has shown that PDT can reduce the risk of visual loss for certain groups of patients who have classic subfoveal choroidal neovascularization due to macular degeneration.

PDT is a two-step process (Fig. 58-17). Verteporfin, a photosensitive dye, is infused intravenously over 10 minutes. Fifteen minutes after the start of the infusion, a diode laser is used to treat the abnormal network of vessels. The dye within the vessels takes up the energy of the diode laser, but the surrounding retina does not, avoiding damage to adjacent areas. Retreatment may be necessary over time.

Nursing Management

Nursing management is primarily educational. Verteporfin is a light-activated dye, and patient education is important preoperatively. The patient should be instructed to bring dark sunglasses,

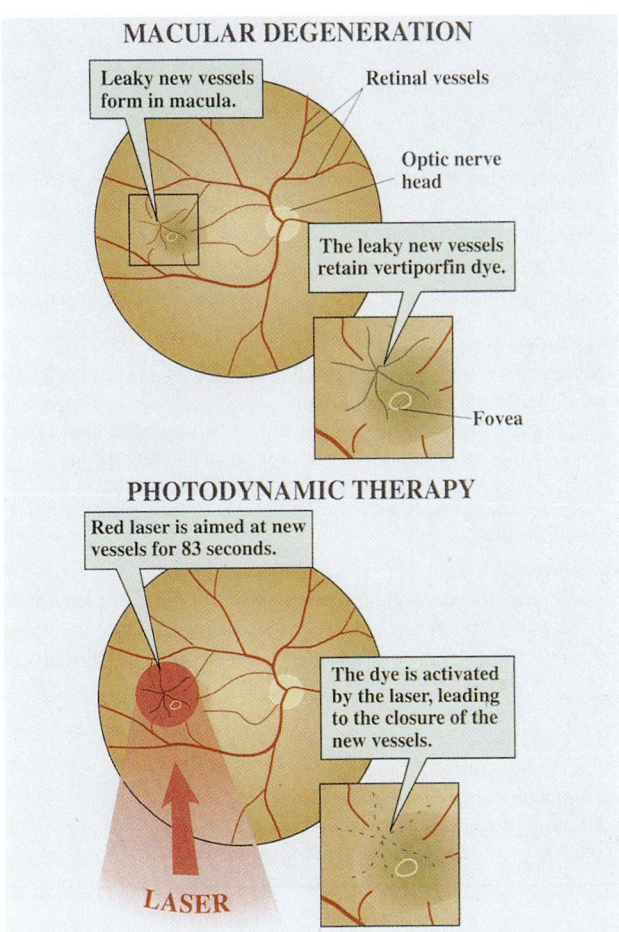

MACULAR DEGENERATION

Leaky new vessels form in macula.

Retinal vessels

Optic nerve head

The leaky new vessels retain vertiporfin dye.

Fovea

PHOTODYNAMIC THERAPY

Red laser is aimed at new vessels for 83 seconds.

The dye is activated by the laser, leading to the closure of the new vessels.

LASER

FIGURE 58-17 Photodynamic therapy (PDT) for slowing progression of age-related macular degeneration. Light-sensitive verteporfin dye is injected into defective vessels. A special laser activates the dye, which releases singlet oxygen that is toxic to endothelial cells, shutting down the vessels without damaging the retina. With permission from Valenz, K. D. (2001). Laser surgery shines as ray of hope. *Helix 18*(3):12–13.

gloves, a wide-brimmed hat, long-sleeved shirt, and slacks to the PDT setting. The patient must be cautioned to avoid exposure to direct sunlight or bright light for 5 days after treatment. The dye within the blood vessels near the surface of the skin could become activated with exposure to strong light. This would include bright sunlight, tanning booths, halogen lights, and the bright lights used in dental offices and operating rooms. Ordinary indoor light is not a problem. If a patient must go outdoors within the first 5 days after treatment, he or she should be counselled to wear long-sleeved shirts and slacks made of tightly woven fabrics. Gloves, shoes, socks, sunglasses, and a wide-brimmed hat should also be worn if the patient has to go outdoors during daylight hours during this period. Inadvertent sunlight exposure can lead to severe blistering of the skin and sunburn that may require plastic surgery.

Macular Translocation

Wet macular degeneration is characterized by the development of an abnormal CNV membrane to the detriment of central vision. One approach to this problem is the surgical procedure known as macular translocation, in which a 360-degree retinal detachment is surgically created and the retina is gently lifted and resettled, placing the macular area a slight distance away from the area of CNV. Laser treatment can then be applied to the abnormal neovascular network with minimal damage occurring to the macula. Pilot studies are evaluating whether this surgical approach is an effective alternative to laser treatments of CNV due to AMD.

Angiogenesis

An important component of the effort against neovascular AMD is the investigation into the causes of the development and progression of angiogenesis (ie, abnormal blood vessel formation). Investigations continue in the laboratory to search for agents that can inhibit angiogenesis. This has implications for ocular neovascularization and treatment of other disorders such as solid tumours.

Management

Most patients benefit from the use of bright lighting and magnification devices and from referral to a low-vision centre. Some low-vision centres send representatives into the patient's home or place of employment to evaluate the living and working conditions and make recommendations to improve lighting, thereby improving vision and promoting safety. The home care nurse can make the same assessment and recommendations.

Amsler grids are given to patients to use in their home to monitor for a sudden onset or distortion of vision. These may provide the earliest sign that macular degeneration is getting worse. Patients should be encouraged to use these grids and to look at them, one eye at a time, several times each week with glasses on. If there is a change in the grid (eg, if the lines or squares appear distorted or faded), the patient should be instructed to notify the ophthalmologist immediately and to arrange to be seen promptly.

The Age-Related Eye Disease Study Group (2001), a multicentre clinical trial, has provided promising information about the prevention and treatment of AMD. The study was designed to determine whether large doses of macronutrients are effective in preventing or slowing the course of AMD. The study revealed that use of antioxidants (ie, vitamin C, vitamin E, and beta-carotene) and minerals (ie, zinc oxide) can slow the progression of AMD and vision loss for people at high risk for developing advanced AMD.

Orbital and Ocular Trauma

Whether affecting the eye or the orbit, trauma to the eye and surrounding structures may have devastating consequences for vision. It is preferable to prevent injury rather than treat it. Chart 58-8 details safety measures to prevent orbital and ocular trauma.

ORBITAL TRAUMA

Injury to the orbit is usually associated with a head injury; hence, the patient's general medical condition must first be stabilized before conducting an ocular examination. Only then is the globe assessed for soft tissue injury. During inspection, the face is meticulously assessed for underlying fractures, which should always be suspected in cases of blunt trauma. To establish the extent of ocular injury, visual acuity is assessed as soon as possible, even if it is only a rough estimate. Soft tissue orbital injuries often result in damage to the optic nerve. Major ocular injuries indicated by a soft globe, prolapsing tissue, ruptured globe, hemorrhage, and loss of red reflex require immediate surgical attention.

Soft Tissue Injury and Hemorrhage

The signs and symptoms of soft tissue injury from blunt or penetrating trauma include tenderness, ecchymosis, lid swelling, **proptosis** (ie, downward displacement of the eyeball), and hemorrhage. Closed injuries lead to contusions with subconjunctival hemorrhage, commonly known as a *black eye*. Blood accumulates in the tissues of the conjunctiva. Hemorrhage may be caused by a soft tissue injury to the eyelid or by an underlying fracture.

Management of soft tissue hemorrhage that does not threaten vision is usually conservative and consists of thorough inspection, cleansing, and repair of wounds. Cold compresses are used in the early phase, followed by warm compresses. Hematomas that appear as swollen, fluctuating areas may be surgically drained or aspirated; if they are causing significant orbital pressure, they may be surgically evacuated.

Penetrating injuries or severe blow to the head can result in severe optic nerve damage. Visual loss can be sudden or delayed and progressive. Immediate loss of vision after an ocular injury is usually irreversible. Delayed visual loss has a better prognosis. Corticosteroid therapy is indicated to reduce optic nerve swelling. Surgery, such as optic nerve decompression, may be performed.

Orbital Fractures

Orbital fractures are detected by facial x-rays. Depending on the orbital structures involved, orbital fractures can be classified as blow-out, zygomatic or tripod, maxillary, midfacial, orbital apex, and orbital roof fractures. Blow-out fractures result from compression of soft tissue and sudden increase in orbital pressure when the force is transmitted to the orbital floor, the area of least resistance.

The inferior rectus and inferior oblique muscles, with their fat and fascial attachments, or the nerve that courses along the inferior oblique muscle may become entrapped, and the globe may be displaced inward (ie, enophthalmos). Computed tomography (CT) can firmly identify the muscle and its auxiliary structures that are entrapped. These fractures are usually caused by blunt small objects, such as a fist, knee, elbow, or tennis or golf balls.

Orbital roof fractures are dangerous because of potential complications to the brain. Surgical management of these fractures requires a neurosurgeon and an ophthalmologist. The most common indications for surgical intervention are displacement of bone fragments disfiguring the normal facial contours, interference with normal binocular vision caused by extraocular muscle entrapment, interference with mastication in zygomatic fracture, and obstruction of the nasolacrimal duct. Surgery is usually nonemergent, and a period of 10 to 14 days gives the ophthalmologist time to assess ocular function, especially the extraocular muscles and the nasolacrimal duct. Emergency surgical repair is usually not performed unless the globe is displaced to the maxillary sinus. Operative repair is primarily directed at freeing the entrapped ocular structures and restoring the integrity of the orbital floor. Cosmetic surgery for deformities of the globe and enophthalmos may follow after 4 to 6 months, but successful repair is usually difficult.

Foreign Bodies

Foreign bodies that enter the orbit are usually tolerated, except for copper, iron, and vegetable materials such as those from plants or trees, which may cause purulent infection. X-rays and

CT scans are used to identify the foreign body. Careful history taking is important, especially if the foreign body has been in the orbit for a period of time and the incident forgotten. It is important to identify metallic foreign bodies because they prohibit the use of magnetic resonance imaging (MRI) as a diagnostic tool.

After the extent of the orbital damage is assessed, the decision is made between conservative treatment and surgical removal. In general, orbital foreign bodies are usually removed if they are superficial and anterior in location, have sharp edges that may affect adjacent orbital structures, or are composed of copper, iron, or vegetable material. The surgical intervention is directed at prevention of further ocular injury and maintaining the integrity of the affected areas. Cultures are usually obtained, and the patient is placed on prophylactic intravenous antibiotics that are later changed to oral antibiotics.

OCULAR TRAUMA

Ocular trauma is the leading cause of blindness among children and young adults, especially male trauma victims. The most common circumstances of ocular trauma are occupational injuries (eg, construction industry), sports (eg, baseball, basketball, hockey, racket sports, boxing), weapons (eg, air guns, BB guns), assault, motor vehicle crashes (eg, broken windshields), and war (eg, blast fragments).

For the nonophthalmic practitioner, initial intervention is performed in only two conditions: chemical burns, for which irrigation of the eye with normal saline solution or even plain tap water must occur immediately, and a foreign body, for which absolutely no attempt is made to remove the foreign material, small or big, or apply pressure or patch to the injured eye. The eye must be protected using a metal shield, if available, or a stiff paper cup (Fig. 58-18). All traumatic eye injuries should be properly shielded.

Assessment and Diagnostic Findings

A thorough history is obtained, particularly assessing the patient's ocular history, such as preinjury vision in the affected eye or past ocular surgery. Details related to the injury that help in the diagnosis and assessment of need for further tests include the nature of the ocular injury (ie, blunt or penetrating trauma), the type of activity causing the injury to determine the nature of the force striking the eye, and whether onset of vision loss was sudden, slow, or progressive. For chemical eye burns, the chemical agent must be identified and tested for pH if a sample is available. The corneal surface is examined for foreign bodies, wounds, and abrasions, after which the other external structures of the eye are examined. Pupillary size, shape, and light reaction of the pupil of the affected eye are compared with the other eye. Ocular motility, which is the ability of the eyes to move synchronously up, down, right, and left, is also assessed.

Medical Management

SPLASH INJURIES

Splash injuries are irrigated with normal saline solution before further evaluation. In cases of ruptured globe, cycloplegic agents (ie, agents that paralyze the ciliary muscle) or topical antibiotics must be deferred because of potential toxicity to exposed intraocular tissues. Further manipulation of the eye must be avoided until the patient is under general anesthesia. Parenteral, broad-spectrum antibiotics are initiated. Tetanus antitoxin is administered, if indicated, as well as analgesics. (Tetanus prophylaxis is recommended for full-thickness ocular and skin wounds.) Any topical medication (eg, anesthetic, dyes) must be sterile.

FOREIGN BODIES AND CORNEAL ABRASIONS

After removal of a foreign body from the surface of the eye, an antibiotic ointment is applied, and the eye is patched. The eye is examined daily for evidence of infection until the wound is completely healed.

Contact lens wear is a common cause of corneal abrasion. The patient experiences severe pain and **photophobia** (ie, ocular pain on exposure to light). Corneal epithelial defects are treated with antibiotic ointment and a pressure patch to immobilize the eyelids. It is of utmost importance that topical anesthetic eye drops are not given to a patient for repeated use after corneal injury because their effects mask further damage, delay healing, and can lead to permanent corneal scarring. Corticosteroids are avoided while the epithelial defect exists.

Penetrating Injuries and Contusions of the Eyeball

Sharp penetrating injury or blunt contusion force can rupture the eyeball. When the eye wall, cornea, and sclera rupture, rapid decompression or herniation of the orbital contents into adjacent sinuses can occur. In general, blunt traumatic injuries (with an increased incidence of retinal detachment, intraocular tissue avulsion, and herniation) have a worse prognosis than penetrating injuries. Most penetrating injuries result in marked loss of vision with the following signs: hemorrhagic **chemosis** (ie, edema of the conjunctiva), conjunctival laceration, shallow anterior chamber with or without an eccentrically placed pupil, **hyphema** (ie, hemorrhage within the chamber), or vitreous hemorrhage.

Hyphema is caused by contusion forces that tear the vessels of the iris and damage the anterior chamber angle. Preventing rebleeding and prolonged increased IOP are the goals of treatment

FIGURE 58-18 Two kinds of eye patches. (**A**) Metal shield. (**B**) Stiff paper cup shield (innovative substitute when metal shield is unavailable). Adapted from MacCumber, M. W. (Ed.). (1997). *Management of ocular injuries and emergencies.* Philadelphia: Lippincott-Raven.

A   B

for hyphema. In severe cases in which patient compliance is questionable, the patient is hospitalized with moderate activity restriction. An eye shield is applied. Topical corticosteroids are prescribed to reduce inflammation. An antifibrinolytic agent, aminocaproic acid (Amicar), stabilizes clot formation at the site of hemorrhage. Aspirin is contraindicated.

A ruptured globe and severe injuries with intraocular hemorrhage require surgical intervention. Vitrectomy is performed for traumatic retinal detachments. Primary **enucleation** (ie, complete removal of the eyeball and part of the optic nerve) is considered only if the globe is irreparable and has no light perception. It is a general rule that enucleation is performed within 2 weeks of the initial injury (in an eye that has no useful vision after sustaining penetrating injury) to prevent the risk of **sympathetic ophthalmia,** an inflammation created in the fellow eye by the affected eye that can result in blindness of the fellow eye.

Intraocular Foreign Bodies

A patient who complains of blurred vision and discomfort should be questioned carefully about recent injuries and exposures. Patients may be injured in a number of different situations and suffer an intraocular foreign body (IOFB). Precipitating circumstances can include working in construction, striking metal against metal, being involved in motor vehicle crashes with facial injury, gunshot wounds, and grinding-wheel work.

IOFB is diagnosed and localized by slit-lamp biomicroscopy and indirect ophthalmoscopy, as well as CT or ultrasonography. MRI is contraindicated because most foreign bodies are metallic and magnetic. It is important to determine the composition, size, and location of the IOFB and affected eye structures. Every effort should be made to identify the type of IOFB and whether it is magnetic. Iron, steel, copper, and vegetable matter cause intense inflammatory reactions. The incidence of endophthalmitis is also high. If the cornea is perforated, tetanus prophylaxis and intravenous antibiotics are administered. The extraction route (ie, surgical incision) of the foreign body depends on its location and composition and associated ocular injuries. Specially designed IOFB forceps and magnets are used to grasp and remove the foreign body. Any damaged area of the retina is treated to prevent retinal detachment.

OCULAR BURNS

Alkali, acid, and other chemically active organic substances, such as mace and tear gas, cause chemical burns. Alkali burns (eg, lye, ammonia) result in the most injury because they penetrate the ocular tissues rapidly and continue to cause damage long after the initial injury is sustained. They also cause an immediate rise in IOP. Acids (eg, bleach, car batteries, refrigerant) generally cause less damage because the precipitated necrotic tissue proteins form a barrier to further penetration and damage. Chemical burns may appear as superficial punctate keratopathy (ie, spotty damage to the cornea), subconjunctival hemorrhage, or complete marbleizing of the cornea.

In treating chemical burns, every minute counts. Immediate tap-water irrigation should be started on site before transport of the patient to an emergency department. Only a brief history and examination are performed. The corneal surfaces and conjunctival fornices are immediately and copiously irrigated with normal saline or any neutral solution. A local anesthetic is instilled, and

a lid speculum is applied to overcome blepharospasm (ie, spasms of the eyelid muscles that result in closure of the lids). Particulate matter must be removed from the fornices using moistened, cotton-tip applicators and minimal pressure on the globe. Irrigation continues until the conjunctival pH normalizes (between 7.3 and 7.6). The pH of the corneal surface is checked by placing a pH paper strip in the fornix. Antibiotics are instilled, and the eye is patched.

The goal of intermediate treatment is to prevent tissue ulceration and promote re-epithelialization. Intense lubrication using nonpreserved (ie, without preservatives to avoid allergic reactions) tears is essential. Re-epithelialization is promoted with patching or therapeutic soft lenses. The patient is usually monitored daily for several days. Prognosis depends on the type of injury and adequacy of the irrigation immediately after exposure. Long-term treatment consists of two phases: restoration of the ocular surface through grafting procedures and surgical restoration of corneal integrity and optical clarity.

Thermal injury is caused by exposure to a hot object (eg, curling iron, tobacco, ash), whereas photochemical injury results from ultraviolet irradiation or infrared exposure (eg, exposure to the reflections from snow, sun gazing, viewing an eclipse of the sun without an adequate filter). These injuries can cause corneal epithelial defect, corneal opacity, conjunctival chemosis and **injection** (ie, congestion of blood vessels), and burns of the eyelids and periocular region. Antibiotics and a pressure patch for 24 hours constitute the treatment of mild injuries. Scarring of the eyelids may require oculoplastic surgery, whereas corneal scarring may require corneal surgery.

Infectious and Inflammatory Conditions

Inflammation and infection of eye structures are common. Eye infection is a leading cause of blindness worldwide. Table 58-7 describes selected common infections and their treatment.

DRY EYE SYNDROME

Dry eye syndrome, or keratoconjunctivitis sicca, is a deficiency in the production of any of the aqueous, mucin, or lipid tear film components; lid surface abnormalities; or epithelial abnormalities related to systemic diseases (eg, thyroid disorders, Parkinson's disease), infection, injury, or complications of medications (eg, antihistamines, oral contraceptives, phenothiazines).

Clinical Manifestations

The most common complaint in dry eye syndrome is a scratchy or foreign body sensation. Other symptoms include itching, excessive mucus secretion, inability to produce tears, a burning sensation, redness, pain, and difficulty moving the lids.

Assessment and Diagnostic Findings

Slit-lamp examination shows an absent or interrupted tear meniscus at the lower lid margin, and the conjunctiva is thickened, edematous, hyperemic, and has lost its luster. A tear meniscus is the crescent-shaped edge of the tear film in the lower lid margin. Chronic dry eyes may result in chronic conjunctival and corneal irritation that can lead to corneal erosion, scarring, ulceration, thinning, or perforation that can seriously threaten vision. Secondary bacterial infection can occur.

Table 58-7 • **Common Infections and Inflammatory Disorders of Eye Structures**

DISORDER	DESCRIPTION	MANAGEMENT
Hordeolum (sty)	Acute suppurative infection of the glands of the eyelids caused by *Staphylococcus aureus.* The lid is red and edematous with a small collection of pus in the form of an abscess. There is considerable discomfort.	Warm compresses are applied directly to the affected lid area three to four times a day for 10 to 15 minutes. If the condition is not improved after 48 hours, incision and drainage may be indicated. Application of topical antibiotics may be prescribed thereafter.
Chalazion	Sterile inflammatory process involving chronic granulomatous inflammation of the meibomian glands; can appear as a single granuloma or multiple granulomas in the upper or lower eyelids.	Warm compresses applied three to four times a day for 10 to 15 minutes may resolve the inflammation in the early stages. Most often, however, surgical excision is indicated. Corticosteroid injection to the chalazion lesion may be used for smaller lesions.
Blepharitis	Chronic bilateral inflammation of the eyelid margins. There are two types: staphylococcal and seborrheic. Staphylococcal blepharitis is usually ulcerative and is more serious due to the involvement of the base of hair follicles. Permanent scarring can result.	The seborrheic type is chronic and is usually resistant to treatment, but the milder cases may respond to lid hygiene. Staphylococcal blepharitis requires topical antibiotic treatment. Instructions on lid hygiene (to keep the lid margins clean and free of exudates) are given to the patient.
Bacterial keratitis	Infection of the cornea by *S. aureus, Streptococcus pneumoniae,* and *Pseudomonas aeruginosa*	Fortified (high-concentration) antibiotic eyedrops are administered every 30 minutes around the clock for the first few days, then every 1–2 hours. Systemic antibiotics may be administered. Cycloplegics are administered to reduce pain caused by ciliary spasm. Corticosteroid therapy and subconjunctival injections of antibiotics are controversial.
Herpes simplex keratitis	Leading cause of corneal blindness. Symptoms are severe pain, tearing, and photophobia. The dendritic ulcer has a branching, linear pattern with feathery edges and terminal bulbs at its ends. Herpes simplex keratitis can lead to recurrent stromal keratitis and persist to 12 months with residual corneal scarring.	Many lesions heal without treatment and residual effects. The treatment goal is to minimize the damaging effect of the inflammatory response and eliminate viral replication within the cornea. Penetrating keratoplasty is indicated for corneal scarring and must be performed when the herpetic disease has been inactive for many months.

Management

Management of dry eye syndrome requires the complete cooperation of the patient with a regimen that needs to be followed at home for a long period, or complete relief of symptoms is unlikely. Instillation of artificial tears during the day and an ointment at night is the usual regimen to hydrate and lubricate the eye through stimulating tears and preserving a moist ocular surface. Anti-inflammatory medications are also used, and moisture chambers (eg, moisture chamber spectacles, swim goggles) may provide additional relief.

Patients may become hypersensitive to chemical preservatives such as benzalkonium chloride and thimerosal. For these patients, preservative-free ophthalmic solutions are used. Management of the dry eye syndrome also includes the concurrent treatment of infections, such as chronic blepharitis and acne rosacea, and treating the underlying systemic disease, such as Sjögren's syndrome (an autoimmune disease).

In advanced cases of dry eye syndrome, surgical treatment that includes punctal occlusion, grafting procedures, and lateral tarsorrhaphy (ie, uniting the edges of the lids) are options. Punctal plugs are made of silicone material for the temporary or permanent occlusion of the puncta. This helps preserve the natural tears and prolongs the effects of artificial tears. Short-term occlusion is performed by inserting punctal or silicone rods in all four puncta. If tearing is induced, the upper plugs are removed, and the remaining lower plugs are removed in another week. Permanent occlusion is performed only in severe cases among adults who do not develop tearing after partial occlusion and who have results on a repeated Schirmer's test of 2 mm or less (filter paper is used to measure tear production).

CONJUNCTIVITIS

Conjunctivitis (ie, inflammation of the conjunctiva) is the most common ocular disease worldwide. It is characterized by a pink appearance (hence the common term *pink eye*) because of subconjunctival blood vessel hemorrhages.

Clinical Manifestations

General symptoms include foreign body sensation, scratching or burning sensation, itching, and photophobia. Conjunctivitis may be unilateral or bilateral, but the infection usually starts in one eye and then spreads to the other eye by hand contact.

Assessment and Diagnostic Findings

The four main clinical features important to evaluate are the type of discharge (ie, watery, mucoid, purulent, or mucopurulent), type of conjunctival reaction (ie, follicular or papillary), presence of pseudomembranes or true membranes, and presence or absence of lymphadenopathy (ie, enlargement of the preauricular and submandibular lymph nodes where the eyelids drain). Pseudomembranes consist of coagulated exudate that adheres to the surface of the inflamed conjunctiva. True membranes form when the exudate adheres to the superficial layer of the conjunctiva, and removal results in bleeding. Follicles are multiple, slightly elevated lesions encircled by tiny blood vessels; they look like grains of rice. Papillae are hyperplastic conjunctival epithelium in numerous projections that are usually seen as a fine mosaic pattern under slit-lamp examination. Diagnosis is based on the distinctive characteristics of ocular signs, acute or chronic presentation, and identification of any precipitating events. Positive results of swab smear preparations and cultures confirm the diagnosis.

Types of Conjunctivitis

Conjunctivitis is classified according to its cause. The major causes are microbial infection, allergy, and irritating toxic stimuli. A wide spectrum of exogenous microbes can cause conjunctivitis, including bacteria (eg, *Chlamydia*), viruses, fungus, and parasites. Conjunctivitis can also result from infection of an existing ocular infection or can be a manifestation of a systemic disease.

MICROBIAL CONJUNCTIVITIS

Bacterial conjunctivitis can be acute or chronic. The acute type can develop into a chronic condition. Signs and symptoms can vary from mild to severe. Chronic bacterial conjunctivitis is usually seen in patients with lacrimal duct obstruction, chronic dacryocystitis, and chronic blepharitis. The most common causative microorganisms are *Streptococcus pneumoniae, Haemophilus influenzae,* and *Staphylococcus aureus.*

Bacterial conjunctivitis manifests with an acute onset of redness, burning, and discharge. There is papillary formation, conjunctival irritation, and injection in the fornices. The exudates are variable but are usually present on waking in the morning. The eyes may be difficult to open because of adhesions caused by the exudate. Purulent discharge occurs in severe acute bacterial infections, whereas mucopurulent discharge appears in mild cases. In gonococcal conjunctivitis, the symptoms are more acute. The exudate is profuse and purulent, and there is lymphadenopathy. Pseudomembranes may be present.

Viral conjunctivitis (Fig. 58-19) can also be acute and chronic. The discharge is watery, and follicles are prominent. Severe cases include pseudomembranes. The common causative organisms are adenovirus and herpes simplex virus. Conjunctivitis caused by adenovirus is highly contagious. The symptoms include extreme tearing, redness, and foreign body sensation that can involve one or both eyes. The condition is usually preceded by symptoms of upper respiratory infection. Corneal involvement causes extreme photophobia. There is lid edema, ptosis, conjunctival **hyperemia** (ie, dilation of the conjunctival blood vessels), watery discharge, follicles, and papillae. These signs and symptoms vary from mild to severe and may last for 2 weeks. Viral conjunctivitis, although self-limited, tends to last longer than bacterial conjunctivitis.

Epidemic keratoconjunctivitis (EKC) is most often accompanied by preauricular lymphadenopathy and occasionally perior-

FIGURE 58-19 Conjunctival hyperemia in viral conjunctivitis.

bital pain. There are marked follicular and papillary formations. EKC can lead to keratopathy. EKC is a highly contagious viral conjunctivitis that is easily transmitted from one person to another among household members, school children, and health care workers. The outbreak of epidemics is seasonal, especially during the summer when people frequent swimming pools.

Chlamydial conjunctivitis includes trachoma and inclusion conjunctivitis. Trachoma is an ancient disease and is the leading cause of preventable blindness in the world. It is prevalent in areas with hot, dry, and dusty climates and in areas with poor living conditions. It is spread by direct contact or fomites, and the vectors can be insects such as flies and gnats.

Trachoma is a bilateral chronic follicular conjunctivitis of childhood that leads to blindness during adulthood, if left untreated. The onset in children is usually insidious, but it can be acute or subacute in adults. The initial symptoms include red inflamed eyes, tearing, photophobia, ocular pain, purulent exudates, preauricular lymphadenopathy, and lid edema. Initial ocular signs include follicular and papillary formations. At the middle stage of the disease, there is an acute inflammation with papillary hypertrophy and follicular necrosis, after which trichiasis (turning inward of hair follicles) and entropion begin to develop. The lashes that are turned in rub against the cornea and, after prolonged irritation, cause corneal erosion and ulceration. The late stage of the disease is characterized by scarred conjunctiva, subepithelial keratitis, abnormal vascularization of the cornea (pannus), and residual scars from the follicles that look like depressions in the conjunctiva (ie, Herbert's pits). Severe corneal ulceration can lead to perforation and blindness.

Inclusion conjunctivitis affects sexually active young people who have genital chlamydial infection. Transmission is by oral-genital sex or hand-to-eye transmission. It has been reported that indirect transmission has been acquired from inadequately chlorinated swimming pools. The eye lesions usually appear a week after exposure and may be associated with a nonspecific urethritis or cervicitis. The discharge is mucopurulent, follicles are present, and there is lymphadenopathy.

ALLERGIC CONJUNCTIVITIS

Immunologic or allergic conjunctivitis is a hypersensitivity reaction as a part of allergic rhinitis (hay fever), or it can be an independent allergic reaction. The patient usually has a history of an allergy to pollens and other environmental allergens. There is extreme itching, epiphora (ie, excessive secretion of tears), injection, and usually severe photophobia. The stringlike mucoid discharge is usually associated with rubbing the eyes because of severe itching. Vernal conjunctivitis is also known as seasonal conjunctivitis because it appears mostly during warm weather. There may be large formations of papillae that have a cobblestone appearance. It is more common in children and young adults. Most affected individuals have a history of asthma or eczema.

TOXIC CONJUNCTIVITIS

Chemical conjunctivitis can be the result of medications, chlorine from swimming pools (more common during the summer), exposure to toxic fumes among industrial workers, or exposure to other irritants such as smoke, hair sprays, acids, and alkalis.

Management

The management of conjunctivitis depends on the type. Most types of mild and viral conjunctivitis are self-limiting, benign conditions that may not require treatment and laboratory procedures. For more severe cases, topical antibiotics, eye drops, or ointment are prescribed.

Patients with gonococcal conjunctivitis require urgent antibiotic therapy. If left untreated, this ocular disease can lead to corneal perforation and blindness. The systemic complications can include meningitis and generalized septicemia.

Acute bacterial conjunctivitis is almost always self-limiting. If left untreated, the disease follows a 2-week course with resolution of symptoms. If treated with appropriate antibiotics, it may last for a few days, with the exception of gonococcal and staphylococcal conjunctivitis. Viral conjunctivitis is not responsive to any treatment. Cold compresses may alleviate some symptoms. It is extremely important to remember that viral conjunctivitis, especially EKC, is highly transmissible. Patients must be made aware of the contagious nature of the disease, and adequate instructions must be given. These instructions should include an emphasis on handwashing and avoiding sharing hand towels, face cloths, and eye drops. Tissues should be directly discarded into a trashcan.

Proper steps must be taken to avoid nosocomial infections. Frequent hand hygiene, procedures for environmental cleaning, and disinfection of equipment used for eye examination must be strictly followed at all times (Chart 58-9). During outbreaks of conjunctivitis caused by adenovirus, it is necessary that health care facilities assign specified areas for treating patients with or suspected of having conjunctivitis caused by adenovirus to prevent spread. All forms of tonometry must be avoided unless medically indicated. All multidose medications must be discarded at the end of each day or when contaminated. Infected employees and others must not be allowed to work or attend school until symptoms have resolved, which can take 3 to 7 days.

Patients with allergic conjunctivitis, especially recurrent vernal or seasonal conjunctivitis, are usually given corticosteroids in ophthalmic preparations. Depending on the severity of the disease, they may be given oral preparations. Use of vasoconstrictors, such as topical epinephrine solution, cold compresses, ice packs, and cool ventilation usually provide comfort by decreasing swelling.

For trachoma, treatment is usually broad-spectrum antibiotics administered topically and systemically. Surgical management includes the correction of trichiasis to prevent conjunctival scarring. Adult inclusion conjunctivitis requires a 1-week course of antibiotics. Prevention of reinfection is important, and affected individuals and their sexual partners must be advised to seek as-

Chart 58-9 • PATIENT EDUCATION
Instructions for Patients With Viral Conjunctivitis

Viral conjunctivitis is a highly contagious eye infection. It can easily spread from one person to another. The symptoms can be alarming, but they are not serious. The following information will help you understand this eye condition and how to take care of yourself and/or your family member at home.

- Your eyes will look red and will have watery discharge, and your lids will be swollen for about a week.
- You will experience eye pain, a sandy sensation in your eye, and sensitivity to light.
- Symptoms will resolve after about 1 week.
- You may use light cold compresses over your eyes for about 10 minutes four to five times a day to soothe the pain.
- You may use artificial tears for the sandy sensation in your eye and mild pain medications such as acetaminophen (Tylenol).
- You need to stay at home. Children must not play outside. You may return to work or school after 7 days when the redness and discharge have cleared. You may obtain a doctor's note to return to work or school.
- Do not share towels, linens, makeup, or toys.
- Wash your hands thoroughly with soap and water frequently, including and before and after you apply artificial tears or cold compresses.
- Use a new tissue every time you wipe the discharge from your eye. You may dampen the tissue with clean water to clean the outside of the eye.
- You may wash your face and take a shower as you normally do.
- Discard all of your makeup articles. You must not apply makeup until the disease is over.
- You may wear dark glasses if bright lights bother you.
- If the discharge from your eye turns yellowish and puslike or you experience changes in your vision, you need to return to the health care provider for an examination.

sessment and treatment for sexually transmitted disease, if indicated.

For conjunctivitis caused by chemical irritants, the eye must be irrigated immediately and profusely with saline or sterile water.

UVEITIS

Inflammation of the uveal tract is called uveitis and can affect the iris, the ciliary body, or the choroid. There are two types of uveitis: nongranulomatous and granulomatous.

The most common type of uveitis is the nongranulomatous type, which manifests as an acute condition with pain, photophobia, and a pattern of conjunctival injection, especially around the cornea. The pupil is small or irregular, and vision is blurred. There may be small, fine precipitates on the posterior corneal surface and cells in the aqueous humour (ie, cell and flare). If severe, a **hypopyon** (ie, accumulation of pus in the anterior chamber) may occur. The condition may be unilateral or bilateral and may be recurrent. Repeated attacks of nongranulomatous anterior uveitis can cause anterior synechia (ie, peripheral iris adheres to the cornea and impedes outflow of aqueous humour). The development of posterior synechia (ie, adherence of the iris and lens) blocks aqueous outflow from the posterior chamber. Secondary glaucoma can result from either anterior or posterior synechia. Cataracts may also occur as a sequela to uveitis.

Granulomatous uveitis can have a more insidious onset and can involve any portion of the uveal tract. It tends to be chronic. Symptoms such as photophobia and pain may be minimal. The keratic precipitate may be large and greyish. Vision is markedly and adversely affected. Conjunctival injection is diffuse, and there may be vitreous clouding. In a severe posterior uveitis, such as chorioretinitis, there may be retinal and choroidal hemorrhages.

Management

Because photophobia is a common complaint, patients should wear dark glasses outdoors. Ciliary spasm and synechia are best avoided through mydriasis; cylopentolate (Cyclogyl) and atropine are commonly used. Local corticosteroid drops, such as Pred Forte 1% and Flarex 0.1%, instilled four to six times a day are also used to decrease inflammation. In very severe cases, systemic corticosteroids, as well as intravitreal corticosteroids, may be used.

If the uveitis is recurrent, a medical workup should be initiated to discover any underlying causes. This evaluation should include a physical examination, complete systems review, and diagnostic tests, including a complete blood cell count, erythrocyte sedimentation rate, antinuclear antibodies (ANA), VDRL, and Lyme disease titer. Underlying causes include toxoplasmosis, herpes zoster virus, ocular candidiasis, histoplasmosis, herpes simplex virus, tuberculosis, and syphilis.

ORBITAL CELLULITIS

Orbital cellulitis is inflammation of the tissues surrounding the eye and may result from bacterial, fungal, or viral inflammatory conditions of contiguous structures, such as the face, oropharynx, dental structures, or intracranial structures. It can also result from foreign bodies and from a preexisting ocular infection, such as dacryocystitis and panophthalmitis, or from generalized septicemia. Infection of the sinuses is the most frequent cause. Infection originating in the sinuses can spread easily to the orbit through the thin bony walls and foramina or by means of the interconnecting venous system of the orbit and sinuses. The most common causative organisms are staphylococci and streptococci in adults and *H. influenzae* in children.

The severe intraorbital tension caused by abscess formation and the impairment of optic nerve function in orbital cellulitis can result in permanent visual loss. Because of the orbit's proximity to the brain, orbital cellulitis can lead to life-threatening complications, such as intracranial abscess and cavernous sinus thrombosis.

Management

Immediate administration of high-dose, broad-spectrum, systemic antibiotics is indicated. Cultures and Gram-stained smears are obtained. Monitoring changes in visual acuity, degree of proptosis, central nervous system function (eg, nausea, vomiting, fever, level of consciousness), displacement of the globe, extraocular movements, pupillary signs, and the fundus is extremely important. Consultation with an otolaryngologist is necessary, especially when sinusitis is suspected. In the event of abscess formation or progressive loss of vision, surgical drainage of the abscess or sinus is performed. Sinusotomy and antibiotic irrigation are also performed.

Orbital and Ocular Tumours

BENIGN TUMOURS OF THE ORBIT

Benign tumours can develop from infancy and grow rapidly or slowly and present themselves in later life. Some benign tumours are superficial and are easily identifiable by external presentation, palpation, and x-rays, but some are deep and may require a CT scan for a more thorough and precise diagnosis. There can be a significant proptosis, and visual function may be jeopardized. Benign tumours are masses characterized by the lack of infiltration in the surrounding tissues. Examples are cystic dermoid cysts and mucocele, hemangiomas, lymphangiomas, lacrimal tumours, and neurofibromas.

Management

To prevent recurrence, benign masses are excised completely when possible. Sometimes, excision is difficult because of the involvement of some portions of the orbital bones, such as deep dermoid cysts, in which dissection of the bone is required. Subtotal resection may be indicated in deep benign tumours that intertwine with other orbital structures, such as optic nerve meningiomas. Complete removal of the tumour may endanger visual function.

BENIGN TUMOURS OF THE EYELID

Benign tumours include a wide variety of neoplasms and increase in frequency with age. Nevi may be unpigmented at birth and may enlarge and darken in adolescence or may never acquire any pigment at all. Hemangiomas are vascular capillary tumours that may be bright, superficial, strawberry-red lesions (ie, strawberry nevus) or bluish and purplish deeper lesions. Milia are small, white, slightly elevated cysts of the eyelid that, when in multiples, create a blemish. Xanthelasma are yellowish, lipoid deposits on both lids near the inner angle of the eye that commonly appear as a result of the aging of the skin or a lipid disorder. Molluscum contagiosum lesions are flat, symmetric growths along the lid margin caused by a virus that can result in conjunctivitis and keratitis after debris gets into the conjunctival sac.

Management

Treatment of benign congenital lid lesions is rarely indicated, except when visual function is affected. Corticosteroid injection to the hemangioma lesion is usually effective, but surgical excision may be performed. Benign lid lesions usually present aesthetic problems rather than visual function problems. Surgical excision, or electrocautery, is primarily performed for cosmetic reasons, except for cases of molluscum contagiosum, for which surgical intervention is performed to prevent an infectious process that may ensue.

BENIGN TUMOURS OF THE CONJUNCTIVA

Conjunctival nevus, a congenital, benign neoplasm, is a flat, slightly elevated, brown spot that becomes pigmented during late childhood or adolescence. This should be differentiated from the pigmented lesion melanosis acquired at middle age, which tends to wax and wane and become malignant melanoma. Keratin- and sebum-containing dermoid cysts are congenital and can be found in the conjunctiva. Dermolipoma is a congenital tumour that manifests as a smooth, rounded growth in the conjunctiva near the lateral canthus. Papillomas are usually soft with irregular surfaces and appear on the lid margins. Treatment consists of surgical excision.

MALIGNANT TUMOURS OF THE ORBIT

Rhabdomyosarcoma is the most common malignant primary orbital tumour in childhood, but it can also develop in elderly persons. The symptoms of rhabdomyosarcoma include sudden painless proptosis of one eye followed by lid swelling, conjunctival chemosis, and impairment of ocular motility. Imaging of these tumours establishes the size, configuration, location, and stage of the disease; delineates the degree of bone destruction; and is useful in estimating the field for radiation therapy, if needed. The most common site of metastasis is the lung.

Management

Management of these primary malignant orbital tumours involves three major therapeutic modalities: surgery, radiation therapy, and adjuvant chemotherapy. The degree of orbital destruction is important in planning the surgical approach. In the orbit, resection often involves removal of the globe. The psychological needs of the patient and family, especially the parents of a pediatric patient, are paramount in planning the management approach.

MALIGNANT TUMOURS OF THE EYELID

Basal cell carcinoma is the most common malignant tumour of the eyelid. Squamous cell carcinoma occurs less frequently but is considered the second most common malignant tumour. Malignant melanoma is rare. Malignant eyelid tumours occur more frequently among people with fair complexion who have a history of chronic exposure to the sun.

Basal cell carcinoma appears as a painless nodule that may ulcerate. The lesion is invasive, spreads to the surrounding tissues, and grows slowly but does not metastasize. It usually appears on the lower lid margin near the inner canthus with a pearly white margin. Squamous cell carcinoma of the eyelids may resemble basal cell carcinoma initially because it also grows slowly and painlessly. It tends to ulcerate and invade the surrounding tissues, but it can metastasize to the regional lymph nodes. Malignant melanoma may not be pigmented and can arise from nevi. It spreads to the surrounding tissues and metastasizes to other organs.

Management

Complete excision of these carcinomas is followed by reconstruction with skin grafting if the surgical excision is extensive. The ocular postoperative site and the graft donor site are monitored for bleeding. Donor graft sites may include the buccal mucosa, the thigh, or the abdomen. The patient is referred to an oncologist for evaluation for the need for radiation therapy treatment and monitoring for metastasis. Early diagnosis and surgical management are the basis of a good prognosis. These conditions have life-threatening consequences, and surgical excisions may result in facial disfigurement. Emotional support and reassurance are important aspects of nursing management.

MALIGNANT TUMOURS OF THE CONJUNCTIVA

Conjunctival carcinoma most often grows in the exposed areas of the conjunctiva. The typical lesions are usually gelatinous and whitish due to keratin formation. They grow gradually, and deep invasion and metastasis are rare. Malignant melanoma is rare but

GENETICS IN NURSING PRACTICE—Genes and the Eye

The mapping of the human genome enhances the opportunity to understand the genetic component of ophthalmic disorders and to develop new methods of prevention and treatment. Apparently more than one gene is involved in any particular condition, making genetic counselling an important part of the care and prevention of inherited diseases. Ocular effects of some genetic conditions follow.

MARFAN'S SYNDROME
Ophthalmic consequences may include amblyopia and dislocation of the lens. Patients are often myopic and may be at increased risk for retinal detachment.

LEBER'S CONGENITAL AMAUROSIS
To date, four genes are implicated in this disorder, which is characterized by decreased vision and onset in childhood, generally before 7 years of age. It accounts for 10% to 18% of congenital blindness (some infants may be blind from birth). Other signs and symptoms include strabismus, nystagmus, photophobia, cataracts, and keratoconus.

RETINOBLASTOMA
A malignant retinal tumour occurring in 1 of every 20,000 live births, it is hereditary in 30% to 40% of cases. All bilateral cases are hereditary. The retinoblastoma gene is found on chromosome 13, region q14. If this gene is inhibited, the growth in retinal cells is unchecked and the retinoblastoma results. Signs and symptoms include an initial leukocoria or "white" pupil with a peculiar light reflection and possibly strabismus as well. Less frequent signs are uveitis, glaucoma, hyphema, nystagmus, and periorbital cellulitis. Treatment for this life-threatening tumour is enucleation, if the tumour is large and unilateral. If the eye is removed before cancer spreads to the optic nerve, the cure rate is greater than 90%.

may arise from a preexisting nevus or acquired melanosis during middle age. Squamous cell carcinoma is also rare but invasive.

Management

The management is surgical incision. Some benign tumours and most malignant tumours recur. To avoid recurrences, patients usually undergo radiation therapy and cryotherapy after the excision of malignant tumours. Cosmetic disfigurement may result from extensive excision when deep invasion by the malignant tumour is involved.

MALIGNANT TUMOUR OF THE GLOBE: OCULAR MELANOMA

A malignant tumour of the retina, retinoblastoma, occurs in childhood, is hereditary, and requires complete enucleation if there is to be a chance for successful outcome. Another cancer that primarily occurs in adults is ocular melanoma. This rare, malignant choroidal tumour is often discovered on a retinal examination. In its early stages, it could be mistaken for a nevus. Many ophthalmologists may practice for decades and never encounter this lesion. For this reason, any patient who is suspected of having ocular melanoma should be immediately referred to an ocular oncologist with experience in this disease.

Although many patients do not have symptoms in the early stages, some patients complain of blurred vision or a change in eye colour. A number of such tumours have been found in people with blindness who have painful eyes. In addition to a complete physical examination to discover any evidence of metastasis (to the liver, lung, and breast), retinal fundus photography, fluorescein angiography, and ultrasonography are performed. The diagnosis is confirmed at biopsy after enucleation.

Management

Tumours are classified according to size (ie, small, medium, and large). Very small tumours are generally monitored, whereas medium and large tumours require treatment. Treatment consists of radiation, enucleation, or both. Radiation therapy is achieved by external beam performed in repeated doses over several days or through the surgical implantation of a radioactive plaque, which is removed after several days.

Surgical Procedures and Enucleation

ORBITAL SURGERIES

Orbital surgeries may be performed to repair fractures, remove a foreign body, or remove benign or malignant growths. Surgical procedures involving the orbit and lids affect facial appearance (ie, cosmesis). The goals are to recover and preserve visual function and to maintain the anatomic relationship of the ocular structures to achieve cosmesis. During the repair of orbital fractures, the orbital bones are realigned to follow the anatomic positions of facial structures.

Orbital surgical procedures involve working around delicate structures of the eye, such as the optic nerve, retinal blood vessels, and ocular muscles. Complications of orbital surgical procedures may include blindness as a result of damage to the optic nerve and its blood supply. Sudden pain and loss of vision may indicate intraorbital hemorrhage or compression of the optic nerve. Ptosis

and diplopia may result from trauma to the extraocular muscles during the surgical procedure, but these conditions typically resolve after a few weeks.

Postoperative Management

Prophylaxis with intravenous antibiotics is the usual postoperative regimen after orbital surgery, especially with repair of orbital fractures and intraorbital foreign body removal. Intravenous corticosteroids are used if there is a concern about optic nerve swelling. Topical ocular antibiotics are typically instilled, and antibiotic ointments are applied externally to the skin suture sites.

For the first 24 to 48 hours postoperatively, ice compresses are applied over the periocular area to decrease periorbital swelling, facial swelling, and hematoma. The head of the patient's bed should be elevated to a comfortable position (30 to 45 degrees).

Discharge teaching should include medication instructions for oral antibiotics, instillation of ophthalmic medications, and application of ocular compresses.

ENUCLEATION

Enucleation is the removal of the entire eye and part of the optic nerve. It may be performed for the following conditions:

- Severe injury resulting in prolapse of uveal tissue or loss of light projection or perception
- An irritated, blind, painful, deformed, or disfigured eye, usually caused by glaucoma, retinal detachment, or chronic inflammation
- An eye without useful vision that is producing or has produced sympathetic ophthalmia in the other eye
- Intraocular tumours that are untreatable by other means

The procedure for enucleation involves the separation and cutting of each of the ocular muscles, dissection of the Tenon's capsule (ie, fibrous membrane covering the sclera), and the cutting of the optic nerve from the eyeball. The insertion of an orbital implant typically follows, and the conjunctiva is closed. A large pressure dressing is applied over the area.

Evisceration involves the surgical removal of the intraocular contents through an incision or opening in the cornea or sclera. The optic nerve, sclera, extraocular muscles, and sometimes, the cornea are left intact. The main advantage of evisceration over enucleation is that the final cosmetic result and motility after fitting the ocular prosthesis are enhanced. This procedure would be more acceptable to a patient whose concept of the alteration of body image is severely threatened. The main disadvantage is the high risk of sympathetic ophthalmia.

Exenteration is the removal of the eyelids, the eye, and various amounts of orbital contents. It is indicated in malignancies in the orbit that are life threatening or when more conservative modalities of treatment have failed or are inappropriate. An example is squamous cell carcinoma of the paranasal sinuses, skin, and conjunctiva with deep orbital involvement. In its most extensive form, exenteration may include the removal of all orbital tissues and resection of the orbital bones.

Ocular Prostheses

Orbital implants and conformers (ie, ocular prostheses usually made of silicone rubber) maintain the shape of the eye after enucleation or evisceration to prevent a contracted sunken appearance. The temporary conformer is placed over the conjunctival closure after the implantation of an orbital implant. A conformer is placed after the enucleation or evisceration procedure to protect the suture line, maintain the fornices, prevent contracture of the socket in preparation for the ocular prosthesis, and promote the integrity of the eyelids.

All ocular prosthetics have limitations in their motility. There are two designs of eye prostheses. The anophthalmic ocular prostheses are used in the absence of the globe. Scleral shells look just like the anophthalmic prosthesis (Fig. 58-20) but are thinner and fit over a globe with intact corneal sensation. An eye prosthesis usually lasts about 6 years, depending on the quality of fit, comfort, and cosmetic appearance. When the anophthalmic socket is completely healed, conformers are replaced with prosthetic eyes.

An ocularist is a specially trained and skilled professional who makes prosthetic eyes. After the ophthalmologist is satisfied that the anophthalmic socket is completely healed and is ready for prosthetic fitting, the patient is referred to an ocularist. The healing period is usually 6 to 8 weeks. It is advisable for the patient to have a consultation with the ocularist before the fitting. Obtaining accurate information and verbalizing concerns can lessen anxiety about wearing an ocular prosthesis.

Medical Management

Removal of an eye has physical, social, and psychological ramifications for any person. The significance of loss of the eye and vision must be addressed in the plan of care. The patient's preparation should include information about the surgical procedure and placement of orbital implants and conformers and the availability of ocular prosthetics to enhance cosmetic appearance. In some cases, patients may choose to see an ocularist before the surgery to discuss ocular prosthetics.

Nursing Management

TEACHING ABOUT POSTSURGICAL AND PROSTHETIC CARE

Patients who undergo eye removal need to know that they will usually have a large ocular pressure dressing, which is typically removed after a week, and that an ophthalmic topical antibiotic ointment is applied in the socket three times daily.

After the removal of an eye, there is a loss of depth perception. Patients must be advised to take extra caution in their ambulation and movement to avoid miscalculations that may result in injury. It may take some time to adjust to monocular vision.

The patient must be advised that conformers may accidentally fall out of the socket. If this happens, the conformer must be

FIGURE 58-20 Eye prostheses. (*Left*) Anophthalmic ocular prosthesis. (*Right*) Scleral shell.

washed, wiped dry, and placed back in the socket. When surgical eye removal is unexpected, such as in severe ocular trauma, leaving no time for the patient and family to prepare for the loss, the nurse's role in providing reassurance and emotional support is crucial.

PROMOTING HOME AND COMMUNITY-BASED CARE

Teaching Patients Self-Care. Patients need to be taught how to insert, remove, and care for the prosthetic eye. Proper hand washing must be observed before inserting and removing an ocular prosthesis. A suction cup may be used if there are problems with manual dexterity. Precautions, such as draping a towel over the sink and closing the sink drain, must be taken to avoid loss of the prosthesis. When instructing patients or family members, a return demonstration is important to assess the level of understanding and ability to perform the procedure.

Before insertion, the inner punctal or outer lateral aspects and the superior and inferior aspects of the prosthesis must be identified by locating the identifying marks, such as a reddish colour in the inner punctal area. For people with low vision, other forms of identifying markers, such as dots or notches, are used. The upper lid is raised high enough to create a space; then the patient learns to slide the prosthesis up, underneath, and behind the upper eyelid. Meanwhile, the patient pulls the lower eyelid down to help put the prosthesis in place and to have its inferior edge fall back gradually to the lower eyelid. The lower eyelid is checked for correct positioning.

To remove the prosthesis, the patient cups one hand on the cheek to catch the prosthesis, places the forefinger of the free hand against the midportion of the lower eyelid, and gazes upward. Gazing upward brings the inferior edge of the prosthesis nearer the inferior eyelid margin. With the finger pushing inward, downward, and laterally against the lower eyelid, the prosthesis slides out, and the cupped hand acts as the receptacle.

Continuing Care. An eye prosthesis can be worn and left in place for several months. Hygiene and comfort are usually maintained with daily irrigation of the prosthesis in place with the use of a balanced salt solution, hard contact lens solution, or artificial tears. In the case of dry eye symptoms, the use of ophthalmic ointment lubricants or oil-based drops, such as vitamin E and mineral oil, can be helpful. Removing crusting and mucous discharge that accumulates overnight is performed with the prosthesis in place. Malpositions may occur when wiping or rubbing the prosthesis in the socket. The prosthesis can be turned back in place with the use of clean fingers. Proper wiping of the prosthesis should be a gentle temporal-to-nasal motion to avoid malpositions.

The prosthesis needs to be removed and cleaned when it becomes uncomfortable and when there is increased mucous discharge. The socket should also be rendered free of mucus and inspected for any signs of infection. Any unusual discomfort, irritation, or redness of the globe or eyelids may indicate excessive wear, debris under the shell, or lack of proper hygiene. Any infection or irritation that does not subside needs medical attention.

Ocular Consequences of Systemic Disease

DIABETIC RETINOPATHY

Of all of the medical disorders that the nurse encounters, diabetes mellitus is one of the most common and one that can have devastating effects on the patient. Diabetes affects every system of the body in a deleterious way and consequently affects the patient's family and society in general. Diabetes causes blindness in approximately 400 Canadians every year and is the leading cause of new cases of blindness in Canada today (Canadian National Institute for the Blind, 2005a). Before the discovery of insulin in the 1920s, diabetic retinopathy was relatively rare. Most people with diabetes did not survive for more than 1 or 2 years; however, with the use of insulin, more and more patients are able to survive and enjoy relatively normal life spans. They are also confronted with the complications of long-term diabetes. One of the most serious complications is retinopathy. Chapter 41 provides a detailed discussion of diabetic retinopathy (Aiello et al., 2001).

CYTOMEGALOVIRUS RETINITIS

Many ophthalmic complications are associated with AIDS. On autopsy, up to 90% of patients have ocular lesions directly related to AIDS. Cytomegalovirus (CMV) is the most common cause of retinal inflammation in patients with AIDS. About 40% of patients who have CMV retinitis lose their central vision in both eyes by the time of death.

Early symptoms of CMV retinitis vary from patient to patient. Some patients complain of floaters or a decrease in peripheral vision. Some patients have a paracentral or central scotoma, whereas others have a fluctuation in vision from macular edema. The retina often becomes thin and atrophic and susceptible to retinal tears and breaks.

CMV retinitis generally takes one of three forms: hemorrhagic, brushfire, or granular. In the hemorrhagic type, large areas of white, necrotic retina may be associated retinal hemorrhage. The brushfire form appears to have a yellow-white margin, which begins at the edge of burned-out atrophic retina. This retinitis expands and, if untreated, involves the entire retina. The granular form of CMV retinitis consists of white, granular lesions in the periphery of the retina that gradually expand. The white, feathery infiltration of the retina destroys sensory retina and leads to necrosis, optic atrophy, and retinal detachment.

Medical Management

PHARMACOLOGIC THERAPY

Pharmacologic agents available for treatment of CMV retinitis include ganciclovir (Cytovene), foscarnet (Foscavir), and cidofovir (Vistide).

Ganciclovir is administered intravenously, orally, or intravitreously in the acute stage of CMV retinitis. A surgically implanted intraocular device has provided a new mode of effective ganciclovir administration. This enables a higher, more effective dose of medication to be administered and is well tolerated by patients. This constant intraocular concentration of ganciclovir lasts for about 6 to 10 months before the inserts must be replaced. Once begun, ganciclovir must be given continuously. A study that combined the use of the intravitreous implant with oral ganciclovir demonstrated a reduction in the risk of new CMV disease as well as a delay in the progression of the retinitis (Martin et al., 1999). This very potent medication, when administered systemically, can cause neutropenia, thrombocytopenia, anemia, and elevated serum creatinine levels. Although the surgically implanted sustained release device enables higher concentrations of ganciclovir to reach the CMV retinitis, there are risks and complications associated with the devices, including endophthalmitis, retinal detachment, and hypotony.

Foscarnet inhibits viral DNA replication. It may be the medication of choice when ganciclovir is ineffective. It may be administered intravenously or locally by intravitreal injections. The combination of foscarnet and ganciclovir has been more effective than either medication alone. Nephrotoxicity may occur with systemic foscarnet, and renal function must be monitored carefully.

Cidofovir impedes CMV replication. This medication is administered intravenously. Cidofovir has been shown to delay the progression of CMV retinitis significantly. Nephrotoxicity, proteinuria, and increased serum creatinine levels are significant side effects of its administration.

HYPERTENSION-RELATED EYE CHANGES

Hypertension, known as the silent killer, can shorten the life span by as many as 20 years. An estimated 5 million Canadians have hypertension, with nearly 43% unaware they have high blood pressure (Canadian Hypertension Society, 2005). End-organ damage affects the heart, brain, kidney, and eye. Hypertension may be manifested in one of two forms: chronic or acute. This differentiation is determined by the rapidity in rise of the blood pressure as well as the degree of elevation. The retinal changes observed with each form are different and have different consequences for the eye.

Chronic hypertension and atherosclerosis go hand in hand, and the associated retinal changes are evidenced by the development of retinal arteriolar changes, such as tortuousness, narrowing, and a change in light reflex. Funduscopic examination reveals a copper or silver colouration of the arterioles and venous compression (arteriovenous nicking) at the arteriolar and venous crossings. Intraretinal hemorrhages from hypertension appear flame shaped because they occur in the nerve fibre layer of the retina.

Acute hypertension can result from pheochromocytoma, acute renal failure, pregnancy-induced hypertension, and malignant essential hypertension. The retinopathy associated with these crisis states is extensive, and the manifestations include cotton-wool spots, retinal hemorrhages, retinal edema, and retinal exudates, often clustered around the macula.

The choroid is also affected by the profound and abrupt rise in blood pressure and resulting vasoconstriction, and ischemia may result in serous retinal detachments and infarction of the retinal pigment epithelium (RPE). Ischemic optic neuropathy and **papilledema** (ie, swelling of the optic disc due to increased IOP) may also result.

Concepts in Ocular Medication Administration

The main objective of ocular medication delivery is to maximize the amount of medication that reaches the ocular site of action in sufficient concentration to produce a beneficial therapeutic effect. This is determined by the dynamics of ocular pharmacokinetics: absorption, distribution, metabolism, and excretion.

Topical administration of ocular medications results in only a 1% to 7% absorption rate by the ocular tissues. Ocular absorption involves the entry of a medication into the aqueous humour through the different routes of ocular drug administration. The rate and extent of aqueous humour absorption are determined by the characteristics of the medication and the barriers imposed by the anatomy and physiology of the eye. The natural barriers of absorption that diminish the efficacy of ocular medications include the following:

- *Limited size of the conjunctival sac.* The conjunctival sac can hold only 50 μL, and any excess is wasted. The volume of

one eye drop from commercial topical ocular solutions typically ranges from 20 to 35 µL.
- *Corneal membrane barriers.* The epithelial, stromal, and endothelial layers are barriers to absorption.
- *Blood–ocular barriers.* Blood–ocular barriers prevent high ocular tissue concentration of most ophthalmic medications because they separate the bloodstream from the ocular tissues and keep foreign substances from entering the eye, thereby limiting a medication's efficacy.
- *Tearing, blinking, and drainage.* Increased tear production and drainage due to ocular irritation or an ocular condition may dilute or wash out an instilled eye drop; blinking expels an instilled eye drop from the conjunctival sac.

Distribution of an ocular medication into the ocular tissues involves partitioning and compartmentalizing of the medication between the tissues of the conjunctiva, cornea, lens, iris, ciliary body, choroid, and vitreous. Medications penetrate the corneal epithelium by diffusion by passing through the cells (intracellular) or by passing between the cells (intercellular). Water-soluble (hydrophilic) medications diffuse through the intracellular route, and fat-soluble (lipophilic) medications diffuse through the intercellular route. Topical administration usually does not reach the retina in significant concentrations. Because the space between the ciliary process and the lens is small, medication diffusion in the vitreous is slow. When high therapeutic medication concentration in the vitreous is required, intraocular injection is often chosen to bypass the natural ocular anatomic and physiologic barriers.

Aqueous solutions are most commonly used for the eye. They are the least expensive medications and interfere least with vision. However, corneal contact time is brief because tears dilute the medication. Ophthalmic ointments have extended retention time in the conjunctival sac and a higher concentration than eye drops. The major disadvantage of ointments is the blurred vision that results after application. In general, eyelids and eyelid margins are best treated with ointments. The conjunctiva, limbus, cornea, and anterior chamber are treated most effectively with instilled solutions or suspensions. Subconjunctival injection may be necessary for better absorption in the anterior chamber. If high medication concentrations are required in the posterior chamber, intravitreal injections or systemically absorbed medications are considered. Contact lenses and collagen shields soaked in antibiotics are alternative delivery methods for treating corneal infections. Of all these delivery methods, the topical route of administration—instilled eye drops and applied ointments—remain the most common. Topical instillation, which is the least invasive method, permits self-administration of medication. It also produces fewer side effects.

Preservatives are commonly used in ocular medications. Benzalkonium chloride, for example, prevents the growth of organisms and enhances the corneal permeability of most medications. Some patients are allergic to this preservative. This may be suspected even if the patient had never before experienced an allergic reaction to systemic use of the medication in question. Eye drops without preservatives can be prepared by pharmacists.

COMMONLY USED OCULAR MEDICATIONS

Common ocular medications include topical anesthetic, mydriatic, and cycloplegic agents that reduce IOP; anti-infective medications, corticosteroids, NSAIDS, antiallergy medications, eye irrigants, and lubricants.

Topical Anesthetics

One to two drops of proparacaine hydrochloride (Ophthaine 0.5%) and tetracaine hydrochloride (Pontocaine 0.5%) are instilled before diagnostic procedures such as tonometry and gonioscopy and in minor ocular procedures such as removal of sutures or conjunctival or corneal scrapings. The nurse must instruct patients not to rub their eyes while anesthetized because this may result in corneal damage. Patients must never be allowed to take topical anesthetics home. Prolonged use can delay wound healing and can lead to permanent corneal opacification and scarring, resulting in visual loss. Topical anesthetic is also used for severe eye pain to allow the patient to open his or her eyes for examination or treatment (eg, eye irrigation for chemical burns). Anesthesia occurs within 20 seconds to 1 minute and lasts 10 to 20 minutes.

Mydriatics and Cycloplegics

Mydriasis, or pupil dilation, is the main objective of the administration of mydriatic and cycloplegic agents (Table 58-8). These two medications function differently and are used in combination to achieve the maximal dilation that is needed during surgery and fundus examinations to give the ophthalmologist a better view of the internal eye structures. Mydriatics potentiate alpha-adrenergic sympathetic effects that result in the relaxation of the ciliary muscle. This causes the pupil to dilate. This sympathetic action alone, however, is not enough to sustain mydriasis because of its short duration of action. The strong light used during an eye examination also stimulates miosis (ie, pupillary contraction). Cycloplegic medications are administered to paralyze the iris sphincter.

Patients are instructed about the temporary effects of mydriasis on vision, such as glare and the inability to focus properly. Patients may not be able to read and should not drive. The effects of the various mydriatics and cycloplegics can last 3 hours to several days. Patients are advised to wear sunglasses (most eye clinics provide protective sunglasses) and to have a responsible adult drive them home.

Mydriatic and cycloplegic agents affect the central nervous system. Their effects are most prominent in children and elderly patients; these patients must be assessed closely for symptoms, such as rise in blood pressure, tachycardia, dizziness, ataxia, confusion, disorientation, incoherent speech, and hallucination. These medications are contraindicated in patients with narrow angles or shallow anterior chambers and in patients taking monoamine oxidase inhibitors or tricyclic antidepressants.

Medications Used to Treat Glaucoma

Therapeutic medications for glaucoma are used to lower IOP by decreasing aqueous production or increasing aqueous outflow. Because glaucoma calls for lifetime therapy, patients must be instructed regarding both the ocular and systemic side effects of the medications.

Most antiglaucoma medications affect the accommodation of the lens and limit light entry through a constricted pupil. Visual acuity and the ability to focus may be affected. Factors to consider in selecting glaucoma medications are efficacy, systemic and ocular side effects, convenience, and cost.

Anti-Infective Medications

Anti-infective medications include antibiotic, antifungal, and antiviral agents. Most are available as drops, ointments, or subconjunctival or intravitreal injections. Antibiotics include peni-

Table 58-8 • Mydriatics and Cycloplegics

DRUG	AVAILABLE PREPARATION/ CONCENTRATION	INDICATION/DOSAGE	PEAK		RECOVERY TIME	
			Mydriasis	Cycloplegia	Mydriasis	Cycloplegia
Phenylephrine	Solution (2.5%, 10%)	Administered with cycloplegics in pupillary dilation for ophthalmoscopy and surgical procedures every 5–10 min ×3 or until the pupils are fully dilated	10–60 min	—	3–6 h	—
Atropine	Ointment (0.5%–2%) Solution (0.5%–3%)	In glaucoma, uveitis, or after surgery, 2× to 4× daily	30–40 min	60–180 min	7–10 d	6–12 d
Scopolamine	Solution (0.25%)	The same as atropine	20–30 min	30–60 min	3–7 d	3–7 d
Homatropine	Solution (5%–2.5%)	The same as atropine and scopolamine	40–60 min	30–60 min	1–3 d	1–3 d
Cyclopentolate	Solution (0.5%–2%)	Administered with mydriatics q 5–10 min ×3 or until the pupils are fully dilated for ophthalmoscopy and surgical procedures	30–60 min	25–75 min	1 d	6–24 h
Tropicamide	Solution (0.25%–1%)		20–40 min	20–35 min	6 h	<6 h

Data on peak and recovery time from *Ophthalmic Drug Facts by Facts and Comparisons* (1998), pp. 45 and 49.
Copyright 1998 by Facts and Comparisons, a Wolters Kluwer Company. Adapted with permission.

cillin, cephalosporins, aminoglycosides, and fluoroquinolones. The main antifungal agent is amphotericin B. Side effects of amphotericin are serious and include severe pain, conjunctival necrosis, iritis, and retinal toxicity. Antiviral medications include acyclovir and ganciclovir. They are used to treat ocular infections associated with herpesvirus and CMV. Patients receiving ocular anti-infective agents are subject to the same side effects and adverse reactions as those receiving oral or parenteral medications.

Corticosteroids and Nonsteroidal Anti-Inflammatory Drugs

The topical preparations of corticosteroids are commonly used in inflammatory conditions of the eyelids, conjunctiva, cornea, anterior chamber, lens, and uvea. In posterior segment diseases that involve the posterior sclera, retina, and optic nerve, the topical agents are less effective, and parenteral and oral routes are preferred. The topical eye drop preparation is prepared in suspension; the patient is instructed to shake the bottle several times to obtain the maximum therapeutic effect of the medication.

The most common ocular side effects of long-term topical corticosteroid administration are glaucoma, cataracts, susceptibility to infection, impaired wound healing, mydriasis, and ptosis. High IOP may develop, which is reversible after corticosteroid use is discontinued. To avoid the side effects of corticosteroids, NSAIDS are used as an alternative in controlling inflammatory eye conditions and postoperatively to reduce inflammation. NSAID therapy in combination with topical and oral preparations is an important adjunct therapy in managing uveitis.

Antiallergy Medications

Ocular hypersensitivity reactions, such as allergic conjunctivitis, are extremely common. These conditions result primarily from responses to environmental allergens. Most allergens are airborne or carried to the eye by the hand or by other means, although allergic reactions may also be drug induced. Corticosteroids are also commonly used as anti-inflammatory and immunosuppressive agents to control ocular hypersensitivity reaction.

Ocular Irrigants

Most irrigating solutions are used to cleanse the external lids to maintain lid hygiene, to irrigate the external corneal surface to regain normal pH (such as in chemical burns), to irrigate the corneal surface to eliminate debris, or to inflate the globe intraoperatively. These solutions have various compositions that include sodium, potassium, magnesium, calcium, bicarbonate, glucose, and glutathione (ie, substance found in the aqueous humour). Sterile irrigating solutions, such as Dacriose, for lid hygiene are available. Irrigating solutions are safe to use with an intact corneal surface; however, the corneal surface should not be irrigated in cases of threatened corneal perforation. For patients with severe corneal ulcer, specific orders must be obtained regarding whether it is safe to irrigate the corneal surface or just to cleanse the external lids. Although it is good practice to promote hygiene, prevention of complications must be the primary concern. Normal saline solutions are commonly used to irrigate the corneal surface when chemical burns occur.

Ocular Lubricants

Lubricants, such as artificial tears, help to alleviate corneal irritation, such as dry eye syndrome. Artificial tears are topical preparations of methyl or hydroxypropyl cellulose that are prepared as eye drop solutions, ointments, or ocular inserts (inserted at the lower conjunctival cul-de-sac once each day). The eye drops can be instilled as often as every hour, depending on the severity of symptoms.

NURSING MANAGEMENT

The objectives in administering ocular medications are to ensure proper administration to maximize the therapeutic effects and to ensure the safety of the patient by monitoring manifestations of possible systemic and local side effects. Absorption of eye drops by the nasolacrimal duct is undesirable because of the potential systemic side effects of ocular medications. To diminish systemic absorption and minimize the side effects, it is important to occlude the puncta (Chart 58-10). This is especially important for patients most vulnerable to medication overdose, including elderly people, children, infants, women who are lactating or are pregnant, and patients with cardiac, pulmonary, hepatic, or renal disease.

A 30-second interval between eye drop instillations has a 45% rate of washout loss. A 1-minute interval between instillation of differing types of ocular drops is recommended (Margolis et al., 2002).

Before the administration of ocular medications, the nurse should warn the patient that blurred vision, stinging, and a burning sensation are symptoms that ordinarily occur after instillation and are temporary. Risk for interactions of the ocular medication with other ocular and systemic medications must be emphasized; therefore, a careful patient interview regarding medications being taken must be obtained.

Chart 58-10 | **Guidelines for Instilling Eye Medications**

Follow these general guidelines when instilling eye medications:

- Shake suspensions or "milky" solutions to obtain the desired medication level.
- Wash hands thoroughly before and after the procedure.
- Ensure adequate lighting.
- Read the label of the eye medication to make sure it is the correct medication.
- Assume a comfortable position.
- Do not touch the tip of the medication container to any part of the eye or face.
- Hold the lower lid down; do not press on the eyeball. Apply gentle pressure to the cheek bone to anchor the finger holding the lid.

- Instill eye drops before applying ointments.
- Apply a 1 cm ribbon of ointment to the lower conjunctival sac.

- Keep the eyelids closed, and apply gentle pressure on the inner canthus (punctal occlusion) near the bridge of the nose for 1 or 2 minutes immediately after instilling eyedrops.
- Using a clean tissue, gently pat skin to absorb excess eyedrops that run onto the cheeks.
- Wait 5 to 10 minutes before instilling another eye medication.

Emphasis must be placed on hand-washing techniques before and after medication instillation. The tip of the eye drop bottle or the ointment tube must never touch any part of the eye. The medication must be recapped immediately after each use. If patients who instill their own medications cannot feel the eye drops when they are instilled, the eye medication may be refrigerated, because a cold drop is easier to detect. A 5-minute interval between successive eye drop administration allows adequate drug retention and absorption. The patient or the caregiver at home should be asked to demonstrate actual eye drop or ointment instillation and punctal occlusion.

Issues in Ophthalmology

Issues that arise in any area of health care usually pose more questions than answers. In ophthalmology, the well-being of the patient physically, emotionally, financially, socially, and spiritually can be at risk when vision is threatened. Patients with a deteriorating eye condition often worry about the impact that visual loss will have on their lives. As they experience visual distortions, scotomas, or gradual visual loss, what was a vague worry can become a consuming preoccupation. The patient may equate a decrease in visual acuity with a loss of independence. The loss of a driver's license may force a patient to relocate his or her home or give up or change careers.

These vulnerable patients may be easy targets for unscrupulous practitioners, who may offer unproven treatments, often at great expense to the patient who is desperate for any treatment that may prove beneficial. Patients travel from one physician to another in search of any treatment that may forestall visual loss. For example, a patient with 20/200 vision may wrongly believe that there is nothing to lose and will submit to invasive surgeries, only to end with a visual acuity of 20/800.

Not all patients who are contemplating ophthalmic surgical procedures are in great distress from a sight-threatening condition. Increasingly, patients are encouraged by friends and family or even by advertisement to have elective procedures such as refractive surgery. Patients are enticed by the thought of being free of eyeglasses or contact lens. Refractive surgery sites are springing up in shopping malls and offering discounts and sales on procedures.

Some cataract surgeons remove cataracts before there is a visual deficit or with the full knowledge that such surgery may offer no increase in vision. Patients should be counselled before such procedures about the potential risk versus the potential benefit. Patients who have an ongoing retinal problem, such as AMD, should be evaluated by both a retinal expert and a cataract surgeon.

Nursing Considerations

Fundamental goals in ophthalmic nursing should include the preservation of vision and the prevention of further visual loss in those patients who have already experienced some degree of loss. The maximal practical use should be sought for any remaining vision.

Skillful listening and interviewing on the part of the nurse or provider are critical tools for the rehabilitation of the distressed patient. The health care provider together with the patient should determine which goals are possible. A referral to a low-vision centre for evaluation may be an appropriate intervention, but for some patients, it may be a signal that all hope of vision restoration is lost.

To be effective, the nurse listens to the patient, tries to determine his or her level of health care need, and makes suggestions

and recommendations that can be of real value to the patient. Lines of communication must be kept open so that the patient is comfortable exploring all treatment modalities without fear of being ridiculed or patronized.

Critical Thinking Exercises

1. You are making a home visit to a 73-year-old patient in an assisted living facility. She has had diabetes mellitus for many years. Her renal function has been deteriorating, and her blood pressure has become increasingly harder to control. She complains that, although her reading vision is better, her distance vision seems to be blurry most of the time. She asks whether she should get her glasses changed (it has been several years since her last eye examination) or wait until her blood pressure medication regimen is settled. How often should a patient with diabetes have a dilated eye examination? What could be the underlying reason for her decrease in distance acuity? How can her fluctuating renal and hypertensive status affect the condition of the retina?

2. A 19-year-old, female student arrives at the college infirmary with scratchy eyes, blurred vision, and photophobia. She has just returned to the campus after spring break. She states that her nose has been running, her eyelids have been stuck together in the mornings, and she has used some eye drops with a red cap that she found in her medicine cabinet at home. She denies any use of other medications. Examination reveals crusting on the lids and lashes, hyperemic conjunctiva, purulent discharge, and fixed, dilated pupils. What should be included in the differential diagnosis? What could account for the photophobia? For the unresponsive pupils? What eyelid hygiene measure will promote ocular comfort? What precautions should be taken to prevent the spread of ocular infection to other students in the dormitory?

REFERENCES AND SELECTED READINGS

Books

Azar, D. T. (2001). *Intraocular lenses in cataract and refractive surgery.* Philadelphia: W. B. Saunders.

Bartlett, J. D., Bennett, E. S., & Fiscella, R. G. (Eds.). (2002). *Ophthalmic drug facts, 2003.* St. Louis: Facts & Comparisons.

Bartlett, J. D., & Siret, D. J. (2001). *Clinical ocular pharmacology* (4th ed.). Boston: Butterworth-Heinemann.

Bickley, L. S., & Szilagyi, P. G. (2003). *Bates guide to physical examination and history taking* (8th ed.). Philadelphia: Lippincott Williams & Wilkins.

Brown, N. A., & Brown, A. J. (1996). *Lens disorders: A clinical manual of cataract diagnosis.* Oxford, UK: Butterworth-Heinemann.

Blasch, B., Wiener, W., & Welsh, R. (Eds.). (1997). *Foundations of orientation and mobility* (2nd ed.). New York: AFB Press.

Corn, A. L., & Koenig, A. J. (Eds.). (2000). *Foundations of low vision.* New York: AFB Press.

Fechner, P. U., & Teichman, K. D. (1998). *Ocular therapeutics: Pharmacology and clinical application.* Thorofare, NJ: Slack.

Fletcher, D. C. (1999). *Low vision rehabilitation: Caring for the whole person.* San Francisco: American Academy of Ophthalmology.

Glaucoma Research Foundation. (1996). *Understanding and living with glaucoma: A reference guide for people with glaucoma and their families.* San Francisco: Glaucoma Research Foundation.

Goldblum, K. (1997). *Core curriculum for ophthalmic nursing.* Dubuque, IA: Kendall/Hunt.

Gottsch, J. D., & Stark, W. J. (1999). Extracapsular cataract extraction. In J. D. Gottsch, W. J. Stark, & M. F. Goldberg (Eds.), *Rob and Smith's operative surgery, ophthalmic surgery* (pp. 175–181). London: Arnold.

Gottsch, J. D., & Stark, W. J. (1999). Phacoemulsification. In J. D. Gottsch, W. J. Stark, & M. F. Goldberg (Eds.), *Rob and Smith's operative surgery, ophthalmic surgery* (pp. 182–196). London: Arnold.

Hersh, P. S., & Wagoner, M. D. (1998). *Excimer laser surgery for corneal disorders.* New York: Thieme.

The Johns Hopkins Hospital. (2001). *Interdisciplinary clinical practice manual: Preventable measures for nosocomial conjunctivitis in the Wilmer Institute* (p. 34). Baltimore: The Johns Hopkins Hospital.

Kanski, J. J. (1999). *Clinical ophthalmology: A systematic approach* (4th ed.). Boston: Butterworth-Heinemann.

Kanski, J., McAllister, J., & Salmon, J. (1996). *Glaucoma: A colour manual of diagnosis and treatment* (2nd ed.). Oxford, UK: Butterworth-Heinemann.

Krachmer, J. H., Mannis, M. J., & Holland, E. J. (1997). *Cornea* (Vol. 3). *Surgery of the cornea and conjunctiva.* St. Louis: C. V. Mosby.

Leibowitz, H. M., & Waring, G. O., III. (1998). *Corneal disorders: Clinical diagnosis and management* (2nd ed.). Philadelphia: W. B. Saunders.

MacCumber, M. W. (Ed.). (1997). *Management of ocular injuries and emergencies.* Philadelphia: Lippincott-Raven.

Margolis, S., Schachat, A. P., & Quigley, H. A. (2002). *Vision: The Johns Hopkins white papers.* New York: Medletter Associates.

Mauger, T. F., & Craig, E. L. (1996). *Mosby's ocular drug handbook.* St. Louis: Mosby.

Moore, J. E., Graves, W. H., & Patterson, J. B. (Eds.). (1997). *Foundations of rehabilitation counseling with persons who are blind or visually impaired.* New York: AFB Press.

Palay, D. A., & Krachmer, J. H. (1997). *Ophthalmology for the primary care physician.* New York: Mosby.

Preshel, N., & Prevent Blindness America. (2002). *Vision problems in the US.* Schaumburg, IL: Prevent Blindness America/National Eye Institute.

Resources for Rehabilitation. (1998). *Living with low vision: A resource guide for people with sight loss* (5th ed.). Lexington, MA: Resources for Rehabilitation.

Rhee, D. J., Pyfer, M. F., & Rhee, D. M. (1999). *The Wills eye manual: Office of emergency room diagnosis and treatment of eye disease* (3rd ed.). Philadelphia: Lippincott Williams & Wilkins.

Ritch, R., Shields, M., & Krupin, T. (1996). *The glaucomas* (Vols. 1–3, 2nd ed.). St. Louis: C. V. Mosby.

Shields, M. B. (1998). *Textbook of glaucoma* (4th ed.). Baltimore: Williams & Wilkins.

Skillen, D. L. & Day, R. A. (Eds.) (2004). *A syllabus for adult health assessment.* Edmonton, AB: Faculty of Nursing, University of Alberta.

Snell, R. S., & Lemp, M. A. (1998). *Clinical anatomy of the eye* (2nd ed.). Malden, MA: Blackwell Science.

Tierney, L. M., McPhee, S. J., & Papadakis, M. A. (2001). *Current medical diagnosis and treatment.* New York: Lange Medical Books/McGraw-Hill.

Tipperman, R. (2000). Cataract surgery 1999. In R. P. Wilson (Ed.), *Yearbook of Ophthalmology 2000* (pp. 1–7). Philadelphia: Mosby.

Traboulsi, E. (Ed.). (1998). *Genetic diseases of the eye.* New York: Oxford University Press.

Varma, R. (Ed.). (1997). *Essentials of eye care: The Johns Hopkins Wilmer handbook.* Philadelphia: Lippincott-Raven.

Vaughn, D. G., Asbury, T., & Riorda-Eva, P. (Eds.). (1999). *General ophthalmology* (15th ed.). Stamford, CT: Appleton & Lange.

Viola, R. S. (2000). Conjunctivitis. In R. Rakel & E. T. Bope (Eds.), *Conn's current therapy* (52nd ed., pp. 67–69). Philadelphia: W. B. Saunders.

Whitcher, J. (1999). Blindness. In D. G. Vaughn, T. Asbury, & P. Riorda-Eva (Eds.), *General ophthalmology* (15th ed., pp. 384–389). Stamford, CT: Appleton & Lange.

Wright, K. (1997). *Textbook of ophthalmology.* Baltimore: Williams & Wilkins.

Zimmerman, G. (1996). Optics and low vision devices. In A. Corn & A. Koenig (Eds.), *Foundations of low vision* (pp. 115–142). New York: AFB Press.

Journals

Adamsons, I. A., Vitale, S., Stark, W. J., & Rubin, G. S. (1996). The association of postoperative subjective visual function with acuity, glare, and contrast sensitivity in patients with early cataract. *Archives of Ophthalmology, 114,* 529–536.

Age-Related Eye Disease Study Research Group. (2000). Risk factors associated with age-related macular degeneration. A case-control study in the age-related eye disease study: Age-related eye disease study report number 3. *Ophthalmology 107*(12), 2224–2232.

Age-Related Eye Disease Study Research Group. (2001). A randomized, placebo-controlled clinical trial of high-dose supplementation with vitamins C and E, beta-carotene, and zinc for age-related macular degeneration and vision loss. *Archives of Ophthalmology, 119*(10), 1439–1452.

Aiello, L. P., Cahill, M. T., & Wong, J. S. (2001). Systemic considerations in the management of diabetic retinopathy. *American Journal of Ophthalmology, 132*(5), 760–776.

Atwood, J. D. (Ed). (1998). What's new in contact lenses. *Review of Ophthalmology, 5*(5), 115–116.

Ayala, M. J., Perez-Santonja, J. J., Artola, A., Claramonte, P., & Alio, J. L. (2001). Laser in situ keratomileusis to correct residual myopia after cataract surgery. *Journal of Refractive Surgery, 17*(1), 12–16.

Azuara-Blanco, A. (1997). Aqueous tube shunts for refractory glaucomas. *Journal of Ophthalmic Nursing and Technology, 16*(3), 103–107.

Barnie, D. C. (2002). Restoring vision in older patients. *RN, 65*(1), 30–36.

Bressler, N. M., & Bressler, S. B. (2000). Photodynamic therapy with verteporfin (Visudyne): Impact on ophthalmology and visual sciences. *Investigative Ophthalmology and Visual Science 41*(3), 624–628.

Calonge, M. (2001). The treatment of dry eye. *Survey of Ophthalmology, 40*(3), 199–208.

Canadian Hypertension Society. (2005). General information on hypertension. Available at: www.hypertension.ca/publicEducation_va.asp. Retrieved June 13, 2005.

Canadian Ophthalmological Society. (2003). Cataracts. Available at: http://eyesite.ca/english/public-information/eye-conditions/pdfs/Cataracts.pdf. Retrieved June 13, 2005.

Davis, E. A., Hardten, D. R., & Lindstrom, R. L. (Eds.). (2000). LASIK complications. *International Ophthalmology Clinics, 40*(3), 67–75.

Duffy, R. (2000). Central island and decentered ablations after LASIK. *International Opthalmology Clinics, 40*(3), 93–101.

Durrie, D. S., & Vande Garde, T. L. (1998). LASIK enhancements. *International Ophthalmology Clinics, 40*(3), 103–110.

Eller, A. W. (1998). Cataract surgery in diabetics: What to consider before you operate. *Review of Ophthalmology, 5*(2), 48–53.

Fechtner, R. D., & Singh, K. (2001). Maximal glaucoma therapy. *Journal of Glaucoma, 10* (Suppl.), S73–S75.

Fine, H. (2000). A randomized controlled trial of intracameral lidocaine during phacoemulsification under topical anesthesia. *Evidence-Based Eyecare, 1*(3), 136–137.

Fishkind, W. J. (1998). A better way to assess cataract patients. *Review of Ophthalmology, 5*(3), 59–66.

Gabelt, B., & Kaufman, P. (1998). A rational approach to adding glaucoma medications. *Review of Ophthalmology, 5*(5), 44–54.

Grehn, F. (2001). World health problem of glaucoma. *Journal of Glaucoma, 10* (Suppl.1), 82–84.

Hannush, S. (Ed.). (1998). What's new in corneal and external disease. *Review of Ophthalmology, 5*(5), 68–74.

Hardten, D. R. (2000). Phakic iris claw artisan intraocular lens for correction of high myopia and hyperopia. *International Ophthalmology Clinics, 40*(3), 209–221.

Higgenbotham, E. J. (2002). "Who's on first?": Considering the options for primary glaucoma therapy. *Archives of Ophthalmology, 120*(2), 191–193.

Holland, S., Mathias, R., Mork, D., Chiu, J., & Slade, S. (2000). Diffuse lamellar keratitis related to endotoxins released from serilizer reservoir biofilms. *Ophthalmology, 107*(7), 1227–1233.

Humayan, M. S., de Juan E., Jr., Weiland, J. D., Dagnelie, G., Katona, S., Greenberg, R., & Satoshi, S. (1999). Pattern electrical stimulation of the human retina. *Vision Research 39*, 2569–2576.

Hurley, M. (2001). Cornea: No sutures needed with transplant technique. *Eye Net, 5*(2), 21–22.

Jampel, H. (1998). Laser trabeculoplasty is the treatment of choice for chronic open-angle glaucoma. *Archives of Ophthalmology, 116*, 240–241.

Lakhanpal, R., Robin, A., Gabelt, B. T., & Kaufman, P. (1998). A global guide to glaucoma medications. *Review of Ophthalmology, 5*(5), 42–57.

Lee, O., & Netland, P. (Ed.). (1998). What's new in glaucoma. *Review of Ophthalmology, 5*(5), 86–95.

Linebarger, E. J., Hardten, R., & Lindstrom, R. L. (2000). Diffuse lamellar keratitis: Identification and management. *International Ophthalmology Clinics, 40*(3), 77–86.

Linebarger, E. J., Song, D., Ruckhofer, J., & Schazlin, D. J. (2000). Intacs: The intrastromal corneal ring. *International Ophthalmology Clinics, 40*(3), 199–208.

Martin, D. F., Kuppermann, B. D., Wolitz, R. A., Palenstine, A. G., Li, H., Robinson, C. A. (1999). Oral ganciclovir for patients with cytomegalovirus retinitis treated with a ganciclovir implant. Roche Ganciclovir Study Group. *New England Journal Medicine, 340*(14), 1063–1070.

Monroe, L. R. (1998). IOLs: The future of refractive surgery? *Eye Net, 2*(8), 20–21.

Peterson, W. C. (2000). Subconjunctival anesthesia for cataract surgery. *Operative Techniques in Cataract and Refractive Surgery, 3*(3), 137–138.

Preshel, N., Hardten, D. R., & Lindstrom, R. L. (2000). LASIK after penetrating keratoplasty. *International Ophthalmology Clinic, 40*(3), 111–123.

Quigley, H. A. (2001). Advances in glaucoma medication during the 1990s and their effects. *Journal of Glaucoma, 10* (Suppl. 1), S71–S72.

Range, L. J. (2001). Cataract: Five anesthesia issues to consider. *Eye Net, 5*(2), 19–20.

Rapuano, C. J. (2000). Amniotic membrane transplantation for bullous keratopathy. *Evidence-Based Practice, 1*(2), 80–81.

Regillo, C. (Ed.). (1998). What's new in retina. *Review of Ophthalmology, 5*(5), 77–82.

Rongé, L. J. (2001). Cornea donation: LASIK shatters assumptions. *Eye Net, 5*(8), 39–42.

Schein, O. D., Katz, J., Bass, E. B., Tielsch, J. M., Lubomski, L. H., Feldman, M. A., et al. (2000). The value of routine postoperative medical testing before cataract surgery. *American Journal of Ophthalmology, 129*(5), 701.

Scherick, K. (1998). How to solve the lens care problem. *Review of Ophthalmology, 5*(1), 57–59.

Stamper, R. L., Wigginton, S. A., & Higgenbotham, E. J. (2002). Primary drug treatments for glaucoma: Beta-blockers versus other medications. *Survey of Ophthalmology, 47*(1), 63–73.

Stein, R. (2000). Photorefractive keratectomy. *International Ophthalmology Clinics, 40*(3), 111–123.

Stonecipher, K. G., & Salz, J. J. (1998). Point-counterpoint: Should we perform bilateral LASIK? *Review of Ophthalmology, 5*(1), 60–76.

Sugar, A., Rapuano, C. J., Culbertson, W. W., Huang, D., Varley, G. A., Agapitos, P. J., et al. (2002). Laser in situ keratomileusis for myopia and astigmatism: Safety and efficacy. A report by the American Academy of Ophthalmology. *Ophthalmology, 109*(1), 175–187.

The Canadian National Institute for the Blind. (2005a). *Diabetes and the eye*. Available at: www.cnib.ca/eng/eye_con/cospubs/diabetes.htm. Retrieved June 13, 2005.

The Canadian National Institute for the Blind. (2005b). *Fast facts*. Available at: www.cnib.ca/eng/media-centre/journalists/facts.htm. Retrieved June 13, 2005.

The Canadian National Institute for the Blind. (2005c). *Glaucoma*. Available at: www.cnib.ca/eng/eye_con. Retrieved June 13, 2005.

The Canadian National Institute for the Blind. (2005d). *Macular degeneration*. Available at: www.cnib.ca/eng/eye_con/cospubs/mclrdegn.htm. Retrieved June 13, 2005.

Treatment of Age-Related Macular Degeneration with Photodynamic Therapy (TAP) Study Group. (1999). Verteporfin (Visudyne) therapy of subfoveal choroidal neovascularization in age-related macular degeneration: One year results of two randomized clinical trials. TAP report no. 1. *Archives of Ophthalmology, 117*, 1329–1345.

Tsai, R. J. F., Li, L. M., & Chen, J. K. (2000). Reconstruction of damaged corneas by transplantation of autologous limbal epithelial cells. *New England Journal of Medicine, 343*(2), 86–97.

West, S. K., Duncan, D. D., Munoz, B., Rubin, G. S., Fried, L. P., Bandeen-Roche, K., & Schein, O. D. (1998). *New England Journal of Medicine, 281*(3), 229–230.

Weinreb, R. N. (2001). Lowering intraocular pressure to minimize glaucoma damage. *Journal of Glaucoma, 10* (Suppl. 1), S76–S77.

RESOURCES AND WEBSITES

Adaptive Technology Resource Centre, J. P. Robarts Library, First floor, University of Toronto, 130 St. George Street, Toronto ON M5S 1A5; (416) 978-4360; www.utoronto.ca.

Alliance for Equality of Blind Canadians, 6-1638 Pandosy Street, Kelowna, BC V1Y 1P8; 1-800-561-4774; www.blindcanadians.ca.

Association for Macular Diseases, Inc., 210 East 64th St., New York, NY 10021; http://www.macular.org.

Canadian Association Disability Service Providers in Post Secondary Education, 4 Cataraqui Street, Suite 310, Kingston, ON K7K 1Z7; (613) 531-9210; www.cacuss.ca.

Canadian Association of Genetic Counsellors (CAGC); www.cagc-accg.ca.

Canadian Association of Independent Living Centres, National Association, 1104-170 Laurier Avenue West, Ottawa, ON K1P 5V5; (613) 563-2581; www.cailc.ca.

Canadian Braille Authority; www.canadianbrailleauthority.ca.

Canadian Cancer Society/Société canadienne du cancer, National Office, Suite 200, 10 Alcorn Avenue, Toronto, ON M4V 3B1; (416) 961-7223; fax: (416) 961-4189; www.cancer.ca.

Canadian Council of the Blind, CCB National Office, 401-396 Cooper Street, Ottawa, ON K2P 2H7; 1-877-304-0968; www.ccbnational.net.

Canadian Council on Social Development, 309 Cooper Street, 5th Floor, Ottawa, ON K2P 0G5; (613) 236-8977; www.ccsd.ca.

Canadian Library Association, 328 Frank Street, Ottawa, ON K2P 0X8; (613) 232-9625; www.cla.ca.

Canadian National Institute for the Blind, National Office, 1929 Bayview Avenue, Toronto, ON M4G 3E8; (416) 486-2500; www.cnib.ca.

Canadian National Society for the Deaf Blind; 519-372-2068; www.cnsdb.ca.

Canadian Organization for Rare Disorders (CORD), PO Box 814, Coaldale, AB T1M 1M7; (403) 345-4544; toll-free: 1-877-302-7273; fax: (403) 345-3948; http://www.cord.ca.

Canadian Ophthalmological Society, 610-1525 Carling Avenue, Ottawa, ON K1Z 8R9; www.eyesite.ca.

Council of Canadians with Disabilities, 926-294 Portage Avenue, Winnipeg, MN R3C 0B9; 204-947-0303; www.ccdonline.ca.

Council on Access to Information for Print-Disabled Canadians, Library and Archives Canada, 395 Wellington Street, Ottawa ON K1A 0N4; (613) 943-8570; www.collectionscanada.ca/accessinfo.

Glaucoma Canada; www.glaucomacanada.com.

Glaucoma Research Foundation, 490 Post St., Suite 830, San Francisco, CA 94102; http://www.glaucoma.org.

Head Cancer Informatics; Ontario Cancer Institute/Princess Margaret Hospital, University Health Network, 610 University Avenue, Toronto, ON M5G 2M9; www.retinoblastoma.ca.

Help the Aged Canada, HTAC head office, 1300 Carling Ave., Unit 205, Ottawa, ON K1Z 7L2; (613) 232-0727; www.helptheaged.ca.

National Educational Association of Disabled Students, 4th Level Unicentre, Carleton University, Ottawa, ON K1S 5B6; www.neads.ca.

Prevent Blindness America, 500 E. Remington Road, Schaumburg, IL 60173; http://www.prevent-blindness.org.

Public Health Agency of Canada, 130 Colonnade Road, AL 6501H, Ottawa, ON K1A 0K9; www.phac-aspc.gc.ca.

Research to Prevent Blindness, 645 Madison Ave., New York, NY 10022-1010. http://www.rpbusa.org.

The Canadian Association of Optometrists, 234 Argyle Ave, Ottawa, ON K2P 1B9; 1-888-263-4676; www.opto.ca.

The Learning Disabilities Association of Canada, National Office, 323 Chapel Street, Ottawa, ON K1N 7Z2; (613) 238-5721; www.ldac-taac.ca.

Veteran Affairs Canada; 10th floor, Trebla Building, 473 Albert Street, Ottawa, ON K1R 5B4; 1-800-883-6094; www.vac-acc.gc.ca.

Vision World Wide, Inc., 5707 Brockton Dr., Suite 302, Indianapolis, IN 46220-5481; http://www.visionww.org.

Assessment and Management of Patients With Hearing and Balance Disorders

Adapted by Tracey Stephen

LEARNING OBJECTIVES

On completion of this chapter, the learner will be able to:

1. Describe methods used to assess hearing and diagnose hearing and balance disorders.
2. List the manifestations that may be exhibited by a person with a hearing disorder.
3. Identify ways to communicate effectively with a hearing-impaired person.
4. Differentiate problems of the external ear from those of the middle ear and inner ear.
5. Compare the various types of surgical procedures used for managing middle ear disorders, including appropriate nursing care.
6. Describe the teaching topics that need to be addressed for patients undergoing middle ear and mastoid surgery.
7. Describe the different types of inner ear disorders, including the clinical manifestations, diagnosis, and management.

The ear is a sensory organ with dual functions—hearing and balance. The sense of hearing is essential for normal development and maintenance of speech and the ability to communicate with others. Balance, or equilibrium, is essential for maintaining body movement, position, and coordination.

The delicate structure and function of the ear make early detection and accurate diagnosis of disorders necessary for preservation of normal hearing and balance. Among the professionals involved in the diagnosis and treatment of these disorders are otolaryngologists, pediatricians, internists, and nurses.

This chapter addresses the assessment and management of hearing and balance disorders common to the adult population. The pediatric otolaryngology literature provides information on otologic disorders pertaining to that population.

Anatomic and Physiologic Overview

The cranium encloses and protects the brain and surrounding structures, providing attachment for various muscles that control head and jaw movements. Eight bones form the cranium: the occipital bone, the frontal bone, two parietal bones, two temporal bones, the sphenoid bone, and the ethmoid bone. Some of these bones contain sinuses, which are cavities lined with mucous membranes and connected to the nasal cavity. The ears are located on either side of the cranium at approximately eye level.

ANATOMY OF THE EXTERNAL EAR

The external ear, housed in the temporal bone, includes the auricle (i.e., pinna) and the external auditory canal (Fig. 59-1). The external ear is separated from the middle ear by a disklike structure called the tympanic membrane (ie, eardrum).

Auricle

The auricle, attached to the side of the head by skin, is composed mainly of cartilage, except for the fat and subcutaneous tissue in the earlobe. The auricle collects the sound waves and directs vibrations into the external auditory canal.

External Auditory Canal

The external auditory canal is approximately 2.5 cm long. The lateral third is an elastic cartilaginous and dense fibrous framework to which thin skin is attached. The medial two thirds is bone lined with thin skin. The external auditory canal ends at the tympanic membrane (Chart 59-1).

The skin of the canal contains hair, sebaceous glands, and ceruminous glands, which secrete a brown, waxlike substance called cerumen (ie, ear wax). The ear's self-cleaning mechanism moves old skin cells and cerumen to the outer part of the ear.

Just anterior to the external auditory canal is the temporomandibular joint. The head of the mandible can be felt by placing a fingertip in the external auditory canal while the patient opens and closes the mouth.

ANATOMY OF THE MIDDLE EAR

The middle ear, an air-filled cavity, includes the tympanic membrane laterally and the otic capsule medially. The middle ear cleft lies between the two. The middle ear is connected by the eustachian tube to the nasopharynx and is continuous with air-filled cells in the adjacent mastoid portion of the temporal bone.

The eustachian tube, which is approximately 1 mm wide and 35 mm long, connects the middle ear to the nasopharynx. Normally, the eustachian tube is closed, but it opens by action of the tensor veli palatini muscle when performing a Valsalva manoeuvre or when yawning or swallowing. The tube serves as a drainage channel for normal and abnormal secretions of the middle ear and equalizes pressure in the middle ear with that of the atmosphere.

Tympanic Membrane

The tympanic membrane (ie, eardrum), about 1 cm in diameter and very thin, is normally pearly grey and translucent. The tympanic membrane consists of three layers of tissue: an outer layer, continuous with the skin of the ear canal; a fibrous middle layer; and an inner mucosal layer, continuous with the lining of the middle ear cavity. Approximately 80% of the tympanic membrane is composed of all three layers and is called the pars

Glossary

acute otitis media: inflammation in the middle ear lasting less than 6 weeks

cholesteatoma: tumour of the middle ear or mastoid, or both, that can destroy structures of the temporal bone

chronic otitis media: repeated episodes of acute otitis media causing irreversible tissue damage and persistent tympanic membrane perforation

conductive hearing loss: loss of hearing in which efficient sound transmission to the inner ear is interrupted by some obstruction or disease process

dizziness: altered sensation of orientation in space

endolymphatic hydrops: dilation of the endolymphatic space of the inner ear; the pathologic correlate of Ménière's disease

exostoses: small, hard, bony protrusions in the lower posterior bony portion of the ear canal

labyrinthitis: inflammation of the labyrinth of the inner ear

Ménière's disease: condition of the inner ear characterized by a triad of symptoms: episodic vertigo, tinnitus, and fluctuating sensorineural hearing loss

middle ear effusion: fluid in the middle ear without evidence of infection

myringotomy (ie, tympanotomy): incision in the tympanic membrane

nystagmus: involuntary rhythmic eye movement

ossiculoplasty: surgical reconstruction of the middle ear bones to restore hearing

otalgia: sensation of fullness or pain in the ear

otitis externa (ie, external otitis): inflammation of the external auditory canal

otorrhea: drainage from the ear

otosclerosis: a condition characterized by abnormal spongy bone formation around the stapes

presbycusis: progressive hearing loss associated with aging

rhinorrhea: drainage from the nose

sensorineural hearing loss: loss of hearing related to damage of the end organ for hearing or cranial nerve VIII, or both

tinnitus: subjective perception of sound with internal origin; unwanted noises in the head or ear

tympanoplasty: surgical repair of the tympanic membrane

vertigo: illusion of movement in which the individual or the surroundings are sensed as moving

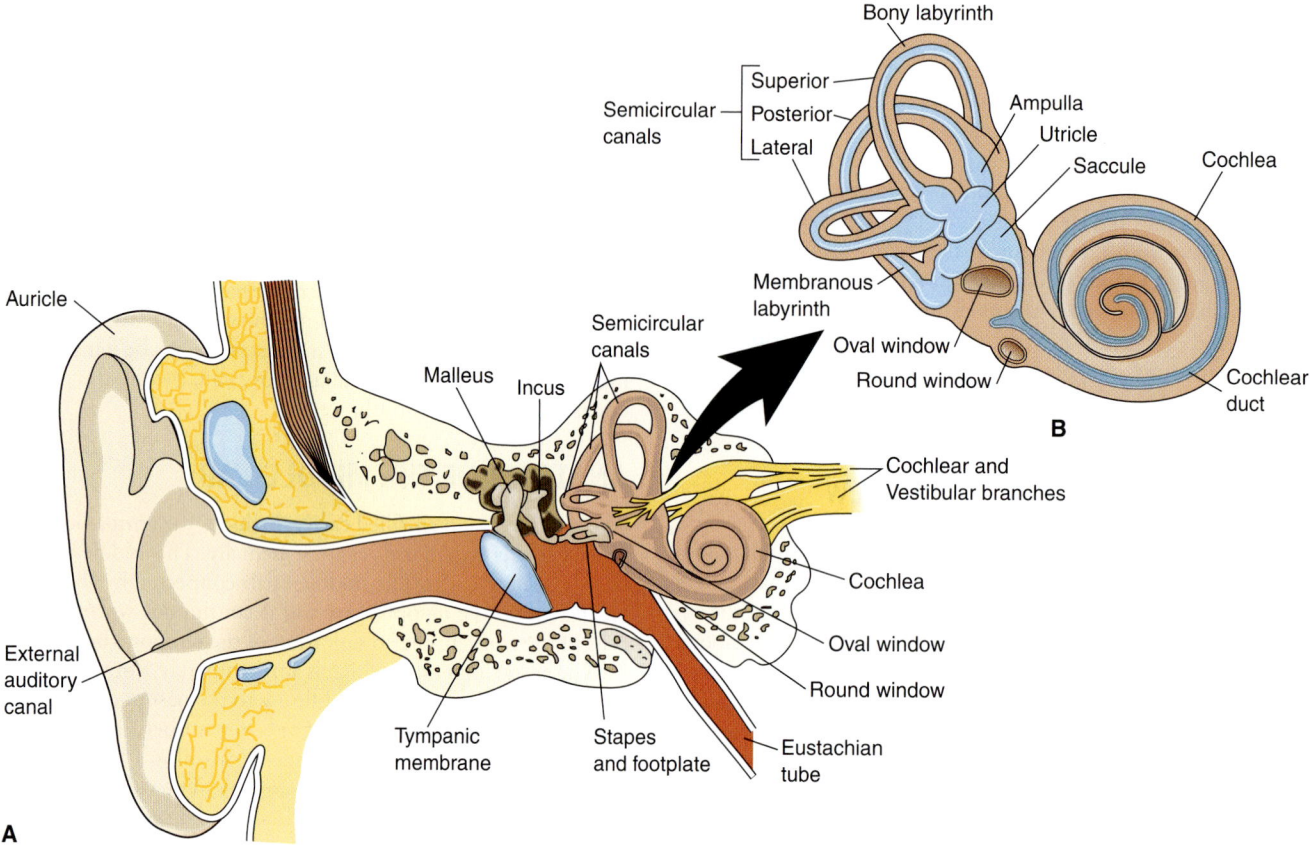

FIGURE 59-1 (**A**) Anatomy of the ear. (**B**) The inner ear.

Chart 59-1 Definition of Terms: Ear Anatomy

Acoustic: pertaining to sound or the sense of hearing

Cerumen: yellow or brown, waxlike secretion found in the external auditory canal

Cochlea: the winding, snail-shaped bony tube that forms a portion of the inner ear and contains the organ of Corti, the transducer for hearing

Cochlear (acoustic) nerve: the division of the eighth cranial (vestibulocochlear) nerve, which goes to the cochlea

Eustachian tube: the 3- to 4-cm tube that extends from the middle ear to the nasopharynx

External auditory canal: the canal leading from the external auditory meatus to the tympanic membrane; about 2.5 cm in length

External ear: the portion of the ear that consists of the auricle and external auditory canal; it is separated from the middle ear by the tympanic membrane

Incus: the second of the three ossicles in the middle ear; it articulates with the malleus and stapes; the anvil

Inner ear: the portion of the ear that consists of the cochlea, vestibule, and semicircular canals

Internal auditory canal: a canal in the petrous portion of the temporal bone, which houses the facial and vestibulocochlear nerves (cranial nerves VII and VIII)

Malleus: the first (most lateral) and largest of the three ossicles in the middle ear; it is connected to the tympanic membrane laterally and articulates with the incus; the hammer

Middle ear: the small, air-filled cavity in the temporal bone that contains the three ossicles

Organ of Corti: the end organ of hearing, located in the cochlea

Ossicle: a small bone; there are three in the middle ear: malleus, incus, and stapes

Oval window: a fenestra (aperture) between the vestibule of the inner ear and the middle ear, occupied by the base of the stapes

Pinna: the outer part of the external ear, which collects and directs sound waves into the external auditory canal; the auricle

Round window: a fenestra between the middle ear and the inner ear at the base of the cochlea, occupied by the round window membrane

Semicircular canals: the superior, posterior, and lateral bony tubes that form part of the inner ear; contain the receptor organs for balance

Stapes: the third (most medial) ossicle of the middle ear; it articulates with the incus, and its footplate fits into the oval window; the stirrup

Temporal bone: a bone on both sides of the skull at its base; composed of the squamous, mastoid, and petrous portions

Tympanic membrane: the membrane that separates the middle ear from the external auditory canal; also referred to as the eardrum

Vestibulocochlear nerve: cranial nerve VIII; cochlear (acoustic) nerve and vestibular nerve tensa. The other 20% of the tympanic membrane lacks the middle layer and is called the pars flaccida. The absence of this fibrous middle layer makes the pars flaccida more vulnerable to pathologic disorders than the pars tensa. Distinguishing landmarks of the tympanic membrane include the annulus, the fibrous border that attaches the eardrum to the temporal bone; the short process of the malleus; the long process of the malleus; the umbo of the malleus, which attaches to the tympanic membrane in the centre; the pars flaccida; and the pars tensa (Fig. 59-2).

The tympanic membrane protects the middle ear and conducts sound vibrations from the external canal to the ossicles. The sound pressure is magnified 22 times as a result of transmission from a larger area to a smaller one.

Ossicles

The middle ear contains the three smallest bones (ie, ossicles) of the body: malleus, incus, and stapes. The ossicles, which are held in place by joints, muscles, and ligaments, assist in the transmission of sound. Two small fenestrae (ie, oval and round windows), located in the medial wall of the middle ear, separate the middle ear from the inner ear. The footplate of the stapes sits in the oval window, secured by a fibrous annulus, or ring-shaped structure. The footplate transmits sound to the inner ear. The round window, covered by a thin membrane, provides an exit for sound vibrations (see Fig. 59-1).

ANATOMY OF THE INNER EAR

The inner ear is housed deep within the temporal bone. The organs for hearing (ie, cochlea) and balance (ie, semicircular canals), as well as cranial nerves VII (ie, facial nerve) and VIII (ie, vestibulocochlear nerve), are all part of this complex anatomy (see Fig. 59-1). The cochlea and semicircular canals are housed in the bony labyrinth. The bony labyrinth surrounds and protects the membranous labyrinth, which is bathed in a fluid called perilymph.

Membranous Labyrinth

The membranous labyrinth is composed of the utricle, the saccule, the cochlear duct, the semicircular canals, and the organ of Corti. The membranous labyrinth contains a fluid called endolymph. The three semicircular canals—posterior, superior, and lateral, which lie at 90-degree angles to one another—contain sensory receptor organs, arranged to detect rotational movement. These receptor end organs are stimulated by changes in the rate or direction of an individual's movement. The utricle and saccule are involved with linear movements.

Organ of Corti

The organ of Corti is located in the cochlea, a snail-shaped, bony tube about 3.5 cm long with two and one-half spiral turns. Membranes separate the cochlear duct (ie, scala media) from the scala vestibuli, and the scala tympani from the basilar membrane. The organ of Corti is located on the basilar membrane stretching from the base to the apex of the cochlea. As sound vibrations enter the perilymph at the oval window and travel along the scala vestibuli, they pass through the scala tympani, enter the cochlear duct, and cause movement of the basilar membrane. The organ of Corti, also called the end organ for hearing, transforms mechanical energy into neural activity and separates sounds into different frequencies. This electrochemical impulse travels through the acoustic nerve to the temporal cortex of the brain to be interpreted as meaningful sound. In the internal auditory canal, the cochlear (acoustic) nerve, arising from the cochlea, joins the vestibular nerve, arising from the semicircular canals, utricle, and saccule, to become the vestibulocochlear nerve (cranial nerve VIII). This canal also houses the facial nerve and the blood supply from the ear to the brain.

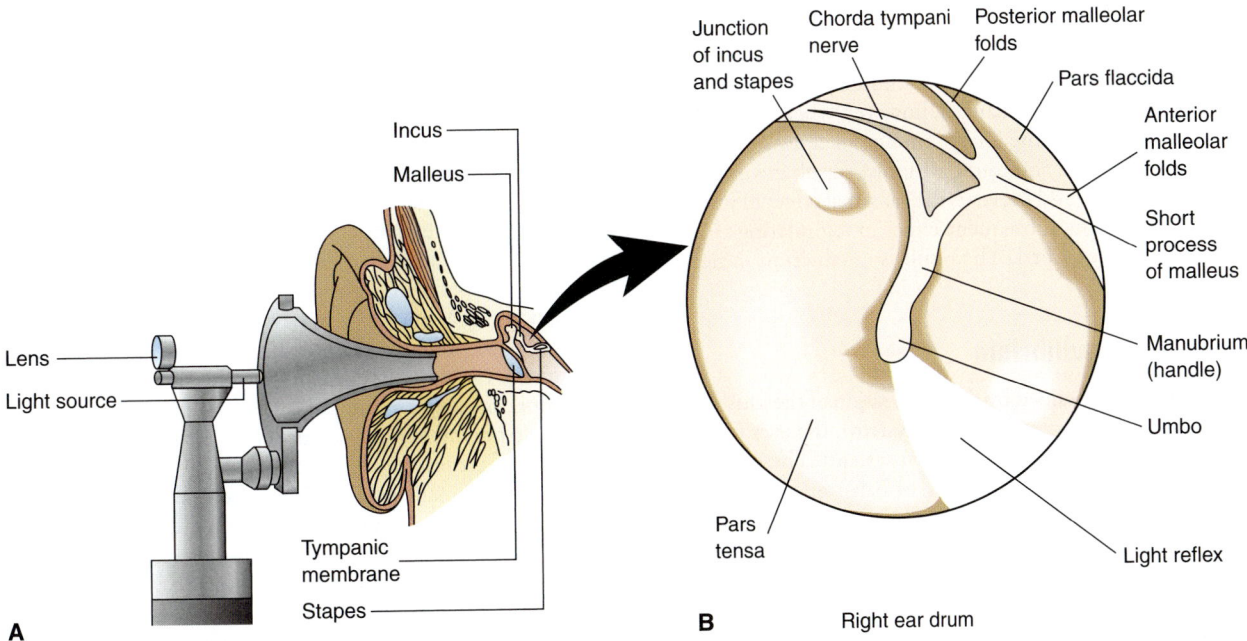

FIGURE 59-2 (**A**) Technique for using the otoscope to see (**B**) the tympanic membrane.

FUNCTION OF THE EARS
Hearing

Hearing is conducted over two pathways: air and bone. Sounds transmitted by air conduction travel over the air-filled external and middle ear through vibration of the tympanic membrane and ossicles. Sounds transmitted by bone conduction travel directly through bone to the inner ear, bypassing the tympanic membrane and ossicles. Normally, air conduction is the more efficient pathway. However, defects in the tympanic membrane or interruption of the ossicular chain disrupt normal air conduction, which results in a loss of the sound-to-pressure ratio and subsequently in a conductive hearing loss.

SOUND CONDUCTION AND TRANSMISSION

Sound enters the ear through the external auditory canal and causes the tympanic membrane to vibrate. These vibrations transmit sound through the lever action of the ossicles to the oval window as mechanical energy. This mechanical energy is then transmitted through the inner ear fluids to the cochlea, stimulating the hair cells, and is subsequently converted to electrical energy. The electrical energy travels through the vestibulocochlear nerve to the central nervous system, where it is analyzed and interpreted in its final form as sound.

Vibrations transmitted by the tympanic membrane to the ossicles of the middle ear are transferred to the cochlea, lodged in the labyrinth of the inner ear. The stapes rocks, causing vibrations (ie, waves) in fluids contained in the inner ear. These fluid waves cause movement of the basilar membrane to occur that then stimulates the hair cells of the organ of Corti in the cochlea to move in a wavelike manner. The movements of the tympanic membrane set up electrical currents that stimulate the various areas of the cochlea. The hair cells set up neural impulses that are encoded and then transferred to the auditory cortex in the brain, where they are decoded into a sound message.

The footplate of the stapes receives impulses transmitted by the incus and the malleus from the tympanic membrane. The round window, which opens on the opposite side of the cochlear duct, is protected from sound waves by the intact tympanic membrane, permitting motion of the inner ear fluids by sound wave stimulation. For example, in the normally intact tympanic membrane, sound waves stimulate the oval window first, and a lag occurs before the terminal effect of the stimulus reaches the round window. This lag phase is changed, however, when a perforation of the tympanic membrane is large enough to allow sound waves to impinge on the oval and round windows simultaneously. This effect cancels the lag and prevents the maximal effect of inner ear fluid motility and its subsequent effect in stimulating the hair cells in the organ of Corti. The result is a reduction in hearing ability (Fig. 59-3).

Balance and Equilibrium

Body balance is maintained by the cooperation of the muscles and joints of the body (ie, proprioceptive system), the eyes (ie, visual system), and the labyrinth (ie, vestibular system). These areas send their information about equilibrium, or balance, to the brain (ie, cerebellar system) for coordination and perception in the cerebral cortex. The brain obtains its blood supply from the heart and arterial system. A problem in any of these areas, such as arteriosclerosis or impaired vision, can cause a balance disturbance. The vestibular apparatus of the inner ear provides feedback regarding the movements and the position of the head and body in space.

Assessment

The external ear is examined by inspection and direct palpation, and the tympanic membrane is inspected with an otoscope and indirect palpation with a pneumatic otoscope. Until the advent of middle ear endoscopy, inspection of the middle ear was impossible. Evaluation of gross auditory acuity also is included in every physical examination.

INSPECTION OF THE EXTERNAL EAR

Inspection of the external ear is a simple procedure, but it is often overlooked. The auricle and surrounding tissues should be inspected for deformities, lesions, and discharge, as well as size, symmetry, and angle of attachment to the head. Manipulation of the auricle does not normally elicit pain. If this manoeuvre is painful, acute external otitis is suspected. Tenderness on palpation in the area of the mastoid may indicate acute mastoiditis or inflammation of the posterior auricular node. Occasionally, sebaceous cysts and tophi (ie, subcutaneous mineral deposits) are present on the pinna. A flaky scaliness on or behind the auricle usually indicates seborrheic dermatitis and can be present on the scalp and facial structures as well.

OTOSCOPIC EXAMINATION

To examine the external auditory canal and tympanic membrane, the otoscope should be held in the examiner's right hand, in a pencil-hold position, with the bottom of the scope pointing up (Fig. 59-4). This position prevents the examiner from inserting the otoscope too far into the external canal. Using the opposite hand, the auricle is grasped and gently pulled back to straighten the canal in the adult. If the canal is not straightened with this technique, the tympanic membrane is harder to visualize because of the canal obstructing the view.

The speculum is slowly inserted into the ear canal, with the examiner's eye held close to the magnifying lens of the otoscope to visualize the canal and tympanic membrane. The largest speculum that the canal can accommodate (usually 5 mm in an adult) is guided gently down into the canal and slightly forward. Because the distal portion of the canal is bony and covered by a sensitive layer of epithelium, only light pressure can be used without causing pain. The examiner looks for any discharge, inflammation, or foreign body in the external auditory canal.

The healthy tympanic membrane is pearly grey and is positioned obliquely at the base of the canal. The landmarks are identified, if visible (see Fig. 59-2): the pars tensa, the umbo, the manubrium of the malleus, and its short process. A slow, circular movement of the speculum allows further visualization of the malleolar folds and periphery. The position and colour of the membrane and any unusual markings or deviations from normal are documented. The presence of fluid, air bubbles, blood, or masses in the middle ear also are noted.

Proper otoscopic examination of the external auditory canal and tympanic membrane requires that the canal be free of large amounts of cerumen. Cerumen is normally present in the external canal, and small amounts should not interfere with otoscopic examination. If the tympanic membrane cannot be visualized because of cerumen, the cerumen may be removed by gently irrigating the external canal with warm water (if there are no contraindications to this). If adherent cerumen is present, a small amount of mineral oil or over-the-counter cerumen softener may be instilled within the ear canal, and the patient is instructed to

FIGURE 59-3 Bone conduction compared to air conduction.

FIGURE 59-4 Proper technique for examining the ear. Hold the otoscope in the right or left hand, in a "pencil hold" position. Steady the hand against the patient's head to avoid inserting the otoscope too far into the external canal.

return for subsequent removal of the cerumen and inspection of the ear. The use of instruments such as a cerumen curette for cerumen removal is reserved for otolaryngologists and nurses with specialized training because of the danger of perforating the tympanic membrane or excoriating the external auditory canal. Cerumen buildup is a common cause of hearing loss and local irritation.

EVALUATION OF GROSS AUDITORY ACUITY

A general estimation of hearing can be made by assessing the patient's ability to hear a whispered phrase or a ticking watch, testing one ear at a time. The Weber and Rinne tests may be used to distinguish conductive loss from sensorineural loss when hearing is impaired. These tests are part of the usual screening physical examination and are useful if a more specific assessment is needed, if hearing loss is detected, or if confirmation of audiometric results is desired.

Whisper Test

To exclude one ear from the testing, the examiner occludes the untested ear by moving a finger or piece of cotton in the patient's ear canal. This produces noise that prevents the untested ear from doing the work for the tested ear. The examiner whispers from a distance of 30 to 60 cm from the nonoccluded ear and out of the patient's sight. The examiner whispers two numbers or words that have equally accented syllables such as "sandbox" or "baseball." The patient is asked to repeat what was whispered to determine gross hearing acuity. If the patient is unable to correctly repeat the whispered words or numbers on the first attempt, the examiner tries again with a slightly louder whisper.

Weber Test

The Weber test uses bone conduction to test lateralization of sound. A tuning fork (ideally, 512 Hz), set in motion by grasping it firmly by its stem and tapping it on the examiner's knee or hand, is placed midline on the patient's head or forehead (Fig. 59-5). A person with

FIGURE 59-5 The Weber test assesses lateralization of hearing. Photo © Day, R. A., Stephen, T., & Day, L. W. 2005. Faculty of Nursing, University of Alberta.

normal hearing will hear the sound equally in both ears or describe the sound as centred in the middle of the head. In cases of **conductive hearing loss**, such as from otosclerosis or otitis media, the sound is heard better in the affected ear. In cases of **sensorineural hearing loss**, resulting from damage to the cochlear or vestibulocochlear nerve, the sound lateralizes to the better-hearing ear. The Weber test is useful for detecting unilateral hearing loss (Table 59-1).

Rinne Test

In the Rinne test (pronounced rin-AY), the examiner shifts the stem of a vibrating tuning fork (preferably 512 Hz) between two positions: against the mastoid bone (ie, for bone conduction) and 4 to 6 cm from the opening of the ear canal (ie, for air conduction) (Fig. 59-6). The examiner places the vibrating tuning fork on the mastoid bone behind the tested ear and asks the patient to indicate when the tone is no longer heard. When the tone is no longer heard, the examiner shifts the tuning fork to the opening of the ear canal and asks the patient if the tone is audible. Sound heard by air conduction is audible longer than sound heard by bone conduction. The Rinne test is useful for distinguishing between conductive and sensorineural hearing losses. With a conductive hearing loss, bone-conducted sound is heard as long as or longer than air-conducted sound, whereas with a sensorineural hearing loss, air-conducted sound is audible longer than bone-conducted sound. In a normal hearing ear, air-conducted sound is louder than bone-conducted sound.

Table 59-1 • **Comparison of Weber and Rinne Tests**

HEARING STATUS	WEBER	RINNE
Normal hearing	Sound is heard equally in both ears.	Air conduction is audible longer than bone conduction.
Conductive hearing loss	Sound heard best in affected ear (hearing loss).	Sound heard as long or longer in affected ear (hearing loss).
Sensorineural hearing loss	Sound heard best in normal hearing ear.	Air conduction is audible longer than bone conduction in affected ear.

Diagnostic Evaluation

Many diagnostic procedures are available to measure the auditory and vestibular systems indirectly. These tests are usually performed by an audiologist or speech-language pathologist who is recognized by the Canadian Association of Speech-Language Pathologists and Audiologists.

FIGURE 59-6 The Rinne test assesses both bone and air conduction of sound. Photo © Day, R. A., Stephen, T., & Day, L. W. 2005. Faculty of Nursing, University of Alberta.

AUDIOMETRY

In detecting hearing loss, audiometry is the single most important diagnostic instrument. Audiometric testing is of two kinds: pure-tone audiometry, in which the sound stimulus consists of a pure or musical tone (the louder the tone before the patient perceives it, the greater the hearing loss), and speech audiometry, in which the spoken word is used to determine the ability to hear and discriminate sounds and words.

When evaluating hearing, three characteristics are important: frequency, pitch, and intensity. *Frequency* refers to the number of sound waves emanating from a source per second, measured as cycles per second, or Hertz (Hz). The normal human ear perceives sounds ranging in frequency from 20 to 20,000 Hz. The frequencies from 500 to 2,000 Hz are important in understanding everyday speech and are referred to as the speech range or speech frequencies. *Pitch* is the term used to describe frequency; a tone with 100 Hz is considered of low pitch, and a tone of 10,000 Hz is considered of high pitch.

The unit for measuring loudness (ie, *intensity* of sound) is the decibel (dB), the pressure exerted by sound. Hearing loss is measured in decibels, a logarithmic function of intensity that is not easily converted into a percentage. The critical level of loudness is approximately 30 dB. The shuffling of papers in quiet surroundings is about 15 dB; a low conversation, 40 dB; and a jet plane 30 metres away, about 150 dB. Sound louder than 80 dB is perceived by the human ear to be harsh and can be damaging to the inner ear. Table 59-2 classifies hearing loss based on decibel level. In surgical treatment of patients with hearing loss, the aim is to improve the hearing level to 30 dB or better within the speech frequencies.

With audiometry, the patient wears earphones and signals to the audiologist when a tone is heard. When the tone is applied directly over the external auditory canal, air conduction is measured. When the stimulus is applied to the mastoid bone, bypassing the conductive mechanism (ie, ossicles), nerve conduction is tested. For accuracy, audiometric evaluations are performed in a soundproof room. Responses are plotted on a graph known as an audiogram, which differentiates conductive

Table 59-2 • **Severity of Hearing Loss**

LOSS IN DECIBELS	INTERPRETATION
0–15	Normal hearing
>15–25	Slight hearing loss
>25–40	Mild hearing loss
>40–55	Moderate hearing loss
>55–70	Moderate to severe hearing loss
>70–90	Severe hearing loss
>90	Profound hearing loss

SPEECH HEARING TESTS					
TEST		R	L	BIN	SF
Sp. Reception Threshold (SRT)		10 db	10 db	db	db
Sp. Discrim. Scores	80 db HL	100%	100%	%	%
(PB)	___ db HL	%	%	%	%
	___ db HL	%	%	%	%

FIGURE 59-7 The speech reception threshold is the sound intensity level at which a patient is just capable of correctly identifying simple speech stimuli. Speech discrimination determines the patient's ability to distinguish different sounds, in the form of words, at a decibel level where sound is heard.

from sensorineural hearing loss. Speech discrimination is also measured (Fig. 59-7).

TYMPANOGRAM

A tympanogram, or impedance audiometry, measures middle ear muscle reflex to sound stimulation and compliance of the tympanic membrane by changing the air pressure in a sealed ear canal. Compliance is impaired with middle ear disease.

AUDITORY BRAIN STEM RESPONSE

The auditory brain stem response is a detectable electrical potential from cranial nerve VIII and the ascending auditory pathways of the brain stem in response to sound stimulation. Electrodes are placed on the patient's forehead. Acoustic stimuli, usually in the form of clicks, are made in the ear. The resulting electrophysiologic measurements can determine at which decibel level a patient hears and whether there are any impairments along the nerve pathways (eg, tumour on cranial nerve VIII).

ELECTRONYSTAGMOGRAPHY

Electronystagmography is the measurement and graphic recording of the changes in electrical potentials created by eye movements during spontaneous, positional, or calorically evoked nystagmus. It is also used to assess the oculomotor and vestibular systems and their corresponding interaction. It helps in diagnosing conditions such as **Ménière's disease** and tumours of the internal auditory canal or posterior fossa. Any vestibular suppressants, such as sedatives, tranquilizers, antihistamines, and alcohol are withheld for 24 hours before testing. Prior to the test the procedure is explained to the patient.

PLATFORM POSTUROGRAPHY

Platform posturography is used to investigate postural control capabilities. The integration of visual, vestibular, and proprioceptive cues (ie, sensory integration) with motor response output and coordination of the lower limbs is tested. The patient stands on a platform, surrounded by a screen, and different conditions such as a moving platform with a moving screen or a stationary platform with a moving screen are presented. The responses from the patient on six different conditions are measured and indicate which of the anatomic systems may be impaired. Preparation for the testing is the same as for electronystagmography.

SINUSOIDAL HARMONIC ACCELERATION

Sinusoidal harmonic acceleration, or a rotary chair, is used to assess the vestibulo-ocular system by analyzing compensatory eye movements in response to the clockwise and counterclockwise rotation of the chair. Although such testing cannot identify the side of the lesion in unilateral disease, it helps identify disease and evaluate the course of recovery. The same patient preparation is required as for electronystagmography.

MIDDLE EAR ENDOSCOPY

With endoscopes with very small diameters and acute angles, the ear can be examined endoscopically by an endoscopist specializing in otolaryngology. Middle ear endoscopy is performed safely and effectively as an office procedure to evaluate suspected perilymphatic fistula and new-onset conductive hearing loss, the anatomy of the round window before transtympanic treatment of Ménière's disease, and the tympanic cavity before ear surgery to treat chronic middle ear and mastoid infections.

The tympanic membrane is anesthetized topically for about 10 minutes. Then, the external auditory canal is irrigated with sterile normal saline solution. With the aid of a microscope, a tympanotomy is created with a laser beam or a myringotomy knife, so that the endoscope can be inserted into the middle ear cavity. Video and photo documentation can be accomplished through the scope.

Hearing Loss

More than 3 million Canadians have some form of hearing impairment. The Canadian Association of the Deaf (2004) estimates that there are 310,000 Canadians who are deaf. Hearing loss affects one in ten Canadians, making it the third most common chronic disability. Many can be helped with medical or surgical therapies or with a hearing aid. Six out of 1000 children are affected by hearing loss and it is the most common birth defect in Canada (The Hearing Foundation of Canada, n.d.). By the year 2026, Canada's population is expected to be approximately 35 million people, with 20% of the population being 65 years or older (Statistics Canada, 2005). Currently, one in three Canadians over age 60 and one in two over age 85 are affected by hearing loss, resulting in increasing numbers of Canadians affected by this chronic condition (Canadian Association of the Deaf, 2004).

Conductive hearing loss usually results from an external ear disorder, such as impacted cerumen, or a middle ear disorder, such as otitis media or otosclerosis. In such instances, the efficient transmission of sound by air to the inner ear is interrupted. A sensorineural loss involves damage to the cochlea or vestibulocochlear nerve.

Mixed hearing loss and functional hearing loss also may occur. The patient with mixed hearing loss has conductive loss and sensorineural loss, resulting from dysfunction of air and bone conduction. A functional (or psychogenic) hearing loss is nonorganic and unrelated to detectable structural changes in the hearing mechanisms; it is usually a manifestation of an emotional disturbance.

Clinical Manifestations

Early manifestations of hearing impairment and loss may include tinnitus, increasing inability to hear in groups, and a need to turn up the volume of the television. Hearing impairment can also trigger changes in attitude, the ability to communicate, the awareness of surroundings, and even the ability to protect oneself, affecting the person's quality of life. In a classroom, a student with impaired hearing may be disinterested and inattentive and have failing grades. A person at home may feel isolated because of an inability to hear the clock chime, the refrigerator hum, the birds sing, or the traffic pass. A hearing-impaired pedestrian may attempt to cross the street and fail to hear an approaching car. Hearing-impaired people may miss parts of a conversation. Many people are unaware of their gradual hearing impairment. Often, it is not the person with the hearing loss, but the people with whom he or she is communicating who recognize the impairment first (see Chart 59-2).

For various reasons, some people with hearing loss refuse to seek medical attention or wear a hearing aid. Others feel self-conscious wearing a hearing aid. Insightful patients generally ask those with whom they are trying to communicate to let them know whether difficulties in communication exist. These attitudes and behaviours should be taken into account when counselling patients who need hearing assistance. The decision to wear a hearing aid is a personal one that is affected by these attitudes and behaviours.

Prevention

Many environmental factors have an adverse effect on the auditory system and, with time, result in permanent sensorineural hearing loss. The World Health Organization (WHO, 2002) estimates

there are 250 million people with disabling hearing impairment and that half of hearing loss and deafness is preventable. Noise exposure is the major preventable cause of hearing impairment.

Noise (ie, unwanted and unavoidable sound) has been identified as one of the environmental hazards of the 21st century. The sheer volume of noise that surrounds us daily has increased from a simple annoyance into a potentially dangerous source of physical and psychological damage.

In terms of physical impact, loud, persistent noise has been found to cause constriction of peripheral blood vessels, increased blood pressure and heart rate (because of increased secretion of adrenalin), and increased gastrointestinal activity. Additional research is needed to address the overall effects of noise on the human body. It seems certain, however, that a quiet environment is more conducive to peace of mind. A person who is ill feels more at ease when noise is kept to a minimum. There are numerous factors that contribute to hearing loss (see Chart 59-3).

The term *noise-induced hearing loss* is used to describe hearing loss that follows a long period of exposure to loud noise (eg, heavy machinery, engines, artillery). *Acoustic trauma* refers to the hearing loss caused by a single exposure to an extremely intense noise, such as an explosion. Usually, noise-induced hearing loss occurs at a high frequency (around 4,000 Hz). However, with continued noise exposure, the hearing loss can become more severe and include adjacent frequencies. The minimum noise level known to cause noise-induced hearing loss, regardless of duration, is about 85 to 90 dB.

In Canadian jurisdictions, the exposure limit to noise for 8 hours per day for 5 days a week is 87 to 90 decibels (Canadian Centre for Occupational Health and Safety [CCOHS], 2004). Several industries (eg, carpentry, plumbing, printing, and mining) and workplaces (eg, shipyards, airports, breweries, and paper mills) have exposures close to or higher than these levels. Musicians and hunters are also at risk. Some equipment, such as power tools, woodworking saws, engines, and compressors, exceeds the exposure limit. For example, the sound levels from woodworking saws can reach 106 decibels (CCOHS, 2004). The Canadian Centre for Occupational Health and Safety (CCOHS) requires that workers wear ear protection to prevent noise-induced hearing loss when exposed to noise above the legal limits. There are no medications that protect against noise-induced hearing loss; hearing loss is permanent because the hair cells in the organ of Corti are destroyed. Ear protection against noise is the most effective preventive measure available.

Gerontologic Considerations

About 30% of people 65 years of age and older and 50% of people 75 years and older have hearing difficulties. The cause is unknown; linkages to diet, metabolism, arteriosclerosis, stress, and heredity have been inconsistent (Cruickshanks et al., 1998).

Chart 59-2 • ASSESSMENT

Symptoms of Hearing Loss

Speech deterioration: The person who slurs words or drops word endings, or produces flat-sounding speech, may not be hearing correctly. The ears guide the voice, both in loudness and in pronunciation.

Fatigue: If a person tires easily when listening to conversation or to a speech, fatigue may be the result of straining to hear. Under these circumstances, the person may become irritable very easily.

Indifference: It is easy for the person who cannot hear what others say to become depressed and disinterested in life in general.

Social withdrawal: Not being able to hear what is going on causes the hearing-impaired person to withdraw from situations that might prove embarrassing.

Insecurity: Lack of self-confidence and fear of mistakes create a feeling of insecurity in many hearing-impaired people. No one likes to say the wrong thing or do anything that might appear foolish.

Indecision and procrastination: Loss of self-confidence makes it increasingly difficult for a hearing-impaired person to make decisions.

Suspiciousness: The hearing-impaired person, who often hears only part of what is being said, may suspect that others are talking about him or her, or that portions of the conversation are deliberately spoken softly so that he or she will not hear them.

False pride: The hearing-impaired person wants to conceal the hearing loss and thus often pretends to be hearing when he or she actually is not.

Loneliness and unhappiness: Although everyone wishes for quiet now and then, *enforced* silence can be boring and even somewhat frightening. People with a hearing loss often feel isolated.

Tendency to dominate the conversation: Many hearing-impaired people tend to dominate the conversation, knowing that as long as it is centred on them and they can control it, they are not so likely to be embarrassed by some mistake.

Chart 59-3
Risk Factors for Hearing Loss

- Family history of sensorineural impairment
- Congenital malformations of the cranial structure (ear)
- Low birth weight (<1500 g)
- Use of ototoxic medications (eg, gentamicin, loop diuretics)
- Recurrent ear infections
- Bacterial meningitis
- Chronic exposure to loud noises
- Perforation of the tympanic membrane

With aging, changes occur in the ear that may eventually lead to hearing deficits. Although few changes occur in the external ear, cerumen tends to become harder and drier, posing a greater chance of impaction. In the middle ear, the tympanic membrane may atrophy or become sclerotic. In the inner ear, cells at the base of the cochlea degenerate. A familial predisposition to sensorineural hearing loss is also seen, manifested by a loss in the ability to hear high-frequency sounds, followed in time by the loss of middle and lower frequencies. The term **presbycusis** is used to describe this progressive hearing loss.

In addition to age-related changes, other factors can affect hearing in the elderly population, such as lifelong exposure to loud noises (eg, jets, guns, heavy machinery, circular saws). Certain medications, such as aminoglycosides and aspirin, have ototoxic effects when renal changes (eg, in the older person) result in delayed medication excretion and increased levels of the medications in the blood. Some older people take quinine for treatment of leg cramps; quinine can cause a hearing loss. Psychogenic factors and other disease processes (eg, diabetes) also may be partially responsible for sensorineural hearing loss.

When a hearing problem occurs, an evaluation is warranted. Even with the best medical care, the person must learn to adjust to various degrees of hearing loss. Care of elderly patients includes recognizing emotional reactions related to hearing loss, such as suspicion of others because of an inability to hear adequately; frustration and anger, with repeated statements such as, "I didn't hear what you said"; and feelings of insecurity because of the inability to hear the telephone or alarms.

Medical Management

If a hearing loss is permanent or untreatable with medical or surgical intervention or if the patient elects not to have surgery, aural rehabilitation (discussed at the end of the chapter) may be beneficial.

GENETICS IN NURSING PRACTICE—Hearing Disorders

SELECTED HEARING DISORDERS INFLUENCED BY GENETIC FACTORS
- Autosomal dominant hearing loss
- Autosomal recessive hearing loss (eg, connexin 26 gene)
- Otosclerosis
- Pendred syndrome
- Usher syndrome
- Waardenburg syndrome

NURSING ASSESSMENTS
FAMILY HISTORY ASSESSMENT
- Assess for other family members in several generations with hearing loss (autosomal dominant hearing loss)
- Inquire about genetic relatedness (eg, individuals who are related, such as first cousins, have a higher chance to share the same recessive genes—autosomal recessive hearing loss)
- Inquire about age at onset of hearing loss

PHYSICAL ASSESSMENT
- Assess for related genetic conditions, such as vision impairment (eg, retinitis pigmentosa in Usher syndrome; thyroid disorder in Pendred syndrome)
- Assess for iris, pigmentary, and hair alterations (white forelock) seen in Waardenburg syndrome

MANAGEMENT ISSUES SPECIFIC TO GENETICS
- Inquire whether DNA gene mutation or other genetic testing has been performed on affected family members.
- If indicated, refer for further genetic counselling and evaluation so that family members can discuss inheritance, risk to other family members, availability of genetic testing, and gene-based interventions.
- Offer appropriate genetics information and resources.
- Assess patient's understanding of genetics information.
- Provide support to families with newly diagnosed genetic-related sensorineural disorders.

- Participate in management and coordination of care of patients with genetic conditions, and individuals predisposed to develop or pass on a genetic condition.

GENETICS RESOURCES
Canadian Association of Genetic Counsellors (CAGC)—a listing of genetic centres across Canada; www.cagc-accg.ca

Canadian Cancer Society—information on genetic factors/risks and genetic testing; www.cancer.ca

Canadian Directory of Genetic Support Groups—resource guide for families and professionals; www.lhsc.on.ca/programs/medgenet

Canadian Genetic Disease Network—its stated mission is to be the primary catalyst in advancing Canada's scientific and commercial competitiveness in genetic research and the application of genetic discoveries to the prevention, diagnosis, and treatment of human disease; www.cgdn.ca

Canadian Organization for Rare Disorders (CORD)—information on over 6,000 rare disorders; links individuals/families together with the same rare disorder; www.cord.ca

Gene Clinics—a listing of common genetic disorders with up-to-date clinical summaries, genetic counselling and testing information; http//www.geneclinics.org

GeneTests—publicly funded medical genetics information resource developed for physicians, other health care providers, and researchers; www.genetests.org

Genetic Alliance—increases the capacity of genetic advocacy groups to achieve their missions and leverages the voices of millions of individuals and families living with genetic conditions; www.geneticalliance.org

The Genetics Society of Canada (GSC)—promotion of research and communication of the results and implications of genetics to the public; http://life.biology.mcmaster.ca/GSC

OMIM: Online Mendelian Inheritance in Man—a catalogue of human genes and genetic disorders; http://www.ncib.nlm.nih.gov/entrez/query.fcgi?db=omim

Nursing Management

The nurse who understands the different types of hearing loss will be more successful in adopting a communication style to fit the patient's needs. Trying to speak in a loud voice to a person who cannot hear high-frequency sounds only makes understanding more difficult. However, strategies such as talking into the less-impaired ear and using gestures and facial expressions can help (see Chart 59-4).

A major issue for many deaf and hearing-impaired people is that they have other health problems that often do not receive attention, in large part because of communication problems with their health care practitioners. To effectively meet the health care needs of these patients, practitioners are legally obligated to make accommodations for the patient's inability to hear. Providing the services of interpreters or those who can communicate through sign language is essential in many situations so that the practitioner can effectively communicate with the patient.

During health care and screening procedures, the practitioner (eg, dentist, physician, nurse) must be aware that patients who are deaf or hearing impaired are unable to read lips, see a signer, or read written materials in dark rooms required during some diagnostic tests. The same situation exists if the practitioner is wearing a mask or not in sight (eg, x-ray studies, magnetic resonance imaging [MRI], colonoscopy).

Nurses and other health care practitioners must work with deaf and hearing-impaired patients and their families to identify workable and effective means of communication. Nurses can serve as catalysts throughout the health care system to ensure that accommodations are made to meet the communication needs of these patients.

Conditions of the External Ear

CERUMEN IMPACTION

Cerumen normally accumulates in the external canal in various amounts and colours. Although wax does not usually need to be removed, impaction occasionally occurs, causing **otalgia**, a sensation of fullness or pain in the ear, with or without a hearing loss. Accumulation of cerumen is especially significant in the geriatric population as a cause of hearing deficit. Attempts to clear the ex-

ternal auditory canal with matches, hairpins, and other implements are dangerous because trauma to the skin, infection, and damage to the tympanic membrane can occur.

Management

Cerumen can be removed by irrigation, suction, or instrumentation. Unless the patient has a perforated eardrum or an inflamed external ear (ie, otitis externa), gentle irrigation usually helps remove impacted cerumen, particularly if it is not tightly packed in the external auditory canal. For successful removal, the water stream must flow behind the obstructing cerumen to move it first laterally and then out of the canal. To prevent injury, the lowest effective pressure should be used. If the eardrum behind the impaction is perforated, however, water can enter the middle ear, producing acute vertigo and infection. If irrigation is unsuccessful, direct visual, mechanical removal can be performed on a cooperative patient by a trained health care provider.

Instilling a few drops of warmed glycerin, mineral oil, or half-strength hydrogen peroxide into the ear canal for 30 minutes can soften cerumen before its removal. Ceruminolytic agents, such as peroxide in glyceryl (Debrox), are available; however, these compounds may cause an allergic dermatitis reaction. Using any softening solution two or three times a day for several days is generally sufficient. If the cerumen cannot be dislodged by these methods, instruments, such as a cerumen curette, aural suction, and a binocular microscope for magnification, can be used.

FOREIGN BODIES

Some objects are inserted intentionally into the ear by adults who may have been trying to clean the external canal or relieve itching or by children who introduce the objects. Other objects, such as insects, peas, beans, pebbles, toys, and beads, may enter or be introduced into the ear canal. In either case, the effects may range from no symptoms to profound pain and decreased hearing.

Management

Removing a foreign body from the external auditory canal can be quite challenging. The three standard methods for removing foreign bodies are the same as those for removing cerumen: irriga-

---

Chart 59-4 **Guidelines for Communicating With the Hearing-Impaired Person**

For the hearing-impaired person whose speech is difficult to understand:
- Devote full attention to what the person is saying. Look and listen—do not try to attend to another task while listening.
- Engage the speaker in conversation when it is possible for you to anticipate the replies. This enables you to become accustomed to any peculiarities in speech patterns.
- Try to determine the essential context of what is being said; you can often fill in the details from context.
- Do not try to appear as if you understand if you do not.
- If you cannot understand at all or have serious doubt about your ability to understand what is being said, have the person write the message rather than risk misunderstanding. Having the person repeat the message in speech, after you know its content, also aids you in becoming accustomed to the person's pattern of speech.

For the hearing-impaired person who speech reads:
- When speaking, always face the person as directly as possible.
- Make sure your face is as clearly visible as possible. Locate yourself so that your face is well lighted; avoid being silhouetted against strong light. Do not obscure the person's view of your mouth in any way; avoid talking with any object held in your mouth.
- Be sure that the patient knows the topic or subject before going ahead with what you plan to say. This enables the person to use contextual clues in speech reading.
- Speak slowly and distinctly, pausing more frequently than you would normally.
- If you question whether some important direction or instruction has been understood, check to be certain that the patient has the full meaning of your message.
- If for any reason your mouth must be covered (as with a mask) and you must direct or instruct the patient, write the message.

tion, suction, and instrumentation. The contraindications for irrigation are also the same. Foreign vegetable bodies and insects tend to swell; thus, irrigation is contraindicated. Usually, an insect can be dislodged by instilling mineral oil, which will kill the insect and allow it to be removed.

Attempts to remove any foreign body from the external canal may be dangerous in unskilled hands. The object may be pushed completely into the bony portion of the canal, lacerating the skin and perforating the tympanic membrane. In difficult cases, the foreign body may have to be extracted in the operating room with the patient under general anesthesia.

EXTERNAL OTITIS (OTITIS EXTERNA)

External otitis, or **otitis externa**, refers to an inflammation of the external auditory canal. Causes include water in the ear canal (ie, swimmer's ear); trauma to the skin of the ear canal, permitting entrance of organisms into the tissues; and systemic conditions, such as vitamin deficiency and endocrine disorders. Bacterial or fungal infections are most frequently encountered. The most common bacterial pathogens associated with external otitis are *Staphylococcus aureus* and *Pseudomonas* species. The most common fungus isolated in both normal and infected ears is *Aspergillus.* External otitis is often caused by a dermatosis such as psoriasis, eczema, or seborrheic dermatitis. Even allergic reactions to hair spray, hair dye, and permanent wave lotions can cause dermatitis, which clears when the offending agent is removed.

Clinical Manifestations

The patient usually reports pain, discharge from the external auditory canal, aural tenderness (usually not present in middle ear infections), and occasionally fever, cellulitis, and lymphadenopathy. Other symptoms may include pruritus and hearing loss or a feeling of fullness. On otoscopic examination, the ear canal is erythematous and edematous. Discharge may be yellow or green and foul smelling. In fungal infections, the hairlike black spores may even be visible.

Medical Management

The principles of therapy are aimed at relieving the discomfort, reducing the swelling of the ear canal, and eradicating the infection. Patients may require analgesics for the first 48 to 92 hours. If the tissues of the external canal are edematous, a wick should be inserted to keep the canal open so that liquid medications (eg, Burow's solution, antibiotic otic preparations) can be introduced. These medications may be administered by dropper at room temperature. Such medications usually combine antibiotic and corticosteroid agents to soothe the inflamed tissues. For cellulitis or fever, systemic antibiotics may be prescribed. For fungal disorders, antifungal agents are prescribed.

Nursing Management

Nurses need to teach patients not to clean the external auditory canal with cotton-tipped applicators, to avoid swimming, and not to allow water to enter the ear when shampooing or showering. A cotton ball can be covered in a water-insoluble gel such as petroleum jelly and placed in the ear as a barrier to water contamination. Infection can be prevented by using antiseptic otic preparations after swimming (eg, Swim Ear, Ear Dry), unless

there is a history of tympanic membrane perforation or a current ear infection.

MALIGNANT EXTERNAL OTITIS

A more serious, although rare, external ear infection is malignant external otitis (ie, temporal bone osteomyelitis). This is a progressive, debilitating, and occasionally fatal infection of the external auditory canal, the surrounding tissue, and the base of the skull. *Pseudomonas aeruginosa* is usually the infecting organism in patients with low resistance to infection (eg, patients with diabetes). Successful treatment includes control of the diabetes, administration of antibiotics (usually intravenously), and aggressive local wound care. Standard parenteral antibiotic treatment includes the combination of an antipseudomonal agent and an aminoglycoside, both of which have potentially serious side effects. Because aminoglycosides are nephrotoxic and ototoxic, serum aminoglycoside levels and renal and auditory function must be monitored during therapy. Local wound care includes limited débridement of the infected tissue, including bone and cartilage, depending on the extent of the infection.

MASSES OF THE EXTERNAL EAR

Exostoses are small, hard, bony protrusions found in the lower posterior bony portion of the ear canal; they usually occur bilaterally. The skin covering the exostosis is normal. Many people think exostoses are caused by an exposure to cold water, as in scuba diving or surfing. The usual treatment, if any, is surgical excision.

Malignant tumours also may be found in the external ear. Most common are basal cell carcinomas on the pinna and squamous cell carcinomas in the ear canal. If untreated, squamous cell carcinoma may spread through the temporal bone, causing facial nerve paralysis and hearing loss. Carcinomas must be treated surgically.

GAPPING EARRING PUNCTURE

Gapping earring puncture results from wearing heavy pierced earrings for a long time or after an infection, or as a reaction from the earring or other impurities in the earring. One or more gapping punctures may result from wearing more than one earring. Whatever its cause, this deformity can only be corrected surgically. The edges of the perforations are excised on the lateral and medial surfaces of the earlobe. Next, the entire tract is removed, joining the above two incisions and resulting in a much larger defect that is closed separately on each surface. Then, an antibiotic dressing is applied.

Conditions of the Middle Ear

TYMPANIC MEMBRANE PERFORATION

Perforation of the tympanic membrane is usually caused by infection or trauma. Sources of trauma include skull fracture, explosive injury, or a severe blow to the ear. Less frequently, perforation is caused by foreign objects (eg, cotton-tipped applicators, bobby pins, keys) that have been pushed too far into the external auditory canal. In addition to tympanic membrane perforation, injury to the ossicles and even the inner ear may result from this type of action. Attempts by patients to clear the external auditory canal should be discouraged. During infection, the tympanic membrane can rupture if the pressure in the middle ear exceeds the atmospheric pressure in the external auditory canal.

Medical Management

Although most tympanic membrane perforations heal spontaneously within weeks after rupture, some may take several months to heal. Some perforations persist because scar tissue grows over the edges of the perforation, preventing extension of the epithelial cells across the margins and final healing. In the case of a head injury or temporal bone fracture, a patient is observed for evidence of cerebrospinal fluid **otorrhea** or **rhinorrhea**—a clear, watery drainage from the ear or nose, respectively. While healing, the ear must be protected from water.

SURGICAL MANAGEMENT

Perforations that do not heal on their own may require surgery. The decision to perform a **tympanoplasty** (ie, surgical repair of the tympanic membrane) is usually based on the need to prevent potential infection from water entering the ear or the desire to improve the patient's hearing. Performed on an outpatient basis, tympanoplasty may involve a variety of surgical techniques. In all techniques, tissue is placed across the perforation to allow healing. Surgery is usually successful in closing the perforation permanently and improving hearing.

ACUTE OTITIS MEDIA

Acute otitis media is an acute infection of the middle ear, usually lasting less than 6 weeks. The primary cause of acute otitis media is usually *Streptococcus pneumoniae, Haemophilus influenzae,* and *Moraxella catarrhalis,* which enter the middle ear after eustachian tube dysfunction caused by obstruction related to upper respiratory infections, inflammation of surrounding structures (eg, sinusitis, adenoid hypertrophy), or allergic reactions (eg, allergic rhinitis). Bacteria can enter the eustachian tube from contaminated secretions in the nasopharynx and the middle ear from a tympanic membrane perforation. A purulent exudate is usually present in the middle ear, resulting in a conductive hearing loss.

Clinical Manifestations

The symptoms of otitis media vary with the severity of the infection. The condition, usually unilateral in adults, may be accompanied by otalgia. The pain is relieved after spontaneous perforation or therapeutic incision of the tympanic membrane. Other symptoms may include drainage from the ear, fever, and hearing loss. On otoscopic examination, the external auditory canal appears normal. The patient reports no pain with movement of the auricle. The tympanic membrane is erythematous and often bulging. Table 59-3 differentiates acute external otitis from acute otitis media.

Medical Management

The outcome of acute otitis media depends on the efficacy of therapy (ie, the prescribed dose of an oral antibiotic and the duration of therapy), the virulence of the bacteria, and the physical status of the patient. With early and appropriate broad-spectrum antibiotic therapy, otitis media may resolve with no serious sequelae. If drainage occurs, an antibiotic otic preparation is usually prescribed. The condition may become subacute (lasting 3 weeks to 3 months), with persistent purulent discharge from the ear. Rarely does permanent hearing loss occur. Secondary complications involving the mastoid and other serious intracranial complications, such as meningitis or brain abscess, although rare, can occur.

SURGICAL MANAGEMENT

An incision in the tympanic membrane is known as **myringotomy** or **tympanotomy**. The tympanic membrane is numbed with a local anesthetic such as phenol or by iontophoresis (ie, electrical current flows through a lidocaine-and-epinephrine solution to numb the ear canal and tympanic membrane). The procedure is painless and takes less than 15 minutes. Under microscopic guidance, an incision is made through the tympanic membrane to relieve pressure and to drain serous or purulent fluid from the middle ear.

Normally, this procedure is unnecessary for treating acute otitis media, but it may be performed if pain persists. Myringotomy also allows the drainage to be analyzed (by culture and sensitivity testing) so that the infecting organism can be identified and appropriate antibiotic therapy prescribed. The incision heals within 24 to 72 hours.

If episodes of acute otitis media recur and there is no contraindication, a ventilating, or pressure-equalizing, tube may be inserted. The ventilating tube, which temporarily takes the place of the eustachian tube in equalizing pressure, is retained for 6 to 18 months. The ventilating tube is then extruded with normal skin migration of the tympanic membrane, with the hole healing in nearly every case. Ventilating tubes are more commonly used to treat recurrent episodes of acute otitis media in children than in adults.

SEROUS OTITIS MEDIA

Serous otitis media (ie, **middle ear effusion**) implies fluid, without evidence of active infection, in the middle ear. In theory, this fluid results from a negative pressure in the middle ear caused by eustachian tube obstruction. This condition is found primarily in children. When it occurs in adults, an underlying cause for the eustachian tube dysfunction must be sought. Middle ear effusion

Table 59-3 • **Clinical Features of Otitis**		
FEATURE	ACUTE OTITIS EXTERNA	ACUTE OTITIS MEDIA
Otorrhea	May or may not be present	Present if tympanic membrane perforates; discharge is profuse
Otalgia	Persistent, may awaken patient at night	Relieved if tympanic membrane ruptures
Aural tenderness	Present on palpation of auricle	Usually absent
Systemic symptoms	Absent	Fever, upper respiratory infection, rhinitis
Edema of external auditory canal	Present	Absent
Tympanic membrane	May appear normal	Erythema, bulging, may be perforated
Hearing loss	Conductive type	Conductive type

is frequently seen in patients after radiation therapy or barotrauma and in patients with eustachian tube dysfunction from a concurrent upper respiratory infection or allergy. Barotrauma results from sudden pressure changes in the middle ear caused by changes in barometric pressure, as in scuba diving or airplane descent. A carcinoma (eg, nasopharyngeal cancer) obstructing the eustachian tube should be ruled out in an adult with persistent unilateral serous otitis media.

Clinical Manifestations

Patients may complain of hearing loss, fullness in the ear or a sensation of congestion, and perhaps even popping and crackling noises, which occur as the eustachian tube attempts to open. The tympanic membrane appears dull on otoscopy, and air bubbles may be visualized in the middle ear. Usually, the audiogram shows a conductive hearing loss.

Management

Serous otitis media need not be treated medically unless infection occurs (ie, acute otitis media). If the hearing loss associated with middle ear effusion is a problem for the patient, a myringotomy can be performed, and a tube may be placed to keep the middle ear ventilated. Corticosteroids in small doses sometimes decrease the edema of the eustachian tube in cases of barotrauma. Decongestants have not proved effective. A Valsalva manoeuvre, which forcibly opens the eustachian tube by increasing nasopharyngeal pressure, may be cautiously performed. Performing the Valsalva manoeuvre may cause worsening pain or perforation of the tympanic membrane.

CHRONIC OTITIS MEDIA

Chronic otitis media is the result of repeated episodes of acute otitis media causing irreversible tissue pathology and persistent perforation of the tympanic membrane. Chronic infections of the middle ear damage the tympanic membrane, destroy the ossicles, and involve the mastoid. Before the discovery of antibiotics, infections of the mastoid were life-threatening. The use of medications in acute otitis media has made acute mastoiditis a rare condition in developed countries.

Clinical Manifestations

Symptoms may be minimal, with varying degrees of hearing loss and the presence of a persistent or intermittent, foul-smelling otorrhea. Pain is not usually experienced, except in cases of acute mastoiditis, when the postauricular area is tender to the touch and may be erythematous and edematous. Otoscopic evaluation of the tympanic membrane may show a perforation, and cholesteatoma can be identified as a white mass behind the tympanic membrane or coming through to the external canal from a perforation.

Cholesteatoma is an ingrowth of the skin of the external layer of the eardrum into the middle ear. It is generally caused by a chronic retraction pocket of the tympanic membrane, creating a persistently high negative pressure of the middle ear. The skin forms a sac that fills with degenerated skin and sebaceous materials. The sac can attach to the structures of the middle ear or mastoid, or both. Cholesteatoma alone usually does not cause pain; however, if treatment or surgery is delayed, the cholesteatoma may destroy structures of the temporal bone. In cases of cholesteatoma, audiometric tests often show a conductive or mixed hearing loss.

Medical Management

Local treatment of chronic otitis media consists of careful suctioning of the ear under microscopic guidance. Instillation of antibiotic drops or application of antibiotic powder is used to treat a purulent discharge. Systemic antibiotics are usually not prescribed except in cases of acute infection.

SURGICAL MANAGEMENT

Surgical procedures, including tympanoplasty, ossiculoplasty, and mastoidectomy, are used after medical treatments are determined to be ineffective. Chronic otitis media can cause chronic mastoiditis and lead to the formation of cholesteatoma. It can occur in the middle ear, mastoid cavity, or both, often dictating the type of surgery to be performed. If untreated, cholesteatoma will continue to enlarge, possibly causing damage to the facial nerve and horizontal canal and destruction of other surrounding structures.

Tympanoplasty. The most common surgical procedure for chronic otitis media is a tympanoplasty, or surgical reconstruction of the tympanic membrane. Reconstruction of the ossicles may also be required. The purposes of a tympanoplasty are to reestablish middle ear function, close the perforation, prevent recurrent infection, and improve hearing.

There are five types of tympanoplasties. The simplest surgical procedure, type I (myringoplasty), is designed to close a perforation in the tympanic membrane. The other procedures, types II through V, involve more extensive repair of middle ear structures. The structures and the degree of involvement can differ, but all tympanoplasty procedures include restoring the continuity of the sound conduction mechanism.

Tympanoplasty is performed through the external auditory canal with a transcanal approach or through a postauricular incision. The contents of the middle ear are carefully inspected, and the ossicular chain is evaluated. Ossicular interruption is most frequent in chronic otitis media, but problems of reconstruction can also occur with malformations of the middle ear and ossicular dislocations due to head injuries. Dramatic improvement in hearing can result from closure of a perforation and reestablishment of the ossicles. Surgery is usually performed in an outpatient environment under moderate sedation or general anesthesia.

Ossiculoplasty. Many people use the term _tympanoplasty_ to include **ossiculoplasty**, or surgical reconstruction of the middle ear bones to restore hearing. Prostheses made of materials such as Teflon, stainless steel, and hydroxyapatite are used to reconnect the ossicles, thereby reestablishing the sound conduction mechanism. However, the greater the damage, the lower the success rate for restoring normal hearing.

Mastoidectomy. The objectives of mastoid surgery are to remove the cholesteatoma, gain access to diseased structures, and create a dry and healthy ear. If possible, the ossicles are reconstructed during the initial surgical procedure. Occasionally, extensive disease dictates that this be performed as part of a planned second-stage operation.

A mastoidectomy is usually performed through a postauricular incision. Infection is eliminated by removing the mastoid air cells. Although infrequently injured, the facial nerve, which runs through the middle ear and mastoid, is at some risk for injury during mastoid surgery. As the patient awakens from anesthesia, any evidence of facial paresis should be reported to the physician. A second mastoidectomy may be necessary to check for recurrent or residual cholesteatoma. The hearing mechanism may be reconstructed at this time. The success rate for correcting this conductive hearing loss is approximately 75%. Surgery is usually performed in an outpatient setting. The patient has a mastoid pressure dressing, which can be removed 24 to 48 hours after surgery.

NURSING PROCESS: THE PATIENT UNDERGOING MASTOID SURGERY

Although several otologic surgical procedures are performed under moderate sedation, mastoid surgery is performed using general anesthesia.

Assessment

The health history includes a complete description of the ear problem, including infection, otalgia, otorrhea, hearing loss, and vertigo. Data are collected about the duration and intensity of the problem, its causes, and previous treatments. Information is obtained about other health problems and all medications that the patient is taking. Medication allergies and family history of ear disease also should be obtained.

Physical assessment includes observation for erythema, edema, otorrhea, lesions, and characteristics such as odour and colour of discharge. The results of the audiogram should be reviewed.

Nursing Diagnoses

Based on the assessment data, the patient's major nursing diagnoses may include the following:

- Anxiety related to surgical procedure, potential loss of hearing, potential taste disturbance, and potential loss of facial movement
- Acute pain related to mastoid surgery
- Risk for infection related to mastoidectomy, placement of grafts, prostheses, electrodes, and surgical trauma to surrounding tissues and structures
- Disturbed auditory sensory perception related to ear disorder, surgery, or packing
- Risk for trauma related to balance difficulties or vertigo during the immediate postoperative period
- Disturbed sensory perception related to potential damage to facial nerve (cranial nerve VII) and chorda tympani nerve
- Impaired skin integrity related to ear surgery, incisions, and graft sites
- Deficient knowledge about mastoid disease, surgical procedure, and postoperative care and expectations

Planning and Goals

The major goals of caring for a patient undergoing mastoidectomy include reduction of anxiety; freedom from pain and discomfort; prevention of infection; stable or improved hearing and communication; absence of injury from vertigo; absence of or adjustment to sensory or perceptual alterations; return of skin integrity; and increased knowledge regarding the disease, surgical procedure, and postoperative care.

Nursing Interventions

REDUCING ANXIETY

Information that the otologic surgeon has discussed with the patient, including anesthesia, the location of the incision (postauricular), and expected surgical results (eg, hearing, balance, taste, facial movement), is reinforced. The patient also is encouraged to discuss any anxieties and concerns about the surgery.

RELIEVING PAIN

Although most patients complain very little about incisional pain after mastoid surgery, they do have some ear discomfort. Aural fullness or pressure after surgery is caused by residual blood or fluid in the middle ear. The prescribed analgesic may be taken for the first 24 hours after surgery and then only as needed. The patient is instructed in the use of and side effects of the medication.

A tympanoplasty may also be performed at the time of the mastoidectomy. A wick or external auditory canal packing is used after a tympanoplasty to stabilize the tympanic membrane. Patients should be informed that they may experience intermittent sharp, shooting pains in the ear for 2 to 3 weeks after surgery as the eustachian tube opens and allows air to enter the middle ear.

PREVENTING INFECTION

Measures are initiated to prevent infection in the operated ear. The external auditory canal wick, or packing, may be impregnated with an antibiotic solution before instillation. Prophylactic antibiotics are administered as prescribed, and the patient is instructed to prevent water from entering the external auditory canal for 6 weeks. A cotton ball or lamb's wool covered with a water-insoluble substance (eg, petroleum jelly) and placed loosely in the ear canal usually prevents water contamination. The postauricular incision should be kept dry for 2 days. Signs of infection such as an elevated temperature and purulent drainage are reported. Some serosanguineous drainage from the external auditory canal is normal after surgery.

IMPROVING HEARING AND COMMUNICATION

Hearing in the operated ear may be reduced for several weeks because of edema, accumulation of blood and tissue fluid in the middle ear, and dressings or packing. Measures are initiated to improve hearing and communication, such as reducing environmental noise, facing the patient when speaking, speaking clearly and distinctly without shouting, providing good lighting if the patient relies on speech reading, and using nonverbal clues (eg, facial expression, pointing, gestures) and other forms of communication. Family members or significant others are instructed about effective ways to communicate with the patient. If the patient uses assistive hearing devices, one can be used in the unaffected ear.

PREVENTING INJURY

Vertigo may occur after mastoid surgery if the semicircular canals or other areas of the inner ear are traumatized. This symptom is relatively uncommon after this type of ear surgery and usually is temporary. Antiemetics or antivertiginous medications (eg, antihistamines) can be prescribed if a balance disturbance or vertigo occurs. The patient should be instructed about the expected effects and potential side effects. Safety measures such as assisted ambulation are implemented to prevent falls. Safety measures must also be implemented at home to prevent falls and injury.

PREVENTING ALTERED SENSORY PERCEPTION

Facial nerve injury is a potential, although rare, complication of mastoid surgery. The patient is instructed to report immediately any evidence of facial nerve (cranial nerve VII) weakness, such as drooping of the mouth on the operated side. A more frequent occurrence is a temporary disturbance in the chorda tympani nerve, a small branch of the facial nerve that runs through the middle ear. Patients experience a taste disturbance and dry mouth on the side of surgery for several months until the nerve regenerates.

PROMOTING WOUND HEALING

The patient is instructed to avoid heavy lifting, straining, exertion, and nose blowing for 2 to 3 weeks after surgery to prevent dislodging the tympanic membrane graft or ossicular prosthesis.

INCREASING KNOWLEDGE

The patient is informed about the surgery and operating room environment. Discussing postoperative expectations helps to decrease anxiety about the unknown. Because postoperative instructions for mastoid surgery vary among otologic surgeons, it is important for the nurse to be aware of the surgeon's preferences when teaching the patient.

PROMOTING HOME AND COMMUNITY-BASED CARE

Teaching Patients Self-Care

Patients require instruction about prescribed medication therapy, such as analgesics, antivertiginous agents, and antihistamines prescribed for balance disturbance. Teaching includes information about the expected effects and potential side effects of the medication. Patients also need instruction about any activity restrictions. Possible complications such as infection, facial nerve weakness, or taste disturbances, including the signs and symptoms to report immediately, should be addressed (see Chart 59-5).

Continuing Care

Some patients, particularly elderly patients, who have had mastoid surgery may require the services of a home care nurse for a few days after returning home. However, most people find that assistance from a family member or a friend is sufficient. The caregiver and patient are cautioned that the patient may experience some vertigo and will therefore require help with ambulation to avoid falling. Any symptoms of complications are to be reported promptly to the surgeon. The importance of scheduling and keeping follow-up appointments is also stressed.

Evaluation

EXPECTED PATIENT OUTCOMES

Expected patient outcomes may include:

1. Demonstrates reduced anxiety about surgical procedure
   a. Verbalizes and exhibits less stress, tension, and irritability
   b. Verbalizes acceptance of the results of surgery and adjustment to possible hearing impairment
2. Remains free of discomfort or pain
   a. Exhibits no facial grimacing, moaning, or crying, and reports absence of pain
   b. Uses analgesics appropriately
3. Demonstrates no signs or symptoms of infection
   a. Has normal vital signs, including temperature
   b. Demonstrates absence of purulent drainage from the external auditory canal

Chart 59-5 • PATIENT EDUCATION
Self-Care After Middle Ear or Mastoid Surgery

Postoperative instructions for patients who have had middle ear and mastoid surgery vary greatly among otolaryngologists. These patient teaching guidelines may require modification for the individual patient.

- Take antibiotics and other medications as prescribed.
- Blow nose gently one side at a time for 1 week after surgery.
- Sneeze and cough with the mouth open for a few weeks after surgery.
- Check with your health care provider about returning to work (usually 2 to 3 days postoperatively). Avoid heavy lifting (>11.4 kg), straining, and bending over for a few weeks after surgery.
- Know that popping and crackling in the operative ear is normal for approximately 3 to 5 weeks after surgery.
- Be aware that packing in the operated ear, as well as blood and fluid in the middle ear after surgery, will cause a hearing loss. You may also feel that you are talking in a well or hearing echoes.
- Remember that minor ear discomfort is normal; use the analgesics prescribed. Report any excessive ear pain to the surgeon.
- Note that some slightly bloody or serosanguineous drainage from the ear is normal after surgery. Report any excessive or purulent ear drainage to the surgeon.
- Change the cotton ball in the ear as needed.
- Check with the surgeon for instructions regarding air travel.
- Avoid getting water in the operated ear for 2 weeks after surgery. You may shampoo the hair 2 to 3 days postoperatively if the ear is protected from water by saturating a cotton ball with petroleum jelly (or some other water-insoluble substance) and loosely placing it in the ear. If the postauricular suture line becomes wet, pat (not rub) the area and cover it with a thin layer of antibiotic ointment.

   c. Describes method for preventing water from contaminating packing
4. Exhibits signs that hearing has stabilized or improved
   a. Describes surgical goal for hearing and judges whether the goal has been met
   b. Verbalizes that hearing has improved
5. Remains free of injury and trauma because of vertigo
   a. Reports absence of vertigo or balance disturbance
   b. Experiences no injury or fall
   c. Modifies environment to avoid falls (eg, night light, no clutter on stairs)
6. Adjusts to or remains free from altered sensory perception
   a. Reports no taste disturbance, mouth dryness, or facial weakness
7. Demonstrates no skin breakdown
   a. Lists ways to prevent dislodging graft or prosthesis
   b. Is aware of limitations in activities (eg, bathing, lifting, air travel) and for how long
8. Verbalizes the reasons for and methods of care and treatment
   a. Shares knowledge with family about treatment protocol
   b. Describes treatment and the time frame for the recovery phase
   c. Discusses the discharge plan formulated with the nurse with regard to rest periods, medication, and activities permitted and restricted

d. Lists symptoms that should be reported to health care personnel
e. Keeps follow-up appointments

OTOSCLEROSIS

Otosclerosis involves the stapes and is thought to result from the formation of new, abnormal spongy bone, especially around the oval window, with resulting fixation of the stapes. The efficient transmission of sound is prevented because the stapes cannot vibrate and carry the sound as conducted from the malleus and incus to the inner ear. More common in women and frequently hereditary, otosclerosis may be worsened by pregnancy.

Clinical Manifestations

The condition can involve one or both ears and manifests as a progressive conductive or mixed hearing loss. The patient may or may not complain of tinnitus. Otoscopic examination usually reveals a normal tympanic membrane. Bone conduction is better than air conduction on Rinne testing. The audiogram confirms conductive hearing loss or mixed loss, especially in the low frequencies.

Medical Management

There is no known nonsurgical treatment for otosclerosis. However, some physicians believe the use of Florical (a fluoride supplement) can mature the abnormal spongy bone growth. Amplification with a hearing aid also may help.

SURGICAL MANAGEMENT

A stapedectomy, performed through the canal, involves removing the stapes superstructure and part of the footplate and inserting a tissue graft and a suitable prosthesis (Fig. 59-8). Some surgeons elect to remove only a small part of the stapes footplate (ie, stapedotomy). Regardless of the method used, the prosthesis bridges the gap between the incus and the inner ear, providing better sound conduction. Stapes surgery is very successful in improving hearing. Balance disturbance or true vertigo, which rarely occurs in other middle ear surgical procedures, can occur for a short time after stapedectomy.

MIDDLE EAR MASSES

Other than cholesteatoma, masses in the middle ear are rare. Glomus jugulare is a tumour that arises from the jugular bulb. A his-

FIGURE 59-8 Stapedectomy for otosclerosis. (**A**) Normal anatomy. (**B**) Arrow points to sclerotic process at the foot of the stapes. (**C**) Stapes broken away surgically from its diseased base. The hole in the footplate provides an area where an instrument can grasp the plate. (**D**) The footplate is removed from its base. Some otosclerotic tissue may remain, and tissue is placed over it. (**E**) Robinson stainless-steel prosthesis in position.

tologically identical tumour that arises from Jacobson's nerve and remains limited to the middle ear is known as a glomus tympanicum. On otoscopy, a red blemish on or behind the tympanic membrane is indicative of a glomus tumour. The treatment for glomus tumours is surgical excision, except in poor surgical candidates, in whom radiation therapy is used.

A facial nerve neuroma is a tumour on cranial nerve VII, the facial nerve. These types of tumours are usually not visible on otoscopic examination but are suspected when a patient presents with a facial nerve paresis. X-ray evaluation is necessary to determine the site of the tumour along the facial nerve. The treatment is surgical removal.

Other less common problems of the middle ear include cholesterin granuloma and tympanosclerosis. Cholesterin granuloma is an immune system reaction to the byproducts of blood (ie, cholesterol crystals) within the middle ear. Tympanosclerosis is a deposit of collagen and minerals within the middle ear that can harden around the ossicles as a result of repeated infections. It can also be found as plaque on the tympanic membrane; this can decrease hearing.

Conditions of the Inner Ear

Disorders of balance and the vestibular system involving the inner ear afflict more than 30 million Americans 17 years of age or older. Falls resulting from these disorders account for more than 100,000 hip fractures in elderly people each year (NIDCD, 1998).

The term **dizziness** is used frequently by patients and health care providers to describe any altered sensation of orientation in space. **Vertigo** is defined as the misperception or illusion of motion of the person or the surroundings. Most people with vertigo describe a spinning sensation or say they feel as though objects are moving around them. Ataxia is a failure of muscular coordination and may be present in patients with vestibular disease. Syncope, fainting, and loss of consciousness are not forms of vertigo, nor are they characteristic of an ear problem; they usually indicate disease in the cardiovascular system.

Nystagmus is an involuntary rhythmic movement of the eyes. Nystagmus occurs normally when a person watches a rapidly moving object (eg, through the side window of a moving car or train). However, pathologically it is an ocular disorder associated with vestibular dysfunction. Nystagmus can be horizontal, vertical, or rotary and can be caused by a disorder in the central or peripheral nervous system.

MOTION SICKNESS

Motion sickness is a disturbance of equilibrium caused by constant motion. For example, it can occur aboard a ship, while riding on a merry-go-round or swing, or in the back seat of a car.

Clinical Manifestations

The syndrome manifests itself in sweating, pallor, nausea, and vomiting caused by vestibular overstimulation. These manifestations may persist for several hours after the stimulation stops.

Management

Over-the-counter antihistamines used to treat vertigo, such as dimenhydrinate (Dramamine) or meclizine hydrochloride (Bonine), provide some relief. Anticholinergic medications, such as scopo-

lamine patches, may be helpful. These must be replaced every few days. Side effects such as dry mouth and drowsiness occur with these medications, which may prove to be more troublesome than helpful. Potentially hazardous activities such as driving a car or operating heavy machinery should be avoided if the patient experiences drowsiness.

MÉNIÈRE'S DISEASE

Ménière's disease is an abnormal inner ear fluid balance caused by a malabsorption in the endolymphatic sac. Evidence indicates that many people with Ménière's disease may have a blockage in the endolymphatic duct. Regardless of the cause, **endolymphatic hydrops**, a dilation in the endolymphatic space, develops. Either increased pressure in the system or rupture of the inner ear membranes occurs, producing symptoms of Ménière's disease.

Ménière's disease affects more than 2.4 million people in the United States. More common in adults, it has an average age of onset in the 40s, with symptoms usually beginning between the ages of 20 and 60 years. However, the disease has been reported in children as young as age 4 years and in adults up to the 90s. Ménière's disease appears to be equally common in both genders. The right and left ears are affected with equal frequency; the disease occurs bilaterally in about 20% of patients. About 20% of the patients have a positive family history for the disease (Knox & McPherson, 1997).

Clinical Manifestations

Ménière's disease involves the following symptoms: fluctuating, progressive sensorineural hearing loss; **tinnitus** or a roaring sound; a feeling of pressure or fullness in the ear; and episodic, incapacitating vertigo, often accompanied by nausea and vomiting. The effects of these symptoms range from a minor nuisance to extreme disability, especially if the attacks of vertigo are severe. At the onset of the disease, perhaps only one or two of the symptoms are manifested.

Some clinicians believe that there are two subsets of the disease, known as atypical Ménière's disease: cochlear and vestibular. Cochlear Ménière's disease is recognized as a fluctuating, progressive sensorineural hearing loss associated with tinnitus and aural pressure in the absence of vestibular symptoms or findings. Vestibular Ménière's disease is characterized as the occurrence of episodic vertigo associated with aural pressure but no cochlear symptoms. In some patients, cochlear or vestibular Ménière's disease develops first. In most patients, however, all of the symptoms develop eventually.

Assessment and Diagnostic Findings

Vertigo is usually the most troublesome complaint. A careful history is taken to determine the frequency, duration, severity, and character of the vertigo attacks. Typically, the patient reports that vertigo lasts minutes to hours, possibly accompanied by nausea or vomiting. Patients also complain of diaphoresis and a persistent feeling of imbalance or disequilibrium, which may last for days. They may complain of attacks that awaken them at night. Between attacks, however, they usually feel well. The hearing loss may fluctuate, with tinnitus and aural pressure waxing and waning with changes in hearing. The tinnitus and feeling of aural pressure may occur only during or before attacks, or they may be constant.

Findings of the physical examination are usually normal, with the exception of the evaluation of cranial nerve VIII. Sounds from a tuning fork (ie, Weber test) may lateralize to the ear opposite the hearing loss, the one affected with Ménière's disease. An audiogram typically reveals a sensorineural hearing loss in the affected ear. This can be in the form of a "Pike's Peak" pattern, which looks like a hill or mountain, or it may show a sensorineural loss in the low frequencies. As the disease progresses, the hearing loss increases. The electronystagmogram may be normal or may show reduced vestibular response. There is, however, no absolute diagnostic test.

Medical Management

Most patients with Ménière's disease can be successfully treated with diet and medication therapy. Many patients can control their symptoms by adhering to a low-sodium (2,000 mg/day) diet. The amount of sodium is one of many factors that regulate the balance of fluid within the body. Sodium and fluid retention disrupts the delicate balance between endolymph and perilymph in the inner ear. Psychological evaluation may be indicated if the patient is anxious, uncertain, fearful, or depressed.

PHARMACOLOGIC THERAPY

Pharmacologic therapy for Ménière's disease consists of antihistamines such as meclizine (Antivert), which suppress the vestibular system. Tranquilizers such as diazepam (Valium) may be used in acute instances to help control vertigo. Antiemetics such as promethazine (Phenergan) suppositories help control the nausea and vomiting and the vertigo because of their antihistamine effect. Diuretic therapy (eg, hydrochlorothiazide) sometimes relieves symptoms by lowering the pressure in the endolymphatic system. Intake of foods containing potassium (eg, bananas, tomatoes, oranges) is necessary if the patient takes a diuretic that causes potassium loss.

Vasodilators, such as nicotinic acid, papaverine hydrochloride (Pavabid), and methantheline bromide (Banthine), have no scientific basis for alleviating the symptoms, but they are often used in conjunction with other therapies.

SURGICAL MANAGEMENT

Although most patients respond well to conservative therapy, some continue to have disabling attacks of vertigo. If these attacks reduce their quality of life, patients may elect to undergo surgery for relief. However, hearing loss, tinnitus, and aural fullness may continue, because the surgical treatment of Ménière's disease is aimed at eliminating the attacks of vertigo.

Endolymphatic Sac Decompression. Endolymphatic sac decompression, or shunting, theoretically equalizes the pressure in the endolymphatic space. A shunt or drain is inserted in the endolymphatic sac through a postauricular incision. This procedure is favoured by many otolaryngologists as a first-line surgical approach to treat the vertigo of Ménière's disease because it is relatively simple and safe and can be performed on an outpatient basis.

Middle and Inner Ear Perfusion. Ototoxic medications, such as streptomycin or gentamicin, can be given to patients by infusion into the middle and inner ear. These medications are used to decrease vestibular function and decrease vertigo. The success rate for eliminating vertigo is high, about 85%, but the risk of significant hearing loss is also high. This procedure of inner ear perfusion usually requires an overnight stay in the hospital. After the procedure, many patients have a period of imbalance that lasts several weeks.

Intraotologic Catheters. In an attempt to deliver medication directly to the inner ear, catheters are being developed to provide a conduit from the outer ear to the inner ear. The route of the catheter is from the external ear canal through or around the tympanic membrane and to the round window niche or membrane. Medicinal fluids can be placed against the round window for a direct route to the inner ear fluids.

Potential uses of these catheters include treatment for sudden hearing loss and various disorders causing intractable vertigo. Future applications may include tinnitus and slowly progressing sensorineural hearing loss. Intratympanic injections of ototoxic medications for round window membrane diffusion can be used to decrease vestibular function. Established surgical techniques can be used for the patient with vertigo who has not responded to medical or physical therapeutic modalities.

Vestibular Nerve Section. Vestibular nerve section provides the greatest success rate (approximately 98%) in eliminating the attacks of vertigo. It can be performed by a translabyrinthine approach (ie, through the hearing mechanism) or in a manner that can conserve hearing (ie, suboccipital or middle cranial fossa), depending on the degree of hearing loss. Most patients with incapacitating Ménière's disease have little or no effective hearing. Cutting the nerve prevents the brain from receiving input from the semicircular canals. This procedure requires a brief hospital stay. Nursing care for the patient with vertigo is presented in Plan of Nursing Care 59-1.

LABYRINTHITIS

Labyrinthitis, an inflammation of the inner ear, can be bacterial or viral in origin. Although rare because of antibiotic therapy, bacterial labyrinthitis usually occurs as a complication of otitis media. The infection can enter the inner ear by penetrating the membranes of the oval or round windows. Viral labyrinthitis is a common medical diagnosis, but little is known about this disorder, which affects hearing and balance. The most commonly identified viral causes are mumps, rubella, rubeola, and influenza. Viral illnesses of the upper respiratory tract and herpetiform disorders of the facial and acoustic nerves (ie, Ramsay Hunt syndrome) also cause labyrinthitis.

Clinical Manifestations

Labyrinthitis is characterized by a sudden onset of incapacitating vertigo, usually with nausea and vomiting, various degrees of hearing loss, and possibly tinnitus. The first episode is usually the worst; subsequent attacks, which usually occur over a period of several weeks to months, are less severe.

Management

Treatment of bacterial labyrinthitis includes intravenous antibiotic therapy, fluid replacement, and administration of a vestibular suppressant, such as meclizine, and antiemetic medications. Treatment of viral labyrinthitis is tailored to the patient's symptoms.

BENIGN PAROXYSMAL POSITIONAL VERTIGO

Benign paroxysmal positional vertigo (BPPV) is a brief period of incapacitating vertigo that occurs when the position of the patient's head is changed with respect to gravity, typically by plac-

(text continues on page 1821)

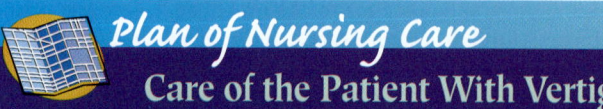

Plan of Nursing Care
Care of the Patient With Vertigo

Nursing Interventions	Rationale	Expected Patient Outcomes

Nursing Diagnosis: Risk for injury related to altered mobility because of gait disturbance and vertigo
Goal: Remains free of any injuries associated with imbalance and/or falls

Nursing Interventions	Rationale	Expected Patient Outcomes
1. Assess for vertigo, including history, onset, description of attacks, duration, frequency, and any associated ear symptoms (hearing loss, tinnitus, aural fullness).	1. History provides basis for interventions.	• Experiences no falls due to balance disturbance • Fear and anxiety are reduced • Performs exercises as prescribed • Takes prescribed medications appropriately • Assumes safe position when vertigo is present • Keeps head still when vertigo is present • Identifies a characteristic fullness or sense of pressure in the ear as occurring before a full-blown attack • Reports measures that help reduce vertigo
2. Assess extent of disability in relation to activities of daily living.	2. Extent of disability indicates risk of falling.	
3. Teach or reinforce vestibular/balance therapy as prescribed.	3. Exercises hasten labyrinthine compensation, which may decrease vertigo and gait disturbance.	
4. Administer, or teach administration of, antivertiginous medications and/or vestibular sedation medication; instruct patient about side effects.	4. Alleviates acute symptoms of vertigo	
5. Encourage patient to sit down when dizzy.	5. Decreases possibility of falling and injury	
6. Place pillow on each side of head to restrict movement.	6. Movement aggravates vertigo.	
7. Assist patient in identifying aura that suggests an impending attack.	7. Recognition of aura may trigger the need to take medication before an attack occurs, thereby minimizing the severity of effects.	
8. Recommend that the patient keep eyes open and stare straight ahead when lying down and experiencing vertigo.	8. Sensation of vertigo decreases and motion decelerates if eyes are kept in a fixed position.	

Nursing Diagnosis: Impaired adjustment related to disability requiring change in lifestyle due to unpredictability of vertigo
Goal: Modifies lifestyle to decrease disability and exert maximum control and independence within limits posed by chronic vertigo

Nursing Interventions	Rationale	Expected Patient Outcomes
1. Encourage patient to identify personal strengths and roles that can still be fulfilled.	1. Maximizes sense of regaining control and independence	• Exerts maximum control of environment and independence within limits imposed by vertigo • Is informed about condition • Family and significant others are included in rehabilitation process • Uses strengths and potentials to engage in the most independent and constructive lifestyle
2. Provide information about vertigo and what to expect.	2. Reduces fear and anxiety	
3. Include family and significant others in rehabilitative process.	3. Perceived beliefs of significant others are important for patient's adherence to medical regimen.	
4. Encourage patient to maintain sense of control by making decisions and assuming more responsibility for care.	4. Reinforces positive psychological and social outcomes	

Nursing Diagnosis: Risk for deficient fluid volume related to increased fluid output, altered intake, and medications
Goal: Maintains a normal fluid-electrolyte balance

Nursing Interventions	Rationale	Expected Patient Outcomes
1. Assess, or have patient assess, intake and output (including emesis, liquid stools, urine, and diaphoresis). Monitor laboratory values.	1. Accurate records provide basis for fluid replacement.	• Laboratory values within normal limits • Alert and oriented; vital signs within normal limits, skin turgor normal; electrolytes normal • Mucous membranes are moist • Vomiting or diarrhea has stopped; usual oral intake resumed
2. Assess indicators of dehydration, including blood pressure (orthostasis), pulse, skin turgor, mucous membranes, and level of consciousness.	2. Prompt recognition of dehydration allows early intervention.	

(continued)

Plan of Nursing Care
Care of the Patient With Vertigo *(Continued)*

Nursing Interventions	Rationale	Expected Patient Outcomes
3. Encourage oral fluids as tolerated; discourage beverages containing caffeine (a vestibular stimulant). 4. Administer, or teach administration of, antiemetics and antidiarrheal medication as prescribed and needed. Instruct patient in side effects.	3. Oral replacement is begun as soon as possible to replace losses. Caffeine may increase diarrhea. 4. Antiemetics reduce nausea and vomiting, reducing fluid losses and improving oral intake. Antidiarrheal medication reduces intestinal motility and fluid losses.	

Nursing Diagnosis: Anxiety related to threat of, or change in, health status and disability effects of vertigo
Goal: Experiences less or no anxiety

1. Assess level of anxiety. Help patient identify coping skills used successfully in the past. 2. Provide information about vertigo and its treatment. 3. Encourage patient to discuss anxieties and explore concerns about vertigo attacks. 4. Teach patient stress management techniques or make appropriate referral. 5. Provide comfort measures and avoid stress-producing activities. 6. Instruct patient in aspects of treatment regimen.	1. Guides therapeutic interventions and participation in self-care. Past coping skills can relieve anxiety. 2. Increased knowledge helps to decrease anxiety. 3. Promotes awareness and understanding of relationship between anxiety level and behaviour 4. Improved stress management can reduce the frequency and severity of some vertiginous attacks. 5. Stressful situations may exacerbate symptoms of the condition. 6. Patient knowledge helps to decrease anxiety.	• Fear and anxiety about attacks of vertigo reduced or eliminated • Acquires knowledge and skills to deal with vertigo • Feels less tension, apprehension, and uncertainty • Uses stress management techniques when needed • Avoids upsetting encounters • Repeats instructions given and verbalizes understanding of treatments

Nursing Diagnosis: Risk for trauma related to impaired balance
Goal: Reduces the risk of trauma by adapting the home environment and by using rehabilitative devices as necessary

1. Assess for balance disturbance and/or vertigo by taking history and by examination for nystagmus, positive Romberg, and inability to perform tandem Romberg. 2. Assist with ambulation when indicated. 3. Assess for visual acuity and proprioceptive deficits. 4. Encourage increased activity level with or without use of assistive devices. 5. Help identify hazards in home environment.	1. Peripheral vestibular disorders cause these signs and symptoms. 2. Abnormal gait can predispose patient to unsteadiness and falls. 3. Balance depends on visual, vestibular, and proprioceptive systems. 4. Increased activity may help retrain balance system. 5. Adaptation of home environment can reduce risk of falls during rehabilitative process.	• Has adapted home environment or uses rehabilitative devices to reduce risk of falling • Ambulates with needed assistance • Visual and proprioceptive risks identified • Activity level increased • Home environment free of hazards

Nursing Diagnosis: Ineffective coping related to personal vulnerability and disabling effects of vertigo
Goal: Develops coping skills necessary to decrease vulnerability and unmet needs and demonstrates effective coping

1. Assess cognitive appraisal of illness and factors that may be contributing to inability to cope. 2. Provide factual information about treatment and future health status.	1. To improve patient's self-image and to enhance coping process 2. To clarify any misinformation or confusion	• Copes effectively with vertigo • Has acquired knowledge and skills to cope with vertigo • Verbalizes less threatening appraisal of situation

(continued)

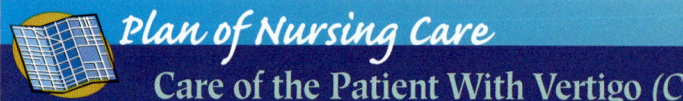

Plan of Nursing Care

Care of the Patient With Vertigo *(Continued)*

Nursing Interventions	Rationale	Expected Patient Outcomes
3. Encourage and help patient to participate in decision making about adjustments in lifestyle.	3. To help patient regain sense of power and control in self-care with activities of daily living	• Is involved in outside activities
4. Encourage patient to maintain diversional or recreational activities, exercise, and social events.	4. Social isolation and avoiding pleasant activities intensify isolation and reduce ability to cope with vertigo.	• Identifies specific strategies for coping
5. Help patient identify personal strengths and develop coping strategies based on previous positive experiences in dealing with stress, and situational supports.	5. To enhance patient's strengths that help maintain hope	• Uses support groups or counselling as appropriate
6. Refer patient to support groups or counselling as indicated.	6. May help patient feel less alone and isolated	

Nursing Diagnosis: Deficient diversional activity related to environmental lack of such activity
Goal: Engages in diversional activities

1. Assess level and type of diversional activity to plan appropriate activities.	1. Boredom may be exhibited as well as depression; helps determine tolerances as well as preferences.	• Verbalizes decreased feelings of boredom and appears alert and animated
2. Discuss usual pattern of diversional activities with patient. Suggest opportunities to continue meaningful diversional activities.	2. To provide information about perceived and actual stressors that influence activity level; to support patient's sense of self-worth and productivity.	• Seeks realistic opportunities for involvement in diversional activities.

Nursing Diagnosis: Self-care deficit: feeding, bathing/hygiene, dressing/grooming, toileting, related to labyrinth dysfunction and episodes of vertigo
Goal: Able to care for self

1. Administer, or teach administration of, antiemetics and other prescribed medications to relieve nausea and vomiting associated with vertigo.	1. Antiemetics and sedative-type medications depress stimuli in the cerebellum.	• Carries out necessary functions during symptom-free periods. Takes medications to relieve nausea or vomiting.
2. Encourage patient to perform self-care when free of vertigo.	2. Spacing activities is important because episodes of vertigo vary in occurrence.	• Carries out daily activities
3. Review diet with patient and caregivers. Offer fluids as necessary.	3. Sodium restriction helps improve an inner ear fluid imbalance in some patients, thereby decreasing vertigo. Fluids help prevent dehydration.	• Accepts dietary plan and reports its effectiveness. • Drinks fluids in sufficient amounts

Nursing Diagnosis: Powerlessness related to illness regimen and being helpless in certain situations due to vertigo/balance disturbance
Goal: Experiences increased sense of control over life and activities despite vertigo/balance disturbance

1. Assess patient's needs, values, attitudes, and readiness to initiate activities.	1. Involving patient in planning activities and care enhances potential for mastery.	• Does not restrict activities unnecessarily due to vertigo
2. Provide opportunities for patient to express feelings about self and illness.	2. Expressing feelings increases understanding of individual coping styles and defense mechanisms.	• Verbalizes positive feelings about own ability to achieve a sense of power and control
3. Help patient identify previous coping behaviours that were successful.	3. Awareness increases understanding of stressors that trigger feeling of powerlessness. Awareness of past successes enhances self-confidence.	• Identifies previous successful coping behaviours

ing the head back with the affected ear turned down. The onset is sudden and followed by a predisposition for positional vertigo, usually for hours to weeks but occasionally for months or years.

It is speculated to be caused by the disruption of debris within the semicircular canal. This debris is formed from small crystals of calcium carbonate from the inner ear structure, the utricle. This is frequently stimulated by head trauma, infection, or other events. In severe cases, vertigo may easily be induced by any head movement. The vertigo is usually accompanied by nausea and vomiting; however, hearing impairment does not generally occur (Hain, 2002).

Bed rest is recommended for patients with acute symptoms. Canalith repositioning procedures (CRP) may be used to provide resolution of vertigo. The Epley procedure is a repositioning technique that is safe, inexpensive, and easy to perform for these patients. However, this procedure is not recommended for patients with acute vertigo or for patients diagnosed with vestibular neuronitis (a paroxysmal attack of severe vertigo).

Patients with acute vertigo may be medicated with meclizine for 1 to 2 weeks. After this time, the meclizine is stopped and the patient is reassessed. Patients who continue to have severe positional vertigo may be premedicated with prochloperazine (Compazine) 1 hour before performing the CRP. The Dix-Hallpike test is used to assess for BPPV. When the Dix-Hallpike test results are positive on the right side, a left-sided CRP is used (Fig. 59-9).

Vestibular rehabilitation can be used in the management of vestibular disorders. This strategy promotes active use of the vestibular system through a multidisciplinary team approach, including medical and nursing care, stress management, biofeedback, vocational rehabilitation, and physical therapy. A physical therapist prescribes balance exercises that help the brain compensate for the impairment to the balance system.

OTOTOXICITY

A variety of medications may have adverse effects on the cochlea, vestibular apparatus, or cranial nerve VIII. All but a few, such as aspirin and quinine, cause irreversible hearing loss. At high doses, aspirin toxicity also can produce tinnitus. Intravenous medications, especially the aminoglycosides, are the most common cause of ototoxicity, and they destroy the hair cells in the organ of Corti (see Chart 59-6).

To prevent loss of hearing or balance, patients receiving potentially ototoxic medications should be counselled about the side effects of these medications. Blood levels of the medications should be monitored and patients receiving long-term intravenous antibiotics should be monitored with an audiogram twice each week during therapy.

ACOUSTIC NEUROMA

An acoustic neuroma is a slow-growing, benign tumour of cranial nerve VIII, usually arising from the Schwann cells of the vestibular portion of the nerve. Most acoustic tumours arise within the internal auditory canal and extend into the cerebellopontine angle to press on the brain stem. Acoustic neuromas account for 5% to 10% of all intracranial tumours and seem to occur with equal frequency in men and women at any age, although most occur during middle age. Most acoustic neuromas are unilateral, except in von Recklinghausen's disease (ie, neurofibromatosis type 2), in which bilateral tumours occur.

Assessment and Diagnostic Findings

The most common findings of assessment of patients with an acoustic neuroma are unilateral tinnitus and hearing loss with or without vertigo or balance disturbance. It is important to identify asymmetry in audiovestibular test results so that further workup can be performed to rule out an acoustic neuroma. MRI with a paramagnetic contrast agent (ie, gadolinium or Magnevist) is the imaging study of choice. If the patient is claustrophobic or cannot tolerate an MRI or if the scan is unavailable, a computed tomography (CT) scan with contrast dye is performed. However, MRI is more sensitive in delineating a small tumour than is CT.

FIGURE 59-9 The Dix-Hallpike manoeuvre is the test used to assess for benign paroxysmal positional vertigo (BPPV). (**A**) The patient sits on the examination table with the head turned to the left at a 45-degree angle. (**B**) The patient is lowered quickly to a supine position with the head turned to one side and slightly lower than the head of the examination table. The patient's eyes should remain open so that the examiner can observe for nystagmus. If the patient has BPPV, vertigo occurs within 5 to 10 seconds and lasts about 30 seconds. Rotary nystagmus and dizziness also occur. The procedure is repeated on the opposite side. Vertigo occurs when the affected ear faces toward the ground.

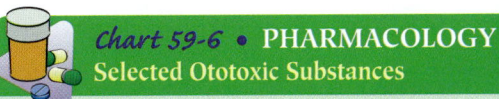

Chart 59-6 • PHARMACOLOGY
Selected Ototoxic Substances

Diuretics: ethacrynic acid, furosemide, acetazolamide
Chemotherapeutic agents: cisplatin, nitrogen mustard
Antimalarial agents: quinine, chloroquine
Anti-inflammatory agents: salicylates (aspirin), indomethacin
Chemicals: alcohol, arsenic
Aminoglycoside antibiotics: amikacin, gentamicin, kanamycin, netilmicin, neomycin, streptomycin, tobramycin
Other antibiotics: erythromycin, minocycline, polymyxin B, vancomycin
Metals: gold, mercury, lead

Management

Surgical removal of acoustic tumours is the treatment of choice because these tumours do not respond well to irradiation or chemotherapy. Because treatment of acoustic tumours crosses several specialties, the multidisciplinary treatment approach involves a neurotologist and a neurosurgeon. The objective of the surgery is to remove the tumour while preserving facial nerve function. Most acoustic tumours have damaged the cochlear portion of cranial nerve VIII, and no serviceable hearing exists before surgery. In these patients, the surgery is performed using a translabyrinthine approach, and the hearing mechanism is destroyed. If hearing is still good before surgery, a suboccipital or middle cranial fossa approach to removing the tumour may be used, and intraoperative monitoring of cranial nerve VIII is performed to save the hearing.

Complications of surgery for acoustic neuroma include facial nerve paralysis, cerebrospinal fluid leak, meningitis, and cerebral edema. Death from acoustic neuroma surgery is rare.

Aural Rehabilitation

If hearing loss is permanent or cannot be treated by medical or surgical means or if the patient elects not to undergo surgery, aural rehabilitation may be beneficial. The purpose of aural rehabilitation is to maximize the hearing-impaired person's communication skills. Aural rehabilitation includes auditory training, speech reading, speech training, and the use of hearing aids and hearing guide dogs.

Auditory training emphasizes listening skills, so the hearing-impaired person concentrates on the speaker. Speech reading (formerly known as lip reading) can help fill the gaps left by missed or misheard words. Speech training attempts to conserve, develop, and prevent deterioration of current skills.

It is important to identify the type of hearing impairment a person has so that rehabilitative efforts can be directed at his or her particular need. Surgical correction may be all that is necessary to treat and improve a conductive hearing loss (Fig. 59-10). With advances in hearing aid technology, amplification for patients with sensorineural hearing loss is more helpful than ever before.

HEARING AIDS

A hearing aid is a device through which speech and environmental sounds are received by a microphone, converted to electrical signals, amplified, and reconverted to acoustic signals. Many aids available for sensorineural hearing loss depress the low frequencies, or tones, and enhance hearing for the high frequencies. A general guideline for assessing the patient's need for a hearing aid

FIGURE 59-10 Management flow chart for conductive hearing loss. The flow chart indicates how the diagnosis determines the management of the patient and predicts the outcome. From Jafek, B. W., & Balkany, T. J. Conductive hearing loss. In B. Eiseman (Ed.). *Prognosis of surgical disease.* Philadelphia: W. B. Saunders.

is a hearing loss exceeding 30 dB in the range of 500 to 2000 Hz in the better-hearing ear.

The evolution in technology has led to the availability of many smaller and more effective hearing aids. It is estimated that 98% of all hearing aids sold today are behind-the-ear, in-the-ear, or in-the-canal types (Table 59-4).

A hearing aid should be fitted according to the patient's needs (eg, type of hearing loss, manual dexterity), rather than the brand name, by a certified audiologist licensed to dispense hearing aids. There are consumer protection laws that allow the hearing aid to be returned after a trial use if the patient is not completely satisfied.

A hearing aid makes sounds louder, but it does not improve a patient's ability to discriminate words or understand speech. People who have low discrimination scores (ie, 20%) on audiograms may derive little benefit from a hearing aid. Hearing aids amplify all sounds, including background noise, which may be disturbing to the wearer. Chart 59-7 identifies additional problems associated with hearing aid use. There are, however, computerized hearing aids available that compensate for background noise or allow amplification at certain programmed frequencies rather than at all frequencies. Occasionally, depending on the type of hearing loss, binaural aids (ie, one for each ear) may be indicated. Chart 59-8 provides tips for hearing aid care.

In Canada, it is not necessary to consult a physician before purchasing a hearing aid. However, in order for people 65 years and older to be eligible for financial assistance for a hearing aid, some provinces require a letter from a physician indicating that "there is no reason not to have a hearing aid." Children must be evaluated by a physician. Health care professionals who dispense hearing aids are required to refer prospective users to a physician if any of the following otologic conditions are evident:

- Visible congenital or traumatic deformity of the ear
- Active drainage from the ear within the previous 90 days
- Sudden or rapidly progressive hearing loss within the previous 90 days
- Complaints of dizziness or tinnitus
- Unilateral hearing loss that occurred suddenly or within the previous 90 days
- Audiometric air–bone gap of 15 dB or more at 500, 1000, and 2000 Hz
- Significant accumulation of cerumen or a foreign body in the external auditory canal
- Pain or discomfort in the ear

Chart 59-7 Hearing Aid Problems

Whistling Noise
Loose ear mold
Improperly made
Improperly worn
Worn out

Improper Aid Selection
Too much power required in aid, with inadequate separation between microphone and receiver
Open mold used inappropriately

Inadequate Amplification
Dead batteries
Wax in ear
Wax or other material in mold
Wires or tubing disconnected from aid
Aid turned off or volume too low
Improper mold
Improper aid for degree of loss

Pain from Mold
Improperly fitted mold
Ear skin or cartilage infection
Middle ear infection
Ear tumour
Unrelated conditions of the temporomandibular joint, throat, or larynx

A user instruction brochure is to accompany every hearing aid device. In this brochure, the following information is presented:

- Notification that any of the eight otologic conditions previously listed should be investigated by a physician before purchase of a hearing aid
- Instructions for proper use, maintenance, and care of the hearing aid, as well as instructions for replacing or recharging the batteries
- Repair service information
- Description of avoidable conditions that could damage the hearing aid
- List of any known side effects that may warrant physician consultation (eg, skin irritation, accelerated cerumen accumulation)

Table 59-4 • Hearing Aids

SITE (AND RANGE OF HEARING LOSS)	ADVANTAGES	DISADVANTAGES
Body (mild–profound)	Separation of receiver and microphone prevents acoustic feedback, allowing high amplification. Generally used in a school setting.	Bulky; requires long wire, which may be cosmetically displeasing; some loss of high-frequency response
Behind the ear (mild–profound)	Larger size permits use of larger components that enable the aid to provide more power and features; most versatile due to size; no long wires	Large size
In the ear (mild–moderately severe)	One-piece custom fit to contour of ear; no tubes or cords; miniature microphone is located in the ear, which is a more natural placement; more cosmetically appealing due to easy concealment	Smaller size limits output; patients who have arthritis or cannot perform tasks requiring good manual dexterity may have difficulty with the small size of aid and/or battery; can require more repair than the behind-the-ear aid
In the canal (mild–moderately severe)	Same as in-the-ear aids; less visible, so more cosmetically pleasing	Even smaller than in-the-ear aids; requires good manual dexterity

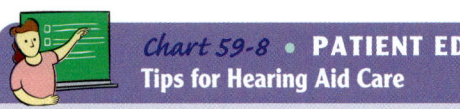

Chart 59-8 • PATIENT EDUCATION
Tips for Hearing Aid Care

Cleaning
The ear mold is the only part of the hearing aid that may be washed frequently (even daily if necessary) with soap and water. The ear mold must be dry before it is snapped into the receiver. The cannula is cleaned with a small pipe cleaner–like device.

Malfunctioning
Inadequate amplification, a whistling noise, or pain from the mold can occur when a hearing aid is not functioning properly. Check for malfunctions: Is the switch on? Are the batteries charged and positioned correctly? If the hearing aid still does not work properly, the hearing aid dealer should be notified. If the unit requires extended time for repair, the dealer may lend the patient a hearing aid until the repair can be accomplished.

Recognizing Complications
When occluded by a hearing aid, the external auditory canal can become moist. Common medical problems among hearing aid wearers include external otitis and pressure ulcers in the external auditory canal or meatus.

IMPLANTED HEARING DEVICES

Three types of implanted hearing devices are commercially available or in the investigational stage: the cochlear implant, the bone conduction device, and the semi-implantable hearing device. Cochlear implants are for patients with little or no hearing. Bone conduction devices, which transmit sound through the skull to the inner ear, are used in patients with a conductive hearing loss if a hearing aid is contraindicated (eg, those with chronic infection). The device is implanted postauricularly under the skin into the skull, and an external device—worn above the ear, not in the canal—transmits the sound through the skin. Semi-implantable hearing aids, although not yet approved except in testing sites, still require the use of an external device. However, research to develop a fully implantable hearing aid continues.

Cochlear Implant

A cochlear implant is an auditory prosthesis used for people with profound sensorineural hearing loss bilaterally who do not benefit from conventional hearing aids. The hearing loss may be congenital or acquired. An implant does not restore normal hearing; rather, it helps the person detect medium to loud environmental sounds and conversation. The implant is designed to provide stimulation directly to the auditory nerve, bypassing the hair cells of the inner ear, which are not functioning. The microphone and signal processor are worn outside the body and transmit electrical stimuli inside the body to the implanted electrodes. The electrical signals stimulate the auditory nerve fibres and then the brain, where they are interpreted.

Candidates for a cochlear implant, who are usually at least 1 year old, are selected after careful screening by otologic history, physical examination, audiologic testing, x-rays, and psychological testing. Several criteria apply for choosing adults who may benefit from a cochlear implant:

- Profound sensorineural hearing loss in both ears
- Inability to hear and recognize speech well with hearing aids
- No medical contraindication to a cochlear implant or general anesthesia
- Indications that being able to hear would enhance the patient's life

The surgery involves implanting a small receiver in the temporal bone through a postauricular incision and placing electrodes into the inner ear (Fig. 59-11). The microphone and transmitter are worn on an external unit. The patient undergoes extensive cochlear rehabilitation with the multidisciplinary team, which includes an audiologist and speech pathologist. Several months may be needed to learn to interpret the sounds heard. Children and adults who lost their hearing before they learned to speak take much longer to acquire speech. There are wide variations of success with cochlear implants, and there is also controversy about their use, especially among the Deaf community. Patients who have had a cochlear implant are cautioned that an MRI will cause the implant to become inactivated; MRI is to be used only when unavoidable.

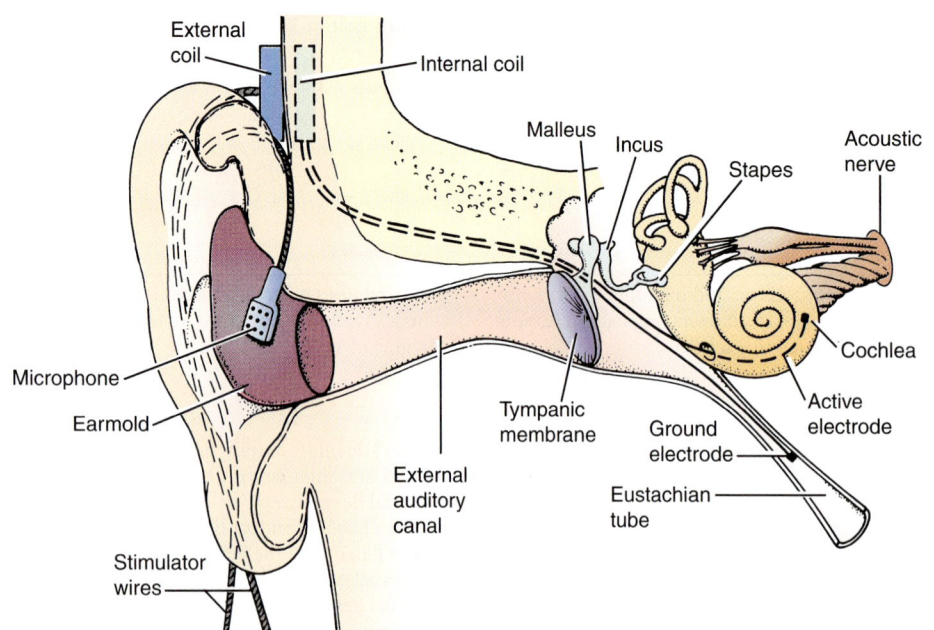

FIGURE 59-11 The cochlear implant. The internal coil has a stranded electrode lead. The electrode is inserted through the round window into the scala tympani of the cochlea. The external coil (the transmitter) is held in alignment with the internal coil (the receiver) by a magnet. The microphone receives the sound. The stimulator wire receives the signal after it has been filtered, adjusted, and modified so that the sound is at a comfortable level for the patient. Sound is passed by the external transmitter to the inner coil receiver by magnetic conduction and is then carried by the electrode to the cochlea.

HEARING GUIDE DOGS

Specially trained dogs are available to assist the person with a hearing loss. People who live alone are eligible to apply for a dog trained by International Hearing Dog, Inc. At home, the dog reacts to the sound of a telephone, a doorbell, an alarm clock, a baby's cry, a knock at the door, a smoke alarm, or an intruder. The dog does not bark but alerts its master by physical contact; the dog then runs to the source of the noise. In public, the dog positions itself between the hearing-impaired person and any potential hazard that the person cannot hear, such as an oncoming vehicle or a loud, hostile person. A hearing-impaired person with a certified hearing guide dog is legally permitted access to public transportation, public eating places, and stores, including food markets.

Critical Thinking Exercises

1. An 82-year-old patient in an extended care facility appears withdrawn and distrustful of others. She does not participate in conversations with other residents. You suspect that she has a hearing loss. Describe the strategies you would use to assess this patient's hearing. What intervention strategies would you implement if your assessment confirms that the woman has a hearing loss? What intervention strategies would you implement if your assessment indicates that she does not have a hearing loss?

2. An antiemetic and a tranquilizer have been prescribed for a patient with Ménière's disease. You realize that safety precautions are indicated. Devise a teaching plan for this patient, and explain the reasons behind each part of the plan.

3. A teenage boy has decided to play the drums in a local band. The music consists of loud, hard rock music. The group practices for 2 to 3 hours each day, approximately 4 nights per week. Describe the teaching plan you would devise for this teenage boy, including rationale.

4. A patient presents with severe vertigo. She lives alone and is afraid of injuring herself because of her dizziness, which is unpredictable. Devise a teaching plan for this patient, including methods to prevent injury. Include interventions and outcomes that will address her fears and anxiety.

5. A patient with severe hearing loss is admitted for abdominal surgery to treat a bowel obstruction. It is anticipated that a colostomy will be created. Explain modifications in preoperative, intraoperative, and postoperative nursing care needed because of her impaired hearing.

REFERENCES AND SELECTED READINGS

Books

Alper, C., Eibling, D., & Myers, E. (2001). *Decision making in ear, nose and throat disorders.* Philadelphia: W. B. Saunders.

Bickley, L. S., & Szilagyi, P. (2003). *Bates's guide to physical examination and history taking* (8th ed.). Philadelphia: Lippincott Williams & Wilkins.

Blitzer, A. (Ed.). (1998). *Office-based surgery in otolaryngology.* New York: Thieme.

Canalis, A., & Lambert, P. (2000). *The ear: Comprehensive otology.* Philadelphia: Lippincott Williams & Wilkins.

Charles, E. (1999). *Introduction to sound: Acoustics for the hearing and speech sciences.* San Diego: Singular Publishing Group.

Franks, J. R. (1996). *Analysis of audiograms for a large cohort of noise-exposed miners.* Cincinnati, OH: HHS Centers for Disease Control & Prevention, NIOSH, Division of Biomedical and Behavioral Science.

Goroll, A., Mulley, A. G., Jr., & May, L. A. (Eds.). (2000). *Primary care medicine: Office evaluation and management of the adult patient.* Philadelphia: Lippincott Williams & Wilkins.

Harris, L. L., & Huntoon, M. B. (1998). *Core curriculum for otorhinolaryngology and head/neck nursing.* New Smyrna Beach, FL: Society of Otorhinolaryngology and Head–Neck Nurses.

National Institute on Deafness and Other Communication Disorders (NIDCD). (1998). *NIDCD national strategic research plan.* Narberth, PA: National Institutes of Health.

Noble, J., Greene, H. L., & Levinson, W. (2001). *Textbook of primary care medicine.* St. Louis: C. V. Mosby.

Patton, K., & Thibodeau, G. (2000). *Mosby's Handbook of anatomy & physiology.* St. Louis: C. V. Mosby.

Society of Otorhinolaryngology–Head and Neck Nurses, Inc. (1996). *Nursing practice guidelines for care of the otorhinolaryngology—head and neck patient.* New Smyrna Beach, FL: Society of Otorhinolaryngology and Head–Neck Nurses.

Woodson, G. (2001). *Ear, nose and throat disorders in primary care.* Philadelphia: Harcourt Health Sciences.

U.S. Public Health Service. (2000). *Healthy People 2010.* Washington, DC: Author.

Journals

Canadian Association of the Deaf. (2004). *Statistics on deaf Canadians.* Available at: http://www.cad.ca/index2.php?lid=e&cid=12&pid=19. Retrieved June 13, 2005.

Canadian Centre for Occupational Health and Safety. (2004). *OSH answers, physical agents, noise.* Available at: www.ccohs.ca/oshanswers/phys_agents/noise_measurement.html. Retrieved June 13, 2005.

Cavenish, R. (1998). Adult hearing loss. *American Journal of Nursing, 98*(8), 50–51.

Cooley, D., Grossan, M., & Hoffman, D. (2002). The ins and outs of common ear problems. In *Patient care for the nurse practitioner: 6.* Montvale, NJ: Medical Economics Company.

Cruickshanks, K. J., Wiley, T. L., Tweed, T. S., Klein, B. E., Klein, R., Mares-Perlman, J. A., & Nondahl, D. M. (1998). Prevalence of hearing loss in order adults in Beaver Dam Wisconsin: The epidemiology of hearing loss study. *American Journal of Epidemiology, 148*(9), 879–886.

Epley, J. M. (1992). The canalith repositioning procedure: For treatment of benign paroxysmal positional vertigo. *Otolaryngology—Head and Neck Surgery, 107*(3), 399–404.

Felis, M. (2000). Acute otitis externa. *Lippincott's Primary Care Practice, 5,* 529–533.

Hain, T. (2002). Benign paroxysmal positional vertigo. Online publication available at http://www.tchain.com/otoneurology/disorders/bppv/bppv.html.

Hannley, M., Denneny, J., & Holzer, S. (2000). Use of ototopical antibiotics in three common ear diseases. *Otolaryngology—Head and Neck Surgery, 122*(6), 934–940.

The Hearing Foundation of Canada (n.d.). *About THFC.* Available at: www.thfc.ca/about.html. Retrieved June 13, 2005.

Kaplan, S. L., Mason, E. O., Wald, E. R., Kim, K. S., Givner, L. B., Bradley, J. S., et al. (2000). Pneumococcal mastoiditis in children. *Pediatrics, 106*(5), 695–699.

Knox, G., & McPherson, A. (1997). Ménière's disease: Differential diagnosis and treatment. *American Family Physician, 55*(4), 1185–1198.

Larson, V. D., Williams, D. W., Henderson, W. G., Luethke, L. E., Beck, L. B., Noffsinger, D., et al. (2000). Efficacy of 3 commonly used hearing aid circuits: A crossover trial. *Journal of the American Medical Association, 284*(14), 1805–1813.

Nobel, W., Ter-Horst, K., & Byrne, D. (1995). Disabilities and handicaps associated with impaired auditory localization. *Journal of the American Academy of Audiology, 6*(2), 129–140.

Rabinowitz, P. (2000). Noise-induced hearing loss. *American Family Physician, 6*(5), 2749–2756, 2759–2760.

Ruckenstein, M. (2000). Vertigo and dysequilibrium with associated hearing loss. *Otolaryngologic Clinics of North America, 33*(3), 535–562.

Statistics Canada. (2005). *Canadian statistics—Population projections.* Available at: www40.statcan.ca/l01/cst01/demo23a.htm?searchstrdisabled=2026&filename=demo23a.htm&lan=eng. Retrieved June 13, 2005.

Weber, P. C., & Klein, A. J. (1999). Hearing loss. *Medical Clinics of North America, 83*(3), 124.

World Health Organization. (2002). Facts about deafness. Available at: www.who.int/pbd/deafness/facts/en. Retrieved June 13, 2005.

RESOURCES AND WEBSITES

Acoustic Neuroma Association of Canada (ANAC), Box 369, Edmonton AB T5J 2J6; 1-800-561-ANAC (2622); www.anac.ca/en.

Balance and Dizziness Disorders Society, #325 - 5525 West Boulevard, Vancouver, BC V6M 3W6; 604-878-8383; www.balanceanddizziness.org.

The Canadian Association of the Deaf, 203-251 Bank Street, Ottawa, ON K2P 1X3; TTY: (613) 565-8882;Voice: (613) 565-2882; www.cad.ca.

Canadian Association of Genetic Counsellors (CAGC); www.cagc-accg.ca.

Canadian Association of Speech-Language Pathologists and Audiologists (CASLPA), 401-200 Elgin Street, Ottawa, ON K2P 1L5; 1-800-259-8519; www.caslpa.ca.

Canadian Cancer Society/Société canadienne du cancer, National Office, Suite 200, 10 Alcorn Avenue, Toronto, ON M4V 3B1; (416) 961-7223; fax: (416) 961-4189; www.cancer.ca.

Canadian Centre for Occupational Health and Safety, 135 Hunter Street East, Hamilton ON L8N 1M5; 1-800-263-8466; www.ccohs.ca.

Canadian Directory of Genetic Support Groups; Support Group Directory, Regional Medical Genetics Centre, Children's Hospital of Western Ontario, 800 Commissioner's Road East, London ON N6C 2V5; 519-685-8453; 1-800-243-8416 (Ontario only); fax: 519-685-8214; e-mail: Database Administrator; http://www.lhsc.on.ca/programs/medgenet.

Canadian Genetic Disease Network, Suite 201, 2150 Western Parkway, Vancouver, BC V6T 1V6; 604-221-7300; fax: 604-221-0778; e-mail: info@cgdn.ca; http://www.cgdn.ca.

Canadian Hard of Hearing Association (CHHA), 2435 Holly Lane, Suite 205, Ottawa, ON K1V 7P2; 1-800-263-8068; www.chha.ca.

The Canadian Hearing Society, 271 Spadina Road, Toronto, ON M5R 2V3; (416) 964-9595; www.chs.ca.

Canadian Organization for Rare Disorders (CORD), PO Box 814, Coaldale, AB T1M 1M7; (403) 345-4544; toll-free: 1-877-302-7273; fax: (403) 345-3948; www.cord.ca.

The Canadian Tinnitus and Hyperacusis Centre, 200 Brock Street North, 2nd Floor, Whitby, ON L1N 4H5; (905) 668-4002; www.canadiantinn.com.

GeneTests, 9725 Third Avenue NE, Suite 602, Seattle, WA 98115; 206-616-4033; fax: 206-221-4679; e-mail: genetests@genetests.org; http://www.genetests.org.

Genetic Alliance, 4301 Connecticut Ave. NW, Suite 404, Washington, DC 20008-2369; 202-966-5557; fax: (202) 966-8553; e-mail: info@geneticalliance.org; http://www.geneticalliance.org.

The Genetics Society of Canada; http://life.biology.mcmaster.ca/GSC.

The Hearing Foundation of Canada, 330 Bay Street, Suite 1402, Toronto, ON M5H 2S8; 1-866-HEAR-YOU or (1-866-432-7968); www.thfc.ca.

Help the Aged Canada, HTAC Head Office, 1300 Carling Avenue, Unit 205, Ottawa, ON K1Z 7L2; (613) 232-0727; www.helptheaged.ca.

I.M.F. International Ménière Federation [directory of member organizations]; www.menieres-disease.net/MemberDetails.html.

International Hearing Dog, Inc., 5901 E. 89th Ave., Henderson, CO 80640; 303-287-3277; http://members.aol.com/ihdi/IHDI.html.

The Learning Disabilities Association of Canada (National Office), 323 Chapel Street, Ottawa, ON K1N 7Z2; (613) 238-5721; www.ldac-taac.ca.

National Educational Association of Disabled Students, 4th Level Unicentre, Carleton University, Ottawa, ON K1S 5B6; www.neads.ca.

National Institute on Deafness and Other Communication Disorders, National Institutes of Health, Building 31, Room 3c35 9000, Rockville Pike, Bethesda, MD 20892; http://www.nidcd.nih.gov.

OMIM Online Mendelian Inheritance in Man; www.ncbi.nlm.nih.gov/entrez/query.fcgi?db=OMIM.

Public Health Agency of Canada, 130 Colonnade Road, AL 6501H, Ottawa, ON K1A 0K9; www.phac-aspc.gc.ca.

Veteran Affairs Canada, Trebla Building, 473 Albert Street, 10th Floor, Ottawa, ON K1R 5B4; 1-800-883-6094; www.vac-acc.gc.ca.

Neurologic Function

Applying Concepts from NANDA, NIC, and NOC

Mr. James is a 54-year-old male with a history of alcohol abuse. On the evening before his admission to the hospital, Mr. James fell down a flight of stairs while intoxicated, hitting the front and left side of his head. He was admitted to the neurologic intensive care unit (NICU) and diagnosed with a traumatic brain injury. After several days in the NICU, which included treatment for alcohol withdrawal, Mr. James was transferred to a general care unit. As his brain injury heals, he still is experiencing limitations. He has expressive aphasia but can say one- or two-word phrases, often offensive in nature. His behaviour seems hostile and he frequently paces about, looking angry and threatening. He cannot focus his attention well, and his wife states that his personality seems completely different. The concept map illustrates the relationships that exist among the nursing diagnoses, interventions, and outcomes for Mr. James's disrupted cognitive and behavioural functioning.

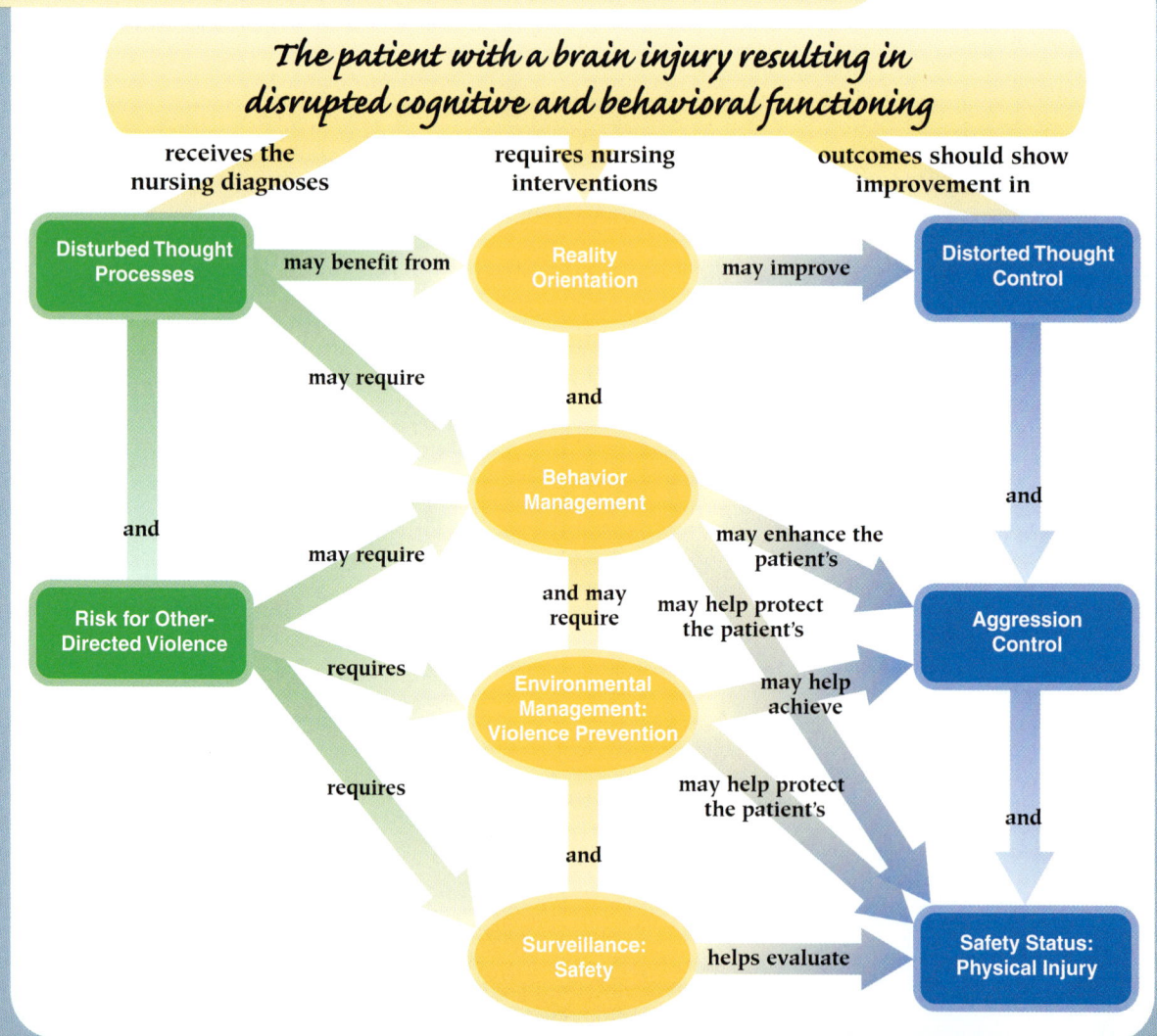

The patient with a brain injury resulting in disrupted cognitive and behavioral functioning

Nursing Classifications and Languages

NANDA
Nursing Diagnoses

Disturbed Thought Processes—Disruption in cognitive operations and activities

Risk for Other-Directed Violence—At risk for behaviours in which an individual demonstrates that he or she can be physically, emotionally, and/or sexually harmful to others

NIC
Nursing Interventions*

Reality Orientation—Promotion of patient's awareness of personal identity, time, and environment

Behaviour Management—Helping a patient manage negative behaviour

Environmental Management: Violence Prevention—Monitoring and manipulation of the physical environment to decrease the potential for violent behaviour directed toward self, others, or environment

Surveillance: Safety—Purposeful and ongoing collection and analysis of information about the patient and the environment for use in promoting and maintaining patient safety

NOC
Nursing Outcomes†

Return to functional baseline status, stabilization of, or improvement in

Distorted Thought Control—Self-restraint or disruption in perception, thought processes, and thought content

Aggression Control—Self restraint of assaultive, combative, or destructive behaviour toward others

Safety Status: Physical Injury—Severity of injuries from trauma

NANDA, North American Nursing Diagnosis Association; NIC, Nursing Interventions Classification; NOC, Nursing Outcomes Classification.

*Iowa Intervention Project © 2000. In McCloskey, J. C., & Bulechek, G. M. (2000). *Nursing interventions classification (NIC)* (3rd ed.). St. Louis: Mosby.

†Iowa Outcomes Project © 2000. In Johnson, M., Maas, M., & Moorhead, S. (2000). *Nursing outcomes classification (NOC)* (3rd ed.). St. Louis: Mosby.

Assessment of Neurologic Function

Adapted by Lynne Esson

On completion of this chapter, the learner will be able to:

1. Describe the structures and functions of the central and peripheral nervous systems.
2. Differentiate between pathologic changes that affect motor control and those that affect sensory pathways.
3. Compare the functioning of the sympathetic and parasympathetic nervous systems.
4. Describe the significance of physical assessment to the diagnosis of neurologic dysfunction.
5. Describe changes in neurologic function associated with aging and their impact on neurologic assessment findings.
6. Describe diagnostic tests used for assessment of suspected neurologic disorders and the related nursing implications.

$\mathcal{N}$urses in many types of practice settings encounter patients with altered neurologic function. Disorders of the nervous system can occur at any time during the life span and can vary from mild, self-limiting symptoms to devastating, life-threatening disorders. The nurse must be skilled in the assessment of the neurologic system whether the assessment is generalized or focused on specific areas of function. Assessment in either case requires knowledge of the anatomy and physiology of the nervous system and an understanding of the array of tests and procedures used to diagnose neurologic disorders. Knowledge about the nursing implications and interventions related to assessment and diagnostic testing is also essential.

Anatomic and Physiologic Overview

The nervous system consists of two divisions: the central nervous system (CNS), including the brain and spinal cord, and the peripheral nervous system, made up of the cranial and spinal nerves. The peripheral nervous system can be further divided into the somatic, or voluntary, nervous system, and the autonomic, or involuntary, nervous system. The function of the nervous system is to control all motor, sensory, autonomic, cognitive, and behavioural activities. The nervous system has approximately 10 million sensory neurons that send information about the internal and external environment to the brain and 500,000 motor neurons that control the muscles and glands. The brain itself contains more than 20 billion nerve cells that link the motor and sensory pathways, monitor the body's processes, respond to the internal and external environment, maintain homeostasis, and direct all psychological, biologic, and physical activity through complex chemical and electrical messages (Bradley, Daroff, Fenichel & Marsden, 2000).

ANATOMY OF THE NERVOUS SYSTEM

Cells of the Nervous System

The basic functional unit of the brain is the neuron (Fig. 60-1). It is composed of a cell body, a dendrite, and an axon. The **dendrite** is a branch-type structure with synapses for receiving electrochemical messages. The **axon** is a long projection that carries impulses away from the cell body. Nerve cell bodies occurring in clusters are called ganglia or nuclei. A cluster of cell bodies with the same function is called a centre (eg, the respiratory centre). Neuroglial cells, another type of nerve cell, support, protect, and nourish neurons.

Neurotransmitters

Neurotransmitters communicate messages from one neuron to another or from a neuron to a specific target tissue. Neurotransmitters are manufactured and stored in synaptic vesicles. They enable conduction of impulses across the synaptic cleft. The neurotransmitter has an affinity for specific receptors in the postsynaptic bulb. When released, the neurotransmitter crosses the synaptic cleft and binds to receptors in the postsynaptic cell membrane. The action of a neurotransmitter is to potentiate, terminate, or modulate a specific action and can either excite or inhibit the target cell's activity. There are usually multiple neurotransmitters at work in the neural synapse. There are various types of neurotransmitters (Bradley et al., 2000; Hickey, 2003); major neurotransmitters are described in Table 60-1.

Many neurologic disorders are due, at least in part, to an imbalance in neurotransmitters—that is, a lack of gamma-aminobutyric acid (GABA) and acetylcholine in Huntington's disease (Bradley et al., 2000), low serotonin levels in some forms of epilepsy (Blows, 2000), and a decrease in dopamine in Parkinson's disease. In fact, probably all brain functions are modulated through neurotransmitter receptor site activity, including memory and other cognitive processes.

There are two types of receptors: direct and indirect. Direct receptors are also known as inotropic because they are linked to ion channels and allow passage of ions when opened. They can be excitatory or inhibitory and are rapid-acting (measured in milliseconds). Indirect receptors affect metabolic processes in the cell, which can take from seconds to hours to occur. Receptor sites are an expanding area of research because they are often the target for the action and development of new medications. These medications either block or stimulate neurotransmitters at receptor sites and thus provide relief from symptoms (Blows, 2000). Receptor sites are also sites for the action of addictive drugs.

Glossary

agnosia: loss of ability to recognize objects through a particular sensory system; may be visual, auditory, or tactile

ataxia: inability to coordinate muscle movements, resulting in difficulty in walking, talking, and performing self-care activities

autonomic nervous system: division of the nervous system that regulates the involuntary body functions

axon: portion of the neuron that conducts impulses away from the cell body

Babinski reflex (sign): a reflex action of the toes, indicative of abnormalities in the motor control pathways leading from the cerebral cortex

clonus: abnormal movement marked by alternating contraction and relaxation of a muscle occurring in rapid succession

delirium: transient loss of intellectual function, usually due to systemic problems

dendrite: portion of the neuron that conducts impulses toward the cell body

dysphagia: difficulty swallowing

flaccid: displaying lack of muscle tone; limp, floppy

myelography (myelogram): x-ray study of the spinal cord after injection of a contrast agent into the subarachnoid space

parasympathetic nervous system: division of the autonomic nervous system active primarily during nonstressful conditions, controlling mostly visceral functions

photophobia: inability to tolerate light

position (postural) sense: awareness of position of parts of the body without looking at them; also referred to as proprioception

rigidity: increase in muscle tone at rest characterized by increased resistance to passive stretch

reflex: an automatic response to stimuli

Romberg test: test for cerebellar dysfunction requiring the patient to stand with feet together, eyes closed and arms extended; inability to maintain the position, with either significant stagger or sway, is a positive test

spasticity: sustained increase in tension of a muscle when it is passively lengthened or stretched

sympathetic nervous system: division of the autonomic nervous system with predominantly excitatory responses, the "fight-or-flight" system

tone: tension present in a muscle at rest

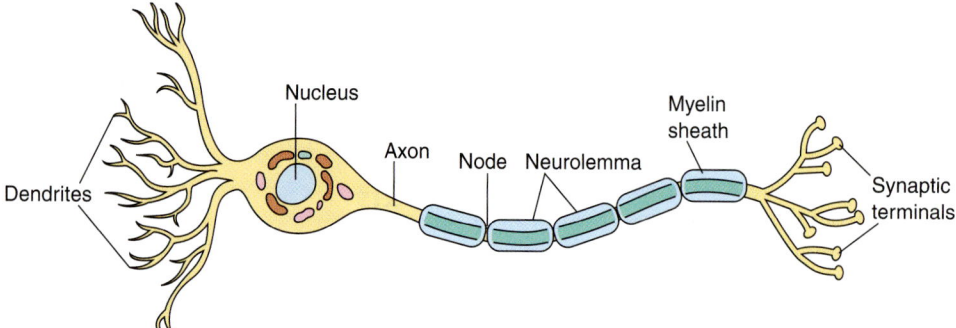

FIGURE 60-1 Neuron.

Another important area of ongoing research is diagnostic testing that can detect abnormal levels of neurotransmitters in the brain. Positron emission tomography (PET), for example, can detect dopamine, serotonin, and acetylcholine (Gjedde et al., 2001). Single photon emission computed tomography (SPECT) is similar to PET. Both PET and SPECT are discussed in more detail later in this chapter.

The Central Nervous System

ANATOMY OF THE BRAIN

The brain is divided into three major areas: the cerebrum, the brain stem, and the cerebellum. The cerebrum is composed of two hemispheres, the thalamus, the hypothalamus, and the basal ganglia. Additionally, connections for the olfactory (cranial nerve I) and optic (cranial nerve III) nerves are found in the cerebrum. The brain stem includes the midbrain, pons, medulla, and connections for cranial nerves II and IV through XII. The cerebellum is located under the cerebrum and behind the brain stem (Fig. 60-2). The brain accounts for approximately 2% of the total body weight; it weighs approximately 1,400 g in an average young adult (Hickey, 2003). In the elderly, the average brain weighs approximately 1,200 g.

Cerebrum. The cerebrum consists of two hemispheres that are incompletely separated by the great longitudinal fissure. This sulcus separates the cerebrum into the right and left hemispheres. The two hemispheres are joined at the lower portion of the fis-

sure by the corpus callosum. The outside surface of the hemispheres has a wrinkled appearance that is the result of many folded layers or convolutions called gyri, which increase the surface area of the brain, accounting for the high level of activity carried out by such a small-appearing organ. The external or outer portion of the cerebrum (the cerebral cortex) is made up of grey matter approximately 2 to 5 mm in depth; it contains billions of neurons/cell bodies, giving it a grey appearance. White matter makes up the innermost layer and is composed of nerve fibres and neuroglia (support tissue) that form tracts or pathways connecting various parts of the brain with one another (transverse and association pathways) and the cortex to lower portions of the brain and spinal cord (projection fibres). The cerebral hemispheres are divided into pairs of frontal, parietal, temporal, and occipital lobes. The four lobes are as follows (see Fig. 60-2):

- Frontal—the largest lobe. The major functions of this lobe are concentration, abstract thought, information storage or memory, and motor function. It also contains Broca's area, critical for motor control of speech. The frontal lobe is also responsible in large part for an individual's affect, judgment, personality, and inhibitions.
- Parietal—a predominantly sensory lobe. The primary sensory cortex, which analyzes sensory information and relays the interpretation of this information to the thalamus and other cortical areas, is located in the parietal lobe. It is also essential to an individual's awareness of the body in space, as well as orientation in space and spatial relations.

Table 60-1 • **Major Neurotransmitters**

NEUROTRANSMITTER	SOURCE	ACTION
Acetylcholine (major transmitter of the parasympathetic nervous system)	Many areas of the brain; autonomic nervous system	Usually excitatory; parasympathetic effects sometimes restrain (stimulation of heart by vagal nerve)
Serotonin	Brain stem, hypothalamus, dorsal horn of the spinal cord	Restraining, helps control mood and sleep, inhibits pain pathways
Dopamine	Substantia nigra and basal ganglia	Usually restrains, affects behaviour (attention, emotions) and fine movement
Norepinephrine (major transmitter of the sympathetic nervous system)	Brain stem, hypothalamus, postganglionic neurons of the sympathetic nervous system	Usually excitatory; affects mood and overall activity
Gamma-aminobutyric acid (GABA)	Spinal cord, cerebellum, basal ganglia, some cortical areas	Excitatory amino acid
Enkephalin, endorphin	Nerve terminals in the spine, brain stem, thalamus and hypothalamus, pituitary gland	Excitatory; pleasurable sensation, inhibits pain transmission

Central fissure (Rolando)

Parietal lobe

Gyri

Frontal
lobe

Occipital
lobe

Lateral
fissure
(Sylvius)

Transverse
fissure

Temporal lobe

Midbrain

Cerebellum

Pons

Medulla
oblongata

Spinal cord

FIGURE 60-2 View of the external surface of the brain showing lobes, cerebellum,
and brain stem.

- Temporal—contains the auditory receptive areas. Contains a vital area called the interpretive area that provides integration of somatization, visual, and auditory areas and plays the most dominant role of any area of the cortex in cerebration.
- Occipital—the posterior lobe of the cerebral hemisphere is responsible for visual interpretation.

The corpus callosum (Fig. 60-3) is a thick collection of nerve fibres that connects the two hemispheres of the brain and is responsible for the transmission of information from one side of the brain to the other. Information transferred includes sensation, memory, and learned discrimination. Right-handed people and some left-handed people have cerebral dominance on the left side of the brain for verbal, linguistic, arithmetical, calculating, and

analytic functions. The nondominant hemisphere is responsible for geometric, spatial, visual, pattern, and musical functions.

The basal ganglia are masses of nuclei located deep in the cerebral hemispheres that are responsible for control of fine motor movements, including those of the hands and lower extremities.

The thalamus (see Fig. 60-3) lies on either side of the third ventricle and acts primarily as a relay station for all sensation except smell. All memory, sensation, and pain impulses also pass through this section of the brain.

The hypothalamus is located anterior and inferior to the thalamus. The hypothalamus lies immediately beneath and lateral to the lower portion of the wall of the third ventricle. It includes the optic chiasm (the point at which the two optic tracts cross) and the mammillary bodies (involved in olfactory reflexes and emotional response to odours). The infundibulum of the hypothalamus connects it to the posterior pituitary gland. The hypothalamus plays an important role in the endocrine system because it regulates the pituitary secretion of hormones that influence metabolism, reproduction, stress response, and urine production. It works with the pituitary to maintain fluid balance and maintains temperature regulation by promoting vasoconstriction or vasodilatation.

The hypothalamus is the site of the hunger centre and is involved in appetite control. It contains centres that regulate the sleep–wake cycle, blood pressure, aggressive and sexual behaviour, and emotional responses (ie, blushing, rage, depression, panic, and fear). The hypothalamus also controls and regulates the autonomic nervous system.

The pituitary gland is located in the sella turcica at the base of the brain and is connected to the hypothalamus. The pituitary is a common site for brain tumours in adults; frequently they are detected by physical signs and symptoms that can be traced to the pituitary, such as hormonal imbalance or visual disturbances

Corpus callosum

Thalamus

Hypothalamus

Pituitary

FIGURE 60-3 Medial view of the brain.

secondary to pressure on the optic chiasm (further information on brain tumours is found later in this unit in Chap. 65).

Nerve fibres from all portions of the cortex converge in each hemisphere and exit in the form of a tight bundle of nerve fibres known as the internal capsule. Having entered the pons and the medulla, each bundle crosses to the corresponding bundle from the opposite side. Some of these axons make connections with axons from the cerebellum, basal ganglia, thalamus, and hypothalamus; some connect with the cranial nerve cells. Other fibres from the cortex and the subcortical centres are channeled through the pons and the medulla into the spinal cord.

Although the various cells in the cerebral cortex are quite similar in appearance, their functions vary widely, depending on location. The topography of the cortex in relation to certain of its functions is shown in Figure 60-4. The posterior portion of each hemisphere (ie, the occipital lobe) is devoted to all aspects of visual perception. The lateral region, or temporal lobe, incorporates the auditory centre. The midcentral zone, or parietal zone, posterior to the fissure of Rolando, is concerned with sensation; the anterior portion is concerned with voluntary muscle movements. The large area behind the forehead (ie, the frontal lobes) contains the association pathways that determine emotional attitudes and responses and contribute to the formation of thought processes. Damage to the frontal lobes as a result of trauma or disease is by no means incapacitating from the standpoint of muscular control or coordination, but it affects a person's personality, as reflected by basic attitudes, sense of humour and propriety, self-restraint, and motivations. (Neurologic trauma and disease states that may result in frontal damage are discussed in later chapters in this unit.)

Brain Stem. The brain stem consists of the midbrain, pons, and medulla oblongata (see Fig. 60-2). The midbrain connects the pons and the cerebellum with the cerebral hemispheres; it contains sensory and motor pathways and serves as the centre for auditory and visual reflexes. Cranial nerves III and IV originate in the midbrain. The pons is situated in front of the cerebellum between the midbrain and the medulla and is a bridge between the two halves of the cerebellum, and between the medulla and the cerebrum. Cranial nerves V through VIII connect to the brain in the pons. The pons contains motor and sensory pathways. Portions of the pons also control the heart, respiration, and blood pressure.

The medulla oblongata contains motor fibres from the brain to the spinal cord and sensory fibres from the spinal cord to the brain. Most of these fibres cross, or decussate, at this level. Cranial nerves IX through XII connect to the brain in the medulla.

Cerebellum. The cerebellum is separated from the cerebral hemispheres by a fold of dura mater, the tentorium cerebelli. The cerebellum has both excitatory and inhibitory actions and is largely responsible for coordination of movement. It also controls fine movement, balance, **position sense** (awareness of where each part of the body is), and integration of sensory input.

STRUCTURES PROTECTING THE BRAIN

The brain is contained in the rigid skull, which protects it from injury. The major bones of the skull are the frontal, temporal, parietal, and occipital bones. These bones join at the suture lines (Fig. 60-5).

The meninges (fibrous connective tissues that cover the brain and spinal cord) provide protection, support, and nourishment to the brain and spinal cord. The layers of the meninges are the dura, arachnoid, and pia mater (Fig. 60-6).

- Dura mater—the outermost layer; covers the brain and the spinal cord. It is tough, thick, inelastic, fibrous, and grey.

FIGURE 60-4 Topography of the cortex as it relates to function.

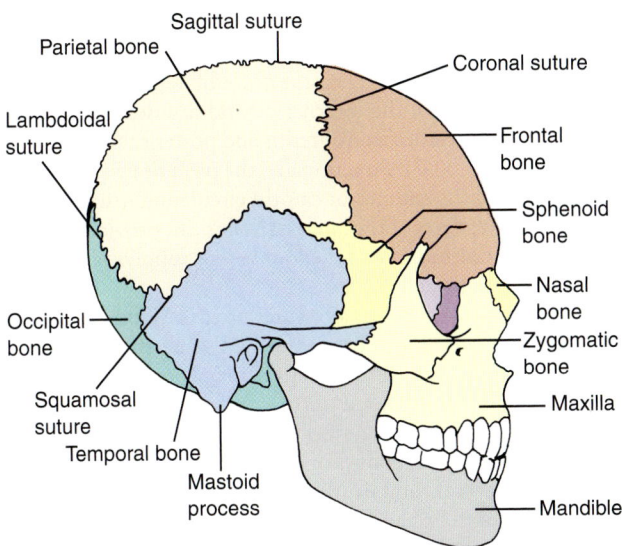

FIGURE 60-5 Bones and sutures of the skull.

There are four extensions of the dura: the falx cerebri, which separates the two hemispheres in a longitudinal plane; the tentorium, which is an infolding of the dura that forms a tough membranous shelf; the falx cerebelli, which is between the two lateral lobes of the cerebellum; and the diaphragm sellae, which provides a "roof" for the sella turcica. The tentorium supports the hemispheres and separates them from the lower part of the brain. When excess pressure occurs in the cranial cavity, brain tissue may be compressed against the tentorium or displaced downward, a process called herniation. Between the dura mater and the skull in the cranium, and between the periosteum and the dura in the vertebral column, is the epidural space, a potential space.

- Arachnoid—the middle membrane; an extremely thin, delicate membrane that closely resembles a spider web (hence the name arachnoid). It appears white because it has no blood supply. The arachnoid layer contains the choroid plexus, which is responsible for the production of cerebrospinal fluid (CSF). This membrane also has unique fingerlike projections, arachnoid villi, that absorb CSF. In the normal adult, approximately 500 mL of CSF is produced each day; all but 125 to 150 mL is absorbed by the villi (Hickey, 2003). When blood enters the system (from trauma or hemorrhagic stroke), the villi become obstructed and hydrocephalus (increased size of ventricles) may result. The subdural space is between the dura and the arachnoid layer, and the subarachnoid space is located between the arachnoid and pia layers and contains the CSF.
- Pia mater—the innermost membrane; a thin, transparent layer that hugs the brain closely and extends into every fold of the brain's surface.

CEREBROSPINAL FLUID

CSF, a clear and colourless fluid with a specific gravity of 1.007, is produced in the ventricles and is circulated around the brain and the spinal cord through the ventricular system. There are four ventricles: the right and left lateral, and the third and fourth ventricles. The two lateral ventricles open into the third ventricle at the interventricular foramen or the foramen of Monro. The third and fourth ventricles connect via the aqueduct of Sylvius. The fourth ventricle supplies CSF to the subarachnoid space and

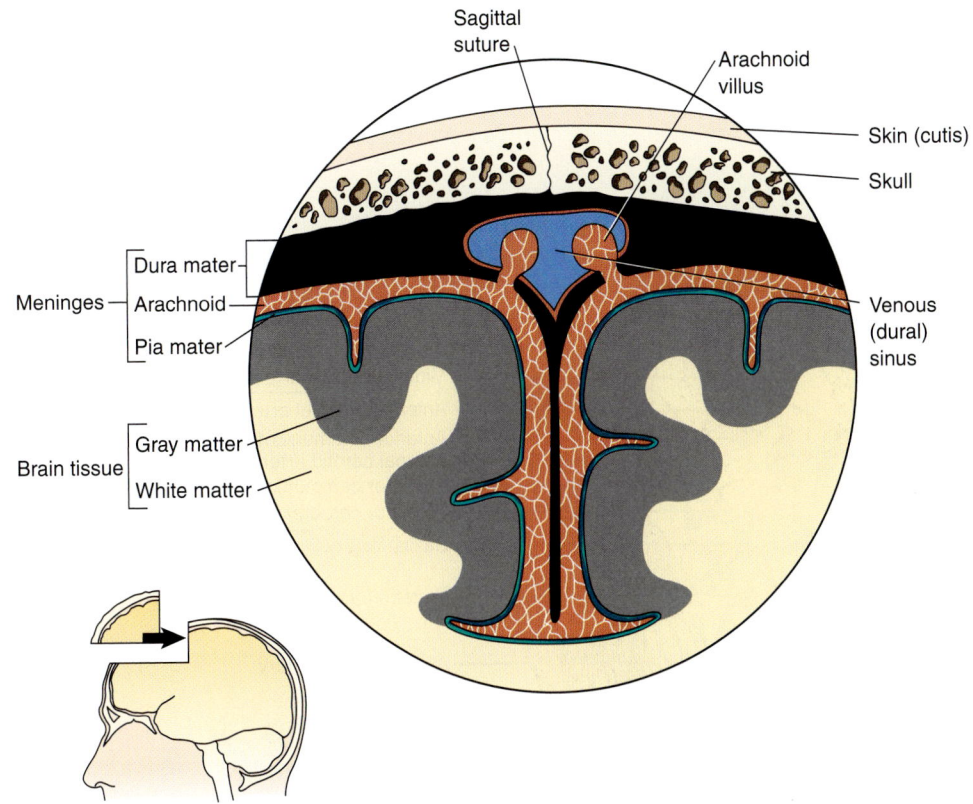

FIGURE 60-6 Meninges and related structures.

down the spinal cord on the dorsal surface. CSF is returned to the brain and is then circulated around the brain, where it is absorbed by the arachnoid villi.

CSF is produced in the choroid plexus of the lateral, third, and fourth ventricles. The ventricular and subarachnoid system contains approximately 125 to 150 mL of fluid, while 15 to 25 mL of CSF is located in each lateral ventricle.

The composition of CSF is similar to other extracellular fluids (such as blood plasma), but the concentrations of the various constituents are different. The analysis and laboratory report of CSF usually contains information on colour, specific gravity, protein count, white blood cell count, glucose, and other electrolyte levels; it may also be tested for immunoglobulins or lactate (Hickey, 2003). Normal CSF contains a minimal number of white blood cells and no red blood cells.

CEREBRAL CIRCULATION

The cerebral circulation receives approximately 15% of the cardiac output, or 750 mL per minute. The brain does not store nutrients and has a high metabolic demand that requires the high blood flow. The brain's blood pathway is unique because it flows against gravity; its arteries fill from below and the veins drain from above. In contrast to other organs that may tolerate decreases in blood flow because of their adequate collateral circulation, the brain lacks additional collateral blood flow, which may result in irreversible tissue damage when blood flow is occluded for even short periods of time.

Arteries. Two internal carotid arteries and two vertebral arteries and their extensive system of branches provide the blood supply to the brain. The internal carotids arise from the bifurcation of the common carotid and supply much of the anterior circulation of the brain. The vertebral arteries branch from the subclavian arteries, flow back and upward on either side of the cervical vertebrae, and enter the cranium through the foramen magnum. The vertebral arteries join to become the basilar artery at the level of the brain stem; the basilar artery divides to form the two branches of the posterior cerebral arteries. The vertebrobasilar arteries supply most of the posterior circulation of the brain.

At the base of the brain surrounding the pituitary gland, a ring of arteries is formed between the vertebral and internal carotid arterial chains. This ring is called the circle of Willis and is formed from the branches of the internal carotid arteries, anterior and middle cerebral arteries, and anterior and posterior communicating arteries (Fig. 60-7). Functionally, the posterior portion of the circulation and the anterior or carotid circulation usually remain separate. The arteries of the circle of Willis can provide collateral circulation if one or more of the four vessels supplying it become occluded or are ligated.

The arterial anastomoses along the circle of Willis are frequent sites of aneurysms. These can be formed when the pressure at a weakened arterial wall causes the artery to balloon out. Aneurysms may be congenital or the result of degenerative changes in the vessel wall associated with arteriosclerotic vascular disease. If an artery with an aneurysm bursts or becomes occluded by vasospasm, an embolus, or a thrombus, the neurons distal to the occlusion are deprived of their blood supply and the cells quickly die. The result is a hemorrhagic stroke (cerebrovascular accident or infarction). The effects of the occlusion depend on which vessels are involved and which areas of the brain these vessels supply. Aneurysms and cerebrovascular accidents are discussed in more detail in Chapter 62.

Veins. Venous drainage for the brain does not follow the arterial circulation as in other body structures. The veins reach the brain's surface, join larger veins, then cross the subarachnoid space and empty into the dural sinuses, which are the vascular channels lying within the tough dura mater (see Fig. 60-6). The network of the sinuses carries venous outflow from the brain and empties into the internal jugular vein, returning the blood to the heart. Cerebral veins and sinuses are unique because, unlike other veins in the body, they do not have valves to prevent blood from flowing backward and depend on both gravity and blood pressure.

BLOOD–BRAIN BARRIER

The CNS is inaccessible to many substances that circulate in the blood plasma (eg, dyes, medications, and antibiotics). After being injected into the blood, many substances cannot reach the neu-

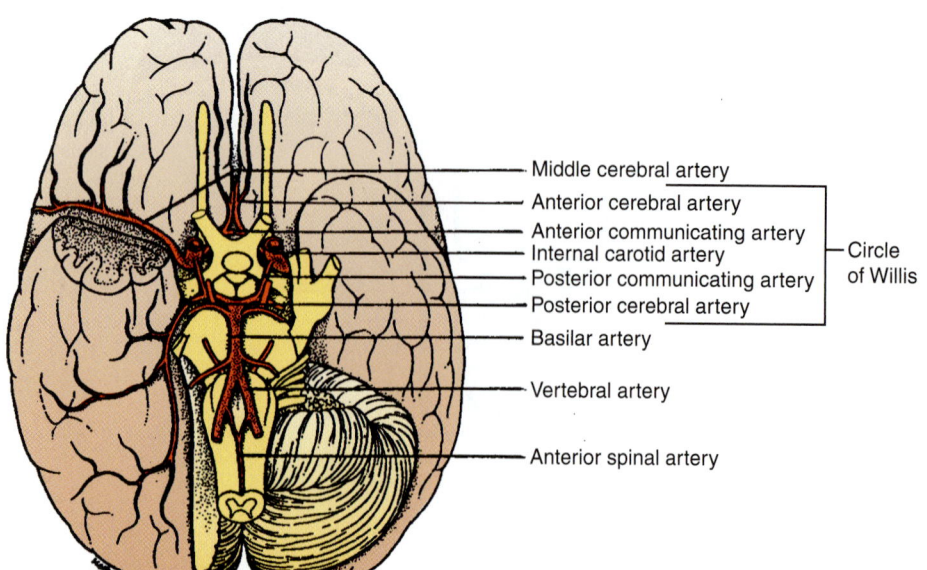

Middle cerebral artery
Anterior cerebral artery
Anterior communicating artery
Internal carotid artery
Posterior communicating artery
Posterior cerebral artery
— Circle of Willis

Basilar artery

Vertebral artery

Anterior spinal artery

FIGURE 60-7 Arterial blood supply of the brain, including the circle of Willis, as viewed from the ventral surface.

rons of the CNS because of the blood–brain barrier. This barrier is formed by the endothelial cells of the brain's capillaries, which form continuous tight junctions, creating a barrier to macromolecules and many compounds. All substances entering the CSF must filter through the capillary endothelial cells and astrocytes (Hickey, 2003). Often altered by trauma, cerebral edema, and cerebral hypoxemia, the blood–brain barrier has implications in the treatment and selection of medication for CNS disorders as well as serving a protective function.

ANATOMY OF THE SPINAL CORD

The spinal cord and medulla form a continuous structure extending from the cerebral hemispheres and serving as the connection between the brain and the periphery. Approximately 45 cm long and about the thickness of a finger, it extends from the foramen magnum at the base of the skull to the lower border of the first lumbar vertebra, where it tapers to a fibrous band called the conus medullaris. Continuing below the second lumbar space are the nerve roots that extend beyond the conus, which are called the cauda equina because they resemble a horse's tail. Similar to the brain, the spinal cord consists of grey and white matter. Grey matter in the brain is external and white matter is internal; in the spinal cord, grey matter is in the centre and is surrounded on all sides by white matter (Fig. 60-8).

The spinal cord is surrounded by the meninges, dura, arachnoid, and pia layers. Between the dura mater and the vertebral canal is the epidural space. The spinal cord is an H-shaped structure with nerve cell bodies (grey matter) surrounded by ascending and descending tracts (white matter) (see Fig. 60-8). The lower portion of the H is broader than the upper portion and corresponds to the anterior horns. The anterior horns contain cells with fibres that form the anterior (motor) root end and are essential for the voluntary and reflex activity of the muscles they innervate. The thinner posterior (upper horns) portion contains cells with fibres that enter over the posterior (sensory) root end and thus serve as a relay station in the sensory/reflex pathway.

The thoracic region of the spinal cord has a projection from each side at the crossbar of the H of grey matter called the lateral horn. It contains the cells that give rise to the autonomic fibres of the sympathetic division. The fibres leave the spinal cord through the anterior roots in the thoracic and upper lumbar segments.

Sensory and Motor Pathways: The Spinal Tracts. The white matter of the cord is composed of myelinated and unmyelinated nerve fibres. The fast-conducting myelinated fibres form bundles that also contain glial cells. Fibre bundles with a common function are called tracts. There are six ascending tracts. Two conduct sensation, principally the perception of touch, pressure, vibration, position, and passive motion from the same side of the body. Before reaching the cerebral cortex, these fibres cross to the opposite side in the medulla. The two spinocerebellar tracts conduct sensory impulses from muscle spindles, providing necessary input for coordinated muscle contraction. They ascend essentially uncrossed and terminate in the cerebellum. The last two spinothalamic tracts are responsible for conduction of pain, temperature, proprioception, fine touch, and vibratory sense from the upper body to the brain. They ascend, cross to the opposite side of the brain, and terminate in the thalamus (Hickey, 2003).

There are eight descending tracts, seven of which are engaged in motor function. The two corticospinal tracts conduct motor impulses to the anterior horn cells from the opposite side of the brain and control voluntary muscle activity. The three vestibulospinal tracts descend uncrossed and are involved in some autonomic functions (sweating, pupil dilation, and circulation) and involuntary muscle control. The corticobulbar tract conducts impulses responsible for voluntary head and facial muscle movement and crosses at the level of the brain stem. The rubrospinal and reticulospinal tracts conduct impulses involved with involuntary muscle movement.

Vertebral Column. The bones of the vertebral column surround and protect the spinal cord and normally consist of 7 cervical, 12 thoracic, and 5 lumber vertebrae, as well as the sacrum (a fused mass of five vertebrae), and terminate in the coccyx. Nerve roots exit from the vertebral column through the intervertebral foramina (openings). The vertebrae are separated by discs, except for the first and second cervical, the sacral, and the coccygeal vertebrae. Each vertebra has a ventral solid body and a dorsal segment or arch, which is posterior to the body. The arch is composed of two pedicles and two laminae supporting seven processes. The vertebral body, arch, pedicles, and laminae all encase the vertebral canal.

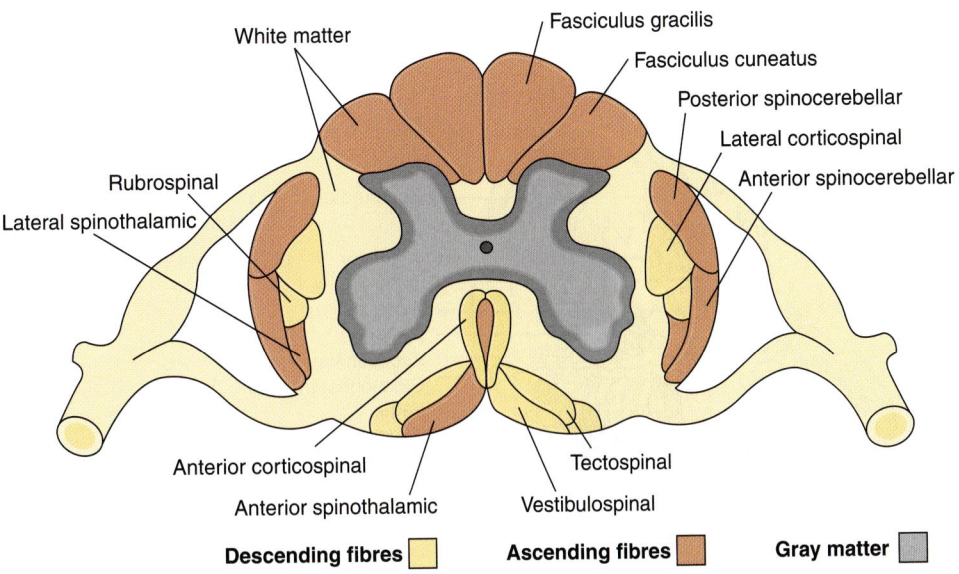

White matter · Fasciculus gracilis · Fasciculus cuneatus · Posterior spinocerebellar · Lateral corticospinal · Anterior spinocerebellar · Rubrospinal · Lateral spinothalamic · Anterior corticospinal · Anterior spinothalamic · Tectospinal · Vestibulospinal

Descending fibres □   **Ascending fibres** ■   **Gray matter** ▨

FIGURE 60-8 Cross-sectional diagram of the spinal cord showing major spinal tracts.

The Peripheral Nervous System

The peripheral nervous system includes the cranial nerves, the spinal nerves, and the autonomic nervous system.

CRANIAL NERVES

There are 12 pairs of cranial nerves that emerge from the lower surface of the brain and pass through the foramina in the skull. Three are entirely sensory (I, II, VIII), five are motor (III, IV, VI, XI, and XII), and four are mixed (V, VII, IX, and X) as they have both sensory and motor functions (Downey & Leigh, 1998; Hickey, 2003). The cranial nerves are numbered in the order in which they arise from the brain. For example, cranial nerves I and II attach in the cerebral hemispheres, whereas cranial nerves IX, X, XI, and XII attach at the medulla (Fig. 60-9). Most cranial nerves innervate the head, neck, and special sense structures. Table 60-2 lists the names and primary functions of the cranial nerves.

SPINAL NERVES

The spinal cord is composed of 31 pairs of spinal nerves: 8 cervical, 12 thoracic, 5 lumbar, 5 sacral, and 1 coccygeal. Each spinal nerve has a ventral root and a dorsal root (Fig. 60-10).

The dorsal roots are sensory and transmit sensory impulses from specific areas of the body known as dermatomes (Fig. 60-11) to the dorsal ganglia. The sensory fibre may be somatic, carrying information about pain, temperature, touch, and position sense (proprioception) from the tendons, joints, and body surfaces; or visceral, carrying information from the internal organs.

The ventral roots are motor and transmit impulses from the spinal cord to the body. These fibres are also either somatic or visceral. The visceral fibres include autonomic fibres that control the cardiac muscles and glandular secretions.

AUTONOMIC NERVOUS SYSTEM

The **autonomic nervous system** regulates the activities of internal organs such as the heart, lungs, blood vessels, digestive organs, and glands. Maintenance and restoration of internal homeostasis is largely the responsibility of the autonomic nervous system. There are two major divisions: the **sympathetic nervous system**, with predominantly excitatory responses, most notably the "fight or flight" response, and the **parasympathetic nervous system**, which controls mostly visceral functions.

The autonomic nervous system innervates most body organs. Although usually considered part of the peripheral nervous system, it is regulated by centres in the spinal cord, brain stem, and

Table 60-2 • Cranial Nerves		
CRANIAL NERVE	**TYPE**	**FUNCTION**
I (olfactory)	Sensory	Sense of smell
II (optic)	Sensory	Visual acuity
III (oculomotor)	Motor	Muscles that move the eye and lid, pupillary constriction, lens accommodation
IV (trochlear)	Motor	Muscles that move the eye
V (trigeminal)	Mixed	Facial sensation, corneal reflex, mastication
VI (abducens)	Motor	Muscles that move the eye
VII (facial)	Mixed	Facial expression and muscle movement, salivation and tearing, taste, sensation in the ear
VIII (acoustic)	Sensory	Hearing and equilibrium
IX (glossopharyngeal)	Mixed	Taste, sensation in pharynx and tongue, pharyngeal muscles
X (vagus)	Mixed	Muscles of pharynx, larynx, and soft palate; sensation in external ear, pharynx, larynx, thoracic and abdominal viscera; parasympathetic innervation of thoracic and abdominal organs
XI (spinal accessory)	Motor	Sternocleidomastoid and trapezius muscles
XII (hypoglossal)	Motor	Movement of the tongue

Name	Location
Optic II	} Cerebral hemisphere
Olfactory I	
Oculomotor III	} Midbrain
Trochlear IV	
Trigeminal V	} Pons
Abducens VI	
Facial VII	
Acoustic VIII	
Glossopharyngeal IX	} Medulla
Vagus X	
Hypoglossal XII	
Spinal accessory XI	

FIGURE 60-9 Diagram of the base of the brain showing entrance or exit of the cranial nerves. The right column shows the anatomic location of the connection of each cranial nerve to the central nervous system.

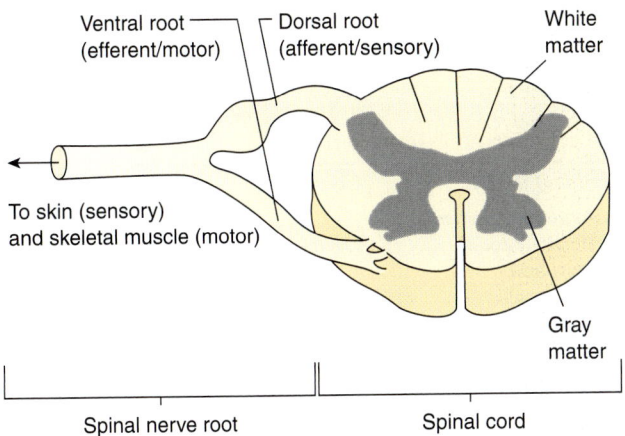

FIGURE 60-10 Cross-section of the spinal cord showing dorsal and ventral roots of a spinal nerve.

hypothalamus. The autonomic nervous system has two neurons in a series extending between the centres in the CNS and the organs innervated. The first neuron, the preganglionic neuron, is located in the brain or spinal cord, and its axon extends to the autonomic ganglia. There, it synapses with the second neuron, the postganglionic neuron, located in the autonomic ganglia, and its axon synapses with the target tissue and innervates the effector

organ. Its regulatory effects are exerted not on individual cells but on large expanses of tissue and on entire organs. The responses elicited do not occur instantaneously but after a lag period. These responses are sustained far longer than other neurogenic responses to ensure maximal functional efficiency on the part of receptor organs, such as blood vessels.

The quality of these responses is explained by the fact that the autonomic nervous system transmits its impulses by way of nerve pathways, enhanced by chemical mediators, resembling in this respect the endocrine system. Electrical impulses, conducted through nerve fibres, stimulate the formation of specific chemical agents at strategic locations within the muscle mass; the diffusion of these chemicals within the muscle is responsible for the contraction.

The hypothalamus is the major subcortical centre for the regulation of visceral and somatic activities, with an inhibitory–excitatory role in the autonomic nervous system. The hypothalamus has connections that link the autonomic system with the thalamus, the cortex, the olfactory apparatus, and the pituitary gland. Located here are the mechanisms for the control of visceral and somatic reactions that were originally important for defense or attack, and are associated with emotional states (eg, fear, anger, anxiety); for the control of metabolic processes, including fat, carbohydrate, and water metabolism; for the regulation of body temperature, arterial pressure, and all muscular and glandular activities of the gastrointestinal tract; for control of genital functions; and for the sleep cycle.

FIGURE 60-11 Dermatome distribution.

The autonomic nervous system is separated into the anatomically and functionally distinct sympathetic and parasympathetic divisions. Most of the tissues and the organs under autonomic control are innervated by both systems. Sympathetic stimuli are mediated by norepinephrine and parasympathetic impulses are mediated by acetylcholine. These chemicals produce opposing and mutually antagonistic effects. Both divisions produce stimulatory and inhibitory effects. For example, the parasympathetic division causes contraction (stimulation) of the urinary bladder muscles and a decrease (inhibition) in heart rate, whereas the sympathetic division produces relaxation (inhibition) of the urinary bladder and an increase (stimulation) in the rate and force of the heartbeat. Table 60-3 compares the sympathetic and the parasympathetic effects on the different systems of the body.

Sympathetic Nervous System. The sympathetic division of the autonomic nervous system is best known for its role in the body's "fight-or-flight" response. Under stress conditions from either physical or emotional causes, sympathetic impulses increase greatly. As a result, the bronchioles dilate for easier gas exchange; the heart's contractions are stronger and faster; the arteries to the heart and voluntary muscles dilate, carrying more blood to these organs; peripheral blood vessels constrict, making the skin feel cool but shunting blood to essential organs; the pupils dilate; the liver releases glucose for quick energy; peristalsis slows; hair stands on end; and perspiration increases. The sympathetic neurotransmitter is norepinephrine (noradrenaline), and this increase in sympathetic discharge is the same as if the body has been given an injection of adrenalin—hence, the term adrenergic is often used to refer to this division.

Sympathetic neurons are located in the thoracic and the lumbar segments of the spinal cord; their axons, or the preganglionic fibres, emerge by way of anterior nerve roots from the eighth cervical or first thoracic segment to the second or third lumbar segment. A short distance from the cord, these fibres diverge to join a chain, composed of 22 linked ganglia, that extends the entire length of the spinal column, adjacent to the vertebral bodies on both sides. Some form multiple synapses with nerve cells within the chain. Others traverse the chain without making connections or losing continuity to join large "prevertebral" ganglia in the thorax, the abdomen, or the pelvis or one of the "terminal" ganglia in the vicinity of an organ, such as the bladder or the rectum (Fig. 60-12). Postganglionic nerve fibres originating in the sympathetic chain rejoin the spinal nerves that supply the extremities and are distributed to blood vessels, sweat glands, and smooth muscle tissue in the skin. Postganglionic fibres from the prevertebral plexuses (eg, the cardiac, pulmonary, splanchnic, and pelvic plexuses) supply structures in the head and neck, thorax, abdomen, and pelvis, respectively, having been joined in these plexuses by fibres from the parasympathetic division.

The adrenal glands, kidneys, liver, spleen, stomach, and duodenum are under the control of the giant celiac plexus, commonly known as the solar plexus. This receives its sympathetic nerve components by way of the three splanchnic nerves, composed of preganglionic fibres from nine segments of the spinal cord (T4 to L1), and is joined by the vagus nerve, representing the parasympathetic division. From the celiac plexus, fibres of both divisions travel along the course of blood vessels to their target organs.

Sympathetic Syndromes. Certain syndromes are distinctive to diseases of the sympathetic nerve trunks. Among these are dilation of the pupil of the eye on the same side as a penetrating wound of the neck (evidence of disturbance of the cervical sympathetic cord); temporary paralysis of the bowel (indicated by the

Table 60-3 • Autonomic Effects of the Nervous System

STRUCTURE OR ACTIVITY	PARASYMPATHETIC EFFECTS	SYMPATHETIC EFFECTS
Pupil of the Eye	Constricted	Dilated
Circulatory System		
Rate and force of heart beat	Decreased	Increased
Blood vessels		
In heart muscle	Constricted	Dilated
In skeletal muscle	*	Dilated
In abdominal viscera and the skin	*	Constricted
Blood pressure	Decreased	Increased
Respiratory System		
Bronchioles	Constricted	Dilated
Rate of breathing	Decreased	Increased
Digestive System		
Peristaltic movements of digestive tube	Increased	Decreased
Muscular sphincters of digestive tube	Relaxed	Contracted
Secretion of salivary glands	Thin, watery saliva	Thick, viscid saliva
Secretions of stomach, intestine, and pancreas	Increased	*
Conversion of liver glycogen to glucose	*	Increased
Genitourinary System		
Urinary bladder		
Muscular walls	Contracted	Relaxed
Sphincters	Relaxed	Contracted
Muscles of the uterus	Relaxed; variable	Contracted under some conditions; varies with menstrual cycle and pregnancy
Blood vessels of external genitalia	Dilated	*
Integumentary System		
Secretion of sweat	*	Increased
Pilomotor muscles	*	Contracted (gooseflesh)
Adrenal Medullae	*	Secretion of epinephrine and norepinephrine

*No direct effect.
From Hickey, J. (2003). *Clinical practice of neurological and neurosurgical nursing* (5th ed.). Philadelphia: Lippincott Williams & Wilkins.

absence of peristaltic waves and the distention of the intestine by gas) after fracture of any one of the lower dorsal or upper lumbar vertebrae with hemorrhage into the base of the mesentery; and the marked variations in pulse rate and rhythm that often follow compression fractures of the upper six thoracic vertebrae.

Parasympathetic Nervous System. The parasympathetic nervous system functions as the dominant controller for most visceral effectors. During quiet, nonstressful conditions, impulses from parasympathetic fibres (cholinergic) predominate. The fibres of the parasympathetic system are located in two sections, one in the

FIGURE 60-12 Anatomy of the autonomic nervous system.

brain stem and the other from spinal segments below L2. Because of the location of these fibres, the parasympathetic system is referred to as the craniosacral division, as distinct from the thoracolumbar (sympathetic) division of the autonomic nervous system.

The parasympathetic nerves arise from the midbrain and the medulla oblongata. Fibres from cells in the midbrain travel with the third oculomotor nerve to the ciliary ganglia, where postganglionic fibres of this division are joined by those of the sympathetic system, creating controlled opposition, with a delicate balance maintained between the two at all times.

Motor and Sensory Functions of the Nervous System

MOTOR SYSTEM FUNCTION

The motor cortex, a vertical band within each cerebral hemisphere, controls the voluntary movements of the body. The exact locations within the brain at which the voluntary movements of the muscles of the face, thumb, hand, arm, trunk, and leg originate are known (Fig. 60-13). To initiate muscle movement, these particular cells must send the stimulus down along their fibres. Stimulation of these cells with an electric current will also result in muscle contraction. En route to the pons, the motor fibres con-

verge into a tight bundle known as the internal capsule. A comparatively small injury to the capsule causes paralysis in more muscles than does a much larger injury to the cortex itself.

Within the medulla, the motor axons from the cortex form the motor pathways or tracts, notably the corticospinal or pyramidal tracts. Here, most of the fibres cross (or decussate) to the opposite side, continuing as a crossed pyramidal tract. The remaining fibres enter the spinal cord on the same side as the direct pyramidal tract. Each fibre in this tract finally crosses to the opposite side of the cord and terminates within the grey matter of the anterior horn on that side, in proximity to a motor nerve cell. Fibres of the crossed pyramidal tract terminate within the anterior horn and make connections with anterior horn cells on the same side. All of the motor fibres of the spinal nerves represent extensions of these anterior horn cells, with each of these fibres communicating with only one particular muscle fibre.

The motor system is complex, and motor function depends on the integrity of the corticospinal tracts, the extrapyramidal system, and cerebellar function. A motor impulse consists of a two-neuron pathway (described below). The motor nerve pathways are contained in the spinal cord. Some represent the pathways of the so-called extrapyramidal system, establishing connections between the anterior horn cells and the automatic control centres located in the basal ganglia and the cerebellum. Others are

FIGURE 60-13 Diagrammatic representation of the cerebrum showing locations for control of motor movement of various parts of the body.

components of reflex arcs, forming synaptic connections between anterior horn cells and sensory fibres that have entered adjacent or neighbouring segments of the cord.

Upper and Lower Motor Neurons. The voluntary motor system consists of two groups of neurons: upper motor neurons and lower motor neurons. Upper motor neurons originate in the cerebral cortex, the cerebellum, and the brain stem and modulate the activity of the lower motor neurons. Upper motor neuron fibres make up the descending motor pathways and are located entirely within the CNS. Lower motor neurons are located either in the anterior horn of the spinal cord grey matter or within cranial nerve nuclei in the brain stem. Axons of both extend through peripheral nerves and terminate in skeletal muscle. Lower motor neurons are located in both the CNS and the peripheral nervous system.

The motor pathways from the brain to the spinal cord, as well as from the cerebrum to the brain stem, are formed by upper motor neurons. They begin in the cortex of one side of the brain, descend through the internal capsule, cross to the opposite side in the brain stem, descend through the corticospinal tract, and synapse with the lower motor neurons in the cord. The lower motor neurons receive the impulse in the posterior part of the cord and run to the myoneural junction located in the peripheral muscle. The clinical features of lesions of upper and lower motor neurons are discussed in the sections that follow and in Table 60-4.

Upper Motor Neuron Lesions. Upper motor neuron lesions can involve the motor cortex, the internal capsule, the spinal cord, and other structures of the brain through which the corticospinal tract descends. If the upper motor neurons are damaged or destroyed, as frequently occurs with stroke or spinal cord injury, paralysis (loss of voluntary movement) results. However, because the inhibitory influences of intact upper motor neurons are now impaired, **reflex** (involuntary) movements are uninhibited, and

hence hyperactive deep tendon reflexes, diminished or absent superficial reflexes, and pathologic reflexes such as a Babinski response occur. Severe leg spasms can occur as the result of an upper motor neuron lesion; the spasms result from the preserved reflex arc, which lacks inhibition along the spinal cord below the level of injury.

There is little or no muscle atrophy, and muscles remain permanently tense, exhibiting spastic paralysis or paresis (weakness). Paralysis associated with upper motor neuron lesions usually affects a whole extremity, both extremities, and an entire half of the body. Hemiplegia (paralysis of an arm and leg on the same side of the body) can be the result of an upper motor neuron lesion. If hemorrhage, an embolus, or a thrombus destroys the fibres from the motor area in the internal capsule, the arm and the leg of the opposite side become stiff and very weak or paralyzed, and the reflexes are hyperactive (further discussion of hemiplegia is found in Chap. 62). When both legs are paralyzed, the condition is called paraplegia; paralysis of all four extremities is quadriplegia (more discussion of these can be found in Chap. 63).

Lower Motor Neuron Lesions. A patient is considered to have lower motor neuron damage if a motor nerve is severed between

Table 60-4 • Comparison of Upper Motor Neuron and Lower Motor Neuron Lesions	
UPPER MOTOR NEURON LESIONS	**LOWER MOTOR NEURON LESIONS**
Loss of voluntary control	Loss of voluntary control
Increased muscle tone	Decreased muscle tone
Muscle spasticity	Flaccid muscle paralysis
No muscle atrophy	Muscle atrophy
Hyperactive and abnormal reflexes	Absent or decreased reflexes

the muscle and the spinal cord. The result of lower motor neuron damage is muscle paralysis. Reflexes are lost, and the muscle becomes **flaccid** (limp) and atrophied from disuse. If the patient has injured the spinal trunk and it can heal, use of the muscles connected to that section of the spinal cord may be regained. If the anterior horn motor cells are destroyed, however, the nerves cannot regenerate and the muscles are never useful again. Flaccid paralysis and atrophy of the affected muscles are the principal signs of lower motor neuron disease. Lower motor neuron lesions can be the result of trauma, infection (poliomyelitis), toxins, vascular disorders, congenital malformations, degenerative processes, and neoplasms. Compression of nerve roots by herniated intervertebral discs is a common cause of lower motor neuron dysfunction.

Coordination of Movement.
The smoothness, accuracy, and strength that characterize the muscular movements of a normal person are attributable to the influence of the cerebellum and the basal ganglia.

The cerebellum (refer to Fig. 60-2), described earlier, is located beneath the occipital lobe of the cerebrum; it is responsible for the coordination, balance, and timing of all muscular movements that originate in the motor centres of the cerebral cortex. Through the action of the cerebellum, the contractions of opposing muscle groups are adjusted in relation to each other to maximal mechanical advantage; muscle contractions can be sustained evenly at the desired tension and without significant fluctuation, and reciprocal movements can be reproduced at high and constant speed, in stereotyped fashion and with relatively little effort.

The basal ganglia, masses of grey matter in the midbrain beneath the cerebral hemispheres, border the lateral ventricles and lie in proximity to the internal capsule. The basal ganglia play an important role in planning and coordinating motor movements and posture. Complex neural connections link the basal ganglia with the cerebral cortex. The major effect of these structures is to inhibit unwanted muscular activity; disorders of the basal ganglia result in exaggerated, uncontrolled movements.

Impaired cerebellar function, which may occur as a result of an intracranial injury or some type of an expanding mass (eg, a hemorrhage, abscess, or tumour), results in loss of muscle tone, weakness, and fatigue. Depending on the area of the brain affected, the patient has different motor symptoms or responses. The patient may demonstrate decorticate, decerebrate, or flaccid posturing, usually as a result of cerebral trauma (Bateman, 2001). For further explanation of this, see Figure 61-1 in Chapter 61. Decortication (decorticate posturing) is the result of lesions of the internal capsule or cerebral hemispheres; the patient has flexion and internal rotation of the arms and wrists and extension, internal rotation, and plantar flexion of the feet. Decerebration (decerebrate posturing), the result of lesions at the midbrain, is more ominous than decortication. The patient has extension and external rotation of the arms and wrists and extension, plantar flexion, and internal rotation of the feet. Flaccid posturing is usually the result of lower brain stem dysfunction; the patient has no motor function, is limp, and lacks motor tone.

Flaccidity preceded by decerebration in a patient with cerebral injury indicates severe neurologic impairment, which may herald brain death. However, before the declaration of brain death, the patient must have spinal cord injury ruled out, the effects of all neuromuscular paralyzing agents must have worn off, and any other possible treatable causes of neurologic impairment must be investigated.

Tumours, infection, or abscess and increased intracranial pressure can all affect the cerebellum. Cerebellar signs, such as ataxia, incoordination, and seizures, as well as CSF obstruction and compression of the brain stem may be seen. Signs of increased intracranial pressure, including vomiting, headache, and changes in vital signs and level of consciousness, are especially common when CSF flow is obstructed.

Destruction or dysfunction of the basal ganglia leads not to paralysis but to muscle rigidity, with disturbances of posture and movement. Such patients tend to have involuntary movements. These may take the form of coarse tremors, most often in the upper extremities, particularly in the distal portions; athetosis, movement of a slow, squirming, writhing, twisting type; or chorea, marked by spasmodic, purposeless, irregular, uncoordinated motions of the trunk and the extremities, and facial grimacing. Disorders due to lesions of the basal ganglia include Parkinson's disease, Huntington's disease (see Chap. 65), and spasmodic torticollis.

SENSORY SYSTEM FUNCTION

Integrating Sensory Impulses.
The thalamus, a major receiving and transmitting centre for the afferent sensory nerves, is a large structure connected to the midbrain. It lies next to the third ventricle and forms the floor of the lateral ventricle (see Fig. 60-3). The thalamus integrates all sensory impulses except olfaction. It plays a role in the conscious awareness of pain and the recognition of variation in temperature and touch. The thalamus is responsible for the sense of movement and position and the ability to recognize the size, shape, and quality of objects.

Receiving Sensory Impulses.
Afferent impulses travel from their points of origin to their destinations in the cerebral cortex via the ascending pathways directly, or they may cross at the level of the spinal cord or in the medulla, depending on the type of sensation that is registered. Sensory information may be integrated at the level of the spinal cord or may be relayed to the brain. Knowledge of these pathways is important for neurologic assessment and for understanding symptoms and their relationship to various lesions.

Sensory impulses enter the spinal cord by way of the posterior root. These axons convey sensations of heat, cold, and pain and enter the posterior grey column of the cord, where they make connections with the cells of secondary neurons. Pain and temperature fibres cross immediately to the opposite side of the cord and course upward to the thalamus. Fibres carrying sensations of touch, light pressure, and localization do not connect immediately with the second neuron but ascend the cord for a variable distance before entering the grey matter and completing this connection. The axon of the secondary neuron crosses the cord and proceeds upward to the thalamus.

Position and vibratory sensation are produced by stimuli arising from muscles, joints, and bones. These stimuli are conveyed, uncrossed, all the way to the brain stem by the axon of the primary neuron. In the medulla, synaptic connections are made with cells of the secondary neurons, whose axons cross to the opposite side and then proceed to the thalamus.

Sensory Losses.
Destruction of a sensory nerve results in total loss of sensation in its area of distribution. Transection of the spinal cord yields complete anesthesia below the level of injury. Selective destruction or degeneration of the posterior columns of the spinal cord is responsible for a loss of position and vibratory sense in segments distal to the lesion, without loss of touch, pain, or temperature perception. A lesion, such as a cyst, in the centre of the spinal cord causes dissociation of sensation—loss of pain

at the level of the lesion. This occurs because the fibres carrying pain and temperature cross within the cord immediately on entering; thus, any lesion that divides the cord longitudinally divides these fibres. Other sensory fibres ascend the cord for variable distances, some even to the medulla, before crossing, thereby bypassing the lesion and avoiding destruction.

Lesions affecting the posterior spinal nerve roots may cause impairment of tactile sensation, including intermittent severe pain that is referred to their areas of distribution. Tingling of the fingers and the toes can be a prominent symptom of spinal cord disease, presumably due to degenerative changes in the sensory fibres that extend to the thalamus (ie, belonging to the spinothalamic tract).

Assessment: The Neurologic Examination

HEALTH HISTORY

An important aspect of the neurologic assessment is the history of the present illness. The initial interview provides an excellent opportunity to systematically explore the patient's current condition and related events while simultaneously observing overall appearance, mental status, posture, movement and affect. Depending on the patient's condition, the nurse may need to rely on yes-or-no answers to questions, on a review of the medical record, or input from the family or a combination of these.

Neurologic disease may be stable or progressive, with both intermittent symptom-free periods as well as times with fluctuations in symptoms. The health history therefore includes details about the onset, character, severity, location, duration, and frequency of symptoms and signs; associated complaints; precipitating, aggravating, and relieving factors; progression, remission, and exacerbation; and the presence or absence of similar symptoms among family members. The nurse may also use the interview to inquire about any family history of genetic diseases. See the Genetics chart for assessment guidelines and Chapter 9 for additional information about genetics.

Included in the health history is a review of the medical history, including a system-by-system evaluation. The nurse should be aware of any history of trauma or falls that may have involved the head or spinal cord. Questions regarding the use of alcohol, medications, and recreational drugs are also included. The history-taking portion of the neurologic examination is critical and, in many cases of neurologic disease, leads to an accurate diagnosis.

CLINICAL MANIFESTATIONS

The clinical manifestations of neurologic disease are as varied as the disease processes themselves. Symptoms can be subtle or intense, fluctuating or permanent, an inconvenience or devastating. An introduction to some of the most common symptoms associ-

GENETICS IN NURSING PRACTICE—Neurologic Disorders

DISEASES AND CONDITIONS INFLUENCED BY GENETIC FACTORS
- Alzheimer's disease
- Amyotrophic lateral sclerosis (ALS)
- Duchenne muscular dystrophy
- Epilepsy
- Friedrich ataxia
- Huntington disease
- Myotonic dystrophy
- Neurofibromatosis type I
- Parkinson's disease
- Spina bifida
- Tourette syndrome

NURSING ASSESSMENTS
FAMILY HISTORY ASSESSMENT
- Assess for other similarly affected relatives with neurologic impairment.
- Inquire about age of onset (eg, present at birth—spina bifida; developed in childhood—Duchenne muscular dystrophy; developed in adulthood—Huntington disease, Alzheimer's disease, amyotrophic lateral sclerosis)
- Inquire about the presence of related conditions such as mental retardation and/or learning disabilities (neurofibromatosis type I).

PHYSICAL ASSESSMENT
- Assess for the presence of other physical features suggestive of an underlying genetic condition, such as skin lesions seen in neurofibromatosis type 1 (café-au-lait spots).
- Assess for other congenital abnormalities (eg, cardiac, ocular).

MANAGEMENT SPECIFIC TO GENETICS
- Inquire whether DNA mutation or other genetic testing has been performed on affected family members.
- If indicated, refer for further genetic counselling and evaluation so that family members can discuss inheritance, risk to other family members, availability of genetic testing and gene-based interventions.
- Offer appropriate genetics information and resources.
- Assess patient's understanding of genetics information.
- Provide support to families with newly diagnosed genetic-related neurologic disorders.
- Participate in management and coordination of care of patients with genetic conditions and individuals predisposed to develop or pass on a genetic condition.

GENETICS RESOURCES FOR NURSES AND THEIR PATIENTS ON THE WEB
Canadian Association of Genetic Counsellors (CAGC)—a listing of genetic centres across Canada; www.cagc-accg.ca
Canadian Directory of Genetic Support Groups—a resource guide for families and professionals; www.lhsc.on.ca/programs/medgenet
Canadian Organization for Rare Disorders (CORD)—information on over 6,000 rare disorders and links individuals/families together with the same rare disorder; www.cord.ca
Organizations for Support Groups and Information—information on hundreds of genetic support groups located in Canada, in the United States, and in other countries; http://www.kumc.edu/gec/support/grouporg.htm;

ated with neurologic disease follows; detailed discussions regarding how specific symptoms relate to a particular disorder will be covered in later chapters in this unit.

Pain

Pain is considered an unpleasant sensory perception and emotional experience associated with actual or potential tissue damage or described in terms of such damage. Pain is therefore considered multidimensional and entirely subjective (Loeser, 2001). Pain can be acute or chronic. In general, acute pain lasts for a relatively short period of time and remits as the pathology resolves. In neurologic disease, this type of pain is often associated with spinal disc disease, trigeminal neuralgia, or other neuropathic pathology (eg, postherpetic neuralgia, or painful neuropathies). In contrast, chronic pain extends for long periods of time and may represent a low level of pathology. This type of pain might also occur with discogenic disease.

Seizures

Seizures are the result of abnormal paroxysmal discharges in the cerebral cortex, which then manifest as an alteration in sensation, behaviour, movement, perception, or consciousness (Hickey, 2003). The alteration may be short, as in a blank stare lasting only a second, or of longer duration, such as a tonic-clonic grand mal seizure that can last several minutes. The type of seizure activity is a direct result of the area of the brain affected. Seizures can occur as isolated events, such as when induced by a high fever, alcohol or drug withdrawal, or hypoglycemia. A seizure may also be the first obvious sign of a brain lesion.

Dizziness

Dizziness is an abnormal sensation of imbalance or movement. It is fairly common in the elderly and one of the most common complaints encountered by health professionals. Dizziness can have a variety of causes, including viral syndromes, hot weather, roller coaster rides, and middle ear infections, to name a few. One difficulty confronting health care providers when assessing dizziness is the vague and varied terms patients use to describe the sensation. *Vertigo,* a specific form of dizziness, is defined as a sensation that is usually a manifestation of vestibular dysfunction. It can be so severe as to result in spatial disorientation, loss of equilibrium, and nausea and vomiting (Greenberg, Aminoff, & Simon, 2002).

Visual Disturbances

Visual defects that cause people to seek health care can range from the decreased visual acuity associated with aging to sudden blindness caused by glaucoma. Normal vision depends upon functioning visual pathways through the retina and optic chiasm and the radiations into the visual cortex in the occipital lobes. Lesions of the eye itself (eg, cataract), lesions along the pathway (eg, tumour), or lesions in the visual cortex (from stroke) interfere with normal visual acuity. Abnormalities of eye movement (as in the nystagmus associated with multiple sclerosis) can also compromise vision by causing diplopia or double vision.

Weakness

Weakness, specifically muscle weakness, is a common manifestation of neurologic disease. Weakness frequently coexists with other symptoms of disease and can affect a variety of muscles, causing a wide range of disability. Weakness can be sudden and permanent, as in stroke, or progressive, as in many neuromuscular diseases such as amyotrophic lateral sclerosis. Any muscle group can be affected.

Abnormal Sensation

Numbness, abnormal sensation, or loss of sensation is a neurologic manifestation of both central and peripheral nervous system disease. Altered sensation can affect small or large areas of the body. It is frequently associated with weakness or pain and is potentially disabling. Both numbness and weakness can significantly affect balance and coordination.

PHYSICAL EXAMINATION

The neurologic examination is a systematic process that includes a variety of clinical tests, observations, and assessments designed to evaluate a complex system. Although the neurologic examination is often limited to a simple screening, the examiner must be able to conduct a thorough neurologic assessment when the patient's history or other physical findings warrant it. Many neurologic rating scales exist; some of the more common ones are discussed here, but an in-depth discussion is beyond the scope of this chapter (see Herndon [1997] and Rapp, Wakefield, Kundrat et al. [2000] for full descriptions of neurologic rating scales).

The brain and spinal cord cannot be examined as directly as other systems of the body. Thus, much of the neurologic examination is an indirect evaluation that assesses the function of the specific body part or parts controlled or innervated by the nervous system. A neurologic assessment is divided into five components: cerebral function, cranial nerves, motor system, sensory system, and reflexes. As in other parts of the physical assessment, the neurologic examination follows a logical sequence and progresses from higher levels of cortical function such as abstract thinking to lower levels of function such as the determination of the integrity of peripheral nerves.

Assessing Cerebral Function

Cerebral abnormalities may cause disturbances in mental status, intellectual functioning, and thought content and in patterns of emotional behaviour. There may also be alterations in perception, motor and language abilities, as well as lifestyle.

MENTAL STATUS

An assessment of mental status begins by observing the patient's appearance and behaviour, noting dress, grooming, and personal hygiene. Posture, gestures, movements, facial expressions, and motor activity often provide important information about the patient. The patient's manner of speech and level of consciousness are also assessed. Is the patient's speech clear and coherent? Is the patient alert and responsive, or drowsy and stuporous?

Assessing orientation to time, place, and person assists in evaluating mental status. Does the patient know what day it is, what year it is, and the name of the Prime Minister of Canada? Is the patient aware of where he or she is? Is the patient aware of who the examiner is and of his or her purpose for being in the room? Is the capacity for immediate memory intact? (See Chart 12-1: Mini-Mental State Examination in Chap. 12.)

INTELLECTUAL FUNCTION

A person with an average IQ can repeat seven digits without faltering and can recite five digits backward. The examiner might ask the patient to count backward from 100 or to subtract 7 from 100, then 7 from that, and so forth (called serial 7s) (Johnson, 2001). The capacity to interpret well-known proverbs tests abstract reasoning, which is a higher intellectual function; for example, does the patient know what is meant by "the early bird catches the worm"? Patients with damage to the frontal cortex appear superficially normal until one or more tests of integrative capacity are performed. Questions designed to assess this capacity might include the ability to recognize similarities: how are a mouse and dog or pen and pencil alike? Can the patient make judgements about situations—for instance, if the patient arrived home without a house key, what alternatives are there?

THOUGHT CONTENT

During the interview, it is important to assess the patient's thought content. Are the patient's thoughts spontaneous, natural, clear, relevant, and coherent? Does the patient have any fixed ideas, illusions, or preoccupations? What are his or her insights into these thoughts? Preoccupation with death or morbid events, hallucinations, and paranoid ideation are examples of unusual thoughts or perceptions that require further evaluation.

EMOTIONAL STATUS

An assessment of cerebral functioning also includes the patient's emotional status. Is the patient's affect (external manifestation of mood) natural and even, or irritable and angry, anxious, apathetic or flat, or euphoric? Does his or her mood fluctuate normally, or does the patient unpredictably swing from joy to sadness during the interview? Is affect appropriate to words and thought content? Are verbal communications consistent with nonverbal cues?

PERCEPTION

The examiner may now consider more specific areas of higher cortical function. **Agnosia** is the inability to interpret or recognize objects seen through the special senses. The patient may see a pencil but not know what it is called or what to do with it. The patient may even be able to describe it but not to interpret its function. The patient may experience auditory or tactile agnosia as well as visual agnosia. Each of the dysfunctions implicates a different part of the cortex (Chart 60-1).

Screening for visual and tactile agnosia provides insight into the patient's cortical interpretation ability. The patient is shown a familiar object and asked to identify it by name. Placing a familiar object (eg, key, coin) in the patient's hand and having him or her identify it with both eyes closed is an easy way to assess tactile interpretation.

MOTOR ABILITY

Assessment of cortical motor integration is carried out by asking the patient to perform a skilled act (throw a ball, move a chair).

Successful performance requires the ability to understand the activity desired and normal motor strength. Failure signals cerebral dysfunction.

LANGUAGE ABILITY

The person with normal neurologic function can understand and communicate in spoken and written language. Does the patient answer questions appropriately? Can he or she read a sentence from a newspaper and explain its meaning? Can the patient write his or her name or copy a simple figure that the examiner has drawn? A deficiency in language function is called aphasia. Different types of aphasia result from injury to different parts of the brain (Chart 60-2). Aphasia is discussed in detail in Chapter 62.

IMPACT ON LIFESTYLE

The nurse assesses the impact the neurologic impairment has on the patient's lifestyle. Issues to consider include the limitations imposed on the patient by any deficit and the patient's role in society, including family and community roles. The plan of care that the nurse develops needs to address and support adaptation to the neurologic deficit and continued function to the extent possible within the patient's support system.

DOCUMENTATION OF FINDINGS

Interpretation and documentation of neurologic abnormalities, particularly mental status abnormalities, should be specific and nonjudgmental. Lengthy descriptions and the use of terms such as "inappropriate" or "demented" should be avoided. Terms such as these often mean different things to different people and are therefore not useful when describing behaviour. The examiner records and reports specific observations regarding orientation, level of consciousness, emotional state, or thought content, all of which permit comparison by others over time. Analysis and the conclusions that may be drawn from these findings usually depend on the examiner's knowledge of neuroanatomy, neurophysiology, and neuropathology.

Examining the Cranial Nerves

Table 60-5 describes how to assess the cranial nerves. Opposite sides of the face and neck are compared throughout the examination.

Examining the Motor System

A thorough examination of the motor system includes an assessment of muscle size, tone, and strength, coordination, and balance. The patient is instructed to walk across the room while the examiner observes posture and gait. The muscles are inspected, and palpated if necessary, for their size and symmetry. Any evidence of atrophy or involuntary movements (tremors, tics) is noted. Muscle **tone** (the tension present in a muscle at rest) is evaluated by palpating various muscle groups at rest and during passive movement. Resistance to these movements is assessed and documented.

Chart 60-1 Types of Agnosia and Corresponding Sites of Lesions

Type of Agnosia	Affected Cerebral Area
Visual	Occipital lobe
Auditory	Temporal lobe (lateral and superior portions)
Tactile	Parietal lobe
Body parts and relationships	Parietal lobe (posteroinferior regions)

Chart 60-2 Types of Aphasia and Region of Brain Involved

Type of Aphasia	Brain Area Involved
Auditory-receptive	Temporal lobe
Visual-receptive	Parietal-occipital area
Expressive speaking	Inferior posterior frontal areas
Expressive writing	Posterior frontal area

Table 60-5 • Assessing Cranial Nerve Function

CRANIAL NERVE	CLINICAL EXAMINATION
I (olfactory)	With eyes closed, the patient identifies familiar odours (coffee, tobacco). Each nostril is tested separately.
II (optic)	Snellen eye chart; visual fields; ophthalmoscopic examination
III (oculomotor) IV (trochlear) VI (abducens)	For cranial nerves III, IV, and VI: test for ocular rotations, conjugate movements, nystagmus. Test for pupillary reflexes, and inspect eyelids for ptosis.
V (trigeminal)	Have patient close the eyes. Touch cotton to forehead, cheeks, and jaw. Sensitivity to superficial pain is tested by using the sharp and dull ends of a broken tongue blade. Alternate between the sharp point and the dull end. Patient reports "sharp" or "dull" with each movement. If responses are incorrect, test for temperature sensation. Test tubes of cold and hot water are used alternately. While the patient looks up, *lightly* touch a wisp of cotton against the temporal surface of each cornea. A blink and tearing are normal responses. Have the patient clench and move the jaw from side to side. Palpate the masseter and temporal muscles, noting strength and equality.
VII (facial)	Observe for symmetry while the patient performs facial movements: smiles, whistles, elevates eyebrows, frowns, tightly closes eyelids against resistance (examiner attempts to open them). Observe face for flaccid paralysis (shallow nasolabial folds). Patient extends tongue. Ability to discriminate between sugar and salt is tested.
VIII (acoustic)	Whisper or watch-tick test Test for lateralization (Weber) Test for air and bone conduction (Rinne)
IX (glossopharyngeal)	Assess patient's ability to discriminate between sugar and salt on posterior third of the tongue.
X (vagus)	Depress a tongue blade on posterior tongue, or stimulate posterior pharynx to elicit gag reflex. Note any hoarseness in voice. Have patient say "ah." Observe for symmetric rise of uvula and soft palate.
XI (spinal accessory)	Palpate and note strength of trapezius muscles while patient shrugs shoulders against resistance. Palpate and note strength of each sternocleidomastoid muscle as patient turns head against opposing pressure of the examiner's hand.
XII (hypoglossal)	While the patient protrudes the tongue, any deviation or tremors are noted. The strength of the tongue is tested by having the patient move the protruded tongue from side to side against a tongue depressor.

Abnormalities in tone include **spasticity** (increased muscle tone), **rigidity** (resistance to passive stretch), and flaccidity.

MUSCLE STRENGTH

Assessing the patient's ability to flex or extend the extremities against resistance tests muscle strength. The function of an individual muscle or group of muscles is evaluated by placing the muscle at a disadvantage. The quadriceps, for example, is a powerful muscle responsible for straightening the leg. Once the leg is straightened, it is exceedingly difficult for the examiner to flex the knee. Conversely, if the knee is flexed and the patient is asked to straighten the leg against resistance, a more subtle disability can be elicited. The evaluation of muscle strength compares the sides of the body to each other. For example, the right upper extremity is compared to the left upper extremity. In this way, subtle differences in muscle strength can be more easily detected and accurately described.

Clinicians use a five-point scale to rate muscle strength (O'Hanlon-Nichols, 1999). A 5 indicates full power of contraction against gravity and resistance or normal muscle strength; 4 indicates fair but not full strength against gravity and a moderate amount of resistance or slight weakness; 3 indicates just sufficient strength to overcome the force of gravity or moderate weakness; 2 indicates the ability to move but not to overcome the force of gravity or severe weakness; 1 indicates minimal contractile power—weak muscle contraction can be palpated but no movement is noted—or very severe weakness; and 0 indicates complete paralysis. A stick figure

may be used to record muscle strength and is a precise form of documenting findings. Distal and proximal strength in both upper and lower extremities is recorded using the five-point scale (Fig. 60-14).

Assessment of muscle strength can be as detailed as necessary. One may quickly test the strength of the proximal muscles of the upper and lower extremities, always comparing both sides. The strength of the finer muscles that control the function of the hand (hand grasp) and the foot (dorsiflexion and plantar flexion) can then be assessed.

BALANCE AND COORDINATION

Cerebellar influence on the motor system is reflected in balance control and coordination. Coordination in the hands and upper extremities is tested by having the patient perform rapid, alternating movements and point-to-point testing. First, the patient is instructed to pat his or her thigh as fast as possible with each hand separately. Then the patient is instructed to alternately pronate and supinate the hand as rapidly as possible. Lastly, the patient is asked to touch each of the fingers with the thumb in a consecutive motion. Speed, symmetry, and degree of difficulty are noted.

In point-to-point testing, the patient touches the examiner's index finger (which is kept in one place) and then his or her own nose (eyes open and then closed). Then (with the patient's eyes open) the examiner's finger moves, requiring the patient's finger to move accordingly. Speed and accuracy are noted (Bickley & Szilagyi, 2004).

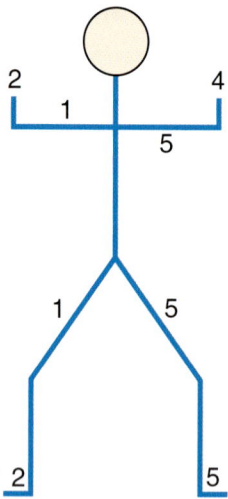

FIGURE 60-14 A stick figure may be used to record muscle strength as follows: 5, full range of motion against gravity and resistance; 4, full range of motion against gravity and a moderate amount of resistance; 3, full range of motion against gravity only; 2, full range of motion when gravity is eliminated; 1, a weak muscle contraction when muscle is palpated, but no movement; and 0, complete paralysis.

Coordination in the lower extremities is tested by having the patient run the heel down the anterior surface of the tibia of the other leg. Each leg is tested in turn. **Ataxia** is defined as incoordination of voluntary muscle action, particularly of the muscle groups used in activities such as walking or reaching for objects. The presence of ataxia or tremors (rhythmic, involuntary movements) during these movements suggests cerebellar disease.

It is not necessary to carry out each of these assessments for coordination. During a routine examination, it is advisable to perform a simple screening of the upper and lower extremities by having the patient perform either rapid, alternating movements or point-to-point testing. When abnormalities are observed, a more thorough examination is indicated.

The **Romberg test** is a screening test for balance. The patient stands with feet together and arms at the side, first with eyes open and then with both eyes closed for 20 to 30 seconds. The examiner stands close to reassure the patient of support if he or she begins to fall. Slight swaying is normal, but a loss of balance is abnormal and is considered a positive Romberg test. Additional cerebellar tests for balance in the ambulatory patient include hopping in place, alternating knee bends, and heel-to-toe walking (both forward and backward).

Examining the Reflexes

The motor reflexes are involuntary contractions of muscles or muscle groups in response to abrupt stretching near the site of the muscle's insertion. The tendon is struck directly with a reflex hammer or indirectly by striking the examiner's thumb, which is placed firmly against the tendon. Testing these reflexes enables the examiner to assess involuntary reflex arcs that depend on the presence of afferent stretch receptors, spinal synapses, efferent motor fibres, and a variety of modifying influences from higher levels. Common reflexes that may be tested include the deep tendon reflexes (biceps, brachioradialis, triceps, patellar, and ankle reflexes) and superficial or cutaneous reflexes (abdominal reflexes and plantar or Babinski response) (Fig. 60-15).

TECHNIQUE

A reflex hammer is used to elicit a deep tendon reflex. The handle of the hammer is held loosely between the thumb and index finger, allowing a full swinging motion. The wrist motion is similar to that used during percussion. The extremity is positioned so that the tendon is slightly stretched. This requires a sound knowledge of the location of muscles and their tendon attachments. The tendon is then struck briskly, and the response is compared with that on the opposite side of the body. A wide variation in reflex response may be considered normal; it is more important, however, that the reflexes be symmetrically equivalent. When the comparison is made, both sides should be equivalently relaxed and each tendon struck with equal force.

Valid findings depend on several factors: proper use of the reflex hammer, proper positioning of the extremity, and a relaxed patient. If the reflexes are symmetrically diminished or absent, the examiner may use reinforcement to increase reflex activity. This involves the isometric contraction of other muscle groups. If lower extremity reflexes are diminished or absent, the patient is instructed to lock the fingers together and pull in opposite directions. Having the patient clench the jaw or press the heels against the floor or examining table may similarly elicit more reliable biceps, triceps, and brachioradialis reflexes.

GRADING THE REFLEXES

The absence of reflexes is significant, although ankle jerks (Achilles reflex) may be normally absent in older people. Deep tendon reflex responses are often graded on a scale of 0 to 4+. A 4+ indicates a hyperactive reflex, often indicating pathology; 3+ indicates a response that is more brisk than average but may be normal or indicative of disease; 2+ indicates an average or normal response; 1+ indicates a hypoactive or diminished response; and 0 indicates no response. As stated previously, scale ratings are highly subjective. Findings can be recorded as a fraction, indicating the scale range (eg, 2/4). Some examiners prefer to use the terms present, absent, and diminished when describing reflexes. As with muscle strength recording, a stick figure such as the one shown in Chart 60-3 may also be used to record numerical findings.

BICEPS REFLEX

The biceps reflex is elicited by striking the biceps tendon of the flexed elbow. The examiner supports the forearm with one arm while placing the thumb against the tendon and striking the thumb with the reflex hammer. The normal response is flexion at the elbow and contraction of the biceps (see Fig. 60-15*A*).

TRICEPS REFLEX

To elicit a triceps reflex, the patient's arm is flexed at the elbow and positioned in front of the chest. The examiner supports the patient's arm and identifies the triceps tendon by palpating 2.5 to 5 cm above the elbow. A direct blow on the tendon normally produces contraction of the triceps muscle and extension of the elbow (see Fig. 60-15*B*).

BRACHIORADIALIS REFLEX

With the patient's forearm resting on the lap or across the abdomen, the brachioradialis reflex is assessed. A gentle strike of the hammer 2.5 to 5 cm above the wrist results in flexion and supination of the forearm.

PATELLAR REFLEX

The patellar reflex is elicited by striking the patellar tendon just below the patella. The patient may be in a sitting or a lying posi-

FIGURE 60-15 Techniques for eliciting major reflexes. (**A**) Biceps reflex. (**B**) Triceps reflex. (**C**) Patellar reflex.
(**D**) Ankle or Achilles reflex. (**E**) Babinski response. From Weber, J. & Kelley, J. (2003). *Health assessment in nursing*
(2nd ed.). Philadelphia: Lippincott Williams & Wilkins. © B. Proud.

tion. If the patient is supine, the examiner supports the legs to facilitate relaxation of the muscles. Contractions of the quadriceps
and knee extension are normal responses (see Fig. 60-15*C*).

ANKLE REFLEX

To elicit an ankle (Achilles) reflex, the foot is dorsiflexed at the
ankle and the hammer strikes the stretched Achilles tendon (see
Fig. 60-15*D*). This reflex normally produces plantar flexion. If
the examiner cannot elicit the ankle reflex and suspects that the
patient cannot relax, the patient is instructed to kneel on a chair
or similar elevated, flat surface. This position places the ankles
in dorsiflexion and reduces any muscle tension in the gastrocnemius. The Achilles tendons are struck in turn, and plantar flexion is usually demonstrated.

CLONUS

When reflexes are very hyperactive, a phenomenon called **clonus**
may be elicited. If the foot is abruptly dorsiflexed, it may continue
to "beat" two or three times before it settles into a position of rest.
Occasionally with central nervous system disease this activity persists and the foot does not come to rest while the tendon is being
stretched but persists in repetitive activity. The unsustained clonus
associated with normal but hyperactive reflexes is not considered
pathologic. Sustained clonus always indicates the presence of central nervous system disease and requires further evaluation.

SUPERFICIAL REFLEXES

The major superficial reflexes include corneal, gag or swallowing,
upper/lower abdominal, cremasteric (men only), plantar, and

Chart 60-3   Documenting Reflexes

Deep tendon reflexes are graded on a scale of 0 to 4:

0	No response
1+	Diminished (hypoactive)
2+	Normal
3+	Increased (may be interpreted as normal)
4+	Hyperactive (hyperreflexia)

The deep tendon responses and plantar reflexes are commonly recorded on stick figures. The arrow points downward if the plantar response is normal and upward if the response is abnormal.

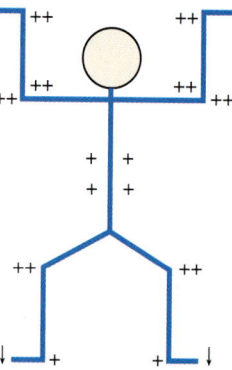

perianal. These reflexes are graded differently than the motor reflexes and are noted to be present (+) or absent (-). Of these, only three are tested commonly. The corneal reflex is tested carefully using a clean wisp of cotton and lightly touching the outer corner of each eye on the sclera. The reflex is present if the action elicits a blink. Conditions such as a cerebrovascular accident or coma might result in loss of this reflex, either unilaterally or bilaterally. Loss of this reflex indicates the need for eye protection and possible lubrication to prevent corneal damage.

The gag reflex is elicited by gently touching the posterior pharynx with a cotton-tipped applicator; first on one side of the uvula and then the other. Positive response is an equal elevation of the uvula and "gag" with stimulation. Absent response on one or both sides can be seen following a cerebrovascular accident and requires careful evaluation and treatment of the resultant swallowing dysfunction to prevent aspiration of food and fluids into the lungs.

The plantar reflex is elicited by stroking the lateral side of the foot with a tongue blade or the handle of a reflex hammer. Stimulation normally causes toe flexion. Toe fanning (positive Babinski) is an abnormal response and is discussed below (O'Hanlon-Nichols, 1999).

BABINSKI RESPONSE

A well-known reflex indicative of central nervous system disease affecting the corticospinal tract is the **Babinski reflex**. In someone with an intact central nervous system, if the lateral aspect of the sole of the foot is stroked, the toes contract and are drawn together (see Fig. 60-15*E*). In patients who have central nervous system disease of the motor system, however, the toes fan out and are drawn back. This is normal in newborns but represents a serious abnormality in adults. Several other reflexes convey similar information. Many of them are interesting but not particularly informative.

Sensory Examination

The sensory system is even more complex than the motor system because sensory modalities are carried in different tracts located in different portions of the spinal cord. The sensory examination is largely subjective and requires the cooperation of the patient. The examiner should be familiar with dermatomes that represent the distribution of the peripheral nerves that arise from the spinal

cord (see Fig. 60-11). Most sensory deficits result from peripheral neuropathy and follow anatomic dermatomes. Exceptions to this include major destructive lesions of the brain; loss of sensation, which may affect an entire side of the body; and the neuropathies associated with alcoholism, which occur in a glove-and-stocking distribution or over the entire hand or foot in areas traditionally covered by a glove or sock.

Assessment of the sensory system involves tests for tactile sensation, superficial pain, vibration, and position sense (proprioception). During the sensory assessment, the patient's eyes are closed. Simple directions and reassurance that the examiner will not hurt or startle the patient encourage the cooperation of the patient.

Tactile sensation is assessed by lightly touching a cotton wisp to corresponding areas on each side of the body. The sensitivity of proximal parts of the extremities is compared with that of distal parts.

Pain and temperature sensations are transmitted together in the lateral part of the spinal cord, so it is unnecessary to test for temperature sense in most circumstances. Determining the patient's sensitivity to a sharp object can assess superficial pain perception. The patient is asked to differentiate between the sharp and dull ends of a broken wooden cotton swab or tongue blade; using a safety pin is inadvisable because it breaks the integrity of the skin. Both the sharp and dull sides of the object are applied with equal intensity at all times, and as with the motor evaluation the two sides are compared.

Vibration and proprioception are transmitted together in the posterior part of the cord. Vibration may be evaluated through the use of a low-frequency (128- or 256-Hz) tuning fork. The handle of the vibrating fork is placed against a bony prominence, and the patient is asked whether he or she feels a sensation and is instructed to signal the examiner when the sensation ceases. Common locations used to test for vibratory sense include the distal joint of the great toe and the proximal thumb joint. If the patient does not perceive the vibrations at the distal bony prominences, the examiner progresses upward with the tuning fork until the patient perceives the vibrations. As with all measurements of sensation, a side-to-side comparison is made.

Position sense or proprioception may be determined by asking the patient to close both eyes and indicate, as the great toe is alternately moved up and down, in which direction movement has taken place. Vibration and position sense are often lost together, frequently in circumstances in which all others remain intact.

Integration of sensation in the brain is evaluated next. This may be performed by testing two-point discrimination—when the patient is touched with two sharp objects simultaneously, are they perceived as two or as one? If touched simultaneously on opposite sides of the body, the patient should normally report being touched in two places. If only one site is reported, the one not being recognized is said to demonstrate extinction. Another test of higher cortical sensory ability is stereognosis. The patient is instructed to close both eyes and identify a variety of objects (eg, keys, coins) that are placed in one hand by the examiner.

 ## Gerontologic Considerations

The nervous system undergoes many changes during the normal aging process and is extremely vulnerable to general systemic illness. Changes throughout the nervous system vary in degree as the person ages. Nerve fibres that connect directly to muscles show little decline in function with age, as do simple neurologic functions that involve a number of connections in the spinal cord. Disease in the elderly often makes it difficult to distinguish normal from abnormal changes. However, it is important for clinicians not to attribute abnormality or dysfunction to aging without appropriate investigation (Kaye & Quinn, 2000).

Structural Changes. There are a number of alterations that occur with increasing age. Brain weight decreases, as does the number of synapses. A loss of neurons occurs in select regions of the brain. There is a reduction in cerebral blood flow and metabolism. Temperature regulation becomes less efficient. In the peripheral nervous system, myelin is lost, resulting in a decrease in conduction velocity in some nerves. There is an overall reduction in muscle bulk and the electrical activity within muscles. Taste buds atrophy and nerve cell fibres in the olfactory bulb degenerate. Nerve cells in the vestibular system of the inner ear, cerebellum, and proprioceptive pathways also degenerate. Deep tendon reflexes can be decreased or in some cases absent. Hypothalamic function is modified such that stage IV sleep is reduced. There is an overall slowing of autonomic nervous system responses. Pupillary responses are reduced or may not appear at all in the presence of cataracts (Kaye & Quinn, 2000).

Motor Alterations. There is an overall reduction in muscle bulk, with atrophy most easily noted in the hands (Kaye & Quinn, 2000). Changes in motor function often result in a flexed posture, shuffling gait, and rigidity of movement. These changes can create difficulties for the older person in maintaining or recovering balance. Strength and agility are diminished, and reaction time and movement time are decreased. Repetitive movements and mild tremours may be noted during an examination and may be of concern to the individual. Observation of gait may reveal a wide-based gait with balance difficulties.

Sensory Alterations. Sensory isolation due to visual and hearing loss can cause confusion, anxiety, disorientation, misinterpretation of the environment, and feelings of inadequacy. Sensory alterations may require modification of the home environment, such as large-print reading materials or sound enhancement for the telephone, as well as extra orientation to new surroundings. Simple explanations of routines, the location of the bathroom, and how to operate the call bell are just a few examples of information the elderly patient needs when hospitalized.

Temperature Regulation and Pain Perception. Other manifestations of neurologic changes are related to temperature regulation and pain. The elderly patient may feel cold more readily than heat and may require extra covering when in bed; a room temperature somewhat higher than usual may be desirable. Reaction to painful stimuli may be decreased with age. Because pain is an important warning signal, caution must be used when hot or cold packs are used. The older patient may be burned or suffer frostbite before being aware of any discomfort. Complaints of pain, such as abdominal discomfort or chest pain, may be more serious than the patient's perception might indicate and thus require careful evaluation.

Taste and Smell Alterations. The acuity of the taste buds decreases with age; along with an altered olfactory sense, this may cause a decreased appetite and subsequent weight loss. Extra seasoning often increases food intake as long as it does not cause gastric irritation. A decreased sense of smell due to atrophy of olfactory organs may present a safety hazard, because elderly people living alone may be unable to detect household gas leaks or fires. Smoke and carbon monoxide detectors, important for all, are critical for the elderly.

Tactile and Visual Alterations. Another neurologic alteration in the elderly patient is the dulling of tactile sensation due to a decrease in the number of areas of the body responding to all stimuli and in the number and sensitivity of sensory receptors. There may be difficulty in identifying objects by touch, and because fewer tactile cues are received from the bottom of the feet, the person may get confused as to body position and location.

These factors, combined with sensitivity to glare, decreased peripheral vision, and a constricted visual field, may result in disorientation, especially at night when there is little or no light in the room. Because the elderly person takes longer to recover visual sensitivity when moving from a light to dark area, night-lights and a safe and familiar arrangement of furniture are essential.

Mental Status. Mental status is evaluated while the history is obtained, and areas of judgment, intelligence, memory, affect, mood, orientation, speech, and grooming are assessed. Family members who bring the patient to the attention of the health care provider may have noticed changes in the patient's mental status. Drug toxicity should always be suspected as a causative factor when the patient has a change in mental status. **Delirium** (mental confusion, usually with delusions and hallucinations) is seen in elderly patients who have underlying central nervous system damage or are experiencing an acute condition such as infection, adverse medication reaction, or dehydration. About 25% of patients over the age of 70 admitted to the hospital have delirium (Johnson, 2001). The cause is often reversible and treatable (as in drug toxicity, vitamin B deficiency, or thyroid disease). Depression may produce impairment of attention and memory. For elderly patients, delirium, which is an acute change in mental status attributable to a treatable medical problem, must be differentiated from dementia, which is a chronic and irreversible deterioration of cognitive status.

Nursing Implications. Nursing care for patients with age-related changes to the nervous system and for patients with long-term neurologic disability who are aging should include the modifications previously described. In addition, the consequences of any neurologic deficit and its impact on overall function such as activities of daily living, use of assistive devices, and individual coping need to be assessed and considered in planning care for patients.

Patient teaching is also affected because the nurse must understand the altered responses and the changing needs of the elderly patient before beginning to teach. When caring for the elderly patient, the nurse adapts activities such as preoperative teaching, diet therapy, and instruction about new medications, their timing, and doses to the patient's needs and capabilities. The nurse considers the presence of decline in fine motor movement and failing vision. When using visual materials for teaching or menu selection, adequate lighting without glare, contrasting colours, and large print are used to offset visual difficulties caused by rigidity and opacity of the lens in the eye and slower pupillary reaction.

Procedures and preparations needed for diagnostic tests are explained, taking into account the possibility of impaired hearing and slowed responses in the elderly. Even with hearing loss, the elderly patient often hears adequately if the speaker uses a low-pitched, clear voice; shouting only makes it harder for the patient to understand the speaker. Providing auditory and visual cues aids understanding; if the patient has a significant hearing or visual loss, assistive devices, a signer, or a translator may be needed.

Teaching at an unrushed pace and using reinforcement enhance learning and retention. Material should be short, concise, and concrete. Vocabulary is matched to the patient's ability, and terms are clearly defined. The elderly patient requires adequate time to receive and respond to stimuli, to learn, and to react. These measures allow comprehension, memory, and formation of association and concepts.

Diagnostic Evaluation

COMPUTED TOMOGRAPHY SCANNING

Computed tomography (CT) makes use of a narrow x-ray beam to scan the head in successive layers. The images provide cross-sectional views of the brain, with distinguishing differences in tissue densities of the skull, cortex, subcortical structures, and ventricles. The brightness of each slice of the brain in the final image is proportional to the degree to which it absorbs x-rays. The image is displayed on an oscilloscope or TV monitor and is photographed and stored digitally (Hinkle, 1999a).

Lesions in the brain are seen as variations in tissue density differing from the surrounding normal brain tissue. Abnormalities of tissue indicate possible tumour masses, brain infarction, displacement of the ventricles, and cortical atrophy. Whole-body CT scanners allow sections of the spinal cord to be visualized. The injection of a water-soluble iodinated contrast agent into the subarachnoid space through lumbar puncture improves the visualization of the spinal and intracranial contents on these images. The CT scan, along with magnetic resonance imaging (MRI), has largely replaced myelography as a diagnostic procedure for the diagnosis of herniated lumbar discs.

CT scanning is usually performed first without contrast material and then with intravenous contrast enhancement. The patient lies on an adjustable table with the head held in a fixed position, while the scanning system rotates around the head and produces cross-sectional images. The patient must lie with the head held perfectly still without talking or moving the face, because head motion will distort the image.

CT scanning is noninvasive and painless and has a high degree of sensitivity for detecting lesions. With advances in CT scan-

ning, the number of disorders and injuries that can be diagnosed is increasing.

Nursing Interventions

Essential nursing interventions include preparation for the procedure and patient monitoring. Preparation includes teaching the patient about the need to lie quietly throughout the procedure. A review of relaxation techniques may be helpful for claustrophobic patients.

Sedation can be used if agitation, restlessness, or confusion will interfere with a successful study (Hinkle, 1999a). Ongoing patient monitoring during sedation is necessary. If a contrast agent is used, the patient must be assessed before the CT scan for an iodine/shellfish allergy, as the contrast agent is iodine-based. An intravenous line for injection of the contrast agent and a period of fasting (usually 4 hours) are required prior to the study. Patients who receive an intravenous or inhalation contrast agent are monitored during and after the procedure for allergic reactions and other side effects, including flushing, nausea, and vomiting.

POSITRON EMISSION TOMOGRAPHY

Positron emission tomography (PET) is a computer-based nuclear imaging technique that produces images of actual organ functioning. The patient either inhales a radioactive gas or is injected with a radioactive substance that emits positively charged particles. When these positrons combine with negatively charged electrons (normally found in the body's cells), the resultant gamma rays can be detected by a scanning device that produces a series of two-dimensional views at various levels of the brain. This information is integrated by a computer and gives a composite picture of the brain at work.

PET permits the measurement of blood flow, tissue composition, and brain metabolism and thus indirectly evaluates brain function. The brain is one of the most metabolically active organs, consuming 80% of the glucose the body uses. PET measures this activity in specific areas of the brain and can detect changes in glucose use.

This test is useful in showing metabolic changes in the brain (Alzheimer's disease), locating lesions (brain tumour, epileptogenic lesions), identifying blood flow and oxygen metabolism in patients with strokes, evaluating new therapies for brain tumours, and revealing biochemical abnormalities associated with mental illness. The isotopes used have a very short half-life and are expensive to produce, requiring specialized equipment for production. PET scanning has been useful in research settings for the last 20 years and is now becoming more available in clinical settings. Improvements in scanning itself and the production of isotopes has increased the availability of PET studies (Gjedde et al., 2001).

Nursing Interventions

Key nursing interventions include patient preparation, which involves explaining the test and teaching the patient about inhalation techniques and the sensations (eg, dizziness, lightheadedness, and headache) that may occur. The intravenous injection of the radioactive substance produces similar side effects. Relaxation exercises may reduce anxiety during the test.

SINGLE PHOTON EMISSION COMPUTED TOMOGRAPHY

Single photon emission computed tomography (SPECT) is a three-dimensional imaging technique that uses radionuclides and instruments to detect single photons. It is a perfusion study that captures a moment of cerebral blood flow at the time of injection of a radionuclide (Huntington, 1999). Gamma photons are emitted from a radiopharmaceutical agent administered to the patient and are detected by a rotating gamma camera or cameras; the image is sent to a minicomputer. This approach allows areas behind overlying structures or background to be viewed, greatly increasing the contrast between normal and abnormal tissue. It is relatively inexpensive, and the duration is similar to that of a CT scan.

SPECT is useful in detecting the extent and location of abnormally perfused areas of the brain, thus allowing detection, localization, and sizing of stroke (before it is visible by CT scan), localization of seizure foci in epilepsy, and evaluation of perfusion before and after neurosurgical procedures. Pregnancy and breastfeeding are contraindications to SPECT.

Nursing Interventions

The nursing interventions for SPECT primarily include patient preparation and patient monitoring. Teaching about what to expect before the test can allay anxiety and ensure patient cooperation during the test. Premenopausal women are advised to practice effective contraception before and for several days after testing, and the woman who is breastfeeding is instructed to stop nursing for the period of time recommended by the nuclear medicine department.

The nurse may need to accompany and monitor the patient during transport to the nuclear medicine department for the scan. Patients are monitored during and after the procedure for allergic reactions to the radiopharmaceutical agent. In a few institutions nurses with special education and training inject the contrast agent before a SPECT scan (Fischbach, 2002; Huntington, 1999).

MAGNETIC RESONANCE IMAGING

Magnetic resonance imaging (MRI) uses a powerful magnetic field to obtain images of different areas of the body (Fig. 60-16). This diagnostic test involves altering hydrogen ions in the body. Placing the patient into a powerful magnetic field causes the hydrogen nuclei (protons) within the body to align like small

magnets in a magnetic field. In combination with radiofrequency pulses, the protons emit signals, which are converted to images. MRI has the potential for identifying a cerebral abnormality earlier and more clearly than other diagnostic tests. It can provide information about the chemical changes within cells, allowing the clinician to monitor a tumour's response to treatment. It is particularly useful in the diagnosis of multiple sclerosis and can describe the activity and extent of disease in the brain and spinal cord. MRI does not involve ionizing radiation.

Several newer MRI techniques, including magnetic resonance angiography (MRA), diffusion-weighted imaging (DWI), perfusion-weighted imaging (PWI), and fluid attenuation inversion recovery (FLAIR), are becoming more widely used (Hinkle, 1999b; Shellock, 2001). The use of MRA allows visualization of the cerebral vasculature without the administration of an arterial contrast agent. A substantial amount of research on the techniques of DWI, PWI, and FLAIR shows promise for clearer visualization and the early diagnosis of ischemic stroke (Hinkle, 1999b). At present MRI is most valuable in the diagnosis of nonacute conditions, as the test takes up to an hour to complete.

Nursing Interventions

Patient preparation should include teaching relaxation techniques and informing the patient that he or she will be able to talk to the staff by means of a microphone located inside the scanner. Many MRI suites provide headphones so patients can listen to the music of their choice during the procedure.

Before the patient enters the room where the MRI is to be performed, all metal objects and credit cards (the magnetic field can erase them) are removed. No metal objects may be brought into the room where the MRI is located (Shellock, 2001): this includes oxygen tanks, traditional ventilators, or even stethoscopes. The magnetic field generated by the unit is so strong that any metal-containing items will be strongly attracted and literally can be pulled away with such force that they fly like projectiles toward the magnet. There is a risk of severe injury and death; furthermore, damage to a very expensive piece of equipment may occur. A patient history is obtained to determine the presence of any metal objects (eg, aneurysm clips, orthopedic hardware, pacemakers, artificial heart valves, intrauterine devices). These objects could malfunction, be dislodged, or heat up as they absorb energy. Cochlear implants will be inactivated by MRI; therefore, other imaging procedures are considered.

! NURSING ALERT For patient safety, the nurse must make sure no patient care equipment (eg, portable oxygen tanks) that contains metal or metal parts enters the room where the MRI is located.

The patient lies on a flat platform that is moved into a tube housing the magnet. The scanning process is painless, but the patient hears loud thumping of the magnetic coils as the magnetic field is being pulsed. Because the MRI scanner is a narrow tube, patients may experience claustrophobia; sedation may be prescribed in these circumstances. Newer versions of MRI machines are less claustrophobic than the earlier devices and are available in some locations. However, the images produced on these machines are not optimal, and the traditional device is preferable for accurate diagnosis.

FIGURE 60-16 Technician explains what to expect during an MRI.

CEREBRAL ANGIOGRAPHY

Cerebral angiography is an x-ray study of the cerebral circulation with a contrast agent injected into a selected artery. Cerebral angiography is a valuable tool to investigate vascular disease, aneurysms, and arteriovenous malformations. It is frequently performed before craniotomy to assess the patency and adequacy of the cerebral circulation and to determine the site, size, and nature of the pathologic processes (Fischbach, 2002; Frizzell, 1998).

Most cerebral angiograms are performed by threading a catheter through the femoral artery in the groin and up to the desired vessel. Alternatively, direct puncture of the carotid or vertebral artery or retrograde injection of a contrast agent into the brachial artery may be performed.

In digital subtraction angiography (DSA), x-ray images of the area in question are obtained before and after the injection of a contrast agent. The computer analyzes the differences between the two images and produces an enhanced image of the carotid and vertebral arterial systems. The injection for a DSA can be given through a peripheral vein (Fischbach, 2002; Rowland, 2000).

Nursing Interventions

The patient should be well hydrated, and clear liquids are usually permitted up to the time of a regular arteriogram or DSA. Before going to the x-ray department, the patient is instructed to void. The locations of the appropriate peripheral pulses are marked with a felt-tip pen. The patient is instructed to remain immobile during the angiogram process and is told to expect a brief feeling of warmth in the face, behind the eyes, or in the jaw, teeth, tongue, and lips, and a metallic taste when the contrast agent is injected.

After the groin is shaved and prepared, a local anesthetic is administered to prevent pain at the insertion site and to reduce arterial spasm. A catheter is introduced into the femoral artery, flushed with heparinized saline, and filled with contrast agent. Fluoroscopy is used to guide the catheter to the appropriate vessels. During injection of the contrast agent, images are made of the arterial and venous phases of circulation through the brain.

Nursing care after cerebral angiography includes observation for signs and symptoms of altered cerebral blood flow. In some instances, patients may experience major or minor arterial blockage due to embolism, thrombosis, or hemorrhage, producing a neurologic deficit. Signs of such an occurrence include alterations in the level of responsiveness and consciousness, weakness on one side of the body, motor or sensory deficits, and speech disturbances. Therefore, it is necessary to observe the patient frequently for these signs and to report them immediately if they occur.

The injection site is observed for hematoma formation (a localized collection of blood), and an ice bag may be applied intermittently to the puncture site to relieve swelling and discomfort. Because a hematoma at the puncture site or embolization to a distant artery affects the peripheral pulses, these pulses are monitored frequently. The colour and temperature of the involved extremity are assessed to detect possible embolism.

MYELOGRAPHY

A **myelogram** is an x-ray of the spinal subarachnoid space taken after the injection of a contrast agent into the spinal subarachnoid space through a lumbar puncture. It outlines the spinal subarachnoid space and shows any distortion of the spinal cord or spinal dural sac caused by tumours, cysts, herniated vertebral discs, or other lesions. Water-based agents have replaced oil-based agents and their use has reduced side effects and complications; these agents disperse upward through the CSF. Myelography is performed less frequently today because of the sensitivity of CT scanning and MRI (Hickey, 2003).

Nursing Interventions

Because many patients have misconceptions about this procedure, the nurse clarifies the explanation given by the physician and answers questions. The patient is informed about what to expect during the procedure and should be aware that changes in position may be made during the procedure. The meal that normally would be eaten before the procedure is omitted. A sedative may be prescribed to help the patient cope with this rather lengthy test. Patient preparation for lumbar puncture is discussed later in this chapter.

After myelography, the patient lies in bed with the head of the bed elevated 30 to 45 degrees. The patient is advised to remain in bed in the recommended position for 3 hours or as prescribed by the physician. The patient is encouraged to drink liberal amounts of fluid for rehydration and replacement of CSF and to decrease the incidence of postlumbar puncture headache. The blood pressure, pulse, respiratory rate, and temperature are monitored, as well as the patient's ability to void. Untoward signs include headache, fever, stiff neck, **photophobia** (sensitivity to light), seizures, and signs of chemical or bacterial meningitis.

NONINVASIVE CAROTID FLOW STUDIES

Noninvasive carotid flow studies use ultrasound imagery and Doppler measurements of arterial blood flow to evaluate carotid and deep orbital circulation. The graph produced indicates blood velocity. Increased blood velocity can indicate stenosis or partial obstruction. These tests are often obtained before arteriography, which carries a higher risk of stroke or death (Fischbach, 2002; Hickey, 2003). Carotid Doppler, carotid ultrasonography, oculoplethysmography, and ophthalmodynamometry are four common noninvasive vascular techniques that permit evaluation of arterial blood flow and detection of arterial stenosis, occlusion, and plaques.

TRANSCRANIAL DOPPLER

Transcranial Doppler uses the same noninvasive techniques as carotid flow studies except that it records the blood flow velocities of the intracranial vessels. Flow velocities of the basal artery can be measured through thin areas of the temporal and occipital bones of the skull. A hand-held Doppler probe emits a pulsed beam; the signal is reflected by the moving red blood cells within the blood vessels (Falyar, 1999). Transcranial Doppler sonography is a noninvasive technique that is helpful in assessing vasospasm (a complication following subarachnoid hemorrhage), altered cerebral blood flow found in occlusive vascular disease or stroke, and other cerebral pathology.

Nursing Interventions

When a carotid flow study or transcranial Doppler is scheduled, the procedure is described to the patient. The patient is informed that this is a noninvasive test, that a hand-held transducer will be placed over the neck and orbits of the eyes, and that some type of water-soluble jelly is used on the transducer. Either one of these low-risk tests can be performed at the patient's bedside.

ELECTROENCEPHALOGRAPHY

An electroencephalogram (EEG) represents a record of the electrical activity generated in the brain. It is obtained through electrodes applied on the scalp or through microelectrodes placed within the brain tissue. It provides a physiologic assessment of cerebral activity.

The EEG is a useful test for diagnosing and evaluating seizure disorders, coma, or organic brain syndrome. Tumours, brain abscesses, blood clots, and infection may cause abnormal patterns in electrical activity. The EEG is also used in making a determination of brain death.

Electrodes are applied to the scalp to record the electrical activity in various regions of the brain. The amplified activity of the neurons between any two of these electrodes is recorded on continuously moving paper; this record is called the encephalogram.

For a baseline recording, the patient lies quietly with both eyes closed. The patient may be asked to hyperventilate for 3 to 4 minutes and then look at a bright, flashing light for photic stimulation. These activation procedures are performed to evoke abnormal electrical discharges, such as seizure potentials. A sleep EEG may be recorded after sedation because some abnormal brain waves are seen only when the patient is asleep. If the epileptogenic area is inaccessible to conventional scalp electrodes, nasopharyngeal electrodes may be used.

Depth recording of EEG is performed by introducing electrodes stereotactically (radiologically placed using instrumentation) into a target area of the brain, as indicated by the patient's seizure pattern and scalp EEG. It is used to identify patients who may benefit from surgical excision of epileptogenic foci.

Special transsphenoidal, mandibular, and nasopharyngeal electrodes can be used, and video recording combined with EEG monitoring and telemetry is used in hospital settings to capture epileptiform abnormalities and their sequelae. Some epilepsy centres provide long-term ambulatory EEG monitoring with portable recording devices.

Nursing Interventions

To increase the chances of recording seizure activity, it is sometimes recommended that the patient be deprived of sleep on the night before the EEG. Antiseizure agents, tranquilizers, stimulants, and depressants should be withheld 24 to 48 hours before an EEG because these medications can alter the EEG wave patterns or mask the abnormal wave patterns of seizure disorders (Hickey, 2003). Coffee, tea, chocolate, and cola drinks are omitted in the meal before the test because of their stimulating effect. The meal is not omitted, however, because an altered blood glucose level can also cause changes in the brain wave patterns.

The patient is informed that the standard EEG takes 45 to 60 minutes, 12 hours for a sleep EEG. The patient is assured that the procedure does not cause an electric shock and that the EEG is a diagnostic test, not a form of treatment. An EEG requires patient cooperation and ability to lie quietly during the test. Sedation is not advisable as it may lower the seizure threshold in patients with a seizure disorder and alter brain wave activity in all patients. Patients with seizures do not stop taking their antiseizure medication prior to testing.

Routine EEGs use a water-soluble lubricant for electrode contact, which at the conclusion of the study can be wiped off and removed by shampooing. Sleep EEGs involve the use of collodion glue for electrode contact, which requires acetone for removal.

EVOKED POTENTIAL STUDIES

In evoked potential studies, electrodes are applied to the scalp and an external stimulus is applied to peripheral sensory receptors to elicit changes in the brain waves. Evoked changes are detected with the aid of computerized devices that extract the signal, display it on an oscilloscope, and store the data on magnetic tape or disc. These studies are based on the concept that any insult or dysfunction that can alter neuronal metabolism or disturb membrane function may change evoked responses in brain waves. In neurologic diagnosis, they reflect conduction times in the peripheral nervous system. In clinical practice, the visual, auditory, and somatosensory systems are most often tested.

In visual evoked responses, the patient looks at a visual stimulus (flashing lights, a checkerboard pattern on a screen). The average of several hundred stimuli is recorded by EEG leads placed over the occiput. The transit time from the retina to the occipital area is measured using computer-averaging methods.

Auditory evoked responses or brain stem evoked responses are measured by applying an auditory stimulus (a repetitive auditory click) and measuring the transit time up the brain stem into the cortex. Specific lesions in the auditory pathway modify or delay the response.

In somatosensory evoked responses, the peripheral nerves are stimulated (electrical stimulation through skin electrodes) and the transit time up the spinal cord to the cortex is measured and recorded from scalp electrodes.

This test is used to detect a deficit in spinal cord conduction and to monitor spinal cord function during operative procedures. Because myelinated fibres conduct impulses at a higher rate of speed, nerves with an intact myelin sheath record the highest velocity. Demyelination of nerve fibres leads to a decrease in speed of conduction, as found in Guillain-Barré syndrome, multiple sclerosis, and polyneuropathies.

Nursing Interventions

There is no specific patient preparation other than to explain the procedure and to reassure the patient and encourage him or her to relax. The patient is advised to remain perfectly still throughout the recording to prevent artefacts (signals not generated by the brain) that interfere with the recording and interpretation of the test.

ELECTROMYOGRAPHY

An electromyogram (EMG) is obtained by introducing needle electrodes into the skeletal muscles to measure changes in the electrical potential of the muscles and the nerves leading to them. The electrical potentials are shown on an oscilloscope and amplified by a loudspeaker so that both the sound and appearance of the waves can be analyzed and compared simultaneously.

An EMG is useful in determining the presence of a neuromuscular disorder and myopathies. They help to distinguish weakness due to neuropathy (functional or pathologic changes in the peripheral nervous system) from weakness due to other causes.

Nursing Interventions

The procedure is explained and the patient is warned to expect a sensation similar to that of an intramuscular injection as the needle is inserted into the muscle. The muscles examined may ache for a short time after the procedure.

NERVE CONDUCTION STUDIES

Nerve conduction studies are performed by stimulating a peripheral nerve at several points along its course and recording the muscle action potential or the sensory action potential that results. Surface or needle electrodes are placed on the skin over the nerve to stimulate the nerve fibres. This test is useful in the study of peripheral neuropathies.

LUMBAR PUNCTURE AND EXAMINATION OF CEREBROSPINAL FLUID

A lumbar puncture (spinal tap) is carried out by inserting a needle into the lumbar subarachnoid space to withdraw CSF. The test may be performed to obtain CSF for examination, to measure and reduce CSF pressure, to determine the presence or absence of blood in the CSF, to detect spinal subarachnoid block, and to administer antibiotics intrathecally (into the spinal canal) in certain cases of infection.

The needle is usually inserted into the subarachnoid space between the third and fourth or fourth and fifth lumbar vertebrae. Because the spinal cord divides into a sheaf of nerves at the first lumbar vertebra, insertion of the needle below the level of the third lumbar vertebra prevents puncture of the spinal cord.

A successful lumbar puncture requires that the patient be relaxed; an anxious patient is tense, and this may increase the pressure reading. CSF pressure with the patient in a lateral recumbent position is normally 70 to 200 mm H_2O. Pressures of more than 200 mm H_2O are considered abnormal.

A lumbar puncture may be risky in the presence of an intracranial mass lesion because intracranial pressure is decreased by the removal of CSF, and the brain may herniate downward through the tentorium and the foramen magnum.

Queckenstedt's Test

A lumbar manometric test (Queckenstedt's test) may be performed by compressing the jugular veins on each side of the neck during the lumbar puncture. The increase in pressure caused by the compression is noted; then the pressure is released and pressure readings are made at 10-second intervals. Normally, CSF pressure rises rapidly in response to compression of the jugular veins and returns quickly to normal when the compression is released. A slow rise and fall in pressure indicates a partial block due to a lesion compressing the spinal subarachnoid pathways. If there is no pressure change, a complete block is indicated. This test is not performed if an intracranial lesion is suspected.

See Chart 60-4 for nursing guidelines for assisting with a lumbar puncture.

Cerebrospinal Fluid Analysis

The CSF should be clear and colourless. Pink, blood-tinged, or grossly bloody CSF may indicate a cerebral contusion, laceration, or subarachnoid hemorrhage. Sometimes with a difficult lumbar puncture, the CSF initially is bloody because of local trauma but then becomes clearer.

Usually, specimens are obtained for cell count, culture, and glucose and protein testing. The specimens should be sent to the laboratory immediately because changes will take place and alter the result if the specimens are allowed to stand. (See Appendix B for the normal values of CSF.)

Post–Lumbar Puncture Headache

A post–lumbar puncture headache, ranging from mild to severe, may appear a few hours to several days after the procedure. This is the most common complication, occurring in 15% to 30% of patients (Connolly, 1999). It is a throbbing bifrontal or occipital headache, dull and deep in character. It is particularly severe on sitting or standing but lessens or disappears when the patient lies down.

The headache is caused by CSF leakage at the puncture site. The fluid continues to escape into the tissues by way of the needle track from the spinal canal. It is then absorbed promptly by the lymphatics. As a result of this leak, the supply of CSF in the cranium is depleted to a point at which it is insufficient to maintain proper mechanical stabilization of the brain. This leakage of CSF allows settling of the brain when the patient assumes an upright position, producing tension and stretching the venous sinuses and pain-sensitive structures. Both traction and pain are lessened and the leakage is reduced when the patient lies down.

Post–lumbar puncture headache may be avoided if a small-gauge needle is used and if the patient remains prone after the procedure. When a large volume of fluid (more than 20 mL) is removed, the patient is positioned prone for 2 hours, then flat in a side-lying position for 2 to 3 hours, and then supine or prone for 6 more hours. Keeping the patient flat overnight may reduce the incidence of headaches.

The postpuncture headache is usually managed by bed rest, analgesic agents, and hydration (Connolly, 1999). Occasionally, if the headache persists, the epidural blood patch technique may be used. Blood is withdrawn from the antecubital vein and injected into the epidural space, usually at the site of the previous spinal puncture. The rationale is that the blood acts as a gelatinous plug to seal the hole in the dura, preventing further loss of CSF.

Other Complications of Lumbar Puncture

Herniation of the intracranial contents, spinal epidural abscess, spinal epidural hematoma, and meningitis are rare but serious complications of lumbar puncture. Other complications include temporary voiding problems, slight elevation of temperature, backache or spasms, and stiffness of the neck.

HOME AND COMMUNITY-BASED CARE
Teaching Patients Self-Care

Many diagnostic tests that were once performed as part of a hospital stay are now carried out in short-procedure units or outpatient testing settings or units. As a result, family members often provide the postprocedure care. Therefore, the patient and family must receive clear verbal and written instructions about precautions to take after the procedure, complications to watch for, and steps to take if complications occur. Because many patients undergoing neurologic diagnostic studies are elderly or have neurologic deficits, provisions must be made to ensure that transportation and postprocedure care and monitoring are available.

Chart 60-4 Guidelines for Assisting with a Lumbar Puncture

A needle is inserted into the subarachnoid space through the third and fourth or fourth and fifth lumbar interface to withdraw spinal fluid.

Preprocedure

1. Determine whether written consent for the procedure has been obtained.
2. Explain the procedure to the patient and describe sensations that are likely during the procedure (ie, a sensation of cold as the site is cleansed with solution, a needle prick when local anesthetic is injected).
3. Determine whether the patient has any questions or misconceptions about the procedure; reassure the patient that the needle will not enter the spinal cord or cause paralysis.
4. Instruct the patient to void before the procedure.

Procedure (performed by the physician)

1. The patient is positioned on one side at the edge of the bed or examining table with back toward the physician; the thighs and legs are flexed as much as possible to increase the space between the spinous processes of the vertebrae, for easier entry into the subarachnoid space.

© B. Proud.

2. A small pillow may be placed under the patient's head to maintain the spine in a horizontal position; a pillow may be placed between the legs to prevent the upper leg from rolling forward.
3. The nurse assists the patient to maintain the position to avoid sudden movement, which can produce a traumatic (bloody) tap.
4. The patient is encouraged to relax and is instructed to breathe normally, because hyperventilation may lower an elevated pressure.

5. The nurse describes the procedure step by step to the patient as it proceeds.
6. The physician cleanses the puncture site with an antiseptic solution and drapes the site.
7. Local anesthetic is injected to numb the puncture site, and then a spinal needle is inserted into the subarachnoid space through the third and fourth or fourth and fifth lumbar interspace.
8. A specimen of CSF is removed and usually collected in three test tubes, labelled in order of collection. A pressure reading may be obtained. The needle is withdrawn.
9. A small dressing is applied to the puncture site.
10. The tubes of CSF are sent to the laboratory immediately.

Postprocedure

1. Instruct the patient to lie prone for 2 to 3 hours to separate the alignment of the dural and arachnoid needle punctures in the meninges, to reduce leakage of CSF.

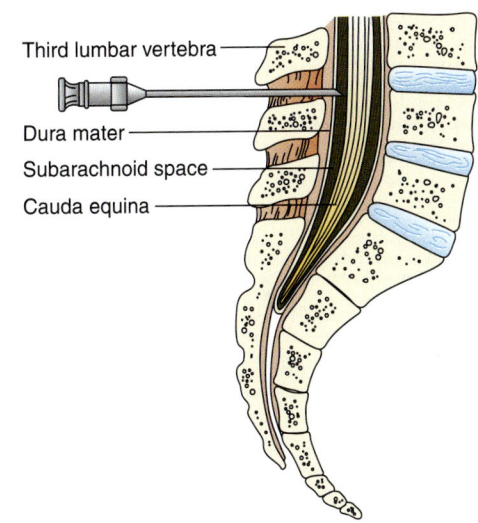

Third lumbar vertebra
Dura mater
Subarachnoid space
Cauda equina

2. Monitor the patient for complications of lumbar puncture; notify physician if complications occur.
3. Encourage increased fluid intake to reduce the risk of postprocedure headache.

Continuing Care

Contacting the patient and family after diagnostic testing enables the nurse to determine whether they have any questions about the procedure or whether the patient had any untoward results. During these phone calls, teaching is reinforced and the patient and family are reminded to make and keep follow-up appointments. Patients, family members, and health care providers are focused on the immediate needs, issues, or deficits that necessitated the diagnostic testing. This is also a good time to remind them of the need for and importance of continuing health promotion and screening practices and make referrals to appropriate health care providers.

 Critical Thinking Exercises

1. A 68-year old patient with a long history of type 1 diabetes is admitted to the hospital to rule out an ischemic stroke and is scheduled for an MRI. Explain why the MRI is indicated for this patient and what, if any, precautions must be taken because this patient is diabetic. What nursing observations and assessments are indicated because of the occurrence of these two disorders? What safety precautions are essential in the MRI suite, and why?

2. Your clinic patient will be having an EEG. Describe the procedure, its duration, and preparation for this test, including medication/diet restrictions, if any. How would the presence of a seizure disorder alter your plan of care?

3. Your patient is scheduled to undergo digital subtraction angiography (DSA). He tells you that he recently had an angiogram. What explanation can you give to the patient and his wife regarding the difference between the two procedures? What additional information will help prepare the patient to undergo this procedure?

REFERENCES AND SELECTED READINGS

Books

Bickley, L. S. & Szilagyi, P. G. (2004). *Bates' guide to physical examination and history taking* (8th ed.). Philadelphia: Lippincott Williams & Wilkins.

Bradley, W., Daroff, R., Fenichel, R., & Marsden, C. (Eds.). (2000). *Neurology in clinical practice* (vol. II, 3d ed.). Boston: Butterworth Heineman.

Fischbach, F. (2002). *Common laboratory and diagnostic tests* (3d ed.). Philadelphia: Lippincott Williams & Wilkins.

Gilman, S. (1999). *Clinical examination of the nervous system.* New York: McGraw-Hill.

Gjedde, A., Hansen, S., Knudsen, G., & Paulson, O. (Eds.). (2001). *Physiological imaging of the brain with PET.* San Diego: Academic Press.

Goetz, C. G., & Pappert, E. J. (1999). *Textbook of clinical neurology.* Philadelphia: W. B. Saunders.

Greenberg, D. A., Aminoff, M., & Simon, R. (2002). *Clinical neurology* (5th ed.). Stamford, CT: Lange Medical Books, McGraw Hill.

Herndon, R. M. (1997). *Handbook of neurological rating scales.* New York: Demos Vermande.

Hickey, J. (2003). *Clinical practice of neurologic and neurosurgical nursing* (5th ed.). Philadelphia: Lippincott Williams & Wilkins.

Joynt, R., Griggs, R., & Haerer, A. (2000). *Baker's clinical neurology on CD-ROM.* Philadelphia: Lippincott Williams & Wilkins.

Kaye, J., & Quinn, J. (2000). Clinical changes associated with normal aging. In C. M. Clark & J. Trojanowski (eds.), *Neurodegenerative dementias.* New York: McGraw-Hill.

Loeser, J., Butler, S. H., Chapman, P. C., et al. (ed.). (2000). *Bonica's management of pain* (3d ed.). Philadelphia: Lippincott Williams & Wilkins.

Lueckenotte, A. (2000). *Gerontological nursing* (2d ed.). St Louis: Mosby.

Rowland, L. (2000). *Merritts' neurology* (10th ed.). Philadelphia: Lippincott Williams & Wilkins.

Shellock, F. (2001). *Magnetic resonance procedures: Health effects and safety.* New York: CRC Press.

Stewart-Amidei, C., & Kunkel, J. (2001). *AANN's neuroscience nursing: Human responses to neurologic dysfunction* (2nd ed.). Philadelphia: W. B. Saunders.

Weiner, L., Levitt, L. P., Rae-Grant, A., & Weiner, H. L. (1999). *Neurology* (6th ed.). Philadelphia: Lippincott Williams & Wilkins.

Journals

Asterisks indicate nursing research articles.

Bateman, D. (2001). Neurological assessment of coma. *Journal of Neurology, Neurosurgery and Psychiatry, 71,* Suppl 1, i13–i17.

Blows, W. (2000). Neurotransmitters of the brain: Serotonin noradrenaline, norepinephrine, and dopamine. *Journal of Neuroscience Nursing, 32*(4), 234–238.

Connolly, M. (1999). Postdural puncture headache. *American Journal of Nursing, 99*(11), 48–49.

Cunning, S. (1999). Preventing secondary brain injuries. *Dimensions in Critical Care Nursing, 18*(5), 20–22.

Downey, D., & Leigh R. (1998). Eye movements: Pathophysiology, examination and clinical importance. *Journal of Neuroscience Nursing, 30*(1), 15–24.

Falyar, C. (1999). Using transcranial Doppler sonography to augment the neurology examination after aneurysmal subarachnoid hemorrhage. *Journal of Neuroscience Nursing, 31*(5), 285–293.

Frizzell, J. (1998). Cerebral angiography. *American Journal of Nursing, 98*(9), 16II–16JJ.

Hinkle, J. (1999a). CT scanning. *American Journal of Nursing, 99*(6), 24AA–24FF.

Hinkle, J. (1999b). Magnetic resonance imaging. *American Journal of Nursing, 99*(11), 24CC–24JJ.

Huntington, N. (1999). The nurse's role in delivery of radioisotope for ictal SPECT scan. *Journal of Neuroscience Nursing, 31*(4), 208–215.

Johnson, M. (2001). Assessing confused patients. *Journal of Neurology, Neurosurgery and Psychiatry, 71,* Suppl. 1, i7–i12.

King, D. (1999). Central nervous system infections: Basic concepts. *Nursing Clinics of North America, 34*(3), 761–771.

O'Hanlon-Nichols, T. (1999). Neurologic assessment. *American Journal of Nursing, 99*(6), 44–50.

*Rapp, C., Wakefield, B., Kundrat, M., et al. (2000). Acute confusion assessment instruments: Clinical versus research usability. *Applied Nursing Research, 13*(1), 37–45.

*Souder, E., & O'Sullivan, P. (2000). Nursing documentation versus standardized assessment of cognitive status in hospitalized medical patients. *Applied Nursing Research, 13*(1), 29–36.

Stewart-Amidei, C. (1998). Neurologic monitoring in the ICU. *Critical Care Nursing Quarterly, 21*(3), 47–60.

Sullivan, J. (1999). Determining brain death. *Critical Care Nursing, 19*(2), 37–46.

Management of Patients With Neurologic Dysfunction

Adapted by Lynne Esson

LEARNING OBJECTIVES

On completion of this chapter, the learner will be able to:

1. Describe the special nursing needs of patients with varied neurologic dysfunction.
2. Describe the multiple needs of the patient with altered level of consciousness.
3. Use the nursing process as a framework for care of the patient with altered level of consciousness.
4. Identify the early and late clinical manifestations of increased intracranial pressure.
5. Use the nursing process as a framework for care of the patient with increased intracranial pressure.
6. Describe the needs of the patient undergoing intracranial or transsphenoidal surgery.
7. Use the nursing process as a framework for care of the patient undergoing intracranial/transsphenoidal surgery.
8. Identify the various types and causes of seizures.
9. Use the nursing process to develop a plan of care for the patient experiencing seizures.
10. Identify the needs of the patient experiencing headaches.

This chapter discusses care of the patient with an altered level of consciousness, the patient with increased **intracranial pressure** (ICP), and the patient undergoing neurosurgical procedures, experiencing seizures, or experiencing headaches. Some of the topics in this chapter, such as headaches and seizures, may be symptoms of dysfunction in another body system. Conversely, headaches and seizures can be quite serious symptoms of a severe disruption of the neurologic system. These disorders can also be diagnosed at times as "idiopathic," or without an identifiable cause. The commonality in these disorders is not in the diagnosis or the medical treatment; it is in the behaviours and needs of the patient and the manner in which nurses can best support the patient through these episodes.

The central nervous system contains a vast network of neurons controlling the body's vital functions. Yet this system is vulnerable, and its optimal function depends on several key factors. First, the neurologic system relies on its own structural integrity for support and homeostasis. Examples of structural disruption include head injury, brain tumour, intracranial hemorrhage, infection, and stroke. As brain tissue expands in the inflexible cranium, ICP rises and cerebral perfusion is impaired. Further expansion places pressure on vital centres, which can cause permanent neurologic deficits or lead to brain death.

Second, the neurologic system also relies on the body's ability to maintain a homeostatic environment. It requires the body to deliver the essential elements of oxygen and glucose and to filter out substrates toxic to the neurons. Sepsis, hypovolemia, myocardial infarction, respiratory arrest, hypoglycemia, electrolyte imbalance, drug and/or alcohol overdose, encephalopathy, and ketoacidosis are all examples of circumstances in which the neurologic system is depressed due to a toxic metabolic effect or due to the body's mechanical inability to provide essential substrates.

Some conditions can be treated and neurologic impairments can be reversed; others result in permanent deficits.

Although neuroscience nursing is a specialty requiring an understanding of neuroanatomy, neurophysiology, neurodiagnostic testing, critical care nursing, and rehabilitation nursing, nurses in all settings care for patients with neurologic disorders. Ongoing assessment of the patient's neurologic function and health needs, identification of problems, mutual goal setting, development and implementation of care plans (including teaching, counselling, and coordinating activities), and evaluation of the outcomes of care are nursing actions integral to the recovery of the patient. The nurse also collaborates with other members of the health care team to provide essential care, offer a variety of solutions to problems, help patients and families gain control of their lives, and explore the educational and supportive resources available in the community. The goals are to achieve as high a level of function as possible and to enhance the quality of life for the patient with neurologic impairment and his or her family.

Altered Level of Consciousness

An **altered level of consciousness** (LOC) is apparent in the patient who is not oriented, does not follow commands, or needs persistent stimuli to achieve a state of alertness. LOC is gauged on a continuum with a normal state of alertness and full cognition (consciousness) on one end and coma on the other end. **Coma** is a clinical state of unconsciousness in which the patient is unaware of self or the environment for prolonged periods (days to months or even years). **Akinetic mutism** is a state of unresponsiveness to the environment in which the patient makes no movement or sound but sometimes opens the eyes. **Persistent vegetative state** is a condition in which the patient is described as wakeful but de-

Glossary

akinetic mutism: unresponsiveness to the environment; the patient makes no movement or sound but sometimes opens the eyes

altered level of consciousness: condition of being less responsive to and aware of environmental stimuli

autoregulation: ability of cerebral blood vessels to dilate or constrict to maintain stable cerebral blood flow despite changes in systemic arterial blood pressure

brain death: irreversible loss of all functions of the entire brain, including the brain stem

coma: prolonged state of unconsciousness

craniotomy: a surgical procedure that involves entry into the cranial vault

craniectomy: a surgical procedure that involves removing a portion of the skull

Cushing's response: brain's attempt to restore blood flow by increasing arterial pressure to overcome the increased intracranial pressure

Cushing's triad: three classic signs—bradycardia, hypertension, and bradypnea—seen with pressure on the medulla as a result of brain stem herniation

decerebration: an abnormal body posture associated with a severe brain injury, char-

acterized by extreme extension of the upper and lower extremities

decortication: an abnormal posture associated with severe brain injury, characterized by abnormal flexion of the upper extremities and extension of the lower extremities

epidural monitor: a sensor placed between the skull and the dura to monitor intracranial pressure

epilepsy: a group of syndromes characterized by paroxysmal transient disturbances of brain function.

fibreoptic monitor: a system that uses light refraction to determine intracranial pressure

herniation: abnormal protrusion of tissue through a defect or natural opening

intracranial pressure: pressure exerted by the volume of the intracranial contents within the cranial vault

migraine headache: a severe, unrelenting headache often accompanied by symptoms such as nausea, vomiting, and visual disturbances

Monro-Kellie hypothesis: theory that states that due to limited space for expansion within the skull, an increase in any one of

the cranial contents—brain tissue, blood, or CSF—causes a change in the volume of the others

persistent vegetative state: condition in which the patient is wakeful but devoid of conscious content, without cognitive or affective mental function

primary headache: a headache for which no specific organic cause can be found

seizures: paroxysmal transient disturbance of the brain resulting from a discharge of abnormal electrical activity

status epilepticus: episode in which the patient experiences multiple seizure bursts with no recovery time in between

secondary headache: headache identified as a symptom of another organic disorder (eg, brain tumour, hypertension)

subarachnoid screw or bolt: device placed into the subarachnoid space to measure intracranial pressure

transsphenoidal: surgical approach to the pituitary via the sphenoid sinuses

ventriculostomy: a catheter placed in one of the lateral ventricles of the brain to measure intracranial pressure and allow for drainage of fluid void of conscious content, without cognitive or affective mental function. The level of responsiveness and consciousness is the most important indicator of the patient's condition.

Pathophysiology

Altered LOC is not a disorder itself; rather, it is a function and symptom of multiple pathophysiologic phenomena. The cause may be neurologic (head injury, stroke), toxicologic (drug overdose, alcohol intoxication), or metabolic (hepatic or renal failure, diabetic ketoacidosis).

The underlying causes of neurologic dysfunction are disruption in the cells of the nervous system, neurotransmitters, or brain anatomy (see Chap. 60).

A disruption in the basic functional units (neurons) or neurotransmitters results in faulty impulse transmission, impeding communication within the brain or from the brain to other parts of the body. These disruptions are caused by cellular edema and other mechanisms such as antibodies disrupting chemical transmission at receptor sites.

Intact anatomic structures of the brain are needed for proper function. The two hemispheres of the cerebrum must communicate, via an intact corpus callosum, and the lobes of the brain (frontal, parietal, temporal, and occipital) must communicate and coordinate their specific functions (see Chap. 60). Additional anatomic structures of importance are the cerebellum and the brain stem. The cerebellum has both excitatory and inhibitory actions and is largely responsible for coordination of movement. The brain stem contains areas that control the heart, respiration, and blood pressure. Disruptions in the anatomic structures are caused by trauma, edema, pressure from tumours as well as other mechanisms such as an increase or decrease in blood or cerebrospinal fluid (CSF) circulation.

Clinical Manifestations

Alterations in LOC occur along a continuum, and the clinical manifestations depend on where the patient is along this continuum. As the patient's state of alertness and consciousness decreases, there will be changes in the pupillary response, eye opening response, verbal response, and motor response. Initial changes may be reflected by subtle behavioural changes such as restlessness or increased anxiety. The pupils, normally round and quickly reactive to light, become sluggish (response is slower); as the patient becomes comatose, the pupils become fixed (no response to light). The patient in a coma does not open the eyes, respond verbally, or move the extremities in response to a request to do so.

Assessment and Diagnostic Findings

The patient with an altered LOC is at risk for alterations in every body system. A complete assessment is performed, with particular attention to the neurologic system. The neurologic examination should be as complete as the LOC allows. It includes an evaluation of mental status, cranial nerve function, cerebellar function (balance and coordination), reflexes, and motor and sensory function. LOC, a sensitive indicator of neurologic function, is assessed based on the criteria in the Glasgow Coma Scale: eye opening, verbal response, and motor response (Bateman, 2001). The patient's responses are rated on a scale from 3 to 15. A score of 3 indicates severe impairment of neurologic function; a score of 15 indicates that the patient is fully responsive (see Chap. 63 for more discussion about the Glasgow Coma Scale).

If the patient is comatose, with localized signs such as abnormal pupillary and motor responses, it is assumed that neurologic disease is present until proven otherwise. If the patient is comatose and pupillary light reflexes are preserved, a toxic or metabolic disorder is suspected.

Procedures used to identify the cause of unconsciousness include scanning, imaging, tomography (eg, computed tomography, magnetic resonance imaging, positron emission tomography), and electroencephalography. Laboratory tests include analysis of blood glucose, electrolytes, serum ammonia, and blood urea nitrogen levels, as well as serum osmolality, calcium level, and partial thromboplastin and prothrombin times. Other studies may be used to evaluate serum ketones and alcohol, drug levels, and arterial blood gas levels.

Complications

Potential complications for the patient with altered LOC include respiratory failure, pneumonia, pressure ulcers, and aspiration. Respiratory failure may develop shortly after the patient becomes unconscious. If the patient cannot maintain effective respirations, supportive care is initiated to provide adequate ventilation. Pneumonia is common in patients receiving mechanical ventilation or in those who cannot maintain and clear the airway. The patient with altered LOC is subject to all the complications associated with immobility, such as pressure ulcers, venous stasis, musculoskeletal deterioration, and disturbed gastrointestinal functioning. Pressure ulcers may become infected and act as a source of sepsis. Aspiration of gastric contents or feedings may occur, precipitating the development of pneumonia or airway occlusion.

Medical Management

The first priority of treatment for the patient with altered LOC is to obtain and maintain a patent airway. The patient may be orally or nasally intubated, or a tracheostomy may be performed. Until the patient's ability to breathe on his or her own is determined, a mechanical ventilator is used to maintain adequate oxygenation. The circulatory status (blood pressure, heart rate) is monitored to ensure adequate perfusion to the body and brain. An intravenous catheter is inserted to provide access for fluids and intravenous medications. Neurologic care focuses on the specific neurologic pathology, if any. Nutritional support, using either a feeding tube or a gastrostomy tube, is initiated as soon as possible. In addition to measures to determine and treat the underlying causes of altered LOC, other medical interventions are aimed at pharmacologic management of complications and strategies to prevent complications.

NURSING PROCESS: THE PATIENT WITH AN ALTERED LEVEL OF CONSCIOUSNESS

Assessment

Where to begin assessing the patient with an altered LOC depends somewhat on each patient's circumstances, but clinicians often start by assessing the verbal response. Determining the patient's orientation to time, person, and place assesses verbal response. The patient is asked to identify the day, date, or season of the year and to identify where he or she is or to identify the clinicians, family members, or visitors present. Other questions such as, "Who is the prime minister?" or "What is the next holiday?"

are also helpful in determining the patient's processing of information in the environment. (Verbal response cannot be evaluated when the patient is intubated or has a tracheostomy, and this should be clearly documented.)

Alertness is measured by the patient's ability to open the eyes spontaneously or to a stimulus. Patients with severe neurologic dysfunction cannot do this. The nurse should assess for periorbital edema or trauma, which may prevent the patient from opening the eyes, and document if this interferes with eye opening.

Motor response includes spontaneous, purposeful movement (eg, the awake patient can move all four extremities with equal strength), movement only in response to noxious stimuli (eg, pressure/pain), or abnormal posturing (Bateman, 2001). If the patient is not responding to commands, the motor response is tested by applying a painful stimulus (firm but gentle pressure) to the nailbed or by squeezing a muscle. If the patient attempts to push away or withdraw, the response is recorded as purposeful or appropriate ("patient withdraws to painful stimuli"). This response is considered purposeful if the patient can cross from one side of the body to the other in response to noxious stimuli. An inappropriate or nonpurposeful response is random and aimless. Posturing may be decorticate or decerebrate (Fig. 61-1; see Chap. 60). The most severe neurologic impairment results in flaccidity. Occasionally, posturing cannot be elicited if the patient has been given pharmacologic paralyzing agents.

In addition to LOC, the nurse monitors parameters such as respiratory status, eye signs, and reflexes on an ongoing basis. Table 61-1 summarizes the assessment and the clinical significance of the findings. Body functions (circulation, respiration, elimination, fluid and electrolyte balance) are examined in a systematic and ongoing manner.

Diagnosis

NURSING DIAGNOSES

Based on the assessment data, the major nursing diagnoses may include the following:

- Ineffective airway clearance related to altered level of consciousness
- Risk of injury related to decreased level of consciousness
- Deficient fluid volume related to inability to take in fluids by mouth

- Impaired oral mucous membranes related to mouth-breathing, absence of pharyngeal reflex, and altered fluid intake
- Risk for impaired skin integrity related to immobility
- Impaired tissue integrity of cornea related to diminished or absent corneal reflex
- Ineffective thermoregulation related to damage to hypothalamic centre
- Impaired urinary elimination (incontinence or retention) related to impairment in neurologic sensing and control
- Bowel incontinence related to impairment in neurologic sensing and control and also related to transitions in nutritional delivery methods
- Disturbed sensory perception related to neurologic impairment
- Interrupted family processes related to health crisis

COLLABORATIVE PROBLEMS/ POTENTIAL COMPLICATIONS

Based on the assessment data, potential complications may include:

- Respiratory distress or failure
- Pneumonia
- Aspiration
- Pressure ulcer
- Deep vein thrombosis

Planning and Goals

The goals of care for the patient with altered LOC include maintenance of a clear airway, protection from injury, attainment of fluid volume balance, achievement of intact oral mucous membranes, maintenance of normal skin integrity, absence of corneal irritation, attainment of effective thermoregulation, and effective urinary elimination. Additional goals include bowel continence, accurate perception of environmental stimuli, maintenance of intact family or support system, and absence of complications (Jacobson & Winslow, 2000).

Because the unconscious patient's protective reflexes are impaired, the quality of nursing care provided literally may mean the difference between life and death. The nurse must assume responsibility for the patient until the basic reflexes (coughing, blinking, and swallowing) return and the patient becomes conscious and oriented. Thus, the major nursing goal is to compensate for the absence of these protective reflexes.

A Plantar flexed | Internally rotated | Flexed | Adducted

B Plantar flexed | Flexed | Pronated | Extended | Adducted

FIGURE 61-1 Abnormal posture response to stimuli. (**A**) Decorticate posturing, involving adduction and flexion of the upper extremities, internal rotation of the lower extremities, and plantar flexion of the feet. (**B**) Decerebrate posturing, involving extension and outward rotation of upper extremities and plantar flexion of the feet.

Table 61-1 • **Nursing Assessment of the Unconscious Patient**

EXAMINATION	CLINICAL ASSESSMENT	CLINICAL SIGNIFICANCE
Level of responsiveness or consciousness	Eye opening; verbal and motor responses; pupils (size, equality, reaction to light)	Obeying commands is a favourable response and demonstrates a return to consciousness.
Pattern of respiration	Respiratory pattern	Disturbances of respiratory centre of brain may result in various respiratory patterns.
	Cheyne-Stokes respiration	Suggests lesions deep in both hemispheres; area of basal ganglia and upper brain stem
	Hyperventilation	Suggests onset of metabolic problem or brain stem damage
	Ataxic respiration with irregularity in depth/rate	Ominous sign of damage to medullary centre
Eyes		
Pupils (size, equality, reaction to light)	Equal, normally reactive pupils	Suggests that coma is toxic or metabolic in origin
	Equal or unequal diameter	Helps determine location of lesion
	Progressive dilation	Indicates increasing ICP
	Fixed dilated pupils	Indicates injury at level of midbrain

Eye movements	Normally, eyes should move from side to side.	Functional and structural integrity of brain stem is assessed by inspection of extraocular movements; usually absent in deep coma.
Corneal reflex	When cornea is touched with a wisp of clean cotton, blink response is present.	Tests cranial nerves V and VII; helps determine location of lesion if unilateral; absent in deep coma

Facial symmetry	Asymmetry (sagging, decrease in wrinkles)	Sign of paralysis
Swallowing reflex	Drooling versus spontaneous swallowing	Absent in coma
		Paralysis of cranial nerves X and XII
Neck	Stiff neck	Subarachnoid hemorrhage, meningitis
	Absence of spontaneous neck movement	Fracture or dislocation of cervical spine
Response of extremity to noxious stimuli	Firm pressure on a joint of the upper and lower extremity	Asymmetric response in paralysis
	Observe spontaneous movements.	Absent in deep coma
Deep tendon reflexes	Tap patellar and biceps tendons.	Brisk response may have localizing value.
		Asymmetric response in paralysis
		Absent in deep coma
Pathologic reflexes	Firm pressure with blunt object on sole of foot, moving along lateral margin and crossing to the ball of foot	Flexion of the toes, especially the great toe, is normal except in newborn. Dorsiflexion of toes (especially great toe) indicates contralateral pathology of corticospinal tract (Babinski reflex). Helps determine location of lesion in brain

Abnormal posture	Observation for posturing (spontaneous or in response to noxious stimuli)	Deep extensive brain lesion
	Flaccidity with absence of motor response	Seen with cerebral hemisphere pathology and in metabolic depression of brain function
	Decorticate posture (flexion and internal rotation of forearms and hands)	Decerebrate posturing indicates deeper and more severe dysfunction than does decorticate posturing; implies brain pathology; poor prognostic sign.
	Decerebrate posture (extension and external rotation)	

Nursing Interventions

MAINTAINING THE AIRWAY

The most important consideration in managing the patient with altered LOC is to establish an adequate airway and ensure ventilation. Obstruction of the airway is a risk because the epiglottis and tongue may relax, occluding the oropharynx, or the patient may aspirate vomitus or nasopharyngeal secretions.

The accumulation of secretions in the pharynx presents a serious problem. Because the patient cannot swallow and lacks pharyngeal reflexes, these secretions must be removed to eliminate the danger of aspiration. Elevating the head of the bed to 30 degrees helps prevent aspiration. Positioning the patient in a lateral or semiprone position will also help as it permits the jaw and tongue to fall forward, thus promoting drainage of secretions.

Positioning alone is not always adequate, however. The patient may require suctioning and oral hygiene. Suctioning is performed to remove secretions from the posterior pharynx and upper trachea. With the suction off, a whistle-tip catheter is lubricated with a water-soluble lubricant and inserted to the level of the posterior pharynx and upper trachea. Continuous suction is applied as the catheter is withdrawn using a twisting motion of the thumb and forefinger. This twisting manoeuvre prevents the suctioning end of the catheter from causing irritation, which increases secretions and causes mucosal trauma and bleeding. Before and after suctioning, the patient is hyperoxygenated and hyperventilated to prevent hypoxia (Hickey, 2003). In addition to these interventions, chest physiotherapy and postural drainage may be initiated to promote pulmonary hygiene, unless contraindicated by the patient's underlying condition. Also, the chest should be auscultated at least every 8 hours to detect adventitious breath sounds or absence of breath sounds.

Despite these measures, or because of the severity of impairment, the patient with altered LOC often requires intubation and mechanical ventilation. Nursing actions for the mechanically ventilated patient include maintaining the patency of the endotracheal tube or tracheostomy, providing frequent oral care, monitoring arterial blood gas measurements, and maintaining ventilator settings (see Chap. 25).

PROTECTING THE PATIENT

For the protection of the patient, padded siderails are provided and raised at all times. Care should be taken to prevent injury from invasive lines and equipment, and other potential sources of injury should be identified (eg, restraints, tight dressings, environmental irritants, damp bedding or dressings, tubes and drains).

> **! NURSING ALERT** If the patient begins to emerge from unconsciousness, every measure that is available and appropriate for calming and quieting him or her should be used. Any form of restraint is likely to be countered by the patient with resistance, leading to self-injury or to a dangerous increase in ICP. Therefore, physical restraints should be avoided if possible; a written order must be obtained if their use is essential for the patient's well-being.

Protection also encompasses the concept of protecting the patient's dignity during altered LOC. Simple measures such as providing privacy and speaking to the patient during nursing care activities preserve the patient's humanity. Not speaking negatively about the patient's condition or prognosis is also important, because patients in a light coma may be able to hear. The comatose patient has an increased need for advocacy, and it is the nurse's responsibility to see that these advocacy needs are met (Elliott & Wright, 1999; Villanueva, 1999).

MAINTAINING FLUID BALANCE AND MANAGING NUTRITIONAL NEEDS

Hydration status is assessed by examining tissue turgor and mucous membranes, assessing intake and output trends, and analyzing laboratory data. Fluid needs are met initially by giving the required fluids intravenously. However, intravenous solutions (and blood transfusions) for patients with intracranial conditions must be administered slowly. If given too rapidly, they may increase ICP. The quantity of fluids administered may be restricted to minimize the possibility of producing cerebral edema.

If the patient does not recover quickly and sufficiently enough to take adequate fluids and calories by mouth, a feeding tube will be inserted for the administration of fluids and enteral feedings (Day, Stotts, Frankfurt et al., 2001).

PROVIDING MOUTH CARE

The mouth is inspected for dryness, inflammation, and crusting. The unconscious patient requires conscientious oral care because there is a risk of parotitis if the mouth is not kept scrupulously clean. The mouth is cleansed and rinsed carefully to remove secretions and crusts and to keep the mucous membranes moist. A thin coating of petrolatum on the lips prevents drying, cracking, and encrustations. If the patient has an endotracheal tube, the tube should be moved to the opposite side of the mouth daily to prevent ulceration of the mouth and lips.

MAINTAINING SKIN AND JOINT INTEGRITY

Preventing skin breakdown requires continuing nursing assessment and intervention. Special attention is given to unconscious patients because they cannot respond to external stimuli. Assessment includes a regular schedule of turning to avoid pressure, which can cause breakdown and necrosis of the skin. Turning also provides kinesthetic (sensation of movement), proprioceptive (awareness of position), and vestibular (equilibrium) stimulation. After turning, the patient is carefully repositioned to prevent ischemic necrosis over pressure areas. Dragging the patient up in bed must be avoided, because this creates a shearing force and friction on the skin surface.

Maintaining correct body position is important; equally important is passive exercise of the extremities to prevent contractures. The use of splints or foam boots aids in the prevention of footdrop and eliminates the pressure of bedding on the toes. Trochanter rolls supporting the hip joints keep the legs in proper alignment. The arms should be in abduction, the fingers lightly flexed, and the hands in slight supination. The heels of the feet should be assessed for pressure areas. Specialty beds, such as fluidized or low-air-loss beds, may be used to decrease pressure on bony prominences.

PRESERVING CORNEAL INTEGRITY

Some unconscious patients have their eyes open and have inadequate or absent corneal reflexes. The cornea is likely to become irritated or scratched, leading to keratitis and corneal ulcers. The eyes may be cleansed with cotton balls moistened with sterile normal saline to remove debris and discharge. If artificial tears are prescribed, they may be instilled every 2 hours. Periocular edema (swelling around the eyes) often occurs after cranial surgery. Cold compresses may be prescribed, and care must be exerted to avoid contact with the cornea. Eye patches should be used cautiously because of the potential for corneal abrasion from the cornea coming in contact with the patch.

ACHIEVING THERMOREGULATION

High fever in the unconscious patient may be caused by infection of the respiratory or urinary tract, drug reactions, or damage to the hypothalamic temperature-regulating centre. A slight elevation of temperature may be caused by dehydration. The environment can be adjusted, depending on the patient's condition, to promote a normal body temperature. If body temperature is elevated, a minimum amount of bedding—a sheet or perhaps only a small drape—is used. The room may be cooled to 18.3°C. However, if the patient is elderly and does not have an elevated temperature, a warmer environment is needed.

> **NURSING ALERT** The body temperature of an unconscious patient is never taken by mouth. Rectal or tympanic (if not contraindicated) temperature measurement is preferred to the less accurate axillary temperature.

Because of damage to the heat-regulating centre in the brain or severe intracranial infection, unconscious patients often develop very high temperatures. Such temperature elevations must be controlled because the increased metabolic demands of the brain can overburden cerebral circulation and oxygenation, resulting in cerebral deterioration (Hickey, 2003). Persistent hyperthermia with no identified clinical source of infection indicates brain stem damage and a poor prognosis.

Strategies for reducing fever include:

- Removing all bedding over the patient (with the possible exception of a light sheet or small drape)
- Administering repeated doses of acetaminophen as prescribed
- Giving a cool sponge bath and allowing an electric fan to blow over the patient to increase surface cooling
- Using a hypothermia blanket

Frequent temperature monitoring is indicated to assess the response to the therapy and to prevent an excessive decrease in temperature and shivering.

PREVENTING URINARY RETENTION

The patient with an altered LOC is often incontinent or has urinary retention. The bladder is palpated or scanned at intervals to determine whether urinary retention is present, because a full bladder may be an overlooked cause of overflow incontinence. A portable bladder ultrasound instrument is a useful tool in bladder management and retraining programs (O'Farrell, Vandervoort, Bisnaire et al., 2001).

If there are signs of urinary retention, initially an indwelling urinary catheter attached to a closed drainage system is inserted. A catheter may be inserted during the acute phase of illness to monitor urinary output. Because catheters are a major factor in causing urinary tract infection, the patient is observed for fever and cloudy urine. The area around the urethral orifice is inspected for drainage. The urinary catheter is usually removed when the patient has a stable cardiovascular system and if no diuresis, sepsis, or voiding dysfunction existed before the onset of coma. Although many unconscious patients urinate spontaneously after catheter removal, the bladder should be palpated or scanned with a portable ultrasound device periodically for urinary retention (O'Farrell et al., 2001). An intermittent catheterization

program may be initiated to ensure complete emptying of the bladder at intervals, if indicated.

An external catheter (condom catheter) for the male patient and absorbent pads for the female patient can be used for the unconscious patient who can urinate spontaneously although involuntarily. As soon as consciousness is regained, a bladder-training program is initiated. The incontinent patient is monitored frequently for skin irritation and skin breakdown. Appropriate skin care is implemented to prevent these complications.

PROMOTING BOWEL FUNCTION

The abdomen is assessed for distention by listening for bowel sounds and measuring the girth of the abdomen with a tape measure. There is a risk of diarrhea from infection, antibiotics, and hyperosmolar fluids. Frequent loose stools may also occur with fecal impaction. Commercial fecal collection bags are available for patients with fecal incontinence.

Immobility and lack of dietary fibre may cause constipation. The nurse monitors the number and consistency of bowel movements and performs a rectal examination for signs of fecal impaction. Stool softeners may be prescribed and can be administered with tube feedings. To facilitate bowel emptying, a glycerine suppository may be indicated. The patient may require an enema every other day to empty the lower colon.

PROVIDING SENSORY STIMULATION

Sensory stimulation is provided at the appropriate time to help overcome the profound sensory deprivation of the unconscious patient. Efforts are made to maintain the sense of daily rhythm by keeping the usual day and night patterns for activity and sleep. The nurse touches and talks to the patient and encourages family members and friends to do so. Communication is extremely important and includes touching the patient and spending enough time with him or her to become sensitive to his or her needs. It is also important to avoid making any negative comments about the patient's status or prognosis in the patient's presence.

The nurse orients the patient to time and place at least once every 8 hours. Sounds from the patient's home and workplace may be introduced using a tape recorder. Family members can read to the patient from a favourite book and may suggest radio and television programs that the patient previously enjoyed as a means of enriching the environment and providing familiar input (Hickey, 2003).

When arousing from coma, many patients experience a period of agitation, indicating that they are becoming more aware of their surroundings but still cannot react or communicate in an appropriate fashion. Although disturbing for many family members, this is actually a good clinical sign. At this time, it is necessary to minimize the stimulation to the patient by limiting background noises, having only one person speak to the patient at a time, giving the patient a longer period of time to respond, and allowing for frequent rest or quiet times.

When the patient has regained consciousness, videotaped family or social events may assist the patient in recognizing family and friends and allow him or her to experience missed events.

MEETING FAMILIES' NEEDS

The family of the patient with altered LOC may be thrown into a sudden state of crisis and go through the process of severe anxiety, denial, anger, remorse, grief, and reconciliation. Depending on the disorder that caused the altered LOC and the extent of the patient's recovery, the family may be unprepared for the changes in the cognitive and physical status of their loved one. If the patient has significant residual deficits, the family may require considerable time, assistance, and support to come to terms with these changes. To help family members mobilize their adaptive capacities, the nurse can reinforce and clarify information about the patient's condition, permit the family to be involved in care, and listen to and encourage ventilation of feelings and concerns while supporting them in their decision-making process about posthospitalization management and placement (Hauber & Testani-Dufour, 2000). Families may benefit from participation in support groups offered through the hospital, rehabilitation facility, or community organizations.

In some circumstances, the family may need to face the death of their loved one. The neurologic patient is often pronounced brain dead before physiologic death occurs. The term **brain death** describes irreversible loss of all functions of the entire brain, including the brain stem. The term may be misleading to the family because although brain function has ceased, the patient appears to be alive, with the heart rate and blood pressure sustained by vasoactive medications, and breathing continues by mechanical ventilation. When discussing a patient who is brain dead with family members, it is important to use the term "dead"; the term "brain dead" may confuse them (Shewmon, 1998). Chart 61-1 discusses ethical issues related to patients with severe neurologic damage. End-of-life care is discussed in Chapter 17.

MONITORING AND MANAGING POTENTIAL COMPLICATIONS

Pneumonia, aspiration, and respiratory failure are potential complications in any patient who has a depressed LOC and who cannot protect the airway or turn, cough, and take deep breaths. The longer the period of unconsciousness, the greater the risk for pulmonary complications.

Vital signs and respiratory function are monitored closely to detect any signs of respiratory failure or distress. Total blood count and arterial blood gas measurements are assessed to determine whether there are adequate red blood cells to carry oxygen and whether ventilation is effective. Chest physiotherapy and suctioning are initiated to prevent respiratory complications such as pneumonia. If pneumonia develops, cultures are obtained to identify the organism so that appropriate antibiotics can be administered.

The patient with altered LOC is monitored closely for evidence of impaired skin integrity, and strategies to prevent skin breakdown and pressure ulcers are continued through all phases of care, including hospital, rehabilitation, and home care. Factors that contribute to impaired skin integrity (eg, incontinence, inadequate dietary intake, pressure on bony prominences, edema) are addressed. If pressure ulcers develop, strategies to promote healing are undertaken. Care is taken to prevent bacterial contamination of pressure ulcers, which may lead to sepsis and septic shock. Assessment and management of pressure ulcers are discussed in Chapter 11.

The patient should also be monitored for signs and symptoms of deep vein thrombosis. Patients who develop deep vein thrombosis are at risk for pulmonary embolism. Prophylaxis such as subcutaneous heparin or low-molecular-weight heparin (Fragmin, Orgaran, Lovenox) should be prescribed (Karch, 2002). Thigh-high elastic compression stockings or pneumatic compression stockings should also be prescribed to reduce the risk for clot formation. Measures to assess for deep vein thrombosis, such as Homans' sign, may be clinically unreliable in this population, and the nurse should observe for redness and swelling in the lower extremities.

Evaluation

EXPECTED PATIENT OUTCOMES

Expected patient outcomes may include:

1. Maintains clear airway and demonstrates appropriate breath sounds
2. Experiences no injuries
3. Attains/maintains adequate fluid status
   a. Has no clinical signs or symptoms of dehydration
   b. Demonstrates normal range of serum electrolytes
   c. Has no clinical signs or symptoms of overhydration
4. Attains/maintains healthy oral mucous membranes
5. Maintains normal skin integrity
6. Has no corneal irritation
7. Attains or maintains thermoregulation
8. Has no urinary retention
9. Has no diarrhea or fecal impaction
10. Receives appropriate sensory stimulation
11. Family members cope with crisis
    a. Verbalize fears and concerns
    b. Participate in patient's care and provide sensory stimulation by talking and touching
12. Is free of complications
    a. Has arterial blood gas values within normal range
    b. Displays no signs or symptoms of pneumonia
    c. Exhibits intact skin over pressure areas
    d. Does not develop deep vein thrombosis

Increased Intracranial Pressure

The rigid cranial vault contains brain tissue (1,400 g), blood (75 mL), and CSF (75 mL) (Hickey, 2003). The volume and pressure of these three components are usually in a state of equi-

Chart 61-1 • Ethics and Related Issues

What Ethical Principles Apply When Treatment Is Withdrawn From the Patient in a Persistent Vegetative State?

Situation
The family of a 55-year-old woman who has been diagnosed as being in a persistent vegetative state wants to withdraw tube feedings and let her die. The nursing staff express concern about removing the feeding tube, relating that the patient has wakeful periods and sometimes seems to move her eyes toward them when they care for her. The family's wishes, however, are honoured and the medical team discontinues all tube feedings and intravenous lines and orders comfort measures only. The patient dies 7 days later.

Dilemma
How do nurses reconcile their ethical obligations of respect for persons and sanctity of life in the face of a decision to withdraw treatment? Is the ethical principle of justice upheld?

Discussion
Is the maintenance of medical treatment obligatory in patients in a persistent vegetative state to provide respect for the patient and the sanctity of life? What mechanisms can the nursing staff use to assist them in resolving these dilemmas?

librium and produce the ICP. ICP is usually measured in the lateral ventricles; normal ICP is 10 to 20 mm Hg (Hickey, 2003).

The **Monro-Kellie hypothesis** states that because of the limited space for expansion within the skull, an increase in any one of the components causes a change in the volume of the others. Because brain tissue has limited space to change, compensation typically is accomplished by displacing or shifting CSF, increasing the absorption of CSF, or decreasing cerebral blood volume. Without such changes, ICP will begin to rise. Under normal circumstances, minor changes in blood volume and CSF volume occur constantly due to alterations in intrathoracic pressure (coughing, sneezing, straining), posture, blood pressure, and systemic oxygen and carbon dioxide levels.

Pathophysiology

Increased ICP is a syndrome that affects many patients with acute neurologic conditions. This is because pathologic conditions alter the relationship between intracranial volume and pressure. Although an elevated ICP is most commonly associated with head injury, it also may be seen as a secondary effect in other conditions, such as brain tumours, subarachnoid hemorrhage, and toxic and viral encephalopathies. Increased ICP from any cause decreases cerebral perfusion, stimulates further swelling (edema), and shifts brain tissue through openings in the rigid dura, resulting in **herniation**, a dire, frequently fatal event.

DECREASED CEREBRAL BLOOD FLOW
Increased ICP may significantly reduce cerebral blood flow, resulting in ischemia and cell death. In the early stages of cerebral ischemia, the vasomotor centres are stimulated and the systemic pressure rises to maintain cerebral blood flow. Usually a slow bounding pulse and respiratory irregularities accompany this. These changes in blood pressure, pulse, and respiration are important clinically because they suggest increased ICP.

The concentration of carbon dioxide in the blood and in the brain tissue also has a role in the regulation of cerebral blood flow. A rise in carbon dioxide partial pressure ($PaCO_2$) causes cerebral vasodilatation, leading to increased cerebral blood flow and increased ICP; a fall in $PaCO_2$ has a vasoconstrictive effect (Young, Ropper & Bolton, 1998). Decreased venous outflow may also increase cerebral blood volume, thus raising ICP.

CEREBRAL EDEMA
Cerebral edema or swelling is defined as an abnormal accumulation of water or fluid in the intracellular space, extracellular space,

or both, associated with an increase in brain tissue volume. Edema can occur in the grey, white, or interstitial matter. As brain tissue swells within the rigid skull, several mechanisms attempt to compensate for the increasing ICP. These mechanisms include autoregulation and decreasing the production and flow of CSF. **Autoregulation** refers to the brain's ability to change the diameter of its blood vessels automatically to maintain a constant cerebral blood flow during alterations in systemic blood pressure.

CEREBRAL RESPONSE TO INCREASED ICP
As ICP rises, compensatory mechanisms in the brain work to maintain blood flow and prevent tissue damage. The brain can maintain a steady perfusion pressure when the arterial systolic blood pressure is 50 to 150 mm Hg and ICP is less than 40 mm Hg. The cerebral perfusion pressure is calculated by subtracting the ICP from the mean arterial pressure. For example, if the mean arterial pressure is 100 and the ICP is 15, then the cerebral perfusion pressure is 85 mm Hg. The normal cerebral perfusion pressure is 70 to 100 mm Hg (Hickey, 2003; Young et al., 1998). As ICP rises, however, and the autoregulatory mechanism of the brain is overwhelmed, cerebral perfusion pressure can rise to greater than 100 mm Hg or fall to less than 50 mm Hg. Patients with a cerebral perfusion pressure less than 50 mm Hg experience irreversible neurologic damage. If ICP equals mean arterial pressure, cerebral circulation ceases (Porth, 2002).

A clinical phenomenon known as the **Cushing's response** (or Cushing's reflex) is seen when cerebral blood flow decreases significantly. When ischemic, the vasomotor centre triggers a rise in arterial pressure in an effort to overcome the increased ICP. A sympathetically mediated response causes a rise in the systolic blood pressure with a widening of the pulse pressure and cardiac slowing. This response, which is mediated by the sympathetic nervous system, is seen clinically as a rise in systolic blood pressure, widening of the pulse pressure, and reflex slowing of the heart rate. This is a sign requiring immediate intervention; however, perfusion may be recoverable if treated rapidly.

At a certain volume or pressure, the brain's ability to autoregulate becomes ineffective and decompensation (ischemia and infarction) begins (Young et al., 1998). When this occurs, the patient exhibits significant changes in mental status and vital signs. The bradycardia, hypertension, and bradypnea associated with this deterioration are known as **Cushing's triad**, a grave sign. At this point, herniation of the brain stem and occlusion of the cerebral blood flow occur if therapeutic intervention is not initiated. Herniation refers to the shifting of brain tissue from an area of high pressure to an area of lower pressure (Fig. 61-2). The herniated

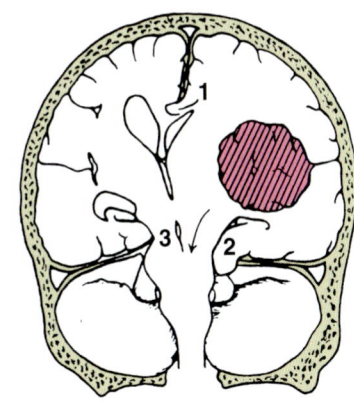

FIGURE 61-2 Cross section of normal brain (*left*) and brain with intracranial shifts from supratentorial lesions (*right*). (1) Herniation of the cingulated gyrus. (2) Herniation of the temporal lobe into the tentorial notch. (3) Downward displacement of the brainstem through the notch.

tissue exerts pressure on the brain area to which it has herniated or shifted, interfering with the blood supply in that area. Cessation of cerebral blood flow results in cerebral ischemia and infarction and brain death.

Clinical Manifestations

When ICP increases to the point at which the brain's ability to adjust has reached its limits, neural function is impaired; this may be manifested by clinical changes first in LOC and later by abnormal respiratory and vasomotor responses.

 NURSING ALERT The earliest sign of increasing ICP is a change in LOC. Slowing of speech and delay in response to verbal suggestions are other early indicators.

Any sudden change in the patient's condition, such as restlessness (without apparent cause), confusion, or increasing drowsiness, has neurologic significance. These signs may result from compression of the brain due to swelling from hemorrhage or edema, an expanding intracranial lesion (hematoma or tumour), or a combination of both.

As ICP increases, the patient becomes stuporous, reacting only to loud auditory or painful stimuli. At this stage, serious impairment of brain circulation is probably taking place, and immediate intervention is required. As neurologic function deteriorates further, the patient becomes comatose and exhibits abnormal motor responses in the form of **decortication**, **decerebration**, or flaccidity (see Fig. 61-1). When the coma is profound, with the pupils dilated and fixed and respirations impaired, death is usually inevitable.

Assessment and Diagnostic Findings

The diagnostic studies used to determine the underlying cause of increased ICP are discussed in detail in Chapter 60. The patient may undergo cerebral angiography, computed tomography (CT) scanning, magnetic resonance imaging (MRI), or positron emission tomography (PET). Transcranial Doppler studies provide information about cerebral blood flow. The patient with increased ICP may also undergo electrophysiologic monitoring to monitor cerebral blood flow indirectly. Evoked potential monitoring measures the electrical potentials produced by nerve tissue in response to external stimulation (auditory, visual, or sensory). Lumbar puncture is avoided in patients with increased ICP because the sudden release of pressure can cause the brain to herniate.

Complications

Complications of increased ICP include brain stem herniation, diabetes insipidus, and syndrome of inappropriate antidiuretic hormone (SIADH).

Brain stem herniation results from an excessive increase in ICP, when the pressure builds in the cranial vault and the brain tissue presses down on the brain stem. This increasing pressure on the brain stem results in the cessation of blood flow to the brain, causing irreversible brain anoxia and brain death.

Diabetes insipidus is the result of decreased secretion of antidiuretic hormone. The patient has excessive urine output, and hyperosmolarity results (Young et al., 1998). Therapy consists of administration of fluid volume, electrolyte replacement, and vasopressin (Pressyn, DDAVP) therapy. Diabetes insipidus is discussed in Chapters 14 and 42.

SIADH is the result of increased secretion of antidiuretic hormone. The patient becomes volume-overloaded, urine output diminishes, and serum sodium concentration becomes dilute. Treatment of SIADH includes fluid restriction, which is usually sufficient to correct the hyponatremia; severe cases call for judicious administration of a 3% hypertonic saline solution (Hickey, 2003). Patients with chronic SIADH may respond to lithium carbonate or demeclocycline, which reduces renal tubule responsiveness to antidiuretic hormone. Further discussion of SIADH is presented in Chapters 14 and 42.

Management

Increased ICP is a true emergency and must be treated promptly. Invasive monitoring of ICP is an important component of management, but immediate management to relieve increased ICP involves decreasing cerebral edema, lowering the volume of CSF, or decreasing cerebral blood volume while maintaining cerebral perfusion (Cunning & Houdek, 1999). These goals are accomplished by administering osmotic diuretics and corticosteroids, restricting fluids, draining CSF, controlling fever, maintaining systemic blood pressure and oxygenation, and reducing cellular metabolic demands. Judicious use of hyperventilation is recommended only if the ICP is refractory to other measures.

MONITORING ICP

The purposes of ICP monitoring are to identify increased pressure early in its course (before cerebral damage occurs), to quantify the degree of elevation, to initiate appropriate treatment, to provide access to CSF for sampling and drainage, and to evaluate the effectiveness of treatment. An intraventricular catheter (ventriculostomy), a subarachnoid bolt, an epidural or subdural catheter, or a fibreoptic transducer-tipped catheter placed in the subdural space or the ventricle can be used to monitor ICP (Fig. 61-3).

When a **ventriculostomy** or ventricular catheter monitoring device is used for monitoring ICP, a fine-bore catheter is inserted into a lateral ventricle, usually in the nondominant hemisphere of the brain (Hickey, 2003). The catheter is connected by a fluid-filled system to a transducer, which records the pressure in the form of an electrical impulse. In addition to obtaining continuous ICP recordings, the ventricular catheter allows CSF to drain, particularly during acute rises in pressure. The ventriculostomy also can be used to drain the ventricle of blood. Also, continuous drainage of ventricular fluid under pressure control is an effective method of treating intracranial hypertension. Another advantage of an indwelling ventricular catheter is the access it provides for the intraventricular administration of medications and the instillation of air or a contrast agent for ventriculography. Complications include ventricular infection, meningitis, ventricular collapse, occlusion of the catheter by brain tissue or blood, and problems with the monitoring system.

The **subarachnoid bolt** (or screw) is a hollow device inserted through the skull and dura mater into the cranial subarachnoid space (Hickey, 2003). It has the advantage of not requiring a ventricular puncture. The subarachnoid screw is attached to a pressure transducer, and the output is recorded on an oscilloscope. The hollow screw technique has the advantage of avoiding complications from brain shift and small ventricle size. Complications include blockage of the screw by clot or brain tissue, which leads to a loss of pressure tracing and a decrease in accuracy at high ICP readings.

An **epidural monitor** uses a pneumatic flow sensor that functions on a nonelectrical basis. This pneumatic epidural ICP mon-

FIGURE 61-3 ICP monitoring. A fibre-optic, transducer-tipped device placed in (**A**) the ventricle or (**B**) the subarachnoid space. These devices connect to a pressure transducer and a display system.

itoring system has a low incidence of infection and complications and appears to read pressures accurately. Calibration of the system is maintained automatically, and abnormal pressure waves trigger an alarm system. One disadvantage of the epidural catheter is the inability to withdraw CSF for analysis.

A **fibreoptic monitor**, or transducer-tipped catheter, is becoming a widely used alternative to standard intraventricular, subarachnoid, and subdural systems (Hickey, 2003). The miniature transducer reflects pressure changes, which are converted to electrical signals in an amplifier and displayed on a digital monitor. The catheter can be inserted into the ventricle, subarachnoid space, subdural space, or brain parenchyma or under a bone flap. If inserted into the ventricle, it can also be used in conjunction with a CSF drainage device.

Waves of high pressure and troughs of relatively normal pressure indicate changes in ICP. Waveforms are captured and recorded on an oscilloscope. These waves have been classified as A waves (plateau waves), B waves, and C waves (Fig. 61-4). The plateau waves (A waves) are transient, paroxysmal, recurring elevations of ICP that may last 5 to 20 minutes and range in amplitude from 50 to 100 mm Hg (Hickey, 2003). Plateau waves have clinical significance and indicate changes in vascular volume within the intracranial compartment that are beginning to compromise cerebral perfusion. A waves may increase in amplitude and frequency, reflecting cerebral ischemia and brain damage that can occur before overt signs and symptoms of raised ICP are seen clinically. B waves are shorter (30 seconds to 2 minutes), with smaller amplitude (up to 50 mm Hg). They have less clinical significance, but if seen in runs in a patient with depressed consciousness, they may precede the appearance of A waves. B waves may be seen in patients with intracranial hypertension and decreased intracranial compliance. C waves are small, rhythmic oscillations with frequencies of approximately six per minute. They

appear to be related to rhythmic variations of the systemic arterial blood pressure and respirations.

DECREASING CEREBRAL EDEMA

Osmotic diuretics (mannitol) may be given to dehydrate the brain tissue and reduce cerebral edema. They act by drawing water across intact membranes, thereby reducing the volume of brain and extracellular fluid. An indwelling urinary catheter is usually inserted to monitor urinary output and to manage the resulting diuresis. When a patient is receiving osmotic diuretics, serum osmolality should be determined to assess hydration status. Corticosteroids (eg, dexamethasone) help reduce the edema

FIGURE 61-4 Intracranial pressure waves. Composite diagram of A (plateau) waves, which indicate cerebral ischemia; B waves, which indicate intracranial hypertension and variations in the respiratory cycle; and C waves, which relate to variations in systemic arterial pressure and respirations.

surrounding brain tumours when a brain tumour is the cause of increased ICP.

Another method for decreasing cerebral edema is fluid restriction (Hickey, 2003). Limiting overall fluid intake leads to dehydration and hemoconcentration, drawing fluid across the osmotic gradient and decreasing cerebral edema. Conversely, overhydration of the patient with increased ICP is avoided, as this will increase cerebral edema.

It has been hypothesized that lowering body temperature will decrease cerebral edema, reduce the oxygen and metabolic requirements of the brain, and protect the brain from continued ischemia. If body metabolism can be reduced by lowering body temperature, the collateral circulation in the brain may be able to provide an adequate blood supply to the brain. The effect of hypothermia on ICP requires more study (Slade, Kerr & Marion, 1999), but as yet induced hypothermia has not been proven to be beneficial in the brain-injured patient (Clifton, Miller, Choi et al., 2001). Inducing and maintaining hypothermia is a major clinical procedure and requires knowledge and skilled nursing observation and management.

MAINTAINING CEREBRAL PERFUSION

The cardiac output may be manipulated to provide adequate perfusion to the brain. Improvements in cardiac output are made using fluid volume and inotropic agents such as dobutamine hydrochloride. The effectiveness of the cardiac output is reflected in the cerebral perfusion pressure, which is maintained at greater than 70 mm Hg (Young et al., 1998). A lower cerebral perfusion pressure indicates that the cardiac output is insufficient to maintain adequate cerebral perfusion.

REDUCING CSF AND INTRACRANIAL BLOOD VOLUME

CSF drainage is frequently performed because the removal of CSF with a ventriculostomy drain may dramatically reduce ICP and restore cerebral perfusion pressure. Caution should be used in draining CSF because excessive drainage may result in collapse of the ventricles.

Hyperventilation, which results in vasoconstriction, has been used for many years in patients with increased ICP. Recent research has demonstrated that hyperventilation may not be as beneficial as once thought (Hickey, 2003). The reduction in the $PaCO_2$ may result in hypoxia, ischemia, and an increase in cerebral lactate levels. Maintaining the $PaCO_2$ at 30 to 35 mm Hg may prove beneficial. Hyperventilation is indicated in patients whose ICP is unresponsive to conventional therapies, but it should be used judiciously.

CONTROLLING FEVER

Preventing a temperature elevation is critical because fever increases cerebral metabolism and the rate at which cerebral edema forms. Strategies to reduce temperature include administration of antipyretic medications, as prescribed, and use of a cooling blanket. Additional strategies for reducing fever are included in the Nursing Process: The Patient With an Altered Level of Consciousness section of this chapter. The patient's temperature is monitored closely, and the patient is observed for shivering, which should be avoided because it increases ICP (Sund-Levander & Wahren, 2000).

MAINTAINING OXYGENATION

Arterial blood gases must be monitored to ensure that systemic oxygenation remains optimal. Hemoglobin saturation can also be optimized to provide oxygen more efficiently at the cellular level.

REDUCING METABOLIC DEMANDS

Cellular metabolic demands may be reduced through the administration of high doses of barbiturates when the patient is unresponsive to conventional treatment. The mechanism by which barbiturates decrease ICP and protect the brain is uncertain, but the resultant comatose state is thought to reduce the metabolic requirements of the brain, thus providing some protection (Greenberg, 2001).

Another method of reducing cellular metabolic demand and improving oxygenation is the administration of pharmacologic paralyzing agents. The patient who receives these agents cannot move, decreasing the metabolic demands and resulting in a decrease in cerebral oxygen demand. Because the patient cannot respond or report pain, sedation and analgesia must be provided because the paralyzing agents do not provide either.

Patients receiving high doses of barbiturates or pharmacologic paralyzing agents require continuous cardiac monitoring, endotracheal intubation, mechanical ventilation, ICP monitoring, and arterial pressure monitoring. Pentobarbital (Nembutal), thiopental (Pentothal), and propofol (Diprivan) are the most common agents used for high-dose barbiturate therapy (Greenberg, 2001). Serum barbiturate levels must be monitored (Hickey, 2003).

The ability to perform serial neurologic assessments on the patient is lost with the use of barbiturates or paralyzing agents (Greenberg, 2001). Therefore, other monitoring tools are needed to assess the patient's status and response to therapy. Important parameters that must be assessed include ICP, blood pressure, heart rate, respiratory rate, and response to ventilator therapy (eg, bucking the ventilator). The level of pharmacologic paralysis is adjusted based on serum levels and the assessed parameters. Potential complications include hypotension due to decreased sympathetic tone and myocardial depression (Greenberg, 2001).

TRENDS IN NEUROLOGIC MONITORING

One controversial trend in cerebral monitoring is the ongoing measurement of venous oxygen saturation in the jugular bulb (SjO_2). Readings taken from a catheter residing in the jugular outflow tract theoretically allow for a comparison of arterial and venous oxygen saturation, and the balance of cerebral oxygen supply and demand is demonstrated. Venous jugular desaturations can reflect early cerebral ischemia, alerting the clinician prior to a rise in ICP. Minimizing elevations in ICP can potentially improve outcome (Clay, 2000). This type of monitoring appears beneficial in the management of patients at risk for cerebral ischemia; however, the invasive nature of this type of monitoring and current limitations in technology mandate caution in its use. More study is needed before SjO_2 monitoring can be considered a valid and reliable tool for the management of cerebral ischemia (Clay, 2000).

NURSING PROCESS: THE PATIENT WITH INCREASED ICP

Assessment

Initial assessment of the patient with increased ICP includes obtaining a history of events leading to the present illness and other subjective data; it may be necessary to obtain this information from family or friends. The neurologic examination should be as complete as the patient's condition allows. It includes an evaluation of mental status, LOC, cranial nerve function, cerebellar function (balance and coordination), reflexes, and motor and sensory function. Because the patient is critically ill, ongoing assessment will be more focused, including pupil checks, assessment of selected cranial nerves, frequent measurements of vital signs and intracranial pressure, and use of the Glasgow Coma Scale. Assessment of the patient with altered LOC is summarized in Table 61-1.

Diagnosis

NURSING DIAGNOSES

Based on the assessment data, the major nursing diagnoses for patients with increased ICP include the following:

- Ineffective airway clearance related to diminished protective reflexes (cough, gag)
- Ineffective breathing patterns related to neurologic dysfunction (brain stem compression, structural displacement)
- Ineffective cerebral tissue perfusion related to the effects of increased ICP
- Deficient fluid volume related to fluid restriction
- Risk for infection related to ICP monitoring system (fibreoptic or intraventricular catheter)

Other relevant nursing diagnoses are included in the section on caring for patients with altered LOC.

COLLABORATIVE PROBLEMS/ POTENTIAL COMPLICATIONS

Based on the assessment data, potential complications include:

- Brain stem herniation
- Diabetes insipidus
- SIADH

Planning and Goals

The goals for the patient include maintenance of a patent airway, normalization of respiration, adequate cerebral tissue perfusion through reduction in ICP, restoration of fluid balance, absence of infection, and absence of complications.

Nursing Interventions

MAINTAINING A PATENT AIRWAY

The patency of the airway is assessed. Secretions obstructing the airway must be suctioned with care, because transient elevations of ICP occur with suctioning (Hickey, 2003). The patient is hyperoxygenated before and after suctioning to maintain adequate oxygenation. Hypoxia caused by poor oxygenation leads to cerebral ischemia and edema. Coughing is discouraged because coughing and straining also increase ICP. The lung fields are auscultated at least every 8 hours to determine the presence of adventitious sounds or any areas of congestion. Elevating the head of the bed may aid in clearing secretions as well as improving venous drainage of the brain.

ACHIEVING AN ADEQUATE BREATHING PATTERN

The patient must be monitored constantly for respiratory irregularities. Increased pressure on the frontal lobes or deep midline structures may result in Cheyne-Stokes respirations, whereas pressure in the midbrain may cause hyperventilation. When the lower portion of the brain stem (the pons and medulla) is involved, respirations become irregular and eventually cease.

If hyperventilation therapy is deemed appropriate to reduce ICP (by causing cerebral vasoconstriction and a decrease in cerebral blood volume), the nurse collaborates with the respiratory

therapist in monitoring PaCO$_2$, which is usually maintained at 35 to 45 mm Hg (Hickey, 2003).

A neurologic observation record (Fig. 61-5) is maintained, and all observations are made in relation to the patient's baseline condition. Repeated assessments of the patient are made (sometimes minute by minute) so that improvement or deterioration may be noted immediately. If the patient's condition deteriorates, preparations are made for surgical intervention.

OPTIMIZING CEREBRAL TISSUE PERFUSION

In addition to ongoing nursing assessment, strategies are initiated to reduce factors contributing to the elevation of ICP (Table 61-2).

Proper positioning helps to reduce ICP. The head is kept in a neutral (midline) position, maintained with the use of a cervical collar if necessary, to promote venous drainage. Elevation of the head is maintained at 0 to 60 degrees to aid in venous drainage unless otherwise prescribed (Sullivan, 2000). Extreme rotation of the neck and flexion of the neck are avoided because compression or distortion of the jugular veins increases ICP. Extreme hip flexion is also avoided because this position causes an increase in intra-abdominal and intrathoracic pressures, which can produce a rise in ICP. Relatively minor changes in position may significantly affect ICP (Sullivan, 2000). If monitoring parameters demonstrate that turning the patient raises ICP, rotating beds, turning sheets, and holding the patient's head during turning may minimize the stimuli that increase ICP.

The Valsalva manoeuvre, which can be produced by straining at defecation or even moving in bed, raises ICP and is to be avoided. Stool softeners may be prescribed. If the patient is alert and able to eat, a diet high in fibre may be indicated. Abdominal distention, which increases intra-abdominal and intrathoracic pressure and ICP, should be noted. Enemas and cathartics are avoided if possible. When moving or being turned in bed, the patient can be instructed to exhale (which opens the glottis) to avoid the Valsalva manoeuvre.

Mechanical ventilation presents unique problems for the patient with increased ICP. Before suctioning, the patient should be preoxygenated and hyperventilated using 100% oxygen on the ventilator (Hickey, 2003). Suctioning should not last longer than 15 seconds. High levels of positive end-expiratory pressure are avoided because they may decrease venous return to the heart and decrease venous drainage from the brain through increased intrathoracic pressure (Hickey, 2003).

Activities that raise ICP, as indicated by changes in waveforms, should be avoided if possible. Spacing nursing interventions may prevent transient increases in ICP. During nursing interventions, the ICP should not rise above 25 mm Hg and should return to baseline levels within 5 minutes. Patients with increased ICP should not demonstrate a significant increase in pressure or change in the ICP waveform. Patients with the potential for a significant increase in ICP should receive sedation or "paralyzation" before initiation of many nursing activities (Hickey, 2003; McConnell, 2001).

Emotional stress and frequent arousal from sleep are avoided. A calm atmosphere is maintained. Environmental stimuli (noise, conversation) should be minimal. Isometric muscle contractions are also contraindicated because they raise the systemic blood pressure and hence the ICP.

MAINTAINING NEGATIVE FLUID BALANCE

The administration of various osmotic and loop diuretics is part of the treatment protocol to reduce ICP. Corticosteroids are used

(text continues on page 1874)

NURSING NEUROLOGICAL CRITICAL CARE FLOWSHEET

		ADDRESSOGRAPH												
	Date													
	Time													
	Initials													
Level of orientation (✓)	Person													
	Place													
	Date and time													
	No orientation													
Awakens to (✓)	Voice													
	Touch													
	Noxious stimuli													
	Painful stimuli													
	No response													
Best verbal response (✓)	Clear and appropriate													
	Clear and inappropriate													
	Difficulty speaking*													
	Perseveration													
	Aphasic expressive (non-fluent)													
	Aphasic receptive (fluent)													
	Sounds no speech													
	No response													
	ETT/TRACH													
Best motor response (✓)	Moves all extremities purposefully													
	Withdraws and lifts to painful stimuli													
	Moves to painful stimuli													
	Triple flexes (spinal reflex)													
	Decorticates (spinal reflex)													
	Decerebrates (spinal reflex)													
	No response													
Best motor strength upper extremities (✓)	No drifts (R/L)	R/L	R/L	R/L	R/L	R/L	R/L	R/L	R/L	R/L	R/L	R/L	R/L
	Drift (R/L)	R/L	R/L	R/L	R/L	R/L	R/L	R/L	R/L	R/L	R/L	R/L	R/L
	Can only lift forearm (R/L)	R/L	R/L	R/L	R/L	R/L	R/L	R/L	R/L	R/L	R/L	R/L	R/L
	Trace movement of hand or arm (R/L)	R/L	R/L	R/L	R/L	R/L	R/L	R/L	R/L	R/L	R/L	R/L	R/L
	Trace movement of fingers only (R/L)	R/L	R/L	R/L	R/L	R/L	R/L	R/L	R/L	R/L	R/L	R/L	R/L
	No response (R/L)	R/L	R/L	R/L	R/L	R/L	R/L	R/L	R/L	R/L	R/L	R/L	R/L
Best strength lower extremities (✓)	Raises leg off bed (R/L)	R/L	R/L	R/L	R/L	R/L	R/L	R/L	R/L	R/L	R/L	R/L	R/L
	Drags heel on bed and lifts knee (R/L)	R/L	R/L	R/L	R/L	R/L	R/L	R/L	R/L	R/L	R/L	R/L	R/L
	Trace movement of foot or leg (R/L)	R/L	R/L	R/L	R/L	R/L	R/L	R/L	R/L	R/L	R/L	R/L	R/L
	Trace movement of toes only (R/L)	R/L	R/L	R/L	R/L	R/L	R/L	R/L	R/L	R/L	R/L	R/L	R/L
	No response (R/L)	R/L	R/L	R/L	R/L	R/L	R/L	R/L	R/L	R/L	R/L	R/L	R/L
Seizure activity (✓)	No seizure activity													
	With loss of consciousness*													
	Without loss of consciousness*													
Ataxia (✓)	Gross ataxia													
	Fine motor ataxia													
	Does not apply													
ICP monitoring	Ventriculostomy mLs													
	ICP mm Hg													
	Not applicable													

*= FURTHER DOCUMENTATION IS REQUIRED TO VALIDATE ASSESSMENT

FIGURE 61-5 A neurological assessment flow sheet.

PUPIL GAUGE (mm)

● ● ● ● ●
2   3   4   5   6

● ● ●
7   8   9

B=Brisk, S=Sluggish, F=Fixed

ADDRESSOGRAPH

Date													
Time													
Initials													

Incision +/–	Dry and intact													
	Drainage													
Pupils refer to gauge (✓) (+)=Present (–)=Absent	Size (R/L)	R/L	R/L	R/L	R/L	R/L	R/L	R/L	R/L	R/L	R/L	R/L
	Regular (R/L)	R/L	R/L	R/L	R/L	R/L	R/L	R/L	R/L	R/L	R/L	R/L
	Irregular* (R/L)	R/L	R/L	R/L	R/L	R/L	R/L	R/L	R/L	R/L	R/L	R/L
	Reaction (R/L) (B) - (S) - (F)	R/L	R/L	R/L	R/L	R/L	R/L	R/L	R/L	R/L	R/L	R/L
	Ptosis (R/L) (+) (–)	R/L	R/L	R/L	R/L	R/L	R/L	R/L	R/L	R/L	R/L	R/L
	Gaze preference (R/L) (+)* (–)	R/L	R/L	R/L	R/L	R/L	R/L	R/L	R/L	R/L	R/L	R/L
Meningeal signs (+)=Present (–)=Absent	Headache													
	Nuchal rigidity													
	Photophobia													
Visual fields (+)=Present (–)=Absent* NA=Not applicable	Right upper outer													
	Right lower outer													
	Left upper outer													
	Left lower outer													
Nystagmus (+)=Present (–)=Absent	Lateral (R/L)	R/L	R/L	R/L	R/L	R/L	R/L	R/L	R/L	R/L	R/L	R/L
	Vertical (R/L)	R/L	R/L	R/L	R/L	R/L	R/L	R/L	R/L	R/L	R/L	R/L
Cranial nerves (+)=Present (–)=Absent	III, IV, VI, Extra occular movements													
	VII – Peripheral facial droop (R/L)	R/L	R/L	R/L	R/L	R/L	R/L	R/L	R/L	R/L	R/L	R/L
	XII – Tongue deviation (R/L)	R/L	R/L	R/L	R/L	R/L	R/L	R/L	R/L	R/L	R/L	R/L
	IX – Gag reflex													
	V, VII – Corneal reflex (R/L)	R/L	R/L	R/L	R/L	R/L	R/L	R/L	R/L	R/L	R/L	R/L
	X, IX – Cough reflex													
	Doll's eyes if appropriate													
Follows commands	Two step verbal command													
	One step verbal command													
	Unable to follow command													

*= FURTHER DOCUMENTATION IS REQUIRED TO VALIDATE ASSESSMENT

Initials	Signature	Title	Initials	Signature	Title

Table 61-2 • Increased ICP and Interventions

FACTOR	PHYSIOLOGY	INTERVENTIONS	RATIONALE
Cerebral edema	Can be caused by contusion, tumour, or abscess; water intoxication (hypo-osmolality); alteration in the blood–brain barrier (protein leaks into the tissue, causing water to follow)	Administer osmotic diuretics as prescribed (monitor serum osmolality). Maintain head of bed elevated 30 degrees. Maintain alignment of the head.	Promotes venous return. Prevents impairment of venous return through the jugular veins
Hypoxia	A decrease in the PaO_2 causes cerebral vasodilation at less than 60 mm Hg.	Maintain PaO_2 greater than 60 mm Hg. Maintain oxygen therapy. Monitor arterial blood gas values. Suction when needed. Maintain a patent airway.	Prevents hypoxia and vasodilation
Hypercapnia (elevated $PaCO_2$)	Causes vasodilation	Maintain $PaCO_2$ (normally 35–45 mm Hg) through hyperventilation.	Decreased $PaCO_2$ prevents vasodilation and thus reduces the cerebral blood volume.
Impaired venous return	Increases the cerebral blood volume	Maintain head alignment. Elevate head of bed 30 degrees.	Hyperextension, rotation, or hyperflexion of the neck causes decreased venous return.
Increase in intrathoracic or abdominal pressure	Increase in these pressures due to coughing, PEEP, Valsalva manoeuvre causes a decrease in venous return.	Monitor arterial blood gas values and keep PEEP as low as possible. Provide humidified oxygen. Administer stool softeners as prescribed.	To keep secretions loose and easy to suction or expectorate. Soft bowel movements will prevent straining or Valsalva manoeuvre.

to reduce cerebral edema, and fluids may be restricted. All of these treatment modalities promote dehydration.

Skin turgor, mucous membranes, and serum and urine osmolality are monitored to assess fluid status. If fluids are given intravenously, the nurse ensures they are administered at a slow to moderate rate with an intravenous infusion pump to prevent too-rapid administration and avoid overhydration. For the patient receiving mannitol, the nurse observes for the possible development of heart failure and pulmonary edema, because the intent of treatment is for fluid to shift from the intracellular compartment to the intravascular system, thus controlling cerebral edema.

For patients undergoing dehydrating procedures, vital signs, including blood pressure, must be monitored to assess fluid volume status. An indwelling urinary catheter is inserted to permit assessment of renal function and fluid status. During the acute phase, urine output should be monitored every hour. An output greater than 200 mL/hr for 2 consecutive hours may indicate the onset of diabetes insipidus (Cruz, 1998). These patients also need careful oral hygiene because mouth dryness is associated with dehydration. Frequently rinsing the mouth, lubricating the lips, and removing encrustations relieve dryness and promote comfort.

PREVENTING INFECTION
Risk for infection is greatest when ICP is monitored with an intraventricular catheter. Most health care facilities have written protocols for managing these systems and maintaining their sterility; strict adherence to them is essential.

The dressing over the ventricular catheter must be kept dry because a wet dressing is conducive to bacterial growth. Aseptic technique must be used when managing the system and changing the ventricular drainage bag. The drainage system is also checked

for loose connections because they cause leakage and contamination of the CSF as well as inaccurate readings of ICP. The nurse should observe the character of the CSF drainage and report observations of increasing cloudiness or blood. The patient is monitored for signs and symptoms of meningitis: fever, chills, nuchal (neck) rigidity, and increasing or persisting headache.

MONITORING AND MANAGING POTENTIAL COMPLICATIONS
The primary complication of increased ICP is brain herniation resulting in death (see Fig. 61-2). Nursing management focuses on detecting early signs of increasing ICP because medical interventions are usually ineffective once later signs develop. Frequent neurologic assessment and documentation and analysis of trends will reveal the subtle changes that may herald rising ICP.

Detecting Early Indications of Increasing ICP
The nurse assesses for and immediately reports any of the following early signs or symptoms of increasing ICP:

- Disorientation, restlessness, increased respiratory effort, purposeless movements, and mental confusion; these are early clinical indications of rising ICP because the brain cells responsible for cognition are extremely sensitive to decreased oxygenation
- Pupillary changes and impaired extraocular movements; these occur as the increasing pressure displaces the brain against the oculomotor and optic nerves (cranial nerves II, III, IV, and VI) arising from the midbrain and brain stem (see Chap. 60)
- Weakness in one extremity or on one side of the body; this occurs as increasing ICP compresses the pyramidal tracts

- Headache that is constant, increasing in intensity, and aggravated by movement or straining; this occurs as increasing ICP causes pressure and stretching of venous and arterial vessels in the base of the brain

Detecting Later Signs of Increased ICP
As ICP rises, the patient's condition worsens, as manifested by the following later signs and symptoms:

- LOC continues to deteriorate until the patient is comatose.
- The pulse rate and respiratory rate decrease or become erratic, and the blood pressure and temperature rise. The pulse pressure (the difference between the systolic and the diastolic pressures) widens. The pulse fluctuates rapidly, varying from bradycardia to tachycardia.
- Altered respiratory patterns develop, including Cheyne-Stokes breathing (rhythmic waxing and waning of rate and depth of respirations alternating with brief periods of apnea) and ataxic breathing (irregular breathing with a random sequence of deep and shallow breaths).
- Projectile vomiting may occur with increased pressure on the reflex centre in the medulla.
- Hemiplegia or decorticate or decerebrate posturing may develop as pressure on the brain stem increases. Bilateral flaccidity occurs before death.
- Loss of brain stem reflexes, including pupillary, corneal, gag, and swallowing reflexes, is an ominous sign.

Monitoring ICP
Because clinical assessment is not always a reliable guide in recognizing increased ICP, especially in comatose patients, ICP monitoring is an essential part of management (Hickey, 2003). ICP is monitored closely for continuous elevation or significant increase over baseline. The trend of ICP measurements over time is an important indication of the patient's underlying status. Vital signs are assessed when the increase in ICP is noted.

Strict aseptic technique is used when handling any part of the monitoring system. The insertion site is inspected for signs of infection. Temperature, pulse, and respirations are closely monitored for systemic signs of infection. All connections and stopcocks are checked for leaks, because even small leaks can distort pressure readings.

When ICP is monitored with a fluid system, the transducer is calibrated at a particular reference point, usually 2.5 cm above the ear with the patient in the supine position; this point corresponds to the level of the foramen of Monro (Fig. 61-6). (CSF pressure readings depend on the patient's position.) For subsequent pressure readings, the head should be in the same position relative to the transducer. Fibreoptic catheters are calibrated before insertion and do not require further referencing; they do not require the head of the bed to be at a specific position to obtain an accurate reading.

Whenever technology is associated with patient management, the nurse must be certain that the technology is functioning properly. The most important concern, however, must be the patient who is attached to the technology. The patient and family must be informed about the technology and the goals of its use. The patient's response is monitored and appropriate comfort measures are implemented to ensure that the patient's stress is minimized.

ICP measurement is only one parameter: repeated neurologic checks and clinical examinations remain important measures. As-

FIGURE 61-6 Location of the foramen of Monro for calibration of intracranial pressure monitoring system.

tute observation, comparison of findings with previous observations, and interventions can assist in preventing life-threatening ICP elevations.

Monitoring for Secondary Complications
The nurse also assesses for complications of increased ICP, including diabetes insipidus and SIADH (see Chaps. 14 and 42). Urine output should be monitored closely. Diabetes insipidus requires fluid and electrolyte replacement, along with the administration of vasopressin, to replace and slow the urine output. Serum electrolyte levels should be monitored for imbalances. SIADH requires fluid restriction and monitoring of serum electrolyte levels.

Evaluation
EXPECTED PATIENT OUTCOMES
Expected patient outcomes may include:

1. Maintains patent airway
2. Attains optimal breathing pattern
   a. Breathes in a regular pattern
   b. Attains or maintains arterial blood gas values within acceptable range
3. Demonstrates optimal cerebral tissue perfusion
   a. Increasingly oriented to time, place, and person
   b. Follows verbal commands; answers questions correctly
4. Attains desired fluid balance
   a. Maintains fluid restriction
   b. Demonstrates serum and urine osmolality values within acceptable range
5. Has no signs or symptoms of infection
   a. Has no fever
   b. Shows no signs of infection at arterial, intravenous, and urinary catheter sites
   c. Has no purulent drainage from invasive intracranial monitoring device

6. Absence of complications
   a. Has ICP values that remain within normal limits
   b. Demonstrates urine output and serum electrolyte levels within acceptable limits

Intracranial Surgery

A **craniotomy** involves opening the skull surgically to gain access to intracranial structures. This procedure is performed to remove a tumour, relieve elevated ICP, evacuate a blood clot, and control hemorrhage. The surgeon cuts the skull to create a bony flap, which can be repositioned after surgery and held in place by periosteal or wire sutures. One of two approaches through the skull is used: (1) above the tentorium (supratentorial craniotomy) into the supratentorial compartment, or (2) below the tentorium into the infratentorial (posterior fossa) compartment. A **transsphenoidal** approach through the mouth and nasal sinuses is used to gain access to the pituitary gland. Table 61-3 compares the three different surgical approaches: supratentorial, infratentorial, and transsphenoidal.

Alternatively, intracranial structures may be approached through burr holes (Fig. 61-7), which are circular openings made in the skull by either a hand drill or an automatic craniotome (which has a self-controlled system to stop the drill when the bone is penetrated). Burr holes are made for exploration or diagnosis. They may be used to determine the presence of cerebral swelling and injury and the size and position of the ventricles. They are also a means of evacuating an intracranial hematoma or abscess and for making a bone flap in the skull and allowing access to the ventricles for decompression, ventriculography, or shunting procedures. Other cranial procedures include **craniectomy** (excision of a portion of the skull) and cranioplasty (repair of a cranial defect using a plastic or metal plate).

Preoperative Management

Preoperative diagnostic procedures may include CT scanning to demonstrate the lesion and show the degree of surrounding brain edema, the ventricular size, and the displacement. MRI provides information similar to that of the CT scan and examines the lesion in other planes (Tornqvist, 2001). Cerebral angiography may be used to study the tumour's blood supply or give information about vascular lesions. Transcranial Doppler flow studies are used to evaluate the blood flow of intracranial blood vessels.

Most patients are placed on an antiseizure medication such as phenytoin (Dilantin) or fosphenytoin (Cerebyx) before surgery to reduce the risk of postoperative **seizures** (paroxysmal transient

Table 61-3 • Comparison of Cranial Surgical Approaches

SUPRATENTORIAL	INFRATENTORIAL	TRANSSPHENOIDAL
		Pituitary tumour / Tip of forceps
Site of Surgery		
Above the tentorium	Below the tentorium, brain stem	Sella turcica
Incision Location		
Incision is made above the area to be operated on; is usually located behind the hairline.	Incision is made at the nape of the neck, around the occipital lobe.	Incision is made beneath the upper lip to gain access into the nasal cavity.
Selected Nursing Interventions		
Maintain head of bed elevated 30 to 45 degrees, with neck in neural alignment. Position patient on either side or back. (Avoid positioning patient on operative side if a large tumour has been removed.)	Maintain neck in straight alignment. Avoid flexion of the neck to prevent possible tearing of the suture line. Position the patient on either side. (Check surgeon's preference for positioning of patient.)	Maintain nasal packing in place and reinforce as needed. Instruct patient to avoid blowing the nose. Provide frequent oral care. Keep head of bed elevated to promote venous drainage and drainage from the surgical site.

FIGURE 61-7 Burr holes may be used in neurosurgical procedures to make a bone flap in the skull, to aspirate a brain abscess, or to evacuate a hematoma.

disturbances of the brain resulting from a discharge of abnormal electrical activity) (Hickey, 2003; Karch, 2002). Before surgery, corticosteroids such as dexamethasone (Decadron) may be administered to reduce cerebral edema. Fluids may be restricted. A hyperosmotic agent (mannitol) and a diuretic agent such as furosemide (Lasix) may be given intravenously immediately before and sometimes during surgery if the patient tends to retain fluid, as do many who have intracranial dysfunction. The patient may be given antibiotics if there is a chance of cerebral contamination; diazepam (Valium) may be prescribed before surgery to allay anxiety.

Preoperative Nursing Management

The preoperative assessment serves as a baseline against which postoperative status and recovery are compared. This assessment includes evaluating LOC and responsiveness to stimuli and identifying any neurologic deficits, such as paralysis, visual dysfunction, alterations in personality or speech, and bladder and bowel disorders. Distal and proximal motor strength in both upper and lower extremities is recorded using the 5-point scale. Testing of motor function is discussed in Chapter 60 (see Fig. 60-14).

The patient's and family's understanding of and reactions to the anticipated surgical procedure and its possible sequelae are assessed, as is the availability of support systems for the patient and family. Adequate preparation for surgery, with attention to the patient's physical and emotional status, can reduce the risk for anxiety, fear, and postoperative complications. The patient is assessed for neurologic deficits and their potential impact after surgery. If there are motor deficits or weakness or paralysis of the arms or legs, trochanter rolls are applied to the extremities and the feet are positioned against a footboard. A patient who can ambulate is encouraged to do so. If the patient is aphasic, writing materials or picture and word cards showing the bedpan, glass of

water, blanket, and other frequently used items may help improve communication.

Preparation of the patient and family includes providing information about what to expect during and after surgery. The surgical site is shaved immediately before surgery (usually in the operating room) so that any resultant superficial abrasions do not have time to become infected. An indwelling urinary catheter is inserted in the operating room to drain the bladder during the administration of diuretics and to permit urinary output to be monitored. The patient may have a central and arterial line placed for fluid administration and monitoring of pressures after surgery. The large head dressing applied after surgery may impair hearing temporarily. Vision may be limited if the eyes are swollen shut. If a tracheostomy or endotracheal tube is in place, the patient will be unable to speak until the tube is removed, so an alternative method of communication should be established.

An altered cognitive state may make the patient unaware of the impending surgery. Even so, encouragement and attention to the patient's needs are necessary. Whatever the state of awareness of the patient, the family needs reassurance and support because they recognize the seriousness of brain surgery.

Postoperative Management

Postoperatively, an arterial line and a central venous pressure line may be in place to monitor and manage blood pressure and central venous pressure. The patient may be intubated and may receive supplemental oxygen therapy. Ongoing postoperative management is aimed at detecting and reducing cerebral edema, relieving pain and preventing seizures, and monitoring ICP.

REDUCING CEREBRAL EDEMA
Medications to reduce cerebral edema include mannitol, which increases serum osmolality and draws free water from areas of the brain (with an intact blood–brain barrier). The fluid is then excreted by osmotic diuresis. Dexamethasone (Decadron) may be administered intravenously every 6 hours for 24 to 72 hours; the route is switched to oral as soon as possible and dosage is tapered over 5 to 7 days (Karch, 2002).

RELIEVING PAIN AND PREVENTING SEIZURES
Acetaminophen is usually prescribed for temperature exceeding 37.5°C and for pain. Commonly, the patient has a headache after a craniotomy, usually as a result of the scalp nerves being stretched and irritated during surgery. Codeine, given parenterally, is often sufficient to relieve headache. Morphine sulfate may also be used in the management of postoperative pain in the craniotomy patient (Leith, 1998).

Antiseizure medication (phenytoin, diazepam) is prescribed for patients who have undergone supratentorial craniotomy because of the high risk of seizures after supratentorial neurosurgical procedures. Serum levels are monitored to keep the medications within the therapeutic range.

MONITORING ICP
A ventricular catheter or other type of drain frequently is inserted in patients undergoing intracranial surgery. The catheter is connected to an external drainage system. The patency of the catheter is noted by the pulsations of the fluid in the tubing. The ICP can be assessed using a stopcock attached to the pressure tubing and transducer. The ICP is measured by turning the three-way stopcock to the appropriate position (Hickey, 2003). Care is required to ensure that the system is tight at all connections and that the

stopcock is in the proper position to avoid drainage of CSF; collapse of the ventricles and brain herniation may result if fluid is removed too rapidly (Hickey, 2003). The catheter is removed when the ventricular pressure is normal and stable. The neurosurgeon must be notified if the catheter appears to be obstructed.

NURSING PROCESS: THE PATIENT UNDERGOING INTRACRANIAL SURGERY

Assessment

After surgery, the frequency of postoperative monitoring is based on the patient's clinical status. Assessing respiratory function is essential because even a small degree of hypoxia can increase cerebral ischemia. The respiratory rate and pattern are monitored, and arterial blood gas values are assessed frequently. Fluctuations in vital signs are carefully monitored and documented because they indicate increased ICP. The patient's temperature is measured at intervals to assess for hyperthermia secondary to damage to the hypothalamus. Neurologic checks are made frequently to detect increased ICP resulting from cerebral edema or bleeding. A change in LOC or response to stimuli may be the first sign of increasing ICP.

The surgical dressing is inspected for evidence of bleeding and CSF drainage. The nurse must be alert to the development of complications; all assessments are carried out with these problems in mind. Chart 61-2 provides an overview of the nursing management of the patient after intracranial surgery. Seizures are a potential complication, and any seizure activity is carefully recorded and reported. Restlessness may occur as the patient becomes more responsive or may be due to pain, confusion, hypoxia, or other stimuli.

Diagnosis

NURSING DIAGNOSES

Based on the assessment data, the patient's major nursing diagnoses after intracranial surgery may include the following:

- Ineffective cerebral tissue perfusion related to cerebral edema
- Potential for ineffective thermoregulation related to damage to the hypothalamus, dehydration, and infection
- Potential for impaired gas exchange related to hypoventilation, aspiration, and immobility
- Disturbed sensory perception related to periorbital edema, head dressing, endotracheal tube, and effects of ICP
- Body image disturbance related to change in appearance or physical disabilities

Other nursing diagnoses may include impaired communication (aphasia) related to insult to brain tissue and high risk for impaired skin integrity related to immobility, pressure, and incontinence. There may be impaired physical mobility related to a neurologic deficit secondary to the neurosurgical procedure or to the underlying disorder.

COLLABORATIVE PROBLEMS/ POTENTIAL COMPLICATIONS

Potential complications include:

- Increased ICP
- Bleeding and hypovolemic shock
- Fluid and electrolyte disturbances

- Infection
- Seizures

Planning and Goals

The major goals for the patient include neurologic homeostasis to improve cerebral tissue perfusion, adequate thermoregulation, normal ventilation and gas exchange, ability to cope with sensory deprivation, adaptation to changes in body image, and absence of complications.

Nursing Interventions

MAINTAINING CEREBRAL TISSUE PERFUSION

Attention to the patient's respiratory status is essential because even slight decreases in the oxygen level (hypoxia) can cause cerebral ischemia and can affect the clinical course and outcome. The endotracheal tube is left in place until the patient shows signs of awakening and has adequate spontaneous ventilation, as evaluated clinically and by arterial blood gas analysis. Secondary brain damage can result from impaired cerebral oxygenation.

Some degree of cerebral edema occurs after brain surgery; it tends to peak 24 to 36 hours after surgery, producing decreased responsiveness on the second postoperative day. The control of cerebral edema is discussed in the earlier section of this chapter on management of increased ICP. Nursing strategies used to control factors that may raise ICP are found earlier in this chapter in Nursing Process: The Patient With Increased ICP. Intraventricular drainage is carefully monitored, using strict asepsis when any part of the system is handled.

Vital signs and neurologic status (LOC and responsiveness, pupillary and motor responses) are assessed every 15 minutes to every 1 hour. Extreme head rotation is avoided because this raises ICP. After supratentorial surgery, the patient is placed on his or her back or side (unoperated side if a large lesion was removed) with one pillow under the head. The head of the bed may be elevated 30 degrees, depending on the level of the ICP and the neurosurgeon's preference. After posterior fossa (infratentorial) surgery, the patient is kept flat on one side (off the back) with the head on a small, firm pillow. The patient may be turned on either side, keeping the neck in a neutral position. When the patient is being turned, the body should be turned as a unit to prevent placing strain on the incision and possibly tearing the sutures. The head of the bed may be elevated slowly as tolerated by the patient.

The patient's position is changed every 2 hours, and skin care is given frequently. During position changes, care is taken to prevent disrupting the ICP monitoring system. A turning sheet placed under the head to the midthigh makes it easier to move and turn the patient safely.

REGULATING TEMPERATURE

Moderate temperature elevation can be expected after intracranial surgery because of the reaction to blood at the operative site or in the subarachnoid space. Injury to the hypothalamic centres that regulate body temperature can occur during surgery. High fever is treated vigorously to combat the effect of an elevated temperature on brain metabolism and function.

Nursing interventions include monitoring the patient's temperature and using the following measures to reduce body temperature: removing blankets, applying ice bags to axilla and groin areas, using a hypothermia blanket as prescribed, and administering prescribed medications to reduce fever.

Overview of Nursing Management for the Patient After Intracranial Surgery

Postoperative Interventions

Nursing Diagnosis: Risk for ineffective breathing pattern related to postoperative cerebral edema

Goal: Achievement of adequate respiratory function

1. Establish proper respiratory exchange to eliminate systemic hypercapnia and hypoxia, which increase cerebral edema.
   a. Unless contraindicated, place the patient in a lateral or a semiprone position to facilitate respiratory gas exchange until consciousness returns.
   b. Suction trachea and pharynx *cautiously* to remove secretions; suctioning can raise ICP.
   c. Maintain patient on controlled ventilation if prescribed to maintain normal ventilatory status; monitor arterial blood gas results to determine respiratory status.
   d. Elevate the head of the bed 30.5 cm after patient is conscious to aid venous drainage of the brain.
   e. Administer nothing by mouth until active coughing and swallowing reflexes are demonstrated, to prevent aspiration.

Nursing Diagnosis: Risk for imbalanced fluid volume related to intracranial pressure or diuretics

Goal: Attainment of fluid and electrolyte balance

1. Monitor for polyuria, especially during first postoperative week; diabetes insipidus may develop in patients with lesions around the pituitary or hypothalamus.
   a. Measure urinary specific gravity at intervals.
   b. Monitor serum and urinary electrolyte levels.
2. Evaluate patient's electrolyte status; patients may retain water and sodium.
   a. Early postoperative weight gain indicates fluid retention; a greater-than-estimated weight loss indicates negative water balance.
   b. Loss of sodium and chloride will produce weakness, lethargy, and coma.
   c. Low potassium levels will cause confusion and decreased level of responsiveness.
3. Weigh patient daily; keep intake and output record.
4. Administer prescribed intravenous fluids cautiously—rate and composition depend on fluid deficit, urine output, and blood loss. Fluid intake and fluid losses should remain relatively equal.

Nursing Diagnosis: Disturbed sensory perception (visual/auditory) related to periorbital edema and head dressings

Goal: Compensate for sensory deprivation; prevention of injury

1. Perform supportive measures until the patient can care for self.
   a. Change position as indicated; position changes can increase ICP.
   b. Administer prescribed analgesics (codeine) that do not mask the level of responsiveness.
2. Use measures prescribed to relieve signs of periocular edema.
   a. Lubricate eyelids and around eyes with petrolatum.
   b. Apply light, cold compresses over eyes at specified intervals.
   c. Observe for signs of keratitis if cornea has no sensation.
3. Put extremities through range-of-motion exercises.
4. Evaluate and support patient during episodes of restlessness.
   a. Evaluate for airway obstruction, distended bladder, meningeal irritation from bloody CSF.
   b. Pad patient's hands and bed rails to prevent injury.
5. Reinforce blood-stained dressings with sterile dressing; blood-soaked dressings act as a culture medium for bacteria.
6. Orient patient frequently to time, place, and person.

Monitor and Manage Complications

1. Cerebral edema
   a. Assess patient's level of responsiveness/consciousness; decreased level of consciousness may be the first sign of increased ICP.

(1) Eye opening (spontaneous, to sound, to pain); pupillary reactions to light
(2) Response to commands
(3) Assessment of spinal motor reflexes (pinch Achilles tendon, arm, or other body site)
(4) Observation of patient's spontaneous activity
   b. Maintain a neurologic flow sheet to assess and document neurologic status, fluid administration, laboratory data, medications, and treatments.
   c. Evaluate for signs and symptoms of increasing ICP, which can lead to ischemia and further impairment of brain function.
     (1) Assess patient minute by minute, hour by hour, for:
        • Diminished response to stimuli
        • Fluctuations of vital signs
        • Restlessness
        • Weakness and paralysis of extremities
        • Increasing headache
        • Changes or disturbances of vision; pupillary changes
     (2) Modify nursing management to prevent further increases in ICP.
   d. Control postoperative cerebral edema as prescribed.
     (1) Administer corticosteroids and osmotic diuretics as prescribed to reduce brain swelling.
     (2) Monitor fluid intake; avoid overhydration.
     (3) Maintain a normal temperature. Temperature control may be impaired in certain neurologic states, and fever increases the metabolic demands of the brain.
        • Monitor rectal temperature at specified intervals. Assess temperature of extremities, which may be cold and dry due to impaired heat-losing mechanisms (vasodilation and sweating).
        • Employ measures as prescribed to reduce fever: ice bags to axillae and groin; hypothermia blanket. Use ECG monitoring to detect dysrhythmias during hypothermia procedures.
     (4) Employ hyperventilation when prescribed and indicated (results in respiratory alkalosis, which causes cerebral vasoconstriction and reduces intracranial pressure).
     (5) Elevate head of bed to reduce ICP and facilitate respirations.
     (6) Avoid excessive stimuli.
     (7) Use ICP monitoring if patient is at risk for intracranial hypertension.
2. Intracranial hemorrhage
   a. Postoperative bleeding may be intraventricular, intracerebellar, subdural, or extradural.
   b. Observe for progressive impairment of state of consciousness and other signs of increasing ICP.
   c. Prepare deteriorating patient for return to surgery for evacuation of hematoma.
3. Seizures (greater risk with supratentorial operations)
   a. Administer prescribed antiseizure agents; monitor antiseizure medication blood levels.
   b. Observe for status epilepticus, which may occur after any intracranial surgery.
4. Infections
   a. Urinary tract infections
   b. Pulmonary infections related to aspiration secondary to depressed level of responsiveness; may result in atelectasis and aspiration pneumonia
   c. CNS infections (postoperative meningitis, CSF shunt infection)
   d. Surgical site infections/septicemia

(continued)

Chart 61-2 — Overview of Nursing Management for the Patient After Intracranial Surgery (Continued)

5. Venous thrombosis
    a. Assess for Homans' sign.
    b. Apply elastic compression stockings.
    c. Administer anticoagulant therapy as prescribed.
6. Leakage of CSF
    a. Differentiate between CSF and mucus.
        (1) Collect fluid on Dextrostix; if CSF is present, the indicator will have a positive reaction, as CSF contains glucose.
        (2) Assess for moderate elevation of temperature and mild neck rigidity.
    b. Caution patient against nose blowing or sniffing.
    c. Elevate head of bed as prescribed.
    d. Assist with insertion of lumbar CSF drainage system if inserted to reduce CSF pressure.
        (1) Ventricular catheters may be inserted in the patient undergoing surgery of the posterior fossa (ventriculostomy); the catheter is connected to a closed drainage system.
        (2) Administer antibiotics as prescribed.
7. Gastrointestinal ulceration; monitor for signs and symptoms of hemorrhage, perforation, or both (probably caused by stress response).

Evaluation
Expected patient outcomes
1. Demonstrates normal breathing pattern
    a. Absence of crackles
    b. Demonstrates active swallowing and coughing reflexes
2. Attains/maintains fluid balance
    a. Takes fluids orally
    b. Maintains weight within expected range
3. Compensates for sensory deprivation
    a. Makes needs known
    b. Demonstrates improvement of vision
4. Exhibits absence of complications
    a. No evidence of increased ICP
    b. Opens eyes on request
    c. Obeys commands
    d. Has appropriate motor responses
    e. Shows increasing alertness
    f. No evidence of rhinorrhea, otorrhea, or CSF leakage
    g. Absence of fever
    h. No evidence of inflammation or infection at surgical site
    i. Absence of seizures

Conversely, hypothermia may be seen after lengthy neurosurgical procedures. Therefore, frequent measurements of rectal temperature are necessary. Rewarming should occur slowly to prevent shivering, which increases cellular oxygen demands.

IMPROVING GAS EXCHANGE

The patient undergoing neurosurgery is at risk for impaired gas exchange and pulmonary infections because of immobility, immunosuppression, decreased LOC, and fluid restriction. Immobility compromises the respiratory system by causing pooling and stasis of secretions in dependent areas and the development of atelectasis. The patient whose fluid intake is restricted may be more vulnerable to atelectasis as a result of inability to expectorate thickened secretions. Pneumonia is frequently seen in neurosurgical patients, possibly related to aspiration and restricted mobility.

The nurse assesses the patient for signs of respiratory infection, which include temperature elevation, increased pulse rate, and changes in respirations, and auscultates the lungs for decreased breath sounds and adventitious sounds.

Repositioning the patient every 2 hours will help to mobilize pulmonary secretions and prevent stasis. When the patient regains consciousness, additional measures to expand collapsed alveoli can be instituted, such as yawning, sighing, deep breathing, incentive spirometry, and coughing (unless contraindicated). If necessary, the oropharynx and trachea are suctioned to remove secretions that cannot be raised by coughing; however, coughing and suctioning increase ICP. Therefore, suctioning should be used cautiously. Increasing the humidity in the oxygen delivery system may help to loosen secretions. The nurse and the respiratory therapist work together to monitor the effects of chest physical therapy.

MANAGING SENSORY DEPRIVATION

Periorbital edema is a common consequence of intracranial surgery because fluid drains into the dependent periorbital areas when the patient has been positioned in a prone position during surgery. A hematoma may form under the scalp and spread down to the orbit, producing an area of ecchymosis (black eye).

Before surgery, the patient and family should be informed that one or both eyes may be edematous temporarily after surgery. After surgery, placing the patient in a head-up position (if not contraindicated) and applying cold compresses over the eyes will help reduce the edema. If periorbital edema increases significantly, the surgeon is notified because it may indicate that a postoperative clot is developing or that there is increasing ICP and poor venous drainage. Health care personnel should announce their presence when entering the room to avoid startling the patient whose vision is impaired due to periorbital edema or neurologic deficits.

Additional factors that can affect sensation include a bulky head dressing, the presence of an endotracheal tube, and effects of increased ICP. The first postoperative dressing change is usually performed by the neurosurgeon. In the absence of bleeding or a CSF leak, every effort is made to minimize the size of the head dressing. If the patient requires an endotracheal tube for mechanical ventilation, every effort is made to extubate the patient as soon as clinical signs indicate it is possible. The patient is monitored closely for the effects of elevated ICP.

ENHANCING SELF-IMAGE

The patient is encouraged to verbalize feelings and frustrations about any change in appearance. Nursing support is based on the patient's reactions and feelings. Factual information may need to be provided if the patient has misconceptions about puffiness about the face, periorbital bruising, and hair loss. Attention to grooming, the use of the patient's own clothing, and covering the head with a turban (and ultimately a wig until hair growth occurs) are encouraged. Social interaction with close friends, family, and hospital personnel may increase the patient's sense of self-worth.

As the patient assumes more responsibility for self-care and participates in more activities, a sense of control and personal competence will develop. The family and social support system can be of assistance while the patient recovers from surgery.

MONITORING AND MANAGING POTENTIAL COMPLICATIONS

Complications that may develop within hours after surgery include increased ICP, bleeding and hypovolemic shock, altered fluid and electrolyte balance (including water intoxication), infection, and seizures. These complications require close collaboration between the nurse and the surgeon.

Monitoring for Increased ICP and Bleeding

Increased ICP and bleeding are life-threatening to the patient who has undergone intracranial neurosurgery. The following must be kept in mind when caring for all patients who undergo such surgery:

- An increase in blood pressure and decrease in pulse with respiratory failure may indicate increased ICP.
- An accumulation of blood under the bone flap (extradural, subdural, intracerebral) may pose a threat to life. A clot must be suspected in any patient who does not awaken as expected or whose condition deteriorates. An intracranial hematoma is suspected if the patient has any new postoperative neurologic deficits (especially a dilated pupil on the operative side). In these events, the patient is returned to the operating room immediately for evacuation of the clot if indicated.
- Cerebral edema, infarction, metabolic disturbances, and hydrocephalus are conditions that may mimic the clinical manifestations of a clot.

The patient is monitored closely for indicators of complications, and early signs and trends in clinical status are reported to the surgeon. Treatments are initiated promptly, and the nurse assists in evaluating the response to treatment. The nurse also provides support to the patient and family.

Should signs and symptoms of increased ICP occur, efforts to decrease the ICP are initiated: alignment of the head in a neutral position without flexion to promote venous drainage, elevation of the head of the bed to 30 degrees, administration of mannitol (an osmotic diuretic), and possible administration of pharmacologic paralyzing agents.

Managing Fluid and Electrolyte Disturbances

Fluid and electrolyte imbalances may occur because of the patient's underlying condition and its management or as complications of surgery. Fluid and electrolyte disturbances can contribute to the development of cerebral edema.

The postoperative fluid regimen depends on the type of neurosurgical procedure and is determined on an individual basis. The volume and composition of fluids are adjusted according to daily serum electrolyte values, along with fluid intake and output.

Sodium retention may occur in the immediate postoperative period. Serum and urine electrolytes, blood urea nitrogen, blood glucose, weight, and clinical status are monitored. Intake and output are measured in view of losses associated with fever, respiration, and CSF drainage. Fluids may have to be restricted in patients with cerebral edema.

Oral fluids are usually resumed after the first 24 hours (Hickey, 2003). The presence of gag and swallowing reflexes must be checked before initiation of oral fluids. Some patients with posterior fossa tumours may have impaired swallowing, so fluids may need to be administered by alternative routes. The patient should be observed for signs and symptoms of nausea and vomiting as the diet is progressed (Hickey, 2003).

Patients undergoing surgery for brain tumours often receive large doses of corticosteroids and thus tend to develop hyperglycemia. Therefore, serum glucose levels are measured every 4 hours. These patients are prone to gastric ulcers, and therefore histamine-2 receptor antagonists (H_2 blockers) are prescribed to suppress the secretion of gastric acid. The patient is monitored for bleeding and assessed for gastric pain.

If the surgical site is near, or causes edema to, the pituitary gland and hypothalamus, the patient may develop symptoms of diabetes insipidus, which is characterized by excessive urinary output. The urine specific gravity is measured hourly, and fluid intake and output are monitored. Fluid replacement must compensate for urine output, and serum potassium levels must be monitored.

SIADH, which results in water retention with hyponatremia and serum hypo-osmolality, occurs in a wide variety of central nervous system disorders (brain tumour, head trauma) causing fluid disturbances. Nursing management includes careful intake and output measurements, specific gravity determinations of urine, and monitoring of serum and urine electrolyte studies, while following directives for fluid restriction. SIADH is usually self-limiting.

Preventing Infection

The patient undergoing neurosurgery is at risk for infection related to the neurosurgical procedure (brain exposure, bone exposure, wound hematomas) and the presence of intravenous and arterial lines for fluid administration and monitoring. Risk for infection is increased in patients who undergo lengthy intracranial operations and those with external ventricular drains in place longer than 48 to 72 hours.

The incision site is monitored for redness, tenderness, bulging, separation, or foul odour. The dressing is often stained with blood in the immediate postoperative period. It is important to reinforce the dressing with sterile pads so that contamination and infection are avoided. (Blood is an excellent culture medium for bacteria.) If the dressing is heavily stained or displaced, this should be reported immediately. (A drain is sometimes placed in the craniotomy incision to facilitate drainage.)

After suboccipital surgical procedures, CSF may leak through the incision. This complication is dangerous because of the possibility of meningitis. Any sudden discharge of fluid from a cranial incision is reported at once because a massive leak requires direct surgical repair. Attention should be paid to the patient who complains of a salty taste, because this can be due to CSF trickling down the throat. The patient is advised to avoid coughing, sneezing, or nose blowing, which may cause CSF leakage by creating pressure on the operative site.

Aseptic technique is used when handling dressings, drainage systems, and intravenous and arterial lines. The patient is monitored carefully for signs and symptoms of infection, and cultures are obtained from the patient with suspected infection. Appropriate antibiotics are administered as prescribed.

Other causes of infection in the patient undergoing intracranial surgery are similar to those in other postoperative patients: pneumonia and urinary tract infections.

Monitoring for Seizure Activity

Seizures and epilepsy may be complications after any intracranial neurosurgical procedure. Preventing seizures is essential to avoid further cerebral edema. Administering the prescribed antiseizure medication before and immediately after surgery may prevent the development of seizures in subsequent months and years. **Status**

epilepticus (prolonged seizures without recovery of consciousness in the intervals between seizures) may occur after craniotomy and also may be related to the development of complications (hematoma, ischemia). The management of status epilepticus is described later in this chapter.

Monitoring and Managing Later Complications
Other complications may occur during the first 2 weeks or later and may threaten the patient's recovery. The most important of these are thromboembolic complications (deep vein thrombosis, pulmonary embolism), pulmonary and urinary tract infection, and pressure ulcers (Warbel, Lewicki & Lupica, 1999). Most of these complications may be avoided with frequent changes of position, adequate suctioning of secretions, assessment for pulmonary complications, observation for urinary complications, and skin care.

PROMOTING HOME AND COMMUNITY-BASED CARE
Teaching Patients Self-Care
The recovery at home of a neurosurgical patient depends on the extent of the surgical procedure and its success. The patient's strengths as well as limitations are explained to the family, along with their part in promoting recovery. Because administration of antiseizure medication is a priority, the patient and family are encouraged to use a check-off system to ensure that the medication is taken as prescribed.

Usually no dietary restrictions are required unless another health problem requiring a special diet exists. Although taking a shower or tub bath is permitted, the scalp should be kept dry until all the sutures have been removed. A clean scarf or cap may be worn until a wig or hairpiece is purchased. If skull bone has been removed, the neurosurgeon may suggest a protective helmet. After a craniotomy, the patient may require rehabilitation, depending on the postoperative level of function. The patient may require physical therapy for residual weakness and mobility issues. Occupational therapy is consulted to assist with self-care issues. If the patient is aphasic, speech therapy may be necessary.

Continuing Care
Barring complications, patients are discharged from the hospital as soon as possible. Patients with severe motor deficits require extensive physical therapy and rehabilitation. Those with postoperative cognitive and speech impairments require psychological evaluation, speech therapy, and rehabilitation. The nurse works collaboratively with the physician and other health care professionals during hospitalization and home care to achieve as complete a rehabilitation as possible.

When tumour, injury, or disease makes the prognosis poor, care is directed toward making the patient as comfortable as possible. With return of the tumour or cerebral compression, the patient becomes less alert and aware. Other possible consequences include paralysis, blindness, and seizures. The home care nurse, hospice nurse, and social worker work with the family to plan for additional home health care or hospice services or placement of the patient in an extended-care facility. (See also the section on cerebral metastases in Chap. 65.) The patient and family are encouraged to discuss end-of-life preferences for care; the patient's end-of-life preferences must be respected (see Chap. 17).

The nurse involved in home and continuing care of patients following cranial surgery needs to remind patients and family

NURSING RESEARCH PROFILE 61-1
Suitability of Printed Patient Education Materials

Murphy, P. W., Chesson, A., Berman, S. A., Arnold, C., & Gallowat, G. (2001). Neurology patient education materials: do our educational aids fit our patients' needs? *Journal of Neuroscience Nursing, 33*(2), 99–112.

Purpose
Nurses often rely on printed patient education materials to supplement patient teaching. The purpose of the study was to assess the suitability of neurology patient education brochures and related information available on the Internet to determine their appropriateness for patients with low literacy skills.

Study Sample and Design
In this descriptive, cross-sectional study, the reading levels of patients and patient education materials were assessed. The Rapid Estimate of Adult Literacy in Medicine tool was used to evaluate a convenience sample of 520 neurology patients. Forty-three patient education materials—35 brochures produced by national organizations and 8 electronic documents from various Internet sources—were assessed using the Fog Index and the Suitability Assessment of Materials Scale. The mean age of patients was 46 years; 40% were African American and 59% Caucasian; 44% were female; the average educational level was 12th grade, with a mean reading level of 7th to 8th grade.

Findings
Patient education materials were classified as not suitable, adequate, or superior for use. Organizations with materials at the suitable level include those of the Epilepsy Foundation of America, the National Multiple Sclerosis Society, and the American Heart Association. The National Stroke Association, the American Academy of Neurology, the American Sleep Medicine, and the Muscular Dystrophy Association had brochures in the adequate range. Overall, only 14% of the materials were considered to have superior suitability, whereas 58% were adequate; 28% were determined not suitable. Of the materials available from the Internet, 88% were not suitable. The authors concluded that readily available neurology patient education aids are not matched to the patient population or to the average reading levels of patients.

Nursing Implications
Nurses should keep in mind that the brochures evaluated in this study represent primarily those available at national meetings and a small sample of those available on the Internet. The study reinforces that there is a need to consider the reading level of the patient when distributing printed material. The last grade attended in school may not reflect reading ability. Nurses should consider modifying existing materials or developing new materials with attention to instructional graphics, simpler words, patient interaction, and cultural sensitivity.

members of the need for health promotion and recommended health screening.

Evaluation
EXPECTED PATIENT OUTCOMES
Expected patient outcomes may include:

1. Achieves optimal cerebral tissue perfusion
   a. Opens eyes on request; uses recognizable words, progressing to normal speech
   b. Obeys commands with appropriate motor responses

2. Attains thermoregulation and normal body temperature
   a. Registers normal body temperature
3. Has normal gas exchange
   a. Has arterial blood gas values within normal ranges
   b. Breathes easily; lung sounds clear without adventitious sounds
   c. Takes deep breaths and changes position as directed
4. Copes with sensory deprivation
5. Demonstrates improving self-concept
   a. Pays attention to grooming
   b. Visits and interacts with others
6. Absence of complications
   a. Exhibits ICP within normal range
   b. Has minimal bleeding at surgical site; surgical incision is healing without evidence of infection
   c. Shows fluid balance and electrolyte levels within desired ranges
   d. Exhibits no evidence of seizures

An overview of care of the patient undergoing intracranial surgery is presented in Chart 61-2.

TRANSSPHENOIDAL SURGERY

Tumours within the sella turcica and small adenomas of the pituitary can be removed through a transsphenoidal approach: an incision is made beneath the upper lip and entry is then gained successively into the nasal cavity, sphenoidal sinus, and sella turcica (see Table 61-3). Although an otorhinolaryngologist may make the initial opening, the neurosurgeon completes the opening into the sphenoidal sinus and exposes the floor of the sella. Microsurgical techniques provide improved illumination, magnification, and visualization so that nearby vital structures can be avoided.

The transsphenoidal approach offers direct access to the sella with minimal risk of trauma and hemorrhage (Greenberg, 2001). It avoids many of the risks of craniotomy, and the postoperative discomfort is similar to that of other transnasal surgical procedures. It may also be used for pituitary ablation (removal) in patients with disseminated breast or prostatic cancer.

Complications

Manipulation of the posterior pituitary gland during surgery may produce transient diabetes insipidus of several days' duration (Greenberg, 2001). It is treated with vasopressin but occasionally persists. Other complications include CSF leakage, visual disturbances, postoperative meningitis, and SIADH.

Preoperative Evaluation

The preoperative workup includes a series of endocrine tests, rhinologic evaluation (to assess the status of the sinuses and nasal cavity), and neuroradiologic studies. Funduscopic examination and visual field determinations are performed, because the most serious effect of pituitary tumour is localized pressure on the optic nerve or chiasm. In addition, the nasopharyngeal secretions are cultured because a sinus infection is a contraindication to an intracranial procedure through this approach. Corticosteroids may be administered before and after surgery (because the surgery involves removal of the pituitary, the source of adrenocorticotropic hormone [ACTH] is removed). Antibiotics may or may not be administered prophylactically (Greenberg, 2001).

Deep breathing is taught before surgery. The patient is instructed that following the surgery he or she will need to avoid vigorous coughing, blowing the nose, sucking through a straw, or sneezing, because these actions may cause a CSF leak (Greenberg, 2001; Hickey, 2003).

Postoperative Management

Because the procedure disrupts the oral and nasal mucous membranes, management focuses on preventing infection and promoting healing. Medications include antimicrobial agents (which are continued until the nasal packing inserted at the time of surgery is removed), corticosteroids, analgesic agents for discomfort, and agents for the control of diabetes insipidus when necessary (Greenberg, 2001).

Nursing Management

Vital signs are measured to monitor hemodynamic, cardiac, and ventilatory status (Eisenberg & Redick, 1998). Because of the anatomic proximity of the pituitary gland to the optic chiasm, visual acuity is assessed at regular intervals. One method is to ask the patient to count the number of fingers held up by the nurse. Evidence of decreasing visual acuity suggests an expanding hematoma.

The head of the bed is raised to decrease pressure on the sella turcica and to promote normal drainage. The patient is cautioned against blowing the nose or engaging in any activity that raises ICP, such as bending over or straining during urination or defecation.

Intake and output are measured as a guide to fluid and electrolyte replacement. The urine specific gravity is measured after each voiding (Greenberg, 2001). Daily weight is monitored. Fluids are generally given when nausea ceases, and the patient then progresses to a regular diet.

The nasal packing inserted during surgery is checked frequently for blood or CSF drainage. The major discomfort is related to the nasal packing and to mouth dryness and thirst from mouth-breathing. Oral care is provided every 4 hours or more frequently. Usually, the teeth are not brushed until the incision above the teeth has healed. The use of warm saline mouth rinses and a cool mist vaporizer is helpful. Petrolatum is soothing when applied to the lips. A room humidifier assists in keeping the mucous membranes moist. The packing is removed in 3 to 4 days, and only then can the area around the nares be cleaned with the prescribed solution to remove crusted blood and moisten the mucous membranes (Hickey, 2003).

Home care considerations include advising the patient to use a room humidifier to keep the mucous membranes moist and to soothe irritation. The head of the bed is elevated for at least 2 weeks after surgery.

Seizure Disorders

SEIZURES

Seizures are episodes of abnormal motor, sensory, autonomic, or psychic activity (or a combination of these) resulting from sudden excessive discharge from cerebral neurons (Greenberg, 2001; Hickey, 2003). A part or all of the brain may be involved. The international classification of seizures differentiates between two main types: partial seizures that begin in one part of the brain, and generalized seizures that involve electrical discharges in the whole brain (Chart 61-3). Most seizures are sudden and transient.

Chart 61-3 International Classification of Seizures

Partial Seizures (seizures beginning locally)

Simple partial seizures (with elementary symptoms, generally without impairment of consciousness)
- With motor symptoms
- With special sensory or somatosensory symptoms
- With autonomic symptoms
- Compound forms

Complex partial seizures (with complex symptoms, generally with impairment of consciousness)
- With impairment of consciousness only
- With cognitive symptoms
- With affective symptoms
- With psychosensory symptoms
- With psychomotor symptoms (automatisms)
- Compound forms

Partial seizures secondarily generalized

Generalized Seizures (convulsive or nonconvulsive, bilaterally symmetric, without local onset)

Tonic-clonic seizures
Tonic seizures
Clonic seizures
Absence seizures
Atonic seizures
Myoclonic seizures (bilaterally massive epileptic)

The underlying cause is an electrical disturbance (dysrhythmia) in the nerve cells in one section of the brain, causing them to emit abnormal, recurring, uncontrolled electrical discharges. The characteristic seizure is a manifestation of this excessive neuronal discharge. There may be associated loss of consciousness, excess movement or loss of muscle tone or movement, and disturbances of behaviour, mood, sensation, and perception.

The specific causes of seizures are varied and can be categorized as idiopathic (genetic, developmental defects) and acquired. Among the causes of acquired seizures are hypoxemia of any cause, including vascular insufficiency, fever (childhood), head injury, hypertension, central nervous system infections, metabolic and toxic conditions (eg, renal failure, hyponatremia, hypocalcemia, hypoglycemia, pesticides), brain tumour, drug and alcohol withdrawal, and allergies (Schumacher, Pruitt & Phillips, 2000). Cerebrovascular disease is the leading cause of seizures in the elderly (Berges, Moulin, Berger et al., 2000).

Nursing Management During a Seizure

A major responsibility of the nurse is to observe and record the sequence of symptoms. The nature of the seizure usually indicates the type of treatment that is required (Wulf, 2000). Before and during a seizure, the following are assessed and documented:

- The circumstances before the seizure (visual, auditory, or olfactory stimuli, tactile stimuli, emotional or psychological disturbances, sleep, hyperventilation)
- The occurrence of an aura (visual, auditory, or olfactory)
- The first thing the patient does in a seizure—where the movements or the stiffness starts, conjugate gaze position, and the position of the head at the beginning of the seizure. This information gives clues to the location of the seizure origin in the brain. (In recording, it is important to state whether the beginning of the seizure was observed.)

- The type of movements in the part of the body involved
- The areas of the body involved (turn back bedding to expose patient)
- The size of both pupils. Are the eyes open? Did the eyes or head turn to one side?
- The presence or absence of automatisms (involuntary motor activity, such as lip smacking or repeated swallowing)
- Incontinence of urine or stool
- Duration of each phase of the seizure
- Unconsciousness, if present, and its duration
- Any obvious paralysis or weakness of arms or legs after the seizure
- Inability to speak after the seizure
- Movements at the end of the seizure
- Whether or not the patient sleeps afterward
- Cognitive status (confused or not confused) after the seizure

In addition to providing data about the seizure, nursing care is directed at preventing injury and supporting the patient. This includes supporting the patient not only physically but also psychologically. Consequences such as distress, embarrassment, fatigue, and depression can be devastating to the patient (Buelow, 2001). Steps to prevent or minimize injury to the patient are presented in Chart 61-4.

Nursing Management After a Seizure

After a patient has a seizure, the nurse's role is to document the events leading to and occurring during the seizure and to prevent complications (eg, aspiration, injury). The patient is at risk for hypoxia, vomiting, and pulmonary aspiration. To prevent complications, the patient is placed in the side-lying position to facilitate drainage of oral secretions and is suctioned, if needed, to maintain a patent airway and prevent aspiration, as described in Chart 61-4. Seizure precautions are maintained, including having available fully functioning suction equipment with a suction catheter and oral airway. The bed is placed in a low position with side rails up and padded if necessary to prevent patient injury. The patient may be drowsy and may wish to sleep after the seizure; he or she may not remember events leading up to the seizure and for a short time thereafter.

THE EPILEPSIES

Epilepsy is a group of syndromes characterized by recurring seizures. Epileptic syndromes are classified by specific patterns of clinical features, including age of onset, family history, and seizure type (Schachter, 2001). Types of epilepsies are differentiated by how the seizure activity manifests (see Chart 61-3), the most common syndromes being those with generalized seizures and those with partial-onset seizures. Epilepsy can be primary (idiopathic) or secondary, when the cause is known and the epilepsy is a symptom of another underlying condition such as a brain tumour (Schachter, 2001).

An estimated 0.6% of the Canadian population has epilepsy, and onset occurs before the age of 18 years in greater than 75% of patients (Epilepsy Canada, 2005). The improved treatment of cerebrovascular disorders, head injuries, brain tumours, meningitis, and encephalitis has increased the number of patients at risk for seizures following recovery from these conditions (Berges et al., 2000). Also, advances in EEG have aided in the diagnosis of

Guidelines for Seizure Care

Chart 61-4

Nursing Care During a Seizure

- Provide privacy and protect the patient from curious on-lookers. (The patient who has an *aura* [warning of an impending seizure] may have time to seek a safe, private place.)
- Ease the patient to the floor, if possible.
- Protect the head with a pad to prevent injury (from striking a hard surface).
- Loosen constrictive clothing.
- Push aside any furniture that may injure the patient during the seizure.
- If the patient is in bed, remove pillows and raise side rails.
- If an aura precedes the seizure, insert an oral airway to reduce the possibility of the tongue or cheek being bitten.
- *Do not attempt to pry open jaws that are clenched in a spasm to insert anything.* Broken teeth and injury to the lips and tongue may result from such an action.
- No attempt should be made to restrain the patient during the seizure because muscular contractions are strong and restraint can produce injury.

- If possible, place the patient on one side with head flexed forward, which allows the tongue to fall forward and facilitates drainage of saliva and mucus. If suction is available, use it if necessary to clear secretions.

Nursing Care After the Seizure

- Keep the patient on one side to prevent aspiration. Make sure the airway is patent.
- There is usually a period of confusion after a grand mal seizure.
- A short apneic period may occur during or immediately after a generalized seizure.
- The patient, on awakening, should be reoriented to the environment.
- If the patient becomes agitated after a seizure (postictal), use calm persuasion and gentle restraint.

epilepsy. The general public has been educated about epilepsy, which has reduced the stigma associated with it; as a result, more people are willing to acknowledge the diagnosis.

Although there is evidence that susceptibility to some types of epilepsy may be inherited, the cause of seizures in many people is unknown. Epilepsy can follow birth trauma, asphyxia neonato-

rum, head injuries, some infectious diseases (bacterial, viral, parasitic), toxicity (carbon monoxide and lead poisoning), circulatory problems, fever, metabolic and nutritional disorders, and drug or alcohol intoxication (Schachter, 2001). It is also associated with brain tumours, abscesses, and congenital malformations. In most cases of epilepsy, the cause is unknown (idiopathic).

Pathophysiology

Messages from the body are carried by the neurons (nerve cells) of the brain by means of discharges of electrochemical energy that sweep along them. These impulses occur in bursts whenever a nerve cell has a task to perform. Sometimes, these cells or groups of cells continue firing after a task is finished. During the period of unwanted discharges, parts of the body controlled by the errant cells may perform erratically. Resultant dysfunction ranges from mild to incapacitating and often causes unconsciousness (Greenberg, 2001; Hickey, 2003). When these uncontrolled, abnormal discharges occur repeatedly, a person is said to have an epileptic syndrome (Schachter, 2001).

Epilepsy is not associated with intellectual level. People with epilepsy without other brain or nervous system disabilities fall within the same intelligence ranges as the overall population. Epilepsy is not synonymous with mental retardation or illness. Many who are developmentally disabled because of serious neurologic damage, however, have epilepsy as well.

Clinical Manifestations

Depending on the location of the discharging neurons, seizures may range from a simple staring episode to prolonged convulsive movements with loss of consciousness. Seizures have been classified according to the area of the brain involved and have been identified as partial, generalized, and unclassified (Greenberg, 2001; Hickey, 2003). Partial seizures are focal in origin and affect only part of the brain. Generalized seizures are nonspecific in origin and affect the entire brain simultaneously. Unclassified seizures are so termed because of incomplete data.

The initial pattern of the seizures indicates the region of the brain in which the seizure originates (see Chart 61-2). In simple partial seizures, only a finger or hand may shake, or the mouth may jerk uncontrollably. The person may talk unintelligibly, may be dizzy, and may experience unusual or unpleasant sights, sounds, odours, or tastes, but without loss of consciousness (Greenberg, 2001; Hickey, 2003).

In complex partial seizures, the person either remains motionless or moves automatically but inappropriately for time and place, or may experience excessive emotions of fear, anger, elation, or irritability. Whatever the manifestations, the person does not remember the episode when it is over.

Generalized seizures, previously referred to as grand mal seizures, involve both hemispheres of the brain, causing both sides of the body to react (Greenberg, 2001; Hickey, 2003). There may be intense rigidity of the entire body followed by alternating muscle relaxation and contraction (generalized tonic–clonic contraction). The simultaneous contractions of the diaphragm and chest muscles may produce a characteristic epileptic cry. The tongue is often chewed, and the patient is incontinent of urine and stool. After 1 or 2 minutes, the convulsive movements begin to subside; the patient relaxes and lies in deep coma, breathing noisily. The respirations at this point are chiefly abdominal. In the postictal state (after the seizure), the patient is often confused and hard to arouse and may sleep for hours. Many patients complain of headache, sore muscles, fatigue, and depression (Buelow, 2001).

Assessment and Diagnostic Findings

The diagnostic assessment is aimed at determining the type of seizures, their frequency and severity, and the factors that precipitate them (Schachter, 2001). A developmental history is taken, including events of pregnancy and childbirth, to seek evidence of preexisting injury. The patient is also questioned about illnesses or head injuries that may have affected the brain. In addition to physical and neurologic evaluations, diagnostic examinations include biochemical, hematologic, and serologic studies. MRI is used to detect lesions in the brain, focal abnormalities, cerebrovascular abnormalities, and cerebral degenerative changes (Schachter, 2001).

The electroencephalogram (EEG) furnishes diagnostic evidence in a substantial proportion of patients with epilepsy and aids in classifying the type of seizure (Schachter, 2001). Abnormalities in the EEG usually continue between seizures or, if not apparent, may be elicited by hyperventilation or during sleep. Microelectrodes can be inserted deep in the brain to probe the action of single brain cells. Some people with seizures have normal EEGs, whereas others who have never had seizures have abnormal EEGs. Telemetry and computerized equipment are used to monitor electrical brain activity while patients pursue their normal activities and to store the readings on computer tapes for analysis. Video recording of seizures taken simultaneously with EEG telemetry is useful in determining the type of seizure as well as its duration and magnitude. This type of intensive monitoring is changing the treatment of severe epilepsy.

Single photon emission computed tomography (SPECT) is an additional tool sometimes used in the diagnostic workup. It is useful for identifying the epileptogenic zone so that the area in the brain giving rise to seizures can be removed surgically (Huntington, 1999).

Women With Epilepsy

Women who have epilepsy face particular needs associated with the syndrome (Schachter, Krishnamurthy & Cantrell, 2000). Women with epilepsy often note an increase in seizure frequency during menses; this has been linked to the increase in sex hormones that alter the excitability of neurons in the cerebral cortex. Women of childbearing age require special care and guidance before, during, and after pregnancy. Many women note a change in the pattern of seizure activity during pregnancy. Fetal malformation has been linked to the use of multiple antiseizure medications (Karch, 2002). The effectiveness of contraceptives is decreased by antiseizure medications. Therefore, patients should be encouraged to discuss family planning with their primary health care provider and to obtain preconception counselling if they are considering childbearing (Liporace, 1997).

Because of bone loss associated with the long-term use of antiseizure medications, patients receiving antiseizure agents should be assessed for low bone mass and osteoporosis. They should be instructed about other strategies to reduce their risks for osteoporosis.

Gerontologic Considerations

Elderly people have a high incidence of new-onset epilepsy (Schachter, 2001). Increased incidence is associated with stroke, head injury, dementia, infection, alcoholism, and aging. Treatment depends on the underlying cause. Because many elderly people have chronic health problems, they may be taking other medications that can interact with medications prescribed for seizure control. In addition, the absorption, distribution, metabolism, and excretion of medications are altered in the elderly as a result of age-related changes in renal and liver function. Therefore, the elderly must be monitored closely for adverse and toxic effects of antiseizure medications and for osteoporosis. The cost of antiseizure medications can lead to poor adherence to the prescribed regimen in elderly patients on fixed incomes.

Prevention

Society-wide efforts are the key to the prevention of epilepsy. The risk for congenital fetal anomaly is two to three times higher in mothers with epilepsy. The effects of maternal seizures, antiseizure medications, and genetic predisposition are all mechanisms that contribute to possible malformation. Because the unborn infants of mothers who take certain antiseizure medications for epilepsy are at risk, these women need careful monitoring, including blood studies to detect the level of antiseizure medications taken throughout pregnancy (Karch, 2002). High-risk mothers (teenagers, women with histories of difficult deliveries, drug use, patients with diabetes or hypertension) should be identified and monitored closely during pregnancy because damage to the fetus during pregnancy and delivery may increase the risk for epilepsy. All of these issues need further study (Schachter, Krishnamurthy & Cantrell, 2000).

Head injury is one of the main causes of epilepsy that can be prevented. Through highway safety programs and occupational safety precautions, lives can be saved and epilepsy due to head injury prevented; these programs are discussed in Chapter 63.

Medical Management

The management of epilepsy is individualized to meet the needs of each patient and not just to manage and prevent seizures. Management differs from patient to patient because some forms of epilepsy arise from brain damage and others are due to altered brain chemistry.

PHARMACOLOGIC THERAPY

Many medications are available to control seizures, although the mechanisms of their actions are still unknown (Karch, 2002). The objective is to achieve seizure control with minimal side effects. Medication therapy controls rather than cures seizures. Medications are selected on the basis of the type of seizure being treated and the effectiveness and safety of the medications (Shafer, 1999a, 1999b; Winkelman, 1999). If properly prescribed and taken, medications control seizures in 50% to 60% of patients with recurring seizures and provide partial control in another 15% to 35%. The condition is not improved by any available medication in 20% and 35% of patients with generalized and partial epilepsy, respectively (Devinsky, 1999).

Treatment is usually started with a single medication. The starting dose and the rate at which the dosage is increased depend on the occurrence of side effects. The medication levels in the blood are monitored because the rate of drug absorption varies among patients. Changing to another medication may be necessary if seizure control is not achieved or if toxicity makes it impossible to increase the dosage. The medication may need to be adjusted because of concurrent illness, weight changes, or increases in stress. Sudden withdrawal of these medications can cause seizures to occur with greater frequency or can precipitate the development of status epilepticus (Greenberg, 2001).

Side effects of antiseizure agents may be divided into three groups: (1) idiosyncratic or allergic disorders, which present primarily as skin reactions; (2) acute toxicity, which may occur when the medication is initially prescribed; or (3) chronic toxicity, which occurs late in the course of therapy.

The manifestations of drug toxicity are variable, and any organ system may be involved. Gingival hyperplasia (swollen and tender gums) can be associated with long-term use of phenytoin (Dilantin), for example (Karch, 2002). Periodic physical and dental examinations and laboratory tests are performed for patients receiving medications known to have hematopoietic, genitourinary, or hepatic effects. Table 61-4 lists the medications in current use.

> **! NURSING ALERT** Nurses must take care when administering lamotrigine (Lamictal), an antiseizure medication. The drug packaging was recently changed in an attempt to reduce medication errors as this medication has been confused with terbinafine (Lamisil), labetalol hydrochloride (Trandate), lamivudine (Epivir), maprotiline (Ludiomil), as well as the combination diphenoxylate and atropine (Lomotil). Any patient given an incorrect medication may suffer adverse effects, and patients with epilepsy are at risk for status epilepticus from having their medication regimen interrupted (Vernarec, 2001).

SURGICAL MANAGEMENT

Surgery is indicated for patients whose epilepsy results from intracranial tumours, abscess, cysts, or vascular anomalies. Some patients have intractable seizure disorders that do not respond to medication. There may be a focal atrophic process secondary to trauma, inflammation, stroke, or anoxia. If the seizures originate in a reasonably well-circumscribed area of the brain that can be excised without producing significant neurologic deficits, the removal of the area generating the seizures may produce long-term control and improvement (Wiebe, Blume, Girvin et al., 2001).

This type of neurosurgery has been aided by several advances, including microsurgical techniques, depth EEGs, improved illumination and hemostasis, and the introduction of neuroleptanalgesic agents (droperidol and fentanyl). These techniques, combined with use of local anesthetic agents, enable the neurosurgeon to perform surgery on an alert and cooperative patient. Using special testing devices, electrocortical mapping, and the patient's response to stimulation, the boundaries of the epileptogenic focus are determined (Huntington, 1999). Any abnormal epileptogenic focus (ie, abnormal area of the brain) is then removed (Wiebe et al., 2001).

As an adjunct to medication and surgery in adolescents and adults with partial seizures, a generator may be implanted under the clavicle. The device is connected to the vagus nerve in the cervical area, where it delivers electrical signals to the brain to control and reduce seizure activity (Kennedy & Schallert, 2001). An external programming system is used by the physician to change stimulator settings. Patients can turn the stimulator on and off with a magnet.

NURSING PROCESS: THE PATIENT WITH EPILEPSY

Assessment

The nurse elicits information about the seizure history. The patient is asked about the factors or events that may precipitate the seizures. Alcohol intake is documented. The nurse determines if the patient has an aura (a premonitory or warning sensation) before an epileptic seizure, which may indicate the origin of the seizure (eg, seeing a flashing light may indicate the seizure originated in the occipital lobe). Observation and assessment during

Table 61-4 • **Major Antiseizure Medication**

MEDICATION	DOSE-RELATED SIDE EFFECTS	TOXIC EFFECTS
carbamazepine (Tegretol)	Dizziness, drowsiness, unsteadiness, nausea and vomiting, diplopia, mild leukopenia	Severe skin rash, blood dyscrasias, hepatitis
clonazepam (Rivotril)	Drowsiness, behaviour changes, headache, hirsutism, alopecia, palpitations	Hepatotoxicity, thrombocytopenia, bone marrow failure, ataxia
ethosuximide (Zarontin)	Nausea and vomiting, headache, gastric distress	Skin rash, blood dyscrasias, hepatitis, lupus erythematosus
gabapentin (Neurotonin)	Dizziness, drowsiness, somnolence, fatigue, ataxia, weight gain, nausea	Leukopenia, hepatotoxicity
lamotrigine (Lamictal)	Drowsiness, tremor, nausea, ataxia, dizziness, headache, weight gain	Severe rash (Stevens-Johnson syndrome)
levetiracetam (Keppra)	Somnolence, dizziness, fatigue	Unknown
oxacarbazepine (Trileptal)	Dizziness, somnolence, double vision, fatigue, nausea, vomiting, loss of coordination, abnormal vision, abdominal pain, tremor, abnormal gait	Hepatotoxicity
phenobarbital (Luminal)	Sedation, irritability, diplopia, ataxia	Skin rash, anemia
phenytoin (Dilantin)	Visual problems, hirsutism, gingival hyperplasia, dysrhythmias, dysarthria, nystagmus	Severe skin reaction, peripheral neuropathy, ataxia, drowsiness, blood dyscrasias
primidone (Mysoline)	Lethargy, irritability, diplopia, ataxia, impotence	Skin rash
topiramate (Topamax)	Fatigue, somnolence, confusion, ataxia, anorexia, depression, weight loss	Nephrolithiasis
valproic acid (Depakene)	Nausea and vomiting, weight gain, hair loss, tremor, menstrual irregularities	Hepatotoxicity, skin rash, blood dyscrasias, nephritis
zonisamide (Zonegran, Excegran)	Somnolence, dizziness, anorexia, headache, nausea, agitation, rash	Leukopenia, hepatotoxicity

and after a seizure assist in identifying the type of seizure and its management.

The effects of epilepsy on the patient's lifestyle are assessed (Buelow, 2001). What limitations are imposed by the seizure disorder? Does the patient have a recreational program? Social contacts? Is the patient working, and is it a positive or stressful experience? What coping mechanisms are used?

Diagnosis

NURSING DIAGNOSES

Based on the assessment data, the patient's major nursing diagnoses may include the following:

- Risk for injury related to seizure activity
- Fear related to the possibility of seizures
- Ineffective individual coping related to stresses imposed by epilepsy
- Deficient knowledge related to epilepsy and its control

COLLABORATIVE PROBLEMS/ POTENTIAL COMPLICATIONS

The major potential complication of patients with epilepsy is as follows:

- Status epilepticus

Planning and Goals

The major goals for the patient may include prevention of injury, control of seizures, achievement of a satisfactory psychosocial adjustment, acquisition of knowledge and understanding about the condition, and absence of complications.

Nursing Interventions

PREVENTING INJURY

Injury prevention for the patient with seizures is a priority. If at risk for injury (depending on the seizure type), the patient should be placed on the floor and any obstructive items should be removed. The patient should never be forced into a position, nor should anyone attempt to insert anything into the patient's mouth once a seizure has begun. Patients on seizure precautions should have pads applied to side rails while in bed.

REDUCING FEAR OF SEIZURES

Fear that a seizure may occur unexpectedly can be reduced by the patient's adherence to the prescribed treatment regimen. Cooperation of the patient and family and their trust in the prescribed regimen are essential for control of seizures (Schachter, 2001). It should be emphasized that the prescribed antiseizure medication must be taken on a continuing basis without fear of drug dependence or addiction. Periodic monitoring is necessary to ensure the adequacy of the treatment regimen and to prevent side effects.

In an effort to control seizures, factors that may precipitate them are identified: emotional disturbances, new environmental stressors, onset of menstruation in female patients, or fever (Greenberg, 2001). The patient is encouraged to follow a regular and moderate routine in lifestyle, diet (avoiding excessive stimulants), exercise, and rest (sleep deprivation may lower the seizure threshold). Moderate activity is therapeutic, but excessive exercise should be avoided.

Photic stimulation (bright flickering lights, television viewing) may precipitate seizures; wearing dark glasses or covering one eye may be preventive. Tension states (anxiety, frustration) induce

NURSING RESEARCH PROFILE 61-2

Nursing Observation and Documentation of Seizures

Wulf, J. A. (2000). Evaluation of seizure observation and documentation. *Journal of Neuroscience Nursing, 32*(1), 27–36.

Purpose

The observation and documentation of seizure activity are challenging yet essential aspects of nursing assessment. Despite their importance, there is a wide variability in nursing observation and documentation skills. The purpose of this study was to evaluate how demographic characteristics and knowledge levels of staff affected seizure documentation skills.

Study Sample and Design

This descriptive study included 58 participants: 38 RNs, 17 certified nursing assistants, and 3 licensed practical nurses or recreational therapists employed at a hospital with an epilepsy centre. All participants had received mandatory seizure observation training within the 2 years preceding the study. Participants observed and documented the same six videotaped seizure events in a randomly ordered sequence over 4 to 6 weeks. Participants used an event record form with observational guidelines similar to those used in the clinical setting. Two raters evaluated and scored the seizure event records, rating each record for detail and quality.

Findings

Seizure event ratings did not vary significantly according to observer characteristics of educational level, employment position, years of employment, or clinical experience with epilepsy. Certified nursing assistants with clinical experience with epilepsy had significantly higher mean seizure rating scores (indicating higher quality and detail) compared to nursing assistants without experience ($p < 0.01$). There were no differences in RNs with and without experience. A master score sheet was developed for each seizure event, and seizures with excess motor activity as an attribute had the highest scores, indicating that a greater number of details about the seizure were observed compared to the master score sheet. Participants missed some details of the seizure events and also documented details not present on the videotapes, such as seizure classification. Opportunities to review videotapes or actual seizures periodically improved observation and documentation skills.

Nursing Implications

The findings of this study suggest that use of a videotape of seizures and a scoring tool is useful for initial training and certification and may assist in periodic retraining of all personnel responsible for seizure observation to maintain quality of observation and documentation. Nurses involved in teaching these skills should keep in mind that observation instruction should emphasize not only predominate seizure features such as motor movements but also less frequently made observations such as responsiveness that may assist in seizure classification. Nurses observing and documenting seizure activity should be cautioned not to include items such as seizure classification that are not direct observations and may be incorrect.

seizures in some patients. Classes in stress management may be of value. Because seizures are known to occur with alcohol intake, alcoholic beverages should be avoided.

IMPROVING COPING MECHANISMS

It has been noted that the social, psychological, and behavioural problems frequently accompanying epilepsy can be more of a handicap than the actual seizures. Epilepsy may be accompanied by feelings of stigmatization, alienation, depression, and uncertainty. The patient must cope with the constant fear of a seizure and its consequences (Buelow, 2001). Children with epilepsy may be ostracized and excluded from school and peer activities. These problems are compounded during adolescence and add to the challenges of dating, not being able to drive, and feeling different. Adults face these problems in addition to the burden of finding employment, concerns about relationships and childbearing, insurance problems, and legal barriers. Alcohol abuse may complicate matters. Family reactions may vary from outright rejection of the person with epilepsy to overprotection. As a result, many people with epilepsy have psychological and behavioural problems.

Counselling assists the individual and family to understand the condition and the limitations imposed by it. Social and recreational opportunities are necessary for good mental health. Nurses can improve the quality of life for patients with epilepsy by educating them and their families about symptoms and their management (Rice, 2000).

PROVIDING PATIENT AND FAMILY EDUCATION

Of all the care contributed by the nurse to the person with epilepsy, perhaps the most valuable facets are education and efforts to modify the attitudes of the patient and family toward the disorder. The person who experiences seizures may consider every seizure a potential source of humiliation and shame. This may result in anxiety, depression, hostility, and secrecy on the part of the patient and family. Ongoing education and encouragement should be given to patients to enable them to overcome these feelings. The patient with epilepsy should carry an emergency medical identification card or wear a medical information bracelet. The patient and family need to be educated about medications as well as care during a seizure.

MONITORING AND MANAGING POTENTIAL COMPLICATIONS

Status epilepticus, the major complication, is described below. Another complication is the toxicity of medications. The patient and family are instructed about side effects and are given specific guidelines to assess and report signs and symptoms indicating medication overdose. Many antiseizure medications require careful monitoring for therapeutic levels. Patients should plan to have serum drug levels drawn at regular intervals. There are also many known drug interactions with antiseizure medications. A complete pharmacologic profile should be reviewed with the patient to avoid interactions either potentiating or inhibiting the effectiveness of the medications.

PROMOTING HOME AND COMMUNITY-BASED CARE

Teaching Patients Self-Care

Thorough oral hygiene after each meal, gum massage, daily flossing, and regular dental care are essential to prevent or control gingival hyperplasia in patients receiving phenytoin (Dilantin). The patient is also instructed to inform all health care providers of the medication being taken because of the possibility of drug interactions. An individual comprehensive teaching plan and written patient education material appropriate to the patient's needs and reading level are required to assist the patient and family to adjust to this chronic disorder (Day, Love, Popowich, et al., 1992). See Chart 61-5 for home care instruction points.

For many, overcoming employment problems is a challenge. Vocational rehabilitation agencies can provide information about

> *Chart 61-5*
> **Home Care Checklist • The Patient With Epilepsy**
>
> *At the completion of the home instruction, the patient and caregiver will be able to:*

	Patient	Caregiver
• Take medications daily as prescribed to keep the drug level constant to prevent seizures. The patient should never discontinue medications, even when there is no seizure activity.	✓	
• Keep a medication and seizure chart, noting when medications are taken and any seizure activity.	✓	✓
• Notify the patient's physician if patient cannot take medications due to illness.	✓	✓
• Have antiseizure serum levels checked regularly. When testing is prescribed, the patient should report to the laboratory for blood sampling before taking morning medication.	✓	
• Avoid activities that require alertness and coordination (driving, operating machinery) until after the effects of the medication have been evaluated.	✓	
• Report signs of toxicity so dosage can be adjusted. Common signs include drowsiness, lethargy, dizziness, difficulty walking, hyperactivity, confusion, inappropriate sleep, and visual disturbances.	✓	✓
• Avoid over-the-counter medications unless approved by the patient's physician.	✓	
• Carry a medical alert bracelet or identification card specifying the name of the patient's antiseizure medication and physician.	✓	
• Avoid seizure triggers, such as alcoholic beverages, electrical shocks, stress, caffeine, constipation, fever, hyperventilation, hypoglycemia.	✓	
• Take showers rather than tub baths to avoid drowning if seizure occurs; never swim alone.	✓	
• Exercise in moderation in a temperature-controlled environment to avoid excessive heat.	✓	
• Develop regular sleep patterns to minimize fatigue and insomnia.	✓	✓
• Identify resources for education and support.	✓	✓

job training. According to the Canadian Human Rights Act, it is illegal for an employer (within federal jurisdiction) to discriminate on the basis of physical or mental disability. However, barriers to employment still exist (Buelow, 2001). Epilepsy Canada, a national organization, works to advocate and lobby for people with disabilities.

People who have uncontrollable seizures accompanied by psychological and social difficulties can be referred to comprehensive epilepsy centres where continuous audio-video and EEG monitoring, specialized treatment, and rehabilitation services are available (Schachter, 2001). Patients and their families need to be reminded of the importance of following the prescribed treatment regimen and keeping follow-up appointments. In addition, they are reminded of the importance of participating in health promotion activities and recommended health screenings to promote a healthy lifestyle. Genetic and preconception counselling is advised.

Evaluation

EXPECTED PATIENT OUTCOMES

Expected patient outcomes may include:

1. Sustains no injury during seizure activity
   a. Complies with treatment regimen and identifies the hazards of stopping the medication
   b. Patient and family can identify appropriate care during seizure
2. Exhibits decreased fear
3. Displays effective individual coping
4. Exhibits knowledge and understanding of epilepsy
   a. Identifies the side effects of medications
   b. Avoids factors or situations that may precipitate seizures (flickering lights, hyperventilation, alcohol)
   c. Follows a healthy lifestyle by getting adequate sleep and eating meals at regular times to avoid hypoglycemia
5. Absence of complications

STATUS EPILEPTICUS

Status epilepticus (acute prolonged seizure activity) is a series of generalized seizures that occur without full recovery of consciousness between attacks (Greenberg, 2001). The term has been broadened to include continuous clinical or electrical seizures lasting at least 30 minutes, even without impairment of consciousness. It is considered a medical emergency. Status epilepticus produces cumulative effects. Vigourous muscular contractions impose a heavy metabolic demand and can interfere with respirations. There is some respiratory arrest at the height of each seizure that produces venous congestion and hypoxia of the brain. Repeated episodes of cerebral anoxia and edema may lead to irreversible and fatal brain damage. Factors that precipitate status epilepticus include withdrawal of antiseizure medication, fever, and concurrent infection.

Medical Management

The goals of treatment are to stop the seizures as quickly as possible, to ensure adequate cerebral oxygenation, and to maintain the patient in a seizure-free state. An airway and adequate oxygenation are established. If the patient remains unconscious and unresponsive, a cuffed endotracheal tube is inserted. Intravenous diazepam (Valium), lorazepam (Ativan), or fosphenytoin (Cerebyx) is given slowly in an attempt to halt seizures immediately. Other medications (phenytoin, phenobarbital) are given later to maintain a seizure-free state.

An intravenous line is established, and blood samples are obtained to monitor serum electrolytes, glucose, and phenytoin levels (Greenberg, 2001). EEG monitoring may be useful in determining the nature of the seizure activity. Vital signs and neurologic signs are monitored on a continuing basis. An intravenous infusion of dextrose is given if the seizure is due to hypoglycemia. If initial treatment is unsuccessful, general anesthesia with a short-acting barbiturate may be used. The serum concentration of the antiseizure medication is measured because a low level suggests that the patient was not taking the medication or that the dosage was too low. Cardiac involvement or respiratory depression may be life-threatening. There is also the potential for postictal cerebral edema.

Nursing Management

The nurse initiates ongoing assessment and monitoring of respiratory and cardiac function because of the risk for delayed depression of respiration and blood pressure secondary to administration of antiseizure medications and sedatives to halt the seizures. Nursing assessment also includes monitoring and documenting the seizure activity and the patient's responsiveness.

The patient is turned to a side-lying position if possible to assist in draining pharyngeal secretions. Suction equipment must be available because of the risk for aspiration. The intravenous line is closely monitored because it may become dislodged during seizures.

A person who has received long-term antiseizure therapy has a significant risk for fractures resulting from bone disease (osteoporosis, osteomalacia, and hyperparathyroidism), a side effect of therapy. Thus, during seizures, the patient should be protected from injury using seizure precautions and monitored closely. No effort should be made to restrain movements. The patient having seizures can inadvertently injure nearby people, so nurses should protect themselves. Other nursing interventions for the person having seizures are presented in Chart 61-4.

Headache

Headache, or cephalgia, is one of the most common of all human physical complaints. Headache is actually a symptom rather than a disease entity; it may indicate organic disease (neurologic or other disease), a stress response, vasodilation (migraine), skeletal muscle tension (tension headache), or a combination of factors. A **primary headache** is one for which no organic cause can be identified. These types of headache include migraine, tension-type, and cluster headaches (Lin, 2001). Cranial arteritis is another common cause of headache. A classification of headaches was issued by the Headache Classification Committee of the International Headache Society in 1988; an abbreviated list is shown in Chart 61-6.

Migraine is a symptom complex characterized by periodic and recurrent attacks of severe headache. The cause of migraine has not been clearly demonstrated, but it is primarily a vascular disturbance that occurs more commonly in women and has a strong familial tendency. The typical time of onset is puberty, and the incidence is highest in adults 20 to 35 years of age. There are seven subtypes of migraine, including migraine with and without aura. Most patients have migraine without an aura.

Tension headaches tend to be more chronic than severe and are probably the most common type of headache. *Cluster headaches* are a severe form of vascular headache. They are seen five times more frequently in men than women (Greenberg, 2001).

Inflammation of the cranial arteries is characterized by a severe headache localized in the region of the temporal arteries. The inflammation may be generalized (in which cranial arteritis is part of a vascular disease) or focal (in which only the cranial arteries are involved). *Cranial arteritis* is a cause of headache in the older population, reaching its greatest incidence in those older than 70 years of age.

A **secondary headache** is a symptom associated with an organic cause, such as a brain tumour or an aneurysm. Most headaches do not indicate serious disease, although persistent headaches require further investigation. Serious disorders related to headache in-

Chart 61-6 International Headache Society Classification of Headache

1. Migraine
2. Tension-type headache
3. Cluster headache and chronic paroxysmal hemicrania
4. Miscellaneous headaches unassociated with structural lesion
5. Headache associated with head trauma
6. Headache associated with vascular disorders
7. Headache associated with nonvascular intracranial disorder
8. Headache associated with substances or their withdrawal
9. Headache associated with noncephalic infection
10. Headache associated with metabolic disorder
11. Headache or facial pain associated with disorder of cranium, neck, eyes, ears, nose, sinuses, teeth, mouth or other facial or cranial structures
12. Cranial neuralgias, nerve trunk pain, and deafferentation pain
13. Headache not classifiable

*Headache classification committee of the International Headache Society. (1988). Classification and diagnostic criteria for headache disorders, cranial neuralgias and facial pain. *Cephalalgia, 8*(Suppl. 7), 13–17.

clude brain tumours, subarachnoid hemorrhage, stroke, severe hypertension, meningitis, and head injuries.

Assessment and Diagnostic Evaluation

The diagnostic evaluation includes a detailed history, a physical assessment of the head and neck, and a complete neurologic examination. Headaches may manifest differently within an individual over the course of a lifetime, and the same type of headache may present differently from patient to patient. The health history focuses on assessing the headache itself, with emphasis on the factors that precipitate or provoke it. Patients are asked to describe headaches in their own words.

Because headache is often the presenting symptom of various physiologic and psychological disturbances, a general health history is an essential component of the patient database. Headache may be a symptom of endocrine, hematologic, gastrointestinal, infectious, renal, cardiovascular, or psychiatric disease. Therefore, questions addressed in the health history should cover major medical and surgical illness as well as a body systems review.

The medication history can provide insight into the patient's overall health status. Antihypertensive agents, diuretic medications, anti-inflammatory agents, and monoamine oxidase inhibitors are a few of the categories of medications that can provoke headaches. Although sometimes exaggerated in importance, emotional factors can play a role in precipitating headaches. Stress is thought to be a major initiating factor in migraine headaches; therefore, sleep patterns, level of stress, recreational interests, appetite, emotional problems, and family stressors are relevant (Cunningham, 2000). There is a strong familial tendency for headache disorders, and a positive family history may help in making a diagnosis.

A direct relationship may exist between exposure to toxic substances and headache. Careful questioning may uncover chemicals to which a worker has been exposed. The Workplace Hazardous Materials Information System (WHMIS) is a national system established in 1988 that provides employees information on hazardous material used in the workplace. Employees have access to the material safety data sheets (commonly referred to as

MSDs) for all the substances with which they come in contact in the workplace. The occupational history also includes assessment of the workplace as a possible source of stress and a possible ergonomic basis for muscle strain and headache.

A complete description of the headache itself is crucial. The age at onset of headache; the headache's frequency, location, and duration; the type of pain; factors that relieve and precipitate the event; and associated symptoms are reviewed. The data obtained should include the patient's own words about the headache in response to the following questions:

- What is the location? Is it unilateral or bilateral? Does it radiate?
- What is the quality—dull, aching, steady, boring, burning, intermittent, continuous, paroxysmal?
- How many headaches occur during a given time?
- What are the precipitating factors, if any (environmental, such as sunlight and weather change; foods; exertion; other)?
- What makes the headache worse (coughing, straining)?
- What time (day or night) does it occur?
- Are there any associated symptoms, such as facial pain, lacrimation (excessive tearing), or scotomas (blind spots in the field of vision)?
- What usually relieves the headache (aspirin, NSAIDs, ergot preparation, food, heat, rest, neck massage)?
- Does nausea, vomiting, weakness, or numbness in the extremities accompany the headache?
- Does the headache interfere with daily activities?
- Do you have any allergies?
- Do you have insomnia, poor appetite, loss of energy?
- Is there a family history of headache?
- What is the relationship of the headache to lifestyle or physical or emotional stress?
- What medications are you taking?

Diagnostic testing is often not helpful in the investigation of headache as there are often few objective findings. In patients who demonstrate abnormalities on the neurologic examination, CT, cerebral angiography, or MRI may be used to detect underlying causes, such as tumour or aneurysm. Electromyography (EMG) may reveal a sustained contraction of the neck, scalp, or facial muscles. Laboratory tests may include complete blood count, erythrocyte sedimentation rate, electrolytes, glucose, creatinine, and thyroid hormone levels.

Pathophysiology

The cerebral signs and symptoms of *migraine* result from dysfunction of the brain stem pathways that normally modulate sensory input (Goadsby, Lipton & Ferrari, 2002). Abnormal metabolism of serotonin, a vasoactive neurotransmitter found in platelets and cells of the brain, plays a major role. The headache is preceded by a rise in plasma serotonin, which dilates the cerebral vessels, but migraines are more than just vascular headaches. The exact mechanism of pain in migraine is not completely understood but is thought to be related to the cranial blood vessels, the innervation of the vessels, and the reflex connections in the brain stem.

Migraines can be triggered by menstrual cycles, bright lights, stress, depression, sleep deprivation, fatigue, overuse of certain medications, and certain foods containing tyramine, monosodium glutamate, nitrites, or milk products. Foods in these categories include aged cheese and many processed foods. Use of oral contraceptives may be associated with increased frequency and severity of attacks in some women.

Emotional or physical stress may cause contraction of the muscles in the neck and scalp, resulting in tension headache. The pathophysiology of cluster headache is not fully understood. One theory is that it is due to dilation of orbital and nearby extracranial arteries. Cranial arteritis is thought to represent an immune vasculitis in which immune complexes are deposited within the walls of affected blood vessels, producing vascular injury and inflammation. A biopsy may be performed on the involved artery to make the diagnosis.

Clinical Manifestations

MIGRAINE

The migraine with aura can be divided into four phases: prodrome, aura, the headache, and recovery (headache termination and postdrome).

Prodrome. The prodrome phase is experienced by 60% of patients with symptoms that occur hours to days before a migraine headache. Symptoms include depression, irritability, feeling cold, food cravings, anorexia, change in activity level, increased urination, diarrhea, or constipation. Patients usually experience the same prodrome with each migraine headache.

Aura Phase. Aura occurs in up to 31% of patients who have migraines (Goadsby et al., 2002). The aura usually lasts less than an hour and may provide enough time for the patient to take the prescribed medication to avert a full-blown attack (described in a later section). This period is characterized by focal neurologic symptoms. Visual disturbances (ie, light flashes and bright spots) are common and may be hemianopic (affecting only half of the visual field). Other symptoms that may follow include numbness and tingling of the lips, face, or hands; mild confusion; slight weakness of an extremity; drowsiness; and dizziness.

This period of aura corresponds to the painless vasoconstriction that is the initial physiologic change characteristic of classic migraine. Cerebral blood flow studies performed during migraine headaches demonstrate that during all phases of the attack, cerebral blood flow is reduced throughout the brain, with subsequent loss of autoregulation and impaired CO_2 responsiveness.

Headache Phase. As vasodilation and a decline in serotonin levels occur, a throbbing headache (unilateral in 60% of patients) intensifies over several hours. This headache is severe and incapacitating and is often associated with photophobia, nausea, and vomiting. Its duration varies, ranging from 4 to 72 hours (Goadsby et al., 2002).

Recovery Phase. In the recovery phase (termination and postdrome), the pain gradually subsides. Muscle contraction in the neck and scalp is common, with associated muscle ache and localized tenderness, exhaustion, and mood changes. Any physical exertion exacerbates the headache pain. During this postheadache phase, patients may sleep for extended periods.

OTHER HEADACHE TYPES

The tension headache is characterized by a steady, constant feeling of pressure that usually begins in the forehead, temple, or back of the neck. It is often bandlike or may be described as "a weight on top of my head."

Cluster headaches are unilateral and come in clusters of one to eight daily, with excruciating pain localized to the eye and orbit and radiating to the facial and temporal regions. The pain is accompanied by watering of the eye and nasal congestion. Each attack lasts 30 to 90 minutes and may have a crescendo–decrescendo pattern

(Greenberg, 2001). The headache is often described as penetrating and steady.

Cranial arteritis often begins with general manifestations, such as fatigue, malaise, weight loss, and fever. Clinical manifestations associated with inflammation (heat, redness, swelling, tenderness, or pain over the involved artery) usually are present. Sometimes a tender, swollen, or nodular temporal artery is visible. Visual problems are caused by ischemia of the involved structures.

Prevention

Prevention begins by having the patient avoid specific triggers that are known to initiate the headache syndrome. Preventive medical management of migraine involves the daily use of one or more agents that are thought to block the physiologic events leading to an attack. Medication therapy should be considered for migraine if attacks occur 3 to 4 days per month (Goadsby et al., 2002). Treatment regimens vary greatly, as do patient responses; thus, close monitoring is indicated.

There are several proven or widely used medications for the prevention of migraine. Two beta-blocking agents, propranolol (Inderal) and metoprolol (Lopressor), inhibit the action of beta-receptors—cells in the heart and brain that control the dilation of blood vessels. This is thought to be a major reason for their antimigraine action. Other medications that are prescribed for migraine prevention include amitriptyline hydrochloride (Elavil), divalproex (Valproate), flunarizine, and several serotonin antagonists (Goadsby et al., 2002).

Calcium antagonists (verapamil HCl) are widely used but may require several weeks at a therapeutic dosage before improvement is noted. Calcium-channel blockers are not as effective as beta-blockers for prevention but may be more appropriate for some patients, such as those with bradycardia, diabetes mellitus, or asthma (Goadsby et al., 2002).

Alcohol, nitrites, vasodilators, and histamines may precipitate cluster headaches. Eliminating these factors helps in preventing the headaches (Silberstein & Rosenberg, 2000). Prophylactic medication therapy may include beta-blockers, ergotamine tartrate (occasionally), lithium, naproxen (Naprosyn), and methysergide (Sansert); such therapy is effective in 20% to 40% of cases (Greenberg, 2001).

Medical Management

Therapy for migraine headache is divided into abortive (symptomatic) and preventive approaches. The abortive approach, best employed in patients who suffer less frequent attacks, is aimed at relieving or limiting a headache at the onset or while it is in progress. The preventive approach is used in patients who experience more frequent attacks at regular or predictable intervals and may have medical conditions that preclude the use of abortive therapies (Evans & Lipton, 2001).

The triptans, serotonin receptor agonists, are the most specific antimigraine agents available. These agents cause vasoconstriction, reduce inflammation, and may reduce pain transmission. The five triptans in routine clinical use include sumatriptan (Imitrex), naratriptan (Amerge), and zolmitriptan (Zomig), (Goadsby et al., 2002). Numerous serotonin receptor agonists are under study.

Ergotamine preparations (taken orally, sublingually, subcutaneously, intramuscularly, by rectum, or by inhalation) may be effective in aborting the headache if taken early in the migraine process. They are low in cost. Ergotamine tartrate acts on smooth muscle, causing prolonged constriction of the cranial blood vessels. Each patient's dosage is based on individual needs. Side effects in-

clude aching muscles, paresthesias (numbness and tingling), nausea, and vomiting. Cafergot, a combination of ergotamine and caffeine, can arrest or reduce the severity of the headache if taken at the first sign of an attack (Karch, 2002).

Perhaps the most widely used triptan is sumatriptan succinate (Imitrex); it is available in oral, intranasal, and subcutaneous preparations and is effective for the treatment of acute migraine and cluster headaches in adults (McAlhany, 2001). The subcutaneous form usually relieves symptoms within an hour and is available in an autoinjector for immediate patient use, although it is expensive in this form. Sumatriptan has been found to be effective in relieving moderate to severe migraines in a large number of adult patients. Sumatriptan may cause chest pain and is contraindicated in patients with ischemic heart disease (Goadsby et al., 2002). Careful administration and dosing instructions to patients are important to prevent adverse reactions such as increased blood pressure, drowsiness, muscle pain, sweating, and anxiety. There are possible interactions when taken in conjunction with St. John's wort (Karch, 2002).

Many of the triptan medications are available in a variety of formulations, such as nasal sprays, inhalers, suppositories, or injections; however, 80% of patients prefer the oral formulations (Goadsby et al., 2002). None of these medications should be taken concurrently with medications containing ergotamine due to the potential for a prolonged vasoactive reaction (Karch, 2002).

The medical management of an acute attack of cluster headaches may include 100% oxygen by face mask for 15 minutes, ergotamine tartrate, sumatriptan, steroids, or a percutaneous sphenopalatine ganglion blockade (Greenberg, 2001).

The medical management of cranial arteritis consists of early administration of a corticosteroid to prevent the possibility of loss of vision due to vascular occlusion or rupture of the involved artery (Greenberg, 2001). The patient is instructed not to stop the medication abruptly because this can lead to relapse. Analgesic agents are prescribed for comfort.

Nursing Management

When migraine or the other types of headaches described above have been diagnosed, the goals of nursing management are to enhance pain relief. It is reasonable to try nonpharmacologic interventions first, but the use of pharmacologic agents should not be delayed. The goal is to treat the acute event of the headache and to prevent recurrent episodes. Prevention involves patient education regarding precipitating factors, possible lifestyle or habit changes that may be helpful, and pharmacologic measures.

RELIEVING PAIN

Individualized treatment depends on the type of headache and differs for migraine, cluster headaches, cranial arteritis, and tension headache (Greenberg, 2001; Silberstein & Rosenberg, 2000). Nursing care is directed toward treatment of the acute episode. A migraine or a cluster headache in the early phase requires abortive medication therapy instituted as soon as possible. Some headaches may be prevented if the appropriate medications are taken before the onset of pain. Nursing care during a fully developed attack includes comfort measures such as a quiet, dark environment and elevation of the head of the bed to 30 degrees. In addition, symptomatic treatment such as antiemetics may be indicated (Goadsby et al., 2002).

Symptomatic pain relief for tension headache may be obtained by application of local heat or massage. Additional strategies may include the use of analgesic agents, antidepressant medications, and muscle relaxants.

Chart 61-7

Home Care Checklist • **The Patient With Migraine Headaches**

At the completion of the home instruction, the patient or caregiver will be able to:	Patient	Caregiver
• Define migraine headaches and describe characteristics and manifestations.	✓	✓

• Identify triggers of migraine headaches and how to avoid such triggers as:
  Foods that contain tyramine, such as chocolate, cheese, coffee, dairy products
  Dietary habits that result in long periods between meals
  Menstruation and ovulation (causes hormone fluctuation)
  Alcohol (causes vasodilation of blood vessels)
  Fatigue and fluctuations in sleep patterns
	✓	✓

• State importance of keeping and how to develop a headache diary.	✓	✓
• State stress management and lifestyle changes to minimize the frequency of headaches.	✓	✓
• State pharmacologic management: acute therapy and prophylaxis, to include medication regimen and side effects.	✓	✓
• Identify comfort measures during headache attacks, such as resting in a quiet and dark environment, applying cold compresses to the painful area, and elevating the head.	✓	✓
• Identify resources for education and support.	✓	✓

HOME AND COMMUNITY-BASED CARE

Teaching Patients Self-Care. Headaches, especially migraines, are more likely to occur when the patient is ill, overly tired, or stressed. Nonpharmacologic therapies are important and include patient education about the type of headache, its mechanism (if known), and appropriate changes in lifestyle to avoid triggers. Regular sleep, meals, exercise, avoidance of peaks and troughs of relaxation, and avoidance of dietary triggers may be helpful in avoiding headaches (Goadsby et al., 2002; Rice, 2000).

The patient with tension headaches needs teaching and reassurance that the headache is not due to a brain tumour. This is a common unspoken fear. Stress reduction techniques, such as biofeedback, exercise programs, and meditation, are examples of nonpharmacologic therapies that may prove helpful. Patients and their families need to be reminded of the importance of following the prescribed treatment regimen for headache and keeping follow-up appointments. In addition, they are reminded of the importance of participating in health promotion activities and recommended health screenings to promote a healthy lifestyle. See Chart 61-7 for a home care checklist for the patient with migraine headaches.

Critical Thinking Exercises

1. Your patient has signs of increased ICP, including disorientation and right-sided weakness. Describe the medical management you would anticipate to control the ICP and the nursing measures that are indicated. How would you determine if your interventions were effective in alleviating the increased ICP? What are signs and symptoms of further deterioration in neurologic status? Explain the physiologic cause of each sign and symptom.

2. Compare and contrast the possible characteristics, causes, prognoses, and nursing interventions for a) the patient who is unconscious, b) the patient in a persistent vegetative state, and c) the patient in coma.

3. A patient is admitted to your unit after undergoing transsphenoidal surgery for a brain tumour. Describe the major complications to assess for, along with the signs and symptoms of each. Describe the nursing measures that are indicated postoperatively. What patient and family teaching is important for the patient and family? How would you modify your teaching and discharge planning if the patient understands little English? If the patient lives alone?

4. You are caring for an 18-year-old patient admitted to the hospital to evaluate the recent onset of seizures and an episode of status epilepticus. He is angry about his situation and states that he has no intention of taking medications or giving up his driver's license. Describe your approach to caring for him. How would your approach differ if the patient is a 28-year-old woman who is 6 months pregnant?

REFERENCES AND SELECTED READINGS

Books

Abram, S. E., & Haddox, J. D. (Eds.). (1999). *The pain clinic manual* (2nd ed.). Philadelphia: Lippincott Williams & Wilkins.

Bickley, L. S., & Szilagyi, P. G. (2003). *Bates' guide to physical examination and history taking* (8th ed.). Philadelphia: Lippincott Williams & Wilkins.

Cruz, J. (Ed.). (1998). *Neurological and neurosurgical emergencies.* Philadelphia: W. B. Saunders.

Epilepsy Canada. (2005). *Epilepsy facts.* Available at: http://www.epilepsy.ca. Retrieved June 15, 2005.

Fischbach, F. (2002). *Common laboratory and diagnostic tests* (3rd ed.). Philadelphia: Lippincott Williams & Wilkins.

Greenberg, M. (2001). *Handbook of neurosurgery* (4th ed.) New York: Thieme Medical Publishers.

Hickey, J. V. (2003). *The clinical practice of neurologic and neurosurgical nursing* (5th ed.). Philadelphia: Lippincott Williams & Wilkins.

Karch, A. (2002). *Lippincott's nursing drug guide.* Philadelphia: Lippincott Williams & Wilkins.

Porth, C. M. (2002). *Pathophysiology: Concepts of altered health states.* Philadelphia: Lippincott Williams & Wilkins.

Rice, V. H. (2000). *Handbook of stress, coping, and health: Implications for nursing research theory and practice.* Thousand Oaks, CA: Sage.

Schachter, S., Krishnamurthy, K., & Cantrell, D. (2000). *The brainstorms woman: Epilepsy in our lives.* Philadelphia: Lippincott Williams & Wilkins.

Stewart-Amidei. Ç, & Kunkel, J. (2001). *AANN's neuroscience nursing: Human responses to neurologic dysfunction* (2nd ed.) Philadelphia: W. B. Saunders.

Young, G., Ropper, A., & Bolton, C. (1998). *Coma and impaired consciousness: A clinical perspective.* New York: McGraw-Hill.

Journals

Asterisks indicate nursing research articles.

General

Bateman, D. (2001). Neurological assessment of coma. *Journal of Neurology, Neurosurgery and Psychiatry, 71*(Suppl 1), i13–i17.

*Day, L., Stotts, N., Frankfurt, A., et al. (2001) Gastric versus duodenal feeding in patients with neurological disease: A pilot study. *Journal of Neuroscience Nursing, 33*(3), 148–159.

Henker, R. (1999). Evidence-based practice: Fever-related interventions. *American Journal of Critical Care, 8*(1), 481–487.

*Murphy, P. W., Chesson, A., Berman S. A., Arnold, C., & Galloway, G. (2001). Neurology patient education materials: Do our educational aids fit our patients' needs? *Journal of Neuroscience Nursing, 33*(2), 99–112.

*O'Farrell, B., Vandervoort, M., Bisnaire, D., et al. (2001). Evaluation of portable bladder ultrasound: Accuracy and effect on nursing practice in an acute care neuroscience unit. *Journal of Neuroscience Nursing, 33*(6), 301–309.

*Richmond, T. (1997). Cerebral resuscitation after global brain ischemia: Linking research to practice. *AACN Clinical Issues, 8*(2), 171–181.

Headache

Cunningham, S. (2000). Migraine: Helping clients choose treatment and identify triggers. *British Journal of Nursing, 8*(22), 1515–1523.

Evans, R., & Lipton, R. (2001). Topics in migraine management. *Neurologic Clinics, 19*(1), 1–20.

Goadsby, P., Lipton, R., & Ferrari, M. (2002). Migraine—current understanding and treatment. *New England Journal of Medicine, 346*(4), 257–270.

Lin, J. (2001). Overview of migraine. *Journal of Neuroscience Nursing, 33*(1), 6–13.

McAlhany, A. (2001). Efficacy of sumatriptan in the treatment of migraine: A review of the literature. *Journal of Neuroscience Nursing, 33*(5), 270–277.

Silberstein, S., & Rosenberg, J. (2000). Multispecialty consensus on diagnosis and treatment of headache. *Neurology, 54,* 1553.

Increased Intracranial Pressure

Clay, H. (2000). Validity and reliability of the SjO₂ catheter in neurologically impaired patients: A critical review of the literature. *Journal of Neuroscience Nursing, 32*(4), 194–203.

Clifton, G., Miller, E., Choi, S., et al. (2001). Lack of effect of induction of hypothermia after acute brain injury. *New England Journal of Medicine, 344*(8), 556–563.

Cunning, S., & Houdek, D. (1999). Preventing secondary brain injuries. *Dimensions of Critical Care Nursing, 18*(5), 20–22.

Hauber, R., & Testani-Dufour, L. (2000). Living in limbo: The low-level brain-injured patient and the patient's family. *Journal of Neuroscience Nursing, 32*(1), 22–26.

Johnson, L. (1999). Factors known to raise intracranial pressure and the associated implications for nursing management. *Nursing in Critical Care, 4*(3), 117–120.

McConnell, E. (2001). Preventing transient increases in ICP. *Nursing, 31*(3), 17.

Shewmon, D. (1998). "Brainstem death", "brain death", and death: A critical re-evaluation of the purported equivalence. *Issues in Law & Medicine, 14*(2), 125–145.

Slade, J., Kerr, M., & Marion, D. (1999). Effect of therapeutic hypothermia on the incidence and treatment of intracranial hypertension. *Journal of Neuroscience Nursing, 31*(5), 264–269.

*Sullivan, J. (2000). Positioning of patients with severe traumatic brain injury: Research-based practice. *Journal of Neuroscience Nursing, 32*(4), 204–209.

*Sund-Levander, M., & Wahren, L. (2000). Assessment and prevention of shivering in patients with severe cerebral injury. A pilot study. *Journal of Clinical Nursing, 9*(1), 55–61.

Winkelman, C. (2000). Effect of backrest position on intracranial and cerebral perfusion pressures in traumatically brain-injured adults. *American Journal of Critical Care, 9*(6), 373–380.

Neurosurgical Care

Eisenberg, A., & Redick, E. (1998). Transsphenoidal resection of pituitary adenoma: Using a critical pathway. *Dimensions of Critical Care Nursing, 17*(6), 306–312.

Leith, B. (1998). Pharmacological management of pain after intracranial surgery. *Journal of Neuroscience Nursing, 30*(4), 220–224.

Rafferty-Mitchell, C., Scanlon, J., & Laskowski-Jones, L. (1999). Gamma knife radiosurgery. *American Journal of Nursing, 99*(10), 52–59.

Tornqvist, A. (2001). Neurosurgery for movement disorders. *Journal of Neuroscience Nursing, 33*(2), 79–82.

Warbel, A., Lewicki, L., & Lupica, K. (1999) Venous thromboembolism: Risk factors in the craniotomy patient population. *Journal of Neuroscience Nursing, 31*(3), 180–186.

Seizures and Epilepsy

Berges, S., Moulin, T., Berger, E., et al. (2000). Seizures and epilepsy following strokes: Recurrence factors. *European Neurology, 43*(3), 3–8.

*Buelow, J. (2001). Epilepsy management issues and techniques. *Journal of Neuroscience Nursing, 33*(5), 260–269.

Day, R. A., Love, S., Popowich, J., & Pilip, V. (1992). Client education in a rehabilitation anticonvulsant outpatient clinic. *Canadian Journal of Rehabilitation, 6*(1), 23–32.

Devinsky, O. (1999). Patients with refractory seizures. *New England Journal of Medicine, 340*(20), 1565–1570.

Huntington, N. (1999). The nurse's role in delivery of radioisotope for ictal SPECT scan. *Journal of Neuroscience Nursing, 31*(4), 208–215.

Kennedy, P., & Schallert, G. (2001). Practical issues and concepts in vagus nerve stimulation: A nursing review. *Journal of Neuroscience Nursing, 33*(2), 105–112.

Liporace, J. D. (1997). Women's issues in epilepsy: Menses, childbearing, and more. *Postgraduate Medicine, 102*(1), 123–138.

Lowenstein, D. H., & Alldredge, B. K. (1998). Current concepts: Status epilepticus. *New England Journal of Medicine, 338*(14), 970–976.

Schumacher, L., Pruitt, J., & Phillips, M. (2000). Identifying patients "at risk" for alcohol withdrawal syndrome and a treatment protocol. *Journal of Neuroscience Nursing, 32*(3), 158–163.

Schachter, S. (2001). Epilepsy. *Neurologic Clinics, 19*(1), 57–78.

Shafer, P. (1999*a*). Epilepsy and seizures. Advances in seizure assessment, treatment, and self-management. *Nursing Clinics of North America, 34*(3), 743–759.

Shafer, P. (1999*b*). New therapies in the management of acute or cluster seizures and seizure emergencies. *Journal of Neuroscience Nursing, 31*(4), 224–230.

Vernarec, E. (2001). Lamictal packaging gets makeover to reduce errors. *RN, 64*(10), 96.

Wiebe, S., Blume, W., Girvin, J., & Eliasziw, M. (2001). A randomized, controlled trial of surgery for temporal-lobe epilepsy. *New England Journal of Medicine, 345*(5), 311–318.

Winkelman, C. (1999). A review of pharmacodynamics and pharmacokinetics in seizure management. *Journal of Neuroscience Nursing, 31*(1), 50–53.

*Wulf, J. (2000). Evaluation of seizure observation and documentation. *Journal of Neuroscience Nursing, 32*(1), 27–36.

Unconsciousness and Coma

*Elliott, R., & Wright, L. (1999). Verbal communication: What do critical care nurses say to their unconscious or sedated patients? *Journal of Advanced Nursing, 29*(6), 12–20.

Jacobson, A., & Winslow, E. (2000). Caring for unconscious patients. *American Journal of Nursing, 100*(1), 69.

*Villanueva, N. (1999). Experiences of critical care nurses caring for unresponsive patients. *Journal of Neuroscience Nursing, 31*(4), 16–23.

RESOURCES AND WEBSITES

BC Brain Injury Association; http://www.bcbia.org.

Brain Injury Association of Alberta; http://www.biaa.ab.ca.

Brain Injury Association of Nova Scotia; http://www3.ns.sympatico.ca/bians1.

Brain Tumour Foundation of Canada; http://www.braintumour.ca.

Canadian Congress of Neurological Sciences; http://www.ccns.org.

Canadian Epilepsy Alliance; http://www.epilepsymatters.com.

Canadian League against Epilepsy; http://www.clae.org.

Canadian Neurological Society; http://www.ccns.org/ccns_information/cns/cns_intro.html.

Council of Canadians with Disabilities; http://www.ccdonline.ca.

Epilepsy Canada; http://www.epilepsy.ca.

Epilepsy Foundation, 4351 Garden City Dr., Landover, MD 20785-2223; (301) 459-3700; http://www.epilepsyfoundation.org.

Help for Headaches; http://www.headache-help.org.

International Bureau for Epilepsy; http://www.ibe-epilepsy.org.

International League against Epilepsy; http://www.ilae-epilepsy.org.

Manitoba Brain Injury Association; http://www.mbia.ca.

National Headache Foundation, 428 W St. James Pl., 2d floor, Chicago, IL 60614-2750; 1-888-NHF-5552; http://www.headaches.org.

Neuro-Patient Resource Center; http://www.mni.mcgill.ca/neuropatient/resource.html.

Newfoundland Brain Injury Association; http://www.nbia.nf.ca.

Ontario Brain Injury Association: http://www.obia.on.ca.

Saskatchewan Brain Injury Association; http://www.sfn.saskatoon.sk.ca/health/shia.

Spina Bifida and Hydrocephalus Association of Canada; http://www.sbhac.ca.

Think First Foundation of Canada; http://www.thinkfirst.ca.

Management of Patients With Cerebrovascular Disorders

Adapted by Lynne Esson

LEARNING OBJECTIVES

On completion of this chapter, the learner will be able to:

1. Describe the incidence and social impact of cerebrovascular disorders.
2. Identify the risk factors for cerebrovascular disorders and related measures for prevention.
3. Compare the various types of cerebrovascular disorders: their causes, clinical manifestations, and medical management.
4. Relate the principles of nursing management to the care of a patient in the acute stage of an ischemic stroke.
5. Use the nursing process as a framework for care of a patient recovering from an ischemic stroke.
6. Use the nursing process as a framework for care of a patient with a cerebral aneurysm.
7. Identify essential elements for family teaching and preparation for home care of the stroke patient.

"Cerebrovascular disorders" is an umbrella term that refers to any functional abnormality of the central nervous system (CNS) that occurs when the normal blood supply to the brain is disrupted. Stroke is the primary cerebrovascular disorder in Canada and in the world. Although preventive efforts have brought about a steady decline in the incidence over the last several years, stroke is still the fourth leading cause of death. Approximately 40,000 to 50,000 people experience a new stroke, and approximately 16,000 die from a stroke each year. More women than men die from strokes. Stroke is the leading cause of neurologic disability in Canada (Heart and Stroke Foundation of Canada, 2002).

In Canada, approximately 300,000 individuals are living with the effects of stroke. The annual cost of stroke care is $2.7 billion. Each stroke costs an average of $27,500 to the acute care system.

Strokes can be divided into two major categories: ischemic (80%), in which vascular occlusion and significant hypoperfusion occur; and hemorrhagic (20%), in which there is extravasation of blood into the brain (Heart and Stroke Foundation of Canada, 2002). Although there are some similarities between the two broad types of stroke, overall the etiology, pathophysiology, medical management, surgical management, and nursing care differ. Table 62-1 reviews the major types of ischemic and hemorrhagic strokes.

Ischemic Stroke

An ischemic stroke, cerebrovascular accident (CVA), or what is now being termed "brain attack" is a sudden loss of function resulting from disruption of the blood supply to a part of the brain. This event is usually the result of long-standing cerebrovascular disease. The term "brain attack" is being used to suggest to health care practitioners and the public that a stroke is an urgent health care issue similar to a heart attack. This change in terms also reflects a similar management strategy in both diseases. Early treatment results in fewer symptoms and less loss of function.

Ischemic strokes are subdivided into five different types according to their cause: large artery thrombosis (20%), small penetrating artery thrombosis (25%), cardiogenic embolic stroke (20%), cryptogenic (30%) and other (5%) (see Table 62-1).

Large artery thrombotic strokes are due to atherosclerotic plaques in the large blood vessels of the brain. Thrombus formation and occlusion at the site of the atherosclerosis result in ischemia and **infarction**.

Small penetrating artery thrombotic strokes affect one or more vessels and are the most common type of ischemic stroke.

Table 62-1 • Major Types of Stroke and Their Causes

CLASSIFICATION	CAUSES
Ischemic	Large artery thrombosis
	Small penetrating artery thrombosis
	Cardiogenic embolic
	Cryptogenic (no known cause)
	Other
Hemorrhagic	Intracerebral hemorrhage
	Subarachnoid hemorrhage
	Cerebral aneurysm
	Arteriovenous malformation

Small artery thrombotic strokes are also called lacunar strokes because of the cavity that is created once the infarcted brain tissue disintegrates.

Cardiogenic embolic strokes are associated with cardiac dysrhythmias, usually atrial fibrillation. Emboli originate from the heart and circulate to the cerebral vasculature, most commonly the left middle cerebral artery, resulting in a stroke. Embolic strokes may be prevented by the use of anticoagulation therapy in patients with atrial fibrillation.

The last two classifications of ischemic strokes are cryptogenic strokes, which have no known cause, and other strokes, from causes such as cocaine use, coagulopathies, migraine, and spontaneous dissection of the carotid or vertebral arteries (Hock, 1999; Schievink, 2001).

Pathophysiology

In an ischemic brain attack, there is disruption of the cerebral blood flow due to obstruction of a blood vessel. This disruption in blood flow initiates a complex series of cellular metabolic events referred to as the ischemic cascade (Fig. 62-1).

The ischemic cascade begins when cerebral blood flow falls to less than 25 mL/100 g/min. At this point, neurons can no longer maintain aerobic respiration. The mitochondria must then switch to anaerobic respiration, which generates large amounts of lactic acid, causing a change in the pH level. This switch to the less efficient anaerobic respiration also renders the neuron incapable of producing sufficient quantities of adenosine triphosphate (ATP) to fuel the depolarization processes. Thus, the membrane

Glossary

agnosia: failure to recognize familiar objects perceived by the senses
aneurysm: a weakening or bulge in an arterial wall
aphasia: inability to express oneself or to understand language
apraxia: inability to perform previously learned purposeful motor acts on a voluntary basis
ataxia: impaired ability to coordinate movement, often seen as a staggering gait or postural imbalance

dysarthria: defects of articulation due to neurologic causes
expressive aphasia: inability to express oneself; often associated with damage to the left frontal lobe area
hemianopsia: blindness of half of the field of vision in one or both eyes
hemiplegia/hemiparesis: weakness/paralysis of one side of the body, or part of it, due to an injury to the motor areas of the brain
infarction: a zone of tissue deprived of blood supply

Korsakoff's syndrome: personality disorder characterized by psychosis, disorientation, delirium, insomnia, and hallucinations
penumbra region: area of low cerebral blood flow
perseveration: continued and automatic repetition of an activity or word or phrase that is no longer appropriate
receptive aphasia: inability to understand what someone else is saying; often associated with damage to the temporal lobe area

Physiology/Pathophysiology

FIGURE 62-1 Processes contributing to ischemic brain cell injury. Courtesy of National Stroke Association, Englewood, Colorado.

pumps that maintain electrolyte balances begin to fail and the cells cease to function.

Early in the cascade, an area of low cerebral blood flow, referred to as the penumbra region, exists around the area of infarction. The **penumbra region** is ischemic brain tissue that can be salvaged with timely intervention. The ischemic cascade threatens cells in the penumbra because membrane depolarization of the cell wall leads to an increase in intracellular calcium and the release of glutamate (Hock, 1999). The penumbra area can be revitalized by administration of tissue plasminogen activator (t-PA), and the influx of calcium can be limited with the use of calcium channel blockers. The influx of calcium and the release of glutamate, if continued, activate a number of damaging pathways that result in the destruction of the cell membrane, the release of more calcium and glutamate, vasoconstriction, and the generation of free radicals. These processes enlarge the area of infarction into the penumbra, extending the stroke.

Each step in the ischemic cascade represents an opportunity for intervention to limit the extent of secondary brain damage caused by a stroke. Medications that protect the brain from secondary injury are called neuroprotectants (Reed, 2000). A number of clinical trials are focusing on calcium channel antagonists that block the calcium influx, glutamate antagonists, antioxidants, and other neuroprotectant strategies that will help prevent secondary complications (NINDS, 1999; Reed, 2000).

Clinical Manifestations

An ischemic stroke can cause a wide variety of neurologic deficits, depending on the location of the lesion (which vessels are obstructed), the size of the area of inadequate perfusion, and the

amount of collateral (secondary or accessory) blood flow. The patient may present with any of the following signs or symptoms:

- Numbness or weakness of the face, arm, or leg, especially on one side of the body
- Confusion or change in mental status
- Trouble speaking or understanding speech
- Visual disturbances
- Difficulty walking, dizziness, or loss of balance or coordination
- Sudden severe headache

Motor, sensory, cranial nerve, cognitive, and other functions may be disrupted. Table 62-2 reviews the neurologic deficits frequently seen in patients with strokes. Table 62-3 compares the symptoms seen in right hemispheric stroke with those seen in left hemispheric stroke. Patients exhibit deficits in specific locations as well as different behaviour.

MOTOR LOSS

A stroke is a lesion of the upper motor neurons and results in loss of voluntary control over motor movements. Because the upper motor neurons decussate (cross), a disturbance of voluntary motor control on one side of the body may reflect damage to the upper motor neurons on the opposite side of the brain. The most common motor dysfunction is **hemiplegia** (paralysis of one side of the body) due to a lesion of the opposite side of the brain. **Hemiparesis**, or weakness of one side of the body, is another sign.

In the early stage of stroke, the initial clinical features may be flaccid paralysis and loss of or decrease in the deep tendon reflexes. When these deep reflexes reappear (usually by 48 hours), increased tone is observed along with spasticity (abnormal increase in muscle tone) of the extremities on the affected side.

COMMUNICATION LOSS

Other brain functions affected by stroke are language and communication. In fact, stroke is the most common cause of aphasia. The following are dysfunctions of language and communication:

- **Dysarthria** (difficulty in speaking), caused by paralysis of the muscles responsible for producing speech
- Dysphasia or **aphasia** (defective speech or loss of speech), which can be **expressive aphasia**, **receptive aphasia**, or global (mixed) aphasia
- **Apraxia** (inability to perform a previously learned action), as may be seen when a patient picks up a fork and attempts to comb his hair with it

PERCEPTUAL DISTURBANCES

Perception is the ability to interpret sensation. Stroke can result in visual-perceptual dysfunctions, disturbances in visual-spatial relations, and sensory loss.

Visual-perceptual dysfunctions are due to disturbances of the primary sensory pathways between the eye and visual cortex. Homonymous **hemianopsia** (loss of half of the visual field) may occur from stroke and may be temporary or permanent. The affected side of vision corresponds to the paralyzed side of the body.

Disturbances in visual-spatial relations (perceiving the relation of two or more objects in spatial areas) are frequently seen in patients with right hemispheric damage.

SENSORY LOSS

The sensory losses from stroke may take the form of slight impairment of touch or may be more severe, with loss of proprio-

Table 62-2 • Neurologic Deficits of Stroke: Manifestations and Nursing Implications

NEUROLOGIC DEFICIT	MANIFESTATION	NURSING IMPLICATIONS/PATIENT TEACHING APPLICATIONS
Visual Field Deficits		
Homonymous hemianopsia (loss of half of the visual field)	• Unaware of persons or objects on side of visual loss • Neglect of one side of the body • Difficulty judging distances	Place objects within intact field of vision. Approach the patient from side of intact field of vision. Instruct/remind the patient to turn head in the direction of visual loss to compensate for loss of visual field. Encourage the use of eyeglasses if available. When teaching the patient, do so within patient's intact visual field.
Loss of peripheral vision	• Difficulty seeing at night • Unaware of objects or the borders of objects	Avoid night driving or other risky activities in the darkness. Place objects in centre of patient's intact visual field. Encourage the use of a cane or other object to identify objects in the periphery of the visual field.
Diplopia	• Double vision	Explain to the patient the location of an object when placing it near the patient. Consistently place patient care items in the same location.
Motor Deficits		
Hemiparesis	• Weakness of the face, arm, and leg on the same side (due to a lesion in the opposite hemisphere)	Place objects within the patient's reach on the nonaffected side. Instruct the patient to exercise and increase the strength on the unaffected side.
Hemiplegia	• Paralysis of the face, arm, and leg on the same side (due to a lesion in the opposite hemisphere)	Encourage the patient to provide range-of-motion exercises to the affected side. Provide immobilization as needed to the affected side. Maintain body alignment in functional position. Exercise unaffected limb to increase mobility, strength, and use.
Ataxia	• Staggering, unsteady gait • Unable to keep feet together; needs a broad base to stand	Support patient during the initial ambulation phase. Provide supportive device for ambulation (walker, cane). Instruct the patient not to walk without assistance or supportive device.
Dysarthria	• Difficulty in forming words	Provide the patient with alternative methods of communicating. Allow the patient sufficient time to respond to verbal communication. Support patient and family to alleviate frustration related to difficulty in communicating.
Dysphagia	• Difficulty in swallowing	Test the patient's pharyngeal reflexes before offering food or fluids. Assist the patient with meals. Place food on the unaffected side of the mouth. Allow ample time to eat.
Sensory Deficits		
Paresthesia (occurs on the side opposite the lesion)	• Numbness and tingling of extremity • Difficulty with proprioception	Instruct the patient to avoid using this extremity as the dominant limb due to altered sensation. Provide range of motion to affected areas and apply corrective devices as needed.
Verbal Deficits		
Expressive aphasia	• Unable to form words that are understandable; may be able to speak in single-word responses	Encourage patient to repeat sounds of the alphabet.
Receptive aphasia	• Unable to comprehend the spoken word; can speak but may not make sense	Speak slowly and clearly to assist the patient in forming the sounds.
Global (mixed) aphasia	• Combination of both receptive and expressive aphasia	Speak clearly and in simple sentences; use gestures or pictures when able. Establish alternative means of communication.
Cognitive Deficits		
	• Short- and long-term memory loss • Decreased attention span • Impaired ability to concentrate • Poor abstract reasoning • Altered judgment	Reorient patient to time, place, and situation frequently. Use verbal and auditory cues to orient patient. Provide familiar objects (family photographs, favourite objects). Use noncomplicated language. Match visual tasks with a verbal cue; holding a toothbrush, simulate brushing of teeth while saying, "I would like you to brush your teeth now." Minimize distracting noises and views when teaching the patient. Repeat and reinforce instructions frequently.
Emotional Deficits	• Loss of self-control • Emotional lability • Decreased tolerance to stressful situations • Depression • Withdrawal • Fear, hostility, and anger • Feelings of isolation	Support patient during uncontrollable outbursts. Discuss with the patient and family that the outbursts are due to the disease process. Encourage patient to participate in group activity. Provide stimulation for the patient. Control stressful situations, if possible. Provide a safe environment. Encourage patient to express feelings and frustrations related to disease process.

Table 62-3 • Comparison of Left and Right Hemispheric Strokes	
LEFT HEMISPHERIC STROKE	**RIGHT HEMISPHERIC STROKE**
Paralysis or weakness on right side of body	Paralysis or weakness on left side of body
Right visual field deficit	Left visual field deficit
Aphasia (expressive, receptive, or global)	Spatial-perceptual deficits
Altered intellectual ability	Increased distractibility
Slow, cautious behaviour	Impulsive behaviour and poor judgment
	Lack of awareness of deficits

Chart 62-1   The Stroke Continuum: Time Course Classification

Strokes are commonly classified using the time course in the following manner: (1) transient ischemic attack (TIA), (2) reversible ischemic neurologic deficit, (3) stroke in evolution, and (4) completed stroke (Hock, 1999).

Transient Ischemic Attack

Temporary episode of neurologic dysfunction manifested by a sudden loss of motor, sensory, or visual function. It may last a few seconds or minutes but not longer than 24 hours. Complete recovery usually occurs between attacks. The symptoms result from temporary impairment of blood flow to a specific region of the brain due to atherosclerosis, obstruction of cerebral microcirculation by a small embolus, a decrease in cerebral perfusion pressure (CPP), or cardiac dysrhythmias.

A TIA may serve as a warning of impending stroke, which has its greatest incidence in the first month after the first attack. Lack of evaluation and treatment of a patient who has experienced previous TIAs may result in a stroke and irreversible deficits.

Reversible Ischemic Neurologic Deficits

Signs and symptoms are consistent with but more pronounced than a TIA and last more than 24 hours. Symptoms resolve in days with no permanent neurologic deficit.

Stroke in Evolution

Worsening of neurologic signs and symptoms over several minutes or hours. This is a progressing stroke.

Completed Stroke

Stabilization of the neurologic signs and symptoms. This indicates no further progression of the hypoxic insult to the brain from this particular ischemic event.

ception (ability to perceive the position and motion of body parts) as well as difficulty in interpreting visual, tactile, and auditory stimuli.

COGNITIVE IMPAIRMENT AND PSYCHOLOGICAL EFFECTS

If damage has occurred to the frontal lobe, learning capacity, memory, or other higher cortical intellectual functions may be impaired. Such dysfunction may be reflected in a limited attention span, difficulties in comprehension, forgetfulness, and a lack of motivation, which cause these patients to become frustrated in their rehabilitation program. Depression is common and may be exaggerated by the patient's natural response to this catastrophic event. Other psychological problems are common and are manifested by emotional lability, hostility, frustration, resentment, and lack of cooperation.

Assessment and Diagnostic Findings

Any patient with neurologic deficits needs a careful history and a complete physical and neurologic examination. Initial assessment will focus on airway patency, which may be compromised by loss of gag or cough reflexes and altered respiratory pattern; cardiovascular status (including blood pressure, cardiac rhythm and rate, carotid bruit), and gross neurologic losses.

Stroke patients may present to the acute care facility at any point along a continuum of neurologic involvement. A system that uses the time course to classify patients along this continuum may be used to guide treatment. Strokes using the time course are commonly classified in the following manner: (1) transient ischemic attack (TIA); (2) reversible ischemic neurologic deficit; (3) stroke in evolution; and (4) completed stroke (Hock, 1999) (Chart 62-1).

The initial diagnostic test for a stroke is a noncontrast computed tomography (CT) scan performed emergently to determine if the event is ischemic or hemorrhagic (which determines treatment). Further diagnostic workup for ischemic stroke involves attempting to identify the source of the thrombi or emboli. A 12-lead electrocardiogram and a carotid ultrasound are standard tests. Other studies may include cerebral angiography, transcranial Doppler flow studies, transthoracic or transesophageal echocardiography, magnetic resonance imaging of the brain and/or neck, xenon CT, and single photon emission CT (Bonnono et al., 2000; Petty et al., 2000).

In a patient with a TIA, a bruit (abnormal sound heard on auscultation resulting from interference with normal blood flow) may be heard over the carotid artery. There are diminished or absent carotid pulsations in the neck. Diagnostic tests for TIA may include carotid phonoangiography; this involves auscultation, direct visualization, and photographic recording of carotid bruits. Oculoplethysmography measures the pulsation of blood flow through the ophthalmic artery. Carotid angiography allows visualization of intracranial and cervical vessels. Digital subtraction angiography is used to define carotid artery obstruction and provides information on patterns of cerebral blood flow.

Prevention

Primary prevention of ischemic stroke is the best approach. Stroke risk screenings are an ideal opportunity to lower stroke risk by identifying high-risk individuals or groups and educating the patients and the community about recognition and prevention of stroke (Lindsey, 2000; Manzella & Galante, 2000).

Advanced age, gender, and race are well-known non-modifiable risk factors for stroke (Heart and Stroke Foundation of Canada, 2002). Specifically, high-risk groups include people over the age of 55, because the incidence of stroke more than doubles in each successive decade, and men, who have a higher rate of stroke than women (due to the higher prevalence of women in the elderly population, however, the absolute numbers of men and women with stroke are similar). Another high-risk group is African Canadians: the incidence of first stroke in African Canadians is almost twice that in Caucasians. African Canadians also suffer more extensive physical impairments and are twice as likely to die from stroke than Caucasians.

Modifiable risk factors for ischemic stroke include hypertension, cardiovascular disease, high cholesterol, obesity, smoking, and diabetes (Chart 62-2). For people at high risk, interventions that alter modifiable factors, such as treating hypertension and hyperglycemia and stopping smoking, will reduce stroke risk. Many health promotion efforts involve encouraging a healthy lifestyle, including eating a low-fat, low-cholesterol diet and increasing exercise. Recent evidence suggests that eating fish two or more times per week reduces the risk of thrombotic stroke for women (Iso et al., 2001).

Several methods of preventing recurrent stroke have been identified for patients with TIAs or mild ischemic stroke. Patients with moderate to severe carotid stenosis are treated with carotid endarterectomy (Wolf et al., 1999). In patients with atrial fibrillation, which increases the risk of emboli, administration of warfarin (Coumadin), an anticoagulant that inhibits clot formation, may prevent both thrombotic and embolic strokes.

> **NURSING ALERT** Many people take herbal remedies and nutritional supplements but do not think of them as "medications" and do not always report their use to health care providers. Patients receiving anticoagulation following a stroke, TIA, or diagnosis of atrial fibrillation need to be cautioned that two herbs, ginkgo and garlic, have demonstrated effects on warfarin (Coumadin). Ginkgo has been associated with increased bleeding times and increased rates of spontaneous hemorrhage and subdural hematomas. Garlic and warfarin taken together can greatly increase the International Normalized Ratio (INR), increasing the risk for bleeding (Evans, 2000).

Medical Management

Patients who have experienced a TIA or mild stroke from atrial fibrillation or from suspected embolic or thrombotic causes are candidates for nonsurgical medical management. Those with

Chart 62-2
Modifiable Risk Factors for Ischemic and Hemorrhagic Stroke

- Hypertension (controlling hypertension, the major risk factor, is the key to preventing stroke)
- Cardiovascular disease (cerebral emboli may originate in the heart)
  - Atrial fibrillation
  - Coronary artery disease
  - Heart failure
  - Left ventricular hypertrophy
  - Myocardial infarction (especially anterior)
  - Rheumatic heart disease
- High cholesterol levels
- Obesity
- Elevated hematocrit (increases the risk of cerebral infarction)
- Diabetes mellitus (associated with accelerated atherogenesis)
- Oral contraceptive use (increases risk, especially with coexisting hypertension, smoking, and high estrogen levels)
- Smoking
- Drug abuse (especially cocaine)
- Excessive alcohol consumption

Hock, 1999; Summers et al., 2000.

atrial fibrillation are treated with dose-adjusted warfarin sodium (Coumadin) unless contraindicated. The INR target is 2.5. When warfarin is contraindicated, aspirin is used in doses between 50 and 325 mg/d (Wolf et al., 1999).

Platelet-inhibiting medications (aspirin, dipyridamole [Persantine], clopidogrel [Plavix], and ticlopidine [Ticlid]) decrease the incidence of cerebral infarction in patients who have experienced TIAs from suspected embolic or thrombotic causes. Currently the most cost-effective antiplatelet regimen is aspirin 50 mg/d and dipyridamole 400 mg/d (Sarasin et al., 2000).

THROMBOLYTIC THERAPY

Thrombolytic agents are used to treat ischemic stroke by dissolving the blood clot that is blocking blood flow to the brain. Recombinant t-PA is a genetically engineered form of t-PA, a thrombolytic substance made naturally by the body. It works by binding to fibrin and converting plasminogen to plasmin, which stimulates fibrinolysis of the atherosclerotic lesion. Rapid diagnosis of stroke and initiation of thrombolytic therapy (within 3 hours) in patients with ischemic stroke leads to a decrease in the size of the stroke and an overall improvement in functional outcome after 3 months (NINDS t-PA Stroke Study Group, 1995). To realize the full potential of thrombolytic therapy, community education directed at recognizing the symptoms of stroke and obtaining appropriate emergency care is necessary to ensure rapid transport to a hospital and initiation of therapy within the 3-hour time frame (Manzella & Galante, 2000). Delays make the patient ineligible for thrombolytic therapy because revascularization of necrotic tissue (which develops after 3 hours) increases the risk for cerebral edema and hemorrhage.

Enhancing Prompt Diagnosis. After being notified by emergency medical service personnel, the emergency department calls the appropriate staff (neurologist, neuroradiologist, radiology department, nursing staff, and electrocardiogram technician) and informs them of the patient's imminent arrival at the hospital. Many institutions have brain attack teams that respond rapidly, ensuring that treatment occurs within the allotted time frame (Alberts et al., 2000; Bonnono et al., 2000).

Initial management requires the definitive diagnosis of an ischemic stroke by CT scanning and determination of whether the patient meets all the criteria for t-PA therapy (Chart 62-3). Some of the contraindications for thrombolytic therapy include symptom onset greater than 3 hours prior to admission, a patient who is anticoagulated, a patient who has had a recent myocardial infarction, or a patient who has had any type of intracranial pathology (eg, stroke, head injury, trauma). Once it is determined that the patient is a candidate for t-PA therapy, no anticoagulants are to be administered in the next 24 hours.

Before receiving t-PA, the patient should be assessed using the National Institutes of Health Stroke Scale (NIHSS), which contains 42 items evaluating neurologic deficits and is useful in differentiating between ischemic strokes and TIAs (Table 62-4). A patient with an NIHSS score of greater than 22 is not eligible to receive t-PA.

Dosage and Administration. The patient is weighed to determine the dose of t-PA. The minimum dose is 0.9 mg/kg; the maximum dose is 90 mg. The loading dose is 10% of the calculated dose and is administered over 1 minute. The remaining dose is administered over 1 hour via an infusion pump. After the infusion is completed, the line is flushed with 20 mL of normal saline solution to ensure that all the medication is administered.

Chart 62-3   Eligibility Criteria for t-PA Administration

Age 18 years or older
Clinical diagnosis of stroke with NIH stroke scale score under 22
Time of onset of stroke known and is 3 hours or less
BP systolic ≤ 185; diastolic ≤ 110
Not a minor stroke or rapidly resolving stroke
No seizure at onset of stroke
Not taking warfarin (Coumadin)
Prothrombin time ≤ 15 seconds or INR ≤ 1.7
Not receiving heparin during the past 48 hours with elevated partial thromboplastin time
Platelet count ≥ 100,000
Blood glucose level between 50 and 400 mg/dL
No acute myocardial infarction
No prior intracranial hemorrhage, neoplasm, arteriovenous malformation, or aneurysm
No major surgical procedures within 14 days
No stroke or serious head injury within 3 months
No gastrointestinal or urinary bleeding within last 21 days
Not lactating or postpartum within last 30 days

The patient is admitted to the intensive care unit, where continuous cardiac monitoring is implemented. Vital signs are obtained every 15 minutes for the first 2 hours, every 30 minutes for the next 6 hours, then every hour for 16 hours. Blood pressure should be maintained with the systolic pressure less than 180 mm Hg and the diastolic pressure less than 100 mm Hg. Airway management is instituted based on the patient's clinical condition and arterial blood gas values.

Side Effects. Bleeding is the most common side effect of t-PA administration, and the patient should be closely monitored for any bleeding (intracranial, intravenous [IV] insertion sites, urinary catheter site, endotracheal tube, nasogastric tube, urine, stool, emesis, other secretions) (Scroggins, 2000). Intracranial bleeding is a major complication that occurs in approximately 6.5% of patients (NINDS t-PA Stroke Study Group, 1995).

THERAPY FOR PATIENTS WITH ISCHEMIC STROKE NOT RECEIVING t-PA

Not all patients are candidates for t-PA therapy. Other treatments include anticoagulant administration (IV heparin or low-molecular-weight heparin) for ischemic strokes and careful maintenance of cerebral hemodynamics to maintain cerebral perfusion. Increased intracranial pressure (ICP) and its associated complications may occur following a large ischemic stroke. Interventions during this period include methods to reduce ICP, such as administering an osmotic diuretic (eg, mannitol), maintaining $PaCO_2$ within the range of 30 to 35 mm Hg, and positioning to avoid hypoxia. Other treatment measures include the following:

- Elevation of the head of the bed to promote venous drainage and to lower increased ICP
- Intubation with an endotracheal tube to establish a patent airway, if necessary
- Continuous hemodynamic monitoring. Systolic pressure should be maintained at less than 180 mm Hg, diastolic pressure at less than 100 mm Hg. Maintaining the blood pressure within this range reduces the potential for additional bleeding or further ischemic damage.

- Neurologic assessment to determine whether the stroke is evolving or whether other acute complications are developing, such as bleeding from anticoagulation or medication-induced bradycardia, which can result in hypotension and subsequent decreases in cardiac output and cerebral perfusion pressure.

See the acute ischemic stroke clinical guidelines in Appendix A.

MANAGING POTENTIAL COMPLICATIONS

Adequate cerebral blood flow is essential for cerebral oxygenation. If cerebral blood flow is inadequate, the amount of oxygen supplied to the brain will decrease and tissue ischemia will result. Therefore, maintaining cardiac output within the normal range of 4 to 8 L/min, or sometimes greater, can improve the cerebral blood flow and oxygen delivery. Adequate oxygenation begins with pulmonary care, maintenance of a patent airway, and administration of supplemental oxygen as needed. The importance of adequate gas exchange cannot be overemphasized in these patients, many of whom are elderly and more prone to developing pneumonia, which can interfere with gas exchange.

ENDARTERECTOMY FOR PREVENTION OF ISCHEMIC STROKE

The main surgical procedure for managing TIAs and small stroke is carotid endarterectomy (Krenzer, 1999). A carotid endarterectomy is the removal of an atherosclerotic plaque or thrombus from the carotid artery to prevent stroke in patients with occlusive disease of the extracranial cerebral arteries (Fig. 62-2). This surgery is indicated for patients with symptoms of TIA or mild stroke found to be due to severe (70% to 99%) carotid artery stenosis or moderate (50% to 69%) stenosis with other significant risk factors (Wolf et al., 1999).

Nursing Management. The primary complications of carotid endarterectomy are stroke, cranial nerve injuries, infection or hematoma at the incision, and carotid artery disruption. It is important to maintain adequate blood pressure levels in the immediate postoperative period. Hypotension is avoided to prevent cerebral ischemia and thrombosis. Uncontrolled hypertension may precipitate cerebral hemorrhage, edema, hemorrhage at the surgical incision, or disruption of the arterial reconstruction. Sodium nitroprusside is commonly used to reduce the blood pressure to previous levels. Close cardiac monitoring is necessary because these patients have a high incidence of coronary artery disease.

A neurologic flow sheet is used to monitor and document all body systems, with particular attention to neurologic status, following carotid endarterectomy. The neurosurgeon is notified immediately if a neurologic deficit develops. Formation of a thrombus at the site of the endarterectomy is suspected if there is a sudden increase in neurologic deficits, such as weakness on one side of the body. The patient should be prepared for repeat endarterectomy.

Difficulty in swallowing, hoarseness, or other signs of cranial nerve dysfunction must be assessed. The nurse should focus on assessment of cranial nerves VI, X, XI, and XII (Krenzer, 1999). Some swelling in the neck after surgery is expected; if large enough, however, swelling and hematoma formation can obstruct the airway. Emergency airway supplies, including those needed for a tracheostomy, must be available. Table 62-5 provides more information about potential complications of carotid surgery.

Table 62-4 • **Summary of NIH Stroke Scale**

CATEGORY	DESCRIPTION	SCORE	BASELINE DATE/TIME	DATE/TIME
1a. Level of Consciousness (Alert, drowsy, etc)	Alert	0		
	Drowsy	1		
	Stuporous	2		
	Coma	3		
1b. LOC Questions (Month, age)	Answers both correctly	0		
	Answers one correctly	1		
	Incorrect	2		
1c. LOC Commands (Open, close eyes, make fist, let go)	Obeys both correctly	0		
	Obeys one correctly	1		
	Incorrect	2		
2. Best Gaze (Eyes open—patient follows examiner's finger or face)	Normal	0		
	Partial Gaze Palsy	1		
	Forced Deviation	2		
3. Visual (Introduce visual stimulus/threat to patient's visual field quadrants)	No Visual Loss	0		
	Partial Hemianopia	1		
	Complete Hemianopia	2		
	Bilateral Hemianopia	3		
4. Facial Palsy (Show teeth, raise eyebrows and squeeze eyes shut)	Normal	0		
	Minor	1		
	Partial	2		
	Complete	3		
5a. Motor Arm—Left (Elevate extremity to 90° and score drift/movement)	No Drift	0		
	Drift	1		
	Can't Resist Gravity	2		
	No Effort Against Gravity	3		
	No Movement	4		
	Amputation, joint fusion (explain)	9		
5b. Motor arm—Right (Elevate extremity to 90° and score drift/movement)	No Drift	0		
	Drift	1		
	Can't Resist Gravity	2		
	No Effort Against Gravity	3		
	No Movement	4		
	Amputation, joint fusion (explain)	9		
6a. Motor leg—Left (Elevate extremity to 30° and score drift/movement)	No Drift	0		
	Drift	1		
	Can't Resist Gravity	2		
	No Effort Against Gravity	3		
	No Movement	4		
	Amputation, joint fusion (explain)	9		
6a. Motor leg—Right (Elevate extremity to 30° and score drift/movement)	No Drift	0		
	Drift	1		
	Can't Resist Gravity	2		
	No Effort Against Gravity	3		
	No Movement	4		
	Amputation, joint fusion (explain)	9		
7. Limb ataxia (Finger-to-nose and heel-to-shin testing)	Absent	0		
	Present in One limb	1		
	Present in Two Limbs	2		
8. Sensory (Pin prick to face, arm, trunk and leg—compare side to side)	Normal	0		
	Partial Loss	1		
	Severe Loss	2		
9. Best Language (Name items, describe a picture and read sentences)	No Aphasia	0		
	Mild to Moderate Aphasia	1		
	Severe Aphasia	2		
	Mute	3		
10. Dysarthria (Evaluate speech clarity by patient repeating words)	Normal Articulation	0		
	Mild to Moderate Dysarthria	1		
	Near to Unintelligible or Worse	2		
	Intubated or Other Physical Barrier	9		
11. Extinction and Inattention (Use information from LOC and motor testing to identify neglect)	No Neglect	0		
	Partial Neglect	1		
	Complete Neglect	2		

Individual Administering Scale: _____

Based on http://www.vh.org/adult/provider/neurology/stroke/Scaledef.html © 1992–2002. University of Iowa and Adams, H., Davis, P., Torner, J., Grimsman, K., & VandaBerg, J.

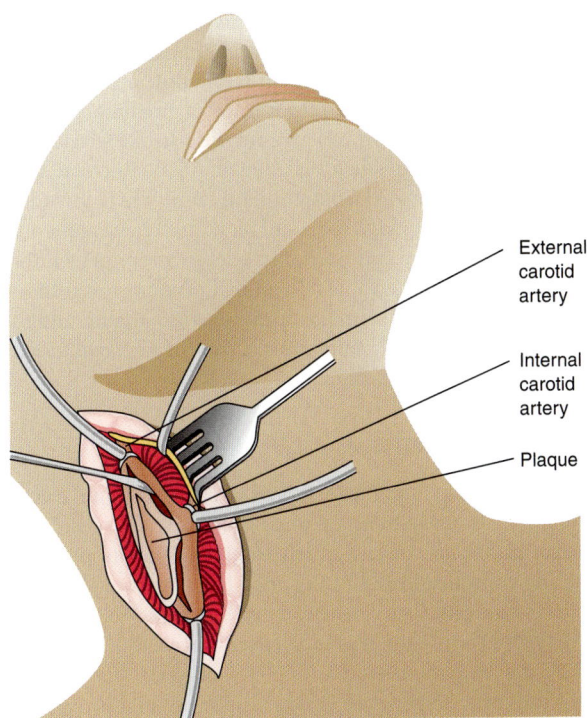

FIGURE 62-2 Plaque, a potential source of emboli in TIA and stroke, is surgically removed from the carotid artery.

NURSING PROCESS: THE PATIENT RECOVERING FROM AN ISCHEMIC STROKE

The acute phase of an ischemic stroke may last 1 to 3 days, but ongoing monitoring of all body systems is essential as long as the patient requires care. The patient who has had a stroke is at risk for multiple complications, including deconditioning and other musculoskeletal problems, swallowing difficulties, bowel and bladder dysfunction, inability to perform self-care, and skin breakdown. After the stroke is complete, management focuses on the prompt initiation of rehabilitation for any deficits.

Assessment

During the acute phase, a neurologic flow sheet is maintained to provide data about the following important measures of the patient's clinical status:

- Change in the level of consciousness or responsiveness as evidenced by movement, resistance to changes of position, and response to stimulation; orientation to time, place, and person
- Presence or absence of voluntary or involuntary movements of the extremities; muscle tone; body posture; and position of the head
- Stiffness or flaccidity of the neck

Table 62-5 • Selected Complications of Carotid Endarterectomy and Nursing Interventions

COMPLICATION	CHARACTERISTICS	NURSING INTERVENTIONS
Incision hematoma	Occurs in 5.5% of patients. Large or rapidly expanding hematomas require emergency treatment. If the airway is obstructed by the hematoma, the incision may be opened at the bedside.	Monitor neck discomfort and wound expansion. Report swelling, subjective feelings of pressure in the neck, difficulty breathing.
Hypertension	Poorly controlled hypertension increases the risk of postoperative complications, including hematoma and hyperperfusion syndrome. There is an increased incidence of neurologic impairment and death due to intracerebral hemorrhage. May be related to surgically induced abnormalities of carotid baroreceptor sensitivity.	Risk is highest in the first 48 hours after surgery. Check blood pressure frequently and report deviations from baseline. Observe for and report new onset of neurologic deficits.
Postoperative hypotension	Occurs in approximately 5% of patients. Treated with fluids and low-dose phenylephrine infusion. Usually resolves in 24 to 48 hours. Patients with hypotension should have serial ECGs to rule out myocardial infarction.	Monitor blood pressure and observe for signs and symptoms of hypotension.
Hyperperfusion syndrome	Occurs when cerebral vessel autoregulation fails. Arteries accustomed to diminished blood flow may be permanently dilated; increased blood flow after endarterectomy coupled with insufficient vasoconstriction leads to capillary bed damage, edema, and hemorrhage.	Observe for severe unilateral headache improved by sitting upright or standing.
Intracerebral hemorrhage	Occurs infrequently, but is often fatal (60%) or results in serious neurologic impairment. Can occur secondary to hyperperfusion syndrome. Increased risk with advanced age, hypertension, presence of high-grade stenosis, poor collateral flow, and slow flow in the region of the middle cerebral artery.	Monitor neurologic status and report any changes in mental status or neurologic functioning immediately.

- Eye opening, comparative size of pupils and pupillary reactions to light, and ocular position
- Colour of the face and extremities; temperature and moisture of the skin
- Quality and rates of pulse and respiration; arterial blood gas values as indicated, body temperature, and arterial pressure
- Ability to speak
- Volume of fluids ingested or administered; volume of urine excreted each 24 hours
- Presence of bleeding
- Maintenance of blood pressure within the desired parameters

After the acute phase, the nurse assesses mental status (memory, attention span, perception, orientation, affect, speech/language), sensation/perception (usually the patient has decreased awareness of pain and temperature), motor control (upper and lower extremity movement), swallowing ability, nutritional and hydration status, skin integrity, activity tolerance, and bowel and bladder function. Ongoing nursing assessment continues to focus on any impairment of function in the patient's daily activities, because the quality of life after stroke is closely related to the patient's functional status.

Diagnosis

NURSING DIAGNOSES
Based on the assessment data, the major nursing diagnoses for a patient with a stroke may include:

- Impaired physical mobility related to hemiparesis, loss of balance and coordination, spasticity, and brain injury
- Acute pain (painful shoulder) related to hemiplegia and disuse
- Self-care deficits (hygiene, toileting, grooming, and feeding) related to stroke sequelae
- Disturbed sensory perception related to altered sensory reception, transmission, and/or integration
- Impaired swallowing
- Incontinence related to flaccid bladder, detrusor instability, confusion, or difficulty in communicating
- Disturbed thought processes related to brain damage, confusion, or inability to follow instructions
- Impaired verbal communication related to brain damage
- Risk for impaired skin integrity related to hemiparesis/hemiplegia, or decreased mobility
- Interrupted family processes related to catastrophic illness and caregiving burdens
- Sexual dysfunction related to neurologic deficits or fear of failure

COLLABORATIVE PROBLEMS/POTENTIAL COMPLICATIONS
Potential complications include:

- Decreased cerebral blood flow due to increased ICP
- Inadequate oxygen delivery to the brain
- Pneumonia

Planning and Goals

Although rehabilitation begins on the day the patient has the stroke, the process is intensified during convalescence and requires a coordinated team effort. It is helpful for the team to know what the patient was like before the stroke: his or her illnesses, abilities, mental and emotional state, behavioural characteristics, and activities of daily living. It is also helpful for clinicians to be knowledgeable about the relative importance of predictors of stroke outcome (age, gender, in order to provide stroke survivors and their families with realistic goals) (Demchuk & Buchan, 2000).

The major goals for the patient (and family) may include improved mobility, avoidance of shoulder pain, achievement of self-care, relief of sensory and perceptual deprivation, prevention of aspiration, continence of bowel and bladder, improved thought processes, achieving a form of communication, maintaining skin integrity, restored family functioning, improved sexual function, and absence of complications.

Nursing Interventions

Nursing care has a significant impact on the patient's recovery. Often many body systems are impaired as a result of the stroke, and conscientious care and timely interventions can prevent debilitating complications. During and after the acute phase, nursing interventions focus on the whole person. In addition to providing physical care, nurses can encourage and foster recovery by listening to patients and asking questions to elicit the meaning of the stroke experience (Eaves, 2000; Pilkington, 1999).

IMPROVING MOBILITY AND PREVENTING JOINT DEFORMITIES
A hemiplegic patient has unilateral paralysis (paralysis on one side). When control of the voluntary muscles is lost, the strong flexor muscles exert control over the extensors. The arm tends to adduct (adductor muscles are stronger than abductors) and to rotate internally. The elbow and the wrist tend to flex, the affected leg tends to rotate externally at the hip joint and flex at the knee, and the foot at the ankle joint supinates and tends toward plantar flexion.

Correct positioning is important to prevent contractures; measures are used to relieve pressure, assist in maintaining good body alignment, and prevent compressive neuropathies, especially of the ulnar and peroneal nerves. Because flexor muscles are stronger than extensor muscles, a posterior splint applied at night to the affected extremity may prevent flexion and maintain correct positioning during sleep. (See Chap. 11 for additional information.)

Preventing Shoulder Adduction
To prevent adduction of the affected shoulder while the patient is in bed, a pillow is placed in the axilla when there is limited external rotation; this keeps the arm away from the chest. A pillow is placed under the arm, and the arm is placed in a neutral (slightly flexed) position, with distal joints positioned higher than the more proximal joints. Thus, the elbow is positoned higher than the shoulder and the wrist higher than the elbow. This helps to prevent edema and the resultant joint fibrosis that will limit range of motion if the patient regains control of the arm (Fig. 62-3).

Positioning the Hand and Fingers
The fingers are positioned so that they are barely flexed. The hand is placed in slight supination (palm faces upward), which is its most functional position. If the upper extremity is flaccid, a volar resting splint can be used to support the wrist and hand in a functional position. If the upper extremity is spastic, a hand roll is not used, because it stimulates the grasp reflex. In this instance a dor-

FIGURE 62-3 Correct positioning to prevent shoulder adduction.

sal wrist splint is useful in allowing the palm to be free of pressure. Every effort is made to prevent hand edema.

Spasticity, particularly in the hand, can be a disabling complication after stroke. Researchers have recently reported that intramuscular injections of botulinum toxin A decreased spasticity in the wrist and fingers and increased functional ability in dressing, washing, and other activities of daily living (Brashear et al., 2002).

Changing Positions

The patient's position should be changed every 2 hours. To place a patient in a lateral (side-lying) position, a pillow is placed between the legs before the patient is turned. To promote venous return and prevent edema, the upper thigh should not be acutely flexed. The patient may be turned from side to side, but the amount of time spent on the affected side should be limited if sensation is impaired.

If possible, the patient is placed in a prone position for 15 to 30 minutes several times a day. A small pillow or a support is placed under the pelvis, extending from the level of the umbilicus to the upper third of the thigh (Fig. 62-4). This helps to promote hyperextension of the hip joints, which is essential for normal gait and helps prevent knee and hip flexion contractures. The prone position also helps to drain bronchial secretions and prevents contractural deformities of the shoulders and knees. During positioning, it is important to reduce pressure and change position frequently to prevent pressure ulcers.

Establishing an Exercise Program

The affected extremities are exercised passively and put through a full range of motion four or five times a day to maintain joint

mobility, regain motor control, prevent contractures in the paralyzed extremity, prevent further deterioration of the neuromuscular system, and enhance circulation. Exercise is helpful in preventing venous stasis, which may predispose the patient to thrombosis and pulmonary embolus.

Repetition of an activity forms new pathways in the CNS and therefore encourages new patterns of motion. At first, the extremities are usually flaccid. If tightness occurs in any area, the range-of-motion exercises should be performed more frequently (see Chap. 11).

The patient is observed for signs and symptoms that may indicate pulmonary embolus or excessive cardiac workload during exercise; these include shortness of breath, chest pain, cyanosis, and increasing pulse rate with exercise. Frequent short periods of exercise always are preferable to longer periods at infrequent intervals. Regularity in exercise is most important. Improvement in muscle strength and maintenance of range of motion can be achieved only through daily exercise.

The patient is encouraged and reminded to exercise the unaffected side at intervals throughout the day. It is helpful to develop a written schedule to remind the patient of the exercise activities. The nurse supervises and supports the patient during these activities. The patient can be taught to put the unaffected leg under the affected one to move it when turning and exercising. Flexibility, strengthening, coordination, endurance, and balancing exercises prepare the patient for ambulation. Quadriceps muscle setting and gluteal setting exercises are started early to improve the muscle strength needed for walking; these are performed at least five times daily for 10 minutes at a time.

Preparing for Ambulation

As soon as possible, the patient is assisted out of bed. Usually, when hemiplegia has resulted from a thrombosis, an active rehabilitation program is started as soon as the patient regains consciousness; a patient who has had a cerebral hemorrhage cannot participate actively until all evidence of bleeding is gone.

The patient is first taught to maintain balance while sitting and then to learn to balance while standing. If the patient has difficulty in achieving standing balance, a tilt table, which slowly brings the patient to an upright position, can be used. Tilt tables are especially helpful for patients who have been on bed rest for prolonged periods and are having orthostatic blood pressure changes.

If the patient needs a wheelchair, the folding type with hand brakes is the most practical because it allows the patient to manipulate the chair. The chair should be low enough to allow the patient to propel it with the uninvolved foot and narrow enough to permit it to be used in the home. When the patient is transferred from the wheelchair, the brakes must be applied and locked on both sides of the chair.

The patient is usually ready to walk as soon as standing balance is achieved. Parallel bars are useful in these first efforts. A chair or wheelchair should be readily available in case the patient suddenly becomes fatigued or feels dizzy.

The training periods for ambulation should be short and frequent. As the patient gains strength and confidence, an adjustable cane can be used for support. Generally, a three- or four-pronged cane provides a stable support in the early phases of rehabilitation.

PREVENTING SHOULDER PAIN

Up to 70% of stroke patients suffer severe pain in the shoulder that prevents them from learning new skills, because shoulder func-

FIGURE 62-4 Prone position with pillow support helps prevent hip flexion.

tion is essential in achieving balance and performing transfers and self-care activities. Three problems can occur: painful shoulder, subluxation of the shoulder, and shoulder–hand syndrome.

A flaccid shoulder joint may be overstretched by the use of excessive force in turning the patient or from overstrenuous arm and shoulder movement. To prevent shoulder pain, the nurse should never lift the patient by the flaccid shoulder or pull on the affected arm or shoulder. If the arm is paralyzed, subluxation (incomplete dislocation) at the shoulder can occur from overstretching the joint capsule and musculature by the force of gravity when the patient sits or stands in the early stages after a stroke. This results in severe pain. Shoulder–hand syndrome (painful shoulder and generalized swelling of the hand) can cause a frozen shoulder and ultimately atrophy of subcutaneous tissues. When a shoulder becomes stiff, it is usually painful.

Medications are helpful in the management of post-stroke pain. Amitriptyline hydrochloride (Elavil) has been used but it can cause cognitive problems, has a sedating effect, and is not effective in all patients. A recent study showed the efficacy of an antiseizure medication lamotrigine (Lamictal) in treating post-stroke pain (Jensen et al., 2001).

Many shoulder problems can be prevented by proper patient movement and positioning. The flaccid arm is positioned on a table or with pillows while the patient is seated. Some clinicians advocate the use of a properly worn sling when the patient first becomes ambulatory to prevent the paralyzed upper extremity from dangling without support. Range-of-motion exercises are important in preventing painful shoulder. Overstrenuous arm movements are avoided. The patient is instructed to interlace the fingers, place the palms together, and push the clasped hands slowly forward to bring the scapulae forward; he or she then raises both hands above the head. This is repeated throughout the day. The patient is instructed to flex the affected wrist at intervals and move all the joints of the affected fingers. He or she is encouraged to touch, stroke, rub, and look at both hands. Pushing the heel of the hand firmly down on a surface is useful. Elevation of the arm and hand is also important in preventing dependent edema of the hand. Patients with continuing pain after movement and positioning have been attempted may require the addition of analgesia to their treatment program.

ENHANCING SELF-CARE

As soon as the patient can sit up, personal hygiene activities are encouraged. The patient is helped to set realistic goals; if feasible, a new task is added daily. The first step is to carry out all self-care activities on the unaffected side. Such activities as combing the hair, brushing the teeth, shaving with an electric razor, bathing, and eating can be carried out with one hand and are suitable for self-care. Although the patient may feel awkward at first, the various motor skills can be learned by repetition, and the unaffected side will become stronger with use. The nurse must be sure that the patient does not neglect the affected side. Assistive devices will help make up for some of the patient's deficits (Chart 62-4). A small towel is easier to control while drying after bathing, and boxed paper tissues are easier to use than a roll of toilet tissue.

Return of functional ability is important to the patient recovering after a stroke. An early baseline assessment of functional ability with an instrument such as the Functional Independence Measure (FIM) is important in team planning and goal setting for the patient. The FIM is a widely used instrument in stroke rehabilitation and also provides valuable functional information during the acute phase of care (Hinkle, 2000, 2001).

Chart 62-4 · **Assistive Devices to Enhance Self-Care After Stroke**

The following list identifies products that may help neurologically impaired patients perform self-care more easily and safely after a stroke or other disorders.

Eating Devices
Nonskid mats to stabilize plates
Plate guards to prevent food from being pushed off plate
Wide-grip utensils to accommodate a weak grasp

Bathing and Grooming Devices
Long-handled bath sponge
Grab bars, nonskid mats, hand-held shower heads
Electric razors with head at 90 degrees to handle
Shower and tub seats, stationary or on wheels

Toileting Aids
Raised toilet seat
Grab bars next to toilet

Dressing Aids
Velcro closures
Elastic shoelaces
Long-handled shoe horn

Mobility Aids
Canes, walkers, wheelchairs
Transfer devices such as transfer boards and belts

The patient's morale will improve if ambulatory activities are carried out in street clothes. The family is instructed to bring in clothing that is preferably a size larger than that normally worn. Clothing fitted with front or side fasteners or Velcro closures is the most suitable. The patient has better balance if most of the dressing activities are done in a seated position.

Perceptual problems may make it difficult for the patient to dress without assistance because of an inability to match the clothing to the body parts. To assist the patient, the nurse can take steps to keep the environment organized and uncluttered, because the patient with a perceptual problem is easily distracted. The clothing is placed on the affected side in the order in which the garments are to be put on. Using a large mirror while dressing promotes the patient's awareness of what he or she is putting on the affected side. Each garment is put on the affected side first. The patient has to make many compensatory movements when dressing; these can produce fatigue and painful twisting of the intercostal muscles. Support and encouragement are provided to prevent the patient from becoming overly fatigued and discouraged. Even with intensive training, not all patients can achieve independence in dressing.

MANAGING SENSORY-PERCEPTUAL DIFFICULTIES

Patients with a decreased field of vision should be approached on the side where visual perception is intact. All visual stimuli (clock, calendar, and television) should be placed on this side. The patient can be taught to turn the head in the direction of the defective visual field to compensate for this loss. The nurse should make eye contact with the patient and draw his or her attention to the affected side by encouraging the patient to move the head. The nurse may also want to stand at a position that encourages the patient to move or turn to visualize who is in the room. Increasing the natural or artificial lighting in the room and providing eyeglasses are important in increasing vision.

The patient with homonymous hemianopsia (loss of half of the visual field) turns away from the affected side of the body and tends to neglect that side and the space on that side; this is called amorphosynthesis. In such instances, the patient cannot see food on half of the tray, and only half of the room is visible. It is important for the nurse to constantly remind the patient of the other side of the body, to maintain alignment of the extremities, and, if possible, to place the extremities where the patient can see them.

MANAGING DYSPHAGIA
Stroke can result in swallowing problems (dysphagia) due to impaired function of the mouth, tongue, palate, larynx, pharynx, or upper esophagus. Patients must be observed for paroxysms of coughing, food dribbling out of or pooling in one side of the mouth, food retained for long periods in the mouth, or nasal regurgitation when swallowing liquids. Swallowing difficulties place the patient at risk for aspiration, pneumonia, dehydration, and malnutrition.

A speech therapist will evaluate the patient's gag reflexes and ability to swallow. Even if partially impaired, swallowing function may return in some patients over time, or the patient may be taught alternative swallowing techniques, advised to take smaller boluses of food, and taught about which foods are easier to swallow. The patient may initially be started on a thick liquid or puréed diet because these foods are easier to swallow than thin liquids. Having the patient sit upright, preferably out of bed in a chair, and instructing him or her to tuck the chin toward the chest as he or she swallows, will help prevent aspiration. The diet may be advanced as the patient becomes more proficient at swallowing. If the patient cannot resume oral intake, a gastrointestinal feeding tube will be placed for ongoing tube feedings.

Managing Tube Feedings
Enteral tubes can be either nasogastric (placed in the stomach) or nasoenteral (placed in the duodenum) to reduce the risk of aspiration. Nursing responsibilities in feeding include elevating the head of the bed at least 30 degrees to prevent aspiration, checking the position of the tube before feeding, ensuring that the cuff of the tracheostomy tube (if in place) is inflated, and giving the tube feeding slowly. The feeding tube is aspirated periodically to ensure that the feedings are passing through the gastrointestinal tract. Retained or residual feedings increase the risk for aspiration. Patients with retained feedings may benefit from the placement of a gastrostomy tube or a percutaneous endoscopic gastrostomy tube. In a patient with a nasogastric tube, the feeding tube should be placed in the duodenum to reduce the risk of aspiration. For long-term feedings, a gastrostomy tube is preferred. Management of patients with tube feedings is discussed in Chapter 36.

ATTAINING BOWEL AND BLADDER CONTROL
After a stroke, the patient may have transient urinary incontinence due to confusion, inability to communicate needs, and inability to use the urinal or bedpan because of impaired motor and postural control. Occasionally after a stroke, the bladder becomes atonic, with impaired sensation in response to bladder filling. Sometimes control of the external urinary sphincter is lost or diminished. During this period, intermittent catheterization with sterile technique is carried out. When muscle tone increases and deep tendon reflexes return, bladder tone increases and spasticity of the bladder may develop. Because the patient's sense of awareness is clouded, persistent urinary incontinence or urinary retention may be symptomatic of bilateral brain damage. The voiding pattern is analyzed and the urinal or bedpan offered on this pattern or schedule. The upright posture and standing position are helpful for male patients during this aspect of rehabilitation.

Patients may also have problems with bowel control or constipation, with constipation being more common. Unless contraindicated, a high-fibre diet and adequate fluid intake (2 to 3 L per day) should be provided and a regular time established (usually after breakfast) for toileting. See Chapter 11 for bowel and bladder retraining programs.

IMPROVING THOUGHT PROCESSES
After a stroke, the patient may have problems with cognitive, behavioural, and emotional deficits related to brain damage. In many instances, however, a considerable degree of function can be recovered because not all areas of the brain are equally damaged; some remain more intact and functional than others.

After assessment that delineates the patient's deficits, the neuropsychologist, in collaboration with the primary care physician, psychiatrist, nurse, and other professionals, structures a training program using cognitive-perceptual retraining, visual imagery, reality orientation, and cueing procedures to compensate for losses.

The role of the nurse is supportive. The nurse reviews the results of neuropsychological testing, observes the patient's performance and progress, gives positive feedback, and, most importantly, conveys an attitude of confidence and hope. Interventions capitalize on the patient's strengths and remaining abilities while attempting to improve performance of affected functions. Other interventions are similar to those for improving cognitive functioning after a head injury (see Chap. 63).

IMPROVING COMMUNICATION
Aphasia, which impairs the patient's ability to understand what is being said and to express himself or herself, may become apparent in various ways. The cortical area responsible for integrating the myriad of pathways required for the comprehension and formulation of language is called Broca's area. It is located in a convolution adjoining the middle cerebral artery. This area is responsible for control of the combinations of muscular movements needed to speak each word. Broca's area is so close to the left motor area that a disturbance in the motor area often affects the speech area. This is why so many patients paralyzed on the right side (due to damage or injury to the left side of the brain) cannot speak, whereas those paralyzed on the left side are less likely to have speech disturbances.

The speech pathologist assesses the communication needs of the stroke patient, describes the precise deficit, and suggests the best overall method of communication. With many language intervention strategies for the aphasic adult, the program can be individually tailored. The patient is expected to take an active part in establishing goals.

A person with aphasia may become depressed because of the inability to talk. The inability to talk on the telephone, answer a question, or participate in conversation causes anger, frustration, fear of the future, and hopelessness. Nursing interventions include doing everything possible to make the atmosphere conducive to communication. This includes being sensitive to the patient's reactions and needs and responding to them in an appropriate manner, always treating the patient as an adult. The nurse provides strong moral support and understanding to allay anxiety.

A common pitfall is for the nurse or other health care team member to complete the thoughts or sentences of the patient.

This should be avoided because it may cause the patient to feel more frustrated at not being allowed to speak and may deter efforts to practice putting thoughts together and completing the sentence. A consistent schedule, routines, and repetitions help the patient to function despite significant deficits. A written copy of the daily schedule, a folder of personal information (birth date, address, names of relatives), checklists, and an audiotaped list help improve the patient's memory and concentration. The patient may also benefit from a communication board, which has pictures of common needs and phrases. The board may be translated into several languages.

When talking with the patient, it is important to have the patient's attention, speak slowly, and keep the language of instruction consistent. One instruction is given at a time, and time is allowed for the patient to process what has been said. The use of gestures may enhance comprehension. Speaking is thinking out loud, and the emphasis is on thinking. The patient must sort out incoming messages and formulate a response. Listening requires mental effort; the patient must struggle against mental inertia and needs time to organize an answer.

In working with the aphasic patient, the nurse must remember to talk to the patient during care activities. This provides social contact for the patient. Chart 62-5 describes points to keep in mind when communicating with the aphasic patient.

MAINTAINING SKIN INTEGRITY

The stroke patient may be at risk for skin and tissue breakdown because of altered sensation and inability to respond to pressure and discomfort by turning and moving. Therefore, preventing skin and tissue breakdown requires frequent assessment of the skin, with emphasis on bony areas and dependent parts of the body. During the acute phase, a specialty bed (eg, low-air-loss bed) may be used until the patient can move independently or assist in moving.

A regular turning and positioning schedule must be followed to minimize pressure and prevent skin breakdown. Pressure-relieving devices may be employed but do not replace regular turning and positioning. The turning schedule (at least every 2 hours) must be adhered to even if pressure-relieving devices are used to prevent tissue and skin breakdown. When the patient is positioned or turned, care must be used to minimize shear and friction forces, which cause damage to tissues and predispose the skin to breakdown.

Chart 62-5 **Communicating With the Aphasic Patient**

- Face the patient and establish eye contact.
- Speak in a normal manner and tone.
- Use short phrases and pause between phrases to allow the patient time to understand what is being said.
- Limit conversation to practical and concrete matters.
- Use gestures, pictures, and objects.
- As the patient uses and handles an object, say what the object is. It helps to match the words with the object or action.
- Be consistent in using the same words and gestures each time you give instructions or ask a question.
- Keep extraneous noises and sounds to a minimum. Too much background noise can distract the patient or make it difficult to sort out the message being spoken.

The patient's skin must be kept clean and dry; gentle massage of healthy (nonreddened) skin and adequate nutrition are other factors that help to maintain normal skin and tissue integrity (see Chap. 11).

IMPROVING FAMILY COPING

Family members play an important role in the patient's recovery. Some type of counselling and support system should be available to them to prevent the care of the patient from taking a significant toll on their health and interfering too radically with their lives. Involving others in the patient's care and teaching stress management techniques and methods for maintaining personal health also facilitate family coping.

The family may have difficulty accepting the patient's disability and may be unrealistic in their expectations. They are given information about the expected outcomes and are counselled to avoid doing for the patient those things that he or she can do. They are assured that their love and interest are part of the patient's therapy.

The family needs to be informed that the rehabilitation of the hemiplegic patient requires many months; progress may be slow. The gains made by the patient in the hospital or rehabilitation unit must be maintained. All should approach the patient with a supportive and optimistic attitude, focusing on the abilities that remain. The rehabilitation team, the medical and nursing team, the patient, and the family all must be involved in developing attainable goals for the patient at home.

Most relatives of stroke patients handle the physical changes better than the emotional aspects of care. The family should be prepared to expect occasional episodes of emotional lability. The patient may laugh or cry easily and may be irritable and demanding or depressed and confused. The nurse can explain to the family that the patient's laughter does not necessarily connote happiness, nor does crying reflect sadness, and that emotional lability usually improves with time.

HELPING THE PATIENT COPE WITH SEXUAL DYSFUNCTION

Sexual functioning can be profoundly altered by stroke. Often stroke is such a catastrophic illness that the patient experiences loss of self-esteem and value as a sexual being. Although research in this area of stroke management is limited, it appears that stroke patients consider sexual function to be important, but most have sexual dysfunction. The combined effects of age and stroke cause a marked decline in many aspects of sexuality (Lipski & Alexander, 1997). In-depth assessments to determine sexual history before and after the stroke should be followed by appropriate interventions. Interventions for the patient and partner focus on providing relevant information, education, reassurance, adjustment of medications, counselling regarding coping skills, suggestions for alternative positions, and a means of sexual expression and satisfaction (Lipski & Alexander, 1997).

PROMOTING HOME AND COMMUNITY-BASED CARE

Teaching Patients Self-Care

Patient and family education is a fundamental component of rehabilitation, and ample opportunity for learning about stroke, its causes and prevention, and the rehabilitation process should be provided (Mumma, 2001). In both acute care and rehabilitation facilities, the focus is on teaching patients to resume as much self-care as possible. This may entail using assistive devices or modifying the home environment to help the patient live with a disability.

An occupational therapist may be helpful in assessing the home environment and recommending modifications to help the patient become more independent. For example, a shower is more convenient than a tub for the hemiplegic patient because most patients do not gain sufficient strength to get up and down from a tub. Sitting on a stool of medium height with rubber suction tips permits the patient to wash with greater ease. A long-handled bath brush with a soap container is helpful to the patient who has only one functional hand. If a shower is not available, a stool may be placed in the tub and a portable shower hose attached to the faucet. Handrails may be attached beside the bathtub and the toilet. Other assistive devices include special utensils for eating, grooming, and dressing (see Chart 62-3).

Continuing Care

The recovery and rehabilitation process after stroke may be prolonged, requiring patience and perseverance on the part of the patient and family. Depending on the specific neurologic deficits resulting from the stroke, the patient at home may require the services of a number of health care professionals. The nurse often coordinates the care of the patient at home. The family (often the spouse) will require assistance in planning and providing care. The caregiver often requires reminders to attend to his or her health problems and well-being.

The family is advised that the patient may tire easily, become irritable and upset by small events, and is likely to show less interest in things. Because a stroke frequently occurs in the later stages of life, there is the possibility of intellectual decline related to dementia.

Emotional problems associated with stroke are often related to speech dysfunction and frustrations about being unable to communicate. A speech therapist who visits the home allows the family to be involved and gives the family practical instructions to help the patient between therapy sessions.

Depression is a common and serious problem in the stroke patient. Antidepressant therapy may help if depression dominates the patient's life. As progress is made in the rehabilitation program, some problems will diminish. The family can help by continuing to support the patient and by giving positive reinforcement for the progress that is being made.

Community-based stroke support groups allow the patient and family to learn from others with similar problems and to share their experiences (Olson, 2001). The patient is encouraged to continue with hobbies, recreational and leisure interests, and contact with friends to prevent social isolation. All nurses coming in contact with the patient should encourage the patient to keep active, adhere to the exercise program, and remain as self-sufficient as possible.

The nurse should recognize the potential effects of caregiving on the family (Teel et al., 2001). Not all families have the adaptive coping skills and psychological functioning necessary for the long-term care of another. The patient's spouse may be elderly, with his or her own health problems; in some instances the stroke patient may have been the provider of care to the spouse. Even healthy caregivers may find it difficult to maintain a schedule that includes being available around the clock. Some effects of sustained caregiving include increased risk for depression and substance abuse, and increased use of health care services by the caregiver (King et al., 2001). Depressed caregivers are more likely to resort to physical or emotional abuse of the patient and are more likely to place the patient in a nursing home. Respite care

(planned short-term care to relieve the family from having to provide continuous 24-hour care) may be available from an adult day care centre. Some hospitals also offer weekend respite care that can provide caregivers with needed time to themselves. Nurses should encourage families to arrange for such services and should provide information to assist them.

The nurse involved in home and continuing care also needs to remind patients and family members of the need for continuing health promotion and screening practices. Patients who have not been involved in these practices in the past are educated about their importance and are referred to appropriate health care providers, if indicated.

NURSING RESEARCH PROFILE 62-1
Caregiving Experience

Teel, C. S., Duncan, P., & Lai, S. M., (2001). Caregiving experiences after stroke. *Nursing Research, 50*(1), 53–60.

Purpose

Family caregiving is often a source of stress for family members. However, despite the high prevalence of stroke, little is known about the experience of family caregiving after stroke. The primary purpose of this study was to examine relationships between patient characteristics, characteristics of the caregiver, and caregiver coping resources with caregiver physical and mental health outcomes at 3 and 6 months following a stroke.

Study Sample and Design

This longitudinal, correlational study was conducted in collaboration with a study of patient outcomes after stroke. The presence of stroke was confirmed by clinical assessment, CT, or MRI; stroke severity was assessed using the Orpington Prognostic Scale. Multiple instruments were used to assess the characteristics of family caregivers as well as their fatigue, vigour, mood disturbances, stress, spirituality, reactions to caregiving situation, coping resources, and physical and mental health status. These instruments were completed at 1, 3, and 6 months after a stroke. The sample for this study consisted of 83 caregivers, the majority of whom were female, Caucasian, and married and had at least a high school education. Their mean age was 57 years.

Findings

The caregivers reported stable perceptions of fatigue, vigour, recurrent sorrow, perceived stress, finances, family support, physical health, and depressive symptoms at 1, 3, and 6 months. Caregivers with more fatigue, sorrow, stress, depression, difficulty with scheduling and finances, and difficulty with family support had more physical health problems. Also less vigour, less importance of spirituality, and less perceived self-esteem (a reaction to caregiving) correlated with more physical health issues at 3 and 6 months.

Nursing Implications

Nurses working with stroke patients and families should note that comprehensive assessments of caregivers of stroke survivors should include physical and mental health components. Early identification of caregivers with more fatigue, sorrow, stress, depression, problems with scheduling and finances, and difficulty with family support may help identify persons at greater risk for physical health issues in the continuing care role. This would permit nurses to provide assistance, support, and referral to social services to family caregivers at greatest risk for physical and mental health issues.

Evaluation

EXPECTED PATIENT OUTCOMES

Expected patient outcomes may include:

1. Achieves improved mobility
   a. Avoids deformities (contractures and footdrop)
   b. Participates in prescribed exercise program
   c. Achieves sitting balance
   d. Uses unaffected side to compensate for loss of function of hemiplegic side
2. Reports absence of shoulder pain
   a. Demonstrates shoulder mobility; exercises shoulder
   b. Elevates arm and hand at intervals
3. Achieves self-care; performs hygiene care; uses adaptive equipment
4. Turns head to see people or objects
5. Demonstrates improved swallowing ability
6. Achieves normal bowel and bladder elimination
7. Participates in cognitive improvement program
8. Demonstrates improved communication
9. Maintains intact skin without breakdown
   a. Demonstrates normal skin turgor
   b. Participates in turning and positioning activities
10. Family members demonstrate a positive attitude and coping mechanisms
    a. Encourage patient in exercise program
    b. Take an active part in rehabilitation process
    c. Contact respite care programs or arrange for other family members to assume some responsibilities for care
11. Has positive attitude regarding alternative approaches to sexual expression

Hemorrhagic Stroke

Hemorrhagic strokes account for 15% of cerebrovascular disorders and are primarily caused by an intracranial or subarachnoid hemorrhage.

Patients generally have more severe deficits and a longer recovery time compared to those with ischemic stroke (AHCPR, 1995).

Hemorrhagic strokes are caused by bleeding into the brain tissue, the ventricles, or the subarachnoid space. Primary intracerebral hemorrhage from a spontaneous rupture of small vessels accounts for approximately 80% of hemorrhagic strokes and is primarily caused by uncontrolled hypertension (Qureshi et al., 2001). Secondary intracerebral hemorrhage is associated with arteriovenous malformations (AVMs), intracranial aneurysms, or certain medications (eg, anticoagulants and amphetamines) (Qureshi et al., 2001).

Pathophysiology

The pathophysiology of hemorrhagic stroke depends on the cause and type of cerebrovascular disorder. Symptoms are produced when an aneurysm or AVM enlarges and presses on nearby cranial nerves or brain tissue or, more dramatically, when an aneurysm or AVM ruptures, causing subarachnoid hemorrhage (hemorrhage into the cranial subarachnoid space). Normal brain metabolism is disrupted by the brain being exposed to blood; by an increase in ICP resulting from the sudden entry of blood into the subarachnoid space, which compresses and injures brain tissue; or by secondary ischemia of the brain resulting from the reduced perfusion pressure and vasospasm that frequently accompany subarachnoid hemorrhage.

INTRACEREBRAL HEMORRHAGE

An intracerebral hemorrhage, or bleeding into the brain substance, is most common in patients with hypertension and cerebral atherosclerosis because degenerative changes from these diseases cause rupture of the vessel. They also may be due to certain types of arterial pathology, brain tumour, and the use of medications (oral anticoagulants, amphetamines, and illicit drugs such as crack and cocaine).

The bleeding is usually arterial and occurs most commonly in the cerebral lobes, basal ganglia, thalamus, brain stem (mostly the pons), and cerebellum (Qureshi et al., 2001). Occasionally, the bleeding ruptures the wall of the lateral ventricle and causes intraventricular hemorrhage, which is frequently fatal.

INTRACRANIAL (CEREBRAL) ANEURYSM

An intracranial (cerebral) **aneurysm** is a dilation of the walls of a cerebral artery that develops as a result of weakness in the arterial wall. The cause of aneurysms is unknown, although research is ongoing. An aneurysm may be due to atherosclerosis, resulting in a defect in the vessel wall with subsequent weakness of the wall; a congenital defect of the vessel wall; hypertensive vascular disease; head trauma; or advancing age.

Any artery within the brain can be the site of cerebral aneurysms, but they usually occur at the bifurcations of the large arteries at the circle of Willis (Fig. 62-5). The cerebral arteries most commonly affected by an aneurysm are the internal carotid artery (ICA), anterior cerebral artery (ACA), anterior communicating artery (ACoA), posterior communicating artery (PCoA), posterior cerebral artery (PCA), and middle cerebral artery (MCA). Multiple cerebral aneurysms are not uncommon.

ARTERIOVENOUS MALFORMATIONS

An AVM is due to an abnormality in embryonal development that leads to a tangle of arteries and veins in the brain without a

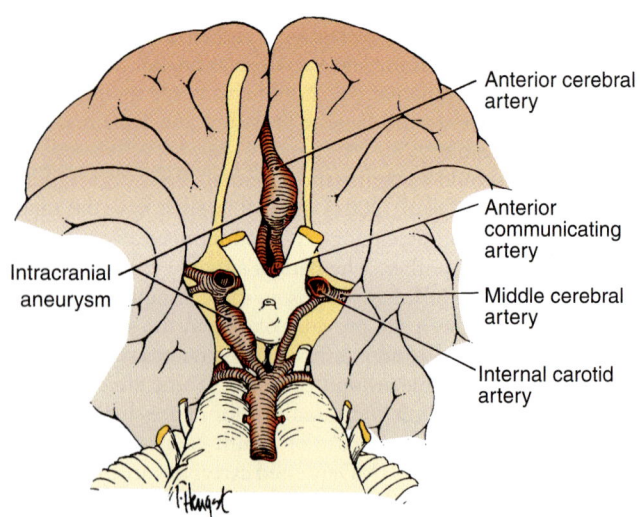

FIGURE 62-5 Intracranial aneurysms.

capillary bed. The absence of a capillary bed leads to dilation of the arteries and veins and eventual rupture. They are commonly a cause of hemorrhage in young people.

SUBARACHNOID HEMORRHAGE

A subarachnoid hemorrhage (hemorrhage into the subarachnoid space) may occur as a result of an AVM, intracranial aneurysm, trauma, or hypertension. The most common cause is a leaking aneurysm in the area of the circle of Willis or a congenital AVM of the brain.

Clinical Manifestations

The patient with a hemorrhagic stroke can present with a wide variety of neurologic deficits, similar to the patient with ischemic stroke. A comprehensive assessment will reveal the extent of the neurologic deficits. Many of the same motor, sensory, cranial nerve, cognitive, and other functions that are disrupted following ischemic stroke are altered following a hemorrhagic stroke. Table 62-2 reviews the neurologic deficits frequently seen in stroke patients. Table 62-3 compares the symptoms seen in right hemispheric stroke with those seen in left hemispheric stroke.

In addition to the neurologic deficits that are similar to ischemic stroke, the patient with an intracranial aneurysm or AVM can have some unique clinical manifestations. Rupture of an aneurysm or AVM usually produces a sudden, unusually severe headache and often loss of consciousness for a variable period. There may be pain and rigidity of the back of the neck (nuchal rigidity) and spine due to meningeal irritation. Visual disturbances (visual loss, diplopia, ptosis) occur when the aneurysm is adjacent to the oculomotor nerve. Tinnitus, dizziness, and hemiparesis may also occur.

At times, an aneurysm or AVM leaks blood, leading to the formation of a clot that seals the site of rupture. In this instance, the patient may show little neurologic deficit. In other cases, severe bleeding occurs, resulting in cerebral damage followed rapidly by coma and death.

Prognosis depends on the neurologic condition of the patient, age, associated diseases, and the extent and location of an intracranial aneurysm. Subarachnoid hemorrhage from an aneurysm is a catastrophic event with significant morbidity and mortality (Pfohman & Criddle, 2001). Chart 62-6 discusses ethical issues related to the patient with a severe hemorrhagic stroke.

Assessment and Diagnostic Findings

Any patient suspected of having a hemorrhagic stroke should undergo CT scanning to determine the size and location of the hematoma as well as the presence or absence of ventricular blood and hydrocephalus (Qureshi et al., 2001). CT scan and cerebral angiography confirm the diagnosis of an intracranial aneurysm or AVM. These tests show the location and size of the lesion and provide information about the affected arteries, veins, adjoining vessels, and vascular branches. Lumbar puncture is performed if there is no evidence of increased ICP, the CT scan results are negative, and subarachnoid hemorrhage must be confirmed. Lumbar puncture in the presence of increased ICP could result in brain stem herniation or rebleeding. In diagnosing a hemorrhagic stroke in a patient younger than 40, some clinicians obtain a toxicology screen for illicit drug use.

The Hunt-Hess classification system guides the physician in diagnosing the severity of subarachnoid hemorrhage after an aneurysmal bleed (Table 62-6). Classifying the patient by severity of neurologic deficit provides a baseline for future comparison.

Chart 62-6 • Ethics and Related Issues DNR Orders in Severe Stroke

Situation

An 85-year-old patient is admitted with a large intracerebral hemorrhage, severe neurologic deficits, and a past medical history of coronary artery bypass graft surgery, hypertension, atrial fibrillation, and gout. The attending physician suggests a do-not-resuscitate (DNR) order to the family.

Dilemma

Does the principle of autonomy include death with dignity, or is beneficence keeping the patient alive at all costs? Does the family have the right to refuse? If the patient goes into cardiac arrest and cardiopulmonary resuscitation (CPR) is not provided, have the health care workers "killed" the patient?

Discussion

What arguments would you pose in favour of the DNR order? What arguments would you pose against the DNR order? Is a DNR order an example of "patient abandonment" by health care workers, or an attempt to limit treatment and avoid CPR in a patient with an anticipated poor outcome?

Prevention

Primary prevention of hemorrhagic stroke is the best approach and includes managing hypertension and ameliorating other significant risk factors (Pfohman & Criddle, 2001). Control of hypertension, especially in individuals over 55 years of age, clearly reduces the risk for hemorrhagic stroke (Qureshi et al., 2001). Additional factors are similar to the risks for ischemic stroke and include smoking, excessive alcohol intake, and high cholesterol (see Chart 62-2). Stroke risk screenings provide an ideal opportunity to lower hemorrhagic stroke risk by identifying high-risk individuals or groups and educating the patients and the community about recognition and prevention (Pfohman & Criddle, 2001).

GRADE	DESCRIPTION
I	Asymptomatic, or mild headache and slight nuchal rigidity
II	Cranial nerve (CN) palsy (eg, oculomotor [CN III], abducens [CN VI], moderate-to-severe headache, nuchal rigidity
III	Mild focal deficit, lethargy, or confusion
IV	Stupor, moderate to severe hemiparesis, early decerebrate rigidity
V	Deep coma, decerebrate rigidity, moribund appearance Add one grade for serious systemic disease (eg, hypertension, chronic obstructive pulmonary disease) or severe vasospasm on angiography Modified classification adds the following:
0	Unrupted aneurysm
1a	No acute meningeal/brain reaction, but with fixed neurological deficit

Table 62-6 • Hunt-Hess Classification of Subarachnoid Hemorrhages

From Hickey, J. V. (2003). *The clinical practice of neurological and neurosurgical nursing* (5th ed., p. 527). Philadelphia: Lippincott Williams & Wilkins.

A prevention effort unique to hemorrhagic stroke is to increase the public's awareness about the association between phenyl-propanolamine (an ingredient found in appetite suppressants as well as cold and cough agents) and hemorrhagic stroke. Recent research has found that phenylpropanolamine is an independent risk factor for hemorrhagic stroke, especially in women (Kernan et al., 2000). Many products have been removed voluntarily from the market, but consumers should continue to look for this ingredient on labels.

Medical Management

The goals of medical treatment of hemorrhagic stroke are to allow the brain to recover from the initial insult (bleeding), to prevent or minimize the risk for rebleeding, and to prevent or treat complications. Management consists of bed rest with sedation to prevent agitation and stress, management of vasospasm, and surgical or medical treatment to prevent rebleeding. Analgesics (codeine, acetaminophen) may be prescribed for head and neck pain. The patient is fitted with elastic compression stockings to prevent deep vein thrombosis, a threat to any patient on bed rest.

COMPLICATIONS

Potential complications include rebleeding; cerebral vasospasm resulting in cerebral ischemia; acute hydrocephalus, which results when free blood obstructs the reabsorption of cerebrospinal fluid (CSF) by the arachnoid villi; and seizures.

Cerebral Hypoxia and Decreased Blood Flow.
Immediate complications of a hemorrhagic stroke include cerebral hypoxia, decreased cerebral blood flow, and extension of the area of injury. Providing adequate oxygenation of blood to the brain minimizes cerebral hypoxia. Brain function is dependent on available oxygen being delivered to the tissues. Administering supplemental oxygen and maintaining the hemoglobin and hematocrit at acceptable levels will assist in maintaining tissue oxygenation.

Cerebral blood flow is dependent on the blood pressure, cardiac output, and integrity of cerebral blood vessels. Adequate hydration (IV fluids) must be ensured to reduce blood viscosity and improve cerebral blood flow. Extremes of hypertension or hypotension need to be avoided to prevent changes in cerebral blood flow and the potential for extending the area of injury.

A seizure can also compromise cerebral blood flow. Seizures occur in approximately 5% of stroke patients (Berges et al., 2000). Observation for and appropriate treatment of seizure activity is an important component of care following a hemorrhagic stroke (Qureshi et al., 2001).

Vasospasm.
The development of cerebral vasospasm (narrowing of the lumen of the involved cranial blood vessel) is a serious complication of subarachnoid hemorrhage and accounts for 40% to 50% of the morbidity and mortality of those who survive the initial intracranial bleed. The mechanism responsible for the spasm is not clear, but vasospasm is associated with increasing amounts of blood in the subarachnoid cisterns and cerebral fissures, as visualized by CT scan.

Vasospasm leads to increased vascular resistance, which impedes cerebral blood flow and causes brain ischemia and infarction. The signs and symptoms reflect the areas of the brain involved. Vasospasm is often heralded by a worsening headache, a decrease in level of consciousness (confusion, lethargy, and dis-

orientation), or a new focal neurologic deficit (aphasia, hemiparesis [partial paralysis affecting one side of the body]).

Vasospasm frequently occurs 4 to 14 days after initial hemorrhage when the clot undergoes lysis (dissolution), increasing the chances of rebleeding.

It is believed that early surgery to clip the aneurysm prevents rebleeding and that removal of blood from the basal cisterns around the major cerebral arteries may prevent vasospasm. The IV administration of the calcium-channel blocker nimodipine during the critical time in which vasospasm may occur may prevent delayed ischemic deterioration. Advances in technology have led to the introduction of interventional neuroradiology for the treatment of aneurysms. Endovascular techniques may be used in selected patients to occlude the artery supplying the aneurysm with a balloon or to occlude the aneurysm itself. As more studies on these techniques are completed, their use will increase.

Management of vasospasm remains difficult and controversial. Based on one theory that vasospasm is caused by an increased influx of calcium into the cell, medication therapy may be used to block or antagonize this action and prevent or reverse the action of vasospasm already present. Calcium-channel blockers may include nimodipine (Nimotop), verapamil (Isoptin), and nifedipine (Adalat). Other therapy for vasospasm is aimed at minimizing the deleterious effects of the associated cerebral ischemia and includes fluid volume expanders and induced arterial hypertension, normotension, or hemodilution.

Increased ICP.
An increase in ICP can follow either an ischemic or hemorrhagic stroke but almost always follows a subarachnoid hemorrhage, usually because of disturbed circulation of CSF caused by blood in the basal cisterns. If the patient shows evidence of deterioration from increased ICP (due to cerebral edema, herniation, hydrocephalus, or vasospasm), CSF drainage may be instituted by cautious lumbar puncture or ventricular catheter drainage, and mannitol is given to reduce ICP. When mannitol is used as a long-term measure to control ICP, dehydration and disturbances in electrolyte balance (hyponatremia or hypernatremia; hypokalemia or hyperkalemia) may occur. Mannitol acts by pulling water out of the brain tissue by osmosis as well as by reducing total-body water through diuresis. The patient is monitored for signs of dehydration and for rebound elevation of ICP.

Systemic Hypertension.
Preventing sudden systemic hypertension is critical in hemorrhagic stroke management. The goal of therapy is to maintain the systolic blood pressure at about 150 mm Hg. If blood pressure is elevated, antihypertensive therapy (labetalol [Trandate], nicardipine [Cardene], nitroprusside [Nipride]) may be prescribed. Hemodynamic monitoring by arterial line during the administration of antihypertensives is important to detect and avoid a precipitous drop in blood pressure, which can produce brain ischemia. Because seizures cause blood pressure elevation, antiseizure agents are administered prophylactically. Stool softeners are used to prevent straining, which can also elevate the blood pressure.

SURGICAL MANAGEMENT

Many patients with a primary intracerebral hemorrhage are not treated surgically. However, surgical evacuation is strongly recommended for the patient with a cerebellar hemorrhage if the diameter exceeds 3 cm and the Glasgow Coma Scale score is below

14 (Qureshi et al., 2001). Surgical evacuation is most frequently accomplished via a craniotomy (see Chap. 61).

The patient with an intracranial aneurysm is prepared for surgical intervention as soon as the condition is considered stable. The Hunt-Hess classification system guides the physician in diagnosing the severity of subarachnoid hemorrhage after an aneurysm bleeds and in timing the surgery (see Table 62-6). Morbidity and mortality from surgery are high if the patient is stuporous or comatose (grade IV or V). Surgical treatment of the patient with an unruptured aneurysm is an option (Pfohman & Criddle, 2001).

The goal of surgery is to prevent bleeding in an unruptured aneurysm and further bleeding in an already ruptured aneurysm. This objective is accomplished by isolating the aneurysm from its circulation or by strengthening the arterial wall. An aneurysm may be excluded from the cerebral circulation by means of a ligature or a clip across its neck. If this is not anatomically possible, the aneurysm can be reinforced by wrapping it with muslin or some other substance to provide support and induce scarring.

An extracranial-intracranial arterial bypass may be performed to establish collateral blood supply to allow surgery on the aneurysm. Alternatively, an extracranial method may be used, whereby the carotid artery is gradually occluded in the neck to reduce pressure within the blood vessel. After ligation of the carotid artery, there is some risk for cerebral ischemia and sudden hemiplegia because during the surgical procedure, there is a temporary occlusion of the blood supply to the brain (unless a temporary bypass shunt is used). In anticipation of these complications, cerebral blood flow and internal carotid pressure may be measured to identify patients at risk for postoperative ischemic episodes.

Several less invasive endovascular treatments are now being used for aneurysms. These procedures are performed by neurosurgeons in neurointerventional radiology suites. Two procedures are endovascular treatment (occlusion of the parent artery) and aneurysm coiling (obstruction of the aneurysm site with a coil). While associated with lower risks than intracranial surgery in general, secondary stroke and rupture of the aneurysm are still potential complications (Pfohman & Criddle, 2001).

Postoperative complications include psychological symptoms (disorientation, amnesia, **Korsakoff's syndrome**, personality changes), intraoperative embolization, postoperative internal artery occlusion, fluid and electrolyte disturbances (from dysfunction of the neurohypophyseal system), and gastrointestinal bleeding.

NURSING PROCESS: THE PATIENT WITH A HEMORRHAGIC STROKE

Assessment

A complete neurologic assessment is performed initially and should include evaluation for the following:

- Altered level of consciousness
- Sluggish pupillary reaction
- Motor and sensory dysfunction
- Cranial nerve deficits (extraocular eye movements, facial droop, presence of ptosis)
- Speech difficulties and visual disturbance
- Headache and nuchal rigidity or other neurologic deficits

All patients should be monitored in the intensive care unit following an intracerebral hemorrhage (Qureshi et al., 2001). Neurologic assessment findings are documented and reported as indicated. The frequency of these assessments varies depending on the patient's condition. Any changes in the patient's condition require reassessment and thorough documentation; changes should be reported immediately.

Alteration in level of consciousness often is the earliest sign of deterioration in a patient with a hemorrhagic stroke. Because nurses have the most frequent contact with patients, they are in the best position to detect what may be subtle changes. Mild drowsiness and slight slurring of speech may be early signs that the level of consciousness is deteriorating. Frequent nursing assessment is crucial in the patient with known or suspected cerebral aneurysm.

Diagnosis

NURSING DIAGNOSES

Based on the assessment data, the patient's major nursing diagnoses may include the following:

- Ineffective cerebral tissue perfusion related to bleeding
- Disturbed sensory perception related to medically imposed restrictions (aneurysm precautions)
- Anxiety related to illness and/or medically imposed restrictions (aneurysm precautions)

COLLABORATIVE PROBLEMS/ POTENTIAL COMPLICATIONS

Based on the assessment data, potential complications that may develop include the following:

- Vasospasm
- Seizures
- Hydrocephalus
- Rebleeding

Planning and Goals

The goals for the patient may include improved cerebral tissue perfusion, relief of sensory and perceptual deprivation, relief of anxiety, and the absence of complications.

Nursing Interventions

OPTIMIZING CEREBRAL TISSUE PERFUSION

The patient is closely monitored for neurologic deterioration occurring from recurrent bleeding, increasing ICP, or vasospasm. A neurologic flow record is maintained. The blood pressure, pulse, level of responsiveness (an indicator of cerebral perfusion), pupillary responses, and motor function are checked hourly. Respiratory status is monitored because a reduction in oxygen in areas of the brain with impaired autoregulation increases the chances of a cerebral infarction. Any changes are reported immediately.

Implementing Aneurysm Precautions

Cerebral aneurysm precautions are implemented for the patient with a diagnosis of aneurysm to provide a nonstimulating environment, prevent increases in ICP pressure, and prevent further bleeding. The patient is placed on immediate and absolute bed rest in a quiet, nonstressful environment because activity, pain, and anxiety elevate the blood pressure, which increases the risk for bleeding. Visitors, except for family, are restricted.

The head of the bed is elevated 15 to 30 degrees to promote venous drainage and decrease ICP. Some neurologists, however, prefer that the patient remain flat to increase cerebral perfusion.

Any activity that suddenly increases the blood pressure or obstructs venous return is avoided. This includes the Valsalva manoeuvre, straining, forceful sneezing, pushing up in bed, acute flexion or rotation of the head and neck (which compromises the jugular veins), and cigarette smoking. Any activity requiring exertion is contraindicated. The patient is instructed to exhale through the mouth during voiding or defecation to decrease strain. No enemas are permitted, but stool softeners and mild laxatives are prescribed. Both prevent constipation, which would cause an increase in ICP, as would enemas. Dim lighting is helpful because photophobia (visual intolerance of light) is common. Coffee and tea, unless decaffeinated, are usually eliminated.

Thigh-high elastic compression stockings or sequential compression boots may be prescribed to decrease the incidence of deep vein thrombosis resulting from immobility. The legs are observed for signs and symptoms of deep vein thrombosis (tenderness, swelling, warmth, discolouration, positive Homans' sign), and abnormal findings are reported.

The nurse administers all personal care. The patient is fed and bathed to prevent any exertion that might raise the blood pressure. External stimuli are kept to a minimum, including no television, no radio, and no reading. Visitors are restricted in an effort to keep the patient as quiet as possible. This precaution must be individualized based on the patient's condition and response to visitors. A sign indicating this restriction should be placed on the door of the room, and the restrictions should be discussed with both patient and family. The purpose of aneurysm precautions should be thoroughly explained to both the patient (if possible) and family.

RELIEVING SENSORY DEPRIVATION AND ANXIETY

Sensory stimulation is kept to a minimum for patients on aneurysm precautions. For patients who are awake, alert, and oriented, an explanation of the restrictions helps reduce the patient's sense of isolation. Reality orientation is provided to help maintain orientation.

Keeping the patient well informed of the plan of care provides reassurance and helps minimize anxiety. Appropriate reassurance also helps relieve the patient's fears and anxiety. The family also requires information and support.

MONITORING AND MANAGING POTENTIAL COMPLICATIONS

Vasospasm

The patient is assessed for signs of possible vasospasm: intensified headaches, a decrease in level of responsiveness (confusion, disorientation, lethargy), or evidence of aphasia or partial paralysis. These signs may develop several days after surgery or on the initiation of treatment and must be reported immediately. If vasospasm is diagnosed, calcium-channel blockers or fluid volume expanders may be prescribed.

Seizures

Seizure precautions are maintained for every patient who may be at risk for seizure activity. Should a seizure occur, maintaining the airway and preventing injury are the primary goals. Medication

therapy is initiated at this time if not already prescribed. The medication of choice is phenytoin (Dilantin) because this agent usually provides adequate antiseizure action while causing no drowsiness at therapeutic levels.

Hydrocephalus

Blood in the subarachnoid space impedes the circulation of CSF, resulting in hydrocephalus. A CT scan that indicates dilated ventricles confirms the diagnosis. Hydrocephalus can occur within the first 24 hours (acute) after subarachnoid hemorrhage or days (subacute) to several weeks (delayed) later. Symptoms vary according to the time of onset and may be nonspecific. Acute hydrocephalus is characterized by sudden onset of stupor or coma and is managed with a ventriculostomy drain to decrease ICP. Symptoms of subacute and delayed hydrocephalus include gradual onset of drowsiness, behavioural changes, and ataxic gait. A ventriculoperitoneal shunt is surgically placed to treat chronic hydrocephalus. Changes in patient responsiveness are reported immediately.

Rebleeding

The rate of recurrent hemorrhage is approximately 2% following a primary intracerebral hemorrhage. Hypertension is the most serious risk factor, suggesting the importance of appropriate antihypertensive treatment (Qureshi et al., 2001).

Aneurysm rebleeding occurs most frequently in the first 2 weeks after the initial hemorrhage and is considered a major complication. Symptoms of rebleeding include sudden severe headache, nausea, vomiting, decreased level of consciousness, and neurologic deficit. A CT scan is performed to confirm rebleeding. Blood pressure is carefully maintained with medications. Antifibrinolytic medications (aminocaproic acid) may be administered to delay the lysis of the clot surrounding the rupture. The most effective preventive treatment is early clipping of the aneurysm if the patient is a candidate for surgery.

PROMOTING HOME AND COMMUNITY-BASED CARE

Teaching Patients Self-Care

The patient and family are provided with information that will enable them to cooperate with the care and restrictions required during the acute phase of hemorrhagic stroke and to prepare them to return home. Patient and family teaching includes information about the causes of hemorrhagic stroke and its possible consequences. In addition, the patient and family are informed about the medical treatments that are implemented, including surgical intervention if warranted, and the importance of interventions taken to prevent and detect complications (ie, aneurysm precautions, close monitoring of the patient). Depending on the presence and severity of neurologic impairment and other complications resulting from the stroke, the patient may be transferred to a rehabilitation unit or centre, where additional patient and family teaching will focus on strategies to regain ability to manage self-care. Teaching may also address the use of assistive devices or modification of the home environment to help the patient live with a disability. Modifications of the home may be required to provide a safe environment (Olson, 2001). (See Nursing Research Profile 62-2.)

Continuing Care

During the acute and rehabilitation phase of care for the patient with a hemorrhagic stroke, the focus is on obvious needs, issues, and deficits. The patient and family are reminded of the impor-

NURSING RESEARCH PROFILE 62-2
The Experience of Stroke for Eight African-American Elders

Eaves, Y. (2000). "What happened to me": Rural African American elders' experiences of stroke. *Journal of Neuro-science Nursing, 32*(1), 37–48.

Purpose
The rate of stroke is higher in African Americans compared to Caucasians, yet little is known about the subjective experiences of stroke in this group and their families. The purpose of this study was to examine the experience of stroke from the perspective of rural African-American elders and their family members.

Study Sample and Design
This descriptive, qualitative study was part of a larger study on caregiving. A purposive sample of eight African-American stroke survivors and their families participated. The survivors had each experienced a stroke in the preceding 4 months, were 55 years or older, and recently had been discharged from a rehabilitation centre. The qualitative method of descriptive narrative analysis was used to explain the stroke experience. Interactive audiotaped interviews and focused observations with written field notes took place in the home of each participant over several sessions. The qualitative text analysis software MARTIN was used for data analysis of the transcribed audiotaped interviews and written field notes.

Findings
The eight stroke survivors ranged in age from 56 to 79 years; primary caregivers ranged in age from 21 to 70 years and secondary caregivers ranged from 8 to 60 years. Five main themes were revealed in this study: (1) discovering stroke, (2) delaying treatment, (3) living with uncertainty, (4) discovering the impact of stroke, and (5) reconstructing life. Each of the five themes revealed at least two patterns; discovering stroke, for example, included stroke signs and explaining stroke. The findings revealed that several of the participants hid their stroke symptoms from family members and delayed seeking treatment for a prolonged time.

Nursing Implications
Nurses in acute care, home care, rehabilitation, and community settings involved with stroke patients and their families can use this information to better understand how African-American elders live through and respond to the experience of stroke. The identified themes of how, when, and why rural African-American elders seek treatment for stroke symptoms can assist nurses in educating this group about signs and symptoms of stroke, stroke prevention, and the emergent nature of stroke. This would permit the development of appropriate strategies to target this high-risk group.

---

tance of following recommendations to prevent further hemorrhagic stroke and keeping follow-up appointments with health care providers for monitoring. Referral for home care may be warranted to assess the home environment and the ability of the patient and to ensure that the patient and family are able to manage at home. The physical and psychological status of the patient and ability of the family to cope with any alterations in the patient's status are monitored during home visits. In addition, the nurse involved in home and continuing care needs to remind patients and family members of the need for continuing health promotion and screening practices. Patients who have not been involved in these practices in the past are educated about their importance and are referred to appropriate health care providers, if indicated. Chart 62-7 lists teaching points for the patient recovering from a stroke.

Evaluation

EXPECTED PATIENT OUTCOMES
Expected patient outcomes may include:

1. Demonstrates intact neurologic status and normal vital signs and respiratory patterns

---

Chart 62-7
Home Care Checklist • The Patient Recovering From A Stroke

At the completion of the home care instruction, the patient or caregiver will be able to:	Patient	Caregiver
• Discuss measures to prevent subsequent strokes.	✓	✓
• Identify signs and symptoms of specific complications.	✓	✓
• Identify potential complications and discuss measures to prevent them (blood clots, aspiration, pneumonia, urinary tract infection, fecal impaction, skin breakdown, contracture).	✓	✓
• Identify psychosocial consequences of stroke and appropriate interventions.	✓	✓
• Identify safety measures to prevent falls.	✓	✓
• State names, doses, indications, and side effects of medications.	✓	✓
• Demonstrate adaptive techniques for accomplishing ADLs.	✓	✓
• Demonstrate swallowing techniques (for patients with dysphagia).	✓	✓
• Demonstrate care of enteric feeding tube, if applicable.	✓	✓
• Demonstrate home exercises, use of splints or orthotics, proper positioning, and need for frequent repositioning.	✓	✓
• Describe procedures for maintaining skin integrity.	✓	✓
• Demonstrate indwelling catheter care, if applicable. Describe a bowel and bladder elimination program as appropriate.	✓	✓
• Identify appropriate recreational or diversional activities, support groups, and community resources.	✓	✓

a. Is alert and oriented to time, place, and person
b. Demonstrates normal speech patterns and intact cognitive processes
c. Demonstrates normal and equal strength, movement, and sensation of all four extremities
d. Exhibits normal deep tendon reflexes and pupillary responses
2. Demonstrates normal sensory perceptions
   a. States rationale for aneurysm precautions
   b. Exhibits clear thought processes
3. Exhibits reduced anxiety level
   a. Is less restless
   b. Exhibits absence of physiologic indicators of anxiety (eg, normal vital signs; normal respiratory rate; absence of excessive, fast speech)
4. Is free of complications
   a. Exhibits absence of vasospasm
   b. Exhibits normal vital signs and neuromuscular activity without seizures
   c. Verbalizes understanding of seizure precautions
   d. Exhibits normal mental status and normal motor and sensory status
   e. Reports no visual changes

Critical Thinking Exercises

1. Your patient had symptoms of an ischemic stroke approximately 2 hours ago and is undergoing a confirmatory CT scan in 30 minutes. You know t-PA must be administered within 3 hours of the symptoms. What actions would you take? What is your rationale for these actions?

2. Your patient has expressive aphasia following an ischemic stroke. How would you explain this phenomenon to the patient and family? Describe appropriate techniques for communicating with a patient with this type of aphasia.

3. Your patient is admitted with hemorrhagic stroke and exhibits homonymous hemianopsia. How would you explain this phenomenon to the patient and family? How would you modify your care for this patient? Describe ways that the patient and family may work together to compensate for this problem.

4. A 50-year-old patient is expected to be discharged to home today following a 5-day stay for an ischemic stroke. He tells you that he lives alone in a small apartment and knows none of his neighbours. He has some residual right-sided weakness. What teaching would be indicated to prevent another stroke? What resources may be needed to enable him to go home as scheduled?

REFERENCES AND SELECTED READINGS

Books

Agency for Health Care Policy and Research, Public Health Service. U.S. Department of Health and Human Services. (1995). *Post-stroke rehabilitation.* Clinical Practice Guideline. AHCPR Publication No. 95-0662. Rockville, MD.

American Heart Association. (2000). *American Heart Association heart and stroke 2000 statistical update.* Dallas: Author.

Cohen, S. (Ed.). (2000). *Management of ischemic stroke.* New York: McGraw-Hill.

Gretzky, W. (2003). *On family, hockey and healing.* Toronto: Seal Books.

Hickey, J. V. (2003). *The clinical practice of neurological and neurosurgical nursing* (5th ed.). Philadelphia: Lippincott Williams & Wilkins.

Lipski, M., & Alexander, C. (1997). *Sexual function in people with disability and chronic illness.* Gaithersburg, MD: Aspen.

Matchar, D. B., & Samsa, G. P. (2000). *Secondary and tertiary prevention of stroke.* Patient Outcomes Research Team (PORT) Final Report, Phase 1. (Prepared by Duke University Medical Center under Contract No. 290-91-0028). AHRQ Pub. No. 00-N001. Rockville, MD: Agency for Healthcare Research and Quality.

National Institute of Neurologic Disorders and Stroke. (1999). *Stroke: Hope through research.* NINDS Office of Communications and Public Liaison. NIH Pub. No. 99-2222. Bethesda, MD: National Institutes of Health.

Journals

Asterisks indicate nursing research articles.

Alberts, M., Hademenos, G., Latchaw, R., et al. (2000). Recommendations for the establishment of primary stroke centers. *Journal of the American Medical Association, 283*(23), 3102–3109.

Bahouth, M., & LaMonte, M. (2000). Update on stroke prevention and initial acute stroke management. *Primary Care Practice, 4*(6), 545–562.

Berges, S., et al. (2000). Seizures and epilepsy following strokes: Recurrence factors. *European Neurology, 43*(3), 3–8.

Bonnono, C., Criddle, L., et al. (2000). Emergi-paths and stroke teams: An emergency department approach to acute ischemic stroke. *Journal of Neuroscience Nursing, 32*(6), 298–305.

Brashear, A., Gordon, M., Elovic, E., et al. (2002). Intramuscular injection of botulinum toxin for the treatment of wrist and finger spasticity after a stroke. *New England Journal of Medicine, 347*(6), 395–400.

Demchuk, A., & Buchan, A. (2000). Predictors of stroke outcome. *Neurologic Clinics, 19*(2), 455–473.

*Eaves, Y. (2000). What happened to me: Rural African American elders' experiences of stroke. *Journal of Neuroscience Nursing, 32*(1), 37–48.

Evans, V. (2000). Herbs and the brain: Friend or foe? *Journal of Neuroscience Nursing, 32*(4), 229–232.

Heart and Stroke Foundation of Canada. (2002). *General information stroke statistics.* Available at: http://ww2.heartandstroke.ca/Page.asp?PageID=33&ArticleID=428&Src=stroke&From=SubCategory.

*Hinkle, J. L. (2001). A descriptive study of function in acute motor stroke. *Western Journal of Nursing Research, 23*(3), 296–312.

Hinkle, J. L. (2000). The use of the FIM instrument in the poststroke population. *Topics in Stroke Rehabilitation, 7*(3), 47–66.

Hock, N. H. (1999). Brain attack: The stroke continuum. *Nursing Clinics of North America, 34*(3), 689–715.

Iso, H., et al. (2001). Intake of fish and omega-3 fatty acids and risk of stroke in women. *Journal of American Medical Association, 285*(3), 304–312.

Kernan, W., Viscoli, C., Brass, L., et al. (2000). Phenylpropanolamine and the risk of hemorrhagic stroke. *New England Journal of Medicine, 343*(25), 1826–1832.

*King, B., Carlson, C., Shade-Zeldow, Y., et al. (2001). Transition to home care after stroke: Depression, physical health, and adaptive processes in support persons. *Research in Nursing & Health, 24*, 307–323.

Krenzer, M. (1999). Unplugging the mystery of carotid endarterectomy patient care. *Critical Care Nursing Clinics of North America, 11*(2), 189–208.

Lindsey, J. (2000). Implementing a stroke risk assessment program in a community setting. *Journal of Neuroscience Nursing, 32*(5), 266–270.

Manzella, S., & Galante, K. (2000). Establishment of stroke treatment plans: One hospital's experience. *Journal of Neuroscience Nursing, 32*(6), 306–310.

Mumma, C. (2001). Rehabilitation and rehabilitation nursing. *Critical Care Nursing Clinics of North America, 13*(3), 335–340.

National Institute of Neurologic Disorders and Stroke (NINDS) rt-PA Stroke Study Group. (1995). Tissue plasminogen activator for acute ischemic stroke. *New England Journal of Medicine, 333*(24), 1581–1587.

Olson, R. (2001). Community re-entry after critical illness. *Critical Care Nursing Clinics of North America, 13*(3), 449–461.

Petty, G. W., Brawn, R. D., Whisnant, J. P., et al. (2000). Ischemic stroke subtypes: A population-based study of functional outcome, survival, and recurrence. *Stroke, 31,* 1062–1068.

Pfohman, M., & Criddle, L. (2001). Epidemiology of intracranial aneurysm and subarachnoid hemorrhage. *Journal of Neuroscience Nursing, 33*(1), 39–41.

*Pilkington, F. B. (1999). A qualitative study of life after stroke. *Journal of Neuroscience Nursing, 31*(6), 336–347.

Qureshi, A., Tuhrim, S., Broderick, J., et al. (2001). Spontaneous intracerebral hemorrhage. *New England Journal of Medicine, 344*(19), 1450–1460.

Reed, S. (2000). Pharmacological therapy for acute stroke. *Current Opinion in Investigational Drugs, 1*(3), 329–339.

Robinson-Smith, G., Johnston, M. V., & Allen, J. (2000). Self-care, self-efficacy, quality of life, and depression after stroke. *Archives of Physical Medicine and Rehabilitation, 81,* 460–464.

Sarasin, F. P., Gaspoz, J. M., & Bounameaux, H. (2000). Cost-effectiveness of new antiplatelet regimens used as secondary prevention of stroke or transient ischemic attack. *Archives of Internal Medicine, 160*(18), 2773–2778.

Schievink, W. (2001). Spontaneous dissection of the carotid and vertebral arteries. *New England Journal of Medicine, 344*(12), 898–906.

Scroggins, N. (2000). Hemorrhagic disorders associated with thrombolytic therapy. *Critical Care Nursing Clinics of North America, 12*(3), 353–363.

Summers, D., Pyle, J., Stahl, M., & Hileman, J. (2000). The heart-brain connection. *Journal of Neuroscience Nursing, 32*(2), 108–116.

*Teel, C., Duncan, P., & Lai, S. (2001). Caregiving experiences after stroke. *Nursing Research, 50*(1), 53–60.

Vestergaard, K., Andersen, G., Gottrup, H., et al. (2001). Lamotrigine for central poststroke pain: A randomized controlled trial. *Neurology, 56*(2), 184–190.

Wolf, P., Clagett, P., Easton, D., et al. (1999). Preventing ischemic stroke in patients with prior stroke and transient ischemic attack. *Stroke, 30,* 1991–1884.

RESOURCES AND WEBSITES

Canadian Health Network; http://www.canadian-health-network.ca.
Canadian Stroke Network; http://www.canadianstrokenetwork.ca.
Health Canada; http://www.hc-sc.gc.ca.
Internet Stroke Center; http://www.strokecenter.org/pat/stats.htm.
Public Health Agency of Canada; http://www.phac-aspc.gc.ca.

Management of Patients With Neurologic Trauma

Adapted by Sue Young

On completion of this chapter, the learner will be able to:

1. Differentiate among patients with head injuries according to mechanism of injury, clinical signs and symptoms, diagnostic testing, and treatment options.

2. Describe the nursing management of head-injured patients.

3. Use the nursing process as a framework for care of patients with brain injury.

4. Identify the population at risk for spinal cord injury.

5. Describe three clinical features of the patient with neurogenic shock.

6. Discuss the pathophysiology of autonomic dysreflexia and describe the appropriate nursing interventions.

7. Use the nursing process as a framework for care of patients with spinal cord injury.

*T*rauma involving the central nervous system can be life-threatening. Even if not life-threatening, brain and spinal cord injury may result in major physical and psychological dysfunction and can alter the patient's life completely. Neurologic trauma affects the patient, the family, the health care system, and society as a whole because of its major sequelae and the costs of acute and long-term care of patients with trauma to the brain and spinal cord.

Head Injuries

Head injury is a broad classification that includes injury to the scalp, skull, or brain. It is the most common cause of death from trauma in Canada. Approximately 150,000 people receive treatment for head injuries every year. Traumatic brain injury is the most serious form of head injury. The most common causes of traumatic brain injury are motor vehicle crashes, violence, and falls. Groups at highest risk for traumatic brain injury are persons age 15 to 19 years and males, who suffer traumatic brain injury at a rate almost twice that of females. The very young (under 5) and the very old (over 75) are also at increased risk. (Canadian Institute for Health Information, 2006). The best approach to head injury is prevention (Chart 63-1).

Pathophysiology

Research suggests that not all brain damage occurs at the moment of impact. Damage to the brain from traumatic injury takes two forms: primary injury and **secondary injury**. Primary injury is the initial damage to the brain that results from the traumatic event. This may include contusions, lacerations, and torn blood vessels from impact, acceleration/deceleration, or foreign object penetration (Blank-Reid & Reid, 2000; Porth, 2002). Secondary injury evolves over the ensuing hours and days after the initial injury and is due primarily to brain swelling or ongoing bleeding.

An injured brain is different from other injured body areas due to its unique characteristics. It resides within the skull, which is a rigid closed compartment (Bader & Palmer, 2000). Unlike an injured ankle, in which the covering skin expands with swelling, the confines of the skull do not allow for the expansion of cranial con-

tents. Thus, any bleeding or swelling within the skull increases the volume of contents within a container of fixed size and so can cause increased intracranial pressure (ICP) (see Chap. 61). If the increased pressure is high enough, it can cause a downward or lateral displacement of the brain through or against the rigid structures of the skull. This causes restriction of blood flow to the brain, decreasing oxygen delivery and waste removal. Cells within the brain become anoxic and cannot metabolize properly, producing ischemia, infarction, irreversible brain damage, and eventually brain death (Fig. 63-1).

SCALP INJURY

Isolated scalp trauma is generally classified as a minor head injury. Because its many blood vessels constrict poorly, the scalp bleeds profusely when injured. Trauma may result in an abrasion (brush wound), contusion, laceration, or hematoma beneath the layers of tissue of the scalp (subgaleal hematoma). Large avulsions (tear-

Chart 63-1 **Head and Spinal Cord Injury Prevention**

The most effective treatment for brain and spinal cord injury is prevention. To decrease the incidence of these devastating and catastrophic injuries, the following steps should be taken:
- Drivers should obey traffic laws, particularly not speeding or driving when under the influence of drugs or alcohol.
- All drivers and passengers should wear seat belts and shoulder harnesses. Children under 12 should be restrained in an age/size-appropriate system in the back seat.
- Passengers should not ride in the back of pick-up trucks.
- Motorcyclists, scooters, bicyclists, skateboarders, and roller skaters should wear helmets.
- Educational programs should be directed toward violence and suicide prevention in the community.
- Water safety instruction should be provided.
- Steps should be taken to prevent falls, particularly in the elderly.
- Athletes should use protective devices; coaches should be educated in proper coaching techniques.
- Owners of firearms should keep them locked in a secure area where children cannot access them.

Glossary

autonomic dysreflexia: a life-threatening emergency in spinal cord injury patients that causes a hypertensive emergency; also called autonomic hyperreflexia

brain injury: an injury to the skull or brain that is severe enough to interfere with normal functioning

brain injury, closed (blunt): occurs when the head accelerates and then rapidly decelerates or collides with another object and brain tissue is damaged, but there is no opening through the skull and dura

brain injury, open: occurs when an object penetrates the skull, enters the brain, and damages the soft brain tissue in its path (penetrating injury), or when blunt trauma to the head is so severe that it opens the scalp, skull, and dura to expose the brain

concussion: a temporary loss of neurologic function with no apparent structural damage to the brain

contusion: bruising of the brain surface

complete spinal cord lesion: a condition that involves total loss of sensation and voluntary muscle control below the lesion

halo vest: a lightweight vest with an attached halo that stabilizes the cervical spine

incomplete spinal cord lesion: a condition where there is preservation of the sensory or motor fibres, or both, below the lesion

neurogenic bladder: bladder dysfunction that results from a disorder or dysfunction of the nervous system; may result in either urinary retention or bladder overactivity

paraplegia: paralysis of the lower extremities with dysfunction of the bowel and bladder from a lesion in the thoracic, lumbar, or sacral regions of the spinal cord

quadriplegia (tetraplegia): paralysis of both arms and legs, with dysfunction of bowel and bladder from a lesion of the cervical segments of the spinal cord

secondary injury: an insult to the brain subsequent to the original traumatic event

spinal cord injury (SCI): an injury to the spinal cord, vertebral column, supporting soft tissue, or intervertebral disks caused by trauma

transection: severing of the spinal cord itself; transection can be complete (all the way through the cord) or incomplete (partially through)

Physiology/Pathophysiology

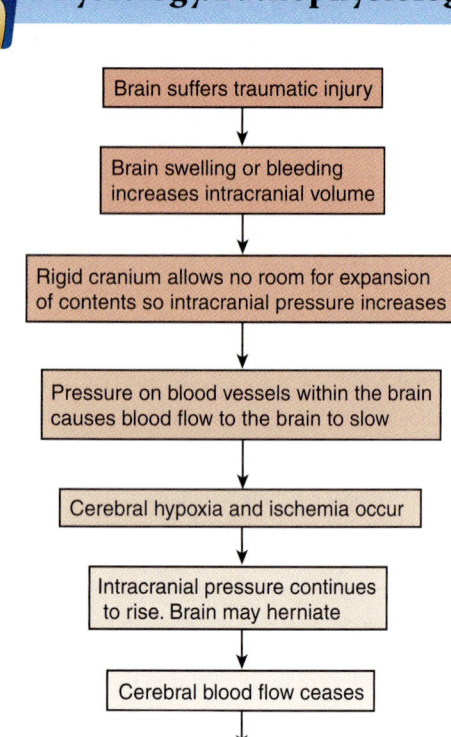

```
Brain suffers traumatic injury
          ↓
Brain swelling or bleeding
increases intracranial volume
          ↓
Rigid cranium allows no room for expansion
of contents so intracranial pressure increases
          ↓
Pressure on blood vessels within the brain
causes blood flow to the brain to slow
          ↓
Cerebral hypoxia and ischemia occur
          ↓
Intracranial pressure continues
to rise. Brain may herniate
          ↓
Cerebral blood flow ceases
          ↓
Neurologic death
```

FIGURE 63-1 Pathophysiology of traumatic brain injury.

FIGURE 63-2 Basilar fractures allow cerebrospinal fluid to leak from the nose and ears. Adapted from Hickey, J. V. (2003). *The clinical practice of neurological and neurosurgical nursing* (5th ed.). Philadelphia: Lippincott Williams & Wilkins.

ing away from a structure) of the scalp may be potentially life-threatening and are true emergencies. Diagnosis of any scalp injury is based on physical examination, inspection, and palpation. Scalp wounds are potential portals of entry of organisms that cause intracranial infections. Therefore, the area is irrigated before the laceration is sutured to remove foreign material and to reduce the risk for infection. Subgaleal hematomas (hematomas below the outer covering of the skull) usually absorb on their own and do not require any specific treatment.

SKULL FRACTURES

A skull fracture is a break in the continuity of the skull caused by forceful trauma. It may occur with or without damage to the brain. Skull fractures are classified as linear, comminuted, depressed, or basilar. A fracture may be open, indicating a scalp laceration or tear in the dura (eg, from a bullet or an ice pick), or closed, in which the dura is intact (Fig. 63-2).

Clinical Manifestations

The symptoms, apart from those of the local injury, depend on the severity and the distribution of brain injury. Persistent, localized pain usually suggests that a fracture is present. Fractures of the cranial vault may or may not produce swelling in the region of the fracture; therefore, an x-ray is needed for diagnosis.

Fractures of the base of the skull (basal skull fractures) tend to traverse the paranasal sinus of the frontal bone or the middle ear located in the temporal bone (see Fig. 63-2). Thus, they frequently produce hemorrhage from the nose, pharynx, or ears, and blood may appear under the conjunctiva. An area of ecchymosis (bruis-

ing) may be seen over the mastoid (Battle's sign). Basal skull fractures are suspected when cerebrospinal fluid escapes from the ears (CSF otorrhea) and the nose (CSF rhinorrhea). A halo sign (a blood stain surrounded by a yellowish stain) may be seen on bed linens or the head dressing and is highly suggestive of a CSF leak. Drainage of CSF is a serious problem because meningeal infection can occur if organisms gain access to the cranial contents through the nose, ear, or sinus through a tear in the dura. Bloody CSF suggests a brain laceration or contusion.

Assessment and Diagnostic Findings

Although a rapid physical examination and evaluation of neurologic status detect the more obvious brain injuries, a computed tomography (CT) scan can detect less apparent abnormalities by the degree to which the soft tissue absorbs the x-rays. It is a fast, accurate, and safe diagnostic study that shows the presence, nature, location, and extent of acute lesions. It is also helpful in the ongoing management of patients with head injury as it can disclose cerebral edema, contusion, intracerebral or extracerebral hematoma, subarachnoid and intraventricular hemorrhage, and late changes (infarction, hydrocephalus). Magnetic resonance imaging (MRI) is used to evaluate patients with head injury when a more accurate picture of the anatomic nature of the injury is warranted and when the patient is stable enough to undergo this longer diagnostic study.

Cerebral angiography may also be used; it identifies supratentorial, extracerebral, and intracerebral hematomas and cerebral contusions. Lateral and anteroposterior views of the skull are obtained.

Medical Management

Nondepressed skull fractures generally do not require surgical treatment; however, close observation of the patient is essential. Nursing personnel may observe the patient in the hospital, but if no underlying brain injury is present, the patient may be allowed to return home. If the patient is discharged home, specific instructions (see the section on concussions below) must be given to the family. Many depressed skull fractures are managed conservatively; only contaminated or deforming fractures require surgery.

If surgery is necessary, the scalp is clipped and cleansed with copious amounts of saline to remove debris. The fracture is then exposed. After the skull fragments are elevated, the area is débrided. Large defects can be repaired immediately with bone or artificial grafts; if significant cerebral edema is present, repair of the defect can be delayed for 3 to 6 months. Penetrating wounds require surgical débridement to remove foreign bodies and devitalized brain tissue and to control hemorrhage (Blank-Reid & Reid, 2000). Antibiotic treatment is instituted immediately, and blood component therapy is administered if indicated.

As stated previously, fractures of the base of the skull are serious because they are usually open (involving the paranasal sinuses or middle or external ear) and result in CSF leakage. The nasopharynx and the external ear should be kept clean. Usually a piece of sterile cotton is placed loosely in the ear, or a sterile cotton pad may be taped loosely under the nose or against the ear to collect the draining fluid. The patient who is conscious is cautioned against sneezing or blowing the nose. The head is elevated 30 degrees to reduce ICP and promote spontaneous closure of the leak (Sullivan, 2000), although some neurosurgeons prefer that the bed be kept flat. Persistent CSF rhinorrhea or otorrhea usually requires surgical intervention.

Brain Injury

The most important consideration in any head injury is whether or not the brain is injured. Even seemingly minor injury can cause significant brain damage secondary to obstructed blood flow and decreased tissue perfusion. The brain cannot store oxygen and glucose to any significant degree. Because the cerebral cells need an uninterrupted blood supply to obtain these nutrients, irreversible brain damage and cell death occur when the blood supply is interrupted for even a few minutes. Clinical manifestations of **brain injury** are listed in Chart 63-2. **Closed (blunt) brain injury** occurs when the head accelerates and then rapidly decelerates or collides with another object (eg, a wall or dashboard of a car) and brain tissue is damaged, but there is no opening through the skull and dura. **Open brain injury** occurs when an object penetrates the skull, enters the brain, and damages the soft brain tissue in its path (penetrating injury), or when blunt trauma to the head is so severe that it opens the scalp, skull, and dura to expose the brain.

Concussion

A cerebral **concussion** after head injury is a temporary loss of neurologic function with no apparent structural damage. A concussion generally involves a period of unconsciousness lasting

Chart 63-2 · Clinical Manifestations of Brain Injury

- Altered level of consciousness
- Confusion
- Pupillary abnormalities (changes in shape, size, and response to light)
- Altered or absent gag reflex
- Absent corneal reflex
- Sudden onset of neurologic deficits (eg, motor weakness or absence)
- Changes in vital signs (altered respiratory pattern, hypertension, bradycardia, tachycardia, hypothermia or hyperthermia)
- Vision and hearing impairment
- Sensory dysfunction
- Spasticity
- Headache
- Vertigo
- Movement disorders
- Seizures
- Behavioural changes

from a few seconds to a few minutes. The jarring of the brain may be so slight as to cause only dizziness and spots before the eyes ("seeing stars"), or it may be severe enough to cause complete loss of consciousness for a time. If the brain tissue in the frontal lobe is affected, the patient may exhibit bizarre irrational behaviour, whereas involvement of the temporal lobe can produce temporary amnesia or disorientation.

The patient may be hospitalized overnight for observation or discharged from the hospital in a relatively short time after a concussion. Treatment involves observing the patient for headache, dizziness, lethargy, irritability, and anxiety. The occurrence of these symptoms after injury is referred to as postconcussion syndrome (PCS). Giving the patient information, explanations, and encouragement may reduce some of the problems of postconcussion syndrome. The patient is advised to resume normal activities slowly, and the family is instructed to observe for the following signs and symptoms and to notify the physician or clinic (or bring the patient to the emergency department) if they occur:

- Difficulty in awakening
- Difficulty in speaking
- Confusion
- Severe headache
- Vomiting
- Weakness of one side of the body

A concussion was once thought of as a minor head injury without significant sequelae. However, studies have demonstrated that there are often disturbing and sometimes residual effects, including headache, lethargy, personality and behaviour changes, attention deficits, difficulty with memory, and disruption in work habits (Ponsford et al., 1999). For example, a late or persistent PCS may persist for more than 6 months (Evans, 2004).

Gerontologic Considerations

Elderly patients must be assessed very carefully. Even given similar mechanisms of injury, an elderly person will often suffer more severe injury than a young person and will often recover more slowly and with more complications (Perdue et al., 1998). The elderly patient with confusion or behavioural disturbances should be assessed for head injury, because unrecognized "minor" head trauma may account for behavioural and confusional episodes in some elderly people (Walshaw, 2000). A misdiagnosed or untreated episode of confusion in an elderly patient may result in long-term disability that might have been avoided if the injury had been detected and treated promptly.

Contusion

Cerebral **contusion** is a more severe injury in which the brain is bruised, with possible surface hemorrhage. The patient is unconscious for more than a few seconds or minutes. Clinical signs and symptoms depend on the size of the contusion and the amount of associated cerebral edema. The patient may lie motionless, with a faint pulse, shallow respirations, and cool, pale skin. Often there is involuntary evacuation of the bowels and the bladder. The patient may be aroused with effort but soon slips back into unconsciousness. The blood pressure and the temperature are subnormal, and the picture is somewhat similar to that of shock.

In general, patients with severe brain injury who have abnormal motor function, abnormal eye movements, and elevated ICP have poor outcomes—that is, brain damage, disability, or death. Conversely, the patient may recover consciousness but pass into a stage of cerebral irritability. In this stage, the patient is conscious and easily disturbed by any form of stimulation such as noises, light, and voices; he or she may become hyperactive at times. Gradually, the pulse, respirations, temperature, and other body functions return to normal, but full recovery can be delayed for months. Residual headache and vertigo are common, and impaired mental function or seizures may occur as a result of irreparable cerebral damage.

Diffuse Axonal Injury

Diffuse axonal injury involves widespread damage to axons in the cerebral hemispheres, corpus callosum, and brain stem. It can be seen in mild, moderate, or severe head trauma and results in axonal swelling and disconnection (Porth, 2002). Clinically, with severe injury, the patient has no lucid intervals and experiences immediate coma, decorticate and decerebrate posturing (see Fig. 61-1 in Chap. 61 and discussion in Chap. 60), and global cerebral edema. Diagnosis is made by clinical signs in conjunction with a CT scan or MRI. Recovery depends on the severity of the axonal injury. Thirty-five percent of deaths from traumatic brain injury are caused by diffuse anoxal injury (Hickey, 2003).

Intracranial Hemorrhage

Hematomas (collections of blood) that develop within the cranial vault are the most serious brain injuries (Porth, 2002). A hematoma may be epidural (above the dura), subdural (below the dura), or intracerebral (within the brain) (Fig. 63-3). Major symptoms are frequently delayed until the hematoma is large enough to cause distortion of the brain and increased ICP. The signs and symptoms of cerebral ischemia resulting from the compression by a hematoma are variable and depend on the speed with which vital areas are affected and the area that is injured. In general, a rapidly developing hematoma, even if small, may be fatal, whereas a larger but slowly developing collection of blood may allow compensation for increases in ICP.

EPIDURAL HEMATOMA (EXTRADURAL HEMATOMA OR HEMORRHAGE)

After a head injury, blood may collect in the epidural (extradural) space between the skull and the dura. This can result from a skull fracture that causes a rupture or laceration of the middle meningeal artery, the artery that runs between the dura and the skull inferior to a thin portion of temporal bone. Hemorrhage from this artery causes rapid pressure on the brain.

Symptoms are caused by the expanding hematoma. Usually, there is a momentary loss of consciousness at the time of injury, followed by an interval of apparent recovery (lucid interval). Although the lucid interval is considered a classic characteristic of an epidural hematoma, no lucid interval has been reported in many patients with this lesion (Servadei, 1997), and thus it should not be considered a critical defining criterion. During the lucid interval, compensation for the expanding hematoma takes place by rapid absorption of CSF and decreased intravascular volume, both of which help maintain a normal ICP. When these mechanisms can no longer compensate, even a small increase in the volume of the blood clot produces a marked elevation in ICP. Then, often suddenly, signs of compression appear (usually deterioration of consciousness and signs of focal neurologic deficits such as dilation and fixation of a pupil or paralysis of an extremity), and the patient deteriorates rapidly.

An epidural hematoma is considered an extreme emergency; marked neurologic deficit or even respiratory arrest can occur within minutes. Treatment consists of making openings through the skull (burr holes) to decrease ICP emergently, remove the clot, and control the bleeding. A craniotomy may be required to remove the clot and control the bleeding. A drain is usually inserted after creation of burr holes or a craniotomy to prevent reaccumulation of blood.

SUBDURAL HEMATOMA

A subdural hematoma is a collection of blood between the dura and the brain, a space normally occupied by a thin cushion of fluid. The most common cause of subdural hematoma is trauma, but it may also occur from coagulopathies or rupture of an aneurysm. A subdural hemorrhage is more frequently venous in

Subdural hematoma

Intracerebral hematoma

Epidural hematoma

FIGURE 63-3 Locations of intracranial hemorrhages.

origin and is due to the rupture of small vessels that bridge the subdural space. A subdural hematoma may be acute, subacute, or chronic, depending on the size of the involved vessel and the amount of bleeding present.

Acute and Subacute Subdural Hematoma.
Acute subdural hematomas are associated with major head injury involving contusion or laceration. Clinical symptoms develop over 24 to 48 hours. Signs and symptoms include changes in the level of consciousness (LOC), pupillary signs, and hemiparesis. There may be minor or even no symptoms with small collections of blood. Coma, increasing blood pressure, decreasing heart rate, and slowing respiratory rate are all signs of a rapidly expanding mass requiring immediate intervention.

Subacute subdural hematomas are the result of less severe contusions and head trauma. Clinical manifestations usually appear between 48 hours and 2 weeks after the injury. Signs and symptoms are similar to those of an acute subdural hematoma.

If the patient can be transported rapidly to the hospital, an immediate craniotomy is performed to open the dura, allowing the subdural clot to be evacuated. Successful outcome also depends on the control of ICP and careful monitoring of respiratory function (see "The Patient Undergoing Intracranial Surgery" in Chap. 61). The mortality rate for patients with acute and subacute subdural hematomas is high because of associated brain damage.

Chronic Subdural Hematoma.
Chronic subdural hematomas can develop from seemingly minor head injuries and are seen most frequently in the elderly. The elderly are prone to this type of head injury secondary to brain atrophy, which is an expected consequence of the aging process. Seemingly minor head trauma may produce enough impact to shift the brain contents abnormally. The time between injury and onset of symptoms may be lengthy (eg, 3 weeks to months), so the actual insult may be forgotten.

A chronic subdural hematoma resembles other conditions and may be mistaken for a stroke. The bleeding is less profuse and there is compression of the intracranial contents. The blood within the brain changes in character in 2 to 4 days, becoming thicker and darker. In a few weeks, the clot breaks down and has the colour and consistency of motor oil. Eventually, calcification or ossification of the clot takes place. The brain adapts to this foreign body invasion, and the clinical signs and symptoms fluctuate. There may be severe headache, which tends to come and go; alternating focal neurologic signs; personality changes; mental deterioration; and focal seizures. Unfortunately, the patient may be labelled neurotic or psychotic if the cause of the symptoms is overlooked.

The treatment of a chronic subdural hematoma consists of surgical evacuation of the clot. The procedure may be carried out through multiple burr holes, or a craniotomy may be performed for a sizable subdural mass that cannot be suctioned or drained through burr holes.

INTRACEREBRAL HEMORRHAGE AND HEMATOMA
Intracerebral hemorrhage is bleeding into the substance of the brain. It is commonly seen in head injuries when force is exerted to the head over a small area (missile injuries or bullet wounds; stab injury). These hemorrhages within the brain may also result from systemic hypertension, which causes degeneration and rupture of a vessel; rupture of a saccular aneurysm; vascular anomalies; intracranial tumours; systemic causes, including bleeding

disorders such as leukemia, hemophilia, aplastic anemia, and thrombocytopenia; and complications of anticoagulant therapy. Nontraumatic causes of intracerebral hemorrhage are discussed in Chapter 62.

The onset may be insidious, beginning with the development of neurologic deficits followed by headache. Management includes supportive care, control of ICP, and careful administration of fluids, electrolytes, and antihypertensive medications. Surgical intervention by craniotomy or craniectomy permits removal of the blood clot and control of hemorrhage but may not be possible because of the inaccessible location of the bleeding or the lack of a clearly circumscribed area of blood that can be removed.

Management of Brain Injuries

Assessment and diagnosis of the extent of injury are accomplished by the initial physical and neurologic examinations. CT and MRI are the primary neuroimaging diagnostic tools and are useful in evaluating soft tissue injuries. Positron emission tomography (PET scan) is available in some trauma centres; this method of scanning examines brain function rather than structure. A flowchart developed by the Brain Trauma Foundation for the initial management of brain-injured patients is presented in Figure 63-4 (Brain Trauma Foundation, 2000).

Any individual with a head injury is presumed to have a cervical spine injury until proven otherwise. From the scene of the injury, the patient is transported on a board with the head and neck maintained in alignment with the axis of the body. A cervical collar should be applied and maintained until cervical spine x-rays have been obtained and the absence of cervical spinal cord injury documented. Special precautions should be taken when turning and positioning the patient until the absence of spinal cord injury is confirmed.

All therapy is directed toward preserving brain homeostasis and preventing secondary brain injury. "Secondary injury" is a term used to describe injury to the brain subsequent to the original traumatic event (Bader & Palmer, 2000). Common causes of secondary injury are cerebral edema, hypotension, and respiratory depression that may lead to hypoxemia and electrolyte imbalance. Treatments to prevent this include stabilization of cardiovascular and respiratory function to maintain adequate cerebral perfusion, control of hemorrhage and hypovolemia, and maintenance of optimal blood gas values (Wong, 2000).

TREATMENT OF INCREASED INTRACRANIAL PRESSURE
As the damaged brain swells with edema or as blood collects within the brain, a rise in ICP occurs; this requires aggressive treatment. See Chapter 61 for a discussion of the relationship of ICP to cerebral perfusion pressure (CPP). If the ICP remains elevated, it can decrease the CPP. Initial management is based on the principle of preventing secondary injury and maintaining adequate cerebral oxygenation (see Fig. 63-4).

Surgery is required for evacuation of blood clots, débridement and elevation of depressed fractures of the skull, and suture of severe scalp lacerations. ICP is monitored closely; if increased, it is managed by maintaining adequate oxygenation, elevating the head of the bed, and maintaining normal blood volume. Devices to monitor ICP or drain CSF can be inserted during surgery or at the bedside using aseptic technique. The patient is cared for in the intensive care unit, where expert nursing care and medical treatment are readily available.

Initial management

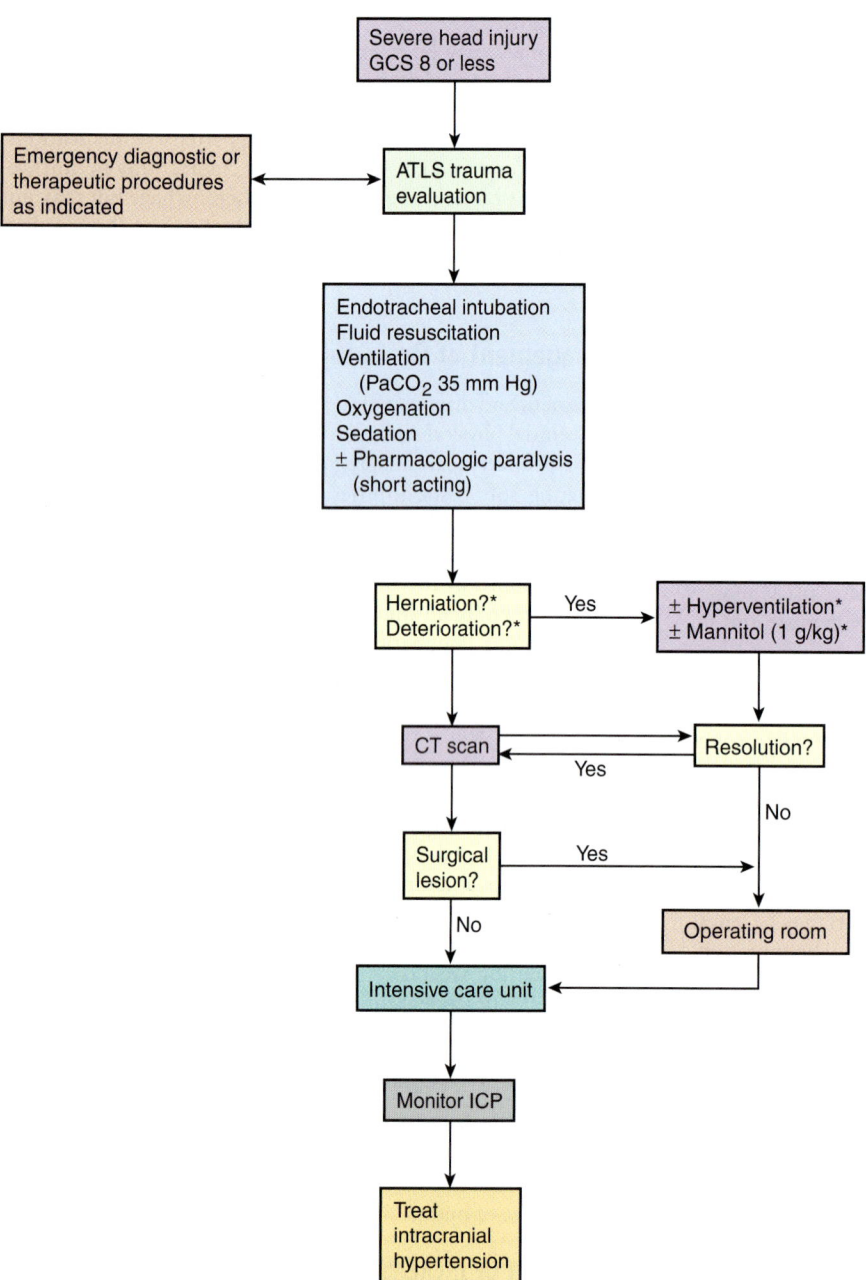

* Only in the presence of signs of herniation or progressive neurologic deterioration not
  attributable to extracranial factors
  (ATLS = Advanced Trauma Life Support).

FIGURE 63-4 Initial management of the severe head injury patient (treatment option). Copyright © 1998 Brain Trauma Foundation, Inc.

SUPPORTIVE MEASURES

Treatment also includes ventilatory support, seizure prevention, fluid and electrolyte maintenance, nutritional support, and pain and anxiety management. Comatose patients are intubated and mechanically ventilated to ensure adequate oxygenation and protect the airway.

Because seizures are common after head injury and can cause secondary brain damage from hypoxia, antiseizure agents may be administered. If the patient is very agitated, benzodiazepines may be prescribed to calm him or her without decreasing LOC. These medications do not affect ICP or CPP, making them good choices for the head-injured patient.

A nasogastric tube may be inserted because reduced gastric motility and reverse peristalsis are associated with head injury, making regurgitation and aspiration common in the first few hours.

NEUROLOGIC DEATH

When a patient has sustained a severe head injury incompatible with life, the physician may conduct a clinical examination to confirm neurologic determination of death (NDD) and assist in the process of organ procurement. In neurologic death, the patient has no neurologic activity upon clinical examination; adjunctive tests such as EEG and cerebral blood flow (CBF) studies are often used to confirm NDD (Lovasik, 2000). Once NDD has been confirmed, many of these patients are potential organ donors; the nurse may provide information to the family, and, in collaboration with the physician and the organ donor coordinator, assist them with the decision-making process about donation.

NURSING PROCESS:
THE PATIENT WITH A BRAIN INJURY

Assessment

Depending on the patient's neurologic status, the nurse may elicit information from the patient, family, or witnesses or from emergency rescue personnel (Munro, 2000). Although it may not be possible to obtain all usual baseline data initially, the immediate health history should include the following questions:

- When did the injury occur?
- What caused the injury? A high-velocity missile? An object striking the head? A fall?
- What was the direction and force of the blow?

Since a history of unconsciousness or amnesia after a head injury indicates a significant degree of brain damage, and since changes that occur minutes to hours after the initial injury can reflect recovery or indicate the development of secondary brain damage, the nurse should try to determine if there was a loss of consciousness, what the duration of the unconscious period was, and if the patient could be aroused.

In addition to questions that establish the nature of the injury and the patient's condition immediately after the injury, the nurse should examine the patient thoroughly. This assessment should include determining the patient's LOC, ability to respond to verbal commands (if conscious), response to tactile stimuli

(if unconscious), pupillary response to light, status of corneal and gag reflexes, motor function, and Glasgow Coma Scale score (Chart 63-4).

Additional detailed neurologic and systems assessments are made initially and at frequent intervals throughout the acute phase of care (Dibsie, 1998). The baseline and ongoing assessments are critical nursing interventions for the brain-injured patient, whose condition can worsen dramatically and irrevocably if subtle signs are overlooked. More information on assessment is provided below and in Figure 63-5 and Table 63-1.

Diagnosis

NURSING DIAGNOSES
Based on the assessment data, the patient's major nursing diagnoses may include the following:

- Ineffective airway clearance and impaired gas exchange related to brain injury
- Ineffective cerebral tissue perfusion related to increased ICP and decreased CPP
- Deficient fluid volume related to decreased LOC and hormonal dysfunction
- Imbalanced nutrition, less than body requirements, related to metabolic changes, fluid restriction, and inadequate intake
- Risk for injury (self-directed and directed at others) related to seizures, disorientation, restlessness, or brain damage
- Risk for imbalanced (increased) body temperature related to damaged temperature-regulating mechanism
- Potential for impaired skin integrity related to bed rest, hemiparesis, hemiplegia, and immobility
- Disturbed thought processes (deficits in intellectual function, communication, memory, information processing) related to brain injury
- Potential for disturbed sleep pattern related to brain injury and frequent neurologic checks
- Potential for compromised family coping related to unresponsiveness of patient, unpredictability of outcome, pro-

---

Chart 63-4 Glasgow Coma Scale

The Glasgow Coma Scale is a tool for assessing a patient's response to stimuli. Scores range from 3 (deep coma) to 15 (normal).

Eye opening response	Spontaneous	4
	To voice	3
	To pain	2
	None	1
Best verbal response	Oriented	5
	Confused	4
	Inappropriate words	3
	Incomprehensible sounds	2
	None	1
Best motor response	Obeys command	6
	Localizes pain	5
	Withdraws	4
	Flexion	3
	Extension	2
	None	1
Total		3 to 15

Chart 63-3 • Ethics and Related Issues

What If a Family Does Not Want Life Support Stopped?

Situation
A 16-year-old involved in a motor vehicle crash suffered a severe closed head injury. Extensive medical tests have determined conclusively that he is brain dead. He remains in the ICU on a mechanical ventilator with multiple medications to keep his heart beating. The patient's medical condition and ultimate physical death cannot be prevented by any medical interventions, yet the family refuses to discontinue any of the medical treatments, hoping for a "miracle."

Dilemma
The family's wish to continue care for their son conflicts with the medical reality of the patient's condition.

Discussion
What arguments could you make in favour of the family's position to continue life support? What arguments could you make in favour of withdrawal of life support?

FIGURE 63-5 Assessment parameters for the patient with a head injury include (**A**) eye opening and responsiveness, (**B**) vital signs, and (**C, D**) motor response reflected in hand strength or response to painful stimulus. Photo © B. Proud.

longed recovery period, and the patient's residual physical and emotional deficit
- Deficient knowledge about recovery and the rehabilitation process

The nursing diagnoses for the unconscious patient and the patient with increased ICP also apply (see Chap. 61).

COLLABORATIVE PROBLEMS/ POTENTIAL COMPLICATIONS

Based on all the assessment data, the major complications include the following:

- Decreased cerebral perfusion
- Cerebral edema and herniation
- Impaired oxygenation and ventilation
- Impaired fluid, electrolyte, and nutritional balance
- Risk of post-traumatic seizures

Planning and Goals

The goals for the patient may include maintenance of a patent airway, adequate CPP, fluid and electrolyte balance, adequate nutritional status, prevention of secondary injury, maintenance of normal body temperature, maintenance of skin integrity, improvement of cognitive function, prevention of sleep deprivation, effective family coping, increased knowledge about the rehabilitation process, and absence of complications.

Nursing Interventions

The nursing interventions for the patient with a head injury are extensive and diverse; they include making nursing assessments, setting priorities for nursing interventions, anticipating needs and complications, and initiating rehabilitation.

MONITORING FOR DECLINING NEUROLOGIC FUNCTION

The importance of ongoing assessment and monitoring of the brain-injured patient cannot be overstated. The following parameters are assessed initially and as frequently as the patient's condition requires. As soon as the initial assessment is made, the use of a neurologic flow chart is started and maintained.

Level of Consciousness

The LOC is regularly assessed because changes in it precede all other changes in vital and neurologic signs. The Glasgow Coma Scale, which is used to assess LOC, is based on the three criteria of eye opening, verbal responses, and motor responses to verbal commands or painful stimuli. It is particularly useful for monitoring changes during the acute phase, the first few days after a head injury. It does not take the place of an in-depth neurologic assessment; rather, it is used to monitor the patient's motor, verbal, and eye-opening responses. The patient's best responses to predetermined stimuli are recorded (see Chart 63-4). Each response is scored (the greater the number the better the functioning), and the sum of these scores

Table 63-1 • Summary of Multisystem Assessment Measures for the Severely Brain-Injured Patient

SYSTEM-SPECIFIC CONSIDERATIONS	ASSESSMENT DATA
Neurologic System • Severe head injury will result in unconsciousness and will alter many neurologic functions. • All body functions must be supported. • Increased ICP and herniation syndromes are life-threatening • Measures are instituted to control elevated ICP.	• Assessment of neurologic signs • Assessment for signs and symptoms of ICP elevation • Calculation of cerebral perfusion pressure if ICP monitor is in place • Monitoring of antiseizure medication blood levels
Integumentary System (Skin and Mucous Membranes) • Immobility secondary to injury and unconsciousness contributes to the development of pressure areas and skin breakdown. • Intubation causes irritation of the mucous membrane.	• Assessment of skin integrity and character of the skin • Assessment of oral mucous membrane
Musculoskeletal System • Immobility contributes to musculoskeletal changes. • Decerebrate or decorticate posturing makes proper positioning difficult. Spasticity leads to the development of contractures.	• Assessment of range of motion of joints and development of deformities or spasticity
Gastrointestinal System • Administration of corticosteroids and stress response places the patient at high risk for GI hemorrhage. • Injury to the GI tract can result in paralytic ileus. • Constipation can result from bed rest, NPO status, fluid restriction, and opioids given for pain control. • Bowel incontinence is related to the patient's unconscious state or altered mental state.	• Assessment of abdomen for bowel sounds and distention • Monitoring for decreased hemoglobin
Genitourinary System • Fluid restriction or use of diuretics can alter the amount of urinary output. • Urinary incontinence is related to the patient's unconscious state.	• Intake and output record
Metabolic (Nutritional) System • The patient receives all fluids intravenously for the first few days until the GI tract is functioning. • A nutritional consultation is initiated within the first 24–48 h; parenteral nutrition may be started.	• Assessment of fluid and electrolyte balance • Recording of weight, if possible • Hematocrit • Electrolyte studies
Respiratory System • Complete or partial airway obstruction will compromise the oxygen supply to the brain. • An altered respiratory pattern can result in cerebral hypoxia. • A short period of apnea at the moment of impact can result in spotty atelectasis. • Systemic disturbances from head injury can cause hypoxemia. • Brain injury can alter brain stem respiratory function. • Shunting of blood to the lungs as a result of a sympathetic discharge at the time of injury can cause neurogenic pulmonary edema.	• Assessment of respiratory function — Auscultate chest for breath sounds. — Note the respiratory pattern if possible (not possible if a ventilator is being used). — Note the respiratory rate — Note whether the cough reflex is intact. • Arterial blood gas levels • Complete blood count • Chest x-ray studies • Sputum cultures • O_2 saturation using pulse oximetry
Cardiovascular System • The patient may develop cardiac dysrhythmias, tachycardia, or bradycardia. • The patient may develop hypotension or hypertension. • Because of immobility and unconsciousness, the patient is at high risk for deep vein thromboses and pulmonary emboli. • Fluid and electrolyte imbalance can be related to several problems, including alterations in antidiuretic hormone (ADH) secretion, the stress response, or fluid restriction. • Specific conditions may occur: — Diabetes insipidus (DI) — Syndrome of inappropriate secretion of ADH (SIADH) — Electrolyte imbalance — Hyperosmolar nonketotic hyperglycemia	• Assessment of vital signs • Monitoring for cardiac dysrhythmias • Assessment for deep vein thromboses of legs • Electrocardiogram • Electrolyte studies • Blood coagulation studies • I^{125} fibrinogen scan of legs • Blood glucose level • Blood acetone level • Blood osmolality • Urine specific gravity
Psychological/Emotional Response • The severely head-injured patient is unconscious. • The family needs emotional support to deal with the crisis.	• Collection of information about the family and the role of the head-injured person within the family • Assessment of the family to determine how functional it was before the injury occurred

gives an indication of the severity of coma and a prediction of possible outcome. The lowest score is 3 (least responsive); the highest is 15 (most responsive). A score of 8 or less is generally accepted as indicating a severe head injury (Teasdale & Jennett, 1974).

Vital Signs

Although a change in LOC is the most sensitive neurologic indication of deterioration of the patient's condition, vital signs are monitored at frequent intervals also to assess the intracranial status. Table 63-1 depicts the general assessment parameters for the patient with a head injury.

Signs of increasing ICP include slowing of the heart rate (bradycardia), increasing systolic blood pressure, and widening pulse pressure. As brain compression increases, respirations become rapid, the blood pressure may decrease, and the pulse slows further. This is an ominous development, as is a rapid fluctuation of vital signs (March, 2000). A rapid rise in body temperature is regarded as unfavourable because hyperthermia increases the metabolic demands of the brain and may indicate brain stem damage, a poor prognostic sign. The temperature is maintained at less than 38°C. Tachycardia and arterial hypotension may indicate that bleeding is occurring elsewhere in the body.

Motor Function

Motor function is assessed frequently by observing spontaneous movements, asking the patient to raise and lower the extremities, and comparing the strength and equality of the hand grasp and pedal push at periodic intervals. To assess the hand grasp, the nurse instructs the patient to squeeze the examiner's fingers tightly. The nurse assesses lower extremity motor strength (pedal push) by placing the hands on the soles of the patient's feet and asking the patient to push down against the examiner's hands. Motor assessment is discussed in Chapter 60 in more detail. The presence or absence of spontaneous movement of each extremity is also noted, and speech and eye signs are assessed.

If the patient does not demonstrate spontaneous movement, responses to painful stimuli are assessed. Motor response to pain is assessed by applying a central stimulus, such as pinching the pectoralis major muscle, to determine the patient's best response. Peripheral stimulation may provide inaccurate assessment data because it may result in a reflex movement rather than a voluntary motor response. Abnormal responses (lack of motor response; extension responses) are associated with a poorer prognosis.

Other Neurologic Signs

In addition to the patient's spontaneous eye opening evaluated with the Glasgow Coma Scale, the size and equality of the pupils and their reaction to light are assessed. A unilaterally dilated and poorly responding pupil may indicate a developing hematoma, with subsequent pressure on the third cranial nerve due to shifting of the brain. If both pupils become fixed and dilated, this indicates overwhelming injury and intrinsic damage to the upper brain stem and is a poor prognostic sign.

The patient with a head injury may develop focal nerve palsies such as anosmia (lack of sense of smell) or eye movement abnormalities and focal neurologic deficits such as aphasia, memory deficits, and post-traumatic seizures or epilepsy. Patients may be left with residual organic psychological deficits (impulsiveness, emotional lability, or uninhibited, aggressive behaviours) and, as a consequence of the impairment, lack insight into their emotional responses (Davis, 2000).

MAINTAINING THE AIRWAY

One of the most important nursing goals in the management of the patient with a head injury is to establish and maintain an adequate airway. The brain is extremely sensitive to hypoxia, and a neurologic deficit can worsen if the patient is hypoxic. Therapy is directed toward maintaining optimal oxygenation to preserve cerebral function. An obstructed airway causes CO_2 retention and hypoventilation, which can produce cerebral vessel dilation and increased ICP.

Interventions to ensure an adequate exchange of air are discussed in Chapter 61 and include the following:

- Keep the unconscious patient in a position that facilitates drainage of oral secretions, with the head of the bed elevated about 30 degrees to decrease intracranial venous pressure (Bader & Palmer, 2000).
- Establish effective suctioning procedures (pulmonary secretions produce coughing and straining, which increase ICP).
- Guard against aspiration and respiratory insufficiency.
- Closely monitor arterial blood gas values to assess the adequacy of ventilation. The goal is to keep blood gas values within the normal range to ensure adequate cerebral blood flow.
- Monitor the patient who is receiving mechanical ventilation.
- Monitor for pulmonary complications such as acute respiratory distress syndrome (ARDS) and pneumonia (Munro, 2000).

MONITORING FLUID AND ELECTROLYTE BALANCE

Brain damage can produce metabolic and hormonal dysfunctions. The monitoring of serum electrolyte levels is important, especially in patients receiving osmotic diuretics, those with inappropriate antidiuretic hormone secretion, and those with post-traumatic diabetes insipidus.

Serial studies of blood and urine electrolytes and osmolality are carried out because head injuries may be accompanied by disorders of sodium regulation. Hyponatremia is common following head injury due to shifts in extracellular fluid, electrolytes, and volume. Hyperglycemia, for example, may cause an increase in extracellular fluid that lowers sodium (Hickey, 2003). Hypernatremia may also occur due to sodium retention that may last several days, followed by sodium diuresis. Increasing lethargy, confusion, and seizures may be due to electrolyte imbalance.

Endocrine function is evaluated by monitoring serum electrolytes, blood glucose values, and intake and output. Urine is tested regularly for acetone. A record of daily weights is maintained, especially if the patient has hypothalamic involvement and is at risk for the development of diabetes insipidus.

PROMOTING ADEQUATE NUTRITION

Head injury results in metabolic changes that increase calorie consumption and nitrogen excretion (Donaldson et al., 2000). There is an increased demand for protein. As soon as possible, nutrition should be provided. Early initiation of nutritional therapy has been shown to improve outcomes in head-injured patients (Bader & Palmer, 2000). Parenteral nutrition via a central line or enteral feedings administered via a nasogastric or nasojejunal feeding tube may be used. If there is discharge of CSF from the nose (CSF rhinorrhea), an oral feeding tube should be inserted in place of a nasal tube.

Laboratory values should be monitored closely in patients receiving parenteral nutrition. Elevating the head of the bed and aspirating the enteral tube for evidence of residual feeding before administering additional feedings can help prevent distention, regurgitation, and aspiration. A continuous-drip infusion or pump may be used to regulate the feeding. The principles and technique of enteral feedings are discussed in Chapter 36. Enteral or parenteral feedings are usually continued until the swallowing reflex returns and the patient can meet caloric requirements orally.

PREVENTING INJURY

As the patient emerges from coma, there is often a period of lethargy and stupor followed by a period of agitation. Each phase is variable and depends on the individual, the location of the injury, the depth and duration of coma, and the patient's age. The patient emerging from a coma may become increasingly agitated toward the end of the day. Restlessness may be due to hypoxia, fever, pain, or a full bladder. It may indicate injury to the brain but may also be a sign that the patient is regaining consciousness. (Some restlessness may be beneficial because the lungs and extremities are exercised.) Agitation may also be due to discomfort from catheters, intravenous lines, restraints, and repeated neurologic checks. Alternatives to restraints must be used whenever possible.

Strategies to prevent injury include the following:

- Assess the patient to ensure that oxygenation is adequate and the bladder is not distended. Check dressings and casts for constriction.
- To protect the patient from self-injury and dislodging of tubes, use padded side rails or wrap the patient's hands in mitts (Fig. 63-6). Restraints are avoided because straining against them can increase ICP or cause other injury. Enclosed or floor-level specialty beds may be indicated.
- Avoid using opioids as a means of controlling restlessness because these medications depress respiration, constrict the pupils, and alter responsiveness.

FIGURE 63-6 Hands of the patient with a head injury may be placed in a Posey mitt to prevent self-injury. This mitt has finger holes so that circulation can be assessed without removing the mitt. Photo courtesy of Sarah Trainer, RN, Roxborough Memorial Hospital, Philadelphia.

- Minimize environmental stimuli by keeping the room quiet, limiting visitors, speaking calmly, and providing frequent orientation information (eg, explaining where the patient is and what is being done).
- Provide adequate lighting to prevent visual hallucinations.
- Minimize disruption of the patient's sleep/wake cycles.
- Lubricate the skin with oil or emollient lotion to prevent irritation due to rubbing against the sheet.
- If incontinence occurs, consider use of an external sheath catheter on a male patient. Because prolonged use of an indwelling catheter inevitably produces infection, the patient may be placed on an intermittent catheterization schedule.

MAINTAINING BODY TEMPERATURE

An increase in body temperature in the head-injured patient can be the result of damage to the hypothalamus, cerebral irritation from hemorrhage, or infection. The nurse monitors the patient's temperature every 4 hours. If the temperature rises, efforts are undertaken to identify the cause and to control it using acetaminophen and cooling blankets as prescribed (Bader & Palmer, 2000). Cooling blankets should be used with caution so as not to induce shivering, which increases ICP. If infection is suspected, potential sites of infection are cultured and antibiotics are prescribed and administered.

MAINTAINING SKIN INTEGRITY

Patients with traumatic head injury often require assistance in turning and positioning because of immobility or unconsciousness. Prolonged pressure on the tissues will decrease circulation and lead to tissue necrosis. Potential areas of breakdown need to be identified early to avoid the development of pressure ulcers. Specific nursing measures include the following:

- Assess all body surfaces and document skin integrity at least every 8 hours.
- Turn and reposition the patient every 2 hours.
- Provide skin care every 4 hours.
- Assist patient to get out of bed to a chair three times a day if physically able.

IMPROVING COGNITIVE FUNCTIONING

Although many patients with head injury survive because of resuscitative and supportive technology, they frequently have significant cognitive sequelae that may not be detected during the acute phase of injury. Cognitive impairment includes memory deficits, decreased ability to focus and sustain attention to a task (distractibility), reduced ability to process information, and slowness in thinking, perceiving, communicating, reading, and writing. Psychiatric or emotional problems develop in as many as 44% of patients with head injury (van Reekum et al., 2000). Resulting psychosocial, behavioural, emotional, and cognitive impairments are devastating to the family as well as to the patient (Davis, 2000; Perlesz, Kinsella, & Crowe, 1999).

These problems require collaboration among many disciplines (Bader & Palmer, 2000). A neuropsychologist (specialist in evaluating and treating cognitive problems) plans a program and initiates therapy or counselling to help the patient reach maximal potential. Cognitive rehabilitation activities help the patient to devise new problem-solving strategies. The retraining is carried out over an extended period and may include the use of sensory stimulation and reinforcement, behaviour modification, reality orientation, computer-training programs, and video games. Assistance from many disciplines is necessary during this phase of recovery. Even if intellectual ability does not improve, social and behavioural abilities may.

The patient recovering from a brain injury may experience fluctuations in the level of cognitive function, with orientation, attention, and memory frequently affected. When pushed to a level greater than the impaired cortical functioning allows, the patient may show symptoms of fatigue, anger, and stress (headache, dizziness). The Rancho Los Amigos Level of Cognitive Function is a scale frequently used to assess cognitive function and evaluate ongoing recovery from head injury. Nursing management and a description of each level are included in Table 63-2.

PREVENTING SLEEP PATTERN DISTURBANCE

Patients who require frequent monitoring of neurologic status may experience sleep deprivation. They are awakened hourly to assess LOC and as a result are deprived of long periods of sleep and rest. In an effort to allow the patient longer times of uninterrupted sleep and rest, the nurse can group nursing care activities so that the patient is disturbed less frequently. Environmental noise is decreased and the room lights are dimmed. Back rubs and other activities to increase comfort can assist in promoting sleep and rest. Clustering nursing care is discouraged for patients with increased ICP. The nurse should monitor the effects of activities on ICP if a monitor is in use (Hickey, 2003).

SUPPORTING FAMILY COPING

Having a loved one sustain a serious head injury can produce a great deal of prolonged stress in the family. This stress can result from the patient's physical and emotional deficits, the unpredictable outcome, and altered family relationships. Families report difficulties in coping with changes in the patient's temperament, behaviour, and personality. Such changes are associated with disruption in family cohesion, loss of leisure pursuits, and loss of work capacity, as well as social isolation of the caretaker. The family may experience anger, grief, guilt, and denial in recurring cycles (Perlesz et al., 1999).

To promote effective coping, the nurse can ask the family how the patient is different at this time: What has been lost? What is most difficult about coping with this situation? Helpful interventions include providing family members with accurate and honest information and encouraging them to continue to set well-defined, mutual, short-term goals. Family counselling helps address the family members' overwhelming feelings of loss and helplessness and gives them guidance for the management of inappropriate behaviours. Support groups help the family members share problems, develop insight, gain information, network, and gain assistance in maintaining realistic expectations and hope. Conversations that are emotionally stimulating may cause increases in the patient's ICP. Such conversations should be held away from the patient's bedside (Hickey, 2003).

The National Head Injury Foundation serves as a clearinghouse for information and resources for patients with head injuries and their families, including specific information on coma, rehabilitation, behavioural consequences of head injury, and family issues. This organization can provide names of facilities and professionals who work with patients with head injuries and can assist families in organizing local support groups. See the end of this chapter for more information on resources.

Many patients with severe head injury die of their injuries, and many of those who survive experience long-term problems that prevent them from resuming their previous roles and functions. During the most acute phase of injury, family members need support and facts from the health care team.

Many individuals with severe head injuries that result in brain death are young and otherwise healthy and are therefore considered for organ donation. Family members of patients with such injuries need support during this extremely stressful time and assistance in making decisions to end life support and permit donation of organs. They need to know that the neurologically-dead patient whose respiratory and cardiovascular systems are maintained through life support is not going to survive and that the severe head injury, not the removal of the patient's organs or the removal of life support, is the cause of patient's death. Bereavement counselors and members of the organ procurement team are often very helpful to family members in making decisions about organ donation and in helping them cope with stress.

MONITORING AND MANAGING POTENTIAL COMPLICATIONS

Decreased Cerebral Perfusion

Maintenance of adequate CPP is important to prevent serious complications of head injury due to decreased cerebral perfusion (Bader & Palmer, 2000; March, 2000). Adequate CPP is greater than 70 mm Hg. Any decrease in this pressure can impair cerebral perfusion and cause brain hypoxia and ischemia, leading to permanent damage. Therapy (eg, elevation of the head of the bed and increased intravenous fluids) is directed toward decreasing cerebral edema and increasing venous outflow from the brain. Systemic hypotension, which causes vasoconstriction and a significant decrease in CPP, is treated with increased intravenous fluids.

Cerebral Edema and Herniation

The patient with a head injury is at risk for additional complications such as increased ICP and brain stem herniation. Cerebral edema is the most common cause of increased ICP in the patient with a head injury, with the swelling peaking approximately 48 to 72 hours after injury. Bleeding also may increase the volume of contents within the rigid closed compartment of the skull, causing increased ICP and herniation of the brain stem and resulting in irreversible brain anoxia and brain death. Measures to control ICP are listed in Chart 63-5 (Zafonte et al., 1999) and discussed in Chapter 61.

Impaired Oxygenation and Ventilation

Impaired oxygen and ventilation may necessitate mechanical ventilatory support. The patient must be monitored for a patent airway, altered breathing patterns, and hypoxemia and pneumonia. Interventions may include endotracheal intubation, mechanical ventilation, and positive end-expiratory pressure. These topics are discussed in further detail in Chapters 25 and 61.

Impaired Fluid, Electrolyte, and Nutritional Balance

Fluid, electrolyte, and nutritional imbalances are common in the patient with a head injury. Common imbalances may include hyponatremia, which is often associated with the syndrome of inappropriate secretion of antidiuretic hormone (see Chaps. 14 and 42), hypokalemia, and hyperglycemia (Hickey, 2003). Modifica-

Table 63-2 • Rancho Los Amigos Scale: Levels of Cognitive Function

COGNITIVE LEVEL	DESCRIPTION	NURSING MANAGEMENT
	For levels I–III, the key approach is to *provide stimulation.*	
I: No response	Completely unresponsive to all stimuli, including painful stimuli	Multiple modalities of sensory input should be used. Examples are listed below, but should be individualized and expanded based on available materials and patient preferences (determined by obtaining information from the family).
II: Generalized response	Nonpurposeful response; responds to pain, but in a nonpurposeful manner	*Olfactory:* perfumes, flowers, shaving lotion *Visual:* family pictures, card, personal items
III: Localized response	Responses more focused: withdraws to pain; turns toward sound; follows moving objects that pass within visual field; pulls on sources of discomfort (eg, tubes, restraints); may follow simple commands but inconsistently and in a delayed manner	*Auditory:* radio, television, tapes of family voices or favourite recordings, talking to patient (nurse, family members). The nurse should tell patient what is going to be done, discuss the environment, provide encouragement. *Tactile:* touching of skin, rubbing various textures on skin *Movement:* range of motion exercises, turning, repositioning, use of water mattress
	For levels IV–VI, the key approach is to *provide structure.*	
IV: Confused, agitated response	Alert, hyperactive state in which patient responds to internal confusion/agitation; behaviour non-purposeful in relation to the environment; aggressive, bizarre behaviour common	For level IV, which lasts 2–4 weeks, interventions are directed at decreasing agitation, increasing environmental awareness, and promoting safety. • Approach patient in a calm manner, and use a soft voice. • Screen patient from environmental stimuli (eg, sounds, sights); provide a quiet, controlled environment. • Remove devices that contribute to agitation (eg, tubes), if possible. • Functional goals cannot be set, because the patient is unable to cooperate.
V: Confused, inappropriate response	When agitation occurs, it is the result of external rather than internal stimuli; focused attention is difficult; memory is severely impaired; responses are fragmented and inappropriate to the situation; there is no carryover of learning from one situation to the other.	For levels V and VI, interventions are directed at decreasing confusion, improving cognitive function, and improving independence in performing ADLs. • Provide supervision. • Use repetition and cues to teach ADLs. Focus the patient's attention and help to increase his or her concentration.
VI: Confused, appropriate response	Follows simple directions consistently but is inconsistently oriented to time and place; short-term memory worse than long-term memory; can perform some ADLs	• Help the patient organize activity. • Clarify misinformation and reorient when confused. • Provide a consistent, predictable schedule (eg, post daily schedule on large poster board).
	For levels VII–X, the key approach is *integration into the community.*	
VII: Automatic, appropriate response	Appropriately responsive and oriented within the hospital setting; needs little supervision in ADLs; some carryover of learning; patient has superficial insight into disabilities; has decreased judgment and problem-solving abilities; lacks realistic planning for future	For levels VII–X, interventions are directed at increasing the patient's ability to function with minimal or no supervision in the community. • Reduce environmental structure. • Help the patient plan for adapting ADLs for self into the home environment. • Discuss and adapt home living skills (eg, cleaning, cooking) to patient's ability.
VIII: Purposeful, appropriate	Alert, oriented, intact memory; has realistic goals for the future. Able to complete familiar tasks for 1 hour in a distracting environment; over-estimates or underestimates abilities, argumentative, easily frustrated, self-centred. Uncharacteristically dependent/independent.	• Provide stand-by assistance as needed for ADLs and home living skills.

(continued)

Table 63-2 • Rancho Los Amigos Scale: Levels of Cognitive Function (Continued)

COGNITIVE LEVEL	DESCRIPTION	NURSING MANAGEMENT
IX: Purposeful, appropriate	Independently shifts back and forth between tasks and completes them accurately for at least two consecutive hours. Uses assistive memory devices to recall schedule and activities. Aware of and acknowledges impairments and disabilities when they interfere with task completion. Depression may continue. May be easily irritable and have a low frustration tolerance.	• Provide assistance on request for adapting ADLs and home living skills.
X: Purposeful, appropriate	Able to handle multiple tasks simultaneously in all environments but may require periodic breaks. Independently initiates and carries out familiar and unfamiliar tasks but may require more than usual amount of time and/or compensatory strategies to complete them. Accurately estimates abilities and independently adjusts to task demands. Periodic periods of depression may occur. Irritability and low frustration tolerance when sick, fatigued and/or under stress.	• Monitor for signs and symptoms of depression. • Help the patient plan, anticipate concerns, and solve problems.

Used with permission from Los Amigos Research and Education Institute, Inc., Downey, CA, 2002.

tions in fluid intake with tube feedings or intravenous fluids may be necessary to treat these imbalances. Insulin administration may be prescribed to treat hyperglycemia.

Undernutrition is also a common problem in response to the increased metabolic needs associated with severe head injury. If the patient cannot eat, enteral feedings or parenteral nutrition may be initiated within 24 hours of injury to provide adequate calories and nutrients.

Post-traumatic Seizures

Patients with head injury are at an increased risk for post-traumatic seizures. Post-traumatic seizures are classified as im-

NURSING RESEARCH PROFILE 63-1

The Experience of Hope for the Relatives of Head-Injured Patients

Gelling, L. (1999). The experience of hope for the relatives of head-injured patients admitted to a neuroscience critical care unit: A phenomenological study. *Nursing in Critical Care, 4*(5), 214–221.

Background

Helping the family members of patients with their emotional needs is a crucial aspect of ICU care. Previous research has demonstrated that meeting needs can be beneficial to both families and patients. One of the most important needs families have identified is to maintain hope. The purpose of this study was to develop a better understanding of what hope means to family members in order to help nurses better meet their needs.

Study Methods and Design

Participants were selected by approaching family members of consecutive patients admitted to a neuroscience ICU. Family members were approached after the patient had been in the ICU at least 48 hours. A total of seven patients had family members who agreed to participate. In this phenomenologic study family members were interviewed about their experiences using a semi-structured format. The interviews were transcribed and returned to the informants for verification of content. Data were analyzed for emergent themes. A summary of the findings was returned to the participants for verification.

Results

Seven themes emerged from analysis of the interview data. The themes that relatives felt most influenced their experience of hope when they had a loved one admitted to the ICU were: 1) Relationships—The positive relationships between the family members and

nurses helped the family members to feel comfortable and safe with the care their loved ones were receiving; 2) Information—Inadequate or poorly delivered information led to uncertainty and difficulty in maintaining hope; 3) The Past—Lack of knowledge and initial negative experiences in the hospital made hope more difficult; 4) The Present—Unfamiliar terminology, devices, and situations needed to be assimilated by the family before they could become hopeful; 5) The future—Goal setting helped the family members have hope for a future for the patient; 6) Loss of control—Relatives felt that though they were asked by the nurses to participate in decisions, they often felt ill equipped to do so, leading to feelings of hopelessness; 7) Emotions—Family members were often so fearful for the patient that it was difficult to have hope.

Nursing Implications

Meeting the needs of families is a key part of nursing care of the patients in a neuroscience unit and furthermore an important component of a holistic nursing approach. Nurses need to be acutely aware of the pivotal role they play in helping the family members to cope and maintain hope in a difficult situation. Nurses should encourage supportive relationships with the families, and maintain an open and honest dialogue. Families need accurate, current information on a level they can understand and assimilate. Nurses need to be cognizant that their care is crucial not just for the patient, but for the entire family.

Chart 63-5 Controlling ICP in Severely Brain-Injured Patients

- Elevate the head of bed 30 degrees.
- Maintain the patient's head and neck in neutral alignment (no twisting).
- Initiate measures to prevent the Valsalva manoeuvre (eg, stool softeners).
- Maintain normal body temperature.
- Administer O_2 to maintain PaO_2 > 90 mm Hg.
- Maintain fluid balance with normal saline solution.
- Avoid noxious stimuli (eg, excessive suctioning, painful procedures).
- Administer sedation to reduce agitation.
- Maintain cerebral perfusion pressure > 70 mm Hg.
- Spread out nursing interventions while monitoring ICP.

mediate (within 24 hours of injury), early (within 1 to 7 days of injury), or late (more than 7 days following injury) (Kado & Patel, 1999). Seizure prophylaxis refers to the practice of administering antiseizure medications to patients following head injury to prevent seizures. It is important to prevent post-traumatic seizures, especially in the immediate and early phase of recovery, as seizures may increase ICP and decrease oxygenation. Many antiseizure medications impair cognitive performance, prolonging the duration of rehabilitation. Therefore, it is important to weigh the overall benefit of these medications against their side effects. Currently, there is no conclusive evidence that long-term antiseizure prophylaxis improves outcomes in patients with head injury. Research evidence supports the use of prophylactic antiseizure agents to prevent immediate and early seizure after head injury, but not for prevention of late seizures (Brain Trauma Foundation, American Association of Neurological Surgeons, Joint Section on Neurotrauma and Critical Care, 2000).

Nurses must assess patients carefully for the development of post-traumatic seizures. Risk factors that increase the likelihood of seizures are brain contusion with subdural hematoma, skull fracture, loss of consciousness or amnesia of 1 day or more, and age over 65 years (Annegers & Coan, 2000). The nursing management of seizures is addressed in Chapter 61.

Other complications after traumatic head injury include systemic infections (pneumonia, urinary tract infection [UTI], septicemia), neurosurgical infections (wound infection, osteomyelitis, meningitis, ventriculitis, brain abscess), and heterotrophic ossification (painful bone overgrowth in weight-bearing joints).

PROMOTING HOME AND COMMUNITY-BASED CARE

Teaching Patients Self-Care

Teaching early in the course of head injury often focuses on reinforcing information given to the family about the patient's condition and prognosis. As the patient's status and expected outcome change over time, family teaching may focus on interpretation and explanation of changes in the patient's physical and psychological responses.

If the patient's physical status allows him or her to be discharged home, the patient and family are instructed about limitations that can be expected and complications that may occur. Monitoring for complications that merit contacting the neurosurgeon is explained to the patient and family verbally and in writing. Depending on the patient's prognosis and physical and cognitive status, the patient may be included in teaching about self-care management strategies.

Because of the risk for post-traumatic seizures, antiseizure medications may be prescribed for 1 to 2 years after injury. The patient and family require instruction about the side effects of these medications and about the importance of continuing to take them as prescribed.

Continuing Care

Rehabilitation of the patient with a head injury begins at the time of injury and extends into the home and community. Depending on the degree of brain damage, the patient may be referred to a rehabilitation setting that specializes in cognitive restructuring of the brain-injured patient. The patient is encouraged to continue the rehabilitation program after discharge because improvement in status may continue 3 or more years after injury. Changes in the head-injured patient and the effects of long-term rehabilitation on the family and their coping abilities need frequent assessment. Teaching and continued support of the patient and family are essential as their needs and the patient's status change. Teaching points to address with the family of the head-injured patient who is about to return home are described in Chart 63-6.

Depending on his or her status, the patient is encouraged to return to normal activities gradually. Referral to local support groups may be warranted.

Chart 63-6 Home Care Checklist • The Patient With a Head Injury

At the completion of the home care instruction, the patient or caregiver will be able to:	Patient	Caregiver
Explain the need for monitoring for changes in neurologic status and for complications	✓	✓
Identify changes in neurologic status and signs and symptoms of complications that should be reported to the neurosurgeon or nurse	✓	✓
Demonstrate safe techniques to assist patient with self-care, hygiene, and ambulation	✓	✓
Demonstrate safe technique for eating, feeding patient, or assisting patient with eating	✓	✓
Explain rationale for taking medications as prescribed	✓	✓
Identify need for close monitoring of behaviour due to changes in cognitive functioning	✓	✓
Describe household modifications needed to ensure safe environment for the patient	✓	✓
Describe strategies for reinforcing positive behaviours		✓
State importance of continuing follow-up by health care team	✓	✓

During the acute and rehabilitation phase of care, the focus of teaching is on obvious needs, issues, and deficits. The nurse needs to remind patients and family members of the need for continuing health promotion and screening practices following these initial phases. Patients who have not been involved in these practices in the past are educated about their importance and are referred to appropriate health care providers.

Evaluation

EXPECTED PATIENT OUTCOMES

Expected patient outcomes may include:

1. Attains or maintains effective airway clearance, ventilation, and brain oxygenation
   a. Achieves normal blood gas values and has normal breath sounds on auscultation
   b. Mobilizes and clears secretions
2. Achieves satisfactory fluid and electrolyte balance
   a. Demonstrates serum electrolytes within normal range
   b. Has no clinical signs of dehydration or overhydration
3. Attains adequate nutritional status
   a. Has less than 50 mL of aspirate in stomach before each tube feeding (bolus feeding)
   b. Is free of gastric distention and vomiting
   c. Shows minimal weight loss
4. Avoids injury
   a. Shows lessening agitation and restlessness
   b. Is oriented to time, place, and person
5. Does not have a fever
6. Demonstrates intact skin integrity
   a. Exhibits no redness or breaks in skin integrity
   b. Exhibits no pressure ulcers. Use barrier cream if incontinent.
7. Shows improvement in cognitive function and improved memory
8. Demonstrates normal sleep/wake cycle
9. Demonstrates absence of complications
   a. Exhibits normal ICP, normal vital signs and body temperature, and increasing orientation to time, place, and person
   b. Demonstrates reduced ICP
10. Patient experiences no post-traumatic seizures
    a. Takes antiseizure medications as prescribed
    b. Identifies side effects/adverse effects of antiseizure medications
11. Demonstrate adaptive coping mechanisms for family members
    a. Join support group
    b. Share feelings with appropriate health care personnel
    c. Make end-of-life decisions, if needed
12. Participate in rehabilitation process as indicated for patient and family members
    a. Take active role in identifying rehabilitation goals and participating in recommended patient care activities
    b. Prepare for discharge of patient

Spinal Cord Injury

Spinal cord injury (SCI) is a major health problem. Approximately 36,000 Canadians live with SCI, with an estimated 1050 new injuries occurring each year (Canadian Paraplegic Association, 2000). According to the Canadian Paraplegic Association, from a 6-year survey of 3000 new spinal cord injuries, vehicular accidents accounted for 54% of the injuries, and industrial accidents and falls for 17% of the injuries. All other causes, such as violence, diving, and sports injuries, accounted for 29%.

The predominant risk factors for SCI include age, gender, and alcohol and drug use. The frequency with which these risk factors are associated with SCI serves to emphasize the importance of primary prevention. The same interventions suggested earlier in this chapter for head injury prevention will serve to decrease the incidence of SCI as well (see Chart 63-1) (CDC, 2001; Elovic & Kirschblum, 1999).

The vertebrae most frequently involved in SCI are the 5th, 6th, and 7th cervical (neck), the 12th thoracic, and the 1st lumbar vertebrae. These vertebrae are the most susceptible because there is a greater range of mobility in the vertebral column in these areas (Dibsie, 1998).

Pathophysiology

Damage to the spinal cord ranges from transient concussion (from which the patient fully recovers) to contusion, laceration, and compression of the cord substance (either alone or in combination), to complete **transection** of the cord (which renders the patient paralyzed below the level of the injury).

SCIs can be separated into two categories: primary injuries and secondary injuries (Porth, 2002). Primary injuries are the result of the initial insult or trauma and are usually permanent. Secondary injuries are usually the result of a contusion or tear injury, in which the nerve fibres begin to swell and disintegrate. A secondary chain of events produces ischemia, hypoxia, edema, and hemorrhagic lesions, which in turn result in destruction of myelin and axons (Hickey, 2003). These secondary reactions, believed to be the principal causes of spinal cord degeneration at the level of injury, are now thought to be reversible 4 to 6 hours after injury. Therefore, if the cord has not suffered irreparable damage, some method of early treatment is needed to prevent partial damage from developing into total and permanent damage (see the section on management) (Zafonte et al., 1999).

Clinical Manifestations

Manifestations depend on the type and level of injury (Chart 63-7). The type of injury refers to the extent of injury to the spinal cord itself. **Incomplete spinal cord lesions** are classified according to the area of spinal cord damage: central, lateral, anterior, or peripheral. The American Spinal Injury Association (ASIA) provides another standard classification of SCI according to the degree of sensory and motor function present after injury (Chart 63-8). "Neurologic level" refers to the lowest level at which sensory and motor functions are normal. Below the neurologic level, there is total sensory and motor paralysis, loss of bladder and bowel control (usually with urinary retention and bladder distention), loss of sweating and vasomotor tone, and marked reduction of blood pressure from loss of peripheral vascular resistance. A **complete spinal cord lesion** can result in **paraplegia** (paralysis of the lower body) or **quadriplegia** (paralysis of all four extremities).

If conscious, the patient usually complains of acute pain in the back or neck, which may radiate along the involved nerve. Absence of pain, however, does not rule out spinal injury, and a careful assessment of the spine should be done in the face of any

Chart 63-7 | **Effects of Spinal Cord Injuries**

Central Cord Syndrome
- Characteristics: Motor deficits (in the upper extremities compared to the lower extremities; sensory loss varies but is more pronounced in the upper extremities); bowel/bladder dysfunction is variable, or function may be completely preserved.
- Cause: Injury or edema of the central cord, usually of the cervical area.

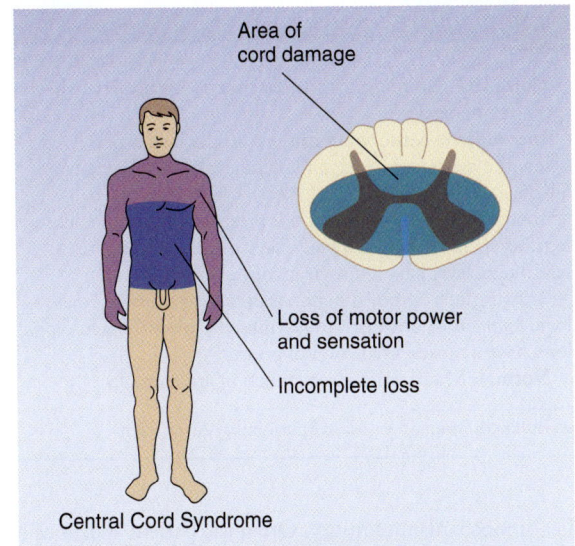

Anterior Cord Syndrome
- Characteristics: Loss of pain, temperature, and motor function is noted below the level of the lesion; light touch, position, and vibration sensation remain intact.
- Cause: The syndrome may be caused by acute disk herniation or hyperflexion injuries associated with fracture-dislocation of vertebra. It also may occur as a result of injury to the anterior spinal artery, which supplies the anterior two thirds of the spinal cord.

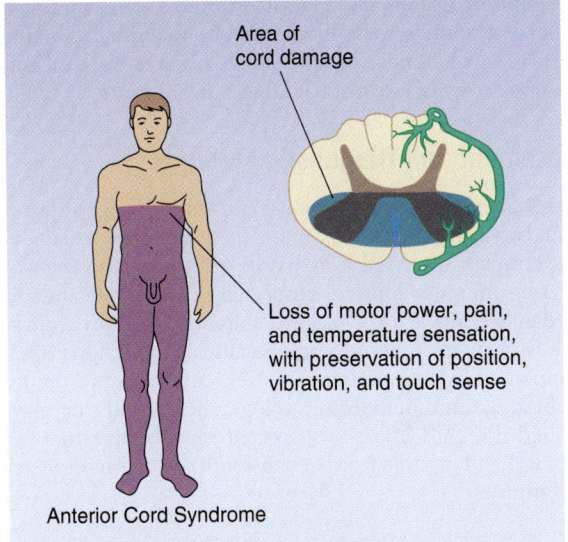

Brown-Sequard Syndrome (Lateral Cord Syndrome)
- Characteristics: Ipsilateral paralysis or paresis is noted, together with ipsilateral loss of touch, pressure, and vibration and contralateral loss of pain and temperature.
- Cause: The lesion is caused by a transverse hemisection of the cord (half of the cord is transected from north to south), usually as a result of a knife or missile injury, fracture-dislocation of a unilateral articular process, or possibly an acute ruptured disk.

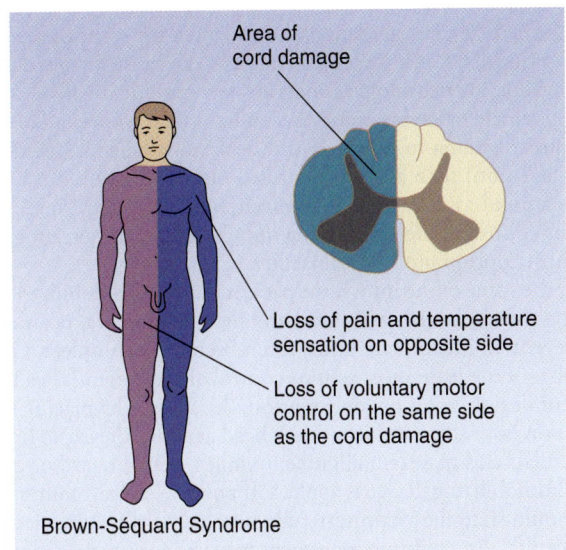

Adapted from Hickey, L. (2003). *The clinical practice of neurological and neurosurgical nursing* (5th ed., pp. 419–421). Philadelphia: Lippincott Williams & Wilkins.

Chart 63-8 ASIA Impairment Scale

A = Complete: No motor or sensory function is preserved in the sacral segments S4-S5.

B = Incomplete: Sensory but not motor function is preserved below the neurologic level, and includes the sacral segments S4-S5.

C = Incomplete: Motor function is preserved below the neurologic level, and more than half of key muscles below the neurologic level have a muscle grade less than 3.

D = Incomplete: Motor function is preserved below the neurologic level, and at least half of key muscles below the neurologic level have a muscle grade of 3 or greater.

E = Normal: Motor and sensory function are normal.

Used with permission of American Spinal Injury Association.

significant mechanism of injury. Often the patient speaks of fear that the neck or back is broken.

Respiratory dysfunction is related to the level of injury. The muscles contributing to respiration are the abdominals and intercostals (T1 to T11) and the diaphragm. In high cervical cord injury, acute respiratory failure is the leading cause of death.

Assessment and Diagnostic Findings

A detailed neurologic examination is performed. Diagnostic x-rays (lateral cervical spine x-rays) and CT scanning are usually performed initially. An MRI scan may be ordered as a further work-up if a ligamentous injury is suspected, since significant spinal cord damage may exist even in the absence of bony injury. A search is made for other injuries, because spinal trauma often is accompanied by concomitant injuries, commonly to the head and chest. Continuous electrocardiographic monitoring may be indicated if a cord injury is suspected since bradycardia (slow heart rate) and asystole (cardiac standstill) are common in acute spinal injuries.

Emergency Management

The immediate management of the patient at the scene of the injury is critical, because improper handling can cause further damage and loss of neurologic function. Any patient involved in a motor vehicle or diving injury, a contact sports injury, a fall, or any direct trauma to the head and neck must be considered to have SCI until such an injury is ruled out. Initial care must include a rapid assessment, immobilization, extrication, stabilization or control of life-threatening injuries, and transportation to the most appropriate medical facility.

At the scene of the injury, the patient must be immobilized on a spinal (back) board, with head and neck in a neutral position, to prevent an incomplete injury from becoming complete. One member of the team must assume control of the patient's head to prevent flexion, rotation, or extension; this is done by placing the hands on both sides of the patient's head at about the ear to limit movement and maintain alignment while a spinal board or cervical immobilizing device is applied. If possible, at least four people should slide the victim carefully onto a board for transfer to the hospital. Any twisting movement may irreversibly damage the spinal cord by causing a bony fragment of the vertebra to cut into, crush, or sever the cord completely.

The patient must be referred to a regional spinal injury or trauma centre because of the multidisciplinary personnel and support services required to counteract the destructive changes that occur in the first few hours after injury. During treatment in the emergency and x-ray departments, the patient is kept on the transfer board. The patient must always be maintained in an extended position. No part of the body should be twisted or turned, nor should the patient be allowed to sit up. Once the extent of the injury has been determined, the patient may be placed on a rotating bed (Fig. 63-7) or in a cervical collar (Fig. 63-8). Later, if SCI and bone instability have been ruled out, the patient can be moved to a conventional bed or the collar removed without harm. If a rotating bed is needed but not available, the patient should be placed in a cervical collar and on a firm mattress with a bedboard under it.

Management of Spinal Cord Injuries (Acute Phase)

The goals of management are to prevent further SCI and to observe for symptoms of progressive neurologic deficits. The patient is resuscitated as necessary, and oxygenation and cardiovascular stability are maintained. Many changes in the treatment of SCI have occurred during the past 20 years. Treatments such as hypothermia, corticosteroids, and naloxone were investigated and used during the 1980s; of these, high-dose corticosteroids have shown the most promise, but their use remains controversial (Short et al., 2000). Currently, regeneration therapy is being investigated; this involves transplanting fetal tissue into the injured spinal cord in hopes of regenerating the damaged tissue (Vacanti et al., 2001). SCI continues to be a devastating event, and new treatment methods are continually being investigated.

PHARMACOLOGIC THERAPY

In some studies, the administration of high-dose corticosteroids, specifically methylprednisolone, has been found to improve motor and sensory outcomes at 6 weeks, 6 months, and 1 year if given within 8 hours of injury (Hickey, 2003). In other studies, little improvement was found (Short et al., 2000). Use of high-dose methylprednisolone, a corticosteroid, is accepted as standard therapy in many countries and remains an established clinical

FIGURE 63-7 Roto Rest® bed. Courtesy of Kinetic Concepts, San Antonio, TX.

FIGURE 63-8 Cervical collar. Courtesy of Aspen Medical Products.

practice in most institutions in the United States and Canada (Bracken, 2000; Hickey, 2003).

RESPIRATORY THERAPY

Oxygen is administered to maintain a high arterial PO$_2$ because hypoxemia can create or worsen a neurologic deficit of the spinal cord. If endotracheal intubation is necessary, extreme care is taken to avoid flexing or extending the patient's neck, which can result in an extension of a cervical injury.

In high cervical spine injuries, spinal cord innervation to the phrenic nerve, which stimulates the diaphragm, is lost. Diaphragmatic pacing (electrical stimulation of the phrenic nerve) attempts to stimulate the diaphragm to help the patient breathe. Diaphragmatic pacing may be considered for the patient with a high cervical lesion but is usually carried out after the acute phase.

SKELETAL FRACTURE REDUCTION AND TRACTION

Management of SCI requires immobilization and reduction of dislocations (restoration of normal position) and stabilization of the vertebral column.

Cervical fractures are reduced and the cervical spine is aligned with some form of skeletal traction, such as skeletal tongs or calipers, or with use of the halo device. Early surgical stabilization has reduced the need for cervical traction in many patients with cervical spine injuries (Gaebler et al., 1999). A variety of skeletal tongs are available, all of which involve fixation in the skull in some manner (Fig. 63-9). The Gardner-Wells tongs require no

FIGURE 63-9 Traction for cervical fractures may be applied with tongs.

predrilled holes in the skull. Crutchfield and Vinke tongs are inserted through holes made in the skull with a special drill under local anesthesia.

Traction is applied to the tongs by weights, the amount depending on the size of the patient and the degree of fracture displacement. The traction force is exerted along the longitudinal axis of the vertebral bodies, with the patient's neck in a neutral position. The traction is then gradually increased by adding more weights. As the amount of traction is increased, the spaces between the intervertebral disks widen and the vertebrae may slip back into position. Reduction usually takes place after correct alignment has been restored. Once reduction is achieved, as verified by cervical spine x-rays and neurologic examination, the weights are gradually removed until the amount of weight needed to maintain the alignment is identified. The weights should hang freely so as not to interfere with the traction. Traction is sometimes supplemented with manual manipulation of the neck by a surgeon to help achieve realignment of the vertebral bodies.

A halo device may be used initially with traction or may be applied after removal of the tongs. It consists of a stainless-steel halo ring that is fixed to the skull by four pins. The ring is attached to a removable **halo vest**, which suspends the weight of the unit circumferentially around the chest. A metal frame connects the ring to the chest. Halo devices provide immobilization of the cervical spine while allowing early ambulation (Fig. 63-10).

Thoracic and lumbar injuries are usually treated with surgical intervention followed by immobilization with a fitted brace. Traction is not indicated either before or after surgery.

Surgical Management

Surgery is indicated in any of the following instances:

- Compression of the cord is evident.
- The injury results in a fragmented or unstable vertebral body.
- The injury involves a wound that penetrates the cord.
- There are bony fragments in the spinal canal.
- The patient's neurologic status is deteriorating.

Surgery is performed to reduce the spinal fracture or dislocation or to decompress the cord. A laminectomy (excision of the posterior arches and spinous processes of a vertebra) may be indicated in the presence of progressive neurologic deficit, suspected epidural hematoma, bony fragments, or penetrating injuries that require surgical débridement, or to permit direct visualization and exploration of the cord. Vertebral bodies may also be surgically fused to create a stable spinal column.

Management of Complications of Spinal Cord Injury

SPINAL AND NEUROGENIC SHOCK

The spinal shock associated with SCI represents a sudden depression of reflex activity in the spinal cord (areflexia) below the level of injury. The muscles innervated by the part of the spinal cord segment below the level of the lesion are without sensation, paralyzed, and flaccid, and the reflexes are absent. In particular, the reflexes that initiate bladder and bowel function are affected. Bowel distention and paralytic ileus can be caused by depression of the reflexes and are treated with intestinal decompression by insertion of a nasogastric tube (Hickey, 2003).

Neurogenic shock develops due to the loss of autonomic nervous system function below the level of the lesion (Hickey, 2003).

A

B

FIGURE 63-10 Halo systems for cervical and thoracic vertebral injuries. (**A**) Halo cervical skeletal traction. Courtesy of Acromed Corp., Cleveland, OH. (**B**) Halo and vest. Courtesy of Bremer Medical, Inc., Darwin Road, Jacksonville, FL.

The vital organs are affected, causing the blood pressure and heart rate to fall. This loss of sympathetic innervation causes a variety of other clinical manifestations, including a decrease in cardiac output, venous pooling in the extremities, and peripheral vasodilation. In addition, the patient does not perspire on the paralyzed portions of the body because sympathetic activity is blocked; therefore, close observation is required for early detection of an abrupt onset of fever. (A discussion of neurogenic shock can be found in Chap. 15.)

> **NURSING ALERT** The patient's vital organ functions and body defenses must be supported and maintained until spinal and neurogenic shock abates and the neurologic system has recovered from the traumatic insult; that can take up to 4 months (Hickey, 2003).

With injuries to the cervical and upper thoracic spinal cord, innervation to the major accessory muscles of respiration is lost and respiratory problems develop. These include decreased vital capacity, retention of secretions, increased $PaCO_2$ levels and decreased oxygen levels, respiratory failure, and pulmonary edema.

> **NURSING ALERT** Special attention also must be directed to the respiratory system. The patient may be unable to generate sufficient intrathoracic pressure to cough effectively. Chest physical therapy and suctioning may assist in clearance of pulmonary secretions.

DEEP VEIN THROMBOSIS

Deep vein thrombosis (DVT) is a potential complication of immobility and is common in patients with SCI. Patients who develop DVT are at risk for pulmonary embolism (PE), a life-threatening complication. One estimate from a meta-analysis of recent studies of the incidence of DVT and PE in SCI patients put the rate at 6.3% for PE and 17.4% for DVT (Velmahos et al., 2000). Manifestations of PE include pleuritic chest pain, anxiety, shortness of breath, and abnormal blood gas values (increased $PaCO_2$ and decreased PaO_2). Thigh and calf measurements are made daily. The patient is evaluated for the presence of DVT if there is a significant increase in the circumference of one extremity. Low-dose anticoagulation therapy usually is initiated to prevent DVT and PE, along with thigh-high elastic compression stockings or pneumatic compression devices. In some cases, permanent indwelling filters (see Chap. 31) may be placed in the vena cava to prevent dislodged clots (emboli) from migrating to the lungs and causing pulmonary emboli (Velmahos et al., 2000).

OTHER COMPLICATIONS

In addition to respiratory complications (respiratory failure, pneumonia) and **autonomic dysreflexia** (characterized by pounding headache, profuse sweating, nasal congestion, piloerection ["goose bumps"], bradycardia, and hypertension), other complications that may occur include pressure ulcers and infection (urinary, respiratory, and local infection at the skeletal traction pin sites) (Sullivan, 1999).

NURSING PROCESS:
THE PATIENT WITH ACUTE
SPINAL CORD INJURY

Assessment

The breathing pattern is observed, the strength of the cough is assessed, and the lungs are auscultated, because paralysis of abdominal and respiratory muscles diminishes coughing and makes it difficult to clear bronchial and pharyngeal secretions. Reduced excursion of the chest also results.

The patient is monitored closely for any changes in motor or sensory function and for symptoms of progressive neurologic damage. It may be impossible in the early stages of SCI to determine whether the cord has been severed, because signs and symptoms of cord edema are indistinguishable from those of cord transection. Edema of the spinal cord may occur with any severe cord injury and may further compromise spinal cord function.

Motor and sensory functions are assessed through careful neurologic examination. These findings are recorded most often on a flow sheet so that changes in the baseline neurologic status can be closely monitored accurately. The American Spinal Injury Association (ASIA) classification is commonly used to describe level of function for SCI patients. Chart 63-7 also gives an example of nursing assessment of spinal cord function.

- Motor ability is tested by asking the patient to spread the fingers, squeeze the examiner's hand, and move the toes or turn the feet.
- Sensation is evaluated by gently pinching the skin or touching it lightly with a small object such as a tongue blade, starting at shoulder level and working down both sides of the extremities. The patient should have both eyes closed so that the examination reveals true findings, not what the patient hopes to feel. The patient is asked where the sensation is felt.
- Any decrease in neurologic function is reported immediately.

The patient is also assessed for spinal shock, a complete loss of all reflex, motor, sensory, and autonomic activity below the level of the lesion that causes bladder paralysis and distention. The lower abdomen is palpated for signs of urinary retention and overdistention of the bladder. Further assessment is made for gastric dilation and ileus due to an atonic bowel, a result of autonomic disruption.

Temperature is monitored because the patient may have periods of hyperthermia as a result of alteration in temperature control due to autonomic disruption.

Diagnosis

NURSING DIAGNOSES

Based on the assessment data, the patient's major nursing diagnoses may include the following:

- Ineffective breathing patterns related to weakness or paralysis of abdominal and intercostal muscles and inability to clear secretions
- Ineffective airway clearance related to weakness of intercostal muscles
- Impaired physical mobility related to motor and sensory impairment
- Disturbed sensory perception related to motor and sensory impairment
- Risk for impaired skin integrity related to immobility and sensory loss

- Urinary retention related to inability to void spontaneously
- Constipation related to presence of atonic bowel as a result of autonomic disruption
- Acute pain and discomfort related to treatment and prolonged immobility

COLLABORATIVE PROBLEMS/
POTENTIAL COMPLICATIONS

Based on the assessment data, potential complications that may develop include:

- DVT
- Orthostatic hypotension
- Autonomic dysreflexia

Planning and Goals

The goals for the patient may include improved breathing pattern and airway clearance, improved mobility, improved sensory and perceptual awareness, maintenance of skin integrity, relief of urinary retention, improved bowel function, promotion of comfort, and absence of complications.

Nursing Interventions

PROMOTING ADEQUATE BREATHING
AND AIRWAY CLEARANCE

Possible impending respiratory failure is detected by observing the patient, measuring vital capacity, monitoring oxygen saturation through pulse oximetry, and monitoring arterial blood gas values. Early and vigorous attention to clearing bronchial and pharyngeal secretions can prevent retention of secretions and atelectasis. Suctioning may be indicated, but caution must be used during suctioning because this procedure can stimulate the vagus nerve, producing bradycardia, which can result in cardiac arrest.

If the patient cannot cough effectively because of decreased inspiratory volume and inability to generate sufficient expiratory pressure, chest physical therapy and assisted coughing may be indicated. Specific breathing exercises are supervised by the nurse to increase the strength and endurance of the inspiratory muscles, particularly the diaphragm. Assisted coughing promotes clearing of secretions from the upper respiratory tract and is similar to using abdominal thrusts to clear an airway (see Chap. 25). It is important to ensure proper humidification and hydration to prevent secretions from becoming thick and difficult to remove even with coughing. The patient is assessed for signs of respiratory infection (cough, fever, dyspnea). Smoking is discouraged because it increases bronchial and pulmonary secretions and impairs ciliary action.

Ascending edema of the spinal cord in the acute phase may cause respiratory difficulty that requires immediate intervention. Therefore, the patient's respiratory status must be monitored frequently.

IMPROVING MOBILITY

Proper body alignment is maintained at all times. The patient is repositioned frequently and is assisted out of bed as soon as the spinal column is stabilized. The feet are prone to footdrop; therefore, various types of splints are used to prevent footdrop. When used, the splints are removed and reapplied every 2 hours. Trochanter rolls, applied from the crest of the ilium to the midthigh of both legs, help prevent external rotation of the hip joints.

Patients with lesions above the midthoracic level have loss of sympathetic control of peripheral vasoconstrictor activity, leading to hypotension. These patients may tolerate changes in position poorly and require monitoring of blood pressure when positions are changed. Usually the patient is turned every 2 hours. If not on a rotating bed, the patient should not be turned unless the spine is stable and the physician has indicated that it is safe to do so.

Contractures develop rapidly with immobility and muscle paralysis. A joint that is immobilized too long becomes fixed as a result of contractures of the tendon and joint capsule. Atrophy of the extremities results from disuse. Contractures and other complications may be prevented by range-of-motion exercises that help preserve joint motion and stimulate circulation. Passive range-of-motion exercises should be implemented as soon as possible after injury. Toes, metatarsals, ankles, knees, and hips should be put through a full range of motion at least four, and ideally five, times daily.

For most patients with a cervical fracture without neurologic deficit, reduction in traction followed by rigid immobilization for about 6 to 8 weeks restores skeletal integrity. These patients are allowed to move gradually to an erect position. A four-poster neck brace or molded collar is applied when the patient is mobilized after traction is removed (see Fig. 63-8).

PROMOTING ADAPTATION TO SENSORY AND PERCEPTUAL ALTERATIONS

The nurse assists the patient to compensate for sensory and perceptual alterations that occur with SCI. The intact senses above the level of the injury are stimulated through touch, aromas, flavorful food and beverages, conversation, and music. Additional strategies include the following:

- Providing prism glasses to enable the patient to see from the supine position
- Encouraging use of hearing aids, if indicated, to enable the patient to hear conversations and environmental sounds
- Providing emotional support to the patient
- Teaching the patient strategies to compensate for or cope with these deficits

MAINTAINING SKIN INTEGRITY

Because the patient with SCI is immobilized and has loss of sensation below the level of the lesion, there is an ever-present, life-threatening risk of pressure ulcers. In areas of local tissue ischemia, where there is continuous pressure and where the peripheral circulation is inadequate as a result of the spinal shock and recumbent position, pressure ulcers have developed within 6 hours. Prolonged immobilization of the patient on a transfer board increases the risk of pressure ulcers. The most common sites are over the ischial tuberosity, the greater trochanter, and the sacrum. In addition, patients who wear cervical collars for prolonged periods may develop breakdown from the pressure of the collar under the chin, on the shoulders, and at the occiput.

The patient's position is changed at least every 2 hours. Turning not only assists in the prevention of pressure ulcers but also prevents the pooling of blood and tissue fluid in the dependent areas.

Careful inspection of the skin is made each time the patient is turned. The skin over the pressure points is assessed for redness or breaks; the perineum is checked for soilage and the catheter is observed for adequate drainage. The patient's general body alignment and comfort are assessed. Special attention should be given to pressure areas in contact with the transfer board.

The patient's skin should be kept clean by washing with a mild soap, rinsed well, and blotted dry. Pressure-sensitive areas should be kept well lubricated and soft with bland cream or lotion. The patient is informed about the danger of pressure ulcers to encourage understanding of the reason for preventive measures. A barrier cream should be used each time the patient is incontinent. See Chapter 11 for other aspects of the prevention of pressure ulcers.

 NURSING ALERT Never massage the calves or thighs due to the danger of dislodging an undetected DVT.

MAINTAINING URINARY ELIMINATION

Immediately after SCI, the urinary bladder becomes atonic and cannot contract by reflex activity. Urinary retention is the immediate result. Because the patient has no sensation of bladder distention, overstretching of the bladder and detrusor muscle may occur, delaying the return of bladder function.

Intermittent catheterization is carried out to avoid overdistention of the bladder and UTI. If this is not feasible, an indwelling catheter is inserted temporarily. At an early stage, family members are shown how to carry out intermittent catheterization and are encouraged to participate in this facet of care, because they will be involved in long-term follow-up and must be able to recognize complications so that treatment can be instituted.

The patient is taught to record fluid intake, voiding pattern, amounts of residual urine after catheterization, characteristics of urine, and any unusual sensations that may occur. The management of a **neurogenic bladder** is discussed in detail in Chapter 11.

IMPROVING BOWEL FUNCTION

Immediately after SCI, a paralytic ileus usually develops due to neurogenic paralysis of the bowel; therefore, a nasogastric tube is often required to relieve distention and prevent aspiration.

Bowel activity usually returns within the first week. As soon as bowel sounds are heard on auscultation, the patient is given a high-calorie, high-protein, high-fibre diet, with the amount of food gradually increased. The nurse administers prescribed stool softeners to counteract the effects of immobility and pain medications. A bowel program is instituted as early as possible.

PROVIDING COMFORT MEASURES

After cervical injury, if pins, tongs, or calipers are in place, the skull is assessed for signs of infection, including drainage. The back of the head is checked periodically for signs of pressure, with care taken not to move the neck. The hair around the tongs usually is shaved to facilitate inspection. Probing under encrusted areas is avoided.

The Patient in Halo Traction

Patients who have been placed in a halo device after cervical stabilization may have a slight headache or discomfort around the skull pins for several days after the pins are inserted. The patient initially may be bothered by the rather startling appearance of this apparatus but usually readily adapts to it because the device provides comfort for the unstable neck. The patient may complain of being caged in and of noise created by any object coming in contact with the steel frame, but he or she can be reassured that adaptation to such annoyances will occur.

The areas around the pin sites are cleansed daily and observed for redness, drainage, and pain. The pins are observed for loosening, which may contribute to infection. If one of the pins becomes detached, the head is stabilized in a neutral position by one person while another notifies the neurosurgeon. A torque screwdriver should be readily available should the screws on the frame need tightening.

The skin under the halo vest is inspected for excessive perspiration, redness, and skin blistering, especially on the bony prominences. The vest is opened at the sides to allow the torso to be washed. The liner of the vest should not become wet, because dampness causes skin excoriation. Powder is not used inside the vest, because it may contribute to the development of pressure ulcers. The liner should be changed periodically to promote hygiene and good skin care. If the patient is to be discharged with the vest, detailed instructions must be given to the family and time allowed for them to return demonstrate the necessary skills (Chart 63-9).

MONITORING AND MANAGING POTENTIAL COMPLICATIONS

Thrombophlebitis

Thrombophlebitis is a relatively common complication in patients after SCI. DVT occurs in a high percentage of SCI patients; thus, they are at risk for PE. The patient must be assessed for symptoms of thrombophlebitis and PE: chest pain, shortness of breath, and changes in arterial blood gas values must be reported promptly to the physician. The circumferences of the thighs and calves are measured and recorded daily; further diagnostic studies will be performed if a significant increase is noted. Patients remain at high risk for thrombophlebitis for several months after the initial injury. Patients with paraplegia or quadriplegia are at increased risk for the rest of their lives. Immobilization and the associated venous stasis, as well as varying degrees of autonomic disruption, contribute to the high risk and susceptibility for DVT (Zafonte et al., 1999).

Anticoagulation is initiated once head and other systemic injuries have been ruled out. Low-dose fractionated or unfractionated heparin may be followed by long-term oral anticoagulation (ie, warfarin) or subcutaneous fractionated heparin injections. Additional measures such as range-of-motion exercises, thigh-high elastic compression stockings, and adequate hydration are important preventive measures. Pneumatic compression devices may also be used to reduce venous pooling and promote venous return. It is also important to avoid external pressure on the lower extremities that may result from flexion of the knees while the patient is in bed.

Orthostatic Hypotension

For the first 2 weeks after SCI, the blood pressure tends to be unstable and quite low. There is a gradual return to preinjury levels, but periodic episodes of severe orthostatic hypotension frequently interfere with efforts to mobilize the patient. Interruption in the reflex arcs that normally produce vasoconstriction in the upright position, coupled with vasodilation and pooling in abdominal and lower extremity vessels, can result in blood pressure readings of 40 mm Hg systolic and 0 mm Hg diastolic. Orthostatic hypotension is a particularly common problem for patients with lesions above T7. In some quadriplegic patients, even slight elevations of the head can result in dramatic changes in blood pressure.

A number of techniques can be used to reduce the frequency of hypotensive episodes. Close monitoring of vital signs before and during position changes is essential. Vasopressor medication can be used to treat the profound vasodilation. Thigh-high elastic compression stockings should be applied to improve venous return from the lower extremities. Abdominal binders may also be used to encourage venous return and provide diaphragmatic support when upright. Activity should be planned in advance and adequate time given for a slow progression of position changes from recumbent to sitting and upright. Tilt tables frequently are helpful in assisting patients to make this transition.

Autonomic Dysreflexia

Autonomic dysreflexia (autonomic hyperreflexia) is an acute emergency that occurs as a result of exaggerated autonomic responses to stimuli that are harmless in normal people. It occurs only after spinal shock has resolved. This syndrome is characterized by a severe, pounding headache with paroxysmal hypertension, profuse diaphoresis (most often of the forehead), nausea, nasal congestion, and bradycardia. It occurs among patients with cord lesions above T6 (the sympathetic visceral outflow level) after spinal shock has subsided. The sudden rise in blood pressure may cause a rupture of one or more cerebral blood vessels or lead to increased ICP. A number of stimuli may trigger this reflex: distended bladder (the most common cause); distention or contraction of the visceral organs, especially the bowel (from constipation, impaction); or stimulation of the skin (tactile, pain, thermal stimuli, pressure ulcer). Because this is an emergency situation, the objective is to remove the triggering stimulus and to avoid the possibly serious complications.

Chart 63-9

Home Care Checklist • The Patient With a Halo Vest

At the completion of the home care instruction, the patient or caregiver will be able to:	Patient	Caregiver
• Describe the rationale for use of the halo vest	✓	✓
• Demonstrate assessment of frame, traction, tongs, and pins	✓	✓
• Describe emergency measures if respiratory or other complications develop while patient is in halo vest or if frame becomes dislodged	✓	✓
• Demonstrate pin care using correct technique		✓
• Identify signs and symptoms of infection	✓	✓
• Assess the skin for reddened or irritated areas and breakdown		✓
• Demonstrate care of skin		✓
• Explain the reasons for and the method for changing the vest liner	✓	✓
• Demonstrate safe techniques to assist patient with self-care, hygiene, and ambulation	✓	✓
• Identify signs and symptoms of complications (deep venous thrombosis, respiratory impairment, urinary tract infection)	✓	✓

The following measures are carried out:

- The patient is placed immediately in a sitting position to lower blood pressure.
- Rapid assessment to identify and alleviate the cause is imperative.
- The bladder is emptied immediately via a urinary catheter. If an indwelling catheter is not patent, it is irrigated or replaced with another catheter.
- The rectum is examined for a fecal mass. If one is present, a topical anesthetic is inserted 10 to 15 minutes before the mass is removed, because visceral distention or contraction can cause autonomic dysreflexia.
- The skin is examined for any areas of pressure, irritation, or broken skin.
- Any other stimulus that can be the triggering event, such as an object on the skin or a draft of cold air, must be removed.
- If these measures do not relieve the hypertension and excruciating headache, a ganglionic blocking agent (hydralazine hydrochloride [Apresoline]) is prescribed and given slowly intravenously.
- The medical record or chart should be labelled with a clearly visible note about the risk for autonomic dysreflexia.
- The patient is instructed about prevention and management measures.
- Any patient with a lesion above the T6 segment is informed that such an episode is possible and may even occur many years after the initial injury.

The rehabilitation of the patient with a SCI (ie, the quadriplegic or paraplegic patient) is discussed below.

PROMOTING HOME AND COMMUNITY-BASED CARE

Teaching Patients Self-Care
In most cases, SCI patients need long-term rehabilitation. The process begins during hospitalization as acute symptoms begin to subside or come under better control and the overall deficits and long-term effects of the injury become clear. The goals begin to shift from merely surviving the injury to learning strategies necessary to cope with the alterations that injury imposes on activities of daily living. The emphasis shifts from ensuring that the patient is stable and free of complications to specific assessment and planning designed to meet the patient's rehabilitation needs. Patient teaching may initially focus on the injury and its effects on mobility, dressing, and bowel, bladder, and sexual function. As the patient and family acknowledge the consequences of the injury, the focus of teaching may broaden to address issues necessary to carry out the tasks of daily living. Teaching begins in the acute phase and continues throughout rehabilitation and throughout the patient's life as changes occur, the patient ages, and problems arise.

Caring for the SCI patient at home may at first seem a daunting task to the family. They will require dedicated nursing support to gradually assume full care of the patient (Craig et al., 1999).

Although maintaining function and preventing complications will remain important, goals regarding self-care and preparation for discharge will assist in a smooth transition to rehabilitation and eventually to the community.

Continuing Care
The ultimate goal of the rehabilitation process is independence. The nurse becomes a support to both the patient and the family, assisting them to assume responsibility for increasing aspects of patient care and management. Care for the SCI patient involves members of all the health care disciplines; these may include nursing, medicine, rehabilitation, respiratory therapy, physical and occupational therapy, case management, social services, and so forth. The nurse often serves as coordinator of the management team and as a liaison with rehabilitation centres and home care agencies. The patient and family often require assistance in dealing with the psychological impact of the injury and its consequences; referral to a psychiatric clinical nurse specialist or other mental health care professional often is helpful.

The nurse should reassure female SCI patients that pregnancy is not contraindicated, but pregnant women with acute or chronic SCI pose unique management challenges. The normal physiologic changes of pregnancy may predispose women with SCI to many potentially life-threatening complications, including autonomic dysreflexia, pyelonephritis, respiratory insufficiency, thrombophlebitis, PE, and unattended delivery (Atterbury & Groome, 1998).

As more patients survive acute SCI, they will face the changes associated with aging with a disability. Thus, teaching in the home and community focuses on health promotion and addresses the need to minimize risk factors (eg, smoking, alcohol and drug abuse, obesity). Home care nurses and others who have contact with patients with SCI are in a position to teach patients about healthy lifestyles, remind them of the need for health screenings, and make referrals as appropriate. Assisting patients to identify accessible health care providers and imaging centres may increase the likelihood that they will participate in health screening (eg, gynecologic examinations, mammograms, etc.).

Evaluation

EXPECTED PATIENT OUTCOMES
Expected patient outcomes may include:

1. Demonstrates improvement in gas exchange and clearance of secretions, as evidenced by normal breath sounds on auscultation
   a. Breathes easily without shortness of breath
   b. Performs hourly deep-breathing exercises, coughs effectively, and clears pulmonary secretions
   c. Is free of respiratory infection (ie, has normal temperature, respiratory rate, and pulse, normal breath sounds, absence of purulent sputum)
2. Moves within limits of the dysfunction and demonstrates completion of exercises within functional limitations
3. Demonstrates adaptation to sensory and perceptual alterations
   a. Uses assistive devices (eg, prism glasses, hearing aids, computers) as indicated
   b. Describes sensory and perceptual alterations as a consequence of injury
4. Demonstrates optimal skin integrity
   a. Exhibits normal skin turgor; skin is free of reddened areas or breaks
   b. Participates in skin care and monitoring procedures within functional limitations
5. Regains urinary bladder function
   a. Exhibits no signs of UTI (ie, has normal temperature; voids clear, dilute urine)
   b. Has adequate fluid intake

c. Participates in bladder training program within functional limitations
6. Regains bowel function
   a. Reports regular pattern of bowel movement
   b. Consumes adequate dietary fibre and oral fluids
   c. Participates in bowel training program within functional limitations
7. Reports absence of pain and discomfort
8. Is free of complications
   a. Demonstrates no signs of thrombophlebitis, DVT, or PE
   b. Exhibits no manifestations of pulmonary embolism (eg, no chest pain or shortness of breath; arterial blood gas values are normal)
   c. Maintains blood pressure within normal limits
   d. Has no lightheadedness with position changes
   e. Exhibits no manifestations of autonomic dysreflexia (ie, no headache, diaphoresis, nasal congestion, bradycardia, or diaphoresis)

Management of the Quadriplegic or Paraplegic Patient

Quadriplegia refers to the loss of movement and sensation in all four extremities and the trunk, associated with injury to the cervical spinal cord. Paraplegia refers to loss of motion and sensation in the lower extremities and all or part of the trunk as a result of damage to the thoracic or lumbar spinal cord or to the sacral root. Both conditions most frequently follow trauma such as falls, injuries, and gunshot wounds, but they may also be the result of spinal cord lesions (intervertebral disk, tumour, vascular lesions), multiple sclerosis, infections and abscesses of the spinal cord, and congenital disorders.

The patient faces a lifetime of great disability, requiring ongoing follow-up and care and the expertise of a number of health professionals, including physicians (specifically a physiatrist), rehabilitation nurses, occupational therapist, physical therapist, psychologist, social worker, rehabilitation engineer, and vocational counselor at different times as the need arises.

As the years go by, these patients also have the same medical problems as others in the aging population. In addition, they face the threat of complications associated with their disability. Usually the patient is encouraged to attend a spinal clinic when complications and other issues arise. Lifetime care includes assessment of the urinary tract at prescribed intervals, because there is the likelihood of continuing alteration in detrusor and sphincter function and the patient is prone to UTI.

Long-term problems and complications of SCI include disuse syndrome, autonomic dysreflexia (discussed earlier), bladder and kidney infections, spasticity, and depression. Pressure ulcers with potential complications of sepsis, osteomyelitis, and fistulas occur in about 10% of patients. Flexor muscle spasms may be particularly disabling and occur in up to 25% of patients (Sullivan, 1999). Heterotopic ossification (overgrowth of bone) in the hips, knees, shoulders, and elbows occurs in up to 30% of SCI patients. This complication is painful and can produce a loss of range of motion (Mitcho & Yanko, 1999; Subbarao & Garrison, 1999). Management includes observing for and addressing any alteration in physiologic status and psychological outlook, and the prevention and treatment of long-term complications. The nursing role involves emphasizing the need for vigilance in self-assessment and care.

NURSING PROCESS: THE PATIENT WITH QUADRIPLEGIA OR PARAPLEGIA

Assessment

Assessment focuses on the patient's general condition, complications, and how the patient is managing at that particular point in time. A head-to-toe assessment and review of systems should be part of the database, with emphasis on the areas prone to problems in this population. A thorough inspection of all areas of the skin for redness or breakdown is critical. It is also important to review with the patient the established bowel and bladder program, because the program must continue uninterrupted. Patients with quadriplegia or paraplegia have varying degrees of loss of motor power, deep and superficial sensation, vasomotor control, bladder and bowel control, and sexual function. They are faced with potential complications related to immobility, skin breakdown and pressure ulcers, recurring UTI, contractures, and psychosocial disruptions. Knowledge about these particular issues can further guide the assessment in any setting. Nurses in all settings, including home care, must be aware of these potential complications in the lifetime management of these patients.

An understanding of the emotional and psychological responses to quadriplegia or paraplegia is achieved by observing the responses and behaviours of the patient and family and by listening to their concerns (see Chart 63-10 for a discussion of ethical issues). Documenting these assessments and reviewing the plan with the entire team on a regular basis provide insight into how both the patient and the family are coping with the changes in lifestyle and body functioning. Additional information frequently can be gathered from the social worker or psychiatric/mental health worker.

Chart 63-10 • Ethics and Related Issues

When the Patient Wants to Die . . .

Situation

A 70-year-old man has been in neurologic intensive care since he suffered a complete C1-C2 cervical fracture 2 weeks ago, which left him quadriplegic and ventilator-dependent. Since his admission, he has asked to be allowed to die. He has a living will and his wife is his designated durable power of attorney for health care. Before his injury, his health was exceptional. He played golf daily and was very active. He is awake, alert, and oriented and can communicate by letter board. He states that he does not want to spend his life unable to do the things he enjoys. He continues to request extubation so that he can die. His family and friends are with him, and he has asked his attorneys to tend to his affairs. With the loving support of his family, the decision to remove the ventilator has been made. Sedatives will be administered to help him deal with hypoxia and anoxia.

Dilemma

What is the nurse's role in caring for this patient at this time?

Discussion

Is the removal of the ventilator an act of assisted suicide? Is it active or passive euthanasia? What is the nurse's role in caring for the patient if this action conflicts with his/her personal beliefs? If no other nurse is available to provide care? If the physician writes the order for the nurse to remove the ventilator?

It takes time for the patient and family to comprehend the magnitude of the disability. They may go through stages of grief, including shock, disbelief, denial, anger, depression, and acceptance. During the acute phase of the injury, denial can be a protective mechanism to shield patients from the overwhelming reality of what has happened. As they realize the permanent nature of paraplegia or quadriplegia, the grieving process may be prolonged and all-encompassing because of the recognition that long-held plans and expectations may be interrupted or permanently altered. A period of depression often follows as the patient experiences a loss of self-esteem in areas of self-identity, sexual functioning, and social and emotional roles. Exploration and assessment of these issues can assist in developing a meaningful plan of care.

Diagnosis

NURSING DIAGNOSES

Based on the assessment data, the major nursing diagnoses of the patient with quadriplegia or paraplegia may include the following:

- Impaired physical mobility related to loss of motor function
- Risk for disuse syndrome
- Risk for impaired skin integrity related to permanent sensory loss and immobility
- Urinary retention related to level of injury
- Constipation related to effects of spinal cord disruption
- Sexual dysfunction related to neurologic dysfunction
- Ineffective coping related to impact of dysfunction on daily living
- Deficient knowledge about requirements for long-term management

COLLABORATIVE PROBLEMS/ POTENTIAL COMPLICATIONS

Based on all the assessment data, potential complications of quadriplegia or paraplegia that may develop include:

- Spasticity
- Infection and sepsis

Planning and Goals

The goals for the patient may include attainment of some form of mobility, maintenance of healthy, intact skin, achievement of bladder management without infection, achievement of bowel control, achievement of sexual expression, strengthening of coping mechanisms, and absence of complications.

Nursing Interventions

The patient requires extensive rehabilitation, which is less difficult if appropriate nursing management has been carried out during the acute phase of the injury or illness. Nursing care is one of the key factors determining the success of the rehabilitation program. The main objective is for the patient to live as independently as possible in the home and community.

INCREASING MOBILITY

Exercise Programs

The unaffected parts of the body are built up to optimal strength to promote maximal self-care. The muscles of the hands, arms, shoulders, chest, spine, abdomen, and neck must be strengthened in the paraplegic patient because he or she must bear full weight on these muscles to ambulate. The triceps and the latissimus dorsi are important muscles used in crutch walking. The muscles of the abdomen and the back also are necessary for balance and for maintaining the upright position.

To strengthen these muscles, the patient can do push-ups when in a prone position and sit-ups when in a sitting position. Extending the arms while holding weights (traction weights can be used) also develops muscle strength. Squeezing rubber balls or crumbling newspaper promotes hand strength.

With encouragement from all members of the rehabilitation team, the paraplegic patient can develop the increased exercise tolerance needed for gait training and ambulation activities. The importance of maintaining cardiovascular fitness is stressed to the patient. Alternative exercises to increase the heart rate to target levels must be designed within the patient's abilities.

Mobilization

When the spine is stable enough to allow the patient to assume an upright posture, mobilization activities are initiated. A brace or vest may be used, depending on the level of the lesion. A patient whose paralysis is due to complete transection of the cord can begin weight-bearing early because no further damage can be incurred. The sooner muscles are used, the less chance there is of disuse atrophy. The earlier the patient is brought to a standing position, the less opportunity for osteoporotic changes to take place in the long bones. Weight-bearing also reduces the possibility of renal calculi and enhances many other metabolic processes.

Braces and crutches enable some paraplegic patients to ambulate for short distances. Ambulation using crutches requires a high expenditure of energy. Motorized wheelchairs and specially equipped vans can provide greater independence and mobility for patients with high-level SCI or other lesions. Every effort should be made to encourage the patient to be as mobile and active as possible.

PREVENTING DISUSE SYNDROME

Patients are at high risk for developing contractures as a result of disuse syndrome due to the musculoskeletal system changes (atrophy) brought about by the loss of motor and sensory functions below the level of injury. Range-of-motion exercises must be provided at least four times a day, and care is taken to stretch the Achilles tendon with exercises (Hickey, 2003). The patient is repositioned frequently and maintained in proper body alignment whether in bed or in a wheelchair (Hickey, 2003).

PROMOTING SKIN INTEGRITY

Because these patients spend a great portion of their lives in wheelchairs, pressure ulcers are an ever-present threat. Contributing factors are permanent sensory loss over pressure areas; immobility, which makes relief of pressure difficult; trauma from bumps (against the wheelchair, toilet, furniture, and so forth) that cause unperceived abrasions and wounds; loss of protective function of the skin from excoriation and maceration due to excessive perspiration and possible urinary and fecal incontinence; and poor general health (anemia, edema, malnutrition), leading to poor tissue perfusion. The prevention and management of pressure ulcers are discussed in detail in Chapter 11.

The person with quadriplegia or paraplegia must take responsibility for monitoring (or directing) his or her skin status. This involves relieving pressure and not remaining in any position for longer than 2 hours, in addition to ensuring that the skin receives meticulous attention and cleansing. The patient is taught that ulcers develop over bony prominences exposed to unrelieved pressure in the lying and sitting positions. The most vulnerable areas are identified. The paraplegic patient is instructed to use mirrors, if possible, to inspect these areas morning and night, observing for redness, slight edema, or any abrasions. While in bed, the patient should turn at 2-hour intervals and then inspect the skin again for redness that does not fade on pressure. The bottom sheet should be checked for wetness and for creases. The quadriplegic or paraplegic patient who cannot perform these activities is encouraged to direct others to check these areas and prevent ulcers from developing.

The patient is taught to relieve pressure while in the wheelchair by doing push-ups, leaning from side to side to relieve ischial pressure, and tilting forward while leaning on a table. The caregiver for the quadriplegic patient will need to perform these activities if the patient cannot do so independently. A wheelchair cushion is prescribed to meet individual needs, which may change in time with changes in posture, weight, and skin tolerance. A referral can be made to a rehabilitation engineer, who can measure pressure levels while the patient is sitting and then tailor the cushion and other necessary aids and assistive devices to the patient's needs.

The diet for the patient with quadriplegia or paraplegia should be high in protein, vitamins, and calories to ensure minimal wasting of muscle and the maintenance of healthy skin, and high in fluids to maintain well-functioning kidneys. Excessive weight gain and obesity should be avoided because they limit mobility.

IMPROVING BLADDER MANAGEMENT

The effect of the spinal cord lesion on the bladder depends on the level of injury, the degree of cord damage, and the length of time after injury. A patient with quadriplegia or paraplegia usually has either a reflex or a nonreflex bladder (see Chaps. 11 and 44). Both bladder types increase the risk of UTI.

The nurse emphasizes the importance of maintaining an adequate flow of urine by encouraging a fluid intake of about 2.5 L daily. The patient should empty the bladder frequently so there is minimal residual urine and should pay attention to personal hygiene, because infection of the bladder and kidneys almost always occurs by the ascending route. The perineum must be kept clean and dry and attention given to the perianal skin after defecation. Underwear should be cotton (more absorbent) and changed at least once a day.

If an external catheter (condom catheter) is used, the sheath is removed nightly; the penis is cleansed to remove urine and is dried carefully, because warm urine on the periurethral skin promotes the growth of bacteria. Attention also is given to the collection bag. The nurse emphasizes the importance of monitoring for indications of UTI: cloudy, foul-smelling urine or hematuria (blood in the urine), fever, or chills.

The female patient who cannot achieve reflex bladder control or self-catheterization may need to wear pads or waterproof undergarments. Surgical intervention may be indicated in some patients to create a urinary diversion.

ESTABLISHING BOWEL CONTROL

The objective of a bowel training program is to establish bowel evacuation through reflex conditioning. This technique is described in Chapter 38. If a cord injury occurs above the sacral segments or nerve roots and there is reflex activity, the anal sphincter may be massaged (digital stimulation) to stimulate defecation. If

the cord lesion involves the sacral segment or nerve roots, anal massage is not performed because the anus may be relaxed and lack tone. Massage is also contraindicated if there is spasticity of the anal sphincter. The anal sphincter is massaged by inserting a gloved finger (which has been adequately lubricated) 2.5 to 3.7 cm into the rectum and moving it in a circular motion or from side to side. It soon becomes apparent which area triggers the defecation response. This procedure should be performed at the same time (usually every 48 hours), after a meal, and at a time that will be convenient for the patient at home. The patient also is taught the symptoms of impaction (frequent loose stools; constipation) and cautioned to watch for hemorrhoids. A diet with sufficient fluids and fibre is essential to a successful bowel training program, avoiding constipation, and decreasing the risk of autonomic dysreflexia.

COUNSELLING ON SEXUAL EXPRESSION

Many paraplegic and quadriplegic patients can have some form of meaningful sexual relationship, although some modifications will be necessary. The patient and partner benefit from counselling about the range of sexual expression possible, special techniques and positions, exploration of body sensations offering sensual feelings, and urinary and bowel hygiene as related to sexual activity. For men with erectile failure, penile prostheses enable them to have and sustain an erection. Sildenafil (Viagra) is an oral smooth muscle relaxant that causes blood to flow into the penis, resulting in an erection (see Chap. 49).

Sexual education and counselling services are included in the rehabilitation services at spinal centres. Small-group meetings in which the patients can share their feelings, receive information, and discuss sexual concerns and practical aspects are helpful in producing effective attitudes and adjustments (Sipski & Alexander, 1997).

ENHANCING COPING MECHANISMS

The impact of the disability and loss becomes marked when patients return home. Each time something new enters their lives (eg, a new relationship, going to work), they are reminded anew of their limitations. Grief reactions and depression are common.

To work through this depression, patients must have some hope for relief in the future. Thus, the nurse can encourage them to feel confident in their ability to achieve self-care and relative independence. The role of the nurse ranges from caretaker during the acute phase to teacher, counsellor, and facilitator as patients gain mobility and independence.

The patient's disability affects not only the patient, but also the entire family. In many cases, family therapy is helpful to help work through issues as they arise.

Adjustment to the disability leads to the development of realistic goals for the future, making the best of the abilities that are left intact and reinvesting in other activities and relationships. Rejection of the disability causes self-destructive neglect and noncompliance with the therapeutic program, which leads to more frustration and depression. Crises for which interventions may be sought include social, psychological, marital, sexual, and psychiatric problems. The family usually requires counselling, social services, and other support systems to help them cope with the changes in their lifestyle and socioeconomic status.

A major goal of nursing management is to help patients overcome their sense of futility and to encourage them in the emotional adjustment that must be made before they are willing to venture into the outside world. However, an excessively sympathetic attitude on the part of the nurse may cause patients to develop an overdependence that defeats the purpose of the entire rehabilitation program. Patients are taught and assisted when necessary, but the nurse should avoid performing activities that patients can do for themselves with a little effort. This approach to care more than repays itself in the satisfaction of seeing a completely demoralized and helpless patient become independent and find meaning in a newly emerging lifestyle. The quadriplegic patient may not be able to use the call bell to reach the nursing staff. The patient should be placed in a room close to the nursing station and set up with a call bell system that can be triggered easily, by means of blowing or by shoulder or arm movement.

MONITORING AND MANAGING POTENTIAL COMPLICATIONS

Spasticity

Muscle spasticity is one of the most problematic complications of quadriplegia and paraplegia. These incapacitating flexor or extensor spasms, which occur below the level of the spinal cord lesion, interfere with both the rehabilitation process and activities of daily living. Spasticity results from an imbalance between the facilitatory and inhibitory effects on neurons that exist normally. The area of the cord distal to the site of injury or lesion becomes disconnected from the higher inhibitory centres located in the brain. Facilitatory impulses, which originate from muscles, skin, and ligaments, thus predominate.

Spasticity is defined as a condition of increased muscle tone in a muscle that is weak. Initial resistance to stretching is quickly followed by sudden relaxation. The stimulus that precipitates spasm can be either obvious, such as movement or a position change, or subtle, such as a slight jarring of the wheelchair. Most patients with quadriplegia or paraplegia have some degree of spasticity. With SCI, the onset of spasticity usually occurs from a few weeks to 6 months after the injury. The same muscles that are flaccid during the period of spinal shock will develop spasticity during recovery. The intensity of spasticity tends to peak around 2 years after the injury, after which the spasms tend to regress.

Management of spasticity is based on the severity of symptoms and the degree of incapacitation. Antispasmodic medications such as diazepam (Valium), baclofen (Lioresal), and dantrolene (Dantrium) are frequently effective in controlling spasm but cause drowsiness, weakness, and vertigo in some patients. Passive range-of-motion exercises and frequent turning and repositioning are helpful because stiffness tends to increase spasticity. These activities also are essential in the prevention of contractures, pressure ulcers, and bowel and bladder dysfunction.

Contractures can complicate day-to-day care, increasing the difficulty with positioning and decreasing mobility. A number of surgical procedures have been tried with varying degrees of success. These techniques are used if more conservative approaches fail. The best treatment is prevention.

Infection and Sepsis

Patients with quadriplegia and paraplegia are at increased risk for infection and sepsis from a variety of sources: urinary tract, respiratory tract, and pressure ulcers. Sepsis remains a major cause of death and complications in these patients. Prevention of infection and sepsis is essential through maintenance of skin integrity, complete emptying of the bladder at regular intervals, and prevention of urinary and fecal incontinence. The risk of respiratory infection can be decreased by avoiding contact with people with symptoms of respiratory infection, performing coughing and deep-breathing exercises to prevent pooling of respiratory se-

cretions, receiving yearly influenza vaccines, and giving up smoking. A high-protein diet is important in maintaining an adequate immune system, as is avoiding factors that may reduce immune system function (eg, excessive stress, drug abuse, excessive alcohol intake).

If infection occurs, the patient requires thorough assessment and prompt treatment. Antibiotic therapy and adequate hydration, in addition to local measures (depending on the site of infection), are initiated immediately.

UTIs are minimized or prevented by:

- Aseptic technique in catheter management
- Adequate hydration
- Bladder training program
- Prevention of overdistention of the bladder and stasis

Skin breakdown and infection are prevented by:

- Maintenance of a turning schedule
- Frequent back care
- Regular assessment of all skin areas
- Regular cleansing and lubrication of the skin
- Passive range-of-motion exercise to prevent contractures
- Pressure relief, particularly over broken skin areas, bony prominences, and heels
- Wrinkle-free bed linen

Pulmonary infections are managed and prevented by:

- Frequent coughing, turning, and deep-breathing exercises and chest physiotherapy
- Aggressive respiratory care and suctioning of the airway if a tracheostomy is present
- Assisted coughing
- Adequate hydration

Infections of any kind can be life-threatening. Therefore, aggressive nursing interventions are key to their prevention and management.

PROMOTING HOME AND COMMUNITY-BASED CARE

Teaching Patients Self-Care

Patients with quadriplegia or paraplegia are at risk for complications for the rest of their lives. Thus, a major aspect of nursing care is teaching patients and their families about these complications and about strategies to minimize this risk. UTIs, contractures, infected pressure ulcers, and sepsis may necessitate hospitalization. Other late complications that may occur include lower extremity edema, joint contractures, respiratory dysfunction, and pain. To avoid these and other complications, the patient and a family member are taught skin care, catheter care, range-of-motion exercises, breathing exercises, and other care techniques. Teaching is initiated as soon as possible and extends into the rehabilitation or long-term care facility and home.

Continuing Care

Referral for home care is often appropriate for assessment of the home setting, patient teaching, and evaluation of the patient's physical and emotional status. During visits by the home care nurse, teaching about strategies to prevent or minimize potential complications is reinforced. The home environment is assessed for adequacy for care and for safety. Environmental modifications are made and specialized equipment is obtained, ideally before the patient goes home.

The home care nurse also assesses the patient's and the family's adherence to recommendations and their use of coping strategies.

The use of inappropriate coping strategies such as drug and alcohol use is assessed and referrals to counselling are made for the patient and family. Appropriate and effective coping strategies are reinforced. The nurse reviews previous teaching and determines the need for further physical or psychological assistance. The patient's self-esteem and body image may be very poor at this time. Because people with high levels of social support often report feelings of well-being despite major physical disability, it is beneficial for the nurse to assess and promote further development of the support system and effective coping strategies of each patient.

The patient requires continuing, life-long follow-up by the physician, physical therapist, and other rehabilitation team members because the neurologic deficit is usually permanent and new deficits and complications can develop. These require prompt attention before they take their toll in additional physical impairment, time, morale, and financial costs. The local counsellor for the Office of Vocational Rehabilitation works with the patient with respect to job placement or additional educational or vocational training.

The nurse is in a good position to remind patients and family members of the need for continuing health promotion and screening practices. Referral to accessible health care providers and imaging centres is important in health promotion.

Evaluation

EXPECTED PATIENT OUTCOMES

Expected patient outcomes may include:

1. Attains some form of mobility
2. Contractures do not develop
3. Maintains healthy, intact skin
4. Achieves bladder control, absence of UTI
5. Achieves bowel control
6. Reports sexual satisfaction
7. Shows improved adaptation to environment and others
8. Exhibits reduction in spasticity
   a. Reports understanding of the precipitating factors
   b. Reports understanding of measures to reduce spasticity
9. Describes long-term management required
10. Exhibits absence of complications

 Critical Thinking Exercises

1. A patient has been brought to the emergency department after he was hit in the head with a bat during a company baseball game. His coworkers report that he was unconscious for about 3 minutes. He now seems alert and oriented. What type of injury has he most likely sustained? What discharge instructions are warranted for this patient's family? How would you modify your discharge instructions if the patient lives alone?

2. A 25-year-old man with paraplegia secondary to SCI is scheduled to return home after an 8-month stay in a rehabilitation facility. What health promotion strategies are relevant to teach the patient prior to discharge? What modifications in patient teaching would be indicated if the patient were a 50-year-old woman?

3. A patient with a T4 SCI has just returned to the nursing unit from physical therapy. He reports a severe, pounding headache and nausea. His blood pressure is very elevated and his pulse is slow. What are the possible causes of these signs and symptoms? What immediate actions should you take? What treatments can you anticipate? What teaching is warranted, and why?

REFERENCES AND SELECTED READINGS

Books

The Brain Trauma Foundation (2000). *Guidelines for the management of severe head injury.* New York: The Brain Trauma Foundation.

The Brain Trauma Foundation (2000). *Guidelines for the pre-hospital management of traumatic brain injury.* New York: The Brain Trauma Foundation.

Cammermeyer, M., & Appledorn, C. (Eds.). (1996). *Core curriculum for neuroscience nurses* (4th ed.). Chicago: American Association of Neuroscience Nurses.

Canadian Institute for Health Information 1996-2002. (2006). National trauma registry: Head injury 1999. Available at: http://secure.cihi.ca/cihiweb/splash.html. Retrieved January 13, 2006.

Consortium for Spinal Cord Medicine. (1998). *Neurogenic bowel management in adults with spinal cord injury.* Clinical Practice Guidelines, Paralyzed Veterans of America, Washington, D.C.

Hickey, J. V. (2003). *The clinical practice of neurological and neurosurgical nursing* (5th ed.). Philadelphia: Lippincott Williams & Wilkins.

Kaye, A. (1997). *Essential neurosurgery* (2nd ed.). New York: Churchill Livingstone.

Porth, C. M. (2002). *Pathophysiology concepts of altered health states* (6th ed.). Philadelphia: Lippincott Williams & Wilkins.

Sipski, M. L., & Alexander, C. J. (1997). *Sexual function in people with disability and chronic illness: A health professional's guide.* Gaithersburg, MD: Aspen.

Young, G. B., Ropper, A. H., & Bolton, C. F. (1998). *Coma and impaired consciousness: A clinical perspective.* New York: McGraw-Hill.

Ylvisaker, M. (1998). *Traumatic brain injury rehabilitation: Children and adolescents* (2nd ed.). Boston: Butterworth-Heinemann.

Journals

Asterisks indicate nursing research articles.

Head Injury

Annegers, J., & Coan, S. (2000). The risks of epilepsy after traumatic brain injury. *Seizure, 9*(7), 453–457.

Bader, M. K., & Palmer, S. (2000). Keeping the brain in the zone: Applying the severe head injury guidelines to practice. *Critical Care Nursing Clinics of North America, 12*(4), 413–427.

Blank-Reid, C. & Reid, P. C. (2000). Penetrating trauma to the head. *Critical Care Nursing Clinics of North America, 12*(4), 477–487.

Bogner, J. A., Corrigan, J. D., Stange, M., & Rabold, D. (1999). Focus on clinical research. Reliability of the agitated behavior scale. *Journal of Head Trauma Rehabilitation, 14*(1), 91–96.

Brain Trauma Foundation, American Association of Neurological Surgeons, Joint Section on Neurotrauma and Critical Care. (2000) Role of antiseizure prophylaxis following head injury. *Journal of Neurotrauma, 17*(6–7), 549–553.

Davis, A. (2000). Cognitive impairments following traumatic brain injury. *Critical Care Nursing Clinics of North America, 12*(4), 447–455.

Evans, R. W. (2004). The post concussion syndrome and whiplash injuries: A question and answer review for primary care physicians. *Primary Care: Clinics in Office Practice, 31*(1), 1–17.

*Faragi, B., & Yu, P. (1998). Serum phenytoin levels of patients on gastrostomy tube feeding. *Journal of Neuroscience Nursing, 30*(1), 55–59.

*Gelling, L. (1999). The experience of hope for the relatives of head injured patients admitted to a neurosciences critical care unit: A phenomenological study. *Nursing in Critical Care, 4*(5), 214–221.

Grzankowski, J. A. (1997). Altered thought processes related to traumatic brain injury and their nursing implications. *Rehabilitation Nursing, 22*(1), 24–31.

Hagen, C., Malkmus, D., & Durham, P. (1972). Communication Disorders Service, Rancho Los Amigos Hospital, Downey CA 1972. Revised 11/15/74 by Danese Malkmus, M. A., and Kathryn Stenderup.

Kado, R., & Patel, A. (1999). Posttraumatic epilepsy prophylaxis in traumatic brain injury. *Journal of Cognitive Rehabilitation, 17*(5), 16–20.

Lovasik, D. (2000). Brain death and organ donation. *Critical Care Nursing Clinics of North America,12*(4), 531–538.

March, K. (2000). Intracranial pressure monitoring and assessing intracranial compliance in brain injury. *Critical Care Nursing Clinics of North America, 12*(4), 429–436.

Mitchell, P. H., & Habermann, B. (1999). Rethinking physiologic stability: Touch and intracranial pressure. *Biological Research for Nursing, 1*(1), 12–19.

National Institutes of Health. (1998). *Consensus statement: Rehabilitation of persons with traumatic brain injury.* October 26–28, 1998.

Patyk, M., Gaynor, S., Kelly, J., & Ott, V. (1998). Touch screen computerized education for patients with brain injuries. *Rehabilitation Nursing, 23*(2), 84–87.

Perdue P., Watts, D., Kaufmann, C., & Trask, A. (1998) Differences in mortality between elderly and younger adult trauma patients: Geriatric status increases risk of delayed death. *Journal of Trauma-Injury Infection & Critical Care, 45*(4), 805–810.

Perlesz, A., Kinsella, G., & Crowe, S. (1999). Impact of traumatic brain injury on the family: A critical review. *Rehabilitation Psychology, 44*(1), 6–35.

Ponsford, J., Willmott, C., Rothwell, A., et al. (1999) Cognitive and behavioral outcome following mild traumatic head injury in children. *Journal of Head Trauma Rehabilitation, 14*(4), 360–372.

Ramritu, P. L., & Croft, G. (1999). Needs of parents of the child hospitalised with acquired brain damage. *International Journal of Nursing Studies, 36*(3), 209–216.

Segatore, M. (1999). Corticosteroids and traumatic brain injury: Status at the end of the decade of the brain. *Journal of Neuroscience Nursing, 31*(4), 239–250.

Servadei, F. (1997). Prognostic factors in severely head injured adult patients with epidural haematomas. *Acta Neurochirurgica, 139*(4), 273–278.

*Sullivan, J. (2000). Positioning of patients with severe traumatic brain injury: Research-based practice. *Journal of Neuroscience Nursing, 32*(4), 204–209.

Teasdale, G. & Jennett, B. (1974). Assessment of coma and impaired consciousness. A practical scale. *Lancet, 2*(7872), 81–84.

van Reekum, R., Cohen, T., & Wong, J. (2000). Can traumatic brain injury cause psychiatric disorders? *Journal of Neuropsychiatry & Clinical Neurosciences, 12*(3), 316–327.

*Villanueva, N. E. (1999). Experiences of critical care nurses caring for unresponsive patients. *Journal of Neuroscience Nursing, 31*(4), 216–223.

Walshaw, L. K. (2000). Assessment of head injuries in a minor injuries unit. *Accident & Emergency Nursing, 8*(4), 210–213.

Wong, F. W. H. (2000). Prevention of secondary brain injury. *Critical Care Nurse, 20*(5), 18–27.

Neurotrauma

Donaldson, J., Borzatta, M. A., & Matossian, D. (2000). Nutrition strategies in neurotrama. *Critical Care Nursing Clinics of North America, 12*(4), 465–473.

Centers for Disease Control and Prevention, National Center for Injury Prevention and Control (2001). Scientific Data, Surveillance, & Injury Statistics: Web-based Injury Statistics Query and Reporting System (WBISQRS) http://www.cdc.gov/ncipc/osp/data.htm; http://

www.cdc.gov/safeusa/home/sci.htm; http://www.cdc.gov/ncipc/dacrrdp/tbi.htm.

Elovic, E., & Kirschblum, S. (1999). Epidemiology of spinal cord injury and traumatic brain injury: The scope of the problem. *Topics in Spinal Cord Injury Rehabilitation, 5*(2), 1–20.

Munro, N. (2000). Pulmonary challenges in neurotrauma. *Critical Care Nursing Clinics of North America, 12*(4), 457–464.

Velmahos, G., Kern, J., Chan, L., et al. (2000). Prevention of venous thromboembolism after injury: an evidence-based report—part II: Analysis of risk factors and evaluation of the role of vena caval filters. *Journal of Trauma-Injury Infection & Critical Care, 49*(1), 140–144.

Zafonte, R. D., Giap, B. T., Coplin, W. M., & Pangilian, P. (1999). Traumatic brain injury and spinal cord injury: Pathophysiology and acute therapeutic strategies. *Topics in Spinal Cord Injury Rehabilitation, 5*(2), 21–40.

Spinal Cord Injury

Atterbury, J. L., & Groome, L. J. (1998). Pregnancy in women with spinal cord injuries. *Nursing Clinics of North America, 33*(4), 603–613.

Bracken, M. B. (2000). Pharmacological interventions for acute spinal cord injury. *Cochrane Database of Systematic Reviews* [computer file]. (2):CD001046.

Canadian Paraplegic Association. (2000). *Spinal cord injury in Canada.* Available at: http://www.canparaplegic.org/national/level2.tpl?var1=resources. Retrieved June 15, 2005.

Craig, A., Hancock, K., & Dickson, H. (1999). Improving the long-term adjustment of spinal cord injured persons. *Spinal Cord, 37*(5), 345–350.

Dibsie, L. G. (1998). Clearing cervical spine injuries: A discussion of the process and the problems. *Critical Care Nursing Quarterly, 21*(2), 36–41.

Gaebler, C., Maier, R., Kutscha-Lissberg, F., et al. (1999). Results of spinal cord decompression and thoracolumbar pedicle stabilisation in relation to the time of operation. *Spinal Cord, 37*(1), 33–39.

Halbert, L. A. (1998). Breastfeeding in the woman with a compromised nervous system. *Journal of Human Lactation, 14*(4), 327–331.

Huston, C. J. (1998). Cervical spine injury. *American Journal of Nursing, 98*(6), 33.

Johnson, R. L., Gerhart, K. A., McGray, J., et al. (1998). Secondary conditions following spinal cord injury in a population-based sample. *Spinal Cord, 36*(1), 45–50.

Kannisto, M., Merikanto, J., & Alaranta, H. (1998). Comparison of health-related quality of life in three subgroups of spinal cord injury patients. *Spinal Cord, 36*(3), 193–199.

Lucke, K. T. (1998). Pulmonary management following acute SCI. *Journal of Neuroscience Nursing, 30*(2), 91–104.

Mitcho, K., & Yanko, J. R. (1999). Acute care management of spinal cord injuries. *Critical Care Nursing Quarterly, 22*(2), 60–79.

Nolan, M., & Nolan, J. (1998). Rehabilitation following spinal injury: The nursing response. *British Journal of Nursing, 7*(2), 97–104.

*Prieto-Fingerhut, T., Banovac, K., & Lynne, C. M. (1997). A study comparing sterile and non-sterile urethral catheterization in patients with spinal cord injury. *Rehabilitation Nursing, 22*(6), 299–302.

Short, D. J., El Masry, W. S., & Jones, P. W. (2000). High-dose methylprednisolone in the management of acute spinal cord injury: A systematic review from a clinical perspective. *Spinal Cord, 38*(5), 273–286.

Subbarao, J., & Garrison, S. (1999). Heterotopic ossification: Diagnosis and management, current concepts and controversies. *Journal of Spinal Cord Medicine, 22*(4), 273–283.

Stillwell, S. B. (2000). When you suspect epidural hematoma. *American Journal of Nursing, 100*(9), 68–76.

*Sullivan, J. (1999). Spinal cord injury research: Review and synthesis. *Critical Care Nursing Quarterly, 22*(2), 80–99.

Travers, P. L. (1999). Autonomic dysreflexia: A clinical rehabilitation problem. *Rehabilitation Nursing, 24*(1), 19–23.

Vacanti, M. P., Leonard, J. L., Dore, B. et al. (2001). Tissue-engineered spinal cord. *Transplantation Proceedings, 33*(1–2), 592–598.

RESOURCES AND WEBSITES

American Association of Neuroscience Nurses (AANN), 4700 W. Lake Ave, Chicago, IL 60025-1485; (847) 375-4733; (888)-557-2266; http://www.aann.org.

American Association of Spinal Cord Injury Nurses (AASCIN), 75-20 Astoria Blvd., Jackson Heights, NY 11370-1177; (718) 803-3782; http://www.aascin.org.

American Paralysis/Spinal Cord Hotline, (800) 526-3456; http://www.scihotline.org.

Association of Rehabilitation Nurses, 5700 Old Orchard Rd., Skokie, IL 60077; (708) 966-8673; http://www.rehabnurse.org.

The Brain Injury Association, Inc., 105 N. Alfred St., Alexandria, VA 22314; (703) 236-6000; family help line: (800) 444-6443; http://www.biausa.org.

The Brain Trauma Foundation 523 East 72d Street, New York, NY 10021; (212) 772-0608; http://www.braintrauma.org.

Canadian Paraplegic Association, 1101 Prince of Wales Drive, Suite 230, Ottawa, ON K2C 3W7; (613) 723-1033; http://canparaplegic.org.

Centers for Disease Control and Prevention, National Center for Injury Prevention and Control, Mailstop K65, 4770 Buford Highway NE, Atlanta, GA 30341-3724; (770) 488-1506; http://www.cdc.gov/ncipc/ncipchm.htm.

Information Center for Individuals with Disabilities, Fort Point Place, 27-43 Wormwood St., Boston, MA 02210-1606; (617) 727-5540; http://www.disability.net.

The Library of Congress, Division of the Blind and Physically Handicapped, 1291 Taylor St., NW, Washington, DC 20542; (202) 707-5100; http://www.loc.gov/access/.

National Head Injury Foundation, 1776 Massachusetts Ave., NW, Suite 100, Washington DC 20036; family help line (800) 444-6443; http://www.healthy.net/pan/cso/cioi/nhif.

National Rehabilitation Information Center, 1010 Wayne Avenue, Suite 800, Silver Spring, MD 20910; (800) 346-2742, TTY (301) 495-5626; http://www.naric.com.

National Spinal Cord Injury Association, 8300 Colesville Rd., Silver Spring, MD 20910; (301) 588-6959; http://www.spinalcord.org.

Paralyzed Veterans of America, 801 18th St., NW, Washington, DC 20006; (202) 872-1300; http://www.pva.org.

Rehabilitation Services Administration, Department of Human Services, 605 G Street, NW, Room 101M, Washington, DC 20001; (202) 727-3211; http://www.ed.gov/offices/OSERS/RSA/rsa.html.

Waiting.com, run by and for the families of traumatic brain injury: http://www.waiting.com.

Management of Patients With Neurologic Infections, Autoimmune Disorders, and Neuropathies

Adapted by Sue Young

LEARNING OBJECTIVES

On completion of this chapter, the learner will be able to:

1. Differentiate among the infectious disorders of the nervous system according to causes, manifestations, medical care, and nursing management.
2. Describe the pathophysiology, clinical manifestations, and medical and nursing management of multiple sclerosis, myasthenia gravis, and Guillain-Barré syndrome.
3. Use the nursing process as a framework for care of patients with multiple sclerosis, myasthenia gravis, and Guillain-Barré syndrome.
4. Describe disorders of the cranial nerves, their manifestations, and indicated nursing interventions.
5. Develop a plan of nursing care for the patient with a cranial nerve disorder.

*T*he diverse group of neurologic disorders that make up infectious and autoimmune disorders, and cranial and peripheral neuropathies present unique challenges for nursing care. Infectious processes of the nervous system sometimes cause death or permanent dysfunction. Autoimmune disorders usually have a slow, progressive course, requiring the nurse to manage symptoms and facilitate patients' and families' understanding of the disease process. Cranial and peripheral nerve disorders may affect the patient's comfort, functional independence, and self-esteem.

The nurse who cares for patients with these disorders must have a clear understanding of the pathologic processes and the clinical outcomes. Some of the issues nurses must help patients and families confront include adaptation to the effects of the disease, potential changes in family dynamics, and, possibly, end-of-life issues.

Infectious Neurologic Disorders

The infectious disorders of the nervous system include meningitis, brain abscesses, various types of encephalitis, and Creutzfeldt-Jakob and new-variant Creutzfeldt-Jakob disease. The clinical manifestations, assessment, and diagnostic findings as well as the medical and nursing management are related to the specific infectious process.

MENINGITIS

Meningitis is an inflammation of the meninges, the protective membranes that surround the brain and spinal cord. Meningitis is classified as aseptic or septic. In aseptic meningitis, bacteria are not the cause of the inflammation; the cause is viral or secondary to lymphoma, leukemia, or brain abscess. Septic meningitis refers to meningitis caused by bacteria, most commonly *Neisseria meningitidis,* although *Haemophilus influenzae* and *Streptococcus pneumoniae* are also causative agents. There are over 1,000 cases of bacterial meningitis each year in Canada (Meningitis Research Foundation of Canada, 2005).

Outbreaks of *N. meningitidis* infection are most likely to occur in dense community groups, such as college campuses and military installations. Though infections occur year round, the peak incidence is in the winter and early spring. Factors that increase the risk for developing bacterial meningitis include tobacco use and viral upper respiratory infection because they increase the amount of droplet production. Otitis media and mastoiditis increase the risk of bacterial meningitis because the bacteria can cross the epithelium membrane and enter the subarachnoid space. Persons with immune system deficiencies are also at greater risk for developing bacterial meningitis. Between 1992 and 1996 there was a 28% increase in the number of new cases reported in the 12-to-

29-year-old age group (Rosenstein, Perkins, Stephens et al., 2001). This increase focused attention on the need to develop a vaccine for high-risk populations.

Pathophysiology

Meningeal infections generally originate in one of two ways: through the bloodstream as a consequence of other infections, or by direct extension, such as might occur after a traumatic injury to the facial bones, or secondary to invasive procedures.

N. meningitidis concentrates in the nasopharynx and is transmitted by secretion or aerosol contamination. Bacterial or meningococcal meningitis also occurs as an opportunistic infection in patients with acquired immunodeficiency syndrome (AIDS) and as a complication of Lyme disease (Chart 64-1). *S. pneumoniae* is the most frequent causative agent of bacterial meningitis associated with AIDS (Rosenstein, Perkins, Stephens et al., 2001).

Once the causative organism enters the bloodstream, it crosses the blood–brain barrier and causes an inflammatory reaction in the meninges. Independent of the causative agent, inflammation of the subarachnoid space and pia mater occurs. Since there is little room for expansion within the cranial vault, the inflammation may cause increased intracranial pressure. Cerebrospinal fluid (CSF) flows in the subarachnoid space, where inflammatory cellular material from the affected meningeal tissue enters and accumulates in the subarachnoid space, thereby increasing the CSF cell count (Coyle, 1999).

The prognosis for bacterial meningitis depends on the causative organism, the severity of the infection and illness, and the timeliness of treatment. In acute fulminant presentations there may be adrenal damage, circulatory collapse, and widespread hemorrhages (Waterhouse-Friderichsen syndrome). This syndrome is the result of endothelial damage and vascular necrosis caused by the bacteria. Complications include visual impairment, deafness, seizures, paralysis, hydrocephalus, and septic shock.

Clinical Manifestations

Headache and fever are frequently the initial symptoms. Fever tends to remain high throughout the course of the illness. The headache is usually severe as a result of meningeal irritation. Meningeal irritation results in a number of other well-recognized signs common to all types of meningitis:

- Nuchal rigidity (stiff neck) is an early sign. Any attempts at flexion of the head are difficult because of spasms in the muscles of the neck. Forceful flexion causes severe pain.
- Positive Kernig's sign: When the patient is lying with the thigh flexed on the abdomen, the leg cannot be completely extended (Fig. 64-1).

Glossary

ataxia: impaired coordination of movements
bulbar paralysis: immobility of muscles innervated by cranial nerves with their cell bodies in the lower portion of the brain stem
diplopia: double vision, or the awareness of two images of the same object occurring in one or both eyes
dyskinesia: impaired ability to execute voluntary movements

dysphagia: difficulty swallowing, causing the patient to be at risk for aspiration
dysphonia: voice impairment or altered voice production
myoclonus: spasms of a single muscle or group of muscles
neuropathy: general term indicating a disorder of the nervous system
paresthesia: a sensation of numbness or tingling or a "pins and needles" sensation

prion: a particle smaller than a virus that is resistant to standard sterilization procedures
spasticity: muscular hypertonicity with increased resistance to stretch often associated with weakness, increased deep tendon reflexes, and diminished superficial reflexes
spongiform: having the appearance or quality of a sponge

Chart 64-1 **Meningitis in Specific Populations**

Meningitis can occur as a complication of other diseases and is an opportunistic infection seen with greater frequency in patients with acquired immunodeficiency syndrome (AIDS)

Meningitis in AIDS Patients

- Aseptic, cryptococcal, and tuberculous forms of meningitis have been reported in patients with AIDS.
- Acute and chronic forms of aseptic meningitis may occur with AIDS; both are accompanied by headache, but signs of meningeal irritation generally occur with the acute form.
- Aseptic meningitis may be accompanied by cranial nerve palsies. The meningitis is thought to be related to direct infection of the central nervous system by human immunodeficiency virus (HIV) because it can be isolated from the cerebrospinal fluid (CSF).
- Cryptococcal meningitis is the most common fungal infection of the central nervous system in patients with AIDS and has a 50% to 60% relapse rate. Patients may experience headache, nausea, vomiting, seizures, confusion, and lethargy. Treatment consists of IV administration of amphotericin B followed by fluconazole. Maintenance therapy with fluconazole may be necessary to prevent relapse.
- Some immunosuppressed patients develop few if any symptoms because of blunted inflammatory responses; others develop atypical features.

Meningitis in Lyme Disease

- Lyme disease is a multisystem inflammatory process caused by the tick-transmitted spirochete *Borrelia burgdorferi.*
- Neurologic abnormalities are seen in later stages (stages 2 or 3). Stage 2 occurs either with the characteristic rash or from 1 to 6 months after it has disappeared.
- Neurologic abnormalities include aseptic meningitis, chronic lymphocytic meningitis, and encephalitis.
- Cranial nerve inflammation, including Bell's palsy and other peripheral neuropathies, is common.
- Stage 3 (the chronic form of the disease) begins years after the initial tick infection and is characterized by arthritis, skin lesions, and neurologic abnormalities.
- Most patients with stage 2 and 3 Lyme disease are treated with intravenous antibiotics, usually ceftriaxone or penicillin G.
- Meningeal and systemic symptoms begin to improve within days, although other symptoms, such as headache, may persist for weeks.

- Positive Brudzinski's sign: When the patient's neck is flexed, flexion of the knees and hips is produced; when passive flexion of the lower extremity of one side is made, a similar movement is seen in the opposite extremity (see Fig. 64-1).
- Photophobia: extreme sensitivity to light; this finding is common, although the cause is unclear.

A rash can be a striking feature of *N. meningitidis* infection, occurring in about half of patients with this type of meningitis. Skin lesions develop, ranging from a petechial rash with purpuric lesions to large areas of ecchymosis.

Disorientation and memory impairment are common early in the course of the illness. The changes depend on the severity of the infection as well as the individual response to the physiologic processes. Behavioural manifestations are also common. As the illness progresses, lethargy, unresponsiveness, and coma may develop.

Seizures and increased intracranial pressure (ICP) are also associated with meningitis. Seizures occur secondary to focal areas of cortical irritability. Intracranial pressure increases secondary to accumulation of purulent exudate. The initial signs of increased ICP include decreased level of consciousness and focal motor deficits. If ICP is not controlled, the uncus of the temporal lobe may herniate through the tentorium into the brain stem. Brain stem herniation is a life-threatening event causing cranial nerve dysfunction and depressing the centres of vital functions, such as the medulla (Rowland, 2000). (See Chap. 61 for discussion of the patient with a change in level of consciousness or increased ICP.)

A fulminating infection occurs in about 10% of patients with meningococcal meningitis, with signs of overwhelming septicemia: an abrupt onset of high fever, extensive purpuric lesions (over the face and extremities), shock, and signs of disseminated intravascular coagulopathy (DIC). Death may occur within a few hours of onset of the infection.

Assessment and Diagnostic Findings

When the clinical presentation points to meningitis, diagnostic testing to identify the causative organism is conducted. Bacterial culture and Gram staining of CSF and blood are key diagnostic tests (Fischbach, 2002). The presence of polysaccharide antigen in CSF further supports the diagnosis of bacterial meningitis (Rosenstein et al., 2001).

Kernig's Sign

Brudzinski's Sign

FIGURE 64-1 Testing for meningeal irritation. (**A**) Kernig's sign. (**B**) Brudzinski's sign.

Prevention

In 1971, the U.S. military began vaccinating all new recruits against meningococcal meningitis, resulting in a dramatic decrease in the incidence. Researchers suggested vaccination of college freshmen as surveillance studies indicated that freshmen living in dormitories were at highest risk for developing meningococcal meningitis. At this time vaccination is not required for college freshmen in the U.S.; however, the American Academy of Pediatrics provides information to college freshmen and their parents about the risk of disease and the availability of vaccination (Bruce et al., 2001; Centers for Disease Control and Prevention [CDC], 2000). Rates of bacterial meningitis are low in Canada due to vaccination of all infants, starting at 2 months of age.

People in close contact with patients with meningococcal meningitis should be treated with antimicrobial chemoprophylaxis using rifampin (Rifadin), ciprofloxacin hydrochloride (Cipro), or ceftriaxone sodium (Rocephin) (CDC, 2000). Therapy should be started as soon as possible after contact; a delay in the initiation of therapy will limit the effectiveness of the prophylaxis (Rosenstein et al., 2001). Vaccination should also be considered as an adjunct to antibiotic chemoprophylaxis for anyone living with a person who develops meningococcal infection. Vaccination for children and at-risk adults should be encouraged to avoid meningitis caused by *H. influenzae* and *S. pneumoniae*.

Medical Management

Successful outcomes depend on the early administration of an antibiotic that crosses the blood–brain barrier into the subarachnoid space in sufficient concentration to halt the multiplication of bacteria. Penicillin antibiotics (eg, ampicillin, piperacillin) or one of the cephalosporins (eg, ceftriaxone sodium, cefotaxime sodium) may be used. Vancomycin hydrochloride alone or in combination with rifampin may be used if resistant strains of bacteria are identified. High doses of the appropriate antibiotic are administered intravenously.

Dexamethasone has been shown to be beneficial as adjunct therapy in the treatment of acute bacterial meningitis and in pneumococcal meningitis if given 15 to 20 minutes before the first dose of antibiotic and every 6 hours for the next 4 days. Studies indicate that dexamethasone improves the outcome in adults and does not increase the risk of gastrointestinal bleeding (de Gans & van de Beek, 2002).

Dehydration and shock are treated with fluid volume expanders. Seizures, which may occur in the early course of the disease, are controlled with phenytoin (Dilantin). Increased ICP is treated as necessary (see Chap. 61).

Nursing Management

The patient may be critically ill; therefore, so many of the nursing interventions are collaborative with those of the physician, respiratory therapist, and other members of the health care team. The patient's prognosis may depend on the supportive care provided.

Neurologic status and vital signs are continually assessed. Pulse oximetry and arterial blood gas values are used to quickly identify the need for respiratory support as the increasing ICP compromises the brain stem. Insertion of a cuffed endotracheal tube (or tracheotomy) and mechanical ventilation may be necessary to maintain adequate tissue oxygenation.

Arterial blood pressures are monitored to assess for incipient shock, which precedes cardiac or respiratory failure. Rapid intra-venous (IV) fluid replacement may be prescribed, but care is taken to prevent fluid overload. Fever also will increase the workload of the heart and cerebral metabolism. ICP will increase in response to increased cerebral metabolic demands. Therefore, measures are taken to reduce body temperature as quickly as possible.

Other important components of nursing care include:

- Monitoring body weight, serum electrolytes, and urine volume, specific gravity, and osmolality, especially if the syndrome of inappropriate antidiuretic hormone (SIADH) secretion is suspected
- Protecting the patient from injury secondary to seizure activity or altered level of consciousness
- Preventing complications associated with immobility, such as pressure ulcers and pneumonia
- Instituting droplet precautions until 24 hours after the initiation of antibiotic therapy (oral and nasal discharge is considered infectious)

Any sudden, critical illness can be devastating to the family. Because the patient's condition is often critical and the prognosis guarded, the family needs to be informed about the patient's condition and permitted to see the patient at intervals, even though the priority is to address the patient's need for immediate and intensive treatment. An important aspect of the nurse's role is to support the patient and to assist the family in identifying others who can be supportive to them during the crisis.

BRAIN ABSCESS

Although brain abscess is relatively rare, it is a complication encountered increasingly in patients whose immune systems have been suppressed either through therapy or disease.

Pathophysiology

A brain abscess is a collection of infectious material within the tissue of the brain. It may occur by direct invasion of the brain from intracranial trauma or surgery; by spread of infection from nearby sites, such as the sinuses, ears, and teeth (paranasal sinus infections, otitis media, dental sepsis); or by spread of infection from other organs (lung abscess, infective endocarditis) (Hickey, 2003). To prevent brain abscess, otitis media, mastoiditis, sinusitis, dental infections, and systemic infections should be treated promptly.

Clinical Manifestations

The clinical manifestations of a brain abscess result from alterations in intracranial dynamics (edema, brain shift), infection, or the location of the abscess (Chart 64-2). Headache, usually worse in the morning, is the most prevailing symptom. Vomiting is also common. Focal neurologic signs (weakness of an extremity, decreasing vision, seizures) may occur, depending on the site of the abscess. There may be a change in mental status, as reflected in lethargic, confused, irritable, or disoriented behaviour. Fever may or may not be present.

Assessment and Diagnostic Findings

Repeated neurologic examinations and continuing assessment of the patient are necessary to determine the location of the abscess. A computed tomography (CT) scan is invaluable in locating the site of the abscess, after the evolution and resolution of suppurative lesions, and in determining the optimal time for surgical inter-

Symptoms of Brain Abscesses

Frontal Lobe
Hemiparesis
Aphasia (expressive)
Seizures
Frontal headache

Temporal Lobe
Localized headache
Changes in vision
Facial weakness
Aphasia

Cerebellar Abscess
Occipital headache
Ataxia (inability to coordinate movements)
Nystagmus (rhythmic, involuntary movements of the eye)

Adapted from Hickey, J. V. (2003). *The clinical practice of neurological and neurosurgical nursing* (5th ed.). Philadelphia: Lippincott Williams & Wilkins.

vention. A magnetic resonance imaging (MRI) scan is useful to obtain images of the brain stem and posterior fossa if an abscess is suspected in these areas.

Medical Management

Brain abscess is treated with antimicrobial therapy and surgical incision or aspiration. If the abscess is encapsulated, CT-guided stereotactic needle aspiration under local anesthesia may be performed. Antimicrobial treatment is prescribed to eliminate the causative organism or reduce its virulence.

Penicillin G (20 million U) and chloramphenicol (Chloromycetin) (4 to 6 g/day given intravenously in divided doses) are usually prescribed because anaerobic streptococci and *Bacterioides* are the most common causative organisms (Hickey, 2003). Large IV doses are usually prescribed preoperatively to penetrate the blood–brain barrier and reach the abscess. The therapy is continued postoperatively. Corticosteroids may be prescribed to help reduce the inflammatory cerebral edema if the patient shows evidence of an increasing neurologic deficit. Antiseizure medications (phenytoin, phenobarbital) may be prescribed to prevent seizures. Multiple abscesses may be treated with appropriate antimicrobial therapy alone, with close monitoring by CT scans.

Nursing Management

Nursing care focuses on ongoing assessment of the neurologic status, administering medications, assessing the response to treatment, and providing supportive care.

Ongoing neurologic assessment alerts the nurse to changes in ICP, which may indicate a need for more aggressive intervention. The nurse also assesses and documents the responses to medications. Blood laboratory test results, specifically blood glucose and serum potassium levels, need to be closely monitored when corticosteroids are prescribed. Medical intervention may be required to return these values to normal or acceptable levels.

Patient safety is also a key nursing responsibility. Injury may result from decreased level of consciousness and falls related to motor weakness or seizures.

The patient with a brain abscess is extremely ill, and neurologic deficits may remain after treatment, such as hemiparesis, seizures, visual deficits, and cranial nerve palsies. Focal seizures are the most common sequelae, occurring in about 30% of patients (Hickey, 2003). The nurse must assess the family's ability to express their distress at the patient's condition, cope with the patient's illness and deficits, and obtain support.

HERPES SIMPLEX VIRUS ENCEPHALITIS

Encephalitis is an acute inflammatory process of the brain tissue. Herpes simplex virus (HSV) is the most common cause of acute encephalitis in the United States (Levitz, 1998). There are two herpes simplex viruses, HSV-1 and HSV-2. HSV-1 typically affects children and adults.

Pathophysiology

There are two possible modes of HSV-1 infection. In most cases, primary HSV-1 infection of the buccal mucosa occurs, followed by retrograde spread along the trigeminal nerve to the brain. It is also believed that latent virus in brain tissue may reactivate and result in encephalitis (Roos, 1999). HSV-2 most commonly affects neonates and is discussed in pediatric textbooks (Gutierrez & Prober, 1998).

Clinical Manifestations

HSV-1 encephalitis causes inflammation and necrosis in the temporal lobe, frontal lobe, and limbic system. The initial symptoms include fever, headache, confusion, and behavioural abnormalities (Roos, 1999). Focal neurologic symptoms reflect the areas of cerebral inflammation and necrosis and include behavioural change, focal seizures, dysphasia, hemiparesis, and altered level of consciousness. Focal symptoms are present within 7 days of infection and progress for 14 to 21 days.

Assessment and Diagnostic Findings

Neuroimaging studies, electroencephalography (EEG), and CSF examination are used to diagnose HSV encephalitis. MRI is the neuroimaging study of choice in the diagnosis of HSV encephalitis as it can help identify lesions in the temporal lobe.

The EEG demonstrates a specific wave pattern in 66% of cases of biopsy-proven HSV encephalitis. CSF reveals a high opening pressure and low glucose and high protein levels. Viral cultures are almost always negative. Since 1996, the polymerase chain reaction (PCR) technique has been used to diagnose HSV encephalitis (Roos, 1999). PCR will identify the DNA bands of the HSV specifically. The validity of PCR is very high between the third and tenth day of symptom onset.

Medical Management

Acyclovir (Zovirax), an antiviral agent, is the medication of choice in HSV treatment (Karch, 2002). The mode of action is the inhibition of viral DNA replication. It is usually well tolerated by the patient. To prevent relapse, treatment should continue for up to 3 weeks. Slow administration over 1 hour will prevent crystallization of the medication in the urine. The usual dose of acyclovir is decreased if the patient has a history of renal insufficiency (Karch, 2002). In the rare case of acyclovir resistance, foscarnet sodium (Foscavir) is prescribed (Roos, 1999).

Nursing Management

Assessment of neurologic function is key to monitoring the progression of disease. Comfort measures to reduce headache include dimming the lights, limiting noise, and administering analgesic agents. Opioid analgesic medications may mask neurologic symptoms; therefore, they are used cautiously. Focal seizures and altered level of consciousness require care directed at injury prevention and safety. Nursing care addressing patient and family anxiety is ongoing throughout the illness. Monitoring of blood chemistry test results and urinary output will alert the nurse to the presence of renal complications related to acyclovir therapy.

ARTHROPOD-BORNE VIRUS ENCEPHALITIS

Arthropod vectors transmit several types of viruses that cause encephalitis. The primary vector in North America is the mosquito. Arbovirus infection occurs in specific geographic areas during the summer and fall. The four types of arboviral encephalitis that occur in North America are LaCrosse encephalitis, St. Louis encephalitis, Western equine encephalitis, and Eastern equine encephalitis (Roos, 1999). The West Nile virus, which may cause encephalitis, was first detected in North America in 1999 and is now present in Canada, the United States, and Mexico (Public Health Agency of Canada, 2005).

Pathophysiology

Viral replication occurs at the site of the mosquito bite. If adequate virus is inoculated, a viremia ensues. The virus gains access to the central nervous system (CNS) via the cerebral capillaries. It spreads from neuron to neuron, predominantly affecting the cortical grey matter, the brain stem, and the thalamus. Meningeal exudates compound the clinical presentation by irritating the meninges and increasing ICP (Roos, 1999).

Clinical Manifestations

All arboviral encephalitis begins with a flu-like prodrome, but specific neurologic manifestations depend on the viral type. LaCrosse encephalitis, for example, may present with focal neurologic symptoms and seizures. Mortality is low but residual seizures may occur. A unique clinical feature of St. Louis encephalitis is SIADH with hyponatremia. The mortality rate is 10% to 20%. The clinical manifestations of Eastern equine encephalitis are acute and carry a high mortality rate of 50% to 75% (Roos, 1999). Although the clinical manifestations of Western equine encephalitis are nonspecific, the morbidity rate is high.

Assessment and Diagnostic Findings

Neuroimaging is not useful in diagnosing many types of encephalitis. In Eastern equine encephalitis, however, CT scan and MRI may reveal lesions in the basal ganglia and thalamus (Roos, 1999). The CSF analysis shows a normal glucose level, elevated protein level, and polymorphonuclear leukocytic pleocytosis. St. Louis, Eastern equine, and Western equine encephalitis viruses are rarely isolated in the CSF (Roos, 1999).

The age of the patient is important information in making a specific viral diagnosis. LaCrosse virus encephalitis is the most common pediatric arboviral encephalitis. St. Louis encephalitis affects adults over 50 years of age; Eastern equine encephalitis is not age-specific (Roos, 1999). Western equine encephalitis can present as pediatric encephalitis but is less prevalent.

Medical Management

There is no specific medication for arboviral encephalitis. Medical management is aimed at controlling seizures and increased ICP (Roos, 1999)

Nursing Management

If the patient is very ill, hospitalization may be required. The nurse carefully assesses neurologic status and identifies improvement or deterioration in the patient's condition. Injury prevention is key in light of the potential for falls or seizures. Arboviral encephalitis may result in death or life-long residual health issues. The family will need support and teaching to cope with these outcomes.

Public education addressing the prevention of arboviral encephalitis is a key nursing role. Clothing that provides coverage and insect repellents should be used in high-risk areas. Community mosquito control is advocated.

FUNGAL ENCEPHALITIS

Fungal infections of the CNS occur rarely in healthy people. The presentation of fungal encephalitis is related to geographic area and a compromised immune system (Leedom & Underman, 2000). The common fungi found around the world that can infect the CNS include *Cryptococcus neoformans, Histoplasma capsulatum, Aspergillus,* and *Candida albicans* (Davis, 1999). Other fungi are found only in certain regions: *Coccidioides immitis,* for example, is found in soil in central California, the southwest United States, northern Mexico, and areas of Argentina (Davis, 1999).

Pathophysiology

The fungal spores enter the body via inhalation. They initially infect the lungs, causing vague respiratory symptoms. In some cases, the fungi may enter the bloodstream, causing a fungemia. If the fungemia overcomes the person's immune system, the fungus may spread to the CNS. The initial presentation is meningitis followed by encephalitis and brain abscesses. In addition to infecting the brain, the fungi may infect the spinal cord, producing an abscess. The abscess will produce symptoms of spinal cord compression (Davis, 1999).

Clinical Manifestations

The common symptoms of fungal encephalitis include fever, malaise, headache, nuchal rigidity, lethargy, and mental status changes (Davis, 1999). *C. neoformans* is the most common fungus to infect the CNS. Symptoms of increased ICP related to hydrocephalus often occur (Go et al., 2000). Vascular changes are associated with *C. immitis* and *Aspergillus* (Leedom & Underman, 2000). Manifestations of vascular change may include arteritis or cerebral infarction.

Assessment and Diagnostic Findings

CNS fungal infections present a diagnostic challenge because their presentations mimic other causes of encephalitis. The symptoms develop over a 2-week period. Fungal infection may also be present in organs such as the lungs or kidney (Davis, 1999). The presence of a compromised immune system and a history of living in or recently having traveled to a geographic area where specific fungi are found in the soil may suggest fungal encephalitis (Davis, 1999; Leedom & Underman, 2000). Laboratory evaluation of blood shows an elevated white cell count and anemia. In some cases, serologic tests may show fungal antibodies in serum (Davis, 1999). The CSF shows an elevated white cell count and protein levels. *C. neoformans* is readily identified in the CSF fungal culture. The CSF culture is positive for other fungi in 50% of cases (Davis, 1999).

Neuroimaging is used to identify CNS changes related to fungal infection and will demonstrate fungal foci in organs initially invaded by the fungus. Although both MRI and CT scan are used in the workup for fungal encephalitis, MRI is more sensitive. The MRI may indicate lesions in the basal ganglia or thalamus, as well as hemorrhage, vascular complications, ischemia, aneurysm formation, or hydrocephalus (Go et al., 2000).

Medical Management

Medical management is directed at the causative fungus and the neurologic consequences of the infection. Seizures are controlled by standard antiseizure medications. Increased ICP is controlled by repeated lumbar punctures or shunting of CSF. In contrast to patients with cryptococcal meningitis, the use of repeated (once or twice daily) lumbar punctures in patients with fungal infections has been an effective strategy to control increased ICP and has been associated with improved survival with fewer neurologic sequelae (Davis, 1999).

Antifungal agents are given for a specific period of time to cure the infection in patients with competent immune systems. Patients with compromised immune systems will receive antifungal therapy until the infection is controlled, after which they will receive a maintenance dose of the medication for an indefinite period of time.

Although the dose and duration of treatment depend on the causative fungi, amphotericin B (Abelcet, AmBisome, Amphocin, Amphotec, Fungizone, and Fungizone IV) is the standard antifungal agent used in treatment (Karch, 2002). Dosing must be high enough to penetrate the blood–brain barrier without causing renal toxicity.

Fluconazole (Diflucan) or flucytosine (5-FC, 5-fluorocytosine, Ancobon) may be administered in conjunction with amphotericin B. Both can be given orally and may be used as maintenance therapy. Potential side effects of fluconazole include nausea, abdominal pain, headache, dizziness, rash, reversible alopecia, and a transient increase in liver enzymes. When flucytosine is prescribed in conjunction with amphotericin B, bone marrow suppression may occur. Therefore, patients receiving these medications in combination should have leukocyte and platelet counts monitored twice a week (Davis, 1999).

Nursing Management

If hydrocephalus develops and inflammation progresses, ICP will rise. Nursing assessment aimed at early identification of increased ICP is necessary to ensure early control and management. (See Chap. 61 for management of the patient with increased ICP.) Patient comfort may be optimized by administering nonopioid analgesics, limiting environmental stimuli, and positioning. Administration of amphotericin B may cause fever, chills, and body aches. Giving diphenhydramine (Benadryl) and acetaminophen (Tylenol) approximately 30 minutes before giving amphotericin B may prevent these side effects. Renal toxicity due to ampho-

tericin B is dose-limiting. Monitoring the serum creatinine and blood urea nitrogen levels may alert the nurse to the development of renal insufficiency and the need to address the patient's renal status.

Providing support will assist the patient and family to cope with the illness. Work-up of the patient for immunodeficiency diseases such as AIDS may put additional stress on the family. The nurse may need to mobilize community support systems for the patient and family.

CREUTZFELDT-JAKOB AND NEW-VARIANT CREUTZFELDT-JAKOB DISEASE

Creutzfeldt-Jakob disease (CJD) and new-variant Creutzfeldt-Jakob (nvCJD) disease belong to a group of degenerative, infectious neurologic disorders called transmissible spongiform encephalopathies (TSE). Although CJD and nvCJD have distinct clinical and histologic differences, they have many features in common. Both are rare and have incubation periods ranging from months to decades. In both, the symptoms are progressive, there is no definitive treatment, and the outcome is fatal.

CJD occurs primarily in adults ages 50 to 70. The incidence of disease is 1 per million worldwide (Weihl & Roos, 1999). nvCJD occurs in younger patients and has a prolonged duration of illness compared to CJD. The risk of nvCJD in the United States is thought to be low as cattle are fed primarily with soy-derived feed (see Pathophysiology, below). Only a few rare cases of TSE have occurred in the United States to date (Weihl & Roos, 1999).

Pathophysiology

Although still debated, the causative agent appears to be a **prion**, a proteinaceous, infectious particle smaller than a virus (Davis & Kennedy, 2000). The prion converts a normal cellular protein to an abnormal form, thus destroying neurons and glial cells. The grey matter takes on a spongy appearance (**spongiform** changes). Lesions, or plaques, also appear in various locations in the CNS (Weihl & Roos, 1999).

In CJD, the method of transmission is frequently unknown; however, direct transmission (by contact with infected animals) of the prion to humans may initiate the degenerative neurologic process. The disease is also heritable, and familial groups account for approximately 15% of cases, clustering in certain parts of the world. Iatrogenic transmission accounts for approximately 5% of cases and is due to contaminated neurosurgical devices and blood transfusions and the use of cadaver-derived growth hormone (growth hormone is now created synthetically) (World Health Organization, 2001).

Based primarily on an outbreak of cases in England in the late 1980s and through the 1990s, it was discovered that in nvCJD, the primary mode of transmission appeared to be the ingestion of CNS tissue of infected cattle. However, in 1998, additional concerns were raised about the safety of the English blood supply. The prion exists in lymphoid tissue and blood in all of the TSEs, but the incidence is higher in nvCJD. In light of the rising incidence of nvCJD, concern arose about the risk of infection through transfusion of blood products. There is no method available to screen blood for infectivity. All blood must be leukocyte-depleted prior to transfusion. In 1998, the use of plasma derived from citizens of the United Kingdom for use in manufacturing blood-derived products was banned in the U.S. and Canada (Weihl & Roos, 1999).

Clinical Manifestations

Many patients with CJD have vague prodromal symptoms prior to specific neurologic changes. Symptoms usually include behavioural changes, dementia, mutism, visual changes, cerebellar, pyramidal, and extrapyramidal signs, and myoclonic jerks. The myoclonic jerks may be spontaneous or precipitated by auditory or tactile stimuli. The **myoclonus** (spasms) may involve a single muscle group, a limb, or the entire body. The symptoms progress until the patient is completely unaware of the environment and immobilized.

Although the same type of agent, a prion, causes nvCJD, there are distinct differences in the clinical manifestations of nvCJD and CJD. In nvCJD, there are more prion-reactive plaques, referred to as florid plaques, surrounding spongiform tissue throughout the cerebrum and cerebellum. The characteristic EEG changes present in CJD are absent in nvCJD. Anxiety, depression, and behavioural changes are the initial symptoms of nvCJD. Cerebellar symptoms occur, with gait changes and **ataxia**. Myoclonus is present in most patients diagnosed with nvCJD. Memory and cognitive impairments occur late in the course of nvCJD. Mutism occurs in both nvCJD and CJD (Almond, 1998).

Assessment and Diagnostic Findings

Historically, sharp waves and spikes on the EEG were the only features available to support the diagnosis of CJD. Recent detection of a polyclonal antibody (protein 14-3-3) in CSF has enabled the diagnosis of CJD (Poser, Mollenhauder, Krab et al., 1999). In addition to the presence of a polyclonal antibody in CSF, a protein increase is demonstrated along with the presence of enzymes indicative of neuronal loss. CT scan is used to rule out disorders that may mimic the symptoms of CJD. MRI scans are useful, identifying lesions in the basal ganglia in most cases of CJD. Definitive diagnosis is made by brain biopsy or at autopsy.

Medical Management

After the onset of specific neurologic symptoms, progression of disease occurs quickly. There is no effective treatment for CJD or nvCJD. The care of the patient is supportive and palliative. Goals of care include prevention of injury related to immobility and dementia, promotion of patient comfort, and provision of support and education for the family. The duration of disease is 4 to 5 months in CJD and 16 months in nvCJD, with death occurring as a result of respiratory failure or sepsis (Weihl & Roos, 1999).

Nursing Management

As with medical management, the nursing care of patients is primarily supportive and palliative. Psychological and emotional support of patients and families throughout the course of the illness is needed This care extends to providing for a dignified death and supporting the family through the processes of grief and loss. Hospice care should be used either at home or at an inpatient facility. (See Chap. 17 for an in-depth discussion of end-of-life issues.)

Prevention of disease transmission is an important part of nursing care. Although patient isolation is not necessary, use of standard precautions is important. Institutional protocols are followed for blood and body fluid exposure and decontamination of equipment. Conventional methods of sterilization do not destroy the prion. The CDC guidelines (based on WHO guidelines) outline the stringent sterilization methods that must be used to destroy the prion on surfaces.

Autoimmune Processes

Autoimmune nervous system disorders include multiple sclerosis, myasthenia gravis, and Guillain-Barré syndrome.

MULTIPLE SCLEROSIS

Multiple sclerosis (MS) is an immune-mediated progressive demyelinating disease of the CNS. Demyelination refers to the destruction of myelin, the fatty and protein material that surrounds certain nerve fibres in the brain and spinal cord; it results in impaired transmission of nerve impulses (Fig. 64-2). MS typically presents in young adults ages 20 to 40, and it affects women more frequently than men (Boyden, 2000).

The cause of MS is an area of ongoing research. Autoimmune activity results in demyelination, but the sensitized antigen has not been identified. Multiple factors play a role in the initiation of the immune process. Geographic prevalence is highest in northern Europe, southern Australia, the northern United States, and southern Canada (Noseworthy, Lucchinetti, Rodriguez et al., 2000). It is believed that an environmental exposure at a young age may play a role in the development of MS later in life.

Genetic predisposition is indicated by the presence of a specific cluster (haplotype) of human leukocyte antigens (HLA) on the cell wall. The presence of this haplotype may promote susceptibility to factors, such as viruses, that trigger the autoimmune response activated in MS. A specific virus capable of initiating the

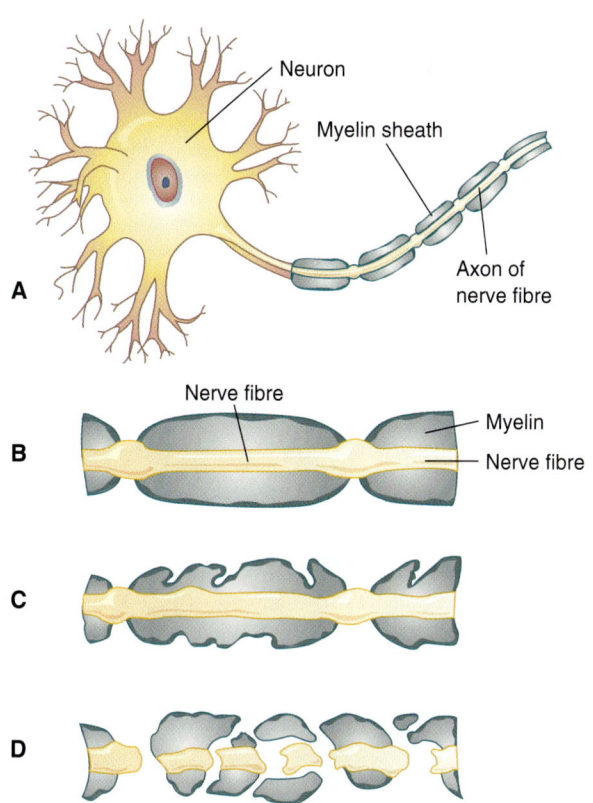

FIGURE 64-2   The process of demyelination. **A** and **B** depict a normal nerve cell and axon with myelin. **C** and **D** show the slow disintegration of myelin, resulting in a disruption in axon function.

autoimmune response has not been identified. It is believed that DNA on the virus mimics the amino acid sequence of myelin, resulting in an immune system cross-reaction in the presence of a defective immune system (Boyden, 2000).

Pathophysiology

Sensitized T cells typically cross the blood–brain barrier; their function is to check the CNS for antigens and then leave. In MS, the sensitized T cells remain in the CNS and promote the infiltration of other agents that damage the immune system. The immune system attack leads to inflammation that destroys myelin (which normally insulates the axon and speeds the conduction of impulses along the axon) and oligodendroglial cells that produce myelin in the CNS.

Plaques of sclerotic tissue appear on demyelinated axons, further interrupting the transmission of impulses. Demyelination interrupts the flow of nerve impulses and results in a variety of manifestations, depending on which nerves are affected. Demyelinated axons are scattered irregularly throughout the CNS (Fig. 64-3). The areas most frequently affected are the optic nerves, chiasm, and tracts; the cerebrum; the brain stem and cerebellum; and the spinal cord. Eventually the axons themselves begin to degenerate, resulting in permanent and irreversible damage (Bashir & Whitaker, 2002; Halper, 2001).

Clinical Manifestations

The course of MS may assume many different patterns (Fig. 64-4). In some patients, the disease follows a benign course, with a normal life span and symptoms so mild that patients do not seek health care and treatment. Eighty percent to 85% of cases of MS begin with a relapsing–remitting course, with complete recovery between clearly defined symptomatic exacerbations (Noseworthy et al., 2000). This form of the disease does not progress between relapses, although the majority of cases with this initial type of course change to a secondary-progressive course after some years (Halper, 2001). Secondary-progressive MS begins as relapsing–remitting disease but changes to a course in which there is not full recovery but rather continued progression between defined relapses. Ten percent to 20% percent of patients have a primary progressive course (Noseworthy et al., 2000; Halper, 2001), in which symptoms progress throughout the disease, with increasing disability. Primary progressive MS is characterized by continuous decline, with the potential development of quadriparesis, cognitive dysfunction, visual loss, and brain stem syndromes.

The signs and symptoms of MS are varied and multiple, reflecting the location of the lesion (plaque) or combination of lesions. The primary symptoms most commonly reported are fatigue, depression, weakness, numbness, difficulty in coordination, loss of balance, and pain. Visual disturbances due to lesions in the optic nerves or their connections may include blurring of vision, **diplopia**, patchy blindness (scotoma), and total blindness.

Fatigue impairs optimal function throughout the course of the disease. Fatigue is exacerbated when febrile illness, environmental temperature, hot showers, and normal circadian rhythms during the afternoon elevate body temperature. Depression may relate to the pathophysiology or may occur as a reaction to the diagnosis. Suicide as the cause of death occurs 7.5 times more frequently among persons diagnosed with MS than among the age-matched general population. If suicide occurs, it is likely to occur within the first 5 years of diagnosis (Walther & Hohlfeld, 1999).

FIGURE 64-3 Multiple sclerosis. (**A**) A CT scan of brain demonstrates an area of demyelination in the periventricular white matter of the right frontal lobe. The plaque is perpendicular to the lateral ventricle, a typical finding in MS. (**B**) An MRI of the spinal cord in the same patient highlights another typical finding: a flame-shaped area of demyelination within the midcervical region of the spinal cord. Courtesy of the Danbury Hospital Department of Radiology.

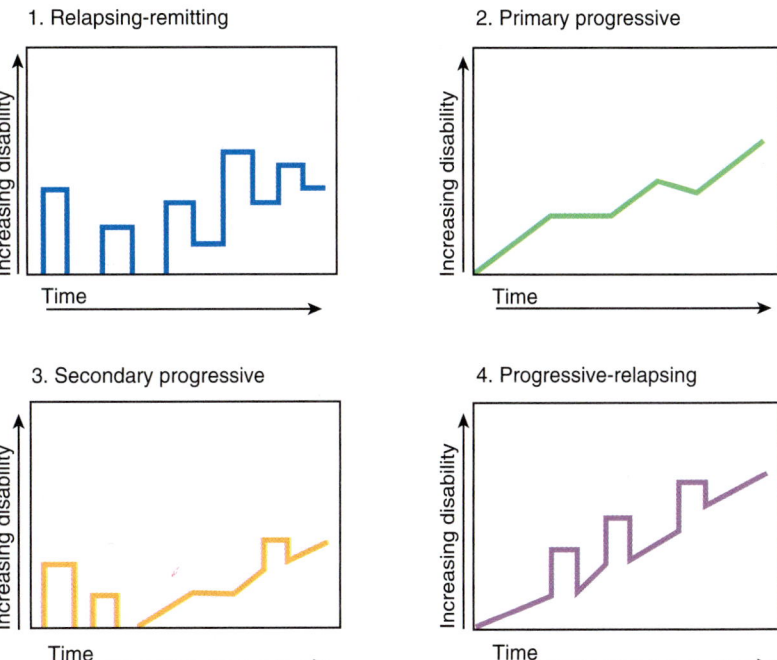

FIGURE 64-4 Types and courses of MS. 1. Relapsing remitting (RR) MS is characterized by clearly acute attacks with full recovery or with sequelae and residual deficit upon recovery. Periods between disease relapses are characterized by lack of disease progression. 2. Primary progressive (PP) MS is characterized by disease showing progression of disability from onset, without plateaus or remissions or with occasional plateaus and temporary minor improvements. 3. Secondary progressive (SP) MS begins with an initial RR course, followed by progression of variable rate, which may also include occasional relapses and minor remissions. 4. Progressive-relapsing (PR) MS shows progression from onset but with clear acute relapses with or without recovery. Lublin, F. D., Reingold, F. C., et al. (1996). Defining the clinical course of multiple sclerosis: Results of an international survey. *Neurology, 46*(64), 907–911. Used with permission from Lippincott Williams & Wilkins.

Pain occurs in 66% of patients with MS. Pain may be due to demyelination of pain fibres, mechanical stress on muscles, bones, and joints due to disability, or treatment measures (Maloni, 2000).

Spasticity (muscle hypertonicity) of the extremities and loss of the abdominal reflexes are due to involvement of the main motor pathways (pyramidal tracts) of the spinal cord. Disruption of the sensory axons may produce sensory dysfunction (paresthesias, pain). Cognitive and psychosocial problems may reflect frontal or parietal lobe involvement; some degree of cognitive change (eg, memory loss, decreased concentration) occurs in about half of patients, but severe cognitive changes with dementia (progressive organic mental disorder) are rare. Involvement of the cerebellum or basal ganglia can produce ataxia (impaired coordination of movements) and tremor. Loss of the control connections between the cortex and the basal ganglia may occur and cause emotional lability and euphoria. Bladder, bowel, and sexual dysfunctions are common.

Secondary complications of MS include urinary tract infections, constipation, pressure ulcers, contracture deformities, dependent pedal edema, pneumonia, reactive depression, and decreased bone mass. Emotional, social, marital, economic, and vocational problems may also be a consequence of the disease.

Exacerbations and remissions are characteristic of MS. During exacerbations, new symptoms appear and existing ones worsen; during remissions, symptoms decrease or disappear. Relapses may be associated with periods of emotional and physical stress. MRI studies demonstrate that many plaques do not produce serious symptoms; however, the disease may be very active, as demonstrated by MRI. There also is evidence that remyelination actually occurs in some patients.

Assessment and Diagnostic Findings

MRI is the primary diagnostic tool for visualizing plaques, documenting disease activity, and evaluating the effect of treatment. Electrophoresis of CSF identifies the presence of oligoclonal banding (several bands of immunoglobulin G bonded together, indicating an immune system abnormality). Evoked potential studies can help define the extent of the disease process and monitor changes. Underlying bladder dysfunction is diagnosed by urodynamic studies. Neuropsychological testing may be indicated to assess cognitive impairment. A sexual history helps to identify changes in sexual function.

Gerontologic Considerations

Due to improved treatment and an increase in the average life span for patients with MS, more individuals are living to become elderly. These patients may have chronic health problems for which they may be taking additional medications that could interact with medications prescribed for MS. The absorption, distribution, metabolism, and excretion of medications are altered in the elderly as a result of age-related changes in renal and liver functions. Therefore, the elderly must be monitored closely for adverse and toxic effects of MS medications and for osteoporosis (particularly with frequent corticosteroid use, which may be required for exacerbations). The cost of medications could lead to poor adherence to the prescribed regimen in elderly patients on fixed incomes.

Elderly MS patients have specific physical and psychosocial challenges. Physical challenges include impaired mobility, spasticity, pain and bladder dysfunction, impaired sleep, and an increased need for assistance with self-care (Klewer et al., 2001). Psychosocial issues include depression and suicidal thoughts (Klewer et al., 2001).

Medical Management

No cure exists for MS. An individualized, organized, and rational treatment program is indicated to relieve the patient's symptoms and provide continuing support, particularly for individuals with cognitive changes (50%), who may need more structure and support. The goals of treatment are to delay the progression of the disease, manage chronic symptoms, and treat acute exacerbations. Many patients with MS have stable disease and require only intermittent treatment, whereas others experience steady progression of their disease. Symptoms requiring intervention include spasticity, fatigue, bladder dysfunction, and ataxia. Management strategies target the various motor and sensory symptoms and effects of immobility that can occur.

PHARMACOLOGIC THERAPY

Three medications, referred to as the "ABC (and R) drugs," are currently the main pharmacologic therapy for MS. The interferons beta-1a (Avonex) and beta-1b (Betaseron) reduce the frequency of relapse by 30% and decrease the appearance of new lesions on MRI by 80% (Tselis & Lisak, 1999). Glatiramer acetate (Copaxone) also reduces the number of lesions on MRI and the relapse rate. In March 2002, the FDA approved a fourth agent, Rebif (a form of interferon beta-1b) for the treatment of relapsing MS (PRISMS Study Group, 2001).

All of these medications have multiple immune activities. The interferons reduce T-cell proliferation; glatiramer acetate inhibits antigen-specific T-cell activation (Noseworthy et al., 2000). All of the disease-modifying medications, the "ABC (and R) drugs," require injections. Interferon beta-1b (Betaseron) is administered subcutaneously every other day, interferon beta-la (Avonex) is given by intramuscular injection once a week, and glatiramer acetate (Copaxone) is administered by subcutaneous injection every day. Rebif is administered subcutaneously three times a week. Seventy-five percent of patients taking one of the interferons experience flu-like symptoms; these symptoms can be controlled with nonsteroidal anti-inflammatory drugs (NSAIDs) and usually resolve after a few months of therapy (Walther & Hohlfeld, 1999). Patients receiving these injectable medications and their families must be instructed in injection technique and must become knowledgeable about site reactions and other possible side effects (Ross, 2001).

Mitoxantrone (Novantrone), which received FDA approval in 2000 (Rolak, 2001), is an antineoplastic agent used primarily to treat leukemia and lymphoma. It received approval to treat secondary progressive MS due to its immunosuppressive qualities (Rolak, 2001). Patients need to have laboratory tests (complete blood count) performed, and the results must be closely monitored due to the potential for leukopenia and cardiac toxicity. A few patients (2% to 3%) will develop signs and symptoms of cardiomyopathy and heart failure due to cardiac toxicity (Rolak, 2001).

Corticosteroids modulate the immune response and are used to limit the severity and duration of exacerbations. These agents suppress the immune response and decrease inflammatory change. Nerve conduction is restored with variable degrees of symptomatic recovery. Typically the patient receives high-dose IV methylprednisolone followed by an oral prednisone taper. The nurse must carefully monitor the patient for side effects related to corticosteroids such as mood changes and fluid and electrolyte alterations and teach the patient and family about side effects.

Researchers continue to investigate other possible treatments for MS. Many agents that have been investigated have proven to be too toxic for clinical use. Researchers are studying strategies that facilitate the proliferation of anti-inflammatory cytokines. T-cell vaccination and agents that inhibit oxygen radicals and proteases are under study (Noseworthy et al., 2000).

Medications are also prescribed for management of specific symptoms. Baclofen (Lioresal), a GABA agonist, is the medication of choice in treating spasms. It can be administered orally or by intrathecal injection. Benzodiazepines (Valium), tizanidine (Zanaflex), and dantrolene (Dantrium) may also be used to treat spasms. Patients with disabling spasms and contractures may re-

quire nerve blocks or surgical intervention. Fatigue that interferes with activities of daily living may be treated with amantadine (Symmetrel), pemoline (Cylert), or fluoxetine (Prozac). Ataxia is a chronic problem most resistant to treatment. Medications used to treat ataxia include beta-adrenergic blockers (Inderal), antiseizure agents (Neurontin), and benzodiazepines (Klonopin).

Various strategies for pain management can be implemented, based on the type of pain that exists. Acute pain may be treated with antidepressants, opiates, or antiseizure medications. Surgical procedures may be required to interrupt the pain pathway. Subacute pain as well as chronic back pain can be effectively treated with NSAIDs. Physical therapy may also benefit the patient by improving posture and strength.

Pain may also be due to osteoporosis (Maloni, 2000). Perimenopausal women with MS are more likely to develop osteoporosis than those without MS. Immobility, corticosteroid therapy, and estrogen loss play a role in the development of osteoporosis in women with MS. Bone mineral density testing is recommended for this high-risk group (Smeltzer, Zimmerman, Capriotti & Fernandes, 2002). Diagnosis and treatment of osteoporosis are discussed at length in Chapter 68.

Management of bladder and bowel control is often among the patient's most difficult problems and a variety of medications (anticholinergics, alpha-adrenergic blockers, or antispasmodic agents) may be prescribed. Nonpharmacologic strategies also assist in establishing effective bowel and bladder elimination (see Nursing Process section).

Urinary tract infection is often superimposed on the underlying neurologic dysfunction. Ascorbic acid (vitamin C) may be prescribed to acidify the urine, making bacterial growth less likely. Antibiotics are prescribed when appropriate.

NURSING PROCESS:
THE PATIENT WITH MULTIPLE SCLEROSIS

Assessment

Nursing assessment addresses actual and potential problems associated with the disease, including neurologic problems, secondary complications, and the impact of the disease on the patient and family. The patient's movements and walking are observed to determine if there is danger of falling. Assessment of function is carried out both when the patient is well rested and when fatigued. The patient is assessed for weakness, spasticity, visual impairment, incontinence, and disorders of swallowing and speech. Additional areas of assessment include the following: How has MS affected the patient's lifestyle? How well is the patient coping? What would the patient like to do better?

Diagnosis

NURSING DIAGNOSES

Based on the assessment data, the patient's major nursing diagnoses may include the following:

- Impaired physical mobility related to weakness, muscle paresis, spasticity
- Risk for injury related to sensory and visual impairment
- Impaired urinary and bowel elimination (urgency, frequency, incontinence, constipation) related to nervous system dysfunction
- Impaired speech and swallowing related to cranial nerve involvement

- Disturbed thought processes (loss of memory, dementia, euphoria) related to cerebral dysfunction
- Ineffective individual coping related to uncertainty of course of MS
- Impaired home maintenance management related to physical, psychological, and social limits imposed by MS
- Potential for sexual dysfunction related to spinal cord involvement or psychological reactions to condition

Planning and Goals

The major goals for the patient may include promotion of physical mobility, avoidance of injury, achievement of bladder and bowel continence, promotion of speech and swallowing mechanisms, improvement of cognitive function, development of coping strengths, improved home maintenance management, and adaptation to sexual dysfunction.

Nursing Interventions

An individualized program of physical therapy, rehabilitation, and education is combined with emotional support. The nursing interventions include face-to-face and telephone interactions that address patient education to enable the person with MS to deal with the physiologic, social, and psychological problems that accompany chronic disease (Madonna & Keating, 1999).

PROMOTING PHYSICAL MOBILITY

Relaxation and coordination exercises promote muscle efficiency. Progressive resistive exercises are used to strengthen weak muscles because diminishing muscle strength is often significant in MS.

Exercises

Walking improves the gait, particularly when there is loss of position sense of the legs and feet. If certain muscle groups are irreversibly affected, other muscles can be trained to take over their actions. Instruction in the use of assistive devices may be needed to ensure their correct and safe use.

Minimizing Spasticity and Contractures

Muscle spasticity is common and, in its later stages, is characterized by severe adductor spasm of the hips with flexor spasm of the hips and knees. If this is not relieved, fibrous contractures of these joints with resultant pressure ulcers over the sacrum and hips (due to diminished sensation and the inability to position the patient properly) occur. Warm packs may be beneficial, but hot baths should be avoided because of risk for burn injury secondary to sensory loss and increasing symptoms that may occur with an elevation of the body temperature.

Daily exercises for muscle stretching are prescribed to minimize joint contractures. Special attention is given to the hamstrings, gastrocnemius muscles, hip adductors, biceps, and wrist and finger flexors. Muscle spasticity is common and interferes with normal function. A stretch–hold–relax routine is helpful for relaxing and treating muscle spasticity. Swimming and stationary bicycling are useful, and progressive weight-bearing can relieve spasticity in the legs. The patient should not be hurried in any of these activities because this often increases spasticity.

Activity And Rest

The patient is encouraged to work to a point just short of fatigue. Very strenuous physical exercise is not advisable because it raises the body temperature and may aggravate symptoms. The patient is advised to take frequent short rest periods, preferably lying down. Extreme fatigue may contribute to the exacerbation of symptoms.

Minimizing Effects of Immobility

Because of the decrease in physical activity that often occurs with MS, complications associated with immobility, including pressure ulcers, expiratory muscle weakness, and accumulation of bronchial secretions, need to be considered and steps taken to prevent them. Measures to prevent such complications include assessment and maintenance of skin integrity and coughing and deep-breathing exercises.

PREVENTING INJURY

If motor dysfunction causes problems of incoordination and clumsiness, or if ataxia is apparent, the patient is at risk for falling. To overcome this disability, the patient is taught to walk with feet wide apart to widen the base of support and to increase walking stability. If there is loss of position sense, the patient is taught to watch the feet while walking. Gait training may require assistive devices (walker, cane, braces, crutches, parallel bars) and instruction about their use by a physical therapist. If the gait remains inefficient, a wheelchair or motorized scooter may be the solution. The occupational therapist is a valuable resource person in suggesting and securing aids to promote independence. If incoordination is a problem and tremor of the upper extremities occurs when voluntary movement is attempted (intention tremor), weighted bracelets or wrist cuffs are helpful. The patient is trained in transfer and activities of daily living.

Because sensory loss may occur in addition to motor loss, pressure ulcers are a continuing threat to skin integrity. Confinement to a wheelchair increases the risk. See Chapter 11 for a discussion of the prevention and treatment of pressure ulcers.

ENHANCING BLADDER AND BOWEL CONTROL

Generally, bladder symptoms fall into the following categories: (1) inability to store urine (hyperreflexic, uninhibited); (2) inability to empty the bladder (hyporeflexic, hypotonic); and (3) a mixture of both types. The patient with urinary frequency, urgency, or incontinence requires special support. The sensation of the need to void must be heeded immediately, so the bedpan or urinal should be readily available. A voiding time schedule is set up (every 1.5 to 2 hours initially, with gradual lengthening of the interval). The patient is instructed to drink a measured amount of fluid every 2 hours and then attempt to void 30 minutes after drinking. Using a timer or wristwatch with an alarm may be helpful for the patient who does not have enough sensation to signal the need to empty the bladder. The nurse encourages the patient to take the prescribed medications to treat bladder spasticity because this allows greater independence. Intermittent self-catheterization has been successful in maintaining bladder control in patients with MS. (See Chap. 11 for a discussion of intermittent self-catheterization.) If the female patient has permanent urinary incontinence, urinary diversion procedures may be considered. The male patient may wear a condom appliance for urine collection.

Bowel problems include constipation, fecal impaction, and incontinence. Adequate fluids, dietary fibre, and a bowel-training program are frequently effective in solving these problems. (See Chap. 11 for a discussion of promoting bowel continence.)

MANAGING SPEECH AND SWALLOWING DIFFICULTIES

When the cranial nerves controlling the mechanisms of speech and swallowing are involved, dysarthrias (defects of articulation) marked by slurring, low volume of speech, and difficulties in phonation may occur. Swallowing disturbances (**dysphagia**) may also occur. A speech therapist evaluates speech and swallowing and instructs the patient, family, and health team members about strategies to compensate for speech and swallowing problems. The nurse reinforces this instruction and encourages the patient and family to adhere to the plan. Impaired swallowing increases the patient's risk for aspiration; therefore, strategies (eg, having suction apparatus available, careful feeding, proper positioning for eating) are needed to reduce that risk (Galvan, 2001).

IMPROVING SENSORY AND COGNITIVE FUNCTION

Measures may be taken if visual defects (the cranial nerves affecting vision may be affected by MS) or changes in cognitive status occur.

Vision

An eye patch or a covered eyeglass lens may be used to block visual impulses of one eye when the patient has diplopia (double vision). Prism glasses may be helpful for the bedridden patient who is having difficulty reading in the supine position. People unable to read regular-print materials are eligible for the free talking book services of the Library of Congress or may obtain large-type books from local libraries.

Cognition and Emotional Responses

Cognitive impairment and emotional lability may occur early in MS in some patients and may impose numerous stresses on the patient and family. Some patients with MS are forgetful and easily distracted and may exhibit emotional lability.

Patients adapt to illness in a variety of ways, which may include denial, depression, withdrawal, and hostility. Emotional support assists patients and their families to adapt to the changes and uncertainties associated with MS and to cope with the disruption in their lives. The patient is assisted to set meaningful and realistic goals to achieve a sense of purpose, to remain as active as possible, and to keep up social interests and activities. Hobbies may help the patient's morale and provide satisfying interests if the disease progresses to the stage in which formerly enjoyed activities can no longer be pursued.

The family should be made aware of the nature and degree of cognitive impairment. The environment is kept structured, and lists and other memory aids are used to help the patient with cognitive changes to maintain a daily routine. The occupational therapist can be helpful in formulating a structured daily routine.

Strengthening Coping Mechanisms

The diagnosis of MS is always distressing to the patient and family. They need to know that no two patients with MS have identical symptoms or courses of illness. Although some patients do experience significant disability early, others have a near-normal life span with minimal disability. Some families, however, face overwhelming frustrations and problems. MS affects people who are often in a productive stage of life and concerned about career and family responsibilities. Family conflict, disintegration, separation, and divorce are not uncommon. Often, very young family members assume the responsibility of caring for a parent with MS. Nursing interventions in this area include alleviating stress and making appropriate referrals for counselling and support to minimize the adverse effects of dealing with chronic illness.

The nurse, mindful of these complex problems, initiates home care and coordinates a network of services, including social services, speech therapy, physical therapy, and homemaker services. To strengthen the patient's coping skills, as much information as possible is provided. People who live with chronic illness need an updated list of the assistive devices, services, and resources that are available.

Coping through problem solving involves helping the patient define the problem and develop alternatives for its management. Careful planning and maintaining flexibility and a hopeful attitude are useful for psychological and physical adaptation.

IMPROVING SELF-CARE ABILITIES

MS can affect every facet of daily living. After certain abilities are lost, they are often impossible to regain. Physical function may vary from day to day. Modifications that allow independence in self-care should be implemented (eg, assistive eating devices, raised toilet seat, bathing aids, telephone modifications, long-handled comb, tongs, modified clothing). Physical and emotional stresses should be avoided as much as possible because these may worsen symptoms and impair performance. Exposure to heat increases fatigue and muscle weakness, so air conditioning in at least one room is recommended. Exposure to extreme cold may increase spasticity.

PROMOTING SEXUAL FUNCTIONING

Patients with MS and their partners face problems that interfere with sexual activity, arising not only as a direct consequence of nerve damage but also from psychological reactions to the disease. Easy fatigability, conflicts arising from dependency and depression, emotional lability, loss of self-esteem, and feelings of low self-worth compound the problem. Erectile and ejaculatory disorders in men and orgasmic dysfunction and adductor spasms of the thigh muscles in women can make sexual intercourse difficult or impossible. Bladder and bowel incontinence and urinary tract infections add to the difficulties.

An experienced sexual counsellor helps bring into focus the patient's or partner's sexual resources and suggests relevant information and supportive therapy (Sipski & Alexander, 1997). Sharing and communicating feelings, planning for sexual activity (to minimize the effects of fatigue), and exploring alternative methods of sexual expression may open up a wide range of sexual enjoyment and experiences.

PROMOTING HOME AND COMMUNITY-BASED CARE

Teaching Patients Self-Care

As the disease progresses, the patient and family need to learn new strategies to maintain optimal independence. Teaching of new self-care techniques may be initiated in the hospital or clinic setting and reinforced in the home. Teaching about self-care may address the use of assistive devices, self-catheterization, and administration of medications that affect the course of the disease or treat complications. Although the disease-modifying medications (the "ABC and R medications") may slow the progression of disease and disability in many persons with MS, they are not effective in all patients. Patients who receive these medications will require teaching and support, while those unable to take them or for whom the medications have not been effective need continued support and assistance in coping with this reality. Exercises that enable the patient to continue some form of activity or that maintain or improve swallowing, speech, or respiratory function may be taught to the patient and family (Chart 64-3).

Continuing Care

After discharge, the home care nurse often provides teaching and reinforcement of these new techniques in the patient's home. Nurses in the home setting assess for changes in the patient's

Chart 64-3
Home Care Checklist • The Patient With Multiple Sclerosis

At the completion of the home care instruction, the patient or caregiver will be able to:	Patient	Caregiver
• State how to access the local chapter of the MS Society of Canada and available resources.	✓	✓
• Discuss the clinical course of MS.	✓	✓
• Identify strategies to manage symptoms (pain, cognitive responses, dysphagia, tremors, visual disturbances).	✓	✓
• State how to prevent complications (pressure ulcers, pneumonia, depression).	✓	✓
• Identify coping strategies.	✓	✓
• Identify ways to minimize fatigue.	✓	✓
• Explain how to prevent injury.	✓	✓
• State ways to adapt to sexual dysfunction.	✓	✓
• Discuss ways to control bowel and bladder function.	✓	✓
• Name benefits of exercise and physical activity.	✓	✓
• Identify ways to minimize immobility and spasticity.	✓	✓
• Describe medication regimen and potential adverse effects.	✓	✓
• Demonstrate correct techniques of administering injectable medications, if prescribed.	✓	✓

physical and emotional status, provide physical care to the patient if required, coordinate outpatient services and resources, and encourage health promotion, appropriate health screenings, and adaptation. If changes in the disease or its course are noted, the home care nurse encourages the patient to contact the primary care provider because treatment of an acute exacerbation or new problem may be indicated. Continuing health care and follow-up are recommended.

The patient with MS is encouraged to contact the local chapter of the Multiple Sclerosis Society of Canada for services, publications, and contact with others with MS. Local chapters also provide direct services to patients. Through group participation, the patient has an opportunity to meet others with similar problems, to share experiences, and to learn self-help methods in a social environment.

Evaluation

EXPECTED PATIENT OUTCOMES

Expected patient outcomes may include:

1. Improved physical mobility
   a. Participates in gait-training and rehabilitation program
   b. Establishes a balanced program of rest and exercise
   c. Uses assistive devices correctly and safely
2. Is free of injury
   a. Uses visual cues to compensate for decreased sense of touch or position
   b. Asks for assistance when necessary
3. Attains or maintains control of bladder and bowel patterns
   a. Monitors self for urine retention and employs intermittent self-catheterization technique, if indicated

NURSING RESEARCH PROFILE 64-1
Quality of Life for People With Multiple Sclerosis

Stuifbergen, A., Seraphine, A., & Roberts, G. (2000). An explanatory model of health promotion and quality of life in chronic disabling conditions. *Nursing Research, 49*(3), 122–129.

Purpose
The purpose of this study was to test an explanatory model of variables influencing health promotion and quality of life in persons with multiple sclerosis (MS). This was the second phase of a project designed to investigate the issues surrounding the health-promotion needs of individuals with chronic disabling conditions and the outcomes associated with the performance of health-promoting behaviours.

Study Sample and Design
This was a one-time cross-sectional design using mailed questionnaires. Participants were recruited for the study using targeted mailings to individuals with MS on the mailing lists of national MS Society chapters. The study sample included 786 persons with MS (630 women and 156 men) who returned surveys. Instruments used included the Incapacity Status Scale (ISS), Barriers to Health Promoting Activities for Disabled Persons Scale, Personal Resource Questionnaire, Acceptance of Illness Scale, Self-Rated Abilities for Health Practices scale, Health Promoting Lifestyle Profile-II (HPLP-II), and the Quality of Life Index (QLI).

Findings
The analysis revealed that the original model was generally well specified, with an adequate fit to the data. The model supported the hypothesis that quality of life is the outcome of a complex interplay between contextual factors (severity of illness), antecedent variables, and health-promoting behaviours. The revised model, with the addition of two paths between personal resources and barriers, had an improved fit of the data compared to the original model. The original and revised models are depicted in the article. Resources, barriers, self-efficacy, and acceptance accounted for 58% of the variance in the frequency of health-promoting behaviours and 66% of the variance in perceived quality of life.

Nursing Implications
Further testing of the model was recommended, especially in samples of differing ethnic and cultural backgrounds. Nurses working with MS patients should be aware that quality of life is the outcome of the interaction of many variables. The authors suggest that nurses can improve health-promoting behaviours and quality of life using interventions that enhance social support, decrease barriers, and increase specific self-efficacy for health behaviours.

b. Identifies the signs and symptoms of urinary tract infection

c. Maintains adequate fluid and fibre intake

4. Participates in strategies to improve speech and swallowing
   a. Practices exercises recommended by speech therapist
   b. Maintains adequate nutritional intake without aspiration

5. Compensates for altered thought processes
   a. Uses lists and other aids to compensate for memory losses
   b. Discusses problems with trusted advisor or friend
   c. Substitutes new activities for those that are no longer possible

6. Demonstrates effective coping strategies
   a. Maintains sense of control
   b. Modifies lifestyle to fit goals and limitations
   c. Verbalizes desire to pursue goals and developmental tasks of adulthood
   d. Adheres to plan for home maintenance management
   e. Uses appropriate self-care techniques to maintain independence
   f. Engages in health promotion activities and health screenings as appropriate

8. Adapts to changes in sexual function
   a. Is able to discuss problem with partner and appropriate health professional
   b. Identifies alternate means of sexual expression

MYASTHENIA GRAVIS

Myasthenia gravis, an autoimmune disorder affecting the myoneural junction, is characterized by varying degrees of weakness of the voluntary muscles. Women tend to develop the disease at an earlier age (20 to 40 years of age) compared to men (60 to 70 years of age), and women are affected more frequently (Heitmiller, 1999).

Pathophysiology

Normally, a chemical impulse precipitates the release of acetylcholine from vesicles on the nerve terminal at the myoneural junction. The acetylcholine attaches to receptor sites on the motor end plate, stimulating muscle contraction. Continuous binding of acetylcholine to the receptor site is required for muscular contraction to be sustained.

In myasthenia gravis, autoantibodies directed at the acetylcholine receptor sites impair transmission of impulses across the myoneural junction. Therefore, fewer receptors are available for stimulation, resulting in voluntary muscle weakness that escalates with continued activity (Fig. 64-5). These antibodies are found in 80% to 90% of the people with myasthenia gravis. Eighty percent of persons with myasthenia gravis have either thymic hyperplasia or a thymic tumour (Roos, 1999), and the thymus gland is believed to be the site of antibody production. In patients who are antibody negative, it is believed that the offending antibody is directed at a portion of the receptor site rather than the whole complex.

Clinical Manifestations

The initial manifestation of myasthenia gravis usually involves the ocular muscles. Diplopia (double vision) and ptosis (drooping of the eyelids) are common. However, the majority of patients also experience weakness of the muscles of the face and throat (bulbar symptoms) and generalized weakness. Weakness of the facial muscles will result in a bland facial expression. Laryngeal involvement produces **dysphonia** (voice impairment) and increases the patient's risk for choking and aspiration. Generalized weakness affects all the extremities and the intercostal muscles, resulting in decreasing vital capacity and respiratory failure. Myasthenia gravis is purely a motor disorder with no effect on sensation or coordination.

Assessment and Diagnostic Findings

An anticholinesterase test is used to diagnose myasthenia gravis. Anticholinesterase agents stop the breakdown of acetylcholine, thereby increasing acetylcholine availability. Edrophonium chloride (Tensilon) is injected intravenously, 2 mg at a time to a total of 10 mg. Thirty seconds after injection, facial muscle weakness and ptosis should resolve for about 5 minutes. This immediate improvement in muscle strength after administration of this agent represents a positive test and usually confirms the diagnosis. Atropine 0.4 mg should be available to control the side effects of edrophonium, which include bradycardia, sweating, and cramping (Roos, 1999).

The acetylcholine receptor antibody titers are elevated as indicated previously. Repetitive nerve stimulation tests record the electrical activity in targeted muscles after nerve stimulation. A 15% decrease in successive action potentials is observed in patients with myasthenia gravis (Heitmiller, 1999). The thymus gland, which is a site of acetylcholine receptor antibody production, is enlarged in myasthenia gravis. MRI demonstrates this enlargement in 90% of cases (Wilkins & Bulkley, 1999).

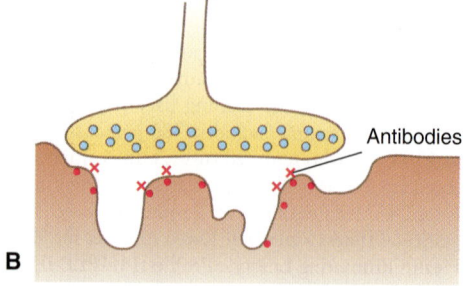

FIGURE 64-5 Myasthenia gravis. (**A**) Normal ACh receptor site. (**B**) ACh receptor site in myasthenia gravis.

Medical Management

Management of myasthenia gravis is directed at improving function and reducing and removing circulating antibodies. Therapeutic modalities include administration of anticholinesterase agents and immunosuppressive therapy, plasmapheresis, and thymectomy.

PHARMACOLOGIC THERAPY

Anticholinesterase agents such as pyridostigmine bromide (Mestinon) and neostigmine bromide (Prostigmin) provide symptomatic relief by increasing the relative concentration of available acetylcholine at the neuromuscular junction. Dosage is increased gradually until maximal benefits (improved strength, less fatigue) are obtained. Adverse effects of anticholinesterase therapy include abdominal pain, diarrhea, nausea, and increased oropharyngeal secretions. Pyridostigmine tends to have fewer side effects (Chart 64-4). Improvement with anticholinesterase therapy is not complete or long-lasting (Heitmiller, 1999).

> **! NURSING ALERT** Maintenance of stable blood levels of anticholinergic medication is imperative to stabilize muscle strength. Therefore, the anticholinesterase medications must be given on time. Any delay in administration of medications may exacerbate muscle weakness and make it impossible for the patient to take medications orally.

The goal of immunosuppressive therapy is to reduce the production of the antibody. Corticosteroids suppress the patient's immune response, thus decreasing the amount of antibody production. As the corticosteroid dosage is gradually increased, the anticholinesterase dosage is lowered. The patient's ability to maintain effective respirations and to swallow is monitored throughout. Prednisone, taken on alternate days to lower the incidence of side effects, appears to be successful in suppressing the disease. The patient sometimes shows a marked decrease in muscle strength right after therapy is started, but this is usually only temporary.

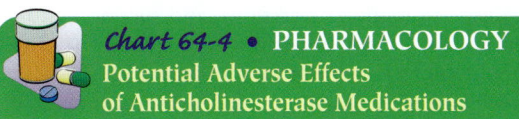

Chart 64-4 • PHARMACOLOGY
Potential Adverse Effects of Anticholinesterase Medications

CNS	Gastrointestinal
Irritability	Abdominal cramps
Anxiety	Nausea
Insomnia	Vomiting
Headache	Diarrhea
Dysarthria	Anorexia
Syncope	Increased salivation
Seizures	**Skeletal Muscles**
Coma	Fasciculations
Diaphoresis	Spasms
	Weakness
Respiratory	**Genitourinary**
Bronchial relaxation	Frequency
Increased bronchial secretions	Urgency
Cardiovascular	**Integumentary**
Tachycardia	Rash
Hypotension	Flushing

Cytotoxic medications have also been used, although the precise mechanism of action in myasthenia is not fully understood. Medications such as azathioprine (Imuran), cyclophosphamide (Cytoxan), and cyclosporine reduce the circulating antiacetylcholine receptor antibody titers. Side effects are significant; therefore, these agents are reserved for patients who do not respond to other forms of therapy.

A number of medications are contraindicated for patients with myasthenia gravis because they worsen myasthenic symptoms. Risks and benefits should be weighed by the physician and the patient before taking any new medications, including antibiotics, cardiovascular medications, antiseizure and psychotropic medications, morphine, quinine and related agents, beta-blockers, and nonprescription medications. Procaine (Novocain) should be avoided, and the patient's dentist is so advised.

PLASMAPHERESIS

Plasma exchange (plasmapheresis) is a technique used to treat exacerbations. The patient's plasma and plasma components are removed through a centrally placed large-bore double-lumen catheter. The blood cells and antibody-containing plasma are separated; then the cells and a plasma substitute are reinfused. Plasma exchange produces a temporary reduction in the titer of circulating antibodies. Plasma exchange improves the symptoms in 75% of patients, although improvement lasts only a few weeks unless plasmapheresis is continued or other forms of treatment such as immunosuppression with corticosteroids are initiated (Bedlack & Sanders, 2000). IV immune globulin (IVIG) has recently been shown to be nearly as effective as plasmapheresis in controlling symptom exacerbation (Qureshi, Choudhry, Akbar et al., 1999). However, neither therapy is a cure as it does not stop the production of the acetylcholine receptor antibodies.

SURGICAL MANAGEMENT

Thymectomy (surgical removal of the thymus gland) can produce antigen-specific immunosuppression and result in clinical improvement. It can decrease or eliminate the need for medication. In one study 92% of post-thymectomy patients had symptomatic improvement, with 50% of them no longer requiring pharmacologic therapy (Wilkins & Bulkley, 1999). The entire gland must be removed for optimal clinical outcomes; therefore, surgeons prefer the transsternal surgical approach. After surgery, the patient is monitored in an intensive care unit, with special attention to respiratory function. After the thymus gland is removed, it may take up to 1 year for the patient to benefit from the procedure due to the long life of circulating T cells (Wilkins & Bulkley, 1999).

Complications: Myasthenic Crisis Versus Cholinergic Crisis

A myasthenic crisis is an exacerbation of the disease process characterized by severe generalized muscle weakness and respiratory and bulbar weakness that may result in respiratory failure. Crisis may result from disease exacerbation or a specific precipitating event. The most common precipitator is infection; others include medication change, surgery, pregnancy, and high environmental temperature (Bella & Chad, 1998).

Symptoms of anticholinergic overmedication (cholinergic crisis) may mimic the symptoms of exacerbation. Differentiation can be achieved with the edrophonium chloride (Tensilon) test. The patient with myasthenic crisis improves immediately following administration of edrophonium, while the patient with cholinergic crisis may experience no improvement or deteriorate. If myasthenic crisis is diagnosed, neostigmine methylsulfate (PMS-Neostigmine, Prostigmin) is administered intramuscularly or intravenously until the patient is able to swallow oral anticholinesterase medications. Plasmapheresis and IVIG, which reduce the antibody load, also may be used to treat myasthenic crisis. If cholinergic crisis is identified, all anticholinesterase medications are stopped. The patient receives atropine (Atropine sulfate), the antidote for the anticholinesterase medications.

Neuromuscular respiratory failure is the critical complication of crisis. Respiratory muscle and bulbar weakness combine to cause respiratory compromise. Weak respiratory muscles will not support inhalation. An inadequate cough and an impaired gag reflex caused by bulbar weakness result in poor airway clearance. Values on two respiratory function tests, the negative inspiratory force and vital capacity, will be the first clinical signs to deteriorate. Careful monitoring of these values enables the nurse to monitor for impending respiratory failure. Respiratory support and airway protection are key interventions for the nurse caring for the patient in crisis. Endotracheal intubation and mechanical ventilation may be needed (see Chap. 25). Nutritional support may be needed if the patient is intubated for a long period.

Nursing Management

Because myasthenia gravis is a chronic disease and most patients are seen on an outpatient basis, much of the nursing care focuses on patient and family teaching. Educational topics for outpatient self-care include medication management, energy conservation, strategies to help with ocular manifestations, and prevention and management of complications.

Medication management is a crucial component of ongoing care. Understanding the action of the medications and taking them on schedule is emphasized, as are the consequences of delaying medication and the signs and symptoms of myasthenic and cholinergic crisis. The patient can determine the best times for daily dosing by keeping a diary to determine fluctuation of symptoms and to learn when the medication is wearing off. The medication schedule can then be manipulated to maximize strength throughout the day.

The patient is also taught srategies to conserve energy. To do this, the nurse helps the patient identify the best times for rest periods throughout the day. If the patient lives in a two-story home, the nurse can suggest that frequently used items such as hygiene products, cleaning products, and snacks be kept on each floor to minimize travel between floors. The patient is encouraged to apply for a handicapped license plate to minimize walking from parking spaces and to schedule activities to coincide with peak energy and strength levels.

To minimize the risk of aspiration, mealtimes should coincide with the peak effects of anticholinesterase medication. In addition, rest before meals is encouraged to reduce muscle fatigue. The patient is advised to sit upright during meals with the neck slightly flexed to facilitate swallowing. Soft foods in gravy or sauces can be swallowed more easily; if choking occurs frequently, the nurse can suggest puréeing food to a pudding consistency. Suction should be available at home and the patient and family instructed in its use. Gastrostomy feedings may be necessary in some patients to ensure adequate nutrition.

Impaired vision results from ptosis of one or both eyelids, decreased eye movement, or double vision. To prevent corneal damage when the eyelids do not close completely, the patient is instructed to tape the eyes closed for short intervals and regularly instill artificial tears. Patients who wear eyeglasses can have "crutches" attached to help lift the eyelids. Patching one eye can help with double vision.

The patient is reminded of the importance of maintaining health promotion practices and of following health care screening recommendations. Factors that will exacerbate symptoms and potentially cause crisis should be noted and avoided: emotional stress, infections (particularly respiratory infections), vigourous physical activity, some medications, and high environmental temperature. The Myasthenia Gravis Foundation of America provides support groups, services, and educational materials for patients, families, and health care providers.

MANAGING MYASTHENIC AND CHOLINERGIC CRISES

Respiratory distress and varying degrees of dysphagia (difficulty swallowing), dysarthria (difficulty speaking), eyelid ptosis, diplopia, and prominent muscle weakness are symptoms of myasthenic and cholinergic crisis. The patient is placed in an intensive care unit for constant monitoring because of associated intense and sudden fluctuations in clinical condition.

IV edrophonium chloride (Tensilon) is used to differentiate the type of crisis. It improves the condition of the patient in myasthenic crisis and temporarily worsens that of the patient in cholinergic crisis. If the patient is in true myasthenic crisis, neostigmine methylsulfate is administered intramuscularly or intravenously. If the edrophonium test is inconclusive or there is increasing respiratory weakness, all anticholinesterase medications are stopped, and atropine sulfate is given to reduce excessive secretions.

Providing ventilatory assistance takes precedence in the immediate management of the patient with myasthenic crisis. Ongoing assessment for respiratory failure is essential. The nurse assesses the respiratory rate, depth, and breath sounds and monitors pulmonary function parameters (vital capacity and negative inspiratory force) to detect pulmonary problems before respiratory dysfunction progresses. Blood is drawn for arterial blood gas analysis. Endotracheal intubation and mechanical ventilation may be needed (see Chap. 25).

When there is severe weakness of the abdominal, intercostal, and pharyngeal muscles, the patient cannot cough, take deep breaths, or clear secretions. Chest physical therapy, including postural drainage to mobilize secretions, and suctioning to remove secretions may have to be performed frequently. (Postural drainage should not be performed for 30 minutes after feeding.)

Assessment strategies and supportive measures include the following:

- Arterial blood gases, serum electrolytes, input and output, and daily weight are monitored.
- If the patient cannot swallow, nasogastric tube feedings may be prescribed.
- Sedatives and tranquilizers are avoided because they aggravate hypoxia and hypercapnia and can cause respiratory and cardiac depression.

GUILLAIN-BARRÉ SYNDROME

Guillain-Barré syndrome is an autoimmune attack of the peripheral nerve myelin. The result is acute, rapid segmental demyelination of peripheral nerves and some cranial nerves, producing ascending weakness with **dyskinesia** (inability to execute voluntary movements), hyporeflexia, and **paresthesias** (numbness). In 66% of cases, there is a predisposing event, most often a respiratory or gastrointestinal infection, although vaccination, pregnancy, and surgery have also been identified as antecedent events (Bella & Chad, 1998). Infection with *Campylobacter jejuni* (a relatively common gastrointestinal bacterial pathogen) precedes Guillain-Barré syndrome in a few cases (Ho & Griffin, 1999; Lindenbaum, Kissel & Mendel, 2001).

The antecedent event usually occurs 2 weeks before symptoms begin. Weakness usually begins in the legs and progresses upward for about 1 month. Maximum weakness varies but usually includes neuromuscular respiratory failure and bulbar weakness. The duration of the symptoms is variable: complete functional recovery may take up to 2 years (Hickey, 2003). Any residual symptoms are permanent and reflect axonal damage from demyelination.

The annual incidence of Guillain-Barré is 0.6 to 1.9 cases per 100,000. Eighty-five percent of patients recover with minimal residual symptoms. Severe residual deficits occur in up to 10% of patients. Residual deficits are most likely in patients with rapid disease progression, those who require mechanical ventilation, or those 60 years of age or older. Death occurs in 3% to 8% of cases, resulting from respiratory failure, autonomic dysfunction, sepsis, or pulmonary emboli (Bella & Chad, 1998).

Pathophysiology

Myelin is a complex substance that covers nerves, providing insulation and speeding the conduction of impulses from the cell body to the dendrites. The cell that produces myelin in the peripheral nervous system is the Schwann cell. In Guillain-Barré the Schwann cell is spared, allowing for remyelination in the recovery phase of the disease.

Guillain-Barré is the result of a cell-mediated immune attack on peripheral nerve myelin proteins (Ho & Griffin, 1999). The best-accepted theory is that an infectious organism contains an amino acid that mimics the peripheral nerve myelin protein. The immune system cannot distinguish between the two proteins and attacks and destroys peripheral nerve myelin. Studies indicate that an exact location within the peripheral nervous system, the ganglioside GM1b, is the most likely target of the immune attack (Yuki, Ang, Koga et al., 2000). With the autoimmune attack there is an influx of macrophages and other immune-mediated agents that attack myelin, cause inflammation and destruction, and leave the axon unable to support nerve conduction.

Clinical Manifestations

Classic Guillain-Barré begins with muscle weakness and diminished reflexes of the lower extremities. Hyporeflexia and weakness progress and may result in quadriplegia. Demyelination of the nerves that innervate the diaphragm and intercostal muscles results in neuromuscular respiratory failure. Twenty-five percent of patients will require mechanical ventilation within 18 days of symptom onset (Bella & Chad, 1998). Sensory symptoms include paresthesias of the hands and feet and pain related to the demyelination of sensory fibres.

Cranial nerve demyelination can result in a variety of clinical manifestations. Optic nerve demyelination may result in blindness. Bulbar muscle weakness related to demyelination of the glossopharyngeal and vagus nerves results in an inability to swallow or clear secretions. Vagus nerve demyelination results in autonomic dysfunction, manifested by instability of the cardiovascular system. The presentation is variable and may include tachycardia, bradycardia, hypertension, or orthostatic hypotension. The symptoms of autonomic dysfunction occur and resolve rapidly. Guillain-Barré does not affect cognitive function or level of consciousness.

While the classic clinical features include areflexia and ascending weakness, variation in presentation occurs. There may be a sensory presentation, with progressive sensory symptoms, an atypical axonal destruction, and the Miller-Fisher variant, which includes paralysis of the ocular muscles, ataxia, and areflexia (Ho & Griffin, 1999).

Assessment and Diagnostic Findings

The patient presents with symmetric weakness, diminished reflexes, and upward progression of motor weakness. A history of a viral illness in the previous few weeks suggests the diagnosis. Changes in vital capacity and negative inspiratory force are assessed to identify impending neuromuscular respiratory failure. Serum laboratory tests are not useful in the diagnosis. However, elevated protein levels are detected in CSF evaluation, without an increase in other cells. Evoked potential studies demonstrate a progressive loss of nerve conduction velocity (Bella & Chad, 1999).

Medical Management

Because of the possibility of rapid progression and neuromuscular respiratory failure, Guillain-Barré is a medical emergency, requiring intensive care unit management. Careful assessment of changes in motor weakness and respiratory function alert the clinician to the physical and respiratory needs of the patient. Respiratory therapy or mechanical ventilation may be necessary to support pulmonary function and adequate oxygenation. Mechanical ventilation may be required for an extended period. The patient is weaned from mechanical ventilation when the respiratory muscles can again support spontaneous respiration and maintain adequate tissue oxygenation.

Other interventions are aimed at preventing the complications of immobility. These may include the use of anticoagulant agents and thigh-high elastic compression stockings or sequential compression boots to prevent thrombosis and pulmonary emboli.

Plasmapheresis and IVIG are used to directly affect the peripheral nerve myelin antibody level. Both therapies decrease circulating antibody levels and reduce the amount of time the patient is immobilized and dependent on mechanical ventilation. Studies indicate that IVIG and plasmapheresis are equally effective in treating Guillain-Barré (Bella & Chad, 1999; Winer, 2002).

The cardiovascular risks posed by autonomic dysfunction require continuous ECG monitoring. Tachycardia and hypertension are treated with short-acting medications such as alpha-adrenergic blocking agents. Hypotension is managed by increasing the amount of IV fluid administered. The use of short-acting agents is important because autonomic dysfunction is very labile.

NURSING PROCESS: THE PATIENT WITH GUILLAIN-BARRÉ SYNDROME

Assessment

Ongoing assessment for disease progression is critical. The patient is monitored for life-threatening complications (respiratory failure, cardiac dysrhythmias, DVTs) so that appropriate interventions can be initiated. Because of the threat to the patient in this sudden, potentially life-threatening disease, the nurse must assess the patient's and family's ability to cope and their use of appropriate coping strategies.

Diagnosis

NURSING DIAGNOSES

Based on the assessment data, the patient's major nursing diagnoses may include the following:

- Ineffective breathing pattern and impaired gas exchange related to rapidly progressive weakness and impending respiratory failure
- Impaired physical mobility related to paralysis
- Imbalanced nutrition, less than body requirements, related to inability to swallow
- Impaired verbal communication related to cranial nerve dysfunction
- Fear and anxiety related to loss of control and paralysis

COLLABORATIVE PROBLEMS/POTENTIAL COMPLICATIONS

Based on the assessment data, potential complications that may develop include the following:

- Respiratory failure
- Autonomic dysfunction

Planning and Goals

The major goals for the patient may include improved respiratory function, increased mobility, improved nutritional status, effective communication, decreased fear and anxiety, and absence of complications.

Nursing Interventions

MAINTAINING RESPIRATORY FUNCTION

Respiratory function can be maximized with incentive spirometry and chest physiotherapy. Monitoring for changes in vital capacity and negative inspiratory force are key to early intervention for neuromuscular respiratory failure. Mechanical ventilation is required if the vital capacity falls, making spontaneous breathing impossible and tissue oxygenation inadequate.

Parameters for determining the appropriate time to begin mechanical ventilation include a vital capacity of 12 to 15 mL/kg, downward vital capacity trend over 4 to 6 hours, and an inability to clear secretions (Bella & Chad, 1999). The potential need for mechanical ventilation should be discussed with the patient and family on admission to provide time for psychological preparation and decision-making. Intubation and mechanical ventilation will result in less anxiety if it is initiated on a nonemergent basis to a well-informed patient. The patient may require mechanical ventilation for a long period. Nursing management of the patient requiring mechanical ventilation is discussed in Chapter 25.

Bulbar weakness that impairs the ability to swallow and clear secretions is another factor in the development of respiratory failure in the patient with Guillain-Barré. Suctioning may be needed to maintain a clear airway.

The nurse assesses the blood pressure and heart rate frequently to identify autonomic dysfunction so that interventions can be initiated quickly if needed. Medications are administered or a temporary pacemaker is placed for clinically significant bradycardia (Winer, 2002).

ENHANCING PHYSICAL MOBILITY

Nursing interventions to enhance physical mobility and prevent the complications of immobility are key to the function and survival of these patients. The paralyzed extremities are supported in functional positions, and passive range-of-motion exercises are performed at least twice daily.

DVT and pulmonary embolism are threats to the paralyzed patient. Nursing interventions are aimed at preventing DVT. Range-of-motion exercises, altering positioning, anticoagulation, thigh-high elastic compression stockings or sequential compression boots, and adequate hydration will decrease the risk for DVT.

Padding may be placed over bony prominences such as the elbows and heels to reduce the risk for pressure ulcers. The need for consistent position changes every 2 hours cannot be overemphasized. The nurse evaluates laboratory test results that may indicate malnutrition or dehydration, both of which increase the risk for pressure ulcers. Collaboration with the physician and dietitian will result in a plan to meet the patient's nutritional and hydration needs.

PROVIDING ADEQUATE NUTRITION

Paralytic ileus may result from insufficient parasympathetic activity. In this event, the nurse administers IV fluids and parenteral nutrition as prescribed and monitors for the return of bowel sounds. If the patient cannot swallow due to **bulbar paralysis** (immobility of muscles), a gastrostomy tube may be placed to administer nutrients. The nurse carefully assesses the return of the gag reflex and bowel sounds before resuming oral nutrition.

IMPROVING COMMUNICATION

Because of paralysis and ventilator management, the patient cannot talk, laugh, or cry and thus has no method for communicating needs or expressing emotion. Establishing some form of communication with picture cards or an eye blink system will provide a means of communication. Collaboration with the speech therapist may be helpful in developing a communication mechanism that is most effective for a specific patient.

DECREASING FEAR AND ANXIETY

The patient and family are faced with a sudden, potentially life-threatening disease, and anxiety and fear are constant themes for them. The impact of disease on the family will depend on the patient's age and role within the family. Referral to a support group may provide information and support to the patient and family.

The family may feel helpless in caring for the patient. Mechanical ventilation and monitoring devices may frighten and intimidate them. Family members often want to participate in physical care; with instruction and support by the nurse, they should be allowed to do so.

In addition to fear, the patient may experience isolation, loneliness, and lack of control. Nursing interventions that increase the patient's sense of control include providing information about the condition, emphasizing a positive appraisal of coping resources, and teaching relaxation exercises and distraction techniques. The positive attitude and atmosphere of the multidisciplinary team are important to promote a sense of well-being.

Diversional activities are encouraged to decrease loneliness and isolation. Encouraging visitors, engaging visitors or volunteers to read to the patient, listening to music or books on tape, and watching television are ways to alleviate the patient's sense of isolation.

MONITORING AND MANAGING POTENTIAL COMPLICATIONS

Thorough assessment of respiratory function at regular intervals is essential because respiratory insufficiency and subsequent failure due to weakness or paralysis of the intercostal muscles and diaphragm may develop quickly. Respiratory failure is the major cause of mortality, which is reported to be as high as 10% to 20%. Vital capacity is monitored frequently and at regular intervals in addition to respiratory rate and the quality of respirations, so that respiratory insufficiency can be anticipated. Decreasing vital capacity associated with weakness of the muscles used in swallowing, which causes difficulty in both coughing and swallowing, indicates impending respiratory failure. Signs and symptoms include breathlessness while speaking, shallow and irregular breathing, use of accessory muscles, tachycardia, and changes in respiratory pattern.

Parameters for determining the onset of respiratory failure are established on admission, allowing intubation and the initiation of mechanical ventilation on a nonemergent basis. This also allows the patient to be prepared for the procedure in a controlled manner, which reduces anxiety and complications.

Other complications include cardiac dysrhythmias, which necessitate ECG monitoring, transient hypertension, orthostatic hypotension, DVT, pulmonary embolism, urinary retention, and other threats to any immobilized and paralyzed patient. These require monitoring and attention to prevent them and prompt treatment if indicated.

PROMOTING HOME AND COMMUNITY-BASED CARE

Teaching Patients Self-Care

Patients with Guillain-Barré syndrome and their families are usually frightened by the sudden onset of life-threatening symptoms and their severity. Therefore, teaching the patient and family about the disorder and its generally favourable prognosis is important (Chart 64-5). During the acute phase of the illness, the patient and family are instructed about strategies they can implement to minimize the effects of immobility and other complications. As function begins to return, family members and other home care providers are instructed about care of the patient and their role in the rehabilitation process. Preparation for discharge is an interdisciplinary effort requiring family or caregiver education by all team members, including the nurse, physician, occupational and physical therapists, speech therapist, and respiratory therapist.

Continuing Care

Most patients with Guillain-Barré syndrome experience complete recovery. Patients who have experienced total or prolonged paralysis require intensive rehabilitation; the extent depends on the patient's needs. Approaches include a comprehensive inpatient program if deficits are significant, an outpatient program if the patient can travel by car, or a home program of physical and occupational therapy. The recovery phase may be long and will require patience as well as involvement on the part of the patient and family.

During acute care the focus is on obvious needs, issues, and deficits. The nurse needs to remind or instruct patients and family members of the need for continuing health promotion and screening practices following this initial phase of care.

Evaluation

EXPECTED PATIENT OUTCOMES

Expected patient outcomes may include:

1. Maintains effective respirations and airway clearance
   a. Has normal breath sounds on auscultation
   b. Demonstrates gradual improvement in respiratory function
2. Shows increasing mobility
   a. Regains use of extremities
   b. Participates in rehabilitation program
   c. Demonstrates no contractures and minimal muscle atrophy
3. Receives adequate nutrition and hydration
   a. Consumes diet adequate to meet nutritional needs
   b. Swallows without aspiration
4. Demonstrates recovery of speech
   a. Can communicate needs through alternative strategies
   b. Practices exercises recommended by the speech therapist
5. Shows lessening fear and anxiety
6. Absence of complications
   a. Breathes spontaneously
   b. Has vital capacity within normal range
   c. Exhibits normal arterial blood gases and oximetry

Chart 64-5
Home Care Checklist • The Patient With Guillain-Barré Syndrome

At the completion of the home care instruction, the patient or caregiver will be able to:	Patient	Caregiver
• Describe the disease process of Guillain-Barré syndrome.	✓	✓
• Manage respiratory needs: tracheostomy care, suctioning.		✓
• Demonstrate proper body mechanics regarding lifting and transfers.		✓
• Practice gait training and strength endurance.	✓	✓
• Perform range-of-motion exercises.	✓	✓
• Perform activities of daily living and manage self-care:		
• Nutrition	✓	✓
• Bowel and bladder management	✓	✓
• Skin care	✓	✓
• Adaptive equipment for bathing, hygiene, grooming, dressing	✓	✓
• Operate and explain function of medical equipment and mobility aids: walkers, wheelchairs, bedside commodes, tub transfer benches, adaptive devices	✓	✓
• Use coping mechanisms and diversional activities appropriately.	✓	✓
• Implement safety measures in the home.	✓	✓
• Know how to contact and use community resources and the Guillain-Barré Syndrome Foundation International.	✓	✓

Cranial Nerve Disorders

Because the brain stem and cranial nerves involve vital motor, sensory, or autonomic functions of the body, these nerves may be affected by conditions arising primarily within these structures or in secondary extension from adjacent disease processes. The cranial nerves (Fig. 64-6) are examined separately and in sequence (see Chap. 60). Some cranial nerve deficits can be detected by observing the patient's face, eye movements, speech, and swallowing. Electromyography (EMG) is used to investigate motor and sensory dysfunction. MRI is used to obtain images of the cranial nerves and brain stem. An overview of disorders that may affect each of the cranial nerves, including clinical manifestations and nursing interventions, is presented in Table 64-1. The following discussion centres on trigeminal neuralgia, a condition affecting the fifth cranial nerve, and Bell's palsy, caused by involvement of the seventh cranial nerve. These are the most common disorders of the cranial nerves.

TRIGEMINAL NEURALGIA (TIC DOULOUREUX)

Trigeminal neuralgia is a condition of the fifth cranial nerve characterized by paroxysms of pain in the area innervated by any of the three branches, but it most commonly occurs in the second and third branches of the trigeminal nerve (Maloni, 2000) (Fig. 64-7). The pain ends as abruptly as it starts and is described as a unilateral shooting and stabbing sensation. The unilateral nature of the pain is an important diagnostic characteristic (Preul, 2001). Associated involuntary contraction of the facial muscles can cause sudden closing of the eye or a twitch of the mouth, hence the name *tic douloureux* (painful twitch). The cause is not certain, but chronic compression or irritation of the trigeminal nerve or de-

generative changes in the gasserian ganglion are suggested causes. Vascular pressure from structural abnormalities (loop of an artery) encroaching on the trigeminal nerve, gasserian ganglion, or root entry zone has also been suggested as a cause.

Trigeminal neuralgia is 400 times more common in patients with MS than in the general population. The pain is more often cyclic and affects men with MS at a higher rate than women with MS (Maloni, 2000).

Early attacks, appearing most often in the fifth decade of life, are usually mild and brief. Pain-free intervals may be measured in terms of minutes, hours, days, or longer. With advancing years, the painful episodes tend to become more frequent and agonizing. The patient lives in constant fear of attacks.

Paroxysms can occur with any stimulation of the terminals of the affected nerve branches, such as washing the face, shaving, brushing the teeth, eating, and drinking. A draft of cold air and direct pressure against the nerve trunk may also cause pain. Certain areas are called trigger points because the slightest touch immediately starts a paroxysm or episode. To avoid stimulating these areas, patients with trigeminal neuralgia try not to touch or wash their faces, shave, chew, or do anything else that might cause an attack. These behaviours are a clue to diagnosis.

Medical Management

PHARMACOLOGIC THERAPY

Antiseizure agents, such as carbamazepine (Tegretol), relieve pain in most patients with trigeminal neuralgia by reducing the transmission of impulses at certain nerve terminals. Carbamazepine is taken with meals. Serum levels must be monitored to avoid toxicity in patients who require high doses to control the pain. Side effects include nausea, dizziness, drowsiness, and aplastic anemia. The patient is monitored for bone marrow depression during long-term therapy. Gabapentin (Neurontin) and baclofen (Lioresal)

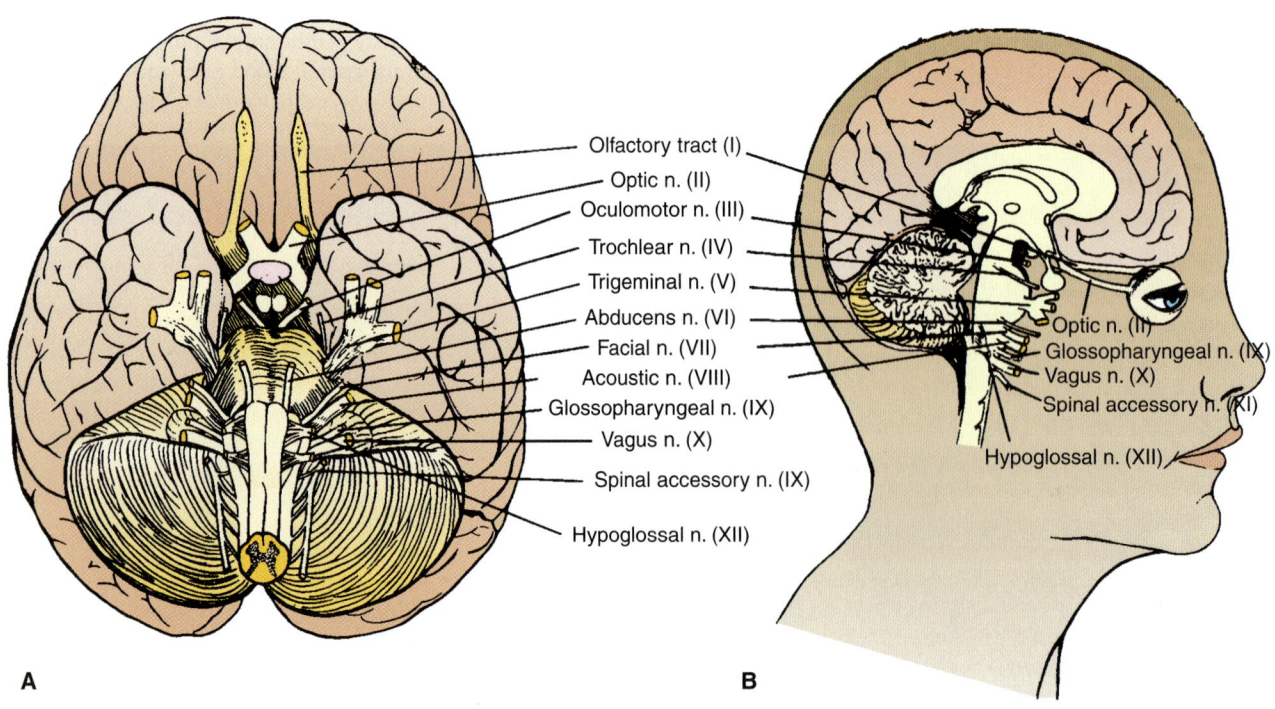

A   **B**

FIGURE 64-6   The cranial nerves. (**A**) Inferior view of the brain showing the cranial nerve. (**B**) Lateral view showing a schematic version of the cranial nerves.

Table 64-1 • **Disorders of Cranial Nerves**

DISORDER	CLINICAL MANIFESTATIONS	NURSING INTERVENTIONS
Olfactory Nerve—I		
Head trauma	Unilateral or bilateral anosmia (temporary or	Assess sense of smell.
Intracranial tumour	persistent)	Assess for cerebrospinal fluid rhinorrhea if
Intracranial surgery	Diminished taste for food	patient has sustained head trauma.
Optic Nerve—II		
Optic neuritis	Lesions of optic tract producing homony-	Assess visual acuity.
Increased intracranial pressure	mous hemianopsia	Restructure environment to prevent injuries.
Pituitary tumour		Teach patient to accommodate for visual loss.
Oculomotor Nerve—III		
Trochlear Nerve—IV		
Abducens Nerve—VI		
Vascular	Dilation of pupil with loss of light reflex on	Assess extraocular movement and for non-
Brain stem ischemia	one side	reactive pupil.
Hemorrhage and infarction	Impairment of ocular movement	
Neoplasm	Diplopia	
Trauma	Gaze palsies	
Infection	Ptosis of eyelid	
Trigeminal Nerve—V		
Trigeminal neuralgia	Pain in face	Assess for pain and triggering mechanisms
Head trauma	Diminished or loss of corneal reflex	for pain.
Cerebellopontine lesion	Chewing dysfunction	Assess for difficulty in chewing.
Sinus tract tumour and metastatic disease		Discuss trigger zones and pain precipitants
Compression of trigeminal root by tumour		with patient.
		Protect cornea from abrasion.
		Ensure good oral hygiene.
		Educate patient about medication regimen.
Facial Nerve—VII		
Bell's palsy	Facial dysfunction; weakness and paralysis	Recognize facial paralysis as emergency;
Facial nerve tumour	Hemifacial spasm	refer for treatment as soon as possible.
Intracranial lesion	Diminished or absent taste	Teach protective care for eyes.
Herpes zoster	Pain	Select easily chewed foods; patient should
		eat and drink from unaffected side of
		mouth.
		Emphasize importance of oral hygiene.
		Provide emotional support for changed
		appearance of face.
Acoustic Nerve—VIII		
Tumours and acoustic neuroma	Tinnitus	Assess pattern of vertigo.
Vascular compression of nerve	Vertigo	Provide for safety measures to prevent falls.
Ménière's syndrome	Hearing difficulties	Ensure that patient can obtain balance
		before ambulating.
		Caution patient to change positions slowly.
		Assist with ambulation.
		Encourage use of activity of daily living aids.
Glossopharyngeal Nerve—IX		
Glossopharyngeal neuralgia from neuro-	Pain at base of tongue	Assess for paroxysmal pain in throat,
vascular compression of cranial nerves IX	Difficulty in swallowing	decreased or absent swallowing, gag
and X	Loss of gag reflex	and cough reflexes.
Trauma	Palatal, pharyngeal, and laryngeal paralysis	Monitor for dysphagia, aspiration, nasal
Inflammatory conditions		dysarthric speech.
Tumour		Position patient upright for eating or tube
Vertebral artery aneurysms		feeding.
Vagus Nerve—X		
Spastic palsy of larynx; bulbar paralysis;	Voice changes (temporary or permanent	Assess for airway obstruction/provide airway
high vagal paralysis	hoarseness)	management.
Guillain-Barré syndrome	Vocal paralysis	Prevent aspiration.
Vagal body tumours	Dysphagia	Support patient having voice reconstruction
Nerve paralysis from malignancy,		procedures.
surgical trauma such as carotid		
endarterectomy		

(continued)

Table 64-1 • **Disorders of Cranial Nerves** (Continued)

DISORDER	CLINICAL MANIFESTATIONS	NURSING INTERVENTIONS
Spinal Accessory Nerve—XI Spinal cord disorder Amyotrophic lateral sclerosis Trauma Guillain-Barré syndrome	Drooping of affected shoulder with limited shoulder movement Weakness or paralysis of head rotation, flexion, extension; shoulder elevation	Support patient undergoing diagnostic tests.
Hypoglossal Nerve—XII Medullary lesions Amyotrophic lateral sclerosis Polio and motor system disease, which may destroy hypoglossal nuclei Multiple sclerosis Trauma	Abnormal movements of tongue Weakness or paralysis of tongue muscles Difficulty in talking, chewing, and swallowing	Observe swallowing ability. Observe speech pattern. Be aware of swallowing or vocal difficulties. Prepare for alternate feeding methods (tube feeding) to maintain nutrition.

are also used for pain control. If pain control is still not achieved, phenytoin (Dilantin) may be used as adjunctive therapy (Rowland, 2000).

Alcohol or phenol injection of the gasserian ganglion and peripheral branches of the trigeminal nerve relieves pain for several months. However, the pain returns with nerve regeneration.

SURGICAL MANAGEMENT
When these methods fail to relieve pain, a number of surgical options are available. The choice of procedure depends on the patient's preference and health status.

Microvascular Decompression of the Trigeminal Nerve. An intracranial approach can be used to decompress the trigeminal nerve. The pain may be caused by vascular compression of the entry zone of the trigeminal root by an arterial loop and occasionally by a vein. With the aid of an operating microscope, the artery loop is lifted from the nerve to relieve the pressure, and a small prosthetic device is inserted to prevent recurrence of impingement on the nerve. This procedure relieves facial pain while preserving normal sensation, but it is a major procedure, involving a craniotomy. The postoperative management is the same as for other intracranial surgeries (see Chap. 61).

Percutaneous Radiofrequency Trigeminal Gangliolysis. Percutaneous radiofrequency interruption of the gasserian ganglion, in which the small unmyelinated and thinly myelinated fibres that conduct pain are thermally destroyed, is the surgical procedure of choice for trigeminal neuralgia (Tronnier, Rasche, Hamer et al., 2001). Use of stereotactic MRI for identification of the trigeminal nerve followed by gamma knife radiosurgery is being used at some centres with good results (Maesawa et al., 2001).

Ophthalmic division (V1)

Trigeminal nerve (V)

Mandibular division (V3)

Maxillary division (V2)

V1

V2

V3

FIGURE 64-7 Distribution of trigeminal nerve branches.

Under local anesthesia, the needle is introduced through the cheek on the affected side. Under fluoroscopic guidance, the needle electrode is guided through the foramen magnum into the gasserian ganglion. The divisions of the gasserian ganglion (mandibular, maxillary, and ophthalmic) are encountered sequentially. The nerve is stimulated with a small current while the patient is awake. The patient reports when a tingling sensation is felt. When the electrode needle is in the desired position, the patient is anesthetized briefly and a radiofrequency current (heating current to destroy the nerve) is passed in a controlled manner to injure the trigeminal ganglion and rootlets thermally. The patient is then awakened from the anesthesia and examined for sensory deficits. This is repeated until the desired effect is achieved. The procedure takes less than 1 hour and provides permanent pain relief in most patients. Touch and proprioceptive functions are left intact.

In the patient with trigeminal neuralgia and MS who is refractory to medical pain management, the surgical treatment of choice is trigeminal rhizotomy (Maloni, 2000). See Chapter 13 for care of the patient following a rhizotomy.

Nursing Management

PREVENTING PAIN

Preoperative management of a patient with trigeminal neuralgia occurs mostly on an outpatient basis and includes recognizing factors that may aggravate excruciating facial pain, such as food that is too hot or too cold or jarring the patient's bed or chair. Even washing the face, combing the hair, or brushing the teeth may produce acute pain. The nurse can assist the patient in preventing or reducing this pain by providing instructions about preventive strategies. Providing cotton pads and room-temperature water for washing the face, instructing the patient to rinse with mouthwash after eating when tooth-brushing causes pain, and performing personal hygiene during pain-free intervals are all effective strategies. The patient is instructed to take food and fluids at room temperature, to chew on the unaffected side, and to ingest soft foods. The nurse recognizes that anxiety, depression, and insomnia often accompany chronic painful conditions and uses appropriate interventions and referrals. (See Chap. 13 for management of patients with chronic pain.)

PROVIDING POSTOPERATIVE CARE

Postoperative neurologic assessments are conducted to evaluate the patient for facial motor and sensory deficits in each of the three branches of the trigeminal nerve. If the surgery results in sensory deficits to the affected side of the face, the patient is instructed not to rub the eye, because pain will not be felt if there is injury. The eye is assessed for irritation or redness. Artificial tears may be prescribed to prevent dryness in the affected eye. The patient is cautioned not to chew on the affected side until numbness has diminished. The patient is observed carefully for any difficulty in eating and swallowing foods of different consistency.

BELL'S PALSY

Bell's palsy (facial paralysis) is due to unilateral inflammation of the seventh cranial nerve, which results in weakness or paralysis of the facial muscles on the affected side (Fig. 64-8). The cause is unknown, although possible causes may include vascular ischemia, viral disease (herpes simplex, herpes zoster), autoimmune disease, or a combination of all of these factors. The incidence is 13 to

Facial nerve

FIGURE 64-8   Distribution of facial nerve.

34 cases per 100,000; it increases with age and among pregnant women in the third trimester (Campbell & Brundage, 2002; Shmorgun, Chan & Ray, 2002).

Bell's palsy is considered by some to represent a type of pressure paralysis. The inflamed, edematous nerve becomes compressed to the point of damage, or its nutrient vessel is occluded, producing ischemic necrosis of the nerve. There is distortion of the face from paralysis of the facial muscles; increased lacrimation (tearing); and painful sensations in the face, behind the ear, and in the eye. The patient may experience speech difficulties and may be unable to eat on the affected side because of weakness or paralysis of the facial muscles.

Management

The objectives of treatment are to maintain the muscle tone of the face and to prevent or minimize denervation. The patient should be reassured that no stroke has occurred and that spontaneous recovery occurs within 3 to 5 weeks in most patients.

Corticosteroid therapy (prednisone) may be prescribed to reduce inflammation and edema; this reduces vascular compression and permits restoration of blood circulation to the nerve. Early administration of corticosteroid therapy appears to diminish the severity of the disease, relieve the pain, and prevent or minimize denervation.

Facial pain is controlled with analgesic agents. Heat may be applied to the involved side of the face to promote comfort and blood flow through the muscles.

Electrical stimulation may be applied to the face to prevent muscle atrophy. Although most patients recover with conservative treatment, surgical exploration of the facial nerve may be indicated in patients who are suspected of having a tumour or for surgical decompression of the facial nerve and for surgical treatment of a paralyzed face.

PROMOTING HOME AND COMMUNITY-BASED CARE

Teaching Patients Self-Care. While the paralysis lasts, the involved eye must be protected. Frequently, the eye does not close completely and the blink reflex is diminished, so the eye is vulnerable to dust and foreign particles. Corneal irritation and ulceration may occur if the eye is unprotected. Distortion of the lower lid alters the proper drainage of tears. To prevent injury, the eye should be covered with a protective shield at night. The eye patch may abrade the cornea, however, because there is some difficulty in keeping the partially paralyzed eyelids closed. The application of eye ointment at bedtime causes the eyelids to adhere to one another and remain closed during sleep. The patient can be taught to close the paralyzed eyelid manually before going to sleep. Wrap-around sunglasses or goggles may be worn to decrease normal evaporation from the eye.

Continuing Care. When the sensitivity of the nerve to touch decreases and the patient can tolerate touching the face, the nurse can suggest massaging the face several times daily, using a gentle upward motion, to maintain muscle tone. Facial exercises, such as wrinkling the forehead, blowing out the cheeks, and whistling, may be performed with the aid of a mirror in an effort to prevent muscle atrophy. Exposure of the face to cold and drafts is avoided.

Disorders of the Peripheral Nervous System

PERIPHERAL NEUROPATHIES

A peripheral **neuropathy** (disorder of the nervous system) is a disorder affecting the peripheral motor, sensory, or autonomic nerves. Peripheral nerves connect the spinal cord and brain to all other organs. They transmit motor impulses from the brain and relay sensory impulses to the brain. A mononeuropathy affects a single peripheral nerve; multiple mononeuropathy or mononeuritis multiplex indicates the involvement of multiple single peripheral nerves or their branches. Polyneuropathies are characterized by bilateral and symmetric disturbance of function, usually beginning in the feet and hands. (Most nutritional, metabolic, and toxic neuropathies take this form.)

The most common causes of peripheral neuropathy are diabetes, alcoholism, and occlusive vascular disease. These disorders result in hypoxia or atrophy of the peripheral nerve. Many bacterial and metabolic toxins and exogenous poisons also cause peripheral neuropathy. Because of the growing use of chemicals in industry, agriculture, and medicine, the number of substances causing peripheral neuropathies and the incidence of peripheral neuropathies have increased. In developing countries, leprosy is a major cause of severe nerve disease because *Mycobacterium leprae* invade the peripheral nervous system.

The major symptoms of peripheral nerve disorders are loss of sensation, muscle atrophy, weakness, diminished reflexes, pain, and paresthesia (numbness, tingling) of the extremities. The patient frequently describes some part of the extremity as numb. Autonomic features include decreased or absent sweating, orthostatic hypotension, nocturnal diarrhea, tachycardia, impotence, and atrophic skin and nail changes.

Peripheral nerve disorders are diagnosed by history, physical examination, EMG, and somatosensory evoked potentials.

MONONEUROPATHY

Mononeuropathy is limited to a single peripheral nerve and its branches. It arises when the trunk of the nerve is compressed or entrapped (as in carpal tunnel syndrome); traumatized, as when bruised by a blow, or overstretched, as in joint dislocation; punctured by a needle used to inject a drug or damaged by the drugs thus injected; or inflamed because an adjacent infectious process extends to the nerve trunk. Mononeuropathy frequently is seen in patients with diabetes.

Pain is seldom a major symptom of mononeuropathy when the condition is due to trauma, but in patients with complicating inflammatory conditions such as arthritis, pain is prominent. Pain is increased by all body movements that tend to stretch, strain, or cause pressure on the injured nerve and by sudden jarring of the body (eg, coughing and sneezing). The skin in the areas supplied by nerves that are injured or diseased may become reddened and glossy; the subcutaneous tissue may become edematous, and the nails and hair in this area become defective. Chemical injuries to a nerve trunk, such as those caused by drugs injected into or near it, are often permanent.

The objective of treatment of mononeuropathy is to remove the cause, if possible, such as by freeing the compressed nerve. Local corticosteroid injections may reduce inflammation and the pressure on the nerve. Aspirin or codeine may be used to relieve pain.

Critical Thinking Exercises

1. A 19-year-old college student is suspected of having meningococcal meningitis. Identify two neurologic changes that may reflect increased ICP. What interventions would be included in your plan of care to protect the patient from injury? The patient's family has many questions about the disease and their risk of contracting meningitis. Develop a teaching plan that would describe meningococcal meningitis and prophylactic therapy for the patient's family and close contacts.

2. Your patient has been receiving one of the injectable interferon medications for the treatment of MS for about 6 months. She reports that she is becoming very discouraged because the medication does not seem to improve her symptoms. In addition, she reports that she has developed skin lesions at the injection sites. Identify the areas of assessment that are of priority at this time. Describe nursing interventions, including teaching and referral, that you would consider at this time. Provide the rationale for your interventions.

3. Your patient has been admitted to the hospital with a diagnosis of possible Guillain-Barré. Identify the priorities of assessment for this patient and the nursing and medical interventions that you would anticipate.

4. Your patient has myasthenia gravis. Although she reports that her condition has been stable and that she has been able to manage without assistance, she reports increasing weakness and fatigue. What nursing assessments and interventions are warranted for her? What discharge plans are indicated if she is to return home to the care of her family? How would your discharge planning change if she lives alone in an apartment on the second floor of a building without an elevator?

5. A 52-year-old man has just been diagnosed with trigeminal neuralgia. Tegretol has been prescribed for pain management. Develop a teaching plan that explains the nature of trigeminal neuralgia, the side effects of Tegretol, and measures he can take to avoid triggering a painful episode. How would you evaluate the outcome of your teaching plan?

REFERENCES AND SELECTED READINGS

Books

Bashir, K., & Whitaker, J. N. (2002). *Handbook of multiple sclerosis.* Philadelphia: Lippincott Williams & Wilkins.

Davis, L. E., & Kennedy, P. G. E. (2000). *Infectious diseases of the nervous system.* Oxford: Butterworth-Heinemann.

Fischbach, F. (2002). *Common laboratory and diagnostic tests* (3rd Ed.). Philadelphia: Lippincott Williams & Wilkins.

Halper, J. (Ed.) (2001). *Advanced concepts in multiple sclerosis nursing care.* New York: Demos Medical Publishing, Inc.

Hickey, J. (2003). *Clinical practice of neurologic and neurosurgical nursing* (4th ed.). Philadelphia: Lippincott Williams & Wilkins.

Karch, A. (2002). *Lippincott's nursing drug guide.* Philadelphia: Lippincott Williams & Wilkins.

Meningitis Research Foundation of Canada. (2005.) *What is meningitis?* Available at: http://www.meningitis.ca. Retrieved June 15, 2005.

Public Health Agency of Canada. (2005). *Disease information: West Nile virus.* Available at: http://www.phac-aspc.gc.ca. Retrieved June 15, 2005.

Ross, A. P. (2001). The evolution of disease management. In J. Halper (Ed.), *Advanced concepts in multiple sclerosis nursing care.* New York: Demos Medical Publishing, Inc.

Rowland, L. (2000). *Merritt's neurology* (10th ed.). Philadelphia: Lippincott Williams & Wilkins.

Sipski, M. L., & Alexander, C. J. (Eds.). (1997). *Sexual function in people with disability and chronic illness: A health professional's guide.* Gaithersburg, MD: Aspen.

Journals

Asterisks indicate nursing research articles.

CNS Infections

Bruce, M. G., Rosenstein, N. E., Capparella, J., et al. (2001). Risk factors for meningococcal disease in college students. *Journal of the American Medical Association, 286*(6), 688–693.

Centers for Disease Control and Prevention. (2000). Prevention and control of meningococcal disease. *MMWR-Morbidity and Mortality Weekly Report, 49*, No. RR-7.

Coyle, P. (1999). Overview of acute and chronic meningitis. *Neurologic Clinics, 17*(4), 691–710.

Davis, L. (1999). Fungal infections of the central nervous system. *Neurologic Clinics, 17*(4), 763–782.

de Gans, J., & van de Beek, D. (2002). Dexamethasone in adults with bacterial meningitis. *New England Journal of Medicine, 347*(20), 1549–1556.

Go, J. L., Kim, P. E., Ahmadi, J., et al. (2000). Fungal infections of the central nervous system. *Neuroimaging Clinics of North America, 10*(2), 409–422.

Gutierrez, K., & Prober, C. (1998). Encephalitis. *Postgraduate Medicine, 103*(3), 123–143.

Leedom, J., & Underman, A. (2000). Epidemiology of central nervous system infections. *Neuroimaging Clinics of North America, 10*(2), 297–307.

Levitz, R. (1998). Herpes simplex encephalitis: A review. *Heart & Lung, 27*(3), 209–211.

Pruitt, A. (1998) Infections of the nervous system. *Neurologic Clinics of North America, 16*(2), 419–433.

Roos, K. (1999). Encephalitis. *Neurologic Clinics, 17*(4), 813–834.

Rubin, L. (2000). Pneumococcal vaccine. *Pediatric Clinics of North America, 47*(2), 269–283.

Rosenstein, N. E., & Perkins, B. (2000). Update on *Haemophilus influenzae* serotype b and meningococcal vaccines. *Pediatric Clinics of North America, 47*(2), 337–348.

Rosenstein, N. E., Perkins, B. A., Stephens, D. S., et al. (2001). Meningococcal disease. *New England Journal of Medicine, 334*(18), 1378–1388.

Spach, D., & Jackson, L. (1999). Bacterial meningitis. *Neurologic Clinics, 17*(4), 711–727.

Creutzfeldt-Jakob Disease

Almond, J. (1998). Bovine spongiform encephalopathy and new variant Creutzfeldt-Jakob disease. *British Medical Bulletin, 54*(3), 749–759.

Brandel, J., Delasneric-Laupretre, N., Laplanche, J. L., et al. (2000). Diagnosis of Creutzfeldt-Jakob disease. *Neurology, 54*(5), 1095–1098.

Johnson, R. T., & Gibbs, C. J. (1998). Creutzfeldt-Jakob disease and related transmissible spongiform encephalopathies. *New England Journal of Medicine, 339*(27), 1994–2004.

Poser, S., Mollenhauder, B., Krab, A., et al. (1999). How to improve the clinical diagnosis of Creutzfeldt-Jakob disease. *Brain, 122*, 2345–2351.

Weihl, C., & Roos, R. (1999). Creutzfeldt-Jakob disease, new variant Creutzfeldt-Jakob disease and bovine spongiform encephalopathy. *Neurologic Clinics, 17*(4), 835–860.

World Health Organization (2002). *Bovine spongiform encephalopathy.* Fact Sheet No. 113; http://www.who.int/mediacentre/factsheets/fs113/en/

Guillain-Barré Syndrome

Bella, I., & Chad, D. (1998). Neuromuscular disorders and acute respiratory failure. *Neurologic Clinics of North America, 16*(2), 391–415.

Ho, T., & Griffin, J. (1999). Guillain-Barré syndrome. *Current Opinion in Neurology, 12*, 389–394.

Lindenbaum, Y., Kissel, J., & Mendel, J. (2001). Treatment approaches for Guillain-Barré syndrome and chronic inflammatory demyelinating polyradiculoneuropathy. *Neurologic Clinics, 19*(1), 187–204.

McMahon-Parkes, K., & Cornock, M. A. (1997). Guillain-Barré syndrome: Biological basis, treatment, and care. *Intensive Critical Care Nursing, 13*(1), 42–48.

Prevots, D. R., & Sutter, R. W. (1997). Assessment of Guillain-Barré syndrome mortality and morbidity in the U.S.: Implications for acute flaccid paralysis surveillance. *Journal of Infectious Diseases, 175*(Suppl 1), S151–S155.

Ross, A. P. (1999). Neurologic degenerative disorders. *Nursing Clinics of North America, 34*(7), 725–741.

Winer, J. B. (2002). Treatment of Guillain-Barré syndrome. *QJM: An International Journal of Medicine, 95*(11), 717–721.

Yuki, N., Wim Ang, C., Koga, M., et al. (2000). Clinical features and response to treatment in Guillain-Barré syndrome associated with antibodies to GM 1b ganglioside. *Annals of Neurology, 47*(3), 314–321.

Multiple Sclerosis

Boyden, K. (2000). The pathophysiology of demyelination and the ionic basis of nerve conduction in multiple sclerosis: An overview. *Journal of Neuroscience Nursing, 32*(1), 49–53.

Clanet, M., & Brassat, D. (2000). The management of multiple sclerosis patients. *Current Opinion in Neurology, 13*, 263–270.

Costello, K., & Conway, K. (1997). Nursing management of MS patients receiving interferon beta-1b therapy. *Rehabilitation Nursing, 22*(2), 62–72.

Galvan, T. J. (2001). Dysphagia: Going down and staying down. *American Journal of Nursing, 101*(1), 37–42.

Halper, J., & Holland, N. (1998). Meeting the challenge of multiple sclerosis. Part I. Treating the person and the disease. *American Journal of Nursing, 98*(10), 26–31.

Halper, J., & Holland, N. (1998). Meeting the challenge of multiple sclerosis. Part II. New strategies, new hope. *American Journal of Nursing, 98*(11), 39–45.

Klewer, J., Pohlau, D., Nippert, I., et al. (2001). Problems reported by elderly patients with multiple sclerosis. *Journal of Neuroscience Nursing, 33*(3), 167–171.

Madonna, M., & Keating, M. (1999). Multiple sclerosis pathways: An innovative nursing role in disease management. *Journal of Neuroscience Nursing, 31*(6), 332–335.

Maloni, H. (2000). Pain in multiple sclerosis: An overview of its nature and management. *Journal of Neuroscience Nursing, 32*(3), 140–144.

Noseworthy, J., Lucchinetti, C., Rodriguez, M., et al. (2000). Multiple sclerosis. *New England Journal of Medicine, 343*(13), 938–949.

Rolak, L. A. (2001). Multiple sclerosis treatment 2001. *Neurologic Clinics, 19*(1), 107–118.

Rudick, R. (1999). Disease-modifying drugs for relapsing-remitting multiple sclerosis and future directions for multiple sclerosis therapeutics. *Archives of Neurology, 56,* 1079–1084.

PRISMS Study Group and the University of British Columbia MS/MRI Analysis Group (2001) PRISMS-4: Long-term efficacy of interferon beta-1-a in relapsing MS. *Neurology, 56*(12), 1628–1636.

*Smeltzer, S. C., & Lavietes, M. H. (1999). Reliability of maximal respiratory pressures in MS. *Chest, 115*(6), 1546–1552.

*Smeltzer, S. C., Zimmerman, V., Capriotti, T., & Fernandes, L. (2002). Osteoporosis risk factors and bone mineral density in women with MS. *International Journal of MS Care, 4*(1), 17–23, 29.

*Smeltzer, S. C. (2002). Reproductive decision making in women with multiple sclerosis. *Journal of Neuroscience Nursing, 34*(3), 145–157.

*Stuifbergen, A., Seraphine, A., & Roberts, G. (2000). An explanatory model of health promotion and quality of life in chronic disabling conditions. *Nursing Research, 49*(3), 122–129.

Sullivan, M., & Sharts-Hopko, N. (2000). Preventing the downward spiral. *American Journal of Nursing, 100*(8), 26–32.

Tselis, A., & Lisak, R. (1999). Multiple sclerosis. *Archives of Neurology, 56,* 277–280.

Walther, E., & Hohlfeld, R. (1999). Multiple sclerosis. *Neurology, 53,* 1622–626.

Myasthenia Gravis

Bedlack, R., & Sanders, D. (2000). How to handle myasthenic crisis. *Postgraduate Medicine, 107*(4), 211–222.

Heitmiller, R. (1999). Myasthenia gravis: Clinical features, pathogenesis, evaluation and medical management. *Seminars in Thoracic and Cardiovascular Surgery, 11*(1), 41–46.

Massey, J. M. (1997). Acquired myasthenia gravis. *Neurologic Clinics, 15*(3), 577–593.

Qureshi, A., Choudhry, M. A., Akbar, M. S., et al. (1999). Plasma exchange versus intravenous immunoglobulin treatment in myasthenic crisis. *Neurology, 52,* 629–632.

Thomas, C. E., Mayer, S. A., Gungor, Y., et al. (1997). Myasthenia crisis: Clinical features, mortality, complications, and risk factors for prolonged intubation. *Neurology, 48*(5), 1253–1260.

Wilkins, K., & Bulkley, G. (1999). Thymectomy in the integrated management of myasthenia gravis. *Advances in Surgery, 32,* 105–133.

Wittbrodt, E. T. (1997). Drugs and myasthenia gravis. *Archives of Internal Medicine, 157,* 399–408.

Trigeminal Neuralgia and Neuropathies

Brown, J. (1997). The trigeminal complex: Anatomy and physiology. *Neurosurgery Clinics of North America, 8*(1), 1–10.

Campbell, K. E., & Brundage, J. F. (2002). Effects of climate, latitude, and season on the incidence of Bell's palsy in the U.S. Armed Forces, October 1997 to September 1999. *American Journal of Epidemiology, 156*(1), 32–39.

Costa, M. E. (1998). Trigeminal neuralgia. *American Journal of Nursing, 98*(6), 42–43.

Maesawa, S., Salame, C., Flickinger, J., et al. (2001). Clinical outcomes after stereotactic radiosurgery for idiopathic trigeminal neuralgia. *Journal of Neurosurgery, 94,* 14–20.

Preul, M. (2001). Historical considerations of the diagnosis and treatment of facial pain. *Neurosurgery Clinics of North America, 12*(1), 111–126.

Shmorgun, D., Chan, W. S., & Ray, J. G. (2002). Association between Bell's palsy in pregnancy and pre-eclampsia. *QJM: An International Journal of Medicine, 95*(6), 359–362.

Tronnier, V., Rasche, D., Hamer, J., et al. (2001) Treatment of idiopathic trigeminal neuralgia: Comparison of long-term outcome after radiofrequency rhizotomy and microvascular decompression. *Neurosurgery, 48*(6), 1261–1266.

RESOURCES AND WEBSITES

Guillain-Barré Syndrome Foundation International, P.O. Box 262, Wynnewood, PA 19096; (610) 667-0131; fax: 610-667-7036; http://www.guillain-barre.com/.

Journal of the American Medical Association Patient Pages: http:/www.ama-assn.org/consumer.htm.

Meningitis Research Foundation of Canada, PO Box 28015, RPO Parkdale, Waterloo, ON N2L 6J8; (519) 746-8306; http://www.meningitis.ca

Multiple Sclerosis Society of Canada, 175 Bloor Street East, Suite 700, North Tower, Toronto, ON M4W 3R8; (416) 922-6065; http://www.mssociety.ca.

Myasthenia Gravis Foundation of America, 222 S. Riverside Plaza, Suite 1540, Chicago, IL 60606; (800) 541-5454; (312) 258-0522; fax: 312-258-0461; http://www.myasthenia.org.

National Multiple Sclerosis Society, 733 Third Avenue, New York, NY 10017; (800) 344-4867; http://www.nmss.org.

Public Health Agency of Canada; http://www.phac-aspc.gc.ca.

The Neuropathy Association: http://www.neuropathy.org/explaining/index.html. (212) 692-0662.

Management of Patients With Oncologic or Degenerative Neurologic Disorders

Adapted by Wanda Pierson

LEARNING OBJECTIVES ●

On completion of this chapter, the learner will be able to:

1. Identify the pathophysiologic processes responsible for oncologic disorders.

2. Describe brain and spinal cord tumours: their classification, clinical manifestations, diagnosis, and medical and nursing management.

3. Use the nursing process as a framework for care of patients with cerebral metastases or inoperable brain tumours.

4. Identify the pathophysiologic processes responsible for various degenerative neurologic disorders.

5. Use the nursing process as a framework for care of patients with degenerative neurologic disorders.

6. Identify resources for patients and families with oncologic and degenerative neurologic disorders.

Disease processes that are oncologic or degenerative produce a unique set of problems when they occur in the neurologic system. Oncologic processes include brain and spinal cord tumours. Degenerative neurologic disorders include Parkinson's disease, Huntington's disease, Alzheimer's disease, amyotrophic lateral sclerosis, muscular dystrophies, and degenerative disc disease. A relatively new phenomenon, post-polio syndrome, may be degenerative in nature and is therefore included in this chapter.

Oncologic Disorders of the Brain and Spinal Cord

Oncologic disorders in the brain and spinal cord include several types of neoplasms, each with its own biology, prognosis, and treatment options. Because of the unique anatomy and physiology of the central nervous system (CNS), this collection of neoplasms is challenging to diagnose and treat. The pathophysiology, clinical manifestations, assessment findings, and medical and nursing management of brain tumours and spinal cord tumours are discussed in the following sections.

PRIMARY BRAIN TUMOURS

A brain tumour is a localized intracranial lesion that occupies space within the skull. Tumours usually grow as a spherical mass, but they can grow diffusely and infiltrate tissue. The effects of neoplasms occur from the compression and infiltration of tissue. A variety of physiologic changes result, causing any or all of the following pathophysiologic events:

- Increased intracranial pressure (ICP) and cerebral edema
- Seizure activity and focal neurologic signs
- Hydrocephalus
- Altered pituitary function

Primary brain tumours originate from cells and structures within the brain. Secondary, or metastatic, brain tumours develop from structures outside the brain and occur in 20% to 40% of all patients with cancer. Brain tumours rarely metastasize outside the CNS, but metastatic lesions to the brain occur commonly from the lung, breast, lower gastrointestinal tract, pancreas, kidney, and skin (melanomas).

The cause of primary brain tumours is unknown. The only known risk factor is exposure to ionizing radiation. Both glial and meningeal neoplasms have been linked to irradiation of the cranium, with a latency period of 10 to 20 years after exposure (DeAngelis, 2001). Additional possible causes have been investigated, but results of studies are conflicting and unconvincing; suggested causes have included use of cellular telephones, exposure to high-tension wires, use of hair dyes, head trauma, dietary exposure to such factors as nitrates (found in some processed and barbecued foods), and other sources (DeAngelis, 2001).

The incidence of brain tumours appears to have increased in the past few decades. Epidemiologic data, however, suggest that this is due more to aggressive and accurate diagnosis rather than to an actual rise in incidence. It is estimated that there are about 17,000 new cases of primary brain tumours per year, 9,600 in men and 7,400 in women in the United States (American Cancer Society, 2002). In Canada, primary brain tumours occur in 6 persons per 100,000 per year (Molson Medical Informatics, 2005). Secondary tumours or metastases to the brain from a systemic primary cancer are more common (DeAngelis, 2001). The highest incidence of brain tumours in adults occurs in the fifth, sixth, and seventh decades, with a slightly higher incidence in men. In adults, most brain tumours originate from glial cells (glial cells make up the structure and support system of the brain and spinal cord) and are supratentorial (located above the covering of the cerebellum). Neoplastic lesions in the brain ultimately cause death by impairing vital functions, such as respiration, or by increasing intracranial pressure (ICP).

Pathophysiology

Brain tumours may be classified into several groups: those arising from the coverings of the brain (eg, dural meningioma), those developing in or on the cranial nerves (eg, acoustic neuroma), those originating within brain tissue (eg, gliomas), and metastatic lesions originating elsewhere in the body. Tumours of the pituitary and pineal glands and of cerebral blood vessels are also types of brain tumours. Relevant clinical considerations include the location and the histologic character of the tumour. Tumours may be benign or malignant. A benign tumour can occur in a vital area and can grow large enough to have effects as serious as those of a malignant tumour.

GLIOMAS

Glial tumours, the most common type of brain neoplasm, are divided into many categories (DeAngelis, 2001). See Chart 65-1 for the classification of brain tumours. Astrocytomas are the most common type of glioma and are graded from I to IV, indicating the degree of malignancy. The grade is based on cellular density, cell mitosis, and appearance. Usually, these tumours spread by infiltrating into the surrounding neural connective tissue and therefore cannot be totally removed without causing considerable damage to vital structures.

Glossary

akathisia: restlessness, urgent need to move around, and agitation

bradykinesia: very slow voluntary movements and speech

chorea: rapid, jerky, involuntary, purposeless movements of the extremities or facial muscles, including facial grimacing

dementia: a progressive organic mental disorder characterized by personality changes, confusion, disorientation, and deterioration of intellect associated with impaired memory and judgment

dyskinesia: impaired ability to execute voluntary movements

dysphonia: abnormal voice quality caused by weakness and incoordination of muscles responsible for speech

micrographia: very minute and often illegible handwriting

neurodegenerative: a disease, process, or condition that leads to deterioration of normal cells or function of the nervous system

papilledema: edema of the optic nerve

paresthesia: a sensation of numbness, tingling, or a "pins and needles" sensation

radiculopathy: disease of a spinal nerve root, often resulting in pain and extreme sensitivity to touch

sciatica: inflammation of the sciatic nerve, resulting in pain and tenderness along the nerve through the thigh and leg

spondylosis: degenerative arthritis or osteoarthritis of the cervical or lumbar vertebrae, resulting in stiffness of the vertebral joint

Chart 65-1

Classification of Adult Brain Tumours

I. Intracerebral Tumours
A. Gliomas—infiltrate any portion of the brain; most common type of brain tumour
   1. Astrocytomas (grades I and II)
   2. Glioblastoma multiforme (astrocytoma grades III and IV)
   3. Oligodendrocytoma (low and high grades)
   4. Ependymoma (grades I to IV)
   5. Medulloblastoma

II. Tumours Arising From Supporting Structures
A. Meningiomas
B. Neuromas (acoustic neuroma, schwannoma)
C. Pituitary adenomas

III. Developmental Tumours
A. Angiomas
B. Dermoid, epidermoid, teroma, craniopharyngioma

IV. Metastatic Lesions

Oligodendroglial tumours are another type of glial tumour, representing 20% of gliomas (DeAngelis, 2001). The histologic distinction between astrocytomas and oligodendrogliomas is difficult to make but important, as recent research shows that oligodendrogliomas are more sensitive to chemotherapy than astrocytomas. These tumours are categorized as low-grade and high-grade (anaplastic).

MENINGIOMAS

Meningiomas, which represent 20% of all primary brain tumours, are common benign encapsulated tumours of arachnoid cells on the meninges (DeAngelis, 2001). They are slow-growing and occur most often in middle-aged adults (more often in women). Meningiomas most often occur in areas proximal to the venous sinuses. Manifestations depend on the area involved and are the result of compression rather than invasion of brain tissue. Standard treatment is surgery with complete removal or partial dissection.

ACOUSTIC NEUROMAS

An acoustic neuroma is a tumour of the eighth cranial nerve, the cranial nerve most responsible for hearing and balance. It usually arises just within the internal auditory meatus, where it frequently expands before filling the cerebellopontine recess.

An acoustic neuroma may grow slowly and attain considerable size before it is correctly diagnosed. The patient usually experiences loss of hearing, tinnitus, and episodes of vertigo and staggering gait. As the tumour becomes larger, painful sensations of the face may occur on the same side as a result of the tumour's compression of the fifth cranial nerve.

With improved imaging techniques and the use of the operating microscope and microsurgical instrumentation, even large tumours can be removed through a relatively small craniotomy. Some of these tumours may be suitable for stereotactic radiotherapy rather than surgery. See the discussion of stereotactic radiotherapy later in this chapter.

PITUITARY ADENOMAS

Pituitary tumours represent about 8% to 12% of all brain tumours and cause symptoms as a result of pressure on adjacent structures or hormonal changes (hyperfunction or hypofunction of the pituitary). The pituitary gland, also called the hypophysis, is a relatively small gland located in the sella turcica. It is attached to the hypothalamus by a short stalk (hypophyseal stalk) and is divided into two lobes: the anterior (adenohypophysis) and the posterior (neurohypophysis).

Pressure Effects of Pituitary Adenomas. Pressure from a pituitary adenoma may be exerted on the optic nerves, optic chiasm, or optic tracts or on the hypothalamus or the third ventricle when the tumour invades the cavernous sinuses or expands into the sphenoid bone. These pressure effects produce headache, visual dysfunction, hypothalamic disorders (eg, disorders of sleep, appetite, temperature and emotions), increased ICP, and enlargement and erosion of the sella turcica.

Hormonal Effects of Pituitary Adenomas. Functioning pituitary tumours can produce one or more hormones normally produced by the anterior pituitary. These hormones may cause prolactin-secreting pituitary adenomas (prolactinomas), growth hormone-secreting pituitary adenomas that produce acromegaly in adults, and adrenocorticotropic hormone (ACTH)-producing pituitary adenomas that result in Cushing's disease. Adenomas that secrete thyroid-stimulating hormone or follicle-stimulating hormone and luteinizing hormone occur infrequently, whereas adenomas that produce both growth hormone and prolactin are relatively common.

The female patient whose pituitary gland is secreting excessive quantities of prolactin presents with amenorrhea or galactorrhea (excessive or spontaneous flow of milk). Male patients with prolactinomas may present with impotence and hypogonadism. Acromegaly, caused by excess growth hormone, produces enlargement of the hands and feet, distortion of the facial features, and pressure on peripheral nerves (entrapment syndromes). The clinical features of Cushing's disease, a condition associated with prolonged overproduction of cortisol, occur with excessive production of ACTH. Manifestations include a form of obesity with redistribution of fat to the facial, supraclavicular, and abdominal areas; hypertension; purple striae and ecchymoses; osteoporosis; elevated blood glucose levels; and emotional disorders.

ANGIOMAS

Brain angiomas (masses composed largely of abnormal blood vessels) are found either in or on the surface of the brain. They occur in the cerebellum in 83% of cases. Some persist throughout life without causing symptoms; others cause symptoms of a brain tumour. Occasionally, the diagnosis is suggested by the presence of another angioma somewhere in the head or by a bruit (an abnormal sound) audible over the skull. Because the walls of the blood vessels in angiomas are thin, these patients are at risk for a cerebral vascular accident (stroke). In fact, cerebral hemorrhage in people younger than 40 years of age should suggest the possibility of an angioma.

Clinical Manifestations

Brain tumours can produce either focal or generalized neurologic signs and symptoms. Generalized symptoms reflect increased ICP, and the most common focal or specific signs and symptoms result from tumours interfering with functions in specific brain regions. Figure 65-1 indicates common tumour sites in the brain.

INCREASING ICP

As discussed in Chapter 61, the skull is a rigid compartment containing essential noncompressible contents: brain matter, intravascular blood, and cerebrospinal fluid (CSF). According to the modified Monro-Kellie hypothesis, if any one of these skull

Corpus callosum
astrocytoma
oligodendroglioma
lipoma

Lateral ventricle
ependymoma
glioblastoma multiforme

Third ventricle and area
ependymoma

Cerebrum
astrocytoma
oligodendroglioma
lymphoma
metastatic tumours

Pineal area
pineocytoma
pineoblastoma

Optic chiasm
astrocytoma

Pituitary area
craniopharyngioma
pituitary adenoma
epidermoid cyst

Acoustic nerve
neuroma

Cerebellum
medulloblastoma
astrocytoma
hemangioblastoma
metastatic tumours

Brain stem
astrocytoma
glioblastoma multiforme
metastatic tumours

Fourth ventricle
ependymoma

FIGURE 65-1 Common brain tumour sites.

components increases in volume, ICP increases unless one of the other components decreases in volume. Consequently, any change in volume occupied by the brain (as occurs with disorders such as brain tumour or cerebral edema) produces signs and symptoms of increased ICP.

Symptoms of increased ICP result from a gradual compression of the brain by the enlarging tumour. The effect is a disruption of the equilibrium that exists between the brain, the CSF, and the cerebral blood, all located within the skull. As the tumour grows, compensatory adjustments may occur through compression of intracranial veins, reduction of CSF volume (by increased absorption or decreased production), a modest decrease of cerebral blood flow, and reduction of intracellular and extracellular brain tissue mass. When these compensatory mechanisms fail, the patient develops signs and symptoms of increased ICP. The three most common signs of increased ICP are headache, nausea and vomiting, and a sixth-nerve palsy (DeAngelis, 2001). Personality changes and a variety of focal deficits, including motor, sensory, and cranial nerve dysfunction, are also common.

Headache. Headache, although not always present, is most common in the early morning and is made worse by coughing, straining, or sudden movement. It is thought to be caused by the tumour invading, compressing, or distorting the pain-sensitive structures or by edema that accompanies the tumour. Headaches are usually described as deep or expanding or as dull but unrelenting. Frontal tumours usually produce a bilateral frontal headache; pituitary gland tumours produce pain radiating between the two temples (bitemporal); in cerebellar tumours, the headache may be located in the suboccipital region at the back of the head.

Vomiting. Vomiting, seldom related to food intake, is usually due to irritation of the vagal centres in the medulla. If the vomiting is of the forceful type, it is described as projectile vomiting.

Visual Disturbances. **Papilledema** (edema of the optic nerve) is present in 70% to 75% of patients and is associated with visual disturbances such as decreased visual acuity, diplopia (double vision), and visual field deficits.

LOCALIZED SYMPTOMS
The most common focal or localized symptoms are hemiparesis, seizures, and mental status changes (DeAngelis, 2001). When specific regions of the brain are affected, additional local signs and symptoms occur, such as sensory and motor abnormalities, visual alterations, alterations in cognition, and language disturbances such as aphasia. The progression of the signs and symptoms is important because it indicates tumour growth and expansion. For example, a rapidly developing hemiparesis is more typical of a highly malignant glioma than a low-grade tumour (DeAngelis, 2001).

Although some tumours are not easily localized because they lie in so-called silent areas of the brain (ie, areas in which functions are not definitely determined), many tumours can be localized by correlating the signs and symptoms to known areas of the brain, as follows:

- A motor cortex tumour produces seizure-like movements localized on one side of the body, called Jacksonian seizures.
- An occipital lobe tumour produces visual manifestations: contralateral homonymous hemianopsia (visual loss in half of the visual field on the opposite side of the tumour) and visual hallucinations.
- A cerebellar tumour causes dizziness, an ataxic or staggering gait with a tendency to fall toward the side of the lesion, marked muscle incoordination, and nystagmus (involuntary rhythmic eye movements), usually in the horizontal direction.
- A frontal lobe tumour frequently produces personality disorders, changes in emotional state and behaviour, and an uninterested mental attitude. The patient often becomes extremely untidy and careless and may use obscene language.
- A cerebellopontine angle tumour usually originates in the sheath of the acoustic nerve and gives rise to a characteristic sequence of symptoms. Tinnitus and vertigo appear first, soon followed by progressive nerve deafness (eighth cranial nerve dysfunction). Numbness and tingling of the face and the tongue occur (due to involvement of the fifth cranial nerve). Later, weakness or paralysis of the face develops (seventh cranial nerve involvement). Finally, because the enlarging tumour presses on the cerebellum, abnormalities in motor function may be present.

FIGURE 65-2 Low-grade glioma. MRI of the brain shows a mass of abnormal density in the right temporal lobe. Courtesy of the Hospital of the University of Pennsylvania, Nuclear Medicine Section, Philadelphia, Pennsylvania.

Assessment and Diagnostic Findings

The history of the illness and the manner and time frame in which the symptoms evolved are key components in the diagnosis of brain tumours. A neurologic examination indicates the areas of the CNS involved. To assist in the precise localization of the lesion, a battery of tests is performed. Computed tomography (CT) scans, enhanced by a contrast agent, can give specific information concerning the number, size, and density of the lesions and the extent of secondary cerebral edema. CT scans can provide information about the ventricular system. Magnetic resonance imaging (MRI) is the most helpful diagnostic tool for detecting brain tumours, particularly smaller lesions, and tumours in the brain stem and pituitary regions, where bone interferes with CT (Fig. 65-2). In a few instances, the appearance of a brain tumour on an MRI is so characteristic that a biopsy is unnecessary, especially when the tumour is located in a part of the brain that is difficult to biopsy (American Cancer Society, 2001).

In centres where positron emission tomography (PET) is available, it is used to supplement MRI. On PET scans, low-grade tumours are associated with hypometabolism and high-grade tumours show hypermetabolism. This information can be useful in treatment decisions (DeAngelis, 2001). Computer-assisted stereotactic (three-dimensional) biopsy is being used to diagnose deep-seated brain tumours and to provide a basis for treatment and prognosis. Cerebral angiography provides visualization of cerebral blood vessels and can localize most cerebral tumours.

An electroencephalogram (EEG) can detect an abnormal brain wave in regions occupied by a tumour and is used to evaluate temporal lobe seizures and assist in ruling out other disorders.

Cytologic studies of the CSF may be performed to detect malignant cells because CNS tumours can shed cells into the CSF.

Gerontologic Considerations

Intracranial tumours can produce personality changes, confusion, speech dysfunction, or disturbances of gait. In elderly patients early signs and symptoms of intracranial tumours can be easily overlooked and incorrectly attributed to cognitive and neurologic changes associated with normal aging. The most frequent tumour types in the elderly are anaplastic astrocytoma, glioblastoma multiforme, and cerebral metastases from other sites. The incidence of primary brain tumours and the likelihood of malignancy increase with age. Signs and symptoms in the elderly must be carefully evaluated because 10% of brain metastases occur in patients with a history of prior cancer (Rude, 2000).

Medical Management

A variety of medical treatment modalities, including chemotherapy and external-beam radiation therapy, are used alone or in combination with surgical resection. Radiation therapy, the cornerstone of treatment of many brain tumours, decreases the incidence of recurrence of incompletely resected tumours. Brachytherapy (the surgical implantation of radiation sources to deliver high doses at a short distance) has had promising results for primary malignancies. It is generally used as an adjunct to conventional radiation therapy or as a rescue measure for recurrent disease.

Intravenous (IV) autologous bone marrow transplantation is used in some patients who will receive chemotherapy or radiation therapy because it has the potential to "rescue" the patient from the bone marrow toxicity associated with high doses of chemotherapy and radiation. A fraction of the patient's bone marrow is aspirated, usually from the iliac crest, and stored. The patient receives large doses of chemotherapy or radiation therapy to destroy large numbers of malignant cells. The marrow is then reinfused intravenously after treatment is completed.

Corticosteroids may be used before and after treatment to reduce cerebral edema and promote a smoother, more rapid recovery. Gene-transfer therapy uses retroviral vectors to carry genes to the tumour, reprogramming the tumour tissue for susceptibility to treatment. This approach is being tested.

A new technique being investigated is photodynamic therapy. This is a treatment of primary malignant brain tumours that delivers a targeted therapy while conserving healthy brain tissue (Goodell & Muller, 2001).

SURGICAL MANAGEMENT

The objective of surgical management is to remove or destroy the entire tumour without increasing the neurologic deficit (paralysis, blindness) or to relieve symptoms by partial removal (decompression). A variety of treatment modalities may be used; the specific approach depends on the type of tumour, its location, and accessibility. In many patients, combinations of these modalities may be used. Most pituitary adenomas are treated by transsphenoidal microsurgical removal (see Chap. 61), whereas the remainder of tumours that cannot be removed completely are treated by radiation. An untreated brain tumour ultimately leads to death, either from increasing ICP or from the damage to brain tissue it causes.

Conventional surgical approaches require an incision into the skull (craniotomy). See Chapter 61 for a discussion of care of the patient following craniotomy. This approach is used in patients with meningiomas, acoustic neuromas, cystic astrocytomas of the cerebellum, colloid cysts of the third ventricle, congenital tumours such as dermoid cyst, and some of the granulomas. For patients with malignant glioma, complete removal of the tumour and cure are not possible, but the rationale for resection includes relieving ICP, removing any necrotic tissue, and reducing the bulk of the tumour, which theoretically leaves behind fewer cells to become resistant to radiation or chemotherapy.

Stereotactic approaches involve use of a three-dimensional frame that allows very precise localization of the tumour; a stereotactic frame and multiple imaging studies (x-rays, CT scans) are used to localize the tumour and verify its position (Fig. 65-3). New brain-mapping technology helps determine how close diseased areas of the brain are to structures essential for normal brain function. Lasers or radiation can be delivered with stereotactic approaches. Radioisotopes such as iodine 131 (^{131}I) can also be implanted directly into the tumour to deliver high doses of radiation to the tumour (brachytherapy) while minimizing effects on surrounding brain tissue.

The use of the gamma knife to perform radiosurgery allows deep, inaccessible tumours to be treated, often in a single session. Precise localization of the tumour is accomplished using the stereotactic approach and by minute measurements and precise positioning of the patient. Multiple narrow beams then deliver a very high dose of radiation. An advantage of this method is that no surgical incision is needed; a disadvantage is the lag time between treatment and the desired result (Rafferty-Mitchell, Scanlon & Laskowski-Jones, 1999).

Nursing Management

The patient with a brain tumour may be at an increased risk for aspiration due to cranial nerve dysfunction. Preoperatively, the gag reflex and ability to swallow are evaluated. In patients with diminished gag response, care includes teaching the patient to direct food and fluids toward the unaffected side, having the patient sit upright to eat, offering a semisoft diet, and having suction readily available. Function should be reassessed postoperatively because changes can occur.

FIGURE 65-3 (**A**) Using stereotactic or "brain-mapping" guided approach, a 3-D computer image fuses the CT and MRI to pinpoint the exact location of the brain tumour. This low-grade astrocytoma is localized adjacent to the brain stem, is nonoperable, and is treated with radiation. Note the optic chasm and optic nerves. (**B**) Computerized image of the prescribed radiation dose.

The effects of increased ICP caused by the tumour mass are reviewed in Chapter 61. The nurse performs neurologic checks, monitors vital signs, maintains a neurologic flow chart, spaces nursing interventions to prevent rapid increase in ICP, and re-orients the patient when necessary to person, time, and place. Patients with changes in cognition caused by the lesion require frequent reorientation and the use of orienting devices (personal possessions, photographs, lists, clock), supervision of and assistance with self-care, and ongoing monitoring and intervention for prevention of injury. Patients with seizures are carefully monitored and protected from injury.

Motor function is checked at intervals because specific motor deficits may occur, depending on the tumour's location. Sensory disturbances are assessed. Speech is evaluated. Eye movement and pupillary size and reaction may be affected by cranial nerve involvement. In one study that examined the experience of brain tumour patients 3 to 5 days postoperatively, the basic needs of patients were met, but changes suggested included minimizing the atmosphere of urgency and hurry, appointing a primary nurse for each patient, and giving more postoperative information (Lepola et al., 2001). The nursing process for patients undergoing neurosurgery is discussed in Chapter 61.

CEREBRAL METASTASES

A significant number of patients with cancer experience neurologic deficits caused by metastasis to the brain. Metastatic lesions to the brain constitute the most common neurologic complication, occurring in 20% to 30% of patients with cancer (Nevidjon & Sowers, 2000). Seventy percent of patients with cerebral metastases have one or two lesions, and 80% of these lesions are located in the cerebral hemispheres (British Columbia Cancer Agency, 2004). This becomes important clinically as more patients with all forms of cancer live longer as a result of improved therapies. Neurologic signs and symptoms include headache, gait disturbances, visual impairment, personality changes, altered mentation (memory loss and confusion), focal weakness, paralysis, aphasia, and seizures. These signs and symptoms can be devastating to both patient and family.

Medical Management

The treatment of metastatic brain cancer is palliative and involves eliminating or reducing serious symptoms. Even when palliation is the goal, distressing signs and symptoms can be relieved, thereby improving the quality of life for both the patient and family. Patients with intracerebral metastases who are not treated have a steady downhill course with a limited survival time, whereas those who are treated may survive for slightly longer periods. The median survival for patients with no treatment for brain metastases is 1 month; with corticosteroid treatment alone it is 2 months; radiation therapy extends the median survival to 3 to 6 months (Nevidjon & Sowers, 2000).

The therapeutic approach includes radiation therapy (the foundation of treatment), surgery (usually for a single intracranial metastasis), and chemotherapy; more often some combination of these treatments is the optimal method. Gamma knife radiosurgery is considered when three or fewer lesions are present.

PHARMACOLOGIC THERAPY

Corticosteroids are useful in relieving headache and alterations in level of consciousness. It is thought that corticosteroids (dexamethasone, prednisone) reduce inflammation around the metastatic deposits and decrease the edema surrounding them. Other medications used include osmotic agents (mannitol, glycerol) to decrease the fluid content of the brain, which leads to a decrease

in ICP. Antiseizure agents (eg, phenytoin) are used to prevent and treat seizures (Nevidjon & Sowers, 2000). Venous thromboembolic events, such as deep vein thrombosis (DVT) and pulmonary embolism (PE), occur in about 15% of patients and are associated with significant morbidity. Anticoagulants are generally not prescribed because of the risk for CNS hemorrhage; however, prophylactic therapy with low-molecular-weight heparin is under investigation.

Chemotherapy plays a small role in managing brain metastasis as a result of poor penetration across the blood–brain barrier. Poor drug penetration and sensitivity of brain cells are two factors that determine the responsiveness of metastatic brain tumours to chemotherapy. Research is being directed at multidrug regimens and drug resistance (American Cancer Society, 2001). Encouraging results have been seen with chemotherapeutic agents such as carmustine (BCNU), lomustine (CCNU), and PCV (a triple-drug combination of procarbazine hydrochloride, lomustine, and vincristine). Promising results have been seen with the use of topotecan (Hycamtin), another chemotherapy agent.

Pain is managed in a stepladder progression in the doses and type of analgesic agents needed for relief. If the patient has severe pain, morphine can be infused into the epidural or subarachnoid space through a spinal needle and a catheter as near as possible to the spinal segment where the pain is projected. Small doses of morphine are administered at prescribed intervals (see Chap. 13).

NURSING PROCESS: THE PATIENT WITH CEREBRAL METASTASES OR INCURABLE BRAIN TUMOUR

Assessment

The nursing assessment includes a baseline neurologic examination and focuses on how the patient is functioning, moving, and walking; adapting to weakness or paralysis and to visual and speech loss; and dealing with seizures. Assessment addresses symptoms that cause distress to the patient, including pain, respiratory problems, bowel and bladder disorders, sleep disturbances, and impairment of skin integrity, fluid balance, and temperature regulation. Tumour invasion, compression, or obstruction may cause these disorders.

Nutritional status is assessed because cachexia (weak and emaciated condition) is common in patients with metastases. The nurse explores changes associated with poor nutritional status (anorexia, pain, weight loss, altered metabolism, muscle weakness, malabsorption, and diarrhea) and asks the patient about altered taste sensations that may be secondary to dysphagia, weakness, and depression and about distortions and impaired sense of smell (anosmia).

The nurse takes a dietary history to assess food intake, intolerance, and preferences. Calculation of body mass index can confirm the loss of subcutaneous fat and lean body mass (see Chap. 5). Biochemical measurements (albumin, transferrin, total lymphocyte count, creatinine index, and urinary tests) are reviewed to assess the degree of malnutrition, impaired cellular immunity, and electrolyte balance. A dietitian assists in determining the caloric needs of the patient.

The nurse works with other members of the health care team to assess the impact of the illness on the family in terms of home care, altered relationships, financial problems, time pressures, and family problems. This information is important in helping family members cope with the diagnosis and changes associated with it.

Diagnosis

NURSING DIAGNOSES

Based on the assessment data, the patient's major nursing diagnoses may include the following:

- Self-care deficit (feeding, bathing, and toileting) related to loss or impairment of motor and sensory function and decreased cognitive abilities
- Imbalanced nutrition, less than body requirements, related to cachexia due to treatment and tumour effects, decreased nutritional intake, and malabsorption
- Anxiety related to fear of dying, uncertainty, change in appearance, altered lifestyle
- Interrupted family processes related to anticipatory grief and the burdens imposed by the care of the person with a terminal illness

Other nursing diagnoses of the patient with cerebral metastases may include acute pain related to tumour compression; impaired gas exchange related to dyspnea; constipation related to decreased fluid and dietary intake and medications; impaired urinary elimination related to reduced fluid intake, vomiting, and reactions to medications; sleep pattern disturbances related to discomfort and fear of dying; impairment of skin integrity related to cachexia, poor tissue perfusion, and decreased mobility; deficient fluid volume related to fever, vomiting, and low fluid intake; and ineffective thermoregulation related to hypothalamic involvement, fever, and chills. See Chapter 16 for assessment and nursing interventions for the patient with cancer.

Planning and Goals

The goals for the patient may include compensating for self-care deficits, improving nutrition, reducing anxiety, enhancing family coping skills, and absence of complications.

Nursing Interventions

COMPENSATING FOR SELF-CARE DEFICITS

The patient may have difficulty participating in goal setting as the tumour metastasizes and affects cognitive function. It is important to encourage the family to keep the patient as independent as possible for as long as possible. Increasing assistance with self-care activities is required. Because the patient with cerebral metastasis and the family live with uncertainty, they are encouraged to plan for each day and to make the most of each day. The tasks and challenges are to assist the patient to find useful coping mechanisms, adaptations, and compensations in solving problems that arise. This helps patients maintain some sense of control. An individualized exercise program helps maintain strength, endurance, and range of motion. Eventually, referral for home or hospice care may be necessary (see Chap. 17).

IMPROVING NUTRITION

Patients with nausea, vomiting, diarrhea, breathlessness, and pain are rarely interested in eating (Wilkes, 2000). These symptoms are managed or controlled through assessment, planning, and care. The nurse teaches the family how to position the patient for comfort during meals. Meals are planned for the times the patient is rested and in less distress from pain or the effects of treatment.

The patient needs to be clean, comfortable, and free of pain for meals, in an environment that is as attractive as possible. Oral hygiene before meals helps to improve intake. Offensive sights, sounds, and odours are eliminated. Creative strategies may be required to make food more palatable, provide enough fluids, and increase opportunities for socialization during meals. The family may be asked to keep a daily weight chart and to record the quantity of food eaten to determine the daily calorie count. Dietary supplements, if acceptable to the patient, can be provided to meet increased caloric needs. If the patient is not interested in most usual foods, those foods preferred by the patient should be offered. When the patient shows marked deterioration as a result of tumour growth and effects, some other form of nutritional support (eg, tube feeding, parenteral nutrition) may be indicated if consistent with the patient's end-of-life preferences. Nursing interventions include assessing the patency of the central and IV line or feeding tube, monitoring the insertion site for infection, checking the infusion rate, monitoring intake and output, and changing the IV tubing and dressing. Family members are instructed in these techniques if they will be providing care at home. Parenteral nutrition can also be provided at home if indicated.

The patient's quality of life may guide the selection, initiation, and maintenance of nutritional support. The nurse and family should not place too much emphasis on eating or on discussions about food as the patient may not desire aggressive nutritional intervention. The subsequent course of action must be congruent with the wishes and choices of the patient and family.

RELIEVING ANXIETY

Patients with cerebral metastases may be restless, with changing moods that may include intense depression, euphoria, paranoia, and severe anxiety. The response of patients to terminal illness reflects their pattern of reaction to other crisis situations. Serious illness imposes additional strains that often bring other unresolved problems to light. The patient's own coping strategies can help deal with anxious and depressed feelings. Caregivers need to be sensitive to the patient's concerns and fears.

Patients need the opportunity to exercise some control over their situation. A sense of mastery can be gained as they learn to understand the disease and its treatment and how to deal with their feelings. The presence of family, friends, a spiritual advisor, and health professionals may be supportive. Support groups such as the Brain Tumour Support Group may provide a feeling of support and strength.

Spending time with patients allows them time to talk and to communicate their fears and concerns. Open communication and acknowledging fears are often therapeutic. Touch is also a form of communication. These patients need reassurance that continuing care will be provided and that they will not be abandoned. The situation becomes more endurable when others share in the experience of dying. If a patient's emotional reactions are very intense or prolonged, additional help from a spiritual advisor, social worker, or mental health professional may be indicated.

ENHANCING FAMILY PROCESSES

The family needs to be reassured that their loved one is receiving optimal care and that attention will be paid to the patient's changing symptoms and to their concerns. When the patient can no longer carry out self-care, the family, additional support systems (social worker, home health aid, home care nurse, hospice nurse) may be needed. A nursing goal is to keep anxiety at a manageable level.

Chart 65-2
Home Care Checklist • The Patient With Cerebral Metastases

At the completion of the home care instruction, the patient or caregiver will be able to:	Patient	Caregiver
• State effects of the tumour according to its location in the brain and type.	✓	✓
• Describe side effects of treatment.	✓	✓
• Identify community resources, including:		
• Home health services	✓	✓
• Hospices	✓	✓
• Support groups	✓	✓
• Identify coping strategies, such as:		
• Taking control, setting daily goals, and staying positive	✓	✓
• Rehabilitation to improve self-care	✓	
• Relaxation techniques	✓	✓
• Family support		✓
• Verbalize an understanding of the treatment plan for:		
• Medications and pain control	✓	✓
• Nutritional needs	✓	✓
• Contacting the health care provider	✓	✓

PROMOTING HOME AND COMMUNITY-BASED CARE

Teaching Patients Self-Care

The patient and family often have major responsibility for care at home. Therefore, teaching includes strategies of pain management, prevention of complications related to treatment strategies, and methods to ensure adequate fluid and food intake (Chart 65-2). Teaching needs of the patient and family regarding care priorities are likely to change as the disease progresses. It is important to assess the changing needs of the patient and the family and to inform them about resources and services early to assist them to deal with changes in the patient's condition.

Continuing Care

Home care nursing and hospice services are valuable resources that should be made available to the patient and the family early in the course of a terminal illness. Anticipating needs before they occur can assist in smooth initiation of services. Home care needs and interventions focus on four major areas: palliation of symptoms and pain control, assistance in self-care, control of treatment complications, and administration of specific forms of treatment, such as parenteral nutrition. The home care nurse assesses pain management, respiratory status, complications of the disorder and its treatment, and the patient's cognitive and emotional status. Additionally, the nurse assesses the family's ability to perform necessary care and notifies the physician about changing needs or complications if indicated.

The patient and family who elect to care for the patient at home as the disease progresses benefit from the care and support provided through hospice services. Steps to initiate hospice care, including discussion of hospice care as an option, should not be postponed until death is imminent. Exploration of hospice care as an option should be initiated at a time when hospice care can provide support and care to the patient and family consistent with their end-of-life decisions and assist in allowing death with dignity. End-of-life care is further described in Chapter 13.

Evaluation

EXPECTED PATIENT OUTCOMES

Expected patient outcomes may include:

1. Engages in self-care activities as long as possible
   a. Uses assistive devices or accepts assistance as needed
   b. Schedules periodic rest periods to permit maximal participation in self-care
2. Maintains as optimal a nutritional status as possible
   a. Eats and accepts food within limits of condition and preferences
   b. Accepts alternative methods of providing nutrition if indicated
3. Reports being less anxious
   a. Is less restless and is sleeping better
   b. Verbalizes concerns and fears about death
   c. Participates in activities of personal importance as long as feasible
4. Family members seek help as needed
   a. Demonstrate ability to bathe, feed, and care for the patient and participate in pain management and prevention of complications
   b. Express feelings and concerns to appropriate health professionals
   c. Discuss and seek hospice care as an option

SPINAL CORD TUMOURS

Tumours within the spine are classified according to their anatomic relation to the spinal cord. They include intramedullary lesions (within the spinal cord), extramedullary-intradural lesions (within or under the spinal dura), and extramedullary-extradural lesions (outside the dural membrane). Tumours occurring within the spinal cord or exerting pressure on it cause symptoms ranging from localized or shooting pains and weakness and loss of reflexes above the tumour level to progressive loss of motor function and paralysis. Usually, sharp pain occurs in the area innervated by the spinal roots that arise from the cord in the region of the tumour. In addition, increasing sensory deficits develop below the level of the lesion.

Assessment and Diagnostic Findings

Neurologic examination and diagnostic studies are used to make the diagnosis. Neurologic examination includes assessment of pain, loss of reflexes, loss of sensation or motor function, and the presence of weakness and paralysis. Helpful diagnostic studies include x-rays, radionuclide bone scans, and MRI. MRI is the most sensitive diagnostic tool and is particularly helpful in detecting epidural spinal cord compression and vertebral bone metastases (Jacobs & Perrin, 2001; Nevidjon & Sowers, 2000).

Medical Management

Treatment of specific intraspinal tumours depends on the type and location of the tumour and the presenting symptoms and physical status of the patient. Surgical intervention is the primary treatment for most spinal cord tumours. Other treatment modalities include partial removal of the tumour, decompression of the spinal cord, chemotherapy, and radiation therapy, particularly for intramedullary tumours and metastatic lesions (Jacobs & Perrin, 2001).

Epidural spinal cord compression occurs in approximately 5% of patients who die of cancer and is considered a neurologic emergency (Nevidjon & Sowers, 2000). In the patient with epidural spinal cord compression resulting from metastatic cancer (most commonly from breast, prostate, or lung), high-dose dexamethasone combined with radiation therapy is effective in relieving pain (Nevidjon & Sowers, 2000).

SURGICAL MANAGEMENT

Tumour removal is desirable but not always possible. The goal is to remove as much tumour as possible while sparing uninvolved portions of the spinal cord. Microsurgical techniques have improved the prognosis for patients with intramedullary tumours. Prognosis is related to the degree of neurologic impairment at the time of surgery, the speed with which symptoms occurred, and the tumour origin. Patients with extensive neurologic deficits before surgery usually do not make significant functional recovery even after successful tumour removal.

Nursing Management

PROVIDING PREOPERATIVE CARE

The objectives of preoperative care include recognition of neurologic changes through ongoing assessments, pain control, and management of altered activities of daily living due to sensory and motor deficits and bowel and bladder dysfunction. The nurse assesses for weakness, muscle wasting, spasticity, sensory changes, bowel and bladder dysfunction, and potential respiratory problems, especially if a cervical tumour is present. The patient is also evaluated for coagulation deficiencies. A history of aspirin intake is obtained and reported because the use of aspirin may impede hemostasis postoperatively. Breathing exercises are taught and demonstrated preoperatively. Postoperative pain management strategies are discussed with the patient before surgery.

ASSESSING THE PATIENT AFTER SURGERY

The patient is monitored for deterioration in neurologic status. A sudden onset of neurologic deficit is an ominous sign and may

be due to vertebral collapse associated with spinal cord infarction. Frequent neurologic checks are carried out, with emphasis on movement, strength, and sensation of the upper and lower extremities. Assessment of sensory function involves pinching the skin of the arms, legs, and trunk to determine if there is loss of feeling and, if so, determining at what level. Vital signs are monitored at regular intervals.

MANAGING PAIN

The prescribed pain medication should be administered in adequate amounts and at appropriate intervals to relieve pain and prevent its recurrence. Pain is the hallmark of spinal metastasis. Patients with sensory root involvement or vertebral collapse may suffer excruciating pain, which requires effective pain management.

The bed is usually kept flat initially. The nurse turns the patient as a unit, keeping shoulders and hips aligned and the back straight. The side-lying position is usually the most comfortable because this position imposes the least pressure on the surgical site. Placement of a pillow between the knees of the patient in a side-lying position helps to prevent extreme knee flexion.

MONITORING AND MANAGING POTENTIAL COMPLICATIONS

If the tumour was in the cervical area, the possibility of postoperative respiratory compromise arises. The nurse monitors the patient for asymmetric chest movement, abdominal breathing, and abnormal breath sounds. For a high cervical lesion, the endotracheal tube remains in place until adequate respiratory function is ensured. The patient is encouraged to perform deep-breathing and coughing exercises.

The area over the bladder is palpated or a bladder scan is performed to assess for urinary retention. The nurse also monitors for incontinence because urinary dysfunction usually implies significant decompensation of spinal cord function. An intake and output record is maintained. Additionally, the abdomen is auscultated for bowel sounds.

Staining of the dressing may indicate leakage of CSF from the surgical site, which may lead to serious infection or to an inflammatory reaction in the surrounding tissues that can cause severe pain in the postoperative period.

PROMOTING HOME AND COMMUNITY-BASED CARE

Teaching Patients Self-Care. In preparation for discharge, patients are assessed for their ability to function independently in the home and for the availability of resources such as family members to assist in caregiving. Patients with residual sensory involvement are cautioned about the dangers of extremes in temperature. They should be alert to the dangers of heating devices (eg, hot water bottles, heating pads, and space heaters). The patient is taught to check skin integrity daily. Patients with impaired motor function related to motor weakness or paralysis may require training in activities of daily living and safe use of assistive devices, such as a cane, walker, or wheelchair.

The patient and family member are instructed about pain management strategies, bowel and bladder management, and assessment for signs and symptoms that should be reported promptly.

Continuing Care. Referral for inpatient or outpatient rehabilitation may be warranted to improve self-care abilities. A home care referral may be indicated and provides the home care nurse with the opportunity to assess the patient's physical and psychological status and the patient's and family's ability to adhere to recommended management strategies. During the home visit, the nurse determines whether changes in neurologic function have occurred. The patient's respiratory and nutritional status is assessed. The adequacy of pain management is assessed, and modifications are made to ensure adequate pain relief. The need for hospice services or placement in an extended-care facility is discussed with the patient and family if warranted, and the patient is asked about preferences for end-of-life care (Chart 65-3). Additionally, social workers may be consulted to assist the patient and family members in identifying support groups and agencies that can provide help in coping with the disease process.

Degenerative Disorders

Neurologic disorders of the central and peripheral nervous system that are degenerative in nature include Parkinson's disease, Huntington's disease, Alzheimer's disease, amyotrophic lateral sclerosis, muscular dystrophies, and degenerative disc disease. A relatively new phenomenon, post-polio syndrome, may be degenerative in nature and is also discussed. A slow onset of signs and symptoms characterizes these disorders. Patients are managed at home for as long as possible and admitted to the acute care setting for exacerbations, treatments, and surgical interventions as needed.

PARKINSON'S DISEASE

Parkinson's disease is a slowly progressing neurologic movement disorder that eventually leads to disability. The degenerative or idiopathic form is the most common; there is also a secondary form with a known or suspected cause. Although the cause of most cases is unknown, research suggests several causative factors, including genetics, atherosclerosis, excessive accumulation of oxygen free radicals, viral infections, head trauma, chronic antipsychotic medication use, and some environmental exposures. Parkinsonian symptoms usually first appear in the fifth decade of life; however, cases have been diagnosed at the age of 30 years. It is the fourth most common **neurodegenerative** disease. Parkinson's disease affects men more frequently than women and nearly 1% of the population older than 60 years of age (Gray & Hildebrand, 2000).

Chart 65-3 • Ethics and Related Issues

What Constitutes Assisted Suicide?

Situation
A 76-year-old man is admitted to the hospital with a metastatic spinal cord tumour. He is in respiratory distress and near death. The patient and family state they want no heroic measures and the physician writes a "do not resuscitate" order on the chart.

Dilemma
What is the nurse's role in caring for this patient at this time?

Discussion
Is the "do not resuscitate" order an act of patient-assisted suicide? Is it active or passive euthanasia? What is the nurse's role in caring for the patient if this action conflicts with his/her personal beliefs? If no other nurse is available to provide care, does the nurse have the right to refuse? Is this patient abandonment?

Pathophysiology

Parkinson's disease is associated with decreased levels of **dopamine** due to destruction of pigmented neuronal cells in the **substantia nigra** in the basal ganglia of the brain (Fig. 65-4). The nuclei of the substantia nigra project fibres or neuronal pathways to the

Physiology/Pathophysiology

Corpus striatum

Substantia nigra

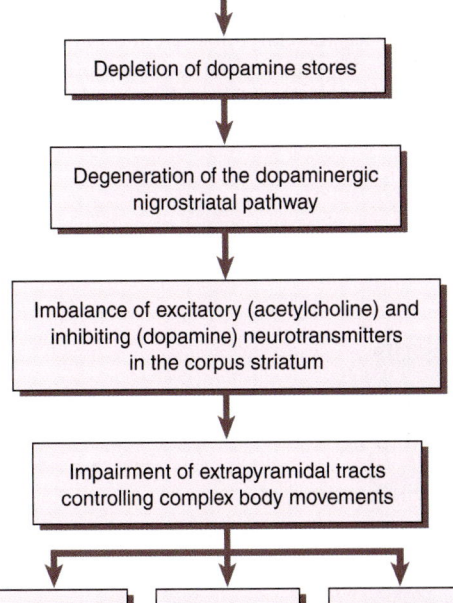

Destruction of dopaminergic neuronal cells in the substantia nigra in the basal ganglia

↓

Depletion of dopamine stores

↓

Degeneration of the dopaminergic nigrostriatal pathway

↓

Imbalance of excitatory (acetylcholine) and inhibiting (dopamine) neurotransmitters in the corpus striatum

↓

Impairment of extrapyramidal tracts controlling complex body movements

↓

Tremors   Rigidity   Bradykinesia

FIGURE 65-4 Pathophysiology of Parkinson's disease. The nuclei in the substantia nigra project fibres to the corpus striatum. The nerve fibres carry dopamine to the corpus striatum. The loss of dopamine nerve cells from the brain's substantia nigra is thought to be responsible for the symptoms of parkinsonism.

corpus striatum, where neurotransmitters are key to control of complex body movements. Through the neurotransmitters acetylcholine (excitatory) and dopamine (inhibitory), striatal neurons relay messages to the higher motor centres that control and refine motor movements. The loss of dopamine stores in this area of the brain results in more excitatory neurotransmitters than inhibitory neurotransmitters, leading to an imbalance that affects voluntary movement.

Basic science research in the past two decades has revealed that more neurotransmitter pathways in the brain than just the dopaminergic system are involved. Parts of the glutamatergic, cholinergic, tryptaminergic, noradrenergic, adrenergic, serotonergic, and peptidergic pathways (responsible for cell metabolism, growth, nutrition, and so forth) show damage in Parkinson's disease (Chase, Oh & Konitsiotis, 2000; Przuntek, 2000; Rascol, 2000).

Clinical symptoms do not appear until 60% of the pigmented neurons are lost and the striatal dopamine level is decreased by 80%. Cellular degeneration impairs the extrapyramidal tracts that control semiautomatic functions and coordinated movements; motor cells of the motor cortex and the pyramidal tracts are not affected.

Clinical Manifestations

Parkinson's disease has a gradual onset and symptoms progress slowly over a chronic, prolonged course. The three cardinal signs are tremor, rigidity, and **bradykinesia** (abnormally slow movements). Other features include hypokinesia, gait disturbances, and postural instability (Gray & Hildebrand, 2000).

TREMOR

Although symptoms are variable, a slow, unilateral, resting tremor is present in 70% of patients at the time of diagnosis. Resting tremor characteristically disappears with purposeful movement but is evident when the extremities are motionless. The tremor may present as a rhythmic, slow turning motion (pronation–supination) of the forearm and the hand and a motion of the thumb against the fingers as if rolling a pill (Fig. 65-5). Tremor is present while the patient is at rest; it increases when the patient is walking, concentrating, or feeling anxious.

RIGIDITY

Resistance to passive limb movement characterizes muscle rigidity. Passive movement of an extremity may cause the limb to move in jerky increments referred to as cogwheeling. Rigidity of the passive extremity increases when another extremity is engaged in voluntary active movement. Stiffness of the neck, trunk, and shoulders is common. Early in the disease, the patient may complain of shoulder pain.

BRADYKINESIA

One of the most common features of Parkinson's disease is bradykinesia. Patients take longer to complete most activities and have difficulty initiating movement, such as rising from a sitting position or turning in bed.

Hypokinesia (abnormally diminished movement) is also common and may appear after the tremor. The freezing phenomenon is a transient inability to perform active movement and is thought to be an extreme form of bradykinesia. Additionally, the patient tends to shuffle and exhibits a decreased arm swing. As dexterity declines, **micrographia** (shrinking, slow handwriting) develops. The face becomes increasingly masklike and expressionless and the frequency of blinking decreases. **Dysphonia** (soft, slurred, low-pitched, and less audible speech) may occur due to weakness and incoordination of the muscles responsible for speech. In many cases, the patient develops dysphagia, begins to drool, and is at risk for choking and aspiration.

The patient commonly develops postural and gait problems. There is a loss of postural reflexes, and the patient stands with the head bent forward and walks with a propulsive gait. The posture is caused by the forward flexion of the neck, hips, knees, and elbows. The patient may walk faster and faster, trying to move the feet forward under the body's centre of gravity (shuffling gait). Difficulty in pivoting and loss of balance (either forward or backward) places the patient at risk for falls.

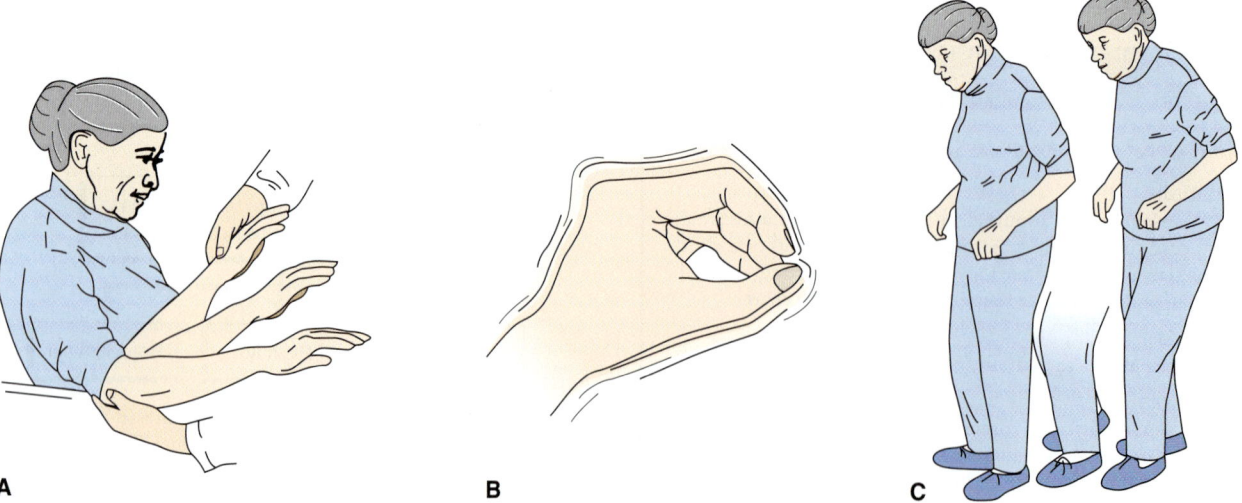

A **B** **C**

FIGURE 65-5 Manifestations of Parkinson's disease: (**A**) "cogwheeling" accompanies passive movement of the hand and arm; (**B**) "pill-rolling" tremor; (**C**) postural instability, forward stoop, shuffling gait.

NURSING RESEARCH PROFILE 65-1
Falls and Risk Factors

Gray, P., & Hildebrand, K. (2000). Fall risk factors in Parkinson's disease. *Journal of Neuroscience Nursing, 32*(4), 222–228.

Purpose
Patients with Parkinson's disease have frequent falls, yet there is little research on identifying risk factors specific to these patients. The purpose of this study was to identify risk factors associated with falls in a group of patients with Parkinson's disease.

Study Sample and Design
The sample for this descriptive, exploratory study was recruited from a hospital-based clinic in Canada. Patients who could stand, walk, and had no other medical conditions that predisposed them to falls were included. The Unified Parkinson's Disease Rating Scale established the degree of symptoms. Multiple instruments were used to assess demographic, environmental, and medical information; participants also completed fall diaries for 12 weeks. The sample consisted of 118 patients; 48 (41%) reported no falls and 70 (59%) reported one or more falls. Participants in the study included 73 (62%) males.

Findings
Demographic, environmental, and medical information and fall diaries were analyzed to identify factors that appeared to increase the risk for falls. A total of 237 falls were reported in the 3-month study period; 59% of the participants reported one or more falls. Males, as well as patients over age 80 years, reported higher rates of falls. Factors associated with a high risk for falls included duration and severity of parkinsonian symptoms including freezing, involuntary movements, and walking and postural difficulties. Postural hypotension and daily intake of alcohol were additional factors associated with a high risk for falls.

Nursing Implications
Nurses, especially home care nurses, can use the findings of this study to help identify patients with risk factors: "freezing," involuntary movements, walking and postural difficulties, postural hypotension, and daily use of alcohol. Patients with these risk factors should be targeted for intervention programs and specific patient and family education to reduce falls. Early identification of risk factors would permit nurses to provide assistance, education, support, and appropriate referrals to patients at high risk for falls.

OTHER MANIFESTATIONS
The effect of Parkinson's disease on the basal ganglia often produces autonomic symptoms that include excessive and uncontrolled sweating, paroxysmal flushing, orthostatic hypotension, gastric and urinary retention, constipation, and sexual disturbances (Herndon et al., 2000).

Psychiatric changes are often interrelated and may be predictive of one another. They include depression, **dementia** (progressive mental deterioration), sleep disturbances, and hallucinations (Herndon et al., 2000). Depression is common; whether it is a reaction to the disorder or is related to a biochemical abnormality remains a question. Mental changes may appear in the form of cognitive, perceptual, and memory deficits, although intellect is not usually affected. A number of psychiatric manifestations (personality changes, psychosis, dementia, and acute confusion) are common among the elderly. The prevalence of dementia is about 25% and the pattern is similar to that of patients with Alzheimer's disease. Although there is no direct documented causal relationship, the rates of depression and dementia are highly correlated in these patients (Herndon et al., 2000).

Approximately 41% of women and 25% of men with Parkinson's disease experience sleep disturbances. This may be connected to depression, dementia, or medications. Auditory and visual hallucinations have been reported in approximately 37% of persons with Parkinson's and may be associated with depression, dementia, lack of sleep, or adverse effects of medications (Herndon et al., 2000).

Complications associated with Parkinson's disease are common and are typically related to disorders of movement. As the disease progresses, patients are at risk for respiratory and urinary tract infection, skin breakdown, and injury from falls. The adverse effects of medications used to treat the symptoms are associated with numerous complications.

Assessment and Diagnostic Findings

Laboratory tests and imaging studies are not helpful in the diagnosis of Parkinson's disease, although PET scanning has been used in evaluating levodopa (precursor of dopamine) uptake and conversion to dopamine in the corpus striatum (Freed et al., 2001). Currently, the disease is diagnosed clinically from the patient's history and the presence of two of the three cardinal manifestations: tremor, muscle rigidity, and bradykinesia.

Early diagnosis can be difficult because the patient can rarely pinpoint when symptoms started. Often a family member notices a change such as stooped posture, a stiff arm, a slight limp, tremor, or slow, small handwriting. The medical history, presenting symptoms, neurologic examination, and response to pharmacologic management are carefully evaluated when making the diagnosis.

Medical Management

Treatment is directed at controlling symptoms and maintaining functional independence because there are no medical or surgical approaches that prevent disease progression. Care is individualized for each patient based on presenting symptoms and social, occupational, and emotional needs. Pharmacologic management is the mainstay of treatment, although advances in research have led to increased interest in surgical interventions. Patients are usually cared for at home and admitted to the hospital only for complications or to initiate new treatments.

PHARMACOLOGIC THERAPY
Antiparkinsonian medications act by 1) increasing striatal dopaminergic activity, 2) reducing the excessive influence of excitatory cholinergic neurons on the extrapyramidal tract, thereby restoring a balance between dopaminergic and cholinergic activities, or 3) acting on neurotransmitter pathways other than the dopaminergic pathway.

Antiparkinsonian Medications. Levodopa (Dopar, Larodopa) is the most effective agent and the mainstay of treatment (Karch, 2002; Obeso et al., 2001). Because levodopa is thought to precipitate oxidation, which further damages the substantia nigra and eventually speeds disease progression, physicians delay prescribing the medication or increasing the dosage for as long as possible (Karch, 2002). Levodopa is converted to dopamine in the basal ganglia, producing symptom relief. The beneficial effects of levodopa are most pronounced in the first few years of treatment. Benefits begin to wane and adverse effects become more severe over time. Confusion, hallucinations, depression, and sleep alterations are associated with prolonged use. Levodopa is usually given in combination with carbidopa (Sinemet), an amino acid decarboxylase inhibitor that helps to maximize the beneficial effects of levodopa by preventing its breakdown outside the brain and reducing its adverse effects (Karch, 2002).

Within 5 to 10 years, most patients develop a response to the medication characterized by **dyskinesia** (abnormal involuntary movements), including facial grimacing, rhythmic jerking movements of the hands, head bobbing, chewing and smacking movements, and involuntary movements of the trunk and extremities. The patient may experience an on–off syndrome in which sudden periods of near immobility ("off effect") are followed by a sudden return of effectiveness ("on effect"). Various adjunctive therapies are used to minimize dyskinesias (Przuntek, 2000; Rascol, 2000).

Budipine, available in Europe but not the United States, is a non-dopaminergic, antiparkinsonian medication that significantly reduces akinesia, rigidity, and tremor. It is non-dopaminergic because the action appears to be on neurotransmitter pathways other than the dopaminergic pathway. It may be used as monotherapy or in conjunction with other available antiparkinsonian medications (Przuntek, 2000; Przuntek et al., 2002). The usual dose of 40 to 60 mg is reached gradually. Nausea and dry mouth are the most common side effects, although 75% of patients experienced no side effects in clinical drug trials (Przuntek, 2000).

Anticholinergic Therapy. Anticholinergic agents (trihexyphenidyl, cycrimine, procyclidine, biperiden, and benztropine mesylate) are effective in controlling tremor and rigidity. They may be used in combination with levodopa. They counteract the action of the neurotransmitter acetylcholine. Because the side effects include blurred vision, flushing, rash, constipation, urinary retention, and acute confusional states, these medications are often poorly tolerated in elderly patients. Intraocular pressure must be closely monitored: these medications are contraindicated in patients with narrow-angle glaucoma. Patients with prostate hyperplasia are monitored for signs of urinary retention.

Antiviral Therapy. Amantadine hydrochloride (Symmetrel) is an antiviral agent used in early Parkinson's treatment to reduce rigidity, tremor, and bradykinesia. It is thought to act by releasing dopamine from neuronal storage sites. Studies suggest it may also have antiglutamatergic properties that affect the glutamatergic pathway, thus improving levodopa-induced dyskinesias (Rascol, 2000). Amantadine has a low incidence of side effects, which include psychiatric disturbances (mood changes, confusion, depression, hallucinations), lower extremity edema, nausea, epigastric distress, urinary retention, headache, and visual impairment.

Dopamine Agonists. Bromocriptine mesylate and pergolide (ergot derivatives) are dopamine receptor agonists and are useful in postponing the initiation of carbidopa or levodopa therapy. Dopamine agonists are often added to the medication regimen when carbidopa or levodopa loses effectiveness. Pergolide (Permax) is 10 times more potent than bromocriptine mesylate (Parlodel), although this provides no therapeutic advantage. Adverse reactions to these medications include nausea, vomiting, diarrhea, lightheadedness, hypotension, impotence, and psychiatric effects.

Two new dopamine agonists, ropinirole hydrochloride (Requip) and pramipexole (Mirapex) (nonergot derivatives), are primarily for patients in the early stages of Parkinson's disease and are not expected to have the potentially serious adverse effects of pergolide and bromocriptine mesylate. Pramipexole (Mirapex) can

be used without levodopa for treatment of early disease and with levodopa in advanced stages. Cabergoline (Dostinex), an ergot alkaloid with a long duration of action, has been approved for use.

Monoamine Oxidase Inhibitors (MAO Inhibitors). Of the MAO inhibitors, selegiline (Eldepryl) is one of the most exciting and controversial developments in the pharmacotherapy of Parkinson's disease (Herndon et al., 2000). This medication inhibits dopamine breakdown and is thought to slow the progression of the disease. Researchers believe this medication may have a neuroprotective effect in the early stages of Parkinson's disease, but this has not been shown in clinical trials. Selegiline is currently used in combination with a dopamine agonist to delay the use of carbidopa or levodopa therapy. Adverse effects are similar to those of levodopa.

Catechol-O-methyltransferase (COMT) Inhibitors. Clinical trials suggest that the COMT inhibitors entacapone (Comtess) and tolcapone (Tasmar) have little effect on parkinsonian symptoms when given alone but can increase the duration of action of carbidopa or levodopa when given in combination with them. COMT inhibitors block an enzyme that metabolizes levodopa, making more levodopa available for conversion to dopamine in the brain. Entacapone and tolcapone reduce motor fluctuations in patients with advanced Parkinson's disease.

Antidepressants. Tricyclic antidepressants may be prescribed to alleviate the depression that is so common in Parkinson's disease. The usual dosage is one-third to one-half the dosage used in depressed patients without Parkinson's disease. Amitriptyline is typically prescribed because of its anticholinergic and antidepressant effect. Serotonin reuptake inhibitors, such as fluoxetine hydrochloride (Prozac) and bupropion hydrochloride (Wellbutrin), are effective for treating depression but may aggravate parkinsonism.

Antihistamines. Diphenhydramine hydrochloride (Benadryl), orphenadrine citrate (Banflex), and phenindamine hydrochloride (Neo-Synephrine) have mild central anticholinergic and sedative effects and may reduce tremors.

SURGICAL MANAGEMENT

The limitations of levodopa therapy, improvements in stereotactic surgery, and new approaches in transplantation have renewed interest in the surgical treatment of Parkinson's disease. In patients with disabling tremor, rigidity, or severe levodopa-induced dyskinesia, surgery may be considered. Although surgery provides some relief in selected patients, it has not been shown to alter the course of the disease or produce permanent improvement.

Stereotactic Procedures. Thalamotomy and pallidotomy are effective in relieving many of the symptoms of Parkinson's disease. Patients eligible for these procedures are those who have had an inadequate response to medical therapy; they must meet strict criteria to be eligible. Candidates eligible for these procedures are patients with idiopathic Parkinson's disease who are taking maximum doses of antiparkinsonian medications. Patients with dementia and atypical Parkinson's disease are usually not considered for stereotactic procedures. Parkinson's disease rating scales and specific neurologic testing are used to identify eligible patients.

The intent of thalamotomy and pallidotomy is to interrupt the nerve pathways and thereby alleviate tremor or rigidity. During thalamotomy, a stereotactic electrical stimulator destroys part of the ventrolateral portion of the thalamus in an attempt to reduce tremor; the most common complications are ataxia and hemiparesis. Pallidotomy involves destroying part of the ventral aspect of the medial globus pallidus through electrical stimulation in patients with advanced disease. The procedure is effective in reducing rigidity, bradykinesia, and dyskinesia, thus improving motor function and activities of daily living in the immediate postoperative course. In small studies, clinical improvements have been demonstrated over 3 to 4 years. The clinical benefit is greater in patients younger than 60 years (Freed et al., 2001). Complications include hemiparesis, stroke, and visual changes.

CT, x-rays, MRI, or angiography is used to localize the appropriate surgical site in the brain. Then the patient's head is positioned in a stereotactic frame (Fig. 65-6). The surgeon makes an incision in the skin and then a burr hole. Next, the surgeon passes an electrode through the burr hole to the target area in the thalamus or globus pallidum. The desired response of the patient to the electrical stimulation is the basis for the final site chosen by the neurosurgeon. Stereotactic procedures are completed on one side of the brain at a time. If rigidity or tremor is bilateral, a 6-month interval is suggested between procedures.

Neural Transplantation. Surgical implantation of adrenal medullary tissue into the corpus striatum is performed in an effort to reestablish normal dopamine release. Preliminary evidence has shown high morbidity and mortality rates, and the implants appear to improve parkinsonian symptoms for only 6 months. Researchers are conducting studies to determine if transplanting human fetal brain cells or genetically engineered cells into the nigrostriatal region is effective (Aminoff, 2000). Legal and ethical issues surrounding the use of fetal brain cells have limited the implementation of this procedure. Recently, fetal pig neuronal cells survived transplantation into a patient with Parkinson's disease; this may provide an alternative to human cell transplants (Aminoff, 2000).

Deep Brain Stimulation. Recently approved by the FDA, pacemaker-like brain implants show promising results in relieving tremors. The stimulation can be bilateral or unilateral, although bilateral stimulation of the subthalamic nucleus is thought to be of greater benefit to patients than results achieved with thalamotomy, pallidotomy, or fetal nigral transplantation (Obeso et al., 2001). In deep brain stimulation, an electrode is placed in the thalamus and connected to a pulse generator implanted in a subcutaneous subclavicular or abdominal pouch. The battery-powered pulse generator sends high-frequency electrical impulses through a wire placed under the skin to a lead anchored to the skull (Fig. 65-7). The electrode blocks nerve pathways in the brain that cause tremors. These devices are not without complications, both from the surgical procedure needed for implantation and from complications (such as lead leakage) of the device itself (Koller et al., 2001; Obeso et al., 2001).

NURSING PROCESS:
THE PATIENT WITH PARKINSON'S DISEASE
Assessment

Assessment focuses on how the disease has affected the patient's activities of daily living and functional abilities. Patients are observed for degree of disability and the functional changes that occur throughout the day, such as responses to medication. Nearly every patient with a movement disorder has some functional alteration and may have some type of behavioural dysfunction. The following questions may be useful to assess alterations:

- Do you have leg or arm stiffness?
- Have you experienced any irregular jerking of your arms or legs?
- Have you ever been "frozen" or rooted to the spot and unable to move?
- Does your mouth water excessively? Have you (or others) noticed yourself grimacing or making faces or chewing movements?
- What specific activities do you have difficulty doing?

During this assessment, the nurse observes the patient for quality of speech, loss of facial expression, swallowing deficits

FIGURE 65-7 Deep brain stimulation is provided by a pulse generator surgically implanted in a pouch beneath the clavicle. The generator sends high-frequency electrical impulses to the thalamus, thereby blocking the nerve pathways associated with tremors in Parkinson's disease.

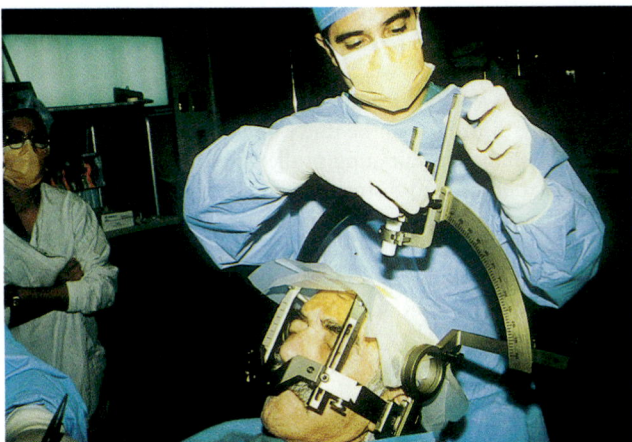

FIGURE 65-6 A stereotactic frame is applied to a patient's head in preparation for pallidotomy. The frame immobilizes the head.

(drooling, poor head control, coughing), tremors, slowness of movement, weakness, forward posture, rigidity, evidence of mental slowness, and confusion. Parkinsonian symptoms, as well as side effects of medications, put these patients at high risk of falls; therefore, a fall risk assessment should be included (Gray & Hildebrand, 2000).

Diagnosis

NURSING DIAGNOSES

Based on the assessment data, the patient's major nursing diagnoses may include the following:

- Impaired physical mobility related to muscle rigidity and motor weakness
- Self-care deficits (feeding, dressing, hygiene, and toileting) related to tremor and motor disturbance
- Constipation related to medication and reduced activity
- Imbalanced nutrition, less than body requirements, related to tremor, slowness in eating, difficulty in chewing and swallowing
- Impaired verbal communication related to decreased speech volume, slowness of speech, inability to move facial muscles
- Ineffective coping related to depression and dysfunction due to disease progression

Other nursing diagnoses may include sleep pattern disturbances, deficient knowledge, risk for injury, risk for activity intolerance, disturbed thought processes, and compromised family coping.

Planning and Goals

The goals for the patient may include improving functional mobility, maintaining independence in activities of daily living, achieving adequate bowel elimination, attaining and maintaining acceptable nutritional status, achieving effective communication, and developing positive coping mechanisms.

Nursing Interventions

IMPROVING MOBILITY

A progressive program of daily exercise will increase muscle strength, improve coordination and dexterity, reduce muscular rigidity, and prevent contractures that occur when muscles are not used. Walking, riding a stationary bicycle, swimming, and gardening are all exercises that help maintain joint mobility. Stretching (stretch–hold–relax) and range-of-motion exercises promote joint flexibility. Postural exercises are important to counter the tendency of the head and neck to be drawn forward and down. A physical therapist may be helpful in developing an individualized exercise program and can provide instruction to the patient and caregiver on exercising safely. Faithful adherence to an exercise and walking program helps to delay the progress of the disease. Warm baths and massage in addition to passive and active exercises help relax muscles and relieve painful muscle spasms that accompany rigidity.

Balance may be adversely affected because of the rigidity of the arms (arm swinging is necessary in normal walking). Special walking techniques must be learned to offset the shuffling gait and the tendency to lean forward. The patient is taught to concentrate on walking erect, to watch the horizon, and to use a wide-based gait (ie, walking with the feet separated). A conscious effort must be made to swing the arms, raise the feet while walking,

and to use a heel-toe placement of the feet with long strides. The patient is advised to practice walking to marching music or to the sound of a ticking metronome because this provides sensory reinforcement. Doing breathing exercises while walking helps to move the rib cage and to aerate parts of the lungs. Frequent rest periods aid in preventing frustration and fatigue.

ENHANCING SELF-CARE ACTIVITIES

Encouraging, teaching, and supporting the patient during activities of daily living promote self-care. See Chapter 11 for rehabilitation techniques.

Environmental modifications are necessary to compensate for functional disabilities. Patients may have severe mobility problems that make normal activities impossible. Adaptive or assistive devices may be useful. A hospital bed at home with bedside rails, an overbed frame with a trapeze, or a rope tied to the foot of the bed can provide assistance in pulling up without help. An occupational therapist can evaluate the patient's needs in the home and make recommendations regarding adaptive devices and teach the patient and caregiver how to improvise.

IMPROVING BOWEL ELIMINATION

The patient may have severe problems with constipation. Among the factors causing constipation are weakness of the muscles used in defecation, lack of exercise, inadequate fluid intake, and decreased autonomic nervous system activity. The medications used for the treatment of the disease also inhibit normal intestinal secretions. A regular bowel routine may be established by encouraging the patient to follow a regular time pattern, consciously increase fluid intake, and eat foods with a moderate fibre content. Laxatives should be avoided. Psyllium, for example, decreases constipation but carries the risk for bowel obstruction (Herndon et al., 2000). A raised toilet seat is useful because the patient has difficulty in moving from a standing to a sitting position.

IMPROVING NUTRITION

Patients may have difficulty maintaining their weight. Eating becomes a very slow process, requiring concentration due to a dry mouth from medications and difficulty chewing and swallowing. They are at risk for aspiration because of impaired swallowing and the accumulation of saliva. They may be unaware that they are aspirating, and subsequently bronchopneumonia may develop.

Monitoring weight on a weekly basis indicates whether caloric intake is adequate. Supplemental feedings increase caloric intake. As the disease progresses, a nasogastric tube or percutaneous endoscopic gastroscopy may be necessary to maintain adequate nutrition. A dietitian can be consulted regarding nutritional needs.

ENHANCING SWALLOWING

Swallowing disorders can be due to poor head control, tongue tremor, hesitancy in initiating swallowing, difficulty in shaping food into a bolus, and disturbances in pharyngeal motility. To offset these problems, the patient should sit in an upright position during mealtime. A semisolid diet with thick liquids is easier to swallow than solids; thin liquids should be avoided. It is helpful for patients to think through the swallowing sequence. The patient is taught to place the food on the tongue, close the lips and teeth, lift the tongue up and then back, and swallow. The patient is encouraged to chew first on one side of the mouth and then on the other. To control the buildup of saliva, the patient is reminded to hold the head upright and make a conscious effort to swallow. Massaging the facial and neck muscles before meals may be beneficial.

Chart 65-4

Home Care Checklist • **The Patient With Parkinson's Disease**

At the completion of the home care instruction, the patient or caregiver will be able to:	Patient	Caregiver
• Define Parkinson's disease and discuss its long-term effects.	✓	✓
• Identify the medication regimen and name adverse effects, and precautions.	✓	✓
• Discuss the risk for injury, prevent falls; implement adaptive measures in the home.	✓	✓
• Describe nutritional needs, dietary restrictions, dysphagia management, and ways to prevent aspiration.	✓	✓
• Manage constipation: fluid intake, bowel routine.	✓	✓
• Manage urinary problems: functional incontinence, retention (Foley catheter care, suprapubic catheter care).	✓	✓
• Explain effects of immobility and define preventive care: skin breakdown (frequent turning, pressure release, skin care), pneumonia (deep breathing, movement), contractures (range-of-motion exercises).	✓	✓
• Define benefits of daily exercise program.	✓	✓
• Walk and balance safely.	✓	
• Demonstrate speech and communication skills: speech exercises, communication techniques, breathing exercises.	✓	
• Name signs and symptoms of infection (urinary and respiratory) and state when health care provider should be notified.	✓	✓
• Describe strategies to promote self-care activities and independence.	✓	✓
• Identify resources: Parkinson Society of Canada has Regional Partners across Canada that can provide specialized programs and support groups.	✓	✓

ENCOURAGING THE USE OF ASSISTIVE DEVICES

An electric warming tray keeps food hot and permits the patient to rest during the prolonged time that it takes to eat. Special utensils also assist at mealtime. A plate that is stabilized, a nonspill cup, and eating utensils with built-up handles are useful self-help devices. The occupational therapist can assist in identifying appropriate adaptive devices.

IMPROVING COMMUNICATION

Speech disorders are present in most patients with Parkinson's disease. Their low-pitched, monotonous, soft speech requires that they make a conscious effort to speak slowly, with deliberate attention to what they are saying. Patients are reminded to face the listener, exaggerate the pronunciation of words, speak in short sentences, and take a few deep breaths before speaking.

A speech therapist may be helpful in designing speech improvement exercises and assisting the family and health care personnel to develop and use a method of communication to meet the patient's needs. A small electronic amplifier is helpful if the patient has difficulty being heard.

SUPPORTING COPING ABILITIES

Support can be given by encouraging the patient and pointing out that activities are being maintained through active participation. A combination of physiotherapy, psychotherapy, medication therapy, and support group participation may help reduce the depression that often occurs.

Patients often feel embarrassed, apathetic, inadequate, bored, and lonely. These feelings may be due, in part, to physical slowness and the great effort that even small tasks require. Patients are assisted and encouraged to set achievable goals (eg, improvement of mobility).

Because parkinsonism tends to lead to withdrawal and depression, patients must be active participants in their therapeutic program, including social and recreational events. There should be a planned program of activity throughout the day to prevent too much daytime sleeping as well as disinterest and apathy.

Every effort should be made to encourage patients to carry out the tasks involved in meeting their own daily needs and to remain independent. Doing things for the patient merely to save time is contrary to the basic goal of improving coping abilities and promoting a positive self-concept.

PROMOTING HOME AND COMMUNITY-BASED CARE

Teaching Patients Self-Care

Patient and family education is important in the management of Parkinson's disease. Teaching needs depend on the severity of symptoms and the stage of the disease. Care must be taken not to overwhelm the patient and family with too much information early in the disease process. The patient's and family's need for information is ongoing as adaptations become necessary. The education plan should include a clear explanation of the disease, assisting the patient to remain functionally independent as long as possible. Every effort is made to explain the nature of the disease and its management to offset disabling anxieties and fears. The patient and family must be taught about the effects and side effects of medications and about the importance of reporting side effects to the physician (Chart 65-4).

Continuing Care

In the early stages patients can be managed well at home. Family members often serve as caregivers, with home care or community services available to assist in meeting health care needs as the disease progresses. The family caregiver may be under considerable stress from living with and caring for a person with a significant disability. Providing information about treatment and care prevents many unnecessary problems. The caregiver is included in the plan and may be advised to learn stress reduction techniques, to include others in the caregiving process, to obtain periodic relief from responsibilities, and to have a yearly health assessment. Allowing family members to express feelings of frustration, anger, and guilt is often helpful to them.

The patient should be evaluated in the home for adaptation and safety needs and compliance with the plan of care. In the advanced stages, patients usually enter long-term care facilities when family support is absent. Periodically, admission to an acute care facility may be necessary for changes in medical management or treatment of complications. Nurses provide support, education, and monitoring of patients over the course of the illness.

The nurse involved in home and continuing care needs to remind patients and family members of the need to address health promotion needs such as screening for hypertension and stroke risk assessments in this predominantly elderly population. Patients who have not been involved in these practices in the past are educated about their importance and are referred to appropriate health care providers. Informational booklets and a newsletter for patient education are published by the National Parkinson's Foundation, Inc. and the American Parkinson's Disease Association.

Evaluation

EXPECTED PATIENT OUTCOMES

Expected patient outcomes may include:

1. Strives toward improved mobility
   a. Participates in exercise program daily
   b. Walks with wide base of support; exaggerates arm swinging when walking
   c. Takes medications as prescribed
2. Progresses toward self-care
   a. Allows time for self-care activities
   b. Uses self-help devices
3. Maintains bowel function
   a. Consumes adequate fluid
   b. Increases dietary intake of fibre
   c. Reports regular pattern of bowel function
4. Attains improved nutritional status
   a. Swallows without aspiration
   b. Takes time while eating
5. Achieves a method of communication
   a. Communicates needs
   b. Practices speech exercises
6. Copes with effects of Parkinson's disease
   a. Sets realistic goals
   b. Demonstrates persistence in meaningful activities
   c. Verbalizes feelings to appropriate person

HUNTINGTON'S DISEASE

Huntington's disease is a chronic, progressive, hereditary disease of the nervous system that results in progressive involuntary choreiform movement and dementia. It affects men and women of all races. Because it is transmitted as an autosomal dominant genetic disorder, each child of a parent with Huntington's disease has a 50% risk of inheriting the illness (Bradley et al., 2000).

Pathophysiology

The basic pathology involves premature death of cells in the striatum (caudate and putamen) of the basal ganglia, the region deep within the brain involved in the control of movement. There is also loss of cells in the cortex, the region of the brain associated with thinking, memory, perception, and judgment, and in the

NURSING RESEARCH PROFILE 65-2
Coping Patterns Following Gene Testing

Williams, J. K., Schutte, D., Evers, C., & Holkup, P. A. (2000). Redefinition: Coping with normal results from predictive gene testing for neurodegenerative disorders. *Research in Nursing & Health, 23,* 260–269.

Purpose
Predictive testing for an inherited neurodegenerative disease is a source of intense stress for adults. The purpose of this study was to describe the psychosocial impact and coping process of normal (negative) results from predictive testing for an inherited neurodegenerative disease.

Study Sample and Design
The study used a qualitative, descriptive design and the constant comparative method of data analysis. Ten adults with normal results of predictive testing for Huntington's disease (HD) or the pallido-pont-nigral degeneration (PPND) gene mutation participated in semistructured interviews 1 and 6 months following gene testing. The sample included 8 females, the age range was 33 to 59 years, 80% were married, and 80% had known they were at risk for one of the diseases for more than 5 years.

Findings
The major descriptive theme identified was redefinition. The redefinition occurred in the following three domains: redefinition of self, relationships with family, and role in society. The process evolved from a personal level at 1 month to a more future-oriented perspective at 6 months following normal gene test results.

Nursing Implications
Nurses working with individuals at risk for HD and PPND should keep in mind that many people prepare for the worst results when undergoing gene testing. The coping process following negative results (ie, absence of gene for the disease) evolves from a personal focus at 1 month to a broader future perspective at 6 months after testing. These components of the redefinition process are important considerations in planning interventions to promote coping with normal gene results within at-risk families during an extremely stressful time.

cerebellum, the area that coordinates voluntary muscle activity. Researchers now believe that a building block for protein called glutamine abnormally collects in the cell nucleus, causing cell death. The reason that the protein destroys only certain brain cells is unknown. The cells' destruction results in a lack of the neurotransmitters gamma-aminobutyric acid (GABA) and acetylcholine, which inhibit nerve action (Bradley et al., 2000). Onset usually occurs between the ages of 35 and 45 years, although about 10% of patients are children. The disease progresses slowly. Despite a ravenous appetite, patients usually become emaciated and exhausted. Patients succumb in 10 to 20 years to heart failure, pneumonia, or infection, or as a result of a fall or choking.

Clinical Manifestations

The most prominent clinical features of the disease are abnormal involuntary movements (**chorea**), intellectual decline, and, often, emotional disturbance. As the disease progresses, a constant writhing, twisting, uncontrollable movement may involve the entire body. These motions are devoid of purpose or rhythm, although patients may try to turn them into purposeful movement. All of the body musculature is involved. Facial movements produce tics and grimaces. Speech is affected, becoming slurred, hesitant, often explosive, and eventually unintelligible. Chewing and swallowing are difficult, and there is a constant danger of choking and aspiration. Choreiform movements persist but diminish during sleep.

As with speech, the gait becomes disorganized to the point that ambulation eventually is impossible. Although independent ambulation should be encouraged for as long as possible, a wheelchair usually becomes necessary. Eventually, the patient is confined to bed when the chorea interferes with walking, sitting, and all other activities. Bladder and bowel control is lost.

Cognitive function is usually affected, with dementia usually occurring. Initially, the patient generally is aware that the disease is responsible for the myriad dysfunctions that are occurring. The mental and emotional changes that occur may be more devastating to the patient and family than the abnormal movements. Personality changes may result in nervous, irritable, or impatient behaviours. In the early stages, patients are particularly subject to uncontrollable fits of anger, profound, often suicidal depression, apathy, anxiety, psychosis, or euphoria (Hofmann, 1999). Judgment and memory are impaired, and dementia eventually ensues. Hallucinations, delusions, and paranoid thinking may precede the appearance of disjointed movements. Emotional symptoms often become less acute as the disease progresses.

Assessment and Diagnostic Findings

The diagnosis is made based on the clinical presentation of characteristic symptoms, a positive family history, and exclusion of other causes. Imaging studies, such as CT and MRI, may show atrophy of the caudate nuclei once the disease is well established (Bradley et al., 2000).

A genetic marker for Huntington's has been identified through the use of recombinant DNA technology. As a result, researchers can now identify presymptomatic individuals who will develop this disease. Although this presymptomatic test can remove the uncertainty, it offers no hope of cure or even specific prediction of the timing of its onset. Researchers continue to study the genetic causes that lead to the death of brain cells (Bradley et al., 2000).

Management

Although no treatment halts or reverses the underlying process, several methods of management have fairly good palliative results (Bradley et al., 2000; Sawle, 1999). Thiothixene hydrochloride (Navane) and haloperidol decanoate (Haldol), which predominantly block dopamine receptors, improve the chorea in many patients (Bradley et al., 2000). Chorea also is lessened by reserpine (depletes presynaptic dopamine) and tetrabenazine (reduces dopaminergic transmission). Motor signs must be assessed and evaluated on an ongoing basis so that optimal therapeutic drug levels can be reached. **Akathisia** (motor restlessness) in the overmedicated patient is dangerous because it may be mistaken for the restless fidgeting of the illness and consequently can be overlooked.

In certain types of the disease, hypokinetic motor impairment resembles parkinsonism. In patients who present with rigidity, some temporary benefit may be obtained from antiparkinson medication, such as levodopa.

Patients who have emotional disturbances, particularly depression, may be helped by antidepressant medications. The threat of suicide is always present. Psychotic symptoms usually respond to antipsychotic medications. Psychotherapy aimed at allaying anxiety and reducing stress may be beneficial (Hofman, 1999). It is imperative that nurses look beyond the disease to focus on the patient's needs and capabilities (Chart 65-5). One study showed improved physical, mental, and social functioning in a small group of patients with Huntington's disease using remotivation therapy and providing a more stimulating environment (Sullivan, Bird, Alpay et al., 2001). Surgically implanted fetal neural allografts are being tested in hopes of improving the functional, motor, and cognitive function of patients (Bachoud-Levi, Remy, Nguyen et al., 2000; Diederich & Goetz, 2000).

PROMOTING HOME AND COMMUNITY-BASED CARE

Teaching Patients Self-Care. The needs of the patient and family for education depend on the nature and severity of physical, cognitive, and psychological changes experienced by the patient. Patients and family members are taught about the medications prescribed and about signs indicating a need for change in medication or dosage. The teaching plan addresses strategies to manage symptoms such as chorea, swallowing problems, limitations in ambulation, and loss of bowel and bladder function. Consultation with a speech therapist may be indicated to assist in identifying alternative communication strategies if speech is affected.

Individuals of child-bearing age often seek information about their risk for transmitting the disease. Even though presymptomatic testing has been offered since 1986, approximately 75% of individuals at risk choose not to be tested (Hayden, 2000). For most people, the benefits of testing are unclear because of ethical and confidentiality issues. Genetic counselling is crucial following testing, and patients and their families may require long-term psychological counselling and emotional, financial, and legal support (Williams, Schutte, Evers et al., 2000).

Continuing Care. A program combining medical, nursing, psychological, social, occupational, speech, and physical rehabilitation services is needed to help the patient and family cope with this severely disabling illness. Huntington's exacts enormous emotional, physical, social, and financial tolls on every member of the patient's family. The family often live under a heavy burden of uncertainty, anxiety, and guilt. Regular follow-up helps to allay the fear of abandonment.

Home care assistance, day care centres, respite care, and eventually skilled long-term care can assist the patient and family in coping with the constant strain of the illness. Although the relentless progression of the disease cannot be halted, families can benefit from supportive care.

Voluntary organizations can be major aids to families and have been largely responsible for bringing the illness to national attention. The Huntington's Disease Foundation of America helps patients and families by providing information, referrals, family and public education, and support for research.

ALZHEIMER'S DISEASE

Alzheimer's disease, or senile dementia of the Alzheimer's type, is a chronic, progressive, and degenerative brain disorder accompanied by profound effects on memory, cognition, and ability for self-care. About 10% of the population older than age 65 are affected, and the prevalence reaches 47% by age 85. Research suggests that inflammation plays a role in the pathophysiology of the

Chart 65-5

Care of the Patient With Huntington's Disease

Nursing Diagnosis

Risk for injury from falls and possible skin breakdown (pressure ulcers, abrasions), resulting from constant movement

Nursing Interventions

Pad the sides and head of the bed; ensure that the patient can see over the sides of bed.

Use padded heel and elbow protectors.

Keep the skin meticulously clean.

Apply emollient cleansing agent and skin lotion frequently.

Use soft sheets and bedding.

Have patient wear football padding or other forms of padding.

Encourage ambulation with assistance to maintain muscle tone.

Secure the patient (only if necessary) in bed or chair with padded protective devices, making sure that they are loosened frequently.

Nursing Diagnosis

Imbalanced nutrition, less than body requirements, due to inadequate intake and dehydration resulting from swallowing or chewing disorders and danger of choking or aspirating food

Nursing Interventions

Administer phenothiazines as prescribed before meals (appears to calm some patients).

Use a warming tray.

Talk to the patient before mealtime to promote relaxation; use mealtime for social interaction. Provide undivided attention. Help the patient enjoy the mealtime experience.

Learn the position that is best for *this* patient. Keep patient as close to upright as possible while feeding. Stabilize patient's head gently with one hand while feeding.

Show the food and tell the patient what the foods are (eg, whether hot or cold).

Encircle the patient with one arm and get as close as possible to provide stability and support. Use pillows and wedges for additional support.

Do not interpret stiffness, turning away, or sudden turning of the head as rejection; these are uncontrollable choreiform movements.

For feeding, use a long-handled spoon (iced-tea spoon). Place spoon on middle of tongue and exert slight pressure.

Place bite-sized food between patient's teeth. Serve stews, casseroles, thick liquids; avoid too many milk drinks (produces mucus).

Disregard messiness. Treat the person with dignity.

Wait for the patient to chew and swallow before introducing another spoonful. Make sure that bite-sized food is small.

Give between-meal feedings. Constant movement expends more calories. Patients often have voracious appetites, particularly for sweets.

Use blenderized meals if patient cannot chew; do not repeatedly give the same strained baby foods; gradually introduce increased textures and consistencies to the diet.

For swallowing difficulties:

Apply gentle deep pressure around the patient's mouth.

Rub fingers in circles on the patient's cheeks.

Rub fingers simultaneously down each side of the patient's throat.

Develop skill in Heimlich manoeuvre (to be used in the event of choking).

Nursing Diagnosis

Anxiety and impaired communication from excessive grimacing and unintelligible speech

Nursing Interventions

Read to the patient.

Employ biofeedback and relaxation therapy to reduce stress.

Consult with speech therapist to help maintain and prolong communication abilities.

Try to devise a communication system, perhaps using cards with words or pictures of familiar objects, before verbal communication becomes too difficult. Patients can indicate correct card by hitting it with hand, grunting, or blinking the eyes.

Learn how this particular patient expresses needs and wants—particularly nonverbal messages (widening of eyes, responses).

Patients can understand even if unable to speak. Do not isolate patients by ceasing to communicate with them.

Nursing Diagnosis

Disturbed thought processes and impaired social interaction

Nursing Interventions

Have clock, calendar, and wall posters to view.

Interact with the patient in a creative manner.

Use every opportunity for one-to-one contact.

Use music for relaxation.

Reorient the patient after awakening.

Have the patient wear an identification bracelet with name, telephone number, and "memory impaired" on it.

Keep the patient in the social mainstream.

Recruit and train volunteers for social interaction. Role model appropriate interactions.

Do not abandon a patient because the disease is eventually terminal. Patients are *living* until the end.

---

disease and that anti-inflammatory agents such as nonsteroidal anti-inflammatory drugs (NSAIDs) may be helpful adjuncts in treatment (Neuroinflammation Working Group, 2000).

Alzheimer's is one of the most feared disorders of modern times because it has catastrophic consequences for the patient and family, who experience what has been termed an endless funeral. Chapter 12 discusses the manifestations, management, and nursing care of the patient with Alzheimer's disease.

AMYOTROPHIC LATERAL SCLEROSIS

Amyotrophic lateral sclerosis (ALS) is a disease of unknown cause in which there is a loss of motor neurons (nerve cells controlling muscles) in the anterior horns of the spinal cord and the motor nuclei of the lower brain stem. As these cells die, the muscle fibres that they supply undergo atrophic changes. Neuronal degeneration may occur in both the upper and lower motor neuron systems. Several theories exist regarding the cause of ALS, including autoimmune disease and free radical damage. The leading theory held by researchers is that overexcitation of nerve cells by the neurotransmitter glutamate leads to cell injury and neuronal degeneration.

Approximately 3000 Canadians live with ALS and 2 to 3 Canadians die each day of ALS (ALS Society of Canada, 2005). ALS affects more men than women, with onset occurring usually in the fifth or sixth decade. It is often referred to as Lou Gehrig's disease after the famous baseball player who suffered from it.

Clinical Manifestations

Clinical manifestations depend on the location of the affected motor neurons, because specific neurons activate specific muscle fibres. The chief symptoms are fatigue, progressive muscle weakness, cramps, fasciculations (twitching), and incoordination (Brown, Meininger & Swash, 2000). Loss of motor neurons in the anterior horns of the spinal cord results in progressive weakness and atrophy of the muscles of the arms, trunk, or legs. Spasticity usually is present, and the deep tendon stretch reflexes become brisk and overactive. Usually, the anal and bladder sphincters are intact because the spinal nerves that control muscles of the rectum and urinary bladder are not affected.

In about 25% of patients, weakness starts in the muscles supplied by the cranial nerves, and there is difficulty talking, swallowing, and ultimately breathing. When the patient ingests liquids, soft palate and upper esophageal weakness causes the liquid to be regurgitated through the nose. Weakness of the posterior tongue and palate impairs the ability to laugh, cough, or even blow the nose. When bulbar muscles are impaired, there is progressive difficulty in speaking and swallowing, and aspiration becomes a risk. The voice assumes a nasal sound, and articulation becomes so disrupted that the speech is unintelligible. Some emotional liability may be present, but intellectual function is not impaired. Eventually, respiratory function is compromised.

The prognosis generally is based on the area of the CNS involved and the speed with which the disease progresses. Death usually occurs as a result of infection, respiratory failure, or aspiration. The average time from onset of the disease to death is about 3 years. A few patients survive for longer periods.

Assessment and Diagnostic Findings

ALS is diagnosed on the basis of the signs and symptoms because no clinical or laboratory tests are specific for this disease. EMG studies of the affected muscles indicate reduction in the number of functioning motor units. MRI may show high signal intensity in the corticospinal tracts; this differentiates it from a multifocal motor neuropathy (Rowland & Shneider, 2001).

Management

There is no specific therapy for ALS. The main focus of medical and nursing management is on interventions to maintain or improve function, well-being, and quality of life (Brown, Meininger & Swash, 2000). One study of 60 patients with ALS found that despite the decline in physical function, quality of life and religiosity change little over time (Robbins, Simmons, Bremer et al., 2001).

The medication riluzole (Rilutek), a glutamate antagonist, slows the deterioration of motor neurons. How riluzole works is not clear, but its pharmacologic properties suggest that it may have a neuroprotective effect in the early stages of ALS. Two randomized drug trials showed a dose of 100 mg riluzole per day to be modestly effective in prolonging survival time for patients with ALS (Miller, Mitchell & Moore, 2001).

Symptomatic treatment and rehabilitative measures are employed to support the patient and improve the quality of life. Baclofen (Lioresal), dantrolene sodium (Dantrium), or diazepam (Valium) may be useful for patients troubled by spasticity, which causes pain and interferes with self-care. Several neurotrophic factors that facilitate nutrition and metabolism for nerve tissue are being investigated (Rowland & Shneider, 2001).

Most patients with ALS are managed at home and in the community, with hospitalization for acute problems. The most common reasons for hospitalization are dehydration and malnutrition, pneumonia, and respiratory failure (Lechtzin, Wiener, Clawson et al., 2001). Recognizing these problems at an earlier stage in the illness will allow for the development of preventive strategies.

A patient experiencing problems with aspiration and swallowing may require enteral feeding. The American Academy of Neurology practice guidelines suggest the placement of a percutaneous endoscopic gastrostomy tube before the forced vital capacity drops below 50% of predicted (Boitano, Jordan & Benditt, 2001). This tube can be safely placed in patients who are using noninvasive positive-pressure ventilation for ventilatory support (Boitano, Jordan & Benditt, 2001).

Mechanical ventilation (using negative-pressure ventilators) is an option when alveolar hypoventilation develops. A small study of patients who used noninvasive positive-pressure ventilation at night showed that hypoventilation and sleep disturbances were at least partially improved, enhancing their cognitive function (Newsom-Davis et al., 2001). The use of noninvasive positive-pressure ventilation also postpones the decision of whether to undergo a tracheotomy for long-term mechanical ventilation (Rowland & Shneider, 2001).

Decisions about life support measures are made by the patient and family and should be based on a thorough understanding of the disease, the prognosis, and the implications of initiating such therapy. Patients are encouraged to complete an advance directive or "living will" to preserve their autonomy in decision-making.

The ALS Association has broad programs of research funding, patient and clinical services, patient information and support, and medical and public information. The *ALS Association Quarterly Newsletter* is a source of practical information.

MUSCULAR DYSTROPHIES

The muscular dystrophies are a group of chronic muscle disorders characterized by progressive weakening and wasting of the skeletal or voluntary muscles. Most of these diseases are inherited. Duchenne muscular dystrophy is the most common and occurs in 1 of every 3,000 male births (Bach, 1999). The pathologic features include degeneration and loss of muscle fibres, variation in muscle fibre size, phagocytosis and regeneration, and replacement of muscle tissue by connective tissue. The common characteristics of these diseases include varying degrees of muscle wasting and weakness, abnormal elevation in blood muscle enzymes, and myopathic findings on EMG and muscle biopsy (Bach, 1999). The differences centre on the pattern of inheritance, the muscles involved, the age of onset, and the rate of progression. The unique needs of these patients, who in the past did not live to adulthood, must be addressed as they live longer as a result of better supportive care (Carson & Hieber, 2001).

Medical Management

Treatment of the muscular dystrophies at this time focuses on supportive care and preventing complications in the absence of a cure or specific pharmacologic interventions (Bach, 1999; Carson & Hieber, 2001). Supportive management aims to keep the patient active and functioning as normally as possible and to minimize functional deterioration. An individualized therapeutic exercise program is prescribed to prevent muscle tightness, contractures, and disuse atrophy. Night splints and stretching exercises are used to delay contractures of the joints, especially the ankles, knees, and hips. Braces may compensate for muscle weakness.

Spinal deformity is a severe problem. Weakness of trunk muscles and spinal collapse occur almost routinely in patients with severe neuromuscular disease. In the battle against spinal deformity, the patient is fitted with an orthotic jacket to improve sitting stability and reduce trunk deformity. This measure also supports cardiovascular status. In time, spinal fusion is performed to maintain spinal stability. Other procedures may be carried out to correct deformities.

Compromised pulmonary function may be due either to progression of the disease or to deformity of the thorax secondary to severe scoliosis. Intercurrent illnesses, upper respiratory infections, and fractures from falls must be vigourously treated in a way that minimizes immobilization because joint contractures become worse when the patient's activities are more restricted than usual.

Other difficulties may be manifested in relation to the underlying disease. Dental and speech problems may result from weakness of the facial muscles, which makes it difficult to attend to dental hygiene and to speak coherently. Gastrointestinal tract problems may include gastric dilation, rectal prolapse, and fecal impaction. Finally, cardiomyopathy appears to be a common complication in all forms of muscular dystrophy.

Genetic counselling is advised for parents and siblings of the patient because of the genetic nature of this disease. The Muscular Dystrophy Association works to combat neuromuscular disease through research, programs of patient services and clinical care, and professional and public education.

Nursing Management

The goals of the patient and the nurse are to maintain function at optimal levels and to enhance the quality of life. Therefore, the patient's physical requirements, which are considerable, are addressed without losing sight of emotional and developmental needs (Carson & Hieber, 2001). The patient and family are actively involved in decision-making, including end-of-life decisions.

During hospitalization for treatment of complications, the knowledge and expertise of the patient and family members responsible for caregiving in the home are assessed. Because the patient and family caregivers often have developed caregiving strategies that work effectively for them, these strategies need to be acknowledged and accepted, and provisions must be made to ensure that they are maintained during hospitalization (Carson & Hieber, 2001).

Families of chronically ill individuals often need assistance to shift the focus of care from pediatric to adult care. Nursing goals include assisting the person with a chronic condition to make the transition to adult values and expectations while providing age-appropriate ongoing care (Carson & Hieber, 2001). The nurse may need to help build the confidence of an older adolescent or adult patient by encouraging him or her to pursue job training to become economically independent. Other nursing interventions might include guidance in accessing adult health care and finding appropriate programs in sex education (Carson & Hieber, 2001).

PROMOTING HOME AND COMMUNITY-BASED CARE

Teaching Patients Self-Care. The management goals are addressed in special rehabilitation programs or in the patient's home and community (Natterlund & Ahlstrom, 1999). Thus, the patient and family require information and instruction about the disorder, its anticipated course, and care and management strategies that will optimize the patient's growth and development and physical and psychological status. Members of a variety of health-related disciplines are involved in patient and family teaching; recommendations are communicated to all members of the health care team so that they may work toward common goals.

Continuing Care. Both the neuromuscular disease and the associated deformities may progress in adolescence and adulthood. Self-help and assistive devices can aid in maintaining maximum independence. Additional self-help devices, recommended by physical and occupational therapists, often become necessary as more muscle groups are affected.

The family is taught to monitor the patient for respiratory problems, as respiratory infection and cardiac failure are the most common causes of death (Carson & Hieber, 2001). As respiratory difficulties develop, patients and their families need information regarding respiratory support. Options currently exist that can provide ventilatory support (negative-pressure devices, positive-pressure ventilators) while allowing mobility (Bach, 1999). Patients can remain relatively independent in a wheelchair, for example, while being maintained on a ventilator at home for many years.

The patient is encouraged to continue with range-of-motion exercises to prevent contractures, which are particularly disabling. Practical adaptations must be made, however, to cope with the effects of chronic neuromuscular disability. The patient at various stages of the disease may require a manual or an electric wheelchair, gait aids, upper and lower extremity and spinal orthoses, seating systems, bathroom equipment, lifts, ramps, and additional assistive devices, all of which require a team approach (Bach, 1999). The home care nurse assesses how the patient and family are managing, makes referrals, and coordinates the activities of the physical therapist, occupational therapist, and social services.

Of great concern to the patient are the issues surrounding the threat of increasing disability and dependence on others, accompanied by a significant deterioration in health-related quality of life (Natterlund, Gunnarsson & Ahlstrom, 2000). The patient is faced with a progressive loss of function, leading eventually to death. Feelings of helplessness and powerlessness are common. Each functional loss is accompanied by grief and mourning. The patient and family are assessed for depression, anger, or denial. The patient and family are assisted to address decisions about end-of-life options before their need arises.

A psychiatric nurse clinician or other mental health professional may assist the patient to cope and adapt to the disease. By understanding and addressing the physical and psychological needs of the patient and family, the nurse provides a hopeful, supportive, and nurturing environment.

DEGENERATIVE DISK DISEASE

Low back pain is a significant public health disorder in the United States (Bigos et al., 1994). It is a challenging disorder to quantify. Current estimates are that between 22% and 65% of individuals have an episode of back pain in any given year, and between 11% and 84% of adults have an episode within their lifetime (Walker, 2000). It is estimated that 90% of Canadians between 20 and 65 will develop back pain (Medbroadcast Canada, 2005). This results in significant economic and social costs. Acute low back pain has a duration of less than 3 months; chronic or degenerative disease has a duration of 3 months or longer. Most back problems are related to disk disease.

Pathophysiology

The intervertebral disk is a cartilaginous plate that forms a cushion between the vertebral bodies (Fig. 65-8A). This tough, fibrous material is incorporated in a capsule. A ball-like cushion in the centre of the disk is called the nucleus pulposus. In herniation of the intervertebral disk (ruptured disk), the nucleus of the disk protrudes into the annulus (the fibrous ring around the disk), with subsequent nerve compression. Protrusion or rupture of the nucleus pulposus usually is preceded by degenerative changes that occur with aging. Loss of protein polysaccharides in the disk decreases the water content of the nucleus pulposus. The development of radiating cracks in the annulus weakens resistance to nucleus herniation. After trauma (falls and repeated minor stresses such as lifting), the cartilage may be injured.

For most patients, the immediate symptoms of trauma are short-lived, and those resulting from injury to the disk do not appear for months or years. Then, with degeneration in the disk, the capsule pushes back into the spinal canal, or it may rupture and allow the nucleus pulposus to be pushed back against the dural sac or against a spinal nerve as it emerges from the spinal column (see Fig. 65-8B). This sequence produces pain due to pressure in the area of distribution of the involved nerve endings (**radiculopathy**). Continued pressure may produce degenerative changes in the involved nerve, such as changes in sensation and deep tendon reflexes.

Clinical Manifestations

A herniated disk with accompanying pain may occur in any portion of the spine: cervical, thoracic (rare), or lumbar. The clinical manifestations depend on the location, the rate of development (acute or chronic), and the effect on the surrounding structures.

Assessment and Diagnostic Findings

A thorough health history and physical examination are important to rule out potentially serious conditions that may present as low back pain, including fracture, tumour, infection, or cauda equina syndrome (Bigos et al., 1994).

MRI has become the diagnostic tool of choice for localizing even small disk protrusions, particularly for lumbar spine disease. If the clinical symptoms are not consistent with the pathology seen on MRI, CT and myelography are then performed. A neurologic examination is carried out to determine if there is reflex, sensory, or motor impairment from root compression and to provide a baseline for future assessment. EMG may be used to localize the specific spinal nerve roots involved.

Medical Management

Herniations of the cervical and the lumbar disks occur most commonly and are usually managed conservatively with bed rest and medication. The specific conservative management strategies, along with surgical interventions for each form of herniation, are discussed next.

SURGICAL MANAGEMENT

In general, surgical excision of a herniated disk is performed when there is evidence of a progressing neurologic deficit (muscle weakness and atrophy, loss of sensory and motor function, loss of sphincter control) and continuing pain and **sciatica** (leg pain resulting from sciatic nerve involvement) that are unresponsive to conservative management. The goal of surgical treatment is to reduce the pressure on the nerve root to relieve pain and reverse neurologic deficits (Hall, 1999). Microsurgical techniques are making it possible to remove only the amount of tissue that is necessary, better preserving the integrity of normal tissue and imposing less trauma on the body. During these procedures, spinal cord function can be monitored electrophysiologically.

To achieve the goal of pain relief, several surgical techniques are used, depending on the type of disk herniation, surgical morbidity, and overall results of surgery:

- Discectomy: removal of herniated or extruded fragments of intervertebral disk

FIGURE 65-8 (**A**) Normal lumbar spine vertebrae, intervertebral disks, and spinal nerve root; (**B**) ruptured vertebral disk.

- Laminectomy: removal of the bone between the spinal process and facet pedicle junction to expose the neural elements in the spinal canal (Hall, 1999); allows the surgeon to inspect the spinal canal, identify and remove pathology, and relieve compression of the cord and roots
- Hemilaminectomy: removal of part of the lamina and part of the posterior arch of the vertebra
- Partial laminectomy or laminotomy: creation of a hole in the lamina of a vertebra (Hall, 1999)
- Discectomy with fusion: a bone graft (from iliac crest or bone bank) is used to fuse the vertebral spinous process; the object of spinal fusion is to bridge over the defective disk to stabilize the spine and reduce the rate of recurrence
- Foraminotomy: removal of the intervertebral foramen to increase the space for exit of a spinal nerve, resulting in reduced pain, compression, and edema

Surgical procedures for herniated cervical disk and lumbar disk are discussed in the sections that follow.

HERNIATION OF A CERVICAL INTERVERTEBRAL DISK

The cervical spine is subjected to stresses that result from disk degeneration (from aging, occupational stresses) and **spondylosis** (degenerative changes occurring in disk and adjacent vertebral bodies). Cervical disk degeneration may lead to lesions that can cause damage to the spinal cord and its roots.

A cervical disk herniation usually occurs at the C5-6 and C6-7 interspaces. Pain and stiffness may occur in the neck, the top of the shoulders, and the region of the scapulae. Sometimes patients interpret these signs as symptoms of heart trouble or bursitis. Pain may also occur in the upper extremities and head, accompanied by **paresthesia** (tingling or a "pins and needles" sensation) and numbness of the upper extremities. Cervical MRI usually confirms the diagnosis.

Medical Management

The goals of treatment are (1) to rest and immobilize the cervical spine to give the soft tissues time to heal and (2) to reduce inflammation in the supporting tissues and the affected nerve roots in the cervical spine. Bed rest (usually 1 to 2 days) is important because it eliminates the stress of gravity and relieves the cervical spine from the need to support the head. It also reduces inflammation and edema in soft tissues around the disk, relieving pressure on the nerve roots. Proper positioning on a firm mattress may bring dramatic relief from pain.

The cervical spine may be rested and immobilized by a cervical collar, cervical traction, or a brace. A collar allows maximal opening of the intervertebral foramina and holds the head in a neutral or slightly flexed position. The patient may have to wear the collar 24 hours a day during the acute phase. The skin under the collar is inspected for irritation. When the patient is free of pain, cervical isometric exercises are started to strengthen the neck muscles.

Cervical traction is accomplished by means of a head halter attached to a pulley and weight. It increases vertebral separation and thus relieves pressure on the nerve roots. The head of the bed is elevated to provide countertraction (see Chap. 67). If the skin becomes irritated, the halter can be padded. Experience has shown that a male patient may suffer more skin irritation if he shaves; the beard offers a natural form of padding.

PHARMACOLOGIC THERAPY

Analgesic agents (NSAIDs, propoxyphene [Darvon], oxycodone [Tylox], or hydrocodone [Vicodin]) are prescribed during the acute phase to relieve pain, and sedatives may be administered to control the anxiety often associated with cervical disk disease. Muscle relaxants (cyclobenzaprine [Flexeril], methocarbamol [Robaxin], metaxalone [Skelaxin]) are administered to interrupt the cycle of muscle spasm and to promote comfort. NSAIDs (aspirin, ibuprofen [Motrin, Advil], naproxen [Naprosyn, Anaprox]) or corticosteroids are prescribed to treat the inflammatory response that usually occurs in the supporting tissues and affected nerve roots. Occasionally, an injection of a corticosteroid into the epidural space may be administered for relief of radicular (spinal nerve root) pain. NSAIDs are given with food and antacids to prevent gastrointestinal irritation. Hot, moist compresses (for 10 to 20 minutes) applied to the back of the neck several times daily increase blood flow to the muscles and help relax the spastic muscles and the patient.

SURGICAL MANAGEMENT

Surgical excision of the herniated disk may be necessary when there is a significant neurologic deficit, progression of the deficit, evidence of cord compression, or pain that either worsens or fails to improve. A cervical discectomy, with or without fusion, may be performed to alleviate symptoms. An anterior surgical approach may be used through a transverse incision to remove disk material that has herniated into the spinal canal and foramina, or a posterior approach may be used at the appropriate level of the cervical spine. Potential complications with the anterior approach include carotid or vertebral artery injury, recurrent laryngeal nerve dysfunction, esophageal perforation, and airway obstruction. Complications of the posterior approach include damage to the nerve root or the spinal cord due to retraction or contusion of either of these structures, resulting in weakness of muscles supplied by the nerve root or cord.

Microsurgery, such as endoscopic microdiscectomy, may be performed in selected patients through a small incision and using magnification techniques. The patient who undergoes microsurgery usually has less tissue trauma and pain and consequently a shorter hospital stay than after conventional surgical approaches.

NURSING PROCESS: THE PATIENT UNDERGOING A CERVICAL DISCECTOMY

Assessment

The patient is asked about past injuries to the neck (whiplash) because unresolved trauma may cause persistent discomfort, pain and tenderness, and symptoms of arthritis in the injured joint of the cervical spine. Assessment includes determining the onset, location, and radiation of pain, paresthesias, limited movement, and diminished function of the neck, shoulders, and upper extremities. It is important to determine whether the symptoms are bilateral because with large herniations, bilateral symptoms may be due to cord compression. The area around the cervical spine is palpated to assess muscle tone and tenderness. Range of motion in the neck and shoulders is evaluated.

The patient is asked about any health concerns that may influence the postoperative course. The nurse determines the patient's need for information about the surgical procedure and reinforces what the physician has explained. Strategies for pain management are discussed with the patient.

Diagnosis

NURSING DIAGNOSES

Based on the assessment data, the patient's major nursing diagnoses may include the following:

- Acute pain related to the surgical procedure
- Impaired physical mobility related to the postoperative surgical regimen
- Deficient knowledge about the postoperative course and home care management

Other nursing diagnoses may include preoperative anxiety, postoperative constipation, urinary retention related to surgical procedure and dehydration, self-care deficits related to neck orthosis, and sleep pattern disturbance related to disruption in lifestyle.

COLLABORATIVE PROBLEMS/ POTENTIAL COMPLICATIONS

Based on all the assessment data, the potential complications may include the following:

- Hematoma at the surgical site, resulting in cord compression and neurologic deficit
- Recurrent or persistent pain after surgery

Planning and Goals

The goals for the patient may include relief of pain, improved mobility, increased knowledge and self-care ability, and prevention of complications.

Nursing Interventions

RELIEVING PAIN

The patient may be kept flat in bed for 12 to 24 hours. If the patient has had a bone fusion with bone removed from the iliac crest, considerable pain may be experienced. Interventions consist of monitoring the donor site for hematoma formation, administering the prescribed postoperative analgesic agent, positioning for comfort, and reassuring the patient that the pain can be relieved. If the patient experiences a sudden reappearance or increase of pain, extrusion of the graft may have occurred, requiring reoperation and surgical repositioning of the graft. This should be promptly reported to the surgeon.

The patient may experience a sore throat, hoarseness, and dysphagia due to temporary edema. These symptoms are relieved by throat lozenges, voice rest, and humidification. A puréed diet may be given if the patient has dysphagia.

IMPROVING MOBILITY

Postoperatively, a cervical collar (neck orthosis) is usually worn, which contributes to limited neck motion and altered mobility. Patients are instructed to turn the body instead of the neck when looking from side to side. The neck should be kept in a neutral (midline) position. Patients are assisted during position changes, making sure that head, shoulders, and thorax are kept aligned. When assisting a patient to a sitting position, the nurse supports the patient's neck and shoulders. Patients should wear shoes when ambulating to increase stability.

MONITORING AND MANAGING POTENTIAL COMPLICATIONS

The patient is evaluated for bleeding and hematoma formation by assessing for excessive pressure in the neck or severe pain in the incision area. The dressing is inspected for serosanguineous drainage, which suggests a dural leak. In this event, meningitis is a threat. A complaint of headache requires careful evaluation. Neurologic checks are made for swallowing deficits and upper and lower extremity weakness because cord compression may produce rapid or delayed onset of paralysis. The patient who has had an anterior cervical discectomy is also assessed for a sudden return of radicular (spinal nerve root) pain, which may indicate instability of the spine.

Throughout the postoperative course, the patient is monitored frequently to detect any signs of respiratory difficulty because retractors during surgery may injure the recurrent laryngeal nerve, resulting in hoarseness and the inability to cough effectively and clear pulmonary secretions. In addition, the blood pressure and pulse are monitored to evaluate cardiovascular status.

Bleeding at the surgical site and subsequent hematoma formation may occur. Severe localized pain not relieved by analgesic agents should be reported to the surgeon. A change in neurologic status (motor or sensory function) should be reported promptly because it suggests hematoma formation that may necessitate surgery to prevent irreversible motor and sensory deficits.

PROMOTING HOME AND COMMUNITY-BASED CARE

Teaching Patients Self-Care

The patient's hospital stay is likely to be short; therefore, the patient and family should understand the care that is important for a smooth recovery. A cervical collar is usually worn for about 6 weeks. The patient is instructed in use and care of the cervical collar. Patients are instructed to alternate tasks in which the body does not move (eg, reading) with tasks that require greater body movement.

The patient is instructed about strategies for pain management and about signs and symptoms that may indicate complications that should be reported to the physician. The nurse assesses the patient's understanding of these management strategies, limitations, and recommendations. Additionally, the nurse assists the patient in identifying strategies to cope with activities of daily living (ie, self-care and childcare) and minimize risks to the surgical site (Chart 65-6).

A discharge teaching plan is developed collaboratively by members of the health care team to decrease the risk for recurrent disk herniation. Topics include those previously discussed as well as proper body mechanics, maintenance of optimal weight, proper exercise techniques, and modifications in activity.

Continuing Care

Patients are instructed to see their physician at prescribed intervals to document the disappearance of old symptoms and for assessment of range of motion of the neck. Recurrent or persistent pain may occur despite removal of the offending disk or disk frag-

> **Chart 65-6**
> **Home Care Checklist • The Patient With Cervical Discectomy and Cervical Collar**

At the completion of the home care instruction, the patient or caregiver will be able to:	Patient	Caregiver
• Care for the surgical incision site.		
• Keep staples or sutures clean and dry and cover with dry dressing.		✓
• Notify physician if any signs or symptoms of infection occur, such as fever, redness or irritation, drainage, increased pain.	✓	✓
• Demonstrate proper body mechanics and prescribed exercise techniques.	✓	
• Modify activity:		
• Avoid sitting or standing for more than 30 minutes.	✓	
• Avoid twisting, flexing, extending, or rotating the neck.	✓	
• Avoid long automobile rides.	✓	
• Avoid sleeping in a prone position or use of pillows, to minimize neck flexion in bed; keep head in a neutral position.	✓	
• Use adequate mattress and chair support.	✓	
• Wear low-heeled shoes.	✓	
• Follow physician's instructions regarding lifting, climbing stairs, driving a car, sexual activity, sports, exercise, and return to work.	✓	
• Practice stress reduction and relaxation techniques.	✓	
• Care of the cervical collar:		
• Wear the collar at all times until directed otherwise by the physician.	✓	
• Wash the neck twice a day with mild soap.	✓	✓
• Keep the neck still while the collar is open.	✓	
• With the assistance of a helper, wash the neck in steps:		
• Lie flat and supine.	✓	
• Open the Velcro tabs on each side of the collar and remove its front portion.		✓
• Gently wash and dry the neck.		✓
• Replace the front part of the collar and refasten the tabs.		✓
• Turn to one side with a thin pillow under the head.	✓	
• Open one tab.	✓	
• Gently wash and dry the back of the neck. Refasten the tab.		✓
• Turn to the other side and wash and dry this side. Refasten the tab.		✓
• Place a wrinkle-free silk scarf under the collar to increase comfort.	✓	✓
• *For men:* Shave without twisting or moving the neck. This may be done with help while lying flat or sitting. Remove only the front part of the collar for shaving.	✓	✓

ments. Patients who undergo discectomy usually have consented to surgery after prolonged pain; they have often undergone repeated courses of ineffective conservative management and previous surgeries to relieve the pain. Therefore, the recurrence or persistence of symptoms postoperatively, including pain and sensory deficits, is often discouraging for the patient and family. The patient who experiences recurrence of symptoms requires emotional support and understanding. Additionally, the patient is assisted in modifying activities and in considering options for subsequent treatment.

The patient with degenerative disk disease tends to focus on obvious needs, issues, and deficits. The nurse needs to remind patients and family members of the need for participating in health promotion and health screening practices.

Evaluation

EXPECTED PATIENT OUTCOMES
Expected patient outcomes may include:

1. Reports decreasing frequency and severity of pain
2. Demonstrates improved mobility

a. Demonstrates progressive participation in self-care activities
b. Identifies prescribed activity limitations and restrictions
c. Demonstrates proper body mechanics
3. Is knowledgeable about postoperative course, medications, and home care management.
   a. Lists the signs and symptoms to be reported postoperatively
   b. Identifies dose, action, and potential side effects of medications
   c. Identifies appropriate home care management activities and any restrictions
4. Absence of complications
   a. Reports no increase in incision pain or sensory symptoms
   b. Demonstrates normal findings on neurologic assessment

HERNIATION OF A LUMBAR DISK

Most lumbar disk herniations occur at the L4-5 or the L5-S1 interspaces (Humphreys & Eck, 1999). A herniated lumbar disk produces low back pain accompanied by varying degrees of sensory and motor impairment.

Clinical Manifestations

The patient complains of low back pain with muscle spasms, followed by radiation of the pain into one hip and down into the leg (sciatica). Pain is aggravated by actions that increase intraspinal fluid pressure (bending, lifting, straining, as in sneezing and coughing) and usually is relieved by bed rest. Usually there is some type of postural deformity, because pain causes an alteration of the normal spinal mechanics. If the patient lies on the back and attempts to raise a leg in a straight position, pain radiates into the leg because this manoeuvre, called the straight leg-raising test, stretches the sciatic nerve. Additional signs include muscle weakness, alterations in tendon reflexes, and sensory loss.

Assessment and Diagnostic Findings

The diagnosis of lumbar disk disease is based on the history and physical findings and the use of imaging techniques such as MRI, CT, and myelography.

Medical Management

The objectives of treatment are to relieve pain, slow disease progression, and increase the patient's functional ability. Bed rest for 1 to 2 days on a firm mattress (to limit spinal flexion) is encouraged to reduce the weight load and gravitational forces, thereby freeing the disk from stress (Humphrey & Eck, 1999). The patient is allowed to assume a comfortable position; usually, a semi-Fowler's position with moderate hip and knee flexion relaxes the back muscles. When the patient is in a side-lying position, a pillow is placed between the legs. To get out of bed, the patient lies on one side while pushing up to a sitting position.

Because muscle spasm is prominent during the acute phase, muscle relaxants are used. NSAIDs and systemic corticosteroids may be administered to counter the inflammation that usually occurs in the supporting tissues and the affected nerve roots. Moist heat and massage help to relax spastic muscles and have a sedative effect. Antidepressant agents appear to help in low back pain that is neuropathic in origin (Fishbain, 2000). See also Nursing Process: The Patient With Low Back Pain in Chapter 13 for nursing interventions.

SURGICAL MANAGEMENT

In the lumbar region, surgical treatment includes lumbar disk excision through a posterolateral laminotomy and the newer techniques of microdiscectomy and percutaneous discectomy. In microdiscectomy, an operating microscope is used to visualize the offending disk and compressed nerve roots; it permits a small incision (2.5 cm) and minimal blood loss and takes about 30 minutes of operating time. Generally, it involves a short hospital stay, and the patient makes a rapid recovery. Percutaneous discectomy is an alternative treatment for herniated intervertebral disks of the lumbar spine at the L4-5 level. One approach in current use is through a 2.5-cm incision just above the iliac crest. A tube, trocar, or cannula is inserted under x-ray guidance through the retroperitoneal space to the involved disk space. Special instruments are used to remove the disk. The operating time is about 15 minutes. Blood loss and postoperative pain are minimal, and the patient is generally discharged within 2 days after surgery. The disadvantage of this procedure is the possibility of damage to structures in the surgical pathway.

Complications of Disk Surgery. A patient undergoing a disk procedure at one level of the vertebral column may have a degenerative process at other levels. A herniation relapse may occur at the same level or elsewhere, so that the patient may become a candidate for another disk procedure. Arachnoiditis (inflammation of the arachnoid membrane) may occur after surgery (and after myelography); it involves an insidious onset of diffuse, frequently burning pain in the lower back, radiating into the buttocks. Disk excision can leave adhesions and scarring around the spinal nerves and dura, which then produce inflammatory changes that create chronic neuritis and neurofibrosis. Disk surgery may relieve pressure on the spinal nerves, but it does not reverse the effects of neural injury and scarring and the pain that results. Failed disk syndrome (recurrence of sciatica after lumbar discectomy) remains a common cause of disability.

Nursing Management

PROVIDING PREOPERATIVE CARE

Most patients fear surgery on any part of the spine and therefore need explanations about the surgery and reassurance that surgery will not weaken the back. When data are being collected for the health history, any reports of pain, paresthesia, and muscle spasm are recorded to provide a baseline for comparison after surgery. Preoperative assessment also includes an evaluation of movement of the extremities as well as bladder and bowel function. To facilitate the postoperative turning procedure, the patient is taught to turn as a unit (called logrolling) as part of the preoperative preparation (Fig. 65-9). Before surgery, the patient is also encouraged to take deep breaths, cough, and perform muscle-setting exercises to maintain muscle tone.

ASSESSING THE PATIENT AFTER SURGERY

After lumbar disk excision, vital signs are checked frequently and the wound is inspected for hemorrhage because vascular injury is a complication of disk surgery. Because postoperative neurologic deficits may occur from nerve root injury, the sensation and motor strength of the lower extremities are evaluated at specified intervals, along with the colour and temperature of the legs and sensation of the toes. It is important to assess for urinary retention, another sign of neurologic deterioration.

In discectomy with fusion, the patient has an additional surgical incision if bone fragments were taken from the iliac crest or fibula to serve as wedges in the spine. The recovery period is longer than for those patients who underwent discectomy without spinal fusion because bony union must take place.

POSITIONING THE PATIENT

To position the patient, a pillow is placed under the head and the knee rest is elevated slightly to relax the back muscles. When the patient is lying on one side, however, extreme knee flexion must be avoided. The patient is encouraged to move from side to side to relieve pressure and is reassured that no injury will result from moving. When the patient is ready to turn, the bed is placed in a flat position and a pillow is placed between the legs. The patient turns as a unit (logrolls), without twisting the back.

To get out of bed, the patient lies on one side while pushing up to a sitting position. At the same time, the nurse or family member eases the patient's legs over the side of the bed. Coming

FIGURE 65-9 Before the patient undergoes laminectomy surgery, the logrolling technique that will be used for turning the patient should be demonstrated. The patient's arms will be crossed and the spine aligned. To avoid twisting the spine, the head, shoulders, knees, and hips are turned at the same time so that the patient rolls over like a log. When in a side-lying position, the patient's back, buttocks, and legs are supported with pillows.

to a sitting or standing posture is accomplished in one long, smooth motion. Most patients walk to the bathroom the same day as surgery. Sitting is discouraged except for defecation.

PROMOTING HOME AND COMMUNITY-BASED CARE

Teaching Patients Self-Care. The patient is advised to gradually increase activity as tolerated because it takes up to 6 weeks for the ligaments to heal. Excessive activity may result in spasm of the paraspinal muscles.

Activities that produce flexion strain on the spine (eg, driving a car) should be avoided until healing has taken place. Heat may be applied to the back to relax muscle spasms. Scheduled rest periods are important, and the patient is advised to avoid heavy work for 2 to 3 months after surgery. Exercises are prescribed to strengthen the abdominal and erector spinal muscles. A back brace or corset may be necessary if back pain persists.

POST-POLIO SYNDROME

Patients who survived the polio epidemic of the 1950s, many now elderly, are developing new symptoms of weakness, fatigue, and musculoskeletal pain. It is estimated that between 60% and 80% of the 640,000 polio survivors are experiencing the phenomenon known as post-polio syndrome. Men and women appear to be equally at risk (Chasens & Umlauf, 2000).

Pathophysiology

The exact cause of post-polio syndrome is not known, but researchers suspect that with aging or muscle overuse the neurons not destroyed originally by the poliovirus cannot continue generating axon sprouts. These new terminal axon sprouts reinnervated the affected muscles following the initial insult but may be more vulnerable as the body ages (Chasens & Umlauf, 2000).

Assessment and Diagnostic Findings

No specific diagnostic test exists for this syndrome. The clinical diagnosis is made on the basis of the history and physical examination and exclusion of other medical conditions that may be causing the new symptoms. Patients report a history of paralytic poliomyelitis with partial or complete recovery of function with a plateau of function for at least 10 years and then the recurrence of symptoms (Chasens & Umlauf, 2000; Chasens, Umlauf, Valappil et al., 2001).

Management

No specific medical or surgical treatment is available for this syndrome, and therefore nursing plays a pivotal role in the team approach to assisting patients and families in dealing with the symptoms of progressive loss of muscle strength and significant fatigue. Other health care professionals who may assist in patient care include physical, occupational, speech, and respiratory therapists. Nursing interventions are aimed at slowing the loss of strength and maintaining the patient's physical, psychological, and social well-being.

Patients need to plan and coordinate activities to conserve energy and reduce fatigue. Rest periods should be planned and assistive devices used to reduce weakness and fatigue. Important activities should be planned for the morning, as fatigue often increases in the afternoon and evening (Chasens & Umlauf, 2000).

One study investigated the barriers (internal and external environmental phenomena) that created further disability in polio survivors (Harrison & Stuifbergen, 2001). Disability, the inability to perform societal roles, was correlated with perceived barriers to health but not with functional limitations, comorbidity, or secondary conditions. Secondary conditions were correlated with the number of years that the patient had lived with the condition.

Pain in muscles and joints may be a problem. Nonpharmacologic techniques such as the application of heat and cold are most appropriate because these patients tend to have strong reactions to medications (Chasens & Umlouf, 2000).

Maintaining a balance between adequate nutritional intake yet avoiding excess calories that can lead to obesity in this sedentary group of patients is a challenge. Pulmonary hygiene and adequate fluid intake can help with airway management. Several interventions can improve sleep, including limiting caffeine intake before bedtime and assessing for nocturia. If nocturia is an issue, the patient needs to be evaluated for obstructive sleep apnea (Chasens et al., 2001). Supportive ventilation may be appropriate with continuous positive airway pressure if sleep apnea is a problem.

Bone density testing in patients with post-polio syndrome has demonstrated low bone mass and osteoporosis. Thus, the importance of identifying risks, preventing falls, and treating osteoporosis must be discussed with patients and families. The nurse also needs to remind patients and family members of the need for health promotion activities and health screening.

Critical Thinking Exercises

1. A 68-year-old patient with known cerebral metastases is admitted to the hospital. He reports a new-onset right-sided weakness and headache. What immediate action should you take? What medical treatments can you anticipate? What surgical treatment (if any) would be anticipated? What teaching for the patient and the family is warranted, and why?

2. A 35-year-old woman with a diagnosis of Huntington's disease is admitted to the nursing unit with pneumonia. Her husband is wondering if he should obtain genetic testing of their two children. What would the risks and benefits of genetic testing be? What type of individual and family supports and counselling services would you anticipate the need for and make referrals to? Explain the rationale for these referrals.

3. A 42-year-old man newly diagnosed with Parkinson's disease asks what type of medication he will be given. What are the possible medications that will be used to treat his disease, and the long-term effects of each? How would your discharge teaching targeted toward medications be modified if the patient lives alone?

4. A 60-year-old patient with post-polio syndrome is having difficulty with fatigue and pain. What interventions and actions would you suggest to assist in the management of these symptoms? What strategies would you advise the patient to avoid? What is the rationale for your suggestions? State the types of health promotion activities you would recommend to this patient and the rationale for your recommendations.

REFERENCES AND SELECTED READINGS

Books

American Cancer Society (2002). *Cancer facts and figures 2002.* Atlanta: American Cancer Society

Bach, J. (1999). *Guide to the evaluation and management of neuromuscular disease.* Philadelphia: Hanley & Belfus Inc.

Bigos, S., Bowyer, O., Braen, G., et al. (1994). *Acute low back problems in adults.* Clinical practice guideline No. 14, AHCPR Publication No. 95-0642. Rockville, MD: Agency for Health Care Policy and Research, Public Health Service, U.S. Department of Health and Human Services.

Bradley, W., Daroff, R., Fenichel, R., & Marsden, C. (Eds.). (2000). *Neurology in clinical practice* (3d ed., vol 2). Boston: Butterworth Heinemann.

British Columbia Cancer Agency. (2004). *Management: Cerebral metastasis.* Available at: http://www.bccancer.bc.ca. Retrieved June 15, 2005.

Brown, R. H., Meininger, V., & Swash, M. (2000). *Amyotrophic lateral sclerosis.* London: Martin Dunitz Ltd.

Karch, A. (2002). *Lippincott's nursing drug guide.* Philadelphia: Lippincott Williams & Wilkins.

Medbroadcast Canada. (2005). *Keeping your back healthy.* Available at: http://www.medbroadcast.com/condition_info_details.asp. Retrieved June 15, 2005.

Nevidjon, B., & Sowers, K. (2000). *A nurse's guide to cancer care.* Philadelphia: Lippincott Williams & Wilkins.

Sawle, G. (Ed.). (1999). *Movement disorders in clinical practice.* Oxford: Isis Medical Media Ltd.

Journals

Asterisks indicate nursing research articles.

Alzheimer's

Neuroinflammation Working Group (2000). Inflammation and Alzheimer's disease. *Neurobiology of Aging, 21,* 383–421.

Aisen, P. (2000). Anti-inflammatory therapy for Alzheimer's disease. *Neurobiology of Aging, 21,* 447–448.

Cooper, N. R., Kalaria, R. N., McGeer, P. L., et al. (2000). Key issues in Alzheimer's disease inflammation. *Neurobiology of Aging, 21,* 451–453.

Roses, A. (2000). Causes or consequences of inflammation and pathological signs of Alzheimer disease. *Neurobiology of Aging, 21,* 423–424.

Thal, L. (2000). Anti-inflammatory drugs and Alzheimer's disease. *Neurobiology of Aging, 21,* 449–450.

Amyotrophic Lateral Sclerosis

Boitano, L., Jordan, T., & Benditt, J. (2001). Noninvasive ventilation allows gastrostomy tube placement in patients with advanced ALS. *Neurology, 56,* 413–414.

Charles, T., & Swash, M. (2001). Amyotrophic lateral sclerosis: Current understanding. *Journal of Neuroscience Nursing, 33*(5), 245–253.

Lechtzin, N., Wiener, C., Clawson, L., et al. (2001). Hospitalization in amyotrophic lateral sclerosis: Causes, costs and outcomes. *Neurology, 56,* 753–757.

Miller, R. G., Mitchell, J. D., & Moore, D. H. (2001). Riluzole for amyotrophic lateral sclerosis (ALS)/motor neuron disease. *The Cochrane Database of Systematic Reviews, 2,* 2–20.

Newsom-Davis, I. C., Lyall, R. A., Leigh, P. N., et al. (2001). The effect of non-invasive positive pressure ventilation (NIPPV) on cognitive function in amyotrophic lateral sclerosis (ALS): A prospective study. *Journal of Neurology Neurosurgery Psychiatry, 71,* 482–487.

Robbins, R., Simmons, Z., Bremer, B., Walsh, et al. (2001). Quality of life in ALS is maintained as physical function declines. *Neurology, 56,* 442–444.

Rowland, L., & Shneider, N. (2001). Amyotrophic lateral sclerosis. *New England Journal of Medicine, 344*(22), 1688–1700.

Degenerative Disk Disease

Fishbain, D. (2000). Evidence-based data on pain relief with antidepressants. *Annals of Medicine, 32,* 305–316.

Hall, H. (1999). Surgery: Indications and options. *Neurological Clinics of North America, 17*(1), 113–130.

Humphreys, S. C., & Eck, J. (1999). Clinical evaluation and treatment for herniated lumbar disc. *American Family Physician, 59*(3), 575–580.

Narrayan, P., & Haid, R. (2001). Treatment of degenerative cervical disc disease. *Neurologic Clinics, 19*(1), 217–229.

Walker, B. F. (2000). The prevalence of low back pain: A systematic review of the literature from 1966 to 1998. *Journal of Spinal Disorders, 13*(3), 205–217.

Huntington's Disease

Bachoud-Levi, A., Remy, P., Nguyen, J. P., et al. (2000). Motor and cognitive improvements in patients with Huntington's disease after neural transplantation. *The Lancet, 356,* 1975–1979.

Diederich, N., & Goetz, C. (2000). Neuropsychological and behavioral aspects of transplants in Parkinson's disease and Huntington's disease. *Brain and Cognition, 42,* 294–306.

Hayden, M. (2000). Predictive testing for Huntington's disease: The calm after the storm. *The Lancet, 356,* 1944–1945.

Hofmann, N. (1999). Understanding the neuropsychiatric symptoms of Huntington's disease. *Journal of Neuroscience Nursing, 31*(5), 309–313.

Sullivan, F., Bird, E., Alpay, M., et al. (2001). Remotivation therapy and Huntington's disease. *Journal of Neuroscience Nursing, 33*(3), 136–142.

*Williams, J. K., Schutte, D., Evers, C., et al. (2000). Redefinition: Coping with normal results from predictive gene testing for neurodegenerative disorders. *Research in Nursing & Health, 23,* 260–269.

Muscular Dystrophy

Carson, A., & Hieber, K. V. (2001). Adult pediatric patients. *American Journal of Nursing, 101*(3), 46–53.

Natterlund, B., & Ahlstrom, G. (1999). Experience of social support in rehabilitation: A phenomenological study. *Journal of Advanced Nursing, 30*(6), 1332–1340.

Natterlund, B., Gunnarsson, L., & Ahlstrom, G. (2000). Disability, coping and quality of life in individuals with muscular dystrophy:

A prospective study over five years. *Disability and Rehabilitation, 22*(17), 776–785.

Oncologic Disorders

American Cancer Society (2001). *What are brain and spinal cord tumors?* Atlanta: American Cancer Society. Available at: http://www3.cancer.org.

DeAngelis, L. M. (2001). Brain tumors. *New England Journal of Medicine, 344*(2), 114–123.

Goodell, T., & Muller, P. (2001) Photodynamic therapy. A novel treatment for primary brain malignancy. *Journal of Neuroscience Nursing, 33*(6), 296–300.

Jacobs, W. B., & Perrin, R. G. (2001). Evaluation and treatment of spinal metastases. An overview. *Neurosurgical Focus, 11*(6), 1–23.

Lepola, I., Toljamo, M., Aho, R., & Louet, T. (2001). Being a brain tumor patient: A descriptive study of patients' experiences. *Journal of Neuroscience Nursing, 33*(3), 143–147.

Molson Medical Informatics Students Projects Site, McGill University. (2005). Brain tumour. Available at: http://sprojects.mmi.mcgill.ca/braintumour.

Rafferty-Mitchell, C., Scanlon, J., & Laskowski-Jones, L. (1999). Gamma knife radiosurgery. *American Journal of Nursing, 99*(10), 52–59.

Rude, M. (2000). Selected neurologic complications in the patient with cancer. *Critical Care Nursing Clinics of North America, 12*(3), 269–278.

Wilkes, G. (2000). Nutrition: The forgotten ingredient in cancer care. *American Journal of Nursing, 100*(4), 46–51.

Parkinson's Disease

Aminoff, M. (2000) Parkinson's disease. *Neurologic Clinics, 19*(1), 119–128.

Chase, T., Oh, J., & Konitsiotis, S. (2000). Antiparkinsonian and antidyskinetic activity of drugs targeting central glutamatergic mechanisms. *Journal of Neurology, 247*(Suppl 2), II/36–II/42.

Freed, C., Greene, P., Breeze, R., et al. (2001). Transplantation of embryonic dopamine neurons for severe Parkinson's disease. *New England Journal of Medicine, 344*(10), 710–719.

*Gray, P., & Hildebrand, K. (2000). Fall risk factors in Parkinson's disease. *Journal of Neuroscience Nursing, 32*(4), 222–228.

Herndon, C. M., Young, K., Herndon, A., & Dole, E. J. (2000). Parkinson's disease revisited. *Journal of Neuroscience Nursing, 32*(4), 216–221.

Koller, W. C., Lyons, K. E., Wilkinson, S. B., et al. (2001). Long-term safety and efficacy of unilateral deep brain stimulation of the thalamus in essential tremor. *Movement Disorders, 16*, 464–468.

Obeso, J., et al. (The Deep-Brain Stimulation for Parkinson's Disease Group). (2001). Deep-brain stimulation of the subthalamic nucleus or the pars interna of the globus pallidus in Parkinson's disease. *New England Journal of Medicine, 345*(13), 956–963.

Przuntek, H. (2000). Non-dopaminergic therapy in Parkinson's disease. *Journal of Neurology, 247*(Suppl 2), II/19–II/24.

Przuntek, H., Bittkau, S., Bliesath, H., et al. (2002). Budipine provides additional benefit in patients with Parkinson disease receiving a stable optimum dopaminergic drug regimen. *Archives of Neurology, 59*(5), 803–806.

Rascol, O. (2000). The pharmacological therapeutic management of levodopa-induced dyskinesias in patients with Parkinson's disease. *Journal of Neurology, 247*(Suppl 2), II/51–II/57.

Post-Polio Syndrome

Chasens, E., & Umlauf, M. (2000). Post-polio syndrome. *American Journal of Nursing, 100*(12), 60–64.

*Chasens, E., Umlauf, M., Valappil, T., & Singh, K. (2001). Nocturnal problems in postpolio syndrome: Sleep apnea symptoms and nocturia. *Rehabilitation Nursing, 26*(2), 66–71.

*Harrison, T., & Stuifbergen, A. (2001). Barriers that further disablement: A study of survivors of polio. *Journal of Neuroscience Nursing, 33*(3), 160–166.

RESOURCES AND WEBSITES

ALS Society of Canada, 265 Yorkland Blvd, Suite 300, Toronto, ON, M2B 1S5; http://www.als.ca.

American Brain Tumor Association, 2720 River Rd., Des Plaines, IL 60018; (847) 827-9910; http://www.abta.org.

American Cancer Society, 1599 Clifton Road NE, Atlanta, Georgia 30329; (800) 227-2345; http://www.cancer.org.

American Parkinson's Disease Association, 1250 Hyland Blvd. Suite 4B, Staten Island, NY 10305-1945; (800) 223-2732; http://www.apdaparkinson.com.

Amyotrophic Lateral Sclerosis Association, 27001 Agoura Road, Suite 150, Calabasas Hills, CA 91301; (800) 782-4747; (818) 880-9007 (patients only); http://www.alsa.org.

Arthritis Society; http://www.arthritis.ca.

British Columbia Cancer Agency; http://www.bccancer.bc.ca.

Huntington's Disease Society of America, 158 W. 29th Street, 7th Floor, New York, NY 10001-5300; (800) 345-4372; (212) 242-1968; http://www.hdsa.org.

Huntington Society of Canada; http://www.hsc-ca.org.

Muscular Dystrophy Association, 3300 East Sunrise Drive, Tucson, AZ 85718; (800) 572-1717; http://www.mdausa.org.

National Parkinson Foundation, Inc., Bob Hope Parkinson Research Center, 1501 NW 9th Ave., Bob Hope Rd., Miami, FL 33136-1494; (800)327-4545; http://www.parkinson.org.

National Brain Tumor Foundation, 414 Thirteenth Street, Suite 700, Oakland, CA 94612-2603; (800) 934-CURE; http://www.braintumor.org.

Ontario Medical Association and Ontario Ministry of Health and Long-term Care: Recommended Clinical Practice Guidelines; http://gacguidelines.ca.

Parkinson Society of Canada; http://www.parkinson.ca.

Société Alzheimer Society Canada; http://www.alzheimer.ca.

Musculoskeletal Function

Applying Concepts from NANDA, NIC, and NOC

Mrs. Jefferson is a 72-year-old woman with severe osteoarthritis of the spine and a recent history of left total hip replacement. She has been attending outpatient physical therapy sessions 3 times a week and uses a wheeled walker at home. She has been admitted to the hospital with a partial small bowel obstruction. The health care team anticipates that the obstruction will resolve with medical treatment, and her expected length of stay is 5 to 7 days. Currently she is allowed nothing by mouth, has a Salem sump tube in place, and is receiving peripheral parenteral nutrition. The nurse is concerned that Mrs. Jefferson's already impaired physical mobility will decline further secondary to her illness and the medical treatments that make independent ambulation difficult. The concept map illustrates the relationships that exist among the nursing diagnoses, interventions, and outcomes for one of Mrs. Jefferson's clinical problems.

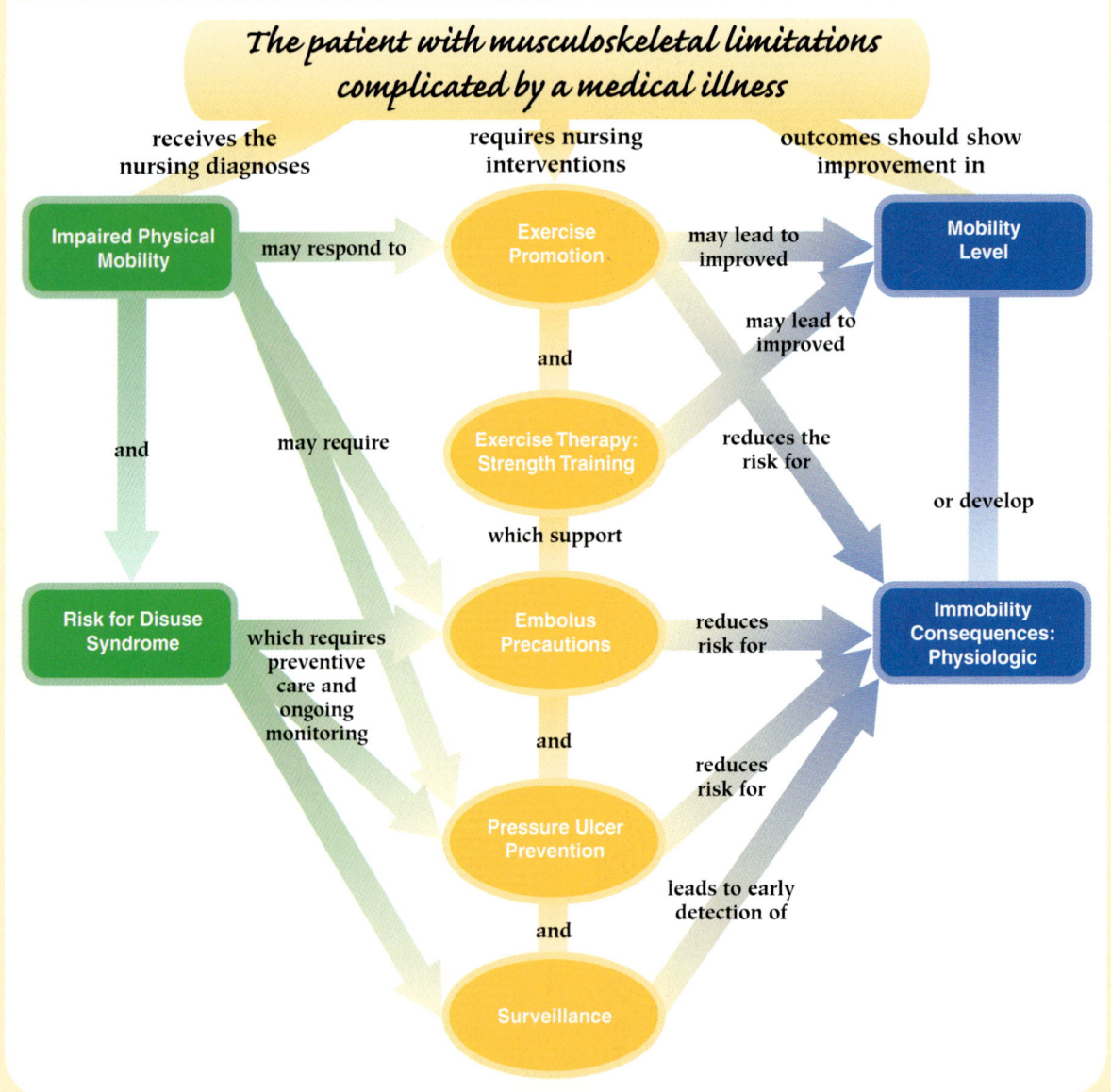

Nursing Classifications and Languages

NANDA
Nursing Diagnoses

Impaired Physical Mobility—Limitation in independent, purposeful physical movement of the body or of one or more extremities

Risk for Disuse Syndrome—At risk for deterioration of body systems as the result of prescribed or unavoidable musculoskeletal incapacity

NIC
Nursing Interventions*

Exercise Promotion—Facilitation of regular physical exercise to maintain or advance a higher degree of fitness

Exercise Therapy: Strength Training—Facilitating regular resistive muscle training to retain or increase muscle strength

Embolus Precautions—Reduction of the risk of embolus in a patient with thrombi or at risk for developing thrombi

Pressure Ulcer Prevention—Prevention of pressure ulcers for a patient at high risk for developing them

Surveillance—Purposeful and ongoing acquisition, interpretation, and synthesis of patient data for clinical decision-making

NOC
Nursing Outcomes†

Return to functional baseline status, stabilization of, or improvement in

Mobility Level—Ability to move purposefully

Immobility Consequences: Physiologic—Extent of compromise in physiologic functioning due to impaired physical mobility

NANDA, North American Nursing Diagnosis Association; NIC, Nursing Interventions Classification; NOC, Nursing Outcomes Classification

*Iowa Intervention Project © 2000. In Dochterman, J. M., & Bulechek, G. M. (2004). *Nursing interventions classification (NIC)* (4th ed.). St. Louis: Mosby.

†Iowa Outcomes Project © 2000. In Johnson, M., Maas, M., & Moorhead, S. (2000). *Nursing outcomes classification (NOC)* (3rd ed.). St. Louis: Mosby.

Assessment of Musculoskeletal Function

Adapted by Bonnie Friesen and Linda Larsen

LEARNING OBJECTIVES

On completion of this chapter, the learner will be able to:

1. Describe the anatomy and physiology of the musculoskeletal system.
2. Discuss the significance of the health history to the assessment of musculoskeletal health.
3. Describe the significance of physical assessment to the diagnosis of musculoskeletal dysfunction.
4. Specify the diagnostic tests used for assessment of musculoskeletal function.
5. Describe physical assessment of the musculoskeletal system.

The musculoskeletal system includes the bones, joints, muscles, tendons, ligaments, and bursae of the body. The problems associated with these structures are common and affect all age groups. Problems with the musculoskeletal system are generally not life-threatening, but they have a significant effect on the patient's normal activities and productivity. Nurses in all practice areas encounter patients with changes in musculoskeletal function.

Anatomic and Physiologic Overview

The health and proper functioning of the musculoskeletal system is interdependent with that of the other body systems. The bony structure provides protection for vital organs, including the brain, heart, and lungs. The bony skeleton provides a sturdy framework to support body structures. The bone matrix stores calcium, phosphorus, magnesium, and fluoride. More than 98% of the total-body calcium is present in bone. In addition, the red bone marrow located within bone cavities produces red and white blood cells in a process called hematopoiesis. Joints hold the bones together and allow the body to move. The muscles attached to the skeleton contract, moving the bones and producing heat, which helps to maintain body temperature.

STRUCTURE AND FUNCTION OF THE SKELETAL SYSTEM

There are 206 bones in the human body, divided into four categories:

- Long bones (eg, femur)
- Short bones (eg, metacarpals)
- Flat bones (eg, sternum)
- Irregular bones (eg, vertebrae)

The shape and construction of a specific bone are determined by its function and the forces exerted on it. Bones are constructed of **cancellous** (trabecular) or **cortical** (compact) bone tissue. Long bones are shaped like rods or shafts with rounded ends (Fig. 66-1). The shaft, known as the **diaphysis**, is primarily cortical bone. The ends of the long bones, called **epiphyses**, are primarily cancellous bone. The epiphyseal plate separates the epiphyses from the diaphysis and is the centre for longitudinal growth in children. In the adult, it is calcified. The ends of long bones are covered at the joints by articular **cartilage**, which is a tough, elastic, avascular tissue. Long bones are designed for weight bearing and movement. Short bones consist of cancellous bone covered by a layer of compact bone. Flat bones are important sites for hematopoiesis and frequently provide vital organ protection. They are made of cancellous bone layered between compact bone. Irregular bones have unique shapes related to their functions. Generally, irregular bone structure is similar to that of flat bones.

Bone is composed of cells, protein matrix, and mineral deposits. The cells are of three basic types—**osteoblasts, osteocytes, and osteoclasts.** Osteoblasts function in bone formation by secreting bone matrix. The matrix, which consists of collagen and ground substances (glycoproteins and proteoglycans), provides a framework in which inorganic mineral salts are deposited. Osteocytes are mature bone cells involved in bone-maintenance functions; they are located in lacunae (bone matrix units). Osteoclasts, located in shallow Howship's lacunae (small pits in bones), are multinuclear cells involved in destroying, resorbing, and remolding bone. The microscopic functioning unit of mature cortical bone is the **osteon** (Haversian system). The centre of the osteon, the Haversian canal, contains a capillary. Around the capillary are circles of mineralized bone matrix called **lamellae**. Within the lamellae are lacunae containing osteocytes. These are nourished

Glossary

atonic: without tone; denervated muscle that atrophies

atrophy: shrinkage-like decrease in the size of a muscle

bursa: fluid-filled sac found in connective tissue, usually in the area of joints

callus: cartilaginous/fibrous tissue at fracture site

cancellous bone: lattice-like bone structure; trabecular bone

cartilage: tough, elastic, avascular tissue at ends of bone

clonus: rhythmic contraction of muscle

contracture: abnormal shortening of muscle or joint, or both; fibrosis

cortical bone: compact bone

crepitus: grating or crackling sound or sensation; may occur with movement of ends of a broken bone or irregular joint surface

diaphysis: shaft of long bone

effusion: excess fluid in joint

endosteum: a thin, vascular membrane covering the marrow cavity of long bones and the spaces in cancellous bone

epiphysis: end of long bone

fascia (epimysium): fibrous tissue that covers, supports, and separates muscles

fasciculation: involuntary twitch of muscle fibres

flaccid: limp; without muscle tone

hypertrophy: enlargement; increase in size of muscle

isometric contraction: muscle tension increased, length unchanged, no joint motion

isotonic contraction: muscle tension unchanged, muscle shortened, joint moved

joint: area where bone ends meet; provides for motion and flexibility

joint capsule: fibrous tissue that encloses bone ends and other joint surfaces

kyphosis: increase in thoracic curvature of the spine

lamellae: mature compact bone structures that form concentric rings of bone matrix; lamellar bone

ligament: fibrous band connecting bones

lordosis: increase in lumbar curvature of the spine

ossification: process in which minerals (calcium) are deposited in bone matrix

osteoarthritis: degenerative joint disease characterized by destruction of the articular cartilage and overgrowth of bone

osteoblast: bone-forming cell

osteoclast: bone resorption cell

osteocyte: mature bone cell

osteogenesis: bone formation

osteoid: pertaining to bone matrix tissue; "pre-bone"

osteon: microscopic functional bone unit

osteoporosis: significant loss of bone mass and strength with increased risk for fracture

paralysis: absence of muscle movement suggesting nerve damage

paresthesia: abnormal sensation (eg, burning, tingling, numbness)

periosteum: fibrous connective tissue covering bone

remodeling: process of reorganizing new bone structure according to function

resorption: removal/destruction of tissue, such as bone

scoliosis: lateral curving of the spine

spastic: having greater than normal muscle tone

synovium: membrane in joint that secretes lubricating fluid

tendon: cord of fibrous tissue connecting muscle to bone

tone (tonus): normal tension (resistance to stretch) in resting muscle

trabeculae: lattice-like bone structure; cancellous bone

Proximal
epiphysis

Cartilage

Growth lines

Spongy bone
(containing red marrow)

Endosteum

Compact bone

Medullary (marrow)
cavity

Yellow marrow

Diaphysis

Periosteum

Artery

Osteocytes

Volkmann's
canal

Periosteum

Distal
epiphysis

Blood vessels

FIGURE 66-1 Structure of a long bone;
composition of compact bone.

through tiny structures, canaliculi (canals), that communicate with adjacent blood vessels within the Haversian system (see Fig. 66-1).

Lacunae in cancellous bone are layered in an irregular lattice network (**trabeculae**). Red bone marrow fills the lattice network. Capillaries nourish the osteocytes located in the lacunae.

Covering the bone is a dense, fibrous membrane known as the **periosteum**. The periosteum nourishes bone and allows for its growth; it also provides for the attachment of tendons and ligaments. The periosteum contains nerves, blood vessels, and lymphatics. The layer closest to the bone contains osteoblasts, which are bone-forming cells.

The **endosteum** is a thin, vascular membrane that covers the marrow cavity of long bones and the spaces in cancellous bone. Osteoclasts, which dissolve bone to maintain the marrow cavity, are located near the endosteum in Howship's lacunae.

Bone marrow is a vascular tissue located in the medullary (shaft) cavity of long bones and in flat bones. Red bone marrow, located mainly in the sternum, ilium, vertebrae, and ribs in adults, is responsible for producing red and white blood cells. In adults, the long bone is filled with fatty, yellow marrow.

Bone tissue is well vascularized. Cancellous bone receives a rich blood supply through metaphyseal and epiphyseal vessels. Periosteal vessels carry blood to compact bone through minute Volkmann's canals. In addition, nutrient arteries penetrate the periosteum and enter the medullary cavity through foramina (small openings). Nutrient arteries supply blood to the marrow and bone. The venous system may accompany arteries or may exit independently.

Bone Formation (Osteogenesis)

Bone begins to form long before birth. **Ossification** is the process by which the bone matrix (collagen fibres and ground substance) is formed and hardening minerals (eg, calcium salts) are deposited on the collagen fibres. The collagen fibres give tensile strength to the bone, and the calcium provides compressional strength.

There are two basic processes of ossification: endochondral and intramembranous. Most bones in the body are formed by endochondral ossification, in which a cartilage-like tissue (**osteoid**) is formed, resorbed, and replaced by bone. Intramembranous ossification occurs when bone develops within membrane, as in the bones of the face and skull.

Bone Maintenance

Bone is a dynamic tissue in a constant state of turnover— **resorption** and formation. The important regulating factors that determine the balance between bone formation and bone resorption include local stress, vitamin D, parathyroid hormone, calcitonin, and blood supply.

Local stress (weight bearing) acts to simulate bone formation and remodeling. Weight-bearing bones are thick and strong. Without weight-bearing or stress, as in prolonged bed rest, the bone loses calcium (resorption) and becomes osteopenic and weak. The weak bone may fracture easily.

Biologically active vitamin D (calcitriol) functions to increase the amount of calcium in the blood by promoting absorption of calcium from the gastrointestinal tract. It also facilitates mineralization of osteoid tissue. A deficiency of vitamin D results in bone mineralization deficit, deformity, and fracture.

Parathyroid hormone and calcitonin are the major hormonal regulators of calcium homeostasis. Parathyroid hormone regulates the concentration of calcium in the blood, in part by promoting movement of calcium from the bone. In response to low calcium levels in the blood, increased levels of parathyroid hormone prompt the mobilization of calcium, the demineralization of bone, and the formation of bone cysts. Calcitonin, secreted by the thyroid gland in response to elevated blood calcium levels, inhibits bone resorption and increases the deposit of calcium in bone.

Blood supply to the bone also affects bone formation. With diminished blood supply or hyperemia (congestion), **osteogenesis** (bone formation) and bone density decrease. Bone necrosis occurs when the bone is deprived of blood.

Bone Healing

Most fractures heal through a combination of intramembranous and endochondral ossification processes. When a bone is fractured, the bone fragments are not merely patched together with scar tissue. Instead, the bone regenerates itself.

Fracture healing occurs in four areas, including:

- Bone marrow, where endothelial cells rapidly undergo transformation and become osteoblastic bone-forming cells
- Bone cortex, where new osteons are formed
- Periosteum, where a hard callus/bone is formed through intramembranous ossification peripheral to the fracture, and where a cartilage model is formed through endochondral ossification adjacent to the fracture site
- External soft tissue, where a bridging **callus** (fibrous tissue) stabilizes the fracture

Buckwalter (2000) summarized the process of fracture healing into six stages stimulated by the release and activation of biologic regulators and signaling molecules:

1. *Hematoma and inflammation:* The body's response is similar to that after injury elsewhere in the body. There is bleeding into the injured tissue and formation of a fracture hematoma. The hematoma is the source of signaling molecules, such as cytokines, transforming growth factor-beta (TGF-β), and platelet-derived growth factor (PDGF), which initiate the fracture healing processes. The fracture fragment ends become devitalized because of the interrupted blood supply. The injured area is invaded by macrophages (large white blood cells), which débride the area. Inflammation, swelling, and pain are present. The inflammatory stage lasts several days and resolves with a decrease in pain and swelling.

2. *Angiogenesis and cartilage formation:* Under the influence of signaling molecules, cell proliferation and differentiation occur. Blood vessels and cartilage overlie the fracture.

3. *Cartilage calcification:* Chondrocytes in the cartilage callus form matrix vesicles, which regulate calcification of the cartilage. Enzymes within these matrix vesicles prepare the cartilage for calcium release and deposit.

4. *Cartilage removal:* The calcified cartilage is invaded by blood vessels and becomes resorbed by chondroblasts and osteoclasts. It is replaced by woven bone similar to that of the growth plate.

5. *Bone formation:* Minerals continue to be deposited until the bone is firmly reunited. With major adult long bone fractures, ossification takes 3 to 4 months.

6. *Remodeling:* The final stage of fracture repair consists of **remodeling** the new bone into its former structural arrangement. Remodeling may take months to years, depending on the extent of bone modification needed, the function of the bone, and the functional stresses on the bone. Cancellous bone heals and remodels more rapidly than does compact cortical bone.

Serial x-ray films are used to monitor the progress of bone healing. The type of bone fractured, the adequacy of blood supply, the surface contact of the fragments, and the general health of the person influence the rate of fracture healing. Adequate immobilization is essential until there is x-ray evidence of bone formation with ossification.

BONE HEALING WITH FRAGMENTS FIRMLY APPROXIMATED

When fractures are treated with open rigid compression plate fixation techniques, the bony fragments can be placed in direct contact. Primary bone healing occurs through cortical bone (Haversian) remodeling. Little or no cartilaginous callus develops. Immature bone develops from the endosteum. There is an intensive regeneration of new osteons, which develop in the fracture line by a process similar to normal bone maintenance. Fracture strength is obtained when the new osteons have become established.

STRUCTURE AND FUNCTION OF THE ARTICULAR SYSTEM

The junction of two or more bones is called a **joint** (articulation). There are three basic kinds of joints: synarthrosis, amphiarthrosis, and diarthrosis joints. Synarthrosis joints are immovable, as exemplified by the skull sutures. Amphiarthrosis joints, such as the vertebral joints and the symphysis pubis, allow limited motion. The bones of amphiarthrosis joints are joined by fibrous cartilage. Diarthrosis joints are freely movable joints (Fig. 66-2).

There are several types of diarthrosis joints:

- *Ball-and-socket* joints, best exemplified by the hip and the shoulder, permit full freedom of movement.
- *Hinge* joints permit bending in one direction only and are best exemplified by the elbow and the knee.
- *Saddle* joints allow movement in two planes at right angles to each other. The joint at the base of the thumb is a saddle, biaxial joint.
- *Pivot* joints are characterized by the articulation between the radius and the ulna. They permit rotation for such activities as turning a doorknob.
- *Gliding* joints allow for limited movement in all directions and are represented by the joints of the carpal bones in the wrist.

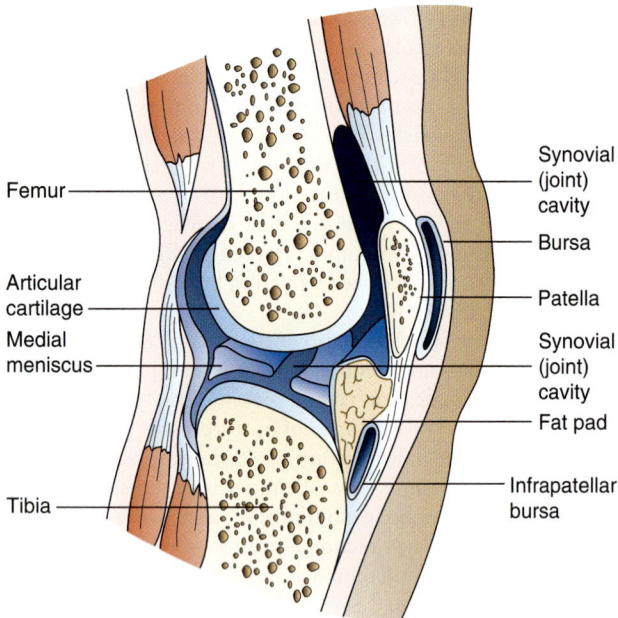

Femur

Articular
cartilage

Medial
meniscus

Tibia

Synovial
(joint)
cavity

Bursa

Patella

Synovial
(joint)
cavity

Fat pad

Infrapatellar
bursa

FIGURE 66-2   Hinge joint of the knee.

The ends of the articulating bones of a typical movable joint are covered with smooth hyaline cartilage. A tough, fibrous sheath called the **joint capsule** surrounds the articulating bones. The capsule is lined with a membrane, the **synovium**, which secretes the lubricating and shock-absorbing synovial fluid into the joint capsule. Therefore, the bone surfaces are not in direct contact. In some synovial joints (eg, the knee), fibrocartilage disks (eg, medial meniscus) are located between the articular cartilage surfaces. These disks provide shock absorption.

Ligaments (fibrous connective tissue bands) bind the articulating bones together. Ligaments and muscle tendons, which pass over the joint, provide joint stability. In some joints, interosseous ligaments (eg, the cruciate ligaments of the knee) are found within the capsule and add stability to the joint.

A **bursa** is a sac filled with synovial fluid that cushions the movement of tendons, ligaments, and bones at a point of friction. Bursae are found at the elbow, shoulder, knee, and some other joints.

STRUCTURE AND FUNCTION OF THE SKELETAL MUSCLE SYSTEM

Muscles are attached by **tendons** (cords of fibrous connective tissue) or aponeuroses (broad, flat sheets of connective tissue) to bones, connective tissue, other muscles, soft tissue, or skin. The muscles of the body are composed of parallel groups of muscle cells (fasciculi) encased in fibrous tissue called **fascia** or **epimysium**. The more fasciculi contained in a muscle, the more precise the movements. Muscles vary in shape and size according to the activities for which they are responsible. Skeletal (striated) muscles are involved in body movement, posture, and heat-production functions. Muscles contract to bring the two points of attachment closer together, resulting in movement.

Skeletal Muscle Contraction

Each muscle cell (also referred to as a muscle fibre) contains myofibrils, which in turn are composed of a series of sarcomeres, the actual contractile units of skeletal muscle. Sarcomeres contain thick myosin and thin actin filaments.

Muscle fibres contract in response to electrical stimulation delivered by an effector nerve cell at the motor end plate. When stimulated, the muscle cell depolarizes and generates an action potential in a manner similar to that described for nerve cells. These action potentials propagate along the muscle cell membrane and lead to the release of calcium ions that are stored in specialized organelles called the sarcoplasmic reticulum. When there is a local increase in calcium ion concentration, the myosin and actin filaments slide across one another. Shortly after the muscle cell membrane is depolarized, it recovers its resting membrane voltage. Calcium is rapidly removed from the sarcomeres by active reaccumulation in the sarcoplasmic reticulum. When calcium concentration in the sarcomere decreases, the myosin and actin filaments cease to interact, and the sarcomere returns to its original resting length (relaxation). Actin and myosin do not interact in the absence of calcium.

Energy is consumed during muscle contraction and relaxation. The primary source of energy for the muscle cells is adenosine triphosphate (ATP), which is generated through cellular oxidative metabolism. At low levels of activity (ie, sedentary activity), the skeletal muscle synthesizes ATP from the oxidation of glucose to water and carbon dioxide. During periods of strenuous activity, when sufficient oxygen may not be available, glucose is metabolized primarily to lactic acid, an inefficient process compared with that of oxidative pathways. Stored muscle glycogen is used to supply glucose during periods of activity. Muscle fatigue is thought to be caused by depletion of glycogen and accumulation of lactic acid. As a result, the cycle of muscle contraction and relaxation cannot continue.

During muscle contraction, the energy released from ATP is not completely used. The excess energy is dissipated in the form of heat. During isometric contraction, almost all of the energy is released in the form of heat; during isotonic contraction, some of the energy is expended in mechanical work. In some situations, such as shivering because of cold, the need to generate heat is the primary stimulus for muscle contraction.

Types of Muscle Contractions

The contraction of muscle fibres can result in either isotonic or isometric contraction of the muscle. In **isometric contraction**, the length of the muscles remains constant but the force generated by the muscles is increased; an example of this is when one pushes against an immovable wall. **Isotonic contraction**, on the other hand, is characterized by shortening of the muscle with no increase in tension within the muscle; an example of this is flexion of the forearm. In normal activities, many muscle movements are a combination of isometric and isotonic contractions. For example, during walking, isotonic contraction results in shortening of the leg, and isometric contraction causes the stiff leg to push against the floor.

The speed of the muscle contraction is variable. Myoglobulin is a hemoglobin-like protein pigment present in striated muscle cells that transports oxygen. Muscles containing large quantities of myoglobulin (red muscles) have been observed to contract slowly and powerfully (eg, respiratory and postural muscles). Muscles containing little myoglobulin (white muscles) contract quickly (eg, extraocular eye muscles). Most muscles contain both red and white muscle fibres.

Muscle Tone

Relaxed muscles demonstrate a state of readiness to respond to contraction stimuli. This state of readiness, known as muscle **tone (tonus),** is produced by the maintenance of some of the muscle fibres in a contracted state. Muscle spindles, which are sense organs in the muscles, monitor muscle tone. Muscle tone is minimal during sleep and is increased when the person is anxious. A muscle that is limp and without tone is described as **flaccid**; a muscle with greater-than-normal tone is described as **spastic**. In conditions characterized by lower motor neuron destruction (eg, polio), denervated muscle becomes **atonic** (soft and flabby) and atrophies.

Muscle Actions

Muscles accomplish movement by contraction. Through the co-ordination of muscle groups, the body is able to perform a wide variety of movements (Chart 66-1). The prime mover is the muscle that causes a particular motion. The muscles assisting the prime mover are known as synergists. The muscles causing movement opposite to that of the prime mover are known as antagonists. An antagonist must relax to allow the prime mover to contract, producing motion. For example, when contraction of the biceps causes flexion of the elbow joint, the biceps is the prime mover, and the triceps is the antagonist. A person with muscle **paralysis**, which is a loss of movement possibly from nerve damage, may be able to retrain functioning muscles within the synergistic group to produce the needed movement. Muscles of the synergistic group then become the prime mover.

Exercise, Disuse, and Repair

Muscles need to be exercised to maintain function and strength. When a muscle repeatedly develops maximum or close to maximum tension over a long time, as in regular exercise with weights, the cross-sectional area of the muscle increases. This enlargement, known as **hypertrophy**, results from an increase in the size of individual muscle fibres without an increase in the number of muscle fibres. Hypertrophy persists only if the exercise is continued. The opposite phenomenon occurs with disuse of muscle over a long period of time. Age and disuse cause loss of muscular function as fibrotic tissue replaces the contractile muscle tissue. The decrease in the size of a muscle is called **atrophy**. Bed rest and immobility cause loss of muscle mass and strength. When immobility is the result of a treatment mode (eg, casting, traction), the patient can decrease the effects of immobility by isometric exercise of the muscles of the immobilized part. Quadriceps setting exercises (tightening the muscles of the thigh) and gluteal setting exercises (tightening of the muscles of the buttocks) help maintain the larger muscle groups that are important in ambulation. Active and weight-resistance exercises of uninjured parts of the body maintain muscle strength. When muscles are injured, they need rest and immobilization until tissue repair occurs. The healed muscle then needs progressive exercise to resume its pre-injury strength and functional ability.

Gerontologic Considerations

Multiple changes in the musculoskeletal system occur with aging (Table 66-1). Bone mass peaks at about 35 years of age, after which there is a universal gradual loss of bone. There is a loss of height due to osteoporosis (abnormal excessive bone loss), kyphosis, thinned intervertebral disks, and flexion of the knees and hips. Numerous metabolic changes, including menopausal withdrawal of estrogen and decreased activity, contribute to osteoporosis. Women lose more bone mass than men do. Additionally, bones change in shape and have reduced strength. Fractures are com-

mon. In the elderly, collagen structures are less able to absorb energy. Ligaments become weak. The articular cartilage degenerates in weight-bearing areas and heals less readily. This contributes to the development of **osteoarthritis**. Joints enlarge and range of motion decreases. Muscle mass and strength are also diminished. There is an actual loss in the size and number of muscle fibres due to myofibril atrophy with fibrous tissue replacement. Increased inactivity, diminished neuron stimulation, and nutritional deficiencies contribute to loss of muscle strength. In addition, remote musculoskeletal problems for which the patient has compensated may become new problems with age-related changes. For example, people who have had polio and who have been able to function normally by using synergistic muscle groups may discover increasing incapacity because of a reduced compensatory ability. Many of the effects of aging, however, can be slowed if the body is kept healthy and active through positive lifestyle behaviours.

Assessment

HEALTH HISTORY

The nursing assessment of the patient with musculoskeletal dysfunction includes an evaluation of the effects of the musculoskeletal problem on the patient. The nurse is concerned with assisting patients who have musculoskeletal problems to maintain their general health, accomplish their activities of daily living, and manage their treatment programs. The nurse ensures systemic homeostasis, encourages optimal nutrition, and prevents problems related to immobility. Through an individualized plan of nursing care, the nurse helps the patient achieve maximum health.

Initial Interview

In the initial interview, the nurse obtains a general impression of the patient's health status, gathering subjective data from the patient concerning the onset of the problem and how it has been managed, as well as the patient's perceptions and expectations related to health. Concurrent health conditions (eg, diabetes, heart disease, chronic obstructive pulmonary disease, infection, preexisting disability) and related problems, such as familial or genetic abnormalities, also need to be considered when developing the plan of care. A history of medication use and response to pain medication aids in designing medication management regimens.

The nurse notes allergies and describes them in terms of the reactions they produce in the patient. The nurse also assesses the patient's use of tobacco, alcohol, and other drugs to evaluate how these agents may affect patient care. Information concerning the patient's learning ability, economic status, and current occupation is needed for rehabilitation and discharge planning. Additions to the initial interview data are made as the nurse interacts with the patient. Such data assist the nurse to adjust the individualized plan of care as needed.

Assessment Data

During the interview and physical assessment, the patient may report pain, tenderness, tightness, and abnormal sensations. The nurse assesses and documents this information.

PAIN

Most patients with diseases and traumatic conditions or disorders of muscles, bones, and joints experience pain. Bone pain is characteristically described as a dull, deep ache that is "boring" in nature,

Chart 66-1 **Body Movements Produced by Muscle Contraction**

Flexion—bending at a joint (eg, elbow)
Extension—straightening at a joint
Abduction—moving away from midline
Adduction—moving toward
   midline
Rotation—turning around a specific
   axis (eg, shoulder joint)
Circumduction—cone-like
   movement
Supination—turning upward
Pronation—turning downward
Inversion—turning inward
Eversion—turning outward
Protraction—pushing forward
Retraction—pulling backward

From Weber, J. W., & Kelley, J. (2003).
Health assessment in nursing (2nd ed.).
Philadelphia: Lippincott Williams & Wilkins.

Abduction

Adduction

Protraction of mandible

Retraction of mandible

Pronation

Supination

Circumduction

Extension

Flexion

Rotation

Inversion

Eversion

Table 66-1 • Age-Related Changes of the Musculoskeletal System			
MUSCULOSKELETAL SYSTEM	**STRUCTURAL CHANGES**	**FUNCTIONAL CHANGES**	**HISTORY AND PHYSICAL FINDINGS**
Bones	Gradual, progressive loss of bone mass after age 35 yr Vertebrae collapse	Bones fragile and prone to fracture: vertebrae, hip, wrist	Loss of height Posture changes Kyphosis Flexion of hips and knees Back pain Osteoporosis Fracture
Muscles	Increase in collagen and resultant fibrosis Muscles diminish in size (atrophy); wasting Tendons less elastic	Loss of strength and flexibility Weakness Fatigue Stumbling Falls	Loss of strength Diminished agility Decreased endurance Prolonged response time (diminished reaction time) Diminished tone Broad base of support History of falls
Joints	Cartilage—progressive deterioration Thinning of intervertebral discs	Stiffness, reduced flexibility, and pain interfere with activities of daily living	Diminished range of motion Loss of flexibility Stiffness Loss of height
Ligaments	Lax ligaments (less than normal strength; weakness)	Postural joint abnormality Weakness	Joint pain on motion; resolves with rest Crepitus Joint swelling/enlargement Degenerative joint disease (osteoarthritis)

whereas muscular pain is described as soreness or aching and is referred to as "muscle cramps." Fracture pain is sharp and piercing and is relieved by immobilization. Sharp pain may also result from bone infection with muscle spasm or pressure on a sensory nerve.

Rest relieves most musculoskeletal pain. Pain that increases with activity may indicate joint sprain or muscle strain, whereas steadily increasing pain points to the progression of an infectious process (osteomyelitis), a malignant tumour, or neurovascular complications. Radiating pain occurs in conditions in which pressure is exerted on a nerve root. Pain is variable, and its assessment and nursing management must be individualized.

Questions that the nurse can ask regarding pain include the following:

How does the patient describe the pain?
Is the pain localized?
Does the pain radiate? If so, in which direction and to which body parts?
Is there pain in any other part of the body?
How intense is the pain on a scale of 0 to 10 (with 10 being the worst possible pain)?
What is the character of the pain (sharp, dull, boring, shooting, throbbing, cramping)?
Is it constant? Is it increasing or decreasing in intensity?
What relieves it?
What makes it worse?
What was the patient doing before the pain occurred?
What was the manner of onset?
Is the body in proper alignment?
Is there pressure from traction, bed linens, a cast, or other appliances?
Is there tension on the skin at a pin site?

Does the patient experience increased discomfort when overly tired from lack of sleep, exciting stimuli, or too much activity?

It is important that the patient's pain and discomfort be managed successfully. Not only is pain exhausting, but, if prolonged, it can force the patient to become increasingly preoccupied and dependent (see Chapter 13).

ALTERED SENSATIONS

Sensory disturbances are frequently associated with musculoskeletal problems. The patient may describe **paresthesias**, which are burning, tingling sensations or numbness. These sensations may be caused by pressure on nerves or by circulatory impairment. Soft tissue swelling or direct trauma to these structures can impair their function. The nurse assesses the neurovascular status of the involved musculoskeletal area.

Questions that the nurse can ask regarding altered sensations include the following:

Is the patient experiencing any abnormal sensations or numbness?
When did this begin? Is it getting worse?
Does the patient also have pain?
Can the patient move the affected part?
What is the colour of the part distal to the affected area? Is it pale? Dusky? Cyanotic?
Does rapid capillary refill occur? (The nurse can gently squeeze a nail until it blanches, then release the pressure. The amount of time for the colour under the nail to return to normal is noted. Colour normally returns within 3 seconds. The return of colour is evidence of capillary refill.)
Is a pulse palpable distal to the affected area?

GENETICS IN NURSING PRACTICE—Musculoskeletal Disorders

When assessing a patient with musculoskeletal complaints, nurses should not overlook the possibility of a genetic component to the patient's problems

MUSCULOSKELETAL IMPAIRMENTS INFLUENCED BY GENETIC FACTORS

- Achondroplasia
- Club foot
- Congenital hip dislocation
- Ehlers-Danlos syndrome
- Marfan syndrome
- Stickler syndrome
- Osteogenesis imperfecta
- Osteoporosis
- Scoliosis

NURSING ASSESSMENTS

FAMILY HISTORY

- Assess for other similarly affected family members
- Assess for the presence of other related genetic conditions (eg, hematologic, cardiac, integumentary conditions)
- Determine the age at onset (eg, fractures present at birth as in osteogenesis imperfecta, or later onset osteoporosis)

PHYSICAL ASSESSMENT

- Assess for other skeletal findings including pectus excavatum, scoliosis, long fingers (Marfan syndrome)
- Assess for signs of blue/grey sclerae, opalescent dentin, hearing impairment (osteogenesis imperfecta)
- Assess stature (unusually short—achondroplasia; unusually tall—Marfan syndrome)
- Assess skin for velvety texture with unusual scarring and/or thin fragile skin (Ehlers-Danlos syndrome)

- Assess for vision impairment (Stickler syndrome, Marfan syndrome)

MANAGEMENT ISSUES SPECIFIC TO GENETICS

- Inquire whether DNA gene mutation or other genetic testing has been performed on affected family members.
- If indicated, refer patient for further genetic counselling and evaluation so that family members can discuss inheritance, risk to other family members, and the availability of genetic testing and gene-based interventions
- Offer appropriate genetics information and resources
- Assess patient's understanding of genetics information
- Provide support to families with newly diagnosed genetic-related digestive disorders
- Participate in management and coordination of care of patients with genetic conditions and individuals predisposed to develop or pass on a genetic condition

GENETICS RESOURCES

Genetic Alliance—a directory of support groups for patients and families with genetic conditions; www.geneticalliance.org

Gene Clinics—a listing of common genetic disorders with up-to-date clinical summaries, genetic counselling and testing information; www.geneclinics.org

National Organization of Rare Disorders—a directory of support groups and information for patients and families with rare genetic disorders; www.rarediseases.org

OMIM: Online Mendelian Inheritance in Man—a complete listing of inherited genetic conditions; http://www.ncbi.nlm.nih.gov/omim/stats/html

---

Is edema present?

Is any constrictive device or clothing causing nerve or vascular compression?

Does elevating the affected part or modifying its position affect the symptoms?

PHYSICAL ASSESSMENT

An examination of the musculoskeletal system ranges from a basic assessment of functional capabilities to sophisticated physical examination manoeuvres that facilitate diagnosis of specific bone, muscle, and joint disorders (Chart 66-2). The extent of assessment depends on the patient's physical complaints, health history, and physical clues that warrant further exploration. The nursing assessment is primarily a functional evaluation, focusing on the patient's ability to perform activities of daily living.

Techniques of inspection and palpation are used to evaluate the patient's posture, gait, bone integrity, joint function, and muscle strength and size. In addition, assessing the skin and neurovascular status is an important part of a complete musculoskeletal assessment. The nurse also should understand and be able to perform correct assessment techniques on patients with musculoskeletal trauma. When specific symptoms or physical findings of musculoskeletal dysfunction are apparent, the nurse carefully

documents the examination findings and shares the information with the physician, who may decide that more extensive examination and diagnostic workup are necessary.

Posture

The normal curvature of the spine is convex through the thoracic portion and concave through the cervical and lumbar portions. Common deformities of the spine include **kyphosis**, an increased forward curvature of the thoracic spine; **lordosis**, or swayback, an exaggerated curvature of the lumbar spine; and **scoliosis**, a lateral curving deviation of the spine (Fig. 66-3). Kyphosis is frequently seen in elderly patients with osteoporosis and in some patients with neuromuscular diseases. Scoliosis may be congenital, idiopathic (without an identifiable cause), or the result of damage to the paraspinal muscles, as in poliomyelitis. Lordosis is frequently seen during pregnancy as the woman adjusts her posture in response to changes in her centre of gravity.

During inspection of the spine, the entire back, buttocks, and legs are exposed. The examiner inspects the spinal curves and trunk symmetry from posterior and lateral views. Standing behind the patient, the examiner notes any differences in the height of the shoulders or iliac crests. The gluteal folds are normally symmetric. Shoulder and hip symmetry, as well as the line of the

Chart 66-2 • ASSESSMENT

Peripheral Nerve Function

Assessment of peripheral nerve function has two key elements: evaluation of sensation and evaluation of motion. The nurse may perform one or all of the following during a musculoskeletal assessment.

Nerve	Test of Sensation	Test of Movement
Peroneal nerve	Prick the skin centred between the great and second toe.	Ask the patient to dorsiflex the ankle and extend the toes.
Tibial nerve	Prick the medial and lateral surface of the sole.	Ask the patient to plantarflex toes and ankle.
Radial nerve	Prick the skin centred between the thumb and second finger.	Ask the patient to stretch out the thumb, then the wrist, and then the fingers at the metacarpal joints.
Ulnar nerve	Prick the fat pad at the top of the small finger.	Ask the patient to spread all fingers.
Median nerve	Prick the top or distal surface of the index finger.	Ask the patient to touch the thumb to the little finger. Also observe whether the patient can flex the wrist.

vertebral column, are inspected with the patient erect and with the patient bending forward (flexion). (Scoliosis is evidenced by an abnormal lateral curve in the spine, shoulders that are not level, an asymmetric waistline, and a prominent scapula, accentuated by bending forward.) Older adults experience a loss in height due to loss of vertebral cartilage and osteoporosis-related vertebral fractures. Therefore, an adult's height should be measured periodically.

Gait

Gait is assessed by having the patient walk away from the examiner for a short distance. The examiner observes the patient's gait for smoothness and rhythm. Any unsteadiness or irregular movements (frequently noted in elderly patients) are considered abnormal. When a limping motion is noted, it is most frequently caused by painful weight bearing. In such instances, the patient can usually pinpoint the area of discomfort, thus guiding further examination. If one extremity is shorter than another, a limp may also be observed as the patient's pelvis drops downward on the affected side with each step. Limited joint motion may affect gait. In addition, a variety of neurologic conditions are associated with abnormal gaits such as a spastic hemiparesis gait (stroke), steppage gait (lower motor neuron disease), and shuffling gait (Parkinson's disease).

Bone Integrity

The bony skeleton is assessed for deformities and alignment. Symmetric parts of the body are compared. Abnormal bony growths due to bone tumours may be observed. Shortened extremities, amputations, and body parts that are not in anatomic alignment are noted. Fracture findings may include abnormal angulation of long bones, motion at points other than joints, and crepitus (a grating sound) at the point of abnormal motion. Movement of fracture fragments must be minimized to avoid additional injury.

Joint Function

The articular system is evaluated by noting range of motion, deformity, stability, and nodular formation. Range of motion is evaluated both actively (the joint is moved by the muscles surrounding the joint) and passively (the joint is moved by the examiner). The examiner is familiar with the normal range of motion of major joints (see Chapter 11). Precise measurement of range of motion can be made by a goniometer (a protractor designed for evaluating joint motion). Limited range of motion may be the result of skeletal deformity, joint pathology, or **contracture** of the surrounding muscles, tendons, and joint capsule. In elderly patients, limitations of range of motion associated with **osteoarthritis** (degenerative joint disease) may reduce their ability to perform activities of daily living.

If joint motion is compromised or the joint is painful, the joint is examined for **effusion** (excessive fluid within the capsule), swelling, and increased temperature that may reflect active inflammation. An effusion is suspected if the joint is swollen and the normal bony landmarks are obscured. The most common site for joint effusion is the knee. If a small amount of fluid is present in the joint spaces beneath the patella, it may be identified by the following manoeuvre. The medial and lateral aspects of the extended knee are milked firmly in a downward motion. This displaces any fluid downward. As pressure is exerted against the

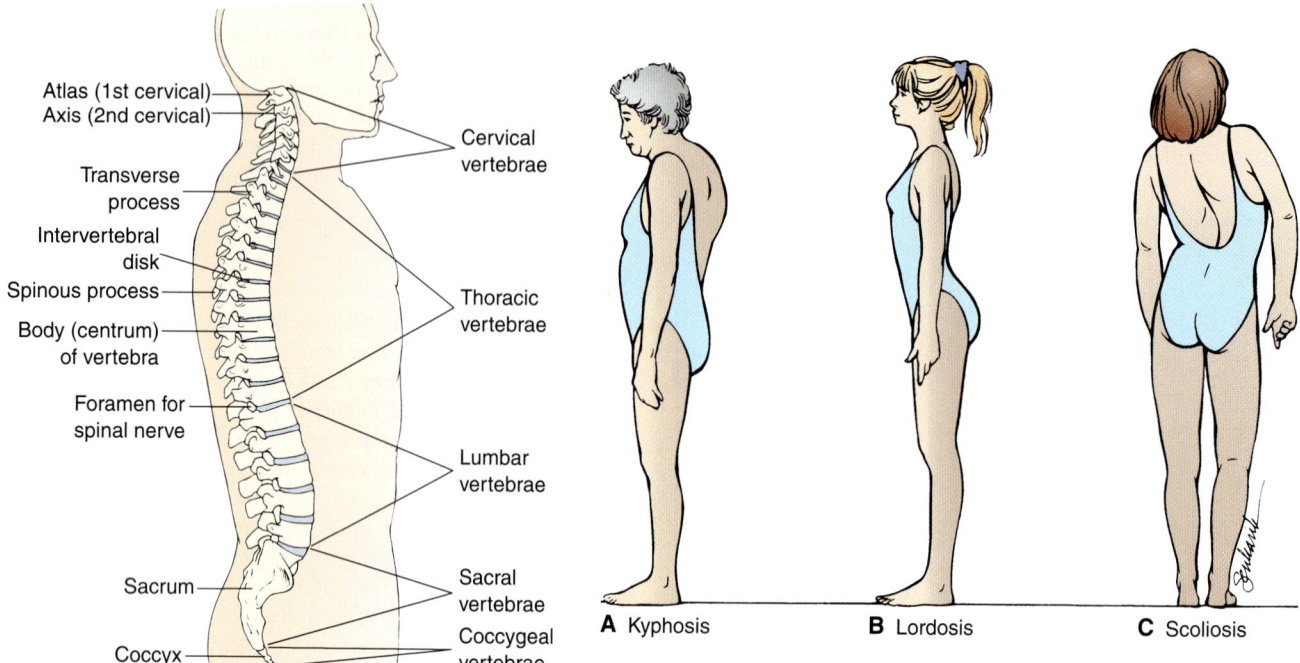

FIGURE 66-3 A normal spine and three abnormalities. (**A**) Kyphosis: an increased convexity or roundness of the spine's thoracic curve. (**B**) Lordosis: swayback; exaggeration of the lumbar spine curve. (**C**) Scoliosis: a lateral curvature of the spine.

medial or lateral side, the examiner observes the opposite side for a bulge below the patella. When larger amounts of fluid are present, the patella becomes elevated from the femur during knee extension and the ballottement test is positive (Fig. 66-4). If inflammation or fluid is suspected in a joint, physician consultation is indicated.

Joint deformity may be caused by contracture (shortening of surrounding joint structures), dislocation (complete separation of joint surfaces), subluxation (partial separation of articular surfaces), or disruption of structures surrounding the joint. Weakness or disruption of joint-supporting structures may result in a weak joint that requires an external supporting appliance (eg, brace).

Palpation of the joint while it is passively moved provides information about the integrity of the joint. Normally, the joint moves smoothly. A snap or crack may indicate that a ligament is slipping over a bony prominence. Slightly roughened surfaces, as in arthritic conditions, result in **crepitus** (grating, crackling sound or sensation) as the irregular joint surfaces move across one another.

The tissues surrounding joints are examined for nodule formation. Rheumatoid arthritis, gout, and osteoarthritis produce characteristic nodules. The subcutaneous nodules of rheumatoid arthritis are soft and occur within and along tendons that provide extensor function to the joints. The nodules of gout are hard and lie within and immediately adjacent to the joint capsule itself.

FIGURE 66-4 (**A**) Technique for ballottement test to detect fluid in the knee (**B**). Photo from Weber, J. W., & Kelley, J. (2003). *Health assessment in nursing* (2nd ed.). Philadelphia: Lippincott Williams & Wilkins.

They may rupture, exuding white uric acid crystals onto the skin surface. Osteoarthritic nodules are hard and painless and represent bony overgrowth that has resulted from destruction of the cartilaginous surface of bone within the joint capsule. They are frequently seen in older adults.

Often, the size of the joint is exaggerated by atrophy of the muscles proximal and distal to that joint. This is seen in rheumatoid arthritis of the knees, in which the quadriceps muscle may atrophy dramatically. In rheumatoid arthritis, joint involvement assumes a symmetric pattern (Fig. 66-5). (See Chapter 54 for further information about rheumatoid arthritis.)

Muscle Strength and Size

The muscular system is assessed by noting the patient's ability to change position, muscular strength and coordination, and the size of individual muscles. Weakness of a group of muscles might indicate a variety of conditions, such as polyneuropathy, electrolyte disturbances (particularly potassium and calcium), myasthenia gravis, poliomyelitis, and muscular dystrophy. By palpating the muscle while passively moving the relaxed extremity, the nurse can determine the muscle tone. The nurse assesses muscle strength by having the patient perform certain manoeuvres with and without added resistance. For example, when the biceps are tested, the patient is asked to extend the arm fully and then to flex it against resistance applied by the nurse. A simple handshake may provide an indication of grasp strength.

The nurse may elicit muscle **clonus** (rhythmic contractions of a muscle) in the ankle or wrist by sudden, forceful, sustained dorsiflexion of the foot or extension of the wrist. **Fasciculations** (involuntary twitching of muscle fibre groups) may be observed.

The nurse measures the girth of an extremity to monitor increased size due to exercise, edema, or bleeding into the muscle. Girth may decrease due to muscle atrophy. The unaffected extremity is measured and used as the reference standard. Measurements are taken at the maximum circumference of the extremity. It is important that the measurements be taken at the same location on the extremity, and with the extremity in the same position, with the muscle at rest. Distance from a specific anatomic landmark (eg, 10 cm below the medial aspect of the knee for measurement of the calf muscle) should be indicated in the patient's record so that subsequent measurements can be made at the same

point. For ease of serial assessment, the nurse may indicate the point of measurement by marking the skin. Variations in size greater than 1 cm are considered significant.

Skin

In addition to assessing the musculoskeletal system, the nurse inspects the skin for edema, temperature, and colour. Palpation of the skin can reveal whether any areas are warmer, suggesting increased perfusion or infection, or cooler, suggesting decreased perfusion, and whether edema is present. Cuts, bruises, skin colour, and evidence of decreased circulation or infection can influence nursing management of musculoskeletal conditions.

Neurovascular Status

It is important for the nurse to perform frequent neurovascular assessments of patients with musculoskeletal disorders (especially of those with fractures) because of the risk of tissue and nerve damage. One complication that the nurse needs to be alert for when assessing the patient is compartment syndrome, which is described in detail later in this unit. This major neurovascular problem is caused by pressure within a muscle compartment that increases to such an extent that microcirculation diminishes, leading to nerve and muscle anoxia and necrosis. Function can be permanently lost if the anoxic situation continues for longer than 6 hours. Assessment of neurovascular status (Chart 66-3) is frequently referred to as assessment of CMS (circulation, motion, and sensation).

The Patient With Musculoskeletal Injury

Special precautions must be taken when assessing a trauma patient. If there is injury to an extremity, it is important to assess for soft tissue trauma, deformity, and neurovascular status. If the patient has a possible cervical spine injury and is wearing a cervical collar, the collar must not be removed until the absence of spinal cord injury is confirmed on x-ray. When the collar is removed, the cervical spine area is gently assessed for swelling, tenderness, and deformity. With pelvic trauma, abdominal organ injuries may occur. The patient is assessed for abdominal pain, tenderness, hematomas, and the presence or absence of femoral pulses. If blood is present at the urinary meatus, the nurse should suspect bladder and urethral injury, and the patient should not

FIGURE 66-5 Rheumatoid arthritis joint deformity with ulnar deviation of fingers and "swan-neck" deformity of fingers (ie, hyperextension of proximal interphalangeal joints with flexion of distal interphalangeal joints).

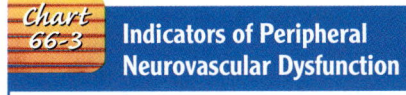

Indicators of Peripheral Neurovascular Dysfunction

Circulation
Colour: Pale or cyanotic
Temperature: Cool
Capillary refill: More than 3 seconds

Motion
Weakness
Paralysis

Sensation
Paresthesia
Unrelenting pain
Pain on passive stretch
Absence of feeling

be catheterized. Instead, such findings should be reported immediately to the primary health care provider.

Diagnostic Evaluation

IMAGING PROCEDURES

X-ray Studies

X-ray studies are important in evaluating patients with musculoskeletal disorders. Bone x-rays determine bone density, texture, erosion, and changes in bone relationships. Multiple x-rays are needed for full assessment of the structure being examined. X-ray study of the cortex of the bone reveals any widening, narrowing, or signs of irregularity. Joint x-rays reveal fluid, irregularity, spur formation, narrowing, and changes in the joint structure. After being positioned for the study, the patient must remain still while the x-rays are taken.

Computed Tomography

A computed tomography (CT) scan shows in detail a specific plane of involved bone and can reveal tumours of the soft tissue or injuries to the ligaments or tendons. It is used to identify the location and extent of fractures in areas that are difficult to evaluate (eg, acetabulum). CT studies, which may be performed with or without the use of contrast agents, last about 1 hour. The patient must remain still during the procedure.

Magnetic Resonance Imaging

Magnetic resonance imaging (MRI) is a noninvasive imaging technique that uses magnetic fields, radio waves, and computers to demonstrate abnormalities (ie, tumours or narrowing of tissue pathways through bone) of soft tissues such as muscle, tendon, cartilage, nerve, and fat. Because an electromagnet is used, patients with any metal implants, clips, or pacemakers are not candidates for MRI.

> **NURSING ALERT** Jewelry, hair clips, hearing aids, credit cards with magnetic strips, and other metal-containing objects must be removed before the MRI is done; otherwise they can become dangerous projectile objects.

To enhance visualization of anatomic structures, contrast media may be injected intravenously. During the procedure, the patient needs to lie still for 1 to 2 hours and will hear a rhythmic knocking sound. Patients who experience claustrophobia may be unable to tolerate the confinement of closed MRI equipment without sedation. Open MRI systems are available, but they use lower-intensity magnetic fields, which reduces the quality of the imaging; repeated imaging may be required. Advantages of open MRI include increased patient comfort, reduced problems with claustrophobic patients, and reduced noise.

Arthrography

Arthrography is useful in identifying acute or chronic tears of the joint capsule or supporting ligaments of the knee, shoulder, ankle, hip, or wrist. A radiopaque substance or air is injected into the joint cavity to outline soft tissue structures and the contour of the joint. The joint is put through its range of motion to distribute the contrast agent while a series of x-rays is obtained. If a tear is present, the contrast agent leaks out of the joint and is evident on the x-ray image.

After an arthrogram, the joint is usually rested for 12 hours, and a compression elastic bandage is applied as prescribed. In addition, the nurse provides comfort measures (mild analgesia, ice) as appropriate. The nurse should explain to the patient that it is normal to experience clicking or crackling in the joint for a day or two after the procedure, until the contrast agent or air is absorbed.

Nursing Interventions

Before the patient undergoes an imaging study, the nurse should assess for conditions that may require special consideration during the study or that may be contraindications to the study (eg, pregnancy; claustrophobia; inability to tolerate required positioning due to age, debility, or disability; metal implants). It is essential that the patient remove all jewelry, hair clips, hearing aids, and other metal before having an MRI. If contrast agents will be used for CT scan, MRI, or arthrography, the nurse should carefully assess the patient for possible allergy.

Bone Densitometry

Bone densitometry is used to estimate bone mineral density (BMD). This can be done through the use of x-rays or ultrasound. Dual-energy x-ray absorptiometry (DEXA) determines bone mineral density at the wrist, hip, or spine to estimate the extent of osteoporosis and to monitor a patient's response to treatment for osteoporosis. Bone sonometry (ultrasound) measures heel bone quantity and quality and is used to estimate BMD and the risk of fracture for people with osteoporosis. Bone density sonography is a cost-effective, readily available screening tool for diagnosing osteoporosis and predicting a person's risk for fracture.

NUCLEAR STUDIES

Bone Scan

A bone scan is performed to detect metastatic and primary bone tumours, osteomyelitis, certain fractures, and aseptic necrosis. A bone-seeking radioisotope is injected intravenously. The scan is performed 2 to 3 hours after the injection. At this point, distribution and concentration of the isotope in the bone are determined. The degree of nuclide uptake is related to the metabolism of the bone. An increased uptake of isotope is seen in primary skeletal disease (osteosarcoma), metastatic bone disease, inflammatory skeletal disease (osteomyelitis), and certain types of fractures.

NURSING INTERVENTIONS

Before the patient undergoes a bone scan, the nurse should inquire about possible allergy to the radioisotope and should assess for any condition that would contraindicate performing the procedure (eg, pregnancy). In addition, it is important to encourage the patient to drink plenty of fluids to help distribute and eliminate the isotope. Before the scan, the nurse asks the patient to empty the bladder, because a full bladder interferes with scanning of the pelvic bones.

ENDOSCOPIC STUDIES

Arthroscopy

Arthroscopy is a procedure that allows direct visualization of a joint to diagnose joint disorders. Treatment of tears, defects, and disease processes may be performed through the arthroscope. The procedure is carried out in the operating room under sterile conditions; injection of a local anesthetic into the joint or general anesthesia is used. A large-bore needle is inserted, and the joint is distended with saline. The arthroscope is introduced, and joint structures, synovium, and articular surfaces are visualized. After the procedure, the puncture wound is closed with adhesive strips or sutures and covered with a sterile dressing. Complications are rare but may include infection, hemarthrosis, neurovascular compromise, thrombophlebitis, stiffness, effusion, adhesions, and delayed wound healing.

NURSING INTERVENTIONS

The joint is wrapped with a compression dressing to control swelling. In addition, ice may be applied to control edema and discomfort. Frequently, the joint is kept extended and elevated to reduce swelling. It is important to monitor neurovascular function. The nurse administers prescribed analgesics to control discomfort. The nurse should explain when the patient can resume activity and what weight-bearing limits to follow, as prescribed by the orthopedic surgeon. The nurse also explains to the patient and family the symptoms (eg, swelling, numbness, cool skin) to watch for in order to determine whether complications are occurring and the importance of notifying the physician of these observations. The physician's prescription for analgesic medication is also explained.

OTHER STUDIES

Arthrocentesis

Arthrocentesis (joint aspiration) is carried out to obtain synovial fluid for purposes of examination or to relieve pain due to effusion. Examination of synovial fluid is helpful in the diagnosis of septic arthritis and other inflammatory arthropathies and reveals the presence of hemarthrosis (bleeding into the joint cavity), which suggests trauma or a bleeding disorder. Normally, synovial fluid is clear, pale, straw-coloured, and scanty in volume. Using aseptic technique, the physician inserts a needle into the joint and aspirates fluid. Anti-inflammatory medications may be injected into the joint. A sterile dressing is applied after aspiration. There is a risk for infection after this procedure.

Electromyography

Electromyography (EMG) provides information about the electrical potential of the muscles and the nerves leading to them. The test is done to evaluate muscle weakness, pain, and disability. The purpose of the procedure is to determine any abnormality of function and to differentiate muscle and nerve problems. Needle electrodes are inserted into selected muscles, and responses to electrical stimuli are recorded on an oscilloscope. Warm compresses may relieve residual discomfort after the study.

Biopsy

Biopsy may be performed to determine the structure and composition of bone marrow, bone, muscle, or synovium to help diagnose specific diseases. The nurse monitors the biopsy site for edema, bleeding, pain, and infection. Ice is applied as prescribed to control bleeding and edema. In addition, analgesics are administered as prescribed for comfort.

LABORATORY STUDIES

Examination of the patient's blood and urine can provide information about a primary musculoskeletal problem (eg, Paget's disease), a developing complication (eg, infection), the baseline

for instituting therapy (eg, anticoagulant therapy), or the response to therapy. The complete blood count includes the hemoglobin level (which is frequently lower after bleeding associated with trauma and surgery) and the white blood cell count (which is elevated in acute infections, trauma, acute hemorrhage, and tissue necrosis). Before surgery, coagulation studies are performed to detect bleeding tendencies (because bone is very vascular tissue).

Blood chemistry studies provide data about a wide variety of musculoskeletal conditions. Serum calcium levels are altered in patients with osteomalacia, parathyroid function, Paget's disease, metastatic bone tumours, or prolonged immobilization. Serum phosphorus levels are inversely related to calcium levels and are diminished in osteomalacia associated with malabsorption syndrome. Acid phosphatase is elevated in Paget's disease and metastatic cancer. Alkaline phosphatase is elevated during early fracture healing and in diseases with increased osteoblastic activity (eg, metastatic bone tumours). Bone metabolism may be evaluated through thyroid studies and determination of calcitonin, parathyroid hormone, and vitamin D levels. Serum enzyme levels of creatine kinase and aspartate aminotransferase become elevated with muscle damage. Aldolase is elevated in muscle diseases (eg, muscular dystrophy, skeletal muscle necrosis). Serum osteocalcin (bone GLA protein) indicates the rate of bone turnover. Urine calcium levels increase with bone destruction (eg, parathyroid dysfunction, metastatic bone tumours, multiple myeloma).

Specific serum biochemical markers can be used to provide information about bone formation; these include bone-specific alkaline phosphatase and osteocalcin from osteoblasts, and procollagen 1 carboxyterminal propeptide and procollagen 1 aminoterminal propeptide from the bone matrix. Specific serum biochemical markers that provide information about bone resorption include tartrate-resistant acid phosphatase and bone sialoprotein from osteoclasts, and aminoterminal telopeptide of type 1 collagen and carboxyterminal telopeptide of type 1 collagen from bone matrix. Biochemical markers of bone resorption in the urine include pyridinoline and deoxypyridinoline crosslinks, aminoterminal telopeptide of type 1 collagen, and hydroxyproline from collagen degradation from bone matrix (Koopman, 2001; Woitge & Seibel, 2001).

Nursing Implications

Determining the patient's functional status and health care needs is an integral part of the nursing assessment. Nursing diagnoses and the care plan are developed and modified according to the patient's needs.

During the period of assessment, the patient requires support and nursing care, including physical and psychological preparation for examinations and tests. Patient education before the tests (what is to be done; why it is being done; what the patient can expect to experience, including tactile, visual, and auditory sensations; and what patient participation is expected) reduces anxiety and enables the patient to be an active participant in care.

The resulting medical diagnosis and prescribed treatment regimen affect the nursing management of the patient. The nursing plan of care includes nursing measures to facilitate the resolution of the patient's health problems and promotion of health. The nursing assessment enables the nurse to identify the health problems that can be improved by nursing interventions. In collaboration with the patient, health goals and nursing strategies are formulated to resolve the identified nursing diagnoses.

Critical Thinking Exercises

1. A young adult patient who experienced multiple fractures of the left tibia is to be confined to non–weight-bearing activity for about 3 months. During a clinic visit 3 weeks after the fracture occurred, he tells the nurse that his left leg is "withering away" and he is afraid that he will have no strength in this leg when he is finally permitted to walk on it. Discuss the nursing interventions to help this patient. What additional assessments and explanations could the nurse make to help this patient deal with the effects of immobility?

2. You are teaching a class on age-associated body changes at a senior centre. Your focus is on the musculoskeletal system. The participants have experienced many of the changes you identify and ask you what they can do about them. What strategies to minimize these changes and maximize musculoskeletal health would you discuss with the participants?

3. An older patient with low back pain is scheduled for a bone scan. She tells the nurse that she just had a bone density study for osteoporosis a month ago and does not understand why the doctor wants her to have another one so soon. What additional assessment should the nurse perform? Discuss the differences in the two procedures.

REFERENCES AND SELECTED READINGS

Books

Bickley, L. S., & Szilagyi, P. G. (2003). *Bates' guide to physical assessment* (8th ed.). Philadelphia: Lippincott Williams & Wilkins.

Buckwalter, J., et al. (2000). *Orthopaedic basic science: Biology and biomechanics of the musculoskeletal system* (2nd ed.). Rosemont, IL: American Academy of Orthopaedic Surgeons.

Bullock, B., & Henze, R. (2000). *Focus on pathophysiology.* Philadelphia: Lippincott Williams & Wilkins.

Fischbach, F. (2004). *A manual of laboratory and diagnostic tests* (7th ed.). Philadelphia: Lippincott Williams & Wilkins.

Kleerekoper, M., et al. (1999). *The bone and mineral manual.* San Diego: Academic Press.

Koopman, W. (2001). *Arthritis and allied conditions* (14th ed.). Philadelphia: Lippincott Williams & Wilkins.

Maher, A., et al. (2002). *Orthopaedic nursing* (3rd ed.). Philadelphia: W. B. Saunders.

Reider, B. (1999). *The orthopaedic physical examination.* Philadelphia: W. B. Saunders.

Rosen, C., et al. (1999). *The aging skeleton.* San Diego: Academic Press.

Ruddy, S. et. al. (2001). *Kelley's textbook of rheumatology* (6th ed.). Philadelphia: W. B. Saunders.

Salter, R. (1999). *Textbook of disorders and injuries of the musculoskeletal system* (3rd ed.). Baltimore: Williams & Wilkins.

Schoen, D. (2000). *Adult orthopaedic nursing.* Philadelphia: Lippincott Williams & Wilkins.

Schoen, D. (Ed.) (2001). *NAON core curriculum for orthopaedic nursing* (4th ed.). Pitman, NJ: National Association of Orthopaedic Nurses.

Weber, J., & Kelley, J. (2003). *Health assessment in nursing* (2nd ed.). Philadelphia: Lippincott Williams & Wilkins.

Journals

Hall, J., & Riley, R. (1999). Nutritional strategies to reduce the risk of osteoporosis. *Medsurg Nursing, 8*(5), 281–293.

Kunkler, C. (1999). Neurovascular assessment. *Orthopaedic Nursing 18*(3), 63–71.

Ludwick, R., et al. (1999). Assessment of the geriatric orthopaedic trauma patient. *Orthopaedic Nursing, 18*(6), 13–18.

Voskey, A. (2001, February 7). Musculoskeletal disorders and orthopedic conditions. *Journal of the American Medical Association, 285*(5), 619–623.

Woitge, H., & Seibel, M. (2001). Biochemical markers to survey bone turnover. *Rheumatic Diseases Clinics of North America, 27*(1), 49–80.

RESOURCES AND WEBSITES

Canadian Institutes of Health Research: Institute of Musculoskeletal Health and Arthritis, 160 Elgin Street, 9th floor, 4809A, Ottawa, ON K1A 0W9; http://www.cihr-irsc.gc.ca/e/13217.html.

Canadian Orthopaedic Association, 1440 St. Catherine Street West, Suite 718, Montreal, QC H3G 1R8; 514-874-9003; www.coa-aco.org.

Canadian Orthopaedic Foundation, PO Box 7029, Innisfail, ON L9S 1A8; 416-410-2341; www.canorth.org.

Canadian Orthopaedic Nurses Association; www.cona-nurse.org.

National Association of Orthopaedic Nurses (NAON), East Holly Avenue, Box 56, Pitman, NJ 08071-0056; 1-856-256-2310; http://www.inurse.com; naon@mail.ajj.com.

National Institute of Arthritis and Musculoskeletal and Skin Diseases, Information Clearing House, National Institutes of Health, 1 AMS Circle, Bethesda, MD 20892-3675; 1-877-22-NIAMS (toll free); 1-301-495-4484.

National Institute of Arthritis and Musculoskeletal and Skin Diseases, Office of Communications and Public Liaison, Bldg. 31/Rm.4C05, 31 Center Drive, MSC 2350, Bethesda, MD 20892-2350; 1-301-496-8190; http://www.nih.gov/niams.

Musculoskeletal Care Modalities

Adapted by Bonnie Friesen and Linda Larsen

LEARNING OBJECTIVES

On completion of this chapter, the learner will be able to:

1. Describe the preventive and health teaching needs of the patient with a cast.
2. Use the nursing process as a framework for care of the patient with a cast.
3. Describe the various types of traction and the principles of effective traction.
4. Identify the preventive nursing care needs of the patient in traction.
5. Use the nursing process as a framework for care of the patient in traction.
6. Compare the nursing needs of the patient undergoing total hip replacement with those of the patient undergoing total knee replacement.
7. Use the nursing process as a framework for care of the patient undergoing orthopedic surgery.

*T*he management of musculoskeletal problems frequently includes the use of casts, traction, artificial joint replacement, and/or surgery. Patient education is essential for optimal outcomes. The nurse prepares the patient for immobilization with casts or traction, for surgery, and for joint replacement when indicated. Nursing care is planned to maximize the effectiveness of these treatment modalities and to prevent potential complications associated with each of the interventions. The patient is taught to manage his or her care at home and how to safely resume activities.

Managing Care of the Patient in a Cast

A **cast** is a rigid external immobilizing device that is molded to the contours of the body. The purposes of a cast are to immobilize a body part in a specific position and to apply uniform pressure on encased soft tissue.

A cast is used specifically to immobilize a reduced **fracture,** to correct a deformity, to apply uniform pressure to underlying soft tissue, or to support and stabilize weakened joints. Generally, casts permit mobilization of the patient while restricting movement of a body part.

The condition being treated influences the type and thickness of the cast applied. Generally speaking, the joints proximal and distal to the area to be immobilized are included in the cast. With some fractures, however, cast construction and molding may allow movement of a joint while immobilizing a fracture (eg, three-point fixation in a patellar tendon weight-bearing cast). Various types of casts include the following:

Short arm cast: Extends from below the elbow to the palmar crease, secured around the base of the thumb. If the thumb is included, it is known as a *thumb spica* or *gauntlet* cast.
Long arm cast: Extends from the upper level of the axillary fold to the proximal palmar crease. The elbow usually is immobilized at a right angle.
Short leg cast: Extends from below the knee to the base of the toes. The foot is flexed at a right angle in a neutral position.
Long leg cast: Extends from the junction of the upper and middle third of the thigh to the base of the toes. The knee may be slightly flexed.
Walking cast: A short or long leg cast reinforced for strength.
Body cast: Encircles the trunk.

Shoulder spica cast: A body jacket that encloses the trunk and the shoulder and elbow.
Hip spica cast: Encloses the trunk and a lower extremity. A double hip spica cast includes both legs.

Figure 67-1 illustrates the long-arm and long-leg cast and areas in which pressure problems commonly occur with these casts.

CASTING MATERIALS

Nonplaster

Generally referred to as fibreglass casts, these water-activated polyurethane materials have the versatility of plaster (see later discussion) but are lighter in weight, stronger, water resistant, and durable. They consist of an open-weave, nonabsorbent fabric impregnated with cool water-activated hardeners that bond and reach full rigid strength in minutes.

Nonplaster casts are porous and therefore diminish skin problems. They do not soften when wet, which allows for hydrotherapy (use of water for treatment) when appropriate. When wet, they are dried with a hair drier on a cool setting; thorough drying is important to prevent skin breakdown. They are used for nondisplaced fractures with minimal swelling and for long-term wear.

Plaster

The traditional cast is made of plaster. Rolls of plaster bandage are wet in cool water and applied smoothly to the body. A crystallizing reaction occurs, and heat is given off (an exothermic reaction). The heat given off during this reaction can be uncomfortable, and the nurse should inform the patient about the sensation of increasing warmth so that the patient does not become alarmed. Additionally, the nurse should explain that the cast needs to be exposed to allow maximum dissipation of the heat and that most casts cool after about 15 minutes.

The crystallization process produces a rigid dressing. The speed of the reaction varies from a few minutes to 15 to 20 minutes. The orthopedist determines the plaster setting speed appropriate for the cast being applied. After the plaster sets, the cast remains wet and somewhat soft. It does not have its full strength

Glossary

abduction: movement away from the centre or median line of the body
adduction: movement toward the centre or median line of the body
arthrodesis: surgical fusion of a joint
arthroplasty: surgical repair of a joint; joint replacement
avascular necrosis: death of tissue due to insufficient blood supply
brace: externally applied device to support body, control movement, and prevent injury
cast: rigid external immobilizing device molded to contours of body part
cast syndrome: psychological (claustrophobic reaction) and physiologic (superior

mesenteric artery syndrome) responses to confinement in body cast
continuous passive motion (CPM) device: a device that promotes range of motion, circulation, and healing
edema: soft tissue swelling due to fluid accumulation
external fixator: external metal frame attached to and stabilizing bone fragments
fasciotomy: surgical procedure to release constricting muscle fascia so as to relieve muscle tissue pressure
fracture: a break in the continuity of the bone
heterotophic ossification: misplaced formation of bone

neurovascular status: neurologic (motor and sensory components) and circulatory functioning of a body part
open reduction with internal fixation (ORIF): surgery to repair and stabilize a fracture
osteomyelitis: infection of the bone
osteotomy: surgical cutting of bone
sling: bandage used to support an arm
splint: device designed specifically to support and immobilize body part in desired position
traction: application of a pulling force to a part of the body
trapeze: overhead patient-helping device to promote patient mobility in bed

FIGURE 67-1 Pressure areas in common types of casts. *Left,* long arm cast; *right,* short leg cast.

until it is dry. While damp, the cast can be dented. Therefore, it must be handled with the palms of the hand and not allowed to rest on hard surfaces or sharp edges. Cast dents may press on the skin causing irritation and skin breakdown. The plaster cast requires 24 to 72 hours to dry completely, depending on its thickness and the environmental drying conditions. A freshly applied cast should be exposed to circulating air to dry and should not be covered with clothing or bed linens. A wet plaster cast appears dull and grey, sounds dull on percussion, feels damp, and smells musty. A dry plaster cast is white and shiny, resonant, odourless, and firm.

NURSING PROCESS:
THE PATIENT IN A CAST

Assessment

Before the cast is applied, the nurse completes an assessment of the patient's general health, presenting signs and symptoms, emotional status, understanding of the need for the cast, and condition of the body part to be immobilized in the cast. Physical assessment of the part to be immobilized must include assessment of the **neurovascular status** (neurologic and circulatory functioning) of the body part, degree and location of swelling, bruising, and skin abrasions.

Diagnosis

NURSING DIAGNOSES

Based on the assessment data, major nursing diagnoses for the patient with a cast may include the following:

- Deficient knowledge related to the treatment regimen
- Acute pain related to the musculoskeletal disorder
- Impaired physical mobility related to the cast
- Self-care deficit: bathing/hygiene, feeding, dressing/grooming, or toileting due to restricted mobility
- Impaired skin integrity related to lacerations and abrasions
- Risk for peripheral neurovascular dysfunction related to physiologic responses to injury and compression effect of cast

COLLABORATIVE PROBLEMS/
POTENTIAL COMPLICATIONS

Based on the assessment data, potential complications that may develop include the following:

- Compartment syndrome
- Pressure ulcer
- Disuse syndrome

Planning and Goals

The major goals for the patient with a cast include knowledge of the treatment regimen, relief of pain, improved physical mobility, achievement of maximum level of self-care, healing of lacerations and abrasions, maintenance of adequate neurovascular function, and absence of complications.

Nursing Interventions

EXPLAINING THE TREATMENT REGIMEN

Before the cast is applied, the patient needs information concerning the pathologic problem and the purpose and expectations of the prescribed treatment regimen. This knowledge promotes the patient's active participation in and adherence to the treatment program. It is important to prepare the patient for the application of the cast by describing the anticipated sights, sounds, and sensations (eg, heat from the hardening reaction of the plaster). The patient needs to know what to expect during application and that the body part will be immobilized after casting (Chart 67-1).

RELIEVING PAIN

The nurse must carefully evaluate pain associated with musculoskeletal problems, asking the patient to indicate the exact site and to describe the character and intensity of the pain to help determine its cause. Most pain can be relieved by elevating the involved part, applying cold as prescribed, and administering usual dosages of analgesics.

Chart 67-1
GUIDELINES FOR Applying a Cast

When applying a cast, the physician or nurse practitioner proceeds as follows:

PROCEDURE	RATIONALE
1. Support extremity or body part to be casted.	1. Minimizes movement; maintains reduction and alignment; increases comfort.
2. Position and maintain part to be casted in position indicated by physician during casting procedure.	2. Facilitates casting; reduces incidence of complications (eg, malunion, nonunion, contracture).
3. Drape patient.	3. Avoids undue exposure; protects other body parts from contact with casting materials.
4. Wash and dry part to be casted.	4. Reduces incidence of skin breakdown.
5. Place knitted material* (eg, stockinette) over part to be casted.	5. Protects skin from casting materials.
• Apply in smooth and nonconstrictive manner.	Protects skin from pressure.
• Allow additional material.	Folds over edges of cast when finishing application; creates smooth, padded edge; protects skin from abrasion.
6. Wrap soft, nonwoven roll padding* smoothly and evenly around part.	6. Protects skin from pressure of cast.
• Use additional padding around bony prominences to protect superficial nerves (eg, head of fibula, olecranon process).	Protects skin at bony prominences. Protects superficial nerves.
7. Apply plaster or nonplaster casting material evenly on body part.	7. Creates smooth, solid, well-contoured cast.
• Choose appropriate width bandage.	Facilitates smooth application.
• Overlap preceding turn by half the width of the bandage.	Creates smooth, solid, immobilizing cast.
• Use continuous motion, maintaining constant contact with body part.	Shapes cast properly for adequate support.
• Use additional casting material (splints) at joints and at points of anticipated cast stress.	Strengthens cast.
8. "Finish" cast:	8. Protects skin from abrasion.
• Smooth edges.	Assures full range of motion of adjacent joints.
• Trim and reshape with cast knife or cutter.	
9. Remove particles of casting materials from skin.	9. Prevents particles from loosening and sliding underneath cast.
10. Support cast during hardening.	10. Casting materials harden in minutes. Maximum hardness of nonplaster cast occurs in minutes. Maximum hardness of plaster cast occurs with drying (24 to 72 hours, depending on environment and thickness of cast).
• Handle hardening casts with palms of hands.	
• Support cast on firm smooth surface.	
• Do not rest cast on hard surfaces or on sharp edges.	
• Avoid pressure on cast.	Avoids denting of cast and development of pressure areas.
11. Promote drying of cast.	11. Facilitates drying.
• Leave cast uncovered and exposed to air.	
• Turn patient every 2 hours supporting major joints.	
• Fans may be used to increase air flow and speed drying.	

*Nonabsorbent materials are used with nonplaster casts.

 NURSING ALERT A patient's unrelieved pain must be immediately reported to the physician to avoid possible paralysis and necrosis.

 NURSING ALERT The nurse must never ignore complaints of pain from the patient in a cast because of the possibility of potential problems, such as impaired tissue perfusion or pressure ulcer formation.

Pain associated with the disease process (eg, fracture) is frequently controlled by immobilization. Pain due to **edema** that is associated with trauma, surgery, or bleeding into the tissues can frequently be controlled by elevation and, if prescribed, intermittent application of cold. Ice bags (one-third to one-half full) or cold application devices are placed on each side of the cast, if prescribed, making sure not to indent the cast.

Pain may be indicative of complications. Pain associated with compartment syndrome is relentless and is not controlled by modalities such as elevation, application of cold if prescribed, and usual dosages of analgesics. Severe pain over a bony prominence warns of an impending pressure ulcer. Pain decreases when ulceration occurs. Discomfort due to pressure on the skin may be relieved by elevation that controls edema or by positioning that alters pressure. It may be necessary, however, to modify the cast or to apply a new cast.

IMPROVING MOBILITY

Every joint that is not immobilized should be exercised and moved through its range of motion to maintain function. If the patient has a leg cast, the nurse encourages toe exercises. If the patient has an arm cast, the nurse encourages finger exercises.

PROMOTING HEALING OF SKIN ABRASIONS

Before the cast is applied, it is important to treat skin lacerations and abrasions to promote healing. The nurse thoroughly cleans the skin and treats it as prescribed. Sterile dressings are used to cover the injured skin. If the skin wounds are extensive, an alternative method (eg, external fixator) may be chosen to immobilize the body part. While the cast is on, the nurse observes the patient for systemic signs of infection, odours from the cast, and purulent drainage staining the cast. It is important to notify the physician if any of these occurs.

MAINTAINING ADEQUATE NEUROVASCULAR FUNCTION

Swelling and edema are natural responses of the tissue to trauma and surgery. The patient may complain that the cast is too tight. Vascular insufficiency and nerve compression due to unrelieved swelling can result in compartment syndrome (see Chap. 69, Management of Patients With Musculoskeletal Trauma). The nurse monitors circulation, motion, and sensation of the affected extremity, assessing the fingers or toes of the casted extremity and comparing them with those of the opposite extremity. Normal findings include minimal swelling, minimal discomfort, pink colour, warm to touch, rapid capillary refill response, normal sensations, and ability to exercise fingers or toes. The nurse encourages the patient to move fingers or toes hourly when awake to stimulate circulation.

It is important to perform frequent, regular assessments of neurovascular status. Early recognition of diminished circulation and nerve function is essential to prevent loss of function. Assessment data including progressive unrelieved pain, pain on passive stretch, paresthesia, motor loss, sensory loss, coolness, paleness, slow capillary refill, and sensation of tightness indicate potential compartment syndrome. The nurse adjusts the extremity so that it is no higher than heart level to enhance arterial perfusion and control edema and notifies the physician at once.

MONITORING AND MANAGING POTENTIAL COMPLICATIONS

Compartment Syndrome

Compartment syndrome occurs when there is increased tissue pressure within a limited space (eg, cast, muscle compartment) that compromises the circulation and the function of the tissue within the confined area. To relieve the pressure, the cast must be bivalved (cut in half longitudinally) while maintaining alignment, and the extremity must be elevated no higher than heart level (Chart 67-2). If pressure is not relieved and circulation is not restored, a **fasciotomy** may be necessary to relieve the pressure within the muscle compartment. The nurse closely monitors the patient's response to conservative and surgical management of compartment syndrome. The nurse records neurovascular responses and promptly reports changes to the physician.

Pressure Ulcers

Pressure of the cast on soft tissues may cause tissue anoxia and pressure ulcers. Lower extremity sites most susceptible to pressure are the heel, malleoli, dorsum of the foot, head of the fibula, and anterior surface of the patella. The main pressure sites on the upper extremity are located at the medial epicondyle of the humerus and the ulnar styloid (see Fig. 67-1).

Usually, the patient with a pressure ulcer reports pain and tightness in the area. A warm area on the cast suggests underlying tissue erythema. The area may break down. The drainage may stain the cast and emit an odour. Even if discomfort does not occur with tissue breakdown and necrosis, there may still be extensive loss of tissue. The nurse must monitor the patient with a cast for pressure ulcer development and report findings to the physician.

To inspect the pressure area, the physician may bivalve the cast or cut an opening (window) in the cast. If the physician elects to create a window to inspect the pressure site, a portion of the cast is cut out. The affected area is inspected and possibly treated. The portion of the cast is replaced and held in place by an elastic compression dressing or tape. This prevents the underlying tissue from swelling through the window and creating pressure areas around its margins.

Disuse Syndrome

While in a cast, the patient needs to learn to tense or contract muscles (eg, isometric muscle contraction) without moving the part. This helps to reduce muscle atrophy and maintain muscle strength. The nurse teaches the patient with a leg cast to "push down" the knee and teaches the patient in an arm cast to "make a fist." Muscle-setting exercises (eg, quadriceps-setting and gluteal-setting exercises) are important in maintaining muscles essential for walking (Chart 67-3). Isometric exercises should be performed hourly while the patient is awake.

PROMOTING HOME AND COMMUNITY-BASED CARE

Teaching the Patient Self-Care

Self-care deficits occur when a portion of the body is immobilized. The nurse encourages the patient to participate actively in personal care and to use assistive devices safely. The nurse must assist the patient in identifying areas of self-care deficit and in developing strategies to achieve independence in activities of daily living (ADLs) (Chart 67-4). The patient's participation in

---

Chart 67-2

GUIDELINES FOR Bivalving a Cast

When cutting a cast in half (bivalving), the physician or nurse practitioner proceeds as follows:

1. With a cast cutter, a longitudinal cut is made to divide the cast in half.
2. The underpadding is cut with scissors.
3. The cast is spread apart with cast spreaders to relieve pressure and to inspect and treat the skin without interrupting the reduction and alignment of the bone.
4. After the pressure is relieved, the anterior and posterior parts of the cast are secured together with an elastic compression bandage to maintain immobilization.
5. To control swelling and promote circulation, the extremity is elevated (but no higher than heart level, to minimize the effect of gravity on perfusion of the tissues).

Chart 67-3 **Muscle-Setting Exercises**

Isometric contractions of the muscle maintain muscle mass and strength and prevent atrophy.

Quadriceps-Setting Exercise
- Position patient supine with leg extended.
- Instruct patient to push knee back onto the mattress by contracting the anterior thigh muscles.
- Encourage patient to hold the position for 5 to 10 seconds.
- Let patient relax.
- Have the patient repeat the exercise 10 times each hour when awake.

Gluteal-Setting Exercise
- Position the patient supine with legs extended, if possible.
- Instruct the patient to contract the muscles of the buttocks.
- Encourage the patient to hold the contraction for 5 to 10 seconds.
- Let the patient relax.
- Have the patient repeat the exercise 10 times each hour when awake.

Chart 67-4
Home Care Checklist • The Patient With a Cast

At the completion of the home care teaching program, the patient or caregiver will be able to:

	Patient	Caregiver
Describe techniques to promote cast drying (eg, do not cover, leave exposed to circulating air; handle damp plaster cast with palms of hands and do not rest the cast on hard surfaces or sharp edges that can dent soft cast)	✓	✓
Describe approaches to controlling swelling and pain (eg, elevate casted extremity to heart level, apply intermittent ice bag if prescribed, take analgesics as prescribed)	✓	✓
Report pain uncontrolled by elevating the casted limb and by analgesics (may be an indicator of impaired tissue perfusion—compartment syndrome or pressure ulcer)	✓	
Demonstrate ability to transfer (eg, from a bed to a chair)	✓	
Use mobility aids safely	✓	
Avoid excessive use of injured extremity; observe prescribed weight-bearing limits	✓	
Manage minor irritations from cast (eg, for skin irritation from cast edge, pad rough edges with tape; to relieve itching, blow cool air from hair drier)	✓	✓
Demonstrate exercises to promote circulation and minimize disuse syndrome	✓	
State indicators of complications to report promptly to physician (eg, uncontrolled swelling and pain; cool, pale fingers or toes; paresthesia; paralysis; purulent drainage staining casts; signs of systemic infection; cast breaks)	✓	✓
Describe care of extremity following cast removal (eg, skin care; gradual resumption of normal activities to protect limb from undue stresses; management of swelling)	✓	✓

planning and accomplishing ADLs is an important aspect of self-care, independence, maintaining control, and avoiding untoward psychological reactions, such as depression.

When the cast is dry, the nurse instructs the patient as follows:

- Move about as normally as possible, but avoid excessive use of the injured extremity and avoid walking on wet, slippery floors or sidewalks.
- Perform prescribed exercises regularly, as scheduled.
- Elevate the casted extremity to heart level frequently to prevent swelling.
- Do not attempt to scratch the skin under the cast. This may cause a break in the skin and result in the formation of a skin ulcer. Cool air from a hair dryer may alleviate an itch.
- Cushion rough edges of the cast with tape.
- Keep the cast dry but do not cover it with plastic or rubber, because this causes condensation, which dampens the cast and skin. Moisture softens a plaster cast. (A wet fibreglass cast must be dried thoroughly with a hair dryer on a cool setting to avoid skin problems.)
- Report any of the following to the physician: persistent pain, swelling that does not respond to elevation, changes in sensation, decreased ability to move exposed fingers or toes, and changes in skin colour and temperature.
- Note odours around the cast, stained areas, warm spots, and pressure areas. Report them to the physician.
- Report a broken cast to the physician; do not attempt to fix it yourself.

The nurse prepares the patient for cast removal or cast changes by explaining what to expect (Chart 67-5). The cast is cut with a cast cutter, which vibrates. The patient can feel the vibration and pressure during its use. The cutter does not penetrate deeply enough to hurt the patient's skin. The cast padding is cut with scissors.

The casted body part is weak from disuse, is stiff, and may appear atrophied. There may be extreme stiffness even after only a few weeks of immobilization. Therefore, support is needed when the cast is removed. The skin, which is usually dry and scaly from accumulated dead skin, is vulnerable to injury from scratching.

The skin needs to be washed gently and lubricated with an emollient lotion.

The nurse and physical therapist teach the patient to resume activities gradually within the prescribed therapeutic regimen. Exercises that are prescribed to help the patient regain joint motion are explained and demonstrated. Because the muscles are weak from disuse, the body part that has been casted cannot withstand normal stresses immediately. In addition, the nurse teaches the patient who has noticeable swelling of the affected extremity after the cast is removed to continue to elevate the extremity to control swelling until normal muscle tone and use are reestablished.

Evaluation

EXPECTED PATIENT OUTCOMES

Expected patient outcomes may include:

1. Understands the therapeutic regimen
   a. Elevates affected extremity
   b. Exercises according to instructions
   c. Keeps cast dry
   d. Reports any problems that develop
   e. Keeps follow-up clinic or physician appointments
2. Reports less pain
   a. Elevates extremity that is in the cast
   b. Repositions self
   c. Uses occasional oral analgesic
3. Demonstrates increased mobility
   a. Uses assistive devices safely
   b. Exercises to increase strength
   c. Changes position frequently
   d. Performs range-of-motion exercises of joints not in the cast
4. Exhibits healing of abrasions and lacerations
   a. Demonstrates no local signs of infection (ie, local discomfort, purulent drainage, cast staining, or odour from cast)
   b. Demonstrates no systemic signs or symptoms of infection
   c. Demonstrates intact skin when cast is removed

Chart 67-5

GUIDELINES FOR Removing a Cast

When removing a cast, the physician or nurse practitioner proceeds as follows:

PROCEDURE	RATIONALE
1. Inform the patient about the procedure.	1. Facilitates cooperation and reduces fear about the procedure.
2. Reassure patient that the electric saw or cast cutter will not cut skin.	2. Reduces anxiety. (Explains that blade oscillates to cut cast and vibrations will be felt.)
3. Wear eye protection (patient and operator of the cast cutter).	3. Protects eyes from flying cast particles.
4. Bivalve cast using a series of alternating pressures and linear movements of blade along the line to be cut.	4. Cuts cast in halves. Avoids burning sensation from prolonged contact of oscillating blade with padding.
5. Cut padding with scissors.	5. Releases all of the casting materials.
6. Support body part as it is removed from the cast.	6. Reduces stresses on body part that has been immobilized.
7. Gently wash and dry area that has been immobilized.* Apply emollient lotion.	7. Removes dead skin that has accumulated during immobilization. Keeps skin supple.
8. Teach patient to avoid rubbing and scratching skin.	8. Prevents skin breakdown.
9. Collaborates with physical therapist to teach patient to resume active use of body part gradually within the guidelines of prescribed therapeutic regimen.	9. Protects weakened part from excessive stress. Progressive exercises reduce stiffness, restore muscle strength and function.
10. Teach patient to control swelling by elevating the extremity or using elastic bandage if prescribed.	10. Facilitates circulation (ie, venous return) and controls fluid pooling.

*If a new cast is to be applied, follow guidelines for application of a cast and associated nursing care.

---

5. Maintains adequate neurovascular function of affected extremity
   a. Exhibits normal skin colour and temperature
   b. Experiences minimal swelling
   c. Exhibits satisfactory capillary refill on testing
   d. Demonstrates active movement of fingers or toes if they are not casted
   e. Reports normal sensations in casted body part
   f. Reports that pain is controllable
6. Exhibits absence of complications
   a. Demonstrates normal neurovascular status of casted extremity
   b. Develops no pressure ulcers
   c. Exhibits minimal muscle wasting
7. Participates in self-care activities
   a. Performs hygiene and grooming activities independently or with minimal assistance
   b. Performs ADLs independently or with minimal assistance
   c. Adheres to prescribed exercise regimen.

Specific Cast Management Considerations

ARM CASTS

The patient whose arm is immobilized in a cast must readjust to many routine tasks. The unaffected arm must assume all the upper extremity activities. The nurse, in consultation with an occupational therapist, suggests devices designed to aid one-handed activities. The patient may experience fatigue due to modified activities and the weight of the cast. Frequent rest periods are necessary.

Nursing Interventions

To control swelling, the nurse elevates the immobilized arm. When the patient is lying down, the arm is elevated so that each joint is positioned higher than the preceding proximal joint (eg, elbow higher than the shoulder, hand higher than the elbow).

A **sling** may be used when the patient ambulates. To prevent pressure on the cervical spinal nerves, the sling should distribute the supported weight over a large area and not on the back of the neck. The nurse encourages the patient to remove the arm from the sling and elevate it frequently.

Circulatory disturbances in the hand may become apparent with signs of cyanosis, swelling, and an inability to move the fingers. One serious effect of impaired circulation in the arm is Volkmann's contracture, a form of compartment syndrome. Contracture of the fingers and wrist occurs as the result of obstructed arterial blood flow to the forearm and hand. The patient is unable to extend the fingers, describes abnormal sensation (eg, unrelenting pain, pain on passive stretch), and exhibits signs of diminished circulation to the hand. Permanent damage develops within a few hours if action is not taken.

This serious complication can be prevented with nursing surveillance and proper care. The nurse makes frequent neurovascular checks (see Chap. 66). Compartment syndrome is managed in part by bivalving (cutting) the cast to release constricting cast and dressings. A fasciotomy may be necessary to improve vascular status.

LEG CASTS

The application of a leg cast imposes a degree of immobility on the patient. The cast may be a short leg cast, extending to the knee, or a long leg cast, extending to the groin. The fresh cast must be handled in a manner that will not cause denting or disruption of the cast.

Nursing Interventions

The nurse supports the patient's leg on pillows to heart level to control swelling and applies ice packs as prescribed over the fracture site for 1 or 2 days. The patient is taught to elevate the casted leg when seated. The patient should also assume a recumbent position several times a day with the casted leg elevated to promote venous return and control swelling.

The nurse assesses circulation by observing the colour, temperature, and capillary refill of the exposed toes. Nerve function is assessed by observing the patient's ability to move the toes and by asking about the sensations in the foot. Numbness, tingling, and burning may be caused by peroneal nerve injury from pressure at the head of the fibula.

 NURSING ALERT Injury to the peroneal nerve as a result of pressure is a cause of footdrop (the inability to maintain the foot in a normally flexed position). Consequently, the patient drags the foot when ambulating.

When the cast is hard and dry, the nurse teaches the patient how to transfer and ambulate safely with assistive devices (eg, crutches, walker). The gait to be used depends on whether the patient is permitted to bear weight. If weight bearing is allowed, the cast is reinforced to withstand the body weight. A cast boot, worn over the casted foot, provides a broad, nonskid walking surface.

BODY OR SPICA CASTS

Casts that encase the trunk (body cast) and portions of one or two extremities (spica cast) require special nursing strategies. Body casts are used to immobilize the spine. Hip spicas are used for some femoral fractures and after some hip joint surgeries, and shoulder spica casts are used for some humeral neck fractures.

Nursing Interventions

Nursing responsibilities include preparing and positioning the patient, assisting with skin care and hygiene, and monitoring for **cast syndrome**. Explaining the procedure helps reduce the patient's apprehension about being encased in a large cast. The nurse reassures the patient that several people will provide care during the application, that support for the injured area will be adequate, and that care providers will be as gentle as possible. Medications for pain relief and relaxation administered before the procedure enable the patient to cooperate during application of the cast.

Cracking or denting of the cast is prevented by supporting the patient on a firm mattress and with flexible, waterproof pillows until the cast dries. The nurse positions the pillows next to each other, because spaces between pillows allow the damp cast to sag, become weak, and possibly break. A pillow is not placed under the head and shoulders of a patient in a body cast while the cast is drying, because doing so causes pressure on the chest.

The nurse turns the patient as a unit toward the uninjured side every 2 hours to relieve pressure and to allow the cast to dry. It is important to avoid twisting the patient's body within the cast. Sufficient personnel (at least three people) are needed when the patient is turned so that the fresh cast can be adequately supported with the palms of the hands at vulnerable points (ie, body joints) to prevent cracking. The nurse encourages the patient to assist in the repositioning, if not contraindicated, by use of the **trapeze** or bed rail. A stabilizing abduction bar incorporated into a spica cast should not be used as a turning device. The nurse adjusts the pillows to provide support without creating areas of pressure.

The nurse turns the patient to a prone position, twice daily if tolerated, to provide postural drainage of the bronchial tree and to relieve pressure on the back. A small pillow under the abdomen enhances comfort. The nurse can either place a pillow lengthwise under the dorsa of the feet or allow the toes to hang over the edge of the bed to prevent the toes from being forced into the mattress.

The nurse inspects the skin around the edges of the cast frequently for signs of irritation. The nurse can inspect some of the skin under the cast by pulling the skin taut and using a flashlight.

The skin can be bathed and massaged by reaching under the cast edges with the fingers.

The perineal opening must be large enough for hygienic care. To protect the cast from soiling, the nurse can insert clean dry plastic sheeting under the cast and over the cast edge before elimination by the patient. Usually, fracture bedpans are easier for patients with a hip spica cast to use than regular bedpans.

Patients immobilized in large casts may develop cast syndrome—psychological and physiologic responses to the confinement. The psychological component is similar to a claustrophobic reaction. The patient exhibits an acute anxiety reaction characterized by behavioural changes and autonomic responses (eg, increased respiratory rate, diaphoresis, dilated pupils, increased heart rate, elevated blood pressure). The nurse needs to recognize the anxiety reaction and provide an environment in which the patient feels secure.

The physiologic cast syndrome responses (superior mesenteric artery syndrome) are associated with immobility in a body cast. With decreased physical activity, gastrointestinal motility decreases, intestinal gases accumulate, intestinal pressure increases, and ileus may occur. The patient exhibits abdominal distention, abdominal discomfort, nausea, and vomiting. As with other instances of adynamic ileus, the patient is treated conservatively with decompression (nasogastric intubation connected to suction) and intravenous fluid therapy until gastrointestinal motility is restored. If the cast restricts the abdomen, the abdominal window must be enlarged. After the ileus resolves and bowel sounds resume, the patient gradually resumes an oral diet. Rarely, the distention places traction on the superior mesenteric artery, reducing the blood supply to the bowel. The bowel may become gangrenous, which requires surgical intervention. The nurse monitors the patient in a large body cast for potential cast syndrome, noting bowel sounds every 4 to 8 hours, and reports distention, nausea, and vomiting to the physician.

The patient with a body or spica cast is often cared for in the home. The nurse teaches family members how to care for the patient, which includes providing hygienic and skin care, ensuring proper positioning, preventing complications, and recognizing symptoms that should be reported to the health care provider.

Managing the Patient With Splints and Braces

Contoured **splints** of plaster or pliable thermoplastic materials may be used for conditions that do not require rigid immobilization, for those in which swelling may be anticipated, and for those that require special skin care. The splint needs to immobilize and support the body part in a functional position. The splint must be well padded to prevent pressure, skin abrasion, and skin breakdown. The splint is overwrapped with an elastic bandage applied in a spiral fashion and with pressure uniformly distributed so that the circulation is not restricted. The nurse frequently assesses the neurovascular status and skin integrity of the splinted extremity.

Soft immobilizers may be used to support an injured body part. Usually, the extremity is wrapped with an elastic bandage and then secured in a padded, contoured, canvas immobilizer. Rigid immobilization is not achieved. The nurse provides skin care and makes adjustments for swelling.

For long-term use, **braces** (orthoses) are used to provide support, control movement, and prevent additional injury. They are custom fitted to various parts of the body. Braces may be constructed of plastic materials, canvas, leather, or metal. The orthotist adjusts the brace for fit, positioning, and motion.

The nurse helps the patient learn to apply the brace and to protect the skin from irritation and breakdown. The nurse also assesses neurovascular integrity and comfort when the patient is wearing the brace, encourages the patient to wear the brace as prescribed, and reassures the patient that minor adjustments of the brace by the orthotist will increase comfort and minimize problems associated with its long-term use.

Managing the Patient With an External Fixator

External fixators are used to manage open fractures with soft tissue damage. They provide stable support for severe comminuted (crushed or splintered) fractures while permitting active treatment of damaged soft tissues (Fig. 67-2). Complicated fractures of the humerus, forearm, femur, tibia, and pelvis are managed with external skeletal fixators. The fracture is reduced, aligned, and immobilized by a series of pins inserted in the bone. Pin position is maintained through attachment to a portable frame. The fixator facilitates patient comfort, early mobility, and active exercise of adjacent uninvolved joints. Complications related to disuse and immobility are minimized.

Nursing Interventions

It is important to prepare the patient psychologically for application of the external fixator. The apparatus looks clumsy and foreign. Reassurance that the discomfort associated with the device is minimal and that early mobility is anticipated promotes acceptance of the device.

After the external fixator is applied, the extremity is elevated to reduce swelling. If there are sharp points on the fixator or pins, they are covered to prevent device-induced injuries. The nurse monitors the neurovascular status of the extremity every 2 to 4 hours and assesses each pin site for redness, drainage, tenderness, pain, and loosening of the pin. Some serous drainage from the pin sites is to be expected. The nurse must be alert for potential problems caused by pressure from the device on the skin, nerves, or blood vessels and for the development of compartment syndrome (see Chap. 69). The nurse carries out pin care as prescribed to prevent pin tract infection. This typically includes cleaning each pin site separately three times a day with cotton-tipped applicators soaked in sterile saline solution. Crusts should not form at the pin site. If signs of infection are present or if the pins or clamps seem loose, the nurse notifies the physician.

 NURSING ALERT The nurse never adjusts the clamps on the external fixator frame. It is the physician's responsibility to do so.

The nurse encourages isometric and active exercises within the limits of tissue damage. When the swelling subsides, the nurse helps the patient to become mobile within the prescribed weight-bearing limits (non–weight bearing to full weight bearing). Adherence to weight-bearing instructions minimizes the chance of loosening of the pins when stress is applied to the bone–pin interface. The fixator is removed after the soft tissue heals. The fracture may require additional stabilization by a cast or molded orthosis while healing.

The Ilizarov external fixator is a special device used to correct angulation and rotational defects, to treat nonunion (failure of bone fragments to heal), and to lengthen limbs. Tension wires are attached to fixator rings, which are joined by telescoping rods. Bone formation is stimulated by prescribed daily adjustment of the telescoping rods. It is important to teach the patient how to adjust the telescoping rods and how to perform skin care. Generally, the nurse can encourage weight bearing. After the desired correction has been achieved, no additional adjustments are made, and the fixator is left in place until the bone heals.

PROMOTING HOME AND COMMUNITY-BASED CARE

Teaching the Patient Self-Care. The nurse teaches the patient to perform pin site care according to the prescribed protocol (clean technique can be used at home [McKenzie, 1999]) and to report promptly any signs of pin site infection: redness, tenderness, increased or purulent pin site drainage, or fever. The nurse also instructs the patient and family to monitor neurovascular status and report any changes promptly. The nurse teaches the patient or family member to check the integrity of the fixator frame daily and to report loose pins or clamps. A physical therapy referral is helpful in teaching the patient how to transfer, use ambulatory aids safely, and adjust to weight-bearing limits and altered gait patterns (Chart 67-6).

Managing the Patient in Traction

Traction is the application of a pulling force to a part of the body. Traction is used to minimize muscle spasms; to reduce, align, and immobilize fractures; to reduce deformity; and to increase space between opposing surfaces. Traction must be applied in the cor-

FIGURE 67-2 External fixation device. Pins are inserted into bone. The fracture is reduced and aligned and then stabilized by attaching the pins to a rigid portable frame. The device facilitates treatment of soft tissue damaged in complex fractures.

At the completion of the home care instruction, the patient or caregiver will be able to:	Patient	Caregiver
• Demonstrate prescribed pin site care	✓	✓
• State signs of pin site infection (eg, redness, tenderness, increased or purulent pin site drainage) to be reported promptly	✓	✓
• Describe approaches to controlling swelling and pain (eg, elevate extremity to heart level, take analgesics as prescribed)	✓	✓
• Report pain uncontrolled by elevation and analgesics (may be an indicator of impaired tissue perfusion, compartment syndrome, or pin tract infection)	✓	
• Demonstrate ability to transfer	✓	
• Use mobility aids safely	✓	
• Avoid excessive use of injured extremity; observe prescribed weight-bearing limits	✓	
• State indicators of complications to report promptly to physician (eg, uncontrolled swelling and pain; cool, pale fingers or toes; paresthesia; paralysis; purulent drainage; signs of systemic infection; loose fixator pins or clamps)	✓	✓
• Describe care of extremity after fixator removal (eg, gradual resumption of normal activities to protect limb from undue stresses)	✓	✓

rect direction and magnitude to obtain its therapeutic effects. As muscle and soft tissues relax, the amount of weight used may be changed to obtain the desired effect.

At times, traction needs to be applied in more than one direction to achieve the desired line of pull. When this is done, one of the lines of pull counteracts the other. These lines of pull are known as the vectors of force. The actual resultant pulling force is somewhere between the two lines of pull (Fig. 67-3). The effects of traction are evaluated with x-ray studies, and adjustments are made if necessary.

Traction is used primarily as a short-term intervention until other modalities, such as external or internal fixation, are possible. This reduces the risk of disuse syndrome and minimizes the length of hospitalization, often allowing the patient to be cared for in the home setting.

PRINCIPLES OF EFFECTIVE TRACTION

Whenever traction is applied, countertraction must be used to achieve effective traction. Countertraction is the force acting in the opposite direction. Usually, the patient's body weight and bed position adjustments supply the needed countertraction.

 NURSING ALERT Countertraction must be maintained for effective traction.

The following are additional principles to follow when caring for the patient in traction:

- Traction must be continuous to be effective in reducing and immobilizing fractures.
- Skeletal traction is *never* interrupted.
- Weights are not removed unless intermittent traction is prescribed.
- Any factor that might reduce the effective pull or alter its resultant line of pull must be eliminated:
  - The patient must be in good body alignment in the centre of the bed when traction is applied.
  - Ropes must be unobstructed.
  - Weights must hang free and not rest on the bed or floor.
  - Knots in the rope or the footplate must not touch the pulley or the foot of the bed.

There are several types of traction. *Straight* or *running traction* applies the pulling force in a straight line with the body part resting on the bed. Buck's extension traction (Fig. 67-4) is an example of straight traction. *Balanced suspension traction* (Fig. 67-5) supports the affected extremity off the bed and allows for some patient movement without disruption of the line of pull.

Traction may be applied to the skin (*skin traction*) or directly to the bony skeleton (*skeletal traction*). The mode of application is determined by the purpose of the traction. Traction can be applied with the hands (*manual traction*). This is temporary traction that may be used when applying a cast, giving skin care under a Buck's extension foam boot, or adjusting the traction apparatus.

SKIN TRACTION

Skin traction is used to control muscle spasms and to immobilize an area before surgery. Skin traction is accomplished by using a weight to pull on traction tape or on a foam boot attached to the skin. The amount of weight applied must not exceed the toler-

FIGURE 67-3 Traction may be applied in different directions to achieve the desired therapeutic line of pull. Adjustments in applied forces may be prescribed over the course of treatment.

FIGURE 67-4 Buck's extension traction. Lower extremity in unilateral Buck's extension traction is aligned in a foam boot and traction applied by the free-hanging weight.

ance of the skin. No more than 2 to 3.5 kg of traction can be used on an extremity. Pelvic traction is usually 4.5 to 9 kg, depending on the weight of the patient.

Types of skin traction used for adults include Buck's extension traction (applied to the lower leg), the cervical head halter (occasionally used to treat neck pain), and the pelvic belt (sometimes used to treat back pain).

Buck's Extension Traction

Buck's extension traction (unilateral or bilateral) is skin traction to the lower leg. The pull is exerted in one plane when partial or temporary immobilization is desired (see Fig. 67-4). It is used to provide immobility after fractures of the proximal femur before surgical fixation.

Before the traction is applied, the nurse inspects the skin for abrasions and circulatory disturbances. The skin and circulation must be in healthy condition to tolerate the traction. The extremity should be clean and dry before the foam boot or traction tape is applied.

To apply Buck's traction, one nurse elevates and supports the extremity under the patient's heel and knee while another nurse

places the foam boot under the leg, with the patient's heel in the heel of the boot. Next, the nurse secures Velcro straps around the leg. Traction tape overwrapped with elastic bandage in a spiral fashion may be used instead of the boot. Excessive pressure is avoided over the malleolus and proximal fibula during application to prevent pressure ulcers and nerve damage. The nurse then passes the rope affixed to the spreader or footplate over a pulley fastened to the end of the bed and attaches the weight—usually 2 to 4 kilograms—to the rope.

Potential Complications

Skin breakdown, nerve pressure, and circulatory impairment are complications that may develop as a result of skin traction. Skin breakdown results from irritation caused by contact of the skin with the tape or foam and shearing forces. Older adults are at greater risk for this complication because of their sensitive, fragile skin.

Nerve pressure results from pressure on the peripheral nerves. Footdrop may occur if pressure is applied to the peroneal nerve at the point at which it passes around the neck of the fibula just below the knee.

Circulatory impairment is manifested by cold skin temperature, decreased peripheral pulses, slow capillary refill time, and bluish skin. Deep vein thrombosis (DVT), a serious circulatory impairment, is manifested by calf tenderness, swelling, and a positive Homans' sign (see Chap. 31).

Nursing Interventions

ENSURING EFFECTIVE TRACTION

To ensure effective skin traction, it is important to avoid wrinkling and slipping of the traction bandage and to maintain countertraction. Proper positioning must be maintained to keep the leg in a neutral position. To prevent bony fragments from moving against one another, the patient should not turn from side to side; however, the patient may shift position slightly with assistance.

MONITORING AND MANAGING POTENTIAL COMPLICATIONS

Skin Breakdown. During the initial assessment, the nurse identifies sensitive, fragile skin (common in older adults). The nurse also closely monitors the reaction of the skin in contact with tape or foam to ensure that shearing forces are avoided. The nurse per-

FIGURE 67-5 Balanced suspension skeletal traction with Thomas leg splint. The patient can move vertically as long as the resultant line of pull is maintained.

forms the following procedures to monitor and prevent skin breakdown:

- Removes the foam boots to inspect the skin, the ankle, and the Achilles tendon three times a day. A second nurse is needed to support the extremity during the inspection and skin care.
- Palpates the area of the traction tapes daily to detect underlying tenderness.
- Provides back care at least every 2 hours to prevent pressure ulcers. The patient who must remain in a supine position is at increased risk for development of a pressure ulcer.
- Uses special mattress overlays (eg, air-filled, high-density foam) to minimize the development of skin ulcers.

Nerve Pressure. Skin traction can place pressure on peripheral nerves. When traction is applied to the lower extremity, care must be taken to avoid pressure on the peroneal nerve at the point at which it passes around the neck of the fibula just below the knee. Pressure at this point can cause footdrop. The nurse questions the patient about sensation and asks the patient to move the toes and foot. Dorsiflexion of the foot demonstrates function of the peroneal nerve. Weakness of dorsiflexion or foot movement and inversion of the foot might indicate pressure on the common peroneal nerve. Plantar flexion demonstrates function of the tibial nerve.

The following are important points to keep in mind when caring for the patient in traction:

- Regularly assess sensation and motion.
- Immediately investigate any complaint of burning sensation under the traction bandage or boot.
- Promptly report altered sensation or motor function.

Circulatory Impairment. After skin traction is applied, the nurse assesses circulation of the foot or hand within 15 to 30 minutes and then every 1 to 2 hours. Circulatory assessment consists of the following:

- Peripheral pulses, colour, capillary refill, and temperature of the fingers or toes
- Indicators of DVT, including calf tenderness, swelling, and a positive Homans' sign

The nurse also encourages the patient to perform active foot exercises every hour when awake.

SKELETAL TRACTION

Skeletal traction is applied directly to the bone. This method of traction is used occasionally to treat fractures of the femur, the tibia, and the cervical spine. The traction is applied directly to the bone by use of a metal pin or wire (eg, Steinmann pin, Kirschner wire) that is inserted through the bone distal to the fracture, avoiding nerves, blood vessels, muscles, tendons, and joints. Tongs applied to the head (eg, Gardner-Wells or Vinke tongs) are fixed in the skull to apply traction that immobilizes cervical fractures.

The orthopedic surgeon applies skeletal traction, using surgical asepsis. The insertion site is prepared with a surgical scrub agent such as povidone-iodine solution. A local anesthetic is administered at the insertion site and periosteum. The surgeon makes a small skin incision and drills the sterile pin or wire through the bone. The patient feels pressure during this procedure and possibly some pain when the periosteum is penetrated.

After insertion, the pin or wire is attached to the traction bow or caliper. The ends of the wire are covered with corks or tape to prevent injury to the patient or caregivers. The weights are attached to the pin or wire bow by a rope-and-pulley system that exerts the appropriate amount and direction of pull for effective traction. Skeletal traction frequently uses 7 to 12 kg to achieve the therapeutic effect. The weights applied initially must overcome the shortening spasms of the affected muscles. As the muscles relax, the traction weight is reduced to prevent fracture dislocation and to promote healing.

Often, skeletal traction is balanced traction, which supports the affected extremity, allows for some patient movement, and facilitates patient independence and nursing care while maintaining effective traction. The Thomas splint with a Pearson attachment is frequently used with skeletal traction for fractures of the femur (see Fig. 67-5). Because upward traction is required, an overbed frame is used.

When skeletal traction is discontinued, the extremity is gently supported while the weights are removed. The pin is cut close to the skin and removed by the physician. Internal fixation, casts, or splints are then used to immobilize and support the healing bone.

Nursing Interventions

MAINTAINING EFFECTIVE TRACTION

When skeletal traction is used, the nurse checks the apparatus to see that the ropes are in the wheel grooves of the pulleys, that the ropes are not frayed, that the weights hang free, and that the knots in the rope are tied securely. The nurse also evaluates the patient's position, because slipping down in bed results in ineffective traction.

 NURSING ALERT The nurse must never remove weights from skeletal traction unless a life-threatening situation occurs. Removal of the weights completely defeats their purpose and may result in injury to the patient.

MAINTAINING POSITIONING

The nurse must maintain alignment of the patient's body in traction as prescribed to promote an effective line of pull. The nurse positions the patient's foot to avoid footdrop (plantar flexion), inward rotation (inversion), and outward rotation (eversion). The patient's foot may be supported in a neutral position by orthopedic devices (eg, foot supports).

PREVENTING SKIN BREAKDOWN

The patient's elbows frequently become sore, and nerve injury may occur if the patient repositions by pushing on the elbows. In addition, patients frequently push on the heel of the unaffected leg when they raise themselves. This digging of the heel into the mattress may injure the tissues. Therefore, the nurse should protect the elbows and heels and inspect them for pressure areas. To encourage movement without using the elbows or heel, the nurse can suspend a trapeze overhead within easy reach of the patient. This apparatus helps the patient to move about in bed and to move on and off the bedpan.

Specific pressure points are assessed for redness and skin breakdown. Areas that are particularly vulnerable to pressure caused by traction apparatus applied to the lower extremity include the ischial tuberosity, popliteal space, Achilles tendon, and heel. If the patient is not permitted to turn on one side or the other, the nurse must make a special effort to provide back care and to keep the bed dry and free of crumbs and wrinkles. The patient can assist by holding the overhead trapeze and raising the hips off the bed. If the patient cannot do this, the nurse can push down on the mattress with one hand to relieve pressure on the back and bony prominences and to provide for some shifting of weight. A pressure-relieving air-filled or high-density foam mattress overlay may reduce the risk of pressure ulcer.

For change of bed linens, the patient raises the torso while nurses on both sides of the bed roll down and replace the upper mattress sheet. Then, as the patient raises the buttocks off the mattress, the nurses slide the sheets under the buttocks. Finally, the nurses replace the lower section of the bed linens while the patient rests on the back. Sheets and blankets are placed over the patient in such a way that the traction is not disrupted.

MONITORING NEUROVASCULAR STATUS

The nurse assesses the neurovascular status of the immobilized extremity at least every hour initially and then every 4 hours. The nurse instructs the patient to report any changes in sensation or movement immediately so that they can be promptly evaluated. DVT is a significant risk for the immobilized patient. The nurse encourages the patient to do active flexion–extension ankle exercises and isometric contraction of the calf muscles (calf-pumping exercises) 10 times an hour while awake to decrease venous stasis. In addition, elastic stockings, compression devices, and anticoagulant therapy may be prescribed to help prevent thrombus formation.

Prompt recognition of a developing neurovascular problem is essential so that corrective measures can be instituted promptly.

PROVIDING PIN SITE CARE

The wound at the pin insertion site requires attention. The goal is to avoid infection and development of **osteomyelitis.** Initially, the site is covered with a sterile dressing. Subsequent care of the pin site is individually prescribed and performed three times a day. The nurse must keep the area clean. Slight serous oozing at the pin site is expected, but crusting should be prevented. The nurse assesses the pin site and drainage for signs of infection, such as redness, tenderness, and purulent drainage. The patient may experience discomfort at the pin site due to traction on the skin caused by an unsupported muscle.

 NURSING ALERT The nurse must inspect the pin site at least every 8 hours for signs of inflammation and evidence of infection.

PROMOTING EXERCISE

Patient exercises, within the therapeutic limits of the traction, assist in maintaining muscle strength and tone and in promoting circulation. Active exercises include pulling up on the trapeze, flexing and extending the feet, and range-of-motion and weight-resistance exercises for noninvolved joints. Isometric exercises of the immobilized extremity (quadriceps-setting and gluteal-setting exercises) are important for maintaining strength in major ambulatory muscles (see Chart 67-3). Without exercise, the patient will lose muscle mass and strength, and rehabilitation will be greatly prolonged.

NURSING PROCESS: THE PATIENT IN TRACTION

Assessment

The nurse must consider the psychological and physiologic impact of the musculoskeletal problem, traction device, and immo-

bility. Traction restricts one's mobility and independence. The equipment often looks threatening, and its application can be frightening. Confusion, disorientation, and behavioural problems may develop in patients who are confined in a limited space for an extended time. Therefore, the nurse must assess and monitor the patient's anxiety level and psychological responses to traction.

It is important to evaluate the body part to be placed in traction and its neurovascular status (ie, colour, temperature, capillary refill, edema, pulses, ability to move, and sensations) and compare it to the unaffected extremity. The nurse also assesses skin integrity along with body system functioning for baseline data. Ongoing assessment is indicated for the patient in traction. Immobility-related problems may include pressure ulcers, stasis pneumonia, constipation, loss of appetite, urinary stasis, urinary tract infections, and venous stasis. Early identification of preexisting or developing problems facilitates prompt interventions to resolve them.

Diagnosis

NURSING DIAGNOSES

Based on the nursing assessment, the patient's major nursing diagnoses related to traction may include the following:

- Deficient knowledge related to the treatment regimen
- Anxiety related to health status and the traction device
- Acute pain related to musculoskeletal disorder
- Self-care deficit: feeding, bathing/hygiene, dressing/grooming, and/or toileting related to traction
- Impaired physical mobility related to musculoskeletal disorder and traction

COLLABORATIVE PROBLEMS/ POTENTIAL COMPLICATIONS

Based on the assessment data, potential complications that may develop include the following:

- Pressure ulcer
- Pneumonia
- Constipation
- Anorexia
- Urinary stasis and infection
- Venous stasis with DVT

Planning and Goals

The major goals for the patient in traction may include understanding of the treatment regimen, reduced anxiety, maximum comfort, maximum level of self-care, maximum mobility within the therapeutic limits of traction, and absence of complications.

Nursing Interventions

PROMOTING UNDERSTANDING OF THE TREATMENT REGIMEN

The patient must understand the problem being treated and the rationale for the traction therapy. The nurse may need to repeat and reinforce the information. With increased understanding of the therapy, the patient becomes an active participant in health care.

REDUCING ANXIETY

Before any traction is applied, the patient needs to be informed about the procedure, its purpose, and its implications. The nurse encourages the patient to participate in decisions that affect care.

Increasing the patient's sense of control reduces feelings of help-lessness, allays apprehension, and fosters coping.

After being in traction for a while, the patient may react to being confined to a limited space. Frequent visits by the nurse can reduce feelings of isolation and confinement. The nurse should encourage family and friends to visit frequently for the same reason. The nurse encourages diversional activities that can be performed within the limits of the traction.

ACHIEVING A MAXIMUM LEVEL OF COMFORT

Because the patient is immobilized in bed, the mattress needs to be firm. Special mattresses or mattress overlays designed to minimize the development of pressure ulcers may be placed on the bed before the traction is applied. The nurse can relieve pressure on dependent body parts by turning and positioning the patient for comfort within the limits of the traction and by making sure the bed linens remain wrinkle-free and dry.

 NURSING ALERT The nurse must promptly investigate every complaint of discomfort expressed by the patient in traction.

ACHIEVING MAXIMUM SELF-CARE

Initially, the patient may require assistance with self-care activities. The nurse helps the patient eat, bathe, dress, and toilet. Convenient arrangement of items such as telephone, tissues, water, and assistive devices (eg, reachers, overbed trapeze) may facilitate self-care. With resumption of self-care activities, the patient feels less dependent and less frustrated and experiences improved self-esteem.

Because some assistance is required throughout the period of immobility, the nurse and the patient can creatively develop routines that maximize the patient's independence.

ATTAINING MAXIMUM MOBILITY WITH TRACTION

During traction therapy, the nurse encourages the patient to exercise muscles and joints that are not in traction to guard against their deterioration. The physical therapist can design bed exercises that minimize loss of muscle strength. During the patient's exercise, the nurse ensures that traction forces are maintained and that the patient is properly positioned to prevent complications resulting from poor alignment.

MONITORING AND MANAGING POTENTIAL COMPLICATIONS

Pressure Ulcers

The nurse examines the patient's skin frequently for evidence of pressure or friction, paying special attention to bony prominences. It is helpful to reposition the patient frequently and to use protective devices (eg, elbow protectors) to relieve pressure. If the risk of skin breakdown is high, as in a patient with multiple trauma or a debilitated elderly patient, use of a specialized bed is considered to prevent skin breakdown. If a pressure ulcer develops, the nurse consults with the physician and the wound care nurse specialist.

Pneumonia

The nurse auscultates the patient's lungs every 4 to 8 hours to determine respiratory status and teaches the patient deep-breathing and coughing exercises to aid in fully expanding the lungs and moving pulmonary secretions. If the patient history and baseline assessment indicate that the patient is at high risk for development of respiratory complications, specific therapies (eg, in-centive spirometer) may be indicated. If a respiratory problem develops, prompt institution of prescribed therapy is needed.

Constipation and Anorexia

Reduced gastrointestinal motility results in constipation and anorexia. A diet high in fibre and fluids may help to stimulate gastric motility. If constipation develops, therapeutic measures might include stool softeners, laxatives, suppositories, and enemas. To improve the patient's appetite, the nurse identifies and includes the patient's food preferences, as appropriate, within the prescribed therapeutic diet.

Urinary Stasis and Infection

Incomplete emptying of the bladder related to positioning in bed can result in urinary stasis and infection. In addition, the patient may find use of the bedpan uncomfortable and may limit fluids to minimize the frequency of urination. The nurse monitors the fluid intake and the character of the urine. The nurse teaches the patient to consume adequate amounts of fluid and to void every 3 to 4 hours. If the patient exhibits signs or symptoms of urinary tract infection, the nurse notifies the physician.

Venous Stasis and Deep Vein Thrombosis

Venous stasis occurs with immobility. The nurse teaches the patient to perform ankle and foot exercises within the limits of the traction therapy every 1 to 2 hours when awake to prevent DVT, which may result from venous stasis. The patient is encouraged to drink fluids to prevent dehydration and associated hemoconcentration, which contribute to stasis. The nurse monitors the patient for signs of DVT, including calf tenderness, warmth, redness, swelling (increased calf circumference), and a positive Homans' sign (discomfort in the calf when the foot is forcibly dorsiflexed). The nurse promptly reports findings to the physician for definitive evaluation and therapy.

Evaluation

EXPECTED PATIENT OUTCOMES

Expected patient outcomes may include:

1. Demonstrates knowledge of traction regimen
   a. Describes purpose of traction
   b. Participates in plan of care
2. Exhibits reduced anxiety
   a. Appears relaxed
   b. Uses effective coping mechanisms
   c. Expresses concerns and feelings
   d. Engages in diversional activities
3. States increased level of comfort
   a. Requests occasional oral analgesia
   b. Repositions self frequently
4. Performs self-care activities
   a. Requires minimal assistance with feeding, bathing/hygiene, dressing/grooming, and/or toileting
   b. Uses assistive devices safely
5. Demonstrates increased mobility
   a. Performs prescribed exercises
   b. Repositions self within limits of traction
6. Experiences no complications
   a. Has intact skin
   b. Has clear lungs
   c. Does not report shortness of breath
   d. Does not have a productive cough
   e. Exhibits a regular bowel evacuation pattern

f. Has a normal appetite
g. Voids clear, yellow, nonconcentrated urine of adequate amount
h. Does not exhibit signs or symptoms of venous stasis

Managing the Patient Undergoing Orthopedic Surgery

Many patients with musculoskeletal dysfunction undergo surgery to correct the problem. Problems that may be corrected by surgery include unstabilized fracture, deformity, joint disease, necrotic or infected tissue, and tumours. Frequent surgical procedures include **open reduction with internal fixation (ORIF)** and closed reduction with internal fixation (fracture fragments are not surgically exposed) for fractures; arthroplasty, meniscectomy, and joint replacement for joint problems; amputation for severe extremity problems (eg, gangrene, massive trauma); bone graft for joint stabilization, defect-filling, or stimulation of bone healing; and tendon transfer for improving motion. The goals include improving function by restoring motion and stability and relieving pain and disability. See Chart 67-7 for descriptions of orthopedic surgeries.

Joint surgery is one the most frequently performed orthopedic surgeries. Joint disease or deformity may necessitate surgical intervention to relieve pain, improve stability, and improve function. Surgical procedures include excision of damaged and diseased tissue, repair of damaged structures (eg, ruptured tendon), removal of loose bodies (débridement), **arthroplasty** (replacement of all or part of the joint surfaces), and **arthrodesis** (immobilizing fusion of a joint).

The procedure is based on the patient's underlying orthopedic condition, general physical health, impact of joint disability on daily activities, and age. Timing of these procedures is important to ensure maximum function. Surgery should be performed before surrounding muscles become contracted and atrophied

and serious structural abnormalities occur. The physician carefully evaluates the patient so that the most appropriate procedure is performed.

Because these are elective procedures, many patients donate their own blood during the weeks preceding their surgery. This blood is used to replace blood lost during surgery. Autologous blood transfusions eliminate many of the risks of transfusion therapy.

Also, during surgery blood is conserved to minimize loss. A pneumatic tourniquet may be applied after exsanguination of the limb with bandages to produce a "bloodless field." Intraoperative blood salvage with reinfusion is used when a large volume of blood loss is anticipated. Postoperative blood salvage with intermittent autotransfusion also reduces the need for blood transfusion.

JOINT REPLACEMENT

Patients with severe joint pain and disability may undergo joint replacement. Conditions contributing to joint degeneration include osteoarthritis (degenerative joint disease), rheumatoid arthritis, trauma, and congenital deformity. Some fractures (eg, femoral neck fracture) may cause disruption of the blood supply and subsequent **avascular necrosis;** management with joint replacement may be elected over ORIF. Joints frequently replaced include the hip, knee (Fig. 67-6), and finger joints. Less fre-

---

Chart 67-7 Orthopedic Surgeries

Open reduction: the correction and alignment of the fracture after surgical dissection and exposure of the fracture

Internal fixation: the stabilization of the reduced fracture by the use of metal screws, plates, nails, and pins

Arthroplasty: the repair of joint problems through the operating arthroscope (an instrument that allows the surgeon to operate within a joint without a large incision) or through open joint surgery

Hemiarthroplasty: the replacement of one of the articular surfaces (eg, in a hip hemiarthroplasty, the femoral head and neck are replaced with a femoral prosthesis—the acetabulum is not replaced)

Joint arthroplasty or *replacement:* the replacement of joint surfaces with metal or synthetic materials

Total joint arthroplasty or *replacement:* the replacement of both articular surfaces within a joint with metal or synthetic materials

Meniscectomy: the excision of damaged joint fibrocartilage

Amputation: the removal of a body part

Bone graft: the placement of bone tissue (autologous or homologous grafts) to promote healing, to stabilize, or to replace diseased bone

Tendon transfer: the movement of tendon insertion to improve function

Fasciotomy: the incision and diversion of the muscle fascia to relieve muscle constriction, as in compartment syndrome, or to reduce fascia contracture

Acetabular (pelvic) component

Femoral (distal) component

Femoral (proximal) component

Tibial component

FIGURE 67-6 Examples of hip and knee replacement.

quently, more complex joints (shoulder, elbow, wrist, ankle) are replaced. The procedure is usually an elective one.

Most joint replacements consist of metal and high-density polyethylene components. Finger prostheses are usually Silastic. The joint implants may be cemented in the prepared bone with polymethyl methacrylate (PMMA), a bone-bonding agent that has properties similar to bone. Loosening of the prosthesis due to cement–bone interface failure is a common reason for prosthesis failure. Press-fit, ingrowth prostheses (porous-coated, cementless artificial joint components) that allow the patient's bone to grow into and securely fix the prosthesis in the bone are alternatives to cemented prostheses. Accurate fitting and the presence of healthy bone with adequate blood supply are important in the use of cementless components. Much progress has been made in reducing prosthesis failure rate through improved techniques, improved materials, and use of bone grafts.

With joint replacement, excellent pain relief is obtained in most patients. Return of motion and function depends on preoperative soft tissue condition, soft tissue reactions, and general muscle strength. Early failure of joint replacement is associated with excessive activity and preoperative joint and bone pathology.

Nursing Interventions

Assessment of the patient and preoperative management are aimed at having the patient in optimal health at the time of surgery. Preoperatively, it is important to evaluate cardiovascular, respiratory, renal, and hepatic functions. Age, obesity, preoperative leg edema, history of DVT, and varicose veins increase the risk of postoperative DVT and pulmonary embolism. These are the most common causes of postoperative mortality for patients older than 60 years of age undergoing total hip replacement. Every effort is made to prevent these complications.

Preoperatively, it is important to assess the neurovascular status of the extremity undergoing joint replacement. Postoperative assessment data are compared with preoperative assessment data to identify changes and deficits. For example, an absent pulse postoperatively is of concern unless the pulse was also absent preoperatively. Nerve palsy could occur as a result of surgery.

PREVENTING INFECTION
Preoperative assessment of the patient for infections, including urinary tract infection, is necessary because of the risk of postoperative infection. Any infection 2 to 4 weeks before planned surgery may result in postponement of surgery. Preoperative skin preparation frequently begins 1 or 2 days before the surgery. Airborne bacteria that contaminate the wound at the time of surgery cause most deep infections. Therefore, as with any surgery, there is strict adherence to aseptic principles and the operating area is controlled and made as bacteria free as possible.

Prophylactic antibiotics are administered perioperatively as a single preoperative or short perioperative course (Rosen et al., 1999). Culture of the joint during surgery, before intraoperative antibiotic therapy is begun, may be important in identifying and treating subsequent infections.

If osteomyelitis develops, it is difficult to treat. Persistent infection at the site of the prosthesis usually requires removal of the implant and joint revision, which is a complex procedure. Also, it is not always possible to achieve a functional joint when the reconstruction procedure has to be repeated.

PROMOTING AMBULATION
Patients with total hip or total knee replacement begin ambulation with a walker or crutches within a day after surgery. The

nurse and the physical therapist assist the patient in achieving the goal of independent ambulation. At first, the patient may only be able to stand for a brief period because of orthostatic hypotension. Specific weight-bearing limits on the prosthesis are determined by the physician and are based on the patient's condition, the procedure, and the fixation method. Usually, patients with cemented prostheses can proceed to weight bearing as tolerated. If the patient has a press-fit, cementless, ingrowth prosthesis, weight bearing immediately after surgery may be limited to minimize micromotion of the prosthesis in the bone. As the patient is able tolerate more activity, the nurse encourages transferring to a chair several times a day for short periods and walking for progressively greater distances.

TOTAL HIP REPLACEMENT

Total hip replacement is the replacement of a severely damaged hip with an artificial joint. Indications for this surgery include arthritis (degenerative joint disease, rheumatoid arthritis), femoral neck fractures, failure of previous reconstructive surgeries (failed prosthesis, **osteotomy**), and problems resulting from congenital hip disease. A variety of total hip prostheses are available. Most consist of a metal femoral component topped by a spherical ball fitted into a plastic acetabular socket (see Fig. 67-6). The surgeon selects the prosthesis that is most suited to the individual patient, considering various factors, including skeletal structure and activity level.

The patient is usually 60 years of age or older and has unremitting pain or irreversibly damaged hip joints. With the advent of improved prosthetic materials and operative techniques, the life of the prosthesis has been extended, and today younger patients with severely damaged and painful hip joints are undergoing total hip replacement.

Nursing Interventions

The nurse must be aware of and monitor for specific potential complications associated with total hip replacement. Complications that may occur include dislocation of the hip prosthesis, excessive wound drainage, thromboembolism, infection, and heel pressure ulcer. Other complications for which the nurse must monitor include those associated with immobility, **heterotophic ossification** (formation of bone in the periprosthetic space), avascular necrosis (bone death caused by loss of blood supply), and loosening of the prosthesis.

PREVENTING DISLOCATION OF THE HIP PROSTHESIS
Maintenance of the femoral head component in the acetabular cup is essential. The nurse teaches the patient about positioning the leg in **abduction,** which helps to prevent dislocation of the prosthesis. The use of an abduction splint, a wedge pillow (Fig. 67-7), or two or three pillows between the legs keeps the hip in abduction. When the nurse turns the patient in bed, it is important to keep the operative hip in abduction. Depending on the surgeon's preference, some patients are not permitted to be turned onto the affected side, whereas others may be turned to either side.

The patient's hip is never flexed more than 90 degrees. To prevent hip flexion, the nurse does not elevate the head of the bed more than 60 degrees. For use of the fracture bedpan, the nurse instructs the patient to flex the unaffected hip and to use the trapeze to lift the pelvis onto the pan. The patient is also reminded not to flex the affected hip.

Limited flexion is maintained during transfers and when sitting. When the patient is initially assisted out of bed, an abduction splint or pillows are kept between the legs. The nurse

FIGURE 67-7 An abduction pillow may be used after a total hip replacement to prevent dislocation of the prosthesis.

encourages the patient to keep the affected hip in extension, instructing the patient to pivot on the unaffected leg with assistance by the nurse, who protects the affected hip from **adduction**, flexion, internal or external rotation, and excessive weight bearing.

High-seat (orthopedic) chairs, semireclining wheelchairs, and raised toilet seats may be used to minimize hip joint flexion. When sitting, the patient's hips should be higher than the knees. The patient's affected leg should not be elevated when sitting. The patient may flex the knee.

The nurse teaches the patient protective positioning, which includes maintaining abduction and avoiding internal and external rotation, hyperextension, and acute flexion. A cradle boot may be used to prevent leg rotation and to support the heel off the bed, preventing development of a pressure ulcer. The patient should use pillows between the legs when in a supine or side-lying position and when turning. Generally, the nurse instructs the patient

not to sleep on the side on which the surgery was performed without consulting the surgeon. At no time should the patient cross his or her legs. The patient must avoid acute flexion of the hip. The patient should not bend at the waist to put on shoes and socks. Occupational therapists can provide the patient with devices to assist with dressing below the waist. Hip precautions are needed for about 4 months after surgery (Chart 67-8).

Dislocation may occur with positioning that exceeds the limits of the prosthesis. The nurse must recognize dislocation of the prosthesis. Indicators are as follows:

- Increased pain at the surgical site, swelling, and immobilization
- Acute groin pain in affected hip or increased discomfort
- Shortening of the leg
- Abnormal external or internal rotation
- Restricted ability or inability to move leg
- Reported "popping" sensation in hip

If a prosthesis becomes dislocated, the nurse (or the patient, if at home) immediately notifies the surgeon, because the hip must be reduced and stabilized promptly so that the leg does not sustain circulatory and nerve damage. After closed reduction, the hip may be stabilized with Buck's traction or a brace to prevent recurrent dislocation. As the muscles and joint capsule heal, the chance of dislocation diminishes. Stresses to the new hip joint should be avoided for the first 3 to 6 months.

MONITORING WOUND DRAINAGE

Fluid and blood accumulating at the surgical site are usually drained with a portable suction device. This prevents accumula-

---

Chart 67-8

Avoiding Hip Dislocation After Replacement Surgery

Until the hip prosthesis stabilizes after hip replacement surgery, the patient needs to learn about proper positioning so that the prosthesis remains in place. Dislocation of the hip is a serious complication of surgery that causes pain and loss of function and necessitates reduction under anesthesia to correct the dislocation. Desirable positions include abduction, neutral rotation, and flexion of less than 90 degrees. When the patient is seated, the knees should be lower than the hip.

Methods for avoiding displacement include the following:
- Keep the knees apart at all times.
- Put a pillow between the legs when sleeping.

- Never cross the legs when seated.
- Avoid bending forward when seated in a chair.
- Avoid bending forward to pick up an object on the floor.
- Use a high-seated chair and a raised toilet seat.
- Do not flex the hip to put on clothing such as pants, stockings, socks or shoes.

Positions to avoid after total hip replacement are illustrated below.

Affected leg should not cross the center of the body

Hip should not bend more than 90 degrees

Affected leg should not turn inward

tion of fluid, which could contribute to discomfort and provide a site for infection. Drainage of 200 to 500 mL in the first 24 hours is expected; by 48 hours postoperatively, the total drainage in 8 hours usually decreases to 30 mL or less, and the suction device is then removed. The nurse promptly notifies the physician of any drainage volumes greater than anticipated.

If extensive blood loss is anticipated after total joint replacement surgery, an autotransfusion drainage system (in which the drained blood is filtered and reinfused into the patient during the immediate postoperative period) may be used to decrease the need for homologous blood transfusions.

PREVENTING DEEP VEIN THROMBOSIS

The risk for thromboembolism is particularly great after reconstructive hip surgery. The incidence of DVT is 45% to 70%. The peak occurrence is 5 to 7 days after surgery. About 20% of patients with DVT develop pulmonary emboli, of which about 1% to 3% of cases are fatal. Therefore, the nurse must institute preventive measures and monitor the patient closely for the development of DVT and pulmonary emboli. Signs of DVT include calf pain, swelling, and tenderness. Measures to promote circulation and decrease venous stasis are priorities for the patient undergoing hip reconstruction. The nurse encourages the patient to consume adequate amounts of fluids, to perform ankle and foot exercises hourly while awake, to use elastic stockings and sequential compression devices

as prescribed, and to transfer out of bed and ambulate with assistance beginning on the first postoperative day. Low-dose heparin, enoxaparin (Lovenox), or dalteparin (Fragmin) is frequently prescribed as prophylaxis for DVT after hip replacement surgery.

PREVENTING INFECTION

Infection, a serious complication of total hip replacement, may necessitate removal of the implant. Patients who are elderly, obese, or poorly nourished and patients who have diabetes, rheumatoid arthritis, concurrent infections (eg, urinary tract infection, dental abscess), or large hematomas are at high risk for infection.

Because total joint infections are so disastrous, all efforts are undertaken to minimize their occurrence. Potential sources of infection are avoided. Prophylactic antibiotics are prescribed. If indwelling urinary catheters or portable wound suction devices are used, they are removed as soon as possible to avoid infection. Prophylactic antibiotics are prescribed if the patient needs any future surgical instrumentation, such as tooth extraction or cystoscopic examination.

Acute infections may occur within 3 months after surgery and are associated with progressive superficial infections or hematomas. Delayed surgical infections may appear 4 to 24 months after surgery and may cause return of discomfort in the hip. Infections occurring more than 2 years after surgery are attributed to the spread of infection through the bloodstream from another site in the body. If

NURSING RESEARCH PROFILE 67-1
Wound Complications After Hip Surgery

Hahn, G., et al. (1999). Wound complications after surgery using a tapeless compressive support. *Orthopaedic Nursing*, 18(3), 43–49.

Purpose
Skin blisters (tape blisters) frequently occur after hip surgery and cause skin breakdown and patient discomfort. This study compared the incidence of blisters and wound drainage with traditional wound taping and with a tapeless compressive (stretch spica) wrap dressing (i.e., cotton stockinette or a commercial single-piece stretch spica wrap).

Study Sample and Design
A total of 499 hip surgeries performed by one surgeon over a 10-year period on 457 patients, whose average age was 65 years, were reviewed. Eighty-seven consecutive hip surgeries with taped dressings (control group) were compared with 368 consecutive hip surgeries with hip wrap dressings (experimental group). The patient characteristics in the two groups were similar. The surgeries were performed for osteoarthritis (60%), fracture (22%), rheumatoid arthritis (8%), and other problems (10%) including osteonecrosis, congenitally dislocated hips, Reiter's syndrome, and Legg-Perthes disease. Surgical procedures performed included hip replacement (67%), revision of hip replacement (25%), and open reduction internal fixation of hip fracture (8%).

A retrospective, descriptive study design was used to compare the incidence of wound drainage, tape blisters, infections, deep vein thrombosis, and pulmonary embolism in the two groups.

Findings
- Wound drainage was difficult to quantify because of the descriptive nature of charting. Twenty-eight (7%) of the spica wrap group and 13 (15%) of the tape group exhibited wound drainage. All drainage was described as slight to moderate with no drainage at the time of discharge from the hospital. The difference in incidence of drainage between groups was statistically significant ($p < .001$).

- Four tape blisters (1%), two from surgical incision adhesive strips and two from taping of the dressing after the spica wrap was discontinued, occurred in the tapeless compressive wrap dressing group, compared with 13 tape blisters (15%) in the tape group. The difference in incidence of blisters between groups was statistically significant ($p < .001$).
- No infections occurred in the spica wrap group, and there was one documented *Staphylococcus aureus* infection in the tape group.
- Thrombotic disease prophylaxis was used for both groups. The incidence of thrombotic disease in the spica wrap group was 12 patients (3%). Because the data recorded for the traditional tape group were insufficient to determine the incidence of thrombotic disease, no comparison with controls could be made. However, the low incidence in the experimental group suggests that the spica wrap does not contribute to an increased incidence of deep vein thrombosis.
- Patients reported that the spica wrap was comfortable and supported the incision well, so that they could move with greater confidence.
- Nurses found the spica wrap easy to apply and easy to unfasten for inspection of the wound. Also, nursing time was not required to care for tape blisters.

Nursing Implications
In this study, the use of a compressive spica wrap dressing, compared with taped dressings, reduced the incidence of wound complications (eg, tape blisters, drainage). Advantages included ease of application and removal for wound inspection. In addition, the hip spica dressing was comfortable for the patient.

Additional studies in other settings and with other patients comparing the use of the hip spica dressing and traditional taped dressings are recommended; randomization of patients to the spica wrap dressing group and to the tape group is also recommended.

an infection occurs, antibiotics are prescribed. Severe infections may require surgical débridement or removal of the prosthesis (Nursing Research Profile 67-1).

PROMOTING HOME AND COMMUNITY-BASED CARE

Teaching the Patient Self-Care. Before the patient prepares to leave the acute care setting, the nurse provides a thorough teaching program to promote continuity of the therapeutic regimen and active participation in the rehabilitation process (Chart 67-9). The nurse advises the patient of the importance of the daily exercise program in maintaining the functional motion of the hip joint and strengthening the abductor muscles of the hip, and reminds the patient that it will take time to strengthen and retrain the muscles.

Assistive devices (crutches, walker, or cane) are used for a time. After sufficient muscle tone has developed to permit a normal gait without discomfort, these devices are not necessary. In general, by 3 months, the patient can resume routine ADLs. Stair climbing is permitted as prescribed and is kept to a minimum for 3 to 6 months. Frequent walks, swimming, and use of a high rocking chair are excellent for hip exercises. Sexual activities should be carried out with the patient in the dependent position (flat on the back) for 3 to 6 months to avoid excessive adduction and flexion of the new hip.

At no time during the first 4 months should the patient cross the legs or flex the hip more than 90 degrees. Assistance in putting on shoes and socks may be needed. The patient should avoid low chairs and sitting for longer than 45 minutes at a time. These precautions minimize hip flexion and the risks for prosthetic dislocation, hip stiffness, and flexion contracture. Traveling long distances should be avoided unless frequent position changes are possible. Other activities to avoid include tub baths, (if no tub seat is available), overexertion, jogging, lifting heavy loads, and excessive bending and twisting (eg, lifting, shoveling snow, forceful turning).

Continuing Care in the Home and Community. The nurse may make a home visit to assess for potential problems and to monitor wound healing (see Chart 67-9). The nurse, physical therapist, or occupational therapist assesses the home environment for physical barriers that may impede the patient's rehabilitation. In addition, the nurse or therapist may need to assist the patient in acquiring devices, such as reachers to help with dressing or toilet seat extenders.

After successful surgery and rehabilitation, the patient can expect a hip joint that is free or almost free of pain, has good motion, is stable, and permits normal or near-normal ambulation (see Plan of Nursing Care).

TOTAL KNEE REPLACEMENT

Total knee replacement surgery is considered for patients who have severe pain and functional disabilities related to joint surfaces destroyed by arthritis (osteoarthritis, rheumatoid arthritis, posttraumatic arthritis) or bleeding into the joint, such as may result from hemophilia. Metal and acrylic prostheses designed to provide the patient with a functional, painless, stable joint may be used. If the patient's ligaments have weakened, a fully constrained (hinged) or semiconstrained prosthesis may be used to provide joint stability. A nonconstrained prosthesis depends on the patient's ligaments for joint stability.

Nursing Interventions

Postoperatively, the knee is dressed with a compression bandage. Ice may be applied to control edema and bleeding. The nurse assesses the neurovascular status of the leg. It is important to encourage active flexion of the foot every hour when the patient is awake. Efforts are directed at preventing complications

(text continues on page 2049)

Chart 67-9 • PATIENT EDUCATION
Providing Home Care After Hip Replacement

Considerations
- Pain management
- Wound care
- Mobility
- Self-care (activities of daily living)
- Potential problems

Nursing Interventions
Discuss with patient methods to reduce pain:
- Periodic rest
- Distraction and relaxation techniques
- Medication therapy (eg, nonsteroidal anti-inflammatory drugs, opioid analgesics): actions of medications, administration, schedule, side effects

Instruct patient in the following:
- Keeping incision clean and dry
- Taking care of the wound and changing the dressing
- Recognizing signs of wound infection (eg, pain, swelling, drainage, fever)

Explain that sutures or staples will be removed 10 to 14 days after surgery.
Teach patient about the following:
- Safe use of assistive devices
- Weight-bearing limits
- How to change positions frequently

- Limitations on hip flexion and adduction (eg, avoid acute flexion and crossing legs)
- How to stand without flexing hip acutely
- Avoidance of low-seated chairs
- Sleeping with pillow between legs to prevent adduction
- Gradual increase in activities and participation in prescribed exercise regimen

Assess home environment for physical barriers.
Instruct patient to use elevated toilet seat and to use reachers to aid in dressing.
Encourage patient to accept assistance with activities of daily living during early convalescence until mobility and strength improve.
Arrange services and accommodations to address the patient's disability or illness, as appropriate.
Assess patient for development of potential problems, and instruct patient to report signs of potential problems:
- Dislocation of prosthesis (eg, increased pain, shortening of leg, inability to move leg, popping sensation in hip, abnormal rotation)
- Deep vein thrombosis (eg, calf pain, swelling)
- Wound infection (eg, swelling, purulent drainage, pain, fever)
- Pulmonary emboli (eg, sudden dyspnea, tachypnea, pleuritic chest pain)

Discuss with patient the need to continue regular health care (routine physical examinations) and screenings.

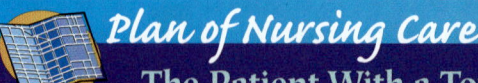

Plan of Nursing Care
The Patient With a Total Hip Replacement

Nursing Interventions	Rationale	Expected Outcomes

Nursing Diagnosis: Pain related to total hip replacement
Goal: Relief of pain

Nursing Interventions	Rationale	Expected Outcomes
1. Assess patient for pain using a standard pain intensity scale.	1. Pain is expected after a surgical procedure because of the surgical trauma and tissue response. Muscle spasms occur after total hip replacements. Immobility causes discomfort at pressure points.	• Patient describes discomfort • Expresses confidence in efforts to control pain • States pain is reduced; pain intensity scores are decreasing • Appears comfortable and relaxed • Uses physical, psychological, and pharmacologic measures to reduce pain and discomfort
2. Ask patient to describe discomfort.	2. Pain characteristics may help to determine the cause of discomfort. Pain may be due to complications (hematoma, infection, dislocation). Pain is an individual experience—it means different things to different people.	
3. Acknowledge existence of pain; inform patient of available analgesics or muscle relaxants.	3. The nurse can reduce the stress experienced by patient by communicating concern and availability of assistance to help the patient deal with the pain	

4. Use pain-modifying techniques.
  a. Use analgesics.
 	
  b. Change position within prescribed limits.
  c. Modify environment.
 	
  d. Notify surgeon about persistent pain.
	4.
	  a. Patient will require parenteral opioids during the first 24–48 hours, and then will progress to oral analgesics.
	  b. Use of pillows to provide adequate support and relief of pressure on bony prominences assists in minimizing pain.
	  c. Interactions with others, distractions, and sensory overload or deprivation may affect pain experience.
	  d. Surgical intervention may be necessary if pain is due to hematoma or excessive edema.	

5. Evaluate and record discomfort and effectiveness of pain-modifying techniques.	5. Effectiveness of action is based on experience; data provide a baseline about pain experiences, management, and pain relief.	

Nursing Diagnosis: Impaired physical mobility related to positioning, weight-bearing, and activity restrictions after hip replacement
Goal: Achieves pain-free, functional, stable hip joint

Nursing Interventions	Rationale	Expected Outcomes
1. Maintain proper positioning of hip joint (abduction, neutral rotation, limited flexion).	1. Prevents dislocation of hip prosthesis.	• Prescribed position maintained • No heel pressure • Patient assists in position changes • Shows increased independence in transfers • Exercises hourly • Participates in progressive ambulation program • Actively participates in exercise regimen • Uses ambulatory aids correctly and safely
2. Keep pressure off heel.	2. Prevents pressure ulcer on heel.	
3. Instruct and assist in position changes and transfers.	3. Encourages patient's active participation while preventing dislocation.	
4. Instruct and supervise isometric quadriceps- and gluteal-setting exercises.	4. Strengthens muscles needed for walking.	
5. In consultation with physical therapist, instruct and supervise progressive safe ambulation within limitations of weight-bearing prescription.	5. Amount of weight-bearing depends on patient's condition and prosthesis; ambulatory aids are used to assist the patient with non–weight-bearing and partial weight-bearing ambulation.	
6. Offer encouragement and support exercise regimen.	6. Reconditioning exercises can be uncomfortable and fatiguing; encouragement helps patient comply with exercise program.	
7. Instruct and supervise safe use of ambulatory aids.	7. Prevents injury from unsafe use.	

(continued)

Plan of Nursing Care

The Patient With a Total Hip Replacement *(Continued)*

Nursing Interventions	Rationale	Expected Outcomes

Collaborative Problems: Hemorrhage; neurovascular compromise; dislocation of prosthesis; deep vein thrombosis; infection related to surgery

Goal: Absence of complications

Hemorrhage

1. Monitor vital signs, observing for shock.

2. Note character and amount of drainage.

3. Notify surgeon if patient develops shock or excessive bleeding and prepare for administration of fluids, blood component therapy, and medications.
4. Monitor hemoglobin and hematocrit values.

1. Changes in pulse, blood pressure, and respirations may indicate development of shock. Blood loss and stress of surgery may contribute to development of shock.
2. Within 48 hours, bloody drainage collected in portable suction device should decrease to 25–30 mL per 8 hours. Excessive drainage (more than 250 mL in first 8 hours after surgery) and bright red drainage may indicate active bleeding.
3. Corrective measures need to be instituted.

4. Anemia due to blood loss may develop. Blood replacement or iron supplementation may be needed.

- Vital signs stabilize within normal limits
- Amount of drainage decreases
- No bright red bloody drainage
- Hematology values are within normal limits

Neurovascular Dysfunction

1. Assess affected extremity for colour and temperature.

2. Assess toes for capillary refill response.

3. Assess extremity for edema and swelling. Report patient complaints of leg tightness.

4. Elevate extremity (keep leg lower than hip when in chair).
5. Assess for deep, throbbing, unrelenting pain.

6. Assess for pain on passive flexion of foot.

7. Assess for change in sensations and numbness.

8. Assess ability to move foot and toes.

9. Assess pedal pulses in both feet.
10. Notify surgeon if altered neurovascular status is noted.

1. The skin becomes pale and feels cool with decreased tissue perfusion. Venous congestion may produce cyanosis.
2. After compression of the nail, rapid return of pink colour indicates good capillary perfusion.
3. The trauma of surgery will cause edema. Excessive swelling and hematoma formation can compromise circulation and function.
4. Minimizes dependent edema.

5. Surgical pain can be controlled; pain due to neurovascular compromise is not relieved by treatment.
6. With nerve ischemia, there will be pain on passive stretch. Additionally, pain may indicate deep vein thrombosis—positive Homans' sign.
7. Diminished pain and sensory function may indicate nerve damage. Sensation in web between great and second toe—peroneal nerve; sensation on sole of foot—tibial nerve.
8. Dorsiflexion of ankle and extension of toes indicate function of peroneal nerve. Plantar flexion of ankle and flexion of toes indicate function of tibial nerve.
9. Indicator of extremity circulation.
10. Function of extremity needs to be preserved.

- Colour normal
- Extremity warm
- Normal capillary refill
- Moderate edema and swelling; tissue not palpably tense
- Pain controllable
- No pain with passive dorsiflexion
- Normal sensations
- No paresthesia
- Normal motor abilities
- No paresis or paralysis
- Pulses strong and equal

(continued)

Plan of Nursing Care

The Patient With a Total Hip Replacement (*Continued*)

Nursing Interventions	Rationale	Expected Outcomes
Dislocation of Prosthesis		
1. Position patient as prescribed.	1. Hip component positioning (femoral component in acetabular component) needs to be maintained.	• Prosthesis not dislocated
2. Use abductor splint or pillows to maintain position and to support extremity.	2. Keep hip in abduction and in a neutral rotation to prevent dislocation.	
3. Support leg and place pillows between legs when patient is turning and side-lying; turn to the unaffected side.	3–5. Prevent dislocation.	
4. Avoid acute flexion of hip (head of bed at 60 degrees or less).		
5. Avoid crossing legs.		
6. Assess for dislocation of prosthesis (extremity shortens, internally or externally rotated, severe hip pain, patient unable to move extremity)	6. Findings may indicate dislocation of prosthesis.	
7. Notify surgeon of possible dislocation.	7. Joint dislocations compromise neurovascular status and future function of extremity.	
Deep Vein Thrombosis		
1. Use elastic compression stocking or sequential compression device as prescribed.	1. Aid in venous blood return and prevent stasis.	• Wears elastic stockings; uses compression device
2. Remove stocking for 20 minutes twice a day and provide skin care.	2. Skin care is necessary to avoid breakdown. Extended removal of stockings defeats purpose of stockings.	• No skin breakdown
3. Assess popliteal, dorsalis pedis, and posterior tibial pulses.	3. Pulses indicate arterial perfusion of extremity.	• Pulses equal and strong • Skin temperature normal
4. Assess skin temperature of legs.	4. Local inflammation will increase local skin temperature.	• Negative Homans' sign
5. Assess for Homans' sign every 8 hours.	5. Pain on dorsiflexion of ankle may indicate deep vein thrombosis.	• Changes position with assistance and supervision
6. Avoid pressure on popliteal blood vessels from equipment (eg, abductor splint straps, sequential compression stockings) or pillows.	6. Compression of blood vessels diminishes blood flow.	• Participates in exercise regimen • Well hydrated • No chest pain; lungs clear to auscultation; no evidence of pulmonary emboli
7. Change position and increase activity as prescribed.	7. Activity promotes circulation and diminishes venous stasis.	
8. Supervise ankle exercises hourly.	8. Muscle exercise promotes circulation.	
9. Monitor body temperature.	9. Body temperature increases with inflammation.	
10. Encourage fluids.	10. Dehydration increases blood viscosity	
Infection		
1. Monitor vital signs.	1. Temperature, pulse, and respirations increase in response to infection. (Magnitude of response may be minimal in an elderly patient.)	• Vital signs normal • Well-approximated incision without drainage or excessive inflammatory response
2. Use aseptic technique for dressing changes and emptying of portable drainage.	2. Avoids introducing organisms.	• Minimal discomfort; no hematoma • Patient tolerates antibiotics
3. Assess wound appearance and character of drainage.	3. Red, swollen, draining incision is indicative of infection.	
4. Assess complaints of pain.	4. Pain may be due to wound hematoma—a possible locus of infection—that needs to be surgically evacuated.	
5. Administer prophylactic antibiotics if prescribed, and observe for side effects.	5. Infected prosthesis is avoided.	

(*continued*)

Plan of Nursing Care
The Patient With a Total Hip Replacement *(Continued)*

Nursing Interventions	Rationale	Expected Outcomes
Nursing Diagnosis: Risk for ineffective health maintenance related to total hip replacement		
Goal: Cares for self at home		
1. Assess home environment for discharge planning.	1. Physical barriers (especially stairs, bathrooms) may limit patient's ability to ambulate and care for self at home.	• Home is accessible for patient at time of discharge.
2. Encourage patient to express concerns about care at home; explore together possible solutions to the problem.	2. Patient may have special problems that need to be identified and resolved.	• Patient appears relaxed and develops strategies to deal with identified problems.
3. Assess availability of physical assistance for health care activities.	3. Because of limitation of mobility and limited hip range of motion, patient may require some assistance in routine health care.	• Personal assistance is available. • Patient demonstrates ability to provide necessary assistance within therapeutic prescription.
4. Teach caregiver home health care regimen.	4. Understanding of rehabilitative regimen is necessary for compliance.	• Patient complies with home care program. • Patient keeps follow-up health care appointments.
5. Instruct patient on posthospital care: a. Activity limitations (hip precautions, weight-bearing limits) b. Exercise instructions c. Safe use of ambulatory aids d. Wound care e. Measures to promote healing f. Medications, if any g. Potential problems h. Continuing health care supervision and management	5. Lack of knowledge and poor preparation for care at home contribute to patient anxiety, insecurity, and nonadherence to therapeutic regimen.	

(thromboembolism, peroneal nerve palsy, infection, limited range of motion).

A wound suction drain removes fluid accumulating in the joint. Drainage ranges from 200 to 400 mL during the first 24 hours after surgery and diminishes to less than 25 mL by 48 hours. Then the surgeon removes the drains. If extensive bleeding is anticipated, an autotransfusion drainage system may be used during the immediate postoperative period. The colour, type, and amount of drainage are documented, and any excessive drainage or change in characteristics of the drainage are promptly reported to the physician.

Frequently, a **continuous passive motion (CPM) device** is used. The patient's leg is placed in this device, which increases circulation and range of motion of the knee joint. The rate and amount of extension and flexion are prescribed. Usually, 10 degrees of extension and 50 degrees of flexion are prescribed initially, increasing to 90 degrees of flexion with full extension (0 degrees) by discharge.

The nurse encourages the patient to use the device most of the time. The physical therapist supervises exercises for strength and range of motion. If satisfactory flexion is not achieved, gentle manipulation of the knee joint under general anesthesia may be necessary about 2 weeks after surgery.

The nurse assists the patient to get out of bed on the evening or the day after surgery. The knee is usually protected with a knee immobilizer (splint, cast, or brace) and is elevated when the patient sits in a chair. The physician prescribes weight-bearing limits. Progressive ambulation, using assistive devices and within the prescribed weight-bearing limits, begins on the day after the surgery.

After discharge from the hospital, the patient may continue to use the CPM device at home and may undergo physical therapy on an outpatient basis. Late complications that may occur include infection and loosening and wear of prosthetic components. Patients usually can achieve a pain-free, functional joint and participate more fully in life activities than before the surgery (Nursing Research Profile 67-2).

NURSING PROCESS: PREOPERATIVE CARE OF THE PATIENT UNDERGOING ORTHOPEDIC SURGERY

Assessment

Assessment of the patient is focused on hydration status, current medication history, and possible infection. Adequate hydration is an important goal for orthopedic patients. Immobilization and bed rest contribute to DVT, to urinary stasis and associated bladder infections, and to kidney stone formation. Adequate hydration decreases blood viscosity and venous stasis and ensures adequate urine flow. To determine preoperative hydration status, the nurse assesses the skin and mucous membranes, vital signs, urinary output, and laboratory values.

The medication history provides information for perioperative management. The patient with chronic illness (eg, rheumatoid arthritis, chronic pulmonary disease, multiple sclerosis, allergies) frequently has received corticosteroid medications to control symptoms. The corticosteroid should be administered preopera-

NURSING RESEARCH PROFILE 67-2
Information Needs of Patients and Spouses After Total Joint Arthroplasty

Showalter, A., et al. (2000). Patients' and their spouses' needs after total joint arthroplasty: A pilot study. *Orthopaedic Nursing*, 19(1), 49–57, 62.

Purpose

Each year almost 250,000 Americans who have arthritis-related disability choose to have total joint arthroplasty in an attempt to reduce pain and improve functional status and mobility. Health care providers need to understand the perceived needs of patients and their families during hospitalization and recovery from total joint arthroplasty so that programs can be developed or modified to meet those needs.

Study Sample and Design

The purposive sample consisted of 5 patients who had recently undergone total joint arthroplasty and their spouses. The mean age of patients was 68.6 years, and the mean age of spouses was 69 years. Three patients had undergone total knee replacement, and two patients had undergone total hip replacement within 4 months of data collection.

Focus group interviews were conducted and videotaped for subsequent analysis. The interviewer used an open-ended interview format to explore the perceptions of patients and spouses regarding what information that was useful before surgery, what information they wished they had received, and what else would have helped them during recovery.

Results

The primary need expressed by this focus group was the need for help in making transitions. The participants expressed problems in mak-

ing situational and role transitions and experienced distress over not being able to resume activities that they had previously enjoyed within an expected time frame. Spouses stated that they felt unprepared for the reality of being a care provider and often felt overwhelmed and insecure about what was expected of them.

In addition, the focus group addressed health and illness transitions and the need to know that each patient progresses toward recovery at his or her own rate. Patients commented that the patient education they received did not prepare them for problems encountered during recovery at home. Pain management was of particular concern. A home visit soon after hospital discharge was suggested as a way to help patients and spouses manage the transitions.

Nursing Implications

Hospital health care professionals need to be sensitive to the needs of patients and their families as they transition to care in their home. The nurse needs to include both the patient and family members in discharge teaching regarding activities and pain management. Knowledge and skills are needed by the patients and families to confidently manage problems that they encounter during recovery at home.

Further research is necessary to explore the needs of patients and families in care after hospitalization.

---

tively, intraoperatively, and postoperatively as prescribed to prevent the occurrence of adrenal insufficiency from suppressed adrenal function. The patient's use of other medications, such as anticoagulants, cardiovascular agents, or insulin, needs to be documented and discussed with the surgeon and anesthesiologist to ensure adequate management.

The nurse asks the patient specifically about the occurrence of colds, dental problems, urinary tract infections, and other infections within the 2 weeks before surgery. Osteomyelitis could develop through hematologous spread. Permanent disability can result if infection occurs within a bone or joint. Preexisting infections must be resolved before elective orthopedic surgery is performed.

Other areas of preoperative assessment are similar to those for any patient undergoing surgery. Intramuscular medications are injected into an uninvolved area, because tissue absorption is better in nontraumatized tissues.

Nursing Diagnosis

Based on the nursing assessment data, the patient's major preoperative nursing diagnoses related to orthopedic status may include the following:

- Acute pain related to fracture, orthopedic problem, swelling, or inflammation
- Risk for peripheral neurovascular dysfunction related to swelling, constricting devices, or impaired venous return
- Risk for ineffective therapeutic regimen management related to insufficient knowledge or lack of available support and resources
- Impaired physical mobility related to pain, swelling, and possible presence of an immobilization device

- Risk for situational low self-esteem: disturbed body image and/or functional impairment related to impact of musculoskeletal disorder

Planning and Goals

The major goals for the patient before orthopedic surgery may include relief of pain, adequate neurovascular function, health promotion, improved mobility, and positive self-esteem.

Nursing Interventions

RELIEVING PAIN

Physical, pharmacologic, and psychological strategies to control pain are useful in the preoperative period. Specific strategies are tailored to the individual patient. Discomfort is decreased with immobilization of a fractured bone or an injured, inflamed joint. Elevation of an edematous extremity promotes venous return and reduces associated discomfort. Ice, if prescribed, relieves swelling and directly reduces discomfort by diminishing nerve stimulation. Analgesics are frequently prescribed to control the acute pain of musculoskeletal injury and associated muscle spasm. During the immediate preoperative period, the nurse needs to discuss and coordinate the administration of analgesic medications with the anesthesiologist and surgeon. Alternative methods of pain control (eg, distraction, focusing, guided imagery, quiet environment, backrubs) may be used to decrease pain perception.

MAINTAINING ADEQUATE NEUROVASCULAR FUNCTION

Trauma, edema, or immobilization devices may interrupt tissue perfusion. The nurse must frequently assess neurovascular status (ie, colour, temperature, capillary refill, pulses, edema, pain, sensation, motion) of the extremity and document the findings. If circulation is compromised, the nurse institutes measures to restore adequate circulation. These include promptly notifying the physician, elevating the extremity, and releasing constricting wraps or casts as prescribed.

PROMOTING HEALTH

The nurse assists the patient in activities that promote health during the perioperative period. The nurse assesses nutritional status and hydration. The preoperative fasting regimen is usually tolerated well. If the patient has diabetes, is elderly and frail, or is the victim of multiple trauma, special fluid and nutritional provisions may be necessary.

The nurse monitors fluid intake, urinary output, urinalysis findings, and complaints of burning on urination. At times, patients may limit their fluid intake to minimize the use of a bedpan. A small fracture pan may be more comfortable for the patient to use. An indwelling catheter should be used only when absolutely necessary to minimize the risk of urinary tract infection. Urinary tract infection must be addressed before surgery.

Coughing, deep breathing, and use of the incentive spirometer are practiced preoperatively for improved respiratory function during the postoperative period. Preoperative teaching facilitates postoperative compliance. Smoking should be stopped during the preoperative period to facilitate optimal respiratory function.

The nurse provides skin care, paying special attention to pressure points. It is important to institute the use of pressure-reducing surfaces (i.e., special mattresses) before surgery for patients at high risk for skin breakdown.

To minimize the risk for infection, the nurse meticulously and gently cleans the skin with soap and water on the day before surgery. If the surgery is elective, the orthopedic surgeon may instruct the patient to use a germicidal soap for several days before hospitalization.

The nurse discusses with the patient and the family the need for assistance with ADLs and the therapeutic regimen during convalescence so that adequate support is available when the patient is discharged. Modification of the home environment may be necessary to accommodate the altered mobility of the patient after surgery. Referral to the social worker and the case manager may be needed to ensure a smooth transition to home care.

IMPROVING MOBILITY

Preoperatively, the patient's mobility may be impaired by pain, swelling, and immobilizing devices (eg, splints, casts, traction). The nurse should elevate and adequately support edematous extremities with pillows. It is important to control pain before an injured part is moved by administering medication in time for it to take effect and by supporting the injured part when it is moved. The nurse encourages movement within the limits of therapeutic immobility. The patient should perform active range-of-motion exercises of uninvolved joints, and, unless contraindicated, the nurse teaches gluteal-setting and quadriceps-setting isometric exercises to maintain the muscles needed for ambulation (see Chart 67-3). The patient who will be using assistive devices postoperatively may exercise to strengthen the upper extremities and shoulders. If the use of assistive devices (eg, crutches, walker, wheelchair) is anticipated, the nurse encourages the patient to practice with them preoperatively to facilitate their safe use and to promote earlier independent mobility.

HELPING THE PATIENT MAINTAIN SELF-ESTEEM

Preoperatively, orthopedic patients may need assistance in accepting changes in body image, diminished self-esteem, or inability to perform their roles and responsibilities. The degree of assistance required in this area varies greatly, depending on the events preceding hospitalization, the surgery and rehabilitation planned, and the temporary or permanent nature of the problems. The nurse promotes a trusting relationship for patients to express concerns and anxieties and helps them examine their feelings about changes in self-concept. The nurse clarifies any misconceptions patients may have and helps them work through modifications needed to adapt to alterations in physical capacity and to reestablish positive self-esteem.

Evaluation

EXPECTED PATIENT OUTCOMES

Expected patient outcomes may include:

1. Reports relief of pain
   a. Uses multiple approaches to reduce pain
   b. States that medication is effective in relieving pain
   c. Moves with increasing comfort
2. Exhibits adequate neurovascular function
   a. Exhibits normal skin colour
   b. Has warm skin
   c. Has normal capillary refill response
   d. Reports normal sensation and demonstrates joint motion
   e. Demonstrates reduced swelling
3. Promotes health
   a. Eats balanced diet appropriate to meet nutritional needs
   b. Maintains adequate hydration
   c. Abstains from smoking
   d. Practices respiratory exercises
   e. Repositions self to relieve skin pressure
   f. Engages in strengthening and preventive exercises
   g. Plans for assistance during convalescence at home
4. Maximizes mobility within the therapeutic limits
   a. Requests assistance when moving
   b. Elevates edematous extremity after transfer
   c. Uses immobilizing devices and assistive devices as prescribed
5. Expresses positive self-esteem
   a. Acknowledges temporary or permanent changes in body image
   b. Discusses role performance changes
   c. Participates in decisions about care

NURSING PROCESS: POSTOPERATIVE CARE OF THE PATIENT UNDERGOING ORTHOPEDIC SURGERY

Assessment

After orthopedic surgery, the nurse continues the preoperative care plan, modifying it to match the patient's current postoperative status. The nurse reassesses the patient's needs in relation to pain, neurovascular status, health promotion, mobility, and self-esteem. Skeletal trauma and surgery performed on bones, muscles, or joints can produce significant pain, especially during the first 1 or 2 postoperative days. Tissue perfusion must be monitored closely, because edema and bleeding into the tissues can compromise circulation and result in compartment syndrome. Inactivity contributes to venous stasis and the development of DVT. General anesthesia, analgesia, and immobility can result in altered functioning of respiratory, gastrointestinal, and urinary systems.

The nurse notes the prescribed limits on mobility and assesses the patient's understanding of the mobility restrictions. The nurse discusses the plan of care with the patient and encourages active participation in the plan.

In addition, the nurse assesses and monitors the patient for potential problems related to the surgery. Frequent assessment of vital signs, level of consciousness, neurovascular status, wound drainage, breath sounds, bowel sounds, fluid balance, and pain provides the nurse with data that may suggest the possible development of complications. The nurse reports abnormal findings to the physician promptly.

With major orthopedic surgery, there is a risk of hypovolemic shock because of blood loss. Muscle dissection frequently produces wounds in which hemostasis is poor. Wounds that are closed under tourniquet control may bleed during the postoperative period. The nurse must be alert for signs of hypovolemic shock.

Changes in the patient's pulse rate, respiratory rate, or colour may indicate pulmonary or cardiovascular complications. Atelectasis and pneumonia are common and may be related to preexisting pulmonary disease, deep anesthesia, decreased activity, analgesics, and reduced respiratory reserve due to advanced age or an underlying musculoskeletal disorder (eg, restrictive lung expansion secondary to kyphosis, rheumatoid arthritis, or osteoporosis).

Voiding in unnatural positions may contribute to urinary retention. In addition, elderly men usually have some degree of prostate enlargement and may already have difficulty voiding. Therefore, it is important to monitor urinary output.

Temperature elevations within the first 48 hours are frequently related to atelectasis or other respiratory problems. Temperature elevations during the next few days are frequently associated with urinary tract infections. Superficial wound infections take 4 to 6 days to develop. Fever from phlebitis usually occurs during the end of the first week through the second week.

Thromboembolic disease (see discussions of deep vein thrombosis in Chap. 31 and pulmonary embolism in Chap. 23) is one of the most common and most dangerous of all complications occurring in the postoperative orthopedic patient. Advanced age, venous stasis, lower extremity orthopedic surgery, and immobilization are significant risk factors. The nurse assesses the patient daily for calf swelling, tenderness, warmth, redness, and a positive Homans' sign. The nurse promptly reports abnormal findings to the physician.

In addition, fat embolus (see Chap. 69) may occur with orthopedic surgery. The nurse must be alert to changes in respiration, behaviour, and level of consciousness that suggest the development of fat embolus.

Nursing Diagnosis

Based on all assessment data, the patient's major nursing diagnoses after orthopedic surgery may include the following:

- Acute pain related to the surgical procedure, swelling, and immobilization
- Risk for peripheral neurovascular dysfunction related to swelling, constricting devices, or impaired circulation
- Risk for ineffective therapeutic regimen management related to insufficient knowledge or available support and resources
- Impaired physical mobility related to pain, edema, or the presence of an immobilizing device (eg, splint, cast, or brace)
- Risk for situational low self-esteem: disturbed body image or role performance related to impact of musculoskeletal problem

COLLABORATIVE PROBLEMS/ POTENTIAL COMPLICATIONS

Based on the assessment data, potential complications may include the following:

- Hypovolemic shock
- Atelectasis; pneumonia
- Urinary retention
- Infection
- Venous stasis and DVT

Planning and Goals

The major goals for the patient after orthopedic surgery may include relief of pain, adequate neurovascular function, health promotion, improved mobility, positive self-esteem, and absence of complications.

Nursing Interventions

RELIEVING PAIN

After orthopedic surgery, pain can be intense. Edema, hematomas, and muscle spasms contribute to the pain experienced. Some patients report that the pain is less than that experienced preoperatively, and only moderate amounts of analgesics are needed. The nurse closely monitors the patient's pain level and response to therapeutic measures and makes every effort to relieve the pain and discomfort.

Multiple pharmacologic approaches to pain management exist. Patient-controlled analgesia (PCA) and epidural analgesia may be prescribed to control the pain. If intramuscular and oral analgesics are prescribed on an as-needed basis (PRN), the nurse instructs the patient to request the analgesic before the pain becomes severe. Alternatively, the nurse can offer the medication at set intervals. The nurse rotates intramuscular injection sites, avoiding the operative hip and thigh. The nurse may administer medications on a preventive basis within the prescribed intervals if the onset of pain can be predicted (eg, 30 minutes before planned activity such as transfer or exercise).

In addition to pharmacologic approaches to controlling pain, elevation of the operative extremity and application of cold, if prescribed, help to control edema and pain. Portable suction of the wound decreases fluid accumulation and hematoma formation. The nurse may find that repositioning, relaxation, distraction, and guided imagery help in reducing the patient's pain.

The nurse should report increasing and uncontrollable pain to the orthopedic surgeon for evaluation. Pain should diminish rapidly after the initial postoperative period. After 2 to 3 days, most patients require only occasional oral analgesia for residual muscle soreness and spasm.

MAINTAINING ADEQUATE NEUROVASCULAR FUNCTION

The nurse continues the preoperative plan of care. The nurse monitors the neurovascular status of the involved body part and notifies the physician promptly of any indications of diminished tissue perfusion. The patient is reminded to perform muscle-setting, ankle, and calf-pumping exercises hourly while awake to enhance circulation.

MAINTAINING HEALTH

The nurse continues the preoperative plan of care. It is important to encourage the patient to participate in the postoperative treatment regimen.

A well-balanced diet with adequate protein and vitamins is needed for wound healing. The patient progresses to a regular diet as soon as possible. Large amounts of milk should not be given to orthopedic patients who are on bed rest, however, because this adds to the calcium pool in the body and requires that the kidneys excrete more calcium, which increases the risk for urinary calculi.

The nurse monitors the patient for pressure ulcers, which are a threat to any patient who must spend an extended time in bed or who is elderly, malnourished, or unable to move without assistance. Turning, washing, and drying the skin and minimizing pressure over bony prominences are necessary to avoid skin breakdown.

IMPROVING PHYSICAL MOBILITY

Patients are frequently reluctant to move after orthopedic surgery. Preoperative education about the planned postoperative treatment regimen promotes patient participation in physical activities. Patients often increase their mobility once they have been reassured that movement within therapeutic limits is beneficial, that the nurse will provide assistance, and that discomfort can be controlled.

Metal pins, screws, rods, and plates used for internal fixation are designed to maintain the position of the bone until ossification occurs. They are not designed to support the body's weight, and they can bend, loosen, or break if stressed. The estimated strength of the bone, the stability of the fracture, reduction and fixation, and the amount of bone healing are important considerations in determining weight-bearing limits. Although the incision may appear healed, the underlying bone requires more time to repair and regain normal strength. Some orthopedic procedures require weight-bearing restrictions. The orthopedic surgeon will prescribe the weight-bearing limits and the use of protective devices (orthoses), if necessary, after surgery.

The physical therapist tailors the exercise program to the individual patient's needs. The goal is the patient's return to the highest level of function in the shortest time possible. Rehabilitation involves progressive increases in the patient's activities and exercises. Assistive devices (crutches, walker) may be used for postoperative mobility. Preoperative practice with assistive devices helps the patient use them postoperatively. The nurse makes sure that the patient uses these devices safely (see discussions of crutch walking and use of a walker in Chap. 11).

MAINTAINING SELF-ESTEEM

The nurse continues the preoperative plan of care. The nurse and the patient set realistic goals. Increased self-care activities within the limits of the therapeutic regimen and resumption of roles facilitate recognition of abilities and promote self-esteem, personal identity, and role performance. Acceptance of altered body image is facilitated by support provided by the nurse, family, and others.

MONITORING AND MANAGING POTENTIAL COMPLICATIONS

Hypovolemic Shock

Excessive loss of blood during or after surgery can result in shock. The nurse monitors the patient for signs and symptoms of hypovolemic shock: increased pulse rate, decreased blood pressure, urine output less than 30 mL per hour, restlessness, change in mentation, thirst, decreased hemoglobin and hematocrit. The nurse reports these findings to the orthopedic surgeon and assists

in appropriate management. (See Chap. 15 for a discussion of managing shock.)

Atelectasis and Pneumonia

The nurse monitors the patient's breath sounds and encourages deep breathing and coughing exercises. Full expansion of the lungs prevents the accumulation of pulmonary secretions and the development of atelectasis and pneumonia. Incentive spirometry, if prescribed, is encouraged. If signs of respiratory problems develop (eg, increased respiratory rate, productive cough, diminished or adventitious breath sounds, fever), the nurse reports the findings to the surgeon.

Urinary Retention

The nurse closely monitors the patient's urinary output after surgery. The nurse encourages the patient to void every 3 to 4 hours to prevent urinary retention and bladder distention. It is important to provide privacy during toileting. Because the patient may need to void in an unusual position, the nurse assists the patient with positioning. Fracture bedpans may be more comfortable than other bedpans. Voiding in the side-lying position may be helpful to the male patient. Some male patients can void only if standing, and clarification with the surgeon of the activity prescription may be needed before the patient is assisted to a standing position. If the patient is unable to void, intermittent catheterizations may be prescribed until the patient is able to void independently. Indwelling urinary catheters are to be used only when absolutely necessary and should be removed as soon as possible.

Infection

Infection is a risk after any surgery, but it is of particular concern for the postoperative orthopedic patient because of the high risk of osteomyelitis. Osteomyelitis often requires prolonged courses of intravenous antibiotics. At times, the infected bone and prosthesis or internal fixation device must be surgically removed. Therefore, prophylactic systemic antibiotics are usually prescribed during the perioperative and immediate postoperative periods. The nurse assesses the patient's response to these antibiotics. When changing dressings and emptying wound drainage devices, aseptic technique is essential. The nurse monitors the patient's vital signs, incision, and drainage. The nurse monitors the patient for signs of urinary tract infection. Prompt assessment for and treatment of infection are essential.

Venous Stasis and Deep Vein Thrombosis

Prevention of DVT requires use of ankle and calf-pumping exercises, elastic compression stockings, and sequential compression devices. Adequate hydration and early mobilization are equally important. Prophylactic warfarin, adjusted-dose heparin, or low-molecular-weight heparin (eg, enoxaparin sodium) may be prescribed. Aspirin has no apparent effect in preventing DVT in the orthopedic patient. The nurse monitors the patient for signs of DVT and promptly reports findings to the physician for management.

PROMOTING HOME AND COMMUNITY-BASED CARE

Teaching the Patient Self-Care

The length of stay in the hospital after orthopedic surgery is usually less than 1 week. Convalescence and rehabilitation take place at home or in a nonacute care setting. The nurse teaches the patient and the family to recognize complications that must be reported promptly to the orthopedic surgeon. The patient must

> ### Chart 67-10
> ### Home Care Checklist • The Patient Who Had Orthopedic Surgery
>
> | At the completion of the home care instruction, the patient or caregiver will be able to: | Patient | Caregiver |
> |---|:---:|:---:|
> | • Describe wound care | ✓ | ✓ |
> | • State indicators of wound infections (eg, redness, swelling, tenderness, purulent drainage, fever) | ✓ | ✓ |
> | • Consume healthy diet to promote wound and bone healing | ✓ | |
> | • Participate in prescribed exercise regimen to promote circulation and mobility | ✓ | |
> | • Use mobility aids safely | ✓ | |
> | • Observe prescribed weight-bearing and activity limits | ✓ | |
> | • Take prescribed therapeutic and prophylactic medications (eg, antibiotics, anticoagulants, analgesics) | ✓ | |
> | • State indicators of complications to report promptly to physician (eg, uncontrolled swelling and pain; cool, pale fingers or toes; paresthesia; paralysis; purulent drainage; signs of systemic infection; signs of deep vein thrombosis or pulmonary emboli) | ✓ | ✓ |
> | • Identify modifications of home environment to promote safe environment and independence during convalescence and rehabilitation | ✓ | ✓ |

understand the prescribed medication regimen. The nurse should demonstrate proper wound care. The patient gradually resumes physical activities and adheres to weight-bearing limits. The patient must be able to perform transfers and to use mobility aids safely. If the patient has a cast or other immobilizing device, family members should be instructed about how to assist the patient in a way that is safe for the patient and for the family member (eg, using proper body mechanics when lifting the patient). Specific exercises need to be taught and practiced before discharge. The nurse discusses recovery and health promotion, emphasizing a healthy lifestyle and diet.

Continuing Care

If special equipment or home modifications are needed for safe care at home, they must be obtained before the patient is discharged home. The nurse, physical therapist, and social worker can assist the patient and family in identifying their needs and in getting ready to care for the patient at home.

Frequently, home health nursing and home physical therapy are part of the discharge plan of care. These referrals provide resources and help the patient and the family cope with the demands of care during convalescence and rehabilitation. The nurse can explore problems that the patient and family identify during the home care visit. The nurse assesses the patient's progress and monitors for possible complications. Regular medical follow-up care after discharge needs to be arranged (Chart 67-10).

Evaluation

EXPECTED PATIENT OUTCOMES

Expected patient outcomes may include:

1. Reports decreased level of pain
   a. Uses multiple approaches to reduce pain
   b. Uses occasional oral medication to control discomfort
   c. Elevates extremity to control edema and discomfort
   d. Moves with greater comfort
2. Exhibits adequate neurovascular function
   a. Exhibits normal colour and temperature of skin
   b. Has warm skin
   c. Has normal capillary refill response
   d. Demonstrates intact sensory and motor function
   e. Demonstrates reduced swelling

3. Promotes health
   a. Eats diet appropriate for nutritional needs
   b. Maintains adequate hydration
   c. Abstains from smoking
   d. Practices respiratory exercises
   e. Repositions self to relieve pressure on skin
   f. Engages in strengthening and preventive exercises
4. Maximizes mobility within the therapeutic limits
   a. Requests assistance when moving
   b. Elevates edematous extremity after transfer
   c. Uses immobilizing devices as prescribed
   d. Complies with prescribed weight-bearing limitation
5. Expresses positive self-esteem
   a. Discusses temporary or permanent changes in body image
   b. Discusses role performances
   c. Views self as capable of assuming responsibilities
   d. Actively participates in planning care and in the therapeutic regimen
6. Exhibits absence of complications
   a. Does not experience shock
   b. Maintains normal vital signs and blood pressure
   c. Has clear lung sounds
   d. Demonstrates wound healing without signs of infection
   e. Does not experience urinary retention
   f. Voids clear urine clear
   g. Exhibits no signs of DVT

 Critical Thinking Exercises

1. You are working in the emergency department of a community hospital. Early this afternoon, an elderly patient who had fallen and broken her right forearm was treated with closed reduction and casting. She was sent home and was told she could call the emergency department if she had any questions or concerns. She has been home for about 7 hours and is calling because she is experiencing extreme pain in her hand and does not know what to do. What information do you need to assess this situation? What potential problems might she be experiencing? What advice would you give? What is the rationale for this advice?

2. You are providing postoperative care to two patients who had elective hip replacements. The 67-year-old patient had a cemented prosthesis. The 52-year-old patient had a press-fit ingrowth prosthesis. Compare and contrast the plans of care for these two patients. How would they be similar? How would they be different?

3. A 48-year-old patient with multiple trauma is placed in balanced skeletal traction to treat his midshaft femoral fracture until his condition is stable for surgical management of the fracture. Discuss the principles of managing a patient in skeletal traction and how these principles can be incorporated into this patient's plan of care. What actions can you take to minimize the effects of immobilization?

4. An 84-year-old woman had an internal fixation for her fractured hip. She complains that her elastic stockings feel tight and hot and asks you to remove them. How would you respond to this request? What is the rationale for your action? Role play your explanation of the purpose of the stockings.

REFERENCES AND SELECTED READINGS

Books

Goldstein, T. (1999). *Geriatric orthopedics: Rehabilitative management of common problems* (2nd ed.). Gaithersburg, MD: Aspen Publishers.

Maher, A., et al. (2002). *Orthopaedic nursing* (3rd ed.). Philadelphia: W. B. Saunders.

Mercier, L. (2000). *Practical orthopedics* (5th ed.). St. Louis: Mosby.

Moehring, H., & Greenspan, A (2000). *Fractures: Diagnosis and treatment.* New York: McGraw-Hill.

Praemer, A., et al. (1999). *Musculoskeletal conditions in the United States.* Rosemont, IL: American Academy of Orthopaedic Surgeons.

Rosen, C., et al. (1999) *The aging skeleton.* San Diego: Academic Press.

Schoen, D. (2000). *Adult orthopaedic nursing.* Philadelphia: Lippincott Williams & Wilkins.

Schoen, D. (Ed.). (2001). *NAON core curriculum for orthopaedic nursing* (4th ed.). Pitman, NJ: National Association of Orthopaedic Nurses.

Steinberg, G., et al. (Eds.). (1999). *Orthopaedics in primary care* (3rd ed.). Philadelphia: Lippincott Williams and Wilkins.

Journals

Asterisks indicate nursing research articles.

Byrne, T. (1999). The setup and care of a patient in Buck's traction. *Orthopaedic Nursing,* 18(2), 79–83.

*Calvin, R., & Lane, P. (1999). Perioperative uncertainty and state of anxiety of orthopaedic surgical patients. *Orthopaedic Nursing,* 18(6), 61–66.

Geier, K. (2000). Improving outcomes in elective orthopaedic surgery: A guide for nurses and total joint arthroplasty patients. *Orthopaedic Nursing,* 19(Suppl.), 4–31.

Graff, M., et al. (2000). Preventing heel breakdown. *Orthopaedic Nursing,* 19(5), 63–69.

*Hahn, G., et al. (1999). Wound complications after hip surgery using a tapeless compressive support. *Orthopaedic Nursing,* 18(3), 43–49.

Harvey, C. (1998). Challenges of traction in critical care: A case study. *Critical Care Nursing Quarterly,* 21(2), 1–13.

Hohlt, T. (2000). Deep-vein thrombosis prevention in orthopaedic patients: Affecting outcomes through interdisciplinary education. *Orthopaedic Nursing,* 19(5), 73–78.

*Kelly, M., & Ackerman, R. (1999). Total joint arthroplasty: A comparison of postacute settings on patient functional outcomes. *Orthopaedic Nursing,* 18(5), 75–83, 84.

Lewis A. (1999). Orthopedic and vascular emergencies. *Nursing 99,* 29(12), 54–56.

McKenzie, L. (1999). In search of a standard for pin site care. *Orthopaedic Nursing,* 18(2), 73–78.

*Milne, C., et al. (1999). Surgical hip dressings: A comparison of taping methods. *Orthopaedic Nursing,* 18(3), 37–42.

*Moon, L., & Backer, J. (2000). Relationships among self-efficacy, outcome expectancy, and postoperative behaviors in total joint replacement patients. *Orthopaedic Nursing,* 19(2), 77–85.

*Neitzel, J., et al. (1999). Improving pain management after total joint replacement surgery. *Orthopaedic Nursing,* 18(4), 37–45, 64.

*Ridge, R., & Goodson, A. (2000). The relationship between multidisciplinary discharge outcomes and functional status after total hip replacement. *Orthopaedic Nursing,* 19(1), 71–82.

*Showalter, A., et al. (2000). Patients' and spouses' needs after total joint arthroplasty. *Orthopaedic Nursing,* 19(1), 49–57, 62.

*Slowikowski, R., & Flaherty, J. (2000). Epidural analgesia for postoperative orthopaedic pain. *Orthopaedic Nursing,* 19(1), 23–32.

*Tarver, H., et al. (2000). Techniques to maintain a bloodless field in lower extremity surgery. *Orthopaedic Nursing,* 19(4), 65–73.

Turkoski, B. (2000). Preventing DVT in orthopaedic patients. *Orthopaedic Nursing,* 19(5), 93–99.

RESOURCES AND WEBSITES

Canadian Institutes of Health Research: Institute of Musculoskeletal Health and Arthritis, 160 Elgin Street, 9th floor, 4809A, Ottawa, ON K1A 0W9; http://www.cihr-irsc.gc.ca/e/13217.html.

Canadian Orthopaedic Association, 1440 St. Catherine Street West, Suite 718, Montreal, QC H3G 1R8; 514-874-9003; www.coa-aco.org.

Canadian Orthopaedic Foundation, PO Box 7029, Innisfail, ON L9S 1A8; 416-410-2341; www.canorth.org.

Canadian Orthopaedic Nurses Association; www.cona-nurse.org.

National Association of Orthopaedic Nurses (NAON), East Holly Avenue, Box 56, Pitman, NJ 08071-0056; 1-800-289-6266; http://www.orthonurses.org; naon@sba.com.

National Institute of Arthritis and Musculoskeletal and Skin Diseases, Information Clearing House, National Institutes of Health, 1 AMS Circle, Bethesda, MD 20892-3675; 1-877-22-NIAMS (toll free); 1-301-495-4484.

National Institute of Arthritis and Musculoskeletal and Skin Diseases, Office of Communications and Public Liaison, Bldg. 31/Rm.4C05, 31 Center Drive, MSC 2350, Bethesda, MD 20892-2350; 1-301-496-8190; http://www.nih.gov/niams.

Management of Patients With Musculoskeletal Disorders

Adapted by Bonnie Friesen, Linda Larsen, and Rene A. Day

LEARNING OBJECTIVES

On completion of this chapter, the learner will be able to:

1. Use the nursing process as a framework for care of the patient with low back pain.
2. Describe the rehabilitation and health education needs of the patient with low back pain.
3. Describe conditions of the upper extremities and nursing care of the patient undergoing surgery of the hand or wrist.
4. Use the nursing process as a framework for care of the patient undergoing foot surgery.
5. Explain the pathophysiology, pathogenesis, prevention, and management of osteoporosis.
6. Identify the causes and related medical management of osteomalacia.
7. Describe the medication therapy program for the patient with Paget's disease.
8. Use the nursing process as a framework for care of the patient with osteomyelitis.
9. Use the nursing process as a framework for care of the patient with a bone tumour.

Musculoskeletal disorders, such as impairment of the back and spine, are leading health problems and causes of disability, particularly in people during their employment years. The limitations imposed on the patient are severe, and the economic cost, in terms of loss of productivity, medical expenses, and other costs that are not compensated, is in the billions of dollars.

Common Musculoskeletal Problems

ACUTE LOW BACK PAIN

The number of medical visits resulting from low back pain is second only to the number of visits for upper respiratory illnesses. Most low back pain is caused by one of many musculoskeletal problems, including acute lumbosacral strain, unstable lumbosacral ligaments and weak muscles, osteoarthritis of the spine, spinal stenosis, intervertebral disk problems, and unequal leg length.

Older patients may experience back pain associated with osteoporotic vertebral fractures or bone metastasis. Other causes include kidney disorders, pelvic problems, retroperitoneal tumours, abdominal aneurysms, and psychosomatic problems.

In addition, obesity, stress, and occasionally depression may contribute to low back pain. Back pain due to musculoskeletal disorders usually is aggravated by activity, whereas pain due to other conditions is not. Patients with chronic low back pain may develop a dependence on alcohol or analgesics in an attempt to cope with and self-treat the pain.

Pathophysiology

The spinal column can be considered as an elastic rod constructed of rigid units (vertebrae) and flexible units (intervertebral disks) held together by complex facet joints, multiple ligaments, and paravertebral muscles. Its unique construction allows for flexibility while providing maximum protection for the spinal cord. The spinal curves absorb vertical shocks from running and jumping. The trunk muscles help to stabilize the spine. The abdominal and thoracic muscles are important in lifting activities. Disuse weakens these supporting structures. Obesity, postural problems, structural problems, and overstretching of the spinal supports may result in back pain.

The intervertebral disks change in character as a person ages. A young person's disks are mainly fibrocartilage with a gelatinous matrix. As a person ages, the disks become dense, irregular fibrocartilage. Disk degeneration is a common cause of back pain. The lower lumbar disks, L4–L5 and L5–S1, are subject to the greatest mechanical stress and the greatest degenerative changes. Disk protrusion (herniated nucleus pulposus) or facet joint changes can cause pressure on nerve roots as they leave the spinal canal, which results in pain that radiates along the nerve. Management of intervertebral disk disease is discussed in Chapter 65.

Clinical Manifestations

The patient complains of either acute back pain or chronic back pain (lasting more than 3 months without improvement) and fatigue. The patient may report pain radiating down the leg, which is known as **radiculopathy** or **sciatica** and which suggests nerve root involvement. The patient's gait, spinal mobility, reflexes, leg length, leg motor strength, and sensory perception may be altered. Physical examination may disclose paravertebral muscle spasm (greatly increased muscle tone of the back postural muscles) with a loss of the normal lumbar curve and possible spinal deformity.

Assessment and Diagnostic Findings

The Agency for Heath Care Policy and Research developed guidelines for assessment and management of acute low back pain (Bigos et al., 1994). These safe, conservative, and cost-effective guidelines have reduced the use of noneffective therapeutic interventions, including prolonged bed rest.

The initial evaluation of acute low back pain includes a focused history and physical examination, including general observation of the patient, back examination, and neurologic testing (reflexes, sensory impairment, straight-leg raising, muscle strength, and muscle atrophy). The findings suggest either nonspecific back symptoms or potentially serious problems, such as sciatica, spine fracture, cancer, infection, or rapidly progressing neurologic deficit. If the initial examination does not suggest a serious condition, no additional testing is performed during the first 4 weeks of symptoms.

The diagnostic procedures described in Chart 68-1 may be indicated for the patient with potentially serious or prolonged low back pain. The nurse prepares the patient for these studies, provides the necessary support during the testing period, and monitors the patient for any adverse responses to the procedures.

Medical Management

Most back pain is self-limited and resolves within 4 weeks with analgesics, rest, stress reduction, and relaxation. Based on initial assessment findings, the patient is reassured that the assessment indicates that the back pain is not due to a serious condition. Management focuses on relief of pain and discomfort, activity modification, and patient education.

Nonprescription analgesics (acetaminophen, ibuprofen) are usually effective in achieving pain relief. At times, a patient may require the addition of muscle relaxants or opioids. Heat or cold therapy frequently provides temporary relief of symptoms. In the absence of symptoms of disease (radiculopathy of the roots of spinal nerves), manipulation may be helpful.

Other physical modalities have no proven efficacy in treating acute low back pain. They include traction, massage, diathermy, ultrasound, cutaneous laser treatment, biofeedback, and transcutaneous electrical nerve stimulation. Likewise, acupuncture and injection procedures have no proven efficacy (Bigos et al., 1994).

Glossary

bursitis: inflammation of a fluid-filled sac in a joint
contracture: abnormal shortening of muscle or fibrosis of joint structures

involucrum: new bone growth around a sequestrum
radiculopathy: disease of a nerve root

sciatica: sciatic nerve pain; pain travels down back of thigh into foot
sequestrum: dead bone in abscess cavity
tendinitis: inflammation of muscle tendons

Chart 68-1   Diagnostic Procedures for Low Back Pain

X-ray of the spine—may demonstrate a fracture, dislocation, infection, osteoarthritis, or scoliosis

Bone scan and blood studies—may disclose infections, tumours, and bone marrow abnormalities

Computed tomography (CT scan)—useful in identifying underlying problems, such as obscure soft tissue lesions adjacent to the vertebral column and problems of vertebral disks

Magnetic resonance imaging (MRI)—permits visualization of the nature and location of spinal pathology

Electromyogram (EMG) and nerve conduction studies—used to evaluate spinal nerve root disorders (radiculopathies)

Most patients need to alter their activity patterns to avoid aggravating the pain. Twisting, bending, lifting, and reaching, all of which stress the back, are avoided. The patient is taught to change position frequently. Sitting should be limited to 20 to 50 minutes based on level of comfort. Bed rest is recommended for 1 to 2 days, with a maximum of 4 days only if pain is severe. A gradual return to activities and low-stress aerobic exercise is recommended. Conditioning exercises for the trunk muscles are begun after about 2 weeks.

If there is no improvement within 1 month, additional assessments for physiologic abnormalities are performed. Management is based on findings.

NURSING PROCESS: THE PATIENT WITH ACUTE LOW BACK PAIN

Assessment

The nurse encourages the patient with low back pain to describe the discomfort (eg, location, severity, duration, characteristics, radiation, associated weakness in the legs). Descriptions of how the pain occurred—with a specific action (eg, opening a garage door) or with an activity in which weak muscles were overused (eg, weekend gardening)—and how the patient has dealt with the pain often suggest areas for intervention and patient teaching.

If back pain is a recurrent problem, information about previous successful pain control methods helps in planning current management. The nurse also asks how the back pain affects the patient's lifestyle. Information about work and recreational activities helps to identify areas for back health education. Because stress and anxiety can evoke muscle spasms and pain, the nurse needs insight into environmental variables, work situations, and family relationships. In addition, the nurse assesses the effect of chronic pain on the emotional well-being of the patient. Referral to a psychiatric nurse clinician for assessment and management of stressors contributing to the low back pain and related depression may be appropriate.

During the interview, the nurse observes the patient's posture, position changes, and gait. Often, the patient's movements are guarded, with the back kept as still as possible. The patient often selects a chair of standard seat height with arms for support. The patient may sit and stand in an unusual position, leaning away from the most painful side, and may ask for assistance when undressing for the physical examination.

On physical examination, the nurse assesses the spinal curve, any leg length discrepancy, and pelvic crest and shoulder symme-

try. The nurse palpates the paraspinal muscles and notes spasm and tenderness. When the patient is in a prone position, the paraspinal muscles relax, and any deformity caused by spasm subsides. The nurse asks the patient to bend forward and then laterally and notes any discomfort or limitations in movement. It is important to determine the effect of these limitations in movement on activities of daily living (ADLs). The nurse evaluates nerve involvement by assessing deep tendon reflexes, sensations (eg, paresthesia), and muscle strength. Back and leg pain on straight-leg raising (with the patient supine, the patient's leg is lifted upward with the knee extended) suggests nerve root involvement. Obesity can contribute to low back pain. If the patient is obese, the nurse completes a nutritional assessment.

Nursing Diagnoses

Based on the assessment data, the patient's major nursing diagnoses may include the following:

- Acute pain related to musculoskeletal problems
- Impaired physical mobility related to pain, muscle spasms, and decreased flexibility
- Deficient knowledge related to back-conserving techniques of body mechanics
- Risk for situational low self-esteem related to impaired mobility, chronic pain, and altered role performance
- Imbalanced nutrition: more than body requirements related to obesity

Planning and Goals

The major goals for the patient may include relief of pain, improved physical mobility, use of back-conserving techniques of body mechanics, improved self-esteem, and weight reduction (Chart 68-2).

Nursing Interventions

RELIEVING PAIN

To relieve pain, the nurse encourages the patient to reduce stress on the back muscles and to change position frequently. Patients are taught to control and modify the perceived pain through behavioural therapies that reduce muscular and psychological tension. Diaphragmatic breathing and relaxation help reduce muscle tension contributing to low back pain. Diverting the patient's attention from the pain to another activity (eg, reading, conversation, watching television) may be helpful in some instances. Guided imagery, in which the relaxed patient learns to focus on a pleasant event, may be used along with other pain-relief strategies (see Chart 68-2).

If medication is prescribed, the nurse assesses the patient's response to each medication. As the acute pain subsides, medications are reduced as prescribed. Self-applied intermittent heat or cold may reduce the pain. The nurse evaluates and notes the patient's response to various pain management modalities.

IMPROVING PHYSICAL MOBILITY

Physical mobility is monitored through continuing assessments. The nurse assesses how the patient moves and stands. As the back pain subsides, self-care activities are resumed with minimal strain on the injured structures. Position changes should be made slowly and carried out with assistance as required. Twisting and jarring motions are avoided. The nurse encourages the patient to alter-

Chart 68-2 • PATIENT EDUCATION
Strategies for the Patient With Low Back Pain

Discuss the following strategies with the patient:

Pain Management
- Limit bed rest; keep knees flexed to decrease strain on back
- *Nonpharmacologic approaches:* distraction, relaxation, imagery, thermal interventions (eg, ice or heat), stress reduction
- *Pharmacologic approaches:* nonsteroidal anti-inflammatory drugs, analgesics, muscle relaxants

Exercise
- Stretch to enhance flexibility, do strengthening exercises
- Perform prescribed back exercises to increase function, emphasizing gradual increases in time and repetitions

Body Mechanics
- Practice good posture
- Avoid twisting body
- Push objects rather than pull them
- Keep load close to body when lifting
- Bend knees and tighten abdominal muscles when lifting

- Avoid overreaching
- Use wide base of support
- Use back brace to protect back

Work Modifications
- Adjust work area to avoid stress on back
- Adjust height of chair or work table
- Use lumbar support in chair
- Avoid prolonged standing and repetitive tasks
- Avoid bending, twisting, and lifting heavy objects
- Avoid work involving continuous vibrations

Stress Reduction
- Discuss with patient the interdependence of stress and anxiety on muscle tension and pain
- Explore effective coping mechanisms
- Teach stress reduction techniques
- Refer patient to back clinic

---

nate lying, sitting, and walking activities frequently and advises the patient to avoid sitting, standing, or walking for long periods. The patient may find that sitting in a chair with arm rests to support some of the body weight and a soft support at the small of the back provides comfort.

With severe pain, the patient limits activity for 1 to 2 days. Extended periods of inactivity are not effective and result in deconditioning. The patient rests in bed on a firm, nonsagging mattress (a bed board may be used). Lumbar flexion is increased by elevating the head and thorax 30 degrees using pillows or a foam wedge and slightly flexing the knees supported on a pillow. Alternatively, the patient assumes a lateral position with knees and hips flexed (curled position) with a pillow between the knees and legs and a pillow supporting the head (Fig. 68-1). A prone position is avoided because it accentuates lordosis. The nurse instructs the patient to get out of bed by rolling to one side and placing the legs down while pushing the torso up, keeping the back straight.

As the patient achieves comfort, activities are gradually resumed, and an exercise program is initiated. Initially, low-stress aerobic exercises, such as short walks or swimming, are suggested. After 2 weeks, conditioning exercises for the abdominal and trunk muscles are started. The physical therapist designs an exercise program for the individual patient to reduce lordosis, increase flexibility, and reduce strain on the back. It may include hyperextension exercises to strengthen the paravertebral muscles, flexion exercises to increase back movement and strength, and isometric flexion exercises to strengthen trunk muscles. Each exercise period begins with relaxation. Exercise begins gradually and increases as the patient recovers.

The nurse encourages the patient to adhere to the prescribed exercise program. Erratic exercising is ineffective. For most exercise programs, it is suggested that the person exercise twice a day, increasing the number of exercises gradually. Some patients may find it difficult to adhere to a program of prescribed exercises for a long period. These patients are encouraged to improve their posture, use good body mechanics on a regular basis, and engage in regular exercise activities (eg, walking, swimming) to maintain a healthy back. Activities should not cause excessive lumbar strain, twisting, or discomfort; for example, activities such as horseback riding and weight-lifting are avoided.

USING PROPER BODY MECHANICS

Good body mechanics and posture are essential to avoid recurrence of back pain. The patient must be taught how to stand, sit, lie, and lift properly (Figs. 68-2 and 68-3). Providing the patient with a list of suggestions helps in making these long-term changes (Chart 68-3). The patient who wears high heels is encouraged to change to low heels. The patient who is required to stand for long periods should shift weight frequently and should rest one foot on a low stool, which decreases lumbar lordosis. The proper posture can be verified by looking in a mirror to see whether the chest is up and the abdomen is tucked in. Locking the knees when standing is avoided, as is bending forward for long periods.

When the patient is sitting, the knees and hips should be flexed, and the knees should be level with the hips or higher to minimize lordosis. The feet should be flat on the floor. The back needs to be supported. The patient should sleep on the side with knees and hips flexed, or supine with knees supported in a flexed position. Sleeping prone should be avoided.

FIGURE 68-1 Positioning to promote lumbar flexion. © B. Proud.

NURSING RESEARCH PROFILE 68-1

Successful Interventions for Back Pain

Reavis, D. (1999). Back injury in primary care: three sides of the coin. *Nurse Practitioner Forum, 10,* 208–212.

Purpose

Low back pain is a common job-related injury. Nurse practitioners managing industrial injuries in primary health care clinics need to design treatment protocols that are effective for the employee and contain costs for the employer.

This study compared the average number of days absent from work for patients treated with various protocols. The conservative treatment consisted of nonsteroidal anti-inflammatory drugs (NSAIDs), muscle relaxants, and rest. The active physical rehabilitation treatment consisted of NSAIDs, muscle relaxants, and referral to an exercise physiologist for muscle strength and range of motion exercise, including ice, electrical stimulation, and/or exercise therapy.

Study Sample and Design

Two primary health care clinics located in different regions of the United States were used. One clinic used a conservative treatment protocol; the other used the active physical rehabilitation protocol. Charts of patients with the appropriate diagnostic code (ie, low-back strain) were reviewed for inclusion criteria (eg, adult age, first-time work-related injury of the back).

The convenience sample consisted of two groups of patients (18 patients in each group). The ages and gender distributions in the two groups were similar. The mean number of days off from work was cal-culated for each of the two treatment groups and compared using the *t* test for independent groups to answer the research question: Do patients with a clinical diagnosis of low back pain differ in their responses to two sets of treatment protocols as measured by number of days absent from work?

Findings

The mean number of days absent from work was 13.3 days for the conservative treatment group and 4.5 days for the active physical rehabilitation group. This was a statistically significant difference ($p < .01$), suggesting active physical rehabilitation is the superior protocol. However, employer costs, including monetary outlay for exercise therapy and loss of productivity due to number of days off from work, were not considered in this study.

Nursing Implications

The findings suggest that active physical rehabilitation may be more effective than conservative treatment; however, additional studies are needed to replicate the findings and should include a cost-benefit analysis and random assignment of subjects.

Prevention of back injury is a primary concern of employee health nurses. Additional studies are warranted to determine effectiveness of health promotion programs before back injury occurs.

FIGURE 68-2 Proper and improper standing postures. (*Left*) Abdominal muscles contracted, giving a feeling of upward pull, and gluteal muscles contracted, giving a downward pull. (*Right*) Slouch position, showing abdominal muscles relaxed and body out of proper alignment.

The nurse instructs the patient in the safe and correct way to lift objects—using the strong quadriceps muscles of the thighs, with minimal use of weak back muscles. With feet placed to provide a wide base of support, the patient should bend the knees, tighten the abdominal muscles, and lift the object close to the body with a smooth motion, avoiding twisting and jerking. To prevent recurrence of acute low back pain, the nurse may instruct the patient to wear a back support when repeated lifting is required and to avoid lifting more than one third of his or her weight without help.

It takes about 6 months for a person to readjust postural habits. Practicing these protective and defensive postures, positions, and body mechanics results in natural strengthening of the back and diminishes the chance that back pain will recur.

IMPROVING SELF-ESTEEM

Because of the immobility associated with low back pain, the patient may depend on others to do various tasks. Dependency may continue beyond physiologic needs and become a way to fulfill psychosocial needs. Assisting both the patient and support people to recognize continued dependency helps the patient identify and cope with the underlying reason for the dependency.

Role-related responsibilities may have been modified with the onset of low back pain. As recovery from acute low back pain and immobility progresses, the patient may resume former role-related responsibilities.

If these activities contributed to the development of low back pain, however, it may be difficult to resume them without chronic low back pain syndrome, with associated disability and depression resulting. If the patient experiences secondary gains associ-

FIGURE 68-3 Proper and improper lifting techniques. (*Left*) Correct position for lifting. This person is using the long and strong muscles of the arms and legs and holding the object so that the line of gravity falls within the base of support. (*Right*) Incorrect position for lifting because pull is exerted on the back muscles and leaning causes the line of gravity to fall outside the base.

ated with low back disability (eg, worker's compensation, easier lifestyle or workload, increased emotional support), a "low back neurosis" may develop. The patient may need help in coping with specific stressors and in learning how to control stressful situations. When people successfully deal with stress, they develop confidence in their abilities to manage other stressful situations. Psychotherapy or counselling may be needed to assist the person in resuming a full, productive life. Back clinics use multidisciplinary approaches to help the patient with pain and with resumption of role-related responsibilities.

MODIFYING NUTRITION FOR WEIGHT REDUCTION

Obesity contributes to back strain by stressing the relatively weak back muscles. Exercises are less effective and more difficult to perform when the patient is overweight. Weight reduction through diet modification may prevent recurrence of back pain. Weight reduction is based on a sound nutritional plan that includes a change in eating habits to maintain desirable weight. Monitoring weight reduction, noting achievement, and providing encouragement and positive reinforcement facilitate adherence. Frequently, back problems resolve as normal weight is achieved.

Chart 68-3
Health Promotion • Activities to Promote a Healthy Back

Standing
- Avoid prolonged standing and walking.
- When standing for any length of time, rest one foot on a small stool or box to relieve lumbar lordosis.
- Avoid forward flexion work positions.
- Avoid high heels.

Sitting
- Avoid sitting for prolonged periods.
- Sit in a straight-back chair with back well supported and arm rests to support some of the body weight; use a footstool to position knees higher than hips if necessary.
- Eradicate the hollow of the back by sitting with the buttocks "tucked under."
- Maintain back support; use a soft support at the small of the back.
- Avoid knee and hip extension. When driving a car, have the seat pushed forward as far as possible for comfort.
- Guard against extension strains—reaching, pushing, sitting with legs straight out.
- Alternate periods of sitting with walking.

Lying
- Rest at intervals; fatigue contributes to spasm of the back muscles.

- Place a firm bed board under the mattress.
- Avoid sleeping in a prone position.
- When lying on the side, place a pillow under the head and one between the legs, with the legs flexed at the hips and knees.
- When supine, use a pillow under the knees to decrease lordosis.

Lifting
- When lifting, keep the back straight and hold the load as close to the body as possible.
- Lift with the large leg muscles, not the back muscles.
- Use trunk muscles to stabilize the spine.
- Squat while keeping the back straight when it is necessary to pick something off the floor.
- Avoid twisting the trunk of the body, lifting above waist level, and reaching up for any length of time.

Exercising
- Daily exercise is important in the prevention of back problems.
- Walking and gradually increasing the distance and pace of walking is recommended.
- Perform prescribed back exercises twice daily, increasing exercise gradually.
- Avoid jumping and jarring activities.

Evaluation

EXPECTED PATIENT OUTCOMES

Expected patient outcomes may include the following:

1. Experiences pain relief
   a. Rests comfortably
   b. Changes positions comfortably
   c. Obtains relief through use of physical modalities, psychological techniques, and medications
   d. Avoids drug dependency
2. Demonstrates resumption of physical mobility
   a. Resumes activities gradually
   b. Avoids positions that cause discomfort and muscle spasm
   c. Plans recumbent rest periods throughout the day
3. Demonstrates back-conserving body mechanics
   a. Improves posture
   b. Positions self to minimize stress on the back
   c. Demonstrates use of good body mechanics
   d. Participates in exercise program
4. Resumes role-related responsibilities
   a. Uses coping techniques to deal with stressful situations
   b. Demonstrates decreased dependence on others for self-care
   c. Resumes role responsibilities as low back pain resolves
   d. Resumes full, productive lifestyle
5. Achieves desired weight
   a. Identifies need to lose weight if appropriate
   b. Sets realistic goals
   c. Participates in development of weight-reduction plan
   d. Complies with weight-reduction regimen

Common Problems of the Upper Extremity

The structures in the upper extremity are frequently the sites of painful syndromes. The structures most frequently affected are the shoulder, wrist, and hand.

BURSITIS AND TENDINITIS

Bursitis and **tendinitis** are inflammatory conditions that commonly occur in the shoulder. Bursae are fluid-filled sacs that prevent friction between joint structures during joint activity. When inflamed, they are painful. Similarly, muscle tendon sheaths become inflamed with repetitive stretching. The inflammation causes proliferation of synovial membrane and pannus formation, which restricts joint movement. Conservative treatment includes rest of the extremity, intermittent ice and heat to the joint, and nonsteroidal anti-inflammatory drugs (NSAIDs) to control the inflammation and pain. Arthroscopic synovectomy may be considered if shoulder pain and weakness persist.

LOOSE BODIES

Loose bodies may occur in a joint as a result of articular cartilage wear and bone erosion. These fragments interfere with joint movement, locking the joint, and cause painful movement. Loose bodies are removed by arthroscopic surgery.

IMPINGEMENT SYNDROME

Overuse (microtrauma) may produce an impingement syndrome in the shoulder. The supraspinatus and biceps tendons become irritated and edematous and press against the acromion process, limiting shoulder motion. The patient experiences pain, shoulder tenderness, limited movement, muscle spasm, and atrophy. The process may progress to a rotator cuff tear. Conservative treatment includes rest, NSAIDs, joint injections, and physical therapy (Chart 68-4). Arthroscopic débridement is used for persistent pain. Gentle joint motion is begun after surgery. (See Chapter 69 for a discussion of rotator cuff injury.)

CARPAL TUNNEL SYNDROME

Carpal tunnel syndrome is an entrapment neuropathy that occurs when the median nerve at the wrist is compressed by a thickened flexor tendon sheath, skeletal encroachment, edema, or a soft tissue mass. The syndrome is commonly caused by repetitive hand activities but may be associated with arthritis, hypothyroidism, or pregnancy. The patient experiences pain, numbness, paresthesia, and possibly weakness along the median nerve (thumb and first two fingers). Tinel's sign may be used to help identify carpal tunnel syndrome (Fig. 68-4). Night pain is common. Treatment is based on cause. Rest splints to prevent hyperextension and prolonged flexion of the wrist, avoidance of repetitive flexion of the wrist (eg, use of ergonomic changes at work to reduce wrist strain), NSAIDs, and carpal canal cortisone injections may relieve the symptoms. Specific yoga postures, relaxation, and acupuncture may provide nontraditional alternatives to relieve carpal tunnel symptoms. Traditional or endoscopic laser surgical release of the transverse carpal ligament may be necessary. The patient wears a hand splint after surgery and limits hand use during healing. The patient may need assistance with personal care and ADLs. Full recovery of motor and sensory function after nerve release surgery may take several weeks or months.

GANGLION

A ganglion, a collection of gelatinous material near the tendon sheaths and joints, appears as a round, firm, cystic swelling, usually on the dorsum of the wrist. It most frequently occurs in women younger than 50 years of age. The ganglion is locally tender and may cause an aching pain. When a tendon sheath is in-

Chart 68-4 • PATIENT EDUCATION
Measures to Promote Shoulder Healing

The nurse provides guidelines for general care and instructs the patient in carrying out measures that will promote shoulder healing. Patient education includes the following points:

- During the acute phase, rest the joint in a position that minimizes stress on the joint structures, to prevent further damage and the development of adhesions.
- Support the affected arm on pillows while sleeping, to keep from turning onto the shoulder.
- For the first 24 to 48 hours of the acute phase, apply cold to reduce swelling and discomfort; then, according to the treatment plan, apply heat intermittently to promote circulation and healing.
- Gradually resume motion and use of the joint. Assistance with dressing and other activities of daily living may be needed.
- Avoid working and lifting above shoulder level or pushing an object against a "locked" shoulder.
- Perform the prescribed daily range-of-motion and strengthening exercises.

FIGURE 68-4 Tinel's sign may be elicited in patients with carpal tunnel syndrome by percussing lightly over the median nerve, located on the inner aspect of the wrist. If the patient reports tingling, numbness, and pain, the test for Tinel's sign is considered positive. From Weber, J. W., & Kelley, J. (2003). *Health assessment in nursing* (2nd ed.). Philadelphia: Lippincott Williams & Wilkins. © B. Proud.

volved, weakness of the finger occurs. Treatment may include aspiration, corticosteroid injection, or surgical excision. After treatment, a compression dressing and immobilization splint are used.

DUPUYTREN'S CONTRACTURE

Dupuytren's deformity is a slowly progressive **contracture** of the palmar fascia, which causes flexion of the fourth and fifth fingers, and frequently the middle finger. This renders the fingers more or less useless (Fig. 68-5). It is caused by an inherited autosomal dominant trait and occurs most frequently in men who are older than 50 years of age and who are of Scandinavian or Celtic origin. It is also associated with arthritis, diabetes, gout, and alcoholism. It starts as a nodule of the palmar fascia. The nodule may not change, or it may progress so that the fibrous thickening extends to involve the skin in the distal palm and produces a contracture of the fingers. The patient may experience dull aching discomfort, morning numbness, cramping, and stiffness in the affected fingers. This condition starts in one hand, but eventually both hands are affected symmetrically. Initially, finger-stretching exercises may prevent contractures. With contracture development, palmar and digital fasciectomies are performed to improve function. Finger exercises are begun on postoperative day 1 or 2.

FIGURE 68-5 Dupuytren's contracture, a flexion deformity caused by an inherited trait, is a slowly progressive contracture of the palmar fascia, which severely impairs the function of the fourth, fifth, and sometimes, the middle fingers.

NURSING PROCESS: THE PATIENT UNDERGOING SURGERY OF THE HAND OR WRIST

Assessment

Surgery of the hand or wrist, unless related to major trauma, is generally an ambulatory surgery procedure. Before surgery, the nurse assesses the patient's level and type of discomfort and limitations in function caused by the ganglion, carpal tunnel syndrome, Dupuytren's contracture, or other condition of the hand.

Nursing Diagnoses

Based on the assessment data, the nursing diagnoses for the patient undergoing surgery of the hand or wrist may include the following:

- Risk for peripheral neurovascular dysfunction related to surgical procedure
- Acute pain related to inflammation and swelling
- Self-care deficit: bathing/hygiene, dressing/grooming, feeding, and/or toileting related to bandaged hands
- Risk for infection related to surgical procedure

Planning and Goals

The goals of the patient may include relief of pain, improved self-care, and absence of infection.

Nursing Interventions

PROMOTING NEUROVASCULAR FUNCTION

Neurovascular assessment of the exposed fingers every hour for the first 24 hours is essential for monitoring function of the nerves and perfusion of the hand. The nurse compares the affected hand with the unaffected hand and the postoperative status with the documented preoperative status. The nurse asks the patient to describe the sensations in the hands and to demonstrate finger mobility. With tendon repairs and nerve, vascular, or skin grafts, motor function is tested only if prescribed. The nurse assesses the temperature of the affected hand. Dressings are to be supportive but nonconstrictive. Pain uncontrolled by analgesics suggests compromised neurovascular functioning.

RELIEVING PAIN

Pain may be related to surgery, edema, hematoma formation, or restrictive bandages. To control swelling that may increase the patient's pain and discomfort, the nurse elevates the hand to heart level with pillows. When higher elevation is prescribed, an elevating sling may be attached to a pole used in intravenous (IV) therapies or to an overhead frame. If the patient is ambulatory, the arm is elevated in a conventional sling with the hand at heart level.

Intermittent ice packs to the surgical area during the first 24 to 48 hours may be prescribed to control swelling. Unless contraindicated, active extension and flexion of the fingers to promote circulation are encouraged, even though movement is limited by the bulky dressing.

Generally, the pain and discomfort can be controlled by oral analgesics. The nurse evaluates the patient's response to analgesics and to other pain-control measures. Patient education concerning analgesics is important.

IMPROVING SELF-CARE

During the first few days after surgery, the patient needs assistance with ADLs because one hand is bandaged and independent self-care is impaired. The patient may need to arrange for assistance with feeding, bathing and hygiene, dressing, grooming, and toileting. Within a few days, the patient develops skills in one-handed ADLs and is usually able to function with minimal assistance and use of assistive devices. The nurse encourages use of the involved hand, unless contraindicated, within the limits of discomfort. As rehabilitation progresses, the patient resumes use of the injured hand. Physical or occupational therapy–directed exercises may be prescribed. The nurse emphasizes adherence to the therapeutic regimen.

PREVENTING INFECTION

As with all surgery, there is a risk for infection. The nurse teaches the patient to monitor temperature and signs and symptoms that suggest an infection. It also is important to instruct the patient to keep the dressing clean and dry and to report any drainage, foul odour, or increased pain and swelling. Patient education includes aseptic wound care as well as education related to prescribed prophylactic antibiotics.

PROMOTING HOME AND COMMUNITY-BASED CARE

Teaching Patients Self-Care

After the patient has undergone hand surgery, the nurse teaches the patient how to monitor neurovascular status and the signs of complications that need to be reported to the surgeon (eg, paresthesia, paralysis, uncontrolled pain, coolness of fingers, extreme swelling, excessive bleeding, purulent drainage, fever). The nurse discusses prescribed medications with the patient. In addition, the nurse teaches the patient to elevate the hand above the elbow and to apply ice (if prescribed) to control swelling. Unless contraindicated, the nurse encourages extension and flexion exercises of the fingers to promote circulation. The use of assistive devices is encouraged if they would be helpful in promoting accomplishment of ADLs. For bathing, the nurse instructs the patient to keep the dressing dry by covering it with a secured plastic bag. Generally, the wound is not redressed until the patient's follow-up visit with the surgeon (Chart 68-5).

Evaluation

EXPECTED PATIENT OUTCOMES

Expected patient outcomes may include:

1. Maintains peripheral tissue perfusion

a. Demonstrates normal skin temperature and capillary refill
b. Exhibits normal sensations
c. Exhibits acceptable motor function
2. Achieves pain relief
a. Reports increased comfort
b. Controls edema through elevation of the hand
c. Experiences no discomfort with movement
3. Demonstrates independent self-care
a. Secures assistance with ADLs during first few days postoperatively
b. Adapts to one-handed ADLs
c. Uses injured hand within its functional capability
4. Demonstrates absence of wound infection
a. Complies with treatment protocol and prevention strategies
b. Reports temperature and pulse within normal limits
c. Experiences no purulent wound drainage
d. Experiences no wound inflammation

Common Foot Problems

Disabilities of the foot are commonly caused by poorly fitting shoes. Fashion, vanity, and eye appeal, rather than function and physiology of the foot, are the determining factors in the design of footwear. Ill-fitting shoes distort normal anatomy while inducing deformity and pain.

Several systemic diseases affect the feet. Patients with diabetes are prone to develop corns and peripheral neuropathies with diminishing sensation, leading to ulcers at pressure points of the foot. Patients with peripheral vascular disease and arteriosclerosis complain of burning and itching feet resulting in scratching and skin breakdown. Foot deformities may occur with rheumatoid arthritis. Dermatology problems commonly affect the feet in the form of fungal infections and plantar warts.

The discomforts of foot strain are treated with rest, elevation, physiotherapy, supportive strappings, and orthotic devices. The patient must inspect the foot and skin under pads and orthotic devices for pressure and skin breakdown daily. If a "window" is cut into shoes to relieve pressure over a bony deformity, the skin must be monitored daily for breakdown from pressure exerted at the "window" area. Active foot exercises promote the circulation and help strengthen the feet. Walking in properly fitting shoes is considered the ideal exercise.

Chart 68-5
Home Care Checklist • Hand Surgery

At the completion of the home care instruction, the patient or caregiver will be able to:	Patient	Caregiver
• Demonstrate how to assess neurovascular status	✓	✓
• State abnormal findings (eg, unrelenting pain; paralysis; paresthesia; cool, nonblanching fingers) to report to physician promptly	✓	✓
• Demonstrate control of edema by elevating hand above elbow and applying ice intermittently if prescribed	✓	✓
• Identify signs and symptoms of infection (eg, elevated temperature, purulent drainage)	✓	✓
• Demonstrate finger exercises to promote circulation, unless contraindicated	✓	
• Describe methods to prevent wound infection (eg, keeping hand dressing clean and dry during activities of daily living)	✓	✓
• Describe use of prescribed medications	✓	✓
• Demonstrate use of assistive devices, if appropriate	✓	

PLANTAR FASCIITIS

Plantar fasciitis, an inflammation of the foot-supporting fascia, presents as an acute onset of heel pain experienced with the first steps in the morning. The pain is localized to the anterior medial aspect of the heel and diminishes with gentle stretching of the foot and Achilles tendon. Management includes stretching exercises, wearing shoes with support and cushioning to relieve pain, orthotic devices (eg, heel cups, arch supports), and NSAIDs. Unresolved plantar fasciitis may progress to fascial tears at the heel and eventual development of heel spurs.

CORN

A corn is an area of hyperkeratosis (overgrowth of a horny layer of epidermis) produced by internal pressure (the underlying bone is prominent because of congenital or acquired abnormality, commonly arthritis) or external pressure (ill-fitting shoes). The fifth toe is most frequently involved, but any toe may be involved.

Corns are treated by soaking and scraping off the horny layer by a podiatrist, by application of a protective shield or pad, or by surgical modification of the underlying offending osseous structure. Soft corns are located between the toes and are kept soft by moisture. Treatment consists of drying the affected spaces and separating the affected toes with lamb's wool or gauze. A wider shoe may be helpful. Usually, a podiatrist is needed to treat the underlying cause.

CALLUS

A callus is a discretely thickened area of the skin that has been exposed to persistent pressure or friction. Faulty foot mechanics usually precede the formation of a callus. Treatment consists of eliminating the underlying causes and having the callus treated by a podiatrist if it is painful. A keratolytic ointment may be applied and a thin plastic cup worn over the heel if the callus is on this area. Felt padding with adhesive backing is also used to prevent and relieve pressure. Orthotic devices can be made to remove the pressure from bony protuberances, or the protuberance may be excised.

INGROWN TOENAIL

An ingrown toenail (onychocryptosis) is a condition in which the free edge of a nail plate penetrates the surrounding skin, either laterally or anteriorly. A secondary infection or granulation tissue may develop. This painful condition is caused by improper self-treatment, external pressure (tight shoes or stockings), internal pressure (deformed toes, growth under the nail), trauma, or infection. Trimming the nails properly (clipping them straight across and filing the corners consistent with the contour of the toe) can prevent this problem. Active treatment consists of washing the foot twice a day, followed by the application of a local antibiotic ointment, and relieving the pain by decreasing the pressure of the nail plate on the surrounding soft tissue. Warm, wet soaks help to drain an infection. A toenail may need to be excised by the podiatrist if there is severe infection.

HAMMER TOE

Hammer toe is a flexion deformity of the interphalangeal joint, which may involve several toes (Fig. 68-6). The condition is usually an acquired deformity. Tight socks or shoes may push an

FIGURE 68-6 Common foot deformities **(A)** Hammer toe, **(B)** Pes cavus (clawfoot), **(C)** Bunion (hallux valgus), **(D)** Site for Morton's neuroma.

Tibial nerve
Medial plantar nerve
Lateral plantar nerve
Site of neurofibroma (Morton's)

overlying toe back into the line of the other toes. The toes usually are pulled upward, forcing the metatarsal joints (ball of the foot) downward. Corns develop on top of the toes, and tender calluses develop under the metatarsal area. The treatment consists of conservative measures: wearing open-toed sandals or shoes that conform to the shape of the foot, carrying out manipulative exercises, and protecting the protruding joints with pads. Surgical correction (osteotomy) is necessary for an established deformity.

HALLUX VALGUS

Hallux valgus (commonly called a bunion) is a deformity in which the great toe deviates laterally (see Fig. 68-6). Associated with this is a marked prominence of the medial aspect of the first metatarsal–phalangeal joint. There is also osseous enlargement (exostosis) of the medial side of the first metatarsal head, over which a bursa may form (secondary to pressure and inflammation). Acute bursitis symptoms include a reddened area, edema, and tenderness.

Factors contributing to bunion formation include heredity, ill-fitting shoes, and gradual lengthening and widening of the foot associated with aging. Osteoarthritis is frequently associated with hallux valgus. Treatment depends on the patient's age, the degree of deformity, and the severity of symptoms. If a bunion deformity is uncomplicated, wearing a shoe that conforms to the shape of the foot or that is molded to the foot to prevent pressure on the protruding portions may be all the treatment that is needed. Corticosteroid injections control acute inflammation. Surgical removal of the bunion (exostosis) and osteotomies to realign the toe may be required to improve function and appearance. Complications related to bunionectomy include limited range of motion, paresthesias, tendon injury, and recurrence of deformity.

Postoperatively, the patient may have intense throbbing pain at the operative site, requiring liberal doses of analgesic medication. The foot is elevated to the level of the heart to decrease edema and pain. The neurovascular status of the toes is assessed. The duration of immobility and initiation of ambulation depend on the procedure used. Toe flexion and extension exercises are initiated to facilitate walking. Shoes that fit the shape and size of the foot are recommended.

PES CAVUS

Pes cavus (clawfoot) refers to a foot with an abnormally high arch and a fixed equinus deformity of the forefoot (see Fig. 68-6). The shortening of the foot and increased pressure produce calluses on the metatarsal area and on the dorsum (bottom) of the foot. Charcot-Marie-Tooth disease (a peripheral neuromuscular disease associated with a familial degenerative disorder), diabetes mellitus, and tertiary syphilis are common causes of pes cavus. Exercises are prescribed to manipulate the forefoot into dorsiflexion and relax the toes. Bracing to protect the foot may be used. In severe cases, arthrodesis (fusion) is performed to reshape and stabilize the foot.

MORTON'S NEUROMA

Morton's neuroma (plantar digital neuroma, neurofibroma) is a swelling of the third (lateral) branch of the median plantar nerve (see Fig. 68-6). The third digital nerve, which is located in the third intermetatarsal (web) space, is most commonly involved. Microscopically, digital artery changes cause an ischemia of the nerve.

The result is a throbbing, burning pain in the foot that is usually relieved when the patient rests. Conservative treatment consists of inserting innersoles and metatarsal pads designed to spread the metatarsal heads and balance the foot posture. Local injections of hydrocortisone and a local anesthetic may provide relief. If these fail, surgical excision of the neuroma is necessary. Pain relief and loss of sensation are immediate and permanent.

FLATFOOT

Flatfoot (pes planus) is a common disorder in which the longitudinal arch of the foot is diminished. It may be caused by congenital abnormalities or associated with bone or ligament injury, muscle and posture imbalances, excessive weight, muscle fatigue, poorly fitting shoes, or arthritis. Symptoms include a burning sensation, fatigue, clumsy gait, edema, and pain.

Exercises to strengthen the muscles and to improve posture and walking habits are helpful. A number of foot orthoses are available to give the foot additional support. Orthopedic surgeons and podiatrists treat severe flatfoot problems.

NURSING PROCESS: THE PATIENT UNDERGOING FOOT SURGERY

Assessment

Surgery of the foot may be necessary because of various conditions, including neuromas and foot deformities (bunion, hammer toe, clawfoot). Generally, foot surgery is performed on an outpatient basis. Before surgery, the nurse assesses the patient's ambulatory ability and balance and the neurovascular status of the foot. Additionally, the nurse considers the availability of assistance at home and the structural characteristics of the home in planning for care during the first few days after surgery. The nurse uses these data, in addition to knowledge of the usual medical management of the condition, to formulate appropriate nursing diagnoses.

Nursing Diagnoses

Based on the assessment data, the nursing diagnoses for the patient undergoing foot surgery may include the following:

- Risk for ineffective peripheral tissue perfusion: related to swelling
- Acute pain related to surgery, inflammation, and swelling
- Impaired physical mobility related to the foot-immobilizing device
- Risk for infection related to the surgical procedure/surgical incision

Planning and Goals

The goals for the patient may include adequate tissue perfusion, relief of pain, improved mobility, and absence of infection.

Nursing Interventions

PROMOTING TISSUE PERFUSION

Neurovascular assessment of the exposed toes every 1 to 2 hours for the first 24 hours is essential to monitor the function of the nerves and the perfusion of the tissues. If the patient is discharged within several hours after the surgery, the nurse teaches the patient and family how to assess for swelling and neurovascular status (circulation, motion, sensation). Compromised neurovascular function can increase the patient's pain. See Chart 66-3 in Chapter 66.

RELIEVING PAIN

Pain experienced by patients who undergo foot surgery is related to inflammation and edema. Formation of a hematoma may contribute to the discomfort. To control the swelling, the foot should be elevated on several pillows when the patient is sitting or lying. Intermittent ice packs applied to the surgical area during the first 24 to 48 hours may be prescribed to control swelling and provide some pain relief. As activity increases, the patient may find that dependent positioning of the foot is uncomfortable. Simply elevating the foot often relieves the discomfort. Oral analgesics may be used to control the pain. The nurse instructs the patient and family about appropriate use of these medications.

IMPROVING MOBILITY

After surgery, the patient will have a bulky dressing on the foot, protected by a light cast or a special protective boot. Limits for weight bearing on the foot will be prescribed by the surgeon. Some patients are allowed to walk on the heel and progress to weight-bearing as tolerated; other patients are restricted to non–weight-bearing activities. Assistive devices (eg, crutches, walker) may be needed. The choice of the devices depends on the patient's general condition and balance and on the weight-bearing prescription. Safe use of the assistive devices must be ensured through adequate patient education and practice before discharge. Strategies to move around the house safely while using assistive devices are discussed with the patient. As healing progresses, the patient gradually resumes ambulation within prescribed limits. The nurse emphasizes adherence to the therapeutic regimen.

PREVENTING INFECTION

Any surgery carries a risk for infection. In addition, percutaneous pins may be used to hold bones in position, and these pins serve as potential sites for infection. Because the foot is on or near the floor, care must be taken to protect it from dirt and moisture. When bathing, the patient can secure a plastic bag over the dressing to prevent it from getting wet. Patient instruction concerning aseptic wound care and pin care may be necessary.

The nurse teaches the patient to monitor for temperature and infection. Drainage on the dressing, foul odour, or increased pain and swelling could indicate infection. The nurse instructs the patient to promptly report any of these findings to the physician. If prophylactic antibiotics are prescribed, the nurse provides instruction about their correct use.

PROMOTING HOME AND COMMUNITY-BASED CARE

Teaching Patients Self-Care

The nurse plans patient teaching for home care, focusing on neurovascular status, pain management, mobility, and wound care (Chart 68-6).

Evaluation

EXPECTED PATIENT OUTCOMES

Expected patient outcomes may include:

1. Maintains peripheral tissue perfusion
   a. Demonstrates normal skin temperature and capillary refill
   b. Exhibits normal sensations
   c. Exhibits acceptable motor function
2. Obtains pain relief
   a. Elevates foot to control edema
   b. Applies ice to foot as prescribed
   c. Uses oral analgesics as needed and prescribed
   d. Reports decreased pain and increased comfort
3. Demonstrates increased mobility
   a. Uses assistive devices safely
   b. Resumes weight-bearing gradually as prescribed
   c. Exhibits diminished disability associated with preoperative condition
4. Develops no infection
   a. Reports temperature and pulse within normal limits
   b. Reports no purulent drainage or signs of wound inflammation
   c. Maintains clean and dry dressing
   d. Takes prophylactic antibiotics as prescribed

Chart 68-6 • PATIENT EDUCATION
Self-care After Foot Surgery

Neurovascular Status
Teach patient indicators of impaired circulation:
- Change in sensation
- Inability to move toes
- Toes or foot cool to touch
- Colour changes

Pain Management
Discuss with patient methods to reduce pain:
- Elevate foot to heart level
- Apply ice as prescribed
- Use analgesics as prescribed
- Report pain that is not relieved

Mobility
- Instruct patient in safe use of assistive devices
- Reinforce prescribed weight-bearing limits
- Encourage patient to wear special protective shoe over wound dressing

Wound Care
- Instruct patient to keep dressing or cast clean and dry
- Instruct patient about signs of wound infection (eg, pain, drainage, fever)
- Discuss prescribed antibiotic regimen with patient
- Explain that the surgeon will perform the initial dressing change

Metabolic Bone Disorders

OSTEOPOROSIS

Osteoporosis is a disease that threatens more than 1.4 million Canadians (Osteoporosis Canada, 2005). One in four women and one in eight men in Canada have osteoporosis (Brown & Josse, 2002). Characteristics of osteoporosis include a reduction of bone density and a change in bone structure, both of which increase susceptibility to fracture. The normal homeostatic bone turnover is altered: the rate of bone resorption is greater than the rate of bone formation, resulting in a reduced total bone mass. Suboptimal bone mass development in children and teens contributes to the development of osteoporosis. With osteoporosis, the bones become progressively porous, brittle, and fragile; they fracture easily under stresses that would not break normal bone ("fragility fracture"). Osteoporosis frequently results in compression fractures (Fig. 68-7) of the thoracic and lumbar spine, fractures of the neck and intertrochanteric region of the femur, and Colles' fractures of the wrist. The risk that a 50-year-old Caucasian woman will experience a hip, vertebra, or wrist fracture during her lifetime is 40% (Brown & Josse, 2002). Men and African Canadians have a lower rate. Multiple compression fractures of the vertebrae result in skeletal deformity. Osteoporosis is a costly disorder in terms of human suffering, pain, disability, decreased independence, and death. It is also very costly in terms of Canadian health care dollars. From 1988 to 1993 the costs of osteoporosis increased from $280 million to $1.3 billion. With the increasing age of the population, within the next 40 years there will be four times more hip fractures in Canada (Papadimitropoulos, Coyte, Josse, et al., 1997).

The gradual collapse of a vertebra may be asymptomatic; it is observed as progressive kyphosis. With the development of kyphosis ("dowager's hump"), there is an associated loss of height (Fig. 68-8).

FIGURE 68-7 Progressive osteoporotic bone loss and compression fractures. From Rubin, E., & Farber, I. L. (1999). *Pathology* (3rd ed.). Philadelphia: Lippincott Williams & Wilkins.

| | 10 yrs. postmenopause | 15 yrs. postmenopause height loss 1.5" | 25 yrs. postmenopause height loss 3.5" |

FIGURE 68-8 Typical loss of height associated with osteoporosis and aging.

Frequently, postmenopausal women lose height from vertebral collapse. The postural changes result in relaxation of the abdominal muscles and a protruding abdomen. The deformity may also produce pulmonary insufficiency. Many patients complain of fatigue.

Prevention

Primary osteoporosis occurs in women after menopause and later in life in men, but it is not merely a consequence of aging. Failure to develop optimal peak bone mass during childhood, adolescence, and young adulthood contributes to the development of osteoporosis without resultant bone loss. Early identification of at-risk teenagers and young adults is important. A prevention program of increased calcium, vitamin D, and protein; participation in regular weight-bearing impact exercise such as walking, gymnastics, soccer, basketball, or baseball, but not long-distance running (Brown & Josse, 2002); modification of lifestyle (eg, reduced use of caffeine, salt, cigarettes, and alcohol) is needed to decrease the risk for development of osteoporosis, fractures, and associated disability later in life. Secondary osteoporosis is the result of medications or other conditions and diseases that affect bone metabolism. Specific disease states (eg, celiac disease, hypogonadism) and medications (eg, corticosteroids, antiseizure medications) that place patients at risk need to be identified and therapies instituted to reverse the development of osteoporosis.

The goal is to prevent the first fracture because a previous fracture leads to more than a twofold increase in risk for additional fractures (Brown & Josse, 2002).

🍂 Gerontologic Considerations

The prevalence of osteoporosis in women older than 80 years of age is 84% (Genant et al., 1997). With the aging of the population, the incidence of hip, vertebra and wrist fractures, pain, and disability associated with osteoporosis is rising. The female lifetime risk (one in six) is considerably greater than the lifetime risk

for breast cancer (one in nine), but hip fractures cause more deaths (Cummings, Black, & Rubin, 1989). Approximately 25,000 hip fractures occur in Canada each year and 70% are osteoporosis related (Osteoporosis Canada, 2005). The mortality rate 1 year after hip fracture is 20% (Osteoporosis Society of Canada), with men twice as likely to die as women (Papadimitropoulos, Coyte & Josse, et al., 1997). For patients with hip fracture, 50% will never regain their prefracture level of functioning and will require assistance with daily activities. Another 20% will need placement in long-term care facilities (Chrischilles, Butler, Davis, et al., 1991).

Elderly people absorb dietary calcium less efficiently and excrete it more readily through their kidneys; therefore, postmenopausal women and the elderly actually need to consume liberal amounts of calcium. As much as 1500 mg daily for postmenopausal women is required. Most residents of long-term care facilities have a low bone mineral density (BMD) and are at risk for fracture. Hip protectors have been found to reduce the incidence of hip fracture in the elderly; however, compliance in wearing these hip protectors is low (Kannus et al., 2000).

Pathophysiology

Normal bone remodeling in the adult results in gradually increased bone mass until the early 30s. Gender, race, genetics, aging, low body weight and body mass index, nutrition, lifestyle choices (eg, smoking, caffeine and alcohol consumption), and physical activity influence peak bone mass and the development of osteoporosis (Fig. 68-9). Although the consequences of osteoporosis (eg, fractures) occur with aging, osteoporosis is not a disease of the elderly. Rather, its onset occurs earlier in life, when bone mass peaks and then begins to decline.

FIGURE 68-9 Pathophysiology of osteoporosis.

Loss of bone mass is a universal phenomenon associated with aging. Age-related loss begins soon after the peak bone mass is achieved (ie, in the fourth decade). Calcitonin, which inhibits bone resorption and promotes bone formation, is decreased. Estrogen, which inhibits bone breakdown, decreases with aging. On the other hand, parathyroid hormone (PTH) increases with aging, increasing bone turnover and resorption. The consequence of these changes is net loss of bone mass over time.

The withdrawal of estrogens at menopause or with oophorectomy causes an accelerated bone resorption that continues during the postmenopausal years. Women develop osteoporosis more frequently and more extensively than men because of lower initial peak bone mass and the effect of estrogen loss during menopause. World Health Organization (WHO) diagnostic categories for osteoporosis are based on BMD scan findings (Walker-Bone et al., 2001).

Secondary osteoporosis is associated with many disease states, nutritional deficiencies, and medications. Coexisting medical conditions (eg, malabsorption syndromes, lactose intolerance, alcohol abuse, renal failure, liver failure, Cushing's syndrome, hyperthyroidism, and hyperparathyroidism) contribute to bone loss and the development of osteoporosis. Medications (eg, cortico-

steroids, antiseizure medications, heparin, tetracycline, aluminum-containing antacids, and thyroid supplements) affect the body's use and metabolism of calcium. The degree of osteoporosis is related to the duration of medication therapy. When the therapy is discontinued or the metabolic problem is corrected, the progression of osteoporosis is halted, but restoration of lost bone mass usually does not occur.

Risk Factors

Risk factors for osteoporosis are not independent but are additive, and need to be examined in relation to age and gender. Whereas small-framed, slender Caucasian and Asian women are at greatest risk for osteoporosis and low BMD, obese women and men can also be at risk due to other factors. African Canadian women, who have a greater bone mass than Caucasian women, are less susceptible to osteoporosis. Men have a greater peak bone mass and do not experience sudden estrogen reduction. As a result, osteoporosis occurs in men at a lower rate and at an older age (about one decade later). At age 50, 19% of men have osteoporosis (Melton, et al., 1998). However, it has been determined that testosterone and estrogen are important in achieving and maintaining bone mass in men.

Nutritional factors contribute to the development of osteoporosis. A balanced diet—including adequate calories and nutrients needed to maintain bone, calcium, and vitamin D—must be consumed. Vitamin D is necessary for calcium absorption and for normal bone mineralization. Dietary calcium and vitamin D must be adequate to maintain bone remodeling and body functions. The best source of calcium and vitamin D is fortified milk. A cup of milk or calcium-fortified orange juice contains about 300 mg of calcium.

The 2002 *Canadian Guidelines for Osteoporosis* contains recommended amounts for calcium and vitamin D by age groups (Brown & Josse, 2002). The recommended adequate intake (AI) level of calcium for 4 to 8 year olds is 800 mg per day. For the age range of puberty to young adulthood (9 to 18 years of age), 1300 mg is required. The goal of this daily level of calcium is to maximize peak bone mass. The AI level for adults 19 to 50 years of age is 1000 mg per day, and the AI level for adults 51 years and older is 1500 mg per day. It is a major health concern that the actual estimated average daily intake of calcium is only 300 to 500 mg per day. Sun exposure in Canada is not enough to eliminate the need for dietary vitamin D. Vitamin D_3 (cholecalciferol) is recommended over D_2. Infants living in northern Canada require 400 IU of vitamin D if bottle-fed and 800 IU if breast-fed. The recommended daily intake for children up to 18 years of age is 200 to 400 IU (Holick, 1998). For 19 to 50 year olds, the recommended vitamin D is 400 IU and could be increased to 600 IU per day. Over 50 years of age, men and women require 800 IU per day (Brown & Josse).

Bone formation is enhanced by the stress of weight and muscle activity. Resistance and impact exercises are most beneficial in developing and maintaining bone mass. Immobility contributes to the development of osteoporosis. When immobilized by casts, general inactivity, paralysis or other disability, the bone is resorbed faster than it is formed, and osteoporosis results. Risk factors for osteoporosis are summarized in Chart 68-7.

Assessment and Diagnostic Findings

Osteoporosis may be identified on routine x-rays when there has been 25% to 40% demineralization. There is radiolucency to the bones. When the vertebrae collapse, the thoracic vertebrae become

Chart 68-7

Risk Factors for Osteoporosis

Individual Risk Factors
- Female, Caucasian, non-Hispanic or Asian
- Increased age
- Low weight and body mass index
- Estrogen deficiency or menopause; testosterone deficiency
- Family history of osteoporosis and/or fractures
- Low initial bone mass
- Contributing, coexisting medical conditions (eg, celiac disease) and medications (eg, corticosteroids, antiseizure medications)

Lifestyle Risk Factors
- Diets low in calcium, vitamin D, and protein
- Cigarette smoking
- Excessive use of salt
- Use of alcohol and/or caffeine (greater than 4 cups of coffee per day)
- Lack of weight-bearing exercise
- Lack of exposure to sunshine

Risk-Lowering Strategies
- Increased dietary calcium, vitamin D, and protein intake
- Smoking cessation
- Reduced salt intake
- Alcohol and caffeine consumption in moderation
- Regular weight-bearing impact exercise regimen
- Walk or exercise outdoors

wedge-shaped and the lumbar vertebrae become biconcave. Osteoporosis is diagnosed by dual-energy x-ray absorptiometry (DEXA), which provides information about BMD at the spine and hip. The DEXA scan data are analyzed and reported as T-scores (the number of standard deviations [SD] above or below the average BMD value for a young, healthy Caucasian woman). A normal BMD is less than 1 SD below the young adult mean value. Osteopenia is diagnosed when the BMD T-score is between 1 and 2.5 SD below the young adult mean value (Walker-Bone, et al., 2001). The WHO defines osteoporosis as being present when the T-score is at least 2.5 SD below the young adult mean value. The WHO has added a fourth category, "severe osteoporosis," for patients with osteoporosis who also have had a fragility fracture (Brown & Josse, 2002). Fracture risk increases progressively as the SD of the T-score falls below the mean value.

Quantitative ultrasound studies (QUS) of the heel also are used to diagnose osteoporosis and to predict the risk of hip and nonvertebral fracture. When standardization of sites and comparability of findings of BMD and QUS are determined, these measurements will become more clinically useful (NIH Consensus Statement, 2000).

Postmenopausal women and men over 50 years of age with risk factors such as vertebral compression fractures, fragility fractures, family history of osteoporosis and/or maternal hip fracture, menopause before age 45, some disease conditions, and certain medications and lifestyle risk factors should have their bone mineral density assessed. All men and women over age 65 years, regardless of the presence of risk factors, should have their BMD measured (Brown & Josse, 2002). These BMD studies are useful in identifying osteopenic and osteoporotic bone and in assessing response to therapy. Through early screening (using both assessment of risk factors and BMD scans), promotion of adequate dietary intake of calcium and vitamin D, encouragement of lifestyle changes, and early institution of preventive medications, bone loss and osteoporosis can be reduced, resulting in a reduced incidence of fracture.

Laboratory studies (eg, serum calcium, serum phosphate, serum alkaline phosphatase, urine calcium excretion, urinary hydroxyproline excretion, hematocrit, erythrocyte sedimentation rate) and x-ray studies are used to exclude other possible medical diagnoses (eg, multiple myeloma, osteomalacia, hyperparathyroidism, malignancy) that contribute to bone loss.

Medical Management

An adequate, balanced diet rich in calcium, vitamin D, and protein throughout life, with an increased calcium intake during adolescence, young adulthood, and the middle years, protects against skeletal demineralization. Such a diet would include three glasses of skim or whole vitamin D–enriched milk or other foods high in calcium (eg, cheese and other dairy products, steamed broccoli, canned salmon with bones), daily. To ensure adequate calcium intake, a calcium supplement (eg, Caltrate, Citracal) may be prescribed and taken with meals or with a beverage high in vitamin C to promote absorption. The recommended daily dose should be split and not taken as a single dose. Common side effects of calcium supplements are abdominal distention and constipation.

Regular weight-bearing impact exercise promotes bone formation. From 20 to 30 minutes of aerobic exercise (eg, walking), 3 days or more a week, is recommended. In addition, muscle strengthening and balance retraining exercises reduce the incidence of falls and fractures (Robertson, et al., 2001) (Chart 68-8).

PHARMACOLOGIC THERAPY

At natural or surgical menopause, HRT with estrogen and progesterone was the mainstay of therapy to retard bone loss and prevent occurrence of fractures. Estrogen replacement decreased bone resorption and increased bone mass, reducing the incidence of osteoporotic fractures. However, recent studies have demonstrated greater risks than previously recognized, leading to a dramatic decrease in the use of HRT for osteoporosis (Chen, Weiss, Newcomb, Barlow & White, 2002).

Selective estrogen receptor modulators (SERMs), such as raloxifene (Evista), reduce the risk for osteoporosis by preserving bone mineral density without estrogenic effects on the uterus. They are indicated for both prevention and treatment of osteoporosis.

Natural estrogens (plant-derived phytoestrogens) have not been shown to be effective in reducing osteoporosis-related fractures (NIH Consensus Statement, 2000).

In Canada, three bisphosphonates are approved for the treatment of osteoporosis: alendronate (Fosamax), risedronate (Actonel), and etidronate (Didrocal). Absorption of bisphosphonates by the oral route is poor, even when taken on an empty stomach. These drugs are considered first-line prevention therapies for low BMD in postmenopausal women and the prevention of glucocorticoid-induced osteoporosis in men and women. They also are first-line treatment therapies for postmenopausal women with osteoporosis and vertebral fractures, for glucocorticoid-induced osteoporosis in both sexes, and for men with low bone mass or osteoporosis (Brown & Josse, 2002). Alendronate offers an alternative to hormone replacement therapy (HRT) and produces increased bone mass (by inhibiting osteoclast function) and decreased bone loss. A weekly dosage strength of alendronate is available and has been shown to be as effective as previously used daily dosing. Adequate calcium and vitamin D intake is needed for maximum effect, but these supplements should not be taken at the same time of day as bisphosphonates. Side effects of alendronate include gastrointestinal symptoms (eg, dyspepsia, nausea, flatulence, diarrhea, constipation). Risedronate can also be

Chart 68-8
Home Care Checklist • Osteoporosis

At the completion of the home care instruction, the patient or caregiver will be able to:	Patient	Caregiver

Adolescents and Young Adults
- List risk factors for osteoporosis — ✓
- Identify calcium- and vitamin D-rich foods — ✓
- Consume diet with adequate calcium (1000–1300 mg/day) and vitamin D (400 IU/day) — ✓
- Engage in weight-bearing exercise daily — ✓
- Modify lifestyle choices—avoid smoking, alcohol, caffeine, carbonated beverages, and salt — ✓

Menopausal and Postmenopausal Women
- List risk factors for osteoporosis — ✓
- Identify calcium- and vitamin D-rich foods — ✓
- Consume diet with adequate calcium (1000–1500 mg/day) and vitamin D (800 IU/day) — ✓
- Discuss calcium supplements — ✓
- Engage in weight-bearing impact exercise at least 3 times weekly — ✓
- Engage in exercise that improves balance and strength to reduce the incidence of falls — ✓
- Demonstrate good body mechanics — ✓
- Modify lifestyle choices—avoid smoking, and use of alcohol, caffeine, salt, and carbonated beverages — ✓
- Participate in screening for osteoporosis (age 50 with risk factors or 65 years of age) — ✓
- Discuss pharmacologic agents to maintain and enhance bone mass — ✓
- Review concurrent medical conditions and medications with health care provider to identify factors that contribute to bone mass loss — ✓ — ✓
- Assess home environment for hazards contributing to falls — ✓ — ✓

Men
- List risk factors associated with osteoporosis in men, including medications (eg, corticosteroids, antiseizure medications, aluminum-containing antacids); chronic diseases (eg, kidney, lung, gastrointestinal); and undiagnosed low testosterone levels — ✓
- Modify lifestyle choices to avoid smoking and excessive intake of alcohol, caffeine, salt, and carbonated beverages — ✓
- Engage in weight-bearing impact exercise daily, such as walking, and exercise to improve balance and strength to limit falls — ✓
- Consume diet with adequate calcium (1500 mg/day) and vitamin D (800 IU/day) — ✓
- Participate in screening for osteoporosis — ✓
- Talk with health care provider about use of medications (eg, alendronate) to enhance bone mass or to correct testosterone deficiency — ✓
- Assess home for hazards contributing to falls — ✓

taken daily or weekly and is well tolerated. Side effects may include headache and diarrhea. Taken daily, risedronate reduces the incidence of hip and vertebral fractures in women with postmenopausal osteoporosis (Brown & Josse, 2002). Alendronate and risedronate are effective in reducing the number of hip and vertebral fractures. Editronate is well tolerated, with diarrhea being the main side effect. The drug is taken in an intermittent pattern of daily for 2 weeks every 3 months. Editronate has produced significant increases in BMD of the lumbar spine with a decrease in vertebral fractures but has not decreased the risk of hip fractures (Brown & Josse).

Calcitonin (Miacalcin) primarily suppresses bone loss through direct action on osteoclasts and reduced bone turnover. Calcitonin is administered daily, primarily by nasal spray and less often by subcutaneous or intramuscular injection. Side effects include nasal irritation, flushing, gastrointestinal disturbances, and urinary frequency. Nasal calcitonin is used to reduce the pain of acute vertebral fractures for postmenopausal women with severe osteoporosis. Calcitonin is effective in the prevention of vertebral fractures but not other types of fractures (Chestnut, et al., 2000). Bone mineral density of the hip and spine is maintained or slightly improved (Downs, et al., 2000). Calcitonin can be used for those on gluco-

corticoid drugs or who have glucocorticoid-induced osteoporosis to maintain or increase BMD (Kotaniemi, et al., 1996).

Recently, in clinical trials, small daily subcutaneous injections of PTH or PTH bioactive fragments (1-34; 1-38), or both, have been found to stimulate bone formation (Neer et al., 2001). In July 2004, the Therapeutic Products Directorate of Health Canada approved PTH (parathyroid hormone; with teriparatide as the active ingredient), under the name Forteo, as a bone formation agent for the treatment of osteoporosis. Route of administration is by subcutaneous injection.

In addition, antilipid medications, such as statins (HMG-CoA reductase inhibitors), reduce the incidence of fractures in patients who take these medications to control their hyperlipidemia. The statins promote bone growth, thereby preventing the development of osteoporosis.

FRACTURE MANAGEMENT
Fractures of the hip are managed surgically by joint replacement or by closed or open reduction with internal fixation (eg, hip pinning). Surgery, early ambulation, intensive physical therapy, and adequate nutrition result in decreased morbidity and improved

outcomes. In addition, patients need to be evaluated for osteoporosis and treated, if indicated.

Osteoporotic compression fractures of the vertebra are managed conservatively. Additional vertebral fractures and progressive kyphosis are common. Pharmacologic and dietary treatments are aimed at increasing vertebral bone density. A new procedure, percutaneous vertebroplasty/kyphoplasty (injection of polymethylmethacrylate bone cement into the fractured vertebra), is reported to provide rapid acute pain relief and improved quality of life. The long-term effect of this procedure is unknown (NIH Consensus Statement, 2000).

NURSING PROCESS: THE PATIENT WITH A SPONTANEOUS VERTEBRAL FRACTURE RELATED TO OSTEOPOROSIS

Assessment

Health promotion, identification of people at risk for osteoporosis, and recognition of problems associated with osteoporosis form the basis for nursing assessment. The health history includes questions concerning the occurrence of osteopenia and osteoporosis and focuses on family history of both conditions and any fractures in parents and grandparents; previous fractures including fragility fractures; dietary consumption of calcium, vitamin D, and protein; exercise patterns; onset of menopause; and use of corticosteroids as well as alcohol, smoking, and salt and caffeine intake. Four main risk factors for fractures related to osteoporosis are low BMD, prior fragility fractures, increasing age, and family history of osteoporosis (Brown & Josse, 2002). Questions are asked about previous falls and risk factors for falling such as reduced muscle strength (seen as problems getting up from a chair unassisted), impaired balance, low body mass, and decreased visual acuity (Cummings, et al., 1995). Any symptoms the patient is experiencing, such as back pain, constipation, or altered body image, are explored.

Physical examination may disclose a fracture, kyphosis of the thoracic spine, or shortened stature. A loss of more than 2 cm in height over 1 year or a total loss of more than 4 cm suggests possible vertebral fractures and the need for x-ray confirmation (Brown & Josse, 2002). Factors that predict a risk of hip fractures can also be assessed: slower gait, difficulty with heel-to-toe walking, and poor visual acuity (Dargent-Molina, et al., 1996). Problems in mobility and breathing may exist as a result of changes in posture and weakened muscles.

Nursing Diagnoses

Based on the assessment data, the major nursing diagnoses for the patient who experiences a spontaneous vertebral fracture related to osteoporosis may include the following:

- Deficient knowledge about the osteoporotic process and treatment regimen
- Acute pain related to fracture and muscle spasm
- Risk for constipation related to immobility or development of ileus (intestinal obstruction)
- Risk for injury: additional fractures related to osteoporosis

Planning and Goals

The major goals for the patient may include knowledge about osteoporosis and the treatment regimen, relief of pain, improved bowel elimination, prevention of falls, and absence of additional fractures.

Nursing Interventions

PROMOTING UNDERSTANDING OF OSTEOPOROSIS AND THE TREATMENT REGIMEN

Patient teaching focuses on factors influencing the development of osteoporosis, interventions to arrest or slow the process, and measures to relieve symptoms. Adequate dietary or supplemental calcium and vitamin D, regular weight-bearing impact exercise, and modification of lifestyle, if necessary (eg, cessation of smoking, reduced use of caffeine, salt, and alcohol), help to maintain bone mass. Diet, exercise, and physical activity are the primary keys to developing high-density bones that are resistant to osteoporosis. It is emphasized that all people continue to need sufficient calcium, vitamin D, sunshine, and weight-bearing impact exercise to slow the progression of osteoporosis.

Patient teaching related to medication therapy is important. Because gastrointestinal symptoms and abdominal distention are frequent side effects of calcium supplements, the nurse instructs the patient to take the calcium supplements with meals. Also, it is important to teach the patient to drink adequate fluids to reduce the risk of renal calculi. If HRT is prescribed, the nurse teaches the patient about the importance of compliance and periodic screening for breast and endometrial cancer. Alendronate requires compliance: it must be taken on an empty stomach with water, and then the patient must not consume foods or liquids or assume a reclining position for 30 to 60 minutes. Nasal calcitonin is administered daily, alternating the nares. An adequate daily intake of dietary calcium and vitamin D is needed along with these prescribed medications.

RELIEVING PAIN

Relief of back pain resulting from compression fracture may be accomplished by resting in bed in a supine or side-lying position several times a day. The mattress should be firm and nonsagging. Knee flexion increases comfort by relaxing back muscles. Nasal calcitonin is the treatment of choice to relieve the pain of vertebral fractures (Lyritis, et al., 1997). Intermittent local heat and back rubs promote muscle relaxation. The nurse instructs the patient to move the trunk as a unit and to avoid twisting. The nurse encourages good posture and teaches body mechanics. When the patient is assisted out of bed, a lumbosacral corset may be worn for temporary support and immobilization, although such a device is frequently uncomfortable and is poorly tolerated by many elderly patients. The patient gradually resumes activities as pain diminishes. Vertebroplasty may be considered for some patients.

IMPROVING BOWEL ELIMINATION

Constipation is a problem related to immobility and medications. Early institution of a high-fibre diet, increased fluids, and the use of prescribed stool softeners help to prevent or minimize constipation. If the vertebral collapse involves the T10–L2 vertebrae, the patient may develop an ileus. The nurse therefore monitors the patient's intake, bowel sounds, and bowel activity.

PREVENTING INJURY

Physical activity is essential to strengthen muscles, improve balance, prevent disuse atrophy, and retard progressive bone demineralization. Isometric exercises can strengthen trunk muscles. The nurse encourages walking, good body mechanics, and good posture. Daily weight-bearing activity, preferably outdoors in the sunshine to enhance the body's ability to produce vitamin D, is encouraged. Sudden bending, jarring, twisting, and strenuous lifting are avoided.

Gerontologic Considerations

Elderly people fall because a hip has fractured (fragility fracture) or as a result of environmental hazards, neuromuscular disorders, diminished senses and cardiovascular responses, and responses to medications. The patient and family need to be included in planning for care and preventive management regimens. For example, the home environment should be assessed for safety and elimination of potential hazards (eg, scatter rugs, cluttered rooms and stairwells, toys on the floor, pets underfoot). A safe environment can then be created (eg, well-lighted staircases with secure hand rails, grab bars in the bathroom, properly fitting footwear). Other safety devices, such as hip protectors (Fig. 68-10), have been used to diminish the impact of a fall and have reduced the hip fracture rate (Kannus et al., 2000).

Evaluation

EXPECTED PATIENT OUTCOMES

Expected patient outcomes may include:

1. Acquires knowledge about osteoporosis and the treatment regimen
   a. States relationship of calcium and vitamin D intake and exercise to bone mass
   b. Consumes adequate dietary calcium, vitamin D, and protein for age group
   c. Increases level of weight-bearing impact exercise
   d. Takes prescribed medication therapy
   e. Complies with prescribed screening and monitoring procedures

2. Achieves pain relief
   a. Experiences pain relief at rest
   b. Experiences minimal discomfort during ADLs
   c. Demonstrates diminished tenderness at fracture site
3. Demonstrates usual bowel elimination
   a. Has active bowel sounds
   b. Reports regular bowel movements
4. Experiences no new fractures
   a. Maintains good posture
   b. Uses good body mechanics
   c. Consumes a diet high in calcium, vitamin D, and protein
   d. Engages in weight-bearing impact exercises (walks daily)
   e. Rests by lying down several times a day
   f. Participates in outdoor activities
   g. Creates a safe home environment
   h. Accepts assistance and supervision as needed

OSTEOMALACIA

Osteomalacia is a metabolic bone disease characterized by inadequate mineralization of bone. As a result of faulty mineralization, there is softening and weakening of the skeleton, causing pain, tenderness to touch, bowing of the bones, and pathologic fractures. On physical examination, skeletal deformities (spinal kyphosis and bowed legs) give patients an unusual appearance and a waddling or limping gait. These patients may be uncomfortable with their appearance. As a result of calcium deficiency, muscle weakness, and unsteadiness, there is an increased risk for falls and fractures.

Pathophysiology

The primary defect in osteomalacia is a deficiency of activated vitamin D (calcitriol), which promotes calcium absorption from the gastrointestinal tract and facilitates mineralization of bone. The supply of calcium and phosphate in the extracellular fluid is low. Without adequate vitamin D, calcium and phosphate are not moved to calcification sites in bones.

Osteomalacia may result from failed calcium absorption (eg, malabsorption syndrome) or from excessive loss of calcium from the body. Gastrointestinal disorders (eg, celiac disease, chronic biliary tract obstruction, chronic pancreatitis, small bowel resection) in which fats are inadequately absorbed are likely to produce osteomalacia through loss of vitamin D (along with other fat-soluble vitamins) and calcium, the latter being excreted in the feces with fatty acids. In addition, liver and kidney diseases can produce a lack of vitamin D because these are the organs that convert vitamin D to its active form.

Severe renal insufficiency results in acidosis. The body uses available calcium to combat the acidosis, and PTH stimulates the release of skeletal calcium in an attempt to reestablish a physiologic pH. During this continual drain of skeletal calcium, bony fibrosis occurs and bony cysts form. Chronic glomerulonephritis, obstructive uropathies, and heavy-metal poisoning result in a reduced serum phosphate level and demineralization of bone.

Hyperparathyroidism leads to skeletal decalcification and thus to osteomalacia by increasing phosphate excretion in the urine. Prolonged use of antiseizure medication (eg, phenytoin, phenobarbital) poses a risk for osteomalacia, as does insufficient vitamin D (dietary, sunlight).

The malnutrition type of osteomalacia (deficiency in vitamin D often associated with poor intake of calcium) is a result of poverty, food faddism, and lack of knowledge about nutrition. It occurs most frequently in parts of the world where vitamin D is not

FIGURE 68-10 HipSaver Slimfit® Hip Protector is designed to prevent fall-induced hip fractures. A pad placed over each trochanter can reduce much of the force transmitted to the vulnerable hip bone when a fall is sustained. Photo courtesy of the HipSaver Company, Canton, MA, www.hipsaver.com.

added to food, where dietary deficiencies exist, and where sunlight is rare.

 ## Gerontologic Considerations

A nutritious diet is particularly important in elderly people. Adequate intake of calcium and vitamin D is promoted. Because sunlight is necessary for synthesizing vitamin D, people should be encouraged to spend some time in the sun. Prevention, identification, and management of osteomalacia in the elderly are essential to reduce the incidence of fractures. When osteomalacia is combined with osteoporosis, the incidence of fracture increases.

Assessment and Diagnostic Findings

On x-ray, generalized demineralization of bone is evident. Studies of the vertebrae may show a compression fracture with indistinct vertebral end-plates. Laboratory studies show low serum calcium and phosphorus levels and a moderately elevated alkaline phosphatase concentration. Urine excretion of calcium and creatinine is low. Bone biopsy demonstrates an increased amount of osteoid.

Medical Management

The underlying cause of osteomalacia is corrected if possible. If osteomalacia is caused by malabsorption, increased doses of vitamin D, along with supplemental calcium, are usually prescribed. Exposure to sunlight for ultraviolet radiation to transform a cholesterol substance (7-dehydrocholesterol) present in the skin into vitamin D may be recommended.

If osteomalacia is dietary in origin, a diet with adequate protein and increased calcium and vitamin D is provided. The patient is instructed about dietary sources of calcium and vitamin D (eg, fortified milk and cereals, eggs, chicken livers). The safe use of supplements is reviewed. Because high doses of vitamin D are toxic and enhance the risk of hypercalcemia, the importance of monitoring serum calcium levels is stressed. Vitamin D raises the concentrations of calcium and phosphorus in the extracellular fluid and thus makes these ions available for mineralization of bone.

Physical, psychological, and pharmaceutical measures are used to reduce the patient's discomfort and pain. When assisting the patient to change positions, the nurse handles the patient gently, and pillows are used to support the body. As the patient responds to therapy, the skeletal discomforts diminish.

Frequently, skeletal problems associated with osteomalacia resolve themselves when the underlying nutritional deficiency or pathologic process is adequately treated. Long-term monitoring of the patient is appropriate to ensure stabilization or reversal of osteomalacia. Some persistent orthopedic deformities may need to be treated with braces or surgery (eg, osteotomy may be performed to correct long bone deformity).

PAGET'S DISEASE

Paget's disease (osteitis deformans) is a disorder of localized rapid bone turnover, most commonly affecting the skull, femur, tibia, pelvic bones, and vertebrae. There is a primary proliferation of osteoclasts, which produces bone resorption. This is followed by a compensatory increase in osteoblastic activity that replaces the bone. As bone turnover continues, a classic mosaic (disorganized) pattern of bone develops. Because the diseased bone in Paget's disease is highly vascularized and structurally weak, pathologic fractures occur. Structural bowing of the legs causes malalignment of the hip, knee, and ankle joints, which contributes to the development of arthritis and back and joint pain.

Paget's disease occurs in about 2% to 3% of the population older than 50 years of age. The incidence is slightly greater in men than in women and increases with aging. A family history has been noted, with siblings developing the disease. The cause of Paget's disease is not known.

Clinical Manifestations

Paget's disease is insidious; most patients never know they have it. Some patients do not experience symptoms but have skeletal deformity. A few patients have symptomatic deformity and pain. The condition is most frequently identified on x-ray during a routine physical examination or in the course of a workup for another problem. Sclerotic changes, skeletal deformities (eg, bowing of femur and tibia, enlargement of the skull, deformity of pelvic bones), and cortical thickening of the long bones occur.

In most patients, skeletal deformity involves the skull or long bones. The skull may thicken, and the patient may report that a hat no longer fits. In some cases of Paget's disease, the cranium, but not the face, is enlarged. This gives the face a small, triangular appearance. Most patients with skull involvement have impaired hearing from cranial nerve compression and dysfunction. Other cranial nerves may also be compressed.

The femurs and tibiae tend to bow, producing a waddling gait. The spine is bent forward and is rigid; the chin rests on the chest. The thorax is compressed and immobile on respiration. The trunk is flexed on the legs to maintain balance; the arms are bent outward and forward and appear long in relation to the shortened trunk, giving the patient an apelike posture.

Pain, tenderness, and warmth over the bones may be noted. The pain is mild to moderate, deep, and aching; it increases with weight bearing if the lower extremities are involved. Pain and discomfort may precede skeletal deformities of Paget's disease by years and are often wrongly attributed by the patient to old age or arthritis.

The temperature of the skin overlying the affected bone increases because of increased bone vascularity. Patients with large, highly vascular lesions may develop high-output cardiac failure because of the increased vascular bed and metabolic demands.

Assessment and Diagnostic Findings

Elevated serum alkaline phosphatase concentration and urinary hydroxyproline excretion reflect increased osteoblastic activity. Higher values suggest more active disease. Patients with Paget's disease have normal blood calcium levels. X-rays confirm the diagnosis of Paget's disease. Local areas of demineralization and bone overgrowth produce characteristic mosaic patterns and irregularities. Bone scans demonstrate the extent of the disease. Bone biopsy may aid in the differential diagnosis.

Medical Management

Pain usually responds to administration of NSAIDs. Gait problems from bowing of the legs are managed with walking aids, shoe lifts, and physical therapy. Weight is controlled to reduce stress on weakened bones and malaligned joints. Asymptomatic patients may be managed with diets adequate in calcium and vitamin D and periodic monitoring.

Fractures, arthritis, and hearing loss are complications of Paget's disease. Fractures are managed according to location. Healing occurs if fracture reduction, immobilization, and stability are adequate. Severe degenerative arthritis may require total joint replacement. Loss of hearing is managed with hearing aids and communication techniques used with the hearing-impaired person (eg, lip reading, body language).

PHARMACOLOGIC THERAPY

Patients with moderate to severe disease may benefit from specific antiosteoclastic therapy. Several medications reduce bone turnover, reverse the course of the disease, relieve pain, and improve mobility.

Calcitonin, a polypeptide hormone, retards bone resorption by decreasing the number and availability of osteoclasts. Calcitonin therapy facilitates remodeling of abnormal bone into normal lamellar bone, relieves bone pain, and helps alleviate neurologic and biochemical signs and symptoms. Calcitonin is administered subcutaneously or by nasal inhalation. Side effects include flushing of the face and nausea. The effect of calcitonin therapy is evident in 3 to 6 months.

Bisphosphonates, such as etidronate disodium (Didronel) and alendronate sodium (Fosamax), produce rapid reduction in bone turnover and relief of pain. They also reduce serum alkaline phosphatase and urinary hydroxyproline levels. Food inhibits absorption of these medications. Adequate daily calcium (1500 mg) and vitamin D (400 to 600 IU) are required during therapy.

Plicamycin (Mithracin), a cytotoxic antibiotic, may be used to control the disease. This medication is reserved for severely affected patients with neurologic compromise and for those whose disease is resistant to other therapy. This medication has dramatic effects on pain reduction and on serum calcium, alkaline phosphatase, and urinary hydroxyproline levels. It is administered by IV infusion and requires that hepatic, renal, and bone marrow function be monitored during therapy. Clinical remissions may continue for months after the medication is discontinued.

 Gerontologic Considerations

Careful assessment of the patient's pain and discomfort is necessary. Patient teaching helps the patient understand the treatment regimen, the need for a diet with adequate calcium and vitamin D, and how to compensate for altered musculoskeletal functioning. The home environment is assessed for safety to prevent falls and to reduce the risk for fracture. Strategies for coping with a chronic health problem and its effect on quality of life need to be developed.

Musculoskeletal Infections

OSTEOMYELITIS

Osteomyelitis is an infection of the bone. The bone becomes infected by one of three modes:

- Extension of soft tissue infection (eg, infected pressure or vascular ulcer, incisional infection)
- Direct bone contamination from bone surgery, open fracture, or traumatic injury (eg, gunshot wound)
- Hematogenous (bloodborne) spread from other sites of infection (eg, infected tonsils, boils, infected teeth, upper respiratory infections). Osteomyelitis resulting from hematogenous spread typically occurs in a bone area of trauma or lowered resistance, possibly from subclinical (nonapparent) trauma.

Patients who are at high risk for osteomyelitis include those who are poorly nourished, elderly, or obese. Also at risk are patients with impaired immune systems, those with chronic illness (eg, diabetes, rheumatoid arthritis), and those receiving long-term corticosteroid therapy.

Postoperative surgical wound infections occur within 30 days after surgery. They are classified as incisional (superficial, located above the deep fascia layer) or deep (involving tissue beneath the deep fascia). If an implant has been used, deep postoperative infections may occur within a year. Deep sepsis after arthroplasty may be classified as follows:

Stage 1, acute fulminating: occurring during the first 3 months after orthopedic surgery; frequently associated with hematoma, drainage, or superficial infection

Stage 2, delayed onset: occurring between 4 and 24 months after surgery

Stage 3, late onset: occurring 2 or more years after surgery, usually as a result of hematogenous spread

Bone infections are more difficult to eradicate than soft tissue infections because the infected bone becomes walled off. Natural body immune responses are blocked, and there is less penetration by antibiotics. Osteomyelitis may become chronic and may affect the patient's quality of life.

Pathophysiology

Staphylococcus aureus causes 70% to 80% of bone infections. Other pathogenic organisms frequently found in osteomyelitis include *Proteus* and *Pseudomonas* species and *Escherichia coli*. The incidence of penicillin-resistant, nosocomial, gram-negative, and anaerobic infections is increasing.

The initial response to infection is inflammation, increased vascularity, and edema. After 2 or 3 days, thrombosis of the blood vessels occurs in the area, resulting in ischemia with bone necrosis. The infection extends into the medullary cavity and under the periosteum and may spread into adjacent soft tissues and joints. Unless the infective process is treated promptly, a bone abscess forms. The resulting abscess cavity contains dead bone tissue (the **sequestrum**), which does not easily liquefy and drain. Therefore, the cavity cannot collapse and heal, as occurs in soft tissue abscesses. New bone growth (the **involucrum**) forms and surrounds the sequestrum. Although healing appears to take place, a chronically infected sequestrum remains and produces recurring abscesses throughout the patient's life. This is referred to as chronic osteomyelitis.

Clinical Manifestations

When the infection is bloodborne, the onset is usually sudden, occurring often with the clinical manifestations of septicemia (eg, chills, high fever, rapid pulse, general malaise). The systemic symptoms at first may overshadow the local signs. As the infection extends through the cortex of the bone, it involves the periosteum and the soft tissues. The infected area becomes painful, swollen, and extremely tender. The patient may describe a constant, pulsating pain that intensifies with movement as a result of the pressure of the collecting pus. When osteomyelitis occurs from spread of adjacent infection or from direct contamination, there are no symptoms of septicemia. The area is swollen, warm, painful, and tender to touch.

The patient with chronic osteomyelitis presents with a continuously draining sinus or experiences recurrent periods of pain, inflammation, swelling, and drainage. The low-grade infection thrives in scar tissue, because it has a reduced blood supply.

Assessment and Diagnostic Findings

In acute osteomyelitis, early x-ray findings demonstrate soft tissue swelling. In about 2 weeks, areas of irregular decalcification, bone necrosis, periosteal elevation, and new bone formation are evident. Radioisotope bone scans, particularly the isotope-labelled white blood cell (WBC) scan, and magnetic resonance imaging (MRI) help with early definitive diagnosis. Blood studies reveal elevated leukocyte levels and an elevated sedimentation rate. Wound and blood culture studies are performed to identify appropriate antibiotic therapy.

With chronic osteomyelitis, large, irregular cavities, raised periosteum, sequestra, or dense bone formations are seen on x-ray. Bone scans may be performed to identify areas of infection. The sedimentation rate and the WBC count are usually normal. Anemia, associated with chronic infection, may be evident. The abscess is cultured to determine the infective organism and appropriate antibiotic therapy.

Prevention

Prevention of osteomyelitis is the goal. Elective orthopedic surgery should be postponed if the patient has a current infection (eg, urinary tract infection, sore throat) or a recent history of infection. During orthopedic surgery, careful attention is paid to the surgical environment and to techniques to decrease direct bone contamination. Prophylactic antibiotics, administered to achieve adequate tissue levels at the time of surgery and for 24 hours after surgery, are helpful. Urinary catheters and drains are removed as soon as possible to decrease the incidence of hematogenous spread of infection.

Treatment of focal infections diminishes hematogenous spread. Aseptic postoperative wound care reduces the incidence of superficial infections and osteomyelitis. Prompt management of soft tissue infections reduces extension of infection to the bone. When patients who have had joint replacement surgery undergo dental procedures or other invasive procedures (eg, cystoscopy), prophylactic antibiotics are frequently recommended.

Medical Management

The initial goal of therapy is to control and halt the infective process. Antibiotic therapy depends on the results of blood and wound cultures. Frequently, the infection is caused by more than one pathogen. General supportive measures (eg, hydration, diet high in vitamins and protein, correction of anemia) should be instituted. The area affected with osteomyelitis is immobilized to decrease discomfort and to prevent pathologic fracture of the weakened bone. Warm wet soaks for 20 minutes several times a day may be prescribed to increase circulation.

PHARMACOLOGIC THERAPY

As soon as the culture specimens are obtained, IV antibiotic therapy begins, based on the assumption that infection results from a staphylococcal organism that is sensitive to a semisynthetic penicillin or cephalosporin. The aim is to control the infection before the blood supply to the area diminishes as a result of thrombosis. Around-the-clock dosing is necessary to achieve a sustained high therapeutic blood level of the antibiotic. An antibiotic to which the causative organism is sensitive is prescribed after results of the culture and sensitivity studies are known. IV antibiotic therapy continues for 3 to 6 weeks. After the infection appears to be controlled, the antibiotic may be administered orally for up to 3 months. To enhance absorption of the orally administered medication, antibiotics should not be administered with food.

SURGICAL MANAGEMENT

If the patient does not respond to antibiotic therapy, the infected bone is surgically exposed, the purulent and necrotic material is removed, and the area is irrigated with sterile saline solution. Antibiotic-impregnated beads may be placed in the wound for direct application of antibiotics for 2 to 4 weeks. IV antibiotic therapy is continued.

In chronic osteomyelitis, antibiotics are adjunctive therapy to surgical débridement. A sequestrectomy (removal of enough involucrum to enable the surgeon to remove the sequestrum) is performed. In many cases, sufficient bone is removed to convert a deep cavity into a shallow saucer (saucerization). All dead, infected bone and cartilage must be removed before permanent healing can occur. A closed suction irrigation system may be used to remove debris. Wound irrigation using sterile physiologic saline solution may be performed for 7 to 8 days.

The wound is either closed tightly to obliterate the dead space or packed and closed later by granulation or possibly by grafting. The débrided cavity may be packed with cancellous bone graft to stimulate healing. With a large defect, the cavity may be filled with a vascularized bone transfer or muscle flap (in which a muscle is moved from an adjacent area with blood supply intact). These microsurgery techniques enhance the blood supply. The improved blood supply facilitates bone healing and eradication of the infection. These surgical procedures may be staged over time to ensure healing. Because surgical débridement weakens the bone, internal fixation or external supportive devices may be needed to stabilize or support the bone to prevent pathologic fracture.

NURSING PROCESS:
THE PATIENT WITH OSTEOMYELITIS

Assessment

The patient reports an acute onset of signs and symptoms (eg, localized pain, swelling, erythema, fever) or recurrent drainage of an infected sinus with associated pain, swelling, and low-grade fever. The nurse assesses the patient for risk factors (eg, older age, diabetes, long-term corticosteroid therapy) and for a history of previous injury, infection, or orthopedic surgery. The patient avoids pressure on the area and guards movement. In acute hematogenous osteomyelitis, the patient exhibits generalized weakness due to the systemic reaction to the infection.

Physical examination reveals an inflamed, markedly swollen, warm area that is tender. Purulent drainage may be noted. The patient has an elevated temperature. With chronic osteomyelitis, the temperature elevation may be minimal, occurring in the afternoon or evening.

Nursing Diagnoses

Based on the nursing assessment data, nursing diagnoses for the patient with osteomyelitis may include the following:

- Acute pain related to inflammation and swelling
- Impaired physical mobility related to pain, use of immobilization devices, and weight-bearing limitations
- Risk for extension of infection: bone abscess formation
- Deficient knowledge related to the treatment regimen

Planning and Goals

The patient's goals may include relief of pain, improved physical mobility within therapeutic limitations, control and eradication of infection, and knowledge of treatment regimen.

Nursing Interventions

RELIEVING PAIN

The affected part may be immobilized with a splint to decrease pain and muscle spasm. The nurse monitors the neurovascular status of the affected extremity. The wounds are frequently very painful, and the extremity must be handled with great care and gentleness. Elevation reduces swelling and associated discomfort. Pain is controlled with prescribed analgesics and other pain-reducing techniques.

IMPROVING PHYSICAL MOBILITY

Treatment regimens restrict activity. The bone is weakened by the infective process and must be protected by immobilization devices and by avoidance of stress on the bone. The patient must understand the rationale for the activity restrictions. The joints above and below the affected part should be gently placed through their range of motion. The nurse encourages full participation in ADLs within the physical limitations to promote general well-being.

CONTROLLING THE INFECTIOUS PROCESS

The nurse monitors the patient's response to antibiotic therapy and observes the IV access site for evidence of phlebitis, infection, or infiltration. With long-term, intensive antibiotic therapy, the nurse monitors the patient for signs of superinfection (eg, oral or vaginal candidiasis, loose or foul-smelling stools).

If surgery was necessary, the nurse takes measures to ensure adequate circulation (wound suction to prevent fluid accumulation, elevation of the area to promote venous drainage, avoidance of pressure on grafted area), to maintain needed immobility, and to comply with weight-bearing restrictions. The nurse changes dressings using aseptic technique to promote healing and to prevent cross-contamination.

The nurse continues to monitor the general health and nutrition of the patient. A diet high in protein and vitamin C ensures a positive nitrogen balance and promotes healing. The nurse encourages adequate hydration as well.

PROMOTING HOME AND COMMUNITY-BASED CARE

Teaching Patients Self-Care

The patient and family must learn and recognize the importance of strictly adhering to the therapeutic regimen of antibiotics and preventing falls or other injuries that could result in bone fracture. The patient needs to know how to maintain and manage the IV access and IV administration equipment in the home. Medication education includes medication name, dosage, frequency, administration rate, safe storage and handling, adverse reactions, and necessary laboratory monitoring. In addition, aseptic dressing and warm compress techniques are taught.

The nurse carefully monitors the patient for the development of additional painful areas or sudden increases in body temperature. The nurse instructs the patient and family to observe and report elevated temperature, drainage, odour, increased inflammation, adverse reactions, and signs of superinfection.

Continuing Care

Management of osteomyelitis, including wound care and IV antibiotic therapy, is usually performed at home. The patient must be medically stable, physically able, and motivated to adhere strictly to the therapeutic regimen of antibiotic therapy. The home care environment needs to be conducive to promotion of health and to the requirements of the therapeutic regimen.

If warranted, the nurse completes a home assessment to determine the patient's and family's abilities regarding continuation of the therapeutic regimen. If the patient's support system is questionable or if the patient lives alone, a home care nurse may be needed to assist with intravenous administration of the antibiotics. The nurse monitors the patient for response to the treatment, signs and symptoms of superinfections, and adverse drug reactions. The nurse stresses the importance of follow-up health care appointments (Chart 68-9).

Evaluation

EXPECTED PATIENT OUTCOMES

Expected patient outcomes may include:

1. Experiences pain relief
   a. Reports decreased pain
   b. Experiences no tenderness at site of previous infection
   c. Experiences no discomfort with movement
2. Increases physical mobility
   a. Participates in self-care activities
   b. Maintains full function of unimpaired extremities
   c. Demonstrates safe use of immobilizing and assistive devices
   d. Modifies environment to promote safety and to avoid falls
3. Shows absence of infection
   a. Takes antibiotic as prescribed

Chart 68-9
Home Care Checklist • Osteomyelitis

At the completion of the home care instruction, the patient or caregiver will be able to:	Patient	Caregiver
Describe osteomyelitis	✓	✓
Relieve pain with pharmacologic and nonpharmacologic interventions	✓	
State weight-bearing and activity restrictions	✓	✓
Demonstrate safe use of ambulatory aids and assistive devices	✓	
Describe use of prescribed medications	✓	✓
Comply with antibiotic regimen	✓	
Promote healing through aseptic dressing changes	✓	✓
Demonstrate proper wound care	✓	✓
Report signs and symptoms of continuing infection or superinfection	✓	✓

b. Reports normal temperature
c. Exhibits no swelling
d. Reports absence of drainage
e. Laboratory results indicate normal white blood cell count and sedimentation rate
f. Wound cultures are negative

4. Complies with therapeutic plan
a. Takes medications as prescribed
b. Protects weakened bones
c. Demonstrates proper wound care
d. Reports signs and symptoms of complications promptly
e. Eats a diet that is high in protein and vitamin C
f. Keeps follow-up health appointments
g. Reports increased strength
h. Reports no elevation of temperature or recurrence of pain, swelling, or other symptoms at the site

SEPTIC (INFECTIOUS) ARTHRITIS

Joints can become infected through spread of infection from other parts of the body (hematogenous spread) or directly through trauma or surgical instrumentation. Previous trauma to joints, joint replacement, coexisting arthritis, and diminished host resistance contribute to the development of an infected joint. *S. aureus* causes most adult joint infections, followed by streptococci and gram-negative organisms. Prompt recognition and treatment of an infected joint are important because accumulating pus results in chondrolysis (destruction of hyaline cartilage).

Clinical Manifestations

The patient with acute septic arthritis usually presents with a warm, painful, swollen joint with decreased range of motion. Systemic chills, fever, and leukocytosis are present. Risk factors include advanced age, diabetes mellitus, rheumatoid arthritis, and preexisting joint disease or joint replacement.

Gerontologic Considerations

Elderly patients and patients taking corticosteroids or immunosuppressive medications may not exhibit typical clinical manifestations of infection. Therefore, they require ongoing assessment to detect infection as early as possible in the infectious process.

Assessment and Diagnostic Findings

An assessment for the source and cause of infection is performed. Diagnostic studies include aspiration, examination, and culture of the synovial fluid. Computed tomography and MRI may disclose damage to the joint lining. Radioisotope scanning may be useful in localizing the infectious process.

Management

Prompt treatment is essential and may save a joint prosthesis for patients who have one. Broad-spectrum IV antibiotics are started promptly and then changed to organism-specific antibiotics after culture results are available. The IV antibiotics are continued until symptoms disappear. The synovial fluid is monitored for sterility and decrease in WBCs.

In addition to prescribing antibiotics, the physician may aspirate the joint with a needle to remove excessive joint fluid, exudate, and debris. This promotes comfort and decreases joint destruction caused by the action of proteolytic enzymes in the purulent fluid. Occasionally, arthrotomy or arthroscopy is used to drain the joint and remove dead tissue.

The inflamed joint is supported and immobilized in a functional position by a splint that increases the patient's comfort. Analgesics, such as codeine, may be prescribed to control pain. After the infection has responded to antibiotic therapy, NSAIDs may be prescribed to limit joint damage. The patient's nutrition and fluid status is monitored. Progressive range-of-motion exercises are prescribed after the infection subsides.

If septic joints are treated promptly, recovery of normal function is expected. The patient is assessed periodically for recurrence. If the articular cartilage was damaged during the inflammatory reaction, joint fibrosis and diminished function may result.

The nurse describes the septic arthritis process to the patient and teaches the patient how to relieve pain using pharmacologic and nonpharmacologic interventions. The nurse also explains the importance of supporting the affected joint, adhering to the prescribed antibiotic regimen, and observing weight-bearing and activity restrictions. Additionally, the nurse demonstrates and encourages the patient to practice safe use of ambulatory aids and assistive devices.

The nurse teaches the patient strategies to promote healing through aseptic dressing changes and proper wound care. The patient is then encouraged to perform range-of-motion exercises after the infection subsides.

Bone Tumours

Neoplasms of the musculoskeletal system are of various types, including osteogenic, chondrogenic, fibrogenic, muscle (rhabdomyogenic), and marrow (reticulum) cell tumours as well as nerve, vascular, and fatty cell tumours. They may be primary tumours or metastatic tumours from primary cancers elsewhere in the body (eg, breast, lung, prostate, kidney). Metastatic bone tumours are more common than primary bone tumours.

BENIGN BONE TUMOURS

Benign tumours of the bone and soft tissue are more common than malignant primary bone tumours. Benign bone tumours generally are slow growing and well circumscribed, present few symptoms, and are not a cause of death.

Benign primary neoplasms of the musculoskeletal system include osteochondroma, enchondroma, bone cyst (eg, aneurysmal bone cyst), osteoid osteoma, rhabdomyoma, and fibroma. Some benign tumours, such as giant cell tumours, have the potential to become malignant.

Osteochondroma is the most common benign bone tumour. It usually occurs as a large projection of bone at the end of long bones (at the knee or shoulder). It develops during growth and then becomes a static bony mass. In fewer than 1% of patients, the cartilage cap of the osteochondroma may undergo malignant transformation after trauma, and a chondrosarcoma or osteosarcoma may develop.

Enchondroma is a common tumour of the hyaline cartilage that develops in the hand, femur, tibia, or humerus. Usually, the only symptom is a mild ache. Pathologic fractures may occur.

Bone cysts are expanding lesions within the bone. Aneurysmal (widening) bone cysts are seen in young adults, who present with a painful, palpable mass of the long bones, vertebrae, or flat bone. Unicameral (single cavity) bone cysts occur in children and cause mild discomfort and possible pathologic fractures of the upper humerus and femur, which may heal spontaneously.

A painful tumour that occurs in children and young adults is the osteoid osteoma. The neoplastic tissue is surrounded by reactive bone formation that assists in its identification by x-ray.

Giant cell tumours (osteoclastomas) are benign for long periods but may invade local tissue and cause destruction. They occur in young adults and are soft and hemorrhagic. Eventually, giant cell tumours may undergo malignant transformation and metastasize.

MALIGNANT BONE TUMOURS

Primary malignant musculoskeletal tumours are relatively rare and arise from connective and supportive tissue cells (sarcomas) or bone marrow elements (multiple myeloma; see Chap. 33). Malignant primary musculoskeletal tumours include osteosarcoma, chondrosarcoma, Ewing's sarcoma, and fibrosarcoma. Soft tissue sarcomas include liposarcoma, fibrosarcoma of soft tissue, and rhabdomyosarcoma. Bone tumour metastasis to the lungs is common.

Osteogenic sarcoma (osteosarcoma) is the most common and most often fatal primary malignant bone tumour. Prognosis depends on whether the tumour has metastasized to the lungs at the time the patient seeks health care. Osteogenic sarcoma appears most frequently in males between the ages of 10 and 25 years (in bones that grow rapidly), in older people with Paget's disease, and as a result of radiation exposure. Clinical manifestations include pain, swelling, limited motion, and weight loss (which is considered an ominous finding). The bony mass may be palpable, tender, and fixed, with an increase in skin temperature over the mass and venous distention. The primary lesion may involve any bone, but the most common sites are the distal femur, the proximal tibia, and the proximal humerus.

Malignant tumours of the hyaline cartilage are called chondrosarcomas. These tumours are the second most common primary malignant bone tumour. They are large, bulky, slow-growing tumours that affect adults. The usual tumour sites include the pelvis, femur, humerus, spine, scapula, and tibia. Metastasis to the lungs occurs in fewer than half of patients. When these tumours are well differentiated, large bloc excision or amputation of the affected extremity results in increased survival rates. These tumours may recur.

METASTATIC BONE DISEASE

Metastatic bone disease (secondary bone tumour) is more common than any primary bone tumour. Tumours arising from tissues elsewhere in the body may invade the bone and produce localized bone destruction (lytic lesions) or bone overgrowth (blastic lesions). The most common primary sites of tumours that metastasize to bone are the kidney, prostate, lung, breast, ovary, and thyroid. Metastatic tumours most frequently attack the skull, spine, pelvis, femur, and humerus and involve more than one bone (polyostotic).

Pathophysiology

A tumour in the bone causes the normal bone tissue to react by osteolytic response (bone destruction) or osteoblastic response (bone formation). Primary tumours cause bone destruction, which weakens the bone, resulting in bone fractures. Adjacent normal bone responds to the tumour by altering its normal pattern of remodeling. The bone's surface changes, and the contours enlarge in the tumour area.

Malignant bone tumours invade and destroy adjacent bone tissue. Benign bone tumours, in contrast, have a symmetric, controlled growth pattern and place pressure on adjacent bone tissue. Malignant invading bone tumours weaken the structure of the bone until it can no longer withstand the stress of ordinary use; pathologic fracture commonly results.

Clinical Manifestations

Patients with metastatic bone tumour may have a wide range of associated clinical manifestations. They may be symptom free or have pain (mild and occasional to constant and severe), varying degrees of disability and, at times, obvious bone growth. Weight loss, malaise, and fever may be present. The tumour may be diagnosed only after pathologic fracture has occurred.

With spinal metastasis, spinal cord compression may occur. It can progress rapidly or slowly. Neurologic deficits (eg, progressive pain, weakness, gait abnormality, paresthesia, paraplegia, urinary retention, loss of bowel or bladder control) must be identified early and treated with decompressive laminectomy to prevent permanent spinal cord injury.

Assessment and Diagnostic Findings

The differential diagnosis is based on the history, physical examination, and diagnostic studies, including computed tomography, bone scans, myelography, arteriography, MRI, biopsy, and biochemical assays of the blood and urine. Serum alkaline phosphatase levels are frequently elevated with osteogenic sarcoma. With metastatic carcinoma of the prostate, serum acid phosphatase levels are elevated. Hypercalcemia is present with breast, lung, or kidney cancer bone metastases. Symptoms of hypercalcemia include muscle weakness, fatigue, anorexia, nausea, vomiting, polyuria, cardiac dysrhythmias, seizures, and coma. Hypercalcemia must be identified and treated promptly. Surgical biopsy is performed for histologic identification. Extreme care is taken during biopsy to prevent seeding and resultant recurrence after excision of the tumour.

Chest x-rays are performed to determine the presence of lung metastasis. Surgical staging of musculoskeletal tumours is based on tumour grade and site (intracompartmental or extracompartmental), as well as on metastasis. Staging is used for planning treatment.

During the diagnostic period, the nurse explains the diagnostic tests and provides psychological and emotional support to the patient and family. The nurse assesses coping behaviours and encourages use of support systems.

Medical Management

PRIMARY BONE TUMOURS

The goal of primary bone tumour treatment is to destroy or remove the tumour. This may be accomplished by surgical excision (ranging from local excision to amputation and disarticulation), radiation therapy if the tumour is radiosensitive, and chemotherapy (preoperative, intraoperative [neoadjuvant], postoperative, and adjunctive for possible micrometastases). Major gains are being made in the use of wide bloc excision with restorative grafting technique. Survival and quality of life are important considerations in procedures that attempt to save the involved extremity.

Limb-sparing (salvage) procedures are used to remove the tumour and adjacent tissue. A customized prosthesis, total joint arthroplasty, or bone tissue from the patient (autograft) or from a cadaver donor (allograft) replaces the resected tissue. Soft tissue and blood vessels may need grafting because of the extent of the excision. Complications may include infection, loosening or dislocation of the prosthesis, allograft nonunion, fracture, devitalization of the skin and soft tissues, joint fibrosis, and recurrence of the tumour. Function and rehabilitation after limb salvage depend on positive encouragement and reducing the risk for complications.

Surgical removal of the tumour may require amputation of the affected extremity, with the amputation extending well above the tumour to achieve local control of the primary lesion (see Nursing Process: The Patient Undergoing an Amputation in Chapter 69.)

Because of the danger of metastasis with malignant bone tumours, combined chemotherapy is started before and continued after surgery in an effort to eradicate micrometastatic lesions. The goal of combined chemotherapy is greater therapeutic effect at a lower toxicity rate with reduced resistance to the medications. There is an improved long-term survival rate when a localized osteosarcoma is removed and chemotherapy is initiated. Soft tissue sarcomas are treated with radiation, limb-sparing excision, and adjuvant chemotherapy (see Chap. 33).

METASTATIC BONE DISEASE

The treatment of metastatic bone cancer is palliative. The therapeutic goal is to relieve the patient's pain and discomfort while promoting quality of life.

If metastatic disease weakens the bone, structural support and stabilization are needed to prevent pathologic fracture. At times, large bones with metastatic lesions are strengthened by prophylactic internal fixation. Internal fixation of pathologic fractures, arthroplasty, or methylmethacrylate (bone cement) reconstruction minimizes associated disability and pain. Patients with metastatic disease are at higher risk for pulmonary congestion, hypoxemia, deep vein thrombosis, and hemorrhage than are other patients after orthopedic surgery.

Hypercalcemia results from breakdown of bone. It needs to be recognized promptly. Treatment includes hydration with IV administration of normal saline solution, diuresis, mobilization, and medications such as bisphosphonates, pamidronate, and calcitonin. Because inactivity leads to loss of bone mass and increased calcium in the blood, the nurse assists the patient to increase activity and ambulation.

Hematopoiesis is frequently disrupted by tumour invasion of the bone marrow or by treatment (chemotherapy or radiation). Blood product transfusions restore hematologic factors. Pain can result from multiple factors, including the osseous metastasis, surgery, chemotherapy or radiation side effects, and arthritis. Pain must be assessed accurately and managed with adequate and appropriate opioid, nonopioid, and nonpharmaceutical interventions. External beam radiation to involved metastasis sites may be used. Patients with multiple bony metastases may achieve pain control with systemically administered "bone-seeking" isotopes (eg, strontium 89). See Chapter 13 for more information about pain management.

Additional therapies are used to treat the original cancer. Radiation and hormonal therapy may be effective in promoting healing of osteolytic lesions. Chemotherapy is used to control the primary disease (see Chap. 33).

NURSING PROCESS:
THE PATIENT WITH A BONE TUMOUR

Assessment

The nurse asks the patient about the onset and course of symptoms. During the interview, the nurse notes the patient's understanding of the disease process, how the patient and the family

have been coping, and how the patient has managed the pain. On physical examination, the nurse gently palpates the mass and notes its size and associated soft tissue swelling, pain, and tenderness. Assessment of the neurovascular status and range of motion of the extremity provides baseline data for future comparisons. The nurse evaluates the patient's mobility and ability to perform ADLs.

Diagnosis

NURSING DIAGNOSES

Based on the nursing assessment data, the major nursing diagnoses for the patient with a bone tumour may include the following:

- Deficient knowledge related to the disease process and the therapeutic regimen
- Acute and chronic pain related to pathologic process and surgery
- Risk for injury: pathologic fracture related to tumour and metastasis
- Ineffective coping related to fear of the unknown, perception of disease process, and inadequate support system
- Risk for situational low self-esteem related to loss of body part or alteration in role performance

COLLABORATIVE PROBLEMS/
POTENTIAL COMPLICATIONS

Potential complications may include the following:

- Delayed wound healing
- Nutritional deficiency
- Infection
- Hypercalcemia

Planning and Goals

The major goals for the patient include knowledge of the disease process and treatment regimen, control of pain, absence of pathologic fractures, effective patterns of coping, improved self-esteem, and absence of complications.

Nursing Interventions

The nursing care of a patient who has undergone excision of a bone tumour is similar in many respects to that of other patients who have had skeletal surgery. Vital signs are monitored; blood loss is assessed; and observations are made to assess for the development of complications such as deep vein thrombosis, pulmonary emboli, infection, contracture, and disuse atrophy. The affected part is elevated to control swelling, and the neurovascular status of the extremity is assessed.

PROMOTING UNDERSTANDING OF THE DISEASE
PROCESS AND TREATMENT REGIMEN

Patient and family teaching about the disease process and diagnostic and management regimens is essential. Explanation of diagnostic tests, treatments (eg, wound care), and expected results (eg, decreased range of motion, numbness, change of body contours) helps the patient deal with the procedures and changes. Cooperation and adherence to the therapeutic regimen are enhanced through understanding. The nurse can most effectively reinforce and clarify information provided by the physician by being present during these discussions.

PROFILE 68-2

Patients' Perceptions of Bone Pain and Pain Control

Coward, D., and Wilkie, D. (2000). Metastatic bone pain: Meanings associated with self-report and self-management decision making. *Cancer Nursing, 23,* 101–108.

Purpose

Patients with cancer and bone metastases experience severe pain, especially when moving. Cancer pain is conceptualized as multidimensional: physiologic, sensory, affective, behavioural, and cognitive. This descriptive study examined the meanings of pain experiences as well as self-disclosure and self-management of pain in both men and women. The study goals were (1) to identify thoughts, feelings, and perceptions reported by patients experiencing metastatic bone pain, (2) to identify methods patients used to tell others about the pain, (3) to describe the process patients used to decide whether to take analgesics, and (4) to describe possible gender-related differences in pain experiences.

Study Sample and Design

A convenience sample consisted of 10 women and 10 men who had pain and objective evidence of bone metastasis. Most of the patients had metastases to the spine and had undergone surgery, chemotherapy, or radiation as cancer treatments before participating in the study.

Data were collected during audiotaped interviews. Interview questions were used to identify the patient's pain-related beliefs, feelings, and actions. The study participants also completed a McGill Pain Questionnaire, a visual analog scale of pain intensity, and a demographic form.

Transcribed tapes were analyzed for themes, and the narrative data were organized into descriptions of the participants' thoughts and feelings about their pain, the impact of pain on their lives, how they disclosed their pain to others, and how they decided to take analgesics.

Results

Participants' reported thoughts and feelings about pain included possible injury, recurrence of cancer, progression of cancer, ineffectiveness of cancer treatments, fright and uncertainty about whether the cancer could be controlled, and the need to work harder to fight the cancer.

Pain interfered with participants' activities, including activities of daily living, work/housework, and pleasure activities. Also, pain interfered with family relationships, causing the participants to be irritable with family members or to isolate themselves from the family.

Most of the participants (7 women and 5 men) preferred not to tell others about their pain because they did not want to disappoint or worry others. Women sought normalcy. Men did not want to complain or saw no purpose in telling others. Those who disclosed their pain (3 women and 5 men) wanted to be honest with their friends and thought it would help health professionals to manage their pain. Only 3 women and 6 men took analgesics on the recommended schedule. Many delayed taking analgesics because the pain reminded them to protect the hurting part and kept them from overexertion. Side effects (eg, gastrointestinal distress, feeling out of control) were a concern for some of the participants (4 women and 5 men). Another reason given for not taking analgesics was to see whether the cancer treatment was working. The sample was too small to draw any conclusions about gender-related differences in pain experiences.

Nursing Implications

Pain means different things to different patients. Nurses need to engage patients with cancer in discussion of their pain and pain management. Disclosure of the characteristics of pain experiences would facilitate development of individualized, effective pain management strategies. If pain is associated with movement, pain management interventions need to be used to encourage movement and participation in activities of daily living and socialization. Alternative activities that bring the patient pleasure can be devised when pain or fear of fracture causes the patient to give up previously pleasurable activities.

For various reasons, a patient may not take analgesics on the recommended schedule; these reasons should be explored by the nurse. If side effects of analgesics are reported, they can be minimized. The nurse needs to discuss with the patient the physiologic benefits of controlling pain.

RELIEVING PAIN

Accurate pain assessment is the foundation for pain management. Pharmacologic and nonpharmacologic pain management techniques are used to relieve pain and increase the patient's comfort level. The nurse works with the patient in designing the most effective pain management regimen, thereby increasing the patient's control over the pain. The nurse prepares the patient and gives support during painful procedures. Prescribed IV or epidural analgesics are used during the early postoperative period. Later, oral or transdermal opioid or nonopioid analgesics are usually adequate to relieve pain. In addition, external radiation or systemic radioisotopes may be used to control pain (see Chapter 13 for further discussion of pain management).

PREVENTING PATHOLOGIC FRACTURE

Bone tumours weaken the bone to a point at which normal activities or even position changes can result in fracture. During nursing care, the affected extremities must be supported and handled gently. External supports (eg, splints) may be used for additional protection. At times, the patient may elect to have surgery (eg, open reduction with internal fixation, joint replacement) in an attempt to prevent pathologic fracture. Prescribed weight-bearing restrictions must be followed. The nurse teaches the patient how to use assistive devices safely and how to strengthen unaffected extremities.

PROMOTING COPING SKILLS

The nurse encourages the patient and family to verbalize their fears, concerns, and feelings. They need to be supported as they deal with the impact of the malignant bone tumour. Feelings of shock, despair, and grief are expected. Referral to a psychiatric nurse liaison, psychologist, counsellor, or spiritual advisor may be indicated for specific psychological help and emotional support.

PROMOTING SELF-ESTEEM

Independence versus dependence is an issue for the patient who has a malignancy. Lifestyle is dramatically changed, at least temporarily. It is important to support the family in working through the adjustments that must be made. The nurse assists the patient in dealing with changes in body image due to surgery and possible amputation. It is helpful to provide realistic reassurance about the future and resumption of role-related activities and to encourage self-care and socialization. The patient participates in planning daily activities. The nurse encourages the patient to be as independent as possible. Involvement of the patient and family throughout treatment encourages confidence, restoration of self-concept, and a sense of being in control of one's life.

MONITORING AND MANAGING POTENTIAL COMPLICATIONS

Delayed Wound Healing

Wound healing may be delayed because of tissue trauma from surgery, previous radiation therapy, inadequate nutrition, or infection. The nurse minimizes pressure on the wound site to promote circulation to the tissues. An aseptic, nontraumatic wound dressing promotes healing. Monitoring and reporting of laboratory findings facilitate initiation of interventions to promote homeostasis and wound healing.

Repositioning the patient at frequent intervals reduces the incidence of skin breakdown due to pressure. Special therapeutic beds may be needed to prevent skin breakdown and to promote wound healing after extensive surgical reconstruction and skin grafting.

Inadequate Nutrition

Because loss of appetite, nausea, and vomiting are frequent side effects of chemotherapy and radiation therapy, it is necessary to provide adequate nutrition for healing and health promotion. Antiemetics and relaxation techniques reduce the gastrointestinal reaction. Stomatitis is controlled with anesthetic or antifungal mouthwash (see Chap. 33). Adequate hydration is essential. Nutritional supplements or total parenteral nutrition may be prescribed to achieve adequate nutrition.

Osteomyelitis and Wound Infections

Prophylactic antibiotics and strict aseptic dressing techniques are used to diminish the occurrence of osteomyelitis and wound infections. During healing, other infections (eg, upper respiratory infections) need to be prevented so that hematogenous spread does not result in osteomyelitis. If the patient is receiving chemotherapy, it is important to monitor the white blood cell count and to instruct the patient to avoid contact with people who have colds or other infections.

Hypercalcemia

Hypercalcemia is a dangerous complication of bone cancer. The symptoms must be recognized and treatment initiated promptly. Symptoms include muscular weakness, incoordination, anorexia, nausea and vomiting, constipation, electrocardiographic changes (eg, shortened QT interval and ST segment, bradycardia, heart blocks), and altered mental states (eg, confusion, lethargy, psychotic behaviour). See Chapter 14 for a full discussion of hypercalcemia and its management.

PROMOTING HOME AND COMMUNITY-BASED CARE

Teaching Patients Self-Care

Preparation for and coordination of continuing health care are begun early as a multidisciplinary effort. Patient teaching addresses medication, dressing, treatment regimens, and the importance of physical and occupational therapy programs. The nurse teaches weight-bearing limitations and special handling to prevent pathologic fractures. It is important that the patient and family know the signs and symptoms of possible complications as well as resources available for continuing care (Chart 68-10).

Continuing Care

Frequently, arrangements are made with a home health care agency for home care supervision and follow-up. The home care nurse assesses the patient's and family's abilities to meet the patient's needs and determines whether the services of other agencies are needed. The nurse advises the patient to have readily available the telephone numbers of people to contact in case concerns arise.

The nurse emphasizes the need for long-term health supervision to ensure cure or to detect tumour recurrence or metastasis. If the patient has metastatic disease, end-of-life issues may need to be explored. Referral for hospice care is made if appropriate.

Evaluation

EXPECTED PATIENT OUTCOMES

Expected patient outcomes may include:

1. Describes disease process and treatment regimen
   a. Describes pathologic condition
   b. States goals of the therapeutic regimen
   c. Seeks clarification of information
2. Achieves control of pain
   a. Uses multiple pain control techniques, including prescribed medications

---

Chart 68-10
Home Care Checklist • Bone Tumour

At the completion of the home care instruction, the patient or caregiver will be able to:	Patient	Caregiver
• Describe tumour process	✓	✓
• Control pain with pharmacologic and nonpharmacologic interventions	✓	✓
• Support affected musculoskeletal area	✓	
• Describe use of prescribed medications	✓	✓
• Comply with medication regimen	✓	✓
• Consume diet to promote healing and health	✓	
• State weight-bearing and activity restrictions	✓	✓
• Demonstrate safe use of ambulatory aids and assistive devices	✓	✓
• Protect affected bone from pathologic fracture	✓	✓
• Identify complications of tumour and therapy	✓	✓
• Report signs and symptoms of complications promptly	✓	✓
• Use effective coping strategies	✓	
• Maintain role performance	✓	✓

b. Experiences no pain or decreased pain at rest, during ADLs, or at surgical sites
3. Experiences no pathologic fracture
   a. Avoids stress to weakened bones
   b. Uses assistive devices safely and appropriately
   c. Strengthens uninvolved extremities with exercise
4. Demonstrates effective coping patterns
   a. Verbalizes feelings
   b. Identifies strengths and abilities
   c. Makes decisions
   d. Requests assistance as needed
5. Demonstrates positive self-concept
   a. Identifies home and family responsibilities that can be accomplished
   b. Exhibits confidence in own abilities
   c. Demonstrates acceptance of altered body image
   d. Demonstrates independence in ADLs
6. Exhibits absence of complications
   a. Demonstrates wound healing
   b. Experiences no skin breakdown
   c. Maintains or increases body weight
   d. Experiences no infections
   e. Does not experience hypercalcemia
   f. Manages side effects of therapies
   g. Reports symptoms of medication toxicity or complications
7. Participates in continuing health care at home
   a. Complies with prescribed regimen (ie, takes prescribed medications, continues physical and occupational therapy programs)
   b. Acknowledges need for long-term health supervision
   c. Keeps follow-up health care appointments
   d. Reports occurrence of symptoms or complications

Critical Thinking Exercises

1. A neighbour, who is a preschool teacher, tells you that she is experiencing low back pain and finds that she is having difficulty working. She asks you for your advice. Describe how you would assess this situation. What information are you seeking? Explain why you need this specific information. How would your critical thinking be redirected if the woman was also pregnant or overweight and postmenopausal? What initial advice would you give her?

2. You are a nurse in an orthopedic clinic. A patient, who is a data entry clerk, will be having same-day carpal tunnel release surgery. What information regarding postoperative care will you include in your preoperative patient education? The patient asks you about returning to work and asks how she can prevent this problem from recurring. What information would you share with her? What is the rationale for this information?

3. Your 18-year-old niece is visiting you for several weeks prior to entering college. Your mother, her grandmother, is suffering from spinal fractures and has experienced a Colles' fracture. You observe your niece's life-style and nutritional habits. What factors would alert you to behaviours which put your niece at risk for the development of osteoporosis? What suggestions would you make to her to optimize her bone density and prevent osteoporosis?

4. A friend has breast cancer. She shares with you that she is experiencing pain in her hips and that the doctors have determined that she has bone metastasis. She asks you if this means that she has a new type of cancer. What additional assessment data would you gather before responding? She asks you how this bony metastasis will affect her. What factors would you consider before responding? What strategies would you discuss with her to (1) control pain, (2) prevent pathologic fracture, (3) promote coping, and (4) promote self-esteem?

REFERENCES AND SELECTED READINGS

Books

Bigos, S., et al. (1994, December). *Acute low back problems in adults: Clinical practice guidelines—Quick reference guide number 14*. (AHCPR Pub. No. 95-0643.) Rockville, MD: U.S. Department of Health and Human Services, Public Health Service, Agency for Health Care Policy and Research.

Bullock, B., & Henze, R. (2000). *Focus on pathophysiology*. Philadelphia: Lippincott Williams & Wilkins.

Childs, S. (Ed.). (1999). *The upper extremity: Traumatic injuries and conditions*. Pitman, NJ: National Association of Orthopaedic Nurses.

Health Canada. (2003). *Arthritis in Canada. An ongoing challenge*. Ottawa: Author.

Kleerekoper, M., et al. (1999). *The bone and mineral manual*. San Diego: Academic Press.

Koopman, W. (Ed.). (2001). *Arthritis and allied conditions* (14th ed.). Philadelphia: Lippincott Williams & Wilkins.

Levesque, J., et al. (1998). *A clinical guide to primary bone tumors*. Baltimore: Williams & Wilkins.

Maher, A., et al. (2003). *Orthopaedic nursing* (3rd ed.). Philadelphia: W. B. Saunders.

Mercier, L. (2000). *Practical orthopedics* (5th ed.). St. Louis: Mosby.

Miaskowski, C., & Buchsel, P. (1999). *Oncology nursing: Assessment and clinical care*. St. Louis: Mosby.

National Institutes of Health. (2000). *Osteoporosis prevention, diagnosis, and therapy: NIH Consensus Statement Online, 17*, 1–36.

National Osteoporosis Foundation. (2000). *Medications and bone loss*. Washington, DC: National Osteoporosis Foundation.

National Osteoporosis Foundation. (2001). *Osteoporosis*. Available at: www.nof.org/osteoporosis/index.htm.

National Osteoporosis Foundation. (1997). *1996 and 2015 osteoporosis prevalence figures: State by state prevalence report*. Washington, DC: National Osteoporosis Foundation.

Osteoporosis Canada. (2005). *About osteoporosis*. Available at: http://www.osteoporosis.ca/english/about%20osteoporosis/default.asp?s=1. Retrieved November 30, 2005.

Praemer, A., et al. (1999). *Musculoskeletal conditions in the United States*. Rosemont, IL: American Academy of Orthopaedic Surgeons.

Rosen, C., et al. (1999). *The aging skeleton*. San Diego: Academic Press.

Rubin, E., & Farber, I. L. (1999). *Pathology* (3rd ed.). Philadelphia: Lippincott Williams & Wilkins.

Schoen, D. C. (Ed.). (2001). NAON *Core curriculum for orthopaedic nursing* (4th ed.). Pitman, NJ: National Association of Orthopaedic Nurses.

Salter, R. (1999). *Textbook of disorders and injuries of the musculoskeletal system* (3rd ed.). Baltimore: Williams & Wilkins.

Schoen, D. (2000). *Adult orthopaedic nursing*. Philadelphia: Lippincott Williams & Wilkins.

Steinberg, G., et al. (Eds.). (1999). *Orthopaedics in primary care* (3rd ed.). Philadelphia: Lippincott Williams & Wilkins.

Yarbro, C., et al. (2000). *Cancer nursing: Principles and practice*s (5th ed.). Boston: Jones & Bartlett Publishers.

Journals

Asterisks indicate nursing research articles.

Adachi, J.D., et al. (1997). Salmon calcitonin nasal spray in the prevention of corticosteroid-induced osteoporosis. *British Journal of Rheumatology, 36*, 255-259.

Amin, S., & Felson, D. (2001) Osteoporosis in men. *Rheumatic Diseases Clinics of North America, 27*(1), 19–40.

Barnett, M. (1999). Hypercalcemia. *Seminar in Oncology Nursing, 15*(3), 190–201.

Barr, J., et al. (2000). Percutaneous vertebroplasty for pain relief and spinal stabilization. *Spine, 25*(8), 923–928.

Brown, J., & Josse, R. G. (2002). Clinical practice guidelines for the diagnosis and management of osteoporosis in Canada. *Canadian Medical Association Journal, 167*(Suppl. 10). S1–S34.

Bryant, J., & Beinlich, N. (1999). Foot care: Focus on the elderly. *Orthopaedic Nursing, 18*(6), 53–60.

Canadian Task Force on Preventive Health Care. (2004). Prevention of osteoporosis and osteoporotic fractures in postmenopausal women. *Canadian Medical Association Journal, 170*(11), 1665–1667.

Chan, K., et al. (2000). Inhibitors of hydoxymethylglutaryl-coenzyme A reductase and risk of fracture among older women. *Lancet, 355*(9222), 2185–2188.

Chen, C. L., Weiss, N. S., Newcome, P., Barlow, W., & White, E. (2002). Hormone replacement therapy in relation to breast cancer. *Journal of the American Medical Association, 287*(6), 734–741.

Chestnut, C. H., et al. (2000). A randomized trial of nasal spray salmon calcitonin in postmenopausal women with established osteoporosis: The prevent recurrence of osteoporotic fractures study. *American Journal of Medicine, 109*, 267–276.

Chrischilles, E. A., Butler, C. D., Davis, C.S., et al. (1991). A model of lifetime osteoporosis impact. *Archives of Internal Medicine, 151,* 2026–2032.

*Cortet, B., et al. (1999). Percutaneous vertebroplasty in the treatment of osteoporotic vertebral compression fractures: An open prospective study. *Journal of Rheumatology, 26*(10), 2222–2228.

*Coward, D., & Wilkie, D. (2000). Metastatic bone pain: Meanings associated with self-report and self-management decision making. *Cancer Nursing, 23*(2), 101–108.

Cummings, S. R., Black, D. M., & Rubin, S.M. (1989). Lifetime risks of hip, Colles', or vertebral fracture and coronary heart disease among white postmenopausal women. *Archives of Internal Medicine, 149,* 2445–2448.

Dargent-Molina, P., et al. (1996). Fall-related factors and risk of hip fracture: The EPIDOS prospective study [published erratum appears in Lancet, 1996, 348–416]. *Lancet, 348,* 145–149.

Dowd, R., & Cavalieri, R. (1999). Help your patient live with osteoporosis. *American Journal of Nursing, 99*(4), 55–60.

Downs, R. W. Jr., et al. (2000). Comparison of alendronate and intranasal calcitonin for treatment of osteoporosis in postmenopausal women. *Journal of Clinical Endocrinology and Metabolism, 85*, 1783–1788.

Dubost, J., et al. (2000). Pyogenic arthritis in adults. *Joint, Bone, and Spine, 67*(1), 11–21.

Glaser, V., et al. (1999). Osteoarthritis, shoulder impingement, cervical radiculopathy, plantar fasciitis. *Patient Care, 33*(12), 176–202.

Genant, H., et al. (1997). Osteoporosis: A treatment approach to long-term care patients. *Nursing Home Medicine, 5,* (Suppl. G), 1G–24G.

Hall, J., & Riley, R. (1999). Nutritional strategies to reduce the risk of osteoporosis. *MedSurg Nursing, 8*(5), 281–293.

Hamel, M. E., Sebaldt, R. J., Siminoski, K., et al. (2005). Influence of fracture history and bone mineral density testing on the treatment of osteoporosis in two nonacademic community centers. *Osteoporosis International, 16*, 208–215.

Heller, H., et al. (1999). Pharmacokinetics of calcium absorption from two commercial calcium supplements. *Journal of Clinical Pharmacology, 39*(11), 1151–1159.

Holick, M. F. (1998). *How much vitamin D is enough?* Available at: http://www.mcmaster.ca/inabis98/atkinson/holick0835/two.html.

Kannus, P., et al. (2000). Prevention of hip fracture in elderly people with use of a hip protector. *New England Journal of Medicine, 343*(21), 1506–1513.

Keen, S., et al. (1999). Individuals with low back pain: How do they view physical activity? *Family Practice, 16*(1), 39–45.

Khan, S. A., de Geus, C., Holroyd, B., et al. (2001). Osteoporosis follow-up after wrist fractures following minor trauma. *Archives of Internal Medicine, 161*, 1309–1312.

Konlian, C. (1999). Aquatic therapy: Making a wave in the treatment of low back injuries. *Orthopaedic Nursing, 18*(1), 11–18.

Kotaniemi, A., et al. (1996). Is continuous intranasal salmon calcitonin effective in treating axial bone loss in patients with active rheumatoid arthritis receiving low dose glucocorticoid therapy? *Journal of Rheumatology, 23*, 1875–1879.

Lane, N. (Ed.). (2001). Osteoporosis. *Rheumatic Diseases Clinics of North America, 27*(1), 1–262.

Lyritis, G.P., et al. (1997). Pain relief from nasal salmon calcitonin in osteoporotic vertebral crush fractures: A double blind, placebo-controlled clinical study. *Acta Orthopaedica Scandinavica. Supplementum, 68*, 112–114.

Mader, J., et al. (2000). Bone and joint infections in the elderly: Practical treatment guidelines. *Drugs and Aging, 16*(1), 67–80.

Marchigiano, G. (1999). Calcium intake in midlife women: One step in preventing osteoporosis. *Orthopaedic Nursing, 18*(5), 11–18.

Melton, L. J., III, Atkinson, E.J., O'Connor, M.K., et al. (1998). Bone density and fracture risk in men. *Journal of Bone and Mineral Research, 13*, 1915–1923.

Neer, R., et al. (2001). Effect of parathyroid hormone (1-34) on fractures and bone mineral density in postmenopausal women with osteoporosis. *New England Journal of Medicine, 344*(19), 1434–1441.

Osteoporosis prevention, diagnosis, and therapy (Consensus Conference). (2001). *Journal of the American Medical Association, 285*(6), 785–794.

Papadimitropoulos, E. A., Coyte, P. C., Josse, R. G., et al. (1997). Current and projected rates of hip fracture in Canada. *Canadian Medical Association Journal, 157*(10), 1357–1363.

Perry, C. (1999). Septic arthritis. *American Journal of Orthopedics, 28*(3), 168–178.

*Reavis, C. (1999). Back injury in primary care: Three sides of the coin. *Nurse Practitioner Forum, 10*(4), 208–212.

Reginato, A., et al. (1999). Musculoskeletal manifestations of osteomalacia. *Seminars in Arthritis and Rheumatism, 28*(5), 287–304.

Robertson, M. C., Devlin, N., Gardner, M. M., et al. (2001). Effectiveness and economic evaluation of a nurse delivered home exercise program to prevent falls. 1: Randomized controlled trial. *British Medical Journal, 322*, 697–701.

Rosen, C. J. (2003). Restoring aging bones. *Scientific American, 288*(3), 71–73.

Rosen, C., & Rackoff, P. (2001). Emerging anabolic treatments for osteoporosis. *Rheumatic Diseases Clinics of North America, 27*(1), 215–234.

*Sedlak, C., et al. (2000). Osteoporosis in older men: Knowledge and health beliefs. *Orthopaedic Nursing, 19*(5), 38–42, 44–46.

*Smeltzer, S. C., Zimmerman, V., Capriotti, T., Fernandes, L. (2002). Osteoporosis risk and bone density screening in women with multiple sclerosis. *International Journal of MS Care, 4*(1):17–23, 29.

Sullivan, M., & Sharts-Hopko, N. (2000). Preventing the downward spiral: Osteoporosis and multiple sclerosis. *American Journal of Nursing, 100*(8), 26–32.

Taft, L., et al. (2000). Osteoporosis: A disease management opportunity. *Orthopaedic Nursing, 19*(2), 67–76.

Tremethick, M., & Wallace, D. (1999). Interdisciplinary teamwork for hip fracture prevention. *Geriatric Nursing, 20*(6), 293–296.

Turner, L., et al. (1999). Osteoporosis diagnosis and fracture. *Orthopaedic Nursing, 18*(5), 21–27.

Walker-Bone, K., et al. (2001). Epidemiology of osteoporosis. *Rheumatic Diseases Clinics of North America, 27*(1), 1–18.

Wang, P., et al. (2000). HMG-CoA reductase inhibitors and the risk of hip fractures in elderly patients. *Journal of the American Medical Association, 283*(24), 3211–3216.

Ward, W., & Peabody, T. (Eds.). (2000). Orthopedic management of metastatic disease [Special issue]. *Orthopedic Clinics of North America, 31(4)*.

RESOURCES AND WEBSITES

American Cancer Society, 1599 Clifton Road NE, Atlanta, GA 30329; 1-800-ACS-2345; http://www.cancer.org.

Arthritis Foundation, P.O. Box 7669, Atlanta, GA 30309; 1-800-283-7800; http://www.arthritis.org.

Canadian Cancer Society, National Office, Suite 200, 10 Alcorn Avenue, Toronto, ON M1V 3B1; 1-416-961-7223; fax: 1-416-961-4189; www.cancer.ca.

Canadian Institutes of Health Research: Institute of Musculoskeletal Health and Arthritis, 160 Elgin Street, 9th floor, 4809A, Ottawa, ON K1A 0W9; http://www.cihr-irsc.gc.ca/e/13217.html.

Canadian Orthopaedic Association, 1440 St. Catherine Street West, Suite 718, Montreal, QC H3G 1R8; 514-874-9003; www.coa-aco.org.

Canadian Orthopaedic Foundation, PO Box 7029, Innisfail, ON L9S 1A8; 416-410-2341; www.canorth.org.

Canadian Rheumatology Association, 912 Tegal Place, Newmarket, ON L3X 1L3; 1-905-952-0698 www.cra-scr.ca.

National Institute of Arthritis and Musculoskeletal and Skin Diseases, Information Clearing House, National Institutes of Health, 1 AMS Circle, Bethesda, MD 20892-3675; 1-877-22-NIAMS (toll free); 1-301-495-4484.

National Institute of Arthritis and Musculoskeletal and Skin Diseases, Office of Communications and Public Liaison, Bldg. 31/Rm.4C05, 31 Center Drive, MSC 2350, Bethesda, MD 20892-2350; 1-301-496-8190; http://www.nih.gov/niams.

National Osteoporosis Foundation, 1232 22nd Street, Washington, DC 20037-1297; 202-223-2226; http://www.nof.org.

Osteoporosis Canada, 1090 Don Mills Road, Suite 301, Toronto, ON M3C 3R6; 416-696-2663; www.osteoporosis.ca.

The Canadian Arthritis Society, Manitoba Division Office, 105-386 Broadway, Winnipeg, MN R3C 3R6; general arthritis help line: 1-800-321-1433; www.arthritis.ca.

The Paget Foundation, 120 Wall Street, Suite 1602, New York, NY 10005; 212-509-5335; http://www.paget.org; PagetFdn@aol.com.

Therapeutic Products Directorate, Health Canada, Holland Cross, Tower B, 1600 Scott Street, 6th floor, AL 3106B, Ottawa, ON K1A 1B6; 1-613-941-0839; drugs product database: http://www.hc-sc.gc.ca/hpfb-dgpsa/tpd-dpt/dpd_index_e.html; approval of Foreo for osteoporosis. http://www.Hc-sc.gc.ca/drug2/product/p73983.html.

Management of Patients With Musculoskeletal Trauma

Adapted by Bonnie Friesen and Linda Larsen

LEARNING OBJECTIVES

On completion of this chapter, the learner will be able to:

1. Differentiate between contusions, strains, sprains, and dislocations.
2. Describe selected sports injuries and their nursing management.
3. Specify the clinical manifestations of a fracture and the emergency management of the patient with a fracture.
4. Describe the principles and methods of fracture reduction, fracture immobilization, and management of open fractures.
5. Use the nursing process as a framework for care of the patient with a simple fracture.
6. Describe the prevention and management of immediate and delayed complications of fractures.
7. Describe the rehabilitative needs of patients with fractures of the clavicle, upper and lower extremities, pelvis, hips, ribs, and thoracolumbar spine.
8. Use the nursing process as a framework for care of the elderly patient with fracture of the hip.
9. Describe the rehabilitative and health education needs of the patient who has had an amputation.
10. Use the nursing process as a framework for care of the patient with an amputation.

*I*njury to one part of the musculoskeletal system usually results in injury or dysfunction of adjacent structures and of structures enclosed or supported by them. If the bone is broken, the muscles cannot function, and blood vessels and nerves in the vicinity of the fracture may be injured. If the nerves do not send impulses to the muscles, as in paralysis, the bones cannot move. If the joint surfaces do not articulate normally, neither the bones nor the muscles can function properly.

Treatment of injury of the musculoskeletal system involves providing support to the injured part until healing is complete. Support may be provided by externally applied bandages, adhesive strapping, splints, or casts. Alternatively, support may be applied directly to the bone in the form of pins or plates. At times, traction must be applied to correct deformity or shortening.

After the immediate and the painful effects of the injury have passed, treatment efforts are focused on preventing fibrosis and stiffness in the injured muscles and joint structures. Proper exercise guards against this disability. In some cases, the support applied permits early activity. Various forms of physical and occupational therapy may hasten the healing process and recovery of function.

Contusions, Strains, and Sprains

A *contusion* is a soft tissue injury produced by blunt force, such as a blow, kick, or fall. Many small blood vessels rupture and bleed into soft tissues (ecchymosis, or bruising). A hematoma develops when the bleeding is sufficient to cause an appreciable collection of blood. Local symptoms (pain, swelling, and discolouration) are controlled with intermittent application of cold. Most contusions resolve in 1 to 2 weeks.

A **strain** is a "muscle pull" caused by overuse, overstretching, or excessive stress. Strains are microscopic, incomplete muscle tears with some bleeding into the tissue. The patient experiences soreness or sudden pain, with local tenderness on muscle use and isometric contraction.

A **sprain** is an injury to the ligaments surrounding a joint that is caused by a wrenching or twisting motion. The function of a ligament is to maintain stability while permitting mobility. A torn ligament loses its stabilizing ability. Blood vessels rupture and edema occurs; the joint is tender, and movement of the joint becomes painful. The degree of disability and pain increases during the first 2 to 3 hours after the injury because of the associated swelling and bleeding. An x-ray should be obtained to rule out bone injury. Avulsion fracture (in which a bone fragment is pulled away by a ligament or tendon) may be associated with a sprain.

Management

Treatment of contusions, strains, and sprains consists of resting and elevating the affected part, applying cold, and using a compression bandage. (The acronym **RICE**—*R*est, *I*ce, *C*ompression, *E*levation—is helpful for remembering treatment interventions.) Rest prevents additional injury and promotes healing. Moist or dry cold applied intermittently for 20 to 30 minutes during the first 24 to 48 hours after injury produces vasoconstriction, which decreases bleeding, edema, and discomfort. Care must be taken to avoid skin and tissue damage from excessive cold. An elastic compression bandage controls bleeding, reduces edema, and provides support for the injured tissues. Elevation controls the swelling. If the sprain is severe (torn muscle fibres and disrupted ligaments), surgical repair or cast immobilization may be necessary so that the joint will not lose its stability. The neurovascular status (circulation, motion, sensation) of the injured extremity is monitored frequently.

After the acute inflammatory stage (eg, 24 to 48 hours after injury), heat may be applied intermittently (for 15 to 30 minutes, four times a day) to relieve muscle spasm and to promote vasodilation, absorption, and repair. Depending on the severity of injury, progressive passive and active exercises may begin in 2 to 5 days. Severe sprains may require 1 to 3 weeks of immobilization before protected exercises are initiated. Excessive exercise early in the course of treatment delays recovery. Strains and sprains take weeks or months to heal. Splinting may be used to prevent reinjury.

Joint Dislocations

A dislocation of a joint is a condition in which the articular surfaces of the bones forming the joint are no longer in anatomic contact. The bones are literally "out of joint." A **subluxation** is a partial dislocation of the articulating surfaces. Traumatic dislocations are orthopedic emergencies because the associated joint structures, blood supply, and nerves are distorted and severely stressed. If the dislocation is not treated promptly, *avascular necrosis* (tissue death due to anoxia and diminished blood supply) and nerve palsy may occur.

Dislocations may be congenital, or present at birth (most often the hip); spontaneous or pathologic, caused by disease of the

Glossary

allograft: tissue harvested from a donor for use in another person

amputation: removal of a body part, usually a limb or part of a limb

arthroscope: surgical instrument used to examine internal joint structures

autograft: tissue harvested from one area of the body and used for transplantation to another area of the body

débridement: surgical removal of contaminated and devitalized tissues and foreign material

dislocation: separation of joint surfaces

fracture: a break in the continuity of a bone

fracture reduction: restoration of fracture fragments into anatomic alignment and rotation

malunion: healing of a fractured bone in a malaligned position

meniscus: crescent-shaped fibrocartilage found in certain joints, such as the knee joint

nonunion: failure of fragments of a fractured bone to heal together

phantom limb pain: pain perceived as being in the amputated limb

RICE: acronym for *R*est, *I*ce, *C*ompression, *E*levation

rotator cuff: shoulder muscles (supraspinatus, subscapularis, infraspinatus, and teres minor) and their tendons

sprain: an injury to ligaments and other soft tissues at a joint

strain: a muscle pull or tear

subluxation: partial separation or dislocation of joint surfaces

tendinitis: inflammation of a tendon

articular or periarticular structures; or traumatic, resulting from injury in which the joint is disrupted by force.

Signs and symptoms of a traumatic dislocation are pain, change in contour of the joint, change in the length of the extremity, loss of normal mobility, and change in the axis of the dislocated bones. X-rays confirm the diagnosis and demonstrate any associated fracture.

Medical Management

The affected joint needs to be immobilized while the patient is transported to the hospital. The dislocation is promptly reduced (ie, displaced parts are brought into normal position) to preserve joint function. Analgesia, muscle relaxants, and possibly anesthesia are used to facilitate closed reduction. The joint is immobilized by bandages, splints, casts, or traction and is maintained in a stable position. Neurovascular status is monitored. After reduction, if the joint is stable, gentle, progressive, active and passive movement is begun to preserve range of motion (ROM) and restore strength. The joint is supported between exercise sessions.

Nursing Management

Nursing care is directed at providing comfort, evaluating the patient's neurovascular status, and protecting the joint during healing. The nurse teaches the patient how to manage the immobilizing devices and how to protect the joint from reinjury.

Sports-Related Injuries

Many people participate in recreational sports. These recreational athletes may push themselves beyond the level of their physical conditioning and incur injuries. Injuries to the musculoskeletal system may be acute (eg, sprains, strains, dislocations, fractures), or they may be gradual, resulting from overuse (eg, chondromalacia patella, tendinitis, stress fractures). Professional athletes are also susceptible to injury, even though their training is supervised closely to minimize the occurrence of injury.

- Contusions result from direct falls or blows. The initial dull pain becomes greater, with edema and stiffness occurring by the next day.
- Sprains commonly occur in fingers, ankles, and knees. If the ligament damage is major, the joint becomes unstable, and surgical repair may be required. In addition, an avulsion fracture may exist.

- Strains manifest with a sharp, stabbing pain caused by bleeding and immediate protective muscle contraction. Tennis players often suffer calf muscle strains; soccer players often experience quadriceps strains; and swimmers, weight lifters, and tennis players often suffer shoulder strains.
- **Tendinitis** (inflammation of a tendon) is caused by overuse and is seen in tennis players (epicondylar tendinitis, or "tennis elbow"), in runners and gymnasts (Achilles tendinitis), and in basketball players (infrapatellar tendinitis).
- Meniscal injuries of the knee occur with excessive rotational stress.
- Dislocations are seen with sports that involve throwing or lifting.
- Fractures occur with falls. Skaters and bikers frequently suffer Colles' fractures of the wrist when they fall on outstretched arms; ballet dancers and track and field athletes may experience metatarsal fractures. Stress fractures occur with repeated bone trauma from activities such as jogging, gymnastics, basketball, and aerobics. The tibias, fibulas, and metatarsals are most vulnerable.

Patients who have experienced a sports-related injury are often highly motivated to return to their previous level of activity. Compliance with restriction of activities and gradual resumption of activities may be a significant problem for these patients. They need to be taught how to avoid further injury or new injury. With recurrence of symptoms, they need to diminish their level and intensity of activity to a comfortable level and to treat the symptoms with RICE. The time required to recover from a sports-related injury can be as short as a few days or longer than 6 weeks.

Prevention

Sports-related injuries can be prevented by the use of proper equipment (eg, running shoes for joggers, wrist guards for skaters) and by effectively training and conditioning of the body. Specific training needs to be tailored to the person and the sport. Warm-up routines generally include walking or slow jogging for about 5 minutes, followed by slow, gradual stretching. The athlete holds the stretch for 10 seconds before relaxing and repeating the stretch (Fig. 69-1). Preparing the body for sports activities increases the person's flexibility and decreases the incidence of strains and sprains.

After exercise, the body needs to cool off to prevent cardiovascular problems such as hypotension, syncope, and dysrhythmias. Changes in activities and stresses should occur gradually. In addition, the athlete needs to be taught to "tune in" to body symptoms

FIGURE 69-1 Stretching exercises. Slow, gradual stretching (after walking to warm the muscles) increases flexibility and decreases the incidence of sprains and strains. Lower extremity stretches include (**A**) quadriceps stretch; (**B**) heel cord stretch; (**C**) hamstring stretch; and (**D**) hamstring and quadriceps stretch.

that indicate stress and to modify activities to minimize injury and to promote healing.

ROTATOR CUFF TEARS

Rotator cuff tears may result from an acute injury or from chronic joint stresses. Patients complain of pain, limited ROM, and some joint dysfunction, including muscle weakness. In many cases, the patient with a rotator cuff tear experiences night pain and is unable to sleep on the involved side. The patient is unable to perform over-the-head activities. The acromioclavicular joint is tender. X-rays are helpful in evaluating the joint. Arthrography and magnetic resonance imaging (MRI) are used to determine soft tissue pathology and the extent of the rotator cuff tear.

Medical Management

Initial conservative management includes use of nonsteroidal anti-inflammatory drugs (NSAIDs) including cyclooxygenase-2 (COX-2) inhibitors, rest with modification of activities, injection of a corticosteroid into the shoulder joint, and progressive stretching, ROM, and strengthening exercises. Some rotator cuff tears require arthroscopic **débridement** (removal of devitalized tissue) or arthroscopic or open acromioplasty with tendon repair. Postoperatively, the shoulder is immobilized for several days to 4 weeks. Physical therapy with shoulder exercises is begun as prescribed, and the patient is instructed in how to perform the exercises at home. Full recovery is expected in 6 to 12 months.

EPICONDYLITIS (TENNIS ELBOW)

Epicondylitis is a chronic, painful condition that is caused by excessive, repetitive extension, flexion, pronation, and supination activities of the forearm. These excessive, repetitious activities result in inflammation (tendinitis) and minor tears in the tendons at the origin of the muscles on the medial or lateral epicondyles. Activities contributing to the development of epicondylitis include tennis, racket sports, pitching, gymnastics, and repetitive use of a screwdriver. The pain characteristically radiates down the extensor (dorsal) surface of the forearm. The patient may have a weakened grasp. Most often, relief is obtained by rest and avoidance of the aggravating activity.

Medical Management

Application of ice after the activity and administration of NSAIDs, including COX-2 inhibitors, usually relieve the pain. In some instances, the arm is immobilized in a molded splint or cast. Because of its degenerative effects on tendons, local injection of a corticosteroid is reserved for patients with severe pain who do not respond to NSAIDs and immobilization. After pain subsides, rehabilitation exercises include gentle and gradually increased stretching of the tendons. A tennis elbow counterforce strap to limit extension of the elbow may be prescribed when activity is resumed. Occasionally, surgery may be needed to release strictures or to débride the joint.

LATERAL AND MEDIAL COLLATERAL LIGAMENT INJURY

Lateral and medial collateral ligaments of the knee (Fig. 69-2) provide stability at the sides of the knee. Injury to these ligaments occurs when the foot is firmly planted and the knee is struck—either medially, causing stretching and tearing injury to the lateral collateral ligament, or laterally, causing stretching and tearing injury to the medial collateral ligament. The patient experiences pain, joint instability, and inability to walk without assistance.

Medical Management

Emergency management includes RICE. The joint is evaluated for fracture. Hemarthrosis (bleeding into the joint) may develop, contributing to the pain. The joint fluid is aspirated to relieve pressure.

The treatment depends on the severity of the sprain. Conservative management includes limited weight bearing and use of protective elastic bandaging or a brace. As pain subsides, ROM exercise is encouraged. The patient's return to full activities, including sports, depends on return of motion, functional stability of the joint, and muscle strength.

If needed, surgical reconstruction may be performed immediately or delayed. Generally, the leg is immobilized, and weight bearing is restricted for 6 to 8 weeks. A progressive rehabilitation program helps to restore the function and strength of the knee. Rehabilitation requires many months, and the patient may need to wear a derotational brace while engaging in sports.

FIGURE 69-2 Knee ligaments. (**A**) Anterolateral view. (**B**) Posterolateral view.

Nursing Management

The nurse provides patient teaching about proper use of ambulatory devices, the healing process, and activity limitation to promote healing. The nurse teaches the surgical patient about pain management, medications (analgesics, antibiotics), brace use, wound care, possible complications (eg, altered neurovascular status, infection, skin breakdown), and self-care.

ANTERIOR AND POSTERIOR CRUCIATE LIGAMENT INJURY

The anterior cruciate ligament (ACL) and the posterior cruciate ligament (PCL) of the knee stabilize forward and backward motion of the femur and tibia (see Fig. 69-2). These ligaments cross in the centre of the knee. Injury occurs when the foot is firmly planted, the knee is hyperextended, and the person twists the torso and femur. The patient reports a pop or tearing sensation with this twisting injury. Usually, the ACL is torn. The patient experiences pain, joint instability, and pain with ambulation.

Medical Management

Emergency management includes RICE. The joint is evaluated for fracture. Joint effusion and hemarthrosis require joint aspiration and wrapping with a compression elastic dressing.

Treatment depends on the severity of the injury and the effect of the injury on daily activities. Conservative treatment involves application of a brace, physical therapy, and avoidance of jumping activities. Surgical ACL reconstruction includes tendon repair with grafting and is performed as ambulatory arthroscopic surgery. After surgery, the patient is taught to control pain with oral opioid analgesics, NSAIDs, COX-2 inhibitors, and cryotherapy (a cooling pad incorporated in a dressing). The patient is taught about monitoring neurovascular status of the leg, wound care, and signs of complications that need to be reported promptly to the surgeon. Exercises (ankle pumps, quadriceps sets, and hamstring sets) are encouraged during the early postoperative period. The nurse reinforces instruction about weight-bearing limits, exercise restrictions, and the use of a knee brace or immobilizer. The patient must protect the graft by complying with exercise restrictions. The physical therapist supervises progressive ROM and weight bearing (as the patient is permitted). Continuous passive motion may be helpful in restoring full ROM. Rehabilitation after surgery typically takes 6 to 12 months.

MENISCAL INJURIES

In the knee, there are two crescent-shaped (semilunar) cartilages, called menisci, attached to the edge of the shallow articulating surface of the head of the tibia (see Fig. 69-2). Each **meniscus** moves slightly backward and forward to accommodate the condyles of the femur when the leg is flexed or extended. Normally, little twisting movement is permitted in the knee joint. In sports or accidents, twisting of the knee or repetitive squatting and impact may result in either tearing or detachment of the cartilage from its attachment to the head of the tibia.

These injuries leave loose cartilage in the knee joint that may slip between the femur and the tibia, preventing full extension of the leg. If this happens during walking or running, patients often describe their leg as "giving way" under them. Patients may hear or feel a click in the knee when they walk, especially when they extend the leg that is bearing weight, as in going upstairs. When the cartilage is attached to the front and back of the knee but torn loose laterally (bucket-handle tear), it may slide between the bones to lie between the condyles and prevent full flexion or extension. As a result, the knee "locks." Meniscal injuries produce pain and disability because the patient never knows when the knee will malfunction. Also, the torn cartilage is an irritant in the joint, causing inflammation, chronic synovitis, and effusion.

Medical Management

Initial conservative treatment includes immobilization of the knee, use of crutches, anti-inflammatory agents, analgesics, and modification of activities to avoid those causing the symptoms. If symptoms persist, the damaged cartilage is surgically removed (meniscectomy) through a procedure in which the surgeon uses an **arthroscope** to visualize and repair the damage. After surgery, a pressure dressing is applied, and a knee-immobilizing splint may be required. The most common complication is an effusion into the knee joint, which produces marked pain. The physician may need to aspirate the joint to remove fluid and relieve the pressure. These patients are taught quadriceps-setting and ROM exercises. Additional exercises help to restore full function, stability, and strength. After arthroscopic meniscectomy, most patients resume activities in a day or two, and sports can be resumed in several weeks, as prescribed by the physician.

RUPTURE OF THE ACHILLES TENDON

Traumatic rupture of the Achilles tendon, generally within the tendon sheath, occurs during activities when there is a sudden contraction of the calf muscle with the foot fixed firmly to the floor or ground. The patient experiences sharp pain and is unable to plantar flex the foot. Immediate surgical repair of complete Achilles tendon ruptures is usually recommended to obtain satisfactory results. After surgery, a cast or brace is used to immobilize the joint. In some situations, conservative management with a plantar-flexed cast for 6 to 8 weeks may be used. After immobilization, a heel lift is worn and progressive physical therapy to promote ankle ROM and strength is begun.

Fractures

A **fracture** is a break in the continuity of bone and is defined according to its type and extent. Fractures occur when the bone is subjected to stress greater than it can absorb. Fractures are caused by direct blows, crushing forces, sudden twisting motions, and even extreme muscle contractions. When the bone is broken, adjacent structures are also affected, resulting in soft tissue edema, hemorrhage into the muscles and joints, joint dislocations, ruptured tendons, severed nerves, and damaged blood vessels. Body organs may be injured by the force that caused the fracture or by the fracture fragments.

Types of Fractures

A *complete fracture* involves a break across the entire cross-section of the bone and is frequently displaced (removed from normal position). In an *incomplete fracture* (eg, greenstick fracture), the break occurs through only part of the cross-section of the bone. A *comminuted* fracture is one that produces several bone fragments. A *closed fracture* (simple fracture) is one that does not cause a break in the skin. An *open fracture* (compound, or complex, fracture) is one in which the skin or mucous membrane wound extends to the fractured bone. Open fractures are graded according to the following criteria:

- Grade I is a clean wound less than 1 cm long.
- Grade II is a larger wound without extensive soft tissue damage.
- Grade III is highly contaminated, has extensive soft tissue damage, and is the most severe.

Fractures may also be described according to the anatomic placement of fragments, particularly if they are displaced or nondisplaced. Specific types of fractures are highlighted in Chart 69-1.

Clinical Manifestations

The clinical manifestations of a fracture are pain, loss of function, deformity, shortening of the extremity, crepitus, and local swelling and discolouration. Not all of these clinical manifestations are present in every fracture. For example, many are not present with linear or fissure fractures or with impacted fractures. The diagnosis of a fracture is based on the patient's symptoms, the physical signs, and the x-ray findings. Usually, the patient reports having sustained an injury to the area.

PAIN

The pain is continuous and increases in severity until the bone fragments are immobilized. The muscle spasm that accompanies fracture is a type of natural splinting designed to minimize further movement of the fracture fragments.

LOSS OF FUNCTION

After a fracture, the extremity cannot function properly, because normal function of the muscles depends on the integrity of the bones to which they are attached. Pain contributes to the loss of function. In addition, abnormal movement (false motion) may be present.

DEFORMITY

Displacement, angulation, or rotation of the fragments in a fracture of the arm or leg causes a deformity (either visible or palpable) that is detectable when the limb is compared with the uninjured extremity. Deformity also results from soft tissue swelling.

SHORTENING

In fractures of long bones, there is actual shortening of the extremity because of the contraction of the muscles that are attached above and below the site of the fracture. The fragments often overlap by as much as 2.5 to 5 cm.

CREPITUS

When the extremity is examined with the hands, a grating sensation, called *crepitus,* can be felt. It is caused by the rubbing of the bone fragments against each other.

 NURSING ALERT Testing for crepitus can produce further tissue damage and should be avoided.

SWELLING AND DISCOLOURATION

Localized swelling and discolouration of the skin (ecchymosis) occurs after a fracture as a result of trauma and bleeding into the tissues. These signs may not develop for several hours after the injury.

Emergency Management of Fractures

Immediately after injury, whenever a fracture is suspected, it is important to immobilize the body part before the patient is moved. If an injured patient must be removed from a vehicle before splints can be applied, the extremity is supported above and below the fracture site to prevent rotation as well as angular motion.

Adequate splinting, including joints adjacent to the fracture, is essential. Movement of fracture fragments causes additional pain, soft tissue damage, and bleeding. Temporary, well-padded splints, firmly bandaged over clothing, serve to immobilize the fracture. Immobilization of the long bones of the lower extremities may be accomplished by bandaging the legs together, with the unaffected extremity serving as a splint for the injured one. In an upper extremity injury, the arm may be bandaged to the chest, or an injured forearm may be placed in a sling. The neurovascular status distal to the injury should be assessed to determine adequacy of peripheral tissue perfusion and nerve function.

With an *open fracture,* the wound is covered with a clean (sterile) dressing to prevent contamination of deeper tissues. No attempt is made to reduce the fracture, even if one of the bone fragments is protruding through the wound. Splints are applied for immobilization.

In the emergency department, the patient is evaluated completely. The clothes are gently removed, first from the uninjured side of the body and then from the injured side. The patient's clothing may be cut away. The fractured extremity is moved as little as possible to avoid more damage.

Medical Management of Fractures

The principles of fracture treatment include reduction, immobilization, and regaining of normal function and strength through rehabilitation.

REDUCTION

Reduction of a fracture ("setting" the bone) refers to restoration of the fracture fragments to anatomic alignment and rotation. Either closed reduction or open reduction may be used to reduce a fracture. The specific method selected depends on the nature of the fracture; however, the underlying principles are the same. Usually, the physician reduces a fracture as soon as possible to prevent loss of elasticity from the tissues through infiltration by edema or hemorrhage. In most cases, **fracture reduction** becomes more difficult as the injury begins healing.

Before fracture reduction and immobilization, the patient is prepared for the procedure; permission for the procedure is obtained, and an analgesic is administered as prescribed. Anesthesia may be administered. The injured extremity must be handled gently to avoid additional damage.

Closed Reduction. In most instances, closed reduction is accomplished by bringing the bone fragments into apposition (ie, placing the ends in contact) through manipulation and manual traction. The extremity is held in the desired position while the physician applies a cast, splint, or other device. Reduction under anesthesia with percutaneous pinning may be used. The immobilizing device maintains the reduction and stabilizes the extremity for bone healing. X-rays are obtained to verify that the bone fragments are correctly aligned.

Traction (skin or skeletal) may be used to effect fracture reduction and immobilization. Traction may be used until the patient is physiologically stable and able to withstand surgical fixation. Use of traction and the nursing management of a patient in traction are discussed more fully in Chapter 67.

Chart 69-1 Specific Types of Fractures

Avulsion: a fracture in which a fragment of bone has been pulled away by a ligament or tendon and its attachment

Comminuted: a fracture in which bone has splintered into several fragments

Compound: a fracture in which damage also involves the skin or mucous membranes; also called an open fracture

Compression: a fracture in which bone has been compressed (seen in vertebral fractures)

Depressed: a fracture in which fragments are driven inward (seen frequently in fractures of skull and facial bones)

Epiphyseal: a fracture through the epiphysis

Greenstick: a fracture in which one side of a bone is broken and the other side is bent

Impacted: a fracture in which a bone fragment is driven into another bone fragment

Oblique: a fracture occurring at an angle across the bone (less stable than a transverse fracture)

Pathologic: a fracture that occurs through an area of diseased bone (eg, osteoporosis, bone cyst, Paget's disease, bony metastasis, tumour); can occur without trauma or a fall

Simple: a fracture that remains contained; does not break the skin

Spiral: a fracture that twists around the shaft of the bone

Stress: a fracture that results from repeated loading without bone and muscle recovery

Transverse: a fracture that is straight across the bone

Simple   Compound or open   Comminuted   Greenstick

Depressed   Avulsion

Oblique   Spiral   Impacted   Transverse   Compression

Open Reduction. Some fractures require open reduction. Through a surgical approach, the fracture fragments are reduced. Internal fixation devices (metallic pins, wires, screws, plates, nails, or rods) may be used to hold the bone fragments in position until solid bone healing occurs. These devices may be attached to the sides of bone, or they may be inserted through the bony fragments or directly into the medullary cavity of the bone (Fig. 63-3). Internal fixation devices ensure firm approximation and fixation of the bony fragments.

IMMOBILIZATION

After the fracture has been reduced, the bone fragments must be immobilized, or held in correct position and alignment, until

FIGURE 69-3 Techniques of internal fixation. (**A**) Plate and six screws for a transverse or short oblique fracture. (**B**) Screws for a long oblique or spiral fracture. (**C**) Screws for a long butterfly fragment. (**D**) Plate and six screws for a short butterfly fragment. (**E**) Medullary nail for a segmental fracture.

union occurs. Immobilization may be accomplished by external or internal fixation. Methods of external fixation include bandages, casts, splints, continuous traction, and external fixators. Metal implants used for internal fixation serve as internal splints to immobilize the fracture.

MAINTAINING AND RESTORING FUNCTION

Reduction and immobilization are maintained as prescribed to promote bone and soft tissue healing. Swelling is controlled by elevating the injured extremity and applying ice as prescribed. Neurovascular status (circulation, movement, sensation) is monitored, and the orthopedic surgeon is notified immediately if signs of neurovascular compromise are identified. Restlessness, anxiety, and discomfort are controlled with a variety of approaches, such as reassurance, position changes, and pain relief strategies, including use of analgesics. Isometric and muscle-setting exercises are encouraged to minimize disuse atrophy and to promote circulation. Participation in activities of daily living (ADLs) is encouraged to promote independent functioning and self-esteem. Gradual resumption of activities is promoted within the therapeutic prescription. With internal fixation, the surgeon determines the amount of movement and weight-bearing stress the extremity can withstand and prescribes the level of activity. (See Nursing Process sections in Chapter 67 for more information about caring for patients who have a cast, are in traction, or are undergoing orthopedic surgery.)

Nursing Management

PATIENTS WITH CLOSED FRACTURES

The nurse encourages patients with closed (simple) fractures to return to their usual activities as rapidly as possible. The nurse teaches patients how to control swelling and pain associated with the fracture and with soft tissue trauma and encourages them to be active within the limits of the fracture immobilization (Chart 69-2). It is important to teach exercises to maintain the health of unaffected

---

Chart 69-2
Home Care Checklist • Closed Fracture

At the completion of the home care instruction, the patient or caregiver will be able to:	Patient	Caregiver
• Describe approaches to controlling swelling and pain (eg, elevate extremity to heart level; take analgesics as prescribed)	✓	✓
• Report pain uncontrolled by elevation and analgesics (may be an indicator of impaired tissue perfusion or compartment syndrome)	✓	✓
• Describe management of immobilizing device or care of incision	✓	
• Consume diet to promote bone healing	✓	
• Demonstrate ability to transfer	✓	
• Use mobility aids safely	✓	
• Avoid excessive use of injured extremity; observe prescribed weight-bearing limits	✓	
• State indicators of complications to report promptly to physician (eg, uncontrolled swelling and pain; cool, pale fingers or toes; paresthesia; paralysis; signs of local and systemic infection; signs of thromboembolism; problems with immobilization device)	✓	✓
• State possible delayed complications of fractures (ie, delayed union; nonunion; avascular necrosis; reaction to internal fixation device; complex regional pain syndrome (CRPS), formally called reflex sympathetic dystrophy syndrome; heterotrophic ossification)	✓	
• Describe gradual resumption of normal activities when medically cleared, and discuss how to protect fracture site from undue stresses	✓	✓

muscles and to increase the strength of muscles needed for transferring and for using assistive devices (eg, crutches, walker, special utensils). The nurse and physical therapist teach patients how to use assistive devices safely. Plans are made to help patients modify their home environment as needed and to secure personal assistance if necessary. Patient teaching includes self-care, medication information, monitoring for potential complications, and the need for continuing health care supervision. Fracture healing and restoration of full strength and mobility may take months.

PATIENTS WITH OPEN FRACTURES

In an open fracture, there is risk of osteomyelitis, tetanus, and gas gangrene. The objectives of management are to prevent infection of the wound, soft tissue, and bone and to promote healing of soft tissue and bone. The nurse administers tetanus prophylaxis if indicated. Serial irrigation and débridement are used to remove anaerobic organisms. Intravenous antibiotics are prescribed to prevent or treat infection.

Prompt, thorough wound irrigation and débridement in the operating room are necessary. The wound is cultured. Devitalized bone fragments are removed. The fracture is carefully reduced and stabilized by external fixation (see Chapter 67) or intramedullary nails. Any damage to blood vessels, soft tissue, muscles, nerves, and tendons is treated.

With open fractures, primary wound closure is usually delayed. Heavily contaminated wounds are left unsutured and dressed with sterile gauze to permit swelling and wound drainage. Wound irrigation and débridement may be repeated, removing infected and devitalized tissue and increasing vascularity in the region. After it has been determined that infection is not present, the wound is closed in 5 to 7 days, and all dead space is obliterated by grafting of autogenous skin or a flap.

The nurse elevates the extremity to minimize edema. It is important to assess neurovascular status frequently. The nurse measures the patient's temperature at regular intervals and monitors the patient for signs of infection. In 4 to 8 weeks, bone grafting may be necessary to bridge bone defects and to stimulate bone healing.

Fracture Healing and Complications (Early and Delayed)

Weeks to months are required for most fractures to heal. Many factors influence the speed with which fractures heal (Chart 69-3). The reduction of fracture fragments must be accurate and maintained to ensure healing. The affected bone must have an adequate blood supply. The type of fracture also affects healing time. In general, fractures of flat bones (pelvis, scapula) heal rapidly. Fractures at the ends of long bones, where the bone is more vascular and cancellous, heal more quickly than do fractures in areas where the bone is dense and less vascular (midshaft). Weight bearing stimulates healing of stabilized fractures of the long bones in the lower extremities.

If fracture healing is disrupted, bone union may be delayed or stopped completely. Factors that can impair fracture healing include inadequate fracture immobilization, inadequate blood supply to the fracture site or adjacent tissue, extensive space between bone fragments, interposition of soft tissue between bone ends, infection, and metabolic problems.

Complications of fractures fall into two categories—early and delayed. Early complications include shock, fat embolism, compartment syndrome, deep vein thrombosis, thromboembolism

Chart 69-3 — Factors That Affect Fracture Healing

Factors That Enhance Fracture Healing
- Immobilization of fracture fragments
- Maximum bone fragment contact
- Sufficient blood supply
- Proper nutrition
- Exercise: weight bearing for long bones
- Hormones: growth hormone, thyroid, calcitonin, vitamin D, anabolic steroids
- Electric potential across fracture

Factors That Inhibit Fracture Healing
- Extensive local trauma
- Bone loss
- Inadequate immobilization
- Space or tissue between bone fragments
- Infection
- Local malignancy
- Metabolic bone disease (eg, Paget's disease)
- Irradiated bone (radiation necrosis)
- Avascular necrosis
- Intra-articular fracture (synovial fluid contains fibrolysins, which lyse the initial clot and retard clot formation)
- Age (elderly persons heal more slowly)
- Corticosteroids (inhibit the repair rate)

(pulmonary embolism), disseminated intravascular coagulopathy, and infection. Delayed complications include delayed union and nonunion, avascular necrosis of bone, reaction to internal fixation devices, complex regional pain syndrome (formerly called reflex sympathetic dystrophy), and heterotrophic ossification.

SHOCK (EARLY)

Hypovolemic or traumatic shock resulting from hemorrhage (both visible and nonvisible blood loss) and from loss of extracellular fluid into damaged tissues may occur in fractures of the extremities, thorax, pelvis, or spine. Because the bone is very vascular, large quantities of blood may be lost as a result of trauma, especially in fractures of the femur and pelvis. Treatment of shock consists of restoring blood volume and circulation, relieving the patient's pain, providing adequate splinting, and protecting the patient from further injury and other complications. (See Chapter 15 for a discussion of shock.)

FAT EMBOLISM SYNDROME (EARLY)

After fracture of long bones or pelvis, multiple fractures, or crush injuries, fat emboli may develop. Fat embolism syndrome occurs most frequently in young adults (typically those 20 to 30 years of age) and elderly adults who experience fractures of the proximal femur. At the time of fracture, fat globules may move into the blood because the marrow pressure is greater than the capillary pressure or because catecholamines elevated by the patient's stress reaction mobilize fatty acids and promote the development of fat globules in the bloodstream. The fat globules (emboli) occlude the small blood vessels that supply the lungs, brain, kidneys, and other organs. The onset of symptoms is rapid, usually occurring within 24 to 72 hours, but may occur up to a week after injury.

Clinical Manifestations

Presenting features include hypoxia, tachypnea, tachycardia, and pyrexia. The respiratory distress response includes tachypnea, dyspnea, crackles, wheezes, precordial chest pain, cough, large amounts of thick white sputum, and tachycardia. Occlusion of a large number of small vessels causes the pulmonary pressure to rise. Edema and hemorrhages in the alveoli impair oxygen transport, leading to hypoxia. Arterial blood gas values show the partial pressure of oxygen (PaO_2) to be less than 60 mm Hg, with an early respiratory alkalosis and later respiratory acidosis. The chest x-ray shows a typical "snowstorm" infiltrate. Eventually, acute pulmonary edema, acute respiratory distress syndrome, and heart failure develop.

Cerebral disturbances (due to hypoxia and the lodging of fat emboli in the brain) are manifested by mental status changes varying from headache, mild agitation, and confusion to delirium and coma.

> **NURSING ALERT** Subtle personality changes, restlessness, irritability, or confusion in a patient who has sustained a fracture are indications for immediate arterial blood gas studies.

With systemic embolization, the patient appears pale. Petechiae, possibly due to a transient thrombocytopenia, are noted in the buccal membranes and conjunctival sacs, on the hard palate, and over the chest and anterior axillary folds. The patient develops a temperature of more than 39.5°C. Free fat may be found in the urine if emboli reach the kidneys. Kidney failure may develop.

Prevention and Management

Immediate immobilization of fractures (including early surgical fixation), minimal fracture manipulation, adequate support for fractured bones during turning and positioning, and maintenance of fluid and electrolyte balance are measures that may reduce the incidence of fat emboli. The nurse monitors high-risk patients (adults between 20 and 30 years of age with long bone, pelvic, or multiple fractures or crush injuries, and elderly patients with femur fractures) to identify this problem. Prompt initiation of respiratory support is essential.

The objectives of management are to support the respiratory system, to prevent respiratory and metabolic acidosis, and to correct homeostatic disturbances. Respiratory failure is the most common cause of death. Respiratory support is provided with oxygen given in high concentrations. Controlled-volume ventilation with positive end-expiratory pressure may be used to prevent or treat pulmonary edema. Corticosteroids may be administered to treat the inflammatory lung reaction and to control cerebral edema. Vasoactive medications to support cardiovascular function are administered to prevent hypotension, shock, and interstitial pulmonary edema. Accurate fluid intake and output records facilitate adequate fluid replacement therapy. Morphine may be prescribed for pain and anxiety for the patient who is on a ventilator. In addition, the nurse provides calm reassurance to allay apprehension. The patient's response to therapy is closely monitored.

Because fat emboli are a major cause of death for patients with fractures, the nurse must recognize early indications of fat embolism syndrome and report them promptly to the physician. Respiratory support must be instituted early.

COMPARTMENT SYNDROME (EARLY)

Compartment syndrome is a complication that develops when tissue perfusion in the muscles is less than that required for tissue viability. The patient complains of deep, throbbing, unrelenting pain, which is not controlled by opioids. This pain can be caused by (1) a reduction in the size of the muscle compartment because the enclosing muscle fascia is too tight or a cast or dressing is constrictive, or (2) an increase in muscle compartment contents because of edema or hemorrhage associated with a variety of problems (eg, fractures, crush injuries). The forearm and leg muscle compartments are involved most frequently. The pressure within a muscle compartment may increase to such an extent as to decrease microcirculation, causing nerve and muscle anoxia and necrosis. Permanent function can be lost if the anoxic situation continues for longer than 6 hours.

Assessment and Diagnostic Findings

Frequent assessment of neurovascular function after fracture is essential. Sensory deficits include paresthesia, unrelenting pain, and hypoesthesia. *Paresthesia* (burning or tingling sensation) and numbness along the involved nerve are early signs of nerve involvement. Motion is evaluated by asking the patient to move fingers or toes distal to the potential problem. Motor weakness may occur as a late sign of nerve ischemia. No movement (*paralysis*) suggests nerve damage.

Peripheral circulation is evaluated by assessing colour, temperature, capillary refill time, swelling, and pulses. Swelling (edema) reduces tissue perfusion. Cyanotic (blue-tinged) nail beds suggest venous congestion. Pale or dusky and cold fingers or toes and prolonged capillary refill time suggest diminished arterial perfusion. Edema may obscure the presence of arterial pulsation, and Doppler ultrasonography may be used to verify a pulse. Pulselessness is a sign of arterial occlusion, not of compartment syndrome, because the tissue pressure would need to be above the systolic blood pressure for major artery occlusion to occur.

As intracompartment pressure increases, the patient complains of deep, throbbing, unrelenting pain, which is greater than expected and not controlled by opioids. Passive stretching of the muscle causes acute pain. With continued nerve ischemia and edema, the patient experiences sensations of hypoesthesia (diminished sensitivity to stimulation) and then absence of feeling. Palpation of the muscle, if possible, reveals it to be swollen and hard. The actual tissue pressure can be measured by inserting a tissue pressure-measuring device into the muscle compartment. (Normal pressure is 8 mm Hg or less.) Nerve and muscle tissues deteriorate as compartment pressure increases. Prolonged pressure of more than 30 mm Hg can result in compromised microcirculation. Nerve tissue is more sensitive than muscle to elevated tissue pressures. Paresthesia generally occurs before paralysis.

Medical Management

Prompt management of acute compartment syndrome is essential. The physician needs to be notified immediately if neurovascular compromise is suspected. Delay may result in permanent nerve and muscle damage or even necrosis.

Compartment syndrome is managed by elevation of the extremity to the heart level, release of restrictive devices (dressings or cast), or both. If conservative measures do not restore tissue perfusion and relieve pain within 1 hour, a fasciotomy (surgical decompression with excision of the fibrous membrane that covers and separates muscles) may be needed to relieve the constrictive muscle fascia. After fasciotomy, the wound is not sutured but instead is left open to permit the muscle tissues to expand; it is covered with moist, sterile saline dressings. The limb is splinted in a functional position and elevated, and prescribed passive ROM exercises are usually performed every 4 to 6 hours. In 3 to 5 days, when the swelling has resolved and tissue perfusion has been restored, the wound is débrided and closed (possibly with skin grafts).

OTHER EARLY COMPLICATIONS

Deep vein thrombosis (DVT), thromboembolism, and pulmonary embolus (PE) are associated with reduced skeletal muscle contractions and bed rest. Patients with fractures of the lower extremities and pelvis are at high risk for thromboembolism. Pulmonary emboli may cause death several days to weeks after injury. (See Chapter 31 for a discussion of DVT; Chapter 30 for discussion of thromboembolism, and Chapter 23 for discussion of PE).

Disseminated intravascular coagulopathy (DIC) includes a group of bleeding disorders with diverse causes, including massive tissue trauma. Manifestations of DIC include ecchymoses, unexpected bleeding after surgery, and bleeding from the mucous membranes, venipuncture sites, and gastrointestinal and urinary tracts. The treatment of DIC is discussed in Chapter 33.

All open fractures are considered contaminated. Surgical internal fixation of fractures carries a risk for infection. The nurse must monitor for and teach the patient to monitor for signs of infection, including tenderness, pain, redness, swelling, local warmth, elevated temperature, and purulent drainage. Infections must be treated promptly. Antibiotic therapy must be appropriate and adequate for prevention and treatment of infection.

DELAYED UNION AND NONUNION (DELAYED)

Delayed union occurs when healing does not occur at a normal rate for the location and type of fracture. Delayed union may be associated with distraction (pulling apart) of bone fragments, systemic or local infection, poor nutrition, or comorbidity (eg, diabetes mellitus; autoimmune disease). Eventually, the fracture heals.

Nonunion results from failure of the ends of a fractured bone to unite. The patient complains of persistent discomfort and abnormal movement at the fracture site. Factors contributing to union problems include infection at the fracture site, interposition of tissue between the bone ends, inadequate immobilization or manipulation that disrupts callus formation, excessive space between bone fragments (bone gap), limited bone contact, and impaired blood supply resulting in avascular necrosis.

In nonunion, fibrocartilage or fibrous tissue exists between the bone fragments; no bone salts have been deposited. A false joint (pseudarthrosis) often develops at the site of the fracture. Nonunion most commonly occurs with fractures of the middle third of the humerus, the lower third of the tibia, and, in elderly people, the neck of the femur.

Medical Management

The physician treats nonunion with internal fixation, bone grafting, electrical bone stimulation, or a combination of these therapies. Internal fixation stabilizes the bone fragments and ensures bone contact.

Bone grafts provide for osteogenesis, osteoconduction, or osteoinduction. *Osteogenesis* (bone formation) occurs after transplantation of bone containing osteoblasts. *Osteoconduction* is provision by

the graft of the structural matrix for ingrowth of blood vessels and osteoblasts. *Osteoinduction* is the stimulation of host stem cells to differentiate into osteoblasts by several growth factors, including bone morphogenic proteins. Bone transplants undergo creeping substitution, a reconstructive process in which the bone transplant is gradually replaced by new bone.

During surgery the bone fragments are trimmed, infection (if present) is removed, and a bone graft is placed in the bony defect. The bone graft may be an **autograft** (tissue harvested from the donor for the donor, frequently from the iliac crest) or an **allograft** (tissue harvested from a donor other than the person who will receive it). The bone graft fills the bone gap, provides a lattice structure for invasion by bone cells, and actively promotes bone growth. The type of bone selected for grafting depends on function: cortical bone for structural strength, cancellous bone for osteogenesis, and corticocancellous bone for strength and rapid incorporation. Bone grafts may be chips, wedges, blocks, bone segments, or demineralized bone matrix. At times, autograft bone, allograft bone, and demineralized cortical matrix are combined to optimize graft incorporation and bone healing. Free vascularized bone autografts are grafted with their own blood supply, allowing for primary fracture healing.

After grafting, immobilization and non–weight bearing are required while the bone graft becomes incorporated and the fracture or defect heals. Depending on the type of bone grafted, healing may take from 6 to 12 months or longer. Bone grafting problems include wound or graft infection, fracture of the graft, and nonunion. Specific autograft problems include a limited quantity of bone available for harvest, increased surgery and anesthesia time, increased blood loss, and donor site pain, hematoma, and infection. Infrequent specific allograft problems include partial acceptance (lack of host and donor histocompatibility, which retards graft incorporation), graft rejection (rapid and complete resorption of the graft), and transmission of disease (rare).

Osteogenesis in nonunion may be stimulated by electrical impulses; the effectiveness is similar to that of bone grafting. Use of electrical impulses is not effective with large bone gaps or synovial pseudarthrosis. The electrical stimulation modifies the tissue environment, making it electronegative, which enhances mineral deposition and bone formation.

In some situations, pins that act as cathodes are inserted percutaneously, directly into the fracture site, and electrical impulses are directed to the fracture continuously. Direct current methods cannot be used when infection is present.

Another method for stimulating osteogenesis is noninvasive inductive coupling. Pulsing electromagnetic fields are delivered to the fracture for approximately 10 hours each day by an electromagnetic coil over the nonunion site (Fig. 69-4). During the electrical stimulation treatment period, which takes 3 to 6 months or longer, rigid fracture fixation with adequate support is needed.

Nursing Management

The patient with a nonunion has experienced an extended time in fracture treatment and frequently becomes frustrated with prolonged therapy. The nurse provides emotional support and encouragement to the patient and encourages compliance with the treatment regimen. The orthopedic surgeon evaluates the progression of bone healing with periodic x-rays.

Nursing care for the patient with a bone graft include pain management, monitoring the patient for signs of infection at the donor and recipient sites, and patient education. The nurse needs to reinforce information concerning the objectives of the bone graft, immobilization, non–weight bearing, wound care, signs of infection, and follow-up care with the orthopedic surgeon.

and stabilization); material failure (faulty or damaged device); corrosion of the device, causing local inflammation; allergic response to the metallic alloy used; and osteoporotic remodeling adjacent to the fixation device (in which stress needed for bone strength is transferred to the device, causing a disuse osteoporosis). If the device is removed, the bone needs to be protected from refracture related to osteoporosis, altered bone structure, and trauma. Bone remodeling reestablishes the bone's structural strength.

COMPLEX REGIONAL PAIN SYNDROME (DELAYED)

Complex regional pain syndrome (CRPS), formerly called reflex sympathetic dystrophy (RSD), is a painful sympathetic nervous system problem. It occurs infrequently. When it does occur, it is most often in an upper extremity after trauma and is seen more often in women. Clinical manifestations of CRPS include severe burning pain, local edema, hyperesthesia, stiffness, discolouration, vasomotor skin changes (ie, fluctuating warm, red, dry and cold, sweaty, cyanotic), and trophic changes (ie, glossy, shiny skin; increased hair and nail growth). This syndrome is frequently chronic, with extension of symptoms to adjacent areas of the body. Disuse muscle atrophy and bone deossification (osteoporosis) occur with persistence of CRPS. Patients may exhibit ineffective individual coping related to the chronic pain.

Management

Prevention may include elevation of the extremity after injury or surgery and selection of an immobilization device (eg, external fixator) that allows for the greatest ROM and functional use of the rest of the extremity. Early effective pain relief is the focus of management. Pain may need to be controlled with analgesics, anesthetic nerve blocks, or intravenous bisphosphonate pamidronate. NSAIDs, corticosteroids, muscle relaxants, and antidepressants are also used. With pain relief, the patient can participate in ROM exercises and functional use of the affected area. The nurse needs to help the patient cope with CRPS manifestations and explore multiple ways to control pain (see Chapter 13). The nurse avoids using the involved extremity for blood pressure measurements and venipunctures.

HETEROTROPHIC OSSIFICATION (DELAYED)

Heterotrophic ossification (myositis ossificans) is the abnormal formation of bone, near bones or in muscle, in response to soft tissue trauma after blunt trauma, fracture, or total joint replacement. The muscle is painful, and normal muscular contraction and movement are limited. Early mobilization has been recommended. Indomethacin (Indocin) may be used prophylactically if deep muscle contusion has occurred. Usually, the bone lesion resorbs over time, but the abnormal bone eventually may need to be excised if symptoms persist.

Fractures of Specific Sites

Injuries to the skeletal structure may vary from a simple linear fracture to a severe crushing injury. The type and location of the fracture and the extent of damage to surrounding structures determine the therapeutic management. Maximum functional recovery is the goal of management.

FIGURE 69-4 Bone healing stimulator applied to the arm. (Courtesy of EBI Medical Systems, Parsippany, NJ)

Nursing care for the patient with electrical bone stimulation focus on patient education that addresses immobilization, weight bearing restrictions, and correct daily use of the stimulator as prescribed.

AVASCULAR NECROSIS OF BONE (DELAYED)

Avascular necrosis occurs when the bone loses its blood supply and dies. It may occur after a fracture with disruption of the blood supply (especially of the femoral neck). It is also seen with dislocations, bone transplantation, prolonged high-dosage corticosteroid therapy, chronic renal disease, sickle cell anemia, and other diseases. The devitalized bone may collapse or reabsorb. The patient develops pain and experiences limited movement. X-rays reveal calcium loss and structural collapse. Treatment generally consists of attempts to revitalize the bone with bone grafts, prosthetic replacement, or arthrodesis (joint fusion).

REACTION TO INTERNAL FIXATION DEVICES (DELAYED)

Internal fixation devices may be removed after bony union has taken place. In most patients, however, the device is not removed unless it produces symptoms. Pain and decreased function are the prime indications that a problem has developed. Problems may include mechanical failure (inadequate insertion

CLAVICLE

Fracture of the clavicle (collar bone) is a common injury that results from a direct blow to the shoulder or a fall. Head or cervical spine injuries may occur with these fractures. The clavicle helps to hold the shoulder upward, outward, and backward from the thorax. Therefore, when the clavicle is fractured, the patient assumes a protective position, slumping the shoulders and immobilizing the arm to prevent shoulder movements. The treatment goal is to align the shoulder in its normal position by means of closed reduction and immobilization.

More than 80% of these fractures occur in the middle third of the clavicle. A clavicular strap, also called a *figure-of-eight bandage* (Fig. 69-5), may be used to pull the shoulders back, reducing and immobilizing the fracture. When a clavicular strap is used, the axillae are well padded to prevent a compression injury to the brachial plexus and the axillary artery. The nurse monitors the circulation and nerve function of both arms. A sling may be used to support the arm and to relieve pain. The patient may be permitted to use the arm for light activities within the range of comfort.

Fracture of the distal third of the clavicle, without displacement and ligament disruption, is treated with a sling and restricted motion of the arm. When a fracture in the distal third is accompanied by a disruption of the coracoclavicular ligament, there is displacement, which may be treated by open reduction and internal fixation.

Complications of clavicular fractures include trauma to the nerves of the brachial plexus, injury to the subclavian vein or artery from a bony fragment, and **malunion** (poorly aligned healing of the fractured bone). Malunion may be a cosmetic problem (eg, when low-neckline clothing is worn).

Nursing Management

The nurse cautions the patient not to elevate the arm above shoulder level until the ends of the bone have united (about 6 weeks) but encourages the patient to exercise the elbow, wrist, and fingers as soon as possible. When prescribed, shoulder exercises (Fig. 69-6) are performed to obtain full shoulder motion. Vigorous activity is limited for 3 months.

HUMERAL NECK

Fractures of the proximal humerus may occur through either the anatomic or the surgical neck of the humerus. The anatomic neck is located just below the humeral head. The surgical neck is the region below the tubercles. Impacted fractures of the surgical neck of the humerus are seen most frequently in older women after a fall on an outstretched arm. These are essentially nondisplaced fractures. Active middle-aged patients who are injured in a fall may suffer severely displaced humeral neck fractures with associated rotator cuff damage.

The patient presents with the affected arm hanging limp at the side and supported by the uninjured hand. Neurovascular assessment of the extremity is essential to evaluate fully the extent of injury and the possible involvement of the neurovascular bundle (nerves and blood vessels) of the arm.

Medical Management

Many impacted fractures of the surgical neck of the humerus are not displaced and do not require reduction. The arm is supported and immobilized by a sling and swathe that secure the supported arm to the trunk (Fig. 69-7). A soft pad is placed in the axilla to absorb moisture and avoid skin breakdown. Limitation of motion and stiffness of the shoulder occur with disuse. Therefore, pendulum exercises are begun as soon as tolerated by the patient. (In pendulum or circumduction exercises, the nurse or physical therapist instructs the patient to lean forward and allow the affected arm to abduct and rotate [see Fig. 69-6].) Early motion of the joint does not displace the fragments if motion is carried out within the limits imposed by pain.

These fractures require 6 to 10 weeks to heal, and the patient should avoid vigorous activity (eg, tennis) for an additional 4 weeks. Residual stiffness, aching, and some limitation of ROM may persist for 6 months or longer.

When a humeral neck fracture is displaced, treatment consists of closed reduction, open reduction with internal fixation, or replacement of the humeral head with a prosthesis. In this type of fracture, exercises are started only after a prescribed period of immobilization.

HUMERAL SHAFT

Fractures of the shaft of the humerus are most frequently caused by (1) direct trauma that results in a transverse, oblique, or comminuted fracture, or (2) an indirect twisting force that results in a spiral fracture. The nerves and brachial blood vessels may be injured with these fractures. Wrist drop is indicative of radial nerve injury. Initial neurovascular assessment is essential to identify nerve or blood vessel injury, which requires immediate attention.

FIGURE 69-5 Fracture of the clavicle. (**A**) Anteroposterior view shows typical displacement in midclavicular fracture. (**B**) Immobilization is accomplished with a clavicular strap.

FIGURE 69-6 Exercises that promote shoulder range of motion include (**A**) pendulum exercise and (**B**) wall climbing. The unaffected arm is used to assist with (**C**) internal rotation, (**D**) external rotation, and (**E**) elevation. In C, D, and E, the unaffected arm is used for power.

Medical Management

Initially, well-padded splints, overwrapped with an elastic bandage, are used to immobilize the upper arm and to support the arm in 90 degrees of flexion at the elbow. A sling or collar and cuff support the forearm. The weight of the hanging arm and splints reduce the

fracture. External fixators are used to treat open fractures of the humeral shaft (see Chapter 67). Open reduction with internal fixation of a fracture of the humerus is necessary with nerve palsy, blood vessel damage, comminuted fracture, or pathologic fracture.

Functional bracing is another form of treatment used for these fractures. A contoured thermoplastic sleeve is secured in

FIGURE 69-7 Immobilizers for proximal humeral fractures. (**A**) Commercial sling with immobilizing strap permits easy removal for hygiene and is comfortable on the neck. (**B**) Conventional sling and swathe. (**C**) Stockinette Velpeau and swathe are used when there is an unstable surgical neck component. This position relaxes the pectoralis major.

FIGURE 69-8   Functional humeral brace with collar and cuff sling.

place with interlocking fabric (Velcro) closures around the upper arm, immobilizing the reduced fracture. As swelling decreases, the sleeve is tightened, and uniform pressure and stability are applied to the fracture. The forearm is supported with a collar and cuff sling (Fig. 69-8). Functional bracing allows active use of muscles, shoulder and elbow motion, and good approximation of fracture fragments. Pendulum shoulder exercises are performed as prescribed to provide active movement of the shoulder, thereby preventing adhesions of the shoulder joint capsule. Isometric exercises may be prescribed to prevent muscle atrophy. The callus that develops is substantial, and the sleeve can be discontinued in about 8 weeks. Complications that are seen with humeral shaft fractures include delayed union and nonunion.

ELBOW

Fractures of the distal humerus result from motor vehicle crashes, falls on the elbow (in the extended or flexed position), or a direct blow. These fractures may result in injury to the median, radial, or ulnar nerves.

The patient is evaluated for paresthesia and signs of compromised circulation in the forearm and hand. The most serious complication of a supracondylar fracture of the humerus is Volkmann's ischemic contracture (a compartment syndrome), which results from antecubital swelling or damage to the brachial artery (Chart 69-4). The nurse needs to monitor the patient regularly for compromised neurovascular status and signs of compartment syndrome.

Chart 69-4	**Volkmann's Contracture**

- Observe the distal extremity for swelling, skin colour, nail bed capillary refill, and temperature. Compare affected and unaffected hands.
- Assess radial pulse.
- Assess for paresthesia (tingling and burning sensations) in the hand, which may indicate nerve injury or impending ischemia.
- Evaluate the patient's ability to move the fingers.
- Explore the intensity and character of the pain.
- Directly measure tissue pressure as prescribed.
- Report indications of diminished nerve function or diminished circulatory perfusion promptly before irreparable damage occurs; fasciotomy may become necessary.

Other potential complications are damage to the joint articular surfaces and hemarthrosis (blood in the joint). If hemarthrosis is present, the physician may aspirate the joint to remove the blood, thereby relieving the pressure and pain.

Management

The goal of therapy is prompt reduction and stabilization of the distal humerus fracture, followed by controlled active motion after swelling has subsided and healing has begun. If the fracture is not displaced, the arm is immobilized in a cast or posterior splint with the elbow at 45 to 90 degrees of flexion and in a sling for 4 to 6 weeks. Then a thermoplastic splint is used to support the fracture and rehabilitation exercises are begun.

Usually, a displaced fracture is treated with open reduction and internal fixation. Excision of bone fragments may be necessary. Additional external support with a splint is then applied. Active finger exercises are encouraged. Gentle ROM exercise of the injured joint is begun about 1 week after internal fixation. Motion promotes healing of injured joints by producing movement of synovial fluid into the articular cartilage. Active exercise of the elbow is performed as prescribed to prevent residual limitation of motion.

RADIAL HEAD

Radial head fractures are common and are usually produced by a fall on the outstretched hand with the elbow extended.

Management

If blood has collected in the elbow joint (hemarthrosis), it is aspirated to relieve pain and to allow early active elbow and forearm ROM. Immobilization for these undisplaced fractures is accomplished with a splint. The patient is instructed not to lift with the arm for approximately 4 weeks. If the fracture is displaced, surgery is required, with excision of the radial head when necessary. Postoperatively, the arm is immobilized in a posterior plaster splint and sling. The patient is encouraged to carry out a program of active motion of the elbow and forearm when prescribed.

RADIAL AND ULNAR SHAFTS

Fractures of the shaft of the bones of the forearm occur most frequently in children. The radius or the ulna may be fractured at any level. Frequently, displacement occurs when both bones are broken. The forearm's unique functions of pronation and supination must be preserved with good anatomic position and alignment.

Management

If the fragments are not displaced, the fracture is treated by closed reduction with a long arm cast applied from the upper arm to the proximal palmar crease. A loop may be incorporated in the cast near the elbow and a sling pulled through it to prevent the cast from sagging against the forearm.

The circulation, motion, and sensation of the hand are assessed after the cast is applied. The arm is elevated to control edema. Frequent finger flexion and extension are encouraged to reduce edema. Active motion of the involved shoulder is essential. The reduction and alignment are monitored closely by x-rays to ensure adequate immobilization. The fracture is immobilized for about 12 weeks; during the last 6 weeks, the arm may be in a functional forearm brace that allows exercise of the wrist and elbow. Lifting and twisting are avoided.

Displaced fractures are managed by open reduction with internal fixation, using a compression plate with screws, intramedullary nails, or rods. The arm is usually immobilized in a plaster splint or cast. Open fractures may be managed with external fixation devices. The arm is elevated to control swelling. Neurovascular status is monitored. Elbow, wrist, and hand exercises are begun as permitted by the immobilization device.

WRIST

Fractures of the distal radius (Colles' fracture) are common and are usually the result of a fall on an open, dorsiflexed hand. This fracture is frequently seen in elderly women with osteoporotic bones and weak soft tissues that do not dissipate the energy of the fall. The patient presents with a deformed wrist, radial deviation, pain, swelling, weakness, limited finger ROM, and numbness.

Management

Treatment usually consists of closed reduction and immobilization with a short arm cast. For fractures with extensive comminution or impaction, open reduction and internal fixation, arthroscopic percutaneous pinning, or external fixation is used to achieve and maintain reduction and to allow for early functional rehabilitation. The wrist and forearm are elevated for 48 hours after reduction to control swelling.

Active motion of the fingers and shoulder should begin promptly. The patient is taught to do the following exercises to reduce swelling and prevent stiffness:

- Hold the hand at the level of the heart.
- Move the fingers from full extension to flexion. Hold and release. (Repeat at least 10 times every hour when awake.)
- Use the hand in functional activities.
- Actively exercise the shoulder and elbow, including complete ROM exercises of both joints.

NURSING RESEARCH PROFILE 69-1
Self-Reported Impact of Wrist Fracture

Morris, N. (2000). Distal radius fracture in adults: Self-reported physical functioning, role functioning, and meaning of injury. *Orthopaedic Nursing, 19*(4), 37–48.

Purpose
Distal radius fracture commonly affects women and their activities of daily living, work productivity, and overall functioning. Having a better understanding of the impact of this injury will enable the nurse to more effectively provide direct care and respond to specific needs of the patient and family.

This study explored (1) differences in physical function, role function, and meaning of injury during the first 3 months of recovery from distal radius fracture; (2) the relationships of age, gender, hand dominance, education, preinjury physical health, and treatment modality to differences in physical function, role function, and meaning of injury; and (3) differences in the patterns of change over time.

Study Sample and Design
A descriptive, prospective, repeated measures design was used to study adults who had sustained fractures of the distal radius. A convenience sample of 60 adults with distal radius fracture completed the study. Seventy-two percent of the subjects were women, and 28% were men. Forty-eight percent were young adults (18 to 44 years of age), 27% were middle-age adults (45 to 64 years), and 25% were older adults (65 to 87 years). Forty-five percent of the subjects were college graduates. Treatment modalities were a surgical approach (53%) and a nonsurgical approach (47%).

Data were collected at the first office visit after fracture, at removal of the immobilizing device, and at the next office visit after device removal.

Several instruments were used to measure the dependent variables of physical function, role function, and meaning of illness/injury (MOI). The relationships of gender, age, education, hand dominance, preinjury physical health, and treatment modality to these dependent variables were analyzed.

Descriptive and inferential statistics were used to analyze the data.

Results
- Over time, there was an improvement in physical function and role function for all subjects. Dependency on others for help with daily activities and injury interference with work and social activities decreased over time.
- Physical function and role function were found to be significantly better among the younger adults ($p < .001$). Middle-age adults experienced greater emotional problems that interfered with work and other daily activities until the immobilizing device was removed. The lower role function observed in middle-age adults may be explained by the multiple demands placed on this age group. The younger and older adults may have had fewer demands on their time. A greater ability to work was observed among those subjects with a higher-level education; they may have had more resources, greater problem-solving abilities, and occupations in which they could work to some extent while their arm was immobilized. Overall, physical function and role function were not affected by gender, hand dominance, education, preinjury physical health, or treatment modality.
- There was a significant change in the MOI score with removal of the immobilization device. This finding suggested that patients were able to acknowledge the disruption and reframe their current situation. There was no significant change in MOI score after this time point.

Nursing Implications
The nurse needs to assess the patient's need for assistance for 6 to 8 weeks while the arm is immobilized. Older adults need greater assistance in meeting self-care needs. Younger adults need less help to perform daily activities while the wrist is immobilized. Middle-age adults may have greater problems in dealing with their usual multiple demands.

The fingers may swell due to diminished venous and lymphatic return. The nurse assesses the sensory function of the median nerve by pricking the distal aspect of the index finger. The motor function is assessed by the patient's ability to touch the thumb to the little finger. Diminished circulation and nerve function must be treated promptly by release of constricting bandages.

HAND

Trauma to the hand often requires extensive reconstructive surgery. The objective of treatment is always to regain maximum function of the hand.

Management

For an undisplaced fracture of the phalanx (finger bone), the finger is splinted for 3 to 4 weeks to relieve pain and to protect the finger from further trauma. Displaced fractures and open fractures may require open reduction with internal fixation, using wires or pins.

The neurovascular status of the injured hand is evaluated. Swelling is controlled by elevation of the hand. Functional use of the uninvolved portion of the hand is encouraged.

PELVIS

The sacrum, ilium, pubis, and ischium bones form the pelvic bone, a fused, stable, bony ring in adults (Fig. 69-9). Falls, motor vehicle crashes, and crush injuries can cause pelvic fractures. Pelvic fractures are serious because at least two thirds of affected patients have significant and multiple injuries. Management of severe, life-threatening pelvic fractures is coordinated with the trauma team. Hemorrhage and thoracic, intra-abdominal, and cranial injuries have priority over treatment of fractures. There is a high mortality rate associated with pelvic fractures, related to hemorrhage, pulmonary complications, fat emboli, intravascular coagulation, thromboembolic complications, and infection.

Pelvic fracture symptoms include ecchymosis; tenderness over the symphysis pubis, anterior iliac spines, iliac crest, sacrum, or coccyx; local swelling; numbness or tingling of pubis, genitals, and proximal thighs; and inability to bear weight without dis-

comfort. Computed tomography of the pelvis helps to determine the extent of injury by demonstrating sacroiliac joint disruption, soft tissue trauma, pelvic hematoma, and fractures. Neurovascular assessment of the lower extremities is completed to detect injury to pelvic blood vessels and nerves.

Hemorrhage and shock are two of the most serious consequences that may occur. Bleeding arises from the cancellous surfaces of the fracture fragments, from laceration of veins and arteries by bone fragments, and possibly from a torn iliac artery. The peripheral pulses of both lower extremities are palpated; absence of pulses may indicate a torn iliac artery or one of its branches. Peritoneal lavage may be performed to detect intra-abdominal hemorrhage. The patient is handled gently to minimize further bleeding and shock.

The nurse assesses for injuries to the bladder, rectum, intestines, other abdominal organs, and pelvic vessels and nerves. To assess for urinary tract injury, the patient's urine is examined for blood. A voiding cystourethrogram and an intravenous urogram may be performed. Laceration of the urethra is suspected in males with anterior fracture of the pelvis and blood at the urethral meatus. (Females rarely experience a lacerated urethra.) A catheter should not be inserted until the status of the urethra is known. Abdominal pain and signs of peritonitis suggest injury to the intestines or abdominal bleeding. Paralytic ileus may accompany pelvic fractures.

Numerous classification systems have been used to describe pelvic fractures in relation to anatomy, stability, and mechanism of injury. Some fractures of the pelvis do not disrupt the pelvic ring; others disrupt the ring, which may be rotationally or vertically unstable. The severity of pelvic fractures varies. Long-term complications of pelvic fractures include malunion, nonunion, residual gait disturbances, and back pain from ligament injury.

Stable Pelvic Fractures

Stable fractures of the pelvis (Fig. 69-10) include fracture of a single pubic or ischial ramus, fracture of ipsilateral pubic and ischial rami, fracture of the pelvic wing of ilium (ie, Duverney's fracture), and fracture of the sacrum or coccyx. Also, if injury results in only a slight widening of the pubic symphysis or the anterior sacroiliac joint and the pelvic ligaments are intact, the disrupted pubic symphysis is likely to heal spontaneously with conservative manage-

FIGURE 69-9 Pelvic bones.

Pelvic wing
(Duverney's)
fracture

Sacral fracture

Simple pubic
ramus fracture

Ipsilateral fractures of
pubic and ischial rami

FIGURE 69-10 Stable pelvic fractures.

ment. Most fractures of the pelvis heal rapidly because the pelvic bones are mostly cancellous bone, which has a rich blood supply.

Stable pelvic fractures are treated with a few days of bed rest and symptom management until the pain and discomfort are controlled. The patient on bed rest is at risk for complications from immobility, including constipation, venous stasis, and pulmonary complications. Fluids, dietary fibre, ankle and leg exercises, elastic compression stockings to aid venous return, log rolling, coughing and deep breathing, and skin care reduce the risk for complications and increase the patient's comfort. The patient with a fractured sacrum is at risk for paralytic ileus, and bowel sounds should be monitored.

The patient with fracture of the coccyx experiences pain on sitting and with defecation. Sitz baths may be prescribed to relieve pain, and stool softeners may be given to prevent the need

to strain on defecation. As pain resolves, activity is gradually resumed with the use of ambulatory aids (eg, crutches, walker) for protected weight bearing. Early mobilization reduces problems related to immobility.

Unstable Pelvic Fractures

Unstable fractures of the pelvis (Fig. 69-11) may result in rotational instability (eg, the open book type, in which a separation occurs at the symphysis pubis with some sacral ligament disruption), vertical instability (eg, the vertical shear type, with superior–inferior displacement), or a combination of both. Lateral or anterior–posterior compression of the pelvis produces rotationally unstable pelvic fractures. Vertically unstable pelvic fractures occur when force is exerted on the pelvis vertically, as when the person falls from a height onto extended legs or is struck from above by a falling object. Vertical shear pelvic fractures involve the anterior and posterior pelvic ring with vertical displacement, usually through the sacroiliac joint. There is generally complete disruption of the posterior sacroiliac, sacrospinous, and sacrotuberous ligaments. Vertical displacement of the hemipelvis is usually evident.

Treatment of unstable pelvic fractures generally involves external fixation or open reduction and internal fixation. This promotes hemostasis, hemodynamic stability, comfort, and early mobilization.

Acetabulum

Fractures of the acetabulum are seen after motor vehicle crashes in which the femur is jammed into the dashboard. Treatment depends on the pattern of fracture. Stable, nondisplaced fractures and fractures that involve minimal articular weight bearing may be managed with traction and protective (toe touch) weight bearing. Displaced and unstable acetabular fractures are treated with open reduction, joint débridement, and internal fixation or arthroplasty. Internal fixation permits early non–weight-bearing ambulation and ROM exercise. Complications seen with acetabular fractures include nerve palsy, heterotopic ossification, and posttraumatic arthritis.

FEMUR

There is a high incidence of hip fracture among elderly people, who have brittle bones from osteoporosis (particularly women) and who tend to fall frequently. Weak quadriceps muscles, gen-

FIGURE 69-11 Unstable pelvic fracture. (**A**) Rotationally unstable fracture: The symphysis pubis is separated and the anterior sacroiliac, sacrotuberous, and sacrospinous ligaments are disrupted. (**B**) Vertically unstable fracture: The hemipelvis is displaced anteriorly and posteriorly through the symphysis pubis, and the sacroiliac joint ligaments are disrupted. (**C**) Undisplaced fracture of the acetabulum.

eral frailty due to age, and conditions that produce decreased cerebral arterial perfusion (transient ischemic attacks, anemia, emboli, cardiovascular disease, effects of medications) contribute to the incidence of falls. The patient who has sustained a hip fracture frequently has a comorbidity (eg, cardiovascular, pulmonary, renal, endocrine). Often, a fractured hip is a catastrophic event that will have a negative impact on the patient's lifestyle and quality of life.

There are two major types of hip fracture. *Intracapsular fractures* are fractures of the neck of the femur. *Extracapsular fractures* are fractures of the trochanteric region (between the base of the neck and the lesser trochanter of the femur) and of the subtrochanteric region (Fig. 69-12). Fractures of the neck of the femur may damage the vascular system that supplies blood to the head and the neck of the femur, and the bone may die. For this reason, nonunion or aseptic necrosis is common in patients with femoral neck fractures.

Extracapsular intertrochanteric fractures have an excellent blood supply and heal readily. However, extensive soft tissue damage

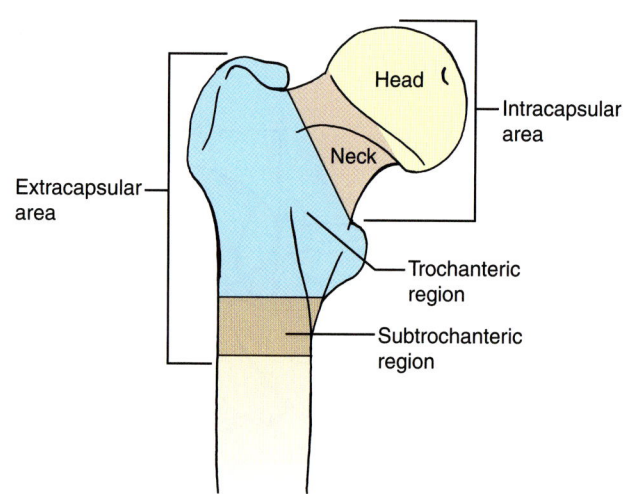

FIGURE 69-12 Regions of the proximal femur.

NURSING RESEARCH PROFILE 69-2
Hip Surgery, Postoperative Pain, and Recovery

Feldt, K., & Oh, H. (2000). Pain and hip fracture outcomes for older adults. *Orthopaedic Nursing, 19*(6), 35–44.

Purpose
Many older adults experience hip fracture. Several factors (eg, age, prefracture functioning, mental status) have been identified as having an effect on functional outcome after surgery. This study focused on postoperative pain as a possible predictor of functional outcome at 2 months after surgery.

Study Sample and Design
A convenience sample of 85 patients, age 65 years or older, who were hospitalized for hip fracture and treated surgically with reduction achieved by screws or pins or with a joint prosthesis, was studied. All patients were able to walk independently (with or without ambulatory aid) before fracture. Almost all of the patients were female (90.6%); most were admitted from home (76.5%) and had used no ambulatory aid (60%).

This descriptive, comparative study included a patient interview on postoperative day 2 or 3 and a second interview at 2 months after surgery to determine functional outcomes.

Variables included demographics, mental status, pain assessment and report, use of analgesics, illness severity (ie, comorbidities, complications), and functional status/dependency as measured by the Functional Status Index.

Results
- Almost half of the patients were identified as cognitively impaired based on the Mini Mental State Examination. These patients were older and had a higher illness severity score.
- Almost two thirds of the patients reported that they had pain. However, significantly more of the cognitively intact patients, compared with cognitively impaired patients (71.1% versus 48.6%, respectively; $p < .05$) responded "Yes" to the question, "Do you have pain?" This finding may suggest that cognitively impaired patients do not remember intermittent pain experienced with movement. When patients were asked to describe their pain, many subjects noted hip pain as well as pain from other sources (eg, osteoarthritis). Comparison of pain at rest and pain with movement was statistically significant

($p < .0001$) for both cognitively intact and cognitively impaired patients.
- There was no difference between cognitively intact and cognitively impaired groups regarding prescribed analgesics and administered analgesics. However, nurses administered less than 25% of the prescribed prn medications to both groups. The study also identified that the mean amount of acetaminophen prescribed was well above the recommended guidelines. Patients were prescribed prn opioid/acetaminophen combination medications as well as prn acetaminophen.
- Functional status declined for patients after hip fracture. Preoperatively, 64% of the cognitively intact patients and 54% of the cognitively impaired patients could walk without any assistive devices; postoperatively, only 29% and 5%, respectively, were able to ambulate without assistive devices. At 2 months after surgery, functional status scores were lower for the cognitively impaired group.
- Stepwise regression analysis showed that age, mental status, illness severity, and report of pain with movement explained 51% of the variance in functional score. Pain with movement accounted for 8% of this variance.

Nursing Implications
Postoperative pain with movement affects functional outcomes for patients with hip fracture. Better management of postoperative pain is required for better functional outcomes.

Pain reported by patients with hip fracture may be intermittent and may be caused by problems other than the hip fracture and surgery (eg, osteoarthritis). Most pain assessments are performed with the patient at rest; however, pain is more intense with movement. Managing pain associated with movement and administering pain medication before moving and before physical therapy sessions may help to improve the outcome.

In addition, the nurse should be aware of the amount of acetaminophen in combination medications and should monitor patients, especially those with liver dysfunction, for intake of acetaminophen that exceeds the recommended maximum daily dose.

may have occurred at the time of injury. It is not uncommon for the fracture to be comminuted and unstable. There is a fairly high mortality rate after intertrochanteric hip fractures, mainly because the patients are usually elderly (70 to 85 years of age) and are poor surgical candidates.

Clinical Manifestations

With fractures of the femoral neck, the leg is shortened, adducted, and externally rotated. The patient complains of pain in the hip and groin or in the medial side of the knee. With most fractures of the femoral neck, the patient is unable to move the leg without a significant increase in pain. The patient is most comfortable with the leg slightly flexed in external rotation. Impacted intracapsular femoral neck fractures cause moderate discomfort (even with movement), may allow the patient to bear weight, and may not demonstrate obvious shortening or rotational changes. With extracapsular femoral fractures of the trochanteric or subtrochanteric regions, the extremity is significantly shortened, externally rotated to a greater degree than intracapsular fractures, exhibits muscle spasm that resists positioning of the extremity in a neutral position, and has an associated large hematoma or area of ecchymosis. The diagnosis of fractured hip is confirmed with x-ray.

Gerontologic Considerations

Hip fractures are a frequent contributor to death after the age of 75 years. Stress and immobility related to the trauma predispose the older adult to pneumonia, sepsis, and reduced ability to cope with other health problems.

Many elderly people hospitalized with hip fracture are confused as a result of the stress of the trauma, unfamiliar surroundings, sleep deprivation, medications, and systemic illness. Preoperative predictors of postoperative delirium include age older than 70 years, alcohol abuse, impaired cognitive status, poor functional status, and markedly abnormal serum sodium, potassium, or glucose concentrations. In addition, confusion that develops in some elderly patients may be caused by mild cerebral ischemia. Other factors associated with confusion include responses to medications and anesthesia, malnutrition, dehydration, infectious processes, mood disturbances, and blood loss.

To prevent complications, the nurse must assess the elderly patient for chronic conditions that require close monitoring. Examination of the legs may reveal edema due to heart failure or peripheral pulselessness from arteriosclerotic vascular disease. Similarly, chronic respiratory problems may be present and may contribute to the possible development of inadequate pulmonary ventilation. Coughing and deep-breathing exercises are encouraged. Frequently, elderly people are taking cardiac, antihypertensive, or respiratory medications that need to be continued. The patient's responses to these medications should be monitored.

Dehydration and poor nutrition may be present. At times, elderly people who live alone are unable to summon help at the time of injury. A day or two may pass before assistance is provided, and as a result, dehydration occurs. Dehydration contributes to hemoconcentration and predisposes to thromboembolism. Therefore, the patient needs to be encouraged to consume adequate fluids and a healthy diet.

Muscle weakness and wasting may have contributed to the fall and fracture in the first place. Bed rest and immobility will cause an additional loss of muscle strength unless the nurse encourages the patient to move all joints except the involved hip and knee. Patients are encouraged to use their arms and the overhead trapeze to reposition themselves. This strengthens the arms and shoulders, which facilitates walking with assistive devices.

Medical Management

Temporary skin traction, Buck's extension, may be applied to reduce muscle spasm, to immobilize the extremity, and to relieve pain. The findings of a recent study (Jerre et al., 2000) suggested that there is no benefit to the routine use of preoperative skin traction for patients with hip fractures and that the use of skin traction should be based on evaluation of the individual patient.

The goal of surgical treatment of hip fractures is to obtain a satisfactory fixation so that the patient can be mobilized quickly and avoid secondary medical complications. Surgical treatment consists of (1) open or closed reduction of the fracture and internal fixation, (2) replacement of the femoral head with a prosthesis (hemiarthroplasty), or (3) closed reduction with percutaneous stabilization for an intracapsular fracture. Surgical intervention is carried out as soon as possible after injury. The preoperative objective is to ensure that the patient is in as favourable a condition as possible for the surgery. Displaced femoral neck fractures may be treated as emergencies, with reduction and internal fixation performed within 12 to 24 hours after fracture. This minimizes the effects of diminished blood supply and reduces the risk for avascular necrosis.

After general or spinal anesthesia, the hip fracture is reduced under x-ray visualization using an image intensifier. A stable fracture is usually fixed with nails, a nail-and-plate combination, multiple pins, or compression screw devices (Fig. 69-13). The orthopedic surgeon determines the specific fixation device based on the fracture site or sites. Adequate reduction is important for fracture healing (the better the reduction, the better the healing).

Hemiarthroplasty (replacement of the head of the femur with a prosthesis) is usually reserved for fractures that cannot be satisfactorily reduced or securely nailed or to avoid complications of nonunion and avascular necrosis of the head of the femur. Total hip replacement (see Chap. 67) may be used in selected patients with acetabular defects.

Postoperative Nursing Management

The immediate postoperative care for a patient with a hip fracture is similar to that for other patients undergoing major surgery (see Care of the Patient Undergoing Orthopedic Surgery in Chap. 20 and Chap. 67). Attention is given to pain management, prevention of secondary medical problems, and early mobilization of the patient so that independent functioning can be restored.

During the first 24 to 48 hours, relief of pain and prevention of complications are priorities. The nurse encourages deep breathing, coughing, and foot flexion exercises every 1 to 2 hours. Thigh-high elastic compression stockings and pneumatic compression devices are used to prevent venous stasis. The nurse administers prescribed intravenous prophylactic antibiotics and monitors the patient's hydration, nutritional status, and urine output. A pillow is placed between the legs to maintain abduction and alignment and to provide needed support when turning the patient.

REPOSITIONING THE PATIENT

The nurse may turn the patient onto the affected or unaffected extremity as prescribed by the physician. The standard method involves placing a pillow between the patient's legs to keep the affected leg in an abducted position. The patient is then turned

Unit 15 MUSCULOSKELETAL FUNCTION

Cannulated screw
fixation

Compression hip screw
and side plate

Blade plate
fixation

FIGURE 69-13 Examples of internal fixation for hip fractures. Internal fixation is achieved through the use of screws and plates specifically designed for stability and fixation.

onto the side while proper alignment and supported abduction are maintained.

PROMOTING STRENGTHENING EXERCISE

The patient is encouraged to exercise as much as possible by means of the overbed trapeze. This device helps strengthen the arms and shoulders in preparation for protected ambulation (eg, toe touch, partial weight bearing). On the first postoperative day, the patient transfers to a chair with assistance and begins assisted ambulation. The amount of weight bearing that can be permitted depends on the stability of the fracture reduction. The physician prescribes the degree of weight bearing and the rate at which the patient can progress to full weight bearing. Physical therapists work with the patient on transfers, ambulation, and the safe use of a walker and crutches.

The patient who has experienced a fractured hip can anticipate discharge to home or to an extended care facility with the use of an ambulatory aid. Some modifications in the home may be needed to permit safe use of walkers and crutches and for the patient's continuing care.

MONITORING AND MANAGING POTENTIAL COMPLICATIONS

Elderly people with hip fractures are particularly prone to complications that may require more vigourous treatment than the fracture. In some instances, shock proves fatal. Achievement of homeostasis after injury and after surgery is accomplished through careful monitoring and collaborative management, including adjustment of therapeutic interventions as indicated.

Neurovascular complications may occur from direct injury to nerves and blood vessels or from increased tissue pressure. With hip fracture, bleeding into the tissues is expected. Excessive swelling may be observed. Therefore, the nurse must monitor the neurovascular status of the affected leg.

Deep vein thrombosis is the most common complication. To prevent DVT, the nurse encourages intake of fluids and ankle and foot exercises. Elastic compression stockings, sequential compression devices, and prophylactic anticoagulant therapy may be prescribed. The nurse assesses the patient's legs at least every 4 hours for signs of DVT.

Pulmonary complications are a threat to elderly patients undergoing hip surgery. Deep-breathing exercises, a change of position at least every 2 hours, and the use of an incentive spirometer help to prevent respiratory complications. The nurse assesses breath sounds at least every 4 to 8 hours to detect adventitious or diminished sounds.

Skin breakdown is often seen in elderly patients with hip fracture. Blisters caused by tape are related to the tension of soft tissue edema under the nonelastic tape. An elastic hip spica wrap dressing (Fig. 69-14) or elastic tape applied in a vertical fashion may reduce the incidence of tape blisters. In addition, patients with hip fractures tend to remain in one position and may develop *pressure ulcers*. Proper skin care, especially on the heels, back, sacrum, and shoulders, helps to relieve pressure. High-density foam, static air, or another type of special mattress may provide protection by distributing pressure more evenly.

Loss of bladder control (incontinence) may occur. In general, the routine use of an indwelling catheter is avoided because of the high risk for urinary tract infection. If a catheter is inserted at the time of surgery, it usually is removed on the morning of the first postoperative day. Because urinary retention is common after surgery, the nurse must assess the patient's voiding patterns. To ensure proper urinary tract function, the nurse encourages liberal fluid intake within the cardiovascular tolerance of the patient.

Delayed complications of hip fractures include infection, nonunion, avascular necrosis of the femoral head (particularly with femoral neck fractures), and fixation device problems (eg, protrusion of the fixation device through the acetabulum, loosening of hardware). Infection is suspected if the patient complains of persistent, moderate discomfort in the hip and has a mildly elevated sedimentation rate. The nursing management of the elderly patient with a hip fracture is summarized in the Plan of Nursing Care.

FIGURE 69-14 Patient using commercial single-piece stretch spica wrap.

HEALTH PROMOTION

Osteoporosis screening of patients who have experienced hip fracture is important for prevention of future fractures. With dual-energy x-ray absorptiometry (DEXA) scan screening, the actual risk for additional fracture can be determined. Specific patient education regarding dietary requirements, lifestyle changes, and exercise to promote bone health is needed. Specific therapeutic interventions need to be initiated to retard additional bone loss and to build bone mineral density. Studies have shown that health care providers caring for patients with hip fractures fail to diagnose or treat these patients for osteoporosis despite the high probability that hip fractures are secondary to osteoporosis (Kamel, et al., 2000). Fall prevention is also important and may be achieved through exercises to improve muscle tone and balance and through the elimination of environmental hazards. In addition, the use of hip protectors that absorb or shunt impact forces may help to prevent an additional hip fracture if the patient were to fall.

FEMORAL SHAFT

Considerable force is required to break the shaft of the femur in adults. Most femoral fractures are seen in young adults who have been involved in a motor vehicle crash or who have fallen from a high place. Frequently, these patients have associated multiple traumas.

The patient presents with an enlarged, deformed, painful thigh and cannot move the hip or the knee. The fracture may be transverse, oblique, spiral, or comminuted. Frequently, the patient de-

velops shock, because the loss of 2 to 3 units of blood into the tissues is common with these fractures. An expanding diameter of the thigh may indicate continued bleeding. Refer to Figure 69-15A for the types of femoral fractures.

Assessment and Diagnostic Findings

Assessment includes checking the neurovascular status of the extremity, especially circulatory perfusion of the lower leg and foot (popliteal, posterior tibial, and pedal pulses and toe capillary refill time). A Doppler ultrasound monitoring device may be needed to assess blood flow. Dislocation of the hip and knee may accompany these fractures. Knee effusion suggests ligament damage and possible instability of the knee joint.

Medical Management

Continued neurovascular monitoring is needed. The fracture is immobilized so that additional soft tissue damage does not occur. Generally, skeletal traction (Fig. 69-15 B and C) or splinting is used to immobilize fracture fragments until the patient is physiologically stable and ready for open reduction and internal fixation procedures.

Internal fixation usually is carried out within a few days after injury. Intramedullary locking nail devices are used for midshaft (diaphyseal) fractures. Depending on the supracondylar fracture pattern, intramedullary nailing or screw plate fixation may be used. Internal fixation permits early mobilization. A thigh cuff orthosis may be used for external support. To preserve muscle strength, the patient is instructed to exercise the lower leg, foot, toes, and hip on a regular basis. Active muscle movement enhances healing by increasing blood supply and electrical potentials at the fracture site. Prescribed weight-bearing limits are based on the fracture pattern. Physical therapy includes ROM and strengthening exercises, safe use of ambulatory aids, and gait training. Functional ambulation stimulates fracture healing. Healing time is 4 to 6 months.

Compression plates and intramedullary nails may need to be removed after 12 to 18 months due to reaction or loosening. After plates are being removed, a thigh cuff orthosis is used for several months to provide support while bone remodeling occurs.

Infrequently, because of patient risks associated with anesthesia and surgery, middle shaft and distal (supracondylar) fractures may be managed with skeletal traction. Between 2 and 4 weeks after injury, when pain and swelling have subsided, the patient is removed from skeletal traction and placed in a cast brace. The cast brace is a total contact device (ie, encircles the limb) and holds the reduced fracture. The muscle, through hydrodynamic compression, stabilizes the bone and stimulates healing. Minimal partial weight bearing is begun and is progressed to full weight bearing as tolerated. The cast brace is worn for 12 to 14 weeks.

An external fixator may be used if the patient has experienced an open fracture, has extensive soft tissue trauma, has lost bone, has an infection, or has hip and tibial fractures.

A common complication after fracture of the femoral shaft is restriction of knee motion. Active and passive knee exercises begin as soon as possible, depending on the management approach and the stability of the fracture and knee ligaments. Other complications include malunion, delayed union or nonunion, pudendal nerve palsy, and infection.

(text continues on page 2113)

Plan of Nursing Care
Care of the Elderly Patient With a Fractured Hip

Nursing Interventions	Rationale	Expected Outcomes

Nursing Diagnosis: Acute pain related to fracture, soft tissue damage, muscle spasm, and surgery
Goal: Relief of pain

Nursing Interventions	Rationale	Expected Outcomes
1. Assess type and location of patient's pain.	1. Pain is expected after fracture; soft tissue damage and muscle spasm contribute to discomfort; pain is subjective and is evaluated through description of characteristics and location, which are important for determining cause of discomfort and for proposing interventions. Continuing pain may indicate development of neurovascular problems.	• Patient describes discomfort • Expresses confidence in efforts to control pain • Expresses little discomfort with position changes • Expresses comfort when leg is positioned and immobilized • Minimizes movement of extremity before reduction and fixation
2. Acknowledge existence of pain; inform patient of available analgesics; record patient's baseline discomfort.	2. Reduces stress experienced by the patient by communicating concern and availability of help in dealing with pain. Documentation provides baseline data.	• Uses physical, psychological, and pharmacologic measures to reduce discomfort • Describes a decrease in pain in 24–48 hours after surgery
3. Handle the affected extremity gently, supporting it with hands or pillow.	3. Movement of bone fragments is painful; muscle spasms occur with movement; adequate support diminishes soft tissue tension.	• Requests pain medications and uses pain relief measures early in pain cycle • States that positioning provides comfort • Appears comfortable and relaxed
4. Apply Buck's traction as prescribed. Use trochanter roll.	4. Immobilizes fracture to decrease pain, muscle spasm, and external rotation of hip.	• Moves with increasing comfort as healing progresses
5. Use pain-modifying strategies.	5. Pain perception can be diminished by distraction and refocusing of attention.	
a. Modify the environment.	a. Interaction with others, distraction, and environmental stimuli may modify pain experiences.	
b. Administer prescribed analgesics as needed.	b. Analgesics reduce the pain; muscle relaxants may be prescribed to decrease discomfort associated with muscle spasm.	
c. Encourage patient to use pain relief measures before pain is "unbearable."	c. Mild pain is easier to control than severe pain.	
d. Evaluate patient's response to medications and other pain-reduction techniques.	d. Assessment of effectiveness of measures provides basis for future management interventions; early identification of adverse reactions is necessary for corrective measures and care plan modifications.	
e. Consult with physician if relief of pain is not obtained.	e. Change in treatment plan may be necessary.	
6. Position for comfort and function.	6. Alignment of body facilitates comfort; positioning for function diminishes stress on musculoskeletal system.	
7. Assist with frequent changes in position.	7. Change of position relieves pressure and associated discomfort.	

Nursing Diagnosis: Impaired physical mobility related to fractured hip
Goal: Achieves pain-free, functional, stable hip

Nursing Interventions	Rationale	Expected Outcomes
1. Maintain neutral positioning of hip.	1. Prevents stress on fixation.	• Patient engages in therapeutic positioning
2. Use trochanter roll.	2. Minimizes external rotation.	• Uses pillow between legs when turning
3. Place pillow between legs when turning.	3. Supports leg; prevents adduction.	• Assists in position changes; shows increased independence in transfers
4. Instruct and assist in position changes and transfers.	4. Encourages patient's active participation while preventing stress on hip fixation.	• Exercises every 2 hours while awake
5. Instruct in and supervise isometric, quadriceps-setting, and gluteal-setting exercises.	5. Strengthens muscles needed for walking.	• Uses trapeze • Participates in progressive ambulation program

(continued)

Plan of Nursing Care
Care of the Elderly Patient With a Fractured Hip *(Continued)*

Nursing Interventions	Rationale	Expected Outcomes
6. Encourage use of trapeze.	6. Strengthens shoulder and arm muscles necessary for use of ambulatory aids.	• Actively participates in exercise regimen
7. In consultation with physical therapist, instruct in and supervise progressive safe ambulation within limitations of weight-bearing prescription.	7. Amount of weight-bearing depends on the patient's condition, fracture stability, and fixation device; ambulatory aids are used to assist the patient with non–weight-bearing and partial–weight-bearing ambulation.	• Uses ambulatory aids correctly and safely
8. Offer encouragement and support exercise regimen.	8. Reconditioning exercises can be uncomfortable and fatiguing; encouragement helps patient comply with the program.	
9. Instruct in and supervise safe use of ambulatory aids.	9. Prevents injury from unsafe use.	

Nursing Diagnosis: Impaired skin integrity related to surgical incision
Goal: Achieves wound healing

1. Monitor vital signs.	1. Temperature, pulse, and respiration increase in response to infection. (Magnitude of response may be minimal in elderly patients.)	• Patient maintains vital signs within normal range
2. Perform aseptic dressing changes.	2. Avoids introducing infectious organisms.	• Exhibits well-approximated incision without drainage or excessive inflammatory response
3. Assess wound appearance and character of drainage.	3. Red, swollen, draining incision is indicative of infection.	• Relates minimal discomfort; demonstrates no hematoma
4. Assess report of pain.	4. Pain may be due to wound hematoma, a possible locus of infection, which needs to be surgically evacuated.	• Tolerates antibiotics; exhibits no evidence of osteomyelitis
5. Administer prophylactic antibiotic if prescribed, and observe for side effects.	5. Antibiotics reduce the risk for infection.	

Nursing Diagnosis: Risk for impaired urinary elimination related to immobility
Goal: Maintains normal urinary elimination patterns

1. Monitor intake and output.	1. Adequate fluid intake ensures hydration; adequate urinary output minimizes urinary stasis.	• Intake and output are adequate; patient exhibits normal voiding patterns
2. Avoid/minimize use of indwelling catheter.	2. Source of bladder infection.	• Demonstrates no evidence of urinary tract infection
3. Perform intermittent catheterization for urinary retention	3. Empties bladder; reduces urinary tract infections	

Nursing Diagnosis: Risk for ineffective coping related to injury, anticipated surgery, and dependence
Goal: Uses effective coping mechanisms to modify stress

1. Encourage patient to express concerns and to discuss the possible impact of fractured hip.	1. Verbalization helps patient deal with problems and feelings. Clarification of thoughts and feelings promotes problem-solving.	• Patient describes feelings concerning fractured hip and implications for lifestyle
2. Support use of coping mechanisms. Involve significant others and support services as needed.	2. Coping mechanisms modify disabling effects of stress; sharing concerns lessens the burden and facilitates necessary modification.	• Uses available resources and coping mechanisms; develops health promotion strategies
3. Contact social services, if needed.	3. Anxiety may be related to financial or social problems; facilitates management of problems associated with continuing care.	• Uses community resources as needed • Participates in development of health care plan
4. Explain anticipated treatment regimen and routines to facilitate positive attitude in relation to rehabilitation.	4. Understanding of plan of care helps to diminish fears of the unknown.	
5. Encourage patient to participate in planning.	5. Participating in care provides for some control of self and environment.	

(continued)

Plan of Nursing Care

Care of the Elderly Patient With a Fractured Hip (Continued)

Nursing Interventions	Rationale	Expected Outcomes

Nursing Diagnosis: Risk for disturbed thought process related to age, stress of trauma, unfamiliar surroundings, and medication therapy

Goal: Remains oriented and participates in decision making

Nursing Interventions	Rationale	Expected Outcomes
1. Assess orientation status.	1. Evaluate presenting orientation of patient; confusion may result from stress of fracture, unfamiliar surroundings, coexisting systemic disease, cerebral ischemia, or other factors. Baseline data are important for determining change.	• Patient establishes effective communication • Demonstrates orientation to time, place, and person • Participates in self-care activities • Remains mentally alert • Avoids episodes of confusion
2. Interview family regarding patient's orientation and cognitive abilities before injury.	2. Provides data for evaluation of current findings.	
3. Assess patient for auditory and visual deficits.	3. Diminished vision and auditory acuity frequently occur with aging; glasses and hearing aid may increase patient's ability to interact with environment.	

a. Assist patient with use of sensory aids (eg, glasses, hearing aid)
  b. Control environmental distractors
	a. Aids must be in good working order and available for use.
	  b. Facilitates communication.	

4. Orient to and stabilize environment
  a. Use orientation activities and aids (eg, clock, calendar, pictures, introduction of self).
  b. Minimize number of staff working with patient.
	4.
	  a. Short-term memory may be faulty in the elderly; frequent reorientation helps.
	  b. Consistency of caregivers promotes trust.	

5. Give simple explanations of procedures and plan of care.	5. Promotes understanding and active participation.	
6. Encourage participation in hygiene and nutritional activities.	6. Participation in routine activities promotes orientation, increases awareness of self.	

7. Provide for safety.
  a. Keep side rails up when patient is in bed.
  b. Keep light on at night.
  c. Have call bell available.
  d. Provide prompt response to requests for assistance.
	7. Side rails decrease chance for additional injury from falls; mechanism for securing assistance is available to patient; independent activities based on faulty judgment may result in injury.	

8. Assess mental responses to medications, especially sedatives and analgesics.	8. Elderly people tend to be more sensitive to medications; abnormal responses (eg, hallucinations, depression) may occur.	

Collaborative Problems: Hemorrhage; peripheral neurovascular dysfunction; deep vein thrombosis; pulmonary complications; pressure ulcers related to surgery and immobility

Goal: Patient experiences an absence of complications

Hemorrhage

Nursing Interventions	Rationale	Expected Outcomes
1. Monitor vital signs, observing for shock.	1. Changes in pulse, blood pressure, and respirations may indicate development of shock; blood loss and stress may contribute to development of shock.	• Vital signs are stabilized within normal limits • Experiences no excessive or bright red drainage • Exhibits hemoglobin and hematocrit values within normal limits
2. Consider preinjury blood pressure values and management of coexisting hypertension, if present.	2. Necessary for interpretation of current blood pressure determinations.	
3. Note character and amount of drainage.	3. Excessive drainage and bright red drainage may indicate active bleeding.	
4. Notify surgeon if patient develops shock or excessive bleeding.	4. Corrective measures need to be instituted.	
5. Note hemoglobin and hematocrit values, and report decreases in values.	5. Anemia due to blood loss may develop; bleeding into tissues after hip fracture may be extensive; blood replacement may be needed.	

(continued)

Plan of Nursing Care
Care of the Elderly Patient With a Fractured Hip *(Continued)*

Nursing Interventions	Rationale	Expected Outcomes
Pulmonary Complications 1. Assess respiratory status: respiratory rate, depth, and duration, breath sounds, sputum. Monitor temperature. 2. Report adventitious and diminished breath sounds and elevated temperature. 3. Supervise deep breathing and coughing exercises. Encourage use of incentive spirometer if prescribed. 4. Administer oxygen as prescribed. 5. Turn and reposition patient at least every 2 hours. Mobilize patient (assist patient out of bed) as soon as possible. 6. Ensure adequate hydration.	1. Anesthesia and bed rest diminish respiratory effort and cause pooling of respiratory secretions. Adventitious breath sounds, pain on respiration, shortness of breath, blood tinged sputum, cough, etc., indicate pulmonary problems. 2. Elevated temperature in the early postoperative period may be due to a respiratory problem. 3. Promote optimal ventilation. Coexisting respiratory conditions diminish lung expansion. 4. Reduced ventilatory efforts may diminish PaO_2 when patient is on room air. 5. Promotes optimal ventilation. Diminishes pooling of respiratory secretions. 6. Liquefies respiratory secretions. Facilitates expectoration.	• Patient has clear breath sounds • Breath sounds present in all fields • Exhibits no shortness of breath, chest pain, or elevated temperature • PaO_2 on room air within normal limits • Performs respiratory exercises; uses incentive spirometer as instructed • Changes position frequently • Consumes adequate fluids
Peripheral Neurovascular Dysfunction 1. Assess affected extremity for colour and temperature. 2. Assess toes for capillary refill response. 3. Assess affected extremity for edema and swelling. 4. Elevate affected extremity. 5. Assess for deep, throbbing, unrelenting pain. 6. Assess for pain on passive flexion of foot. 7. Assess for sensations and numbness. 8. Assess ability to move foot and toes. 9. Assess pedal pulses in both feet. 10. Notify surgeon if diminished neurovascular status occurs.	1. The skin becomes pale and feels cool with decreased tissue perfusion. Venous congestion may cause cyanosis. 2. After compression of the nail, rapid return of pink colour indicates good capillary perfusion. 3. The trauma of surgery will cause swelling; excessive swelling and hematoma formation can compromise circulation and function; edema may be due to coexisting cardiovascular disease. 4. Minimizes dependent edema. 5. Surgical pain can be controlled; pain due to neurovascular compromise is refractory to treatment with analgesics. 6. With nerve ischemia, there will be pain on passive stretch. 7. Diminished pain and paresthesia may indicate nerve damage. Sensation in web between great and second toe—peroneal nerve; sensation on sole of foot—tibial nerve. 8. Dorsiflexion of ankle and extension of toes indicate function of peroneal nerve. Plantar flexion of ankle and flexion of toes indicate functioning of tibial nerve. 9. Indicates circulatory status of extremities. 10. Function of extremity needs to be preserved.	• Patient has normal colour and the extremity is warm • Demonstrates normal capillary refill response • Exhibits moderate swelling; tissue not palpably tense • States pain is controllable • Reports no pain with passive dorsiflexion • Reports normal sensations and no paresthesia • Demonstrates normal motor abilities and no paresis or paralysis • Has strong and equal pulses
Deep Vein Thrombosis 1. Apply thigh-high elastic compression stockings and/or sequential compression device as prescribed. 2. Remove stockings for 20 minutes twice a day, and provide skin care. 3. Assess popliteal, dorsalis pedis, and posterior tibial pulses.	1. Compression aids venous blood return and prevents stasis. 2. Skin care is necessary to avoid skin breakdown. Extended removal of stocking or device defeats purpose. 3. Pulses indicate arterial perfusion of extremity. With coexisting arteriosclerotic	• Wears thigh-high elastic compression stockings • Uses sequential compression device • Experiences no skin breakdown • Experiences no more warmth than usual in skin areas • Exhibits no increase in calf circumference • Demonstrates a negative Homans' sign

(continued)

Plan of Nursing Care
Care of the Elderly Patient With a Fractured Hip *(Continued)*

Nursing Interventions	Rationale	Expected Outcomes
	vascular disease, pulses may be diminished or absent.	• Changes position with assistance and supervision
4. Assess skin temperature of legs.	4. Local inflammation increases local skin temperature.	• Participates in exercise regimen
5. Assess for Homans' sign every 4 hours.	5. Pain in calf on dorsiflexion of ankle may indicate deep vein thrombosis.	• Experiences no chest pain; has lungs clear to auscultation; presents no evidence of pulmonary emboli
6. Measure calf circumference twice daily.	6. Increased calf circumference indicates edema or altered perfusion.	• Exhibits no signs of dehydration; has normal hematocrit
7. Avoid pressure on popliteal blood vessels from appliances or pillows.	7. Compression of blood vessels diminishes blood flow.	• Maintains normal body temperature
8. Change patient's position and increase activity as prescribed.	8. Activity promotes circulation and diminishes venous stasis.	
9. Supervise ankle exercises hourly while patient is awake.	9. Muscle exercise promotes circulation.	
10. Ensure adequate hydration.	10. Elderly people may become dehydrated because of low fluid intake, resulting in hemoconcentration.	
11. Monitor body temperature.	11. Body temperature increases with inflammation (magnitude of response minimal in elderly people).	
Pressure Ulcers		
1. Monitor condition of skin at pressure points (eg, heels, sacrum, shoulders); inspect heels at least twice a day.	1. Elderly patients are subject to skin breakdown at points of pressure because of diminished subcutaneous tissue.	• Patient exhibits no signs of skin breakdown
2. Reposition patient at least every 2 hours. Avoid skin shearing.	2. Avoids prolonged pressure and trauma to the skin.	• Skin remains intact
3. Administer skin care, especially to pressure points.	3. Immobility causes pressure at bony prominences; position changes relieve pressure.	• Repositions self frequently
4. Use special care mattress and other protective devices (eg, heel protectors); support heel off the mattress.	4. Devices minimize pressure on skin at bony prominences.	• Uses protective devices
5. Institute care according to protocol at first indication of potential skin breakdown.	5. Early interventions prevent tissue destruction and prolonged rehabilitation.	

Nursing Diagnosis: Risk for ineffective health maintenance related to fractured hip and impaired mobility
Goal: Exhibits health maintenance/promotion behaviours

1. Assess home environment for discharge planning.	1. Physical barriers (especially stairs, bathrooms) may limit patient's ability to ambulate and care for self at home.	• Home is accessible for patient at time of discharge
2. Encourage patient to express concerns about care at home; explore with patient possible solutions to problems.	2. Patient may have special problems that need to be identified and dealt with.	• Patient appears relaxed and develops strategies to deal with identified problems
3. Assess availability of physical assistance for ADLs and health care activities.	3. Because of limitation of mobility, patient requires some assistance in ADLs and routine health care.	• Has personal assistance available • Demonstrates ability to use necessary assistance within therapeutic prescription
4. Teach caregiver the home health care regimen.	4. Understanding of rehabilitative regimen is necessary for compliance.	• Complies with home care program; keeps follow-up health care appointments

5. Instruct patient in posthospital care:
  a. Activity limitations
  b. Reinforce exercise instructions
  c. Safe use of ambulatory aids
  d. Wound care
  e. Measures to promote healing (nutrition, wound care)
  f. Medications, if any
  g. Potential problems
  h. Continuing health care supervision
	5. Lack of knowledge and poor preparation for care at home contribute to patient anxiety, insecurity, and nonadherence to therapeutic regimen.	

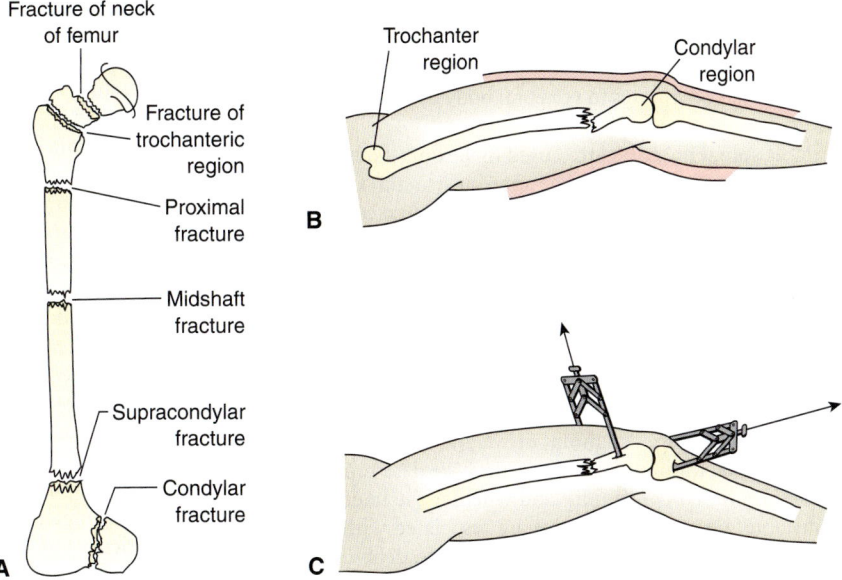

FIGURE 69-15 (**A**) Types of femoral fractures. One method of correction for a fracture of the femur in the distal third is two-wire skeletal traction. (**B**) Example of deformity on admission to hospital. (**C**) Adequate reduction is achieved when additional wire is inserted in the lower femoral fragment, and vertical lift is secured.

TIBIA AND FIBULA

The most common fracture below the knee is one of the tibia (and fibula) that results from a direct blow, falls with the foot in a flexed position, or a violent twisting motion. Fractures of the tibia and fibula often occur in association with each other. The patient presents with pain, deformity, obvious hematoma, and considerable edema. Frequently, these fractures are open and involve severe soft tissue damage because there is little subcutaneous tissue in the area.

Assessment and Diagnostic Findings

Peroneal nerve damage is assessed. If nerve function is impaired, the patient is unable to dorsiflex the great toe and has diminished sensation in the first web space. Tibial artery damage is assessed by evaluating pulses, skin temperature, and colour and by testing the capillary refill response. Hemiarthrosis or ligament damage may occur with fracture near the joint.

The patient is monitored for an anterior compartment syndrome. Symptoms include pain unrelieved by medications and increasing with plantar flexion, tense and tender muscle lateral to tibial crest, and paresthesia.

Medical Management

Most closed tibial fractures are treated with closed reduction and initial immobilization in a long leg walking cast or a patellar tendon–bearing cast. Reduction must be relatively accurate in relation to angulation and rotation. As with other lower extremity fractures, the leg should be elevated to control edema. Partial weight bearing is usually prescribed after 7 to 10 days. Activity decreases edema and increases circulation. The cast is changed to a short leg cast or brace in 3 to 4 weeks, which allows for knee motion. Fracture healing takes 6 to 10 weeks. At times it is difficult to maintain reduction, and percutaneous pins may be placed in the bone and held in position by an external fixator.

Comminuted fractures may be treated with skeletal traction, internal fixation with intramedullary nails or plates and screws, or external fixation. External support may be used with internal fixation. Hip, foot, and knee exercises are encouraged within the limits of the immobilizing device. Partial weight bearing is begun when prescribed and is progressed as the fracture heals in 4 to 8 weeks.

Open fractures are treated with external fixation. Distal fractures with extensive soft tissue damage heal slowly and may require bone grafting.

Continued neurovascular evaluation is needed. The development of compartment syndrome requires prompt recognition and resolution to prevent permanent functional deficit. Other complications include delayed union, infection, impaired wound edge healing due to limited soft tissue, and loosening of the internal fixation hardware.

RIB

Uncomplicated fractures of the ribs occur frequently in adults and usually result in no impairment of function. Because these fractures produce painful respiration, the patient tends to decrease respiratory excursions and refrains from coughing. As a result, tracheobronchial secretions are not mobilized, aeration of the lung is diminished, and a predisposition to *pneumonia* and *atelectasis* results. To help the patient cough and take deep breaths, the nurse may splint the chest with her hands. Occasionally, the physician administers intercostal nerve blocks to relieve pain and to permit productive coughing.

Chest strapping to immobilize the rib fracture is *not* used, because decreased chest expansion may result in pneumonia and atelectasis. The pain associated with rib fracture diminishes significantly in 3 or 4 days, and the fracture heals within 6 weeks. In addition to pneumonia and atelectasis, complications may include a *flail chest, pneumothorax,* and *hemothorax.* The management of patients with these conditions is discussed in Chapter 23.

THORACOLUMBAR SPINE

Fractures of the thoracolumbar spine may involve (1) the vertebral body, (2) the laminae and articulating processes, and (3) the spinous processes or transverse processes. The T12 to L2 area of the spine is most vulnerable to fracture. Fractures generally result from indirect trauma caused by excessive loading, sudden muscle contraction, or excessive motion beyond physiologic limits. Osteoporosis contributes to vertebral body collapse (compression fracture).

Stable spinal fractures are caused by flexion, extension, lateral bending, or vertical loading. The anterior structural column (vertebral bodies and disks) or the posterior structural column (neural arch, articular processes, ligaments) has been disrupted. Unstable fractures occur with fracture-dislocations and exhibit disruption of both anterior and posterior structural columns. The potential for neural damage exists.

The patient with a spinal fracture presents with acute tenderness, swelling, paravertebral muscle spasm, and change in the normal curves or in the gap between spinous processes. Pain is greater with moving, coughing, or weight bearing. Immobilization is essential until initial assessments have determined whether there is any spinal cord injury and whether the fracture is stable or unstable. Few spinal fractures are associated with neurologic deficits. If spinal cord injury with neurologic deficit does occur, it usually requires immediate surgery (laminectomy with spinal fusion) to decompress the spinal cord.

Medical Management

Stable spinal fractures are treated conservatively with limited bed rest. The head of the bed is elevated less than 30 degrees until the acute pain subsides (several days). Analgesics are prescribed for pain relief. The patient is monitored for a transient *paralytic ileus* caused by associated retroperitoneal hemorrhage. Sitting is avoided until the pain subsides. A spinal brace or plastic thoracolumbar orthosis may be applied for support during progressive ambulation and resumption of activities.

The patient with an unstable fracture is treated with bed rest, possibly with the use of a special turning device (eg, Stryker frame) to maintain spinal alignment. Neurologic status is monitored closely during the preoperative and postoperative periods. Within 24 hours after fracture, open reduction, decompression, and fixation with spinal fusion and instrument stabilization are usually accomplished. Postoperatively, the patient may be cared for on the turning device or in a bed with a firm mattress. Progressive ambulation is begun a few days after surgery, with the patient using a body brace orthosis. Patient teaching emphasizes good posture, good body mechanics, and, after healing is sufficient, back-strengthening exercises. (Spinal cord injury is discussed in Chapter 63.)

Amputation

Amputation is the removal of a body part, usually an extremity. Amputation of a lower extremity is often made necessary by progressive peripheral vascular disease (often a sequela of diabetes mellitus), fulminating gas gangrene, trauma (crushing injuries, burns, frostbite, electrical burns), congenital deformities, chronic osteomyelitis, or malignant tumour. Of all these causes, peripheral vascular disease accounts for most amputations of lower extremities. (See Chapter 31 for more information.)

Amputation is used to relieve symptoms, improve function, and save or improve the patient's quality of life. If the health care team communicates a positive attitude, the patient adjusts to the amputation more readily and actively participates in the rehabilitative plan, learning how to modify activities and how to use assistive devices for ADLs and mobility.

Levels of Amputation

Amputation is performed at the most distal point that will heal successfully. The site of amputation is determined by two factors: circulation in the part, and functional usefulness (ie, meets the requirements for the use of the prosthesis).

The circulatory status of the extremity is evaluated through physical examination and specific studies. Muscle and skin perfusion is important for healing. Doppler flowmetry, segmental blood pressure determinations, and transcutaneous partial pressure of oxygen (PaO$_2$) are valuable diagnostic aids. Angiography is performed if revascularization is considered an option.

The objective of surgery is to conserve as much extremity length as possible. Preservation of knee and elbow joints is desired. Figure 69-16 shows the levels at which an extremity may be amputated. Almost any level of amputation can be fitted with a prosthesis.

The amputation of toes and portions of the foot causes minor changes in gait and balance. A Syme amputation (modified ankle disarticulation amputation) is performed most frequently for extensive foot trauma and produces a painless, durable extremity end that can withstand full weight-bearing. Below-knee amputations are preferred to above-knee amputations because of the importance of the knee joint and the energy requirements for walking. Knee disarticulations are most successful with young, active patients who are able to develop precise control of the prosthesis. When above-knee amputations are performed, all possible length is preserved, muscles are stabilized and shaped, and hip contractures are prevented for maximum ambulatory potential. Most people who have a hip disarticulation amputation must rely on a wheelchair for mobility.

Upper extremity amputations are performed to preserve the maximum functional length. The prosthesis is fitted early for maximum function.

A *staged amputation* may be used when gangrene and infection exist. Initially, a guillotine amputation is performed to remove the necrotic and infected tissue. The wound is débrided and allowed to drain. Sepsis is treated with systemic antibiotics. In a few days, after the infection has been controlled and the patient's condition has stabilized, a definitive amputation with skin closure is performed.

Complications

Complications that may occur with amputation include *hemorrhage, infection, skin breakdown, phantom limb pain,* and *joint contracture.* Because major blood vessels have been severed, massive bleeding may occur. Infection is a risk with all surgical procedures. The risk for infection increases with contaminated wounds after traumatic amputation. Skin irritation caused by the prosthesis may result in skin breakdown. **Phantom limb pain** is caused by the severing of peripheral nerves. Joint contracture is caused by positioning and a protective flexion withdrawal pattern associated with pain and muscle imbalance.

Medical Management

The objective of treatment is to achieve healing of the amputation wound, the result being a nontender residual limb (stump) with healthy skin for prosthesis use. Healing is enhanced by gentle handling of the residual limb, control of residual limb edema through rigid or soft compression dressings, and use of aseptic technique in wound care to avoid infection.

FIGURE 69-16 Levels of amputation are determined by circulatory adequacy, type of prosthesis, function of the part, and muscle balance. (**A**) Levels of amputation of upper extremity. (**B**) Levels of amputation of lower extremity.

A *closed rigid cast dressing* is frequently used to provide uniform compression, to support soft tissues, to control pain, and to prevent joint contractures. Immediately after surgery, a sterilized residual limb sock is applied to the residual limb. Felt pads are placed over pressure-sensitive areas. The residual limb is wrapped with elastic plaster-of-paris bandages while firm, even pressure is maintained. Care is taken not to constrict circulation.

For the patient with a lower extremity amputation, the plaster cast may be equipped to attach a temporary prosthetic extension (pylon) and an artificial foot. This rigid dressing technique is used as a means of creating a socket for immediate postoperative prosthetic fitting. The length of the prosthesis is tailored to the individual patient. Early minimal weight bearing on the residual limb with a rigid cast dressing and a pylon attached produces little discomfort. The cast is changed in about 10 to 14 days. Elevated body temperature, severe pain, or a loose-fitting cast may necessitate earlier replacement.

A *removable rigid dressing* may be placed over a soft dressing to control edema, to prevent joint flexion contracture, and to protect the residual limb from unintentional trauma during transfer activities. This rigid dressing is removed several days after surgery for wound inspection and is then replaced to control edema. The dressing facilitates residual limb shaping.

A *soft dressing* with or without compression may be used if there is significant wound drainage and frequent inspection of the residual limb (stump) is desired. An immobilizing splint may be incorporated in the dressing. Stump (wound) hematomas are controlled with wound drainage devices to minimize infection.

Rehabilitation

Patients who require amputation because of severe trauma are usually, but not always, young and healthy, heal rapidly, and participate in a vigourous rehabilitation program. Because the amputation is the result of an injury, the patient needs psychological support in accepting the sudden change in body image and in dealing with the stresses of hospitalization, long-term rehabilitation, and modification of lifestyle. Patients who undergo amputation need support as they grieve the loss, and they need time to work through their feelings about their permanent loss and change in body image. Their reactions are unpredictable and can include anger, bitterness, and hostility.

The multidisciplinary rehabilitation team (patient, nurse, physician, social worker, psychologist, prosthetist, vocational rehabilitation worker) helps the patient achieve the highest possible level of function and participation in life activities (Fig. 69-17). Prosthetic clinics and amputee support groups facilitate this rehabilitation process. Vocational counselling and job retraining may be necessary to help patients return to work.

Psychological problems (eg, denial, withdrawal) may be influenced by the type of support the patient receives from the rehabilitation team and by how quickly ADLs and use of the

FIGURE 69-17 Many amputees receive prostheses soon after surgery and begin learning how to use them with the help and support of the rehabilitation team, which includes nurses, physicians, physical therapists, and others.

prosthesis are learned. Knowing the full options and capabilities available with the various prosthetic devices can give the patient a sense of control over the disability.

NURSING PROCESS: THE PATIENT UNDERGOING AN AMPUTATION

Assessment

Before surgery, the nurse must evaluate the neurovascular and functional status of the extremity through history and physical assessment. If the patient has experienced a traumatic amputation, the nurse assesses the function and condition of the residual limb. The nurse also assesses the circulatory status and function of the unaffected extremity. If infection or gangrene develops, the patient may have associated enlarged lymph nodes, fever, and purulent drainage. A culture is taken to determine the appropriate antibiotic therapy.

The nurse evaluates the patient's nutritional status and creates a plan for nutritional care, if indicated. For wound healing, a balanced diet with adequate protein and vitamins is essential.

Any concurrent health problems (eg, dehydration, anemia, cardiac insufficiency, chronic respiratory problems, diabetes mellitus) need to be identified and treated so that the patient is in the best possible condition to withstand the trauma of surgery. The use of corticosteroids, anticoagulants, vasoconstrictors, or vasodilators may influence management and wound healing.

The nurse assesses the patient's psychological status. Determination of the patient's emotional reaction to amputation is essential for nursing care. Grief response to a permanent alteration in body image is normal. An adequate support system and professional counselling can help the patient cope in the aftermath of amputation surgery.

Diagnosis

NURSING DIAGNOSES
Based on the assessment data, the patient's major nursing diagnoses may include the following:

- Acute pain related to amputation
- Risk for disturbed sensory perception: phantom limb pain related to amputation
- Impaired skin integrity related to surgical amputation
- Disturbed body image related to amputation of body part
- Ineffective coping, related to failure to accept loss of body part
- Risk for anticipatory and/or dysfunctional grieving related to loss of body part
- Self-care deficit: feeding, bathing/hygiene, dressing/grooming, or toileting, related to loss of extremity
- Impaired physical mobility related to loss of extremity

COLLABORATIVE PROBLEMS/ POTENTIAL COMPLICATIONS
Based on the assessment data, potential complications that may develop include the following:

- Postoperative hemorrhage
- Infection
- Skin breakdown

Planning and Goals

The major goals of the patient may include relief of pain, absence of altered sensory perceptions, wound healing, acceptance of altered body image, resolution of the grieving process, independence in self-care, restoration of physical mobility, and absence of complications.

Nursing Interventions

RELIEVING PAIN
Surgical pain can be effectively controlled with opioid analgesics, nonpharmaceutical interventions, or evacuation of the hematoma or accumulated fluid. Pain may be incisional or may be caused by inflammation, infection, pressure on a bony prominence, or hematoma. Muscle spasms may add to the patient's discomfort. Changing the patient's position or placing a light sandbag on the residual limb to counteract the muscle spasm may improve the patient's level of comfort. Evaluation of the patient's pain and responses to interventions is an important part of the nurse's role in pain management. The pain may be an expression of grief and alteration of body image.

MINIMIZING ALTERED SENSORY PERCEPTIONS
Amputees may experience phantom limb pain soon after surgery or 2 to 3 months after amputation. It occurs more frequently may in above-knee amputations. The patient describes pain or unusual sensations, such as numbness, tingling, or muscle cramps, as well as a feeling that the extremity is present, crushed, cramped, or twisted in an abnormal position. When a patient describes phantom pains or sensations, the nurse acknowledges these feelings and helps the patient modify these perceptions.

Phantom sensations diminish over time. The pathogenesis of the phantom limb phenomenon is unknown. Keeping the patient active helps decrease the occurrence of phantom limb pain. Early intensive rehabilitation and stump desensitization with kneading massage brings relief. Distraction techniques and activity are helpful. Transcutaneous electrical nerve stimulation (TENS), ultrasound, or local anesthetics may provide relief for some patients. In addition, beta-blockers may relieve dull, burning discomfort; antiseizure medications control stabbing and cramping pain; and tricyclic antidepressants are used to improve mood and coping ability.

PROMOTING WOUND HEALING

The residual limb must be handled gently. Whenever the dressing is changed, aseptic technique is required to prevent wound infection and possible osteomyelitis.

> **NURSING ALERT** If the cast or elastic dressing inadvertently comes off, the nurse must immediately wrap the residual limb with an elastic compression bandage. If this is not done, excessive edema will develop in a short time, resulting in a delay in rehabilitation. The nurse notifies the surgeon if a cast dressing comes off, so that another cast can be applied.

Residual limb shaping is important for prosthesis fitting. The nurse instructs the patient and family in wrapping the residual limb with elastic dressings (Figs. 69-18 and 69-19). After the incision is healed, the nurse teaches the patient to care for the residual limb.

ENHANCING BODY IMAGE

Amputation is a reconstructive procedure that alters the patient's body image. The nurse who has established a trusting relationship with the patient is better able to communicate acceptance of the patient who has experienced an amputation. The nurse encourages the patient to look at, feel, and then care for the residual limb. It is important to identify the patient's strength and resources to facilitate rehabilitation. The nurse assists the patient to regain the previous level of independent functioning. The patient who is accepted as a whole person is more readily able to resume responsibility for self-care; self-concept improves, and body-image changes are accepted. Even with highly motivated patients, this process may take months.

FIGURE 69-18 Wrapping the residual leg after an above-knee amputation. Elastic bandaging minimizes edema and shapes the stump in a firm conical form to fit a prosthesis.

FIGURE 69-19 Wrapping the residual arm after an above-elbow amputation. Passing the bandage wrap across the back and shoulders may augment security.

HELPING THE PATIENT TO RESOLVE GRIEVING

The loss of an extremity (or part of one) may come as a shock even if the patient was prepared preoperatively. The patient's behaviour (eg, crying, withdrawal, apathy, anger) and expressed feelings (eg, depression, fear, helplessness) will reveal how the patient is coping with the loss and working through the grieving process. The nurse acknowledges the loss by listening and providing support.

The nurse creates an accepting and supportive atmosphere in which the patient and family are encouraged to express and share their feelings and work through the grief process. The support from family and friends promotes the patient's acceptance of the loss. The nurse helps the patient deal with immediate needs and become oriented to realistic rehabilitation goals and future independent functioning. Mental health and support group referrals may be appropriate.

PROMOTING INDEPENDENT SELF-CARE

Amputation of an extremity affects the patient's ability to provide adequate self-care. The patient is encouraged to be an active participant in self-care. The patient needs time to accomplish these tasks and must not be rushed. Practicing an activity with consistent, supportive supervision in a relaxed environment enables the patient to learn self-care skills. The patient and the nurse need to maintain positive attitudes and to minimize fatigue and frustration during the learning process.

Independence in dressing, toileting, and bathing (shower or tub) depends on balance, transfer abilities, and physiologic tolerance of the activities. The nurse works with the physical therapist and occupational therapist to teach and supervise the patient in these self-care activities.

The patient with an upper extremity amputation has self-care deficits in feeding, bathing, and dressing. Assistance is provided only as needed; the nurse encourages the patient to learn to do these tasks, using feeding and dressing aids when needed. The nurse, therapists, and prosthetist work with the patient to achieve maximum independence.

HELPING THE PATIENT TO ACHIEVE PHYSICAL MOBILITY

Positioning assists in preventing the development of hip or knee joint contracture in the patient with a lower extremity amputation. Abduction, external rotation, and flexion of the lower extremity are avoided. Depending on the surgeon's preference, the residual limb may be placed in an extended position or elevated for a brief period after surgery. The foot of the bed is raised to elevate the residual limb.

 NURSING ALERT The residual limb should not be placed on a pillow, because a flexion contracture of the hip may result.

The nurse encourages the patient to turn from side to side and to assume a prone position, if possible, to stretch the flexor muscles and to prevent flexion contracture of the hip. The nurse discourages sitting for prolonged periods, to prevent flexion contracture. The legs should remain close together to prevent an abduction deformity.

Postoperative ROM exercises are started early, because contracture deformities develop rapidly. ROM exercises include hip and knee exercises for below-knee amputations and hip exercises for above-knee amputations. It is important that the patient understand the importance of exercising the residual limb.

The upper extremities, trunk, and abdominal muscles are exercised and strengthened. The extensor muscles in the arm and the depressor muscles in the shoulder play an important part in crutch walking. The patient uses an overhead trapeze to change position and strengthen the biceps. The patient may flex and extend the arms while holding weights. Doing push-ups while seated strengthens the triceps muscles. Exercises, such as hyperextension of the residual limb, conducted under the supervision of the physical therapist or occupational therapist, also aid in strengthening muscles as well as increasing circulation, reducing edema, and preventing atrophy.

Because an upper extremity amputee uses both shoulders to operate the prosthesis, the muscles of both shoulders are exercised. A patient with an above-the-elbow amputation or shoulder disarticulation is likely to develop a postural abnormality caused by loss of the weight of the amputated extremity. Postural exercises are helpful.

Strength and endurance are assessed, and activities are increased gradually to prevent fatigue. As the patient progresses to independent use of the wheelchair, use of ambulatory aids, or ambulation with a prosthesis, the nurse emphasizes safety considerations. Environmental barriers (eg, steps, inclines, doors, wet surfaces) are identified, and methods of managing them are practiced. It is important to anticipate, identify and manage problems associated with the use of the mobility aids (eg, pressure on the axillae from crutches, skin irritation of the hands from wheelchair use, residual limb irritation from a prosthesis).

Amputation of the leg changes the centre of gravity; therefore, the patient may need to practice position changes (eg, standing from sitting, standing on one foot). The patient is taught transfer techniques early and is reminded to maintain good posture when getting out of bed. A well-fitting shoe with a nonskid sole should be worn. During position changes, the patient should be guarded and stabilized with a transfer belt at the waist to prevent falling.

As soon as possible, the patient with a lower extremity amputation is assisted to stand between parallel bars to allow extension of the temporary prosthesis to the floor with minimal weight bearing. How soon after surgery the patient is allowed to touch down the artificial foot depends on the patient's physical status and wound healing. As endurance increases and balance is achieved, ambulation is started with the use of parallel bars or crutches. The patient learns to use a normal gait, with the residual limb moving back and forth while the patient is walking with the crutches. To prevent a permanent flexion deformity from occurring, the residual limb should *not* be held up in a flexed position.

The patient with an upper extremity amputation is taught how to carry out the ADLs with one arm. The patient is started on one-handed self-care activities as soon as possible. The use of a temporary prosthesis is encouraged. The patient who learns to use the prosthesis soon after the amputation is less dependent on one-handed self-care activities.

A patient with an upper extremity amputation may wear a cotton T-shirt to prevent contact between the skin and shoulder harness and to promote absorption of perspiration. The prosthetist advises about cleaning the washable portions of the harness. Periodically, the prosthesis is inspected for potential problems.

The residual limb must be conditioned and shaped into a conical form to permit accurate fit, maximum comfort, and function of the prosthetic device. Elastic bandages, an elastic residual limb shrinker, or an air splint is used to condition and shape the residual limb. The nurse teaches the patient or a member of the family the correct method of bandaging.

Bandaging supports the soft tissue and minimizes the formation of edema while the residual limb is in a dependent position. The bandage is applied in such a manner that the remaining muscles required to operate the prosthesis are as firm as possible, whereas those muscles that are no longer useful atrophy. An im-

properly applied elastic bandage contributes to circulatory problems and a poorly shaped residual limb.

Effective preprosthetic care is important to ensure proper fitting of the prosthesis. The major problems that can delay prosthetic fitting during this period are (1) flexion deformities, (2) nonshrinkage of the residual limb, and (3) abduction deformities of the hip.

The physician usually prescribes activities to condition or "toughen" the residual limb in preparation for a prosthesis. The patient begins by pushing the residual limb into a soft pillow, then into a firmer pillow, and finally against a hard surface. The patient is taught to massage the residual limb to mobilize the surgical incision site, decrease tenderness, and improve vascularity. Massage is usually started once healing has occurred and is first done by the physical therapist. Skin inspection and preventive care are taught.

The prosthesis socket is custom molded to the residual limb by the prosthetist. Prostheses are designed for specific activity levels and patient abilities. Types of prostheses include hydraulic, pneumatic, biofeedback-controlled, myoelectrically controlled, and synchronized prostheses.

Adjustments of the prosthetic socket are made by the prosthetist to accommodate the residual limb changes that occur during the first 6 months to 1 year after surgery. A light plaster cast, an elastic bandage, or a shrinking sock is used to limit edema during periods when the patient is not wearing the permanent prosthesis.

Some patients are not candidates for a prosthesis and are thus *nonambulatory amputees.* If use of a prosthesis is not possible, the patient is instructed in the use of a wheelchair to achieve independence. A special wheelchair designed for patients who have had amputations is recommended. Because of the decreased weight in the front, a regular wheelchair may tip backward when the patient sits in it. In an amputee wheelchair, the rear axle is set back about 5 cm to compensate for the change in weight distribution.

MONITORING AND MANAGING POTENTIAL COMPLICATIONS

After any surgery, efforts are made to reestablish homeostasis and to prevent problems related to surgery, anesthesia, and immobility. The nurse assesses body systems (eg, respiratory, gastrointestinal, genitourinary) for problems associated with immobility (eg, pneumonia, anorexia, constipation, urinary stasis) and institutes corrective management. Avoiding problems associated with immobility and restoring physical activity are necessary for maintenance of health.

Massive *hemorrhage* due to a loosened suture is the most threatening problem. The nurse monitors the patient for any signs or symptoms of bleeding. It is also important to monitor the patient's vital signs and to observe the suction drainage.

> **! NURSING ALERT** Immediate postoperative bleeding may develop slowly or may take the form of a massive hemorrhage resulting from a loosened suture. A large tourniquet should be in plain sight at the patient's bedside so that, if severe bleeding occurs, it can be applied to the residual limb to control the hemorrhage. The nurse immediately notifies the surgeon in the event of excessive bleeding.

Infection is a frequent complication of amputation. Patients who have undergone traumatic amputation have a contaminated wound. The nurse administers antibiotics as prescribed. It is important to monitor the incision, dressing, and drainage for indications of infection (eg, change in colour, odour, or consistency of drainage; increasing discomfort). The nurse also monitors for systemic indicators of infection (eg, elevated temperature) and promptly reports indications of infection to the surgeon.

Skin breakdown may result from immobilization or from pressure from various sources. The prosthesis may cause pressure areas to develop. The nurse and the patient assess for breaks in the skin. Careful skin hygiene is essential to prevent skin irritation, infection, and breakdown. The healed residual limb is washed and dried (gently) at least twice daily. The skin is inspected for pressure areas, dermatitis, and blisters. If they are present, they must be treated before further skin breakdown occurs. Usually, a residual limb sock is worn to absorb perspiration and to prevent direct contact between the skin and the prosthetic socket. The sock is changed daily and must fit smoothly to prevent irritation caused by wrinkles. The socket of the prosthesis is washed with a mild detergent, rinsed, and dried thoroughly with a clean cloth. The nurse advises the patient that the socket must be thoroughly dry before the prosthesis is applied.

PROMOTING HOME AND COMMUNITY-BASED CARE

Teaching the Patient to Manage Self-Care

Before discharge to the home or to a rehabilitation facility, the nurse encourages the patient and family to become active participants in care. They participate, as appropriate, in skin care and residual limb care and in the management of the prosthesis. The patient receives ongoing instructions and practice sessions in learning how to transfer and how to use mobility aids and other assistive devices safely. The nurse explains the signs and symptoms of complications that must be reported to the physician (Chart 69-5).

Continuing Care in the Home and Community

After the patient has achieved physiologic homeostasis and has demonstrated achievement of major health care goals, rehabilitation continues either in a rehabilitation facility or at home. Continued support and supervision by the home care nurse are essential.

Before the patient's discharge to the home, the nurse should assess the home environment. Modifications are made to ensure the patient's continuing care, safety, and mobility. An overnight or weekend experience at home may be tried to identify problems that were not identified on the assessment visit. Physical therapy and occupational therapy may continue in the home or on an outpatient basis. Transportation to continuing health care appointments must be arranged. The social service department of the hospital or the community agency managing continued health care may be of great assistance in securing personal assistance and transportation services.

During follow-up health visits, the nurse evaluates the patient's physical and psychosocial adjustment. Periodic preventive health assessments are necessary. Frequently, an elderly spouse is unable to provide the assistance required, and additional help at home is needed. Modifications in the plan of care are made on the basis of such findings. Often, the patient and family find involvement in an amputee support group to be of value; here, they are able to share problems, solutions, and resources. Talking with those who have successfully dealt with a similar problem may help the patient develop a satisfactory solution.

Because patients and their family members and health care providers tend to focus on the most obvious needs and issues, the nurse reminds the patient and family about the importance of continuing health promotion and screening practices, such as regular physical examinations and diagnostic screening tests. Those patients who have not been involved in these practices in the past are instructed in their importance and are referred to appropriate health care providers.

Evaluation

EXPECTED PATIENT OUTCOMES

Expected patient outcomes may include:

1. Experiences absence of pain
   a. Appears relaxed
   b. Verbalizes comfort
   c. Uses measures to increase comfort
   d. Participates in self-care and rehabilitative activities

---

Chart 69-5

Home Care Checklist • Amputation

At the completion of the home care instruction, the patient or caregiver will be able to:	Patient	Caregiver
• Describe approaches to controlling pain (eg, take analgesics as prescribed; use nonpharmacologic interventions)	✓	✓
• Report pain that is uncontrolled by analgesics and other pain management techniques	✓	
• Describe care of residual limb and conditioning for prosthesis	✓	✓
• Consume healthy diet to promote wound healing	✓	
• Demonstrate ability to transfer	✓	
• Use mobility and activity aids safely	✓	
• Participate in rehabilitation program to regain functional independence	✓	✓
• State indicators of complication to report promptly to physician (eg, uncontrolled pain; signs of local or systemic infection; residual limb skin breakdown)	✓	✓
• Identify professionals and community agencies to help with transition to home	✓	✓
• Identify support group to facilitate rehabilitation	✓	
• Describe effects of amputation on self-image	✓	
• Acknowledge grieving as part of coping process	✓	
• Identify modifications of home environment to promote safe environment and independence during rehabilitation	✓	✓

2. Experiences absence of phantom limb pain
   a. Reports diminished phantom sensations
   b. Uses distraction techniques
   c. Performs stump desensitization massage
3. Achieves wound healing
   a. Controls residual limb edema
   b. Achieves healed, nontender, nonadherent scar
   c. Demonstrates residual limb care
4. Demonstrates improved body image and effective coping
   a. Acknowledges change in body image
   b. Participates in self-care activities
   c. Demonstrates increasing independence
   d. Projects self as a whole person
   e. Resumes role-related responsibilities
   f. Reestablishes social contacts
   g. Demonstrates confidence in abilities
5. Exhibits resolution of grieving
   a. Expresses grief
   b. Works through feelings with family and friends
   c. Focuses on future functioning
   d. Participates in support group
6. Achieves independent self-care
   a. Asks for assistance when needed
   b. Uses aids and assistive devices to facilitate self-care
   c. Verbalizes satisfaction with abilities to perform ADLs
7. Achieves maximum independent mobility
   a. Avoids positions contributing to contracture development
   b. Demonstrates full active ROM
   c. Maintains balance when sitting and transferring
   d. Increases strength and endurance
   e. Demonstrates safe transferring technique
   f. Achieves functional use of prosthesis
   g. Overcomes environmental barriers to mobility
   h. Uses community services and resources as needed
8. Exhibits absence of complications of hemorrhage, infection, skin breakdown
   a. Does not experience excessive bleeding
   b. Maintains normal blood values
   c. Is free of local or systemic signs of infection
   d. Repositions self frequently
   e. Is free of pressure-related problems
   f. Reports any skin discomfort and irritations promptly

Critical Thinking Exercises

1. Your church is participating in a women's soccer league and asks you to help out with first aid on the field. Common injuries you would expect include sprains, strains, and, possibly, dislocations and fractures. What specific assessment would you make to differentiate these problems? Discuss the emergency management for each of these problems. Explain your rationale for these emergency interventions.

2. A 46-year-old man experiences an open fracture of his right ankle while skiing. The orthopedic surgeon recommends surgery and external fixation. The patient asks why surgery is needed—a lot of his friends have broken their ankles, have not had surgery, and have just had a cast put on for a couple of weeks. What would you include in your discussion of the need for surgery and external fixation? Describe the anticipated postoperative care, monitoring to prevent complications, and activity restrictions.

3. A middle-aged patient who had been hospitalized for 3 days with a fractured pelvis is making plans for discharge. His wife approaches you and expresses concern that he has become very irritable and that he "just doesn't seem to be himself." Analyze this information and identify the possible causes for this behaviour. Describe additional data that you would seek to further assess the situation.

4. You make a home health care visit to a middle-aged patient with type 2 diabetes who had a partial foot amputation 4 days ago because of peripheral vascular disease and gangrene. What is the rationale for the assessment data you gather to assist you in determining the patient's progress? What findings might suggest that the patient is developing a problem? Describe your plan of action for each of these potential problems. What home environment factors would you include in your assessment of the home care situation?

REFERENCES AND SELECTED READINGS

Books

Bullock, B., & Henze, R. (2000). *Focus on pathophysiology*. Philadelphia: Lippincott Williams & Wilkins.

Childs, S. (Ed.). (1999). *The upper extremity: Traumatic injuries and conditions*. Pitman, NJ: National Association of Orthopaedic Nurses.

Childs, S., & Holmes, S. (1999). *NAON guidelines for orthopaedic nursing: Adult trauma*. Pitman, NJ: National Association of Orthopaedic Nurses.

Cree, M. (2000). *Treatment of variations of femoral neck fractures in Alberta*. Edmonton, AB: Institute of Health Economics.

Goldstein, T. (1999). *Geriatric orthopedics. Rehabilitative management of common problems* (2nd ed.). Gaithersburg, MD: Aspen Publishers.

Kleerekoper, M., et al. (1999). *The bone and mineral manual*. San Diego: Academic Press.

Lusardi, M., & Nielsen, C. (2000). *Orthotics and prosthetics in rehabilitation*. Boston. Butterworth Heinemann.

Maher, A., et al. (2003). *Orthopaedic nursing* (3rd ed.). Philadelphia: W. B. Saunders.

Mercier, L. (2000). *Practical orthopedics* (5th ed.). St. Louis: Mosby.

Moehring, H., & Greenspan, A. (2000). *Fractures: Diagnosis and treatment*. New York: McGraw-Hill.

Rosen, C., et al. (1999). *The aging skeleton*. San Diego: Academic Press.

Salter, R. (1999). *Textbook of disorders and injuries of the musculoskeletal system* (3rd ed.). Baltimore: Williams & Wilkins.

Schoen, D. (2000). *Adult orthopaedic nursing*. Philadelphia: Lippincott Williams & Wilkins.

Schoen, D. C. (Ed.). (2001). *NAON core curriculum for orthopaedic nursing* (4th ed.). Pitman, NJ: National Association of Orthopaedic Nurses.

Simon, R., & Koenigsknecht, S. (2001). *Emergency orthopedics: The extremities* (4th ed.). New York: McGraw-Hill.

Steinberg, G., et al. (Eds.). (1999). *Orthopaedics in primary care* (3rd ed.). Philadelphia: Lippincott Williams & Wilkins.

Wiss, D. (1998). *Fractures*. Philadelphia: Lippincott-Raven.

Journals

Asterisks indicate nursing research articles.

Arcuni, S. (2000). Rotator cuff pathology and subacromial impingement. *Nurse Practitioner, 25*(5), 58–78.

Berg, E. (2000). Deep muscle contusion complicated by myositis ossificans (a.k.a. heterotopic bone). *Orthopaedic Nursing, 19*(6), 66–67.

Cortet, R., et al. (1997). Treatment of severe, recalcitrant reflex sympathetic dystrophy: Assessment of efficacy and safety of the second generation bisphosphonate pamidronate. *Clinical Rheumatology, 16*(1), 51–56.

Cypher, T. J., & Grossman, J. P. (1996). Biological principles of bone graft healing. *Journal of Foot and Ankle Surgery, 35*(5), 413–417.

DeLong, W., et al. (1999). Aggressive treatment of 119 open fracture wounds. *Journal of Trauma, 46*(6), 1049–1054.

*Feldt, K., & Oh, H. (2000). Pain and hip fracture outcomes for older adults. *Orthopaedic Nursing, 19*(6), 35–44.

Feinberg, S. (2000). Complex regional pain syndrome. *American Journal of Nursing, 100*(12), 23–24.

Frye, K., & Luterman, A. (1999). Burns and fractures. *Orthopaedic Nursing, 18*(1), 30–35.

Jerre, R., et al. (2000). Preoperative skin traction in patients with hip fractures is not useful. *Clinical Orthopaedics and Related Research, 378*, 169–173.

Kamel, H. K., Hussain, M. S., Tarig, S., Perry, H. M., Morley, J. E. (2000). Failure to diagnose and treat osteoporosis in elderly patients hospitalized with hip fracture. *American Journal of Medicine, 109*, 326–328.

Koval, K., et al. (1999). The effects of nutritional status on outcome after hip fracture. *Journal of Orthopaedic Trauma, 13*(3), 164–169.

*Morris, N. (2000). Distal radius fracture in adults: Self-reported physical functioning, role functioning, and meaning of injury. *Orthopaedic Nursing, 19*(4), 37–48.

Morrison, C. (2000). A practical approach to stress fractures. *Orthopaedic Nursing, 19*(6), 23–27.

Mortensen, H., et al. (1999). Early motion of the ankle after operative treatment of a rupture of the Achilles tendon. *Journal of Bone and Joint Surgery, American Volume, 81*(7), 983–990.

Ocelus, S. (2000). Autologous cultured chondrocytes for the treatment of knee cartilage injury. *Orthopaedic Nursing, 19*(4), 19–27.

Patterson, M. (2000). What's the buzz on external bone growth stimulators? *Nursing 2000, 30*(6), 44–45.

Shell, J., & Miller, M. (1999). The cancer amputee and sexuality. *Orthopaedic Nursing, 18*(5), 53–57, 62–64.

Yarnold, B. (1999). Hip fracture: Caring for a fragile population. *American Journal of Nursing, 99*(2), 36–40.

RESOURCES AND WEBSITES

Amputee Resources for the Canadian Amputee; www.amputee.ca.

Canadian Orthopaedic Association, 1440 St. Catherine Street West, Suite 718, Montreal, QC H3G 1R8; 514-874-9003; www.coa-aco.org.

Canadian Orthopaedic Foundation, PO Box 7029, Innisfail, ON L9S 1A8; 416-410-2341; www.canorth.org.

Easter Seal Society of Canada, c/o The Easter Seals/March of Dimes National Council, 90 Eglinton East, Suite 511, Toronto, ON M4P 2Y3; 416-932-8382; www.easterseals.ca.

National Institute of Arthritis and Musculoskeletal and Skin Diseases, Information Clearing House, National Institutes of Health, 1 AMS Circle, Bethesda, MD 20892-3675; (877) 22-NIAMS (toll free); (301) 495-4484.

National Institute of Arthritis and Musculoskeletal and Skin Diseases, Office of Communications and Public Liaison, Bldg. 31/Rm. 4C05, 31 Center Drive, MSC 2350, Bethesda, MD 20892-2350; (301) 496-8190; http://www.nih.gov/niams.

Reflex Sympathetic Dystrophy Syndrome Association of America (RSDSA). 116 Haddonfield Ave, Suite D, Haddonfield, NJ. 08033-2306. (609) 795-8845. http://www.rsds.org.

The War Amps, 1 Maybrook Drive, Scarborough, ON M1V 5K9; 800-250-3030; www.waramps.ca.

Other Acute Problems

Applying Concepts from NANDA, NIC, and NOC

Rescue personnel bring 19-year-old Mia Kim to the Emergency Department (ED) after a motorcycle crash. She has facial contusions and lacerations, a fractured sternum, three fractured ribs, a hemothorax, a dislocated hip and fractured pelvis, and multiple minor lacerations. She is moaning, but responds to her name. Initial findings include an unobstructed airway with absent breath sounds in the right basilar lung field, tachypnea with 32 shallow respirations per minute, and ABG values as follows: pH 7.29; pCO_2 48; SaO_2 90%; HCO_3 24. Blood pressure is 94/70; skin is cool and clammy; heart rate is 100, and peripheral pulses are intact. After a preliminary survey and placement of IV access lines, a chest tube is inserted. Immediately 300 mL of bloody fluid drain into the collection chamber. Grossly bloody fluid continues to drain from the chest tube at a rate of 20 mL every 15 minutes. The concept map illustrates the relationships among selected nursing diagnoses, interventions, and outcomes for one of Ms. Kim's clinical problems.

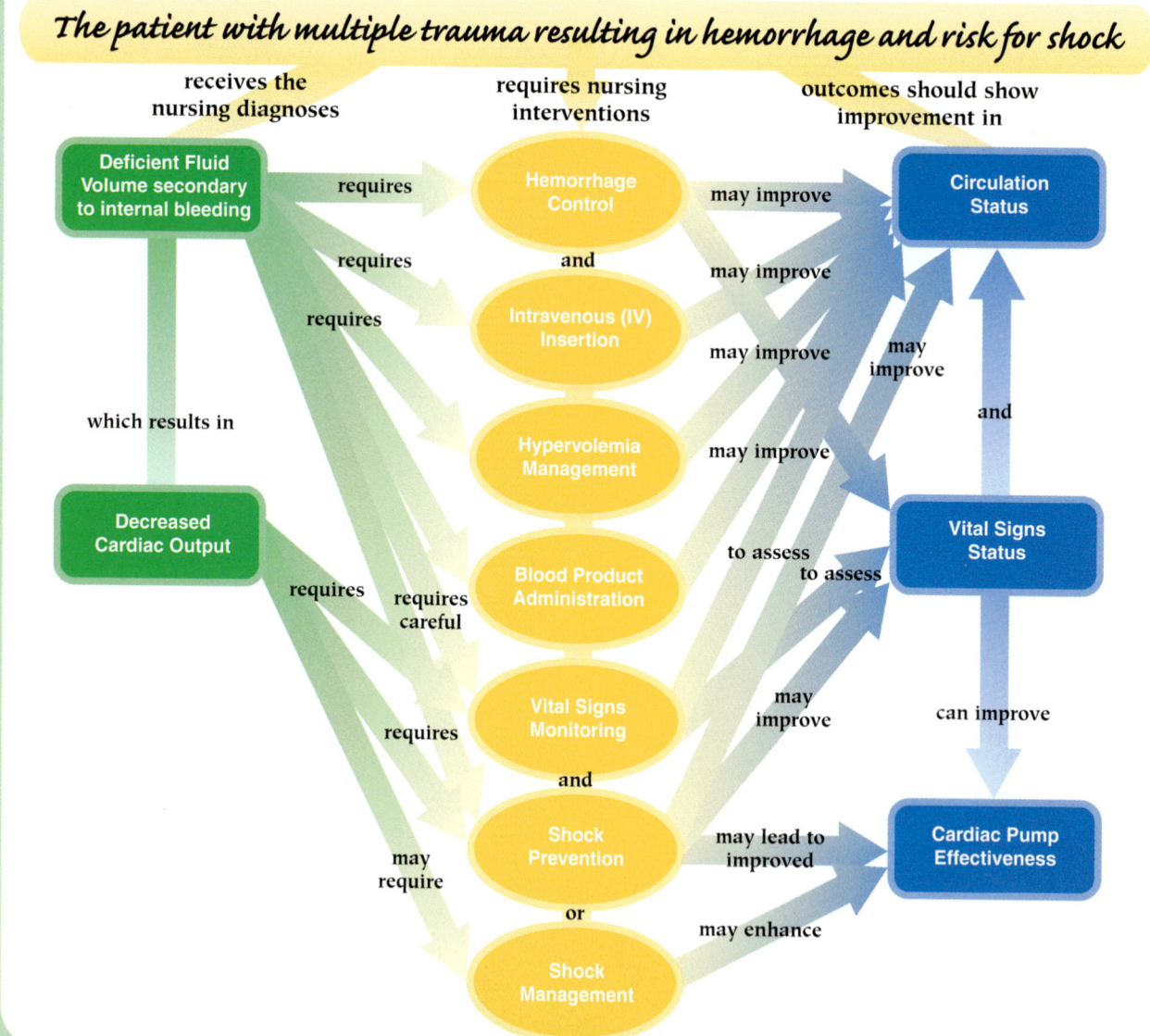

The patient with multiple trauma resulting in hemorrhage and risk for shock

Nursing Classifications and Languages

NANDA
Nursing Diagnoses

Deficient Fluid Volume— Decreased intravascular, interstitial, and/or intracellular fluid

Decreased Cardiac Output— Inadequate blood pumped by the heart to meet metabolic demands of the body

NIC
Nursing Interventions*

Hemorrhage Control—Reduction or elimination of rapid and excessive blood loss

IV Insertion—Insertion of a needle into a peripheral or central vein for the purpose of administering fluids, blood, or medications

Hypovolemic Management— Expansion of intravascular fluid volume in a patient who is volume depleted

Blood Products Administration— Administration of blood or blood products and monitoring of patient's response

Vital Signs Monitoring— Collection and analysis of cardiovascular, respiratory, and body temperature data to determine and prevent complications

Shock Prevention—Detecting and treating a patient at risk for impending shock

Shock Management—Facilitation of the delivery of oxygen and nutrients to systemic tissue with removal of cellular waste products in a patient with severely altered tissue perfusion

NOC
Nursing Outcomes†

Return to functional baseline status, stabilization of, or improvement in

Circulation Status—Extent to which blood flows unobstructed, unidirectionally, and at an appropriate pressure through large vessels of the systemic and pulmonary circuits

Vital Signs Status—Temperature, pulse, respirations, and blood pressure within expected range for the individual

Cardiac Pump Effectiveness— Extent to which blood is ejected from the left ventricle per minute to support systolic perfusion pressure

NANDA, North American Nursing Diagnosis Association; NIC, Nursing Interventions Classification; NOC, Nursing Outcomes Classification

*Iowa Intervention Project © 2000. In McCloskey, J. C., & Bulechek, G. M. (2000). *Nursing interventions classification (NIC)* (3rd ed.). St. Louis: Mosby.

†Iowa Outcomes Project © 2000. In Johnson, M., Maas, M., & Moorhead, S. (2000). *Nursing outcomes classification (NOC)* (3rd ed.). St. Louis: Mosby.

Management of Patients With Infectious Diseases

Adapted by Audrey Groeneveld

On completion of this chapter, the learner will be able to:

1. Differentiate between colonization, infection, and disease.
2. Use information obtained from the microbiology report to interpret infectious disease evidence.
3. Identify federal and local resources available to the nurse seeking information about infectious diseases.
4. Identify the merit of vaccines recommended for health care workers.
5. Identify the reasons for Routine Practices and Additional Precautions and discuss recommended behaviours.
6. Describe the concept of emerging infectious diseases and factors that lead to the development of these diseases.
7. List potential biological warfare agents and describe recommended precautions
8. Use the nursing process as a framework for care of patients with sexually transmitted disease.
9. Describe home health care measures that reduce the risk for infection.
10. Use the nursing process as a framework for care of patients with infectious diseases.

An infectious disease is any disease caused by the growth of pathogenic microbes in the body. It may or may not be communicable (ie, contagious). Modern science has controlled, eradicated, or decreased the incidence of many infectious diseases. However, increases in other infections, such as those caused by antibiotic-resistant organisms and emerging infectious diseases, are of great concern. Examples of these types of infectious diseases are highlighted in this chapter. Other infectious diseases are discussed in the appropriate chapters, such as the information on tuberculosis (TB) found in Chapter 23.

It is important to understand infectious causes and treatment for contagious, serious, and common infections. Table 70-1 presents an overview of many infectious diseases, their causative organisms, mode of transmission, and usual **incubation periods** (ie, time between contact and development of the first signs and symptoms).

The nurse has an important role in infection control and prevention activities. Educating patients may decrease their risk of becoming infected or may decrease the sequelae of infection. Using appropriate barrier precautions, observing prudent hand hygiene, and ensuring aseptic care of intravenous catheters and other interventional equipment also assists in reducing infections.

The Infectious Process

A complete chain of events is necessary for infection to occur. Figure 70-1 illustrates the elements of the chain and identifies weak links where health care workers' interventions can interrupt the chain. The necessary elements of infection include the following:

- A causative organism
- A reservoir of available organisms
- A portal or mode of exit from the reservoir
- A mode of transmission from reservoir to host
- A susceptible host
- A mode of entry to host

ELEMENTS OF INFECTION

Causative Organism

The types of microorganisms that cause infections are bacteria, rickettsiae, viruses, protozoa, fungi, and helminths.

Reservoir

Reservoir is the term used for any person, plant, animal, substance, or location that provides nourishment for microorganisms and enables further dispersal of the organism. Infections may be prevented by eliminating the causative organisms from the reservoir.

Mode of Exit

The organism must have a mode of exit from a reservoir. An infected host must shed organisms to another or to the environment before transmission can occur. Organisms exit through the

Glossary

Additional Precautions: precautions used in addition to Routine Practices when contagious or epidemiologically significant organisms are recognized. The three types of Additional Precautions are Airborne, Droplet, and Contact Precautions. Note that the CDC uses the term *Transmission-Based Precautions* for this category.

bacteremia: laboratory-proven presence of bacteria in the bloodstream

carrier: person who carries an organism without apparent signs and symptoms; one who is able to transmit an infection to others

Centers for Disease Control and Prevention (CDC): American federal agency responsible for monitoring endemic and epidemic disease, for recommending strategies to decrease disease incidence, and for developing guidelines to reduce risk to patients and health care workers in the U.S.A.

colonization: microorganisms present in or on a host, without host interference or interaction and without eliciting symptoms in the host

disease: state in which the infected host displays a decline in health due to the infection

emerging infectious diseases: human infectious diseases with incidence increased within the past two decades or potential increase in the near future

fungemia: a bloodstream infection caused by a fungal organism

Health Canada: federal governmental department responsible for national leadership to develop health policy, enforce health regulations, promote disease prevention, and enhance healthy living for all Canadians

high-level disinfection: removal of all microorganisms, with the possible exception of spores. This level of disinfection is appropriate for instruments that come in contact with mucous membranes but that cannot be sterilized because of mechanical issues.

host: person who provides living conditions to support a microorganism

immune: person with protection from a previous infection or immunization who resists reinfection when re-exposed to the same agent

incubation period: time between contact and onset of signs and symptoms

infection: condition in which the host interacts physiologically and immunologically with a microorganism

latency: time interval after primary infection when a microorganism lives within the host without producing clinical evidence

methicillin-resistant *Staphylococcus aureus* (MRSA): *Staphylococcus aureus* bacterium that is not susceptible to extended-penicillin antibiotic formulas, such as methicillin, oxacillin, or nafcillin

normal flora: persistent nonpathogenic organisms colonizing a host

nosocomial infection: infection acquired in the hospital that was not present or incubating at the time of hospital admission

Public Health Agency of Canada (PHAC): federal agency responsible for emergency preparedness and response, infectious and chronic disease prevention and control, and injury prevention

reservoir: any person, plant, animal, substance, or location that provides living conditions for microorganisms and that enables further dispersal of the organism

Routine Practices: strategy of assuming all patients may carry infectious agents and using appropriate barrier precautions for all health care worker–patient interactions Note that the CDC uses the term *Standard Precautions* for this category.

sterilization: complete removal of all microorganisms

susceptible: not possessing immunity to a particular pathogen

transient flora: organisms that have been recently acquired and are likely to be shed in a relatively short period

vancomycin-resistant *Staphylococcus aureus* (VRSA): *Staphylococcus aureus* bacterium that is not susceptible to vancomycin

vancomycin-resistant *Enterococcus* (VRE): *Enterococcus* bacterium that is resistant to the antibiotic vancomycin

virulence: degree of pathogenicity of an organism

Table 70-1 • Infectious Diseases, Causative Organisms, Modes of Transmission, and Usual Incubation Period

DISEASE OR CONDITION	ORGANISM	USUAL MODE OF TRANSMISSION	USUAL INCUBATION PERIOD (INFECTION TO FIRST SYMPTOM)
Acquired immuno-deficiency syndrome (AIDS)	Human immunodeficiency virus (HIV)	Sexual; percutaneous; perinatal	Median of 10 yr
Amebiasis	*Entamoeba histolytica*	Contaminated water	2–4 wk
Anthrax	*Bacillus anthracis*	Airborne or contact	2–60 days
Chancroid	*Haemophilus ducreyi*	Sexual	3–5 days
Chickenpox	Varicella zoster	Airborne or contact	About 14 days
Cholera	*Vibrio cholerae*	Ingestion of water contaminated with human waste	A few hours to 5 days
Cryptococcosis	*Cryptococcus neoformans*	Probably by inhalation	Unknown
Cryptosporidiosis	*Cryptosporidium* species	Ingestion of contaminated water; direct contact with carrier	Probably 1–12 days
Cytomegalovirus (CMV) infection	Cytomegalovirus	Transfusion and transplantation; sexual; perinatal	Highly variable: 3–8 wk after transfusion, 3–12 wk after delivery of newborn
Diarrheal disease (common causes)	*Campylobacter* species	Ingestion of contaminated food	3–5 days
	Clostridium difficile	Fecal–oral	Variable; in part related to the influence of antibiotics
	Salmonella species	Ingestion of contaminated food or drink	12–36 hr
	Shigella species	Ingestion of contaminated food or drink; direct contact with carrier	1–3 days
	Yersinia species	Ingestion of contaminated food or drink; direct contact with carrier	1–3 days
Ebola	Ebola virus	Contact with blood or body fluids	2–21 days
Gonorrhea	*Neisseria gonorrhoeae*	Sexual; perinatal	2–7 days
Hand, foot, and mouth disease	Coxsackievirus	Direct contact with nose and throat secretions and with feces of infected people	3–5 days
Hantavirus pulmonary syndrome (HPS)	Sin nombre virus	Contact (direct or indirect) with rodents	Unclear
Foodborne hepatitis	Hepatitis A virus	Ingestion of contaminated food or drink; direct contact with carrier	15–50 days
	Hepatitis E virus	Ingestion of contaminated food or drink; direct contact with carrier	Unclear
Bloodborne hepatitis	Hepatitis B virus	Sexual; perinatal; percutaneous	45–160 days
	Hepatitis C virus	Sexual; perinatal; percutaneous	6–9 mo
	Hepatitis D	Sexual; perinatal; percutaneous	Unclear
	Hepatitis G	Percutaneous	Unclear
Herpangina	Coxsackievirus	Direct contact with nose and throat secretions and feces of infected people	3–5 days
Herpes simplex	Human herpesvirus 1 and 2	Contact with mucous membrane secretions	2–12 days
Histoplasmosis	*Histoplasma capsulatum*	Inhalation of airborne spores	5–18 days
Hookworm disease	*Necator americanus; Ancyclostoma duodenale*	Contact with soil contaminated with human feces	A few weeks to many months
Impetigo	*Staphylococcus aureus*	Contact with *S. aureus* carrier	4–10 days
Influenza	Influenza virus A, B, or C	Droplet spread	24–72 hr
Lassa fever	Lassa virus	Contact with animal droppings; direct contact with blood or body fluids	7–21 days
Legionnaires' disease	*Legionella pneumophila*	Airborne from water source	2–10 days
Listeriosis	*Listeria monocytogenes*	Foodborne; perinatal	Unclear; probably 3–70 days
Lyme disease	*Borrelia burgdorferi*	Tick bite	14–23 days
Lymphogranuloma venereum	*Chlamydia inguinale*	Sexual	Weeks to years
Malaria	*Plasmodium vivax; Plasmodium malariae; Plasmodium falciparum; Plasmodium ovale*	Bite from *Anopheles* species mosquito	12–30 days
Meningococcal meningitis or bacteremia	*Neisseria meningitidis*	Contact with pharyngeal secretions; perhaps airborne	2–10 days

(continued)

Table 70-1 • Infectious Diseases, Causative Organisms, Modes of Transmission, and Usual Incubation Period (Continued)

DISEASE OR CONDITION	ORGANISM	USUAL MODE OF TRANSMISSION	USUAL INCUBATION PERIOD (INFECTION TO FIRST SYMPTOM)
Mononucleosis	Epstein-Barr virus	Contact with pharyngeal secretions	4–6 weeks
Mycobacterial diseases (nontuberculosis *Mycobacterium* species)	*Mycobacterium avium; Mycobacterium kansasii; Mycobacterium fortuitum; Mycobacterium gordonae;* other *Mycobacterium* species	Variable; probably contact with soil, water, or other environmental source; none is transmissible person-to-person	Variable
Mycoplasmal pneumonia	*Mycoplasma pneumoniae*	Droplet inhalation	14–21 days
Pediculosis	*Pediculus humanus capitis* (head louse); *Phthirus pubis* (crab louse)	Direct contact	1–2 wk
Pinworm disease	*Enterobius vermicularis*	Direct contact with egg-contaminated articles	4- to 6-wk life cycle; often takes months of infection before recognition
Pneumocystis carinii pneumonia	*Pneumocystis carinii*	Unknown; not transmitted person-to-person	Infants: 1–2 mo; adults: unclear
Pneumococcal pneumonia	*Streptococcus pneumoniae*	Droplet spread	Probably 1–3 days
Rabies	Rabies virus	Bite from rabid animal	2–8 wk
Respiratory syncytial disease	Respiratory syncytial virus	Self-inoculation by mouth or nose after contact with infectious respiratory secretions	3–7 days
Ringworm	*Microsporum* species; *Trychophyton* species	Direct and indirect contact with lesions	4–10 days
Rocky mountain spotted fever	*Rickettsia rickettsii*	Bite from infected tick	3–14 days
Roseola infantum	Human herpes virus 6	Saliva	10–15 days
Rotavirus gastroenteritis	Rotavirus	Fecal–oral route	About 48 hr
Rubella	Rubella virus	Droplet spread; direct contact	14–21 days
Scabies	*Sarcoptes scabei*	Direct skin contact	2–6 wk
Smallpox	*Variola major*	Airborne and contact	7–14 days
Syphilis	*Treponema pallidum*	Sexual; perinatal	10 days to 10 wk
Tetanus	*Clostridium tetani*	Puncture wound	4–21 days
Trichinosis	*Trichinella spiralis*	Ingestion of insufficiently cooked foods, especially pork and beef	10–14 days
Tuberculosis	*Mycobacterium tuberculosis*	Airborne	4–12 wk to the formation of primary lesion

respiratory tract, the gastrointestinal tract, the genitourinary tract, and the blood.

Route of Transmission

A route of transmission is necessary to connect the infectious source with its new host. Organisms may be transmitted through sexual contact, skin-to-skin contact, percutaneous injection, or infectious particles carried in the air. A person who carries, or transmits, an organism and who does not have apparent signs and symptoms of infection is called a **carrier**.

It is important to recognize that different organisms require specific routes of transmission for infection to occur. For example, *Mycobacterium tuberculosis* is almost always transmitted by the airborne route. Health care providers do not "carry" *M. tuberculosis* bacteria on their hands or clothing. In contrast, bacteria such as *Staphylococcus aureus* are easily transmitted from patient to patient on the hands of health care providers.

When appropriate, the nurse should explain routes of disease transmission to patients. For example, a nurse may explain that sharing a room with a patient who is infected with human immuno-

deficiency virus (HIV) does not pose a risk because intimate contact (ie, sexual or parenteral) is necessary for transmission to occur.

Susceptible Host

For infection to occur, the **host** must be **susceptible** (ie, not possessing immunity to a particular pathogen). Previous infection or vaccine administration may render the host **immune** (ie, not susceptible) to further infection with an agent. Many infections are prevented because of the powerful human immune defense. Although exposure to potentially infectious microorganisms occurs essentially on a constant basis, our elaborate immune systems generally prevent infection from occurring. The immune-suppressed person has much greater susceptibility than the normal, healthy host.

Portal of Entry

A portal of entry is needed for the organism to gain access to the host. For example, airborne *M. tuberculosis* does not cause disease when it settles on the skin of an exposed host. The only entry route for the bacterium that is of concern is through the respiratory system.

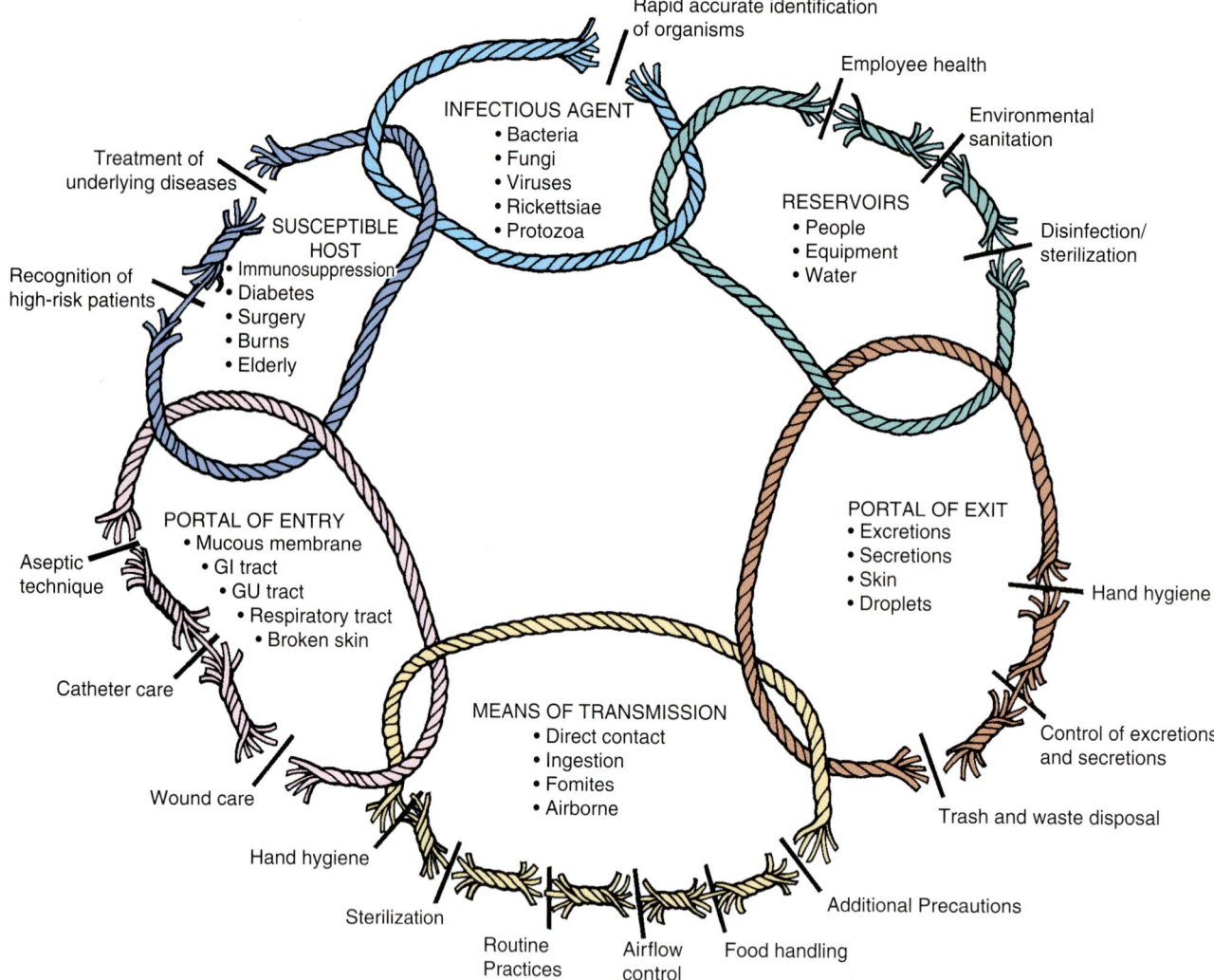

FIGURE 70-1 Health care workers' interventions used to break the chain of infection transmission.

COLONIZATION, INFECTION, AND DISEASE

Relatively few anatomic sites (eg, brain, blood, bone, heart, vascular system) are sterile. Bacteria found throughout the body usually provide beneficial **normal flora** to compete with potential pathogens, to facilitate digestion, or to work in other ways symbiotically with the host.

Colonization

The term **colonization** is used to describe microorganisms present without host interference or interaction. Understanding the principle of colonization facilitates interpretation of microbiologic reports. Organisms reported in microbiology results often reflect colonization rather than infection.

Infection

Infection indicates a host interaction with an organism. A patient colonized with *S. aureus* may have staphylococci on the skin without any skin interruption or irritation. If the patient had an incision, *S. aureus* could enter the wound, with an immune system reaction

of local inflammation and routing of white cells to the site. Clinical evidence of redness, heat, and pain and laboratory evidence of white cells on the wound specimen smear suggest infection. In this example, the host identifies the staphylococci as *foreign*. Infection is recognized by the host reaction and by organism identification.

Disease

It is important to recognize the difference between infection and **disease**. Infectious disease is the state in which the infected host displays a decline in wellness due to the infection. When the host interacts immunologically with an organism but remains symptom free, the definition of disease has not been met. *M. tuberculosis* is an example of an organism that often persists as infection without producing disease. The host may become infected after exposure to the tubercle bacillus. The person is *infected* when bacteria are first detected by nonspecific immunologic recognition and later as newly sensitized T cells propagate daughter lines of TB-specific protective cells. After this initial infection, the untreated host has a low probability of actually becoming ill. About 90% of hosts infected with the *M. tuberculosis* do not develop TB, the disease. Figure 70-2 depicts responses to bacterial infection at the cellular level and at the host level.

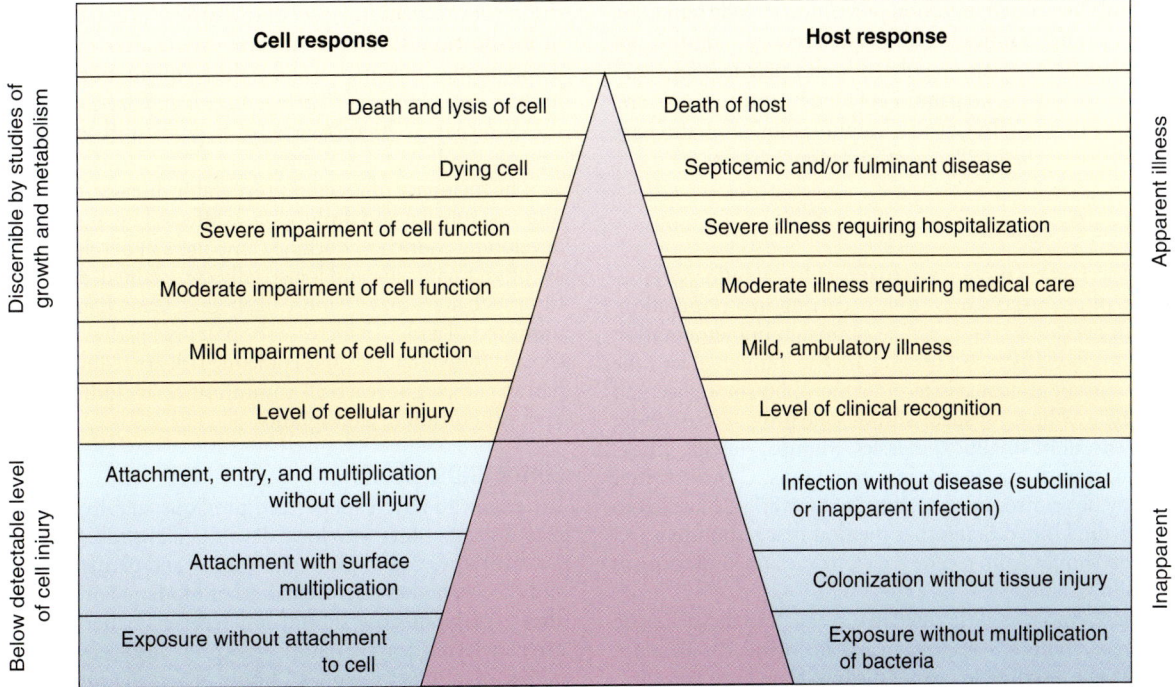

Cell response	Host response		
Death and lysis of cell	Death of host		Apparent illness
Dying cell	Septicemic and/or fulminant disease		
Severe impairment of cell function	Severe illness requiring hospitalization		
Moderate impairment of cell function	Moderate illness requiring medical care		
Mild impairment of cell function	Mild, ambulatory illness		
Level of cellular injury	Level of clinical recognition		
Attachment, entry, and multiplication without cell injury	Infection without disease (subclinical or inapparent infection)		Inapparent
Attachment with surface multiplication	Colonization without tissue injury		
Exposure without attachment to cell	Exposure without multiplication of bacteria		

Left side label: Discernible by studies of growth and metabolism / Below detectable level of cell injury

FIGURE 70-2 Biologic spectrum of response to bacterial infection at the cellular level (*left*) and of the intact host (*right*). Redrawn from Evans, A. S., & Brachman, P. S. (1998). *Bacterial infections in humans.* New York: Plenum.

MICROBIOLOGY REPORT

The primary source of information about most bacterial infections is the microbiology report. The microbiology report should be viewed as a tool to be used along with clinical indicators to determine whether a patient is colonized, infected, or diseased.

When specimens are sent to the laboratory for culture, results usually show three components: the smear and stain, the culture and organism identification, and the antimicrobial susceptibility (ie, sensitivity). As a marker for the likelihood of infection, the smear and stain generally provides the most helpful information because it describes the mix of cells present at the site at the time of specimen collection. Culture and sensitivity processes specify which organisms are recognized and which antibiotics inhibit growth.

Infection Control and Prevention

ORGANIZATIONS INVOLVED IN INFECTION PREVENTION

Health Canada and the Public Health Agency of Canada (PHAC) are federal agencies involved in controlling and preventing infection.

Health Canada and the Public Health Agency of Canada

The impact of infectious diseases changes through time as microorganisms mutate, as human behaviour patterns shift, or as therapeutic options change. **Health Canada** and the **Public Health Agency of Canada (PHAC)** serve an important function in providing timely scientific recommendations about many of the situations that a nurse may face when caring for or teaching a patient with an infectious disease. Health Canada and PHAC routinely publish recommendations, guidelines, and summaries. Through their Internet sites (http://www.hc-sc.gc.ca and http://www.phac-aspc.

gc.ca) and the biweekly journal, the *Canada Communicable Diseases Report* (CCDR), Health Canada and PHAC report significant cases, outbreaks, environmental hazards, or other public health problems. Examples of important Health Canada and PHAC guidelines and summaries are *Hand Washing, Cleaning, Disinfection and Sterilization in Health Care* (Health Canada, 1998b); *Preventing the Spread of Vancomycin-Resistant Enterococci (VRE) in Canada* (Public Health Agency of Canada, 1997a); and *Preventing the Transmission of Bloodborne Pathogens in Health Care and Public Service Settings* (Public Health Agency of Canada, 1997b).

Occupational Health and Safety

In Canada, responsibility for occupational health and safety, including prevention of infections, is shared between the federal and provincial/territorial governments. The Canadian Centre for Occupational Health and Safety (CCOHS) is a key information source about safe and healthy work environments. Health Canada and PHAC publish a variety of occupational health infection control guidelines including *Prevention and Control of Occupational Infections in Health Care* (2002). Each province and territory has occupational and safety legislation that mandates specific practices. Nurses should be familiar with the details of occupational health and safety in their specific institutions, including immunization programs, what to do in the event of a needle stick injury, and fit testing equipment (i.e., determining appropriate mask size) for respiratory protection.

PREVENTING INFECTION IN THE COMMUNITY

Prevention and control of infection in the community are goals shared by Health Canada, PHAC, provincial/territorial, and local public health departments. Much of public health emphasis is placed on prevention to avoid outbreaks and other situations that require control. Methods of infection prevention include sanitation techniques (eg, water purification, disposal of sewage and other potentially infectious materials), regulated health practices (eg, handling, storage, packaging, preparation of food by institutions), and immunization programs. In Canada, immunization programs have markedly decreased the incidence of infectious diseases.

Vaccination Programs

The goal of vaccination programs is to use wide scale efforts to prevent specific infectious diseases from occurring in a population. Public health decisions about vaccine campaign implementation efforts are complex. Risks and benefits for the individual and the community must be evaluated in terms of morbidity, mortality, and financial benefit. The most successful vaccine programs are those for the prevention of smallpox, measles, mumps, rubella, chickenpox, polio, diphtheria, pertussis, and tetanus. Concerns that smallpox may be reintroduced as an act of biowarfare have led to a decision in the United States that medical first responders and selected others should again receive smallpox vaccine. Bioterrorism is addressed in Chapter 72.

More than 25 vaccines are licensed in Canada. Vaccines are made of antigen preparations in a suspension and are intended to produce a human immune response to protect the host from future encounters with the organism. No vaccine is completely safe for all recipients. Some people are allergic to the antigen or the carrier substance. When live organisms are used as antigen, the actual disease (often with a modified course) may follow. Contraindications on package inserts of a vaccine must be heeded. These guidelines detail studied experience with allergy and other complications and provide crucial information about refrigeration, storage, dosage, and administration. Variations to the recommended vaccination schedule should be made on a case-by-case basis, depending on the patient's risk factors and ability to return for follow-up vaccinations at the appointed time. For example, although the first dose of measles vaccine is recommended at the age of 12 to 15 months, babies in developing countries (where measles contributes significantly to childhood morbidity and mortality) should be vaccinated at 9 months.

The standard recommended vaccination schedule for infants, children, and youth as developed by the National Advisory Committee on Immunization (NACI) is shown in Table 70-2. The schedule is revised as epidemiologic evidence warrants, and nurses are advised to consult the NACI to determine the most recent schedule.

Vaccine recommendations for adults are designed to protect those with underlying diseases that increase infection risk, those with potential for occupational exposure, and those who may be exposed to infectious agents during travel. Immunosuppressed adults (including those who have had splenectomy) should be vaccinated for pneumococcus (*Streptococcus pneumoniae*), meningococcus (*Neisseria meningitidis*), and *Haemophilus influenzae*. Health care workers should be immune to measles, mumps, rubella, hepatitis B, and varicella. It is strongly recommended that all of the previously described adult groups and those with asthma or other chronic respiratory conditions receive annual influenza vaccine.

Information about individual vaccines or the most current vaccine schedules may be found on the Internet (http://www.phac-aspc.gc.ca/naci-ccni) as is advice about optimal vaccination for travelers (http://www.TravelHealth.gc.ca). Publicly funded immunization programs may vary by province or territory.

Nurses should ask parents or adult vaccine recipients to provide information about any problems encountered after vaccination. A Report of a Vaccine-Associated Adverse Event form should be completed with the following information: type of vaccine received,

timing of vaccination, onset of the adverse event, current illnesses or medication, history of adverse events after vaccination, and demographic information about the recipient. Forms are available in the *Compendium of Pharmaceuticals and Specialties* or through the Internet at http://www.hc-sc.gc.ca/hpfb-dgpsa/tpd-dpt/adverse_e.pdf.

The incidence of vaccine-preventable diseases, such as measles, mumps, rubella, and diphtheria, is affected by immigration from developing countries. Vaccine campaigns in developing countries are often financially and logistically constrained, and immigrants from such areas may be more likely than Canadian residents to be unprotected and may increase the potential pathways for epidemic spread. Individual risk and epidemic risk are reduced when vaccination campaigns reach all communities, including those with a high proportion of immigrants.

CONTRAINDICATIONS

Patients who have experienced previous anaphylaxis or similar reactions; patients who have developed encephalopathy within 7 days of a previous diphtheria, tetanus, and pertussis (DTP) dose; and those who have developed other moderate or severe sequelae after a previous dose should not receive further doses. DTP is often deferred for the child who previously developed a fever higher than 40°C within 48 hours of vaccination or who had a seizure or developed a shocklike state within 3 days of previous vaccination. Live vaccines usually are not indicated for patients, or for close contacts of patients, with severe immunosuppression (eg, HIV infection, leukemia, lymphoma, generalized malignancy, significant corticosteroid use, use of immunosuppressive medications to prevent transplant rejection). The measles, mumps, and rubella vaccine should not be administered to pregnant women.

MEASLES, MUMPS, AND RUBELLA VACCINE

Since the measles, mumps, and rubella (MMR) vaccines were licensed, reported cases of these diseases have decreased substantially in Canada (ie, fewer than 60 cases per year in 2003; PHAC, 2004). All public health departments are encouraged to vigorously promote vaccination for all children and for susceptible adults unless contraindicated. Routine MMR vaccination should be given to children at 12 to 15 months of age, with repeat dosing at 18 months or at 4 to 6 years of age (NACI, 2005). All who work in health care should demonstrate immunity to these three viruses by one of the following: birth date before 1970, documented administration of two doses of vaccine, laboratory evidence of immunity, or documentation of physician-diagnosed measles or mumps.

Side Effects. Epidemiologic evidence supports that the risk for side effects is greater in nonimmune vaccine recipients than in those receiving repeat doses. Patients should be advised that fever, transient lymphadenopathy, or hypersensitivity reaction might occur. Antipyretics may be used to decrease the risk for fever, but aspirin should be avoided in infants and children because of the risk for Reye's syndrome.

VARICELLA (CHICKENPOX) VACCINE

Varicella zoster is the causative viral agent of chickenpox and herpes zoster. In its natural state, the varicella virus attacks most individuals as children, causing disseminated disease in the form of chickenpox. Chickenpox is often more severe in adults. Transmission occurs by the airborne and contact routes. With rare exception, varicella infects an individual only once. The incubation period is about 2 weeks (range, 10 to 21 days). During a pro-

Table 70-2 • Recommended Immunization Schedule for Infants, Children and Youth, Canada, 2005

Age at vaccination	DTaP-IPV	Hib	MMR	Var	Hep B	Pneu-C	Men-C	dTap	Flu
Birth					Infancy 3 doses ★				
2 months	○	✳				◆	◗		
4 months	○	✳				◆	◗		
6 months	○	✳				◆	◗ or		6–23 months
12 months			■	❖		◆ 12–15 months	◗ if not yet given		◆ 1–2 doses
18 months	○	✳	■ or		or				
4–6 years	○		■						
14–16 years					Pre-teen/teen 2–3 doses if not yet given		◗ if not yet given	♠	

This is an update of the NACI Recommended Routine Immunization Schedule for Infants and Children published in the *Canadian Immunization Guide–6th Edition*, 2002 (Table 1, page 56). Publicly funded immunization programs may vary by province and territory. For more information on specific vaccines and on the NACI recommended immunization schedules for children who did not commence their immunization in early infancy, please consult the *Canadian Immunization Guide–6th Edition, 2002* (http://www.phac-aspc.gc.ca/publicat/cig-gci/index.html) and the vaccine manufacturer's package insert.

○ **Diphtheria, Tetanus, acellular Pertussis and inactivated Polio virus vaccine (DTaP-IPV)**: DTaP-IPV vaccine is the preferred vaccine for all doses in the vaccination series, including completion of the series in children who have received = one dose of DPT (whole cell) vaccine (e.g., recent immigrants).

✳ **Haemophilus influenzae type b conjugate vaccine (Hib)**: Hib schedule shown is the haemophilus b capsular polysaccharide–PRP conjugated to tetanus toxoid (Act-HIB™) or the Haemophilus b oligosaccharide conjugate–HbOC (HibTITER™) vaccines.

■ **Measles, Mumps and Rubella vaccine (MMR)**: A second dose of MMR is recommended, at least 1 month after the first dose for the purpose of better measles protection. For convenience, options include giving it with the next scheduled vaccination at 18 months of age or at school entry (4–6 years) (depending on the provincial/territorial policy), or at any intervening age that is practical. The need for a second dose of mumps and rubella vaccine is not established but may benefit (given for convenience as MMR). The second dose of MMR should be given at the same visit as DTaP-IPV (± Hib) to ensure high uptake rates.

❖ **Varicella vaccine (Var)**: Children aged 12 months to 12 years should receive one dose of varicella vaccine. Individuals = 13 years of age should receive two doses at least 28 days apart.

◆ **Influenza vaccine (Flu)**: Previously unvaccinated children in the 6–23 month age group require two doses with an interval of at least 4 weeks. The second dose is not required if the child has received one or more doses of influenza vaccine during the previous immunization season.

★ **Hepatitis B vaccine (Hep B)**: Hepatitis B vaccine can be routinely given to infants or preadolescents, depending on the provincial/territorial policy. For infants born to chronic carrier mothers, the first dose should be given at birth (with hepatitis B immunoglobin); otherwise, the first dose can be given at 2 months of age to fit more conveniently with other routine infant immunization visits. The second dose should be administered at least 1 month after the first dose, and the third at least 2 months after the second dose, but again may fit more conveniently into the 4 and 6 month immunization visits. A two-dose schedule for adolescents is an option.

◆ **Pneumococcal conjugate vaccine–7-valent (Pneu-C)**: Recommended schedule, number of doses and subsequent use of 23 valent polysaccharide pneumococcal vaccine depend on the age of the child when vaccination is begun.

◗ **Meningococcal C conjugate vaccine (Men-C)**: Recommended schedule and number of doses of meningococcal vaccine depends on the age of the child. If the provincial/territorial policy is to give Men-C after 12 months of age, one dose is sufficient.

♠ **Diphtheria, Tetanus, accellular Pertussis vaccine–adult/adolescent formulation (dTap)**: a combined adsorbed "adult type" preparation for use in people = 7 years of age, contains less diphtheria toxoid and pertussis antigens than preparations given to younger children and is less likely to cause reactions in older people.

drome of general malaise (often noticed about 2 days before the rash develops), the newly infected host is capable of transmitting the virus to other susceptible contacts. Typically, the rash is vesicular and pustular and spreads rapidly from a few to many lesions in a matter of hours. New lesion formation continues for 2 to 3 days, with lesions appearing at different stages throughout this time. By the fourth symptomatic day, the lesions begin to dry, and new lesions usually do not develop. Fever is common during the 4 to

6 days of rash progression. When the lesions have crusted, the patient is no longer contagious to others.

Herpes zoster, also known as shingles, is a localized rash caused by recurrent varicella. Vesicles are restricted to areas supplied by single associated nerve groups. Varicella may be transmitted from the rash of those with shingles to people who are susceptible to varicella.

The varicella vaccine was first recommended as part of the routine vaccine schedule in Canada in 1998. The vaccine is effective in preventing chickenpox in approximately 85% of those vaccinated and significantly reduces the severity in almost all those who get the disease despite vaccination (Atkinson, et al., 2002). The vaccine should not be given to those who have depressed immune function, are pregnant, have received blood products in the past 6 months, or have demonstrated allergy to varicella vaccine.

INFLUENZA VACCINE

Influenza is an acute viral disease that predictably and periodically causes worldwide epidemics. Epidemics occur every 2 to 3 years, with a highly variable degree of severity. Surveillance of influenza in Canada is coordinated through the FluWatch program at the PHAC. The goals of FluWatch include early detection of influenza outbreaks and monitoring of the circulating strains of influenza virus.

Each year, a new vaccine is available. It is composed of the three virus strains (usually two type A influenza and one type B influenza strains) considered most likely to occur in the coming season. When the presumed influenza agents have been correctly anticipated and included in that year's vaccine, vaccine offers approximately 70% to 90% protection for healthy children and young adults. Although less effective in the elderly (as low as 30% to 40% in the frail elderly), it decreases the severity of illness in those who do get infected, is 50% to 70% effective in preventing pneumonia and hospitalization, and is 80% effective in preventing death. In extended care facilities, risk of transmission is greatly reduced by vaccination of all residents (CDC, 2001d).

The NACI recommends annual influenza vaccinations for the following groups at risk for influenza complications: those 65 years of age or older, residents of extended care facilities, those with chronic pulmonary or cardiovascular diseases, and those with diabetes, immunosuppression, or renal dysfunction. Vaccination is also advised for children (eg, those with juvenile rheumatoid arthritis) who require long-term aspirin therapy to reduce the likelihood of developing Reye's syndrome. Health care providers and household members of those in high-risk groups should receive the vaccine to reduce the risk of transmission to those vulnerable to influenza sequelae. Vaccine campaigns among health care workers and patients should be intensified when there is evidence of community influenza disease. Vaccination of healthy persons aged 2 to 64 years is also encouraged (PHAC, 2005a).

PREVENTING INFECTION IN THE HOSPITAL

Nurses specializing in infection control are responsible for agency-wide policy development and program direction. Infection risk is significantly increased as patient care equipment becomes more complex and as more devices that disrupt naturally protective anatomic barriers are used. Staff nurses play an important role in risk reduction by paying careful attention to hand hygiene, by ensuring careful administration of prescribed antibiotics, and by following procedures to reduce the risks associated with patient care devices.

The Canadian Adverse Events Study estimated that 7.5% of patients admitted to acute care hospitals in Canada in 2000 experienced one or more adverse events, including **nosocomial infections** (Baker, et al., 2004).

The CDC estimates that approximately one third of all nosocomial infections could be prevented with effective infection control programs. An effective program includes the following components: a program of surveillance for nosocomial infections and vigourous control efforts, at least one infection control practitioner for every 250 hospital beds, a trained hospital epidemiologist, and feedback to surgeons about individual surgical site infections. Unfortunately, a Canadian study of infection control

resources demonstrated that many hospitals have not introduced all four required aspects. For example, only 37% of hospitals in the study reported surgical site infection rates to individual surgeons. The study concluded that greater investment in resources is needed to meet recommended standards and thereby reduce morbidity, mortality, and expense associated with nosocomial infections and antibiotic-resistant pathogens (Zoutman, et al., 2003).

Specific Organisms With Nosocomial Infection Potential

CLOSTRIDIUM DIFFICILE

Clostridium difficile is a spore-forming bacterium with significant nosocomial potential. Infection is usually preceded by antibiotics that disrupt normal intestinal flora and allow the antibiotic-resistant *C. difficile* spores to proliferate within the intestine.

The organism causes pathology by releasing toxins into the lumen of the bowel. In pseudomembranous colitis, the most extreme form of *C. difficile* infection, debris from the injured lumen of the bowel and from white blood cells accumulate in the form of pseudomembranes or studded areas of the colon. The destruction of such a large anatomic area can produce profound sepsis.

Because antibiotics are used so extensively in the hospital setting, most hospitalized patients are at risk for infection with *C. difficile*. The nosocomial potential is increased because the spore is relatively resistant to disinfectants and can be spread on the hands of health care providers after contact with equipment that has previously been contaminated with *C. difficile*. Control is best achieved by intensifying cleaning, using Contact Precautions for infected patients, and stressing glove use and hand hygiene for all care workers.

METHICILLIN-RESISTANT *STAPHYLOCOCCUS AUREUS*

Methicillin-resistant *S. aureus* (MRSA) is a common nosocomial infection in hospitals and extended care facilities. Rates of MRSA reported in Canada in 2005 were ten times higher than rates reported in 1995 (PHAC, 2005b). MRSA refers to *S. aureus* organisms that are resistant to methicillin or its comparable pharmaceutical agents, oxacillin and nafcillin. Because of the pathogenicity of *S. aureus*, there has been concern about antibiotic resistance since the discovery of penicillin in the 1940s. Soon after penicillin was introduced, *S. aureus* became all but universally penicillin resistant. Fortunately, alternative therapies in the form of cephalosporins and, more importantly, synthetic penicillin solutions such as methicillin, were introduced. It was not until the late 1970s that *S. aureus* showed resistance to methicillin. At that time, the prevalence of the organism was originally linked epidemiologically to the IV/injecting drug use community. Since the late 1960s, however, MRSA has become increasingly more prevalent, and transmission within hospitals and nursing homes has been well documented.

Vancomycin is the preferred alternative treatment for serious MRSA infection. However, there is concern that MRSA will eventually also become resistant to this medication because it is used so commonly. For the first time, in April 2002, a patient in Michigan, USA was diagnosed with an *S. aureus* infection that was fully resistant to vancomycin (ie, **vancomycin-resistant *S. aureus* [VRSA]**). The CDC and other professional organizations have focused preventive efforts against the threat of transmission of this strain and the development of similar strains in other patients. The threat of the growth of VRSA is considered a public health catastrophe because many patients with *S. aureus* infections are likely to have a poor outcome (CDC, 2002b). So far, no cases of VRSA have been reported in Canada.

Health care providers often transmit MRSA to patients because *S. aureus* easily colonizes skin. Because colonization is seldom recognized, the health care provider must assume that *every* patient contact offers the possibility of MRSA exposure. Although there is no evidence that MRSA is more virulent than other strains of staphylococci, the colonized patient faces the likelihood of infection with MRSA when invasive procedures, such as intravenous therapy, respiratory therapy, or surgery, are performed. The patient colonized with MRSA also serves as a reservoir of resistant organisms to be transmitted to others. MRSA acquired in the hospital may persist as normal flora in the patient in the future.

VANCOMYCIN-RESISTANT *ENTEROCOCCUS*

Enterococcus is a gram-positive bacterium that is part of the normal flora of the gastrointestinal tract. It can produce significant disease when allowed to infect blood, wounds, or urine.

Enterococcus has several traits that make it an ideal nosocomial organism. The host carries an abundance of the organism even in a noninfected state; the organism is bile resistant and can withstand harsh anatomic sites, such as the intestine; *Enterococcus* has the potential for resistance to many antibiotics, so that therapeutic agents reducing local bacterial competition may leave it to replicate freely; and the organism endures well on the hands of health care providers and on environmental objects.

As a relatively resistant organism at baseline, therapy for *Enterococcus* has been essentially limited to penicillin formulations (eg, ampicillin) or vancomycin in combination with an aminoglycoside (eg, gentamicin). In the 1980s, resistance to all of these agents was first reported. Between 1994 and 1999, the CDC recorded a more than 40% increase in the percentage of cases of **vancomycin-resistant *Enterococcus* (VRE)** infections in intensive care unit patients (CDC, 2001c). The first outbreak of VRE in Canada occurred in 1995 on a renal unit in an Ontario hospital (Health Canada, 1996).

This rapidly growing problem has serious implications. Because many strains of VRE are resistant to all other antimicrobial therapies, clinicians are left without effective therapy for what was once seen as a relatively common infection. VRE infections may serve as a reservoir of genes coded for vancomycin resistance that may be transferred to the even more prevalent and virulent *S. aureus.* The first case of a patient infected with VRSA, illustrates this concern, as that patient was infected with VRE and VRSA. The gene that commonly causes resistance in VRE was found in both organisms, which strongly suggested genetic transfer between species (CDC, 2002b).

Preventing Nosocomial Bloodstream Infections (Bacteremia and Fungemia)

Reducing the risk of nosocomial bloodstream infections requires preventive activities (in addition to Routine Practices and Additional Precautions, which are discussed later). If a nosocomial bloodstream infection occurs, early diagnosis is important to prevent complications, such as endocarditis and brain abscess. Mortality rates may be as high as 25% for infection with some organisms. The estimated cost attributed to catheter-related bloodstream infections is U.S. $3,700 to U.S. $29,000 per case (Mermel, 2000).

Bacteremia is defined as laboratory-proven presence of bacteria in the bloodstream. **Fungemia** is a bloodstream infection caused by a fungal organism. Any vascular access device (VAD) can serve as the source for a bloodstream infection. Contamination can occur from the patient's own flora traversing the exterior of a catheter or by contamination of internal tubing during manipulation. The intravenous fluid itself can become contaminated and serve as a source of infection. Most hospitalized patients receive VADs, and increasingly, long-term central catheters are used to provide intravenous therapy to outpatients in a clinic or home setting. In all instances, the nurse must use appropriate care to re-

duce the risk of bacteremia and to be alert for signs of bacteremia. Chart 70-1 identifies conditions that suggest the presence of nosocomial VAD-related bacteremia or fungemia.

DISINFECTING SKIN

During the insertion of all VADs, there must be strict attention to aseptic technique. Those inserting VADs must vigorously wash or decontaminate their hands before insertion. Those inserting central catheters should use surgical technique, including sterile gloves, sterile gowns with long sleeves, masks, and a large drape over the patient. The preferred solution to disinfect the insertion site is chlorhexidine gluconate. Alternative solutions are povidone iodine or alcohol. Triple-antibiotic ointment should not be used on the insertion site because it has been shown to lead to increased colonization with *Candida* species (Mermel, 2000).

There is no apparent difference in risk or benefit when comparing the use of transparent polyurethane dressings or gauze dressings. However, if blood is oozing from the catheter insertion site, a gauze dressing should be used. The most important aspects for either material are that the dressing should be applied using aseptic technique and that the dressing should be sealed along its entire perimeter (Mermel, 2000).

USING GUIDE WIRES

Guide wires should not be used routinely when replacing central venous catheters. However, they may be used if there is no evidence of infection and insertion risk is unacceptably high, as when the patient has a coagulopathy or is obese.

CHANGING INFUSION SETS, CAPS, AND SOLUTIONS

Infusion sets and stopcock caps should be changed at 72-hour intervals, unless an infusion set is used for the delivery of blood or lipid solutions. Infusion sets and tubing for blood or blood products should be changed as soon as possible after administration, and lipid emulsions should be changed within 24 hours of initiating the infusion. Solutions other than blood, blood components, lipids, or those with time-limited stability should be completely used or discarded at the time of delivery system change (72 hours). Injection ports should be cleaned with 70% alcohol or an iodophor before accessing the system (Health Canada, 1997a).

Nurses have an important role in the prevention of bloodstream infections as they assess patients for evidence of infection, make daily VAD site inspections, and monitor the interval of line changes. Signs of sepsis in patients with indwelling vascular lines should be promptly assessed and treated.

Chart 70-1 — **Conditions That Suggest the Presence of Nosocomial Vascular Access Device-Related Bacteremia or Fungemia**

- The patient has catheter in place, appears septic, but has no obvious reason to suggest predisposition to sepsis.
- There is no infection at another body site to indicate probable source of sepsis.
- The site of vascular line insertion is red, swollen, or draining (especially purulent drainage).
- The patient has a central vascular line in place at the onset of sepsis.
- The bloodstream infection is caused by *Candida* species or by common skin organisms such as coagulase-negative staphylococci, *Bacillus* species, or *Corynebacterium* species.
- The patient remains septic after appropriate therapy without removal of the vascular access device.

Isolation Precautions

Isolation precautions are guidelines created to prevent transmission of microorganisms in hospitals. In 1999, Health Canada implemented two tiers of isolation precautions. The first tier, called Routine Practices, was designed for the care of *all* patients in the hospital and is the primary strategy for preventing nosocomial infections. The second tier, called Additional Precautions, was designed for care of patients with known or suspected infectious diseases spread by airborne, droplet, or contact routes.

ROUTINE PRACTICES

The tenets of **Routine Practices** are that all patients are colonized or infected with microorganisms, whether or not there are signs or symptoms, and that a uniform level of caution should be used in the care of all patients. The elements of Routine Practices include hand hygiene, use of gloves and other barriers (eg, mask, eye protection, face shield, gown), handling of patient care equipment and linen, environmental control, and patient placement. Hand hygiene, glove use, needlestick prevention, and avoidance of splash or spray of body fluids are discussed in the following sections. Chart 52-3 in Chapter 52 describes Routine Practices (referred to as Standard Precautions) in detail.

Hand Hygiene. The most frequent cause of infection outbreaks in health care institutions is transmission by the hands of health care workers. Hands should be washed or decontaminated frequently during patient care. Table 70-3 describes the recommended situations for hand hygiene.

When hands are visibly dirty or contaminated with biologic material from patient care, hands should be washed with soap and water. In intensive care units and other locations in which virulent or resistant organisms are likely to be present, antimicrobial agents (eg, chlorhexidine gluconate, iodophors, chloroxylenol, triclosan) may be used. Effective hand washing requires at least *15 seconds of vigourous scrubbing* with special attention to the area around nail beds and between fingers, where there is high bacterial burden. Hands should be thoroughly rinsed after this washing.

Table 70-3 • Comparing Hand Hygiene Methods

Hand Decontamination with Alcohol-Based Product
- After contact with body fluids, excretions, mucous membranes, nonintact skin, or wound dressings as long as hands are not visibly soiled
- After contact with a patient's intact skin (as after taking pulse or blood pressure or lifting a patient)
- In patient care, when moving from a contaminated body site to a clean body site
- After contact with inanimate objects in the patient's immediate vicinity
- Before caring for patients with severe neutropenia or other forms of severe immune suppression
- Before donning sterile gloves when inserting central catheters
- Before inserting urinary catheters or other devices that do not require a surgical procedure
- After removing gloves

Hand Washing
- When hands are visibly dirty or contaminated with biologic material from patient care
- When health care workers do not tolerate waterless alcohol product

---

If hands are not visibly soiled, health care providers are strongly encouraged to use alcohol-based, waterless antiseptic agents for routine hand decontamination. These solutions are superior to soap or antimicrobial handwashing agents in their speed of action and effectiveness against bacteria and viruses. Because they are formulated with emollients, they are usually better tolerated than other agents, and because they can be used without sinks and towels, health care workers have been found to be more compliant with their use. Nurses working in home health care or other settings where they are relatively mobile should carry pocket-sized containers of alcohol-based solutions (Zaragoza et al., 1999).

Normal skin flora usually consist of coagulase-negative staphylococci or diphtheroids. In the health care setting, employees may temporarily carry bacteria (ie, **transient flora**) such as *S. aureus, Pseudomonas aeruginosa,* and other organisms with strong pathogenic potential. Generally, transient flora are superficially attached and are shed with hand hygiene and skin regeneration.

Hand washing or disinfection reduces the amount of benign normal flora and transient bacteria and decreases the risk of transfer to other patients. All health care settings should have programs to evaluate compliance with hand disinfection by all who care for patients.

Nurses should not wear artificial fingernails or extenders when providing patient care. These items have been epidemiologically linked to several significant outbreaks of infections. Natural nails should be kept less than 0.6-cm long, and nail polish should be removed when chipped, because it can support increased bacterial growth (CDC, 2002a).

Glove Use. Gloves provide an effective barrier for hands from the microflora associated with patient care. Gloves should be worn when a health care worker has contact with any patient's secretions or excretions and must be discarded after each patient care contact. Because hospital organisms colonizing health care workers' hands can proliferate in the warm, moist environment provided by gloves, hands must be thoroughly washed or decontaminated after gloves are removed. As patient advocates, nurses have an important role in promoting hand washing and glove use by other hospital workers, such as laboratory personnel, technicians, and others who have contact with patients.

Latex gloves are often preferred over vinyl gloves because of greater comfort and fit and because some studies indicate that they afford greater protection from exposure. Their increased use in recent years, however, has been accompanied by increased reports of allergic reactions to latex among health care workers. Reactions range from local skin irritation to more severe reactions, including generalized dermatitis, conjunctivitis, asthma, angioedema, and anaphylaxis (see Chap. 53).

The nurse who experiences irritation or allergic reaction associated with exposure to latex should report symptoms to an occupational health specialist or private physician. Suggested methods for reducing the incidence of such reactions include use of vinyl gloves, powder-free gloves, or "low-protein" latex gloves.

Avoidance of Spray and Splash Exposure. When the health care provider is involved in an activity in which body fluids may be sprayed or splashed, appropriate barriers must be used. If a splash to the face may occur, goggles and facemask are warranted. If the health care worker is handling material that may soil clothing or is involved in a procedure in which clothing may be splashed with biologic material, a cover gown should be worn.

Accommodations and Patient Care Equipment. Single rooms are generally not required for routine patient care. In the acute care setting, patients who visibly soil the environment or for whom appropriate hygiene cannot be maintained should be placed in a single room with dedicated toileting facilities. Where possible, dedicated patient care equipment that will not be shared between patients should be considered. Reusable equipment that has been in direct contact with a patient should be cleaned and reprocessed before use in the care of another patient.

ADDITIONAL PRECAUTIONS

Some microbes are so contagious or epidemiologically significant that precautions in addition to the Routine Practices should be used when such organisms are recognized. Health Canada recommends a second tier of precautions, called Additional Precautions. The additional safety measures are called Airborne, Droplet, and Contact Precautions (Health Canada, 1999).

Airborne Precautions are required for patients with presumed or proven pulmonary TB or chickenpox. Airborne Precautions are also advised if, as a victim of bioterrorism, a patient is suspected of having smallpox. When hospitalized, patients should be put in rooms with negative air pressure; the door should remain closed, and health care providers should wear an N-95 respirator (ie, protective mask) at all times while in the patient's room.

Droplet Precautions are used for organisms that can be transmitted by close, face-to-face contact, such as influenza or meningococcal meningitis. While taking care of a patient requiring Droplet Precautions, the nurse should wear a surgical/procedure mask if within 1 metre of the patient, but because the risk of transmission is limited to close contact, the door may remain open.

Contact Precautions are used for organisms that are spread by skin-to-skin contact, such as antibiotic-resistant organisms or *C. difficile.* Contact Precautions are designed to emphasize cautious technique for organisms that have serious epidemiologic consequences or those easily transmitted by contact between health care worker and patient. The principles of transmission control used in the Routine Practices are accentuated. When possible, the patient requiring contact isolation is placed in a private room to facilitate hand hygiene and protection of garments from environmental contamination. Masks are not needed, and doors do not need to be closed (Chart 70-2).

Emerging Infectious Diseases

As defined by the CDC, **emerging infectious diseases** are diseases of infectious origin with human incidences that have increased within the past two decades or that are likely to increase in the near future (CDC, 1994). Examples of emerging infectious diseases are presented within this section: West Nile virus, Legionnaires' disease, Lyme disease, hantavirus pulmonary syndrome, Ebola and

---

Chart 70-2 **Synopsis of Types of Precautions and Patients Requiring the Precautions**

Routine Practices
Use Routine Practices for the care of all patients.

Airborne Precautions
In addition to Routine Practices, use Airborne Precautions for patients known or suspected to have serious illnesses transmitted by airborne droplet nuclei. Examples of such illnesses include the following:
    Measles
    Varicella (including disseminated zoster)*
    Tuberculosis

Droplet Precautions
In addition to Routine Practices, use Droplet Precautions for patients known or suspected to have serious illnesses transmitted by large particle droplets. Examples of such illnesses include:
    Invasive *Haemophilus influenzae* type b disease, including meningitis, pneumonia, epiglottitis, and sepsis
    Invasive *Neisseria meningitidis* disease, including meningitis, pneumonia, and sepsis
    Other serious bacterial respiratory infections spread by droplet transmission, including:
        Diphtheria (pharyngeal)
        Primary atypical pneumonia (*Mycoplasma pneumoniae*)
        Pertussis
        Pneumonic plague
        Streptococcal (group A) pharyngitis, pneumonia, or scarlet fever in infants and young children
    Serious viral infections spread by droplet transmission, including:
        Adenovirus*
        Influenza
        Mumps
        Parvovirus B19
        Rubella

Contact Precautions
In addition to Routine Practices, use Contact Precautions for patients known or suspected to have serious illnesses easily transmitted by direct patient contact or by contact with items in the patient's environment. Examples of such illnesses include:
    Gastrointestinal, respiratory, skin, or wound infections or colonization with multidrug-resistant bacteria judged by the infection control program, based on current provincial/territorial, regional, or national recommendations, to be of special clinical and epidemiologic significance
    Enteric infections with a low infectious dose or prolonged environmental survival, including:
        Clostridium difficile
        For diapered or incontinent patients: enterohemorrhagic *Escherichia coli* O157:H7, *Shigella* species, hepatitis A, or rotavirus
    Respiratory syncytial virus, parainfluenza virus, or enteroviral infections in infants and young children
    Skin infections that are highly contagious or that may occur on dry skin, including:
        Diphtheria (cutaneous)
        Herpes simplex virus (neonatal or mucocutaneous)
        Impetigo
        Major (noncontained) abscesses, cellulitis, or pressure ulcers
        Pediculosis
        Scabies
        Staphylococcal furunculosis in infants and young children
        Zoster (disseminated or in the immunocompromised host)*
    Viral and hemorrhagic conjunctivitis
    Viral hemorrhagic infections (Ebola, Lassa, or Marburg)

Note that precautions vary for adult and pediatric patient populations.
*Certain infections require more than one type of precaution.
From Health Canada, 1999.

Marburg viruses, and Severe Acute Respiratory Syndrome (SARS). Table 70-1 provides an overview of infectious diseases, including emerging infectious diseases.

Many factors contribute to newly emerging or re-emerging infectious diseases. These include travel, globalization of food supply and central processing of food, population growth and increased urban crowding, population movements (eg, war, famine, disaster), ecologic changes, human behaviour (eg, risky sexual behaviour, IV/injection drug use), antimicrobial resistance, environmental sources, and breakdown in public health measures.

These diseases are important from an epidemiologic standpoint because their incidence has not yet stabilized. As physicians and scientists are learning about the pattern of disease in a community, patients and their families often have increased anxiety about these diseases. During times of increased concern about bioterrorism, whether triggered by actual events or by hoaxes, nurses have an increased responsibility to rationally separate facts from fears. In discussions with patients and other caregivers, it is important to keep the focus on what is known and to clarify the plan for diagnosis, treatment, and containment.

WEST NILE VIRUS

The West Nile virus was first recognized in the 1930s in Africa and first seen in humans in the United States in 1999. The 1999 epidemic was distressing as residents of New York City reported to hospitals with initially undiagnosable meningitis. Most human infections are asymptomatic. When symptoms are present, headache and fever are most frequently reported. Less than 1% of those infected develop more severe illness, including meningitis (CDC, 2001e).

The incubation period (ie, from mosquito bite to onset of symptoms) is between 5 and 15 days. There is no treatment for West Nile virus infection. Patients are supported by fluid replacement, airway management, and standard nursing care when meningitis symptoms are present.

Birds are the natural reservoir for the virus and as of 2002, West Nile virus has been found in five provinces (Nova Scotia, Quebec, Ontario, Manitoba, and Saskatchewan). Mosquitoes become infected when feeding on birds and can transmit the virus to animals and humans. Most communities in central and western Canada have developed a public health surveillance system to estimate the prevalence in birds and mosquitoes. There is no human-to-human transmission of the virus and no evidence of transfer from infected birds to humans. However, as a precaution, it is wise to teach people in affected areas to wear gloves if handling a dead bird. The Public Health Agency of Canada publishes information about West Nile virus on the Internet at http://www.phac-aspc.gc.ca/wn-no/.

LEGIONNAIRES' DISEASE

Legionnaires' disease is a multisystem illness that usually includes pneumonia and is caused by the gram-negative bacteria, *Legionella pneumophila.* Named after an outbreak of the disease among people attending a convention of the American Legion in 1976, its potential to cause outbreaks has been demonstrated numerous times in hospitals and other settings. *Legionella* organisms are found in many man-made and naturally occurring water sources. Although the organisms may initially be introduced in low numbers, growth is enhanced by water storage, scaling (biofilm) on the inside of water towers, temperatures ranging from 25° to 42°C, and certain amoebae frequently present in water that can support intracellular growth of legionellae.

Pathophysiology

L. pneumophila is transmitted by an aerosolized route from an environmental source to an individual's respiratory tract. It is not transmitted from person to person. In hospitals, patients may be exposed to aerosols created by cooling towers, water sources from plumbing, and respiratory therapy equipment. Because underlying medical conditions can increase host susceptibility and subsequent severity of disease and because hospital plumbing systems are often very complex, outbreaks occur in hospitals more frequently than at other centres within the community. Mortality rates among hospitalized patients are about twofold greater than those for people with community-acquired *Legionella* pneumonia (CDC, 2002e).

Risk Factors

Risk factors strongly associated with *Legionella* infection include diseases that lead to severe immunosuppression, such as acquired immunodeficiency syndrome (AIDS), hematologic malignancy, end-stage renal disease, or use of immunosuppressive agents. Other factors associated with increased risk include advanced age, diabetes, alcohol abuse, smoking, and other pulmonary diseases.

Clinical Manifestations

The lungs are the principal organs of infection; however, disease without pulmonary involvement has been reported. Other organs may also be involved. The incubation period ranges from 2 to 10 days. Early symptoms may include malaise, myalgias, headache, and dry cough. With disease progression, the patient develops increased pulmonary symptoms, including productive cough, dyspnea, and chest pain. Patients are usually febrile, and body temperatures may reach 39.4°C and higher. Diarrhea and other gastrointestinal complaints commonly accompany the array of pulmonary symptoms. In severe cases, multiorgan involvement and failure may follow.

Assessment and Diagnostic Findings

Laboratory tests available for the diagnosis of *Legionella* include culture (ie, using special microbiologic methods and media), immunofluorescent microscopy, antibody titer interpretation, and urinary antigen detection. Diagnosis of *Legionella* by antibody titer requires evidence that titers have increased at least fourfold over time. A single elevated titer is not sufficient to determine current disease. The urinary antigen test (for *L. pneumophila* serotype 1, the most prevalent subspecies) is helpful because urine is easy to obtain and the test remains positive after initial antibiotic treatment. This persistent marker especially aids in the diagnosis of community-acquired pneumonia as patients are frequently treated empirically. *Legionella* cultures rapidly become negative after antibiotic treatment, even when the patient's condition is deteriorating. Frequently, more than one laboratory test is used in the diagnosis of *Legionella* because no one test is 100% sensitive. The diagnostic approach generally involves accumulation of information obtained from the history, physical examination, x-rays, laboratory findings, and assessment of therapeutic effectiveness. Chest x-ray abnormalities may vary in severity and in location of the diseased site.

Medical Management

Azithromycin (Zithromax) is considered the antibiotic of choice. Other options include clarithromycin (Biaxin), erythromycin, and levofloxacin (Levaquin).

Nursing Management

The nursing management described for the patient with any pneumonia (see Chap. 23) should form the basis of care for the patient with *Legionella* pneumonia. Special isolation techniques are not used for these patients because there is no evidence of transmission between humans.

LYME DISEASE

Lyme disease, caused by the spirochete *Borrelia burgdorferi,* is transmitted to humans by ticks. It is more common in the Northeast and Mid-Atlantic United States, where the deer tick (*Ixodes dammini*) is prevalent. Ticks may feed on infected white-tailed deer or white-footed mice and then serve as a vector to transmit disease to humans. Lyme disease is less common in the western U.S. states, where the California black-legged tick (*Ixodes pacificus*), capable of transmitting Lyme disease, prefers to feed on reptiles, which do not carry *B. burgdorferi*. In Canada, diagnosis of Lyme disease is usually epidemiologically linked to travel or exposure in endemic areas of the United States (NACI, 2000).

Lyme disease can be manifested by a wide range of symptoms and severity. In its early form, a rash is often present and may be accompanied by regional lymphadenopathy. In later stages, neurologic manifestations ranging from Bell's palsy to Guillain-Barré–like syndrome or dementia are possible. Other sites that may be affected include skin, joints, heart, and eyes.

Assessment and Diagnostic Findings

The rash frequently associated with Lyme disease, known as erythema migrans, is often described as having an expanding bull's-eye appearance. It may be confused with a spider bite. The diagnosis may be made when a patient has this typical rash and at least one late manifestation (eg, arthritis, facial palsy, meningitis, carditis) along with laboratory confirmation of infection.

Medical Management

Doxycycline, ceftriaxone (Rocephin), and azithromycin are among the commonly used antibiotics. Treatment regimens are usually for 3 to 4 weeks. Patients should be encouraged to complete the full course of therapy and to report changes in symptoms during therapy, because the regimen may need to be altered if treatment appears to be failing.

HANTAVIRUS PULMONARY SYNDROME

Hantavirus pulmonary syndrome (HPS) is caused by a member of the Hantavirus family of viruses. In Canada, the Sin Nombre hantavirus causes severe cardiopulmonary illness with a case mortality rate of approximately 38%. Cases occur most frequently in the western provinces, but the rodents known to carry the virus are found throughout the country (PHAC, 2000).

The diagnosis of HPS should be suspected in patients who live in rural areas, who may have had exposure to rodents, and who report fever, aching muscles, and nausea. Thrombocytopenia and hemoconcentration are also common.

Although no specific treatment for HPS has been approved, early treatment with ribavirin (Virazole) may reduce mortality. Early identification, assessment, and maintenance of respiratory status are the most important aspects of care for these patients.

Intake and output should be monitored closely, because overhydration is possible with resultant cardiopulmonary compromise.

Reduction of risk requires strategies to reduce human contact with rodents and their droppings. Public health programs and clinics in rural areas should regularly teach people to eliminate food sources of rodents in areas close to humans. Openings in walls or cabinets should be sealed. Traps should be used in areas such as sheds and barns in which rodents may enter and in which humans work. Gloves should be worn when removing the animal from the trap. The trap should be disinfected with a 1:10 bleach solution. People entering such areas should be taught to avoid stirring up dust or breathing potentially contaminated dust. Brooms and vacuum cleaners should not be used; areas that may emit dust while being cleaned should be first dampened with a bleach solution to reduce viral contaminants and the potential for dust dispersion.

EBOLA AND MARBURG VIRUSES

The Ebola and Marburg viruses are known as filoviruses. Since the 1960s, they have been the source for approximately 20 outbreaks. Both viruses have been prepared as biological weapons and cause great concern because of the extreme virulence and high mortality rates associated with infection.

The clinical course differs among patients, but often includes fever, rash, and encephalitis. Symptoms usually occur rapidly, and with both viruses, the course of the illness often progresses rapidly to profound hemorrhage, organ destruction, and shock. The mortality rate approaches 90%. When patients survive, the recovery period is often prolonged, with weakness, malaise, and cachexia common.

Despite aggressive research, the natural reservoirs for filoviruses have not yet been found, but it is thought that humans are infected only incidentally after exposure to an unrecognized host or by insect bite. Human-to-human transmission usually occurs after exposure to blood or other body fluid. When transmission is percutaneous, it appears that a very low inoculum of contaminated blood is required for transmission to occur. The virus can also be spread by mucous membrane exposure. Although airborne transmission does not appear to be a likely mode of transmission, the possibility has not been entirely eliminated. All involved in caring for patients with filoviruses must adhere to strict infection control measures. It is advisable that systems be set up to have objective monitors to ensure that each nurse or other health care worker wears complete protective equipment in the form of goggles, masks, gown, and gloves (Health Canada, 1997b).

Because there have been no cases diagnosed in Canada, it is likely that early signs of disease may be initially misclassified. The diagnosis should be considered in a patient who has a febrile, hemorrhagic illness after traveling to Asia or Africa or who has handled animals or animal carcasses from those parts of the world. Because neither hospital nor local public health laboratories would be able to confirm a diagnosis, the local Medical Officer of Health should be contacted immediately when Ebola and Marburg viruses are suspected to be the cause of illness. For more information nurses should refer to the Canadian Contingency Plan for Viral Hemorrhagic Fevers and Other Related Diseases (Health Canada, 1997b).

No antivirals have been approved or show promise against Ebola and Marburg. Treatment is largely supportive maintenance of the circulatory system and respiratory systems. It is likely that the infected patient would need ventilator and dialysis support through the acute phases of illness.

Supportive care for a patient with such a devastating disease requires psychological support for the patient and family. The natural fear of an untreatable, aggressive disease would likely be intensified because of the rarity of the disease. The patient, his family, health care workers, and others in the community will need substantial, coordinated education about the known and unknown elements. Intervention may be required from those trained to provide psychological support for traumatic or terrorist events.

SEVERE ACUTE RESPIRATORY SYNDROME (SARS)

In March 2003, the World Health Organization issued a global warning about the appearance of a newly recognized type of pnemonia, Severe Acute Respiratory Syndrome (SARS). SARS is an influenza-like disease, with patients presenting with fever and cough. A minority will progress to experience respiratory distress. The disease was first recognized in China, with a second generation of cases erupting quickly in Hong Kong, Vietnam, and over 17 other countries including Canada in a number of weeks.

The pattern of worldwide dissemination was largely attributed to travel because of strong epidemiologic evidence that patients from many countries had shared common exposures. SARS serves as an example of how suddenly benign microorganisms, especially viruses, can mutate to become important human pathogens. The epidemic illustrates important principles of public health and infection control. Before the disease came to the attention of the WHO, transmission to nurses and other health care professionals occured frequently. Once patients were appropriately isolated, with health care workers using barrier precautions and cleaning contaminated surfaces carefully, transmission was effectively reduced or prevented.

TRAVEL AND IMMIGRATION

Historically, migration of populations has often led to epidemics of disease in countries where people have no immunity to the disease. Because of trade, immigration, and wars, yellow fever, malaria, hookworm, leprosy, smallpox, measles, mumps, syphilis, and many other infectious diseases have been brought to the Western Hemisphere. More recently, the HIV epidemic was transmitted worldwide by means of travel and immigration.

Few diseases carried by travelers spread efficiently in the Canadian environment because of enforced vaccination, clean water, and insect and rodent control. However, there is growing concern that vector-borne diseases, such as dengue, may be transmitted by mosquitoes if a reservoir of infected humans is established. Health Canada and the Public Health Agency of Canada maintain an active surveillance system to prospectively monitor and halt the incidence of many diseases.

Immigration and Acquired Immunodeficiency Disease Syndrome

The fact that AIDS reached pandemic proportions in less than a decade after its recognition attests to the efficiency of world travel in spreading disease. The significance of such rapid transmission rates is especially dramatic in that HIV essentially requires intimate contact between two people through sexual activity or sharing blood through needles.

HIV and AIDS surveillance data from Canada are presented regularly in Health Canada's semi-annual report *HIV and AIDS in Canada*. At the end of 2002, an estimated 56,000 people in Canada were living with HIV infection (including AIDS) (PHAC, 2003).

HIV-1 was probably first introduced to North America in the 1970s when asymptomatically infected travelers returned to the United States after having acquired the virus in other countries. HIV-2, which is similar to HIV-1 in causing immunodeficiency but less contagious in the early stages, is most prevalent in West Africa. The public health challenge is to set up surveillance and control mechanisms for this disease so that undiagnosed HIV infections can be detected. Because HIV-2 is rare, patients with signs of immune dysfunction do not need to be routinely tested for it. However, patients with immunodeficiency should be tested for HIV-2 if they have negative HIV-1 confirmatory test results or have traveled from countries where HIV-2 is prevalent. All donated blood must be screened for HIV-2 (Grant & DeCock, 2001)

Immigration and Tuberculosis

Although there are substantive plans to eliminate TB in Canada, it remains a growing epidemic in developing nations. Immigration has always been an important influence in the dynamic epidemiology of TB in Canada. In 2002, TB among foreign-born individuals accounted for 67% of all reported cases in Canada (PHAC, 2005c).

The association between immigration and transmission risk is greatest in urban areas because these locations are frequently heavily populated and visited by foreign-born people. These locales are also often the epicentres of the HIV epidemic, a population with suppressed immunity to TB. The combination of social, financial, and immunologic risks makes the goal of TB elimination very challenging.

A positive purified protein derivative (PPD) skin test establishes that TB infection has occurred at some time in a person's life. Because it does not provide information about current infectivity, it cannot be used to determine transmission potential. The complexity of PPD interpretation is increased because of the common use of the bacillus Calmette-Guérin (BCG) vaccine in many foreign countries. After receiving BCG, individuals are often PPD positive for a prolonged time, decreasing the ability of the PPD to serve as a TB screen.

Immigration and Vector-Borne Diseases

Malaria, yellow fever, and dengue are diseases that cause significant morbidity and mortality throughout the developing world. These diseases are spread by infected mosquitoes. Many other vector-borne parasitic diseases in developing countries rely on mosquitoes and other organisms to complete their life cycles and transmit disease.

Dengue fever is an example of the risk of imported vector-borne disease. The disease is caused by a virus that is spread through human populations by the *Aedes aegypti* mosquito. The mosquitoes thrive in tropical zones and breed in stagnant water sources. Travelers, immigrants, and returning military personnel can serve as reservoirs of infection. A recent increase of dengue virus in the Caribbean has caused concern that outbreaks may occur in the United States in areas where there are vector mosquitoes. Travelers should investigate the risk of infectious disease prior to leaving home.

Infection from dengue produces flulike symptoms of fever, chills, eye pain, joint pain, and sometimes, a hyperpigmented rash. Symptoms often wax and wane and are generally self-limited. A small proportion of patients may develop hemorrhagic disease, which can be life-threatening in extreme forms. There is no specific treatment for this infection. Control efforts rely on local effective mosquito control.

DIARRHEAL DISEASES

In developing countries of the world, infectious diarrhea kills about 4 million people per year. In the United States, it is estimated that children younger than 5 years of age experience more than 20 million episodes of diarrheal diseases each year, with about 400 deaths per year attributed to such episodes. Dehydration is the most important factor for the morbidity and mortality associated with diarrheal disease. Dehydration is largely controllable by using rehydration therapy (Guerrant & Steiner, 2000).

Transmission

The portal of entry of all diarrheal pathogens is oral ingestion. Although the food we eat is far from sterile, the high acidity of the stomach and the antibody-producing cells of the small bowel generally serve to decrease the potential of pathogens. If the number of organisms is large enough, or if the food neutralizes the acidic environment, infection can occur. Decreased gastric acidity with disruption of normal bowel flora (as occurs after surgery), use of antimicrobial agents, and the immune dysfunction of AIDS all decrease intestinal defenses.

Specific Causes

There are many viral, bacterial, and parasitic causes for diarrheal diseases. Rotavirus is the most significant viral cause of diarrhea in young children. Common causes of bacterial infection include *Escherichia coli* and *Salmonella, Shigella, Campylobacter,* and *Yersinia* species. Parasitic infections of importance include *Giardia* and *Cryptosporidium* species and *Entamoeba histolytica.*

ESCHERICHIA COLI

E. coli is the most common aerobic organism colonizing the large bowel. When *E. coli* organisms are cultured from fecal specimens, the results seldom suggest pathology, but rather reflect normal flora. However, certain strains of *E. coli* with increased **virulence** (ie, degree of pathogenicity of an organism) have been responsible for significant outbreaks in recent years. These stronger pathologic strains are subgrouped as enterotoxigenic *E. coli* (ETEC) because of their production of enterotoxins. ETEC strains often cause cholera-like disease, with rapid, severe dehydration and an increased risk of death.

Recent outbreaks of an *E. coli* species, 0157:H7, have often been linked to the ingestion of undercooked beef. This bacterium lives in the intestines of cattle and can be introduced into meat at the time of slaughter. Prevention of disease from this strain of *E. coli* is aimed at teaching the public to cook ground beef thoroughly (ie, until the meat is no longer pink and the juices run clear).

SALMONELLA INFECTION

Salmonella is a gram-negative bacillus with many species, including the very pathogenic *Salmonella typhi* (ie, typhoid fever). Of the nontyphi species, most organisms are prevalent in animal food sources. It is estimated that *Salmonella* species contaminate more

than 50% of commercially available chicken products and are frequently found in eggs (intact and with broken shells), in raw milk, and occasionally in beef (Crump et al., 2002). Approximately 40% of the deaths caused by *Salmonella* occur in nursing home residents. The high mortality rate reflects the seriousness of the infection in the elderly, who often have weakened immune systems (CDC, 2000a).

There is great variability of symptoms associated with *Salmonella* species infection, including an asymptomatic carrier state, gastroenteritis, and systemic infection. Diarrhea with gastroenteritis is common. Disseminated disease and bacteremia, whether accompanied by diarrhea or not, is less common.

The person with *Salmonella*-caused diarrhea can be a source for transmission to others. The importance of good hygiene should be emphasized, and health care workers should use special care when handling bedpans, stool specimens, or other objects that may have fecal contamination. Hand hygiene is imperative after any contact with a person with *Salmonella* diarrhea. Patients with gastroenteritis generally are not treated with antibiotics because antibiotic use may increase the period of time that the patient carries the bacteria while not improving the clinical outcome. However, those with systemic salmonellosis require antimicrobial therapy.

SHIGELLA INFECTION

The *Shigella* species is a gram-negative organism that invades the lumen of the intestine and causes disease and severe watery (possibly bloody) diarrhea. *Shigella* species spread through the fecal-oral route, with easy transmission from one person to another. Small numbers of organisms are needed to cause disease. Because transmission occurs easily with improper hygiene, it is not surprising that *Shigella* organisms disproportionately affect pediatric populations. Disease in the very young may infrequently be complicated by pulmonary or neurologic symptoms.

Antimicrobial therapy should be instituted early. Frequently, initial therapy choices must be altered when final microbiologic testing reveals the organism's sensitivity.

CAMPYLOBACTER INFECTIONS

In the United States, diarrheal disease attributed to *Campylobacter* species surpasses that recorded for *Salmonella* and *Shigella* species. The organism is found abundantly in animal food sources. It is especially common in poultry but can also be found in beef and pork. Transmission appears to be almost entirely by the fecal-oral route, with food sources representing the reservoir of organism. Direct person-to-person transmission appears to be less common than for other enteric pathogens, such as *Shigella*.

Cooking and storing food at appropriate temperatures protects against *Campylobacter*. It is important that kitchen utensils used in meat preparation be kept away from other food to prevent *Campylobacter* transmission.

After a person is infected, the organism directly attacks the lumen of the intestine and may cause disease through enterotoxin release. Symptoms can range from mild abdominal cramping and minimal diarrhea to severe disease with profuse watery bloody diarrhea and debilitating abdominal cramping. Antimicrobial therapy is recommended only for those who are seriously ill.

GIARDIA LAMBLIA

Giardia lamblia is a protozoan. Transmission occurs when food or drink is contaminated with viable cysts of the organism. People often become infected while traveling to endemic areas in industrialized and nonindustrialized countries of the world or by drinking contaminated water from mountain streams within Canada and the United States. The organism can be transmitted by close contact, as occurs in day care settings. Transmission by sexual contact has also been documented.

Frequently, the infection goes unnoticed. Infection is often recognized more easily in children than in adults. In extreme cases, the patient may experience abdominal pain and chronic diarrhea, usually described as containing mucus and fat but not blood. Microscopic examination of stool specimens reveals the trophozoite or cyst stages of the parasitic life cycle.

Metronidazole (Flagyl) is commonly used to treat *Giardia,* but success rates for this and alternative therapies are inconsistent. Patients with *Giardia* infections should be instructed that the organism can be easily transmitted in family or group settings. Personal hygiene measures should be reinforced, and those who travel or camp where water is not treated and filtered should be advised to avoid local water supplies unless water is purified before drinking or used in cooking.

VIBRIO CHOLERA

Although reported cases of cholera have been rare in Canada, no discussion of infectious diarrhea is complete without mention of this very serious infectious disease. Historically, epidemics of cholera have influenced all aspects of life—from medical to political—and infection rates have been significant enough to destroy governments and armies. Cholera is always a concern when wars or natural disasters result in inadequately processed wastewater. *Vibrio cholera* also may be found naturally in brackish rivers and coastal waters.

The *V. cholera* organism is a gram-negative organism with several different serotypes. The type usually associated with epidemics is toxigenic *V. cholera* 01. The organism is transmitted by contaminated food or water. Travelers should be aware that most recent cases in the United States have been from contaminated shellfish found in the Gulf of Mexico or by visitors who have brought contaminated shellfish into the United States.

Cholera causes disease with a very rapid onset of copious diarrhea in which up to 1 L of fluid per hour can be lost. Dehydration, with subsequent cardiopulmonary collapse may cause rapid progression from onset of signs and symptoms to death. The principal therapy is rehydration. Rehydration efforts should be vigourous and sustained. If oral rehydration cannot be accomplished, the patient should be hospitalized for intravenous therapy support.

In North America, cholera should be suspected in patients who have watery diarrhea after eating shellfish harvested from the Gulf of Mexico. Confirmation of the causative organism can be made by stool culture. It is imperative that all cases are reported to local public health authorities. People traveling to areas where cholera occurs regularly should remember the simple rule of thumb: "boil it, cook it, peel it, or forget it."

NURSING PROCESS: THE PATIENT WITH INFECTIOUS DIARRHEA

Assessment

The most important element of assessment in the patient with diarrhea is to determine hydration status. The goal of rehydration is to correct the dehydration. Assessment includes evaluation for

thirst, oral mucous membrane dryness, sunken eyes, a weakened pulse, and loss of skin turgor. Careful observation for these signs is especially important in cases of rapidly dehydrating diseases (most notably cholera) and in younger children.

Intake and output measurements are crucial in determining fluid balance. Liquid stool should be measured and recorded along with a record of the frequency of stools. It is important to note the consistency and appearance of stool as key indicators of the type and severity of the diarrheal disease. The presence of mucus or blood should also be documented.

When conducting a health history, the nurse must determine whether the patient has recently traveled, whether the patient is being treated with antibiotics, whether the patient has been in contact with anyone who has recently had diarrheal disease, and what the patient has recently eaten. Frequently, patients attribute the most recent meals eaten as the cause of symptoms. However, the incubation period for most diarrheal conditions is longer than the time interval between meals, and the nurse needs to get detailed information about the meal preceding the illness and about all food intake in the previous 3 to 4 days. When eliciting this kind of history, it is helpful to ask the patient to list every food tasted. The nurse also asks patients if they are employed in a food preparation service, because the local public health departments should be notified about any patient with infectious diarrhea who works in the food industry.

Diagnosis

NURSING DIAGNOSES

Based on the assessment data, the patient's major nursing diagnoses may include the following:

- Deficient fluid volume related to fluid lost through diarrhea
- Deficient knowledge about the infection and the risk of transmission to others

COLLABORATIVE PROBLEMS/POTENTIAL COMPLICATIONS

Based on the assessment data, potential complications that may develop include the following:

- Bacteremia
- Hypovolemic shock

Planning and Goals

The most important goals are maintenance of fluid and electrolyte balance, increased knowledge about the disease and risk of transmission, and absence of complications.

Nursing Interventions

CORRECTING DEHYDRATION ASSOCIATED WITH DIARRHEA

The patient is assessed to determine the degree of dehydration. This assessment helps determine the amount and route of rehydration needed. Oral therapy can rehydrate most patients. Oral rehydration therapy is a strategy used to reduce the severe complications of diarrheal disease regardless of causative agent. It is inexpensive and effective, but it is often underused because of sustained cultural beliefs discouraging oral intake during episodes of diarrhea. After much refinement of the formula, the World Health Organization (WHO) and the United Nation's International Children's Emergency Fund (UNICEF) agreed on the makeup of a single solution for treatment of dehydration and electrolyte imbalance associated with cholera and other forms of diarrheal disease. The solution contains (in millimoles per litre) sodium, 90; potassium, 20; chloride, 80; citrate, 10; and glucose, 111.

Mild Dehydration

The patient exhibits dry mucous membranes of the mouth and increased thirst. The rehydration goal at this level is to deliver about 50 mL of oral rehydration solution (ORS) per 1 kg of weight over a 4-hour interval.

Moderate Dehydration

Sunken eyes, loss of skin turgor, and dry oral mucous membranes are common manifestations. An infant may have a sunken fontanel. The rehydration goal is about 100 mL/kg over 4 hours for the patient with moderate dehydration.

Severe Dehydration

The patient with severe dehydration shows signs of shock (ie, rapid thready pulse, cyanosis, cold extremities, rapid breathing, lethargy, or coma) and should receive intravenous replacement until hemodynamic and mental status return to normal. When improvement is evident, the patient can be treated with ORS.

ADMINISTERING REHYDRATION THERAPY

In Canada, commercially available preparations, such as Pedialyte, have been effective fluid and electrolyte replacements for children with viral diarrheal disorders common in this country. When diarrheal losses are very high (>10 mL/kg per hour), however, the lower sodium concentrations of these formulas make them less appropriate than the WHO formula.

For the hospitalized child, diarrheal fluid loss should be weighed, and ORS should be administered at a rate of 1 mL for each gram of diarrheal stool. Stool losses can be estimated so that the patient receives about 10 mL/kg ORS for each diarrheal stool.

It is important for children and adults suffering from acute diarrheal symptoms to maintain caloric intake. Infants who are breastfed should continue to feed on demand; those who are receiving formula should receive full-strength, lactose-free or lactose-reduced formulas immediately after rehydration. Children who normally eat semisolid or solid food should have that food offered. Recommended foods include starches, cereals, yogurt, fruits, and vegetables. Foods that are high in simple sugars, such as undiluted apple juice or gelatin, should be avoided.

Because diarrheal episodes are often accompanied by vomiting, rehydration and refeeding can be difficult. Oral rehydration therapy should be delivered frequently in small amounts. When vomiting is persistent, small children often require frequent administration of fluids by spoonfuls rather than by drinking from a bottle or a cup. Intravenous therapy is necessary for the patient who is severely dehydrated or in shock.

INCREASING KNOWLEDGE AND PREVENTING SPREAD OF INFECTION

Public health nurses, school nurses, and others who are involved in patient teaching should emphasize principles of safe food preparation, with special attention to meat preparation and cooking. Ground beef should be cooked until no longer pink, and all meat should be maintained at temperatures below 4.4°C or above 60°C. In planning events for groups of people, adequate provision for storage and reheating to meet temperature thresholds is important. When preparing food, it is important to use different surfaces, knives, and other equipment for meat and nonmeat items.

Diarrheal diseases discussed in this section must be reported to local public health departments. The goal of reporting is to provide information that will be used to assess disease incidence trends and to identify at the earliest point if there is a restaurant or other food preparation establishment that has served contaminated food.

The need for rehydration and refeeding should be taught to parents of children with diarrheal disease. Beliefs about illness and food patterns may have a traditional or cultural basis, and any teaching of health facts requires cultural sensitivity.

Good hygiene in the health care delivery and home settings must be a focus when caring for patients with infectious diarrheal diseases. The principles of hand hygiene and glove use that are emphasized with Routine Practices are important aspects of disease control.

MONITORING AND MANAGING POTENTIAL COMPLICATIONS

Bacteremia

E. coli and *Salmonella* and *Shigella* species are all organisms that can be introduced into the bloodstream and disseminated to other organs. Blood cultures should be done for the acutely febrile patient with diarrhea. If initial smear results reveal gram-negative organisms, antibiotic therapy is instituted.

Hypovolemic Shock

Shock associated with diarrheal diseases demands accurate intake and output assessment and vigourous fluid replacement. In rare instances, patients with severe fluid imbalance require intensive care nursing support with aggressive hemodynamic monitoring.

Evaluation

EXPECTED PATIENT OUTCOMES

Expected patient outcomes may include the following:

1. Attains fluid balance
   a. Output approximates intake
   b. Mucous membranes appear moist
   c. Normal skin turgor
   d. Adequate amounts of fluids and calories ingested
   e. Absence of vomiting
   f. Stools of normal colour and consistency
2. Acquires knowledge and understanding about infectious diarrhea and transmission potential
   a. Takes proper precautions to prevent spread of infection to others
   b. Describes principles and techniques of safe food storage, preparation, and cooking
3. Absence of complications
   a. Temperature within normal range
   b. Negative blood culture reports
   c. Achieves fluid balance

Sexually Transmitted Diseases

A sexually transmitted disease (STD) is a disease acquired through sexual contact with an infected person. Table 70-4 identifies diseases that can be classified as STDs.

Other organisms can be transmitted during sexual contact, although they are generally not considered to be STDs. For example, *G. lamblia*, usually associated with contaminated water, can also be transmitted through sexual exposure.

Table 70-4 • Conditions Classified as Sexually Transmitted Diseases (STDs) and Their Routes of Transmission

DISEASE	ROUTE(S) OF TRANSMISSION
Chancroid, *Lymphogranuloma venereum*, and *Granuloma inguinale*	Sexual
Chlamydia	Sexual
Cytomegalovirus (CMV)	Sexual, less intimate contact
Gonorrhea	Sexual, perinatal
Hepatitis B (HBV)	Sexual, percutaneous, perinatal
Hepatitis C (HCV)	Percutaneous, probably sexual, probably perinatal
Herpes simplex	Sexual
HIV infection/AIDS	Sexual, percutaneous, perinatal
Human papillomavirus (HPV)	Sexual
Syphilis	Sexual, perinatal

STDs are common infectious diseases in Canada and are epidemic in most parts of the world (Chart 70-3). Portals of entry of STD microorganisms and sites of infection include the skin and mucosal linings of the urethra, cervix, vagina, rectum, and oropharynx.

In June 2001, U.S. Surgeon General Satcher published a document entitled, *The Surgeon General's Call to Action to Promote Sexual Health and Responsible Sexual Behavior.* This document discusses the public health impact of sexually transmitted diseases and other problems associated with lack of sexual responsibility. The Surgeon General reports that approximately 12 million Americans become infected with an STD each year. He encourages educators and health care providers to study methods of influencing irresponsible behaviour and to provide education and services appropriate to the communities they serve (Satcher, 2001). STDs (eg, human papillomavirus, herpesvirus, *Chlamydia*, gonorrhea) are also discussed in Chapter 47.

Prevention

Education about prevention of STDs includes information about risk factors and behaviours that can lead to infection. Included in this education is information about the relative value of condoms in reducing risk for infection.

The use of a condom to provide a protective barrier from transmission of STD-related organisms has been broadly pro-moted, especially since the recognition of HIV/AIDS. At first referred to as a method to ensure *safe sex,* the use of condoms has been shown to reduce but not eliminate the risk of transmission of HIV and other venereal diseases. The term *safer sex* more appropriately connotes the public health message to be used when promoting the use of condoms.

Significance

STDs provide a unique set of challenges for nurses, physicians, and public health officials. Because of perceived stigma and possible threat to emotional relationships, those with symptoms of STDs are often reluctant to seek health care in a timely fashion. Similar to many other infectious diseases, STDs may progress without symptoms. A delay in diagnosis and treatment is potentially harmful because the risk of complications for the infected individual and the risk of transmission to others increase over time.

Infection with one STD suggests the possibility of infection with other organisms as well. After one STD is identified, diagnostic evaluation for others should be performed. The possibility of HIV infection should be pursued when any STD is diagnosed.

HUMAN IMMUNODEFICIENCY VIRUS

HIV is the causative agent of AIDS. The definition of AIDS, as determined by the CDC, has changed several times since the syndrome was first recognized in 1981. In general, the definition sets a point in the continuum of HIV pathogenesis in which the host has clinically demonstrated profound immune dysfunction. Many opportunistic infections and neoplasms serve as markers for immunosuppression severity. Since 1993, the AIDS definition has also included a CD4-positive (CD4+) cell count of less than 200 as a threshold criterion. CD4+ cells are a subset of lymphocytes and one of the targets of HIV infection.

HIV is transmitted through sexual contact, percutaneous injection of contaminated blood, or perinatally from infected mother to fetus. Most people infected by the percutaneous route are intravenous or injecting drug users who share contaminated needles, but transmission is also remotely possible through contaminated blood transfusion. Since 1985, all blood transfusions have been screened, and transfusion-related transmission of HIV is now extremely unlikely. Additional information on HIV is provided in Chapter 52.

Risk to Health Care Workers

NEEDLESTICK INJURIES
Health care workers can be infected through the percutaneous route if needlestick or other injury from a sharp object introduces contaminated blood. Prospective studies of this risk demonstrate that less than 1% of such occupational exposures (in which the source patient is infected with HIV) lead to transmission (CDC 2001a). Despite the rarity of transmission, health care workers are advised to take extreme care to avoid needlestick or mucous membrane exposure to blood of all patients. In most provinces and territories, health care institutions are required to provide devices designed to reduce the risk of needlestick and other injury when such devices are found to be beneficial. Since 1996, the CDC has recommended postexposure prophylaxis for significant occupational exposures to HIV. Counselling about the advisability of prophylaxis and appropriate medication and dose selection

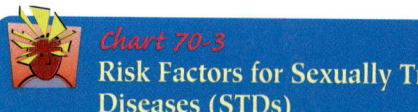

Chart 70-3
Risk Factors for Sexually Transmitted Diseases (STDs)

The risk for acquiring STDs increases for individuals who engage in the following high-risk behaviours:
- Having sexual relations with infected individuals, with multiple partners, or with prostitutes
- Engaging in oral or anal sex
- Using IV/injection drugs

In addition, the rising incidence of STDs in adolescents reflects an increase in sexual activity among individuals in that age group.

Table 70-5 • Recommended Algorithm to Determine Post Exposure Prophylaxis (PEP)

EXPOSURE TYPE	SOURCE HIV POSITIVE ASYMPTOMATIC OR VIRAL LOAD <1,500 RNA COPIES/ML	SOURCE HIV POSITIVE SYMPTOMATIC OR KNOWN HIGH VIRAL LOAD	SOURCE WITH UNKNOWN HIV STATUS	UNKNOWN SOURCE	SOURCE HIV NEGATIVE
Less severe percutaneous exposure (solid needle and superficial injury)	Basic two-drug regimen*	Basic two-drug regimen* and one drug from expanded drug list†	Generally, no PEP warranted, but consider basic two-drug regimen* if source has HIV risk factors	Generally, no PEP warranted, but consider basic two-drug regimen* in settings where exposure to HIV-infected persons is likely	No prophylaxis is warranted
More severe percutaneous exposure (large-bore hollow needle, deep puncture, visible blood on device, needle used in patient's artery or vein)	Basic two-drug regimen* and one drug from expanded drug list†	Basic two-drug regimen* and one drug from expanded drug list†	Same as above	Same as above	Same as above
Small-volume mucous membrane exposure or nonintact skin exposure (a few drops)	Basic two-drug regimen*	Basic two-drug regimen*	Same as above	Same as above	Same as above
Large volume mucous membrane exposure or nonintact skin exposure (large volume splash or spray)	Basic two-drug regimen*	Basic two-drug regimen* and one drug from expanded drug list†	Same as above	Same as above	Same as above

d4T, stavudine (Zerit); ddI, didanosine (Videx™); 3TC, lamivudine (Heptovir); ZDV, zidovudine (Retrovir [AZT])
*Basic two-drug regimen = (ZDV and 3TC) *or* (3TC and d4T) *or* (d4T and ddI).
†Expanded drug list: indinavir (Crixivan), nelfinavir (Viracept), abacavir (Ziagen), efavirenz (Sustiva)
Recommendations based on: Centers for Disease Control and Prevention. (2001). Updated U.S. Public Health Service guidelines for the management of occupational exposures to HBV, HCV, and HIV and recommendations for postexposure prophylaxis. *Morbidity and Mortality Weekly Report, 50* (RR-11), 1–42.

should be made on a case-by-case basis. Table 70-5 provides the recommended algorithm to determine which combination of antiretroviral drugs should be offered to the exposed health care worker. Similar recommendations are made in Canada. All health care workers should understand the need to report a needlestick or other percutaneous exposure immediately (CDC, 2001f).

SYPHILIS

Syphilis is an acute and chronic infectious disease caused by the spirochete *Treponema pallidum*. It is acquired through sexual contact or may be congenital in origin.

Stages of Syphilis

In the untreated person, the course of syphilis can be divided into three stages: primary, secondary, and tertiary. These stages reflect the time from infection and the clinical manifestations observed in that period, and are the basis for treatment decisions.

Primary syphilis occurs 2 to 3 weeks after initial inoculation with the organism. A painless lesion at the site of infection is called a *chancre*. Untreated, these lesions usually resolve spontaneously within about 2 months.

Secondary syphilis occurs when the hematogenous spread of organisms from the original chancre leads to generalized infection.

The rash of secondary syphilis generally occurs about 2 to 8 weeks after the chancre and involves the trunk and the extremities, including the palms of the hands and the soles of the feet. Transmission of the organism can occur through contact with these lesions. Generalized signs of infection may include lymphadenopathy, arthritis, meningitis, hair loss, fever, malaise, and weight loss.

After the secondary stage, there is a period of **latency**, during which the infected person has no signs or symptoms of syphilis. Latency can be interrupted by a recurrence of secondary syphilis.

Tertiary syphilis is the final stage in the natural history of the disease. It is estimated that between 20% and 40% of those infected do not exhibit signs and symptoms of this final stage. In this stage, syphilis presents as a slowly progressive, inflammatory disease with the potential to affect multiple organs. The most common manifestations at this level are aortitis and neurosyphilis, as evidenced by dementia, psychosis, paresis, stroke, or meningitis.

Assessment and Diagnostic Findings

Because syphilis shares symptoms with many diseases, clinical history and laboratory evaluation are important. The conclusive diagnosis of syphilis can be made by direct identification of the spirochete obtained from the chancre lesions of primary syphilis. Serologic tests used in the diagnosis of secondary and tertiary syphilis require clinical correlation in interpretation. The serologic tests are summarized as follows:

- *Nontreponemal* or *reagin tests,* such as the Venereal Disease Research Laboratory (VDRL) or the rapid plasma reagin circle card test (RPR-CT), are generally used for screening and diagnosis. After adequate therapy, the test result is expected to decrease quantitatively until it is read as negative, usually about 2 years after therapy is completed.
- *Treponemal tests,* such as the fluorescent treponemal antibody absorption test (FTA-ABS) and the microhemagglutination test (MHA-TP), are used to verify that the screening test did not represent a false-positive result. Positive results usually are positive for life and therefore are not appropriate to determine therapeutic effectiveness.

Medical Management

Treatment of all stages of syphilis is administration of antibiotics. Penicillin G benzathine is the medication of choice for early syphilis or latent syphilis of less than 1 year's duration but in Canada this drug can only be obtained through the Special Access Program of the Therapeutics Product Directorate of Health Canada. It is administered by intramuscular injection at a single session. The same therapy is recommended for patients with early latent syphilis. Patients with late latent or latent syphilis of unknown duration should receive three injections at 1-week intervals. Patients who are allergic to penicillin are usually treated with doxycycline. The patient treated with penicillin is monitored for 30 minutes after the injection to observe for a possible allergic reaction.

Treatment guidelines established by Health Canada are updated on a regular basis. Recommendations provide special guidelines for treatment in the settings of pregnancy, allergy, HIV infection, pediatric infection, congenital infection, and neurosyphilis (Health Canada, 1998a).

Nursing Management

Syphilis is a reportable communicable disease. In any health care facility, a mechanism should be in place to ensure that all patients who are diagnosed are reported to the state or local public health department to ensure community follow-up. The public health department is responsible for interviewing the patient to determine sexual contacts, so that contact notification and screening can be initiated.

Lesions of primary and secondary syphilis may be highly infective. Gloves are worn when having direct contact with lesions, and hands are decontaminated after gloves are removed. Isolation in a private room is not required (Chart 70-4).

Chart 70-4 • PATIENT EDUCATION
Treating and Preventing the Spread of Syphilis

- The patient is instructed to complete the full course of therapy if multiple penicillin injections are required.
- The patient with primary or secondary syphilis is assured that with proper treatment, skin lesions and other sequelae of infection will improve, and serology eventually will reflect cure.
- The patient is instructed to refrain from sexual contact with previous or current partners until they have been treated.

GONORRHEA

N. gonorrhoeae is a gram-negative bacterium that is transmitted primarily through sexual contact. Infection can also occur in neonates as a result of contact during birth. *N. gonorrhoeae* can cause mucosal, local, or disseminated infection. Asymptomatic infection is somewhat common.

Clinical Manifestations

Gonorrhea most frequently manifests with local manifestations. In men, urethritis and epididymitis are the most common symptoms. Gonorrhea is more likely to be asymptomatic in women than in men. The uterine cervix is the primary site of local infection, and symptoms often include urinary tract infection, increased vaginal discharge, and itching. The most common complication of localized gonococcal infection in women is pelvic inflammatory disease (PID), in which the organism infects the uterus, fallopian tubes, or peritoneal fluid. A complication of gonococcal PID is increased risk for ectopic pregnancy and bilateral tubal occlusion, which results in infertility.

In rare circumstances, the organism may disseminate in untreated, infected people. Other systemic signs, such as arthritis or dermatitis, can accompany bacteremia. In rare instances, valves of the heart can be infected with *N. gonorrhoeae,* or gonococcal meningitis can develop.

Assessment and Diagnostic Findings

The patient is assessed for fever; for urethral, vaginal, and rectal discharge; and for signs of arthritis. Culture and sensitivity studies are the usual and preferred methods of diagnosing and verifying effectiveness of therapy. In the male patient, specimens are obtained from the urethra, anal canal, and pharynx. In the female patient, cultures are obtained from the endocervix, pharynx, and anal canal. When obtaining these cultures, the nurse should wear disposable gloves and decontaminate hands thoroughly after glove removal. Lubricating jelly is not used for the vaginal examination because it may contain substances that inhibit growth or kill some pathogens, decreasing the microbiologic test accuracy. Instead, water is used as the lubricant. Because *N. gonorrhoeae* organisms are susceptible to environmental changes, specimens must be delivered to the laboratory immediately after they are obtained.

Medical Management

The Health Canada–recommended treatment (1998) for gonorrheal infections is administration of cefixime (Suprax) (or ceftriaxone [Rocephin], ciprofloxacin [Cipro], or ofloxacin [Floxin]) along with azithromycin or doxycycline. Azithromycin or doxycycline is added to first-line therapy to treat presumptive *Chlamydia trachomatis,* which commonly causes coinfection in patients with gonorrhea. Patients with uncomplicated gonorrhea who are treated with recommended therapy do not routinely need to return for a proof-of-cure visit. If the patient reports a new episode of symptoms or tests reveal gonorrhea again, the most likely explanation is reinfection rather than treatment failure. Serologic testing for syphilis and HIV should be offered to patients with gonorrhea, because any STD increases the risk for other STD infections.

Nursing Management

Gonorrhea is a reportable communicable disease. In any health care facility, a mechanism should be in place to ensure that all patients diagnosed with gonorrhea are reported to the local public health department to ensure follow-up of the patient. The public health department also is responsible for interviewing the patient to identify sexual contacts, so that contact notification and screening can be initiated.

CHLAMYDIA TRACHOMATIS

C. trachomatis is a bacterium that requires attachment to the host cell, invasion, intracellular growth, and replication. This requirement for intracellular growth, which is similar to that of viruses, has made the identification and laboratory testing more difficult than for organisms that grow and replicate independently, but advances have made diagnosis and screening much more available.

Clinical Manifestations

In women, the most frequent clinical manifestation is PID, but symptoms often are so subtle that pathologic progression can occur without detection. Long-term effects may include chronic pain, increased risk for ectopic pregnancy, postpartum endometritis, and infertility.

Transmission of infection from an infected pregnant woman to her vaginally born infant is common. About 20% to 50% of infected infants develop chlamydial conjunctivitis, and about 20% develop chlamydial pneumonia (Schacter & Grossman, 2001).

Although men infected with *Chlamydia* are frequently asymptomatic, they easily transmit the infection to their sexual partners. Urethritis is the most common illness associated with infection in the heterosexual man with symptoms. Among homosexual men, the rectum is the common site of infection.

Assessment and Diagnostic Findings

Chlamydia should be suspected in cases of gonorrhea, nongonorrheal urethritis, PID, and epididymitis. Diagnostic tools include cell culture techniques and a relatively wide range of nonculture techniques, including immunologic assays, DNA probes, and enzyme-sensitive tests.

Medical Management

Treatment of chlamydial infection is usually administration of doxycycline or azithromycin. Neither of these antibiotics is recommended during pregnancy. Health Canada (1998a) guidelines should be used to determine alternative therapy for the patient who is pregnant or allergic or who has complicated chlamydial infection. The patient and the sexual partner must be treated.

Prevention and Patient Education

The target group for preventive patient teaching about *C. trachomatis* is the adolescent and young adult population. Abstinence, postponing the age of initial sexual exposure, limiting the number of sexual partners, and use of condoms for barrier protection should be promoted. It should also be stressed that screening for *Chlamydia* and treating infection at an early stage are important to decrease disease progression common to women and to decrease the likelihood of infection in infants.

NURSING PROCESS: THE PATIENT WITH A SEXUALLY TRANSMITTED DISEASE

Assessment

The patient should be asked to describe the onset and progression of symptoms and to characterize any lesions by location and by describing drainage, if present. Protecting confidentiality is important when discussing sexual issues. When a detailed sexual history is necessary, it is important to respect the patient's right to privacy. Brief explanations of why the information is asked are often helpful. Clarification of terms may be necessary if the patient or nurse uses words unfamiliar to the other. Asking specific information about sexual contacts usually should be done only when the nurse is part of a team that will contact the partners for follow-up. In the history-taking process, discussion about the patient's understanding of responsibility to inform sexual partners may be helpful in determining patient teaching goals.

During physical examination, the examiner looks for rashes, lesions, drainage, discharge, or swelling. Inguinal nodes are palpated to elicit tenderness and to assess swelling. Women are examined for abdominal or uterine tenderness. The mouth and throat are examined for signs of inflammation or exudate. The nurse wears gloves while examining the mucous membranes, and gloves are changed and replaced after vaginal or rectal examination.

Diagnosis

NURSING DIAGNOSES

Based on assessment data, the patient's major nursing diagnoses may include the following:

- Deficient knowledge about the disease and risk for spread of infection and reinfection
- Anxiety related to anticipated stigmatization and to prognosis and complications
- Noncompliance with treatment

COLLABORATIVE PROBLEMS/ POTENTIAL COMPLICATIONS

Based on assessment data, potential complications that may develop include the following:

- Increased risk for ectopic pregnancy
- Infertility
- Transmission of infection to fetus resulting in congenital abnormalities and other outcomes
- Neurosyphilis
- Gonococcal meningitis
- Gonococcal arthritis
- Syphilitic aortitis
- HIV-related complications

Planning and Goals

Major goals are increased patient understanding of the natural history and treatment of the infection, reduction in fear, increased compliance with therapeutic and preventive goals, and absence of complications.

Nursing Interventions

INCREASING KNOWLEDGE AND PREVENTING SPREAD OF DISEASE

Education about and prevention of the spread of STDs to others is often accomplished simultaneously. Discussion about risk factors should emphasize that the same behaviours that led to infection with one STD may introduce risk for any other STD, including HIV. Methods used to contact sexual partners should be discussed. The patient should understand that, until the partner has been treated, continued sexual exposure to the same person may lead to reinfection. Patients may need help in planning discussion with partners. If the patient is especially apprehensive about this aspect, referral to a social worker or other specialist may be appropriate. Such support is especially important when the patient has newly diagnosed HIV infection.

The relative value of condoms in reducing the risk for infection with STDs should be addressed. When appropriate, the patient should be encouraged to discuss any reasons for resistance to condom use, so that decision making about this preventive method can be facilitated.

The infected patient should be told what the causative organism is and should receive an explanation of the usual course of the infection (including interval of potential communicability to others) and possible complications. The nurse should stress the importance of following therapy as prescribed and the need to report any therapeutic side effects or symptom progression.

REDUCING ANXIETY

When appropriate, the patient is encouraged to discuss anxieties and fear associated with the diagnosis, therapy, or prognosis. By individualizing teaching efforts, factual information applied to specific needs may offer reassurance. For example, patients with HIV should be encouraged to participate in well-coordinated programs in which support, education, counselling, and therapeutic goals are combined. Such programs are designed to offer coordinated care throughout the course of disease progression.

INCREASING COMPLIANCE

In group settings (eg, offered in an outpatient obstetric setting) or in a one-on-one setting, open discussion about STD information facilitates patient teaching. Discomfort can be reduced by factual explanation of causes, consequences, treatments, prevention, and responsibilities. Because most communities have expanded STD prevention resources, referrals to appropriate agencies can complement individual educational efforts and ensure that later questions or uncertainties can be addressed by experts.

MONITORING AND MANAGING POTENTIAL COMPLICATIONS

Infertility and Increased Risk for Ectopic Pregnancy

STDs may lead to PID and, with it, increased risk for ectopic pregnancy and infertility.

Congenital Infections

All STDs can be transmitted to infants in utero or at the time of birth. Complications of congenital infection can range from localized infection (eg, throat infection with *N. gonorrhoeae*) to congenital abnormalities (eg, stunting of growth or deafness from congenital syphilis), to life-threatening disease (eg, congenital herpes simplex virus).

Neurosyphilis, Gonococcal Meningitis, Gonococcal Arthritis, Syphilitic Aortitis

STDs can cause disseminated infection. The central nervous system may be infected, as seen in cases of neurosyphilis or gonococcal meningitis. Gonorrhea that infects the skeletal system may result in gonococcal arthritis. Syphilis can infect the cardiovascular system by forming vegetative lesions on the mitral or aortic valves.

Human Immunodeficiency Virus–Related Complications

HIV, which is primarily spread as an STD, leads to the profound immunosuppression of AIDS. Complications of HIV infection include many opportunistic infections, including *Pneumocystis carinii, Cryptococcus neoformans,* cytomegalovirus, and *Mycobacterium avium.*

Evaluation

EXPECTED PATIENT OUTCOMES

Expected patient outcomes may include the following:

1. Acquires knowledge and understanding of STDs
2. Demonstrates a less anxious demeanor
   a. Discusses anxieties and goals for treatment
   b. Inspects self for lesions, rashes, and discharge
   c. Accepts support education, and counselling when indicated
   d. Assists with sharing information about infection to sexual partners
   e. Discusses risk-reduction behaviours and safer sex practices
3. Complies with treatment
   a. Achieves effective treatment
   b. Reports for follow-up examination if necessary
4. Absence of complications

Home-Based Care of the Patient With an Infectious Disease

REDUCING RISK

The nurse who cares for the patient in the home should provide infection risk prevention for the patient, the family, and the caregiver (Chart 70-5).

Reducing Risk to the Patient

Patients requiring home care are often those with immunosuppression from underlying conditions, such as HIV infection or cancer, or those who have therapy-induced immunosuppression, as occurs with many antineoplastic agents. Careful assessment for signs of infection is important.

HAND HYGIENE

Hand washing or use of an alcohol-based hand disinfectant in the home is an important preventive strategy. Whether a treatment is performed by the nurse, the family, or the patient, appropriate hand hygiene reduces the risk of transient flora.

EQUIPMENT CARE

Health care equipment increases infection risk because it is complex and invasive. All caregivers must be taught to pay careful attention to disinfection and aseptic technique. The nurse and the

---

Chart 70-5
Home Care Checklist • **Prevention of Infection in the Home Care Setting**

At the completion of the home care instruction, the patient or caregiver will be able to:	**Patient**	**Caregiver**
• Demonstrate aseptic technique in the care of technical equipment such as intravenous catheter, indwelling urinary catheter.	✓	✓
• Demonstrate thorough hand washing after patient care.	✓	✓
• Provide assurance of compliance with antibiotic regimen or with completion of vaccination series.	✓	✓
• State the rationale for thoroughly cooking all foods and storing meat products separate from other food groups.	✓	✓
• Use separate eating utensils and towels.	✓	✓
• Avoid contact with someone who has a known infectious disease.	✓	✓

---

family members should be alert for any redness, swelling, or drainage around a catheter insertion site. Catheter-related sepsis should be suspected in a patient who has unexplained fever.

There is no recommended interval for the changing of indwelling urinary catheters. The nurse should promptly report to the patient's physician signs of urinary tract infection or of generalized sepsis.

PATIENT TEACHING

When assessing the immune-suppressed patient in the home environment for infectious risk, it is important to realize that intrinsic colonizing bacteria and latent viral infections present a greater risk than do extrinsic environmental contaminants. The patient and family need reassurance that their home should be clean but not sterile. Common-sense approaches to cleanliness and risk reduction are helpful. The severely neutropenic patient should refrain from eating uncooked fruits and vegetables. For patients with neutropenia or with T-cell dysfunction (eg, patients with AIDS), it is wise to restrict visits of people with potentially contagious illnesses.

Reducing Risk to Household Members

ESTABLISHING BARRIERS AND PRECAUTIONS

Establishing careful barriers to infection transmission in the household is an important part of home care. The route of transmission of the organism in question must first be determined. The nurse can then teach household members strategies to reduce their risk of becoming infected. If the patient has active pulmonary TB, the public health department should be contacted to provide screening and treatment for family members. If a patient has shingles (herpes zoster), family members who have had varicella vaccine or who have previously had chickenpox are considered immune and need no precautions. However, if a family member is immunosuppressed or otherwise susceptible to varicella, maintaining physical separation may be an important strategy during the time when the patient has draining lesions.

FOOD PREPARATION AND PERSONAL HYGIENE

Organisms transmitted by the fecal-oral route may be readily spread in a household setting unless careful attention to food preparation and personal hygiene is maintained. Family caregivers may be vulnerable to acquiring organisms such as *Shigella* species and *C. difficile* when assisting in personal care. Hands should be thoroughly disinfected after such contact. The family should be reassured that common household disinfectants are effective in killing environmental sources of such organisms.

BLOODBORNE INFECTION RISK

Family members who assist in the care of a patient with a bloodborne infection such as HIV or hepatitis C should be alert for the potential of transmission if sharp objects contaminated with blood are handled. Family teaching may be designed to discuss the need for caution when shaving the patient, performing dressing changes, or administering any intravenous, intramuscular, or subcutaneous medication. It is important to set up an impenetrable container for the collection of needles, syringes, and vascular access equipment.

The nurse should also teach the family about infections that are and are not contagious to family members. With the exception of TB, the opportunistic infections associated with AIDS do not pose a risk to the healthy family member. Family members should be reassured that dishes are safe to use after being washed with hot water and that linens and clothing are safe to use after being washed in a hot-water cycle.

Reducing Risk to the Caregiver

Recognizing that a health history may not identify all active or latent infections, the caregiver should carefully follow Routine Practices in the home. Setting up a work environment in which hand disinfection and aseptic technique can be accomplished as carefully as they are in a hospital setting is important.

It is important for the home caregiver to receive annual influenza vaccine. This is especially true if the caregiver or the patient is older than 50 years of age, has underlying cardiac or pulmonary disease, or has underlying immunosuppression.

NURSING PROCESS: THE PATIENT WITH AN INFECTIOUS DISEASE

Assessment

Symptoms of infectious diseases vary significantly between and within diseases. For some infections, such as chickenpox (varicella), widely disseminated rash represents the first suggestion of infection, and it occurs in most newly infected people. In other infections, such as TB and HIV, latency is prolonged, and most of those infected do not have symptoms; instead, infection is determined through diagnostic procedures.

History taking, physical examination, and the use of diagnostic tests are important for determining the presence of infection and infectious diseases. The goals of eliciting the history are to establish the likelihood and probable source of infection and the degree of associated pathology and symptoms. The patient's previous medical record is reviewed when possible. In obtaining a health history, some of the following questions may be asked:

- Does the patient have a history of previous or recurrent infections? Is the patient aware of infection with an organism associated with prolonged latency, such as HIV, herpesvirus, or TB?
- Has there been fever? How high has the patient's temperature been? What is the fever pattern? Is the temperature constant, or does it rise and fall? Has fever been associated with chills? Has the patient taken medication to relieve fever?
- Is there cough? Is the cough chronic or acute? Is it associated with shortness of breath? Does the cough produce sputum? Is the sputum bloody? Has the patient had a PPD test performed recently? If so, what were the results? Has the patient been given isoniazid (INH) prophylaxis for TB infection? Has the patient been treated for TB in the past?
- Is there pain? Where is the pain? What is the nature of the pain? Does the patient have sore throat, headache, myalgias, or arthralgias? Is there pain on urination or other activity?
- Is there swelling? Is there drainage associated with the swelling? Is the swollen area warm to touch?
- Is there a draining site? Is the drainage associated with trauma or a previous procedure? Is the drainage purulent or clear?
- Does the patient have diarrhea, vomiting, or abdominal pain?
- Is there rash? What is the nature of the rash—is it flat, raised, red, crusted, purulent, or lacelike?
- What is the patient's vaccination history?
- Has the patient taken medications that could induce rash?
- Has there been exposure to another person who has an identified infectious disease or rash?
- Has there been an insect or animal bite? Has there been an animal scratch or other exposure to pets, farm animals, or experimental animals?
- What medications are used? Have antibiotics been taken recently or long-term? Is the patient being treated with corticosteroids, immunosuppressing agents, or chemotherapy?
- Is there a history of substance abuse?
- Has the patient been treated in the past for other infectious diseases? Has the patient been hospitalized for infectious diseases?
- If sexual history is pertinent, has there been sexual exposure to another person with a known STD? Has the patient been treated for STDs in the past? Is the patient pregnant, or has she recently been pregnant? Has the patient been tested for HIV?
- Has the patient traveled to or from a developing country or abroad? What was the immunization or antimicrobial prophylaxis used for protection while traveling?
- What is the patient's occupation?

Because infection may occur in any body system, physical examination may reveal signs of infection at any body site. Generalized signs of chronic infection may include significant weight loss or pallor associated with anemia of chronic diseases. Acute infection may manifest with fever, chills, lymphadenopathy, or rash. Localized signs vary significantly according to the source of infection. Purulence, pain, swelling, and redness are strongly associated with localized infection. Cough and shortness of breath may be caused by influenza, pneumonia, or TB, as well as many noninfectious causes.

Diagnosis

NURSING DIAGNOSES

Based on assessment data, the patient's major nursing diagnoses related specifically to infection may include the following:

- Risk for infection transmission
- Deficient knowledge about the disease, cause of infection, treatment, and prevention measures
- Risk for imbalanced body temperature (fever) related to the presence of infection

Infection may interrupt normal function of any affected body system. These system alterations can be reviewed through the nursing diagnoses for body systems listed in the appropriate chapters.

COLLABORATIVE PROBLEMS/POTENTIAL COMPLICATIONS

Based on the assessment data, potential complications that may develop include the following:

- Septicemia, bacteremia, or sepsis
- Septic shock
- Dehydration
- Abscess formation
- Endocarditis
- Infectious disease–related cancers
- Infertility
- Congenital abnormalities

Planning and Goals

Major goals for the patient may include prevention of spread of infection, increased knowledge about the infection and its treatment, control of fever and related discomforts, and absence of complications.

Nursing Interventions

PREVENTING INFECTION TRANSMISSION

Preventing the spread of infection requires an understanding of the usual routes of transmission of the organism. The hospitalized patient may serve as a risk for transmission to other patients if the patient's disease was spread by the airborne route or if infected by an organism such as *C. difficile,* which can be spread directly to others by persistence of spores in the environment. In these situations, strict adherence to isolation measures is important in reducing the opportunity for spread. Preventing transmission of organisms from patient to patient usually requires participation of the health care team. Transmission of organisms on the hands and gloves of health care workers remains a common source of cross-infection in the hospital or clinic setting.

Nurses serve an important role in preventing the transfer of organisms in two ways. First, as the health professionals who often spend the most time with patients, nurses have a greater opportunity for spreading organisms. It is imperative that nurses disinfect their hands before and after contact with patients and

(text continues on page 2156)

Plan of Nursing Care
Care of the Patient With An Infectious Disease

Nursing Interventions	Rationale	Expected Outcomes

Nursing Diagnosis: Risk for infection transmission
Goal: Preventing transmission of infectious agents

1. Prevent patient-to-patient infection spread

   a. Provide isolation according to Health Canada guidelines and Routine Practices

   b. Ensure that patients with airborne infections remain in private rooms during hospital stay. If they must leave their rooms, arrangements should be made to decrease the likelihood of contact with other patients. Rooms should be ventilated according to Health Canada criteria. Personal protective equipment in the form of N95 respirators should be worn as indicated.

   The N95 respirator is the minimal level of personal protection for tuberculosis control. The "N" indicates the filter resistance to oil aerosols; and the "95" indicates that the respirator has 95% effectiveness in filtering test particles (CDC, 1998c).

   In any care setting where patients may have increased risk for the sequelae of influenza, annual influenza vaccination should be encouraged for personnel and patients.

   c. Ensure that patients with highly transmissible, nonairborne organisms such as *Clostridium difficile* and *Shigella* species are physically separated from other patients if hygiene or institutional policy dictates.

2. Prevent health care worker's transfer of organisms from patient to patient

   a. Perform hand hygiene (by hand washing or by use of alcohol-based solution) consistently and thoroughly, disinfecting hands before and after each patient contact, and after procedures that offer contamination risk while caring for an individual patient

   b. Use gloves when handling any body fluid from any patient. Change gloves between patient care activities, and disinfect hands after gloves are removed.

   c. Avoid wearing artificial fingernails or extenders when providing patient care. Keep natural nails less than 0.6 cm long

1. Organisms that are spread through an airborne route or are very contagious through direct contact can be transmitted in a health care setting.

   a. Health Canada isolation strategies are developed to reduce the likelihood of transmission from patient to patient.

   b. Engineering controls are important in the prevention of airborne diseases. Influenza vaccine safely reduces risk of illness associated with this highly communicable, and frequently virulent, condition.

   c. Increased prevention strategies are needed when the organism has high epidemic potential.

2. Transfer of organisms on the hands of health care workers is a common route of transmission. Hospital organisms colonizing the hands of health care workers may be virulent.

   a. Hand hygiene is important in reducing transient flora on outer epidermal layers of skin. Alcohol-based hand disinfectants are effective methods to reduce transient flora.

   b. Gloves provide effective barrier protection. Gloves quickly become contaminated and then become a potential vehicle for the transfer of organisms between patients. Microflora on hands are likely to proliferate while gloves are worn.

- No evidence of patient-to patient transmission of infection
- No evidence of transmission via health care workers
- No occupationally acquired infections in nurses and other health care workers
- No evidence of transmission due to contaminated equipment
- Absence of bacteremia, septicemia, and sepsis
- Absence of urinary tract infections
- Absence of pneumonia

(continued)

Plan of Nursing Care
Care of the Patient With An Infectious Disease *(Continued)*

Nursing Interventions	Rationale	Expected Outcomes
d. Monitor the hand hygiene and glove use behaviours of health care professionals caring for the patient.	d. Poor compliance with hand hygiene among health care workers has been well documented and should be anticipated. It is important for the nurse as the patient's advocate to communicate protective behaviour.	
3. Prevent patient-to-health care worker transmission of infection.	3. Health care workers may acquire infections occupationally due to close contact with patients.	
a. Avoid risk of infection with tuberculosis	a. The most important element in the reduction of tuberculosis is early identification. Many of the symptoms of tuberculosis are subtle, and may be first observed by the nurse who has prolonged contact with the patient.	
(1) Participate in the early identification of patients with active disease. Patients will be asked about risk factors, symptoms, previous exposure, and PPD status.	(1) Identification of patients at risk can help to prevent exposure.	
(2) Expedite diagnostic work-up with chest x-ray, sputum analysis for organisms, and PPD administration as appropriate.	(2) Confirmation of diagnosis facilitates development of an appropriate treatment plan, including prevention of spread of infection.	
(3) Maintain engineering controls. Keep the patient in a private room with a closed door.	(3) Confining airflow to the immediate vicinity of the patient and exhausting air to the outside reduce the likelihood of transmission to health care workers in areas outside of the patient room.	
(4) Use protection in isolation room or when participating in procedures that are likely to generate cough, such as suctioning, intubation, or administering nebulized medications.	(4) N95 respirators are designed to reduce health care worker risk.	
b. Avoid risk of transmission of blood-borne diseases such as hepatitis B, hepatitis C, and the human immunodeficiency virus	b. Health care workers can contract blood-borne diseases via percutaneous injury such as needlestick or by contact with blood or bloody body fluids to mucous membranes, such as eyes and mouth.	
(1) Get hepatitis B vaccination	(1) Hepatitis B vaccine should be administered to reduce risk from this contagious bloodborne virus.	
(2) Use Routine Practices as defined by Health Canada	(2) Routine Practices are based on the recognition that most patients are not identified as infected by physical assessment or history taking. Health care workers must assume that all patients may be infected with bloodborne or other infection and must use barrier precautions appropriately for *all* patients.	
(3) Use "needleless" syringes and other injury-preventing devices	(3) Use of injury-preventing devices decreases risk of transmission of blood-borne diseases.	

(continued)

Plan of Nursing Care
Care of the Patient With An Infectious Disease *(Continued)*

Nursing Interventions	Rationale	Expected Outcomes

c. Avoid risk of airborne diseases.
   (1) Get influenza vaccination annually.
   (2) Get vaccinated or produce proof of immunity to measles, mumps, rubella, and varicella.
4. Prevent patient exposure to contaminated medical equipment.
 	
a. Ensure that equipment that is inserted through intact skin is sterilized between patient uses.
b. Ensure that equipment that has contact with mucous membranes is sterilized or receives "high-level disinfection" between patient uses.
c. Ensure that equipment used against intact skin is thoroughly cleaned and receives "low-level disinfection" between patient uses.
 	
5. Follow established guidelines for the routine removal and replacement of intravenous devices.
6. Remove urinary catheters at the earliest time possible.
 	
7. Remove endotracheal and nasogastric tubes as soon as possible.
	c. Influenza vaccine is recommended for health care workers to reduce the likelihood of transmission in health care settings where immunocompromised patients can become exposed.
	4. Technologic advances offer increased opportunity for invasive procedures. Equipment may be complex and difficult to clean.
	a. Sterilization renders equipment free of all microorganisms.
	
	b. High-level disinfection renders an object free of all microorganisms with the possible exception of spore-producing organisms.
	c. The disinfection goal for low-level disinfection is to reduce the load of microorganisms to a level that is not threatening to the host with intact skin.
	5. Indwelling intravascular devices can serve as a conduit for organisms to migrate into the bloodstream.
	6. The risk of urinary tract infections is directly proportional to the length of time that a urinary catheter remains in place.
	7. The risk for pneumonia is increased as the duration of indwelling equipment increases.	

Nursing Diagnosis: Deficient knowledge about disease, cause of infection, and preventive measures
Goal: Acquisition of knowledge about the infectious process

1. Listen carefully to what the patient says about illness and previous treatment.
 	
2. Provide pertinent explanations about:
   a. Organism and route of transmission
   b. Treatment goals
   c. Follow-up schedule
   d. Prevention of transmission to others
3. Allow opportunities for questions and discussions
4. Teach the patient and family about:
   a. Prophylaxis or immunization, if recommended
   b. Community resources, if necessary
   c. Means of preventing transmission within the home
	1. Listening facilitates detection of misunderstanding and misinformation and provides opportunity for education.
	2. Knowledge about specific diagnoses and treatments may increase compliance.
	
	3. The patient's questions indicate issues that need clarification.
	4. Understanding of the risks and precautions associated with an infectious disease may reduce the opportunity for further spread.
		• Patient actively participates in treatment.
		• Patient complies with infection control measures

Nursing Diagnosis: Risk for imbalanced body temperature (fever) related to the presence of infection
Goal: Patient comfort and return of normal temperature

1. Monitor temperature, pulse, and respirations at regular intervals	1. Graph fever curve to help evaluate when fever occurs, how long it lasts, and whether it responds to therapy.	• Body temperature within normal limits • Maintenance of fluid and electrolyte balance • Patient comfortable

(continued)

Plan of Nursing Care
Care of the Patient With An Infectious Disease *(Continued)*

Nursing Interventions	Rationale	Expected Outcomes

Collaborative Problems: Among potential complications are septicemia, bacteremia, or sepsis, septic shock, dehydration, abscess formation, endocarditis, infectious disease–related cancers, and infertility.

Goal: Absence of complications

Septicemia, Bacteremia, Sepsis

1. Monitor patient for evidence of infection at any location.

2. Assess treatment effectiveness of all identified infections.

3. Administer antibiotics as prescribed with first dose given at the earliest time possible.

1. Vigilance for bacterial or fungal infection at any site promotes early recognition and treatment and reduces the likelihood of secondary infections.

2. The natural course of some infections may be rapid unless antibiotics are administered promptly.

3. Prompt treatment will improve outcomes.

- No episode of infection
- Effective treatment of identified bacterial and fungal infections without progression to bloodstream infection
- Early improvement in septic course

Septic Shock

1. Routinely, and as warranted, monitor vital signs for patients with recognized infections and severely immune suppressed patients at risk for shock. In particular, be alert for signs of:
   a. Fever
   b. Tachycardia (more than 90 bpm)
   c. Tachypnea (more than 20 breaths/min)
   d. Evidence of decreased perfusion or dysfunction of vital organs in the form of
      (1) Change of mental status
      (2) Hypoxemia as measured by arterial blood gases
      (3) Elevated lactate levels
      (4) Urine output (less than 30 mL/h)

2. Administer antibiotics, fluid replacement, vasopressors, and oxygen as prescribed.

1. Early recognition of the signs and prompt treatment of impending shock may reduce the associated severity or mortality.

2. Therapeutic maintenance of hemodynamic and respiratory status is necessary until infection is effectively treated with antimicrobial regimen.

- Absence of symptoms of septic shock
- Hemodynamic and respiratory status within normal range

Dehydration

1. Assess for dehydration (thirst, dryness of mucous membranes, loss of skin turgor, reduced peripheral pulses, urine output less than 30 mL/h).

2. Monitor weight.

3. Monitor intake and output and serum electrolyte levels.

4. Replace fluids as needed. If the patient can tolerate oral fluids, offer fluids every 2–4 hours. Administer intravenous fluids as prescribed.

1. Signs of dehydration provide a basis for fluid replacement and suggest possible further complications of circulatory collapse.

2. Rapid changes in weight indicate fluid volume changes.

3. Dehydration produces a deficit in some electrolytes. Decreased urine production may indicate hypovolemia and decreased renal perfusion.

4. When possible, oral hydration is preferable because the patient can select the beverage, control the rate and interval of replacement, and care for self at home. Additionally, the risks associated with vascular devices are avoided. If intravenous fluid is required, intravenous solutions are formulated to facilitate intestinal reabsorption of fluid and electrolytes.

- Attains fluid balance (output approximates intake: body weight unchanged)
- Mucous membranes appear moist; normal skin turgor
- Serum electrolytes are within normal limits

(continued)

Plan of Nursing Care
Care of the Patient With An Infectious Disease (Continued)

Nursing Interventions	Rationale	Expected Outcomes
Abscess Formation 1. Assess vascular access sites, wound sites, pressure ulcers, and other appropriate sites for apparent collections of purulent material.	1. Collections of purulent material often require drainage before antimicrobial therapy is effective.	• Absence of abscess • Takes antibiotics as prescribed.
2. Assess the patient who has had abdominal surgery or trauma to abdominal area for localized signs of intra-abdominal abscess. These signs include: a. Low-grade fever b. Elevated peripheral white blood cell count c. Localized pain d. Abdominal tenderness e. Visible or palpable mass f. Postoperative diarrhea g. GI bleeding	2. Intra-abdominal abscess formation is most common following traumatic or surgical disruption of the GI tract. Signs are often initially subtle.	
3. Assess patient who has had percutaneous abscess drainage to determine whether drainage has been successful. Be alert for all of the above signs and symptoms.	3. After percutaneous drainage, recurrent or persistent signs of abscess may indicate the need for surgical treatment.	
4. Administer antibiotics as prescribed	4. Antibiotics, along with drainage, are the most important elements of intra-abdominal abscess management.	
Endocarditis *Prevention* 1. Teach patients with the following conditions about the value of antibiotic prophylaxis for events and procedures that may introduce the risk of endocarditis: a. Valvular disease b. Congenital heart disease c. Intracardiac prosthesis d. Previous endocarditis	1. Patients with underlying valvular disease and other cardiac abnormalities are at increased risk for "seeding" of the cardiac valves during procedures that can cause bacteremia.	• Informs health care professionals of cardiac conditions that require antibiotic prophylaxis before invasive procedures • Takes prophylactic antibiotics as prescribed
Management 1. Obtain blood cultures as prescribed; carefully record results. Note persistent bloodstream infections with a particular organism.	1. A definitive diagnosis of endocarditis requires blood culture confirmation.	• Endocarditis is diagnosed, treated, and cured.
2. Obtain a detailed history about the duration of fever in the absence of well-recognized cause.	2. Endocarditis should be suspected in patients who report an unexplained fever of more than 1 week's duration	
3. Administer intravenous antibiotic therapy at prescribed time schedule.	3. Intravenous therapy is usually required for cure. The goal of therapy is complete eradication of all organisms. Careful adherence to following the scheduled administration is therefore essential.	

Infectious Disease-Related Cancers and Infertility
These potential complications of infectious diseases are prevented by primary avoidance of infection. Management of them is directed toward treating each of them as a non-infectious entity. For example, the management of cancer secondary to hepatitis B is handled as an oncology issue, not as an infectious disease issue.

after performing a potentially hand-contaminating activity. Hands must be decontaminated each time gloves are removed. For example, the nurse who has performed endotracheal suctioning should remove gloves and decontaminate hands before performing wound care on the same patient.

The second way that nurses reduce hand-to-hand spread is to serve as patient advocates. With the number of health care workers involved in patient care each day, there is a significant opportunity for breaks in hand-hygiene technique. To the degree feasible, the nurse should observe the hand-hygiene activities of other professionals and discuss them when lapses in technique are observed.

TEACHING ABOUT THE INFECTIOUS PROCESS

For infectious diseases, interruption of transmission requires diagnosis and patient compliance with the treatment regimen. The nurse's role is to educate and, in some situations, to report the case to public health officials for contact tracing and verification of follow-up.

The nurse must stress the importance of immunization to parents of young children and to others for whom vaccines are recommended, such as patients who are elderly, are immunosuppressed, or have chronic illnesses. Nurses should recognize their personal responsibility to receive hepatitis B and annual influenza vaccines to reduce potential transmission to self and vulnerable patient groups.

Infectious diseases often seem mysterious and frequently are socially stigmatizing. Patient teaching efforts require empathy and sensitivity. For example, in the past, TB was considered a stigmatized disease. The nurse may need to provide core information to the patient who needs INH prophylaxis in order to promote understanding and allay guilt that the patient may feel.

CONTROLLING FEVER AND ACCOMPANYING DISCOMFORTS

Fever must always be investigated to determine whether infection is the source. There is evidence that fever, mediated by the hypothalamus, may potentiate beneficial functions in the syndrome of reactions known as *acute-phase reaction*. These reactions include changes in liver protein synthesis; alterations in serum metals, such as iron; and increased production of certain classes of white blood cells and other immune system cells. Most fevers are physiologically controlled to stay below 41°C. However, severe fever, as occurs with meningococcal meningitis, may cause heat stroke and other complications. Even milder fevers accompanied by fatigue, chills, and diaphoresis are often uncomfortable for the patient. The physician makes decisions regarding fever control. Whether fever is treated or untreated, adequate fluid intake is important during febrile episodes.

NURSING ALERT Because fever offers clues about infection severity and success of antibiotic therapy, outpatients with fever should be taught to obtain accurate temperature readings. Frequently, parents know that a child has warm skin but do not disturb the child by taking a temperature reading. Body temperature information can be very helpful in adjusting therapy or in reevaluating a preliminary diagnosis.

MONITORING AND MANAGING POTENTIAL COMPLICATIONS

The patient with a rapidly progressive infectious disease should have vital signs and level of consciousness closely monitored. X-ray findings and microbiologic, immunologic, hematologic,

cytologic, and parasitologic laboratory values must be interpreted in the context of other clinical findings to assess the infectious disease course.

Antibiotic therapy is frequently complex, with modifications necessary because of sensitivity test results and disease progression. It is important to initiate antibiotic therapy as soon as it is prescribed, rather than waiting until routine medication scheduling times. This ensures that therapeutic blood levels can be attained as quickly as possible. The Plan of Nursing Care describes nursing interventions for specific complications of infection.

Evaluation

EXPECTED PATIENT OUTCOMES

Expected patient outcomes may include the following:

1. Uses appropriate methods to prevent the spread of infection
2. Acquires knowledge about the infectious process
3. Exhibits absence of elevated body temperature

Critical Thinking Exercises

1. Several patients on your nursing unit have become infected with the same bacteria. The staff wants to develop a campaign to reduce the risk of bacterial transmission between patients. What issues should be stressed? What products should be available? How can the situation be monitored? What outcome measures can be used to determine success of the campaign?

2. You are supervising a patient care technician who is preparing to perform a venipuncture. The equipment that he has brought into the patient's room does not include gloves. How would you evaluate this situation, and what action would you take? Explain the rationale for your decision.

3. An elderly patient with cardiac disease and diabetes asks you why her physician suggested that she receive influenza and pneumococcal vaccinations. She states that she is afraid the vaccinations will "make me sick." How would you respond to her and explain the situation? Describe the line of reasoning you would follow to persuade her to get the vaccine. If she rejects your explanation, examine the different courses of action you could take and the pros and cons of each strategy.

REFERENCES AND SELECTED READINGS

Books

Atkinson, W., Wolfe, C., & Centers for Disease Control and Prevention (Eds.). (2002). *Epidemiology and prevention of vaccine preventable diseases* (7th ed., pp. 97–113). Atlanta: Centers for Disease Control and Prevention.

Centers for Disease Control and Prevention. (2000b). Tracking the hidden epidemics: Trends in STDs in the United States [on-line]. Available: http://www.cdc.gov/nchstp/dstd/stats_trends2000.pdf.

Chin, J. (2000). *Control of communicable diseases in man.* Washington, DC: American Public Health Association

Gorbach, S. L., Bartlett, J., & Blacklow, N. R. (1998). *Infectious diseases.* Philadelphia: W. B. Saunders.

Guerrant, R. L., & Steiner, T. S. (2000). Principles and syndromes of enteric infection. In Mandell, G. L., Douglas, R. G., & Bennett, J. E. (Eds.), *Principles and practice of infectious diseases.* New York: Churchill Livingstone.

Jenson, H. B., & Baltimore, R. S. (2001). *Pediatric infectious diseases.* New York: Churchill Livingstone.

Long, S. S., Pickering, L. K., & Prober, C. G. (1997). *Principles and practice of pediatric infectious diseases.* New York: Churchill Livingstone.

Mayhall, G. (1999). *Hospital epidemiology and infection control.* Baltimore: Williams & Wilkins.

Miller, J., Engelberg, S., & Broad, W. (2001). *Germs, biological weapons and America's secret war.* New York: Simon & Schuster.

Satcher, D. (2001, June). *The Surgeon General's call to action to promote sexual health and responsible sexual behavior* [on-line]. Available: http://www.surgeongeneral.gov/library/sexualhealth.

Schacter, J., & Grossman, M. (2001). *Chlamydia.* In Remington, J. S., & Klein, J. O. (Eds.), *Infectious diseases of the fetus and newborn infant.* Philadelphia: W. B. Saunders.

Wenzel, R. (1997). *Prevention and control of nosocomial infections.* Baltimore: Williams & Wilkins.

Journals

Asterisks indicate nursing research articles.

Baker, G. R., Norton, P. G., Flintoft, V., et al. (2004). The Canadian adverse events study: The incidence of adverse events among hospital patients in Canada. *Canadian Medical Association Journal, 170*(11), 1678–1686.

Borio, L., Inglesby, T., Peters, C. J., Schmaljohn, A. L., Hughes, J. M., Jahrling, P. B., Ksiazek, T., Johnson, K. M., Meyerhoff, A., O'Toole, T., Ascher, M. S., Bartlett, J., Breman, J. G., Eitzen, E. M., Jr., Hamburg, M., Hauer, J., Henderson, D. A., Johnson, R. T., Kwik, G., Layton, M., Lillibridge, S., Nabel, G. J., Osterholm, M. T., Perl, T. M., Russell, P., Tonat, K., & The Working Group on Civilian Biodefense. (2002). Hemorrhagic fever viruses as biological weapons. *Journal of the American Medical Association, 287,* 2391–2405.

*Byers, J. F. (2000). Analysis of factors related to the development of ventilator-associated pneumonia: Use of existing databases. *American Journal of Critical Care, 9*(5), 344–351.

Campbell, A., & Dreher, H. M. (2002). A new transcontinental disease: The West Nile virus. *MedSurg Nursing 11*(3), 112–119.

Centers for Disease Control and Prevention. (1992). The management of acute diarrhea in children: Oral rehydration, maintenance, and nutritional therapy. *Morbidity and Mortality Weekly Report: CDC Surveillance Summaries, 41,* (RR-16), 1–20.

Centers for Disease Control and Prevention. (1997). Immunization of health-care workers: Recommendations of the Advisory Committee on Immunization Practices (ACIP) and the Hospital Infection Control Advisory Committee. *Morbidity and Mortality Weekly Report: CDC Surveillance Summaries, 47,* (RR-18), 1–42.

Centers for Disease Control and Prevention. (1998a). Guideline for infection control in healthcare personnel, 1998. *Infection Control and Hospital Epidemiology, 19*(6), 407–463.

Centers for Disease Control and Prevention. (1998b). Measles, mumps, and rubella: Vaccine use and strategies for elimination of measles, rubella, congenital rubella syndrome and control of mumps. Recommendations of the Advisory Committee on Immunization Practices. *Morbidity and Mortality Weekly Report: CDC Surveillance Summaries, 47,* (RR-8), 1–57.

Centers for Disease Control and Prevention. (1998c). Laboratory performance evaluation of N95 filtering facepiece respirators, 1996. *Morbidity and Mortality Weekly Report, 47*(48), 1045–1049.

Centers for Disease Control and Prevention. (2000a). Surveillance for foodborne disease outbreaks—United States, 1993–1997. *Morbidity and Mortality Weekly Report, 49,* (SS-01), 1–51.

Centers for Disease Control and Prevention. (2001a). Updated U.S. Public Health Service guidelines for the management of occupational exposures to HBV, HCV, and HIV and recommendations for post-exposure prophylaxis. *Morbidity and Mortality Weekly Report, 50,* (RR-11), 1–42.

Centers for Disease Control and Prevention. (2001b). Recommendations for preventing transmission of infections among chronic hemodialysis patients. *Morbidity and Mortality Weekly Report, 50,* (RR05), 1–43.

Centers for Disease Control and Prevention. (2001c). National Nosocomial Infections Surveillance System report: Data summary, from January 1992–June 2001, issued August 2001. *American Journal of Infection Control, 29*(6), 404–421.

Centers for Disease Control and Prevention. (2001d). Prevention and control of influenza: Recommendations of the Advisory Committee on Immunization Practices. *Morbidity and Mortality Weekly Report: CDC Surveillance Summaries, 50,* (RR-4), 1–46.

Centers for Disease Control and Prevention. (2001e). Epidemic/epizootic West Nile virus control in the United States: Revised guidelines for prevention, surveillance and control. 1–99. Available: http://www.cdc.gov/nchstp/tb/surv/surv.htm.

Centers for Disease Control and Prevention. (2001f). Management of occupational exposures to hepatitis B, hepatitis C, and HIV and recommendations for postexposure prophylaxis. Updated U.S. Public Health Service Guidelines, 2001. *Morbidity and Mortality Weekly Report, 50,* (RR-11), 1–42.

Centers for Disease Control and Prevention. (2001g). Surveillance reports: Reported tuberculosis in the United States, 2001. Available: http://www.cdc.gov/nchstp/tb/surv/surv.htm.

Centers for Disease Control and Prevention. (2002a). Guideline for hand hygiene in health care settings. *Morbidity and Mortality Weekly Report, 51* (RR-16), 1–56.

Centers for Disease Control and Prevention. (2002b). *Staphylococcus aureus* resistant to vancomycin—United States, 2002. *Morbidity and Mortality Weekly Report, 51*(26), 565–567.

Centers for Disease Control and Prevention. (2002c). West Nile virus—2001. *Morbidity and Mortality Weekly Report, 51*(23), 497–501.

Centers for Disease Control and Prevention. (2002d). Sexually transmitted diseases: Treatment guidelines, 2002. *Morbidity and Mortality Weekly Report, 51,* (RR-6), 1–80.

Centers for Disease Control and Prevention. (2002e). Healthcare Infection Control Practices Advisory Committee: Draft guideline for prevention of healthcare-associated pneumonia.

Crump, J. A., Griffin, P. M., & Angulo, F. (2002). Bacterial contamination of animal feed and its relationship to human foodborne illness. *Clinical Infectious Diseases, 35,* 859–865.

Drinka, P., Faulks, J. T., Gauerke, C., Goodman, B., Stemper, M., & Reed, K. (2001). Adverse events associated with methicillin-resistant *Staphylococcus aureus* in a nursing home. *Archives of Internal Medicine, 161*(19), 2371–2377.

Doyle, T. J., Bryan, R. T., & Peters, C. J. (1998). Viral hemorrhagic fevers and hantavirus infections in the Americas. *Infectious Disease Clinics of North America, 12,* 95–110.

Fleming, S. (2001). Preventing needlesticks. *Job Safety and Health Quarterly, 12*(4), 12–14.

Force, M. V. (1999). Living with Lyme disease. *MedSurg Nursing, 8*(3), 184–190.

Grant, A. D., & DeCock, K. M. (2001). HIV infection and AIDS in the developing world. Clinical review: ABC of AIDS. *British Medical Journal, 322,* 1475–1478.

*Harris, J. R., & Miller, T. H. (2000). Preventing nosocomial pneumonia: Evidence-based practice. *Critical Care Nurse, 20,* 51–66.

Health Canada. (1996). Vancomycin-resistant enterococci on a renal ward in an Ontario hospital. *Canada Communicable Disease Report, 22*–15. Available at: http://www.phac-aspc.gc.ca/publicat/ccdr-rmtc/index.html.

Health Canada. (1997a). Preventing infections associated with indwelling intravascular access devices. *Canada Communicable Disease Report, 23S8.* Available at: http://www.phac-aspc.gc.ca/publicat/ccdr-rmtc/index.html.

Health Canada. (1997b). Canadian contingency plan for viral hemorrhagic fevers and other related diseases. *Canada Communicable Disease Report, 23S1.* Available at: http://www.phac-aspc.gc.ca/publicat/ccdr-rmtc/index.html.

Health Canada. (1998a). Canadian STD guidelines. Available at: http://www.phac-aspc.gc.ca/publicat/std-mts98/index.html.

Health Canada. (1998b). Hand washing, cleaning, disinfection and sterilization in health care. *Canada Communicable Disease Report, 24S8*. Avaiable at: http://www.phac-aspc.gc.ca/publicat/ccdr-rmtc/index.html.

Health Canada. (1999). Routine practices and additional precautions for preventing the transmission of infection in health care. *Canada Communicable Disease Report, 25S4*, 1–142. Available at: http://www.phac-aspc.gc.ca/publicat/ccdr-rmtc/index.html.

Health Canada. (2002). Prevention and control of occupational infections in health care. *Canada Communicable Disease Report, 28S1*. Available at: http://www.phac-aspc.gc.ca/publicat/ccdr-rmtc/index.html.

Health Canada. (2004). Statement on influenza vaccination for the 2004–2005 season. *Canada Communicable Disease Report, 30*, ACS-3. Available at: http://www.phac-aspc.gc.ca/publicat/ccdr-rmtc/index.html.

Inglesby, T. V., Dennis, D. T., Henderson, D. A., Bartlett, J. G., Ascher, M. S., Eitzen, E., Fine, A. D., Friedlander, A. M., Hauer, J., Koerner, J. F., Layton, M., McDade, J., Osterholm, M. T., O'Toole, T., Parker, G., Perl, T. M., Russell, P. K., Schoch-Spana, M., Tonat, K., & the Working Group on Civilian Biodefense. (2002). Plague as a biological weapon. *Journal of the American Medical Association, 283*, 2281–2290.

*Larson, E., Silberger, M., Jakob, K., Whittier, S., Lai, L., Della Latta, P., & Saiman, L. (2000). Assessment of alternative hand hygiene regimens to improve skin health among neonatal intensive care unit nurses. *Heart & Lung, 29*(1), 136–142.

Mangram, A. J., Horan, T. C., Pearson, M. L., Silver, L. C., & Jarvis, W. R. (1999). Guideline for the prevention of surgical site infection, 1999. *Infection Control and Hospital Epidemiology, 20*(4), 250–278.

Mermel, L. A., Farr, B. M., Sherertz, R. J., & Raad, I. I. (2001). Guidelines for the management of intravascular catheter-related infections. *Journal of Intravenous Nursing 24*(3), 180–207.

Mermel, L. A. (2000). Prevention of intravascular catheter-related infections. *Annals of Internal Medicine, 132*(5), 391–402.

Michael, P. A. (2002). Preventing and treating meningococcal meningitis. *MedSurg Nursing, 11*(1), 9–12.

National Advisory Committee on Immunization. (2000). Statement on immunization for Lyme disease. *Canada Communicable Disease Report, 26*, ACS-3. Available at: http://www.phac-aspc.gc.ca/publicat/ccdr-rmtc/index.html.

National Advisory Committee on Immunization. (2002). *Canadian immunization guide* (6th ed.). Available at: http://www.phac-aspc.gc.ca/publicat/cig-gci/index.html.

National Advisory Committee on Immunization. (2005). *Update to Canadian immunization guide* (6th ed.). Available at: http://www.phac-aspc.gc.ca/naci-ccni/is-si/index-icy.html.

Occupational Safety and Health Administration (OSHA). (2001). Occupational exposure to bloodborne pathogens: Needlestick and other sharps injuries. Final rule. *Federal Register, 66*, 5317–5325.

Public Health Agency of Canada. (1997a). Preventing the spread of vancomycin-resistant enterococci (VRE) in Canada. *Canada Communicable Disease Report, 23S8*. Available at: http://www.phac-aspc.gc.ca/publicat/ccdr-rmtc/index.html.

Public Health Agency of Canada. (1997b). Preventing the transmission of bloodborne pathogens in health care and public service settings. *Canada Communicable Disease Report, 23S3*. Available at: http://www.phac-aspc.gc.ca/publicat/ccdr-rmtc/index.html.

Public Health Agency of Canada. (2000). Hantavirus pulmonary syndrome in Canada, 1989–1999. *Canada Communicable Disease Report, 26-08*. Available at: http://www.phac-aspc.gc.ca/publicat/ccdr-rmtc/index.html.

Public Health Agency of Canada. (2003). Estimates of HIV prevalence and incidence in Canada, 2002. *Canada Communicable Disease Report, 29-23*. Available at: http://www.phac-aspc.gc.ca/publicat/ccdr-rmtc/index.html.

Public Health Agency of Canada (2004). Notifiable disease summary. *Canada Communicable Disease Report, 30-21*. Available at: http://www.phac-aspc.gc.ca/publicat/ccdr-rmtc/index.html.

Public Health Agency of Canada. (2005a). Influenza in Canada: 2003-2004 season. *Canada Communicable Disease Report, 31-01*. Available at: http://www.phac-aspc.gc.ca/publicat/ccdr-rmtc/index.html.

Public Health Agency of Canada. (2005b). Surveillance for methicillin-resistant *Staphylococcus aureus* in Canadian hospitals: A report update from the Canadian Nosocomial Infection Surveillance Program. *Canada Communicable Disease Report, 31-03*. Available at: http://www.phac-aspc.gc.ca/publicat/ccdr-rmtc/index.html.

Public Health Agency of Canada. (2005c). Tuberculosis in Canada 2002: Executive summary. *Canada Communicable Disease Report, 31-04*. Available at: http://www.phac-aspc.gc.ca/publicat/ccdr-rmtc/index.html.

Scheckler, W. E., Brimhall, D., Buck, A. S., Farr, B. M., Friedman, C., Garibaldi, R. A., Gross, P. A., Harris, J. A., Hierholzer, W. J., Jr., Martone, W. J., McDonald, L. L., & Solomon, S. L. (1998). Requirements for infrastructure and essential activities in infection control and epidemiology in hospitals: A consensus panel report. *Infection Control and Hospital Epidemiology, 19*, 114–124.

Shlaes, D. M., Gerding, D. N., John, J. F., Jr., Craig, W. A., Bornstein, D. L., Duncan, R. A., Eckman, M. R., Farrer, W. E., Greene, W. H., Lorian, V., Levy, S., McGowan, J. E., Jr., Paul, S. M., Ruskin, J., Tenover, F. C., & Watanakunakorn, C. (1997). Society for Healthcare Epidemiology of America and the Infectious Diseases Society of America Joint Committee on the Prevention of Antimicrobial Resistance. Guidelines for the prevention of antimicrobial resistance in hospitals. *Infection Control and Hospital Epidemiology, 18*, 275–291.

Shay, L. E., & Freifeld, A. G. (1999). The current state of infectious disease: A clinical perspective on antimicrobial resistance. *Lippincott's Primary Care Practice, 3*(1), 1–17.

Society for Healthcare Epidemiology of America Long Term Care Committee. (1996). Antimicrobial resistance in long term care facilities. *Infection Control and Hospital Epidemiology, 17*, 129–140.

Tablan, O. C., Anderson, L. J., Arden, N. H., Breiman, R. F., Butler, J. C., & McNeil, M. M. (1994). Guideline for prevention of nosocomial pneumonia. *American Journal of Infection Control, 22*, 247–292.

Zaragoza, M., Salles, M., Gomez, J., Bayas, J. M., & Trilla, A. (1999). Handwashing with soap or alcoholic solutions? A randomized clinical trial of its effectiveness. *American Journal of Infection Control, 27*, 258–261.

Zoutman, D. E., Ford, B. D., Bryce, E., et al. (2003). The state of infection surveillance and control in Canadian acute care hospitals. *American Journal of Infection Control, 31*(5), 266–272.

RESOURCES AND WEBSITES

American Lung Association, 1740 Broadway, New York, NY 10019; (800) 586-4872; http://www.lungusa.org.

American Public Health Association, 1015 Fifteenth St. NW, Washington, DC 20005; (302) 777-2742; http://www.apha.org.

Association for Professionals in Infection Control and Epidemiology, Inc., 1016 Sixteenth St. NW, Washington, DC 20036; (202) 789-1870; http://www.apic.org.

Canadian Centre for Occupational Health and Safety; http://www.ccohs.ca.

Centers for Disease Control and Prevention (Center for Prevention Services, Center for Environmental Health, Center for Health Promotion and Education, Center for Infectious Diseases), 1600 Clifton Road NE, Atlanta, GA 30333; (404) 639-3311; http://www.cdc.gov/nicdod.hip/hip.htm.

Health Canada; http://www.hc-sc.gc.ca.

National Advisory Committee on Immunization; http://www.phac-aspc.gc.ca/naci-ccni.

Public Health Agency of Canada; http://www.phac-aspc.gc.ca.

Public Health Agency of Canada: West Nile virus website; http://www.phac-aspc.gc.ca/wn-no/.

Society for Healthcare Epidemiology of America (SHEA), 875 Kings Highway, Suite 200, Woodbury, NJ 08096; (856) 423-0087; http://www.sheaonline.org.

World Health Organization, Avenue Appia 20, 1211 Geneva 27, Switzerland; (4 122) 791-222; http://www.who.int/home-page.

Emergency Nursing

Adapted by Glenn Donnelly

On completion of this chapter, the learner will be able to:

1. Explain emergency care as a collaborative, holistic approach that includes the patient, the family, and significant others.

2. Discuss priority emergency measures instituted for any patient with an emergency condition.

3. Describe the emergency management of patients with intra-abdominal injuries.

4. Identify the priorities of care for the patient with multiple injuries.

5. Compare and contrast the emergency management of patients with heat stroke, frostbite, and hypothermia.

6. Specify the similarities and differences for the emergency management of patients with swallowed or inhaled poisons, skin contamination, and food poisoning.

7. Discuss the emergency management of patients with drug overdose and with acute alcohol intoxication.

8. Describe the significance of crisis intervention in the care of the rape victim.

9. Differentiate between the emergency care of patients who are overactive, those who are violent, those who are depressed, and those who are suicidal.

The term *emergency management* traditionally refers to care given to patients with urgent and critical needs. Because many people lack access to health care, however, the emergency department (ED) is increasingly used for non-urgent problems. Therefore, the philosophy of emergency management has broadened to include the concept that an emergency is whatever the patient or the family considers it to be.

Large numbers of people seek emergency care for serious life-threatening cardiac conditions, such as myocardial infarction, acute heart failure, pulmonary edema, and cardiac dysrhythmias. Priorities for managing these cardiac conditions are discussed in Chapters 27, 28, and 30. Emergency management of trauma and other conditions not found elsewhere in this book are discussed in this chapter. It is assumed that care and treatment are provided under the direction of a physician or emergency nurse practitioner.

Scope and Practice of Emergency Nursing

The emergency nurse has had specialized education, training, and experience to gain expertise in assessing and identifying patients' health care problems in crisis situations. In addition, the emergency nurse establishes priorities, monitors and continuously assesses acutely ill and injured patients, supports and attends to families, supervises allied health personnel, and teaches patients and families within a time-limited, high-pressured care environment. Nursing interventions are accomplished interdependently, in consultation with a licensed physician or nurse practitioner. The strengths of nursing and medicine are complementary in an emergency situation. Appropriate nursing and medical interventions are anticipated based on assessment data. The emergency health care staff members work as a team in performing the highly technical, hands-on skills required to care for patients in an emergency situation.

The nursing process provides a logical framework for problem solving in this environment. Patients in the ED have a wide variety of actual or potential problems, and their condition may change constantly. Therefore, nursing assessment must be continuous, and nursing diagnoses change with the patient's condition. Although a patient may have several diagnoses at a given time, the focus is on the most life-threatening ones; often, both independent and interdependent nursing interventions are required.

ISSUES IN EMERGENCY NURSING CARE

Emergency nursing is demanding because of the diversity of conditions and situations that, if not unique to the ED, certainly present a challenge (Chart 71-1). These issues include legal issues, occupational health and safety risks for ED staff, and the challenge of providing holistic care in the context of a fast-paced, technology-driven environment in which serious illness and death are confronted on a daily basis. Another dimension of emergency nursing is nursing in disasters. With the increasing use of weapons of terror and mass destruction, the emergency nurse must expand his or her knowledge base to encompass recognizing and treating patients exposed to biologic and other terror weapons and anticipate nursing care in the event of a mass casualty incident. See Chapter 72 for a full discussion of nursing care in disasters, including caring for victims of terrorism.

Documentation of Consent

Consent to examine and treat the patient is part of the ED record. The patient must consent to invasive procedures (eg, angiography, lumbar puncture) unless he or she is unconscious or in critical condition and unable to make decisions. If the patient is unconscious and brought to the ED without family or friends, this fact should be documented. Monitoring of the patient's condition, as well as all instituted treatments and the times at which they were performed, must be documented. After treatment, a notation is made on the record about the patient's condition on discharge or transfer and about instructions given to the patient and family for follow-up care.

Limiting Exposure to Health Risks

Because of the increasing numbers of people infected with hepatitis B and with human immunodeficiency virus (HIV), health care providers are at an increased risk for exposure to communicable diseases through blood or other body fluids. This risk is further compounded in the ED because of the common use of invasive treatments in addition to the wide range of patient conditions. All emergency health care providers should adhere strictly to standard precautions for minimizing exposure.

The reemergence of tuberculosis, a major health problem, is complicated by multidrug-resistant tuberculosis and by tuberculosis concomitant with HIV infection. The rates of methicillin-

Glossary

antivenin: antitoxin manufactured from venom of poisonous snakes to assist the patient's immune system response to an envenomation
carboxyhemoglobin: hemoglobin that is bound to carbon monoxide and therefore is unable to bind with oxygen, resulting in hypoxemia
corrosive poison: alkaline or acidic agent, causes tissue destruction after contact
cricothyroidotomy: surgical opening of the cricothyroid membrane to obtain an airway that is maintained with a tracheostomy or endotracheal tube

diagnostic peritoneal lavage: instillation of lactated Ringer's or normal saline solution into the abdominal cavity to detect red blood cells, white blood cells, bile, bacteria, amylase, or gastrointestinal contents indicative of abdominal injury
emergent: triage category signifying life-threatening or potentially life-threatening injuries or illnesses requiring immediate treatment
evenomation: injection of a poisonous material by sting, spine, bite, or other means
fasciotomy: surgical incision of the extremity to the level of the fascia to relieve pres-

sure and restore neurovascular function to the extremity
Hare traction: portable in-line traction applied to the lower extremity to manage femur or hip fractures or dislocations
non-urgent: triage category signifying episodic or minor injury or illness in which treatment may be delayed several hours or longer without increased morbidity
triage: process of assessing patients to determine management priorities
urgent: triage category signifying serious illness or injury that is not immediately life-threatening

resistant *staphylococcus aureus* (MRSA) and vancomycin-resistant *enterococci* (VRE) have both increased (Health Canada, 2005; Health Canada, 1997). Severe acute respiratory syndrome (SARS), a new atypical type of pneumonia associated with the coronavirus, has the potential for large outbreaks (Public Health Agency of Canada, 2004). Early identification and adherence to transmission-based precautions for patients who are potentially infectious is crucial. Nurses in the ED are usually fitted with a personal high-efficiency particulate air (HEPA)-filter mask apparatus to use when treating patients with airborne diseases.

The potential for exposure to highly contagious organisms, hazardous chemicals or gases, and radiation related to acts of terrorism or natural or manmade disasters present additional risks to ED staff. Refer to Chapter 72 for information about decontamination procedures.

Providing Holistic Care

Sudden illness or trauma is a stress to physiologic and psychological homeostasis that requires physiologic and psychological healing. Patients and families experiencing sudden injury or illness often are overwhelmed by anxiety because they have not had time to adapt to the crisis. They experience real and terrifying fear of death, mutilation, immobilization, and other assaults on their personal identity and body integrity. When confronted with trauma, severe disfigurement, severe illness, or sudden death, the family experiences several stages of crisis. The stages begin with anxiety and progress through denial, remorse and guilt, anger, grief, and reconciliation. The initial goal for the patient and family is anxiety reduction, a prerequisite to recovering the ability to cope.

Assessment of the patient and family's psychological function includes evaluating emotional expression, degree of anxiety, and cognitive functioning. Possible nursing diagnoses include anxiety related to uncertain potential outcomes of the illness or trauma and ineffective individual coping related to acute situational crisis. In addition to anxiety, possible nursing diagnoses for the family include anticipatory grieving and alterations in family processes related to acute situational crises.

PATIENT-FOCUSED INTERVENTIONS

Those caring for the patient should act confidently and competently to relieve anxiety. Reacting and responding to the patient in a warm manner promotes a sense of security. Explanations

should be given on a level that the patient can understand, because an informed patient is better able to cope positively with stress. Human contact and reassuring words reduce the panic of the severely injured person and aid in dispelling fear of the unknown.

The unconscious patient should be treated as if conscious. That is, the patient should be touched, called by name, and given an explanation of every procedure that is performed. As the patient regains consciousness, the nurse should orient the patient by stating his or her name, the date, and the location. This basic information should be provided repeatedly, as needed, in a reassuring way.

FAMILY-FOCUSED INTERVENTIONS

The family is kept informed about where the patient is, how he or she is doing, and the care that is being given. Allowing the family to stay with the patient, when possible, also helps allay their anxieties. Additional interventions are based on the assessment of the stage of crisis that the family is experiencing. Measures to help family members cope with sudden death are presented in Chart 71-2.

Anxiety and Denial. During these stages, family members are encouraged to recognize and talk about their feelings of anxiety. Asking questions is encouraged. Honest answers given at the level of the family's understanding must be provided. Although denial is an ego-defense mechanism that protects one from recognizing painful and disturbing aspects of reality, prolonged denial is not encouraged or supported. The family must be prepared for the reality of what has happened and what may come.

Remorse and Guilt. Expressions of remorse and guilt may be heard, with family members accusing themselves (or each other) of negligence or minor omissions. Family members are urged to verbalize their feelings until they realize that there was probably little that they could have done to prevent the injury or illness.

Anger. Expressions of anger, common in crisis situations, are a way of handling anxiety and fear. Anger is frequently directed at the patient, but it is also often expressed toward the physician, the nurse, or admitting personnel. The therapeutic approach is to allow the anger to be ventilated, then assist the family to identify their feelings of frustration.

Grief. Grief is a complex emotional response to anticipated or actual loss. The key nursing intervention is to help family members work through their grief and to support their coping mechanisms, letting them know that it is normal and acceptable for them to cry, feel pain, and express loss. The hospital chaplain and social services staff both serve as invaluable members of the team when assisting families to work through their grief.

EMERGENCY NURSING AND THE CONTINUUM OF CARE

As stated previously, one principle underlying emergency care is that the patient will be rapidly assessed, treated, and referred to the appropriate setting for ongoing care. This makes the ED a very temporary point on the continuum of care. Most patients who receive emergency care are discharged directly from the ED to their homes, and emergency nurses must plan and facilitate the patient's safe discharge and follow-up care in the home and the community.

Discharge Planning

Before discharge, instructions for continuing care are given to the patient and the family or significant others. All instructions should be given not only verbally but also in writing, so that the patient can refer to them later. Many EDs have preprinted standard instruction sheets for the more common conditions. These instructions are then individualized for each patient. These instructions may be available in a variety of languages. If they are not available in the language that the patient needs, an interpreter should be used. Instructions should include information about prescribed medications, treatments, diet, activity, and when to contact a health care provider or schedule follow-up appointments. It is imperative that instructions are written legibly, use simple language, and are clear in their teaching. When providing discharge instructions, the nurse also considers any special needs the patient may have related to hearing or visual deficits.

Community Services

Before discharge, some patients require the services of a social worker to help them meet continuing health care needs. For patients and families who cannot provide care at home, community agencies (eg, Home Care Nursing Services, Visiting Nurse Association) may be contacted before discharge to arrange services. This is particularly important for elderly patients who need assistance. Identifying continuing health care needs and making arrangements for meeting these needs can prevent return visits to the ED and readmission to the hospital.

For patients who are returning to extended care facilities and for those who already rely on community agencies for continuing health care, communication about the patient's condition and any changes in health care needs that have occurred must be provided to the appropriate facilities or agencies. This communication is essential to promote continuity of care and to ensure ongoing care to meet the patient's changing health care needs.

 Gerontologic Considerations

The ED is a common point of entry into the health care system for patients 65 years of age and older. Elderly patients typically arrive with one or more presenting conditions involving the skin, cardiovascular system, or abdomen. Nonspecific symptoms, such as weakness and fatigue, episodes of falling, incontinence, and change in mental status, may be manifestations of acute, potentially life-threatening illness in the elderly person. Emergencies in this age group may be more difficult to manage because elderly patients may have

- An atypical presentation
- An altered response to treatment
- A greater risk of developing complications

The elderly patient may perceive the emergency as a crisis signaling the end of an independent lifestyle or even resulting in death. The nurse should give attention to the patient's feelings of anxiety and fear.

The older patient may have fewer sources of social and financial support in addition to frail health. The nurse should assess the psychosocial resources of the patient (and of the caregiver, if necessary) and anticipate discharge needs. Referrals for support services (eg, to the social service department or a gerontologic nurse specialist) may be necessary.

Principles of Emergency Care

By definition, emergency care is care that must be rendered without delay. In a hospital ED, several patients with diverse health problems—some life-threatening, some not—may present to the ED simultaneously. One of the first principles of emergency care is triage.

TRIAGE

The word **triage** comes from the French word *trier,* meaning "to sort." In the daily routine of the ED, triage is used to sort patients into groups based on the severity of their health problems and the immediacy with which these problems must be treated.

The Canadian Triage and Acuity Scale (CTAS) is a five-level triage score developed in the emergency care setting to determine which patients require most urgent attention from emergency department nurses and physicians. Presenting acuity is measured using a nationally recognized standardized triage scoring system. The triage nurse assigns each patient a priority level, which allows for best practice. The five-level triage scores are Level 1, Resuscitation; Level 2, Emergent; Level 3, Urgent; Level 4, Semi or Less Urgent; and Level 5, Non Urgent (Beveridge, Clarke, Janes, et al. 1998).

Triage is an advanced skill; emergency nurses spend many hours learning to classify different illnesses and injuries to ensure that patients most in need of care do not wait to receive it. Protocols may be followed to initiate laboratory or x-ray studies from the triage area while the patient waits for a bed in the ED. Collaborative protocols are developed and used by the triage nurse based on his or her level of experience. Also, nurses in the triage area collect crucial initial data: vital signs and history, neurologic assessment findings, and diagnostic data if necessary. The following questions reflect the minimum information that should be obtained from the patient or from the person who accompanied the patient to the ED. Of course, all answers are documented for reference by other health care providers.

- What were the circumstances, precipitating events, location, and time of the injury or illness?
- When did the symptoms appear?
- Was the patient unconscious after the injury or onset of illness?
- How did the patient get to the hospital?
- What was the health status of the patient before the injury or illness?
- Is there a medical or surgical history? A history of admissions to the hospital?
- Is the patient currently taking any medications, especially hormones, insulin, digitalis, anticoagulants?
- Does the patient have any allergies? If so, what are they?
- Does the patient have any bleeding tendencies?
- When was the last meal eaten? (This is important if general anesthesia is to be given or if the patient is unconscious.)
- Is the patient under a physician's care? What are the name and location of the physician?
- What was the date of the patient's most recent tetanus immunization?

Routine ED triage protocols differ significantly from the triage protocols used in disasters and mass casualty incidents (field triage). Routine hospital triage directs all available resources to the patients who are most critically ill, regardless of potential outcome. In field triage (or hospital triage during a disaster), scarce resources must be used to benefit the most people possible. This distinction affects triage decisions. Refer to Chapter 72 for a complete discussion of triage in mass casualty situations.

ASSESS AND INTERVENE

For the patient with an emergent or urgent health problem, stabilization, provision of critical treatments, and prompt transfer to the appropriate setting (intensive care unit, operating room, general care unit) are the priorities of emergency care. Although treatment is initiated in the ED, ongoing definitive treatment of the underlying problem is provided in other settings, and the sooner the patient is stabilized and moved to that area, the better.

A systematic approach to effectively establishing and treating health priorities is the primary survey/secondary survey approach. The primary survey focuses on stabilizing life-threatening conditions. The ED staff work collaboratively and follow the ABCD (**a**irway, **b**reathing, **c**irculation, **d**isability) method:

- Establish a patent airway.
- Provide adequate ventilation, employing resuscitation measures when necessary. (Trauma patients must have the cervical spine protected and chest injuries assessed first.)
- Evaluate and restore cardiac output by controlling hemorrhage, preventing and treating shock, and maintaining or restoring effective circulation.

- Determine neurologic disability by assessing neurologic function using the Glasgow Coma Scale (see Chapter 65).

After these priorities have been addressed, the ED team proceeds with the secondary survey. This includes

- A complete health history and head-to-toe assessment
- Diagnostic and laboratory testing
- Insertion or application of monitoring devices such as electrocardiogram (ECG) electrodes, arterial lines, or urinary catheters
- Splinting of suspected fractures
- Cleaning and dressing of wounds
- Performance of other necessary interventions based on the individual patient's condition

Once the patient has been assessed, stabilized, and tested, appropriate medical and nursing diagnoses are formulated, initial important treatment is started, and plans for the proper disposition of the patient are made. Many emergent and urgent conditions and priority emergency interventions are discussed in detail in the remaining sections of this chapter.

Airway Obstruction

Acute upper airway obstruction is a life-threatening medical emergency. The airway may be partially or completely occluded. If the airway is completely obstructed, permanent brain damage or death will occur within 3 to 5 minutes secondary to hypoxia. Partial obstruction of the airway can lead to progressive hypoxia, hypercarbia, and respiratory and cardiac arrest.

Pathophysiology

Upper airway obstruction has a number of causes, including aspiration of foreign bodies, anaphylaxis, viral or bacterial infection, trauma, and inhalation or chemical burns. In adults, aspiration of a bolus of meat is the most common cause of airway obstruction. In children, small toys, buttons, coins, and other objects are commonly aspirated in addition to food. Peritonsillar abscesses, epiglottitis, and other acute infectious processes of the posterior pharynx can result in airway obstruction.

Clinical Manifestations

Common signs and symptoms include choking, apprehensive appearance, inspiratory and expiratory stridor, laboured breathing, use of accessory muscles (suprasternal and intercostal retraction), flaring nostrils, increasing anxiety, restlessness, and confusion. Cyanosis and loss of consciousness develop as hypoxia worsens.

Assessment and Diagnostic Findings

Assessment of the patient who has a foreign object occluding the airway may involve simply asking the person whether he or she is choking and requires help. If the person is unconscious, inspection of the oropharynx may reveal the offending object. X-rays, laryngoscopy, or bronchoscopy also may be performed.

 Gerontologic Considerations

For elderly patients, especially those in extended care facilities, sedatives and hypnotic medications, diseases affecting motor coordination (eg, Parkinson's disease), and mental dysfunction (eg, dementia, mental retardation) are risk factors for asphyxiation by food. Nursing staff involved in the care of elderly patients must be aware of the symptoms of upper airway obstruction and be skillful in performing the Heimlich manoeuvre. Typically, the victim with a foreign body airway obstruction cannot speak, breathe, or cough. The patient may clutch the neck between the thumb and fingers (*universal distress signal*). The first response is to ask this person whether he or she is choking.

If the patient can breathe and cough spontaneously, a partial obstruction should be suspected. The victim is encouraged to cough forcefully and to persist with spontaneous coughing and breathing efforts as long as good air exchange exists. There may be some wheezing between coughs. If the patient demonstrates a weak, ineffective cough, high-pitched noise while inhaling, increased respiratory difficulty, or cyanosis, the patient should be managed as if there were complete airway obstruction.

After the obstruction is removed, rescue breathing is initiated. If the patient has no pulse, cardiac compressions are instituted. These measures provide oxygen to the brain, heart, and other vital organs until definitive medical treatment can restore and support normal heart and ventilatory activity.

Management

Establishing an airway may be as simple as repositioning the patient's head to prevent the tongue from obstructing the pharynx. Alternatively, other manoeuvres, such as abdominal thrusts, the head-tilt–chin-lift manoeuvre, the jaw-thrust manoeuvre, or insertion of specialized equipment may be needed to open the airway, remove a foreign body, or maintain the airway (Chart 71-3). In all manoeuvres, the cervical spine must be protected from injury.

HEAD-TILT–CHIN-LIFT MANOEUVRE

The patient is placed supine on a firm, flat surface. If the patient is lying face down, the body is turned as a unit so that the head, shoulders, and torso move simultaneously with no twisting. Next, the airway is opened using either the head-tilt–chin-lift manoeuvre or the jaw-thrust manoeuvre. In the head-tilt–chin-lift manoeuvre, one hand is placed on the victim's forehead, and firm backward pressure is applied with the palm to tilt the head back. The fingers of the other hand are placed under the bony part of the lower jaw near the chin and lifted up. The chin and the teeth are brought forward almost to occlusion to support the jaw.

 NURSING ALERT The head-tilt–chin-lift manoeuvre, which helps to tilt the head back, should be used only if it is determined that the patient's cervical spine is not injured.

JAW-THRUST MANOEUVRE

After one hand is placed on each side of the patient's jaw, the angles of the victim's lower jaw are grasped and lifted, displacing the mandible forward. This is a safe approach to opening the airway of a victim with suspected neck injury because it can be accomplished without extending the neck.

OROPHARYNGEAL AIRWAY INSERTION

An oropharyngeal airway is a semicircular tube or tubelike plastic device that is inserted over the back of the tongue into the lower posterior pharynx in a patient who is breathing spontaneously but unconscious (Chart 71-4). This type of airway pre-

vents the tongue from falling back against the posterior pharynx and obstructing the airway. It also allows health care providers to suction secretions.

ENDOTRACHEAL INTUBATION

The purpose of endotracheal intubation is to establish and maintain the airway in patients with respiratory insufficiency or hypoxia. Endotracheal intubation is indicated for the following reasons: (1) to establish an airway for patients who cannot be adequately ventilated with an oropharyngeal airway, (2) to bypass an upper airway obstruction, (3) to prevent aspiration, (4) to permit connection of the patient to a resuscitation bag or mechanical ventilator, and (5) to facilitate the removal of tracheobronchial secretions (Fig. 71-1). Because the procedure requires skill, endotracheal intubation is performed only by those who have had extensive training. These include physicians, nurse anesthetists, respiratory therapists, flight nurses, and nurse practitioners. The emergency nurse, however, is commonly called upon to assist with intubation.

ALTERNATIVE INTUBATION METHOD

If the patient is outside the hospital and cannot be intubated in the field, the emergency medical personnel may insert a Combitube. The tube rapidly provides pharyngeal ventilation. When the tube is inserted into the trachea, it functions like an endotracheal tube.

One of the two balloons around the tube can be inflated. One balloon is large (100 mL) and occludes the oropharynx. This could effectively provide for ventilation through forced air by way of the larynx. The smaller balloon is inflated with 15 mL of air and can effectively occlude the trachea if placed there. Breath sounds are auscultated to make sure that the oropharyngeal cuff does not obstruct the glottis. Patients can be ventilated through either port of the tube, depending on its placement.

CRICOTHYROIDOTOMY (CRICOTHYROID MEMBRANE PUNCTURE)

Cricothyroidotomy is the opening of the cricothyroid membrane to establish an airway. This procedure is used in emergency situations in which endotracheal intubation is either not possible or contraindicated, as in airway obstruction from extensive maxillofacial trauma, cervical spine injuries, laryngospasm, laryngeal edema (after an allergic reaction), hemorrhage into neck tissue, or obstruction of the larynx.

After these manoeuvres are performed, the patient is assessed for breathing by watching for chest movement and listening and feeling for air movement.

In such a case, nursing diagnoses would include ineffective airway clearance due to obstruction of the tongue, object, or fluids (blood, saliva). The nursing diagnosis may also be ineffective breathing pattern due to obstruction or injury.

Hemorrhage

Only a few conditions, such as obstructed airway or a sucking wound of the chest, take precedence over the immediate control of hemorrhage. Stopping bleeding is essential to the care and survival of patients in an emergency or disaster situation. Hemorrhage that results in the reduction of circulating blood volume is a primary cause of shock. Minor bleeding, which is usually venous, generally stops spontaneously unless the patient has a bleeding disorder or has been taking anticoagulants.

Chart 71-3

GUIDELINES FOR Managing a Foreign Body Airway Obstruction

ACTION	RATIONALE/AMPLIFICATION
ASSESS FOR INDICATIONS OF AIRWAY OBSTRUCTION • Victim may clutch the neck between thumb and fingers • Weak, ineffective cough; high-pitched noises on inspiration • Increased respiratory distress • Inability to speak, breathe, or cough • Collapse	Air movement is absent in the presence of *complete airway obstruction.* Oxygen saturation in the blood decreases rapidly because the obstructed airway prevents entry of air into the lungs. Oxygen deficit occurs in the brain, resulting in unconsciousness, with death following rapidly.
HEIMLICH MANOEUVRE (subdiaphragmatic abdominal thrusts) **For standing or sitting conscious patient:** Stand behind the patient; wrap your arms around the patient's waist, and proceed as follows: 1. Make a fist with one hand, placing the thumb side of the fist against the patient's abdomen, in the midline slightly above the umbilicus and well below the xiphoid process. Grasp the fist with the other hand. 2. Press your fist into the patient's abdomen with a quick inward and upward thrust. Each new thrust should be a separate and distinct manoeuvre.	The term *Heimlich manoeuvre* is used for the sake of uniformity. The terms *subdiaphragmatic abdominal thrusts* and *abdominal thrusts* are used interchangeably, depending on the circumstances. A subdiaphragmatic abdominal thrust, by elevating the diaphragm, can force air from the lungs to create an artificial cough intended to move and expel an obstructing foreign body from the airway.
For patient lying (unconscious): 1. Position patient on the back. 2. Kneel astride the patient's thighs, facing the head. 3. Place the heel of one hand against the patient's abdomen, in the midline slightly above the umbilicus and well below the tip of the xiphoid; place the second hand directly on top of the first. 4. Press into the abdomen with a quick upward thrust.	
Finger sweep: 1. Open the adult patient's mouth by grasping both the tongue and lower jaw between the thumb and fingers and lifting the mandible (tongue–jaw lift). 2. Insert the index finger of the other hand down along the inside of the cheek and scrape across the back of the throat. 3. Use a hooking action to dislodge the foreign body and manoeuvre it into the mouth for removal.	This manoeuvre is to be used *only in the unconscious adult patient.* This action draws the tongue away from the back of the throat and away from the foreign body that may be lodged there. Care is used to avoid forcing the object deeper into the throat.
Chest thrusts with conscious patient standing or sitting: 1. Stand behind patient with arms under patient's axillae to encircle patient's chest. 2. Place thumb side of your fist on middle of patient's sternum, taking care to avoid xiphoid process and margins of rib cage. 3. Grasp your fist with the other hand and perform backward thrusts until the foreign body is expelled or patient becomes unconscious.	This technique is to be used *only in the patient in advanced stages of pregnancy or in the markedly obese person.* Each thrust should be administered with the intent of relieving the obstruction.
Chest thrust with patient lying (unconscious): 1. Place the patient on the back and kneel close to the side of the patient's body. 2. Place the heel of your hand on the lower half of the sternum. 3. Deliver each chest thrust slowly and distinctly with the intent of relieving the obstruction.	This manoeuvre is *used only in the patient in advanced stages of pregnancy or when the rescuer cannot apply the Heimlich manoeuvre effectively to the unconscious, markedly obese person.*

Adapted from *Cardiopulmonary resuscitation (CPR).* Tulsa, OK: CPR Publishers, 2001.

The patient is assessed for signs and symptoms of shock: cool, moist skin (resulting from poor peripheral perfusion), falling blood pressure, increasing heart rate, delayed capillary refill, and decreasing urine volume (a late sign) (Chart 71-5). The goals of emergency management are to control the bleeding, maintain an adequately circulating blood volume for tissue oxygenation, and prevent shock. Patients who hemorrhage are at risk for cardiac arrest caused by hypovolemia with secondary anoxia. Nursing interventions are carried out collaboratively with other members of the emergency health care team.

Management

FLUID REPLACEMENT

Whenever a patient is experiencing hemorrhage—whether external or internal—a loss of circulating blood results in a fluid volume deficit and decreased cardiac output. Therefore, fluid replacement is imperative to maintain circulation. Typically, two large-bore intravenous cannulae are inserted to provide a means for fluid and blood replacement, and blood samples are obtained for analysis, typing, and cross-matching. Replacement fluids are

Chart 71-4   Inserting an Oropharyngeal Airway

1. Measure the oral airway alongside the head. The airway should reach from lip to ear.
2. Extend the patient's head by placing one hand under the bony chin (*only if the cervical spine is uninjured*). With the other hand, tilt the head backward by applying pressure to the forehead while simultaneously lifting the chin forward.
3. Open the patient's mouth.

4. (**A**) Insert the oropharyngeal airway with the tip facing up toward the roof of the mouth until it passes the uvula. (**B**) Rotate the tip 180 degrees so that the tip is pointed down toward the pharynx. This displaces the tongue anteriorly, and the patient then breathes through and around the airway.
5. The distal end of the oropharyngeal airway is in the hypopharynx, and the flange is approximately at the patient's lips. Make sure that the tongue has not been pushed into the airway.

A

B

administered as prescribed, depending on clinical estimates of the type and volume of fluid lost. Replacement fluids may include isotonic electrolyte solutions (lactated Ringer's, normal saline), colloid, and blood component therapy.

Packed red blood cells are infused when there is massive blood loss. In emergencies, O-negative blood is used for women of childbearing age and O-positive blood is used for men and for postmenopausal women. In an emergent situation, there is

not time to type and cross-match or type and screen blood. O-negative blood provides safe administration of blood immediately without sensitizing an Rh-negative woman to Rh-positive blood. Sensitization can result in difficulties during pregnancy later.

Additional platelets and clotting factors are given when large amounts of blood are needed, because replacement blood is deficient in clotting factors.

A   **B**

FIGURE 71-1 Endotracheal intubation in a patient without a cervical spine injury. (**A**) The primary glottic landmarks for tracheal intubation as visualized with proper placement of the laryngoscope. (**B**) Positioning the endotracheal tube.

Signs and Symptoms of Hypovolemic Shock

Chart 71-5

Decreasing arterial pressure
Increasing pulse rate
Cold, moist skin
Delayed capillary refill
Pallor
Thirst
Diaphoresis
Altered sensorium
Oliguria
Metabolic acidosis
Hyperpnea

! NURSING ALERT The infusion rate is determined by the severity of the blood loss and the clinical evidence of hypovolemia. If massive blood replacement is necessary, the blood must be warmed in a commercial blood warmer, because administration of large amounts of blood that has been refrigerated has a core cooling effect that may lead to cardiac arrest.

CONTROL OF EXTERNAL HEMORRHAGE

If a patient is hemorrhaging externally (eg, from a wound), a rapid physical assessment is performed as the patient's clothing is cut away in an attempt to identify the area of hemorrhage. Direct, firm pressure is applied over the bleeding area or the involved artery (Fig. 71-2). Most bleeding can be stopped or at least controlled by application of direct pressure. Otherwise, unchecked arterial bleeding results in death. A firm pressure dressing is applied, and the injured part is elevated to stop venous and capillary bleeding if possible. If the injured area is an extremity, the extremity is immobilized to control blood loss.

Tourniquets. A tourniquet is applied to an extremity only as a *last resort* when the external hemorrhage cannot be controlled in any other way. Care must be taken when applying a tourniquet because of the risk of loss of the extremity. The tourniquet is applied just proximal to the wound and tied tightly enough to control arterial blood flow. The patient is tagged with a skin-marking pencil or on adhesive tape on the forehead with a "T," stating the location of the tourniquet and the time applied. Periodically, the tourniquet is loosened to prevent irreparable vascular or neurologic damage. If there is arterial bleeding, the tourniquet is removed and a pressure dressing is applied. If the patient has suffered a traumatic amputation with uncontrollable hemorrhage, the tourniquet remains in place until the patient is in the operating room.

CONTROL OF INTERNAL BLEEDING

If the patient shows no external signs of bleeding but exhibits tachycardia, falling blood pressure, thirst, apprehension, cool and

FIGURE 71-2 Pressure points for control of hemorrhage.

moist skin, or delayed capillary refill, internal hemorrhage is suspected. Typically, packed red blood cells (O-negative) are administered at a rapid rate, and the patient is prepared for more definitive treatment (eg, surgery, pharmacologic therapy). Additionally, arterial blood specimens are obtained to evaluate pulmonary function and tissue perfusion and to establish baseline hemodynamic parameters, which are then used as an index for determining the amount of fluid replacement the patient can tolerate and the response to therapy. The patient is maintained in the supine position and monitored closely until hemodynamic or circulatory parameters improve, or until transport to the operating room or intensive care.

Hypovolemic Shock

Shock is a condition in which there is loss of effective circulating blood volume. Inadequate organ and tissue perfusion follow, ultimately resulting in cellular metabolic derangements. In any emergency situation, the onset of shock should be anticipated by assessing all injured people immediately. The underlying cause of shock (hypovolemic, cardiogenic, neurogenic, or septic) must be determined. Of these, hypovolemia is the most common cause (see Chap. 14).

Altered tissue perfusion related to failing circulation, impaired gas exchange related to a ventilation–perfusion imbalance, and decreased cardiac output related to decreased circulating blood volume are possible problems associated with hypovolemic shock. Therefore, the goals of treatment are to restore and maintain tissue perfusion and to correct physiologic abnormalities.

Management

For the patient experiencing hypovolemic shock, ensuring a patent airway and maintaining breathing are crucial. Additional ventilatory assistance is given as required. A rapid physical examination is performed to determine the cause of shock.

Restoration of the circulating blood volume is accomplished with rapid fluid and blood replacement as prescribed based on the patient's response to therapy. Blood component therapy helps to optimize cardiac preload, correct hypotension, and maintain tissue perfusion.

Large-gauge intravenous needles or catheters are inserted into peripheral veins. Two or more catheters are necessary for rapid fluid replacement and reversal of hemodynamic instability. The emphasis is on volume replacement. If it is suspected that a major vessel in the chest or abdomen has been disrupted, intravenous lines may be established in both upper and lower extremities.

A central venous pressure (CVP) catheter also may be inserted (in or near the right atrium) to serve as a guide for fluid replacement. Continuous CVP readings give the direction and degree of change from baseline readings. The catheter is also a vehicle for emergency fluid volume replacement.

Intravenous fluids are infused at a rapid rate until systolic blood pressure or CVP rises to a satisfactory level above the baseline measurement or until there is improvement in the patient's clinical condition. Infusion of lactated Ringer's solution is useful initially because it approximates plasma electrolyte composition and osmolality, allows time for blood typing and screening, restores circulation, and serves as an adjunct to blood component therapy.

Blood component therapy may also be prescribed, especially if blood loss has been severe or if the patient continues to hemorrhage. Measures to control hemorrhage are instituted because

hemorrhage compounds the shock state. Serial hematocrit values are obtained if continued bleeding is suspected. Also, the feet are elevated slightly to improve cerebral circulation and promote venous return to the heart. However, this position is contraindicated for patients with head injuries. Unnecessary movement is also avoided.

An indwelling urinary catheter is inserted to record urinary output every hour. Urine volume indicates the adequacy of kidney perfusion. However, fluid replacement should not be delayed.

Ongoing nursing surveillance of the *total patient* is maintained. Blood pressure, heart and respiratory rates, skin temperature, colour, pulse oximetry, neurologic status, CVP, arterial blood gases, ECG recordings, hematocrit, hemoglobin, coagulation profile, electrolytes, and urinary output are monitored serially to assess patient response to treatment. Commonly, a flow sheet is used to document these parameters, providing an analysis of trends rather than single values to reveal improvement or deterioration of the patient's condition.

Additionally, the body's defense mechanisms should be supported. The patient should be reassured and comforted. Sedation may be necessary to relieve apprehension. Analgesics are used cautiously to relieve pain. Body temperature is maintained within normal limits to prevent increasing metabolic demands that the body may be unable to meet.

Resuscitation of the patient goes well beyond a normal blood pressure and visual evidence of perfusion. Lactic acidosis is a common side effect of hemorrhage and injury. It is associated with poor cardiac performance and higher rates of morbidity and mortality. Base deficit and lactate are measures of successful and complete resuscitation. End points for resuscitation include a serum lactic acid level lower than 2.5 mmol/L within 24 hours after injury and normalizing vital signs without ongoing hemorrhage.

Wounds

Wounds involving injury to soft tissues can vary from minor tears to severe crushing injuries. The types of wounds that may occur are defined in Chart 71-6. The primary goal is to restore the physical integrity and function of the injured tissue, with minimal scarring and without infection. Proper documentation of the wound, using precise descriptions and correct terminology, is essential. Such information may be needed in the future for

Chart 71-6	**Definition of Terms: Wounds**

Laceration: skin tear with irregular edges and vein bridging
Avulsion: tearing away from supporting structures
Abrasion: denuded skin
Ecchymosis/contusion: blood trapped under the surface of the skin
Hematoma: tumourlike mass of blood trapped under the skin
Stab: incision of the skin with well-defined edges, usually caused by a sharp instrument; a stab wound is typically deeper than long
Cut: incision of the skin with well-defined edges, usually longer than deep
Patterned: wound representing the outline of the object (eg, steering wheel) causing the wound

forensic evidence. Photographs are helpful because they provide an accurate, visible description of the wound.

Determining *when* and *how* the wound occurred is important, because a treatment delay exceeding 3 hours increases infection risk. Using aseptic technique, the clinician inspects the wound to determine the extent of damage to underlying structures. Sensory, motor, and vascular function are evaluated for changes that might indicate complications.

Management

WOUND CLEANSING

Hair around the wound may be clipped or shaved (only as directed) if it is anticipated that the hairs will interfere with wound closure. Typically, the area around the wound is cleaned with normal saline solution or a polymer agent (eg, SureClens). Antibacterial agents, such as povidone-iodine (Betadine) or hydrogen peroxide, should not be allowed to get deep into the wound without thorough rinsing. These agents are used only for the initial cleansing because they injure exposed and healthy tissue, resulting in further cell injury.

If indicated, the area is infiltrated with a local intradermal anesthetic through the wound margins or by regional block. Patients with soft tissue injuries usually have localized pain at the site of injury. The nurse then assists the physician, nurse practitioner, or physician's assistant in cleaning and débriding the wound.

The wound is irrigated gently and copiously with sterile isotonic saline solution to remove surface dirt. Devitalized tissue and foreign matter are removed because they impede healing and may encourage infection. Any small bleeding vessels are clamped or tied. Alternatively, hemostasis may be achieved with cauterization. After wound treatment, a nonadherent dressing is commonly applied to protect the wound. The dressing may serve as a splint and also as a reminder to the patient that the area is injured.

PRIMARY CLOSURE

The decision to suture a wound depends on the nature of the wound, the time since the injury was sustained, the degree of contamination, and the vascularity of tissues. If primary closure is indicated, the wound is sutured, usually by the physician, with the patient receiving a form of anesthesia known as moderate sedation. Wound closure begins when subcutaneous fat is brought together loosely with a few sutures to close off the dead space. The subcuticular layer is then closed, and finally the epidermis is closed. Sutures are placed near the wound edge, with the skin edges leveled carefully to promote optimal healing. Instead of sutures, sterile strips of reinforced microporous tape or a bonding agent (skin glue) may be used to close clean, superficial wounds.

DELAYED PRIMARY CLOSURE

Delayed primary closure may be indicated if tissue has been lost or there is a high potential for infection.

A thin layer of gauze (to ensure drainage and prevent pooling of exudate), covered by an occlusive dressing, may be used. Other options include split-thickness cadaver or porcine xenografts to simulate the function of epithelium. The wound is splinted in a functional position to prevent motion and decrease the possibility of contracture.

If there are no signs of suppuration, the wound may be sutured (with the patient receiving a local anesthetic). Use of antibiotics to prevent infection depends on factors such as how the

injury occurred, the age of the wound, and the risk for contamination. The site is immobilized and elevated to limit accumulation of fluid in the interstitial spaces of the wound.

Tetanus prophylaxis is administered as prescribed, based on the condition of the wound and the patient's immunization status. The patient is instructed about signs and symptoms of infection and is told to contact the health care provider or clinic if there is sudden or persistent pain, fever or chills, bleeding, rapid swelling, foul odour, drainage, or redness surrounding the wound.

Trauma

Trauma, the unintentional or intentional wound or injury inflicted on the body from a mechanism against which the body cannot protect itself, is the fourth leading cause of death in the United States. Trauma is the leading cause of death in children and in adults younger than 44 years of age (McQuillan, VonReuden, Hartsock, Flynn, & Whalen, 2002). The incidence is increasing in adults older than 44 years of age. Alcohol and drug abuse are often implicated as factors in both blunt and penetrating trauma.

Collection of Forensic Evidence

In assessing and managing any patient with an emergency condition, but especially the patient experiencing trauma, documentation of all that occurs is essential. Included in documentation are descriptions of all wounds, mechanism of injury, time of events, and collection of evidence. In trauma care, the nurse must be exceedingly careful with all potential evidence, handling and documenting it properly.

The basics of care management for patients with traumatic injury include an understanding that trauma in any patient (living or dead) has potential legal, or forensic, implications. Hence, proper management from both a medical and forensic perspective is essential.

When clothing is removed from the patient who has experienced trauma, the nurse must be careful not to cut through or disrupt any tears, holes, blood stains, or dirt present on the clothing. Each piece of clothing should be placed in an individual paper bag. If the clothing is wet, it should be hung to dry. Clothing should not be given to families. Valuables should be placed in the hospital safe or clearly documented as to which family member they were given. If a police officer is present to collect clothing or any other items from the patient, each item is labelled. The transfer of custody to the officer, the officer's name, the date, and the time are documented.

If suicide or homicide is suspected in a deceased trauma patient, the medical examiner will examine the body on site or have the body moved to the coroner's office for autopsy. All tubes and lines must remain in place. The patient's hands must be covered with paper bags to protect evidence on the hands or under the fingernails. In the surviving patient, tissue specimens may be swabbed from the hands and nails as potential evidence. Photographs of wounds or clothing are essential and should include a reference ruler in one photo and one without the ruler.

Documentation should also include any statements made by the patient in the patient's own words and surrounded by quotation marks. A chain of evidence is essential. If the patient's case is adjudicated in the future, clear documentation will assist the judicial process and help to identify the activities that occurred in the ED.

Injury Prevention

Any discussion of trauma management must include a discussion of injury prevention. A component of the emergency nurse's daily role is to provide injury prevention information to every patient with whom there is contact, including patients admitted for reasons other than injury. The only way to reduce the incidence of trauma is to prevent the injuries in the first place. Everyone can benefit from injury prevention information. Using the information after leaving the ED or other health care site is the patient's responsibility. However, the information must be provided.

The key to decreasing the incidence of trauma and saving the lives of productive members of society and children is injury prevention. The emergency nurse should make injury prevention part of daily nursing practice.

There are three components of injury prevention. The first is education. Providing information and materials to help prevent violence and to maintain safety at home and in vehicles is important. Involvement in local injury prevention organizations, nursing organizations, and health fairs promotes wellness and safety. In practice, nursing and other health care professionals should avoid using the word "accident," because trauma events are *preventable* and should be viewed as such rather than as "fate" or "happenstance." Responsibility and accountability must be assigned to traumatic incidents, particularly because of the high rate of trauma recidivism. Those who are at risk for trauma and repeated trauma should be identified and provided with education and counselling directed toward altering risky behaviours and preventing further trauma.

The second component of injury prevention is legislation. Nurses should be actively involved in safety legislation at the local, provincial/territorial, and federal levels. Such legislation is meant to provide universal safety measures, not to infringe on rights.

The third component is automatic protection. Airbags and automatic safety belts are in this category. These mechanisms provide for safety without requiring personal intervention.

INTRA-ABDOMINAL INJURIES

Intra-abdominal injuries are categorized as penetrating or blunt trauma. *Penetrating* abdominal injuries (ie, gunshot wounds, stab wounds) are serious and usually require surgery. Penetrating abdominal trauma results in a high incidence of injury to hollow organs, particularly the small bowel. The liver is the most frequently injured solid organ. In gunshot wounds, the most important factor is the velocity at which the missile enters the body. High-velocity missiles (bullets) create extensive tissue damage. All abdominal gunshot wounds that cross the peritoneum or are associated with peritoneal signs require surgical exploration. Stab wounds may be managed nonoperatively.

Blunt trauma to the abdomen may result from motor vehicle crashes, falls, blows, or explosions. Blunt trauma is commonly associated with extra-abdominal injuries to the chest, head, or extremities. Patients with blunt trauma are a challenge because of injuries that may be hidden and difficult to detect. The incidence of delayed and trauma-related complications is greater than for penetrating injuries. This is especially true of blunt injuries involving the liver, kidneys, spleen, or blood vessels, which can lead to massive blood loss into the peritoneal cavity.

Assessment and Diagnostic Findings

In conjunction with the history, the abdomen is inspected for obvious signs of injury, including penetrating injuries, bruises, and abrasions. Abdominal assessment continues with auscultation of bowel sounds to provide baseline data from which changes can be noted. Absence of bowel sounds may be an early sign of intraperitoneal involvement, although stress can also decrease or eliminate bowel sounds. Further abdominal assessment may reveal progressive abdominal distention, involuntary guarding, tenderness, pain, muscular rigidity, or rebound tenderness along with changes in bowel sounds, all of which are signs of peritoneal irritation. Hypotension and signs and symptoms of shock may also be noted. Additionally, the chest and other body systems are assessed for injuries that frequently accompany intra-abdominal injuries.

Laboratory studies that aid in assessment include the following:

- Urinalysis to detect hematuria (indicative of a urinary tract injury)
- Serial hematocrit levels to evaluate trends reflecting the presence or absence of bleeding
- White blood cell count to detect elevation (generally associated with trauma)
- Serum amylase analysis to detect rising levels, which suggest pancreatic injury or perforation of the gastrointestinal tract

INTERNAL BLEEDING

Hemorrhage frequently accompanies abdominal injury, especially if the liver or spleen has been traumatized. Therefore, the patient is assessed continuously for signs and symptoms of external and internal bleeding. The front of the body, flanks, and back are inspected for bluish discolouration, asymmetry, abrasion, and contusion. Abdominal CT scans permit detailed evaluation of abdominal contents and retroperitoneal examination. Abdominal ultrasound studies can rapidly assess hemodynamically unstable patients to detect intraperitoneal bleeding and pericardial tamponade. This is referred to as the FAST (Focused Assessment for Sonographic Examination of the Trauma Patient) examination. Pain in the left shoulder is common in a patient with bleeding from a ruptured spleen, whereas pain in the right shoulder can result from laceration of the liver. Even though the patient complains of pain, administration of opioids is avoided during the observation period because their effect may obscure the clinical picture.

INTRAPERITONEAL INJURY

The abdomen is assessed for tenderness, rebound tenderness, guarding, rigidity, spasm, increasing distention, and pain. Referred pain is a significant finding because it suggests intraperitoneal injury. To determine whether there is intraperitoneal injury and bleeding, the patient is usually prepared for diagnostic procedures, such as peritoneal lavage, abdominal ultrasonography, or abdominal computed tomography (CT) scanning. **Diagnostic peritoneal lavage** involves the instillation of 1 L of warmed lactated Ringer's or normal saline solution into the abdominal cavity. After a minimum of 400 mL has been returned, a fluid specimen is sent to the laboratory for analysis. Positive laboratory findings include a red blood cell count higher than $100,000/mm^3$, a white blood cell count exceeding $500/mm^3$, or the presence of bile, feces, or food.

In patients with stab wounds, sinography may be performed to detect peritoneal penetration. With this procedure, a purse-string suture is placed around the wound, and a small catheter is introduced through the wound. A contrast agent is then introduced through the catheter, and x-rays are taken to identify any peritoneal penetration.

GENITOURINARY INJURY

A rectal or vaginal examination is performed to determine any injury to the pelvis, bladder, and intestinal wall. To decompress the bladder and monitor urine output, an indwelling catheter is inserted after a rectal examination (not before). In the male patient, a high-riding prostate gland (abnormal position) discovered during a rectal examination indicates a potential urethral injury.

> **! NURSING ALERT** Urethral catheter insertion with a possible urethral injury is contraindicated; a urology consultation and further evaluation of the urethra are required.

Management

As indicated by the patient's condition, resuscitation procedures (restoration of airway, breathing, and circulation) are initiated. A patent airway is maintained, and attempts to stabilize the respiratory, circulatory, and nervous systems are made. Bleeding is controlled by application of direct pressure to any external bleeding wounds and by occlusion of any chest wounds. Circulating blood volume is maintained with intravenous fluid replacement, including blood component therapy. The patient is monitored for signs and symptoms of shock after an initial response to transfusion therapy, because these are often the first signs of internal hemorrhage.

With blunt trauma, the patient is kept on a stretcher to immobilize the spine. A backboard may be used for transporting the patient to the x-ray department, to the operating room, or to the intensive care unit. Cervical spine immobilization is maintained until cervical x-rays have been obtained and cervical spine injury ruled out.

Knowing the mechanism of injury (eg, penetrating force from a gunshot or knife, blunt force from a blow), is essential to determining the type of management needed. All wounds are located, counted, and documented. If abdominal viscera protrude, the area is covered with sterile, moist saline dressings to keep the viscera from drying.

Typically, oral fluids are withheld in anticipation of surgery, and the stomach contents are aspirated with a nasogastric tube to reduce the risk of aspiration. Nasogastric aspiration also decompresses the stomach in preparation for diagnostic procedures.

Trauma predisposes the patient to infection by disruption of mechanical barriers, exposure to exogenous bacteria from the environment at the time of injury, and diagnostic and therapeutic procedures (nosocomial infection). Tetanus prophylaxis and broad-spectrum antibiotics are administered as prescribed.

Throughout the stay in the ED, the patient's condition is continuously monitored for changes. If there is continuing evidence of shock, blood loss, free air under the diaphragm, evisceration, hematuria, or suspected or known abdominal injury, the patient is rapidly transported to surgery. In most cases, blunt liver and spleen injuries are managed nonoperatively.

CRUSH INJURIES

Crush injuries occur when a person is caught between objects, run over by a moving vehicle, or compressed by machinery.

Assessment and Diagnostic Findings

The patient is observed for the following:

- Hypovolemic shock resulting from extravasation of blood and plasma into injured tissues after compression has been released
- Paralysis of a body part
- Erythema and blistering of skin
- Damaged body part (usually an extremity) appearing swollen, tense, and hard
- Renal dysfunction (prolonged hypotension causes kidney damage and acute renal insufficiency; myoglobinuria secondary to muscle damage can cause acute renal failure)

Management

In conjunction with maintaining the airway, breathing, and circulation, the patient is observed for acute renal insufficiency. Injury to the back can cause severe kidney damage. Severe muscular damage causes a significant release of myoglobin, which can result in acute tubular necrosis. Additionally, major soft tissue injuries are splinted early to control bleeding and pain. Again, the serum lactic acid concentration is monitored; a decrease to less than 2.5 mmol/L is an indication of successful resuscitation (Blow, Magliore, Claridge, Butler, & Young, 1999).

If an extremity is involved, it is elevated to relieve swelling and pressure. To restore neurovascular function, the physician may perform a **fasciotomy** (surgical incision to the level of the fascia). Medications for pain and anxiety are then administered as prescribed, and the patient is quickly transported to the operating suite for wound débridement and fracture repair. Then, a hyperbaric chamber (if one is available) can be used for hyperoxygenation of the crushed tissue, if indicated.

MULTIPLE INJURIES

Care of the patient with multiple injuries requires a team approach, with one person responsible for coordinating the treatment. Immediately after injury, the body is hypermetabolic, hypercoagulable, and severely stressed. Mortality in patients with multiple injuries is related to the severity of the injuries and the number of systems and organs involved.

Multiple trauma potentially affects every body system. The nursing staff assumes responsibility for assessing and monitoring the patient, ensuring intravenous access, administering prescribed medications, collecting laboratory specimens, and documenting activities and the patient's response.

Assessment and Diagnostic Findings

Gross evidence of trauma may be slight or absent. The injury regarded as the least significant in appearance may be the most lethal. For example, the pelvis fracture not identified until x-ray may be the injury from which the patient is exsanguinating into the pelvic cavity. Another example is a pneumothorax that is insidiously increasing in size, affecting both the heart and lungs, while the staff are focused on the treatment of external lacerations. An obvious amputation of the arm may have already stopped bleeding from the body's normal response of vasoconstriction, despite being obvious and a devastating injury; meanwhile, the patient may be dying from an internal, not so visible, injury.

Management

The goals of treatment are to determine the extent of injuries and to establish priorities of treatment. Any injury interfering with a vital physiologic function (eg, airway, breathing, circulation) is an immediate threat to life and has the highest priority for immediate treatment. Essential life-saving procedures are performed simultaneously by the emergency team. As soon as the pa-

tient is resuscitated, clothes are usually cut off, and a rapid physical assessment is performed. Transfer from field management to the ED must be orderly and controlled, with attention given to the verbal report from emergency medical services. Treatment in a level I trauma centre is appropriate for patients experiencing major trauma. Treatment priorities are illustrated in Figure 71-3.

FRACTURES

Immediate management of a fracture may determine the patient's outcome and may mean the difference between recovery and disability. When the patient is being examined for fracture, the body part is handled gently and as little as possible. Clothing is cut off

1 Establish airway and ventilation.

2 Control of hemorrhage

3 Prevent and treat hypovolemic shock. Monitor urine output.

4 Assess for head and neck injuries. Maintain spine immobilization.

5 Evaluate for other injuries — reassess head and neck, chest; assess abdomen, back, and extremities.

6 Splint fractures

7 Carry out a more thorough and ongoing examination and assessment.

FIGURE 71-3 Management of the patient with multiple injuries.

to visualize the body. Assessment is conducted for pain over or near a bone, swelling (from blood, lymph, and exudate infiltrating the tissue), and circulatory disturbance. The patient is assessed for ecchymosis, tenderness, and crepitation. The nurse must remember that the patient may have multiple fractures accompanied by head, chest, spine, or abdominal injuries.

Management

Immediate attention is given to the patient's general condition. Assessment of airway, breathing, and circulation (which includes pulses in the extremities) is conducted. The patient is also evaluated for neurologic or abdominal injuries before the extremity is treated, unless a pulseless extremity is detected.

If a pulseless extremity is identified, repositioning of the extremity to proper alignment is required. If the pulseless extremity involves a fractured hip or femur, **Hare traction** (a portable in-line traction device) may be applied to assist with alignment. If repositioning is ineffective in restoring the pulse, a rapid total-body assessment should be completed, followed by transfer of the patient to the operating room for arteriography and possible arterial repair.

After the initial evaluation has been completed, all injuries identified are evaluated and treated. The fractured body part is inspected. Using a systematic head-to-toe approach, the clinician inspects the entire body, observing for lacerations, swelling, and deformities, including angulation (bending), shortening, rotation, and asymmetry. All peripheral pulses, especially those distal to the fractured extremity, are palpated. The extremity is also assessed for coolness, blanching, and decreased sensation and motor function, which are indicative of injury to the extremity's neurovascular supply.

A splint is applied before the patient is moved. Splinting immobilizes the joint above and below the fracture, relieves pain, restores or improves circulation, prevents further tissue injury, and prevents a closed fracture from becoming an open one. To splint an extremity, one hand is placed distal to the fracture and some traction is applied while the other hand is placed beneath the fracture for support. The splints should extend beyond the joints adjacent to the fracture. Upper extremities must be splinted in a functional position. If the fracture is open, a moist, sterile dressing is applied.

After splinting, the vascular status of the extremity is checked by assessing colour, temperature, pulse, and blanching of the nail bed. If there is evidence of neurovascular compromise, the splint is removed and reapplied. In addition, any complaints of pain or pressure are investigated. (See Chap. 69 for a complete description of fracture management.)

Environmental Emergencies

HEAT STROKE

Heat stroke is an acute medical emergency caused by failure of the heat-regulating mechanisms of the body. It usually occurs during extended heat waves, especially when they are accompanied by high humidity. People at risk are those not acclimatized to heat, elderly and very young people, those unable to care for themselves, those with chronic and debilitating diseases, and those taking certain medications (eg, major tranquilizers, anticholinergics, diuretics, beta-adrenergic blocking agents). Exertional heat stroke occurs in healthy individuals during sports or work activities (eg, exercising in extreme heat and humidity). Hyperthermia

results because of inadequate heat loss. This type of heat stroke can also cause death. See Chart 71-7 for prevention strategies.

Gerontologic Considerations

Most heat-related deaths occur in the elderly, because their circulatory systems are unable to compensate for stress imposed by heat. Elderly people have a decreased ability to perspire as well as a decreased thirst mechanism to compensate for heat.

Assessment and Diagnostic Findings

Heat stroke causes thermal injury at the cellular level, resulting in widespread damage to the heart, liver, kidney, and blood coagulation. Recent patient history reveals exposure to elevated ambient temperature or excessive exercise during extreme heat. When assessing the patient, the nurse notes the following symptoms: profound central nervous system (CNS) dysfunction (manifested by confusion, delirium, bizarre behaviour, coma); elevated body temperature (40.6°C or higher); hot, dry skin; and usually anhidrosis (absence of sweating), tachypnea, hypotension, and tachycardia.

Management

The primary goal is to reduce the high temperature as quickly as possible, because mortality is directly related to the duration of hyperthermia. Simultaneous treatment focuses on stabilizing oxygenation using the ABCs of basic life support.

After the patient's clothing is removed, the core (internal) temperature is reduced to 39°C as rapidly as possible. One or more of the following methods may be used as directed:

- Cool sheets and towels or continuous sponging with cool water
- Ice applied to the neck, groin, chest, and axillae while spraying with tepid water
- Cooling blankets
- Iced saline lavage of the stomach or colon if the temperature does not decrease
- Immersion of the patient in a cold water bath (if possible)

During cooling, the patient is massaged to promote circulation and maintain cutaneous vasodilation. An electric fan is positioned so that it blows on the patient to augment heat dissipation by convection and evaporation. The patient's temperature is con-

Chart 71-7
Health Promotion • Preventing Heat Stroke

- Advise the patient to avoid immediate reexposure to high temperatures; hypersensitivity to high temperatures may remain for a considerable time.
- Emphasize the importance of maintaining adequate fluid intake, wearing loose clothing, and reducing activity in hot weather.
- Advise athletes to monitor fluid losses and weight loss during workout activities or exercise and to replace fluids.
- Advise the patient to use a gradual approach to physical conditioning, allowing sufficient time for acclimatization.
- Direct frail elderly patients living in urban settings with high environmental temperatures to places where air conditioning is available (eg, shopping mall, library, church).

stantly monitored with a thermistor placed in the rectum, bladder, or esophagus to evaluate core temperature. Caution is used to avoid hypothermia and to prevent hyperthermia, which may recur spontaneously within 3 to 4 hours.

Throughout treatment, the patient's status is monitored carefully, including vital signs, ECG findings (for possible myocardial ischemia, myocardial infarction, and dysrhythmias), CVP, and level of responsiveness, all of which may change with rapid alterations in body temperature. A seizure may be followed by recurrence of hyperthermia. To meet tissue needs exaggerated by the hypermetabolic condition, 100% oxygen is administered. The patient may require endotracheal intubation and mechanical ventilation to support failing cardiopulmonary systems.

Intravenous infusion therapy of normal saline or lactated Ringer's solution is initiated as directed to replace fluid losses and maintain adequate circulation. Fluids are administered carefully because of the dangers of myocardial injury from high body temperature and poor renal function. Cooling redistributes fluid volume from the periphery to the core.

Urine output is also measured frequently, because acute tubular necrosis is a complication of heat stroke from rhabdomyolysis (myoglobin in the urine). Blood specimens are obtained for serial testing to detect bleeding disorders, such as disseminated intravascular coagulopathy, and for serial enzyme studies to estimate thermal hypoxic injury to the liver, heart, and muscle tissue. Permanent liver, cardiac, and CNS damage may occur.

Additional supportive care may include dialysis for renal failure, antiseizure agents to control seizures, potassium for hypokalemia, and sodium bicarbonate to correct metabolic acidosis. Benzodiazepines or chlorpromazine may be prescribed to suppress seizure activity. Patient education regarding the prevention of heat stroke (ie, adequate fluid intake, staying out of the sun especially between 10 AM and 2 PM) is also important to prevent a recurrence of heat stroke.

FROSTBITE

Frostbite is trauma from exposure to freezing temperatures and actual freezing of the tissue fluids in the cell and intercellular spaces. It results in cellular and vascular damage. Body parts most frequently affected by frostbite include the feet, hands, nose, and ears. Frostbite ranges from first degree (redness and erythema) to fourth degree (full-depth tissue destruction).

Assessment and Diagnostic Findings

A frozen extremity may be hard, cold, and insensitive to touch and may appear white or mottled blue-white. The extent of injury from exposure to cold is not always initially known. The history of the patient should include environmental temperature, duration of exposure, humidity, and the presence of wet conditions.

Management

The goal of management is to restore normal body temperature. Constrictive clothing and jewelry that could impair circulation are removed. If the lower extremities are involved, the patient should not be allowed to ambulate.

> **! NURSING ALERT** If the patient requires transport, do not initiate rewarming. During transport, rewarming procedures may not be able to be maintained. In addition, any further cooling or freezing experience will cause significant damage to the already frozen body part.

Controlled yet rapid rewarming is instituted. The extremity is usually placed in a 37° to 40°C circulating bath for 30- to 40-minute spans. This treatment is repeated until circulation is effectively restored. Early rewarming appears to decrease the amount of ultimate tissue loss. During rewarming, an analgesic for pain is administered as prescribed, because the rewarming process may be very painful. To avoid further mechanical injury, the body part is not handled. Massage is contraindicated.

Once rewarmed, the part is protected from further injury and is elevated to help control swelling. Sterile gauze or cotton is placed between affected fingers or toes to prevent maceration. A foot cradle may be used to prevent contact with bedclothes if the feet are involved. Blebs, which develop 1 hour to a few days after rewarming, are left intact and not ruptured, especially if they are hemorrhagic.

A physical assessment is conducted with rewarming to observe for concomitant injury, such as soft tissue injury, dehydration, alcohol coma, or fat embolism. Problems such as dehydration, hyperkalemia, and hypovolemia, which occur frequently in people with frostbite, are corrected. Risk for infection is also great; therefore, strict aseptic technique is used during dressing changes, and tetanus prophylaxis is administered as indicated. Anti-inflammatory medication is also prescribed.

Additional measures that may be carried out when appropriate include the following:

- Whirlpool bath for the affected extremity to aid circulation, debride necrotic tissue, and help prevent infection
- Escharotomy (incision through the eschar) to prevent further tissue damage, allow for normal circulation, and permit joint motion
- Fasciotomy to treat compartment syndrome

After rewarming, hourly active motion of the affected digits is encouraged to promote maximal restoration of function and to prevent contractures. Refreezing is avoided. The patient is also encouraged to avoid tobacco, alcohol, and caffeine because of their vasoconstrictive effects, which further reduce the already deficient blood supply to injured tissues.

HYPOTHERMIA

Hypothermia is a condition in which the core (internal) temperature is 35°C or less as a result of exposure to cold. Hypothermia occurs when a patient loses the ability to maintain body temperature. Urban hypothermia (extreme exposure to cold in an urban setting) is associated with a high mortality rate; elderly people, infants, people with concurrent illnesses, and the homeless are particularly susceptible. Alcohol ingestion increases susceptibility because it causes systemic vasodilation. Trauma victims are also at risk for hypothermia resulting from treatment with cold fluids, unwarmed oxygen, and exposure during examination. The patient may also have frostbite, but the hypothermia takes precedence in treatment.

Assessment and Diagnostic Findings

Hypothermia leads to physiologic changes in all organ systems. There is progressive deterioration, with apathy, poor judgment, ataxia, dysarthria, drowsiness, pulmonary edema, acid-base abnormalities, coagulopathy, and eventual coma. Shivering may be suppressed below a temperature of 32.2°C, because the body's self-warming mechanisms become ineffective. The heartbeat and blood pressure may be so weak that peripheral pulses become undetectable. Cardiac irregularities may also occur. Other physiologic abnormalities include hypoxemia and acidosis.

Management

Management consists of continuous monitoring, rewarming, removal of wet clothing, insulation, and supportive care.

MONITORING

The ABCs of basic life support are a priority. The patient's vital signs, CVP, urine output, arterial blood gas levels, blood chemistry determinations (blood urea nitrogen, creatinine, glucose, electrolytes), and chest x-rays are evaluated frequently. Body temperature is monitored with an esophageal, bladder, or rectal thermistor. Continuous ECG monitoring is performed, because cold-induced myocardial irritability leads to conduction disturbances, especially ventricular fibrillation. An arterial line is inserted and maintained to record blood pressure and to facilitate blood sampling.

REWARMING

Rewarming methods include active core (internal) rewarming, active external rewarming, and passive or spontaneous rewarming.

Core rewarming methods include cardiopulmonary bypass, warm fluid administration, warm humidified oxygen by ventilator, and warmed peritoneal lavage. Core rewarming is recommended for severe hypothermia. Monitoring for ventricular fibrillation as the patient passes through 31° to 32°C is essential.

Passive external rewarming includes the use of warm blankets or over-the-bed heaters. Passive rewarming of the extremities increases blood flow to the acidotic, anaerobic extremities. The cold blood with high lactic acid levels returning to the core has significant effects on the core temperature and metabolic response, possibly causing cardiac dysrhythmias and electrolyte disturbances.

SUPPORTIVE CARE

Supportive care during rewarming includes the following as directed:

- External cardiac compression (only as directed in the very cold patient)
- Defibrillation of ventricular fibrillation. Patients whose temperature is less than 32°C will experience spontaneous ventricular fibrillation if moved or touched. Defibrillation is ineffective in patients with temperatures lower than 31°C.
- Mechanical ventilation with positive end-expiratory pressure (PEEP) and heated humidified oxygen to maintain tissue oxygenation
- Administration of warmed intravenous fluids to correct hypotension and maintain urine output and core rewarming, as described previously
- Administration of sodium bicarbonate to correct metabolic acidosis if necessary
- Administration of antiarrhythmic medications
- Insertion of an indwelling urinary catheter to monitor fluid status

NEAR-DROWNING

Near-drowning is survival for at least 24 hours after submersion. The most common consequence is hypoxemia. Drowning is one of the leading causes of unintentional death in children younger than 14 years of age. An estimated 7000 drownings and 90,000 near-drownings occur yearly in the United States. There are approximately 1000 deaths by drowning of children every year. Children younger than 4 years of age account for 40% of drownings (Suominen et al., 2002).

Factors associated with drowning and near-drowning include alcohol ingestion, inability to swim, diving injuries, hypothermia, and exhaustion. Efforts to save the victim should not be abandoned prematurely. Successful resuscitation with full neurologic recovery has occurred in near-drowning victims after prolonged submersion in cold water. This is possible because of a decrease in metabolic demands or the diving reflex.

After resuscitation, hypoxia and acidosis, the primary problems of a victim who has nearly drowned, require immediate intervention in the ED. Resultant pathophysiologic changes and pulmonary injury depend on the type of fluid (fresh or salt water) and the volume aspirated. Fresh water aspiration results in a loss of surfactant, hence an inability to expand the lungs. Salt water aspiration leads to pulmonary edema from the osmotic effects of the salt within the lung. After a person survives submersion, acute respiratory distress syndrome resulting in hypoxia, hypercarbia, and respiratory or metabolic acidosis can occur.

Management

Therapeutic goals include maintaining cerebral perfusion and adequate oxygenation to prevent further damage to vital organs. Immediate cardiopulmonary resuscitation is the factor with the greatest influence on survival. The treatment goal, prevention of hypoxia, is accomplished by ensuring an adequate airway and respiration, thus improving ventilation (which helps to correct respiratory acidosis) and oxygenation. Arterial blood gas analyses are performed to evaluate oxygen, carbon dioxide, and bicarbonate levels and pH. These parameters determine the type of ventilatory support needed. Use of endotracheal intubation with positive-pressure ventilation (with PEEP) improves oxygenation, prevents aspiration, and corrects intrapulmonary shunting and ventilation–perfusion abnormalities (caused by aspiration of water). If the patient is breathing spontaneously, supplemental oxygen may be administered by mask. However, an endotracheal tube is necessary if the patient does not breathe spontaneously.

Because of submersion, the patient is usually hypothermic. A rectal probe is used to determine the degree of hypothermia. Prescribed rewarming procedures (eg, extracorporeal warming, warmed peritoneal dialysis, inhalation of warm aerosolized oxygen, torso warming) are started during resuscitation. The choice is determined by the severity and duration of hypothermia and available resources. Intravascular volume expansion and inotropic agents are used to manage hypotension and impaired tissue perfusion. ECG monitoring is initiated, because dysrhythmias frequently occur. An indwelling urinary catheter is inserted to measure urine output. Hypothermia and accompanying metabolic acidosis may compromise renal function. Nasogastric intubation is used to decompress the stomach and to prevent the patient from aspirating gastric contents.

In case the patient appears deceptively healthy, close monitoring continues with serial vital signs, serial arterial blood gas values, ECG monitoring, intracranial pressure assessments, serum electrolyte levels, intake and output, and serial chest x-rays. After a near-drowning, the patient is at risk for complications, such as hypoxic or ischemic cerebral injury, acute respiratory distress syndrome, pulmonary damage secondary to aspiration, and life-threatening cardiac arrest.

DECOMPRESSION SICKNESS

Decompression sickness (DCS), also called "the bends," occurs in patients who have engaged in diving, high-altitude flying, or flying in commercial aircraft within 24 hours after diving. Although DCS occurs in relatively few divers compared with the number of dives worldwide, its effects can be hazardous. Being aware of DCS and assessing the patient properly will ensure proper management and result in the least morbidity possible.

DCS results from nitrogen bubbles trapped in the body. They may occur in joint or muscle spaces, resulting in musculoskeletal pain, numbness, or hypesthesia. More significantly, nitrogen bubbles can become air emboli in the bloodstream and thereby produce stroke, paralysis, or death. Taking a rapid history about the events preceding the symptoms is essential. Recompression is necessary as soon as possible and may necessitate a low-altitude flight to the nearest hyperbaric chamber.

Assessment and Diagnostic Findings

To identify DCS, a detailed history is obtained from the patient or diving buddy. Evidence of rapid ascent, loss of air in the tank, buddy breathing, recent alcohol intake or lack of sleep, or a flight within 24 hours after diving suggests the potential for DCS. Note that some patients describe a perfect dive yet still have the signs and symptoms of DCS and must be treated as such.

Signs and symptoms include joint or extremity pain, numbness, hypesthesia, and loss of range of motion. Neurologic symptoms mimicking those of a stroke or spinal cord injury could indicate an air embolus. Cardiopulmonary arrest can also occur with severe cases of DCS. Because of hypoxia, these patients seldom survive. Any neurologic symptoms should be rapidly assessed. All patients with DCS need rapid transfer to a hyperbaric chamber.

Management

A patent airway and adequate ventilation are established as described previously, and 100% oxygen is administered throughout treatment and transport. A chest x-ray is obtained to identify aspiration, and at least one intravenous line is started with lactated Ringer's or normal saline solution.

The cardiopulmonary and neurologic systems are supported as needed. If an air embolus is suspected, the head of the bed should be lowered. The patient's wet clothing is removed, and the patient is kept warm. Transfer to the closest hyperbaric chamber capable of treating DCS is initiated. If air transport is necessary, low-altitude flight (below 1000 feet) is required. However, the patient who is awake and alert without central neurologic deficits may be able to travel by ground ambulance or by automobile, depending on the severity of symptoms. Throughout treatment, the patient is continually assessed, and changes are documented. If aspiration is suspected, antibiotics and other treatment may be prescribed.

Canadian hyperbaric facilities and diving medicine centres are located in Vancouver, Esquimalt, Edmonton, Calgary, Moose Jaw, Winnipeg, Tobermory, Hamilton, Toronto, Ottawa, Montreal, Halifax, Shearwater, and St. John's (Allan & Kenny, 2003).

ANAPHYLACTIC REACTION

An anaphylactic reaction is an acute systemic hypersensitivity reaction that occurs within seconds or minutes after exposure to certain foreign substances, such as medications (eg, penicillin, iodinated contrast material), and other agents, such as insect stings (eg, bee, wasp, yellow jacket, hornet) or foods (eg, eggs, peanuts). Repeated administration of parenteral or oral therapeutic agents (eg, repeated exposures to penicillin) may also precipitate an anaphylactic reaction when initially only a mild allergic response occurred. See Chart 71-8 for anaphylaxis prevention strategies.

An anaphylactic reaction is the result of an antigen–antibody interaction in a sensitized individual who, as a consequence of previous exposure, has developed a special type of antibody (immunoglobulin) that is specific for that particular allergen. The antibody immunoglobulin E (IgE) is responsible for most of the immediate types of human allergic responses. The individual becomes sensitive to a particular antigen after production of IgE to that antigen. A second exposure to the same antigen results in a more severe and more rapid response (see Chap. 53).

Anaphylactic reaction produces a wide range of clinical manifestations, especially respiratory symptoms (difficulty breathing and stridor secondary to laryngeal edema), fainting, itching, swelling of mucous membranes, and a sudden drop in blood pressure secondary to massive vasodilation (see Chart 71-9 and Chapters 15 and 53 for additional discussion).

Management

With an anaphylactic reaction, establishing a patent airway and ventilation is essential. (This is performed while another person administers epinephrine.) Early endotracheal tube intubation is essential to avoid loss of the airway, and oropharyngeal suction

---

Chart 71-8

Preventing Anaphylactic Reactions

- Be aware of the danger of anaphylactic reactions and the early signs of anaphylaxis.
- Ask the patient about previous allergies to medications, foods, stings, latex, pollen, and so on.
- Before giving a foreign serum or other type of antigenic agent, ask the patient or caregiver whether the agent was received at some earlier time.
- Ask about allergies to eggs.
- Avoid giving medications to patients with hay fever, asthma, or other allergic disorders unless absolutely necessary.
- Avoid giving parenteral medications unless absolutely necessary, because anaphylactic reactions are more likely to occur when the agent is given parenterally.
- Perform a skin test before administration of certain materials known to produce anaphylactic reactions (eg, horse serum). Remember that negative skin test results do not always indicate safety and that skin testing can precipitate anaphylaxis in highly sensitive individuals. Have epinephrine, intravenous infusions, and intubation and tracheostomy equipment available as precautionary measures.
- If the patient is an outpatient, keep him or her in the office, hospital, or clinic for at least 30 minutes after injection of any agent. Caution the patient to return if symptoms develop.
- Caution patients who are highly sensitive (eg, to insect bites and stings) to carry kits equipped to treat insect stings (epinephrine). Instruct the patient, family, and significant others in the use of the emergency supplies.
- Encourage patients with allergies to wear medical identification tags or bracelets.

Signs and Symptoms of Anaphylaxis

Respiratory Signs
- Nasal congestion
- Itching
- Sneezing and coughing
- Possible respiratory distress that progresses rapidly (caused by bronchospasm or edema of the larynx)
- Chest tightness
- Other respiratory difficulties, such as wheezing, dyspnea, and cyanosis

Skin Manifestations
- Flushing with a sense of warmth and diffuse erythema
- Generalized itching over the entire body (indicates developing general systemic reaction)
- Urticaria (hives)
- Massive facial angioedema possible with accompanying upper respiratory edema

Cardiovascular Manifestations
- Tachycardia or bradycardia
- Peripheral vascular collapse as indicated by
  - Pallor
  - Imperceptible pulse
  - Decreasing blood pressure
  - Circulatory failure, leading to coma and death

Gastrointestinal Problems
- Nausea
- Vomiting
- Colicky abdominal pains
- Diarrhea

- Aminophylline by slow intravenous infusion for severe bronchospasm and wheezing refractory to other treatment
- Albuterol inhalers or humidified treatments to decrease bronchoconstriction; crystalloids, colloids, or vasopressors to treat prolonged hypotension
- Isoproterenol or dopamine for reduced cardiac output; oxygen to enhance tissue perfusion
- Intravenous benzodiazepines for control of seizures, and corticosteroids for prolonged reaction with persistent hypotension or bronchospasm

After the acute symptoms have been treated, the patient is usually admitted to the hospital for observation. The patient should be informed about ways to prevent anaphylactic reactions. See Chart 71-10 for strategies to limit exposure to stinging insects.

LATEX ALLERGY

Another allergy situation with which emergency nurses are dealing on a daily basis is latex allergy. The number of products that contain latex is staggering. Nurses must be aware of latex allergy (health care providers have died from anaphylaxis related to latex allergy) and the potential for patients to react to latex.

There is an increased awareness among manufacturers of the need for products that are latex free. Latex-free gloves are provided for nurses who have latex allergy or who have signs of allergy, such as itching, redness, or rash associated with use of a latex product. Severe anaphylaxis can occur even on first exposure; therefore, recognition of the signs and symptoms of anaphylaxis is essential. Treatment must be rapid, and the latex product must be removed promptly. See Chapters 19 and 53 for more information about latex allergy.

---

may be necessary to remove excessive secretions. Resuscitative measures are used, especially for patients with stridor and progressive pulmonary edema. If glottal edema occurs, a cricothyroidotomy is used to provide an airway.

Simultaneously with airway management, aqueous epinephrine is administered as prescribed to provide rapid relief of the hypersensitivity reaction. Epinephrine may be administered again, if necessary and as prescribed. Judgment is used in choosing the route of administration, as follows:

- Subcutaneous injection for mild, generalized symptoms
- Intramuscular injection when the reaction is more severe and progressive, and with concern that vascular collapse will inhibit absorption
- Intravenous route (aqueous epinephrine diluted in saline solution and administered *slowly*), used in rare instances in which there is complete loss of consciousness and severe cardiovascular collapse. This method may precipitate cardiac dysrhythmias. ECG monitoring with a readily available defibrillator is necessary. This method is controversial and is not usually recommended because it can lead to more distress than is initially present. An intravenous infusion of saline solution is initiated to provide for emergency access to a vein and to treat hypotension.

Additional treatments may include

- Antihistamines to block further histamine binding at target cells

Limiting Exposure to Stinging Insects

- Avoid places where stinging insects congregate, such as camp and picnic sites, and insect feeding areas, such as flower beds, ripe fruit orchards, garbage, and fields of clover.
- Wear covering on the feet, and avoid going barefoot outdoors, because yellow jackets nest and pollinate on the ground.
- Avoid perfumes, scented soaps, and bright colours, which attract bees.
- Keep car windows closed.
- Spray garbage cans with quick-acting insecticide.
- Secure a professional exterminator to dispose of wasp and hornet nests or beehives in the home area.
- Remain motionless if an insect is buzzing around. Motion, especially running, increases the likelihood of being stung.
- If allergic, carry a self-treatment kit containing injectable and inhalant forms of epinephrine, an oral antihistamine, and written instructions. Carry it with you at all times.

If Stung, Do the Following:
1. Inject self immediately with epinephrine if allergy is known or allergic response occurs.
2. Remove the stinger with one quick scrape of the fingernail. *Do not* squeeze the venom sac because this may cause injection of additional venom.
3. Clean the area with soapy water, and apply ice.
4. Report to the nearest health care facility for further examination if allergic response or allergy is suspected.

INJECTED POISONS: STINGING INSECTS

A person may have an extreme sensitivity to the venoms of the Hymenoptera (bees, hornets, yellow jackets, fire ants, and wasps). Venom allergy is thought to be an IgE-mediated reaction, and it constitutes an acute emergency. Although stings in any area of the body can trigger anaphylaxis, stings of the head and neck are especially serious.

Clinical manifestations range from generalized urticaria, itching, malaise, and anxiety due to laryngeal edema to severe bronchospasm, shock, and death. Generally, the shorter the time between the sting and the onset of severe symptoms, the worse the prognosis.

Management

Management includes stinger removal if the bite is from a bee, because the venom is associated with sacs around the barb of the stinger itself. Wound care with soap and water is sufficient for stings. Scratching is avoided because it results in a histamine response. Ice application reduces swelling and also decreases venom absorption. An oral antihistamine and analgesic will decrease the itching and pain.

In the case of an anaphylactic or severe allergic response, epinephrine (aqueous) is injected subcutaneously (*not intravenously*), and the injection site is massaged to hasten absorption. The patient is assessed for signs and symptoms of anaphylactic reaction and treated as necessary (see previous discussion and also Chap. 15). Desensitization therapy should be given to people who have had systemic or significant local reactions.

Patient and family education is an important measure in preventing exposure to stinging insects.

SNAKE BITES

Venomous (poisonous) snakes cause 7000 to 8000 bites in the United States each year and result in 12 to 15 deaths. Children between the ages of 1 and 9 years are the most likely victims. The greatest number of bites occur through the daylight hours into early evening during summer months. The most frequent poisonous snake bite occurs from pit vipers. The most common site is the upper extremity. Of these bites, only 20% to 25% result in **envenomation** (injection of a poisonous material by sting, spine, bite, or other means). Venomous snake bites are medical emergencies (Moon & Galvan, 2000).

Nineteen different species of venomous snakes are found in every part of the United States, with different parts of the country and the world having different types of snakes. Rattlesnakes, also known as pit vipers, are the only venomous snakes found in the wild in Canada. Instances of snake bite are very rare in this country (The Canadian Encyclopedia Online, 2005). Because snake bites are medical emergencies, nurses should be familiar with the types of snakes that are common to the geographic region in which they practice. Snake venom consists primarily of proteins with a broad range of physiologic effects. Multiple organ systems, especially the neurologic, cardiovascular, and respiratory systems, may be affected.

Management

Initial first aid at the site of the snake bite includes having the victim lie down, removing constrictive items such as rings, providing warmth, cleansing the wound, covering the wound with a light sterile dressing, and immobilizing the injured body part below the level of the heart. Ice or a tourniquet *is not* applied. Initial evaluation in the ED is performed quickly and includes information about the following:

- Whether the snake was venomous or nonvenomous; if the snake is dead, it should be transported to the ED with the patient for identification
- Where and when the bite occurred and the circumstances of the bite
- Sequence of events, signs and symptoms (fang punctures, pain, edema, and erythema of the bite and nearby tissues)
- Severity of poisonous effects
- Vital signs
- Circumference of the bitten extremity or area at several points; the circumference of the extremity that was bitten is compared with the circumference of the opposite extremity
- Laboratory data (complete blood count, urinalysis, and clotting studies)

The course and prognosis of snake bite injuries depend on the kind and amount of venom injected, where on the body the bite occurred, and the general health, age, and size of the victim. There is no one specific protocol for treatment of snake bites. Generally, ice, tourniquets, heparin, and corticosteroids are not used during the acute stage. Corticosteroids are contraindicated in the first 6 to 8 hours after the bite, because they may depress antibody production and hinder the action of **antivenin** (antitoxin manufactured from the snake venom and used to treat snake bites).

Parenteral fluids may be used to treat hypotension. If vasopressors are used to treat hypotension, their use should be short-term. Surgical exploration of the bite is rarely indicated. Typically, the patient is observed closely for at least 6 hours. The patient is *never* left unattended.

ADMINISTRATION OF ANTIVENIN (ANTITOXIN)

Although envenomation is rare, it can occur with snake bites. An assessment of progressive signs and symptoms is essential before considering administration of antivenin, which is most effective if administered within 12 hours after the snake bite. The dosage depends on the type of snake and the estimated severity of the bite. Children may require more antivenin than adults because their smaller bodies are more susceptible to toxic effects of venom. A skin or eye test should be performed before the initial dose to detect allergy to the antivenin. However, because even the skin test can cause an anaphylactic reaction, patients should not be tested unless antivenin is to be given.

Before administering antivenin and every 15 minutes thereafter, the circumference of the affected part is measured proximally. Premedication with diphenhydramine and cimetidine decreases the allergic response to antivenin. Antivenin is administered as an intravenous infusion whenever possible, although intramuscular administration can be used. Depending on the severity of the bite, the antivenin is diluted in 500 to 1000 mL of normal saline solution; the fluid volume may be reduced for children. The infusion is started slowly, and the rate is increased after 10 minutes if there is no reaction. The total dose should be infused during the first 4 to 6 hours after poisoning. The initial dose is repeated until symptoms decrease. After the symptoms decrease, the circumference of the affected part should be measured every 30 to 60 minutes for the next 48 hours to detect symptoms of compartment syndrome (swelling, loss of pulse, increased pain, and paresthesias).

The most common cause of allergic reaction to the antivenin is its too-rapid infusion, although about 3% of patients with negative skin test results develop reactions not related to infusion rate. Reactions may consist of a feeling of fullness in the face, urticaria, pruritus, malaise, and apprehension. These symptoms may be followed by tachycardia, shortness of breath, hypotension, and shock. In this situation, the infusion should be stopped immediately and intravenous diphenhydramine (Benadryl) administered. Vasopressors are used for patients in shock, and resuscitation equipment must be on standby while antivenin is infusing.

Poisoning

A poison is any substance that, when ingested, inhaled, absorbed, applied to the skin, or produced within the body in relatively small amounts, injures the body by its chemical action. Poisoning from inhalation and ingestion of toxic materials, both intentional and unintentional, constitutes a major health hazard and an emergency situation. Emergency treatment is initiated with the following goals:

- To remove or inactivate the poison before it is absorbed
- To provide supportive care in maintaining vital organ systems
- To administer a specific antidote to neutralize a specific poison
- To implement treatment that hastens the elimination of the absorbed poison

INGESTED (SWALLOWED) POISONS

Swallowed poisons may be corrosive. **Corrosive poisons** include alkaline and acid agents that can cause tissue destruction after coming in contact with mucous membranes. Alkaline products include lye, drain cleaners, toilet bowl cleaners, bleach, nonphosphate detergents, oven cleaners, and button batteries (batteries used to power watches, calculators, or cameras). Acid products include toilet bowl cleaners, pool cleaners, metal cleaners, rust removers, battery acid.

Management

Control of the airway, ventilation, and oxygenation are essential. In the absence of cerebral or renal damage, the patient's prognosis depends largely on successful management of respiration and circulation. Measures are instituted to stabilize cardiovascular and other body functions. ECG, vital signs, and neurologic status are monitored closely for changes. Shock, which may result from the cardiodepressant action of the substance ingested, from venous pooling in lower extremities, or from reduced circulating blood volume resulting from increased capillary permeability, is treated. An indwelling urinary catheter is inserted to monitor renal function. Blood specimens are obtained to test for concentration of drug or poison.

Efforts are initiated to determine what substance was taken; the amount; time since ingestion; signs and symptoms, such as pain or burning sensations, any evidence of redness or burn in the mouth or throat, pain on swallowing or an inability to swallow, vomiting, or drooling; age and weight of the patient; and pertinent health history.

Measures are instituted to remove the toxin or decrease its absorption. The patient who has ingested a corrosive poison is given

 NURSING ALERT The area poison control centre should be called if an unknown toxic agent has been taken or if it is necessary to identify an antidote for a known toxic agent.

water or milk to drink for dilution. However, dilution is not attempted if the patient has acute airway edema or obstruction or if there is clinical evidence of esophageal, gastric, or intestinal burn or perforation. The following gastric emptying procedures may be used as prescribed:

- Syrup of ipecac to induce vomiting in the alert patient.
- Gastric lavage for the obtunded patient (Chart 71-11). Gastric aspirate is saved and sent to the laboratory for testing (toxicology screens)
- Activated charcoal administration if poison is one that is absorbed by charcoal
- Cathartic, when appropriate

NURSING ALERT Vomiting is never induced after ingestion of caustic substances (acid or alkaline) or petroleum distillates.

The specific chemical or physiologic antagonist (antidote) is administered as early as possible, to reverse or diminish the effects of the toxin. If these measures are ineffective, procedures are initiated to remove the ingested substance. These procedures include administration of multiple doses of charcoal, diuresis (for substances excreted by the kidneys), dialysis, and hemoperfusion. Hemoperfusion involves detoxification of the blood by processing it through an extracorporeal circuit and an adsorbent cartridge containing charcoal or resin, after which the cleaned blood is returned to the patient.

Throughout detoxification, the patient's vital signs, CVP, and fluid and electrolyte balance are monitored closely. Hypotension and cardiac dysrhythmias are possible. Seizures are also possible because of CNS excitement from the poison or from oxygen deprivation. If the patient complains of pain, analgesics are administered cautiously. Severe pain causes vasomotor collapse and reflex inhibition of normal physiologic functions.

After the patient's condition has stabilized and discharge is imminent, written material indicating the signs and symptoms of potential problems related to the poison ingested and signs or symptoms requiring evaluation by a physician should be given to the patient. If poisoning was determined to be a suicide attempt, a psychiatric consultation should be requested before the patient is discharged. In cases of inadvertent poison ingestion, poison prevention and home poison-proofing instructions should be provided to the patient and family.

INHALED POISONS: CARBON MONOXIDE POISONING

Carbon monoxide poisoning may occur as a result of industrial or household incidents or attempted suicide. It is implicated in more deaths than any other toxin except alcohol. Carbon monoxide exerts its toxic effect by binding to circulating hemoglobin and thereby reducing the oxygen-carrying capacity of the blood. Hemoglobin absorbs carbon monoxide 200 times more readily than it absorbs oxygen. Carbon monoxide–bound hemoglobin, called **carboxyhemoglobin**, does not transport oxygen.

Because the CNS has a critical need for oxygen, CNS symptoms predominate with carbon monoxide toxicity. A person suffering from carbon monoxide poisoning may appear intoxicated (from cerebral hypoxia). Other signs and symptoms include headache, muscular weakness, palpitation, dizziness, and confusion, which can progress rapidly to coma. Skin colour, which can range from pink or cherry-red to cyanotic and pale, is not a reliable sign. Pulse oximetry is also not valid, because the hemoglobin

Chart 71-11

GUIDELINES FOR Assisting With Gastric Lavage

Gastric lavage is the aspiration of stomach contents and washing out of the stomach by means of a large-bore gastric tube. Gastric lavage is contraindicated after acid or alkali ingestion, in the presence of seizures, or after ingestion of hydrocarbons or petroleum distillates. It is particularly dangerous after ingestion of strong corrosive agents.

Purposes:
- For urgent removal of ingested substance to decrease systemic absorption
- To empty the stomach before endoscopic procedures
- To diagnose gastric hemorrhage and to arrest hemorrhage

Equipment:
Large-bore Levin tubes or large-bore Ewald tube
Large irrigating syringe with adapter
Large plastic funnel with adapter to fit tube
Water-soluble lubricant
Tap water or appropriate antidote (milk, saline solution, sodium
   bicarbonate solution, fruit juice, activated charcoal)
Container for aspirate; suction apparatus
Nasotracheal or endotracheal tubes with inflatable cuffs
Containers for specimens

During gastric lavage, the patient is positioned on the left side, which allows the gastric contents to pool and decreases the passage of fluid into the duodenum during lavage.

PROCEDURE	RATIONALE/AMPLIFICATION
1. Remove dentures and inspect the oral cavity for loose teeth.	1. This will prevent aspiration of teeth.
2. Measure the distance between the bridge of the nose and the xiphoid process. Mark the tube with indelible pencil or tape.	2. This distance is a rule-of-thumb measurement of the distance the tube must be passed to reach the stomach. This avoids curling and kinking of excess tubing in the stomach.
3. Lubricate the tube with water-soluble lubricant.	3. Lubrication eases insertion of the tube.
4. If comatose, the patient is intubated with a cuffed nasotracheal or endotracheal tube before placement of the nasogastric tube.	4. A cuffed nasotracheal or endotracheal tube decreases the risk of aspiration of gastric contents.
5. Place the patient in a left lateral position with the head lowered about 15 degrees.	5. This position decreases passage of gastric contents into the duodenum during lavage.
6. Pass the tube orally while keeping the patient's head in a neutral position. Pass the tube to the adhesive marking or about 50 cm. Encourage patient to swallow to assist with passage of the tube. Then lower the head of the stretcher or bed. Have standby suction available.	6. The depth of insertion of the tube varies according to the size of the patient. If the tube enters the trachea instead of the esophagus, the patient will experience coughing, dyspnea, stridor, and cyanosis. Positive confirmation of tube placement is accomplished by x-ray.
7. Aspirate the stomach contents with the syringe attached to the tube before instilling water or an antidote. Save the specimen for analysis. Ensure correct placement before installation.	7. Aspiration is carried out to determine that the tube is in the stomach and to remove the stomach contents. Positive confirmation of tube placement is accomplished by x-ray.
8. Remove the syringe. Attach the funnel to the end of the tube, or use a 50-mL syringe to instill solution in the gastric tube. The volume of fluid placed in the stomach should be small.	8. Overfilling of the stomach may cause regurgitation and aspiration or force the stomach contents through the pylorus.
9. Elevate the funnel above the patient's head and pour 150 to 200 mL of solution into the funnel.	9. Gravity allows the solution to flow into the tube.
10. Lower the funnel and siphon the gastric contents into the container or connect to suction.	10. The fluid should flow in freely and drain by gravity.
11. Save samples of the first two washings.	11. Keep the first washing sample isolated from other washings for toxicologic analysis.
12. Repeat the lavage procedure until the returns are relatively clear and no particulate matter is seen.	12. This usually requires a total volume of at least 2 L; some clinicians advocate the use of 5 to 20 L.
13. At the completion of lavage:	13.
a. The stomach may be left empty.	a. The stomach is kept empty if no further medications are required.
b. An adsorbent (powder form of activated charcoal mixed with water to form a liquid the consistency of thick soup) may be instilled in the tube and allowed to remain in the stomach.	b. Activated charcoal reduces absorption by adsorbing (attaching to its surface) a wide range of substances; it renders the poison inaccessible to the circulation, thereby reducing its toxicity.
c. A saline cathartic may be instilled in the tube.	c. A cathartic may be given to hasten the elimination of remaining ingested material.
14. Pinch off the tube during removal or maintain suction while the tube is being withdrawn. Keep the patient's head lower than the body.	14. Pinching off the tube prevents aspiration and the initiation of the gag reflex. Keeping the patient's head lower than the body also helps to prevent initiation of the gag reflex.
15. Warn the patient that his stools will turn black from the charcoal.	

is well saturated. It is not saturated with oxygen, but the pulse oximeter reads the saturation as such and presents the false impression that the patient is well oxygenated and in no danger. Exposure to carbon monoxide requires immediate treatment.

Management

Goals of management are to reverse cerebral and myocardial hypoxia and to hasten elimination of carbon monoxide. Whenever a patient inhales a poison, the following general measures apply:

- Carry the patient to fresh air immediately; open all doors and windows.
- Loosen all tight clothing.
- Initiate cardiopulmonary resuscitation if required; administer oxygen.
- Prevent chilling; wrap the patient in blankets.
- Keep the patient as quiet as possible.
- Do not give alcohol in any form.

In addition, for the patient with carbon monoxide poisoning, carboxyhemoglobin levels are analyzed on arrival at the ED and before treatment with oxygen if possible. Then 100% oxygen is administered at atmospheric or hyperbaric pressures to reverse hypoxia and accelerate the elimination of carbon monoxide. Oxygen is administered until the carboxyhemoglobin level is less than 5%. The patient is monitored continuously. Psychoses, spastic paralysis, ataxia, visual disturbances, and deterioration of mental status and behaviour may persist after resuscitation and may be symptoms of permanent brain damage.

When unintentional carbon monoxide poisoning occurs, the health department should be contacted, so that the dwelling or building in question can be inspected. A psychiatric consultation is warranted if poisoning was determined to be a suicide attempt.

SKIN CONTAMINATION POISONING (CHEMICAL BURNS)

Skin contamination injuries from exposure to chemicals are challenging because of the large number of offending agents with diverse actions and metabolic effects. The severity of a chemical burn is determined by the mechanism of action, the penetrating strength and concentration, and the amount and duration of exposure of the skin to the chemical.

Management

The skin should be drenched immediately with running water from a shower, hose, or faucet.

 NURSING ALERT Water should not be applied to burns from lye or white phosphorus because of the potential for an explosion or for deepening of the burn. All evidence of these chemicals should be brushed off the patient before any flushing.

A constant stream of water should continue as the patient's clothing is being removed. The skin of health care personnel assisting the patient should be appropriately protected if the burn is extensive or if the agent is significantly toxic or is still present. Prolonged lavage with generous amounts of tepid water is important.

In the meantime, attempts to determine the identity and characteristics of the chemical agent are necessary for future treat-

ment. The standard burn treatment appropriate for the size and location of the wound (antimicrobial treatment, débridement, tetanus prophylaxis as prescribed) is instituted. The patient may require plastic surgery for further wound management. The patient is instructed to have the affected area reexamined at 24 and 72 hours and in 7 days because of the risk for underestimating the extent and depth of these types of injuries.

FOOD POISONING

Food poisoning is a sudden illness that occurs after ingestion of contaminated food or drink. Botulism is a serious form of food poisoning that requires continual surveillance. See Chart 71-12 for assessment questions.

Management

The key to treatment is determining the source and type of food poisoning. If possible, the suspected food should be brought to the medical facility and a history obtained from the patient or family.

Food, gastric contents, vomitus, serum, and feces are collected for examination. The patient's respirations, blood pressure, sensorium, CVP (if indicated), and muscular activity are monitored closely. Measures are instituted to support the respiratory system. Death from respiratory paralysis can occur with botulism, fish poisoning, and other food poisonings.

Because large volumes of electrolytes and water are lost by vomiting and diarrhea, fluid and electrolyte balance is also an important area to assess. Severe vomiting produces alkalosis, and severe diarrhea produces acidosis. Hypovolemic shock may also occur from severe fluid and electrolyte losses. The patient is assessed for signs and symptoms of fluid and electrolyte imbalances, including lethargy, rapid pulse rate, fever, oliguria, anuria, hypotension, and delirium. Weight and serum electrolyte levels are obtained for future comparisons.

Measures to control nausea are also important to prevent vomiting, which could further exacerbate fluid and electrolyte imbalances. An antiemetic medication is administered parenterally as prescribed if the patient cannot tolerate fluids or medications by mouth. For mild nausea, the patient is encouraged to take sips of weak tea, carbonated drinks, or tap water. After nausea and

Chart 71-12 Food Poisoning

Use the following questions to elicit information about the circumstances surrounding the possibility of food poisoning:
- How soon after eating did the symptoms occur? (Immediate onset suggests chemical, plant, or animal poisoning.)
- What was eaten in the previous meal? Did the food have an unusual odour or taste? (Most foods causing bacterial poisoning *do not* have unusual odour or taste.)
- Did anyone else become ill from eating the same food?
- Did vomiting occur? What was the appearance of the vomitus?
- Did diarrhea occur? (Diarrhea is usually absent with botulism and with shellfish or other fish poisoning.)
- Are any neurologic symptoms present? (These occur in botulism and in chemical, plant, and animal poisoning.)
- Does the patient have a fever? (Fever is characteristic in salmonella, ingestion of fava beans, and some fish poisoning.)
- What is the patient's appearance?

vomiting subside, clear liquids are usually prescribed for 12 to 24 hours, and the diet is gradually progressed to a low-residue, bland diet.

Substance Abuse

Substance abuse is the misuse of specific substances to alter mood or behaviour; drug and alcohol abuse are two examples of substance abuse. Drug abuse is the use of drugs for other than legitimate medical purposes. People who use drugs often take a variety of drugs simultaneously (such as alcohol, barbiturates, opioids, and tranquilizers), and the combination may have additive and addictive effects. IV/injecting drug users are at increased risk for HIV infection, acquired immunodeficiency syndrome (AIDS), and hepatitis B and are the most frequent victims of tetanus in the United States.

Clinical manifestations vary with the substance used, but the underlying principles of management are essentially the same. Table 71-1 identifies commonly abused drugs, listing their clinical manifestations and therapeutic management. Treatment goals for a patient suffering from drug overdose are to support the respiratory and cardiovascular functions, to enhance clearance of the agent, and to provide for safety of the patient and staff.

ACUTE ALCOHOL INTOXICATION

Alcohol is a psychotropic drug that affects mood, judgment, behaviour, concentration, and consciousness. Many heavy drinkers are young adults or people older than 60 years of age. There is a high prevalence of alcoholism among ED patients. Because patients who abuse alcohol return frequently to the ED, they often frustrate and tax the patience of the health care professionals who care for them. Their management requires patience and thoughtful, accurate, long-term treatment.

Alcohol, or ethanol, is a direct multisystem toxin and CNS depressant that causes drowsiness, incoordination, slurring of speech, sudden mood changes, aggression, belligerence, grandiosity, and uninhibited behaviour. In excess, it also can cause stupor, coma, and death. In the ED, the patient is assessed for head injury, hypoglycemia (which mimics intoxication), and other health problems. Possible nursing diagnoses include ineffective breathing pattern related to CNS depression and risk for violence (self-directed or directed at others) related to severe intoxication from alcohol.

Management

Treatment involves detoxification of the acute poisoning, recovery, and rehabilitation. Commonly, the patient uses mechanisms of denial and defensiveness. The nurse should approach the patient in a nonjudgmental manner, using a firm, consistent, accepting, and reasonable attitude. Speaking in a calm and slow manner is helpful because alcohol interferes with thought processes. If the patient appears intoxicated, hypoxia, hypovolemia, and neurologic impairment must be ruled out before it is assumed that the patient is intoxicated. Typically, a blood specimen is obtained for analysis of the blood alcohol level.

If drowsy, the patient should be allowed to sleep off the state of alcoholic intoxication. During this time, maintenance of a patent airway and observation for symptoms of CNS depression are essential. The patient should be undressed and kept warm with blankets. On the other hand, if the patient is noisy or belligerent, sedation may be necessary. If sedation is used, the patient should

be monitored carefully for hypotension and decreased level of consciousness.

Additionally, the patient is examined for alcohol withdrawal delirium and also for injuries and organic disease, such as head injury, seizures, pulmonary infections, hypoglycemia, and nutritional deficiencies, that may be masked by alcoholic intoxication. People with alcoholism suffer more injuries than the general population. Also, acute alcohol intoxication is the cause of trauma for many nonalcoholic patients. Pulmonary infections are also more common in patients with alcoholism, resulting from respiratory depression, an impaired defense system, and a tendency toward aspiration of gastric contents. The patient may show little increase in temperature or white blood cell count. The patient may be hospitalized or admitted to a detoxification centre in an effort to examine problems underlying substance abuse.

ALCOHOL WITHDRAWAL SYNDROME/DELIRIUM TREMENS

Alcohol withdrawal syndrome (AWS) is an acute toxic state that occurs as a result of sudden cessation of alcohol intake after a bout of heavy drinking or, more usually, after prolonged intake of alcohol. Severity of symptoms depends on how much alcohol was ingested and for how long. Delirium tremens may be precipitated by acute injury or infection (pneumonia, pancreatitis, hepatitis) and is the most severe form of AWS.

Patients with AWS show signs of anxiety, uncontrollable fear, tremor, irritability, agitation, insomnia, and incontinence. They are talkative and preoccupied and experience visual, tactile, olfactory, and auditory hallucinations that often are terrifying. Autonomic overactivity occurs and is evidenced by tachycardia, dilated pupils, and profuse perspiration. Usually, all vital signs are elevated in the alcoholic toxic state. Delirium tremens is a life-threatening condition and carries a high mortality rate.

Management

The goals of management are to give adequate sedation and support to allow the patient to rest and recover without danger of injury or peripheral vascular collapse. A physical examination is performed to identify preexisting or contributing illnesses or injuries (eg, head injury, pneumonia). A drug history is obtained to elicit information that may facilitate adjustment of any sedative requirements. Baseline blood pressure is determined, because the patient's subsequent treatment may depend on blood pressure changes.

Usually, the patient is sedated as directed with a sufficient dosage of benzodiazepines to establish and maintain sedation, which reduces agitation, prevents exhaustion, prevents seizures, and promotes sleep. The patient should be calm, able to respond, and able to maintain an airway safely on his or her own. A variety of medications and combinations of medications are used (for example, chlordiazepoxide [Librium], lorazepam, and clonidine). Haloperidol or droperidol may be administered for severe acute AWS. Dosages are adjusted according to the patient's symptoms (agitation, anxiety) and blood pressure response.

The patient is placed in a calm, nonstressful environment (usually a private room) and observed closely. The room remains lighted to minimize the potential for illusions and hallucinations. Homicidal or suicidal responses may result from hallucinations. Closet and bathroom doors are closed to eliminate shadows. Someone is designated to stay with the patient as much as possible. The presence of another person has a reassuring and calming effect,

(text continues on page 2186)

Table 71-1 • Emergency Management of Drug Abuse Patients and Patients with Drug Overdose

DRUG	CLINICAL MANIFESTATIONS	THERAPEUTIC MANAGEMENT

Narcotics
Cocaine
  Intranasally ("snorting"): inhaled into nostrils through straws
  By smoking ("freebasing"): cocaine hydrochloride dissolved in ether to yield a pure cocaine alkaloid base (called "crack"); smoking in a small pipe delivers large quantities of cocaine to lungs
  Intravenously
	Cocaine is a central nervous system (CNS) stimulant that can increase heart rate and blood pressure and cause hyperpyrexia, seizures, and ventricular dysrhythmias. It produces intense euphoria, then anxiety, sadness, insomnia, and sexual indifference; cocaine hallucinations with delusions; psychosis with extreme paranoia and ideas of persecution; and hypervigilance. Chronic psychotic symptoms may persist.	1. Ensure airway and ventilation.
		2. Control seizures.
		3. Monitor cardiovascular effects; have lidocaine and defibrillator available.
		4. Treat for hyperthermia.
		5. If cocaine was ingested, use charcoal to treat.
		6. Refer for psychiatric evaluation and treatment in an inpatient unit that eliminates access to the drug. Include drug rehabilitation counselling.

Heroin Opium or paregoric Morphine, codeine, OxyContin, synthetic derivatives (methadone, meperidine) Fentanyl (Sublimaze)	Acute intoxication (overdose) Pinpoint pupils (may be dilated with severe hypoxia); decreased blood pressure Marked respiratory depression Stupor → coma Fresh needle marks along course of any superficial vein; skin abscesses	1. Support respiratory and cardiovascular functions. 2. Establish an intravenous (IV) line; obtain blood for chemical and toxicologic analysis. Patient may be given bolus of glucose to eliminate possibility of hypoglycemia. 3. Give narcotic antagonist (naloxone hydrochloride [Narcan]) as prescribed to reverse severe respiratory depression and coma. 4. Continue to monitor level of responsiveness and respirations, pulse, and blood pressure. Duration of action of naloxone hydrochloride is shorter than that of heroin; repeated dosages may be necessary. 5. Send urine for analysis; opiates can be detected in urine. 6. Obtain an electrocardiogram. 7. Do not leave patient unattended; he or she may lapse back into coma rapidly. Clinical status may change from minute to minute. Hemodialysis may be indicated for severe drug intoxication. 8. Monitor for pulmonary edema, which is frequently seen in patients who abuse/overdose on narcotics. 9. Refer patient for psychiatric and drug rehabilitation evaluation before discharge.

Barbiturates
Pentobarbital (Nembutal)
Secobarbital (Seconal)
Amobarbital (Amytal)
	Acute intoxication (may mimic alcohol intoxication):
	• Respiratory depression
	• Flushed face
	• Decreased pulse rate; decreased blood pressure
	• Increasing nystagmus
	• Depressed deep tendon reflexes
	• Decreasing mental alertness
	• Difficulty in speaking
	• Poor motor coordination
	• Coma, death
		1. Maintain airway and provide respiratory support.
		2. Endotracheal intubation or tracheostomy is considered if there is any doubt about the adequacy of airway exchange.
		  a. Check airway frequently.
		  b. Perform suctioning as necessary.
		3. Support cardiovascular and respiratory functions; most deaths result from respiratory depression or shock.
		4. Start infusion through large-gauge needle or IV catheter to support blood pressure; coma and dehydration result in hypotension and respond to infusion of intravenous fluids with elevation of blood pressure. Sodium bicarbonate may be prescribed to alkalinize urine; it promotes excretion of barbiturates.
		5. Evacuate stomach contents or lavage as soon as possible to prevent absorption; repeated doses of activated charcoal may be administered.

(continued)

Table 71-1 • Emergency Management of Drug Abuse Patients and Patients with Drug Overdose (Continued)

DRUG	CLINICAL MANIFESTATIONS	THERAPEUTIC MANAGEMENT
		6. Assist with hemodialysis for severely over-dosed patient. 7. Maintain neurologic and vital sign flow sheet. 8. Patient awakening from overdose may demonstrate combative behaviour. 9. Refer for psychiatric and drug rehabilitation consultation/rehabilitation to evaluate suicide potential and drug abuse.
Amphetamine-Type Drugs (Pep Pills, "Uppers," "Speed," "Crystal," "Meth") Amphetamine (Benzedrine) Dextroamphetamine (Dexedrine) Methamphetamine (Desoxyn) MDMA ("Ecstasy," "Adam") MDEA ("Eve") MDA	Nausea, vomiting, anorexia, palpitations, tachycardia, increased blood pressure, tachypnea, anxiety, nervousness, diaphoresis, mydriasis Repetitive or stereotyped behaviour Irritability, insomnia, agitation Visual misperceptions, auditory hallucinations Fearful anxiety/depression, cold, distant hostility, paranoia Hyperactivity, rapid speech, euphoria Seizures, coma, hyperthermia, cardiovascular collapse, rhabdomyolysis	1. Provide airway support, ventilation, cardiac monitoring; insert IV line. 2. Employ gastrointestinal (GI) decontamination in cases of oral overdose; activated charcoal, gastric lavage. 3. Keep in calm, cool, quiet environment; elevated temperature potentiates amphetamine toxicity. 4. Use small doses of diazepam (IV) or haloperidol as prescribed for CNS and muscular hyperactivity. 5. Administer appropriate pharmacologic therapy as prescribed for severe hypertension and ventricular dysrhythmias. 6. Treat seizures with benzodiazepines. 7. Treat sympathetic stimulation with beta-blocker agents. 8. Try to communicate with patient if delusions or hallucinations are present. 9. Place in a protective environment (preferably psychiatric security room with video monitoring) to observe for suicide attempt. 10. Refer for psychiatric and drug rehabilitation evaluation.

Hallucinogens or Psychedelic-Type Drugs
Lysergic acid diethylamide (LSD)
Phencyclidine HCl (PCP, "angel dust")
Mescaline, psilocybin
Cannabinoids (marijuana)
	Nystagmus
	Mild hypertension
	Marked confusion bordering on panic
	Incoherence, hyperactivity
	Withdrawn
	Combative behaviour; delirium, mania, self-injury
	Hallucinations, body image distortion
	Hypertension, hyperthermia, renal failure
	Flashback: recurrence of LSD-like state without having taken the drug; may occur weeks or months after drug was taken
		Emergency Management
		1. Evaluate and maintain patient's airway, breathing, and circulation.
		2. Determine by urine or serum drug screen whether the patient has ingested hallucinogenic drug or has a toxic psychosis.
		3. Try to communicate with and reassure the patient.
		  a. "Talking down" involves understanding the process through which the patient is proceeding and helping him overcome his fears while establishing contact with reality.
		  b. Remind the patient that fear is common with this problem.
		  c. Reassure the patient that he is not losing his mind but is experiencing the effect of drugs and that this will wear off.
		  d. Instruct the patient to keep the eyes open; this reduces the intensity of reaction.
		  e. Reduce sensory stimuli: minimize noise, lights, movement, tactile stimulation.
		4. Sedate the patient as prescribed if hyperactivity cannot be controlled; diazepam (Valium) or a barbiturate may be prescribed.

(continued)

DRUG	CLINICAL MANIFESTATIONS	THERAPEUTIC MANAGEMENT
		5. Search for evidence of trauma; hallucinogen users have a tendency to "act out" their hallucinations.
		6. Manage seizures.
		7. Observe patient closely; patient's behaviour may become hazardous. Have safety officers stationed near the patient's room.
		8. Monitor for hypertensive crisis if patient has prolonged psychosis due to drug ingestion.
		9. Place patient in a protected environment under proper medical supervision to prevent self-inflicted bodily harm.
		Management for Phencyclidine Abusers
		1. Place patient in a calm, supportive environment to minimize stimuli; protect from self-injury.
		2. Avoid talking down.
		3. Do not leave patient unobserved. Treat symptoms as they occur.
		a. Drug effects are unpredictable and prolonged.
		b. Symptoms are likely to exacerbate; patient becomes out of control.
		4. Refer all patients in this category for psychiatric and drug evaluation/rehabilitation.
Drugs Producing Sedation, Intoxication, or Psychological and Physical Dependence (Nonbarbiturate Sedatives)		

Diazepam (Valium)
Chlordiazepoxide (Librium)
Oxazepam (Serax)
Lorazepam (Ativan)
Midazolam (Versed)
	Seizures, coma, circulatory collapse, death
	Acute intoxication:
	• Respiratory depression
	• Decreasing mental alertness
	• Confusion
	• Slurred speech, decreased blood pressure
	• Ataxia
	• Pulmonary edema
	• Coma, death
		Management
		1. Endotracheal tube is inserted as a precaution; use assisted ventilation to stabilize and correct respiratory depression. Observe for sudden apnea and laryngeal spasm (especially in patients dependent on glutethimide [Doriden]).
		2. Assess for hypotension
		   a. Insert indwelling urinary catheter for comatose patient; decreased urinary volume is an index of reduced renal flow associated with reduced intravascular volume or vascular collapse.
		   b. Start volume expansion with saline or dextrose as prescribed.
		3. Evacuate stomach contents; emesis; lavage; activated charcoal; cathartic.
		4. Start ECG monitoring. Observe for dysrhythmias.
		5. Administer flumazenil (Romazicon), the benzodiazepine antagonist (reversal agent)
		6. Refer patient for psychiatric evaluation (potential suicide intent).

Salicylate Poisoning Aspirin (present in compound analgesic tablets)	Restlessness, tinnitus, deafness, blurring of vision Hyperpnea, hyperpyrexia, sweating Epigastric pain, vomiting, dehydration Respiratory and metabolic acidosis Disorientation, coma, cardiovascular collapse	1. Treat respiratory depression. 2. Induce gastric emptying by lavage. 3. Give activated charcoal to adsorb aspirin; a cathartic may be administered with charcoal to help ensure intestinal cleansing. 4. Support patient with IV infusions as prescribed to establish hydration and correct electrolyte imbalances. 5. Enhance elimination of salicylates as directed by forced diuresis, alkalinization of urine, peritoneal dialysis, or hemodialysis, according to severity of intoxication.

(continued)

Table 71-1 • **Emergency Management of Drug Abuse Patients and Patients with Drug Overdose** (Continued)		
DRUG	**CLINICAL MANIFESTATIONS**	**THERAPEUTIC MANAGEMENT**
		6. Monitor serum salicylate level for efficacy of treatment. 7. Administer specific prescribed pharmacologic agent for bleeding and other problems. 8. Refer patient for psychiatric evaluation (potential suicide intent).
Acetaminophen (present in prescription and nonprescription analgesics, antipyretics, and cold remedies)	Lethargy to encephalopathy and death GI upset, diaphoresis Right upper quadrant pain Abnormal liver function tests, prolonged prothrombin time, increased bilirubin Hepatomegaly leading to liver failure	1. Maintain airway 2. Obtain acetaminophen level. Levels ≥ 140 mg/kg are toxic. 3. Laboratory studies—liver function tests, prothrombin time/partial thromboplastin time, complete blood count, blood urea nitrogen, creatinine 4. Administer syrup of ipecac and follow emesis with activated charcoal. 5. Prepare for possible hemodialysis, which clears acetaminophen but does not halt liver damage. 6. Administer *N*-acetylcysteine (NAC, Mucomyst) as soon as possible. NAC replenishes essential liver enzymes and requires a total of 18 doses every 4 hr. Charcoal absorbs NAC; do not administer together. Repeat NAC dose if patient vomits. 7. Refer patient for psychiatric evaluation (potential suicide intent).
Tricyclic Antidepressants (TCA) Amitriptyline Doxepin Nortriptyline Imipramine	Dysrhythmia: ventricular fibrillation/tachycardia, tachycardia Hypotension Pulmonary edema, hypoxemia, acidosis Confusion, agitation, coma Visual hallucinations Clonus, hyperactive reflexes, nystagmus, myoclonic jerking Seizures Blurred vision, flushing, hyperthermia	1. Provide airway support, ventilation, cardiac monitoring; insert IV line with normal saline solution. 2. If within 1 hr after overdose, insert a nasogastric tube and instill activated charcoal with sorbitol every 4 hr ×3. 3. Administer a sodium bicarbonate drip to decrease dysrhythmias; the alkaline environment increases the protein binding of the metabolite. 4. Administer vasopressors 5. Use only Class IB antiarrhythmics (eg, lidocaine), as some other types of antiarrhymics have the same effect as TCA. 6. Manage seizure activity 7. Refer patient for psychiatric evaluation for potential suicide intent and evaluation of medication regimen for effectiveness.

which helps the patient maintain contact with reality. Any visual misrepresentations (illusions) are explained, to orient the patient to reality.

> **NURSING ALERT** Restraints are used as prescribed, if necessary, if the client is aggressive or violent, but only when other alternatives have been unsuccessful. The least restrictive device that will prevent the patient from injuring self or others is used. Caution is taken to ensure that restraints are applied properly and that they are not impairing circulation to any part of the body or interfering with respirations. Restraints must be released according to protocol. Physical observation (eg, skin integrity, circulatory status, respiratory status) is ongoing, and the patient's response is documented.

Fluid losses may result from gastrointestinal losses (vomiting), profuse perspiration, and respiration (hyperventilation). In addition, the patient may be dehydrated as a result of alcohol's effect of decreasing antidiuretic hormone. The oral or intravenous route is used to restore fluid and electrolyte balance.

Temperature, pulse, respiration, and blood pressure are recorded frequently (every 30 minutes in severe forms of delirium) in anticipation of peripheral circulatory collapse or hyperthermia (the two most lethal complications). Phenytoin (Dilantin) or other antiseizure medications may be prescribed to prevent or control repeated withdrawal seizures.

Frequently seen complications include infections (eg, pneumonia), trauma, hepatic failure, hypoglycemia, and cardiovascular problems. Hypoglycemia may accompany alcohol withdrawal, because alcohol depletes liver glycogen stores and impairs gluco-neogenesis; many patients with alcoholism also are malnourished. Parenteral dextrose may be prescribed if the liver glycogen level is depleted. Orange juice, Gatorade, or other forms of carbohydrates are given to stabilize the blood glucose level and counteract tremulousness. Supplemental vitamin therapy and a high-protein diet are provided as prescribed to counteract vitamin deficiency. The patient should be referred to an alcoholic treatment centre for follow-up care and rehabilitation.

Violence, Abuse, and Neglect

FAMILY VIOLENCE, ABUSE, AND NEGLECT

EDs are often the first place where victims of family violence, abuse, or neglect go to seek help. In Canada, trends in self-reported spousal violence indicate that each year, 653,000 women and 546,000 men are either physically or sexually abused by their current or previous partners. However, violence against women continues to be of a more serious nature. In 2004, 44% of women who have been in violent situations reported injuries, whereas only 11% of the men in such situation reported injuries (Mihorean, 2005). Although it remains a significant issue, it must be noted that in the last 30 years, the number of spousal homicides has significantly decreased in Canada. For female victims, the rate dropped from 16.5 per 1 million in 1974 to 7.5 per 1 million in 2003, whereas for male victims it fell from 4.4 in 1974 to 1.7 in 2003 (Beattie, 2005a). Children and older individuals are also affected by violence. In 2003, "the rate of all police-reported assault against children and youth was 1,099 per 100,000 under the age of 18" (Beattie, 2005b, p. 69). "In 2003, just under 4,000 incidents of violence against older persons were reported to the police" (AuCoin, 2005, p. 79). There are reasons to believe that family violence against older adults is underestimated as elders may be more hesitant than younger adults to report incidents affecting them. Data reveals that older women are more likely than older men to be abused by family members. In 2003, 4 out of 10 older female victims and 2 out of 10 male victims had been victimized by a family member (AuCoin, 2005). Elder abuse takes many forms, including physical and psychological abuse, neglect, violation of personal rights, and financial abuse. Emergency nurses must be aware that individuals of all age groups and of both genders may be victims of abuse and should include questions to this effect in their evaluations of clients.

Clinical Manifestations

When victims of abuse seek treatment, they may present with physical injuries or with health problems, such as anxiety, insomnia, or gastrointestinal symptoms, that are related to stress. They usually do not identify their abuser.

The possibility of abuse should be investigated whenever a person presents with multiple injuries that are in various stages of healing, when injuries are unexplained, and when the explanation does not fit the physical picture (Chart 71-13). The possibility of neglect should be investigated whenever a dependent person with adequate resources and a designated care provider shows evidence of inattention to hygiene, to nutrition, or to known medical needs (eg, unfilled medication prescriptions, missed appointments with health care providers). In the ED, the most common physical injuries seen are unexplained bruises, lacerations, abrasions, head injuries, or fractures. The most common clinical manifestations of neglect are malnutrition and dehydration.

Chart 71-13 | **Abuse, Maltreatment, and Neglect**

The following questions may be helpful when assessing a patient for abuse, maltreatment, and neglect:

- I noticed that you have a number of bruises. Can you tell me how they happened? Has anyone hurt you?
- You seem frightened. Has anyone ever hurt you?
- Sometimes patients tell me that they have been hurt by someone at home or at work. Could this be happening to you?
- Are you afraid of anyone at home or work? Or of anyone with whom you come in contact?
- Has anyone failed to help you to take care of yourself when you needed help?
- Has anyone prevented you from seeing friends or other people whom you wish to see?
- Have you signed any papers that you did not understand or did not wish to sign?
- Has anyone forced you to sign papers against your will?

Assessment and Diagnostic Findings

Nurses in EDs are in an ideal position to provide early detection and interventions for victims of domestic violence. This requires an acute awareness of the signs of possible abuse, maltreatment, and neglect. Nurses must be skilled in interviewing techniques that are likely to elicit accurate information. A careful history is crucial in the screening process. Asking questions in private—away from others—may be helpful in eliciting information about abuse, maltreatment, and neglect.

Whenever evidence leads one to suspect abuse or neglect, an evaluation with careful documentation of descriptions of events and drawings or photos of injuries is important, because the medical record may be used as part of a legal document. Assessment of the patient's general appearance and interactions with significant others, an examination of the entire surface area of the body, and a mental status examination are crucial.

Management

Whenever abuse, maltreatment, or neglect is suspected, the health care worker's primary concern should be the safety and welfare of the patient. Treatment focuses on the consequences of the abuse, violence, or neglect and on prevention of further injury. Protocols of most EDs require that a multidisciplinary approach be used. Nurses, physicians, social workers, and community agencies work collaboratively to develop and implement a plan for meeting the patient's needs.

If in immediate danger, the patient should be separated from the abusing or neglecting person whenever possible. On the basis of this danger, or on the basis of injuries or neglected medical conditions, hospitalization is justified until alternative plans are made. However, it must be remembered that third-party payers may not approve hospitalization that is based solely on abuse or neglect.

When abuse or neglect is considered to be the result of stress experienced by a caregiver who is no longer able to cope with the burden of caring for an elderly person or a person with chronic disease or a disability, respite services may be necessary. Support groups may be helpful to these caregivers. When mental illness of the abuser or neglecter is responsible for the situation, alternative living arrangements may be required.

Nurses must be mindful that competent adults are free to accept or refuse the help that is offered to them. Some patients will insist on remaining in the home environment where the abuse or neglect is occurring. The wishes of patients who are competent and not cognitively impaired should be respected. However, all possible alternatives and available resources should be explored with the patient.

Mandatory reporting laws in most states require health care workers to report *suspected* abuse to an official agency, usually Adult (or Child) Protective Services. All that is required for reporting is the suspicion of abuse. The health care worker is not required to prove anything. Likewise, health care workers who report suspected abuse are immune to civil or criminal liability if the report is made in good faith. Subsequent home visits resulting from the report of suspected abuse are a part of gathering information about the patient in the home environment. In addition, many states have resource hotlines for use by health care workers and by patients who seek answers to questions about abuse and neglect.

SEXUAL ASSAULT

The definition of *rape* is forced sexual acts, especially vaginal or anal penetration. Perpetrators and victims may be either male or female. The feminist movement has focused on the rights and care of rape victims, and law enforcement agencies are becoming increasingly sensitive and aggressive in managing these crimes. Rape crisis centres offer support, educate victims, and help them through the subsequent courtroom experience.

The manner in which the patient is received and treated in the ED is important to his or her future psychological well-being. Crisis intervention should begin when the patient enters the health care facility. The patient should be seen immediately. Most hospitals have a written protocol that reflects consideration for the victim's physical and emotional needs as well as forensic evidence collection that is required.

The Sexual Assault Nurse Examiner

In the United States, there is the opportunity for emergency nurses to become trained sexual assault nurse examiners (SANEs). The role allows for specific training in forensic evidence collection, history taking, documentation, and ways to approach the patient and family. Specialized training also includes proper photography and the use of colposcopy. Colposcopy increases assessment by examination for microtrauma through magnification. Evidence is collected through photography, videography, and analysis of specimens. Another tool useful to SANEs is the light-staining microscope, which enables the examiner to identify motile and nonmotile sperm and infection. This tool saves time and also enhances assessment. SANEs complement the ED staff and can spend more time with both the patient and police officers investigating the incident.

Assessment and Diagnostic Findings

The patient's reaction to rape has been termed *rape trauma syndrome* and is seen as an acute stress reaction to a life-threatening situation. The nurse performing the assessment is aware that the patient may go through several phases of psychological reactions (Dole, 1996; Ritchie, 1998):

- An acute disorganization phase, which may manifest as an expressed state in which shock, disbelief, fear, guilt, humilia-

tion, anger, and other such emotions are encountered or as a controlled state in which feelings are masked or hidden and the victim appears composed
- A phase of denial and unwillingness to talk about the incident, followed by a phase of heightened anxiety, fear, flashbacks, sleep disturbances, hyperalertness, and psychosomatic reactions
- A phase of reorganization, in which the incident is put into perspective. Some victims never fully recover and go on to develop chronic stress disorders and phobias.

Management

The goals of management are to give sympathetic support, to reduce the emotional trauma of the patient, and to gather available evidence for possible legal proceedings. All of the interventions have the ultimate goal of having the patient regain control over his or her life.

Throughout the patient's stay in the ED, the patient's privacy and sensitivity must be respected. The patient may exhibit a wide range of emotional reactions, such as hysteria, stoicism, or feelings of being overwhelmed. Support and caring are crucial. The patient should be reassured that anxiety is natural and asked whether a support person may be called. Appropriate support is available from professional and community resources. The Rape Victim Companion Program, if available in the community, can be contacted, and services of a volunteer can be requested. The patient should never be left alone.

PHYSICAL EXAMINATION

A written, witnessed informed consent must be obtained from the patient (or parent or guardian if the patient is a minor) for examination, for taking of photographs, and for release of findings to police. A history is obtained only if the patient has not already talked to a police officer, social worker, or crisis intervention worker. The patient should not be asked to repeat the history. Any history of the event that is obtained should be recorded in the patient's own words. The patient is asked whether he or she has bathed, douched, brushed teeth, changed clothes, urinated, or defecated since the attack, because these actions may alter interpretation of subsequent findings. The time of admission, time of examination, date and time of the alleged rape, and the patient's emotional state and general appearance (including any evidence of trauma, such as discolouration, bruises, lacerations, secretions, or torn and bloody clothing) are documented.

For the physical examination, the patient is helped to undress and is draped properly. Each item of clothing is placed in a separate paper bag. Plastic bags are not used because they retain moisture; moisture may promote mold and mildew formation, which can destroy evidence. The bags are labelled and given to appropriate law enforcement authorities.

The patient is examined (from head to toe) for injuries, especially injuries to the head, neck, breast, thighs, back, and buttocks. Body diagrams and photographs aid in documenting the evidence of trauma. The physical examination focuses on the following:

- External evidence of trauma (bruises, contusions, lacerations, stab wounds)
- Dried semen stains (appearing as crusted, flaking areas) on the patient's body or clothes
- Broken fingernails and body tissue and foreign materials under nails (if found, samples are taken)

- Oral examination, including a specimen of saliva and prescribed cultures of gum and tooth areas

Pelvic and rectal examinations are also performed. The perineum and other areas are examined with a Wood lamp or other filtered ultraviolet light. Areas that appear fluorescent may indicate semen stains. The colour and consistency of any discharge present is noted. A water-moistened rather than a lubricated vaginal speculum is used for the examination. Lubricant contains chemicals that may interfere with later forensic testing of specimens and acid phosphatase determinations. The rectum is examined for signs of trauma, blood, and semen. During the examination, the patient should be advised of the nature and necessity of each procedure and given the rationale for each question asked.

SPECIMEN COLLECTION
During the physical examination, numerous laboratory specimens may be collected, including the following:

- Vaginal aspirate, examined for presence or absence of motile and nonmotile sperm
- Secretions (obtained with a sterile swab) from the vaginal pool for acid phosphatase, blood group antigen of semen, and precipitin test against human sperm and blood
- Separate smears from the oral, vaginal, and anal areas
- Culture of body orifices for gonorrhea
- Blood serum for syphilis and HIV testing; a sample of serum for syphilis may be frozen and saved for future testing
- Pregnancy test if there is a possibility that the patient may be pregnant
- Any foreign material (leaves, grass, dirt), which is placed in a clean envelope
- Pubic hair samples obtained by combing or trimming. Several pubic hairs with follicles are placed in separate containers and identified as the patient's hairs.

To preserve the chain of evidence, each specimen is labelled with the name of the patient, the date and time of collection, the body area from which the specimen was obtained, and the names of personnel collecting specimens. Then the specimens are given to a designated person (eg, crime laboratory technician), and an itemized receipt is obtained.

TREATING POTENTIAL CONSEQUENCES OF RAPE
After the initial physical examination is completed and specimens have been obtained, any associated injuries are treated as indicated. The patient is given the option of prophylaxis against sexually transmitted disease. Ceftriaxone (Rocephin), administered intramuscularly with 1% lidocaine (Xylocaine), may be prescribed as prophylaxis for gonorrhea. Doxycycline (Vibramycin) taken for 10 days may be prescribed as prophylaxis for syphilis and chlamydia.

Antipregnancy measures may be considered if the patient is of childbearing age, is not using contraceptives, and is at high risk in her menstrual cycle. A postcoital contraceptive medication, such as Ovral, which contains estrogen ethinyl estradiol and progestin norgestrel, may be prescribed after a pregnancy test. To promote effectiveness, Ovral should be administered within 12 to 24 hours and no later than 72 hours after intercourse. The 21-day package rather than the 28-day package is prescribed, so that the patient does not take the inert tablets by mistake. An antiemetic may be administered as prescribed to decrease discomfort from side effects. A cleansing douche, mouthwash, and fresh clothing are usually offered.

FOLLOW-UP CARE
The patient is informed of counselling services to prevent long-term psychological effects. Counselling services should be made available to both the patient and the family. A referral is made to the Rape Victim Companion Program, if available. Appointments for follow-up surveillance for pregnancy, sexually transmitted disease, and HIV testing also are made.

The patient is encouraged to return to his or her previous level of functioning as soon as possible. When leaving the health care facility, the patient should be accompanied by a family member or friend.

VIOLENCE IN THE EMERGENCY DEPARTMENT

Not only do ED staff members encounter patients who are violent from substance abuse, injury, or other emergencies, but they may also encounter violent situations in the rest of the environment. Patients and families waiting for assistance are increasingly volatile. Often, waiting rooms are the site for dissatisfaction, fear, and anger to be acted out in violence. Some EDs assign security officers to the area and have installed metal detectors to identify weapons and protect patients, families, and staff. It is not unusual for a patient to come to the ED armed. Nurses and other personnel must be prepared to deal with such circumstances.

Management

Safety is the first priority. Protecting the ED on a daily basis will prevent any untoward events from occurring. Protection of the department provides protection for the patients, families, and staff. It is essential that all nurses be aware of the environment in which they are working.

Metal detectors, silent alarm systems, and secured entry into the department assist in maintaining safety. Members of gangs and feuding families need to be separated in the ED, in the waiting room, and later in the inpatient nursing unit to avoid angry confrontations. Security officers should be ready to assist at all times. The department should be able to be locked against entry if security is at all in question.

Patients from prison and those who are under guard need to be shackled to the bed with appropriate assessment. The same assessment and care that are provided to patients with hand or ankle restraints are provided to patients with handcuffs. In addition, the following precautions are taken:

- Never release the hand or ankle restraint (handcuff).
- Always have a guard present in the room.
- Place the patient face down on the stretcher to avoid injury from head-butting, spitting, or biting.
- Use restraints on any violent patient as needed.
- Administer medication if necessary to control violent behaviour until definitive treatment can be obtained.

In the case of gunfire in the ED, self-protection is a priority. There is no advantage to protecting others if the caregivers are also injured. Security officers and police must gain control of the situation first; then care is provided to the injured.

Psychiatric Emergencies

A psychiatric emergency is an urgent, serious disturbance of behaviour, affect, or thought that makes the patient unable to cope with life situations and interpersonal relationships. A patient presenting with a psychiatric emergency may display overactive or violent, underactive or depressed, or suicidal behaviours.

The most important concern of the ED personnel is determining whether the patient is at risk for injuring self or others. The aim is to try to maintain the patient's self-esteem (and life, if necessary) while providing care. Determining whether the patient is currently under psychiatric treatment is important so that contact can be made with the therapist or physician who works with the patient.

OVERACTIVE PATIENTS

Patients who display disturbed, uncooperative, and paranoid behaviour and those who feel anxious and panicky may be prone to assaultive and destructive impulses and abnormal social behaviour. Intense nervousness, depression, and crying are evident in some patients. Disturbed and noisy behaviour may be exacerbated or compounded by alcohol or drug intoxication.

Management

A reliable source is needed to identify events leading to the crisis, and a history is obtained. Past mental illness, hospitalizations, injuries, serious illnesses, use of alcohol or drugs, crises in interpersonal relationships, or intrapsychic conflicts are explored. Because abnormal thoughts and behaviour may be manifestations of an underlying physical disorder, such as hypoglycemia, stroke, epilepsy, head injury, or drug or alcohol toxicity, a physical assessment is performed when possible.

The immediate goal is to gain control of the situation. If the patient is potentially violent, security or local police should be nearby. Restraints are used as a *last* resort and as prescribed. Approaching the patient with a calm, confident, and firm manner is therapeutic and has a calming effect. Helpful interventions include the following:

- Introduce yourself by name.
- Tell the patient, "I am here to help you."
- Repeat the patient's name from time to time.
- Speak in one-thought sentences and be consistent.
- Give the patient space and time to slow down.
- Show interest in, listen to, and encourage the patient to talk about personal thoughts and feelings.
- Offer appropriate and honest explanations.

A psychotropic agent (ie, one that exerts an effect on the mind) may be prescribed for emergency management of functional psychosis. However, personality disorders cannot and should not be treated with psychotropic medications; nor are psychotropic medications used if the patient's behaviour results from use of hallucinogens (eg, lysergic acid diethylamide [LSD]).

Agents such as chlorpromazine (Thorazine) and haloperidol (Haldol) act specifically against psychotic symptoms of thought fragmentation and perceptual and behavioural aberrations. The initial dosage depends on the patient's body weight and the severity of the symptoms. After administration of the initial dose, the patient is observed closely to determine the degree of change in psychotic behaviour. Subsequent dosages depend on the patient's response.

Typically, after stabilization, the patient is transferred to a psychiatric unit or psychiatric outpatient treatment is arranged.

VIOLENT BEHAVIOUR

Violent and aggressive behaviour, usually episodic, is a means of expressing feelings of anger, fear, or hopelessness about a situation. Usually, the patient has a history of outbursts of rage, temper tantrums, or impulsive behaviour. People with a tendency for violence frequently lose control when intoxicated with alcohol or drugs. Family members are the most frequent victims of their aggression (see earlier discussion). Patients with a propensity for violence include those intoxicated by drugs or alcohol; those going through drug or alcohol withdrawal; and those diagnosed with acute paranoid schizophrenic state, acute organic brain syndrome, acute psychosis, paranoid character, borderline personality, or antisocial personality disorders.

Management

The goal of treatment is to bring the violence under control. A specially designated room with at least two exits should be used for the interview. The door of the room should be kept open, and the nurse should remain in clear view of the staff, *staying between the patient and the door.* However, the patient's exit to the door must not be blocked, because the patient may feel trapped and threatened. No objects that could be used as weapons should be in sight, in the room, or carried in with health care personnel. If the interviewer feels anxious or uneasy about the patient's response, security staff, a family member, or another health care worker should be asked to remain in the hall nearby in the event that additional help is needed. The patient should never be left alone, because this may be interpreted as rejection or provide an opportunity for self-harm.

To bring the violence under control, it is crucial to use a calm, noncritical approach while remaining in control of the situation. Sudden movements are avoided. External calm and structure in conjunction with providing the patient some space may help the patient gain control. If the patient is carrying a weapon, the emergency health care provider should ask that it be surrendered. If the patient is unwilling to surrender the weapon, the security staff is called. If necessary, the security staff may seek further assistance from the local police department.

The patient's violent behaviour is a crisis situation for the patient and the ED. Crisis intervention, achieved by talking and listening to the patient, is best accomplished by expressing an interest in the patient's well-being while attempting to tune in to the patient and remain firm. The patient's agitated state is acknowledged by statements such as, "I want to work with you to relieve your distress."

The patient is allowed the opportunity to ventilate anger verbally. If the patient is delusional, challenging the patient is avoided. Trying to hear what the patient is saying, conveying an expectation of appropriate behaviour, and making the patient aware that help is available are key. The patient should be informed that violent behaviour may be frightening others and that violence is not acceptable. Help that is available in crisis situations (from a clinic, ED, or mental health facility) should be described and offered. Often, the offer of protection by hospitalization is welcomed by the patient, who fears losing control or harming self or others. If the patient does not calm down, security personnel or police intervention may be necessary.

If these measures fail to alleviate the patient's tension, medication may be prescribed (rapid sedation with haloperidol, diazepam, or chlorpromazine) to reduce tension, anxiety, and hyperactivity. Restraints must be prescribed by a physician. They are applied with a minimum of force and only when necessary and when other alternatives have been unsuccessful.

> **NURSING ALERT** The least restrictive device to prevent the patient from injuring self or others is used. Caution is taken to ensure that restraints are applied properly. Restraints should be used with verbal intervention to calm the patient and promote compliance. Appropriate personnel must be available when applying restraints (in such a way that they do not impair circulation to any part of the body or interfere with breathing). Physical observation (eg, skin integrity, circulatory status, respiratory status) is ongoing, and the patient's response is documented.

After combativeness, agitation, and fear have decreased, the patient is referred for further mental health treatment.

POSTTRAUMATIC STRESS DISORDER

Posttraumatic stress disorder (PTSD) is the development of characteristic symptoms after a psychologically stressful event that is considered outside the range of normal human experience (eg, rape, combat, motor vehicle crash, natural catastrophe, terrorist attack). Symptoms of this disorder include intrusive thoughts and dreams, phobic avoidance reaction (avoidance of activities that arouse recollection of the traumatic event), heightened vigilance, exaggerated startle reaction, generalized anxiety, and societal withdrawal. PTSD may be acute, chronic, or delayed.

Assessment and Diagnostic Findings

Assessment includes an evaluation of the patient's pretrauma history, the trauma itself, and posttrauma functioning. PTSD often presents as multiple readmissions to the ED for minor or recurring complaints without evidence of injury. The patient is allowed to discuss the traumatic event and permitted to grieve.

Management

The patient's goal is to organize and begin to integrate the experience so that he or she can return to the pretrauma level of functioning as soon as possible. Emergency management focuses on the patient's presenting behaviours. A wide range of interventions are carried out, including crisis intervention strategies, establishing a trusting and sharing relationship, and educating the patient and family about stress management and support services available in the community. Psychiatric support may be useful to the patient.

UNDERACTIVE OR DEPRESSED PATIENTS

In the ED, depression may be seen as the primary condition bringing the patient to the health care facility, or it may be masked by anxiety and somatic complaints. The depressed person has a mood disturbance.

Clinical manifestations may include sadness, apathy, feelings of worthlessness, self-blame, suicidal thoughts, desire to escape, avoidance of simple problems, anorexia and weight loss, decreased interest in sex, sleeplessness, and ceaseless activity or reduction in activity. The agitated depressed individual may exhibit motor restlessness and severe anxiety.

Management

The depressed patient benefits from ventilating personal feelings and should be provided an opportunity to talk about personal problems while emergency health care personnel listen in a calm, unhurried manner. Information about a perceived or real illness or a sudden worsening of depression is an important clue. Any patient who is depressed may be at risk for suicide.

Attempts are made to find out whether the patient has thought about or attempted suicide. Questions such as, "Have you ever thought about taking your own life?" may be helpful. Generally, the patient is relieved to have an opportunity to discuss personal feelings. If the patient is seriously depressed, relatives should be notified. The patient should never be left alone, because suicide is usually committed in solitude.

The patient needs to understand that depression is treatable. Antidepressant and antianxiety agents may be prescribed. Crisis and supportive services in the community, including mental health centres, telephone counselling and referral, suicide prevention centres, group therapy, and marital and family counselling, should be offered to the patient and family. Usually, the patient is referred for psychiatric consultation or to a psychiatric facility.

SUICIDAL PATIENTS

Attempted suicide is an act that stems from depression (eg, loss of a loved one, loss of body integrity or status, poor self-image) and can be viewed as a cry for help and intervention. Males are at greater risk than females. Others at risk are elderly people; young adults; people who are enduring unusual loss or stress; those who are unemployed, divorced, widowed, or living alone; those showing signs of significant depression (eg, weight loss, sleep disturbances, somatic complaints, suicidal preoccupation); and those with a history of a previous suicide attempt, suicide in the family, or psychiatric illness.

Being aware of people at risk and assessing for specific factors that predispose a person to suicide are key management strategies. Specific signs and symptoms of potential suicide include the following:

- Communication of *suicidal intent*, such as preoccupation with death or talking of someone else's suicide (eg, "I'm tired of living. I've put my affairs in order. I'm better off dead. I'm a burden to my family")
- History of a previous suicide attempt (the risk is much greater in these cases)
- Family history of suicide
- Loss of a parent at an early age
- Specific plan for suicide
- A means to carry out the plan

Management

Emergency management focuses on treating the consequences of the suicide attempt (eg, gunshot wound, drug overdose) and preventing further self-injury. A patient who has made a suicidal gesture may do so again. Crisis intervention is employed to determine suicidal potential, to discover areas of depression and conflict, to find out about the patient's support system, and to determine whether hospitalization or psychiatric referral is necessary. Depending on the patient's potential for suicide, the patient may be admitted to the intensive care unit, referred for follow-up care, or admitted to the psychiatric unit.

Critical Thinking Exercises

1. A young woman arrives at the ED by ambulance after a car crash. She is immobilized on a backboard with a cervical collar. An oxygen mask is in place. You note shallow, slow respirations and no movement of the left chest wall. She complains of pain in her abdomen, and it is tense. Her left leg is angulated. How would you prioritize the patient's needs? Develop an assessment strategy, identify diagnostic studies that will benefit the patient, and describe the patient's treatment needs.

2. A man who was out ice fishing all day, wearing sneakers instead of his boots, comes to the ED for treatment of frostbite of his feet. His friends have been massaging his feet en route to the ED. The patient insists that his feet be placed in a pan of hot water. Describe how you would respond and the explanation you would give to this patient. How would you proceed with managing this patient's care? Describe the treatment dilemmas for this type of injury.

3. A young woman with a toddler in her arms waits her turn in line at the triage desk of the ED. The child is crying and rubbing her eyes and face. You overhear the mother telling another patient that the child has had an allergic reaction to her first soft-cooked egg, which the child smeared on her face. While waiting, the child becomes quiet and pale in colour. Analyze this information. What is your immediate response? What action would you take and what is the rationale for your decision?

4. An elderly patient is brought to the ED by her son. She is complaining of pain in her hip, and the son says that she tripped over her oxygen tubing and fell. On initial assessment you notice that the patient has many bruises on her body in varying stages of resolution. What conclusions might you draw from these findings, and how might you proceed to evaluate the situation to determine your course of action?

REFERENCES AND SELECTED READINGS

Books

American College of Surgeons. (1997). *Advanced trauma life support* (6th ed.). Chicago: American College of Surgeons.

AuCoin, K. (2005). Family violence against older adults. In K. AuCoin (Ed.), *Family violence in Canada: A statistical profile* (pp. 78–84). Ottawa: Canadian Centre for Justice Statistics–Statistics Canada.

Auerbach, P. S., Donner, H. S., & Weiss, E. H. (1999). *Field guide to wilderness medicine.* St. Louis: C. V. Mosby.

Beattie, K. (2005a). Family homicides. In K. AuCoin (Ed.), *Family violence in Canada: A statistical profile* (pp. 48–59). Ottawa: Canadian Centre for Justice Statistics–Statistics Canada.

Beattie, K. (2005b). Family violence against children and youth. In K. AuCoin (Ed.), *Family violence in Canada: A statistical profile* (pp. 68–77). Ottawa: Canadian Centre for Justice Statistics–Statistics Canada.

Berner, A. R. (2001). Triage. In A. Harwood-Nuss (Ed.), *The clinical practice of emergency medicine* (3rd ed.). Philadelphia: Lippincott Williams & Wilkins.

Beveridge, R., Clarke, B., Janes, L., et al. (1998). *Implementation Guidelines for the Canadian ED Triage and Acuity Scale (CTSA).* Ottawa: Canadian Association of Emergency Physicians, National Emer-gency Nurses Affiliation of Canada, and L'Association des médecins d'urgence du Québec.

Bove, A. A., & Davis, J. C. (1997). *Diving medicine.* Philadelphia: W. B. Saunders.

Bullock, B. L. (1996). *Pathophysiology.* Philadelphia: Lippincott-Raven.

Emergency Nurses Association. (2000). *Emergency nursing core curriculum* (5th ed.). Philadelphia: W. B. Saunders.

Handysides, G. (1996). *Triage in emergency practice.* St. Louis: C. V. Mosby.

Holleran, R. S. (1996). *Flight nursing principles and practice* (2nd ed.). St. Louis: C. V. Mosby.

McQuillan, K., VonReuden, K., Hartsock, R., Flynn, M. B., & Whalen, E. (2002). *Trauma nursing: Resuscitation through rehabilitation* (3rd ed.). Philadelphia: W. B. Saunders.

Mihorean, K. (2005). Trends in self-reported spousal violence. In K. AuCoin (Ed.), *Family violence in Canada: A statistical profile* (pp. 13–32). Ottawa: Canadian Centre for Justice Statistics–Statistics Canada.

Mohan, D., & Tiwari, G. (2000). *Injury prevention and control.* London: Taylor and Francis.

Public Health Agency of Canada. (2004). *Update: Health Canada activities with respect to SARS.* Ottawa: Author.

Sheehy, S. B. (1998). *Emergency nursing principles and practice* (4th ed.). St. Louis: C. V. Mosby.

Journals

Abramson, D., Scalea, T. M., Hitchcock, R., Trooskin, S. Z., Henry, S. M., & Greenspan, J. (1993). Lactate clearance and survival following injury. *Journal of Trauma, 35*(4), 584–588.

Adams, M. H., Lammon, C. B., & Stover, L. M. (1999). Responding to tricyclic antidepressant overdose. *Nursing 99, 29*(10), 32cc1-2,4,6.

Allan, M. G., & Kenny, D. (2003). High-altitude decompression illness: Case report and discussion. *Canadian Medical Association Journal, 169*(8), 803–807.

American Academy of Pediatrics. (2000). Diagnostic imaging of child abuse. *Pediatrics, 105*(6), 1345–1348.

American Public Health Association. (2001). Effective public health assessment, prevention, response, and training for emerging and reemerging infectious diseases, including bioterrorism. *American Journal of Public Health, 91*(3), 500–501.

Bernardo, L. M. (2002). Emergency nurses' role in pediatric injury and prevention. *Nursing Clinics of North America, 37*(1), 135–143.

Bernstein, M. L. (1998). Latex safe emergency cart products list. *Journal of Emergency Nursing, 24*(1), 58–61.

Blanchard, J. C., & Curtis, K. M. (1999). Violence in the emergency department. *Emergency Medicine Clinics of North America, 17*(3), 717–731.

Blank-Reid, C. (1996). The incidence, etiology, and management of anaphylaxis presenting to an accident and emergency department. *Quarterly Journal of Medicine, 89*(11), 859–864.

Blenkiron, P, House, A., & Milnes, D. (2000). The timing of acts of deliberate self-harm: Is there any relation with suicidal intent, mental disorder or psychiatric management? *Journal of Psychosomatic Research, 49*(1), 3–6.

Blow, O., Magliore, L, Claridge, J. A., Butler, K., Young, J. S. (1999). The golden hour and the silver day: Detection and correction of occult hypoperfusion within 24 hours improves outcome from major trauma. *Journal of Trauma, 47*(5), 964–969.

Brown, A. F., McKinnon, D., & Chu, K. (2001). Emergency department anaphylaxis: A review of 142 patients in a single year. *Journal of Allergy and Clinical Immunology, 108*(5), 861–866.

Buhr, V. (2000). Screening patients for latex allergies. *Journal of American Academy of Nurse Practitioners, 12*(9), 384–386.

Campbell, J. C. (1999). If I can't have you no one can. *Reflections, 3rd quarter,* 8–12.

Catallozzi, M., Pletcher, J. R., Schwartz, D. F. (2001). Prevention of suicide in adolescents. *Current Opinion in Pediatrics, 13*(5), 417–422.

Caywood, M. J. (2000). Near-fatal rattlesnake envenomation. *Journal of Emergency Nursing, 26*(2), 113–116.

Claridge, J. A., Crabtree, T. D., Pelletier, S. J., Butler, K., Sawyer, R. G., & Young, J. S. (2000). Persistent occult hypoperfusion is associated with a significant increase in infection rate and mortality in major trauma patients. *Journal of Trauma, 48*(1), 8–14.

Crowl, A. C., Young, J. S., Kahler, D. M., Claridge, J. A., Chrzanowski, D. S., & Pomphrey, M. (2000). Occult hypoperfusion is associated with increased morbidity in patients undergoing early femur fracture fixation. *Journal of Trauma, 48*(2), 260–267.

DeBoer, S. L. (1997). Neurological outcomes after near drowning. *Critical Care Nurse, 17*(4), 19–25.

Dole, P. J. (1996). Centering: Reducing rape trauma syndrome anxiety during a gynecologic examination. *Journal of Psychosocial Nursing and Mental Health Services, 34*(10), 32–37.

Eberhard, L. W., Morabito, D. J., Matthay, M. A., Mackersie, R. C., Campbell, A. R., Marks, J. D., Alonso, J. A., & Pittet, J. F. (2000). Initial severity of metabolic acidosis predicts the development of acute lung injury in severely traumatized patients. *Critical Care Medicine, 28*(1), 125–131.

Frick, E. J., Jr., Pasquale, M. D., & Cipolle, M. D. (1999). Small-bowel and mesentery injuries in blunt trauma. *Journal of Trauma, 46*(5), 920–926.

Galea, S. (2002). Psychological sequelae of the September 11 terrorist attacks in New York City. *New England Journal of Medicine, 346*(13), 982–987.

Ghuran, A., Van der Wieken, L. R., & Nolan, J. (2001). Cardiovascular complications of recreational drugs: An important cause of morbidity and mortality. *British Medical Journal, 323*(7311), 464–466.

Glow, S. D. (1997). Acutely agitated patients: A comparison of the use of haloperidol and droperidol in the emergency department. *Journal of Emergency Nursing, 23*(6), 626–628.

Gray-Vickrey, P. (2000). Protecting the older adult. *Nursing 2000, 30*(7), 34–38.

Grossman, M. D., Miller, D., Scaff, D. W., & Arcona, S. (2002) When is elder old? Effect of preexisting conditions on mortality on geriatric trauma. *Journal of Trauma, 52*(2), 242–246.

Guth, A. A., & Pachter, H. L. (2000). Domestic violence and the trauma surgeon. *American Journal of Surgery, 179*(2), 134–140.

Hagstad, D. (2000). Emergency: Bioterrorism. *American Journal of Nursing, 100*(12), 33–35.

Hansen, K. A. (1998). It's no accident. . . . it's preventable. *Journal of Emergency Nursing, 24*(1), 101–103.

Harrahil, M. (1997). Strategies for improving trauma documentation. *Journal of Emergency Nursing, 23*(2), 187–188.

Harrell, R., Toronjo, C. H., McLaughlin, J., Pavlik, V. N., Hyman, D. J., & Bitondo, D. (2002). How geriatricians identify elder abuse and neglect. *American Journal of Medical Sciences, 323*(1), 34–38.

Hart, B. G., & Trickett, D. (1995). Alcohol and trauma in the emergency department. *Journal of Emergency Nursing, 21*(5), 426–429.

Health Canada. (1997). *Canada Communicable Disease Report, Supplement Volume 23*, S8.

Health Canada. (2005). *Canada Communicable Disease Report, 31*(3).

Hoag-Apel, C. M. (1998). Violence in the emergency department. *Nursing Management, 29*(7), 60–62.

Hoak, S., & Koestner, A. (1997). Esophageal tracheal Combitube in the emergency department. *Journal of Emergency Nursing, 23*(4), 347–350.

Hollingsworth, H. (1997). Preventing insect sting anaphylaxis. *Journal of the American Medical Association, 277*(15), 1196–1197.

Hopkins, A. G. (1994). The trauma nurse's role with families in crisis. *Critical Care Nurse, 14*(2), 35–43.

Insect stings. (2000). *RN, 63*(6), (Suppl.), 9–10.

Judkins, D., & Neff, J. (1995). Innovations in care: The cutting edge—fluids and blood warming systems. *Journal of Trauma Nursing, 2*(4), 105–109.

Jurewicz, M. A. (2000). Anaphylaxis: When the body overreacts. *Nursing 2000, 30*(7), 58–61.

Kanzenbach, T. L., & Dexter, W. W. (1999). Cold injuries: Protecting your patients from the dangers of hypothermia and frostbite. *Postgraduate Medicine, 105*(1), 72–78.

Kulig, K. (1992). Initial management of ingestions of toxic substances. *New England Journal of Medicine, 326*(25), 1677–1681.

Laskowski-Jones, L. (1999). Responding to winter emergencies. *Dimensions of Critical Care Nursing, 18*(6), 13–22.

Ledray, L. E. (2000). Is the SANE role within the scope of nursing practice? On pelvics, colposcopy, and dispensing of medications. *Journal of Emergency Nursing, 26*(1), 79–81.

Leiding, L. (2001). Domestic violence. *On the Edge, 7,* 1, 3.

Lenehan, G. (1995). An ED forensic kit. *Journal of Emergency Nursing, 21*(5), 440–444.

Leske, J. S. (1998). Treatment for family members in crisis after critical injury. *AACN Clinical Issues 9*(1), 129–139.

Linden, J. A. (1999). Sexual assault. *Emergency Medicine Clinics of North America 17*(3), 685–697.

Lisanti, P. (1998). Barbiturate overdose. *American Journal of Nursing, 98*(10), 38.

Luci, T. S., & Merrell, J. C. (1995). Perceived dangerousness of recreational drugs. *Journal of Drug Education, 25*(4), 297–306.

Ludwig, R., Dieckman, B., Snelson, C. M. (1999). Assessment of the geriatric orthopaedic trauma patient. *Orthopaedic Nursing, 18*(6), 13–18.

MacConnachie, A. M. (1997). Ecstasy poisoning. *Intensive and Critical Care Nursing, 13*(6), 365–366.

Management of poisoning. (1996). *Nursing Times, 92* (11, Suppl. 1), 13–19.

Mayer, B. W., Smith, F. B., & King, C. A. (1999). Factors associated with victimization of personnel in emergency departments. *Journal of Emergency Nursing, 25*(5), 361–366.

McMahon, M. M. (2003). ED triage: Is a five-level triage system best? *American Journal of Nursing, 103*(3), 61–63.

Moon, M. D., & Galvan, T. J. (2000). Management of a 36 year old man with a pit viper envenomation. *Journal of Emergency Nursing, 26*(2), 108–112.

Moskowitz, H., Griffith, J. L., DiScala, C., & Sege, R. D. (2001). Serious injuries and deaths of adolescent girls resulting from interpersonal violence: Characteristics and trends from the United States, 1989–1998. *Archives of Pediatrics and Adolescent Medicine, 155*(8), 903–908.

Mulryan, K., Cathers, P., & Fagin, A. (2000). Protecting the child. *Nursing 2000, 30*(7), 39–43.

Murphy, J. V., Banwell, P. E., Roberts, A. H., & McGrouther, D. A. (2000). Frostbite: Pathogenesis and treatment. *Journal of Trauma, 48*(1), 171–178.

Nayduch, D. A. (1999). Trauma wound management. *Nursing Clinics of North America, 34*(4), 895–906.

O'Brien, C. (1997). Improved forensic documentation of genital injuries with colposcopy. *Journal of Emergency Nursing, 23*(5), 461–462.

O'Brien, C. (1998). Light staining microscope: Clinical experience in a sexual assault nurse examiner (SANE) program. *Journal of Emergency Nursing, 24*(1), 95–97.

Pakieser, R. A., Lenaghan, P. A., & Muelleman, R. L. (1998). Battered women: Where they go for help. *Journal of Emergency Nursing, 24*(1), 16–19.

Powell, A. H. (1999). Alcohol withdrawal in critical care. *Dimensions of Critical Care Nursing, 18*(6), 24–28.

Project Team of the Resuscitation Council. (2001). Update on the emergency medical treatment of anaphylactic reactions for the first medical responders and for community areas. *Emergency Medicine Journal, 18*(5), 393–395.

Pudalek, B. (2002). Geriatric trauma: Special needs for a special population. *AACN Clinical Issues, 13*(1), 61–72.

Ringland, R., & Early, S. (1997). Conscious sedation: Documenting the procedure. *Journal of Emergency Nursing, 23*(6), 611–617.

Rintamaki, H. (2000). Predisposing factors and prevention of frostbite. *International Journal of Circumpolar Health, 59*(2), 114–121.

Ritchie, E. C. (1998). Reactions to rape: A military forensic psychiatrist's perspective. *Military Medicine, 163*(8), 505–509.

Rogers, F. B., Osler, T. M., Shackford, S. R., Morrow, P. L., Sartorelli, K. H., Camp, L., Healey, M. A., & Martin, F. (2001). A population-based study of geriatric trauma in a rural state. *Journal of Trauma, 50*(5), 604–611.

Sachdeva, R. C. (1999). Near drowning. *Critical Care Clinics, 15*(2), 281–289.

Selig, C. (2000). Sexual assault nurse examiner and sexual assault response team (SANE/SART) program. *Nursing Clinics of North America, 35*(2), 311–319.

Somerson, J. J., Husted, C. W., Somerson, S. W., & Sicilia, M. R. (1996). Mastering emergency airway management. *American Journal of Nursing, 96*(5), 24–30.

Stamatos, C. A. (1994). Geriatric trauma patients: Initial assessment and management of shock. *Journal of Trauma Nursing, 1*(2), 45–56.

Sterling, D. A., O'Connor, J. A., & Bonadies, J. (2001). Geriatric falls: Injury severity is high and disproportionate to mechanism. *Journal of Trauma, 50*(1), 116–119.

Suominen, P., Baillie, C., Korpela, R., Rautanen, S., Ranta, S., & Olkkola, K. T. (2002). Impact of age, submersion time, and water temperature on outcome in near-drowning. *Resuscitation, 52*(3), 247–254.

Swanson, E. R., Seaberg, D. C., & Mathias, S. (1996). The use of propofol in the emergency department. *Academic Emergency Medicine 3*(3), 234–238.

Terriff, C. M., & Tee, A. M. (2001). Citywide pharmaceutical preparation for bioterrorism. *American Journal of Health-System Pharmacy, 58*(3), 233–237.

Thanel, F. (1998). Near drowning: Rescuing patients through education as well as treatment. *Postgraduate Medicine, 103*(6), 141–144, 149–153.

The Canadian Encyclopedia Online. (2005). Available at: http://www.thecanadianencyclopedia.com.

Thurlow, K. L. (2001). Latex allergies: Management and clinical responsibilities. *Home Healthcare Nurse, 19*(6), 369–375.

Tumbarello, C. (1998). Ultrasound evaluation of abdominal trauma in the emergency department. *Journal of Trauma Nursing, 5*(3), 67–72.

Vernon, D. D., & Gleich, M. C. (1997). Poisoning and drug overdose. *Critical Care Clinics, 13*(3), 646–677.

Verzosa, J. D. (1997). Methemoglobinemia: Cyanosis and street methamphetamines. *Journal of the American Board of Family Practice, 10*(2), 137–140.

Weesner, B. W., Jr. (1997). Latex allergies and adverse reactions: A review of the literature. *Journal of the Tennessee Dental Association, 77*(2), 21–26.

White, G. L., Stewart, J. S., & Murdock, R. T. (2001). Hymenoptera stings: Treatment and prevention. *Physician Assistant, 25*(2), 15–24.

Wright, J. A. (1997). Seven abdominal assessment signs every emergency nurse should know. *Journal of Emergency Nursing, 23*(5), 446–450.

Young, P. A., & Kendall, J. M. (2001). Sedation for children requiring wound repair: A randomized controlled double blind comparison of oral midazolam and oral ketamine. *Emergency Medicine Journal, 18*(1), 30–33.

Zametkin, A. J., Alter, M. R., & Yemini, T. (2001). Suicide in teenagers: Assessment, management, and prevention. *Journal of the American Medical Association, 286*(24), 3120–3125.

Zook, R. (2001). Developing a crisis response team. *Journal for Nurses in Staff Development, 17*(3), 125–130.

RESOURCES AND WEBSITES

American Heart Association, 4217 Park Place Ct., Glen Allen, VA, 23060; (804) 747-8334; http://www.americanheart.org.

Centers for Disease Control and Prevention, 1600 Clifton Road, NE, Atlanta, GA 30333; (404) 639-3311; http://www.cdc.gov.

Emergency Nurses Association, 915 Lee Street, Des Plaines, IL 60016-6560; (800) 900-9159; http://www.ena.org.

National Emergency Nurses' Affiliation; http://www.nena.ca.

Disaster, Mass Casualty, Epidemics/Pandemics, and Terrorism Nursing

Adapted by Rene A. Day, Cathy Giblin, and Eric Bone

LEARNING OBJECTIVES

On completion of this chapter, the learner will be able to:

1. Identify the necessary components of an emergency operations plan.

2. Discuss how triage in a disaster differs from triage in an emergency.

3. Develop a plan of care for a patient experiencing short- or long-term psychological effects after a disaster.

4. Describe conditions necessary for an influenza pandemic to occur.

5. Describe isolation precautions necessary for biological agents.

6. Evaluate the different levels of personal protection and decontamination procedures that may be necessary during an event involving mass casualties or weapons of mass destruction.

7. Identify the differences among the various chemical agents used in terrorist events, their effects, and the decontamination and treatment procedures that are necessary.

8. Determine the injuries associated with varying levels of radiation or chemical exposure and the associated decontamination processes.

The contemporary Canadian health care provider needs to be prepared to deal with mass casualties from natural disasters, radiation leaks or other industrial accidents, dangerous infectious diseases, terrorism, and biological warfare. Airplane crashes, train crashes, and toxic substance spillages are examples of manmade disasters that can result in casualties and tax the resources of health care organizations and their communities. Natural phenomena such as floods, tornadoes, fires, forest fires, blizzards, ice storms, earthquakes, hurricanes, and tsunamis result in deaths and injuries worldwide.

The possibility and reality of mass casualties associated with disasters, terrorism, and biological warfare are not new to human history; nor is the concept of using **weapons of mass destruction (WMDs).** The use of WMDs dates as far back as the 6th century BC for biological weapons and the year 436 BC for chemical weapons (U.S. Army Medical Research Institute of Infectious Disease, 1996; U.S. Army Medical Research Institute of Chemical Defense, 1999). However, geopolitical forces and interests, religious differences, the "shrinking globe," and the availability of destructive technology have brought the possibility of more terrorist events close to home. Examples include the bombing of subway trains and a double-decker bus in London (July 7, 2005); bombing of commuter trains in Spain (March 11, 2004); the nightclub bombing in Bali (October 12, 2002); the total destruction of the World Trade Center towers (New York) and the damage to the Pentagon (Washington, D.C.) (September 11, 2001); the release of anthrax in the United States in 2001; release of Saran nerve gas in Japan (March 19, 1995); and the 1993 bombing of the World Trade Center in New York City. Terrorism has become increasingly sophisticated, organized, and therefore effective. It is no longer a question of *whether* it will happen again, but *when* it will happen again. Canada is the one remaining country on a list of possible Al-Queda targets that has not yet been attacked.

Following the September 11, 2001 attacks, the United States government created the Department of Homeland Security to coordinate federal and state efforts to combat terrorist activity. In 2001–2002, all acute care facilities across the U.S. were asked to present detailed plans for their health departments on how they would handle situations involving weapons of mass destruction (WMDs).

Canadians expect that all levels of government (municipal, provincial/territorial, and federal) will protect them from health crises. The Canadian health care organizations must be prepared for any and all types of emergencies. The focus of this chapter is on emergency preparedness and the process of responding to disasters, mass casualties, epidemics/pandemics, and terrorism.

EMERGENCY PREPAREDNESS
Federal, Provincial/Territorial, and Local Responses

There are many resources available at the federal, provincial/territorial, and local levels to assist in the management of disasters and emergencies. Disasters are often assigned levels, which indicate the anticipated level of response (Chart 72-1). A list of the local resources with specific instructions about how and when to contact them should be readily available and frequently reviewed for needed updates. The following are a few of the resources that may be of assistance during a **mass casualty incident (MCI)** or a disaster.

FEDERAL AGENCIES

There are many federal resources that can be accessed through a process of requests. The provincial/territorial authorities must request the federalization of resources through the proper channels. This request for federal resources generally is made when local resources have become or are in the process of becoming depleted.

Federal resources include Health Canada, the Public Health Agency of Canada (PHAC), the Department of Public Safety and Emergency Preparedness Canada (PSEPC), and the Department of National Defense (DND)–Canadian Forces. See Chart 72-2.

Under the Public Health Agency of Canada is the Centre for Emergency Preparedness and Response (CEPR) that coordinates planning and response to national emergencies.

In 2004 the Department of Public Safety and Emergency Preparedness Canada (PSEPC) was created to fulfill the role of government in securing the public's safety and security. PSEPC administers the Joint Emergency Preparedness Program (JEPP). The goal of JEPP is to assist provincial/territorial governments to be prepared to respond to all types of emergencies in a national standardized way. Funds are available to support developmental activities.

DART (Disaster Assistance Response Team) can be deployed by Canadian Forces to provide medical care and to make large quantities of safe water. DART has recently been deployed following the tsunami in Southeast Asia (December 2004) and the earthquake in Pakistan (October 2005). The Office of Critical

Glossary

antigenic shift: a sudden change in the antigen or protein substances on the surface of a virus, usually as a result of genetic mutation.

biological warfare: use of a biological agent, such as anthrax, as a WMD

chemical warfare: use of a chemical agent, such as chlorine, as a WMD

decontamination: process of removing, or rendering harmless, contaminants that have accumulated on personnel, patients, and equipment

epidemic: an outbreak of a disease or illness that spreads rapidly throughout a segment of a human population, affecting a signifi-

cantly large number of people at the same time.

mass casualty incident (MCI): situation in which the number of casualties exceeds the number of resources

nuclear warfare: use of nuclear contamination as a WMD

pandemic: outbreak of a disease over a wide geographic area or worldwide, and affecting an exceptionally high proportion of the population.

personal protective equipment (PPE): equipment beyond standard precautions; may include level A, B, C, and D equipment.

vaccination: any injection of attenuated or killed microorganisms given to induce immunity or to reduce the effects of associated infectious diseases.

vaccine: a suspension of attenuated or killed microorganisms administered orally or by injection to induce active immunity to infectious agents.

weapons of mass destruction (WMDs): weapons used to cause widespread death and destruction

Chart 72-1 Disaster Levels

Disasters are often classified by the resultant anticipated necessary response:

Level I: Local emergency response personnel and organizations can contain and effectively manage the disaster and its aftermath.

Level II: Regional efforts and aid from surrounding communities are sufficient to manage the effects of the disaster.

Level III: Local and regional assets are overwhelmed; provincial/territorial or federal assistance is required.

Infrastructure Protection and Emergency Procedures (OCIPEP) under PCEPC helps civilian authorities and others handle crises by providing assistance and advice during emergencies.

Health Canada takes the lead role in managing the Federal Nuclear Emergency Plan (FNEP). The Plan includes:

- Accidents at Canadian nuclear facilities, those on the Canadian/American border, and facilities outside of Canada
- Accidents in nuclear-powered vessels in Canadian waters
- Other events related to the uncontrolled release of radioactivity

PROVINCIAL/TERRITORIAL AND LOCAL AGENCIES

An example at the provincial level is Emergency Management Alberta, which works with municipalities, First Nations, and industry to develop plans of how to respond to emergencies or disasters and then how to recover from these situations (Emergency Management Alberta, 2005).

Chart 72-2 Federal Agencies

Health Canada
  Public Health Agency of Canada (PHAC)
    Centre for Emergency Preparedness and Response (CEPR)
      Office of Emergency Preparedness, Planning, and Training
      Office of Emergency Response Services (OERS)
        National Emergency Stockpile System (NESS)
      Emergency Social Services (ESS)
        Registration and Inquiry Services
        Emergency Clothing Service
        Emergency Lodging Service
        Personal Services
        Emergency Food Services
        Reception Centre Service
      Global Public Health Intelligence Network (GPHIN)
    Canadian Science Centre for Human and Animal Health
      National Microbiology Laboratory
    Canadian Bioterrorism Lab Response Network
  Federal Nuclear Emergency Plan (FNEP)
Public Safety and Emergency Preparedness Canada (PSEPC)
  Office of Critical Infrastructure Protection and Emergency Preparedness (OCIPEP)
  Joint Emergency Preparedness Program (JEPP)
  Canadian Emergency Preparedness College (CEPC)
  National Exercise Program (NEP)
Department of National Defense (DND)
  Canadian Forces
    Disaster Assistance Response Team (DART)

Its role includes:

- Coordinating a provincial response to a major emergency or disaster
- Working with the federal government plans
- Developing and maintaining standards for disaster services training
- Managing disaster recovery programs
- Assisting provincial government departments to ensure they have plans to sustain continuity of programs and services during and following a disaster
- Coordinating and directing counter-terrorism plans and preparedness

Within communities, existing social service agencies are responsible for developing the Emergency Social Services (ESS) planning. Agencies such as municipal and provincial departments of social services, public health, mental health, family and children's services, service clubs, church groups, and business and professional associations are involved. ESS is a planned response that provides six basic services for the well-being of individuals and families during a disaster (see Chart 72-1). Other resources may include the Canadian Red Cross, poison control centres, and other local volunteers.

THE INCIDENT COMMAND SYSTEM

The Incident Command System (ICS) is a management tool for organizing personnel, facilities, equipment, and communication for any emergency situation. For example, in Alberta, Capital Health (a large health region that includes Edmonton) is moving toward an Incident Command System. This is a structure with well-defined roles and responsibilities that other agencies recognize. The goal is to maximize use of limited resources and monitor the length of time to respond (Hill, 2005). Under this structure, one person is designated as incident commander. This person must be continuously informed of all activities and informed about any deviation from the established plan (Currance & Bronstein, 1999; Lewis & Aghababian, 1996; Londorf, 1995). Whereas the ICS is primarily a field structure and process, aspects of it are used at the level of an individual hospital's or health care organization's emergency response plan as well.

Health Care Emergency Preparedness Plans

Health care organizations are required by the Canadian Council on Health Services Accreditation (CCHSA) to create and test a plan for emergency preparedness. Generally, health care organizations develop and test emergency preparedness plans through the oversight of a senior administrator and/or Emergency Preparedness Officer.

Before the basic emergency operations plan (EOP) can be developed, the planning committee of the organization first evaluates the community to anticipate the types of natural and manmade disasters that might occur. This information can be gathered by questioning local law enforcement and fire departments and assessing the amount of air or train traffic, automobile traffic, transportation of dangerous goods by truck or train, and flood, earthquake, tornado, blizzard, or hurricane activity. Consideration is given to special situations such as proximity to chemical plants, oil refineries, nuclear facilities, or military bases that may enhance the community's potential for manmade disasters. Federal, judicial, or financial buildings, schools, and any places where large groups of people gather can be considered high-risk areas.

Based on the needs assessment, the planning committee must identify what supplies are necessary. A stockpile of drugs should include the top 10 critical medications used during normal day-to-day operations, those that might be required in a disaster or MCI, and those necessary for treating specific biological and chemical agents such as antibiotics and cyanide kits (Anteau, 1997; Stopford, 2000). Another scenario that might be anticipated is the dispersal of a pulmonary intoxicant or choking agent. This requires the planners to find out the numbers and types of personal protective equipment (PPE) required and available to protect health care providers as well as how many ventilators would be available for patients within the organization and in the community. The committee might also outline how staff within an organization would triage and assign priority to patients when the number of ventilators is limited. Information should be available about local resources for stocking and restocking any of the basic and special supplies, how those supplies are requested, and the time required to receive those supplies. Food and water also need to be stockpiled for use by staff, patients' families, and others who may be at health care facilities for an extended period. Multiple factors influence an organization's ability to respond effectively to a sudden influx of injured patients, and the committee must anticipate various scenarios to improve its preparedness.

COMPONENTS OF EMERGENCY OPERATIONS PLAN

Once the initial assessment is complete, the facility develops the EOP. Essential components of the plan are as follows:

- *An activation response:* The EOP activation response of a health care facility or organization should define where, how, and when the response is initiated.
- *An internal/external communication plan:* Communication is critical for all parties involved, including communication to and from the prehospital arena (Heightman, 1999; Lewis & Aghababian, 1996; Mickelson, Burno, & Schario, 1999).
- *A plan for coordinated patient care:* A response is planned for coordinated patient care into and out of the facility, including transfers to other facilities. The site of the disaster can determine where the greater number of patients may self-refer. (For example, in the Edmonton Tornado in 1987, the wounded from a badly damaged trailer park began arriving at a hospital for persons with mental illnesses [the nearest facility] before the institution even knew there was a disaster.)
- *Security plans:* A coordinated security plan involving facility or organization and community agencies is key to the control of an otherwise chaotic situation.
- *Identification of external resources:* External resources are identified, including local, provincial/territorial, and federal resources and information about how to activate these resources.
- *A plan for people management and traffic flow:* "People management" includes strategies to manage the patients, the public, the media, and personnel. Specific areas are assigned, and a designated person is delegated to manage each of these areas (Anteau, 1997; Lewis & Aghababian, 1996).
- *A data management strategy:* A data management plan for every aspect of the disaster will save time at every step. If a computerized system is used for charting, tracking, and staffing, a backup system is necessary.

- *Deactivation response:* Deactivation of the response is as important as activation; resources should not be overused. The person who decides when the facility is able to go from the disaster response back to daily activities is clearly identified. Any possible residual effects of a disaster must be considered before this decision is made (Anteau, 1997).
- *A post-incident response:* Post-incident response must include a critique and a debriefing for all parties involved, immediately and again at a later date. Often facilities see increased volumes of patients up to 3 months after an incident.
- *A plan for practice drills:* Practice drills that include community participation allow for troubleshooting any issues before a real-life incident occurs. Similar experiences can be used to prepare health care personnel to respond to a variety of patient care situations both in a health care facility and at a disaster site.
- *Mass casualty incident planning:* MCI planning includes such issues as mass fatality and morgue readiness.
- *An educational plan for all of the above:* A strong educational plan for all personnel regarding each step of the plan allows for improved readiness and additional input for fine-tuning of the EOP (Howard, 2001; Kotzmann, 1999; Anteau, 1997; Burgess et al., 1999; Lewis & Aghababian, 1996; Heightman, 2000; Levitin & Siegelson, 1996).

The EOP should also include a structure that defines roles for all employees in each emergency situation. The most common structure is the ICS described earlier, but applied at the level of the health care organization itself instead of at the site of the disaster. For example, an administrator, possibly the nurse executive, will act as Incident Commander and coordinate all aspects of the implementation of the plan. Other personnel will be designated to perform key roles, such as resource manager or patient disposition coordinator. Such a predetermined organization is essential to minimize confusion, ensure that all key operations are directed, and promote a well-coordinated response.

INITIATING THE EMERGENCY OPERATIONS PLAN

Notification of a disaster situation to a health care organization varies with each situation. Generally, the notification to the organization comes from outside sources unless the initial incident occurred at the facility. The disaster activation plan should clearly state how the EOP is to be initiated. If communication is functioning, field incident command will give notice of the approximate number of arriving patients, although the number of self-referring patients will not be known.

Identifying Patients and Documenting Patient Information

Patient tracking is a critical component of casualty management. Disaster tags, which are numbered and include triage priority, name, address, age, location and description of injuries, and treatments or medications given, are used to communicate patient information. The tag should be securely placed on the patient and remain with the patient at all times. The tag number and the patient's name are recorded in a disaster log. The log is used by the command centre to track patients, assign beds, and provide families with information.

Triage

Triage is the sorting of casualties to determine priority of health care needs and the proper site for treatment. In nondisaster situations, health care workers assign a high priority and allocate the most resources to those who are the most critically ill. For example, a young man who has a chest injury and is in full cardiac arrest would receive advanced cardiopulmonary resuscitation, including medications, chest tubes, intravenous fluids, blood, possibly even emergency surgery in an effort to restore life. The Canadian Triage and Acuity Scale (CTAS) is a tool used in emergency departments to triage (rank) patients based on the seriousness of presenting signs and symptoms to be sure that the sickest patients are seen first, and that patients are reassessed during their time in an emergency department. The scale includes triage levels, time to nurse and physician assessment, usual presentation of the patient, and a sentinel diagnosis. The time from arrival to assessment is an objective and does not necessarily represent standards of care. All Canadian hospital emergency departments are mandated to determine the triage level by using the CTAS criteria for each patient seen and report the information to the Canadian Institutes for Health Information. Examples from the CTAS are in Table 72-1. In a disaster, however, when health care providers are faced with a large number of casualties, the fundamental principle guiding resource allocation is to do the greatest good for the greatest number of people. Decisions are based on the likelihood of survival and consumption of available resources. Therefore, this same patient, and others with conditions associated with a high mortality rate, would be assigned a low triage priority in a disaster situation, even if the person is conscious. Although this may sound uncaring, from an ethical standpoint the expenditure of limited resources on individuals with a low chance of survival, and denial of those resources to others with serious but treatable conditions, cannot be justified.

TRIAGE CATEGORIES IN DISASTER SITUATIONS

At the disaster site, Simple Triage & Rapid Treatment (START) is an organized approach that first responders such as fire/rescue squads, school and industrial safety personnel, or medical professionals can use in an emergency situation. Also available is a Multiple Victim Incident (MVI) Plan that prepares responders to improve the medical management of patients through knowledge of field management, organization, communication, and documentation. The MVI has a relationship with an Incident Command System and can accommodate a mass casualty incident. Training packages are available for both the START approach (www.start-triage.com/START_TRIAGE.htm) and the MVI Plan (www.start-triage.com/MVI.htm).

The triage officer rapidly assesses those injured at the disaster scene. Victims are immediately tagged and transported or given life-saving interventions. One person performs the initial triage while other emergency services personnel perform life-saving measures (eg, intubation) and transport patients. Although emergency medical services personnel carry out initial field triage, secondary and continuous triage at all subsequent levels of care is essential.

Table 72-1 • **Examples from the Canadian Triage and Acuity Scale for Emergency Departments**

TRIAGE LEVEL	TIME TO ASSESSMENT	USUAL PRESENTATION	SENTINEL DIAGNOSIS
I—RESUSCITATION	IMMEDIATE (Nurse and Physician)	CODE/ARREST	Acute myocardial infarction with complications/ Congestive heart failure/Low blood pressure
		MAJOR TRAUMA	Pneumothorax—traumatic/tension
		ALTERED MENTAL STATUS (unconscious, delirious)	Head injury—major/unconscious
II—EMERGENT	IMMEDIATE (Nurse)	CHEMICAL EXPOSURE (eyes)	Alkaline/Caustic – ocular burns
	WITHIN 15 MINUTES (Physician)	MODERATE/ SEVERE DYSPNEA (difficulty breathing)	COPD, croup
		FEVER (age < 3 months, temp > 38° C [rectal])	Epiglottitis, meningitis, sepsis
III—URGENT	WITHIN 30 MINUTES (Nurse and Physician)	HEAD INJURY (alert, no vomiting)	Head injury
		SIGNS OF INFECTION	Pyelonephritis
		GI BLEED (normal vital signs)	GI bleed, no complications
IV—LESS URGENT	WITHIN 60 MINUTES (Nurse and Physician)	MINOR TRAUMA	Colles' fracture, ankle sprain
		ABDOMINAL PAIN (acute)	Appendicitis, cholecystitis
		ALLERGIC REACTION (minor)	Urticaria
V—NON URGENT	WITHIN 120 MINUTES (Nurse and Physician)	SORE THROAT (no respiratory symptoms)	Upper respiratory infection
		DIARRHEA (alone, no dehydration)	Gastroenteritis
		ABDOMINAL PAIN (chronic)	Constipation

Triage categories separate patients according to severity of injury and use a colour-coded tagging system so that the triage category is immediately obvious. There are several triage systems in use across the country, and every nurse should be aware of the system used by his or her facility and community. The North Atlantic Treaty Organization (NATO) triage system is one that is widely used and is presented here. It consists of four colours—red, yellow, green, and black. Each colour signifies a different level of priority. Table 72-2 describes each category and gives examples of how different injuries would be classified. If the situation requires additional resources, provincial/territorial agencies are contacted (eg, Emergency Management Alberta) and, if necessary, the Centre for Emergency Preparedness and Response (CEPR) of the Public Health Agency of Canada can be contacted. The CEPR immediately sends out two field hospitals along with extra cots and bedding for shelters. These supplies along with medical supplies and medications are part of Canada's National Emergency Stockpile System (NESS). If needed, CEPR can send a field medical response team that can provide medical services, counselling, and mental health services (Centre for Emergency Preparedness and Response, 2001).

Managing Internal Problems

Staff should control all entrances to the acute care facility so that incoming patients are directed to the triage area first. The triage area may be outside the entry or just at the door of the ED. This allows all patients, including those arriving by medical transport and those who walk in, to be triaged. Some patients already seen in the field will be reclassified in the triage area, based on their current presentation.

Communicating With the Media and Family

Communication is a key component of disaster management. Communication within the vast team of disaster responders is paramount; however, effective, informative communication with the media and worried family members is also crucial.

MANAGING MEDIA REQUESTS FOR INFORMATION

Although the media have an obligation to report the news and can play a significant positive role in communication, the number of reporters, newscasters, and their support teams can be overwhelming, possibly compromising operations and patient confidentiality. A clearly defined process for managing the media, which includes a designated spokesperson, a site for the dissemination of information (away from patient care areas), and a regular schedule for providing updates should be part of the disaster plan.

Such a plan helps to prevent the release of contradictory or inaccurate information. Initial statements should focus on current efforts and what is being done to better understand the scope and impact of the situation. Information about casualties should not be released. Security staff should not allow media personnel access to patient care areas.

CARING FOR FAMILIES

Friends and family members converging on the scene must be cared for by the facility. They may be feeling intense anxiety, shock, or grief and should be provided with information and updates about their loved ones as soon as possible and regularly thereafter. There is often a need to "see" the loved one and this should be permitted, if possible. Ideally, family members and friends are in a designated area away from the triage and treatment area that is staffed by available social workers, counsellors, therapists, or clergy. Access to this area should be controlled to prevent families from being disturbed. See Chart 72-3 for a discussion of cultural variables to consider when coping with disaster-related injuries and death.

The Role of Nursing in Disaster Response Plans

The role of the nurse during a disaster varies. In rural or remote settings where there are few providers, the nurse may be asked to perform outside his or her area of expertise and may take on re-

Table 72-2 • Triage Categories			
TRIAGE CATEGORY	**PRIORITY**	**COLOUR**	**TYPICAL CONDITIONS**
Immediate: Injuries are life-threatening but survivable with minimal intervention. Individuals in this group can progress rapidly to expectant if treatment is delayed.	1	Red	Sucking chest wound, airway obstruction secondary to mechanical cause, shock, hemothorax, tension pneumothorax, asphyxia, unstable chest and abdominal wounds, incomplete amputations, open fractures of long bones, and 2nd/3rd degree burns of 15–40% total body surface area.
Delayed: Injuries are significant and require medical care, but can wait hours without threat to life or limb. Individuals in this group receive treatment only after immediate casualties are treated.	2	Yellow	Stable abdominal wounds without evidence of significant hemorrhage; soft tissue injuries; maxillofacial wounds without airway compromise; vascular injuries with adequate collateral circulation; genitourinary tract disruption; fractures requiring open reduction, débridement, and external fixation; most eye and CNS injuries.
Minimal: Injuries are minor and treatment can be delayed hours to days. Individuals in this group should be moved away from the main triage area.	3	Green	Upper extremity fractures, minor burns, sprains, small lacerations without significant bleeding, behavioural disorders or psychological disturbances.
Expectant: Injuries are extensive and chances of survival are unlikely even with definitive care. Persons in this group should be separated from other casualties, but not abandoned. Comfort measures should be provided when possible	4	Black	Unresponsive patients with penetrating head wounds, high spinal cord injuries, wounds involving multiple anatomical sites and organs, 2nd/3rd degree burns in excess of 60% of body surface area, seizures or vomiting within 24 hr after radiation exposure, profound shock with multiple injuries, agonal respirations; no pulse, no BP, pupils fixed and dilated.

Chart 72-3 Cultural Considerations

Any disaster or mass casualty incident can be expected to involve members of diverse religious and ethnic groups or may be targeted at and predominately affect a specific religious or ethnic group. Health care providers likewise include members of all religious and ethnic backgrounds and should bear in mind that victims may have

- Language difficulties that increase fears and frustrations
- Specific religious practices related to medical treatment, hygiene, or diet
- Specific places/times for prayer
- Rituals about handling the dead
- Timing of funeral services

Some religious communities have plans for emergencies and disasters, and organizations should integrate these plans to the extent possible into their emergency operations plans.

Chart 72-4 Caring for Persons with Disabilities During a Disaster

When disaster occurs, the multiple agencies involved attempt to provide food, water, and shelter to all of those affected. People with disabilities have specific needs that require attention. It is recommended that persons with disabilities have a personal support network to check on them after a disaster and to assist them with any needs. Organizations need to be aware that service animals are also affected during a disaster and may be brought to shelters with their companions.

Evacuation assistance is imperative for those with disabilities. Directions to personal equipment (eg, communication devices, medications, oxygen) should be available to rescue personnel. In a rapid evacuation, mobility devices, oxygen, suction, and medications will be needed at the shelters. Persons skilled in sign language are also valuable resources during a disaster. On their website, the American Red Cross provides a handbook for disaster preparedness for people with disabilities: http://www.redcross.org/services/disaster/beprepared/disability.html.

sponsibilities normally held by physicians or advanced practice nurses. For example, a critical care nurse may intubate a patient or even insert chest tubes. Wound débridement or suturing may be performed by staff registered nurses. A nurse may serve as the triage officer.

Although the exact role of a nurse in disaster management depends on the specific needs of the facility at the time, it should be clear which nurse or physician is in charge of a given patient care area and which procedures each individual nurse may or may not perform. Assistance can be obtained through the incident command centre, and nonmedical personnel can provide services where possible. For example, where appropriate, family members can provide nonskilled interventions for their loved ones. Nurses should remember that nursing care in a disaster focuses on essential care from a perspective of what is best for all patients.

New settings and atypical roles for nurses arise during a disaster: the nurse may provide shelter care in a temporary housing area, or bereavement support and assistance with identification of deceased loved ones. Individuals may require crisis intervention, or the nurse may participate in counselling other staff members and in critical incident stress management (CISM). At-risk populations may also require special considerations during a disaster (Chart 72-4).

CONSIDERING ETHICAL CONFLICTS

Disasters represent a disparity between the resources of the health care organization and the needs of the victims. This generates ethical dilemmas for the nurses and other providers of care. Issues include conflicts related to

- Rationing care
- Futile therapy
- Consent
- Duty
- Confidentiality
- Resuscitation
- Assisted suicide

Nurses may find it difficult to not provide medical care to the dying, or to withhold information to avoid spreading fear and panic. Clinical scenarios that are unimaginable in normal circumstances, confront the nurse in extreme instances. Other ethical dilemmas may arise out of health care providers' instinct for self-protection and protection of their families. For example, what should a pregnant nurse do when incoming disaster victims have been exposed to radiation, yet too few nurses are available?

Nurses can plan for the ethical dilemmas they will face during disasters by establishing a framework for evaluating ethical questions before they arise and by identifying and exploring possible responses to difficult clinical situations. They can refer to the *Code of Ethics for Registered Nurses* (Canadian Nurses Association, 2002). (See Chapter 3.) They can consider how the fundamental ethical principles of utilitarianism, beneficence, and justice will influence their decisions and care in disaster response.

MANAGING BEHAVIOURAL ISSUES

Although most people pull together and function during a disaster, both individuals and communities suffer immediate and sometimes long-term psychological trauma. Common responses to disaster include

- Depression
- Anxiety
- Somatization (fatigue, general malaise, headaches, gastrointestinal disturbances, skin rashes)
- Posttraumatic stress disorder
- Substance abuse
- Interpersonal conflicts
- Impaired performance

Factors that influence an individual's response to disaster include the degree and nature of the exposure to the disaster, loss of friends and loved ones, existing coping strategies, available resources and support, and the personal meaning attached to the event. Other factors, such as loss of home and valued possessions, extended exposure to danger, and exposure to toxic contamination, also influence response and increase the risk of adjustment problems. Those exposed to the dead and injured, eyewitnesses and those endangered by the event, the elderly, children, emergency first-responders, and medical personnel caring for victims are considered to be at higher risk for emotional sequelae.

Nurses can assist disaster victims by providing active listening and emotional support, giving information, and referring patients to a therapist or social worker. Health care workers must refer individuals to mental health care services, because experience has shown that while few disaster victims seek these services, early intervention minimizes psychological consequences. Nurses can also discourage victims from subjecting themselves to repeated exposure to the event through media replays and news articles, and encourage them to return to normal activities and social roles when appropriate.

Critical Incident Stress Management (CISM)

CISM is an approach to preventing and treating the emotional trauma that can affect emergency responders and others as a consequence of their jobs and that can also occur to anyone involved in a disaster or MCI. Critical incident stress management is handled by CISM teams that are available to the OEM and health care organizations. All branches of emergency services have CISM teams, as do the military, health care organizations, and many industries (eg, airline industry).

Components of a management plan include education before an incident about critical incident stress and coping strategies; field support (ensuring that staff get adequate rest, food and fluids, and rotating work loads) during an incident; and defusings, debriefings, demobilization, and follow-up care after the incident.

Defusing is a process by which the individual receives education about recognition of stress reactions and management strategies for handling stress. Debriefing is a more complicated intervention; it involves a 2- to 3-hour process during which participants are asked about their emotional reactions to the incident, what symptoms they may be experiencing (eg, flashbacks, difficulty sleeping, intrusive thoughts), and other psychological ramifications. In follow-up, members of the CISM team contact the participants of a debriefing and schedule a follow-up meeting if necessary. People with ongoing stress reactions should be referred to mental health specialists, but this is not mandatory (Gans & Kennedy, 1996).

EMERGENCY DEBRIEFING

Just as planning for a disaster, or mass casualty incident is critical, debriefing after the event is equally important. Debriefing provides the opportunity to examine what went well and what went wrong. For example, in the days and weeks following Hurricane Katrina and Hurricane Rita in the United States (2005), television and print sources provided details of the lack of preparedness to respond to a major disaster. Offers to provide aid came from around the world, including third world countries.

An example of an Alberta natural disaster follows. A tornado hit a campground at Pine Lake Alberta at 1700 hours on a sunny summer weekend in 2000. Winds of 300 km/hr tossed cars, trailers, trees, and people into the air and some into the lake. Survivors immediately began searching and rescuing others; other survivors left the scene. The first responders were the RCMP (Royal Canadian Mounted Police) and emergency medical services (EMS) personnel. Other EMS units, the Shock Trauma Air Rescue Society (STARS) helicopter system, and the Red Deer Regional Hospital (RDH) were all notified. STARS immediately initiated their disaster plan, sent two helicopters, and updated the Red Deer Regional Hospital and large hospitals in Edmonton and Calgary. Meanwhile, the first responders set up a triage centre, a helipad, and a morgue.

Some patients were treated at nearby local hospitals. Stable "green" category patients (see Table 72-2) were evaluated and treated by EMS personnel at a local community centre. Others

with more serious injuries were sent to RDH. Once additional physicians arrived from Edmonton, a staging centre (like a mini emergency room) was established in an empty hangar at the Red Deer airport. There, patients received blood transfusions, reduction of fractures, intubations, and placement of chest tubes. RDH activated its emergency plan and expected a large number of category "red" or "yellow" patients. One hospital in Calgary and two in Edmonton implemented full disaster plans. By the end of the first night, over 130 people were injured and nine were dead. Three more victims died of their injuries in ICUs. Most injuries were from blunt trauma to the head, torso, and extremities. Critical incident stress debriefing was offered to rescue workers and personnel.

What went wrong:

- The disaster response grew out of control with too many ambulances lined up trying to get into the campground, leaving surrounding communities without service.
- All phone communication failed between the disaster site and receiving hospitals. Although communication was sent via STARS, hospitals waited for other confirmation before acting. A mobile communication vehicle was needed.
- Regional receiving hospitals overreacted and fully activated their disaster plans rather than a staged response.

What went right:

- Survivors helped each other.
- The first STARS physician to arrive at the site became the "triage master."
- Physicians functioned well at the site and at the staging centre to complement EMS personnel.
- Patients were classified according to colour coding (see Table 72-2) and received treatment from appropriate personnel.
- Following changes due to regionalization, Red Deer Regional Hospital had recently revised its disaster plan.

PREPARING FOR EPIDEMICS/PANDEMICS

An **epidemic** means that the number of people with a disease in a specific geographical area is higher than usual (Valanis, 1992). Even one case of smallpox or polio in Canada would be an epidemic since it is believed that both diseases have been eradicated. The danger of smallpox has been eliminated worldwide and **vaccination** against the disease is no longer required. Canada was declared free of polio in 1977. This status has been achieved by an extensive program of immunization, and this level must be maintained to prevent polio from recurring.

A recent example of an epidemic was the outbreak of severe acute respiratory syndrome (SARS) that began in November 2002 in China, and by March 2003, had rapidly spread to Hong Kong, Singapore, Vietnam, Taiwan, Toronto, and other areas. Initially, there was a lack of information about cases of a novel form of atypical pneumonia in China in November/December 2002. The second problem was difficulty in determining the causative organism, which later was identified as a zoonosis caused by a different coronavirus. This organism is highly infectious by close contacts through airborne and droplet spread. It then took time to develop a laboratory test to confirm a diagnosis, and even when the test was available, it was not possible to get a rapid confirmation of disease in individuals in a pre-symptom or early stage of the disease.

Naylor, Chantler, and Griffiths (2004) identified what was learned from SARS outbreaks in Hong Kong and Toronto. The key findings included problems with capacity, preparedness, co-ordination, and communication (Chart 72-5). Despite the problems, public health and health care personnel accepted the challenge and contained the SARS outbreak.

Following the SARS epidemic, several researchers have examined the effects of the crisis on health care personnel. In a study of staff of a Toronto hospital that maintained high alert precautions but had few cases of SARS, nurses experienced a greater impact on morale and job satisfaction, depended more on peer support, felt less informed, and felt less involved in decision making than physicians. More nurses reported that infection control procedures were not strict enough (Tolomiczenko, Kahan, Ricci, et al., 2005). In a study in Hong Kong on work-related risk for nurses during the SARS outbreak, the importance of support systems and occupational health policies to promote nurse well-being during the outbreak were identified (Chan, Leung, Tiwari, et al., 2005). In Taiwan, three groups of nurses involved in the SARS outbreak were studied: those in low-risk areas (N = 45), on units with high risk of exposure to SARS (N = 65), and those conscripted to units with a high risk of exposure (N = 21). The level of stress among the nurses was moderate, but 11% were identified as having stress reaction syndrome (anxiety, depression, hostility, and somatization). Nurses working in high-risk units had the highest rate of stress reaction syndrome, but those nurses who were conscripted to high-risk areas experienced the most severe distress (Chen, Wu, Yang, et al., 2005). In Hong Kong, using a phenomenology approach, 10 nursing students were interviewed to examine perceptions of professional identity and the SARS outbreak. Three central themes emerged: appreciation and sharing of the nursing identity, a sense of moral duty and a change in their worldview, and feelings of self-growth (Heung, Wong, Kwong, et al., 2005).

Influenza

Influenza is an example of a disease that can occur as an epidemic or as a **pandemic**. Influenza is an acute viral disease of the respiratory tract. Major signs and symptoms include fever, sore muscles, rhinitis, cough, sore throat, headaches, and fatigue. After 2 to 3 days the individual's symptoms improve, although the cough and fatigue may persist for several weeks (Nicholson, 1998). The primary complications of influenza are bacterial pneumonia (which can be fatal) and viral pneumonia.

There are three types of influenza virus: Type A, Type B, and Type C. Type A occurs each year in humans, avians, and animals such as pigs and horses and can cause epidemics and pandemics. Type B also occurs each year, primarily in humans, but usually causes a milder illness. Type C has a more local distribution and may even be asymptomatic (Springhouse Corporation, 2001).

The influenza virus also contains the antigens haemogglutinin (with subtypes H1, H2, and H3) and neuraminidase (with subtypes N1 and N2). These antigens sit on the surface of the virus and are responsible for the virus's ability to change (**antigenic shift**). Antibodies produced against one subtype of antigen are ineffective against another subtype. This is the reason influenza occurs each year and that WHO recommends the influenza **vaccine** for each year is based on the previous year's virus and antigens as well as several current and new strains. The National Advisory Committee on Immunization Practices makes the final decision on the vaccine composition by taking into account Canadian data (Public Health Agency of Canada, 2005).

Influenza tends to occur as seasonal epidemics globally each year. It occurs between November and March in the northern hemisphere and May to September in the southern hemisphere (WHO, 1999). Those most affected by influenza are the very young, the elderly, and those with co-morbidities.

When influenza occurs worldwide, does not follow seasonal variations, occurs primarily in healthy adults 20 to 50 years old, and accounts for millions of deaths, it is considered a pandemic. Pandemics occur when the influenza virus has changed so dramatically, often through interactions with animal strains, that very few individuals have immunity.

HISTORY OF PANDEMIC INFLUENZA

One of the early pandemics occurred in 1918: Spanish flu (H1N1). The end result was up to 40 million deaths, with healthy adults between 20 and 50 years of age being most affected.

Chart 72-5 Key Findings Learned from SARS

Capacity
- Lack of investment in public health infrastructure and leadership
- Lack of acute hospital beds in single negative pressure rooms
- Lack of infection control areas in emergency departments
- Shortage of infection control personnel (80% of Canadian hospitals are unable to meet the Canadian Standard of one infection control practitioner for 175 acute care beds [Detsky & Naylor, 2003; Zoutman, Ford, Bryce, et al, 2003])

Preparedness
- Slow alert system in Canada
- No plan for an infectious disease outbreak
- Serious lack of knowledge of basic principles of infection control
- Deficiency in providing personal protection equipment
- Failure of surveillance, which allowed SARS cases to go undetected, leading to a secondary outbreak of SARS
- Lack of frontline preparedness
- Difficulties in mounting a large quarantine operation
- No international consensus on travel screening and border controls

Coordination
- Poor linkages between public health and health care systems
- Lack of agreement to share public health and clinical personnel, which led to shortage of specialized personnel in acute care institutions
- Lack of linkages between hospital and public health diagnostic laboratories
- Initial shutdown of all elective procedures at all 28 Toronto hospitals (which led to a massive backlog) followed by containing SARS cases to four hospitals

Communication
- Confused lines of authority among leaders for health care, public health, and general emergency response, which led to tensions and no single spokesperson
- Risk information to health care personnel and the public was uneven
- Nurses alerted officials of problems in containing the spread of SARS but were ignored
- Poor communication between Toronto, Hong Kong, and other centres prevented personnel from learning from each other (Naylor, Chantler, & Griffiths, 2004).

In 1957, the Asian flu (H2N2) pandemic occurred due to a dual infection with human and avian influenza. In North America, initial outbreaks affected children and young adults, with a second wave affecting adults older than 65 years of age. A vaccine was not ready until July 1957, so only 7 million were immunized. In total, over 1 million deaths occurred worldwide, primarily due to secondary bacterial pneumonia.

In 1968, the Hong Kong flu (H3N2) resulted in more than 1 million deaths worldwide, with those older than age 65 most affected. In 1997, Hong Kong reported the first known occurrences of transmission of avian flu (H5N1) from birds to humans. There were 18 cases and six deaths.

Concerns about a pandemic are rising because of an unprecedented increase in the number of countries with avian flu H5N1 in chickens (Hong Kong) and other poultry in Thailand, Vietnam, Cambodia, Indonesia, Russia, and Europe.

WHAT TO EXPECT

It is not a question of *if* an influenza pandemic will occur, it is a question of *when* it will occur. Influenza pandemics occur three to four times in a 100-year period. Once cases are reported, it will take from 1 to 5 months to reach a full-scale pandemic. There will be simultaneous outbreaks with multiple waves and up to 50% of populations will be clinically ill (including health care professionals). There will be severe shortages of vaccine, drugs, hospital beds, and ventilators. It will likely be at least 3 to 4 months before a vaccine is available. It is expected that two doses of the vaccine, 1 month apart, will be required. Health Canada will establish priority groups to receive the vaccine. Once the vaccine is available, vaccine administration will become the priority, taking health care workers away from direct care services. Issues will include finding additional personnel (eg, nursing students, nursing faculty members, and retired nurses) as well as space for vaccine administration.

POTENTIAL IMPACT

The potential of a pandemic impact in Alberta (2003 population was 3,134,337 [Health Surveillance. Alberta Health and Wellness, 2005]) includes the following (Hill, 2005):

- 0.5 to 1.3 million will be ill
- 264,000 to 617,000 will require outpatient care
- 5,600 to 13,000 will require hospitalization
- 1,100 to 2,600 deaths will occur
- Continuing intense media and public scrutiny
- Devastating societal impact

When estimating the potential impact on a health region compared to a usual influenza season, Capital Health (includes Edmonton and surrounding area) predicts the following (Hill, 2005):

- 3.7 to 7.4 times as many outpatient visits
- 3.9 to 6.9 times as many hospitalizations
- 8.2 to 20.3 times as many deaths

Economists are speculating that the global impact of an influenza pandemic could result in a situation similar to the Great Depression. "Travel would cease, transportation of goods and exports would stop, and tourism and hospitality sectors would disappear and financial panic would occur" (Branswell, 2005).

PANDEMIC PREPAREDNESS

The overall goals of planning for a pandemic are to minimize serious illness, the number of deaths, and the degree of societal disruption. Planning is occurring at federal, provincial/territorial, and local levels, and agreement has been reached to have a common committee structure and common planning assumptions. Included within the Operational Pandemic Plan are five committees: Surveillance, Vaccine and Antiviral, Health Services, Emergency Preparedness, and Communication.

At a regional level, Capital Health has undertaken the following activities (Hill, 2005):

- Completion of a community resources assessment
- Completion of a plan for Regional Pandemic Triage Centres
- Planning for vaccination centres
- Development of a regional nontraditional care site
- Identifying the requirements for a Regional Centralized Communication and Control Centre
- Planning for consolidation of health services

Next steps include a Tabletop Exercise to test the Pandemic Plan and a Triage Centre Pilot during the 2005–2006 flu season. Lessons learned from these activities will be used to update the Pandemic Plan.

Individual nurses can play a role in planning for a pandemic by

- Yearly flu vaccination and other self care
- Being flexible and prepared to do some things differently

Countries such as Canada and the United States are beginning to stockpile antivirals such as Tamiflu (oseltamivir), which is in pill form. With recent reports of a strain of avian flu that is resistant to Tamiflu, stockpiling of a second antiviral, Relenza (zanamivir), which is a powder that is inhaled, may be required. It is thought that antivirals may be useful to slow the spread of influenza during a pandemic until an effective vaccine can be developed.

Laboratories around the world are being pressured to increase production capabilities to keep up with current demands for the yearly flu vaccines and antivirals and to be ready to begin development and production of a vaccine once a pandemic begins.

DISASTER/EMERGENCY PREPAREDNESS

The Canadian Red Cross recommends preparing a plan, building a disaster kit, and getting trained in preparation for a possible disaster. The disaster kit consists of six basic categories of supplies for your home and vehicle: water, food, first aid supplies, tools/emergency supplies, clothing/bedding, and special items. The Red Cross disaster preparations are outlined on their web site (www.redcross.ca/prepare).

The Canadian Automobile Association, on their web site (www.caa.ca/english/automotive/auto%20tips/survival.html), recommends having emergency items in your vehicle and always having at least half a tank of gas.

NURSES AND INFLUENZA VACCINATION

In a study in British Columbia, 25% of health care workers were infected with influenza virus during the winter months, meaning they could pass the virus to others (Skowronski, Parker & Strang, 2000). Nurses are in a unique position: they can transmit the influenza virus to vulnerable patients through close personal contact and can influence patients and other health care personnel to be vaccinated or not. Nurses make up the largest group of health care providers and have been identified as being the most reluctant to be vaccinated against influenza (O'Rorke, Bourke, & Bedford, 2003). The National Advisory Committee on Immunization (NACI) in Canada reported in 2002 that influenza vaccination rates for health care personnel working in hospitals was 26%, whereas for those working in long-term care facilities the rate was 61%. Because most immunization programs for influenza aim for at least a 70% vaccination rate, the previous results are cause for concern (NACI, 2002).

As the possibility of an influenza pandemic increases, many health care facilities encourage staff participation by providing influenza vaccination on site. Slogan campaigns such as "Influenza doesn't work here—THE BUG STOPS HERE" may be useful (Capital Health and Caritas Health Group, 2005). Hospital visitors are alerted not to visit if they are feeling "under the weather."

Nursing students are encouraged to receive the influenza vaccination but are often required to do so if they will be working in long-term care or with other vulnerable patient populations. Their only alternative is to take antiviral medication for the duration of the clinical experience. It is hoped that the nursing students of today who are immunized as students will continue to receive influenza vaccination as graduates. There is an ethical element to this discussion as nurses should not be putting their patients at risk of contracting influenza.

Nursing students in parts of Canada are participating in giving influenza vaccination to health care personnel and to seniors. This practice has several benefits: students learn about the efficacy of the influenza vaccine and how immunity develops; they learn how to screen prospective participants; they gain practice in administering the vaccine as an intramuscular injection; and they provide health information postvaccination.

Government Agencies/Facilities

Canada has the first facility in the world where diseases in both humans and animals can be studied (also managed by the Public Health Agency of Canada). Located within the Canadian Centre for Human and Animal Health in Winnipeg is the National Microbiology Laboratory. This laboratory contains Canada's first biosafety Level 4 laboratories where scientists work with the most dangerous human and animal diseases and pathogens such as hepatitis and influenza, and hemorrhagic viruses such as Ebola and Lassa fever. These organisms are particularly dangerous as they are transmitted by air and there are no treatments or vaccines available. The National Microbiology Laboratories also contain laboratories for biosafety Levels 1, 2, and 3, each of which requires different levels of protection for workers depending on mode of transmission of the organisms. Security is vital; one system controls admission to the laboratories and another controls the biological safety of workers and the surrounding community. The Level 4 laboratory is central to the establishment of the new Canadian Bioterrorism Lab Response Network. This network of local and provincial/territorial laboratories across Canada will be capable of testing and identifying unknown agents. Canada also works closely with the Center for Disease Control in Atlanta, Georgia. In 2001, Canada helped to establish the Global Health Security Action Group (the United States, France, Germany, Italy, Japan, Mexico, the United Kingdom, and the European Union) to fight terrorism on an international level. In addition, CEPR manages the Global Public Health Intelligence Network (GPHIN). This network was developed in a partnership between Health Canada and the World Health Organization. GPHIN uses the World Wide Web to track events such as disease outbreaks, infectious diseases, contaminated food and water, bioterrorism, natural disasters, and issues related to the safety of products, drugs and medical devices (Public Health Agency of Canada, 2001). Information collected by CEPR, both in Canada and internationally, is used to update activities. "The result is a continuous effort to assess and be ready to act on threats to the

health and safety of Canadians" (Public Health Agency of Canada, 2001).

The Public Health Agency of Canada includes the following threats on their Emergency Preparedness web page: anthrax, botulism, viral hemorrhagic fevers, plague, smallpox, and ricin (www.phac-aspc.gc.ca/ep-mu/index.html). Other examples pertinent to Canada include brucellosis, cholera, Q fever, Venezuelan equine encephalitis, staphylococcal enterotoxin B, and mycotoxins.

PREPARING FOR TERRORISM
Recognition and Awareness

Being prepared for terrorism as a health care provider includes awareness of the potential for covert use of WMDs, self-protection, and early detection, containment, or decontamination of substances and agents that may affect others by secondary exposure. The strength of many toxins, today's mobile society, and long incubation periods for some substances can result in an epidemic that can quickly and silently spread across the entire country. For example, there must be awareness that the healthy person with a rapid onset of flu-like symptoms can have an ominous illness such as SARS (2002–2003) and as occurred with the anthrax exposures in 2001.

Health care personnel should have a heightened awareness for trends that may suggest the beginning of an epidemic/pandemic or a deliberate dispersal of toxic or infectious agents (Howard, 2001). The following are some general principles of awareness that should raise suspicion:

- Be aware of an unusual increase in the number of people seeking care for fever or respiratory or gastrointestinal complaints.
- Take note of an unusual illness for the time of year. Clusters of patients from a single location should raise suspicion. Clusters can be from a specific geographical location, such as a city, or from a single sporting or entertainment event.
- A large number of rapidly fatal cases should raise suspicion, especially when death occurs within 72 hours after hospital admission.
- Any increase in disease incidence in a normally healthy population should also raise suspicion. These cases should be reported to the local or provincial/territorial medical officer of health (Chettle, 2001).

An extensive patient history is taken in an attempt to identify the agent involved. This history includes an occupational, work, and environmental assessment in addition to the regular admission history. An exposure history contains, at a minimum, information about current and past exposures to possible hazards and an assessment of the patient's typical day and any deviations in routines. The work history includes, at a minimum, a description of all previous jobs, including short-term, seasonal, and part-time employment and any military service. The environmental history includes assessment of present and previous home locations, water supply, and any hobbies, to name a few factors. The admission history should include such information as recent travel and contact with others who have been ill or have recently died of a fatal illness. This is just a brief review of the extensive history that may need to be obtained to identify an exposure agent. This type of history should become a universal part of admission processes at all health care facilities (Agency for Toxic Substances and Disease Registry, 2000).

Suspicions or findings are reported to the appropriate resources in the facility and to proper authorities in the community. Resources can include the Infection Control Department, the local or provincial/territorial medical officer of health, the Public Health Agency of Canada, the local poison control centre, and many Internet sites (Chettle, 2001). Reporting furnishes data elements to those agencies responsible for epidemiology and response. Reporting also allows for sharing of information among facilities and jurisdictions and can help determine the source of infections or exposure and prevent further exposures and even deaths.

Personal Protective Equipment

Another component of preparedness and response involves the protection of the health care provider by additional **personal protective equipment (PPE)**. Chemical or biological agents and radiation are silent killers and are generally colourless and odourless. The purpose of PPE is to shield individuals from the chemical, physical, and biological hazards that may exist when caring for contaminated patients. The U.S. Environmental Protection Agency (EPA) has divided protective clothing and respiratory protection into four categories, level A through level D:

- Level A protection is worn when the highest level of respiratory, skin, eye, and mucous membrane protection is required. Briefly, this includes a self-contained breathing apparatus (SCBA) available in the prehospital arena. This also includes a fully encapsulating, vapor-tight, chemical-resistant suit with chemical-resistant gloves and boots.
- Level B is similar to level A and is selected when the situation requires the highest level of respiratory protection but a lesser level of skin and eye protection. This level of protection includes the SCBA and a chemical-resistant suit (Currance & Bronstein, 1999).
- Level C protection requires the air-purified respirator (APR), which uses filters or sorbent materials to remove harmful substances from the air. A chemical-resistant coverall with splash hood, chemical-resistant gloves, and boots are included in level C protection.
- Level D protection is basically the work uniform.

Level C and Level D PPE are the levels most often used in hospital facilities (Currance & Bronstein, 1999).

Protective equipment must be donned before contact with a contaminated patient. The acute care facility's standard precaution PPE (level D or C) generally is not adequate for protection from a contaminated patient. The health care provider must use equipment that is capable of providing protection against the agent involved. This may mean using a splash suit along with a full-face positive- or negative-pressure respirator (a filter-type gas mask) or even an SCBA for medical personnel in the field (Burgess et al., 1999; Currance & Bronstein, 1999).

No single combination of PPE is capable of protecting against all hazards. Under no circumstances should responders wear any PPE without proper training, practice, and fit testing of respirator masks as necessary. For example, since SARS (2002 to 2003), nursing students in Edmonton and surrounding areas must be fit tested for masks before beginning any acute care clinical placement.

Decontamination

Decontamination, the process of removing accumulated contaminants, is critical to the health and safety of health care providers by preventing secondary contamination. The decontamination plan should establish procedures and educate employees about decontamination procedures, identify the equipment needed and methods to be used, and establish methods for disposal of contaminated materials (Currance & Bronstein, 1999).

Although many principles and theories surround decontamination of a patient, authorities agree that, to be effective, decontamination must include a minimum of two steps. The first step is removal of the patient's clothing and jewelry and then rinsing the patient with water. Depending on the type of exposure, this step alone can remove a large amount of the contamination and decrease secondary contamination (Burgess et al., 1999). The second step consists of a thorough soap-and-water wash and rinse. When patients arrive at the facility from a prehospital provider, it should not be assumed that they have been thoroughly decontaminated.

WEAPONS OF TERROR
Biological Weapons

Biological weapons are weapons that spread disease among the general population or the military. Use of biological weapons dates far back into history, but improved production techniques and genetic engineering have expanded the potential for widespread casualties as a result of biological weaponry.

EFFECTS OF BIOLOGICAL WEAPONS

Biological warfare is a covert method of severely affecting the target. Overall, biological weapons are easily obtained and easily disseminated, and they result in significant mortality and morbidity. The potential use of biological agents calls for continuous increased surveillance by health care organizations and ministries of health and an increased index of suspicion by clinicians. Many biological weapons result in signs and symptoms similar to those of common disease processes.

Biological agents are delivered in either a liquid or dry state, applied to foods or water, or vaporized for inhalation or direct contact. Vaporization may be accomplished through spray or explosives loaded with the agent. With increased travel, an agent could be released in one city and affect people in other cities thousands of miles away. The vector can be an insect, animal, or person, or there may be direct contact with the agent itself.

The following is a discussion of two of the agents most likely to be used or weaponized. Table 72-3 describes other easily weaponized biological agents.

ANTHRAX

Bacillus anthracis is a naturally occurring gram-positive, encapsulated rod that lives in the soil in the spore state throughout the world. The bacterium sporulates (is liberated) when exposed to air and is infective only in the spore form. Contact with infected animal products (raw meat) or inhalation of the spores results in infection. Cattle and other herbivores are vaccinated against anthrax to prevent transmission through contaminated meat.

It is believed that approximately 8000 to 50,000 spores must be inhaled to put a person at risk. As an aerosol, anthrax is odourless and invisible and can travel a great distance before disseminating; hence, the site of release and the site of infection can be miles apart.

Anthrax is recognized as the most likely weaponized biological agent available. Anthrax has been known as a highly debilitating agent for centuries. It is believed that the plague in 1500 BC Egypt was caused by anthrax (Spencer, Whitman & Morton, 2001). In 1979, Sverdlosk, Russia, experienced the intentional release of

Table 72-3 • Examples of Biological Agents That Can Be Used as Weapons

AGENT/ORGANISM	CONTAGION	DECONTAMINATION AND PROTECTIVE EQUIPMENT	SIGNS AND SYMPTOMS	TREATMENT (MORTALITY RATE)
Tularemia—*Francisella tularensis:* gram-negative coccobacillus, one of the most infectious bacteria known	Direct contact with infected animals or aerosolized as a bioterror weapon; bites Not contagious through human-to-human contact	Standard barrier precautions Clothing and linens should be laundered under the usual hospital protocol	*Initial:* Abrupt onset of fever, fatigue, chills, headache, lower backache, malaise, rigour, coryza, dry cough, and sore throat without adenopathy. Nausea and vomiting or diarrhea possible. *As disease progresses:* Sweating, fever, progressive weakness, anorexia, and weight loss demonstrate continued illness. *Mortality secondary to:* pneumonitis (if inhalation is the source) with copious watery or purulent sputum, hemoptysis, respiratory insufficiency, sepsis, and shock.	Streptomycin or gentamicin/aminoglycoside for 10–14 days. Inhalation tularemia must be treated within 48 hours of onset. In mass casualty situations, doxycycline or ciprofloxacin is recommended. For persons exposed to tularemia, tetracycline or doxycycline is recommended for 14 days. (Mortality rate = 2%)
Botulism—*Clostridium botulinum:* Botulinum blocks acetylcholine-containing vesicles from fusing with the terminal membranes of the motor-neuron endplate, resulting in a flaccid paralysis.	Direct contact Not contagious through human-to-human contact	Any exposure to the botulism toxin can be treated with soap and water or a 0.1% hypochlorite solution. Standard precautions are used when treating patients with botulism.	*Gastrointestinal botulism:* abdominal cramps, nausea, vomiting, and diarrhea. *Inhalation botulism:* fever; symmetric descending flaccid paralysis with multiple cranial nerve palsies. Classic signs and symptoms include diplopia, dysphagia, dry mouth, lack of fever, and alert mental status. Other possible symptoms include ptosis of the eyelids, blurred vision, enlarged sluggish pupils, dysarthria, and dysphonia. *Mortality secondary to:* airway obstruction and inadequate tidal volume.	Supportive ventilatory therapy is necessary if respiratory infection occurs. Aminoglycosides and clindamycin are contraindicated because they exacerbate neuromuscular blockage. Equine antitoxin is used to minimize subsequent nerve damage. There is a 2% rate of anaphylaxis to the antitoxin; therefore, diphenhydramine (Benadryl) and epinephrine must be immediately available for use. Supportive care—mechanical ventilation, nutrition, fluids, prevention of complications (Mortality rate = 5%)
Plague—*Yersinia pestis:* nonsporulating gram-negative coccobacillus. The bacterium causes destruction and necrosis of the lymph nodes.	Contagious *Bubonic plague:* transmitted through flea bites with no person-to-person transmission *Pneumonic plague:* transmitted through respiratory droplet contact	Isolation barrier precautions with full face respirators. The patient should wear a mask. Rooms should receive a terminal cleaning. Clothing and linens with body fluids on them should be cleaned with the usual disinfectant. Routine precautions should be used in the case of death.	*Bubonic plague:* Sudden fever and chills, weakness, a swollen and tender lymph node (bubo) in the groin, axilla, or cervical area. The resultant bacteremia progresses to septicemia from the endotoxin and, finally, shock and death. *Primary septicemic plague:* Disseminated intravascular coagulopathy (DIC), necrosis of small vessels, purpura, and gangrene of the digits and nose (black death). *Pneumonic plague:* Severe bronchospasm, chest pain, dyspnea, cough, and hemoptysis. There is a 100% mortality associated with pneumonic plague if not treated within the first 24 hours.	Streptomycin or gentamicin for 10–14 days. Tetracycline or doxycycline is an acceptable alternative if an aminoglycoside cannot be given. People with close contact exposure (<2 meters) require prophylaxis with doxycycline for 7 days. (Mortality rate = 50%)

anthrax, with widespread mortality and morbidity. Anthrax was released with the sarin gas attack in Tokyo, Japan, in 1995; however, the method of release chosen was poorly designed for effect.

Anthrax is caused by replicating bacteria that release toxin resulting in hemorrhage, edema, and necrosis. The incubation period is from 1 to 6 days. There are three primary methods of infection: skin contact, inhalation, and gastrointestinal ingestion. Skin lesions (the most common infection) cause edema with pruritis and macule or papule formation resulting in ulceration with 1- to 3-mm vesicles. A painless eschar develops, which falls off in 1 to 2 weeks.

Ingestion of anthrax results in fever, nausea and vomiting, abdominal pain, bloody diarrhea, and occasionally ascites. If massive diarrhea develops, decreased intravascular volume becomes the primary treatment concern. The bacterium affects the terminal ileum and cecum. Sepsis can occur. Treatment is fluoroquinolones or tetracycline.

The inhalation form of anthrax is the most severe. Its symptoms mimic those of the flu, and usually treatment is sought only when the second stage of severe respiratory distress occurs. At this point, even antibiotic therapy will not halt the progress of the disease. The inhalation form can have an incubation period of up to 60 days, making it difficult to identify the source of the bacterium. Initial signs and symptoms include cough, headache, fever, vomiting, chills, weakness, mild chest discomfort, dyspnea, and syncope, without rhinorrhea or nasal congestion.

Most patients have a brief recovery period followed by the second stage within 1 to 3 days, characterized by fever, severe respiratory distress, stridor, hypoxia, cyanosis, diaphoresis, hypotension, and shock. These patients require optimization of oxygenation, correction of electrolyte imbalances, and ventilatory and hemodynamic support. More than 50% of these patients have hemorrhagic mediastinitis on chest x-ray (a hallmark sign) (Spencer, Whitman, & Morton 2001; Altman, 2002; Inglesby et al., 1999). The disease can also progress to include meningitis with subarachnoid hemorrhage. Death results in approximately 24 to 36 hours after the onset of severe respiratory distress. The mortality rate nears 100%.

Treatment. Presently anthrax is penicillin sensitive; however, the Russian government has been involved in the production of penicillin-resistant anthrax. Recommended treatment includes penicillin, erythromycin, chloramphenicol, gentamicin, or doxycycline. If antibiotic treatment begins within 24 hours after exposure, death can be prevented (Franz & Zajtchuk, 2000). In a mass casualty situation, ciprofloxacin or doxycycline is recommended. Treatment is continued for 60 days. For patients who have been directly exposed to anthrax but have no signs and symptoms of disease, ciprofloxacin or doxycycline is used for prophylaxis for 60 days.

When caring for a patient infected with anthrax, standard precautions are all that are necessary. The patient is not contagious, and the disease cannot be spread from person to person. Equipment should be cleaned using standard hospital disinfectant. After death, cremation is recommended because the spores can survive for decades and represent a threat to morticians and forensic medicine personnel.

SMALLPOX

Variola is classified as a DNA virus. It has an incubation period of approximately 12 days. It is extremely contagious and is spread by direct contact, contact with clothing or linens, or by droplets from person to person only after the fever has decreased and the rash phase has begun (Inglesby et al., 1999). There is an associated 30% case-fatality rate. Aerosolization of the virus would result in widespread dissemination. The World Health Organization (WHO) declared smallpox eradicated in 1977 and stopped worldwide vaccination in 1980. In Canada, the last children were vaccinated in the 1970s. Therefore, a large portion of the current population has no immunity to the virus. Recently, plans have been instituted in the U.S. for smallpox vaccination, with health care personnel being the first to receive the vaccine.

Smallpox was used as biowarfare during the French and Indian War in 1754–1767, when blankets from smallpox patients were sent into the Indian camps, resulting in greater than 50% fatality rates (Inglesby et al., 1999). Smallpox virus survives for up to 24 hours in cool temperatures and low humidity.

Signs and symptoms include high fever, malaise, headache, backache, and prostration. After 1 to 2 days, a maculopapular rash appears, evolving at the same rate and beginning on the face, mouth and pharynx, and forearms (Fig. 72-1). Only then does the rash progress to the trunk and also become vesicular to pustular (Inglesby et al., 1999; Hagstad, 2000; Franz & Zajtchuk, 2000). There is a large amount of the virus in the saliva and pustules. Smallpox (variola) is contagious only after the appearance of the rash. Variola major has a 30% case fatality rate. Hemorrhagic smallpox includes all of the above signs and symptoms with the addition of a dusky erythema and petechiae to frank hemorrhage of the skin and mucous membranes, resulting in death by day 5 or 6. Variola minor produces fewer constitutional symptoms and a sparse rash.

Treatment. Treatment includes supportive care with antibiotics for any additional infection. The patient must be isolated with the use of transmission precautions. Laundry and biological wastes should be autoclaved before being washed with hot water and bleach. Standard decontamination of the room is effective. All persons who have household or face-to-face contact with the patient after the fever begins should be vaccinated within 4 days

FIGURE 72-1 Comparison of progression of smallpox rash and chickenpox rash. From World Health Organization. (2001). WHO slide set on the diagnosis of smallpox. Reproduced by permission of the World Health Organization. Available at: http://www.who.int/emc/diseases/smallpox/slides/index.htm.

to prevent infection and death (Franz & Zajtchuk, 2000; Inglesby et al., 1999). A patient with a temperature of 38°C or higher within 17 days after exposure requires isolation. Postvaccination encephalitis occurs in approximately 1 of every 300,000 patients and has a 25% fatality rate. Cremation is preferred for all deaths, because the virus can survive in scabs for up to 13 years.

Chemical Weapons

Agents that may potentially be used in **chemical warfare** are overt agents in that the effects are more apparent and occur more quickly than those caused by biological weapons. Agents are available and well-known, result in major mortality and morbidity, and cause panic and social disruption. There are many agents, including those that affect nerves (sarin, soman, and tabun), those that affect blood (cyanide), those that are vesicants (lewisite, nitrogen and sulfur mustard, phosgene), heavy metals (arsenic, lead), volatile toxins (benzene, chloroform), pulmonary agents (chlorine), and corrosive acids (nitric acid, sulfuric acid) (Table 72-4). Chlorine, phosgene, and cyanide are widely used in industry and therefore are readily available.

CHARACTERISTICS OF CHEMICALS

Volatility. Volatility is the tendency for a chemical to become a vapor. The most volatile agents are phosgene and cyanide. Most chemicals are heavier than air, except for hydrogen cyanide. Therefore, in the presence of most chemicals, the victim should stand up to avoid heavy exposure (because the chemical will sink toward the floor or ground).

Persistence. Persistence means that the chemical is less likely to vaporize and disperse. More volatile chemicals do not evaporate very quickly. Most industrial chemicals are not very persistent. Weaponized agents (chemicals developed as weapons by the mil-

itary) are more likely than industrial chemicals to penetrate and cause secondary exposure as well.

Toxicity. Toxicity is the potential of an agent to cause injury to the body. The median lethal dose (LD50) is the amount of the chemical that will cause death in 50% of those who are exposed. The median effective dose (ED50) is the amount of the chemical that will cause signs and symptoms in 50% of those who are exposed. The concentration time (CT) is the concentration released multiplied by the time exposed (mg/min). For example, if 1000 mg of a chemical were released and the time of exposure to this amount of chemical was 10 minutes, then the concentration time would be 10,000 mg/min.

Latency. Latency is the time from absorption to the appearance of symptoms. Sulfur mustards and pulmonary agents have the longest latency, whereas vesicants, nerve agents, and cyanide produce symptoms within seconds.

LIMITING EXPOSURE

Evacuation is essential, as are removal of clothing and decontamination as close to the scene as possible and before transport of the person exposed. Soap and water are effective means of decontamination in most cases. Staff involved in decontamination efforts must wear PPE and contain the runoff after decontamination procedures.

VESICANTS

Vesicants are chemicals that cause blistering and result in burning, conjunctivitis, bronchitis, pneumonia, hematopoietic suppression, and death. Examples of vesicants include lewisite, phosgene, nitrogen mustard, and sulfur mustard. In World War I and in the Iran–Iraq conflict of 1980–1988, vesicants were used to disable the opponent. Vesicants were the primary incapacitating agents, resulting in minimal (less than 5%) death but large numbers of injured (Brennan, Waeckerle, Sharp, & Lillibridge, 1999). Liquid

Table 72-4 • **Common Chemical Agents**

AGENT	ACTION	SIGNS AND SYMPTOMS	DECONTAMINATION AND TREATMENT
Nerve Agents Sarin Soman organophosphates Tabun	Inhibition of cholinesterase	Increased secretions, gastrointestinal motility, diarrhea, bronchospasm	Soap and water Supportive care Benzodiazepine Pralidoxime Atropine
Blood Agent Cyanide and derived compounds (hydrocyanic acid, hydrogen cyanide, and cyanogen chloride)	Inhibition of aerobic metabolism	Inhalation—tachypnea, tachycardia, coma, seizures. Can progress to respiratory arrest, respiratory failure, cardiac arrest, death.	Sodium nitrite Sodium thiocyanate Amyl nitrate Hydroxycobalamin
Vesicant Agents Lewisite Sulfur mustard Nitrogen mustard Phosgene	Blistering agents	Superficial to partial-thickness burn with vesicles that coalesce	Soap and water Blot; do not rub dry
Pulmonary Agents Phosgene Chlorine	Separation of alveoli from capillary bed	Pulmonary edema, bronchospasm	Airway management Ventilatory support Bronchoscopy

sulfur mustard was the most frequently used vesicant in these conflicts. It is an oily liquid with a garlic odour, has a long latent period, and penetrates the skin if not rapidly removed. The skin damage is irreversible but is seldom fatal (2% to 3% mortality).

The initial presentation after exposure to a vesicant is similar to that of a large superficial to partial-thickness burn in the warm and moist areas of the body (ie, perineum, axillae, antecubital spaces). There is stinging and erythema for approximately 24 hours, followed by pruritus, painful burning, and small vesicle formation after 2 to 18 hours. These vesicles can coalesce into large, fluid-filled bullae. Lewisite and phosgene result in immediate pain after exposure. Tissue damage occurs within minutes.

If the eye is exposed, there is pain, photophobia, lacrimation, and decreased vision. This progresses to conjunctivitis, blepharospasm, corneal ulcer, and corneal edema.

Respiratory effects are more serious and often are the cause of mortality with vesicant exposure. Purulent fibrinous pseudomembrane discharge leads to obstruction of the airways. Gastrointestinal exposure includes nausea and vomiting, leukopenia, and upper gastrointestinal bleeding.

Appropriate decontamination includes soap and water. Scrubbing and the use of hypochlorite solutions should be avoided, because they increase penetration. Once the substance has penetrated, it cannot be removed. Eye exposure requires copious irrigation. For respiratory exposure, intubation and bronchoscopy to remove necrotic tissue are essential. With lewisite exposure, dimercaprol (BAL in oil) is administered intravenously for systemic toxicity and topically for skin lesions. All persons with sulfur mustard exposures should be monitored for 24 hours for delayed (latent) effects.

NERVE AGENTS

The most toxic agents in existence are the nerve agents such as sarin, soman, tabun, VX, and organophosphates (pesticides). They are inexpensive, effective in small quantities, and easily dispersed. In the liquid form, nerve agents evaporate into a colourless, odourless vapor. Organophosphates are similar in nature to the nerve agents used in warfare and are readily available. Nerve agents can be inhaled or absorbed percutaneously or subcutaneously. These agents bond with acetylcholinesterase, so that acetylcholine is not removed; the adverse result is continuous stimulation (hyperstimulation) of the nerve endings. Carbamates, which are insecticides originally extracted from the Calabar bean, are derivatives of carbamic acid; they are nerve agents that specifically inhibit acetylcholinesterase for several hours and then spontaneously become unbound from the acetylcholinesterase. Organophosphates, however, require the formation of new enzyme (acetylcholinesterase) before function can be restored.

A very small drop of agent is enough to result in sweating and twitching at the site of exposure. A larger amount results in more systemic symptoms. Effects can begin anywhere from 30 minutes up to 18 hours after exposure. The more common organophosphates and carbamates that are used in agriculture (sevin and malathion) result in less severe symptoms than do those used in warfare.

Signs and symptoms of nerve gas exposure are those of cholinergic crisis and include bilateral miosis, visual disturbances, increased gastrointestinal motility, nausea and vomiting, diarrhea, substernal spasm, indigestion, bradycardia and atrioventricular block, bronchoconstriction, laryngeal spasm, weakness, fasciculations, and incontinence. The patient must be examined in a dark area to truly identify miosis. Neurologic responses include insomnia, forgetfulness, impaired judgment, depression, and ir-

ritability. A lethal dose results in loss of consciousness, seizures, copious secretions, fasciculations, flaccid muscles, and apnea.

Decontamination with copious amounts of soap and water or saline solution for 8 to 20 minutes is essential. The water is blotted, not wiped, off. Fresh 0.5% hypochlorite solution can also be used. The airway is maintained, and suctioning is frequently required. One must be aware that plastic airway equipment will absorb sarin gas, resulting in continued exposure to the agent.

Treatment. Intravenous atropine 2 to 4 mg is administered, followed by 2 mg every 3 to 8 minutes for up to 24 hours of treatment. Alternatively, intravenous atropine 1 to 2 mg/hr may be administered until clear signs of anticholinergic activity have returned (decreased secretions, tachycardia, and decreased gastrointestinal motility). Another medication is pralidoxime; which allows cholinesterase to become active against acetylcholine. Pralidoxime 1 to 2 g in 100 to 150 mL of normal saline solution should be administered over 15 to 30 minutes. Pralidoxime has no effect on secretions and may have any of the following side effects: hypertension, tachycardia, weakness, dizziness, blurred vision, and diplopia.

Diazepam (Valium) or other benzodiazepines should be administered for seizures, to decrease fasciculations, and to alleviate apprehension and agitation. The military provides all military personnel with Mark I autoinjectors, which contain 2 mg atropine and 600 mg pralidoxime chloride. Diazepam is administered by a partner.

BLOOD AGENTS

Blood agents have a direct effect on cellular metabolism, resulting in asphyxiation through alterations in hemoglobin. Examples include hydrogen cyanide and cyanogen chloride. Cyanide is an agent that has profound systemic effects. It is commonly used in the mining of gold and silver and in the plastics and dye industries. In 1984, the Union Carbide pesticide plant in Bhopal, India, released large amounts of cyanide in an industrial disaster, and hundreds of deaths occurred.

A cyanide release is often associated with the odour of bitter almonds. In house fires, cyanide is released during the combustion of plastics, rugs, silk, furniture, and other construction materials. There is a significant correlation between blood cyanide and carbon monoxide levels in fire victims, and most often the cause of death is cyanide.

Cyanide can be ingested, inhaled, or absorbed through the skin and mucous membranes.

Cyanide is protein bound and inhibits aerobic metabolism, leading to respiratory muscle failure, respiratory arrest, cardiac arrest, and death. Inhalation of cyanide results in flushing, tachypnea, tachycardia, nonspecific neurologic symptoms, stupor, coma, and seizure preceding respiratory arrest.

Emergency Treatment. Rapid administration of the following medications is essential to the successful management of cyanide exposure: amyl nitrate, sodium nitrite, and sodium thiosulfate. First, the patient is intubated and placed on a ventilator. Next, amyl nitrate pearls are crushed and placed in the ventilator reservoir to induce methemoglobinemia. Cyanide has a 20% to 25% higher affinity for methemoglobin than it does for hemoglobin; it binds methemoglobin to form either cyanomethemoglobin or sulfmethemoglobin. The cyanomethemoglobin is then detoxified in the liver by the enzyme rhodanase. Next, sodium nitrite is administered intravenously, also to induce the rapid formation of methemoglobin. Sodium thiosulfate is then administered intravenously; it has a higher affinity for cyanide than methemoglobin does and stimulates the conversion of cyanide to sodium thiocyanate, which can be renally excreted. There are side effects of these emergency medications: sodium nitrite can result in severe hypotension, and thiocyanate can cause vomiting, psychosis, arthralgia, and myalgia.

The production of methemoglobin is contraindicated in patients with smoke inhalation, because they already have decreased oxygen-carrying capacity secondary to the carboxyhemoglobin produced by smoke inhalation. An alternative suggested treatment for cyanide poisoning is hydroxycobalamin (vitamin B_{12}a). Hydroxyocobalamin binds cyanide to form cyanocobalamin (vitamin B_{12}). It must be administered intravenously in large doses. Administration of vitamin B_{12}a can result in transient pink discolouration of mucous membranes, skin, and urine. In high doses, tachycardia and hypertension can occur, but they usually resolve within 48 hours.

PULMONARY AGENTS

Pulmonary agents such as phosgene and chlorine destroy the pulmonary membrane that separates the alveolus from the capillary bed. Hence, the person exposed cannot release carbon dioxide or acquire oxygen. Capillary leak results in fluid-filled alveoli. Phosgene and chlorine both vaporize, rapidly causing this pulmonary injury. Phosgene has the odour of fresh-mown hay.

Signs and symptoms include pulmonary edema with shortness of breath, especially during exertion. Cough starts as a hacking cough followed by frothy sputum production. A mask is the only protection required. Phosgene does not injure the eyes.

Nuclear Radiation Exposure

The threat of **nuclear warfare** or radiation exposure is very real with the availability of nuclear material and easily concealed simple devices, such as the so-called dirty bomb, for dispersal. A dirty bomb is a conventional explosive (eg, dynamite) that is packaged with radioactive material that scatters when the bomb is detonated. It disperses radioactive material and may be called a radiologic weapon, but is not a nuclear weapon, which is a complex nuclear fission reaction that is thousands of times more devastating than the dirty bomb.

Sources of radioactive material include not only nuclear weapons but reactors and simple radioactive samples, such as weapons-grade plutonium or uranium, freshly spent nuclear fuel, or medical supplies (eg, radium, certain cesium isotopes) used in cancer treatments and radiography machines. Exposure of a large number of people can be accomplished by placing a radioactive sample in a public place. Thousands may be exposed this way; some may be immediately affected, and others may require health monitoring for many years to assess long-term effects.

History has demonstrated the effectiveness of these weapons in the devastating results of the bombings of Hiroshima and Nagasaki in World War II. The effects of radiation exposure also were felt by the inhabitants of a small town in Brazil, who in 1987 found and opened a small canister of cesium 137 and rubbed the blue powder on themselves; 249 people were sickened, and 4 died (Jagminas & Suner, 2001). In 1983, a hospital sample was stolen in Mexico, resulting in the release of radioactive material among some scrap metal. A year later, the radiation contamination was detected when the scrap metal was inadvertently transported into the Los Alamos National Laboratory and triggered a Geiger counter.

On a larger scale, nuclear reactor incidents have occurred in the Chernobyl (1986) and Three Mile Island (1979) nuclear fa-

cilities. There were 31 official deaths on the day of the Chernobyl incident, which involved a core meltdown and explosion, releasing radiation throughout the community. The long-term effects of this incident, including increased incidence of thyroid cancers and leukemia, continue to be evaluated. Reactors, however, follow very strict security measures and protocols for prevention of core meltdown. These measures decrease the possibility of a radiation incident from a reactor.

TYPES OF RADIATION

Atoms consist of protons, neutrons, and electrons. The protons and neutrons are in balance in the nucleus. The protons repel each other, because they are all positively charged. The number of protons is specific for each element in the periodic table. There is a specific ratio of protons and neutrons for each different atom, and the result is element stability. When an element is radioactive, there is an imbalance in the nucleus resulting from an excess of neutrons.

To achieve stability, a radioactive nuclide can eject particles until the most stable number (an even number) of protons and neutrons exists. A proton can become a neutron by ejecting a positron; conversely, a neutron can become a proton by ejecting a negative electron. An alpha particle is released when two protons and two electrons are ejected.

Alpha particles cannot penetrate the skin. A thin layer of paper or clothing is all that is necessary to protect the skin from alpha-radiation. However, this low-level radiation can enter the body through inhalation, ingestion, or injection (open wound). Only localized damage will occur.

Beta particles have the ability to moderately penetrate the skin to the layer in which skin cells are being produced. This high-energy radiation can cause skin damage if the skin is exposed for a prolonged period and can cause injury if beta particles become internal by penetrating the skin.

Gamma-radiation is a short-wavelength electromagnetic energy that is emitted when there is excess core nucleus energy. Gamma particles are penetrating. It is difficult to shield against gamma-radiation. X-rays are an example of gamma-radiation. Gamma-radiation often accompanies both alpha- and beta-particle emissions.

MEASUREMENT AND DETECTION

Radiation is measured in several different units. The *rad* is the basic unit of measurement. A rad is equivalent to 0.01 joule of energy per kilogram of tissue. To determine the damaging effect of the rad, a conversion to the *rem* (Roentgen equivalent man) is necessary. The rem reflects the type of radiation absorbed and the potential for damage. For example, 200,000 mrem will result in mild radiation sickness (1 rem = 1000 millirem) (Jagminas & Suner, 2001). Typical natural yearly exposure for an individual is 360 mrem. Another important concept is *half-life*. The half-life of a radioactive product is the time it takes to lose one half of its radioactivity.

Radiation is invisible. The only means of detection is through a device that determines the exposure per minute. There are various devices for this purpose. The Geiger counter (or Geiger-Mueller survey meter) can measure background radiation quickly through detection of gamma- and some beta-radiation. With high-level radiation, the Geiger counter may underestimate exposure. Other devices include the ionization chamber survey meter, alpha monitors, and dose-rate meters. Personal dosimeters are simple tools to identify radiation exposure and are worn by radiology personnel.

EXPOSURE

Exposure is affected by time, distance, and shielding. The longer a person is within the radiation area, the higher the exposure. Also, the larger the amount of radioactive material in the area, the greater the exposure. The farther away the person is from the radiation source, the lower the exposure. Shielding from the radiation source also decreases exposure. One should never touch radioactive materials directly.

Three types of radiation-induced injury can occur: external irradiation, contamination with radioactive materials, and incorporation of radioactive material into body cells, tissues, or organs.

External irradiation exposure occurs when all or part of the body is exposed to radiation that penetrates or passes completely through the body. In this type of exposure, the patient is not radioactive and does not require special isolation or decontamination measures. Irradiation does not necessarily constitute a medical emergency.

Contamination occurs when the body is exposed to radioactive gases, liquids, or solids either externally or internally. If internal, the contaminant can be deposited within the body. Contamination requires immediate medical management to prevent incorporation.

Incorporation is the actual uptake of radioactive material into the cells, tissues, and susceptible organs. The organs involved are usually the kidneys, bone, liver, and thyroid.

Sequelae of contamination and incorporation can occur days to years later. The thyroid gland can be largely protected from radiation exposure by administration of stable iodine (potassium iodide, or KI) before or promptly after the intake of radioactive iodine (WHO, 1999).

Priorities in the treatment of any type of radiation exposure are always treatment of life-threatening injuries and illnesses first, followed by measures to limit exposure, contamination control, and finally decontamination.

DECONTAMINATION

Hospital and countywide disaster plans should be in effect when managing a radiation disaster. Access restriction is essential to prevent contamination of other areas of the hospital. Triage outside the hospital is the most effective means of preventing contamination of the facility itself. Floors are covered to prevent tracking of contaminants throughout the treatment areas. Strict isolation precautions should be in effect. Waste is controlled through double-bagging and the use of plastic-lined containers outside of the facility.

Staff are required to wear protective clothing, such as water-resistant gowns, two pairs of gloves, masks, caps, goggles, and booties. Dosimetry devices should be worn by all staff members participating in patient care. The radiation safety officer in the hospital should be notified immediately to assist with surveys (using a radiation survey meter) of the incoming patients and to provide dosimeters to all staff personnel involved with patient care of exposed victims. There is minimal risk to staff if the patients are properly surveyed and decontaminated. The majority of patients can be safely decontaminated with soap and water.

Each patient arriving at the hospital should be first surveyed with the radiation survey meter for external contamination and then directed toward the decontamination area as needed. Decontamination occurs outside of the Emergency Department with a shower, collection pool, tarp, and collection containers for patient belongings, as well as soap, towels, and disposable paper gowns for patients. Water runoff needs to be contained. Patients who are uninjured can perform self-decontamination with the use of handheld showers. After the patient has showered, a resur-

vey should be conducted to determine whether the radioactive contaminants have been removed. Additional washings should occur until the patient is free of contamination. It is important to ensure during showers that previously clean areas are not contaminated with runoff from the washed contaminated areas (eg, hair should be washed in the bent-over position to protect the body from contamination).

Biologic samples should be taken through nasal and throat swabs, and a complete blood count with differential should be obtained. Wounds should be irrigated and then covered with a water-resistant dressing prior to total body decontamination.

Internal contamination or incorporation requires decontamination through catharsis and/or gastric lavage with chelating agents (agents that bind with radioactive substances and are then excreted). Samples of urine, feces, and vomitus are surveyed to determine internal contamination levels.

ACUTE RADIATION SYNDROME

Acute radiation syndrome (ARS) can occur after exposure to radiation. It is the dose rather than the source that determines whether ARS develops. Factors that determine whether the patient's response to exposure will result in ARS include a high dose (minimum 100 rad) and rate of radiation with total body exposure and penetrating-type radiation. Age, medical history, and genetics also affect the outcome after exposure. The effects follow a predictable course. Table 72-5 identifies the phases of ARS.

Each body system is affected differently in ARS. Systems with cells that rapidly reproduce are the most affected. The effects on the hematopoietic system include decreased numbers of lymphocytes, granulocytes, thrombocytes, and reticulocytes. It is the first system affected and serves as an indicator of the severity of radiation exposure (Jarrett, 2001; Jagminas & Suner, 2001). A marker of outcome is the absolute lymphocyte count at 48 hours after exposure. A significant exposure would be indicated by lymphocyte counts of 300 to 1200 per cubic millimeter of blood (the normal lymphocyte count is 1500 to 3000/mm³). Barrier precautions should be implemented to protect the patient from infection. Neutrophils decrease within 1 week, platelets decrease within 2 weeks, and red blood cells decrease within 3 weeks. Hemorrhagic complications, fever, and sepsis are common.

The gastrointestinal system, with its rapidly producing cells, is also readily affected by radiation. Doses of radiation required to produce symptoms are approximately 600 rad or higher (Jagminas & Suner, 2001). The gastrointestinal symptoms usually occur at the same time as the changes in the hematopoietic system. Nausea and vomiting occur within 2 hours after exposure. Sepsis, fluid and electrolyte imbalance, and opportunistic infections can occur as complications. An ominous sign is the presence of high fever and bloody diarrhea; these typically appear on day 10 after exposure.

The central nervous system is affected with doses greater than 1000 rad (Jagminas & Suner, 2001). The symptoms occur when damage to the blood vessels of the brain results in fluid leakage. Signs and symptoms include cerebral edema, nausea, vomiting, headache, and increased intracranial pressure. Increased intracranial pressure heralds a poor outcome and imminent death. Central nervous system injury with this amount of exposure is irreversible and occurs before hematopoietic or gastrointestinal system symptoms appear. Cardiovascular collapse is usually seen in conjunction with these injuries.

Depending on the dose, skin effects can also occur. With exposure of 600 to 1000 rad, erythema occurs; it can disappear within hours, and then reappear. The exposed patient must be

Table 72-5 • Phases of Effects of Radiation Exposure

PHASE	TIME OF OCCURRENCE	SIGNS AND SYMPTOMS
Prodromal phase (presenting symptoms)	48–72 hr after exposure	Nausea, vomiting, loss of appetite, diarrhea, fatigue High-dose radiation—fever, respiratory distress, and increased excitability
Latent phase (a symptom-free period)	After resolution of prodromal phase; can last up to 3 wk With high-dose radiation—latent period is shorter	Decreasing lymphocytes, leukocytes, thrombocytes, red blood cells
Illness phase	After latent period phase	Infection, fluid and electrolyte imbalance, bleeding, diarrhea, shock, and altered level of consciousness
Recovery phase OR	After illness phase	Can take weeks to months for full recovery
Death	After illness phase	Increased intracranial pressure is a sign of impending death

evaluated hourly for the presence of erythema. With exposures greater than 1000 rad, desquamation (radiation dermatitis) of the skin occurs. Necrosis becomes evident within a few days to months at doses greater than 5000 rad. Skin signs are an indication of the dose of radiation exposure.

Secondary injury can occur when the radiation exposure occurs during a traumatic event such as a blast or burn. Trauma in addition to radiation exposure increases patient mortality. Attention must first be directed toward the primary assessment for trauma. Airway, breathing, circulation, and fracture reduction require immediate attention. All definitive treatments must occur within the first 48 hours. Thereafter, all surgical procedures should be delayed for 2 to 3 months because of the potential for delayed wound healing and the possible development of opportunistic infections several weeks after exposure.

SURVIVAL
There are three categories of predicted survival after radiation exposure: probable, possible, and improbable. Triage of victims at the scene, after decontamination, is conducted with the routine system for disaster triage. Presenting signs and symptoms determine the potential for survival and therefore the category of predicted survival during triage.

Probable survival victims have either no initial symptoms or only minimal symptoms (eg, nausea and vomiting), or these symptoms resolve within a few hours. These patients should receive a complete blood count and may be discharged with instructions to return if any symptoms recur.

Possible survivors are those who present with nausea and vomiting that persists for 24 to 48 hours. They will experience a latent period, during which leukopenia, thrombocytopenia, and lymphocytopenia occur. Barrier precautions and protective isolation are implemented if the patient's lymphocyte count is less than 1200/mm³. Supportive treatment includes administration of blood products, prevention of infection, and provision of enhanced nutrition.

The improbable survival group is composed of those who have received more than 800 rad of total body penetrating irradiation. Acutely, people in this group demonstrate vomiting, diarrhea, and shock. Any neurologic symptoms suggest a lethal dose of radiation (Jarrett, 2001). These patients still require decontamination, to prevent contamination of the area. Personal protection is essen-

tial, because it is virtually impossible to fully decontaminate these patients since all of their internal organs have been irradiated. The survival time is variable; however, death usually ensues swiftly due to shock. If there are no neurologic symptoms, the patient may be alert and oriented, similar to a patient with extensive burns. In a mass casualty situation, the nurse should expect to triage these patients into the black category, where they will receive comfort measures and emotional support. If it is not a mass casualty situation, aggressive fluid and electrolyte therapy are essential.

Although radiation, biological, and chemical events are not everyday events, when they do occur every facility and every nurse will need to know the basics of caring for affected patients.

Any terrorist-sponsored or unintentional radiation release can be sizeable and may require the entire hospital and prehospital staff to be prepared, recognize signs and symptoms of exposure, and rapidly treat victims without contamination of personnel, visitors, patients, or the facility itself.

 Critical Thinking Exercises

1. You are the triage nurse at the receiving facility for casualties after a tornado. Five patients arrive at the same time. Together with the surgeon on duty, you must identify the patients' needs. You are presented with an elderly man with a respiratory rate of 8 breaths per minute, colour ashen, tense abdomen, and only carotid pulses present; a 7-year-old child with a bleeding scalp laceration who has a Glasgow Coma Score of 8 and needs intubation; the 30-year-old mother of the child, who is crying hysterically, is walking, and appears to have no pain or visible injuries; a 15-year-old girl who complains of pain in her left leg, with obvious deformity at the calf but good pulses in the foot; and a 65-year-old woman who arrives in a police car holding her right wrist, which is cool, ecchymotic, and painful with good pulses. How would you classify these patients using triage categories?

Family members, members of the press, and city officials begin arriving at the hospital in large numbers. How would you expect these people to be managed? How will the family members be cared for?

2. A patient arrives at the triage desk complaining of sudden onset of high fever and respiratory flu-like symptoms. What are the signs and symptoms that you should identify if considering an infection disease or a biological warfare agent? Which organisms/agents cause pneumonia-like signs and symptoms? What precautions would be taken to protect staff?

3. Multiple patients begin arriving at the Emergency Department complaining of burning eyes and difficulty breathing. All of these persons work at the railroad, where there are often tanker trucks transporting chemical agents. What should you do first? Where do you find information about chemical agents and their treatment?

4. You are a member of the disaster committee at your hospital. What are the elements of the disaster plan that you will be sure to include? How will you plan for triage? What types of PPE will you purchase?

5. A nursing colleague remarks, "I'm not getting a flu shot this year. They are not effective and may harm my immune system." Discuss your response in terms of the facts about influenza immunization and the responsibility to protect patients, colleagues, and citizens.

REFERENCES AND SELECTED READINGS

Books and Internet Readings

Agency for Toxic Substances and Disease Registry. (2000). *Taking an exposure history.* Atlanta: U.S. Department of Health and Human Services.

American Red Cross Disaster Services. (2001). *Disaster preparedness for people with disabilities.* Available at: http://www.americanredcross.com.

Canadian Council on Health Services Accreditation. (2002). *2005 Accreditation recognition guidelines.* Ottawa: Author. Available at: www.cchsa.ca/pdf/SurveyGuidelines2005.pdf. Retrieved June 29, 2005.

Canadian Nurses Association (2002). *Code of ethics for registered nurses.* Ottawa: Author.

Canadian Red Cross Disaster Services. (2005). *Together we prepare.* Available at: www.redcross.ca/prepare. Retrieved October 21, 2005.

Canadian Red Cross Disaster Services. (2005). *Expect the unexpected program.* Available at: www.redcross.ca/article.asp?id=009874&tid=028. Retrieved October 21, 2005.

Canadian Red Cross Disaster Services. (2005). *Facing fear.* Available at: www.redcross.ca/article.asp?id=009899&tid=025. Retrieved October 21, 2005.

Capital Health and Caritas Health Group. (2005). *Influenza doesn't work here—THE BUG STOPS HERE.* Edmonton, AB: Author.

Centers for Disease Control and Prevention. (2004). *Six common misconceptions about vaccination and how to respond to them.* Available at: www.cdc.gov/nip/publications/6mishome.htm. Retrieved October 21, 2005.

Centre for Emergency Preparedness and Response. (2001). *Two scenarios offer examples of how the Centre delivers results for Canadians.* Ottawa: Author. Available at: www.phac-aspc.gc.ca/cepr-cmiu/scenario_e.html.Retrieved June 29, 2005.

Currance, P., & Bronstein, A., C. (1999). *Hazardous materials for EMS: Practices and procedures.* St. Louis: Mosby.

Emergency Management Alberta. (2005). *Emergency management Alberta.* Edmonton, AB: Author. Available at: www.municipalaffairs.gov.ab.ca/ema. Retrieved June 29, 2005.

Federal Nuclear Emergency Plan (FNEP) (2005). Available at: www.hc-sc.gc.ca/ed-ud/fedplan/index_e.html. Retrieved June 29, 2005.

Health Canada. (2003). *Learning from SARS: Renewal of public health in Canada.* Ottawa: Author.

Health Surveillance, Alberta Health and Wellness. (2005). *Population projections for Alberta and its health regions 2004–2033.* Edmonton, AB: Author. Available at: www.health.gov.ab.ca/resources/publications/pdf/PopProject05.pdf. Retrieved October 21, 2005.

Hill, W. (2005). *Pandemic planning.* [Presentation]. Edmonton, AB: Regional Nursing Affairs, Capital Health. Available at: http://www.capitalhealth.ca/default.htm.

Institute of Medicine and National Research Council. (1999). *Chemical and biological terrorism: Research and development to improve civilian medical response.* Washington, DC: National Academy Press.

Jagminas, L., & Suner, S. (2001). *Weapons of terrorism handout.* Baltimore, MD: International Trauma Anesthesia and Critical Care Society.

National CTAS Working Group. (2004). *The Canadian triage & acuity scale (CTAS) for emergency departments.* Ottawa: Canadian Association of Emergency Physicians.

Nicholson, K. (1998). Human influenza. In K. Nicholson, R. Webster, & A. Hays (Eds.), *Textbook of influenza* (pp. 219–264). London: Blackwell Science Ltd.

Ontario Ministry of Health and Long-Term Care. For the public's health: *A plan of action. Final report of the Ontario Expert Panel on SARS and Infectious Disease Control April 2004.* Available at: www.health.gov.on.ca/english/public/pub/ministry_reports/walker04/walker04_mn.html. Retrieved October 21, 2005.

Public Health Agency of Canada. (2001). *Two scenarios offer examples of how the Centre delivers results for Canadians.* Available at: www.phac-aspc.gc.ca/cepr-cmiu/scenario_e.html. Retrieved October 21, 2005.

Public Health Agency of Canada. (2005). *National Advisory Committee on Immunization (NACI). About NACI.* Available at: www.phac-aspc.gc.ca/naci-ccni/index.html. Retrieved October 21, 2005.

Sidell, F. R., Patrick, W. C., & Dashiell, T. R. (2000). *Jane's chem-bio handbook.* Alexandria, VA: Jane's Information Group.

Springhouse Corporation. (2001). *Handbook of infectious diseases.* Springhouse, PA: Author.

U.S. Army Medical Research Institute of Infectious Disease. (1996). *Medical management of biological casualties handbook.* Fort Detrick, MD: U.S. Army.

U.S. Army Medical Research Institute of Chemical Defense. (1999). *Medical management of chemical casualties handbook.* Fort Detrick, MD: Aberdeen Proving Ground.

Valanis, B. (1992). *Epidemiology in nursing and health care.* Stamford, CT: Appleton & Lange.

World Health Organization. *Summary of probable SARS cases with onset of illness from 1 November 2002 to 31 July 2003.* Available at: www.who.int/csr/sars/country/table2004_04_21/en/index.html. Retrieved October 21, 2005.

World Health Organization. (1999). *Guidelines for iodine prophylaxis following nuclear accidents.* Geneva: Author.

World Health Organization. (2003). *Influenza (Fact sheet No. 21). Revised March 2003.* Available at: www.who.int/mediacentre/factsheets/fs211/en/index.html. Retrieved October 21, 2005.

Journals

Altman, G. B. (2002). Invisible threats. *Nursing Management, 33,* 43, 45–47.

Anteau, C. M., & Williams, L. A. (1997). The Oklahoma bombing: Lessons learned. *Critical Care Nursing Clinics of North America, 9*(2), 231–236.

Arnon, S. S., Schechter, R., Inglesby, T. V., et al., (2001). Botulinum toxin as a biological weapon. *Journal of the American Medical Association 285,* 1059–1070.

Bonner, S. (Ed.). (1996). *Managing hazardous materials in the ED.* ED Management, 1*(9).*

Branswell, H. (2005, August 17). Pandemic could trigger new Depression. *Edmonton Journal*, p. G7.

Brennan, R. J., Waeckerle, J. F., Sharp, T. W., & Lillibridge, S. R. (1999). Chemical warfare agents: EMS and emergency public health issues. *Annals of Emergency Medicine, 34*(2), 191–204.

Burgess, J. L., Kirk, M. B., Burron, S. W., & Cisek, J. (1999). Emergency department hazarrdous materials protocol for contaminated patients. *Annals of Emergency Medicine, 34*(2), 205–212.

Centers for Disease Control and Prevention Strategic Planning Workgroup. (2000). Biological and chemical terrorism: Strategic plan for preparedness and response. *Morbidity and Mortality Weekly Report, 49,* 1–14.

Chan, S. S. C., Leung, G. M., Tiwari, A. F. Y., et al. (2005). The impact of work-related risk on nurses during the SARS outbreak in Hong Kong. *Family & Community Health, 28*(3), 274–287.

Chen, C., Wu, H., Yang, P., et al. (2005). Psychological distress of nurses in Taiwan who worked during the outbreak of SARS. *Psychiatric Services* 56(1), 76–79.

Chettle, C. C. (2001, November). Recognizing bioterrorism. *Nurse-Week,* 28–29. Available at: http://www.nurseweek.com/ce/ce71a.html. Accessed February, 2002.

Davis, K. G., Aspera, G. (2001). Exposure to liquid sulfur mustard. *Annals of Emergency Medicine, 37,* 653–656.

Dennis, D. T., Inglesby, T. V., Henderson, D. A., et al., (2001). Tularemia as a biological weapon. *Journal of the American Medical Association, 285,* 2763–2773.

Detsky, A. S., & Naylor, C. D. (2003). Canada's health care system—reform delayed. *New England Journal of Medicine, 349*(8), 804–810.

Franz, D. R., & Zajtchuk, R. (2000). Biological terrorism: Understanding the threat, preparation, and medical response. *Disease-a-month, 46,* 125–192.

Gans, L., & Kennedy, T. (1996). Management of unique clinical entities in disaster medicine. *Emergency Medicine Clinics of North America, 14*(2), 301–306.

Hagstad, D. (2000). Bioterrorism. *American Journal of Nursing, 100,* 33–35.

Hauer, J., Layton, M., McDade, J. (1999). Smallpox as a biological weapon. *Journal of the American Medical Association, 281,* 2127–2137.

Heightman, A. J. (1999). Assault on Columbine. *Journal of Emergency Medical Services, 24*(9), 32–46.

Heightman, A. J. (2000). TIPS for MCI management. *Journal of Emergency Medical Services, 25*(6), 30–40.

Heung, Y. Y. J., Wong, K. Y. F., Kwong, W. Y. E., et al. (2005). Severe acute respiratory syndrome outbreak promotes a strong sense of professional identity among nursing students. *Nurse Education Today, 25*(2), 112–118.

Hogarth, W. D., & Neil, G. F. (2001). Tornado at Pine Lake, Alberta–July 14, 2000. Anatomy of a disaster: One hospital's experience and recommendations. *Canadian Journal of Emergency Medicine, 3*(1), 38–40.

Howard, A. (2001, November). On the frontlines. *NurseWeek,* 19–20.

Inglesby, T. V., Dennis, D. T., Henderson, D. A. et al., Plague as a biological weapon. *Journal of the American Medical Association 283,* 2281–2290.

Inglesby, T. V., Henderson, D. A., Bartlett, J. G. (1999). Anthrax as a biological weapon. *Journal of the American Medical Association 281,* 1735–1745.

Jarrett, D. G. (2001). Medical aspects of ionizing radiation weapons. *Military Medicine, 166,* (Supp. 12), 6–8.

Kotzmann, K. (1999). Preparedness without panic. *Nursing Spectrum* [On-line]. Available: http://www.nursingspectrum.com. Accessed February 2002.

Lee, T., Saskin, R., McArthur, M., et al. (2005). Beliefs and practice of Ontario midwives about influenza immunization. *Vaccine,* 23(13), 1574–1578.

Lewis, P. C., & Aghababian, R. V. (1996). Disaster planning: Part I. Overview of hospital and emergency department planning for inter-nal and external disasters. *Emergency Medicine Clinics of North America, Disaster Medicine, 14*(2), 439–453.

Levitin, H. W., & Siegelson, H. J. (1996). Hazardous materials, disaster medical planning and response. *Emergency Medicine Clinics of North America, 14*(2), 327–349.

Londorf, D. (1995). Hospital application of the incident management system. *Prehospital and Disaster Medicine, 10*(3), 184–188.

Mickelson, A. S., Bruno, L., & Schario, M. E. (1999). The City of New Orleans Amtrak train disaster: One emergency department's experience. *Journal of Emergency Nursing, 25*(5), 367–371.

National Advisory Committee on Immunization (NACI). (2002). Statement on influenza vaccination for the 2002–2003 season. *Canada Communicable Disease Report, 28*(ACS-5), 1–20. Available at: www.phac-aspc.gc.ca/publicat/ccdr-rmtc/02pdf/acs-dcc-5.pdf. Retrieved October 21, 2005.

National Advisory Committee on Immunization (NACI). (2004). Statement on influenza vaccination for the 2004–2005 season. *Canada Communicable Disease Report, 30*(ACS-3), 1–32. Available at: www.phac-aspc.gc.ca/publicat/ccdr-rmtc/04pdf/acs-dcc-30-3.pdf. Retrieved October 21, 2005.

Naylor, C. D., Chantler, C., & Griffiths, S. (2004). Learning from SARS in Hong Kong and Toronto. *Journal of the American Medical Association,* 291(20), 2483–2487.

O'Rorke, C., Bourke, W., & Bedford, D. (2003). Uptake of influenza vaccine by health care workers in an acute hospital in Ireland. *Irish Medical Journal,* 96(7), 207–209.

Pfaff, B. L. (1998). Emergency department management of nerve agent exposure. *IJTN,* 4, 71–78.

Richards, C. F., Burstein, J. L., Waeckerle, J. F., & Hutson, H. R. (1999). Emergency physicians and biological terrorism. *Annals of Emergency Medicine, 34*(2), 183–190.

Sauer, S. W., & Keim, M. E. (2001). Hydroxycobalamin: Improved public health readiness for cyanide disasters. *Annals of Emergency Medicine, 37*(6), 635–641.

Seto, W. H., Tsang, D., Yung, R. W. H., et al. (2003). Effectiveness of precautions against droplets and contact in prevention of nosocomial transmission of severe acute respiratory syndrome (SARS). *Lancet,* 361(9368), 1519–1520.

Skowronski, D., Parker, R., & Strang, R. (2000). The importance of influenza immunization for health care workers. *British Columbia Medical Journal,* 42(2), 91–93.

Sookram, S., Borkent, H., Powell, G., et al. (2001). Tornado at Pine Lake, Alberta–July 14, 2000. Assessment of the emergency response to a disaster. *Canadian Journal of Emergency Medicine On-Line, 3*(1). Available at: www.caep.ca.login.ezproxy.library.ualberta.ca/004.cjem-jcmu/004-00.cjem/vol-3.2001/v31-034.htm. Retrieved June 29, 2005.

Spencer, D. A., Whitman, K. M., & Morton, P. G. (2001). Inhalational anthrax. *MedSurg Nursing, 10,* 308–312.

Stopford, B. M. (2000). Are you prepared? Tips for counter terrorism. *ENA connection, Official Newsletter of the ENA, Emergency Nurses Association, June 2000,* 24(5), 1, 5–6.

Tolomiczenko, G. S., Kahan, M., Ricci, M., et al. (2005). SARS: Coping with the impact at a community hospital. *Journal of Advanced Nursing,* 50(1), 101–110.

Tur-Kaspa, I., Lev, E. I., Hendler, I., Siebner, R., Shapira, Y., & Shemer, J. (1999). Preparing hospitals for toxicological mass casualties events. *Critical Care Medicine,* 27(5), 1004–1008.

Vollman, A. R., & Pierrynowski-Gallant, D. M. (2004). Influenza vaccination choices: Do nurses and other healthcare professionals make the right choices about influenza vaccination? Should we be taking a second look at the impact of our choices? *Canadian Nurse,* 100(2), 16–21.

Yergler, M. (2002). Emergency: Mass casualty. Nerve gas attack. *American Journal of Nursing,* 102(7), 57–60.

Zoutman, D. E., Ford, B. D., Bryce, E., et al. (2003). The state of infection surveillance and control in Canadian acute care hospitals. AJIC: *American Journal of Infection Control,* 31(5), 266–273.

RESOURCES AND WEBSITES

Canadian Association of Emergency Physicians: www.caep.ca.

Canadian Red Cross: www.redcross.ca.

Centers for Disease Control and Prevention, 1600 Clifton Road NE, Atlanta, GA 30333; (404) 639-3311; http://www.cdc.gov.

Centre for Emergency Preparedness and Response: www.phac-aspc.gc.ca/cepr-cmiu.

Health Canada: www.hc-sc.gc.ca.

National CTAS Working Group: www.caep.ca/002.policies/002-022.ctas.htm.

National Emergency Nurses Affiliation: www.nena.ca

National Microbiology Laboratory: www.nml.ca.

Public Safety and Emergency Preparedness Canada: www.ocipep.gc.ca.

The Public Health Agency of Canada: www.phac-aspc.gc.ca/new_e.html.

US Homeland Security; (800) BE-READY; http://www.dhs.gov/dhspublic/theme_home2.jsp.

World Health Organization: www.who.int.

Understanding Clinical Pathways

Adapted by Deborah Michalyk and Cathy Giblin

*C*linical pathways (also called critical pathways or care paths) are care plans developed collaboratively by physicians, nurses, physiotherapists, occupational therapists, pharmacists, speech therapists, case managers, technicians, and other staff members involved in patient care. Nurses are instrumental in ensuring the successful use of clinical pathways and can best contribute by gaining a thorough understanding of why and how pathways are used.

UNDERSTANDING AND USING CLINICAL PATHWAYS IN PATIENT CARE

Clinical pathways grew out of financial upheaval in the health care industry. They represent a significant change in how patient care is managed. In the past (and currently for many patients), each health care discipline developed its own plan of care and used the patient's chart (medical record) as the primary communication tool. Each care provider needed to read the notes written by other care providers of other disciplines to get a complete picture of the plan of care and the patient's progress. Although there was probably general agreement about how patient progress would be facilitated and measured, individual steps in the processes of care and outcomes to be achieved were not usually specifically articulated. The physician managed the case and most patients remained in the hospital until they required very little care or could be transferred to a convalescent centre. The length of hospital stay was not an issue; 2 to 3 weeks in an acute care facility was not unusual.

COST AND EFFECTS

Although this system worked for decades, it was expensive. Not including charges for diagnostic tests or treatments, each day in the hospital could easily cost $800 or more. The federal government and provincial/territorial governments balked at paying these costs when highly skilled care was no longer needed. So they determined how many days of hospitalization a patient with a specific diagnosis required and decided to reimburse the health care organizations or facilities only for that number of days. At the same time, hospitals tried to obtain meaningful financial data about the costs of hospital-based patient care—where the greatest costs were generated and how they could be reduced. Decreasing the length of stay was seen as one way to save money. As hospital stays became shorter and shorter, nurses and physicians began to express concerns about the quality of care. Patients were discharged to home or rehabilitation centres much sooner than before. They were weaker, had relatively fresh incisions, or often could not perform even minimal self-care independently. Regulatory agencies and consumers shared these concerns and demands arose for hard data demonstrating that patients were not being harmed.

This scenario compelled health care administrators and clinicians to develop a new way to measure and manage costs, quality, and outcomes. Thoughtful examination of how patient care was provided exposed inefficiencies and highlighted the lack of face-to-face communication among disciplines. It became apparent that patient care could be managed more cost-effectively, possibly saving hundreds of thousands or millions of dollars yearly. Organizations adopted a system known as case management to address these issues.

CASE MANAGEMENT

Under case management, care is planned collaboratively so that important events, such as initiation of physiotherapy, home care consultation, or discontinuation of invasive treatments, occur on a schedule that clinicians, through experience or research, have identified as optimum for enhancing recovery. Care is mapped out by day or by other pivotal time intervals and goals or desired outcomes are specified for each time frame. When the patient has met all the goals, he or she is ready for discharge to home or to the next level of care. Responsibility for monitoring an individual patient's progress and tracking variance or deviation from the pathway is given to the case manager who usually, but not always, is a nurse. The tool on which all this information is contained is the clinical pathway. The purposes of a clinical pathway are to

- Promote quality care and improve clinical outcomes
- Standardize important aspects of care
- Reduce unnecessary delays in care
- Reduce costs

ELEMENTS OF A CLINICAL PATHWAY

Clinical pathways are now used in a variety of settings and cover diverse diagnoses and conditions. They are often developed by individual organizations and, although the format varies from institution to institution, clinical pathways have major features in common.

Patient Population

The first important element of the clinical pathway is the patient population (Fig. AP-1*A*). Each pathway clearly specifies the patients appropriate for inclusion on the pathway. Pathways tend to cover patient groups in which the treatment and recovery are relatively predictable. Institutions typically use a diagnosis-related group (DRG) to identify patients, but qualifiers may be added. For example, a pathway for community-acquired pneumonia may exclude patients with *Pneumocystis carinii* pneumonia or underlying obstructive pulmonary disease because those patients require highly individualized treatment plans and may not respond as quickly to intervention as patients without these underlying disorders.

Time Frames

All pathways are divided into useful time frames (Fig. AP-1*B*). The identified time frame may be minutes, hours, days, weeks, or phases. Conditions requiring emergency treatment (myocardial infarction, head injury, stroke) might be divided into 15-minute intervals, whereas conditions requiring chronic care (chronic pain, spinal cord injury rehabilitation) may be divided into weekly or monthly intervals. An example of interventions by phases might be seen in postanesthesia care pathways.

Interventional Categories

Interventional categories consist of the groups of activities that make up a comprehensive treatment plan and are shown in the left-hand column of the pathway (Fig. AP-1*C*). Although the order in which they are listed varies, these categories typically include

- Tests
- Treatments and nursing interventions
- Consultations
- Medications
- Diet
- Activity
- Patient and family education
- Discharge planning

Clinical pathway teams begin working with a blank grid and fill in the appropriate interventions. The discipline responsible for the intervention recommends the optimal timing.

In many organizations, pre-printed patient care order (PPCO) forms are used in support of clinical pathways. The PPCO is developed by all disciplines involved in the care of the patient population and is the mechanism by which patient care orders are initiated and carried out. The content of the PPCO mirrors the pathway but focuses specifically on patient care orders.

Outcomes

Defined outcomes provide the focus for patient care activities and unify the various disciplines. All well-written pathways include outcomes identified for each time interval (Fig. AP-1*D*). They should be realistic, reflect incremental progress, and ideally be achievable by 100% of the population. Pathway outcomes are similar in content and language to the goals or expected outcomes written into nursing plans of care; physiologic, psychological, social, and educational outcomes are included to capture all elements of complete recovery.

Variance Record

The variance record (Fig. AP-2) is an extremely important part of the pathway and represents the mechanism through which improvements in patient care can be accomplished. Variance is defined as any deviation from the pathway. Because all events on the pathway are critical to recovery, deviations can have a negative impact on outcomes. If the pathway calls for a specific test or treatment on day 2 and it is not carried out on day 2, a variance has occurred. If the patient is to ambulate 3 times a day and ambulates only once, a variance has occurred. The variance and the causes are recorded. Some variance records require a written note and others use code numbers (see Fig. AP-2). Many hospitals have developed or purchased software so that variances can be recorded electronically.

Case managers collect and analyze the variance data to identify trends in patient care and outcomes. For example, a pneumonia pathway may specify that the first dose of antibiotics be given within 3 hours of admission to the hospital (delays in administration of the first dose of an antibiotic are associated with increased morbidity and mortality). The case manager reviews the variance records and determines that only 40% of pneumonia patients are receiving the antibiotic in that time frame. Assessment of the problem reveals that delays are a result of the length of time it takes for the medication order to be taken off the chart and delivered to the pharmacy, and the length of time it takes for the medication to be delivered. The pneumonia pathway team discusses this problem and determines

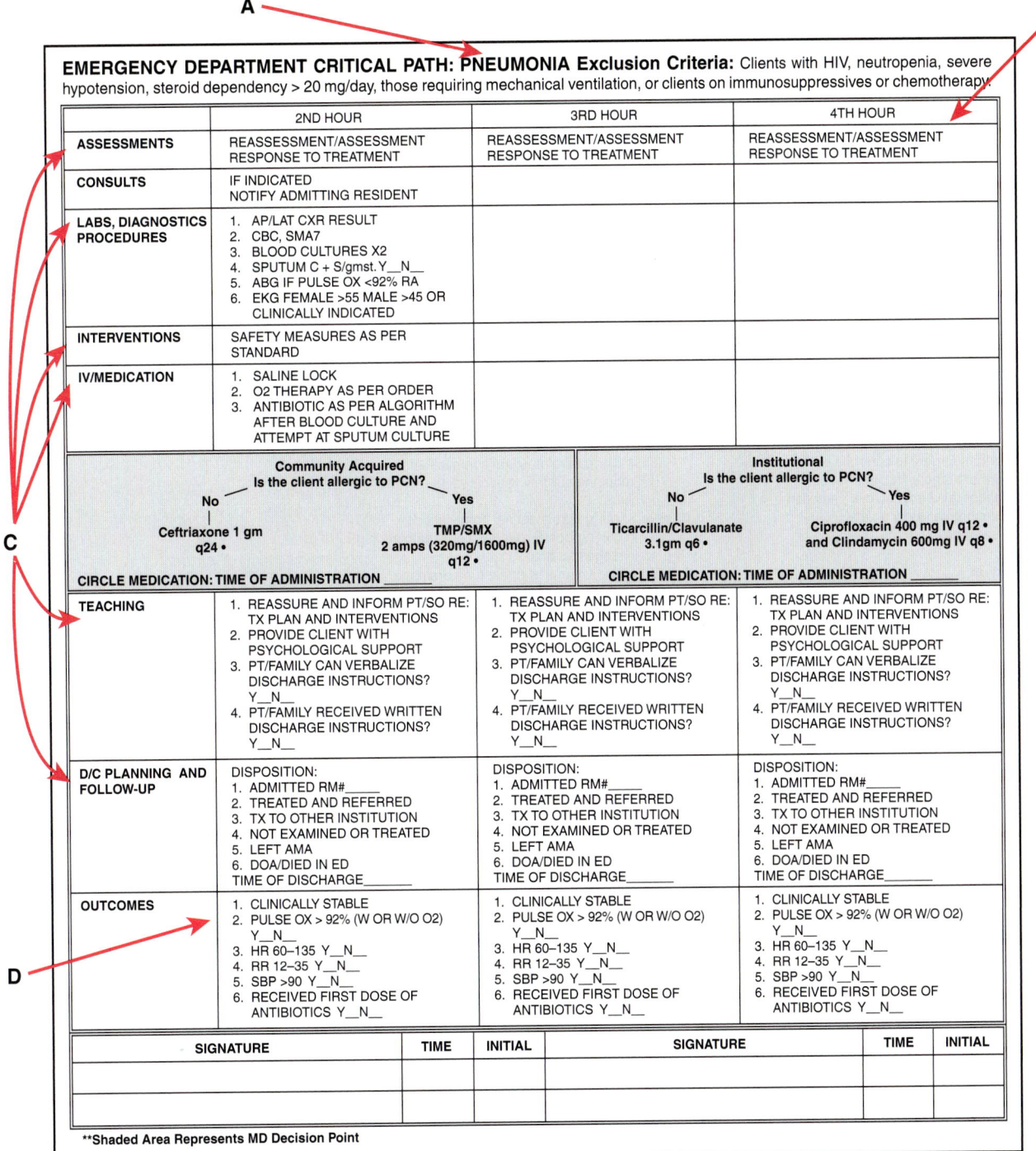

FIGURE AP-1 Key elements of a clinical pathway. (**A**) Patient population clearly defined. (**B**) Clinically meaningful time frames. (**C**) Interventional categories. (**D**) Outcomes for each time frame should be specific and measurable. Reproduced with permission from Graduate Hospital, Philadelphia, Pennsylvania.

that the first dose of medication should be given in the emergency department since the emergency department stocks these medications. The pathway is revised to reflect this change in care. At the next review, the case manager reports that 92% of pneumonia patients on the clinical pathway received their antibiotics within 1 to 2 hours of admission. This scenario illustrates how pathway use and variance data collection provide the forum for assessing a problem, determining a plan of action, implementing the plan, and evaluating the effectiveness of the plan.

THE NURSE'S ROLE

Nurses have a key role in all aspects of clinical pathway use. Participating in the development of the pathway is the first step. Because they begin and end the chain of staff involved in delivering care, nurses possess a unique perspective in how health care systems work to enhance or impede the delivery of care. In the above example about antibiotic administration, staff nurses were able to identify the problem quickly and suggest solutions. Other staff

A

Clinical Pathway: _____
(Department Name)

Patient's Name: _____   MedRecNo: _ _ _ _ _ _

(Please list each code separately)

Date	Path Day #	Variance Code	Comment / Action Taken
__ / __ / __			
__ / __ / __			
__ / __ / __			
__ / __ / __			
__ / __ / __			

A

B

VARIANCE CODES

Patient's Condition/Problem

A1. Operative
A1a. Further surgery to control bleeding
A1b. Further surgery for other reason
A1c. Perioperative myocardial infarction
A1d. Tamponade (early or late)
A1e. Dissection

A2. Infection
A2a. Sternum, requiring debridement
A2b. Sternum, superficial (antibiotics and dressings only)
A2c. Leg
A2d. Urinary tract infection
A2e. Sepsis

A3. Neurological
A3a. Stroke, temporary or permanent deficit
A3b. Delirium
A3c. Coma
A3d. Confusion or agitation

A4. Respiratory
A4a. Prolonged ventilation
A4b. Acute respiratory distress syndrome
A4c. Respiratory failure, reintubation
A4d. Pneumonia
A4e. Atelectasis

A5. Renal
A5a. Renal failure
A5b. Dialysis

A6. Cardiac
A6a. Atrial arrhythmia
A6b. Ventricular arrhythmia
A6c. Heart block with or without pacemaker implantation
A6d. Heart failure
A6e. Cardiac arrest
A6f. Hemodynamic instability
A6g. Unable to wean off inotropic agents

A7. Vascular
A7a. Deep vein thrombosis
A7b. Limb ischemia

Other Condition/Problem

A8. Other
A8a. Major gastrointestinal complication requiring surgery (eg, bleeding, perforation, ileus)
A8b. Minor gastrointestinal complication requiring bowel rest (eg, ileus, nausea, high nasogastric output)
A8c. Large volume of chest-tube drainage
A8d. Poor wound healing (ie, significant sterile drainage from leg or chest wound)
A8e. Pulmonary embolism
A8f. Anticoagulant complication
A8g. Thromboembolism
A8h. Activity intolerance
A8i. Medication reaction
A8j. Altered skin integrity

B: Practitioner Related
B1. Practitioner unavailability
B2. Transcription error
B3. Incorrect sequencing of therapy
B4. Delay in consult or referral
B5. Incomplete discharge planning
B6. Delay or cancel test or procedure
B7. Discharge day delay
B8. Other

C: Hospital/System
C1. Bed unavailable (state issue)
C2. Equipment or supplies not available
C3. Results not available
C4. Unable to schedule test, procedure, or therapy
C5. Case, test, procedure, or therapy delayed
C6. Preoperative teaching not documented
C7. Follow-up after discharge not documented

D: Family/Placement
D1. Extended care not available
D2. Homecare not available
D3. Patient or family delaying discharge planning
D4. Financial issues
D5. Other

Form used at Westchester County Medical Center for tracking variances from clinical pathway for cardiac surgery (CABG).

B

FIGURE AP-2 Variance record. (**A**) Blank pages for recording variance. (**B**) Variance codes. Reproduced with permission from *Critical Care Nurse, 17*(16), December 1997, pp. 29–30.

from other disciplines, being single links in the chain, cannot supply this global view of the problem.

Nurses are also responsible for initiating the pathway on appropriate patients and ensuring that the various events occur as planned. In some care settings or conditions, case managers who are advanced practice nurses closely follow pathway patients; in others, staff nurses or community-based nurses function as case managers. In any environment, enhancing and monitoring outcome achievement is a nursing activity. Patients are often given a printed patient pathway for reference. The pathway describes the care plan in simple language and pictures. The nurse discusses the pathway with the patient and focuses on achieving specific outcomes.

Nurses are also responsible for completing required documentation. Practices vary, but well-designed pathways strive for simplicity and should not duplicate documentation required elsewhere. For example, a separate nursing plan of care is not necessary when using a clinical pathway. The outcome section of the pathway usually requires documentation; other areas may need to be checked off or initialed so that other providers can readily see what has been accomplished. Documenting variance and initiating steps to address the variance are equally important as is participating in redesigning care practices to promote the highest quality of cost-effective care.

PATHWAYS IN PRACTICE

Several pathways are provided in the following pages to demonstrate the variety of formats the nurse may encounter. Figure AP-3 is a pathway used at Medical College of Ohio for patients with acute ischemic stroke. The time frame (3 to 5 days) is identified at the top of the pathway and in the Expected Outcomes portion. The pathway provides clear expected outcomes as well as a variety of checklists identifying all significant and sequential aspects of patient care. Figure APA-4 is a clinical pathway used by Capital Health (a health region in Alberta that includes Edmonton and surrounding area) for a patient having a radical prostatectomy. The pathway begins at the pre-admission clinic, continues through to the fourth post-operative day, and ends with a discharge summary sheet.

Whatever format is used or condition treated, clinical pathways are documents in transition; they will change as research suggests better treatment strategies and as variance data are analyzed. Nurses' participation in these processes is essential for the successful implementation of clinical pathways and, ultimately, the opportunity to improve patient care.

ACUTE ISCHEMIC STROKE
CLINICAL GUIDELINES
EXPECTED LOS: 3-5 Days (check box to initiate order)
ORDERS (*) ARE 24 HOURS ORDERS AND MUST BE ASSESSED DAILY

	ADDRESSOGRAPH

	ADMISSION DAY: Day 1 Date: _____ Time: _____
ADMIT TO:	❒ ICU ❒ Unit _____ ❒ Tag/Order Clinical Practice Guideline "Acute Ischemic Stroke" in Care Manager ❒ **Patient not appropriate for Clinical Practice Guideline because:** _____ _____
ATTENDING PHYSICIAN	Dr. _____ Admitting Resident _____ Pager # _____
DIAGNOSIS	❒ Ischemic Stroke
CONDITION OF PATIENT	❒ Good ❒ Fair ❒ Critical ❒ Other _____
CATEGORY OF CARE	❒ Full Support ❒ Category of Care Order Form ❒ (Total support except Advance Life support, DNRCC-Arrest, DNRCC)
ALLERGIES	❒ NKA ❒ _____
***NUTRITION (24 hour order)**	❒ NPO Completely ❒ NPO except for medications ❒ Other_____
***ACTIVITY (24 hour order)**	❒ Complete bedrest (elevate head of bed 30°), reposition q 2 hours if needed ❒ Other _____
CONSULTS	❒ Speech Therapy for bedside dysphagia screening exam ❒ Speech Therapy for Speech and Language Evaluation and Treatment ❒ Physical Therapy Evaluation and Treatment (ROM) ❒ Occupational Therapy Evaluation and Treatment ❒ Other

NURSING	❒ *Cardiac monitor
	❒ *Continuous pulse ox for, call if $SpO_2 < 94$
	❒ Seizure precautions
	❒ No lifting or pulling of limbs on affected side
	❒ I & O
	❒ EPC cuffs
	❒ ROM q 4 hours
	❒ *No invasive procedures except venous blood draws for 24 hours
	    until _____ (date/time) *if given tPA*
	❒ Vital signs and Neuro assessments q 30 min x 6 hours, then
	    q 1 hour x 16 hours, then q 4 hours *(recommended for patients post tPA)*
	                OR
	❒ Vital signs and Neuro Assessments q 2 hours x 8 hours,
	    then q 4 hours
	❒ *Foley to dependent drainage
	❒ Evaluate stool, urine, emesis or other secretions for signs of blood. Hemoccult testing if there is evidence of bleeding. *(recommended for patients post tPA)*
	❒ Weight on admission
	❒ O_2 @ 2L per NC
	
	☑ **Call MD immediately for:**
	
	SBP ≥ 185 < 120
	DBP ≥ 105 or < 60
	Pulse < 50 or > 120
	RR > 30
	T > 101°F / 38.5° C
	
	❒ neuro status
	change in mental status
	headache, vomiting
	evidence of bleeding
	❒ language or motor deficit

MD/DO SIGNATURE	
(PRINT NAME)	

9/2001   Guidelines do not replace clinical judgement and should be modified according to individual patient needs

FIGURE AP-3 This clinical guideline for patients with acute ischemic stroke includes space for 24-hour orders.
Reproduced with permission of Medical College of Ohio, Toledo, Ohio. (Continued)

ACUTE ISCHEMIC STROKE
CLINICAL GUIDELINES

EXPECTED LOS: 3-5 Days (check box to initiate order)
ORDERS (*) ARE 24 HOURS ORDERS AND MUST BE ASSESSED DAILY

ADDRESSOGRAPH

	ADMISSION Day Orders (Continued) DAY 1 Date: _____ Time: _____
LABS	☐ CBC in a.m. x 1 ☐ *Glucose finger stick q 6 hours ☐ Fasting Lipid Profile in a.m. x 1 ☐ Other _____
I.V.	☐ I.V. 0.45 NaCl @ _____ cc/hr ☐ I.V. other _____
MEDICATIONS	Stroke Prevention Medications if no tPA and other medications should be ordered below.
CARE COORDINATION	☐ Contact Care Coordinator for discharge planning
PATIENT/FAMILY EDUCATION	☐ Stroke Education Folder, Specific material as needed ☐ Education Record – Patient/Caregiver – Stroke/TIA Form # 49812 (Please include in medical record) ☐ The Brain at Risk, Stroke (Story of Treatment and Recovery)
EXPECTED OUTCOMES	• **Day 1** – Appropriate consult/studies ordered. D/C planning related to placement started. • **Day 2** – Consults completed, OOB/Chair, nutritional route established - tube feeding/diet started – PO fluids tolerated. • **Day 3** – Advanced activity, order consult for PEG if appropriate. Expected D/C date determined. • **Day 4** – Final D/C arrangements made. Care Coordinator to make arrangements for home Lovenox until INR therapeutic on Coumadin (if applicable). • **Day 5** - D/C to home/ECF/Rehab. Neurologically stable last 24 hours. If not D/C'd document reason in medical record.
MD/DO SIGNATURE	
(PRINT NAME)	

ADDITIONS/CHANGES - *PLEASE NOTE: ASA , antiplatelet agents, Coumadin or heparin not recommended for 24 hours if tPA was given* Date & time it can be started: _____

TIME	ORDER	MD/DO SIGNATURE

9/2001   Guidelines do not replace clinical judgement and should be modified according to individual patient needs

FIGURE AP-3 (Continued)

ACUTE ISCHEMIC STROKE
CLINICAL GUIDELINES
EXPECTED LOS: 3-5 Days (check box to initiate order)
ORDERS (*) ARE 24 HOURS ORDERS AND MUST BE ASSESSED DAILY

---

24 HOUR ORDERS THAT MUST BE ASSESSED DAILY
If not checked will continue for another 24 hours

Date _____ Time: _____

Activity _____

❑ Diet _____

❑ IV _____

D/C GLUCOSE FINGERSTICK	YES ❑	NO ❑	N/A ❑
D/C FOLEY	YES ❑	NO ❑	N/A ❑
D/C CARDIAC MONITOR	YES ❑	NO ❑	N/A ❑
D/C PULSE OX/O$_2$	YES ❑	NO ❑	N/A ❑

CONSULTS NEEDED _____

_____
(Consider Rehab evaluation, PEG, etc)

Reminder-Should be on medication to prevent recurrent stroke.
If patient to be D/C'd complete NIHSS

Signature _____ MD/DO
(Use additional physician order sheets as needed)

Discharge plan ❑ home ❑ Rehab ❑ ECF ❑ Other:

---

24 HOUR ORDERS THAT MUST BE ASSESSED DAILY
If not checked will continue for another 24 hours

Date _____ Time: _____

Activity _____

❑ Diet _____

❑ IV _____

D/C GLUCOSE FINGERSTICK	YES ❑	NO ❑	N/A ❑
D/C FOLEY	YES ❑	NO ❑	N/A ❑
D/C CARDIAC MONITOR	YES ❑	NO ❑	N/A ❑
D/C PULSE OX/O$_2$	YES ❑	NO ❑	N/A ❑

CONSULTS NEEDED _____

_____
(Consider Rehab evaluation, PEG, etc)

Reminder-Should be on medication to prevent recurrent stroke
If patient to be D/C'd complete NIHSS

Signature _____ MD/DO
(Use additional physician order sheets as needed)

Discharge plan ❑ home ❑ Rehab ❑ ECF ❑ Other:

---

24 HOUR ORDERS THAT MUST BE ASSESSED DAILY
If not checked will continue for another 24 hours

Date _____ Time: _____

Activity _____

❑ Diet _____

❑ IV _____

D/C GLUCOSE FINGERSTICK	YES ❑	NO ❑	N/A ❑
D/C FOLEY	YES ❑	NO ❑	N/A ❑
D/C CARDIAC MONITOR	YES ❑	NO ❑	N/A ❑
D/C PULSE OX/O$_2$	YES ❑	NO ❑	N/A ❑

CONSULTS NEEDED _____

_____
(Consider Rehab evaluation, PEG, etc)

Reminder-Should be on medication to prevent recurrent stroke
If patient to be D/C'd complete NIHSS

Signature _____ MD/DO
(Use additional physician order sheets as needed)

Discharge plan ❑ home ❑ Rehab ❑ ECF ❑ Other:

---

24 HOUR ORDERS THAT MUST BE ASSESSED DAILY
If not checked will continue for another 24 hours

Date _____ Time: _____

Activity _____

❑ Diet _____

❑ IV _____

D/C GLUCOSE FINGERSTICK	YES ❑	NO ❑	N/A ❑
D/C FOLEY	YES ❑	NO ❑	N/A ❑
D/C CARDIAC MONITOR	YES ❑	NO ❑	N/A ❑
D/C PULSE OX/O$_2$	YES ❑	NO ❑	N/A ❑

CONSULTS NEEDED _____

_____
(Consider Rehab evaluation, PEG, etc)

Reminder-Should be on medication to prevent recurrent stroke
If patient to be D/C'd complete NIHSS

Signature _____ MD/DO
(Use additional physician order sheets as needed)

Discharge plan ❑ home ❑ Rehab ❑ ECF ❑ Other:

9/2001 Guidelines do not replace clinical judgement and should be modified according to individual patient needs

FIGURE AP-3 (Continued)

MEDICAL COLLEGE OF OHIO
STROKE DATA SUMMARY

ADDRESSOGRAPH

Clinical Diagnosis (Check all that apply)

	Anterior R	**L**	**Posterior**
☐ TIA	☐	☐	☐
☐ Ischemic Stroke	☐	☐	☐
☐ Cerebral Hemorrhage	☐	☐	☐

Mechanism of Stroke

- ☐ Small Vessel Occlusive
- ☐ Cardioembolic
- ☐ Large Vessel Atherosclerotic
- ☐ Tandem Lesion Stroke (Artery to Artery embolus)
- ☐ Vasculitis
- ☐ Hypercoagulable State (specify defect) _____
- ☐ Other identified cause (specify) _____
- ☐ Cryptogenic (unidentified cause) _____
- ☐ Hemorrhagic Transformation of Ischemic Stroke
- ☐ Hypertensive Hemorrhage
- ☐ Lobar Hemorrhage
- ☐ Ruptured Aneurysm
- ☐ Ruptured AVM

Clinical Manifestations

Presenting Deficits	*Residual Deficits*
☐ Aphasia	☐ Aphasia
☐ Ataxia	☐ Ataxia
☐ Dysarthria	☐ Dysarthria
☐ Dysphagia	☐ Dysphagia
☐ Numbness/Tingling	☐ Numbness/Tingling
☐ Weakness	☐ Weakness
☐ Visual loss	☐ Visual loss
☐ Others:	☐ Others:
☐ NIHSS _____	☐ NIHSS _____ (at D/C)

Location of Infarcts

☐ Cerebral Cortex:	☐ Subcortical Areas
☐ Lt. hemisphere	☐ Subcortical white
☐ Rt. hemisphere	matter
☐ Frontal Lobe	☐ Internal capsule
☐ Parietal Lobe	☐ Basal ganglia
☐ Occipital Lobe	☐ Thalamus
☐ Temporal Lobe	☐ Brainstem
☐ ACA	☐ Cerebellum (VB)
☐ PCA	☐ Spinal Cord
☐ MCA	☐ Unknown

Risk Factors Identified and Modified (Circle)

Hypertension   Diabetes   Hyperlipidemia   Smoking
ETOH   A-Fib   prior CVA/TIA   PFO/ASD   Migraines
PVD   CHF   CAD
Other: _____

Complications (Circle)
DVT   Pneumonia   UTI   Death   Other _____

Diagnostic Procedure Results

- ☐ **CT Results:** ☐ Hemorrhage ☐ Ischemic Infarction
- ☐ **TEE Results (Circle)**
  1. Negative   4. Cardiac thrombus
  2. PFO   5. LVEF
  3. Left atrial enlargement 6. Other: _____
- ☐ **TTE Results: (Circle)**
  1. Negative   3. Positive Lt. Ventricular
  2. Positive for   Hypertrophy
      intra-ventricular clot   4. Other: _____
- ☐ **MRI Results:** ☐ Normal ☐ Infarct
          ☐ Diffuse microvascular disease ☐ Other
- ☐ **DWI** ☐ Normal ☐ Acute infarct
- ☐ **MRA Results:** ☐ Normal ☐ Infarct
          ☐ Intracranial stenosis ☐ Other
- ☐ **Carotid Duplex Results: (Circle)**
  1. Negative
  2. R Carotid Stenosis > 60%
  3. L Carotid Stenosis > 60%
- ☐ **Angiogram:** Results: _____
- ☐ **EKG** ☐ NSR ☐ A-Fib ☐ Other
- ☐ **Labs:**
  Total cholesterol: _____ LDL: _____ HDL: _____
  Other Coag. Studies: _____
  Other: _____

Stroke Treatment/Prevention

Acute therapy
- ☐ Thrombolysis: ☐ IV ☐ IA
- ☐ Neurology Consult
- ☐ Stroke Study Enrollment: (specify which study) _____

Prevention therapy

Pre-admission	*Discharge*
☐ ASA (dose ____ mg)	☐ ASA (dose ____ mg)
☐ Aggrenox	☐ Aggrenox
☐ Warfarin	☐ Warfarin
☐ Ticlopidine	☐ Ticlopidine
☐ Clopidogrel	☐ Clopidogrel
☐ C. Endarterectomy/ Stent	☐ C. Endarter./Stent
☐ Cholesterol Lowering Agent	☐ Chol. Lower. Agent
☐ No Therapy	☐ No Therapy
☐ LMWH	☐ LMWH

Discharge Destination: _____

Date of Stroke _____ #of days in hospital ___

Attending Signature: _____
                            (Date/Time)

Resident Signature: _____
                            (Date/Time)

(9/2001)

FIGURE AP-3 (Continued)

Regional Radical Prostatectomy – Clinical Pathway, April 2002

		Pre-Admission Clinic	Day 0 – Admission/Pre operative	Day 0 - Post-operative
	Date			
Consults		As ordered		
Tests / Diagnostics		EKG Type and Screen CBC, Sodium, Potassium, CR, Chloride, CO_2 and urinalysis		CBC at 2000 h
Interventions		Two day bowel prep. NPO after midnight, night before surgery	Start IV with #18 catheter, give Normal Saline bolus 500 mL / h x 2, then run at 150 mL / h Antiembolic stockings Oxygen saturation on room air Pre-op checklist completed	Routine post-operative vital signs In and out q2h overnight Indwelling catheter care IV Normal Saline at 150 mL / h Pneumatic stockings Incentive spirometer q1h while awake Monitor Jackson Pratt (JP) drainage Dressing
Medications			Heparin sc if ordered Cefazolin Sodium 1g IV or if allergy check Patient Care Orders	Heparin sc if ordered For patients receiving intraspinal morphine in O.R. follow protocol on "<u>Intraspinal Analgesia</u>" orders For patients using PCA follow "Standing Patient Care Orders" for <u>Patient Controlled Analgesia</u>
Diet			NPO	Sips - clear fluids
Activity		Activity as tolerated (AAT)	AAT	
Teaching		Deep breathing and coughing "Before And After Your Radical Prostatectomy" booklet Leg exercises	Reinforce deep breathing and coughing exercises, leg exercises	Deep breathing and coughing Use of inspirometer PCA pump use

FIGURE AP-4 This clinical pathway for patients having a radical prostatectomy begins with the pre-admission clinic and ends with discharge on post-operative day four. Reproduced with permission of Capital Health, Edmonton, Alberta. (Continued)

Capital Health: Radical Prostatectomy

	Day 1 - Post-operative	INITIAL	Day 2 - Post-operative	INITIAL
Date				
Consults			Home care referral, if required Social worker, if required	
Tests / Diagnostics	CBC, Sodium, Potassium, Chloride, CO$_2$			
Interventions	Routine vital signs In and out q shift Indwelling catheter care Decrease IV to 100 mL / h Discontinue pneumatic stockings, remove antiembolic stockings bid for skin care, and reapply Incentive spirometer q1h while awake Monitor JP drainage Remove dressing - leave incision open to air		Routine vital signs In and out q shift Teach patient to change urometer bag to leg bag during day Indwelling catheter care Discontinue IV if drinking well Remove antiembolic stockings bid for skin care, then reapply Remove one JP drain if drainage < 20 mL in 8 h Check incision - wound care	
Medications	Heparin sc if ordered Administer analgesics as required / monitor PCA pump Monitor pain control		Heparin sc if ordered Discontinue PCA pump / administer analgesics as required Monitor pain control Bowel routine as ordered	
Diet	Clear fluids		Full fluids Regular diet if passing flatus	
Activity	Mobilize qid		AAT	
Teaching	Deep breathing and coughing		Catheter care Application and care of leg bag Kegel exercises	

FIGURE AP-4 (Continued)

Capital Health: Radical Prostatectomy

	Day 3 - Post-operative	INITIAL	Day 4 - Post-operative	INITIAL
Date				
Consults	Pharmacy - re: discharge medications			
Tests / Diagnostics			Discharge	
Interventions	Routine vital signs In and out q shift Indwelling catheter care / Leg bag on during day Remove antiembolic stockings bid for skin care / discontinue if ambulating well Remove second JP drain if drainage < 20 mL in 8 h Check incision - wound care		Routine vital signs In and out q shift Indwelling catheter care / Leg bag on during the day Make arrangements for staple removal	
Medications	Discontinue Heparin sc if ambulating well Bowel routine as ordered Administer oral analgesics as required for pain control		Bowel routine as ordered Administer oral analgesics as required	
Diet	Diet as tolerated (DAT)		DAT	
Activity	AAT		AAT	
Teaching	Reinforce teaching Discharge teaching Review 'Before and After Your Radical Prostatectomy' booklet with patient		Discharge teaching Follow-up appointment Prescription	

FIGURE AP-4 (Continued)

Capital Health

Standard Discharge Summary for Uncomplicated Radical Prostatectomy Patients

PRINT FIRMLY AND NEATLY TO ENSURE ALL COPIES ARE LEGIBLE

☐ UAH   ☐ RAH   ☐ Leduc   ☐ Sturgeon

Referring Physician _____   ☐ Faxed   ☐ Mailed

Address _____

Family Physician _____   ☐ Faxed   ☐ Mailed

Address _____

Additional copies to _____   ☐ Faxed   ☐ Mailed

Address _____

Admission date _____   Discharge date _____

Procedure performed: (**PROSTATECTOMY**)   ☐ Retropubic   ☐ Laparoscopic   ☐ Perineal

Course in hospital _____

_____

_____

_____

Condition on discharge _____

_____

_____

_____

_____

☐ Indwelling Catheter in situ   ☐ Jackson Pratt drain in   ☐ Staples in   ☐ Dressing

☐ Home Care referral: a)   catheter care _____

  b)   staple removal _____

  c)   wound care _____

  d)   Jackson Pratt care _____

Prescriptions on discharge:

  ☐ Pain control _____

  ☐ Bowel routine _____

  ☐ Antibiotic _____

  ☐ Other _____

☐ Follow-up appointment   a)   Indwelling catheter removal _____

  b)   Physician's visit _____

Physician *(signature)* _____ MD.

FIGURE AP-4 (Continued)

Diagnostic Studies and Interpretation

TEST VALUE STUDIED

Reference Ranges—Hematology
Reference Ranges—Serum, Plasma, and Whole Blood Chemistries
Reference Ranges—Immunodiagnostic Tests
Reference Ranges—Urine Chemistry
Reference Ranges—Cerebrospinal Fluid (CSF)
Miscellaneous Values

SELECTED ABBREVIATIONS USED IN REFERENCE RANGES

Conventional Units

kg = kilogram
gm = gram
mg = milligram
μg = microgram
μμg = micromicrogram
ng = nanogram
pg = picogram
dL = 100 millilitres
mL = millilitre
mm³ = cubic millimetre
fL = femtolitre
mM = millimole
nM = nanomole
mOsm = milliosmole
mm = millimetre
μm = micron or micrometer
mm Hg = millimetres of mercury
U = unit

mU = milliunit
μU = microunit
mEq = milliequivalent
IU = International Unit
mIU = milliInternational Unit

SI Units

g = gram
L = litre
d = day
h = hour
mol = mole
mmol = millimole
μmol = micromole
nmol = nanomole
pmol = picomole

Table B-1 • **Reference Ranges—Hematology***

	REFERENCE RANGE		
DETERMINATION	**SI Units**	**Conventional Units**	**CLINICAL SIGNIFICANCE**
A_2 hemoglobin	Mass fraction: 0.015–0.035 of total hemoglobin	2.0%–3.2% of total hemoglobin	Increased in certain types of thalassemia
Bleeding time	1.5–9.5 min	1.5–9.5 min	Prolonged in thrombocytopenia, defective platelet function, and aspirin therapy
Factor V assay (pro-accelerin factor)		60%–140%	
Factor VIII assay (anti-hemophiliac factor)		60%–140%	Deficient in classical hemophilia
Factor IX assay (plasma thromboplastin component)		60%–140%	Deficient in Christmas disease (pseudohemophilia)
Factor X (Stuart factor)		60%–140%	Deficient in Stuart clotting defect
Fibrinogen	2–4 g/dL	200–400 mg/dL	Increased in pregnancy, infections accompanied by leukocytosis, nephrosis. Decreased in severe liver disease, abruptio placentae
Fibrin split (degradation) products	<5 µg/mL	<5 µg/mL	Increased in disseminated intravascular coagulation
Fibrinolysins (whole blood clot lysis time)		No lysis in 24 h	Increased activity associated with massive hemorrhage, extensive surgery, transfusion reactions
Partial thromboplastin time (activated)		Lower limit of normal: 20–25 sec; Upper limit of normal: 32–39 sec	Prolonged in deficiency of fibrinogen, factors II, V, VIII, IX, X, XI, and XII, and in heparin therapy
Prothrombin consumption		Lower limit of normal: 10 sec Lower limit of normal: 14 sec	Impaired in deficiency of factors VIII, IX, and X
Prothrombin time		9.5–12 sec	Prolonged by deficiency of factors I, II, V, VII, and X, fat malabsorption, severe liver disease, coumarin anticoagulant therapy.
INR		1.0	
		2–3 for therapy in atrial fibrillation, deep vein thrombosis, and pulmonary embolism. 2.5–3.5 for therapy in prosthetic heart valves	INR used to standardize the prothrombin time and anticoagulation therapy
Erythrocyte count	$4.6–6.2 \times 10^{12}$/L $4.2–5.4 \times 10^{12}$/L	Males: 4,600,000–6,200,000/cu mm Females: 4,200,000–5,400,000/cu mm	Increased in severe diarrhea and dehydration, polycythemia, acute poisoning, pulmonary fibrosis. Decreased in all anemias in leukemia, and after hemorrhage, when blood volume has been restored
Erythrocyte indices			
Mean corpuscular volume (MCV)	84–96 fL	84–96 cu µm	Increased in macrocytic anemias; decreased in microcytic anemia
Mean corpuscular hemoglobin (MCH)	28–33 pg	28–33 µµg/cell	Increased in macrocytic anemias; decreased in microcytic anemia
Mean corpuscular hemoglobin concentration (MCHC)	Concentration fraction: 0.33–0.35	33%–35%	Decreased in severe hypochromic anemia
Reticulocytes	Number fraction: 0.005–0.015	0.5%–1.5% of red cells	Increased with any condition stimulating increase in bone marrow activity (ie, infection, blood loss [acute and chronically following iron therapy in iron deficiency anemia], polycythemia rubra vera). Decreased with any condition depressing bone marrow activity, acute leukemia, late stage of severe anemias

(continued)

DETERMINATION	REFERENCE RANGE		CLINICAL SIGNIFICANCE
	SI Units	Conventional Units	
Erythrocyte sedimentation rate (ESR)—Westergren method	<15 mm/h <20 mm/h <25 mm/h <30 mm/h	Males under 50 yr: <15 mm/h Males over 50 yr: <20 mm/h Females under 50 yr: <25 mm/h Females over 50 yr: <30 mm/h	Increased in tissue destruction, whether inflammatory or degenerative; during menstruation and pregnancy; and in acute febrile diseases
Erythrocyte sedimentation ratio—Zeta centrifuge	Volume fraction: <0.55 0.40–0.60	<50 years: <55% 50–80 years: 40%–60%	Significance similar to ESR
Hematocrit	Volume fraction: 0.42–0.52 Volume fraction: 0.35–0.47	Males: 42%–52% Females: 35%–47%	Decreased in severe anemias, anemia of pregnancy, acute massive blood loss Increased in erythrocytosis of any cause, and in dehydration or hemoconcentration associated with shock
Hemoglobin	2.02–2.79 mmol/L 1.86–2.48 mmol/L	Males: 13–18 gm/dL Females: 12–16 gm/dL	Decreased in various anemias, pregnancy, severe or prolonged hemorrhage, and with excessive fluid intake Increased in polycythemia, chronic obstructive pulmonary disease, failure of oxygenation because of congestive heart failure, and normally in people living at high altitudes
Hemoglobin F	Mass fraction: <0.02	Less than 2% of total hemoglobin	Increased in infants and children, and in thalassemia and many anemias
Leukocyte alkaline phosphatase		Score of 15–130 (varies among labs)	Increased in polycythemia vera, myelofibrosis, and infections Decreased in chronic granulocytic leukemia, paroxysmal nocturnal hemoglobinuria, hypoplastic marrow, and viral infections, particularly infectious mononucleosis
Leukocyte count 　Neutrophils 　Eosinophils 　Basophils 　Lymphocytes 　Monocytes	4.5–11 × 10^9/L Number fraction: 0.45–0.73 Number fraction: 0.00–0.04 Number fraction: 0.00–0.01 Number fraction: 0.2–0.4 Number fraction: 0.02–0.08	Total: 4,500–11,000/cu mm 45%–73% 0%–4% 0%–1% 20%–40% 2%–8%	Neutrophils increased with acute infections, trauma or surgery, leukemia, malignant disease, necrosis; decreased with viral infections, bone marrow suppression, primary bone marrow disease Eosinophils increased in allergy, parasitic disease, collagen disease, subacute infections; decreased with stress, use of some medications (ACTH, epinephrine, thyroxine) Basophils increased with acute leukemia and following surgery or trauma; decreased with allergic reactions, stress, allergy, parasitic disease, use of corticosteroids Lymphocytes increased with infectious mononucleosis, viral and some bacterial infections, hepatitis; decreased with aplastic anemia, SLE, immunodeficiency including AIDS Monocytes increased with viral infections, parasitic disease, collagen and hemolytic disorders; decreased with use of corticosteroids, RA, HIV infection
Platelet count	0.15–0.45 × 10^{12}/L	150,000–450,000/cu mm	Increased in malignancy, myeloproliferative disease, rheumatoid arthritis, and postoperatively; about 50% of patients with unexpected increase of platelet count will be found to have a malignancy Decreased in thrombocytopenic purpura, acute leukemia, aplastic anemia, and during cancer chemotherapy.

*Laboratory values may vary according to the techniques used in different laboratories.

Table B-2 • **Reference Ranges—Serum, Plasma, and Whole Blood Chemistries**

DETERMINATION	NORMAL ADULT REFERENCE RANGE		CLINICAL SIGNIFICANCE	
	SI Units	Conventional Units	Increased	Decreased
Acetoacetate	19.6–98 μmol/L	0.2–1.0 mg/dL	Diabetic acidosis Fasting	
Acetone	51.6–344.0/μmol/L	0.3–2.0 mg/dL	Diabetic ketoacidosis Toxemia of pregnancy Carbohydrate-free diet High-fat diet	
Acid, total phos-phatase	Males: 2–12 UL Females: 0.3–9.2 UL	Males: 2–12 UL Females: 0.3–9.2 UL	Carcinoma of prostate Advanced Paget's disease Hyperparathyroidism Gaucher's disease	
Acid, phosphatase, prostatic—RIA	2.5–3.37 μg/L	2.5–3.37 ng/mL	Carcinoma of prostate	
Alkaline phosphatase	50–120 UL	Adults: 50–120 UL	Conditions reflecting increased osteoblastic activity of bone Rickets Hyperparathyroidism Hepatic disease Bone disease	
Alkaline phos-phatase, ther-mostable fraction		Hepatic: >25% Combined: 10%–25% Skeletal: <10%		
Adrenocorticotropic hormone (ACTH) (plasma)—RIA*	<50 ng/L	<50 pg/mL	Pituitary-dependent Cushing's syndrome Ectopic ACTH syndrome Primary adrenal atrophy	Adrenocortical tumour Adrenal insufficiency secondary to hypo-pituitarism
Aldolase	22–59 mU/L at 37°C	3–8 Sibley-Lehninger U/dL at 37°C	Hepatic necrosis Granulocytic leukemia Myocardial infarction Skeletal muscle disease	
Aldosterone (plasma)—RIA	0.08–0.30 nmol/L 0.14–0.90 nmol/L 5.54–22.16 nmol/L	Supine: 3–10 ng/dL Upright: 5–30 ng/dL Adrenal vein: 200–800 ng/dL	Primary aldosteronism Secondary aldosteronism	Addison's disease
Alpha-1-antitrypsin	1.1–1.4 g/L	110–140 mg/dL		Certain forms of chronic lung and liver disease in young adults
Alpha-1-fetoprotein	<15 μg/L	<15 ng/mL	Hepatocarcinoma Metastatic carcinoma of liver Germinal cell carcinoma of the testicle or ovary Fetal neural tube defects—elevation in maternal serum	
Alpha-hydroxy-butyric dehydroge-nase	<140 U/L	<140 U/L	Myocardial infarction Granulocytic leukemia Hemolytic anemias Muscular dystrophy	
Ammonia (plasma)	11–32/μmol/L	15–45, μg/dL (varies with method	Severe liver disease Hepatic decompensation	
Amylase	111–296U/L	60–160 Somogyi U/dL	Acute pancreatitis Mumps Duodenal ulcer Carcinoma of head of pancreas Prolonged elevation with pseudo-cyst of pancreas Increased by medications that constrict pancreatic duct sphincters: morphine, codeine, cholinergics	Chronic pancreatitis Pancreatic fibrosis and atrophy Cirrhosis of liver Pregnancy (2nd and 3rd trimesters)

(continued)

Table B-2 • Reference Ranges—Serum, Plasma, and Whole Blood Chemistries (Continued)

DETERMINATION	NORMAL ADULT REFERENCE RANGE		CLINICAL SIGNIFICANCE	
	SI Units	Conventional Units	Increased	Decreased
Arsenic	<0.93–2.6 µmol/L; poisoning: 133–6.65 µmol/L	<70 µg/dL; poisoning: 100–150 µg/dL	Intentional or unintentional poisoning Excessive occupational exposure	
Ascorbic acid (vitamin C)	23–85 µmol/L	0.4–1.5 mg/dL	Large doses of ascorbic acid as a prophylactic against the common cold	
ALT (alanine aminotransferase), formerly SGPT	Males: 0.17–0.68 µkat/L Females: 0.14–0.60 µkat/L	Males: 10–40 U/mL Females: 8–35 U/mL	Same conditions as AST (SGOT), but increase is more marked in liver disease than AST (SGOT)	
AST (aspartate aminotransferase), formerly SGOT	Males: 0.34–0.68 µkat/L Females: 0.25–0.51 µkat/L	Males: 10–40 U/L Females: 15–30 U/L	Myocardial infarction Skeletal muscle disease Liver disease	
Bilirubin	5–17µmol/L 1.7–3.7/µmol/L 3.4–11.2 µmol/L	Total: 0.3–1.0 mg/dL Direct: 0.1–0.4 mg/dL Indirect: 0.1–0.4 mg/dL	Hemolytic anemia (indirect) Biliary obstruction and disease Hepatocellular damage (hepatitis) Pernicious anemia Hemolytic disease of newborn	
Blood gases Oxygen, arterial (whole blood): Partial pressure (PaO_2)	10.64–12.64 kPa	85–95 mm Hg	Polycythemia	Anemia Cardiac or pulmonary disease
Saturation (SaO_2)	Volume fraction: 0.95–0.99	95%–99%		Cardiac decompensation Chronic obstructive lung disease
Carbon dioxide, arterial (whole blood) partial pressure ($PaCO_2$)	4.66–5.99 kPa	35–45 mm Hg	Respiratory acidosis Metabolic alkalosis	Respiratory alkalosis Metabolic acidosis
pH (whole blood, arterial)	7.35–7.45	7.35–7.45	Vomiting Hyperventilation Fever Intestinal obstruction	Uremia Diabetic acidosis Hemorrhage Nephritis
Calcitonin	19 ng/L <350 ng/L <100 ng/L	Basal: <19 pg/mL Stimulation test Males: <350 pg/mL Females: <100 pg/mL	Medullary carcinoma of the thyroid Some nonthyroid tumours Zollinger-Ellison syndrome	
Calcium	2.15–2.55 mmol/L	8.6–10.2 mg/dL	Tumour or hyperplasia of parathyroid Hypervitaminosis D Multiple myeloma Nephritis with uremia Malignant tumours Sarcoidosis Hyperthyroidism Skeletal immobilization Excess calcium intake:milk alkali syndrome	Hypoparathyroidism Diarrhea Celiac disease Vitamin D deficiency Acute pancreatitis Nephrosis After parathyroidectomy
CO_2, venous	24–32 mmol/L 18–24 mmol/L	Adults 24–32 mEq/L Infants: 18–24 mEq/L	Tetany Respiratory disease Intestinal obstruction Vomiting	Acidosis Nephritis Eclampsia Diarrhea Anesthesia

(continued)

Table B-2 • Reference Ranges—Serum, Plasma, and Whole Blood Chemistries (Continued)

DETERMINATION	NORMAL ADULT REFERENCE RANGE SI Units	Conventional Units	CLINICAL SIGNIFICANCE Increased	Decreased
Catecholamines (plasma)—RIA	<540 pmol/L	Epinephrine: <100 pg/mL	Pheochromocytoma	
	<2360 pmol/L	Norepinephrine: <400 pg/mL		
	<935 pmol/L	Dopamine: <143 pg/mL		
Ceruloplasmin	1.26–2.52 µmol/L	20–40 mg/dL		Wilson's disease (hepatolenticular degeneration)
Chloride	97–107 mmol/L	97–107 mEq/L	Nephrosis Nephritis Urinary obstruction Cardiac decompensation Anemia	Diabetes mellitus Diarrhea Vomiting Pneumonia Heavy metal poisoning Cushing's syndrome Intestinal obstruction Febrile conditions
Cholesterol	3.9–5.2 mmol/L	150–200 mg/dL	Lipemia Obstructive jaundice Diabetes Hypothyroidism	Pernicious anemia Hemolytic anemia Hyperthyroidism Severe infection Terminal states of debilitating disease
Cholesterol esters	Fraction of total cholesterol 0.6–0.7	60%–70% of total		The esterified fraction decreases in liver diseases
Cholinesterase	0.6–1.6 U 0.6–1 U	Serum: 0.6–1.6 delta pH Red cells-0.6–1 delta pH	Nephrosis Exercise	Nerve gas exposure (greater effect on red cell activity) Insecticide poisoning
Chorionic gonadotropin, beta subunit	0–5 IU/L	0–5 IU/L	Pregnancy Hydatidiform mole Choriocarcinoma	Threatened abortion Ectopic pregnancy
Complement, C₃	0.8–1.7 g/L	80–170 mg/dL	Some inflammatory diseases, acute myocardial infarction, cancer	Acute glomerulonephritis Disseminated lupus erythematosus with renal involvement
Complement C₄	180–510 mg/L	18–51 mg/dL	Some inflammatory diseases, acute myocardial infarction, cancer	Often decreased in immunologic disease, especially with active systemic lupus erythematosus Hereditary angioneurotic edema
Complement, total (hemolytic)	25–70 U/mL	90%–94% complement	Some inflammatory diseases	Acute glomerulonephritis Epidemic meningitis Subacute bacterial endocarditis
Copper	11–24 µmol/L	70–150 µg/dL	Cirrhosis of liver Pregnancy	Wilson's disease
Cortisol-RIA	138–690 nmol/L 83–442 nmol/L	8 AM: 5–25/µg/dL 4 PM: 3–16 µg/dL	Stress: infectious disease, surgery, burns, etc. Pregnancy Cushing's syndrome Pancreatitis Eclampsia	Addison's disease Anterior pituitary hypofunction
C-peptide reactivity	0.9–4.0 µg/L	0.9–4.0 ng/mL	Insulinoma	Diabetes mellitus

(continued)

Table B-2 • **Reference Ranges—Serum, Plasma, and Whole Blood Chemistries** (Continued)

DETERMINATION	NORMAL ADULT REFERENCE RANGE		CLINICAL SIGNIFICANCE	
	SI Units	Conventional Units	Increased	Decreased
Creatine	15.3–61 µmol/L	0.2–0.8 mg/mL	Pregnancy Skeletal muscle necrosis or atrophy Starvation Hyperthyroidism	
Creatine phosphoki- nase (CPK)	50–325 U/L 50–250 U/L	Males: 50–325 mU/mL Females: 50–250 mU/mL	Myocardial infarction Skeletal muscle diseases Intramuscular injections Crush syndrome Hypothyroidism Alcohol withdrawal delirium Alcoholic myopathy Cerebrovascular disease	
Creatine phosphoki- nase isoenzymes		MM band present (skele- tal muscle)-MB band absent (heart muscle)	MB band increased in myocardial infarction, ischemia	
Creatinine	62–124 µmol/L	0.7–1.4 mg/dL	Nephritis Chronic renal disease	
Creatinine clearance	1.42–2.08 mL/s 1.25–1.92 mL/s	Males: 85–125 mL/min Females: 75–115 mL/min		Kidney diseases
Cryoglobulins, qual- itative		Negative	Multiple myeloma Chronic lymphocytic leukemia Lymphosarcoma Systemic lupus erythematosus Rheumatoid arthritis Infective subacute endocarditis Some malignancies Scleroderma	
11-Deoxycortisol	<0.029 µmol/L	1/µg/dL	Hypertensive form of virilizing adrenal hyperplasia due to an 11-β-hydroxylase defect	
Dibucaine number		Normal: 70%–85% inhibition Heterozygote: 50%–65% inhibition Homozygote: 16%–25% inhibition		Important in detecting carriers of abnormal cholinesterase activity who are susceptible to succinylcholine anesthetic shock
Dihydrotestosterone	1.72–7.22 nmol/L	Males: 50–210 ng/dL Females: none detectable		Testicular feminization syndrome
Estradiol—RIA	 37–370 pmol/L 367–1835 pmol/L 184–881 pmol/L	Females: Follicular: 10–90 pg/mL Midcycle: 100–500 pg/mL Luteal: 50–240 pg/mL Follicular phase: 2–20 ng/dL Midcycle: 12–40 ng/dL Luteal phase: 10-30 ng/dL Postmenopausal: 1–5 ng/dL Males: 0.5–5 ng/dL	Pregnancy	Depressed or failure to peak—ovarian failure
Estriol—RIA	<1.75 nmol/L Up to 3.5 nmol/L 2.8–24.3 nmol/L 17.4–86.8 nmol/L	Nonpregnant females: <0.5 ng/mL Pregnant females: 1st trimester: up to 1 ng/mL 2nd trimester: 0.8–7 ng/mL 3rd trimester: 5–25 ng/mL	Pregnancy	Depressed or failure to peak—ovarian failure

(continued)

Table B-2 • Reference Ranges—Serum, Plasma, and Whole Blood Chemistries (Continued)

DETERMINATION	NORMAL ADULT REFERENCE RANGE SI Units	Conventional Units	CLINICAL SIGNIFICANCE Increased	Decreased
Estrogens, total—RIA	61–394 ng/L 122–437 ng/L 156–350 ng/L 40–115 ng/L	Females: cycle days: Day 1–10: 61–394 pg/mL Day 11–20: 122–437 pg/mL Day 21–30: 156–350 pg/mL Males: 40–115 pg/mL	Pregnancy Measured on a daily basis, can be used to evaluate response of hypogonadotrophic, hypoestrogenic women to human menopausal or pituitary gonadotropin	Fetal distress Ovarian failure
Estrone—RIA	15.9–66.6 pmol/L 27.8–72.5 pmol/L 48.1–74 pmol/L 9.3–27.8 pmol/L	Females: Day 1–10: 4.3–18 ng/dL Day 11–20: 7.5–19.6 ng/dL Day 21–30: 13–20 ng/dL Males: 2.5–7.5 ng/dL		Depressed or failure to peak—ovarian failure
Ferritin—RIA	20–250 µg/L 12–250 µg/L	Males: 20–250 ng/mL Females: 12–250 ng/mL	Nephritis Hemochromatosis Certain neoplastic diseases Acute myelogenous leukemia Multiple myeloma	Iron deficiency
Folic acid—RIA	6–46 nmol/L	2.5–20 ng/mL		Megaloblastic anemias of infancy and pregnancy Inadequate diet Liver disease Malabsorption syndrome Severe hemolytic anemia
Follicle stimulating hormone (FSH)—RIA	5–20 IU/L 12–30 IU/L 5–15 IU/L 40–200 IU/L	Males: 2–10 mIU/mL Females: Follicular phase: 5–20 mIU/mL Peak of middle cycle: 12–30 mIU/mL Luteinic phase: 5–15 mIU/mL Menopausal females: 40–200 mIU/mL	Menopause and primary ovarian failure	Pituitary failure
Galactose	<0.28 mmol/L	<5 mg/dL		Galactosemia
Gamma glutamyl transpeptidase	0.03–0.5/µkat/L 0.02–0.4/µkat/L	Males: 20–30U/L Females: 1–24U/L	Hepatobiliary disease Drug toxicity Myocardial infarction Renal infarction Zollinger-Ellison syndrome	
Gastrin—RIA	50–155 ng/L 80–170 ng/L	Fasting: 50–155 pg/mL Postprandial: 80–170 pg/mL	Peptic ulceration of the duodenum Pernicious anemia	
Glucose	3.3–6.05 mmol/L 3.58–7.7 mmol/L	Fasting: 60–110 mg/dL Postprandial (2 h): 65–140 mg/dL	Diabetes mellitus Nephritis Hyperthyroidism Early hyperpituitarism Cerebral lesions Infections Pregnancy Uremia	Hyperinsulinism Hypothyroidism Late hyperpituitarism Pernicious vomiting Addison's disease Extensive hepatic damage

(continued)

Table B-2 • Reference Ranges—Serum, Plasma, and Whole Blood Chemistries (Continued)

DETERMINATION	NORMAL ADULT REFERENCE RANGE		CLINICAL SIGNIFICANCE	
	SI Units	Conventional Units	Increased	Decreased
Glucose tolerance (oral)		Features of a normal response:	Two-hour value >200 mg/dL (11.1 mmol/L) is diagnostic for diabetes mellitus	Decreased 2 and 3 hour values may occur with hypoglycemia mellitus
	3.3–6.05 mmol/L	1. Normal fasting between 60–110 mg/dL 2. No sugar in urine 3. Upper limits of normal:		
	6.88 mmol/L 10.45 mmol/L 7.70 mmol/L 6.88 mmol/L	Fasting = 125 1 hour = 190 2 hours = 140 3 hours = 125		
Glucose-6-phosphate dehydrogenase (red cells)	1860–2500 U/L	Screening: Decolourization in 20–100 min Quantitative: 1.86–2.5 IU/mL RBC		Drug-induced hemolytic anemia Hemolytic disease of newborn
Glycoprotein (alpha-1-acid)	0.5–1.2 g/L	50–120 mg/dL	Neoplasm Tuberculosis Diabetes complicated by degenerative vascular disease Pregnancy Rheumatoid arthritis Rheumatic fever Infectious liver disease Lupus erythematosus	
Growth hormone—RIA	0.4 μg/L 0–18 μg/L	Males: 0–4 ng/mL Females: 0–18 ng/mL	Acromegaly	Failure to stimulate with arginine or insulin—hypopituitarism
Haptoglobin	0.3–2.0 g/L	30–200 mg/dL	Pregnancy Estrogen therapy Chronic infections Various inflammatory conditions	Hemolytic anemia Hemolytic blood transfusion reaction
Hemoglobin (plasma)	5–50 mg/L	0.5–5 mg/dL	Transfusion reactions Paroxysmal nocturnal hemoglobinuria Intravascular hemolysis	Anemia, pregnancy, chronic renal failure
Glycohemoglobin (GHB, hemoglobin A$_{1c}$, hemoblobin A1)		Nondiabetics and diabetics with good control: 4.4%–6.4%	Suboptimal glucose control	
Hexosaminidase, total Hexosaminidase A	333–375 μmol/L/h Fraction of total: 0.49–0.68 0.26–0.45 0–0.04 0.39–0.59	Controls: 333–375 nM/mL/h Controls: 49%–68% of total Heterozygotes: 26%–45% of total Tay-Sachs disease: 0%–4% of total Diabetics: 39%–59% of total	Sandhoff's disease	Tay-Sachs disease and heterozygotes
High-density lipoprotein cholesterol (HDL cholesterol)	0.91–1.81 mmol/L 0.91–2.20 mmol/L	Males: 35–70 mg/dL Females: 35–85 mg/dL		HDL cholesterol is lower in patients with increased risk for coronary heart disease
17 Hydroxy-progesterone—RIA	1.5–6.0 nmol/L 0.6–9.0 nmol/L <3.0 nmol/L	Males: 0.5–2.0 ng/mL Females: 0.2–3.0 ng/mL Children: <1.0 ng/mL	Congenital adrenal hyperplasia Pregnancy Some cases of adrenal or ovarian adenomas	

(continued)

Table B-2 • **Reference Ranges—Serum, Plasma, and Whole Blood Chemistries** (Continued)

DETERMINATION	NORMAL ADULT REFERENCE RANGE		CLINICAL SIGNIFICANCE	
	SI Units	Conventional Units	Increased	Decreased
Immunoglobulin A	0.85–3.85 g/L	Adults: 85–385 mg/dL (in children the normals are lower and vary with age)	Gamma A myeloma Wiskott-Aldrich syndrome Autoimmune disease Hepatic cirrhosis	Ataxia telangiectasis Agammaglobulinemia Hypogammaglobuline-mia, transient Dysgammaglobulinemia Protein-losing enteropathies
Immunoglobulin D	0–140 mg/L	0–14 mg/dL	IgD multiple myeloma Some patients with chronic infec-tious diseases	
Immunoglobulin E	100–700 µg/L	100–700 ng/mL	Allergic patients and those with parasitic infections	
Immunoglobulin G	6.35–14 g/L	Adults: 565–1765 mg/dL	IgG myeloma Following hyperimmunization Autoimmune disease states Chronic infections	Congenital and ac-quired hypogamma-globulinemia IgA myelomas, Waldenstrom's (IgM) macroglobulinemia Some malabsorption syndromes Extensive protein loss
Immunoglobulin M	0.4–2.8 g/L	Adults: 55–375 mg/dL	Waldenström's macroglobu-linemia Parasitic infections Hepatitis	Agammaglobulinemias Some IgG and IgA myelomas Chronic lymphatic leukemia
Insulin—RIA	0.2–1 µg/L	5–25 µU/mL	Insulinoma Acromegaly	Diabetes mellitus
Iron	9–29 µmol/L	50–160/µg/dL	Pernicious anemia Aplastic anemia Hemolytic anemia Hepatitis Hemochromatosis	Iron deficiency anemia
Iron-binding capacity	45–63 µmol/L 45–85 µmol/L Fraction of total iron-binding capacity: 0.2-0.5	IBC: 250–350 µg/dL TIBC: 250–475 µg/dL % Saturation: 20–50	Iron deficiency anemia Acute and chronic blood loss Hepatitis	Chronic infectious diseases Cirrhosis
Isocitric dehydro-genase	0.83–3 UIL	50–180 U	Hepatitis, cirrhosis Obstructive jaundice Metastatic carcinoma of the liver Megaloblastic anemia	
Lactic acid (whole blood)	0.5–1.7 mmol/L 0.36–1.25 mmol/L	Venous: 5–15 mg/dL Arterial: 3–11 mg/dL	Increased muscular activity Congestive heart failure Hemorrhage Shock Lactic acidosis Some febrile infections May be increased in severe liver disease	
Lactic dehydroge-nase (LDH)	90–176 U/L	90–176 mU/mL	Untreated pernicious anemia Myocardial infarction Pulmonary infarction Liver disease	
*Lactic dehydroge-nase isoenzymes Total lactic dehy-drogenase LDH-1 LDH-2 LDH-3 LDH-4 LDH-5	90–176 U/L Fraction of total LDH: 0.2–0.36 0.35–0.46 0.13–0.26 0.03–0.10 0.02–0.12	90–176 mU/mL 22%–36% 35%–46% 13%–26% 3%–10% 2%–12%	LDH-1 and LDH-2 are increased in myocardial infarction, mega-loblastic anemia, and hemolytic anemia LDH-4 and LDH-5 are increased in pulmonary infarction, congestive heart failure, and liver disease	

(continued)

Table B-2 • **Reference Ranges—Serum, Plasma, and Whole Blood Chemistries** (Continued)

DETERMINATION	NORMAL ADULT REFERENCE RANGE		CLINICAL SIGNIFICANCE	
	SI Units	Conventional Units	Increased	Decreased
Lead (whole blood)	Up to 2 µmol/L	Up to 40 µg/dL	Lead poisoning	
Leucine amino-peptidase	19.2–48 U/L	80–200 U/mL	Liver or bilary tract diseases Pancreatic disease Metastatic carcinoma of liver and pancreas Biliary obstruction	
†Lipase	<200 U/L	<200 U/mL	Acute and chronic pancreatitis Biliary obstruction Cirrhosis Hepatitis Peptic ulcer	
Lipids, total	4–8 g/L	400–800 mg/dL	Hypothyroidism Diabetes mellitus Nephrosis Glomerulonephritis Hyperlipoproteinemias	Hyperthyroidism
Low-density lipoprotein cholesterol (LDL cholesterol)		mg/dL desirable levels: <160 if no coronary artery disease (CAD) and <2 risk factors <130 if no CAD and 2 or more risk factors <100 if CAD present	LDL cholesterol is higher in patients with increased risk for coronary heart disease	

Luteinizing hormone—RIA	1.5–9.3 U/L
	
	1.9–12.5 U/L
	
	8.7–76.3 U/L
		Males: 1.5–9.3 mU/mL
		Females:
		  Follicular phase:
		    1.9–12.5 mU/mL
		  Midcycle:
		    8.7–76.3 mU/mL
			Pituitary tumour
			Ovarian failure
				Depressed or failure to peak—pituitary failure

Lysozyme (muramidase)	0.28–1.10 µmol/L	4.0–15.6 µg/mL	Certain types of leukemia (acute monocytic leukemia) Inflammatory states and infections	Acute lymphocytic leukemia
Magnesium	0.62–0.95 mmol/L	1.3–2.3 mg/dL	Excess ingestion of magnesium-containing antacids	Chronic alcoholism Severe renal disease Diarrhea Defective growth
Mercury	<50 µmol/L	<10 µg/L	Mercury poisoning	
Myoglobin—RIA	5–70 µg/mL	5–70 ng/mL	Myocardial infarction Muscle necrosis	
5′ Nucleotidase	3.2–11.6 U/L	3.2–11.6 IU/L	Hepatobiliary disease	
Osmolality	275–300 mmol/L	275–300 mOsm/kg	Diabetes insipidus, osmotic diuresis	Inappropriate secretion of ADH Addison's disease
Parathyroid hormone	10–65 ng/L	10–65 pg/mL	Hyperparathyroidism	Chronic renal failure Hypoparathyroidism
Phenylalanine	0.07–0.21 mmol/L 0.04–0.21 mmol/L	1.2–3.5 mg/dL 1st week 0.7–3.5 mg/dL thereafter	Phenylketonuria	
Phosphohexose isomerase	20–90 U/L	20–90 IU/L	Malignancy Disease of heart, liver, and skeletal muscles	
Phospholipids	1.25–3 g/L	125–300 mg/dL	Diabetes mellitus Nephritis	
Phosphorus, inorganic	0.8–1.45 mmol/L	2.5–4.5 mg/dL	Chronic nephritis Hypoparathyroidism	
Potassium	3.5–5 mmol/L	3.5–5 mEq/L	Renal Failure Acidosis Cell lysis Tissue breakdown or hemolysis	Hyperparathyroidism Vitamin D deficiency GI losses Diuretic administration

(continued)

Table B-2 • **Reference Ranges—Serum, Plasma, and Whole Blood Chemistries** (Continued)

DETERMINATION	NORMAL ADULT REFERENCE RANGE		CLINICAL SIGNIFICANCE	
	SI Units	Conventional Units	Increased	Decreased
Progesterone—RIA	2.5 nmol/L	Follicular phase: up to 0.8 ng/mL	Useful in evaluation of menstrual disorders and infertility and in the evaluation of placental function during pregnancies complicated by toxemia, diabetes mellitus, or threatened miscarriage	
	31.8–63.6 nmol/L	Luteal phase: 10–20 ng/mL		
	<3 nmol/L	End of cycle: <1 ng/mL		
	Up to 160 nmol/L	Pregnant: up to 50 ng/mL in 20th week		
Prolactin—RIA	4–30 µg/L	4–30 ng/mL	Pregnancy	
			Functional or structural disorders of the hypothalamus	
			Pituitary stalk section	
			Pituitary tumours	
Prostate-specific antigen		<4 ng/mL	Prostatic cancer, benign prostatic hyperplasia, prostatitis	
Protein, total	60–80 g/L	6–8 gm/dL	Hemoconcentration	Malnutrition
Albumin	40–55 g/L	4–5.5 g/dL	Shock	Hemorrhage
Globulin	17–33 g/L	1.7–3.3 g/dL	Globulin fraction increased in multiple myeloma, chronic infection, liver disease	Loss of plasma from burns
				Proteinuria
Protein Electrophoresis	35–50 g/L			
Albumin	40–55 g/L	4.0–5.5 g/dL		
Alpha-1 globulin	1.5–2.5 g/L	0.15–0.25 g/dL		
Alpha-2 globulin	4.3–7.5 g/L	0.43–0.75 g/dL		
Beta globulin	5–10 g/L	0.5–1.0 g/dL		
Gamma globulin	6–13 g/L	0.6–1.3 g/dL		
Protoporphyrin erythrocyte (whole blood)	0.20–0.80 µmol/L	Males: 11–45 µg/dL	Lead toxicity	
	0.34–0.92 µmol/L	Females: 19–52 µg/dL	Erythropoietic porphyria	
Pyridoxine	20–1.21 nmol/L	5–30 ng/mL		A wide spectrum of clinical conditions, such as mental depression, peripheral neuropathy, anemia, neonatal seizures, and reactions to certain drug therapies
Pyruvic acid (whole blood)	34–102 µmol/L	0.3–0.9 mg/dL	Diabetes mellitus	
			Severe thiamine deficiency	
			Acute phase of some infections, possibly secondary to increased glycogenolysis and glycolysis	
Renin (plasma)—RLA		Normal diet:	Renovascular hypertension	Frank primary aldosteronism
	0.08–0.52 ng/L/S	Supine: 0.3–1.9 ng/mL/h	Malignant hypertension	
			Untreated Addison's disease	Increased salt intake
	0.16–1.00 µg/L/S	Upright: 0.6–3.6 ng/mL/h	Primary salt-losing nephropathy	Salt–retaining steroid therapy
		Low salt diet:	Low-salt diet	Antidiuretic hormone therapy
	0.25–1.25 µg/L/S	Supine: 0.9–4.5 ng/mL/h	Diuretic therapy	
			Hemorrhage	Blood transfusion
	1.13–2.53 µg/L/S	Upright: 4.1–9.1 ng/mL/h		
Sodium	135–145 mmol/L	135–145 mEq/L	Hemoconcentration	Alkali deficit
			Nephritis	Addison's disease
			Pyloric obstruction	Myxedema
Sulfate (inorganic)	0.05–0.15 mmol/L	0.5–1.5 mg/dL	Nephritis	
			Nitrogen retention	

Table B-2 • **Reference Ranges—Serum, Plasma, and Whole Blood Chemistries** (Continued)

DETERMINATION	NORMAL ADULT REFERENCE RANGE		CLINICAL SIGNIFICANCE	
	SI Units	Conventional Units	Increased	Decreased
Testosterone—RIA	0.7–2.8 nmol/L 18.3–41.8 nmol/L	Females: 20–80 ng/dL Males: 240–1200 ng/dL	Females: Polycystic ovary Virilizing tumours	Males Orchidectomy for neoplastic disease of the prostate or breast Estrogen therapy Klinefelter's syndrome Hypopituitarism Hypogonadism Hepatic cirrhosis Hypothyroidism
T_3 (triiodothyronine) uptake	Relative uptake fraction: 0.24–0.34	24%–34%	Hyperthyroidism Thyroxine-binding globulin (TBG) deficiency Androgens and anabolic steroids	Pregnancy TBG excess Estrogens and anti-ovulatory drugs Hypothyroidism
T_3 total circulating—RIA	1.08–3.14 nmol/L	70–204 ng/dL	Pregnancy Hyperthyroidism	
T_4 (thyroxine)—RIA	65–138 nmol/L	5–11 μg/dL	Hyperthyroidism Thyroiditis Elevated thyroxine-binding proteins caused by oral contraceptives Pregnancy	Primary and pituitary hypothyroidism Idiopathic involvement Cases of diminished thyroxine-binding proteins caused by androgenic and anabolic steroids Hypoproteinemia Nephrotic syndrome
T_4, free	10.3–35 pmol/L	0.8–2.7 ng/dL	Euthyroid patients with normal free thyroxine levels may have abnormal T3 and T4 levels caused by drug preparations Hypothyroidism	Hyperthyroidism
Thyroid-stimulating hormone (TSH)—RIA	0.4–4.2 mIU/L			
Thyroid-binding globulin	100–260/μg/L	10–26 μg/dL	Hypothyroidism Pregnancy Estrogen therapy Oral contraceptive use Genetic and idiopathic liver disease	Use of androgens and anabolic steroids Nephrotic syndrome Marked hypoproteinemia
Transferrin	2.3–3.2 g/L	200–380 mg/dL	Pregnancy Iron deficiency anemia due to hemorrhaging Acute hepatitis Polycythemia Oral contraceptive use	Pernicious anemia in relapse Thalassemic and sickle cell anemia Chromatosis Neoplastic and hepatic diseases
Triglycerides	1.13–3.8 mmol/L	100–200 mg/dL		
Tryptophan	68.6–147 nmol/L	1.4–3 mg/dL		Tryptophan-specific malabsorption syndrome
Tyrosine	27.6–220.8 mmol/L	0.5–4 mg/dL	Tyrosinosis	
Urea nitrogen (BUN)	3.6–7.2 mmol/L	10–20 mg/dL	Acute glomerulonephritis Obstructive uropathy Mercury poisoning Nephrotic syndrome	Severe hepatic failure Pregnancy
Uric acid	0.15–0 mmol/L	2.5–8 mg/dL	Gouty arthritis Acute leukemia Lymphomas treated by chemotherapy Toxemia of pregnancy	Defective tubular reabsorption

(continued)

Table B-2 • Reference Ranges—Serum, Plasma, and Whole Blood Chemistries (Continued)

DETERMINATION	NORMAL ADULT REFERENCE RANGE		CLINICAL SIGNIFICANCE	
	SI Units	Conventional Units	Increased	Decreased
Viscosity		1.4–1.8 relative to water at 37°C (98.6°F)	Patients with marked increases of the gamma globulins	
Vitamin A	1.05–4.20 µmol/L	30–120 µg/dL	Hypervitaminosis A	Vitamin A deficiency Celiac disease Sprue Obstructive jaundice Giardiasis Parenchymal hepatic disease
Vitamin B, (thiamine)	47.4–135.7 nmol/L	1.6–4 µg/dL		Anorexia Beriberi Polyneuropathy Cardiomyopathies
Vitamin B$_6$ (pyridoxal phosphate)	20–121 nmol/L	5–30 ng/mL		Chronic alcoholism Malnutrition Uremia Neonatal seizures Malabsorption, such as celiac syndrome
Vitamin B$_{12}$—RIA	148–666 pmol/L	200–900 pg/mL	Hepatic cell damage and in association with the myeloproliferative disorders (the highest levels are encountered in myeloid leukemia)	Strict vegetarianism Alcoholism Pernicious anemia Total or partial gastrectomy Ileal resection Sprue and celiac disease Fish tapeworm infestation
Vitamin E	12–42 µmol/L	0.5–1.8 mg/dL		Vitamin E deficiency
Xylose absorption test	2–3.35 mmol/L	2 hr, 30–50 mg/dL		Malabsorption syndrome
Zinc	7.65–22.95 µmol/L	55–150/µg/dL	Coronary artery disease Arteriosclerosis Industrial exposure	Metastatic liver disease Tuberculosis Sprue

*By radioimmunoassay.
†Varies among methods.

Table B-3 • Reference Ranges—Immunodiagnostic Tests

DETERMINATION	NORMAL VALUE	CLINICAL SIGNIFICANCE
Acetylcholine receptor binding antibody	Negative or <0.03 nmol/L	Considered to be diagnostic for myasthenia gravis in patients with symptoms.
Anti-ds-DNA antibody	<70 U by enzyme-linked immunosorbent assay (ELISA) <1:20 by indirect fluorescence	Valuable in supporting diagnosis or monitoring disease activity and prognosis of systemic lupus erythematosus (SLE).
Antiglomerular basement membrane antibody	Negative or less than 5εUL	Primarily used in the differential diagnosis of glomerular nephritis induced by antiglomerular basement membrane antibodies from other types of glomerular nephritis.
Anti-insulin antibody	<3% binding of labelled beef and pork insulin by patient's serum; or <9 mIU/L	Helpful in determining the best therapeutic agent in diabetics and the cause of allergic manifestations. Also used to identify insulin resistance.
Antinuclear antibody	Negative, <1:40	Increased in SLE, chronic hepatitis, scleroderma, leukemia, and mononucleosis.
Anti-parietal cell antibody	Negative	Helpful in diagnosing chronic gastric disease and differentiating autoimmune pernicious anemia from other megaloblastic anemias.
Antiribonucleoprotein antibody	Negative	Helpful in differential diagnosis of systemic rheumatic disease.
Antiscleroderma antibody	Negative	Highly diagnostic for scleroderma.
Anti-Smith antibody	Negative	Highly diagnostic of SLE.
Anti-SS-A/anti-SS-B antibody	Negative	SS-A antibodies are found in Sjögren's syndrome alone or associated with lupus. SS-B antibodies are associated with primary Sjögren's syndrome.
Antithyroglobulin and antimicrosomal antibodies	<1:100 titer by gelatin or hemagglutination	Presence and concentration is important in evaluation and treatment of various thyroid disorders, such as Hashimoto's thyroiditis and Graves' disease. May indicate previous antoimmune disorders.
CA 15-3 tumour marker	<30 IU/mL	Increased in metastatic breast cancer.
CA 19-9 tumour marker	<37 IU/mL	Increased in pancreatic, hepatobiliary, gastric, and colorectal cancer, gallstones.
CA 125	0–35 IU/mL	Increased in colon, upper gastrointestinal (GI), ovarian, and other gynecologic cancers: pregnancy, peritonitis.
Carcinoembryonic antigen (CEA)—RLK	0–2.5 µg/L (nonsmoker) 0–5/µg/L (smoker)	The repeatedly high incidence of this antigen in cancers of the colon, rectum, pancreas, and stomach suggests that CEA levels may be useful in the therapeutic monitoring of these conditions, but it is not a screening test
Cold agglutinins	Negative or <1:32	Increased in mycoplasma pneumonia, viral illness, mononucleosis, multiple myeloma, scleroderma.
C-reactive protein	<0.8 mg/dL	Increase indicates active inflammation.
Cytomegalovirus antibodies (CMV IgG)	Negative: <0.9 units/mL	Positive >1:0 unit/mL if exposed to CMV at anytime. Acute and convalescent specimens can help identify acute infection.
Cytomegalovirus antibodies (CMV IgM)	Negative: <0:79 Equivocal: 0:80–1.20	Positive >1:20 usually indicates acute infection. Repeat specimen in 1–2 weeks for equivocal result.
Epstein-Barr virus serology (viral capsid antigen IgG and IgM, early antigen IgG, and nuclear antigen IgG)	Negative: <1:20 or <1:20 for each individual test	Differentiation of acute from chronic or old infection by interpretation of table below.
Hepatitis A virus antibodies, IgM (HAV-Ab/IgM)	Negative	Positive in acute-stage hepatitis A; develops early in disease.

EBV INTERPRETATION

	VCA-IgG	VCA-IgM	EA-IgG	EBV-NA
Susceptible	−	−	−	−
Acute infection	+	+	±	−
Convalescent phase	+	±	±	+
Chronic or reactivated	+	−	+	±
Old infection	±	−	−	+

Antibody present: +
Antibody absent: −
VCA, viral capsid antigen; EA, early antigen; EBV-NA, Epstein Barr virus-nuclear antigen

(continued)

Table B-3 • **Reference Ranges—Immunodiagnostic Tests** (Continued)

DETERMINATION	NORMAL VALUE	CLINICAL SIGNIFICANCE
Hepatitis A virus antibodies, IgG (HAV-Ab/IgG)	Negative	Positive if previous exposure and immunity to hepatitis A.
Hepatitis B surface antigen (HBsAg)	Negative	Positive in acute-stage hepatitis B.
Hepatitis B surface antibody (HBsAb)	Negative	Positive if previous exposure and immunity to hepatitis B.
Hepatitis C virus antibodies	Negative	Positive in exposure to hepatitis C virus; may indicate acute, chronic, or cleared infection.
Hepatitis C virus RNA	Negative	Positive in hepatitis C infection, can be quantitative
Infectious mononucleosis tests (monospot, monotest, heterophile antigen test, Epstein-Barr virus (EBV), antiviral capsid antigen IgM and IgG)	Negative	Positive monospot and monotest are presumptive, positive EBV IgM and IgG indicate acute and recent or past infection, respectively.
Lyme disease titer	Negative, <1:256 by indirect fluorescent antibody method; nonreactive by ELISA	Positive results help diagnose Lyme disease. False positive may occur with high rheumatoid factor titers or syphilis. Positive ELISA confirmed by Western blot test.
Pyroglobulin test	Negative	These abnormal proteins may be associated with myeloma, lymphoma, polycythemia vera, and SLE.
Rheumatoid factor	Negative or less than 40 IU/mL	Elevated in rheumatoid arthritis, lupus endocarditis, tuberculosis, syphilis, sarcoidosis, cancer.
T and B cell lymphocyte surface markers T-helper/T-suppressor ratio	T and B cell lymphocyte surface markers: Percent T cells (CD2) 60–88% Percent helper cells (CD4) 34–67% Percent suppressor cells (CD8) 10–42% Percent B cells (CD19) 3–21% Absolute counts: Lymphocytes 0.66–4.60 thou/mL T cells 644–2201 cells/mL Helper cells 493–1191 cells/mL Suppressor T cells 182–785 cells/mL B cells 92–392 cells/mL Lymphocyte ratio: T_H/T_S ratio > 1	Used to evaluate immune system by identifying the specific cells involved in the immune response. Valuable in diagnosis of lymphocytic leukemia, lymphoma, and immunodeficiency diseases including acquired immunodeficiency syndrome, and in the assessment of patient response to chemotherapy and radiation.

Table B-4 • **Reference Ranges—Urine Chemistry**

DETERMINATION	NORMAL ADULT REFERENCE RANGE		CLINICAL SIGNIFICANCE	
	SI Units	Conventional Units	Increased	Decreased
Acetone and acetoacetate		Zero	Diabetic ketoacidosis Starvation	
Aldosterone	11.1–55.5 nmol/24h 27.7–111 nmol/24 h 55.4–277 nmol/24 h	With normal salt diet: Normal: 4–20 µg/24 h Renovascular: 10–40 µg/24 h Tumour: 20–100 µg/24 h	Primary aldosteronism (adrenocortical tumour) Secondary aldosteronism Salt depletion Potassium loading ACTH in large doses Cardiac failure Cirrhosis with ascites formation Nephrosis Pregnancy	
Alpha amino nitrogen	3.6–14.3 nmol/24 h	50–200 mg/24 h	Leukemia Phenylketonuria Other metabolic diseases	
Amylase	6.5–48.1 U/h	35–260 units excreted per h	Acute pancreatitis	
Arylsulfatase A		>2.4 U/mL		
Bence-Jones protein		None detected	Myeloma	Metachromatic leukodystrophy
Calcium	2.5–6.2 mmol/24 h	100–250 mg/24 h	Hyperparathyroidism Vitamin D intoxication Fanconi's syndrome	Hypoparathyroidism Vitamin D deficiency
Catecholamines	0–275 µg/24 h Fraction total: 0.10–8.4 Fraction total: 0.60–0.90	Total: 0–275 µg/24 h Epinephrine: 10%–40% Norepinephrine: 60%–90%	Pheochromocytoma Neuroblastoma	
Chorionic gonadotrophin, qualitative (pregnancy test)		Negative	Pregnancy Chorionepithelioma Hydatidiform mole	
Copper	0.22–0.9 µmol/24 h	15–60 µg/24 h	Wilson's disease Cirrhosis Nephrosis Poliomyelitis	
Coproporphyrin	0.075–0.45 µmol/24 h	50–300 µg/24 h	Lead poisoning Porphyria	
Cortisol, free	55.2–248.4 nmol/d	20–90 µg/24 h	Cushing's syndrome	
Creatinine	8.8–17.7 mmol/24 h 7.1–15.9 mmol/24 h	Males: 1–2 g/24 h Females: 0.8–1.8 g/24 h	Muscular dystrophy Fever Carcinoma of liver Pregnancy Hyperthyroidism Myositis	
Creatine	0–2.05 mmol/24 h	0–270 mg/24 h	Typhoid fever Salmonella infections Tetanus	Muscular atrophy Anemia Advanced degeneration of kidneys Leukemia Renal diseases
Creatinine clearance	1.42–2.08 mL/s 1.25–1.92 mL/s	Males: 85–125 mL/min Females: 75–115 mL/min		
Cystine and cysteine	0.08–0.83 mmol/24 h	10–100 mg/24 h	Cystinuria	
Delta aminolevulimic acid	0–40/µmol/L	0–0.54 mg/dL	Lead poisoning Porphyria hepatica Hepatitis Hepatic carcinoma	
11-Desoxycortisol	0.6–2.9/µmol/d	20–100 µg/24 h	Hypertensive form of virilizing adrenal hyperplasia due to an 11-beta hydroxylase defect	

(continued)

Table B-4 • **Reference Ranges—Urine Chemistry** (Continued)

DETERMINATION	NORMAL ADULT REFERENCE RANGE		CLINICAL SIGNIFICANCE	
	SI Units	Conventional Units	Increased	Decreased
Estriol (placental)	μm/24 h mmol/24 h <1 <3.5 2–7 7–24.5 4–9 14–32 6–13 21–45.5 8–22 28–77 12–43 42–150 14–45 49–158 19–46 66.5–160	Weeks of pregnancy 12 16 20 24 28 32 36 40		Decreased values occur with fetal distress of many conditions, including preeclampsia, placental insufficiency, and poorly controlled diabetes mellitus
Estrogens, total (fluorometric)	4–25 μg/24 h 28–100 μg/24 h 22–105 μg/24 h 1.4–19.6 μg/24 h 5–18 μg/24 h	Females: Onset of menstruation: 4–25 μg/24 h Ovulation peak: 28–100 μg/24 h Luteal peak: 22–105 μg/24 h Menopausal: 1.4–19.6 μg/24 h Males: 5–18 μg/24 h	Hyperestrogenism due to gonadal or adrenal neoplasm	Primary or secondary amenorrhea
Etiocholanolone	6.5–20.6 μmol/24 h 1.7–13.8 μmol/24 h	Males: 1.9–6 mg/24 h Females: 0.5–4 mg/24 h	Adrenogenital syndrome Idiopathic hirsutism	
Follicle-stimulating hormone—RIA	5–20 IU/d 5–15 IU/d 15–60 IU/d 50–100 IU/d 5–25 IU/d	Females: Follicular: 5–20 IU/24 h Luteal: 5–15 IU/24 h Midcycle: 15–60 IU/24 h Menopausal: 50–100 IU/24 h Males: 5–25 IU/24 h	Menopause and primary ovarian failure	Pituitary failure
Glucose		Negative	Diabetes mellitus Pituitary disorders Increased ICP Lesion in floor of 4th ventricle	
Hemoglobin and myoglobin		Negative	Extensive burns Transfusion of incompatible blood Myoglobin increased in severe crushing injuries to muscles	
Homovanillic acid	<44 μmol/24h		Neuroblastoma	
17-hydroxycorticosteroids	5.5–27.5 μmol/d	8 mg/24 h 2–10 mg/24 h	Cushing's disease	Addison's disease Anterior pituitary hypofunction
5-Hydroxyindoleacetic acid, qualitative		Negative	Malignant carcinoid tumours	
17-ketosteroids, total	35–76 μmol/24h 21–55 μmol/24h	Males: 10–22 mg/24 h Females: 6–16 mg/24 h	Interstitial cell tumour of testes Simple hirsutism, occasionally Adrenal hyperplasia Cushing's syndrome Adrenal cancer, virilism Adrenoblastoma	Thyrotoxicosis Female hypogonadism Diabetes mellitus Hypertension Debilitating disease of mild to moderate severity Eunuchoidism Addison's disease Panhypopituitarism Myxedema Nephrosis
Lead	<60 μmol/24 h	<125 μg/24 h	Lead poisoning	
Luteinizing hormone		Males: 5–18 IU/24 h	Pituitary tumour Ovarian failure	Depressed or failure to peak—pituitary failure

(continued)

Table B-4 • **Reference Ranges—Urine Chemistry** (Continued)

DETERMINATION	NORMAL ADULT REFERENCE RANGE		CLINICAL SIGNIFICANCE	
	SI Units	Conventional Units	Increased	Decreased
	2–25 IU/d	Females: Follicular phase: 2–25 IU/24 h		
	30–95 IU/d	Ovulatory peak: 30–95 IU/24 h		
	2–20 IU/d	Luteal phase: 2–20 IU/24 h		
Metanephrines, total	40–110 IU/d <7 μmol/24h	Postmenopausal: 40–110 IU/24 h <1.4 mg/24 h	Pheochromocytoma; a few patients with pheochromocytoma may have elevated urinary metanephines but normal catecholamines and vanillylmandelic acid (VMA)	
Osmolality	250–900 mmol/kg	250–900 mOsm/kg	Useful in the study of electrolyte and water balance	
Oxalate	Up to 500/μmol/24 h	Up to 45 mg/24 h	Primary hyperoxaluria	
Phenylpyruvic acid qualitative		Negative	Phenylketonuria	
Phosphorus, inorganic	29–42 mmol/24 h	0.9–1.3 g/24 h	Hypoparathyroidism Vitamin D intoxication Paget's disease Metastatic neoplasm to bone Chronic lead poisoning	Hypoparathyroidism Vitamin D deficiency
Porphobilinogen, qualitative		Negative	Acute porphyria Liver disease	
Porphobilinogen quantitative	0–4.4 μmol/24 h	0–1 mg/24 h	Acute porphyria Liver disease	
Porphyrins, qualitative		Negative	See porphyrins, quantitative	
Porphyrins, quantitative (coproporphyrin and uroporphyrin)	0.075–0.24 μmol/24h Up to 0.06 μmol/24 h	Coproporphyrin: 50–160 μg/24 h Uroporphyrin: up to 50 μ/24 h	Porphyria Lead poisoning (only coproporphyrin increased)	
Potassium	26–123 mmol/24 h	26–123 mEq/24 h	Hemolysis Chronic renal failure Acidosis Cushing's disease Corpus luteum cysts	Diarrhea Adrenocortical insufficiency
Pregnanediol	1.6–4.8 μmol/24 h 6–22 μmol/24 h 0.6–3.1 μmol/24 h	Females: Proliferative phase: 0.5–1.5 mg/24 h Luteal phase: 2–7 mg/24 h Menopause: 0.2–1 mg/24 h	When placental tissue remains in the uterus following parturition Some cases of adrenocortical tumours	Placental dysfunction Threatened abortion Intrauterine death
Pregnancy: Weeks of gestation 10–12 12–18 18–24 24–28 28–32	μmol/24 h 15.6–47 15.6–78.0 47.0–103.0 62.4–131.0 84.2–146.6	mg/24 h 5–15 5–25 15–33 20–42 27–47		

(continued)

Table B-4 • **Reference Ranges—Urine Chemistry** (Continued)

DETERMINATION	NORMAL ADULT REFERENCE RANGE		CLINICAL SIGNIFICANCE	
	SI Units	Conventional Units	Increased	Decreased
Pregnanetriol	0.3–6.5 μmol/24 h 1.2–7.5 μmol/24 h	Females: 0.1–2.2 mg/24 h Males: 0.4–2.5 mg/24 h	Congenital adrenal an- drogenic hyperplasia	
Protein	<150 mg/24 h	<150 mg/24 h	Nephritis Cardiac failure Mercury poisoning Bence-Jones protein in multiple myeloma Febrile states Hematuria	
Sodium	75–200 mmol/24 h	75–200 mEq/24 h	Useful in detecting gross changes in water and salt balance	Metabolic alkalosis
Titratable acidity	20–40 mmol/24 h	20–40 mEq/24 h	Metabolic acidosis	Impaired kidney
Urea nitrogen	0.32–0.57 mol/L	9–16 gm/24 h	Excessive protein catabolism	function Nephritis
Uric acid	1.48–4.43 mmol/24 h	250–750 mg/24 h	Gout	Complete or nearly
Urobilinogen	<0.42 mol/24 h	Random urine: <0.25 mg/dL	Liver and biliary tract disease	complete biliary obstruction
	Up to 6.76 μmol/24 h	24-hour urine: up to 4 mg/24 h	Hemolytic anemias	Diarrhea Renal insufficiency
Vanillylmandelic acid (VMA)	3.5–34.3 μmol/24 h	0.7–6.8 mg/24 h	Pheochromocytoma Neuroblastoma Ingestion of coffee, tea, aspirin, bananas, and several different drugs	
Xylose absorption test (5-hour)	Fraction absorbed: 0.16–0.33	16%–33% of ingested xylose		
Zinc	2.3–18.4 μmol/24h	0.15–1.2 mg/24 h		Malabsorption syndromes

Table B-5 • **Reference Ranges—Cerebrospinal Fluid (CSF)**

DETERMINATION	NORMAL ADULT REFERENCE RANGE		CLINICAL SIGNIFICANCE	
	SI Units	Conventional Units	Increased	Decreased
Albumin	150–300 mg/L	15–30 mg/dL	Certain neurologic disorders Lesion in the choroid plexus or blockage of the flow of CSF Damage to the blood–brain barrier	
Cell count (white blood cells)	0–5 × 10⁶/L	0–5 cells per cu mm	Bacterial meningitis Neurosyphilis Anterior poliomyelitis Encephalitis lethargica	
Chloride	120–130 mmol/L	120–130 mEq/L	Uremia	Acute generalized meningitis Tuberculous meningitis
Glucose	2.75–4.13 mmol/L	50–75 mg/dL; 50%–80% of blood glucose value	Diabetes mellitus Diabetic coma Epidemic encephalitis Uremia	Acute meningitis Tuberculous meningitis Insulin shock Subarachnoid hemorrhage
Glutamine	0.41–1 mmol/L	6–15 mg/dL	Hepatic encephalopathies, including Reye's syndrome Hepatic coma Cirrhosis	
IgG	<50 mg/L	<5 mg/dL	Damage to the blood–brain barrier Multiple sclerosis Neurosyphilis Subacute sclerosing panencephalitis Chronic phases of CNS infections	
Lactic acid	0.5–3.2 mmol/L	4.5–28.8 mg/dL	Bacterial meningitis Hypocapnia Hydrocephalus Brain abscesses Cerebral ischemia Fungal meningitis	
Lactate dehydrogenase	Activity fraction: 0.1 of serum	¹⁄₁₀ that of serum level	CNS disease Acute meningitis	
Protein	150–450 mg/L	15–45 mg/dL	Tubercular meningitis Neurosyphilis Poliomyelitis Guillain-Barré syndrome Subdural hematoma Brain tumour Multiple sclerosis	

Table B-6 • **Miscellaneous Values**

DETERMINATIONS	NORMAL VALUE	CLINICAL SIGNIFICANCE	
		SI Units	Conventional Units
Acetaminophen	Zero	10–30 mg/L	Therapeutic level = 10–30 µg/mL
Aminophylline (theophylline)	Zero	10–20 mg/L	Therapeutic level = 10–20/µg/mL
Bromide	Zero	50–500 mg/L	Therapeutic level = 5–50 mg/dL
Carbamazepine	Zero	34–51 µmol/L	Therapeutic level = 8–12 mg/mL
Carbon monoxide	0%–2%		Symptoms with 10%–30% saturation
Chlordiazepoxide	Zero	0.7–1.0 mg/L	Therapeutic level = 0.7–1.0 µg/mL
Diazepam	Zero	0.2–1.0 mg/L	Therapeutic level = 0.2–1.0 µg/mL
Digitoxin	Zero	18–35 µg/L	Therapeutic level = 18–35 ng/mL
Digoxin	Zero	0.8–2/µg/L	Therapeutic level = 0.8–2 ng/mL
Ethanol	0%–0.01%		Legal intoxication level = 0.10% or above
			0.3%–0.4% = marked intoxication
			0.4%–0.5% = alcoholic stupor
Gentamicin	Zero	4–10 mg/L	Therapeutic level = 4–10 µg/mL
Lithium	Zero	0.6–1.2 mmol/L	Therapeutic level = 0.6–1.2 mEq/L
Methanol	Zero	100 mg/L	May be fatal in concentration as low as 10 mg/dL
Phenobarbital	Zero	20–40 mg/L	Therapeutic level = 20–40 µg/mL
Phenytoin	Zero	10–20 mg/L	Therapeutic level = 10–20 µg/mL
Primidone	Zero	5–12 mg/L	Therapeutic level = 5–12 µg/mL
Quinidine	Zero	2–5 mg/L	Therapeutic level = 0.2–0.5 mg/dL
Salicylate	Zero	20–250 mg/L	Therapeutic level = 2–25 mg/dL
		300 mg/L	Toxic level = >30 mg/dL
Vancomycin	Zero		Therapeutic peak 20–40 µg/mL
			Therapeutic trough 5–10 µg/mL
Amitriptyline	Zero	289–722 nmol/L	Therapeutic level 80–200 ng/mL
Doxepin	Zero	540–900 nmol/L	Therapeutic level 150–250 ng/mL (includes metabolites)
Imipramine	Zero	360–1070 nmol/L	Therapeutic level 100–300 ng/mL (includes metabolites)
Lidocaine	Zero	6.4–21.4 µmol/L	Therapeutic level 1.5–5 µg/mL
Methotrexate	Zero	1000 mmol/L	Toxic (48 hr. after high dose) 454 mg/mL
Propranolol	Zero	193–386 nmol/L	Therapeutic level 50–100 ng/mL
Valproic acid	Zero	347–693 µmol/L	Therapeutic level 50–100 µg/mL

References
1. *Jacobs and Demott's Laboratory Test Handbook.* 5th ed. Lexi-Comp. Inc. Hudson (OH), 2001.
2. Traub SL. *Basic Skills in Interpreting Laboratory Data.* 2nd ed. American Society of Health-Systems Pharmacy, Bethesda, MD, 1996.
3. www.bioscientia.de
4. http://www.gpnotebook.co.uk/simplepage.cfm?ID=429195241&linkID=8734
5. www.bloodbook.com/ranges.html
6. http://www.buymedicals.com/MedicalInfo/2-urine.asp
7. http://thailabonline.com/lab-normalrange1.htm
8. Directory of Services and Interpretive Guide. LabCorp. 2001.

Index

Letters following page numbers indicate the following: c - chart, f - figure, t - table.

Drug(s). *See also* Medication(s)
abuse of. *See* Substance abuse
administration of, culturally competent, 119–120
anaphylactic reaction to, 2176–2177
aplastic anemia caused by, 887, 887c
cellular injury caused by, 91
effective metabolizers of, 139
with hemolytic effects, in glucose-6-phosphate dehydrogenase (G6PD) deficiency, 895
metabolism of
genetic factors affecting, 138–139
in liver, 1082
overdose, emergency management of, 2183t–2186t
and platelet function, 917, 918c
poor metabolizers of, 139
ultra-rapid or rapid metabolizers of, 139
Drug resistance
multidrug, 539
primary, 539
secondary (acquired), 539
in tuberculosis, 539
Drusen, 1777, 1777f
Dry eye syndrome, 1782–1783
assessment of, 1782
clinical manifestations of, 1782
diagnosis of, 1782
management of, 1783
Dry mouth, 970
in older persons, 965
D4t. *See* Stavudine (Zerit)
DTP vaccine, contraindications to, 2132
Dual-energy x-ray absorptiometry, 2024
for osteoporosis, 2107
in osteoporosis, 2070
Dubin-Johnson syndrome, 1088
Dubos, Rene Jules, 82
Duchenne muscular dystrophy, genetics of, 128, 131t
Duct(s), of breast, 1452, 1453f
Ductal carcinoma, infiltrating, 1463
Ductal carcinoma in situ, 1462–1463
comedo, 1463
definition of, 1452
noncomedo, 1463
Ductal lavage, 1462
Ductule(s), of breast, 1453f
Dullness, on percussion, 67
Dumping syndrome
definition of, 990, 1015, 1030
after gastric surgery, 1030
in tube feeding, 996–997, 999t, 1000–1001
confirmation of, 1000–1001
prevention of, 1001c
Duodenal ulcers, 1019–1025, 1019t. *See also* Peptic ulcer disease
Duodenum, 945, 946f, 1019
definition of, 990, 1015
feeding tubes in, 990
function of, 947–948
tube feeding into, 991
DuoDerm, for burn grafts, 1732
Dupuytren's contracture, 2063, 2063f
Durable power of attorney, 194
medical, 380c
Dura mater, 1834–1835
Duramorph. *See* Morphine sulfate (Duramorph, Astramorph)
Duverney's fracture, 2102
DVT. *See* Deep vein thrombosis
Dwarfism, 1213
definition of, 1217
Dying. *See* Death and dying
Dynamic orthoses, 176
Dysarthria
definition of, 1898
ischemic stroke and, 1899, 1900t
in multiple sclerosis, 1963–1964
Dysautonomia, mitral valve prolapse and, 769
Dysfibrinogenemia, 924t
Dyskinesia
definition of, 1953, 1980
in Guillain-Barré syndrome, 1968
in Parkinson's disease, 1992
Dyslipidemia
definition of, 859
hypertension and, 859
Dysmenorrhea, 1378, 1397
assessment in, 1397
definition of, 1375
diagnosis of, 1397
management of, 1397
primary, 1397
secondary, 1397
Dyspareunia, 1378, 1398
definition of, 1375
in menopausal women, 1393
Dysphagia, 976
in achalasia, 976
definition of, 497, 963, 1831, 1953
esophageal cancer and, 984
with esophageal spasm, 980
after gastric surgery, 1029

gerontologic considerations in, 199
ischemic stroke and, 1900t, 1909
in laryngeal cancer, 510–511
in multiple sclerosis, 1964
with peritonsillar abscess, 504
Dysphonia
definition of, 1953, 1980
in myasthenia gravis, 1966
in Parkinson's disease, 1990
Dysplasia, 89t, 90
of blood cells, 889–890
definition of, 81, 323, 872, 1417
Dyspnea, 475–476
in alpha₁-antitrypsin deficiency, management of, nursing research on, 580
assessment of, 66
in asthma, 592–593
in cardiovascular disease, assessment of, 659, 663t
in chronic obstructive pulmonary disease, 575
clinical significance of, 476
definition of, 467, 475
on exertion
definition of, 792
in heart failure, 798
in laryngeal cancer, 510–511
in lung cancer, 559
nursing interventions for, 561
mitral stenosis and, 771
nursing interventions for, 388c
with pulmonary embolism, 552–553
relief measures for, 476
self-management of, nursing research on, 477
in terminal illness, 387–388
assessment of, 387–388
nursing interventions for, 387–388
Dysreflexia, autonomic, 1940
definition of, 1921
spinal cord injury and, 1943–1944
Dysrhythmia(s), cardiac, 659, 667, 687–703
ablation of, 712
assessment for, 702
atrial, 693–696
after cardiac surgery, 755t
in cardiogenic shock, 313, 314, 811
classification of
by mechanisms of formation or conduction, 687c
by site of origin, 687c
complications of, 703
definition of, 687
electrophysiologic testing with, 712–713
expected outcomes with, 703
in heart failure, 798
hemochromatosis and, 897
in hemodialysis, 1293
hypothyroidism and, 1221
incidence of, factors affecting, 688
junctional, 696–697
management of. *See also* Antiarrhythmic agents
adjunctive modalities for, 703–713
monitoring with, 703
myocarditis and, 786
nursing diagnoses related to, 702–703
nursing management of, 703
nursing process with, 702–703
planning and goals with, 703
postoperative, 444, 641
sinus node, 692–693
after thoracic surgery, 641
types of, 691–702
ventricular, 697–698
Dysuria, 1261, 1263, 1264t
definition of, 1255

E

Eagle-Barrett syndrome, 1279
Ear. *See also* Balance; Equilibrium; Hearing
anatomy of, 1799–1802, 1800f
assessment of, 1802–1804
external
anatomy of, 1799
definition of, 1800c
foreign bodies in, 1809–1810
inspection of, 1802
masses of, 1810
functions of, 1802
infection of, 503
inner
anatomy of, 1800f, 1801
conditions of, 1816–1822
definition of, 1800c
perfusion, 1817
middle
anatomy of, 1799–1801
definition of, 1800c
effusion, 1799
endoscopy, 1806
infection of, 503
masses of, 1815–1816
perfusion, 1817

otoscopic examination of, 1802–1804, 1804f
physiology of, 1799–1802
Eardrum. *See* Tympanic membrane
Earring puncture, gapping, 1810
Eastern equine encephalitis, 1957
Easter Seal Society of Canada, contact information for, 2122
Eating disorder(s)
and amenorrhea, 1397
resources and websites on, 113
EBCT. *See* Electron-beam computed tomography
Ebola virus, 2139–2140
incubation period of, 2128t
transmission of, 2128t
ECCE. *See* Extracapsular cataract extraction
Ecchymosis, 666, 1649t, 1658c
in acute myeloid leukemia, 903
definition of, 872, 2168c
ECF-A. *See* Eosinophil chemotactic factor of anaphylaxis
ECG. *See* Electrocardiogram/electrocardiography
Echocardiography, 676–677, 677f
in aortic stenosis, 772
in heart failure, 800
nursing interventions in, 677
with pulmonary hypertension, 550
Economics, and health care, 8
Ecstasy (drug). *See* MDMA (Ecstasy, Adam)
Ectopic pregnancy, 1408–1411
assessment in, 1409, 1410
causes of, 1408
clinical manifestations of, 1408–1409
complications of, 1410
continuing care for, 1411
diagnosis of, 1409, 1410
expected outcomes in, 1411
home and community-based care for, 1411
incidence of, 1408
medical management of, 1409–1410
nursing diagnoses related to, 1410
nursing interventions for, 1410–1411
nursing process with, 1410–1411
pelvic inflammatory disease and, 1426
pharmacologic treatment of, 1409–1410
planning and goals for, 1410
sexually transmitted infection and, 2148
sites of, 1408, 1410f
surgical treatment of, 1409
Ectropion, 1762t
Eczema herpeticum, 1680
Eczema Society of Canada, contact information for, 1661, 1710
ED. *See* Emergency department; Erectile dysfunction
Edema, 823, 824. *See also* Cerebral edema; Lymphedema; Pulmonary edema
in acute glomerulonephritis, 1323
angioneurotic, 509–510, 1545t, 1549
definition of, 1544, 1589
of breast, 1455c
breast cancer surgery and, 1469
in cardiovascular disease, assessment of, 663t
cerebral, brain injury and, 1932
in chronic renal failure, 1332
in cirrhosis, 1109
definition of, 2028
dependent, in heart failure, 799
drugs causing, 268
with fractures, 2030
in heart failure, 799, 799f, 805
laryngeal, 509–510
in liver disease, 1099
in nephrotic syndrome, 1325–1326
patient teaching about, 268
peripheral, 671
pitting, 799, 799f
and pressure ulcers, 177
pulmonary, burns and, 1740, 1743
and wound healing, 455t
Edrophonium (Tensilon)
in cholinergic vs. myasthenic crisis diagnosis, 1967
in myasthenia gravis diagnosis, 1966
Education
of nurses, 12
patient. *See* Patient teaching
EEG. *See* Electroencephalography
Efavirenz (Sustiva), for HIV infection, 1563t
Effector stage, of immune response, 1531
Effusion, 2021–2022. *See also* Pericardial effusion; Pleural effusions
joint, 1615
definition of, 1614, 2013
middle ear, definition of, 1799
EGD. *See* Esophagogastroduodenoscopy
Egophony, 485
in pneumonia, 531
EIA. *See* Enzyme immunoassay
Ejaculation
inhibited, 1497
premature, 1497
problems with, 1497
retrograde, 1406, 1497